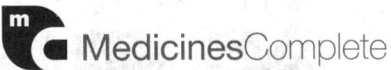
MedicinesComplete

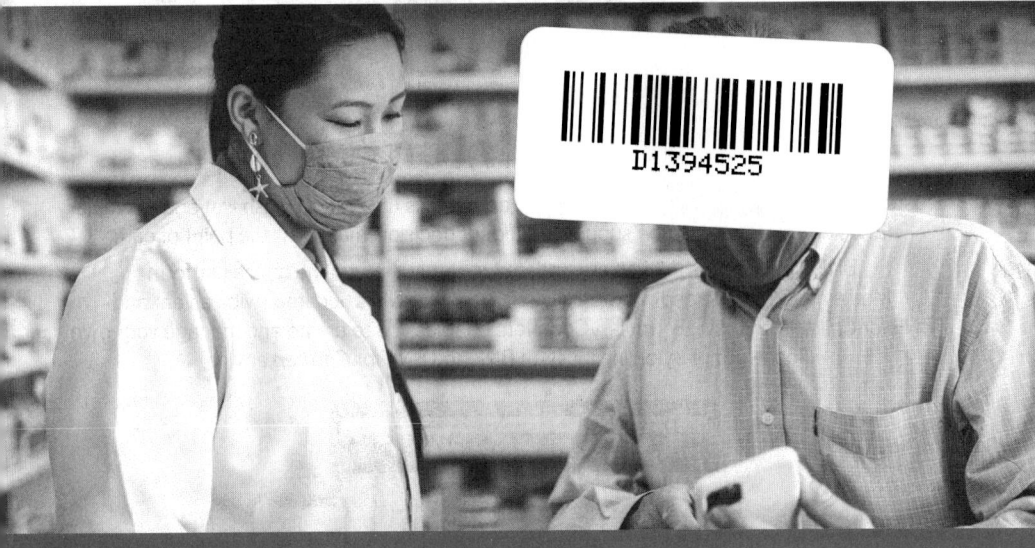

COMMUNITY PHARMACIST SPECIAL OFFER

Instant access to essential medicines information

As a community pharmacist, we know you strive to provide safe and effective patient care. Subscribe now for instant access to essential resources at a reduced rate subscription to MedicinesComplete. Resources include: **Stockley's Drug Interactions**, **Stockley's Interactions Checker**, **Martindale: The Complete Drug Reference**, **Martindale's ADR Checker**, **British National Formulary** and **BNF** *for Children*.

MedicinesComplete makes it easy for healthcare professionals to access essential medicines information at the point of care.

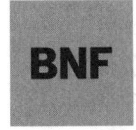
British National
Formulary (BNF)

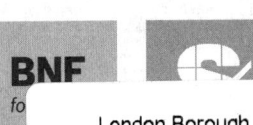

The
Drug
e

Martindale's
ADR Checker

Find out more at
about.medicinescomplete.com/sector/pharmacy/England-Wales

Offers also available to Ireland and Rest of World

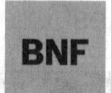
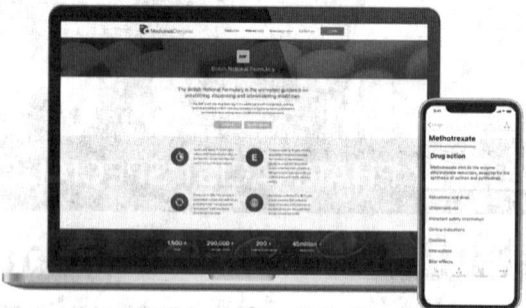

BNF

81

March –
September 2021

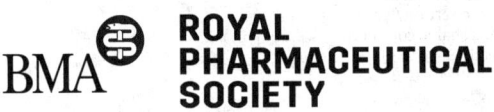

Published jointly by
BMJ Group
Tavistock Square, London, WC1H 9JP, UK
and

Pharmaceutical Press
Pharmaceutical Press is the publishing division of the Royal Pharmaceutical Society.
66-68 East Smithfield, London E1W 1AW, UK

Copyright © BMJ Group and the Royal Pharmaceutical Society of Great Britain 2021.

ISBN: 978 0 85711 410 5

ISBN: 978 0 85711 408 2 (ePDF)

Printed by GGP Media GmbH, Pößneck, Germany

Typeset by Data Standards Ltd, UK

Text design by Peter Burgess

A catalogue record for this book is available from the British Library.

Requesting copies of BNF Publications
Paper copies may be obtained through any bookseller or direct from:

Pharmaceutical Press
c/o Macmillan Distribution (MDL)
Hampshire International Business Park
Lime Tree Way
Basingstoke
Hampshire
RG24 8YJ
Tel: +44 (0) 1256 302 699
Fax: +44 (0) 1256 812 521
direct@macmillan.co.uk

or via our website www.pharmpress.com/

For all bulk orders of more than 20 copies:
Tel: +44 (0) 207 572 2266
pharmpress-support@rpharms.com

The BNF is available as a mobile app, online (bnf.nice.org.uk/) and also through MedicinesComplete; a PDA version is also available. In addition, BNF content can be integrated into a local formulary by using BNF on FormularyComplete; see www.bnf.org for details.

Distribution of printed BNFs
In **England**, NICE purchases print editions of the BNF (September editions only) for distribution within the NHS. For details of who is eligible to receive a copy and further contact details, please refer to the NICE website: www.nice.org.uk/about/what-we-do/evidence-services/british-national-formulary. If you are entitled to a shared copy of the BNF, please call (0)1268 495 609 or email: BNF@wilmingtonhealthcare.com.

In **Scotland**, email:
nss.psd-bnf@nhs.net

In **Wales**, email:
nwssp-primarycareservices@wales.nhs.uk

In **Northern Ireland**:
Primary care: contact the Business Services Organisation
Secondary care: contact your local Trust pharmacy department

About BNF content
The BNF is designed as a digest for rapid reference and it may not always include all the information necessary for prescribing and dispensing. Also, less detail is given on areas such as obstetrics, malignant disease, and anaesthesia since it is expected that those undertaking treatment will have specialist knowledge and access to specialist literature. BNF *for Children* should be consulted for detailed information on the use of medicines in children. The BNF should be interpreted in the light of professional knowledge and supplemented as necessary by specialised publications and by reference to the product literature. Information is also available from Medicines Information Services.

Please refer to digital versions of BNF for the most up-to-date content. BNF is published in print but interim updates are issued and published in the digital versions of BNF. The publishers work to ensure that the information is as accurate and up-to-date as possible at the date of publication, but knowledge and best practice in this field change regularly. BNF's accuracy and currency cannot be guaranteed and neither the publishers nor the authors accept any responsibility for errors or omissions. While considerable efforts have been made to check the material in this publication, it should be treated as a guide only. Prescribers, pharmacists and other healthcare professionals are advised to check www.bnf.org/ for information about key updates and corrections.

Pharmaid
Numerous requests have been received from developing countries for BNFs. The Pharmaid scheme of the Commonwealth Pharmacists Association will dispatch old BNFs to certain Commonwealth countries. For more information on this scheme see commonwealthpharmacy.org/what-we-do/pharmaid/. If you would like to donate your copy email: admin@commonwealthpharmacy.org

Preface

The BNF is a joint publication of the British Medical Association and the Royal Pharmaceutical Society. It is published under the authority of a Joint Formulary Committee which comprises representatives of the two professional bodies, the UK Health Departments, the Medicines and Healthcare products Regulatory Agency, and a national guideline producer. The Dental Advisory Group oversees the preparation of advice on the drug management of dental and oral conditions; the Group includes representatives of the British Dental Association and a representative from the UK Health Departments. The Nurse Prescribers' Advisory Group advises on the content relevant to nurses and includes representatives from different parts of the nursing community and from the UK Health Departments.

The BNF aims to provide prescribers, pharmacists, and other healthcare professionals with sound up-to-date information about the use of medicines.

The BNF includes key information on the selection, prescribing, dispensing and administration of medicines. Medicines generally prescribed in the UK are covered and those considered less suitable for prescribing are clearly identified. Little or no information is included on medicines promoted for purchase by the public.

Information on drugs is drawn from the manufacturers' product literature, medical and pharmaceutical literature, UK health departments, regulatory authorities, and professional bodies. Advice is constructed from clinical literature and reflects, as far as possible, an evaluation of the evidence from diverse sources. The BNF also takes account of authoritative national guidelines and emerging safety concerns. In addition, the editorial team receives advice on all therapeutic areas from expert clinicians; this ensures that the BNF's recommendations are relevant to practice.

The BNF is designed as a digest for rapid reference and it may not always include all the information necessary for prescribing and dispensing. Also, less detail is given on areas such as obstetrics, malignant disease, and anaesthesia since it is expected that those undertaking treatment will have specialist knowledge and access to specialist literature. Similarly, little or no information is included on medicines for very rare conditions. *BNF for Children* should be consulted for detailed information on the use of medicines in children. The BNF should be interpreted in the light of professional knowledge and supplemented as necessary by specialised publications and by reference to the product literature. Information is also available from medicines information services, see Medicines Information Services (see inside front cover).

It is **important** to use the most recent BNF information for making clinical decisions. The print edition of the BNF is updated in March and September each year. Monthly updates are provided online via Medicines Complete and the NHS Evidence portal. The more important changes are listed under Changes; changes listed online are cumulative (from one print edition to the next), and can be printed off each month to show the main changes since the last print edition as an aide memoire for those using print copies.

The BNF Publications website (www.bnf.org) includes additional information of relevance to healthcare professionals. Other digital formats of the BNF—including versions for mobile devices and integration into local formularies—are also available.

BNF Publications welcomes comments from healthcare professionals. Comments and constructive criticism should be sent to:

British National Formulary,
Royal Pharmaceutical Society,
66–68 East Smithfield
London
E1W 1AW
editor@bnf.org

The contact email for manufacturers or pharmaceutical companies wishing to contact BNF Publications is manufacturerinfo@bnf.org

Contents

Acknowledgements

The Joint Formulary Committee is grateful to individuals and organisations that have provided advice and information to the BNF.

Contributors for this update were:

K.W. Ah-See, M.N. Badminton, A.K. Bahl, D. Bilton, M.F. Bultitude, I.F. Burgess, C.E. Dearden, D.W. Denning, D.A.C. Elliman, P. Emery, A. Freyer, N.J.L. Gittoes, M. Gupta, T.L. Hawkins, S.P. Higgins, T.H. Lee, A. Lekkas, D.N.J. Lockwood, A.M. Lovering, M.G. Lucas, P.D. Mason, D.A. McArthur, L.M. Melvin, R.M. Mirakian, P. Morrison, S.M.S. Nasser, C. Nelson-Piercy, D.J. Nutt, R. Patel, A.B. Provan, A.S.C. Rice, D.J. Rowbotham, S.E. Slater, J. Soar, M.D. Stewart, S. Thomas, A.D. Weeks, A. Wilcock.

Expert advice on the management of oral and dental conditions was kindly provided by A. Crighton, C. Scully, R.A. Seymour, and R. Welbury. S. Kaur provided valuable advice on dental prescribing policy.

Valuable advice has been provided by the following expert groups: Advisory Committee on Malaria Prevention, Association of British Neurologists, British Association of Dermatologists' Therapy & Guidelines Sub-committee, British Geriatrics Society, British Menopause Society, British Society for Allergy & Clinical Immunology, British Society for Antimicrobial Chemotherapy, British Society of Gastroenterology, British Society of Rheumatology, College of Mental Health Pharmacy, ENT UK, Faculty of Sexual and Reproductive Healthcare, National Poisons Information Service & TOXBASE, Public Health England, Renal Association, Royal College of Anaesthetists, Royal College of Obstetricians and Gynaecologists, Royal College of Ophthalmologists, Royal College of Physicians, Royal College of Psychiatrists, Society for Endocrinology, UK Teratology Information Service, Vascular Society.

The MHRA have provided valuable assistance.

Correspondents in the pharmaceutical industry have provided information on new products and commented on products in the BNF.

Numerous doctors, pharmacists, nurses, and others have sent comments and suggestions.

The BNF team are grateful for the support and access to in-house expertise at Pharmaceutical Press and acknowledge the assistance of K. Baxter, A. Naylor, J. Macdonald, N. Potter and their teams.

This edition of the BNF carries a rainbow in recognition of the work and dedication of all frontline healthcare workers throughout the COVID-19 pandemic.

BNF Staff

Joint Formulary Committee

CHAIR
Fraz A. Mir
BSc, MA, MBBS, FRCP

COMMITTEE MEMBERS
Andy Burman (lay member)
CMgr, FCMI, FRSA, FIAM

Daniel Burrage
MRCP, MSc, PhD, FHEA

Jo Lyn Chooi
BMedSc, BM BS, FRCA

Carmel M. Darcy
BSc, MSc, IP, MPSNI, MRPharmS

Andrew Evans
BPharm, MPH, DipClinPharm, MRPharmS

Sue Faulding
BPharm, MSc, FRPharmS

Tracy Hall
BSc, MSc, RN, DN, NIP, Dip N, Cert N, QN

Lynn Haygarth
BPharm, MEd, FFRPS, FRPharmS, FCMHP

Simon Hurding
MB, ChB, MRCGP

Sandeep Kapur
BSc(Hons), MB BS, MRCGP(Dist)

Mark P. Lythgoe
MB BS, MRPharmS

Louise Picton
BSc, DipCommPharm, MSc, MRPharmS

Bernadette Rae
Pg Cert Ed, Fellow HEA, MSc Nursing, Pg CertANP, BSc(Hons), Grad Cert NMP, RGN

Muhammad Magdi Yaqoob
MD, FRCP

Dental Advisory Group

CHAIR
Sarah Manton
BDS, FDSRCS Ed, FHEA, PhD, FDFTEd

COMMITTEE MEMBERS
Andrew K. Brewer
BSc, BchD, MFDS (Glas)

Alexander Crighton
BDS, MB, ChB, FDS, OM

Michelle Moffat
BDS MFDS RCS Ed, M Paed Dent RCPS, FDS (Paed Dent) RCS Ed

Barbara Okpala
MPharm, PGDipHospPharm

Wendy Thompson
BSc(Hons), BDS, PhD, MFGDP, MCGDent

Kate Towers
BPharm (AU), GCClinPharm (AU)

SECRETARY
Arianne J. Matlin
MA, MSci, PhD

ADVICE ON DENTAL PRACTICE
The **British Dental Association** has contributed to the advice on medicines for dental practice through its representatives on the Dental Advisory Group.

Nurse Prescribers' Advisory Group

CHAIR
Molly Courtenay
PhD, MSc, Cert Ed, BSc, RGN

COMMITTEE MEMBERS
Penny M. Franklin
RN, RCN, RSCPHN(HV), MA, PGCE

Matt Griffiths
BA(Hons), FAETC, RGN, Cert A&E, NISP, PHECC

Tracy Hall
BSc, MSc, RN, DN, NIP, Dip N, Cert N, QN

Joan Myers
MSc, BSc, RGN, RSCN, Dip DN

Fiona Peniston-Bird
BSc(Hons), NIP, RHV, RGN

Kathy Radley
BSc, RGN

Kate Towers
BPharm (AU), GCClinPharm (AU)

How BNF Publications are constructed

Overview

The BNF is an independent professional publication that addresses the day-to-day prescribing information needs of healthcare professionals. Use of this resource throughout the health service helps to ensure that medicines are used safely, effectively, and appropriately.

Hundreds of changes are made between print editions, and are published monthly in a number of digital formats. The most clinically significant updates are listed under Changes p. xvi.

The BNF is unique in bringing together authoritative, independent guidance on best practice with clinically validated drug information. Validation of information follows a standardised process, reviewing emerging evidence, best-practice guidelines, and advice from a network of clinical experts. Where the evidence base is weak, further validation is undertaken through a process of peer review. The process and its governance are outlined in greater detail in the sections that follow.

Joint Formulary Committee

The Joint Formulary Committee (JFC) is responsible for the content of the BNF. The JFC includes pharmacy, medical, nursing and lay representatives; there are also representatives from the Medicines and Healthcare products Regulatory Agency (MHRA), the UK Health Departments, and a national guideline producer. The JFC decides on matters of policy and reviews amendments to the BNF in the light of new evidence and expert advice.

Dental Advisory Group

The Dental Advisory Group oversees the preparation of advice on the drug management of dental and oral conditions; the group includes representatives from the British Dental Association and a representative from the UK Health Departments.

Nurse Prescribers' Advisory Group

The Nurse Prescribers' Advisory Group oversees the list of drugs approved for inclusion in the Nurse Prescribers' Formulary; the group includes representatives from a range of nursing disciplines and stakeholder organisations.

Expert advisers

The BNF uses about 60 expert clinical advisers (including doctors, pharmacists, nurses, and dentists) throughout the UK to help with clinical content. The role of these expert advisers is to review existing text and to comment on amendments drafted by the clinical writers. These clinical experts help to ensure that the BNF remains reliable by:

- commenting on the relevance of the text in the context of best clinical practice in the UK;
- checking draft amendments for appropriate interpretation of any new evidence;
- providing expert opinion in areas of controversy or when reliable evidence is lacking;
- providing independent advice on drug interactions, prescribing in hepatic impairment, renal impairment, pregnancy, breast-feeding, children, the elderly, palliative care, and the emergency treatment of poisoning.

In addition to consulting with regular advisers, the BNF calls on other clinical specialists for specific developments when particular expertise is required.

The BNF works closely with a number of expert bodies that produce clinical guidelines. Drafts or pre-publication copies of guidelines are often received for comment and assimilation into the BNF.

Editorial team

BNF clinical writers have all worked as pharmacists or possess a pharmacy degree and a further, relevant post-graduate qualification, and have a sound understanding of how drugs are used in clinical practice. As a team, the clinical writers are responsible for editing, maintaining, and updating BNF content. They follow a systematic prioritisation process in response to updates to the evidence base in order to ensure the most clinically important topics are reviewed as quickly as possible. In parallel the team of clinical writers undertakes a process of rolling revalidation, aiming to review all of the content in the BNF over a 3- to 4-year period.

Amendments to the text are drafted when the clinical writers are satisfied that any new information is reliable and relevant. A set of standard criteria define when content is referred to expert advisers, the Joint Formulary Committee or other advisory groups, or submitted for peer review.

Clinical writers prepare the text for publication and undertake a number of validation checks on the knowledge at various stages of the production process.

Sources of BNF information

The BNF uses a variety of sources for its information; the main ones are shown below.

Summaries of product characteristics

The BNF reviews summaries of product characteristics (SPCs) of all new products as well as revised SPCs for existing products. The SPCs are the principal source of product information and are carefully processed. Such processing involves:

- verifying the approved names of all relevant ingredients including 'non-active' ingredients (the BNF is committed to using approved names and descriptions as laid down by the Human Medicine Regulations 2012);
- comparing the indications, cautions, contra-indications, and side-effects with similar existing drugs. Where these are different from the expected pattern, justification is sought for their inclusion or exclusion;
- seeking independent data on the use of drugs in pregnancy and breast-feeding;
- incorporating the information into the BNF using established criteria for the presentation and inclusion of the data;
- checking interpretation of the information by a second clinical writer before submitting to a content manager; changes relating to doses receive a further check;
- identifying potential clinical problems or omissions and seeking further information from manufacturers or from expert advisers;
- constructing, with the help of expert advisers, a comment on the role of the drug in the context of similar drugs.

Much of this processing is applicable to the following sources as well.

Literature

Clinical writers monitor core medical and pharmaceutical journals. Research papers and reviews relating to drug therapy are carefully processed. When a difference between the advice in the BNF and the paper is noted, the new information is assessed for reliability (using tools based on SIGN methodology) and relevance to UK clinical practice. If necessary, new text is drafted and discussed with expert advisers and the Joint Formulary Committee. The BNF enjoys a close working relationship with a number of national information providers.

In addition to the routine process, which is used to identify 'triggers' for changing the content, systematic literature searches are used to identify the best quality evidence available to inform an update. Clinical writers receive training in critical appraisal, literature evaluation, and search strategies.

Consensus guidelines

The advice in the BNF is checked against consensus guidelines produced by expert bodies. The quality of the guidelines is assessed using adapted versions of the AGREE II tool. A number of bodies make drafts or pre-publication copies of the guidelines available to the BNF; it is therefore possible to ensure that a consistent message is disseminated. The BNF routinely processes guidelines from the National Institute for Health and Care Excellence (NICE), the All Wales Medicines Strategy Group (AWMSG), the Scottish Medicines Consortium (SMC), and the Scottish Intercollegiate Guidelines Network (SIGN).

Reference sources

Textbooks and reference sources are used to provide background information for the review of existing text or for the construction of new text. The BNF team works closely with the editorial team that produces *Martindale: The Complete Drug Reference*. The BNF has access to *Martindale* information resources and each team keeps the other informed of significant developments and shifts in the trends of drug usage.

Peer review
Although every effort is made to identify the most robust data available, inevitably there are areas where the evidence base is weak or contradictory. While the BNF has the valuable support of expert advisers and the Joint Formulary Committee, the recommendations made may be subject to a further level of scrutiny through peer review to ensure they reflect best practice.

Content for peer review is posted on bnf.org and interested parties are notified via a number of channels, including the BNF e-newsletter.

Statutory information
The BNF routinely processes relevant information from various Government bodies including Statutory Instruments and regulations affecting the Prescriptions only Medicines Order. Official compendia such as the British Pharmacopoeia and its addenda are processed routinely to ensure that the BNF complies with the relevant sections of the Human Medicines Regulations 2012.

The BNF maintains close links with the Home Office (in relation to controlled drug regulations) and the Medicines and Healthcare products Regulatory Agency (including the British Pharmacopoeia Commission). Safety warnings issued by the Commission on Human Medicines (CHM) and guidelines on drug are issued by the UK health departments are processed as a matter of routine.

Relevant professional statements issued by the Royal Pharmaceutical Society are included in the BNF as are guidelines from bodies such as the Royal College of General Practitioners.

Medicines and devices
NHS Prescription Services (from the NHS Business Services Authority) provides non-clinical, categorical information (including prices) on the medicines and devices included in the BNF.

Comments from readers
Readers of the BNF are invited to send in comments. Numerous letters and emails are received by the BNF team. Such feedback helps to ensure that the BNF provides practical and clinically relevant information. Many changes in the presentation and scope of the BNF have resulted from comments sent in by users.

Comments from industry
Close scrutiny of BNF by the manufacturers provides an additional check and allows them an opportunity to raise issues about BNF's presentation of the role of various drugs; this is yet another check on the balance of BNF's advice. All comments are looked at with care and, where necessary, additional information and expert advice are sought.

Market research
Market research is conducted at regular intervals to gather feedback on specific areas of development.

Assessing the evidence
From January 2016, recommendations made in BNF publications have been evidence graded to reflect the strength of the recommendation. The addition of evidence grading is to support clinical decision making based on the best available evidence.

The BNF aims to revalidate all content over a rolling 3- to 4-year period and evidence grading will be applied to recommendations as content goes through the revalidation process. Therefore, initially, only a small number of recommendations will have been graded.

Recommendations from summaries of product characteristics
Recommendations from summaries of product characteristics (SPCs) and other product literature are either preceded by "manufacturer advises" or have the symbol M (manufacturer information) displayed next to the recommendation within the text.

Grading system
The BNF has adopted a five level grading system from A to E, based on the former SIGN grading system. This grade is displayed next to the recommendation within the text.

Evidence used to make a recommendation is assessed for validity using standardised methodology tools based on AGREE II and assigned a level of evidence. The recommendation is then given a grade that is extrapolated from the level of evidence, and an assessment of the body of evidence and its applicability.

Evidence assigned a level 1- or 2- score has an unacceptable level of bias or confounding and is not used to form recommendations.

Levels of evidence
- **Level 1++**
  High quality meta-analyses, systematic reviews of randomised controlled trials (RCTs), or RCTs with a very low risk of bias.

- **Level 1+**
  Well-conducted meta-analyses, systematic reviews, or RCTs with a low risk of bias.

- **Level 1-**
  Meta-analyses, systematic reviews, or RCTs with a high risk of bias.

- **Level 2++**
  High quality systematic reviews of case control or cohort studies; or high quality case control or cohort studies with a very low risk of confounding or bias and a high probability that the relationship is causal.

- **Level 2+**
  Well-conducted case control or cohort studies with a low risk of confounding or bias and a moderate probability that the relationship is causal.

- **Level 2-**
  Case control or cohort studies with a high risk of confounding or bias and a significant risk that the relationship is not causal.

- **Level 3**
  Non-analytic studies, e.g. case reports, case series.

- **Level 4**
  Expert advice or clinical experience from respected authorities.

Grades of recommendation
- **Grade A: High strength**
  NICE-accredited guidelines; or guidelines that pass AGREE II assessment; or at least one meta-analysis, systematic review, or RCT rated as 1++, and directly applicable to the target population; or a body of evidence consisting principally of studies rated as 1+, directly applicable to the target population, and demonstrating overall consistency of results.

- **Grade B: Moderate strength**
  A body of evidence including studies rated as 2++, directly applicable to the target population, and demonstrating overall consistency of results; or extrapolated evidence from studies rated as 1++ or 1+.

- **Grade C: Low strength**
  A body of evidence including studies rated as 2+, directly applicable to the target population and demonstrating overall consistency of results; or extrapolated evidence from studies rated as 2++.

- **Grade D: Very low strength**
  Evidence level 3; or extrapolated evidence from studies rated as 2+; or tertiary reference source created by a transparent, defined methodology, where the basis for recommendation is clear.

- **Grade E: Practice point**
  Evidence level 4.

How to use BNF Publications in print

How to use the BNF

This edition of the BNF continues to display the fundamental change to the structure of the content that was first shown in BNF 70. The changes were made to bring consistency and clarity to BNF content, and to the way that the content is arranged within print and digital products, increasing the ease with which information can be found.

For reference, the most notable changes to the structure of the content include:

- Drug monographs – where possible, all information that relates to a single drug is contained within its drug monograph, moving information previously contained in the prescribing notes. Drug monographs have also changed structurally: additional sections have been added, ensuring greater regularity around where information is located within the publication.
- Drug class monographs – where substantial amounts of information are common to all drugs within a drug class (e.g. macrolides p. 568), a drug class monograph has been created to contain the common information.
- Medicinal forms – categorical information about marketed medicines, such as price and pack size, continues to be sourced directly from the Dictionary of Medicines and Devices provided by the NHS Business Services Authority. However, clinical information curated by the BNF team has been clearly separated from the categorical pricing and pack size information and is included in the relevant section of the drug monograph.
- Section numbering – the BNF section numbering has been removed. This section numbering tied the content to a rigid structure and enforced the retention of defunct classifications, such as mercurial diuretics, and hindered the relocation of drugs where therapeutic use had altered. It also caused constraints between the BNF and BNF *for Children*, where drugs had different therapeutic uses in children.
- Appendix 4 – the content has been moved to individual drug monographs. The introductory notes have been replaced with a new guidance section, Guidance on intravenous infusions p. 16.

Introduction

In order to achieve the safe, effective, and appropriate use of medicines, healthcare professionals must be able to use the BNF effectively, and keep up to date with significant changes in the BNF that are relevant to their clinical practice. This *How to Use the BNF* is key in reinforcing the details of the new structure of the BNF to all healthcare professionals involved with prescribing, monitoring, supplying, and administering medicines, as well as supporting the learning of students training to join these professions.

Structure of the BNF

This BNF edition continues to broadly follows the high-level structure of earlier editions of the BNF (i.e. those published before BNF 70):

Front matter, comprising information on how to use the BNF, the significant content changes in each edition, and guidance on various prescribing matters (e.g. prescription writing, the use of intravenous drugs, particular considerations for special patient populations).

Chapters, containing drug monographs describing the uses, doses, safety issues and other considerations involved in the use of drugs; drug class monographs; and treatment summaries, covering guidance on the selection of drugs. Monographs and treatment summaries are divided into chapters based on specific aspects of medical care, such as Chapter 5, Infections, or Chapter 16, Emergency treatment

of poisoning; or drug use related to a particular system of the body, such as Chapter 2, Cardiovascular.

Within each chapter, content is organised alphabetically by therapeutic use (e.g. Airways disease, obstructive), with the treatment summaries first, (e.g. asthma), followed by the monographs of the drugs used to manage the conditions discussed in the treatment summary. Within each therapeutic use, the drugs are organised alphabetically by classification (e.g. Antimuscarinics, Beta$_2$-agonist bronchodilators) and then alphabetically within each classification (e.g. Aclidinium bromide, Glycopyrronium bromide, Ipratropium bromide).

Appendices, covering interactions, borderline substances, cautionary and advisory labels, and woundcare.

Back matter, covering the lists of medicines approved by the NHS for Dental and Nurse Practitioner prescribing, proprietary and specials manufacturers' contact details, and the index. Yellow cards are also included, to facilitate the reporting of adverse events, as well as quick reference guides for life support and key drug doses in medical emergencies, for ease of access.

Navigating the BNF

The contents page provides the high-level layout of information within the BNF; and in addition, each chapter begins with a small contents section, describing therapeutic uses covered within that chapter. Once in a chapter, location is guided by the side of the page showing the chapter number (the *thumbnail*), alongside the chapter title. The top of the page includes the therapeutic use (the *running head*) alongside the page number.

Once on a page, visual cues aid navigation: treatment summary information is in black type, with therapeutic use titles similarly styled in black, whereas the use of colour indicates drug-related information, including drug classification titles, drug class monographs, and drug monographs.

Although navigation is possible by browsing, primarily access to the information is via the index, which covers the titles of drug class monographs, drug monographs, and treatment summaries. The index also includes the names of branded medicines and other topics of relevance, such as abbreviations, guidance sections, tables, and images.

Content types

Treatment summaries

Treatment summaries are of three main types;

- an overview of delivering a drug to a particular body system (e.g. Skin conditions, management p. 1264)
- a comparison between a group or groups of drugs (e.g. beta-adrenoceptor blockers (systemic) p. 161)
- an overview of the drug management or prophylaxis of common conditions intended to facilitate rapid appraisal of options (e.g. Hypertension p. 153, or Malaria, prophylaxis p. 646).

In order to select safe and effective medicines for individual patients, information in the treatment summaries must be used in conjunction with other prescribing details about the drugs and knowledge of the patient's medical and drug history.

Monographs

Overview

In earlier editions (i.e. before BNF 70), a systemically administered drug with indications for use in different body systems was split across the chapters relating to those body systems. So, for example, codeine phosphate p. 475 was found in chapter 1, for its antimotility effects and chapter 4 for its analgesic effects. However, the monograph in chapter

1 contained only the dose and some selected safety precautions.

Now, all of the information for the systemic use of a drug is contained within one monograph, so codeine phosphate p. 475 is now included in chapter 4. This carries the advantage of providing all of the information in one place, so the user does not need to flick back and forth across several pages to find all of the relevant information for that drug. Cross references are included in chapter 1, where the management of diarrhoea is discussed, to the drug monograph to assist navigation.

Where drugs have systemic and local uses, for example, chloramphenicol, and the considerations around drug use are markedly different according to the route of administration, the monograph is split, as with earlier editions, into the relevant chapters.

This means that the majority of drugs are still placed in the same chapters and sections as earlier editions, and although there may be some variation in order, all of the relevant information will be easier to locate.

One of the most significant changes to the monograph structure is the increased granularity, with a move from around 9 sections to over 20 sections; sections are only included when relevant information has been identified. The following information describes these sections and their uses in more detail.

Nomenclature
Monograph titles follow the convention of recommended international non-proprietary names (rINNs), or, in the absence of a rINN, British Approved Names. Relevant synonyms are included below the title and, in some instances a brief description of the drug action is included. Over future editions these drug action statements will be rolled out for all drugs.

In some monographs, immediately below the nomenclature or drug action, there are a number of cross references or flags used to signpost the user to any additional information they need to consider about a drug. This is most common for drugs formulated in combinations, where users will be signposted to the monographs for the individual ingredients (e.g. senna with ispaghula husk p. 68) or for drugs that are related to a drug class monograph (see Drug class monographs, below).

Indication and dose
User feedback has highlighted that one of the main uses of the BNF is identifying indications and doses of drugs. Therefore, indication and dose information has been promoted to the top of the monograph and highlighted by a coloured panel to aid quick reference.

The indication and dose section is more highly structured than in earlier editions, giving greater clarity around which doses should be used for which indications and by which route. In addition, if the dose varies with a specific preparation or formulation, that dosing information has been moved out of the preparations section and in to the indication and dose panel, under a heading of the preparation name.

Doses are either expressed in terms of a definite frequency (e.g. 1 g 4 times daily) or in the total daily dose format (e.g. 6 g daily in 3 divided doses); the total daily dose should be divided into individual doses (in the second example, the patient should receive 2 g 3 times daily).

Doses for specific patient groups (e.g. the elderly) may be included if they are different to the standard dose. Doses for children can be identified by the relevant age range and may vary according to their age or body-weight.

In earlier editions of the BNF, age ranges and weight ranges overlapped. For clarity and to aid selection of the correct dose, wherever possible these age and weight ranges now do not overlap. When interpreting age ranges it is important to understand that a patient is considered to be 64 up until the point of their 65th birthday, meaning that an age

range of adult 18 to 64 is applicable to a patient from the day of their 18th birthday until the day before their 65th birthday. All age ranges should be interpreted in this way. Similarly, when interpreting weight ranges, it should be understood that a weight of up to 30 kg is applicable to a patient up to, but not including, the point that they tip the scales at 30 kg and a weight range of 35 to 59 kg is applicable to a patient as soon as they tip the scales at 35 kg right up until, but not including, the point that they tip the scales at 60 kg. All weight ranges should be interpreted in this way.

In all circumstances, it is important to consider the patient in question and their physical condition, and select the dose most appropriate for the individual.

Other information relevant to Indication and dose
The dose panel also contains, where known, an indication of **pharmacokinetic considerations** that may affect the choice of dose, and **dose equivalence** information, which may aid the selection of dose when switching between drugs or preparations.

The BNF includes **unlicensed use** of medicines when the clinical need cannot be met by licensed medicines; such use should be supported by appropriate evidence and experience. When the BNF recommends an unlicensed medicine or the 'off-label' use of a licensed medicine, this is shown below the indication and dose panel in the unlicensed use section.

Minimising harm and drug safety
The drug chosen to treat a particular condition should minimise the patient's susceptibility to adverse effects and, where co-morbidities exist, have minimal detrimental effects on the patient's other diseases. To achieve this, the *Contra-indications*, *Cautions* and *Side-effects* of the relevant drug should be reviewed.

The information under Cautions can be used to assess the risks of using a drug in a patient who has co-morbidities that are also included in the Cautions for that drug—if a safer alternative cannot be found, the drug may be prescribed while monitoring the patient for adverse-effects or deterioration in the co-morbidity. Contra-indications are far more restrictive than Cautions and mean that the drug should be avoided in a patient with a condition that is contra-indicated.

The impact that potential side-effects may have on a patient's quality of life should also be assessed. For instance, in a patient who has difficulty sleeping, it may be preferable to avoid a drug that frequently causes insomnia.

The *Important safety advice* section in the BNF, delineated by a coloured outline box, highlights important safety concerns, often those raised by regulatory authorities or guideline producers. Safety warnings issued by the Commission on Human Medicines (CHM) or Medicines and Healthcare products Regulatory Agency (MHRA) are found here.

Drug selection should aim to minimise drug interactions. If it is necessary to prescribe a potentially serious combination of drugs, patients should be monitored appropriately. The mechanisms underlying drug interactions are explained in Appendix 1, followed by details of drug interactions.

Use of drugs in specific patient populations
Drug selection should aim to minimise the potential for drug accumulation, adverse drug reactions, and exacerbation of pre-existing hepatic or renal disease. If it is necessary to prescribe drugs whose effect is altered by hepatic or renal disease, appropriate drug dose adjustments should be made, and patients should be monitored adequately. The general principles for prescribing are outlined under Prescribing in hepatic impairment p. 23, and Prescribing in renal impairment p. 23. Information about drugs that should be avoided or used with caution in hepatic disease or renal impairment can be found in drug monographs under *Hepatic impairment* and *Renal impairment* (e.g. fluconazole p. 634).

Typical layout of a monograph and associated medicinal forms

❶ Class Monographs and drug monographs

In most cases, all information that relates to an individual drug is contained in its drug monograph and there is no symbol. Class monographs have been created where substantial amounts of information are common to all drugs within a drug class, these are indicated by a flag symbol in a circle: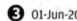

Drug monographs with a corresponding class monograph are indicated by a tab with a flag symbol: **⚑ 1234**

The page number of the corresponding class monograph is indicated within the tab. For further information, see How to use BNF Publications

❷ Drug classifications

Used to inform users of the class of a drug and to assist in finding other drugs of the same class. May be based on pharmacological class (e.g. opioids) but can also be associated with the use of the drug (e.g. cough suppressants)

❸ Review date

The date of last review of the content

❹ Specific preparation name

If the dose varies with a specific preparation or formulation it appears under a heading of the preparation name

---

Class monograph ❶

CLASSIFICATION ❷
⚑ 1234

| Drug monograph ❶   ❸ 01-Jun-2016

(Synonym) another name by which a drug may be known

- DRUG ACTION how a drug exerts its effect in the body

- **INDICATIONS AND DOSE**
  Indications are the clinical reasons a drug is used. The dose of a drug will often depend on the indications

  Indication
  ‣ ROUTE
  ‣ Age groups: [Child/Adult/Elderly]
  Dose and frequency of administration (max. dose)
  SPECIFIC PREPARATION NAME ❹
  Indication
  ‣ ROUTE
  ‣ Age groups: [Child/Adult/Elderly]
  Dose and frequency of administration (max. dose)
  DOSE ADJUSTMENTS DUE TO INTERACTIONS dosing information when used concurrently with other drugs
  DOSES AT EXTREMES OF BODY-WEIGHT dosing information for patients who are overweight or underweight
  DOSE EQUIVALENCE AND CONVERSION information around the bioequivalence between formulations of the same drug, or equivalent doses of drugs that are members of the same class
  PHARMACOKINETICS how the body affects a drug (absorption, distribution, metabolism, and excretion)
  POTENCY a measure of drug activity expressed in terms of the concentration required to produce an effect of given intensity

- UNLICENSED USE describes the use of medicines outside the terms of their UK licence (off-label use), or use of medicines that have no licence for use in the UK

> IMPORTANT SAFETY INFORMATION
> Information produced and disseminated by drug regulators often highlights serious risks associated with the use of a drug, and may include advice that is mandatory

- CONTRA-INDICATIONS circumstances when a drug should be avoided
- CAUTIONS details of precautions required
- INTERACTIONS when one drug changes the effects of another drug; the mechanisms underlying drug interactions are explained in Appendix 1
- SIDE-EFFECTS listed in order of frequency, where known, and arranged alphabetically
- ALLERGY AND CROSS-SENSITIVITY for drugs that carry an increased risk of hypersensitivity reactions
- CONCEPTION AND CONTRACEPTION potential for a drug to have harmful effects on an unborn child when prescribing for a woman of childbearing age or for a man trying to father a child; information on the effect of drugs on the efficacy of latex condoms or diaphragms

- PREGNANCY advice on the use of a drug during pregnancy
- BREAST FEEDING EvGr advice on the use of a drug during breast feeding ⟨A⟩ ❺
- HEPATIC IMPAIRMENT advice on the use of a drug in hepatic impairment
- RENAL IMPAIRMENT advice on the use of a drug in renal impairment
- PRE-TREATMENT SCREENING covers one off tests required to assess the suitability of a patient for a particular drug
- MONITORING REQUIREMENTS specifies any special monitoring requirements, including information on monitoring the plasma concentration of drugs with a narrow therapeutic index
- EFFECTS ON LABORATORY TESTS for drugs that can interfere with the accuracy of seemingly unrelated laboratory tests
- TREATMENT CESSATION specifies whether further monitoring or precautions are advised when the drug is withdrawn
- DIRECTIONS FOR ADMINISTRATION practical information on the preparation of intravenous drug infusions; general advice relevant to other routes of administration
- PRESCRIBING AND DISPENSING INFORMATION practical information around how a drug can be prescribed and dispensed including details of when brand prescribing is necessary
- HANDLING AND STORAGE includes information on drugs that can cause adverse effects to those who handle them before they are taken by, or administered to, a patient; advice on storage conditions
- PATIENT AND CARER ADVICE for drugs with a special need for counselling
- PROFESSION SPECIFIC INFORMATION provides details of the restrictions certain professions such as dental practitioners or nurse prescribers need to be aware of when prescribing on the NHS
- NATIONAL FUNDING/ACCESS DECISIONS references to NICE Technology Appraisals, SMC advice and AWMSG advice
- LESS SUITABLE FOR PRESCRIBING preparations that are considered by the Joint Formulary Committee to be less suitable for prescribing
- EXCEPTION TO LEGAL CATEGORY advice and information on drugs which may be sold without a prescription under specific conditions

- MEDICINAL FORMS
  Form
  CAUTIONARY AND ADVISORY LABELS if applicable
  EXCIPIENTS clinically important but not comprehensive [consult manufacturer information for full details]
  ELECTROLYTES if clinically significant quantities occur
  ▸ Preparation name (Manufacturer/Non-proprietary)
    Drug name and strength pack sizes PoM ❻ Prices

  Combinations available this indicates a combination preparation is available and a cross reference page number is provided to locate this preparation

❺ Evidence grading

Evidence grading to reflect the strengths of recommendations will be applied as content goes through the revalidation process. A five level evidence grading system based on the former SIGN grading system has been adopted. The grades ⟨A⟩ ⟨B⟩ ⟨C⟩ ⟨D⟩ ⟨E⟩ are displayed next to the recommendations within the text, and are preceded by the symbol: EvGr

The symbol ⟨M⟩ indicates manufacturer information

For further information, see How BNF Publications are constructed

❻ Legal categories

PoM This symbol has been placed against those preparations that are available only on a prescription issued by an appropriate practitioner. For more detailed information see *Medicines, Ethics and Practice*, London, Pharmaceutical Press (always consult latest edition)

CD1 CD2 CD3 CD4-1 CD4-2 CD5 These symbols indicate that the preparations are subject to the prescription requirements of the Misuse of Drugs Act

For regulations governing prescriptions for such preparations, see Controlled Drugs and Drug Dependence

Not all monographs include all possible sections; sections are only included when relevant information has been identified

Similarly, drug selection should aim to minimise harm to the fetus, nursing infant, and mother. The infant should be monitored for potential side-effects of drugs used by the *mother during pregnancy or breast-feeding*. The general principles for prescribing are outlined under Prescribing in pregnancy p. 27 and Prescribing in breast-feeding p. 27. The Treatment Summaries provide guidance on the drug treatment of common conditions that can occur during pregnancy and breast-feeding (e.g. Asthma, acute p. 256). Information about the use of specific drugs during pregnancy and breast-feeding can be found in their drug monographs under *Pregnancy*, and *Breast-feeding* (e.g. fluconazole p. 634).

A section, *Conception and contraception*, containing information around considerations for females of childbearing potential or men who might father a child (e.g. isotretinoin p. 1314) has been included.

Administration and monitoring
When selecting the most appropriate drug, it may be necessary to screen the patient for certain genetic markers or metabolic states. This information is included within a section called *Pre-treatment screening* (e.g. abacavir p. 685). This section covers one-off tests required to assess the suitability of a patient for a particular drug.

Once the drug has been selected, it needs to be given in the most appropriate manner. A *Directions for administration* section contains the information about intravenous administration previously located in Appendix 4. This provides practical information on the preparation of intravenous drug infusions, including compatibility of drugs with standard intravenous infusion fluids, method of dilution or reconstitution, and administration rates. In addition, general advice relevant to other routes of administration is provided within this section (e.g. fentanyl p. 478).

After selecting and administering the most appropriate drug by the most appropriate route, patients should be monitored to ensure they are achieving the expected benefits from drug treatment without any unwanted side-effects. The *Monitoring* section specifies any special monitoring requirements, including information on monitoring the plasma concentration of drugs with a narrow therapeutic index (e.g. theophylline p. 289). Monitoring may, in certain cases, be affected by the impact of a drug on laboratory tests (e.g. hydroxocobalamin p. 1072), and this information is included in *Effects on laboratory tests*.

In some cases, when a drug is withdrawn, further monitoring or precautions may be advised (e.g. clonidine hydrochloride p. 159): these are covered under *Treatment cessation*.

Choice and supply
The prescriber and the patient should agree on the health outcomes that the patient desires and on the strategy for achieving them (see *Taking Medicines to Best Effect*). Taking the time to explain to the patient (and carers) the rationale and the potential adverse effects of treatment may improve adherence. For some medicines there is a special need for counselling (e.g. appropriate posture during administration of doxycycline p. 601); this is shown in *Patient and carer advice*.

Other information contained in the latter half of the monograph also helps prescribers and those dispensing medicines choose medicinal forms (by indicating information such as flavour or when branded products may not be interchangeable (e.g. diltiazem hydrochloride p. 171), assess the suitability of a drug for prescribing, understand the NHS funding status for a drug (e.g. sildenafil p. 860), or assess when a patient may be able to purchase a drug without prescription (e.g. loperamide hydrochloride p. 72).

Medicinal forms
In the BNF, preparations follow immediately after the monograph for the drug that is their main ingredient.

In earlier editions, when a particular preparation had safety information, dose advice or other clinical information specific to the product, it was contained within the preparations section. This information has been moved to the relevant section in the main body of the monograph under a heading of the name of the specific medicinal form (e.g. peppermint oil p. 52).

The medicinal forms (formerly preparations) section provides information on the type of formulation (e.g. tablet), the amount of active drug in a solid dosage form, and the concentration of active drug in a liquid dosage form. The legal status is shown for prescription-only medicines and controlled drugs, as well as pharmacy medicines and medicines on the general sales list. Practitioners are reminded, by a statement under the heading of "Medicinal Forms" that not all products containing a specific drug ingredient may be similarly licensed. To be clear on the precise licensing status of specific medicinal forms, practitioners should check the product literature for the particular product being prescribed or dispensed.

Details of all medicinal forms available on the dm+d for each drug in BNF Publications appears online on MedicinesComplete. In print editions, due to space constraints, only certain branded products are included in detail. Where medicinal forms are listed they should not be inferred as equivalent to the other brands listed under the same form heading. For example, all the products listed under a heading of "Modified release capsule" will be available as modified release capsules, however, the brands listed under that form heading may have different release profiles, the available strengths may vary and/or the products may have different licensing information. As with earlier editions of the BNF, practitioners must ensure that the particular product being prescribed or dispensed is appropriate.

As medicinal forms are derived from dm+d data, some drugs may appear under names derived from that data; this may vary slightly from those in previous BNF versions, e.g. sodium acid phosphate, is now sodium dihydrogen phosphate anhydrous.

Patients should be prescribed a preparation that complements their daily routine, and that provides the right dose of drug for the right indication and route of administration. When dispensing liquid preparations, a sugar-free preparation should always be used in preference to one containing sugar. Patients receiving medicines containing cariogenic sugars should be advised of appropriate dental hygiene measures to prevent caries.

In earlier editions, the BNF only included excipients and electrolyte information for proprietary medicines. This information is now covered at the level of the dose form (e.g. tablet). It is not possible to keep abreast of all of the generic products available on the UK market, and so this information serves as a reminder to the healthcare professional that, if the presence of a particular excipient is of concern, they should check the product literature for the particular product being prescribed or dispensed.

Cautionary and advisory labels that pharmacists are recommended to add when dispensing are included in the medicinal forms section. Details of these labels can be found in Appendix 3, Guidance for cautionary and advisory labels p. 1656. As these labels have now been applied at the level of the dose form, a full list of medicinal products with their relevant labels would be extensive. This list has therefore been removed, but the information is retained within the monograph.

In the case of compound preparations, the prescribing information for all constituents should be taken into account.

Prices in the BNF
Basic NHS **net prices** are given in the BNF to provide an indication of relative cost. Where there is a choice of suitable

preparations for a particular disease or condition the relative cost may be used in making a selection. Cost-effective prescribing must, however, take into account other factors (such as dose frequency and duration of treatment) that affect the total cost. The use of more expensive drugs is justified if it will result in better treatment of the patient, or a reduction of the length of an illness, or the time spent in hospital.

Prices are regularly updated using the Drug Tariff and proprietary price information published by the NHS dictionary of medicines and devices (dm+d, www.nhsbsa.nhs.uk/pharmacies-gp-practices-and-appliance-contractors/dictionary-medicines-and-devices-dmd). The weekly updated dm+d data (including prices) can be accessed using the dm+d browser of the NHS Business Services Authority (apps.nhsbsa.nhs.uk/DMDBrowser/DMDBrowser.do). Prices have been calculated from the net cost used in pricing NHS prescriptions and generally reflect whole dispensing packs. Prices for extemporaneously prepared preparations are not provided in the BNF as prices vary between different manufacturers. In Appendix 4, prices stated are per dressing or bandage.

BNF prices are not suitable for quoting to patients seeking private prescriptions or contemplating over-the-counter purchases because they do not take into account VAT, professional fees, and other overheads.

A fuller explanation of costs to the NHS may be obtained from the Drug Tariff. Separate drug tariffs are applicable to England and Wales (www.ppa.org.uk/ppa/edt_intro.htm), Scotland (www.isdscotland.org/Health-Topics/Prescribing-and-Medicines/Scottish-Drug-Tariff/), and Northern Ireland (www.hscbusiness.hscni.net/services/2034.htm); prices in the different tariffs may vary.

Drug class monographs

In earlier editions of the BNF, information relating to a class of drugs sharing the same properties (e.g. tetracyclines p. 600), was contained within the prescribing notes. In the updated structure, drug class monographs have been created to contain the common information; this ensures such information is easier to find, and has a more regularised structure.

For consistency and ease of use, the class monograph follows the same structure as a drug monograph. Class monographs are indicated by the presence of a flag ⊝ (e.g. beta-adrenoceptor blockers (systemic) p. 161). If a drug monograph has a corresponding class monograph, that needs to be considered in tandem, in order to understand the full information about a drug, the monograph is also indicated by a flag ◢⬛1234 (e.g. metoprolol tartrate p. 169). Within this flag, the page number of the drug class monograph is provided (e.g. 1234), to help navigate the user to this information. This is particularly useful where occasionally, due to differences in therapeutic use, the drug monograph may not directly follow the drug class monograph (e.g. sotalol hydrochloride p. 116).

Other content

Nutrition

Appendix 2, Borderline substances p. 1622, includes tables of ACBS-approved enteral feeds and nutritional supplements based on their energy and protein content. There are separate tables for specialised formulae for specific clinical conditions. Classified sections on foods for special diets and nutritional supplements for metabolic diseases are also included.

Wound dressings

A table on wound dressings in Appendix 4, Wound management products and elasticated garments p. 1659, allows an appropriate dressing to be selected based on the appearance and condition of the wound. Further information about the dressing can be found by following the cross-reference to the relevant classified section in the Appendix.

Advanced wound contact dressings have been classified in order of increasing absorbency.

Other useful information

Finding significant changes in the BNF

- **Changes**, provides a list of significant changes, dose changes, classification changes, new names, and new preparations that have been incorporated into the BNF, as well as a list of preparations that have been discontinued and removed from the BNF. Changes listed online are cumulative (from one print edition to the next), and can be printed off each month to show the main changes since the last print edition as an aide memoire for those using print copies. So many changes are made for each update of the BNF, that not all of them can be accommodated in the *Changes* section. We encourage healthcare professionals to regularly review the prescribing information on drugs that they encounter frequently;

- **Changes to the Dental Practioners' Formulary**, are located at the end of the Dental List;

- **E-newsletter**, the BNF & BNF *for Children* e-newsletter service is available free of charge. It alerts healthcare professionals to details of significant changes in the clinical content of these publications and to the way that this information is delivered. Newsletters also review clinical case studies, provide tips on using these publications effectively, and highlight forthcoming changes to the publications. To sign up for e-newsletters go to www.bnf.org.

Using other sources for medicines information

The BNF is designed as a digest for rapid reference. Less detail is given on areas such as obstetrics, malignant disease, and anaesthesia since it is expected that those undertaking treatment will have specialist knowledge and access to specialist literature. BNF *for Children* should be consulted for detailed information on the use of medicines in children. The BNF should be interpreted in the light of professional knowledge and supplemented as necessary by specialised publications and by reference to the product literature. Information is also available from medicines information services.

Changes

Monthly updates are provided online via Medicines Complete and the NHS Evidence portal. The changes listed below are cumulative (from one print edition to the next).

Significant changes

Significant changes that appear in the print edition of BNF 81 (March – September 2021):

- Aflibercept p. 1054: Systemically administered VEGF pathway inhibitors: risk of aneurysm and artery dissection [MHRA/CHM advice].
- Amisulpride p. 414: Clozapine and other antipsychotics: monitoring blood concentrations for toxicity [MHRA/CHM advice].
- Amphotericin: name change to amphotericin B p. 632.
- Amphotericin B p. 632: Liposomal and lipid-complex formulations: name change to reduce medication errors [MHRA/CHM advice].
- Andexanet alfa p. 131 for adults treated with apixaban or rivaroxaban when reversal of anticoagulation is needed due to life-threatening or uncontrolled bleeding [SMC guidance].
- Andexanet alfa p. 131 (*Ondexxya®*): Commercial anti-FXa activity assays are unsuitable for measuring anti-FXa activity following administration of andexanet alfa [MHRA/CHM advice].
- Antibacterials, use for prophylaxis p. 529: updated guidance for the prevention of secondary *Haemophilus influenzae* type b disease.
- Apixaban p. 136: Direct-acting oral anticoagulants (DOACs): reminder of bleeding risk, availability of reversal agents [MHRA/CHM advice].
- Aripiprazole p. 415: Clozapine and other antipsychotics: monitoring blood concentrations for toxicity [MHRA/CHM advice].
- Atezolizumab p. 907 (*Tecentriq®*) in combination with carboplatin and etoposide, is indicated for the first-line treatment of adult patients with extensive-stage small cell lung cancer [SMC guidance].
- Atezolizumab p. 907 (*Tecentriq®*) in combination with nab-paclitaxel for the treatment of adult patients with unresectable locally advanced or metastatic triple-negative breast cancer whose tumours have PD-L1 expression at a level of 1 % or more and who have not received prior chemotherapy for metastatic disease [SMC guidance].
- Atezolizumab p. 907 (*Tecentriq®*) with carboplatin and etoposide for untreated extensive-stage small-cell lung cancer [NICE guidance].
- Atezolizumab p. 907 (*Tecentriq®*) with nab-paclitaxel for untreated PD-L1-positive, locally advanced or metastatic, triple-negative breast cancer [NICE guidance].
- Avatrombopag p. 1079 for treating thrombocytopenia in people with chronic liver disease needing a planned invasive procedure [NICE guidance].
- Avelumab p. 908 (*Bavencio®*) in combination with axitinib for the first-line treatment of adult patients with advanced renal cell carcinoma [SMC guidance].
- Avelumab p. 908 with axitinib p. 1013 for untreated advanced renal cell carcinoma [NICE guidance].
- Axitinib p. 1013: Systemically administered VEGF pathway inhibitors: risk of aneurysm and artery dissection [MHRA/CHM advice].
- Baricitinib p. 1152 (*Olumiant®* ▼): increased risk of diverticulitis, particularly in patients with risk factors [MHRA/CHM advice].
- Bedaquiline p. 622 in combination regimen for multiple-drug resistant pulmonary tuberculosis [AWMSG guidance].
- Bevacizumab p. 909: Systemically administered VEGF pathway inhibitors: risk of aneurysm and artery dissection [MHRA/CHM advice].

- Bisacodyl p. 65: Stimulant laxatives (bisacodyl, senna and sennosides, sodium picosulfate) available over-the-counter: new measures to support safe use [MHRA/CHM advice].
- BNF updates for Community Practitioner Nurse Prescribers: For *BNF app and online versions of the BNF*- list of medicinal preparations (renamed as Approved list for prescribing by Community Practitioner Nurse Prescribers (NPF) p. 1685) updated with indications for use by Community Practitioner Nurse Prescribers and links to BNF monographs; general guidance and treatment summaries for use by Community Practitioner Nurse Prescribers have also been added. For *BNF print editions*- list of medicinal preparations (Nurse Prescribers' Formulary (NPF)) updated with indications for use by Community Practitioner Nurse Prescribers and cross-references to BNF monographs. For further information, see *How to use the NPF* above the list of medicinal preparations.
- Brentuximab vedotin p. 911 in combination for untreated systemic anaplastic large cell lymphoma [NICE guidance].
- Brolucizumab p. 1234 for the treatment of adults with neovascular (wet) age-related macular degeneration [SMC guidance].
- Budesonide p. 48 (*Jorveza®*) for the treatment of eosinophilic oesophagitis in adults [SMC guidance].
- Bupropion hydrochloride p. 520 (*Zyban®*): risk of serotonin syndrome with use with other serotonergic drugs [MHRA/CHM advice].
- Cabozantinib p. 1016: Systemically administered VEGF pathway inhibitors: risk of aneurysm and artery dissection [MHRA/CHM advice].
- Cannabidiol p. 326 with clobazam for therapy of seizures associated with Dravet syndrome [SMC guidance].
- Cannabidiol p. 326 with clobazam for therapy of seizures associated with Lennox-Gastaut syndrome [SMC guidance].
- Capecitabine p. 950: Fluorouracil (i.v.), capecitabine and tegafur containing products: Pre-treatment testing to identify DPD-deficient patients at increased risk of severe and fatal toxicity [MHRA/CHM advice].
- Caplacizumab p. 1080 for the treatment of adults with acquired thrombotic thrombocytopenic purpura [SMC guidance].
- Carfilzomib p. 1007 for previously treated multiple myeloma [NICE guidance].
- Carfilzomib p. 1007 (*Kyprolis®*) in combination with lenalidomide and dexamethasone for the treatment of adult patients with multiple myeloma who have received at least one prior therapy [for patients who have received only one prior therapy] [SMC guidance].
- Cariprazine p. 416 for the treatment of schizophrenia [AWMSG guidance].
- Clozapine p. 417: Clozapine and other antipsychotics: monitoring blood concentrations for toxicity [MHRA/CHM advice].
- Cyproterone acetate p. 812: new advice to minimise risk of meningioma [MHRA/CHM advice].
- Cyproterone acetate p. 812: Restrictions in use of cyproterone acetate due to risk of meningioma (letter) [MHRA/CHM advice].
- Cytarabine p. 953: Liposomal and lipid-complex formulations: name change to reduce medication errors [MHRA/CHM advice].
- Dabigatran etexilate p. 148: Direct-acting oral anticoagulants (DOACs): reminder of bleeding risk, availability of reversal agents [MHRA/CHM advice].
- Daratumumab p. 913 (*Darzalex®*) subcutaneous injection as monotherapy, for the treatment of adult patients with

relapsed and refractory multiple myeloma, whose prior therapy included a proteasome inhibitor and an immunomodulatory agent and have demonstrated disease progression on the last therapy [SMC guidance].

- Daratumumab p. 913 (*Darzalex*®) subcutaneous injection in combination with lenalidomide and dexamethasone, or bortezomib and dexamethasone, for the treatment of adult patients with multiple myeloma who have received at least one prior therapy [SMC guidance].

- Darolutamide p. 991 (*Nubeqa*®) for the treatment of adult men with non-metastatic castration-resistant prostate cancer who are at high risk of developing metastatic disease [SMC guidance].

- Darolutamide p. 991 with androgen deprivation therapy for treating hormone-relapsed non-metastatic prostate cancer [NICE guidance].

- Darunavir with cobicistat p. 695 (*Rezolsta*®) in combination with other antiretroviral medicinal products for the treatment of human immunodeficiency virus-1 (HIV-1) infection in adults and adolescents (aged 12 years and older with body weight at least 40 kg) [AWMSG guidance].

- Daunorubicin p. 944: Liposomal and lipid-complex formulations: name change to reduce medication errors [MHRA/CHM advice].

- Daunorubicin with cytarabine p. 945: Liposomal and lipid-complex formulations: name change to reduce medication errors [MHRA/CHM advice].

- Denosumab p. 774 60 mg (*Prolia*®): increased risk of multiple vertebral fractures after stopping or delaying ongoing treatment [MHRA/CHM advice].

- Dolutegravir p. 680 (*Tivicay*® ▼, *Triumeq*® ▼, *Juluca*® ▼): updated advice on increased risk of neural tube defects [MHRA/CHM advice].

- Doravirine p. 683 in combination with other antiretroviral drugs for the treatment of adults infected with HIV-1 [AWMSG guidance].

- Doxorubicin hydrochloride p. 946: Liposomal and lipid-complex formulations: name change to reduce medication errors [MHRA/CHM advice].

- Edoxaban p. 137: Direct-acting oral anticoagulants (DOACs): reminder of bleeding risk, availability of reversal agents [MHRA/CHM advice].

- Emtricitabine with tenofovir disoproxil p. 690 for pre-exposure prophylaxis to reduce the risk of sexually acquired HIV-1 infection [AWMSG guidance].

- Entrectinib p. 1023 for treating NTRK fusion-positive solid tumours [NICE guidance].

- Entrectinib p. 1023 for treating ROS1-positive advanced non-small-cell lung cancer [NICE guidance].

- Esketamine p. 1393 for adults with treatment-resistant major depressive disorder [SMC guidance].

- Eye p. 1203: updated guidance for expiration of eye preparations.

- Fentanyl p. 478 transdermal patches for non-cancer pain: do not use in opioid-naive patients [MHRA/CHM advice].

- Ferric carboxymaltose p. 1067 (*Ferinject*® ▼): risk of symptomatic hypophosphataemia leading to osteomalacia and fractures [MHRA/CHM advice].

- Flucytosine p. 639 (*Ancotil*®): new contra-indication in patients with DPD deficiency [MHRA/CHM advice].

- Flucytosine p. 639: Updated recommendations for the use in patients with dihydropyrimidine dehydrogenase (DPD) deficiency [MHRA/CHM advice].

- Fluocinolone acetonide p. 1236 for prevention of relapse in recurrent non-infectious uveitis affecting the posterior segment of the eye [SMC guidance].

- 5-Fluorouracil (intravenous), capecitabine, tegafur: DPD testing recommended before initiation to identify patients at increased risk of severe and fatal toxicity [MHRA/CHM advice] (advice in fluorouracil p. 955, capecitabine p. 950, and tegafur with gimeracil and oteracil p. 961).

- Fremanezumab p. 498 for preventing migraine [NICE guidance].

- Galcanezumab p. 498 for preventing migraine [NICE guidance].

- Genital system infections, antibacterial therapy p. 536: updated guidance for the management of uncomplicated gonorrhoea.

- Gilteritinib p. 1027 for the treatment of adults who have relapsed or refractory acute myeloid leukaemia with a FLT3 mutation [SMC guidance].

- Gilteritinib p. 1027 for treating relapsed or refractory acute myeloid leukaemia [NICE guidance].

- Haemophilus influenzae type b conjugate vaccine p. 1344: updated guidance in-line with Public Health England recommendations.

- Hepatitis A vaccine p. 1345: updated guidance in-line with Public Health England recommendations.

- Hydroxycarbamide p. 977 for the prevention of vaso-occlusive complications of sickle-cell disease in patients over 2 years of age [AWMSG guidance].

- Hydroxycarbamide p. 977 for the prevention of vaso-occlusive complications of sickle-cell disease in patients over 2 years of age [SMC guidance].

- Hyperthyroidism p. 813: updated guidance on management.

- Hypothyroidism p. 816: updated guidance on management.

- Ibrutinib p. 1027 (*Imbruvica*®) in combination with rituximab for the treatment of adult patients with Waldenström's macroglobulinaemia [SMC guidance].

- Immunisation schedule p. 1341: updated National flu immunisation programme in-line with Public Health England recommendations.

- Immunoglobulins p. 1331: updated guidance in-line with Public Health England recommendations for the use of normal immunoglobulin for protection against hepatitis A infection.

- Immunoglobulins p. 1331: updated guidance on the use of varicella-zoster immunoglobulin in-line with Public Health England recommendations.

- Influenza p. 699: updated guidance on management.

- Influenza vaccine p. 1348: updated guidance in-line with Public Health England recommendations.

- Insulins (all types): risk of cutaneous amyloidosis at injection site [MHRA/CHM advice] (advice in biphasic insulin aspart, biphasic insulin lispro, biphasic isophane insulin, insulin, insulin aspart, insulin degludec, insulin detemir, insulin glargine, insulin glulisine, insulin lispro, isophane insulin; see Insulins p. 752).

- Interactions: drugs that cause myelosuppression: pharmacodynamic effects drug group revalidated and updated.

- Introduction of a new symbol to indicate manufacturer information: the symbol M (manufacturer information) will be used within text to indicate when recommendations are based on summaries of product characteristics; see How BNF Publications are constructed p. viii.

- Irinotecan hydrochloride p. 970: Liposomal and lipid-complex formulations: name change to reduce medication errors [MHRA/CHM advice].

- Isatuximab p. 918 with pomalidomide and dexamethasone for treating relapsed and refractory multiple myeloma [NICE guidance].

- Isotretinoin p. 1314 (*Roaccutane*® ▼): reminder of important risks and precautions [MHRA/CHM advice].

- Ketotifen p. 1205 for the symptomatic treatment of seasonal allergic conjunctivitis [AWMSG guidance].

- Lamivudine with tenofovir disoproxil and doravirine p. 692 for the treatment of adults infected with HIV-1 [AWMSG guidance].

- Larotrectinib p. 1031 for treating NTRK fusion-positive solid tumours [NICE guidance].
- Lenalidomide p. 1001: Immunomodulatory drugs and pregnancy prevention: temporary advice for management during coronavirus (COVID-19) [MHRA/CHM advice].
- Lenalidomide p. 1001 (*Revlimid*®) as monotherapy for the maintenance treatment of adult patients with newly diagnosed multiple myeloma who have undergone autologous stem cell transplantation [SMC guidance].
- Lenalidomide p. 1001 (*Revlimid*®) in combination with rituximab (anti-CD20 antibody) for the treatment of adult patients with previously treated follicular lymphoma (Grade 1 to 3a) [SMC guidance].
- Lenvatinib p. 1031: Systemically administered VEGF pathway inhibitors: risk of aneurysm and artery dissection [MHRA/CHM advice].
- Lorlatinib p. 1033 for previously treated ALK-positive advanced non-small-cell lung cancer [NICE guidance].
- Meropenem with vaborbactam p. 550 (*Vaborem*®) for the treatment of: complicated urinary tract infection; complicated intra-abdominal infection; hospital-acquired pneumonia; bacteraemia that occurs in association with, or is suspected to be associated with, any of these infections; infections due to aerobic Gram-negative organisms in adults with limited treatment options [AWMSG and SMC guidance].
- Methotrexate p. 957 once-weekly for autoimmune diseases: new measures to reduce risk of fatal overdose due to inadvertent daily instead of weekly dosing [MHRA/CHM advice].
- Modafinil p. 513 (*Provigil*®): increased risk of congenital malformations if used during pregnancy [MHRA/CHM advice].
- Naldemedine p. 70 for treating opioid-induced constipation [NICE guidance].
- National funding decisions: advice from NICE, SMC, and AWMSG now briefly referenced in relevant monographs— funding body website should be accessed for full details; see Guidance on prescribing p. 1.
- Neratinib p. 1034 for the extended adjuvant treatment of adult patients with early-stage hormone receptor positive HER2-overexpressed/amplified breast cancer [SMC guidance].
- Nintedanib p. 1036: Systemically administered VEGF pathway inhibitors: risk of aneurysm and artery dissection [MHRA/CHM advice].
- Niraparib p. 1050 (*Zejula*® ▼): reports of severe hypertension and posterior reversible encephalopathy syndrome (PRES), particularly in early treatment [MHRA/CHM advice].
- Nivolumab p. 920 for advanced squamous non-small-cell lung cancer after chemotherapy [NICE guidance].
- Obinutuzumab p. 922 with bendamustine for treating follicular lymphoma after rituximab [NICE guidance].
- Olanzapine p. 419: Clozapine and other antipsychotics: monitoring blood concentrations for toxicity [MHRA/CHM advice].
- Olanzapine embonate p. 425: Clozapine and other antipsychotics: monitoring blood concentrations for toxicity [MHRA/CHM advice].
- Opioids: risk of dependence and addiction [MHRA/CHM advice] (advice in alfentanil, buprenorphine, co-codamol, codeine phosphate, co-phenotrope, diamorphine hydrochloride, dihydrocodeine tartrate, fentanyl, hydromorphone hydrochloride, kaolin with morphine, meptazinol, methadone hydrochloride, morphine, oxycodone hydrochloride, pentazocine, pethidine hydrochloride, remifentanil, tapentadol, tramadol hydrochloride; see Opioids p. 467).
- Osimertinib p. 1037 for treating EGFR T790M mutation-positive advanced non-small-cell lung cancer [NICE guidance].
- Osimertinib p. 1037 for untreated EGFR mutation-positive non-small-cell lung cancer [NICE guidance].
- Osteoporosis p. 765: updated guidance on management.
- Patiromer calcium p. 1104 (*Veltassa*®) for the treatment of hyperkalaemia in adults [SMC guidance].
- Pazopanib p. 1039: Systemically administered VEGF pathway inhibitors: risk of aneurysm and artery dissection [MHRA/CHM advice].
- Pembrolizumab p. 923 for the treatment of metastatic or unresectable recurrent head and neck squamous cell carcinoma [SMC guidance].
- Pembrolizumab p. 923 for untreated metastatic or unresectable recurrent head and neck squamous cell carcinoma [NICE guidance].
- Pembrolizumab p. 923 with axitinib for first-line treatment of advanced renal cell carcinoma [SMC guidance].
- Pembrolizumab p. 923 with axitinib p. 1013 for untreated advanced renal cell carcinoma [NICE guidance].
- Peri-operative analgesia p. 1392: updated guidance for the management of postoperative pain.
- Pertuzumab p. 925 in combination with trastuzumab and chemotherapy for the treatment of adults with HER2-positive early breast cancer [SMC guidance].
- Pirfenidone p. 314 (*Esbriet*®): risk of serious liver injury; updated advice on liver function testing [MHRA/CHM advice].
- Poisoning, emergency treatment p. 1413: updated guidance on the management of paracetamol poisoning in-line with TOXBASE recommendations.
- Polatuzumab vedotin p. 926 with rituximab and bendamustine for the treatment of relapsed or refractory diffuse large B-cell lymphoma [NICE and SMC guidance].
- Pomalidomide p. 1003: Immunomodulatory drugs and pregnancy prevention: temporary advice for management during coronavirus (COVID-19) [MHRA/CHM advice].
- Ponatinib p. 1040: Systemically administered VEGF pathway inhibitors: risk of aneurysm and artery dissection [MHRA/CHM advice].
- Psoriasis p. 1283: updated guidance on management.
- Quetiapine p. 422: Clozapine and other antipsychotics: monitoring blood concentrations for toxicity [MHRA/CHM advice].
- Rabies vaccine p. 1355: updated guidance in-line with Public Health England recommendations.
- Ramucirumab p. 926: Systemically administered VEGF pathway inhibitors: risk of aneurysm and artery dissection [MHRA/CHM advice].
- Regorafenib p. 1041: Systemically administered VEGF pathway inhibitors: risk of aneurysm and artery dissection [MHRA/CHM advice].
- Risperidone p. 423: Clozapine and other antipsychotics: monitoring blood concentrations for toxicity [MHRA/CHM advice].
- Rivaroxaban p. 139: Direct-acting oral anticoagulants (DOACs): reminder of bleeding risk, availability of reversal agents [MHRA/CHM advice].
- Romosozumab p. 776 (*Evenity*®) for the treatment of severe osteoporosis in postmenopausal women at high risk of fracture [SMC guidance].
- Semaglutide p. 741 (*Rybelsus*® ▼) for the treatment of adults with insufficiently controlled type 2 diabetes mellitus [SMC guidance].
- Senna p. 67: Stimulant laxatives (bisacodyl, senna and sennosides, sodium picosulfate) available over-the-counter: new measures to support safe use [MHRA/CHM advice].
- Siponimod p. 902 for treating secondary progressive multiple sclerosis [NICE guidance].
- Siponimod p. 902 (*Mayzent*®) for the treatment of adult patients with secondary progressive multiple sclerosis (SPMS) with active disease evidenced by relapses or imaging features of inflammatory activity [SMC guidance].

- Skin infections, antibacterial therapy p. 541: new guidance for the management of insect bites and stings.
- Smallpox vaccine p. 1356: updated guidance in-line with Public Health England recommendations.
- Sodium picosulfate p. 68: Stimulant laxatives (bisacodyl, senna and sennosides, sodium picosulfate) available over-the-counter: new measures to support safe use [MHRA/CHM advice].
- Sodium valproate p. 345: Valproate Pregnancy Prevention Programme: temporary advice for management during coronavirus (COVID-19) [MHRA/CHM advice].
- Sodium zirconium cyclosilicate p. 1105 for the treatment of adults with hyperkalaemia [SMC guidance].
- Sorafenib p. 1043: Systemically administered VEGF pathway inhibitors: risk of aneurysm and artery dissection [MHRA/CHM advice].
- Steroid Emergency Card to support early recognition and treatment of adrenal crisis in adults [NHS Improvement Patient Safety Alert] (see Corticosteroids, general use p. 709).
- Sulpiride p. 409: Clozapine and other antipsychotics: monitoring blood concentrations for toxicity [MHRA/CHM advice].
- Sunitinib p. 1044: Systemically administered VEGF pathway inhibitors: risk of aneurysm and artery dissection [MHRA/CHM advice].
- Tegafur with gimeracil and oteracil p. 961: Fluorouracil (i.v.), capecitabine and tegafur containing products: Pre-treatment testing to identify DPD-deficient patients at increased risk of severe and fatal toxicity [MHRA/CHM advice].
- Thalidomide p. 1004: Immunomodulatory drugs and pregnancy prevention: temporary advice for management during coronavirus (COVID-19) [MHRA/CHM advice].
- Tick-borne encephalitis vaccine p. 1357: updated guidance in-line with Public Health England recommendations.
- Tivozanib p. 1046: Systemically administered VEGF pathway inhibitors: risk of aneurysm and artery dissection [MHRA/CHM advice].
- Trabectedin p. 965 (*Yondelis* ®) for the treatment of adult patients with advanced soft tissue sarcoma, after failure of anthracyclines and ifosfamide, or who are unsuited to receive these agents [SMC guidance].
- Trastuzumab emtansine p. 931 for adjuvant treatment of HER2-positive early breast cancer [NICE guidance].
- Trastuzumab emtansine p. 931 (*Kadcyla* ®) as a single agent, for the adjuvant treatment of adult patients with HER2-positive early breast cancer who have residual invasive disease, in the breast and/or lymph nodes, after neoadjuvant taxane-based and HER2-targeted therapy [SMC guidance].
- Treosulfan p. 943 with fludarabine for malignant disease before allogeneic stem cell transplant [NICE guidance].
- Ustekinumab p. 1151 for treating moderately to severely active ulcerative colitis [NICE guidance].
- Vaccination, general principles p. 1339: updated guidance.
- Valproic acid p. 373: Valproate Pregnancy Prevention Programme: temporary advice for management during coronavirus (COVID-19) [MHRA/CHM advice].
- Vandetanib p. 1048: Systemically administered VEGF pathway inhibitors: risk of aneurysm and artery dissection [MHRA/CHM advice].
- Varicella-zoster vaccine p. 1358: updated guidance in-line with Public Health England recommendations.
- Vedolizumab p. 50 for the treatment of adults with moderately to severely active Crohn's disease [SMC guidance].
- Vedolizumab p. 50 for the treatment of adults with moderately to severely active ulcerative colitis [SMC guidance].
- Venous thromboembolism p. 125: updated guidance for the treatment of venous thromboembolism.

- Volanesorsen p. 223 for treating familial chylomicronaemia syndrome [NICE guidance].
- Warfarin and other anticoagulants: monitoring of patients during the COVID-19 pandemic [MHRA/CHM advice] (advice in acenocoumarol, apixaban, dabigatran etexilate, edoxaban, phenindione, rivaroxaban, warfarin sodium; see example in Vitamin K antagonists p. 151).

Dose changes

Changes in dose statements that appear in the print edition of BNF 81 (March — September 2021):

- Atovaquone with proguanil hydrochloride p. 654 [update to dosing for prophylaxis of malaria].
- Avelumab p. 908 [dosing information updated].
- Azithromycin p. 568 [update to dosing for uncomplicated gonorrhoea].
- Cefixime p. 556 [update to dosing for uncomplicated gonorrhoea].
- Ceftriaxone p. 558 [update to dosing for gonococcal infections].
- Chloroquine p. 655 [update to dosing for prophylaxis of malaria].
- Ciprofloxacin p. 593 [update to dosing for gonococcal infections].
- *Clinorette* ® (estradiol with norethisterone p. 804) [update to dosing].
- *Elleste-Duet* ®Conti (estradiol with norethisterone p. 804) [update to dosing].
- Escitalopram p. 384 [elderly dosing for panic disorder updated].
- *Evorel* ®Conti (estradiol with norethisterone p. 804) [update to dosing].
- *Evorel* ®Sequi (estradiol with norethisterone p. 804) [update to dosing].
- *Gaviscon infant* ® (alginic acid p. 74) [update to dosing for management of gastro-oesophageal reflux disease].
- Hydrocortisone p. 716 [dosing updated].
- Influenza vaccine p. 1373 [update to dosing for immunisation].
- Isotretinoin p. 1314 [indication updated].
- *Kliofem* ® (estradiol with norethisterone p. 804) [update to dosing].
- *Kliovance* ® (estradiol with norethisterone p. 804) [update to dosing].
- Mefloquine p. 656 [update to dosing for prophylaxis of malaria].
- Mercaptamine p. 1110 [update to dosing for nephropathic cystinosis].
- *Novofem* ® (estradiol with norethisterone p. 804) [update to dosing].
- Ofloxacin p. 597 [update to dosing for complicated skin and soft-tissue infections].
- Ofloxacin p. 597 [update to dosing for complicated urinary-tract infections].
- Ofloxacin p. 597 [update to dosing for lower respiratory-tract infections].
- Ofloxacin p. 597 [update to dosing for urinary-tract infections].
- Omeprazole p. 86 [update to dosing for acid reflux disease].
- Oseltamivir p. 701 [update to dosing for treatment and prevention of influenza].
- Pembrolizumab p. 923 [dosing information updated].
- Proguanil hydrochloride p. 658 [update to dosing for prophylaxis of malaria].
- *Subgam* ® (normal immunoglobulin p. 1335) [update to dosing for hepatitis A prophylaxis].
- Sumatriptan p. 502 [update to dosing for treatment of acute migraine].
- *Trisequens* ® (estradiol with norethisterone p. 804) [update to dosing].
- Zanamivir p. 702 [update to dosing for treatment of influenza].

New monographs

New monographs that appear in the print edition of BNF 81 (March — September 2021):

- *Atectura Breezhaler*® [indacaterol with mometasone furoate p. 282].
- *Ayvakyt*® ▼ [avapritinib p. 1012].
- *Calquence*® ▼ [acalabrutinib p. 1010].
- Cefazolin p. 553.
- *Daurismo*® [glasdegib p. 1049].
- *Doptelet*® [avatrombopag p. 1079].
- *Enerzair Breezhaler*® [mometasone furoate with glycopyrronium bromide and indacaterol p. 282].
- *Fetcroja*® [cefiderocol p. 561].
- *Jyseleca*® [filgotinib p. 1153].
- *Kaftrio*® [tezacaftor with ivacaftor and elexacaftor p. 311].
- *Myopridin*® [pridinol p. 1174].
- *Nilemdo*® [bempedoic acid p. 221].
- *Nubeqa*® [darolutamide p. 991].
- *Nustendi*® [bempedoic acid with ezetimibe p. 221].
- *Otigo*® [phenazone with lidocaine p. 1243].
- *Piqray*® [alpelisib p. 1012].
- *Quofenix*® [delafloxacin p. 595].
- *Recarbrio*® [imipenem with cilastatin and relebactam p. 549].
- *Rozlytrek*® [entrectinib p. 1023].
- *Sarclisa*® [isatuximab p. 918].
- *Sunosi*® [solriamfetol p. 514].
- *Tavlesse*® [fostamatinib p. 1081].
- *Veklury*® [remdesivir p. 661].
- *Zeposia*® [ozanimod p. 901].

New preparations

New preparations that appear in the print edition of BNF 81 (March — September 2021):

- *Lecicarbon A*® [sodium acid phosphate with sodium bicarbonate p. 68].
- *Lecicarbon C*® [sodium acid phosphate with sodium bicarbonate p. 68].
- *Lenzetto*® [estradiol p. 798].
- *Medabon*® [mifepristone and misoprostol p. 872].
- *Remsima*® solution for injection in pre-filled pens or syringes [infliximab p. 1162].
- *Rybelsus*® ▼ [semaglutide p. 741].
- *Spravato*® [esketamine p. 1393].
- *Symbicort*® 100 micrograms/3 micrograms per actuation pressurised inhalation [budesonide with formoterol p. 276].
- *Trecondi*® [treosulfan p. 943].

Deleted monographs

Deleted monographs since the print edition of BNF 80 (September 2020 — March 2021):

- Collagenase.
- Conjugated oestrogens with bazedoxifene acetate.
- Fenticonazole nitrate.
- Nedocromil sodium.
- Pergolide.
- Rolapitant.
- Sodium stibogluconate.
- Stavudine.
- Telbivudine.
- Ticarcillin with clavulanic acid.

Deleted preparations

Deleted preparations since the print edition of BNF 80 (September 2020 — March 2021):

- *Climagest*® 1 mg [estradiol with norethisterone p. 804].
- *Climagest*® 2 mg [estradiol with norethisterone p. 804].
- *Climesse*® [estradiol with norethisterone p. 804].
- *Esmya*® [ulipristal acetate p. 851].

Guidance on prescribing

General guidance

Medicines should be prescribed only when they are necessary, and in all cases the benefit of administering the medicine should be considered in relation to the risk involved. This is particularly important during pregnancy, when the risk to both mother and fetus must be considered.

It is important to discuss treatment options carefully with the patient to ensure that the patient is content to take the medicine as prescribed. In particular, the patient should be helped to distinguish the adverse effects of prescribed drugs from the effects of the medical disorder. When the beneficial effects of the medicine are likely to be delayed, the patient should be advised of this.

For guidance on medicines optimisation, see Medicines optimisation p. 18.

Never Events Never events are serious and avoidable medical errors for which there should be preventative measures in place to stop their occurrence.

The NHS Never Events policy and framework can be viewed at: improvement.nhs.uk/documents/2265/Revised_Never_Events_policy_and_framework_FINAL.pdf.

For never events related to single drugs or drug classes, BNF Publications contain information within the monographs, in the important safety information section.

Prescribing competency framework The Royal Pharmaceutical Society has published a Prescribing Competency Framework that includes a common set of competencies that form the basis for prescribing, regardless of professional background. The competencies have been developed to help healthcare professionals to be safe and effective prescribers, with the aim of supporting patients to get the best outcomes from their medicines. It is available at www.rpharms.com/resources/frameworks/prescribers-competency-framework.

Biological medicines

Biological medicines are medicines that are made by or derived from a biological source using biotechnology processes, such as recombinant DNA technology. The size and complexity of biological medicines, as well as the way they are produced, may result in a degree of natural variability in molecules of the same active substance, particularly in different batches of the medicine. This variation is maintained within strict acceptable limits. Examples of biological medicines include insulins and monoclonal antibodies. EvGr Biological medicines must be prescribed by brand name and the brand name specified on the prescription should be dispensed in order to avoid inadvertent switching. Automatic substitution of brands at the point of dispensing is not appropriate for biological medicines. ⟨A⟩

Biosimilar medicines

A **biosimilar medicine** is a biological medicine that is highly similar and clinically equivalent (in terms of quality, safety, and efficacy) to an existing biological medicine that has already been authorised in the European Union (known as the reference biological medicine or originator medicine). The active substance of a biosimilar medicine is similar, but not identical, to the originator biological medicine. Once the patent for a biological medicine has expired, a biosimilar medicine may be authorised by the European Medicines Agency (EMA). A biosimilar medicine is not the same as a generic medicine, which contains a simpler molecular structure that is identical to the originator medicine.

Therapeutic equivalence EvGr Biosimilar medicines should be considered to be therapeutically equivalent to the originator biological medicine within their authorised indications. ⟨A⟩ Biosimilar medicines are usually licensed for all the indications of the originator biological medicine, but this depends on the evidence submitted to the EMA for authorisation and must be scientifically justified on the basis of demonstrated or extrapolated equivalence.

Prescribing and dispensing The choice of whether to prescribe a biosimilar medicine or the originator biological medicine rests with the clinician in consultation with the patient. EvGr Biological medicines (including biosimilar medicines) must be prescribed by brand name and the brand name specified on the prescription should be dispensed in order to avoid inadvertent switching. Automatic substitution of brands at the point of dispensing is not appropriate for biological medicines. ⟨A⟩

Safety monitoring Biosimilar medicines are subject to a black triangle status (▼) at the time of initial authorisation. EvGr It is important to report suspected adverse reactions using the Yellow Card Scheme (see Adverse reactions to drugs p. 12). For all biological medicines, adverse reaction reports should clearly state the brand name and the batch number of the suspected medicine. ⟨A⟩

UK Medicines Information centres have developed a validated tool to determine potential safety issues associated with all new medicines. These 'in-use product safety assessment reports' will be published for new biosimilar medicines as they become available, see www.sps.nhs.uk/home/medicines/.

National funding/access decisions The Department of Health has confirmed that, in England, NICE can decide to apply the same remit, and the resulting technology appraisal guidance, to relevant biosimilar medicines which appear on the market subsequent to their originator biological medicine. In other circumstances, where a review of the evidence for a particular biosimilar medicine is necessary, NICE will consider producing an evidence summary (see *Evidence summary: new medicines*, www.nice.org.uk/about/what-we-do/our-programmes/nice-advice/evidence-summaries-new-medicines).

National information In England, see www.nice.org.uk/Media/Default/About/what-we-do/NICE-guidance/NICE-technology-appraisals/biosimilars-statement.pdf.

In Northern Ireland, see niformulary.hscni.net/managed-entry/biosimilars/.

In Scotland, see www.scottishmedicines.org.uk/About_SMC/Policy_statements/Biosimilar_Medicines.

In Wales, see www.wales.nhs.uk/sites3/Documents/814/BIOSIMILARS-ABUHBpositionStatement%5BNov2015%5D.pdf.

Availability The following drugs are available as a biosimilar medicine:

- Adalimumab p. 1157
- Bevacizumab p. 909
- Enoxaparin sodium p. 144
- Epoetin alfa p. 1059
- Epoetin zeta p. 1061
- Etanercept p. 1159
- Filgrastim p. 1076
- Follitropin alfa p. 786
- Infliximab p. 1162
- Insulin glargine p. 758
- Insulin lispro p. 755
- Rituximab p. 927
- Somatropin p. 789

- Teriparatide p. 774
- Trastuzumab p. 930

Complementary and alternative medicine

An increasing amount of information on complementary and alternative medicine is becoming available. The scope of the BNF is restricted to the discussion of conventional medicines but reference is made to complementary treatments if they affect conventional therapy (e.g. interactions with St John's wort). Further information on herbal medicines is available at www.mhra.gov.uk.

Abbreviation of titles

In general, titles of drugs and preparations should be written in full. Unofficial abbreviations should not be used as they may be misinterpreted.

Non-proprietary titles

Where non-proprietary ('generic') titles are given, they should be used in prescribing. This will enable any suitable product to be dispensed, thereby saving delay to the patient and sometimes expense to the health service. The only exception is where there is a demonstrable difference in clinical effect between each manufacturer's version of the formulation, making it important that the patient should always receive the same brand; in such cases, the brand name or the manufacturer should be stated. Non-proprietary titles should not be invented for the purposes of prescribing generically since this can lead to confusion, particularly in the case of compound and modified-release preparations.

Titles used as headings for monographs may be used freely in the United Kingdom but in other countries may be subject to restriction.

Many of the non-proprietary titles used in this book are titles of monographs in the European Pharmacopoeia, British Pharmacopoeia, or British Pharmaceutical Codex 1973. In such cases the preparations must comply with the standard (if any) in the appropriate publication, as required by the Human Medicines Regulations 2012.

Proprietary titles

Names followed by the symbol ® are or have been used as proprietary names in the United Kingdom. These names may in general be applied only to products supplied by the owners of the trade marks.

Marketing authorisation and BNF advice

In general the *doses, indications, cautions, contra-indications,* and *side-effects* in the BNF reflect those in the manufacturers' data sheets or Summaries of Product Characteristics (SPCs) which, in turn, reflect those in the corresponding marketing authorisations (formerly known as Product Licences). The BNF does not generally include proprietary medicines that are not supported by a valid Summary of Product Characteristics or when the marketing authorisation holder has not been able to supply essential information. When a preparation is available from more than one manufacturer, the BNF reflects advice that is the most clinically relevant regardless of any variation in the marketing authorisations. Unlicensed products can be obtained from 'special-order' manufacturers or specialist importing companies.

Where an unlicensed drug is included in the BNF, this is indicated in the unlicensed use section of the drug monograph. When the BNF suggests a use that is outside the terms defined by the licence ('off-label' use), this too is indicated. Unlicensed or off-label use may be necessary if the clinical need cannot be met by licensed medicines; such use should be supported by appropriate evidence and experience.

The doses stated in the BNF are intended for general guidance and represent, unless otherwise stated, the usual range of doses that are generally regarded as being suitable for adults.

Prescribing unlicensed medicines

Prescribing medicines outside the recommendations of their marketing authorisation alters (and probably increases) the prescriber's professional responsibility and potential liability. The prescriber should be able to justify and feel competent in using such medicines, and also inform the patient or the patient's carer that the prescribed medicine is unlicensed.

Oral syringes

An **oral syringe** is supplied when oral liquid medicines are prescribed in doses other than multiples of 5 mL. The oral syringe is marked in 0.5 mL divisions from 1 to 5 mL to measure doses of less than 5 mL (other sizes of oral syringe may also be available). It is provided with an adaptor and an instruction leaflet. The 5–*mL spoon* is used for doses of 5 mL (or multiples thereof).

Important To avoid inadvertent intravenous administration of oral liquid medicines, only an appropriate oral or enteral syringe should be used to measure an oral liquid medicine (if a medicine spoon or graduated measure cannot be used); these syringes should not be compatible with intravenous or other parenteral devices. Oral or enteral syringes should be clearly labelled 'Oral' or 'Enteral' in a large font size; it is the healthcare practitioner's responsibility to label the syringe with this information if the manufacturer has not done so.

Excipients

Branded oral liquid preparations that do not contain *fructose, glucose,* or *sucrose* are described as 'sugar-free' in the BNF. Preparations containing hydrogenated glucose syrup, mannitol, maltitol, sorbitol, or xylitol are also marked 'sugar-free' since there is evidence that they do not cause dental caries. Patients receiving medicines containing cariogenic sugars should be advised of appropriate dental hygiene measures to prevent caries. Sugar-free preparations should be used whenever possible.

Where information on the presence of *aspartame, gluten, sulfites, tartrazine, arachis (peanut) oil* or *sesame oil* is available, this is indicated in the BNF against the relevant preparation.

Information is provided on selected excipients in skin preparations, in vaccines, and on *selected preservatives* and *excipients* in eye drops and injections.

The presence of *benzyl alcohol* and *polyoxyl castor oil* (polyethoxylated castor oil) in injections is indicated in the BNF. Benzyl alcohol has been associated with a fatal toxic syndrome in preterm neonates, and therefore, parenteral preparations containing the preservative should not be used in neonates. Polyoxyl castor oils, used as vehicles in intravenous injections, have been associated with severe anaphylactoid reactions.

The presence of *propylene glycol* in oral or parenteral medicines is indicated in the BNF; it can cause adverse effects if its elimination is impaired, e.g. in renal failure, in neonates and young children, and in slow metabolisers of the substance. It may interact with disulfiram p. 517 and metronidazole p. 575.

The *lactose* content in most medicines is too small to cause problems in most lactose-intolerant patients. However in severe lactose intolerance, the lactose content should be determined before prescribing. The amount of lactose varies according to manufacturer, product, formulation, and strength.

Electrolytes

The *sodium* content of medicines should be considered for all patients, especially those with cardiovascular disease or on a reduced sodium diet, or those requiring long-term or regular medication.

Some formulations of medicines, especially those that are effervescent, dispersible or soluble, can contain high levels of sodium as an excipient and this may be associated with an increased risk of cardiovascular events, including hypertension.

The sodium content of a medicine is provided in the product literature for all medicines containing ≥ 1 mmol sodium per dose; below this level is considered essentially sodium-free. Medicines containing ≥ 17 mmol sodium in the total daily dose are considered to have a high sodium content and this is highlighted for medicines intended to be taken regularly (repeated use for more than 2 days every week) or long-term (continuous daily use for more than 1 month). 17 mmol sodium is approximately 20% of the WHO recommended maximum daily dietary intake of sodium for an adult.

Important In the absence of information on excipients or electrolytes in the BNF and in the product literature (available at www.medicines.org.uk/emc), contact the manufacturer (see Index of Manufacturers) if it is essential to check details.

Extemporaneous preparation
A product should be dispensed extemporaneously only when no product with a marketing authorisation is available.

The BP direction that a preparation must be *freshly prepared* indicates that it must be made not more than 24 hours before it is issued for use. The direction that a preparation should be *recently prepared* indicates that deterioration is likely if the preparation is stored for longer than about 4 weeks at 15–25° C.

The term **water** used without qualification means either potable water freshly drawn direct from the public supply and suitable for drinking or freshly boiled and cooled purified water. The latter should be used if the public supply is from a local storage tank or if the potable water is unsuitable for a particular preparation (Water for injections).

Drugs and driving
Prescribers and other healthcare professionals should advise patients if treatment is likely to affect their ability to perform skilled tasks (e.g. driving). This applies especially to drugs with sedative effects; patients should be warned that these effects are increased by alcohol. General information about a patient's fitness to drive is available from the Driver and Vehicle Licensing Agency at www.gov.uk/government/organisations/driver-and-vehicle-licensing-agency.

A new offence of driving, attempting to drive, or being in charge of a vehicle, with certain specified controlled drugs in excess of specified limits, came into force on 2nd March 2015. This offence is an addition to the existing rules on drug impaired driving and fitness to drive, and applies to two groups of drugs—commonly abused drugs, including amfetamines, cannabis, cocaine, and ketamine p. 1399, and drugs used mainly for medical reasons, such as opioids and benzodiazepines. Anyone found to have any of the drugs (including related drugs, for example, apomorphine hydrochloride p. 438) above specified limits in their blood will be guilty of an offence, whether their driving was impaired or not. This also includes prescribed drugs which metabolise to those included in the offence, for example, selegiline hydrochloride p. 447. However, the legislation provides a statutory "medical defence" for patients taking drugs for medical reasons in accordance with instructions, *if their driving was not impaired*—it continues to be an offence to drive if actually impaired. Patients should therefore be advised to continue taking their medicines as prescribed, and when driving, to carry suitable evidence that the drug was prescribed, or sold, to treat a medical or dental problem, and that it was taken according to the instructions given by the

prescriber, or information provided with the medicine (e.g. a repeat prescription form or the medicine's patient information leaflet). Further information is available from the Department for Transport at www.gov.uk/government/collections/drug-driving.

Patents
In the BNF, certain drugs have been included notwithstanding the existence of actual or potential patent rights. In so far as such substances are protected by Letters Patent, their inclusion in this Formulary neither conveys, nor implies, licence to manufacture.

Health and safety
When handling chemical or biological materials particular attention should be given to the possibility of allergy, fire, explosion, radiation, or poisoning. Substances such as corticosteroids, some antimicrobials, phenothiazines, and many cytotoxics, are irritant or very potent and should be handled with caution. Contact with the skin and inhalation of dust should be avoided.

Safety in the home
Patients must be warned to keep all medicines out of the reach of children. All solid dose and all oral and external liquid preparations must be dispensed in a reclosable *child-resistant container* unless:

- the medicine is in an original pack or patient pack such as to make this inadvisable;
- the patient will have difficulty in opening a child-resistant container;
- a specific request is made that the product shall not be dispensed in a child-resistant container;
- no suitable child-resistant container exists for a particular liquid preparation.

All patients should be advised to dispose of *unwanted medicines* by returning them to a supplier for destruction.

Labelling of prescribed medicines
There is a legal requirement for the following to appear on the label of any prescribed medicine:

- name of the patient;
- name and address of the supplying pharmacy;
- date of dispensing;
- name of the medicine;
- directions for use of the medicine;
- precautions relating to the use of the medicine.

The Royal Pharmaceutical Society recommends that the following also appears on the label:

- the words 'Keep out of the sight and reach of children';
- where applicable, the words 'Use this medicine only on your skin'.

A pharmacist can exercise professional skill and judgement to amend or include more appropriate wording for the name of the medicine, the directions for use, or the precautions relating to the use of the medicine.

Non-proprietary names of compound preparations
Non-proprietary names of **compound preparations** which appear in the BNF are those that have been compiled by the British Pharmacopoeia Commission or another recognised body; whenever possible they reflect the names of the active ingredients.

Prescribers should avoid creating their own compound names for the purposes of generic prescribing; such names do not have an approved definition and can be misinterpreted.

Special care should be taken to avoid errors when prescribing compound preparations; in particular the hyphen in the prefix 'co-' should be retained.

Special care should also be taken to avoid creating generic names for **modified-release** preparations where the use of these names could lead to confusion between formulations with different lengths of action.

EEA and Swiss prescriptions

Pharmacists can dispense prescriptions issued by doctors, dentists, and nurse prescribers from the European Economic Area (EEA) or Switzerland (except prescriptions for controlled drugs in Schedules 1, 2, or 3, or for drugs without a UK marketing authorisation). Prescriptions should be written in ink or otherwise so as to be indelible, should be dated, should state the name of the patient, should state the address of the prescriber, should contain particulars indicating whether the prescriber is a doctor, dentist, or nurse, and should be signed by the prescriber.

Security and validity of prescriptions

The Councils of the British Medical Association and the Royal Pharmaceutical Society have issued a joint statement on the security and validity of prescriptions.

In particular, prescription forms should:

- not be left unattended at reception desks;
- not be left in a car where they may be visible; and
- when not in use, be kept in a locked drawer within the surgery and at home.

Where there is any doubt about the authenticity of a prescription, the pharmacist should contact the prescriber. If this is done by telephone, the number should be obtained from the directory rather than relying on the information on the prescription form, which may be false.

Patient group direction (PGD)

In most cases, the most appropriate clinical care will be provided on an individual basis by a prescriber to a specific individual patient. However, a Patient Group Direction for supply and administration of medicines by other healthcare professionals can be used where it would benefit patient care without compromising safety.

A Patient Group Direction is a written direction relating to the supply and administration (or administration only) of a licensed prescription-only medicine (including some Controlled Drugs in specific circumstances) by certain classes of healthcare professionals; the Direction is signed by a doctor (or dentist) and by a pharmacist. Further information on Patient Group Directions is available in Health Service Circular HSC 2000/026 (England), HDL (2001) 7 (Scotland), and WHC (2000) 116 (Wales); see also the Human Medicines Regulations 2012.

NICE, Scottish Medicines Consortium and All Wales Medicines Strategy Group

Advice issued by the National Institute for Health and Care Excellence (NICE), the Scottish Medicines Consortium (SMC) and the All Wales Medicines Strategy Group (AWMSG) is referenced in the BNF when relevant. Full details of this advice together with updates can be obtained from the funding body websites: www.nice.org.uk, www.scottishmedicines.org.uk and awmsg.nhs.wales/.

Specialised commissioning decisions

NHS England develops specialised commissioning policies that define access to specialised services for particular groups of patients to ensure consistency in access to treatments nationwide. For further information, see www.england.nhs.uk/specialised-commissioning-document-library/routinely-commissioned-policies/.

Prescription writing

Shared care

In its guidelines on responsibility for prescribing (circular EL (91) 127) between hospitals and general practitioners, the Department of Health has advised that legal responsibility for prescribing lies with the doctor who signs the prescription.

Requirements

Prescriptions should be written legibly in ink or otherwise so as to be indelible (it is permissible to issue carbon copies of NHS prescriptions as long as they are signed in ink), should be dated, should state the name and address of the patient, the address of the prescriber, an indication of the type of prescriber, and should be signed in ink by the prescriber (computer-generated facsimile signatures do not meet the legal requirement). The age and the date of birth of the patient should preferably be stated, and it is a legal requirement in the case of prescription-only medicines to state the age for children under 12 years. These recommendations are acceptable for **prescription-only medicines**. Prescriptions for controlled drugs have additional legal requirements.

Wherever appropriate the prescriber should state the current weight of the child to enable the dose prescribed to be checked. Consideration should also be given to including the dose per unit mass e.g. mg/kg or the dose per m² body-surface area e.g. mg/m² where this would reduce error.

The following should be noted:

- The strength or quantity to be contained in capsules, lozenges, tablets etc. should be stated by the prescriber. In particular, strength of liquid preparations should be clearly stated (e.g. 125 mg/5 mL).
- The unnecessary use of decimal points should be avoided, e.g. 3 mg, not 3.0 mg. Quantities of 1 gram or more should be written as 1 g etc. Quantities less than 1 gram should be written in milligrams, e.g. 500 mg, not 0.5 g. Quantities less than 1 mg should be written in micrograms, e.g. 100 micrograms, not 0.1 mg. When decimals are unavoidable a zero should be written in front of the decimal point where there is no other figure, e.g. 0.5 mL, not .5 mL. Use of the decimal point is acceptable to express a range, e.g. 0.5 to 1 g.
- 'Micrograms' and 'nanograms' should **not** be abbreviated. Similarly 'units' should **not** be abbreviated.
- The term 'millilitre' (ml or mL) is used in medicine and pharmacy, and cubic centimetre, c.c., or cm³ should not be used. (The use of capital 'L' in mL is a printing convention throughout the BNF; both 'mL' and 'ml' are recognised SI abbreviations).
- Dose and dose frequency should be stated; in the case of preparations to be taken 'as required' a **minimum dose interval** should be specified. Care should be taken to ensure children receive the correct dose of the active drug. Therefore, the dose should normally be stated in terms of the mass of the active drug (e.g. '125 mg 3 times daily'); terms such as '5 mL' or '1 tablet' should be avoided except for compound preparations. When doses other than multiples of 5 mL are prescribed for *oral liquid preparations* the dose-volume will be provided by means of an **oral syringe**, (except for preparations intended to be measured with a pipette). Suitable quantities:
  - Elixirs, Linctuses, and Paediatric Mixtures (5-mL dose), 50, 100, or 150 mL
  - Adult Mixtures (10 mL dose), 200 or 300 mL
  - Ear Drops, Eye drops, and Nasal Drops, 10 mL (or the manufacturer's pack)
  - Eye Lotions, Gargles, and Mouthwashes, 200 mL
- The names of drugs and preparations should be written clearly and **not** abbreviated, using approved titles **only**;

avoid creating generic titles for modified-release preparations.

- The quantity to be supplied may be stated by indicating the number of days of treatment required in the box provided on NHS forms. In most cases the exact amount will be supplied. This does not apply to items directed to be used as required—if the dose and frequency are not given then the quantity to be supplied needs to be stated. When several items are ordered on one form the box can be marked with the number of days of treatment provided the quantity is added for any item for which the amount cannot be calculated.
- Although directions should preferably be in **English without abbreviation**, it is recognised that some Latin abbreviations are used.

Sample prescription

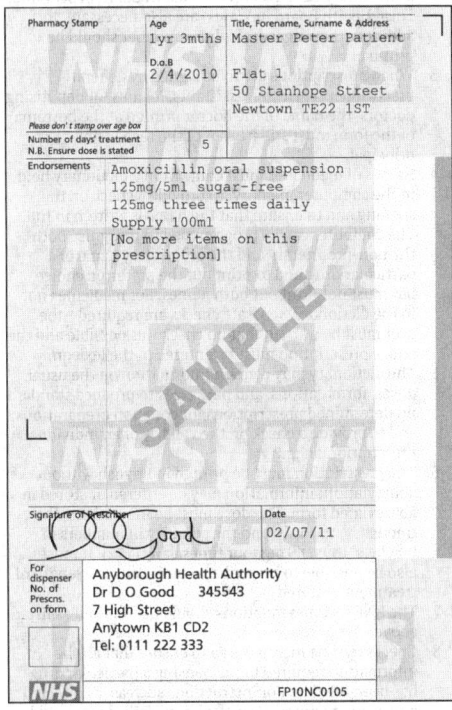

Prescribing by dentists

Until new prescribing arrangements are in place for NHS prescriptions, dentists should use form FP10D (GP14 in Scotland, WP10D in Wales) to prescribe only those items listed in the Dental Practitioners' Formulary. The Human Medicines Regulations 2012 does not set any limitations upon the number and variety of substances which the dentist may administer to patients in the surgery or may order by private prescription—provided the relevant legal requirements are observed the dentist may use or order whatever is required for the clinical situation. There is no statutory requirement for the dentist to communicate with a patient's medical practitioner when prescribing for dental use. There are, however, occasions when this would be in the patient's interest and such communication is to be encouraged. For legal requirements relating to prescriptions of Controlled Drugs, see Controlled drugs and drug dependence p. 8.

Computer-issued prescriptions

For computer-issued prescriptions the following advice, based on the recommendations of the Joint GP Information Technology Committee, should also be noted:

1. The computer must print out the date, the patient's surname, one forename, other initials, and address, and may also print out the patient's title and date of birth. The age of children under 12 years and of adults over 60 years must be printed in the box available; the age of children under 5 years should be printed in years and months. A facility may also exist to print out the age of patients between 12 and 60 years.

2. The doctor's name must be printed at the bottom of the prescription form; this will be the name of the doctor responsible for the prescription (who will normally sign it). The doctor's surgery address, reference number, and Primary Care Trust (PCT, Health Board in Scotland, Local Health Board in Wales) are also necessary. In addition, the surgery telephone number should be printed.

3. When prescriptions are to be signed by general practitioner registrars, assistants, locums, or deputising doctors, the name of the doctor printed at the bottom of the form must still be that of the responsible principal.

4. Names of medicines must come from a dictionary held in the computer memory, to provide a check on the spelling and to ensure that the name is written in full. The computer can be programmed to recognise both the non-proprietary and the proprietary name of a particular drug and to print out the preferred choice, but must not print out both names. For medicines not in the dictionary, separate checks are required—the user must be warned that no check was possible and the entire prescription must be entered in the lexicon.

5. The dictionary may contain information on the usual doses, formulations, and pack sizes to produce standard predetermined prescriptions for common preparations, and to provide a check on the validity of an individual prescription on entry.

6. The prescription must be printed in English without abbreviation; information may be entered or stored in abbreviated form. The dose must be in numbers, the frequency in words, and the quantity in numbers in brackets, thus: 40 mg four times daily (112). It must also be possible to prescribe by indicating the length of treatment required.

7. The BNF recommendations should be followed as listed above.

8. Checks may be incorporated to ensure that all the information required for dispensing a particular drug has been filled in. For instructions such as 'as directed' and 'when required', the maximum daily dose should normally be specified.

9. Numbers and codes used in the system for organising and retrieving data must never appear on the form.

10. Supplementary warnings or advice should be written in full, should not interfere with the clarity of the prescription itself, and should be in line with any warnings or advice in the BNF; numerical codes should not be used.

11. A mechanism (such as printing a series of nonspecific characters) should be incorporated to cancel out unused space, or wording such as 'no more items on this prescription' may be added after the last item. Otherwise the doctor should delete the space manually.

12. To avoid forgery the computer may print on the form the number of items to be dispensed (somewhere separate from the box for the pharmacist). The number of items per form need be limited only by the ability of the printer to produce clear and well-demarcated instructions with sufficient space for each item and a spacer line before each fresh item.

13. Handwritten alterations should only be made in exceptional circumstances—it is preferable to print out a new prescription. Any alterations must be made in the doctor's own handwriting and countersigned; computer records should be updated to fully reflect any alteration. Prescriptions for drugs used for contraceptive purposes (but which are not promoted as contraceptives) may need to be marked in handwriting with the symbol ♀, (or endorsed in another way to indicate that the item is prescribed for contraceptive purposes).

14. Prescriptions for controlled drugs can be printed from the computer, but the prescriber's signature must be handwritten (See Controlled Drugs and Drug Dependence; the prescriber may use a date stamp).

15. The strip of paper on the side of the FP10SS (GP10SS in Scotland, WP10SS in Wales) may be used for various purposes but care should be taken to avoid including confidential information. It may be advisable for the patient's name to appear at the top, but this should be preceded by 'confidential'.

16. In rural dispensing practices prescription requests (or details of medicines dispensed) will normally be entered in one surgery. The prescriptions (or dispensed medicines) may then need to be delivered to another surgery or location; if possible the computer should hold up to 10 alternatives.

17. Prescription forms that are reprinted or issued as a duplicate should be labelled clearly as such.

Emergency supply of medicines

Emergency supply requested by member of the public

Pharmacists are sometimes called upon by members of the public to make an emergency supply of medicines. The Human Medicines Regulations 2012 allows exemptions from the Prescription Only requirements for emergency supply to be made by a person lawfully conducting a retail pharmacy business provided:

a) that the pharmacist has interviewed the person requesting the prescription-only medicine and is satisfied:

   i) that there is immediate need for the prescription-only medicine and that it is impracticable in the circumstances to obtain a prescription without undue delay;

   ii) that treatment with the prescription-only medicine has on a previous occasion been prescribed for the person requesting it;

   iii) as to the dose that it would be appropriate for the person to take;

b) that no greater quantity shall be supplied than will provide 5 days' treatment of phenobarbital p. 353, *phenobarbital sodium*, or Controlled Drugs in Schedules 4 or 5 (doctors, dentists, or nurse prescribers from the European Economic Area and Switzerland, or their patients, cannot request an emergency supply of Controlled Drugs in Schedules 1, 2, or 3, or drugs that do not have a UK marketing authorisation) or 30 days' treatment for other prescription-only medicines, except when the prescription-only medicine is:

   i) insulin, an ointment or cream, or a preparation for the relief of asthma in an aerosol dispenser when the smallest pack can be supplied;

   ii) an oral contraceptive when a full cycle may be supplied;

   iii) an antibiotic in liquid form for oral administration when the smallest quantity that will provide a full course of treatment can be supplied;

c) that an entry shall be made by the pharmacist in the prescription book stating:

   i) the date of supply;

   ii) the name, quantity and, where appropriate, the pharmaceutical form and strength;

   iii) the name and address of the patient;

   iv) the nature of the emergency;

d) that the container or package must be labelled to show:

   i) the date of supply;

   ii) the name, quantity and, where appropriate, the pharmaceutical form and strength;

   iii) the name of the patient;

   iv) the name and address of the pharmacy;

   v) the words 'Emergency supply';

   vi) the words 'Keep out of the reach of children' (or similar warning);

e) that the prescription-only medicine is not a substance specifically excluded from the emergency supply provision, and does not contain a Controlled Drug specified in Schedules 1, 2, or 3 to the Misuse of Drugs Regulations 2001 except for phenobarbital p. 353 or *phenobarbital sodium* for the treatment of epilepsy: for details see *Medicines, Ethics and Practice,* London, Pharmaceutical Press (always consult latest edition). Doctors, dentists, or nurse prescribers from the European Economic Area and Switzerland, or their patients, cannot request an emergency supply of Controlled Drugs in Schedules 1, 2, or 3, or drugs that do not have a UK marketing authorisation.

Emergency supply requested by prescriber

Emergency supply of a prescription-only medicine may also be made at the request of a doctor, a dentist, a supplementary prescriber, a community practitioner nurse prescriber, a nurse, pharmacist, physiotherapist, therapeutic radiographer, optometrist, podiatrist or paramedic independent prescriber; or a doctor, dentist, or nurse prescriber from the European Economic Area or Switzerland, provided:

a) that the pharmacist is satisfied that the prescriber by reason of some emergency is unable to furnish a prescription immediately;

b) that the prescriber has undertaken to furnish a prescription within 72 hours;

c) that the medicine is supplied in accordance with the directions of the prescriber requesting it;

d) that the medicine is not a Controlled Drug specified in Schedules 1, 2, or 3 to the Misuse of Drugs Regulations 2001 except for phenobarbital p. 353 or *phenobarbital sodium* for the treatment of epilepsy: for details see *Medicines, Ethics and Practice,* London, Pharmaceutical Press (always consult latest edition); (Doctors, dentists, or nurse prescribers from the European Economic Area and Switzerland, or their patients, cannot request an emergency supply of Controlled Drugs in Schedules 1, 2, or 3, or drugs that do not have a UK marketing authorisation;

e) that an entry shall be made in the prescription book stating:

   i) the date of supply;

   ii) the name, quantity and, where appropriate, the pharmaceutical form and strength;

   iii) the name and address of the practitioner requesting the emergency supply;

   iv) the name and address of the patient;

   v) the date on the prescription;

   vi) when the prescription is received the entry should be amended to include the date on which it is received.

Royal Pharmaceutical Society's guidelines

1. The pharmacist should consider the medical consequences of not supplying a medicine in an emergency.

2. If the pharmacist is unable to make an emergency supply of a medicine the pharmacist should advise the patient how to obtain essential medical care.

For conditions that apply to supplies made at the request of a patient see Medicines, Ethics and Practice, London Pharmaceutical Press, (always consult latest edition).

Controlled drugs and drug dependence

Regulations and classification

The Misuse of Drugs Act, 1971 as amended prohibits certain activities in relation to 'Controlled Drugs', in particular their manufacture, supply, and possession (except where permitted by the 2001 Regulations or under licence from the Secretary of State). The penalties applicable to offences involving the different drugs are graded broadly according to the *harmfulness attributable to a drug when it is misused* and for this purpose the drugs are defined in the following three classes:

- **Class A** includes: alfentanil p. 1397, cocaine, diamorphine hydrochloride p. 476 (heroin), dipipanone hydrochloride, fentanyl p. 478, lysergide (LSD), methadone hydrochloride p. 524, 3, 4-methylenedioxymethamfetamine (MDMA, 'ecstasy'), morphine p. 483, opium, oxycodone hydrochloride p. 486, pethidine hydrochloride p. 489, phencyclidine, remifentanil p. 1398, and class B substances when prepared for injection.
- **Class B** includes: oral amfetamines, barbiturates, cannabis, *Sativex*®, codeine phosphate p. 475, dihydrocodeine tartrate p. 477, ethylmorphine, glutethimide, ketamine p. 1399, nabilone p. 450, pentazocine, phenmetrazine, and pholcodine p. 313.
- **Class C** includes: certain drugs related to the amfetamines such as benzfetamine and chlorphentermine, buprenorphine p. 468, mazindol, meprobamate, pemoline, pipradrol, most benzodiazepines, tramadol hydrochloride p. 491, zaleplon, zolpidem tartrate, zopiclone, androgenic and anabolic steroids, clenbuterol, chorionic gonadotrophin (HCG), non-human chorionic gonadotrophin, somatotropin, somatrem, somatropin p. 789, gabapentin p. 332, and pregabalin.

The Misuse of Drugs (Safe Custody) Regulations 1973 as amended details the storage and safe custody requirements for Controlled Drugs.

The Misuse of Drugs Regulations 2001 (and subsequent amendments) defines the classes of person who are authorised to supply and possess Controlled Drugs while acting in their professional capacities and lays down the conditions under which these activities may be carried out. In the 2001 regulations, drugs are divided into five Schedules, each specifying the requirements governing such activities as import, export, production, supply, possession, prescribing, and record keeping which apply to them.

- **Schedule 1** includes drugs not used medicinally such as hallucinogenic drugs (e.g. LSD), ecstasy-type substances, raw opium, and cannabis. A Home Office licence is generally required for their production, possession, or supply. A Controlled Drug register must be used to record details of any Schedule 1 Controlled Drugs received or supplied by a pharmacy.
- **Schedule 2** includes opiates (e.g. diamorphine hydrochloride p. 476 (heroin), morphine p. 483, methadone hydrochloride p. 524, oxycodone hydrochloride p. 486, pethidine hydrochloride p. 489), major stimulants (e.g. amfetamines), quinalbarbitone (secobarbital), cocaine, ketamine p. 1399, and cannabis-based products for medicinal use in humans. Schedule 2 Controlled Drugs are subject to the full Controlled Drug requirements relating to prescriptions, safe custody (except for quinalbarbitone (secobarbital) and some liquid preparations), and the need to keep a Controlled Drug register, (unless exempted in Schedule 5). Possession, supply and procurement is authorised for pharmacists and other classes of persons named in the 2001 Regulations.

- **Schedule 3** includes the barbiturates (except secobarbital, now Schedule 2), buprenorphine p. 468, gabapentin p. 332, mazindol, meprobamate, midazolam p. 358, pentazocine, phentermine, pregabalin, temazepam p. 509, and tramadol hydrochloride p. 491. They are subject to the special prescription requirements. Safe custody requirements do apply, except for any 5,5 disubstituted barbituric acid (e.g. phenobarbital), gabapentin p. 332, mazindol, meprobamate, midazolam p. 358, pentazocine, phentermine, pregabalin, tramadol hydrochloride p. 491, or any stereoisomeric form or salts of the above. Records in registers do not need to be kept (although there are requirements for the retention of invoices for 2 years).
- **Schedule 4** includes in Part I drugs that are subject to minimal control, such as benzodiazepines (except temazepam p. 509 and midazolam p. 358, which are in Schedule 3), non-benzodiazepine hypnotics (zaleplon, zolpidem tartrate, and zopiclone) and *Sativex*®. Part II includes androgenic and anabolic steroids, clenbuterol, chorionic gonadotrophin (HCG), non-human chorionic gonadotrophin, somatotropin, somatrem, and somatropin p. 789. Controlled drug prescription requirements do not apply and Schedule 4 Controlled Drugs are not subject to safe custody requirements. Records in registers do not need to be kept (except in the case of *Sativex*®).
- **Schedule 5** includes preparations of certain Controlled Drugs (such as codeine, pholcodine p. 313 or morphine p. 483) which due to their low strength, are exempt from virtually all Controlled Drug requirements other than retention of invoices for two years.

Since the Responsible Pharmacist Regulations were published in 2008, standing operation procedures for the management of Controlled Drugs, are required in registered pharmacies.

The Health Act 2006 introduced the concept of the 'accountable officer' with responsibility for the management of Controlled Drugs and related governance issues in their organisation. Most recently, in 2013 The Controlled Drugs (Supervision of Management and Use) Regulations were published to ensure good governance concerning the safe management and use of Controlled Drugs in England and Scotland.

Prescriptions

Preparations in Schedules 1, 2, 3, 4 and 5 of the Misuse of Drugs Regulations 2001 (and subsequent amendments) are identified throughout the BNF and BNF *for children* using the following symbols:

CD1	for preparations in Schedule 1
CD2	for preparations in Schedule 2
CD3	for preparations in Schedule 3
CD4-1	for preparations in Schedule 4 (Part I)
CD4-2	for preparations in Schedule 4 (Part II)
CD5	for preparations in Schedule 5

The principal legal requirements relating to medical prescriptions are listed below (see also Department of Health Guidance at www.gov.uk/dh).

Prescription requirements Prescriptions for Controlled Drugs that are subject to prescription requirements (all preparations in Schedules 2 and 3) must be indelible, must be *signed* by the prescriber, include the *date* on which they were signed, and specify the prescriber's *address* (must be within the UK). A machine-written prescription is acceptable, but the prescriber's signature must be handwritten. Advanced electronic signatures can be accepted for Schedule 2 and 3 Controlled Drugs where the Electronic Prescribing Service (EPS) is used. All prescriptions for Controlled Drugs that are subject to the prescription requirements must always state:

- the name and address of the patient (use of a PO Box is not acceptable);
- in the case of a preparation, the form (the dosage form e.g. tablets must be included on a Controlled Drugs prescription irrespective of whether it is implicit in the proprietary name e.g. *MST Continus*, or whether only one form is available), and, where appropriate, the strength of the preparation (when more than one strength of a preparation exists the strength required must be specified); to avoid ambiguity, where a prescription requests multiple strengths of a medicine, each strength should be prescribed separately (i.e. separate dose, total quantity, etc);
- for liquids, the total volume in millilitres (in both words and figures) of the preparation to be supplied; for dosage units (tablets, capsules, ampoules), state the total number (in both words and figures) of dosage units to be supplied (e.g. 10 tablets [of 10 mg] rather than 100 mg total quantity);
- the dose, which must be clearly defined (i.e. the instruction 'one as directed' constitutes a dose but 'as directed' does not); it is not necessary that the dose is stated in both words and figures;
- the words 'for dental treatment only' if issued by a dentist.

A pharmacist is **not** allowed to dispense a Controlled Drug unless all the information required by law is given on the prescription. In the case of a prescription for a Controlled Drug in Schedule 2 or 3, a pharmacist can amend the prescription *if* it specifies the total quantity only in words or in figures or if it contains minor typographical errors, provided that such amendments are indelible and clearly attributable to the pharmacist (e.g. name, date, signature and GPhC registration number). The prescription should be marked with the date of supply at the time the Controlled Drug supply is made.

 The Department of Health and the Scottish Government have issued a strong recommendation that the maximum quantity of Schedule 2, 3 or 4 Controlled Drugs prescribed should not exceed 30 days; exceptionally, to cover a justifiable clinical need and after consideration of any risk, a prescription can be issued for a longer period, but the reasons for the decision should be recorded on the patient's notes.

 A prescription for a Controlled Drug in Schedules 2, 3, or 4 is valid for 28 days from the date stated thereon (the prescriber may forward-date the prescription; the start date may also be specified in the body of the prescription). Schedule 5 prescriptions are valid for 6 months from the appropriate date.

 Medicines that are not Controlled Drugs should not be prescribed on the same form as a Schedule 2 or 3 Controlled Drug.

See sample prescription:

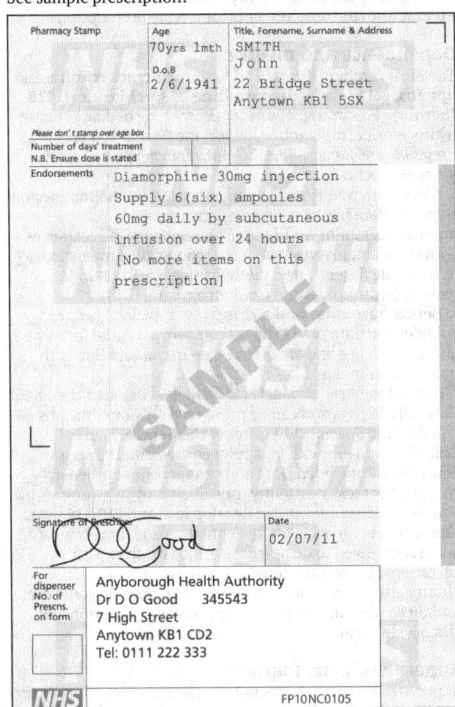

Instalments and repeatable prescriptions

Prescriptions for Schedule 2 or 3 Controlled Drugs can be dispensed by instalments. An instalment prescription must have an instalment direction including both the dose and the instalment amount specified separately on the prescription, and it must also state the interval between each time the medicine can be supplied.

 The first instalment must be dispensed within 28 days of the appropriate day (i.e. date of signing unless the prescriber indicates a date before which the Controlled Drug should not be dispensed) and the remainder should be dispensed in accordance with the instructions on the prescription. The prescription must be marked with the date of each supply.

 The instalment direction is a legal requirement and needs to be complied with, however, for certain situations (e.g. if a pharmacy is closed on the day an instalment is due) the Home Office has approved specific wording which provides pharmacists some flexibility for supply. For details, see Medicines, Ethics and Practice, London, Pharmaceutical Press (always consult latest edition) or see Home Office approved wording for instalment prescribing (Circular 027/2015), available at www.gov.uk/.

 Repeatable prescriptions are prescriptions which contain a direction that they can be dispensed more than once (e.g. repeat × 3). Only Schedule 4 and 5 Controlled Drugs are permitted on repeatable prescriptions.

Private prescriptions

Private prescriptions for Controlled Drugs in Schedules 2 and 3 must be written on specially designated forms which are provided by local NHS England area teams in England (form FP10PCD), local NHS Health Boards in Scotland (form PPCD) and Wales (form W10PCD); in addition, prescriptions must specify the *prescriber's identification number* (or a NHS prescriber code in Scotland).

Prescriptions to be supplied by a pharmacist in hospital are exempt from the requirements for private prescriptions.

Dependence and misuse

The most common drugs of addiction are **crack cocaine** and **opioids**, particularly **diamorphine hydrochloride p. 476 (heroin)** . For arrangements for prescribing of diamorphine hydrochloride, dipipanone, or cocaine for addicts, see *Prescribing of diamorphine (heroin), dipipanone, and cocaine for addicts* below.

Along with traditional stimulants, such as amfetamine and cocaine, there has been an emerging use of methamphetamine and a range of psychoactive substances with stimulant, depressant or hallucinogenic properties such as lysergide (lysergic acid diethylamide, LSD), ketamine or gamma-hydroxybutyrate (sodium oxybate, GHB).

Benzodiazepines and z-drugs (i.e. zopiclone p. 512, zolpidem tartrate p. 511) have their own potential for misuse and dependence and are often taken in combination with opiates or stimulants.

Cannabis-based products for medicinal use are Schedule 2 Controlled Drugs and can be prescribed only by clinicians listed on the Specialist Register of the General Medical Council. Cannabis with no approved medicinal use is a Schedule 1 Controlled Drug and cannot be prescribed. It remains the most frequently used illicit drug by young people and dependence can develop in around 10% of users. Cannabis use can exacerbate depression and it may cause an acute short-lived toxic psychosis which resolves with cessation, however paranoid symptoms may persist in chronic users; withdrawal symptoms can occur in some users and these can contribute to sleep problems, agitation and risk of self-harm.

Supervised consumption

Supervised consumption is not a legal requirement under the 2001 Regulations. Nevertheless, when supervised consumption is directed on the prescription, the Department of Health recommends that any deviation from the prescriber's intended method of supply should be documented and the justification for this recorded.

Individuals prescribed opioid substitution therapy can take their daily dose under the supervision of a doctor, nurse, or pharmacist during the dose stabilisation phase (usually the first 3 months of treatment), after a relapse or period of instability, or if there is a significant increase in the dose of methadone. Supervised consumption should continue (in accordance with local protocols) until the prescriber is confident that the patient is compliant with their treatment. It is good practice for pharmacists to alert the prescriber when a patient has missed consecutive daily doses.

Prescribing drugs likely to cause dependence or misuse

The prescriber has three main responsibilities:
- To avoid creating dependence by introducing drugs to patients without sufficient reason. In this context, the proper use of the morphine-like drugs is well understood. The dangers of other Controlled Drugs are less clear because recognition of dependence is not easy and its effects, and those of withdrawal, are less obvious.
- To see that the patient does not gradually increase the dose of a drug, given for good medical reasons, to the point where dependence becomes more likely. This tendency is seen especially with hypnotics and anxiolytics. The prescriber should keep a close eye on the amount prescribed to prevent patients from accumulating stocks. A minimal amount should be prescribed in the first instance, or when seeing a patient for the first time.
- To avoid being used as an unwitting source of supply for addicts and being vigilant to methods for obtaining

medicines. Methods include visiting more than one doctor, fabricating stories, and forging prescriptions.

Patients under temporary care should be given only small supplies of drugs unless they present an unequivocal letter from their own doctor. Doctors should also remember that their own patients may be attempting to collect prescriptions from other prescribers, especially in hospitals. It is sensible to reduce dosages steadily or to issue weekly or even daily prescriptions for small amounts if it is apparent that dependence is occurring.

Prescribers are responsible for the security of prescription forms once issued to them. The stealing and misuse of prescription forms could be minimised by the following precautions:
- records of serial numbers received and issued should be retained for at least three years;
- blank prescriptions should never be pre-signed;
- prescription forms should not be left unattended and should be locked in a secure drawer, cupboard, or carrying case when not in use;
- doctors', dentists' and surgery stamps should be kept in a secure location separate from the prescription forms;
- alterations are best avoided but if any are made and the prescription is to be used, best practice is for the prescriber to cross out the error, initial and date the error, then write the correct information;
- if an error made in a prescription cannot be corrected, best practice for the prescriber is to put a line through the script and write 'spoiled' on the form, or destroy the form and start writing a new prescription;
- prescribers and pharmacists dispensing drugs prone to abuse should ensure compliance with all relevant legal requirements specially when dealing with prescriptions for Controlled Drugs (see *Prescription requirements* and *Instalments* above);
- at the time of dispensing, prescriptions should be stamped with the pharmacy stamp and endorsed by the pharmacist or pharmacy technician with what has been supplied; where loss or theft is suspected, the police should be informed immediately.

Travelling abroad

Prescribed drugs listed in Schedule 4 Part II (CD Anab) for self-administration and Schedule 5 of the Misuse of Drugs Regulations 2001 (and subsequent amendments) are not subject to export or import licensing. A personal import/export licence is required for patients travelling abroad with Schedules 2, 3, or 4 Part I (CD Benz) and Part II (CD Anab) Controlled Drugs if, they are carrying more than 3 months' supply or are travelling for 3 calendar months or more. A Home Office licence is required for any amount of a Schedule 1 Controlled Drug imported into the UK for personal use regardless of the duration of travel. Further details can be obtained at www.gov.uk/guidance/controlled-drugs-licences-fees-and-returns or from the Home Office by contacting DFLU.ie@homeoffice.gsi.gov.uk. In cases of emergency, telephone (020) 7035 6330.

Applications for obtaining a licence must be supported by a cover letter signed by the prescribing doctor or drug worker, which must confirm:
- the patient's name and address;
- the travel itinerary;
- the names of the prescribed Controlled Drug(s), doses and total amounts to be carried.

Applications for licences should be sent to the Home Office, Drugs & Firearms Licensing Unit, Fry Building, 2 Marsham Street, London, SW1P 4DF.

Alternatively, completed application forms can be emailed to DFLU.ie@homeoffice.gsi.gov.uk. A minimum of 10 days should be allowed for processing the application.

Patients travelling for less than 3 months or carrying less than 3 months supply of Controlled Drugs do not require a personal export/import licence, but are advised to carry a cover letter signed by the prescribing doctor or drug worker. Those travelling for more than 3 months are advised to make arrangements to have their medication prescribed by a practitioner in the country they are visiting.

Doctors who want to take Controlled Drugs abroad while accompanying patients may similarly be issued with licences. Licences are not normally issued to doctors who want to take Controlled Drugs abroad solely in case a family emergency should arise.

Personal export/import licences do not have any legal status outside the UK and are issued only to comply with the Misuse of Drugs Act 2001 and to facilitate passage through UK Customs and Excise control. For clearance in the country to be visited it is necessary to approach that country's consulate in the UK.

Notification of patients receiving structured drug treatment for substance dependence

In **England**, doctors should report cases where they are providing structured drug treatment for substance dependence to their local National Drug Treatment Monitoring System (NDTMS) Team. General information about NDTMS can be found at www.gov.uk/government/collections/alcohol-and-drug-misuse-prevention-and-treatment-guidance.

Enquiries about NDTMS, and how to submit data, should initially be directed to:

- EvidenceApplicationteam@phe.gov.uk

In **Scotland**, doctors should report cases to the Substance Drug Misuse Database. General information about the Scottish Drug Misuse Database can be found in www.isdscotland.org/Health-Topics/Drugs-and-Alcohol-Misuse/Drugs-Misuse/Scottish-Drug-Misuse-Database/. Enquiries about reporting can be directed to:

- nss.isdsubstancemisuse@nhs.net

In **Northern Ireland**, the Misuse of Drugs (Notification of and Supply to Addicts) (Northern Ireland) Regulations 1973 require doctors to send particulars of persons whom they consider to be addicted to certain Controlled Drugs to the Chief Medical Officer of the Ministry of Health and Social Services. The Northern Ireland contact is:

Public Health Information & Research Branch
Department of Health
Annexe 2
Castle Buildings
Stormont
Belfast
BT4 3SQ
028 9052 2340
phirb@health-ni.gov.uk

Public Health Information & Research Branch also maintains the Northern Ireland Drug Misuse Database (NIDMD) which collects detailed information on those presenting for treatment, on drugs misused and injecting behaviour; participation is not a statutory requirement.

In **Wales**, doctors should report cases where they are providing structured drug treatment for substance dependence on the Welsh National Database for Substance Misuse; enquiries should be directed to: substancemisuse-queries@wales.nhs.uk.

Prescribing of diamorphine (heroin), dipipanone, and cocaine for addicts

The Misuse of Drugs (Supply to Addicts) Regulations 1997 require that **only** medical practitioners who hold a special licence issued by the Home Secretary (or Scottish Government's Chief Medical Officer) may prescribe, administer, or supply diamorphine hydrochloride p. 476, dipipanone, or cocaine for *the treatment of drug addiction*.

Medical prescribers, pharmacists independent prescribers, nurses independent prescribers and supplementary prescribers do not require a special licence for prescribing diamorphine hydrochloride p. 476, dipipanone, or cocaine for patients (including addicts) for relieving pain from organic disease or injury.

Adverse reactions to drugs

Yellow card scheme

Any drug may produce unwanted or unexpected adverse reactions. Rapid detection and recording of adverse drug reactions is of vital importance so that unrecognised hazards are identified promptly and appropriate regulatory action is taken to ensure that medicines are used safely. Healthcare professionals and coroners are urged to report suspected adverse drug reactions directly to the Medicines and Healthcare products Regulatory Agency (MHRA) through the Yellow Card Scheme using the electronic form at www.mhra. gov.uk/yellowcard. Alternatively, prepaid Yellow Cards for reporting are available from the address below and are also bound in the inside back cover of the BNF.

Send Yellow Cards to:

FREEPOST YELLOW CARD
(No other address details required).
0800 731 6789

Suspected adverse drug reactions to any therapeutic agent should be reported, including drugs (self-medication as well as those prescribed), blood products, vaccines, radiographic contrast media, complementary and herbal products. For biosimilar medicines and vaccines, adverse reaction reports should clearly state the brand name and the batch number of the suspected medicine or vaccine.

Suspected adverse drug reactions should be reported through the Yellow Card Scheme at www.mhra.gov.uk/ yellowcard. Yellow Cards can be used for reporting suspected adverse drug reactions to medicines, vaccines, herbal or complementary products, whether self-medicated or prescribed. This includes suspected adverse drug reactions associated with misuse, overdose, medication errors or from use of unlicensed and off-label medicines. Yellow Cards can also be used to report medical device incidents, defective medicines, and suspected fake medicines.

Spontaneous reporting is particularly valuable for recognising possible new hazards rapidly. An adverse reaction should be reported even if it is not certain that the drug has caused it, or if the reaction is well recognised, or if other drugs have been given at the same time. Reports of overdoses (deliberate or accidental) can complicate the assessment of adverse drug reactions, but provide important information on the potential toxicity of drugs.

A freephone service is available to all parts of the UK for advice and information on suspected adverse drug reactions; contact the National Yellow Card Information Service at the MHRA on 0800 731 6789. Outside office hours a telephone-answering machine will take messages.

The following Yellow Card Centres can be contacted for further information:

Yellow Card Centre North West
2nd Floor
70 Pembroke Place
Liverpool
L69 3GF
(0151) 794 8117
YCCNorthwest@rlbuht.nhs.net

Yellow Card Centre Wales
All Wales Therapeutics and Toxicology Centre
Academic Building
University Hospital Llandough
Penlan Road
Penarth
Vale of Glamorgan
CF64 2XX
(029) 2184 5831
CAV_YCCWales@wales.nhs.uk

Yellow Card Centre Northern & Yorkshire
Regional Drug and Therapeutics Centre
16/17 Framlington Place
Newcastle upon Tyne
NE2 4AB
(0191) 213 7855

Yellow Card Centre West Midlands
City Hospital
Dudley Road
Birmingham
B18 7QH
(0121) 507 5672

Yellow Card Centre Scotland
CARDS, Royal Infirmary of Edinburgh
51 Little France Crescent
Old Dalkeith Road
Edinburgh
EH16 4SA
(0131) 242 2919
YCCScotland@luht.scot.nhs.uk

The MHRA's database facilitates the monitoring of adverse drug reactions. More detailed information on reporting and a list of products currently under additional monitoring can be found on the MHRA website: www.mhra.gov.uk.

MHRA Drug Safety Update *Drug Safety Update* is a monthly newsletter from the MHRA and the Commission on Human Medicines (CHM); it is available at www.gov.uk/drug-safety-update.

Self-reporting

Patients and their carers can also report suspected adverse drug reactions to the MHRA. Reports can be submitted directly to the MHRA through the Yellow Card Scheme using the electronic form at www.mhra.gov.uk/yellowcard, by telephone on 0808 100 3352, or by downloading the Yellow Card form from www.mhra.gov.uk. Alternatively, patient Yellow Cards are available from pharmacies and GP surgeries. Information for patients about the Yellow Card Scheme is available in other languages at www.mhra.gov.uk/ yellowcard.

Prescription-event monitoring

In addition to the MHRA's Yellow Card Scheme, an independent scheme monitors the safety of new medicines using a different approach. The Drug Safety Research Unit identifies patients who have been prescribed selected new medicines and collects data on clinical events in these patients. The data are submitted on a voluntary basis by general practitioners on green forms. More information about the scheme and the Unit's educational material is available from www.dsru.org.

Newer drugs and vaccines

Only limited information is available from clinical trials on the safety of new medicines. Further understanding about the safety of medicines depends on the availability of information from routine clinical practice.

The black triangle symbol identifies newly licensed medicines that require additional monitoring by the European Medicines Agency. Such medicines include new active substances, biosimilar medicines, and medicines that the European Medicines Agency consider require additional monitoring. The black triangle symbol also appears in the Patient Information Leaflets for relevant medicines, with a brief explanation of what it means. Products usually retain a black triangle for 5 years, but this can be extended if required.

Spontaneous reporting is particularly valuable for recognising possible new hazards rapidly. For medicines showing the black triangle symbol, the MHRA asks that **all** suspected reactions (including those considered not to be serious) are reported through the Yellow Card Scheme. An adverse reaction should be reported even if it is not certain that the drug has caused it, or if the reaction is well recognised, or if other drugs have been given at the same time.

Established drugs and vaccines

Healthcare professionals and coroners are asked to report all suspected reactions to established drugs (including over-the-counter, herbal, and unlicensed medicines and medicines used off-label) and vaccines that are **serious, medically significant, or result in harm**. Serious reactions include those that are fatal, life-threatening, disabling, incapacitating, or which result in or prolong hospitalisation, or a congenital abnormality; they should be reported even if the effect is well recognised. Examples include anaphylaxis, blood disorders, endocrine disturbances, effects on fertility, haemorrhage from any site, renal impairment, jaundice, ophthalmic disorders, severe CNS effects, severe skin reactions, reactions in pregnant women, and any drug interactions. Reports of serious adverse reactions are required to enable comparison with other drugs of a similar class. Reports of overdoses (deliberate or accidental) can complicate the assessment of adverse drug reactions, but provide important information on the potential toxicity of drugs.

For established drugs there is no need to report well-known, relatively minor side-effects, such as dry mouth with tricyclic antidepressants or constipation with opioids.

Medication errors

Adverse drug reactions where harm occurs as a result of a medication error are reportable as a Yellow Card or through the local risk management systems into the National Reporting and Learning System (NRLS). If reported to the NRLS, these will be shared with the MHRA. If the NRLS is not available and harm occurs, report using a Yellow Card.

Adverse reactions to medical devices

Suspected adverse reactions to medical devices including dental or surgical materials, intra-uterine devices, and contact lens fluids should be reported. Information on reporting these can be found at: www.mhra.gov.uk.

Side-effects in the BNF

The BNF includes clinically relevant side-effects for most drugs; an exhaustive list is not included for drugs that are used by specialists (e.g. cytotoxic drugs and drugs used in anaesthesia). Where causality has not been established, side-effects in the manufacturers' literature may be omitted from the BNF.

Recognising that hypersensitivity reactions (including anaphylactic and anaphylactoid reactions) can occur with virtually all drugs, this effect is not generally listed, unless the drug carries an increased risk of such reactions or specific management advice is provided by the manufacturer. Administration site reactions have been omitted from the BNF (e.g. pain at injection site). The BNF also omits effects that are likely to have little clinical consequence (e.g. transient increase in liver enzymes). Drugs that are applied locally or topically carry a theoretical or low risk of systemic absorption and therefore systemic side-effects for these drugs are not listed in the BNF unless they are associated with a high risk to patient safety. Infections are a known complication of treatment with drugs that affect the immune system (e.g. corticosteroids or immunosuppressants); this side-effect is listed in the BNF as 'increased risk of infection'.

Symptoms of drug withdrawal reactions are not individually listed, but are collectively termed 'withdrawal syndrome'.

Side-effects are generally listed alphabetically in order of frequency. In the product literature the frequency of side-effects is generally described as follows:

Description of the frequency of side-effects	
Very common	greater than 1 in 10
Common	1 in 100 to 1 in 10
Uncommon [formerly 'less commonly' in BNF publications]	1 in 1000 to 1 in 100
Rare	1 in 10 000 to 1 in 1000
Very rare	less than 1 in 10 000
Frequency not known	frequency is not defined by product literature or the side-effect has been reported from post-marketing surveillance data

For consistency, the terms used to describe side-effects are standardised using a defined vocabulary across all of the drug monographs in the BNF (e.g. postural hypotension is used for the term orthostatic hypotension).

Special problems

Delayed drug effects Some reactions (e.g. cancers, chloroquine retinopathy, and retroperitoneal fibrosis) may become manifest months or years after exposure. Any suspicion of such an association should be reported directly to the MHRA through the Yellow Card Scheme.

The elderly Particular vigilance is required to identify adverse reactions in the elderly.

Congenital abnormalities When an infant is born with a congenital abnormality or there is a malformed aborted fetus doctors are asked to consider whether this might be an adverse reaction to a drug and to report all drugs (including self-medication) taken during pregnancy.

Children Particular vigilance is required to identify and report adverse reactions in children, including those resulting from the unlicensed use of medicines; **all** suspected reactions should be reported directly to the MHRA through the Yellow Card Scheme (see also Adverse Drug Reactions in Children).

Prevention of adverse reactions

Adverse reactions may be prevented as follows:

- never use any drug unless there is a good indication. If the patient is pregnant do not use a drug unless the need for it is imperative;
- allergy and idiosyncrasy are important causes of adverse drug reactions. Ask if the patient had previous reactions to the drug or formulation;
- ask if the patient is already taking other drugs including self-medication drugs, health supplements, complementary and alternative therapies; interactions may occur;
- age and hepatic or renal disease may alter the metabolism or excretion of drugs, so that much smaller doses may be needed. Genetic factors may also be responsible for variations in metabolism, and therefore for the adverse effect of the drug; notably of isoniazid p. 624 and the tricyclic antidepressants;
- prescribe as few drugs as possible and give very clear instructions to the elderly or any patient likely to misunderstand complicated instructions;
- whenever possible use a familiar drug; with a new drug, be particularly alert for adverse reactions or unexpected events;

- consider if excipients (e.g. colouring agents) may be contributing to the adverse reaction. If the reaction is minor, a trial of an alternative formulation of the same drug may be considered before abandoning the drug;
- warn the patient if serious adverse reactions are liable to occur.

Drug allergy (suspected or confirmed)

Suspected drug allergy is any reaction caused by a drug with clinical features compatible with an immunological mechanism. All drugs have the potential to cause adverse drug reactions, but not all of these are allergic in nature. A reaction is more likely to be caused by drug allergy if:

- The reaction occurred while the patient was being treated with the drug, or
- The drug is known to cause this pattern of reaction, or
- The patient has had a similar reaction to the same drug or drug-class previously.

A suspected reaction is less likely to be caused by a drug allergy if there is a possible non-drug cause or if there are only gastro-intestinal symptoms present.

The following signs, allergic patterns and timing of onset can be used to help decide whether to suspect drug allergy:

Immediate, rapidly-evolving reactions (onset usually less than 1 hour after drug exposure)

- Anaphylaxis, with erythema, urticaria or angioedema, and hypotension and/or bronchospasm. See also Antihistamines, allergen immunotherapy and allergic emergencies p. 292
- Urticaria or angioedema without systemic features
- Exacerbation of asthma e.g. with non-steroidal anti-inflammatory drugs (NSAIDs)

*Non-immediate reactions, **without** systemic involvement* (onset usually 6–10 days after first drug exposure or 3 days after second exposure)

- Cutaneous reactions, e.g. widespread red macules and/or papules, or, fixed drug eruption (localised inflamed skin)

*Non-immediate reactions, **with** systemic involvement* (onset may be variable, usually 3 days to 6 weeks after first drug exposure, depending on features, or 3 days after second exposure)

- Cutaneous reactions with systemic features, e.g. drug reaction with eosinophilia and systemic signs (DRESS) or drug hypersensitivity syndrome (DHS), characterised by widespread red macules, papules or erythroderma, fever, lymphadenopathy, liver dysfunction or eosinophilia
- Toxic epidermal necrolysis or Stevens–Johnson syndrome
- Acute generalised exanthematous pustulosis (AGEP)

EvGr Suspected drug allergy information should be clearly and accurately documented in clinical notes and prescriptions, and shared among all healthcare professionals. Patients should be given information about which drugs and drug-classes to avoid and encouraged to share their drug allergy status.

If a drug allergy is suspected, consider stopping the suspected drug and advising the patient or carer to avoid this drug in future. Symptoms of the acute reaction should be treated, in hospital if severe. Patients presenting with a suspected anaphylactic reaction, or a severe or non-immediate cutaneous reaction, should be referred to a specialist drug allergy service. Patients presenting with a suspected drug allergic reaction or anaphylaxis to NSAIDs, and local and general anaesthetics may also need to be referred to a specialist drug allergy service, e.g. in cases of anaphylactoid reactions or to determine future treatment options. Patients presenting with a suspected drug allergic reaction or anaphylaxis associated with beta-lactam antibiotics should be referred to a specialist drug allergy service if their disease or condition can only be treated by a beta-lactam antibiotic or they are likely to need beta-lactam

antibiotics frequently in the future (e.g. immunodeficient patients). ⒶFor further information see Drug allergy: diagnosis and management. NICE Clinical Guideline 183 (September 2014) www.nice.org.uk/guidance/cg183.

Oral side-effects of drugs

Drug-induced disorders of the mouth may be due to a local action on the mouth or to a systemic effect manifested by oral changes. In the latter case urgent referral to the patient's medical practitioner may be necessary.

Oral mucosa Medicaments left in contact with or applied directly to the oral mucosa can lead to inflammation or ulceration; the possibility of allergy should also be borne in mind.

Aspirin tablets p. 132 allowed to dissolve in the sulcus for the treatment of toothache can lead to a white patch followed by ulceration.

Flavouring agents, particularly **essential oils**, may sensitise the skin, but mucosal swelling is not usually prominent.

The oral mucosa is particularly vulnerable to ulceration in patients treated with cytotoxic drugs, e.g. methotrexate p. 957. Other drugs capable of causing oral ulceration include **ACE inhibitors, gold, nicorandil p. 227, NSAIDs, pancreatin p. 104, penicillamine p. 1146, proguanil hydrochloride p. 658,** and **protease inhibitors.**

Erythema multiforme or Stevens-Johnson syndrome may follow the use of a wide range of drugs including **antibacterials, antiretrovirals, sulfonamide derivatives,** and **anticonvulsants**; the oral mucosa may be extensively ulcerated, with characteristic target lesions on the skin. Oral lesions of toxic epidermal necrolysis have been reported with a similar range of drugs.

Lichenoid eruptions are associated with **ACE inhibitors, NSAIDs,** methyldopa p. 159, chloroquine p. 655, **oral antidiabetics, thiazide diuretics,** and **gold.**

Candidiasis can complicate treatment with **antibacterials** and **immunosuppressants** and is an occasional side-effect of **corticosteroid inhalers.**

Teeth and jaw *Brown staining* of the teeth frequently follows the use of chlorhexidine mouthwash, spray or gel, p. 1255 but can readily be removed by polishing. **Iron** salts in liquid form can stain the enamel black. Superficial staining has been reported rarely with co-amoxiclav suspension p. 585.

Intrinsic staining of the teeth is most commonly caused by **tetracyclines.** They will affect the teeth if given at any time from about the fourth month *in utero* until the age of twelve years; they are contra-indicated during pregnancy, in breast-feeding women, and in children under 12 years. All tetracyclines can cause permanent, unsightly staining in children, the colour varying from yellow to grey.

Excessive ingestion of **fluoride** leads to *dental fluorosis* with mottling of the enamel and areas of hypoplasia or pitting; fluoride supplements occasionally cause mild mottling (white patches) if the dose is too large for the child's age (taking into account the fluoride content of the local drinking water and of toothpaste).

The risk of *osteonecrosis of the jaw* is substantially greater for patients receiving intravenous bisphosphonates in the treatment of cancer than for patients receiving oral bisphosphonates for osteoporosis or Paget's disease. All patients receiving bisphosphonates should have a dental check-up (and any necessary remedial work should be performed) before bisphosphonate treatment, or as soon as possible after starting treatment. Patients with cancer receiving bevacizumab p. 909 or sunitinib p. 1044 may also be at risk of osteonecrosis of the jaw.

Periodontium *Gingival overgrowth* (gingival hyperplasia) is a side-effect of phenytoin p. 340 and sometimes of ciclosporin p. 884 or of nifedipine p. 176 (and some other calcium-channel blockers).

Thrombocytopenia may be drug related and may cause bleeding at the gingival margins, which may be spontaneous or may follow mild trauma (such as toothbrushing).

Salivary glands The most common effect that drugs have on the salivary glands is to *reduce flow* (xerostomia). Patients with a persistently dry mouth may have poor oral hygiene; they are at an increased risk of dental caries and oral infections (particularly candidiasis). Many drugs have been implicated in xerostomia, particularly **antimuscarinics** (anticholinergics), **antidepressants** (including tricyclic antidepressants, and selective serotonin re-uptake inhibitors), **alpha-blockers, antihistamines, antipsychotics, baclofen p. 1173, bupropion hydrochloride p. 520, clonidine hydrochloride p. 159, 5HT$_1$ agonists, opioids**, and tizanidine p. 1175. Excessive use of **diuretics** can also result in xerostomia.

Some drugs (e.g. clozapine p. 417, neostigmine p. 1170) can *increase saliva production* but this is rarely a problem unless the patient has associated difficulty in swallowing.

Pain in the salivary glands has been reported with some **antihypertensives** (e.g. clonidine hydrochloride p. 159, methyldopa p. 159) and with **vinca alkaloids**.

Swelling of the salivary glands can occur with **iodides, antithyroid drugs, phenothiazines**, and **sulfonamides**.

Taste There can be *decreased* taste acuity or *alteration* in taste sensation. Many drugs are implicated, including amiodarone hydrochloride p. 113, **calcitonin, ACE inhibitors**, carbimazole p. 814, clarithromycin p. 569, **gold**, griseofulvin p. 640, **lithium salts**, metformin hydrochloride p. 732, metronidazole p. 575, penicillamine p. 1146, phenindione p. 153, propafenone hydrochloride p. 112, **protease inhibitors**, terbinafine p. 1279, and zopiclone p. 512.

Defective medicines

During the manufacture or distribution of a medicine an error or accident may occur whereby the finished product does not conform to its specification. While such a defect may impair the therapeutic effect of the product and could adversely affect the health of a patient, it should **not** be confused with an Adverse Drug Reaction where the product conforms to its specification.

The Defective Medicines Report Centre assists with the investigation of problems arising from licensed medicinal products thought to be defective and co-ordinates any necessary protective action. Reports on suspect defective medicinal products should include the brand or the non-proprietary name, the name of the manufacturer or supplier, the strength and dosage form of the product, the product licence number, the batch number or numbers of the product, the nature of the defect, and an account of any action already taken in consequence. The Centre can be contacted at:

The Defective Medicines Report Centre
Medicines and Healthcare products Regulatory Agency
151 Buckingham Palace Road
London
SW1W 9SZ
(020) 3080 6574
dmrc@mhra.gsi.gov.uk

Guidance on intravenous infusions

Intravenous additives policies

A local policy on the addition of drugs to intravenous fluids should be drawn up by a multi-disciplinary team and issued as a document to the members of staff concerned.

Centralised additive services are provided in a number of hospital pharmacy departments and should be used in preference to making additions on wards.

The information that follows should be read in conjunction with local policy documents.

Guidelines

- Drugs should only be added to infusion containers when constant plasma concentrations are needed or when the administration of a more concentrated solution would be harmful.
- In general, only one drug should be added to any infusion container and the components should be compatible. Ready-prepared solutions should be used whenever possible. Drugs should not normally be added to blood products, mannitol, or sodium bicarbonate. Only specially formulated additives should be used with fat emulsions or amino-acid solutions.
- Solutions should be thoroughly mixed by shaking and checked for absence of particulate matter before use.
- Strict asepsis should be maintained throughout and in general the giving set should not be used for more than 24 hours (for drug admixtures).
- The infusion container should be labelled with the patient's name, the name and quantity of additives, and the date and time of addition (and the new expiry date or time). Such additional labelling should not interfere with information on the manufacturer's label that is still valid. When possible, containers should be retained for a period after use in case they are needed for investigation.
- It is good practice to examine intravenous infusions from time to time while they are running. If cloudiness, crystallisation, change of colour, or any other sign of interaction or contamination is observed the infusion should be discontinued.

Problems

Microbial contamination The accidental entry and subsequent growth of micro-organisms converts the infusion fluid pathway into a potential vehicle for infection with micro-organisms, particularly species of *Candida*, *Enterobacter*, and *Klebsiella*. Ready-prepared infusions containing the additional drugs, or infusions prepared by an additive service (when available) should therefore be used in preference to making extemporaneous additions to infusion containers on wards etc. However, when this is necessary strict aseptic procedure should be followed.

Incompatibility Physical and chemical incompatibilities may occur with loss of potency, increase in toxicity, or other adverse effect. The solutions may become opalescent or precipitation may occur, but in many instances there is no visual indication of incompatibility. Interaction may take place at any point in the infusion fluid pathway, and the potential for incompatibility is increased when more than one substance is added to the infusion fluid.

Common incompatibilities Precipitation reactions are numerous and varied and may occur as a result of pH, concentration changes, 'salting-out' effects, complexation or other chemical changes. Precipitation or other particle formation must be avoided since, apart from lack of control of dosage on administration, it may initiate or exacerbate adverse effects. This is particularly important in the case of drugs which have been implicated in either thrombophlebitis

(e.g. diazepam) or in skin sloughing or necrosis caused by extravasation (e.g. sodium bicarbonate and certain cytotoxic drugs). It is also especially important to effect solution of colloidal drugs and to prevent their subsequent precipitation in order to avoid a pyrogenic reaction (e.g. amphotericin B).

It is considered undesirable to mix beta-lactam antibiotics, such as semi-synthetic penicillins and cephalosporins, with proteinaceous materials on the grounds that immunogenic and allergenic conjugates could be formed.

A number of preparations undergo significant loss of potency when added singly or in combination to large volume infusions. Examples include ampicillin in infusions that contain glucose or lactates. The breakdown products of dacarbazine have been implicated in adverse effects.

Blood Because of the large number of incompatibilities, drugs should not normally be added to blood and blood products for infusion purposes. Examples of incompatibility with blood include hypertonic mannitol solutions (irreversible crenation of red cells), dextrans (rouleaux formation and interference with cross-matching), glucose (clumping of red cells), and oxytocin (inactivated).

If the giving set is not changed after the administration of blood, but used for other infusion fluids, a fibrin clot may form which, apart from blocking the set, increases the likelihood of microbial growth.

Intravenous fat emulsions These may break down with coalescence of fat globules and separation of phases when additions such as antibacterials or electrolytes are made, thus increasing the possibility of embolism. Only specially formulated products such as *Vitlipid N*® may be added to appropriate intravenous fat emulsions.

Other infusions Infusions that frequently give rise to incompatibility include amino acids, mannitol, and sodium bicarbonate.

Bactericides Bactericides such as chlorocresol 0.1% or phenylmercuric nitrate 0.001% are present in some injection solutions. The total volume of such solutions added to a container for infusion on one occasion should not exceed 15 mL.

Method

Ready-prepared infusions should be used whenever available. **Potassium chloride** is usually available in concentrations of 20, 27, and 40 mmol/litre in sodium chloride intravenous infusion (0.9%), glucose intravenous infusion (5%) or sodium chloride and glucose intravenous infusion. **Lidocaine hydrochloride** is usually available in concentrations of 0.1 or 0.2% in glucose intravenous infusion (5%).

When addition is required to be made extemporaneously, any product reconstitution instructions such as those relating to concentration, vehicle, mixing, and handling precautions should be strictly followed using an aseptic technique throughout. Once the product has been reconstituted, addition to the infusion fluid should be made immediately in order to minimise microbial contamination and, with certain products, to prevent degradation or other formulation change which may occur; e.g. reconstituted ampicillin injection degrades rapidly on standing, and also may form polymers which could cause sensitivity reactions.

It is also important in certain instances that an infusion fluid of specific pH be used (e.g. **furosemide** injection requires dilution in infusions of pH greater than 5.5).

When drug additions are made it is important to mix thoroughly; additions should not be made to an infusion container that has been connected to a giving set, as mixing is hampered. If the solutions are not thoroughly mixed a concentrated layer of the additive may form owing to differences in density. **Potassium chloride** is particularly prone to this 'layering' effect when added without adequate mixing to infusions packed in non-rigid infusion containers; if such a mixture is administered it may have a serious effect on the heart.

A time limit between addition and completion of administration must be imposed for certain admixtures to guarantee satisfactory drug potency and compatibility. For admixtures in which degradation occurs without the formation of toxic substances, an acceptable limit is the time taken for 10% decomposition of the drug. When toxic substances are produced stricter limits may be imposed. Because of the risk of microbial contamination a maximum time limit of 24 hours may be appropriate for additions made elsewhere than in hospital pharmacies offering central additive service.

Certain injections must be protected from light during continuous infusion to minimise oxidation, e.g. dacarbazine and sodium nitroprusside.

Dilution with a small volume of an appropriate vehicle and administration using a motorised infusion pump is advocated for preparations such as unfractionated heparin where strict control over administration is required. In this case the appropriate dose may be dissolved in a convenient volume (e.g. 24–48 mL) of sodium chloride intravenous infusion (0.9%).

Information provided in the *BNF*

The *BNF* gives information about preparations given by three methods:

- continuous infusion;
- intermittent infusion;
- addition via the drip tubing.

Drugs for **continuous infusion** must be diluted in a large volume infusion. Penicillins and cephalosporins are not usually given by continuous infusion because of stability problems and because adequate plasma and tissue concentrations are best obtained by intermittent infusion. Where it is necessary to administer them by continuous infusion, detailed literature should be consulted.

Drugs that are both compatible and clinically suitable may be given by **intermittent infusion** in a relatively small volume of infusion over a short period of time, e.g. 100 mL in 30 minutes. The method is used if the product is incompatible or unstable over the period necessary for continuous infusion; the limited stability of ampicillin or amoxicillin in large volume glucose or lactate infusions may be overcome in this way.

Intermittent infusion is also used if adequate plasma and tissue concentrations are not produced by continuous infusion as in the case of drugs such as dacarbazine, gentamicin, and ticarcillin.

An in-line burette may be used for intermittent infusion techniques in order to achieve strict control over the time and rate of administration, especially for infants and children and in intensive care units. Intermittent infusion may also make use of the 'piggy-back' technique provided that no additions are made to the primary infusion. In this method the drug is added to a small secondary container connected to a Y-type injection site on the primary infusion giving set; the secondary solution is usually infused within 30 minutes.

Addition *via* the drip tubing is indicated for a number of cytotoxic drugs in order to minimise extravasation. The preparation is added aseptically via the rubber septum of the injection site of a fast-running infusion. In general, drug preparations intended for a bolus effect should be given directly into a separate vein where possible. Failing this, administration may be made via the drip tubing provided that the preparation is compatible with the infusion fluid when given in this manner.

Drugs given by intravenous infusion The BNF includes information on addition to *Glucose intravenous infusion* 5 and 10%, and *Sodium chloride intravenous infusion* 0.9%. Compatibility with glucose 5% and with sodium chloride 0.9% indicates compatibility with *Sodium chloride and glucose intravenous infusion*. Infusion of a large volume of hypotonic solution should be avoided therefore care should be taken if water for injections is used. The information relates to the proprietary preparations indicated; for other preparations suitability should be checked with the manufacturer.

Medicines optimisation

Overview

Medicines are the most common intervention in healthcare for the prevention, treatment and/or management of many illnesses. As life expectancy increases and as the population ages, more people are living with several long-term conditions that are being managed with an increasing number of medicines. Medicines use can be complex and how patients can take their medicines safely and effectively is a challenge for the health service.

Multimorbidity (the presence of 2 or more long-term conditions) is associated with a greater use of health services, higher mortality, higher treatment burden (due to polypharmacy or multiple appointments), and reduced quality of life. The risk of patients suffering harm from their medicines increases with polypharmacy, and treatment regimens (including non-pharmacological treatments) can very easily become burdensome for patients with multimorbidity and can lead to care becoming fragmented and uncoordinated. Prescribers should consider the risks and benefits of treatments recommended from guidance for single health conditions, as the evidence for these recommendations is regularly drawn from patients without multimorbidity and who are taking fewer prescribed regular medicines. The management of risk factors for future disease can also be a major treatment burden for patients with multimorbidity and should be taken into consideration.

Medicines optimisation encompasses many aspects of medicines use and helps to ensure that they are taken as intended, thus supporting the management of long-term conditions, multimorbidities, and appropriate polypharmacy. Through the adoption of a patient-focused approach to safe and effective medicines use, medicines optimisation changes the way patients are supported to get the best possible outcomes from their medicines. The use of shared decision-making informed by the best available evidence to guide decisions, ensures all patients have the opportunity to be involved in decisions about their medicines, taking into account their needs, preferences and values.

To reduce the risk of harm, ensure patients taking multiple medicines are receiving the most appropriate treatments for their needs, and to manage the spend on medicines, the Department of Health and Social Care are reviewing over-prescribing in the NHS.

Optimisation tools

Medicines optimisation includes aspects of care such as clinical assessment, clinical audits, disease prevention, health education, individual reviews and monitoring, and risk management. Having effective processes and systems in place can minimise the risk of preventable medicines-related problems (such as interactions with other medicines or comorbidities, and side-effects). Health and social care organisations should consider the use of multiple methods for identifying medicines-related patient safety incidents; learning from these incidents is important for guiding practice and minimising patient harm.

When optimising patient care, areas of intervention to consider include: deprescribing; medicines reconciliation; reviews and repeat prescribing; problematic polypharmacy; reducing medication waste and errors; and self-management plans. Self-management plans can be patient or health professional led and vary in their content depending on the individual needs of the patient, with the aim of supporting both their involvement and empowerment in managing their condition.

Medication reviews involve a structured critical examination of a patient's medicines to optimise treatment, minimise the number of medication-related problems, and reduce waste. These should be led by an appropriate health professional with effective communication skills, technical knowledge in the processes for managing medicines, and therapeutic knowledge on medicines use. Reviews can be carried out in different care settings, such as Primary Care Networks utilising pharmacists within the GP practice. For further information on review services available from community pharmacists, such as the 'New Medicines Service' and 'Medicines Use Review', see *Advanced pharmacy services*.

To support the medicines optimisation agenda, The Royal Pharmaceutical Society have produced good practice guidance for health professionals, which details four guiding principles for medicines optimisation. These are:

- Aim to understand the patient's experience;
- Evidence-based choice of medicines;
- Ensure medicines use is as safe as possible;
- Make medicines optimisation part of routine practice.

For further guidance around medicines optimisation and tools to use, NHS England have compiled useful links as part of **RightCare**; NICE have produced guidelines on **Medicines optimisation**, **Medicines adherence**, and **Multimorbidity**; and the Scottish Government have produced a guideline on **Polypharmacy**, see *Useful resources*.

Advanced Pharmacy Services Advanced Services are provided as part of the NHS Community Pharmacy Contractual Framework, and include services such as the New Medicines Service and Medicines Use Review service. These services are provided by accredited community pharmacists, with the aim of targeting specific patients to help manage their medicines more effectively, improve adherence, and reduce medicines wastage.

New Medicines Service The New Medicines Service (NMS) provides education and support to patients who are newly prescribed a medicine to manage a long-term condition. The service is split into three stages; patient engagement, intervention and follow-up. As of 2018, this service is available for patients living in England who have either been prescribed a new medicine for one of the following conditions – asthma, chronic obstructive pulmonary disease (COPD), type 2 diabetes or hypertension, or have been prescribed a new antiplatelet or anticoagulant. Patients can be offered the service by prescriber referral, or opportunistically by the community pharmacy. For further information, see: psnc.org.uk/services-commissioning/advanced-services/nms/.

Medicines Use Review The Medicines Use Review (MUR) service consists of structured adherence-centred reviews with patients on multiple medicines, particularly those receiving medicines for long-term conditions. The service is undertaken periodically, not usually more than once a year, and can also be prompted when an adherence issue is identified during the dispensing service.

The pharmacist providing the MUR service must ensure that at least 70% of all MURs undertaken in a year are for patients who fall within the two national target groups. The national target groups for MURs in England are:

- patients taking high-risk medicines (NSAIDs, anticoagulants (including low molecular weight heparin), antiplatelets, or diuretics);
- patients recently discharged from hospital who have had changes made to their medicines while they were in hospital.

For further information, see: psnc.org.uk/services-commissioning/advanced-services/murs/.

Wales, Northern Ireland, and Scotland have variations on this service, including different national target groups.

In Wales, see: www.cpwales.org.uk/Contract-support-and-IT/Advanced-Services.aspx.

In Northern Ireland, see: www.hscbusiness.hscni.net/services/2427.htm.

In Scotland, see: www.cps.scot/nhs-services/core/medicines-care-review/.

Communication

As health professionals from various disciplines and specialties may be caring for the same patient at the same time, good communication is required between health professionals in order to avoid fragmentation of care. Medication reviews may be carried out by health professionals other than the prescriber, therefore the prescriber should be informed of the review and its outcome—particularly if difficulties with adherence were discussed and further review is required.

There is a greater risk of poor communication and unintended medication changes when patients transfer between different care providers (such as when a person is admitted to or discharged from hospital). To support high-quality care when moving from one care setting to another, relevant information about medicines should be shared with patients, their family members/carers (if appropriate), and between health and social care practitioners using robust and transparent processes. Information should be securely shared between health and social care practitioners ideally within 24 hours of patient transfer.

Good communication between health professionals and patients, and their family members/carers (if appropriate) is needed for shared decision-making and supporting adherence. Information about their condition and possible treatments should be provided in a format that meets a patient's (and carer's) individual needs and preferences. The use of patient decision aids during consultations can help support a shared decision-making approach, and ensure patients and their family members/carers (where appropriate) are able to make well-informed choices that are consistent with their values and preferences.

For further guidance around communication between health professionals and patients (and carers), NICE have produced guidelines on **Medicines optimisation, Medicines adherence**, and **Supporting adult carers** (see *Useful resources*).

Organisations such as the 'NHS Specialist Pharmacy Service' help support medicines optimisation across the NHS by joining health professionals together through online networks (e.g. Regional Medicines Optimisation Committees and the English Deprescribing Network). This is available at: www.sps.nhs.uk/home/networks/.

Useful resources

Medicines optimisation: the safe and effective use of medicines to enable the best possible outcomes. National Institute for Health and Care Excellence. NICE guideline 5. March 2015.
www.nice.org.uk/guidance/ng5

Multimorbidity: clinical assessment and management. National Institute for Health and Care Excellence. NICE guideline 56. September 2016.
www.nice.org.uk/guidance/ng56

Medicines adherence: involving patients in decisions about prescribed medicines and supporting adherence. National Institute for Health and Care Excellence. Clinical guideline 76. January 2009.
www.nice.org.uk/guidance/cg76

Medicines Optimisation. NHS RightCare. NHS England.
www.england.nhs.uk/rightcare/useful-links/medicines-optimisation/

Polypharmacy Guidance, Realistic Prescribing. Scottish Government Polypharmacy Model of Care Group. 3rd Edition. 2018.
www.therapeutics.scot.nhs.uk/wp-content/uploads/2018/09/Polypharmacy-Guidance-2018.pdf

Supporting adult carers. National Institute for Health and Care Excellence. NICE Guideline 150. January 2020.
www.nice.org.uk/guidance/ng150

Medicines Optimisation: Helping patients to make the most of medicines. Royal Pharmaceutical Society. May 2013.
www.rpharms.com/resources/pharmacy-guides/medicines-optimisation-hub

Antimicrobial stewardship

Overview

Effective antimicrobials are required for preventive and curative measures, protecting patients from potentially fatal diseases, and ensuring that complex procedures can be provided at low risk of infection. Antimicrobial resistance (AMR) is the loss of antimicrobial effectiveness, and although it evolves naturally, this process is accelerated by the inappropriate or incorrect use of antimicrobials. Direct consequences of infection with resistant microorganisms can be severe and affect all areas of health, such as prolonged illnesses and hospital stays, increased costs and mortality, and reduced protection for patients undergoing operations or procedures. AMR is an international problem with an increasing prevalence that has consequences for the whole of society. The UK Government has recognised AMR as a significant area of concern and have committed global action to address this as a priority. For information and resources on the UK's plans for AMR, see the Public Health England (PHE) collection: **Antimicrobial resistance** (www.gov.uk/ government/collections/antimicrobial-resistance-amr-information-and-resources).

Antimicrobial stewardship (AMS) refers to an organisational or healthcare system-wide approach to promoting and monitoring judicious use of antimicrobials to preserve their future effectiveness. Addressing AMR through improving stewardship is a national medicines optimisation priority, led by NHS England and supported by PHE.

AMR can be managed by a combination of interventions that address:

- A political commitment to prioritise AMR;
- Monitoring antimicrobial use and resistance in microbes;
- Development of new drugs, treatments, and diagnostics;
- Individuals' behaviour relating to infection prevention and control, antimicrobial use, and AMR;
- Healthcare professionals' prescribing decisions.

Guidance for organisations (commissioners and providers)

Commissioners (clinical commissioning groups and local authorities) and providers (e.g. hospitals, GPs, out-of-hours services, dentists, and social enterprises) of health or social care services should establish an AMS programme, taking into account the resources needed to support AMS across all care settings. An AMS programme should take into consideration monitoring and evaluating antimicrobial prescribing, regular feedback to individual prescribers, education and training for health and social care staff, and integrating audits into existing quality improvement programmes.

Commissioners should work collaboratively to provide consistent information and advice to the public and health professionals that reduces inappropriate antimicrobial demand and use, and limits the spread of infection. Local authority public health teams should ensure that information and resources (such as posters, leaflets and digital resources) are made available through multiple routes to provide a coordinated system of information. Information should include simple and practical steps such as scrupulous personal and safe food hygiene practices.

Organisations should involve local health and social care staff in establishing processes for developing, reviewing, updating, and implementing local antimicrobial guidelines in line with national guidance and informed by local prescribing data and resistance patterns.

Organisations should also consider establishing processes for reviewing national horizon scanning to plan for the availability of new antimicrobials and to use an existing local decision-making group to consider the introduction of new antimicrobials locally.

Guidance for health and social care staff

Health and social care staff should assist with the implementation of local or national guidelines and recognise the significance of them for AMS.

Health professionals should be familiar with current AMS campaigns and programmes. For further information, see PHE and Health Education England's e-learning session **All Our Health: Antimicrobial Resistance** (portal.e-lfh.org.uk/ Component/Details/571263), PHE guidance **Health matters: antimicrobial resistance** (www.gov.uk/government/ publications/health-matters-antimicrobial-resistance), and the PHE campaigns **Antibiotic Guardian** (antibioticguardian.com/) and **Keep Antibiotics Working** (campaignresources.phe.gov. uk/resources/campaigns/58-keep-antibiotics-working).

Health professionals should be aware of resources and services that can help individuals minimise infections such as travel vaccination clinics, screening programmes, sexual health services, immunisation programmes, and other local referral pathways or schemes. The benefits of good hygiene, vaccination, and other preventative measures to reduce the risk of acquiring infections should be discussed with individuals, and individuals referred to further information or services if necessary.

Those involved in providing care should be educated about the standard principles of infection prevention and control. They should be trained in hand decontamination, the use of personal protective equipment, and the safe use and disposal of sharps. For further information, see NICE guideline: **Healthcare-associated infections** (see *Useful resources*).

Guidance on antimicrobial prescribing

National antimicrobial prescribing and stewardship competencies have been developed to improve the quality of antimicrobial treatment and stewardship. For further information, see Antimicrobial Resistance and Healthcare Associated Infections and PHE guidance: **Antimicrobial prescribing and stewardship competencies** (see *Useful resources*).

National toolkits to support the implementation of AMS best practice include the Royal College of General Practitioners' **TARGET antibiotics toolkit** (www.rcgp.org.uk/ TARGETantibiotics) for primary care, and PHE's **Start smart – then focus** (www.gov.uk/government/publications/ antimicrobial-stewardship-start-smart-then-focus) for secondary care, and **Dental antimicrobial stewardship: toolkit** (www.gov.uk/guidance/dental-antimicrobial-stewardship-toolkit) for dentists.

Clinical syndrome-specific guidance and advice to help slow the development of AMR have been developed by NICE, in collaboration with PHE, and are available at www.nice.org. uk/.

Considerations for antimicrobial prescribing When deciding whether or not to prescribe an antimicrobial, undertake a clinical assessment and consider the risk of AMR for individual patients and the population as a whole. An immediate antimicrobial prescription for a patient who is likely to have a self-limiting condition is not recommended.

Document in the patient's records (electronically wherever possible) the decisions related to antimicrobial use, including the plan as discussed with the patient, and their family and/or carers (if appropriate), and reason for prescribing/not prescribing an antimicrobial.

In hospital, microbiological samples should be taken before initiating an antimicrobial for patients with suspected infection. In primary care, consider taking microbiological samples when prescribing an antimicrobial for patients with recurrent or persistent infections. The choice of antimicrobial should be reviewed when microbiological results are available. For non-severe infections, consider taking microbiological samples before making a decision about prescribing an antimicrobial, providing it is safe to withhold treatment until the results are available.

Follow local or national guidelines on prescribing the shortest effective course and most appropriate dose and route of administration. Review intravenous antimicrobials within 48 hours (taking into account response to treatment and microbiological results) and consider stepping down to oral antimicrobials where possible. If prescribing outside of local or national guidelines, document in the patient's records the reasons for the decision.

Patients on antimicrobial treatment should be appropriately monitored to reduce side-effects and be assessed on the continued need for treatment. Repeat antimicrobial prescriptions are not recommended, unless needed for a particular clinical condition or indication. Avoid issuing a repeat prescription for longer than 6 months without review.

Advice for patients and their family and/or carers

Prescribers, primary care and community pharmacy teams should provide patients with resources educating them about not asking for antimicrobials as a preventive measure against becoming ill or as a stand-by measure, unless the patient has a specific condition or a specific risk that requires antimicrobial prophylaxis.

Prescribers should discuss with patients, and their family and/or carers (if appropriate) the likely nature of the condition, their views on antimicrobials, benefits and harms of antimicrobial prescribing, and why prescribing an antimicrobial may not always be the best option. Information should be provided about what to do if their symptoms worsen or if problems arise as a result of treatment. Written information should be provided if needed.

If antimicrobial treatment is not the most appropriate option, prescribers should advise patients, and their family and/or carers (if appropriate) about other options (as appropriate), such as self-care with over-the-counter preparations, back-up (delayed) prescribing, or other non-pharmacological interventions. Prescribers, primary care and community pharmacy teams should verbally emphasise and provide written advice about managing self-limiting infections.

If antimicrobials are prescribed or supplied, prescribers, primary care and community pharmacy teams should provide patients with verbal and written information on the correct use of antimicrobials. Advice should encourage people to:

- Take, or use antimicrobials only when recommended by a suitably qualified health professional;
- Obtain antimicrobials only from a health professional;
- Take, or use antimicrobials as instructed (right dose for the duration specified and via the right route);
- Return any unused antimicrobials to a pharmacy for safe disposal.

Useful resources

Antimicrobial prescribing and stewardship competencies. Antimicrobial Resistance and Healthcare Associated Infections (ARHAI) and Public Health England guideline. October 2013.
www.gov.uk/government/publications/antimicrobial-prescribing-and-stewardship-competencies

Antimicrobial resistance (AMR): applying All Our Health. Public Health England guideline. April 2015 (updated June 2019).
www.gov.uk/government/publications/antimicrobial-resistance-amr-applying-all-our-health

Antimicrobial stewardship: systems and processes for effective antimicrobial medicine use. National Institute for Health and Care Excellence. NICE guideline 15. August 2015.
www.nice.org.uk/guidance/NG15

Antimicrobial stewardship: changing risk-related behaviours in the general population. National Institute for Health and Care Excellence. NICE guideline 63. January 2017.
www.nice.org.uk/guidance/NG63

Healthcare-associated infections: prevention and control in primary and community care. National Institute for Health and Care Excellence. Clinical guideline 139. March 2012 (updated February 2017).
www.nice.org.uk/guidance/cg139

Prescribing in children

Overview

For detailed advice on medicines used for children, consult BNF *for Children*.

Children, and particularly neonates, differ from adults in their response to drugs. Special care is needed in the neonatal period (first 28 days of life) and doses should always be calculated with care. At this age, the risk of toxicity is increased by reduced drug clearance and differing target organ sensitivity.

Whenever possible, intramuscular injections should be **avoided** in children because they are painful.

Where possible, medicines for children should be prescribed within the terms of the marketing authorisation (product licence). However, many children may require medicines not specifically licensed for paediatric use.

Although medicines cannot be promoted outside the limits of the licence, the Human Medicines Regulations 2012 does not prohibit the use of unlicensed medicines. It is recognised that the informed use of unlicensed medicines or of licensed medicines for unlicensed applications ('off-label' use) is often necessary in paediatric practice.

Adverse drug reactions in children

Suspected adverse drug reactions in children and young adults under 18 years should be reported through the Yellow Card Scheme. Yellow cards can be used for reporting suspected adverse drug reactions to medicines, vaccines, herbal or complementary products, whether self-medicated or prescribed. This includes suspected adverse drug reactions associated with misuse, overdose, medication errors or from use of unlicensed and off-label medicines. Yellow Cards can also be used to report medical device incidents, defective medicines, and suspected fake medicines.

Report all suspected adverse drug reactions that are:

- **serious, medically significant or result in harm.** Serious events are fatal, life-threatening, a congenital abnormality, disabling or incapacitating, or resulting in hospitalisation;
- associated with **newer drugs and vaccines;** the most up to date list of black triangle medicines is available at: www.mhra.gov.uk/blacktriangle

If in doubt whether to report a suspected adverse drug reaction, please complete a Yellow Card.

The identification and reporting of adverse reactions to drugs in children and neonates is particularly important because:

- the action of the drug and its pharmacokinetics in children (especially in the very young) may be different from that in adults;
- drugs may not have been extensively tested in children;
- many drugs are not specifically licensed for use in children and are used either 'off-label' or as unlicensed products;
- drugs may affect the way a child grows and develops or may cause delayed adverse reactions which do not occur in adults;
- suitable formulations may not be available to allow precise dosing in children or they may contain excipients that should be used with caution in children;
- the nature and course of illnesses and adverse drug reactions may differ between adults and children.

Even if reported through the British Paediatric Surveillance Unit's Orange Card Scheme, any identified suspected adverse drug reactions should also be submitted to the Yellow Card Scheme.

Adverse drug reactions where harm occurs as a result of a medication error are reportable as a Yellow Card or through the local risk management systems into the National Reporting and Learning System (NRLS). If reported to the NRLS, these will be shared with the MHRA. If the NRLS is not available and harm occurs, report using a Yellow Card.

Prescription writing

Prescriptions should be written according to the guidelines in Prescription Writing. Inclusion of age is a legal requirement in the case of prescription-only medicines for children under 12 years of age, but it is preferable to state the age for **all** prescriptions for children.

It is particularly important to state the strengths of capsules or tablets. Although liquid preparations are particularly suitable for children, they may contain sugar which encourages dental decay. Sugar-free medicines are preferred for long-term treatment.

Many children are able to swallow tablets or capsules and may prefer a solid dose form; involving the child and parents in choosing the formulation is helpful.

When a prescription for a liquid oral preparation is written and the dose ordered is smaller than 5 mL an **oral syringe** will be supplied. Parents should be advised not to add any medicines to the infant's feed, since the drug may interact with the milk or other liquid in it; moreover the ingested dosage may be reduced if the child does not drink all the contents.

Parents must be warned to keep **all** medicines out of reach of children.

Rare paediatric conditions

Information on substances such as *biotin* and *sodium benzoate* used in rare metabolic conditions is included in BNF *for Children*; further information can be obtained from:

Alder Hey Children's Hospital
Drug Information Centre
Liverpool
L12 2AP
(0151) 252 5381

Great Ormond Street Hospital for Children
Pharmacy
Great Ormond St
London
WC1N 3JH
(020) 7405 9200

Dosage in children

Children's doses in the BNF are stated in the individual drug entries.

Doses are generally based on body-weight (in kilograms) or specific age ranges. In the BNF and BNF *for Children*, the term neonate is used to describe a newborn infant aged 0–28 days. The terms child or children are used generically to describe the entire range from infant to adolescent (1 month–17 years). An age range is specified when the dose information applies to a narrower age range than a child from 1 month–17 years.

Dose calculation

Many children's doses are standardised by **weight** (and therefore require multiplying by the body-weight in kilograms to determine the child's dose); occasionally, the doses have been standardised by **body surface area** (in m^2). These methods should be used rather than attempting to calculate a child's dose on the basis of doses used in adults.

For most drugs the adult maximum dose should not be exceeded. For example if the dose is stated as 8 mg/kg (max. 300 mg), a child weighing 10 kg should receive 80 mg but a child weighing 40 kg should receive 300 mg (rather than 320 mg).

Young children may require a higher dose per kilogram than adults because of their higher metabolic rates. Other problems need to be considered. For example, calculation by body-weight in the overweight child may result in much higher doses being administered than necessary; in such cases, dose should be calculated from an ideal weight, related to height and age.

Body surface area (BSA) estimates are sometimes preferable to body-weight for calculation of paediatric doses since many physiological phenomena correlate better with body surface area. Body surface area can be estimated from weight. For more information, refer to BNF *for Children*.

Where the dose for children is not stated, prescribers should consult BNF *for Children* or seek advice from a medicines information centre.

Dose frequency
Antibacterials are generally given at regular intervals throughout the day. Some flexibility should be allowed in children to avoid waking them during the night. For example, the night-time dose may be given at the child's bedtime.

Where new or potentially toxic drugs are used, the manufacturers' recommended doses should be carefully followed.

Prescribing in hepatic impairment

Overview
Liver disease may alter the response to drugs in several ways as indicated below, and drug prescribing should be kept to a minimum in all patients with severe liver disease. The main problems occur in patients with jaundice, ascites, or evidence of encephalopathy.

Impaired drug metabolism
Metabolism by the liver is the main route of elimination for many drugs, but hepatic reserve is large and liver disease has to be severe before important changes in drug metabolism occur. Routine liver-function tests are a poor guide to the capacity of the liver to metabolise drugs, and in the individual patient it is not possible to predict the extent to which the metabolism of a particular drug may be impaired.

A few drugs, e.g. rifampicin p. 619 and fusidic acid p. 608, are excreted in the bile unchanged and can accumulate in patients with intrahepatic or extrahepatic obstructive jaundice.

Hypoproteinaemia
The hypoalbuminaemia in severe liver disease is associated with reduced protein binding and increased toxicity of some highly protein-bound drugs such as phenytoin p. 340 and prednisolone p. 718.

Reduced clotting
Reduced hepatic synthesis of blood-clotting factors, indicated by a prolonged prothrombin time, increases the sensitivity to oral anticoagulants such as warfarin sodium p. 153 and phenindione p. 153.

Hepatic encephalopathy
In severe liver disease many drugs can further impair cerebral function and may precipitate hepatic encephalopathy. These include all sedative drugs, opioid analgesics, those diuretics that produce hypokalaemia, and drugs that cause constipation.

Fluid overload
Oedema and ascites in chronic liver disease can be exacerbated by drugs that give rise to fluid retention e.g. NSAIDs and corticosteroids.

Hepatotoxic drugs
Hepatotoxicity is either dose-related or unpredictable (idiosyncratic). Drugs that cause dose-related toxicity may do so at lower doses in the presence of hepatic impairment than in individuals with normal liver function, and some drugs that produce reactions of the idiosyncratic kind do so more frequently in patients with liver disease. These drugs should be avoided or used very carefully in patients with liver disease.

Where care is needed when prescribing in hepatic impairment, this is indicated under the relevant drug in the BNF.

Prescribing in renal impairment

Issues encountered in renal impairment
The use of drugs in patients with reduced renal function can give rise to problems for several reasons:

- reduced renal excretion of a drug or its metabolites may cause toxicity;
- sensitivity to some drugs is increased even if elimination is unimpaired;
- many side-effects are tolerated poorly by patients with renal impairment;
- some drugs are not effective when renal function is reduced.

Many of these problems can be avoided by reducing the dose or by using alternative drugs.

If even mild renal impairment is considered likely on clinical grounds, renal function should be checked before prescribing any drug which requires dose modification.

General guidance
Where care is needed when prescribing in renal impairment, this is indicated under the relevant drug monograph in the BNF.

When both efficacy and toxicity are closely related to plasma-drug concentration, recommended regimens should be regarded only as a guide to initial treatment; subsequent doses must be adjusted according to clinical response and plasma-drug concentration.

Dose recommendations are based on the severity of renal impairment. The total daily maintenance dose of a drug can be reduced either by reducing the size of the individual doses or by increasing the interval between doses.

For some drugs, although the size of the maintenance dose is reduced it is important to give a loading dose if an immediate effect is required. This is because it takes about five times the half-life of the drug to achieve steady-state plasma concentrations. Because the plasma half-life of drugs excreted by the kidney is prolonged in renal impairment it can take many doses for the reduced dosage to achieve a therapeutic plasma concentration.

For information and advice on the prevention, detection, and management of acute kidney injury, see NICE clinical guideline: **Acute Kidney Injury** (www.nice.org.uk/guidance/ng148).

Important: dosage adjustment advice in the BNF Clinical laboratories routinely report renal function in adults based on *estimated glomerular filtration rate* (eGFR) normalised to a body surface area of 1.73 m^2—this is derived from either the Chronic Kidney Disease Epidemiology Collaboration (CKD-EPI) formula or the Modification of Diet in Renal disease (MDRD) formula.

However, in product literature, the effects of renal impairment on drug elimination is usually stated in terms of *creatinine clearance* as a surrogate for GFR.

The information on dosage adjustment in the BNF is *usually* expressed in terms of eGFR. Exceptions to the use of eGFR include toxic drugs, in elderly patients and in patients at extremes of muscle mass (see *Estimating renal function in patients at extremes of muscle mass* and *Estimating renal function in elderly patients*, below) where calculation of CrCl is recommended. Although these two measures of renal function are not interchangeable, for most drugs and for most adult patients of average build and height, eGFR (rather than CrCl) can be used to determine dosage adjustments.

MHRA/CHM advice: Prescribing medicines in renal impairment: using the appropriate estimate of renal function to avoid the risk of adverse drug reactions (October 2019) For cases where creatinine clearance (CrCl), calculated using the Cockcroft and Gault formula, should be used to determine renal dose adjustments, see *Important: dosage adjustment advice in the BNF*, above. In addition, the MHRA advises that CrCl should be used as an estimate of renal function for direct-acting oral anticoagulants (DOACs), and drugs with a narrow therapeutic index that are mainly renally excreted.

If dose adjustment based on CrCl is important and no advice is provided in the relevant BNF drug monograph, prescribers should consult product literature.

Renal function and drug dosing should be reassessed in situations where eGFR and/or CrCl change rapidly, such as in patients with acute kidney injury (AKI).

Nephrotoxic drugs Nephrotoxic drugs should, if possible, be avoided in patients with renal disease because the consequences of nephrotoxicity are likely to be more serious when renal reserve is already reduced. During intercurrent illness the risk of acute kidney injury is increased in patients with an eGFR of less than 60 mL/min/1.73 m^2; potentially nephrotoxic or renally excreted drugs may require dose reduction or temporary discontinuation.

Renal replacement therapy and transplantation For prescribing in patients who have received a renal transplant or who are on renal replacement therapy (peritoneal dialysis or haemodialysis), consult specialist literature.

Estimating renal function

Direct measure of Glomerular filtration rate (GFR) using plasma or urinary clearance is considered the best overall index of renal function. However, this is difficult to do in practice.

As an alternative, the *estimated* Glomerular filtration rate (eGFR) based on serum creatinine is used to assess renal function. Creatinine clearance (CrCl) is also used as an estimate of GFR.

Various equations for estimating glomerular filtration rate exist, however there is no compelling evidence to support the superiority of any given method for drug dosing in *all* patient populations or clinical situations. There is also insufficient evidence to provide *definitive* guidance about dosage adjustment of all drugs in patients with reduced renal function. Therefore, an understanding of drug pharmacokinetics is necessary in order to make appropriate dosing decisions.

Using serum creatinine to derive eGFR has a number of limitations; serum creatinine levels are dependent on muscle mass and diet, therefore estimates should be interpreted with caution in certain individuals (such as the elderly, body builders, amputees, in muscle-wasting disorders and vegans)—estimates will be higher or lower than the true value. Creatinine-derived measurements are also **not** useful in periods of rapidly changing renal function or in patients with AKI.

Estimated glomerular filtration rate Chronic Kidney Disease Epidemiology Collaboration (CKD-EPI) formula The CKD-EPI formula is the recommended method for estimating GFR and calculating drug doses in **most** patients with renal impairment.

CKD-EPI is adjusted for body surface area (BSA) and utilises serum creatinine, age, sex and race as variables. Clinical laboratories should use the CKD-EPI formula to routinely report eGFR.

CKD-EPI equation

$$\text{eGFR (ml/min/1.73 m}^2) = 141 \times \min(S_{Cr}/K, 1)^{\alpha} \times \max (S_{Cr}/K, 1)^{-1.209} \times 0.993^{Age}[\times 1.018 \text{ if female}] [\times 1.159 \text{ if black}]$$

Where:

- S_{Cr}= serum creatinine in mg/dL;
- K = 0.7 for females and 0.9 for males;
- α = -0.329 for females and -0.411 for males;
- $\min(S_{Cr}/K, 1)$ indicates the minimum of S_{Cr}/K or 1;
- $\max(S_{Cr}/K, 1)$ indicates the maximum of S_{Cr}/K or 1.

Modification of Diet in Renal Disease (MDRD) The MDRD formula, like CKD-EPI, is expressed in terms of body surface area. It is less accurate than the CKD-EPI formula when eGFR is greater than 60 mL/min/1.73 m^2. It also overestimates GFR in elderly patients.

Estimated creatinine clearance Cockcroft and Gault The Cockcroft and Gault formula is the preferred method for estimating renal function or calculating drug doses in patients with renal impairment who are elderly or at extremes of muscle mass (see below); it provides an estimate of CrCl (which is not equivalent to eGFR).

$$\text{Estimated Creatinine Clearance in mL/minute} = \frac{(140 - \text{Age}) \times \text{Weight} \times \text{Constant}}{\text{Serum creatinine}}$$

- Age in years
- Weight in kilograms (use ideal body weight where fat is likely to be the major contributor to body mass)
- Serum creatinine in micromol/litre
- Constant = 1.23 for men; 1.04 for women

Estimating renal function in patients at extremes of muscle mass In patients at both extremes of muscle mass, eGFR should be interpreted with caution. Reduced muscle mass will lead to overestimation of GFR and increased muscle mass will lead to underestimation of the GFR.

Creatinine clearance or *absolute glomerular filtration rate* should be used to adjust drug doses in patients with a BMI less than 18 kg/m^2 or greater than 40 kg/m^2.

Ideal body weight should be used to calculate the CrCl. Where the patient's actual body weight is less than their ideal body weight, actual body weight should be used instead.

The absolute glomerular filtration rate is determined by removing the normalisation for BSA from the eGFR using the following formula:

GFR (Absolute) = eGFR × (individual's body surface area / 1.73)

The ideal body weight is calculated as follows:

Ideal body weight (kilograms) = Constant + 0.91 (Height - 152.4)

Where:

- Constant = 50 for men; 45.5 for women
- Height in centimetres

Estimating renal function in elderly patients The Cockcroft and Gault formula is the preferred method for estimating renal function in elderly patients aged 75 years and over.

Chronic kidney disease

For recommendations on the management of patients with chronic kidney disease during the COVID-19 pandemic, see NICE rapid guidelines: **Chronic kidney disease** (available at: www.nice.org.uk/guidance/ng176). For further information on COVID-19, see COVID-19 p. 660.

Classification of chronic kidney disease using GFR and ACR categories Chronic kidney disease is classified using a combination of GFR and albumin:creatinine ratio (ACR). A decreased GFR and an increased ACR is associated with an increased risk of adverse outcomes.

For example, a person with an eGFR of 25 ml/min/1.73 m^2 and an ACR of 15 mg/mmol has a CKD classification of G4A2.

Advanced Pharmacy Services

Patients with renal impairment may be eligible for the Medicines Use Review service provided by a community pharmacist. For further information, see *Advanced Pharmacy Services* in Medicines optimisation p. 18.

Classification of chronic kidney disease using GFR and ACR categories

GFR and ACR categories and risk of adverse outcomes			ACR categories (mg/mmol), description and range		
			<3 Normal to mild increase	3–30 Moderate increase	>30 Severe increase
			A1	A2	A3
GFR categories (ml/min/1.73m²), description and range	≥90 Normal or high	G1	No CKD in the absence of markers of kidney damage		
	60–89 Mild reduction relative to normal range for a young adult	G2			
	45–59 Mild-moderate reduction	G3a			
	30–44 Moderate-severe reduction	G3b			
	15–29 Severe reduction	G4			
	<15 Kidney failure	G5			

Increasing risk →

↓ Increasing risk

Abbreviations: ACR, albumin:creatinine ratio; CKD, chronic kidney disease; GFR, glomerular filtration rate

Adapted with the kind permission of the Kidney Disease: Improving Global Outcomes (KDIGO) CKD Work Group, 2013.

Prescribing in pregnancy

Overview

Drugs can have harmful effects on the embryo or fetus at any time during pregnancy. It is important to bear this in mind when prescribing for a woman of *childbearing age* or for men *trying* to *father* a child.

During the *first trimester* drugs can produce congenital malformations (teratogenesis), and the period of greatest risk is from the third to the eleventh week of pregnancy.

During the *second* and *third trimesters* drugs can affect the growth or functional development of the fetus, or they can have toxic effects on fetal tissues.

Drugs given shortly before term or during labour can have adverse effects on labour or on the neonate after delivery.

Not all the damaging effects of intra-uterine exposure to drugs are obvious at birth, some may only manifest later in life. Such late-onset effects include malignancy, e.g. adenocarcinoma of the vagina after puberty in females exposed to diethylstilbestrol in the womb, and adverse effects on intellectual, social, and functional development.

The BNF and *BNF for Children* identify drugs which:

- may have harmful effects in pregnancy and indicate the trimester of risk
- are not known to be harmful in pregnancy

The information is based on human data, but information from *animal* studies has been included for some drugs when its omission might be misleading. Maternal drug doses may require adjustment during pregnancy due to changes in maternal physiology but this is beyond the scope of the *BNF* and *BNF for Children*.

Where care is needed when prescribing in pregnancy, this is indicated under the relevant drug in the BNF and *BNF for Children*.

Important

Drugs should be prescribed in pregnancy only if the expected benefit to the mother is thought to be greater than the risk to the fetus, and all drugs should be avoided if possible during the first trimester. Drugs which have been extensively used in pregnancy and appear to be usually safe should be prescribed

in preference to new or untried drugs; and the smallest effective dose should be used. Few drugs have been shown conclusively to be teratogenic in humans, but no drug is safe beyond all doubt in early pregnancy. Screening procedures are available when there is a known risk of certain defects.

Absence of information does not imply safety. It should be noted that the BNF and *BNF for Children* provide independent advice and may not always agree with the product literature.

Information on drugs and pregnancy is also available from the UK Teratology Information Service. www.uktis.org
Tel: 0344 892 0909 (09.00–17:00 Monday to Friday; urgent enquiries only outside these hours).

MHRA/CHM advice: Medicines with teratogenic potential: what is effective contraception and how often is pregnancy testing needed? (March 2019)

Guidance is available on contraceptive methods and frequency of pregnancy testing to reduce inadvertent exposures during pregnancy in a woman taking a medicine of teratogenic potential. When using these medicines, a woman should be advised of the risks and encouraged to use the most effective contraceptive method taking into account her personal circumstances. The likelihood of pregnancy should be assessed before each prescription of a medicine with known teratogenic potential, by performing a pregnancy test if required. If pregnancy cannot be excluded, the decision to start or continue treatment will depend on individual circumstances, such as the urgency for treatment and alternative treatment options. If feasible, treatment with a medicine with teratogenic potential should be delayed until pregnancy has been excluded by a repeat test.

Information on pregnancy testing and contraception for pregnancy prevention during treatment with medicines of teratogenic potential is available at: www.gov.uk/drug-safety-update/medicines-with-teratogenic-potential-what-is-effective-contraception-and-how-often-is-pregnancy-testing-needed#download-print-and-use-new-table

Prescribing in breast-feeding

Overview

Breast-feeding is beneficial; the immunological and nutritional value of breast milk to the infant is greater than that of formula feeds.

Although there is concern that drugs taken by the mother might affect the infant, there is very little information on this. In the absence of evidence of an effect, the potential for harm to the infant can be inferred from:

- the amount of drug or active metabolite of the drug delivered to the infant (dependent on the pharmacokinetic characteristics of the drug in the mother);
- the efficiency of absorption, distribution, and elimination of the drug by the infant (infant pharmacokinetics);
- the nature of the effect of the drug on the infant (pharmacodynamic properties of the drug in the infant).

The amount of drug transferred in breast milk is rarely sufficient to produce a discernible effect on the infant. This applies particularly to drugs that are poorly absorbed and need to be given parenterally. However, there is a theoretical possibility that a small amount of drug present in breast milk can induce a hypersensitivity reaction.

A clinical effect can occur in the infant if a pharmacologically significant quantity of the drug is present in milk. For some drugs (e.g. fluvastatin p. 217), the ratio

between the concentration in milk and that in maternal plasma may be high enough to expose the infant to adverse effects. Some infants, such as those born prematurely or who have jaundice, are at a slightly higher risk of toxicity.

Some drugs inhibit the infant's sucking reflex (e.g. phenobarbital p. 353) while others can affect lactation (e.g. bromocriptine p. 440).

The BNF identifies drugs:

- that should be used with caution or are contra-indicated in breast-feeding;
- that can be given to the mother during breast-feeding because they are present in milk in amounts which are too small to be harmful to the infant;
- that might be present in milk in significant amount but are not known to be harmful.

Where care is needed when prescribing in breast-feeding, this is indicated under the relevant drug in the BNF.

Important

For many drugs insufficient evidence is available to provide guidance and it is advisable to administer only essential drugs to a mother during breast-feeding. Because of the inadequacy of information on drugs in breast-feeding, absence of information does not imply safety.

Prescribing in palliative care

Overview

Palliative care is an approach that improves the quality of life of patients and their families facing life-threatening illness, through the prevention and relief of suffering by means of early identification and impeccable assessment and treatment of pain and other problems, physical, psychosocial, and spiritual. Careful assessment of symptoms and needs of the patient should be undertaken by a multidisciplinary team.

Specialist palliative care is available in most areas as day hospice care, home-care teams (often known as Macmillan teams), in-patient hospice care, and hospital teams. Many acute hospitals and teaching centres now have consultative, hospital-based teams.

Hospice care of terminally ill patients has shown the importance of symptom control and psychosocial support of the patient and family. Families should be included in the care of the patient if they wish.

Many patients wish to remain at home with their families. Although some families may at first be afraid of caring for the patient at home, support can be provided by community nursing services, social services, voluntary agencies and hospices together with the general practitioner. The family may be reassured by the knowledge that the patient will be admitted to a hospital or hospice if the family cannot cope.

Drug treatment The number of drugs should be as few as possible, for even the taking of medicine may be an effort. Oral medication is usually satisfactory unless there is severe nausea and vomiting, dysphagia, weakness, or coma, when parenteral medication may be necessary.

Pain

Pain management in palliative care is focused on achieving control of pain by administering the right drug in the right dose at the right time. Analgesics can be divided into three broad classes: non-opioid (paracetamol p. 464, NSAID), opioid (e.g. codeine phosphate p. 475 'weak', morphine p. 483 'strong') and adjuvant (e.g. antidepressants, antiepileptics). Drugs from the different classes are used alone or in combination according to the type of pain and response to treatment. Analgesics are more effective in preventing pain than in the relief of established pain; it is important that they are given regularly.

Paracetamol or a **NSAID** given regularly will often be sufficient to manage mild pain. If non-opioid analgesics alone are not sufficient, then an opioid analgesic alone or in combination with a non-opioid analgesic at an adequate dosage, may be helpful in the control of moderate pain. Codeine phosphate or tramadol hydrochloride p. 491 can be considered for moderate pain. If these preparations do not control the pain then morphine p. 483 is the most useful opioid analgesic. Alternatives to morphine p. 483, including transdermal buprenorphine p. 468, transdermal fentanyl p. 478, hydromorphone hydrochloride p. 482, methadone hydrochloride p. 524, or oxycodone hydrochloride p. 486, should be initiated by those with experience in palliative care. Initiation of an opioid analgesic should not be delayed by concern over a theoretical likelihood of psychological dependence (addiction).

Bone metastases In addition to the above approach, radiotherapy, **bisphosphonates**, and radioactive isotopes of strontium chloride (*Metastron*® available from GE Healthcare) may be useful for pain due to bone metastases.

Neuropathic pain Patients with **neuropathic pain** may benefit from a trial of a tricyclic antidepressant. An antiepileptic may be added or substituted if pain persists; gabapentin p. 332 and pregabalin p. 342 are licensed for neuropathic pain. Ketamine p. 1399 is sometimes used under specialist supervision for neuropathic pain that responds poorly to opioid analgesics. Pain due to nerve compression may be reduced by a corticosteroid such as dexamethasone p. 714, which reduces oedema around the tumour, thus reducing compression. Nerve blocks or regional anaesthesia techniques (including the use of epidural and intrathecal catheters) can be considered when pain is localised to a specific area.

Pain management with opioids

Oral route Treatment with morphine p. 483 is given by mouth as immediate-release or modified-release preparations. During the titration phase the initial dose is based on the previous medication used, the severity of the pain, and other factors such as presence of renal impairment, increasing age, or frailty. The dose is given either as an immediate-release preparation 4-hourly or as a modified-release preparation 12-hourly, in addition to rescue doses.

If pain occurs between regular doses of morphine ('breakthrough pain'), an additional dose ('rescue dose') of immediate-release morphine should be given. An additional dose should also be given 30 minutes before an activity that causes pain, such as wound dressing. The standard dose of a strong opioid for breakthrough pain is usually one-tenth to one-sixth of the regular 24-hour dose, repeated every 2–4 hours as required (up to hourly may be needed if pain is severe or in the last days of life). Review pain management if rescue analgesic is required frequently (twice daily or more). Each patient should be assessed on an individual basis. Formulations of fentanyl p. 478 that are administered nasally, buccally or sublingually are also licensed for breakthrough pain.

When adjusting the dose of morphine, the number of rescue doses required and the response to them should be taken into account; increments of morphine should not exceed one-third to one-half of the total daily dose every 24 hours. Thereafter, the dose should be adjusted with careful assessment of the pain, and the use of adjuvant analgesics should also be considered. Upward titration of the dose of morphine stops when either the pain is relieved or unacceptable adverse effects occur, after which it is necessary to consider alternative measures.

Morphine immediate-release 30mg 4-hourly (or modified-release 100 mg 12-hourly) is usually adequate for most patients; some patients require morphine immediate-release up to 200mg 4-hourly (or modified-release 600 mg 12-hourly), occasionally more is needed.

Once their pain is controlled, patients started on 4-hourly immediate-release morphine can be transferred to the same total 24-hour dose of morphine given as the modified-release preparation for 12-hourly or 24-hourly administration. The first dose of the modified-release preparation is given with, or within 4 hours of, the last dose of the immediate-release preparation. For preparations suitable for 12-hourly or 24-hourly administration see modified-release preparations under morphine. Increments should be made to the dose, not to the frequency of administration. The patient must be monitored closely for efficacy and side-effects, particularly constipation, and nausea and vomiting. A suitable laxative should be prescribed routinely.

Oxycodone hydrochloride p. 486 can be used in patients who require an opioid but cannot tolerate morphine. If the patient is already receiving an opioid, oxycodone hydrochloride should be started at a dose equivalent to the current analgesic (see p. 29). Oxycodone hydrochloride immediate-release preparations p. 486 can be given for breakthrough pain.

Equivalent doses of opioid analgesics.

This table is only an **approximate** guide (doses may not correspond with those given in clinical practice); patients should be carefully monitored after any change in medication and dose titration may be required.

Analgesic/Route	Dose
Codeine: PO	100 mg
Diamorphine: IM, IV, SC	3 mg
Dihydrocodeine: PO	100 mg
Hydromorphone: PO	2 mg
Morphine: PO	10 mg
Morphine: IM, IV, SC	5 mg
Oxycodone: PO	6.6 mg
Tramadol: PO	100 mg

PO = by mouth; IM = intramuscular; IV = intravenous; SC = subcutaneous

Parenteral route The equivalent parenteral dose of morphine p. 483 (subcutaneous, intramuscular, or intravenous) is about half of the oral dose. If the patient becomes unable to swallow, generally morphine is administered as a continuous subcutaneous infusion (for details, see Continuous Subcutaneous Infusions p. 30). Diamorphine hydrochloride p. 476 is sometimes preferred, because being more soluble, it can be given in a smaller volume. The equivalent subcutaneous dose of diamorphine hydrochloride is about one-third of the oral dose of morphine.

If the patient can resume taking medicines by mouth, then oral morphine may be substituted for subcutaneous infusion of morphine or diamorphine hydrochloride, see table above of approximate equivalent doses of morphine and diamorphine hydrochloride. The infusion is discontinued when the first oral dose of morphine is given.

Rectal route Morphine p. 483 is also available for rectal administration as suppositories; alternatively oxycodone hydrochloride p. 486 can be obtained on special order.

Transdermal route Transdermal preparations of fentanyl p. 478 and buprenorphine p. 468 are available, they are not suitable for acute pain or in patients whose analgesic requirements are changing rapidly because the long time to steady state prevents rapid titration of the dose. Prescribers should ensure that they are familiar with the correct use of transdermal preparations, see under buprenorphine and fentanyl (inappropriate use has caused fatalities). Immediate-release morphine can be given for breakthrough pain.

The following 24-hour oral doses of morphine are considered to be *approximately* equivalent to the buprenorphine and fentanyl patches shown, however when switching due to possible opioid-induced hyperalgesia, reduce the calculated equivalent dose of the new opioid by one-quarter to one-half.

Buprenorphine patches are *approximately* equivalent to the following 24-hour doses of oral morphine

morphine salt 12 mg daily	≡ buprenorphine '5' patch
morphine salt 24 mg daily	≡ buprenorphine '10' patch
morphine salt 36 mg daily	≡ buprenorphine '15' patch
morphine salt 48 mg daily	≡ buprenorphine '20' patch
morphine salt 84 mg daily	≡ buprenorphine '35' patch
morphine salt 126 mg daily	≡ buprenorphine '52.5' patch
morphine salt 168 mg daily	≡ buprenorphine '70' patch

Formulations of transdermal patches are available as 72-hourly, 96-hourly and 7-day patches, for further information see buprenorphine p. 468. Conversion ratios vary and these figures are a guide only. Morphine equivalences for transdermal opioid preparations have been approximated to allow comparison with available preparations of oral morphine.

72-hour Fentanyl patches are *approximately* equivalent to the following 24-hour doses of oral morphine

morphine salt 30 mg daily	≡ fentanyl '12' patch
morphine salt 60 mg daily	≡ fentanyl '25' patch
morphine salt 120 mg daily	≡ fentanyl '50' patch
morphine salt 180 mg daily	≡ fentanyl '75' patch
morphine salt 240 mg daily	≡ fentanyl '100' patch

Fentanyl equivalences in this table are for patients on well-tolerated opioid therapy for long periods; for patients who are opioid naive or who have been stable on oral morphine or other immediate release opioid for only several weeks, see Transdermal Route. Conversion ratios vary and these figures are a guide only. Morphine equivalences for transdermal opioid preparations have been approximated to allow comparison with available preparations of oral morphine.

Symptom control

Several recommendations in this section involve unlicensed indications or routes.

Anorexia Anorexia may be helped by prednisolone p. 718 or dexamethasone p. 714.

Bowel colic and excessive respiratory secretions Bowel colic and excessive respiratory secretions may be reduced by a subcutaneous injection of hyoscine hydrobromide p. 458, hyoscine butylbromide p. 93, or glycopyrronium bromide p. 1387. These antimuscarinics are generally given every 4 hours when required, but hourly use is occasionally necessary, particularly in excessive respiratory secretions. If symptoms persist, they can be given regularly via a continuous infusion device. Care is required to avoid the discomfort of dry mouth.

Capillary bleeding Capillary bleeding can be treated with tranexamic acid p. 118 by mouth; treatment is usually discontinued one week after the bleeding has stopped, or, if necessary, it can be continued at a reduced dose. Alternatively, gauze soaked in tranexamic acid 100 mg/mL p. 118 or adrenaline/epinephrine solution 1 mg/mL (1 in 1000) p. 238 can be applied to the affected area.

Vitamin K may be useful for the treatment and prevention of bleeding associated with prolonged clotting in liver disease. In severe chronic cholestasis, absorption of vitamin K may be impaired; either parenteral or water-soluble oral vitamin K (see phytomenadione p. 1138 and menadiol sodium phosphate p. 1138) should be considered.

Constipation Constipation is a common cause of distress and is almost invariable after administration of an opioid analgesic. It should be prevented if possible by the regular administration of laxatives; a faecal softener with a peristaltic stimulant (e.g. co-danthramer p. 66) or lactulose solution p. 60 with a senna preparation p. 67 should be used. Methylnaltrexone bromide p. 69 is licensed for the treatment of opioid-induced constipation.

Convulsions Patients with cerebral tumours or uraemia may be susceptible to convulsions. Prophylactic treatment with phenytoin p. 340 or carbamazepine p. 327 should be considered. When oral medication is no longer possible, diazepam p. 362 given rectally, or phenobarbital p. 353 by injection is continued as prophylaxis. For the use of midazolam p. 358 by subcutaneous infusion using a continuous infusion device see below.

Dry mouth Dry mouth may be relieved by good mouth care and measures such as chewing sugar-free gum, sucking ice or pineapple chunks, or the use of artificial saliva,dry mouth associated with candidiasis can be treated by oral preparations of nystatin p. 1263 or miconazole p. 1262, alternatively, fluconazole p. 634 can be given by mouth. Dry mouth may be caused by certain medications including opioids, antimuscarinic drugs (e.g. hyoscine), antidepressants and some antiemetics; if possible, an alternative preparation should be considered.

Dysphagia A corticosteroid such as dexamethasone p. 714 may help, temporarily, if there is an obstruction due to tumour. See also *Dry mouth*, above.

Dyspnoea Breathlessness at rest may be relieved by regular oral morphine p. 483 in carefully titrated doses. Diazepam p. 362 may be helpful for dyspnoea associated with anxiety. A corticosteroid, such as dexamethasone p. 714, may also be helpful if there is bronchospasm or partial obstruction.

Fungating tumours Fungating tumours can be treated by regular dressing and antibacterial drugs; systemic treatment with metronidazole p. 575 is often required to reduce malodour but topical metronidazole p. 1275 is also used.

Gastro-intestinal pain The pain of bowel colic may be reduced by loperamide hydrochloride p. 72. Hyoscine hydrobromide p. 458 may also be helpful, given sublingually as *Kwells* ® tablets. Subcutaneous injections of hyoscine butylbromide p. 93, hyoscine hydrobromide p. 458, and glycopyrronium bromide p. 1387 can also be used to treat bowel colic.

Gastric distension pain due to pressure on the stomach may be helped by a preparation incorporating an antacid with an antiflatulent and a prokinetic such as domperidone p. 451 before meals.

Hiccup Hiccup due to gastric distension may be helped by a preparation incorporating an antacid with an antiflatulent. If this fails, metoclopramide hydrochloride p. 451 by mouth or by subcutaneous or intramuscular injection can be added; if this also fails, baclofen p. 1173, or nifedipine p. 176, or chlorpromazine hydrochloride p. 404 can be tried.

Insomnia Patients with advanced cancer may not sleep because of discomfort, cramps, night sweats, joint stiffness, or fear. There should be appropriate treatment of these problems before hypnotics are used. Benzodiazepines, such as temazepam p. 509, may be useful.

Intractable cough Intractable cough may be relieved by moist inhalations or by regular administration of oral morphine p. 483. Methadone hydrochloride linctus p. 524 should be avoided because it has a long duration of action and tends to accumulate.

Muscle spasm The pain of muscle spasm can be helped by a muscle relaxant such as diazepam p. 362 or baclofen p. 1173.

Nausea and vomiting Nausea and vomiting are common in patients with advanced cancer. Ideally, the cause should be determined before treatment with an antiemetic is started. A prokinetic antiemetic may be a preferred choice for first-line therapy.

Nausea and vomiting may occur with opioid therapy particularly in the initial stages but can be prevented by giving an antiemetic such as haloperidol p. 405 or metoclopramide hydrochloride p. 451. An antiemetic is usually necessary only for the first 4 or 5 days and therefore combined preparations containing an opioid with an antiemetic are not recommended because they lead to unnecessary antiemetic therapy (and associated side-effects when used long-term).

Metoclopramide hydrochloride p. 451 has a prokinetic action and is used by mouth for nausea and vomiting associated with gastritis, gastric stasis, and functional bowel obstruction. Drugs with antimuscarinic effects antagonise prokinetic drugs and, if possible, should not be used concurrently.

Haloperidol p. 405 is used by mouth for most metabolic causes of vomiting (e.g. hypercalcaemia, renal failure).

Cyclizine p. 449 is given by mouth. It is used for nausea and vomiting due to mechanical bowel obstruction, raised intracranial pressure, and motion sickness.

Levomepromazine p. 459 is used as an antiemetic; it is given by mouth or by subcutaneous injection at bedtime. For the dose by subcutaneous infusion see below.

Dexamethasone p. 714 by mouth can be used as an adjunct.

Antiemetic therapy should be reviewed every 24 hours; it may be necessary to substitute the antiemetic or to add another one.

For the administration of antiemetics by subcutaneous infusion using a continuous infusion device, see below.

For the treatment of nausea and vomiting associated with cancer chemotherapy see Cytotoxic drugs p. 932.

Pruritus Pruritus, even when associated with obstructive jaundice, often responds to simple measures such as application of emollients. In the case of obstructive jaundice, further measures include administration of colestyramine p. 212.

Raised intracranial pressure Headache due to raised intracranial pressure often responds to a high dose of a corticosteroid, such as dexamethasone p. 714 and should be given before 6 p.m. to reduce the risk of insomnia.

Restlessness and confusion Restlessness and confusion may require treatment with an antipsychotic, e.g. haloperidol p. 405 or levomepromazine p. 459, by mouth or by subcutaneous injection, both repeated every 2 hours if required. The dose and frequency is adjusted according to the level of patient distress and the response. A regular maintenance dose should also be considered, given twice daily either by mouth or by subcutaneous injection; alternatively use a continuous infusion device.

Levomepromazine p. 459 is licensed to treat pain in palliative care—this use is reserved for distressed patients with severe pain unresponsive to other measures (seek specialist advice).

Continuous subcutaneous infusions

Although drugs can usually be administered *by mouth* to control the symptoms of advanced cancer, the parenteral route may sometimes be necessary. Repeated administration of *intramuscular injections* can be difficult in a cachectic patient. This has led to the use of portable continuous infusion devices, such as syringe drivers, to give a *continuous subcutaneous infusion*, which can provide good control of symptoms with little discomfort or inconvenience to the patient.

Indications for the **parenteral route** are:
- the patient is unable to take medicines by mouth owing to *nausea and vomiting, dysphagia, severe weakness*, or *coma*

- there is *malignant bowel obstruction* in patients for whom further surgery is inappropriate (avoiding the need for an intravenous infusion or for insertion of a nasogastric tube)
- occasionally when the patient *does not wish* to take regular medication by mouth.

Syringe driver rate settings Staff using syringe drivers should be **adequately trained** and different rate settings should be **clearly identified** and **differentiated**; incorrect use of syringe drivers is a common cause of medication errors.

Bowel colic and excessive respiratory secretions Hyoscine hydrobromide p. 458 effectively reduces respiratory secretions and bowel colic and is sedative (but occasionally causes paradoxical agitation).

Hyoscine butylbromide p. 93 is used for bowel colic and for excessive respiratory secretions, and is less sedative than hyoscine hydrobromide p. 458.

Glycopyrronium bromide p. 1387 may also be used to treat bowel colic or excessive respiratory secretions.

Confusion and restlessness Haloperidol p. 405 has little sedative effect.

Levomepromazine p. 459 has a sedative effect.

Midazolam p. 358 is a sedative and an antiepileptic that may be used in addition to an antipsychotic drug in a very restless patient. Midazolam p. 358 is also used for myoclonus.

Convulsions If a patient has previously been receiving an antiepileptic drug *or* has a primary or secondary cerebral tumour *or* is at risk of convulsion (e.g. owing to uraemia) antiepileptic medication should not be stopped. Midazolam p. 358 is the benzodiazepine antiepileptic of choice for *continuous subcutaneous infusion.*

Nausea and vomiting Haloperidol p. 405 and levomepromazine p. 459 can both be given as a *subcutaneous infusion* but sedation can limit the dose of levomepromazine p. 459.

Cyclizine is particularly likely to precipitate if mixed with diamorphine or other drugs (see under Mixing and Compatibility, below)

Metoclopramide hydrochloride p. 451 can cause skin reactions.

Octreotide p. 993, which stimulates water and electrolyte absorption and inhibits water secretion in the small bowel, can be used by subcutaneous infusion to reduce intestinal secretions and to reduce vomiting due to bowel obstruction.

Pain control Diamorphine hydrochloride p. 476 is the preferred opioid since its high solubility permits a large dose to be given in a small volume (see under Mixing and Compatibility, below). The table shows approximate equivalent doses of morphine p. 483 and diamorphine hydrochloride.

Mixing and compatibility The general principle that injections should be given into separate sites (and should not be mixed) does not apply to the use of syringe drivers in palliative care. Provided that there is evidence of compatibility, selected injections can be mixed in syringe drivers. Not all types of medication can be used in a subcutaneous infusion. In particular, chlorpromazine hydrochloride p. 404, prochlorperazine p. 408, and diazepam p. 362 are **contra-indicated** as they cause skin reactions at the injection site; to a lesser extent cyclizine p. 449 and levomepromazine p. 459 also sometimes cause local irritation.

In theory injections dissolved in water for injections are more likely to be associated with pain (possibly owing to their hypotonicity). The use of physiological saline (sodium chloride 0.9% p. 1089) however increases the likelihood of precipitation when more than one drug is used; moreover subcutaneous infusion rates are so slow (0.1– 0.3 mL/hour)

that pain is not usually a problem when water is used as a diluent.

Compatibility with diamorphine Diamorphine can be given by *subcutaneous infusion* in a strength of up to 250 mg/mL; up to a strength of 40 mg/mL either *water for injections* or *physiological saline* (sodium chloride 0.9%) is a suitable diluent—above that strength only *water for injections* is used (to avoid precipitation).

The following can be mixed with *diamorphine*:

- **Cyclizine,** may precipitate at concentrations above 10 mg/mL *or* in the presence of sodium chloride 0.9% *or* as the concentration of diamorphine relative to cyclizine increases; mixtures of diamorphine and cyclizine are also likely to precipitate after 24 hours.
- **Dexamethasone,** special care is needed to avoid precipitation of dexamethasone when preparing it.
- **Haloperidol,** mixtures of haloperidol and diamorphine are likely to precipitate after 24 hours if haloperidol concentration is above 2 mg/mL.
- **Hyoscine butylbromide**
- **Hyoscine hydrobromide**
- **Levomepromazine**
- **Metoclopramide,** under some conditions infusions containing metoclopramide become discoloured; such solutions should be discarded.
- **Midazolam**

Subcutaneous infusion solution should be monitored regularly both to check for precipitation (and discolouration) and to ensure that the infusion is running at the correct rate.

Problems encountered with syringe drivers The following are problems that may be encountered with syringe drivers and the action that should be taken:

- if the subcutaneous infusion runs *too quickly* check the rate setting and the calculation;
- if the subcutaneous infusion runs *too slowly* check the start button, the battery, the syringe driver, the cannula, and make sure that the injection site is not inflamed;
- if there is an *injection site reaction* make sure that the site does not need to be changed—firmness or swelling at the site of injection is not in itself an indication for change, but pain or obvious inflammation is.

Prescribing in palliative care

Equivalent doses of morphine sulfate and diamorphine hydrochloride given over 24 hours

These equivalences are *approximate only* and should be adjusted according to response

ORAL MORPHINE	PARENTERAL MORPHINE	PARENTERAL DIAMORPHINE
Oral morphine sulfate **over 24 hours**	Subcutaneous infusion of morphine sulfate **over 24 hours**	Subcutaneous infusion of diamorphine hydrochloride **over 24 hours**
30 mg	15 mg	10 mg
60 mg	30 mg	20 mg
90 mg	45 mg	30 mg
120 mg	60 mg	40 mg
180 mg	90 mg	60 mg
240 mg	120 mg	80 mg
360 mg	180 mg	120 mg
480 mg	240 mg	160 mg
600 mg	300 mg	200 mg
780 mg	390 mg	260 mg
960 mg	480 mg	320 mg
1200 mg	600 mg	400 mg

If breakthrough pain occurs give a subcutaneous (preferable) or intramuscular injection equivalent to one-tenth to one-sixth of the total 24-hour subcutaneous infusion dose. It is kinder to give an intermittent bolus injection *subcutaneously*–absorption is smoother so that the risk of adverse effects at peak absorption is avoided (an even better method is to use a subcutaneous butterfly needle). To minimise the risk of infection no individual subcutaneous infusion solution should be used for longer than 24 hours.

Prescribing in the elderly

Overview
Old people, especially the very old, require special care and consideration from prescribers. *Medicines for Older People*, a component document of the National Service Framework for Older People (Department of Health. National Service Framework for Older People. London: Department of Health, March 2001), describes how to maximise the benefits of medicines and how to avoid excessive, inappropriate, or inadequate consumption of medicines by older people.

Appropriate prescribing
Elderly patients often receive multiple drugs for their multiple diseases. This greatly increases the risk of drug interactions as well as adverse reactions, and may affect compliance. The balance of benefit and harm of some medicines may be altered in the elderly. Therefore, elderly patients' medicines should be reviewed regularly and medicines which are not of benefit should be stopped.

Non-pharmacological measures may be more appropriate for symptoms such as headache, sleeplessness, and light-headedness when associated with social stress as in widowhood, loneliness, and family dispersal.

In some cases prophylactic drugs are inappropriate if they are likely to complicate existing treatment or introduce unnecessary side-effects, especially in elderly patients with poor prognosis or with poor overall health. However, elderly patients should not be denied medicines which may help them, such as anticoagulants or antiplatelet drugs for atrial fibrillation, antihypertensives, statins, and drugs for osteoporosis.

STOPP/START criteria STOPP/START criteria are evidence-based criteria used to review medication regimens in elderly people. STOPP (Screening Tool of Older Persons' potentially inappropriate Prescriptions) aims to reduce the incidence of medicines-related adverse events from potentially inappropriate prescribing and polypharmacy. START (Screening Tool to Alert to Right Treatment) can be used to prevent omissions of indicated, appropriate medicines in older patients with specific conditions.

For STOPP criteria related to single drugs or drug classes, BNF Publications contain information within the monographs, in the cautions section. Where criteria relate to a drug class without a class monograph, information is outlined in the relevant treatment summaries. START criteria are not included within the monographs, however further information can be found in:

- Gallagher, P. et al. (2008). STOPP (Screening Tool of Older Persons' Prescriptions) and START (Screening Tool to Alert Doctors to Right Treatment): Consensus Validation. Int J Clin Pharmacol Ther 46(2):72-83.
- O'Mahony, D. et al. (2015). STOPP/START criteria for potentially inappropriate prescribing in older people: version 2. Age Ageing 44(2):213-8.

Form of medicine
Frail elderly patients may have difficulty swallowing tablets; if left in the mouth, ulceration may develop. They should always be encouraged to take their tablets or capsules with enough fluid, and whilst in an upright position to avoid the possibility of oesophageal ulceration. It can be helpful to discuss with the patient the possibility of taking the drug as a liquid if available.

Manifestations of ageing
In the very old, manifestations of normal ageing may be mistaken for disease and lead to inappropriate prescribing. In addition, age-related muscle weakness and difficulty in maintaining balance should not be confused with neurological disease. Disorders such as light-headedness not associated with postural or postprandial hypotension are unlikely to be helped by drugs.

Sensitivity
The nervous system of elderly patients is more sensitive to many commonly used drugs, such as opioid analgesics, benzodiazepines, antipsychotics, and antiparkinsonian drugs, all of which must be used with caution. Similarly, other organs may also be more susceptible to the effects of drugs such as anti-hypertensives and NSAIDs.

Pharmacokinetics
Pharmacokinetic changes can markedly increase the tissue concentration of a drug in the elderly, especially in debilitated patients.

The most important effect of age is reduced renal clearance. Many aged patients thus *excrete drugs slowly*, and are *highly susceptible to nephrotoxic drugs*. Acute illness can lead to rapid reduction in renal clearance, especially if accompanied by dehydration. Hence, a patient stabilised on a drug with a narrow margin between the therapeutic and the toxic dose (e.g. digoxin p. 117) can rapidly develop adverse effects in the aftermath of a myocardial infarction or a respiratory-tract infection. The hepatic metabolism of lipid soluble drugs is reduced in elderly patients because there is a reduction in liver volume. This is important for drugs with a narrow therapeutic window.

Adverse reactions
Adverse reactions often present in the elderly in a vague and non-specific fashion. *Confusion* is often the presenting symptom (caused by almost any of the commonly used drugs). Other common manifestations are *constipation* (with antimuscarinics and many tranquillisers) and postural *hypotension* and *falls* (with diuretics and many psychotropics).

Hypnotics
Many hypnotics with long half-lives have serious hangover effects, including drowsiness, unsteady gait, slurred speech, and confusion. Hypnotics with short half-lives should be used but they too can present problems. Short courses of hypnotics are occasionally useful for helping a patient through an acute illness or some other crisis but every effort must be made to avoid dependence. Benzodiazepines impair balance, which can result in falls.

Diuretics
Diuretics are overprescribed in old age and should **not** be used on a long-term basis to treat simple gravitational oedema which will usually respond to increased movement, raising the legs, and support stockings. A few days of diuretic treatment may speed the clearing of the oedema but it should rarely need continued drug therapy.

NSAIDs
Bleeding associated with aspirin and other NSAIDs is more common in the elderly who are more likely to have a fatal or serious outcome. NSAIDs are also a special hazard in patients with cardiac disease or renal impairment which may again place older patients at particular risk.

Owing to the *increased susceptibility of the elderly* to the *side-effects of NSAIDs* the following recommendations are made:

- for *osteoarthritis, soft-tissue lesions,* and *back pain*, first try measures such as weight reduction (if obese), warmth, exercise, and use of a walking stick;

Drugs and sport

- for *osteoarthritis, soft-tissue lesions, back pain*, and *pain in rheumatoid arthritis*, paracetamol p. 464 should be used first and can often provide adequate pain relief;
- alternatively, a low-dose NSAID (e.g. ibuprofen p. 1186 up to 1.2 g daily) may be given;
- for pain relief when either drug is inadequate, paracetamol in a full dose plus a low-dose NSAID may be given;
- if necessary, the NSAID dose can be increased or an opioid analgesic given with paracetamol p. 464;
- do not give two NSAIDs at the same time.

Prophylaxis of NSAID-induced peptic ulcers may be required if continued NSAID treatment is necessary. For further information, see Peptic ulcer disease p. 77.

Other drugs

Other drugs which commonly cause adverse reactions are *antiparkinsonian drugs, antihypertensives, psychotropics*, and digoxin p. 117. The usual maintenance dose of digoxin p. 117 in very old patients is 125 micrograms daily (62.5 micrograms in those with renal disease); lower doses are often inadequate but toxicity is common in those given 250 micrograms daily.

Drug-induced blood disorders are much more common in the elderly. Therefore drugs with a tendency to cause bone marrow depression (e.g. co-trimoxazole p. 598, mianserin hydrochloride p. 391) should be avoided unless there is no acceptable alternative.

The elderly generally require a lower maintenance dose of warfarin sodium p. 153 than younger adults; once again, the outcome of bleeding tends to be more serious.

Guidelines

Always consider whether a drug is indicated at all.

Limit range It is a sensible policy to prescribe from a limited range of drugs and to be thoroughly familiar with their effects in the elderly.

Reduce dose Dosage should generally be substantially lower than for younger patients and it is common to start with about 50% of the adult dose. Some drugs (e.g. long-acting antidiabetic drugs such as glibenclamide p. 749) should be avoided altogether.

Review regularly Review repeat prescriptions regularly. In many patients it may be possible to stop some drugs, provided that clinical progress is monitored. It may be necessary to reduce the dose of some drugs as renal function declines.

Simplify regimens Elderly patients benefit from simple treatment regimens. Only drugs with a clear indication should be prescribed and whenever possible given once or twice daily. In particular, regimens which call for a confusing array of dosage intervals should be avoided.

Explain clearly Write full instructions on every prescription (*including* repeat prescriptions) so that containers can be properly labelled with full directions. Avoid imprecisions like 'as directed'. Child-resistant containers may be unsuitable.

Repeats and disposal Instruct patients what to do when drugs run out, and also how to dispose of any that are no longer necessary. Try to prescribe matching quantities.

If these guidelines are followed most elderly people will cope adequately with their own medicines. If not then it is essential to enrol the help of a third party, usually a relative or a friend.

Drugs and sport

Anti-doping

UK Anti-Doping, the national body responsible for the UK's anti-doping policy, advises that athletes are personally responsible should a prohibited substance be detected in their body. Information regarding the use of medicines in sport is available from:

UK Anti-doping
Fleetbank House
2-6 Salisbury Square
London
EC4Y 8AE
(020) 7842 3450
ukad@ukad.org.uk
www.ukad.org.uk

Information about the prohibited status of specific medications based on the current World Anti-Doping Agency Prohibited List is available from Global Drug Reference Online: www.globaldro.com/UK/search

General Medical Council's advice

Doctors who prescribe or collude in the provision of drugs or treatment with the intention of improperly enhancing an individual's performance in sport contravene the GMC's guidance, and such actions would usually raise a question of a doctor's continued registration. This does not preclude the provision of any care or treatment where the doctor's intention is to protect or improve the patient's health.

Prescribing in dental practice

General guidance

Advice on the drug management of dental and oral conditions has been integrated into the main text. For ease of access, guidance on such conditions is usually identified by means of a relevant heading (e.g. Dental and Orofacial Pain) in the appropriate sections of the BNF.

The following is a list of topics of particular relevance to dentists.

- Prescribing by dentists, see Prescription writing p. 5
- Oral side-effects of drugs, see Adverse reactions to drugs p. 12
- Medical emergencies in dental practice, see below
- Medical problems in dental practice, see below

Drug management of dental and oral conditions

Dental and orofacial pain

- Neuropathic pain p. 504
- Non-opioid analgesics and compound analgesic preparations, see Analgesics p. 462
- Opioid analgesics, see Analgesics p. 462
- Non-steroidal anti-inflammatory drugs p. 1176

Oral infections

Bacterial infections, see Antibacterials, principles of therapy p. 527

- Phenoxymethylpenicillin p. 581
- Broad-spectrum penicillins (amoxicillin p. 582 and ampicillin p. 584)
- Cephalosporins (cefalexin p. 552 and cefradine p. 554)
- Tetracyclines p. 600
- Macrolides (clarithromycin p. 569, erythromycin p. 572 and azithromycin p. 568)
- Clindamycin p. 566
- Metronidazole p. 575
- Fusidic acid p. 608

Fungal infections, see Antifungals, systemic use p. 629

- Local treatment, see Oropharyngeal fungal infections p. 1262
- Systemic treatment, see Antifungals, systemic use p. 629

Viral infections

- Herpetic gingivostomatitis, local treatment, see Oropharyngeal viral infections p. 1263
- Herpetic gingivostomatitis, systemic treatment, see Oropharyngeal viral infections p. 1263 and Herpesvirus infections p. 671
- Herpes labialis, see Skin infections p. 1272

Anaesthetics, anxiolytics and hypnotics

- Sedation, anaesthesia, and resuscitation in dental practice p. 1381
- Hypnotics, see Hypnotics and anxiolytics p. 505
- Sedation for dental procedures, see Hypnotics and anxiolytics p. 505
- Anaesthesia (local) p. 1401

Minerals

- Fluoride p. 1256

Oral ulceration and inflammation p. 1257
Mouthwashes, gargles and dentifrices, see
Mouthwashes and other preparations for oropharyngeal use p. 1254
Dry mouth, see Dry mouth p. 1252
Aromatic inhalations, see Aromatic inhalations, cough preparations and systemic nasal decongestants p. 312
Nasal decongestants, see Aromatic inhalations, cough preparations and systemic nasal decongestants p. 312

Dental Practitioners' Formulary p. 1683

Medical emergencies in dental practice

This section provides guidelines on the management of the more common medical emergencies which may arise in dental practice. Dentists and their staff should be familiar with standard resuscitation procedures, but in all circumstances it is advisable to summon medical assistance as soon as possible. See also **algorithm** of the procedure for Cardiopulmonary resuscitation p. 237.

The drugs referred to in this section include:

- Adrenaline/epinephrine Injection p. 238, adrenaline 1 in 1000, (adrenaline 1 mg/mL as acid tartrate), 1 mL amps
- Aspirin Dispersible Tablets 300 mg p. 132
- Glucagon Injection, glucagon (as hydrochloride), 1- unit vial (with solvent) p. 764
- Glucose p. 1090 (for administration by mouth)
- Glyceryl trinitrate Spray p. 233
- Midazolam Oromucosal Solution p. 358
- Oxygen
- Salbutamol Aerosol Inhalation, salbutamol 100 micrograms/metered inhalation p. 269

Adrenal insufficiency

Adrenal insufficiency may follow prolonged therapy with corticosteroids and can persist for years after stopping. A patient with adrenal insufficiency may become hypotensive under the stress of a dental visit (important: see individual monographs for details of corticosteroid cover before dental surgical procedures under general anaesthesia).

Management

- Lay the patient flat
- Give **oxygen**
- Transfer patient urgently to hospital

Anaphylaxis

A severe allergic reaction may follow oral or parenteral administration of a drug. Anaphylactic reactions in dentistry may follow the administration of a drug or contact with substances such as latex in surgical gloves. In general, the more rapid the onset of the reaction the more profound it tends to be. Symptoms may develop within minutes and rapid treatment is essential.

Anaphylactic reactions may also be associated with *additives* and *excipients* in foods and medicines. Refined arachis (peanut) oil, which may be present in some medicinal products, is unlikely to cause an allergic reaction—nevertheless it is wise to check the full formula of preparations which may contain allergens (including those for topical application, particularly if they are intended for use in the mouth or for application to the nasal mucosa).

Symptoms and signs

- Paraesthesia, flushing, and swelling of face
- Generalised itching, especially of hands and feet
- Bronchospasm and laryngospasm (with wheezing and difficulty in breathing)
- Rapid weak pulse together with fall in blood pressure and pallor; finally cardiac arrest

Management

First-line treatment includes securing the airway, restoration of blood pressure (laying the patient flat and raising the feet, or in the recovery position if unconscious or nauseous and at risk of vomiting), and administration of adrenaline/epinephrine injection p. 238. This is given **intramuscularly** in a dose of 500 micrograms (0.5 mL adrenaline injection 1 in 1000); a dose of 300 micrograms (0.3 mL adrenaline injection 1 in 1000) may be appropriate for immediate self-administration. The dose is repeated if

Prescribing in dental practice

necessary at 5-minute intervals according to blood pressure, pulse, and respiratory function. **Oxygen** administration is also of primary importance. Arrangements should be made to transfer the patient to hospital urgently.

Asthma

Patients with asthma may have an attack while at the dental surgery. Most attacks will respond to 2 puffs of the patient's short-acting beta$_2$ agonist inhaler such as salbutamol 100 micrograms/puff p. 269; further puffs are required if the patient does not respond rapidly. If the patient is unable to use the inhaler effectively, further puffs should be given through a large-volume spacer device (or, if not available, through a plastic or paper cup with a hole in the bottom for the inhaler mouthpiece). If the response remains unsatisfactory, or if further deterioration occurs, then the patient should be transferred urgently to hospital. Whilst awaiting transfer, **oxygen** should be given with salbutamol 5 mg or terbutaline sulfate 10 mg by nebuliser p. 271; if a nebuliser is unavailable, then 2–10 puffs of salbutamol 100 micrograms/metered inhalation should be given (preferably by a large-volume spacer), and repeated every 10–20 minutes if necessary. If asthma is part of a more generalised anaphylactic reaction, an intramuscular injection of adrenaline/epinephrine p. 238 (as detailed under Anaphylaxis) should be given.

Patients with severe chronic asthma or whose asthma has deteriorated previously during a dental procedure may require an increase in their prophylactic medication before a dental procedure. This should be discussed with the patient's medical practitioner and may include increasing the dose of inhaled or oral corticosteroid.

Cardiac emergencies

If there is a history of *angina* the patient will probably carry glyceryl trinitrate spray or tablets p. 233 (or isosorbide dinitrate tablets p. 235) and should be allowed to use them. Hospital admission is not necessary if symptoms are mild and resolve rapidly with the patient's own medication. See also Coronary Artery Disease below.

Arrhythmias may lead to a sudden reduction in cardiac output with loss of consciousness. Medical assistance should be summoned. For advice on pacemaker interference, see also Pacemakers below.

The pain of *myocardial infarction* is similar to that of angina but generally more severe and more prolonged. For general advice see also Coronary Artery Disease below.

Symptoms and signs of myocardial infarction:

- Progressive onset of severe, crushing pain across front of chest; pain may radiate towards the shoulder and down arm, or into neck and jaw
- Skin becomes pale and clammy
- Nausea and vomiting are common
- Pulse may be weak and blood pressure may fall
- Breathlessness

Initial management of myocardial infarction:

Call immediately for medical assistance and an ambulance, as appropriate.

Allow the patient to rest in the position that feels most comfortable; in the presence of breathlessness this is likely to be sitting position, whereas the syncopal patient should be laid flat; often an intermediate position (dictated by the patient) will be most appropriate. **Oxygen** may be administered.

Sublingual glyceryl trinitrate p. 233 may relieve pain. Intramuscular injection of drugs should be avoided because absorption may be too slow (particularly when cardiac output is reduced) and pain relief is inadequate. Intramuscular injection also increases the risk of local bleeding into the muscle if the patient is given a thrombolytic drug.

Reassure the patient as much as possible to relieve further anxiety. If available, aspirin p. 132 in a single dose of 300 mg should be given. A note (to say that aspirin has been given) should be sent with the patient to the hospital. For further details on the initial management of myocardial infarction, see Management of ST-Segment Elevation Myocardial Infarction.

If the patient collapses and loses consciousness attempt standard resuscitation measures. See also **algorithm** of the procedure for Cardiopulmonary resuscitation p. 237.

Epileptic seizures

Patients with epilepsy must continue with their normal dosage of anticonvulsant drugs when attending for dental treatment. It is not uncommon for epileptic patients not to volunteer the information that they are epileptic but there should be little difficulty in recognising a tonic-clonic (grand mal) seizure.

Symptoms and signs

- There may be a brief warning (but variable)
- Sudden loss of consciousness, the patient becomes rigid, falls, may give a cry, and becomes cyanotic (tonic phase)
- After 30 seconds, there are jerking movements of the limbs; the tongue may be bitten (clonic phase)
- There may be frothing from mouth and urinary incontinence
- The seizure typically lasts a few minutes; the patient may then become flaccid but remain unconscious. After a variable time the patient regains consciousness but may remain confused for a while

Management

During a convulsion try to ensure that the patient is not at risk from injury but make no attempt to put anything in the mouth or between the teeth (in mistaken belief that this will protect the tongue). Give **oxygen** to support respiration if necessary.

Do not attempt to restrain convulsive movements.

After convulsive movements have subsided place the patient in the coma (recovery) position and check the airway.

After the convulsion the patient may be confused ('post-ictal confusion') and may need reassurance and sympathy. The patient should not be sent home until fully recovered. Seek medical attention or transfer the patient to hospital if it was the first episode of epilepsy, or if the convulsion was atypical, prolonged (or repeated), or if injury occurred.

Medication should only be given if convulsive seizures are prolonged (convulsive movements lasting 5 minutes or longer) or repeated rapidly.

Midazolam oromucosal solution p. 358 can be given by the buccal route in adults as a single dose of 10 mg [unlicensed]. For further details on the management of status epilepticus, including details of paediatric doses of midazolam p. 358, see Drugs used in status epilepticus (Epilepsy p. 321).

Focal seizures similarly need very little active management (in an automatism only a minimum amount of restraint should be applied to prevent injury). Again, the patient should be observed until post-ictal confusion has completely resolved.

Hypoglycaemia

Insulin-treated diabetic patients attending for dental treatment under local anaesthesia should inject insulin and eat meals as normal. If food is omitted the blood glucose will fall to an abnormally low level (hypoglycaemia). Patients can often recognise the symptoms themselves and this state responds to sugar in water or glucose tablets. Children may not have such prominent changes but may appear unduly lethargic.

Symptoms and signs

Hypoglycaemia should be excluded in any person with diabetes who is acutely unwell, drowsy, unconscious, unable to co-operate, or presenting with aggressive behaviour or seizures. Symptoms of hypoglycaemia in the young include shakiness, pounding heart, sweatiness, headache, drowsiness, and difficulty concentrating. In young children, behavioural changes such as irritability, agitation, quietness, and tantrums, may be prominent.

Management of adults

EvGr Any patient with a blood-glucose concentration less than 4 mmol/litre, with or without symptoms, and who is **conscious and able to swallow**, should have 15–20 g of fast-acting carbohydrate. This is available in approximately 3–4 heaped teaspoonfuls of sugar dissolved in water, 4–7 glucose tablets, or 150–200 mL pure fruit juice. Orange juice should not be given to patients following a low-potassium diet due to chronic kidney disease, and sugar dissolved in water will not be effective in patients taking acarbose. E Proprietary products of fast-acting carbohydrate, as glucose 40% gel (e.g. *Glucogel®*, *Dextrogel®*, or *Rapilose gel®*) are also available; EvGr 2 tubes should be taken.

If necessary, repeat treatment after 10–15 minutes, up to a maximum of 3 treatments in total. Once blood-glucose concentration is above 4 mmol/litre and the patient has recovered, a snack providing a long-acting carbohydrate should be given to prevent blood-glucose concentration from falling again (e.g. two biscuits, one slice of bread, 200–300 mL milk (not soya or other forms of 'alternative' milk, e.g. almond or coconut), or a normal carbohydrate-containing meal if due).

If hypoglycaemia is unresponsive, or the oral route cannot be used, intramuscular glucagon 1 mg p. 764 should be given. Once blood-glucose concentration is above 4 mmol/litre and the patient has recovered, a snack providing a long-acting carbohydrate should be given. Patients who have received glucagon p. 764 require a larger portion of long-acting carbohydrate to replenish glycogen stores (e.g. four biscuits, two slices of bread, 400–600 mL of milk (not soya or other forms of 'alternative' milk, e.g. almond or coconut) or a normal carbohydrate containing meal if due).

Glucagon may be less effective in patients taking a sulfonylurea or under the influence of alcohol; in these cases, intravenous glucose 10% will be required. If glucagon is unsuitable or ineffective after 10 minutes, the patient should be transferred urgently to hospital. E The patient must also be admitted to hospital if hypoglycaemia is caused by an oral antidiabetic drug.

Management of children

EvGr Non-severe hypoglycaemia in children who **are able to swallow**, should be treated with 10–20 g of fast-acting carbohydrate by mouth, preferably in liquid form, which may be taken more easily. Oral glucose solutions p. 1090 should not be used if consciousness is reduced as this could be dangerous (risk of choking). 10–20 g is available from approximately 2–4 teaspoonfuls of sugar added to a cup of water, or 3–6 glucose tablets. A

Blood-glucose concentrations should rise within 5–15 minutes; EvGr if hypoglycaemia persists after 15 minutes, repeat the fast-acting glucose p. 1090. As symptoms improve or normoglycaemia is restored, a long-acting carbohydrate snack (e.g. two biscuits, one banana) or a meal, can be given to prevent blood-glucose concentration from falling again. A

EvGr Severe hypoglycaemia may be treated with concentrated oral glucose solution, as long as the child is **conscious and able to swallow**. E Proprietary products of fast-acting carbohydrate, as glucose 40% gel (e.g. *Glucogel®*, *Dextrogel®*, or *Rapilose gel®*) are available for use in severe hypoglycaemia.

EvGr If hypoglycaemia is unresponsive, or the oral route cannot be used, intramuscular glucagon p. 764 should be given. Children aged 8 years and under *or* who weigh less than 25 kg should be given 500 micrograms; children aged

9 years and above *or* who weigh 25 kg and over should be given 1 mg of glucagon p. 764. As symptoms improve or normoglycaemia is restored, and the child is sufficiently awake, a long-acting carbohydrate snack (e.g. two biscuits, one banana) or a meal should be given. A

EvGr Glucagon may be less effective in patients taking a sulfonylurea or under the influence of alcohol; in these cases, intravenous glucose 10% will be required. E EvGr If glucagon p. 764 is unsuitable or ineffective after 10 minutes, the child should be transferred urgently to hospital. A The child must also be admitted to hospital if hypoglycaemia is caused by an oral antidiabetic drug.

Syncope

Insufficient blood supply to the brain results in loss of consciousness. The commonest cause is a vasovagal attack or simple faint (syncope) due to emotional stress.

Symptoms and signs

- Patient feels faint
- Low blood pressure
- Pallor and sweating
- Yawning and slow pulse
- Nausea and vomiting
- Dilated pupils
- Muscular twitching

Management

- Lay the patient as flat as is reasonably comfortable and, in the absence of associated breathlessness, raise the legs to improve cerebral circulation
- Loosen any tight clothing around the neck
- Once consciousness is regained, give sugar in water or a cup of sweet tea

Other possible causes Postural hypotension can be a consequence of rising abruptly or of standing upright for too long; antihypertensive drugs predispose to this. When rising, susceptible patients should take their time. Management is as for a vasovagal attack.

Under stressful circumstances, some patients hyperventilate. This gives rise to feelings of faintness but does not usually result in syncope. In most cases reassurance is all that is necessary; rebreathing from cupped hands or a bag may be helpful but calls for careful supervision.

Adrenal insufficiency or arrhythmias are other possible causes of syncope.

Medical problems in dental practice

Individuals presenting at the dental surgery may also suffer from an unrelated medical condition; this may require modification to the management of their dental condition. If the patient has systemic disease or is taking other medication, the matter may need to be discussed with the patient's general practitioner or hospital consultant.

Allergy

Patients should be asked about any history of allergy; those with a history of atopic allergy (asthma, eczema, hay fever, etc.) are at special risk. Those with a history of a severe allergy or of anaphylactic reactions are at high risk—it is essential to confirm that they are not allergic to any medication, or to any dental materials or equipment (including latex gloves). See also Anaphylaxis above.

Arrhythmias

Patients, especially those who suffer from heart failure or who have sustained a myocardial infarction, may have irregular cardiac rhythm. Atrial fibrillation is a common arrhythmia even in patients with normal hearts and is of little concern except that dentists should be aware that such patients may be receiving anticoagulant therapy. The patient's medical practitioner should be asked whether any special precautions are necessary. Premedication (e.g. with temazepam p. 509) may be useful in some instances for very anxious patients.

See also Cardiac emergencies above, and Dental Anaesthesia (Anaesthesia (local) p. 1401).

Cardiac prostheses

For an account of the risk of infective endocarditis in patients with prosthetic heart valves, see Infective Endocarditis below. For advice on patients receiving anticoagulants, see Thromboembolic disease below.

Coronary artery disease

Patients are vulnerable for at least 4 weeks following a myocardial infarction or following any sudden increase in the symptoms of angina. It would be advisable to check with the patient's medical practitioner before commencing treatment. See also Cardiac Emergencies above.

Treatment with low-dose aspirin (75 mg daily), clopidogrel p. 134, or dipyridamole p. 135 should not be stopped routinely nor should the dose be altered before dental procedures.

A Working Party of the British Society for Antimicrobial Chemotherapy has not recommended antibiotic prophylaxis for patients following coronary artery bypass surgery.

Cyanotic heart disease

Patients with cyanotic heart disease are at risk in the dental chair, particularly if they have pulmonary hypertension. In such patients a syncopal reaction increases the shunt away from the lungs, causing more hypoxia which worsens the syncopal reaction—a vicious circle that may prove fatal. The advice of the cardiologist should be sought on any patient with congenital cyanotic heart disease. Treatment in hospital is more appropriate for some patients with this condition.

Hypertension

Patients with hypertension are likely to be receiving antihypertensive drugs. Their blood pressure may fall dangerously low under general anaesthesia, see also under Dental Anaesthesia (Anaesthesia (local) p. 1401).

Immunosuppression and indwelling intraperitoneal catheters

Advice of a Working Party of the British Society for Antimicrobial Chemotherapy is that patients who are immunosuppressed (including transplant patients) and patients with indwelling intraperitoneal catheters do not require antibiotic prophylaxis for dental treatment provided there is no other indication for prophylaxis.

The Working Party has commented that there is little evidence that dental treatment is followed by infection in immunosuppressed and immunodeficient patients nor is there evidence that dental treatment is followed by infection in patients with indwelling intraperitoneal catheters.

Infective endocarditis

While almost any dental procedure can cause bacteraemia, there is no clear association with the development of infective endocarditis. Routine daily activities such as tooth brushing also produce a bacteraemia and may present a greater risk of infective endocarditis than a single dental procedure.

Antibacterial prophylaxis and chlorhexidine mouthwash p. 1255 are **not** recommended for the prevention of endocarditis in patients undergoing dental procedures. Such prophylaxis may expose patients to the adverse effects of antimicrobials when the evidence of benefit has not been proven.

Reduction of oral bacteraemia Patients at risk of endocarditis including those with valve replacement, acquired valvular heart disease with stenosis or

regurgitation, structural congenital heart disease (including surgically corrected or palliated structural conditions, but excluding isolated atrial septal defect, fully repaired ventricular septal defect, fully repaired patent ductus arteriosus, and closure devices considered to be endothelialised), hypertrophic cardiomyopathy, or a previous episode of infective endocarditis, should be advised to maintain the highest possible standards of oral hygiene in order to reduce the:

- need for dental extractions or other surgery;
- chances of severe bacteraemia if dental surgery is needed;
- possibility of 'spontaneous' bacteraemia.

Postoperative care Patients at risk of endocarditis including those with valve replacement, acquired valvular heart disease with stenosis or regurgitation, structural congenital heart disease (including surgically corrected or palliated structural conditions, but excluding isolated atrial septal defect, fully repaired ventricular septal defect, fully repaired patent ductus arteriosus, and closure devices considered to be endothelialised), hypertrophic cardiomyopathy, or a previous episode of infective endocarditis, should be warned to report to the doctor or dentist any unexplained illness that develops after dental treatment.

Any infection in patients at risk of endocarditis should be investigated promptly and treated appropriately to reduce the risk of endocarditis.

Patients on anticoagulant therapy

For general advice on dental surgery in patients receiving oral anticoagulant therapy see Thromboembolic Disease below.

Joint prostheses

Advice of a Working Party of the British Society for Antimicrobial Chemotherapy is that patients with prosthetic joint implants (including total hip replacements) do not require antibiotic prophylaxis for dental treatment. The Working Party considers that it is unacceptable to expose patients to the adverse effects of antibiotics when there is no evidence that such prophylaxis is of any benefit, but that those who develop any intercurrent infection require prompt treatment with antibiotics to which the infecting organisms are sensitive.

The Working Party has commented that joint infections have rarely been shown to follow dental procedures and are even more rarely caused by oral streptococci.

Pacemakers

Pacemakers prevent asystole or severe bradycardia. Some ultrasonic scalers, electronic apex locators, electro-analgesic devices, and electrocautery devices interfere with the normal function of pacemakers (including shielded pacemakers) and should not be used. The manufacturer's literature should be consulted whenever possible. If severe bradycardia occurs in a patient fitted with a pacemaker, electrical equipment should be switched off and the patient placed supine with the legs elevated. If the patient loses consciousness and the pulse remains slow or is absent, cardiopulmonary resuscitation may be needed. Call immediately for medical assistance and an ambulance, as appropriate.

A Working Party of the British Society for Antimicrobial Chemotherapy does not recommend antibacterial prophylaxis for patients with pacemakers.

Thromboembolic disease

Patients receiving a **heparin** or an oral anticoagulant such as warfarin sodium p. 153, acenocoumarol p. 152 (nicoumalone), phenindione p. 153, apixaban p. 136, dabigatran etexilate p. 148 or rivaroxaban p. 139 may be liable to excessive bleeding after extraction of teeth or other dental surgery. Often dental surgery can be delayed until the anticoagulant therapy has been completed.

For a patient requiring long-term therapy with warfarin sodium p. 153, the patient's medical practitioner should be consulted and the International Normalised Ratio (INR) should be assessed 72 hours before the dental procedure. This allows sufficient time for dose modification if necessary. In those with an unstable INR (including those who require weekly monitoring of their INR, or those who have had some INR measurements greater than 4.0 in the last 2 months), the INR should be assessed within 24 hours of the dental procedure. Patients requiring minor dental procedures (including extractions) who have an INR below 4.0 may continue warfarin sodium p. 153 without dose adjustment. There is no need to check the INR for a patient requiring a non-invasive dental procedure.

If it is necessary to remove several teeth, a single extraction should be done first; if this goes well further teeth may be extracted at subsequent visits (two or three at a time). Measures should be taken to minimise bleeding during and after the procedure. This includes the use of sutures and a haemostatic such as oxidised cellulose, collagen sponge or resorbable gelatin sponge. Scaling and root planing should initially be restricted to a limited area to assess the potential for bleeding.

For a patient on long-term warfarin sodium p. 153, the advice of the clinician responsible for the patient's anticoagulation should be sought if:

- the INR is unstable, or if the INR is greater than 4.0;
- the patient has thrombocytopenia, haemophilia, or other disorders of haemostasis, or suffers from liver impairment, alcoholism, or renal failure;
- the patient is receiving antiplatelet drugs, cytotoxic drugs or radiotherapy.

Intramuscular injections are *contra-indicated* in patients taking anticoagulants with an INR above the therapeutic range, and in those with any disorder of haemostasis. In patients taking anticoagulants who have a stable INR within the therapeutic range, intramuscular injections should be avoided if possible; if an intramuscular injection is necessary, the patient should be informed of the increased risk of localised bleeding and monitored carefully.

A local anaesthetic containing a vasoconstrictor should be given by infiltration, or by intraligamentary or mental nerve injection if possible. If regional nerve blocks cannot be avoided the local anaesthetic should be given cautiously using an aspirating syringe.

Drugs which have potentially serious interactions with anticoagulants include aspirin and other NSAIDs, carbamazepine p. 327, imidazole and triazole antifungals (including miconazole p. 1262), erythromycin p. 572, clarithromycin p. 569, and metronidazole p. 575; for details of these and other interactions with anticoagulants, see Appendix 1 (dabigatran etexilate, heparins, phenindione, rivaroxaban, and coumarins).

Although studies have failed to demonstrate an interaction, common experience in anticoagulant clinics is that the INR can be altered following a course of an oral broad-spectrum antibiotic, such as ampicillin p. 584 or amoxicillin p. 582.

Information on the treatment of patients who take anticoagulants is available at www.npsa.nhs.uk/patientsafety/alerts-and-directives/alerts/anticoagulant.

Liver disease

Liver disease may alter the response to drugs and drug prescribing should be kept to a minimum in patients with severe liver disease. Problems are likely mainly in patients with *jaundice, ascites,* or evidence of *encephalopathy*.

For guidance on prescribing for patients with hepatic impairment, see Prescribing in hepatic impairment p. 23. Where care is needed when prescribing in hepatic

impairment, this is indicated under the relevant drug in the BNF.

Renal impairment

The use of drugs in patients with reduced renal function can give rise to many problems. Many of these problems can be avoided by reducing the dose or by using alternative drugs.

Special care is required in renal transplantation and immunosuppressed patients; if necessary such patients should be referred to specialists.

For guidance on prescribing in patients with renal impairment, see Prescribing in renal impairment p. 23. Where care is needed when prescribing in renal impairment, this is indicated under the relevant drug in the BNF.

Pregnancy

Drugs taken during pregnancy can be harmful to the fetus and should be prescribed only if the expected benefit to the mother is thought to be greater than the risk to the fetus; all drugs should be avoided if possible during the first trimester.

For guidance on prescribing in pregnancy, see Prescribing in pregnancy p. 27. Where care is needed when prescribing in pregnancy, this is indicated under the relevant drug in the BNF.

Breast-feeding

Some drugs taken by the mother whilst breast-feeding can be transferred to the breast milk, and may affect the infant.

For guidance on prescribing in breast-feeding, see Prescribing in breast-feeding p. 27. Where care is needed when prescribing in breast-feeding, this is indicated under the relevant drug in the BNF.

Chapter 1
Gastro-intestinal system

CONTENTS

1   Chronic bowel disorders
1.1   Coeliac disease

Coeliac disease
25-Jul-2016

Description of condition

Coeliac disease is an autoimmune condition which is associated with chronic inflammation of the small intestine. Dietary proteins known as gluten, which are present in wheat, barley and rye, activate an abnormal immune response in the intestinal mucosa, which can lead to malabsorption of nutrients.

Aims of treatment

The management of coeliac disease is aimed at eliminating symptoms (such as diarrhoea, bloating and abdominal pain) and reducing the risk of complications, including those resulting from malabsorption.

Non-drug treatment

EvGr The only effective treatment for coeliac disease is a strict, life-long, gluten-free diet. A range of gluten-free products is available for prescription (see *Borderline substances*). ⟨A⟩

Drug treatment

EvGr Patients who have coeliac disease are at an increased risk of malabsorption of key nutrients (such as calcium and vitamin D). Their risk of osteoporosis and the need for active treatment of bone disease should form part of the ongoing management of coeliac disease. Supplementation of key nutrients may be required if dietary intake is insufficient.

Patients who have coeliac disease should be advised **not** to self-medicate with over-the-counter vitamins or mineral supplements. Initiation of supplementation should involve a discussion with a member of the patient's healthcare team in order to identify the individual needs of the patient and to allow for appropriate ongoing monitoring.

Confirmed cases of refractory coeliac disease should be referred to a specialist centre. Treatment with prednisolone p. 718 can be considered for initial management while awaiting specialist advice. ⟨A⟩

Useful Resources

Coeliac disease: recognition, assessment and management. National Institute for Health and Care Excellence. Clinical guideline 20. September 2015.
www.nice.org.uk/guidance/ng20

1.2   Diverticular disease and diverticulitis

Diverticular disease and diverticulitis
20-Feb-2020

Description of condition

Diverticulosis is an asymptomatic condition characterised by the presence of diverticula (small pouches protruding from the walls of the large intestine). Its prevalence is difficult to determine but it is age dependent, with the majority of patients aged 40 years and over.

Diverticular disease is a condition where diverticula are present with symptoms such as abdominal tenderness and/or mild, intermittent lower abdominal pain with constipation, diarrhoea, or occasional large rectal bleeds. Symptoms of diverticular disease may overlap with other conditions such as Irritable bowel syndrome p. 51, colitis (bowel inflammation related to Crohn's disease p. 41, Ulcerative colitis p. 43, ischaemia or microscopic colitis), and malignancy.

Acute diverticulitis occurs when diverticula suddenly become inflamed or infected. Signs and symptoms include constant lower abdominal pain (usually severe) together with features such as fever, a sudden change in bowel habits and significant rectal bleeding, lower abdominal tenderness, or a palpable abdominal mass. **Complicated acute diverticulitis** refers to diverticulitis associated with complications such as abscess, bowel perforation and peritonitis, fistula, intestinal obstruction, haemorrhage, or sepsis. For further information on signs and symptoms of acute diverticulitis or complicated acute diverticulitis, see NICE clinical guideline: **Diverticular disease** (see *Useful resources*).

Aims of treatment

Treatment aims to relieve symptoms of diverticular disease, improve quality of life, manage episodes of acute diverticulitis, and reduce the risk of recurrence and complications.

Non drug management

EvGr Patients and their family and/or carers, where appropriate, should be provided with information about diet and lifestyle changes, the course of the disease and likelihood of progression, symptoms and symptom management, investigations and treatment options, and when and how to seek further medical advice.

Patients with diverticulosis or diverticular disease should be advised to eat a healthy, balanced diet including whole grains, fruit and vegetables. In patients with constipation and on a low fibre diet, a gradual increase of dietary fibre may minimise flatulence and bloating. Patients increasing dietary fibre should be advised to drink an adequate amount of fluid, especially if dehydration is a risk. Advice should also be given about the benefits of exercise, weight loss (if overweight or obese), and Smoking cessation p. 519, in reducing the risk of symptomatic disease and acute diverticulitis.

Patients with diverticular disease should also be informed that it may take several weeks for the benefits of increasing fibre in their diet to be achieved and that if a high-fibre diet is tolerated, it should be continued for life.

In patients with complicated acute diverticulitis, emergency or elective surgical management may be required. ⒶFor information on surgical management, see NICE clinical guideline: **Diverticular disease** (see *Useful resources*).

Drug treatment

Diverticulosis

EvGr As diverticulosis is an asymptomatic condition, specific treatments are not recommended. Bulk-forming laxatives can be considered for patients with constipation. Ⓐ

Diverticular disease

EvGr Antibacterials are not recommended for patients with diverticular disease.

Bulk-forming laxatives should be considered when a high-fibre diet is unsuitable, or for patients with persistent constipation or diarrhoea.

Consider the use of simple analgesia such as paracetamol p. 464 in patients with ongoing abdominal pain, and antispasmodics in those with abdominal cramps. Non-steroidal anti-inflammatory drugs and opioid analgesics are not recommended as their use may increase the risk of diverticular perforation.

For patients with persistent symptoms or symptoms that do not respond to treatment, consider an alternative diagnosis. Ⓐ

Acute diverticulitis

EvGr Offer simple analgesia such as paracetamol to patients with acute diverticulitis who are systemically well. Consider a watchful waiting and a no antibacterial prescribing strategy, and advise patients to re-present if symptoms persist or worsen. Ⓐ

For guidance on antibacterial management, see *Diverticulitis, acute* in Gastro-intestinal system infections, antibacterial therapy p. 535.

EvGr Patients with persistent or worsening symptoms should be reassessed in primary care and considered for referral to hospital for further assessment.

Refer patients with suspected complicated acute diverticulitis and uncontrolled abdominal pain for same-day hospital assessment. Those presenting with significant rectal bleeding should be referred to hospital urgently.

Treatment with aminosalicylates or prophylactic antibacterials are not recommended to prevent recurrent acute diverticulitis. Ⓐ

Useful Resources

Diverticular disease: diagnosis and management. National Institute for Health and Care Excellence. NICE guideline 147. November 2019.
www.nice.org.uk/guidance/ng147

1.3   Inflammatory bowel disease

Inflammatory bowel disease

Chronic inflammatory bowel diseases include Crohn's disease below and Ulcerative colitis p. 43.

Drugs used in chronic bowel disorders

Aminosalicylates

Sulfasalazine p. 47 is a combination of 5-aminosalicylic acid ('5-ASA') and sulfapyridine; sulfapyridine acts only as a carrier to the colonic site of action but still causes side-effects. In the newer aminosalicylates, mesalazine p. 45 (5-aminosalicylic acid), balsalazide sodium p. 44 (a pro-drug of 5-aminosalicylic acid) and olsalazine sodium p. 47 (a dimer of 5-aminosalicylic acid which cleaves in the lower bowel), the sulfonamide-related side-effects of sulfasalazine are avoided, but 5-aminosalicylic acid alone can still cause side-effects including blood disorders and lupus-like syndrome also seen with sulfasalazine.

Drugs affecting the immune response

Folic acid p. 1071 should be given to reduce the possibility of methotrexate p. 957 toxicity [unlicensed indication]. Folic acid is usually given once weekly on a different day to the methotrexate; alternative regimens may be used in some settings.

Cytokine modulators

Infliximab p. 1162, adalimumab p. 1157, and golimumab p. 1161 are monoclonal antibodies which inhibit the pro-inflammatory cytokine, tumour necrosis factor alpha. They should be used under specialist supervision.

Crohn's disease   20-Dec-2016

Description of condition

Crohn's disease is a chronic, inflammatory bowel disease that mainly affects the gastro-intestinal tract. It is characterised by thickened areas of the gastro-intestinal wall with inflammation extending through all layers, deep ulceration and fissuring of the mucosa, and the presence of granulomas; affected areas may occur in any part of the gastro-intestinal tract, interspersed with areas of relatively normal tissue. Crohn's disease may present as recurrent attacks, with acute exacerbations combined with periods of remission or less active disease. Symptoms depend on the site of disease but may include abdominal pain, diarrhoea, fever, weight loss and rectal bleeding.

Complications of Crohn's disease include intestinal strictures, abscesses in the wall of the intestine or adjacent structures, fistulae, anaemia, malnutrition, colorectal and small bowel cancers, and growth failure and delayed puberty in children. Crohn's disease may also be associated with extra-intestinal manifestation: the most common are arthritis and abnormalities of the joints, eyes, liver and skin.

Crohn's disease is also a cause of secondary osteoporosis and those at greatest risk should be monitored for osteopenia and assessed for the risk of fractures.

Fistulating Crohn's disease

Fistulating Crohn's disease is a complication that involves the formation of a fistula between the intestine and adjacent structures, such as perianal skin, bladder, and vagina. It occurs in about one quarter of patients, mostly when the disease involves the ileocolonic area.

Aims of treatment

Treatment is largely directed at the induction and maintenance of remission and the relief of symptoms. Active treatment of acute Crohn's disease should be distinguished from preventing relapse. The aims of drug treatment are to reduce symptoms and maintain or improve quality of life, while minimising toxicity related to drugs over both the short and long term.

In fistulating Crohn's disease, surgery and medical treatment aim to close and maintain closure of the fistula.

Non-drug treatment

EvGr In addition to drug treatment, management options for Crohn's disease include Smoking cessation p. 519 and attention to nutrition, which plays an important role in supportive care. Surgery may be considered in certain patients with early disease limited to the distal ileum and in severe or chronic active disease. ⟨A⟩

Drug treatment

Treatment of acute disease
Monotherapy
EvGr A corticosteroid (either prednisolone p. 718 or methylprednisolone p. 717 or intravenous hydrocortisone p. 716), is used to induce remission in patients with a first presentation or a single inflammatory exacerbation of Crohn's disease in a 12-month period.

In patients with distal ileal, ileocaecal or right-sided colonic disease, in whom a conventional corticosteroid is unsuitable or contra-indicated, budesonide p. 48 may be considered. Budesonide is less effective but may cause fewer side-effects than other corticosteroids, as systemic exposure is limited. Aminosalicylates (such as sulfasalazine p. 47 and mesalazine p. 45) are an alternative option in these patients. They are less effective than a corticosteroid or budesonide, but may be preferred because they have fewer side-effects. Aminosalicylates and budesonide are not appropriate for severe presentations or exacerbations. ⟨A⟩

Add-on treatment
EvGr Add on treatment is prescribed if there are two or more inflammatory exacerbations in a 12-month period, or the corticosteroid dose cannot be reduced.

Azathioprine p. 882 or mercaptopurine p. 956 [unlicensed indications] can be added to a corticosteroid or budesonide to induce remission. In patients who cannot tolerate azathioprine or mercaptopurine or in whom thiopurine methyltransferase (TPMT) activity is deficient, methotrexate p. 957 can be added to a corticosteroid.

Under specialist supervision, the tumour necrosis factor-alpha inhibitors adalimumab p. 1157 and infliximab p. 1162 are options for the treatment of severe, active Crohn's disease, following inadequate response to conventional therapies or in those who are intolerant of or have contra-indications to conventional therapy. Vedolizumab p. 50 is recommended for moderate to severely active Crohn's disease when therapy with adalimumab or infliximab is unsuccessful, is contra-indicated or not tolerated. Ustekinumab p. 1151 is recommended for moderate to severely active Crohn's disease when conventional therapy or therapy with adalimumab or infliximab is unsuccessful, is contra-indicated or not tolerated. See also *National*

funding/access decisions for adalimumab, infliximab, ustekinumab p. 1151, and vedolizumab.

Adalimumab and infliximab can be used as monotherapy or combined with an immunosuppressant although there is uncertainty about the comparative effectiveness and long-term side-effects of therapy. ⟨A⟩

Maintenance of remission
EvGr Patients who choose not to receive maintenance treatment during remission should be made aware of the symptoms that may suggest a relapse (most frequently unintended weight loss, abdominal pain, diarrhoea and general ill-health). For those who choose not to receive maintenance treatment during remission, a suitable follow up plan should be agreed upon and information provided on how to access healthcare if a relapse should occur.

Azathioprine or mercaptopurine [unlicensed indications] as monotherapy can be used to maintain remission when previously used with a corticosteroid to induce remission. They may also be used in patients who have not previously received these drugs (particularly those with adverse prognostic factors such as early age of onset, perianal disease, corticosteroid use at presentation, and severe presentations). Methotrexate can be used to maintain remission only in patients who required methotrexate to induce remission, or who are intolerant of or are not suitable for azathioprine or mercaptopurine for maintenance. Corticosteroids or budesonide should not be used. ⟨A⟩

Maintaining remission following surgery
EvGr Azathioprine in combination with up to 3 months' postoperative metronidazole p. 575 [unlicensed indication] should be considered to maintain remission in patients with ileocolonic Crohn's disease who have had complete macroscopic resection within the previous 3 months. Azathioprine alone should be considered for patients who cannot tolerate metronidazole p. 575. ⟨A⟩ Aminosalicylates are no longer recommended due to the lack of clinical efficacy. NICE do not consider mercaptopurine to be a cost-effective treatment and do not recommend its use.

EvGr Biologic therapies should no longer be used to maintain remission after complete macroscopic resection of ileocolonic Crohn's disease because of limited evidence. Budesonide should also not be used in these patients. ⟨A⟩

Other treatments
EvGr Loperamide hydrochloride p. 72 or codeine phosphate p. 475 can be used to manage diarrhoea associated with Crohn's disease in those who do not have colitis. ⟨A⟩ Colestyramine p. 212 is licensed for the relief of diarrhoea associated with Crohn's disease. See also Diarrhoea (acute) p. 71.

Fistulating Crohn's disease
Perianal fistulae are the most common occurrence in patients with fistulating Crohn's disease. EvGr Treatment may not be necessary for simple, asymptomatic perianal fistulae. When fistulae are symptomatic, local drainage and surgery may be required in conjunction with the medical therapy.

Metronidazole p. 575 or ciprofloxacin p. 593 [unlicensed indications], alone or in combination, can improve symptoms of fistulating Crohn's disease but complete healing occurs rarely. Metronidazole p. 575 is usually given for 1 month, but no longer than 3 months because of concerns about peripheral neuropathy. Other antibacterials should be given if specifically indicated (e.g. in sepsis associated with fistulae and perianal disease) and for managing bacterial overgrowth in the small bowel.

Either azathioprine p. 882 or mercaptopurine p. 956 [unlicensed indications] is used to control the inflammation in fistulating Crohn's disease and they are continued for maintenance.

Infliximab p. 1162 is recommended for patients with active fistulating Crohn's disease who have not responded to conventional therapy (including antibacterials, drainage and immunosuppressive treatments), or who are intolerant of or have contra-indications to conventional therapy. Infliximab should be used after ensuring that all sepsis is actively draining.

Abscess drainage, fistulotomy, and seton insertion may be appropriate, particularly before infliximab treatment.

Azathioprine, mercaptopurine, or infliximab should be continued as maintenance treatment for at least one year.

For the management of non-perianal fistulating Crohn's disease (including entero-gynaecological and enterovesical fistulae) surgery is the only recommended approach. ⒶⒷ

Useful Resources

Crohn's disease: management. National Institute for Health and Care Excellence. Clinical guideline 129. May 2019. www.nice.org.uk/guidance/ng129

Ulcerative colitis

20-Feb-2017

Description of condition

Ulcerative colitis is a chronic inflammatory condition, characterised by diffuse mucosal inflammation—it has a relapsing-remitting pattern. It is a life-long disease that is associated with significant morbidity. It most commonly presents between the ages of 15 and 25 years, although diagnosis can be made at any age.

The pattern of inflammation is continuous, extending from the rectum upwards to a varying degree. Inflammation of the rectum is referred to as **proctitis**, and inflammation of the rectum and sigmoid colon as **proctosigmoiditis**. **Left-sided colitis** refers to disease involving the colon distal to the splenic flexure. **Extensive colitis** affects the colon proximal to the splenic flexure, and includes pan-colitis, where the whole colon is involved. Common symptoms of active disease or relapse include bloody diarrhoea, an urgent need to defaecate, and abdominal pain.

Complications associated with ulcerative colitis include an increased risk of colorectal cancer, secondary osteoporosis, venous thromboembolism, and toxic megacolon.

Aims of treatment

Treatment is focused on treating active disease to manage symptoms and to induce and maintain remission.

Drug treatment

Overview

Management of ulcerative colitis is dependent on factors such as clinical severity, extent of disease, and patient preference. Clinical and laboratory investigations are used to determine the extent and severity of disease and to guide treatment. Severity is classified as mild, moderate or severe by using the Truelove and Witts' Severity Index to assess bowel movements, heart rate, erythrocyte sedimentation rate and the presence of pyrexia, melaena or anaemia—see the NICE guideline for Ulcerative Colitis for further information (see *Useful resources*).

ᴇᵛᴳʳ The extent of disease should be considered when choosing the route of administration for aminosalicylates and corticosteroids; whether oral treatment, topical treatment or both are to be used. If the inflammation is distal, a rectal preparation is adequate but if the inflammation is extended, systemic medication is required. Either suppositories or enemas can be offered, taking into account the patient's preferences. ⒶⒷ

ᴇᵛᴳʳ Rectal foam preparations and suppositories can be used when patients have difficulty retaining liquid enemas.

Diarrhoea associated with ulcerative colitis is sometimes treated with anti-diarrhoeal drugs (such as loperamide hydrochloride p. 72 or codeine phosphate p. 475) on the advice of a specialist; however their use is contra-indicated

in acute ulcerative colitis as they can increase the risk of toxic megacolon.

A macrogol-containing osmotic laxative (such as macrogol 3350 with potassium chloride, sodium bicarbonate and sodium chloride p. 61) may be useful for proximal faecal loading in proctitis. ⒺⒷ

Oral aminosalicylates for the treatment of ulcerative colitis are available in different preparations and release forms. ᴇᵛᴳʳ The preparation and dosing schedule should be chosen taking into account the delivery characteristics and suitability for the patient. When used to maintain remission, single daily doses of oral aminosalicylates can be more effective than multiple daily dosing, but may result in more side-effects.

The duration of corticosteroid course (usually 4 to 8 weeks) depends on the corticosteroid chosen. ⒶⒷ

Treatment of acute mild-to-moderate ulcerative colitis

Proctitis

ᴇᵛᴳʳ A topical aminosalicylate is recommended as first-line treatment for patients with a mild-to-moderate initial presentation or inflammatory exacerbation of proctitis. If remission is not achieved within 4 weeks, adding an oral aminosalicylate should be considered. If response remains inadequate, consider addition of a topical or an oral corticosteroid for 4 to 8 weeks.

Monotherapy with an oral aminosalicylate can be considered for patients who prefer not to use enemas or suppositories, although this may not be as effective. If remission is not achieved within 4 weeks, adding a topical or an oral corticosteroid for 4 to 8 weeks should be considered.

A topical or an oral corticosteroid for 4 to 8 weeks should be considered for patients in whom aminosalicylates are unsuitable. ⒶⒷ

Proctosigmoiditis and left-sided ulcerative colitis

ᴇᵛᴳʳ A topical aminosalicylate is recommended as first-line treatment for patients with a mild-to-moderate initial presentation or inflammatory exacerbation of proctosigmoiditis or left-sided ulcerative colitis. If remission is not achieved within 4 weeks, consider adding a high-dose oral aminosalicylate, or switching to a high-dose oral aminosalicylate and 4 to 8 weeks of a topical corticosteroid. If response remains inadequate, stop topical treatment and offer an oral aminosalicylate and 4 to 8 weeks of an oral corticosteroid.

Monotherapy with a high-dose oral aminosalicylate can be considered for patients who prefer not to use enemas or suppositories, although this may not be as effective. If remission is not achieved within 4 weeks, an oral corticosteroid for 4 to 8 weeks in addition to the high-dose aminosalicylate should be offered.

A topical or an oral corticosteroid for 4 to 8 weeks should be considered for patients in whom aminosalicylates are unsuitable. ⒶⒷ

Extensive ulcerative colitis

ᴇᵛᴳʳ A topical aminosalicylate and a high-dose oral aminosalicylate are recommended as first-line treatment for patients with a mild-to-moderate initial presentation or inflammatory exacerbation of extensive ulcerative colitis. If remission is not achieved within 4 weeks, stop topical aminosalicylate treatment and offer a high-dose oral aminosalicylate and 4 to 8 weeks of an oral corticosteroid. An oral corticosteroid for 4 to 8 weeks should be considered for patients in whom aminosalicylates are unsuitable. ⒶⒷ

Treatment of acute moderate-to-severe ulcerative colitis

ᴇᵛᴳʳ The biological drugs adalimumab p. 1157, golimumab p. 1161, infliximab p. 1162, vedolizumab p. 50, and the Janus kinase inhibitor tofacitinib p. 1154 can be used to treat moderate-to-severe active ulcerative colitis following an inadequate response to conventional treatment options, or if conventional treatment options are not tolerated or contra-indicated. Treatment with these agents is continued into the

1

Gastro-intestinal system

maintenance phase, if effective and tolerated. See *National funding/access decisions* for infliximab p. 1162, adalimumab p. 1157, golimumab p. 1161, vedolizumab p. 50, and tofacitinib p. 1154. Ⓐ

Treatment of acute severe ulcerative colitis

Acute severe ulcerative colitis of any extent can be life-threatening and is regarded as a medical emergency. EvGr Immediate hospital admission is required for treatment.

Intravenous corticosteroids (such as hydrocortisone p. 716 or methylprednisolone p. 717) should be given to induce remission in patients with acute severe ulcerative colitis (at first presentation or an exacerbation) while assessing the need for surgery. If intravenous corticosteroids are contra-indicated, declined or cannot be tolerated, then intravenous ciclosporin p. 884 [unlicensed indication] or surgery should be considered. A combination of intravenous ciclosporin with intravenous corticosteroids, or surgery is second line therapy for patients who have little or no improvement within 72 hours of starting intravenous corticosteroids or whose symptoms worsen despite treatment.

Infliximab p. 1162 can be used to treat acute exacerbations of severely active ulcerative colitis if ciclosporin p. 884 is contra-indicated or clinically inappropriate. Ⓐ

EvGr In patients who experience an initial response to steroids followed by deterioration, stool cultures should be taken to exclude the presence of pathogens; cytomegalovirus activation should be considered. Ⓔ

Maintaining remission in mild, moderate or severe ulcerative colitis

EvGr To reduce the chances of relapse occurring, maintenance therapy with an aminosalicylate is recommended in most patients. Corticosteroids are **not** suitable for maintenance treatment because of their side-effects.

After a mild-to-moderate inflammatory exacerbation of *proctitis* or *proctosigmoiditis*, a rectal aminosalicylate can be started alone or in combination with an oral aminosalicylate, administered daily or as part of an intermittent regimen (such as twice to three times weekly or the first seven days of each month). An oral aminosalicylate can be used alone in patients who prefer not to use enemas or suppositories, although this may not be as effective.

A low-dose of oral aminosalicylate is given to maintain remission in patients after a mild-to-moderate inflammatory exacerbation of left-sided or extensive ulcerative colitis.

When used to maintain remission, single daily doses of oral aminosalicylates can be more effective than multiple daily dosing, but may result in more side-effects.

Oral azathioprine p. 882 or mercaptopurine p. 956 [unlicensed indications] can be considered to maintain remission, if there has been two or more inflammatory exacerbations in a 12-month period that required treatment with systemic corticosteroids, or if remission is not maintained by aminosalicylates, or following a single acute severe episode. Ⓐ

There is no evidence to support the use of methotrexate p. 957 to induce or maintain remission in ulcerative colitis, though its use is common in clinical practice.

Biological drugs and Janus Kinase inhibitors for maintaining remission of ulcerative colitis

EvGr Treatment with these agents is continued into the maintenance phase, if effective and tolerated in acute disease. See also *National funding/access decisions* for adalimumab p. 1157, golimumab p. 1161, infliximab, vedolizumab p. 50, and tofacitinib p. 1154. Ⓐ

Non-drug treatment

EvGr Surgery may be necessary as emergency treatment for severe ulcerative colitis that does not respond to drug treatment. Patients can also choose to have elective surgery

for unresponsive or frequently relapsing disease that is affecting their quality of life. Ⓐ

Useful Resources

Ulcerative colitis: management. National Institute for Health and Care Excellence. Clinical guideline 130. May 2019. www.nice.org.uk/guidance/NG130

AMINOSALICYLATES

Aminosalicylates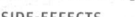

- **SIDE-EFFECTS**
  - ‣ **Common or very common** Arthralgia · cough · diarrhoea · dizziness · fever · gastrointestinal discomfort · headache · leucopenia · nausea · skin reactions · vomiting
  - ‣ **Uncommon** Alopecia · depression · dyspnoea · myalgia · photosensitivity reaction · thrombocytopenia
  - ‣ **Rare or very rare** Agranulocytosis · bone marrow disorders · cardiac inflammation · hepatitis · neutropenia · pancreatitis · peripheral neuropathy · renal impairment · respiratory disorders
  - ‣ **Frequency not known** Angioedema · eosinophilia · haemolytic anaemia · nephritis tubulointerstitial · oligozoospermia (reversible) · ulcerative colitis aggravated

  SIDE-EFFECTS, FURTHER INFORMATION A blood count should be performed and the drug stopped immediately if there is suspicion of a blood dyscrasia.
- **ALLERGY AND CROSS-SENSITIVITY** EvGr Contra-indicated in salicylate hypersensitivity Ⓜ.
- **RENAL IMPAIRMENT**
  Monitoring Renal function should be monitored more frequently in renal impairment.
- **MONITORING REQUIREMENTS** Renal function should be monitored before starting an oral aminosalicylate, at 3 months of treatment, and then annually during treatment.
- **PATIENT AND CARER ADVICE**
  Blood disorders Patients receiving aminosalicylates, and their carers, should be advised to report any unexplained bleeding, bruising, purpura, sore throat, fever or malaise that occurs during treatment.

▸ above

Balsalazide sodium

29-Apr-2020

- **INDICATIONS AND DOSE**
  Treatment of mild to moderate ulcerative colitis, acute attack
  - ‣ BY MOUTH
    - ‣ Adult: 2.25 g 3 times a day until remission occurs or for up to maximum of 12 weeks

  Maintenance of remission of ulcerative colitis
  - ‣ BY MOUTH
    - ‣ Adult: 1.5 g twice daily (max. per dose 3 g), adjusted according to response; maximum 6 g per day

- **CAUTIONS** History of asthma
- **INTERACTIONS** → Appendix 1: balsalazide
- **SIDE-EFFECTS** Blood disorder · cholelithiasis · lupus-like syndrome
- **PREGNANCY** Manufacturer advises avoid.
- **BREAST FEEDING** Diarrhoea may develop in the infant.
  Monitoring Monitor breast-fed infants for diarrhoea.
- **HEPATIC IMPAIRMENT** Manufacturer advises caution; avoid in severe impairment (no information available).
- **RENAL IMPAIRMENT** Manufacturer advises avoid in moderate to severe impairment.

● MEDICINAL FORMS There can be variation in the licensing of different medicines containing the same drug.

Capsule
CAUTIONARY AND ADVISORY LABELS 21, 25
▸ Colazide (Almirall Ltd)
Balsalazide disodium 750 mg Colazide 750mg capsules |
130 capsule PoM £30.42 DT = £30.42

F 44

Mesalazine
23-Jul-2020

● **INDICATIONS AND DOSE**
DOSE EQUIVALENCE AND CONVERSION
There is no evidence to show that any one oral preparation of mesalazine is more effective than another; however, the delivery characteristics of oral mesalazine preparations may vary.

ASACOL® MR 400MG TABLETS
Treatment of mild to moderate ulcerative colitis, acute attack
▸ BY MOUTH
  ▸ Child 12-17 years: 800 mg 3 times a day
  ▸ Adult: 2.4 g daily in divided doses

Maintenance of remission of ulcerative colitis and Crohn's ileo-colitis
▸ BY MOUTH
  ▸ Child 12-17 years: 400-800 mg 2-3 times a day
  ▸ Adult: 1.2-2.4 g daily in divided doses

ASACOL® MR 800MG TABLETS
Treatment of mild to moderate ulcerative colitis, acute attack
▸ BY MOUTH
  ▸ Adult: 2.4-4.8 g daily in divided doses

Maintenance of remission of ulcerative colitis
▸ BY MOUTH
  ▸ Adult: Up to 2.4 g once daily, alternatively up to 2.4 g daily in divided doses

Maintenance of remission of Crohn's ileo-colitis
▸ BY MOUTH
  ▸ Adult: Up to 2.4 g daily in divided doses

ASACOL® FOAM ENEMA
Treatment of acute attack of mild to moderate ulcerative colitis affecting the rectosigmoid region
▸ BY RECTUM
  ▸ Adult: 1 g daily for 4-6 weeks, to be administered into the rectum

Treatment of acute attack of mild to moderate ulcerative colitis, affecting the descending colon
▸ BY RECTUM
  ▸ Adult: 2 g once daily for 4-6 weeks, to be administered into the rectum

ASACOL® SUPPOSITORIES
Treatment of acute attack of mild to moderate ulcerative colitis and maintenance of remission
▸ BY RECTUM
  ▸ Adult: 0.75-1.5 g daily in divided doses, last dose to be administered at bedtime

MEZAVANT® XL
Treatment of mild to moderate ulcerative colitis, acute attack
▸ BY MOUTH
  ▸ Adult: 2.4 g once daily, increased if necessary to 4.8 g once daily, review treatment at 8 weeks

Maintenance of remission of ulcerative colitis
▸ BY MOUTH
  ▸ Adult: 2.4 g once daily

OCTASA®
Treatment of mild to moderate ulcerative colitis, acute attack
▸ BY MOUTH
  ▸ Adult: 2.4-4.8 g once daily, alternatively 2.4-4.8 g daily in divided doses, dose over 2.4 g daily in divided doses only

Maintenance of remission of ulcerative colitis and Crohn's ileo-colitis
▸ BY MOUTH
  ▸ Adult: 1.2-2.4 g once daily, alternatively daily in divided doses

PENTASA® GRANULES
Treatment of mild to moderate ulcerative colitis, acute attack
▸ BY MOUTH
  ▸ Child 5-17 years (body-weight up to 40 kg): 10-20 mg/kg 3 times a day
  ▸ Child 5-17 years (body-weight 40 kg and above): 1-2 g twice daily, total daily dose may alternatively be given in 3-4 divided doses
  ▸ Adult: Up to 4 g once daily, alternatively up to 4 g daily in 2-4 divided doses

Maintenance of remission of ulcerative colitis
▸ BY MOUTH
  ▸ Child 5-17 years (body-weight up to 40 kg): 7.5-15 mg/kg twice daily, total daily dose may alternatively be given in 3 divided doses
  ▸ Child 5-17 years (body-weight 40 kg and above): 2 g once daily
  ▸ Adult: 2 g once daily

PENTASA® RETENTION ENEMA
Treatment of acute attack of mild to moderate ulcerative colitis or maintenance of remission
▸ BY RECTUM
  ▸ Adult: 1 g once daily, dose to be administered at bedtime

Treatment of acute attack of mild to moderate ulcerative colitis affecting the rectosigmoid region
▸ BY RECTUM
  ▸ Child 12-17 years: 1 g once daily, dose to be administered at bedtime

PENTASA® SUPPOSITORIES
Treatment of acute attack, ulcerative proctitis
▸ BY RECTUM
  ▸ Adult: 1 g daily for 2-4 weeks

Maintenance, ulcerative proctitis
▸ BY RECTUM
  ▸ Adult: 1 g daily

PENTASA® TABLETS
Treatment of mild to moderate ulcerative colitis, acute attack
▸ BY MOUTH
  ▸ Adult: Up to 4 g once daily, alternatively up to 4 g daily in 2-3 divided doses

Maintenance of remission of ulcerative colitis
▸ BY MOUTH
  ▸ Adult: 2 g once daily

SALOFALK® ENEMA
Treatment of acute attack of mild to moderate ulcerative colitis or maintenance of remission
▸ BY RECTUM
  ▸ Adult: 2 g once daily, dose to be administered at bedtime

continued →

SALOFALK ® GRANULES

Treatment of mild to moderate ulcerative colitis, acute attack
▸ BY MOUTH
▸ Child 5-17 years (body-weight up to 40 kg): 30–50 mg/kg once daily, dose preferably given in the morning, alternatively 10–20 mg/kg 3 times a day
▸ Child 5-17 years (body-weight 40 kg and above): 1.5–3 g once daily, dose preferably given in the morning, alternatively 0.5–1 g 3 times a day
▸ Adult: 1.5–3 g once daily, dose preferably taken in the morning, alternatively 0.5–1 g 3 times a day

Maintenance of remission of ulcerative colitis
▸ BY MOUTH
▸ Child 5-17 years (body-weight up to 40 kg): 7.5–15 mg/kg twice daily, total daily dose may alternatively be given in 3 divided doses
▸ Child 5-17 years (body-weight 40 kg and above): 500 mg 3 times a day
▸ Adult: 500 mg 3 times a day

SALOFALK ® RECTAL FOAM

Treatment of mild ulcerative colitis affecting sigmoid colon and rectum
▸ BY RECTUM
▸ Child 12-17 years: 2 g once daily, dose to be administered into the rectum at bedtime, alternatively 2 g daily in 2 divided doses
▸ Adult: 2 g once daily, dose to be administered into the rectum at bedtime, alternatively 2 g daily in 2 divided doses

SALOFALK ® SUPPOSITORIES

Treatment of acute attack of mild to moderate ulcerative colitis affecting the rectum, sigmoid colon and descending colon
▸ BY RECTUM
▸ Adult: 0.5–1 g 2–3 times a day, adjusted according to response, dose to be given using 500 mg suppositories

Treatment of acute attack of mild to moderate ulcerative colitis affecting the rectum
▸ BY RECTUM
▸ Adult: 1 g daily, preferably at bedtime, dose to be given using 1 g suppositories

SALOFALK ® TABLETS

Treatment of mild to moderate ulcerative colitis, acute attack
▸ BY MOUTH
▸ Child 5-17 years (body-weight up to 40 kg): 10–20 mg/kg 3 times a day
▸ Child 5-17 years (body-weight 40 kg and above): 0.5–1 g 3 times a day
▸ Adult: 0.5–1 g 3 times a day

Maintenance of remission of ulcerative colitis
▸ BY MOUTH
▸ Child 5-17 years (body-weight up to 40 kg): 7.5–15 mg/kg twice daily, total daily dose may alternatively be given in 3 divided doses
▸ Child 5-17 years (body-weight 40 kg and above): 500 mg 3 times a day
▸ Adult: 500 mg 3 times a day

● UNLICENSED USE
▸ With oral use in children *Asacol* ® (all preparations) not licensed for use in children under 18 years. *Pentasa* ® granules and *Salofalk* ® tablets and granules not licensed for use in children under 6 years.
▸ With rectal use in children *Salofalk* ® rectal foam no dose recommendations for children (age range not specified by manufacturer).

● CONTRA-INDICATIONS
▸ With oral use Blood clotting abnormalities
● CAUTIONS Elderly · maintain adequate fluid intake · pulmonary disease
● INTERACTIONS → Appendix 1: mesalazine
● SIDE-EFFECTS
GENERAL SIDE-EFFECTS
▸ **Rare or very rare** Cholestasis exacerbated · drug fever · flatulence · nephritis
SPECIFIC SIDE-EFFECTS
▸ **Rare or very rare**
▸ With rectal use Constipation
● PREGNANCY Negligible quantities cross placenta.
● BREAST FEEDING Diarrhoea reported in breast-fed infants, but negligible amounts of mesalazine detected in breast milk.
Monitoring Monitor breast-fed infant for diarrhoea.
● HEPATIC IMPAIRMENT Manufacturer advises caution in mild to moderate impairment; avoid in severe impairment.
● RENAL IMPAIRMENT
▸ In adults Use with caution. Avoid if eGFR less than 20 mL/minute/1.73 m^2.
▸ In children Use with caution. Avoid if estimated glomerular filtration rate less than 20 mL/minute/1.73 m^2.
● DIRECTIONS FOR ADMINISTRATION
PENTASA ® TABLETS Manufacturer advises tablets may be halved, quartered, or dispersed in water, but should not be chewed.
PENTASA ® GRANULES Manufacturer advises granules should be placed on tongue and washed down with water or orange juice without chewing.
▸ In children Expert sources advise contents of one sachet should be weighed and divided immediately before use; discard any remaining granules.
SALOFALK ® GRANULES Manufacturer advises granules should be placed on tongue and washed down with water without chewing.
● PRESCRIBING AND DISPENSING INFORMATION There is no evidence to show that any one oral preparation of mesalazine is more effective than another; however, the delivery characteristics of oral mesalazine preparations may vary.
   Flavours of granule formulations of *Salofalk* ® may include vanilla.
● PATIENT AND CARER ADVICE If it is necessary to switch a patient to a different brand of mesalazine, the patient should be advised to report any changes in symptoms. Some products may require special administration advice; patients and carers should be informed.
Medicines for Children leaflet: Mesalazine (oral) for inflammatory bowel disease www.medicinesforchildren.org.uk/mesalazine-oral-inflammatory-bowel-disease
Medicines for Children leaflet: Mesalazine foam enema for inflammatory bowel disease www.medicinesforchildren.org.uk/mesalazine-foam-enema-inflammatory-bowel-disease
Medicines for Children leaflet: Mesalazine liquid enema for inflammatory bowel disease www.medicinesforchildren.org.uk/mesalazine-liquid-enema-inflammatory-bowel-disease

● MEDICINAL FORMS There can be variation in the licensing of different medicines containing the same drug.
Modified-release tablet
CAUTIONARY AND ADVISORY LABELS 21(does not apply to Pentasa ® tablets), 25 (does not apply to Pentasa ® tablets)
▸ Mezavant XL (Shire Pharmaceuticals Ltd)
   Mezalazine 1.2 gram Mezavant XL 1200mg tablets | 60 tablet [PoM] £42.95 DT = £42.95
▸ Pentasa (Ferring Pharmaceuticals Ltd)
   Mesalazine 500 mg Pentasa 500mg modified-release tablets | 100 tablet [PoM] £30.74 DT = £30.74

Mesalazine 1 gram Pentasa 1g modified-release tablets | 60 tablet PoM £36.89 DT = £36.89

Foam
EXCIPIENTS: May contain Cetostearyl alcohol (including cetyl and stearyl alcohol), disodium edetate, hydroxybenzoates (parabens), polysorbates, propylene glycol, sodium metabisulfite
▸ Salofalk (Dr. Falk Pharma UK Ltd)
    Mesalazine 1 gram per 1 application Salofalk 1g/application foam enema | 14 dose PoM £30.17 DT = £30.17

Gastro-resistant tablet
CAUTIONARY AND ADVISORY LABELS 5(does not apply to Octasa ®), 25
▸ Asacol MR (Allergan Ltd)
    Mesalazine 400 mg Asacol 400mg MR gastro-resistant tablets | 84 tablet PoM £27.45 DT = £27.45 | 168 tablet PoM £54.90
    Mesalazine 800 mg Asacol 800mg MR gastro-resistant tablets | 84 tablet PoM £54.90 DT = £54.90
▸ Octasa MR (Tillotts Pharma Ltd)
    Mesalazine 400 mg Octasa 400mg MR gastro-resistant tablets | 90 tablet PoM £16.58 DT = £16.58 | 120 tablet PoM £22.10
    Mesalazine 800 mg Octasa 800mg MR gastro-resistant tablets | 90 tablet PoM £40.38 | 180 tablet PoM £80.75 DT = £80.75
▸ Salofalk (Dr. Falk Pharma UK Ltd)
    Mesalazine 250 mg Salofalk 250mg gastro-resistant tablets | 100 tablet PoM £16.19 DT = £16.19
    Mesalazine 500 mg Salofalk 500mg gastro-resistant tablets | 100 tablet PoM £32.38 DT = £32.38

Suppository
▸ Pentasa (Ferring Pharmaceuticals Ltd)
    Mesalazine 1 gram Pentasa 1g suppositories | 28 suppository PoM £40.01 DT = £40.01
▸ Salofalk (Dr. Falk Pharma UK Ltd)
    Mesalazine 500 mg Salofalk 500mg suppositories | 30 suppository PoM £14.81 DT = £14.81
    Mesalazine 1 gram Salofalk 1g suppositories | 30 suppository PoM £29.62

Modified-release granules
CAUTIONARY AND ADVISORY LABELS 25 (does not apply to Pentasa ® granules)
EXCIPIENTS: May contain Aspartame
▸ Pentasa (Ferring Pharmaceuticals Ltd)
    Mesalazine 1 gram Pentasa 1g modified-release granules sachets sugar-free | 50 sachet PoM £30.74 DT = £30.74
    Mesalazine 2 gram Pentasa 2g modified-release granules sachets sugar-free | 60 sachet PoM £73.78 DT = £73.78
▸ Salofalk (Dr. Falk Pharma UK Ltd)
    Mesalazine 1 gram Salofalk 1g gastro-resistant modified-release granules sachets sugar-free | 50 sachet PoM £28.74 DT = £28.74
    Mesalazine 1.5 gram Salofalk 1.5g gastro-resistant modified-release granules sachets sugar-free | 60 sachet PoM £48.85 DT = £48.85
    Mesalazine 3 gram Salofalk 3g gastro-resistant modified-release granules sachets sugar-free | 60 sachet PoM £97.70 DT = £97.70

Enema
▸ Pentasa (Ferring Pharmaceuticals Ltd)
    Mesalazine 10 mg per 1 ml Pentasa Mesalazine 1g/100ml enema | 7 enema PoM £17.73 DT = £17.73
▸ Salofalk (Dr. Falk Pharma UK Ltd)
    Mesalazine 33.9 mg per 1 ml Salofalk 2g/59ml enema | 7 enema PoM £29.92 DT = £29.92

⚑ 44

Olsalazine sodium
12-Aug-2020

● **INDICATIONS AND DOSE**
Treatment of acute attack of mild ulcerative colitis
▸ BY MOUTH
▸ **Adult:** 1 g daily in divided doses, doses to be taken after meals, then increased if necessary up to 3 g daily in divided doses (max. per dose 1 g), dose to be increased over 1 week

Maintenance of remission of mild ulcerative colitis
▸ BY MOUTH
▸ **Adult:** Maintenance 500 mg twice daily, dose to be taken after food

● **SIDE-EFFECTS**
▸ **Uncommon** Paraesthesia · tachycardia
▸ **Frequency not known** Palpitations · vision blurred

● **PREGNANCY** Manufacturer advises avoid unless potential benefit outweighs risk.
● **BREAST FEEDING**
    Monitoring Monitor breast-fed infants for diarrhoea.
● **RENAL IMPAIRMENT** Use with caution; manufacturer advises avoid in significant impairment.
● **DIRECTIONS FOR ADMINISTRATION** Expert sources advise capsules can be opened and contents sprinkled on food.

● **MEDICINAL FORMS** There can be variation in the licensing of different medicines containing the same drug. Forms available from special-order manufacturers include: oral suspension, oral solution

Tablet
CAUTIONARY AND ADVISORY LABELS 21
▸ Olsalazine sodium (Non-proprietary)
    Olsalazine sodium 500 mg Olsalazine 500mg tablets | 60 tablet PoM £161.00 DT = £161.00

Capsule
CAUTIONARY AND ADVISORY LABELS 21
▸ Olsalazine sodium (Non-proprietary)
    Olsalazine sodium 250 mg Olsalazine 250mg capsules | 112 capsule PoM £144.00 DT = £144.00

⚑ 44

Sulfasalazine
29-Apr-2020

(Sulphasalazine)

● **INDICATIONS AND DOSE**
Treatment of acute attack of mild to moderate and severe ulcerative colitis | Active Crohn's disease
▸ BY MOUTH
▸ **Adult:** 1–2 g 4 times a day until remission occurs, corticosteroids may also be given, if necessary
▸ BY RECTUM
▸ **Adult:** 0.5–1 g twice daily, administered alone or in conjunction with oral therapy, morning and night after a bowel movement

Maintenance of remission of mild to moderate and severe ulcerative colitis
▸ BY MOUTH
▸ **Adult:** 500 mg 4 times a day
▸ BY RECTUM
▸ **Adult:** 0.5–1 g twice daily, administered alone or in conjunction with oral therapy, morning and night after a bowel movement

Active rheumatoid arthritis (administered on expert advice)
▸ BY MOUTH
▸ **Adult:** Initially 500 mg daily, increased in steps of 500 mg every week, increased to 2–3 g daily in divided doses, enteric coated tablets to be administered

---
IMPORTANT SAFETY INFORMATION
SAFE PRACTICE
Sulfasalazine has been confused with sulfadiazine; care must be taken to ensure the correct drug is prescribed and dispensed.

● **CAUTIONS** Acute porphyrias p. 1107 · G6PD deficiency · history of allergy · history of asthma · maintain adequate fluid intake · risk of haematological toxicity · risk of hepatic toxicity · slow acetylator status
● **INTERACTIONS** → Appendix 1: sulfasalazine
● **SIDE-EFFECTS**
▸ **Common or very common** Insomnia · stomatitis · taste altered · tinnitus · urine abnormalities
▸ **Uncommon** Face oedema · seizure · vasculitis · vertigo
▸ **Frequency not known** Anaemia · appetite decreased · ataxia · cyanosis · encephalopathy · haematuria · hallucination · hepatic failure · hypoprothrombinaemia ·

lymphadenopathy · macrocytosis · meningitis aseptic · methaemoglobinaemia · nephrotic syndrome · parotitis · periorbital oedema · pseudomembranous enterocolitis · serum sickness · severe cutaneous adverse reactions (SCARs) · smell disorders · systemic lupus erythematosus (SLE) · yellow discolouration of body fluids

SIDE-EFFECTS, FURTHER INFORMATION Incidence of side-effects increases with higher doses.

> **Blood disorders** Haematological abnormalities occur usually in the first 3 to 6 months of treatment—discontinue if these occur.

● PREGNANCY Theoretical risk of neonatal haemolysis in third trimester; adequate folate supplements should be given to mother.

● BREAST FEEDING Small amounts in milk (1 report of bloody diarrhoea); theoretical risk of neonatal haemolysis especially in G6PD-deficient infants.

● HEPATIC IMPAIRMENT Manufacturer advises caution.

● RENAL IMPAIRMENT Risk of toxicity, including crystalluria, in moderate impairment—ensure high fluid intake. Avoid in severe impairment.

● MONITORING REQUIREMENTS

▸ Blood disorders Close monitoring of full blood counts (including differential white cell count and platelet count) is necessary initially, and at monthly intervals during the first 3 months.

▸ Renal function Although the manufacturer recommends renal function tests in rheumatic diseases, evidence of practical value is unsatisfactory.

▸ Liver function Liver function tests should be performed at monthly intervals for first 3 months.

● PATIENT AND CARER ADVICE

Contact lenses Some soft contact lenses may be stained.

● MEDICINAL FORMS There can be variation in the licensing of different medicines containing the same drug. Forms available from special-order manufacturers include: oral suspension

Oral suspension
CAUTIONARY AND ADVISORY LABELS 14
EXCIPIENTS: May contain Alcohol
▸ Sulfasalazine (Non-proprietary)
  Sulfasalazine 50 mg per 1 ml Sulfasalazine 250mg/5ml oral suspension sugar free sugar-free | 500 ml [PoM] £63.56 DT = £57.09

Gastro-resistant tablet
CAUTIONARY AND ADVISORY LABELS 5, 14, 25
▸ Sulfasalazine (Non-proprietary)
  Sulfasalazine 500 mg Sulfasalazine 500mg gastro-resistant tablets | 112 tablet [PoM] £12.83 DT = £10.06
▸ Salazopyrin EN (Pfizer Ltd)
  Sulfasalazine 500 mg Salazopyrin EN-Tabs 500mg | 112 tablet [PoM] £8.43 DT = £10.06
▸ Sulazine EC (Genesis Pharmaceuticals Ltd)
  Sulfasalazine 500 mg Sulazine EC 500mg tablets | 112 tablet [PoM] £6.74 DT = £10.06

Tablet
CAUTIONARY AND ADVISORY LABELS 14
▸ Sulfasalazine (Non-proprietary)
  Sulfasalazine 500 mg Sulfasalazine 500mg tablets | 112 tablet [PoM] £8.94 DT = £6.15
▸ Salazopyrin (Pfizer Ltd)
  Sulfasalazine 500 mg Salazopyrin 500mg tablets | 112 tablet [PoM] £6.97 DT = £6.15

Suppository
CAUTIONARY AND ADVISORY LABELS 14
▸ Salazopyrin (Pfizer Ltd)
  Sulfasalazine 500 mg Salazopyrin 500mg suppositories | 10 suppository [PoM] £3.30 DT = £3.30

CORTICOSTEROIDS

☞ 711

Beclometasone dipropionate
25-Sep-2020

(Beclomethasone dipropionate)

● INDICATIONS AND DOSE

Adjunct to aminosalicylates in acute mild to moderate ulcerative colitis
▸ BY MOUTH
  ▸ Adult: 5 mg daily maximum duration of treatment of 4 weeks, dose to be taken in the morning

● INTERACTIONS → Appendix 1: corticosteroids

● SIDE-EFFECTS
▸ **Uncommon** Constipation · idiopathic intracranial hypertension · muscle cramps

● HEPATIC IMPAIRMENT Manufacturer advises avoid in severe impairment (no information available).

● MEDICINAL FORMS There can be variation in the licensing of different medicines containing the same drug.
Modified-release tablet
CAUTIONARY AND ADVISORY LABELS 25
▸ Clipper (Chiesi Ltd)
  Beclometasone dipropionate 5 mg Clipper 5mg gastro-resistant modified-release tablets | 30 tablet [PoM] £56.56 DT = £56.56

☞ 711

Budesonide
12-Nov-2020

● DRUG ACTION Budesonide is a glucocorticoid, which exerts significant local anti-inflammatory effects.

● INDICATIONS AND DOSE

BUDENOFALK ® CAPSULES
Mild to moderate Crohn's disease affecting the ileum or ascending colon
▸ BY MOUTH
  ▸ Adult: 9 mg once daily for 8 weeks, to be taken in the morning, alternatively 3 mg 3 times a day for 8 weeks, reduce dose gradually over two weeks following treatment

Collagenous colitis
▸ BY MOUTH
  ▸ Adult: 9 mg once daily for 8 weeks, to be taken in the morning, reduce dose gradually over two weeks following treatment

Autoimmune hepatitis, induction of remission
▸ BY MOUTH
  ▸ Adult: 3 mg 3 times a day

Autoimmune hepatitis, maintenance
▸ BY MOUTH
  ▸ Adult: 3 mg twice daily

BUDENOFALK ® GRANULES
Mild to moderate Crohn's disease affecting the ileum or ascending colon | Collagenous colitis
▸ BY MOUTH
  ▸ Adult: 9 mg once daily for 8 weeks, to be taken in the morning about 30 minutes before breakfast, reduce dose gradually over two weeks following treatment

BUDENOFALK ® RECTAL FOAM
Ulcerative colitis affecting sigmoid colon and rectum
▸ BY RECTUM
  ▸ Adult: 1 metered application once daily for up to 8 weeks

DOSE EQUIVALENCE AND CONVERSION
▸ For *Budenofalk* ® rectal foam: 1 metered application is equivalent to budesonide 2 mg.

CORTIMENT ®

Induction of remission of mild-to-moderate active ulcerative colitis
▸ BY MOUTH
▸ Adult: 9 mg once daily for up to 8 weeks, dose to be taken in the morning

ENTOCORT ® CAPSULES

Active microscopic colitis
▸ BY MOUTH
▸ Adult: 9 mg once daily, to be taken in the morning

Mild to moderate Crohn's disease affecting the ileum or ascending colon
▸ BY MOUTH
▸ Adult: 9 mg once daily for up to 8 weeks; reduce dose for the last 2–4 weeks of treatment, to be taken in the morning

ENTOCORT ® ENEMA

Ulcerative colitis involving rectal and recto-sigmoid disease
▸ BY RECTUM
▸ Adult: 1 enema daily for 4 weeks, to be administered at bedtime

JORVEZA ®

Eosinophilic oesophagitis (initiated by a specialist)
▸ BY MOUTH
▸ Adult: 1 mg twice daily for 6 weeks; treatment may be extended to up to 12 weeks if required, to be taken after food

● CAUTIONS Autoimmune hepatitis
● INTERACTIONS → Appendix 1: corticosteroids
● SIDE-EFFECTS
▸ Common or very common
▸ With oral use Muscle twitching · oedema · oral disorders
▸ With rectal use Diarrhoea · gastrointestinal disorders
● HEPATIC IMPAIRMENT For *Budenofalk* ® manufacturer advises avoid in cirrhosis (risk of increased exposure, limited information available).
JORVEZA ® Manufacturer advises avoid (no information available).
● RENAL IMPAIRMENT
JORVEZA ® Manufacturer advises caution in mild to moderate impairment; avoid in severe impairment (no information available).
● MONITORING REQUIREMENTS Manufacturer advises when used in autoimmune hepatitis, liver function tests should be monitored every 2 weeks for 1 month, then at least every 3 months.
● DIRECTIONS FOR ADMINISTRATION
▸ With oral use Manufacturer advises granules should be placed on tongue and washed down with water without chewing.
JORVEZA ® Manufacturer advises the tablet should be placed on the tip of the tongue, gently pressed against the roof of the mouth to dissolve, and the dissolved material swallowed with saliva as the tablet disintegrates. Patients should avoid eating, drinking or performing oral hygiene for at least 30 minutes after taking the tablet. Oral solutions, sprays or chewable tablets should be avoided for at least 30 minutes before and after taking the tablet.
● PRESCRIBING AND DISPENSING INFORMATION
▸ With oral use Flavours of granule formulations may include lemon.

ENTOCORT ® CAPSULES
▸ With oral use Dispense modified-release capsules in original container (contains desiccant).
● PATIENT AND CARER ADVICE
▸ With oral use Patients or carers should be given advice on how to administer budesonide granules.
JORVEZA ® Manufacturer advises patients or carers should be given advice on how to administer orodispersible tablets.
● NATIONAL FUNDING/ACCESS DECISIONS
For full details see funding body website
Scottish Medicines Consortium (SMC) decisions
▸ Budesonide (*Jorveza* ®) for the treatment of eosinophilic oesophagitis in adults (October 2020) SMC No. SMC2158 Recommended with restrictions
CORTIMENT ® For full details see funding body website
Scottish Medicines Consortium (SMC) decisions
▸ Budesonide (*Cortiment* ®) in adults for induction of remission in patients with mild to moderate active ulcerative colitis (UC) where aminosalicylate (5-ASA) treatment is not sufficient (October 2016) SMC No. 1093/15 Recommended with restrictions
BUDENOFALK ® CAPSULES For full details see funding body website
Scottish Medicines Consortium (SMC) decisions
▸ Budesonide 3 mg gastro-resistant capsules (*Budenofalk* ®) for autoimmune hepatitis (May 2015) SMC No. 1043/15 Recommended with restrictions

● MEDICINAL FORMS There can be variation in the licensing of different medicines containing the same drug.
Modified-release tablet
CAUTIONARY AND ADVISORY LABELS 25
▸ Cortiment (Ferring Pharmaceuticals Ltd)
  Budesonide 9 mg Cortiment 9mg modified-release tablets | 30 tablet PoM £75.00 DT = £75.00
Gastro-resistant capsule
CAUTIONARY AND ADVISORY LABELS 5, 10, 22, 25
▸ Budenofalk (Dr. Falk Pharma UK Ltd)
  Budesonide 3 mg Budenofalk 3mg gastro-resistant capsules | 100 capsule PoM £75.05 DT = £75.05
Foam
EXCIPIENTS: May contain Cetostearyl alcohol (including cetyl and stearyl alcohol), disodium edetate, propylene glycol, sorbic acid
▸ Budenofalk (Dr. Falk Pharma UK Ltd)
  Budesonide 2 mg per 1 actuation Budenofalk 2mg foam enema | 14 dose PoM £57.11 DT = £57.11
Modified-release capsule
CAUTIONARY AND ADVISORY LABELS 5, 10, 25
▸ Entocort CR (Tillotts Pharma Ltd)
  Budesonide 3 mg Entocort CR 3mg capsules | 50 capsule PoM £37.53 | 100 capsule PoM £75.05 DT = £75.05
Gastro-resistant granules
CAUTIONARY AND ADVISORY LABELS 5, 10, 22, 25
▸ Budenofalk (Dr. Falk Pharma UK Ltd)
  Budesonide 9 mg Budenofalk 9mg gastro-resistant granules sachets | 60 sachet PoM £135.00 DT = £135.00
Orodispersible tablet
CAUTIONARY AND ADVISORY LABELS 10
ELECTROLYTES: May contain Sodium
▸ Jorveza (Dr. Falk Pharma UK Ltd)
  Budesonide 1 mg Jorveza 1mg orodispersible tablets sugar-free | 90 tablet PoM £323.00 DT = £323.00
Enema
▸ Entocort (Tillotts Pharma Ltd)
  Budesonide 20 microgram per 1 ml Entocort 2mg/100ml enema | 7 enema PoM £33.66 DT = £33.66

1

Gastro-intestinal system

IMMUNOSUPPRESSANTS > MONOCLONAL ANTIBODIES, ANTI-LYMPHOCYTE

Vedolizumab

04-Nov-2020

- **DRUG ACTION** Vedolizumab is a monoclonal antibody that binds specifically to the $\alpha_4\beta_7$ integrin, which is expressed on gut homing T helper lymphocytes and causes a reduction in gastrointestinal inflammation.

- **INDICATIONS AND DOSE**

Ulcerative colitis (under expert supervision)
▶ BY INTRAVENOUS INFUSION
▶ Adult: Initially 300 mg, then 300 mg after 2 weeks, followed by 300 mg after 4 weeks, followed by 300 mg every 8 weeks, dose to be given over 30 minutes, if treatment is interrupted or response decreases, dosing frequency may be increased—consult product literature; review treatment if no response within 10 weeks of initial dose
▶ BY SUBCUTANEOUS INJECTION
▶ Adult: Maintenance 108 mg every 2 weeks, following at least 2 intravenous infusions; the first subcutaneous dose should be administered in place of the next scheduled intravenous dose

Crohn's disease (under expert supervision)
▶ BY INTRAVENOUS INFUSION
▶ Adult: Initially 300 mg, then 300 mg after 2 weeks, followed by 300 mg after 4 weeks, followed by 300 mg every 8 weeks, dose to be given over 30 minutes, if no response is observed, an additional dose of 300 mg may be given 10 weeks after initial dose; if treatment is interrupted or response decreases, dosing frequency may be increased—consult product literature; review treatment if no response within 14 weeks of initial dose
▶ BY SUBCUTANEOUS INJECTION
▶ Adult: Maintenance 108 mg every 2 weeks, following at least 2 intravenous infusions; the first subcutaneous dose should be administered in place of the next scheduled intravenous dose

- **CONTRA-INDICATIONS** Severe active infection
- **CAUTIONS** Controlled chronic severe infection · history of recurring severe infection · previous treatment with natalizumab (wait at least 12 weeks between natalizumab use and initiation of vedolizumab unless potential benefit outweighs risk) · previous treatment with rituximab
  CAUTIONS, FURTHER INFORMATION
  ▶ Risk of infection Patients must be screened for tuberculosis before starting treatment; if latent tuberculosis is diagnosed, appropriate treatment must be initiated prior to vedolizumab treatment; if tuberculosis is diagnosed during treatment, discontinue vedolizumab until infection is resolved.
  Patients should be brought up to date with current immunisation schedule before initiating treatment.
- **INTERACTIONS** → Appendix 1: monoclonal antibodies
- **SIDE-EFFECTS**
▶ **Common or very common** Arthralgia · constipation · cough · fatigue · fever · gastrointestinal discomfort · gastrointestinal disorders · headache · hypertension · increased risk of infection · muscle spasms · muscle weakness · nasal congestion · nausea · night sweats · oropharyngeal pain · pain · paraesthesia · skin reactions
▶ **Uncommon** Chills · feeling cold · infusion related reaction
▶ **Rare or very rare** Hypersensitivity · vision blurred
▶ **Frequency not known** Meningitis listeria · sepsis
  SIDE-EFFECTS, FURTHER INFORMATION Infusion-related and hypersensitivity reactions have been reported. Patients should be observed continuously during each infusion for signs and symptoms of acute hypersensitivity

reactions; they should also be observed for 2 hours after the initial two infusions, and for 1 hour after subsequent infusions. Discontinue treatment if a severe infusion-related or other severe reaction occurs and initiate appropriate treatment (e.g. adrenaline and antihistamines); if a mild to moderate infusion-related reaction occurs, interrupt infusion or reduce infusion rate and initiate appropriate treatment (if reaction subsides the infusion may be continued)—consider pretreatment with an antihistamine, hydrocortisone, and/or paracetamol prior to subsequent infusions in patients who experience mild to moderate infusion-related reactions.

- **CONCEPTION AND CONTRACEPTION** Manufacturer advises effective contraception required during and for at least 18 weeks after treatment.
- **PREGNANCY** Manufacturer advises use only if potential benefit outweighs risk.
- **BREAST FEEDING** EvGr Specialist sources indicate use with caution—present in milk. ⓓ
- **MONITORING REQUIREMENTS**
▶ Manufacturer advises monitor closely for infection before, during and after treatment—potential increased risk of opportunistic infection.
▶ Manufacturer advises monitor for new onset or worsening neurological signs and symptoms (withhold treatment if progressive multifocal leukoencephalopathy (PML) is suspected).
- **DIRECTIONS FOR ADMINISTRATION** For *intravenous infusion* (*Entyvio®*), manufacturer advises give intermittently in Sodium chloride 0.9%; allow vial to reach room temperature then reconstitute with 4.8 mL of water for injection (using a syringe with a 21–25 gauge needle); gently swirl vial for at least 15 seconds, do not shake vigorously or invert; allow to stand for up to 20 minutes (gently swirl vial if needed), leave for an additional 10 minutes if not dissolved; gently invert vial three times, withdraw 5 mL of reconstituted solution (using a syringe with a 21–25 gauge needle), and add to 250 mL of infusion fluid; gently mix and give over 30 minutes.
- **PRESCRIBING AND DISPENSING INFORMATION** Vedolizumab is a biological medicine. Biological medicines must be prescribed and dispensed by brand name, see *Biological medicines* and *Biosimilar medicines*, under Guidance on prescribing p. 1; manufacturer advises to record the brand name and batch number after each administration.
- **PATIENT AND CARER ADVICE**
  Self-administration
▶ With subcutaneous use Manufacturer advises patients and their carers should be given training in subcutaneous injection technique if appropriate.
  Alert card Patients should be provided with a patient alert card.
- **NATIONAL FUNDING/ACCESS DECISIONS**
  For full details see funding body website
  NICE decisions
▶ Vedolizumab for treating moderately to severely active Crohn's disease after prior therapy (August 2015) NICE TA352 Recommended with restrictions
▶ Vedolizumab for treating moderately to severely active ulcerative colitis (June 2015) NICE TA342 Recommended
  Scottish Medicines Consortium (SMC) decisions
▶ Vedolizumab powder for concentrate for solution for infusion (*Entyvio®*) for the treatment of adult patients with moderately to severely active Crohn's disease who have had an inadequate response with, lost response to, or were intolerant to either conventional therapy or a tumour necrosis factor-alpha antagonist (July 2015) SMC No. 1064/15 Recommended with restrictions

▸ Vedolizumab solution for injection (*Entyvio*®) for the treatment of adult patients with moderately to severely active Crohn's disease who have had an inadequate response with, lost response to, or were intolerant to either conventional therapy or a tumour necrosis factor-alpha antagonist (August 2020) SMC No. SMC2277 Recommended with restrictions

▸ Vedolizumab powder for concentrate for solution for infusion (*Entyvio*®) for the treatment of adult patients with moderately to severely active ulcerative colitis who had an inadequate response with, lost response to, or were intolerant to either conventional therapy or a tumour necrosis factor-alpha antagonist (May 2015) SMC No. 1045/15 Recommended

▸ Vedolizumab solution for injection (*Entyvio*®) for the treatment of adult patients with moderately to severely active ulcerative colitis who have had an inadequate response with, lost response to, or were intolerant to either conventional therapy or a tumour necrosis factor-alpha antagonist (August 2020) SMC No. SMC2276 Recommended

● MEDICINAL FORMS There can be variation in the licensing of different medicines containing the same drug.

Solution for injection
CAUTIONARY AND ADVISORY LABELS 10
EXCIPIENTS: May contain Polysorbates
▸ Entyvio (Takeda UK Ltd)
Vedolizumab 158.82 mg per 1 ml Entyvio 108mg/0.68ml solution for injection pre-filled pens | 1 pre-filled disposable injection PoM £512.50 (Hospital only) | 2 pre-filled disposable injection PoM £1,025.00 (Hospital only)
Entyvio 108mg/0.68ml solution for injection pre-filled syringes | 1 pre-filled disposable injection PoM £512.50 (Hospital only) | 2 pre-filled disposable injection PoM £1,025.00 (Hospital only)

Powder for solution for infusion
CAUTIONARY AND ADVISORY LABELS 10
EXCIPIENTS: May contain Polysorbates
▸ Entyvio (Takeda UK Ltd)
Vedolizumab 300 mg Entyvio 300mg powder for concentrate for solution for infusion vials | 1 vial PoM £2,050.00 (Hospital only)

1.4 Irritable bowel syndrome

Irritable bowel syndrome

02-May-2020

Description of condition

Irritable bowel syndrome (IBS) is a common, chronic, relapsing, and often life-long condition, mainly affecting people aged between 20 and 30 years. It is more common in women. Symptoms include abdominal pain or discomfort, disordered defaecation (either diarrhoea, or constipation with straining, urgency, and incomplete evacuation), passage of mucus, and bloating. Symptoms are usually relieved by defaecation. Obtaining an accurate clinical diagnosis of IBS prior to treatment is crucial.

Aims of treatment

The treatment of IBS is focused on symptom control, in order to improve quality of life.

Non-drug treatment

EvGr Diet and lifestyle changes are important for effective self-management of IBS. Patients should be encouraged to increase physical activity, and advised to eat regularly, without missing meals or leaving long gaps between meals. Dietary advice should also include, limiting fresh fruit consumption to no more than 3 portions per day. The fibre intake of patients with IBS should be reviewed. If an increase in dietary fibre is required, soluble fibre such as ispaghula husk p. 58, or foods high in soluble fibre such as oats, are recommended. Intake of insoluble fibre (e.g. bran) and 'resistant starch' should be reduced or discouraged as they may exacerbate symptoms. Fluid intake (mostly water)

should be increased to at least 8 cups each day and the intake of caffeine, alcohol and fizzy drinks reduced. The artificial sweetener sorbitol should be avoided in patients with diarrhoea. Where probiotics are being used, continue for at least 4 weeks while monitoring the effect.

If a patient's symptoms persist following lifestyle and dietary advice, single food avoidance and exclusion diets may be an option under the supervision of a dietitian or medical specialist. Ⓐ

Drug treatment

EvGr The choice of drug treatment depends on the nature and severity of the symptoms. Many drug treatment options for IBS are available over-the-counter.

Antispasmodic drugs (such as alverine citrate p. 94, mebeverine hydrochloride p. 94 and peppermint oil p. 52) can be taken in addition to dietary and lifestyle changes. A laxative (excluding lactulose p. 60 as it may cause bloating) can be used to treat constipation. Patients who have not responded to laxatives from the different classes and who have had constipation for at least 12 months, can be treated with linaclotide p. 52. Loperamide hydrochloride p. 72 is the first-line choice of anti-motility drug for relief of diarrhoea. Patients with IBS should be advised how on to adjust their dose of laxative or anti-motility drug according to stool consistency, with the aim of achieving a soft, well-formed stool. Ⓐ See Constipation p. 57, for information on other drugs used for chronic constipation.

EvGr A low-dose tricyclic antidepressant, such as amitriptyline hydrochloride p. 392 [unlicensed indication], can be used for abdominal pain or discomfort as a second-line option in patients who have not responded to antispasmodics, anti-motility drugs, or laxatives. A selective serotonin reuptake inhibitor may be considered in those who do not respond to a tricyclic antidepressant [unlicensed indication].

Psychological intervention can be offered to patients who have no relief of IBS symptoms after 12 months of drug treatment. Ⓐ

Useful Resources

Irritable bowel syndrome in adults: diagnosis and management. National Institute for Health and Care Excellence. Clinical guideline 61. February 2008 (updated April 2017).
www.nice.org.uk/guidance/cg61

ANTISPASMODICS

Mebeverine with ispaghula husk

09-Nov-2020

The properties listed below are those particular to the combination only. For the properties of the components please consider, mebeverine hydrochloride p. 94, ispaghula husk p. 58.

● INDICATIONS AND DOSE
Irritable bowel syndrome
▸ BY MOUTH
  ▸ **Child 12-17 years:** 1 sachet twice daily, in water, morning and evening, 30 minutes before food and 1 sachet daily if required, taken 30 minutes before midday meal
  ▸ **Adult:** 1 sachet twice daily, in water, morning and evening, 30 minutes before food and 1 sachet daily if required, taken 30 minutes before midday meal

● DIRECTIONS FOR ADMINISTRATION Manufacturer advises contents of one sachet should be stirred into a glass (approx. 150 mL) of cold water and drunk immediately.

- PATIENT AND CARER ADVICE Patients or carers should be given advice on how to administer ispaghula husk with mebeverine granules.

- MEDICINAL FORMS There can be variation in the licensing of different medicines containing the same drug.
Effervescent granules
CAUTIONARY AND ADVISORY LABELS 13, 22
EXCIPIENTS: May contain Aspartame
ELECTROLYTES: May contain Potassium
‣ Fybogel Mebeverine (Reckitt Benckiser Healthcare (UK) Ltd)
Mebeverine hydrochloride 135 mg, Ispaghula husk
3.5 gram Fybogel Mebeverine effervescent granules sachets orange sugar-free | 10 sachet P £5.44 DT = £5.44

Peppermint oil

19-Nov-2020

- INDICATIONS AND DOSE
COLPERMIN ®

Relief of abdominal colic and distension, particularly in irritable bowel syndrome
▸ BY MOUTH
‣ Child 15-17 years: 1-2 capsules 3 times a day for up to 3 months if necessary, capsule to be swallowed whole with water
‣ Adult: 1-2 capsules 3 times a day for up to 3 months if necessary, capsule to be swallowed whole with water
MINTEC ®

Relief of abdominal colic and distension, particularly in irritable bowel syndrome
▸ BY MOUTH
‣ Adult: 1-2 capsules 3 times a day for up to 2-3 months if necessary, dose to be taken before meals, swallowed whole with water

- CAUTIONS Sensitivity to menthol
- INTERACTIONS → Appendix 1: peppermint
- SIDE-EFFECTS Ataxia · bradycardia · gastrointestinal discomfort · gastrooesophageal reflux disease · headache · nausea · paraesthesia · rash erythematous · tremor · vomiting
- PREGNANCY Not known to be harmful.
- BREAST FEEDING Significant levels of menthol in breast milk unlikely.
- DIRECTIONS FOR ADMINISTRATION Manufacturer advises capsules should not be broken or chewed because peppermint oil may irritate mouth or oesophagus.

- MEDICINAL FORMS There can be variation in the licensing of different medicines containing the same drug.
Gastro-resistant capsule
CAUTIONARY AND ADVISORY LABELS 5, 22, 25
‣ Mintec (Almirall Ltd)
Peppermint oil 200 microlitre Mintec 0.2ml gastro-resistant capsules | 84 capsule GSL £7.04 DT = £7.04
Modified-release capsule
CAUTIONARY AND ADVISORY LABELS 5, 22, 25
EXCIPIENTS: May contain Arachis (peanut) oil
‣ Colpermin (Johnson & Johnson Ltd)
Peppermint oil 200 microlitre Colpermin IBS Relief gastro-resistant modified-release capsules | 20 capsule GSL £3.94 | 100 capsule GSL £14.97 DT = £14.97

LAXATIVES > GUANYLATE CYCLASE-C RECEPTOR AGONISTS

Linaclotide

10-Nov-2020

- INDICATIONS AND DOSE

Moderate to severe irritable bowel syndrome with constipation
▸ BY MOUTH
‣ Adult: 290 micrograms once daily, dose to be taken at least 30 minutes before meals, review treatment if no response after 4 weeks

- CONTRA-INDICATIONS Gastro-intestinal obstruction · inflammatory bowel disease
- CAUTIONS Predisposition to fluid and electrolyte disturbances
- SIDE-EFFECTS
▸ Common or very common Diarrhoea · dizziness · gastrointestinal discomfort · gastrointestinal disorders
▸ Uncommon Appetite decreased · dehydration · haemorrhage · hypokalaemia · nausea · postural hypotension · vomiting
▸ Frequency not known Rash

SIDE-EFFECTS, FURTHER INFORMATION Manufacturer advises if diarrhoea severe or prolonged, consider suspending treatment.

- PREGNANCY Manufacturer advises avoid.
- BREAST FEEDING Unlikely to be present in milk in significant amounts, but manufacturer advises avoid.
- PRESCRIBING AND DISPENSING INFORMATION Dispense capsules in original container (contains desiccant); discard any capsules remaining 18 weeks after opening.
- NATIONAL FUNDING/ACCESS DECISIONS
For full details see funding body website
Scottish Medicines Consortium (SMC) decisions
‣ Linaclotide (*Constella* ®) for the symptomatic treatment of moderate to severe irritable bowel syndrome with constipation (IBS-C) in adults (June 2013) SMC No. 869/13 Recommended with restrictions

- MEDICINAL FORMS There can be variation in the licensing of different medicines containing the same drug.
Capsule
CAUTIONARY AND ADVISORY LABELS 22
‣ Constella (Allergan Ltd)
Linaclotide 290 microgram Constella 290microgram capsules | 28 capsule PoM £37.56 DT = £37.56

1.5 Short bowel syndrome

Short bowel syndrome

31-Aug-2016

Description of condition

Patients with a shortened bowel due to large surgical resection (with or without stoma formation) may require medical management to ensure adequate absorption of nutrients and fluid. Absorption of oral medication is also often impaired.

Aims of treatment

The management of short bowel syndrome focuses on ensuring adequate nutrition and drug absorption, thereby reducing the risk of complications resulting from these effects.

Drug treatment

Nutritional deficiencies

EvGr Patients with a short bowel may require replacement of vitamins and minerals depending on the extent and position of the bowel resection. Deficiencies in vitamins A, B_{12}, D, E, and K, essential fatty acids, zinc, and selenium can occur.

Hypomagnesaemia is common and is treated with oral or intravenous magnesium supplementation (see Magnesium imbalance p. 1098), though administration of oral magnesium may cause diarrhoea. Occasionally the use of oral alfacalcidol p. 1132 and correction of sodium depletion may be useful. Nutritional support can range from oral supplements to parenteral nutrition, depending on the severity of intestinal failure. A

Diarrhoea and high output stomas

Diarrhoea is common in short bowel syndrome and can be due to multiple factors. EvGr The use of oral rehydration salts can be considered in order to promote adequate hydration. Oral intake influences the volume of stool passed, so reducing food intake will lessen diarrhoea, but will also exacerbate the problems of undernutrition. A patient may require parenteral nutrition to allow them to eat less, if the extent of diarrhoea is unacceptable.

Pharmacological treatment may be necessary, with the choice of drug depending on the potential for side-effects and the degree of resection. A

Antimotility drugs

EvGr Loperamide hydrochloride p. 72 and codeine phosphate p. 475 reduce intestinal motility and thus exert antidiarrhoeal actions. Loperamide hydrochloride is preferred as it is not sedative and does not cause dependence or fat malabsorption. High doses of loperamide hydrochloride [unlicensed] may be required in patients with a short bowel due to disrupted enterohepatic circulation and rapid gastrointestinal transit time. If the desired response is not obtained with loperamide hydrochloride, codeine phosphate may be added to therapy.

Co-phenotrope p. 71 has traditionally been used alone or in combination with other medications to help decrease faecal output. Co-phenotrope crosses the blood–brain barrier and can produce central nervous system side-effects, which may limit its use; the potential for dependence and anticholinergic effects may also restrict its use. A

Colestyramine

EvGr In patients with an intact colon and less than 100 cm of ileum resected, colestyramine p. 212 can be used to bind the unabsorbed bile salts and reduce diarrhoea. When colestyramine is given to these patients, it is important to monitor for evidence of fat malabsorption (steatorrhoea) or fat-soluble vitamin deficiencies. A

Antisecretory drugs

EvGr Drugs that reduce gastric acid secretion reduce jejunostomy output. Omeprazole p. 86 is readily absorbed in the duodenum and upper small bowel, but if less than 50 cm of jejunum remains, it may need to be given intravenously. Use of a proton pump inhibitor alone does not eliminate the need for further intervention for fluid control (such as antimotility agents, intravenous fluids, or oral rehydration salts).

Octreotide [unlicensed indication] reduces ileostomy diarrhoea and large volume jejunostomy output by inhibiting multiple pro-secretory substances. There is insufficient evidence to establish its role in the management of short bowel syndrome. A

Growth factors

Growth factors can be used to facilitate intestinal adaptation after surgery in patients with short bowel syndrome, thus enhancing fluid, electrolyte, and micronutrient absorption.

Teduglutide below is an analogue of endogenous human glucagon-like peptide 2 (GLP-2) which is licensed for use in the management of short bowel syndrome. It may be considered after a period of stabilisation following surgery, during which intravenous fluids and nutritional support should have been optimised.

Drug absorption

For *Prescribing in patients with stoma*, see Stoma care p. 105.

EvGr Many drugs are incompletely absorbed by patients with a short bowel and may need to be prescribed in much higher doses than usual (such as levothyroxine, warfarin, oral contraceptives, and digoxin) or may need to be given intravenously. A

Several factors can alter the absorption of drugs taken by mouth in patients with a compromised gastrointestinal system. The most important factors are the length of intestine available for drug absorption, and which section has been removed. The small intestine, with its large surface area and high blood flow, is the most important site of drug absorption. The larger the amount of the small intestine that has been removed, the higher the possibility that drug absorption will be affected. Other factors, such as gastric emptying and gastric transit time, also affect drug handling.

EvGr Enteric-coated and modified-release preparations are unsuitable for use in patients with short bowel syndrome, particularly in patients with an ileostomy, as there may not be sufficient release of the active ingredient.

Dosage forms with quick dissolution (soluble tablets) should be used. Uncoated tablets and liquid formulations may also be suitable. A EvGr Before prescribing liquid formulations, prescribers should consider the osmolarity, excipient content and volume required. Hyperosmolar liquids and some excipients (such as sorbitol) can result in fluid loss. The calorie density of oral supplements should also be considered, as it will influence the volume to be taken. E

> **Other drugs used for Short bowel syndrome** Cimetidine, p. 79

AMINO ACIDS AND DERIVATIVES

Teduglutide

18-Nov-2020

● **DRUG ACTION** Teduglutide is an analogue of human glucagon-like peptide-2 (GLP-2), which preserves mucosal integrity by promoting growth and repair of the intestine.

● **INDICATIONS AND DOSE**

Short bowel syndrome (initiated under specialist supervision)

▶ BY SUBCUTANEOUS INJECTION

▸ Adult: 0.05 mg/kg once daily, dose to be administered to alternating quadrants of the abdomen; alternatively the thigh can be used, for optimal injection volume per body weight, consult product literature. Review treatment after 6 months

● **CONTRA-INDICATIONS** Active or suspected malignancy · history of gastro-intestinal malignancy (in previous 5 years)

● **CAUTIONS** Abrupt withdrawal of parenteral support (reduce gradually with concomitant monitoring of fluid status) · cardiac insufficiency · cardiovascular disease · colo-rectal polyps · hypertension

● **SIDE-EFFECTS**

▶ **Common or very common** Anxiety · appetite decreased · congestive heart failure · cough · dyspnoea · fluid imbalance · gallbladder disorders · gastrointestinal discomfort · gastrointestinal disorders · gastrointestinal stoma complication · headache · influenza like illness · insomnia · nausea · pancreatitis · peripheral oedema · respiratory tract infection · vomiting

▶ **Uncommon** Syncope

- ALLERGY AND CROSS-SENSITIVITY Manufacturer advises caution in patients with tetracycline hypersensitivity.
- PREGNANCY EvGr Specialist sources indicate use if necessary—no human data available. ◇
- BREAST FEEDING Manufacturer advises avoid—toxicity in *animal* studies.
- RENAL IMPAIRMENT
  Dose adjustments Manufacturer advises use half the daily dose in moderate or severe impairment and end-stage renal disease.
- MONITORING REQUIREMENTS Manufacturer advises monitoring of small bowel function, gall bladder, bile ducts and pancreas during treatment.
- TREATMENT CESSATION Caution when discontinuing treatment—risk of dehydration.
- PATIENT AND CARER ADVICE Patients with cardiovascular disease should seek medical attention if they notice sudden weight gain, swollen ankles or dyspnoea—may indicate increased fluid absorption.
- NATIONAL FUNDING/ACCESS DECISIONS
  For full details see funding body website
  Scottish Medicines Consortium (SMC) decisions
  ▸ Teduglutide (*Revestive*®) for the treatment of adults with short bowel syndrome (SBS). Patients should be stable following a period of intestinal adaptation after surgery (February 2020) SMC No. SMC2225 Recommended

- MEDICINAL FORMS There can be variation in the licensing of different medicines containing the same drug.
  Powder and solvent for solution for injection
  ▸ Revestive (Shire Pharmaceuticals Ltd) ▼
    Teduglutide 1.25 mg Revestive 1.25mg powder and solvent for solution for injection vials | 28 vial [PoM] £7,307.70
    Teduglutide 5 mg Revestive 5mg powder and solvent for solution for injection vials | 28 vial [PoM] £14,615.39

2 Constipation and bowel cleansing

2.1 Bowel cleansing

Other drugs used for Bowel cleansing Bisacodyl, p. 65 · Docusate sodium, p. 64 · Magnesium sulfate, p. 1099

LAXATIVES 〉 OSMOTIC LAXATIVES

Citric acid with magnesium carbonate

02-Sep-2020

(Formulated as a bowel cleansing preparation)

- INDICATIONS AND DOSE

Bowel evacuation for surgery, colonoscopy or radiological examination
▸ BY MOUTH
▸ Child 5–9 years: One-third of a sachet to be given at 8 a.m. the day before the procedure and, one-third of a sachet to be given between 2 and 4 p.m. the day before the procedure
▸ Child 10–17 years: 0.5–1 sachet, given at 8 a.m. the day before the procedure and 0.5–1 sachet, given between 2 and 4 p.m. the day before the procedure
▸ Adult: 1 sachet, given at 8 a.m. the day before the procedure and 1 sachet, given between 2 and 4 p.m. the day before the procedure, use half the dose in frail elderly patients

- CONTRA-INDICATIONS Acute intestinal or gastric ulceration · acute severe colitis · gastric retention · gastro-intestinal obstruction · gastro-intestinal perforation · toxic megacolon
- CAUTIONS Debilitated · elderly (in adults) · hypovolaemia (should be corrected before administration of bowel cleansing preparations) · patients with fluid and electrolyte disturbances
  CAUTIONS, FURTHER INFORMATION Adequate hydration should be maintained during treatment.
- INTERACTIONS → Appendix 1: bowel cleansing preparations
- SIDE-EFFECTS
  ▸ **Common or very common** Gastrointestinal discomfort · nausea · vomiting
  ▸ **Uncommon** Dehydration · dizziness · electrolyte imbalance · headache
  SIDE-EFFECTS, FURTHER INFORMATION Abdominal pain is usually transient and can be reduced by taking preparation more slowly.
- PREGNANCY Use with caution.
- BREAST FEEDING Use with caution.
- RENAL IMPAIRMENT
  ▸ In adults Avoid if eGFR less than 30 mL/minute/1.73 m² — risk of hypermagnesaemia.
  ▸ In children Avoid if estimated glomerular filtration rate less than 30 mL/minute/1.73 m² — risk of hypermagnesaemia.
- MONITORING REQUIREMENTS Renal function should be measured before starting treatment in patients at risk of fluid and electrolyte disturbances.
- DIRECTIONS FOR ADMINISTRATION Manufacturer advises one sachet should be reconstituted with 200 mL of hot water; the solution should be allowed to cool for approx. 30 minutes before drinking.
- PRESCRIBING AND DISPENSING INFORMATION Reconstitution of one sachet containing 11.57 g magnesium carbonate and 17.79 g anhydrous citric acid produces a solution containing magnesium citrate with 118 mmol Mg²⁺.
  Flavours of oral powders may include lemon and lime.
- PATIENT AND CARER ADVICE Low residue or fluid only diet (e.g. water, fruit squash, clear soup, black tea or coffee) recommended before procedure (according to prescriber's advice) and copious intake of clear fluids recommended until procedure. Patient or carers should be given advice on how to administer oral powder.

- MEDICINAL FORMS There can be variation in the licensing of different medicines containing the same drug.
  Effervescent powder
  CAUTIONARY AND ADVISORY LABELS 13, 10
  ELECTROLYTES: May contain Magnesium
  ▸ Citramag (Sanochemia Diagnostics UK Ltd)
    Magnesium carbonate heavy 11.57 gram, Citric acid anhydrous 17.79 gram Citramag effervescent powder sachets sugar-free | 10 sachet [P] £20.50 DT = £20.50

Macrogol 3350 with anhydrous sodium sulfate, ascorbic acid, potassium chloride, sodium ascorbate and sodium chloride   01-Mar-2018

(Polyethylene glycols)

● **INDICATIONS AND DOSE**

MOVIPREP ®

Bowel cleansing [before any procedure requiring a clean bowel]
▶ BY MOUTH
  ▶ Adult: 1 litre daily for 2 doses; first dose of reconstituted solution taken on the evening before procedure and the second dose on the morning of procedure, alternatively 2 litres daily for 1 dose; reconstituted solution to be taken on the evening before the procedure, or on the morning of the procedure, treatment should be completed at least 1 hour before clinical procedures conducted without general anaesthesia, and at least 2 hours before clinical procedures conducted under general anaesthesia

PLENVU ®

Bowel cleansing [before any procedure requiring a clean bowel]
▶ BY MOUTH
  ▶ Adult: 500 mL daily for 2 doses; first dose of reconstituted solution taken on the evening before procedure and the second dose on the morning of procedure, alternatively 1 litre daily in 2 divided doses, reconstituted solution to be taken either on the evening before the procedure, or in the morning of the procedure—separate doses by at least 1 hour, treatment should be completed at least 1 hour before clinical procedures conducted without general anaesthesia, and at least 2 hours before clinical procedures conducted under general anaesthesia

● CONTRA-INDICATIONS Disorders of gastric emptying · G6PD deficiency · gastro-intestinal obstruction · gastro-intestinal perforation · ileus · toxic megacolon
● CAUTIONS Debilitated patients · dehydration (correct before administration) · impaired consciousness · impaired gag reflex or possibility of regurgitation or aspiration · moderate-to-severe cardiac impairment · patients at risk of arrhythmia (including those with thyroid disease or electrolyte imbalance) · severe acute inflammatory bowel disease
● INTERACTIONS → Appendix 1: bowel cleansing preparations
● SIDE-EFFECTS
▶ **Common or very common** Chills · dehydration · dizziness · fever · gastrointestinal discomfort · headaches · hunger · malaise · nausea · sleep disorder · thirst · vomiting
▶ **Uncommon** Arrhythmias · asthenia · drowsiness · dry mouth · dry throat · dysphagia · electrolyte imbalance · hot flush · pain · palpitations · temperature sensation altered
▶ **Frequency not known** Flatulence · hyponatraemic seizure
  SIDE-EFFECTS, FURTHER INFORMATION Abdominal pain is usually transient and can be reduced by taking preparation more slowly.
● PREGNANCY Manufacturer advises use only if essential—no or limited information available.
● BREAST FEEDING Manufacturer advises use only if essential—no information available.
● RENAL IMPAIRMENT Manufacturer advises caution if eGFR less than 30 mL/minute/1.73 m^2.

● MONITORING REQUIREMENTS Manufacturer advises consider monitoring baseline and post-treatment electrolytes, renal function and ECG as appropriate, in debilitated patients, those with significant renal impairment, arrhythmia, or at risk of electrolyte imbalance.
● DIRECTIONS FOR ADMINISTRATION
  PLENVU ® Manufacturer advises the contents of the single sachet for Dose 1 should be made up to 500 mL with water and taken over 30 minutes; the contents of the 2 sachets (A and B) for Dose 2 should be made up to 500 mL with water and taken over 30 minutes. Each dose should be followed by 500 mL of clear fluid taken over 30 minutes.
  MOVIPREP ® Manufacturer advises one pair of sachets (A and B) should be made up to 1 litre with water and taken over 1–2 hours; 1 litre of other clear fluid should also be taken during treatment.
● PRESCRIBING AND DISPENSING INFORMATION
  PLENVU ® Dose 1 (single sachet) when reconstituted up to 500 mL with water provides Na$^+$ 160.9 mmol, K$^+$ 13.3 mmol, Cl$^-$ 47.6 mmol; Dose 2 (sachets A and B) when reconstituted up to 500 mL with water provides Na$^+$ 297.6 mmol, K$^+$ 16.1 mmol, Cl$^-$ 70.9 mmol.
  MOVIPREP ® 1 pair of sachets (A+B) when reconstituted up to 1 litre with water provides Na$^+$ 181.6 mmol (Na$^+$ 56.2 mmol absorbable), K$^+$ 14.2 mmol, Cl$^-$ 59.8 mmol.
● PATIENT AND CARER ADVICE Manufacturer advises solid food should not be taken during treatment until procedure completed.
● MEDICINAL FORMS There can be variation in the licensing of different medicines containing the same drug.
  Form unstated
  CAUTIONARY AND ADVISORY LABELS 10, 13
  EXCIPIENTS: May contain Aspartame
  ELECTROLYTES: May contain Chloride, potassium, sodium
  ▶ Moviprep (Forum Health Products Ltd)
    Moviprep oral powder sachets sugar-free | 4 sachet ℗ £10.36
  ▶ Plenvu (Forum Health Products Ltd)
    Plenvu oral powder sachets sugar-free | 3 sachet ℗ £12.43

Macrogol 3350 with anhydrous sodium sulfate, potassium chloride, sodium bicarbonate and sodium chloride   16-Nov-2020

(Formulated as a bowel cleansing preparation)

● **INDICATIONS AND DOSE**

Bowel cleansing before radiological examination, colonoscopy, or surgery
▶ INITIALLY BY MOUTH
  ▶ Adult: Initially 2 litres daily for 2 doses: first dose of reconstituted solution taken on the evening before procedure and the second dose on the morning of procedure, alternatively (by mouth) initially 250 mL every 10–15 minutes, reconstituted solution to be administered, alternatively (by nasogastric tube) initially 20–30 mL/minute, starting on the day before procedure until 4 litres have been consumed

● CONTRA-INDICATIONS Acute severe colitis · gastric retention · gastro-intestinal obstruction · gastro-intestinal perforation · toxic megacolon
● CAUTIONS Colitis · debilitated patients · fluid and electrolyte disturbances · heart failure (avoid if moderate to severe) · hypovolaemia (should be corrected before administration of bowel cleansing preparations) · impaired gag reflex or possibility of regurgitation or aspiration

- INTERACTIONS → Appendix 1: bowel cleansing preparations
- SIDE-EFFECTS Angioedema · arrhythmia · chills · confusion · dehydration · dizziness · dyspnoea · electrolyte imbalance · fever · flatulence · gastrointestinal discomfort · headache · malaise · nausea · palpitations · seizure · skin reactions · thirst · vomiting

  SIDE-EFFECTS, FURTHER INFORMATION Abdominal pain is usually transient and can be reduced by taking preparation more slowly.
- PREGNANCY Manufacturers advise use only if essential—no information available.
- BREAST FEEDING Manufacturers advise use only if essential—no information available.
- MONITORING REQUIREMENTS Renal function should be measured before starting treatment in patients at risk of fluid and electrolyte disturbances.
- DIRECTIONS FOR ADMINISTRATION EvGr 1 sachet should be reconstituted with 1 litre of water. After reconstitution the solution should be kept in a refrigerator and discarded if unused after 24 hours. Ⓜ
- PRESCRIBING AND DISPENSING INFORMATION Each *Klean-Prep* ® sachet provides Na+ 125 mmol, K+ 10 mmol, Cl− 35 mmol and HCO3 − 20mmol when reconstituted with 1 litre of water.
- PATIENT AND CARER ADVICE Solid food should not be taken for 2 hours before starting treatment. Adequate hydration should be maintained during treatment. Treatment can be stopped if bowel motions become watery and clear.

- MEDICINAL FORMS There can be variation in the licensing of different medicines containing the same drug.

Powder

CAUTIONARY AND ADVISORY LABELS 10, 13
EXCIPIENTS: May contain Aspartame
ELECTROLYTES: May contain Bicarbonate, chloride, potassium, sodium
- Klean-Prep (Forum Health Products Ltd)
  Potassium chloride 742.5 mg, Sodium chloride 1.465 gram, Sodium bicarbonate 1.685 gram, Sodium sulfate anhydrous 5.685 gram, Polyethylene glycol 3350 59 gram Klean-Prep oral powder 69g sachets sugar-free | 4 sachet P £10.48

LAXATIVES 〉 STIMULANT LAXATIVES

Magnesium citrate with sodium picosulfate
27-Jul-2020

(Formulated as a bowel cleansing preparation)

- **INDICATIONS AND DOSE**

CITRAFLEET ® SACHETS

Bowel evacuation on day before radiological examination, endoscopy, or surgery
- BY MOUTH
  - Adult: 1 sachet taken before 8 a.m, then 1 sachet after 6–8 hours
PHARMACOKINETICS
- For *CitraFleet* ®: Acts within 3 hours of first dose.
PICOLAX ® SACHETS

Bowel evacuation on day before radiological procedure, endoscopy, or surgery
- BY MOUTH
  - Child 1 year: 0.25 sachet taken before 8 a.m, then 0.25 sachet after 6–8 hours
  - Child 2-3 years: 0.5 sachet taken before 8 a.m, then 0.5 sachet after 6–8 hours
  - Child 4-8 years: 1 sachet taken before 8 a.m, then 0.5 sachet after 6–8 hours

- Child 9-17 years: 1 sachet taken before 8 a.m, then 1 sachet after 6–8 hours
- Adult: 1 sachet taken before 8 a.m, then 1 sachet after 6–8 hours
PHARMACOKINETICS
- For *Picolax* ®: Acts within 3 hours of first dose.

- CONTRA-INDICATIONS Acute severe colitis · ascites · congestive cardiac failure · gastric retention · gastro-intestinal obstruction · gastro-intestinal perforation · gastro-intestinal ulceration · toxic megacolon
- CAUTIONS Cardiac disease · children · colitis · debilitated patients · elderly · fluid and electrolyte disturbances (avoid in severe dehydration or hypermagnesaemia) · hypovolaemia (should be corrected before administration) · recent gastro-intestinal surgery
- INTERACTIONS → Appendix 1: bowel cleansing preparations
- SIDE-EFFECTS
  - **Common or very common** Gastrointestinal discomfort · headache · nausea
  - **Uncommon** Confusion · electrolyte imbalance · gastrointestinal disorders · seizures · skin reactions · vomiting
- PREGNANCY Caution.
- BREAST FEEDING Caution.
- HEPATIC IMPAIRMENT Avoid in hepatic coma if risk of renal failure.
- RENAL IMPAIRMENT
  - In adults Avoid if eGFR less than 30 mL/minute/1.73 m2—risk of hypermagnesaemia.
  - In children Avoid if estimated glomerular filtration rate less than 30 mL/minute/1.73 m2—risk of hypermagnesaemia.
- DIRECTIONS FOR ADMINISTRATION Manufacturer advises one sachet of sodium picosulfate with magnesium citrate powder should be reconstituted with 150 mL (approx. half a glass) of cold water; patients should be warned that heat is generated during reconstitution and that the solution should be allowed to cool before drinking.
- PRESCRIBING AND DISPENSING INFORMATION Flavours of oral powder formulations may include lemon.
  PICOLAX ® SACHETS One reconstituted sachet contains K+ 5 mmol and Mg2+ 87 mmol.
  CITRAFLEET ® SACHETS One reconstituted sachet contains K+ 5 mmol and Mg2+ 86 mmol.
- PATIENT AND CARER ADVICE Low residue diet recommended on the day before procedure and copious intake of water or other clear fluids recommended during treatment. Patients and carers should be given advice on how to administer oral powder; they should be warned that heat is generated during reconstitution and that the solution should be allowed to cool before drinking.

- MEDICINAL FORMS There can be variation in the licensing of different medicines containing the same drug.
Powder
CAUTIONARY AND ADVISORY LABELS 10, 13
ELECTROLYTES: May contain Magnesium, potassium
- CitraFleet (Casen Recordati S.L.)
  Sodium picosulfate 10 mg, Magnesium oxide light 3.5 gram, Citric acid anhydrous 10.97 gram CitraFleet oral powder 15.08g sachets sugar-free | 2 sachet PoM £3.25
- Picolax (Ferring Pharmaceuticals Ltd)
  Sodium picosulfate 10 mg, Magnesium oxide 3.5 gram, Citric acid anhydrous 12 gram Picolax oral powder 16.1g sachets sugar-free | 2 sachet P £3.39

2.2 Constipation

Constipation
06-Jun-2017

Description of condition

Constipation is defaecation that is unsatisfactory because of infrequent stools, difficult stool passage, or seemingly incomplete defaecation. It can occur at any age and is commonly seen in women, the elderly, and during pregnancy.

It is important for those who complain of constipation to understand that bowel habit can vary considerably in frequency without doing harm. Some people erroneously consider themselves constipated if they do not have a bowel movement each day.

New onset constipation, especially in patients over 50 years of age, or accompanying symptoms such as anaemia, abdominal pain, weight loss, or overt or occult blood in the stool should provoke urgent investigation because of the risk of malignancy or other serious bowel disorder. In those patients with secondary constipation caused by a drug, the drug should be reviewed.

Overview

EvGr In all patients with constipation, an increase in dietary fibre, adequate fluid intake and exercise is advised. Diet should be balanced and contain whole grains, fruits and vegetables. Fibre intake should be increased gradually (to minimise flatulence and bloating). The effects of a high-fibre diet may be seen in a few days although it can take as long as 4 weeks. Adequate fluid intake is important (particularly with a high-fibre diet or fibre supplements), but can be difficult for some people (for example, the frail or elderly). Fruits high in fibre and sorbitol, and fruit juices high in sorbitol, can help prevent and treat constipation. ⟨A⟩

Misconceptions about bowel habits have led to excessive laxative use. Laxative abuse may lead to hypokalaemia. Before prescribing laxatives it is important to be sure that the patient is constipated and that the constipation is not secondary to an underlying undiagnosed complaint.

Laxatives

Bulk-forming laxatives

Bulk-forming laxatives include bran, ispaghula husk p. 58, methylcellulose p. 59 and sterculia p. 59. They are of particular value in adults with small hard stools if fibre cannot be increased in the diet. Onset of action is up to 72 hours. Symptoms of flatulence, bloating, and cramping may be exacerbated. Adequate fluid intake must be maintained to avoid intestinal obstruction.

Methylcellulose, ispaghula husk and sterculia may be used in patients who cannot tolerate bran. Methylcellulose also acts as a faecal softener.

Stimulant laxatives

Stimulant laxatives include bisacodyl p. 65, sodium picosulfate p. 68, and members of the anthraquinone group (senna p. 67, co-danthramer p. 66 and co-danthrusate p. 66). Stimulant laxatives increase intestinal motility and often cause abdominal cramp; manufacturer advises they should be avoided in intestinal obstruction.

The use of co-danthramer and co-danthrusate is limited to constipation in terminally ill patients because of potential carcinogenicity (based on animal studies) and evidence of genotoxicity.

Docusate sodium p. 64 is believed to act as both a stimulant laxative and as a faecal softener (below). Glycerol suppositories act as a lubricant and as a rectal stimulant by virtue of the mildly irritant action of glycerol.

Faecal softeners

Faecal softeners are claimed to act by decreasing surface tension and increasing penetration of intestinal fluid into the faecal mass. Docusate sodium and glycerol suppositories p. 67 have softening properties. Enemas containing arachis oil p. 64 (ground-nut oil, peanut oil) lubricate and soften impacted faeces and promote a bowel movement. Liquid paraffin p. 65 has also been used as a lubricant for the passage of stools but manufacturer advises that it should be used with caution because of its adverse effects, which include anal seepage and the risks of granulomatous disease of the gastro-intestinal tract or of lipoid pneumonia on aspiration.

Osmotic laxatives

Osmotic laxatives increase the amount of water in the large bowel, either by drawing fluid from the body into the bowel or by retaining the fluid they were administered with. Lactulose p. 60 is a semi-synthetic disaccharide which is not absorbed from the gastro-intestinal tract. It produces an osmotic diarrhoea of low faecal pH, and discourages the proliferation of ammonia-producing organisms. It is therefore useful in the treatment of hepatic encephalopathy. Macrogols (such as macrogol 3350 with potassium chloride, sodium bicarbonate and sodium chloride p. 61) are inert polymers of ethylene glycol which sequester fluid in the bowel; giving fluid with macrogols may reduce the dehydrating effect sometimes seen with osmotic laxatives.

Other drugs used in constipation

Linaclotide p. 52 is a guanylate cyclase-C receptor agonist that is licensed for the treatment of moderate to severe irritable bowel syndrome associated with constipation. It increases intestinal fluid secretion and transit, and decreases visceral pain.

Prucalopride p. 64 is a selective serotonin $5HT_4$-receptor agonist with prokinetic properties. It is licensed for the treatment of chronic constipation in adults, when other laxatives have failed to provide an adequate response.

Bowel cleansing preparations

Bowel cleansing preparations are used before colonic surgery, colonoscopy or radiological examination to ensure the bowel is free of solid contents; examples include macrogol 3350 with anhydrous sodium sulfate, potassium chloride, sodium bicarbonate and sodium chloride p. 55, citric acid with magnesium carbonate p. 54, magnesium citrate with sodium picosulfate p. 56 and sodium acid phosphate with sodium phosphate p. 63. Bowel cleansing treatments are not treatments for constipation.

Management

Short-duration constipation

EvGr In the management of short-duration constipation (where dietary measures are ineffective) treatment should be started with a bulk-forming laxative, ensuring adequate fluid intake. If stools remain hard, add or switch to an osmotic laxative. If stools are soft but difficult to pass or the person complains of inadequate emptying, a stimulant laxative should be added. ⟨A⟩

Opioid-induced constipation

See also *Constipation* under Prescribing in palliative care p. 28. EvGr In patients with opioid-induced constipation, an osmotic laxative (or docusate sodium to soften the stools) and a stimulant laxative is recommended. Bulk-forming laxatives should be avoided.

Naloxegol p. 70 is recommended for the treatment of opioid-induced constipation when response to other laxatives is inadequate. ⟨A⟩

Methylnaltrexone bromide p. 69 is licensed for the treatment of opioid-induced constipation when response to other laxatives is inadequate. Manufacturer advises that in patients receiving palliative care, methylnaltrexone bromide should be used as an adjunct to existing laxative therapy.

Gastro-intestinal system

1

Faecal impaction

The treatment of faecal impaction depends on the stool consistency. EvGr In patients with hard stools, a high dose of an oral macrogol (such as macrogol 3350 with potassium chloride, sodium bicarbonate and sodium chloride) may be considered. In those with soft stools, or with hard stools after a few days treatment with a macrogol, an oral stimulant laxative should be started or added to the previous treatment. If the response to oral laxatives is inadequate, for soft stools consider rectal administration of bisacodyl, and for hard stools rectal administration of glycerol alone, or glycerol plus bisacodyl. Alternatively, a docusate sodium or sodium citrate enema p. 833 may be tried.

If the response is still insufficient, a sodium acid phosphate with sodium phosphate or arachis oil retention enema may be necessary. For hard faeces it can be helpful to give the arachis oil enema p. 64 overnight before giving a sodium acid phosphate with sodium phosphate p. 63 or sodium citrate enema p. 833 the following day. Enemas may need to be repeated several times to clear hard impacted faeces. Ⓐ

Chronic constipation

EvGr In the management of chronic constipation, treatment should be started with a bulk-forming laxative, whilst ensuring good hydration. If stools remain hard, add or change to an osmotic laxative such as a macrogol. Lactulose p. 60 is an alternative if macrogols are not effective, or not tolerated. If the response is inadequate, a stimulant laxative can be added. The dose of laxative should be adjusted gradually to produce one or two soft, formed stools per day.

If at least two laxatives (from different classes) have been tried at the highest tolerated recommended doses for at least 6 months, the use of prucalopride p. 64 (in women only) should be considered. If treatment with prucalopride is not effective after 4 weeks, the patient should be re-examined and the benefit of continuing treatment reconsidered.

Laxatives can be slowly withdrawn when regular bowel movements occur without difficulty, according to the frequency and consistency of the stools. If a combination of laxatives has been used, reduce and stop one laxative at a time; if possible, the stimulant laxative should be reduced first. However, it may be necessary to also adjust the dose of the osmotic laxative to compensate. Ⓐ

Constipation in pregnancy and breast-feeding

EvGr If dietary and lifestyle changes fail to control constipation in pregnancy, fibre supplements in the form of bran or wheat are likely to help women experiencing constipation in pregnancy, and raise no serious concerns about side-effects to the mother or fetus.

A bulk-forming laxative is the first choice during pregnancy if fibre supplements fail. An osmotic laxative, such as lactulose, can also be used. Bisacodyl p. 65 or senna p. 67 may be suitable if a stimulant effect is necessary but use of senna should be avoided near term or if there is a history of unstable pregnancy. Stimulant laxatives are more effective than bulk-forming laxatives but are more likely to cause side-effects (diarrhoea and abdominal discomfort), reducing their acceptability to patients. Docusate sodium p. 64 and glycerol suppositories p. 67 can also be used.

A bulk-forming laxative is the first choice during breast-feeding, if dietary measures fail. Lactulose or a macrogol may be used if stools remain hard. As an alternative, a short course of a stimulant laxative such as bisacodyl or senna can be considered. Ⓐ

Constipation in children

Early identification of constipation and effective treatment can improve outcomes for children. Without early diagnosis and treatment, an acute episode of constipation can lead to anal fissure and become chronic.

EvGr The first-line treatment for children with constipation requires the use of a laxative in combination with dietary modification or with behavioural interventions. Diet modification alone is not recommended as first-line treatment.

In children an increase in dietary fibre, adequate fluid intake, and exercise is advised. Diet should be balanced and contain fruits, and vegetables, high-fibre bread, baked beans, and wholegrain breakfast cereals. Unprocessed bran (which may cause bloating and flatulence and reduces the absorption of micronutrients) is **not** recommended.

If faecal impaction is not present (or has been treated), the child should be treated promptly with a laxative. A macrogol (such as macrogol 3350 with potassium chloride, sodium bicarbonate and sodium chloride p. 61) is preferred as first-line management. If the response is inadequate, add a stimulant laxative or change to a stimulant laxative if the first-line therapy is not tolerated. If stools remain hard, lactulose or another laxative with softening effects, such as docusate sodium can be added.

In children with chronic constipation, laxatives should be continued for several weeks after a regular pattern of bowel movements or toilet training is established. The dose of laxatives should then be tapered gradually, over a period of months, according to response. Some children may require laxative therapy for several years.

A shorter duration of laxative treatment may be possible in some children with a short history of constipation.

Laxatives should be administered at a time that produces an effect that is likely to fit in with the child's toilet routine. Ⓐ

Faecal impaction in children

EvGr Treatment of faecal impaction may initially increase symptoms of soiling and abdominal pain. In children over 1 year of age with faecal impaction, an oral preparation containing a macrogol (such as macrogol 3350 with potassium chloride, sodium bicarbonate and sodium chloride) is used to clear faecal mass and to establish and maintain soft well-formed stools, using an escalating dose regimen depending on symptoms and response. If disimpaction does not occur after 2 weeks, a stimulant laxative can be added or if stools are hard, used in combination with an osmotic laxative such as lactulose. Long-term regular use of laxatives is essential to maintain well-formed stools and prevent recurrence of faecal impaction; intermittent use may provoke relapses. Ⓐ

LAXATIVES ⟩ BULK-FORMING LAXATIVES

Ispaghula husk

27-Jul-2020

- **DRUG ACTION** Bulk-forming laxatives relieve constipation by increasing faecal mass which stimulates peristalsis.

- **INDICATIONS AND DOSE**

  Constipation
  - ▶ BY MOUTH
    - ▶ Child 1 month-5 years: 2.5–5 mL twice daily, dose to be taken only when prescribed by a doctor, as half or whole level spoonful in water, preferably after meals, morning and evening
    - ▶ Child 6–11 years: 2.5–5 mL twice daily, dose to be given as a half or whole level spoonful in water, preferably after meals, morning and evening
    - ▶ Child 12–17 years: 1 sachet twice daily, dose to be given in water preferably after meals, morning and evening
    - ▶ Adult: 1 sachet twice daily, dose to be given in water preferably taken after food, morning and evening

Constipation (dose approved for use by community practitioner nurse prescribers)

▶ BY MOUTH

▸ Child 6-11 years: 2.5–5 mL twice daily, dose to be given as a half or whole level spoonful in water, preferably after meals, morning and evening

▸ Child 12-17 years: 1 sachet twice daily, dose to be given in water preferably after meals, morning and evening

▸ Adult: 1 sachet twice daily, dose to be given in water preferably taken after food, morning and evening

DOSE EQUIVALENCE AND CONVERSION

▶ 1 sachet equivalent to 2 level 5 ml spoonsful.

● CONTRA-INDICATIONS Colonic atony · faecal impaction · intestinal obstruction · reduced gut motility · sudden change in bowel habit that has persisted more than two weeks · undiagnosed rectal bleeding

● CAUTIONS Adequate fluid intake should be maintained to avoid oesophageal or intestinal obstruction

● SIDE-EFFECTS Abdominal distension · bronchospasm · conjunctivitis · gastrointestinal disorders · hypersensitivity · rhinitis · skin reactions

● DIRECTIONS FOR ADMINISTRATION Manufacturer advises dose to be taken with at least 150 mL liquid.

● PRESCRIBING AND DISPENSING INFORMATION Flavours of soluble granules formulations may include plain, lemon, or orange.

● HANDLING AND STORAGE Ispaghula husk contains potent allergens. Individuals exposed to the product (including those handling the product) can develop hypersensitivity reactions such as rhinitis, conjunctivitis, bronchospasm and in some cases, anaphylaxis.

● PATIENT AND CARER ADVICE Manufacturer advises that preparations that swell in contact with liquid should always be carefully swallowed with water and should not be taken immediately before going to bed. Patients and their carers should be advised that the full effect may take some days to develop and should be given advice on how to administer ispaghula husk.

● MEDICINAL FORMS There can be variation in the licensing of different medicines containing the same drug.

Effervescent granules

CAUTIONARY AND ADVISORY LABELS 13

EXCIPIENTS: May contain Aspartame

▸ Fybogel (Reckitt Benckiser Healthcare (UK) Ltd)
Ispaghula husk 3.5 gram Fybogel 3.5g effervescent granules sachets plain SF sugar-free | 30 sachet GSL £2.83 DT = £2.83
Fybogel Orange 3.5g effervescent granules sachets SF sugar-free | 30 sachet GSL £2.83 DT = £2.83
Fybogel Lemon 3.5g effervescent granules sachets SF sugar-free | 30 sachet GSL £2.83 DT = £2.83

▸ Fybogel Hi-Fibre (Reckitt Benckiser Healthcare (UK) Ltd)
Ispaghula husk 3.5 gram Fybogel Hi-Fibre Orange 3.5g effervescent granules sachets sugar-free | 10 sachet GSL £2.26 sugar-free | 30 sachet GSL £4.85 DT = £2.83
Fybogel Hi-Fibre Lemon 3.5g effervescent granules sachets sugar-free | 10 sachet GSL £2.26

▸ Ispagel (Bristol Laboratories Ltd)
Ispaghula husk 3.5 gram Ispagel Orange 3.5g effervescent granules sachets sugar-free | 10 sachet GSL £1.92 sugar-free | 30 sachet GSL £2.45 DT = £2.83

Granules

CAUTIONARY AND ADVISORY LABELS 13

EXCIPIENTS: May contain Aspartame

▸ Ispaghula husk (Non-proprietary)
Ispaghula husk 3.5 gram Ispaghula husk 3.5g granules sachets gluten free | 30 sachet GSL £2.83

Combinations available: *Senna with ispaghula husk,* p. 68

Methylcellulose
27-Jul-2020

● DRUG ACTION Bulk-forming laxatives relieve constipation by increasing faecal mass which stimulates peristalsis.

● INDICATIONS AND DOSE

Constipation | Diarrhoea

▶ BY MOUTH USING TABLETS

▸ Adult: 3–6 tablets twice daily

● CONTRA-INDICATIONS Colonic atony · difficulty in swallowing · faecal impaction · infective bowel disease · intestinal obstruction · severe dehydration

● CAUTIONS Adequate fluid intake should be maintained to avoid oesophageal or intestinal obstruction

CAUTIONS, FURTHER INFORMATION It may be necessary to supervise elderly or debilitated patients or those with intestinal narrowing or decreased motility to ensure adequate fluid intake.

● SIDE-EFFECTS Abdominal distension · gastrointestinal disorders

● DIRECTIONS FOR ADMINISTRATION Manufacturer advises, for constipation the dose should be taken with at least 300 mL liquid; for diarrhoea avoid liquid intake for 30 minutes before and after dose.

● PATIENT AND CARER ADVICE Patients and their carers should be advised that the full effect may take some days to develop. Preparations that swell in contact with liquid should always be carefully swallowed with water and should not be taken immediately before going to bed.

● MEDICINAL FORMS There can be variation in the licensing of different medicines containing the same drug.

Tablet

▸ Celevac (Advanz Pharma)
Methylcellulose "450" 500 mg Celevac 500mg tablets | 112 tablet GSL £3.22 DT = £3.22

Sterculia
12-Aug-2020

● DRUG ACTION Sterculia is a bulk-forming laxative. It relieves constipation by increasing faecal mass which stimulates peristalsis.

● INDICATIONS AND DOSE

Constipation

▶ BY MOUTH

▸ Child 6-11 years: 0.5–1 sachet 1–2 times a day, alternatively, half to one heaped 5 mL spoonful once or twice a day; washed down without chewing with plenty of liquid after meals

▸ Child 12-17 years: 1–2 sachets 1–2 times a day, alternatively, one to two heaped 5 mL spoonfuls once or twice a day; washed down without chewing with plenty of liquid after meals

▸ Adult: 1–2 sachets 1–2 times a day, alternatively, one to two heaped 5 mL spoonfuls once or twice a day; washed down without chewing with plenty of liquid after meals

● CONTRA-INDICATIONS Colonic atony · difficulty swallowing · faecal impaction · intestinal obstruction

● CAUTIONS Adequate fluid intake should be maintained to avoid oesophageal or intestinal obstruction

CAUTIONS, FURTHER INFORMATION
It may be necessary to supervise elderly or debilitated patients or those with intestinal narrowing or decreased motility to ensure adequate fluid intake.

● SIDE-EFFECTS Diarrhoea · gastrointestinal discomfort · gastrointestinal disorders · nausea

- DIRECTIONS FOR ADMINISTRATION Manufacturer advises may be mixed with soft food (e.g. yoghurt) before swallowing, followed by plenty of liquid.
- PATIENT AND CARER ADVICE Patients and their carers should be advised that the full effect may take some days to develop. Preparations that swell in contact with liquid should always be carefully swallowed with water and should not be taken immediately before going to bed.

- MEDICINAL FORMS There can be variation in the licensing of different medicines containing the same drug.

  Granules
  CAUTIONARY AND ADVISORY LABELS 25, 27
  - Normacol (Forum Health Products Ltd)
    Sterculia 620 mg per 1 gram Normacol granules 7g sachets | 60 sachet GSL £6.67 DT = £6.67
    Normacol granules | 500 gram GSL £7.92 DT = £7.92

Sterculia with frangula

The properties listed below are those particular to the combination only. For the properties of the components please consider, sterculia p. 59.

- INDICATIONS AND DOSE
  After haemorrhoidectomy
  ▶ BY MOUTH
  ▸ Adult: 1–2 sachets 1–2 times a day, alternatively, 1–2 heaped 5 mL spoonfuls once or twice a day; washed down without chewing with plenty of liquid after meals
  Constipation
  ▶ BY MOUTH
  ▸ Adult: 1–2 sachets 1–2 times a day, alternatively, 1–2 heaped 5 mL spoonfuls once or twice a day; washed down without chewing with plenty of liquid after meals

- PREGNANCY Manufacturer advises avoid.
- BREAST FEEDING Manufacturer advises avoid.
- PATIENT AND CARER ADVICE Patients and their carers should be advised that the full effect may take some days to develop. Preparations that swell in contact with liquid should always be carefully swallowed with water and should not be taken immediately before going to bed.

- MEDICINAL FORMS There can be variation in the licensing of different medicines containing the same drug.

  Granules
  - Normacol Plus (Forum Health Products Ltd)
    Frangula 80 mg per 1 gram, Sterculia 620 mg per 1 gram Normacol Plus granules 7g sachets | 60 sachet GSL £7.12 DT = £7.12
    Normacol Plus granules | 500 gram GSL £8.45 DT = £8.45

LAXATIVES > OSMOTIC LAXATIVES

Lactulose

10-Mar-2020

- INDICATIONS AND DOSE
  Constipation
  ▶ BY MOUTH
  ▸ Child 1–11 months: 2.5 mL twice daily, adjusted according to response
  ▸ Child 1–4 years: 2.5–10 mL twice daily, adjusted according to response
  ▸ Child 5–17 years: 5–20 mL twice daily, adjusted according to response
  ▸ Adult: Initially 15 mL twice daily, adjusted according to response

Hepatic encephalopathy (portal systemic encephalopathy)
▶ BY MOUTH
▸ Adult: Adjusted according to response to 30–50 mL 3 times a day, subsequently adjusted to produce 2–3 soft stools per day

Constipation (dose approved for use by community practitioner nurse prescribers)
▶ BY MOUTH
▸ Child 1–11 months: 2.5 mL twice daily, adjusted according to response
▸ Child 1–4 years: 5 mL twice daily, adjusted according to response
▸ Child 5–10 years: 10 mL twice daily, adjusted according to response
▸ Child 11–17 years: Initially 15 mL twice daily, adjusted according to response
▸ Adult: Initially 15 mL twice daily, adjusted according to response

PHARMACOKINETICS
▸ Lactulose may take up to 48 hours to act.

- UNLICENSED USE
  ▶ In adults Lactulose doses in the BNF may differ from those in product literature.

- CONTRA-INDICATIONS Galactosaemia · gastro-intestinal obstruction · gastro-intestinal perforation · risk of gastro-intestinal perforation
- CAUTIONS Lactose intolerance
- SIDE-EFFECTS
  ▶ Common or very common Abdominal pain · diarrhoea · flatulence · nausea · vomiting
  ▶ Uncommon Electrolyte imbalance
- PREGNANCY Not known to be harmful.
- PATIENT AND CARER ADVICE
  Medicines for Children leaflet: Lactulose for constipation www.medicinesforchildren.org.uk/lactulose-constipation

- MEDICINAL FORMS There can be variation in the licensing of different medicines containing the same drug.
  Oral solution
  - Lactulose (Non-proprietary)
    Lactulose 666.667 mg per 1 ml Lactulose 10g/15ml oral solution 15ml sachets sugar free sugar-free | 10 sachet P £2.51 DT = £2.51
    Lactulose 10g/15ml oral solution 15ml sachets sugar free unflavoured sugar-free | 10 sachet P £2.50 DT = £2.51
    Lactulose 10g/15ml oral solution 15ml sachets sugar free plum sugar-free | 10 sachet P £2.60 DT = £2.51
    Lactulose 680 mg per 1 ml Lactulose 3.1-3.7g/5ml oral solution | 300 ml P £1.37-£5.00 | 500 ml P £6.00 DT = £3.62
  - Duphalac (Mylan)
    Lactulose 680 mg per 1 ml Duphalac 3.35g/5ml oral solution | 200 ml P £1.92 | 300 ml P £2.88 | 500 ml P £4.80 DT = £3.62

Macrogol 3350

21-Aug-2017

- INDICATIONS AND DOSE
  Chronic constipation
  ▶ BY MOUTH
  ▸ Adult: 2 sachets once daily usually for up to 2 weeks, dose to be taken preferably in the morning
  PHARMACOKINETICS
  ▸ Onset of action 24–48 hours.

- CONTRA-INDICATIONS Ileus · intestinal obstruction · intestinal perforation · risk of intestinal perforation · severe inflammatory bowel disease · toxic megacolon
- SIDE-EFFECTS
  ▶ Common or very common Flatulence · gastrointestinal discomfort · nausea · vomiting
  ▶ Uncommon Anaemia · angioedema · appetite disorder · dehydration · dizziness · fatigue · hiccups · hypertension ·

hypoglycaemia · hypothyroidism · increased risk of infection · local swelling · migraine · muscle twitching · neuritis · oedema · pain · pelvic pain · sinus congestion · skin reactions · tachycardia · taste altered

- ● PREGNANCY Limited data, but manufacturer advises no effects anticipated as systemic exposure is negligible.
- ● DIRECTIONS FOR ADMINISTRATION Manufacturer advises contents of each sachet to be dissolved in half a glass (approx. 100 mL) of water just before administration.

- ● MEDICINAL FORMS There can be variation in the licensing of different medicines containing the same drug.

Powder
CAUTIONARY AND ADVISORY LABELS 13
▸ TransiSoft (HFA Healthcare Products Ltd)
Macrogol '3350' 85 gram per 1 litre TransiSoft oral powder 8.5g sachets sugar-free | 28 sachet P £49.85 DT = £49.85

Macrogol 3350 with potassium chloride, sodium bicarbonate and sodium chloride   18-Apr-2018

- ● INDICATIONS AND DOSE

Chronic constipation (dose for 'paediatric' sachets) | Prevention of faecal impaction (dose for 'paediatric' sachets)
▸ BY MOUTH
▸ Child 2-5 years: 1 sachet daily, adjust dose to produce regular soft stools; maximum 4 sachets per day
▸ Child 6-11 years: 2 sachets daily, adjust dose to produce regular soft stools; maximum 4 sachets per day

Faecal impaction (dose for 'paediatric' sachets)
▸ BY MOUTH
▸ Child 5-11 years: 4 sachets on first day, then increased in steps of 2 sachets daily, total daily dose to be taken over a 12-hour period, after disimpaction, switch to maintenance laxative therapy; maximum 12 sachets per day

Chronic constipation (dose for 'half-strength' sachets)
▸ BY MOUTH
▸ Child 12-17 years: 2-6 sachets daily in divided doses usually for up to 2 weeks; maintenance 2-4 sachets daily
▸ Adult: 2-6 sachets daily in divided doses usually for up to 2 weeks; maintenance 2-4 sachets daily

Faecal impaction (dose for 'half-strength' sachets)
▸ BY MOUTH
▸ Child 12-17 years: 8 sachets on first day, then increased in steps of 4 sachets daily, total daily dose to be drunk within a 6 hour period, after disimpaction, switch to maintenance laxative therapy if required; maximum 16 sachets per day
▸ Adult: 8 sachets on first day, then increased in steps of 4 sachets daily, total daily dose to be drunk within a 6 hour period, after disimpaction, switch to maintenance laxative therapy if required; maximum 16 sachets per day

Chronic constipation (dose for 'full-strength' sachets)
▸ BY MOUTH
▸ Child 12-17 years: 1-3 sachets daily in divided doses usually for up to 2 weeks; maintenance 1-2 sachets daily
▸ Adult: 1-3 sachets daily in divided doses usually for up to 2 weeks; maintenance 1-2 sachets daily

Faecal impaction (dose for 'full-strength' sachets)
▸ BY MOUTH
▸ Child 12-17 years: 4 sachets on first day, then increased in steps of 2 sachets daily, total daily dose to be drunk within a 6 hour period, after disimpaction, switch to

maintenance laxative therapy if required; maximum 8 sachets per day
▸ Adult: 4 sachets on first day, then increased in steps of 2 sachets daily, total daily dose to be drunk within a 6 hour period, after disimpaction, switch to maintenance laxative therapy if required; maximum 8 sachets per day

DOSE EQUIVALENCE AND CONVERSION
▸ Each 'paediatric' sachet contains 6.563 g of macrogol 3350; each 'half-strength' sachet contains 6.563 g of macrogol 3350; each 'full-strength' sachet contains 13.125 g of macrogol 3350.

MOVICOL® READY TO TAKE SACHETS

Chronic constipation
▸ BY MOUTH
▸ Child 12-17 years: 1-3 sachets daily in divided doses usually for up to 2 weeks; maintenance 1-2 sachets daily
▸ Adult: 1-3 sachets daily in divided doses usually for up to 2 weeks; maintenance 1-2 sachets daily

Faecal impaction
▸ BY MOUTH
▸ Child 12-17 years: 4 sachets on first day, then increased in steps of 2 sachets daily, total daily dose to be drunk within a 6 hour period; patients should also take an additional 1 litre of fluid daily, after disimpaction, switch to maintenance laxative therapy if required; maximum 8 sachets per day
▸ Adult: 4 sachets on first day, then increased in steps of 2 sachets daily, total daily dose to be drunk within a 6 hour period; patients should also take an additional 1 litre of fluid daily, after disimpaction, switch to maintenance laxative therapy if required; maximum 8 sachets per day

MOVICOL® LIQUID

Chronic constipation
▸ BY MOUTH
▸ Child 12-17 years: 25 mL 1-3 times a day usually for up to 2 weeks; maintenance 25 mL 1-2 times a day
▸ Adult: 25 mL 1-3 times a day usually for up to 2 weeks; maintenance 25 mL 1-2 times a day

VISTAPREP® ORAL POWDER

Bowel cleansing before colonoscopy
▸ BY MOUTH
▸ Adult: 3-4 litres, reconstituted solution taken over 4 hours, generally on the day of procedure; alternatively, it can be taken on the evening before procedure or started on the evening before procedure and completed on the morning of procedure

- ● UNLICENSED USE
▸ In children Macrogol 3350 with potassium chloride, sodium bicarbonate and sodium chloride may be used as detailed below, although these situations are considered outside the scope of its licence:
  - ● EvGr dose for chronic constipation/prevention of faecal impaction in children aged 6 years;
  - ● dose titration schedule for faecal impaction in children aged 12-17 years Ⓐ.
▸ In adults Macrogol 3350 with potassium chloride, sodium bicarbonate and sodium chloride may be used as detailed below, although this is considered outside the scope of its licence: EvGr dose titration schedule for faecal impaction Ⓔ

- ● CONTRA-INDICATIONS Intestinal obstruction · intestinal perforation · paralytic ileus · severe inflammatory conditions of the intestinal tract (including Crohn's disease, ulcerative colitis and toxic megacolon) · use of 'paediatric' sachets for faecal impaction in impaired cardiovascular function (no information available) (in children)

VISTAPREP ® ORAL POWDER Impaired consciousness · impaired swallowing reflex · moderate-to-severe heart failure—limited safety information available · risk of regurgitation or aspiration · severe dehydration—limited safety information available

- CAUTIONS Cardiovascular impairment (should not take more than 2 'full-strength' sachets or 4 'half-strength' sachets in any one hour) · impaired consciousness (with high doses) · impaired gag reflex (with high doses) · reflux oesophagitis (with high doses)

VISTAPREP ® ORAL POWDER Chronic inflammatory bowel disease · elderly · heart rhythm abnormalities · reflux oesophagitis

- SIDE-EFFECTS Electrolyte imbalance (discontinue if symptoms occur) · flatulence · gastrointestinal discomfort · nausea · vomiting

- PREGNANCY Manufacturers advise may be used—limited data available.

- HEPATIC IMPAIRMENT

VISTAPREP ® ORAL POWDER Manufacturer advises avoid (limited information available).

- RENAL IMPAIRMENT

‣ In children Manufacturers advise avoid use of 'paediatric' sachets for faecal impaction—no information available.

VISTAPREP ® ORAL POWDER Manufacturer advises avoid— limited safety information available.

- DIRECTIONS FOR ADMINISTRATION Manufacturers advise dissolve contents of each 'half-strength' sachet of oral powder in 62.5 mL of water, and each 'full-strength' sachet of oral powder in 125 mL of water; after reconstitution the solution should be kept in a refrigerator—for further information consult product literature.

‣ In children Manufacturers advise dissolve contents of each 'paediatric' sachet of oral powder in 62.5 mL of water; after reconstitution the solution should be kept in a refrigerator—for further information consult product literature.

MOVICOL ® LIQUID Manufacturer advises dilute 25 mL of oral concentrate with 100 mL of water; after dilution the solution should be discarded if unused after 24 hours.

VISTAPREP ® ORAL POWDER Manufacturer advises dissolve the contents of each sachet in 1 L water; if not consumed immediately, the reconstituted solution should be kept in a refrigerator and discarded if unused after 48 hours.

- PATIENT AND CARER ADVICE Patients or carers should be counselled on how to take the oral powder and oral solution.

Medicines for Children leaflet: Movicol for constipation
www.medicinesforchildren.org.uk/movicol-constipation

VISTAPREP ® ORAL POWDER Manufacturer advises treatment can be stopped if bowel motions become watery and clear.

- MEDICINAL FORMS There can be variation in the licensing of different medicines containing the same drug.

Oral solution
CAUTIONARY AND ADVISORY LABELS 13
ELECTROLYTES: May contain Bicarbonate, chloride, potassium, sodium
‣ Movicol (Forum Health Products Ltd)
Macrogol '3350' 105 gram per 1 litre, Potassium 5.4 mmol per 1 litre, Bicarbonate 17 mmol per 1 litre, Chloride 53 mmol per 1 litre, Sodium 65 mmol per 1 litre Movicol Liquid sugar-free | 500 ml P £5.41 DT = £5.41
Macrogol '3350' 13.125 gram, Potassium 27 mmol per 1 litre, Bicarbonate 85 mmol per 1 litre, Chloride 267 mmol per 1 litre, Sodium 325 mmol per 1 litre Movicol Ready to Take oral solution 25ml sachets sugar-free | 30 sachet P £7.72 DT = £7.72

Powder
CAUTIONARY AND ADVISORY LABELS 10, 13
ELECTROLYTES: May contain Bicarbonate, chloride, potassium, sodium
‣ Macrogol 3350 with potassium chloride, sodium bicarbonate and sodium chloride (Non-proprietary)
Macrogol '3350' 105 gram per 1 litre, Potassium 5.4 mmol per 1 litre, Bicarbonate 17 mmol per 1 litre, Chloride 53 mmol per 1 litre, Sodium 65 mmol per 1 litre Macrogol compound oral powder sachets sugar free sugar-free | 20 sachet P £2.63-£4.45 sugar-free | 30 sachet P £6.68 DT = £3.94
Macrogol compound oral powder sachets sugar free plain sugar-free | 20 sachet P £3.71 sugar-free | 30 sachet P £4.54 DT = £3.94
Macrogol compound oral powder sachets sugar free citrus sugar-free | 30 sachet P £4.38 DT = £3.94
‣ CosmoCol (Stirling Anglian Pharmaceuticals Ltd)
Macrogol '3350' 105 gram per 1 litre, Potassium 5.4 mmol per 1 litre, Bicarbonate 17 mmol per 1 litre, Chloride 53 mmol per 1 litre, Sodium 65 mmol per 1 litre CosmoCol Paediatric oral powder 6.9g sachets sugar-free | 30 sachet PoM £2.99 DT = £4.38
CosmoCol Orange Flavour oral powder sachets sugar-free | 20 sachet P £2.85 sugar-free | 30 sachet P £4.10 DT = £3.94
CosmoCol Lemon and Lime Flavour oral powder sachets sugar-free | 20 sachet P £2.85 sugar-free | 30 sachet P £4.10 DT = £3.94
CosmoCol Half oral powder 6.9g sachets sugar-free | 30 sachet P £4.10 DT = £4.38
CosmoCol Orange Lemon and Lime oral powder sachets sugar-free | 30 sachet P £4.10 DT = £3.94
CosmoCol Plain oral powder sachets sugar-free | 30 sachet P £4.10 DT = £3.94
‣ Laxido (Galen Ltd)
Macrogol '3350' 105 gram per 1 litre, Potassium 5.4 mmol per 1 litre, Bicarbonate 17 mmol per 1 litre, Chloride 53 mmol per 1 litre, Sodium 65 mmol per 1 litre Laxido Orange oral powder sachets sugar free sugar-free | 20 sachet P £2.85 sugar-free | 30 sachet P £4.10 DT = £3.94
Laxido Paediatric Plain oral powder 6.9g sachets sugar-free | 30 sachet PoM £2.99 DT = £4.38
‣ Molaxole (Mylan)
Macrogol '3350' 105 gram per 1 litre, Potassium 5.4 mmol per 1 litre, Bicarbonate 17 mmol per 1 litre, Chloride 53 mmol per 1 litre, Sodium 65 mmol per 1 litre Molaxole oral powder sachets sugar-free | 20 sachet P £3.78 sugar-free | 30 sachet P £5.68 DT = £3.94
‣ Movicol (Forum Health Products Ltd, Norgine Pharmaceuticals Ltd)
Macrogol '3350' 105 gram per 1 litre, Potassium 5.4 mmol per 1 litre, Bicarbonate 17 mmol per 1 litre, Chloride 53 mmol per 1 litre, Sodium 65 mmol per 1 litre Movicol Chocolate oral powder 13.9g sachets sugar-free | 30 sachet P £8.11 DT = £3.94
Movicol-Half oral powder 6.9g sachets sugar-free | 20 sachet P £3.54 sugar-free | 30 sachet P £5.31 DT = £4.38
Movicol Paediatric Plain oral powder 6.9g sachets sugar-free | 30 sachet PoM £4.38 DT = £4.38
Movicol oral powder 13.8g sachets lemon & lime sugar-free | 20 sachet P £5.41 sugar-free | 30 sachet P £8.11 DT = £3.94 sugar-free | 50 sachet P £13.49
Movicol Paediatric Chocolate oral powder 6.9g sachets sugar-free | 30 sachet PoM £4.38 DT = £4.38
Movicol Plain oral powder 13.7g sachets sugar-free | 30 sachet P £8.11 DT = £3.94 sugar-free | 50 sachet P £13.49
‣ VistaPrep (Tillotts Pharma Ltd)
Macrogol '3350' 105 gram per 1 litre, Potassium 5.4 mmol per 1 litre, Bicarbonate 17 mmol per 1 litre, Chloride 53 mmol per 1 litre, Sodium 65 mmol per 1 litre VistaPrep oral powder 110g sachets sugar-free | 4 sachet P £7.92

Magnesium hydroxide
22-Jun-2020

- INDICATIONS AND DOSE

Constipation

‣ BY MOUTH

‣ Child 3-11 years: 5–10 mL as required, dose to be given mixed with water at bedtime

‣ Child 12-17 years: 30–45 mL as required, dose to be given mixed with water at bedtime

‣ Adult: 30–45 mL as required, dose to be given mixed with water at bedtime

- CONTRA-INDICATIONS Acute gastro-intestinal conditions

● **CAUTIONS** Debilitated patients · elderly

● **INTERACTIONS** → Appendix 1: magnesium

● **HEPATIC IMPAIRMENT** Avoid in hepatic coma if risk of renal failure.

● **RENAL IMPAIRMENT** Increased risk of toxicity in renal impairment.
Dose adjustments Avoid or reduce dose.

● **PRESCRIBING AND DISPENSING INFORMATION** When prepared extemporaneously, the BP states Magnesium Hydroxide Mixture, BP consists of an aqueous suspension containing about 8% hydrated magnesium oxide.

● **MEDICINAL FORMS** There can be variation in the licensing of different medicines containing the same drug.
Oral suspension
▸ Magnesium hydroxide (Non-proprietary)
Magnesium hydroxide 79 mg per 1 ml Magnesium hydroxide 7.45-8.35% oral suspension BP | 500 ml GSL £5.31
Magnesium hydroxide 80 mg per 1 ml Magnesium hydroxide 8% oral suspension | 500 ml GSL £8.05 DT = £8.05
▸ Brands may include Phillips' Milk of Magnesia

Sodium acid phosphate with sodium phosphate

26-Oct-2020

● **INDICATIONS AND DOSE**

Constipation (using Phosphates Enema BP Formula B) | Bowel evacuation before abdominal radiological procedures, endoscopy, and surgery (using Phosphates Enema BP Formula B)
▸ BY RECTUM
▸ Child 3-6 years: 45–65 mL once daily
▸ Child 7-11 years: 65–100 mL once daily
▸ Child 12-17 years: 100–128 mL once daily
▸ Adult: 128 mL daily

Constipation, using Phosphates Enema BP Formula B (dose approved for use by community practitioner nurse prescribers)
▸ BY RECTUM
▸ Child 3-17 years: Reduced according to body-weight
▸ Adult: 128 mL daily

Constipation, using Phosphates Enema (Cleen Ready-to-Use) (dose approved for use by community practitioner nurse prescribers)
▸ BY RECTUM
▸ Child 3-11 years: On doctor's advice only
▸ Child 12-17 years: 118 mL
▸ Adult: 118 mL

FLEET® READY-TO-USE ENEMA
Constipation | Bowel evacuation before abdominal radiological procedures | Bowel evacuation before endoscopy | Bowel evacuation before surgery
▸ BY RECTUM
▸ Adult: 118 mL

FLEET® PHOSPHO-SODA
Bowel evacuation before colonic surgery | Bowel evacuation before colonoscopy | Bowel evacuation before radiological examination
▸ BY MOUTH
▸ Adult: 45 mL twice daily, each dose must be diluted with half a glass (120 mL) of cold water, followed by one full glass (240 mL) of cold water, timing of doses is dependent on the time of the procedure, for morning procedure, the first dose should be taken at 7 a.m. and second at 7 p.m. on day before the procedure.; for afternoon procedure, first dose should be taken at 7 p.m. on day before and second dose at 7 a.m. on day of the procedure

PHARMACOKINETICS
▸ For *Fleet*® *Phospho-soda* : onset of action is within half to 6 hours of first dose.

● **CONTRA-INDICATIONS**
▸ With oral use Acute severe colitis · ascites · congestive cardiac failure · gastric retention · gastro-intestinal obstruction · gastro-intestinal perforation · toxic megacolon
▸ With rectal use conditions associated with increased colonic absorption · gastro-intestinal obstruction · inflammatory bowel disease

● **CAUTIONS**
▸ With oral use Cardiac disease · colitis · debilitated patients · elderly · fluid and electrolyte disturbances · hypovolaemia (should be corrected before administration)
▸ With rectal use Ascites · congestive heart failure · debilitated patients · elderly · fluid and electrolyte disturbances · uncontrolled hypertension

● **INTERACTIONS** → Appendix 1: bowel cleansing preparations

● **SIDE-EFFECTS**
GENERAL SIDE-EFFECTS
▸ **Common or very common** Chills · gastrointestinal discomfort · nausea · vomiting
▸ **Uncommon** Dehydration
▸ **Rare or very rare** Electrolyte imbalance · metabolic acidosis

SPECIFIC SIDE-EFFECTS
▸ **Common or very common**
▸ With oral use Asthenia · chest pain · dizziness · headache
▸ **Rare or very rare**
▸ With oral use Allergic dermatitis · arrhythmia · hypotension · loss of consciousness · muscle cramps · myocardial infarction · nephrocalcinosis · paraesthesia · renal impairment · tetany
▸ With rectal use Pain

● **PREGNANCY**
▸ With oral use Caution.

● **BREAST FEEDING**
▸ With oral use Caution.

● **RENAL IMPAIRMENT**
▸ With oral use Avoid if eGFR less than 60 mL/minute/1.73 m^2.
▸ With rectal use Use with caution.

● **MONITORING REQUIREMENTS**
▸ With oral use Renal function should be measured before starting treatment in patients at risk of fluid and electrolyte disturbances.

● **DIRECTIONS FOR ADMINISTRATION**
FLEET® PHOSPHO-SODA Manufacturer advises copious intake of water or other clear fluids (e.g. clear soup, strained fruit juice without pulp, black tea or coffee) recommended until midnight before morning procedure and until 8 a.m. before afternoon procedure. At least one glass (approx 240 mL) of water or other clear fluid should also be taken immediately before each dose.

● **PRESCRIBING AND DISPENSING INFORMATION** When prepared extemporaneously, the BP states Phosphates Enema BP Formula B consists of sodium dihydrogen phosphate dihydrate 12.8 g, disodium phosphate dodecahydrate 10.24 g, purified water, freshly boiled and cooled, to 128 mL.

● **PATIENT AND CARER ADVICE**
FLEET® PHOSPHO-SODA Intake of solid food should be stopped for at least 6 hours before starting treatment and until procedure completed.
Patients or carers should be advised that adequate hydration should be maintained during treatment.
Patients or carers should be given advice on administration of *Fleet*® *Phospho-soda* oral solution.

● MEDICINAL FORMS There can be variation in the licensing of different medicines containing the same drug.

Oral solution

CAUTIONARY AND ADVISORY LABELS 10

ELECTROLYTES: May contain Phosphate, sodium

▸ Fleet Phospho-soda (Casen Recordati S.L.)
**Disodium hydrogen phosphate dodecahydrate 240 mg per 1 ml,
Sodium dihydrogen phosphate dihydrate 542 mg per
1 ml** Phospho-soda 24.4g/10.8g oral solution sugar-free | 90 ml P
£4.79

Enema

▸ Sodium acid phosphate with sodium phosphate (Non-proprietary)
**Disodium hydrogen phosphate dodecahydrate 80 mg per 1 ml,
Sodium dihydrogen phosphate dihydrate 100 mg per
1 ml** Phosphates enema (Formula B) 128ml long tube | 1 enema P
£27.93 DT = £27.93
Phosphates enema (Formula B) 128ml standard tube | 1 enema P
£27.93 DT = £27.93

▸ Fleet Ready-to-use (Casen Recordati S.L.)
**Disodium hydrogen phosphate dodecahydrate 80 mg per 1 ml,
Sodium dihydrogen phosphate dihydrate 181 mg per 1 ml** Cleen
Ready-to-use 133ml enema | 1 enema P £1.95 DT = £1.95

LAXATIVES ❭ SELECTIVE 5-HT₄ RECEPTOR
AGONISTS

Prucalopride

31-Aug-2020

● DRUG ACTION A selective serotonin 5HT₄-receptor agonist with prokinetic properties.

● INDICATIONS AND DOSE

Chronic constipation when other laxatives fail to provide an adequate response
▸ BY MOUTH
▸ **Adult:** 2 mg once daily, review treatment if no response after 4 weeks
▸ **Elderly:** Initially 1 mg once daily, increased if necessary to 2 mg once daily, review treatment if no response after 4 weeks

● CONTRA-INDICATIONS Crohn's disease · intestinal obstruction · intestinal perforation · toxic megacolon · ulcerative colitis

● CAUTIONS History of arrhythmias · history of ischaemic heart disease

● SIDE-EFFECTS
▸ **Common or very common** Appetite decreased · diarrhoea · dizziness · fatigue · gastrointestinal discomfort · gastrointestinal disorders · headache · nausea · vomiting
▸ **Uncommon** Anorectal haemorrhage · fever · malaise · palpitations · tremor · urinary frequency increased

SIDE-EFFECTS, FURTHER INFORMATION Side-effects generally occur at the start of treatment and are usually transient.

● CONCEPTION AND CONTRACEPTION Manufacturer recommends effective contraception during treatment.

● PREGNANCY Manufacturer advises avoid—limited data available.

● BREAST FEEDING Manufacturer advises avoid—present in milk.

● HEPATIC IMPAIRMENT Manufacturer advises caution in severe impairment (risk of increased exposure, limited information available).
Dose adjustments Manufacturer advises initial dose of 1 mg once daily in severe impairment; if tolerated this may be increased to 2 mg once daily.

● RENAL IMPAIRMENT
Dose adjustments Manufacturer recommends a reduced dose of 1 mg daily if eGFR less than 30 mL/minute/1.73 m².

● PATIENT AND CARER ADVICE
Driving and skilled tasks Manufacturer advises that dizziness and fatigue may initially affect ability to drive or operate machinery.

● NATIONAL FUNDING/ACCESS DECISIONS
For full details see funding body website

NICE decisions
▸ Prucalopride for the treatment of chronic constipation in women (December 2010) NICE TA211 Recommended with restrictions

Scottish Medicines Consortium (SMC) decisions
▸ Prucalopride (*Resolor*®) for chronic constipation (July 2011) SMC No. 653/10 Not recommended

● MEDICINAL FORMS There can be variation in the licensing of different medicines containing the same drug.

Tablet

▸ Resolor (Shire Pharmaceuticals Ltd)
Prucalopride (as Prucalopride succinate) 1 mg Resolor 1mg
tablets | 28 tablet PoM £38.69 DT = £38.69
Prucalopride (as Prucalopride succinate) 2 mg Resolor 2mg
tablets | 28 tablet PoM £59.52 DT = £59.52

LAXATIVES ❭ SOFTENING LAXATIVES

Arachis oil

18-Nov-2020

● INDICATIONS AND DOSE

To soften impacted faeces
▸ BY RECTUM
▸ **Adult:** 130 mL as required

● CONTRA-INDICATIONS Inflammatory bowel disease (except under medical supervision)

● CAUTIONS Hypersensitivity to soya · intestinal obstruction

● ALLERGY AND CROSS-SENSITIVITY EvGr Contra-indicated if hypersensitivity to arachis oil or peanuts. ⓜ

● DIRECTIONS FOR ADMINISTRATION Manufacturer advises warm enema in warm water before use.

● MEDICINAL FORMS There can be variation in the licensing of different medicines containing the same drug.

Enema

▸ Arachis oil (Non-proprietary)
Arachis oil 1 ml per 1 ml Arachis oil 130ml enema | 1 enema P
£47.50 DT = £47.50

Docusate sodium

30-Jul-2020

(Dioctyl sodium sulphosuccinate)

● INDICATIONS AND DOSE

Chronic constipation
▸ BY MOUTH
▸ **Child 6-23 months:** 12.5 mg 3 times a day, adjusted according to response, use paediatric oral solution
▸ **Child 2-11 years:** 12.5–25 mg 3 times a day, adjusted according to response, use paediatric oral solution
▸ **Child 12-17 years:** Up to 500 mg daily in divided doses, adjusted according to response
▸ **Adult:** Up to 500 mg daily in divided doses, adjusted according to response
▸ BY RECTUM
▸ **Child 12-17 years:** 120 mg for 1 dose
▸ **Adult:** 120 mg for 1 dose

Adjunct in abdominal radiological procedures
▸ BY MOUTH
▸ **Adult:** 400 mg, to be administered with barium meal

▶ BY RECTUM
▶ Adult: 120 mg for 1 dose

PHARMACOKINETICS
▶ With oral use or rectal use
  ▶ Oral preparations act within 1–2 days; response to rectal administration usually occurs within 20 minutes.

● UNLICENSED USE
▶ With oral use in children *Adult oral solution and capsules* not licensed for use in children under 12 years.

● CONTRA-INDICATIONS Avoid in intestinal obstruction

● CAUTIONS Do not give with liquid paraffin · excessive use of stimulant laxatives can cause diarrhoea and related effects such as hypokalaemia
▶ With rectal use rectal preparations not indicated if haemorrhoids or anal fissure

● INTERACTIONS → Appendix 1: docusate sodium

● SIDE-EFFECTS
▶ **Rare or very rare**
▶ With oral use Abdominal cramps · nausea · rash

● PREGNANCY Not known to be harmful—manufacturer advises caution.

● BREAST FEEDING
▶ With oral use Manufacturer advises caution—present in milk following oral administration.
▶ With rectal use Rectal administration not known to be harmful.

● DIRECTIONS FOR ADMINISTRATION
▶ With oral use in children For administration *by mouth*, manufacturer advises solution may be mixed with milk or squash.

● MEDICINAL FORMS There can be variation in the licensing of different medicines containing the same drug.

Oral solution
▶ Docusate sodium (Non-proprietary)
  Docusate sodium 2.5 mg per 1 ml Docusate 12.5mg/5ml oral solution sugar free sugar-free | 300 ml P £8.96 DT = £8.96
  Docusate sodium 10 mg per 1 ml Docusate 50mg/5ml oral solution sugar free sugar-free | 300 ml P £9.19 DT = £9.19
▶ Docusol (Typharm Ltd)
  Docusate sodium 2.5 mg per 1 ml Docusol Paediatric 12.5mg/5ml oral solution sugar-free | 125 ml P £4.46

Enema
▶ Norgalax (Essential Pharma Ltd)
  Docusate sodium 12 mg per 1 gram Norgalax 120mg/10g enema | 6 enema P £28.00 DT = £28.00

Capsule
▶ Dioctyl (UCB Pharma Ltd)
  Docusate sodium 100 mg Dioctyl 100mg capsules | 30 capsule P £2.09 DT = £2.09 | 100 capsule P £6.98

Combinations available: *Co-danthrusate*, p. 66

Liquid paraffin
01-May-2020

● INDICATIONS AND DOSE

Constipation
▶ BY MOUTH
  ▶ Adult: 10–30 mL daily if required, to be administered at night

● CAUTIONS Avoid prolonged use

● SIDE-EFFECTS Anal irritation · contact dermatitis · granuloma · pneumonia lipoid · rectal discharge of drug

● PATIENT AND CARER ADVICE Oral emulsion should not be taken immediately before going to bed.

● MEDICINAL FORMS There can be variation in the licensing of different medicines containing the same drug.

Liquid
▶ Liquid paraffin (Non-proprietary)
  Liquid paraffin 1 ml per 1 ml Liquid paraffin liquid | 150 ml P £1.37–£1.51 DT = £1.37

LAXATIVES > STIMULANT LAXATIVES

Bisacodyl
10-Sep-2020

● INDICATIONS AND DOSE

Constipation
▶ BY MOUTH
  ▶ Child 4–17 years: 5–20 mg once daily, adjusted according to response, dose to be taken at night
  ▶ Adult: 5–10 mg once daily; increased if necessary up to 20 mg once daily, dose to be taken at night
▶ BY RECTUM
  ▶ Child 2–17 years: 5–10 mg once daily, adjusted according to response
  ▶ Adult: 10 mg once daily, dose to be taken in the morning

Bowel clearance before radiological procedures and surgery
▶ INITIALLY BY MOUTH
  ▶ Adult: 10 mg twice daily, dose to be taken in the morning and evening on the day before procedure and (by rectum) 10 mg, to be administered 1–2 hours before procedure the following day

Constipation (dose approved for use by community practitioner nurse prescribers)
▶ BY MOUTH
  ▶ Child 4–17 years: 5–20 mg once daily, adjusted according to response, dose to be taken at night (on doctor's advice only)
  ▶ Adult: 5–10 mg once daily; increased if necessary up to 20 mg once daily, dose to be taken at night
▶ BY RECTUM
  ▶ Child 4–9 years: 5 mg once daily, adjusted according to response
  ▶ Child 10–17 years: 10 mg once daily, dose to be taken in the morning
  ▶ Adult: 10 mg once daily, dose to be taken in the morning

PHARMACOKINETICS
▶ Tablets act in 10–12 hours; suppositories act in 20–60 minutes.

● UNLICENSED USE
▶ With rectal use in children EvGr Bisacodyl may be used in children aged under 10 years for the management of constipation, ⒶA but the higher dose option is not licensed in this age group.
▶ With oral use in children EvGr Bisacodyl may be used in children for the management of constipation, ⒶA but the higher dose option is not licensed.

> **IMPORTANT SAFETY INFORMATION**
>
> MHRA/CHM ADVICE: STIMULANT LAXATIVES (BISACODYL, SENNA AND SENNOSIDES, SODIUM PICOSULFATE) AVAILABLE OVER-THE-COUNTER: NEW MEASURES TO SUPPORT SAFE USE (AUGUST 2020)
> Following a national safety review and concerns over misuse and abuse, the MHRA has introduced new pack size restrictions, revised recommended ages for use, and new safety warnings for over-the-counter stimulant laxatives (administered orally and rectally). Patients should be advised that dietary and lifestyle measures should be used first-line for relieving short-term occasional constipation, and that stimulant laxatives should only be used if these measures and other laxatives (bulk-forming and osmotic) are ineffective.
>   Smaller packs will remain available for general sale for

the treatment of short-term, occasional constipation in adults only, and will be limited to a pack size of two short treatment courses. Stimulant laxatives should not be used in children under 12 years of age without advice from a prescriber; in children aged 12 to 17 years, products can be supplied under the supervision of a pharmacist.

- CONTRA-INDICATIONS Acute abdominal conditions · acute inflammatory bowel disease · intestinal obstruction · severe dehydration
- CAUTIONS Excessive use of stimulant laxatives can cause diarrhoea and related effects such as hypokalaemia · prolonged use may harm intestinal function · risk of electrolyte imbalance with prolonged use
- SIDE-EFFECTS
- **Common or very common** Gastrointestinal discomfort · nausea
- **Uncommon** Haematochezia · vomiting
- **Rare or very rare** Angioedema · colitis · dehydration
- PREGNANCY May be suitable for constipation in pregnancy, if a stimulant effect is necessary.

- MEDICINAL FORMS There can be variation in the licensing of different medicines containing the same drug. Forms available from special-order manufacturers include: oral suspension, suppository

Gastro-resistant tablet

CAUTIONARY AND ADVISORY LABELS 5, 25
- Bisacodyl (Non-proprietary)
  Bisacodyl 5 mg Bisacodyl 5mg gastro-resistant tablets | 60 tablet ℗ £3.32 DT = £2.20 | 100 tablet ℗ £3.45–£5.40 | 500 tablet ℗ £18.33–£50.00 | 1000 tablet ℗ £36.67–£100.00
- Dulco-Lax (bisacodyl) (Sanofi)
  Bisacodyl 5 mg Dulcolax 5mg gastro-resistant tablets | 40 tablet ℗ £2.44 | 100 tablet ℗ £3.60

Suppository
- Bisacodyl (Non-proprietary)
  Bisacodyl 10 mg Bisacodyl 10mg suppositories | 12 suppository ℗ £3.53 DT = £3.53
- Dulco-Lax (bisacodyl) (Sanofi)
  Bisacodyl 5 mg Dulcolax 5mg suppositories for children | 5 suppository ℗ £1.04 DT = £1.04
  Bisacodyl 10 mg Dulcolax 10mg suppositories | 12 suppository ℗ £2.35 DT = £3.53

Co-danthramer

16-Mar-2020

- INDICATIONS AND DOSE

Constipation in palliative care (standard strength capsules)
- BY MOUTH USING CAPSULES
- Child 6–11 years: 1 capsule once daily, dose should be taken at night
- Child 12–17 years: 1–2 capsules once daily, dose should be taken at night
- Adult: 1–2 capsules once daily, dose should be taken at night

Constipation in palliative care (strong capsules)
- BY MOUTH USING CAPSULES
- Child 12–17 years: 1–2 capsules once daily, dose should be given at night
- Adult: 1–2 capsules once daily, dose should be given at night

Constipation in palliative care (standard strength suspension)
- BY MOUTH USING ORAL SUSPENSION
- Child 2–11 years: 2.5–5 mL once daily, dose should be taken at night
- Child 12–17 years: 5–10 mL once daily, dose should be taken at night

- Adult: 5–10 mL once daily, dose should be taken at night

Constipation in palliative care (strong suspension)
- BY MOUTH USING ORAL SUSPENSION
- Child 12–17 years: 5 mL once daily, dose should be taken at night
- Adult: 5 mL once daily, dose should be taken at night

DOSE EQUIVALENCE AND CONVERSION
- Co-danthramer (standard strength) capsules contain dantron 25 mg with poloxamer '188' 200 mg per capsule.
- Co-danthramer (standard strength) oral suspension contains dantron 25 mg with poloxamer '188' 200 mg per 5 mL.
- Co-danthramer **strong** capsules contain dantron 37.5 mg with poloxamer '188' 500 mg.
- Co-danthramer **strong** oral suspension contains dantron 75 mg with poloxamer '188' 1 g per 5 mL.
- Co-danthramer suspension 5 mL = one co-danthramer capsule, **but** strong co-danthramer suspension 5 mL = two strong co-danthramer capsules.

- CONTRA-INDICATIONS Acute abdominal conditions · acute inflammatory bowel disease · intestinal obstruction · severe dehydration
- CAUTIONS Excessive use of stimulant laxatives can cause diarrhoea and related effects such as hypokalaemia · may cause local irritation · *rodent* studies indicate potential carcinogenic risk

CAUTIONS, FURTHER INFORMATION
- Local irritation Avoid prolonged contact with skin (incontinent patients or infants wearing nappies—risk of irritation and excoriation).
- SIDE-EFFECTS Abdominal cramps · asthenia · gastrointestinal disorders · hypermagnesaemia · skin reactions · urine red
- PREGNANCY Manufacturers advise avoid—limited information available.
- BREAST FEEDING Manufacturers advise avoid—no information available.
- PRESCRIBING AND DISPENSING INFORMATION

Palliative care For further information on the use of co-danthramer in palliative care, see www.medicinescomplete.com/#/content/palliative/stimulant-laxatives.

- MEDICINAL FORMS There can be variation in the licensing of different medicines containing the same drug.

Oral suspension

CAUTIONARY AND ADVISORY LABELS 14 (urine red)
- Co-danthramer (Non-proprietary)
  Dantron 5 mg per 1 ml, Poloxamer 188 40 mg per 1 ml Co-danthramer 25mg/200mg/5ml oral suspension sugar free sugar-free | 300 ml PoM £180.00 DT = £180.00
  Dantron 15 mg per 1 ml, Poloxamer 188 200 mg per 1 ml Co-danthramer 75mg/1000mg/5ml oral suspension sugar free sugar-free | 300 ml PoM £367.50 DT = £367.50

Co-danthrusate

16-Mar-2020

- INDICATIONS AND DOSE

Constipation in palliative care
- BY MOUTH USING ORAL SUSPENSION
- Child 6–11 years: 5 mL once daily, to be taken at night
- Child 12–17 years: 5–15 mL once daily, to be taken at night
- Adult: 5–15 mL once daily, to be taken at night

DOSE EQUIVALENCE AND CONVERSION
- Co-danthrusate suspension contains dantron 50 mg and docusate sodium 60 mg per 5 mL.

- CONTRA-INDICATIONS Acute abdominal conditions · acute inflammatory bowel disease · intestinal obstruction · severe dehydration
- CAUTIONS Excessive use of stimulant laxatives can cause diarrhoea and related effects such as hypokalaemia · may cause local irritation · *rodent* studies indicate potential carcinogenic risk

  CAUTIONS, FURTHER INFORMATION
  ▸ Local irritation Avoid prolonged contact with skin (incontinent patients—risk of irritation and excoriation).
- INTERACTIONS → Appendix 1: docusate sodium
- SIDE-EFFECTS Gastrointestinal disorders · skin reactions · urine orange
- PREGNANCY Manufacturers advise avoid—limited information available.
- BREAST FEEDING Manufacturers advise avoid—no information available.

- MEDICINAL FORMS There can be variation in the licensing of different medicines containing the same drug.

  Oral suspension
  CAUTIONARY AND ADVISORY LABELS 14 (urine orange)
  ▸ Co-danthrusate (Non-proprietary)
  Dantron 10 mg per 1 ml, Docusate sodium 12 mg per 1 ml Co-danthrusate 50mg/60mg/5ml oral suspension sugar free sugar-free | 200 ml [PoM] £202.50 DT = £202.50

Glycerol
05-Aug-2020

(Glycerin)

- INDICATIONS AND DOSE

  Constipation
  ▸ BY RECTUM
    ▸ Child 1-11 months: 1 g as required
    ▸ Child 1-11 years: 2 g as required
    ▸ Child 12-17 years: 4 g as required
    ▸ Adult: 4 g as required

- DIRECTIONS FOR ADMINISTRATION Manufacturer advises moisten suppositories with water before insertion.
- PRESCRIBING AND DISPENSING INFORMATION When prepared extemporaneously, the BP states Glycerol Suppositories, BP consists of gelatin 140 mg, glycerol 700 mg, purified water to 1 g.
- PATIENT AND CARER ADVICE
  Medicines for Children leaflet: Glycerin (glycerol) suppositories for constipation www.medicinesforchildren.org.uk/glycerin-glycerol-suppositories-constipation

- MEDICINAL FORMS There can be variation in the licensing of different medicines containing the same drug. Forms available from special-order manufacturers include: suppository
  Suppository
  ▸ Glycerol (Non-proprietary)
    Glycerol 700 mg Glycerol 1g suppositories | 12 suppository [GSL] £2.65 DT = £2.18
    Glycerol 1400 mg Glycerol 2g suppositories | 12 suppository [GSL] £2.91 DT = £2.25
    Glycerol 2800 mg Glycerol 4g suppositories | 12 suppository [GSL] £1.73 DT = £1.61

Senna
10-Sep-2020

- DRUG ACTION Senna is a stimulant laxative. After metabolism of sennosides in the gut the anthrone component stimulates peristalsis thereby increasing the motility of the large intestine.

- INDICATIONS AND DOSE

  Constipation
  ▸ BY MOUTH USING TABLETS
    ▸ Child 6-17 years: 7.5–30 mg once daily, adjusted according to response
    ▸ Adult: 7.5–15 mg daily (max. per dose 30 mg daily), dose usually taken at bedtime; initial dose should be low then gradually increased, higher doses may be prescribed under medical supervision
  ▸ BY MOUTH USING SYRUP
    ▸ Child 1 month-3 years: 3.75–15 mg once daily, adjusted according to response
    ▸ Child 4-17 years: 3.75–30 mg once daily, adjusted according to response
    ▸ Adult: 7.5–15 mg once daily (max. per dose 30 mg daily), dose usually taken at bedtime, higher doses may be prescribed under medical supervision

  Constipation (dose approved for use by community practitioner nurse prescribers)
  ▸ BY MOUTH USING TABLETS
    ▸ Child 6-17 years: 7.5–30 mg once daily, adjusted according to response
    ▸ Adult: 15–30 mg daily, dose usually taken at night; initial dose should be low then gradually increased
  ▸ BY MOUTH USING SYRUP
    ▸ Child 2-3 years: 3.75–15 mg once daily, adjusted according to response
    ▸ Child 4-17 years: 3.75–30 mg once daily, adjusted according to response
    ▸ Adult: 15–30 mg once daily, dose usually taken at bedtime

  PHARMACOKINETICS
  ▸ Onset of action 8–12 hours.

- UNLICENSED USE *Syrup* not licensed for use in children under 2 years.
  Doses in BNF adhere to national guidelines and may differ from those in product literature.

  IMPORTANT SAFETY INFORMATION
  MHRA/CHM ADVICE: STIMULANT LAXATIVES (BISACODYL, SENNA AND SENNOSIDES, SODIUM PICOSULFATE) AVAILABLE OVER-THE-COUNTER: NEW MEASURES TO SUPPORT SAFE USE (AUGUST 2020)
  Following a national safety review and concerns over misuse and abuse, the MHRA has introduced new pack size restrictions, revised recommended ages for use, and new safety warnings for over-the-counter stimulant laxatives (administered orally and rectally). Patients should be advised that dietary and lifestyle measures should be used first-line for relieving short-term occasional constipation, and that stimulant laxatives should only be used if these measures and other laxatives (bulk-forming and osmotic) are ineffective.
  Smaller packs will remain available for general sale for the treatment of short-term, occasional constipation in adults only, and will be limited to a pack size of two short treatment courses. Stimulant laxatives should not be used in children under 12 years of age without advice from a prescriber; in children aged 12 to 17 years, products can be supplied under the supervision of a pharmacist.

- CONTRA-INDICATIONS Atony · intestinal obstruction · undiagnosed abdominal pain

- SIDE-EFFECTS Albuminuria · diarrhoea · electrolyte imbalance · fluid imbalance · gastrointestinal discomfort · haematuria · pseudomelanosis coli · skin reactions · urine discolouration

  SIDE-EFFECTS, FURTHER INFORMATION Prolonged or excessive use can cause hypokalaemia.
- PREGNANCY EvGr Specialist sources indicate suitable for use in pregnancy. ⓓ
- BREAST FEEDING EvGr Specialist sources indicate suitable for use in breast-feeding in infants over 1 month. ⓓ
- PATIENT AND CARER ADVICE
  Medicines for Children leaflet: Senna for constipation
  www.medicinesforchildren.org.uk/senna-constipation
- NATIONAL FUNDING/ACCESS DECISIONS
  NHS restrictions Senokot® tablets are not prescribable in NHS primary care.
- EXCEPTIONS TO LEGAL CATEGORY Senna is on sale to the public for use in children over 12 years; doses on packs may vary from those in BNF Publications.
- MEDICINAL FORMS There can be variation in the licensing of different medicines containing the same drug.

  Oral solution
  ▸ Senokot (Forum Health Products Ltd, Reckitt Benckiser Healthcare (UK) Ltd)
    Sennoside B (as Sennosides) 1.5 mg per 1 ml Senokot 7.5mg/5ml Syrup Pharmacy sugar free sugar-free | 500 ml Ⓟ £5.98 DT = £5.98

  Tablet
  ▸ Senna (Non-proprietary)
    Sennoside B (as Sennosides) 7.5 mg Senokot 7.5mg tablets 12 Years Plus | 60 tablet Ⓟ £4.20 DT = £2.20
    Senna 7.5mg tablets | 20 tablet Ⓟ £1.00 | 24 tablet Ⓟ £0.55 | 60 tablet Ⓟ £3.51 DT = £2.20 | 100 tablet Ⓟ £2.15
    Sennoside B (as Sennosides) 15 mg Senokot Max Strength tablets Adult | 10 tablet GSL £1.93
  ▸ Senokot (Reckitt Benckiser Healthcare (UK) Ltd, Forum Health Products Ltd)
    Sennoside B (as Sennosides) 7.5 mg Senokot 7.5mg tablets | 500 tablet Ⓟ £12.50
    Sennoside B (as Sennosides) 15 mg Senokot Max Strength 15mg tablets | 24 tablet GSL £3.23 | 48 tablet GSL £5.69 DT = £5.69

Senna with ispaghula husk

11-Nov-2020

The properties listed below are those particular to the combination only. For the properties of the components please consider, senna p. 67, ispaghula husk p. 58.

- INDICATIONS AND DOSE

Constipation
▸ BY MOUTH
  ▸ Child 12-17 years: 5–10 g once daily, to be taken at night, up to 2–3 times a week
  ▸ Adult: 5–10 g once daily, to be taken at night, up to 2–3 times a week

DOSE EQUIVALENCE AND CONVERSION
▸ 5 g equivalent to one level spoonful of granules.

- PREGNANCY Manufacturer advises avoid during first trimester. To be used only intermittently and only if dietary and lifestyle changes fail.
- DIRECTIONS FOR ADMINISTRATION EvGr Take at night with at least 150 mL liquid. ⓜ
- MEDICINAL FORMS There can be variation in the licensing of different medicines containing the same drug.

  Granules
  CAUTIONARY AND ADVISORY LABELS 25
  EXCIPIENTS: May contain Sucrose
  ▸ Manevac (Mylan)
    Senna fruit 124 mg per 1 gram, Ispaghula 542 mg per 1 gram Manevac granules | 250 gram Ⓟ £6.30

Sodium acid phosphate with sodium bicarbonate

03-Dec-2020

The properties listed below are those particular to the combination only. For the properties of the components please consider, sodium bicarbonate p. 1086.

- INDICATIONS AND DOSE

LECICARBON A ®

Constipation | Bowel evacuation [before diagnostic or therapeutic procedures in the rectum]
▸ BY RECTUM
  ▸ Child 12-17 years: 1 suppository as required, dose may be repeated after 30–60 minutes
  ▸ Adult: 1 suppository as required, dose may be repeated after 30–60 minutes

PHARMACOKINETICS
▸ Onset of action 15–30 minutes.

LECICARBON C ®

Constipation | Bowel evacuation [before diagnostic or therapeutic procedures in the rectum]
▸ BY RECTUM
  ▸ Child 1-11 years: 1 suppository as required, dose may be repeated after 30–60 minutes

PHARMACOKINETICS
▸ Onset of action 15–30 minutes.

- CONTRA-INDICATIONS Anal and rectal region diseases (risk of excessive absorption of carbon dioxide, particularly in infants and children) · ileus · toxic megacolon (except with explicit permission of the physician)
- INTERACTIONS → Appendix 1: bowel cleansing preparations · sodium bicarbonate
- ALLERGY AND CROSS-SENSITIVITY EvGr Contra-indicated in patients with peanut or soya hypersensitivity. ⓜ
- PREGNANCY EvGr Use only if potential benefit outweighs risk—effect of the expanding volume of carbon dioxide may be negligible. ⓜ
- BREAST FEEDING EvGr Suitable for use in breast-feeding— the developed carbon dioxide will not be excreted in milk. ⓜ
- DIRECTIONS FOR ADMINISTRATION EvGr Moisten suppositories with water before insertion if needed. ⓜ
- MEDICINAL FORMS There can be variation in the licensing of different medicines containing the same drug.

  Suppository
  ▸ Lecicarbon A (Aspire Pharma Ltd)
    Sodium bicarbonate 500 mg, Sodium dihydrogen phosphate anhydrous 680 mg Lecicarbon A suppositories | 10 suppository Ⓟ £8.20 DT = £8.20
  ▸ Lecicarbon C (Aspire Pharma Ltd)
    Sodium bicarbonate 250 mg, Sodium dihydrogen phosphate anhydrous 340 mg Lecicarbon C suppositories | 10 suppository Ⓟ £8.20 DT = £8.20

Sodium picosulfate

10-Sep-2020

(Sodium picosulphate)

- DRUG ACTION Sodium picosulfate is a stimulant laxative. After metabolism in the colon it stimulates the mucosa thereby increasing the motility of the large intestine.

- INDICATIONS AND DOSE

Constipation
▸ BY MOUTH
  ▸ Child 1 month-3 years: 2.5–10 mg once daily, adjusted according to response

- Child 4-17 years: 2.5–20 mg once daily, adjusted according to response
- Adult: 5–10 mg once daily, dose to be taken at bedtime

Constipation (dose approved for use by community practitioner nurse prescribers)
▸ BY MOUTH
- Child 1 month-3 years: 250 micrograms/kg once daily (max. per dose 5 mg), adjusted according to response, (on doctor's advice only); dose to be taken at night
- Child 4-10 years: 2.5–5 mg once daily, adjusted according to response, (on doctor's advice only); dose to be taken at night
- Child 11-17 years: 5–10 mg once daily, adjusted according to response, dose to be taken at night
- Adult: 5–10 mg once daily, dose to be taken at night

PHARMACOKINETICS
▸ Onset of action 6–12 hours.

- UNLICENSED USE Sodium picosulfate doses in BNF Publications adhere to national guidelines and may differ from those in product literature.

IMPORTANT SAFETY INFORMATION
MHRA/CHM ADVICE: STIMULANT LAXATIVES (BISACODYL, SENNA AND SENNOSIDES, SODIUM PICOSULFATE) AVAILABLE OVER-THE-COUNTER: NEW MEASURES TO SUPPORT SAFE USE (AUGUST 2020)
Following a national safety review and concerns over misuse and abuse, the MHRA has introduced new pack size restrictions, revised recommended ages for use, and new safety warnings for over-the-counter stimulant laxatives (administered orally and rectally). Patients should be advised that dietary and lifestyle measures should be used first-line for relieving short-term occasional constipation, and that stimulant laxatives should only be used if these measures and other laxatives (bulk-forming and osmotic) are ineffective.
Smaller packs will remain available for general sale for the treatment of short-term, occasional constipation in adults only, and will be limited to a pack size of two short treatment courses. Stimulant laxatives should not be used in children under 12 years of age without advice from a prescriber; in children aged 12 to 17 years, products can be supplied under the supervision of a pharmacist.

- CONTRA-INDICATIONS Intestinal obstruction · undiagnosed abdominal pain
- INTERACTIONS → Appendix 1: sodium picosulfate
- SIDE-EFFECTS
▸ **Common or very common** Diarrhoea · gastrointestinal discomfort
▸ **Uncommon** Dizziness · nausea · vomiting
▸ **Frequency not known** Angioedema · skin reactions · syncope
SIDE-EFFECTS, FURTHER INFORMATION Prolonged or excessive use can cause diarrhoea and related effects such as hypokalaemia.
- PREGNANCY Manufacturer states evidence limited but not known to be harmful.
- BREAST FEEDING EvGr Specialist sources indicate suitable for use in breast-feeding in infants over 1 month—not known to be present in milk. ◎
- PATIENT AND CARER ADVICE
Medicines for Children leaflet: Sodium picosulfate for constipation www.medicinesforchildren.org.uk/sodium-picosulfate-constipation

- MEDICINAL FORMS There can be variation in the licensing of different medicines containing the same drug.
Oral solution
EXCIPIENTS: May contain Alcohol
▸ Sodium picosulfate (Non-proprietary)
Sodium picosulfate 1 mg per 1 ml Sodium picosulfate 5mg/5ml oral solution sugar free sugar-free | 100 ml P £2.69 sugar-free | 300 ml P £8.08 DT = £8.08
▸ Laxoberal (Sanofi)
Sodium picosulfate 1 mg per 1 ml Dulcolax Pico 5mg/5ml liquid sugar-free | 300 ml P £4.62 DT = £8.08

OPIOID RECEPTOR ANTAGONISTS

Methylnaltrexone bromide   29-Jul-2020

- DRUG ACTION Methylnaltrexone bromide is a peripherally acting opioid-receptor antagonist. It therefore blocks the gastro-intestinal (constipating) effects of opioids without altering their central analgesic effects.

- INDICATIONS AND DOSE
Opioid-induced constipation in patients with chronic pain (except palliative care patients with advanced illness)
▸ BY SUBCUTANEOUS INJECTION
- Adult: 12 mg once daily if required, to be given as 4–7 doses weekly

Adjunct to other laxatives in opioid-induced constipation in palliative care
▸ BY SUBCUTANEOUS INJECTION
- Adult (body-weight up to 38 kg): 150 micrograms/kg once daily on alternate days for maximum duration of treatment 4 months, two consecutive doses may be given 24 hours apart if no response to treatment on the preceding day
- Adult (body-weight 38-61 kg): 8 mg once daily on alternate days for maximum duration of treatment 4 months, two consecutive doses may be given 24 hours apart if no response to treatment on the preceding day
- Adult (body-weight 62-114 kg): 12 mg once daily on alternate days for maximum duration of treatment 4 months, two consecutive doses may be given 24 hours apart if no response to treatment on the preceding day
- Adult (body-weight 115 kg and above): 150 micrograms/kg once daily on alternate days for maximum duration of treatment 4 months, two consecutive doses may be given 24 hours apart if no response to treatment on the preceding day

PHARMACOKINETICS
▸ May act within 30–60 minutes.

- CONTRA-INDICATIONS Acute surgical abdominal conditions · gastro-intestinal obstruction
- CAUTIONS Diverticular disease (when active) · faecal impaction · gastro-intestinal tract lesions (known or suspected) · patients with colostomy · patients with peritoneal catheter
- SIDE-EFFECTS
▸ **Common or very common** Abdominal pain · diarrhoea · dizziness · gastrointestinal disorders · nausea · opioid withdrawal-like syndrome · vomiting

Overdose Symptoms of overdosage include orthostatic hypotension.

- PREGNANCY Manufacturer advises avoid unless essential—toxicity at high doses in *animal* studies.
- BREAST FEEDING Manufacturer advises use only if potential benefit outweighs risk—present in milk in *animal* studies.
- HEPATIC IMPAIRMENT Manufacturer advises avoid in severe impairment (no information available).

1

Gastro-intestinal system

- **RENAL IMPAIRMENT**
  Dose adjustments If eGFR less than 30 mL/minute/1.73 m², reduce dose as follows: body-weight under 62 kg, 75 micrograms/kg on alternate days; body-weight 62–114 kg, 8 mg on alternate days; body-weight over 114 kg, 75 micrograms/kg on alternate days.
- **DIRECTIONS FOR ADMINISTRATION** Rotate injection site.
- **PRESCRIBING AND DISPENSING INFORMATION**
  Palliative care For further information on the use of methylnaltrexone in palliative care, see www.medicinescomplete.com/#/content/palliative/opioid-antagonists-therapeutic-target-outside-the-cns.
- **HANDLING AND STORAGE** Protect from light.

- **MEDICINAL FORMS** There can be variation in the licensing of different medicines containing the same drug.
  Solution for injection
  ‣ Relistor (Bausch & Lomb UK Ltd)
  Methylnaltrexone bromide 20 mg per 1 ml Relistor 12mg/0.6ml solution for injection vials | 1 vial [PoM] £21.05 | 7 vial [PoM] £147.35

Naldemedine
10-Dec-2020

- **DRUG ACTION** Naldemedine is a peripherally acting opioid receptor antagonist. It therefore decreases the constipating effects of opioids without altering their central analgesic effects.

- **INDICATIONS AND DOSE**
  Opioid-induced constipation [previous treatment with a laxative]
  ‣ BY MOUTH
  ‣ Adult: 200 micrograms once daily

- **CONTRA-INDICATIONS** Increased risk of recurrent obstruction (risk of gastro-intestinal perforation) · known or suspected gastro-intestinal obstruction (risk of gastro-intestinal perforation)
- **CAUTIONS** Conditions with impaired integrity of the gastro-intestinal wall (risk of gastro-intestinal perforation) · treatment initiation in patients aged 75 years and over (limited information available)
  CAUTIONS, FURTHER INFORMATION
  ‣ Disruptions to blood-brain barrier Manufacturer advises caution in patients with clinically important disruptions to the blood-brain barrier (e.g. advanced Alzheimer's disease, active multiple sclerosis, primary brain malignancies)—risk of opioid withdrawal or reduced analgesia.
  ‣ Cardiovascular disorders Safety and efficacy has not been established in patients with these conditions.
- **INTERACTIONS** → Appendix 1: naldemedine
- **SIDE-EFFECTS**
  ‣ Common or very common Diarrhoea · gastrointestinal discomfort · nausea · vomiting
- **PREGNANCY** Manufacturer advises avoid unless potential benefit outweighs risk— animal studies do not indicate toxicity; risk of opioid withdrawal in fetus.
- **BREAST FEEDING** Manufacturer advises avoid—present in milk in animal studies; theoretical risk of opioid withdrawal in breast-fed neonate.
- **HEPATIC IMPAIRMENT** Manufacturer advises avoid in severe impairment (no information available).
- **PATIENT AND CARER ADVICE** Manufacturer advises patients and carers to report severe, persistent or worsening gastro-intestinal effects (such as abdominal pain) to their prescriber. Manufacturer advises patients and carers should be counselled on the risk of opioid withdrawal syndrome and to seek medical advice if this occurs.

- **NATIONAL FUNDING/ACCESS DECISIONS**
  For full details see funding body website
  NICE decisions
  ‣ Naldemedine for treating opioid-induced constipation (September 2020) NICE TA651 Recommended
  Scottish Medicines Consortium (SMC) decisions
  ‣ Naldemedine (Rizmoic®) for the treatment of opioid-induced constipation (OIC) in adult patients who have previously been treated with a laxative (April 2020) SMC No. SMC2242 Recommended

- **MEDICINAL FORMS** There can be variation in the licensing of different medicines containing the same drug.
  Tablet
  ‣ Naldemedine (non-proprietary) ▼
  Naldemedine (as Naldemedine tosylate) 200 microgram Rizmoic 200microgram tablets | 28 tablet [PoM] £41.72

Naloxegol
04-Aug-2020

- **DRUG ACTION** Naloxegol is a peripherally acting opioid receptor antagonist. It therefore decreases the constipating effects of opioids without altering their central analgesic effects.

- **INDICATIONS AND DOSE**
  Opioid-induced constipation when response to laxatives inadequate
  ‣ BY MOUTH
  ‣ Adult: 25 mg once daily, to be taken in the morning
  DOSE ADJUSTMENTS DUE TO INTERACTIONS
  ‣ Manufacturer advises reduce initial dose to 12.5 mg daily with concurrent use of moderate inhibitors of CYP3A4, increasing to 25 mg daily if well tolerated.

- **CONTRA-INDICATIONS** Gastro-intestinal or peritoneum malignancy (risk of gastro-intestinal perforation) · known or suspected gastro-intestinal obstruction · patients at risk of recurrent gastro-intestinal obstruction · recurrent or advanced ovarian cancer (risk of gastro-intestinal perforation) · vascular endothelial growth factor (VEGF) inhibitor treatment (risk of gastro-intestinal perforation)
- **CAUTIONS** Alzheimer's disease (advanced) · cardiovascular disease · CNS metastases · congestive heart failure (symptomatic) · Crohn's disease · diverticulitis (active or recurrent) · multiple sclerosis (active) · peptic ulcer disease (severe) · primary brain malignancies · QT interval over 500 milliseconds · recent history of myocardial infarction (within 6 months)
  CAUTIONS, FURTHER INFORMATION
  ‣ Disruptions to blood-brain barrier Manufacturer advises caution in patients with clinically important disruptions to the blood-brain barrier (e.g. advanced Alzheimer's disease, active multiple sclerosis, primary brain malignancies)—risk of uptake into the CNS.
  ‣ Cardiovascular disorders Safety and efficacy has not been established in patients with these conditions.
- **INTERACTIONS** → Appendix 1: naloxegol
- **SIDE-EFFECTS**
  ‣ Common or very common Abdominal pain · diarrhoea · flatulence · headache · hyperhidrosis · nasopharyngitis · nausea · vomiting
  ‣ Uncommon Withdrawal syndrome
  SIDE-EFFECTS, FURTHER INFORMATION Manufacturer advises that gastrointestinal side-effects typically occur shortly after initiation of treatment — consider reducing the dose.
- **PREGNANCY** Manufacturer advises avoid—limited data available but toxicity at high doses in animal studies; theoretical risk of opioid withdrawal in fetus.

- BREAST FEEDING Manufacturer advises avoid—present in milk in *animal* studies and theoretical risk of opioid withdrawal in breast-fed infants.
- HEPATIC IMPAIRMENT Manufacturer advises avoid in severe impairment (no information available).
- RENAL IMPAIRMENT
  Dose adjustments Manufacturer advises lower initial dose in moderate to severe impairment—initially 12.5 mg daily, increase to 25 mg if well tolerated.
- DIRECTIONS FOR ADMINISTRATION Manufacturer advises tablets can be crushed, mixed with 120 mL of water and taken immediately if patients are unable to swallow tablets whole. The mixture may be administered via a nasogastric tube, if required.
- PATIENT AND CARER ADVICE Manufacturer advises patients report severe, persistent or worsening gastro-intestinal effects (such as abdominal pain) to their prescriber.
- NATIONAL FUNDING/ACCESS DECISIONS
  For full details see funding body website
  NICE decisions
  ▸ **Naloxegol for treating opioid-induced constipation (July 2015)** NICE TA345 Recommended

- MEDICINAL FORMS There can be variation in the licensing of different medicines containing the same drug.
  Tablet
  CAUTIONARY AND ADVISORY LABELS 23
  ▸ Moventig (Kyowa Kirin Ltd)
  Naloxegol (as Naloxegol oxalate) 12.5 mg Moventig 12.5mg tablets | 30 tablet [PoM] £55.20 DT = £55.20
  Naloxegol (as Naloxegol oxalate) 25 mg Moventig 25mg tablets | 30 tablet [PoM] £55.20 DT = £55.20

3   Diarrhoea

Diarrhoea (acute)   01-Aug-2017

Description of condition

Diarrhoea is the abnormal passing of loose or liquid stools, with increased frequency, increased volume, or both. Acute diarrhoea is that which lasts less than 14 days, but symptoms usually improve within 2–4 days. It can result from infection, as a side-effect of a drug, or as an acute symptom of a chronic gastro-intestinal disorder (such as Inflammatory bowel disease p. 41 or Irritable bowel syndrome p. 51). It may also result from the accumulation of non-absorbed osmotically active solutes in the gastro-intestinal lumen (e.g. in lactase deficiency) or from the gastro-intestinal effects of secretory stimuli (other than the enterotoxins from an infection). It may also occur when intestinal motility or morphology is altered.

Prompt investigation is required to identify or exclude any serious underlying cause if the patient has any red flag symptoms such as unexplained weight loss, rectal bleeding, persistent diarrhoea, a systemic illness, has received recent hospital treatment or antibiotic treatment, or following foreign travel (other than to Western Europe, North America, Australia or New Zealand).

Aims of treatment

The priority of acute diarrhoea treatment, as in gastro-enteritis, is the prevention or reversal of fluid and electrolyte depletion and the management of dehydration when it is present. This is particularly important in infants, frail and elderly patients, when excessive water and electrolyte loss and dehydration can be life-threatening.

Treatment

Most episodes of acute diarrhoea will settle spontaneously without the need for any medical treatment. [EvGr] Oral rehydration therapy (ORT, such as disodium hydrogen citrate with glucose, potassium chloride and sodium chloride p. 1091; potassium chloride with sodium chloride p. 1089; potassium chloride with rice powder, sodium chloride and sodium citrate p. 1091) is the mainstay of treatment for acute diarrhoea to prevent or correct diarrhoea dehydration and to maintain the appropriate fluid intake once rehydration is achieved—see Fluids and electrolytes p. 1084.

However, in patients with severe dehydration and in those unable to drink, immediate admission to hospital and urgent replacement treatment with an intravenous rehydration fluid is recommended—see Fluids and electrolytes p. 1084.

The antimotility drug loperamide hydrochloride p. 72 is usually considered to be the standard treatment when rapid control of symptoms is required. It can also be used for mild-to-moderate travellers' diarrhoea (e.g. where toilet amenities are limited or unavailable) but should be avoided in bloody or suspected inflammatory diarrhoea (febrile patients) and in cases of significant abdominal pain (which also suggests inflammatory diarrhoea).

Loperamide hydrochloride is also the first-line treatment for patients with faecal incontinence [unlicensed indication] after the underlying cause of incontinence has been addressed. Ⓐ

Racecadotril is licensed as an adjunct to rehydration for the symptomatic treatment of uncomplicated acute diarrhoea in adults and children over 3 months.

There is insufficient evidence to recommend adsorbent preparations (such as kaolin) in acute diarrhoea.

Antibacterial drugs for acute diarrhoea

[EvGr] Ciprofloxacin p. 593 is occasionally used for prophylaxis against travellers' diarrhoea, but routine use is **not** recommended. Ⓐ See also Gastro-intestinal system infections, antibacterial therapy p. 535.

Related drugs

Other drugs used for diarrhoea: codeine phosphate p. 475, co-phenotrope below, methylcellulose p. 59, rifaximin p. 612.

> **Other drugs used for Diarrhoea** Colesevelam hydrochloride, p. 211 · Colestyramine, p. 212

ANTIDIARRHOEALS ›
ANTIPROPULSIVES

> ▣ 467

Co-phenotrope   25-Nov-2020

- INDICATIONS AND DOSE

  Adjunct to rehydration in acute diarrhoea
  ▸ BY MOUTH
  - Child 4-8 years: 1 tablet 3 times a day
  - Child 9-11 years: 1 tablet 4 times a day
  - Child 12-15 years: 2 tablets 3 times a day
  - Child 16-17 years: Initially 4 tablets, followed by 2 tablets every 6 hours until diarrhoea controlled
  - Adult: Initially 4 tablets, followed by 2 tablets every 6 hours until diarrhoea controlled

  Control of faecal consistency after colostomy or ileostomy
  ▸ BY MOUTH
  - Child 4-8 years: 1 tablet 3 times a day
  - Child 9-11 years: 1 tablet 4 times a day
  - Child 12-15 years: 2 tablets 3 times a day
  - Child 16-17 years: Initially 4 tablets, then 2 tablets 4 times a day
  - Adult: Initially 4 tablets, then 2 tablets 4 times a day

- CONTRA-INDICATIONS Antibiotic-associated colitis ·
gastro-intestinal obstruction · intestinal atony ·
myasthenia gravis (but some antimuscarinics may be used
to decrease muscarinic side-effects of anticholinesterases)
· paralytic ileus · prostatic enlargement (in adults) · pyloric
stenosis · severe ulcerative colitis · significant bladder
outflow obstruction · toxic megacolon · urinary retention
- CAUTIONS Presence of subclinical doses of atropine may
give rise to atropine side-effects in susceptible individuals
or in overdosage · young children are particularly
susceptible to **overdosage**—symptoms may be delayed
and observation is needed for at least 48 hours after
ingestion
- INTERACTIONS → Appendix 1: atropine · opioids
- SIDE-EFFECTS Abdominal discomfort · angioedema · angle
closure glaucoma · appetite decreased · cardiac disorder ·
depression · dysuria · fever · gastrointestinal disorders ·
malaise · mucosal dryness · mydriasis · restlessness · vision
disorders
- PREGNANCY Manufacturer advises caution.
- BREAST FEEDING May be present in milk.
- HEPATIC IMPAIRMENT Manufacturer advises caution; avoid
in jaundice.
- DIRECTIONS FOR ADMINISTRATION Expert sources advise
for administration *by mouth* tablets may be crushed.
- PRESCRIBING AND DISPENSING INFORMATION A mixture of
diphenoxylate hydrochloride and atropine sulfate in the
mass proportions 100 parts to 1 part respectively.
- EXCEPTIONS TO LEGAL CATEGORY Co-phenotrope
2.5/0.025 can be sold to the public for adults and children
over 16 years (provided packs do not contain more than
20 tablets) as an adjunct to rehydration in acute diarrhoea
(max. daily dose 10 tablets).

- MEDICINAL FORMS There can be variation in the licensing of
different medicines containing the same drug. Forms available
from special-order manufacturers include: tablet
Tablet
▸ Co-phenotrope (Imported)
**Atropine sulfate 25 microgram, Diphenoxylate hydrochloride
2.5 mg** Lomotil 2.5mg/25microgram tablets |
100 tablet [PoM] [⚠] [CD5]
Lofenoxal 2.5mg/25microgram tablets | 20 tablet [PoM] [⚠] [CD5]

[F 467]

Kaolin with morphine
25-Nov-2020

- INDICATIONS AND DOSE
Acute diarrhoea
▸ BY MOUTH
▸ Adult: 10 mL every 6 hours, dose to be given in water

- CONTRA-INDICATIONS Acute abdomen · delayed gastric
emptying · heart failure secondary to chronic lung disease ·
phaeochromocytoma
- CAUTIONS Cardiac arrhythmias · pancreatitis · severe cor
pulmonale
- INTERACTIONS → Appendix 1: kaolin · opioids
- BREAST FEEDING Therapeutic doses unlikely to affect
infant.
- RENAL IMPAIRMENT Avoid use or reduce dose; opioid
effects increased and prolonged, and increased cerebral
sensitivity occurs.
- PRESCRIBING AND DISPENSING INFORMATION When
prepared extemporaneously, the BP states Kaolin and
Morphine Mixture, BP consists of light kaolin or light
kaolin (natural) 20%, sodium bicarbonate 5%, and
chloroform and morphine tincture 4% in a suitable
vehicle. Contains anhydrous morphine
550–800 micrograms/10 mL.

- LESS SUITABLE FOR PRESCRIBING Kaolin and Morphine
Mixture, BP (Kaolin and Morphine Oral Suspension) is less
suitable for prescribing.

- MEDICINAL FORMS There can be variation in the licensing of
different medicines containing the same drug.
Oral suspension
▸ Kaolin with morphine (Non-proprietary)
**Morphine hydrochloride 91.6 mg per 1 litre, Sodium bicarbonate
50 gram per 1 litre, Kaolin light 200 gram per 1 litre, Chloroform
5 ml per 1 litre** Kaolin and Morphine mixture | 200 ml [P] £1.71 DT =
£1.71 [CD5]

Loperamide hydrochloride
10-Mar-2020

- INDICATIONS AND DOSE
Symptomatic treatment of acute diarrhoea
▸ BY MOUTH
▸ Child 4-7 years: 1 mg 3–4 times a day for up to 3 days
only
▸ Child 8-11 years: 2 mg 4 times a day for up to 5 days
▸ Child 12-17 years: Initially 4 mg, followed by 2 mg for up
to 5 days, dose to be taken after each loose stool; usual
dose 6–8 mg daily; maximum 16 mg per day
▸ Adult: Initially 4 mg, followed by 2 mg for up to 5 days,
dose to be taken after each loose stool; usual dose
6–8 mg daily; maximum 16 mg per day
Chronic diarrhoea
▸ BY MOUTH
▸ Adult: Initially 4–8 mg daily in divided doses, adjusted
according to response; maintenance up to 16 mg daily
in 2 divided doses
Faecal incontinence
▸ BY MOUTH
▸ Adult: Initially 500 micrograms daily, adjusted
according to response, maximum daily dose to be given
in divided doses; maximum 16 mg per day
Pain of bowel colic in palliative care
▸ BY MOUTH
▸ Adult: 2–4 mg 4 times a day

- UNLICENSED USE *Capsules* not licensed for use in children
under 8 years.
▸ In adults Use for faecal incontinence is an unlicensed
indication.

┌───┐
│ IMPORTANT SAFETY INFORMATION
│ MHRA/CHM ADVICE: REPORTS OF SERIOUS CARDIAC ADVERSE
│ REACTIONS WITH HIGH DOSES OF LOPERAMIDE ASSOCIATED WITH
│ ABUSE OR MISUSE (SEPTEMBER 2017)
│ Serious cardiovascular events (such as QT prolongation,
│ torsades de pointes, and cardiac arrest), including
│ fatalities, have been reported in association with large
│ overdoses of loperamide.
│ Healthcare professionals are reminded that if
│ symptoms of overdose occur, naloxone can be given as
│ an antidote. The duration of action of loperamide is
│ longer than that of naloxone (1–3 hours), so repeated
│ treatment with naloxone might be indicated; patients
│ should be monitored closely for at least 48 hours to
│ detect possible CNS depression.
│ Pharmacists should remind patients not to take more
│ than the recommended dose on the label.
└───┘

- CONTRA-INDICATIONS Active ulcerative colitis · antibiotic-
associated colitis · bacterial enterocolitis · conditions
where abdominal distension develops · conditions where
inhibition of peristalsis should be avoided
- CAUTIONS Not recommended for children under 12 years
- INTERACTIONS → Appendix 1: loperamide

- **SIDE-EFFECTS**
- ▶ **Common or very common** Gastrointestinal disorders · headache · nausea
- ▶ **Uncommon** Dizziness · drowsiness · dry mouth · gastrointestinal discomfort · skin reactions · vomiting
- ▶ **Rare or very rare** Angioedema · consciousness impaired · coordination abnormal · fatigue · miosis · muscle tone increased · severe cutaneous adverse reactions (SCARs) · urinary retention
- **PREGNANCY** Manufacturers advise avoid—no information available.
- **BREAST FEEDING** Amount probably too small to be harmful.
- **HEPATIC IMPAIRMENT** Manufacturer advises caution—risk of reduced first pass metabolism leading to central nervous system toxicity.
- **PRESCRIBING AND DISPENSING INFORMATION**
  Palliative care ▶ In adults For further information on the use of loperamide in palliative care, see www.medicinescomplete.com/#/content/palliative/loperamide.
- **PATIENT AND CARER ADVICE**
  Medicines for Children leaflet: Loperamide for diarrhoea www.medicinesforchildren.org.uk/loperamide-diarrhoea
- **EXCEPTIONS TO LEGAL CATEGORY** Loperamide can be sold to the public, for use in adults and children over 12 years, provided it is licensed and labelled for the treatment of acute diarrhoea.
  - ▶ In adults Loperamide can be sold to the public, provided it is licensed and labelled for the treatment of acute diarrhoea associated with irritable bowel syndrome (after initial diagnosis by a doctor) in adults over 18 years of age.
- **MEDICINAL FORMS** There can be variation in the licensing of different medicines containing the same drug. Forms available from special-order manufacturers include: oral suspension, oral solution

Tablet
- ▶ Loperamide hydrochloride (Non-proprietary)
  Loperamide hydrochloride 2 mg Loperamide 2mg tablets | 30 tablet [PoM] £1.46 DT = £1.46
- ▶ Norimode (Tillomed Laboratories Ltd)
  Loperamide hydrochloride 2 mg Norimode 2mg tablets | 30 tablet [PoM] £2.15 DT = £1.46

Oral solution
- ▶ Imodium (Janssen-Cilag Ltd)
  Loperamide hydrochloride 200 microgram per 1 ml Imodium 1mg/5ml oral solution sugar-free | 100 ml [PoM] £1.17 DT = £1.17

Capsule
- ▶ Loperamide hydrochloride (Non-proprietary)
  Loperamide hydrochloride 2 mg Loperamide 2mg capsules | 30 capsule [PoM] £2.99 DT = £1.11

Orodispersible tablet
- ▶ Imodium (McNeil Products Ltd)
  Loperamide hydrochloride 2 mg Imodium Instant Melts 2mg orodispersible tablets sugar-free | 12 tablet [P] £4.60 sugar-free | 18 tablet [P] £6.15 DT = £6.15

┃ Loperamide with simeticone   24-Apr-2020

The properties listed below are those particular to the combination only. For the properties of the components please consider, loperamide hydrochloride p. 72, simeticone p. 77.

- **INDICATIONS AND DOSE**
  Acute diarrhoea with abdominal colic
  - ▶ BY MOUTH
    - ▶ **Child 12–17 years:** Initially 1 tablet, then 1 tablet, after each loose stool, for up to 2 days; maximum 4 tablets per day
    - ▶ **Adult:** Initially 2 tablets, then 1 tablet, after each loose stool, for up to 2 days; maximum 4 tablets per day

- **INTERACTIONS** → Appendix 1: loperamide

- **MEDICINAL FORMS** There can be variation in the licensing of different medicines containing the same drug.
  Tablet
  - ▶ Imodium Plus (McNeil Products Ltd)
    Loperamide hydrochloride 2 mg, Dimeticone (as Simeticone) 125 mg Imodium Plus caplets | 12 tablet [P] £4.40 DT = £4.40

4 Disorders of gastric acid and ulceration

4.1 Dyspepsia

Dyspepsia   31-Oct-2019

Description of condition

Dyspepsia describes a range of upper gastro-intestinal symptoms, which are typically present for 4 or more weeks. Symptoms include but are not limited to upper abdominal pain or discomfort, heartburn, gastric reflux, bloating, nausea and/or vomiting. Symptoms can be attributed to an underlying cause (e.g. Gastro-oesophageal reflux disease p. 89, Peptic ulcer disease p. 77, gastro-oesophageal malignancy, or side effects from drugs), but the majority of patients are likely to have functional dyspepsia, where an underlying cause cannot be identified and endoscopy findings are normal. Uninvestigated dyspepsia describes symptoms in patients who have not had an endoscopy.

Dyspepsia symptoms in pregnancy are commonly due to gastro-oesophageal reflux disease (GORD), for management see *GORD in pregnancy* in Gastro-oesophageal reflux disease p. 89.

Aims of treatment

The aim of treatment is to manage symptoms, and where possible, to treat the underlying cause of dyspepsia.

Non-drug treatment

[EvGr] Lifestyle measures, such as healthy eating, weight loss (if obese), avoiding any trigger foods, eating smaller meals, eating the evening meal 3–4 hours before going to bed, raising the head of the bed, Smoking cessation p. 519, and reducing alcohol consumption may improve symptoms. Assess the patient for stress, anxiety, or depression, as these conditions may exacerbate symptoms.

Urgent endoscopic investigation is required for patients with dysphagia, significant acute gastrointestinal bleeding, or in those aged 55 years and over with unexplained weight loss and symptoms of upper abdominal pain, reflux or dyspepsia. Ⓐ

Drug treatment

[EvGr] Drugs that may cause dyspepsia, such as alpha-blockers, antimuscarinics, aspirin, benzodiazepines, beta-blockers, bisphosphonates, calcium-channel blockers, corticosteroids, nitrates, non-steroidal anti-inflammatory drugs (NSAIDs), theophyllines, and tricyclic antidepressants, should be reviewed. The lowest effective dose should be used and if possible, stopped.

Antacids and/or alginates may be used for short-term symptom control, but long-term, continuous use is not recommended. Ⓐ

Initial management
Uninvestigated dyspepsia
[EvGr] A proton pump inhibitor should be taken for 4 weeks. Patients with dyspepsia should be tested for *Helicobacter pylori (H. pylori)* infection, and treated if positive. Ⓐ Public Health England recommends that patients who are at high

risk for *H. pylori* infection should be tested for *H. pylori* first, or in parallel with a course of proton pump inhibitor. For treatment regimens, see Helicobacter pylori infection p. 90.

Functional dyspepsia

EvGr Patients should be tested for *H. pylori* infection and treated if positive. Ⓐ See Helicobacter pylori infection p. 90 for testing and management of *H. pylori* infection. EvGr In patients not infected with *H. pylori*, a proton pump inhibitor or a histamine$_2$-receptor antagonist (H$_2$-receptor antagonist) should be taken for 4 weeks. Ⓐ

Follow up management

Uninvestigated and functional dyspepsia

EvGr For patients with refractory dyspepsia symptoms, new alarm symptoms should be assessed and alternative diagnoses should be considered. The patient's adherence to initial management should be checked and lifestyle advice reinforced.

If symptoms persist or recur following initial management, a proton pump inhibitor or H$_2$-receptor antagonist therapy should be used at the lowest dose needed to control symptoms. The patient may use the treatment on an 'as-needed' basis.

In patients with uninvestigated dyspepsia taking an NSAID and unable to stop the drug, consider reducing the NSAID dose and using long-term gastro-protection with acid suppression therapy, or switching to an alternative to the NSAID, such as paracetamol p. 464 or a selective cyclo-oxygenase (COX)-2 inhibitor (but see *Cardiovascular Events* under Non-steroidal anti-inflammatory drugs p. 1176).

In patients with uninvestigated dyspepsia taking aspirin and unable to stop the drug, consider switching from aspirin to an alternative antiplatelet drug.

Patients treated with *H. pylori* eradication therapy do not require routine retesting. Ⓐ There are specific situations where retesting may be appropriate, see *Retesting for Helicobacter pylori*, under Helicobacter pylori infection p. 90. EvGr If retesting is positive, second-line eradication therapy should be prescribed.

An annual review should be performed for patients with dyspepsia to assess their symptoms and treatment. A 'step down' approach, or stopping treatment, should be encouraged if possible and clinically appropriate. A return to self-treatment with antacid and/or alginate therapy may be appropriate.

Referral to a specialist for further investigations should occur in patients of any age with gastro-oesophageal symptoms that are unexplained or non-responsive to treatment, or in patients with *H. pylori* infection that has not responded to second-line eradication therapy—see Helicobacter pylori infection p. 90. Ⓐ

Useful Resources

Gastro-oesophageal reflux disease and dyspepsia in adults: investigation and management. National Institute for Health and Care Excellence. NICE guideline 184. September 2014, reviewed October 2019.
www.nice.org.uk/guidance/cg184

ANTACIDS

Antacids

Overview

Antacids (usually containing aluminium or magnesium compounds) can often relieve symptoms in *ulcer dyspepsia* and in *non-erosive gastro-oesophageal reflux*; they are also sometimes used in functional (non-ulcer) dyspepsia but the evidence of benefit is uncertain. Antacids are best given when symptoms occur or are expected, usually between meals and at bedtime, although additional doses may be required. Conventional doses of liquid magnesium–

aluminium antacids promote ulcer healing, but less well than antisecretory drugs; proof of a relationship between healing and neutralising capacity is lacking. Liquid preparations are more effective than tablet preparations.

Aluminium- and **magnesium-containing** antacids (e.g. aluminium hydroxide, magnesium carbonate p. 76, co-magaldrox p. 75 and magnesium trisilicate p. 76), being relatively insoluble in water, are long-acting if retained in the stomach. They are suitable for most antacid purposes. Magnesium-containing antacids tend to be laxative whereas aluminium-containing antacids may be constipating; antacids containing both magnesium and aluminium may reduce these colonic side-effects. Aluminium accumulation does not appear to be a risk if renal function is normal.

The acid-neutralising capacity of preparations that contain more than one antacid may be the same as simpler preparations. Complexes such as **hydrotalcite** confer no special advantage.

Sodium bicarbonate p. 1086 should no longer be prescribed alone for the relief of dyspepsia but it is present as an ingredient in many indigestion remedies. However, it retains a place in the management of urinary-tract disorders and acidosis.

Bismuth-containing antacids (unless chelates) are not recommended because absorbed bismuth can be neurotoxic, causing encephalopathy; they tend to be constipating. **Calcium-containing** antacids can induce rebound acid secretion: with modest doses the clinical significance is doubtful, but prolonged high doses also cause hypercalcaemia and alkalosis, and can precipitate the milk-alkali syndrome.

Simeticone

Simeticone p. 77 (activated dimeticone) is added to an antacid as an antifoaming agent to relieve flatulence. These preparations may be useful for the relief of hiccup in palliative care.

Alginates

Alginates taken in combination with an antacid increases the viscosity of stomach contents and can protect the oesophageal mucosa from acid reflux. Some alginate-containing preparations form a viscous gel ('raft') that floats on the surface of the stomach contents, thereby reducing symptoms of reflux.

The amount of additional ingredient or antacid in individual preparations varies widely, as does their sodium content, so that preparations may not be freely interchangeable.

ANTACIDS > ALGINATE

Alginic acid   26-Aug-2020

● **INDICATIONS AND DOSE**

GAVISCON INFANT ® POWDER SACHETS

Management of gastro-oesophageal reflux disease

▶ BY MOUTH

▸ Child 1-23 months (body-weight up to 4.5 kg): 1 sachet as required, to be mixed with feeds (or water, for breast-fed infants); maximum 6 sachets per day

▸ Child 1-23 months (body-weight 4.5 kg and above): 2 sachets as required, to be mixed with feeds (or water, for breast-fed infants); maximum 12 sachets per day

● CONTRA-INDICATIONS Intestinal obstruction · preterm neonates · where excessive water loss likely (e.g. fever, diarrhoea, vomiting, high room temperature)

GAVISCON INFANT ® POWDER SACHETS Concurrent use of preparations containing thickening agents

- RENAL IMPAIRMENT In patients with fluid retention, avoid antacids containing large amounts of sodium.

- MEDICINAL FORMS There can be variation in the licensing of different medicines containing the same drug.
Powder
ELECTROLYTES: May contain Sodium
▸ Gaviscon Infant (Forum Health Products Ltd)
Magnesium alginate 87.5 mg, Sodium alginate 225 mg Gaviscon Infant oral powder sachets sugar-free | 30 sachet P £5.32 DT = £5.32

Sodium alginate with potassium bicarbonate

The properties listed below are those particular to the combination only. For the properties of the components please consider, alginic acid p. 74.

- INDICATIONS AND DOSE
Management of mild symptoms of dyspepsia and gastro-oesophageal reflux disease
▶ BY MOUTH USING CHEWABLE TABLETS
▸ Child 6–11 years (under medical advice only): 1 tablet, to be chewed after meals and at bedtime
▸ Child 12–17 years: 1–2 tablets, to be chewed after meals and at bedtime
▸ Adult: 1–2 tablets, to be chewed after meals and at bedtime
▶ BY MOUTH USING ORAL SUSPENSION
▸ Child 2–11 years (under medical advice only): 2.5–5 mL, to be taken after meals and at bedtime
▸ Child 12–17 years: 5–10 mL, to be taken after meals and at bedtime
▸ Adult: 5–10 mL, to be taken after meals and at bedtime

- PRESCRIBING AND DISPENSING INFORMATION Flavours of oral liquid formulations may include aniseed or peppermint.

- MEDICINAL FORMS There can be variation in the licensing of different medicines containing the same drug.
Oral suspension
ELECTROLYTES: May contain Potassium, sodium
▸ Acidex Advance (Wockhardt UK Ltd)
Potassium bicarbonate 20 mg per 1 ml, Sodium alginate 100 mg per 1 ml Acidex Advance oral suspension peppermint sugar-free | 250 ml P £1.92 sugar-free | 500 ml P £3.84 DT = £5.12
Acidex Advance oral suspension aniseed sugar-free | 250 ml P £1.92 sugar-free | 500 ml P £3.84 DT = £5.12
▸ Gaviscon Advance (Reckitt Benckiser Healthcare (UK) Ltd)
Potassium bicarbonate 20 mg per 1 ml, Sodium alginate 100 mg per 1 ml Gaviscon Advance oral suspension aniseed sugar-free | 150 ml P £3.88 sugar-free | 250 ml P £2.56 sugar-free | 300 ml P £6.46 sugar-free | 500 ml P £5.12 DT = £5.12 sugar-free | 600 ml P £10.35
Gaviscon Advance oral suspension peppermint sugar-free | 250 ml P £2.56 sugar-free | 300 ml P £6.46 sugar-free | 500 ml P £5.12 DT = £5.12

Chewable tablet
EXCIPIENTS: May contain Aspartame
ELECTROLYTES: May contain Potassium, sodium
▸ Gaviscon Advance (Reckitt Benckiser Healthcare (UK) Ltd)
Potassium bicarbonate 100 mg, Sodium alginate 500 mg Gaviscon Advance Mint chewable tablets sugar-free | 24 tablet GSL £4.46 sugar-free | 60 tablet GSL £3.07 DT = £3.07

ANTACIDS ⟩ ALUMINIUM AND MAGNESIUM

Co-magaldrox 15-Dec-2020

The properties listed below are those particular to the combination only. For the properties of the components please consider, magnesium hydroxide p. 62.

- INDICATIONS AND DOSE
MAALOX ®
Dyspepsia
▶ BY MOUTH
▸ Child 14–17 years: 10–20 mL, to be taken 20–60 minutes after meals, and at bedtime or when required
▸ Adult: 10–20 mL, to be taken 20–60 minutes after meals, and at bedtime or when required
MUCOGEL ®
Dyspepsia
▶ BY MOUTH
▸ Child 12–17 years: 10–20 mL 3 times a day, to be taken 20–60 minutes after meals, and at bedtime, or when required
▸ Adult: 10–20 mL 3 times a day, to be taken 20–60 minutes after meals, and at bedtime, or when required

- INTERACTIONS → Appendix 1: aluminium hydroxide · magnesium

- SIDE-EFFECTS
▶ **Uncommon** Constipation · diarrhoea
▶ **Rare or very rare** Electrolyte imbalance
▶ **Frequency not known** Abdominal pain · hyperaluminaemia

- RENAL IMPAIRMENT There is a risk of accumulation and aluminium toxicity with antacids containing aluminium salts. Absorption of aluminium from aluminium salts is increased by citrates, which are contained in many effervescent preparations (such as effervescent analgesics).

- PRESCRIBING AND DISPENSING INFORMATION Co-magaldrox is a mixture of aluminium hydroxide and magnesium hydroxide; the proportions are expressed in the form x/y where x and y are the strengths in milligrams per unit dose of magnesium hydroxide and aluminium hydroxide respectively.
MAALOX ® Maalox ® suspension is low in sodium.
MUCOGEL ® Mucogel ® suspension is low in sodium.

- MEDICINAL FORMS There can be variation in the licensing of different medicines containing the same drug.
Oral suspension
▸ Maalox (Sanofi)
Aluminium hydroxide 35 mg per 1 ml, Magnesium hydroxide 40 mg per 1 ml Maalox 175mg/200mg/5ml oral suspension sugar-free | 250 ml GSL £2.33 DT = £2.33
▸ Mucogel (Chemidex Pharma Ltd)
Magnesium hydroxide 39 mg per 1 ml, Aluminium hydroxide gel dried 44 mg per 1 ml Mucogel oral suspension sugar-free | 500 ml GSL £2.99 DT = £2.99

Co-simalcite 17-Apr-2020

- INDICATIONS AND DOSE
Dyspepsia
▶ BY MOUTH
▸ Child 8–11 years: 5 mL, to be taken between meals and at bedtime
▸ Child 12–17 years: 10 mL, to be taken between meals and at bedtime
▸ Adult: 10 mL, to be taken between meals and at bedtime

Gastro-intestinal system

● CONTRA-INDICATIONS Infants · neonates

CONTRA-INDICATIONS, FURTHER INFORMATION
▸ Aluminium-containing antacids Aluminium-containing antacids should not be used in neonates and infants because accumulation may lead to increased plasma-aluminium concentrations.

● RENAL IMPAIRMENT
▸ In adults There is a risk of accumulation and aluminium toxicity with antacids containing aluminium salts. Absorption of aluminium from aluminium salts is increased by citrates, which are contained in many effervescent preparations (such as effervescent analgesics).
▸ In children Aluminium-containing antacids should not be used in children with renal impairment, because accumulation may lead to increased plasma-aluminium concentrations.
Dose adjustments Antacids containing magnesium salts should be avoided or used at a reduced dose because there is an increased risk of toxicity.

● PRESCRIBING AND DISPENSING INFORMATION *Altacite Plus ®* is low in Na⁺.

● MEDICINAL FORMS There can be variation in the licensing of different medicines containing the same drug.

Oral suspension
▸ Altacite Plus (Peckforton Pharmaceuticals Ltd)
Simeticone 25 mg per 1 ml, Hydrotalcite 100 mg per 1 ml Altacite Plus oral suspension sugar-free | 100 ml Ⓟ £4.00 sugar-free | 500 ml Ⓟ £5.20 DT = £5.20

Simeticone with aluminium hydroxide and magnesium hydroxide

04-May-2020

The properties listed below are those particular to the combination only. For the properties of the components please consider, simeticone p. 77.

● **INDICATIONS AND DOSE**

Dyspepsia
▸ BY MOUTH
▸ Child 12–17 years: 5–10 mL 4 times a day, to be taken after meals and at bedtime, or when required
▸ Adult: 5–10 mL 4 times a day, to be taken after meals and at bedtime, or when required

● INTERACTIONS → Appendix 1: aluminium hydroxide · antacids · magnesium

● SIDE-EFFECTS
▸ **Uncommon** Constipation · diarrhoea
▸ **Rare or very rare** Electrolyte imbalance
▸ **Frequency not known** Abdominal pain · hyperaluminaemia

● RENAL IMPAIRMENT There is a risk of accumulation and aluminium toxicity with antacids containing aluminium salts. Absorption of aluminium from aluminium salts is increased by citrates, which are contained in many effervescent preparations (such as effervescent analgesics).

● MEDICINAL FORMS There can be variation in the licensing of different medicines containing the same drug.

Oral suspension
▸ Maalox Plus (Sanofi)
Simeticone 5 mg per 1 ml, Magnesium hydroxide 39 mg per 1 ml, Aluminium hydroxide gel dried 44 mg per 1 ml Maalox Plus oral suspension sugar-free | 250 ml GSL £2.91

ANTACIDS > MAGNESIUM

Magnesium carbonate

● **INDICATIONS AND DOSE**

Dyspepsia
▸ BY MOUTH USING ORAL SUSPENSION
▸ Adult: 10 mL 3 times a day, dose to be taken in water

● CONTRA-INDICATIONS Hypophosphataemia

● INTERACTIONS → Appendix 1: magnesium

● SIDE-EFFECTS Diarrhoea

● HEPATIC IMPAIRMENT In patients with fluid retention, avoid antacids containing large amounts of sodium. Avoid antacids containing magnesium salts in hepatic coma if there is a risk of renal failure.

● RENAL IMPAIRMENT Magnesium carbonate mixture has a high sodium content; avoid in patients with fluid retention.
Dose adjustments Avoid or use at a reduced dose; increased risk of toxicity.

● PRESCRIBING AND DISPENSING INFORMATION When prepared extemporaneously, the BP states Aromatic Magnesium Carbonate Mixture, BP consists of light magnesium carbonate 3%, sodium bicarbonate 5%, in a suitable vehicle containing aromatic cardamom tincture.

● MEDICINAL FORMS No licensed medicines listed.

Magnesium trisilicate

● **INDICATIONS AND DOSE**

Dyspepsia
▸ BY MOUTH USING CHEWABLE TABLETS
▸ Adult: 1–2 tablets as required

● CONTRA-INDICATIONS Hypophosphataemia

● INTERACTIONS → Appendix 1: magnesium

● SIDE-EFFECTS Diarrhoea · nephrolithiasis (long term use)

● HEPATIC IMPAIRMENT Avoid in hepatic coma; risk of renal failure.

● RENAL IMPAIRMENT
Dose adjustments Avoid or used at a reduced dose (increased risk of toxicity).

● MEDICINAL FORMS No licensed medicines listed.

Magnesium trisilicate with magnesium carbonate and sodium bicarbonate

22-Apr-2020

The properties listed below are those particular to the combination only. For the properties of the components please consider, magnesium trisilicate above, magnesium carbonate above, sodium bicarbonate p. 1086.

● **INDICATIONS AND DOSE**

Dyspepsia
▸ BY MOUTH
▸ Child 5–11 years: 5–10 mL 3 times a day, alternatively as required, dose to be made up with water
▸ Child 12–17 years: 10–20 mL 3 times a day, alternatively as required, dose to be made up with water
▸ Adult: 10–20 mL 3 times a day, alternatively as required, dose to be made up with water

● CONTRA-INDICATIONS Hypophosphataemia · Severe renal failure

- CAUTIONS Heart failure · hypermagnesaemia · hypertension · metabolic alkalosis · respiratory alkalosis
- INTERACTIONS → Appendix 1: magnesium · sodium bicarbonate
- HEPATIC IMPAIRMENT In patients with fluid retention avoid antacids containing large amounts of sodium. Avoid antacids containing magnesium salts in hepatic coma if there is a risk of renal failure.
- RENAL IMPAIRMENT Magnesium trisilicate and magnesium carbonate mixtures have high sodium content; avoid in patients with fluid retention.
- PRESCRIBING AND DISPENSING INFORMATION When prepared extemporaneously, the BP states Magnesium Trisilicate Mixture, BP consists of 5% each of magnesium trisilicate, light magnesium carbonate, and sodium bicarbonate in a suitable vehicle with a peppermint flavour.
- MEDICINAL FORMS There can be variation in the licensing of different medicines containing the same drug.

Oral suspension

▸ Magnesium trisilicate with magnesium carbonate and sodium bicarbonate (Non-proprietary)

    Magnesium carbonate light 50 mg per 1 ml, Magnesium trisilicate 50 mg per 1 ml, Sodium bicarbonate 50 mg per 1 ml Magnesium trisilicate oral suspension | 200 ml GSL £1.65 DT = £1.65

ANTIFOAMING DRUGS

Simeticone

                                   05-Jun-2020

(Activated dimeticone)

- DRUG ACTION Simeticone (activated dimeticone) is an antifoaming agent.

- INDICATIONS AND DOSE

DENTINOX®

Colic | Wind pains
▸ BY MOUTH
  ▸ Child 1 month-1 year: 2.5 mL, to be taken with or after each feed; may be added to bottle feed; maximum 6 doses per day

INFACOL®

Colic | Wind pains
▸ BY MOUTH
  ▸ Child 1 month-1 year: 0.5–1 mL, to be taken before feeds

- PRESCRIBING AND DISPENSING INFORMATION

DENTINOX® The brand name *Dentinox*® is also used for other preparations including teething gel.

- PATIENT AND CARER ADVICE

INFACOL® Patients or carers should be given advice on use of the *Infacol*® dropper.

- LESS SUITABLE FOR PRESCRIBING

INFACOL® *Infacol*® is less suitable for prescribing (evidence of benefit in infantile colic uncertain).

DENTINOX® *Dentinox*® colic drops are less suitable for prescribing (evidence of benefit in infantile colic uncertain).

- MEDICINAL FORMS There can be variation in the licensing of different medicines containing the same drug.

Oral suspension

▸ Infacol (Teva UK Ltd)

    Simeticone 40 mg per 1 ml Infacol 40mg/ml oral suspension sugar-free | 55 ml GSL £3.20 DT = £3.20 sugar-free | 85 ml GSL £4.66 DT = £4.66

Oral drops

▸ Dentinox Infant (Dendron Ltd)

    Simeticone 8.4 mg per 1 ml Dentinox Infant colic drops | 100 ml GSL £2.01 DT = £2.01

Combinations available: *Co-simalcite*, p. 75 · *Simeticone with aluminium hydroxide and magnesium hydroxide*, p. 76

4.2 Gastric and duodenal ulceration

Peptic ulcer disease

                                   31-Oct-2019

Description of condition

Peptic ulcer disease includes gastric or duodenal ulceration, which is a breach in the epithelium of the gastric or duodenal mucosa. The main symptom of peptic ulcer disease is upper abdominal pain but other less common symptoms include nausea, indigestion, heartburn, loss of appetite, weight loss and a bloated feeling. Non-steroidal anti-inflammatory drugs p. 1176 (NSAIDs) use and *Helicobacter pylori* (*H. pylori*) infection are the most common causes of peptic ulcer disease. Smoking, alcohol consumption, and stress may also contribute to the development of peptic ulcer disease.

    NSAIDs may have an additive effect if there is co-existent *H. pylori* infection, further increasing the risk of peptic ulceration. The risk of upper gastro-intestinal side-effects varies between individual NSAIDs and is influenced by the dose and duration of use. For recommendations on individual NSAID choice, see under *NSAIDs and gastro-intestinal events* in Non-steroidal anti-inflammatory drugs p. 1176.

    Complications of peptic ulcer disease include gastric outlet obstruction and potentially life-threatening gastro-intestinal perforation and haemorrhage. Patients at high risk of developing gastro-intestinal complications with an NSAID include those with a history of complicated peptic ulcer, or those with more than 2 of the following risk factors:

- age over 65 years;
- high dose NSAIDs;
- other drugs that increase the risk of gastro-intestinal adverse-effects (e.g. anticoagulants, corticosteroids, selective serotonin reuptake inhibitors);
- serious co-morbidity (e.g. cardiovascular disease, hypertension, diabetes, renal or hepatic impairment);
- heavy smoker;
- excessive alcohol consumption;
- previous adverse reaction to NSAIDs;
- prolonged requirement for NSAIDs.

Aims of treatment

The aims of treatment are to promote ulcer healing, manage symptoms, treat *H. pylori* infection if detected and reduce the risk of ulcer complications and recurrence.

Non-drug treatment

EvGr Lifestyle measures, such as healthy eating, weight loss (if obese), avoiding trigger foods, eating smaller meals, eating the evening meal 3–4 hours before going to bed, raising the head of the bed, smoking cessation, and reducing alcohol consumption may improve symptoms. Assess the patient for stress, anxiety, or depression, as these conditions may exacerbate symptoms.

    Urgent endoscopic investigation is required for patients with dysphagia, significant acute gastrointestinal bleeding, or in those aged 55 years and over with unexplained weight loss and symptoms of upper abdominal pain, reflux or dyspepsia. Ⓐ

Initial management

EvGr Drugs that induce peptic ulcers, such as NSAIDs, aspirin, bisphosphonates, immunosuppressive agents (e.g. corticosteroids), potassium chloride, selective serotonin reuptake inhibitors (SSRIs) and recreational drugs such as crack cocaine should be reviewed and stopped, if clinically appropriate. Antacids and/or alginates may be used for short-term symptom control, but long-term, continuous use is not recommended.

The treatment strategy in peptic ulcer disease can vary depending on whether a patient has *H. pylori* infection, or has recently taken NSAIDs.

EvGr The patient should be tested for *H. pylori* infection. Ⓐ See *Testing for Helicobacter pylori* in Helicobacter pylori infection p. 90.

EvGr In patients who have tested positive for *H. pylori* and have no history of NSAID use, Helicobacter pylori infection p. 90 infection should be eradicated.

If the ulcer is associated with NSAID use, a proton pump inhibitor or H$_2$-receptor antagonist should be used for 8 weeks, followed by Helicobacter pylori infection p. 90 eradication treatment if the patient has tested positive for *H. pylori*.

In patients who have tested negative for *H. pylori* and have no history of NSAID use, a proton pump inhibitor or histamine$_2$-receptor antagonist (H$_2$-receptor antagonist) should be used for 4–8 weeks. Ⓐ

Follow-up management

EvGr Patients with peptic ulcers (gastric or duodenal) who tested positive for *H. pylori* should be reviewed 6–8 weeks after starting eradication treatment and re-tested, depending on the size of the lesion. Patients with a gastric ulcer who tested positive for *H. pylori* should also have a repeat endoscopy 6–8 weeks after treatment to confirm ulcer healing, depending on the size of the lesion.

If the ulcer is healed and the patient is to continue taking NSAIDs, the potential harm from NSAID treatment should be discussed. The need for NSAIDs should be reviewed at least every 6 months, and use on a limited, 'as-needed' basis trialled. Consider reducing the dose, substituting the NSAID with paracetamol p. 464, or use of an alternative analgesic or low dose ibuprofen.

In patients with previous ulceration, for whom NSAID continuation is necessary, or those at high risk of gastro-intestinal side effects, consider a cyclo-oxygenase (COX)-2 inhibitor instead of a standard NSAID (but see *Cardiovascular Events* under Non-steroidal anti-inflammatory drugs p. 1176). Gastro-protection with acid suppression therapy should always be co-prescribed. A proton pump inhibitor is the preferred choice for gastro-protection; other options include a H$_2$-receptor antagonist or misoprostol, but the side effects of misoprostol limit its use.

If symptoms recur after initial treatment, a proton pump inhibitor may be taken at the lowest dose possible to control symptoms. Treatment should be used on an 'as-needed' basis with patients managing their own symptoms.

In cases where there are persistent symptoms or an unhealed ulcer, the patient's adherence to initial management should be checked and lifestyle advice reinforced. Other causes, such as malignancy, failure to detect *H. pylori*, inadvertent NSAID use, other ulcer-inducing medication, and rare causes such as Zollinger-Ellison syndrome or Crohn's disease should be considered.

Switching to an alternative acid suppression therapy, e.g. H2-receptor antagonists p. 79 may be beneficial if the response to proton pump inhibitor therapy is inadequate.

Referral to a specialist for investigations and management should occur in refractory or recurrent peptic ulcer cases with gastro-oesophageal symptoms that are unexplained, or non-responsive to treatment.

Patients with peptic ulcer disease who are on long-term treatment should receive an annual review of their symptoms and treatment. A step down approach, or stopping treatment, should be encouraged if possible and clinically appropriate. Ⓐ

Useful Resources

Gastro-oesophageal reflux disease and dyspepsia in adults: investigation and management. National Institute for Health and Care Excellence. NICE guideline 184. September 2014, reviewed October 2019.
www.nice.org.uk/guidance/cg184

ANTACIDS

Bismuth subsalicylate

26-Nov-2019

● **INDICATIONS AND DOSE**

Helicobacter pylori **eradication [in combination with other drugs (see Helicobacter pylori infection p. 90)]**
▸ BY MOUTH
▸ Adult: 525 mg 4 times a day for 7 days for first- and second-line eradication therapy; 10 days for third-line eradication therapy

● **UNLICENSED USE** EvGr Bismuth subsalicylate is used for the eradication of *Helicobacter pylori*, Ⓐ but is not licensed for this indication.

● **CONTRA-INDICATIONS** Children under 16 years (risk of Reye's syndrome)

● **CAUTIONS** Blood clotting disorders · gout

● **INTERACTIONS** → Appendix 1: bismuth

● **SIDE-EFFECTS**
▸ **Common or very common** Black faeces · black tongue

Overdose The main features of salicylate poisoning are hyperventilation, tinnitus, deafness, vasodilatation, and sweating. Bismuth overdose may present as acute encephalopathy with confusion, myoclonus, tremor, dysarthria and gait disturbances. Gastrointestinal disturbances, skin reactions, discolouration of mucous membranes and renal impairment may also be present.

● **ALLERGY AND CROSS-SENSITIVITY** Contra-indicated in patients with a history of hypersensitivity to aspirin or other salicylates.

● **PREGNANCY** Manufacturer advises avoid unless essential—no information available.

● **BREAST FEEDING** Manufacturer advises avoid unless essential—no information available.

● **MEDICINAL FORMS** There can be variation in the licensing of different medicines containing the same drug.

Oral suspension
CAUTIONARY AND ADVISORY LABELS 12
▸ Pepto-Bismol (Procter & Gamble (Health & Beauty Care) Ltd)
 Bismuth subsalicylate 17.5 mg per 1 ml Pepto-Bismol 17.5mg/1ml oral suspension sugar-free | 120 ml Ⓟ 🅢

Chewable tablet
CAUTIONARY AND ADVISORY LABELS 12, 24
▸ Pepto-Bismol (Procter & Gamble (Health & Beauty Care) Ltd)
 Bismuth subsalicylate 262.5 mg Pepto-Bismol 262.5mg chewable tablets sugar-free | 12 tablet Ⓟ 🅢

GASTROPROTECTIVE COMPLEXES AND CHELATORS

Chelates and complexes

Overview

Sucralfate p. 79 may act by protecting the mucosa from acid-pepsin attack in gastric and duodenal ulcers. It is a complex of aluminium hydroxide and sulfated sucrose but has minimal antacid properties.

Sucralfate

16-Nov-2020

● **INDICATIONS AND DOSE**

Benign gastric ulceration | Benign duodenal ulceration

▸ BY MOUTH

▸ Child 15–17 years: 2 g twice daily, dose to be taken on rising and at bedtime, alternatively 1 g 4 times a day for 4–6 weeks, or in resistant cases up to 12 weeks, dose to be taken 1 hour before meals and at bedtime; maximum 8 g per day

▸ Adult: 2 g twice daily, dose to be taken on rising and at bedtime, alternatively 1 g 4 times a day for 4–6 weeks, or in resistant cases up to 12 weeks, dose to be taken 1 hour before meals and at bedtime; maximum 8 g per day

Chronic gastritis

▸ BY MOUTH

▸ Adult: 2 g twice daily, dose to be taken on rising and at bedtime, alternatively 1 g 4 times a day for 4–6 weeks or in resistant cases up to 12 weeks, dose to be taken 1 hour before meals and at bedtime; maximum 8 g per day

Prophylaxis of stress ulceration in child under intensive care

▸ BY MOUTH

▸ Child 15–17 years: 1 g 6 times a day; maximum 8 g per day

Prophylaxis of stress ulceration

▸ BY MOUTH

▸ Adult: 1 g 6 times a day; maximum 8 g per day

● **UNLICENSED USE**

▸ In children Tablets not licensed for prophylaxis of stress ulceration.

● **CAUTIONS** Patients under intensive care (**Important:** reports of bezoar formation)

CAUTIONS, FURTHER INFORMATION

▸ Bezoar formation Following reports of bezoar formation associated with sucralfate, caution is advised in seriously ill patients, especially those receiving concomitant enteral feeds or those with predisposing conditions such as delayed gastric emptying.

● **INTERACTIONS** → Appendix 1: sucralfate

● **SIDE-EFFECTS**

▸ **Common or very common** Constipation

▸ **Uncommon** Dry mouth · nausea

▸ **Rare or very rare** Bezoar · rash

▸ **Frequency not known** Back pain · bone disorders · diarrhoea · dizziness · drowsiness · encephalopathy · flatulence · headache · vertigo

● **PREGNANCY** No evidence of harm; absorption from gastro-intestinal tract negligible.

● **BREAST FEEDING** Amount probably too small to be harmful.

● **RENAL IMPAIRMENT** Use with caution; aluminium is absorbed and may accumulate.

● **DIRECTIONS FOR ADMINISTRATION** Expert sources advise administration of sucralfate and enteral feeds should be separated by 1 hour. ⟨EvGr⟩ For administration by *mouth*, sucralfate should be given 1 hour before meals. ⟨M⟩ *Oral suspension* blocks fine-bore feeding tubes. Expert sources advise crushed *tablets* may be dispersed in water.

● **PRESCRIBING AND DISPENSING INFORMATION** Flavours of oral liquid formulations may include aniseed and caramel.

● **MEDICINAL FORMS** There can be variation in the licensing of different medicines containing the same drug. Forms available from special-order manufacturers include: tablet, oral suspension

Tablet

CAUTIONARY AND ADVISORY LABELS 5

▸ Sucralfate (Imported)

Sucralfate 1 gram Sulcrate 1g tablets | 100 tablet ⟨N⟩ Carafate 1g tablets | 100 tablet ⟨N⟩

Oral suspension

CAUTIONARY AND ADVISORY LABELS 5

▸ Sucralfate (Non-proprietary)

Sucralfate 100 mg per 1 ml Carafate 1g/10ml oral suspension sugar-free | 420 ml ⟨N⟩

Sucralfate 200 mg per 1 ml Sucralfate 1g/5ml oral suspension sugar free sugar-free | 200 ml ⟨PoM⟩ £73.75 DT = £73.75

H₂-RECEPTOR ANTAGONISTS

H₂-receptor antagonists

Overview

Histamine H₂-receptor antagonists heal *gastric and duodenal ulcers* by reducing gastric acid output as a result of histamine H₂-receptor blockade; they are also used to relieve symptoms of *gastro-oesophageal reflux disease*. H₂-receptor antagonists should not normally be used for *Zollinger-Ellison syndrome* because proton pump inhibitors are more effective.

Treatment with a H₂-receptor antagonist has not been shown to be beneficial in haematemesis and melaena, but prophylactic use reduces the frequency of bleeding from *gastroduodenal erosions in hepatic coma*, and possibly in other conditions requiring intensive care. H₂- receptor antagonists also reduce the risk of *acid aspiration* in obstetric patients at delivery (Mendelson's syndrome).

H₂-receptor antagonists

● **CAUTIONS** Signs and symptoms of gastric cancer (in adults)

CAUTIONS, FURTHER INFORMATION

▸ Gastric cancer

▸ In adults H₂-receptor antagonists might mask symptoms of gastric cancer; particular care is required in patients presenting with 'alarm features' in such cases gastric malignancy should be ruled out before treatment.

● **SIDE-EFFECTS**

▸ **Common or very common** Constipation · diarrhoea · dizziness · fatigue · headache · myalgia · skin reactions

▸ **Uncommon** Confusion · depression · erectile dysfunction · gynaecomastia · hallucination · hepatic disorders · leucopenia · nausea · tachycardia

▸ **Rare or very rare** Agranulocytosis · alopecia · arthralgia · atrioventricular block · fever · galactorrhoea · pancytopenia · thrombocytopenia · vasculitis

⌐ above

Cimetidine

13-May-2020

● **INDICATIONS AND DOSE**

Benign duodenal ulceration

▸ BY MOUTH

▸ Adult: 400 mg twice daily for at least 4 weeks, to be taken with breakfast and at night, alternatively 800 mg once daily for at least 4 weeks, to be taken at night; increased if necessary up to 400 mg 4 times a day; maintenance 400 mg once daily, to be taken at night, alternatively maintenance 400 mg twice daily, to be taken in the morning and at night

continued →

Benign gastric ulceration
▸ BY MOUTH
▹ Adult: 400 mg twice daily for 6 weeks, to be taken with breakfast and at night, alternatively 800 mg daily for 6 weeks, to be taken at night; increased if necessary up to 400 mg 4 times a day; maintenance 400 mg once daily, to be taken at night, alternatively maintenance 400 mg twice daily, to be taken in the morning and at night

NSAID-associated ulceration
▸ BY MOUTH
▹ Adult: 400 mg twice daily for 8 weeks, to be taken with breakfast and at night, alternatively 800 mg daily for 8 weeks, to be taken at night; increased if necessary up to 400 mg 4 times a day; maintenance 400 mg daily, to be taken at night, alternatively maintenance 400 mg twice daily, to be taken in the morning and at night

Reflux oesophagitis
▸ BY MOUTH
▹ Adult: 400 mg 4 times a day for 4–8 weeks

Prophylaxis of stress ulceration
▸ BY MOUTH
▹ Adult: 200–400 mg every 4–6 hours

Gastric acid reduction in obstetrics
▸ BY MOUTH
▹ Adult: Initially 400 mg, to be administered at start of labour, then increased if necessary up to 400 mg every 4 hours, do not use syrup in prophylaxis of acid aspiration; maximum 2.4 g per day

Gastric acid reduction during surgical procedures
▸ BY MOUTH
▹ Adult: 400 mg, to be given 90–120 minutes before induction of general anaesthesia

Short-bowel syndrome
▸ BY MOUTH
▹ Adult: 400 mg twice daily, adjusted according to response, to be taken with breakfast and at bedtime

To reduce degradation of pancreatic enzyme supplements
▸ BY MOUTH
▹ Adult: 0.8–1.6 g daily in 4 divided doses, dose to be taken 1–1½ hours before meals

● INTERACTIONS → Appendix 1: H2 receptor antagonists
● SIDE-EFFECTS
▸ Rare or very rare Anaphylactic reaction · aplastic anaemia · nephritis tubulointerstitial · pancreatitis · sinus bradycardia
● PREGNANCY Manufacturer advises avoid unless essential.
● BREAST FEEDING Significant amount present in milk—not known to be harmful but manufacturer advises avoid.
● HEPATIC IMPAIRMENT Increased risk of confusion.
  Dose adjustments Reduce dose.
● RENAL IMPAIRMENT Occasional risk of confusion.
  Dose adjustments Reduce dose to 200 mg 4 times daily if eGFR 30–50 mL/minute/1.73 m^2.
  Reduce dose to 200 mg 3 times daily if eGFR 15–30 mL/minute/1.73 m^2.
  Reduce dose to 200 mg twice daily if eGFR less than 15 mL/minute/1.73 m^2.
● EXCEPTIONS TO LEGAL CATEGORY Cimetidine can be sold to the public for adults and children over 16 years (provided packs do not contain more than 2 weeks' supply) for the short-term symptomatic relief of heartburn, dyspepsia, and hyperacidity (max. single dose 200 mg, max. daily dose 800 mg), and for the prophylactic management of nocturnal heartburn (single night-time dose 100 mg).

● MEDICINAL FORMS There can be variation in the licensing of different medicines containing the same drug. Forms available from special-order manufacturers include: oral suspension

Oral solution
EXCIPIENTS: May contain Propylene glycol
▹ Cimetidine (Non-proprietary)
  Cimetidine 40 mg per 1 ml Cimetidine 200mg/5ml oral solution sugar free sugar-free | 300 ml [PoM] £34.17 DT = £34.17
▹ Tagamet (Essential Pharma Ltd)
  Cimetidine 40 mg per 1 ml Tagamet 200mg/5ml syrup | 600 ml [PoM] £28.49 DT = £28.49

Tablet
▹ Cimetidine (Non-proprietary)
  Cimetidine 200 mg Cimetidine 200mg tablets | 60 tablet [PoM] £40.00 DT = £18.52
  Cimetidine 400 mg Cimetidine 400mg tablets | 60 tablet [PoM] £17.84 DT = £15.91
  Cimetidine 800 mg Cimetidine 800mg tablets | 30 tablet [PoM] £21.25 DT = £21.25

▶ 79

Famotidine

13-May-2020

● INDICATIONS AND DOSE
Treatment of benign gastric and duodenal ulceration
▸ BY MOUTH
▹ Adult: 40 mg once daily for 4–8 weeks, dose to be taken at night

Maintenance treatment of duodenal ulceration
▸ BY MOUTH
▹ Adult: 20 mg once daily, dose to be taken at night

Reflux oesophagitis
▸ BY MOUTH
▹ Adult: 20–40 mg twice daily for 6–12 weeks; maintenance 20 mg twice daily

● INTERACTIONS → Appendix 1: H2 receptor antagonists
● SIDE-EFFECTS
▸ Uncommon Appetite decreased · dry mouth · taste altered · vomiting
▸ Rare or very rare Anxiety · chest tightness · drowsiness · insomnia · interstitial pneumonia · libido decreased · muscle cramps · neutropenia · paraesthesia · psychiatric disorder · seizures · severe cutaneous adverse reactions (SCARs)
● PREGNANCY Manufacturer advises avoid unless potential benefit outweighs risk.
● BREAST FEEDING Present in milk—not known to be harmful but manufacturer advises avoid.
● RENAL IMPAIRMENT Seizures reported very rarely.
  Dose adjustments Use normal dose every 36–48 hours or use half normal dose if eGFR less than 50 mL/minute/1.73 m^2.
● EXCEPTIONS TO LEGAL CATEGORY Famotidine can be sold to the public for adults and children over 16 years (provided packs do not contain more than 2 weeks' supply) for the short-term symptomatic relief of heartburn, dyspepsia, and hyperacidity, and for the prevention of these symptoms when associated with consumption of food or drink including when they cause sleep disturbance (max. single dose 10 mg, max. daily dose 20 mg).

● MEDICINAL FORMS There can be variation in the licensing of different medicines containing the same drug.
Tablet
▹ Famotidine (Non-proprietary)
  Famotidine 20 mg Famotidine 20mg tablets | 28 tablet [PoM] £22.50 DT = £22.20
  Famotidine 40 mg Famotidine 40mg tablets | 28 tablet [PoM] £39.00 DT = £38.99

Nizatidine

⚑ 79

13-May-2020

- ● **INDICATIONS AND DOSE**

Benign gastric, duodenal or NSAID-associated ulceration
- ▶ BY MOUTH
  - ‣ Adult: 300 mg once daily for 4–8 weeks, dose to be taken in the evening, alternatively 150 mg twice daily for 4–8 weeks; maintenance 150 mg once daily, dose to be taken at night

Gastro-oesophageal reflux disease
- ▶ BY MOUTH
  - ‣ Adult: 150–300 mg twice daily for up to 12 weeks

- ● INTERACTIONS → Appendix 1: H2 receptor antagonists
- ● SIDE-EFFECTS
- ▶ **Rare or very rare** Anaemia · hyperuricaemia · serum sickness
- ▶ **Frequency not known** Hyperhidrosis
- ● PREGNANCY Manufacturer advises avoid unless essential.
- ● BREAST FEEDING Amount too small to be harmful.
- ● HEPATIC IMPAIRMENT Manufacturer advises caution.
- ● RENAL IMPAIRMENT
  Dose adjustments Use half normal dose if eGFR 20–50 mL/minute/1.73 m^2.
  Use one-quarter normal dose if eGFR less than 20 mL/minute/1.73 m^2.
- ● EXCEPTIONS TO LEGAL CATEGORY Nizatidine can be sold to the public for the prevention and treatment of symptoms of food-related heartburn and meal-induced indigestion in adults and children over 16 years; max. single dose 75 mg, max. daily dose 150 mg for max. 14 days.

- ● MEDICINAL FORMS There can be variation in the licensing of different medicines containing the same drug. Forms available from special-order manufacturers include: oral suspension, oral solution
  Capsule
  - ‣ Nizatidine (Non-proprietary)
    Nizatidine 150 mg Nizatidine 150mg capsules | 30 capsule PoM
    £18.00 DT = £7.59
    Nizatidine 300 mg Nizatidine 300mg capsules | 30 capsule PoM
    £19.50 DT = £18.89

Ranitidine

⚑ 79

11-Aug-2020

- ● **INDICATIONS AND DOSE**

Benign gastric ulceration | Duodenal ulceration
- ▶ BY MOUTH
  - ‣ Child 1–5 months: 1 mg/kg 3 times a day (max. per dose 3 mg/kg 3 times a day)
  - ‣ Child 6 months–2 years: 2–4 mg/kg twice daily
  - ‣ Child 3–11 years: 2–4 mg/kg twice daily (max. per dose 150 mg)
  - ‣ Child 12–17 years: 150 mg twice daily, alternatively 300 mg once daily, dose to be taken at night
  - ‣ Adult: 150 mg twice daily for 4–8 weeks, alternatively 300 mg once daily for 4–8 weeks, dose to be taken at night

Chronic episodic dyspepsia
- ▶ BY MOUTH
  - ‣ Adult: 150 mg twice daily for 6 weeks, alternatively 300 mg once daily for 6 weeks, dose to be taken at night

NSAID-associated gastric ulceration
- ▶ BY MOUTH
  - ‣ Adult: 150 mg twice daily for up to 8 weeks, alternatively 300 mg once daily for up to 8 weeks, dose to be taken at night

NSAID-associated duodenal ulcer
- ▶ BY MOUTH
  - ‣ Adult: 300 mg twice daily for 4 weeks, to achieve a higher healing rate

Prophylaxis of NSAID-associated gastric ulcer |
Prophylaxis of NSAID-associated duodenal ulcer
- ▶ BY MOUTH
  - ‣ Adult: 300 mg twice daily

Gastro-oesophageal reflux disease
- ▶ BY MOUTH
  - ‣ Adult: 150 mg twice daily for up to 8 weeks or if necessary 12 weeks, alternatively 300 mg once daily for up to 8 weeks or if necessary 12 weeks, dose to be taken at night

Moderate to severe gastro-oesophageal reflux disease
- ▶ BY MOUTH
  - ‣ Adult: 600 mg daily in 2–4 divided doses for up to 12 weeks

Long-term treatment of healed gastro-oesophageal reflux disease
- ▶ BY MOUTH
  - ‣ Adult: 150 mg twice daily

Gastric acid reduction (prophylaxis of acid aspiration) in obstetrics
- ▶ BY MOUTH
  - ‣ Adult: 150 mg, dose to be given at onset of labour, then 150 mg every 6 hours

Gastric acid reduction (prophylaxis of acid aspiration) in surgical procedures
- ▶ INITIALLY BY INTRAMUSCULAR INJECTION, OR BY SLOW INTRAVENOUS INJECTION
  - ‣ Adult: 50 mg, to be given 45–60 minutes before induction of anaesthesia, intravenous injection diluted to 20 mL and given over at least 2 minutes, alternatively (by mouth) 150 mg, to be given 2 hours before induction of anaesthesia and also when possible on the preceding evening

Prophylaxis of stress ulceration
- ▶ INITIALLY BY SLOW INTRAVENOUS INJECTION
  - ‣ Adult: 50 mg every 8 hours, dose to be diluted to 20 mL and given over at least 2 minutes, then (by mouth) 150 mg twice daily, may be given when oral feeding commences

Reflux oesophagitis and other conditions where gastric acid reduction is beneficial
- ▶ BY MOUTH
  - ‣ Child 1–5 months: 1 mg/kg 3 times a day (max. per dose 3 mg/kg 3 times a day)
  - ‣ Child 6 months–2 years: 2–4 mg/kg twice daily
  - ‣ Child 3–11 years: 2–4 mg/kg twice daily (max. per dose 150 mg); increased to up to 5 mg/kg twice daily (max. per dose 300 mg), dose increase for severe gastro-oesophageal disease
  - ‣ Child 12–17 years: 150 mg twice daily, alternatively 300 mg once daily, dose to be taken at night, then increased if necessary to 300 mg twice daily for up to 12 weeks in moderate to severe gastro-oesophageal reflux disease, alternatively increased if necessary to 150 mg 4 times a day for up to 12 weeks in moderate to severe gastro-oesophageal reflux disease

Conditions where reduction of gastric acidity is beneficial and oral route not available
- ▶ BY INTRAMUSCULAR INJECTION
  - ‣ Adult: 50 mg every 6–8 hours
- ▶ BY SLOW INTRAVENOUS INJECTION
  - ‣ Adult: 50 mg, dose to be diluted to 20 mL and given over at least 2 minutes; may be repeated every 6–8 hours

1

Gastro-intestinal system

● UNLICENSED USE
▸ In children *Oral* preparations not licensed for use in children under 3 years.
▸ In adults Doses given for prophylaxis of NSAID-associated gastric or duodenal ulcer, and prophylaxis of stress ulceration, are not licensed.

● INTERACTIONS → Appendix 1: H2 receptor antagonists

● SIDE-EFFECTS

GENERAL SIDE-EFFECTS
▸ **Rare or very rare** Bone marrow depression · bradycardia · breast conditions · dyskinesia · nephritis acute interstitial · pancreatitis acute · vision blurred
▸ **Frequency not known** Dyspnoea

SPECIFIC SIDE-EFFECTS
▸ **Rare or very rare**
▸ With parenteral use Anaphylactic shock · cardiac arrest

● PREGNANCY Manufacturer advises avoid unless essential, but not known to be harmful.

● BREAST FEEDING Significant amount present in milk, but not known to be harmful.

● RENAL IMPAIRMENT
Dose adjustments ▸ In adults Use half normal dose if egFR less than 50 mL/minute/1.73 m².
▸ In children Use half normal dose if estimated glomerular filtration rate less than 50 mL/minute/1.73 m².

● DIRECTIONS FOR ADMINISTRATION For *intravenous infusion* (*Zantac*®), manufacturer advises give intermittently in Glucose 5% or Sodium Chloride 0.9%.

● PATIENT AND CARER ADVICE In fat malabsorption syndrome, give oral doses 1–2 hours before food to enhance effects of pancreatic enzyme replacement.
Medicines for Children leaflet: Ranitidine for acid reflux www.medicinesforchildren.org.uk/ranitidine-acid-reflux

● EXCEPTIONS TO LEGAL CATEGORY Ranitidine can be sold to the public for adults and children over 16 years (provided packs do not contain more than 2 weeks' supply) for the short-term symptomatic relief of heartburn, dyspepsia, and hyperacidity, and for the prevention of these symptoms when associated with consumption of food or drink (max. single dose 75 mg, max. daily dose 300 mg).

● MEDICINAL FORMS There can be variation in the licensing of different medicines containing the same drug. Forms available from special-order manufacturers include: oral suspension, oral solution, infusion

Tablet
▸ Ranitidine (Non-proprietary)
Ranitidine (as Ranitidine hydrochloride) 75 mg Ranitidine 75mg tablets | 12 tablet GSL £0.30–£0.80
Ranitidine (as Ranitidine hydrochloride) 150 mg Ranitidine 150mg tablets | 60 tablet PoM £0.90–£1.09
Ranitidine (as Ranitidine hydrochloride) 300 mg Ranitidine 300mg tablets | 30 tablet PoM £0.90–£1.07
▸ Gavilast (Reckitt Benckiser Healthcare (UK) Ltd)
Ranitidine (as Ranitidine hydrochloride) 75 mg Gavilast 75mg tablets | 12 tablet GSL £2.79
▸ Ranicalm (Bristol Laboratories Ltd)
Ranitidine (as Ranitidine hydrochloride) 75 mg Ranicalm 75mg tablets | 12 tablet GSL £2.25
Solution for injection
▸ Ranitidine (Non-proprietary)
Ranitidine (as Ranitidine hydrochloride) 25 mg per 1 ml Ranitidine 50mg/2ml solution for injection ampoules | 5 ampoule PoM £2.69 DT = £3.99
Effervescent tablet
CAUTIONARY AND ADVISORY LABELS 13
ELECTROLYTES: May contain Sodium
▸ Ranitidine (Non-proprietary)
Ranitidine (as Ranitidine hydrochloride) 150 mg Ranitidine 150mg effervescent tablets | 60 tablet PoM £35.00 DT = £35.00
Ranitidine (as Ranitidine hydrochloride) 300 mg Ranitidine 300mg effervescent tablets | 30 tablet PoM £35.00 DT = £35.00

Oral solution
EXCIPIENTS: May contain Alcohol
▸ Ranitidine (Non-proprietary)
Ranitidine (as Ranitidine hydrochloride) 15 mg per 1 ml Ranitidine 75mg/5ml oral solution sugar free sugar-free | 300 ml PoM £21.55 DT = £4.22

PROSTAGLANDINS AND ANALOGUES

Misoprostol
20-Apr-2020

● DRUG ACTION Misoprostol is a synthetic prostaglandin analogue that has antisecretory and protective properties, promoting healing of gastric and duodenal ulcers.

● INDICATIONS AND DOSE

CYTOTEC ®

Benign gastric ulcer | Benign duodenal ulcer | NSAID-induced peptic ulcer
▸ BY MOUTH
▸ Adult: 400 micrograms twice daily, alternatively 200 micrograms 4 times a day continued for at least 4 weeks or may be continued for up to 8 weeks if required, dose to be taken with breakfast (or main meals) and at bedtime

Prophylaxis of NSAID-induced peptic ulcer
▸ BY MOUTH
▸ Adult: 200 micrograms 2–4 times a day

● CAUTIONS

CYTOTEC ® Conditions where hypotension might precipitate severe complications (e.g. cerebrovascular disease, cardiovascular disease) · conditions which predispose to diarrhoea (e.g. inflammatory bowel disease)

● SIDE-EFFECTS

GENERAL SIDE-EFFECTS
▸ **Common or very common** Nausea · rash · vomiting
▸ **Uncommon** Uterine rupture

SPECIFIC SIDE-EFFECTS
▸ **Common or very common** Constipation · diarrhoea · dizziness · flatulence · gastrointestinal discomfort · headache
▸ **Uncommon** Fever · haemorrhage · menstrual cycle irregularities · postmenopausal haemorrhage · uterine cramps
▸ **Frequency not known** Chills

SIDE-EFFECTS, FURTHER INFORMATION Diarrhoea may occasionally be severe and require withdrawal, reduced by giving single doses not exceeding 200 micrograms and by avoiding magnesium-containing antacids.

● CONCEPTION AND CONTRACEPTION

CYTOTEC ® Manufacturer advises do not use in women of childbearing potential unless pregnancy has been excluded; patients must use effective contraception during treatment, and be informed of the risks of taking misoprostol if pregnant.

● PREGNANCY

CYTOTEC ® Manufacturer advises avoid—induces uterine contractions, and associated with abortion and birth defects; teratogenic in first trimester.

● BREAST FEEDING Manufacturer advises avoid—present in milk, and may cause diarrhoea in nursing infants. EvGr Tertiary sources state present in milk but amount probably too small to be harmful; to further reduce risk following termination of pregnancy, consider interrupting breastfeeding for 5 hours after a dose. ◈

● PATIENT AND CARER ADVICE
Driving and skilled tasks Manufacturer advises patients should be cautioned on the effects on driving and performance of skilled tasks—increased risk of dizziness.

- MEDICINAL FORMS There can be variation in the licensing of different medicines containing the same drug.

Tablet
CAUTIONARY AND ADVISORY LABELS 21
- Cytotec (Pfizer Ltd)
  Misoprostol 200 microgram Cytotec 200microgram tablets | 60 tablet PoM £10.03 DT = £10.03

PROTON PUMP INHIBITORS

Proton pump inhibitors

Overview

Proton pump inhibitors are effective short-term treatments for *gastric* and *duodenal ulcers*; they are also used in combination with antibacterials for the eradication of *Helicobacter pylori* (see specific regimens). Following endoscopic treatment of severe peptic ulcer bleeding, an intravenous, high-dose proton pump inhibitor reduces the risk of rebleeding and the need for surgery. Proton pump inhibitors can be used for the treatment of *dyspepsia* and *gastro-oesophageal reflux disease*.

Proton pump inhibitors are also used for the prevention and treatment of NSAID-associated ulcers. In patients who need to continue NSAID treatment after an ulcer has healed, the dose of proton pump inhibitor should normally not be reduced because asymptomatic ulcer deterioration may occur.

A proton pump inhibitor can be used to reduce the degradation of pancreatic enzyme supplements in patients with cystic fibrosis. They can also be used to control excessive secretion of gastric acid in *Zollinger–Ellison syndrome*; high doses are often required.

Proton pump inhibitors   🄿

- DRUG ACTION Proton pump inhibitors inhibit gastric acid secretion by blocking the hydrogen-potassium adenosine triphosphatase enzyme system (the 'proton pump') of the gastric parietal cell.

> **IMPORTANT SAFETY INFORMATION**
>
> MHRA ADVICE: PROTON PUMP INHIBITORS (PPIS): VERY LOW RISK OF SUBACUTE CUTANEOUS LUPUS ERYTHEMATOSUS (SEPTEMBER 2015)
>
> Very infrequent cases of subacute cutaneous lupus erythematosus (SCLE) have been reported in patients taking PPIs. Drug-induced SCLE can occur weeks, months or even years after exposure to the drug.
>
> If a patient treated with a PPI develops lesions—especially in sun-exposed areas of the skin—and it is accompanied by arthralgia:
> - advise them to avoid exposing the skin to sunlight;
> - consider SCLE as a possible diagnosis;
> - consider discontinuing PPI treatment unless it is imperative for a serious acid-related condition; a patient who develops SCLE with a particular PPI may be at risk of the same reaction with another;
> - in most cases, symptoms resolve on PPI withdrawal; topical or systemic steroids might be necessary for treatment of SCLE only if there are no signs of remission after a few weeks or months.

- CAUTIONS Can increase the risk of fractures (particularly when used at high doses for over a year in the elderly) · may increase the risk of gastro-intestinal infections (including *Clostridioides difficile* infection) · may mask the symptoms of gastric cancer (in adults) · patients at risk of osteoporosis

CAUTIONS, FURTHER INFORMATION
- Risk of osteoporosis Patients at risk of osteoporosis should maintain an adequate intake of calcium and vitamin D, and if necessary, receive other preventative therapy.
- Gastric cancer
- In adults Particular care is required in those presenting with 'alarm features', in such cases gastric malignancy should be ruled out before treatment.
- Elderly Prescription potentially inappropriate (STOPP criteria) for uncomplicated peptic ulcer disease or erosive peptic oesophagitis at full therapeutic dosage for longer than 8 weeks (dose reduction or earlier discontinuation indicated). See also Prescribing in the elderly p. 33.

- SIDE-EFFECTS
- **Common or very common** Abdominal pain · constipation · diarrhoea · dizziness · dry mouth · gastrointestinal disorders · headache · insomnia · nausea · skin reactions · vomiting
- **Uncommon** Arthralgia · bone fractures · confusion · depression · drowsiness · leucopenia · malaise · myalgia · paraesthesia · peripheral oedema · thrombocytopenia · vertigo · vision disorders
- **Rare or very rare** Agranulocytosis · alopecia · gynaecomastia · hallucination · hepatic disorders · hyperhidrosis · hyponatraemia · nephritis tubulointerstitial · pancytopenia · photosensitivity reaction · severe cutaneous adverse reactions (SCARs) · stomatitis · taste altered
- **Frequency not known** Hypomagnesaemia (more common after 1 year of treatment, but sometimes after 3 months of treatment) · subacute cutaneous lupus erythematosus

- MONITORING REQUIREMENTS Measurement of serum-magnesium concentrations should be considered before and during prolonged treatment with a proton pump inhibitor, especially when used with other drugs that cause hypomagnesaemia or with digoxin.

- PRESCRIBING AND DISPENSING INFORMATION A proton pump inhibitor should be prescribed for appropriate indications at the lowest effective dose for the shortest period; the need for long-term treatment should be reviewed periodically.

🄵 above

Esomeprazole   24-Nov-2020

- INDICATIONS AND DOSE

Peptic ulcer disease
- BY MOUTH
  - Adult: 20 mg once daily for 4–8 weeks

NSAID-associated gastric ulcer
- BY MOUTH
  - Adult: 20 mg once daily for 4–8 weeks
- BY INTRAVENOUS INJECTION, OR BY INTRAVENOUS INFUSION
  - Adult: 20 mg daily continue until oral administration possible, injection to be given over at least 3 minutes

Prophylaxis of NSAID-associated gastric ulcer in patients with an increased risk of gastroduodenal complications who require continued NSAID treatment
- BY MOUTH
  - Adult: 20 mg daily

Prophylaxis of NSAID-associated gastric or duodenal ulcer
- BY INTRAVENOUS INJECTION, OR BY INTRAVENOUS INFUSION
  - Adult: 20 mg daily continue until oral administration possible, injection to be given over at least 3 minutes

Gastro-oesophageal reflux disease (in the presence of erosive reflux oesophagitis)
- BY MOUTH
  - Child 1–11 years (body-weight 10–19 kg): 10 mg once daily for 8 weeks

continued →

▸ Child 1-11 years (body-weight 20 kg and above): 10–20 mg once daily for 8 weeks
▸ Child 12-17 years: Initially 40 mg once daily for 4 weeks, continued for further 4 weeks if not fully healed or symptoms persist; maintenance 20 mg daily
▸ BY INTRAVENOUS INJECTION, OR BY INTRAVENOUS INFUSION
▸ Adult: 40 mg daily continue until oral administration possible, injection to be given over at least 3 minutes

Severe oesophagitis
▸ BY MOUTH
▸ Adult: 40 mg once daily for 8 weeks, continue as maintenance treatment if appropriate

Severe oesophagitis, refractory to initial treatment
▸ BY MOUTH
▸ Adult: 40 mg twice daily

Gastro-oesophageal reflux disease (in the absence of oesophagitis)
▸ BY MOUTH
▸ Child 1-11 years (body-weight 10 kg and above): 10 mg once daily for up to 8 weeks
▸ Child 12-17 years: 20 mg once daily for up to 4 weeks
▸ Adult: 20 mg once daily 4 or 8 weeks, then 20 mg daily if required
▸ BY INTRAVENOUS INJECTION, OR BY INTRAVENOUS INFUSION
▸ Adult: 20 mg once daily continue until oral administration is possible, injection to be given over at least 3 minutes

Uninvestigated dyspepsia
▸ BY MOUTH
▸ Adult: 20 mg once daily for 4 weeks

Zollinger–Ellison syndrome
▸ BY MOUTH
▸ Adult: Initially 40 mg twice daily, adjusted according to response; usual dose 80–160 mg daily, daily doses above 80 mg should be given in 2 divided doses

Severe peptic ulcer bleeding (following endoscopic treatment)
▸ INITIALLY BY INTRAVENOUS INFUSION
▸ Adult: Initially 80 mg, to be given over 30 minutes, then (by continuous intravenous infusion) 8 mg/hour for 72 hours, then (by mouth) 40 mg once daily for 4 weeks

Helicobacter pylori **eradication [in combination with other drugs (see Helicobacter pylori infection p. 90)]**
▸ BY MOUTH
▸ Adult: 20 mg twice daily for 7 days for first- and second-line eradication therapy; 10 days for third-line eradication therapy

● UNLICENSED USE
▸ In adults EvGr Combination regimens and durations for *Helicobacter pylori* eradication may differ from product literature but adhere to national guidelines. ⒶSee Helicobacter pylori infection p. 90 for further information. Esomeprazole may be used as detailed below, although these situations are considered outside the scope of its licence:
● EvGr treatment of peptic ulcer disease, Ⓐ see Peptic ulcer disease p. 77 for further information;
● EvGr treatment of severe oesophagitis, refractory to initial treatment, Ⓐ see Gastro-oesophageal reflux disease p. 89 for further information;
● EvGr treatment of uninvestigated dyspepsia, Ⓐ see Dyspepsia p. 73 for further information.
▸ With oral use in adults EvGr Duration of treatment of gastro-oesophageal reflux disease (in the absence of oesophagitis) differs from product literature but adheres to national guidelines. Ⓐ See Gastro-oesophageal reflux disease p. 89 for further information.

● INTERACTIONS → Appendix 1: proton pump inhibitors

● SIDE-EFFECTS
GENERAL SIDE-EFFECTS
▸ **Uncommon** Encephalopathy
▸ **Rare or very rare** Aggression · agitation · bronchospasm · increased risk of infection · muscle weakness
SPECIFIC SIDE-EFFECTS
▸ **Rare or very rare**
▸ With parenteral use Renal failure
▸ **Frequency not known**
▸ With parenteral use Electrolyte imbalance · vitamin B12 deficiency

● PREGNANCY Manufacturer advises caution—no information available.

● BREAST FEEDING Manufacturer advises avoid—no information available.

● HEPATIC IMPAIRMENT Manufacturer advises caution in severe impairment.
Dose adjustments ▸ With oral use in adults Manufacturer advises max. 20 mg daily in severe impairment.
▸ With intravenous use in adults Manufacturer advises for gastro-oesophageal reflux disease, max. 20 mg daily in severe impairment.
▸ With intravenous use in adults Manufacturer advises for bleeding ulcers, by intravenous infusion, initially 80 mg, then 4 mg/hour for 72 hours in severe impairment.
▸ In children Manufacturer advises in children 1–11 years, max. 10 mg daily in severe impairment. Manufacturer advises in children 12–17 years, max. 20 mg daily in severe impairment.

● RENAL IMPAIRMENT Manufacturer advises caution in severe renal insufficiency.

● DIRECTIONS FOR ADMINISTRATION
▸ With intravenous use For *intravenous infusion* (*Nexium* ®), give continuously *or* intermittently in Sodium Chloride 0.9%; reconstitute 40–80 mg with up to 100 ml infusion fluid; for intermittent infusion, give requisite dose over 10–30 minutes; stable for 12 hours in Sodium Chloride 0.9%.
▸ With oral use EvGr Do not chew or crush capsules; swallow whole *or* mix capsule contents in water and drink within 30 minutes. Do not crush or chew tablets; swallow whole *or* disperse in water and drink within 30 minutes. Disperse the contents of each sachet of gastro-resistant granules in approx. 15 mL water. Stir and leave to thicken for a few minutes; stir again before administration and use within 30 minutes; rinse container with 15 mL water to obtain full dose. ⓂFor administration through a gastric tube, consult product literature.

● PATIENT AND CARER ADVICE
▸ With oral use Counselling on administration of gastro-resistant capsules, tablets, and granules advised.

● MEDICINAL FORMS There can be variation in the licensing of different medicines containing the same drug. Forms available from special-order manufacturers include: oral suspension
Gastro-resistant capsule
▸ Esomeprazole (Non-proprietary)
Esomeprazole (as Esomeprazole magnesium dihydrate)
20 mg Esomeprazole 20mg gastro-resistant capsules |
28 capsule [PoM] £12.95 DT = £3.09
Esomeprazole (as Esomeprazole magnesium dihydrate)
40 mg Esomeprazole 40mg gastro-resistant capsules |
28 capsule [PoM] £17.63 DT = £2.80
▸ Emozul (Consilient Health Ltd)
Esomeprazole (as Esomeprazole magnesium dihydrate)
20 mg Emozul 20mg gastro-resistant capsules | 28 capsule [PoM] £5.30 DT = £3.09
Esomeprazole (as Esomeprazole magnesium dihydrate)
40 mg Emozul 40mg gastro-resistant capsules | 28 capsule [PoM] £6.37 DT = £2.80

▹ Ventra (Ethypharm UK Ltd)
Esomeprazole (as Esomeprazole magnesium dihydrate)
20 mg Ventra 20mg gastro-resistant capsules | 28 capsule PoM
£2.55 DT = £3.09
Esomeprazole (as Esomeprazole magnesium dihydrate)
40 mg Ventra 40mg gastro-resistant capsules | 28 capsule PoM
£2.97 DT = £2.80

Gastro-resistant tablet
▹ Esomeprazole (Non-proprietary)
Esomeprazole 20 mg Esomeprazole 20mg gastro-resistant tablets |
28 tablet PoM £18.50 DT = £2.83
Esomeprazole 40 mg Esomeprazole 40mg gastro-resistant tablets |
28 tablet PoM £25.19 DT = £3.70
▹ Nexium (Grunenthal Ltd, GlaxoSmithKline Consumer Healthcare)
Esomeprazole 20 mg Nexium 20mg gastro-resistant tablets |
28 tablet PoM £18.50 DT = £2.83
Esomeprazole 40 mg Nexium 40mg gastro-resistant tablets |
28 tablet PoM £25.19 DT = £3.70

Powder for solution for injection
▹ Esomeprazole (Non-proprietary)
Esomeprazole (as Esomeprazole sodium) 40 mg Esomeprazole
40mg powder for solution for injection vials | 1 vial PoM £3.07-£3.13
(Hospital only)
▹ Nexium (Grunenthal Ltd)
Esomeprazole (as Esomeprazole sodium) 40 mg Nexium I.V 40mg
powder for solution for injection vials | 10 vial PoM £42.50 (Hospital
only)

Gastro-resistant granules
CAUTIONARY AND ADVISORY LABELS 25
▹ Nexium (Grunenthal Ltd)
Esomeprazole (as Esomeprazole magnesium trihydrate)
10 mg Nexium 10mg gastro-resistant granules sachets |
28 sachet PoM £25.19 DT = £25.19

▶ 83

Lansoprazole
14-Aug-2020

● **INDICATIONS AND DOSE**

Helicobacter pylori eradication [in combination with other drugs (see Helicobacter pylori infection p. 90)]
▸ BY MOUTH
▹ **Adult:** 30 mg twice daily for 7 days for first- and second-line eradication therapy; 10 days for third-line eradication therapy

Benign gastric ulcer
▸ BY MOUTH
▹ **Adult:** 30 mg once daily for 8 weeks, dose to be taken in the morning

Duodenal ulcer
▸ BY MOUTH
▹ **Adult:** 30 mg once daily for 4 weeks, dose to be taken in the morning; maintenance 15 mg once daily

NSAID-associated duodenal ulcer | NSAID-associated gastric ulcer
▸ BY MOUTH
▹ **Adult:** 30 mg once daily for 4 weeks, continued for further 4 weeks if not fully healed

Prophylaxis of NSAID-associated duodenal ulcer | Prophylaxis of NSAID-associated gastric ulcer
▸ BY MOUTH
▹ **Adult:** 15-30 mg once daily

Zollinger-Ellison syndrome (and other hypersecretory conditions)
▸ BY MOUTH
▹ **Adult:** Initially 60 mg once daily, adjusted according to response, daily doses of 120 mg or more given in two divided doses

Gastro-oesophageal reflux disease
▸ BY MOUTH
▹ **Adult:** 30 mg once daily for 4 weeks, continued for further 4 weeks if not fully healed; maintenance 15-30 mg once daily, doses to be taken in the morning

Severe oesophagitis
▸ BY MOUTH
▹ **Adult:** 30 mg once daily for 8 weeks, continue as maintenance treatment if appropriate

Severe oesophagitis, refractory to initial treatment
▸ BY MOUTH
▹ **Adult:** 30 mg twice daily

Functional dyspepsia
▸ BY MOUTH
▹ **Adult:** 15 mg once daily for 4 weeks

Uninvestigated dyspepsia
▸ BY MOUTH
▹ **Adult:** 30 mg once daily for 4 weeks

● UNLICENSED USE Lansoprazole doses in BNF may differ from those in product literature. Lansoprazole may be used as detailed below, although these situations are considered outside the scope of its licence:
  ● EvGr treatment of severe oesophagitis, refractory to initial treatment, Ⓐ see Gastro-oesophageal reflux disease p. 89 for further information;
  ● EvGr treatment of functional and uninvestigated dyspepsia, Ⓐ see Dyspepsia p. 73 for further information.

● INTERACTIONS → Appendix 1: proton pump inhibitors

● SIDE-EFFECTS
▸ **Common or very common** Dry throat · fatigue
▸ **Uncommon** Eosinophilia · oedema
▸ **Rare or very rare** Anaemia · angioedema · appetite decreased · erectile dysfunction · fever · glossitis · oesophageal candidiasis · pancreatitis · restlessness · tremor

● PREGNANCY Manufacturer advises avoid.

● BREAST FEEDING Avoid—present in milk in *animal* studies.

● HEPATIC IMPAIRMENT Manufacturer advises caution in moderate to severe impairment (risk of increased exposure).
Dose adjustments Manufacturer advises dose reduction of 50% in moderate to severe impairment.

● DIRECTIONS FOR ADMINISTRATION Manufacturer advises orodispersible tablets should be placed on the tongue, allowed to disperse and swallowed, or may be swallowed whole with a glass of water. Alternatively, tablets can be dispersed in a small amount of water and administered by an oral syringe or nasogastric tube.

● PATIENT AND CARER ADVICE Counselling on administration of orodispersible tablet advised.

● PROFESSION SPECIFIC INFORMATION
Dental practitioners' formulary
Lansoprazole capsules may be prescribed.

● MEDICINAL FORMS There can be variation in the licensing of different medicines containing the same drug. Forms available from special-order manufacturers include: oral suspension, oral solution, powder

Gastro-resistant capsule
CAUTIONARY AND ADVISORY LABELS 5, 22, 25
▹ Lansoprazole (Non-proprietary)
Lansoprazole 15 mg Lansoprazole 15mg gastro-resistant capsules |
28 capsule PoM £12.93 DT = £1.04
Lansoprazole 30 mg Lansoprazole 30mg gastro-resistant capsules |
28 capsule PoM £23.63 DT = £1.35

Orodispersible tablet
CAUTIONARY AND ADVISORY LABELS 5, 22
EXCIPIENTS: May contain Aspartame
▹ Lansoprazole (Non-proprietary)
Lansoprazole 15 mg Lansoprazole 15mg orodispersible tablets |
28 tablet PoM £4.73 DT = £3.22
Lansoprazole 30 mg Lansoprazole 30mg orodispersible tablets |
28 tablet PoM £5.76 DT = £4.88

1

Gastro-intestinal system

▶ **Zoton FasTab** (Pfizer Ltd)
Lansoprazole 15 mg Zoton FasTab 15mg | 28 tablet PoM £2.99 DT
= £3.22
Lansoprazole 30 mg Zoton FasTab 30mg | 28 tablet PoM £5.50 DT
= £4.88

▶ 83

Omeprazole
16-Nov-2020

● **INDICATIONS AND DOSE**

Helicobacter pylori eradication [in combination with other drugs (see Helicobacter pylori infection p. 90)]
▶ BY MOUTH
  ▸ Adult: 20–40 mg twice daily for 7 days for first- and second-line eradication therapy; 10 days for third-line eradication therapy

Benign gastric ulceration
▶ BY MOUTH
  ▸ Adult: 20 mg once daily for 8 weeks, increased if necessary to 40 mg once daily, in severe or recurrent cases

Duodenal ulceration
▶ BY MOUTH
  ▸ Adult: 20 mg once daily for 4 weeks, increased if necessary to 40 mg once daily, in severe or recurrent cases

Prevention of relapse in gastric ulcer
▶ BY MOUTH
  ▸ Adult: 20 mg once daily, increased if necessary to 40 mg once daily

Prevention of relapse in duodenal ulcer
▶ BY MOUTH
  ▸ Adult: 20 mg once daily, dose may range between 10–40 mg daily

NSAID-associated duodenal ulcer | NSAID-associated gastric ulcer | NSAID-associated gastroduodenal erosions
▶ BY MOUTH
  ▸ Adult: 20 mg once daily for 4 weeks, continued for a further 4 weeks if not fully healed

Prophylaxis in patients with a history of NSAID-associated duodenal ulcer who require continued NSAID treatment | Prophylaxis in patients with a history of NSAID-associated gastric ulcer who require continued NSAID treatment | Prophylaxis in patients with a history of NSAID-associated gastroduodenal lesions who require continued NSAID treatment | Prophylaxis in patients with a history of NSAID-associated dyspeptic symptoms who require continued NSAID treatment
▶ BY MOUTH
  ▸ Adult: 20 mg once daily

Zollinger–Ellison syndrome
▶ BY MOUTH
  ▸ Adult: Initially 60 mg once daily; usual dose 20–120 mg daily, total daily doses greater than 80 mg should be given in 2 divided doses
▶ BY INTRAVENOUS INFUSION
  ▸ Adult: Initially 60 mg once daily, adjusted according to response, total daily doses greater than 60 mg should be given in 2 divided doses, infusion to be given over 20–30 minutes

Gastro-oesophageal reflux disease
▶ BY MOUTH
  ▸ Adult: 20 mg once daily for 4 or 8 weeks

Severe oesophagitis
▶ BY MOUTH
  ▸ Adult: 40 mg once daily for 8 weeks, continue as maintenance treatment if appropriate

Severe oesophagitis, refractory to initial treatment
▶ BY MOUTH
  ▸ Adult: 40 mg twice daily

Acid reflux disease (long-term management)
▶ BY MOUTH
  ▸ Adult: 10 mg once daily, increased if necessary up to 40 mg once daily, dose only increased if symptoms return

Functional dyspepsia
▶ BY MOUTH
  ▸ Adult: 10 mg once daily for 4 weeks

Uninvestigated dyspepsia
▶ BY MOUTH
  ▸ Adult: 20 mg once daily for 4 weeks

Treatment and prevention of benign gastric ulcers | Treatment and prevention of duodenal ulcers | Treatment and prevention of NSAID-associated ulcers | Treatment and prevention of gastro-oesophageal reflux disease
▶ BY INTRAVENOUS INFUSION
  ▸ Adult: 40 mg once daily until oral administration possible, infusion to be given over 20–30 minutes

Major peptic ulcer bleeding (following endoscopic treatment)
▶ INITIALLY BY INTRAVENOUS INFUSION
  ▸ Adult: Initially 80 mg, to be given over 40–60 minutes, then (by continuous intravenous infusion) 8 mg/hour for 72 hours, subsequent dose then changed to oral therapy

● **UNLICENSED USE**
▶ With oral use EvGr Duration of treatment for gastro-oesophageal reflux disease differs from product literature and adheres to national guidelines. ⚠ See Gastro-oesophageal reflux disease p. 89 for further information.
  Omeprazole may be used as detailed below, although these situations are considered outside the scope of its licence:
  ● EvGr treatment of severe oesophagitis, refractory to initial treatment, ⚠ see Gastro-oesophageal reflux disease p. 89 for further information;
  ● EvGr treatment of functional and uninvestigated dyspepsia, ⚠ see Dyspepsia p. 73 for further information;
  ● treatment of major peptic ulcer bleeding (following endoscopic treatment).
  Oral suspension not licensed for use in Zollinger-Ellison syndrome.

● **INTERACTIONS** → Appendix 1: proton pump inhibitors

● **SIDE-EFFECTS**
▶ **Rare or very rare** Aggression · agitation · bronchospasm · encephalopathy · gastrointestinal candidiasis · muscle weakness

● **PREGNANCY** Not known to be harmful.

● **BREAST FEEDING** Present in milk but not known to be harmful.

● **HEPATIC IMPAIRMENT**
  Dose adjustments Not more than 20 mg daily should be needed.

● **DIRECTIONS FOR ADMINISTRATION** For administration by *mouth* using tablets or capsules:
  ● Tablets (*Losec MUPS*®, *Mezzopram*®) or capules (*Losec*®) containing enteric-coated pellets can be dispersed in non-carbonated water or a slightly acidic liquid e.g. fruit juice or apple sauce; do **not** use milk or carbonated water. The dispersion should be stirred just before drinking and taken immediately, rinsed down with half a glass of water. The enteric-coated pellets must not be chewed.
  ● Enteric-coated tablets (*Dexcel*) or capsules containing an enteric-coated tablet (*Mepradec*®) must be swallowed whole and not chewed or crushed.

For instructions on reconstitution of oral suspension, consult product literature.

▸ With intravenous use [EvGr] For *continuous or intermittent intravenous infusion*, reconstitute each 40 mg vial with infusion fluid and dilute to 100 mL with Glucose 5% or Sodium Chloride 0.9%; for *intermittent infusion* give 40 mg over 20–30 minutes; stable for 6 hours in Glucose 5% or 12 hours in Sodium Chloride 0.9%. ⟨⟩

● PATIENT AND CARER ADVICE
▸ With oral use Counselling on administration advised.

● PROFESSION SPECIFIC INFORMATION

Dental practitioners' formulary
Gastro-resistant omeprazole capsules may be prescribed.

● EXCEPTIONS TO LEGAL CATEGORY
▸ With oral use Omeprazole 10 mg tablets can be sold to the public for the short-term relief of reflux-like symptoms (e.g. heartburn) in adults over 18 years, max. daily dose 20 mg for max. 4 weeks, and a pack size of 28 tablets.

● MEDICINAL FORMS There can be variation in the licensing of different medicines containing the same drug. Forms available from special-order manufacturers include: oral suspension, oral solution

Gastro-resistant capsule
CAUTIONARY AND ADVISORY LABELS 25
▸ Omeprazole (Non-proprietary)
Omeprazole 10 mg Omeprazole 10mg gastro-resistant capsules | 28 capsule [PoM] £9.30 DT = £1.08
Omeprazole 20 mg Omeprazole 20mg gastro-resistant capsules | 28 capsule [PoM] £13.36 DT = £1.10 | 250 capsule [PoM] £8.50–£9.82
Omeprazole 40 mg Omeprazole 40mg gastro-resistant capsules | 7 capsule [PoM] £6.96 DT = £0.82 | 28 capsule [PoM] £2.48–£26.72
▸ Losec (AstraZeneca UK Ltd)
Omeprazole 10 mg Losec 10mg gastro-resistant capsules | 28 capsule [PoM] £11.16 DT = £1.08
Omeprazole 20 mg Losec 20mg gastro-resistant capsules | 28 capsule [PoM] £16.70 DT = £1.10
Omeprazole 40 mg Losec 40mg gastro-resistant capsules | 7 capsule [PoM] £8.35 DT = £0.82

Gastro-resistant tablet
CAUTIONARY AND ADVISORY LABELS 25
▸ Omeprazole (Non-proprietary)
Omeprazole 10 mg Omeprazole 10mg gastro-resistant tablets | 28 tablet [PoM] £18.91 DT = £7.90
Omeprazole 20 mg Omeprazole 20mg gastro-resistant tablets | 28 tablet [PoM] £28.56 DT = £6.71
Omeprazole 40 mg Omeprazole 40mg gastro-resistant tablets | 7 tablet [PoM] £14.28 DT = £6.89
▸ Losec MUPS (AstraZeneca UK Ltd)
Omeprazole (as Omeprazole magnesium) 10 mg Losec MUPS 10mg gastro-resistant tablets | 28 tablet [PoM] £9.30 DT = £9.30
Omeprazole (as Omeprazole magnesium) 20 mg Losec MUPS 20mg gastro-resistant tablets | 28 tablet [PoM] £13.92 DT = £13.92
Omeprazole (as Omeprazole magnesium) 40 mg Losec MUPS 40mg gastro-resistant tablets | 7 tablet [PoM] £6.96 DT = £6.96
▸ Mezzopram (Sandoz Ltd)
Omeprazole (as Omeprazole magnesium) 10 mg Mezzopram 10mg dispersible gastro-resistant tablets | 28 tablet [PoM] £6.58 DT = £9.30
Omeprazole (as Omeprazole magnesium) 20 mg Mezzopram 20mg dispersible gastro-resistant tablets | 28 tablet [PoM] £9.86 DT = £13.92
Omeprazole (as Omeprazole magnesium) 40 mg Mezzopram 40mg dispersible gastro-resistant tablets | 7 tablet [PoM] £4.93 DT = £6.96

Oral suspension
▸ Omeprazole (Non-proprietary)
Omeprazole 2 mg per 1 ml Omeprazole 10mg/5ml oral suspension sugar free sugar-free | 75 ml [PoM] £92.17 DT = £92.17
Omeprazole 4 mg per 1 ml Omeprazole 20mg/5ml oral suspension sugar free sugar-free | 75 ml [PoM] £178.35 DT = £178.35

Powder for solution for infusion
▸ Omeprazole (Non-proprietary)
Omeprazole (as Omeprazole sodium) 40 mg Omeprazole 40mg powder for solution for infusion vials | 5 vial [PoM] £6.50–£32.48 DT = £26.00 (Hospital only)

F 83

Pantoprazole

15-Sep-2020

● INDICATIONS AND DOSE

Helicobacter pylori eradication [in combination with other drugs (see Helicobacter pylori infection p. 90)]
▸ BY MOUTH
▸ Adult: 40 mg twice daily for 7 days for first- and second-line eradication therapy; 10 days for third-line eradication therapy

Benign gastric ulcer
▸ BY MOUTH
▸ Adult: 40 mg daily for 8 weeks; increased if necessary up to 80 mg daily, dose increased in severe cases

Gastric ulcer
▸ BY INTRAVENOUS INJECTION, OR BY INTRAVENOUS INFUSION
▸ Adult: 40 mg daily until oral administration can be resumed, injection to be given over at least 2 minutes

Duodenal ulcer
▸ BY MOUTH
▸ Adult: 40 mg daily for 4 weeks; increased if necessary up to 80 mg daily, dose increased in severe cases
▸ BY INTRAVENOUS INJECTION, OR BY INTRAVENOUS INFUSION
▸ Adult: 40 mg daily until oral administration can be resumed, injection to be given over at least 2 minutes

NSAID-associated peptic ulcer disease
▸ BY MOUTH
▸ Adult: 40 mg once daily for 8 weeks

Prophylaxis of NSAID-associated gastric ulcer in patients with an increased risk of gastroduodenal complications who require continued NSAID treatment | Prophylaxis of NSAID-associated duodenal ulcer in patients with an increased risk of gastroduodenal complications who require continued NSAID treatment
▸ BY MOUTH
▸ Adult: 20 mg daily

Gastro-oesophageal reflux disease
▸ BY MOUTH
▸ Adult: 40 mg once daily for 4 or 8 weeks
▸ BY INTRAVENOUS INJECTION, OR BY INTRAVENOUS INFUSION
▸ Adult: 40 mg daily until oral administration can be resumed, injection to be given over at least 2 minutes

Severe oesophagitis
▸ BY MOUTH
▸ Adult: 40 mg once daily for 8 weeks, continue as maintenance treatment if appropriate

Severe oesophagitis, refractory to initial treatment
▸ BY MOUTH
▸ Adult: 40 mg twice daily

Functional dyspepsia
▸ BY MOUTH
▸ Adult: 20 mg once daily for 4 weeks

Uninvestigated dyspepsia
▸ BY MOUTH
▸ Adult: 40 mg once daily for 4 weeks

Zollinger–Ellison syndrome (and other hypersecretory conditions)
▸ BY MOUTH
▸ Adult: Initially 80 mg daily (max. per dose 80 mg), adjusted according to response
▸ BY INTRAVENOUS INJECTION, OR BY INTRAVENOUS INFUSION
▸ Adult: Initially 80 mg, alternatively 160 mg in 2 divided doses, if rapid acid control required, then 80 mg once daily (max. per dose 80 mg), adjusted according to response

● UNLICENSED USE
▸ With oral use [EvGr] Dose for the treatment of gastro-oesophageal reflux disease differs from product literature and adheres to national guidelines. ⟨A⟩

Gastro-intestinal system

1

Pantoprazole may be used as detailed below, although these situations are considered outside the scope of its licence:

- EvGr treatment of severe oesophagitis, refractory to initial treatment, ⒶⒶ see Gastro-oesophageal reflux disease p. 89 for further information;
- EvGr treatment of NSAID-associated peptic ulcer disease, Ⓐ see Peptic ulcer disease p. 77 for further information;
- EvGr treatment of functional and uninvestigated dyspepsia, Ⓐ see Dyspepsia p. 73 for further information.

- INTERACTIONS → Appendix 1: proton pump inhibitors
- SIDE-EFFECTS

GENERAL SIDE-EFFECTS
- **Uncommon** Asthenia · gastrointestinal discomfort · sleep disorder
- **Rare or very rare** Angioedema · hyperlipidaemia · weight change

SPECIFIC SIDE-EFFECTS
- With intravenous use Electrolyte imbalance · muscle spasms
- PREGNANCY Manufacturer advises avoid unless potential benefit outweighs risk—fetotoxic in *animals*.
- BREAST FEEDING Manufacturer advises avoid unless potential benefit outweighs risk—small amount present in milk.
- HEPATIC IMPAIRMENT Manufacturer advises caution in severe impairment (increased half-life)—monitor liver function and discontinue if deterioration.
  Dose adjustments Manufacturer advises maximum dose of 20 mg daily in severe impairment.
- RENAL IMPAIRMENT
  Dose adjustments Max. oral dose 40 mg daily.
- DIRECTIONS FOR ADMINISTRATION For *intravenous infusion* (*Protium*®), manufacturer advises give intermittently in Glucose 5% or Sodium chloride 0.9%; reconstitute 40 mg with 10 mL sodium chloride 0.9% and dilute with 100 mL of infusion fluid; give 40 mg over 15 minutes.
- EXCEPTIONS TO LEGAL CATEGORY Pantoprazole 20 mg tablets can be sold to the public for the short-term treatment of reflux symptoms (e.g. heartburn) in adults over 18 years, max. daily dose 20 mg for max. 4 weeks.

- MEDICINAL FORMS There can be variation in the licensing of different medicines containing the same drug. Forms available from special-order manufacturers include: oral suspension

Gastro-resistant tablet
CAUTIONARY AND ADVISORY LABELS 25
- Pantoprazole (Non-proprietary)
  Pantoprazole (as Pantoprazole sodium sesquihydrate)
  20 mg Pantoprazole 20mg gastro-resistant tablets | 28 tablet PoM £12.11 DT = £2.26
  Pantoprazole (as Pantoprazole sodium sesquihydrate)
  40 mg Pantoprazole 40mg gastro-resistant tablets | 28 tablet PoM £20.57 DT = £2.47

Powder for solution for injection
- Pantoprazole (Non-proprietary)
  Pantoprazole (as Pantoprazole sodium sesquihydrate)
  40 mg Pantoprazole 40mg powder for solution for injection vials | 1 vial PoM £5.00 DT = £5.00 | 5 vial PoM £22.50 DT = £22.50 (Hospital only) | 5 vial PoM Ⓧ DT = £22.50
- Protium (Takeda UK Ltd)
  Pantoprazole (as Pantoprazole sodium sesquihydrate)
  40 mg Protium I.V. 40mg powder for solution for injection vials | 5 vial PoM £25.53 DT = £22.50

Rabeprazole sodium

⌑ 83
14-Sep-2020

- INDICATIONS AND DOSE
Benign gastric ulcer
▸ BY MOUTH
▹ Adult: 20 mg daily for 8 weeks, dose to be taken in the morning

Duodenal ulcer
▸ BY MOUTH
▹ Adult: 20 mg daily for 4 weeks, dose to be taken in the morning

NSAID-associated peptic ulcer disease
▸ BY MOUTH
▹ Adult: 20 mg once daily for 8 weeks

Gastro-oesophageal reflux disease
▸ BY MOUTH
▹ Adult: 20 mg once daily for 4-8 weeks; maintenance 10–20 mg daily

Gastro-oesophageal reflux disease (symptomatic treatment in the absence of oesophagitis)
▸ BY MOUTH
▹ Adult: 10 mg daily for up to 4 weeks, then 10 mg daily if required

Severe oesophagitis
▸ BY MOUTH
▹ Adult: 20 mg once daily for 8 weeks, continue as maintenance treatment if appropriate

Severe oesophagitis, refractory to initial treatment
▸ BY MOUTH
▹ Adult: 20 mg twice daily

Functional dyspepsia
▸ BY MOUTH
▹ Adult: 10 mg once daily for 4 weeks

Uninvestigated dyspepsia
▸ BY MOUTH
▹ Adult: 20 mg once daily for 4 weeks

Zollinger–Ellison syndrome
▸ BY MOUTH
▹ Adult: Initially 60 mg once daily, adjusted according to response, doses above 100 mg daily given in 2 divided doses; maximum 120 mg per day

***Helicobacter pylori* eradication [in combination with other drugs (see Helicobacter pylori infection p. 90)]**
▸ BY MOUTH
▹ Adult: 20 mg twice daily for 7 days for first- and second-line eradication therapy; 10 days for third-line eradication therapy

- UNLICENSED USE Rabeprazole may be used as detailed below, although these situations are considered outside the scope of its licence:
  - EvGr treatment of NSAID-associated peptic ulcer disease, Ⓐ see Peptic ulcer disease p. 77 for further information;
  - EvGr treatment of severe oesophagitis and severe oesophagitis, refractory to initial treatment, Ⓐ see Gastro-oesophageal reflux disease p. 89 for further information;
  - EvGr treatment of functional and uninvestigated dyspepsia, Ⓐ see Dyspepsia p. 73 for further information.
  EvGr Combination regimens and durations for *Helicobacter pylori* eradication may differ from product literature but adhere to national guidelines. Ⓐ See Helicobacter pylori infection p. 90 for further information.

- INTERACTIONS → Appendix 1: proton pump inhibitors
- SIDE-EFFECTS
▸ **Common or very common** Asthenia · cough · increased risk of infection · influenza like illness · pain

▶ **Uncommon** Burping · dyspepsia · leg cramps · nervousness
▶ **Rare or very rare** Appetite decreased · hepatic encephalopathy · leucocytosis · neutropenia · weight increased
▶ **Frequency not known** Chest pain · chills · fever
● PREGNANCY Manufacturer advises avoid—no information available.
● BREAST FEEDING Manufacturer advises avoid—no information available.
● HEPATIC IMPAIRMENT Manufacturer advises caution in severe impairment (no information available).

● MEDICINAL FORMS There can be variation in the licensing of different medicines containing the same drug.

Gastro-resistant tablet
CAUTIONARY AND ADVISORY LABELS 25
▶ Rabeprazole sodium (Non-proprietary)
Rabeprazole sodium 10 mg Rabeprazole 10mg gastro-resistant tablets | 28 tablet [PoM] £11.56 DT = £1.46
Rabeprazole sodium 20 mg Rabeprazole 20mg gastro-resistant tablets | 28 tablet [PoM] £19.55 DT = £1.65
▶ Pariet (Eisai Ltd)
Rabeprazole sodium 10 mg Pariet 10mg gastro-resistant tablets | 28 tablet [PoM] £5.78 DT = £1.46
Rabeprazole sodium 20 mg Pariet 20mg gastro-resistant tablets | 28 tablet [PoM] £11.34 DT = £1.65

4.3 Gastro-oesophageal reflux disease

Gastro-oesophageal reflux disease

31-Oct-2019

Description of condition

Gastro-oesophageal reflux disease (GORD) is usually a chronic condition where there is reflux of gastric contents (particularly acid, bile, and pepsin) back into the oesophagus, causing symptoms of heartburn and acid regurgitation. Less common symptoms such as chest pain, hoarseness, cough, wheezing, asthma and dental erosions can also occur if acid reflux reaches the oropharynx and/or respiratory tract.

GORD can be classified as non-erosive when a person has symptoms of GORD but the endoscopy is normal or erosive oesophagitis when oesophageal inflammation and mucosal erosions are seen at endoscopy.

Certain factors may contribute to the risk of developing GORD. These include consumption of trigger and fatty foods, pregnancy, hiatus hernia, family history of GORD, increased intra-gastric pressure from straining and coughing, stress, anxiety, obesity, drug side-effects, smoking and alcohol consumption.

Complications of GORD include oesophageal inflammation (oesophagitis), ulceration, haemorrhage and stricture formation, anaemia due to chronic blood loss, aspiration pneumonia, and Barrett's oesophagus.

Aims of treatment

The aim of treatment is to manage the symptoms of GORD and reduce the risk of recurrence and complications associated with the disease.

Non-drug treatment

[EvGr] Lifestyle measures, such as healthy eating, weight loss (if obese), avoiding trigger foods, eating smaller meals, eating the evening meal 3–4 hours before going to bed, raising the head of the bed, Smoking cessation p. 519, and reducing alcohol consumption may improve symptoms.

Assess the patient for stress and anxiety as these conditions may exacerbate symptoms.

Urgent endoscopic investigation is required for patients with dysphagia, significant acute gastrointestinal bleeding, or in those aged 55 years and over with unexplained weight loss and symptoms of upper abdominal pain, reflux or dyspepsia. Endoscopy can be considered to diagnose Barrett's oesophagus if the patient has GORD. Patient preference and individual risk factors should be taken into account. ⟨A⟩

Drug treatment

Initial management

[EvGr] Drugs that may cause or exacerbate the symptoms of GORD, such as alpha-blockers, anticholinergics, benzodiazepines, beta-blockers, bisphosphonates, calcium-channel blockers, corticosteroids, non-steroidal anti-inflammatory drugs (NSAIDs), nitrates, theophyllines, and tricyclic antidepressants should be reviewed. The lowest effective dose should be used and if appropriate, stopped.

Long term continuous use of antacids is not recommended for the treatment of GORD.

Patients with uninvestigated symptoms which suggest GORD should be managed as uninvestigated Dyspepsia p. 73.

In patients with an endoscopy confirmed diagnosis of GORD, a proton pump inhibitor (PPI), should be offered for 4 or 8 weeks. ⟨A⟩ If there is no response to a PPI, then offer a histamine₂-receptor antagonist (H₂-receptor antagonist).

[EvGr] Severe oesophagitis should be treated with a PPI for 8 weeks, taking into consideration patient preference and factors such as underlying health conditions and possible interactions with other drugs. ⟨A⟩

Follow up management

[EvGr] For patients with refractory GORD, new alarm symptoms should be assessed and alternate diagnoses considered. Other options include prescribing a further course of the initial PPI dose for 1 month, double the initial PPI dose for 1 month or the addition of a H₂-receptor antagonist at bedtime for nocturnal symptoms or for short term use. The patient's adherence to initial management should also be checked and lifestyle advice reinforced.

For patients diagnosed with GORD in whom symptoms recur after initial treatment, a PPI should be given at the lowest dose that can achieve symptom control and self management on an "as-needed" basis should be discussed.

If treatment for severe oesophagitis fails, a higher dose of the same PPI should be used or switching to another PPI should be considered taking into account patient preference, tolerability, underlying health conditions and possible interactions with other drugs.

For patients with severe oesophagitis that fail to respond to long term maintenance PPI therapy a clinical review and switching to another PPI can be considered and/or specialist advice can be sought.

Patients with severe oesophagitis or who have had dilatation of an oesophageal stricture should remain on long-term PPI therapy taking into consideration the factors mentioned above. ⟨A⟩

GORD in pregnancy

[EvGr] Heartburn and acid reflux are symptoms of Dyspepsia p. 73 in pregnancy commonly caused by GORD. Dietary and lifestyle advice should be given as first-line management. If this approach fails to control symptoms, an antacid or an alginate can be used. If this is ineffective or symptoms are severe omeprazole p. 86 or ranitidine p. 81 (unlicensed) may help to control symptoms. ⟨A⟩

Useful Resources

Gastro-oesophageal reflux disease and dyspepsia in adults: investigation and management. National Institute for Health

1

Gastro-intestinal system

and Care Excellence. NICE clinical guideline 184. September 2014, updated October 2019.
www.nice.org.uk/guidance/cg184

NICE Patient Decision Aid: Option grid to help people make decisions about long term heartburn treatment
www.nice.org.uk/about/what-we-do/our-programmes/nice-guidance/nice-guidelines/shared-decision-making

---

Other drugs used for Gastro-oesophageal reflux disease
Cimetidine, p. 79 · Esomeprazole, p. 83 · Famotidine, p. 80 · Lansoprazole, p. 85 · Nizatidine, p. 81 · Pantoprazole, p. 87 · Rabeprazole sodium, p. 88

ANTACIDS > ALGINATE

Sodium alginate with calcium carbonate and sodium bicarbonate

24-Apr-2020

The properties listed below are those particular to the combination only. For the properties of the components please consider, alginic acid p. 74, sodium bicarbonate p. 1086, calcium carbonate p. 1095.

● **INDICATIONS AND DOSE**

Gastro-oesophageal reflux disease
▸ BY MOUTH
  ▸ Child 6-11 years: 5–10 mL, to be taken after meals and at bedtime
  ▸ Child 12-17 years: 10–20 mL, to be taken after meals and at bedtime
  ▸ Adult: 10–20 mL, to be taken after meals and at bedtime

● **INTERACTIONS** → Appendix 1: calcium salts · sodium bicarbonate

● **PRESCRIBING AND DISPENSING INFORMATION** Flavours of oral liquid formulations may include aniseed or peppermint.

● **PATIENT AND CARER ADVICE**
Medicines for Children leaflet: Gaviscon for gastro-oesophageal reflux disease www.medicinesforchildren.org.uk/gaviscon-gastro-oesophageal-reflux-disease

● **MEDICINAL FORMS** There can be variation in the licensing of different medicines containing the same drug.
Oral suspension
ELECTROLYTES: May contain Sodium
  ▸ Acidex (Pinewood Healthcare)
    Calcium carbonate 16 mg per 1 ml, Sodium bicarbonate 26.7 mg per 1 ml, Sodium alginate 50 mg per 1 ml Acidex oral suspension aniseed sugar-free | 500 ml GSL £2.56 DT = £1.95
    Acidex oral suspension peppermint sugar-free | 150 ml GSL £1.21 DT = £2.58 sugar-free | 500 ml GSL £2.56 DT = £1.95
  ▸ Entrocalm Heartburn and Indigestion Relief (Galpharm International Ltd)
    Calcium carbonate 16 mg per 1 ml, Sodium bicarbonate 26.7 mg per 1 ml, Sodium alginate 50 mg per 1 ml Entrocalm Heartburn and Indigestion Relief oral suspension sugar-free | 150 ml GSL ⚚ DT = £2.58
  ▸ Gaviscon (Reckitt Benckiser Healthcare UK Ltd)
    Calcium carbonate 16 mg per 1 ml, Sodium bicarbonate 26.7 mg per 1 ml, Sodium alginate 50 mg per 1 ml Gaviscon Original Aniseed Relief sugar-free | 150 ml GSL £2.58 DT = £2.58 sugar-free | 300 ml GSL £4.33 DT = £4.33 sugar-free | 600 ml GSL £7.11 DT = £7.11
  ▸ Gaviscon Liquid Relief (Reckitt Benckiser Healthcare (UK) Ltd)
    Calcium carbonate 16 mg per 1 ml, Sodium bicarbonate 26.7 mg per 1 ml, Sodium alginate 50 mg per 1 ml Gaviscon Peppermint Liquid Relief sugar-free | 150 ml GSL £2.58 DT = £2.58 sugar-free | 300 ml GSL £4.33 DT = £4.33 sugar-free | 600 ml GSL £7.11 DT = £7.11

▸ Peptac (Teva UK Ltd)
  Calcium carbonate 16 mg per 1 ml, Sodium bicarbonate 26.7 mg per 1 ml, Sodium alginate 50 mg per 1 ml Peptac liquid peppermint sugar-free | 500 ml GSL £1.95 DT = £1.95
  Peptac liquid aniseed sugar-free | 500 ml GSL £1.95 DT = £1.95
▸ Rennie (Bayer Plc)
  Calcium carbonate 16 mg per 1 ml, Sodium bicarbonate 26.7 mg per 1 ml, Sodium alginate 50 mg per 1 ml Rennie Liquid Heartburn Relief oral suspension sugar-free | 150 ml GSL £2.52 DT = £2.58 sugar-free | 250 ml GSL £3.47

4.4 Helicobacter pylori infection

Helicobacter pylori infection
31-Oct-2019

Description of condition

Helicobacter pylori (*H. pylori*) infection is one of the most common causes of peptic ulcer disease, with 95% of duodenal and 70–80% of gastric ulcers associated with it. The use of non-steroidal anti-inflammatory drugs (NSAIDs) may have an additive effect if there is co-existent *H. pylori* infection, further increasing the risk of peptic ulceration and bleeding. *H. pylori* is also associated with acute and chronic gastritis, gastric cancer, and gastric mucosa associated lymphoid tissue (MALT) lymphoma.

Aims of treatment

Treatment aims to eradicate *H. pylori*, reduce the risk of peptic ulcer disease, ulcer bleeding and gastric malignancy, and the recurrence of gastritis and peptic ulcers.

Testing for *Helicobacter pylori*

EvGr The presence of *H. pylori* should be confirmed before starting eradication treatment ('test and treat' strategy). Ⓐ
Testing for *H. pylori* is recommended in the following patients in line with Public Health England (PHE) Guidance:
● Patients with uncomplicated dyspepsia and no alarm symptoms who are unresponsive to lifestyle changes and antacids, following a single one month treatment course with a proton pump inhibitor;
● Patients considered to be at high risk of *H. pylori* infection (such as older people, individuals of North African ethnicity, and those living in a known high risk area) should be tested for *H. pylori* first, or in parallel with a course of a proton pump inhibitor;
● Previously untested patients with a history of peptic ulcers or bleeds;
● Prior to initiating NSAIDs in patients with a prior history of peptic ulcers or bleeds;
● Patients with unexplained iron-deficiency anaemia after endoscopic investigation has excluded malignancy, and other causes have been investigated.

EvGr The urea (13C) p. 91 breath test, Stool Helicobacter Antigen Test (SAT), or laboratory-based serology where its performance has been locally validated, are recommended for the diagnosis of gastro-duodenal infection with *H. pylori*. Ⓐ PHE advise that the urea (13C) breath test and SAT should not be performed within 2 weeks of treatment with a proton pump inhibitor or within 4 weeks of antibacterial treatment, as this can lead to false negatives.

EvGr Office based serological tests for *H. pylori* are not recommended due to their inadequate performance. Ⓐ

Retesting for *Helicobacter pylori*

EvGr In patients with functional dyspepsia, routine retesting after *H. pylori* eradication is not recommended. Retesting may be considered in patients who would value the information. Ⓐ
PHE recommend retesting in the following circumstances:
● If compliance is poor, or there are high local resistance rates;

- The patient has persistent symptoms and the initial test was performed within 2 weeks of treatment with a proton pump inhibitor, or within 4 weeks of antibacterial treatment;
- In patients with an associated peptic ulcer, MALT lymphoma, or after resection of an early gastric carcinoma;
- Patients taking aspirin without concomitant treatment with a proton pump inhibitor;
- Patients with severe persistent or recurrent symptoms, particularly if not typical of gastro-oesophageal reflux disease.

Retesting should be performed at least 4 weeks (ideally 8 weeks) after treatment. In patients requiring gastric acid suppression H2-receptor antagonists p. 79 should be used. [EvGr] The urea (13C) breath test should be used for retesting. [A]

Drug treatment

Treatment of *H. pylori* usually involves a triple-therapy regimen that comprises a proton pump inhibitor **and** 2 antibacterials. PHE advise that the choice of antibacterials should take into consideration the patient's antibacterial treatment history, as each additional course of clarithromycin, metronidazole, or quinolone increases the risk of resistance.

[EvGr] Consider referral to a specialist in patients who remain *H. pylori* positive after second-line eradication therapy. [A] PHE also advise that patients should be referred for an endoscopy, culture and susceptibility testing if the choice of antibacterial treatment is reduced due to hypersensitivity, there are known high local resistance rates, or patients have previously received treatment with clarithromycin, metronidazole, and a quinolone.

PHE advise that if diarrhoea develops, *Clostridioides difficile* infection should be considered and the need for treatment reviewed. [EvGr] The importance of adherence to treatment should be discussed and emphasised to the patient. [A]

Choice of treatment regimen
No penicillin allergy

- **Oral** first line for 7 days:
    - [EvGr] A proton pump inhibitor, plus amoxicillin p. 582, and *either* clarithromycin p. 569 or metronidazole p. 575 (treatment choice should take into account previous treatment with clarithromycin or metronidazole). [A]
- **Oral** second line for 7 days (if ongoing symptoms after first line treatment):
    - [EvGr] A proton pump inhibitor, plus amoxicillin, and *either* clarithromycin or metronidazole (whichever was not used first line). [A]
- **Oral** alternative second line for 7 days (for patients who have received previous treatment with clarithromycin and metronidazole):
    - [EvGr] A proton pump inhibitor, plus amoxicillin, and tetracycline p. 604 [unlicensed] (or, if a tetracycline cannot be used, levofloxacin p. 595 [unlicensed]). [A]
- **Oral** third line for 10 days **on specialist advice only** in line with PHE Guidance:
    - A proton pump inhibitor, plus bismuth subsalicylate p. 78 [unlicensed], and *either* 2 antibacterials from those mentioned above not previously used, or rifabutin p. 612 [unlicensed], or furazolidone [unlicensed].

Penicillin allergy

- **Oral** first line for 7 days:
    - [EvGr] A proton pump inhibitor, plus clarithromycin, and metronidazole. [A]

- **Oral** alternative first line for 7 days (for patients previously treated with clarithromycin):
    - [EvGr] A proton pump inhibitor, plus bismuth subsalicylate [unlicensed], plus metronidazole, and tetracycline [unlicensed]. [A]
- **Oral** second line for 7 days (if ongoing symptoms after first line treatment in patients who have **not** received previous treatment with a fluoroquinolone):
    - [EvGr] A proton pump inhibitor, plus metronidazole, and levofloxacin [unlicensed]. [A]
- **Oral** alternative second line for 7 days (in patients who have received previous treatment with a fluoroquinolone):
    - [EvGr] A proton pump inhibitor, plus bismuth subsalicylate [unlicensed], plus metronidazole, and tetracycline [unlicensed]. [A]
- **Oral** third line for 10 days **on specialist advice only** in line with PHE Guidance:
    - A proton pump inhibitor, plus bismuth subsalicylate [unlicensed], and *either* rifabutin [unlicensed] or furazolidone [unlicensed].

For any advice, consult a local microbiologist or the Helicobacter Reference Laboratory at: www.gov.uk/guidance/gbru-reference-and-diagnostic-services.

For additional information on the management of patients with *H. pylori* infection and peptic ulcer disease or dyspepsia, see Peptic ulcer disease p. 77 and Dyspepsia p. 73.

Useful Resources

Gastro-oesophgeal reflux disease and dyspepsia in adults: investigation and management. National Institute for Health and Care Excellence. NICE guideline 184. September 2014, updated October 2019.
www.nice.org.uk/guidance/cg184

Test and treat for *Helicobacter pylori* (HP) in dyspepsia; Quick reference guide for primary care: For consultation and local adaptation. Public Health England. July 2017, updated August 2019.
www.gov.uk/government/publications/helicobacter-pylori-diagnosis-and-treatment

DIAGNOSTIC AGENTS

▌Urea (13C)

- ● **INDICATIONS AND DOSE**
  Diagnosis of gastro-duodenal *Helicobacter pylori* infection
  ▶ BY MOUTH
    ▹ **Adult:** (consult product literature)

- ● **MEDICINAL FORMS** There can be variation in the licensing of different medicines containing the same drug.
  Soluble tablet
  ▶ Pylobactell (Torbet Laboratories Ltd)
    Urea [13-C] 100 mg Pylobactell breath test kit | 1 kit [PoM] £20.75
    DT = £20.75
  Powder
  ▶ Helicobacter Test INFAI (INFAI UK Ltd)
    Urea [13-C] 45 mg Helicobacter Test INFAI for children breath test kit sugar-free | 1 kit [PoM] £15.00 DT = £19.10
    Urea [13-C] 75 mg Helicobacter Test INFAI breath test kit sugar-free | 1 kit [PoM] £17.00 DT = £21.70 sugar-free | 50 kit [PoM] £724.00
  Tablet
  ▶ Diabact UBT (HFA Healthcare Products Ltd)
    Urea [13-C] 50 mg diabact UBT 50mg tablets | 1 tablet [PoM] £21.25
    DT = £21.25 | 10 tablet [PoM] £78.75 (Hospital only)

1

Gastro-intestinal system

5   Food allergy

Food allergy

15-Dec-2016

Description of condition

Food allergy is an adverse immune response to a food, commonly associated with cutaneous and gastro-intestinal reactions, and less frequently associated with respiratory reactions and anaphylaxis. It is distinct from food intolerance which is non-immunological. Cow's milk, hen's eggs, soy, wheat, peanuts, tree nuts, fish, and shellfish are the most common allergens. Cross-reactivity between similar foods can occur (e.g. allergy to other mammalian milk in patients with cow's milk allergy).

Management of food allergy

EvGr Allergy caused by specific foods should be managed by strict avoidance of the causal food. Sodium cromoglicate p. 286 is licensed as an adjunct to dietary avoidance in patients with food allergy. Educating patients about appropriate nutrition, food preparation, and the risks of accidental exposure is recommended, such as food and drinks to avoid, ensuring adequate nutritional intake, and interpreting food labels. ⟨A⟩

Drug treatment

EvGr There is low quality evidence to support the use of antihistamines to treat acute, **non-life-threatening** symptoms (such as flushing and urticaria) if accidental ingestion of allergenic food has occurred (see *Antihistamines*, under Antihistamines, allergen immunotherapy and allergic emergencies p. 292). Chlorphenamine maleate p. 299 is licensed for the symptomatic control of food allergy. In case of food-induced anaphylaxis, adrenaline/epinephrine p. 238 is the first-line immediate treatment (see also *Allergic emergencies*, under Antihistamines, allergen immunotherapy and allergic emergencies p. 292). Patients who are at risk of anaphylaxis should be trained to use self-injectable adrenaline/epinephrine. ⟨A⟩

6   Gastro-intestinal smooth muscle spasm

Antispasmodics

02-May-2020

Overview

Antispasmodics can be divided into two main classifications: antimuscarinics and smooth muscle relaxants. Antimuscarinics (formerly termed 'anticholinergics') reduce intestinal motility and are used for gastro-intestinal smooth muscle spasm. They include the tertiary amines atropine sulfate p. 1210 and dicycloverine hydrochloride below, and the quaternary ammonium compounds propantheline bromide p. 94 and hyoscine butylbromide p. 93. The quaternary ammonium compounds are less lipid soluble than tertiary amines and are less likely to cross the blood–brain barrier; therefore have a lower risk for central nervous system side-effects. They are also less well absorbed from the gastro-intestinal tract.

Dicycloverine hydrochloride has a much less marked antimuscarinic action than atropine sulfate and may also have some direct action on smooth muscle. Hyoscine butylbromide is advocated as a gastro-intestinal antispasmodic, but is poorly absorbed.

Alverine citrate p. 94, mebeverine hydrochloride p. 94, and peppermint oil p. 52 are direct-acting intestinal smooth muscle relaxants and may relieve abdominal pain or spasm in Irritable bowel syndrome p. 51.

ANTIMUSCARINICS

⚑ 821

Dicycloverine hydrochloride

23-Apr-2020

(Dicyclomine hydrochloride)

● **INDICATIONS AND DOSE**

Symptomatic relief of gastro-intestinal disorders characterised by smooth muscle spasm
▸ BY MOUTH
  ▸ Child 6–23 months: 5–10 mg 3–4 times a day, dose to be taken 15 minutes before feeds
  ▸ Child 2–11 years: 10 mg 3 times a day
  ▸ Child 12–17 years: 10–20 mg 3 times a day
  ▸ Adult: 10–20 mg 3 times a day

● CONTRA-INDICATIONS Child under 6 months
● INTERACTIONS → Appendix 1: dicycloverine
● SIDE-EFFECTS Appetite decreased · fatigue · thirst
● PREGNANCY Not known to be harmful; manufacturer advises use only if essential.
● BREAST FEEDING Avoid—present in milk; apnoea reported in infant.
● EXCEPTIONS TO LEGAL CATEGORY Dicycloverine hydrochloride can be sold to the public provided that max. single dose is 10 mg and max. daily dose is 60 mg.
● MEDICINAL FORMS There can be variation in the licensing of different medicines containing the same drug.

Oral solution
  ▸ Dicycloverine hydrochloride (Non-proprietary)
  Dicycloverine hydrochloride 2 mg per 1 ml Dicycloverine 10mg/5ml oral solution | 120 ml PoM £196.36 DT = £174.21

Tablet
  ▸ Dicycloverine hydrochloride (Non-proprietary)
  Dicycloverine hydrochloride 10 mg Dicycloverine 10mg tablets | 100 tablet PoM £215.60 DT = £215.14
  Dicycloverine hydrochloride 20 mg Dicycloverine 20mg tablets | 84 tablet PoM £229.22 DT = £228.86

Dicycloverine hydrochloride with aluminium hydroxide, magnesium oxide and simeticone

28-Apr-2020

The properties listed below are those particular to the combination only. For the properties of the components please consider, dicycloverine hydrochloride above, simeticone p. 77.

● **INDICATIONS AND DOSE**

Symptomatic relief of gastro-intestinal disorders characterised by smooth muscle spasm
▸ BY MOUTH
  ▸ Child 12–17 years: 10–20 mL every 4 hours as required
  ▸ Adult: 10–20 mL every 4 hours as required

● INTERACTIONS → Appendix 1: aluminium hydroxide · antacids · dicycloverine · magnesium
● SIDE-EFFECTS Anticholinergic syndrome
● RENAL IMPAIRMENT There is a risk of accumulation and aluminium toxicity with antacids containing aluminium salts. Absorption of aluminium from aluminium salts is increased by citrates, which are contained in many effervescent preparations (such as effervescent analgesics).

● MEDICINAL FORMS There can be variation in the licensing of different medicines containing the same drug.

Oral suspension
▸ Kolanticon (Peckforton Pharmaceuticals Ltd)
Dicycloverine hydrochloride 500 microgram per 1 ml, Simeticone 4 mg per 1 ml, Magnesium oxide light 20 mg per 1 ml, Aluminium hydroxide dried 40 mg per 1 ml Kolanticon gel sugar-free | 200 ml ℗ £4.00 sugar-free | 500 ml ℗ £6.00

⌑ 821

Hyoscine butylbromide

25-Nov-2020

● INDICATIONS AND DOSE

Symptomatic relief of gastro-intestinal or genito-urinary disorders characterised by smooth muscle spasm
▸ BY MOUTH
▸ Child 6-11 years: 10 mg 3 times a day
▸ Child 12-17 years: 20 mg 4 times a day
▸ Adult: 20 mg 4 times a day

Irritable bowel syndrome
▸ BY MOUTH
▸ Adult: 10 mg 3 times a day; increased if necessary up to 20 mg 4 times a day

Acute spasm | Spasm in diagnostic procedures
▸ INITIALLY BY INTRAMUSCULAR INJECTION, OR BY SLOW INTRAVENOUS INJECTION
▸ Adult: 20 mg, then (by intramuscular injection or by slow intravenous injection) 20 mg after 30 minutes if required, dose may be repeated more frequently in endoscopy; maximum 100 mg per day

Excessive respiratory secretions in palliative care
▸ BY MOUTH
▸ Child 1 month-1 year: 300–500 micrograms/kg 3–4 times a day (max. per dose 5 mg)
▸ Child 2-4 years: 5 mg 3–4 times a day
▸ Child 5-11 years: 10 mg 3–4 times a day
▸ Child 12-17 years: 10–20 mg 3–4 times a day
▸ BY INTRAMUSCULAR INJECTION, OR BY INTRAVENOUS INJECTION
▸ Child 1 month-4 years: 300–500 micrograms/kg 3–4 times a day (max. per dose 5 mg)
▸ Child 5-11 years: 5–10 mg 3–4 times a day
▸ Child 12-17 years: 10–20 mg 3–4 times a day
▸ BY SUBCUTANEOUS INJECTION
▸ Adult: 20 mg every 4 hours if required, adjusted according to response to up to 20 mg every 1 hour
▸ BY SUBCUTANEOUS INFUSION
▸ Adult: 20–120 mg/24 hours

Bowel colic in palliative care
▸ BY MOUTH
▸ Child 1 month-1 year: 300–500 micrograms/kg 3–4 times a day (max. per dose 5 mg)
▸ Child 2-4 years: 5 mg 3–4 times a day
▸ Child 5-11 years: 10 mg 3–4 times a day
▸ Child 12-17 years: 10–20 mg 3–4 times a day
▸ BY INTRAMUSCULAR INJECTION, OR BY INTRAVENOUS INJECTION
▸ Child 1 month-4 years: 300–500 micrograms/kg 3–4 times a day (max. per dose 5 mg)
▸ Child 5-11 years: 5–10 mg 3–4 times a day
▸ Child 12-17 years: 10–20 mg 3–4 times a day
▸ BY SUBCUTANEOUS INJECTION
▸ Adult: 20 mg every 4 hours if required, adjusted according to response to up to 20 mg every 1 hour
▸ BY SUBCUTANEOUS INFUSION
▸ Adult: 60–300 mg/24 hours

PHARMACOKINETICS
▸ Administration by mouth is associated with poor absorption.

● UNLICENSED USE
▸ In children *Tablets* not licensed for use in children under 6 years. *Injection* not licensed for use in children (age range not specified by manufacturer).

IMPORTANT SAFETY INFORMATION
MHRA/CHM ADVICE: HYOSCINE BUTYLBROMIDE (*BUSCOPAN*®) INJECTION: RISK OF SERIOUS ADVERSE EFFECTS IN PATIENTS WITH UNDERLYING CARDIAC DISEASE (FEBRUARY 2017)
The MHRA advises that hyoscine butylbromide injection can cause serious adverse effects including tachycardia, hypotension, and anaphylaxis; several reports have noted that anaphylaxis is more likely to be fatal in patients with underlying coronary heart disease. Hyoscine butylbromide injection is contra-indicated in patients with tachycardia and should be used with caution in patients with cardiac disease; the MHRA recommends that these patients are monitored and that resuscitation equipment and trained personnel are readily available.

● CONTRA-INDICATIONS
▸ With intramuscular use or intravenous use or subcutaneous use Tachycardia
● INTERACTIONS → Appendix 1: hyoscine
● SIDE-EFFECTS
GENERAL SIDE-EFFECTS
Dyspnoea
SPECIFIC SIDE-EFFECTS
▸ With parenteral use Feeling hot · hypotension · mydriasis · sweat changes
● PREGNANCY Manufacturer advises avoid.
● BREAST FEEDING Amount too small to be harmful.
● DIRECTIONS FOR ADMINISTRATION
▸ With oral use in children For administration by *mouth*, expert sources advise injection solution may be used; content of ampoule may be stored in a refrigerator for up to 24 hours after opening.
▸ With intravenous use in children For *intravenous injection*, expert sources advise may be diluted with Glucose 5% or Sodium Chloride 0.9%; give over at least 1 minute.
● PRESCRIBING AND DISPENSING INFORMATION
Palliative care For further information on the use of hyoscine butylbromide in palliative care, see www.medicinescomplete.com/#/content/palliative/hyoscine-butylbromide.
● EXCEPTIONS TO LEGAL CATEGORY Hyoscine butylbromide tablets can be sold to the public for medically confirmed irritable bowel syndrome, provided single dose does not exceed 20 mg, daily dose does not exceed 80 mg, and pack does not contain a total of more than 240 mg.

● MEDICINAL FORMS There can be variation in the licensing of different medicines containing the same drug. Forms available from special-order manufacturers include: oral suspension, oral solution

Solution for injection
▸ Hyoscine butylbromide (Non-proprietary)
Hyoscine butylbromide 20 mg per 1 ml Hyoscine butylbromide 20mg/1ml solution for injection ampoules | 10 ampoule PoM £2.92 DT = £2.92 (Hospital only)
▸ Buscopan (Sanofi)
Hyoscine butylbromide 20 mg per 1 ml Buscopan 20mg/1ml solution for injection ampoules | 10 ampoule PoM £2.92 DT = £2.92

Tablet
▸ Buscopan (Sanofi)
Hyoscine butylbromide 10 mg Buscopan 10mg tablets | 56 tablet PoM £3.00 DT = £3.00 | 100 tablet PoM £5.35

1

Gastro-intestinal system

Propantheline bromide

F 821

● **INDICATIONS AND DOSE**

Adult enuresis | Hyperhidrosis | Symptomatic relief of gastro-intestinal disorders characterised by smooth muscle spasm
▸ BY MOUTH
  ▸ Adult: 15 mg 3 times a day, dose to be taken at least one hour before food and 30 mg, dose to be taken at bedtime; maximum 120 mg per day

● INTERACTIONS → Appendix 1: propantheline
● SIDE-EFFECTS Arrhythmias · bronchial secretion decreased · mydriasis
● PREGNANCY Manufacturer advises avoid unless essential—no information available.
● BREAST FEEDING May suppress lactation.
● HEPATIC IMPAIRMENT Manufacturer advises caution.
● RENAL IMPAIRMENT Manufacturer advises caution.

● MEDICINAL FORMS There can be variation in the licensing of different medicines containing the same drug. Forms available from special-order manufacturers include: oral suspension, oral solution

Tablet
CAUTIONARY AND ADVISORY LABELS 23
▸ Pro-Banthine (Kyowa Kirin Ltd)
  Propantheline bromide 15 mg Pro-Banthine 15mg tablets | 112 tablet [PoM] £20.74 DT = £20.74

ANTISPASMODICS

Alverine citrate

28-Aug-2020

● **INDICATIONS AND DOSE**

Symptomatic relief of gastro-intestinal disorders characterised by smooth muscle spasm | Dysmenorrhoea
▸ BY MOUTH
  ▸ Child 12-17 years: 60–120 mg 1–3 times a day
  ▸ Adult: 60–120 mg 1–3 times a day

● CONTRA-INDICATIONS Intestinal obstruction · paralytic ileus
● SIDE-EFFECTS Dizziness · dyspnoea · headache · jaundice (reversible on discontinuation) · nausea · skin reactions · wheezing
● PREGNANCY Manufacturer advises avoid—limited information available
● BREAST FEEDING Manufacturer advises avoid—limited information available.
● PATIENT AND CARER ADVICE
  Driving and skilled tasks Dizziness may affect performance of skilled tasks (e.g. driving).

● MEDICINAL FORMS There can be variation in the licensing of different medicines containing the same drug.
Capsule
▸ Alverine citrate (Non-proprietary)
  Alverine citrate 60 mg Alverine 60mg capsules | 100 capsule [PoM] £10.74-£19.49 DT = £8.59
  Alverine citrate 120 mg Alverine 120mg capsules | 60 capsule [PoM] £10.50 DT = £10.28

Mebeverine hydrochloride

03-Nov-2020

● **INDICATIONS AND DOSE**

Adjunct in gastro-intestinal disorders characterised by smooth muscle spasm
▸ BY MOUTH USING IMMEDIATE-RELEASE MEDICINES
  ▸ Child 10-17 years: 135–150 mg 3 times a day, dose preferably taken 20 minutes before meals
  ▸ Adult: 135–150 mg 3 times a day, dose preferably taken 20 minutes before meals
Irritable bowel syndrome
▸ BY MOUTH USING MODIFIED-RELEASE MEDICINES
  ▸ Child 12-17 years: 200 mg twice daily
  ▸ Adult: 200 mg twice daily

● UNLICENSED USE
  ▸ In children Tablets and modified-release capsules not licensed for use in children.
● CONTRA-INDICATIONS Paralytic ileus
● SIDE-EFFECTS Angioedema · face oedema · skin reactions
● PREGNANCY Not known to be harmful—manufacturers advise avoid.
● BREAST FEEDING Manufacturers advise avoid—no information available.
● PATIENT AND CARER ADVICE Patients or carers should be given advice on the timing of administration of mebeverine hydrochloride tablets and oral suspension. Medicines for Children leaflet: Mebeverine for intestinal spasms www.medicinesforchildren.org.uk/mebeverine-intestinal-spasms

● EXCEPTIONS TO LEGAL CATEGORY
  ▸ In adults Mebeverine hydrochloride can be sold to the public for symptomatic relief of irritable bowel syndrome provided that max. single dose is 135 mg and max. daily dose is 405 mg; for uses other than symptomatic relief of irritable bowel syndrome provided that max. single dose is 100 mg and max. daily dose is 300 mg.

● MEDICINAL FORMS There can be variation in the licensing of different medicines containing the same drug. Forms available from special-order manufacturers include: oral suspension
Oral suspension
▸ Mebeverine hydrochloride (Non-proprietary)
  Mebeverine hydrochloride (as Mebeverine pamoate) 10 mg per 1 ml Mebeverine 50mg/5ml oral suspension sugar free sugar-free | 300 ml [PoM] £237.15 DT = £186.60
Modified-release capsule
CAUTIONARY AND ADVISORY LABELS 25
▸ Mebeverine hydrochloride (Non-proprietary)
  Mebeverine hydrochloride 200 mg Mebeverine 200mg modified-release capsules | 60 capsule [PoM] £9.89 DT = £9.88
▸ Aurobeverine MR (Milpharm Ltd)
  Mebeverine hydrochloride 200 mg Aurobeverine MR 200mg capsules | 60 capsule [PoM] £6.92 DT = £9.88
▸ Colofac MR (Mylan)
  Mebeverine hydrochloride 200 mg Colofac MR 200mg capsules | 60 capsule [PoM] £6.92 DT = £9.88
Tablet
▸ Mebeverine hydrochloride (Non-proprietary)
  Mebeverine hydrochloride 135 mg Mebeverine 135mg tablets | 100 tablet [PoM] £20.00 DT = £4.76
▸ Colofac (Mylan)
  Mebeverine hydrochloride 135 mg Colofac 135mg tablets | 100 tablet [PoM] £9.02 DT = £4.76

1

7 Liver disorders and related conditions

7.1 Biliary disorders

Cholestasis
01-May-2017

Description of condition

Cholestasis is an impairment of bile formation and/or bile flow, which may clinically present with fatigue, pruritus, dark urine, pale stools and, in its most overt form, jaundice and signs of fat soluble vitamin deficiencies.

Treatment of cholestatic pruritus

Several drugs are used to relieve cholestatic pruritus, even if evidence to support their use is limited.

[EvGr] Colestyramine p. 212 is the drug of choice for treating cholestatic pruritus. It is an anion-exchange resin that is not absorbed from the gastro-intestinal tract. It relieves pruritus by forming an insoluble complex in the intestine with bile acids and other compounds—the reduction of serum bile acid levels reduces excess deposition in the dermal tissue with a resultant decrease in pruritus. ⟨A⟩

[EvGr] Ursodeoxycholic acid p. 97 has a small and variable impact on cholestatic pruritus. ⟨E⟩

[EvGr] Rifampicin p. 619 [unlicensed indication] can be used as an alternative treatment for pruritus, but should be used with caution in patients with pre-existing liver disease because of possible hepatotoxicity. ⟨A⟩

[EvGr] Where previous therapy has proved ineffective or was not tolerated, other drugs including sertraline p. 387 [unlicensed indication] and naltrexone hydrochloride p. 519 [unlicensed indication], may be used to treat cholestatic pruritus. However, their use is limited due to significant side-effects. ⟨E⟩

Intrahepatic cholestasis in pregnancy

[EvGr] Ursodeoxycholic acid is effective for the treatment of pruritus associated with intrahepatic cholestasis in pregnancy. ⟨E⟩

Intrahepatic cholestasis usually occurs in late pregnancy and is associated with adverse fetal outcomes. [EvGr] There is no evidence that ursodeoxycholic acid used in late pregnancy affects birth weight in the infant or the risk of preterm delivery. There is limited data about the effect of fetal exposure during the first trimester. ⟨D⟩

Gallstones
01-May-2017

Description of condition

Gallstones (cholelithiases) occur when hard mineral or fatty deposits form in the gallbladder. Gallstone disease is a general term that describes the presence of one or more stones in the gallbladder or in the bile duct, and the symptoms and complications that they may cause.

The majority of patients with gallstones remain asymptomatic. When the stones irritate the gallbladder or block part of the biliary system, the patient can experience symptoms such as pain, or infection and inflammation that if left untreated, can lead to severe complications such as biliary colic, acute cholecystitis, cholangitis, pancreatitis, and obstructive jaundice.

Non-drug treatment

[EvGr] Asymptomatic gallbladder stones do not need to be treated unless symptoms develop.

The definitive treatment of symptomatic gallstones (and all bile duct stones) is surgical removal by laparoscopic cholecystectomy. ⟨A⟩

Drug treatment

[EvGr] Analgesia should be offered to control pain symptoms. Paracetamol p. 464 or a nonsteroidal anti-inflammatory drug (see Non-steroidal anti-inflammatory drugs p. 1176) is recommended for intermittent mild-to-moderate pain. Intramuscular diclofenac sodium p. 1181 can be given for severe pain or, if not suitable, an intramuscular opioid (such as morphine p. 483 or pethidine hydrochloride p. 489). ⟨A⟩

Although ursodeoxycholic acid p. 97 has been used for the management of gallstone disease, there is no evidence to support its use.

Useful Resources

Gallstone disease: diagnosis and management. National Institute for Health and Care Excellence. Clinical guideline 188. October 2014.
www.nice.org.uk/guidance/cg188

Inborn errors of primary bile acid synthesis
27-Apr-2018

Description of condition

Inborn errors of primary bile acid synthesis are a group of diseases in which the liver does not produce enough primary bile acids due to enzyme deficiencies. These acids are the main components of the bile, and include cholic acid and chenodeoxycholic acid.

Treatment

Cholic acid p. 96 is licensed for the treatment of inborn errors in primary bile acid synthesis due to an inborn deficiency of two specific liver enzymes. It acts by replacing some of the missing bile acids, therefore relieving the symptoms of the disease.

Chenodeoxycholic acid p. 96 is licensed for the treatment of inborn errors of primary bile acid synthesis due to a deficiency of one specific enzyme in the bile acid synthesis pathway when presenting as cerebrotendinous xanthomatosis.

Ursodeoxycholic acid p. 97 [unlicensed indication] has been used to treat inborn errors of primary bile acid synthesis, but there is an absence of evidence to recommend its use.

Primary biliary cholangitis
30-May-2017

Description of condition

Primary biliary cholangitis (or primary biliary cirrhosis) is a chronic cholestatic disease which develops due to progressive destruction of small and intermediate bile ducts within the liver, subsequently evolving to fibrosis and cirrhosis.

Treatment

[EvGr] Ursodeoxycholic acid p. 97 is recommended for the management of primary biliary cholangitis, including those with asymptomatic disease. It slows disease progression, but the effect on overall survival is uncertain. Liver transplantation can be considered in patients with advanced primary biliary cholangitis. ⟨A⟩

BILE ACIDS

Chenodeoxycholic acid

05-Apr-2018

- **INDICATIONS AND DOSE**

Cerebrotendinous xanthomatosis (specialist use only)
▶ BY MOUTH
 ▪ Adult: Initially 750 mg daily in 3 divided doses, increased if necessary up to 1000 mg daily in divided doses

- **CONTRA-INDICATIONS** Non-functioning gall bladder · radio-opaque stones
- **INTERACTIONS** → Appendix 1: chenodeoxycholic acid
- **SIDE-EFFECTS** Constipation
- **PREGNANCY** Manufacturer advises avoid—fetotoxicity reported in *animal* studies.
- **HEPATIC IMPAIRMENT** Manufacturer advises monitor—no information available.
- **RENAL IMPAIRMENT** Manufacturer advises monitor—no information available.
- **MONITORING REQUIREMENTS** Manufacturer advises to monitor serum cholestanol levels and/or urine bile alcohols every 3 months during the initiation of therapy and dose adjustment, and then at least annually; liver function should also be monitored during initiation of therapy and then at least annually; additional or more frequent investigations may need to be undertaken to monitor therapy during periods of fast growth or concomitant disease.
- **DIRECTIONS FOR ADMINISTRATION** For administration *by mouth* in patients who are unable to swallow capsules and/or need to take a dose below 250 mg, manufacturer advises to add capsule contents to sodium bicarbonate solution 8.4%—for further information, consult product literature.
- **MEDICINAL FORMS** There can be variation in the licensing of different medicines containing the same drug.

Capsule
 ▶ Chenodeoxycholic acid (non-proprietary) ▼
  Chenodeoxycholic acid 250 mg Chenodeoxycholic acid 250mg capsules | 100 capsule PoM £14,000.00 DT = £9,999.99

Cholic acid

04-Sep-2020

- **DRUG ACTION** Cholic acid is the predominant primary bile acid in humans, which can be used to provide a source of bile acid in patients with inborn deficiencies in bile acid synthesis.

- **INDICATIONS AND DOSE**

Inborn errors of primary bile acid synthesis (initiated by a specialist)
▶ BY MOUTH
 ▪ Adult: Usual dose 5–15 mg/kg daily; increased in steps of 50 mg daily in divided doses if required, dose to be given with food at the same time each day; Usual maximum 500 mg/24 hours

- **INTERACTIONS** → Appendix 1: cholic acid
- **SIDE-EFFECTS** Cholelithiasis (long term use) · diarrhoea · pruritus
 SIDE-EFFECTS, FURTHER INFORMATION Patients presenting with pruritus and/or persistent diarrhoea should be investigated for potential overdose by a serum and/or urine bile acid assay.
- **PREGNANCY** Limited data available—not known to be harmful, manufacturer advises continue treatment.
 Monitoring Manufacturer advises monitor patient parameters more frequently in pregnancy.

- **BREAST FEEDING** Present in milk but not known to be harmful.
- **HEPATIC IMPAIRMENT** Manufacturer advises caution and stop treatment if there are signs of severe hepatic failure—limited information available (no experience with impairment from causes not related to inborn errors of primary bile acid synthesis).
 Dose adjustments Manufacturer advises adjust dose as the degree of impairment improves during treatment.
- **MONITORING REQUIREMENTS** Manufacturer advises monitor serum and/or urine bile-acid concentrations every 3 months for the first year, then every 6 months for three years, then annually; monitor liver function tests at the same or greater frequency.
- **DIRECTIONS FOR ADMINISTRATION** Manufacturer advises capsules may be opened and the content added to infant formula, juice, fruit compote, or yoghurt for administration.
- **PATIENT AND CARER ADVICE** Counselling advised on administration.
- **MEDICINAL FORMS** There can be variation in the licensing of different medicines containing the same drug.

Capsule
CAUTIONARY AND ADVISORY LABELS 25
 ▶ Orphacol (Laboratoires CTRS) ▼
  Cholic acid 50 mg Orphacol 50mg capsules | 30 capsule PoM £1,860.00
  Cholic acid 250 mg Orphacol 250mg capsules | 30 capsule PoM £6,630.00

Obeticholic acid

26-Aug-2020

- **DRUG ACTION** Obeticholic acid is a selective farnesoid X receptor agonist, which decreases circulating bile acid.

- **INDICATIONS AND DOSE**

Primary biliary cholangitis in combination with ursodeoxycholic acid when response to ursodeoxycholic acid has been inadequate, or as monotherapy in patients intolerant of ursodeoxycholic acid
▶ BY MOUTH
 ▪ Adult: Initially 5 mg once daily for 6 months, then increased to 10 mg once daily if necessary and if tolerated, for dose adjustments due to severe pruritus, consult product literature

> **IMPORTANT SAFETY INFORMATION**
>
> MHRA/CHM ADVICE: OBETICHOLIC ACID (*OCALIVA*®): RISK OF SERIOUS LIVER INJURY IN PATIENTS WITH PRE-EXISTING MODERATE OR SEVERE HEPATIC IMPAIRMENT; REMINDER TO ADJUST DOSING ACCORDING TO LIVER FUNCTION MONITORING (APRIL 2018)
>
> The MHRA is aware of reports of serious liver injuries and deaths in patients with primary biliary cholangitis with pre-existing moderate or severe liver impairment who were not adequately dose-adjusted. Follow dose reduction and monitoring advice in these patients to reduce the risk of serious liver injury; for further information, see *Hepatic impairment* and *Monitoring*.

- **CONTRA-INDICATIONS** Complete biliary obstruction
- **INTERACTIONS** → Appendix 1: obeticholic acid
- **SIDE-EFFECTS**
 ▶ **Common or very common** Arthralgia · constipation · dizziness · fatigue · fever · gastrointestinal discomfort · oropharyngeal pain · palpitations · peripheral oedema · skin reactions
 ▶ **Frequency not known** Hepatic failure

- PREGNANCY
  Dose adjustments No evidence of harm but manufacturer advises avoid.
- BREAST FEEDING Not known to be harmful but manufacturer advises avoid.
- HEPATIC IMPAIRMENT Manufacturer advises caution in moderate to severe impairment or decompensated cirrhosis (risk of increased exposure).
  Dose adjustments Manufacturer advises initial dose reduction to 5 mg once weekly in moderate to severe impairment or decompensated cirrhosis; titrate dose according to alkaline phosphatase and/or total bilirubin level—consult product literature.
- MONITORING REQUIREMENTS Manufacturer advises assess hepatic status before treatment initiation and then monitor for progression of primary biliary cholangitis with laboratory and clinical assessment to evaluate the need for dose reduction; patients at an increased risk of hepatic decompensation, including those with laboratory evidence of worsening liver function and/or progression to cirrhosis, should be monitored more closely.
- NATIONAL FUNDING/ACCESS DECISIONS
  For full details see funding body website
  NICE decisions
  ▸ Obeticholic acid for treating primary biliary cholangitis (April 2017) NICE TA443 Recommended with restrictions
  Scottish Medicines Consortium (SMC) decisions
  ▸ Obeticholic acid (*Ocaliva*®) for the treatment of primary biliary cholangitis in combination with ursodeoxycholic acid in adults with an inadequate response to ursodeoxycholic acid or as monotherapy in adults unable to tolerate ursodeoxycholic acid (June 2017) SMC No. 1232/17 Recommended

- MEDICINAL FORMS There can be variation in the licensing of different medicines containing the same drug.
  Tablet
  ▸ Ocaliva (Intercept Pharma UK & Ireland Ltd) ▼
    Obeticholic acid 5 mg Ocaliva 5mg tablets | 30 tablet [PoM]
    £2,384.04 (Hospital only)
    Obeticholic acid 10 mg Ocaliva 10mg tablets | 30 tablet [PoM]
    £2,384.04 (Hospital only)

Ursodeoxycholic acid

02-Sep-2020

- **INDICATIONS AND DOSE**
  Dissolution of gallstones
  ▸ BY MOUTH
  ▸ **Adult:** 8–12 mg/kg once daily, dose to be taken at bedtime, alternatively 8–12 mg/kg daily in 2 divided doses for up to 2 years; treatment is continued for 3–4 months after stones dissolve

  Primary biliary cirrhosis
  ▸ BY MOUTH
  ▸ **Adult:** 12–16 mg/kg daily in 3 divided doses for 3 months, then 12–16 mg/kg once daily, dose to be taken at bedtime

  Gall reflux gastritis
  ▸ BY MOUTH
  ▸ **Adult (body-weight 47 kg and above):** 250 mg once daily for 10–14 days, dose to be taken at bedtime

- CONTRA-INDICATIONS Acute inflammation of the gall bladder · frequent episodes of biliary colic · inflammatory diseases and other conditions of the colon, liver or small intestine which interfere with enterohepatic circulation of bile salts · non-functioning gall bladder · radio-opaque stones
- INTERACTIONS → Appendix 1: ursodeoxycholic acid
- SIDE-EFFECTS
- **Common or very common** Diarrhoea · pale faeces

▸ **Rare or very rare** Abdominal pain upper · cholelithiasis calcification · hepatic cirrhosis exacerbated · skin reactions
▸ **Frequency not known** Nausea · vomiting
- PREGNANCY No evidence of harm but manufacturer advises avoid.
- BREAST FEEDING Not known to be harmful but manufacturer advises avoid.
- HEPATIC IMPAIRMENT Avoid in chronic liver disease (but used in primary biliary cirrhosis).
- MONITORING REQUIREMENTS In primary biliary cirrhosis, monitor liver function every 4 weeks for 3 months, then every 3 months.
- PATIENT AND CARER ADVICE Patients should be given dietary advice (including avoidance of excessive cholesterol and calories).

- MEDICINAL FORMS There can be variation in the licensing of different medicines containing the same drug. Forms available from special-order manufacturers include: oral suspension, oral solution
  Oral suspension
  CAUTIONARY AND ADVISORY LABELS 21
  ▸ Ursofalk (Dr. Falk Pharma UK Ltd)
    Ursodeoxycholic acid 50 mg per 1 ml Ursofalk 250mg/5ml oral suspension sugar-free | 250 ml [PoM] £26.98 DT = £26.98
  Tablet
  CAUTIONARY AND ADVISORY LABELS 21
  ▸ Ursodeoxycholic acid (Non-proprietary)
    Ursodeoxycholic acid 150 mg Ursodeoxycholic acid 150mg tablets | 60 tablet [PoM] £19.02 DT = £19.02
    Ursodeoxycholic acid 300 mg Ursodeoxycholic acid 300mg tablets | 60 tablet [PoM] £55.72 DT = £55.98
  ▸ Cholurso (HFA Healthcare Products Ltd)
    Ursodeoxycholic acid 250 mg Cholurso 250mg tablets | 60 tablet [PoM] £18.00 DT = £18.00
    Ursodeoxycholic acid 500 mg Cholurso 500mg tablets | 60 tablet [PoM] £45.00
  ▸ Destolit (Norgine Pharmaceuticals Ltd)
    Ursodeoxycholic acid 150 mg Destolit 150mg tablets | 60 tablet [PoM] £19.02 DT = £19.02
  ▸ Ursofalk (Dr. Falk Pharma UK Ltd)
    Ursodeoxycholic acid 500 mg Ursofalk 500mg tablets | 100 tablet [PoM] £80.00 DT = £80.00
  ▸ Ursonorm (PRO.MED.CS Praha a.s.)
    Ursodeoxycholic acid 500 mg Ursonorm 500mg tablets | 60 tablet [PoM] £45.00 | 100 tablet [PoM] £79.00 DT = £80.00
  Capsule
  CAUTIONARY AND ADVISORY LABELS 21
  ▸ Ursodeoxycholic acid (Non-proprietary)
    Ursodeoxycholic acid 250 mg Ursodeoxycholic acid 250mg capsules | 60 capsule [PoM] £29.00 DT = £11.80 | 100 capsule [PoM] £27.10
  ▸ Ursofalk (Dr. Falk Pharma UK Ltd)
    Ursodeoxycholic acid 250 mg Ursofalk 250mg capsules | 60 capsule [PoM] £30.17 DT = £11.80 | 100 capsule [PoM] £31.88
  ▸ Ursonorm (PRO.MED.CS Praha a.s.)
    Ursodeoxycholic acid 250 mg Ursonorm 250mg capsules | 60 capsule [PoM] £29.00 DT = £11.80

TERPENES

Borneol with camphene, cineole, menthol, menthone and pinene

- **INDICATIONS AND DOSE**
  Biliary disorders
  ▸ BY MOUTH
  ▸ **Adult:** 1–2 capsules 3 times a day, to be taken before food

- LESS SUITABLE FOR PRESCRIBING *Rowachol*® is less suitable for prescribing.

1

Gastro-intestinal system

● MEDICINAL FORMS There can be variation in the licensing of different medicines containing the same drug.

Gastro-resistant capsule

CAUTIONARY AND ADVISORY LABELS 22

▸ Rowachol (Meadow Laboratories Ltd)

Cineole 2 mg, Borneol 5 mg, Camphene 5 mg, Menthone 6 mg, Pinene 17 mg, Menthol 32 mg Rowachol gastro-resistant capsules | 50 capsule PoM £7.35

7.2   Oesophageal varices

Other drugs used for Oesophageal varices Vasopressin, p. 708

PITUITARY AND HYPOTHALAMIC HORMONES AND ANALOGUES ⟩VASOPRESSIN AND ANALOGUES

Terlipressin acetate

● INDICATIONS AND DOSE

GLYPRESSIN ® INJECTION

Bleeding from oesophageal varices

▸ BY INTRAVENOUS INJECTION

▸ **Adult (body-weight up to 50 kg):** Initially 2 mg every 4 hours until bleeding controlled, then reduced to 1 mg every 4 hours if required, maximum duration 48 hours

▸ **Adult (body-weight 50 kg and above):** Initially 2 mg every 4 hours until bleeding controlled, reduced if not tolerated to 1 mg every 4 hours, maximum duration 48 hours

VARIQUEL ® INJECTION

Bleeding from oesophageal varices

▸ BY INTRAVENOUS INJECTION

▸ **Adult (body-weight up to 50 kg):** Initially 1 mg, then 1 mg every 4–6 hours for up to 72 hours, to be administered over 1 minute

▸ **Adult (body-weight 50–69 kg):** Initially 1.5 mg, then 1 mg every 4–6 hours for up to 72 hours, to be administered over 1 minute

▸ **Adult (body-weight 70 kg and above):** Initially 2 mg, then 1 mg every 4–6 hours for up to 72 hours, to be administered over 1 minute

● CAUTIONS Arrhythmia · elderly · electrolyte and fluid disturbances · heart disease · history of QT-interval prolongation · respiratory disease · septic shock · uncontrolled hypertension · vascular disease

● SIDE-EFFECTS

▸ **Common or very common** Abdominal cramps · arrhythmias · diarrhoea · headache · hypertension · hypotension · pallor · peripheral ischaemia · vasoconstriction

▸ **Uncommon** Chest pain · cyanosis · fluid overload · heart failure · hot flush · hyponatraemia · intestinal ischaemia · ischaemic heart disease · lymphangitis · myocardial infarction · nausea · pulmonary oedema · respiratory disorders · seizure · skin necrosis · uterine disorders · vomiting

▸ **Rare or very rare** Dyspnoea · hyperglycaemia · stroke

● PREGNANCY Avoid unless benefits outweigh risk—uterine contractions and increased intra-uterine pressure in early pregnancy, and decreased uterine blood flow reported.

● BREAST FEEDING Avoid unless benefits outweigh risk—no information available.

● RENAL IMPAIRMENT Use with caution in chronic renal failure.

● MEDICINAL FORMS There can be variation in the licensing of different medicines containing the same drug.

Solution for injection

▸ Glypressin (Ferring Pharmaceuticals Ltd)

Terlipressin acetate 120 microgram per 1 ml Glypressin 1mg/8.5ml solution for injection ampoules | 5 ampoule PoM ⬭

▸ Variquel (Alliance Pharmaceuticals Ltd)

Terlipressin acetate 200 microgram per 1 ml Variquel 1mg/5ml solution for injection vials | 5 vial PoM £89.98 (Hospital only)

8   Obesity

Obesity

01-Jun-2016

Description of condition

Obesity is directly linked to many health problems including cardiovascular disease, type 2 diabetes, fatty liver disease, gallstones, and gastro-oesophageal reflux disease. It is also linked to psychological and psychiatric morbidities.

In adults, obesity is generally classified as a body mass index (BMI) of ≥ 30 kg/m^2, though BMI should be interpreted with caution as it is not a direct measure of adiposity, particularly in patients who are very muscular or have muscle weakness or atrophy.

Waist circumference should also be considered as it may provide an indication of total body fat and a risk of obesity-related health problems. Men with a waist circumference ≥ 94 cm (≥ 90 cm for Asian men), and women with a waist circumference of ≥ 80 cm are at increased risk of obesity-related health problems. A waist circumference of ≥ 102 cm in men and ≥ 88 cm in women indicates a very high risk of obesity-related health problems.

Aims of treatment

Management should be aimed at modest, sustainable weight loss and maintenance of a healthy weight, to reduce the risk factors associated with obesity.

Overview

EvGr Obesity should be managed in an appropriate setting by staff who have been trained in the management of obesity. Patients should be monitored for changes in weight, as well as changes in blood pressure and blood lipids, and for other associated conditions.

An initial assessment should consider potential underlying causes (e.g. hypothyroidism) and a review of the appropriateness of current medications which are known to cause weight gain, e.g. atypical antipsychotics, beta-adrenoceptor blocking drugs, insulin (when used in the treatment of type 2 diabetes), lithium carbonate, lithium citrate, sodium valproate, sulphonylureas, thiazolidinediones, and tricyclic antidepressants. ⒶGr

Lifestyle changes

EvGr Patients should be encouraged to engage in a sustainable weight management programme which includes strategies to change behaviour, increase physical activity, and improve diet and eating behaviour. ⒶGr

Drug treatment

EvGr Drug treatment should **never** be used as the sole element of treatment and should be used as part of an overall weight management plan. An anti-obesity drug should be considered only for those with a BMI of ≥ 30 kg/m^2, in whom diet, exercise and behaviour changes fail to achieve a realistic reduction in weight. In the presence of associated risk factors, it may be appropriate to prescribe an anti-obesity drug to individuals with a BMI of ≥ 28 kg/m^2. A vitamin and mineral supplement may also be considered if there is concern about inadequate micronutrient intake, particularly for vulnerable groups such as in the elderly and younger patients.

The effect of management should be monitored on a regular basis with reinforcement of supporting lifestyle advice. Rates of weight loss may be slower in patients with type 2 diabetes, so less strict goals than in those without diabetes may be appropriate.

Orlistat below, is the only drug currently available in the UK that is recommended specifically for the management of obesity; it acts by reducing the absorption of dietary fat.

Orlistat is licensed for use as an adjunct in the management of obesity in patients with a BMI of $\geq 30 \text{ kg/m}^2$, or, in individuals with a BMI of $\geq 28 \text{ kg/m}^2$ in the presence of other risk factors. Treatment with orlistat may also be used to maintain weight loss rather than to continue to lose weight. Discontinuation of treatment with orlistat should be considered after 12 weeks if weight loss has not exceeded 5% since the start of treatment. ⒶⒶ

Drugs which produce a feeling of satiety (such as methylcellulose p. 59 and sterculia p. 59 [unlicensed indications]) have been used in an attempt to control appetite, but there is little evidence for their efficacy. Various centrally acting appetite suppressants, including stimulants and serotonergic drugs (such as dexfenfluramine, fenfluramine, sibutramine, and rimonabant), have been used in the management of obesity but have been withdrawn or are no longer recommended due to serious safety concerns or their addictive potential.

Surgery

EvGr Bariatric surgery may be considered for patients who have a BMI of $\geq 40 \text{ kg/m}^2$ (Obesity III, morbid obesity), or between 35–39.9 kg/m^2 (Obesity II) and a significant disease (such as type 2 diabetes or high blood pressure) which could be improved with weight loss, and if all appropriate non-surgical measures have been tried but clinically beneficial weight loss has not been achieved or maintained. ⒶⒶ

Useful Resources

Obesity: identification, assessment and management. Clinical Guideline 189. National Institute for Health and Care Excellence. November 2014.
www.nice.org.uk/guidance/cg189

> **Other drugs used for Obesity** Liraglutide, p. 739

ANTIDEPRESSANTS ⟩ SEROTONIN AND NORADRENALINE RE-UPTAKE INHIBITORS

▍Naltrexone with bupropion   10-Sep-2019

The properties listed below are those particular to the combination only. For the properties of the components please consider, bupropion hydrochloride p. 520, naltrexone hydrochloride p. 519.

- ● **INDICATIONS AND DOSE**

   Adjunct in obesity (in conjunction with dietary measures and increased physical activity in individuals with a body mass index (BMI) of 30 kg/m^2 or more or in individuals with a BMI of 27 kg/m^2 or more in the presence of one or more weight related co-morbidity)
   ▸ BY MOUTH
   ▸ Adult 18–75 years: Initially 1 tablet daily for 7 days, then increased to 1 tablet twice daily for 7 days, then increased to 3 tablets daily in divided doses for 7 days, two tablets to be taken in the morning, and one tablet to be taken in the evening, then maintenance 2 tablets twice daily, review treatment after 16 weeks and then annually

---

DOSE EQUIVALENCE AND CONVERSION
▸ Each tablet contains 8 mg naltrexone with 90 mg bupropion.

IMPORTANT SAFETY INFORMATION

MHRA/CHM ADVICE: NALTREXONE/BUPROPION (*MYSIMBA*®): RISK OF ADVERSE REACTIONS THAT COULD AFFECT ABILITY TO DRIVE (AUGUST 2019)
An EU cumulative review of worldwide data has found naltrexone with bupropion to be commonly associated with dizziness or somnolence, and rarely with loss of consciousness or seizure. These can affect the ability of patients to drive, operate machinery, or perform dangerous tasks, particularly at the start of treatment or during the dose titration phase. Healthcare professionals are advised to inform patients of these adverse effects and to avoid such tasks until they are resolved.

- ● CONTRA-INDICATIONS Uncontrolled hypertension
- ● CAUTIONS History of mania · hypertension
- ● INTERACTIONS → Appendix 1: bupropion · naltrexone
- ● HEPATIC IMPAIRMENT Manufacturer advises avoid (no information available).
- ● RENAL IMPAIRMENT Manufacturer advises avoid in moderate-to-severe impairment—limited information available.
- ● PRESCRIBING AND DISPENSING INFORMATION Prescribers should consult the *Mysimba*® *Physician Prescribing Checklist* provided by the manufacturer, before initiation of treatment.
- ● NATIONAL FUNDING/ACCESS DECISIONS
   For full details see funding body website
   NICE decisions
   ▸ **Naltrexone–bupropion for managing overweight and obesity (December 2017) NICE TA494 Not recommended**
- ● MEDICINAL FORMS There can be variation in the licensing of different medicines containing the same drug.
   Modified-release tablet
   CAUTIONARY AND ADVISORY LABELS 21, 25
   ▸ Mysimba (Orexigen Therapeutics Ireland Ltd) ▼
      Naltrexone hydrochloride 8 mg, Bupropion hydrochloride 90 mg Mysimba 8mg/90mg modified-release tablets |
      112 tablet PoM £73.00 DT = £73.00

PERIPHERALLY ACTING ANTIOBESITY PRODUCTS ⟩ LIPASE INHIBITORS

▍Orlistat

- ● DRUG ACTION Orlistat, a lipase inhibitor, reduces the absorption of dietary fat.

- ● **INDICATIONS AND DOSE**

   Adjunct in obesity (in conjunction with a mildly hypocaloric diet in individuals with a body mass index (BMI) of 30 kg/m^2 or more or in individuals with a BMI of 28 kg/m^2 or more in the presence of other risk factors such as type 2 diabetes, hypertension, or hypercholesterolaemia)
   ▸ BY MOUTH
   ▸ Adult: 120 mg up to 3 times a day, dose to be taken immediately before, during, or up to 1 hour after each main meal, continue treatment beyond 12 weeks only if weight loss since start of treatment exceeds 5% (target for initial weight loss may be lower in patients with type 2 diabetes), if a meal is missed or contains no fat, the dose of orlistat should be omitted

- ● CONTRA-INDICATIONS Cholestasis · chronic malabsorption syndrome

- CAUTIONS Chronic kidney disease · may impair absorption of fat-soluble vitamins · volume depletion

  CAUTIONS, FURTHER INFORMATION Vitamin supplementation (especially of vitamin D) may be considered if there is concern about deficiency of fat-soluble vitamins.
- INTERACTIONS → Appendix 1: orlistat
- SIDE-EFFECTS
- ▶ **Common or very common** Abdominal pain (may be minimised by reduced fat intake) · anxiety · diarrhoea · gastrointestinal disorders
- ▶ **Frequency not known** Anorectal haemorrhage · bullous dermatitis · cholelithiasis · diverticulitis · hepatitis · oxalate nephropathy · pancreatitis · renal failure
- PREGNANCY Use with caution.
- BREAST FEEDING Avoid—no information available.

- MEDICINAL FORMS There can be variation in the licensing of different medicines containing the same drug.

  Capsule
- ▶ Orlistat (Non-proprietary)
  Orlistat 120 mg Orlistat 120mg capsules | 84 capsule PoM £30.05 DT = £25.28
- ▶ Alli (GlaxoSmithKline Consumer Healthcare)
  Orlistat 60 mg Alli 60mg capsules | 84 capsule P £30.70 DT = £30.70
- ▶ Beacita (Actavis UK Ltd)
  Orlistat 120 mg Beacita 120mg capsules | 84 capsule PoM £21.95 DT = £25.28
- ▶ Orlos (Crescent Pharma Ltd)
  Orlistat 60 mg Orlos 60mg capsules | 84 capsule P £16.95 DT = £30.70
- ▶ Xenical (Cheplapharm Arzneimittel GmbH)
  Orlistat 120 mg Xenical 120mg capsules | 84 capsule PoM £31.63 DT = £25.28

9 Rectal and anal disorders

Other drugs used for Rectal and anal disorders Diltiazem hydrochloride, p. 171

9.1 Anal fissures

Anal fissure

31-Aug-2016

Description of condition

An anal fissure is a tear or ulcer in the lining of the anal canal, immediately within the anal margin. Clinical features of anal fissure include bleeding and persistent pain on defecation, and a linear split in the anal mucosa.

Aims of treatment

The aim of treatment is to relieve pain and promote healing of the fissure.

Drug treatment

Acute anal fissure

EvGr Initial management of acute anal fissures (present for less than 6 weeks) should focus on ensuring that stools are soft and easily passed. Bulk-forming laxatives (such as ispaghula husk p. 58) are recommended and an osmotic laxative (such as lactulose p. 60) can be considered as an alternative—see also Constipation p. 57, for further information about these laxatives. Short-term use of a topical preparation containing a local anaesthetic (such as lidocaine hydrochloride p. 1406) or a simple analgesic (such as paracetamol p. 464 or ibuprofen p. 1186) may be offered for prolonged burning pain following defecation. If these

measures are inadequate, the patient should be referred for specialist treatment in hospital. ◁Ⓐ▷

Chronic anal fissure

EvGr Chronic anal fissures (present for 6 weeks or longer), and associated pain, may be treated with glyceryl trinitrate rectal ointment 0.4% or 0.2% p. 233 [unlicensed] (available from Special-order manufacturers p. 1696 or specialist importing companies). Limited evidence suggests that the strength used does not influence the effectiveness, but that the higher strength potentially increases the incidence of side-effects. Healing rates with topical glyceryl trinitrate are marginally superior to placebo, but the incidence of headache as an adverse effect is quite high (about 20-30% of patients). Recurrence of the fissure after treatment is common.

As an alternative to glyceryl trinitrate rectal ointment, chronic anal fissure may also be treated with topical diltiazem hydrochloride p. 171 2% [unlicensed] or nifedipine p. 176 0.2-0.5% [unlicensed] (available from Special-order manufacturers p. 1696 or specialist importing companies), which have a lower incidence of adverse effects than topical glyceryl trinitrate. Oral nifedipine [unlicensed indication] and oral diltiazem hydrochloride [unlicensed indication] may be as effective as topical treatment, but the incidence of adverse effects are likely to be higher and topical preparations are preferred.

Patients who do not respond to first-line treatment may be referred to a specialist for local injection of botulinum toxin type A [unlicensed indication]. ◁Ⓐ▷

Non-drug treatment

EvGr Surgery is an effective option for the management of chronic anal fissure in adults but is generally reserved for those who do not respond to drug treatment. ◁Ⓐ▷

9.2 Haemorrhoids

Haemorrhoids

01-Dec-2016

Description of condition

Haemorrhoids, or piles, are abnormal swellings of the vascular mucosal anal cushions around the anus. Internal haemorrhoids arise above the dentate line and are usually painless unless they become strangulated. External haemorrhoids originate below the dentate line and can be itchy or painful. Women are predisposed to developing haemorrhoids during pregnancy.

Aims of treatment

The aims of treatment are to reduce the symptoms (pain, bleeding and swelling), promote healing, and prevent recurrence.

Non-drug treatment

EvGr Stools should be kept soft and easy to pass (to minimise straining) by increasing dietary fibre and fluid intake. Advice about perianal hygiene is helpful to aid healing and reduce irritation and itching. ◁Ⓐ▷

Drug treatment

EvGr If constipation is reported, it should be treated. A bulk-forming laxative can be prescribed (see Constipation p. 57)

A simple analgesic such as paracetamol p. 464 can be used for pain relief. Opioid analgesics should be avoided as they can cause constipation, and NSAIDs should be avoided if rectal bleeding is present. ◁Ⓐ▷

Topical preparations that contain a combination of local anaesthetics, corticosteroids, astringents, lubricants, and antiseptics are available—see *Related drugs* below. EvGr They can offer symptomatic relief of local pain and itching but evidence does not suggest that any preparation is more effective than any other.

Topical preparations containing local anaesthetics (lidocaine, benzocaine, cinchocaine and pramocaine) should only be used for a few days as they may cause sensitisation of the anal skin. Local anaesthetics can be absorbed through the rectal mucosa (with a theoretical risk of systemic side effects) and very rarely may cause increased irritation; therefore excessive application should be **avoided**. Ⓐ

Topical preparations combining corticosteroids with local anaesthetics and soothing agents are available for the management of haemorrhoids. They may ameliorate local perianal inflammation, but no data suggest that they actually reduce haemorrhoidal swelling, bleeding, or protrusion.

EvGr Topical corticosteroids are suitable for occasional short-term use (no more than 7 days) after exclusion of infections (such as perianal streptococcal infection, *herpes simplex* or perianal thrush). Long-term use of corticosteroid creams can cause ulceration or permanent damage due to thinning of the perianal skin and should be avoided. ⒶA Continuous or excessive use carries a risk of adrenal suppression and systemic corticosteroid effects.

EvGr Recurrent symptoms, should be referred to secondary care for further investigation and management.

Treatments available from *specialists* include rubber band ligation, injection sclerotherapy (using phenol p. 103 in oil), infrared coagulation/photocoagulation, bipolar diathermy and direct-current electrotherapy, haemorrhoidectomy, stapled haemorrhoidectomy, and haemorrhoidal artery ligation. ⒶA

Pregnancy

EvGr Bulk forming laxatives are not absorbed, and are therefore safe for use in pregnant women (see Pregnancy, under Constipation p. 57). ⒶA No topical haemorrhoidal preparations are licensed for use during pregnancy.

EvGr If treatment with a topical haemorrhoidal preparation is required, a soothing preparation containing simple, soothing products (**not** local anaesthetics or corticosteroids) can be considered. ⒶA

Related drugs

Topical preparations used for haemorrhoids: lidocaine hydrochloride p. 1406, benzyl benzoate with bismuth oxide, bismuth subgallate, hydrocortisone acetate, peru balsam and zinc oxide below, cinchocaine hydrochloride with fluocortolone caproate and fluocortolone pivalate below, cinchocaine with hydrocortisone p. 102, cinchocaine with prednisolone p. 102.

CORTICOSTEROIDS

Benzyl benzoate with bismuth oxide, bismuth subgallate, hydrocortisone acetate, peru balsam and zinc oxide

25-Sep-2020

● **INDICATIONS AND DOSE**

Haemorrhoids | **Pruritus ani**

▸ BY RECTUM USING OINTMENT

▸ Adult: Apply twice daily for no longer than 7 days, to be applied morning and night, an additional dose should be applied after a bowel movement

▸ BY RECTUM USING SUPPOSITORIES

▸ Adult: 1 suppository twice daily for no longer than 7 days, to be inserted night and morning, additional dose after a bowel movement

IMPORTANT SAFETY INFORMATION

MHRA/CHM ADVICE: CORTICOSTEROIDS: RARE RISK OF CENTRAL SEROUS CHORIORETINOPATHY WITH LOCAL AS WELL AS SYSTEMIC ADMINISTRATION (AUGUST 2017)
See Corticosteroids, general use p. 709.

NHS IMPROVEMENT PATIENT SAFETY ALERT: STEROID EMERGENCY CARD TO SUPPORT EARLY RECOGNITION AND TREATMENT OF ADRENAL CRISIS IN ADULTS (AUGUST 2020)
See Corticosteroids, general use p. 709.

● CONTRA-INDICATIONS Tubercular, fungal or viral lesions

● SIDE-EFFECTS Skin reactions · vision disorders

● PREGNANCY Manufacturer advises avoid—toxicity in animal studies.

● BREAST FEEDING Manufacturer advises avoid.

● PRESCRIBING AND DISPENSING INFORMATION A proprietary brand *Anusol Plus HC*® (ointment and suppositories) is on sale to the public.

● MEDICINAL FORMS There can be variation in the licensing of different medicines containing the same drug.

Ointment

▸ Anusol-Hc (Church & Dwight UK Ltd)
Hydrocortisone acetate 2.5 mg per 1 gram, Bismuth oxide 8.75 mg per 1 gram, Benzyl benzoate 12.5 mg per 1 gram, Peru Balsam 18.75 mg per 1 gram, Bismuth subgallate 22.5 mg per 1 gram, Zinc oxide 107.5 mg per 1 gram Anusol HC ointment | 30 gram PoM £2.49

Suppository

▸ Anusol-Hc (Church & Dwight UK Ltd)
Hydrocortisone acetate 10 mg, Bismuth oxide 24 mg, Benzyl benzoate 49 mg, Peru Balsam 49 mg, Bismuth subgallate 59 mg, Zinc oxide 296 mg Anusol HC suppositories | 12 suppository PoM £1.74

Cinchocaine hydrochloride with fluocortolone caproate and fluocortolone pivalate

25-Sep-2020

● **INDICATIONS AND DOSE**

Haemorrhoids | **Pruritus ani**

▸ BY RECTUM USING OINTMENT

▸ Adult: Apply twice daily for 5–7 days, apply 3–4 times a day if required, on the first day of treatment, then apply once daily for a few days after symptoms have cleared

▸ BY RECTUM USING SUPPOSITORIES

▸ Adult: Initially 1 suppository daily for 5–7 days, to be inserted after a bowel movement, then 1 suppository once daily on alternate days for 1 week

Haemorrhoids (severe cases) | **Pruritus ani (severe cases)**

▸ BY RECTUM USING SUPPOSITORIES

▸ Adult: Initially 1 suppository 2–3 times a day for 5–7 days, then 1 suppository once daily on alternate days for 1 week

IMPORTANT SAFETY INFORMATION

MHRA/CHM ADVICE: CORTICOSTEROIDS: RARE RISK OF CENTRAL SEROUS CHORIORETINOPATHY WITH LOCAL AS WELL AS SYSTEMIC ADMINISTRATION (AUGUST 2017)
See Corticosteroids, general use p. 709.

NHS IMPROVEMENT PATIENT SAFETY ALERT: STEROID EMERGENCY CARD TO SUPPORT EARLY RECOGNITION AND TREATMENT OF ADRENAL CRISIS IN ADULTS (AUGUST 2020)
See Corticosteroids, general use p. 709.

1

Gastro-intestinal system

- CAUTIONS Local anaesthetic component can be absorbed through the rectal mucosa (avoid excessive application) · local anaesthetic component may cause sensitisation (use for short periods only—no longer than a few days)

- MEDICINAL FORMS There can be variation in the licensing of different medicines containing the same drug.

Ointment
- Ultraproct (Meadow Laboratories Ltd)
  Fluocortolone pivalate 920 microgram per 1 gram, Fluocortolone caproate 950 microgram per 1 gram, Cinchocaine hydrochloride 5 mg per 1 gram Ultraproct ointment | 30 gram PoM £8.27

Suppository
- Ultraproct (Meadow Laboratories Ltd)
  Fluocortolone pivalate 610 microgram, Fluocortolone caproate 630 microgram, Cinchocaine hydrochloride 1 mg Ultraproct suppositories | 12 suppository PoM £4.06

Cinchocaine with hydrocortisone

21-Dec-2017

- INDICATIONS AND DOSE

PROCTOSEDYL® OINTMENT

Haemorrhoids | Pruritus ani
▸ TO THE SKIN, OR BY RECTUM
- Child: Apply twice daily, to be administered morning and night and after a bowel movement. Apply externally or by rectum. Do not use for longer than 7 days
- Adult: Apply twice daily, to be administered morning and night and after a bowel movement. Apply externally or by rectum. Do not use for longer than 7 days

PROCTOSEDYL® SUPPOSITORIES

Haemorrhoids | Pruritus ani
▸ BY RECTUM
- Child 12-17 years: 1 suppository, insert suppository night and morning and after a bowel movement. Do not use for longer than 7 days
- Adult: 1 suppository, insert suppository night and morning and after a bowel movement. Do not use for longer than 7 days

UNIROID-HC® OINTMENT

Haemorrhoids | Pruritus ani
▸ TO THE SKIN, OR BY RECTUM
- Child 12-17 years: Apply twice daily, and apply after a bowel movement, apply externally or by rectum, do not use for longer than 7 days
- Adult: Apply twice daily, and apply after a bowel movement, apply externally or by rectum, do not use for longer than 7 days

UNIROID-HC® SUPPOSITORIES

Haemorrhoids | Pruritus ani
▸ BY RECTUM
- Child 12-17 years: 1 suppository, insert twice daily and after a bowel movement. Do not use for longer than 7 days
- Adult: 1 suppository, insert twice daily and after a bowel movement. Do not use for longer than 7 days

> IMPORTANT SAFETY INFORMATION
> MHRA/CHM ADVICE: CORTICOSTEROIDS: RARE RISK OF CENTRAL SEROUS CHORIORETINOPATHY WITH LOCAL AS WELL AS SYSTEMIC ADMINISTRATION (AUGUST 2017)
> See Corticosteroids, general use p. 709.
>
> NHS IMPROVEMENT PATIENT SAFETY ALERT: STEROID EMERGENCY CARD TO SUPPORT EARLY RECOGNITION AND TREATMENT OF ADRENAL CRISIS IN ADULTS (AUGUST 2020)
> See Corticosteroids, general use p. 709.

- CAUTIONS Local anaesthetic component can be absorbed through the rectal mucosa (avoid excessive application, particularly in children and infants) · local anaesthetic component may cause sensitisation (use for short periods only—no longer than a few days)

- SIDE-EFFECTS Adrenal suppression · skin reactions · vision disorders

- MEDICINAL FORMS There can be variation in the licensing of different medicines containing the same drug.

Ointment
- Proctosedyl (Sanofi)
  Cinchocaine hydrochloride 5 mg per 1 gram, Hydrocortisone 5 mg per 1 gram Proctosedyl ointment | 30 gram PoM £10.34 DT = £10.34
- Uniroid HC (Chemidex Pharma Ltd)
  Cinchocaine hydrochloride 5 mg per 1 gram, Hydrocortisone 5 mg per 1 gram Uniroid HC ointment | 30 gram PoM £5.63 DT = £10.34

Suppository
- Proctosedyl (Sanofi)
  Cinchocaine hydrochloride 5 mg, Hydrocortisone 5 mg Proctosedyl suppositories | 12 suppository PoM £5.08 DT = £5.08
- Uniroid HC (Chemidex Pharma Ltd)
  Cinchocaine hydrochloride 5 mg, Hydrocortisone 5 mg Uniroid HC suppositories | 12 suppository PoM £2.54 DT = £5.08

Cinchocaine with prednisolone

25-Sep-2020

- INDICATIONS AND DOSE

Haemorrhoids | Pruritus ani
▸ BY RECTUM USING OINTMENT
- Adult: Apply twice daily for 5–7 days, apply 3–4 times a day on the first day if necessary, then apply once daily for a few days after symptoms have cleared
▸ BY RECTUM USING SUPPOSITORIES
- Adult: 1 suppository daily for 5–7 days, to be inserted after a bowel movement

Haemorrhoids (severe cases) | Pruritus ani (severe cases)
▸ BY RECTUM USING SUPPOSITORIES
- Adult: Initially 1 suppository 2–3 times a day, then 1 suppository daily for a total of 5–7 days, to be inserted after a bowel movement

> IMPORTANT SAFETY INFORMATION
> MHRA/CHM ADVICE: CORTICOSTEROIDS: RARE RISK OF CENTRAL SEROUS CHORIORETINOPATHY WITH LOCAL AS WELL AS SYSTEMIC ADMINISTRATION (AUGUST 2017)
> See Corticosteroids, general use p. 709.
>
> NHS IMPROVEMENT PATIENT SAFETY ALERT: STEROID EMERGENCY CARD TO SUPPORT EARLY RECOGNITION AND TREATMENT OF ADRENAL CRISIS IN ADULTS (AUGUST 2020)
> See Corticosteroids, general use p. 709.

- CAUTIONS Local anaesthetic component can be absorbed through the rectal mucosa (avoid excessive application) · local anaesthetic component may cause sensitisation (use for short periods only—no longer than a few days)

- MEDICINAL FORMS There can be variation in the licensing of different medicines containing the same drug.

Ointment
- Scheriproct (LEO Pharma)
  Prednisolone hexanoate 1.9 mg per 1 gram, Cinchocaine hydrochloride 5 mg per 1 gram Scheriproct ointment | 30 gram PoM £3.23 DT = £3.23

Suppository
- Scheriproct (LEO Pharma)
  Cinchocaine hydrochloride 1 mg, Prednisolone hexanoate 1.3 mg Scheriproct suppositories | 12 suppository PoM £1.52 DT = £1.52

Gastro-intestinal system

Hydrocortisone with lidocaine 25-Sep-2020

- **INDICATIONS AND DOSE**

Haemorrhoids | Pruritus ani
▸ BY RECTUM USING AEROSOL SPRAY
▸ Adult: 1 spray up to 3 times a day for no longer than 7 days without medical advice, spray once over the affected area
▸ BY RECTUM USING OINTMENT
▸ Adult: Apply several times daily, for short term use only

IMPORTANT SAFETY INFORMATION

MHRA/CHM ADVICE: CORTICOSTEROIDS: RARE RISK OF CENTRAL SEROUS CHORIORETINOPATHY WITH LOCAL AS WELL AS SYSTEMIC ADMINISTRATION (AUGUST 2017)
See Corticosteroids, general use p. 709.

NHS IMPROVEMENT PATIENT SAFETY ALERT: STEROID EMERGENCY CARD TO SUPPORT EARLY RECOGNITION AND TREATMENT OF ADRENAL CRISIS IN ADULTS (AUGUST 2020)
See Corticosteroids, general use p. 709.

- CAUTIONS Local anaesthetic component can be absorbed through the rectal mucosa (avoid excessive application) · local anaesthetic component may cause sensitisation (use for short periods only—no longer than a few days)
- SIDE-EFFECTS Adrenal suppression · paraesthesia · skin reactions · vision disorders
- MEDICINAL FORMS There can be variation in the licensing of different medicines containing the same drug.

Ointment
▸ Xyloproct (Aspen Pharma Trading Ltd)
Hydrocortisone acetate 2.75 mg per 1 gram, Lidocaine 50 mg per 1 gram Xyloproct 5%/0.275% ointment | 20 gram [PoM] £4.19 DT = £4.19

Spray
▸ Perinal (Dermal Laboratories Ltd)
Hydrocortisone 2 mg per 1 gram, Lidocaine hydrochloride 10 mg per 1 gram Perinal spray | 30 ml [P] £6.11 DT = £6.11

Hydrocortisone with pramocaine

25-Sep-2020

- **INDICATIONS AND DOSE**

Haemorrhoids | Proctitis
▸ BY RECTUM
▸ Adult: 1 applicatorful 2–3 times a day and 1 applicatorful, after a bowel movement, do not use for longer than 7 days; maximum 4 applicatorfuls per day

---

IMPORTANT SAFETY INFORMATION

MHRA/CHM ADVICE: CORTICOSTEROIDS: RARE RISK OF CENTRAL SEROUS CHORIORETINOPATHY WITH LOCAL AS WELL AS SYSTEMIC ADMINISTRATION (AUGUST 2017)
See Corticosteroids, general use p. 709.

NHS IMPROVEMENT PATIENT SAFETY ALERT: STEROID EMERGENCY CARD TO SUPPORT EARLY RECOGNITION AND TREATMENT OF ADRENAL CRISIS IN ADULTS (AUGUST 2020)
See Corticosteroids, general use p. 709.

- CAUTIONS Local anaesthetic component can be absorbed through the rectal mucosa (avoid excessive application) · local anaesthetic component may cause sensitisation (use for short periods only—no longer than a few days)
- SIDE-EFFECTS Anxiety · behaviour abnormal · cognitive impairment · confusion · Cushing's syndrome · delusions · hallucination · infection · memory loss · mood altered · paraesthesia · psychiatric disorder · psychosis · skin

reactions · sleep disorder · suppression of the hypothalamic-pituitary-adrenal axis · vision disorders

- MEDICINAL FORMS No licensed medicines listed.

SCLEROSANTS

Phenol

- **INDICATIONS AND DOSE**

Haemorrhoids (particularly when unprolapsed)
▸ BY SUBMUCOSAL INJECTION
▸ Adult: 2–3 mL, dose (using phenol 5%) to be injected into the submucosal layer at the base of the pile; several injections may be given at different sites, max. total injected 10 mL at any one time

- SIDE-EFFECTS Abdominal sepsis · abscess · dizziness · erectile dysfunction · fever · hepatitis · increased risk of infection · injection site necrosis · ulcer · urinary disorders
- PRESCRIBING AND DISPENSING INFORMATION When prepared extemporaneously, the BP states Oily Phenol Injection, BP consists of phenol 5% in a suitable fixed oil.

- MEDICINAL FORMS There can be variation in the licensing of different medicines containing the same drug. Forms available from special-order manufacturers include: solution for injection

Solution for injection
▸ Phenol (Non-proprietary)
Phenol 50 mg per 1 ml Oily phenol 5% solution for injection 5ml ampoules | 10 ampoule [PoM] £85.27 DT = £81.21

10   Reduced exocrine secretions

Exocrine pancreatic insufficiency

10-Dec-2020

Description of condition

Exocrine pancreatic insufficiency is characterised by reduced secretion of pancreatic enzymes into the duodenum.

The main clinical manifestations are maldigestion and malnutrition, associated with low circulating levels of micronutrients, fat-soluble vitamins and lipoproteins. Patients also present with gastro-intestinal symptoms such as diarrhoea, abdominal cramps and steatorrhoea.

Exocrine pancreatic insufficiency can result from chronic pancreatitis, cystic fibrosis, obstructive pancreatic tumours, coeliac disease, Zollinger-Ellison syndrome, and gastro-intestinal or pancreatic surgical resection.

Aims of treatment

The aim of treatment is to relieve gastro-intestinal symptoms and to achieve a normal nutritional status.

Drug treatment

Pancreatic enzyme replacement therapy with pancreatin p. 104 is the mainstay of treatment for exocrine pancreatic insufficiency.

Pancreatin contains the three main groups of digestive enzymes: lipase, amylase and protease. These enzymes respectively digest fats, carbohydrates and proteins into their basic components so that they can be absorbed and utilised by the body. [EvGr] Pancreatin should be administered with meals and snacks. The dose should be adjusted, as necessary, to the lowest effective dose according to the symptoms of maldigestion and malabsorption. ⟨A⟩

Fibrosing colonopathy has been reported in patients with cystic fibrosis taking high dose pancreatic enzyme replacement therapy (in excess of 10 000 units/kg/day of lipase). Possible risk factors are gender (in children, boys are at greater risk than girls), more severe cystic fibrosis, and concomitant use of laxatives. The peak age for developing fibrosing colonopathy is between 2 and 8 years. Manufacturers of *Pancrease HL*® and *Nutrizym 22*® recommend that the total dose of pancreatin used in patients with cystic fibrosis should not usually exceed 10 000 units/kg/day of lipase. Manufacturers of pancreatin recommend that if a patient taking pancreatin develops new abdominal symptoms (or any change in existing abdominal symptoms) the patient should be reviewed to exclude the possibility of colonic damage.

There is limited evidence that acid suppression may improve the effectiveness of pancreatin. EvGr Acid-suppressing drugs (proton pump inhibitors or H_2-receptor antagonists) may be trialled in patients who continue to experience symptoms despite high doses of pancreatin.

Levels of fat-soluble vitamins and micronutrients (such as zinc and selenium) should be routinely assessed and supplementation advised whenever necessary. Ⓐ

Pancreatin preparations

Preparation	Protease units	Amylase units	Lipase units
Creon® 10 000 capsule, e/c granules	600	8000	10 000
Creon® Micro e/c granules (per 100 mg)	200	3600	5000
Pancrex V® capsule, powder	430	9000	8000
Pancrex V '125'® capsule, powder	160	3300	2950
Pancrex V® powder (per gram)	1400	30 000	25 000

Higher-strength pancreatin preparations

Preparation	Protease units	Amylase units	Lipase units
Creon® 25 000 capsule, e/c pellets	1000	18 000	25 000
Nutrizym 22® capsule, e/c minitablets	1100	19 800	22 000
Pancrease HL® capsule, e/c minitablets	1250	22 500	25 000

Non-drug treatment

EvGr Dietary advice should be provided. Food intake should be distributed between three main meals per day, and two or three snacks. Food that is difficult to digest should be avoided, such as legumes (peas, beans, lentils) and high-fibre foods. Alcohol should be avoided completely. Reduced fat diets are not recommended. Ⓐ

Medium-chain triglycerides (see MCT oil, in *Borderline substances*), which are directly absorbed by the intestinal mucosa, were thought to be useful in some patients. However evidence has shown that MCT-enriched preparations offer no advantage over a normal balanced diet.

PANCREATIC ENZYMES

Pancreatin

05-Aug-2020

- **DRUG ACTION** Supplements of pancreatin are given to compensate for reduced or absent exocrine secretion. They assist the digestion of starch, fat, and protein.

- **INDICATIONS AND DOSE**

CREON® 10000

Pancreatic insufficiency
▸ BY MOUTH
- Child: Initially 1–2 capsules, dose to be taken with each meal either taken whole or contents mixed with acidic fluid or soft food (then swallowed immediately without chewing)
- Adult: Initially 1–2 capsules, dose to be taken with each meal either taken whole or contents mixed with acidic fluid or soft food (then swallowed immediately without chewing)

CREON® 25000

Pancreatic insufficiency
▸ BY MOUTH
- Child 2-17 years: Initially 1–2 capsules, dose to be taken with each meal either taken whole or contents mixed with acidic fluid or soft food (then swallowed immediately without chewing)
- Adult: Initially 1–2 capsules, dose to be taken with each meal either taken whole or contents mixed with acidic fluid or soft food (then swallowed immediately without chewing)

CREON® 40000

Pancreatic insufficiency
▸ BY MOUTH
- Child 2-17 years: Initially 1–2 capsules, dose to be taken with each meal either taken whole or contents mixed with acidic fluid or soft food (then swallowed immediately without chewing)
- Adult: Initially 1–2 capsules, dose to be taken with each meal either taken whole or contents mixed with acidic fluid or soft food (then swallowed immediately without chewing)

CREON® MICRO

Pancreatic insufficiency
▸ BY MOUTH
- Child: Initially 100 mg, for administration advice, see *Directions for administration*
- Adult: Initially 100 mg, for administration advice, see *Directions for administration*

DOSE EQUIVALENCE AND CONVERSION
- For *Creon*® *Micro* : 100 mg granules = one measured scoopful (scoop supplied with product).

NUTRIZYM 22® GASTRO-RESISTANT CAPSULES

Pancreatic insufficiency
▸ BY MOUTH
- Adult: Initially 1–2 capsules, dose to be taken with meals and 1 capsule as required, dose to be taken with snacks, doses should be swallowed whole or contents taken with water, or mixed with acidic fluid or soft food (then swallowed immediately without chewing)

PANCREASE HL®

Pancreatic insufficiency
▸ BY MOUTH
- Child 15-17 years: Initially 1–2 capsules, dose to be taken during each meal and 1 capsule, to be taken with snacks, all doses either taken whole or contents mixed with slightly acidic liquid or soft food (then swallowed immediately without chewing)

‣ **Adult:** Initially 1–2 capsules, dose to be taken during each meal and 1 capsule, to be taken with snacks, all doses either taken whole or contents mixed with slightly acidic liquid or soft food (then swallowed immediately without chewing)

PANCREX ® V

Pancreatic insufficiency

‣ BY MOUTH

‣ **Child 1-11 months:** 1–2 capsules, contents of capsule to be mixed with feeds

‣ **Child 1-17 years:** 2–6 capsules, dose to be taken with each meal either swallowed whole or sprinkled on food

‣ **Adult:** 2–6 capsules, dose to be taken with each meal either swallowed whole or sprinkled on food

PANCREX ® V POWDER

Pancreatic insufficiency

‣ BY MOUTH

‣ **Child:** 0.5–2 g, to be taken before or with meals, washed down or mixed with milk or water

‣ **Adult:** 0.5–2 g, to be taken before or with meals, washed down or mixed with milk or water

● CAUTIONS Can irritate the perioral skin and buccal mucosa if retained in the mouth · excessive doses can cause perianal irritation

● INTERACTIONS → Appendix 1: pancreatin

● SIDE-EFFECTS

‣ **Common or very common** Abdominal distension · constipation · nausea · vomiting

‣ **Uncommon** Skin reactions

‣ **Frequency not known** Fibrosing colonopathy

● PREGNANCY Not known to be harmful.

● DIRECTIONS FOR ADMINISTRATION Pancreatin is inactivated by gastric acid therefore manufacturer advises pancreatin preparations are best taken with food (or immediately before or after food). Since pancreatin is inactivated by heat, excessive heat should be avoided if preparations are mixed with liquids or food; manufacturer advises the resulting mixtures should not be kept for more than one hour and any left-over food or liquid containing pancreatin should be discarded. Enteric-coated preparations deliver a higher enzyme concentration in the duodenum (provided the capsule contents are swallowed whole without chewing). Manufacturer advises gastro-resistant granules should be mixed with slightly acidic soft food or liquid such as apple juice, and then swallowed immediately without chewing. Capsules containing enteric-coated granules can be opened and the granules administered in the same way. For infants, *Creon® Micro* granules can be mixed with a small amount of milk on a spoon and administered immediately—granules should not be added to the baby's bottle. Manufacturer advises *Pancrex® V* powder may be administered via nasogastric tube or gastrostomy tube—consult local and national official guidelines.

● PRESCRIBING AND DISPENSING INFORMATION Preparations may contain pork pancreatin—consult product literature.

● HANDLING AND STORAGE Hypersensitivity reactions have occasionally occurred in those handling the powder.

● PATIENT AND CARER ADVICE Patients or carers should be given advice on administration. It is important to ensure adequate hydration at all times in patients receiving higher-strength pancreatin preparations.

Medicines for Children leaflet: Pancreatin for pancreatic insufficiency www.medicinesforchildren.org.uk/pancreatin-pancreatic-insufficiency

● MEDICINAL FORMS There can be variation in the licensing of different medicines containing the same drug.

Gastro-resistant capsule

‣ Creon (Mylan)

Protease 600 unit, Amylase 8000 unit, Lipase 10000 unit Creon 10000 gastro-resistant capsules | 100 capsule Ⓟ £12.93

Protease 1000 unit, Amylase 18000 unit, Lipase 25000 unit Creon 25000 gastro-resistant capsules | 100 capsule PoM £28.25

‣ Nutrizym (Zentiva)

Protease 1100 unit, Amylase 19800 unit, Lipase 22000 unit Nutrizym 22 gastro-resistant capsules | 100 capsule PoM £33.33

‣ Pancrease (Janssen-Cilag Ltd)

Protease 1250 unit, Amylase 22500 unit, Lipase 25000 unit Pancrease HL gastro-resistant capsules | 100 capsule PoM £40.38

Gastro-resistant granules

CAUTIONARY AND ADVISORY LABELS 25

‣ Creon (Mylan)

Protease 200 unit, Amylase 3600 unit, Lipase 5000 unit Creon Micro Pancreatin 60.12mg gastro-resistant granules | 20 gram Ⓟ £31.50

Powder

‣ Pancrex (Essential Pharmaceuticals Ltd)

Protease 1400 unit, Lipase 25000 unit, Amylase 30000 unit Pancrex V oral powder sugar-free | 300 gram Ⓟ £224.00

Capsule

‣ Pancrex (Essential Pharmaceuticals Ltd)

Protease 430 unit, Lipase 8000 unit, Amylase 9000 unit Pancrex V capsules | 300 capsule Ⓟ £53.20

11 Stoma care

Stoma care

24-Feb-2016

Description of condition

A stoma is an artificial opening on the abdomen to divert flow of faeces or urine into an external pouch located outside of the body. This procedure may be temporary or permanent. Colostomy and ileostomy are the most common forms of stoma but a gastrostomy, jejunostomy, duodenostomy or caecostomy may also be performed. Understanding the type and extent of surgical intervention in each patient is crucial in managing the patient's pharmaceutical needs correctly.

Overview

Prescribing for patients with stoma calls for special care due to modifications in drug delivery, resulting in a higher risk of sub-optimal absorption. The following is a brief account of some of the main points to be borne in mind.

Enteric-coated and modified-release medicines are **unsuitable**, particularly in patients with an ileostomy, as there may not be sufficient release of active ingredient. Soluble tablets, liquids, capsules or uncoated tablets are more suitable due to their quicker dissolution. When a solid-dose form such as a capsule or a tablet is given, the contents of the ostomy bag should be checked for any remnants.

Preparations containing sorbitol as an excipient should be avoided, due to its laxative side-effects.

Analgesics

Opioid analgesics may cause troublesome constipation in colostomy patients. When a non-opioid analgesic is required, paracetamol is usually suitable. Anti-inflammatory analgesics may cause gastric irritation and bleeding; faecal output should be monitored for traces of blood.

Antacids

The tendency to diarrhoea from magnesium salts or constipation from aluminium or calcium salts may be increased in patients with stoma.

Antisecretory drugs

The gastric acid secretion often increases stoma output. Proton pump inhibitors and somatostatin analogues (octreotide p. 993 and lanreotide p. 993) are often used to reduce this risk.

Antidiarrhoeal drugs

Loperamide hydrochloride p. 72 and codeine phosphate p. 475 reduce intestinal motility and decrease water and sodium output from an ileostomy. Loperamide hydrochloride circulates through the enterohepatic circulation, which is disrupted in patients with a short bowel; high doses of loperamide hydrochloride may be required. Codeine phosphate can be added if response with loperamide hydrochloride alone is inadequate.

Digoxin

Patients with a stoma are particularly susceptible to hypokalaemia if taking digoxin p. 117, due to fluid and sodium depletion. Potassium supplements or a potassium-sparing diuretic may be advisable with monitoring for early signs of toxicity.

Diuretics

Diuretics should be used with caution in patients with an ileostomy or with urostomy as they may become excessively dehydrated and potassium depletion may easily occur. It is usually advisable to use a potassium-sparing diuretic.

Iron preparations

Iron preparations may cause loose stools and sore skin in these patients. If this is troublesome and if iron is definitely indicated, an intramuscular iron preparation should be used. Modified-release preparations should be avoided for the reasons given above.

Laxatives

Laxatives should not be used in patients with an ileostomy where possible as they may cause rapid and severe loss of water and electrolytes.

Colostomy patients may suffer from constipation and whenever possible should be treated by increasing fluid intake or dietary fibre. Bulk-forming drugs can be tried. If they are insufficient, as small a dose as possible of a stimulant laxative such as senna p. 67 can be used with caution.

Potassium supplements

Liquid formulations are preferred to modified-release formulations. The daily dose should be split to avoid osmotic diarrhoea.

Care of stoma

Patients and their carers are usually given advice about the use of cleansing agents, protective creams, lotions, deodorants, or sealants whilst in hospital, either by the surgeon or by stoma care nurses. Voluntary organisations offer help and support to patients with stoma.

Chapter 2
Cardiovascular system

CONTENTS

1   Arrhythmias

Arrhythmias
06-May-2020

Overview

Management of an arrhythmia requires precise diagnosis of the type of arrhythmia, and electrocardiography is essential; underlying causes such as heart failure require appropriate treatment.

For recommendations on the management of acute myocardial injury and its cardiac complications in adults with known or suspected COVID-19 but without known pre-existing cardiovascular disease, see NICE rapid guidelines: **Acute myocardial injury** (available at: www.nice.org.uk/guidance/ng171). For further information on COVID-19, see COVID-19 p. 660.

Ectopic beats

If ectopic beats are spontaneous and the patient has a normal heart, treatment is rarely required and reassurance to the patient will often suffice. If they are particularly troublesome, beta-blockers are sometimes effective and may be safer than other suppressant drugs.

Atrial fibrillation

Treatment of patients with atrial fibrillation aims to reduce symptoms and prevent complications, especially stroke. All patients with atrial fibrillation should be assessed for their risk of stroke and thromboembolism. Atrial fibrillation can be managed by either controlling the ventricular rate ('rate control') or by attempting to restore and maintain sinus rhythm ('rhythm control'). At any stage if treatment fails to control symptoms, or, if symptoms reoccur after cardioversion and specialised management is required, referral should be made within 4 weeks. If drug treatment fails to control the symptoms of atrial fibrillation or is unsuitable, ablation strategies can be considered. Review anticoagulation, stroke, and bleeding risk at least annually in all patients with atrial fibrillation.

Acute presentation

All patients with life-threatening haemodynamic instability caused by new-onset atrial fibrillation should undergo emergency electrical cardioversion without delaying to achieve anticoagulation. In patients presenting acutely but without life-threatening haemodynamic instability, rate or rhythm control can be offered if the onset of arrhythmia is less than 48 hours; rate control is preferred if onset is more than 48 hours or uncertain. Consideration of pharmacological or electrical cardioversion should be based on clinical circumstances. If pharmacological cardioversion has been agreed, intravenous amiodarone hydrochloride p. 113, or alternatively flecainide acetate p. 111, can be used (amiodarone hydrochloride is preferred if there is structural heart disease). If urgent rate control is required, a beta-blocker or verapamil hydrochloride p. 178 can be given intravenously.

Cardioversion

Sinus rhythm can be restored by electrical cardioversion, or pharmacological cardioversion with an oral or intravenous antiarrhythmic drug e.g. flecainide acetate or amiodarone hydrochloride. If atrial fibrillation has been present for more than 48 hours, electrical cardioversion is preferred and should not be attempted until the patient has been fully anticoagulated for at least 3 weeks; if this is not possible, parenteral anticoagulation should be commenced, and a left atrial thrombus ruled out immediately before cardioversion; oral anticoagulation should be given after cardioversion and continued for at least 4 weeks; prior to cardioversion, offer rate control as appropriate.

Drug treatment

Rate control is the preferred first-line drug treatment strategy for atrial fibrillation except in patients with new-onset atrial fibrillation, atrial flutter suitable for an ablation strategy, atrial fibrillation with a reversible cause, or if rhythm control is more suitable based on clinical judgement. Ventricular rate can be controlled with a standard beta-blocker (not sotalol hydrochloride p. 116) or a rate-limiting calcium channel blocker such as diltiazem hydrochloride p. 171 [unlicensed indication], or verapamil hydrochloride as monotherapy. Choice of drug should be based on individual symptoms, heart rate, comorbidities, and patient preference. Digoxin p. 117 is usually only effective for controlling the ventricular rate at rest, and should therefore only be used as monotherapy in predominantly sedentary patients with non-paroxysmal atrial fibrillation. When a single drug fails to adequately control the ventricular rate, a combination of two drugs including a beta-blocker, digoxin, or diltiazem hydrochloride can be used. If symptoms are not controlled with a combination of two drugs, a rhythm-control strategy should be considered. If ventricular function is diminished, the combination of a beta-blocker (that is licensed for use in heart failure) and digoxin is preferred. Digoxin is also used when atrial fibrillation is accompanied by congestive heart failure.

If drug treatment is required to maintain sinus rhythm ('rhythm control') post-cardioversion, a standard beta-blocker is used. If a standard beta-blocker is not appropriate or is ineffective, consider an oral anti-arrhythmic drug such as sotalol hydrochloride, flecainide acetate, propafenone hydrochloride p. 112, or amiodarone hydrochloride; dronedarone p. 114 may be considered in paroxysmal or persistent atrial fibrillation (see NICE guidance). If necessary, amiodarone hydrochloride can be started 4 weeks before and continuing for up to 12 months after electrical cardioversion to increase success of the procedure, and to maintain sinus rhythm. Flecainide acetate or propafenone hydrochloride should not be given when there is known ischaemic or structural heart disease. Consider amiodarone hydrochloride in patients with left ventricular impairment or heart failure.

Paroxysmal atrial fibrillation
In symptomatic paroxysmal atrial fibrillation, ventricular rhythm is controlled with a standard beta-blocker. Alternatively, if symptoms persist or a standard beta-blocker is not appropriate, an oral anti-arrhythmic drug such as dronedarone (see NICE guidance), sotalol hydrochloride, flecainide acetate, propafenone hydrochloride, or amiodarone hydrochloride can be given (see also Paroxysmal supraventricular tachycardia and Supraventricular arrhythmias). In selected patients with infrequent episodes of symptomatic paroxysmal atrial fibrillation, sinus rhythm can be restored using the 'pill-in-the-pocket' approach; this involves the patient taking oral flecainide acetate or propafenone hydrochloride to self-treat an episode of atrial fibrillation when it occurs.

Stroke prevention
All patients with atrial fibrillation should be assessed for their risk of stroke and the need for thromboprophylaxis; this needs to be balanced with the patient's risk of bleeding; a NICE guideline (NICE clinical guideline 180 (June 2014). Atrial fibrillation: The management of atrial fibrillation) recommends using the CHA_2DS_2-VASc assessment tool for stroke risk and the HAS-BLED tool for bleeding risk prior to and during anticoagulation. Risk factors for stroke taken into account by CHA_2DS_2-VASc include prior ischaemic stroke, transient ischaemic attacks, or thromboembolic events, heart failure, left ventricular systolic dysfunction, vascular disease, diabetes, hypertension, females, and patients over 65 years. Patients with a very low risk of stroke (CHA_2DS_2-VASc score of 0 for men or 1 for women) do not require an antithrombotic for stroke prevention. Parenteral anticoagulation should be offered to patients with new-onset atrial fibrillation who are receiving subtherapeutic or no anticoagulation therapy until assessment is made, and appropriate anticoagulation is started. Oral anticoagulation should be offered to patients with confirmed diagnosis of atrial fibrillation in whom sinus rhythm has not been successfully restored within 48 hours of onset, patients who have had, or are at high risk of recurrence of atrial fibrillation such as those with structural heart disease, prolonged history of atrial fibrillation (more than 12 months), a history of failed attempts at cardioversion, and patients whom the risk of stroke outweighs the risk of bleeding. Anticoagulation treatment should not be withheld solely because of the risk of falls, and choice of treatment should be based on clinical features and patient preferences. Oral anticoagulation may be with a vitamin K antagonist (e.g. warfarin sodium p. 153), or in non-valvular atrial fibrillation with apixaban p. 136, dabigatran etexilate p. 148, edoxaban p. 137, or rivaroxaban p. 139. Anticoagulants are also indicated during

cardioversion procedures. Aspirin p. 132 is less effective than warfarin sodium at preventing emboli; the modest benefit is offset by the risk of bleeding, and aspirin should not be offered as monotherapy solely for stroke prevention in atrial fibrillation. If anticoagulant treatment is contra-indicated or not tolerated, left atrial appendage occlusion can be considered.

Atrial flutter
Like atrial fibrillation, treatment options for atrial flutter involve either controlling the ventricular rate or attempting to restore and maintain sinus rhythm. However, atrial flutter generally responds less well to drug treatment than atrial fibrillation.

Control of the ventricular rate is usually an interim measure pending restoration of sinus rhythm. Ventricular rate can be controlled by administration of a beta-blocker, diltiazem hydrochloride p. 171 [unlicensed indication], or verapamil hydrochloride p. 178; an intravenous beta-blocker or verapamil hydrochloride is preferred for rapid control. Digoxin p. 117 can be added if rate control remains inadequate, and may be particularly useful in those with heart failure.

Conversion to sinus rhythm can be achieved by electrical cardioversion (by cardiac pacing or direct current), pharmacological cardioversion, or catheter ablation. If the duration of atrial flutter is unknown, or it has lasted for over 48 hours, cardioversion should not be attempted until the patient has been fully anticoagulated for at least 3 weeks; if this is not possible, parenteral anticoagulation should be commenced and a left atrial thrombus ruled out immediately before cardioversion; oral anticoagulation should be given after cardioversion and continued for at least 4 weeks.

Direct current cardioversion is usually the treatment of choice when rapid conversion to sinus rhythm is necessary (e.g. when atrial flutter is associated with haemodynamic compromise); catheter ablation is preferred for the treatment of recurrent atrial flutter. There is a limited role for anti-arrhythmic drugs as their use is not always successful. Flecainide acetate p. 111 or propafenone hydrochloride p. 112 can slow atrial flutter, resulting in 1:1 conduction to the ventricles, and should therefore be prescribed in conjunction with a ventricular rate controlling drug such as a beta-blocker, diltiazem hydrochloride [unlicensed indication], or verapamil hydrochloride. Amiodarone hydrochloride p. 113 can be used when other drug treatments are contra-indicated or ineffective.

All patients should be assessed for their risk of stroke and the need for thromboprophylaxis; the choice of anticoagulant is based on the same criteria as for atrial fibrillation.

Paroxysmal supraventricular tachycardia
This will often terminate spontaneously or with reflex vagal stimulation such as a Valsalva manoeuvre, immersing the face in ice-cold water, or carotid sinus massage; such manoeuvres should be performed with ECG monitoring.

If the effects of reflex vagal stimulation are transient or ineffective, or if the arrhythmia is causing severe symptoms, intravenous adenosine p. 115 should be given. If adenosine is ineffective or contra-indicated, intravenous verapamil hydrochloride is an alternative, but it should be avoided in patients recently treated with beta-blockers.

Failure to terminate paroxysmal supraventricular tachycardia with reflex vagal stimulation or drug treatment may suggest an arrhythmia of atrial origin, such as focal atrial tachycardia or atrial flutter.

Treatment with direct current cardioversion is needed in haemodynamically unstable patients or when the above measures have failed to restore sinus rhythm (and an alternative diagnosis has not been found).

Recurrent episodes of paroxysmal supraventricular tachycardia can be treated by catheter ablation, or prevented with drugs such as diltiazem hydrochloride, verapamil hydrochloride, beta-blockers including sotalol hydrochloride p. 116, flecainide acetate or propafenone hydrochloride.

Arrhythmias after myocardial infarction

In patients with a paroxysmal tachycardia or rapid irregularity of the pulse it is best not to administer an anti-arrhythmic until an ECG record has been obtained. Bradycardia, particularly if complicated by hypotension, should be treated with an intravenous dose of atropine sulfate p. 1386 the dose may be repeated if necessary. If there is a risk of asystole, or if the patient is unstable and has failed to respond to atropine sulfate, adrenaline/epinephrine p. 238 should be given by intravenous infusion, and the dose adjusted according to response.

For further advice, refer to the most recent recommendations of the Resuscitation Council (UK) available at www.resus.org.uk.

Ventricular tachycardia

Pulseless ventricular tachycardia or ventricular fibrillation should be treated with immediate defibrillation (see Cardiopulmonary resuscitation).

Patients with unstable sustained ventricular tachycardia, who continue to deteriorate with signs of hypotension or reduced cardiac output, should receive direct current cardioversion to restore sinus rhythm. If this fails, intravenous amiodarone hydrochloride should be administered and direct current cardioversion repeated. Patients with sustained ventricular tachycardia who are haemodynamically stable can be treated with intravenous anti-arrhythmic drugs. Amiodarone hydrochloride is the preferred drug. Flecainide acetate, propafenone hydrochloride, and, although less effective, lidocaine hydrochloride p. 111 have all been used. If sinus rhythm is not restored, direct current cardioversion or pacing should be considered. Catheter ablation is an alternative if cessation of the arrhythmia is not urgent. Non-sustained ventricular tachycardia can be treated with a beta-blocker.

All patients presenting with ventricular tachycardia should be referred to a specialist. Following restoration of sinus rhythm, patients who remain at high risk of cardiac arrest will require maintenance therapy. Most patients will be treated with an implantable cardioverter defibrillator. Beta-blockers or sotalol hydrochloride (in place of a standard beta-blocker), or amiodarone hydrochloride (in combination with a standard beta-blocker), can be used in addition to the device in some patients; alternatively, they can be used alone when use of an implantable cardioverter defibrillator is not appropriate.

Torsade de pointes

Torsade de pointes is a form of ventricular tachycardia associated with a long QT syndrome (usually drug-induced, but other factors including hypokalaemia, severe bradycardia, and genetic predisposition are also implicated). Episodes are usually self-limiting, but are frequently recurrent and can cause impairment or loss of consciousness. If not controlled, the arrhythmia can progress to ventricular fibrillation and sometimes death. Intravenous infusion of magnesium sulfate p. 1099 is usually effective. A beta-blocker (but not sotalol hydrochloride) and atrial (or ventricular) pacing can be considered. Anti-arrhythmics can further prolong the QT interval, thus worsening the condition.

Anti-arrhythmic drugs

Anti-arrhythmic drugs can be classified clinically into those that act on supraventricular arrhythmias (e.g. verapamil hydrochloride), those that act on both supraventricular and ventricular arrhythmias (e.g. amiodarone hydrochloride),

and those that act on ventricular arrhythmias (e.g. lidocaine hydrochloride).

Anti-arrhythmic drugs can also be classified according to their effects on the electrical behaviour of myocardial cells during activity (the Vaughan Williams classification) although this classification is of less clinical significance:

- Class I: membrane stabilising drugs (e.g. lidocaine, flecainide)
- Class II: beta-blockers
- Class III: amiodarone; sotalol (also Class II)
- Class IV: calcium-channel blockers (includes verapamil but not dihydropyridines)

The negative inotropic effects of anti-arrhythmic drugs tend to be additive. Therefore special care should be taken if two or more are used, especially if myocardial function is impaired. Most drugs that are effective in countering arrhythmias can also provoke them in some circumstances; moreover, hypokalaemia enhances the arrhythmogenic (pro-arrhythmic) effect of many drugs.

Supraventricular arrhythmias

Adenosine p. 115 is usually the treatment of choice for terminating paroxysmal supraventricular tachycardia. As it has a very short duration of action (half-life only about 8 to 10 seconds, but prolonged in those taking dipyridamole p. 135), most side-effects are short lived. Unlike verapamil hydrochloride p. 178, adenosine can be used after a beta-blocker. Verapamil hydrochloride may be preferable to adenosine in asthma.

Oral administration of a **cardiac glycoside** (such as digoxin p. 117) slows the ventricular response in cases of atrial fibrillation and atrial flutter. However, intravenous infusion of digoxin is rarely effective for rapid control of ventricular rate. Cardiac glycosides are contra-indicated in supraventricular arrhythmias associated with accessory conducting pathways (e.g. Wolff- Parkinson-White syndrome).

Verapamil hydrochloride is usually effective for supraventricular tachycardias. An initial intravenous dose (**important:** serious beta-blocker interaction hazard) may be followed by oral treatment; hypotension may occur with large doses. It should not be used for tachyarrhythmias where the QRS complex is wide (i.e. broad complex) unless a supraventricular origin has been established beyond reasonable doubt. It is also contra-indicated in atrial fibrillation or atrial flutter associated with accessory conducting pathways (e.g. Wolff-Parkinson-White syndrome). It should not be used in children with arrhythmias without specialist advice; some supraventricular arrhythmias in childhood can be accelerated by verapamil hydrochloride with dangerous consequences.

Intravenous administration of a **beta-blocker** such as esmolol hydrochloride p. 168 or propranolol hydrochloride p. 164, can achieve rapid control of the ventricular rate.

Drugs for both supraventricular and ventricular arrhythmias include amiodarone hydrochloride p. 113, **beta-blockers**, disopyramide p. 110, flecainide acetate p. 111, **procainamide** (available from 'special-order' manufacturers or specialist importing companies), and propafenone hydrochloride p. 112.

Supraventricular and ventricular arrhythmias

Amiodarone hydrochloride is used in the treatment of arrhythmias, particularly when other drugs are ineffective or contra-indicated. It can be used for paroxysmal supraventricular, nodal and ventricular tachycardias, atrial fibrillation and flutter, and ventricular fibrillation. It can also be used for tachyarrhythmias associated with Wolff-Parkinson-White syndrome. It should be initiated only under hospital or specialist supervision. Amiodarone hydrochloride may be given by intravenous infusion as well as by mouth, and has the advantage of causing little or no myocardial depression. Unlike oral amiodarone hydrochloride, intravenous amiodarone hydrochloride acts relatively rapidly.

Intravenous injection of amiodarone hydrochloride can be used in cardiopulmonary resuscitation for ventricular fibrillation or pulseless tachycardia unresponsive to other interventions.

Amiodarone hydrochloride has a very long half-life (extending to several weeks) and only needs to be given once daily (but high doses can cause nausea unless divided). Many weeks or months may be required to achieve steady-state plasma-amiodarone concentration; this is particularly important when drug interactions are likely.

Beta-blockers act as anti-arrhythmic drugs principally by attenuating the effects of the sympathetic system on automaticity and conductivity within the heart. Sotalol hydrochloride p. 116 has a role in the management of ventricular arrhythmias.

Disopyramide can be given by intravenous injection to control arrhythmias after myocardial infarction (including those not responding to lidocaine hydrochloride p. 111), but it impairs cardiac contractility. Oral administration of disopyramide is useful, but it has an antimuscarinic effect which limits its use in patients susceptible to angle-closure glaucoma or with prostatic hyperplasia.

Flecainide acetate belongs to the same general class as lidocaine hydrochloride and may be of value for serious symptomatic ventricular arrhythmias. It may also be indicated for junctional re-entry tachycardias and for paroxysmal atrial fibrillation. However, it can precipitate serious arrhythmias in a small minority of patients (including those with otherwise normal hearts).

Propafenone hydrochloride is used for the prophylaxis and treatment of ventricular arrhythmias and also for some supraventricular arrhythmias. It has complex mechanisms of action, including weak beta-blocking activity (therefore caution is needed in obstructive airways disease—contra-indicated if severe).

Drugs for supraventricular arrhythmias include adenosine, **cardiac glycosides**, and verapamil hydrochloride. Drugs for ventricular arrhythmias include lidocaine hydrochloride.

Mexiletine and procainamide are both available from 'special-order' manufacturers or specialist importing companies. Mexiletine can be used for life-threatening ventricular arrhythmias; procainamide is given by intravenous injection to control ventricular arrhythmias.

Ventricular arrhythmias

Intravenous lidocaine hydrochloride can be used for the treatment of ventricular tachycardia in haemodynamically stable patients, and ventricular fibrillation and pulseless ventricular tachycardia in cardiac arrest refractory to defibrillation, however it is no longer the anti-arrhythmic drug of first choice.

Drugs for both supraventricular and ventricular arrhythmias include amiodarone hydrochloride, **beta-blockers**, disopyramide, flecainide acetate, **procainamide** (available from 'special- order' manufacturers or specialist importing companies), and propafenone hydrochloride.

Mexiletine is available from 'special-order' manufacturers or specialist importing companies for treatment of life-threatening ventricular arrhythmias.

Advanced Pharmacy Services

Patients with an arrhythmia may be eligible for the New Medicines Service / Medicine Use Review service provided by a community pharmacist. For further information, see *Advanced Pharmacy Services* in Medicines optimisation p. 18.

Useful resources

Patient decision aid: Atrial fibrillation: medicines to help reduce your risk of a stroke—what are the options? National Institute for Health and Care Excellence. June 2014.
www.nice.org.uk/about/what-we-do/our-programmes/nice-guidance/nice-guidelines/shared-decision-making

Other drugs used for Arrhythmias Acebutolol, p. 166 · Metoprolol tartrate, p. 169 · Nadolol, p. 164

ANTIARRHYTHMICS ⟩ CLASS IA

Disopyramide

05-Jul-2019

● **INDICATIONS AND DOSE**

Prevention and treatment of ventricular and supraventricular arrhythmias, including after myocardial infarction | Maintenance of sinus rhythm after cardioversion

▸ BY MOUTH USING IMMEDIATE-RELEASE MEDICINES
▸ Adult: 300–800 mg daily in divided doses
▸ BY MOUTH USING MODIFIED-RELEASE MEDICINES
▸ Adult: 250–375 mg every 12 hours

● CONTRA-INDICATIONS Bundle-branch block associated with first-degree AV block · pre-existing long QT syndrome · second- and third-degree AV block or bifascicular block (unless pacemaker fitted) · severe heart failure (unless secondary to arrhythmia) · severe sinus node dysfunction

● CAUTIONS Atrial flutter or atrial tachycardia with partial block · avoid in Acute porphyrias p. 1107 · elderly · heart failure (avoid if severe) · myasthenia gravis · prostatic enlargement · structural heart disease · susceptibility to angle-closure glaucoma

● INTERACTIONS → Appendix 1: antiarrhythmics

● SIDE-EFFECTS Abdominal pain · appetite decreased · arrhythmias · cardiac conduction disorders · cardiogenic shock · cognitive disorder · constipation · diarrhoea · dizziness · dry mouth · erectile dysfunction · headache · heart failure · hyperhidrosis · hypoglycaemia · hypotension · jaundice cholestatic · nausea · neutropenia · psychotic disorder · QT interval prolongation · rash · urinary disorders · vision disorders · vomiting

● PREGNANCY Manufacturer advises use only if potential benefit outweighs risk; may induce labour if used in third trimester.

● BREAST FEEDING Present in milk—use only if essential.
Monitoring Monitor infant for antimuscarinic effects.

● HEPATIC IMPAIRMENT For *immediate-release capsules*, manufacturer advises caution (risk of increased half-life). For *modified-release tablets*, manufacturer advises avoid.
Dose adjustments For *immediate-release capsules*, manufacturer advises consider dose reduction.

● RENAL IMPAIRMENT Avoid modified-release preparation.
Dose adjustments Reduce dose by increasing dose interval; adjust according to response.

● MONITORING REQUIREMENTS
▸ Monitor for hypotension, hypoglycaemia, ventricular tachycardia, ventricular fibrillation or torsade de pointes (discontinue if occur).
▸ Monitor serum potassium.

● MEDICINAL FORMS There can be variation in the licensing of different medicines containing the same drug. Forms available from special-order manufacturers include: capsule, oral suspension, oral solution

Modified-release tablet
CAUTIONARY AND ADVISORY LABELS 25
▸ Rythmodan Retard (Neon Healthcare Ltd)
Disopyramide (as Disopyramide phosphate) 250 mg Rythmodan Retard 250mg tablets | 60 tablet [PoM] £32.08 DT = £32.08

Capsule
▸ Disopyramide (Non-proprietary)
Disopyramide 100 mg Disopyramide 100mg capsules | 84 capsule [PoM] £26.51 DT = £26.51
Disopyramide 150 mg Disopyramide 150mg capsules | 84 capsule [PoM] £33.40 DT = £33.09

▸ Rythmodan (Neon Healthcare Ltd)
Disopyramide 100 mg Rythmodan 100mg capsules |
84 capsule PoM £14.14 DT = £26.51

ANTIARRHYTHMICS › CLASS IB

Lidocaine hydrochloride   10-Nov-2020
(Lignocaine hydrochloride)

● **INDICATIONS AND DOSE**

Cardiopulmonary resuscitation (as an alternative if amiodarone is not available)
▸ BY INTRAVENOUS INJECTION
▸ **Adult:** 1 mg/kg, do not exceed 3 mg/kg over the first hour

Ventricular arrhythmias, especially after myocardial infarction in patients without gross circulatory impairment
▸ INITIALLY BY INTRAVENOUS INJECTION
▸ **Adult:** 100 mg, to be given as a bolus dose over a few minutes, followed immediately by (by intravenous infusion) 4 mg/minute for 30 minutes, then (by intravenous infusion) 2 mg/minute for 2 hours, then (by intravenous infusion) 1 mg/minute, reduce concentration further if infusion continued beyond 24 hours (ECG monitoring and specialist advice for infusion), following intravenous injection lidocaine has a short duration of action (lasting for 15–20 minutes). If an intravenous infusion is not immediately available the initial intravenous injection of 100 mg can be repeated if necessary once or twice at intervals of not less than 10 minutes

Ventricular arrhythmias, especially after myocardial infarction in lighter patients or those whose circulation is severely impaired
▸ INITIALLY BY INTRAVENOUS INJECTION
▸ **Adult:** Initially 50 mg, to be given as a bolus dose over a few minutes, followed immediately by (by intravenous infusion) 4 mg/minute for 30 minutes, then (by intravenous infusion) 2 mg/minute for 2 hours, then (by intravenous infusion) 1 mg/minute, reduce concentration further if infusion continued beyond 24 hours (ECG monitoring and specialist advice for infusion), following intravenous injection lidocaine has a short duration of action (lasting for 15–20 minutes). If an intravenous infusion is not immediately available the initial intravenous injection of 50 mg can be repeated if necessary once or twice at intervals of not less than 10 minutes

● CONTRA-INDICATIONS All grades of atrioventricular block · severe myocardial depression · sino-atrial disorders
● CAUTIONS Acute porphyrias p. 1107 (consider infusion with glucose for its anti-porphyrinogenic effects) · congestive cardiac failure (consider lower dose) · post cardiac surgery (consider lower dose)
● INTERACTIONS → Appendix 1: antiarrhythmics
● SIDE-EFFECTS Anxiety · arrhythmias · atrioventricular block · cardiac arrest · circulatory collapse · confusion · dizziness · drowsiness · euphoric mood · headache · hypotension (may lead to cardiac arrest) · loss of consciousness · methaemoglobinaemia · muscle twitching · myocardial contractility decreased · nausea · neurological effects · nystagmus · pain · psychosis · respiratory disorders · seizure · sensation abnormal · temperature sensation altered · tinnitus · tremor · vision blurred · vomiting

SIDE-EFFECTS, FURTHER INFORMATION
Methaemoglobinaemia Methylthioninium chloride is licensed for the acute symptomatic treatment of drug-induced methaemoglobinaemia.

● PREGNANCY Crosses the placenta but not known to be harmful in *animal* studies—use if benefit outweighs risk.
● BREAST FEEDING Present in milk but amount too small to be harmful.
● HEPATIC IMPAIRMENT Manufacturer advises caution (risk of increased exposure).
Dose adjustments Manufacturer advises slower infusion rate.
● RENAL IMPAIRMENT Possible accumulation of lidocaine and active metabolite; caution in severe impairment.
● MONITORING REQUIREMENTS Monitor ECG and have resuscitation facilities available.

● MEDICINAL FORMS There can be variation in the licensing of different medicines containing the same drug. Forms available from special-order manufacturers include: solution for injection

Solution for injection
▸ Lidocaine hydrochloride (Non-proprietary)
Lidocaine hydrochloride 5 mg per 1 ml Lidocaine 50mg/10ml (0.5%) solution for injection ampoules | 10 ampoule PoM £7.00
Lidocaine hydrochloride 10 mg per 1 ml Lidocaine 100mg/10ml (1%) solution for injection ampoules | 10 ampoule PoM £5.00 DT = £5.00
Lidocaine 200mg/20ml (1%) solution for injection vials | 10 vial PoM £22.00 DT = £22.00
Lidocaine 200mg/20ml (1%) solution for injection ampoules | 10 ampoule PoM £10.00-£11.00 DT = £11.00
Lidocaine 50mg/5ml (1%) solution for injection ampoules | 10 ampoule PoM £3.00-£12.00 DT = £3.00
Lidocaine 20mg/2ml (1%) solution for injection ampoules | 10 ampoule PoM £12.00 DT = £2.50
Lidocaine hydrochloride 20 mg per 1 ml Lidocaine 100mg/5ml (2%) solution for injection ampoules | 10 ampoule PoM £3.20-£12.00 DT = £3.20
Lidocaine 400mg/20ml (2%) solution for injection vials | 10 vial PoM £23.00 DT = £23.00
Lidocaine 200mg/10ml (2%) solution for injection Mini-Plasco ampoules | 20 ampoule PoM £14.95 DT = £14.95
Lidocaine 40mg/2ml (2%) solution for injection ampoules | 10 ampoule PoM £12.00 DT = £2.70
Lidocaine 400mg/20ml (2%) solution for injection ampoules | 10 ampoule PoM £11.00-£11.40 DT = £11.40

ANTIARRHYTHMICS › CLASS IC

Flecainide acetate   12-Oct-2020

● **INDICATIONS AND DOSE**

Supraventricular arrhythmias (initiated under direction of hospital consultant)
▸ BY MOUTH
▸ **Adult:** Initially 50 mg twice daily, increased if necessary up to 300 mg daily

Ventricular arrhythmias (initiated under direction of hospital consultant)
▸ BY MOUTH
▸ **Adult:** Initially 100 mg twice daily for 3–5 days, maximum 400 mg daily reserved for rapid control or in heavily built patients; for maintenance, reduce to the lowest dose that controls the arrhythmia

DOSE ADJUSTMENTS DUE TO INTERACTIONS
▸ Manufacturer advises reduce dose by half with concurrent use of amiodarone.

● CONTRA-INDICATIONS Abnormal left ventricular function · atrial conduction defects (unless pacing rescue available) · bundle branch block (unless pacing rescue available) · distal block (unless pacing rescue available) · haemodynamically significant valvular heart disease · heart failure · history of myocardial infarction and either asymptomatic ventricular ectopics or asymptomatic non-sustained ventricular tachycardia · long-standing atrial fibrillation where conversion to sinus rhythm not attempted · second-degree or greater AV block (unless

pacing rescue available) · sinus node dysfunction (unless pacing rescue available)
- CAUTIONS Atrial fibrillation following heart surgery · elderly (accumulation may occur) · patients with pacemakers (especially those who may be pacemaker dependent because stimulation threshold may rise appreciably)
- INTERACTIONS → Appendix 1: antiarrhythmics
- SIDE-EFFECTS
  - **Common or very common** Arrhythmias · asthenia · dizziness · dyspnoea · fever · oedema · vision disorders
  - **Uncommon** Alopecia · appetite decreased · constipation · diarrhoea · flatulence · gastrointestinal discomfort · nausea · skin reactions · vomiting
  - **Rare or very rare** Anxiety · confusion · corneal deposits · depression · drowsiness · flushing · hallucination · headache · hepatic disorders · hyperhidrosis · inflammation · insomnia · memory loss · movement disorders · peripheral neuropathy · photosensitivity reaction · respiratory disorders · seizure · sensation abnormal · syncope · tinnitus · tremor · vertigo
  - **Frequency not known** Altered pacing threshold · atrioventricular block · cardiac arrest · chest pain · heart failure · hypotension · palpitations · QT interval prolongation
- PREGNANCY Used in pregnancy to treat maternal and fetal arrhythmias in specialist centres; toxicity reported in animal studies; infant hyperbilirubinaemia also reported.
- BREAST FEEDING Significant amount present in milk but not known to be harmful.
- HEPATIC IMPAIRMENT
  Dose adjustments Avoid or reduce dose in severe impairment.
- RENAL IMPAIRMENT
  Dose adjustments Reduce initial oral dose to max. 100 mg daily if eGFR less than 35 mL/minute/1.73 m^2.

- MEDICINAL FORMS There can be variation in the licensing of different medicines containing the same drug. Forms available from special-order manufacturers include: oral suspension, oral solution

Tablet
- Flecainide acetate (Non-proprietary)
  Flecainide acetate 50 mg Flecainide 50mg tablets | 60 tablet [PoM] £7.68 DT = £3.45
  Flecainide acetate 100 mg Flecainide 100mg tablets | 60 tablet [PoM] £8.06 DT = £4.20
- Tambocor (Teva UK Ltd)
  Flecainide acetate 50 mg Tambocor 50mg tablets | 60 tablet [PoM] £11.57 DT = £3.45

▌Propafenone hydrochloride   03-Feb-2020

- INDICATIONS AND DOSE

Ventricular arrhythmias (specialist supervision in hospital) | Paroxysmal supraventricular tachyarrhythmias which include paroxysmal atrial flutter or fibrillation and paroxysmal re-entrant tachycardias involving the AV node or accessory pathway, where standard therapy ineffective or contra-indicated (specialist supervision in hospital)
- BY MOUTH
  - **Adult:** Initially 150 mg 3 times a day, dose to be taken after food, monitor ECG and blood pressure, if QRS interval prolonged by more than 20%, reduce dose or discontinue until ECG returns to normal limits; increased if necessary to 300 mg twice daily (max. per dose 300 mg 3 times a day), dose to be increased at intervals of at least 3 days, reduce total daily dose for patients under 70 kg

  - **Elderly:** Initially 150 mg 3 times a day, dose to be taken after food, monitor ECG and blood pressure, if QRS interval prolonged by more than 20%, reduce dose or discontinue until ECG returns to normal limits; increased if necessary to 300 mg twice daily (max. per dose 300 mg 3 times a day), dose to be increased at intervals of at least 5 days, reduce total daily dose for patients under 70 kg

- CONTRA-INDICATIONS Atrial conduction defects (unless adequately paced) · Brugada syndrome · bundle branch block (unless adequately paced) · cardiogenic shock (except arrhythmia induced) · distal block (unless adequately paced) · electrolyte disturbances · marked hypotension · myasthenia gravis · myocardial infarction within last 3 months · second degree or greater AV block (unless adequately paced) · severe bradycardia · severe obstructive pulmonary disease (due to weak beta-blocking activity) · sinus node dysfunction (unless adequately paced) · uncontrolled congestive heart failure with left ventricular ejection fraction less than 35%
- CAUTIONS Elderly · heart failure · mild to moderate obstructive airways disease owing to beta-blocking activity · pacemaker patients · potential for conversion of paroxysmal atrial fibrillation to atrial flutter with 2:1 conduction block or 1:1 conduction
- INTERACTIONS → Appendix 1: antiarrhythmics
- SIDE-EFFECTS
  - **Common or very common** Anxiety · arrhythmias · asthenia · cardiac conduction disorder · chest pain · constipation · diarrhoea · dizziness · dry mouth · dyspnoea · fever · gastrointestinal discomfort · headache · hepatic disorders · nausea · palpitations · sleep disorders · taste altered · vision blurred · vomiting
  - **Uncommon** Appetite decreased · erectile dysfunction · gastrointestinal disorders · hypotension · movement disorders · paraesthesia · skin reactions · syncope · thrombocytopenia · vertigo
  - **Frequency not known** Agranulocytosis · confusion · granulocytopenia · heart failure · leucopenia · lupus-like syndrome · seizure
- PREGNANCY Use only if potential benefit outweighs risk.
- BREAST FEEDING Use with caution—present in milk.
- PATIENT AND CARER ADVICE
  Driving and skilled tasks May affect performance of skilled tasks e.g. driving.

- MEDICINAL FORMS There can be variation in the licensing of different medicines containing the same drug. Forms available from special-order manufacturers include: oral suspension, oral solution

Tablet
CAUTIONARY AND ADVISORY LABELS 21, 25
- Propafenone hydrochloride (Non-proprietary)
  Propafenone hydrochloride 150 mg Propafenone 150mg tablets | 90 tablet [PoM] £7.37 DT = £7.37
  Propafenone hydrochloride 300 mg Propafenone 300mg tablets | 60 tablet [PoM] £9.34 DT = £9.34
- Arythmol (Mylan)
  Propafenone hydrochloride 150 mg Arythmol 150mg tablets | 90 tablet [PoM] £7.37 DT = £7.37
  Propafenone hydrochloride 300 mg Arythmol 300mg tablets | 60 tablet [PoM] £9.34 DT = £9.34

ANTIARRHYTHMICS 〉 CLASS III

▌ Amiodarone hydrochloride   16-Nov-2020

● **INDICATIONS AND DOSE**

Treatment of arrhythmias, particularly when other drugs are ineffective or contra-indicated (including paroxysmal supraventricular, nodal and ventricular tachycardias, atrial fibrillation and flutter, ventricular fibrillation, and tachyarrhythmias associated with Wolff-Parkinson-White syndrome) (initiated in hospital or under specialist supervision)
▸ BY MOUTH
▸ Adult: 200 mg 3 times a day for 1 week, then reduced to 200 mg twice daily for a further week, followed by maintenance dose, usually 200 mg daily or the minimum dose required to control arrhythmia
▸ BY INTRAVENOUS INFUSION
▸ Adult: Initially 5 mg/kg, to be given over 20–120 minutes with ECG monitoring, subsequent infusions given if necessary according to response; maximum 1.2 g per day

Ventricular fibrillation or pulseless ventricular tachycardia refractory to defibrillation (for cardiopulmonary resuscitation)
▸ INITIALLY BY INTRAVENOUS INJECTION
▸ Adult: Initially 300 mg, dose to be considered after administration of adrenaline, dose should be given from a pre-filled syringe or diluted in 20 mL Glucose 5%, then (by intravenous injection) 150 mg if required, followed by (by intravenous infusion) 900 mg/24 hours

> **IMPORTANT SAFETY INFORMATION**
> MHRA/CHM ADVICE: SOFOSBUVIR WITH DACLATASVIR; SOFOSBUVIR AND LEDIPASVIR (MAY 2015); SIMEPREVIR WITH SOFOSBUVIR (AUGUST 2015): RISK OF SEVERE BRADYCARDIA AND HEART BLOCK WHEN TAKEN WITH AMIODARONE
> Avoid concomitant use unless other antiarrhythmics cannot be given.

● **CONTRA-INDICATIONS**
GENERAL CONTRA-INDICATIONS Avoid in severe conduction disturbances (unless pacemaker fitted) · avoid in sinus node disease (unless pacemaker fitted) · iodine sensitivity · sino-atrial heart block (except in cardiac arrest) · sinus bradycardia (except in cardiac arrest) · thyroid dysfunction
SPECIFIC CONTRA-INDICATIONS
▸ With intravenous use Avoid bolus injection in cardiomyopathy · avoid bolus injection in congestive heart failure · avoid in circulatory collapse · avoid in severe arterial hypotension · avoid in severe respiratory failure
● **CAUTIONS**
GENERAL CAUTIONS Acute porphyrias p. 1107 · conduction disturbances (in excessive dosage) · elderly · heart failure · hypokalaemia · severe bradycardia (in excessive dosage)
SPECIFIC CAUTIONS
▸ With intravenous use moderate and transient fall in blood pressure (circulatory collapse precipitated by rapid administration or overdosage) · severe hepatocellular toxicity
CAUTIONS, FURTHER INFORMATION
▸ Elderly Prescription potentially inappropriate (STOPP criteria) as first-line antiarrhythmic therapy in supraventricular tachyarrhythmias (higher risk of side-effects than beta-blockers, digoxin, verapamil or diltiazem). See also Prescribing in the elderly p. 33.
● INTERACTIONS → Appendix 1: antiarrhythmics

● **SIDE-EFFECTS**
GENERAL SIDE-EFFECTS
▸ Common or very common Arrhythmias · hepatic disorders · hyperthyroidism · nausea · respiratory disorders · skin reactions
▸ Rare or very rare Bronchospasm (in patients with severe respiratory failure) · headache · idiopathic intracranial hypertension · nerve disorders · SIADH
▸ Frequency not known Angioedema · confusion · delirium · pancreatitis · severe cutaneous adverse reactions (SCARs)
SPECIFIC SIDE-EFFECTS
▸ Common or very common
▸ With oral use Constipation · corneal deposits · hypothyroidism · movement disorders · photosensitivity reaction · sleep disorders · taste altered · vomiting
▸ With parenteral use Hypotension (following rapid injection)
▸ Uncommon
▸ With oral use Cardiac conduction disorders · dry mouth · myopathy (usually reversible on discontinuation) · peripheral neuropathy (usually reversible on discontinuation)
▸ Rare or very rare
▸ With oral use Alopecia · aplastic anaemia · epididymo-orchitis · erectile dysfunction · haemolytic anaemia · pulmonary haemorrhage · thrombocytopenia · vertigo
▸ With parenteral use Hot flush · hyperhidrosis
▸ Frequency not known
▸ With oral use Altered smell sensation · appetite decreased · parkinsonism · vasculitis
▸ With parenteral use Agranulocytosis · libido decreased · neutropenia
SIDE-EFFECTS, FURTHER INFORMATION **Corneal microdeposits** Patients taking amiodarone may develop corneal microdeposits (reversible on withdrawal of treatment). However, if vision is impaired or if optic neuritis or optic neuropathy occur, amiodarone must be stopped to prevent blindness and expert advice sought.
    Thyroid function Amiodarone contains iodine and can cause disorders of thyroid function; both hypothyroidism and hyperthyroidism can occur. Hypothyroidism can be treated with replacement therapy without withdrawing amiodarone if it is essential; careful supervision is required.
    Hepatotoxicity Amiodarone is also associated with hepatotoxicity and treatment should be discontinued if severe liver function abnormalities or clinical signs of liver disease develop.
    Pulmonary toxicity Pneumonitis should always be suspected if new or progressive shortness of breath or cough develops in a patient taking amiodarone.
● PREGNANCY Possible risk of neonatal goitre; use only if no alternative.
● BREAST FEEDING Avoid; present in milk in significant amounts; theoretical risk of neonatal hypothyroidism from release of iodine.
● **MONITORING REQUIREMENTS**
▸ Thyroid function tests should be performed before treatment and then every 6 months. Clinical assessment of thyroid function alone is unreliable. Thyroxine (T4) may be raised in the absence of hyperthyroidism; therefore tri-iodothyronine (T3), T4, and thyroid-stimulating hormone (thyrotrophin, TSH) should all be measured. A raised T3 and T4 with a very low or undetectable TSH concentration suggests the development of thyrotoxicosis.
▸ Liver function tests required before treatment and then every 6 months.
▸ Serum potassium concentration should be measured before treatment.
▸ Chest x-ray required before treatment.
▸ If concomitant use of amiodarone with sofosbuvir and daclatasvir, simeprevir and sofosbuvir, or sofosbuvir and

2

Cardiovascular system

ledipasvir cannot be avoided because other anti-arrhythmics are not tolerated or contra-indicated, patients should be closely monitored, particularly during the first weeks of treatment. Patients at high risk of bradycardia should be monitored continuously for 48 hours in an appropriate clinical setting after starting concomitant treatment. Patients who have stopped amiodarone within the last few months and need to start sofosbuvir and daclatasvir, simeprevir and sofosbuvir, or sofosbuvir and ledipasvir should be monitored.

▸ With intravenous use ECG monitoring and resuscitation facilities must be available. Monitor liver transaminases closely.

● DIRECTIONS FOR ADMINISTRATION
▸ With intravenous use For *intravenous infusion* (*Cordarone X*®), manufacturer advises give continuously or intermittently in Glucose 5%. Suggested initial infusion volume 250 mL given over 20–120 minutes; for repeat infusions up to 1.2 g in max. 500 mL; should not be diluted to less than 600 micrograms/mL. See cardio-pulmonary resuscitation for details of infusion in extreme emergency. Incompatible with Sodium Chloride infusion fluids; avoid equipment containing the plasticizer di-2-ethylhexphthalate (DEHP).
▸ With oral use For administration *by mouth*, expert sources advise tablets may be crushed and dispersed in water; injection solution should **not** be given orally (irritant).

● PATIENT AND CARER ADVICE
Phototoxicity Because of the possibility of phototoxic reactions, patients should be advised to shield the skin from light during treatment and for several months after discontinuing amiodarone; a wide-spectrum sunscreen to protect against both long-wave ultraviolet and visible light should be used.
Concurrent sofosbuvir-containing regimens If taking amiodarone with concurrent sofosbuvir-containing regimens, patients and their carers should be told how to recognise signs and symptoms of bradycardia and heart block and advised to seek immediate medical attention if symptoms such as shortness of breath, light-headedness, palpitations, fainting, unusual tiredness or chest pain develop.
Driving and skilled tasks Patients and carers should be cautioned on the effects on driving and performance of skilled tasks—corneal microdeposits may be associated with blurred vision (see *Side-effects, further information*).

● MEDICINAL FORMS There can be variation in the licensing of different medicines containing the same drug. Forms available from special-order manufacturers include: oral suspension, oral solution

Tablet
CAUTIONARY AND ADVISORY LABELS 11
▸ Amiodarone hydrochloride (Non-proprietary)
  Amiodarone hydrochloride 100 mg Amiodarone 100mg tablets | 28 tablet PoM £4.25 DT = £2.16
  Amiodarone hydrochloride 200 mg Amiodarone 200mg tablets | 28 tablet PoM £7.80 DT = £2.46
▸ Cordarone X (Zentiva)
  Amiodarone hydrochloride 100 mg Cordarone X 100 tablets | 28 tablet PoM £4.28 DT = £2.16
  Amiodarone hydrochloride 200 mg Cordarone X 200 tablets | 28 tablet PoM £6.99 DT = £2.46

Solution for injection
EXCIPIENTS: May contain Benzyl alcohol
▸ Amiodarone hydrochloride (Non-proprietary)
  Amiodarone hydrochloride 30 mg per 1 ml Amiodarone 300mg/10ml solution for injection pre-filled syringes | 1 pre-filled disposable injection PoM £14.68–£15.41 DT = £14.68
  Amiodarone hydrochloride 50 mg per 1 ml Amiodarone 150mg/3ml concentrate for solution for injection ampoules | 5 ampoule PoM £7.75 (Hospital only) | 10 ampoule PoM £17.00 (Hospital only)

▸ Cordarone X (Sanofi)
  Amiodarone hydrochloride 50 mg per 1 ml Cordarone X 150mg/3ml solution for injection ampoules | 6 ampoule PoM £9.60 (Hospital only)

Dronedarone
02-Sep-2020

● DRUG ACTION Dronedarone is a multi-channel blocking anti-arrhythmic drug.

● INDICATIONS AND DOSE
Maintenance of sinus rhythm after cardioversion in clinically stable patients with paroxysmal or persistent atrial fibrillation, when alternative treatments are unsuitable (initiated under specialist supervision)
▸ BY MOUTH
▸ Adult: 400 mg twice daily

● CONTRA-INDICATIONS Atrial conduction defects · bradycardia · complete bundle branch block · distal block · existing or previous heart failure or left ventricular systolic dysfunction · haemodynamically unstable patients · liver toxicity associated with previous amiodarone use · lung toxicity associated with previous amiodarone use · permanent atrial fibrillation · prolonged QT interval · second- or third- degree AV block · sick sinus syndrome (unless pacemaker fitted) · sinus node dysfunction

● CAUTIONS Coronary artery disease · correct hypokalaemia and hypomagnesaemia before starting and during treatment

● INTERACTIONS → Appendix 1: antiarrhythmics

● SIDE-EFFECTS
▸ **Common or very common** Asthenia · bradycardia · congestive heart failure · diarrhoea · gastrointestinal discomfort · nausea · QT interval prolongation · skin reactions · vomiting
▸ **Uncommon** Photosensitivity reaction · respiratory disorders · taste altered
▸ **Rare or very rare** Hepatic disorders · vasculitis

SIDE-EFFECTS, FURTHER INFORMATION **Liver injury** Liver injury including life-threatening acute liver failure reported rarely; discontinue treatment if 2 consecutive alanine aminotransferase concentrations exceed 3 times upper limit of normal.
Heart failure New onset or worsening heart failure reported. If heart failure or left ventricular systolic dysfunction develops, discontinue treatment.
Pulmonary toxicity Interstitial lung disease, pneumonitis and pulmonary fibrosis reported. Investigate if symptoms such as dyspnoea or dry cough develop and discontinue if confirmed.

● PREGNANCY Manufacturer advises avoid—toxicity in *animal* studies.

● BREAST FEEDING Manufacturer advises avoid—present in milk in *animal* studies.

● HEPATIC IMPAIRMENT Manufacturer advises avoid in severe impairment.

● RENAL IMPAIRMENT Avoid if eGFR less than 30 mL/minute/1.73 m^2.

● MONITORING REQUIREMENTS
▸ Ongoing monitoring should occur under specialist supervision.
▸ Monitor for heart failure.
▸ Perform ECG at least every 6 months—consider discontinuation if atrial fibrillation reoccurs.
▸ Measure serum creatinine before treatment and 7 days after initiation—if raised, measure again after a further 7 days and consider discontinuation if creatinine continues to rise.
▸ Monitor liver function before treatment, 1 week and 1 month after initiation of treatment, then monthly for

6 months, then every 3 months for 6 months and periodically thereafter.

● PATIENT AND CARER ADVICE
Heart failure Patients or their carers should be told how to recognise signs of heart failure and advised to seek prompt medical attention if symptoms such as weight gain, dependent oedema, or dyspnoea develop or worsen.
Hepatic disorders Patients or their carers should be told how to recognise signs of liver disorder and advised to seek prompt medical attention if symptoms such as abdominal pain, anorexia, nausea, vomiting, fever, malaise, itching, dark urine, or jaundice develop.

● NATIONAL FUNDING/ACCESS DECISIONS
For full details see funding body website

NICE decisions
▶ **Dronedarone for the treatment of non-permanent atrial fibrillation (updated December 2012)** NICE TA197
Recommended

● MEDICINAL FORMS There can be variation in the licensing of different medicines containing the same drug.
Tablet
CAUTIONARY AND ADVISORY LABELS 21
▶ Dronedarone (Non-proprietary)
Dronedarone (as Dronedarone hydrochloride)
400 mg Dronedarone 400mg tablets | 20 tablet PoM £22.49–£22.50 DT = £22.50 | 60 tablet PoM £67.49–£67.50
▶ Multaq (Sanofi)
Dronedarone (as Dronedarone hydrochloride) 400 mg Multaq 400mg tablets | 20 tablet PoM £22.50 DT = £22.50 | 60 tablet PoM £67.50

ANTIARRHYTHMICS > OTHER

Adenosine
28-Jul-2020

● INDICATIONS AND DOSE

Rapid reversion to sinus rhythm of paroxysmal supraventricular tachycardias, including those associated with accessory conducting pathways (e.g. Wolff-Parkinson-White syndrome) | Used to aid to diagnosis of broad or narrow complex supraventricular tachycardias
▶ BY RAPID INTRAVENOUS INJECTION
▶ Adult: Initially 6 mg, administer into central or large peripheral vein and give over 2 seconds, cardiac monitoring required, followed by 12 mg after 1–2 minutes if required, then 12 mg after 1–2 minutes if required, increments should not be given if high level AV block develops at any particular dose

Rapid reversion to sinus rhythm of paroxysmal supraventricular tachycardias, including those associated with accessory conducting pathways (e.g. Wolff-Parkinson-White syndrome) in patients with a heart transplant | Aid to diagnosis of broad or narrow complex supraventricular tachycardias in patients with a heart transplant
▶ BY RAPID INTRAVENOUS INJECTION
▶ Adult: Initially 3 mg, administer into a central or large peripheral vein and give over 2 seconds, followed by 6 mg after 1–2 minutes if required, then 12 mg after 1–2 minutes if required, patients with a heart transplant are very sensitive to the effects of adenosine

Used in conjunction with radionuclide myocardial perfusion imaging in patients who cannot exercise adequately or for whom exercise is inappropriate
▶ BY INTRAVENOUS INFUSION
▶ Adult: (consult product literature)

● UNLICENSED USE Adenosine doses in the BNF may differ from those in the product literature.

● CONTRA-INDICATIONS Asthma · chronic obstructive lung disease · decompensated heart failure · long QT syndrome · second- or third-degree AV block and sick sinus syndrome (unless pacemaker fitted) · severe hypotension

● CAUTIONS Atrial fibrillation · atrial fibrillation with accessory pathway (conduction down anomalous pathway may increase) · atrial flutter · atrial flutter with accessory pathway (conduction down anomalous pathway may increase) · autonomic dysfunction · bundle branch block · first-degree AV block · heart transplant · left main coronary artery stenosis · left to right shunt · pericardial effusion · pericarditis · QT-interval prolongation · recent myocardial infarction · severe heart failure · stenotic carotid artery disease with cerebrovascular insufficiency · stenotic valvular heart disease · uncorrected hypovolaemia

● INTERACTIONS → Appendix 1: antiarrhythmics

● SIDE-EFFECTS
▶ **Common or very common** Abdominal discomfort · arrhythmias · atrioventricular block · chest discomfort · chest pain (discontinue) · dizziness · dry mouth · dyspnoea · flushing · headache · hypotension (discontinue if severe) · pain · paraesthesia · throat discomfort
▶ **Uncommon** Asthenia · back discomfort · bradycardia (discontinue if asystole or severe bradycardia occur) · hyperhidrosis · limb discomfort · nervousness · taste metallic
▶ **Rare or very rare** Drowsiness · nasal congestion · nipple tenderness · respiratory disorders · respiratory failure (discontinue) · tinnitus · tremor · urinary urgency · vision blurred
▶ **Frequency not known** Apnoea · cardiac arrest · loss of consciousness · nausea · seizure · syncope · vomiting

● PREGNANCY Large doses may produce fetal toxicity; manufacturer advises use only if potential benefit outweighs risk.

● BREAST FEEDING No information available—unlikely to be present in milk owing to short half-life.

● MONITORING REQUIREMENTS Monitor ECG and have resuscitation facilities available.

● DIRECTIONS FOR ADMINISTRATION For *rapid intravenous injection*, expert sources advise give over 2 seconds into central or large peripheral vein followed by rapid Sodium Chloride 0.9% flush; injection solution may be diluted with Sodium Chloride 0.9% if required.

● MEDICINAL FORMS There can be variation in the licensing of different medicines containing the same drug. Forms available from special-order manufacturers include: solution for injection, infusion, solution for infusion
Solution for injection
ELECTROLYTES: May contain Sodium
▶ Adenosine (Non-proprietary)
Adenosine 3 mg per 1 ml Adenosine 6mg/2ml solution for injection pre-filled syringes | 10 pre-filled disposable injection PoM 🅢 (Hospital only)
Adenosine 6mg/2ml solution for injection vials | 5 vial PoM £4.90–£20.00 (Hospital only) | 6 vial PoM £26.70–£29.24 (Hospital only)
Adenosine 12mg/4ml solution for injection pre-filled syringes | 10 pre-filled disposable injection PoM 🅢 (Hospital only)
▶ Adenocor (Sanofi)
Adenosine 3 mg per 1 ml Adenocor 6mg/2ml solution for injection vials | 6 vial PoM £6.45 (Hospital only)
Solution for infusion
ELECTROLYTES: May contain Sodium
▶ Adenosine (Non-proprietary)
Adenosine 3 mg per 1 ml Adenosine 30mg/10ml solution for infusion vials | 5 vial PoM £12.50–£30.00 (Hospital only) | 6 vial PoM £70.00–£85.57 (Hospital only)
▶ Adenoscan (Sanofi)
Adenosine 3 mg per 1 ml Adenoscan 30mg/10ml solution for infusion vials | 6 vial PoM £16.05 (Hospital only)

Vernakalant

15-Jul-2019

- **DRUG ACTION** Vernakalant is an anti-arrhythmic drug that blocks potassium and sodium channels in the atria, thereby restoring normal heart rhythm.

- **INDICATIONS AND DOSE**

Rapid conversion of recent onset atrial fibrillation to sinus rhythm (specialist supervision in hospital)
▸ BY INTRAVENOUS INFUSION
▸ Adult: Initially 3 mg/kg (max. per dose 339 mg), followed by 2 mg/kg (max. per dose 226 mg), if conversion to sinus rhythm does not occur within 15 minutes after the end of initial infusion, maximum 5 mg/kg per 24 hours; maximum 565 mg per day
DOSE EQUIVALENCE AND CONVERSION
▸ Doses expressed as vernakalant hydrochloride.

- **CONTRA-INDICATIONS** Acute coronary syndrome within the last 30 days · baseline QT interval 440 milliseconds or greater · congestive heart failure with left ventricular ejection fraction ≤ 35% · heart failure (New York Heart Association class III/IV) · second- or third-degree heart block (unless pacemaker fitted) · severe aortic stenosis · severe bradycardia · sinus node dysfunction · systolic blood pressure less than 100 mmHg

- **CAUTIONS** Haemodynamically stable patients with congestive heart failure (increased risk of hypotension and ventricular arrhythmia) · patients receiving oral anti-arrhythmics (class I or III) (risk of atrial flutter) · valvular heart disease (increased incidence of ventricular arrhythmia)

- **INTERACTIONS** → Appendix 1: antiarrhythmics

- **SIDE-EFFECTS**
▸ **Common or very common** Arrhythmias · cough · dizziness · feeling hot · headache · hypotension · nasal complaints · nausea · oral disorders · sensation abnormal · skin reactions · sweat changes · taste altered · vomiting
▸ **Uncommon** Altered smell sensation · cardiac conduction disorders · cardiogenic shock · chest discomfort · choking sensation · defaecation urgency · diarrhoea · drowsiness · dry mouth · dyspnoea · excessive tearing · eye irritation · fatigue · malaise · pain in extremity · pallor · palpitations · QT interval prolongation · suffocation feeling · syncope · throat irritation · vasodilation · visual impairment
SIDE-EFFECTS, FURTHER INFORMATION Discontinue and initiate appropriate treatment if hypotension, bradycardia, ECG changes, or a sudden drop in blood pressure or heart rate occur.

- **PREGNANCY** Manufacturer advises avoid—no information available.

- **BREAST FEEDING** Manufacturer advises caution—no information available.

- **MONITORING REQUIREMENTS** Manufacturer advises monitor blood pressure and ECG during and for at least 15 minutes after completion of the infusion.

- **DIRECTIONS FOR ADMINISTRATION** Manufacturer advises for *intermittent intravenous infusion* in patients with body-weight up to and including 100 kg, dilute to a concentration of 4 mg/mL with 100 mL of Glucose 5% *or* Sodium Chloride 0.9% *or* Lactated Ringer's Solution; give over 10 minutes. Manufacturer advises for *intermittent intravenous infusion* in patients with body-weight more than 100 kg, dilute to a concentration of 4 mg/mL with 120 mL of Glucose 5% *or* Sodium Chloride 0.9% *or* Lactated Ringer's Solution; give over 10 minutes.

- **PRESCRIBING AND DISPENSING INFORMATION** The manufacturer of *Brinavess*® has provided a *Pre-infusion Checklist* and a *Healthcare Professional Card*.

- **PATIENT AND CARER ADVICE**
Driving and skilled tasks Manufacturer advises patients and carers should be counselled on the effects on driving and performance of skilled tasks—increased risk of dizziness.

- **MEDICINAL FORMS** There can be variation in the licensing of different medicines containing the same drug.
Solution for infusion
ELECTROLYTES: May contain Sodium
▸ Brinavess (Correvio UK Ltd)
Vernakalant hydrochloride 20 mg per 1 ml Brinavess 500mg/25ml concentrate for solution for infusion vials | 1 vial [PoM] £290.00 (Hospital only)

BETA-ADRENOCEPTOR BLOCKERS ›
NON-SELECTIVE

⚑ 161

Sotalol hydrochloride

21-Jul-2020

- **INDICATIONS AND DOSE**

Symptomatic non-sustained ventricular tachyarrhythmias | Prophylaxis of paroxysmal atrial tachycardia or fibrillation, paroxysmal AV re-entrant tachycardias (both nodal and involving accessory pathways), and paroxysmal supraventricular tachycardia after cardiac surgery | Maintenance of sinus rhythm following cardioversion of atrial fibrillation or flutter
▸ BY MOUTH
▸ Adult: Initially 80 mg daily in 1–2 divided doses, then increased to 160–320 mg daily in 2 divided doses, dose to be increased gradually at intervals of 2–3 days

Life-threatening arrhythmias including ventricular tachyarrhythmias
▸ BY MOUTH
▸ Adult: Initially 80 mg daily in 1–2 divided doses, then increased to 160–320 mg daily in 2 divided doses, dose to be increased gradually at intervals of 2–3 days, higher doses of 480–640 mg daily may be required for life-threatening ventricular arrhythmias (under specialist supervision)

IMPORTANT SAFETY INFORMATION
Sotalol may prolong the QT interval, and it occasionally causes life threatening ventricular arrhythmias (**important**: manufacturer advises particular care is required to avoid hypokalaemia in patients taking sotalol—electrolyte disturbances, particularly hypokalaemia and hypomagnesaemia should be corrected before sotalol started and during use).
    Manufacturer advises reduce dose or discontinue if corrected QT interval exceeds 550 msec.

- **CONTRA-INDICATIONS** Long QT syndrome (congenital or acquired) · torsade de pointes

- **CAUTIONS** Diarrhoea (severe or prolonged)

- **INTERACTIONS** → Appendix 1: beta blockers, non-selective

- **SIDE-EFFECTS**
▸ **Common or very common** Anxiety · arrhythmia · chest pain · dyspepsia · fever · flatulence · hearing impairment · mood altered · muscle spasms · oedema · palpitations · sexual dysfunction · taste altered · torsade de pointes (increased risk in females)

- **BREAST FEEDING** Water soluble beta-blockers such as sotalol are present in breast milk in greater amounts than other beta blockers.

- **RENAL IMPAIRMENT** Manufacturer advises avoid if creatinine clearance less than 10 mL/minute.
Dose adjustments Manufacturer advises use half normal dose if creatinine clearance 30–60 mL/minute; use one-quarter normal dose if creatinine clearance 10–30 mL/minute.

● MONITORING REQUIREMENTS Measurement of corrected QT interval, and monitoring of ECG and electrolytes required; correct hypokalaemia, hypomagnesaemia, or other electrolyte disturbances.

● MEDICINAL FORMS There can be variation in the licensing of different medicines containing the same drug. Forms available from special-order manufacturers include: oral suspension, oral solution

Tablet

CAUTIONARY AND ADVISORY LABELS 8

▸ Sotalol hydrochloride (Non-proprietary)
  Sotalol hydrochloride 40 mg Sotalol 40mg tablets |
  28 tablet PoM £1.26 DT = £1.26
  Sotalol hydrochloride 80 mg Sotalol 80mg tablets |
  28 tablet PoM £3.75 DT = £1.38
  Sotalol hydrochloride 160 mg Sotalol 160mg tablets |
  28 tablet PoM £5.93 DT = £4.69
▸ Beta-Cardone (Advanz Pharma)
  Sotalol hydrochloride 200 mg Beta-Cardone 200mg tablets |
  28 tablet PoM £2.40 DT = £2.40
▸ Sotacor (Cheplapharm Arzneimittel GmbH)
  Sotalol hydrochloride 80 mg Sotacor 80mg tablets |
  30 tablet PoM £3.28

CARDIAC GLYCOSIDES

Cardiac glycosides

Digoxin-specific antibody

Serious cases of digoxin toxicity should be discussed with the National Poisons Information Service (see further information, under Poisoning, emergency treatment p. 1413). Digoxin-specific antibody fragments p. 1423 are indicated for the treatment of known or strongly suspected life-threatening digoxin toxicity associated with ventricular arrhythmias or bradyarrhythmias unresponsive to atropine sulfate p. 1386 and when measures beyond the withdrawal of digoxin below and correction of any electrolyte abnormalities are considered necessary.

Digoxin

Digoxin is most useful for controlling ventricular response in persistent and permanent atrial fibrillation and atrial flutter. Digoxin also has a role in heart failure.

For management of atrial fibrillation the maintenance dose of digoxin can usually be determined by the ventricular rate at rest, which should not usually be allowed to fall persistently below 60 beats per minute.

Digoxin is now rarely used for rapid control of heart rate (see management of supraventricular arrhythmias). Even with intravenous administration, response may take many hours; persistence of tachycardia is therefore not an indication for exceeding the recommended dose. The intramuscular route is **not** recommended.

In patients with heart failure who are in sinus rhythm a loading dose is not required, and a satisfactory plasma-digoxin concentration can be achieved over a period of about a week.

Digoxin has a long half-life and maintenance doses need to be given only once daily (although higher doses may be divided to avoid nausea); renal function is the most important determinant of digoxin dosage.

Unwanted effects depend both on the concentration of digoxin in the plasma and on the sensitivity of the conducting system or of the myocardium, which is often increased in heart disease. It can sometimes be difficult to distinguish between toxic effects and clinical deterioration because symptoms of both are similar. The plasma concentration alone cannot indicate toxicity reliably, but the likelihood of toxicity increases progressively through the range 1.5 to 3 micrograms/litre for digoxin. Digoxin should

be used with special care in the elderly, who may be particularly susceptible to digitalis toxicity.

Regular monitoring of plasma-digoxin concentration during maintenance treatment is not necessary unless problems are suspected. Hypokalaemia predisposes the patient to digitalis toxicity; it is managed by giving a potassium-sparing diuretic or, if necessary, potassium supplementation.

If toxicity occurs, digoxin should be withdrawn; serious manifestations require urgent specialist management. Digoxin-specific antibody fragments are available for reversal of life-threatening overdosage.

Digoxin   02-Sep-2020

● DRUG ACTION Digoxin is a cardiac glycoside that increases the force of myocardial contraction and reduces conductivity within the atrioventricular (AV) node.

● INDICATIONS AND DOSE

Rapid digitalisation, for atrial fibrillation or flutter
▸ BY MOUTH
▸ Adult: 0.75–1.5 mg in divided doses, dose to be given over 24 hours, reduce dose in the elderly

Maintenance, for atrial fibrillation or flutter
▸ BY MOUTH
▸ Adult: Maintenance 125–250 micrograms daily, dose according to renal function and initial loading dose, reduce dose in the elderly

Heart failure (for patients in sinus rhythm)
▸ BY MOUTH
▸ Adult: 62.5–125 micrograms once daily, reduce dose in the elderly

Emergency loading dose, for atrial fibrillation or flutter
▸ INITIALLY BY INTRAVENOUS INFUSION
▸ Adult: Loading dose 0.75–1 mg, to be given over at least 2 hours, then (by mouth) maintenance, loading dose is rarely necessary, maintenance dose to be started on the day following the loading dose, reduce dose in the elderly

DOSE ADJUSTMENTS DUE TO INTERACTIONS
▸ Manufacturer advises reduce dose by half with concurrent use of amiodarone, dronedarone and quinine.

DOSE EQUIVALENCE AND CONVERSION
▸ Dose may need not to be reduced if digoxin (or another cardiac glycoside) has been given in the preceding 2 weeks.
▸ When switching from intravenous to oral route may need to increase dose by 20–33% to maintain the same plasma-digoxin concentration.

● UNLICENSED USE Digoxin doses in the BNF may differ from those in product literature.

● CONTRA-INDICATIONS Constrictive pericarditis (unless to control atrial fibrillation or improve systolic dysfunction—but use with caution) · hypertrophic cardiomyopathy (unless concomitant atrial fibrillation and heart failure—but use with caution) · intermittent complete heart block · myocarditis · second degree AV block · supraventricular arrhythmias associated with accessory conducting pathways e.g. Wolff-Parkinson-White syndrome (although can be used in infancy) · ventricular tachycardia or fibrillation

● CAUTIONS Hypercalcaemia (risk of digitalis toxicity) · hypokalaemia (risk of digitalis toxicity) · hypomagnesaemia (risk of digitalis toxicity) · hypoxia (risk of digitalis toxicity) · recent myocardial infarction · severe respiratory disease · sick sinus syndrome · thyroid disease

CAUTIONS, FURTHER INFORMATION
▸ **Elderly** Prescription potentially inappropriate (STOPP criteria):
  ● in heart failure with normal systolic ventricular function (no clear evidence of benefit)
  ● at a long-term dose greater than 125 micrograms daily if eGFR less than 30 mL/minute/1.73 m^2 (risk of digoxin toxicity if plasma levels not measured)
  See also Prescribing in the elderly p. 33.
● **INTERACTIONS** → Appendix 1: digoxin
● **SIDE-EFFECTS**
▸ **Common or very common** Arrhythmias · cardiac conduction disorder · cerebral impairment · diarrhoea · dizziness · eosinophilia · nausea · skin reactions · vision disorders · vomiting
▸ **Uncommon** Depression
▸ **Rare or very rare** Appetite decreased · asthenia · confusion · gastrointestinal disorders · gynaecomastia · headache · malaise · psychosis · thrombocytopenia
  Overdose If toxicity occurs, digoxin should be withdrawn; serious manifestations require urgent specialist management.
● **PREGNANCY**
  Dose adjustments May need dosage adjustment.
● **BREAST FEEDING** Amount too small to be harmful.
● **RENAL IMPAIRMENT**
  Dose adjustments Reduce dose.
  Monitoring Monitor plasma-digoxin concentration in renal impairment.
● **MONITORING REQUIREMENTS**
▸ For plasma-digoxin concentration assay, blood should be taken at least 6 hours after a dose.
▸ Monitor serum electrolytes and renal function. Toxicity increased by electrolyte disturbances.
● **DIRECTIONS FOR ADMINISTRATION**
▸ With intravenous use Avoid rapid intravenous administration (risk of hypertension and reduced coronary flow). For *intravenous infusion (Lanoxin®)*, give intermittently in Glucose 5% or Sodium chloride 0.9%; dilute to a concentration of not more than 62.5 micrograms/mL. To be given over at least 2 hours.
▸ With oral use For *oral* administration, oral solution must **not** be diluted.
● **PATIENT AND CARER ADVICE** Patient counselling is advised for digoxin elixir (use pipette).

● **MEDICINAL FORMS** There can be variation in the licensing of different medicines containing the same drug. Forms available from special-order manufacturers include: oral suspension, oral solution, solution for injection

Tablet
▸ Digoxin (Non-proprietary)
  Digoxin 62.5 microgram Digoxin 62.5microgram tablets | 28 tablet [PoM] £9.99 DT = £1.56
  Digoxin 125 microgram Digoxin 125microgram tablets | 28 tablet [PoM] £4.99 DT = £1.55
  Digoxin 250 microgram Digoxin 250microgram tablets | 28 tablet [PoM] £4.99 DT = £1.55
▸ Lanoxin (Aspen Pharma Trading Ltd)
  Digoxin 62.5 microgram Lanoxin PG 62.5microgram tablets | 500 tablet [PoM] £8.09
  Digoxin 125 microgram Lanoxin 125 tablets | 500 tablet [PoM] £8.09
  Digoxin 250 microgram Lanoxin 250microgram tablets | 500 tablet [PoM] £8.09
Solution for infusion
▸ Digoxin (Non-proprietary)
  Digoxin 250 microgram per 1 ml Digoxin 500micrograms/2ml solution for infusion ampoules | 10 ampoule [PoM] £7.00
▸ Lanoxin (Aspen Pharma Trading Ltd)
  Digoxin 250 microgram per 1 ml Lanoxin 500micrograms/2ml solution for infusion ampoules | 5 ampoule [PoM] £3.30

Oral solution
▸ Lanoxin (Aspen Pharma Trading Ltd)
  Digoxin 50 microgram per 1 ml Lanoxin PG 50micrograms/ml elixir | 60 ml [PoM] £5.35 DT = £5.35

2 Bleeding disorders

Antifibrinolytic drugs and haemostatics

Overview
Fibrin dissolution can be impaired by the administration of tranexamic acid below, which inhibits fibrinolysis. It can be used to prevent bleeding or to treat bleeding associated with excessive fibrinolysis (e.g. in surgery, dental extraction, obstetric disorders, and traumatic hyphaema) and in the management of menorrhagia. Tranexamic acid may also be used in hereditary angioedema, epistaxis, and in thrombolytic overdose.

Desmopressin p. 706 is used in the management of mild to moderate haemophilia and von Willebrand's disease. It is also used for fibrinolytic response testing.

Etamsylate reduces capillary bleeding in the presence of a normal number of platelets; it does not act by fibrin stabilisation, but probably by correcting abnormal adhesion. Etamsylate is less effective than other treatments in the management of heavy menstrual bleeding and its use is no longer recommended.

ANTIHAEMORRHAGICS ❭ ANTIFIBRINOLYTICS

Tranexamic acid
17-Aug-2020

● **INDICATIONS AND DOSE**
  Local fibrinolysis
▸ BY MOUTH
  ▸ Adult: 1–1.5 g 2–3 times a day, alternatively 15–25 mg/kg 2–3 times a day
▸ INITIALLY BY SLOW INTRAVENOUS INJECTION
  ▸ Adult: 0.5–1 g 2–3 times a day, to be administered at a rate not exceeding 100 mg/minute, followed by (by continuous intravenous infusion) 25–50 mg/kg if required, dose to be given over 24 hours
  Menorrhagia
▸ BY MOUTH
  ▸ Adult: 1 g 3 times a day for up to 4 days, to be initiated when menstruation has started; maximum 4 g per day
  Hereditary angioedema
▸ BY MOUTH
  ▸ Adult: 1–1.5 g 2–3 times a day, for short-term prophylaxis of hereditary angioedema, tranexamic acid is started several days before planned procedures which may trigger an acute attack of hereditary angioedema (e.g. dental work) and continued for 2–5 days afterwards
  Epistaxis
▸ BY MOUTH
  ▸ Adult: 1 g 3 times a day for 7 days
  General fibrinolysis
▸ BY SLOW INTRAVENOUS INJECTION
  ▸ Adult: 1 g every 6–8 hours, alternatively 15 mg/kg every 6–8 hours, dose to be given at a rate not exceeding 100 mg/minute

Prevention and treatment of significant haemorrhage following trauma

▶ INITIALLY BY SLOW INTRAVENOUS INJECTION
▶ **Adult:** Loading dose 1 g to be given over 10 minutes, treatment should commence within 8 hours of injury, followed by (by intravenous infusion) 1 g to be given over 8 hours

● UNLICENSED USE Use of tranexamic acid by continuous intravenous infusion for treatment of local fibrinolysis is an unlicensed route of administration.
  [EvGr] Not licensed for prevention and treatment of significant haemorrhage following trauma. ⟨A⟩

● CONTRA-INDICATIONS Fibrinolytic conditions following disseminated intravascular coagulation (unless predominant activation of fibrinolytic system with severe bleeding) · history of convulsions · thromboembolic disease

● CAUTIONS Irregular menstrual bleeding (establish cause before initiating therapy) · massive haematuria (avoid if risk of ureteric obstruction) · patients receiving oral contraceptives (increased risk of thrombosis)

CAUTIONS, FURTHER INFORMATION
▶ Menorrhagia Before initiating treatment for menorrhagia, exclude structural or histological causes or fibroids causing distortion of uterine cavity.

● INTERACTIONS → Appendix 1: tranexamic acid

● SIDE-EFFECTS
GENERAL SIDE-EFFECTS
▶ **Common or very common** Diarrhoea (reduce dose) · nausea · vomiting
▶ **Uncommon** Allergic dermatitis
▶ **Rare or very rare** Colour vision change (discontinue) · embolism and thrombosis
▶ **Frequency not known** Seizure (more common at high doses) · visual impairment (discontinue)
SPECIFIC SIDE-EFFECTS
▶ With intravenous use Hypotension · malaise (on rapid intravenous injection)

● PREGNANCY No evidence of teratogenicity in *animal* studies; manufacturer advises use only if potential benefit outweighs risk—crosses the placenta.

● BREAST FEEDING Small amount present in milk—antifibrinolytic effect in infant unlikely.

● RENAL IMPAIRMENT
  Dose adjustments Reduce dose—consult product literature for details.

● MONITORING REQUIREMENTS Regular liver function tests in long-term treatment of hereditary angioedema.

● DIRECTIONS FOR ADMINISTRATION For *intravenous infusion* (*Cyklokapron®*), manufacturer advises give in Glucose 5% or Sodium chloride 0.9%.

● MEDICINAL FORMS There can be variation in the licensing of different medicines containing the same drug. Forms available from special-order manufacturers include: oral suspension, oral solution

Tablet
▶ Tranexamic acid (Non-proprietary)
  Tranexamic acid 500 mg Tranexamic acid 500mg tablets | 60 tablet [PoM] £35.43 DT = £9.10
▶ Cyklokapron (Mylan)
  Tranexamic acid 500 mg Cyklokapron 500mg tablets | 60 tablet [PoM] £14.30 DT = £9.10

Solution for injection
▶ Tranexamic acid (Non-proprietary)
  Tranexamic acid 100 mg per 1 ml Tranexamic acid 500mg/5ml solution for injection ampoules | 5 ampoule [PoM] £7.50 DT = £7.50 (Hospital only) | 10 ampoule [PoM] £15.47 DT = £15.47 (Hospital only)

▶ Cyklokapron (Pfizer Ltd)
  Tranexamic acid 100 mg per 1 ml Cyklokapron 500mg/5ml solution for injection ampoules | 10 ampoule [PoM] £15.47 DT = £15.47 (Hospital only)

ANTIHAEMORRHAGICS ⟩ HAEMOSTATICS

Emicizumab   09-May-2018

● DRUG ACTION Emicizumab is a monoclonal antibody that bridges activated factor IX and factor X to restore function of missing activated factor VIII, which is needed for haemostasis.

● INDICATIONS AND DOSE
Prophylaxis of haemorrhage in haemophilia A (initiated by a specialist)
▶ BY SUBCUTANEOUS INJECTION
▶ **Adult:** Initially 3 mg/kg once weekly for 4 weeks, then maintenance 1.5 mg/kg once weekly, alternatively maintenance 3 mg/kg every 2 weeks, alternatively maintenance 6 mg/kg every 4 weeks

● CAUTIONS Concomitant bypassing agent · risk factors for thrombotic microangiopathy

CAUTIONS, FURTHER INFORMATION
▶ Concomitant bypassing agent Manufacturer advises discontinue bypassing agents the day before starting emicizumab; if a bypassing agent is required—consult product literature.

● SIDE-EFFECTS
▶ **Common or very common** Arthralgia · diarrhoea · fever · headache · myalgia
▶ **Uncommon** Cavernous sinus thrombosis · embolism and thrombosis · skin necrosis · thrombotic microangiopathy

● CONCEPTION AND CONTRACEPTION Manufacturer advises effective contraception during and for 6 months after treatment in women of childbearing potential.

● PREGNANCY Manufacturer advises use only if potential benefit outweighs risk—no information available.

● BREAST FEEDING Manufacturer advises avoid—no information available.

● EFFECT ON LABORATORY TESTS Manufacturer advises to avoid intrinsic pathway clotting-based laboratory tests or use with caution as results may be misinterpreted—consult product literature.

● DIRECTIONS FOR ADMINISTRATION Manufacturer advises max. 2 mL per injection site; rotate injection site and avoid skin that is tender, damaged or scarred. Patients or their caregivers may self-administer *Hemlibra®* after appropriate training.

● PRESCRIBING AND DISPENSING INFORMATION Emicizumab is a biological medicine. Biological medicines must be prescribed and dispensed by brand name, see *Biological medicines* and *Biosimilar medicines*, under Guidance on prescribing p. 1; manufacturer advises to record the brand name and batch number after each administration.

● PATIENT AND CARER ADVICE
  Missed doses Manufacturer advises if a dose is missed, the missed dose may be taken up to a day before the next scheduled dose. The next dose should then be taken on the usual scheduled dosing day.

● MEDICINAL FORMS There can be variation in the licensing of different medicines containing the same drug.
  Solution for injection
▶ Hemlibra (Roche Products Ltd) ▼
  Emicizumab 30 mg per 1 ml Hemlibra 30mg/1ml solution for injection vials | 1 vial [PoM] £2,415.30
  Emicizumab 150 mg per 1 ml Hemlibra 150mg/1ml solution for injection vials | 1 vial [PoM] £12,076.50

Cardiovascular system

Hemlibra 105mg/0.7ml solution for injection vials | 1 vial PoM
£8,453.55

Hemlibra 60mg/0.4ml solution for injection vials | 1 vial PoM
£4,830.60

2.1 Coagulation factor deficiencies

BLOOD AND RELATED PRODUCTS >
COAGULATION PROTEINS

Dried prothrombin complex

20-Nov-2020

(Human prothrombin complex)

- ● INDICATIONS AND DOSE
Treatment and peri-operative prophylaxis of haemorrhage in patients with congenital deficiency of factors II, VII, IX, or X if purified specific coagulation factors not available | Treatment and peri-operative prophylaxis of haemorrhage in patients with acquired deficiency of factors II, VII, IX, or X (e.g. during warfarin treatment)
  - ▸ BY INTRAVENOUS INFUSION
  - ▸ Adult: (consult haematologist)

Major bleeding in patients on warfarin following phytomenadione (initiated under specialist supervision)
  - ▸ BY INTRAVENOUS INFUSION
  - ▸ Adult: 25–50 units/kg

- ● CONTRA-INDICATIONS History of heparin induced thrombocytopenia · myocardial infarction within the last 3 months (no information available) · unstable angina within the last 3 months (no information available)
- ● CAUTIONS Disseminated intravascular coagulation · history of myocardial infarction or coronary heart disease · postoperative use · risk of thrombosis · vaccination against hepatitis A and hepatitis B may be required
- ● SIDE-EFFECTS
  - ▸ Common or very common Embolism and thrombosis
  - ▸ Uncommon Anxiety · device thrombosis · haemorrhage · hepatic function abnormal · hypertension · respiratory disorders
  - ▸ Frequency not known Cardiac arrest · chills · circulatory collapse · disseminated intravascular coagulation · dyspnoea · heparin-induced thrombocytopenia · hypotension · nausea · skin reactions · tachycardia · tremor
- ● HEPATIC IMPAIRMENT Manufacturer advises caution (risk of thromboembolic complications).
  Monitoring Monitor closely in hepatic impairment (risk of thromboembolic complications).
- ● PRESCRIBING AND DISPENSING INFORMATION Dried prothrombin complex is prepared from human plasma by a suitable fractionation technique, and contains factor IX, together with variable amounts of factors II, VII, and X.
- ● MEDICINAL FORMS There can be variation in the licensing of different medicines containing the same drug.
  Powder and solvent for solution for injection
  - ▸ Beriplex P/N (CSL Behring UK Ltd)
    Factor VII 175 unit, Protein S 195 unit, Factor IX 255 unit, Protein C 300 unit, Factor II 340 unit, Factor X 410 unit Beriplex P/N 250 powder and solvent for solution for injection vials | 1 vial PoM £150.00
    Factor VII 350 unit, Protein S 390 unit, Factor IX 510 unit, Protein C 600 unit, Factor II 680 unit, Factor X 820 unit Beriplex P/N 500 powder and solvent for solution for injection vials | 1 vial PoM £300.00
    Factor VII 700 unit, Protein S 1000 unit, Factor IX 1020 unit, Protein C 1200 unit, Factor II 1360 unit, Factor X

1640 unit Beriplex P/N 1,000 powder and solvent for solution for injection vials | 1 vial PoM £600.00
- ▸ Prothromplex Total (Shire Pharmaceuticals Ltd)
  Factor VII 500 unit, Factor II 600 unit, Factor IX 600 unit, Factor X 600 unit Prothromplex Total 600 powder and solvent for solution for injection vials | 1 vial PoM £306.00

Powder and solvent for solution for infusion
- ▸ Octaplex (Octapharma Ltd)
  Octaplex 1,000unit powder and solvent for solution for infusion vials | 1 vial PoM £416.50 (Hospital only)
  Factor VII 330 unit, Protein C 380 unit, Protein S 390 unit, Factor X 480 unit, Factor II 490 unit, Factor IX 500 unit Octaplex 500unit powder and solvent for solution for infusion vials | 1 vial PoM £245.00

Factor VIIa (recombinant)

30-Jan-2020

(Eptacog alfa (activated))

- ● INDICATIONS AND DOSE
Treatment and prophylaxis of haemorrhage in patients with haemophilia A or B with inhibitors to factors VIII or IX, acquired haemophilia, factor VII deficiency, or Glanzmann's thrombasthenia
  - ▸ BY INTRAVENOUS INJECTION
  - ▸ Adult: (consult haematologist)

- ● CAUTIONS Disseminated intravascular coagulation · risk of thrombosis
- ● SIDE-EFFECTS
  - ▸ Uncommon Embolism and thrombosis · fever · hepatic disorders · intestinal ischaemia · skin reactions
  - ▸ Rare or very rare Angina pectoris · cerebrovascular insufficiency · coagulation disorders · headache · myocardial infarction · nausea · peripheral ischaemia
  - ▸ Frequency not known Angioedema · flushing

- ● MEDICINAL FORMS There can be variation in the licensing of different medicines containing the same drug.
  Powder and solvent for solution for injection
  - ▸ NovoSeven (Novo Nordisk Ltd)
    Eptacog alfa activated 50000 unit NovoSeven 1mg (50,000units) powder and solvent for solution for injection pre-filled syringes | 1 pre-filled disposable injection PoM £525.20 (Hospital only) NovoSeven 1mg (50,000units) powder and solvent for solution for injection vials | 1 vial PoM £525.20 (Hospital only)
    Eptacog alfa activated 100000 unit NovoSeven 2mg (100,000units) powder and solvent for solution for injection vials | 1 vial PoM £1,050.40 (Hospital only)
    NovoSeven 2mg (100,000units) powder and solvent for solution for injection pre-filled syringes | 1 pre-filled disposable injection PoM £1,050.40 (Hospital only)
    Eptacog alfa activated 250000 unit NovoSeven 5mg (250,000units) powder and solvent for solution for injection pre-filled syringes | 1 pre-filled disposable injection PoM £2,626.00 (Hospital only)
    NovoSeven 5mg (250,000units) powder and solvent for solution for injection vials | 1 vial PoM £2,626.00 (Hospital only)
    Eptacog alfa activated 400000 unit NovoSeven 8mg (400,000units) powder and solvent for solution for injection vials | 1 vial PoM £4,201.60 (Hospital only)
    NovoSeven 8mg (400,000units) powder and solvent for solution for injection pre-filled syringes | 1 pre-filled disposable injection PoM £4,201.60 (Hospital only)

Factor VIII fraction, dried

05-Feb-2020

(Human coagulation factor VIII, dried)

- ● INDICATIONS AND DOSE
Treatment and prophylaxis of haemorrhage in congenital factor VIII deficiency (haemophilia A), acquired factor VIII deficiency | Von Willebrand's disease
  - ▸ BY INTRAVENOUS INJECTION, OR BY INTRAVENOUS INFUSION, OR BY CONTINUOUS INTRAVENOUS INFUSION
  - ▸ Adult: (consult haematologist)

- CAUTIONS Risk of intravascular haemolysis after large or frequently repeated doses in patients with blood groups A, B, or AB (in products containing isoagglutinins) · vaccination against hepatitis A and hepatitis B may be required (consult product literature)
- SIDE-EFFECTS
- ▸ Rare or very rare Fever
- ▸ Frequency not known Hypersensitivity
- MONITORING REQUIREMENTS Monitor for development of factor VIII inhibitors.
- PRESCRIBING AND DISPENSING INFORMATION Dried factor VIII fraction is prepared from human plasma by a suitable fractionation technique; it may also contain varying amounts of von Willebrand factor. *Optivate*®, *Fanhdi*®, and *Octanate*® are not indicated for use in von Willebrand's disease.
  Recombinant human coagulation factor VIII including octocog alfa, moroctocog alfa, and simoctocog alfa are not indicated for use in von Willebrand's disease.

- MEDICINAL FORMS There can be variation in the licensing of different medicines containing the same drug.

Powder and solvent for solution for injection
▸ Factor viii fraction, dried (Non-proprietary)
   Factor VIII 500 unit Dried Factor VIII Fraction type 8Y 500unit powder and solvent for solution for injection vials | 1 vial [PoM] £210.00

   Factor VIII high purity 2000 unit, von Willebrand factor 2400 unit Alphanate 2,000unit powder and solvent for solution for injection vials | 1 vial [PoM] £780.00
   Efmoroctocog alfa 4000 unit Elocta 4,000unit powder and solvent for solution for injection vials | 1 vial [PoM] [℟] (Hospital only)
▸ Advate (Shire Pharmaceuticals Ltd)
   Octocog alfa 250 unit Advate 250unit powder and 2ml solvent for solution for injection vials | 1 vial [PoM] £177.50
   Advate 250unit powder and 5ml solvent for solution for injection vials | 1 vial [PoM] £177.50
   Octocog alfa 500 unit Advate 500unit powder and 5ml solvent for solution for injection vials | 1 vial [PoM] £355.00
   Advate 500unit powder and 2ml solvent for solution for injection vials | 1 vial [PoM] £355.00
   Octocog alfa 1000 unit Advate 1,000unit powder and solvent for solution for injection vials | 1 vial [PoM] £710.00
   Octocog alfa 2000 unit Advate 2,000unit powder and solvent for solution for injection vials | 1 vial [PoM] £1,420.00
▸ Alphanate (Grifols UK Ltd)
   Factor VIII high purity 1000 unit, von Willebrand factor 1200 unit Alphanate 1,000unit powder and solvent for solution for injection vials | 1 vial [PoM] £390.00
   Factor VIII high purity 1500 unit, von Willebrand factor 1800 unit Alphanate 1,500unit powder and solvent for solution for injection vials | 1 vial [PoM] £585.00
▸ Elocta (Swedish Orphan Biovitrum Ltd)
   Efmoroctocog alfa 250 unit Elocta 250unit powder and solvent for solution for injection vials | 1 vial [PoM] [℟] (Hospital only)
   Efmoroctocog alfa 500 unit Elocta 500unit powder and solvent for solution for injection vials | 1 vial [PoM] [℟] (Hospital only)
   Efmoroctocog alfa 750 unit Elocta 750unit powder and solvent for solution for injection vials | 1 vial [PoM] [℟] (Hospital only)
   Efmoroctocog alfa 1000 unit Elocta 1,000unit powder and solvent for solution for injection vials | 1 vial [PoM] [℟] (Hospital only)
   Efmoroctocog alfa 1500 unit Elocta 1,500unit powder and solvent for solution for injection vials | 1 vial [PoM] [℟] (Hospital only)
   Efmoroctocog alfa 2000 unit Elocta 2,000unit powder and solvent for solution for injection vials | 1 vial [PoM] [℟] (Hospital only)
   Efmoroctocog alfa 3000 unit Elocta 3,000unit powder and solvent for solution for injection vials | 1 vial [PoM] [℟] (Hospital only)
▸ Fanhdi (Grifols UK Ltd)
   Factor VIII high purity 500 unit Fanhdi 500unit powder and solvent for solution for injection vials | 1 vial [PoM] £165.00 (Hospital only)
   Factor VIII high purity 1000 unit Fanhdi 1,000unit powder and solvent for solution for injection vials | 1 vial [PoM] £330.00 (Hospital only)
   Factor VIII high purity 1500 unit Fanhdi 1,500unit powder and solvent for solution for injection vials | 1 vial [PoM] £495.00

▸ Haemoctin (Biotest (UK) Ltd)
   Factor VIII high purity 250 unit Haemoctin 250unit powder and solvent for solution for injection vials | 1 vial [PoM] £150.00 (Hospital only)
   Factor VIII high purity 500 unit Haemoctin 500unit powder and solvent for solution for injection vials | 1 vial [PoM] £300.00 (Hospital only)
   Factor VIII high purity 1000 unit Haemoctin 1,000unit powder and solvent for solution for injection vials | 1 vial [PoM] £600.00 (Hospital only)
▸ Nuwiq (Octapharma Ltd)
   Simoctocog alfa 250 unit Nuwiq 250unit powder and solvent for solution for injection vials | 1 vial [PoM] £190.00
   Simoctocog alfa 500 unit Nuwiq 500unit powder and solvent for solution for injection vials | 1 vial [PoM] £380.00
   Simoctocog alfa 1000 unit Nuwiq 1,000unit powder and solvent for solution for injection vials | 1 vial [PoM] £760.00
   Simoctocog alfa 2000 unit Nuwiq 2,000unit powder and solvent for solution for injection vials | 1 vial [PoM] £1,520.00
▸ Octanate LV (Octapharma Ltd)
   Factor VIII high purity 500 unit Octanate LV 500unit powder and solvent for solution for injection vials | 1 vial [PoM] £300.00 (Hospital only)
   Factor VIII high purity 1000 unit Octanate LV 1,000unit powder and solvent for solution for injection vials | 1 vial [PoM] £600.00 (Hospital only)
▸ ReFacto (Pfizer Ltd)
   Moroctocog alfa 250 unit ReFacto AF 250unit powder and solvent for solution for injection vials | 1 vial [PoM] £125.55 (Hospital only)
   ReFacto AF 500unit powder and solvent for solution for injection pre-filled syringes | 1 pre-filled disposable injection [PoM] £251.10 (Hospital only)
   ReFacto AF 250unit powder and solvent for solution for injection pre-filled syringes | 1 pre-filled disposable injection [PoM] £125.55 (Hospital only)
   Moroctocog alfa 500 unit ReFacto AF 500unit powder and solvent for solution for injection vials | 1 vial [PoM] £251.10 (Hospital only)
   Moroctocog alfa 1000 unit ReFacto AF 1,000unit powder and solvent for solution for injection vials | 1 vial [PoM] £502.20 (Hospital only)
   ReFacto AF 1,000unit powder and solvent for solution for injection pre-filled syringes | 1 pre-filled disposable injection [PoM] £502.20 (Hospital only)
   Moroctocog alfa 2000 unit ReFacto AF 2,000unit powder and solvent for solution for injection pre-filled syringes | 1 pre-filled disposable injection [PoM] £1,004.40 (Hospital only)
   ReFacto AF 2,000unit powder and solvent for solution for injection vials | 1 vial [PoM] £1,004.40 (Hospital only)
   Moroctocog alfa 3000 unit ReFacto AF 3,000unit powder and solvent for solution for injection pre-filled syringes | 1 pre-filled disposable injection [PoM] £1,506.60 (Hospital only)
▸ Voncento (CSL Behring UK Ltd)
   Factor VIII 500 unit, von Willebrand factor 1200 unit Voncento 500unit/1,200unit powder and solvent for solution for injection vials | 1 vial [PoM] £385.00
   Factor VIII 1000 unit, von Willebrand factor 2400 unit Voncento 1,000unit/2,400unit powder and solvent for solution for injection vials | 1 vial [PoM] £770.00

Powder and solvent for solution for infusion
▸ Advate (Shire Pharmaceuticals Ltd)
   Octocog alfa 1500 unit Advate 1,500unit powder and solvent for solution for infusion vials | 1 vial [PoM] £1,065.00
   Octocog alfa 3000 unit Advate 3,000unit powder and solvent for solution for infusion vials | 1 vial [PoM] £2,130.00
▸ Optivate (Bio Products Laboratory Ltd)
   Factor VIII 250 unit, von Willebrand factor 430 unit Optivate 250unit powder and solvent for solution for infusion vials | 1 vial [PoM] £90.00
▸ Wilate 1000 (Octapharma Ltd)
   Factor VIII 1000 iu, von Willebrand factor 1000 iu Wilate 1000 powder and solvent for solution for infusion vials | 1 vial [PoM] £500.00
▸ Wilate 500 (Octapharma Ltd)
   Factor VIII 500 iu, von Willebrand factor 500 iu Wilate 500 powder and solvent for solution for infusion vials | 1 vial [PoM] £250.00

2

Cardiovascular system

Factor IX fraction, dried
30-Jan-2020

● **INDICATIONS AND DOSE**

Treatment and prophylaxis of haemorrhage in congenital factor IX deficiency (haemophilia B)

▸ BY INTRAVENOUS INJECTION, OR BY CONTINUOUS INTRAVENOUS INFUSION

▸ Adult: (consult haematologist)

● CONTRA-INDICATIONS Disseminated intravascular coagulation

● CAUTIONS Risk of thrombosis—principally with low purity products · vaccination against hepatitis A and hepatitis B may be required (consult product literature)

● SIDE-EFFECTS

▸ **Common or very common** Anxiety · back pain · dyspnoea · hypersensitivity · nausea · sensation abnormal · skin reactions · vasodilation

▸ **Rare or very rare** Angioedema · cardiac discomfort · chills · disseminated intravascular coagulation · embolism and thrombosis · headache · hypotension · lethargy · myocardial infarction · tachycardia · vomiting · wheezing

▸ **Frequency not known** Nephrotic syndrome

● PRESCRIBING AND DISPENSING INFORMATION Dried factor IX fraction is prepared from human plasma by a suitable fractionation technique; it may also contain clotting factors II, VII, and X.

● MEDICINAL FORMS There can be variation in the licensing of different medicines containing the same drug.

Powder and solvent for solution for injection

▸ Haemonine (Biotest (UK) Ltd)

Factor IX high purity 500 unit Haemonine 500unit powder and solvent for solution for injection vials | 1 vial PoM £300.00 (Hospital only)

Factor IX high purity 1000 unit Haemonine 1,000unit powder and solvent for solution for injection vials | 1 vial PoM £600.00 (Hospital only)

▸ Replenine-VF (Bio Products Laboratory Ltd)

Factor IX high purity 500 unit Replenine-VF 500unit powder and solvent for solution for injection vials | 1 vial PoM £180.00 (Hospital only)

Factor IX high purity 1000 unit Replenine-VF 1,000unit powder and solvent for solution for injection vials | 1 vial PoM £360.00 (Hospital only)

Powder and solvent for solution for infusion

▸ BeneFIX (Pfizer Ltd)

Nonacog alfa 250 unit BeneFIX 250unit powder and solvent for solution for infusion vials | 1 vial PoM £151.80 (Hospital only)

Nonacog alfa 500 unit BeneFIX 500unit powder and solvent for solution for infusion vials | 1 vial PoM £303.60 (Hospital only)

Nonacog alfa 1000 unit BeneFIX 1,000unit powder and solvent for solution for infusion vials | 1 vial PoM £607.20 (Hospital only)

Nonacog alfa 2000 unit BeneFIX 2,000unit powder and solvent for solution for infusion vials | 1 vial PoM £1,214.40 (Hospital only)

Nonacog alfa 3000 unit BeneFIX 3,000unit powder and solvent for solution for infusion vials | 1 vial PoM £1,821.60 (Hospital only)

Factor XIII fraction, dried
30-Jan-2020

(Human fibrin-stabilising factor, dried)

● **INDICATIONS AND DOSE**

Congenital factor XIII deficiency

▸ BY INTRAVENOUS INJECTION, OR BY INTRAVENOUS INFUSION

▸ Adult: (consult haematologist)

● CAUTIONS Vaccination against hepatitis A and hepatitis B may be required

● SIDE-EFFECTS

▸ **Rare or very rare** Anaphylactoid reaction · dyspnoea · skin reactions

● MEDICINAL FORMS There can be variation in the licensing of different medicines containing the same drug.

Powder and solvent for solution for injection

▸ Fibrogammin P (CSL Behring UK Ltd)

Factor XIII 250 unit Fibrogammin 250unit powder and solvent for solution for injection vials | 1 vial PoM £106.58

Factor XIII 1250 unit Fibrogammin 1,250unit powder and solvent for solution for injection vials | 1 vial PoM £532.90

Fibrinogen, dried
30-Jan-2020

(Human fibrinogen)

● **INDICATIONS AND DOSE**

Treatment of haemorrhage in congenital hypofibrinogenaemia or afibrinogenaemia

▸ BY INTRAVENOUS INJECTION, OR BY INTRAVENOUS INFUSION

▸ Adult: (consult haematologist)

● CAUTIONS Risk of thrombosis · vaccination against hepatitis A and hepatitis B may be required

● SIDE-EFFECTS

▸ **Common or very common** Fever · thromboembolism

▸ **Frequency not known** Chest pain · chills · cough · dyspnoea · nausea · skin reactions · tachycardia · vomiting

● PREGNANCY Manufacturer advises not known to be harmful—no information available.

● BREAST FEEDING Manufacturer advises avoid—no information available.

● PRESCRIBING AND DISPENSING INFORMATION Fibrinogen is prepared from human plasma.

● MEDICINAL FORMS There can be variation in the licensing of different medicines containing the same drug.

Powder for solution for infusion

▸ Riastap (CSL Behring UK Ltd)

Human fibrinogen 1 gram Riastap 1g powder for solution for infusion vials | 1 vial PoM £400.00

Protein C concentrate
30-Jan-2020

● **INDICATIONS AND DOSE**

Congenital protein C deficiency

▸ BY INTRAVENOUS INJECTION

▸ Adult: (consult haematologist)

● CAUTIONS Hypersensitivity to heparins · vaccination against hepatitis A and hepatitis B may be required

● SIDE-EFFECTS

▸ **Rare or very rare** Dizziness · fever · skin reactions

▸ **Frequency not known** Haemothorax · hyperhidrosis · restlessness

● PRESCRIBING AND DISPENSING INFORMATION Protein C is prepared from human plasma.

● MEDICINAL FORMS There can be variation in the licensing of different medicines containing the same drug.

Powder and solvent for solution for injection

▸ Ceprotin (Shire Pharmaceuticals Ltd)

Protein C 500 unit Ceprotin 500unit powder and solvent for solution for injection vials | 1 vial PoM £2,000.00

Protein C 1000 unit Ceprotin 1000unit powder and solvent for solution for injection vials | 1 vial PoM £1,000.00

BLOOD AND RELATED PRODUCTS 〉
HAEMOSTATIC PRODUCTS

Factor VIII inhibitor bypassing fraction
30-Jan-2020

- **INDICATIONS AND DOSE**
  Treatment and prophylaxis of haemorrhage in patients with congenital factor VIII deficiency (haemophilia A) and factor VIII inhibitors | Treatment of haemorrhage in non-haemophiliac patients with acquired factor VIII inhibitors
  ▶ BY INTRAVENOUS INFUSION, OR BY INTRAVENOUS INJECTION
  ▶ Adult: (consult haematologist)

- **CONTRA-INDICATIONS** Disseminated intravascular coagulation

- **CAUTIONS** Risk of thrombosis · vaccination against hepatitis A and hepatitis B may be required

- **SIDE-EFFECTS**
  ▶ **Common or very common** Dizziness · headache · hypersensitivity · hypotension · skin reactions
  ▶ **Frequency not known** Abdominal discomfort · anamnestic reaction · angioedema · chest discomfort · chills · cough · diarrhoea · disseminated intravascular coagulation · drowsiness · dyspnoea · embolism and thrombosis · fever · flushing · hypertension · ischaemic stroke · malaise · myocardial infarction · nausea · paraesthesia · respiratory disorders · restlessness · tachycardia · taste altered · vomiting

- **PRESCRIBING AND DISPENSING INFORMATION** Preparations with factor VIII inhibitor bypassing activity are prepared from human plasma.

- **MEDICINAL FORMS** There can be variation in the licensing of different medicines containing the same drug.
  Powder and solvent for solution for injection
  ▶ FEIBA Imuno (Shire Pharmaceuticals Ltd)
  Factor VIII inhibitor bypassing fraction 500 unit FEIBA 500unit powder and solvent for solution for injection vials | 1 vial [PoM] £390.00
  Powder and solvent for solution for infusion
  ▶ FEIBA Imuno (Shire Pharmaceuticals Ltd)
  Factor VIII inhibitor bypassing fraction 1000 unit FEIBA 1,000unit powder and solvent for solution for infusion vials | 1 vial [PoM] £780.00

BLOOD AND RELATED PRODUCTS 〉 PLASMA PRODUCTS

Fresh frozen plasma
30-Jan-2020

- **INDICATIONS AND DOSE**
  Replacement of coagulation factors or other plasma proteins where their concentration or functional activity is critically reduced
  ▶ BY INTRAVENOUS INFUSION
  ▶ Adult: (consult haematologist)
  Major bleeding in patients on warfarin following phytomenadione (if dried prothrombin complex is unavailable)
  ▶ Adult: 15 mL/kilogram

- **CONTRA-INDICATIONS** Avoid use as a volume expander · IgA deficiency with confirmed antibodies to IgA

- **CAUTIONS** Cardiac decompensation · pulmonary oedema · risk of thrombosis · severe protein S deficiency (avoid products with low protein S activity e.g. *OctaplasLG*®) · vaccination against hepatitis A and hepatitis B may be required

- **SIDE-EFFECTS**
  ▶ **Common or very common** Skin reactions
  ▶ **Uncommon** Fever · hypersensitivity · hypoxia · nausea · sensation abnormal · vomiting
  ▶ **Rare or very rare** Abdominal pain · anxiety · arrhythmias · back pain · cardiac arrest · chest discomfort · chills · circulatory collapse · citrate toxicity · dizziness · dyspnoea · flushing · haemolytic anaemia · haemorrhage · hyperhidrosis · hypertension · hypotension · localised oedema · malaise · procedural complications · pulmonary oedema · respiratory disorders · thromboembolism

- **PRESCRIBING AND DISPENSING INFORMATION** Fresh frozen plasma is prepared from the supernatant liquid obtained by centrifugation of one donation of whole blood.
  A preparation of solvent/detergent treated human plasma (frozen) from pooled donors is available from Octapharma (*OctaplasLG*®).

- **MEDICINAL FORMS** There can be variation in the licensing of different medicines containing the same drug.
  Infusion
  ▶ OctaplasLG (Octapharma Ltd)
  Human plasma proteins 57.5 mg per 1 ml OctaplasLG Blood Group A infusion 200ml bags | 1 bag [PoM] £75.00
  OctaplasLG Blood Group B infusion 200ml bags | 1 bag [PoM] £75.00
  OctaplasLG Blood Group AB infusion 200ml bags | 1 bag [PoM] £75.00
  OctaplasLG Blood Group O infusion 200ml bags | 1 bag [PoM] £75.00

2.2 Subarachnoid haemorrhage

CALCIUM-CHANNEL BLOCKERS
Ⓕ 170

Nimodipine
14-Feb-2020

- **DRUG ACTION** Nimodipine is a dihydropyridine calcium-channel blocker.

- **INDICATIONS AND DOSE**
  Prevention of ischaemic neurological defects following aneurysmal subarachnoid haemorrhage
  ▶ BY MOUTH
  ▶ Adult: 60 mg every 4 hours, to be started within 4 days of aneurysmal subarachnoid haemorrhage and continued for 21 days
  Treatment of ischaemic neurological defects following aneurysmal subarachnoid haemorrhage
  ▶ BY INTRAVENOUS INFUSION
  ▶ Adult (body-weight up to 70 kg): Initially up to 0.5 mg/hour, increased after 2 hours if no severe fall in blood pressure; increased to 2 mg/hour and continue for at least 5 days (max. 14 days); if surgical intervention during treatment, continue for at least 5 days after surgery; max. total duration of nimodipine use 21 days, to be given via central catheter
  ▶ Adult (body-weight 70 kg and above): Initially 1 mg/hour, increased after 2 hours if no severe fall in blood pressure; increased to 2 mg/hour and continue for at least 5 days (max. 14 days); if surgical intervention during treatment, continue for at least 5 days after surgery; max. total duration of nimodipine use 21 days, to be given via central catheter
  Treatment of ischaemic neurological defects following aneurysmal subarachnoid haemorrhage in patients with unstable blood pressure
  ▶ BY INTRAVENOUS INFUSION
  ▶ Adult: Initially up to 0.5 mg/hour, increased after 2 hours if no severe fall in blood pressure; increased to 2 mg/hour and continue for at least 5 days (max. 14 days); if surgical intervention during treatment, continue for at least 5 days after surgery; continued →

2

Cardiovascular system

max. total duration of nimodipine use 21 days, to be given via central catheter

---

IMPORTANT SAFETY INFORMATION
SAFE PRACTICE
Nimodipine has been confused with amlodipine; care must be taken to ensure the correct drug is prescribed and dispensed.

- CONTRA-INDICATIONS Unstable angina · within 1 month of myocardial infarction
- CAUTIONS Cerebral oedema · hypotension · severely raised intracranial pressure
- INTERACTIONS → Appendix 1: calcium channel blockers
- SIDE-EFFECTS
  - **Uncommon** Thrombocytopenia · vasodilation
  - **Rare or very rare** Bradycardia · ileus
- PREGNANCY Manufacturer advises use only if potential benefit outweighs risk.
- BREAST FEEDING Manufacturer advises avoid—present in milk.
- HEPATIC IMPAIRMENT
  - With oral use Manufacturer advises consider avoiding in severe impairment.
  Dose adjustments ▸ With oral use Manufacturer advises dose reduction, if used in severe impairment.
- RENAL IMPAIRMENT
  Monitoring ▸ With intravenous use Manufacturer advises monitor renal function closely in renal impairment.
- DIRECTIONS FOR ADMINISTRATION Avoid concomitant administration of nimodipine infusion and tablets.
  ▸ With oral use For administration *by mouth*, tablets may be crushed or halved but are light sensitive—administer immediately.
  ▸ With intravenous use For *intravenous infusion*, give via drip tubing in Glucose 5% or Sodium chloride 0.9%. Not to be added to infusion container; administer via an infusion pump through a Y-piece into a central catheter; incompatible with polyvinyl chloride giving sets or containers; protect infusion from light.
  ▸ With intravenous use Polyethylene, polypropylene, or glass apparatus should be used.

- MEDICINAL FORMS There can be variation in the licensing of different medicines containing the same drug. Forms available from special-order manufacturers include: oral suspension
  Solution for infusion
  ▸ Nimotop (Bayer Plc)
  Nimodipine 200 microgram per 1 ml Nimotop 0.02% solution for infusion 50ml vials | 1 vial [PoM] £13.60 (Hospital only)
  Tablet
  ▸ Nimotop (Bayer Plc)
  Nimodipine 30 mg Nimotop 30mg tablets | 100 tablet [PoM] £40.00 DT = £40.00

---

3   Blood clots

3.1   Blocked catheters and lines

Other drugs used for Blocked catheters and lines Heparin (unfractionated), p. 145 · Urokinase, p. 150

PROSTAGLANDINS AND ANALOGUES

Epoprostenol

28-Jul-2020

(Prostacyclin)

- DRUG ACTION Epoprostenol is a prostaglandin and a potent vasodilator. It is also a powerful inhibitor of platelet aggregation.

- **INDICATIONS AND DOSE**
  Inhibition of platelet aggregation during renal dialysis when heparins are unsuitable or contra-indicated | Treatment of primary pulmonary hypertension resistant to other treatments, usually with oral anti-coagulation (initiated by a specialist)
  ▸ BY CONTINUOUS INTRAVENOUS INFUSION
  ▸ Adult: (consult product literature)
  PHARMACOKINETICS
  ▸ Short half-life of approximately 3 minutes, therefore it must be administered by continuous intravenous infusion.

- CONTRA-INDICATIONS Severe left ventricular dysfunction
- CAUTIONS Avoid abrupt withdrawal when used for primary pulmonary hypertension (risk of rebound pulmonary hypertension) · extreme caution in coronary artery disease · haemorrhagic diathesis · pulmonary veno-occlusive disease · reconstituted solution highly alkaline—avoid extravasation (irritant to tissues) · risk of pulmonary oedema (dose titration for pulmonary hypertension should be in hospital)
- INTERACTIONS → Appendix 1: epoprostenol
- SIDE-EFFECTS
  ▸ **Common or very common** Abdominal pain · anxiety · arrhythmias · arthralgia · chest discomfort · diarrhoea · flushing · haemorrhage · headache · intracranial haemorrhage · nausea · pain · rash · sepsis · vomiting
  ▸ **Uncommon** Dry mouth · hyperhidrosis
  ▸ **Rare or very rare** Fatigue · hyperthyroidism · intravenous catheter occlusion · local infection · pallor
  ▸ **Frequency not known** Ascites · pulmonary oedema (avoid chronic use if occurs during dose titration) · spleen abnormalities
- PREGNANCY Use if potential benefit outweighs risk.
- BREAST FEEDING Manufacturer advises avoid—no information available.
- MONITORING REQUIREMENTS Anticoagulant monitoring required when given with anticoagulants.
- TREATMENT CESSATION Avoid abrupt withdrawal when used for primary pulmonary hypertension (risk of rebound pulmonary hypertension).
- DIRECTIONS FOR ADMINISTRATION Directions for administration vary depending on the preparation used— consult product literature.

- MEDICINAL FORMS There can be variation in the licensing of different medicines containing the same drug.
  Powder for solution for infusion
  ▸ Epoprostenol (Non-proprietary)
  Epoprostenol (as Epoprostenol sodium)
  500 microgram Epoprostenol 500microgram powder (pH12) for solution for infusion vials | 1 vial [PoM] ⓢ (Hospital only)
  Epoprostenol (as Epoprostenol sodium) 1.5 mg Epoprostenol 1.5mg powder (pH12) for solution for infusion vials | 1 vial [PoM] ⓢ (Hospital only)
  ▸ Veletri (Janssen-Cilag Ltd)
  Epoprostenol (as Epoprostenol sodium) 500 microgram Veletri 500microgram powder for solution for infusion vials | 1 vial [PoM] £24.44
  Epoprostenol (as Epoprostenol sodium) 1.5 mg Veletri 1.5mg powder for solution for infusion vials | 1 vial [PoM] £49.24

Powder and solvent for solution for infusion
ELECTROLYTES: May contain Sodium
▸ Epoprostenol (Non-proprietary)

Epoprostenol (as Epoprostenol sodium)
500 microgram Epoprostenol 500microgram powder and solvent
(pH10.5) for solution for infusion vials | 1 vial [PoM] £58.95
Epoprostenol (as Epoprostenol sodium) 1.5 mg Epoprostenol
1.5mg powder and solvent (pH10.5) for solution for infusion vials |
1 vial [PoM] £118.75
▸ Flolan (GlaxoSmithKline UK Ltd)

Epoprostenol (as Epoprostenol sodium) 500 microgram Flolan
500microgram powder and solvent (pH12) for solution for infusion
vials | 1 vial [PoM] £22.22
Epoprostenol (as Epoprostenol sodium) 1.5 mg Flolan 1.5mg
powder and solvent (pH12) for solution for infusion vials | 1 vial [PoM]
£44.76

3.2 Thromboembolism

Venous thromboembolism   14-Dec-2020

Description of condition
Venous thromboembolism (VTE) includes both deep-vein
thrombosis (DVT) and pulmonary embolism (PE), and refers
to a blood clot that forms in a vein which partially or
completely obstructs blood flow. Hospital-acquired venous
thromboembolism refers to a VTE that occurs within 90 days
of hospital admission. It is a common and potentially
preventable problem.

Risk factors for VTE include surgery, trauma, significant
immobility, malignancy, obesity, acquired or inherited
hypercoagulable states, pregnancy and the postpartum
period, and hormonal therapy (combined hormonal
contraception or hormone replacement therapy).

A DVT, the most common form of VTE, usually occurs in
the deep veins of the legs or pelvis but may affect other sites
such as the upper limbs, and the intracranial and splanchnic
veins. Symptoms of a DVT include unilateral localised pain,
swelling, tenderness, skin changes, and/or vein distension.

A PE most commonly occurs when a thrombus, usually
from a DVT, travels in the blood (embolus) and obstructs
blood flow to the lungs causing respiratory dysfunction.
Symptoms of a PE include chest pain, shortness of breath,
and/or haemoptysis.

Venous thromboembolism prophylaxis
For recommendations on reducing the risk of venous
thromboembolism in individuals with COVID-19
pneumonia, see the National Institute of Health and Care
Excellence (NICE) rapid guideline: **Reducing the risk of
venous thromboembolism in over 16s with COVID-19**
(available at: www.nice.org.uk/guidance/ng186). The Scottish
Intercollegiate Guidelines Network have issued a position
statement for the **Prevention and management of
thromboembolism in hospitalised patients with COVID-
19-related disease**, available at: www.sign.ac.uk/media/1691/
sg_prevention_of_thromboembolism_in_hospitalised_patients.pdf.
For further information on COVID-19, see COVID-19 p. 660.

[EvGr] All patients should undergo a risk assessment to
identify their risk of venous thromboembolism (VTE) and
bleeding on admission to hospital. ⒶCommonly used risk
assessment tools can be found at www.nice.org.uk/guidance/
ng89/resources.

There are two methods of thromboprophylaxis:
mechanical and pharmacological. Options for mechanical
prophylaxis are anti-embolism stockings that provide
graduated compression and produce a calf pressure of
14–15 mmHg, and intermittent pneumatic compression.
[EvGr] Anti-embolism stockings should be worn day and night
until the patient is sufficiently mobile; they should not be
offered to patients admitted with acute stroke or those with

conditions such as peripheral arterial disease, peripheral
neuropathy, severe leg oedema, or local conditions (e.g.
gangrene, dermatitis).

When using pharmacological prophylaxis, in most cases, it
should start as soon as possible or within 14 hours of
admission. Patients with risk factors for bleeding (e.g. acute
stroke, thrombocytopenia, acquired or untreated inherited
bleeding disorders) should only receive pharmacological
prophylaxis when their risk of VTE outweighs their risk of
bleeding. Patients receiving anticoagulant treatment who
are at high risk of VTE should be considered for prophylaxis
if their anticoagulant treatment is interrupted, for example
during the peri-operative period. ⒶFor full guidance on the prophylaxis of VTE, see NICE
guideline: **Venous thromboembolism in over 16s** (see
Useful resources).

Surgical patients
[EvGr] To reduce the risk of VTE in surgical patients, regional
anaesthesia over general anaesthesia should be used if
possible.

Mechanical prophylaxis (e.g. anti-embolism stockings or
intermittent pneumatic compression) should be offered to
patients with major trauma, or undergoing cranial,
abdominal, bariatric, thoracic, maxillofacial, ear, nose, and
throat, cardiac or elective spinal surgery. Prophylaxis should
continue until the patient is sufficiently mobile or
discharged from hospital (or for 30 days in spinal injury,
elective spinal surgery or cranial surgery). ⒶChoice of
mechanical prophylaxis depends on factors such as the type
of surgery, suitability for the patient, and their condition.

[EvGr] Pharmacological prophylaxis should be considered in
patients undergoing general or orthopaedic surgery when
the risk of VTE outweighs the risk of bleeding. ⒶThe
choice of prophylaxis will depend on the type of surgery,
suitability for the patient, and local policy. [EvGr] A low
molecular weight heparin is suitable in all types of general
and orthopaedic surgery; heparin (unfractionated) p. 145 is
preferred in patients with renal impairment. Fondaparinux
sodium p. 138 is an option for patients undergoing
abdominal, bariatric, thoracic or cardiac surgery, or for
patients with lower limb immobilisation or fragility fractures
of the pelvis, hip or proximal femur.

Pharmacological prophylaxis in general surgery should
usually continue for at least 7 days post-surgery, or until
sufficient mobility has been re-established. Pharmacological
prophylaxis should be extended to 28 days after major cancer
surgery in the abdomen, and to 30 days in spinal surgery.

Mechanical prophylaxis with intermittent pneumatic
compression should be considered when pharmacological
prophylaxis is contra-indicated in patients undergoing lower
limb amputation, or those with major trauma or fragility
fractures of the pelvis, hip or proximal femur.

Patients undergoing an *elective hip replacement* should be
given thromboprophylaxis with either a low molecular
weight heparin administered for 10 days followed by low-
dose aspirin p. 132 for a further 28 days, or a low molecular
weight heparin administered for 28 days in combination with
anti-embolism stockings until discharge, or rivaroxaban
p. 139. If these options are unsuitable, apixaban p. 136 or
dabigatran etexilate p. 148 can be considered as alternatives.
If pharmacological prophylaxis is contra-indicated, anti-
embolism stockings can be used until discharge.

Patients undergoing an *elective knee replacement* should be
given thromboprophylaxis with either low-dose aspirin
p. 132 for 14 days, or a low molecular weight heparin
administered for 14 days in combination with anti-embolism
stockings until discharge, or rivaroxaban. If these options are
unsuitable, apixaban or dabigatran etexilate can be
considered as alternatives. If pharmacological prophylaxis is
contra-indicated, intermittent pneumatic compression can
be used until the patient is mobile. Ⓐ

Medical patients
The choice of prophylaxis will depend on the medical condition, suitability for the patient, and local policy. [EvGr] Acutely ill medical patients who are at high risk of VTE should be offered pharmacological prophylaxis. Patients should be given either a low molecular weight heparin as a first-line option, or fondaparinux sodium as an alternative, for a minimum of 7 days. Patients with renal impairment should be given either a low molecular weight heparin or heparin (unfractionated) and the dose should be adjusted as necessary.

Mechanical prophylaxis can be considered when pharmacological prophylaxis is contra-indicated; their use should be continued until the patient is sufficiently mobile. In patients admitted with acute stroke, mechanical prophylaxis with intermittent pneumatic compression should be considered, as anti-embolism stockings are unsuitable in these patients; their use should be started within 3 days of the acute stroke and continued for 30 days, or until the patient is sufficiently mobile or discharged from hospital. Ⓐ

Thromboprophylaxis in pregnancy
[EvGr] All pregnant women (who are not in active labour), or women who have given birth, had a miscarriage or termination of pregnancy during the past 6 weeks, with a risk of VTE that outweighs the risk of bleeding should be considered for pharmacological prophylaxis with a low molecular weight heparin during hospital admission. In pregnant women, prophylaxis should be continued until there is no longer a risk of VTE, or until discharge from hospital. Women who have given birth, had a miscarriage or termination of pregnancy during the past 6 weeks, should start thromboprophylaxis with a low molecular weight heparin 4–8 hours after the event, unless contra-indicated, and continue for a minimum of 7 days.

Additional mechanical prophylaxis should be considered for women who are likely to be immobilised or have significantly reduced mobility and continued until the woman is sufficiently mobile or discharged from hospital. Intermittent pneumatic compression should be used as the first-line option and anti-embolism stockings as an alternative. Ⓐ

Venous thromboembolism treatment

The Scottish Intercollegiate Guidelines Network have issued a position statement for the **Prevention and management of thromboembolism in hospitalised patients with COVID-19-related disease**, available at: www.sign.ac.uk/media/1691/sg_prevention_of_thromboembolism_in_hospitalised_patients.pdf. For further information on COVID-19, see COVID-19 p. 660.

For full guidance on assessment and diagnostic investigations for a deep-vein thrombosis (DVT) or a pulmonary embolism (PE), see NICE guideline: **Venous thromboembolic diseases** (see *Useful resources*).

[EvGr] Immediately refer patients for hospital admission if they have a suspected PE and signs of haemodynamic instability (including pallor, tachycardia, hypotension, shock, and collapse). Ⓐ

Non-drug treatment
[EvGr] Elastic graduated compression stockings may be used to manage leg symptoms after a DVT. Patients should be given information about their correct use, duration of application, and replacement. Elastic graduated compression stockings are not recommended to prevent post-thrombotic syndrome or venous thromboembolism (VTE) recurrence after a DVT.

Mechanical interventions (such as inferior vena caval filters or percutaneous mechanical thrombectomy) can be considered in certain patients. For further information, see NICE guideline: **Venous thromboembolic diseases** (see *Useful resources*). Ⓐ

Drug treatment
[EvGr] Thrombolytic treatment may be appropriate for selected patients with a symptomatic iliofemoral DVT or a PE with haemodynamic instability. For full guidance, see NICE guideline: **Venous thromboembolic diseases** (see *Useful resources*).

Offer interim therapeutic anticoagulation [unlicensed use for some options] to patients in whom diagnostic investigations cannot be completed or results obtained within the required time frame. If possible, the choice of interim therapeutic anticoagulant should be one that can be continued if a proximal DVT and/or PE is confirmed.

When offering anticoagulation treatment, take into account comorbidities, contra-indications, and the patient's preferences. When starting treatment, carry out baseline blood tests (including full blood count, renal and hepatic function, prothrombin time and activated partial thromboplastin time).

Offer either apixaban p. 136 or rivaroxaban p. 139 for patients with a confirmed proximal DVT or PE (see below for guidance on specific population groups). If apixaban or rivaroxaban are unsuitable, offer either a:

- low molecular weight heparin (LMWH) for at least 5 days followed by dabigatran etexilate p. 148 or edoxaban p. 137; **or**
- LMWH given concurrently with a vitamin K antagonist for at least 5 days or until the INR is at least 2.0 for 2 consecutive readings, followed by a vitamin K antagonist on its own.

The use of heparin (unfractionated) p. 145 with a vitamin K antagonist to treat a confirmed proximal DVT or PE is not routinely recommended, unless the patient has renal impairment, established renal failure, or an increased risk of bleeding.

For renally impaired patients (estimated creatinine clearance between 15–50 ml/min) with a confirmed proximal DVT or PE, follow locally agreed protocols, or advice from a specialist or multidisciplinary team, and offer one of the following options:

- Apixaban;
- Rivaroxaban;
- LMWH for at least 5 days followed by either dabigatran etexilate (if estimated creatinine clearance is 30 ml/min or above) or edoxaban;
- LMWH or heparin (unfractionated), given concurrently with a vitamin K antagonist for at least 5 days or until the INR is at least 2.0 for 2 consecutive readings, followed by a vitamin K antagonist on its own. Ⓐ

For guidance on anticoagulation treatment for patients with established renal failure (estimated creatinine clearance less than 15 ml/min), see NICE guideline: **Venous thromboembolic diseases** (see *Useful resources*).

For further information on anticoagulation treatment for patients at extremes of body weight (less than 50 kg or more than 120 kg), and for guidance on anticoagulation treatment in those with active cancer, triple positive antiphospholipid syndrome, or confirmed PE with haemodynamic instability, see NICE guideline: **Venous thromboembolic diseases** (see *Useful resources*).

[EvGr] Provide patients initiated on anticoagulation treatment with verbal and written information. This should include how to take anticoagulants and for how long, possible side-effects, interactions, monitoring requirements, affect on activities (such as sports or travel) and on dental treatments, and when and how to seek medical help. In addition, women should be provided with advice on the use of anticoagulants if planning a pregnancy or they become pregnant. An 'anticoagulant alert card' that is specific to the patient's treatment should also be provided—advise patients to carry this at all times.

If anticoagulation treatment fails, assess adherence and other potential sources of hypercoagulability; increase the dose of the anticoagulant or change to an anticoagulant with a different mode of action as appropriate. Ⓐ

Duration of anticoagulation treatment and long-term anticoagulation for secondary prevention

EvGr Patients with a confirmed proximal DVT or PE should be offered anticoagulation treatment for at least 3 months (3 to 6 months for those with active cancer). The benefits and risks of continuing, stopping, or changing anticoagulation treatment should be assessed and discussed with the patient after this duration.

Consider stopping anticoagulation treatment 3 months (3 to 6 months for those with active cancer) after a provoked DVT or PE if the provoking factor is no longer present and the clinical course has been uncomplicated. Patients should be given advice about the risk of recurrence; written information on symptoms or signs to look out for; and who to contact to discuss any new signs, symptoms or other concerns.

For patients with an unprovoked DVT or PE, consider continuing anticoagulation beyond 3 months (beyond 6 months for those with active cancer). Discuss with the patient their preferences, and risk of VTE recurrence and bleeding—explain to patients with low bleeding risk that the benefits of continuing anticoagulation treatment are likely to outweigh the risks. If there is a plan to stop anticoagulation treatment, consider testing for hereditary thrombophilia in patients who have a first-degree relative who has had a DVT or PE, and testing for antiphospholipid antibodies—these tests can be affected by anticoagulants and specialist advice may be needed.

Consider the patient's preferences and their clinical situation when selecting an anticoagulant for long-term treatment. Predictive risk tools (such as HAS-BLED score) can be considered to assess whether long-term anticoagulation is appropriate, but relying on them solely is not recommended.

Offer continued treatment with the anticoagulant used for initial treatment if it is well tolerated for patients who do not have renal impairment, active cancer, established triple positive antiphospholipid syndrome, or are not at extremes of body weight. If the current treatment is not well tolerated, or the clinical situation or patient's preferences has changed, consider switching to apixaban p. 136 if the current treatment is a direct-acting anticoagulant other than apixaban.

For patients with renal impairment, active cancer, established triple positive antiphospholipid syndrome, or are at extremes of body weight, consider continuing current anticoagulation treatment if it is well tolerated.

Consider aspirin p. 132 [unlicensed] for patients who decline continued anticoagulation treatment.

Patients on long-term anticoagulation or aspirin treatment should be reviewed at least once a year for general health, risk of VTE recurrence, bleeding risk, and treatment preferences. Ⓐ

Venous thromboembolism treatment in pregnancy

EvGr Women with a suspected deep-vein thrombosis (DVT) and/or pulmonary embolism (PE) who are pregnant or who have given birth during the past 6 weeks, should be referred immediately to hospital for assessment and management.

Before initiating pharmacological anticoagulation treatment for venous thromboembolism (VTE), carry out baseline blood tests (including full blood count, coagulation screen, urea and electrolytes, and liver function tests).

A low molecular weight heparin (LMWH) should be started immediately for suspected VTE (until VTE has been excluded) and be continued as maintenance treatment in patients with confirmed DVT or PE. Routine measurements of peak anti-Xa activity is recommended for women on LMWH who are at extremes of body weight (less than 50 kg

or 90 kg or more) or those with complicating factors (such as renal impairment or recurrent VTE).

In the initial management of a DVT, an elastic graduated compression stocking should be applied on the affected leg as an additional treatment to manage symptoms such as pain and swelling.

Women considered to be at high risk of haemorrhage and in whom continued heparin treatment is essential, should be treated with intravenous heparin (unfractionated) p. 145 until the risk factors for haemorrhage have resolved. If VTE occurs at term, consider using intravenous heparin (unfractionated).

Pregnant women who develop heparin-induced thrombocytopenia or are heparin allergic should be managed with an alternative anticoagulant under specialist advice. Ⓐ

For further guidance on anticoagulation treatment during pregnancy and labour or prior to planned delivery; and for full guidance on anticoagulation treatment postnatally, and duration of treatment, see Royal College of Obstetricians and Gynaecologists guideline: **Thromboembolic Disease in Pregnancy and the Puerperium** (see *Useful resources*).

Extracorporeal circuits

Heparin (unfractionated) is also used in the maintenance of extracorporeal circuits in cardiopulmonary bypass and haemodialysis.

Haemorrhage

If haemorrhage occurs, it is usually sufficient to withdraw unfractionated or low molecular weight heparin, but if rapid reversal of the effects of the heparin is required, protamine sulfate p. 1423 is a specific antidote (but only partially reverses the effects of low molecular weight heparins).

Advanced Pharmacy Services

Patients with, or at risk of venous thromboembolism may be eligible for the New Medicines Service/Medicines Use Review service provided by a community pharmacist. For further information, see *Advanced Pharmacy Services* in Medicines optimisation p. 18.

Useful Resources

Thromboembolic Disease in Pregnancy and the Puerperium: Acute Management. Royal College of Obstetricians and Gynaecologists guidelines. Green-top Guideline 37b. April 2015.
www.rcog.org.uk/en/guidelines-research-services/guidelines/gtg37b/

Venous thromboembolic diseases: diagnosis, management and thrombophilia testing. National Institute for Health and Care Excellence. NICE guideline 158. March 2020.
www.nice.org.uk/guidance/ng158

Venous thromboembolism in over 16s: reducing the risk of hospital-acquired deep vein thrombosis or pulmonary embolism. National Institute for Health and Care Excellence. NICE guideline 89. March 2018 (updated August 2019).
www.nice.org.uk/guidance/ng89

Stroke   16-May-2017

Overview

Stroke is associated with a significant risk of morbidity and mortality. Patients presenting with acute symptoms should be immediately transferred to hospital for accurate diagnosis of stroke type, and urgent initiation of appropriate treatment; patients should be managed by a specialist multidisciplinary stroke team.

The following section gives an overview of the initial and long-term management of transient ischaemic attack, ischaemic stroke, and intracerebral haemorrhage.

Transient ischaemic attack

EvGr Patients suspected of having a transient ischaemic attack should immediately receive aspirin p. 132. Patients with aspirin hypersensitivity, or those intolerant of aspirin despite the addition of a proton pump inhibitor, should receive a suitable alternative antiplatelet. Following a confirmed diagnosis, patients should receive treatment for secondary prevention (see Long-term Management, under Ischaemic Stroke). ⟨A⟩

Ischaemic stroke

Initial management

EvGr Alteplase p. 231 is recommended in the treatment of acute ischaemic stroke if it can be administered within 4.5 hours of symptom onset and if intracranial haemorrhage has been excluded by appropriate imaging techniques. It should be given by medical staff experienced in the administration of thrombolytics and the treatment of acute stroke, preferably within a specialist stroke centre. Provided that intracranial haemorrhage has been excluded, treatment with aspirin should be initiated as soon as possible within 24 hours of symptom onset; a proton pump inhibitor should be considered for patients with a history of dyspepsia associated with aspirin. Patients with aspirin hypersensitivity, or those intolerant of aspirin despite the addition of a proton pump inhibitor, should receive an alternative antiplatelet.

Anticoagulants are not recommended as an alternative to antiplatelet drugs in acute ischaemic stroke in patients who are in sinus rhythm. However, parenteral anticoagulants may be indicated in patients who are symptomatic of, or at high risk of developing, deep vein thrombosis or pulmonary embolism. ⟨A⟩

Warfarin sodium p. 153 should not be given in the acute phase of an ischaemic stroke.

EvGr Patients with a disabling ischaemic stroke and atrial fibrillation should receive aspirin for 2 weeks before being considered for anticoagulant treatment. Patients already receiving anticoagulation for a prosthetic heart valve who experience a disabling ischaemic stroke and are at significant risk of haemorrhagic transformation, should have their anticoagulant treatment stopped for 7 days and substituted with aspirin.

Treatment of hypertension in the acute phase of ischaemic stroke can result in reduced cerebral perfusion, and should therefore only be instituted in the event of a hypertensive emergency, or in those patients considered for thrombolysis. ⟨A⟩

Long-term management

EvGr Patients should receive long-term treatment following a transient ischaemic attack or an ischaemic stroke to reduce the risk of further cardiovascular events.

Following a *transient ischaemic attack* or an *ischaemic stroke* (not associated with atrial fibrillation), long-term treatment with clopidogrel p. 134 [unlicensed in transient ischaemic attack] is recommended. If clopidogrel is contra-indicated or not tolerated, patients can receive modified-release dipyridamole p. 135 in combination with aspirin; if both aspirin and clopidogrel are contra-indicated or not tolerated, then modified-release dipyridamole alone is recommended; if both modified-release dipyridamole and clopidogrel are contra-indicated or not tolerated, then aspirin alone is recommended.

Patients with ischaemic stroke or transient ischaemic attack associated with atrial fibrillation should be reviewed for long-term anticoagulant treatment (for stroke, see also Initial Management under Ischaemic Stroke).

Anticoagulants are not routinely recommended in the long-term prevention of recurrent stroke, except when atrial fibrillation or other indications (such as a cardiac source of embolism, cerebral venous thrombosis or arterial dissection) are present.

A high-intensity statin (such as atorvastatin p. 217), should be initiated 48 hours after stroke symptom onset in patients not already taking a statin, irrespective of the patient's serum-cholesterol concentration. See Dyslipidaemias p. 210 for further information. Patients with acute stroke who are already taking a statin can continue statin treatment.

Following the acute phase of ischaemic stroke, blood pressure should be measured and treatment initiated to achieve a target blood pressure of <130/80 mmHg. Beta-blockers should not be used in the management of hypertension following a stroke, unless they are indicated for a co-existing condition.

All patients should be advised to make lifestyle modifications that include beneficial changes to diet, exercise, weight, alcohol intake, and Smoking cessation p. 519. ⟨A⟩

Intracerebral haemorrhage

Initial Management

EvGr Surgical intervention may be required following intracerebral haemorrhage to remove the haematoma and relieve intracranial pressure.

Patients presenting within 6 hours of symptom onset should be given rapid blood pressure lowering therapy if they have a systolic blood pressure between 150 and 220 mmHg and they do not fit any exclusion criteria. A systolic blood pressure target of 130 to 140 mmHg should be aimed to be attained within 1 hour of starting treatment and maintained for at least 7 days. Rapid blood pressure lowering should also be considered for patients presenting beyond 6 hours of symptom onset or who have a systolic blood pressure greater than 220 mmHg.

Rapid blood pressure lowering should not be given to patients who have an underlying structural cause, have a score on the Glasgow Coma Scale of below 6, are going to have early neurosurgery to evacuate the haematoma or have a massive haematoma with a poor expected prognosis.

Patients taking anticoagulants should have this treatment stopped and reversed. Anticoagulant therapy has, however, been used in patients with intracerebral haemorrhage who are symptomatic of deep vein thrombosis or pulmonary embolism; placement of a caval filter is an alternative in this situation. ⟨A⟩

Long-term management

EvGr Specialist advice should be sought for patients with atrial fibrillation and those at a high risk of ischaemic stroke or cardiac ischaemic events as aspirin and anticoagulant therapy are not normally recommended following an intracerebral haemorrhage. Blood pressure should be measured and treatment initiated where appropriate, taking care to avoid hypoperfusion. Statins should be avoided following intracerebral haemorrhage, however they can be used with caution when the risk of a vascular event outweighs the risk of further haemorrhage. ⟨A⟩

Advanced Pharmacy Services

Patients at risk of, or patients with a history of stroke or transient ischaemic attack, may be eligible for the New Medicines Service / Medicines Use Review service provided by a community pharmacist. For further information, see *Advanced Pharmacy Services* in Medicines optimisation p. 18.

Useful resources

Stroke and transient ischaemic attack in over 16s: diagnosis and initial management. National Institute for Health and Care Excellence guideline NG128. May 2019.
www.nice.org.uk/guidance/ng128

Oral anticoagulants

27-May-2020

Overview

The main use of anticoagulants is to prevent thrombus formation or extension of an existing thrombus in the slower-moving venous side of the circulation, where the thrombus consists of a fibrin web enmeshed with platelets and red cells. For further information on prevention and treatment of venous thromboembolism, see Venous thromboembolism p. 125.

Anticoagulants are of less use in preventing thrombus formation in arteries, for in faster-flowing vessels thrombi are composed mainly of platelets with little fibrin.

Vitamin K antagonists

The oral anticoagulants warfarin sodium p. 153, acenocoumarol p. 152 and phenindione p. 153, antagonise the effects of vitamin K, and take at least 48 to 72 hours for the anticoagulant effect to develop fully; warfarin sodium is the drug of choice. If an immediate effect is required, unfractionated or low molecular weight heparin must be given concomitantly.

These oral anticoagulants should not be used in cerebral artery thrombosis or peripheral artery occlusion as first-line therapy; aspirin p. 132 is more appropriate for reduction of risk in transient ischaemic attacks. Unfractionated or a low molecular weight heparin (see under Parenteral anticoagulants p. 130) is usually preferred for the prophylaxis of venous thromboembolism in patients undergoing surgery; alternatively, warfarin sodium can be continued in selected patients currently taking long-term warfarin sodium and who are at high risk of thromboembolism (seek expert advice).

Dose

The base-line prothrombin time should be determined but the initial dose should not be delayed whilst awaiting the result.

Target INR

The following indications and target INRs for adults for warfarin take into account recommendations of the British Society for Haematology guidelines on oral anticoagulation with warfarin—fourth edition. Br J Haematol 2011; **154**: 311–324:

An INR which is within 0.5 units of the target value is generally satisfactory; larger deviations require dosage adjustment. Target values (rather than ranges) are now recommended.

INR 2.5 for:

- treatment of deep-vein thrombosis or pulmonary embolism (including those associated with antiphospholipid syndrome or for recurrence in patients no longer receiving warfarin sodium)
- atrial fibrillation
- cardioversion—target INR should be achieved at least 3 weeks before cardioversion and anticoagulation should continue for at least 4 weeks after the procedure (higher target values, such as an INR of 3, can be used for up to 4 weeks before the procedure to avoid cancellations due to low INR)
- dilated cardiomyopathy
- mitral stenosis or regurgitation in patients with either atrial fibrillation, a history of systemic embolism, a left atrial thrombus, or an enlarged left atrium
- bioprosthetic heart valves in the mitral position (treat for 3 months), or in patients with a history of systemic embolism (treat for at least 3 months), or with a left atrial thrombus at surgery (treat until clot resolves), or with other risk factors (e.g. atrial fibrillation or a low ventricular ejection fraction)
- acute arterial embolism requiring embolectomy (consider long-term treatment)
- myocardial infarction

INR 3.5 for:

- recurrent deep-vein thrombosis or pulmonary embolism in patients currently receiving anticoagulation and with an INR above 2;

Mechanical prosthetic heart valves:

- the recommended target INR depends on the type and location of the valve, and patient-related risk factors
- consider increasing the INR target or adding an antiplatelet drug, if an embolic event occurs whilst anticoagulated at the target INR.

Duration

The risks of thromboembolism recurrence and anticoagulant-related bleeding should be considered when deciding the duration of anticoagulation.

The British Society for Haematology (Guidelines on Oral Anticoagulation with Warfarin—fourth edition. Br J Haematol 2011; **154**: 311–324) recommend 6 weeks of warfarin sodium for isolated calf-vein deep-vein thrombosis.

For information on duration of anticoagulant treatment following a confirmed proximal deep-vein thrombosis or pulmonary embolism, see Venous thromboembolism p. 125.

Haemorrhage

The main adverse effect of all oral anticoagulants is haemorrhage. Checking the INR and omitting doses when appropriate is essential; if the anticoagulant is stopped but not reversed, the INR should be measured 2–3 days later to ensure that it is falling. The cause of an elevated INR should be investigated. The following recommendations (which take into account the recommendations of the British Society for Haematology Guidelines on Oral Anticoagulation with Warfarin—fourth edition. Br J Haematol 2011; **154**: 311–324) are based on the result of the INR and whether there is major or minor bleeding; the recommendations apply to adults taking warfarin:

- Major bleeding—stop warfarin sodium; give phytomenadione p. 1138 (vitamin K_1) by slow intravenous injection; give dried prothrombin complex p. 120 (factors II, VII, IX, and X); if dried prothrombin complex unavailable, fresh frozen plasma can be given but is less effective; recombinant factor VIIa is not recommended for emergency anticoagulation reversal
- INR >8.0, minor bleeding—stop warfarin sodium; give phytomenadione (vitamin K_1) by slow intravenous injection; repeat dose of phytomenadione if INR still too high after 24 hours; restart warfarin sodium when INR <5.0
- INR >8.0, no bleeding—stop warfarin sodium; give phytomenadione (vitamin K_1) by mouth using the intravenous preparation orally [unlicensed use]; repeat dose of phytomenadione if INR still too high after 24 hours; restart warfarin when INR <5.0
- INR 5.0–8.0, minor bleeding—stop warfarin sodium; give phytomenadione (vitamin K_1) by slow intravenous injection; restart warfarin sodium when INR <5.0
- INR 5.0–8.0, no bleeding—withhold 1 or 2 doses of warfarin sodium and reduce subsequent maintenance dose
- Unexpected bleeding at therapeutic levels—always investigate possibility of underlying cause e.g. unsuspected renal or gastro-intestinal tract pathology

Peri-operative anticoagulation

Warfarin sodium should usually be stopped 5 days before elective surgery; phytomenadione (vitamin K_1) by mouth (using the intravenous preparation orally [unlicensed use]) should be given the day before surgery if the INR is ≥1.5. If haemostasis is adequate, warfarin sodium can be resumed at the normal maintenance dose on the evening of surgery or the next day.

Patients stopping warfarin sodium prior to surgery who are considered to be at high risk of thromboembolism (e.g. those with a venous thromboembolic event within the last

2

Cardiovascular system

3 months, atrial fibrillation with previous stroke or transient ischaemic attack, or mitral mechanical heart valve) may require interim therapy ('bridging') with a low molecular weight heparin (using treatment dose). The low molecular weight heparin should be stopped at least 24 hours before surgery; if the surgery carries a high risk of bleeding, the low molecular weight heparin should not be restarted until at least 48 hours after surgery.

Patients on warfarin sodium who require emergency surgery that can be delayed for 6–12 hours can be given intravenous phytomenadione p. 1138 (vitamin K_1) to reverse the anticoagulant effect. If surgery cannot be delayed, dried prothrombin complex p. 120 can be given in addition to intravenous phytomenadione (vitamin K_1) and the INR checked before surgery.

Combined anticoagulant and antiplatelet therapy

Existing antiplatelet therapy following an acute coronary syndrome or percutaneous coronary intervention should be continued for the necessary duration according to the indication being treated. The addition of warfarin sodium p. 153, when indicated (e.g. for venous thromboembolism or atrial fibrillation) should be considered following an assessment of the patient's risk of bleeding and discussion with a cardiologist. The duration of treatment with dual therapy (e.g. aspirin p. 132 and warfarin sodium) or triple therapy (e.g. aspirin with clopidogrel p. 134 and warfarin sodium) should be kept to a minimum where possible. The risk of bleeding with aspirin and warfarin sodium dual therapy is lower than with clopidogrel and warfarin sodium. Depending on the indications being treated and the patient's risk of thromboembolism, it may be possible to withhold antiplatelet therapy while warfarin sodium therapy is complete, or vice versa (on specialist advice) in order to reduce the length of time on dual or triple therapy.

Advanced Pharmacy Services

Patients taking oral anticoagulants may be eligible for the New Medicines Service / Medicines Use Review service provided by a community pharmacist. For further information, see *Advanced Pharmacy Services* in Medicines optimisation p. 18.

Parenteral anticoagulants   27-May-2020

Overview

The main use of anticoagulants is to prevent thrombus formation or extension of an existing thrombus in the slower-moving venous side of the circulation, where the thrombus consists of a fibrin web enmeshed with platelets and red cells. For information on the prevention and treatment of venous thromboembolism, see Venous thromboembolism p. 125.

Anticoagulants are of less use in preventing thrombus formation in arteries, for in faster-flowing vessels thrombi are composed mainly of platelets with little fibrin.

Heparin

Heparin initiates anticoagulation rapidly but has a short duration of action. It is often referred to as **'standard'** or heparin (unfractionated) p. 145 to distinguish it from the **low molecular weight heparins**, which have a longer duration of action. Although a low molecular weight heparin is generally preferred for routine use, heparin (unfractionated) can be used in those at high risk of bleeding because its effect can be terminated rapidly by stopping the infusion.

Low molecular weight heparins

Low molecular weight heparins (dalteparin sodium p. 143, enoxaparin sodium p. 144, and tinzaparin sodium p. 146) are

usually preferred over heparin (unfractionated) in the *prevention* of venous thromboembolism because they are as effective and they have a lower risk of heparin-induced thrombocytopenia. The standard prophylactic regimen does not require anticoagulant monitoring. The duration of action of low molecular weight heparins is longer than that of heparin (unfractionated) and *once-daily subcutaneous* administration is possible for some indications, making them convenient to use.

Low molecular weight heparins are generally preferred over heparin (unfractionated) in the *treatment* of deep vein thrombosis and pulmonary embolism, and are also used in the treatment of myocardial infarction, unstable coronary artery disease (see under Acute coronary syndromes p. 228) and for the prevention of clotting in extracorporeal circuits.

Heparinoids

Danaparoid sodium p. 142 is a heparinoid used for prophylaxis of deep-vein thrombosis in patients undergoing general or orthopaedic surgery. Providing there is no evidence of cross-reactivity, it also has a role in patients who develop heparin-induced thrombocytopenia.

Argatroban

An oral anticoagulant can be given with argatroban monohydrate p. 147, but it should only be started once thrombocytopenia has substantially resolved.

Hirudins

Bivalirudin, a hirudin analogue, is a thrombin inhibitor which is licensed for unstable angina or non-ST-segment elevation myocardial infarction in patients planned for urgent or early intervention, and as an anticoagulant for patients undergoing percutaneous coronary intervention (including patients with ST-segment elevation myocardial infarction undergoing primary percutaneous coronary intervention—see also Management of ST-segment elevation myocardial infarction (STEMI) in Acute coronary syndromes p. 228).

Heparin flushes

The use of heparin flushes should be kept to a minimum. For maintaining patency of peripheral venous catheters, sodium chloride injection 0.9% is as effective as heparin flushes. The role of heparin flushes in maintaining patency of arterial and central venous catheters is unclear.

Epoprostenol

Epoprostenol (prostacyclin) can be given to inhibit platelet aggregation during renal dialysis when heparins are unsuitable or contra-indicated. It is also licensed for the treatment of primary pulmonary hypertension resistant to other treatment, usually with oral anticoagulation; it should be initiated by specialists in pulmonary hypertension. Epoprostenol is a potent vasodilator. It has a short half-life of approximately 3 minutes and therefore must be administered by continuous intravenous infusion.

Fondaparinux

Fondaparinux sodium is a synthetic pentasaccharide that inhibits activated factor X.

> **Other drugs used for Thromboembolism** Streptokinase, p. 232

ANTIDOTES AND CHELATORS

Andexanet alfa
02-Nov-2020

- **DRUG ACTION** Andexanet alfa is a recombinant form of human factor X_a protein which binds specifically to apixaban or rivaroxaban, thereby reversing their anticoagulant effects.

- **INDICATIONS AND DOSE**

Reversal of apixaban or rivaroxaban in life-threatening or uncontrolled bleeding (specialist supervision in hospital)
▸ BY INTRAVENOUS INFUSION
 ▸ Adult: (consult product literature)

IMPORTANT SAFETY INFORMATION
MRHA/CHM ADVICE: *ONDEXXYA®* (ANDEXANET ALFA): COMMERCIAL ANTI-FXA ACTIVITY ASSAYS ARE UNSUITABLE FOR MEASURING ANTI-FXA ACTIVITY FOLLOWING ADMINISTRATION OF ANDEXANET ALFA (JULY 2020)
Treatment monitoring after administration of andexanet alfa should not be based on anti-FXa activity assays. In these assays, the FXa inhibitor dissociates from andexanet alfa, resulting in the detection of falsely elevated anti-FXa activity levels, and consequently a substantial underestimation of the reversal activity of andexanet alfa. Healthcare professionals are advised to monitor treatment using clinical parameters indicative of appropriate response (i.e. achievement of haemostasis), lack of efficacy (i.e. re-bleeding), and adverse events (i.e. thromboembolic events).

- **CAUTIONS** Risk of thrombosis
 CAUTIONS, FURTHER INFORMATION Manufacturer advises to consider re-starting anticoagulant therapy as soon as medically appropriate to reduce the risk of thrombosis.

- **SIDE-EFFECTS**
▸ **Common or very common** Back pain · cerebrovascular insufficiency · chest discomfort · cough · dizziness postural · dry mouth · dyspnoea · feeling hot · fever · flushing · gastrointestinal discomfort · headache · hyperhidrosis · muscle spasms · nausea · palpitations · peripheral coldness · skin reactions · taste altered
▸ **Uncommon** Cardiac arrest · embolism and thrombosis · iliac artery occlusion · myocardial infarction

- **PREGNANCY** Manufacturer advises avoid—no information available.

- **BREAST FEEDING** Manufacturer advises discontinue breast-feeding—no information available.

- **HANDLING AND STORAGE** Manufacturer advises store in a refrigerator (2–8°C)—consult product literature about storage after reconstitution.

- **NATIONAL FUNDING/ACCESS DECISIONS**
 For full details see funding body website
 Scottish Medicines Consortium (SMC) decisions
 ▸ Andexanet alfa (*Ondexxya®*) for adult patients treated with a direct factor Xa (FXa) inhibitor (apixaban or rivaroxaban) when reversal of anticoagulation is needed due to life-threatening or uncontrolled bleeding (September 2020) SMC No. SMC2273 Recommended

- **MEDICINAL FORMS** There can be variation in the licensing of different medicines containing the same drug.
 Powder for solution for infusion
 EXCIPIENTS: May contain Polysorbates, sucrose
 ▸ Ondexxya (Portola Pharma UK Ltd) ▼
  Andexanet alfa 200 mg Ondexxya 200mg powder for solution for infusion vials | 4 vial PoM £11,100.00 (Hospital only)

Idarucizumab
31-Aug-2020

- **DRUG ACTION** Idarucizumab is a humanised monoclonal antibody fragment that binds specifically to dabigatran and its metabolites, thereby reversing the anticoagulant effect.

- **INDICATIONS AND DOSE**

Rapid reversal of dabigatran for emergency procedures, or in life-threatening or uncontrolled bleeding (specialist supervision in hospital)
▸ BY INTRAVENOUS INJECTION, OR BY INTRAVENOUS INFUSION
 ▸ Adult: 5 g, followed by 5 g if required

- **CAUTIONS** Risk of thrombosis
 CAUTIONS, FURTHER INFORMATION Manufacturer advises to consider re-starting anticoagulant therapy as soon as medically appropriate to reduce the risk of thrombosis. Dabigatran can be re-started 24 hours after administration of idarucizumab; other anticoagulant therapy can be started at any time.

- **PREGNANCY** Manufacturer advises use only if potential benefit outweighs risk—no information available.

- **DIRECTIONS FOR ADMINISTRATION** Manufacturer advises that one dose of *Praxbind®* is administered as either two consecutive intravenous infusions, each given over 5–10 minutes, *or* as a bolus injection.

- **HANDLING AND STORAGE** Manufacturer advises store in a refrigerator at 2–8°C.

- **NATIONAL FUNDING/ACCESS DECISIONS**
 For full details see funding body website
 Scottish Medicines Consortium (SMC) decisions
 ▸ Idarucizumab (*Praxbind®*) is a specific reversal agent for dabigatran and is indicated in adult patients treated with dabigatran etexilate when rapid reversal of its anticoagulant effects is required for emergency surgery/urgent procedures or in life-threatening or uncontrolled bleeding (September 2016) SMC No. 1178/16 Recommended

- **MEDICINAL FORMS** There can be variation in the licensing of different medicines containing the same drug.
 Solution for infusion
 EXCIPIENTS: May contain Polysorbates, sorbitol
 ELECTROLYTES: May contain Sodium
 ▸ Praxbind (Boehringer Ingelheim Ltd)
  Idarucizumab 50 mg per 1 ml Praxbind 2.5g/50ml solution for infusion vials | 2 vial PoM £2,400.00 (Hospital only)

ANTITHROMBOTIC DRUGS › ANTIPLATELET DRUGS

Antiplatelet drugs
12-Jan-2018

Overview

Antiplatelet drugs decrease platelet aggregation and inhibit thrombus formation in the arterial circulation, because in faster-flowing vessels, thrombi are composed mainly of platelets with little fibrin.

EvGr Use of aspirin p. 132 in primary prevention of cardiovascular disease, in patients with or without diabetes, or hypertension, is not recommended. Long-term use of low-dose aspirin is recommended in patients with established cardiovascular disease (secondary prevention); Ⓐ unduly high blood pressure must be controlled before aspirin is given. If the patient is at a high risk of gastro-intestinal bleeding, a proton pump inhibitor can be added. For full guidance on the assessment and prevention of cardiovascular disease risk, see Cardiovascular disease risk assessment and prevention p. 203.

Aspirin is given following coronary bypass surgery. It is also used in atrial fibrillation, for intermittent claudication,

2

Cardiovascular system

for stable angina and acute coronary syndromes, for use following placement of coronary stents and for use in stroke.

Clopidogrel p. 134 is used for the prevention of atherothrombotic events in patients with a history of symptomatic ischaemic disease (e.g. ischaemic stroke). EvGr In patients with non-ST elevation acute coronary syndromes, clopidogrel, should be given for three months in addition to long-term low-dose aspirin. In patients with ST elevation acute coronary syndromes, clopidogrel, should be given up to four weeks in addition to long-term low-dose aspirin. ⒶⒶ

Clopidogrel is also used, in combination with low-dose aspirin, for the prevention of atherothrombotic and thromboembolic events in patients with atrial fibrillation (and at least one risk factor for a vascular event), and for whom warfarin sodium p. 153 is unsuitable.

Use of clopidogrel with aspirin increases the risk of bleeding. Clopidogrel monotherapy may be an alternative when aspirin is contra-indicated, for example in patients with aspirin hypersensitivity, or when aspirin is not tolerated despite the addition of a proton pump inhibitor.

Dipyridamole p. 135 is used by mouth as an adjunct to oral anticoagulation for prophylaxis of thromboembolism associated with prosthetic heart valves. Modified-release preparations are licensed for secondary prevention of ischaemic stroke and transient ischaemic attacks.

Prasugrel p. 230, in combination with aspirin, is licensed for the prevention of atherothrombotic events in patients with acute coronary syndrome undergoing percutaneous coronary intervention; the combination is usually given for up to 12 months.

Ticagrelor p. 230, in combination with aspirin, is licensed for the prevention of atherothrombotic events in patients with acute coronary syndrome; the combination is usually given for up to 12 months.

Cangrelor p. 224, in combination with aspirin, is licensed for the reduction of thrombotic cardiovascular events in patients with coronary artery disease undergoing percutaneous coronary intervention (PCI) who have not received treatment with oral clopidogrel, prasugrel or ticagrelor prior to the procedure and in whom oral therapy with these drugs is not suitable. Cangrelor is to be used under expert supervision only.

Antiplatelet drugs and coronary stents
Patients selected for percutaneous coronary intervention, with the placement of a coronary stent, will require dual antiplatelet therapy with aspirin and either cangrelor, clopidogrel, prasugrel, or ticagrelor [unlicensed]. Aspirin therapy should continue indefinitely. EvGr Following percutaneous coronary intervention in patients with stable angina, clopidogrel is recommended in addition to aspirin for at least 1 month after placement of a bare-metal stent, and for at least 6 months if a drug-eluting stent is used. ⒶⒶ Clopidogrel should not be discontinued prematurely in patients with a drug-eluting stent—there is an increased risk of stent thrombosis as a result of the eluted drug slowing the re-endothelialisation process. Patients considered to be at high-risk of developing late stent thrombosis with a drug-eluting stent may require a longer duration of treatment with clopidogrel combined with aspirin. Prasugrel or ticagrelor are alternatives to clopidogrel in certain patients undergoing percutaneous coronary intervention.

Glycoprotein IIb/IIIa inhibitors
Glycoprotein IIb/IIIa inhibitors prevent platelet aggregation by blocking the binding of fibrinogen to receptors on platelets. Abciximab is a monoclonal antibody which binds to four glycoprotein IIb/IIIa receptors and to other related sites; it is licensed as an adjunct to heparin (unfractionated) p. 145 and aspirin for the prevention of ischaemic complications in high-risk patients undergoing percutaneous transluminal coronary intervention. Abciximab should be used once only (to avoid additional risk

of thrombocytopenia). Eptifibatide p. 225 (in combination with heparin (unfractionated) and aspirin) and tirofiban p. 225 (in combination with heparin (unfractionated), aspirin, and clopidogrel) also inhibit glycoprotein IIb/IIIa receptors; they are licensed for use to prevent early myocardial infarction in patients with unstable angina or non-ST-segment-elevation myocardial infarction. Tirofiban is also licensed for use in combination with heparin (unfractionated), aspirin, and clopidogrel, for the reduction of major cardiovascular events in patients with ST-segment elevation myocardial infarction intended for primary percutaneous coronary intervention. Abciximab, eptifibatide and tirofiban should be used by specialists only.

Epoprostenol p. 124 is also used to inhibit platelet aggregation during renal dialysis when heparins are unsuitable or contra-indicated.

Advanced Pharmacy Services

Patients taking antiplatelet drugs may be eligible for the New Medicines Service / Medicines Use Review service provided by a community pharmacist. For further information, see *Advanced Pharmacy Services* in Medicines optimisation p. 18.

Aspirin

20-Nov-2020

(Acetylsalicylic Acid)

● **INDICATIONS AND DOSE**

Cardiovascular disease (secondary prevention)
▶ BY MOUTH
▸ Adult: 75 mg daily

Secondary prevention of deep-vein thrombosis (in patients who decline continued anticoagulation treatment) | Secondary prevention of pulmonary embolism (in patients who decline continued anticoagulation treatment)
▶ BY MOUTH
▸ Adult: 75 mg daily, alternatively 150 mg daily

Management of unstable angina and non-ST-segment elevation myocardial infarction (NSTEMI) | Management of ST-segment elevation myocardial infarction (STEMI)
▶ BY MOUTH
▸ Adult: 300 mg, chewed or dispersed in water

Suspected transient ischaemic attack
▶ BY MOUTH
▸ Adult: 300 mg once daily until diagnosis established

Transient ischaemic attack (long-term treatment in combination with dipyridamole) | Ischaemic stroke not associated with atrial fibrillation (in combination with dipyridamole if clopidogrel contra-indicated or not tolerated) | Ischaemic stroke not associated with atrial fibrillation (used alone if clopidogrel and dipyridamole contra-indicated or not tolerated)
▶ BY MOUTH
▸ Adult: 75 mg once daily

Acute ischaemic stroke
▶ BY MOUTH
▸ Adult: 300 mg once daily for 14 days, to be initiated 24 hours after thrombolysis or as soon as possible within 48 hours of symptom onset in patients not receiving thrombolysis

Atrial fibrillation following a disabling ischaemic stroke (before being considered for anticoagulant treatment)
▶ BY MOUTH
▸ Adult: 300 mg once daily for 14 days

Following disabling ischaemic stroke in patients receiving anticoagulation for a prosthetic heart valve and who are at significant risk of haemorrhagic transformation
▸ BY MOUTH
▸ Adult: 300 mg once daily, anticoagulant treatment stopped for 7 days and to be substituted with aspirin

Following coronary by-pass surgery
▸ BY MOUTH
▸ Adult: 75–300 mg daily

Mild to moderate pain | Pyrexia
▸ BY MOUTH
▸ Adult: 300–900 mg every 4–6 hours as required; maximum 4 g per day
▸ BY RECTUM
▸ Adult: 450–900 mg every 4 hours; maximum 3.6 g per day

Acute migraine
▸ BY MOUTH
▸ Adult: 900 mg for 1 dose, to be taken as soon as migraine symptoms develop

Prevention of pre-eclampsia in women at moderate or high risk
▸ BY MOUTH
▸ Adult: 75–150 mg once daily from 12 weeks gestation until the birth of the baby

Mild to moderate pain (dose approved for use by community practitioner nurse prescribers) | Pyrexia (dose approved for use by community practitioner nurse prescribers)
▸ BY MOUTH
▸ Child 16-17 years: 300–600 mg every 4–6 hours as required, maximum 2.4 g per day without doctor's advice
▸ Adult: 300–600 mg every 4–6 hours as required, maximum 2.4 g per day without doctor's advice

● UNLICENSED USE
▸ With oral use in adults Aspirin may be used as detailed below, although these situations are considered unlicensed:
  ● EvGr secondary prevention of deep-vein thrombosis in patients who decline continued anticoagulation treatment
  ● secondary prevention of pulmonary embolism in patients who decline continued anticoagulation treatment
  ● prevention of pre-eclampsia in women at moderate or high risk Ⓐ

● CONTRA-INDICATIONS Active peptic ulceration · bleeding disorders · children under 16 years (risk of Reye's syndrome) · haemophilia · previous peptic ulceration (analgesic dose) · severe cardiac failure (analgesic dose)

CONTRA-INDICATIONS, FURTHER INFORMATION
▸ Reye's syndrome Owing to an association with Reye's syndrome, manufacturer advises aspirin-containing preparations should not be given to children under 16 years, unless specifically indicated, e.g. for Kawasaki disease.

● CAUTIONS Allergic disease · anaemia · asthma · dehydration · elderly · G6PD deficiency · hypertension · may mask symptoms of infection · preferably avoid during fever or viral infection in children (risk of Reye's syndrome) · previous peptic ulceration (but manufacturers may advise avoidance of aspirin in history of peptic ulceration) · thyrotoxicosis

CAUTIONS, FURTHER INFORMATION
▸ Elderly Prescription potentially inappropriate (STOPP criteria):
  ● at long-term doses greater than 160 mg daily (increased risk of bleeding, no evidence for increased efficacy)

● with a past history of peptic ulcer disease without concomitant proton pump inhibitor use (risk of recurrent peptic ulcer)
● with concurrent significant bleeding risk, such as uncontrolled severe hypertension, bleeding diathesis or recent non-trivial spontaneous bleeding (high risk of bleeding)
● when used with clopidogrel as secondary stroke prevention unless the patient has a coronary stent(s) inserted in the previous 12 months, or concurrent acute coronary syndrome,or has a high grade symptomatic carotid arterial stenosis (no evidence of added benefit over clopidogrel monotherapy)
● when used with vitamin K antagonists, direct thrombin inhibitors or factor Xa inhibitors in patients with chronic atrial fibrillation (no added benefit from aspirin)
See also Prescribing in the elderly p. 33.

● INTERACTIONS → Appendix 1: aspirin

● SIDE-EFFECTS
GENERAL SIDE-EFFECTS
▸ Rare or very rare Asthmatic attack · bronchospasm
SPECIFIC SIDE-EFFECTS
▸ Common or very common
▸ With oral use Dyspepsia · haemorrhage
▸ Uncommon
▸ With oral use Dyspnoea · rhinitis · severe cutaneous adverse reactions (SCARs) · skin reactions
▸ Rare or very rare
▸ With oral use Aplastic anaemia · erythema nodosum · gastrointestinal haemorrhage (severe) · granulocytosis · haemorrhagic vasculitis · intracranial haemorrhage · menorrhagia · nausea · thrombocytopenia · vomiting
▸ Frequency not known
▸ With oral use Fluid retention · gastrointestinal disorders · headache · hearing loss · hepatic failure · hyperuricaemia · iron deficiency anaemia · renal impairment · sodium retention · tinnitus · vertigo

Overdose The main features of salicylate poisoning are hyperventilation, tinnitus, deafness, vasodilatation, and sweating. Coma is uncommon but indicates very severe poisoning.
  For specific details on the management of poisoning, see Aspirin, under Emergency treatment of poisoning p. 1413.

● ALLERGY AND CROSS-SENSITIVITY EvGr Aspirin is **contra-indicated** in history of hypersensitivity to aspirin or any other NSAID—which includes those in whom attacks of asthma, angioedema, urticaria, or rhinitis have been precipitated by aspirin or any other NSAID. ⒶⒷ

● PREGNANCY Use antiplatelet doses with caution during third trimester; impaired platelet function and risk of haemorrhage; delayed onset and increased duration of labour with increased blood loss; avoid analgesic doses if possible in last few weeks (low doses probably not harmful); high doses may be related to intra-uterine growth restriction, teratogenic effects, closure of fetal ductus arteriosus in utero and possibly persistent pulmonary hypertension of newborn; kernicterus may occur in jaundiced neonates.

● BREAST FEEDING Avoid—possible risk of Reye's syndrome; regular use of high doses could impair platelet function and produce hypoprothrombinaemia in infant if neonatal vitamin K stores low.

● HEPATIC IMPAIRMENT Manufacturer advises use with caution in mild-to-moderate impairment; avoid in severe impairment.

● RENAL IMPAIRMENT Use with caution; avoid in severe impairment; sodium and water retention; deterioration in renal function; increased risk of gastro-intestinal bleeding.

2

Cardiovascular system

• PRESCRIBING AND DISPENSING INFORMATION
‣ In adults BP directs that when no strength is stated the 300 mg strength should be dispensed, and that when soluble aspirin tablets are prescribed, dispersible aspirin tablets shall be dispensed.

• PROFESSION SPECIFIC INFORMATION

Dental practitioners' formulary
Aspirin Dispersible Tablets 300 mg may be prescribed.

• EXCEPTIONS TO LEGAL CATEGORY
Can be sold to the public provided packs contain no more than 32 capsules or tablets; pharmacists can sell multiple packs up to a total quantity of 100 capsules or tablets in justifiable circumstances.

• MEDICINAL FORMS There can be variation in the licensing of different medicines containing the same drug. Forms available from special-order manufacturers include: capsule, oral suspension, oral solution

Gastro-resistant tablet
CAUTIONARY AND ADVISORY LABELS 5, 25, 32
‣ Aspirin (Non-proprietary)
   Aspirin 75 mg Aspirin 75mg gastro-resistant tablets | 28 tablet [P] £1.53 DT = £1.53 | 56 tablet [P] £2.40–£3.06
   Aspirin 300 mg Aspirin 300mg gastro-resistant tablets | 100 tablet [PoM] £25.29 DT = £25.29
‣ Nu-Seals (Alliance Pharmaceuticals Ltd)
   Aspirin 75 mg Nu-Seals 75 gastro-resistant tablets | 56 tablet [P] £3.12

Tablet
CAUTIONARY AND ADVISORY LABELS 21, 32
‣ Aspirin (Non-proprietary)
   Aspirin 75 mg Aspirin 75mg tablets | 28 tablet [PoM] £3.50 DT = £1.38
   Aspirin 300 mg Aspirin 300mg tablets | 32 tablet [P] £3.42 DT = £3.42 | 32 tablet [GSL] £0.23 DT = £3.42 | 100 tablet [PoM] £10.68 DT = £10.68

Suppository
CAUTIONARY AND ADVISORY LABELS 32
‣ Aspirin (Non-proprietary)
   Aspirin 150 mg Aspirin 150mg suppositories | 10 suppository [P] £21.57 DT = £20.54
   Aspirin 300 mg Aspirin 300mg suppositories | 10 suppository [P] £39.48–£41.45 DT = £39.48

Dispersible tablet
CAUTIONARY AND ADVISORY LABELS 13, 21, 32
‣ Aspirin (Non-proprietary)
   Aspirin 75 mg Aspirin 75mg dispersible tablets | 28 tablet [P] £1.06 DT = £1.07 | 100 tablet [P] £0.28–£3.82 DT = £3.82 | 1000 tablet [PoM] £38.20
   Aspirin 300 mg Aspirin 300mg dispersible tablets | 32 tablet [P] £1.24 DT = £1.24 | 100 tablet [PoM] [✕] DT = £3.88
‣ Danamep (Ecogen Europe Ltd)
   Aspirin 75 mg Danamep 75mg dispersible tablets | 28 tablet [PoM] £0.50 DT = £1.07
‣ Disprin (Reckitt Benckiser Healthcare (UK) Ltd)
   Aspirin 300 mg Disprin 300mg dispersible tablets | 32 tablet [P] £1.94 DT = £1.24

Clopidogrel

20-Nov-2020

• INDICATIONS AND DOSE

Prevention of atherothrombotic events in percutaneous coronary intervention (adjunct with aspirin) in patients not already on clopidogrel
‣ BY MOUTH
‣ **Adult:** Loading dose 300 mg, to be taken prior to the procedure, alternatively loading dose 600 mg, higher dose may produce a greater and more rapid inhibition of platelet aggregation

Transient ischaemic attack for patients with aspirin hypersensitivity, or those intolerant of aspirin despite the addition of a proton pump inhibitor | Acute ischaemic stroke for patients with aspirin hypersensitivity, or those intolerant of aspirin despite the addition of a proton pump inhibitor
‣ BY MOUTH
‣ **Adult:** 75 mg once daily

Prevention of atherothrombotic events in peripheral arterial disease or within 35 days of myocardial infarction, or within 6 months of ischaemic stroke
‣ BY MOUTH
‣ **Adult:** 75 mg once daily

Prevention of atherothrombotic events in acute coronary syndrome without ST-segment elevation (given with aspirin)
‣ BY MOUTH
‣ **Adult:** Initially 300 mg, then 75 mg daily for up to 12 months

Prevention of atherothrombotic events in acute myocardial infarction with ST-segment elevation (given with aspirin)
‣ BY MOUTH
‣ **Adult 18–75 years:** Initially 300 mg, then 75 mg for at least 4 weeks
‣ **Adult 76 years and over:** 75 mg daily for at least 4 weeks

Prevention of atherothrombotic and thromboembolic events in patients with atrial fibrillation and at least one risk factor for a vascular event (with aspirin) and for whom warfarin is unsuitable
‣ BY MOUTH
‣ **Adult:** 75 mg once daily

• UNLICENSED USE 600 mg loading dose prior to percutaneous coronary intervention is an unlicensed dose. Use in transient ischaemic attack or acute ischaemic stroke, in patients with aspirin hypersensitivity or intolerant of aspirin, is unlicensed.

• CONTRA-INDICATIONS Active bleeding

• CAUTIONS Discontinue 7 days before elective surgery if antiplatelet effect not desirable · patients at risk of increased bleeding from trauma, surgery, or other pathological conditions

CAUTIONS, FURTHER INFORMATION
‣ Elderly Prescription potentially inappropriate (STOPP criteria) with concurrent significant bleeding risk, such as uncontrolled severe hypertension, bleeding diathesis or recent non-trivial spontaneous bleeding (high risk of bleeding). See also Prescribing in the elderly p. 33.

• INTERACTIONS → Appendix 1: clopidogrel

• SIDE-EFFECTS
‣ **Common or very common** Diarrhoea · gastrointestinal discomfort · haemorrhage · skin reactions
‣ **Uncommon** Constipation · dizziness · eosinophilia · gastrointestinal disorders · headache · intracranial haemorrhage · leucopenia · nausea · paraesthesia · thrombocytopenia · vomiting
‣ **Rare or very rare** Acquired haemophilia · agranulocytosis · anaemia · angioedema · arthralgia · arthritis · bone marrow disorders · confusion · fever · glomerulonephritis · gynaecomastia · hallucination · hepatic disorders · hypersensitivity · hypotension · myalgia · neutropenia · pancreatitis · respiratory disorders · severe cutaneous adverse reactions (SCARs) · stomatitis · taste altered · ulcerative colitis · vasculitis · vertigo · wound haemorrhage
‣ **Frequency not known** Kounis syndrome

• ALLERGY AND CROSS-SENSITIVITY [EvG] Caution with history of hypersensitivity reactions to thienopyridines (e.g. prasugrel). ⓜ

- **PREGNANCY** Manufacturer advises avoid—no information available.
- **BREAST FEEDING** Manufacturer advises avoid.
- **HEPATIC IMPAIRMENT** Manufacturer advises caution in moderate impairment in patients with an increased risk of bleeding—limited information available; avoid in severe impairment.
- **RENAL IMPAIRMENT** Manufacturer advises caution.
- **NATIONAL FUNDING/ACCESS DECISIONS** For full details see funding body website

NICE decisions
▸ Clopidogrel and modified-release dipyridamole for the prevention of occlusive vascular events (December 2010) NICE TA210 Recommended

Scottish Medicines Consortium (SMC) decisions
▸ Clopidogrel (*Plavix*®) for the prevention of atherothrombotic events in acute coronary syndrome (without ST-segment elevation) in combination with aspirin (March 2004) SMC No. 88/04 Recommended with restrictions
▸ Clopidogrel (*Plavix*®) for ST-segment elevation myocardial infarction (STEMI), in combination with aspirin (August 2007) SMC No. 390/07 Recommended with restrictions

- **MEDICINAL FORMS** There can be variation in the licensing of different medicines containing the same drug. Forms available from special-order manufacturers include: oral suspension, oral solution

Tablet
▸ Clopidogrel (Non-proprietary)
  Clopidogrel 75 mg Clopidogrel 75mg tablets | 28 tablet [PoM] £35.31 DT = £1.60 | 30 tablet [PoM] £1.71–£36.95
▸ Plavix (Sanofi)
  Clopidogrel 75 mg Plavix 75mg tablets | 30 tablet [PoM] £35.64
  Clopidogrel (as Clopidogrel hydrogen sulfate) 300 mg Plavix 300mg tablets | 30 tablet [PoM] £142.54 DT = £142.54

Dipyridamole

04-Jun-2020

- **INDICATIONS AND DOSE**

Secondary prevention of ischaemic stroke (not associated with atrial fibrillation) and transient ischaemic attacks (used alone or with aspirin) | Adjunct to oral anticoagulation for prophylaxis of thromboembolism associated with prosthetic heart valves
▸ BY MOUTH USING MODIFIED-RELEASE MEDICINES
▸ Adult: 200 mg twice daily, to be taken preferably with food

Adjunct to oral anticoagulation for prophylaxis of thromboembolism associated with prosthetic heart valves
▸ BY MOUTH USING IMMEDIATE-RELEASE MEDICINES
▸ Adult: 300–600 mg daily in 3–4 divided doses

- **CAUTIONS** Aortic stenosis · coagulation disorders · heart failure · hypotension · left ventricular outflow obstruction · may exacerbate migraine · myasthenia gravis (risk of exacerbation) · rapidly worsening angina · recent myocardial infarction

CAUTIONS, FURTHER INFORMATION
▸ Elderly Prescription potentially inappropriate (STOPP criteria) with concurrent significant bleeding risk, such as uncontrolled severe hypertension, bleeding diathesis or recent non-trivial spontaneous bleeding (high risk of bleeding). See also Prescribing in the elderly p. 33.

- **INTERACTIONS** → Appendix 1: dipyridamole
- **SIDE-EFFECTS**
▸ **Common or very common** Angina pectoris · diarrhoea · dizziness · headache · myalgia · nausea · skin reactions · vomiting

- **Frequency not known** Angioedema · bronchospasm · haemorrhage · hot flush · hypotension · tachycardia · thrombocytopenia
- **PREGNANCY** Not known to be harmful.
- **BREAST FEEDING** Manufacturers advise use only if essential—small amount present in milk.
- **PRESCRIBING AND DISPENSING INFORMATION** Modified-release capsules should be dispensed in original container (pack contains a desiccant) and any capsules remaining should be discarded 6 weeks after opening.
- **NATIONAL FUNDING/ACCESS DECISIONS** For full details see funding body website

NICE decisions
▸ Clopidogrel and modified-release dipyridamole for the prevention of occlusive vascular events (December 2010) NICE TA210 Recommended with restrictions

- **MEDICINAL FORMS** There can be variation in the licensing of different medicines containing the same drug. Forms available from special-order manufacturers include: oral suspension, oral solution

Oral suspension
▸ Dipyridamole (Non-proprietary)
  Dipyridamole 10 mg per 1 ml Dipyridamole 50mg/5ml oral suspension sugar free sugar-free | 150 ml [PoM] £43.01 DT = £42.96
  Dipyridamole 40 mg per 1 ml Dipyridamole 200mg/5ml oral suspension sugar free sugar-free | 150 ml [PoM] £133.53 DT = £133.53

Modified-release capsule
CAUTIONARY AND ADVISORY LABELS 21, 25
▸ Attia (Dr Reddy's Laboratories (UK) Ltd)
  Dipyridamole 200 mg Attia 200mg modified-release capsules | 60 capsule [PoM] £13.15 DT = £13.15
▸ Ofcram PR (Advanz Pharma)
  Dipyridamole 200 mg Ofcram PR 200mg capsules | 60 capsule [PoM] £10.06 DT = £13.15

Tablet
CAUTIONARY AND ADVISORY LABELS 22
▸ Dipyridamole (Non-proprietary)
  Dipyridamole 25 mg Dipyridamole 25mg tablets | 84 tablet [PoM] £9.20 DT = £7.93
  Dipyridamole 100 mg Dipyridamole 100mg tablets | 84 tablet [PoM] £12.50 DT = £5.42

Dipyridamole with aspirin

The properties listed below are those particular to the combination only. For the properties of the components please consider, dipyridamole above, aspirin p. 132.

- **INDICATIONS AND DOSE**

Secondary prevention of ischaemic stroke and transient ischaemic attacks
▸ BY MOUTH USING MODIFIED-RELEASE MEDICINES
▸ Adult: 25/200 mg twice daily

- **INTERACTIONS** → Appendix 1: aspirin · dipyridamole
- **PRESCRIBING AND DISPENSING INFORMATION** Dispense in original container (pack contains a desiccant) and discard any capsules remaining 6 weeks after opening.

- **MEDICINAL FORMS** There can be variation in the licensing of different medicines containing the same drug.

Modified-release capsule
CAUTIONARY AND ADVISORY LABELS 21, 25, 32
▸ Molita (Dr Reddy's Laboratories (UK) Ltd)
  Aspirin 25 mg, Dipyridamole 200 mg Molita 200mg/25mg modified-release capsules | 60 capsule [PoM] £13.50 DT = £13.50

2

Cardiovascular system

ANTITHROMBOTIC DRUGS > FACTOR XA INHIBITORS

Apixaban

17-Nov-2020

- **DRUG ACTION** Apixaban is a direct inhibitor of activated factor X (factor Xa).

- **INDICATIONS AND DOSE**

Prophylaxis of venous thromboembolism following knee replacement surgery
▶ BY MOUTH
▷ Adult: 2.5 mg twice daily for 10–14 days, to be started 12–24 hours after surgery

Prophylaxis of venous thromboembolism following hip replacement surgery
▶ BY MOUTH
▷ Adult: 2.5 mg twice daily for 32–38 days, to be started 12–24 hours after surgery

Treatment of deep-vein thrombosis | Treatment of pulmonary embolism
▶ BY MOUTH
▷ Adult: Initially 10 mg twice daily for 7 days, then maintenance 5 mg twice daily

Prophylaxis of recurrent deep-vein thrombosis | Prophylaxis of recurrent pulmonary embolism
▶ BY MOUTH
▷ Adult: 2.5 mg twice daily, following completion of 6 months anticoagulant treatment

Prophylaxis of stroke and systemic embolism in non-valvular atrial fibrillation and at least one risk factor (such as previous stroke or transient ischaemic attack, symptomatic heart failure, diabetes mellitus, hypertension, or age 75 years and over)
▶ BY MOUTH
▷ Adult: 5 mg twice daily, reduce dose to 2.5 mg twice daily in patients with at least two of the following characteristics: age 80 years and over, body-weight less than 61 kg, or serum creatinine 133 micromol/litre and over

DOSE EQUIVALENCE AND CONVERSION
▶ For information on changing from, or to, other anticoagulants, consult product literature.

IMPORTANT SAFETY INFORMATION
MHRA/CHM ADVICE: DIRECT-ACTING ORAL ANTICOAGULANTS (DOACS): INCREASED RISK OF RECURRENT THROMBOTIC EVENTS IN PATIENTS WITH ANTIPHOSPHOLIPID SYNDROME (JUNE 2019)
A clinical trial has shown an increased risk of recurrent thrombotic events associated with rivaroxaban compared with warfarin, in patients with antiphospholipid syndrome and a history of thrombosis. There may be a similar risk associated with other DOACs. Healthcare professionals are advised that DOACs are not recommended in patients with antiphospholipid syndrome, particularly high-risk patients who test positive for all three antiphospholipid tests—lupus anticoagulant, anticardiolipin antibodies, and anti-beta$_2$ glycoprotein I antibodies. Continued treatment should be reviewed in these patients to determine if appropriate, and switching to a vitamin K antagonist such as warfarin should be considered.

MHRA/CHM ADVICE: DIRECT-ACTING ORAL ANTICOAGULANTS (DOACS): REMINDER OF BLEEDING RISK, INCLUDING AVAILABILITY OF REVERSAL AGENTS (JUNE 2020)
The MHRA reminds healthcare professionals to remain vigilant for signs and symptoms of bleeding complications during treatment with apixaban after ongoing reports of serious, potentially fatal bleeds associated with the use of DOACs. Healthcare professionals are also advised to use apixaban with

caution in patients with increased bleeding risk, and to ensure that those with renal impairment are dosed appropriately and their renal function monitored during treatment. Patients should be counselled on the signs and symptoms of bleeding, and encouraged to read the patient information leaflet. The apixaban reversal agent andexanet alfa (*Ondexxya*®) is available if required; its reversal effects should be monitored using clinical parameters, as anti-FXa assay results may not be reliable.

MHRA/CHM ADVICE: WARFARIN AND OTHER ANTICOAGULANTS: MONITORING OF PATIENTS DURING THE COVID-19 PANDEMIC (OCTOBER 2020)
Healthcare professionals are reminded that:
- direct-acting oral anticoagulants (DOACs), such as apixaban, may interact with other medicines (including antibacterials and antivirals)—advice in product literature should be followed to minimise the risk of potential interactions;
- if patients are switched from warfarin to apixaban, warfarin treatment should be stopped before apixaban treatment is started to reduce the risk of over-anticoagulation and bleeding.

- **CONTRA-INDICATIONS** Active, clinically significant bleeding · antiphospholipid syndrome (increased risk of recurrent thrombotic events) · risk factors for major bleeding
CONTRA-INDICATIONS, FURTHER INFORMATION
▶ Risk factors for major bleeding Manufacturer advises avoid in conditions with significant risk factors for major bleeding, including current or recent gastrointestinal ulceration, malignant neoplasms at high risk of bleeding, recent brain or spinal injury, recent brain, spinal or ophthalmic surgery, recent intracranial haemorrhage, known or suspected oesophageal varices, arteriovenous malformations, vascular aneurysms or major intraspinal or intracerebral vascular abnormalities.

- **CAUTIONS** Anaesthesia with postoperative indwelling epidural catheter (risk of paralysis—monitor neurological signs and wait 20–30 hours after apixaban dose before removing catheter and do not give next dose until at least 5 hours after catheter removal) · prosthetic heart valve (efficacy not established) · risk of bleeding
CAUTIONS, FURTHER INFORMATION
▶ Elderly For factor Xa inhibitors, prescription potentially inappropriate (STOPP criteria):
- with concurrent significant bleeding risk, such as uncontrolled severe hypertension, bleeding diathesis or recent non-trivial spontaneous bleeding (high risk of bleeding)
- for first deep venous thrombosis without continuing provoking risk factors (e.g. thrombophilia) for greater than 6 months (no proven added benefit)
- for first pulmonary embolus without continuing provoking risk factors for greater than 12 months (no proven added benefit)
- as part of dual therapy with an antiplatelet agent in patients with stable coronary, cerebrovascular or peripheral arterial disease, without a clear indication for anticoagulant therapy (no added benefit)
- if eGFR less than 15 ml/min/1.73 m^2 (risk of bleeding)
See also Prescribing in the elderly p. 33.

- **INTERACTIONS** → Appendix 1: factor XA inhibitors
- **SIDE-EFFECTS**
▶ **Common or very common** Anaemia · haemorrhage · nausea · skin reactions
▶ **Uncommon** CNS haemorrhage · hypotension · post procedural haematoma · thrombocytopenia · wound complications

- **PREGNANCY** Manufacturer advises avoid—no information available.
- **BREAST FEEDING** Manufacturer advises avoid—present in milk in *animal* studies.
- **HEPATIC IMPAIRMENT** Manufacturer advises caution in mild to moderate impairment (or if hepatic transaminases greater than 2 times the upper limit of normal, or if bilirubin is equal or greater than 1.5 times the upper limit of normal); avoid in severe impairment or impairment associated with coagulopathy and clinically relevant bleeding risk.
- **RENAL IMPAIRMENT** Manufacturer advises avoid if creatinine clearance less than 15 mL/minute—no information available. When used for *prophylaxis of venous thromboembolism following knee or hip replacement surgery, prophylaxis of recurrent deep-vein thrombosis or pulmonary embolism, and treatment of deep-vein thrombosis or pulmonary embolism*, use with caution if creatinine clearance 15–29 mL/minute.
  Dose adjustments When used for *prophylaxis of stroke and systemic embolism in non-valvular atrial fibrillation*, reduce dose to 2.5 mg twice daily if serum-creatinine 133 micromol/litre and over is associated with age 80 years and over or body-weight less than 61 kg; reduce dose to 2.5 mg twice daily if creatinine clearance 15–29 mL/minute.
- **MONITORING REQUIREMENTS**
  - Patients should be monitored for signs of bleeding or anaemia; treatment should be stopped if severe bleeding occurs.
  - No routine anticoagulant monitoring required (INR tests are unreliable).
- **PRESCRIBING AND DISPENSING INFORMATION** Duration of treatment should be determined by balancing the benefit of treatment with the bleeding risk; shorter duration of treatment (at least 3 months) should be based on transient risk factors i.e recent surgery, trauma, immobilisation.
  Apixaban should not be used as an alternative to unfractionated heparin in pulmonary embolism in patients with haemodynamic instability, or who may receive thrombolysis or pulmonary embolectomy.
- **PATIENT AND CARER ADVICE** Patients should be provided with an alert card and advised to keep it with them at all times.
- **NATIONAL FUNDING/ACCESS DECISIONS**
  For full details see funding body website
  NICE decisions
  - Apixaban for the prevention of venous thromboembolism after total hip or knee replacement in adults (January 2012) NICE TA245 Recommended
  - Apixaban for preventing stroke and systemic embolism in people with non-valvular atrial fibrillation (February 2013) NICE TA275 Recommended
  - Apixaban for the treatment and secondary prevention of deep vein thrombosis and/or pulmonary embolism (June 2015) NICE TA341 Recommended

- **MEDICINAL FORMS** There can be variation in the licensing of different medicines containing the same drug.
  Tablet
  CAUTIONARY AND ADVISORY LABELS 10
  - Eliquis (Bristol-Myers Squibb Pharmaceuticals Ltd)
    Apixaban 2.5 mg Eliquis 2.5mg tablets | 10 tablet [PoM] £9.50 | 20 tablet [PoM] £19.00 | 60 tablet [PoM] £57.00 DT = £57.00
    Apixaban 5 mg Eliquis 5mg tablets | 28 tablet [PoM] £26.60 | 56 tablet [PoM] £53.20 DT = £53.20

Edoxaban

17-Nov-2020

- **DRUG ACTION** Edoxaban is a direct and reversible inhibitor of activated factor X (factor Xa), which prevents conversion of prothrombin to thrombin and prolongs clotting time, thereby reducing the risk of thrombus formation.

- **INDICATIONS AND DOSE**

  Prophylaxis of stroke and systemic embolism in non-valvular atrial fibrillation, in patients with at least one risk factor (such as congestive heart failure, hypertension, aged 75 years and over, diabetes mellitus, previous stroke or transient ischaemic attack)
  - BY MOUTH
    - Adult (body-weight up to 61 kg): 30 mg once daily
    - Adult (body-weight 61 kg and above): 60 mg once daily

  Treatment of deep-vein thrombosis | Prophylaxis of recurrent deep-vein thrombosis | Treatment of pulmonary embolism | Prophylaxis of recurrent pulmonary embolism
  - BY MOUTH
    - Adult (body-weight up to 61 kg): 30 mg once daily, duration of treatment adjusted according to risk factors—consult product literature, treatment should follow initial use of parenteral anticoagulant for at least 5 days
    - Adult (body-weight 61 kg and above): 60 mg once daily, duration of treatment adjusted according to risk factors—consult product literature), treatment should follow initial use of parenteral anticoagulant for at least 5 days

  DOSE ADJUSTMENTS DUE TO INTERACTIONS
  - Manufacturer advises max. dose of 30 mg once daily with concurrent ciclosporin, dronedarone, erythromycin, or ketoconazole.

  DOSE EQUIVALENCE AND CONVERSION
  - For information on changing from, or to, other anticoagulants, consult product literature.

IMPORTANT SAFETY INFORMATION

MHRA/CHM ADVICE: DIRECT-ACTING ORAL ANTICOAGULANTS (DOACS): INCREASED RISK OF RECURRENT THROMBOTIC EVENTS IN PATIENTS WITH ANTIPHOSPHOLIPID SYNDROME (JUNE 2019)
A clinical trial has shown an increased risk of recurrent thrombotic events associated with rivaroxaban compared with warfarin, in patients with antiphospholipid syndrome and a history of thrombosis. There may be a similar risk associated with other DOACs. Healthcare professionals are advised that DOACs are not recommended in patients with antiphospholipid syndrome, particularly high-risk patients who test positive for all three antiphospholipid tests—lupus anticoagulant, anticardiolipin antibodies, and anti-beta$_2$ glycoprotein I antibodies. Continued treatment should be reviewed in these patients to determine if appropriate, and switching to a vitamin K antagonist such as warfarin should be considered.

MHRA/CHM ADVICE: DIRECT-ACTING ORAL ANTICOAGULANTS (DOACS): REMINDER OF BLEEDING RISK, INCLUDING AVAILABILITY OF REVERSAL AGENTS (JUNE 2020)
The MHRA reminds healthcare professionals to remain vigilant for signs and symptoms of bleeding complications during treatment with edoxaban after ongoing reports of serious, potentially fatal bleeds associated with the use of DOACs. Healthcare professionals are also advised to use edoxaban with caution in patients with increased bleeding risk, and to ensure that those with renal impairment are dosed appropriately and their renal function monitored during treatment. Patients should be counselled on the signs and symptoms of bleeding, and encouraged to read the

2

Cardiovascular system

2

Cardiovascular system

patient information leaflet. There is currently no specific authorised reversal agent available for edoxaban.

MHRA/CHM ADVICE: WARFARIN AND OTHER ANTICOAGULANTS: MONITORING OF PATIENTS DURING THE COVID-19 PANDEMIC (OCTOBER 2020)

Healthcare professionals are reminded that:
● direct-acting oral anticoagulants (DOACs), such as edoxaban, may interact with other medicines (including antibacterials and antivirals)—advice in product literature should be followed to minimise the risk of potential interactions;
● if patients are switched from warfarin to edoxaban, warfarin treatment should be stopped before edoxaban treatment is started to reduce the risk of over-anticoagulation and bleeding.

● CONTRA-INDICATIONS Active bleeding · antiphospholipid syndrome (increased risk of recurrent thrombotic events) · arteriovenous malformations · current or recent gastro-intestinal ulceration · hepatic disease (associated with coagulopathy and clinically relevant bleeding risk) · known or suspected oesophageal varices · major intraspinal or intracerebral vascular abnormalities · presence of malignant neoplasms at high risk of bleeding · recent brain or spinal injury · recent brain, spinal or ophthalmic surgery · recent intracranial haemorrhage · uncontrolled severe hypertension · vascular aneurysms

CONTRA-INDICATIONS, FURTHER INFORMATION
▸ Risk for major bleeding Edoxaban treatment is contra-indicated in patients with significant risk factors for major bleeding, these include those listed above.

● CAUTIONS Moderate to severe mitral stenosis (safety and efficacy not established) · prosthetic heart valve (safety and efficacy not established) · risk of bleeding · surgery

CAUTIONS, FURTHER INFORMATION
▸ Surgery Manufacturer recommends to discontinue treatment at least 24 hours before a surgical procedure; the risk of bleeding should be weighed against the urgency of the intervention—consult product literature.
▸ Elderly For factor Xa inhibitors, prescription potentially inappropriate (STOPP criteria):
  ● with concurrent significant bleeding risk, such as uncontrolled severe hypertension, bleeding diathesis or recent non-trivial spontaneous bleeding (high risk of bleeding)
  ● for first deep venous thrombosis without continuing provoking risk factors (e.g. thrombophilia) for greater than 6 months (no proven added benefit)
  ● for first pulmonary embolus without continuing provoking risk factors for greater than 12 months (no proven added benefit)
  ● as part of dual therapy with an antiplatelet agent in patients with stable coronary, cerebrovascular or peripheral arterial disease, without a clear indication for anticoagulant therapy (no added benefit)
  ● if eGFR less than 15 ml/min/1.73 m² (risk of bleeding) See also Prescribing in the elderly p. 33.

● INTERACTIONS → Appendix 1: factor XA inhibitors
● SIDE-EFFECTS
▸ Common or very common Abdominal pain · anaemia · dizziness · haemorrhage · headache · nausea · skin reactions
▸ Uncommon CNS haemorrhage · thrombocytopenia

SIDE-EFFECTS, FURTHER INFORMATION Should a bleeding complication arise in a patient receiving edoxaban, the manufacturer recommends to delay the next dose or treatment should be discontinued as appropriate.

● PREGNANCY Manufacturer advises avoid—toxicity in *animal* studies.

● BREAST FEEDING Manufacturer advises avoid—present in milk in *animal* studies.

● HEPATIC IMPAIRMENT Manufacturer advises caution in mild to moderate impairment, or if liver transaminases greater than 2 times the upper limit of normal, or total bilirubin 1.5 times the upper limit of normal or greater; avoid in severe impairment or hepatic disease associated with coagulopathy and clinically relevant bleeding risk.

● RENAL IMPAIRMENT Manufacturer advises avoid if creatinine clearance less than 15 mL/minute.
Dose adjustments Manufacturer advises use a dose of 30 mg once daily if creatinine clearance 15–50 mL/minute.

● MONITORING REQUIREMENTS
▸ Manufacturer advises monitor renal function before treatment and when clinically indicated during treatment; monitor hepatic function before treatment and repeat periodically if treatment duration longer than 1 year.
▸ Manufacturer advises monitor for signs of mucosal bleeding and anaemia in patients at increased risk; treatment should be stopped if severe bleeding occurs.
▸ No routine anticoagulant monitoring required (INR tests are unreliable).

● PATIENT AND CARER ADVICE Patients should be provided with an alert card and advised to keep it with them at all times.

● NATIONAL FUNDING/ACCESS DECISIONS
For full details see funding body website
NICE decisions
▸ Edoxaban for treating and preventing deep vein thrombosis and pulmonary embolism (August 2015) NICE TA354 Recommended
▸ Edoxaban for preventing stroke and systemic embolism in people with non-valvular atrial fibrillation (September 2015) NICE TA355 Recommended

● MEDICINAL FORMS There can be variation in the licensing of different medicines containing the same drug.
Tablet
CAUTIONARY AND ADVISORY LABELS 10
▸ Lixiana (Daiichi Sankyo UK Ltd) ▼
  Edoxaban (as Edoxaban tosilate) 15 mg Lixiana 15mg tablets | 10 tablet [PoM] £17.50 DT = £17.50
  Edoxaban (as Edoxaban tosilate) 30 mg Lixiana 30mg tablets | 28 tablet [PoM] £49.00 DT = £49.00
  Edoxaban (as Edoxaban tosilate) 60 mg Lixiana 60mg tablets | 28 tablet [PoM] £49.00 DT = £49.00

Fondaparinux sodium   11-Nov-2020

● DRUG ACTION Fondaparinux sodium is a synthetic pentasaccharide that inhibits activated factor X.

● INDICATIONS AND DOSE
Prophylaxis of venous thromboembolism in patients after undergoing major orthopaedic surgery of the hip or leg, or abdominal surgery
▸ BY SUBCUTANEOUS INJECTION
▸ Adult: Initially 2.5 mg, dose to be given 6 hours after surgery, then 2.5 mg once daily

Prophylaxis of venous thromboembolism in medical patients immobilised because of acute illness
▸ BY SUBCUTANEOUS INJECTION
▸ Adult: 2.5 mg once daily

Treatment of superficial-vein thrombosis
▸ BY SUBCUTANEOUS INJECTION
▸ Adult (body-weight 50 kg and above): 2.5 mg once daily for at least 30 days (max. 45 days if high risk of thromboembolic complications), treatment should be stopped 24 hours before surgery and restarted at least 6 hours post operatively

Treatment of unstable angina and non-ST-segment elevation myocardial infarction
▸ BY SUBCUTANEOUS INJECTION
▸ Adult: 2.5 mg once daily for up to 8 days (or until hospital discharge if sooner), treatment should be stopped 24 hours before coronary artery bypass graft surgery (where possible) and restarted 48 hours post operatively

Treatment of ST-segment elevation myocardial infarction
▸ INITIALLY BY INTRAVENOUS INJECTION, OR BY INTRAVENOUS INFUSION
▸ Adult: Initially 2.5 mg daily for the first day, then (by subcutaneous injection) 2.5 mg once daily for up to 8 days (or until hospital discharge if sooner), treatment should be stopped 24 hours before coronary artery bypass graft surgery (where possible) and restarted 48 hours post operatively

Treatment of deep-vein thrombosis and pulmonary embolism
▸ BY SUBCUTANEOUS INJECTION
▸ Adult (body-weight up to 50 kg): 5 mg every 24 hours, an oral anticoagulant (usually warfarin) is started at the same time as fondaparinux (fondaparinux should be continued for at least 5 days and until INR ≥ 2 for at least 24 hours)
▸ Adult (body-weight 50-100 kg): 7.5 mg every 24 hours, an oral anticoagulant (usually warfarin) is started at the same time as fondaparinux (fondaparinux should be continued for at least 5 days and until INR ≥ 2 for at least 24 hours)
▸ Adult (body-weight 101 kg and above): 10 mg every 24 hours, an oral anticoagulant (usually warfarin) is started at the same time as fondaparinux (fondaparinux should be continued for at least 5 days and until INR ≥ 2 for at least 24 hours)

● CONTRA-INDICATIONS Active bleeding · bacterial endocarditis
● CAUTIONS Active gastro-intestinal ulcer disease · bleeding disorders · brain surgery · elderly patients · low body-weight · ophthalmic surgery · recent intracranial haemorrhage · risk of catheter thrombus during percutaneous coronary intervention · spinal or epidural anaesthesia (risk of spinal haematoma—avoid if using treatment doses) · spinal surgery
● INTERACTIONS → Appendix 1: factor XA inhibitors
● SIDE-EFFECTS
▸ Common or very common Anaemia · haemorrhage
▸ Uncommon Chest pain · coagulation disorder · dyspnoea · fever · hepatic function abnormal · nausea · oedema · platelet abnormalities · skin reactions · thrombocytopenia · vomiting · wound secretion
▸ Rare or very rare Anxiety · confusion · constipation · cough · diarrhoea · dizziness · drowsiness · fatigue · gastritis · gastrointestinal discomfort · genital oedema · headache · hyperbilirubinaemia · hypersensitivity · hypokalaemia · hypotension · leg pain · post procedural infection · syncope · vasodilation · vertigo
● PREGNANCY Manufacturer advises avoid unless potential benefit outweighs possible risk—no information available.
● BREAST FEEDING Present in milk in *animal* studies—manufacturer advises avoid.
● HEPATIC IMPAIRMENT
▸ When used for Venous thromboembolism, unstable angina, non-ST-segment elevation myocardial infarction and ST-segment elevation myocardial infarction Manufacturer advises caution in severe impairment (increased risk of bleeding complications).
▸ When used for Superficial-vein thrombosis Manufacturer advises avoid in severe impairment (no information available).

● RENAL IMPAIRMENT Increased risk of bleeding in renal impairment.
▸ When used for treatment of acute coronary syndromes or prophylaxis of venous thromboembolism and treatment of superficial-vein thrombosis Avoid if eGFR less than 20 mL/minute/1.73 m².
▸ When used for treatment of venous thromboembolism Use with caution if eGFR 30–50 mL/minute/1.73 m², avoid if eGFR less than 30 mL/minute/1.73 m².
Dose adjustments
▸ When used for prophylaxis of venous thromboembolism and treatment of superficial-vein thrombosis Reduce dose to 1.5 mg daily if eGFR 20–50 mL/minute/1.73 m².
● DIRECTIONS FOR ADMINISTRATION For *intravenous infusion* (*Arixtra*®), give intermittently in Sodium chloride 0.9%. For ST-segment elevation myocardial infarction, add requisite dose to 25-50 mL infusion fluid and give over 1-2 minutes.

● MEDICINAL FORMS There can be variation in the licensing of different medicines containing the same drug.
Solution for injection
▸ Fondaparinux sodium (Non-proprietary)
Fondaparinux sodium 5 mg per 1 ml Fondaparinux sodium 2.5mg/0.5ml solution for injection pre-filled syringes | 10 pre-filled disposable injection PoM £62.79 DT = £62.79
Fondaparinux sodium 12.5 mg per 1 ml Fondaparinux sodium 5mg/0.4ml solution for injection pre-filled syringes | 10 pre-filled disposable injection PoM £110.70 DT = £116.53
Fondaparinux sodium 10mg/0.8ml solution for injection pre-filled syringes | 10 pre-filled disposable injection PoM £110.70 DT = £116.53
Fondaparinux sodium 7.5mg/0.6ml solution for injection pre-filled syringes | 10 pre-filled disposable injection PoM £110.70 DT = £116.53 (Hospital only)
▸ Arixtra (Aspen Pharma Trading Ltd)
Fondaparinux sodium 5 mg per 1 ml Arixtra 2.5mg/0.5ml solution for injection pre-filled syringes | 10 pre-filled disposable injection PoM £62.79 DT = £62.79 (Hospital only)
Arixtra 1.5mg/0.3ml solution for injection pre-filled syringes | 10 pre-filled disposable injection PoM £62.79 DT = £62.79 (Hospital only)
Fondaparinux sodium 12.5 mg per 1 ml Arixtra 7.5mg/0.6ml solution for injection pre-filled syringes | 10 pre-filled disposable injection PoM £116.53 DT = £116.53 (Hospital only)
Arixtra 5mg/0.4ml solution for injection pre-filled syringes | 10 pre-filled disposable injection PoM £116.53 DT = £116.53 (Hospital only)
Arixtra 10mg/0.8ml solution for injection pre-filled syringes | 10 pre-filled disposable injection PoM £116.53 DT = £116.53 (Hospital only)

Rivaroxaban

17-Nov-2020

● DRUG ACTION Rivaroxaban is a direct inhibitor of activated factor X (factor Xa).

● INDICATIONS AND DOSE
Prophylaxis of venous thromboembolism following knee replacement surgery
▸ BY MOUTH
▸ Adult: 10 mg once daily for 2 weeks, to be started 6–10 hours after surgery

Prophylaxis of venous thromboembolism following hip replacement surgery
▸ BY MOUTH
▸ Adult: 10 mg once daily for 5 weeks, to be started 6–10 hours after surgery

Treatment of deep-vein thrombosis | Treatment of pulmonary embolism
▸ BY MOUTH
▸ Adult: Initially 15 mg twice daily for 21 days, then maintenance 20 mg once daily, to be taken with food, for duration of treatment, consult product literature

continued →

Cardiovascular system

2

Prophylaxis of recurrent deep-vein thrombosis | Prophylaxis of recurrent pulmonary embolism
▸ BY MOUTH
▸ Adult: 10 mg once daily, following completion of at least 6 months of anticoagulant treatment, to be taken with food, consider 20 mg once daily in those at high risk of recurrence (such as complicated comorbidities, or previous recurrence with rivaroxaban 10 mg once daily)

Prophylaxis of stroke and systemic embolism in patients with non-valvular atrial fibrillation and with at least one of the following risk factors: congestive heart failure, hypertension, previous stroke or transient ischaemic attack, age ≥ 75 years, or diabetes mellitus
▸ BY MOUTH
▸ Adult: 20 mg once daily, to be taken with food

Prophylaxis of atherothrombotic events following an acute coronary syndrome (in combination with aspirin alone or aspirin and clopidogrel)
▸ BY MOUTH
▸ Adult: 2.5 mg twice daily usual duration 12 months

Prophylaxis of atherothrombotic events in patients with coronary artery disease or symptomatic peripheral artery disease at high risk of ischaemic events (in combination with aspirin)
▸ BY MOUTH
▸ Adult: 2.5 mg twice daily

DOSE EQUIVALENCE AND CONVERSION
▸ For information on changing from, or to, other anticoagulants—consult product literature.

IMPORTANT SAFETY INFORMATION
MHRA/CHM ADVICE: DIRECT-ACTING ORAL ANTICOAGULANTS (DOACS): INCREASED RISK OF RECURRENT THROMBOTIC EVENTS IN PATIENTS WITH ANTIPHOSPHOLIPID SYNDROME (JUNE 2019)
A clinical trial has shown an increased risk of recurrent thrombotic events associated with rivaroxaban compared with warfarin, in patients with antiphospholipid syndrome and a history of thrombosis. There may be a similar risk associated with other DOACs. Healthcare professionals are advised that DOACs are not recommended in patients with antiphospholipid syndrome, particularly high-risk patients who test positive for all three antiphospholipid tests—lupus anticoagulant, anticardiolipin antibodies, and anti-beta$_2$ glycoprotein I antibodies. Continued treatment should be reviewed in these patients to determine if appropriate, and switching to a vitamin K antagonist such as warfarin should be considered.

MHRA/CHM ADVICE: RIVAROXABAN (*XARELTO*®): REMINDER THAT 15 MG AND 20 MG TABLETS SHOULD BE TAKEN WITH FOOD (JULY 2019)
The MHRA has received a small number of reports suggesting a lack of efficacy (thromboembolic events) in patients taking 15 mg or 20 mg rivaroxaban tablets on an empty stomach. Healthcare professionals are advised to remind patients to take rivaroxaban 15 mg or 20 mg tablets with food. In those who have difficulty swallowing, these tablets can be crushed and mixed with water or apple puree immediately before, and followed by food immediately after, ingestion.

MHRA/CHM ADVICE: DIRECT-ACTING ORAL ANTICOAGULANTS (DOACS): REMINDER OF BLEEDING RISK, INCLUDING AVAILABILITY OF REVERSAL AGENTS (JUNE 2020)
The MHRA reminds healthcare professionals to remain vigilant for signs and symptoms of bleeding complications during treatment with rivaroxaban after ongoing reports of serious, potentially fatal bleeds associated with the use of DOACs. Healthcare professionals are also advised to use rivaroxaban with

caution in patients with increased bleeding risk, and to ensure that those with renal impairment are dosed appropriately and their renal function monitored during treatment. Patients should be counselled on the signs and symptoms of bleeding, and encouraged to read the patient information leaflet. The rivaroxaban reversal agent andexanet alfa (*Ondexxya*®) is available if required; its reversal effects should be monitored using clinical parameters, as anti-FXa assay results may not be reliable.

MHRA/CHM ADVICE: WARFARIN AND OTHER ANTICOAGULANTS: MONITORING OF PATIENTS DURING THE COVID-19 PANDEMIC (OCTOBER 2020)
Healthcare professionals are reminded that:
- direct-acting oral anticoagulants (DOACs), such as rivaroxaban, may interact with other medicines (including antibacterials and antivirals)—advice in product literature should be followed to minimise the risk of potential interactions;
- if patients are switched from warfarin to rivaroxaban, warfarin treatment should be stopped before rivaroxaban treatment is started to reduce the risk of over-anticoagulation and bleeding.

● CONTRA-INDICATIONS
GENERAL CONTRA-INDICATIONS
Active bleeding · antiphospholipid syndrome (increased risk of recurrent thrombotic events) · malignant neoplasms at high risk of bleeding · oesophageal varices · recent brain surgery · recent gastro-intestinal ulcer · recent intracranial haemorrhage · recent ophthalmic surgery · recent spine surgery · significant risk of major bleeding · vascular aneurysm

SPECIFIC CONTRA-INDICATIONS
▸ When used for Prophylaxis of atherothrombotic events following an acute coronary syndrome Previous stroke · transient ischaemic attack
▸ When used for Prophylaxis of atherothrombotic events in patients with coronary artery disease or symptomatic peripheral artery disease Previous stroke (no information available—consult product literature)

● CAUTIONS
GENERAL CAUTIONS Anaesthesia with postoperative indwelling epidural catheter (risk of paralysis—monitor neurological signs and wait at least 18 hours after rivaroxaban dose before removing catheter and do not give next dose until at least 6 hours after catheter removal) · bronchiectasis · elderly · prosthetic heart valve (efficacy not established) · risk of bleeding · rivaroxaban should not be used as an alternative to unfractionated heparin in pulmonary embolism in patients with haemodynamic instability, or who may receive thrombolysis or pulmonary embolectomy · severe hypertension · vascular retinopathy

SPECIFIC CAUTIONS
▸ When used for Prophylaxis of atherothrombotic events following an acute coronary syndrome Body-weight less than 60 kg
▸ When used for Prophylaxis of atherothrombotic events in patients with coronary artery disease or symptomatic peripheral artery disease Body-weight less than 60 kg

CAUTIONS, FURTHER INFORMATION
▸ Elderly For factor Xa inhibitors, prescription potentially inappropriate (STOPP criteria):
- with concurrent significant bleeding risk, such as uncontrolled severe hypertension, bleeding diathesis or recent non-trivial spontaneous bleeding (high risk of bleeding)
- for first deep venous thrombosis without continuing provoking risk factors (e.g. thrombophilia) for greater than 6 months (no proven added benefit)

- for first pulmonary embolus without continuing provoking risk factors for greater than 12 months (no proven added benefit)
- as part of dual therapy with an antiplatelet agent in patients with stable coronary, cerebrovascular or peripheral arterial disease, without a clear indication for anticoagulant therapy (no added benefit)
- if eGFR less than 15 ml/min/1.73 m² (risk of bleeding)
  See also Prescribing in the elderly p. 33.

- INTERACTIONS → Appendix 1: factor XA inhibitors
- SIDE-EFFECTS
▸ **Common or very common** Anaemia · asthenia · constipation · diarrhoea · dizziness · fever · gastrointestinal discomfort · haemorrhage · headache · hypotension · menorrhagia · nausea · oedema · pain in extremity · post procedural anaemia · renal impairment · skin reactions · vomiting · wound complications
▸ **Uncommon** Angioedema · dry mouth · hepatic disorders · hypersensitivity · intracranial haemorrhage · malaise · syncope · tachycardia · thrombocytopenia · thrombocytosis
▸ **Rare or very rare** Severe cutaneous adverse reactions (SCARs) · vascular pseudoaneurysm
- PREGNANCY Manufacturer advises avoid—toxicity in *animal* studies.
- BREAST FEEDING Manufacturer advises avoid—present in milk in *animal* studies.
- HEPATIC IMPAIRMENT Manufacturer advises avoid in hepatic disease with coagulopathy and clinically-relevant bleeding risk including patients with moderate to severe cirrhosis.
- RENAL IMPAIRMENT Manufacturer advises caution if creatinine clearance 15–29 mL/minute; avoid if creatinine clearance less than 15 mL/minute. Use with caution if concomitant use of drugs that increase plasma-rivaroxaban concentration (consult product literature).
  Dose adjustments
  ▸ When used for Treatment of deep-vein thrombosis or pulmonary embolism Following the first 21 days of treatment for deep-vein thrombosis or pulmonary embolism, the usual dose of 20 mg once daily can be given, but manufacturer advises consider reducing to 15 mg once daily if creatinine clearance 15–49 mL/minute and the risk of bleeding outweighs the risk of recurrent deep-vein thrombosis or pulmonary embolism.
  ▸ When used for Prophylaxis of recurrent deep-vein thrombosis or pulmonary embolism When the recommended dose is 20 mg once daily, manufacturer advises consider reducing to 15 mg once daily if creatinine clearance 15–49 mL/minute and the risk of bleeding outweighs the risk of recurrent deep-vein thrombosis or pulmonary embolism.
  ▸ When used for Prophylaxis of stroke and systemic embolism in patients with non-valvular atrial fibrillation Manufacturer advises reduce dose to 15 mg once daily if creatinine clearance 15–49 mL/minute.
- MONITORING REQUIREMENTS
▸ Patients should be monitored for signs of bleeding or anaemia; treatment should be stopped if severe bleeding occurs.
▸ No routine anticoagulant monitoring required (INR tests are unreliable).
- DIRECTIONS FOR ADMINISTRATION Manufacturer advises tablets may be crushed and mixed with water or apple puree just before administration.
- PRESCRIBING AND DISPENSING INFORMATION Low-dose rivaroxaban, in combination with aspirin alone *or* aspirin and clopidogrel, is licensed for the prevention of atherothrombotic events following an acute coronary syndrome with elevated cardiac biomarkers. Treatment should be started as soon as possible after the patient has been stabilised following the acute coronary event, at the

earliest 24 hours after admission to hospital, and at the time when parenteral anticoagulation therapy would normally be discontinued; the usual duration of treatment is 12 months.

- PATIENT AND CARER ADVICE Patients should be provided with an alert card and advised to keep it with them at all times.
- NATIONAL FUNDING/ACCESS DECISIONS
  For full details see funding body website
  NICE decisions
  ▸ Rivaroxaban for the prevention of venous thromboembolism after total hip or total knee replacement in adults (April 2009) NICE TA170 Recommended
  ▸ Rivaroxaban for the prevention of stroke and systemic embolism in people with atrial fibrillation (May 2012) NICE TA256 Recommended
  ▸ Rivaroxaban for the treatment of deep-vein thrombosis and prevention of recurrent deep-vein thrombosis and pulmonary embolism (July 2012) NICE TA261 Recommended
  ▸ Rivaroxaban for treating pulmonary embolism and preventing recurrent venous thromboembolism (June 2013) NICE TA287 Recommended
  ▸ Rivaroxaban for preventing adverse outcomes after acute management of acute coronary syndrome (March 2015) NICE TA335 Recommended
  ▸ Rivaroxaban for preventing atherothrombotic events in people with coronary or peripheral artery disease (October 2019) NICE TA607 Recommended
  Scottish Medicines Consortium (SMC) decisions
  ▸ Rivaroxaban (*Xarelto*®) for the prevention of venous thromboembolism in elective hip or knee replacement surgery (December 2008) SMC No. 519/08 Recommended
  ▸ Rivaroxaban (*Xarelto*®) for the prevention of stroke and systemic embolism in patients with atrial fibrillation (February 2012) SMC No. 756/12 Recommended with restrictions
  ▸ Rivaroxaban (*Xarelto*®) for the treatment of deep-vein thrombosis (DVT) and prevention of recurrent DVT and pulmonary embolism following acute DVT in adults (February 2012) SMC No. 755/12 Recommended
  ▸ Rivaroxaban (*Xarelto*®) for the treatment of pulmonary embolism (PE), and prevention of recurrent deep-vein thrombosis (DVT) and PE in adults (March 2013) SMC No. 852/13 Recommended
  ▸ Rivaroxaban (*Xarelto*®) co-administered with acetylsalicylic acid [aspirin] for the prevention of atherothrombotic events in adult patients with coronary artery disease or symptomatic peripheral artery disease at high risk of ischaemic events (February 2019) SMC No. SMC2128 Recommended with restrictions

- MEDICINAL FORMS There can be variation in the licensing of different medicines containing the same drug.
  Tablet
  CAUTIONARY AND ADVISORY LABELS 21 (15 and 20 mg tablets)
  ▸ Xarelto (Bayer Plc) ▼
    Rivaroxaban 2.5 mg Xarelto 2.5mg tablets | 56 tablet PoM £50.40 DT = £50.40
    Rivaroxaban 10 mg Xarelto 10mg tablets | 10 tablet PoM £18.00 | 30 tablet PoM £54.00 DT = £54.00 | 100 tablet PoM £180.00
    Rivaroxaban 15 mg Xarelto 15mg tablets | 14 tablet PoM £25.20 | 28 tablet PoM £50.40 DT = £50.40 | 42 tablet PoM £75.60 | 100 tablet PoM £180.00
    Rivaroxaban 20 mg Xarelto 20mg tablets | 28 tablet PoM £50.40 DT = £50.40 | 100 tablet PoM £180.00

2

Cardiovascular system

ANTITHROMBOTIC DRUGS 〉 HEPARINOIDS

Danaparoid sodium

07-Aug-2020

● INDICATIONS AND DOSE

Prevention of deep-vein thrombosis in general or orthopaedic surgery
▸ BY SUBCUTANEOUS INJECTION
▸ Adult: 750 units twice daily for 7–10 days, initiate treatment before operation, with last pre-operative dose 1–4 hours before surgery

Thromboembolic disease in patients with history of heparin-induced thrombocytopenia
▸ INITIALLY BY INTRAVENOUS INJECTION
▸ Adult (body-weight up to 55 kg): Initially 1250 units, then (by continuous intravenous infusion) 400 units/hour for 2 hours, then (by continuous intravenous infusion) 300 units/hour for 2 hours, then (by continuous intravenous infusion) 200 units/hour for 5 days
▸ Adult (body-weight 55–89 kg): Initially 2500 units, then (by continuous intravenous infusion) 400 units/hour for 2 hours, then (by continuous intravenous infusion) 300 units/hour for 2 hours, then (by continuous intravenous infusion) 200 units/hour for 5 days
▸ Adult (body-weight 90 kg and above): Initially 3750 units, then (by continuous intravenous infusion) 400 units/hour for 2 hours, then (by continuous intravenous infusion) 300 units/hour for 2 hours, then (by continuous intravenous infusion) 200 units/hour for 5 days

● CONTRA-INDICATIONS Active peptic ulcer (unless this is the reason for operation) · acute bacterial endocarditis · diabetic retinopathy · epidural anaesthesia (with treatment doses) · haemophilia and other haemorrhagic disorders · recent cerebral haemorrhage · severe uncontrolled hypertension · spinal anaesthesia (with treatment doses) · thrombocytopenia (unless patient has heparin-induced thrombocytopenia)

● CAUTIONS Antibodies to heparins (risk of antibody-induced thrombocytopenia) · body-weight over 90 kg · recent bleeding · risk of bleeding

● INTERACTIONS → Appendix 1: danaparoid

● SIDE-EFFECTS
▸ **Common or very common** Haemorrhage · heparin-induced thrombocytopenia · skin reactions · thrombocytopenia
▸ **Uncommon** Post procedural haematoma
▸ **Rare or very rare** Anastomotic haemorrhage

● PREGNANCY Manufacturer advises avoid—limited information available but not known to be harmful.

● BREAST FEEDING Amount probably too small to be harmful but manufacturer advises avoid.

● HEPATIC IMPAIRMENT Manufacturer advises caution in moderate impairment with impaired haemostasis—increased risk of bleeding; avoid in severe hepatic failure unless patient has heparin-induced thrombocytopenia and no alternative available.

● RENAL IMPAIRMENT Use with caution in moderate impairment. Avoid in severe impairment unless patient has heparin-induced thrombocytopenia and no alternative available.
Monitoring Increased risk of bleeding in renal impairment, monitor anti-Factor Xa activity.

● MONITORING REQUIREMENTS Monitor anti factor Xa activity in patients with body-weight over 90 kg.

● DIRECTIONS FOR ADMINISTRATION Manufacturer advises for *intravenous infusion*, give continuously in Glucose 5% or Sodium chloride 0.9%.

● MEDICINAL FORMS There can be variation in the licensing of different medicines containing the same drug.
Solution for injection
▸ Danaparoid sodium (Non-proprietary)
  Danaparoid sodium 1250 unit per 1 ml Danaparoid sodium 750units/0.6ml solution for injection ampoules | 10 ampoule [PoM] £599.99 (Hospital only)

ANTITHROMBOTIC DRUGS 〉 HEPARINS

Heparins

● CONTRA-INDICATIONS Acute bacterial endocarditis · after major trauma · Avoid injections containing benzyl alcohol in neonates · epidural anaesthesia with treatment doses · haemophilia or other haemorrhagic disorders · peptic ulcer · recent cerebral haemorrhage · recent surgery to eye · recent surgery to nervous system · spinal anaesthesia with treatment doses · thrombocytopenia (including history of heparin-induced thrombocytopenia)

● CAUTIONS Elderly · severe hypertension

● SIDE-EFFECTS
▸ **Common or very common** Haemorrhage · heparin-induced thrombocytopenia · skin reactions · thrombocytopenia · thrombocytosis
▸ **Uncommon** CNS haemorrhage
▸ **Rare or very rare** Alopecia · hyperkalaemia · osteoporosis (following long term use) · priapism
▸ **Frequency not known** Hypoaldosteronism

SIDE-EFFECTS, FURTHER INFORMATION **Haemorrhage** If haemorrhage occurs it is usually sufficient to withdraw unfractionated or low molecular weight heparin, but if rapid reversal of the effects of the heparin is required, protamine sulfate is a specific antidote (but only partially reverses the effects of low molecular weight heparins).

Heparin-induced thrombocytopenia Clinically important heparin-induced thrombocytopenia is immune-mediated and can be complicated by thrombosis. Signs of heparin-induced thrombocytopenia include a 30% reduction of platelet count, thrombosis, or skin allergy. If heparin-induced thrombocytopenia is strongly suspected or confirmed, the heparin should be stopped and an alternative anticoagulant, such as danaparoid, should be given. Ensure platelet counts return to normal range in those who require warfarin.

Hyperkalaemia Inhibition of aldosterone secretion by unfractionated or low molecular weight heparin can result in hyperkalaemia; patients with diabetes mellitus, chronic renal failure, acidosis, raised plasma potassium or those taking potassium-sparing drugs seem to be more susceptible. The risk appears to increase with duration of therapy.

● ALLERGY AND CROSS-SENSITIVITY Hypersensitivity to unfractionated or low molecular weight heparin.

● MONITORING REQUIREMENTS
▸ **Heparin-induced thrombocytopenia** Platelet counts should be measured just before treatment with unfractionated or low molecular weight heparin, and regular monitoring of platelet counts may be required if given for longer than 4 days. See the British Society for Haematology's Guidelines on the diagnosis and management of heparin-induced thrombocytopenia: second edition. *Br J Haematol* 2012; **159**: 528–540.
▸ **Hyperkalaemia** Plasma-potassium concentration should be measured in patients at risk of hyperkalaemia before starting the heparin and monitored regularly thereafter, particularly if treatment is to be continued for longer than 7 days.

▶ 142

Dalteparin sodium

04-Nov-2020

● **INDICATIONS AND DOSE**

FRAGMIN ®

Treatment of deep-vein thrombosis | Treatment of pulmonary embolism

▶ BY SUBCUTANEOUS INJECTION

▸ Adult: 200 units/kg daily (max. per dose 18 000 units) until adequate oral anticoagulation with vitamin K antagonist established (at least 5 days of combined treatment is usually required)

Treatment of deep-vein thrombosis (in patients at increased risk of haemorrhage) | Treatment of pulmonary embolism (in patients at increase risk of haemorrhage)

▶ BY SUBCUTANEOUS INJECTION

▸ Adult: 100 units/kg twice daily until adequate oral anticoagulation with vitamin K antagonist established (at least 5 days of combined treatment is usually required)

Unstable coronary artery disease

▶ BY SUBCUTANEOUS INJECTION

▸ Adult: 120 units/kg every 12 hours (max. per dose 10 000 units twice daily) for 5–8 days

Prevention of clotting in extracorporeal circuits

▶ TO THE DEVICE AS A FLUSH

▸ Adult: (consult product literature)

FRAGMIN ® GRADUATED SYRINGES

Unstable coronary artery disease (including non-ST-segment-elevation myocardial infarction)

▶ BY SUBCUTANEOUS INJECTION

▸ Adult: 120 units/kg every 12 hours (max. per dose 10 000 units twice daily) for up to 8 days

Patients with unstable coronary artery disease (including non-ST-segment-elevation myocardial infarction) awaiting angiography or revascularisation and having already had 8 days treatment with dalteparin

▶ BY SUBCUTANEOUS INJECTION

▸ Adult (body-weight up to 70 kg and male): 5000 units every 12 hours until the day of the procedure (max. 45 days).

▸ Adult (body-weight up to 80 kg and female): 5000 units every 12 hours until the day of the procedure (max. 45 days).

▸ Adult (body-weight 70 kg and above and male): 7500 units every 12 hours until the day of the procedure (max. 45 days).

▸ Adult (body-weight 80 kg and above and female): 7500 units every 12 hours until the day of the procedure (max. 45 days).

FRAGMIN ® SINGLE-DOSE SYRINGES

Prophylaxis of deep-vein thrombosis in surgical patients— moderate risk

▶ BY SUBCUTANEOUS INJECTION

▸ Adult: Initially 2500 units for 1 dose, dose to be given 1–2 hours before surgery, then 2500 units every 24 hours

Prophylaxis of deep-vein thrombosis in surgical patients— high risk

▶ BY SUBCUTANEOUS INJECTION

▸ Adult: Initially 2500 units for 1 dose, dose to be administered 1–2 hours before surgery, followed by 2500 units after 8–12 hours, then 5000 units every 24 hours, alternatively initially 5000 units for 1 dose, dose to be given on the evening before surgery, followed by 5000 units after 24 hours, then 5000 units every 24 hours

Prophylaxis of deep-vein thrombosis in medical patients

▶ BY SUBCUTANEOUS INJECTION

▸ Adult: 5000 units every 24 hours

Treatment of deep-vein thrombosis | Treatment of pulmonary embolism

▶ BY SUBCUTANEOUS INJECTION

▸ Adult (body-weight up to 46 kg): 7500 units once daily until adequate oral anticoagulation with vitamin K antagonist established (at least 5 days of combined treatment is usually required)

▸ Adult (body-weight 46-56 kg): 10 000 units once daily until adequate oral anticoagulation with vitamin K antagonist established (at least 5 days of combined treatment is usually required)

▸ Adult (body-weight 57-68 kg): 12 500 units once daily until adequate oral anticoagulation with vitamin K antagonist established (at least 5 days of combined treatment is usually required)

▸ Adult (body-weight 69-82 kg): 15 000 units once daily until adequate oral anticoagulation with vitamin K antagonist established (at least 5 days of combined treatment is usually required)

▸ Adult (body-weight 83 kg and above): 18 000 units once daily until adequate oral anticoagulation with vitamin K antagonist established (at least 5 days of combined treatment is usually required)

Extended treatment of venous thromboembolism and prevention of recurrence in patients with solid tumours

▶ BY SUBCUTANEOUS INJECTION

▸ Adult (body-weight 40-45 kg): 7500 units once daily for 30 days, then 7500 units once daily for a further 5 months, interrupt treatment or reduce dose in chemotherapy-induced thrombocytopenia—consult product literature

▸ Adult (body-weight 46-56 kg): 10 000 units once daily for 30 days, then 7500 units once daily for a further 5 months, interrupt treatment or reduce dose in chemotherapy-induced thrombocytopenia—consult product literature

▸ Adult (body-weight 57-68 kg): 12 500 units once daily for 30 days, then 10 000 units once daily for a further 5 months, interrupt treatment or reduce dose in chemotherapy-induced thrombocytopenia—consult product literature

▸ Adult (body-weight 69-82 kg): 15 000 units once daily for 30 days, then 12 500 units once daily for a further 5 months, interrupt treatment or reduce dose in chemotherapy-induced thrombocytopenia—consult product literature

▸ Adult (body-weight 83-98 kg): 18 000 units once daily for 30 days, then 15 000 units once daily for a further 5 months, interrupt treatment or reduce dose in chemotherapy-induced thrombocytopenia—consult product literature

▸ Adult (body-weight 99 kg and above): 18 000 units once daily for 30 days, then 18 000 units once daily for a further 5 months, interrupt treatment or reduce dose in chemotherapy-induced thrombocytopenia—consult product literature

Treatment of venous thromboembolism in pregnancy

▶ BY SUBCUTANEOUS INJECTION

▸ Adult (body-weight up to 50 kg): 5000 units twice daily, use body-weight in early pregnancy to calculate the dose

▸ Adult (body-weight 50-69 kg): 6000 units twice daily, use body-weight in early pregnancy to calculate the dose

▸ Adult (body-weight 70-89 kg): 8000 units twice daily, use body-weight in early pregnancy to calculate the dose

▸ Adult (body-weight 90 kg and above): 10 000 units twice daily, use body-weight in early pregnancy to calculate the dose

2

Cardiovascular system

2

Cardiovascular system

- UNLICENSED USE Not licensed for treatment of venous thromboembolism in pregnancy.
- INTERACTIONS → Appendix 1: low molecular-weight heparins
- SIDE-EFFECTS Epidural haematoma · prosthetic cardiac valve thrombosis
- PREGNANCY Not known to be harmful, low molecular weight heparins do not cross the placenta. Multidose vial contains benzyl alcohol—manufacturer advises avoid.
- BREAST FEEDING Due to the relatively high molecular weight and inactivation in the gastro-intestinal tract, passage into breast-milk and absorption by the nursing infant are likely to be negligible, however manufacturers advise avoid.
- HEPATIC IMPAIRMENT Manufacturer advises caution in severe impairment (increased risk of bleeding complications).
  Dose adjustments Manufacturer advises consider dose reduction in severe impairment.
- RENAL IMPAIRMENT Use of unfractionated heparin may be preferable.
  Dose adjustments Risk of bleeding may be increased—dose reduction may be required.
- MONITORING REQUIREMENTS
  ▸ For monitoring during treatment of deep-vein thrombosis and of pulmonary embolism, blood should be taken 3–4 hours after a dose (recommended plasma concentration of anti-Factor Xa 0.5–1 unit/mL); monitoring not required for once-daily treatment regimen and not generally necessary for twice-daily regimen.
  ▸ Routine monitoring of anti-Factor Xa activity is not usually required during treatment with dalteparin, but may be necessary in patients at increased risk of bleeding (e.g. in renal impairment and those who are underweight or overweight).
- NATIONAL FUNDING/ACCESS DECISIONS
  For full details see funding body website
  Scottish Medicines Consortium (SMC) decisions
  ▸ Dalteparin (*Fragmin®*) for use in patients with solid tumours: extended treatment of symptomatic VTE and prevention of recurrence (March 2011) SMC No. 683/11 Recommended with restrictions

- MEDICINAL FORMS There can be variation in the licensing of different medicines containing the same drug.
  Solution for injection
  EXCIPIENTS: May contain Benzyl alcohol
  ▸ Fragmin (Pfizer Ltd)
  Dalteparin sodium 2500 unit per 1 ml Fragmin 10,000units/4ml solution for injection ampoules | 10 ampoule [PoM] £51.22 DT = £51.22
  Dalteparin sodium 10000 unit per 1 ml Fragmin 10,000units/1ml solution for injection pre-filled syringes | 5 pre-filled disposable injection [PoM] £28.23 DT = £28.23
  Fragmin 10,000units/1ml solution for injection ampoules | 10 ampoule [PoM] £51.22 DT = £51.22
  Dalteparin sodium 12500 unit per 1 ml Fragmin 2,500units/0.2ml solution for injection pre-filled syringes | 10 pre-filled disposable injection [PoM] £18.58 DT = £18.58
  Dalteparin sodium 25000 unit per 1 ml Fragmin 18,000units/0.72ml solution for injection pre-filled syringes | 5 pre-filled disposable injection [PoM] £50.82 DT = £50.82
  Fragmin 15,000units/0.6ml solution for injection pre-filled syringes | 5 pre-filled disposable injection [PoM] £42.34 DT = £42.34
  Fragmin 5,000units/0.2ml solution for injection pre-filled syringes | 10 pre-filled disposable injection [PoM] £28.23 DT = £28.23
  Fragmin 12,500units/0.5ml solution for injection pre-filled syringes | 5 pre-filled disposable injection [PoM] £35.29 DT = £35.29
  Fragmin 7,500units/0.3ml solution for injection pre-filled syringes | 10 pre-filled disposable injection [PoM] £42.34 DT = £42.34
  Fragmin 100,000units/4ml solution for injection vials | 1 vial [PoM] £48.66 DT = £48.66
  Fragmin 10,000units/0.4ml solution for injection pre-filled syringes | 5 pre-filled disposable injection [PoM] £28.23 DT = £28.23

▶ 142

Enoxaparin sodium

06-Aug-2020

- INDICATIONS AND DOSE
  Treatment of venous thromboembolism in pregnancy
  ▸ BY SUBCUTANEOUS INJECTION
  ▸ Adult (body-weight up to 50 kg): 40 mg twice daily, dose based on early pregnancy body-weight
  ▸ Adult (body-weight 50–69 kg): 60 mg twice daily, dose based on early pregnancy body-weight
  ▸ Adult (body-weight 70–89 kg): 80 mg twice daily, dose based on early pregnancy body-weight
  ▸ Adult (body-weight 90 kg and above): 100 mg twice daily, dose based on early pregnancy body-weight
  Prophylaxis of deep-vein thrombosis, especially in surgical patients—moderate risk
  ▸ BY SUBCUTANEOUS INJECTION
  ▸ Adult: 20 mg for 1 dose, dose to be given approximately 2 hours before surgery, then 20 mg every 24 hours
  Prophylaxis of deep-vein thrombosis, especially surgical patients—high risk (e.g. orthopaedic surgery)
  ▸ BY SUBCUTANEOUS INJECTION
  ▸ Adult: 40 mg for 1 dose, dose to be given 12 hours before surgery, then 40 mg every 24 hours
  Prophylaxis of deep-vein thrombosis in medical patients
  ▸ BY SUBCUTANEOUS INJECTION
  ▸ Adult: 40 mg every 24 hours
  Treatment of deep-vein thrombosis in uncomplicated patients with low risk of recurrence | Treatment of pulmonary embolism in uncomplicated patients with low risk of recurrence
  ▸ BY SUBCUTANEOUS INJECTION
  ▸ Adult: 1.5 mg/kg every 24 hours until adequate oral anticoagulation established
  Treatment of deep-vein thrombosis in patients with risk factors such as obesity, cancer, recurrent VTE, or proximal thrombosis | Treatment of pulmonary embolism in patients with risk factors such as obesity, symptomatic pulmonary embolism, cancer, or recurrent VTE
  ▸ BY SUBCUTANEOUS INJECTION
  ▸ Adult: 1 mg/kg every 12 hours until adequate oral anticoagulation established
  Treatment of acute ST-segment elevation myocardial infarction (patients not undergoing percutaneous coronary intervention)
  ▸ INITIALLY BY INTRAVENOUS INJECTION
  ▸ Adult 18–74 years: Initially 30 mg, followed by (by subcutaneous injection) 1 mg/kg for 1 dose, then (by subcutaneous injection) 1 mg/kg every 12 hours (max. per dose 100 mg) for up to 8 days, maximum dose applies for the first two subcutaneous doses only
  ▸ BY SUBCUTANEOUS INJECTION
  ▸ Adult 75 years and over: 750 micrograms/kg every 12 hours (max. per dose 75 mg), maximum dose applies for the first two doses only
  Treatment of acute ST-segment elevation myocardial infarction (patients undergoing percutaneous coronary intervention)
  ▸ INITIALLY BY INTRAVENOUS INJECTION
  ▸ Adult 18–74 years: Initially 30 mg, followed by (by subcutaneous injection) 1 mg/kg for 1 dose, then (by subcutaneous injection) 1 mg/kg every 12 hours (max. per dose 100 mg) for up to 8 days, maximum dose applies for the first two subcutaneous doses only, then (by intravenous injection) 300 micrograms/kg for 1 dose, dose to be given at the time of procedure if the last subcutaneous dose was given more than 8 hours previously

▸ INITIALLY BY SUBCUTANEOUS INJECTION
▸ **Adult 75 years and over:** 750 micrograms/kg every 12 hours (max. per dose 75 mg), maximum dose applies for the first two doses only, then (by intravenous injection) 300 micrograms/kg for 1 dose, dose to be given at the time of procedure if the last subcutaneous dose was given more than 8 hours previously

Unstable angina | Non-ST-segment-elevation myocardial infarction
▸ BY SUBCUTANEOUS INJECTION
▸ **Adult:** 1 mg/kg every 12 hours usually for 2–8 days (minimum 2 days)

Prevention of clotting in extracorporeal circuits
▸ TO THE DEVICE AS A FLUSH
▸ **Adult:** (consult product literature)
DOSE EQUIVALENCE AND CONVERSION
▸ 1 mg equivalent to 100 units.

● UNLICENSED USE Not licensed for treatment of venous thromboembolism in pregnancy.
● CAUTIONS Low body-weight (increased risk of bleeding)
● INTERACTIONS → Appendix 1: low molecular-weight heparins
● SIDE-EFFECTS
▸ **Common or very common** Haemorrhagic anaemia · headache · hypersensitivity
▸ **Uncommon** Hepatic disorders · injection site necrosis
▸ **Rare or very rare** Cutaneous vasculitis · eosinophilia
● PREGNANCY Not known to be harmful, low molecular weight heparins do not cross the placenta. Multidose vial contains benzyl alcohol—avoid.
● BREAST FEEDING Manufacturer advises suitable for use during breast feeding—passage into breast milk and absorption by the nursing infant considered to be negligible due to the relatively high molecular weight of enoxaparin and inactivation in the gastro-intestinal tract.
● HEPATIC IMPAIRMENT Manufacturer advises caution—no information available.
● RENAL IMPAIRMENT Risk of bleeding increased; use of unfractionated heparin may be preferable. Manufacturer advises avoid if creatinine clearance less than 15 mL/minute.
Dose adjustments Manufacturer advises reduce dose if creatinine clearance 15–30 mL/minute—consult product literature for details.
● MONITORING REQUIREMENTS Routine monitoring of anti-Factor Xa activity is not usually required during treatment with enoxaparin, but may be necessary in patients at increased risk of bleeding (e.g. in renal impairment and those who are underweight or overweight).
● DIRECTIONS FOR ADMINISTRATION When administered in conjunction with a thrombolytic, manufacturer advises enoxaparin should be given between 15 minutes before and 30 minutes after the start of thrombolytic therapy.
● PRESCRIBING AND DISPENSING INFORMATION Enoxaparin sodium is a biological medicine. Biological medicines must be prescribed and dispensed by brand name, see *Biological medicines* and *Biosimilar medicines*, under Guidance on prescribing p. 1.

● MEDICINAL FORMS There can be variation in the licensing of different medicines containing the same drug.

Solution for injection
EXCIPIENTS: May contain Benzyl alcohol
▸ Arovi (ROVI Biotech Ltd) ▼
   Enoxaparin sodium 100 mg per 1 ml Arovi 20mg/0.2ml solution for injection pre-filled syringes | 10 pre-filled disposable injection [PoM] £15.65 DT = £20.86
   Arovi 60mg/0.6ml solution for injection pre-filled syringes | 10 pre-filled disposable injection [PoM] £29.45 DT = £39.26

Arovi 40mg/0.4ml solution for injection pre-filled syringes | 10 pre-filled disposable injection [PoM] £22.70 DT = £30.27
Arovi 80mg/0.8ml solution for injection pre-filled syringes | 10 pre-filled disposable injection [PoM] £41.35 DT = £55.13
Arovi 100mg/1ml solution for injection pre-filled syringes | 10 pre-filled disposable injection [PoM] £54.23 DT = £72.30
Enoxaparin sodium 150 mg per 1 ml Arovi 150mg/1ml solution for injection pre-filled syringes | 10 pre-filled disposable injection [PoM] £74.93 DT = £99.91
Arovi 120mg/0.8ml solution for injection pre-filled syringes | 10 pre-filled disposable injection [PoM] £65.95 DT = £87.93
▸ Clexane (Sanofi)
   Enoxaparin sodium 100 mg per 1 ml Clexane 60mg/0.6ml solution for injection pre-filled syringes | 10 pre-filled disposable injection [PoM] £39.26 DT = £39.26
   Clexane 300mg/3ml solution for injection multidose vials | 1 vial [PoM] £21.33 DT = £21.33
   Clexane 80mg/0.8ml solution for injection pre-filled syringes | 10 pre-filled disposable injection [PoM] £55.13 DT = £55.13
   Clexane 40mg/0.4ml solution for injection pre-filled syringes | 10 pre-filled disposable injection [PoM] £30.27 DT = £30.27
   Clexane 100mg/1ml solution for injection pre-filled syringes | 10 pre-filled disposable injection [PoM] £72.30 DT = £72.30
   Clexane 20mg/0.2ml solution for injection pre-filled syringes | 10 pre-filled disposable injection [PoM] £20.86 DT = £20.86
   Enoxaparin sodium 150 mg per 1 ml Clexane Forte 120mg/0.8ml solution for injection pre-filled syringes | 10 pre-filled disposable injection [PoM] £87.93 DT = £87.93
   Clexane Forte 150mg/1ml solution for injection pre-filled syringes | 10 pre-filled disposable injection [PoM] £99.91 DT = £99.91
▸ Inhixa (Techdow Pharma England Ltd) ▼
   Enoxaparin sodium 100 mg per 1 ml Inhixa 40mg/0.4ml solution for injection pre-filled syringes | 10 pre-filled disposable injection [PoM] £30.27 DT = £30.27
   Inhixa 80mg/0.8ml solution for injection pre-filled syringes | 10 pre-filled disposable injection [PoM] £55.13 DT = £55.13
   Inhixa 60mg/0.6ml solution for injection pre-filled syringes | 10 pre-filled disposable injection [PoM] £39.26 DT = £39.26
   Inhixa 100mg/1ml solution for injection pre-filled syringes | 10 pre-filled disposable injection [PoM] £72.30 DT = £72.30
   Inhixa 20mg/0.2ml solution for injection pre-filled syringes | 10 pre-filled disposable injection [PoM] £20.86 DT = £20.86
   Inhixa 300mg/3ml solution for injection multidose vials | 1 vial [PoM] £21.33 DT = £21.33
   Enoxaparin sodium 150 mg per 1 ml Inhixa 120mg/0.8ml solution for injection pre-filled syringes | 10 pre-filled disposable injection [PoM] £87.93 DT = £87.93
   Inhixa 150mg/1ml solution for injection pre-filled syringes | 10 pre-filled disposable injection [PoM] £99.91 DT = £99.91

◀ 142

Heparin (unfractionated)   05-May-2017

● INDICATIONS AND DOSE
Treatment of mild to moderate pulmonary embolism | Treatment of unstable angina | Treatment of acute peripheral arterial occlusion
▸ INITIALLY BY INTRAVENOUS INJECTION
▸ **Adult:** Loading dose 5000 units, alternatively (by intravenous injection) loading dose 75 units/kg, followed by (by continuous intravenous infusion) 18 units/kg/hour, laboratory monitoring essential—preferably on a daily basis, and dose adjusted accordingly

Treatment of severe pulmonary embolism
▸ INITIALLY BY INTRAVENOUS INJECTION
▸ **Adult:** Loading dose 10 000 units, followed by (by continuous intravenous infusion) 18 units/kg/hour, laboratory monitoring essential—preferably on a daily basis, and dose adjusted accordingly

Treatment of deep-vein thrombosis
▸ INITIALLY BY INTRAVENOUS INJECTION
▸ **Adult:** Loading dose 5000 units, alternatively (by intravenous injection) loading dose 75 units/kg, followed by (by continuous intravenous infusion) 18 units/kg/hour, alternatively (by subcutaneous injection) 15 000 units every 12 hours,   continued →

2

Cardiovascular system

laboratory monitoring essential—preferably on a daily basis, and dose adjusted accordingly

Thromboprophylaxis in medical patients

▸ BY SUBCUTANEOUS INJECTION

▸ Adult: 5000 units every 8–12 hours

Thrombophylaxis in surgical patients

▸ BY SUBCUTANEOUS INJECTION

▸ Adult: 5000 units for 1 dose, to be taken 2 hours before surgery, then 5000 units every 8–12 hours

Thromboprophylaxis during pregnancy

▸ BY SUBCUTANEOUS INJECTION

▸ Adult: 5000–10 000 units every 12 hours, to be administered with monitoring, **Important**: prevention of prosthetic heart-valve thrombosis in pregnancy calls for **specialist management**

Haemodialysis

▸ INITIALLY BY INTRAVENOUS INJECTION

▸ Adult: Initially 1000–5000 units, followed by (by continuous intravenous infusion) 250–1000 units/hour

Prevention of clotting in extracorporeal circuits

▸ TO THE DEVICE AS A FLUSH

▸ Adult: (consult product literature)

To maintain patency of catheters, cannulas, other indwelling intravenous infusion devices

▸ TO THE DEVICE AS A FLUSH

▸ Adult: 10–200 units, to be flushed through every 4–8 hours, not for therapeutic use

● INTERACTIONS → Appendix 1: heparin

● SIDE-EFFECTS Adrenal insufficiency · hypokalaemia · rebound hyperlipidaemia

● PREGNANCY Does not cross the placenta; maternal osteoporosis reported after prolonged use; multidose vials may contain benzyl alcohol—some manufacturers advise avoid.

● BREAST FEEDING Not excreted into milk due to high molecular weight.

● HEPATIC IMPAIRMENT Manufacturer advises caution; consider avoiding in severe impairment (increased risk of bleeding complications).
Dose adjustments Manufacturer advises consider dose reduction if used in severe impairment.

● RENAL IMPAIRMENT
Dose adjustments Risk of bleeding increased in severe impairment—dose may need to be reduced.

● DIRECTIONS FOR ADMINISTRATION For *intravenous infusion*, give continuously in Glucose 5% or Sodium chloride 0.9%; administration with a motorised pump is advisable.

● PRESCRIBING AND DISPENSING INFORMATION Doses listed take into account the guidelines of the British Society for Haematology.

● MEDICINAL FORMS There can be variation in the licensing of different medicines containing the same drug. Forms available from special-order manufacturers include: solution for injection, solution for infusion

Solution for injection
EXCIPIENTS: May contain Benzyl alcohol
▸ Heparin (unfractionated) (Non-proprietary)
Heparin sodium 1000 unit per 1 ml Heparin sodium 1,000units/1ml solution for injection ampoules | 10 ampoule [PoM] £14.85 DT = £14.85
Heparin sodium 5,000units/5ml solution for injection vials | 10 vial [PoM] £16.50–£37.41 DT = £16.50
Heparin sodium 20,000units/20ml solution for injection ampoules | 10 ampoule [PoM] £70.88 DT = £70.88
Heparin sodium 5,000units/5ml solution for injection ampoules | 10 ampoule [PoM] £37.47 DT = £37.47
Heparin sodium 10,000units/10ml solution for injection ampoules | 10 ampoule [PoM] £64.59 DT = £64.59

Heparin sodium 5000 unit per 1 ml Heparin sodium 5,000units/1ml solution for injection ampoules | 10 ampoule [PoM] £29.04 DT = £29.04
Heparin sodium 25,000units/5ml solution for injection vials | 10 vial [PoM] £45.00–£84.60 DT = £45.00
Heparin sodium 25,000units/5ml solution for injection ampoules | 10 ampoule [PoM] £28.90–£75.78 DT = £75.78
Heparin calcium 25000 unit per 1 ml Heparin calcium 5,000units/0.2ml solution for injection ampoules | 10 ampoule [PoM] £44.70 DT = £44.70
Heparin sodium 25000 unit per 1 ml Heparin sodium 25,000units/1ml solution for injection ampoules | 10 ampoule [PoM] £76.95 DT = £76.95
Heparin sodium 5,000units/0.2ml solution for injection ampoules | 10 ampoule [PoM] £37.35 DT = £37.35

Intravenous flush
EXCIPIENTS: May contain Benzyl alcohol
▸ Heparin (unfractionated) (Non-proprietary)
Heparin sodium 10 unit per 1 ml Heparin sodium 50units/5ml patency solution ampoules | 10 ampoule [PoM] £14.96 DT = £14.96
Heparin sodium 50units/5ml I.V. flush solution ampoules | 10 ampoule [PoM] £14.96 DT = £14.96
Heparin sodium 100 unit per 1 ml Heparin sodium 200units/2ml I.V. flush solution ampoules | 10 ampoule [PoM] £15.68 DT = £15.68
Heparin sodium 200units/2ml patency solution ampoules | 10 ampoule [PoM] £15.68 DT = £15.68

Infusion
▸ Heparin (unfractionated) (Non-proprietary)
Heparin sodium 1 unit per 1 ml Heparin sodium 500units/500ml infusion Viaflex bags | 1 bag [PoM] [🅂]
Heparin sodium 2 unit per 1 ml Heparin sodium 1,000units/500ml infusion Viaflex bags | 1 bag [PoM] [🅂]
Heparin sodium 2,000units/1litre infusion Viaflex bags | 1 bag [PoM] [🅂]
Heparin sodium 5 unit per 1 ml Heparin sodium 5,000units/1litre infusion Viaflex bags | 1 bag [PoM] [🅂]

🠖 142

Tinzaparin sodium

06-Aug-2018

● INDICATIONS AND DOSE

INNOHEP ® 10,000 UNITS/ML

Prophylaxis of deep-vein thrombosis (general surgery)

▸ BY SUBCUTANEOUS INJECTION

▸ Adult: 3500 units for 1 dose, dose to be given 2 hours before surgery, then 3500 units every 24 hours

Prophylaxis of deep-vein thrombosis (orthopaedic surgery)

▸ BY SUBCUTANEOUS INJECTION

▸ Adult: Initially 50 units/kg for 1 dose, dose to be given 2 hours before surgery, then 50 units/kg every 24 hours, alternatively initially 4500 units for 1 dose, dose to be given 12 hours before surgery, then 4500 units every 24 hours

Prevention of clotting in extracorporeal circuits

▸ TO THE DEVICE AS A FLUSH

▸ Adult: (consult product literature)

INNOHEP ® 20,000 UNITS/ML

Extended treatment of venous thromboembolism and prevention of recurrence in patients with active cancer

▸ BY SUBCUTANEOUS INJECTION

▸ Adult: 175 units/kg once daily for 6 months; the benefit of continued treatment beyond 6 months should be evaluated

Treatment of deep-vein thrombosis | Treatment of pulmonary embolism

▸ BY SUBCUTANEOUS INJECTION

▸ Adult: 175 units/kg once daily until adequate oral anticoagulation established, treatment regimens do not require anticoagulation monitoring

Treatment of venous thromboembolism in pregnancy
▶ BY SUBCUTANEOUS INJECTION
▸ **Adult:** 175 units/kg once daily, dose based on early pregnancy body-weight, treatment regimens do not require anticoagulation monitoring

● UNLICENSED USE Not licensed for the treatment of venous thromboembolism in pregnancy.

● INTERACTIONS → Appendix 1: low molecular-weight heparins

● SIDE-EFFECTS
▸ **Common or very common** Anaemia
▸ **Rare or very rare** Angioedema · Stevens-Johnson syndrome

● PREGNANCY Not known to be harmful, low molecular weight heparins do not cross the placenta. Vials contain benzyl alcohol—manufacturer advises avoid.

● BREAST FEEDING Due to the relatively high molecular weight of tinzaparin and inactivation in the gastro-intestinal tract, passage into breast-milk and absorption by the nursing infant are likely to be negligible; however manufacturer advise avoid.

● RENAL IMPAIRMENT Risk of bleeding may be increased. Unfractionated heparin may be preferable. Manufacturer advises caution if eGFR less than 30 mL/minute/1.73 m^2.
Monitoring In renal impairment monitoring of anti-Factor Xa may be required if eGFR less than 30 mL/minute/1.73 m^2.

● MONITORING REQUIREMENTS Routine monitoring of anti-Factor Xa activity is not usually required during treatment with tinzaparin, but may be necessary in patients at increased risk of bleeding (e.g. in renal impairment and those who are underweight or overweight).

● MEDICINAL FORMS There can be variation in the licensing of different medicines containing the same drug.
Solution for injection
EXCIPIENTS: May contain Benzyl alcohol, sulfites
▸ Innohep (LEO Pharma)
  Tinzaparin sodium 10000 unit per 1 ml Innohep 20,000units/2ml solution for injection vials | 10 vial PoM £105.66 DT = £105.66
  Tinzaparin sodium 20000 unit per 1 ml Innohep 18,000units/0.9ml solution for injection pre-filled syringes | 6 pre-filled disposable injection PoM £64.25 | 10 pre-filled disposable injection PoM £107.08 DT = £107.08
  Innohep 40,000units/2ml solution for injection vials | 1 vial PoM £34.20 DT = £34.20 | 10 vial PoM £342.00
  Innohep 14,000units/0.7ml solution for injection pre-filled syringes | 6 pre-filled disposable injection PoM £49.98 | 10 pre-filled disposable injection PoM £83.30 DT = £83.30
  Innohep 10,000units/0.5ml solution for injection pre-filled syringes | 6 pre-filled disposable injection PoM £35.70 | 10 pre-filled disposable injection PoM £59.50 DT = £59.50

ANTITHROMBOTIC DRUGS ⟩ THROMBIN INHIBITORS, DIRECT

Argatroban monohydrate   21-Aug-2018

● INDICATIONS AND DOSE
Anticoagulation in patients with heparin-induced thrombocytopenia type II who require parenteral antithrombotic treatment
▶ INITIALLY BY CONTINUOUS INTRAVENOUS INFUSION
▸ **Adult:** Initially 2 micrograms/kg/minute, dose to be adjusted according to activated partial thromboplastin time, (by intravenous infusion) increased to up to 10 micrograms/kg/minute maximum duration of treatment 14 days

Anticoagulation in patients with heparin-induced thrombocytopenia type II who require parenteral antithrombotic treatment (for dose in cardiac surgery, percutaneous coronary intervention, or critically ill patients)
▶ BY CONTINUOUS INTRAVENOUS INFUSION
▸ **Adult:** (consult product literature)

Anticoagulation in patients with heparin-induced thrombocytopenia type II who require parenteral antithrombotic treatment (when initiating concomitant warfarin treatment)
▶ BY CONTINUOUS INTRAVENOUS INFUSION
▸ **Adult:** Reduced to 2 micrograms/kg/minute, dose should be temporarily reduced and INR measured after 4–6 hours; warfarin should be initiated at intended maintenance dose (do not give loading dose of warfarin); consult product literature for further details

● CAUTIONS Bleeding disorders · diabetic retinopathy · gastro-intestinal ulceration · immediately after lumbar puncture · major surgery (especially of brain, spinal cord, or eye) · risk of bleeding · severe hypertension · spinal anaesthesia

● INTERACTIONS → Appendix 1: thrombin inhibitors

● SIDE-EFFECTS
▸ **Common or very common** Anaemia · haemorrhage · nausea · skin reactions
▸ **Uncommon** Alopecia · appetite decreased · arrhythmias · cardiac arrest · confusion · constipation · deafness · diarrhoea · dizziness · dysphagia · dyspnoea · fatigue · fever · gastritis · headache · hepatic disorders · hiccups · hyperbilirubinaemia · hyperhidrosis · hypertension · hypoglycaemia · hyponatraemia · hypotension · hypoxia · increased risk of infection · leucopenia · muscle tone decreased · muscle weakness · myalgia · myocardial infarction · pain · pericardial effusion · peripheral ischaemia · peripheral oedema · pleural effusion · renal failure · shock · speech disorder · stroke · syncope · thrombocytopenia · tongue disorder · visual impairment · vomiting · wound secretion

● PREGNANCY Manufacturer advises avoid unless essential—limited information available.

● BREAST FEEDING Avoid—no information available.

● HEPATIC IMPAIRMENT Manufacturer advises caution in mild to moderate impairment—monitor aPTT; avoid in severe impairment or in patients with impairment undergoing percutaneous coronary intervention.
Dose adjustments Manufacturer advises reduce initial dose to 0.5 micrograms/kg/minute in moderate impairment; adjust dose according to aPTT and as clinically indicated—consult product literature.

● MONITORING REQUIREMENTS Determine activated partial thromboplastin time 2 hours after start of treatment, then 2 or 4 hours after infusion rate altered (consult product literature), and at least once daily thereafter.

● DIRECTIONS FOR ADMINISTRATION For *intravenous infusion* (*Exembol - Ready to use*®), manufacturer advises administer 1 mg/mL solution via a syringe driver. For *intravenous infusion* (*Exembol - Multidose*®), manufacturer advises give continuously in Glucose 5%, Sodium chloride 0.9% or Sodium lactate intravenous infusion compound; dilute to a concentration of 1 mg/mL prior to use.

● MEDICINAL FORMS There can be variation in the licensing of different medicines containing the same drug.
Solution for infusion
EXCIPIENTS: May contain Ethanol
▸ Argatroban monohydrate (Non-proprietary)
  Argatroban monohydrate 1 mg per 1 ml Argatroban 50mg/50ml solution for infusion vials | 1 vial PoM £49.69 (Hospital only)

▸ Exembol (Mitsubishi Tanabe Pharma Europe Ltd)
Argatroban monohydrate 1 mg per 1 ml Exembol 50mg/50ml solution for infusion vials | 4 vial $\boxed{\text{PoM}}$ £198.80 (Hospital only)
Argatroban monohydrate 100 mg per 1 ml Exembol Multidose 250mg/2.5ml concentrate for solution for infusion vials | 1 vial $\boxed{\text{PoM}}$ £248.50

Bivalirudin
03-Nov-2020

● DRUG ACTION Bivalirudin, a hirudin analogue, is a thrombin inhibitor.

● INDICATIONS AND DOSE

Unstable angina or non-ST-segment elevation myocardial infarction in patients planned for urgent or early intervention (in addition to aspirin and clopidogrel)

▸ INITIALLY BY INTRAVENOUS INJECTION
▸ Adult: Initially 100 micrograms/kg, then (by intravenous infusion) 250 micrograms/kg/hour (for up to 72 hours in medically managed patients)

Unstable angina or non-ST-segment elevation myocardial infarction (in addition to aspirin and clopidogrel) in patients proceeding to percutaneous coronary intervention or coronary artery bypass surgery without cardiopulmonary bypass

▸ INITIALLY BY INTRAVENOUS INJECTION
▸ Adult: Initially 100 micrograms/kg for 1 dose, then (by intravenous injection) 500 micrograms/kg for 1 dose, then (by intravenous infusion) 1.75 mg/kg/hour for duration of procedure; (by intravenous infusion) reduced to 250 micrograms/kg/hour for 4–12 hours as necessary following percutaneous coronary intervention, for patients proceeding to coronary artery bypass surgery with cardiopulmonary bypass, discontinue intravenous infusion 1 hour before procedure and treat with unfractionated heparin

Anticoagulation in patients undergoing percutaneous coronary intervention including patients with ST-segment elevation myocardial infarction undergoing primary percutaneous coronary intervention (in addition to aspirin and clopidogrel)

▸ INITIALLY BY INTRAVENOUS INJECTION
▸ Adult: Initially 750 micrograms/kg, followed immediately by (by intravenous infusion) 1.75 mg/kg/hour during procedure and for up to 4 hours after procedure, then (by intravenous infusion) reduced to 250 micrograms/kg/hour for a further 4–12 hours if necessary

● CONTRA-INDICATIONS Bleeding (active) · bleeding disorders · hypertension (severe) · subacute bacterial endocarditis

● CAUTIONS Brachytherapy procedures · previous exposure to lepirudin (theoretical risk from lepirudin antibodies)

● INTERACTIONS → Appendix 1: thrombin inhibitors

● SIDE-EFFECTS
▸ **Common or very common** Procedural complications · skin reactions
▸ **Uncommon** Anaemia · headache · hypersensitivity · hypotension · nausea · shock · thrombocytopenia
▸ **Rare or very rare** Arrhythmias · cardiac tamponade · chest pain · compartment syndrome · dyspnoea · embolism and thrombosis · intracranial haemorrhage · pain · vascular disorders · vomiting

● PREGNANCY Manufacturer advises avoid unless potential benefit outweighs risk—no information available.

● BREAST FEEDING Manufacturer advises caution—no information available.

● RENAL IMPAIRMENT Avoid if eGFR less than 30 mL/minute/1.73 m^2.

Dose adjustments
▸ When used for percutaneous coronary intervention Reduce rate of infusion to 1.4 mg/kg/hour if eGFR 30–60 mL/minute/1.73 m^2 and monitor blood clotting parameters.

● DIRECTIONS FOR ADMINISTRATION For *intravenous infusion*, manufacturer advises give continuously in Glucose 5% or Sodium chloride 0.9%. Reconstitute each 250-mg vial with 5 mL water for injections then withdraw 5 mL and dilute to 50 mL with infusion fluid.

● NATIONAL FUNDING/ACCESS DECISIONS
For full details see funding body website

NICE decisions
▸ Bivalirudin for the treatment of ST-segment elevation myocardial infarction (July 2011) NICE TA230 Recommended

Scottish Medicines Consortium (SMC) decisions
▸ Bivalirudin (Angiox®) for acute coronary syndromes (December 2008) SMC No. 516/08 Recommended with restrictions
▸ Bivalirudin (Angiox®) as an anticoagulant in adult patients undergoing PCI, including patients with ST-segment elevation myocardial infarction (STEMI) undergoing primary PCI (September 2010) SMC No. 638/10 Recommended with restrictions

● MEDICINAL FORMS There can be variation in the licensing of different medicines containing the same drug.

Powder for solution for infusion
▸ Bivalirudin (Non-proprietary)
Bivalirudin 250 mg Bivalirudin 250mg powder for concentrate for solution for infusion vials | 1 vial $\boxed{\text{PoM}}$ £175.00 (Hospital only) | 5 vial $\boxed{\text{PoM}}$ £875.00 (Hospital only)

Dabigatran etexilate
17-Nov-2020

● DRUG ACTION Dabigatran etexilate is a direct thrombin inhibitor with a rapid onset of action.

● INDICATIONS AND DOSE

Prophylaxis of venous thromboembolism following total knee replacement surgery

▸ BY MOUTH
▸ Adult 18–74 years: 110 mg, to be taken 1–4 hours after surgery, followed by 220 mg once daily for 10 days, to be taken on the first day after surgery
▸ Adult 75 years and over: 75 mg, to be taken 1–4 hours after surgery, followed by 150 mg once daily for 10 days, to be taken on the first day after surgery

Prophylaxis of venous thromboembolism following total knee replacement surgery in patients receiving concomitant treatment with amiodarone or verapamil

▸ BY MOUTH
▸ Adult 18–74 years: 75 mg, to be taken 1–4 hours after surgery, followed by 150 mg once daily for 10 days, to be taken on the first day after surgery
▸ Adult 75 years and over: 75 mg, to be taken 1–4 hours after surgery, followed by 150 mg once daily for 10 days, to be taken on the first day after surgery

Prophylaxis of venous thromboembolism following total hip replacement surgery

▸ BY MOUTH
▸ Adult 18–74 years: 110 mg, to be taken 1–4 hours after surgery, followed by 220 mg once daily for 28–35 days, to be taken on the first day after surgery
▸ Adult 75 years and over: 75 mg, to be taken 1–4 hours after surgery, followed by 150 mg once daily for 28–35 days, to be taken on the first day after surgery

Cardiovascular system

Prophylaxis of venous thromboembolism following total hip replacement surgery in patients receiving concomitant treatment with amiodarone or verapamil
▶ BY MOUTH
▹ Adult 18-74 years: 75 mg, to be taken 1-4 hours after surgery, followed by 150 mg once daily for 28-35 days, to be taken on the first day after surgery
▹ Adult 75 years and over: 75 mg, to be taken 1-4 hours after surgery, followed by 150 mg once daily for 28-35 days, to be taken on the first day after surgery

Treatment of deep-vein thrombosis | Treatment of pulmonary embolism | Prophylaxis of recurrent deep-vein thrombosis | Prophylaxis of recurrent pulmonary embolism
▶ BY MOUTH
▹ Adult 18-74 years: 150 mg twice daily, following at least 5 days treatment with a parenteral anticoagulant
▹ Adult 75-79 years: 110-150 mg twice daily, following at least 5 days treatment with a parenteral anticoagulant
▹ Adult 80 years and over: 110 mg twice daily, following at least 5 days treatment with a parenteral anticoagulant

Treatment of deep-vein thrombosis in patients with moderate renal impairment | Treatment of deep-vein thrombosis in patients at increased risk of bleeding | Treatment of pulmonary embolism in patients with moderate renal impairment | Treatment of pulmonary embolism in patients at increased risk of bleeding | Prophylaxis of recurrent deep-vein thrombosis in patients with moderate renal impairment | Prophylaxis of recurrent deep-vein thrombosis in patients at increased risk of bleeding | Prophylaxis of recurrent pulmonary embolism in patients with moderate renal impairment | Prophylaxis of recurrent pulmonary embolism in patients at increased risk of bleeding
▶ BY MOUTH
▹ Adult: 110-150 mg twice daily, following at least 5 days treatment with a parenteral anticoagulant

Treatment of deep-vein thrombosis in patients receiving concomitant treatment with verapamil | Treatment of pulmonary embolism in patients receiving concomitant treatment with verapamil | Prophylaxis of recurrent deep-vein thrombosis in patients receiving concomitant treatment with verapamil | Prophylaxis of recurrent pulmonary embolism in patients receiving concomitant treatment with verapamil
▶ BY MOUTH
▹ Adult: 110 mg twice daily, following at least 5 days treatment with a parenteral anticoagulant

Prophylaxis of stroke and systemic embolism in non-valvular atrial fibrillation and with one or more risk factors such as previous stroke or transient ischaemic attack, symptomatic heart failure, age ≥ 75 years, diabetes mellitus, or hypertension
▶ BY MOUTH
▹ Adult 18-74 years: 150 mg twice daily
▹ Adult 75-79 years: 110-150 mg twice daily
▹ Adult 80 years and over: 110 mg twice daily

Prophylaxis of stroke and systemic embolism in non-valvular atrial fibrillation and with one or more risk factors such as previous stroke or transient ischaemic attack, symptomatic heart failure, age ≥ 75 years, diabetes mellitus, or hypertension in patients receiving concomitant treatment with verapamil
▶ BY MOUTH
▹ Adult: 110 mg twice daily

Prophylaxis of stroke and systemic embolism in non-valvular atrial fibrillation and with one or more risk factors such as previous stroke or transient ischaemic attack, symptomatic heart failure, age ≥ 75 years, diabetes mellitus, or hypertension, in patients at increased risk of bleeding | Prophylaxis of stroke and systemic embolism in non-valvular atrial fibrillation and with one or more risk factors such as previous stroke or transient ischaemic attack, symptomatic heart failure, age ≥ 75 years, diabetes mellitus, or hypertension, in patients with moderate renal impairment
▶ BY MOUTH
▹ Adult: 110-150 mg twice daily

DOSE EQUIVALENCE AND CONVERSION
▶ For information on changing from, or to, other anticoagulants, consult product literature.

IMPORTANT SAFETY INFORMATION

MHRA/CHM ADVICE: DIRECT-ACTING ORAL ANTICOAGULANTS (DOACS): INCREASED RISK OF RECURRENT THROMBOTIC EVENTS IN PATIENTS WITH ANTIPHOSPHOLIPID SYNDROME (JUNE 2019)
A clinical trial has shown an increased risk of recurrent thrombotic events associated with rivaroxaban compared with warfarin, in patients with antiphospholipid syndrome and a history of thrombosis. There may be a similar risk associated with other DOACs. Healthcare professionals are advised that DOACs are not recommended in patients with antiphospholipid syndrome, particularly high-risk patients who test positive for all three antiphospholipid tests—lupus anticoagulant, anticardiolipin antibodies, and anti-beta$_2$ glycoprotein I antibodies. Continued treatment should be reviewed in these patients to determine if appropriate, and switching to a vitamin K antagonist such as warfarin should be considered.

MHRA/CHM ADVICE: DIRECT-ACTING ORAL ANTICOAGULANTS (DOACS): REMINDER OF BLEEDING RISK, INCLUDING AVAILABILITY OF REVERSAL AGENTS (JUNE 2020)
The MHRA reminds healthcare professionals to remain vigilant for signs and symptoms of bleeding complications during treatment with dabigatran after ongoing reports of serious, potentially fatal bleeds associated with the use of DOACs. Healthcare professionals are also advised to use dabigatran with caution in patients with increased bleeding risk, and to ensure that those with renal impairment are dosed appropriately and their renal function monitored during treatment. Patients should be counselled on the signs and symptoms of bleeding, and encouraged to read the patient information leaflet. The dabigatran reversal agent idarucizumab (*Praxbind®*) is available if required.

MHRA/CHM ADVICE: WARFARIN AND OTHER ANTICOAGULANTS: MONITORING OF PATIENTS DURING THE COVID-19 PANDEMIC (OCTOBER 2020)
Healthcare professionals are reminded that:
- direct-acting oral anticoagulants (DOACs), such as dabigatran, may interact with other medicines (including antibacterials and antivirals)—advice in product literature should be followed to minimise the risk of potential interactions;
- if patients are switched from warfarin to dabigatran, warfarin treatment should be stopped before dabigatran treatment is started to reduce the risk of over-anticoagulation and bleeding.

● CONTRA-INDICATIONS Active bleeding · antiphospholipid syndrome (increased risk of recurrent thrombotic events) · do not use as anticoagulant for prosthetic heart valve · malignant neoplasms · oesophageal varices · recent brain surgery · recent gastro-intestinal ulcer · recent intracranial haemorrhage · recent ophthalmic surgery · recent spine

2

Cardiovascular system

surgery · significant risk of major bleeding · vascular aneurysm
- CAUTIONS Anaesthesia with postoperative indwelling epidural catheter (risk of paralysis—give initial dose at least 2 hours after catheter removal and monitor neurological signs) · bacterial endocarditis · bleeding disorders · body-weight less than 50 kg · elderly · gastritis · gastro-oesophageal reflux · oesophagitis · recent biopsy · recent major trauma · thrombocytopenia

CAUTIONS, FURTHER INFORMATION
▸ Elderly For direct thrombin inhibitors, prescription potentially inappropriate (STOPP criteria):
  - with concurrent significant bleeding risk, such as uncontrolled severe hypertension, bleeding diathesis or recent non-trivial spontaneous bleeding (high risk of bleeding)
  - for first deep venous thrombosis without continuing provoking risk factors (e.g. thrombophilia) for greater than 6 months (no proven added benefit)
  - for first pulmonary embolus without continuing provoking risk factors for greater than 12 months (no proven added benefit)
  - as part of dual therapy with an antiplatelet agent in patients with stable coronary, cerebrovascular or peripheral arterial disease, without a clear indication for anticoagulant therapy (no added benefit)
  - if eGFR less than 30 ml/min/1.73 m² (risk of bleeding)
  See also Prescribing in the elderly p. 33.
- INTERACTIONS → Appendix 1: thrombin inhibitors
- SIDE-EFFECTS
▸ **Common or very common** Hepatic function abnormal
▸ **Uncommon** Anaemia · diarrhoea · haemorrhage · hyperbilirubinaemia · nausea · post procedural complications · vomiting · wound complications
▸ **Rare or very rare** Angioedema · dysphagia · gastrointestinal discomfort · gastrointestinal disorders · intracranial haemorrhage · post procedural drainage · skin reactions · thrombocytopenia · wound drainage
▸ **Frequency not known** Bronchospasm
- PREGNANCY Manufacturer advises avoid unless essential—toxicity in *animal* studies.
- BREAST FEEDING Manufacturer advises avoid—no information available.
- HEPATIC IMPAIRMENT Manufacturer advises avoid in severe impairment; consider avoiding in those with liver enzymes greater than 2 times the upper limit of normal (no information available).
- RENAL IMPAIRMENT Manufacturer advises avoid if creatinine clearance less than 30 mL/minute.
  Dose adjustments When used for *prophylaxis of venous thromboembolism following knee or hip replacement surgery*, reduce initial dose to 75 mg and subsequent doses to 150 mg once daily if creatinine clearance 30–50 mL/minute; consider reducing dose to 75 mg once daily if creatinine clearance 30–50 mL/minute and patient receiving concomitant treatment with verapamil.
  When used for *treatment of deep-vein thrombosis and pulmonary embolism, prophylaxis of recurrent deep-vein thrombosis and pulmonary embolism, prophylaxis of stroke and systemic embolism in non-valvular atrial fibrillation*, consider reduced dose of 110–150 mg twice daily if creatinine clearance 30–50 mL/minute, based on individual assessment of thromboembolic risk and risk of bleeding.
  Monitoring In renal impairment monitor renal function at least annually (manufacturer recommends Cockroft and Gault formula to calculate creatinine clearance).
- MONITORING REQUIREMENTS
▸ Patients should be monitored for signs of bleeding or anaemia; treatment should be stopped if severe bleeding occurs.

▸ No routine anticoagulant monitoring required (INR tests are unreliable).
▸ Assess renal function (manufacturer recommends Cockroft and Gault formula to calculate creatinine clearance) before treatment in all patients and at least annually in elderly.
- DIRECTIONS FOR ADMINISTRATION Ⓔⱽᴳ When dose reduction recommended due to concurrent amiodarone or verapamil, doses should be taken at the same time ◁Ⓜ▷(see *Indications and dose*).
- PRESCRIBING AND DISPENSING INFORMATION Dabigatran etexilate, is given orally for prophylaxis of venous thromboembolism in adults after total hip replacement or total knee replacement surgery; it is also licensed for the treatment of deep-vein thrombosis and pulmonary embolism, and prophylaxis of recurrent deep-vein thrombosis and pulmonary embolism in adults. Duration of treatment should be determined by balancing the benefit of treatment with the bleeding risk; shorter duration of treatment (at least 3 months) should be based on transient risk factors i.e recent surgery, trauma, immobilisation, and longer duration of treatment should be based on permanent risk factors, or idiopathic deep-vein thrombosis or pulmonary embolism.
- PATIENT AND CARER ADVICE Patients should be provided with an alert card and advised to keep it with them at all times.
- NATIONAL FUNDING/ACCESS DECISIONS
  For full details see funding body website
  NICE decisions
  ▸ Dabigatran etexilate for the prevention of venous thromboembolism after hip or knee replacement surgery in adults (September 2008) NICE TA157 Recommended
  ▸ Dabigatran etexilate for the prevention of stroke and systemic embolism in atrial fibrillation (March 2012) NICE TA249 Recommended
  ▸ Dabigatran etexilate for the treatment and secondary prevention of deep vein thrombosis and/or pulmonary embolism (December 2014) NICE TA327 Recommended

- MEDICINAL FORMS There can be variation in the licensing of different medicines containing the same drug.
  Capsule
  CAUTIONARY AND ADVISORY LABELS 10, 25
  ▸ Pradaxa (Boehringer Ingelheim Ltd)
    Dabigatran etexilate (as Dabigatran etexilate mesilate)
    75 mg Pradaxa 75mg capsules | 10 capsule ᴾᵒᴹ £8.50 |
    60 capsule ᴾᵒᴹ £51.00 DT = £51.00
    Dabigatran etexilate (as Dabigatran etexilate mesilate)
    110 mg Pradaxa 110mg capsules | 10 capsule ᴾᵒᴹ £8.50 |
    60 capsule ᴾᵒᴹ £51.00 DT = £51.00
    Dabigatran etexilate (as Dabigatran etexilate mesilate)
    150 mg Pradaxa 150mg capsules | 60 capsule ᴾᵒᴹ £51.00 DT = £51.00

ANTITHROMBOTIC DRUGS ›TISSUE PLASMINOGEN ACTIVATORS

🖙 231

Urokinase

24-Nov-2020

- INDICATIONS AND DOSE

Deep-vein thrombosis (thromboembolic occlusive vascular disease)
▸ BY INTRAVENOUS INFUSION
▸ **Adult:** Initially 4400 units/kg, to be given over 10–20 minutes, followed by 100 000 units/hour for 2–3 days

Pulmonary embolism (thromboembolic occlusive vascular disease)
▶ BY INTRAVENOUS INFUSION
▶ Adult: Initially 4400 units/kg, to be given over 10–20 minutes, followed by 4400 units/kg/hour for 12 hours

Occlusive peripheral arterial disease (thromboembolic occlusive vascular disease)
▶ BY INTRA-ARTERIAL INFUSION
▶ Adult: (consult product literature)

Occluded central venous catheters (blocked by fibrin clots)
▶ TO THE DEVICE AS A FLUSH
▶ Adult: Instil directly into occluded catheter **only**, to be dissolved in sodium chloride 0.9% to a concentration of 5000 units/mL; use a volume sufficient to fill the catheter lumen; leave for 20–60 minutes then aspirate the lysate; repeat if necessary

Occluded arteriovenous haemodialysis shunts (blocked by fibrin clots)
▶ TO THE DEVICE AS A FLUSH
▶ Adult: (consult product literature)

SYNER-KINASE ®

Deep-vein thrombosis (thromboembolic occlusive vascular disease)
▶ BY INTRAVENOUS INFUSION
▶ Adult: Initially 4400 units/kg, to be given over 10 minutes, dose to be made up in 15 mL sodium chloride 0.9%, followed by 4400 units/kg/hour for 12–24 hours

Pulmonary embolism (thromboembolic occlusive vascular disease)
▶ INITIALLY BY INTRAVENOUS INFUSION
▶ Adult: Initially 4400 units/kg, to be given over 10 minutes, dose to be made up in 15 mL sodium chloride 0.9%, followed by (by intravenous infusion) 4400 units/kg/hour for 12 hours, alternatively (by intra-arterial injection) initially 15 000 units/kg, to be injected into pulmonary artery, subsequent doses adjusted according to response; maximum 3 doses per day

Occlusive peripheral arterial disease
▶ BY INTRA-ARTERIAL INFUSION
▶ Adult: (consult product literature)

Occluded intravascular catheters and cannulas (blocked by fibrin clots)
▶ TO THE DEVICE AS A FLUSH
▶ Adult: 5000–25 000 units, instil directly into catheter or cannula lumen **only**, dose dissolved in suitable volume of sodium chloride 0.9% to fill the catheter or cannula lumen; leave for 20–60 minutes then aspirate the lysate; repeat if necessary, alternatively up to 250 000 units, instil directly into the catheter or cannula lumen **only**, dose dissolved in sodium chloride 0.9% to a concentration of 1000–2500 units/mL and infused over 90–180 minutes into the catheter or cannula

● CAUTIONS Cavernous pulmonary disease
● INTERACTIONS → Appendix 1: urokinase
● SIDE-EFFECTS
▶ **Common or very common** Artery dissection · embolism and thrombosis · stroke
▶ **Uncommon** Renal failure
▶ **Rare or very rare** Vascular pseudoaneurysm
● BREAST FEEDING Manufacturer advises avoid—no information available.
● HEPATIC IMPAIRMENT Manufacturer advises caution in mild to moderate impairment.

Dose adjustments Manufacturer advises consider dose reduction in mild to moderate impairment.
● RENAL IMPAIRMENT
Dose adjustments Dose reduction may be required.
● DIRECTIONS FOR ADMINISTRATION For *intravenous infusion* (*Syner-KINASE®*), give continuously or intermittently in Sodium chloride 0.9%.

● MEDICINAL FORMS There can be variation in the licensing of different medicines containing the same drug.
Powder for solution for injection
▶ Syner-KINASE (Syner-Med (Pharmaceutical Products) Ltd)
Urokinase 10000 unit Syner-KINASE 10,000unit powder for solution for injection vials | 1 vial PoM £35.95 (Hospital only)
Urokinase 25000 unit Syner-KINASE 25,000unit powder for solution for injection vials | 1 vial PoM £45.95 (Hospital only)
Urokinase 100000 unit Syner-KINASE 100,000unit powder for solution for injection vials | 1 vial PoM £112.95 (Hospital only)
Urokinase 250000 unit Syner-KINASE 250,000unit powder for solution for injection vials | 1 vial PoM 🅢 (Hospital only)
Urokinase 500000 unit Syner-KINASE 500,000unit powder for solution for injection vials | 1 vial PoM 🅢 (Hospital only)

ANTITHROMBOTIC DRUGS ⟩ VITAMIN K ANTAGONISTS

Vitamin K antagonists

IMPORTANT SAFETY INFORMATION
MHRA/CHM ADVICE: DIRECT-ACTING ANTIVIRALS TO TREAT CHRONIC HEPATITIS C: RISK OF INTERACTION WITH VITAMIN K ANTAGONISTS AND CHANGES IN INR (JANUARY 2017)
A EU-wide review has identified that changes in liver function, secondary to hepatitis C treatment with direct-acting antivirals, may affect the efficacy of vitamin K antagonists; the MHRA has advised that INR should be monitored closely in patients receiving concomitant treatment.

MHRA/CHM ADVICE: WARFARIN AND OTHER ANTICOAGULANTS: MONITORING OF PATIENTS DURING THE COVID-19 PANDEMIC (OCTOBER 2020)
Healthcare professionals are reminded that:
● acute illness (including COVID-19 infection) may exaggerate the effect of warfarin and necessitate a dose reduction;
● continued INR monitoring is important in patients taking warfarin or other vitamin K antagonists if they have suspected or confirmed COVID-19 infection, so they can be clinically managed at an early stage to reduce the risk of bleeding;
● vitamin K antagonists may interact with other medicines (including antibacterials and antivirals)—advice in product literature, such as INR monitoring in patients taking vitamin K antagonists who have recently started new medicines, should be followed to minimise the risk of potential interactions;
● if patients are switched from warfarin to a direct-acting oral anticoagulant (DOAC), warfarin treatment should be stopped before DOAC treatment is started to reduce the risk of over-anticoagulation and bleeding.
Patients on vitamin K antagonists should be reminded to carefully follow instructions for use (including the patient information leaflet) and advised to notify their GP or healthcare team if they:
● have symptoms of, or confirmed, COVID-19 infection;
● are otherwise unwell with sickness or diarrhoea, or have lost their appetite;
● have changed their diet, smoking habits, or alcohol consumption;
● are taking any new medicines or supplements;
● are unable to attend their next scheduled blood test for any reason.

2

Cardiovascular system

Cardiovascular system

- CONTRA-INDICATIONS Avoid use within 48 hours postpartum · haemorrhagic stroke · significant bleeding
- CAUTIONS Bacterial endocarditis (use only if warfarin otherwise indicated) · conditions in which risk of bleeding is increased · history of gastrointestinal bleeding · hyperthyroidism · hypothyroidism · peptic ulcer · postpartum (delay warfarin until risk of haemorrhage is low—usually 5–7 days after delivery) · recent ischaemic stroke · recent surgery · uncontrolled hypertension
- CAUTIONS, FURTHER INFORMATION
  ‣ Elderly Prescription potentially inappropriate (STOPP criteria):
    - with concurrent significant bleeding risk, such as uncontrolled severe hypertension, bleeding diathesis or recent non-trivial spontaneous bleeding (high risk of bleeding)
    - as part of dual therapy with an antiplatelet agent in patients with stable coronary, cerebrovascular or peripheral arterial disease, without a clear indication for anticoagulant therapy (no added benefit)
    - for first deep venous thrombosis without continuing provoking risk factors (e.g. thrombophilia) for longer than 6 months (no proven added benefit)
    - for first pulmonary embolus without continuing provoking risk factors for longer than 12 months (no proven added benefit)
    See also Prescribing in the elderly p. 33.
- SIDE-EFFECTS
  ‣ **Common or very common** Haemorrhage
  ‣ **Rare or very rare** Alopecia · nausea · vomiting
  ‣ **Frequency not known** Blue toe syndrome · CNS haemorrhage · diarrhoea · fever · haemothorax · jaundice · pancreatitis · skin necrosis (increased risk in patients with protein C or protein S deficiency) · skin reactions
- CONCEPTION AND CONTRACEPTION Women of child-bearing age should be warned of the danger of teratogenicity.
- PREGNANCY Should not be given in the first trimester of pregnancy. Warfarin, acenocoumarol, and phenindione cross the placenta with risk of congenital malformations, and placental, fetal, or neonatal haemorrhage, especially during the last few weeks of pregnancy and at delivery. Therefore, if at all possible, they should be avoided in pregnancy, especially in the first and third trimesters (difficult decisions may have to be made, particularly in women with prosthetic heart valves, atrial fibrillation, or with a history of recurrent venous thrombosis or pulmonary embolism). Stopping these drugs before the sixth week of gestation may largely avoid the risk of fetal abnormality.
- HEPATIC IMPAIRMENT In general, manufacturers advise caution in mild to moderate impairment; avoid in severe impairment.
- MONITORING REQUIREMENTS
  ‣ The base-line prothrombin time should be determined but the initial dose should not be delayed whilst awaiting the result.
  ‣ It is essential that the INR be determined daily or on alternate days in early days of treatment, then at longer intervals (depending on response), then up to every 12 weeks.
  ‣ Change in patient's clinical condition, particularly associated with liver disease, intercurrent illness, or drug administration, necessitates more frequent testing.
- PATIENT AND CARER ADVICE Anticoagulant treatment booklets should be issued to all patients or their carers; these booklets include advice for patients on anticoagulant treatment, an alert card to be carried by the patient at all times, and a section for recording of INR results and dosage information. In **England**, **Wales**, and **Northern Ireland**, they are available for purchase from:

3M Security Print and Systems Limited
Gorse Street, Chadderton
Oldham
OL9 9QH
Tel: 0845 610 1112

GP practices can obtain supplies through their Local Area Team stores. NHS Trusts can order supplies from www.nhsforms.co.uk or by emailing nhsforms@spsl.uk.com.

In **Scotland**, treatment booklets and starter information packs can be obtained by emailing stockorders.DPPAS@apsgroup.co.uk or by fax on (0131) 6299 967

Electronic copies of the booklets and further advice are also available at www.npsa.nhs.uk/nrls/alerts-and-directives/alerts/anticoagulant.

F 151

Acenocoumarol
(Nicoumalone)

11-Sep-2018

- **INDICATIONS AND DOSE**
  Prophylaxis of embolisation in rheumatic heart disease and atrial fibrillation | Prophylaxis after insertion of prosthetic heart valve | Prophylaxis and treatment of venous thrombosis and pulmonary embolism | Transient ischaemic attacks
  ‣ BY MOUTH
    ‣ Adult: Initially 2–4 mg once daily for 2 days, alternatively initially 6 mg on day 1, then 4 mg on day 2; maintenance 1–8 mg daily, adjusted according to response, dose to be taken at the same time each day, lower doses may be required in patients over 65 years, severe heart failure with hepatic congestion, and malnutrition
- CAUTIONS Patients over 65 years
- INTERACTIONS → Appendix 1: coumarins
- SIDE-EFFECTS
  ‣ **Rare or very rare** Appetite decreased · liver injury · skin necrosis haemorrhagic (increased risk in patients with protein C or protein S deficiency) · vasculitis
- BREAST FEEDING Risk of haemorrhage; increased by vitamin K deficiency—manufacturer recommends prophylactic vitamin K for the infant (consult product literature).
- HEPATIC IMPAIRMENT
  Dose adjustments Manufacturer advises consider dose reduction in mild to moderate impairment.
- RENAL IMPAIRMENT Caution in mild to moderate impairment. Avoid in severe impairment.
- PATIENT AND CARER ADVICE Anticoagulant card to be provided.

- MEDICINAL FORMS There can be variation in the licensing of different medicines containing the same drug.
  Tablet
  CAUTIONARY AND ADVISORY LABELS 10
  ‣ Sinthrome (Norgine Pharmaceuticals Ltd)
    Acenocoumarol 1 mg Sinthrome 1mg tablets | 100 tablet [PoM] £4.62 DT = £4.62

➤ 151

Phenindione

● **INDICATIONS AND DOSE**

Prophylaxis of embolisation in rheumatic heart disease and atrial fibrillation | Prophylaxis after insertion of prosthetic heart valve | Prophylaxis and treatment of venous thrombosis and pulmonary embolism
▸ BY MOUTH
▸ Adult: Initially 200 mg on day 1, then 100 mg on day 2, then, adjusted according to response; maintenance 50–150 mg daily

● INTERACTIONS → Appendix 1: phenindione

● SIDE-EFFECTS Agranulocytosis · albuminuria · eosinophilia · hepatitis · increased leucocytes · kidney injury · leucopenia · lymphadenopathy · pancytopenia · renal tubular necrosis · taste altered

● BREAST FEEDING Avoid. Risk of haemorrhage; increased by vitamin K deficiency.

● RENAL IMPAIRMENT Caution in mild to moderate impairment. Avoid in severe impairment.

● PATIENT AND CARER ADVICE Patient counselling is advised for phenindione tablets (may turn urine pink or orange). Anticoagulant card to be provided.

● MEDICINAL FORMS There can be variation in the licensing of different medicines containing the same drug.
Tablet
CAUTIONARY AND ADVISORY LABELS 10, 14
▸ Phenindione (Non-proprietary)
Phenindione 10 mg Phenindione 10mg tablets | 28 tablet PoM £600.00 DT = £600.00
Phenindione 25 mg Phenindione 25mg tablets | 28 tablet PoM £600.00 DT = £600.00

➤ 151

Warfarin sodium

10-Oct-2016

● **INDICATIONS AND DOSE**

Prophylaxis of embolisation in rheumatic heart disease and atrial fibrillation | Prophylaxis after insertion of prosthetic heart valve | Prophylaxis and treatment of venous thrombosis and pulmonary embolism | Transient ischaemic attacks
▸ BY MOUTH
▸ Adult: Initially 5–10 mg, to be taken on day 1; subsequent doses dependent on the prothrombin time, reported as INR (international normalised ratio), a lower induction dose can be given over 3–4 weeks in patients who do not require rapid anticoagulation, elderly patients to be given a lower induction dose; maintenance 3–9 mg daily, to be taken at the same time each day

IMPORTANT SAFETY INFORMATION

MHRA/CHM ADVICE: WARFARIN: REPORTS OF CALCIPHYLAXIS (JULY 2016)

An EU-wide review has concluded that on rare occasions, warfarin use may lead to calciphylaxis—patients should be advised to consult their doctor if they develop a painful skin rash; if calciphylaxis is diagnosed, appropriate treatment should be started and consideration should be given to stopping treatment with warfarin. The MHRA has advised that calciphylaxis is most commonly observed in patients with known risk factors such as end-stage renal disease, however cases have also been reported in patients with normal renal function.

● INTERACTIONS → Appendix 1: coumarins

● SIDE-EFFECTS Calciphylaxis · hepatic function abnormal

● PREGNANCY Babies of mothers taking warfarin at the time of delivery need to be offered immediate prophylaxis with intramuscular phytomenadione (vitamin K_1).

● BREAST FEEDING Not present in milk in significant amounts and appears safe. Risk of haemorrhage which is increased by vitamin K deficiency.

● RENAL IMPAIRMENT Use with caution in mild to moderate impairment.
Monitoring In severe renal impairment, monitor INR more frequently.

● PATIENT AND CARER ADVICE Anticoagulant card to be provided.

● MEDICINAL FORMS There can be variation in the licensing of different medicines containing the same drug. Forms available from special-order manufacturers include: oral suspension, oral solution

Oral suspension
CAUTIONARY AND ADVISORY LABELS 10
▸ Warfarin sodium (Non-proprietary)
Warfarin sodium 1 mg per 1 ml Warfarin 1mg/ml oral suspension sugar free sugar-free | 150 ml PoM £124.50 DT = £117.50
Tablet
CAUTIONARY AND ADVISORY LABELS 10
▸ Warfarin sodium (Non-proprietary)
Warfarin sodium 500 microgram Warfarin 500microgram tablets | 28 tablet PoM £1.70 DT = £1.44
Warfarin sodium 1 mg Warfarin 1mg tablets | 28 tablet PoM £1.16 DT = £0.88 | 500 tablet PoM £9.46
Warfarin sodium 3 mg Warfarin 3mg tablets | 28 tablet PoM £1.20 DT = £0.94 | 500 tablet PoM £11.07
Warfarin sodium 5 mg Warfarin 5mg tablets | 28 tablet PoM £1.29 DT = £1.11 | 500 tablet PoM £26.79

4   Blood pressure conditions

4.1 Hypertension

Hypertension

01-Dec-2020

Description of condition

Hypertension is defined as persistently raised arterial blood pressure and is one of the most important treatable causes of premature morbidity and mortality. It is a major risk factor for stroke, myocardial infarction, heart failure, chronic kidney disease, cognitive decline and premature death. Hypertension is more common in advancing age, in women aged between 65–74 years and in people of black African or African-Caribbean origin. Other risk factors include social deprivation, lifestyle factors, anxiety, and emotional stress.

Aims of treatment

Treatment aims to reduce the risk of cardiovascular morbidity and mortality, including myocardial infarction and stroke, by lowering blood pressure.

Non-drug treatment

EvGr In patients with suspected or diagnosed hypertension, offer lifestyle advice and support to enable patients to make healthy lifestyle changes.
  Give advice about the benefits of regular exercise, a healthy diet, low dietary sodium intake, and reduced alcohol intake (if excessive) as these changes can reduce blood pressure.
  Discourage excessive consumption of coffee and other caffeine-rich products, and offer advice to help smokers to stop smoking (see Smoking cessation p. 519). Ⓐ

Cardiovascular system

Hypertension thresholds for treatment

Recommendations on the management of hypertension and blood pressure thresholds are from the *National Institute for Health and Care Excellence (NICE)—Hypertension in adults: diagnosis and management guidelines (NG136, August 2019), and Scottish Intercollegiate Guidelines Network (SIGN)—A national clinical guideline: Risk estimation and the prevention of cardiovascular disease (SIGN 149, June 2017)*. These recommendations differ slightly. Recommendations are based on NICE guidelines, and differences with SIGN (2017) have been highlighted.

For blood pressure thresholds, targets, and the management of hypertension in renal, diabetic or pregnant hypertensive patients, see *Hypertension in renal disease, Hypertension in diabetes*, and *Hypertension in pregnancy*.

[EvGr] Patients presenting with a blood pressure of 140/90 mmHg or higher when measured in a clinic setting, should be offered ambulatory blood pressure monitoring (ABPM), or home blood pressure monitoring if ABPM is unsuitable, to confirm the diagnosis and stage of hypertension. ⟨Ⓐ⟩

Stage 1 hypertension is a clinic blood pressure of between 140/90 mmHg and 160/100 mmHg, and ambulatory daytime average or home blood pressure average of 135/85 mmHg or higher.

[EvGr] Discuss treatment options with patients aged under 80 years who have stage 1 hypertension if they have one or more of the following: target-organ damage (for example left ventricular hypertrophy, chronic kidney disease or hypertensive retinopathy), established cardiovascular disease, renal disease, diabetes, or a 10 year cardiovascular risk ≥10%.

Consider antihypertensive drug treatment in addition to lifestyle advice for adults aged under 60 with stage 1 hypertension and an estimated 10 year cardiovascular risk below 10%.

Consider antihypertensive drug treatment in addition to lifestyle advice for patients aged over 80 years with a clinic blood pressure of over 150/90 mmHg.

For patients aged under 40 years with stage 1 hypertension consider seeking specialist advice for evaluation of secondary causes of hypertension.

SIGN (2017) recommend antihypertensive drug treatment be offered to patients at high cardiovascular risk or with evidence of cardiovascular disease, and a sustained clinic systolic blood pressure over 140 mmHg and/or diastolic blood pressure over 90 mmHg regardless of age. For information about cardiovascular disease risk assessment, see Cardiovascular disease risk assessment and prevention p. 203. SIGN (2017) also recommend antihypertensive drug treatment should be offered to patients who have had a haemorrhagic or ischaemic stroke, or transient ischaemic attack even when their baseline blood pressure is at a level that would be considered conventionally normotensive. ⟨Ⓐ⟩

Stage 2 hypertension is a clinic blood pressure of between 160/100 mmHg and 180/120 mmHg, and ambulatory daytime average or home blood pressure average of 150/95 mmHg or higher.

[EvGr] Treat all patients who have stage 2 hypertension, regardless of age. ⟨Ⓐ⟩

Severe hypertension is a clinic systolic blood pressure of 180 mmHg or higher, or a clinic diastolic blood pressure of 120 mmHg or higher.

[EvGr] Treat severe hypertension promptly (see *Same-day specialist referral*). ⟨Ⓐ⟩

Same-day specialist referral

[EvGr] If a patient has severe hypertension but no symptoms or signs indicating same-day referral *(see below)*, carry out investigations for target organ damage as soon as possible. If target organ damage is identified, consider starting antihypertensive drug treatment immediately, without waiting for the results of ambulatory or home blood pressure monitoring. If no target organ damage is identified, repeat clinic blood pressure measurement within 7 days.

Refer patients for specialist assessment, carried out on the same day, if they have a clinic blood pressure of 180/120 mmHg and higher with signs of retinal haemorrhage or papilloedema (accelerated hypertension), or life-threatening symptoms for example new onset confusion, chest pain, signs of heart failure, or acute kidney injury.

Refer patients for specialist assessment, carried out on the same day, if they have suspected phaeochromocytoma (for example labile or postural hypotension, headache, palpitations, pallor, abdominal pain, or diaphoresis). ⟨Ⓐ⟩

Assessment of cardiovascular risk

[EvGr] Cardiovascular risk should be estimated and assessed for all patients with confirmed hypertension using clinic blood pressure measurements. In these patients, glycated haemoglobin, electrolytes, creatinine, estimated glomular filtration rate, total and HDL cholesterol should be measured, tests for the presence of proteinuria, haematuria, and hypertensive retinopathy undertaken, and a 12-lead ECG performed.

Aspirin reduces the risk of cardiovascular events and myocardial infarction, however high blood pressure must be controlled before aspirin is given. Unless contra-indicated, aspirin is recommended for all patients with established cardiovascular disease. ⟨Ⓐ⟩

For full guidance on the risk assessment and prevention of cardiovascular disease, see Cardiovascular disease risk assessment and prevention p. 203.

Hypertension targets for treatment

For blood pressure thresholds, targets, and the management of hypertension in renal, diabetic or pregnant hypertensive patients, see *Hypertension in renal disease, Hypertension in diabetes*, and *Hypertension in pregnancy*.

[EvGr] A target clinic blood pressure below 140/90 mmHg is suggested for patients aged under 80 years; whilst a target clinic blood pressure below 150/90 mmHg is suggested for patients aged over 80 years. For ambulatory or home blood pressure monitoring (during the patient's waking hours), a target average of below 135/85 mmHg is suggested for patients aged under 80 years; whilst a target average of below 145/85 mmHg is suggested for patients aged over 80 years. SIGN (2017) instead recommend a target clinic blood pressure below 140/90 mmHg regardless of age, whilst patients with high cardiovascular risk and target organ damage should aim for a clinic blood pressure below 135/85 mmHg. These figures are a general guide and may be adapted depending on tolerability, especially in the frail or elderly. ⟨Ⓐ⟩

Drugs for hypertension

A single antihypertensive drug is often inadequate in the management of hypertension and additional antihypertensive drugs are usually added in a step-wise manner until control is achieved. [EvGr] Clinicians should ensure antihypertensive drugs are titrated to the optimum or maximum tolerated dose at each step of treatment along with support and discussions around adherence throughout treatment. Response to drug treatment may be affected by age and ethnicity.

Discuss treatment options, preferences for treatment and individual cardiovascular disease risk with the patient. Continue to offer lifestyle advice and support (see *Non-drug treatment*), whether or not they choose to start antihypertensive drug treatment.

Clinical judgement should be used for all patients with frailty or multimorbidity when starting antihypertensive drug treatment.

Cardiovascular system

For women with diagnosed hypertension who are considering pregnancy or who are pregnant or breastfeeding, manage hypertension in line with the recommendations in the *Hypertension in pregnancy* section.

If an angiotensin-converting enzyme (ACE) inhibitor is not tolerated, for example because of cough, offer an angiotensin II receptor blocker (ARB) to treat hypertension.

The use of an ACE inhibitor with an ARB is not recommended in the treatment of hypertension.

When choosing antihypertensive drug treatment for adults of black African or African–Caribbean family origin, consider an ARB, in preference to an ACE inhibitor.

If a calcium channel blocker is not tolerated, for example because of oedema, offer a thiazide-like diuretic to treat hypertension.

If starting or changing diuretic treatment for hypertension, offer a thiazide-like diuretic such as indapamide p. 181 in preference to conventional thiazide diuretics, for example bendroflumethiazide p. 180 or hydrochlorothiazide p. 180. Continue current treatment in patients with hypertension who already have stable, well-controlled blood pressure whilst on bendroflumethiazide or hydrochlorothiazide. Ⓐ

For blood pressure thresholds, targets, and the management of hypertension in renal and diabetic patients, see *Hypertension in renal disease* and *Hypertension in diabetes*.

Isolated systolic hypertension

EvGr Offer patients with isolated systolic hypertension (systolic blood pressure of160 mmHg or more) the same treatment as patients with both raised systolic and diastolic blood pressure. Ⓐ

Hypertension with type 2 diabetes in all patients (any age or origin), or hypertension without type 2 diabetes in those aged 55 years or below and not of black African or African-Caribbean origin

EvGr **Step 1:** Offer an ACE inhibitor or ARB.

Step 2: In addition to an ACE inhibitor or ARB, add in a calcium channel blocker or thiazide-like diuretic. Offer a thiazide-like diuretic if there is evidence of heart failure. ⒶFor full guidance on the management of chronic heart failure, see Chronic heart failure p. 206.

EvGr **Step 3:** Offer an ACE inhibitor or ARB, a calcium channel blocker and a thiazide-like diuretic.

Step 4: Before considering further treatment for a person with resistant hypertension, confirm elevated clinic blood pressure measurements using ambulatory or home blood pressure recordings, assess for postural hypotension and discuss adherence. If further treatment is required, consider seeking specialist advice, or the addition of low dose spironolactone [unlicensed indication] if potassium is 4.5 mmol/litre or less; or an alpha blocker or a beta blocker if potassium is greater than 4.5 mmol/litre.

When using further diuretic therapy for step 4 treatment of resistant hypertension, monitor blood sodium, potassium and renal function within 1 month of starting treatment and repeat as needed thereafter.

Seek specialist advice if blood pressure remains uncontrolled despite taking optimal tolerated doses of 4 drugs. Ⓐ

Hypertension without type 2 diabetes in patients aged 55 and over, or all ages of black African or African-Caribbean origin patients without type 2 diabetes

EvGr **Step 1:** Offer a calcium channel blocker.

Step 2: In addition to a calcium channel blocker offer an ACE inhibitor, ARB or a thiazide-like diuretic.

Step 3: Offer an ACE inhibitor or ARB, a calcium channel blocker and a thiazide-like diuretic.

Step 4: Before considering further treatment for a person with resistant hypertension, confirm elevated clinic blood pressure measurements using ambulatory or home blood pressure recordings, assess for postural hypotension and

discuss adherence. If further treatment is required, consider seeking specialist advice, or consider low dose spironolactone [unlicensed indication] if potassium is 4.5 mmol/litre or less; or an alpha blocker or a beta blocker if potassium is greater than 4.5 mmol/litre.

When using further diuretic therapy for step 4 treatment of resistant hypertension, monitor blood sodium, potassium, and renal function within 1 month of starting treatment and repeat as needed thereafter.

Seek specialist advice if blood pressure remains uncontrolled despite taking optimal tolerated doses of 4 drugs. Ⓐ

Hypertension in diabetes

EvGr Hypertension in diabetic patients should be treated aggressively with lifestyle modification and drug treatment. Lowering blood pressure in patients with diabetes reduces the risk of macrovascular and microvascular complications. Ⓐ

Hypertension in type 1 diabetes

EvGr In **type 1 diabetes**, aim for a clinic blood pressure of 135/85 mmHg or less unless the adult with type 1 diabetes has albuminuria or 2 or more features of metabolic syndrome, in which case it should be 130/80 mmHg or less.

If drug treatment is required start a trial of a renin–angiotensin system blocking drug as first-line treatment for hypertension in adults with type 1 diabetes. Potential side effects should not prevent the use of a particular class of drug in order to control blood pressure, unless the side effects become symptomatic or otherwise clinically significant. In particular:

- selective beta-blockers should not be avoided where indicated for adults on insulin;
- low-dose thiazides may be used in combination with beta-blockers;
- calcium channel blockers (use only long-acting preparations). Ⓐ

Hypertension in type 2 diabetes

Recommendations on the management of hypertension and blood pressure thresholds are from the *National Institute for Health and Care Excellence (NICE)—Hypertension in adults: diagnosis and management guidelines (NG136, August 2019), Scottish Intercollegiate Guidelines Network (SIGN)—A national clinical guideline: Risk estimation and the prevention of cardiovascular disease (SIGN 149, June 2017), and Scottish Intercollegiate Guidelines Network (SIGN)—A national clinical guideline: the management of diabetes (SIGN 116, updated November 2017)*. These recommendations differ slightly. Recommendations are based on NICE guidelines, and differences with SIGN (2017) have been highlighted.

EvGr SIGN (June 2017) recommend that regardless of age, patients with high cardiovascular disease risk should be offered antihypertensive drug treatment if clinic systolic blood pressure is above 140 mmHg. Antihypertensive drug treatment should also be considered even if clinic systolic blood pressure is below 140 mmHg, with treatment targeted at individuals thought to be at greatest risk of complications.

In type 2 diabetic patients with hypertension, NICE recommend a clinic blood pressure below 140/90 mmHg in those aged under 80 years, and below 150/90 mmHg in those aged 80 years and over. SIGN (November 2017) recommend a clinic blood pressure of 130/80 mmHg. SIGN (June 2017) recommend a clinic blood pressure below 135/85 mmHg regardless of age if the patient has established cardiovascular disease. Ⓐ

For the management of hypertension in patients with type 2 diabetes, see **Hypertension with type 2 diabetes in all patients (any age or origin), or hypertension without type 2 diabetes in those aged 55 years or below and not of black African or African-Caribbean origin** in *Drugs for hypertension*.

2

Cardiovascular system

Hypertension in renal disease

Recommendations on the management of hypertension and blood pressure thresholds are from the *National Institute for Health and Care Excellence (NICE)—Hypertension in adults: diagnosis and management guidelines (NG136, August 2019)*, and *Scottish Intercollegiate Guidelines Network (SIGN)—A national clinical guideline: Risk estimation and the prevention of cardiovascular disease (SIGN 149, June 2017)*. These recommendations differ slightly. Recommendations are based on NICE guidelines, and differences with SIGN (2017) have been highlighted.

EvGr SIGN (2017) recommend that all people with stage 3 or higher chronic kidney disease, or micro- or macroalbuminuria, or who are on dialysis should be offered blood pressure-lowering treatment.

A target clinic blood pressure below 140/90 mmHg is suggested in patients with renal disease (chronic kidney disease). A blood pressure below 130/80 mmHg is advised in patients with chronic kidney disease and diabetes, or if urine albumin to creatinine ratio (ACR) exceeds 70 mg/mmol). SIGN (2017) recommend a blood pressure below 135/85 mmHg should be considered in patients with established cardiovascular disease and chronic kidney disease.

If possible, offer treatment with drugs taken only once a day. ⒶFor guidance on the choice of antihypertensive agent in patients with chronic kidney disease, see NICE clinical guideline: **Chronic kidney disease in adults** (see *Useful resources*).

Hypertension in pregnancy

Hypertensive disorders during pregnancy affect approximately 8% to 10% of all pregnant women and the complications can be associated with significant morbidity and mortality to the mother and baby. Hypertension can exist before pregnancy or it can be diagnosed in the first 20 weeks of gestation (known as chronic hypertension), it can occur as new-onset of hypertension after 20 weeks gestation (gestational hypertension) or it can occur after 20 weeks gestation with features of multi-organ involvement (pre-eclampsia). EvGr Pregnant women with chronic hypertension, gestational hypertension or pre-eclampsia should be referred to a specialist. ⒶSymptoms of pre-eclampsia include severe headache, problems with vision, severe pain below ribs, vomiting and sudden swelling of hands, feet or face accompanied with significant proteinuria and blood pressure greater than 140/90 mmHg.

EvGr Pregnant women are at high risk of developing pre-eclampsia if they have chronic kidney disease, diabetes mellitus, autoimmune disease, chronic hypertension, or if they have had hypertension during a previous pregnancy; these women are advised to take aspirin p. 132 [unlicensed indication] from week 12 of pregnancy until the baby is born. Women with more than one moderate risk factor for developing pre-eclampsia (first pregnancy, greater than 40 years of age, pregnancy interval of greater than 10 years, BMI above 35 kg/m² at first visit, multiple pregnancy, or family history of pre-eclampsia) are also advised to take aspirin [unlicensed indication] from week 12 of pregnancy until the baby is born.

Pregnant women with chronic hypertension who are already receiving antihypertensive treatment should be referred to a specialist and have their drug therapy reviewed. Stop ACE inhibitors, ARBs, thiazide or thiazide-like diuretics due to an increased risk of congenital abnormalities.

Women with pre-eclampsia, gestational or chronic hypertension who present with a sustained blood pressure of 140/90 mmHg or higher should be offered antihypertensive treatment. First-line treatment is with oral labetalol hydrochloride p. 163 to achieve a target blood pressure of less than 135/85 mmHg. If labetalol is unsuitable, consider nifedipine modified-release [unlicensed] p. 176 and if

nifedipine and labetalol are both unsuitable consider methyldopa p. 159 [unlicensed].

Women with a blood pressure of greater than 160/110 mmHg who require critical care during pregnancy or after birth should receive immediate treatment with either oral or intravenous labetalol hydrochloride, intravenous hydralazine hydrochloride p. 194, or oral nifedipine modified-release to achieve a target blood pressure of 135/85 mmHg or less.

Give intravenous magnesium sulfate p. 1099 to women in a critical care setting with severe hypertension or severe pre-eclampsia or if they have or have previously had an eclamptic fit. Consider intravenous magnesium sulfate in severe pre-eclampsia if birth is planned within 24 hours.

In women with pre-eclampsia where early birth is considered likely within 7 days, consider a course of antenatal corticosteroids for fetal lung maturation.

Appropriate antihypertensive treatment should be continued if required after birth (with dose adjustment according to blood pressure).

Women who have been managed with methyldopa during pregnancy should discontinue treatment within 2 days of the birth and switch to an alternative antihypertensive.

Post-birth, advise women with hypertension that the need to take antihypertensives does not prevent them from breastfeeding should they wish to do so, although very low levels of antihypertensive medicines can pass into breast milk and most medicines are not tested in pregnant or breastfeeding women. For women who decide to breastfeed, offer enalapril maleate p. 182 first-line to treat hypertension during the post-natal period, and monitor maternal renal function and serum potassium. In women of black African or African-Caribbean family origin consider nifedipine or amlodipine p. 170 first line. If blood pressure is not controlled with a single drug consider a combination of nifedipine (or amlodipine) and enalapril. If this combination is not tolerated or ineffective consider either adding labetalol hydrochloride or atenolol p. 166 to the combination treatment or swapping one of the medicines being used for atenolol or labetalol. Blood pressure monitoring should be considered in babies born to mothers taking antihypertensives who are breastfeeding, and women should be advised to monitor their babies for any adverse reactions (for example: drowsiness, lethargy, pallor, cold peripheries or poor feeding).

Women with hypertension in the postnatal period who are not and do not plan to breastfeed should be treated the same way as patients in the section *Drugs for hypertension*.

Following birth, women remaining on antihypertensives should have their treatment reviewed 2 weeks after the birth. Women treated for hypertension during pregnancy should have a medical review 6-8 weeks after birth with their GP or specialist. Ⓐ

Advanced Pharmacy Services

Patients with hypertension may be eligible for the New Medicines Service / Medicines Use Review service provided by a community pharmacist. For further information, see *Advanced Pharmacy Services* in Medicines optimisation p. 18.

Useful Resources

Hypertension in pregnancy: diagnosis and management. National Institute for Health and Care Excellence guideline NG133. June 2019. www.nice.org.uk/guidance/ng133

Hypertension in adults: diagnosis and management. National Institute for Health and Care Excellence guideline NG136. August 2019. www.nice.org.uk/guidance/ng136

Chronic kidney disease in adults: assessment and management. National Institute for Health and Care Excellence guideline CG182. July 2014 (updated January 2015). www.nice.org.uk/guidance/cg182

Risk estimation and the prevention of cardiovascular disease. Scottish Intercollegiate Guidelines Network. Clinical guideline 149. June 2017. www.sign.ac.uk/sign-149-risk-estimation-and-the-prevention-of-cardiovascular-disease.html

Management of diabetes. Scottish Intercollegiate Guidelines Network. Clinical guideline 116. March 2010 (updated November 2017). www.sign.ac.uk/sign-116-and-154-diabetes.html

Antihypertensive drugs

Vasodilator antihypertensive drugs

Vasodilators have a potent hypotensive effect, especially when used in combination with a beta-blocker and a thiazide. **Important:** see Hypertension (hypertension crises) for a warning on the hazards of a very rapid fall in blood pressure.

Hydralazine hydrochloride p. 194 is given by mouth as an adjunct to other antihypertensives for the treatment of resistant hypertension but is rarely used; when used alone it causes tachycardia and fluid retention.

Sodium nitroprusside p. 196 [unlicensed] is given by intravenous infusion to control severe hypertensive emergencies when parenteral treatment is necessary.

Minoxidil p. 195 should be reserved for the treatment of severe hypertension resistant to other drugs. Vasodilatation is accompanied by increased cardiac output and tachycardia and the patients develop fluid retention. For this reason the addition of a beta-blocker and a diuretic (usually furosemide p. 243, in high dosage) are mandatory. Hypertrichosis is troublesome and renders this drug unsuitable for females.

Prazosin p. 829, doxazosin p. 827, and terazosin p. 830 have alpha-blocking and vasodilator properties.

Ambrisentan p. 197, bosentan p. 197, iloprost p. 199, macitentan p. 198, sildenafil p. 860, and tadalafil p. 861 are licensed for the treatment of pulmonary arterial hypertension and should be used under specialist supervision. Epoprostenol p. 124 can be used in patients with primary pulmonary hypertension resistant to other treatments. Bosentan is also licensed to reduce the number of new digital ulcers in patients with systemic sclerosis and ongoing digital ulcer disease. Riociguat p. 198 is licensed for the treatment of pulmonary arterial hypertension and chronic thromboembolic pulmonary hypertension; it should be used under specialist supervision.

Sitaxentan has been withdrawn from the market because the benefit of treatment does not outweigh the risk of severe hepatotoxicity.

Centrally acting antihypertensive drugs

Methyldopa p. 159 is a centrally acting antihypertensive; it may be used for the management of hypertension in pregnancy.

Clonidine hydrochloride p. 159 has the disadvantage that sudden withdrawal of treatment may cause severe rebound hypertension.

Moxonidine p. 160, a centrally acting drug, is licensed for mild to moderate essential hypertension. It may have a role when thiazides, calcium-channel blockers, ACE inhibitors, and beta-blockers are not appropriate or have failed to control blood pressure.

Adrenergic neurone blocking drugs

Adrenergic neurone blocking drugs prevent the release of noradrenaline from postganglionic adrenergic neurones. These drugs do not control supine blood pressure and may cause postural hypotension. For this reason they have largely fallen from use, but may be necessary with other therapy in resistant hypertension.

Guanethidine monosulfate, which also depletes the nerve endings of noradrenaline, is licensed for rapid control of blood pressure, however alternative treatments are preferred.

Alpha-adrenoceptor blocking drugs

Prazosin has post-synaptic alpha-blocking and vasodilator properties and rarely causes tachycardia. It may, however, reduce blood pressure rapidly after the first dose and should be introduced with caution. Doxazosin, indoramin p. 828, and terazosin have properties similar to those of prazosin.

Alpha-blockers can be used with other antihypertensive drugs in the treatment of resistant hypertension.

Prostatic hyperplasia

Alfuzosin hydrochloride p. 827, doxazosin, indoramin, prazosin, tamsulosin hydrochloride p. 829, and terazosin are indicated for benign prostatic hyperplasia.

Drugs affecting the renin-angiotensin system

Angiotensin-converting enzyme inhibitors

Angiotensin-converting enzyme inhibitors (ACE inhibitors) inhibit the conversion of angiotensin I to angiotensin II. They have many uses and are generally well tolerated. The main indications of ACE inhibitors are shown below.

Heart failure

ACE inhibitors are used in all grades of heart failure, usually combined with a beta-blocker. Potassium supplements and potassium-sparing diuretics should be discontinued before introducing an ACE inhibitor because of the risk of hyperkalaemia. However, a low dose of spironolactone p. 208 may be beneficial in severe heart failure and can be used with an ACE inhibitor provided serum potassium is monitored carefully. Profound first-dose hypotension may occur when ACE inhibitors are introduced to patients with heart failure who are already taking a high dose of a loop diuretic (e.g. furosemide p. 243 80 mg daily or more). Temporary withdrawal of the loop diuretic reduces the risk, but may cause severe rebound pulmonary oedema. Therefore, for patients on high doses of loop diuretics, the ACE inhibitor may need to be initiated under specialist supervision. An ACE inhibitor can be initiated in the community in patients who are receiving a low dose of a diuretic or who are not otherwise at risk of serious hypotension; nevertheless, care is required and a very low dose of the ACE inhibitor is given initially.

Hypertension

An ACE inhibitor may be the most appropriate initial drug for hypertension in younger Caucasian patients; Afro-Caribbean patients, those aged over 55 years, and those with primary aldosteronism respond less well. ACE inhibitors are particularly indicated for hypertension in patients with type 1 diabetes with nephropathy. They may reduce blood pressure very rapidly in some patients particularly in those receiving diuretic therapy.

Diabetic nephropathy

ACE inhibitors have a role in the management of diabetic nephropathy.

Prophylaxis of cardiovascular events

ACE inhibitors are used in the early and long-term management of patients who have had a myocardial infarction. ACE inhibitors may also have a role in preventing cardiovascular events.

Initiation under specialist supervision

ACE inhibitors should be initiated under specialist supervision and with careful clinical monitoring in those with severe heart failure or in those:

- receiving multiple or high-dose diuretic therapy (e.g. more than 80 mg of furosemide daily or its equivalent);
- receiving concomitant angiotensin-II receptor antagonist or aliskiren;
- with hypovolaemia;
- with hyponatraemia (plasma-sodium concentration below 130 mmol/litre);
- with hypotension (systolic blood pressure below 90 mmHg);
- with unstable heart failure;
- receiving high-dose vasodilator therapy;
- known renovascular disease.

Renal effects
Renal function and electrolytes should be checked before starting ACE inhibitors (or increasing the dose) and monitored during treatment (more frequently if features mentioned below present); hyperkalaemia and other side-effects of ACE inhibitors are more common in those with impaired renal function and the dose may need to be reduced. Although ACE inhibitors now have a specialised role in some forms of renal disease, including chronic kidney disease, they also occasionally cause impairment of renal function which may progress and become severe in other circumstances (at particular risk are the elderly). A specialist should be involved if renal function is significantly reduced as a result of treatment with an ACE inhibitor.

Concomitant treatment with NSAIDs increases the risk of renal damage, and potassium-sparing diuretics (or potassium-containing salt substitutes) increase the risk of hyperkalaemia.

In patients with severe bilateral renal artery stenosis (or severe stenosis of the artery supplying a single functioning kidney), ACE inhibitors reduce or abolish glomerular filtration and are likely to cause severe and progressive renal failure. They are therefore not recommended in patients known to have these forms of critical renovascular disease.

ACE inhibitor treatment is unlikely to have an adverse effect on overall renal function in patients with severe unilateral renal artery stenosis and a normal contralateral kidney, but glomerular filtration is likely to be reduced (or even abolished) in the affected kidney and the long-term consequences are unknown.

ACE inhibitors are therefore best avoided in patients with known or suspected renovascular disease, unless the blood pressure cannot be controlled by other drugs. If ACE inhibitors are used, they should be initiated only under specialist supervision and renal function should be monitored regularly.

ACE inhibitors should also be used with particular caution in patients who may have undiagnosed and clinically silent renovascular disease. This includes patients with peripheral vascular disease or those with severe generalised atherosclerosis.

ACE inhibitors in combination with other drugs
See also, *Concomitant use of drugs affecting the renin-angiotensin system*, below.

Concomitant diuretics
ACE inhibitors can cause a very rapid fall in blood pressure in volume-depleted patients; treatment should therefore be initiated with very low doses. If the dose of diuretic is greater than 80 mg furosemide or equivalent, the ACE inhibitor should be initiated under close supervision and in some patients the diuretic dose may need to be reduced or the diuretic discontinued at least 24 hours beforehand (may not be possible in heart failure—risk of pulmonary oedema). If high-dose diuretic therapy cannot be stopped, close observation is recommended after administration of the first dose of ACE inhibitor, for at least 2 hours or until the blood pressure has stabilised.

Combination products
Products incorporating an ACE inhibitor with a thiazide diuretic or a calcium-channel blocker are available for the management of hypertension. Use of these combination products should be reserved for patients whose blood pressure has not responded adequately to a single antihypertensive drug and who have been stabilised on the individual components of the combination in the same proportions.

Angiotensin-II receptor antagonists

Azilsartan medoxomil p. 188, candesartan cilexetil p. 189, eprosartan p. 189, irbesartan p. 189, losartan potassium p. 190, olmesartan medoxomil p. 191, telmisartan p. 192, and valsartan p. 193 are angiotensin-II receptor antagonists with many properties similar to those of the ACE inhibitors. However, unlike ACE inhibitors, they do not inhibit the breakdown of bradykinin and other kinins, and thus are less likely to cause the persistent dry cough which can complicate ACE inhibitor therapy. They are therefore a useful alternative for patients who have to discontinue an ACE inhibitor because of persistent cough.

An angiotensin-II receptor antagonist may be used as an alternative to an ACE inhibitor in the management of heart failure or diabetic nephropathy. Candesartan cilexetil and valsartan are also licensed as adjuncts to ACE inhibitors under specialist supervision, in the management of heart failure when other treatments are unsuitable.

Renal effects
Angiotensin-II receptor antagonists should be used with caution in renal artery stenosis (see also Renal effects under Angiotensin-converting enzyme inhibitors, above).

Renin inhibitor

Aliskiren is a renin inhibitor that is licensed for the treatment of hypertension.

Concomitant use of drugs affecting the renin-angiotensin system

Combination therapy with two drugs affecting the renin-angiotensin system (ACE inhibitors, angiotensin-II receptor antagonists, and aliskiren p. 193 is not recommended due to an increased risk of hyperkalaemia, hypotension, and renal impairment, compared to use of a single drug. Patients with diabetic nephropathy are particularly susceptible to developing hyperkalaemia and should not be given an ACE inhibitor with an angiotensin-II receptor antagonist. There is some evidence that the benefits of combination use of an ACE inhibitor with candesartan or valsartan may outweigh the risks in selected patients with heart failure for whom other treatments are unsuitable, however, the concomitant use of this combination, together with an aldosterone antagonist or a potassium-sparing diuretic is not recommended.

For patients currently taking combination therapy, the need for continued combined therapy should be reviewed. If combination therapy is considered essential, it should be carried out under specialist supervision, with close monitoring of blood pressure, renal function, and electrolytes (particularly potassium); monitoring should be considered at the start of treatment, then monthly, and also after any change in dose or during intercurrent illness.

> **Other drugs used for Hypertension** Amiloride hydrochloride, p. 245 · Chlortalidone, p. 246 · Co-triamterzide, p. 247 · Metolazone, p. 247 · Torasemide, p. 244 · Triamterene with chlortalidone, p. 246 · Xipamide, p. 247

ANTIHYPERTENSIVES, CENTRALLY ACTING

| Clonidine hydrochloride

04-Sep-2020

● **INDICATIONS AND DOSE**

Hypertension
▸ BY MOUTH
▸ **Adult:** Initially 50–100 micrograms 3 times a day, increase dose every second or third day, usual maximum dose 1.2 mg daily

Prevention of recurrent migraine | Prevention of vascular headache | Menopausal symptoms, particularly flushing and vasomotor conditions
▸ BY MOUTH
▸ **Adult:** Initially 50 micrograms twice daily for 2 weeks, then increased if necessary to 75 micrograms twice daily

● CONTRA-INDICATIONS Severe bradyarrhythmia secondary to second- or third-degree AV block or sick sinus syndrome

● CAUTIONS Cerebrovascular disease · constipation · heart failure · history of depression · mild to moderate bradyarrhythmia · polyneuropathy · Raynaud's syndrome or other occlusive peripheral vascular disease
CAUTIONS, FURTHER INFORMATION
▸ Elderly For centrally-acting antihypertensives, prescription potentially inappropriate (STOPP criteria), unless clear intolerance of, or lack of efficacy with, other classes of antihypertensives (generally less well tolerated by older people).
See also Prescribing in the elderly p. 33.

● INTERACTIONS → Appendix 1: clonidine

● SIDE-EFFECTS
▸ **Common or very common** Constipation · depression · dizziness · dry mouth · fatigue · headache · nausea · postural hypotension · salivary gland pain · sedation · sexual dysfunction · sleep disorders · vomiting
▸ **Uncommon** Delusions · hallucination · malaise · paraesthesia · Raynaud's phenomenon · skin reactions
▸ **Rare or very rare** Alopecia · atrioventricular block · dry eye · gynaecomastia · intestinal pseudo-obstruction · nasal dryness
▸ **Frequency not known** Accommodation disorder · arrhythmias · confusion

● PREGNANCY May lower fetal heart rate. Avoid oral use unless potential benefit outweighs risk. Avoid using injection.

● BREAST FEEDING Avoid—present in milk.

● RENAL IMPAIRMENT
Dose adjustments Use with caution in severe impairment—reduce initial dose and increase gradually.

● TREATMENT CESSATION In hypertension, must be withdrawn gradually to avoid severe rebound hypertension.

● PATIENT AND CARER ADVICE
Driving and skilled tasks Drowsiness may affect performance of skilled tasks (e.g. driving); effects of alcohol may be enhanced.

● LESS SUITABLE FOR PRESCRIBING Clonidine is less suitable for prescribing.

● MEDICINAL FORMS There can be variation in the licensing of different medicines containing the same drug. Forms available from special-order manufacturers include: oral suspension, oral solution, solution for injection

Tablet
CAUTIONARY AND ADVISORY LABELS 3, 8
▸ Clonidine hydrochloride (Non-proprietary)
  Clonidine hydrochloride 25 microgram Clonidine 25microgram tablets | 112 tablet [PoM] £18.75 DT = £18.59

▸ Catapres (Boehringer Ingelheim Ltd)
  Clonidine hydrochloride 100 microgram Catapres 100microgram tablets | 100 tablet [PoM] £8.04 DT = £8.04
Oral solution
▸ Clonidine hydrochloride (Non-proprietary)
  Clonidine hydrochloride 10 microgram per 1 ml Clonidine 50micrograms/5ml oral solution sugar free sugar-free | 100 ml [PoM] £97.13 DT = £86.69

| Methyldopa

20-Jan-2020

● **INDICATIONS AND DOSE**

Hypertension
▸ BY MOUTH
▸ **Adult:** Initially 250 mg 2–3 times a day, dose should be increased gradually at intervals of at least 2 days; maximum 3 g per day
▸ **Elderly:** Initially 125 mg twice daily, dose should be increased gradually; maximum 2 g per day

● CONTRA-INDICATIONS Acute porphyrias p. 1107 · depression · paraganglioma · phaeochromocytoma

● CAUTIONS History of hepatic impairment
CAUTIONS, FURTHER INFORMATION
▸ Elderly For centrally-acting antihypertensives, prescription potentially inappropriate (STOPP criteria), unless clear intolerance of, or lack of efficacy with, other classes of antihypertensives (generally less well tolerated by older people).
See also Prescribing in the elderly p. 33.

● INTERACTIONS → Appendix 1: methyldopa

● SIDE-EFFECTS Abdominal distension · amenorrhoea · angina pectoris · angioedema · arthralgia · asthenia · atrioventricular block · bone marrow failure · bradycardia · breast enlargement · cardiac inflammation · carotid sinus syndrome · cerebrovascular insufficiency · choreoathetosis · cognitive impairment · constipation · depression · diarrhoea · dizziness · dry mouth · eosinophilia · facial paralysis · fever · gastrointestinal disorders · granulocytopenia · gynaecomastia · haemolytic anaemia · headache · hepatic disorders · hyperprolactinaemia · lactation disorder · leucopenia · lupus-like syndrome · myalgia · nasal congestion · nausea · nightmare · oedema · pancreatitis · paraesthesia · parkinsonism · postural hypotension · psychiatric disorder · psychosis · sedation · sexual dysfunction · sialadenitis · skin reactions · thrombocytopenia · tongue burning · tongue discolouration · toxic epidermal necrolysis · vomiting
SIDE-EFFECTS, FURTHER INFORMATION Side-effects are minimised if the daily dose is kept below 1g; discontinue permanently if fever or hepatic disorders occur.

● PREGNANCY Not known to be harmful.

● BREAST FEEDING Amount too small to be harmful.

● HEPATIC IMPAIRMENT Manufacturer advises avoid in active disease.

● RENAL IMPAIRMENT Increased sensitivity to hypotensive and sedative effect.
Dose adjustments Start with small dose.

● MONITORING REQUIREMENTS Monitor blood counts and liver-function before treatment and at intervals during first 6–12 weeks or if unexplained fever occurs.

● EFFECT ON LABORATORY TESTS Interference with laboratory tests. Positive direct Coombs' test in up to 20% of patients (may affect blood cross-matching).

● PATIENT AND CARER ADVICE
Driving and skilled tasks Drowsiness may affect performance of skilled tasks (e.g. driving); effects of alcohol may be enhanced.

2

Cardiovascular system

2

Cardiovascular system

- MEDICINAL FORMS There can be variation in the licensing of different medicines containing the same drug. Forms available from special-order manufacturers include: oral suspension, oral solution

Tablet

CAUTIONARY AND ADVISORY LABELS 3, 8

▸ Methyldopa (Non-proprietary)

Methyldopa anhydrous 125 mg Methyldopa 125mg tablets | 56 tablet [PoM] £102.54 DT = £102.28

Methyldopa anhydrous 250 mg Methyldopa 250mg tablets | 56 tablet [PoM] £25.03 DT = £23.79

Methyldopa anhydrous 500 mg Methyldopa 500mg tablets | 56 tablet [PoM] £17.91 DT = £17.91

▸ Aldomet (Aspen Pharma Trading Ltd)

Methyldopa anhydrous 250 mg Aldomet 250mg tablets | 60 tablet [PoM] £6.15

Methyldopa anhydrous 500 mg Aldomet 500mg tablets | 30 tablet [PoM] £4.55

Moxonidine

16-Jan-2020

- **INDICATIONS AND DOSE**

Mild to moderate essential hypertension

▸ BY MOUTH

▸ Adult: 200 micrograms once daily for 3 weeks, dose to be taken in the morning, then increased if necessary to 400 micrograms daily in 1–2 divided doses (max. per dose 400 micrograms), maximum daily dose to be given in 2 divided doses; maximum 600 micrograms per day

- CONTRA-INDICATIONS Bradycardia · second- or third-degree AV block · severe heart failure · sick sinus syndrome · sino-atrial block

- CAUTIONS First-degree AV block · moderate heart failure · severe coronary artery disease · unstable angina

CAUTIONS, FURTHER INFORMATION

▸ Elderly For centrally-acting antihypertensives, prescription potentially inappropriate (STOPP criteria), unless clear intolerance of, or lack of efficacy with, other classes of antihypertensives (generally less well tolerated by older people).

See also Prescribing in the elderly p. 33.

- INTERACTIONS → Appendix 1: moxonidine

- SIDE-EFFECTS

▸ Common or very common Asthenia · diarrhoea · dizziness · drowsiness · dry mouth · dyspepsia · headache · insomnia · nausea · pain · skin reactions · vertigo · vomiting

▸ Uncommon Angioedema · bradycardia · nervousness · oedema · syncope · tinnitus

- PREGNANCY Manufacturer advises avoid—no information available.

- BREAST FEEDING Present in milk—manufacturer advises avoid.

- RENAL IMPAIRMENT Avoid if egFR less than 30 mL/minute/1.73 m².

Dose adjustments Max. single dose 200 micrograms and max. daily dose 400 micrograms if eGFR 30–60 mL/minute/1.73 m².

- TREATMENT CESSATION Avoid abrupt withdrawal (if concomitant treatment with beta-blocker has to be stopped, discontinue beta-blocker first, then moxonidine after a few days).

- MEDICINAL FORMS There can be variation in the licensing of different medicines containing the same drug.

Tablet

CAUTIONARY AND ADVISORY LABELS 3

▸ Moxonidine (Non-proprietary)

Moxonidine 200 microgram Moxonidine 200microgram tablets | 28 tablet [PoM] £10.48 DT = £1.34

Moxonidine 300 microgram Moxonidine 300microgram tablets | 28 tablet [PoM] £11.92 DT = £1.42

Moxonidine 400 microgram Moxonidine 400microgram tablets | 28 tablet [PoM] £13.75 DT = £1.41

▸ Physiotens (Mylan)

Moxonidine 200 microgram Physiotens 200microgram tablets | 28 tablet [PoM] £9.72 DT = £1.34

Moxonidine 300 microgram Physiotens 300microgram tablets | 28 tablet [PoM] £11.49 DT = £1.42

Moxonidine 400 microgram Physiotens 400microgram tablets | 28 tablet [PoM] £13.26 DT = £1.41

BETA-ADRENOCEPTOR BLOCKERS

Beta-adrenoceptor blocking drugs

13-Dec-2019

Overview

Beta-adrenoceptor blocking drugs (beta-blockers) block the beta-adrenoceptors in the heart, peripheral vasculature, bronchi, pancreas, and liver.

Many beta-blockers are now available and in general they are all equally effective. There are, however, differences between them, which may affect choice in treating particular diseases or individual patients.

Intrinsic sympathomimetic activity (ISA, partial agonist activity) represents the capacity of beta-blockers to stimulate as well as to block adrenergic receptors. Celiprolol hydrochloride p. 168, pindolol p. 164, acebutolol p. 166, and oxprenolol hydrochloride have intrinsic sympathomimetic activity; they tend to cause less bradycardia than the other beta-blockers and may also cause less coldness of the extremities.

Some beta-blockers are lipid soluble and some are water soluble. Water-soluble beta-blockers (such as atenolol p. 166, celiprolol hydrochloride, nadolol p. 164, and sotalol hydrochloride p. 116) are less likely to enter the brain, and may therefore cause less sleep disturbance and nightmares. Water-soluble beta-blockers are excreted by the kidneys and dosage reduction is often necessary in renal impairment.

Beta-blockers with a relatively short duration of action have to be given two or three times daily. Many of these are, however, available in modified-release formulations so that administration once daily is adequate for hypertension. For angina twice-daily treatment may sometimes be needed even with a modified-release formulation. Some beta-blockers, such as atenolol, bisoprolol fumarate p. 167, celiprolol hydrochloride, and nadolol, have an intrinsically longer duration of action and need to be given only once daily.

Beta-blockers slow the heart and can depress the myocardium; they are contra-indicated in patients with second- or third-degree heart block. Beta-blockers should also be avoided in patients with worsening unstable heart failure; care is required when initiating a beta-blocker in those with stable heart failure.

Labetalol hydrochloride p. 163, celiprolol hydrochloride, carvedilol p. 162, and nebivolol p. 169 are beta-blockers that have, in addition, an arteriolar vasodilating action, by diverse mechanisms, and thus lower peripheral resistance. There is no evidence that these drugs have important advantages over other beta-blockers in the treatment of hypertension.

Beta-blockers can precipitate bronchospasm and should therefore usually be avoided in patients with a history of asthma. When there is no suitable alternative, it may be necessary for a patient with well-controlled asthma, or chronic obstructive pulmonary disease (without significant reversible airways obstruction), to receive treatment with a beta-blocker for a co-existing condition (e.g. heart failure or following myocardial infarction). In this situation, a cardioselective beta-blocker should be selected and initiated at a low dose by a specialist; the patient should be closely monitored for adverse effects. Atenolol, bisoprolol fumarate, metoprolol tartrate p. 169, nebivolol, and (to a lesser extent) acebutolol, have less effect on the beta₂(bronchial) receptors and are, therefore, relatively *cardioselective*, but they are not *cardiospecific*. They have a lesser effect on airways resistance but are not free of this side-effect.

Beta-blockers are also associated with fatigue, coldness of the extremities (may be less common with those with ISA), and sleep disturbances with nightmares (may be less common with the water-soluble beta-blockers).

Beta-blockers can affect carbohydrate metabolism, causing hypoglycaemia or hyperglycaemia in patients with or without diabetes; they can also interfere with metabolic and autonomic responses to hypoglycaemia, thereby masking symptoms such as tachycardia. However, beta-blockers are not contra-indicated in diabetes, although the cardioselective beta-blockers may be preferred. Beta-blockers should be avoided altogether in those with frequent episodes of hypoglycaemia. Beta-blockers, especially when combined with a thiazide diuretic, should be avoided for the routine treatment of uncomplicated hypertension in patients with diabetes or in those at high risk of developing diabetes.

Hypertension

The mode of action of beta-blockers in hypertension is not understood, but they reduce cardiac output, alter baroceptor reflex sensitivity, and block peripheral adrenoceptors. Some beta-blockers depress plasma renin secretion. It is possible that a central effect may also partly explain their mode of action.

Beta-blockers are effective for reducing blood pressure but other antihypertensives are usually more effective for reducing the incidence of stroke, myocardial infarction, and cardiovascular mortality, especially in the elderly. Other antihypertensives are therefore preferred for routine initial treatment of uncomplicated hypertension.

In general, the dose of a beta-blocker does not have to be high.

Beta-blockers can be used to control the pulse rate in patients with *phaeochromocytoma*. However, they should never be used alone as beta-blockade without concurrent alpha-blockade may lead to a hypertensive crisis. For this reason phenoxybenzamine hydrochloride p. 195 should always be used together with the beta-blocker.

Angina

By reducing cardiac work beta-blockers improve exercise tolerance and relieve symptoms in patients with *angina* (see management of stable angina and acute coronary syndromes for further details). As with hypertension there is no good evidence of the superiority of any one drug, although occasionally a patient will respond better to one beta-blocker than to another. There is some evidence that sudden withdrawal may cause an exacerbation of angina and therefore gradual reduction of dose is preferable when beta-blockers are to be stopped. There is a risk of precipitating heart failure when beta-blockers and verapamil are used together in established ischaemic heart disease.

Myocardial infarction

For specific comments see management of ST-segment elevation myocardial infarction and non-ST-segment elevation myocardial infarction.

Several studies have shown that some beta-blockers can reduce the recurrence rate of *myocardial infarction*. However, uncontrolled heart failure, hypotension, bradyarrhythmias, and obstructive airways disease render beta-blockers unsuitable in some patients following a myocardial infarction. Atenolol and metoprolol tartrate may reduce early mortality after intravenous and subsequent oral administration in the acute phase, while acebutolol, metoprolol tartrate, propranolol hydrochloride p. 164, and

timolol maleate p. 165 have protective value when started in the early convalescent phase. The evidence relating to other beta-blockers is less convincing; some have not been tested in trials of secondary prevention.

Arrhythmias

Beta-blockers act as *anti-arrhythmic drugs* principally by attenuating the effects of the sympathetic system on automaticity and conductivity within the heart. They can be used in conjunction with digoxin to control the ventricular response in atrial fibrillation, especially in patients with thyrotoxicosis. Beta-blockers are also useful in the management of supraventricular tachycardias, and are used to control those following myocardial infarction.

Esmolol hydrochloride p. 168 is a relatively cardioselective beta-blocker with a very short duration of action, used intravenously for the short-term treatment of supraventricular arrhythmias, sinus tachycardia, or hypertension, particularly in the peri-operative period. It may also be used in other situations, such as acute myocardial infarction, when sustained beta-blockade might be hazardous.

Sotalol hydrochloride p. 116, a non-cardioselective beta-blocker with additional class III anti-arrhythmic activity, is used for prophylaxis in paroxysmal supraventricular arrhythmias. It also suppresses ventricular ectopic beats and non-sustained ventricular tachycardia. It has been shown to be more effective than lidocaine in the termination of spontaneous sustained ventricular tachycardia due to coronary disease or cardiomyopathy. However, it may induce torsade de pointes in susceptible patients.

Heart failure

Beta-blockers may produce benefit in heart failure by blocking sympathetic activity. Bisoprolol fumarate p. 167 and carvedilol p. 168 reduce mortality in any grade of stable heart failure; nebivolol p. 169 is licensed for stable mild to moderate heart failure in patients over 70 years. Ideally, treatment should be initiated by those experienced in the management of heart failure.

Thyrotoxicosis

Beta-blockers are used in pre-operative preparation for thyroidectomy. Administration of propranolol hydrochloride p. 164 can reverse clinical symptoms of *thyrotoxicosis* within 4 days. Routine tests of increased thyroid function remain unaltered. The thyroid gland is rendered less vascular thus making surgery easier.

Other uses

Beta-blockers have been used to alleviate some symptoms of *anxiety*; probably patients with palpitation, tremor, and tachycardia respond best. Beta-blockers are also used in the *prophylaxis of migraine*. Betaxolol p. 1224, levobunolol hydrochloride p. 1224, and timolol maleate p. 165 are used topically in *glaucoma*.

Beta-adrenoceptor blockers (systemic)

- ● CONTRA-INDICATIONS Asthma · cardiogenic shock · hypotension · marked bradycardia · metabolic acidosis · phaeochromocytoma (apart from specific use with alpha-blockers) · Prinzmetal's angina · second-degree AV block · severe peripheral arterial disease · sick sinus syndrome · third-degree AV block · uncontrolled heart failure

  CONTRA-INDICATIONS, FURTHER INFORMATION
- ▸ **Bronchospasm** Beta-blockers, including those considered to be cardioselective, should usually be avoided in patients with a history of asthma, bronchospasm or a history of obstructive airways disease. However, when there is no

Cardiovascular system

2

alternative, a cardioselective beta-blocker can be given to these patients with caution and under specialist supervision. In such cases the risk of inducing bronchospasm should be appreciated and appropriate precautions taken.

● CAUTIONS Diabetes · first-degree AV block · history of obstructive airways disease (introduce cautiously) · myasthenia gravis · portal hypertension (risk of deterioration in liver function) · psoriasis · symptoms of hypoglycaemia may be masked · symptoms of thyrotoxicosis may be masked

CAUTIONS, FURTHER INFORMATION

▸ Elderly Prescription potentially inappropriate (STOPP criteria):
  ● in combination with verapamil or diltiazem (risk of heart block)
  ● with bradycardia (heart rate less than 50 beats per minute), type II heart block or complete heart block (risk of complete heart block, asystole)
  ● in diabetes mellitus patients with frequent hypoglycaemic episodes (risk of suppressing hypoglycaemic symptoms)
  ● if prescribed a **non-selective** beta-blocker (including topical beta-blockers) in a history of asthma requiring treatment (risk of increased bronchospasm)
  See also Prescribing in the elderly p. 33.

● SIDE-EFFECTS
▸ **Common or very common** Abdominal discomfort · bradycardia · confusion · depression · diarrhoea · dizziness · dry eye (reversible on discontinuation) · dyspnoea · erectile dysfunction · fatigue · headache · heart failure · nausea · paraesthesia · peripheral coldness · peripheral vascular disease · rash (reversible on discontinuation) · sleep disorders · syncope · visual impairment · vomiting
▸ **Uncommon** Atrioventricular block · bronchospasm
▸ **Rare or very rare** Hallucination

SIDE-EFFECTS, FURTHER INFORMATION With administration by intravenous injection, excessive bradycardia can occur and may be countered with **intravenous injection** of atropine sulfate.

Overdose Therapeutic overdosages with beta-blockers may cause lightheadedness, dizziness, and possibly syncope as a result of bradycardia and hypotension; heart failure may be precipitated or exacerbated. With administration by intravenous injection, excessive bradycardia can occur and may be countered with intravenous injection of atropine sulfate.

For details on the management of poisoning, see Beta-blockers, under Emergency treatment of poisoning p. 1413.

● ALLERGY AND CROSS-SENSITIVITY Caution is advised in patients with a history of hypersensitivity—may increase sensitivity to allergens and result in more serious hypersensitivity response. Furthermore beta-adrenoceptor blockers may reduce response to adrenaline (epinephrine).

● PREGNANCY Beta-blockers may cause intra-uterine growth restriction, neonatal hypoglycaemia, and bradycardia; the risk is greater in severe hypertension.

● BREAST FEEDING With systemic use in the mother, infants should be monitored as there is a risk of possible toxicity due to beta-blockade. However, the amount of most beta-blockers present in milk is too small to affect infants.

● MONITORING REQUIREMENTS Monitor lung function (in patients with a history of obstructive airway disease).

● TREATMENT CESSATION Avoid abrupt withdrawal especially in ischaemic heart disease. Sudden cessation of a beta-blocker can cause a rebound worsening of myocardial ischaemia and therefore gradual reduction of dose is preferable when beta-blockers are to be stopped.

BETA-ADRENOCEPTOR BLOCKERS ❯
ALPHA- AND BETA-ADRENOCEPTOR BLOCKERS

◀ 161

Carvedilol

10-Mar-2020

● **INDICATIONS AND DOSE**

Hypertension
▸ BY MOUTH
  ▸ Adult: Initially 12.5 mg once daily for 2 days, then increased to 25 mg once daily; increased if necessary up to 50 mg daily, dose to be increased at intervals of at least 2 weeks and can be given as a single dose or in divided doses
  ▸ Elderly: Initially 12.5 mg daily, initial dose may provide satisfactory control

Angina
▸ BY MOUTH
  ▸ Adult: Initially 12.5 mg twice daily for 2 days, then increased to 25 mg twice daily

Adjunct to diuretics, digoxin, or ACE inhibitors in symptomatic chronic heart failure
▸ BY MOUTH
  ▸ Adult: Initially 3.125 mg twice daily, dose to be taken with food, then increased to 6.25 mg twice daily, then increased to 12.5 mg twice daily, then increased to 25 mg twice daily, dose should be increased at intervals of at least 2 weeks up to the highest tolerated dose, max. 25 mg twice daily in patients with severe heart failure or body-weight less than 85 kg; max. 50 mg twice daily in patients over 85 kg

● CONTRA-INDICATIONS Acute or decompensated heart failure requiring intravenous inotropes

● INTERACTIONS → Appendix 1: beta blockers, non-selective

● SIDE-EFFECTS
▸ **Common or very common** Anaemia · asthma · dyspepsia · eye irritation · fluid imbalance · genital oedema · hypercholesterolaemia · hyperglycaemia · hypoglycaemia · increased risk of infection · oedema · postural hypotension · pulmonary oedema · renal impairment · urinary disorders · weight increased
▸ **Uncommon** Alopecia · angina pectoris · constipation · hyperhidrosis · skin reactions
▸ **Rare or very rare** Dry mouth · hypersensitivity · leucopenia · nasal congestion · severe cutaneous adverse reactions (SCARs) · thrombocytopenia

● PREGNANCY Information on the safety of carvedilol during pregnancy is lacking. If carvedilol is used close to delivery, infants should be monitored for signs of alpha-blockade (as well as beta-blockade).

● BREAST FEEDING Infants should be monitored as there is a risk of possible toxicity due to alpha-blockade (in addition to beta-blockade).

● HEPATIC IMPAIRMENT Manufacturer advises avoid in severe impairment.
  Dose adjustments Manufacturer advises dose adjustment may be required in moderate impairment.

● MONITORING REQUIREMENTS Monitor renal function during dose titration in patients with heart failure who also have renal impairment, low blood pressure, ischaemic heart disease, or diffuse vascular disease.

● MEDICINAL FORMS There can be variation in the licensing of different medicines containing the same drug. Forms available from special-order manufacturers include: oral suspension
  Tablet
  CAUTIONARY AND ADVISORY LABELS 8
  ▸ Carvedilol (Non-proprietary)
    Carvedilol 3.125 mg Carvedilol 3.125mg tablets | 28 tablet [PoM]
    £3.00 DT = £1.18

Carvedilol 6.25 mg Carvedilol 6.25mg tablets | 28 tablet [PoM]
£2.20 DT = £1.29
Carvedilol 12.5 mg Carvedilol 12.5mg tablets | 28 tablet [PoM] £4.55
DT = £1.72
Carvedilol 25 mg Carvedilol 25mg tablets | 28 tablet [PoM] £5.99 DT
= £1.98

◄ 161

Labetalol hydrochloride   10-Mar-2020

● **INDICATIONS AND DOSE**

Controlled hypotension in anaesthesia
▸ BY INTRAVENOUS INFUSION, OR BY INTRAVENOUS INJECTION
▸ Adult: (consult product literature or local protocols)

Hypertension of pregnancy
▸ BY INTRAVENOUS INFUSION
▸ Adult: Initially 20 mg/hour, then increased if necessary
to 40 mg/hour after 30 minutes, then increased if
necessary to 80 mg/hour after 30 minutes, then
increased if necessary to 160 mg/hour after 30 minutes,
adjusted according to response; Usual maximum
160 mg/hour
▸ BY MOUTH
▸ Adult: Use dose for hypertension

Hypertension following myocardial infarction
▸ BY INTRAVENOUS INFUSION
▸ Adult: 15 mg/hour, then increased to up to
120 mg/hour, dose to be increased gradually

Hypertensive emergencies
▸ BY INTRAVENOUS INJECTION
▸ Adult: 50 mg, to be given over at least 1 minute, then
50 mg every 5 minutes if required until a satisfactory
response occurs; maximum 200 mg per course
▸ BY INTRAVENOUS INFUSION
▸ Adult: Initially 2 mg/minute until a satisfactory
response is achieved, then discontinue; usual dose
50–200 mg

Hypertension
▸ BY MOUTH
▸ Adult: Initially 100 mg twice daily, dose to be increased
at intervals of 14 days; usual dose 200 mg twice daily,
increased if necessary up to 800 mg daily in 2 divided
doses, to be taken with food, higher doses to be given
in 3–4 divided doses; maximum 2.4 g per day
▸ Elderly: Initially 50 mg twice daily, dose to be increased
at intervals of 14 days; usual dose 200 mg twice daily,
increased if necessary up to 800 mg daily in 2 divided
doses, to be taken with food, higher doses to be given
in 3–4 divided doses; maximum 2.4 g per day
▸ BY INTRAVENOUS INJECTION
▸ Adult: 50 mg, dose to be given over at least 1 minute,
then 50 mg after 5 minutes if required; maximum
200 mg per course
▸ BY INTRAVENOUS INFUSION
▸ Adult: Initially 2 mg/minute until a satisfactory
response is achieved, then discontinue; usual dose
50–200 mg

● CAUTIONS Liver damage
● INTERACTIONS → Appendix 1: beta blockers, non-selective
● SIDE-EFFECTS
GENERAL SIDE-EFFECTS
▸ **Common or very common** Drug fever · ejaculation failure ·
hypersensitivity · urinary disorders
▸ **Rare or very rare** Hepatic disorders · systemic lupus
erythematosus (SLE) · toxic myopathy · tremor
▸ **Frequency not known** Alopecia · cyanosis · hyperhidrosis ·
hyperkalaemia · interstitial lung disease · lethargy · muscle
cramps · nasal congestion · peripheral oedema · postural
hypotension · psychosis · skin reactions ·
thrombocytopenia

SPECIFIC SIDE-EFFECTS
▸ With intravenous use Fever · hypoglycaemia masked ·
thyrotoxicosis masked
▸ With oral use Photosensitivity reaction
● PREGNANCY The use of labetalol in maternal hypertension
is not known to be harmful, except possibly in the first
trimester. If labetalol is used close to delivery, infants
should be monitored for signs of alpha-blockade (as well as
beta blockade).
● BREAST FEEDING Infants should be monitored as there is a
risk of possible toxicity due to alpha-blockade (in addition
to beta-blockade).
● HEPATIC IMPAIRMENT Manufacturer advises caution (risk
of slow metabolism).
Dose adjustments Manufacturer advises consider dose
reduction.
● RENAL IMPAIRMENT
Dose adjustments Dose reduction may be required.
● MONITORING REQUIREMENTS
▸ Liver damage Severe hepatocellular damage reported after
both short-term and long-term treatment. Appropriate
laboratory testing needed at first symptom of liver
dysfunction and if laboratory evidence of damage (or if
jaundice) labetalol should be stopped and not restarted.
● EFFECT ON LABORATORY TESTS Interferes with laboratory
tests for catecholamines.
● DIRECTIONS FOR ADMINISTRATION For *intravenous
infusion*, give intermittently *in* Glucose 5% *or* Sodium
chloride and glucose. Dilute to a concentration of
1 mg/mL; suggested volume 200 mL; adjust rate with in-
line burette. Avoid upright position during and for 3 hours
after intravenous administration.

● MEDICINAL FORMS There can be variation in the licensing of
different medicines containing the same drug. Forms available
from special-order manufacturers include: oral suspension, oral
solution

Solution for injection
▸ Labetalol hydrochloride (Non-proprietary)
Labetalol hydrochloride 5 mg per 1 ml Labetalol 50mg/10ml
solution for injection ampoules | 10 ampoule [PoM] **⅀** (Hospital only)
Labetalol 100mg/20ml solution for injection ampoules |
5 ampoule [PoM] £123.06 DT = £123.06 (Hospital only) |
5 ampoule [PoM] £126.45 DT = £123.06

Tablet
CAUTIONARY AND ADVISORY LABELS 8, 21
▸ Labetalol hydrochloride (Non-proprietary)
Labetalol hydrochloride 100 mg Labetalol 100mg tablets |
56 tablet [PoM] £7.52 DT = £6.15
Labetalol hydrochloride 200 mg Labetalol 200mg tablets |
56 tablet [PoM] £10.10 DT = £8.72
Labetalol hydrochloride 400 mg Labetalol 400mg tablets |
56 tablet [PoM] £21.12 DT = £19.64
▸ Trandate (RPH Pharmaceuticals AB)
Labetalol hydrochloride 50 mg Trandate 50mg tablets |
56 tablet [PoM] £3.79 DT = £3.79
Labetalol hydrochloride 100 mg Trandate 100mg tablets |
56 tablet [PoM] £4.64 DT = £6.15 | 250 tablet [PoM] £15.62
Labetalol hydrochloride 200 mg Trandate 200mg tablets |
56 tablet [PoM] £7.41 DT = £8.72 | 250 tablet [PoM] £24.76
Labetalol hydrochloride 400 mg Trandate 400mg tablets |
56 tablet [PoM] £10.15 DT = £19.64

2

Cardiovascular system

Cardiovascular system

2

Nadolol

● **INDICATIONS AND DOSE**

Hypertension
▸ BY MOUTH
▸ Adult: Initially 80 mg once daily, then increased in steps of up to 80 mg every week if required, doses higher than the maximum are rarely necessary; maximum 240 mg per day

Angina
▸ BY MOUTH
▸ Adult: Initially 40 mg once daily, then increased if necessary up to 160 mg daily, doses should be increased at weekly intervals, maximum dose rarely is used; maximum 240 mg per day

Arrhythmias
▸ BY MOUTH
▸ Adult: Initially 40 mg once daily, then increased if necessary up to 160 mg once daily, doses should be increased at weekly intervals; reduced to 40 mg daily if bradycardia occurs

Migraine prophylaxis
▸ BY MOUTH
▸ Adult: Initially 40 mg once daily, then increased in steps of 40 mg every week, adjusted according to response; maintenance 80–160 mg once daily

Thyrotoxicosis (adjunct)
▸ BY MOUTH
▸ Adult: 80–160 mg once daily

● INTERACTIONS → Appendix 1: beta blockers, non-selective

● SIDE-EFFECTS
▸ **Uncommon** Appetite decreased · behaviour abnormal · constipation · cough · dry mouth · dyspepsia · facial swelling · flatulence · hyperhidrosis · nasal congestion · sedation · sexual dysfunction · skin reactions · speech slurred · tinnitus · vision blurred · weight increased
▸ **Frequency not known** Alopecia · hypoglycaemia

● BREAST FEEDING Water soluble beta-blockers such as nadolol are present in breast milk in greater amounts than other beta blockers.

● HEPATIC IMPAIRMENT Manufacturer advises caution.

● RENAL IMPAIRMENT
Dose adjustments Increase dosage interval if eGFR less than 50 mL/minute/1.73 m².

● MEDICINAL FORMS There can be variation in the licensing of different medicines containing the same drug. Forms available from special-order manufacturers include: tablet, oral suspension, oral solution
Tablet
CAUTIONARY AND ADVISORY LABELS 8
▸ Corgard (Sanofi)
  Nadolol 80 mg Corgard 80mg tablets | 28 tablet [PoM] £6.00 DT = £6.00

F 161

Pindolol

● **INDICATIONS AND DOSE**

Hypertension
▸ BY MOUTH
▸ Adult: Initially 5 mg 2–3 times a day, alternatively 15 mg once daily, doses to be increased as required at weekly intervals; maintenance 15–30 mg daily; maximum 45 mg per day

Angina
▸ BY MOUTH
▸ Adult: 2.5–5 mg up to 3 times a day

● INTERACTIONS → Appendix 1: beta blockers, non-selective

● SIDE-EFFECTS Agranulocytosis · arrhythmia · arthralgia · constipation · cutaneous lupus erythematosus · diabetes mellitus · dry mouth · dyspepsia · gastrointestinal disorders · glycosuria · hyperglycaemia · hyperhidrosis · hyperpyrexia · hypoglycaemia · hypoglycaemia masked · keratoconjunctivitis · muscle complaints · myasthenia gravis · psychosis · sexual dysfunction · skin reactions · thrombocytopenia · thyrotoxicosis masked · toxic epidermal necrolysis · tremor · vasculitis necrotising · vision blurred

● RENAL IMPAIRMENT May adversely affect renal function in severe impairment—manufacturer advises avoid.

● MEDICINAL FORMS There can be variation in the licensing of different medicines containing the same drug.
Tablet
CAUTIONARY AND ADVISORY LABELS 8
▸ Pindolol (Non-proprietary)
  Pindolol 5 mg Pindolol 5mg tablets | 100 tablet [PoM] £15.00 DT = £8.05

F 161

Propranolol hydrochloride
28-Jul-2020

● **INDICATIONS AND DOSE**

Thyrotoxicosis (adjunct)
▸ BY MOUTH
▸ Adult: 10–40 mg 3–4 times a day

Thyrotoxic crisis
▸ BY INTRAVENOUS INJECTION
▸ Adult: 1 mg, to be given over 1 minute, dose may be repeated if necessary at intervals of 2 minutes, maximum total dose is 5 mg in anaesthesia; maximum 10 mg per course

Hypertension
▸ BY MOUTH
▸ Adult: Initially 80 mg twice daily, dose should be increased at weekly intervals as required; maintenance 160–320 mg daily

Prophylaxis of variceal bleeding in portal hypertension
▸ BY MOUTH
▸ Adult: Initially 40 mg twice daily, then increased to 80 mg twice daily (max. per dose 160 mg twice daily), dose to be adjusted according to heart rate

Phaeochromocytoma (only with an alpha-blocker) in preparation for surgery
▸ BY MOUTH
▸ Adult: 60 mg daily for 3 days before surgery

Phaeochromocytoma (only with an alpha-blocker) in patients unsuitable for surgery
▸ BY MOUTH
▸ Adult: 30 mg daily

Angina
▸ BY MOUTH
▸ Adult: Initially 40 mg 2–3 times a day; maintenance 120–240 mg daily

Hypertrophic cardiomyopathy | Anxiety tachycardia
▸ BY MOUTH
▸ Adult: 10–40 mg 3–4 times a day

Anxiety with symptoms such as palpitation, sweating and tremor
▸ BY MOUTH
▸ Adult: 40 mg once daily, then increased if necessary to 40 mg 3 times a day

Prophylaxis after myocardial infarction
▶ BY MOUTH
▶ Adult: Initially 40 mg 4 times a day for 2–3 days, then 80 mg twice daily, start treatment 5 to 21 days after infarction

Essential tremor
▶ BY MOUTH
▶ Adult: Initially 40 mg 2–3 times a day; maintenance 80–160 mg daily

Migraine prophylaxis
▶ BY MOUTH
▶ Adult: 80–240 mg daily in divided doses

Arrhythmias
▶ BY MOUTH
▶ Adult: 10–40 mg 3–4 times a day
▶ BY INTRAVENOUS INJECTION
▶ Adult: 1 mg, to be given over 1 minute, dose may be repeated if necessary at intervals of 2 minutes, maximum 10 mg per course (5 mg in anaesthesia)

IMPORTANT SAFETY INFORMATION

SAFE PRACTICE

Propranolol has been confused with prednisolone; care must be taken to ensure the correct drug is prescribed and dispensed.

● INTERACTIONS → Appendix 1: beta blockers, non-selective

● SIDE-EFFECTS
▶ **Rare or very rare** Alopecia · memory loss · mood altered · neuromuscular dysfunction · postural hypotension · psychosis · skin reactions · thrombocytopenia
▶ **Frequency not known** Hypoglycaemia

Overdose Severe overdosages with propranolol may cause cardiovascular collapse, CNS depression, and convulsions.

● HEPATIC IMPAIRMENT Manufacturer advises caution (increased risk of hepatic encephalopathy; risk of increased half-life).
Dose adjustments ▶ With oral use Manufacturer advises consider dose reduction.

● RENAL IMPAIRMENT
Dose adjustments Manufacturer advises caution; dose reduction may be required.

● PRESCRIBING AND DISPENSING INFORMATION Modified-release preparations can be used for once daily administration.

● MEDICINAL FORMS There can be variation in the licensing of different medicines containing the same drug. Forms available from special-order manufacturers include: oral suspension, oral solution

Oral solution
CAUTIONARY AND ADVISORY LABELS 8
▶ Propranolol hydrochloride (Non-proprietary)
Propranolol hydrochloride 1 mg per 1 ml Propranolol 5mg/5ml oral solution sugar free sugar-free | 150 ml [PoM] £23.51 DT = £23.51
Propranolol hydrochloride 2 mg per 1 ml Propranolol 10mg/5ml oral solution sugar free sugar-free | 150 ml [PoM] £28.45 DT = £28.45
Propranolol hydrochloride 8 mg per 1 ml Propranolol 40mg/5ml oral solution sugar free sugar-free | 150 ml [PoM] £36.51 DT = £36.51
Propranolol hydrochloride 10 mg per 1 ml Propranolol 50mg/5ml oral solution sugar free sugar-free | 150 ml [PoM] £38.51 DT = £38.51

Modified-release capsule
CAUTIONARY AND ADVISORY LABELS 8, 25
▶ Bedranol SR (Sandoz Ltd, Almus Pharmaceuticals Ltd)
Propranolol hydrochloride 80 mg Bedranol SR 80mg capsules | 28 capsule [PoM] £4.16 DT = £4.95
Propranolol hydrochloride 160 mg Bedranol SR 160mg capsules | 28 capsule [PoM] £4.59–£5.09 DT = £4.88
▶ Beta-Prograne (Actavis UK Ltd, Teva UK Ltd, Tillomed Laboratories Ltd)
Propranolol hydrochloride 160 mg Beta-Prograne 160mg modified-release capsules | 28 capsule [PoM] £4.88–£6.11 DT = £4.88

▶ Half Beta-Prograne (Actavis UK Ltd, Tillomed Laboratories Ltd, Teva UK Ltd)
Propranolol hydrochloride 80 mg Half Beta-Prograne 80mg modified-release capsules | 28 capsule [PoM] £4.95 DT = £4.95

Tablet
CAUTIONARY AND ADVISORY LABELS 8
▶ Propranolol hydrochloride (Non-proprietary)
Propranolol hydrochloride 10 mg Propranolol 10mg tablets | 28 tablet [PoM] £7.00 DT = £1.84
Propranolol hydrochloride 40 mg Propranolol 40mg tablets | 28 tablet [PoM] £7.00 DT = £1.77
Propranolol hydrochloride 80 mg Propranolol 80mg tablets | 56 tablet [PoM] £5.23 DT = £2.72
Propranolol hydrochloride 160 mg Propranolol 160mg tablets | 56 tablet [PoM] £5.88 DT = £5.88
▶ Bedranol (Ennogen Pharma Ltd)
Propranolol hydrochloride 10 mg Bedranol 10mg tablets | 28 tablet [PoM] £1.54 DT = £1.84
Propranolol hydrochloride 40 mg Bedranol 40mg tablets | 28 tablet [PoM] £1.38 DT = £1.77
Propranolol hydrochloride 80 mg Bedranol 80mg tablets | 56 tablet [PoM] £0.95 DT = £2.72
Propranolol hydrochloride 160 mg Bedranol 160mg tablets | 56 tablet [PoM] £4.70 DT = £5.88

F 161

Timolol maleate
31-Jul-2019

● INDICATIONS AND DOSE

Hypertension
▶ BY MOUTH
▶ Adult: Initially 10 mg daily in 1–2 divided doses, then increased if necessary up to 60 mg daily, doses to be increased gradually. Doses above 30 mg daily given in divided doses, usual maintenance 10–30 mg daily; maximum 60 mg per day

Angina
▶ BY MOUTH
▶ Adult: Initially 5 mg twice daily, then increased in steps of 10 mg daily (max. per dose 30 mg twice daily), to be increased every 3–4 days

Prophylaxis after myocardial infarction
▶ BY MOUTH
▶ Adult: Initially 5 mg twice daily for 2 days, then increased if tolerated to 10 mg twice daily

Migraine prophylaxis
▶ BY MOUTH
▶ Adult: 10–20 mg daily in 1–2 divided doses

● INTERACTIONS → Appendix 1: beta blockers, non-selective

● SIDE-EFFECTS
▶ **Rare or very rare** Arthralgia · retroperitoneal fibrosis · skin reactions
▶ **Frequency not known** Cyanosis · drowsiness · dyspepsia · psychosis · vertigo

● BREAST FEEDING Manufacturer advises avoidance.

● HEPATIC IMPAIRMENT Manufacturer advises caution.
Dose adjustments Manufacturer advises consider dose reduction.

● RENAL IMPAIRMENT
Dose adjustments Manufacturer advises caution—dose reduction may be required.

● MEDICINAL FORMS There can be variation in the licensing of different medicines containing the same drug.
Tablet
CAUTIONARY AND ADVISORY LABELS 8
▶ Timolol maleate (Non-proprietary)
Timolol maleate 10 mg Timolol 10mg tablets | 30 tablet [PoM] £39.89 DT = £39.89

Timolol with amiloride and hydrochlorothiazide

The properties listed below are those particular to the combination only. For the properties of the components please consider, timolol maleate p. 165, amiloride hydrochloride p. 245, hydrochlorothiazide p. 180.

● **INDICATIONS AND DOSE**

Hypertension
▸ BY MOUTH
  ▸ Adult: 1–2 tablets daily

● **INTERACTIONS** → Appendix 1: beta blockers, non-selective · potassium-sparing diuretics · thiazide diuretics

● **MEDICINAL FORMS** There can be variation in the licensing of different medicines containing the same drug.

Tablet
CAUTIONARY AND ADVISORY LABELS 8
▸ Timolol with amiloride and hydrochlorothiazide (Non-proprietary)
  Amiloride hydrochloride 2.5 mg, Timolol maleate 10 mg, Hydrochlorothiazide 25 mg Timolol 10mg / Amiloride 2.5mg / Hydrochlorothiazide 25mg tablets | 28 tablet [PoM] £29.87

Timolol with bendroflumethiazide

The properties listed below are those particular to the combination only. For the properties of the components please consider, timolol maleate p. 165, bendroflumethiazide p. 180.

● **INDICATIONS AND DOSE**

Hypertension
▸ BY MOUTH
  ▸ Adult: 1–2 tablets daily; maximum 4 tablets per day

● **INTERACTIONS** → Appendix 1: beta blockers, non-selective · thiazide diuretics

● **MEDICINAL FORMS** There can be variation in the licensing of different medicines containing the same drug.

Tablet
CAUTIONARY AND ADVISORY LABELS 8
▸ Timolol with bendroflumethiazide (Non-proprietary)
  Bendroflumethiazide 2.5 mg, Timolol maleate 10 mg Timolol 10mg / Bendroflumethiazide 2.5mg tablets | 30 tablet [PoM] £23.75–£63.08 DT = £63.08

BETA-ADRENOCEPTOR BLOCKERS ❯
SELECTIVE

Acebutolol

● **INDICATIONS AND DOSE**

Hypertension
▸ BY MOUTH
  ▸ Adult: Initially 400 mg daily for 2 weeks, alternatively initially 200 mg twice daily for 2 weeks, then increased if necessary to 400 mg twice daily; maximum 1.2 g per day

Angina
▸ BY MOUTH
  ▸ Adult: Initially 400 mg daily, alternatively initially 200 mg twice daily; maximum 1.2 g per day

Arrhythmias
▸ BY MOUTH
  ▸ Adult: 0.4–1.2 g daily in 2–3 divided doses

Severe angina
▸ BY MOUTH
  ▸ Adult: Initially 300 mg 3 times a day; maximum 1.2 g per day

● **INTERACTIONS** → Appendix 1: beta blockers, selective

● **SIDE-EFFECTS**
▸ **Common or very common** Gastrointestinal disorder
▸ **Frequency not known** Cyanosis · hepatic disorders · lupus-like syndrome · nervous system disorder · psychosis · respiratory disorders · sexual dysfunction

● **BREAST FEEDING** Acebutolol and water soluble beta-blockers are present in breast milk in greater amounts than other beta-blockers.

● **RENAL IMPAIRMENT**
Dose adjustments Halve dose if eGFR 25–50 mL/minute/1.73 m^2; use quarter dose if eGFR less than 25 mL/minute/1.73 m^2; do not administer more than once daily.

● **MEDICINAL FORMS** There can be variation in the licensing of different medicines containing the same drug.

Tablet
CAUTIONARY AND ADVISORY LABELS 8
▸ Sectral (Sanofi)
  Acebutolol (as Acebutolol hydrochloride) 400 mg Sectral 400mg tablets | 28 tablet [PoM] £18.62 DT = £18.62

Capsule
CAUTIONARY AND ADVISORY LABELS 8
▸ Sectral (Sanofi)
  Acebutolol (as Acebutolol hydrochloride) 100 mg Sectral 100mg capsules | 84 capsule [PoM] £14.97 DT = £14.97
  Acebutolol (as Acebutolol hydrochloride) 200 mg Sectral 200mg capsules | 56 capsule [PoM] £19.18 DT = £19.18

Atenolol

24-Jul-2020

● **INDICATIONS AND DOSE**

Hypertension
▸ BY MOUTH
  ▸ Adult: 25–50 mg daily, higher doses are rarely necessary

Angina
▸ BY MOUTH
  ▸ Adult: 100 mg daily in 1–2 divided doses

Arrhythmias
▸ BY MOUTH
  ▸ Adult: 50–100 mg daily
▸ BY INTRAVENOUS INJECTION
  ▸ Adult: 2.5 mg every 5 minutes if required, to be given at a rate of 1 mg/minute, treatment course may be repeated every 12 hours if required; maximum 10 mg per course
▸ BY INTRAVENOUS INFUSION
  ▸ Adult: 150 micrograms/kg every 12 hours if required, to be given over 20 minutes

Migraine prophylaxis
▸ BY MOUTH
  ▸ Adult: 50–200 mg daily in divided doses

Early intervention within 12 hours of myocardial infarction
▸ INITIALLY BY INTRAVENOUS INJECTION
  ▸ Adult: 5–10 mg, to be given at a rate of 1 mg/minute, followed by (by mouth) 50 mg after 15 minutes, then (by mouth) 50 mg after 12 hours, then (by mouth) 100 mg after 12 hours, then (by mouth) 100 mg once daily

- UNLICENSED USE Use of atenolol for migraine prophylaxis is an unlicensed indication.

IMPORTANT SAFETY INFORMATION

SAFE PRACTICE
Atenolol has been confused with amlodipine; care must be taken to ensure the correct drug is prescribed and dispensed.

- INTERACTIONS → Appendix 1: beta blockers, selective
- SIDE-EFFECTS
▸ **Common or very common** Gastrointestinal disorder
▸ **Rare or very rare** Alopecia · dry mouth · hepatic disorders · mood altered · postural hypotension · psychosis · skin reactions · thrombocytopenia
▸ **Frequency not known** Hypersensitivity · lupus-like syndrome
- BREAST FEEDING Water soluble beta-blockers such as atenolol are present in breast milk in greater amounts than other beta blockers.
- RENAL IMPAIRMENT
Dose adjustments ▸ With oral use Max. 50 mg daily if eGFR 15–35 mL/minute/1.73 m^2; max. 25 mg daily or 50 mg on alternate days if eGFR less than 15 mL/minute/1.73 m^2.
▸ With intravenous use Max. 10 mg on alternate days if eGFR 15–35 mL/minute/1.73 m^2; max.10 mg every 4 days if eGFR less than 15 mL/minute/1.73 m^2.
- DIRECTIONS FOR ADMINISTRATION For *intravenous infusion* (*Tenormin*®), manufacturer advises give intermittently in Glucose 5% or Sodium chloride 0.9%. Suggested infusion time 20 minutes.

- MEDICINAL FORMS There can be variation in the licensing of different medicines containing the same drug. Forms available from special-order manufacturers include: oral suspension, oral solution

Solution for injection
▸ Tenormin (AstraZeneca UK Ltd)
  Atenolol 500 microgram per 1 ml Tenormin 5mg/10ml solution for injection ampoules | 10 ampoule [PoM] £34.45 (Hospital only)

Oral solution
CAUTIONARY AND ADVISORY LABELS 8
▸ Atenolol (Non-proprietary)
  Atenolol 5 mg per 1 ml Atenolol 25mg/5ml oral solution sugar free sugar-free | 300 ml [PoM] £73.00 DT = £6.86

Tablet
CAUTIONARY AND ADVISORY LABELS 8
▸ Atenolol (Non-proprietary)
  Atenolol 25 mg Atenolol 25mg tablets | 28 tablet [PoM] £1.39 DT = £0.76
  Atenolol 50 mg Atenolol 50mg tablets | 28 tablet [PoM] £1.44 DT = £0.78
  Atenolol 100 mg Atenolol 100mg tablets | 28 tablet [PoM] £1.74 DT = £0.86
▸ Tenormin (AstraZeneca UK Ltd)
  Atenolol 50 mg Tenormin LS 50mg tablets | 28 tablet [PoM] £10.22 DT = £0.78

Atenolol with nifedipine

The properties listed below are those particular to the combination only. For the properties of the components please consider, atenolol p. 166, nifedipine p. 176.

- INDICATIONS AND DOSE

Hypertension
▸ BY MOUTH
▸ Adult: 1 capsule daily, increased if necessary to 1 capsule twice daily
▸ Elderly: 1 capsule daily

Angina
▸ BY MOUTH
▸ Adult: 1 capsule twice daily

- INTERACTIONS → Appendix 1: beta blockers, selective · calcium channel blockers
- PRESCRIBING AND DISPENSING INFORMATION Only indicated when calcium-channel blocker or beta-blocker alone proves inadequate.
- MEDICINAL FORMS There can be variation in the licensing of different medicines containing the same drug.
Modified-release capsule
CAUTIONARY AND ADVISORY LABELS 8, 25
▸ Tenif (AstraZeneca UK Ltd)
  Nifedipine 20 mg, Atenolol 50 mg Tenif 50mg/20mg modified-release capsules | 28 capsule [PoM] £15.30 DT = £15.30

F 161

Bisoprolol fumarate
07-Jun-2018

- INDICATIONS AND DOSE

Hypertension | Angina
▸ BY MOUTH
▸ Adult: 5–10 mg once daily; maximum 20 mg per day

Adjunct in heart failure
▸ BY MOUTH
▸ Adult: Initially 1.25 mg once daily for 1 week, dose to be taken in the morning, then increased if tolerated to 2.5 mg once daily for 1 week, then increased if tolerated to 3.75 mg once daily for 1 week, then increased if tolerated to 5 mg once daily for 4 weeks, then increased if tolerated to 7.5 mg once daily for 4 weeks, then increased if tolerated to 10 mg once daily; maximum 10 mg per day

---

- CONTRA-INDICATIONS Acute or decompensated heart failure requiring intravenous inotropes · sino–atrial block
- CAUTIONS Ensure heart failure not worsening before increasing dose
- INTERACTIONS → Appendix 1: beta blockers, selective
- SIDE-EFFECTS
▸ **Common or very common** Constipation
▸ **Uncommon** Muscle cramps · muscle weakness · postural hypotension
▸ **Rare or very rare** Allergic rhinitis · alopecia · auditory disorder · conjunctivitis · flushing · hepatitis · hypersensitivity · pruritus
- HEPATIC IMPAIRMENT Manufacturer advises caution.
Dose adjustments
▸ When used for angina or hypertension Manufacturer advises consider maximum dose of 10 mg once daily in severe impairment—consult product literature.
▸ When used for heart failure Manufacturer advises caution when titrating dose (no information available).
- RENAL IMPAIRMENT
Dose adjustments Reduce dose if eGFR less than 20 mL/minute/1.73 m^2 (max. 10 mg daily).

- MEDICINAL FORMS There can be variation in the licensing of different medicines containing the same drug. Forms available from special-order manufacturers include: oral suspension, oral solution
Tablet
CAUTIONARY AND ADVISORY LABELS 8
▸ Bisoprolol fumarate (Non-proprietary)
  Bisoprolol fumarate 1.25 mg Bisoprolol 1.25mg tablets | 28 tablet [PoM] £7.43 DT = £0.98 | 100 tablet [PoM] £3.50-£6.79
  Bisoprolol fumarate 2.5 mg Bisoprolol 2.5mg tablets | 28 tablet [PoM] £4.39 DT = £0.91 | 100 tablet [PoM] £3.25-£6.39
  Bisoprolol fumarate 3.75 mg Bisoprolol 3.75mg tablets | 28 tablet [PoM] £4.89 DT = £1.17
  Bisoprolol fumarate 5 mg Bisoprolol 5mg tablets | 28 tablet [PoM] £5.89 DT = £0.91 | 100 tablet [PoM] £3.25-£4.25
  Bisoprolol fumarate 7.5 mg Bisoprolol 7.5mg tablets | 28 tablet [PoM] £5.89 DT = £1.22
  Bisoprolol fumarate 10 mg Bisoprolol 10mg tablets | 28 tablet [PoM] £1.02 DT = £1.02 | 100 tablet [PoM] £3.64-£4.50

2

Cardiovascular system

▸ Cardicor (Merck Serono Ltd)
Bisoprolol fumarate 1.25 mg Cardicor 1.25mg tablets |
28 tablet [PoM] £2.35 DT = £0.98
Bisoprolol fumarate 2.5 mg Cardicor 2.5mg tablets |
28 tablet [PoM] £2.35 DT = £0.91
Bisoprolol fumarate 3.75 mg Cardicor 3.75mg tablets |
28 tablet [PoM] £4.90 DT = £1.17
Bisoprolol fumarate 5 mg Cardicor 5mg tablets | 28 tablet [PoM]
£5.90 DT = £0.91
Bisoprolol fumarate 7.5 mg Cardicor 7.5mg tablets |
28 tablet [PoM] £5.90 DT = £1.22
Bisoprolol fumarate 10 mg Cardicor 10mg tablets | 28 tablet [PoM]
£5.90 DT = £1.02

⚑ 161

Celiprolol hydrochloride
25-Jun-2018

● **INDICATIONS AND DOSE**

Mild to moderate hypertension
▸ BY MOUTH
▸ **Adult:** 200 mg once daily, dose to be taken in the
morning, then increased if necessary to 400 mg once
daily

● INTERACTIONS → Appendix 1: beta blockers, selective

● SIDE-EFFECTS Alveolitis allergic · dermatitis psoriasiform ·
drowsiness · hypoglycaemia masked · palpitations ·
thyrotoxicosis masked · tremor

● BREAST FEEDING Manufacturers advise avoidance.

● HEPATIC IMPAIRMENT Manufacturer advises caution.
Dose adjustments Manufacturer advises consider dose
reduction.

● RENAL IMPAIRMENT Avoid if eGFR less than
15 mL/minute/1.73 m².
Dose adjustments Reduce dose by half if eGFR
15–40 mL/minute/1.73 m².

● MEDICINAL FORMS There can be variation in the licensing of
different medicines containing the same drug. Forms available
from special-order manufacturers include: oral suspension
Tablet
CAUTIONARY AND ADVISORY LABELS 8, 22
▸ Celiprolol hydrochloride (Non-proprietary)
Celiprolol hydrochloride 200 mg Celiprolol 200mg tablets |
28 tablet [PoM] £8.96 DT = £6.13
Celiprolol hydrochloride 400 mg Celiprolol 400mg tablets |
28 tablet [PoM] £13.17 DT = £9.33
▸ Celectol (Neon Healthcare Ltd)
Celiprolol hydrochloride 200 mg Celectol 200mg tablets |
28 tablet [PoM] £19.83 DT = £6.13
Celiprolol hydrochloride 400 mg Celectol 400mg tablets |
28 tablet [PoM] £39.65 DT = £9.33

⚑ 161

Co-tenidone

● **INDICATIONS AND DOSE**

Hypertension
▸ BY MOUTH
▸ **Adult:** 50/12.5 mg daily, alternatively increased if
necessary to 100/25 mg daily, doses higher than 50 mg
atenolol rarely necessary

DOSE EQUIVALENCE AND CONVERSION
▸ A mixture of atenolol and chlortalidone in mass
proportions corresponding to 4 parts of atenolol and
1 part chlortalidone.

● INTERACTIONS → Appendix 1: beta blockers, selective ·
thiazide diuretics

● SIDE-EFFECTS
▸ **Common or very common** Gastrointestinal disorder ·
glucose tolerance impaired
▸ **Rare or very rare** Alopecia · hepatic disorders · mood
altered · neutropenia · psychosis

▸ **Frequency not known** Lupus-like syndrome

● PREGNANCY Avoid. Diuretics not used to treat
hypertension in pregnancy.

● BREAST FEEDING Atenolol present in milk in greater
amounts than some other beta-blockers. Possible toxicity
due to beta-blockade—monitor infant. Large doses of
chlortalidone may suppress lactation.

● RENAL IMPAIRMENT Avoid if eGFR less than
30 mL/minute/1.73 m²—consider alternative treatment.

● MEDICINAL FORMS There can be variation in the licensing of
different medicines containing the same drug. Forms available
from special-order manufacturers include: oral suspension, oral
solution
Tablet
CAUTIONARY AND ADVISORY LABELS 8
▸ Co-tenidone (Non-proprietary)
Chlortalidone 12.5 mg, Atenolol 50 mg Co-tenidone 50mg/12.5mg
tablets | 28 tablet [PoM] £4.85 DT = £1.69
Chlortalidone 25 mg, Atenolol 100 mg Co-tenidone 100mg/25mg
tablets | 28 tablet [PoM] £4.85 DT = £1.89
▸ Tenoret (AstraZeneca UK Ltd)
Chlortalidone 12.5 mg, Atenolol 50 mg Tenoret 50mg/12.5mg
tablets | 28 tablet [PoM] £10.36 DT = £1.69
▸ Tenoretic (AstraZeneca UK Ltd)
Chlortalidone 25 mg, Atenolol 100 mg Tenoretic 100mg/25mg
tablets | 28 tablet [PoM] £10.36 DT = £1.89

⚑ 161

Esmolol hydrochloride
28-Jul-2020

● **INDICATIONS AND DOSE**

**Short-term treatment of supraventricular arrhythmias
(including atrial fibrillation, atrial flutter, sinus
tachycardia) | Tachycardia and hypertension in peri-
operative period**
▸ BY INTRAVENOUS INFUSION
▸ **Adult:** 50–200 micrograms/kg/minute, consult product
literature for details of dose titration and doses during
peri-operative period

● INTERACTIONS → Appendix 1: beta blockers, selective

● SIDE-EFFECTS
▸ **Common or very common** Anxiety · appetite decreased ·
concentration impaired · drowsiness · hyperhidrosis
▸ **Uncommon** Arrhythmias · chills · constipation ·
costochondritis · dry mouth · dyspepsia · fever · flushing ·
nasal congestion · oedema · pain · pallor · pulmonary
oedema · respiratory disorders · seizure · skin reactions ·
speech disorder · taste altered · thinking abnormal · urinary
retention
▸ **Rare or very rare** Cardiac arrest · extravasation necrosis ·
thrombophlebitis
▸ **Frequency not known** Angioedema · coronary vasospasm ·
hyperkalaemia · metabolic acidosis

● BREAST FEEDING Manufacturer advises avoidance.

● RENAL IMPAIRMENT Manufacturer advises caution.

● MEDICINAL FORMS There can be variation in the licensing of
different medicines containing the same drug.
Solution for injection
▸ Esmolol hydrochloride (Non-proprietary)
Esmolol hydrochloride 10 mg per 1 ml Esmolol hydrochloride
100mg/10ml solution for injection vials | 5 vial [PoM] £38.95 (Hospital
only)
Esmolol hydrochloride 100mg/10ml solution for injection vials | 10 vial [PoM]
£100.00 (Hospital only)
▸ Brevibloc (Baxter Healthcare Ltd)
Esmolol hydrochloride 10 mg per 1 ml Brevibloc Premixed
100mg/10ml solution for injection vials | 5 vial [PoM] [▣]

Solution for infusion
▸ Brevibloc (Baxter Healthcare Ltd)
  Esmolol hydrochloride 10 mg per 1 ml Brevibloc Premixed
  2.5g/250ml infusion bags | 1 bag [PoM] £89.69

F 161

Metoprolol tartrate

● **INDICATIONS AND DOSE**

Hypertension
▸ BY MOUTH USING IMMEDIATE-RELEASE MEDICINES
▸ Adult: Initially 100 mg daily, increased if necessary to
  200 mg daily in 1–2 divided doses, high doses are rarely
  required; maximum 400 mg per day
▸ BY MOUTH USING MODIFIED-RELEASE MEDICINES
▸ Adult: 200 mg once daily

Angina
▸ BY MOUTH USING IMMEDIATE-RELEASE MEDICINES
▸ Adult: 50–100 mg 2–3 times a day
▸ BY MOUTH USING MODIFIED-RELEASE MEDICINES
▸ Adult: 200–400 mg daily

Arrhythmias
▸ BY MOUTH USING IMMEDIATE-RELEASE MEDICINES
▸ Adult: Usual dose 50 mg 2–3 times a day, then
  increased if necessary up to 300 mg daily in divided
  doses
▸ BY INTRAVENOUS INJECTION
▸ Adult: Up to 5 mg, dose to be given at a rate of
  1–2 mg/minute, then up to 5 mg after 5 minutes if
  required, total dose of 10–15 mg

Migraine prophylaxis
▸ BY MOUTH USING IMMEDIATE-RELEASE MEDICINES
▸ Adult: 100–200 mg daily in divided doses
▸ BY MOUTH USING MODIFIED-RELEASE MEDICINES
▸ Adult: 200 mg daily

Hyperthyroidism (adjunct)
▸ BY MOUTH USING IMMEDIATE-RELEASE MEDICINES
▸ Adult: 50 mg 4 times a day

In surgery
▸ BY SLOW INTRAVENOUS INJECTION
▸ Adult: Initially 2–4 mg, given at induction or to control
  arrhythmias developing during anaesthesia, then 2 mg,
  repeated if necessary; maximum 10 mg per course

Early intervention within 12 hours of infarction
▸ INITIALLY BY INTRAVENOUS INJECTION
▸ Adult: Initially 5 mg every 2 minutes, to a max. of
  15 mg, followed by (by mouth) 50 mg every 6 hours for
  48 hours, to be taken 15 minutes after intravenous
  injection; (by mouth) maintenance 200 mg daily in
  divided doses

● INTERACTIONS → Appendix 1: beta blockers, selective
● SIDE-EFFECTS
  GENERAL SIDE-EFFECTS
▸ **Common or very common** Constipation · palpitations ·
  postural disorders
▸ **Uncommon** Chest pain · drowsiness · dystrophic skin lesion
  · hyperhidrosis · muscle cramps · oedema · skin reactions ·
  weight increased
▸ **Rare or very rare** Alopecia · arrhythmia · conjunctivitis · dry
  mouth · eye irritation · gangrene · hepatitis · rhinitis ·
  sexual dysfunction · thrombocytopenia
  SPECIFIC SIDE-EFFECTS
▸ **Uncommon**
▸ With intravenous use Cardiogenic shock · concentration
  impaired
▸ **Rare or very rare**
▸ With intravenous use Anxiety · arthralgia · atrioventricular
  block exacerbated · memory loss · photosensitivity reaction
  · taste altered · tinnitus

▸ With oral use Alertness decreased · arthritis · auditory
  disorder · personality disorder
▸ **Frequency not known**
▸ With oral use Peyronie's disease · retroperitoneal fibrosis
● HEPATIC IMPAIRMENT Manufacturer advises caution in
  severe impairment (bioavailability may be increased in
  patients with liver cirrhosis).
  Dose adjustments Manufacturer advises consider dose
  reduction in severe impairment.

● MEDICINAL FORMS There can be variation in the licensing of
  different medicines containing the same drug. Forms available
  from special-order manufacturers include: capsule, oral
  suspension, oral solution
  Tablet
  CAUTIONARY AND ADVISORY LABELS 8
  ▸ Metoprolol tartrate (Non-proprietary)
    Metoprolol tartrate 50 mg Metoprolol 50mg tablets |
    28 tablet [PoM] £3.40 DT = £2.85 | 56 tablet [PoM] £5.70
    Metoprolol tartrate 100 mg Metoprolol 100mg tablets |
    28 tablet [PoM] £4.40 DT = £2.94 | 56 tablet [PoM] £5.68
  Solution for injection
  ▸ Betaloc (Recordati Pharmaceuticals Ltd)
    Metoprolol tartrate 1 mg per 1 ml Betaloc I.V. 5mg/5ml solution for
    injection ampoules | 5 ampoule [PoM] £5.02 (Hospital only)

F 161

Nebivolol

● **INDICATIONS AND DOSE**

Essential hypertension
▸ BY MOUTH
▸ Adult: 5 mg daily
▸ Elderly: Initially 2.5 mg daily, then increased if
  necessary to 5 mg daily

Hypertension in patient with renal impairment
▸ BY MOUTH
▸ Adult: Initially 2.5 mg once daily, then increased if
  necessary to 5 mg once daily

Adjunct in stable mild to moderate heart failure
▸ BY MOUTH
▸ Adult 70 years and over: Initially 1.25 mg once daily for
  1–2 weeks, then increased if tolerated to 2.5 mg once
  daily for 1–2 weeks, then increased if tolerated to 5 mg
  once daily for 1–2 weeks, then increased if tolerated to
  10 mg once daily

● CONTRA-INDICATIONS Acute or decompensated heart
  failure requiring intravenous inotropes
● INTERACTIONS → Appendix 1: beta blockers, selective
● SIDE-EFFECTS
▸ **Common or very common** Constipation · oedema · postural
  hypertension
▸ **Uncommon** Dyspepsia · flatulence · skin reactions
● BREAST FEEDING Manufacturers advise avoidance.
● HEPATIC IMPAIRMENT Manufacturer advises avoid (limited
  information available).
● RENAL IMPAIRMENT Manufacturer advises avoid in heart
  failure if serum creatinine greater than 250 micromol/litre.

● MEDICINAL FORMS There can be variation in the licensing of
  different medicines containing the same drug.
  Tablet
  CAUTIONARY AND ADVISORY LABELS 8
  ▸ Nebivolol (Non-proprietary)
    Nebivolol (as Nebivolol hydrochloride) 1.25 mg Nebivolol 1.25mg
    tablets | 28 tablet [PoM] £16.56–£30.18
    Nebivolol (as Nebivolol hydrochloride) 2.5 mg Nebivolol 2.5mg
    tablets | 28 tablet [PoM] £69.84 DT = £11.84
    Nebivolol (as Nebivolol hydrochloride) 5 mg Nebivolol 5mg tablets
    | 28 tablet [PoM] £9.23 DT = £2.02
    Nebivolol (as Nebivolol hydrochloride) 10 mg Nebivolol 10mg
    tablets | 28 tablet [PoM] £27.92 DT = £27.39

2

Cardiovascular system

▸ Nebilet (A. Menarini Farmaceutica Internazionale SRL)
Nebivolol (as Nebivolol hydrochloride) 5 mg Nebilet 5mg tablets |
28 tablet [PoM] £9.23 DT = £2.02

CALCIUM-CHANNEL BLOCKERS

Calcium-channel blockers

Overview

Calcium-channel blockers differ in their predilection for the various possible sites of action and, therefore, their therapeutic effects are disparate, with much greater variation than those of beta-blockers. There are important differences between verapamil hydrochloride p. 178, diltiazem hydrochloride p. 171, and the dihydropyridine calcium-channel blockers (amlodipine below, felodipine p. 174, lacidipine p. 174, lercanidipine hydrochloride p. 175, nicardipine hydrochloride p. 175, nifedipine p. 176, and nimodipine p. 123). [EvGr] Calcium channel blockers, with the exception of amlodipine, should be avoided in heart failure as they can further depress cardiac function and exacerbate symptoms. ⓐ For further guidance on the management of heart failure, see Chronic heart failure p. 206. With the exception of amlodipine, they can also increase mortality after myocardial infarction in patients with left ventricular dysfunction and pulmonary congestion.

Verapamil hydrochloride is used for the treatment of angina, hypertension, and arrhythmias. It is a highly negatively inotropic calcium channel-blocker and it reduces cardiac output, slows the heart rate, and may impair atrioventricular conduction. It may precipitate heart failure, exacerbate conduction disorders, and cause hypotension at high doses and should be **not** be used with beta-blockers. Constipation is the most common side-effect.

Nifedipine relaxes vascular smooth muscle and dilates coronary and peripheral arteries. It has more influence on vessels and less on the myocardium than does verapamil hydrochloride, and unlike verapamil hydrochloride has no anti-arrhythmic activity. It rarely precipitates heart failure because any negative inotropic effect is offset by a reduction in left ventricular work.

Nicardipine hydrochloride has similar effects to those of nifedipine and may produce less reduction of myocardial contractility. Amlodipine and felodipine also resemble nifedipine and nicardipine hydrochloride in their effects and do not reduce myocardial contractility and they do not produce clinical deterioration in heart failure. They have a longer duration of action and can be given once daily. Nifedipine, nicardipine hydrochloride, amlodipine, and felodipine are used for the treatment of angina or hypertension. All are valuable in forms of angina associated with coronary vasospasm. Side-effects associated with vasodilatation such as flushing and headache (which become less obtruse after a few days), and ankle swelling (which may respond only partially to diuretics) are common.

Intravenous nicardipine hydrochloride is licensed for the treatment of acute life-threatening hypertension, for example in the event of malignant arterial hypertension or hypertensive encephalopathy; aortic dissection, when a short-acting beta-blocker is not suitable, or in combination with a beta-blocker when beta-blockade alone is not effective; severe pre-eclampsia, when other intravenous anti-hypertensives are not recommended or are contra-indicated; and for treatment of postoperative hypertension.

Lacidipine and lercanidipine hydrochloride have similar effects to those of nifedipine and nicardipine hydrochloride; they are indicated for hypertension only.

Nimodipine is related to nifedipine but the smooth muscle relaxant effect preferentially acts on cerebral arteries. Its use is confined to prevention and treatment of vascular spasm following aneurysmal subarachnoid haemorrhage.

Diltiazem hydrochloride is effective in most forms of angina; the longer-acting formulation is also used for hypertension. It may be used in patients for whom beta-blockers are contra-indicated or ineffective. It has a less negative inotropic effect than verapamil hydrochloride and significant myocardial depression occurs rarely. Nevertheless because of the risk of bradycardia it should be used with caution in association with beta-blockers.

Unstable angina

Calcium-channel blockers do not reduce the risk of myocardial infarction in unstable angina. The use of diltiazem hydrochloride or verapamil hydrochloride should be reserved for patients resistant to treatment with beta-blockers.

Calcium-channel blockers

● DRUG ACTION Calcium-channel blockers (less correctly called 'calcium-antagonists') interfere with the inward displacement of calcium ions through the slow channels of active cell membranes. They influence the myocardial cells, the cells within the specialised conducting system of the heart, and the cells of vascular smooth muscle. Thus, myocardial contractility may be reduced, the formation and propagation of electrical impulses within the heart may be depressed, and coronary or systemic vascular tone may be diminished.

● CAUTIONS
▸ Elderly Prescription potentially inappropriate (STOPP criteria) with persistent postural hypotension i.e. recurrent drop in systolic blood pressure ≥ 20 mmHg (risk of syncope and falls).
　See also Prescribing in the elderly p. 33.

● SIDE-EFFECTS
▸ Common or very common Abdominal pain · dizziness · drowsiness · flushing · headache · nausea · palpitations · peripheral oedema · skin reactions · tachycardia · vomiting
▸ Uncommon Angioedema · depression · erectile dysfunction · gingival hyperplasia · myalgia · paraesthesia · syncope

Overdose Features of calcium-channel blocker poisoning include nausea, vomiting, dizziness, agitation, confusion, and coma in severe poisoning. Metabolic acidosis and hyperglycaemia may occur. In overdose, the dihydropyridine calcium-channel blockers cause severe hypotension secondary to profound peripheral vasodilatation. For details on the management of poisoning, see Calcium-channel blockers, under Emergency treatment of poisoning

● HEPATIC IMPAIRMENT In general, manufacturers advise caution (risk of increased exposure).

● TREATMENT CESSATION There is some evidence that sudden withdrawal of calcium-channel blockers may be associated with an exacerbation of myocardial ischaemia.

◤ **above**

Amlodipine
22-Jul-2020

● DRUG ACTION Amlodipine is a dihydropyridine calcium-channel blocker.

● INDICATIONS AND DOSE
Prophylaxis of angina
▸ BY MOUTH
▸ Adult: Initially 5 mg once daily; maximum 10 mg per day
Hypertension
▸ BY MOUTH
▸ Adult: Initially 5 mg once daily; maximum 10 mg per day

Amlodipine **10 mg** Istin 10mg tablets | 28 tablet `PoM` £16.55 DT = £0.92

Combinations available: *Olmesartan with amlodipine,* p. 191 · *Olmesartan with amlodipine and hydrochlorothiazide,* p. 191

DOSE EQUIVALENCE AND CONVERSION

▸ Tablets from various suppliers may contain different salts (e.g. amlodipine besilate, amlodipine maleate, and amlodipine mesilate) but the strength is expressed in terms of amlodipine (base); tablets containing different salts are considered interchangeable.

IMPORTANT SAFETY INFORMATION

SAFE PRACTICE
Amlodipine has been confused with nimodipine and atenolol; care must be taken to ensure the correct drug is prescribed and dispensed.

● CONTRA-INDICATIONS Cardiogenic shock · significant aortic stenosis · unstable angina

● INTERACTIONS → Appendix 1: calcium channel blockers

● SIDE-EFFECTS

▸ **Common or very common** Asthenia · constipation · diarrhoea · dyspepsia · dyspnoea · gastrointestinal disorders · joint disorders · muscle cramps · oedema · vision disorders

▸ **Uncommon** Alopecia · anxiety · arrhythmias · chest pain · cough · dry mouth · gynaecomastia · hyperhidrosis · hypotension · insomnia · malaise · mood altered · numbness · pain · rhinitis · taste altered · tinnitus · tremor · urinary disorders · weight changes

▸ **Rare or very rare** Confusion · hepatic disorders · hyperglycaemia · hypersensitivity · leucopenia · muscle tone increased · myocardial infarction · pancreatitis · peripheral neuropathy · photosensitivity reaction · Stevens-Johnson syndrome · thrombocytopenia · vasculitis

▸ **Frequency not known** Extrapyramidal symptoms · pulmonary oedema

● PREGNANCY No information available—manufacturer advises avoid, but risk to fetus should be balanced against risk of uncontrolled maternal hypertension.

● BREAST FEEDING Manufacturer advises avoid—no information available.

● HEPATIC IMPAIRMENT
Dose adjustments Manufacturer advises initiate at low dose and titrate slowly (limited information available).

● DIRECTIONS FOR ADMINISTRATION Expert sources advise tablets may be dispersed in water.

● MEDICINAL FORMS There can be variation in the licensing of different medicines containing the same drug. Forms available from special-order manufacturers include: oral suspension, oral solution

Oral solution
▸ Amlodipine (Non-proprietary)
Amlodipine **1 mg per 1 ml** Amlodipine 5mg/5ml oral solution sugar free sugar-free | 150 ml `PoM` £75.78 DT = £75.78
Amlodipine **2 mg per 1 ml** Amlodipine 10mg/5ml oral solution sugar free sugar-free | 150 ml `PoM` £115.73 DT = £115.73

Oral suspension
▸ Amlodipine (Non-proprietary)
Amlodipine **1 mg per 1 ml** Amlodipine 5mg/5ml oral suspension sugar free sugar-free | 150 ml `PoM` £70.00 DT = £70.00

Tablet
▸ Amlodipine (Non-proprietary)
Amlodipine **2.5 mg** Amlodipine 2.5mg tablets | 28 tablet `PoM` £4.50–£6.09
Amlodipine **5 mg** Amlodipine 5mg tablets | 28 tablet `PoM` £9.99 DT = £0.89 | 500 tablet `PoM` £9.87–£18.00
Amlodipine **10 mg** Amlodipine 10mg tablets | 28 tablet `PoM` £14.07 DT = £0.92 | 500 tablet `PoM` £10.17–£22.50
▸ Istin (Upjohn UK Ltd)
Amlodipine **5 mg** Istin 5mg tablets | 28 tablet `PoM` £11.08 DT = £0.89

Amlodipine with valsartan

The properties listed below are those particular to the combination only. For the properties of the components please consider, amlodipine p. 170, valsartan p. 193.

● INDICATIONS AND DOSE

Hypertension in patients stabilised on the individual components in the same proportions
▸ BY MOUTH
▸ **Adult:** (consult product literature)

● INTERACTIONS → Appendix 1: angiotensin-II receptor antagonists · calcium channel blockers

● MEDICINAL FORMS There can be variation in the licensing of different medicines containing the same drug.

Tablet
▸ Exforge (Novartis Pharmaceuticals UK Ltd)
Amlodipine (as Amlodipine besilate) 5 mg, Valsartan **80 mg** Exforge 5mg/80mg tablets | 28 tablet `PoM` £20.11 DT = £20.11
Amlodipine (as Amlodipine besilate) 10 mg, Valsartan **160 mg** Exforge 10mg/160mg tablets | 28 tablet `PoM` £26.51 DT = £26.51
Amlodipine (as Amlodipine besilate) 5 mg, Valsartan **160 mg** Exforge 5mg/160mg tablets | 28 tablet `PoM` £26.51 DT = £26.51

◀ 170

Diltiazem hydrochloride

14-Feb-2020

● INDICATIONS AND DOSE

Prophylaxis and treatment of angina
▸ BY MOUTH
▸ **Adult:** Initially 60 mg 3 times a day, adjusted according to response; maximum 360 mg per day
▸ **Elderly:** Initially 60 mg twice daily, adjusted according to response; maximum 360 mg per day

Chronic anal fissure
▸ BY RECTUM USING CREAM, OR BY RECTUM USING OINTMENT
▸ **Adult:** Apply twice daily until pain stops. Max. duration of use 8 weeks, apply to the anal canal, using 2% topical preparation
▸ BY MOUTH
▸ **Adult:** 60 mg twice daily until pain stops. Max. duration of use 8 weeks

ADIZEM-SR ® CAPSULES

Mild to moderate hypertension
▸ BY MOUTH
▸ **Adult:** 120 mg twice daily, dose form not appropriate for initial dose titration

Angina
▸ BY MOUTH
▸ **Adult:** Initially 90 mg twice daily; increased if necessary to 180 mg twice daily, dose form not appropriate for initial dose titration in the elderly

ADIZEM-XL ®

Angina | Mild to moderate hypertension
▸ BY MOUTH
▸ **Adult:** Initially 240 mg once daily, increased if necessary to 300 mg once daily
▸ **Elderly:** Initially 120 mg once daily, increased if necessary up to 300 mg once daily

continued →

Cardiovascular system

2

ANGITIL ® SR

Angina | Mild to moderate hypertension

▸ BY MOUTH
▸ Adult: Initially 90 mg twice daily; increased if necessary to 120–180 mg twice daily

ANGITIL ® XL

Angina | Mild to moderate hypertension

▸ BY MOUTH
▸ Adult: Initially 240 mg once daily; increased if necessary to 300 mg once daily, dose form not appropriate for initial dose titration in the elderly

DILCARDIA ® SR

Angina | Mild to moderate hypertension

▸ BY MOUTH
▸ Adult: Initially 90 mg twice daily; increased if necessary to 180 mg twice daily
▸ Elderly: Initially 60 mg twice daily; increased if necessary to 90 mg twice daily

DILZEM ® SR

Angina | Mild to moderate hypertension

▸ BY MOUTH
▸ Adult: Initially 90 mg twice daily; increased if necessary up to 180 mg twice daily
▸ Elderly: Initially 60 mg twice daily; increased if necessary up to 180 mg twice daily

DILZEM ® XL

Angina | Mild to moderate hypertension

▸ BY MOUTH
▸ Adult: Initially 180 mg once daily; increased if necessary to 360 mg once daily
▸ Elderly: Initially 120 mg once daily; increased if necessary to 360 mg once daily

SLOZEM ®

Angina | Mild to moderate hypertension

▸ BY MOUTH
▸ Adult: Initially 240 mg once daily; increased if necessary to 360 mg once daily
▸ Elderly: Initially 120 mg once daily; increased if necessary to 360 mg once daily

TILDIEM RETARD ®

Mild to moderate hypertension

▸ BY MOUTH
▸ Adult: Initially 90–120 mg twice daily; increased if necessary to 360 mg daily in divided doses
▸ Elderly: Initially 120 mg once daily; increased if necessary to 120 mg twice daily

Angina

▸ BY MOUTH
▸ Adult: Initially 90–120 mg twice daily; increased if necessary to 480 mg daily in divided doses
▸ Elderly: Up to 120 mg twice daily, dose form not appropriate for initial dose titration

TILDIEM ® LA

Angina | Mild to moderate hypertension

▸ BY MOUTH
▸ Adult: Initially 200 mg once daily, to be taken with or before food, increased if necessary to 300–400 mg once daily; maximum 500 mg per day
▸ Elderly: Initially 200 mg once daily, increased if necessary to 300 mg once daily

VIAZEM ® XL

Angina | Mild to moderate hypertension

▸ BY MOUTH
▸ Adult: Initially 180 mg once daily, adjusted according to response to 240 mg once daily; maximum 360 mg per day

▸ Elderly: Initially 120 mg once daily, adjusted according to response

ZEMTARD ®

Angina

▸ BY MOUTH
▸ Adult: 180–300 mg once daily, increased if necessary to 480 mg once daily
▸ Elderly: Initially 120 mg once daily, increased if necessary to 480 mg once daily

Mild to moderate hypertension

▸ BY MOUTH
▸ Adult: 180–300 mg once daily, increased if necessary to 360 mg once daily
▸ Elderly: Initially 120 mg once daily, increased if necessary to 360 mg once daily

● UNLICENSED USE [EvGr] Diltiazem is used for the treatment of chronic anal fissures, Ⓔ but it is not licensed for this indication.

● CONTRA-INDICATIONS
▸ With systemic use Acute porphyrias p. 1107 · cardiogenic shock · heart failure (with reduced ejection fraction) · left ventricular failure with pulmonary congestion · second- or third-degree AV block (unless pacemaker fitted) · severe bradycardia · sick sinus syndrome · significant aortic stenosis

CONTRA-INDICATIONS, FURTHER INFORMATION Systemic absorption following rectal use is unknown, therefore consider the possibility of contra-indications listed for systemic use.

● CAUTIONS
▸ With systemic use Bradycardia (avoid if severe) · first degree AV block · prolonged PR interval · significantly impaired left ventricular function

CAUTIONS, FURTHER INFORMATION Systemic absorption following rectal use is unknown, therefore consider the possibility of cautions listed for systemic use.
▸ Elderly Prescription potentially inappropriate (STOPP criteria) in patients with NYHA Class III or IV heart failure (may worsen heart failure). See also Prescribing in the elderly p. 33.

● INTERACTIONS → Appendix 1: calcium channel blockers

● SIDE-EFFECTS
▸ **Common or very common** Cardiac conduction disorders · constipation · gastrointestinal discomfort · malaise
▸ **Uncommon** Arrhythmias · diarrhoea · insomnia · nervousness · postural hypotension
▸ **Rare or very rare** Dry mouth
▸ **Frequency not known** Cardiac arrest · congestive heart failure · extrapyramidal symptoms · fever · gynaecomastia · hepatitis · hyperglycaemia · hyperhidrosis · mood altered · photosensitivity reaction · severe cutaneous adverse reactions (SCARs) · thrombocytopenia · vasculitis

SIDE-EFFECTS, FURTHER INFORMATION Systemic absorption following rectal use is unknown, therefore consider the possibility of side-effects listed for oral use.

Overdose ▸ With oral use In overdose, diltiazem has a profound cardiac depressant effect causing hypotension and arrhythmias, including complete heart block and asystole.

● PREGNANCY
▸ With systemic use Avoid.

● BREAST FEEDING
▸ With systemic use Significant amount present in milk—no evidence of harm but avoid unless no safer alternative.

● HEPATIC IMPAIRMENT

Dose adjustments ▸ With systemic use In general, manufacturers advise initial dose reduction to 60 mg twice daily (or 120 mg daily if using a once daily formulation), increased gradually as required.

TILDIEM RETARD ® For *treatment of angina*, dose form not appropriate for initial titration; manufacturer advises maximum 120 mg twice daily.

For *mild to moderate hypertension*, manufacturer advises initial dose reduction to 120 mg once daily; maximum 120 mg twice daily.

ANGITIL ® SR Dose form not appropriate for initial dose titration.

ADIZEM-SR ® CAPSULES Dose form not appropriate for initial dose titration.

DILCARDIA ® SR Dose form not appropriate for initial titration; manufacturer advises maximum 90 mg twice daily in hypertension.

ANGITIL ® XL Dose form not appropriate for initial dose titration.

TILDIEM ® LA Manufacturer advises initial dose 200 mg daily; maximum 300 mg daily.

● RENAL IMPAIRMENT
Dose adjustments ▸ With systemic use Start with smaller dose.

TILDIEM RETARD ® Dose for mild to moderate hypertension—initially 120 mg once a day; increased if necessary to 120 mg twice a day.

For treatment of angina, dose form not appropriate for initial titration; up to 120 mg twice a day may be required.

ADIZEM-XL ® Dose for angina and mild to moderate hypertension—initially 120 mg once daily.

DILZEM ® XL Dose for angina and mild to moderate hypertension—initially 120 mg once daily.

ZEMTARD ® Dose for angina and mild to moderate hypertension—initially 120 mg once daily.

DILCARDIA ® SR Dose for angina and mild to moderate hypertension—initially 60 mg twice a day; maximum 90 mg twice a day.

ANGITIL ® XL Dose form not appropriate for initial dose titration.

SLOZEM ® Dose for angina and mild to moderate hypertension—initially 120 mg once daily.

TILDIEM ® LA Dose for angina and mild to moderate hypertension—initially 200 mg daily; increased if necessary to 300 mg daily.

VIAZEM ® XL Dose for angina and mild to moderate hypertension—initially 120 mg once daily, adjusted according to response.

● PRESCRIBING AND DISPENSING INFORMATION
▸ With systemic use The standard formulations containing 60 mg diltiazem hydrochloride are licensed as generics and there is no requirement for brand name dispensing. Although their means of formulation has called for the strict designation 'modified-release', their duration of action corresponds to that of tablets requiring administration more frequently. Different versions of modified-release preparations containing more than 60 mg diltiazem hydrochloride may not have the same clinical effect. To avoid confusion between these different formulations of diltiazem, prescribers should specify the brand to be dispensed.

● PATIENT AND CARER ADVICE
TILDIEM RETARD ® Tablet membrane may pass through gastro-intestinal tract unchanged, but being porous has no effect on efficacy.

● MEDICINAL FORMS There can be variation in the licensing of different medicines containing the same drug. Forms available from special-order manufacturers include: oral suspension, oral solution

Modified-release tablet
CAUTIONARY AND ADVISORY LABELS 25
▸ Diltiazem hydrochloride (Non-proprietary)
   Diltiazem hydrochloride 60 mg Diltiazem 60mg modified-release tablets | 84 tablet [PoM] £42.93 DT = £42.93 | 100 tablet [PoM] £51.10–£51.11
▸ Retalzem (Kent Pharmaceuticals Ltd)
   Diltiazem hydrochloride 60 mg Retalzem 60 modified-release tablets | 84 tablet [PoM] £7.43 DT = £42.93
▸ Tildiem (Sanofi)
   Diltiazem hydrochloride 60 mg Tildiem 60mg modified-release tablets | 90 tablet [PoM] £7.96
▸ Tildiem Retard (Sanofi)
   Diltiazem hydrochloride 90 mg Tildiem Retard 90mg tablets | 56 tablet [PoM] £7.27 DT = £7.27
   Diltiazem hydrochloride 120 mg Tildiem Retard 120mg tablets | 56 tablet [PoM] £7.15 DT = £7.15

Modified-release capsule
CAUTIONARY AND ADVISORY LABELS 25
▸ Adizem-SR (Napp Pharmaceuticals Ltd)
   Diltiazem hydrochloride 90 mg Adizem-SR 90mg capsules | 56 capsule [PoM] £8.50 DT = £8.50
   Diltiazem hydrochloride 120 mg Adizem-SR 120mg capsules | 56 capsule [PoM] £9.45 DT = £9.45
   Diltiazem hydrochloride 180 mg Adizem-SR 180mg capsules | 56 capsule [PoM] £14.15 DT = £14.15
▸ Adizem-XL (Napp Pharmaceuticals Ltd)
   Diltiazem hydrochloride 120 mg Adizem-XL 120mg capsules | 28 capsule [PoM] £9.14 DT = £9.14
   Diltiazem hydrochloride 180 mg Adizem-XL 180mg capsules | 28 capsule [PoM] £10.37 DT = £10.37
   Diltiazem hydrochloride 200 mg Adizem-XL 200mg capsules | 28 capsule [PoM] £6.30 DT = £6.29
   Diltiazem hydrochloride 240 mg Adizem-XL 240mg capsules | 28 capsule [PoM] £11.52 DT = £11.52
   Diltiazem hydrochloride 300 mg Adizem-XL 300mg capsules | 28 capsule [PoM] £9.14 DT = £9.01
▸ Angitil SR (Ethypharm UK Ltd)
   Diltiazem hydrochloride 90 mg Angitil SR 90 capsules | 56 capsule [PoM] £7.03 DT = £8.50
   Diltiazem hydrochloride 120 mg Angitil SR 120 capsules | 56 capsule [PoM] £6.91 DT = £9.45
   Diltiazem hydrochloride 180 mg Angitil SR 180 capsules | 56 capsule [PoM] £13.27 DT = £14.15
▸ Angitil XL (Ethypharm UK Ltd)
   Diltiazem hydrochloride 240 mg Angitil XL 240 capsules | 28 capsule [PoM] £7.94 DT = £11.52
   Diltiazem hydrochloride 300 mg Angitil XL 300 capsules | 28 capsule [PoM] £6.98 DT = £9.01
▸ Dilcardia SR (Mylan)
   Diltiazem hydrochloride 90 mg Dilcardia SR 90mg capsules | 56 capsule [PoM] £9.61 DT = £8.50
   Diltiazem hydrochloride 120 mg Dilcardia SR 120mg capsules | 56 capsule [PoM] £10.69 DT = £9.45
▸ Slozem (Zentiva)
   Diltiazem hydrochloride 120 mg Slozem 120mg capsules | 28 capsule [PoM] £5.49 DT = £9.14
   Diltiazem hydrochloride 180 mg Slozem 180mg capsules | 28 capsule [PoM] £5.58 DT = £10.37
   Diltiazem hydrochloride 240 mg Slozem 240mg capsules | 28 capsule [PoM] £5.67 DT = £11.52
   Diltiazem hydrochloride 300 mg Slozem 300mg capsules | 28 capsule [PoM] £6.03 DT = £9.01
▸ Tildiem LA (Sanofi)
   Diltiazem hydrochloride 200 mg Tildiem LA 200 capsules | 28 capsule [PoM] £6.29 DT = £6.29
   Diltiazem hydrochloride 300 mg Tildiem LA 300 capsules | 28 capsule [PoM] £9.01 DT = £9.01
▸ Uard XL (Ennogen Healthcare Ltd)
   Diltiazem hydrochloride 120 mg Uard 120XL capsules | 28 capsule [PoM] £7.31 DT = £9.14
   Diltiazem hydrochloride 180 mg Uard 180XL capsules | 28 capsule [PoM] £8.30 DT = £10.37
   Diltiazem hydrochloride 240 mg Uard 240XL capsules | 28 capsule [PoM] £9.22 DT = £11.52

2

Cardiovascular system

Diltiazem hydrochloride 300 mg Uard 300XL capsules |
28 capsule [PoM] £7.21 DT = £9.01
▸ **Viazem XL (Thornton & Ross Ltd)**
Diltiazem hydrochloride 120 mg Viazem XL 120mg capsules |
28 capsule [PoM] £6.60 DT = £9.14
Diltiazem hydrochloride 180 mg Viazem XL 180mg capsules |
28 capsule [PoM] £7.36 DT = £10.37
Diltiazem hydrochloride 240 mg Viazem XL 240mg capsules |
28 capsule [PoM] £7.74 DT = £11.52
Diltiazem hydrochloride 300 mg Viazem XL 300mg capsules |
28 capsule [PoM] £8.03 DT = £9.01
Diltiazem hydrochloride 360 mg Viazem XL 360mg capsules |
28 capsule [PoM] £13.85 DT = £13.85
▸ **Zemret XL (Tillomed Laboratories Ltd)**
Diltiazem hydrochloride 180 mg Zemret 180 XL capsules |
28 capsule [PoM] £7.00 DT = £10.37
Diltiazem hydrochloride 240 mg Zemret 240 XL capsules |
28 capsule [PoM] £7.00 DT = £11.52
Diltiazem hydrochloride 300 mg Zemret 300 XL capsules |
28 capsule [PoM] £7.00 DT = £9.01
▸ **Zemtard XL (Galen Ltd)**
Diltiazem hydrochloride 120 mg Zemtard 120 XL capsules |
28 capsule [PoM] £6.10 DT = £9.14
Diltiazem hydrochloride 180 mg Zemtard 180 XL capsules |
28 capsule [PoM] £6.20 DT = £10.37
Diltiazem hydrochloride 240 mg Zemtard 240 XL capsules |
28 capsule [PoM] £6.30 DT = £11.52
Diltiazem hydrochloride 300 mg Zemtard 300 XL capsules |
28 capsule [PoM] £6.70 DT = £9.01

F 170

Felodipide Felodipine

24-Feb-2020

● DRUG ACTION Felodipine is a dihydropyridine calcium-channel blocker.

● **INDICATIONS AND DOSE**
Prophylaxis of angina
▸ BY MOUTH
▸ **Adult:** Initially 5 mg once daily; increased if necessary to 10 mg once daily, to be taken in the morning
▸ **Elderly:** Initially 2.5 mg once daily; increased if necessary to 10 mg once daily, to be taken in the morning

Hypertension
▸ BY MOUTH
▸ **Adult:** Initially 5 mg once daily; usual maintenance 5–10 mg once daily, to be taken in the morning, doses above 20 mg daily rarely needed
▸ **Elderly:** Initially 2.5 mg daily; usual maintenance 5–10 mg daily, to be taken in the morning, doses above 20 mg daily rarely needed

● CONTRA-INDICATIONS Cardiac outflow obstruction · significant cardiac valvular obstruction (e.g. aortic stenosis) · uncontrolled heart failure · unstable angina · within 1 month of myocardial infarction

● CAUTIONS Predisposition to tachycardia · severe left ventricular dysfunction

CAUTIONS, FURTHER INFORMATION Manufacturer advises discontinue if ischaemic pain occurs or existing pain worsens shortly after initiating treatment.

● INTERACTIONS → Appendix 1: calcium channel blockers

● SIDE-EFFECTS
▸ **Uncommon** Fatigue
▸ **Rare or very rare** Arthralgia · gingivitis · hypersensitivity vasculitis · photosensitivity reaction · sexual dysfunction · urinary frequency increased

● PREGNANCY Avoid; toxicity in *animal* studies; may inhibit labour.

● BREAST FEEDING Present in milk but amount probably too small to be harmful.

● HEPATIC IMPAIRMENT
Dose adjustments Manufacturer advises consider dose reduction.

● MEDICINAL FORMS There can be variation in the licensing of different medicines containing the same drug. Forms available from special-order manufacturers include: oral solution
Modified-release tablet
CAUTIONARY AND ADVISORY LABELS 25
▸ Felodipine (Non-proprietary)
Felodipine 5 mg Vascalpha 5mg modified-release tablets |
28 tablet [PoM] £1.99 DT = £5.66
Felodipine 10 mg Vascalpha 10mg modified-release tablets |
28 tablet [PoM] £1.99 DT = £5.66
▸ Cardioplen XL (Chiesi Ltd)
Felodipine 2.5 mg Cardioplen XL 2.5mg tablets | 28 tablet [PoM]
£5.68 DT = £5.68
Felodipine 5 mg Cardioplen XL 5mg tablets | 28 tablet [PoM] £3.87
DT = £4.21
Felodipine 10 mg Cardioplen XL 10mg tablets | 28 tablet [PoM]
£4.81 DT = £5.66
▸ Felendil XL (Teva UK Ltd)
Felodipine 2.5 mg Folpik XL 2.5mg tablets | 28 tablet [PoM] £6.31
DT = £5.68
Felodipine 5 mg Folpik XL 5mg tablets | 28 tablet [PoM] £4.21 DT =
£4.21
Felodipine 10 mg Folpik XL 10mg tablets | 28 tablet [PoM] £7.21 DT
= £5.66
▸ Felotens XL (Thornton & Ross Ltd)
Felodipine 2.5 mg Felotens XL 2.5mg tablets | 28 tablet [PoM] £5.11
DT = £5.68
▸ Parmid XL (Sandoz Ltd)
Felodipine 2.5 mg Parmid XL 2.5mg tablets | 28 tablet [PoM] £5.36
DT = £5.68
▸ Plendil (AstraZeneca UK Ltd)
Felodipine 2.5 mg Plendil 2.5mg modified-release tablets |
98 tablet [PoM] £22.08
Felodipine 5 mg Plendil 5mg modified-release tablets |
28 tablet [PoM] £4.21 DT = £4.21
Felodipine 10 mg Plendil 10mg modified-release tablets |
28 tablet [PoM] £5.66 DT = £5.66
▸ Vascalpha (Accord Healthcare Ltd)
Felodipine 5 mg Vascalpha 5mg modified-release tablets |
28 tablet [PoM] £1.99 DT = £4.21
Felodipine 10 mg Vascalpha 10mg modified-release tablets |
28 tablet [PoM] £1.99 DT = £5.66

Combinations available: *Ramipril with felodipine,* p. 187

F 170

Lacidipine

14-Feb-2020

● DRUG ACTION Lacidipine is a dihydropyridine calcium-channel blocker.

● **INDICATIONS AND DOSE**
Hypertension
▸ BY MOUTH
▸ **Adult:** Initially 2 mg daily; increased if necessary to 4 mg daily, then increased if necessary to 6 mg daily, dose increases should occur at intervals of 3–4 weeks, to be taken preferably in the morning

● CONTRA-INDICATIONS Acute porphyrias p. 1107 · aortic stenosis · avoid within 1 month of myocardial infarction · cardiogenic shock · unstable angina

● CAUTIONS Cardiac conduction abnormalities · poor cardiac reserve

● INTERACTIONS → Appendix 1: calcium channel blockers

● SIDE-EFFECTS
▸ **Common or very common** Abdominal discomfort · asthenia · polyuria
▸ **Uncommon** Ischaemic heart disease
▸ **Rare or very rare** Muscle cramps · tremor

● PREGNANCY Manufacturer advises avoid; may inhibit labour.

- **BREAST FEEDING** Manufacturer advises avoid—no information available.
- **HEPATIC IMPAIRMENT**
  Dose adjustments Manufacturer advises consider dose reduction if hypotension occurs.

- **MEDICINAL FORMS** There can be variation in the licensing of different medicines containing the same drug.
  Tablet
  - Lacidipine (Non-proprietary)
    Lacidipine 2 mg Lacidipine 2mg tablets | 28 tablet PoM £6.85 DT = £2.10
    Lacidipine 4 mg Lacidipine 4mg tablets | 28 tablet PoM £6.85 DT = £2.30
    Lacidipine 6 mg Lacidipine 6mg tablets | 28 tablet PoM £5.75
  - Molap (Rivopharm (UK) Ltd)
    Lacidipine 4 mg Molap 4mg tablets | 28 tablet PoM £2.90 DT = £2.30
  - Motens (GlaxoSmithKline UK Ltd)
    Lacidipine 2 mg Motens 2mg tablets | 28 tablet PoM £2.95 DT = £2.10
    Lacidipine 4 mg Motens 4mg tablets | 28 tablet PoM £3.10 DT = £2.30

F 170

Lercanidipine hydrochloride
14-Feb-2020

- **DRUG ACTION** Lercanidipine is a dihydropyridine calcium-channel blocker.

- **INDICATIONS AND DOSE**
  Mild to moderate hypertension
  - BY MOUTH
  - Adult: Initially 10 mg once daily; increased if necessary to 20 mg daily, dose can be adjusted after 2 weeks

- **CONTRA-INDICATIONS** Aortic stenosis · uncontrolled heart failure · unstable angina · within 1 month of myocardial infarction
- **CAUTIONS** Left ventricular dysfunction · sick sinus syndrome (if pacemaker not fitted)
- **INTERACTIONS** → Appendix 1: calcium channel blockers
- **SIDE-EFFECTS**
  - **Rare or very rare** Angina pectoris · asthenia · chest pain · diarrhoea · dyspepsia · urinary disorders
- **PREGNANCY** Manufacturer advises avoid—no information available.
- **BREAST FEEDING** Manufacturer advises avoid.
- **HEPATIC IMPAIRMENT** Manufacturer advises avoid in severe impairment.
- **RENAL IMPAIRMENT** Avoid if eGFR less than 30 mL/minute/1.73 m².

- **MEDICINAL FORMS** There can be variation in the licensing of different medicines containing the same drug.
  Tablet
  CAUTIONARY AND ADVISORY LABELS 22
  - Lercanidipine hydrochloride (Non-proprietary)
    Lercanidipine hydrochloride 10 mg Lercanidipine 10mg tablets | 28 tablet PoM £12.99 DT = £2.09
    Lercanidipine hydrochloride 20 mg Lercanidipine 20mg tablets | 28 tablet PoM £15.99 DT = £2.35
  - Zanidip (Recordati Pharmaceuticals Ltd)
    Lercanidipine hydrochloride 10 mg Zanidip 10mg tablets | 28 tablet PoM £5.70 DT = £2.09
    Lercanidipine hydrochloride 20 mg Zanidip 20mg tablets | 28 tablet PoM £10.82 DT = £2.35

F 170

Nicardipine hydrochloride
30-Jul-2020

- **DRUG ACTION** Nicardipine is a dihydropyridine calcium-channel blocker.

- **INDICATIONS AND DOSE**
  Prophylaxis of angina
  - BY MOUTH USING IMMEDIATE-RELEASE MEDICINES
  - Adult: Initially 20 mg 3 times a day, then increased to 30 mg 3 times a day, dose increased after at least 3 days; usual dose 60–120 mg daily
  Mild to moderate hypertension
  - BY MOUTH USING IMMEDIATE-RELEASE MEDICINES
  - Adult: Initially 20 mg 3 times a day, then increased to 30 mg 3 times a day, dose increased after at least 3 days; usual dose 60–120 mg daily
  Life-threatening hypertension (specialist use only) | Post-operative hypertension (specialist use only)
  - BY CONTINUOUS INTRAVENOUS INFUSION
  - Adult: Initially 3–5 mg/hour for 15 minutes, increased in steps of 0.5–1 mg every 15 minutes, adjusted according to response, maximum rate 15 mg/hour, reduce dose gradually when target blood pressure achieved; maintenance 2–4 mg/hour
  - Elderly: Initially 1–5 mg/hour, then adjusted in steps of 500 micrograms/hour after 30 minutes, adjusted according to response, maximum rate 15 mg/hour
  Life-threatening hypertension in patients with hepatic or renal impairment (specialist use only) | Postoperative hypertension in patients with hepatic or renal impairment (specialist use only)
  - BY CONTINUOUS INTRAVENOUS INFUSION
  - Adult: Initially 1–5 mg/hour, then adjusted in steps of 500 micrograms/hour after 30 minutes, adjusted according to response, maximum rate 15 mg/hour
  Acute life-threatening hypertension in pregnancy (specialist use only)
  - BY CONTINUOUS INTRAVENOUS INFUSION
  - Adult: Initially 1–5 mg/hour, then adjusted in steps of 500 micrograms/hour after 30 minutes, adjusted according to response, usual maximum rate 4 mg/hour in treatment of pre-eclampsia (maximum rate 15 mg/hour)

- **CONTRA-INDICATIONS**
  GENERAL CONTRA-INDICATIONS Acute porphyrias p. 1107 · cardiogenic shock · significant or advanced aortic stenosis · unstable or acute attacks of angina
  SPECIFIC CONTRA-INDICATIONS
  - With intravenous use avoid within 8 days of myocardial infarction · compensatory hypertension
  - With oral use avoid within 1 month of myocardial infarction
- **CAUTIONS**
  GENERAL CAUTIONS Congestive heart failure · elderly · increased risk of serious hypotension · ischaemic heart disease · pulmonary oedema · significantly impaired left ventricular function · stroke
  SPECIFIC CAUTIONS
  - With intravenous use Elevated intracranial pressure · portal hypertension
  CAUTIONS, FURTHER INFORMATION Manufacturer advises discontinue if ischaemic pain occurs or existing pain worsens within 30 minutes of initiating treatment or increasing dose.
- **INTERACTIONS** → Appendix 1: calcium channel blockers
- **SIDE-EFFECTS**
  GENERAL SIDE-EFFECTS
  - **Common or very common** Hypotension

2

Cardiovascular system

▶ **Frequency not known** Pulmonary oedema · thrombocytopenia

SPECIFIC SIDE-EFFECTS
▶ **With intravenous use** Atrioventricular block · hepatic disorders · ischaemic heart disease · paralytic ileus
▶ **With oral use** Abdominal distress · angina pectoris exacerbated · asthenia · dyspnoea · feeling hot · hepatic function abnormal · insomnia · nervous system disorder · renal impairment · tinnitus · urinary frequency increased

SIDE-EFFECTS, FURTHER INFORMATION Systemic hypotension and reflex tachycardia with rapid reduction of blood pressure may occur — during intravenous use consider stopping infusion or decreasing dose by half.

● PREGNANCY May inhibit labour. Not to be used in multiple pregnancy (twins or more) unless there is no other acceptable alternative. Toxicity in *animal* studies. Risk of severe maternal hypotension and fatal fetal hypoxia—avoid excessive decrease in blood pressure. For treatment of acute life-threatening hypertension only.

● BREAST FEEDING Manufacturer advises avoid—present in breast milk.

● HEPATIC IMPAIRMENT
Dose adjustments ▶ With oral use Manufacturer advises consider using lowest initial dose and extending dosing interval according to individual response.
▶ With intravenous use See Indications and dose section.

● RENAL IMPAIRMENT
Dose adjustments ▶ With oral use Consider using lowest initial dose and extending dosing interval according to individual response.
▶ With intravenous use Use with caution—use lower initial dose.

● MONITORING REQUIREMENTS Monitor blood pressure and heart rate at least every 5 minutes during intravenous infusion, and then until stable, and continue monitoring for at least 12 hours after end of infusion.

● DIRECTIONS FOR ADMINISTRATION Intravenous nicardipine should only be administered under the supervision of a specialist and in a hospital or intensive care setting in which patients can be closely monitored.
▶ With intravenous use For *intravenous infusion*, manufacturer advises give continuously *in* Glucose 5%; dilute dose in infusion fluid to a final concentration of 100–200 micrograms/mL (undiluted solution *via* central venous line only) and give *via* volumetric infusion pump or syringe driver; protect from light; risk of adsorption on to plastic of infusion set in the presence of saline solutions; incompatible with bicarbonate or alkaline solutions—consult product literature. To minimise peripheral venous irritation, expert sources advise change site of infusion every 12 hours.

● MEDICINAL FORMS There can be variation in the licensing of different medicines containing the same drug. Forms available from special-order manufacturers include: oral suspension, oral solution

Solution for infusion
▶ Nicardipine hydrochloride (Non-proprietary)
Nicardipine hydrochloride 1 mg per 1 ml Nicardipine 10mg/10ml solution for injection ampoules | 5 ampoule [PoM] £50.00
▶ Cardene (Imported (United States))
Nicardipine hydrochloride 2.5 mg per 1 ml Cardene I.V. 25mg/10ml solution for infusion ampoules | 10 ampoule [PoM] [S]

Capsule
▶ Nicardipine hydrochloride (Non-proprietary)
Nicardipine hydrochloride 20 mg Nicardipine 20mg capsules | 56 capsule [PoM] £8.38 DT = £7.65
Nicardipine hydrochloride 30 mg Nicardipine 30mg capsules | 56 capsule [PoM] £9.73 DT = £9.57
▶ Cardene (Astellas Pharma Ltd)
Nicardipine hydrochloride 20 mg Cardene 20mg capsules | 56 capsule [PoM] £6.00 DT = £7.65

Nicardipine hydrochloride 30 mg Cardene 30mg capsules | 56 capsule [PoM] £6.96 DT = £9.57

◀ 170

Nifedipine

10-Mar-2020

● **INDICATIONS AND DOSE**
Raynaud's syndrome
▶ BY MOUTH USING IMMEDIATE-RELEASE MEDICINES
▶ **Adult:** Initially 5 mg 3 times a day, then adjusted according to response to 20 mg 3 times a day

Angina prophylaxis (not recommended)
▶ BY MOUTH USING IMMEDIATE-RELEASE MEDICINES
▶ **Adult:** Initially 5 mg 3 times a day, then adjusted according to response to 20 mg 3 times a day

Postponement of premature labour
▶ BY MOUTH USING IMMEDIATE-RELEASE MEDICINES
▶ **Adult:** Initially 20 mg, followed by 10–20 mg 3–4 times a day, adjusted according to uterine activity

Hiccup in palliative care
▶ BY MOUTH USING IMMEDIATE-RELEASE MEDICINES
▶ **Adult:** 10 mg 3 times a day

Chronic anal fissure
▶ BY RECTUM USING OINTMENT
▶ **Adult:** Apply 2–3 times a day until pain stops. Max. duration of use 8 weeks, apply to anal canal, using 0.2%–0.5% topical preparation
▶ BY MOUTH USING MODIFIED-RELEASE MEDICINES
▶ **Adult:** 20 mg twice daily until pain stops. Max. duration of use 8 weeks

ADIPINE ® MR
Hypertension | Angina prophylaxis
▶ BY MOUTH
▶ **Adult:** 10 mg twice daily, adjusted according to response to 40 mg twice daily

ADIPINE ® XL
Hypertension | Angina prophylaxis
▶ BY MOUTH
▶ **Adult:** 30 mg daily, increased if necessary up to 90 mg daily

CORACTEN ® SR
Hypertension | Angina prophylaxis
▶ BY MOUTH
▶ **Adult:** Initially 10 mg twice daily, increased if necessary up to 40 mg twice daily

CORACTEN ® XL
Hypertension | Angina prophylaxis
▶ BY MOUTH
▶ **Adult:** Initially 30 mg daily, increased if necessary up to 90 mg daily

FORTIPINE ® LA 40
Hypertension | Angina prophylaxis
▶ BY MOUTH
▶ **Adult:** Initially 40 mg once daily, increased if necessary to 80 mg daily in 1–2 divided doses

NIFEDIPRESS ® MR
Hypertension | Angina prophylaxis
▶ BY MOUTH
▶ **Adult:** 10 mg twice daily, adjusted according to response to 40 mg twice daily

TENSIPINE ® MR
Hypertension | Angina prophylaxis
▶ BY MOUTH
▶ **Adult:** Initially 10 mg twice daily, adjusted according to response to 40 mg twice daily

Cardiovascular system

VALNI ® XL

Severe hypertension | Prophylaxis of angina
▸ BY MOUTH
▸ Adult: 30 mg once daily, increased if necessary up to 90 mg once daily

● UNLICENSED USE
▸ With systemic use Not licensed for use in postponing premature labour.

     EvGr Nifedipine is used for the treatment of chronic anal fissure, ⟨E⟩ but is not licensed for this indication.

● CONTRA-INDICATIONS
▸ With systemic use Acute attacks of angina · cardiogenic shock · significant aortic stenosis · unstable angina · within 1 month of myocardial infarction

CONTRA-INDICATIONS, FURTHER INFORMATION
Systemic absorption following rectal use is unknown, therefore consider the possibility of contra-indications listed for systemic use.

● CAUTIONS
▸ With systemic use Diabetes mellitus · elderly · heart failure · ischaemic pain · poor cardiac reserve · severe hypotension · short-acting formulations are not recommended for angina or long-term management of hypertension (their use may be associated with large variations in blood pressure and reflex tachycardia) · significantly impaired left ventricular function (heart failure deterioration observed)

CAUTIONS, FURTHER INFORMATION Systemic absorption following rectal use is unknown, therefore consider the possibility of cautions listed for systemic use.
▸ Ischaemic pain Manufacturer advises discontinue if ischaemic pain occurs or existing pain worsens shortly after initiating treatment.

VALNI ® XL Dose form not appropriate for use where there is a history of oesophageal or gastro-intestinal obstruction, decreased lumen diameter of the gastro-intestinal tract, inflammatory bowel disease, or ileostomy after proctocolectomy.

● INTERACTIONS → Appendix 1: calcium channel blockers

● SIDE-EFFECTS
▸ **Common or very common** Constipation · malaise · oedema · vasodilation
▸ **Uncommon** Allergic oedema · anxiety · chills · diarrhoea · dry mouth · epistaxis · gastrointestinal discomfort · gastrointestinal disorders · hypotension · joint disorders · laryngeal oedema · migraine · muscle complaints · nasal congestion · pain · sleep disorders · tremor · urinary disorders · vertigo · vision disorders
▸ **Rare or very rare** Appetite decreased · burping · cardiovascular disorder · fever · hyperhidrosis · mood altered · sensation abnormal
▸ **Frequency not known** Agranulocytosis · bezoar · cerebral ischaemia · chest pain · dysphagia · dyspnoea · eye pain · gingival disorder · gynaecomastia (following long term use) · hepatic disorders · hyperglycaemia · ischaemic heart disease · leucopenia · myasthenia gravis aggravated · photoallergic reaction · pulmonary oedema · telangiectasia · toxic epidermal necrolysis · weight decreased

SIDE-EFFECTS, FURTHER INFORMATION Systemic absorption following rectal use is unknown therefore consider the possibility of side-effects listed for oral use.

● PREGNANCY
▸ With systemic use May inhibit labour; manufacturer advises avoid before week 20, but risk to fetus should be balanced against risk of uncontrolled maternal hypertension. Use only if other treatment options are not indicated or have failed.

● BREAST FEEDING
▸ With systemic use Amount too small to be harmful but manufacturers advise avoid.

● HEPATIC IMPAIRMENT
▸ With oral use For *once-daily* preparations, manufacturers advise dose form not appropriate (owing to the duration of action of the formulation).
Dose adjustments ▸ With oral use Manufacturer advises consider dose reduction in severe impairment.

● DIRECTIONS FOR ADMINISTRATION
FORTIPINE ® LA 40 Take with or just after food, or a meal.

● PRESCRIBING AND DISPENSING INFORMATION Different versions of modified-release preparations may not have the same clinical effect. To avoid confusion between these different formulations of nifedipine, prescribers should specify the brand to be dispensed.

Palliative care For further information on the use of nifedipine in palliative care, see www.medicinescomplete. com/#/content/palliative/nifedipine.

● MEDICINAL FORMS There can be variation in the licensing of different medicines containing the same drug. Forms available from special-order manufacturers include: oral suspension, oral drops

Modified-release tablet
CAUTIONARY AND ADVISORY LABELS 25
▸ Nifedipine (Non-proprietary)
    Nifedipine 30 mg Nifedipine 30mg modified-release tablets | 28 tablet [PoM] ⟨S⟩ DT = £4.70
    Nifedipine 60 mg Nifedipine 60mg modified-release tablets | 28 tablet [PoM] ⟨S⟩ DT = £7.10
▸ Adanif XL (Advanz Pharma)
    Nifedipine 30 mg Adanif XL 30mg tablets | 28 tablet [PoM] £9.70 DT = £4.70
    Nifedipine 60 mg Adanif XL 60mg tablets | 28 tablet [PoM] £11.20 DT = £7.10
▸ Adipine MR (Chiesi Ltd)
    Nifedipine 10 mg Adipine MR 10 tablets | 56 tablet [PoM] £3.73 DT = £9.23
    Nifedipine 20 mg Adipine MR 20 tablets | 56 tablet [PoM] £5.21 DT = £10.06
▸ Adipine XL (Chiesi Ltd)
    Nifedipine 30 mg Adipine XL 30mg tablets | 28 tablet [PoM] £4.70 DT = £4.70
    Nifedipine 60 mg Adipine XL 60mg tablets | 28 tablet [PoM] £7.10 DT = £7.10
▸ Fortipine LA (Advanz Pharma)
    Nifedipine 40 mg Fortipine LA 40 tablets | 30 tablet [PoM] £14.40 DT = £14.40
▸ Nidef (Morningside Healthcare Ltd)
    Nifedipine 30 mg Nidef 30mg modified-release tablets | 28 tablet [PoM] £6.85 DT = £4.70
    Nifedipine 60 mg Nidef 60mg modified-release tablets | 28 tablet [PoM] £9.03 DT = £7.10
▸ Nifedipress MR (Dexcel-Pharma Ltd)
    Nifedipine 10 mg Nifedipress MR 10 tablets | 56 tablet [PoM] £9.23 DT = £9.23
    Nifedipine 20 mg Nifedipress MR 20 tablets | 56 tablet [PoM] £10.06 DT = £10.06
▸ Tensipine MR (Genus Pharmaceuticals Ltd)
    Nifedipine 10 mg Tensipine MR 10 tablets | 56 tablet [PoM] £4.30 DT = £9.23
    Nifedipine 20 mg Tensipine MR 20 tablets | 56 tablet [PoM] £5.49 DT = £10.06
▸ Valni Retard (Tillomed Laboratories Ltd)
    Nifedipine 20 mg Valni 20 Retard tablets | 56 tablet [FoM] £10.06 DT = £10.06
▸ Valni XL (Zentiva)
    Nifedipine 30 mg Valni XL 30mg tablets | 28 tablet [PoM] £6.85 DT = £4.70
    Nifedipine 60 mg Valni XL 60mg tablets | 28 tablet [PoM] £9.03 DT = £7.10

2

Cardiovascular system

Modified-release capsule

CAUTIONARY AND ADVISORY LABELS 25

▸ Coracten SR (UCB Pharma Ltd)

Nifedipine 10 mg Coracten SR 10mg capsules | 60 capsule [PoM] £3.90 DT = £3.90

Nifedipine 20 mg Coracten SR 20mg capsules | 60 capsule [PoM] £5.41 DT = £5.41

▸ Coracten XL (UCB Pharma Ltd)

Nifedipine 30 mg Coracten XL 30mg capsules | 28 capsule [PoM] £4.89 DT = £4.89

Nifedipine 60 mg Coracten XL 60mg capsules | 28 capsule [PoM] £7.34 DT = £7.34

Oral drops

▸ Nifedipin-ratiopharm (Imported (Germany))

Nifedipine 20 mg per 1 ml Nifedipin-ratiopharm 20mg/ml oral drops | 30 ml [PoM] [⅃]

Capsule

▸ Nifedipine (Non-proprietary)

Nifedipine 5 mg Nifedipine 5mg capsules | 90 capsule [PoM] £51.95 DT = £51.95

Nifedipine 10 mg Nifedipine 10mg capsules | 90 capsule [PoM] £65.63 DT = £65.63

Combinations available: *Atenolol with nifedipine*, p. 167

F 170

Verapamil hydrochloride

17-Jul-2020

● **INDICATIONS AND DOSE**

Treatment of supraventricular arrhythmias

▸ BY MOUTH USING IMMEDIATE-RELEASE MEDICINES

▸ Adult: 40–120 mg 3 times a day

▸ BY SLOW INTRAVENOUS INJECTION

▸ Adult: 5–10 mg, to be given over 2 minutes, preferably with ECG monitoring

▸ Elderly: 5–10 mg, to be given over 3 minutes, preferably with ECG monitoring

Paroxysmal tachyarrhythmias

▸ BY SLOW INTRAVENOUS INJECTION

▸ Adult: Initially 5–10 mg, followed by 5 mg after 5–10 minutes if required, to be given over 2 minutes, preferably with ECG monitoring

▸ Elderly: Initially 5–10 mg, followed by 5 mg after 5–10 minutes if required, to be given over 3 minutes, preferably with ECG monitoring

Angina

▸ BY MOUTH USING IMMEDIATE-RELEASE MEDICINES

▸ Adult: 80–120 mg 3 times a day

Hypertension

▸ BY MOUTH USING IMMEDIATE-RELEASE MEDICINES

▸ Adult: 240–480 mg daily in 2–3 divided doses

Prophylaxis of cluster headache (initiated under specialist supervision)

▸ BY MOUTH USING IMMEDIATE-RELEASE MEDICINES

▸ Adult: 240–960 mg daily in 3–4 divided doses

HALF SECURON ® SR

Hypertension (in patients new to verapamil)

▸ BY MOUTH

▸ Adult: Initially 120 mg daily, increased if necessary up to 480 mg daily, doses above 240 mg daily as 2 divided doses

Hypertension

▸ BY MOUTH

▸ Adult: 240 mg daily, increased if necessary up to 480 mg daily, doses above 240 mg daily as 2 divided doses

Angina

▸ BY MOUTH

▸ Adult: 240 mg twice daily, may sometimes be reduced to once daily

Prophylaxis after myocardial infarction where beta-blockers not appropriate

▸ BY MOUTH

▸ Adult: 360 mg daily in divided doses, started at least 1 week after infarction, given as either 240 mg in the morning and 120 mg in the evening *or* 120 mg 3 times daily

SECURON ® SR

Hypertension (in patients new to verapamil)

▸ BY MOUTH

▸ Adult: Initially 120 mg daily, increased if necessary up to 480 mg daily, doses above 240 mg daily as 2 divided doses

Hypertension

▸ BY MOUTH

▸ Adult: 240 mg daily, increased if necessary up to 480 mg daily, doses above 240 mg daily as 2 divided doses

Angina

▸ BY MOUTH

▸ Adult: 240 mg twice daily, may sometimes be reduced to once daily

Prophylaxis after myocardial infarction where beta-blockers not appropriate

▸ BY MOUTH

▸ Adult: 360 mg daily in divided doses, started at least 1 week after infarction, given as either 240 mg in the morning and 120 mg in the evening *or* 120 mg 3 times daily

VERAPRESS ® MR

Hypertension

▸ BY MOUTH

▸ Adult: 240 mg daily, increased if necessary to 240 mg twice daily

Angina

▸ BY MOUTH

▸ Adult: 240 mg twice daily, may sometimes be reduced to once daily

VERTAB ® SR 240

Mild to moderate hypertension

▸ BY MOUTH

▸ Adult: 240 mg daily, increased if necessary to 240 mg twice daily

Angina

▸ BY MOUTH

▸ Adult: 240 mg twice daily, may sometimes be reduced to once daily

● **UNLICENSED USE**

Prophylaxis of cluster headaches is an unlicensed indication.

● **CONTRA-INDICATIONS** Acute porphyrias p. 1107 · atrial flutter or fibrillation associated with accessory conducting pathways (e.g. Wolff-Parkinson-White-syndrome) · bradycardia · cardiogenic shock · heart failure (with reduced ejection fraction) · history of significantly impaired left ventricular function (even if controlled by therapy) · hypotension · second- and third-degree AV block · sick sinus syndrome · sino-atrial block

● **CAUTIONS** Acute phase of myocardial infarction (avoid if bradycardia, hypotension, left ventricular failure) · first-degree AV block · neuromuscular disorders

CAUTIONS, FURTHER INFORMATION

▸ Elderly Prescription potentially inappropriate (STOPP criteria) in patients with NYHA Class III or IV heart failure (may worsen heart failure). See also Prescribing in the elderly p. 33.

● **INTERACTIONS** → Appendix 1: calcium channel blockers

● SIDE-EFFECTS

GENERAL SIDE-EFFECTS

▶ **Common or very common** Hypotension

▶ **Frequency not known** Atrioventricular block · extrapyramidal symptoms · gynaecomastia · Stevens-Johnson syndrome · vertigo

SPECIFIC SIDE-EFFECTS

▶ **Common or very common**

▶ With intravenous use Bradycardia

▶ **Frequency not known**

▶ With intravenous use Cardiac arrest · hepatic impairment · hyperhidrosis · myocardial contractility decreased · nervousness · seizure

▶ With oral use Abdominal discomfort · alopecia · arrhythmias · arthralgia · constipation · erythromelalgia · fatigue · galactorrhoea · heart failure · ileus · muscle weakness · tinnitus · tremor

Overdose In overdose, verapamil has a profound cardiac depressant effect causing hypotension and arrhythmias, including complete heart block and asystole.

● PREGNANCY May reduce uterine blood flow with fetal hypoxia. Manufacturer advises avoid in first trimester unless absolutely necessary. May inhibit labour.

● BREAST FEEDING Amount too small to be harmful.

● HEPATIC IMPAIRMENT

Dose adjustments ▶ With oral use Manufacturer advises dose reduction.

● MEDICINAL FORMS There can be variation in the licensing of different medicines containing the same drug. Forms available from special-order manufacturers include: oral suspension, oral solution

Modified-release tablet

CAUTIONARY AND ADVISORY LABELS 25

▶ Half Securon (Mylan)
Verapamil hydrochloride 120 mg Half Securon SR 120mg tablets | 28 tablet PoM £7.71 DT = £7.71

▶ Securon SR (Mylan)
Verapamil hydrochloride 240 mg Securon SR 240mg tablets | 28 tablet PoM £5.55 DT = £5.55

▶ Vera-Til SR (Tillomed Laboratories Ltd, Actavis UK Ltd)
Verapamil hydrochloride 120 mg Vera-Til SR 120mg tablets | 28 tablet PoM £6.98 DT = £7.71
Verapamil hydrochloride 240 mg Vera-Til SR 240mg tablets | 28 tablet PoM £10.00 DT = £5.55

▶ Verapress MR (Dexcel-Pharma Ltd)
Verapamil hydrochloride 240 mg Verapress MR 240mg tablets | 28 tablet PoM £9.90 DT = £5.55

▶ Vertab SR (Chiesi Ltd)
Verapamil hydrochloride 240 mg Vertab SR 240 tablets | 28 tablet PoM £5.45 DT = £5.55

Tablet

▶ Verapamil hydrochloride (Non-proprietary)
Verapamil hydrochloride 40 mg Verapamil 40mg tablets | 84 tablet PoM £2.40 DT = £1.95
Verapamil hydrochloride 80 mg Verapamil 80mg tablets | 84 tablet PoM £3.07 DT = £2.46
Verapamil hydrochloride 120 mg Verapamil 120mg tablets | 28 tablet PoM £4.45 DT = £4.45
Verapamil hydrochloride 160 mg Verapamil 160mg tablets | 56 tablet PoM £33.84 DT = £29.47

Solution for injection

▶ Securon (Mylan)
Verapamil hydrochloride 2.5 mg per 1 ml Securon IV 5mg/2ml solution for injection ampoules | 5 ampoule PoM £5.41

Oral solution

▶ Verapamil hydrochloride (Non-proprietary)
Verapamil hydrochloride 8 mg per 1 ml Verapamil 40mg/5ml oral solution sugar free sugar-free | 150 ml PoM £44.92 DT = £44.74

DIURETICS ❭ THIAZIDES AND RELATED DIURETICS

Thiazides and related diuretics

● CONTRA-INDICATIONS Addison's disease · hypercalcaemia · hyponatraemia · refractory hypokalaemia · symptomatic hyperuricaemia

● CAUTIONS Diabetes · gout · risk of hypokalaemia · systemic lupus erythematosus

CAUTIONS, FURTHER INFORMATION

▶ Existing conditions Thiazides and related diuretics can exacerbate diabetes, gout, and systemic lupus erythematosus.

▶ Potassium loss Hypokalaemia can occur with thiazides and related diuretics.

Hypokalaemia is dangerous in severe cardiovascular disease and in patients also being treated with cardiac glycosides. Often the use of potassium-sparing diuretics avoids the need to take potassium supplements.

In hepatic impairment, hypokalaemia caused by diuretics can precipitate encephalopathy.

▶ Elderly Manufacturer advises lower initial doses of diuretics may be necessary in the elderly because they are particularly susceptible to the side-effects. The dose should then be adjusted according to renal function.

Prescription potentially inappropriate (STOPP criteria):

● with current significant hypokalaemia (serum potassium less than 3 mmol/L), hyponatraemia (serum sodium less than 130 mmol/L) or hypercalcaemia (corrected serum calcium greater than 2.65 mmol/L)—hypokalaemia, hyponatraemia and hypercalcaemia can be precipitated by a thiazide diuretic

● with a history of gout (gout can be precipitated by a thiazide diuretic)

See also Prescribing in the elderly p. 33.

● SIDE-EFFECTS

▶ **Common or very common** Alkalosis hypochloraemic · constipation · diarrhoea · dizziness · dry mouth · electrolyte imbalance · erectile dysfunction · fatigue · headache · hyperglycaemia · hyperuricaemia · nausea · postural hypotension · skin reactions

▶ **Uncommon** Agranulocytosis · aplastic anaemia · leucopenia · pancreatitis · photosensitivity reaction · thrombocytopenia · vomiting

▶ **Rare or very rare** Paraesthesia

● PREGNANCY Thiazides and related diuretics should not be used to treat gestational hypertension. They may cause neonatal thrombocytopenia, bone marrow suppression, jaundice, electrolyte disturbances, and hypoglycaemia; placental perfusion may also be reduced. Stimulation of labour, uterine inertia, and meconium staining have also been reported.

● HEPATIC IMPAIRMENT In general, manufacturer advises caution in mild to moderate impairment; avoid in severe impairment.

● RENAL IMPAIRMENT Thiazides and related diuretics are ineffective if eGFR is less than 30 mL/minute/1.73 m^2 and should be avoided. Metolazone remains effective if eGFR is less than 30 mL/minute/1.73 m^2 but is associated with a risk of excessive diuresis.

Monitoring Electrolytes should be monitored in renal impairment.

● MONITORING REQUIREMENTS Electrolytes should be monitored, particularly with high doses and long-term use.

2

Cardiovascular system

Bendroflumethiazide

ᴼ ⏆179

(Bendrofluazide)

● **INDICATIONS AND DOSE**

Oedema
▸ BY MOUTH
▸ **Adult:** Initially 5–10 mg once daily or on alternate days, dose to be taken in the morning, then maintenance 5–10 mg 1–3 times a week

Hypertension
▸ BY MOUTH
▸ **Adult:** 2.5 mg daily, dose to be taken in the morning, higher doses are rarely necessary

● INTERACTIONS → Appendix 1: thiazide diuretics

● SIDE-EFFECTS Blood disorder · cholestasis · gastrointestinal disorder · gout · neutropenia · pneumonitis · pulmonary oedema · severe cutaneous adverse reactions (SCARs)

● BREAST FEEDING The amount present in milk is too small to be harmful. Large doses may suppress lactation.

● MEDICINAL FORMS There can be variation in the licensing of different medicines containing the same drug. Forms available from special-order manufacturers include: oral suspension, oral solution

Tablet
▸ Bendroflumethiazide (Non-proprietary)
   Bendroflumethiazide 2.5 mg Bendroflumethiazide 2.5mg tablets | 28 tablet ⟦PoM⟧ £0.76 DT = £0.76 | 500 tablet ⟦PoM⟧ £10.71
   Bendroflumethiazide 5 mg Bendroflumethiazide 5mg tablets | 28 tablet ⟦PoM⟧ £1.30 DT = £1.30
▸ Neo-Naclex (Advanz Pharma)
   Bendroflumethiazide 2.5 mg Neo-Naclex 2.5mg tablets | 28 tablet ⟦PoM⟧ £0.33 DT = £0.76

Combinations available: *Timolol with bendroflumethiazide*, p. 166

Co-amilozide

23-Sep-2020

The properties listed below are those particular to the combination only. For the properties of the components please consider, hydrochlorothiazide below.

● **INDICATIONS AND DOSE**

Hypertension
▸ BY MOUTH
▸ **Adult:** Initially 2.5/25 mg daily, increased if necessary up to 5/50 mg daily

Congestive heart failure
▸ BY MOUTH
▸ **Adult:** Initially 2.5/25 mg daily; increased if necessary up to 10/100 mg daily, reduce dose for maintenance if possible

Oedema and ascites in cirrhosis of the liver
▸ BY MOUTH
▸ **Adult:** Initially 5/50 mg daily; increased if necessary up to 10/100 mg daily, reduce dose for maintenance if possible

DOSE EQUIVALENCE AND CONVERSION
▸ A mixture of amiloride hydrochloride and hydrochlorothiazide in the mass proportions of 1 part amiloride hydrochloride to 10 parts hydrochlorothiazide.

● CONTRA-INDICATIONS Anuria · hyperkalaemia
● CAUTIONS Diabetes mellitus · elderly
● INTERACTIONS → Appendix 1: potassium-sparing diuretics · thiazide diuretics

● SIDE-EFFECTS Angina pectoris · appetite abnormal · arrhythmias · arthralgia · asthenia · chest pain · confusion · constipation · depression · diarrhoea · dizziness · drowsiness · dyspnoea · electrolyte imbalance · erectile dysfunction · flatulence · flushing · gastrointestinal discomfort · gastrointestinal haemorrhage · gout · headache · hiccups · hyperhidrosis · insomnia · malaise · muscle cramps · nasal congestion · nausea · nervousness · pain · paraesthesia · postural hypotension · renal impairment · skin reactions · stupor · syncope · taste unpleasant · urinary disorders · vertigo · visual impairment · vomiting

● BREAST FEEDING Avoid—no information regarding amiloride component available. Amount of hydrochlorothiazide in milk probably too small to be harmful. Large doses of hydrochlorothiazide may suppress lactation.

● RENAL IMPAIRMENT Manufacturers advise avoid in severe impairment.
   Monitoring Monitor plasma-potassium concentration (high risk of hyperkalaemia in renal impairment).

● MONITORING REQUIREMENTS Monitor electrolytes.

● MEDICINAL FORMS There can be variation in the licensing of different medicines containing the same drug. Forms available from special-order manufacturers include: oral solution

Tablet
▸ Co-amilozide (Non-proprietary)
   Amiloride hydrochloride 2.5 mg, Hydrochlorothiazide 25 mg Co-amilozide 2.5mg/25mg tablets | 28 tablet ⟦PoM⟧ £12.14 DT = £9.33
   Amiloride hydrochloride 5 mg, Hydrochlorothiazide 50 mg Co-amilozide 5mg/50mg tablets | 28 tablet ⟦PoM⟧ £2.81 DT = £2.28
▸ Moduretic (Merck Sharp & Dohme Ltd)
   Amiloride hydrochloride 5 mg, Hydrochlorothiazide 50 mg Moduretic 5mg/50mg tablets | 28 tablet ⟦PoM⟧ £1.29 DT = £2.28

Hydrochlorothiazide

⏆179

03-Dec-2018

● **INDICATIONS AND DOSE**

Indications listed in combination monographs (available in the UK only in combination with other drugs)
▸ BY MOUTH
▸ **Adult:** Doses listed in combination monographs

IMPORTANT SAFETY INFORMATION

MHRA/CHM ADVICE: HYDROCHLOROTHIAZIDE: RISK OF NON-MELANOMA SKIN CANCER, PARTICULARLY IN LONG-TERM USE (NOVEMBER 2018)

The MHRA advises healthcare professionals to:
● inform patients taking hydrochlorothiazide-containing products of the cumulative, dose-dependent increased risk of non-melanoma skin cancer, particularly in long-term use, and advise patients to regularly check for and report any new or changed skin lesions or moles;
● advise patients to limit exposure to sunlight and UV rays and use adequate sun protection;
● reconsider the use of hydrochlorothiazide in patients who have had previous skin cancer;
● examine all suspicious moles or skin lesions (potentially including histological examination of biopsies).

● INTERACTIONS → Appendix 1: thiazide diuretics

● SIDE-EFFECTS
▸ **Uncommon** Appetite decreased · epigastric discomfort · fever · gastrointestinal spasm · glycosuria · haemolytic anaemia · insomnia · jaundice cholestatic · muscle cramps · nephritis tubulointerstitial · pulmonary oedema · renal

impairment · respiratory disorders · sialadenitis · toxic epidermal necrolysis · vasculitis · vision disorders
► **Frequency not known** Basal cell carcinoma (particularly in long term use) · cutaneous lupus erythematosus · restlessness · squamous cell carcinoma (particularly in long term use)

● MEDICINAL FORMS Forms available from special-order manufacturers include: tablet, oral suspension, oral solution

Combinations available: *Enalapril with hydrochlorothiazide,* p. 183 · *Irbesartan with hydrochlorothiazide,* p. 190 · *Lisinopril with hydrochlorothiazide,* p. 185 · *Losartan with hydrochlorothiazide,* p. 191 · *Olmesartan with amlodipine and hydrochlorothiazide,* p. 191 · *Olmesartan with hydrochlorothiazide,* p. 192 · *Quinapril with hydrochlorothiazide,* p. 186 · *Telmisartan with hydrochlorothiazide,* p. 192 · *Timolol with amiloride and hydrochlorothiazide,* p. 166 · *Valsartan with hydrochlorothiazide,* p. 193

⬛ 179

Indapamide
24-Nov-2020

● DRUG ACTION Indapamide is a thiazide-like diuretic with antihypertensive effects. At lower doses, vasodilatation is more prominent than diuresis; the diuretic effect becomes more apparent with higher doses.

● INDICATIONS AND DOSE
Essential hypertension
► BY MOUTH USING IMMEDIATE-RELEASE MEDICINES
► Adult: 2.5 mg daily, dose to be taken in the morning
► BY MOUTH USING MODIFIED-RELEASE MEDICINES
► Adult: 1.5 mg daily, dose to be taken preferably in the morning

● CAUTIONS Acute porphyrias p. 1107
● INTERACTIONS → Appendix 1: thiazide diuretics
● SIDE-EFFECTS
► **Common or very common** Hypersensitivity
► **Rare or very rare** Angioedema · arrhythmias · haemolytic anaemia · hepatic disorders · renal failure · severe cutaneous adverse reactions (SCARs) · vertigo
► **Frequency not known** Hepatic encephalopathy · QT interval prolongation · syncope · systemic lupus erythematosus exacerbated · vision disorders

● ALLERGY AND CROSS-SENSITIVITY EvGr Contra-indicated if history of hypersensitivity to sulfonamides. ⬥Ⓜ⬥

● BREAST FEEDING Present in milk—manufacturer advises avoid.

● MEDICINAL FORMS There can be variation in the licensing of different medicines containing the same drug. Forms available from special-order manufacturers include: oral suspension
Modified-release tablet
CAUTIONARY AND ADVISORY LABELS 25
► Alkapamid XL (HBS Healthcare Ltd, Rivopharm (UK) Ltd)
Indapamide 1.5 mg Alkapamid XL 1.5mg tablets | 30 tablet PoM £2.20–£3.40 DT = £3.40
► Cardide SR (Teva UK Ltd)
Indapamide 1.5 mg Cardide SR 1.5mg tablets | 30 tablet PoM £4.32 DT = £3.40
► Indipam XL (Accord Healthcare Ltd)
Indapamide 1.5 mg Indipam XL 1.5mg tablets | 30 tablet PoM £1.99 DT = £3.40
► Lorvacs XL (Torrent Pharma (UK) Ltd)
Indapamide 1.5 mg Lorvacs XL 1.5mg tablets | 30 tablet PoM £4.32 DT = £3.40
► Natrilix SR (Servier Laboratories Ltd)
Indapamide 1.5 mg Natrilix SR 1.5mg tablets | 30 tablet PoM £3.40 DT = £3.40
► Rawel XL (Consilient Health Ltd)
Indapamide 1.5 mg Rawel XL 1.5mg tablets | 30 tablet PoM £2.89 DT = £3.40

► Tensaid XL (Mylan)
Indapamide 1.5 mg Tensaid XL 1.5mg tablets | 30 tablet PoM £3.40 DT = £3.40
Tablet
► Indapamide (Non-proprietary)
Indapamide hemihydrate 2.5 mg Indapamide 2.5mg tablets | 28 tablet PoM £6.34 DT = £3.12 | 56 tablet PoM £4.02–£12.68
► Natrilix (Servier Laboratories Ltd)
Indapamide hemihydrate 2.5 mg Natrilix 2.5mg tablets | 30 tablet PoM £3.40 | 60 tablet PoM £6.80

Combinations available: *Perindopril arginine with indapamide,* p. 185

DRUGS ACTING ON THE RENIN-ANGIOTENSIN SYSTEM ⟩ ACE INHIBITORS

Angiotensin-converting enzyme inhibitors
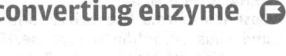

● CONTRA-INDICATIONS Hereditary or idiopathic angioedema · history of angioedema associated with prior ACE inhibitor therapy · the combination of an ACE inhibitor with aliskiren is contra-indicated in patients with an eGFR less than 60 mL/minute/1.73 m^2 · the combination of an ACE inhibitor with aliskiren is contra-indicated in patients with diabetes mellitus

● CAUTIONS Afro-Caribbean patients (may respond less well to ACE inhibitors) · concomitant diuretics · diabetes (may lower blood glucose) · first dose hypotension (especially in patients taking high doses of diuretics, on a low-sodium diet, on dialysis, dehydrated, or with heart failure) · peripheral vascular disease or generalised atherosclerosis (risk of clinically silent renovascular disease) · primary aldosteronism (patients may respond less well to ACE inhibitors) · the risk of agranulocytosis is possibly increased in collagen vascular disease (blood counts recommended) · use with care in patients with hypertrophic cardiomyopathy · use with care in patients with severe or symptomatic aortic stenosis (risk of hypotension)

CAUTIONS, FURTHER INFORMATION
► **Anaphylactoid reactions** To prevent anaphylactoid reactions, ACE inhibitors should be avoided during dialysis with high-flux polyacrylonitrile membranes and during low-density lipoprotein apheresis with dextran sulfate; they should also be withheld before desensitisation with wasp or bee venom.
► **Elderly** Prescription potentially inappropriate (STOPP criteria):
  ● with hyperkalaemia
  ● with persistent postural hypotension i.e. recurrent drop in systolic blood pressure ≥ 20 mmHg (risk of syncope and falls)
  See also Prescribing in the elderly p. 33.

● SIDE-EFFECTS
► **Common or very common** Alopecia · angina pectoris · angioedema (may be delayed; more common in Afro-Caribbean patients) · arrhythmias · asthenia · chest pain · constipation · cough · diarrhoea · dizziness · drowsiness · dry mouth · dyspnoea · electrolyte imbalance · gastrointestinal discomfort · headache · hypotension · myalgia · nausea · palpitations · paraesthesia · renal impairment · rhinitis · skin reactions · sleep disorder · syncope · taste altered · tinnitus · vertigo · vomiting
► **Uncommon** Arthralgia · confusion · eosinophilia · erectile dysfunction · fever · haemolytic anaemia · hyperhidrosis · myocardial infarction · pancreatitis · peripheral oedema · photosensitivity reaction · respiratory disorders · stroke
► **Rare or very rare** Agranulocytosis · hepatitis · leucopenia · neutropenia · pancytopenia · Stevens-Johnson syndrome · thrombocytopenia

2

Cardiovascular system

Cardiovascular system

2

SIDE-EFFECTS, FURTHER INFORMATION In light of reports of cholestatic jaundice, hepatitis, fulminant hepatic necrosis, and hepatic failure, ACE inhibitors should be discontinued if marked elevation of hepatic enzymes or jaundice occur.

- ALLERGY AND CROSS-SENSITIVITY ACE inhibitors are contra-indicated in patients with hypersensitivity to ACE inhibitors (including angioedema).
- PREGNANCY ACE inhibitors should be avoided in pregnancy unless essential. They may adversely affect fetal and neonatal blood pressure control and renal function; skull defects and oligohydramnios have also been reported.
- BREAST FEEDING Information on the use of ACE inhibitors in breast-feeding is limited.
- RENAL IMPAIRMENT
  Dose adjustments Use with caution, starting with low dose, and adjust according to response. Hyperkalaemia and other side-effects of ACE inhibitors are more common in those with impaired renal function and the dose may need to be reduced.
- MONITORING REQUIREMENTS Renal function and electrolytes should be checked before starting ACE inhibitors (or increasing the dose) and monitored during treatment (more frequently if side effects mentioned are present).
- DIRECTIONS FOR ADMINISTRATION For hypertension the first dose should preferably be given at bedtime.

F 181

Captopril

10-Mar-2020

- INDICATIONS AND DOSE
Hypertension
▸ BY MOUTH
▸ Adult: Initially 12.5–25 mg twice daily, then increased if necessary up to 150 mg daily in 2 divided doses, doses to be increased at intervals of at least 2 weeks, once-daily dosing may be appropriate if other concomitant antihypertensive drugs taken
▸ Elderly: Initially 6.25 mg twice daily, then increased if necessary up to 150 mg daily in 2 divided doses, doses to be increased at intervals of at least 2 weeks, once-daily dosing may be appropriate if other concomitant antihypertensive drugs taken

Essential hypertension if used in volume depletion, cardiac decompensation, or renovascular hypertension
▸ BY MOUTH
▸ Adult: Initially 6.25–12.5 mg for 1 dose (under close medical supervision), then 6.25–12.5 mg twice daily; increased if necessary up to 100 mg daily in 1–2 divided doses, doses to be increased at intervals of at least 2 weeks, once-daily dosing may be appropriate if other concomitant antihypertensive drugs taken

Heart failure
▸ BY MOUTH
▸ Adult (under close medical supervision): Initially 6.25–12.5 mg 2–3 times a day, then increased if tolerated to up to 150 mg daily in divided doses, dose to be increased gradually at intervals of at least 2 weeks

Short-term treatment within 24 hours of onset of myocardial infarction in clinically stable patients
▸ BY MOUTH
▸ Adult: Initially 6.25 mg, then increased to 12.5 mg after 2 hours, followed by 25 mg after 12 hours; increased if tolerated to 50 mg twice daily for 4 weeks

Prophylaxis of symptomatic heart failure after myocardial infarction in clinically stable patients with asymptomatic left ventricular dysfunction (starting 3–16 days after infarction) (under close medical supervision)
▸ BY MOUTH
▸ Adult: Initially 6.25 mg daily, then increased to 12.5 mg 3 times a day for 2 days, then increased if tolerated to 25 mg 3 times a day, then increased if tolerated to 75–150 mg daily in 2–3 divided doses, doses exceeding 75 mg per day to be increased gradually

Diabetic nephropathy in type 1 diabetes mellitus
▸ BY MOUTH
▸ Adult: 75–100 mg daily in divided doses

- INTERACTIONS → Appendix 1: ACE inhibitors
- SIDE-EFFECTS
- **Common or very common** Insomnia · peptic ulcer
- **Uncommon** Appetite decreased · flushing · malaise · pallor · Raynaud's phenomenon
- **Rare or very rare** Anaemia · aplastic anaemia · autoimmune disorder · cardiac arrest · cardiogenic shock · cerebrovascular insufficiency · depression · gynaecomastia · hepatic disorders · hypoglycaemia · lymphadenopathy · nephrotic syndrome · oral disorders · proteinuria · urinary disorders · vision blurred
- BREAST FEEDING Avoid in first few weeks after delivery, particularly in preterm infants—risk of profound neonatal hypotension; can be used in mothers breast-feeding older infants if essential but monitor infant's blood pressure.
- RENAL IMPAIRMENT
  Dose adjustments Reduce dose; max. initial dose 50 mg if eGFR above 40 mL/minute/1.73 m^2; max. initial dose 25 mg daily (do not exceed 100 mg daily) if eGFR 20–40 mL/minute/1.73 m^2; max. initial dose 12.5 mg daily (do not exceed 75 mg daily) if eGFR 10–20 mL/minute/1.73 m^2; max. initial dose 6.25 mg daily (do not exceed 37.5 mg daily) if eGFR less than 10 mL/minute/1.73 m^2.

- MEDICINAL FORMS There can be variation in the licensing of different medicines containing the same drug. Forms available from special-order manufacturers include: tablet, capsule, oral suspension, oral solution
Tablet
▸ Captopril (Non-proprietary)
  Captopril 12.5 mg Captopril 12.5mg tablets | 56 tablet [PoM] £1.54 DT = £1.54
  Captopril 25 mg Captopril 25mg tablets | 56 tablet [PoM] £1.75 DT = £1.75
  Captopril 50 mg Captopril 50mg tablets | 56 tablet [PoM] £1.51 DT = £1.51
Oral solution
ELECTROLYTES: May contain Sodium
▸ Captopril (Non-proprietary)
  Captopril 1 mg per 1 ml Captopril 5mg/5ml oral solution sugar free sugar-free | 100 ml [PoM] £98.21 DT = £93.63
  Captopril 5 mg per 1 ml Captopril 25mg/5ml oral solution sugar free sugar-free | 100 ml [PoM] £108.94 DT = £103.55
▸ Noyada (Martindale Pharmaceuticals Ltd)
  Captopril 1 mg per 1 ml Noyada 5mg/5ml oral solution sugar-free | 100 ml [PoM] £98.21 DT = £93.63
  Captopril 5 mg per 1 ml Noyada 25mg/5ml oral solution sugar-free | 100 ml [PoM] £108.94 DT = £103.55

F 181

Enalapril maleate

10-Mar-2020

- INDICATIONS AND DOSE
Hypertension
▸ BY MOUTH
▸ Adult: Initially 5 mg once daily, lower initial doses may be required when used in addition to diuretic or in

renal impairment; maintenance 20 mg once daily; maximum 40 mg per day

Heart failure
▶ BY MOUTH
▶ Adult (under close medical supervision): Initially 2.5 mg once daily, increased if tolerated to 10–20 mg twice daily, dose to be increased gradually over 2–4 weeks

Prevention of symptomatic heart failure in patients with asymptomatic left ventricular dysfunction
▶ BY MOUTH
▶ Adult (under close medical supervision): Initially 2.5 mg once daily, increased if tolerated to 10–20 mg twice daily, dose to be increased gradually over 2–4 weeks

● INTERACTIONS → Appendix 1: ACE inhibitors

● SIDE-EFFECTS
▶ **Common or very common** Depression · hypersensitivity · vision blurred
▶ **Uncommon** Anaemia · appetite decreased · asthma · bone marrow disorders · flushing · gastrointestinal disorders · hoarseness · hypoglycaemia · malaise · muscle cramps · nervousness · proteinuria · rhinorrhoea · sleep disorders · throat pain
▶ **Rare or very rare** Autoimmune disorder · gynaecomastia · hepatic disorders · lymphadenopathy · oral disorders · Raynaud's phenomenon · toxic epidermal necrolysis
▶ **Frequency not known** Arthritis · leucocytosis · myositis · serositis · SIADH · vasculitis

● BREAST FEEDING Avoid in first few weeks after delivery, particularly in preterm infants—risk of profound neonatal hypotension; can be used in mothers breast-feeding older infants if essential but monitor infant's blood pressure.

● HEPATIC IMPAIRMENT Enalapril is a prodrug.

● RENAL IMPAIRMENT
Dose adjustments Max. initial dose 2.5 mg daily if eGFR less than 30 mL/minute/1.73 m^2.

● DIRECTIONS FOR ADMINISTRATION Tablets may be crushed and suspended in water immediately before use.

● MEDICINAL FORMS There can be variation in the licensing of different medicines containing the same drug. Forms available from special-order manufacturers include: oral suspension, oral solution
Tablet
▶ Enalapril maleate (Non-proprietary)
   Enalapril maleate 2.5 mg Enalapril 2.5mg tablets | 28 tablet [PoM] £7.39 DT = £7.04
   Enalapril maleate 5 mg Enalapril 5mg tablets | 28 tablet [PoM] £4.13 DT = £1.61
   Enalapril maleate 10 mg Enalapril 10mg tablets | 28 tablet [PoM] £5.64 DT = £1.88
   Enalapril maleate 20 mg Enalapril 20mg tablets | 28 tablet [PoM] £11.05 DT = £2.22
▶ Innovace (Merck Sharp & Dohme Ltd)
   Enalapril maleate 2.5 mg Innovace 2.5mg tablets | 28 tablet [PoM] £5.35 DT = £7.04
   Enalapril maleate 5 mg Innovace 5mg tablets | 28 tablet [PoM] £7.51 DT = £1.61
   Enalapril maleate 10 mg Innovace 10mg tablets | 28 tablet [PoM] £10.53 DT = £1.88
   Enalapril maleate 20 mg Innovace 20mg tablets | 28 tablet [PoM] £12.51 DT = £2.22

Enalapril with hydrochlorothiazide

The properties listed below are those particular to the combination only. For the properties of the components please consider, enalapril maleate p. 182, hydrochlorothiazide p. 180.

● INDICATIONS AND DOSE
Mild to moderate hypertension in patients stabilised on the individual components in the same proportions
▶ BY MOUTH
▶ Adult: (consult product literature)

● INTERACTIONS → Appendix 1: ACE inhibitors · thiazide diuretics

● MEDICINAL FORMS There can be variation in the licensing of different medicines containing the same drug.
Tablet
▶ Enalapril with hydrochlorothiazide (Non-proprietary)
   Hydrochlorothiazide 12.5 mg, Enalapril maleate 20 mg Enalapril 20mg / Hydrochlorothiazide 12.5mg tablets | 28 tablet [PoM] £19.99 DT = £19.99
▶ Innozide (Merck Sharp & Dohme Ltd)
   Hydrochlorothiazide 12.5 mg, Enalapril maleate 20 mg Innozide 20mg/12.5mg tablets | 28 tablet [PoM] £13.90 DT = £19.99

F 181

Fosinopril sodium

23-Jul-2018

● INDICATIONS AND DOSE
Hypertension
▶ BY MOUTH
▶ Adult: Initially 10 mg daily for 4 weeks, then increased if necessary up to 40 mg daily, doses over 40 mg not shown to increase efficacy

Congestive heart failure (adjunct) (under close medical supervision)
▶ BY MOUTH
▶ Adult: Initially 10 mg once daily, then increased if tolerated to 40 mg once daily, doses to be increased gradually

● INTERACTIONS → Appendix 1: ACE inhibitors

● SIDE-EFFECTS
▶ **Common or very common** Eye disorder · increased risk of infection · mood altered · oedema · pain · sexual dysfunction · urinary disorder · visual impairment
▶ **Frequency not known** Appetite abnormal · arthritis · balance impaired · behaviour abnormal · cardiac arrest · cardiac conduction disorder · cerebrovascular insufficiency · depression · dysphagia · dysphonia · ear pain · flatulence · flushing · gout · haemorrhage · hypertensive crisis · lymphadenopathy · memory loss · muscle weakness · oral disorders · prostatic disorder · tremor · weight changes

● BREAST FEEDING Not recommended; alternative treatment options, with better established safety information during breast-feeding, are available.

● HEPATIC IMPAIRMENT Fosinopril is a prodrug. Manufacturer advises caution (risk of increased exposure).

● MEDICINAL FORMS There can be variation in the licensing of different medicines containing the same drug. Forms available from special-order manufacturers include: oral suspension, oral solution
Tablet
▶ Fosinopril sodium (Non-proprietary)
   Fosinopril sodium 10 mg Fosinopril 10mg tablets | 28 tablet [PoM] £6.78 DT = £4.23
   Fosinopril sodium 20 mg Fosinopril 20mg tablets | 28 tablet [PoM] £7.00 DT = £1.62

2

Cardiovascular system

Imidapril hydrochloride

F 181

● **INDICATIONS AND DOSE**

Essential hypertension
▸ BY MOUTH
▸ Adult: Initially 5 mg daily, increased if necessary to 10 mg daily, dose to be taken before food, doses to be increased at intervals of at least 3 weeks; maximum 20 mg per day
▸ Elderly: Initially 2.5 mg daily, increased if necessary to 10 mg daily, dose to be taken before food, doses to be increased at intervals of at least 3 weeks

Essential hypertension in patients with heart failure, angina or cerebrovascular disease
▸ BY MOUTH
▸ Adult: Initially 2.5 mg daily, increased if necessary to 10 mg daily, dose to be taken before food, dose to be increased at intervals of at least 3 weeks; maximum 20 mg per day

● **INTERACTIONS** → Appendix 1: ACE inhibitors

● **SIDE-EFFECTS**
▸ **Uncommon** Cerebrovascular disorder · increased risk of infection · joint swelling · limb pain · oedema
▸ **Rare or very rare** Anaemia

● **BREAST FEEDING** Not recommended; alternative treatment options, with better established safety information during breast-feeding, are available.

● **HEPATIC IMPAIRMENT** Imidapril is a prodrug. Manufacturer advises caution (risk of increased exposure). **Dose adjustments** Manufacturer advises initial dose of 2.5 mg daily.

● **RENAL IMPAIRMENT** Avoid if eGFR less than 30 mL/minute/1.73 m^2. **Dose adjustments** Initial dose 2.5 mg daily if eGFR 30–80 mL/minute/1.73 m^2.

● **MEDICINAL FORMS** There can be variation in the licensing of different medicines containing the same drug.
Tablet
▸ Tanatril (Mitsubishi Tanabe Pharma Europe Ltd)
Imidapril hydrochloride 5 mg Tanatril 5mg tablets | 28 tablet PoM £6.40 DT = £6.40
Imidapril hydrochloride 10 mg Tanatril 10mg tablets | 28 tablet PoM £7.22 DT = £7.22
Imidapril hydrochloride 20 mg Tanatril 20mg tablets | 28 tablet PoM £8.67 DT = £8.67

Lisinopril

F 181

10-Mar-2020

● **INDICATIONS AND DOSE**

Hypertension
▸ BY MOUTH
▸ Adult: Initially 10 mg once daily; usual maintenance 20 mg once daily; maximum 80 mg per day

Hypertension, when used in addition to diuretic, in cardiac decompensation or in volume depletion
▸ BY MOUTH
▸ Adult: Initially 2.5–5 mg once daily; usual maintenance 20 mg once daily; maximum 80 mg per day

Short-term treatment following myocardial infarction in haemodynamically stable patients—systolic blood pressure over 120 mmHg
▸ BY MOUTH
▸ Adult: Initially 5 mg, taken within 24 hours of myocardial infarction, followed by 5 mg, to be taken 24 hours after initial dose, then 10 mg, to be taken 24 hours after second dose, then 10 mg once daily for 6 weeks (or continued if heart failure), temporarily

reduce maintenance dose to 5 mg and if necessary 2.5 mg daily if systolic blood pressure 100 mmHg or less during treatment; withdraw if prolonged hypotension occurs during treatment (systolic blood pressure less than 90 mmHg for more than 1 hour)

Short-term treatment following myocardial infarction in haemodynamically stable patients—systolic blood pressure 100–120 mmHg
▸ BY MOUTH
▸ Adult: Initially 2.5 mg once daily, maintenance 5 mg once daily, increase to maintenance dose only after at least 3 days of the initial dose, should not be started after myocardial infarction if systolic blood pressure less than 100 mmHg, temporarily reduce maintenance dose to 2.5 mg daily if systolic blood pressure 100 mmHg or less during treatment; withdraw if prolonged hypotension occurs (systolic blood pressure less than 90 mmHg for more than 1 hour)

Renal complications of diabetes mellitus
▸ BY MOUTH
▸ Adult: Initially 2.5–5 mg once daily, adjusted according to response; usual dose 10–20 mg once daily

Heart failure (adjunct) (under close medical supervision)
▸ BY MOUTH
▸ Adult: Initially 2.5 mg once daily; increased in steps of up to 10 mg at least every 2 weeks; maximum 35 mg per day

● **INTERACTIONS** → Appendix 1: ACE inhibitors

● **SIDE-EFFECTS**
▸ **Common or very common** Postural disorders
▸ **Uncommon** Hallucination · mood altered · Raynaud's phenomenon
▸ **Rare or very rare** Anaemia · autoimmune disorder · azotaemia · bone marrow depression · gynaecomastia · hepatic disorders · hypersensitivity · hypoglycaemia · lymphadenopathy · olfactory nerve disorder · SIADH · sinusitis · toxic epidermal necrolysis
▸ **Frequency not known** Depressive symptom · leucocytosis · vasculitis

● **BREAST FEEDING** Not recommended; alternative treatment options, with better established safety information during breast-feeding, are available.

● **RENAL IMPAIRMENT** **Dose adjustments** Max. initial doses 5–10 mg daily if eGFR 30–80 mL/minute/1.73 m^2 (max. 40 mg daily); 2.5–5 mg daily if eGFR 10–30 mL/minute/1.73 m^2 (max. 40 mg daily); 2.5 mg daily if eGFR less than 10 mL/minute/1.73 m^2.

● **MEDICINAL FORMS** There can be variation in the licensing of different medicines containing the same drug. Forms available from special-order manufacturers include: oral suspension, oral solution
Oral solution
▸ Lisinopril (Non-proprietary)
Lisinopril 1 mg per 1 ml Lisinopril 5mg/5ml oral solution sugar free sugar-free | 150 ml PoM £154.11 DT = £154.11
Tablet
▸ Lisinopril (Non-proprietary)
Lisinopril 2.5 mg Lisinopril 2.5mg tablets | 28 tablet PoM £0.80 DT = £0.80 | 500 tablet PoM £11.84–£14.29
Lisinopril 5 mg Lisinopril 5mg tablets | 28 tablet PoM £7.54 DT = £0.85 | 500 tablet PoM £10.93–£15.18
Lisinopril 10 mg Lisinopril 10mg tablets | 28 tablet PoM £11.81 DT = £0.95 | 500 tablet PoM £10.78–£16.96
Lisinopril 20 mg Lisinopril 20mg tablets | 28 tablet PoM £10.42 DT = £1.04 | 500 tablet PoM £15.72–£18.57
▸ Zestril (AstraZeneca UK Ltd)
Lisinopril 5 mg Zestril 5mg tablets | 28 tablet PoM £9.42 DT = £0.85
Lisinopril 10 mg Zestril 10mg tablets | 28 tablet PoM £14.76 DT = £0.95
Lisinopril 20 mg Zestril 20mg tablets | 28 tablet PoM £13.02 DT = £1.04

Lisinopril with hydrochlorothiazide

The properties listed below are those particular to the combination only. For the properties of the components please consider, lisinopril p. 184, hydrochlorothiazide p. 180.

● **INDICATIONS AND DOSE**

Mild to moderate hypertension in patients stabilised on the individual components in the same proportions
▸ BY MOUTH
▸ Adult: (consult product literature)

● INTERACTIONS → Appendix 1: ACE inhibitors · thiazide diuretics

● MEDICINAL FORMS There can be variation in the licensing of different medicines containing the same drug.
Tablet
▸ Lisinopril with hydrochlorothiazide (Non-proprietary)
Lisinopril 10 mg, Hydrochlorothiazide 12.5 mg Lisinopril 10mg / Hydrochlorothiazide 12.5mg tablets | 28 tablet [PoM] £2.32 DT = £2.31
Hydrochlorothiazide 12.5 mg, Lisinopril 20 mg Lisinopril 20mg / Hydrochlorothiazide 12.5mg tablets | 28 tablet [PoM] £2.50 DT = £2.29
▸ Zestoretic (AstraZeneca UK Ltd)
Lisinopril 10 mg, Hydrochlorothiazide 12.5 mg Zestoretic 10 tablets | 28 tablet [PoM] £13.62 DT = £2.31
Hydrochlorothiazide 12.5 mg, Lisinopril 20 mg Zestoretic 20 tablets | 28 tablet [PoM] £13.82 DT = £2.29

◀ 181

Perindopril arginine

● **INDICATIONS AND DOSE**

Hypertension
▸ BY MOUTH
▸ Adult: Initially 5 mg once daily for 1 month, dose to be taken in the morning, then, adjusted according to response; maximum 10 mg per day
▸ Elderly: Initially 2.5 mg once daily for 1 month, dose to be taken in the morning, then, adjusted according to response; maximum 10 mg per day

Hypertension, if used in addition to diuretic, or in cardiac decompensation or volume depletion
▸ BY MOUTH
▸ Adult: Initially 2.5 mg once daily for 1 month, dose to be taken in the morning, then, adjusted according to response; maximum 10 mg per day

Symptomatic heart failure (adjunct) (under close medical supervision)
▸ BY MOUTH
▸ Adult: Initially 2.5 mg once daily for 2 weeks, then increased if tolerated to 5 mg once daily, dose to be taken in the morning

Prophylaxis of cardiac events following myocardial infarction or revascularisation in stable coronary artery disease
▸ BY MOUTH
▸ Adult: Initially 5 mg once daily for 2 weeks, then increased if tolerated to 10 mg once daily, dose to be taken in the morning
▸ Elderly: Initially 2.5 mg once daily for 1 week, then increased if tolerated to 5 mg once daily for 1 week, then increased if tolerated to 10 mg once daily, dose to be taken in the morning

● INTERACTIONS → Appendix 1: ACE inhibitors

● SIDE-EFFECTS
▸ **Common or very common** Muscle cramps · visual impairment
▸ **Uncommon** Fall · hypoglycaemia · malaise · mood altered · vasculitis
▸ **Rare or very rare** Cholestasis

● HEPATIC IMPAIRMENT Perindopril is a prodrug.
● RENAL IMPAIRMENT
Dose adjustments Max. initial dose 2.5 mg once daily if eGFR 30–60 mL/minute/1.73 m^2; 2.5 mg once daily on alternate days if eGFR 15–30 mL/minute/1.73 m^2.

● MEDICINAL FORMS There can be variation in the licensing of different medicines containing the same drug.
Tablet
CAUTIONARY AND ADVISORY LABELS 22
▸ Coversyl Arginine (Servier Laboratories Ltd)
Perindopril arginine 2.5 mg Coversyl Arginine 2.5mg tablets | 30 tablet [PoM] £4.43 DT = £4.43
Perindopril arginine 5 mg Coversyl Arginine 5mg tablets | 30 tablet [PoM] £6.28 DT = £6.28
Perindopril arginine 10 mg Coversyl Arginine 10mg tablets | 30 tablet [PoM] £10.65 DT = £10.65

Perindopril arginine with indapamide

The properties listed below are those particular to the combination only. For the properties of the components please consider, perindopril arginine above, indapamide p. 181.

● **INDICATIONS AND DOSE**

Hypertension not adequately controlled by perindopril alone
▸ BY MOUTH
▸ Adult: (consult product literature)

● INTERACTIONS → Appendix 1: ACE inhibitors · thiazide diuretics

● MEDICINAL FORMS There can be variation in the licensing of different medicines containing the same drug.
Tablet
CAUTIONARY AND ADVISORY LABELS 22
▸ Coversyl Arginine Plus (Servier Laboratories Ltd)
Indapamide 1.25 mg, Perindopril arginine 5 mg Coversyl Arginine Plus 5mg/1.25mg tablets | 30 tablet [PoM] £9.51 DT = £9.51

◀ 181

Perindopril erbumine

● **INDICATIONS AND DOSE**

Hypertension
▸ BY MOUTH
▸ Adult: Initially 4 mg once daily for 1 month, dose to be taken in the morning, then, adjusted according to response; maximum 8 mg per day
▸ BY MOUTH
▸ Elderly: Initially 2 mg once daily for 1 month, dose to be taken in the morning, then, adjusted according to response; maximum 8 mg per day

Hypertension, if used in addition to diuretic, or in cardiac decompensation or volume depletion
▸ BY MOUTH
▸ Adult: Initially 2 mg once daily for 1 month, dose to be taken in the morning, then, adjusted according to response; maximum 8 mg per day

Heart failure (adjunct) (under close medical supervision)
▸ BY MOUTH
▸ Adult: Initially 2 mg once daily for at least 2 weeks, dose to be taken in the morning, then increased if tolerated to 4 mg once daily

continued →

Prophylaxis of cardiac events following myocardial infarction or revascularisation in stable coronary artery disease
▶ BY MOUTH
  ▶ Adult: Initially 4 mg once daily for 2 weeks, dose to be taken in the morning, then increased if tolerated to 8 mg once daily
  ▶ Elderly: Initially 2 mg once daily for 1 week, then increased if tolerated to 4 mg once daily for 1 week, then increased if tolerated to 8 mg once daily

● INTERACTIONS → Appendix 1: ACE inhibitors
● SIDE-EFFECTS
▶ **Common or very common** Muscle cramps · visual impairment
▶ **Uncommon** Fall · hypoglycaemia · malaise · mood altered · vasculitis
▶ **Rare or very rare** Cholestasis
● BREAST FEEDING Not recommended; alternative treatment options, with better established safety information during breast-feeding, are available.
● HEPATIC IMPAIRMENT Perindopril is a prodrug.
● RENAL IMPAIRMENT
  Dose adjustments Max. initial dose 2 mg once daily if eGFR 30–60 mL/minute/1.73 m^2; 2 mg once daily on alternate days if eGFR 15–30 mL/minute/1.73 m^2.

● MEDICINAL FORMS There can be variation in the licensing of different medicines containing the same drug. Forms available from special-order manufacturers include: oral suspension, oral solution
Tablet
CAUTIONARY AND ADVISORY LABELS 22
  ▶ Perindopril erbumine (Non-proprietary)
    Perindopril erbumine 2 mg Perindopril erbumine 2mg tablets | 30 tablet [PoM] £10.95 DT = £2.85 | 56 tablet [PoM] £3.34 | 60 tablet [PoM] £13.90
    Perindopril erbumine 4 mg Perindopril erbumine 4mg tablets | 30 tablet [PoM] £12.99 DT = £4.49 | 56 tablet [PoM] £3.38 | 60 tablet [PoM] £27.80
    Perindopril erbumine 8 mg Perindopril erbumine 8mg tablets | 30 tablet [PoM] £12.99 DT = £5.25 | 56 tablet [PoM] £3.88 | 60 tablet [PoM] £40.00

F 181

Quinapril

● INDICATIONS AND DOSE
Essential hypertension
▶ BY MOUTH
  ▶ Adult: Initially 10 mg once daily; maintenance 20–40 mg daily in up to 2 divided doses; maximum 80 mg per day
  ▶ Elderly: Initially 2.5 mg once daily; maintenance 20–40 mg daily in up to 2 divided doses; maximum 80 mg per day

Essential hypertension if used in addition to diuretic
▶ BY MOUTH
  ▶ Adult: Initially 2.5 mg once daily; maintenance 20–40 mg daily in up to 2 divided doses; maximum 80 mg per day

Heart failure (adjunct) (under close medical supervision)
▶ BY MOUTH
  ▶ Adult: Initially 2.5 mg daily, increased if tolerated to 10–20 mg daily in 1–2 divided doses, doses to be increased gradually; maximum 40 mg per day

● INTERACTIONS → Appendix 1: ACE inhibitors
● SIDE-EFFECTS
▶ **Common or very common** Back pain · increased risk of infection · insomnia

▶ **Uncommon** Depression · dry throat · gastrointestinal disorders · generalised oedema · nervousness · proteinuria · transient ischaemic attack · vasodilation · vision disorders
▶ **Rare or very rare** Balance impaired · glossitis
▶ **Frequency not known** Arthritis · hypersensitivity · jaundice cholestatic · leucocytosis · pulmonary oedema · serositis · toxic epidermal necrolysis · vasculitis necrotising
● BREAST FEEDING Avoid in the first few weeks after delivery, particularly in preterm infants, due to the risk of profound neonatal hypotension; if essential, may be used in mothers breast-feeding older infants—the infant's blood pressure should be monitored.
● HEPATIC IMPAIRMENT Quinapril is a prodrug. Manufacturer advises caution when used in combination with a diuretic.
● RENAL IMPAIRMENT
  Dose adjustments Max. initial dose 2.5 mg once daily if eGFR less than 40 mL/minute/1.73 m^2.

● MEDICINAL FORMS There can be variation in the licensing of different medicines containing the same drug.
Tablet
  ▶ Quinapril (Non-proprietary)
    Quinapril (as Quinapril hydrochloride) 5 mg Quinapril 5mg tablets | 28 tablet [PoM] [S] DT = £8.60
  ▶ Accupro (Pfizer Ltd)
    Quinapril (as Quinapril hydrochloride) 5 mg Accupro 5mg tablets | 28 tablet [PoM] £8.60 DT = £8.60
    Quinapril (as Quinapril hydrochloride) 10 mg Accupro 10mg tablets | 28 tablet [PoM] £8.60 DT = £8.60
    Quinapril (as Quinapril hydrochloride) 20 mg Accupro 20mg tablets | 28 tablet [PoM] £10.79 DT = £10.79
    Quinapril (as Quinapril hydrochloride) 40 mg Accupro 40mg tablets | 28 tablet [PoM] £9.75 DT = £9.75

Quinapril with hydrochlorothiazide

The properties listed below are those particular to the combination only. For the properties of the components please consider, quinapril above, hydrochlorothiazide p. 180.

● INDICATIONS AND DOSE
Hypertension in patients stabilised on the individual components in the same proportions
▶ BY MOUTH
  ▶ Adult: (consult product literature)

● INTERACTIONS → Appendix 1: ACE inhibitors · thiazide diuretics

● MEDICINAL FORMS There can be variation in the licensing of different medicines containing the same drug.
Tablet
  ▶ Quinapril with hydrochlorothiazide (Non-proprietary)
    Quinapril (as Quinapril hydrochloride) 10 mg, Hydrochlorothiazide 12.5 mg Quinapril 10mg / Hydrochlorothiazide 12.5mg tablets | 28 tablet [PoM] £11.75 DT = £11.75
  ▶ Accuretic (Pfizer Ltd)
    Quinapril (as Quinapril hydrochloride) 10 mg, Hydrochlorothiazide 12.5 mg Accuretic 10mg/12.5mg tablets | 28 tablet [PoM] £11.75 DT = £11.75

F 181

Ramipril

17-Aug-2020

● INDICATIONS AND DOSE
Hypertension
▶ BY MOUTH
  ▶ Adult: Initially 1.25–2.5 mg once daily, increased if necessary up to 10 mg once daily, dose to be increased at intervals of 2–4 weeks

Symptomatic heart failure (adjunct) (under close medical supervision)
▸ BY MOUTH
▸ Adult: Initially 1.25 mg once daily, increased if tolerated to 10 mg daily, preferably taken in 2 divided doses, increase dose gradually at intervals of 1–2 weeks

Prophylaxis after myocardial infarction in patients with clinical evidence of heart failure (started at least 48 hours after infarction)
▸ BY MOUTH
▸ Adult: Initially 2.5 mg twice daily for 3 days, then increased to 5 mg twice daily

Prophylaxis after myocardial infarction in patients with clinical evidence of heart failure (started at least 48 hours after infarction) when initial dose not tolerated
▸ BY MOUTH
▸ Adult: 1.25 mg twice daily for 2 days, then increased to 2.5 mg twice daily, then increased to 5 mg twice daily, withdraw treatment if dose cannot be increased to 2.5 mg twice daily

Prevention of cardiovascular events in patients with atherosclerotic cardiovascular disease or with diabetes mellitus and at least one additional risk factor for cardiovascular disease
▸ BY MOUTH
▸ Adult: Initially 2.5 mg once daily for 1–2 weeks, then increased to 5 mg once daily for a further 2–3 weeks, then increased to 10 mg once daily

Nephropathy (consult product literature)
▸ BY MOUTH
▸ Adult: Initially 1.25 mg once daily for 2 weeks, then increased to 2.5 mg once daily for a further 2 weeks, then increased if tolerated to 5 mg once daily

● INTERACTIONS → Appendix 1: ACE inhibitors
● SIDE-EFFECTS
▸ **Common or very common** Gastrointestinal disorders · increased risk of infection · muscle spasms
▸ **Uncommon** Anxiety · appetite decreased · asthma exacerbated · depressed mood · flushing · libido decreased · myocardial ischaemia · nasal congestion · proteinuria aggravated · vision disorders
▸ **Rare or very rare** Conjunctivitis · hearing impairment · hepatic disorders · hypoperfusion · movement disorders · onycholysis · oral disorders · tremor · vascular stenosis · vasculitis
▸ **Frequency not known** Altered smell sensation · bone marrow failure · cerebrovascular insufficiency · concentration impaired · enanthema · gynaecomastia · hypersensitivity · Raynaud's phenomenon · SIADH · toxic epidermal necrolysis

● BREAST FEEDING Not recommended; alternative treatment options, with better established safety information during breast-feeding, are available.

● HEPATIC IMPAIRMENT Ramipril is a prodrug. Manufacturer advises caution.
Dose adjustments Manufacturer advises maximum 2.5 mg daily.

● RENAL IMPAIRMENT
Dose adjustments Max. daily dose 5 mg if eGFR 30–60 mL/minute/1.73 m^2; max. initial dose 1.25 mg once daily (do not exceed 5 mg daily) if eGFR less than 30 mL/minute/1.73 m^2.

● MEDICINAL FORMS There can be variation in the licensing of different medicines containing the same drug. Forms available from special-order manufacturers include: oral suspension, oral solution

Oral solution
▸ Ramipril (Non-proprietary)
Ramipril 500 microgram per 1 ml Ramipril 2.5mg/5ml oral solution sugar free sugar-free | 150 ml [PoM] £130.00 DT = £113.10

Tablet
▸ Ramipril (Non-proprietary)
Ramipril 1.25 mg Ramipril 1.25mg tablets | 28 tablet [PoM] £5.00 DT = £1.65
Ramipril 2.5 mg Ramipril 2.5mg tablets | 28 tablet [PoM] £6.76 DT = £1.56
Ramipril 5 mg Ramipril 5mg tablets | 28 tablet [PoM] £9.42 DT = £1.55
Ramipril 10 mg Ramipril 10mg tablets | 28 tablet [PoM] £12.81 DT = £1.59
▸ Tritace (Sanofi)
Ramipril 1.25 mg Tritace 1.25mg tablets | 28 tablet [PoM] £5.09 DT = £1.65
Ramipril 2.5 mg Tritace 2.5mg tablets | 28 tablet [PoM] £7.22 DT = £1.56
Ramipril 5 mg Tritace 5mg tablets | 28 tablet [PoM] £10.05 DT = £1.55
Ramipril 10 mg Tritace 10mg tablets | 28 tablet [PoM] £13.68 DT = £1.59

Capsule
▸ Ramipril (Non-proprietary)
Ramipril 1.25 mg Ramipril 1.25mg capsules | 28 capsule [PoM] £2.00 DT = £1.15
Ramipril 2.5 mg Ramipril 2.5mg capsules | 28 capsule [PoM] £5.78 DT = £1.01
Ramipril 5 mg Ramipril 5mg capsules | 28 capsule [PoM] £10.94 DT = £1.03
Ramipril 10 mg Ramipril 10mg capsules | 28 capsule [PoM] £10.94 DT = £1.11

Ramipril with felodipine

The properties listed below are those particular to the combination only. For the properties of the components please consider, ramipril p. 186, felodipine p. 174.

● INDICATIONS AND DOSE
Hypertension in patients stabilised on the individual components in the same proportions
▸ BY MOUTH
▸ Adult: (consult product literature)

● INTERACTIONS → Appendix 1: ACE inhibitors · calcium channel blockers

● MEDICINAL FORMS There can be variation in the licensing of different medicines containing the same drug.
Modified-release tablet
CAUTIONARY AND ADVISORY LABELS 25
▸ Triapin (Sanofi)
Felodipine 2.5 mg, Ramipril 2.5 mg Triapin 2.5mg/2.5mg modified-release tablets | 28 tablet [PoM] £24.55 DT = £24.55
Felodipine 5 mg, Ramipril 5 mg Triapin 5mg/5mg modified-release tablets | 28 tablet [PoM] £16.13 DT = £16.13

F 181

Trandolapril

05-Aug-2018

● INDICATIONS AND DOSE
Mild to moderate hypertension
▸ BY MOUTH
▸ Adult: Initially 500 micrograms once daily; increased to 1–2 mg once daily, dose to be increased at intervals of 2–4 weeks; maximum 4 mg per day

Prophylaxis after myocardial infarction in patients with left ventricular dysfunction (starting as early as 3 days after infarction)
▸ BY MOUTH
▸ Adult: Initially 500 micrograms once daily, then increased to up to 4 mg once daily, doses to be increased gradually

● INTERACTIONS → Appendix 1: ACE inhibitors

- SIDE-EFFECTS
- ▶ **Uncommon** Feeling abnormal · gastrointestinal disorders · hot flush · increased risk of infection · insomnia · libido decreased · malaise · muscle spasms · pain · rhinorrhoea
- ▶ **Rare or very rare** Anaemia · anxiety · appetite abnormal · azotaemia · cerebrovascular insufficiency · depression · enzyme abnormality · eye disorder · eye inflammation · gout · haemorrhage · hallucination · hyperbilirubinaemia · hyperglycaemia · hypersensitivity · hyperuricaemia · migraine · movement disorders · myocardial ischaemia · oedema · osteoarthritis · platelet disorder · throat irritation · urinary disorders · vascular disorders · visual impairment · white blood cell disorder
- ▶ **Frequency not known** Atrioventricular block · cardiac arrest · jaundice · proteinuria · toxic epidermal necrolysis

  SIDE-EFFECTS, FURTHER INFORMATION If symptomatic hypotension develops during titration, do not increase dose further; if possible, reduce dose of any adjunctive treatment and if this is not effective or feasible, reduce dose of trandolapril.

- BREAST FEEDING Not recommended; alternative treatment options, with better established safety information during breast-feeding, are available.
- HEPATIC IMPAIRMENT Trandolapril is a prodrug. Manufacturer advises caution.

  Dose adjustments Manufacturer advises initiate under close supervision and adjust dose according to blood pressure response in severe impairment.

- RENAL IMPAIRMENT

  Dose adjustments Max. 2 mg daily if eGFR less than 10 mL/minute/1.73 m^2.

- MEDICINAL FORMS There can be variation in the licensing of different medicines containing the same drug. Forms available from special-order manufacturers include: oral suspension

  Capsule
  - ▶ Trandolapril (Non-proprietary)
    Trandolapril 500 microgram Trandolapril 500microgram capsules | 14 capsule PoM £1.68 DT = £1.68
    Trandolapril 1 mg Trandolapril 1mg capsules | 28 capsule PoM £20.20 DT = £20.20
    Trandolapril 2 mg Trandolapril 2mg capsules | 28 capsule PoM £3.18 DT = £2.65
    Trandolapril 4 mg Trandolapril 4mg capsules | 28 capsule PoM £13.39 DT = £13.39

DRUGS ACTING ON THE RENIN-ANGIOTENSIN SYSTEM > ANGIOTENSIN II RECEPTOR ANTAGONISTS

Angiotensin II receptor antagonists

- CONTRA-INDICATIONS The combination of an angiotensin-II receptor antagonist with aliskiren is contra-indicated in patients with an eGFR less than 60 mL/minute/1.73 m^2 · the combination of an angiotensin-II receptor antagonist with aliskiren is contra-indictated in patients with diabetes mellitus
- CAUTIONS Afro-Caribbean patients—particularly those with left ventricular hypertrophy (may not benefit from an angiotensin-II receptor antagonist) · aortic or mitral valve stenosis · elderly (lower initial doses may be appropriate) · hypertrophic cardiomyopathy · patients with a history of angioedema · patients with primary aldosteronism (may not benefit from an angiotensin-II receptor antagonist) · renal artery stenosis

  CAUTIONS, FURTHER INFORMATION
  - ▶ Elderly Prescription potentially inappropriate (STOPP criteria):
    - with hyperkalaemia

- with persistent postural hypotension i.e. recurrent drop in systolic blood pressure $\geq$ 20 mmHg (risk of syncope and falls)

  See also Prescribing in the elderly p. 33.

- SIDE-EFFECTS
- ▶ **Common or very common** Abdominal pain · asthenia · back pain · cough · diarrhoea · dizziness · headache · hyperkalaemia · hypotension · nausea · postural hypotension (more common in patients with intravascular volume depletion, e.g. those taking high-dose diuretics) · renal impairment · vertigo · vomiting
- ▶ **Uncommon** Angioedema · myalgia · skin reactions · thrombocytopenia
- ▶ **Rare or very rare** Arthralgia · hepatic function abnormal
- PREGNANCY Angiotensin-II receptor antagonists should be avoided in pregnancy unless essential. They may adversely affect fetal and neonatal blood pressure control and renal function; neonatal skull defects and oligohydramnios have also been reported.
- BREAST FEEDING Information on the use of angiotensin-II receptor antagonists in breast-feeding is limited. They are not recommended in breast-feeding and alternative treatment options, with better established safety information during breast-feeding, are available.
- HEPATIC IMPAIRMENT In general, manufacturers advise caution in mild to moderate impairment (limited information available); avoid in severe impairment (no information available).
- RENAL IMPAIRMENT

  Dose adjustments Use with caution, starting with low dose, and adjust according to response.

- MONITORING REQUIREMENTS Monitor plasma-potassium concentration, particularly in the elderly and in patients with renal impairment.

⬛ above

Azilsartan medoxomil

05-Jun-2018

- INDICATIONS AND DOSE

  Hypertension
  - ▶ BY MOUTH
  - ▶ **Adult 18–74 years:** Initially 40 mg once daily, increased if necessary to 80 mg once daily
  - ▶ **Adult 75 years and over:** Initially 20–40 mg once daily, increased if necessary to 80 mg once daily

  Hypertension with intravascular volume depletion
  - ▶ BY MOUTH
  - ▶ **Adult:** Initially 20–40 mg daily, increased if necessary to 80 mg daily

- CAUTIONS Heart failure
- INTERACTIONS → Appendix 1: angiotensin-II receptor antagonists
- SIDE-EFFECTS
- ▶ **Uncommon** Hyperuricaemia · muscle spasms · peripheral oedema
- HEPATIC IMPAIRMENT

  Dose adjustments Manufacturer advises consider initial dose of 20 mg in mild to moderate impairment.
  Monitoring Manufacturer advises monitor closely in mild to moderate hepatic impairment (limited information available).

- RENAL IMPAIRMENT Manufacturer advises caution in severe impairment—no information available.

- MEDICINAL FORMS There can be variation in the licensing of different medicines containing the same drug.
  Tablet
  - ▶ Edarbi (Takeda UK Ltd)
    Azilsartan medoxomil 20 mg Edarbi 20mg tablets | 28 tablet PoM £16.80 DT = £16.80

Azilsartan medoxomil 40 mg Edarbi 40mg tablets | 28 tablet PoM
£16.80 DT = £16.80
Azilsartan medoxomil 80 mg Edarbi 80mg tablets | 28 tablet PoM
£19.95 DT = £19.95

F 188

Candesartan cilexetil
29-Jul-2019

● **INDICATIONS AND DOSE**

Hypertension
► BY MOUTH
► Adult: Initially 8 mg once daily, increased if necessary
up to 32 mg once daily, doses to be increased at
intervals of 4 weeks; usual dose 8 mg once daily

Hypertension with intravascular volume depletion
► BY MOUTH
► Adult: Initially 4 mg once daily, increased if necessary
up to 32 mg daily, doses to be increased at intervals of
4 weeks; usual dose 8 mg once daily

**Heart failure with impaired left ventricular systolic
function when ACE inhibitors are not tolerated | Heart
failure with impaired left ventricular systolic function in
conjunction with an ACE inhibitor (under expert
supervision)**
► BY MOUTH
► Adult: Initially 4 mg once daily, increased at intervals
of at least 2 weeks to 'target' dose of 32 mg once daily
or to maximum tolerated dose; maximum 32 mg per
day

Migraine prophylaxis
► BY MOUTH
► Adult: 16 mg once daily

● UNLICENSED USE EvGr Candesartan is used for migraine
prophylaxis, ⟨A⟩ but is not licensed for this indication.

● CONTRA-INDICATIONS Cholestasis

● INTERACTIONS → Appendix 1: angiotensin-II receptor
antagonists

● SIDE-EFFECTS
► **Common or very common** Increased risk of infection
► **Rare or very rare** Agranulocytosis · hepatitis ·
hyponatraemia · leucopenia · neutropenia

● HEPATIC IMPAIRMENT Manufacturer advises avoid in
severe impairment or cholestasis.
Dose adjustments Manufacturer advises initial dose
reduction to 4 mg once daily in mild to moderate
impairment; adjust according to response.

● RENAL IMPAIRMENT Use with caution if eGFR less than
15 mL/minute/1.73 m^2—limited experience.
Dose adjustments Initially 4 mg daily.

● MEDICINAL FORMS There can be variation in the licensing of
different medicines containing the same drug. Forms available
from special-order manufacturers include: oral suspension, oral
solution
Tablet
► Candesartan cilexetil (Non-proprietary)
Candesartan cilexetil 2 mg Candesartan 2mg tablets |
7 tablet PoM £16.13 DT = £1.27
Candesartan cilexetil 4 mg Candesartan 4mg tablets |
7 tablet PoM £3.88 DT = £0.81 | 28 tablet PoM £0.49-£9.78
Candesartan cilexetil 8 mg Candesartan 8mg tablets |
28 tablet PoM £9.89 DT = £1.58
Candesartan cilexetil 16 mg Candesartan 16mg tablets |
28 tablet PoM £12.72 DT = £1.66
Candesartan cilexetil 32 mg Candesartan 32mg tablets |
28 tablet PoM £16.13 DT = £2.15
► Amias (Takeda UK Ltd)
Candesartan cilexetil 2 mg Amias 2mg tablets | 7 tablet PoM
£3.58 DT = £1.27
Candesartan cilexetil 4 mg Amias 4mg tablets | 7 tablet PoM
£3.88 DT = £0.81 | 28 tablet PoM £9.78
Candesartan cilexetil 8 mg Amias 8mg tablets | 28 tablet PoM
£9.89 DT = £1.58

Candesartan cilexetil 16 mg Amias 16mg tablets | 28 tablet PoM
£12.72 DT = £1.66
Candesartan cilexetil 32 mg Amias 32mg tablets | 28 tablet PoM
£16.13 DT = £2.15

F 188

Eprosartan
14-Jul-2018

● **INDICATIONS AND DOSE**

Hypertension
► BY MOUTH
► Adult: 600 mg once daily

● INTERACTIONS → Appendix 1: angiotensin-II receptor
antagonists

● SIDE-EFFECTS
► **Common or very common** Gastrointestinal disorder ·
rhinitis

● RENAL IMPAIRMENT
Dose adjustments Caution if eGFR less than
30 mL/minute/1.73 m^2.

● MEDICINAL FORMS There can be variation in the licensing of
different medicines containing the same drug. Forms available
from special-order manufacturers include: oral suspension, oral
solution
Tablet
CAUTIONARY AND ADVISORY LABELS 21
► Eprosartan (Non-proprietary)
Eprosartan (as Eprosartan mesilate) 300 mg Eprosartan 300mg
tablets | 28 tablet PoM £7.31 DT = £7.31
Eprosartan (as Eprosartan mesilate) 400 mg Eprosartan 400mg
tablets | 56 tablet PoM £23.39 DT = £23.39
Eprosartan (as Eprosartan mesilate) 600 mg Eprosartan 600mg
tablets | 28 tablet PoM £18.16 DT = £18.16
► Teveten (Mylan)
Eprosartan (as Eprosartan mesilate) 300 mg Teveten 300mg
tablets | 28 tablet PoM £7.31 DT = £7.31
Eprosartan (as Eprosartan mesilate) 600 mg Teveten 600mg
tablets | 28 tablet PoM £14.31 DT = £18.16

F 188

Irbesartan

● **INDICATIONS AND DOSE**

Hypertension
► BY MOUTH
► Adult 18-74 years: Initially 150 mg once daily, increased
if necessary to 300 mg once daily
► Adult 75 years and over: Initially 75-150 mg once daily,
increased if necessary to 300 mg once daily

Hypertension in patients receiving haemodialysis
► BY MOUTH
► Adult: Initially 75-150 mg once daily, increased if
necessary to 300 mg once daily

Renal disease in hypertensive type 2 diabetes mellitus
► BY MOUTH
► Adult 18-74 years: Initially 150 mg once daily, increased
if tolerated to 300 mg once daily
► Adult 75 years and over: Initially 75-150 mg once daily,
increased if tolerated to 300 mg once daily

**Renal disease in hypertensive type 2 diabetes mellitus in
patients receiving haemodialysis**
► BY MOUTH
► Adult: Initially 75-150 mg once daily, increased if
tolerated to 300 mg once daily

● INTERACTIONS → Appendix 1: angiotensin-II receptor
antagonists

● SIDE-EFFECTS
► **Common or very common** Musculoskeletal pain
► **Uncommon** Chest pain · dyspepsia · flushing · hepatic
disorders · sexual dysfunction · tachycardia

▸ **Frequency not known** Hypersensitivity vasculitis · muscle cramps · taste altered · tinnitus

● MEDICINAL FORMS There can be variation in the licensing of different medicines containing the same drug. Forms available from special-order manufacturers include: oral suspension

Tablet

▸ Irbesartan (Non-proprietary)
Irbesartan 75 mg Irbesartan 75mg tablets | 28 tablet PoM £8.24 DT = £2.85
Irbesartan 150 mg Irbesartan 150mg tablets | 28 tablet PoM £10.06 DT = £7.54
Irbesartan 300 mg Irbesartan 300mg tablets | 28 tablet PoM £13.54 DT = £5.40
▸ Aprovel (Sanofi)
Irbesartan 75 mg Aprovel 75mg tablets | 28 tablet PoM £9.69 DT = £2.85
Irbesartan 150 mg Aprovel 150mg tablets | 28 tablet PoM £11.84 DT = £7.54
Irbesartan 300 mg Aprovel 300mg tablets | 28 tablet PoM £15.93 DT = £5.40
▸ Ifirmasta (Consilient Health Ltd)
Irbesartan 75 mg Ifirmasta 75mg tablets | 28 tablet PoM £8.23 DT = £2.85
Irbesartan 150 mg Ifirmasta 150mg tablets | 28 tablet PoM £10.06 DT = £7.54
Irbesartan 300 mg Ifirmasta 300mg tablets | 28 tablet PoM £13.54 DT = £5.40

Irbesartan with hydrochlorothiazide

The properties listed below are those particular to the combination only. For the properties of the components please consider, irbesartan p. 189, hydrochlorothiazide p. 180.

● **INDICATIONS AND DOSE**

Hypertension not adequately controlled with irbesartan alone

▸ BY MOUTH
▸ Adult: (consult product literature)

● INTERACTIONS → Appendix 1: angiotensin-II receptor antagonists · thiazide diuretics

● MEDICINAL FORMS There can be variation in the licensing of different medicines containing the same drug.

Tablet

▸ Irbesartan with hydrochlorothiazide (Non-proprietary)
Hydrochlorothiazide 12.5 mg, Irbesartan 150 mg Irbesartan 150mg / Hydrochlorothiazide 12.5mg tablets | 28 tablet PoM £11.44 DT = £10.30
Hydrochlorothiazide 25 mg, Irbesartan 300 mg Irbesartan 300mg / Hydrochlorothiazide 25mg tablets | 28 tablet PoM £8.24 DT = £7.72
Hydrochlorothiazide 12.5 mg, Irbesartan 300 mg Irbesartan 300mg / Hydrochlorothiazide 12.5mg tablets | 28 tablet PoM £10.37 DT = £4.95
▸ CoAprovel (Sanofi)
Hydrochlorothiazide 12.5 mg, Irbesartan 150 mg CoAprovel 150mg/12.5mg tablets | 28 tablet PoM £11.84 DT = £10.30
Hydrochlorothiazide 25 mg, Irbesartan 300 mg CoAprovel 300mg/25mg tablets | 28 tablet PoM £15.93 DT = £7.72
Hydrochlorothiazide 12.5 mg, Irbesartan 300 mg CoAprovel 300mg/12.5mg tablets | 28 tablet PoM £15.93 DT = £4.95

◤ 188

Losartan potassium

03-Aug-2018

● **INDICATIONS AND DOSE**

Diabetic nephropathy in type 2 diabetes mellitus

▸ BY MOUTH
▸ Adult 18–75 years: Initially 50 mg once daily for several weeks, then increased if necessary to 100 mg once daily
▸ Adult 76 years and over: Initially 25 mg once daily for several weeks, then increased if necessary to 100 mg once daily

Chronic heart failure when ACE inhibitors are unsuitable or contra-indicated

▸ BY MOUTH
▸ Adult: Initially 12.5 mg once daily, increased if tolerated to up to 150 mg once daily, doses to be increased at weekly intervals

Hypertension (including reduction of stroke risk in hypertension with left ventricular hypertrophy)

▸ BY MOUTH
▸ Adult 18–75 years: Initially 50 mg once daily for several weeks, then increased if necessary to 100 mg once daily
▸ Adult 76 years and over: Initially 25 mg once daily for several weeks, then increased if necessary to 100 mg once daily

Hypertension with intravascular volume depletion

▸ BY MOUTH
▸ Adult 18–75 years: Initially 25 mg once daily for several weeks, then increased if necessary up to 100 mg once daily

● CAUTIONS Severe heart failure

● INTERACTIONS → Appendix 1: angiotensin-II receptor antagonists

● SIDE-EFFECTS

▸ **Common or very common** Anaemia · hypoglycaemia · postural disorders
▸ **Uncommon** Angina pectoris · constipation · drowsiness · dyspnoea · oedema · palpitations · sleep disorder
▸ **Rare or very rare** Atrial fibrillation · hepatitis · hypersensitivity · paraesthesia · stroke · syncope · vasculitis
▸ **Frequency not known** Depression · erectile dysfunction · hyponatraemia · influenza like illness · malaise · migraine · pancreatitis · photosensitivity reaction · rhabdomyolysis · taste altered · tinnitus · urinary tract infection

● HEPATIC IMPAIRMENT

Dose adjustments Manufacturer advises consider dose reduction if history of impairment (risk of increased plasma concentrations).

● PRESCRIBING AND DISPENSING INFORMATION Flavours of oral liquid formulations may include berry-citrus.

● MEDICINAL FORMS There can be variation in the licensing of different medicines containing the same drug. Forms available from special-order manufacturers include: oral suspension, oral solution

Tablet

▸ Losartan potassium (Non-proprietary)
Losartan potassium 12.5 mg Losartan 12.5mg tablets | 28 tablet PoM £30.00 DT = £5.59
Losartan potassium 25 mg Losartan 25mg tablets | 28 tablet PoM £16.18 DT = £1.54
Losartan potassium 50 mg Losartan 50mg tablets | 28 tablet PoM £12.80 DT = £1.71 | 500 tablet PoM £30.36–£34.82
Losartan potassium 100 mg Losartan 100mg tablets | 28 tablet PoM £16.18 DT = £2.07
▸ Cozaar (Merck Sharp & Dohme Ltd)
Losartan potassium 12.5 mg Cozaar 12.5mg tablets | 28 tablet PoM £9.70 DT = £5.59
Losartan potassium 25 mg Cozaar 25mg tablets | 28 tablet PoM £16.18 DT = £1.54
Losartan potassium 50 mg Cozaar 50mg tablets | 28 tablet PoM £12.80 DT = £1.71
Losartan potassium 100 mg Cozaar 100mg tablets | 28 tablet PoM £16.18 DT = £2.07

Losartan with hydrochlorothiazide

The properties listed below are those particular to the combination only. For the properties of the components please consider, losartan potassium p. 190, hydrochlorothiazide p. 180.

● **INDICATIONS AND DOSE**

Hypertension not adequately controlled with losartan alone
▸ BY MOUTH
▸ Adult: (consult product literature)

● INTERACTIONS → Appendix 1: angiotensin-II receptor antagonists · thiazide diuretics

● MEDICINAL FORMS There can be variation in the licensing of different medicines containing the same drug.

Tablet
▸ Losartan with hydrochlorothiazide (Non-proprietary)
Hydrochlorothiazide 12.5 mg, Losartan potassium 50 mg Losartan 50mg / Hydrochlorothiazide 12.5mg tablets | 28 tablet [PoM] £12.80 DT = £1.57
Hydrochlorothiazide 25 mg, Losartan potassium 100 mg Losartan 100mg / Hydrochlorothiazide 25mg tablets | 28 tablet [PoM] £16.18 DT = £1.85
Hydrochlorothiazide 12.5 mg, Losartan potassium 100 mg Losartan 100mg / Hydrochlorothiazide 12.5mg tablets | 28 tablet [PoM] £16.18 DT = £12.60
▸ Cozaar-Comp (Merck Sharp & Dohme Ltd)
Hydrochlorothiazide 12.5 mg, Losartan potassium 50 mg Cozaar-Comp 50mg/12.5mg tablets | 28 tablet [PoM] £12.80 DT = £1.57
Hydrochlorothiazide 25 mg, Losartan potassium 100 mg Cozaar-Comp 100mg/25mg tablets | 28 tablet [PoM] £16.18 DT = £1.85
Hydrochlorothiazide 12.5 mg, Losartan potassium 100 mg Cozaar-Comp 100mg/12.5mg tablets | 28 tablet [PoM] £16.18 DT = £12.60

◤ 188

Olmesartan medoxomil

● **INDICATIONS AND DOSE**

Hypertension
▸ BY MOUTH
▸ Adult: Initially 10 mg daily, increased if necessary to 20 mg daily; maximum 40 mg per day

● CONTRA-INDICATIONS Biliary obstruction

● INTERACTIONS → Appendix 1: angiotensin-II receptor antagonists

● SIDE-EFFECTS
▸ **Common or very common** Arthritis · bone pain · chest pain · dyspepsia · haematuria · hypertriglyceridaemia · hyperuricaemia · increased risk of infection · influenza like illness · oedema
▸ **Uncommon** Angina pectoris · malaise
▸ **Rare or very rare** Lethargy · muscle spasms · sprue-like enteropathy

● HEPATIC IMPAIRMENT Manufacturer advises caution in moderate impairment; avoid in severe impairment (no information available).
Dose adjustments Manufacturer advises maximum 20 mg daily in moderate impairment.

● RENAL IMPAIRMENT Avoid if eGFR less than 20 mL/minute/1.73 m^2.
Dose adjustments Max. 20 mg daily if eGFR 20–60 mL/minute/1.73 m^2.

● MEDICINAL FORMS There can be variation in the licensing of different medicines containing the same drug. Forms available from special-order manufacturers include: oral suspension, oral solution

Tablet
▸ Olmesartan medoxomil (Non-proprietary)
Olmesartan medoxomil 10 mg Olmesartan medoxomil 10mg tablets | 28 tablet [PoM] £10.95 DT = £2.16
Olmesartan medoxomil 20 mg Olmesartan medoxomil 20mg tablets | 28 tablet [PoM] £12.95 DT = £2.17
Olmesartan medoxomil 40 mg Olmesartan medoxomil 40mg tablets | 28 tablet [PoM] £17.50 DT = £2.35
▸ Olmetec (Daiichi Sankyo UK Ltd)
Olmesartan medoxomil 10 mg Olmetec 10mg tablets | 28 tablet [PoM] £10.95 DT = £2.16
Olmesartan medoxomil 20 mg Olmetec 20mg tablets | 28 tablet [PoM] £12.95 DT = £2.17
Olmesartan medoxomil 40 mg Olmetec 40mg tablets | 28 tablet [PoM] £17.50 DT = £2.35

Olmesartan with amlodipine

The properties listed below are those particular to the combination only. For the properties of the components please consider, olmesartan medoxomil above, amlodipine p. 170.

● **INDICATIONS AND DOSE**

Hypertension in patients stabilised on the individual components in the same proportions
▸ BY MOUTH
▸ Adult: (consult product literature)

● INTERACTIONS → Appendix 1: angiotensin-II receptor antagonists · calcium channel blockers

● MEDICINAL FORMS There can be variation in the licensing of different medicines containing the same drug.
Tablet
▸ Sevikar (Daiichi Sankyo UK Ltd)
Amlodipine (as Amlodipine besilate) 5 mg, Olmesartan medoxomil 20 mg Sevikar 20mg/5mg tablets | 28 tablet [PoM] £16.95 DT = £16.95
Amlodipine (as Amlodipine besilate) 10 mg, Olmesartan medoxomil 40 mg Sevikar 40mg/10mg tablets | 28 tablet [PoM] £16.95 DT = £16.95
Amlodipine (as Amlodipine besilate) 5 mg, Olmesartan medoxomil 40 mg Sevikar 40mg/5mg tablets | 28 tablet [PoM] £16.95 DT = £16.95

Olmesartan with amlodipine and hydrochlorothiazide

The properties listed below are those particular to the combination only. For the properties of the components please consider, olmesartan medoxomil above, amlodipine p. 170, hydrochlorothiazide p. 180.

● **INDICATIONS AND DOSE**

Hypertension in patients stabilised on the individual components in the same proportions, or for hypertension not adequately controlled with olmesartan and amlodipine
▸ BY MOUTH
▸ Adult: (consult product literature)

● INTERACTIONS → Appendix 1: angiotensin-II receptor antagonists · calcium channel blockers · thiazide diuretics

2

Cardiovascular system

2

Cardiovascular system

- MEDICINAL FORMS There can be variation in the licensing of different medicines containing the same drug.

Tablet
▸ Sevikar HCT (Daiichi Sankyo UK Ltd)
Amlodipine besilate 5 mg, Hydrochlorothiazide 12.5 mg, Olmesartan medoxomil 20 mg Sevikar HCT 20mg/5mg/12.5mg tablets | 28 tablet [PoM] £16.95
Amlodipine besilate 5 mg, Hydrochlorothiazide 25 mg, Olmesartan medoxomil 40 mg Sevikar HCT 40mg/5mg/25mg tablets | 28 tablet [PoM] £16.95
Amlodipine besilate 10 mg, Hydrochlorothiazide 25 mg, Olmesartan medoxomil 40 mg Sevikar HCT 40mg/10mg/25mg tablets | 28 tablet [PoM] £16.95
Amlodipine besilate 5 mg, Hydrochlorothiazide 12.5 mg, Olmesartan medoxomil 40 mg Sevikar HCT 40mg/5mg/12.5mg tablets | 28 tablet [PoM] £16.95
Amlodipine besilate 10 mg, Hydrochlorothiazide 12.5 mg, Olmesartan medoxomil 40 mg Sevikar HCT 40mg/10mg/12.5mg tablets | 28 tablet [PoM] £16.95

Olmesartan with hydrochlorothiazide

The properties listed below are those particular to the combination only. For the properties of the components please consider, olmesartan medoxomil p. 191, hydrochlorothiazide p. 180.

- **INDICATIONS AND DOSE**

Hypertension not adequately controlled with olmesartan alone
▸ BY MOUTH
▸ Adult: (consult product literature)

- INTERACTIONS → Appendix 1: angiotensin-II receptor antagonists · thiazide diuretics

- MEDICINAL FORMS There can be variation in the licensing of different medicines containing the same drug.

Tablet
▸ Olmesartan with hydrochlorothiazide (Non-proprietary)
Hydrochlorothiazide 12.5 mg, Olmesartan medoxomil 20 mg Olmesartan medoxomil 20mg / Hydrochlorothiazide 12.5mg tablets | 28 tablet [PoM] £12.50-£12.95 DT = £12.95
Olmesartan medoxomil 20 mg, Hydrochlorothiazide 25 mg Olmesartan medoxomil 20mg / Hydrochlorothiazide 25mg tablets | 28 tablet [PoM] £12.95 DT = £12.95
Hydrochlorothiazide 12.5 mg, Olmesartan medoxomil 40 mg Olmesartan medoxomil 40mg / Hydrochlorothiazide 12.5mg tablets | 28 tablet [PoM] £17.50 DT = £17.50
▸ Olmetec Plus (Daiichi Sankyo UK Ltd)
Hydrochlorothiazide 12.5 mg, Olmesartan medoxomil 20 mg Olmetec Plus 20mg/12.5mg tablets | 28 tablet [PoM] £12.95 DT = £12.95
Olmesartan medoxomil 20 mg, Hydrochlorothiazide 25 mg Olmetec Plus 20mg/25mg tablets | 28 tablet [PoM] £12.95 DT = £12.95
Hydrochlorothiazide 12.5 mg, Olmesartan medoxomil 40 mg Olmetec Plus 40mg/12.5mg tablets | 28 tablet [PoM] £17.50 DT = £17.50

[▶ 188]

Telmisartan

- **INDICATIONS AND DOSE**

Hypertension
▸ BY MOUTH
▸ Adult: Initially 20–40 mg once daily for at least 4 weeks, increased if necessary up to 80 mg once daily

Prevention of cardiovascular events in patients with established atherosclerotic cardiovascular disease, or type 2 diabetes mellitus with target-organ damage
▸ BY MOUTH
▸ Adult: 80 mg once daily

- CONTRA-INDICATIONS Biliary obstructive disorders · cholestasis

- INTERACTIONS → Appendix 1: angiotensin-II receptor antagonists

- SIDE-EFFECTS
▸ **Uncommon** Anaemia · arrhythmias · chest pain · cystitis · depression · dyspnoea · flatulence · gastrointestinal discomfort · hyperhidrosis · increased risk of infection · insomnia · muscle spasms · sciatica · syncope
▸ **Rare or very rare** Anxiety · drowsiness · dry mouth · eosinophilia · hypoglycaemia · influenza like illness · interstitial lung disease · liver disorder · pain in extremity · sepsis · taste altered · tendon pain · visual impairment

- HEPATIC IMPAIRMENT
Dose adjustments Manufacturer advises maximum 40 mg daily in mild to moderate impairment.

- RENAL IMPAIRMENT
Dose adjustments Manufacturer advises initial dose of 20 mg once daily in severe impairment.

- MEDICINAL FORMS There can be variation in the licensing of different medicines containing the same drug.

Tablet
▸ Telmisartan (Non-proprietary)
Telmisartan 20 mg Telmisartan 20mg tablets | 28 tablet [PoM] £11.10 DT = £2.87
Telmisartan 40 mg Telmisartan 40mg tablets | 28 tablet [PoM] £13.61 DT = £3.76
Telmisartan 80 mg Telmisartan 80mg tablets | 28 tablet [PoM] £17.00 DT = £4.59
▸ Micardis (Boehringer Ingelheim Ltd)
Telmisartan 20 mg Micardis 20mg tablets | 28 tablet [PoM] £11.10 DT = £2.87
Telmisartan 40 mg Micardis 40mg tablets | 28 tablet [PoM] £13.61 DT = £3.76
Telmisartan 80 mg Micardis 80mg tablets | 28 tablet [PoM] £17.00 DT = £4.59
▸ Tolura (Consilient Health Ltd)
Telmisartan 20 mg Tolura 20mg tablets | 28 tablet [PoM] £11.10 DT = £2.87
Telmisartan 40 mg Tolura 40mg tablets | 28 tablet [PoM] £13.61 DT = £3.76
Telmisartan 80 mg Tolura 80mg tablets | 28 tablet [PoM] £17.00 DT = £4.59

Telmisartan with hydrochlorothiazide

The properties listed below are those particular to the combination only. For the properties of the components please consider, telmisartan above, hydrochlorothiazide p. 180.

- **INDICATIONS AND DOSE**

Hypertension not adequately controlled by telmisartan alone
▸ BY MOUTH
▸ Adult: (consult product literature)

- INTERACTIONS → Appendix 1: angiotensin-II receptor antagonists · thiazide diuretics

- MEDICINAL FORMS There can be variation in the licensing of different medicines containing the same drug.

Tablet
▸ Telmisartan with hydrochlorothiazide (Non-proprietary)
Hydrochlorothiazide 12.5 mg, Telmisartan 40 mg Telmisartan 40mg / Hydrochlorothiazide 12.5mg tablets | 28 tablet [PoM] £13.61 DT = £13.61
Hydrochlorothiazide 25 mg, Telmisartan 80 mg Telmisartan 80mg / Hydrochlorothiazide 25mg tablets | 28 tablet [PoM] £24.38 DT = £20.57
Hydrochlorothiazide 12.5 mg, Telmisartan 80 mg Telmisartan 80mg / Hydrochlorothiazide 12.5mg tablets | 28 tablet [PoM] £17.00 DT = £16.97

▸ Actelsar HCT (Accord Healthcare Ltd, Actavis UK Ltd)
Hydrochlorothiazide 12.5 mg, Telmisartan 40 mg Actelsar HCT
40mg/12.5mg tablets | 28 tablet [PoM] £13.61 DT = £13.61
Hydrochlorothiazide 25 mg, Telmisartan 80 mg Actelsar HCT
80mg/25mg tablets | 28 tablet [PoM] £17.00 DT = £20.57

▸ MicardisPlus (Boehringer Ingelheim Ltd)
Hydrochlorothiazide 12.5 mg, Telmisartan 40 mg MicardisPlus
40mg/12.5mg tablets | 28 tablet [PoM] £13.61 DT = £13.61
Hydrochlorothiazide 12.5 mg, Telmisartan 80 mg MicardisPlus
80mg/12.5mg tablets | 28 tablet [PoM] £17.00 DT = £16.97

▸ MicardisPlus 80/25 (Boehringer Ingelheim Ltd)
Hydrochlorothiazide 25 mg, Telmisartan 80 mg MicardisPlus
80mg/25mg tablets | 28 tablet [PoM] £17.00 DT = £20.57

▸ Tolucombi (Consilient Health Ltd)
Hydrochlorothiazide 12.5 mg, Telmisartan 40 mg Tolucombi
40mg/12.5mg tablets | 28 tablet [PoM] £13.61 DT = £13.61
Hydrochlorothiazide 25 mg, Telmisartan 80 mg Tolucombi
80mg/25mg tablets | 28 tablet [PoM] £17.00 DT = £20.57
Hydrochlorothiazide 12.5 mg, Telmisartan 80 mg Tolucombi
80mg/12.5mg tablets | 28 tablet [PoM] £17.00 DT = £16.97

F 188

Valsartan

● **INDICATIONS AND DOSE**

Hypertension
▸ BY MOUTH
▸ Adult: Initially 80 mg once daily, increased if necessary
up to 320 mg daily, doses to be increased at intervals of
4 weeks

Hypertension with intravascular volume depletion
▸ BY MOUTH
▸ Adult: Initially 40 mg once daily, increased if necessary
up to 320 mg daily, doses to be increased at intervals of
4 weeks

**Heart failure when ACE inhibitors cannot be used, or in
conjunction with an ACE inhibitor when a beta-blocker
cannot be used | Heart failure, in conjunction with an ACE
inhibitor when a beta-blocker cannot be used (under
expert supervision)**
▸ BY MOUTH
▸ Adult: Initially 40 mg twice daily, increased to up to
160 mg twice daily, doses to be increased at intervals of
at least 2 weeks

**Myocardial infarction with left ventricular failure or left
ventricular systolic dysfunction (adjunct)**
▸ BY MOUTH
▸ Adult: Initially 20 mg twice daily, increased if necessary
up to 160 mg twice daily, doses to be increased over
several weeks if tolerated

● **CONTRA-INDICATIONS** Biliary cirrhosis · cholestasis
● **INTERACTIONS** → Appendix 1: angiotensin-II receptor
antagonists
● **SIDE-EFFECTS**
▸ **Uncommon** Heart failure · syncope
▸ **Frequency not known** Neutropenia · serum sickness ·
vasculitis
● **HEPATIC IMPAIRMENT**
Dose adjustments Manufacturer advises maximum 80 mg
daily in mild to moderate impairment.
● **RENAL IMPAIRMENT** Use with caution if eGFR less than
10 mL/minute/1.73 m^2—no information available.

● **MEDICINAL FORMS** There can be variation in the licensing of
different medicines containing the same drug. Forms available
from special-order manufacturers include: oral suspension, oral
solution
Oral solution
▸ Diovan (Novartis Pharmaceuticals UK Ltd)
Valsartan 3 mg per 1 ml Diovan 3mg/1ml oral solution |
160 ml [PoM] £7.20 DT = £7.20

Tablet
▸ Valsartan (Non-proprietary)
Valsartan 40 mg Valsartan 40mg tablets | 7 tablet [PoM] £7.78 DT =
£7.78
Valsartan 80 mg Valsartan 80mg tablets | 28 tablet [PoM] £9.41-
£13.69
Valsartan 160 mg Valsartan 160mg tablets | 28 tablet [PoM]
£13.69-£14.69 DT = £14.69
Valsartan 320 mg Valsartan 320mg tablets | 28 tablet [PoM] £20.23
DT = £18.17
Capsule
▸ Valsartan (Non-proprietary)
Valsartan 40 mg Valsartan 40mg capsules | 28 capsule [PoM]
£13.97 DT = £5.48
Valsartan 80 mg Valsartan 80mg capsules | 28 capsule [PoM]
£13.97 DT = £9.08
Valsartan 160 mg Valsartan 160mg capsules | 28 capsule [PoM]
£18.41 DT = £11.88

Combinations available: *Amlodipine with valsartan*, p. 171

Valsartan with hydrochlorothiazide

The properties listed below are those particular to the
combination only. For the properties of the components
please consider, valsartan above, hydrochlorothiazide p. 180.

● **INDICATIONS AND DOSE**

**Hypertension not adequately controlled by valsartan
alone**
▸ BY MOUTH
▸ Adult: (consult product literature)

● **INTERACTIONS** → Appendix 1: angiotensin-II receptor
antagonists · thiazide diuretics

● **MEDICINAL FORMS** There can be variation in the licensing of
different medicines containing the same drug.
Tablet
▸ Valsartan with hydrochlorothiazide (Non-proprietary)
Hydrochlorothiazide 12.5 mg, Valsartan 80 mg Valsartan 80mg /
Hydrochlorothiazide 12.5mg tablets | 28 tablet [PoM] £21.38 DT =
£21.28
Hydrochlorothiazide 25 mg, Valsartan 160 mg Valsartan 160mg /
Hydrochlorothiazide 25mg tablets | 28 tablet [PoM] £28.17 DT =
£28.04
Hydrochlorothiazide 12.5 mg, Valsartan 160 mg Valsartan 160mg
/ Hydrochlorothiazide 12.5mg tablets | 28 tablet [PoM] £18.41 DT =
£12.64
▸ Co-Diovan (Novartis Pharmaceuticals UK Ltd)
Hydrochlorothiazide 12.5 mg, Valsartan 80 mg Co-Diovan
80mg/12.5mg tablets | 28 tablet [PoM] £16.76 DT = £21.28
Hydrochlorothiazide 25 mg, Valsartan 160 mg Co-Diovan
160mg/25mg tablets | 28 tablet [PoM] £22.09 DT = £28.04
Hydrochlorothiazide 12.5 mg, Valsartan 160 mg Co-Diovan
160mg/12.5mg tablets | 28 tablet [PoM] £22.09 DT = £12.64

DRUGS ACTING ON THE RENIN-ANGIOTENSIN
SYSTEM ⟩ RENIN INHIBITORS

Aliskiren
31-Aug-2020

● **DRUG ACTION** Renin inhibitors inhibit renin directly; renin
converts angiotensinogen to angiotensin I.

● **INDICATIONS AND DOSE**

**Essential hypertension either alone or in combination
with other antihypertensives**
▸ BY MOUTH
▸ Adult: 150 mg once daily, increased if necessary to
300 mg once daily

● **CONTRA-INDICATIONS** Concomitant treatment with an
ACE inhibitor or an angiotensin-II receptor antagonist in
patients with an eGFR less than 60 mL/minute/1.73 m^2 ·
concomitant treatment with an ACE inhibitor or an
angiotensin-II receptor antagonist in patients with

2

Cardiovascular system

diabetes mellitus · hereditary angioedema · idiopathic angioedema

- CAUTIONS Combination treatment with an ACE inhibitor · combination treatment with an angiotensin-II receptor antagonist · concomitant use of diuretics (first doses may cause hypotension—initiate with care) · history of angioedema · moderate to severe congestive heart failure · patients at risk of renal impairment · salt depletion (first doses may cause hypotension—initiate with care) · volume depletion (first doses may cause hypotension—initiate with care)

CAUTIONS, FURTHER INFORMATION
▸ Concomitant use of drugs affecting the renin-angiotensin system Combination therapy with two drugs affecting the renin-angiotensin system (ACE inhibitors, angiotensin-II receptor antagonists, and aliskiren) is not recommended due to an increased risk of hyperkalaemia, hypotension, and renal impairment, compared to use of a single drug. Patients with diabetic nephropathy are particularly susceptible to developing hyperkalaemia and should not be given an ACE inhibitor with an angiotensin-II receptor antagonist. There is some evidence that the benefits of combination use of an ACE inhibitor with candesartan or valsartan may outweigh the risks in selected patients with heart failure for whom other treatments are unsuitable, however, the concomitant use of this combination, together with an aldosterone antagonist or a potassium-sparing diuretic is not recommended. For patients currently taking combination therapy, the need for continued combined therapy should be reviewed. If combination therapy is considered essential, it should be carried out under specialist supervision, with close monitoring of blood pressure, renal function, and electrolytes (particularly potassium); monitoring should be considered at the start of treatment, then monthly, and also after any change in dose or during intercurrent illness.

- INTERACTIONS → Appendix 1: aliskiren
- SIDE-EFFECTS
  ▸ **Common or very common** Arthralgia · diarrhoea · dizziness · electrolyte imbalance
  ▸ **Uncommon** Cough · oral disorder · palpitations · peripheral oedema · renal impairment · severe cutaneous adverse reactions (SCARs) · skin reactions
  ▸ **Rare or very rare** Angioedema · hypersensitivity
  ▸ **Frequency not known** Dyspnoea · hepatic disorders · nausea · vertigo · vomiting

SIDE-EFFECTS, FURTHER INFORMATION If diarrhoea is severe or persistent discontinue treatment.

- PREGNANCY Manufacturer advises avoid—no information available; other drugs acting on the renin-angiotensin system have been associated with fetal malformations and neonatal death.
- BREAST FEEDING Present in milk in *animal* studies—manufacturer advises avoid.
- RENAL IMPAIRMENT Avoid if eGFR is less than 30 mL/minute/1.73 m^2— no information available. Use with caution in renal artery stenosis—no information available.
  Monitoring Monitor plasma-potassium concentration in renal impairment.
- MONITORING REQUIREMENTS Monitor patients with a history of angioedema closely during treatment.
- NATIONAL FUNDING/ACCESS DECISIONS
  For full details see funding body website
  Scottish Medicines Consortium (SMC) decisions
  ▸ Aliskiren (*Rasilez*®) for essential hypertension (February 2010) SMC No. 462/08 Not recommended

- MEDICINAL FORMS There can be variation in the licensing of different medicines containing the same drug.
  Tablet
  CAUTIONARY AND ADVISORY LABELS 21
  ▸ Rasilez (Noden Pharma DAC)
  Aliskiren (as Aliskiren hemifumarate) 150 mg Rasilez 150mg tablets | 28 tablet PoM £28.51 DT = £28.51
  Aliskiren (as Aliskiren hemifumarate) 300 mg Rasilez 300mg tablets | 28 tablet PoM £34.27 DT = £34.27

VASODILATORS ⟩ VASODILATOR ANTIHYPERTENSIVES

| Hydralazine hydrochloride
04-Feb-2020

- INDICATIONS AND DOSE
  Moderate to severe hypertension (adjunct)
  ▸ BY MOUTH
  ▸ **Adult:** Initially 25 mg twice daily, increased if necessary up to 50 mg twice daily
  Heart failure (with long acting nitrate) (initiated in hospital or under specialist supervision)
  ▸ BY MOUTH
  ▸ **Adult:** Initially 25 mg 3–4 times a day, subsequent doses to be increased every 2 days if necessary; usual maintenance 50–75 mg 4 times a day
  Hypertensive emergencies (including during pregnancy) | Hypertension with renal complications
  ▸ BY INTRAVENOUS INFUSION
  ▸ **Adult:** Initially 200–300 micrograms/minute; usual maintenance 50–150 micrograms/minute
  ▸ BY SLOW INTRAVENOUS INJECTION
  ▸ **Adult:** 5–10 mg, to be diluted with 10 mL sodium chloride 0.9%; dose may be repeated after 20–30 minutes

- CONTRA-INDICATIONS Acute porphyrias p. 1107 · cor pulmonale · dissecting aortic aneurysm · high output heart failure · idiopathic systemic lupus erythematosus · myocardial insufficiency due to mechanical obstruction · severe tachycardia
- CAUTIONS Cerebrovascular disease · coronary artery disease (may provoke angina, avoid after myocardial infarction until stabilised) · occasionally blood pressure reduction too rapid even with low parenteral doses
- INTERACTIONS → Appendix 1: hydralazine
- SIDE-EFFECTS
  ▸ **Common or very common** Angina pectoris · diarrhoea · dizziness · flushing · gastrointestinal disorders · headache · hypotension · joint disorders · lupus-like syndrome (after long-term therapy with over 100 mg daily (or less in women and in slow acetylator individuals)) · myalgia · nasal congestion · nausea · palpitations · tachycardia · vomiting
  ▸ **Rare or very rare** Acute kidney injury · agranulocytosis · anaemia · anxiety · appetite decreased · conjunctivitis · depression · dyspnoea · eosinophilia · eye disorders · fever · glomerulonephritis · haematuria · haemolytic anaemia · hallucination · heart failure · hepatic disorders · leucocytosis · leucopenia · lymphadenopathy · malaise · nerve disorders · neutropenia · oedema · pancytopenia · paradoxical pressor response · paraesthesia · pleuritic pain · proteinuria · skin reactions · splenomegaly · thrombocytopenia · urinary retention · vasculitis · weight decreased

SIDE-EFFECTS, FURTHER INFORMATION The incidence of side-effects is lower if the dose is kept below 100mg daily, but systemic lupus erythematosus should be suspected if there is unexplained weight loss, arthritis, or any other unexplained ill health.

- PREGNANCY Neonatal thrombocytopenia reported, but risk should be balanced against risk of uncontrolled maternal hypertension. Manufacturer advises avoid before third trimester.
- BREAST FEEDING Present in milk but not known to be harmful.
  Monitoring Monitor infant in breast-feeding.
- HEPATIC IMPAIRMENT Manufacturer advises caution (risk of accumulation).
  Dose adjustments Manufacturer advises adjust dose or dosing interval according to clinical response.
- RENAL IMPAIRMENT
  Dose adjustments Reduce dose if eGFR less than 30 mL/minute/1.73 m^2.
- MONITORING REQUIREMENTS Manufacturer advises test for antinuclear factor and for proteinuria every 6 months and check acetylator status before increasing dose above 100 mg daily, but evidence of clinical value unsatisfactory.
- DIRECTIONS FOR ADMINISTRATION For *intravenous infusion* (*Apresoline*®) give continuously in Sodium chloride 0.9%. Suggested infusion volume 500 mL.

- MEDICINAL FORMS There can be variation in the licensing of different medicines containing the same drug. Forms available from special-order manufacturers include: tablet, oral suspension, oral solution
  Tablet
  EXCIPIENTS: May contain Gluten, propylene glycol
  ▸ Hydralazine hydrochloride (Non-proprietary)
  Hydralazine hydrochloride 10 mg Apo-Hydralazine 10mg tablets | 100 tablet PoM ⚠
  Hydralazine hydrochloride 25 mg Hydralazine 25mg tablets | 56 tablet PoM £7.37 DT = £5.62 | 84 tablet PoM £14.00
  Hydralazine hydrochloride 50 mg Hydralazine 50mg tablets | 56 tablet PoM £15.46 DT = £7.50
  ▸ Apresoline (Advanz Pharma)
  Hydralazine hydrochloride 25 mg Apresoline 25mg tablets | 84 tablet PoM £3.38
  Powder for solution for injection
  ▸ Hydralazine hydrochloride (Non-proprietary)
  Hydralazine hydrochloride 20 mg Hydralazine 20mg powder for concentrate for solution for injection ampoules | 5 ampoule PoM £74.17

Minoxidil
07-Sep-2020

- **INDICATIONS AND DOSE**
Severe hypertension, in addition to a diuretic and a beta-blocker
  ▸ BY MOUTH
  ▸ Adult: Initially 5 mg daily in 1–2 divided doses, then increased in steps of 5–10 mg, increased at intervals of at least 3 days; maximum 100 mg per day
  ▸ Elderly: Initially 2.5 mg daily in 1–2 divided doses, then increased in steps of 5–10 mg, increased at intervals of at least 3 days; maximum 100 mg per day

- CONTRA-INDICATIONS Phaeochromocytoma
- CAUTIONS Acute porphyrias p. 1107 · after myocardial infarction (until stabilised) · angina
- INTERACTIONS → Appendix 1: minoxidil
- SIDE-EFFECTS
  ▸ **Common or very common** Fluid retention · hair changes · oedema · pericardial disorders · pericarditis · tachycardia
  ▸ **Rare or very rare** Leucopenia · skin reactions · Stevens-Johnson syndrome · thrombocytopenia
  ▸ **Frequency not known** Angina pectoris · breast tenderness · gastrointestinal disorder · pleural effusion · sodium retention · weight increased
- PREGNANCY Avoid—possible toxicity including reduced placental perfusion. Neonatal hirsutism reported.

- BREAST FEEDING Present in milk but not known to be harmful.
- RENAL IMPAIRMENT Use with caution in significant impairment.

- MEDICINAL FORMS There can be variation in the licensing of different medicines containing the same drug.
  Tablet
  ▸ Loniten (Pfizer Ltd)
  Minoxidil 2.5 mg Loniten 2.5mg tablets | 60 tablet PoM £8.88 DT = £8.88
  Minoxidil 5 mg Loniten 5mg tablets | 60 tablet PoM £15.83 DT = £15.83
  Minoxidil 10 mg Loniten 10mg tablets | 60 tablet PoM £30.68 DT = £30.68

4.1a Hypertension associated with phaeochromocytoma

> **Other drugs used for Hypertension associated with phaeochromocytoma** Propranolol hydrochloride, p. 164

VASODILATORS > PERIPHERAL VASODILATORS

Phenoxybenzamine hydrochloride
28-Jul-2020

- **INDICATIONS AND DOSE**
Hypertension in phaeochromocytoma
  ▸ BY MOUTH
  ▸ Adult: Initially 10 mg daily, increased in steps of 10 mg daily until hypertension controlled or treatment not tolerated; maintenance 1–2 mg/kg daily in 2 divided doses

- CONTRA-INDICATIONS During recovery period after myocardial infarction (usually 3–4 weeks) · history of cerebrovascular accident
- CAUTIONS Avoid in Acute porphyrias p. 1107 · carcinogenic in *animals* · cerebrovascular disease · congestive heart failure · elderly · severe ischaemic heart disease
- SIDE-EFFECTS Abdominal distress · dizziness · ejaculation failure · fatigue · miosis · nasal congestion · postural hypotension · reflex tachycardia
- PREGNANCY Hypotension may occur in newborn.
- BREAST FEEDING May be present in milk.
- RENAL IMPAIRMENT Use with caution.
- HANDLING AND STORAGE Owing to risk of contact sensitisation healthcare professionals should avoid contamination of hands.

- MEDICINAL FORMS There can be variation in the licensing of different medicines containing the same drug. Forms available from special-order manufacturers include: oral suspension, oral solution
  Capsule
  ▸ Phenoxybenzamine hydrochloride (Non-proprietary)
  Phenoxybenzamine hydrochloride 10 mg Phenoxybenzamine 10mg capsules | 30 capsule PoM £118.00 DT = £118.00

4.1b Hypertensive crises

> **Other drugs used for Hypertensive crises** Hydralazine hydrochloride, p. 194 · Labetalol hydrochloride, p. 163

VASODILATORS ❯ VASODILATOR ANTIHYPERTENSIVES

Sodium nitroprusside
03-Aug-2020

- **INDICATIONS AND DOSE**
Hypertensive emergencies
  ▶ BY INTRAVENOUS INFUSION
  ▸ Adult: Initially 0.5–1.5 micrograms/kg/minute, adjusted in steps of 500 nanograms/kg/minute every 5 minutes, usual dose 0.5–8 micrograms/kg/minute, use lower doses if already receiving other antihypertensives, stop if response unsatisfactory with max. dose in 10 minutes, lower initial dose of 300 nanograms/kg/minute has been used

Maintenance of blood pressure at 30–40% lower than pretreatment diastolic blood pressure
  ▶ BY INTRAVENOUS INFUSION
  ▸ Adult: 20–400 micrograms/minute, use lower doses for patients being treated with other antihypertensives

Controlled hypotension in anaesthesia during surgery
  ▶ BY INTRAVENOUS INFUSION
  ▸ Adult: Up to 1.5 micrograms/kg/minute

Acute or chronic heart failure
  ▶ BY INTRAVENOUS INFUSION
  ▸ Adult: Initially 10–15 micrograms/minute, increased every 5–10 minutes as necessary; usual dose 10–200 micrograms/minute normally for max. 3 days

- **UNLICENSED USE** Not licensed for use in the UK.
- **CONTRA-INDICATIONS** Compensatory hypertension · impaired cerebral circulation · Leber's optic atrophy · severe vitamin B$_{12}$ deficiency
- **CAUTIONS** Elderly · hyponatraemia · hypothermia · hypothyroidism · ischaemic heart disease
- **INTERACTIONS** → Appendix 1: nitroprusside
- **SIDE-EFFECTS** Abdominal pain · anaemia · arrhythmias · chest discomfort · cyanide toxicity · dizziness · flushing · headache · hyperhidrosis · hypothyroidism · hypovolaemia · ileus · intracranial pressure increased · methaemoglobinaemia · muscle twitching · nausea · palpitations · rash · thiocyanate toxicity

  SIDE-EFFECTS, FURTHER INFORMATION Side-effects associated with over rapid reduction in blood pressure: Headache, dizziness, nausea, retching, abdominal pain, perspiration, palpitation, anxiety, retrosternal discomfort—reduce infusion rate if any of these side-effects occur.

  Overdose Side-effects caused by excessive plasma concentration of the cyanide metabolite include tachycardia, sweating, hyperventilation, arrhythmias, marked metabolic acidosis (discontinue and give antidote, see cyanide in Emergency treatment of poisoning p. 1413).

- **PREGNANCY** Avoid prolonged use—potential for accumulation of cyanide in fetus.
- **BREAST FEEDING** No information available. Caution advised due to thiocyanate metabolite.
- **HEPATIC IMPAIRMENT** Use with caution. Avoid in hepatic failure—cyanide or thiocyanate metabolites may accumulate.
- **RENAL IMPAIRMENT** Avoid prolonged use—cyanide or thiocyanate metabolites may accumulate.
- **MONITORING REQUIREMENTS** Monitor blood pressure (including intra-arterial blood pressure) and blood-cyanide concentration, and if treatment exceeds 3 days, also blood thiocyanate concentration.
- **TREATMENT CESSATION** Avoid sudden withdrawal— terminate infusion over 15–30 minutes.

- **DIRECTIONS FOR ADMINISTRATION** For *continuous intravenous infusion* in Glucose 5%, manufacturer advises infuse *via* infusion device to allow precise control. For further details, consult product literature. Protect infusion from light.

- **MEDICINAL FORMS** There can be variation in the licensing of different medicines containing the same drug.
  Powder and solvent for solution for infusion
  ▸ Sodium nitroprusside (Non-proprietary)
    Sodium nitroprusside dihydrate 50 mg Sodium nitroprusside 50mg powder and solvent for solution for infusion vials | 1 vial PoM ▶

4.1c Pulmonary hypertension

Other drugs used for Pulmonary hypertension
Epoprostenol, p. 124 · Sildenafil, p. 860 · Tadalafil, p. 861

ANTITHROMBOTIC DRUGS ❯ ANTIPLATELET DRUGS

Selexipag
19-Aug-2020

- **DRUG ACTION** Selexipag is a selective prostacyclin (IP) receptor agonist.

- **INDICATIONS AND DOSE**
Pulmonary arterial hypertension either as combination therapy (if insufficiently controlled with an endothelin receptor antagonist and/or a phosphodiesterase type-5 inhibitor), or as monotherapy (initiated under specialist supervision)
  ▶ BY MOUTH
  ▸ Adult: Initially 200 micrograms twice daily, increased in steps of 200 micrograms twice daily at weekly intervals up to the highest tolerated dose, usual maintenance 200–1600 micrograms twice daily, initial dose and first dose after each dose increase should be taken in the evening; maximum 3200 micrograms per day

  DOSE ADJUSTMENTS DUE TO INTERACTIONS
  ▸ Manufacturer advises reduce dose frequency to once daily with concurrent use of clopidogrel or moderate CYP2C8 inhibitors.

- **CONTRA-INDICATIONS** Cerebrovascular event (within the last 3 months) · congenital or acquired valvular defects with myocardial function disorders (not related to pulmonary hypertension) · decompensated cardiac failure (unless under close medical supervision) · myocardial infarction (within last 6 months) · severe arrhythmias · severe coronary heart disease · unstable angina
- **CAUTIONS** Elderly (limited information available)
- **INTERACTIONS** → Appendix 1: selexipag
- **SIDE-EFFECTS**
  ▶ Common or very common Abdominal pain · anaemia · appetite decreased · arthralgia · diarrhoea · flushing · headache · hyperthyroidism · hypotension · myalgia · nasal congestion · nasopharyngitis · nausea · pain · skin reactions · vomiting · weight decreased
  ▶ Uncommon Sinus tachycardia
- **PREGNANCY** Manufacturer advises avoid—no information available.
- **BREAST FEEDING** Manufacturer advises avoid—present in milk in *animal* studies.
- **HEPATIC IMPAIRMENT** Manufacturer advises caution in moderate impairment (risk of increased exposure); avoid in severe impairment (no information available).
  Dose adjustments Manufacturer advises initial dose reduction to 200 micrograms once daily in moderate

impairment, increased in steps of 200 micrograms once daily at weekly intervals up to the highest tolerated dose.

- RENAL IMPAIRMENT Manufacturer advises caution with dose titration in severe impairment.
- PATIENT AND CARER ADVICE
Missed doses Manufacturer advises if a dose is more than 6 hours late, the missed dose should not be taken and the next dose should be taken at the normal time; if a dose is missed for 3 days or more, treatment should be restarted at a lower dose and then increased—consult product literature.
- NATIONAL FUNDING/ACCESS DECISIONS
For full details see funding body website
Scottish Medicines Consortium (SMC) decisions
 ▸ Selexipag (*Uptravi*®) for the long-term treatment of pulmonary arterial hypertension (PAH) in adult patients with WHO functional class (FC) II-III, either as combination therapy in patients insufficiently controlled with an endothelin receptor antagonist (ERA) and/or a phosphodiesterase type-5 (PDE-5) inhibitor, or as monotherapy in patients who are not candidates for these therapies (May 2018) SMC No. 1235/17 Recommended with restrictions
All Wales Medicines Strategy Group (AWMSG) decisions
 ▸ Selexipag (*Uptravi*®) for long-term treatment of pulmonary arterial hypertension (PAH) in adult patients with WHO functional class (FC) II-III, either as combination therapy in patients insufficiently controlled with an endothelin receptor antagonist (ERA) and/or a phosphodiesterase type-5 (PDE-5) inhibitor, or as monotherapy in patients who are not candidates for these therapies (June 2018) AWMSG No. 700 Recommended with restrictions

- MEDICINAL FORMS There can be variation in the licensing of different medicines containing the same drug.
Tablet
CAUTIONARY AND ADVISORY LABELS 21, 25
 ▸ Uptravi (Janssen-Cilag Ltd) ▼
Selexipag 200 microgram Uptravi 200microgram tablets | 60 tablet [PoM] £3,000.00 | 140 tablet [PoM] £7,000.00
Selexipag 400 microgram Uptravi 400microgram tablets | 60 tablet [PoM] £3,000.00
Selexipag 600 microgram Uptravi 600microgram tablets | 60 tablet [PoM] £3,000.00
Selexipag 800 microgram Uptravi 800microgram tablets | 60 tablet [PoM] £3,000.00
Selexipag 1 mg Uptravi 1,000microgram tablets | 60 tablet [PoM] £3,000.00
Selexipag 1.2 mg Uptravi 1,200microgram tablets | 60 tablet [PoM] £3,000.00
Selexipag 1.4 mg Uptravi 1,400microgram tablets | 60 tablet [PoM] £3,000.00
Selexipag 1.6 mg Uptravi 1,600microgram tablets | 60 tablet [PoM] £3,000.00

ENDOTHELIN RECEPTOR ANTAGONISTS

| Ambrisentan
02-Nov-2020

- INDICATIONS AND DOSE
Pulmonary arterial hypertension (initiated under specialist supervision)
 ▸ BY MOUTH
 ▸ Adult: 5 mg once daily, increased if necessary to 10 mg once daily
DOSE ADJUSTMENTS DUE TO INTERACTIONS
 ▸ Manufacturer advises max. dose 5 mg daily and close monitoring with concurrent use of ciclosporin.

- CONTRA-INDICATIONS Idiopathic pulmonary fibrosis
- CAUTIONS Not to be initiated in significant anaemia · pulmonary veno-occlusive disease
- INTERACTIONS → Appendix 1: endothelin receptor antagonists

- SIDE-EFFECTS
 ▸ **Common or very common** Abdominal pain · anaemia · asthenia · constipation · diarrhoea · dizziness · epistaxis · flushing · headaches · hypersensitivity · increased risk of infection · nasal congestion · nausea · palpitations · skin reactions · syncope · tinnitus · vision disorders · vomiting
 ▸ **Uncommon** Hepatic disorders · sudden hearing loss
- CONCEPTION AND CONTRACEPTION Exclude pregnancy before treatment and ensure effective contraception during treatment. Monthly pregnancy tests advised.
- PREGNANCY Avoid (teratogenic in *animal studies*).
- BREAST FEEDING Manufacturer advises avoid—no information available.
- HEPATIC IMPAIRMENT Manufacturer advises avoid in severe impairment or if baseline serum transaminases exceed 3 times the upper limit of normal.
- RENAL IMPAIRMENT Use with caution if eGFR less than 30 mL/minute/1.73 m^2.
- MONITORING REQUIREMENTS
 ▸ Monitor haemoglobin concentration or haematocrit after 1 month and 3 months of starting treatment, and periodically thereafter (reduce dose or discontinue treatment if significant decrease in haemoglobin concentration or haematocrit observed).
 ▸ Monitor liver function before treatment, and monthly thereafter—discontinue if liver enzymes raised significantly or if symptoms of liver impairment develop.
- PATIENT AND CARER ADVICE
Alert card A patient alert card should be provided.
- NATIONAL FUNDING/ACCESS DECISIONS
For full details see funding body website
Scottish Medicines Consortium (SMC) decisions
 ▸ Ambrisentan (*Volibris*®) for pulmonary arterial hypertension (November 2008) SMC No. 511/08 Recommended with restrictions

- MEDICINAL FORMS There can be variation in the licensing of different medicines containing the same drug.
Tablet
 ▸ Ambrisentan (Non-proprietary)
Ambrisentan 5 mg Ambrisentan 5mg tablets | 30 tablet [PoM] £1,375.37 DT = £1,618.08 | 30 tablet [PoM] £1,618.08 DT = £1,618.08 (Hospital only)
Ambrisentan 10 mg Ambrisentan 10mg tablets | 30 tablet [PoM] £1,375.37 DT = £1,618.08 | 30 tablet [PoM] £1,618.08 DT = £1,618.08 (Hospital only)
 ▸ Volibris (GlaxoSmithKline UK Ltd)
Ambrisentan 5 mg Volibris 5mg tablets | 30 tablet [PoM] £1,618.08 DT = £1,618.08
Ambrisentan 10 mg Volibris 10mg tablets | 30 tablet [PoM] £1,618.08 DT = £1,618.08

| Bosentan
05-Feb-2020

- INDICATIONS AND DOSE
Pulmonary arterial hypertension (initiated under specialist supervision)
 ▸ BY MOUTH
 ▸ Adult: Initially 62.5 mg twice daily for 4 weeks, then increased to 125 mg twice daily (max. per dose 250 mg); maximum 500 mg per day
Systemic sclerosis with ongoing digital ulcer disease (to reduce number of new digital ulcers)
 ▸ BY MOUTH
 ▸ Adult: Initially 62.5 mg twice daily for 4 weeks, then increased to 125 mg twice daily

- CONTRA-INDICATIONS Acute porphyrias p. 1107
- CAUTIONS Not to be initiated if systemic systolic blood pressure is below 85 mmHg · pulmonary veno-occlusive disease

- INTERACTIONS → Appendix 1: endothelin receptor antagonists
- SIDE-EFFECTS
  ▸ **Common or very common** Anaemia · diarrhoea · flushing · gastrooesophageal reflux disease · headache · nasal congestion · palpitations · skin reactions · syncope
  ▸ **Uncommon** Hepatic disorders · leucopenia · neutropenia · thrombocytopenia
  ▸ **Rare or very rare** Angioedema
  ▸ **Frequency not known** Vision blurred
- CONCEPTION AND CONTRACEPTION Effective contraception required during administration (hormonal contraception not considered effective). Monthly pregnancy tests advised.
- PREGNANCY Avoid (teratogenic in *animal* studies).
- BREAST FEEDING Manufacturer advises avoid—no information available.
- HEPATIC IMPAIRMENT Manufacturer advises avoid in moderate-to-severe impairment or if baseline serum transaminases exceed 3 times the upper limit of normal.
- MONITORING REQUIREMENTS
  ▸ Monitor haemoglobin before and during treatment (monthly for first 4 months, then 3-monthly).
  ▸ Monitor liver function before treatment, at monthly intervals during treatment, and 2 weeks after dose increase (reduce dose or suspend treatment if liver enzymes raised significantly)—discontinue if symptoms of liver impairment.
- TREATMENT CESSATION Avoid abrupt withdrawal—withdraw treatment gradually.
- MEDICINAL FORMS There can be variation in the licensing of different medicines containing the same drug.
  Tablet
  ▸ Bosentan (Non-proprietary)
  Bosentan (as Bosentan monohydrate) 62.5 mg Bosentan 62.5mg tablets | 56 tablet [PoM] £112.50 (Hospital only) | 56 tablet [PoM] £1,359.19–£1,510.21
  Bosentan (as Bosentan monohydrate) 125 mg Bosentan 125mg tablets | 56 tablet [PoM] £112.50 (Hospital only) | 56 tablet [PoM] £101.25–£1,510.21
  ▸ Stayveer (Advanz Pharma)
  Bosentan (as Bosentan monohydrate) 125 mg Stayveer 125mg tablets | 56 tablet [PoM] £208.34
  ▸ Tracleer (Janssen-Cilag Ltd)
  Bosentan (as Bosentan monohydrate) 62.5 mg Tracleer 62.5mg tablets | 56 tablet [PoM] £1,510.21
  Bosentan (as Bosentan monohydrate) 125 mg Tracleer 125mg tablets | 56 tablet [PoM] £1,510.21

Macitentan

10-Nov-2020

- INDICATIONS AND DOSE
  Pulmonary arterial hypertension (initiated under specialist supervision)
  ▸ BY MOUTH
  ▸ Adult: 10 mg daily
- CONTRA-INDICATIONS Severe anaemia
- CAUTIONS Patients over 75 years · pulmonary veno-occlusive disease
- INTERACTIONS → Appendix 1: endothelin receptor antagonists
- SIDE-EFFECTS
  ▸ **Common or very common** Anaemia · headache · increased risk of infection · nasal congestion
- CONCEPTION AND CONTRACEPTION Manufacturer advises exclude pregnancy before treatment and ensure effective contraception during and for one month after stopping treatment. Monthly pregnancy tests advised.
- PREGNANCY Toxicity in *animal* studies.

- BREAST FEEDING Manufacturer advises avoid—present in milk in *animal* studies.
- HEPATIC IMPAIRMENT Manufacturer advises avoid in severe impairment or if hepatic transaminases are greater than 3 times the upper limit of normal.
- RENAL IMPAIRMENT Manufacturer advises caution in severe impairment and avoid in patients undergoing dialysis (no information available).
  Monitoring In renal impairment consider monitoring blood pressure (risk of hypotension).
- MONITORING REQUIREMENTS
  ▸ Monitor liver function before treatment, then monthly thereafter (discontinue if unexplained persistent raised serum transaminases or signs of hepatic injury—can restart on advice on hepatologist if liver function tests return to normal and no hepatic injury).
  ▸ Monitor haemoglobin concentration before treatment and then as indicated.
- PATIENT AND CARER ADVICE Patients should be told how to recognise signs of liver disorder and advised to seek immediate medical attention if symptoms such as dark urine, nausea, vomiting, fatigue, abdominal pain, or pruritus develop.
  Patient card should be provided.
- NATIONAL FUNDING/ACCESS DECISIONS
  For full details see funding body website
  Scottish Medicines Consortium (SMC) decisions
  ▸ **Macitentan (*Opsumit®*), as monotherapy or in combination, for the long-term treatment of pulmonary arterial hypertension in adult patients of World Health Organisation Functional Class II to III (April 2014)** SMC No. 952/14 Recommended with restrictions
- MEDICINAL FORMS There can be variation in the licensing of different medicines containing the same drug.
  Tablet
  CAUTIONARY AND ADVISORY LABELS 25
  ▸ Opsumit (Janssen-Cilag Ltd)
  Macitentan 10 mg Opsumit 10mg tablets | 30 tablet [PoM] £2,306.00

GUANYLATE CYCLASE STIMULATORS

Riociguat

14-Dec-2020

- INDICATIONS AND DOSE
  Chronic thromboembolic pulmonary hypertension that is recurrent or persistent following surgery, or is inoperable (initiated under specialist supervision) | Monotherapy or in combination with an endothelin receptor antagonist for idiopathic or hereditary pulmonary arterial hypertension, or pulmonary arterial hypertension associated with connective tissue disease (initiated under specialist supervision)
  ▸ BY MOUTH
  ▸ Adult: Initially 1 mg 3 times a day for 2 weeks, increased in steps of 0.5 mg 3 times a day, dose to be increased every 2 weeks, increased to up to 2.5 mg 3 times a day (max. per dose 2.5 mg 3 times a day), increase up to maximum dose only if systolic blood pressure ≥ 95 mmHg and no signs of hypotension, if treatment interrupted for 3 or more days, restart at 1 mg three times daily for 2 weeks and titrate as before, during titration, reduce dose by 0.5 mg three times daily if systolic blood pressure falls below 95 mmHg and patient shows signs of hypotension
  DOSE ADJUSTMENTS DUE TO INTERACTIONS
  ▸ Manufacturer advises consider initial dose of 0.5 mg 3 times daily in those stable on a strong multi-pathway cytochrome P450 and P-glycoprotein (P-gp)/breast cancer resistance protein (BCRP) inhibitor.

IMPORTANT SAFETY INFORMATION

MHRA/CHM ADVICE: PULMONARY HYPERTENSION ASSOCIATED WITH IDIOPATHIC INTERSTITIAL PNEUMONIAS (PH-IIP) (AUGUST 2016)

Interim results from a terminated study to investigate the efficacy and safety of riociguat in patients with symptomatic PH-IIP, showed increased mortality and increased risk of serious adverse events in the riociguat group compared with the placebo group. The MHRA has advised that use of riociguat is contra-indicated in these patients and that existing treatment for this unauthorised indication should be discontinued.

- **CONTRA-INDICATIONS** History of serious haemoptysis · previous bronchial artery embolisation · pulmonary hypertension associated with idiopathic interstitial pneumonias · pulmonary veno-occlusive disease
- **CAUTIONS** Autonomic dysfunction · elderly (risk of hypotension) · hypotension (do not initiate if systolic blood pressure below 95 mmHg) · hypovolaemia · severe left ventricular outflow obstruction

  CAUTIONS, FURTHER INFORMATION
  ‣ Smoking Smoking cessation advised (response possibly reduced); dose adjustment may be necessary if smoking started or stopped during treatment.
- **INTERACTIONS** → Appendix 1: riociguat
- **SIDE-EFFECTS**
  ‣ Common or very common Anaemia · constipation · diarrhoea · dizziness · dysphagia · gastroenteritis · gastrointestinal discomfort · gastrointestinal disorders · haemorrhage · headache · hypotension · nasal congestion · nausea · palpitations · peripheral oedema · vomiting
- **CONCEPTION AND CONTRACEPTION** Effective contraception required during treatment. Monthly pregnancy tests advised.
- **PREGNANCY** Avoid—toxicity in *animal* studies.
- **BREAST FEEDING** Manufacturer advises avoid—present in milk in *animal* studies.
- **HEPATIC IMPAIRMENT** Manufacturer advises caution in moderate impairment; avoid in severe impairment (no information available).
  Dose adjustments Manufacturer advises cautious dose titration in moderate impairment.
- **RENAL IMPAIRMENT** Manufacturer advises avoid if eGFR less than 30 mL/minute/1.73 m² —limited information available.
  Dose adjustments Titrate dose cautiously—risk of hypotension.
- **DIRECTIONS FOR ADMINISTRATION** Manufacturer advises tablets may be crushed and mixed with water or soft foods and swallowed immediately.
- **PATIENT AND CARER ADVICE** Smoking cessation advised (response possibly reduced).
- **NATIONAL FUNDING/ACCESS DECISIONS**
  For full details see funding body website
  Scottish Medicines Consortium (SMC) decisions
  ‣ Riociguat (*Adempas*®) for chronic thromboembolic pulmonary hypertension (CTEPH) treatment in adult patients with World Health Organisation functional class II to III with inoperable CTEPH, persistent or recurrent CTEPH after surgical treatment, to improve exercise capacity (December 2014) SMC No. 1001/14 Recommended with restrictions
  ‣ Riociguat (*Adempas*®) for pulmonary arterial hypertension (PAH) as monotherapy or in combination with endothelin receptor antagonists, for the treatment of adult patients with PAH with World Health Organisation Functional Class II to III to improve exercise capacity (July 2015) SMC No. 1056/15 Recommended with restrictions

- **MEDICINAL FORMS** There can be variation in the licensing of different medicines containing the same drug.

Tablet

CAUTIONARY AND ADVISORY LABELS 5
‣ Adempas (Merck Sharp & Dohme Ltd)
  Riociguat 500 microgram Adempas 0.5mg tablets | 42 tablet [PoM] £997.36 DT = £997.36
  Riociguat 1 mg Adempas 1mg tablets | 42 tablet [PoM] £997.36 DT = £997.36
  Riociguat 1.5 mg Adempas 1.5mg tablets | 42 tablet [PoM] £997.36 DT = £997.36
  Riociguat 2 mg Adempas 2mg tablets | 42 tablet [PoM] £997.36 DT = £997.36 | 84 tablet [PoM] £1,994.72
  Riociguat 2.5 mg Adempas 2.5mg tablets | 42 tablet [PoM] £997.36 DT = £997.36 | 84 tablet [PoM] £1,994.72

PROSTAGLANDINS AND ANALOGUES

Iloprost
09-Nov-2020

- **INDICATIONS AND DOSE**

Idiopathic or familial pulmonary arterial hypertension (initiated under specialist supervision)
‣ BY INHALATION OF NEBULISED SOLUTION
‣ Adult: Initially 2.5 micrograms for 1 dose, increased to 5 micrograms for 1 dose, increased if tolerated to 5 micrograms 6–9 times a day, adjusted according to response; reduced if not tolerated to 2.5 micrograms 6–9 times a day, reduce to lower maintenance dose if high dose not tolerated

Severe Raynaud's phenomenon in patients with progressive trophic disorders
‣ BY INTRAVENOUS INFUSION
‣ Adult: Initially 0.5 nanogram/kg/minute for 30 minutes, then increased, if tolerated, in steps of 0.5 nanogram/kg/minute every 30 minutes (max. per dose 2 nanograms/kg/minute); usual dose 1.5–2 nanograms/kg/minute given over 6 hours daily for 5 days, repeat cycles should take place at intervals of at least 4 weeks (preferably 6–12 weeks)

Severe chronic lower limb ischaemia
‣ BY INTRAVENOUS INFUSION
‣ Adult: Initially 0.5 nanogram/kg/minute for 30 minutes, then increased, if tolerated, in steps of 0.5 nanogram/kg/minute every 30 minutes (max. per dose 2 nanograms/kg/minute); usual dose 0.5–2 nanograms/kg/minute given over 6 hours daily for up to 4 weeks

- **CONTRA-INDICATIONS**

  GENERAL CONTRA-INDICATIONS
  Conditions which increase risk of haemorrhage · congenital or acquired valvular defects with myocardial function disorders (not related to pulmonary hypertension) · decompensated heart failure (unless under close medical supervision) · severe arrhythmias · severe coronary heart disease · unstable angina · within 3 months of cerebrovascular events · within 6 months of myocardial infarction

  SPECIFIC CONTRA-INDICATIONS
  ‣ When used by inhalation Pulmonary veno-occlusive disease · systolic blood pressure below 85 mmHg · unstable pulmonary hypertension with advanced right heart failure
  ‣ With intravenous use acute or chronic congestive heart failure (NYHA II-IV) · pulmonary oedema

2

Cardiovascular system

- **CAUTIONS**

  GENERAL CAUTIONS Hypotension

  SPECIFIC CAUTIONS
  ▸ When used by inhalation Acute pulmonary infection · chronic obstructive pulmonary disease · severe asthma
  ▸ With intravenous use Significant heart disease

- **INTERACTIONS** → Appendix 1: iloprost

- **SIDE-EFFECTS**

  GENERAL SIDE-EFFECTS
  ▸ Common or very common Cough · diarrhoea · dizziness · dyspnoea · haemorrhage · hypotension · nausea · pain · palpitations · syncope · vomiting
  ▸ Uncommon Taste altered · thrombocytopenia

  SPECIFIC SIDE-EFFECTS
  ▸ Common or very common
  ▸ When used by inhalation Chest discomfort · headache · oral disorders · rash · tachycardia · throat complaints · vasodilation
  ▸ With intravenous use Angina pectoris · anxiety · appetite decreased · arrhythmias · arthralgia · asthenia · bradyphrenia · chills · confusion · drowsiness · feeling hot · fever · flushing · gastrointestinal discomfort · headaches · hyperhidrosis · muscle complaints · sensation abnormal · thirst · vertigo
  ▸ Uncommon
  ▸ With intravenous use Asthma · cerebrovascular insufficiency · constipation · depression · dry mouth · dysphagia · dysuria · embolism and thrombosis · eye discomfort · hallucination · heart failure · hepatic impairment · myocardial infarction · pruritus · pulmonary oedema · renal pain · seizure · tetany · tremor · vision blurred
  ▸ Frequency not known
  ▸ When used by inhalation Respiratory disorders

- **PREGNANCY**
  ▸ When used by inhalation Use if potential benefit outweighs risk.
  ▸ With intravenous use Manufacturer advises avoid—toxicity in *animal* studies.

- **BREAST FEEDING** Manufacturer advises avoid—no information available.

- **HEPATIC IMPAIRMENT** Manufacturer advises caution (risk of increased exposure).
  Dose adjustments ▸ When used by inhalation Manufacturer advises initial dose reduction to 2.5 micrograms at intervals of 3–4 hours (max. 6 times daily), adjusted according to response—consult product literature.
  ▸ With intravenous use Manufacturer advises initial dose reduction in severe impairment, consider half the normal dose.

- **MONITORING REQUIREMENTS**
  ▸ With intravenous use Manufacturer advises monitor blood pressure and heart rate at the start of the infusion and at every dose increase.

- **DIRECTIONS FOR ADMINISTRATION**
  ▸ With intravenous use For *intravenous infusion* dilute to a concentration of 200 nanograms/mL with Glucose 5% or Sodium Chloride 0.9%; alternatively, may be diluted to a concentration of 2 micrograms/mL and given via syringe driver.
  ▸ When used by inhalation To minimise accidental exposure use only with nebulisers listed in product literature in a well ventilated room.

- **PRESCRIBING AND DISPENSING INFORMATION**
  ▸ When used by inhalation Delivery characteristics of nebuliser devices may vary—only switch devices under medical supervision.
  ▸ With intravenous use Concentrate for infusion available on a named patient basis from Bayer Schering in 0.5 mL and 1 mL ampoules.

- **HANDLING AND STORAGE** Manufacturer advises avoid contact with skin and eyes.

- **PATIENT AND CARER ADVICE**
  Driving and skilled tasks Manufacturer advises patients and carers should be counselled on the effects on driving and performance of skilled tasks—increased risk of dizziness.

- **NATIONAL FUNDING/ACCESS DECISIONS**
  For full details see funding body website
  Scottish Medicines Consortium (SMC) decisions
  ▸ Iloprost trometamol (*Ventavis*®) for primary pulmonary hypertension (December 2005) SMC No. 219/05 Recommended with restrictions

- **MEDICINAL FORMS** There can be variation in the licensing of different medicines containing the same drug.

  Solution for infusion
  EXCIPIENTS: May contain Ethanol
  ▸ Iloprost (Non-proprietary)
  Iloprost (as Iloprost trometamol) 100 microgram per 1 ml Iloprost 50micrograms/0.5ml concentrate for solution for infusion ampoules | 1 ampoule PoM £75.00 (Hospital only) | 5 ampoule PoM £300.00 (Hospital only)
  ▸ Ilomedin (Imported (Greece))
  Iloprost (as Iloprost trometamol) 100 microgram per 1 ml Ilomedin 100micrograms/1ml solution for infusion ampoules | 1 ampoule PoM ⓧ

  Nebuliser liquid
  EXCIPIENTS: May contain Ethanol
  ▸ Iloprost (Non-proprietary)
  Iloprost (as Iloprost trometamol) 10 microgram per 1 ml Iloprost 10micrograms/1ml nebuliser liquid ampoules | 30 ampoule PoM £300.00 | 160 ampoule PoM £1,700.00
  Ventavis 10micrograms/ml nebuliser solution 1ml ampoules with Breelib | 168 ampoule PoM £2,241.08
  Iloprost (as Iloprost trometamol) 20 microgram per 1 ml Ventavis 20micrograms/ml nebuliser solution 1ml ampoules with Breelib | 168 ampoule PoM £2,241.08
  ▸ Ventavis (Bayer Plc)
  Iloprost (as Iloprost trometamol) 10 microgram per 1 ml Ventavis 10micrograms/ml nebuliser solution 1ml ampoules | 42 ampoule PoM £560.27 | 168 ampoule PoM £2,241.08
  Iloprost (as Iloprost trometamol) 20 microgram per 1 ml Ventavis 20micrograms/ml nebuliser solution 1ml ampoules | 42 ampoule PoM £560.27

4.2 Hypotension and shock

Sympathomimetics

Inotropic sympathomimetics

Shock

Shock is a medical emergency associated with a high mortality. The underlying causes of shock such as haemorrhage, sepsis, or myocardial insufficiency should be corrected. The profound hypotension of shock must be treated promptly to prevent tissue hypoxia and organ failure. Volume replacement is essential to correct the hypovolaemia associated with haemorrhage and sepsis but may be detrimental in cardiogenic shock. Depending on haemodynamic status, cardiac output may be improved by the use of sympathomimetic inotropes such as adrenaline/epinephrine p. 238, dobutamine p. 237 or dopamine hydrochloride p. 201. In septic shock, when fluid replacement and inotropic support fail to maintain blood pressure, the vasoconstrictor noradrenaline/norepinephrine p. 202 may be considered. In cardiogenic shock peripheral resistance is frequently high and to raise it further may worsen myocardial performance and exacerbate tissue ischaemia.

The use of sympathomimetic inotropes and vasoconstrictors should preferably be confined to the intensive care setting and undertaken with invasive haemodynamic monitoring.

See also advice on the management of anaphylactic shock in Antihistamines, allergen immunotherapy and allergic emergencies p. 292.

Vasoconstrictor sympathomimetics

Vasoconstrictor sympathomimetics raise blood pressure transiently by acting on alpha-adrenergic receptors to constrict peripheral vessels. They are sometimes used as an emergency method of elevating blood pressure where other measures have failed.

The danger of vasoconstrictors is that although they raise blood pressure they also reduce perfusion of vital organs such as the kidney.

Spinal and epidural anaesthesia may result in sympathetic block with resultant hypotension. Management may include intravenous fluids (which are usually given prophylactically), oxygen, elevation of the legs, and injection of a pressor drug such as ephedrine hydrochloride p. 287. As well as constricting peripheral vessels ephedrine hydrochloride also accelerates the heart rate (by acting on beta receptors). Use is made of this dual action of ephedrine hydrochloride to manage associated bradycardia (although intravenous injection of atropine sulfate p. 1386 may also be required if bradycardia persists).

SYMPATHOMIMETICS ⟩ INOTROPIC

▌Dopamine hydrochloride

- **DRUG ACTION** Dopamine is a cardiac stimulant which acts on beta$_1$ receptors in cardiac muscle, and increases contractility with little effect on rate.

- **INDICATIONS AND DOSE**
Cardiogenic shock in infarction or cardiac surgery
  - ▶ BY INTRAVENOUS INFUSION
  - ▶ Adult: Initially 2–5 micrograms/kg/minute

- **CONTRA-INDICATIONS** Phaeochromocytoma · tachyarrhythmia

- **CAUTIONS** Correct hypovolaemia · hypertension (may raise blood pressure) · hyperthyroidism · low dose in shock due to acute myocardial infarction

- **INTERACTIONS** → Appendix 1: sympathomimetics, inotropic

- **SIDE-EFFECTS** Angina pectoris · anxiety · arrhythmias · azotaemia · cardiac conduction disorder · dyspnoea · gangrene · headache · hypertension · mydriasis · nausea · palpitations · piloerection · polyuria · tremor · vasoconstriction · vomiting

- **PREGNANCY** No evidence of harm in *animal* studies—manufacturer advises use only if potential benefit outweighs risk.

- **BREAST FEEDING** May suppress lactation—not known to be harmful.

- **DIRECTIONS FOR ADMINISTRATION** Dopamine concentrate for intravenous infusion to be diluted before use.
For *intravenous infusion* give continuously in Glucose 5% or Sodium chloride 0.9%. Dilute to max. concentration of 3.2 mg/mL; incompatible with bicarbonate.

- **MEDICINAL FORMS** There can be variation in the licensing of different medicines containing the same drug. Forms available from special-order manufacturers include: solution for infusion
Solution for infusion
  - ▶ Dopamine hydrochloride (Non-proprietary)
    Dopamine hydrochloride 40 mg per 1 ml Dopamine 200mg/5ml solution for infusion ampoules | 5 ampoule [PoM] £20.00 (Hospital only) | 10 ampoule [PoM] £9.04 | 10 ampoule [PoM] £9.04 (Hospital only)

Dopamine 200mg/5ml concentrate for solution for infusion ampoules | 10 ampoule [PoM] Ⓢ (Hospital only)
Dopamine hydrochloride 160 mg per 1 ml Dopamine 800mg/5ml solution for infusion ampoules | 10 ampoule [PoM] Ⓢ

SYMPATHOMIMETICS ⟩ VASOCONSTRICTOR

▌Metaraminol

28-Apr-2020

- **INDICATIONS AND DOSE**
Emergency treatment of acute hypotension
  - ▶ INITIALLY BY INTRAVENOUS INJECTION
  - ▶ Adult: Initially 0.5–5 mg, then (by intravenous infusion) 15–100 mg, adjusted according to response
Acute hypotension
  - ▶ BY INTRAVENOUS INFUSION
  - ▶ Adult: 15–100 mg, adjusted according to response

- **CAUTIONS** Cirrhosis · coronary vascular thrombosis · diabetes mellitus · elderly · extravasation at injection site may cause necrosis · following myocardial infarction · hypercapnia · hypertension · hyperthyroidism · hypoxia · mesenteric vascular thrombosis · peripheral vascular thrombosis · Prinzmetal's variant angina · uncorrected hypovolaemia

  CAUTIONS, FURTHER INFORMATION
  - ▶ Hypertensive response Metaraminol has a longer duration of action than noradrenaline, and an excessive vasopressor response may cause a prolonged rise in blood pressure.

- **INTERACTIONS** → Appendix 1: sympathomimetics, vasoconstrictor

- **SIDE-EFFECTS**
  - ▶ **Common or very common** Headache · hypertension
  - ▶ **Rare or very rare** Skin exfoliation · soft tissue necrosis
  - ▶ **Frequency not known** Abscess · arrhythmias · nausea · palpitations · peripheral ischaemia

- **PREGNANCY** May reduce placental perfusion—manufacturer advises use only if potential benefit outweighs risk.

- **BREAST FEEDING** Manufacturer advises caution—no information available.

- **MONITORING REQUIREMENTS** Monitor blood pressure and rate of flow frequently.

- **DIRECTIONS FOR ADMINISTRATION** For *intravenous infusion*, give continuously or via drip tubing in Glucose 5% or Sodium chloride 0.9%. Suggested volume 500 mL.

- **MEDICINAL FORMS** There can be variation in the licensing of different medicines containing the same drug. Forms available from special-order manufacturers include: solution for injection
Solution for injection
  - ▶ Metaraminol (Non-proprietary)
    Metaraminol (as Metaraminol tartrate) 500 microgram per 1 ml Metaraminol 2.5mg/5ml solution for injection ampoules | 10 ampoule £37.40
    Metaraminol 5mg/10ml solution for injection ampoules | 10 ampoule [PoM] £76.10
    Metaraminol (as Metaraminol tartrate) 10 mg per 1 ml Metaraminol 10mg/1ml solution for injection ampoules | 10 ampoule [PoM] £21.50

2

Cardiovascular system

2

Cardiovascular system

Midodrine hydrochloride

01-Apr-2016

- DRUG ACTION Midodrine hydrochloride is a pro-drug of desglymidodrine. Desglymidodrine is a sympathomimetic agent, which acts on peripheral alpha-adrenergic receptors to increase arterial resistance, resulting in an increase in blood pressure.

● INDICATIONS AND DOSE

Severe orthostatic hypotension due to autonomic dysfunction when corrective factors have been ruled out and other forms of treatment are inadequate
▸ BY MOUTH
▸ Adult: Initially 2.5 mg 3 times a day, increased if necessary up to 10 mg 3 times a day, dose to be increased at weekly intervals, according to blood pressure measurements; usual maintenance 10 mg 3 times a day, avoid administration at night; the last daily dose should be taken at least 4 hours before bedtime

- CONTRA-INDICATIONS Aortic aneurysm · blood vessel spasm · bradycardia · cardiac conduction disturbances · cerebrovascular occlusion · congestive heart failure · hypertension · hyperthyroidism · myocardial infarction · narrow-angle glaucoma · phaeochromocytoma · proliferative diabetic retinopathy · serious obliterative blood vessel disease · serious prostate disorder · urinary retention

- CAUTIONS Atherosclerotic cardiovascular disease (especially with symptoms of intestinal angina or claudication of the legs) · autonomic dysfunction · elderly (manufacturer recommends cautious dose titration) · prostate disorders

- INTERACTIONS → Appendix 1: sympathomimetics, vasoconstrictor

- SIDE-EFFECTS
▸ **Common or very common** Chills · flushing · gastrointestinal discomfort · headache · nausea · paraesthesia · piloerection · scalp pruritus · skin reactions · stomatitis · supine hypertension (dose-dependent) · urinary disorders
▸ **Uncommon** Anxiety · arrhythmias · irritability · sleep disorders
▸ **Rare or very rare** Hepatic function abnormal · palpitations
▸ **Frequency not known** Confusion · diarrhoea · vomiting

  SIDE-EFFECTS, FURTHER INFORMATION Manufacturer advises that treatment must be stopped if supine hypertension is not controlled by reducing the dose.

- CONCEPTION AND CONTRACEPTION Manufacturer recommends effective contraception during treatment in women of childbearing potential.

- PREGNANCY Manufacturer advises avoid—toxicity in *animal* studies.

- BREAST FEEDING Manufacturer advises avoid—no information available.

- RENAL IMPAIRMENT Manufacturer advises avoid in severe or acute impairment.

- MONITORING REQUIREMENTS
▸ Manufacturer advises measure hepatic and renal function before treatment and at regular intervals during treatment.
▸ Manufacturer advises regular monitoring of supine and standing blood pressure due to the risk of hypertension in the supine position.

- PATIENT AND CARER ADVICE Manufacturer advises that patients report symptoms of supine hypertension (such as chest pain, palpitations, shortness of breath, headache and blurred vision) immediately. The risk of supine hypertension at night can be reduced by raising the head of the bed.

- MEDICINAL FORMS There can be variation in the licensing of different medicines containing the same drug.

Tablet
▸ Midodrine hydrochloride (Non-proprietary)
  Midodrine hydrochloride 2.5 mg Midodrine 2.5mg tablets |
  100 tablet [PoM] £69.90 DT = £55.05
  Midodrine hydrochloride 5 mg Midodrine 5mg tablets |
  100 tablet [PoM] £96.33 DT = £75.05
▸ Bramox (Brancaster Pharma Ltd)
  Midodrine hydrochloride 2.5 mg Bramox 2.5mg tablets |
  100 tablet [PoM] £55.05 DT = £55.05
  Midodrine hydrochloride 5 mg Bramox 5mg tablets |
  100 tablet [PoM] £75.05 DT = £75.05

Noradrenaline/norepinephrine

13-May-2020

● INDICATIONS AND DOSE

Acute hypotension [initial and on-going treatment]
▸ BY INTRAVENOUS INFUSION
▸ Adult: Initially 0.16–0.33 mL/minute, adjusted according to response, dose applies to a solution containing noradrenaline 40 micrograms(base)/mL only; dilute the 1 mg/mL concentrate for infusion for this solution—consult product literature

On-going treatment of acute hypotension [with escalating dose requirements]
▸ BY INTRAVENOUS INFUSION
▸ Adult (body-weight 50 kg and above): Use the 0.08 mg/mL or 0.16 mg/mL solution for infusion (consult product literature)

DOSE EQUIVALENCE AND CONVERSION
▸ 1 mg of noradrenaline base is equivalent to 2 mg of noradrenaline acid tartrate. **Doses expressed as the base.**

IMPORTANT SAFETY INFORMATION
ASSOCIATION OF NORADRENALINE/NOREPINEPHRINE 0.08 MG/ML (4 MG IN 50 ML) AND 0.16 MG/ML (8 MG IN 50 ML) SOLUTION FOR INFUSION WITH POTENTIAL RISK OF MEDICATION ERRORS

Healthcare professionals should be aware of the differences in strength and presentation between noradrenaline/norepinephrine products—manufacturer advises noradrenaline 0.08 mg/mL solution for infusion and noradrenaline 0.16 mg/mL solution for infusion must **not** be diluted before use and should only be used for the on-going treatment of patients already established on noradrenaline therapy, whose dose requirements are clinically confirmed to be escalating.

- CONTRA-INDICATIONS Hypertension

- CAUTIONS Coronary vascular thrombosis · diabetes mellitus · elderly · extravasation at injection site may cause necrosis · following myocardial infarction · hypercapnia · hyperthyroidism · hypoxia · mesenteric vascular thrombosis · peripheral vascular thrombosis · Prinzmetal's variant angina · uncorrected hypovolaemia

- INTERACTIONS → Appendix 1: sympathomimetics, vasoconstrictor

- SIDE-EFFECTS Acute glaucoma · anxiety · arrhythmias · asthenia · cardiomyopathy · confusion · dyspnoea · extravasation necrosis · gangrene · headache · heart failure · hypovolaemia · hypoxia · injection site necrosis · insomnia · ischaemia · myocardial contractility increased · nausea · palpitations · peripheral ischaemia · psychotic disorder · respiratory failure · tremor · urinary retention · vomiting

- PREGNANCY Manufacturer advises use if potential benefit outweighs risk—may reduce placental perfusion and induce fetal bradycardia.

- MONITORING REQUIREMENTS Monitor blood pressure and rate of flow frequently.
- DIRECTIONS FOR ADMINISTRATION For *intravenous infusion* using a solution containing noradrenaline 40 micrograms (base)/mL, manufacturer advises give continuously in Glucose 5% or Sodium Chloride and Glucose via a controlled infusion device. For administration via syringe pump, dilute 2 mg (2 mL of 1 mg/mL concentrate for infusion) noradrenaline base with 48 mL infusion fluid. For administration via drip counter dilute 20 mg (20 mL of 1 mg/mL concentrate for infusion) noradrenaline base with 480 mL infusion fluid; give through a central venous catheter; incompatible with alkalis.
- PRESCRIBING AND DISPENSING INFORMATION For a period of time, preparations on the UK market may be described as either noradrenaline base or noradrenaline acid tartrate; doses in the BNF are expressed as the base.

- MEDICINAL FORMS There can be variation in the licensing of different medicines containing the same drug. Forms available from special-order manufacturers include: infusion, solution for infusion

Solution for infusion
▸ Noradrenaline/norepinephrine (Non-proprietary)
  Noradrenaline (as Noradrenaline acid tartrate) 80 microgram per 1 ml Noradrenaline (base) 4mg/50ml solution for infusion vials | 10 vial [PoM] [⊠]
  Noradrenaline (as Noradrenaline acid tartrate) 1 mg per 1 ml Noradrenaline (base) 1mg/1ml concentrate for solution for infusion ampoules | 10 ampoule [PoM] [⊠] (Hospital only)
  Noradrenaline (base) 8mg/8ml concentrate for solution for infusion ampoules | 10 ampoule [PoM] £116.00
  Noradrenaline (base) 2mg/2ml solution for infusion ampoules | 5 ampoule [PoM] £12.00 (Hospital only)
  Noradrenaline (base) 4mg/4ml concentrate for solution for infusion ampoules | 5 ampoule [PoM] £22.00 (Hospital only) | 10 ampoule [PoM] £58.00 (Hospital only)
  Noradrenaline (base) 10mg/10ml concentrate for solution for infusion ampoules | 10 ampoule [PoM] [⊠] (Hospital only)
▸ Sinora (Sintetica Ltd)
  Noradrenaline (as Noradrenaline acid tartrate) 80 microgram per 1 ml Sinora 4mg/50ml solution for infusion vials | 1 vial [PoM] £9.97
  Noradrenaline (as Noradrenaline acid tartrate) 160 microgram per 1 ml Sinora 8mg/50ml solution for infusion vials | 1 vial [PoM] £14.22

Phenylephrine hydrochloride

- INDICATIONS AND DOSE
Acute hypotension
▸ BY SUBCUTANEOUS INJECTION, OR BY INTRAMUSCULAR INJECTION
▸ Adult: Initially 2–5 mg, followed by 1–10 mg, after at least 15 minutes if required
▸ BY SLOW INTRAVENOUS INJECTION
▸ Adult: 100–500 micrograms, repeated as necessary after at least 15 minutes
▸ BY INTRAVENOUS INFUSION
▸ Adult: Initially up to 180 micrograms/minute, reduced to 30–60 micrograms/minute, adjusted according to response

- CONTRA-INDICATIONS Hypertension · severe hyperthyroidism
- CAUTIONS Coronary disease · coronary vascular thrombosis · diabetes · elderly · extravasation at injection site may cause necrosis · following myocardial infarction · hypercapnia · hyperthyroidism · hypoxia · mesenteric vascular thrombosis · peripheral vascular thrombosis · Prinzmetal's variant angina · susceptibility to angle-closure glaucoma · uncorrected hypovolaemia

CAUTIONS, FURTHER INFORMATION
▸ Hypertensive response Phenylephrine has a longer duration of action than noradrenaline (norepinephrine), and an excessive vasopressor response may cause a prolonged rise in blood pressure.
- INTERACTIONS → Appendix 1: sympathomimetics, vasoconstrictor
- SIDE-EFFECTS Angina pectoris · arrhythmias · cardiac arrest · dizziness · dyspnoea · flushing · glucose tolerance impaired · headache · hyperhidrosis · hypersalivation · hypotension · intracranial haemorrhage · metabolic change · mydriasis · palpitations · paraesthesia · peripheral coldness · pulmonary oedema · soft tissue necrosis · syncope · urinary disorders · vomiting
- PREGNANCY Avoid if possible; malformations reported following use in first trimester; fetal hypoxia and bradycardia reported in late pregnancy and labour.
- MONITORING REQUIREMENTS Contra-indicated in hypertension—monitor blood pressure and rate of flow frequently.
- DIRECTIONS FOR ADMINISTRATION For *intravenous infusion* give intermittently in Glucose 5% or Sodium chloride 0.9%. Dilute 10 mg in 500 mL infusion fluid.

- MEDICINAL FORMS There can be variation in the licensing of different medicines containing the same drug. Forms available from special-order manufacturers include: solution for injection, eye drops

Solution for injection
▸ Phenylephrine hydrochloride (Non-proprietary)
  Phenylephrine (as Phenylephrine hydrochloride) 50 microgram per 1 ml Phenylephrine 500micrograms/10ml solution for injection pre-filled syringes | 1 pre-filled disposable injection [PoM] £15.00 | 10 pre-filled disposable injection [PoM] £150.00
  Phenylephrine hydrochloride 100 microgram per 1 ml Phenylephrine 1mg/10ml solution for injection ampoules | 10 ampoule [PoM] £42.00
  Phenylephrine hydrochloride 10 mg per 1 ml Phenylephrine 10mg/1ml solution for injection ampoules | 10 ampoule [PoM] £99.12
  Phenylephrine 10mg/1ml concentrate for solution for injection ampoules | 10 ampoule [PoM] £99.12

---

5   Cardiovascular risk assessment and prevention

Cardiovascular disease risk assessment and prevention   29-Nov-2019

Description of condition
Cardiovascular disease (CVD) is a term that describes a group of disorders of the heart and blood vessels caused by atherosclerosis and thrombosis, which includes coronary heart disease, stroke, peripheral arterial disease, and aortic disease.

The risk of CVD is greater in men, patients with a family history of CVD, and in certain ethnic backgrounds such as South Asians. CVD risk is also greater in patients aged over 50 years and increases with age; patients aged 85 years and over are at particularly high risk. CVD has several important and potentially modifiable risk factors such as hypertension, abnormal lipids, obesity, diabetes mellitus, and psychosocial factors such as depression, anxiety, and social isolation. Low physical activity, poor diet, smoking, and excessive alcohol intake are also modifiable risk factors.

Aims of treatment
The overall aim of treatment is to prevent the occurrence of a cardiovascular event by reducing modifiable risk factors through lifestyle changes and drug management.

2

Cardiovascular system

Cardiovascular disease risk assessment

Recommendations on cardiovascular disease (CVD) risk assessment are from the *National Institute for Health and Care Excellence (NICE)—Cardiovascular disease: risk assessment and reduction, including lipid modification guideline (CG181, 2016)*, and *Scottish Intercollegiate Guidelines Network (SIGN)—Risk estimation and the prevention of cardiovascular disease guideline (SIGN 149, 2017)*. SIGN 149 uses risk assessment strategies outlined by the *Joint British Society (JBS)—Joint British Societies' consensus recommendations for the prevention of cardiovascular disease (2014)*. Recommendations where NICE and SIGN differ have been highlighted.

EvGr NICE (2016) recommend that for primary prevention of CVD in primary care, a systematic approach be used to identify those who are likely to be at high risk. Patients should be prioritised based on an estimate of their CVD risk using risk factors already recorded in their medical records, before a full formal risk assessment. Priority for a full formal risk assessment should be given to patients with an estimated 10-year risk of 10% or more. Patients aged over 40 years should have their estimate of CVD risk reviewed on an ongoing basis. SIGN (2017) instead recommend that CVD risk assessments are offered at least every 5 years to all patients aged 40 years and over with no history of CVD, familial hypercholesterolaemia, chronic kidney disease or diabetes and who are not receiving treatment to reduce blood pressure or lipids. As well as to patients with a first-degree relative who has premature atherosclerotic CVD or familial dyslipidaemia, regardless of their age.

Risk assessment with a calculator is not required in patients who are at increased or high risk of CVD. This includes those with established CVD, chronic kidney disease stage 3 or higher (eGFR <60 mL/minute/1.73 m^2), albuminuria, or familial hypercholesterolaemia. In addition to these patients, NICE (2016) do not recommend the use of a risk calculator in patients with other hereditary disorders of lipid metabolism, or type 1 diabetes mellitus. Whereas SIGN (2017) do not recommend the use of a risk calculator in patients with diabetes mellitus aged 40 years and over, and in those aged under 40 years with diabetes mellitus who have either had it for more than 20 years, present with target organ damage (such as proteinuria, albuminuria, proliferative retinopathy, or autonomic neuropathy), or have other significantly elevated cardiovascular risk factors. Ⓐ

Risk calculators

Cardiovascular risk assessment calculators are used to predict the approximate likelihood of a cardiovascular event occurring over a given period of time. EvGr Standard risk scores may be underestimated in patients with additional risk due to existing conditions or medications that can cause dyslipidaemia (e.g. antipsychotics, corticosteroids, or immunosuppressants). CVD risk may also be underestimated in patients who are already taking antihypertensives or lipid-regulating drugs, or who have recently stopped smoking. Interpretation of risk scores as well as the need for further management of risk factors in those who fall below the CVD risk threshold, should always reflect informed clinical judgement. Ⓐ

QRISK® 2 and JBS3

QRISK® 2 and JBS3 risk calculators are used to assess CVD risk for patients in England and Wales. Both tools assess cardiovascular risk of coronary heart disease (angina and myocardial infarction), stroke, and transient ischaemic attack. This is based on lipid profile, systolic blood pressure, gender, age, ethnicity, smoking status, BMI, chronic kidney disease (stage 4 or above), diabetes mellitus, atrial fibrillation, treated hypertension, rheumatoid arthritis, social deprivation, or a family history of premature CVD.

The QRISK® 2 risk calculator (www.qrisk.org/) is recommended by *NICE clinical guideline* 181, and the JBS3

risk calculator (www.jbs3risk.com/pages/risk_calculator.htm) is endorsed by the Joint British Society.

QRISK® 3 is an updated version of the QRISK® 2 risk calculator. It considers additional risk factors such as chronic kidney disease (stage 3 or above), migraine, corticosteroid use, systemic lupus erythematosus, atypical antipsychotics use, severe mental illness, erectile dysfunction, and a measure of systolic blood pressure variability.

The JBS3 calculator is not only able to estimate short term (10-year) risk, but also lifetime risk of CVD events. Patients with a 10-year risk of CVD of less than 10% may benefit from an assessment of their lifetime risk using the JBS3 tool, and a discussion on the impact of lifestyle interventions and, if necessary, drug therapy.

ASSIGN

The ASSIGN cardiovascular risk assessment calculator is tailored to the Scottish population and uses factors such as age, sex, smoking, systolic blood pressure, lipid profile, family history of premature CVD, diabetes mellitus, rheumatoid arthritis, and social deprivation to estimate cardiovascular risk. EvGr Other risk factors not included in this CVD risk assessment calculator (such as ethnicity, BMI, atrial fibrillation, psychological wellbeing, and physical inactivity) should also be taken into account when assessing and managing the patient's overall risk.

SIGN (2017) recommend that asymptomatic patients without established CVD (or other conditions that are automatically associated with a high CVD risk) should be considered at high risk if they are assessed as having a 20% or more risk of a first cardiovascular event within 10 years. Ⓐ

The online calculator tool can be found at www.assign-score.com/estimate-the-risk/. Full details can be found in the *SIGN 149 clinical guideline* (see *Useful resources*).

Cardiovascular disease prevention

Recommendations on cardiovascular disease (CVD) prevention are from the *National Institute for Health and Care Excellence (NICE)—Cardiovascular disease: risk assessment and reduction, including lipid modification guideline (CG181, 2016)*, and *Scottish Intercollegiate Guidelines Network (SIGN)—Risk estimation and the prevention of cardiovascular disease guideline (SIGN 149, 2017)*. SIGN 149 uses strategies outlined by the *Joint British Society (JBS)—Joint British Societies' consensus recommendations for the prevention of cardiovascular disease (2014)*. Recommendations where NICE and SIGN differ have been highlighted.

EvGr All patients at any risk of CVD should be advised to make lifestyle modifications that may include beneficial changes to diet (such as increasing fruit and vegetable consumption, reducing saturated fat and dietary salt intake), increasing physical exercise, weight management, reducing alcohol consumption, and Smoking cessation p. 519. An annual review should be considered to discuss lifestyle modification, medication adherence and risk factors. The frequency of review may be tailored to the individual.

Further preventative measures with drug treatment should be taken in individuals with a high risk of developing CVD (primary prevention), and to prevent recurrence of events in those with established CVD (secondary prevention). Ⓐ

Primary prevention

Antiplatelet therapy

EvGr Aspirin p. 132 is not recommended for *primary prevention* of CVD due to the limited benefit gained versus risk of side-effects such as bleeding. Ⓐ

Antihypertensive therapy

EvGr Antihypertensive drug treatment should be offered to patients who are at high risk of CVD and have a sustained elevated systolic blood pressure over 140 mmHg and/or diastolic blood pressure over 90 mmHg. For further guidance on prescribing antihypertensive drugs in patients without symptomatic CVD and for specific groups at high cardiovascular risk, see Hypertension p. 153. ⒶⒶ

Lipid-lowering therapy

EvGr A statin is recommended as the lipid-lowering drug of choice for primary prevention of CVD. All modifiable risk factors, comorbidities and secondary causes of dyslipidaemia (e.g. uncontrolled diabetes mellitus, hepatic disease, nephrotic syndrome, excessive alcohol consumption, and hypothyroidism) should be managed before starting treatment with a statin. Factors such as polypharmacy, frailty, and comorbidities should be taken into account before starting statin therapy.

NICE (2016) recommend low-dose atorvastatin p. 217 for patients who have a 10% or greater 10-year risk of developing CVD (using the QRISK2 calculator), and for patients with chronic kidney disease. Low-dose atorvastatin p. 217 should be considered in all patients with type 1 diabetes mellitus, and be offered to patients with type 1 diabetes who are either aged over 40 years, have had diabetes for more than 10 years, have established nephropathy, or have other CVD risk factors. Patients aged 85 years and over may also benefit from low-dose atorvastatin p. 217 to reduce their risk of non-fatal myocardial infarction. SIGN (2017) recommend low-dose atorvastatin p. 217 for patients who are considered to be at high risk of CVD and not on dialysis.

Patients taking statins should have an annual medication review to discuss medication adherence, lifestyle modification, CVD risk factors, and non-fasting, non-HDL cholesterol concentration (if testing deemed appropriate). Total cholesterol, HDL-cholesterol, and non-HDL-cholesterol concentrations should be checked 3 months after starting treatment with a high-intensity statin. For statin intensity categorisation, see Dyslipidaemias p. 210.

Aiming for a reduction in non-HDL-cholesterol concentration of greater than 40% is recommended. If this is not achieved, adherence to drug treatment should be checked and lifestyle modifications optimised. In patients deemed to be at a higher risk due to comorbidities, risk score, or clinical judgement, an increase in the statin dose should be considered. NICE (2016) recommend that the use of higher doses in those with chronic kidney disease with an eGFR less than 30ml/minute/1.73 m2 should be discussed with a renal specialist.

Specialist advice should be sought regarding treatment options in patients at high risk of CVD who are intolerant of three different statins.

SIGN (2017) recommend that ezetimibe p. 212 and bile acid sequestrants such as colestyramine p. 212 and colestipol hydrochloride p. 212 only be considered for primary prevention in patients with an elevated cardiovascular risk in whom statin therapy is contra-indicated, and in patients with familial hypercholesterolaemia. However, NICE (2016) recommend that ezetimibe p. 212 be considered for primary hypercholesterolaemia in line with National funding/access decisions for ezetimibe p. 212, and do not recommend bile acid sequestrants.

Although fibrates are not routinely recommended for primary prevention of CVD, SIGN (2017) recommend that they be considered in patients with a combination of high CVD risk, marked hypertriglyceridaemia and low HDL-cholesterol concentration.

If cholesterol remains above the target concentration despite other tolerated lipid-lowering therapy in patients at high risk of vascular events, the use of PCSK9 inhibitors, such as alirocumab p. 221 and evolocumab p. 222 should be considered. ⒶⒶ

Lipid-lowering therapy recommendations from Joint British Societies' consensus (2014), NICE Clinical guideline 181 (2016), and SIGN Clinical guideline 149 (2017) all differ in certain respects for prevention of CVD in patients with diabetes mellitus—see individual guidelines for further details.

For further information on lipid-lowering therapy and familial hypercholesterolaemia, see Dyslipidaemias p. 210.

Secondary prevention
Antiplatelet therapy

EvGr Antiplatelet therapy with low-dose daily aspirin p. 132 should be offered to patients with established atherosclerotic disease. Alternatively, clopidogrel p. 134 can be considered in patients who are intolerant to *aspirin* or in whom it is contra-indicated.

Clopidogrel p. 134 or a combination of dipyridamole with aspirin p. 135 should be considered to prevent recurrence of stroke and other vascular events in all patients with a history of stroke or transient ischaemic attack who are in sinus rhythm. ⒶⒶ For further information, see Stroke p. 127.

Antihypertensive therapy

EvGr Antihypertensive drug treatment is recommended in patients with established CVD and a sustained elevated systolic blood pressure over 140 mmHg and/or diastolic blood pressure over 90 mmHg. For further guidance on prescribing antihypertensive drugs in patients with CVD, see Hypertension p. 153. ⒶⒶ

Lipid-lowering therapy

EvGr A statin is recommended as the lipid-lowering drug of choice for secondary prevention of CVD. Factors such as polypharmacy, frailty, and comorbidities should be taken into account before starting statin therapy.

Treatment with high-dose atorvastatin p. 217 should be offered to patients with established atherosclerotic disease. However, a lower dose can be used if the patient is at an increased risk of side-effects or drug interactions. NICE (2016) recommend that low-dose atorvastatin p. 217 be offered to patients with established CVD and chronic kidney disease.

High-dose simvastatin p. 219 is generally avoided due to the risk of myopathy, unless the patient has been stable on this regimen for at least one year. ⒶⒶ Furthermore, the MHRA advise that high-dose simvastatin p. 219 only be considered for patients who have not achieved their treatment goals with lower doses and have severe hypercholesterolaemia and high risk of cardiovascular complications; benefits should outweigh risks.

EvGr Patients taking statins should have an annual medication review to discuss medication adherence, lifestyle modification, CVD risk factors, and non-fasting, non-HDL-cholesterol concentrations (if testing deemed appropriate). Total cholesterol, HDL-cholesterol, and non-HDL-cholesterol concentrations should be checked 3 months after starting treatment with a high-intensity statin. Patients who are stable on a low or medium-intensity statin should discuss the benefits and risks of switching to a high-intensity statin at their next medication review. For statin intensity categorisation, see Dyslipidaemias p. 210.

Aiming for a reduction in non-HDL-cholesterol concentration of greater than 40% is recommended. ⒶⒶ JBS3 instead recommend a target non-HDL-cholesterol concentration below 2.5 mmol/litre. EvGr If these targets are not achieved, adherence to drug treatment should be checked and lifestyle modifications optimised. In patients judged to be at a higher risk because of comorbidities, risk score, or clinical judgement, an increase in the statin dose (if started on less than maximum atorvastatin p. 217 dose) should be considered. NICE (2016) recommend that the use of higher doses in those with chronic kidney disease with an eGFR less than 30ml/minute/1.73 m^2 be discussed with a renal specialist.

Specialist advice should be sought regarding treatment options in patients with existing CVD who are intolerant of three different statins.

If LDL-cholesterol remains inadequately controlled, SIGN (2017) recommend that ezetimibe p. 212 and bile acid sequestrants such as colestyramine p. 212 and colestipol hydrochloride p. 212, can be considered for use in

2

Cardiovascular system

combination with a statin at the maximum tolerated dose. However, NICE (2016) do not recommend bile acid sequestrants for the secondary prevention of CVD.

Although fibrates are not routinely recommended for secondary prevention of CVD, SIGN (2017) recommend that they be considered in patients with both marked hypertriglyceridaemia and low HDL-cholesterol concentrations. ⒶA

For further information on lipid-lowering therapy and familial hypercholesterolaemia, see Dyslipidaemias p. 210.

Psychological risk factors

EvGr Psychological treatment should be considered in patients with mood and anxiety disorders and comorbid CVD; complex patients may require referral to mental health services for assessment and delivery of high-intensity or specialist treatments. Selective serotonin re-uptake inhibitors (SSRIs) should be considered for treatment in patients with depression and coronary heart disease. ⒶA For guidance on prescribing of antidepressant drugs see Antidepressant drugs p. 378.

Advanced Pharmacy Services

Patients with or at risk of cardiovascular disease, may be eligible for the New Medicines Service / Medicines Use Review service provided by a community pharmacist. For further information, see *Advanced Pharmacy Services* in Medicines optimisation p. 18.

Useful Resources

Risk estimation and the prevention of cardiovascular disease. Scottish Intercollegiate Guidelines Network. Clinical guideline 149. June 2017.
www.sign.ac.uk/sign-149-risk-estimation-and-the-prevention-of-cardiovascular-disease.html

Cardiovascular disease: risk assessment and reduction, including lipid modification. National Institute for Health and Care Excellence. Clinical guideline CG181. July 2014 (updated September 2016).
www.nice.org.uk/guidance/cg181

Joint British Societies' consensus recommendations for the prevention of cardiovascular disease (JBS3). April 2014.
www.jbs3risk.com/pages/report.htm

6   Heart failure

Chronic heart failure
23-Oct-2018

Description of condition

Heart failure is a progressive clinical syndrome caused by structural or functional abnormalities of the heart, resulting in reduced cardiac output. It is characterised by symptoms such as shortness of breath, persistent coughing or wheezing, ankle swelling, reduced exercise tolerance, and fatigue. These symptoms may be accompanied by signs such as elevated jugular venous pressure, pulmonary crackles, and pulmonary oedema.

The risk of heart failure is greater in men, smokers and diabetic patients, and increases with age.

The most common cause of heart failure is coronary heart disease, however, patients of African or Afro-Caribbean origin are more likely to develop heart failure secondary to hypertension. In addition to coronary heart disease, heart failure often co-exists with other co-morbidities such as chronic kidney disease, atrial fibrillation, hypertension, dyslipidaemia, obesity, diabetes mellitus, and chronic obstructive pulmonary disease. Patients with co-morbidities have a worse prognosis, and the presence of atrial fibrillation or chronic kidney disease affects the management of heart failure in these patients. Complications of heart failure

include chronic kidney disease, atrial fibrillation, depression, cachexia, sexual dysfunction, and sudden cardiac death.

Heart failure can be defined as either having a reduced or preserved ejection fraction. Both conditions present with signs and symptoms of heart failure. In heart failure with reduced ejection fraction, the left ventricle loses its ability to contract normally and therefore presents with an ejection fraction of less than 40%. In heart failure with preserved ejection fraction, the left ventricle loses its ability to relax normally therefore the ejection fraction is normal or only mildly reduced.

The New York Heart Association (NYHA) functional classification tool is used to define the progression of chronic heart failure according to severity of symptoms and limitation to physical activity. Heart failure is considered to be stable or chronic when symptoms remain unchanged for at least one month despite optimal management.

Aims of treatment

The aims of treatment are to reduce mortality, relieve symptoms, improve exercise tolerance, and reduce the incidence of acute exacerbations.

Non-drug treatment

EvGr Patients with heart failure should be advised to make lifestyle changes to reduce the risk of progression of their heart failure and associated co-morbidities. These include Smoking cessation p. 519, reducing alcohol consumption, increasing physical exercise if appropriate, weight control, and dietary changes such as increasing fruit and vegetable consumption and reducing saturated fat intake. Patients should be encouraged to weigh themselves daily at a set time of day and to report any weight gain of more than 1.5–2.0 kg in 2 days to their GP or heart failure specialist. Salt and fluid intake should only be restricted if these are high, and a salt intake of less than 6 g per day is advised. Patients with dilutional hyponatraemia should only restrict their fluid intake. Salt substitutes containing potassium should be avoided to reduce the risk of hyperkalaemia.

Contraception and pregnancy should be discussed with women of childbearing potential and heart failure. Advice from a heart failure specialist and an obstetrician should be sought if pregnancy occurs or is being considered.

Patients should be given the opportunity to join a personalised rehabilitation programme including education, psychological support, and exercise when appropriate.

Implantable cardioverter defibrillators and cardiac resynchronisation therapy are treatment options recommended in patients with heart failure and a reduced ejection fraction of less than 35%. If symptoms remain severe and unresponsive despite optimal drug treatment, specialist referral should be considered. ⒶA

Drug treatment

EvGr The treatment of heart failure should include management of symptoms, risk factors and underlying causes and complications. Patients should have their medication reviewed, and any drugs that may cause or worsen their heart failure should be stopped if appropriate.

Vaccination against pneumococcal disease, and annual influenza vaccination is recommended. ⒶA

Chronic heart failure with reduced ejection fraction

EvGr Rate-limiting calcium-channel blockers (verapamil hydrochloride p. 178, and diltiazem hydrochloride p. 171) and short-acting dihydropyridines (e.g. nifedipine p. 176, or nicardipine hydrochloride p. 175) should be avoided in patients who have heart failure with reduced ejection fraction as these drugs reduce cardiac contractility. Patients with heart failure and angina may safely be treated with amlodipine p. 170.

Diuretics are recommended for the relief of breathlessness and oedema in patients with fluid retention. Loop diuretics such as furosemide p. 243, bumetanide p. 242, or torasemide p. 244 are usually the diuretics of choice. Thiazide diuretics may only be of benefit in patients with mild fluid retention and an eGFR greater than 30 mL/minute/1.73 m². Diuretic doses should be titrated according to clinical response and adjusted if needed following the initiation of subsequent heart failure treatments, to minimise the risk of dehydration, renal impairment or hypotension. If symptoms persist despite optimal titration, advice from a heart failure specialist should be sought.

An angiotensin-converting enzyme (ACE) inhibitor (e.g. perindopril, ramipril p. 186, captopril p. 182, enalapril maleate p. 182, lisinopril p. 184, quinapril p. 186 or fosinopril sodium p. 183) and a beta-blocker licensed for heart failure (e.g. bisoprolol fumarate p. 167, carvedilol p. 162, or nebivolol p. 169) should be given as first-line treatment to reduce morbidity and mortality. Treatment with a beta-blocker should not be withheld because of age or the presence of diabetes, chronic obstructive pulmonary disease, peripheral vascular disease, erectile dysfunction, or interstitial pulmonary disease. Patients who are already taking a beta-blocker for co-morbidities (e.g. angina or hypertension) and whose condition is stable should be switched to a beta-blocker licensed for heart failure. Clinical judgement should be used when deciding whether to start an ACE inhibitor or beta blocker first. The additional drug should only be initiated when the patient is stable on their existing treatment. Treatment should be initiated at a low dose and slowly titrated up to the maximum tolerated dose. An angiotensin II receptor blocker (ARB) licensed for heart failure (e.g. candesartan cilexetil p. 189, losartan potassium p. 190, or valsartan p. 193) can be considered if ACE inhibitors are not tolerated.

If heart failure symptoms persist or worsen despite optimal first-line treatment, an aldosterone antagonist such as spironolactone p. 208 or eplerenone p. 208 should be offered as add-on therapy unless contra-indicated (e.g. due to hyperkalaemia or renal impairment). Hydralazine hydrochloride p. 194 combined with a nitrate can be considered under the advice of a heart failure specialist in patients who are intolerant of both ACE inhibitors and ARBs (in particular those of African or Caribbean origin with moderate to severe heart failure).

If symptoms persist despite optimal treatment, advice from a heart failure specialist should be sought on the use of amiodarone hydrochloride p. 113, digoxin p. 117, sacubitril with valsartan p. 209, or ivabradine p. 227.

For patients in sinus rhythm, digoxin is recommended as add-on therapy in worsening or severe heart failure despite optimal treatment. Although digoxin does not reduce mortality, it may decrease symptoms and hospitalisation due to acute exacerbations. Routine monitoring of serum levels is not recommended in patients with heart failure. Anticoagulation should also be considered for patients in sinus rhythm with heart failure if they have a history of thromboembolism, left ventricular aneurysm or intracardiac thrombus. ⟨A⟩ For guidance in patients with atrial fibrillation see Arrhythmias p. 107.

Monitoring drug treatment
EvGr When initiating ACE inhibitors, ARBs and aldosterone antagonists, serum potassium and sodium, renal function, and blood pressure should be checked prior to starting treatment, 1-2 weeks after starting treatment, and at each dose increment. Once the target, or maximum tolerated dose is achieved, treatment should be monitored monthly for 3 months and then at least every 6 months, and if the patient becomes acutely unwell.

When initiating beta blockers, heart rate, blood pressure and symptom control should be assessed at the start of treatment and after each dose change.

In patients with chronic kidney disease, lower doses and slower dose titrations of ACE inhibitors, ARBs, aldosterone

antagonists and digoxin should be considered. Advice from a renal specialist should be considered where appropriate. ⟨A⟩

Chronic heart failure with preserved ejection fraction
EvGr Patients with heart failure and preserved ejection fraction should be managed under the care of a heart failure specialist. For the relief of fluid retention symptoms, a low to medium dose loop diuretic should be prescribed. If the patient fails to respond to treatment, advice from a heart failure specialist should be sought. ⟨A⟩

Advanced heart failure
Breathlessness is a common symptom in advanced heart failure and may occur even with optimal management and in the absence of clinical pulmonary oedema. EvGr Long-term oxygen therapy is not recommended in advanced heart failure, although it may be considered in patients with heart failure and additional co-morbidities that would benefit from oxygen therapy such as chronic obstructive pulmonary disease. ⟨A⟩

Advanced Pharmacy Services
Patients with heart failure may be eligible for the Medicines Use Review service provided by a community pharmacist. For further information, see *Advanced Pharmacy Services* in Medicines optimisation p. 18.

Useful Resources

Chronic heart failure in adults: diagnosis and management. National Institute of Health and Care Excellence. Clinical guideline 106. September 2018.
www.nice.org.uk/guidance/ng106

Management of chronic heart failure. Scottish Intercollegiate Guidelines Network. Clinical guideline 147. March 2016. www.sign.ac.uk/assets/sign1472.pdf

> **Other drugs used for Heart failure** Bendroflumethiazide, p. 180 · Chlortalidone, p. 246 · Co-amilozide, p. 180 · Glyceryl trinitrate, p. 233 · Isosorbide dinitrate, p. 235 · Isosorbide mononitrate, p. 236 · Metoprolol tartrate, p. 169 · Perindopril arginine, p. 185 · Perindopril erbumine, p. 185 · Prazosin, p. 829 · Sodium nitroprusside, p. 196

DIURETICS > POTASSIUM-SPARING DIURETICS > ALDOSTERONE ANTAGONISTS

Co-flumactone

The properties listed below are those particular to the combination only. For the properties of the components please consider, spironolactone p. 208.

● **INDICATIONS AND DOSE**
Congestive heart failure
▶ BY MOUTH
▶ Adult: Initially 100/100 mg daily; maintenance 25/25–200/200 mg daily, maintenance dose not recommended because spironolactone generally given in lower dose

● INTERACTIONS → Appendix 1: aldosterone antagonists · thiazide diuretics

● LESS SUITABLE FOR PRESCRIBING Co-flumactone tablets are less suitable for prescribing.

● MEDICINAL FORMS There can be variation in the licensing of different medicines containing the same drug.
Tablet
▶ Aldactide (Pfizer Ltd)
  Hydroflumethiazide 25 mg, Spironolactone 25 mg Aldactide 25 tablets | 100 tablet [PoM] £20.23 DT = £20.23
  Hydroflumethiazide 50 mg, Spironolactone 50 mg Aldactide 50 tablets | 28 tablet [PoM] £10.70 | 100 tablet [PoM] £38.23 DT = £38.23

Eplerenone

11-Dec-2020

● INDICATIONS AND DOSE

Adjunct in stable patients with left ventricular ejection fraction ≤40% with evidence of heart failure, following myocardial infarction (start therapy within 3–14 days of event) | Adjunct in chronic mild heart failure with left ventricular ejection fraction ≤30%

▸ BY MOUTH
▸ Adult: Initially 25 mg daily, then increased to 50 mg daily, increased within 4 weeks of initial treatment

DOSE ADJUSTMENTS DUE TO INTERACTIONS
▸ Manufacturer advises max. dose 25 mg daily with concurrent use of amiodarone or moderate inhibitors of CYP3A4.

● CONTRA-INDICATIONS Hyperkalaemia

● CAUTIONS
▸ Elderly For aldosterone antagonists, prescription potentially inappropriate (STOPP criteria) with concurrent potassium-conserving drugs without monitoring of serum potassium (risk of dangerous hyperkalaemia).
    See also Prescribing in the elderly p. 33.

● INTERACTIONS → Appendix 1: aldosterone antagonists

● SIDE-EFFECTS
▸ **Common or very common** Arrhythmias · asthenia · constipation · cough · diarrhoea · dizziness · dyslipidaemia · electrolyte imbalance · headache · insomnia · muscle spasms · nausea · pain · renal impairment · skin reactions · syncope · vomiting
▸ **Uncommon** Angioedema · arterial thrombosis · cholecystitis · eosinophilia · flatulence · gynaecomastia · hyperhidrosis · hypothyroidism · increased risk of infection · malaise · numbness · postural hypotension

● PREGNANCY Manufacturer advises caution—no information available.

● BREAST FEEDING Manufacturer advises use only if potential benefit outweighs risk.

● HEPATIC IMPAIRMENT Manufacturer advises avoid in severe impairment (no information available).

● RENAL IMPAIRMENT Avoid if eGFR less than 30 mL/minute/1.73 m^2.
Dose adjustments Initially 25 mg on alternate days if eGFR 30–60 mL/minute/1.73 m^2, adjust dose according to serum-potassium concentration—consult product literature.
Monitoring Increased risk of hyperkalaemia in renal impairment—close monitoring required.

● MONITORING REQUIREMENTS Monitor plasma-potassium concentration before treatment, during initiation, and when dose changed.

● MEDICINAL FORMS There can be variation in the licensing of different medicines containing the same drug.
Tablet
▸ Eplerenone (Non-proprietary)
    Eplerenone 25 mg Eplerenone 25mg tablets | 28 tablet [PoM]
    £42.72 DT = £4.55 | 30 tablet [PoM] £24.95
    Eplerenone 50 mg Eplerenone 50mg tablets | 28 tablet [PoM]
    £42.72 DT = £5.25 | 30 tablet [PoM] £24.95
▸ Inspra (Upjohn UK Ltd)
    Eplerenone 25 mg Inspra 25mg tablets | 28 tablet [PoM] £42.72 DT
    = £4.55
    Eplerenone 50 mg Inspra 50mg tablets | 28 tablet [PoM] £42.72 DT
    = £5.25

Spironolactone

11-Dec-2020

● INDICATIONS AND DOSE

Oedema | Ascites in cirrhosis of the liver
▸ BY MOUTH
▸ Adult: 100–400 mg daily, adjusted according to response

Malignant ascites
▸ BY MOUTH
▸ Adult: Initially 100–200 mg daily, then increased if necessary to 400 mg daily, maintenance dose adjusted according to response

Nephrotic syndrome
▸ BY MOUTH
▸ Adult: 100–200 mg daily

Oedema in congestive heart failure
▸ BY MOUTH
▸ Adult: Initially 100 mg daily, alternatively initially 25–200 mg daily, dose may be taken as a single dose or divided doses, maintenance dose adjusted according to response

Moderate to severe heart failure (adjunct)
▸ BY MOUTH
▸ Adult: Initially 25 mg once daily, then adjusted according to response to 50 mg once daily

Resistant hypertension (adjunct)
▸ BY MOUTH
▸ Adult: 25 mg once daily

Primary hyperaldosteronism in patients awaiting surgery
▸ BY MOUTH
▸ Adult: 100–400 mg daily, may be used for long-term maintenance if surgery inappropriate, use lowest effective dose

● UNLICENSED USE Resistant hypertension (adjunct) unlicensed indication.

● CONTRA-INDICATIONS Addison's disease · anuria · hyperkalaemia

● CAUTIONS Acute porphyrias p. 1107 · elderly · *rodent* studies indicate potential carcinogenic risk

CAUTIONS, FURTHER INFORMATION
▸ Elderly For aldosterone antagonists, prescription potentially inappropriate (STOPP criteria) with concurrent potassium-conserving drugs without monitoring of serum potassium (risk of dangerous hyperkalaemia).
    See also Prescribing in the elderly p. 33.

● INTERACTIONS → Appendix 1: aldosterone antagonists

● SIDE-EFFECTS Acidosis hyperchloraemic · acute kidney injury · agranulocytosis · alopecia · breast neoplasm benign · breast pain · confusion · dizziness · electrolyte imbalance · gastrointestinal disorder · gynaecomastia · hepatic function abnormal · hyperkalaemia (discontinue) · hypertrichosis · leg cramps · leucopenia · libido disorder · malaise · menstrual disorder · nausea · severe cutaneous adverse reactions (SCARs) · skin reactions · thrombocytopenia

● PREGNANCY Use only if potential benefit outweighs risk—feminisation of male fetus in *animal* studies.

● BREAST FEEDING Metabolites present in milk, but amount probably too small to be harmful.

● RENAL IMPAIRMENT Avoid in acute renal insufficiency or severe impairment.
Monitoring Monitor plasma-potassium concentration (high risk of hyperkalaemia in renal impairment).

● MONITORING REQUIREMENTS Monitor electrolytes—discontinue if hyperkalaemia occurs (in *severe heart failure* monitor potassium and creatinine 1 week after initiation and after any dose increase, monthly for first 3 months, then every 3 months for 1 year, and then every 6 months).

- MEDICINAL FORMS There can be variation in the licensing of different medicines containing the same drug. Forms available from special-order manufacturers include: oral suspension, oral solution

Tablet

CAUTIONARY AND ADVISORY LABELS 21

- Spironolactone (Non-proprietary)

Spironolactone 25 mg Spironolactone 25mg tablets | 28 tablet [PoM] £1.95 DT = £1.44 | 500 tablet [PoM] £25.54

Spironolactone 50 mg Spironolactone 50mg tablets | 28 tablet [PoM] £9.99 DT = £4.40 | 250 tablet [PoM] £39.20

Spironolactone 100 mg Spironolactone 100mg tablets | 28 tablet [PoM] £2.96 DT = £2.36 | 250 tablet [PoM] £20.98

- Aldactone (Pfizer Ltd)

Spironolactone 25 mg Aldactone 25mg tablets | 100 tablet [PoM] £8.89

Spironolactone 50 mg Aldactone 50mg tablets | 100 tablet [PoM] £17.78

Spironolactone 100 mg Aldactone 100mg tablets | 28 tablet [PoM] £9.96 DT = £2.36 | 100 tablet [PoM] £35.56

DRUGS ACTING ON THE RENIN-ANGIOTENSIN SYSTEM > ANGIOTENSIN II RECEPTOR ANTAGONISTS

Sacubitril with valsartan   06-Feb-2019

The properties listed below are those particular to the combination only. For the properties of the components please consider, valsartan p. 193.

- DRUG ACTION Sacubitril (a prodrug) inhibits the breakdown of natriuretic peptides resulting in varied effects including increased diuresis, natriuresis, and vasodilation.

● **INDICATIONS AND DOSE**

Symptomatic chronic heart failure with reduced ejection fraction (in patients not currently taking an ACE inhibitor or angiotensin II receptor antagonist, or stabilised on low doses of either of these agents)
▸ BY MOUTH
▸ Adult: Initially 24/26 mg twice daily for 3–4 weeks, increased if tolerated to 49/51 mg twice daily for 3–4 weeks, then increased if tolerated to 97/103 mg twice daily

Symptomatic chronic heart failure with reduced ejection fraction (in patients currently stabilised on an ACE inhibitor or angiotensin II receptor antagonist)
▸ BY MOUTH
▸ Adult: Initially 49/51 mg twice daily for 2–4 weeks, increased if tolerated to 97/103 mg twice daily, consider a starting dose of 24/26 mg if systolic blood pressure less than 110 mmHg

DOSE EQUIVALENCE AND CONVERSION
- *Entresto*® tablets contain sacubitril and valsartan; the proportions are expressed in the form x/y where x and y are the strength in milligrams of sacubitril and valsartan respectively. Valsartan, in this formulation, is more bioavailable than other tablet formulations— 26 mg, 51 mg, and 103 mg valsartan is equivalent to 40 mg, 80 mg and 160 mg, respectively. Furthermore, note that the 24/26 mg, 49/51 mg and 97/103 mg strengths are sometimes referred to as a total of both drug strengths, that is, 50 mg, 100 mg and 200 mg, respectively.

- CONTRA-INDICATIONS Concomitant use with an ACE inhibitor (do not initiate until at least 36 hours after discontinuing ACE inhibitor—risk of angioedema) · concomitant use with an angiotensin II receptor antagonist · systolic blood pressure less than 100 mmHg
- INTERACTIONS → Appendix 1: angiotensin-II receptor antagonists · sacubitril

- SIDE-EFFECTS
▸ **Common or very common** Anaemia · asthenia · cough · diarrhoea · dizziness · electrolyte imbalance · gastritis · headache · hypoglycaemia · hypotension · nausea · renal impairment · syncope · vertigo
▸ **Uncommon** Angioedema · skin reactions
- PREGNANCY Manufacturer advises avoid—toxicity with sacubitril in *animal* studies.
- BREAST FEEDING Manufacturer advises avoid—present in milk in *animal* studies.
- HEPATIC IMPAIRMENT Manufacturer advises caution in moderate impairment or if hepatic transaminases exceed 2 times the upper limit of normal (limited information available); avoid in severe impairment, biliary cirrhosis or cholestasis (no information available).
  Dose adjustments Manufacturer advises initial dose reduction to 24/26 mg twice daily in moderate impairment or if hepatic transaminases exceed 2 times the upper limit of normal.
- RENAL IMPAIRMENT
  Dose adjustments Manufacturer recommends a starting dose of 24/26 mg twice daily if eGFR less than 30 mL/minute/1.73m^2. Also consider this starting dose if eGFR 30 to 60 mL/minute/1.73m^2.
- NATIONAL FUNDING/ACCESS DECISIONS
  For full details see funding body website
  NICE decisions
▸ Sacubitril valsartan for treating symptomatic chronic heart failure with reduced ejection fraction (April 2016) NICE TA388 Recommended with restrictions

- MEDICINAL FORMS There can be variation in the licensing of different medicines containing the same drug.
Tablet
▸ Entresto (Novartis Pharmaceuticals UK Ltd)
  Sacubitril 24 mg, Valsartan 26 mg Entresto 24mg/26mg tablets | 28 tablet [PoM] £45.78 DT = £45.78
  Sacubitril 49 mg, Valsartan 51 mg Entresto 49mg/51mg tablets | 28 tablet [PoM] £45.78 | 56 tablet [PoM] £91.56 DT = £91.56
  Sacubitril 97 mg, Valsartan 103 mg Entresto 97mg/103mg tablets | 56 tablet [PoM] £91.56 DT = £91.56

PHOSPHODIESTERASE TYPE-3 INHIBITORS

Enoximone   10-Mar-2020

- DRUG ACTION Enoximone is a phosphodiesterase type-3 inhibitor that exerts most effect on the myocardium; it has positive inotropic properties and vasodilator activity.

● **INDICATIONS AND DOSE**

Congestive heart failure where cardiac output reduced and filling pressures increased
▸ BY SLOW INTRAVENOUS INJECTION
▸ Adult: Initially 0.5–1 mg/kg, rate not exceeding 12.5 mg/minute, then 500 micrograms/kg every 30 minutes until satisfactory response or total of 3 mg/kg given; maintenance, initial dose of up to 3 mg/kg may be repeated every 3–6 hours as required
▸ BY INTRAVENOUS INFUSION
▸ Adult: Initially 90 micrograms/kg/minute, dose to be given over 10–30 minutes, followed by 5–20 micrograms/kg/minute, dose to be given as either a continuous or intermittent infusion; maximum 24 mg/kg per day

- CAUTIONS Heart failure associated with hypertrophic cardiomyopathy, stenotic or obstructive valvular disease or other outlet obstruction
- SIDE-EFFECTS
▸ **Common or very common** Headache · hypotension · insomnia

Cardiovascular system

▶ **Uncommon** Arrhythmias · diarrhoea · dizziness · nausea · vomiting
▶ **Rare or very rare** Chills · fever · fluid retention · myalgia · oliguria · urinary retention
● PREGNANCY Manufacturer advises use only if potential benefit outweighs risk.
● BREAST FEEDING Manufacturer advises caution—no information available.
● RENAL IMPAIRMENT
Dose adjustments Consider dose reduction.
● MONITORING REQUIREMENTS Monitor blood pressure, heart rate, ECG, central venous pressure, fluid and electrolyte status, renal function, platelet count and hepatic enzymes.
● DIRECTIONS FOR ADMINISTRATION Incompatible with glucose solutions. Use only plastic containers or syringes; crystal formation if glass used. Avoid extravasation.
    For *intravenous infusion* (*Perfan*®), give continuously or intermittently in Sodium chloride 0.9% or Water for injections; dilute to a concentration of 2.5 mg/mL.
● PRESCRIBING AND DISPENSING INFORMATION Sustained haemodynamic benefit has been observed after administration of phosphodiesterase type-3 inhibitors, but there is no evidence of any beneficial effect on survival.

● MEDICINAL FORMS There can be variation in the licensing of different medicines containing the same drug.
Solution for injection
EXCIPIENTS: May contain Alcohol, propylene glycol
▶ Perfan (Carinopharm GmbH)
Enoximone 5 mg per 1 ml Perfan 100mg/20ml solution for injection ampoules | 10 ampoule PoM ⟨S⟩ (Hospital only)

Milrinone

27-Jan-2020

● DRUG ACTION Milrinone is a phosphodiesterase type-3 inhibitor that exerts most effect on the myocardium; it has positive inotropic properties and vasodilator activity.

● INDICATIONS AND DOSE
Short-term treatment of severe congestive heart failure unresponsive to conventional maintenance therapy (not immediately after myocardial infarction) | Acute heart failure, including low output states following heart surgery
▶ INITIALLY BY INTRAVENOUS INJECTION
▶ Adult: Initially 50 micrograms/kg, given over 10 minutes, followed by (by intravenous infusion) 375–750 nanograms/kg/minute usually given following surgery for up to 12 hours or in congestive heart failure for 48-72 hours; maximum 1.13 mg/kg per day

● CONTRA-INDICATIONS Severe hypovolaemia
● CAUTIONS Correct hypokalaemia · heart failure associated with hypertrophic cardiomyopathy, stenotic or obstructive valvular disease or other outlet obstruction
● SIDE-EFFECTS
▶ **Common or very common** Arrhythmia supraventricular (increased risk in patients with pre-existing arrhythmias) · arrhythmias · headache · hypotension
▶ **Uncommon** Angina pectoris · chest pain · hypokalaemia · thrombocytopenia · tremor
▶ **Rare or very rare** Anaphylactic shock · bronchospasm · skin eruption
▶ **Frequency not known** Renal failure
● PREGNANCY Manufacturer advises use only if potential benefit outweighs risk.
● BREAST FEEDING Manufacturer advises avoid—no information available.

● RENAL IMPAIRMENT
Dose adjustments Reduce dose and monitor response if eGFR less than 50 mL/minute/1.73 m² —consult product literature for details.
● MONITORING REQUIREMENTS Monitor blood pressure, heart rate, ECG, central venous pressure, fluid and electrolyte status, renal function, platelet count and hepatic enzymes.
● DIRECTIONS FOR ADMINISTRATION Avoid extravasation.
    For *intravenous injection*, may be given either undiluted or diluted before use.
    For *intravenous infusion* (*Primacor*®) give continuously in Glucose 5% or Sodium chloride 0.9%; dilute to a suggested concentration of 200 micrograms/mL.
● PRESCRIBING AND DISPENSING INFORMATION Sustained haemodynamic benefit has been observed after administration of phosphodiesterase type-3 inhibitors, but there is no evidence of any beneficial effect on survival.

● MEDICINAL FORMS There can be variation in the licensing of different medicines containing the same drug. Forms available from special-order manufacturers include: solution for infusion
Solution for infusion
▶ Milrinone (Non-proprietary)
Milrinone 1 mg per 1 ml Milrinone 10mg/10ml solution for infusion ampoules | 5 ampoule PoM £35.00 | 10 ampoule PoM £199.06
Milrinone 10mg/10ml concentrate for solution for infusion ampoules | 10 ampoule PoM ⟨S⟩
▶ Primacor (Sanofi)
Milrinone 1 mg per 1 ml Primacor 10mg/10ml solution for injection ampoules | 10 ampoule PoM £199.06

7   Hyperlipidaemia

Dyslipidaemias

23-Mar-2018

Hypercholesterolaemia and hypertriglyceridaemia

Statins are the drugs of first choice for treating hypercholesterolaemia and moderate hypertriglyceridaemia. Severe hypercholesterolaemia or hypertriglyceridaemia not adequately controlled with a maximal dose of a statin may require the use of an additional lipid-regulating drug such as ezetimibe p. 212; such treatment should generally be supervised by a specialist.

A number of conditions, some familial, are characterised by very high LDL-cholesterol concentration, high triglyceride concentration, or both. Although statins are more effective than other lipid-regulating drugs at lowering LDL-cholesterol concentration, they are less effective than fibrates in reducing triglyceride concentration. Fenofibrate p. 214 may be added to statin therapy if triglycerides remain high even after the LDL-cholesterol concentration has been reduced adequately.

Familial hypercholesterolaemia

Patients with familial hypercholesterolaemia are at high risk of premature coronary heart disease. EvGr Lifelong lipid-modifying therapy and advice on lifestyle changes should be offered to all patients with familial hypercholesterolaemia.

A high-intensity statin, defined as the dose at which a reduction in LDL-cholesterol of greater than 40% is achieved, is recommended as first-line therapy in all patients with familial hypercholesterolaemia. The dose of the statin should be titrated to achieve a reduction in LDL-cholesterol concentration of greater than 50% from baseline.

Patients with primary *heterozygous familial hypercholesterolaemia* who have contra-indications to, or are intolerant of statins, can be considered for treatment with ezetimibe as monotherapy. A combination of a statin and ezetimibe is recommended if the maximum tolerated dose of a statin alone fails to provide adequate control of LDL-cholesterol, or a switch to an alternative statin is being considered. Treatment with a fibrate or a bile acid sequestrant (such as colestyramine p. 212 or colestipol hydrochloride p. 212) can be considered under specialist advice, in patients for whom statins or ezetimibe are inappropriate.

The combination of a statin with a fibrate carries an increased risk of muscle-related side-effects (including rhabdomyolysis) and should be used under specialist supervision. The concomitant administration of gemfibrozil with a statin increases the risk of rhabdomyolysis considerably—this combination should not be used.

Alirocumab p. 221 and evolocumab p. 222 can be considered for patients with primary heterozygous familial hypercholesterolaemia whose LDL-cholesterol has not been adequately controlled on maximum tolerated lipid-lowering therapy. ⟨A⟩ See National funding/access decisions information for alirocumab p. 221 and evolocumab p. 222.

[EvGr] The prescribing of drug therapy in *homozygous familial hypercholesterolaemia* should be undertaken in a specialist centre. ⟨A⟩

Reduction in low-density lipoprotein cholesterol

Therapy intensity	Drug	Daily dose (reduction in LDL cholesterol)
High-intensity	Atorvastatin	20 mg (43%)
		40 mg (49%)
		80 mg (55%)
	Rosuvastatin	10 mg (43%)
		20 mg (48%)
		40 mg (53%)
	Simvastatin	80 mg (42%)
Medium-intensity	Atorvastatin	10 mg (37%)
	Fluvastatin	80 mg (33%)
	Rosuvastatin	5 mg (38%)
	Simvastatin	20 mg (32%)
		40 mg (37%)
Low-intensity	Fluvastatin	20 mg (21%)
		40 mg (27%)
	Pravastatin	10 mg (20%)
		20 mg (24%)
		40 mg (29%)
	Simvastatin	10 mg (27%)

Advice from the MHRA: there is an increased risk of myopathy associated with high-dose (80 mg) simvastatin. The 80 mg dose should be considered only in patients with severe hypercholesterolaemia and high risk of cardiovascular complications who have not achieved their treatment goals on lower doses, when the benefits are expected to outweigh the potential risks.

Other drugs used for Hyperlipidaemia Inositol nicotinate, p. 248

LIPID MODIFYING DRUGS 〉 BILE ACID SEQUESTRANTS

Bile acid sequestrants

- **DRUG ACTION** Bile acid sequestrants act by binding bile acids, preventing their reabsorption; this promotes hepatic conversion of cholesterol into bile acids; the resultant increased LDL-receptor activity of liver cells increases the clearance of LDL-cholesterol from the plasma.

- **CAUTIONS** Interference with the absorption of fat-soluble vitamins (supplements of vitamins A, D, K, and folic acid may be required when treatment is prolonged).

- **SIDE-EFFECTS**
- ► **Common or very common** Constipation · gastrointestinal discomfort · headache · nausea · vomiting
- ► **Uncommon** Appetite decreased · diarrhoea · gastrointestinal disorders

- **PREGNANCY** Bile acid sequestrants should be used with caution as although the drugs are not absorbed, they may cause fat-soluble vitamin deficiency on prolonged use.

- **BREAST FEEDING** Bile acid sequestrants should be used with caution as although the drugs are not absorbed, they may cause fat-soluble vitamin deficiency on prolonged use.

⌐ above

Colesevelam hydrochloride   04-Feb-2020

- **INDICATIONS AND DOSE**

Primary hypercholesterolaemia as an adjunct to dietary measures [monotherapy]
- ► BY MOUTH
  - ► Adult: 3.75 g daily in 1–2 divided doses; maximum 4.375 g per day

Primary hypercholesterolaemia as an adjunct to dietary measures [in combination with a statin] | Primary and familial hypercholesterolaemia [in combination with ezetimibe, either with or without a statin]
- ► BY MOUTH
  - ► Adult: 2.5–3.75 g daily in 1–2 divided doses, may be taken at the same time as the statin and ezetimibe

Bile acid malabsorption
- ► BY MOUTH
  - ► Adult: 1.25–3.75 g daily in 2–3 divided doses

- **UNLICENSED USE** [EvGr] Colesevelam is used for the treatment of bile acid malabsorption, ⟨D⟩ but is not licensed for this indication.

- **CONTRA-INDICATIONS** Biliary obstruction · bowel obstruction

- **CAUTIONS** Gastro-intestinal motility disorders · inflammatory bowel disease · major gastro-intestinal surgery

- **INTERACTIONS** → Appendix 1: colesevelam

- **SIDE-EFFECTS**
- ► **Uncommon** Dysphagia · myalgia
- ► **Rare or very rare** Pancreatitis

- **HEPATIC IMPAIRMENT** Manufacturer advises caution in hepatic failure (no information available).

- **MONITORING REQUIREMENTS** Patients receiving ciclosporin should have their blood-ciclosporin concentration monitored before, during, and after treatment with colesevelam.

- **PATIENT AND CARER ADVICE** Patient counselling on administration is advised for colesevelam hydrochloride tablets (avoid other drugs at same time).

- **MEDICINAL FORMS** There can be variation in the licensing of different medicines containing the same drug.

Tablet
CAUTIONARY AND ADVISORY LABELS 21
- ► Cholestagel (Sanofi)
  Colesevelam hydrochloride 625 mg Cholestagel 625mg tablets | 180 tablet [PoM] £115.32 DT = £115.32

Colestipol hydrochloride

F 211

20-Jul-2020

- **INDICATIONS AND DOSE**

Hyperlipidaemias, particularly type IIa, in patients who have not responded adequately to diet and other appropriate measures
- ▸ BY MOUTH
- ▸ Adult: Initially 5 g 1–2 times a day, increased in steps of 5 g every month if required, total daily dose may be given in 1–2 divided doses; maximum 30 g per day

- **INTERACTIONS** → Appendix 1: colestipol
- **SIDE-EFFECTS** Angina pectoris · arthralgia · arthritis · asthenia · burping · chest pain · dizziness · dyspnoea · gallbladder disorders · headaches · inflammation · insomnia · pain · peptic ulcer haemorrhage · tachycardia
- **DIRECTIONS FOR ADMINISTRATION** Manufacturer advises the contents of each sachet should be mixed with at least 100 mL of water or other suitable liquid such as fruit juice or skimmed milk; alternatively it can be mixed with thin soups, cereals, yoghurt, or pulpy fruits ensuring at least 100 mL of liquid is provided.
- **PATIENT AND CARER ADVICE** Patient counselling on administration is advised for colestipol hydrochloride granules (avoid other drugs at same time).

- **MEDICINAL FORMS** There can be variation in the licensing of different medicines containing the same drug. Forms available from special-order manufacturers include: tablet

Granules
CAUTIONARY AND ADVISORY LABELS 13
- ▸ Colestid (Pfizer Ltd)
  Colestipol hydrochloride 5 gram Colestid 5g granules sachets plain sugar-free | 30 sachet [PoM] £15.05 DT = £15.05
  Colestid Orange 5g granules sachets sugar-free | 30 sachet [PoM] £15.05 DT = £15.05

Tablet
- ▸ Colestid (Imported (Canada))
  Colestipol hydrochloride 1 gram Colestid 1g tablets | 120 tablet [PoM] 🚫

Colestyramine

F 211

20-Jul-2020

(Cholestyramine)

- **INDICATIONS AND DOSE**

Hyperlipidaemias, particularly type IIa, in patients who have not responded adequately to diet and other appropriate measures | Primary prevention of coronary heart disease in men aged 35–59 years with primary hypercholesterolaemia who have not responded to diet and other appropriate measures
- ▸ BY MOUTH
- ▸ Adult: Initially 4 g daily, increased in steps of 4 g every week; increased to 12–24 g daily in 1–4 divided doses, adjusted according to response; maximum 36 g per day

Pruritus associated with partial biliary obstruction and primary biliary cirrhosis
- ▸ BY MOUTH
- ▸ Adult: 4–8 g once daily

Diarrhoea associated with Crohn's disease, ileal resection, vagotomy, diabetic vagal neuropathy, and radiation
- ▸ BY MOUTH
- ▸ Adult: Initially 4 g daily, increased in steps of 4 g every week; increased to 12–24 g daily in 1–4 divided doses, adjusted according to response, if no response within 3 days an alternative therapy should be initiated; maximum 36 g per day

Accelerated elimination of teriflunomide
- ▸ BY MOUTH
- ▸ Adult: 8 g 3 times a day for 11 days; reduced to 4 g 3 times a day, dose should only be reduced if not tolerated

Accelerated elimination of leflunomide (washout procedure)
- ▸ BY MOUTH
- ▸ Adult: 8 g 3 times a day for 11 days

- **CONTRA-INDICATIONS** Complete biliary obstruction (not likely to be effective)
- **INTERACTIONS** → Appendix 1: colestyramine
- **SIDE-EFFECTS**
- ▸ **Uncommon** Bleeding tendency · hypoprothrombinaemia · night blindness · osteoporosis · skin reactions · tongue irritation · vitamin deficiencies
- **DIRECTIONS FOR ADMINISTRATION** Manufacturer advises the contents of each sachet should be mixed with at least 150 mL of water or other suitable liquid such as fruit juice, skimmed milk, thin soups, and pulpy fruits with a high moisture content.
- **PATIENT AND CARER ADVICE** Patient counselling on administration is advised for colestyramine powder (avoid other drugs at same time).

- **MEDICINAL FORMS** There can be variation in the licensing of different medicines containing the same drug. Forms available from special-order manufacturers include: oral suspension, oral solution

Powder
CAUTIONARY AND ADVISORY LABELS 13
EXCIPIENTS: May contain Aspartame, sucrose
- ▸ Colestyramine (Non-proprietary)
  Colestyramine anhydrous 4 gram Colestyramine 4g oral powder sachets sugar free sugar-free | 50 sachet [PoM] £33.30 DT = £33.28
- ▸ Questran (Cheplapharm Arzneimittel GmbH)
  Colestyramine anhydrous 4 gram Questran 4g oral powder sachets | 50 sachet [PoM] £10.76 DT = £10.76
- ▸ Questran Light (Cheplapharm Arzneimittel GmbH)
  Colestyramine anhydrous 4 gram Questran Light 4g oral powder sachets sugar-free | 50 sachet [PoM] £16.15 DT = £33.28

LIPID MODIFYING DRUGS > CHOLESTEROL ABSORPTION INHIBITORS

Ezetimibe

08-Feb-2019

- **DRUG ACTION** Ezetimibe inhibits the intestinal absorption of cholesterol. If used alone, it has a modest effect on lowering LDL-cholesterol, with little effect on other lipoproteins.

- **INDICATIONS AND DOSE**

Adjunct to dietary measures and statin treatment in primary hypercholesterolaemia | Adjunct to dietary measures and statin in homozygous familial hypercholesterolaemia | Primary hypercholesterolaemia (if statin inappropriate or not tolerated) | Adjunct to dietary measures in homozygous sitosterolaemia
- ▸ BY MOUTH
- ▸ Adult: 10 mg daily

- **INTERACTIONS** → Appendix 1: ezetimibe
- **SIDE-EFFECTS**
- ▸ **Common or very common** Asthenia · diarrhoea · gastrointestinal discomfort · gastrointestinal disorders
- ▸ **Uncommon** Appetite decreased · arthralgia · chest pain · cough · hot flush · hypertension · muscle complaints · nausea · pain
- ▸ **Frequency not known** Constipation · depression · dizziness · dyspnoea · hepatitis · myopathy · pancreatitis · paraesthesia · skin reactions · thrombocytopenia

- PREGNANCY Manufacturer advises use only if potential benefit outweighs risk—no information available.
- BREAST FEEDING Manufacturer advises avoid—present in milk in *animal* studies.
- HEPATIC IMPAIRMENT Manufacturer advises avoid in moderate to severe impairment.
- NATIONAL FUNDING/ACCESS DECISIONS
  For full details see funding body website
  NICE decisions
- ▸ **Ezetimibe for treating primary heterozygous-familial and non-familial hypercholesterolaemia (February 2016)** NICE TA385
  Recommended with restrictions

- MEDICINAL FORMS There can be variation in the licensing of different medicines containing the same drug.
  Tablet
  - ▸ Ezetimibe (Non-proprietary)
    Ezetimibe 10 mg Ezetimibe 10mg tablets | 28 tablet PoM £26.31 DT = £2.69
  - ▸ Ezetrol (Merck Sharp & Dohme Ltd)
    Ezetimibe 10 mg Ezetrol 10mg tablets | 28 tablet PoM £26.31 DT = £2.69

  Combinations available: *Bempedoic acid with ezetimibe*, p. 221 · *Simvastatin with ezetimibe*, p. 220

LIPID MODIFYING DRUGS ❭ FIBRATES

Bezafibrate

15-Jan-2020

- DRUG ACTION Fibrates act by decreasing serum triglycerides; they have variable effect on LDL-cholestrol.

- ● INDICATIONS AND DOSE

  Adjunct to diet and other appropriate measures in mixed hyperlipidaemia if statin contra-indicated or not tolerated | Adjunct to diet and other appropriate measures in severe hypertriglyceridaemia
  - ▸ BY MOUTH USING IMMEDIATE-RELEASE MEDICINES
  - ▸ Adult: 200 mg 3 times a day
  - ▸ BY MOUTH USING MODIFIED-RELEASE MEDICINES
  - ▸ Adult: 400 mg once daily, modified-release dose form is not appropriate in patients with renal impairment

- CONTRA-INDICATIONS Gall bladder disease · hypoalbuminaemia · nephrotic syndrome · photosensitivity to fibrates
- CAUTIONS Correct hypothyroidism before initiating treatment · risk factors for myopathy
- INTERACTIONS → Appendix 1: fibrates
- SIDE-EFFECTS
- ▸ **Common or very common** Appetite decreased · gastrointestinal disorder
- ▸ **Uncommon** Acute kidney injury · alopecia · cholestasis · constipation · diarrhoea · dizziness · erectile dysfunction · gastrointestinal discomfort · headache · muscle complaints · muscle weakness · nausea · photosensitivity reaction · skin reactions
- ▸ **Rare or very rare** Cholelithiasis · depression · insomnia · interstitial lung disease · pancreatitis · pancytopenia · paraesthesia · peripheral neuropathy · rhabdomyolysis (increased risk in renal impairment) · severe cutaneous adverse reactions (SCARs) · thrombocytopenic purpura
- PREGNANCY Manufacturers advise avoid—no information available.
- BREAST FEEDING Manufacturer advises avoid—no information available.
- HEPATIC IMPAIRMENT Manufacturer advises avoid in significant impairment (except in fatty liver disease).
- RENAL IMPAIRMENT Avoid *immediate-release* preparations if eGFR less than 15 mL/minute/1.73 m^2.

Avoid *modified-release* preparations if eGFR less than 60 mL/minute/1.73 m^2.
Myotoxicity Special care needed in patients with renal disease, as progressive increases in serum creatinine concentration or failure to follow dosage guidelines may result in myotoxicity (rhabdomyolysis); discontinue if myotoxicity suspected or creatine kinase concentration increases significantly.
Dose adjustments Reduce dose to 400 mg daily if eGFR 40–60 mL/minute/1.73 m^2.
Reduce dose to 200 mg every 1–2 days if eGFR 15–40 mL/minute/1.73 m^2.

- MONITORING REQUIREMENTS Consider monitoring of liver function and creatine kinase when fibrates used in combination with a statin.
- PRESCRIBING AND DISPENSING INFORMATION Fibrates are mainly used in those whose serum-triglyceride concentration is greater than 10 mmol/litre or in those who cannot tolerate a statin (specialist use).
- MEDICINAL FORMS There can be variation in the licensing of different medicines containing the same drug. Forms available from special-order manufacturers include: oral suspension
  Modified-release tablet
  CAUTIONARY AND ADVISORY LABELS 21, 25
  - ▸ Bezalip Mono (Teva UK Ltd)
    Bezafibrate 400 mg Bezalip Mono 400mg modified-release tablets | 30 tablet PoM £7.63 DT = £7.63
  - ▸ Fibrazate XL (Sandoz Ltd)
    Bezafibrate 400 mg Fibrazate XL 400mg tablets | 30 tablet PoM £6.87 DT = £6.87
  Tablet
  CAUTIONARY AND ADVISORY LABELS 21
  - ▸ Bezalip (Teva UK Ltd)
    Bezafibrate 200 mg Bezalip 200mg tablets | 100 tablet PoM £8.63 DT = £8.63

Ciprofibrate

15-Jan-2020

- DRUG ACTION Fibrates act by decreasing serum triglycerides; they have variable effect on LDL-cholestrol.

- ● INDICATIONS AND DOSE

  Adjunct to diet and other appropriate measures in mixed hyperlipidaemia if statin contra-indicated or not tolerated | Adjunct to diet and other appropriate measures in severe hypertriglyceridaemia
  - ▸ BY MOUTH
  - ▸ Adult: 100 mg daily

- CONTRA-INDICATIONS Gall bladder disease · hypoalbuminaemia · nephrotic syndrome · photosensitivity to fibrates
- CAUTIONS Correct hypothyroidism before initiating treatment · risk factors for myopathy
- INTERACTIONS → Appendix 1: fibrates
- SIDE-EFFECTS
- ▸ **Common or very common** Alopecia · diarrhoea · dizziness · drowsiness · fatigue · gastrointestinal discomfort · headache · myalgia · nausea · skin reactions · vertigo · vomiting
- ▸ **Frequency not known** Cholelithiasis · erectile dysfunction · hepatic disorders · leucopenia · myopathy · photosensitivity reaction · respiratory disorders · rhabdomyolysis (increased risk in renal impairment) · thrombocytopenia
- PREGNANCY Manufacturers advise avoid—toxicity in *animal* studies.
- BREAST FEEDING Manufacturer advises avoid—present in milk in *animal* studies.

2

Cardiovascular system

● HEPATIC IMPAIRMENT Manufacturer advises use with caution in mild-to-moderate impairment; avoid in severe impairment

● RENAL IMPAIRMENT Avoid in severe impairment. Myotoxicity Special care needed in patients with renal disease, as progressive increases in serum creatinine concentration or failure to follow dosage guidelines may result in myotoxicity (rhabdomyolysis); discontinue if myotoxicity suspected or creatine kinase concentration increases significantly.
Dose adjustments Reduce dose to 100 mg on alternate days in moderate impairment.

● MONITORING REQUIREMENTS
▶ Liver function tests recommended every 3 months for first year (discontinue treatment if significantly raised).
▶ Consider monitoring liver function and creatine kinase when fibrates used in combination with a statin.

● PRESCRIBING AND DISPENSING INFORMATION Fibrates are mainly used in those whose serum-triglyceride concentration is greater than 10 mmol/litre or in those who cannot tolerate a statin (specialist use).

● MEDICINAL FORMS There can be variation in the licensing of different medicines containing the same drug.
Tablet
▶ Ciprofibrate (Non-proprietary)
Ciprofibrate 100 mg Ciprofibrate 100mg tablets | 28 tablet PoM
£134.21 DT = £122.53

Fenofibrate

15-Jan-2020

● DRUG ACTION Fibrates act by decreasing serum triglycerides; they have variable effect on LDL-cholesterol.

● INDICATIONS AND DOSE

Adjunct to diet and other appropriate measures in mixed hyperlipidaemia if statin contra-indicated or not tolerated | Adjunct to diet and other appropriate measures in severe hypertriglyceridaemia | Adjunct to statin in mixed hyperlipidaemia if triglycerides and HDL-cholesterol inadequately controlled in patients at high cardiovascular risk
▶ BY MOUTH USING CAPSULES
▶ Adult: Initially 200 mg daily, then increased if necessary to 267 mg daily, maximum 200 mg daily with concomitant statin, 267 mg capsules not appropriate for initial dose titration
▶ BY MOUTH USING TABLETS
▶ Adult: 160 mg daily

DOSE ADJUSTMENTS DUE TO INTERACTIONS
▶ Manufacturer advises max. dose 200 mg daily with concurrent use of a statin.

● CONTRA-INDICATIONS Gall bladder disease · pancreatitis (unless due to severe hypertriglyceridaemia) · photosensitivity to fibrates · photosensitivity to ketoprofen

● CAUTIONS Correct hypothyroidism before initiating treatment · risk factors for myopathy

● INTERACTIONS → Appendix 1: fibrates

● SIDE-EFFECTS
▶ **Common or very common** Abdominal pain · diarrhoea · flatulence · nausea · vomiting
▶ **Uncommon** Cholelithiasis · embolism and thrombosis · headache · muscle complaints · muscle weakness · myopathy · pancreatitis · sexual dysfunction · skin reactions
▶ **Rare or very rare** Alopecia · hepatic disorders · photosensitivity reaction

▶ **Frequency not known** Fatigue · interstitial lung disease · rhabdomyolysis (increased risk in renal impairment) · severe cutaneous adverse reactions (SCARs)

● PREGNANCY Avoid—embryotoxicity in *animal* studies.

● BREAST FEEDING Manufacturers advise avoid—no information available.

● HEPATIC IMPAIRMENT Manufacturer advises avoid —no information available.

● RENAL IMPAIRMENT Manufacturer advises use with caution in mild-to-moderate impairment; avoid if eGFR less than 30 mL/minute/1.73 m^2.
Myotoxicity Special care needed in patients with renal disease, as progressive increases in serum creatinine concentration or failure to follow dosage guidelines may result in myotoxicity (rhabdomyolysis); discontinue if myotoxicity suspected or creatine kinase concentration increases significantly.
Dose adjustments Manufacturer advises max. 67 mg daily if eGFR 30–59 mL/minute/1.73 m^2.

● MONITORING REQUIREMENTS Manufacturer advises monitor hepatic transaminases every 3 months during the first 12 months of treatment and periodically thereafter—discontinue treatment if levels increase to more than 3 times the upper limit of normal; monitor serum creatinine levels during the first 3 months of treatment and periodically thereafter—interrupt treatment if creatinine level is 50% above the upper limit of normal.

● PRESCRIBING AND DISPENSING INFORMATION Fibrates are mainly used in those whose serum-triglyceride concentration is greater than 10 mmol/litre or in those who cannot tolerate a statin (specialist use).

● MEDICINAL FORMS There can be variation in the licensing of different medicines containing the same drug.
Tablet
CAUTIONARY AND ADVISORY LABELS 21
▶ Fenofibrate (Non-proprietary)
Fenofibrate micronised 160 mg Fenofibrate micronised 160mg tablets | 28 tablet PoM £10.00 DT = £3.98
▶ Supralip (Mylan)
Fenofibrate micronised 160 mg Supralip 160mg tablets | 28 tablet PoM £6.69 DT = £3.98
Capsule
CAUTIONARY AND ADVISORY LABELS 21
▶ Fenofibrate (Non-proprietary)
Fenofibrate micronised 67 mg Fenofibrate micronised 67mg capsules | 90 capsule PoM £23.30 DT = £23.23
Fenofibrate micronised 200 mg Fenofibrate micronised 200mg capsules | 28 capsule PoM £11.98 DT = £3.37
Fenofibrate micronised 267 mg Fenofibrate micronised 267mg capsules | 28 capsule PoM £21.75 DT = £3.67
▶ Lipantil Micro (Mylan)
Fenofibrate micronised 67 mg Lipantil Micro 67 capsules | 90 capsule PoM £23.30 DT = £23.23
Fenofibrate micronised 200 mg Lipantil Micro 200 capsules | 28 capsule PoM £14.23 DT = £3.37
Fenofibrate micronised 267 mg Lipantil Micro 267 capsules | 28 capsule PoM £21.75 DT = £3.67

Combinations available: *Simvastatin with fenofibrate*, p. 220

Gemfibrozil

05-Feb-2020

- **DRUG ACTION** Fibrates act by decreasing serum triglycerides; they have variable effect on LDL-cholesterol.

- ● **INDICATIONS AND DOSE**

  Adjunct to diet and other appropriate measures in mixed hyperlipidaemia if statin contra-indicated or not tolerated | Adjunct to diet and other appropriate measures in primary hypercholesterolaemia if statin contra-indicated or not tolerated | Adjunct to diet and other appropriate measures in severe hypertriglyceridaemia | Adjunct to diet and other appropriate measures in primary prevention of cardiovascular disease in men with hyperlipidaemias if statin contra-indicated or not tolerated
  - ▸ BY MOUTH
  - ▸ Adult: 1.2 g daily in 2 divided doses, maintenance 0.9–1.2 g daily

- ● **CONTRA-INDICATIONS** History of gall-bladder or biliary tract disease including gallstones · photosensitivity to fibrates

- ● **CAUTIONS** Correct hypothyroidism before initiating treatment · elderly · risk factors for myopathy

- ● **INTERACTIONS** → Appendix 1: fibrates

- ● **SIDE-EFFECTS**
  - ▸ **Common or very common** Constipation · diarrhoea · fatigue · flatulence · gastrointestinal discomfort · headache · nausea · skin reactions · vertigo · vomiting
  - ▸ **Uncommon** Atrial fibrillation
  - ▸ **Rare or very rare** Alopecia · anaemia · angioedema · appendicitis · bone marrow failure · depression · dizziness · drowsiness · eosinophilia · gallbladder disorders · hepatic disorders · joint disorders · laryngeal oedema · leucopenia · muscle weakness · myalgia · myopathy · pain in extremity · pancreatitis · paraesthesia · peripheral neuropathy · photosensitivity reaction · sexual dysfunction · thrombocytopenia · vision blurred

- ● **PREGNANCY** Manufacturers advise avoid unless essential— toxicity in *animal* studies.

- ● **BREAST FEEDING** Manufacturer advises avoid—no information available.

- ● **HEPATIC IMPAIRMENT** Manufacturer advises avoid.

- ● **RENAL IMPAIRMENT** Avoid if eGFR less than 30 mL/minute/1.73 m^2.
  Myotoxicity Special care needed in patients with renal disease, as progressive increases in serum creatinine concentration or failure to follow dosage guidelines may result in myotoxicity (rhabdomyolysis); discontinue if myotoxicity suspected or creatine kinase concentration increases significantly.
  Dose adjustments Initially 900 mg daily if eGFR 30–80 mL/minute/1.73 m^2.

- ● **MONITORING REQUIREMENTS**
  - ▸ Monitor blood counts for first year.
  - ▸ Monitor liver-function (discontinue treatment if abnormalities persist).
  - ▸ Consider monitoring creatine kinase if used in combination with a statin.

- ● **PRESCRIBING AND DISPENSING INFORMATION** Fibrates are mainly used in those whose serum-triglyceride concentration is greater than 10 mmol/litre or in those who cannot tolerate a statin (specialist use).

- ● **MEDICINAL FORMS** There can be variation in the licensing of different medicines containing the same drug.
  Tablet
  CAUTIONARY AND ADVISORY LABELS 22
  - ▸ Gemfibrozil (Non-proprietary)
    Gemfibrozil 600 mg Gemfibrozil 600mg tablets | 56 tablet [PoM] £45.38 DT = £45.38

  - ▸ Lopid (Pfizer Ltd)
    Gemfibrozil 600 mg Lopid 600mg tablets | 56 tablet [PoM] £35.57 DT = £45.38
  Capsule
  CAUTIONARY AND ADVISORY LABELS 22
  - ▸ Lopid (Pfizer Ltd)
    Gemfibrozil 300 mg Lopid 300mg capsules | 100 capsule [PoM] £31.76 DT = £31.76

LIPID MODIFYING DRUGS › NICOTINIC ACID DERIVATIVES

Acipimox

20-Jul-2020

- ● **INDICATIONS AND DOSE**

  Adjunct or alternative treatment in hyperlipidaemias of types IIb and IV in patients who have not responded adequately to other lipid-regulating drugs such as a statin or fibrate, and lifestyle changes (including diet, exercise, and weight reduction)
  - ▸ BY MOUTH
  - ▸ Adult: 250 mg 2–3 times a day

- ● **CONTRA-INDICATIONS** Peptic ulcer

- ● **SIDE-EFFECTS**
  - ▸ **Common or very common** Asthenia · gastrointestinal discomfort · headache · skin reactions · vasodilation
  - ▸ **Uncommon** Angioedema · arthralgia · feeling hot · malaise · myalgia · myositis · nausea
  - ▸ **Frequency not known** Bronchospasm · diarrhoea · dry eye · eye disorder · eyes gritty

- ● **PREGNANCY** Manufacturer advises avoid—no information available.

- ● **BREAST FEEDING** Manufacturer advises avoid—no information available.

- ● **RENAL IMPAIRMENT** Avoid if eGFR less than 30 mL/minute/1.73 m^2.
  Dose adjustments Reduce dose to 250 mg 1–2 times daily if eGFR 30–60 mL/minute/1.73 m^2.

- ● **MONITORING REQUIREMENTS** Monitor hepatic and renal function.

- ● **MEDICINAL FORMS** There can be variation in the licensing of different medicines containing the same drug.
  Capsule
  CAUTIONARY AND ADVISORY LABELS 21
  - ▸ Olbetam (Pfizer Ltd)
    Acipimox 250 mg Olbetam 250mg capsules | 90 capsule [PoM] £46.33 DT = £46.33

Nicotinic acid

07-Feb-2020

- ● **DRUG ACTION** In doses of 1.5 to 3 g daily, it lowers both cholesterol and triglyceride concentrations by inhibiting synthesis; it also increases HDL-cholesterol.

- ● **INDICATIONS AND DOSE**

  Adjunct to statin in dyslipidaemia or used alone if statin not tolerated
  - ▸ BY MOUTH
  - ▸ Adult: (consult product literature)

- ● **CONTRA-INDICATIONS** Active peptic ulcer disease · arterial bleeding

- ● **CAUTIONS** Acute myocardial infarction · diabetes mellitus · gout · history of peptic ulceration · unstable angina

- ● **INTERACTIONS** → Appendix 1: nicotinic acid

- ● **SIDE-EFFECTS** Angioedema · arrhythmias · asthenia · burping · cough aggravated · diarrhoea · dizziness · dyspnoea · flushing · gastrointestinal disorders · gout · hepatic disorders · hyperhidrosis · hypotension · insomnia ·

macular oedema · migraine · myalgia · myopathy · nausea · nervousness · oedema · palpitations · paraesthesia · respiratory disorders · skin reactions · syncope · tongue oedema · vision blurred · vomiting

SIDE-EFFECTS, FURTHER INFORMATION Prostaglandin-mediated flushing is common, typically within an hour of dosing and lasting for 15–30 minutes (particularly with the initial doses). Taking after a meal or taking asprin before dosing minimises flushing.

● PREGNANCY No information available—manufacturer advises avoid unless potential benefit outweighs risk.

● BREAST FEEDING Present in milk—avoid.

● HEPATIC IMPAIRMENT Avoid in severe impairment. Discontinue if severe abnormalities in liver function tests. **Monitoring** Manufacturer advises monitor liver function in mild to moderate hepatic impairment.

● RENAL IMPAIRMENT Manufacturer advises use with caution—no information available.

● MEDICINAL FORMS There can be variation in the licensing of different medicines containing the same drug. Forms available from special-order manufacturers include: tablet, modified-release tablet, capsule

Capsule
▸ Solgar Niacin (Solgar Vitamin and Herb)
  Nicotinic acid 500 mg Solgar Niacin 500mg capsules | 100 capsule ⓢ

LIPID MODIFYING DRUGS ⟩ STATINS

Statins 🅟

● DRUG ACTION Statins competitively inhibit 3-hydroxy-3-methylglutaryl coenzyme A (HMG CoA) reductase, an enzyme involved in cholesterol synthesis, especially in the liver.

● CAUTIONS Elderly · high alcohol intake · history of liver disease · hypothyroidism · known genetic polymorphisms—consult product literature · patients at increased risk of muscle toxicity, including myopathy or rhabdomyolysis (e.g. those with a personal or family history of muscular disorders, previous history of muscular toxicity and a high alcohol intake)

CAUTIONS, FURTHER INFORMATION
▸ Muscle effects Muscle toxicity can occur with all statins, however the likelihood increases with higher doses and in certain patients (see below). Statins should be used with caution in patients at increased risk of muscle toxicity, including those with a personal or family history of muscular disorders, previous history of muscular toxicity, a high alcohol intake, renal impairment or hypothyroidism.

In patients at increased risk of muscle effects, a statin should not usually be started if the baseline creatine kinase concentration is more than 5 times the upper limit of normal (some patients may present with an extremely elevated baseline creatine kinase concentration, for example because of a physical occupation or rigorous exercise—specialist advice should be sought regarding consideration of statin therapy in these patients).

▸ Hypothyroidism Hypothyroidism should be managed adequately before starting treatment with a statin.

● SIDE-EFFECTS
▸ **Common or very common** Asthenia · constipation · diarrhoea · dizziness · flatulence · gastrointestinal discomfort · headache · myalgia · nausea · sleep disorders · thrombocytopenia

▸ **Uncommon** Alopecia · hepatic disorders · memory loss · pancreatitis · paraesthesia · sexual dysfunction · skin reactions · vomiting

▸ **Rare or very rare** Myopathy · peripheral neuropathy · tendinopathy

▸ **Frequency not known** Depression · diabetes mellitus (in those at risk) · interstitial lung disease

SIDE-EFFECTS, FURTHER INFORMATION **Muscle effects** The risk of myopathy, myositis, and rhabdomyolysis associated with statin use is rare. Although myalgia has been reported commonly in patients receiving statins, muscle toxicity truly attributable to statin use is rare. When a statin is suspected to be the cause of myopathy, and creatine kinase concentration is markedly elevated or if muscular symptoms are severe, treatment should be discontinued. If symptoms resolve and creatine kinase concentrations return to normal, the statin should be reintroduced at a lower dose and the patient monitored closely. Statins should not be discontinued if there is an increase in the blood-glucose concentration as the benefits continue to outweigh the risks.

Interstitial lung disease If patients develop symptoms such as dyspnoea, cough, and weight loss, they should seek medical attention.

● CONCEPTION AND CONTRACEPTION Adequate contraception is required during treatment and for 1 month afterwards.

● PREGNANCY Statins should be avoided in pregnancy (discontinue 3 months before attempting to conceive) as congenital anomalies have been reported and the decreased synthesis of cholesterol possibly affects fetal development.

● HEPATIC IMPAIRMENT In general, manufacturers advise caution (risk of increased exposure); avoid in active disease or unexplained persistent elevations in serum transaminases.

● MONITORING REQUIREMENTS
▸ Before starting treatment with statins, at least one full lipid profile (non-fasting) should be measured, including total cholesterol, HDL-cholesterol, non-HDL-cholesterol (calculated as total cholesterol minus HDL-cholesterol), and triglyceride concentrations, thyroid-stimulating hormone, and renal function should also be assessed.

▸ Liver function There is little information available on a rational approach to liver-function monitoring; however, NICE suggests that liver enzymes should be measured before treatment, and repeated within 3 months and at 12 months of starting treatment, unless indicated at other times by signs or symptoms suggestive of hepatotoxicity (NICE clinical guideline 181 (July 2014). Lipid Modification—Cardiovascular risk assessment and the modification of blood lipids for the primary and secondary prevention of cardiovascular disease).

Those with serum transaminases that are raised, but less than 3 times the upper limit of the reference range, should **not** be routinely excluded from statin therapy. Those with serum transaminases of more than 3 times the upper limit of the reference range should discontinue statin therapy.

▸ Creatine kinase Before initiation of statin treatment, creatine kinase concentration should be measured in patients who have had persistent, generalised, unexplained muscle pain (whether associated or not with previous lipid-regulating drugs); if the concentration is more than 5 times the upper limit of normal, a repeat measurement should be taken after 7 days. If the repeat concentration remains above 5 times the upper limit, statin treatment should not be started; if concentrations are still raised but less than 5 times the upper limit, the statin should be started at a lower dose.

▸ Diabetes Patients at high risk of diabetes mellitus should have fasting blood-glucose concentration or HbA_{1C} checked before starting statin treatment, and then repeated after 3 months.

- **PRESCRIBING AND DISPENSING INFORMATION**
Patient decision aid Taking a statin to reduce the risk of coronary heart disease and stroke. National Institute for Health and Care Excellence. November 2014.
www.nice.org.uk/about/what-we-do/our-programmes/nice-guidance/nice-guidelines/shared-decision-making
- **PATIENT AND CARER ADVICE** Advise patients to report promptly unexplained muscle pain, tenderness, or weakness.

☞ 216

Atorvastatin
05-Feb-2020

- **INDICATIONS AND DOSE**

Primary hypercholesterolaemia in patients who have not responded adequately to diet and other appropriate measures | Combined (mixed) hyperlipidaemia in patients who have not responded adequately to diet and other appropriate measures
▸ BY MOUTH
▸ Adult: Usual dose 10 mg once daily; increased if necessary up to 80 mg once daily, dose to be increased at intervals of at least 4 weeks

Heterozygous familial hypercholesterolaemia in patients who have not responded adequately to diet and other appropriate measures | Homozygous familial hypercholesterolaemia in patients who have not responded adequately to diet and other appropriate measures
▸ BY MOUTH
▸ Adult: Initially 10 mg once daily, then increased to 40 mg once daily, dose to be increased at intervals of at least 4 weeks; maximum 80 mg per day

Primary prevention of cardiovascular events in patients at high risk of a first cardiovascular event
▸ BY MOUTH
▸ Adult: 20 mg once daily, dose can be increased if necessary

Secondary prevention of cardiovascular events
▸ BY MOUTH
▸ Adult: 80 mg once daily

DOSE ADJUSTMENTS DUE TO INTERACTIONS
▸ Manufacturer advises if concurrent use of ciclosporin is unavoidable, max. dose cannot exceed 10 mg daily.
▸ Manufacturer advises max. dose 40 mg daily when combined with anion-exchange resin for heterozygous familial hypercholesterolaemia.
▸ Manufacturer advises max. dose 20 mg daily with concurrent use of elbasvir with grazoprevir.
▸ Manufacturer advises max. dose 20 mg daily with concurrent use of letermovir without ciclosporin.
▸ Manufacturer advises max. dose 20 mg daily with concurrent use of sofosbuvir with velpatasvir and voxilaprevir.

- **UNLICENSED USE** EvGr Not licensed for secondary prevention of cardiovascular events. Starting dose of 20 mg once daily is not licensed for the primary prevention of cardiovascular events. ⚠
- **CAUTIONS** Haemorrhagic stroke
- **INTERACTIONS** → Appendix 1: statins
- **SIDE-EFFECTS**
▸ **Common or very common** Epistaxis · hyperglycaemia · hypersensitivity · joint disorders · laryngeal pain · muscle complaints · nasopharyngitis · pain
▸ **Uncommon** Appetite decreased · burping · chest pain · fever · hypoglycaemia · malaise · numbness · peripheral oedema · taste altered · tinnitus · vision disorders · weight increased
▸ **Rare or very rare** Angioedema · gynaecomastia · hearing loss · severe cutaneous adverse reactions (SCARs)

- **BREAST FEEDING** Manufacturer advises avoid—no information available.
- **RENAL IMPAIRMENT**
Dose adjustments In chronic kidney disease, for primary and secondary prevention of cardiovascular events [unlicensed starting dose in *primary* prevention; unlicensed in *secondary* prevention], initially 20 mg once daily, increased if necessary (on specialist advice if eGFR < 30 mL/minute/1.73 m²); max. 80 mg once daily.
- **PATIENT AND CARER ADVICE** Patient counselling is advised for atorvastatin tablets (muscle effects).

- **MEDICINAL FORMS** There can be variation in the licensing of different medicines containing the same drug. Forms available from special-order manufacturers include: oral suspension, oral solution

Tablet
▸ Atorvastatin (Non-proprietary)
Atorvastatin (as Atorvastatin calcium trihydrate)
10 mg Atorvastatin 10mg tablets | 28 tablet [PoM] £13.00 DT = £0.93 | 90 tablet [PoM] £41.78 | 500 tablet [PoM] £9.72
Atorvastatin (as Atorvastatin calcium trihydrate)
20 mg Atorvastatin 20mg tablets | 28 tablet [PoM] £24.64 DT = £1.20 | 90 tablet [PoM] £79.20 | 500 tablet [PoM] £11.69
Atorvastatin (as Atorvastatin calcium trihydrate)
30 mg Atorvastatin 30mg tablets | 28 tablet [PoM] £24.51 DT = £24.51
Atorvastatin (as Atorvastatin calcium trihydrate)
40 mg Atorvastatin 40mg tablets | 28 tablet [PoM] £24.64 DT = £1.31 | 90 tablet [PoM] £79.20 | 500 tablet [PoM] £14.42
Atorvastatin (as Atorvastatin calcium trihydrate)
60 mg Atorvastatin 60mg tablets | 28 tablet [PoM] £28.01 DT = £28.01
Atorvastatin (as Atorvastatin calcium trihydrate)
80 mg Atorvastatin 80mg tablets | 28 tablet [PoM] £28.21 DT = £1.94 | 90 tablet [PoM] £90.67
▸ Lipitor (Upjohn UK Ltd)
Atorvastatin (as Atorvastatin calcium trihydrate) 10 mg Lipitor 10mg tablets | 28 tablet [PoM] £13.00 DT = £0.93
Atorvastatin (as Atorvastatin calcium trihydrate) 20 mg Lipitor 20mg tablets | 28 tablet [PoM] £24.64 DT = £1.20
Atorvastatin (as Atorvastatin calcium trihydrate) 40 mg Lipitor 40mg tablets | 28 tablet [PoM] £24.64 DT = £1.31
Atorvastatin (as Atorvastatin calcium trihydrate) 80 mg Lipitor 80mg tablets | 28 tablet [PoM] £28.21 DT = £1.94

Chewable tablet
CAUTIONARY AND ADVISORY LABELS 24
▸ Lipitor (Upjohn UK Ltd)
Atorvastatin (as Atorvastatin calcium trihydrate) 10 mg Lipitor 10mg chewable tablets sugar-free | 30 tablet [PoM] £13.80 DT = £13.80
Atorvastatin (as Atorvastatin calcium trihydrate) 20 mg Lipitor 20mg chewable tablets sugar-free | 30 tablet [PoM] £26.40 DT = £26.40

☞ 216

Fluvastatin
10-Dec-2020

- **INDICATIONS AND DOSE**

Adjunct to diet in primary hypercholesterolaemia or combined (mixed) hyperlipidaemia (types IIa and IIb)
▸ BY MOUTH USING IMMEDIATE-RELEASE MEDICINES
▸ Adult: Initially 20–40 mg daily, dose to be taken in the evening, increased if necessary up to 80 mg daily in 2 divided doses, dose to be adjusted at intervals of at least 4 weeks
▸ BY MOUTH USING MODIFIED-RELEASE MEDICINES
▸ Adult: 80 mg daily, dose form is not appropriate for initial dose titration

Prevention of coronary events after percutaneous coronary intervention
▸ BY MOUTH USING IMMEDIATE-RELEASE MEDICINES
▸ Adult: 80 mg daily

continued →

▸ BY MOUTH USING MODIFIED-RELEASE MEDICINES
▸ **Adult:** 80 mg daily, dose form is not appropriate for initial dose titration

DOSE ADJUSTMENTS DUE TO INTERACTIONS
▸ Max. dose 20 mg daily with concomitant elbasvir with grazoprevir.

● INTERACTIONS → Appendix 1: statins
● SIDE-EFFECTS
▸ **Rare or very rare** Angioedema · face oedema · lupus-like syndrome · muscle weakness · sensation abnormal · vasculitis
● BREAST FEEDING Manufacturer advises avoid—no information available.
● RENAL IMPAIRMENT
Dose adjustments Manufacturer advises doses above 40 mg daily should be initiated with caution if eGFR less than 30 mL/minute/1.73 m^2.
● PATIENT AND CARER ADVICE Patient counselling is advised for fluvastatin tablets/capsules (muscle effects).
● NATIONAL FUNDING/ACCESS DECISIONS
For full details see funding body website
Scottish Medicines Consortium (SMC) decisions
▸ Fluvastatin (*Lescol*®) for the secondary prevention of coronary events after percutaneous coronary intervention (February 2004) SMC No. 76/04 Recommended with restrictions

● MEDICINAL FORMS There can be variation in the licensing of different medicines containing the same drug.
Modified-release tablet
CAUTIONARY AND ADVISORY LABELS 25
▸ Dorisin XL (Aspire Pharma Ltd)
Fluvastatin (as Fluvastatin sodium) 80 mg Dorisin XL 80mg tablets | 28 tablet [PoM] £19.20 DT = £19.20
▸ Lescol XL (Novartis Pharmaceuticals UK Ltd)
Fluvastatin (as Fluvastatin sodium) 80 mg Lescol XL 80mg tablets | 28 tablet [PoM] £19.20 DT = £19.20
▸ Nandovar XL (Sandoz Ltd)
Fluvastatin (as Fluvastatin sodium) 80 mg Nandovar XL 80mg tablets | 28 tablet [PoM] £16.32 DT = £19.20
Capsule
▸ Fluvastatin (Non-proprietary)
Fluvastatin (as Fluvastatin sodium) 20 mg Fluvastatin 20mg capsules | 28 capsule [PoM] £6.96 DT = £2.97
Fluvastatin (as Fluvastatin sodium) 40 mg Fluvastatin 40mg capsules | 28 capsule [PoM] £7.42 DT = £3.45

F 216

Pravastatin sodium

05-Dec-2020

● INDICATIONS AND DOSE
Adjunct to diet for primary hypercholesterolaemia or combined (mixed) hyperlipidaemias in patients who have not responded adequately to dietary control
▸ BY MOUTH
▸ **Adult:** 10–40 mg daily, dose to be taken at night, dose to be adjusted at intervals of at least 4 weeks

Prevention of cardiovascular events in patients with previous myocardial infarction or unstable angina | Adjunct to diet to prevent cardiovascular events in patients with hypercholesterolaemia
▸ BY MOUTH
▸ **Adult:** 40 mg daily, dose to be taken at night

Reduction of hyperlipidaemia in patients receiving immunosuppressive therapy following solid-organ transplantation
▸ BY MOUTH
▸ **Adult:** Initially 20 mg daily, then increased if necessary up to 40 mg daily, dose to be taken at night, close medical supervision is required if dose is increased to maximum dose

DOSE ADJUSTMENTS DUE TO INTERACTIONS
▸ Manufacturer advises reduce dose by half with concurrent use of ombitasvir with paritaprevir and ritonavir.
▸ Manufacturer advises max. 20 mg daily with concurrent use of glecaprevir with pibrentasvir.
▸ Manufacturer advises max. 40 mg daily with concurrent use of sofosbuvir with velpatasvir and voxilaprevir.

● INTERACTIONS → Appendix 1: statins
● SIDE-EFFECTS
▸ **Uncommon** Hair abnormal · scalp abnormal · urinary disorders · vision disorders
● BREAST FEEDING Manufacturer advises avoid—small amount of drug present in breast milk.
● HEPATIC IMPAIRMENT
Dose adjustments Manufacturer advises initial dose reduction to 10 mg daily; adjust according to response.
● RENAL IMPAIRMENT
Dose adjustments Manufacturer advises initial dose of 10 mg once daily in moderate to severe impairment.
● PATIENT AND CARER ADVICE Patient counselling is advised for pravastatin tablets (muscle effects).

● MEDICINAL FORMS There can be variation in the licensing of different medicines containing the same drug. Forms available from special-order manufacturers include: oral suspension, oral solution
Tablet
▸ Pravastatin sodium (Non-proprietary)
Pravastatin sodium 10 mg Pravastatin 10mg tablets | 28 tablet [PoM] £2.68 DT = £1.02
Pravastatin sodium 20 mg Pravastatin 20mg tablets | 28 tablet [PoM] £3.05 DT = £1.24
Pravastatin sodium 40 mg Pravastatin 40mg tablets | 28 tablet [PoM] £3.82 DT = £1.55

F 216

Rosuvastatin

05-Dec-2020

● INDICATIONS AND DOSE
Primary hypercholesterolaemia (type IIa including heterozygous familial hypercholesterolaemia), mixed dyslipidaemia (type IIb), or homozygous familial hypercholesterolaemia in patients who have not responded adequately to diet and other appropriate measures
▸ BY MOUTH
▸ **Adult 18–69 years:** Initially 5–10 mg once daily, then increased if necessary up to 20 mg once daily, dose to be increased gradually at intervals of at least 4 weeks
▸ **Adult (patients of Asian origin):** Initially 5 mg once daily, then increased if necessary up to 20 mg once daily, dose to be increased gradually at intervals of at least 4 weeks.
▸ **Adult 70 years and over:** Initially 5 mg once daily, then increased if necessary up to 20 mg once daily, dose to be increased gradually at intervals of at least 4 weeks

Primary hypercholesterolaemia (type IIa including heterozygous familial hypercholesterolaemia), mixed dyslipidaemia (type IIb), or homozygous familial hypercholesterolaemia in patients who have not responded adequately to diet and other appropriate measures and who have risk factors for myopathy or rhabdomyolysis
▸ BY MOUTH
▸ **Adult:** Initially 5 mg once daily, then increased if necessary up to 20 mg once daily, dose to be increased gradually at intervals of at least 4 weeks

Severe primary hypercholesterolaemia (type IIa including heterozygous familial hypercholesterolaemia), mixed dyslipidaemia (type IIb), or homozygous familial hypercholesterolaemia in patients with high cardiovascular risk who have not responded adequately to diet and other appropriate measures (specialist use only)
▸ BY MOUTH
▸ Adult 18–69 years: Initially 5–10 mg once daily, then increased if necessary up to 40 mg once daily, dose to be increased gradually at intervals of at least 4 weeks
▸ Adult (patients of Asian origin): Initially 5 mg once daily, then increased if necessary up to 20 mg once daily, dose to be increased gradually at intervals of at least 4 weeks.
▸ Adult 70 years and over: Initially 5 mg once daily, then increased if necessary up to 40 mg once daily, dose to be increased gradually at intervals of at least 4 weeks

Severe primary hypercholesterolaemia (type IIa including heterozygous familial hypercholesterolaemia), mixed dyslipidaemia (type IIb), or homozygous familial hypercholesterolaemia in patients with high cardiovascular risk who have not responded adequately to diet and other appropriate measures, and who have risk factors for myopathy or rhabdomyolysis (specialist use only)
▸ BY MOUTH
▸ Adult: Initially 5 mg once daily, then increased if necessary up to 20 mg once daily, dose to be increased gradually at intervals of at least 4 weeks

Prevention of cardiovascular events in patients at high risk of a first cardiovascular event
▸ BY MOUTH
▸ Adult 18–69 years: 20 mg once daily
▸ Adult (patients of Asian origin): Initially 5 mg once daily, then increased if tolerated to 20 mg once daily, dose to be increased gradually at intervals of at least 4 weeks.
▸ Adult 70 years and over: Initially 5 mg once daily, then increased if tolerated to 20 mg once daily, dose to be increased gradually at intervals of at least 4 weeks

Prevention of cardiovascular events in patients at high risk of a first cardiovascular event and with risk factors for myopathy or rhabdomyolysis
▸ BY MOUTH
▸ Adult: Initially 5 mg once daily, then increased if tolerated to 20 mg once daily, dose to be increased gradually at intervals of at least 4 weeks

DOSE ADJUSTMENTS DUE TO INTERACTIONS
▸ Manufacturer advises initially 5 mg daily with concurrent use of bezafibrate, ciprofibrate, and fenofibrate—40 mg dose is contra-indicated.
▸ Manufacturer advises initially 5 mg daily with concurrent use of clopidogrel—max. dose 20 mg daily.
▸ Manufacturer advises initially 5 mg daily with concurrent use of simeprevir—max. dose 10 mg daily.
▸ Manufacturer advises max. dose 5 mg daily with concurrent ombitasvir, paritaprevir, and ritonavir given with dasabuvir, but max. 10 mg dose with concurrent ombitasvir, paritaprevir, and ritonavir given without dasabuvir.
▸ Manufacturer advises max. dose 10 mg daily with concurrent use of sofosbuvir with velpatasvir, or elbasvir with grazoprevir.
▸ Manufacturer advises reduce dose by half with concurrent use of teriflunomide.
▸ Manufacturer advises max. 5 mg daily with concurrent use of glecaprevir with pibrentasvir.

● INTERACTIONS → Appendix 1: statins

● SIDE-EFFECTS
▸ **Rare or very rare** Arthralgia · gynaecomastia · haematuria · polyneuropathy
▸ **Frequency not known** Cough · dyspnoea · oedema · proteinuria · Stevens-Johnson syndrome · tendon disorders
● BREAST FEEDING Manufacturer advises avoid—no information available.
● RENAL IMPAIRMENT Avoid if eGFR less than 30 mL/minute/1.73 m^2.
  Dose adjustments Initially 5 mg once daily (do not exceed 20 mg daily) if eGFR 30–60 mL/minute/1.73 m^2.
● MONITORING REQUIREMENTS Manufacturer advises consider routine monitoring of renal function when using 40 mg daily dose.
● PATIENT AND CARER ADVICE Patient counselling is advised for rosuvastatin tablets (muscle effects).

● MEDICINAL FORMS There can be variation in the licensing of different medicines containing the same drug. Forms available from special-order manufacturers include: oral suspension

Tablet
▸ Rosuvastatin (Non-proprietary)
  Rosuvastatin (as Rosuvastatin calcium) 5 mg Rosuvastatin 5mg tablets | 28 tablet [PoM] £18.03 DT = £1.52
  Rosuvastatin (as Rosuvastatin calcium) 10 mg Rosuvastatin 10mg tablets | 28 tablet [PoM] £18.03 DT = £1.60
  Rosuvastatin (as Rosuvastatin calcium) 20 mg Rosuvastatin 20mg tablets | 28 tablet [PoM] £26.02 DT = £2.42
  Rosuvastatin (as Rosuvastatin calcium) 40 mg Rosuvastatin 40mg tablets | 28 tablet [PoM] £29.69 DT = £2.38
▸ Crestor (AstraZeneca UK Ltd)
  Rosuvastatin (as Rosuvastatin calcium) 5 mg Crestor 5mg tablets | 28 tablet [PoM] £18.03 DT = £1.52
  Rosuvastatin (as Rosuvastatin calcium) 10 mg Crestor 10mg tablets | 28 tablet [PoM] £18.03 DT = £1.60
  Rosuvastatin (as Rosuvastatin calcium) 20 mg Crestor 20mg tablets | 28 tablet [PoM] £26.02 DT = £2.42
  Rosuvastatin (as Rosuvastatin calcium) 40 mg Crestor 40mg tablets | 28 tablet [PoM] £29.69 DT = £2.38

F 216

Simvastatin   22-Oct-2020

● INDICATIONS AND DOSE
Primary hypercholesterolaemia, or combined (mixed) hyperlipidaemia in patients who have not responded adequately to diet and other appropriate measures
▸ BY MOUTH
▸ Adult: 10–20 mg once daily, then increased if necessary up to 80 mg once daily, adjusted at intervals of at least 4 weeks, dose to be taken at night; 80 mg dose only for those with severe hypercholesterolaemia and at high risk of cardiovascular complications

Homozygous familial hypercholesterolaemia in patients who have not responded adequately to diet and other appropriate measures
▸ BY MOUTH
▸ Adult: Initially 40 mg once daily, then increased if necessary up to 80 mg once daily, adjusted at intervals of at least 4 weeks, dose to be taken at night; 80 mg dose only for those with severe hypercholesterolaemia and at high risk of cardiovascular complications

Prevention of cardiovascular events in patients with atherosclerotic cardiovascular disease or diabetes mellitus
▸ BY MOUTH
▸ Adult: Initially 20–40 mg once daily, increased if necessary up to 80 mg once daily, adjusted at intervals of at least 4 weeks, dose to be taken at night; 80 mg dose only for those with severe hypercholesterolaemia and at high risk of cardiovascular complications

continued →

DOSE ADJUSTMENTS DUE TO INTERACTIONS
▸ Manufacturer advises max. 10 mg daily with concurrent use of bezafibrate or ciprofibrate.
▸ Manufacturer advises max. 20 mg daily with concurrent use of amiodarone, amlodipine, or ranolazine.
▸ Manufacturer advises reduce dose with concurrent use of some moderate inhibitors of CYP3A4 (max. 20 mg daily with verapamil and diltiazem).
▸ Manufacturer advises max. 40 mg daily with concurrent use of lomitapide or ticagrelor.
▸ Manufacturer advises max. 20 mg daily with concurrent use of elbasvir with grazoprevir.
▸ Manufacturer advises usual max. 20 mg daily with concurrent use of bempedoic acid or bempedoic acid with ezetimibe; max. dose 40 mg daily in patients with severe hypercholesterolaemia and at high risk of cardiovascular complications.

● INTERACTIONS → Appendix 1: statins
● SIDE-EFFECTS
▸ **Rare or very rare** Acute kidney injury · anaemia · muscle cramps
▸ **Frequency not known** Cognitive impairment
● BREAST FEEDING Manufacturer advises avoid—no information available.
● RENAL IMPAIRMENT Doses above 10 mg daily should be used with caution if eGFR less than 30 mL/minute/1.73 m^2.
● PATIENT AND CARER ADVICE Patient counselling is advised for simvastatin tablets/oral suspension (muscle effects).
● EXCEPTIONS TO LEGAL CATEGORY Simvastatin 10 mg tablets can be sold to the public to reduce risk of first coronary event in individuals at moderate risk of coronary heart disease (approx. 10–15 % risk of major event in 10 years), max. daily dose 10 mg and pack size of 28 tablets; treatment should form part of a programme to reduce risk of coronary heart disease.

● MEDICINAL FORMS There can be variation in the licensing of different medicines containing the same drug. Forms available from special-order manufacturers include: oral suspension, oral solution
Oral suspension
EXCIPIENTS: May contain Propylene glycol
▸ Simvastatin (Non-proprietary)
Simvastatin 4 mg per 1 ml Simvastatin 20mg/5ml oral suspension sugar free sugar-free | 150 ml [PoM] £153.04 DT = £153.04
Simvastatin 8 mg per 1 ml Simvastatin 40mg/5ml oral suspension sugar free sugar-free | 150 ml [PoM] £233.78 DT = £233.78
Tablet
▸ Simvastatin (Non-proprietary)
Simvastatin 10 mg Simvastatin 10mg tablets | 28 tablet [PoM] £14.42 DT = £0.95 | 500 tablet [PoM] £15.71
Simvastatin 20 mg Simvastatin 20mg tablets | 28 tablet [PoM] £23.75 DT = £1.07 | 500 tablet [PoM] £8.04
Simvastatin 40 mg Simvastatin 40mg tablets | 28 tablet [PoM] £23.75 DT = £1.19
Simvastatin 80 mg Simvastatin 80mg tablets | 28 tablet [PoM] £6.00 DT = £1.64
▸ Simvador (Dexcel-Pharma Ltd)
Simvastatin 10 mg Simvador 10mg tablets | 28 tablet [PoM] £0.65 DT = £0.95
Simvastatin 20 mg Simvador 20mg tablets | 28 tablet [PoM] £0.77 DT = £1.07
Simvastatin 40 mg Simvador 40mg tablets | 28 tablet [PoM] £0.88 DT = £1.19
▸ Zocor (Merck Sharp & Dohme Ltd)
Simvastatin 10 mg Zocor 10mg tablets | 28 tablet [PoM] £18.03 DT = £0.95
Simvastatin 20 mg Zocor 20mg tablets | 28 tablet [PoM] £29.69 DT = £1.07
Simvastatin 40 mg Zocor 40mg tablets | 28 tablet [PoM] £29.69 DT = £1.19

Simvastatin with ezetimibe
10-Dec-2020

The properties listed below are those particular to the combination only. For the properties of the components please consider, simvastatin p. 219, ezetimibe p. 212.

● INDICATIONS AND DOSE
Homozygous familial hypercholesterolaemia, primary hypercholesterolaemia, and mixed hyperlipidaemia in patients over 10 years stabilised on the individual components in the same proportions, or for patients not adequately controlled by statin alone
▸ BY MOUTH
▸ Adult: (consult product literature)

● INTERACTIONS → Appendix 1: ezetimibe · statins

● MEDICINAL FORMS There can be variation in the licensing of different medicines containing the same drug.
Tablet
▸ Inegy (Merck Sharp & Dohme Ltd)
Ezetimibe 10 mg, Simvastatin 20 mg Inegy 10mg/20mg tablets | 28 tablet [PoM] £33.42 DT = £33.42
Ezetimibe 10 mg, Simvastatin 40 mg Inegy 10mg/40mg tablets | 28 tablet [PoM] £38.98 DT = £38.98
Ezetimibe 10 mg, Simvastatin 80 mg Inegy 10mg/80mg tablets | 28 tablet [PoM] £41.21 DT = £41.21

Simvastatin with fenofibrate
05-Dec-2020

The properties listed below are those particular to the combination only. For the properties of the components please consider, simvastatin p. 219, fenofibrate p. 214.

● INDICATIONS AND DOSE
Adjunct to diet and exercise in mixed dyslipidaemia, when LDL-cholesterol levels are adequately controlled with the corresponding dose of simvastatin monotherapy (in patients at high cardiovascular risk)
▸ BY MOUTH
▸ Adult: 20/145 mg once daily, alternatively 40/145 mg once daily, dose should be based on previous simvastatin monotherapy dose

● CAUTIONS History of pulmonary embolism
● INTERACTIONS → Appendix 1: fibrates · statins
● RENAL IMPAIRMENT Manufacturer advises avoid if eGFR less than 60 mL/minute/1.73 m^2; use with caution if eGFR 60–89 mL/minute/1.73 m^2.

● MEDICINAL FORMS There can be variation in the licensing of different medicines containing the same drug.
Tablet
CAUTIONARY AND ADVISORY LABELS 25
EXCIPIENTS: May contain Butylated hydroxyanisole, lecithin
▸ Cholib (Mylan)
Simvastatin 20 mg, Fenofibrate 145 mg Cholib 145mg/20mg tablets | 30 tablet [PoM] £7.71 DT = £7.71
Simvastatin 40 mg, Fenofibrate 145 mg Cholib 145mg/40mg tablets | 30 tablet [PoM] £8.33 DT = £8.33

LIPID MODIFYING DRUGS > OTHER

Alirocumab
03-Nov-2020

- ● DRUG ACTION Alirocumab binds to a pro-protein involved in the regulation of LDL receptors on liver cells; receptor numbers are increased, which results in increased uptake of LDL-cholesterol from the blood.

- ● INDICATIONS AND DOSE

Primary hypercholesterolaemia or mixed dyslipidaemia in patients who have not responded adequately to other appropriate measures [in combination with a statin, or with a statin and other lipid-lowering therapies, or with other lipid-lowering therapies or alone if a statin contra-indicated or not tolerated] | Established atherosclerotic cardiovascular disease [in combination with the maximum tolerated dose of a statin with or without other lipid-lowering therapies, or with other lipid-lowering therapies or alone if a statin contra-indicated or not tolerated]
- ▸ BY SUBCUTANEOUS INJECTION
- ▸ Adult: Initially 75 mg every 2 weeks; increased if necessary to 150 mg every 2 weeks, alternatively 300 mg every 4 weeks, patients requiring an LDL-C reduction of greater than 60% may be initiated on 150 mg every 2 weeks or 300 mg every 4 weeks, dose adjustments should be made at 4 to 8 weekly intervals

- ● SIDE-EFFECTS
- ▸ **Common or very common** Nasal complaints · oropharyngeal pain · pulmonary reaction · skin reactions
- ▸ **Rare or very rare** Hypersensitivity · hypersensitivity vasculitis
- ▸ **Frequency not known** Angioedema · influenza like illness
- ● PREGNANCY Manufacturer advises avoid unless clinical condition requires treatment—maternal toxicity in *animal* studies.

- ● BREAST FEEDING Manufacturer advises avoid—no information available.

- ● HEPATIC IMPAIRMENT Manufacturer advises use with caution in severe impairment—no information available.

- ● RENAL IMPAIRMENT Manufacturer advises use with caution in severe impairment—no information available.

- ● HANDLING AND STORAGE Manufacturer advises store in a refrigerator (2–8 °C)—consult product literature for further information regarding storage outside refrigerator.

- ● NATIONAL FUNDING/ACCESS DECISIONS
For full details see funding body website
NICE decisions
- ▸ **Alirocumab for treating primary hypercholesterolaemia and mixed dyslipidaemia** (June 2016) NICE TA393 Recommended with restrictions
Scottish Medicines Consortium (SMC) decisions
- ▸ **Alirocumab** (*Praluent*®) for primary hypercholesterolaemia or mixed dyslipidaemia, as an adjunct to diet: in combination with a statin or statin with other lipid lowering therapies in patients unable to reach LDL-C goals with the maximum tolerated dose of a statin or, alone or in combination with other lipid-lowering therapies in patients who are statin-intolerant, or for whom a statin is contra-indicated (August 2016) SMC No. 1147/16 Recommended with restrictions

- ● MEDICINAL FORMS There can be variation in the licensing of different medicines containing the same drug.
Solution for injection
EXCIPIENTS: May contain Polysorbates
- ▸ Praluent (Sanofi)
Alirocumab 75 mg per 1 ml Praluent 75mg/1ml solution for injection pre-filled pens | 1 pre-filled disposable injection PoM £168.00 | 2 pre-filled disposable injection PoM £336.00 DT = £336.00

Alirocumab 150 mg per 1 ml Praluent 150mg/1ml solution for injection pre-filled pens | 1 pre-filled disposable injection PoM £168.00 | 2 pre-filled disposable injection PoM £336.00 DT = £336.00

Bempedoic acid
18-Sep-2020

- ● DRUG ACTION Bempedoic acid is an adenosine triphosphate citrate lyase (ACL) inhibitor which inhibits cholesterol synthesis in the liver, thereby lowering LDL-cholesterol.

- ● INDICATIONS AND DOSE

Primary hypercholesterolaemia or mixed dyslipidaemia in patients who have not responded adequately to other appropriate measures [in combination with a statin, or with a statin and other lipid-lowering therapies, or with other lipid-lowering therapies or alone if a statin contra-indicated or not tolerated]
- ▸ BY MOUTH
- ▸ Adult: 180 mg daily

- ● INTERACTIONS → Appendix 1: bempedoic acid
- ● SIDE-EFFECTS
- ▸ **Common or very common** Anaemia · gout · hyperuricaemia · pain in extremity
- ▸ **Frequency not known** Diarrhoea · muscle spasms · nausea
SIDE-EFFECTS, FURTHER INFORMATION **Hepatic enzyme changes** Manufacturer advises discontinue treatment if transaminase levels at least 3 time the upper limit of normal, and persist.
Hyperuricaemia Manufacturer advises discontinue treatment if hyperuricaemia accompanied with symptoms of gout occur.

- ● PREGNANCY Manufacturer advises avoid—toxicity in *animal* studies.

- ● BREAST FEEDING Manufacturer advises avoid—no information available.

- ● MEDICINAL FORMS There can be variation in the licensing of different medicines containing the same drug.
Tablet
- ▸ Nilemdo (Daiichi Sankyo UK Ltd) ▼
Bempedoic acid 180 mg Nilemdo 180mg tablets | 28 tablet PoM £55.44

Bempedoic acid with ezetimibe
18-Sep-2020

The properties listed below are those particular to the combination only. For the properties of the components please consider, bempedoic acid above, ezetimibe p. 212.

- ● INDICATIONS AND DOSE

Primary hypercholesterolaemia or mixed dyslipidaemia in patients who have not responded adequately to other appropriate measures [in combination with a statin, or alone if a statin is contra-indicated or not tolerated] | Primary hypercholesterolaemia or mixed dyslipidaemia in patients already taking bempedoic acid and ezetimibe as separate tablets with or without statin
- ▸ BY MOUTH
- ▸ Adult: 180/10 mg daily

DOSE EQUIVALENCE AND CONVERSION
- ▸ Dose expressed as x/y mg bempedoic acid/ezetimibe.

- ● INTERACTIONS → Appendix 1: bempedoic acid · ezetimibe

- ● MEDICINAL FORMS There can be variation in the licensing of different medicines containing the same drug.
Tablet
- ▸ Nustendi (Daiichi Sankyo UK Ltd) ▼
Ezetimibe 10 mg, Bempedoic acid 180 mg Nustendi 180mg/10mg tablets | 28 tablet PoM £55.44

Evolocumab

05-Nov-2020

- DRUG ACTION Evolocumab binds to a pro-protein involved in the regulation of LDL receptors on liver cells; receptor numbers are increased, which results in increased uptake of LDL-cholesterol from the blood.

● INDICATIONS AND DOSE

Primary hypercholesterolaemia or mixed dyslipidaemia in patients who have not responded adequately to other appropriate measures (in combination with a statin, or with a statin and other lipid-lowering therapies, or with other lipid-lowering therapies or alone if a statin contra-indicated or not tolerated) | Established atherosclerotic cardiovascular disease (in combination with the maximum tolerated dose of a statin with or without other lipid-lowering therapies, or with other lipid-lowering therapies or alone if a statin contra-indicated or not tolerated)

- ▸ BY SUBCUTANEOUS INJECTION
- ▸ Adult: 140 mg every 2 weeks, alternatively 420 mg every month, to be administered into the thigh, abdomen or upper arm

Homozygous familial hypercholesterolaemia (in combination with other lipid-lowering therapies)
- ▸ BY SUBCUTANEOUS INJECTION
- ▸ Adult: Initially 420 mg every month; increased if necessary to 420 mg every 2 weeks, if inadequate response after 12 weeks of treatment, to be administered into the thigh, abdomen or upper arm

Homozygous familial hypercholesterolaemia in patients on apheresis (in combination with other lipid-lowering therapies)
- ▸ BY SUBCUTANEOUS INJECTION
- ▸ Adult: 420 mg every 2 weeks, to correspond with apheresis schedule, to be administered into the thigh, abdomen or upper arm

- SIDE-EFFECTS
- ▸ **Common or very common** Arthralgia · back pain · hypersensitivity · increased risk of infection · nausea · skin reactions
- ▸ **Uncommon** Influenza like illness
- ▸ **Rare or very rare** Angioedema
- PREGNANCY Manufacturer advises avoid unless essential—limited information available.
- BREAST FEEDING Manufacturer advises avoid—no information available.
- HEPATIC IMPAIRMENT Manufacturer advises caution in moderate to severe impairment (risk of reduced efficacy; no information available in severe impairment).
- RENAL IMPAIRMENT Manufacturer advises caution if eGFR less than 30 mL/minute/1.73 m² —no information available.
- HANDLING AND STORAGE Manufacturer advises store in a refrigerator (2–8°C)—consult product literature for further information regarding storage outside refrigerator.
- PATIENT AND CARER ADVICE Patients and their carers should be given training in subcutaneous injection technique.
- NATIONAL FUNDING/ACCESS DECISIONS
  For full details see funding body website

  NICE decisions
- ▸ Evolocumab for treating primary hypercholesterolaemia and mixed dyslipidaemia (June 2016) NICE TA394 Recommended with restrictions

  Scottish Medicines Consortium (SMC) decisions
- ▸ Evolocumab (*Repatha®*) for use in adults with primary hypercholesterolaemia (heterozygous familial hypercholesterolaemia and non-familial) or mixed

dyslipidaemia (February 2017) SMC No. 1148/16 Recommended with restrictions

- MEDICINAL FORMS There can be variation in the licensing of different medicines containing the same drug.
  Solution for injection
  - ▸ Repatha SureClick (Amgen Ltd)
    Evolocumab 140 mg per 1 ml Repatha SureClick 140mg/1ml solution for injection pre-filled pens | 2 pre-filled disposable injection [PoM] £340.20 DT = £340.20

Lomitapide

15-Jan-2020

- DRUG ACTION Lomitapide, an inhibitor of microsomal triglyceride transfer protein (MTP), reduces lipoprotein secretion and circulating concentrations of lipoprotein-borne lipids such as cholesterol and triglycerides.

● INDICATIONS AND DOSE

Adjunct to dietary measures and other lipid-regulating drugs with or without low-density lipoprotein apheresis in homozygous familial hypercholesterolaemia (under expert supervision)
- ▸ BY MOUTH
- ▸ Adult: Initially 5 mg daily for 2 weeks, dose to be taken at least 2 hours after evening meal, then increased if necessary to 10 mg daily, for at least 4 weeks, then increased to 20 mg daily for at least 4 weeks, then increased in steps of 20 mg daily, adjusted at intervals of at least 4 weeks; maximum 60 mg per day

- CONTRA-INDICATIONS Significant or chronic bowel disease
- CAUTIONS Concomitant use of hepatotoxic drugs · lomitapide can interfere with the absorption of fat-soluble nutrients and supplementation of vitamin E and fatty acids is required · patients over 65 years
- INTERACTIONS → Appendix 1: lomitapide
- SIDE-EFFECTS
- ▸ **Common or very common** Aerophagia · appetite abnormal · asthenia · burping · constipation · diarrhoea · dizziness · gastrointestinal discomfort · gastrointestinal disorders · haemorrhage · headaches · hepatic disorders · increased risk of infection · muscle complaints · nausea · skin reactions · vomiting · weight decreased
- ▸ **Uncommon** Anaemia · chest pain · chills · dehydration · drowsiness · dry mouth · eye swelling · fever · gait abnormal · hyperhidrosis · joint disorders · malaise · pain in extremity · paraesthesia · throat lesion · upper-airway cough syndrome · vertigo
- ▸ **Frequency not known** Alopecia

  SIDE-EFFECTS, FURTHER INFORMATION Reduce dose if serum transaminases raised during treatment (consult product literature).
- CONCEPTION AND CONTRACEPTION Manufacturer advises exclude pregnancy before treatment and ensure effective contraception used.
- PREGNANCY Avoid—teratogenicity and embryotoxicity in *animal* studies.
- BREAST FEEDING Manufacturer advises avoid—no information available.
- HEPATIC IMPAIRMENT Manufacturer advises avoid in moderate to severe impairment, or if unexplained persistent abnormal liver function tests.
  Dose adjustments Manufacturer advises max. 40 mg daily in mild impairment.
- RENAL IMPAIRMENT
  Dose adjustments Max. 40 mg daily in end-stage renal disease.
- MONITORING REQUIREMENTS
- ▸ Monitor liver function tests before treatment, then at least monthly and before each dose increase for first year, then

at least every 3 months and before each dose increase thereafter.
▸ Screen for hepatic steatosis and fibrosis before treatment, then annually thereafter.

● MEDICINAL FORMS There can be variation in the licensing of different medicines containing the same drug.

Capsule
▸ Lojuxta (Amryt Pharma) ▼
Lomitapide 5 mg Lojuxta 5mg capsules | 28 capsule [PoM] £17,765.00
Lomitapide 10 mg Lojuxta 10mg capsules | 28 capsule [PoM] £17,765.00
Lomitapide 20 mg Lojuxta 20mg capsules | 28 capsule [PoM] £17,765.00

Omega-3-acid ethyl esters   26-Aug-2020

● INDICATIONS AND DOSE

Adjunct to diet and statin in type IIb or III hypertriglyceridaemia | Adjunct to diet in type IV hypertriglyceridaemia
▸ BY MOUTH
▸ Adult: Initially 2 capsules daily, dose to be taken with food, increased if necessary to 4 capsules daily

Adjunct in secondary prevention in those who have had a myocardial infarction in the preceding 3 months
▸ BY MOUTH
▸ Adult: 1 capsule daily, dose to be taken with food

● CAUTIONS Anticoagulant treatment (bleeding time increased) · haemorrhagic disorders
● INTERACTIONS → Appendix 1: omega-3-acid ethyl esters
● SIDE-EFFECTS
▸ **Common or very common** Burping · constipation · diarrhoea · gastrointestinal discomfort · gastrointestinal disorders · nausea · vomiting
▸ **Uncommon** Dizziness · gout · haemorrhage · headache · hyperglycaemia · hypotension · skin reactions · taste altered
▸ **Rare or very rare** Liver disorder
● PREGNANCY Manufacturers advise use only if potential benefit outweighs risk—no information available.
● BREAST FEEDING Manufacturers advise avoid—no information available.
● NATIONAL FUNDING/ACCESS DECISIONS
For full details see funding body website
Scottish Medicines Consortium (SMC) decisions
▸ Omega-3-acid ethyl esters (*Omacor*®) for hypertriglyceridaemia (November 2002) SMC No. 16/02 Not recommended

● MEDICINAL FORMS There can be variation in the licensing of different medicines containing the same drug.
Capsule
CAUTIONARY AND ADVISORY LABELS 21
▸ Omega-3-acid ethyl esters (Non-proprietary)
Eicosapentaenoic acid 60 mg, Docosahexaenoic acid 300 mg Omega-3 600mg capsules | 28 capsule [Ⓔ]
Docosahexaenoic acid 380 mg, Eicosapentaenoic acid 460 mg Eicosapentaenoic acid 460mg / Docosahexaenoic acid 380mg capsules | 28 capsule £14.24 DT = £14.24
AceOmeg 1000mg capsules | 28 capsule £6.97 DT = £14.24
▸ Omacor (Mylan)
Docosahexaenoic acid 380 mg, Eicosapentaenoic acid 460 mg Omacor capsules | 28 capsule [P] £14.24 DT = £14.24 | 100 capsule [P] £50.84
▸ Teromeg (Advanz Pharma)
Docosahexaenoic acid 380 mg, Eicosapentaenoic acid 460 mg Teromeg 1000mg capsules | 28 capsule [PoM] £11.39 DT = £14.24 | 100 capsule [PoM] £40.67

Volanesorsen   11-Nov-2020

● DRUG ACTION Volanesorsen is an antisense oligonucleotide which inhibits the formation of the apolipoprotein apoC–III, thereby lowering serum triglycerides.

● INDICATIONS AND DOSE

Familial chylomicronaemia syndrome (specialist use only)
▸ BY SUBCUTANEOUS INJECTION
▸ Adult: Initially 285 mg once weekly for 3 months, then reduced to 285 mg every 2 weeks, review and adjust dosing based on serum triglycerides—consult product literature

● CONTRA-INDICATIONS Chronic or unexplained thrombocytopenia (platelet count less than 140×10^9/litre)
● CAUTIONS Body-weight less than 70 kg (increased risk of thrombocytopenia)
● INTERACTIONS → Appendix 1: volanesorsen
● SIDE-EFFECTS
▸ **Common or very common** Arthritis · asthenia · chills · cough · diabetes mellitus · diarrhoea · dizziness · dry mouth · dyspnoea · eosinophilia · facial swelling · feeling hot · fever · gastrointestinal discomfort · haemorrhage · headaches · hot flush · hypersensitivity · hypertension · immunisation reaction · influenza like illness · insomnia · joint disorders · leucopenia · malaise · muscle complaints · myositis · nasal congestion · nausea · numbness · oedema · oral disorders · pain · polymyalgia rheumatica · proteinuria · skin reactions · sweat changes · syncope · throat oedema · thrombocytopenia · tremor · vision blurred · vomiting · wheezing
▸ **Frequency not known** Nephrotoxicity
● PREGNANCY Manufacturer advises avoid—limited information; *animal* studies do not indicate toxicity.
● BREAST FEEDING Manufacturer advises avoid—present in very low levels in milk in *animal* studies.
● MONITORING REQUIREMENTS
▸ Manufacturer advises monitor platelet count before treatment and then at least every 2 weeks during treatment.
▸ Manufacturer advises monitor liver function, erythrocyte sedimentation rate, and urine dipstick every 3 months during treatment.
● DIRECTIONS FOR ADMINISTRATION Manufacturer advises administer injection into the upper thigh or abdomen, or upper arm (if not self-administered). Patients may self-administer *Waylivra*® after appropriate training in subcutaneous injection technique.
● HANDLING AND STORAGE Manufacturer advises store in a refrigerator (2°C–8°C) and protect from light—consult product literature about storage outside refrigerator.
● PATIENT AND CARER ADVICE Manufacturer advises patients should immediately report any signs of bleeding, neck stiffness, or atypical severe headache.
Missed doses Manufacturer advises if a dose is more than 48 hours late, the missed dose should be omitted and the next dose given at the normal time.
● NATIONAL FUNDING/ACCESS DECISIONS
For full details see funding body website
NICE decisions
▸ **Volanesorsen for treating familial chylomicronaemia syndrome (October 2020)** NICE HST13 Recommended

Cardiovascular system

2

● MEDICINAL FORMS There can be variation in the licensing of different medicines containing the same drug.

Solution for injection

▸ Waylivra (Akcea Therapeutics UK Ltd) ▼

Volanesorsen (as Volanesorsen sodium) 190 mg per 1 ml Waylivra 285mg/1.5ml solution for injection pre-filled syringes | 1 pre-filled disposable injection [PoM] 🅢

8 Myocardial ischaemia

Stable angina

Description of condition

Stable angina is characterised by predictable chest pain or pressure, often precipitated by physical exertion or emotional stress causing an increase in myocardial oxygen demand. Although pain typically occurs in the front of the chest, it may also radiate to the neck, shoulders, jaw or arms; the pain is relieved with rest. Stable angina usually results from atherosclerotic plaques in the coronary arteries that restrict blood flow and oxygen supply to the heart; it can lead to cardiovascular complications such as stroke, unstable angina, myocardial infarction, and sudden cardiac death. For information about *unstable angina* and *myocardial infarction*, see Acute coronary syndromes.

Prinzmetal's or vasospastic angina is a rare form of angina caused by narrowing or occlusion of proximal coronary arteries due to spasm, in which pain is experienced at rest rather than during activity.

Aims of treatment

Antianginal drug therapy and revascularisation aims to prevent or minimise angina symptoms, in order to improve quality of life and long-term morbidity and mortality. The aim of drug therapy for secondary prevention is to minimise the risk of cardiovascular events such as myocardial infarction and stroke.

Drug treatment

Antianginal drug therapy

[EvGr] Acute attacks of stable angina should be managed with sublingual glyceryl trinitrate p. 233, which can also be used as a preventative measure immediately before performing activities that are known to bring on an attack.

For long-term prevention of chest pain in patients with stable angina, a beta-blocker (such as atenolol p. 166, bisoprolol fumarate p. 167, metoprolol tartrate p. 169 or propranolol hydrochloride p. 164) should be given as first-line therapy. A rate-limiting calcium-channel blocker (such as verapamil hydrochloride p. 178 or diltiazem hydrochloride p. 171) should be considered as an alternative if beta-blockers are contra-indicated, for example in patients with Prinzmetal's angina or decompensated heart failure. Dihydropyridine derivative calcium-channel blockers (such as amlodipine p. 170) may be effective in patients with Prinzmetal's angina.

If a beta-blocker alone fails to control symptoms adequately, a combination of a beta-blocker and a calcium-channel blocker should be considered. If this combination is not appropriate due to intolerance of, or contra-indication to, either beta-blockers or calcium-channel blockers, NICE CG126 recommends to consider addition of either a long-acting nitrate, ivabradine p. 227, nicorandil p. 227, or ranolazine p. 226.

A long-acting nitrate, ivabradine p. 227, nicorandil p. 227, or ranolazine p. 226, should also be considered as monotherapy in patients who cannot tolerate beta-blockers and calcium-channel blockers, if both are contra-indicated, or when they both fail to adequately control angina symptoms.

Response to treatment should be assessed every 2–4 weeks following initiation or change of drug therapy; drug doses should be titrated to the maximum tolerated effective dose.

If a combination of two drugs at a maximum therapeutic dose fails to control angina symptoms, patients should be considered for referral to a specialist. ⟨A⟩

Secondary prevention of cardiovascular events

All patients with angina are assumed to be at high-risk for cardiovascular events. The occurrence of cardiovascular events can be prevented by management of cardiovascular risk factors through lifestyle changes (such as smoking cessation, weight management, increased physical activity), psychological support, and drug treatment.

[EvGr] All patients with stable angina due to atherosclerotic disease should be given long-term treatment with low-dose aspirin p. 132 and a statin. Treatment with an ACE inhibitor should also be considered, particularly if the patient has diabetes. ⟨A⟩ See also *Secondary prevention* in Cardiovascular disease risk assessment and prevention p. 203 for further information.

Non-drug treatment

[EvGr] Revascularisation by coronary artery bypass graft or percutaneous coronary intervention should be considered for patients with stable angina who remain symptomatic whilst on optimal drug therapy. ⟨A⟩ See also *Antiplatelet drugs and coronary stents* in Antiplatelet drugs p. 131.

Advanced Pharmacy Services

Patients with stable angina may be eligible for the New Medicines Service / Medicines Use Review service provided by a community pharmacist. For further information, see *Advanced Pharmacy Services* in Medicines optimisation p. 18.

Useful Resources

Management of stable angina. Scottish Intercollegiate Guidelines Network. A national clinical guideline 151. April 2018. www.sign.ac.uk/assets/sign151.pdf

Stable angina: management. National Institute for Health and Care Excellence. Clinical guideline 126. July 2011 (updated August 2016). www.nice.org.uk/guidance/cg126

> **Other drugs used for Myocardial ischaemia** Acebutolol, p. 166 · Bivalirudin, p. 148 · Carvedilol, p. 162 · Felodipine, p. 174 · Fondaparinux sodium, p. 138 · Nadolol, p. 164 · Nicardipine hydrochloride, p. 175 · Nifedipine, p. 176 · Pindolol, p. 164 · Timolol maleate, p. 165

ANTITHROMBOTIC DRUGS 〉 ANTIPLATELET DRUGS

Cangrelor

07-Aug-2020

● DRUG ACTION Cangrelor is a direct $P2Y_{12}$ platelet receptor antagonist that blocks adenosine diphosphate induced platelet activation and aggregation.

● INDICATIONS AND DOSE

In combination with aspirin for the reduction of thrombotic cardiovascular events in patients with coronary artery disease undergoing percutaneous coronary intervention (PCI) who have not received an oral $P2Y_{12}$ inhibitor (e.g. clopidogrel, prasugrel, ticagrelor) prior to the PCI procedure and in whom oral therapy with a $P2Y_{12}$ inhibitor is not suitable (under expert supervision)

▸ INITIALLY BY INTRAVENOUS INJECTION

▸ Adult: Initially 30 micrograms/kg, to be given as a bolus dose, followed immediately by (by intravenous infusion) 4 micrograms/kg/minute, start treatment before percutaneous coronary intervention and continue infusion for at least 2 hours or for the duration of intervention if longer; maximum duration of infusion 4 hours

- CONTRA-INDICATIONS Active bleeding · history of stroke · history of transient ischaemic attack · patients at increased risk of bleeding (e.g. impaired haemostasis, irreversible coagulation disorders, major surgery or trauma, uncontrolled severe hypertension)
- CAUTIONS Disease states associated with increased bleeding risk
- INTERACTIONS → Appendix 1: cangrelor
- SIDE-EFFECTS
- ▶ **Common or very common** Dyspnoea · haemorrhage · skin reactions
- ▶ **Uncommon** Cardiac tamponade · haemodynamic instability · renal impairment · retroperitoneal haemorrhage (including fatal cases)
- ▶ **Rare or very rare** Anaemia · haematoma infection · intracranial haemorrhage · menorrhagia · skin neoplasm haemorrhage · stroke · thrombocytopenia · vascular pseudoaneurysm · wound haemorrhage
- PREGNANCY Manufacturer advises avoid—toxicity in *animal* studies.
- BREAST FEEDING Manufacturer advises potential risk to infant —no information available.
- RENAL IMPAIRMENT Manufacturer advises caution in severe renal impairment—increased risk of bleeding.
- DIRECTIONS FOR ADMINISTRATION For *intravenous bolus injection* and *intravenous infusion*, manufacturer advises reconstitute each 50 mg vial with 5 mL of water for injection and gently swirl, do not shake vigorously. Withdraw 5 mL of reconstituted solution, add to 250 mL of either Sodium Chloride 0.9% *or* Glucose 5% and mix thoroughly. The bolus injection and infusion should be administered from the infusion solution.

- MEDICINAL FORMS There can be variation in the licensing of different medicines containing the same drug.

Powder for solution for injection
- ▶ Kengrexal (Chiesi Ltd)
  Cangrelor (as Cangrelor tetrasodium) 50 mg Kengrexal 50mg powder for concentrate for solution for injection / infusion vials | 10 vial [PoM] £2,500.00 (Hospital only)

ANTITHROMBOTIC DRUGS > GLYCOPROTEIN IIB/IIIA INHIBITORS

Eptifibatide

26-Jun-2019

- INDICATIONS AND DOSE

In combination with aspirin and unfractionated heparin for the prevention of early myocardial infarction in patients with unstable angina or non-ST-segment-elevation myocardial infarction and with last episode of chest pain within 24 hours (specialist use only)
- ▶ INITIALLY BY INTRAVENOUS INJECTION
- ▶ Adult: Initially 180 micrograms/kg, then (by intravenous infusion) 2 micrograms/kg/minute for up to 72 hours (up to 96 hours if percutaneous coronary intervention during treatment)

- CONTRA-INDICATIONS Abnormal bleeding within 30 days · haemorrhagic diathesis · history of haemorrhagic stroke · increased INR · increased prothrombin time · intracranial disease · major surgery or severe trauma within 6 weeks · severe hypertension · stroke within last 30 days · thrombocytopenia
- CAUTIONS Discontinue if emergency cardiac surgery necessary · discontinue if intra-aortic balloon pump necessary · discontinue if thrombolytic therapy necessary ·

risk of bleeding—discontinue immediately if uncontrolled serious bleeding
- INTERACTIONS → Appendix 1: eptifibatide
- SIDE-EFFECTS
- ▶ **Common or very common** Arrhythmias · atrioventricular block · cardiac arrest · congestive heart failure · haemorrhage · hypotension · intracranial haemorrhage · procedural complications · shock
- ▶ **Uncommon** Cerebral ischaemia · thrombocytopenia
- ▶ **Rare or very rare** Rash
- PREGNANCY Manufacturer advises use only if potential benefit outweighs risk—no information available.
- BREAST FEEDING Manufacturer advises avoid—no information available.
- HEPATIC IMPAIRMENT Manufacturer advises caution; avoid in significant impairment (increased risk of bleeding complications, limited information available).
- RENAL IMPAIRMENT Avoid if eGFR less than 30 mL/minute/1.73 m^2.
  Dose adjustments Reduce infusion to 1 microgram/kg/minute if eGFR 30–50 mL/minute/1.73 m^2.
- MONITORING REQUIREMENTS
- ▶ Measure baseline prothrombin time, activated partial thromboplastin time, platelet count, haemoglobin, haematocrit and serum creatinine.
- ▶ Monitor haemoglobin, haematocrit and platelets within 6 hours after start of treatment, then at least once daily.

- MEDICINAL FORMS There can be variation in the licensing of different medicines containing the same drug.
Solution for injection
- ▶ Eptifibatide (Non-proprietary)
  Eptifibatide 2 mg per 1 ml Eptifibatide 20mg/10ml solution for injection vials | 1 vial [PoM] [▨] (Hospital only)
- ▶ Integrilin (GlaxoSmithKline UK Ltd)
  Eptifibatide 2 mg per 1 ml Integrilin 20mg/10ml solution for injection vials | 1 vial [PoM] £13.61 (Hospital only)
Solution for infusion
- ▶ Eptifibatide (Non-proprietary)
  Eptifibatide 750 microgram per 1 ml Eptifibatide 75mg/100ml solution for infusion vials | 1 vial [PoM] [▨] (Hospital only)
- ▶ Integrilin (GlaxoSmithKline UK Ltd)
  Eptifibatide 750 microgram per 1 ml Integrilin 75mg/100ml solution for infusion vials | 1 vial [PoM] £42.79 (Hospital only)

Tirofiban

06-Aug-2020

- INDICATIONS AND DOSE

In combination with unfractionated heparin, aspirin, and clopidogrel for prevention of early myocardial infarction in patients with unstable angina or non-ST-segment-elevation myocardial infarction (NSTEMI) and with last episode of chest pain within 12 hours (with angiography planned for 4–48 hours after diagnosis) (initiated under specialist supervision)
- ▶ BY INTRAVENOUS INFUSION
- ▶ Adult: Initially 400 nanograms/kg/minute for 30 minutes, then 100 nanograms/kg/minute for at least 48 hours (continue during and for 12–24 hours after percutaneous coronary intervention), maximum duration of treatment 108 hours continued →

In combination with unfractionated heparin, aspirin, and clopidogrel for prevention of early myocardial infarction in patients with unstable angina or non-ST-segment-elevation myocardial infarction (NSTEMI) and with last episode of chest pain within 12 hours (with angiography within 4 hours of diagnosis) (initiated under specialist supervision)
▶ INITIALLY BY INTRAVENOUS INJECTION
▶ Adult: 25 micrograms/kg, to be given over 3 minutes at start of percutaneous coronary intervention, then (by intravenous infusion) 150 nanograms/kg/minute for 12–24 hours, maximum duration of treatment 48 hours

In combination with unfractionated heparin, aspirin, and clopidogrel for reduction of major cardiovascular events in patients with ST-segment elevation myocardial infarction (STEMI) intended for primary percutaneous coronary intervention (PCI) (initiated under specialist supervision)
▶ INITIALLY BY INTRAVENOUS INJECTION
▶ Adult: 25 micrograms/kg, to be given over 3 minutes at start of percutaneous coronary intervention, then (by intravenous infusion) 150 nanograms/kg/minute for 12–24 hours, maximum duration of treatment 48 hours

● CONTRA-INDICATIONS Abnormal bleeding within 30 days · history of haemorrhagic stroke · history of intracranial disease · increased INR · increased prothrombin time · severe hypertension · stroke within 30 days · thrombocytopenia

● CAUTIONS Active peptic ulcer (within 3 months) · acute pericarditis · anaemia · aortic dissection · cardiogenic shock · discontinue if intra-aortic balloon pump necessary · discontinue if thrombolytic therapy necessary · discontinue immediately if serious or uncontrollable bleeding occurs · discontiue if emergency cardiac surgery necessary · elderly · faecal occult blood · haematuria · haemorrhagic retinopathy · low body-weight · major surgery within 3 months (avoid if within 6 weeks) · organ biopsy or lithotripsy within last 2 weeks · puncture of non-compressible vessel within 24 hours · risk of bleeding (within 3 months) · severe heart failure · severe trauma within 3 months (avoid if within 6 weeks) · traumatic or protracted cardiopulmonary resuscitation within last 2 weeks · uncontrolled severe hypertension · vasculitis

● INTERACTIONS → Appendix 1: tirofiban

● SIDE-EFFECTS
▶ **Common or very common** Ecchymosis · fever · haemorrhage · headache · nausea · thrombocytopenia
▶ **Frequency not known** Intracranial haemorrhage

● PREGNANCY Manufacturer advises use only if potential benefit outweighs risk—no information available.

● BREAST FEEDING Manufacturer advises avoid—no information available.

● HEPATIC IMPAIRMENT Manufacturer advises caution in mild to moderate hepatic failure; avoid in severe hepatic failure (no information available).

● RENAL IMPAIRMENT Increased risk of bleeding.
Dose adjustments Use half normal dose if eGFR less than 30 mL/minute/1.73 m².
Monitoring Monitor carefully if eGFR less than 60 mL/minute/1.73 m².

● MONITORING REQUIREMENTS Monitor platelet count, haemoglobin and haematocrit before treatment, 2–6 hours after start of treatment and then at least once daily.

● DIRECTIONS FOR ADMINISTRATION For *intravenous infusion* (*Aggrastat*®), manufacturer advises give continuously in Glucose 5% or Sodium chloride 0.9%. Withdraw 50 mL infusion fluid from 250 mL bag and replace with 50 mL tirofiban concentrate (250 micrograms/mL) to give a final concentration of 50 micrograms/mL.

● MEDICINAL FORMS There can be variation in the licensing of different medicines containing the same drug.
Solution for infusion
ELECTROLYTES: May contain Sodium
▶ Aggrastat (Correvio UK Ltd)
Tirofiban 250 microgram per 1 ml Aggrastat 12.5mg/50ml concentrate for solution for infusion vials | 1 vial [PoM] £146.11 (Hospital only)
Infusion
ELECTROLYTES: May contain Sodium
▶ Tirofiban (Non-proprietary)
Tirofiban 50 microgram per 1 ml Tirofiban 12.5mg/250ml infusion bags | 1 bag [PoM] £159.00-£160.72 (Hospital only)
▶ Aggrastat (Correvio UK Ltd)
Tirofiban 50 microgram per 1 ml Aggrastat 12.5mg/250ml infusion bags | 1 bag [PoM] £160.72 (Hospital only)

PIPERAZINE DERIVATIVES

Ranolazine

23-Nov-2020

● INDICATIONS AND DOSE
As adjunctive therapy in the treatment of stable angina in patients inadequately controlled or intolerant of first-line antianginal therapies
▶ BY MOUTH
▶ Adult: Initially 375 mg twice daily for 2–4 weeks, then increased to 500 mg twice daily, then adjusted according to response to 750 mg twice daily; reduced if not tolerated to 375–500 mg twice daily

● CAUTIONS Body-weight less than 60 kg · elderly · moderate to severe congestive heart failure · QT interval prolongation

● INTERACTIONS → Appendix 1: ranolazine

● SIDE-EFFECTS
▶ **Common or very common** Asthenia · constipation · headache · vomiting
▶ **Uncommon** Anxiety · appetite decreased · confusion · cough · dehydration · dizziness postural · drowsiness · dry mouth · gastrointestinal discomfort · gastrointestinal disorders · haemorrhage · hallucination · hot flush · hypotension · insomnia · joint swelling · muscle cramps · muscle weakness · pain in extremity · peripheral oedema · QT interval prolongation · sensation abnormal · skin reactions · syncope · tinnitus · tremor · urinary disorders · urine discolouration · vertigo · vision disorders · weight decreased
▶ **Rare or very rare** Acute kidney injury · altered smell sensation · angioedema · consciousness impaired · coordination abnormal · erectile dysfunction · gait abnormal · hearing impairment · hyponatraemia · memory loss · oral hypoaesthesia · pancreatitis · peripheral coldness

● PREGNANCY Manufacturer advises avoid unless essential—no information available.

● BREAST FEEDING Manufacturer advises avoid—no information available.

● HEPATIC IMPAIRMENT Manufacturer advises caution in mild impairment; avoid in moderate to severe impairment (risk of increased exposure).
Dose adjustments Manufacturer advises careful dose titration in mild impairment.

● RENAL IMPAIRMENT Use with caution if eGFR 30–80 mL/minute/1.73 m²; avoid if eGFR less than 30 mL/minute/1.73 m².

● NATIONAL FUNDING/ACCESS DECISIONS
For full details see funding body website
Scottish Medicines Consortium (SMC) decisions
▶ Ranolazine (*Ranexa*®) as add-on therapy for the symptomatic treatment of patients with stable angina pectoris who are inadequately controlled or intolerant to first-line antianginal

therapies (such as beta-blockers and/or calcium antagonists) (November 2012) SMC No. 565/09 Not recommended

● MEDICINAL FORMS There can be variation in the licensing of different medicines containing the same drug.

Modified-release tablet

CAUTIONARY AND ADVISORY LABELS 25

▸ Ranexa (A. Menarini Farmaceutica Internazionale SRL)
 Ranexa 375 mg Ranexa 375mg modified-release tablets |
 60 tablet [PoM] £48.98 DT = £48.98
 Ranolazine 500 mg Ranexa 500mg modified-release tablets |
 60 tablet [PoM] £48.98 DT = £48.98
 Ranolazine 750 mg Ranexa 750mg modified-release tablets |
 60 tablet [PoM] £48.98 DT = £48.98

SELECTIVE SINUS NODE I$_F$ INHIBITORS

Ivabradine

09-Nov-2020

● INDICATIONS AND DOSE

Treatment of angina in patients in normal sinus rhythm
▸ BY MOUTH
▸ Adult 18–74 years: Initially 2.5–5 mg twice daily for 3–4 weeks, then increased if necessary up to 7.5 mg twice daily, dose to be increased gradually; reduced if not tolerated to 2.5–5 mg twice daily, heart rate at rest should not be allowed to fall below 50 beats per minute, discontinue treatment if no improvement in symptoms within 3 months
▸ Adult 75 years and over: Initially 2.5 mg twice daily for 3–4 weeks, then increased if necessary up to 7.5 mg twice daily, dose to be increased gradually; reduced if not tolerated to 2.5–5 mg twice daily, heart rate at rest should not be allowed to fall below 50 beats per minute, discontinue treatment if no improvement in symptoms within 3 months

Mild to severe chronic heart failure
▸ BY MOUTH
▸ Adult 18–74 years: Initially 5 mg twice daily for 2 weeks, then increased if necessary to 7.5 mg twice daily; reduced if not tolerated to 2.5–5 mg twice daily, heart rate at rest should not be allowed to fall below 50 beats per minute
▸ Adult 75 years and over: Initially 2.5 mg twice daily for 2 weeks, then increased if necessary up to 7.5 mg twice daily, dose to be increased gradually; reduced if not tolerated to 2.5–5 mg twice daily, heart rate at rest should not be allowed to fall below 50 beats per minute

DOSE ADJUSTMENTS DUE TO INTERACTIONS
▸ Manufacturer advises reduce initial dose to 2.5 mg twice daily with concurrent use of moderate CYP3A4 inhibitors (except diltiazem, erythromycin and verapamil where concurrent use is contra-indicated).

● CONTRA-INDICATIONS Acute myocardial infarction · cardiogenic shock · congenital QT syndrome · do not initiate for angina if heart rate below 70 beats per minute · do not initiate for chronic heart failure if heart rate below 75 beats per minute · immediately after cerebrovascular accident · patients dependent on pacemaker · second- and third-degree heart block · severe hypotension · sick-sinus syndrome · sino-atrial block · unstable angina · unstable or acute heart failure

● CAUTIONS Atrial fibrillation or other arrhythmias (treatment ineffective) · elderly · in angina, consider stopping if there is no or limited symptom improvement after 3 months · intraventricular conduction defects · mild to moderate hypotension (avoid if severe) · retinitis pigmentosa

● INTERACTIONS → Appendix 1: ivabradine

● SIDE-EFFECTS
▸ Common or very common Arrhythmias · atrioventricular block · dizziness · headache · hypertension · vision disorders
▸ Uncommon Abdominal pain · angioedema · constipation · diarrhoea · eosinophilia · hyperuricaemia · hypotension · muscle cramps · nausea · QT interval prolongation · skin reactions · syncope · vertigo

● PREGNANCY Manufacturer advises avoid— *toxicity* in animal studies.

● BREAST FEEDING Present in milk in *animal* studies— manufacturer advises avoid.

● HEPATIC IMPAIRMENT Manufacturer advises caution in moderate impairment; avoid in severe impairment—no information available.

● RENAL IMPAIRMENT Manufacturer advises use with caution if eGFR less than 15 mL/minute/1.73 m^2—no information available.

● MONITORING REQUIREMENTS
▸ Monitor regularly for atrial fibrillation (consider benefits and risks of continued treatment if atrial fibrillation occurs).
▸ Monitor for bradycardia, especially after any dose increase, and discontinue if resting heart rate persistently below 50 beats per minute or continued symptoms of bradycardia despite dose reduction.

● NATIONAL FUNDING/ACCESS DECISIONS
For full details see funding body website
NICE decisions
▸ Ivabradine for the treatment of chronic heart failure (November 2012) NICE TA267 Recommended with restrictions
Scottish Medicines Consortium (SMC) decisions
▸ Ivabradine (*Procoralan®*) for chronic heart failure New York Heart Association (NYHA) II to IV class with systolic dysfunction, in patients in sinus rhythm and whose heart rate is ≥75 beats per minute (bpm), in combination with standard therapy including beta-blocker therapy or when beta-blocker therapy is contra-indicated or not tolerated (October 2012) SMC No. 805/12 Recommended with restrictions

● MEDICINAL FORMS There can be variation in the licensing of different medicines containing the same drug.

Tablet

▸ Ivabradine (Non-proprietary)
 Ivabradine (as Ivabradine hydrochloride) 2.5 mg Ivabradine 2.5mg tablets | 56 tablet [PoM] £93.56 DT = £93.56
 Ivabradine (as Ivabradine hydrochloride) 5 mg Ivabradine 5mg tablets | 56 tablet [PoM] £40.17 DT = £4.81
 Ivabradine (as Ivabradine hydrochloride) 7.5 mg Ivabradine 7.5mg tablets | 56 tablet [PoM] £40.17 DT = £4.70
▸ Procoralan (Servier Laboratories Ltd)
 Ivabradine (as Ivabradine hydrochloride) 5 mg Procoralan 5mg tablets | 56 tablet [PoM] £40.17 DT = £4.81
 Ivabradine (as Ivabradine hydrochloride) 7.5 mg Procoralan 7.5mg tablets | 56 tablet [PoM] £40.17 DT = £4.70

VASODILATORS > POTASSIUM-CHANNEL OPENERS

Nicorandil

06-Feb-2020

● INDICATIONS AND DOSE

Prophylaxis and treatment of stable angina (second-line)
▸ BY MOUTH
▸ Adult: Initially 5–10 mg twice daily, then increased if tolerated to 40 mg twice daily; usual dose 10–20 mg twice daily, use lower initial dose regimen if patient susceptible to headache

● CONTRA-INDICATIONS Acute pulmonary oedema · hypovolaemia · left ventricular dysfunction with low filling

Cardiovascular system

2

pressure or cardiac decompensation · severe hypotension · shock (including cardiogenic shock)

- CAUTIONS Diverticular disease (risk of fistula formation or bowel perforation) · G6PD deficiency · heart failure (class III–IV) · hyperkalaemia
- INTERACTIONS → Appendix 1: nicorandil
- SIDE-EFFECTS
- ▸ Common or very common Asthenia · dizziness · haemorrhage · headache (more common on initiation, usually transitory) · nausea · vasodilation · vomiting
- ▸ Rare or very rare Abdominal pain · angioedema · conjunctivitis · eye disorders · gastrointestinal disorders · genital ulceration · hepatic disorders · hyperkalaemia · mucosal ulceration · myalgia · oral disorders · skin reactions · skin ulcer
- ▸ Frequency not known Diplopia

SIDE-EFFECTS, FURTHER INFORMATION Nicorandil can cause serious skin, mucosal, and eye ulceration; including gastrointestinal ulcers, which may progress to perforation, haemorrhage, fistula or abscess. Stop treatment if ulceration occurs and consider an alternative.

- PREGNANCY Manufacturer advises use only if potential benefit outweighs risk—no information available.
- BREAST FEEDING No information available—manufacturer advises avoid.
- PATIENT AND CARER ADVICE
  Driving and skilled tasks Patients should be warned not to drive or operate machinery until it is established that their performance is unimpaired.

- MEDICINAL FORMS There can be variation in the licensing of different medicines containing the same drug.
  Tablet
  ▸ Nicorandil (Non-proprietary)
    Nicorandil 10 mg Nicorandil 10mg tablets | 60 tablet [PoM] £7.71 DT = £3.39
    Nicorandil 20 mg Nicorandil 20mg tablets | 60 tablet [PoM] £14.64 DT = £4.50
  ▸ Ikorel (Sanofi)
    Nicorandil 10 mg Ikorel 10mg tablets | 60 tablet [PoM] £7.71 DT = £3.39
    Nicorandil 20 mg Ikorel 20mg tablets | 60 tablet [PoM] £14.64 DT = £4.50

8.1 Acute coronary syndromes

Acute coronary syndromes

06-May-2020

Overview

Acute coronary syndromes encompass a spectrum of conditions which include unstable angina, and myocardial infarction with or without ST-segment elevation. Patients with different acute coronary syndromes may present similarly; definitive diagnosis is made on the basis of clinical presentation, ECG changes, and measurement of biochemical cardiac markers.

For recommendations on the management of acute myocardial injury and its cardiac complications in adults with known or suspected COVID-19 but without known pre-existing cardiovascular disease, see NICE rapid guidelines: **Acute myocardial injury** (available at: www.nice.org.uk/guidance/ng171). For further information on COVID-19, see COVID-19 p. 660.

Unstable angina and non-ST-segment elevation myocardial infarction (NSTEMI)

These are related acute coronary syndromes that fall between the classifications of stable angina and ST-segment elevation myocardial infarction (STEMI). They usually occur as a result of atheromatous plaque rupture, and are often characterised by stable angina that suddenly worsens, recurring or prolonged angina at rest, or new onset of severe angina. Patients with unstable angina have no evidence of myocardial necrosis, whereas in NSTEMI, myocardial necrosis (less significant than with STEMI) will be evident. There is a risk of progression to STEMI or sudden death, particularly in patients who experience pain at rest.

Management of unstable angina and non-ST-segment elevation myocardial infarction (NSTEMI)

These conditions are managed similarly; the aims of management are to provide supportive care and pain relief during the acute attack and to prevent further cardiac events and death. For advice on the management of patients with acute ST-segment elevation myocardial infarction (STEMI), see below.

Initial management

Oxygen should be administered if there is evidence of hypoxia, pulmonary oedema, or continuing myocardial ischaemia; hyperoxia should be avoided and particular care is required in patients with chronic obstructive airways disease.

Nitrates are used to relieve ischaemic pain. If sublingual glyceryl trinitrate p. 233 is not effective, intravenous or buccal glyceryl trinitrate or intravenous isosorbide dinitrate p. 235 is given. If pain continues, diamorphine hydrochloride p. 476 or morphine p. 483 can be given by slow intravenous injection; an antiemetic such as metoclopramide hydrochloride p. 451 should also be given.

Aspirin p. 132 (chewed or dispersed in water) is given for its antiplatelet effect. If aspirin is given before arrival at hospital, a note saying that it has been given should be sent with the patient. Clopidogrel p. 134 should also be given. Prasugrel p. 230 is an alternative to clopidogrel in certain patients undergoing percutaneous coronary intervention (see NICE guidance). Ticagrelor p. 230 is also an alternative to clopidogrel (see NICE guidance). Patients should also receive either heparin (unfractionated) p. 145, a **low molecular weight heparin**, or fondaparinux sodium p. 138.

Patients without contra-indications should receive **beta-blockers** which should be continued indefinitely. In patients without left ventricular dysfunction and in whom beta-blockers are inappropriate, diltiazem hydrochloride p. 171 or verapamil hydrochloride p. 178 can be given.

The glycoprotein IIb/IIIa inhibitors eptifibatide p. 225 (in combination with heparin (unfractionated) and aspirin) and tirofiban p. 225 (in combination with heparin (unfractionated), aspirin, and clopidogrel) can be used for unstable angina or for NSTEMI in patients at a high risk of either myocardial infarction or death.

In intermediate- and high-risk patients, abciximab or eptifibatide (in combination with heparin (unfractionated) and aspirin), or tirofiban (in combination with heparin (unfractionated), aspirin, and clopidogrel) can also be used in patients undergoing percutaneous coronary intervention, to reduce the immediate risk of vascular occlusion. In intermediate- and high-risk patients in whom early intervention is planned, bivalirudin p. 148 can be considered as an alternative to the combination of a glyocprotein IIb/IIIa inhibitor plus a heparin.

Revascularisation procedures are often appropriate for patients with unstable angina or NSTEMI; see Antiplatelet drugs p. 131 for the use of antiplatelet drugs in patients undergoing coronary stenting.

Long-term management

The need for long-term angina treatment or for coronary angiography should be assessed. Most patients will require standard angina treatment to prevent recurrence of symptoms.

ST-segment elevation myocardial infarction (STEMI)

This is an acute coronary syndrome where atheromatous plaque rupture leads to thrombosis and myocardial ischaemia, with irreversible necrosis of the heart muscle, often leading to long-term complications. STEMI can also occasionally occur as a result of coronary spasm or embolism, arteritis, spontaneous thrombosis, or sudden severe elevation in blood pressure.

Management of ST-segment elevation myocardial infarction (STEMI)

These notes give an overview of the initial and long-term management of myocardial infarction with ST segment elevation (STEMI). For advice on the management of non-ST-segment elevation myocardial infarction (NSTEMI) and unstable angina, see above. The aims of management of STEMI are to provide supportive care and pain relief, to promote reperfusion and to reduce mortality. Oxygen, nitrates, and diamorphine hydrochloride or morphine can provide initial support and pain relief; aspirin and percutaneous coronary intervention or thrombolytics promote reperfusion; anticoagulants help to reduce re-occlusion and systemic embolisation; long-term use of aspirin, beta-blockers, ACE inhibitors, and statins help to reduce mortality further.

Local guidelines for the management of myocardial infarction should be followed where they exist.

Initial management

Oxygen should be administered if there is evidence of hypoxia, pulmonary oedema, or continuing myocardial ischaemia; hyperoxia should be avoided and particular care is required in patients with chronic obstructive airways disease.

The pain (and anxiety) of myocardial infarction is managed with slow intravenous injection of diamorphine hydrochloride or morphine; an antiemetic such as metoclopramide hydrochloride (or, if left ventricular function is not compromised, cyclizine p. 449) by intravenous injection should also be given.

Aspirin (chewed or dispersed in water) is given for its antiplatelet effect. If aspirin is given before arrival at hospital, a note saying that it has been given should be sent with the patient. Clopidogrel, should also be given. Prasugrel, is an alternative to clopidogrel in certain patients undergoing percutaneous coronary intervention (see NICE guidance). Ticagrelor, is also an alternative to clopidogrel (see NICE guidance).

Patency of the occluded artery can be restored by percutaneous coronary intervention or by giving a **thrombolytic drug**, unless contra-indicated. Percutaneous coronary intervention is the preferred method; a **glycoprotein IIb/IIIa inhibitor** can be used to reduce the risk of immediate vascular occlusion in intermediate- and high-risk patients. Patients undergoing percutaneous coronary intervention should also receive either heparin (unfractionated) or a low molecular weight heparin (e.g. enoxaparin sodium p. 144); bivalirudin is an alternative to the combination of a glycoprotein IIb/IIIa inhibitor plus a heparin (see also NICE guidance). In patients who cannot be offered percutaneous coronary intervention within 90 minutes of diagnosis, a thrombolytic drug should be administered along with either low molecular weight heparin (for maximum 2 days), a low molecular weight heparin (e.g. enoxaparin sodium p. 144), or fondaparinux sodium p. 138. See use of antiplatelet drugs in patients undergoing coronary stenting in Antiplatelet drugs p. 131.

Patients who do not receive reperfusion therapy (with percutaneous coronary intervention or a thrombolytic) should be treated with either fondaparinux sodium, enoxaparin sodium, or heparin (unfractionated) p. 145. Prescribers should consult product literature and local protocols (where they exist) for details of anticoagulant dose and duration.

Nitrates are used to relieve ischaemic pain. If sublingual glyceryl trinitrate p. 233 is not effective, intravenous glyceryl trinitrate or isosorbide dinitrate p. 235 is given.

Early administration of some **beta-blockers** has been shown to be of benefit and should be given to patients without contra-indications.

ACE inhibitors, and angiotensin-II receptor antagonists if an ACE inhibitor cannot be used, are also of benefit to patients who have no contra-indications; in hypertensive and normotensive patients treatment with an ACE inhibitor, or an angiotensin-II receptor antagonist, can be started within 24 hours of the myocardial infarction and continued for at least 5–6 weeks (see below for long-term treatment).

All patients should be closely monitored for hyperglycaemia; those with diabetes or raised blood-glucose concentration should receive insulin p. 753.

Long-term management

Long-term management following STEMI involves the use of several drugs which should ideally be started before the patient is discharged from hospital.

Aspirin p. 132 should be given to all patients, unless contra-indicated. The addition of clopidogrel p. 134 has been shown to reduce morbidity and mortality. Prasugrel p. 230 or ticagrelor p. 230 are alternatives to clopidogrel in certain patients. For those intolerant of clopidogrel, and who are at low risk of bleeding, the combination of warfarin sodium p. 153 and aspirin should be considered. In those intolerant of both aspirin and clopidogrel, warfarin sodium alone can be used. Warfarin sodium should be continued for those who are already being treated for another indication, such as atrial fibrillation, with the addition of aspirin if there is a low risk of bleeding. The combination of aspirin with clopidogrel or warfarin sodium increases the risk of bleeding. Low-dose rivaroxaban p. 139, in combination with aspirin alone *or* aspirin and clopidogrel, is licensed for the prevention of atherothrombotic events following STEMI—see Prevention of cardiovascular events. For details of antiplatelet drug duration following coronary stenting—see also Antiplatelet drugs and coronary stents in Antiplatelet drugs p. 131.

Beta-blockers should be given to all patients in whom they are not contra-indicated. Acebutolol p. 166, metoprolol tartrate p. 169, propranolol hydrochloride p. 164 and timolol maleate p. 165 are suitable; for patients with left ventricular dysfunction, carvedilol p. 162, bisoprolol fumarate p. 167, or long-acting metoprolol tartrate may be appropriate

Diltiazem hydrochloride p. 171 [unlicensed] or verapamil hydrochloride p. 178 can be considered if a beta-blocker cannot be used; however, they are contra-indicated in those with left ventricular dysfunction. Other calcium-channel blockers have no place in routine long-term management after a myocardial infarction.

An **ACE inhibitor** should be considered for all patients, especially those with evidence of left ventricular dysfunction. If an ACE inhibitor cannot be used, an angiotensin-II receptor antagonist may be used for patients with heart failure. A relatively high dose of either the ACE inhibitor or angiotensin-II receptor antagonist may be required to produce benefit.

Nitrates are used for patients with angina. Eplerenone p. 208 is licensed for use following a myocardial infarction in those with left ventricular dysfunction and evidence of heart failure.

See also the role of **statins** in preventing recurrent cardiovascular events in Dyslipidaemias p. 210.

Prevention of cardiovascular events

Patients with stable angina, unstable angina, or NSTEMI should be given advice and treatments to reduce their cardiovascular risk. The importance of life-style changes, especially stopping smoking, should be emphasised.

Cardiovascular system

2

Aspirin should be given indefinitely. Antihypertensive treatment should be initiated if appropriate, and a **statin** should also be given.

In patients with stable angina, addition of an **ACE inhibitor** should be considered for patients with diabetes (and should be continued if indicated for a co-morbidity).

In patients with unstable angina or NSTEMI, clopidogrel is given, in combination with aspirin, for up to 12 months—most benefit occurs during the first 3 months. Prasugrel or ticagrelor are alternatives to clopidogrel in certain patients. An ACE inhibitor should also be given.

Low-dose rivaroxaban, in combination with aspirin alone *or* aspirin and clopidogrel, is licensed for the prevention of atherothrombotic events following an acute coronary syndrome with elevated cardiac biomarkers.

Advanced Pharmacy Services

Patients with a history of acute coronary syndrome may be eligible for the New Medicines Service / Medicines Use Review service provided by a community pharmacist. For further information, see *Advanced Pharmacy Services* in Medicines optimisation p. 18.

Other drugs used for Acute coronary syndromes
Captopril, p. 182 · Dalteparin sodium, p. 143 · Lisinopril, p. 184 · Perindopril arginine, p. 185 · Perindopril erbumine, p. 185 · Ramipril, p. 186 · Trandolapril, p. 187 · Valsartan, p. 193

ANTITHROMBOTIC DRUGS > ANTIPLATELET DRUGS

Prasugrel
02-Dec-2020

● **INDICATIONS AND DOSE**

In combination with aspirin for the prevention of atherothrombotic events in patients with acute coronary syndrome undergoing percutaneous coronary intervention
▸ BY MOUTH
▸ Adult 18-74 years (body-weight up to 60 kg): Initially 60 mg for 1 dose, then 5 mg once daily usually for up to 12 months
▸ Adult 18-74 years (body-weight 60 kg and above): Initially 60 mg for 1 dose, then 10 mg once daily usually for up to 12 months
▸ Adult 75 years and over: Initially 60 mg for 1 dose, then 5 mg once daily usually for up to 12 months

Patients undergoing coronary angiography within 48 hours of admission for unstable angina or NSTEMI
▸ BY MOUTH
▸ Adult: Loading dose 60 mg, not to be administered until the time of percutaneous coronary intervention in order to minimise the risk of bleeding, maintenance dose of 10 mg or 5 mg daily should then be selected as appropriate based on age and weight

● CONTRA-INDICATIONS Active bleeding · history of stroke or transient ischaemic attack
● CAUTIONS Body-weight less than 60 kg · discontinue at least 7 days before elective surgery if antiplatelet effect not desirable · elderly · patients at increased risk of bleeding (e.g. from recent trauma, surgery, gastro-intestinal bleeding, or active peptic ulcer disease)
● INTERACTIONS → Appendix 1: prasugrel
● SIDE-EFFECTS
▸ **Common or very common** Anaemia · haemorrhage · skin reactions
▸ **Rare or very rare** Thrombocytopenia

● ALLERGY AND CROSS-SENSITIVITY EvGr Caution in patients with history of hypersensitivity reactions to thienopyridines (e.g. clopidogrel). ⓜ
● PREGNANCY Manufacturer advises use only if potential benefit outweighs risk.
● BREAST FEEDING Manufacturer advises avoid—no information available.
● HEPATIC IMPAIRMENT Manufacturer advises caution in moderate impairment (increased risk of bleeding, limited information available); avoid in severe impairment (no information available).
● RENAL IMPAIRMENT Use with caution—increased risk of bleeding.
● NATIONAL FUNDING/ACCESS DECISIONS
For full details see funding body website
NICE decisions
▸ Prasugrel with percutaneous coronary intervention for treating acute coronary syndromes (July 2014) NICE TA317 Recommended
Scottish Medicines Consortium (SMC) decisions
▸ Prasugrel (*Efient*®) for the prevention of atherothrombotic events in acute coronary syndrome (September 2009) SMC No. 562/09 Recommended with restrictions

● MEDICINAL FORMS There can be variation in the licensing of different medicines containing the same drug.
Tablet
▸ Prasugrel (Non-proprietary)
Prasugrel 5 mg Prasugrel 5mg tablets | 28 tablet PoM £47.56 DT = £11.09
Prasugrel 10 mg Prasugrel 10mg tablets | 28 tablet PoM £47.56 DT = £5.87
▸ Efient (Daiichi Sankyo UK Ltd)
Prasugrel 5 mg Efient 5mg tablets | 28 tablet PoM £47.56 DT = £11.09
Prasugrel 10 mg Efient 10mg tablets | 28 tablet PoM £47.56 DT = £5.87

Ticagrelor
19-Oct-2018

● DRUG ACTION Ticagrelor is a $P2Y_{12}$ receptor antagonist that prevents ADP-mediated $P2Y_{12}$ dependent platelet activation and aggregation.

● **INDICATIONS AND DOSE**

Prevention of atherothrombotic events in patients with acute coronary syndrome [in combination with aspirin]
▸ BY MOUTH
▸ Adult: Initially 180 mg for 1 dose, then 90 mg twice daily usually for up to 12 months

Prevention of atherothrombotic events in patients with a history of myocardial infarction and a high risk of an atherothrombotic event [in combination with aspirin]
▸ BY MOUTH
▸ Adult: 60 mg twice daily, extended treatment may be started without interruption after the initial 12-month therapy for acute coronary syndrome. Treatment may also be initiated up to 2 years from the myocardial infarction, or within 1 year after stopping previous ADP receptor inhibitor treatment. There are limited data on the efficacy and safety of extended treatment beyond 3 years

● CONTRA-INDICATIONS Active bleeding · history of intracranial haemorrhage
● CAUTIONS Asthma · bradycardia (unless pacemaker fitted) · chronic obstructive pulmonary disease · discontinue 5 days before elective surgery if antiplatelet effect not desirable · history of hyperuricaemia · patients at increased risk of bleeding (e.g. from recent trauma, surgery, gastro-intestinal bleeding, or coagulation disorders) · second- or

third-degree AV block (unless pacemaker fitted) · sick sinus syndrome (unless pacemaker fitted)

● INTERACTIONS → Appendix 1: ticagrelor

● SIDE-EFFECTS
▶ **Common or very common** Constipation · diarrhoea · dizziness · dyspepsia · dyspnoea · gout · gouty arthritis · haemorrhage · headache · hyperuricaemia · hypotension · nausea · skin reactions · syncope · vertigo
▶ **Uncommon** Angioedema · confusion · intracranial haemorrhage · tumour haemorrhage
▶ **Frequency not known** Thrombotic thrombocytopenic purpura

● PREGNANCY Manufacturer advises avoid—toxicity in *animal* studies.

● BREAST FEEDING Manufacturer advises avoid—present in milk in *animal* studies.

● HEPATIC IMPAIRMENT Manufacturer advises caution in moderate impairment (limited information available); avoid in severe impairment (no information available).

● MONITORING REQUIREMENTS Manufacturer advises monitor renal function 1 month after initiation in patients with acute coronary syndrome.

● NATIONAL FUNDING/ACCESS DECISIONS
For full details see funding body website
NICE decisions
▶ **Ticagrelor for the treatment of acute coronary syndromes (October 2011)** NICE TA236 Recommended
▶ **Ticagrelor for preventing atherothrombotic events after myocardial infarction (December 2016)** NICE TA420 Recommended

● MEDICINAL FORMS There can be variation in the licensing of different medicines containing the same drug.
Orodispersible tablet
▶ Brilique (AstraZeneca UK Ltd)
Ticagrelor 90 mg Brilique 90mg orodispersible tablets sugar-free | 56 tablet PoM £54.60 DT = £54.60
Tablet
▶ Brilique (AstraZeneca UK Ltd)
Ticagrelor 60 mg Brilique 60mg tablets | 56 tablet PoM £54.60 DT = £54.60
Ticagrelor 90 mg Brilique 90mg tablets | 56 tablet PoM £54.60 DT = £54.60

ANTITHROMBOTIC DRUGS > TISSUE PLASMINOGEN ACTIVATORS

Fibrinolytic drugs

Overview

The value of thrombolytic drugs for the treatment of *myocardial infarction* has been established. Streptokinase p. 232 and alteplase below have been shown to reduce mortality. Reteplase and tenecteplase p. 233 are also licensed for acute myocardial infarction. Thrombolytic drugs are indicated for any patient with acute myocardial infarction for whom the benefit is likely to outweigh the risk of treatment. Trials have shown that the benefit is greatest in those with ECG changes that include ST segment elevation (especially in those with anterior infarction) and in patients with bundle branch block. Patients should not be denied thrombolytic treatment on account of age alone because mortality in the elderly is high and the reduction in mortality is the same as in younger patients. Alteplase should be given within 6–12 hours of symptom onset, reteplase and streptokinase within 12 hours of symptom onset, but ideally all should be given within 1 hour; use after 12 hours requires specialist advice. Tenecteplase should be given as early as possible and usually within 6 hours of symptom onset.

Alteplase, streptokinase and urokinase p. 150 can be used for other thromboembolic disorders such as deep-vein

thrombosis and pulmonary embolism. Alteplase is also used for acute ischaemic stroke.

Urokinase is also licensed to restore the patency of occluded intravenous catheters and cannulas blocked with fibrin clots.

Fibrinolytics

● DRUG ACTION Fibrinolytic drugs act as thrombolytics by activating plasminogen to form plasmin, which degrades fibrin and so breaks up thrombi.

● CONTRA-INDICATIONS Acute pancreatitis · aneurysm · aortic dissection · arteriovenous malformation · bacterial endocarditis · bleeding diatheses · coagulation defects · coma · heavy vaginal bleeding · history of cerebrovascular disease (especially recent events or with any residual disability) · neoplasm with risk of haemorrhage · oesophageal varices · pericarditis · recent gastro-intestinal ulceration · recent haemorrhage · recent surgery (including dental extraction) · recent trauma · severe hypertension

● CAUTIONS Conditions in which thrombolysis might give rise to embolic complications such as enlarged left atrium with atrial fibrillation (risk of dissolution of clot and subsequent embolisation) · elderly · external chest compression · hypertension · risk of bleeding (including that from venepuncture or invasive procedures)

● SIDE-EFFECTS
▶ **Common or very common** Anaphylactic reaction · angina pectoris · cardiac arrest · cardiogenic shock · chills · CNS haemorrhage · ecchymosis · fever · haemorrhage · haemorrhagic stroke · heart failure · hypotension · ischaemia recurrent (when used in myocardial infarction) · nausea · pericarditis · pulmonary oedema · vomiting
▶ **Uncommon** Aphasia · mitral valve incompetence · myocardial rupture · pericardial disorders · reperfusion arrhythmia (when used in myocardial infarction) · seizure
SIDE-EFFECTS, FURTHER INFORMATION Serious bleeding calls for discontinuation of the thrombolytic and may require administration of coagulation factors and antifibrinolytic drugs.

● PREGNANCY Thrombolytic drugs can possibly lead to premature separation of the placenta in the first 18 weeks of pregnancy. There is also a risk of maternal haemorrhage throughout pregnancy and post-partum, and also a theoretical risk of fetal haemorrhage throughout pregnancy.

● HEPATIC IMPAIRMENT Manufacturers advise avoid in severe impairment.

⬆ above

Alteplase
20-Nov-2020

(rt-PA; Tissue-type plasminogen activator)

● INDICATIONS AND DOSE
Acute myocardial infarction, accelerated regimen
▶ INITIALLY BY INTRAVENOUS INJECTION
▶ Adult (body-weight up to 65 kg): Initially 15 mg, to be initiated within 6 hours of symptom onset, followed by (by intravenous infusion) 0.75 mg/kg, to be given over 30 minutes, then (by intravenous infusion) 0.5 mg/kg, to be given over 60 minutes, maximum total dose of 100 mg administered over 90 minutes
▶ Adult (body-weight 65 kg and above): Initially 15 mg, to be initiated within 6 hours of symptom onset, followed by (by intravenous infusion) 50 mg, to be given over 30 minutes, then (by intravenous infusion) 35 mg, to be given over 60 minutes, maximum total dose of 100 mg administered over 90 minutes continued →

2

Cardiovascular system

2

Cardiovascular system

Acute myocardial infarction

▸ INITIALLY BY INTRAVENOUS INJECTION
▸ Adult: Initially 10 mg, to be initiated within 6–12 hours of symptom onset, followed by (by intravenous infusion) 50 mg, to be given over 60 minutes, then (by intravenous infusion) 10 mg for 4 infusions, each 10 mg infusion dose to be given over 30 minutes, total dose of 100 mg over 3 hours; maximum 1.5 mg/kg in patients less than 65 kg

Pulmonary embolism

▸ INITIALLY BY INTRAVENOUS INJECTION
▸ Adult: Initially 10 mg, to be given over 1–2 minutes, followed by (by intravenous infusion) 90 mg, to be given over 2 hours, maximum 1.5 mg/kg in patients less than 65 kg

Acute ischaemic stroke (under specialist neurology physician only)

▸ BY INTRAVENOUS INFUSION
▸ Adult 18-79 years: Initially 900 micrograms/kg (max. per dose 90 mg), treatment **must** begin within 4.5 hours of symptom onset, to be given over 60 minutes, the initial 10% of dose is to be administered by intravenous injection and the remainder by intravenous infusion

ACTILYSE CATHFLO ®

Thrombolytic treatment of occluded central venous access devices (including those used for haemodialysis)

▸ BY INTRAVENOUS INJECTION
▸ Adult: (consult product literature)

● CONTRA-INDICATIONS
GENERAL CONTRA-INDICATIONS
Recent delivery

SPECIFIC CONTRA-INDICATIONS
▸ When used for acute ischaemic stroke Convulsion accompanying stroke · history of stroke in patients with diabetes · hyperglycaemia · hypoglycaemia · severe stroke · stroke in last 3 months

● INTERACTIONS → Appendix 1: alteplase

● SIDE-EFFECTS
▸ **Uncommon** Haemothorax
▸ **Rare or very rare** Agitation · confusion · delirium · depression · epilepsy · psychosis · speech disorder
▸ **Frequency not known** Brain oedema (caused by reperfusion)

● ALLERGY AND CROSS-SENSITIVITY EvGr Contra-indicated if history of hypersensitivity to gentamicin (residue from manufacturing process). ◄

● MONITORING REQUIREMENTS
▸ When used for acute ischaemic stroke Monitor for intracranial haemorrhage, and monitor blood pressure (antihypertensive recommended if systolic above 180 mmHg or diastolic above 105 mmHg).

● DIRECTIONS FOR ADMINISTRATION For *intravenous infusion* (*Actilyse*®), manufacturer advises give intermittently in Sodium chloride 0.9%; dissolve in water for injections to a concentration of 1 mg/mL or 2 mg/mL and infuse intravenously; alternatively dilute the solution further in the infusion fluid to a concentration of not less than 200 micrograms/mL; not to be infused in glucose solution.

● NATIONAL FUNDING/ACCESS DECISIONS
For full details see funding body website

NICE decisions

▸ **Alteplase for treating acute ischaemic stroke (September 2012)** NICE TA264 Recommended

● MEDICINAL FORMS There can be variation in the licensing of different medicines containing the same drug. Forms available from special-order manufacturers include: solution for injection

Powder and solvent for solution for injection

▸ Actilyse (Boehringer Ingelheim Ltd)
Alteplase 10 mg Actilyse 10mg powder and solvent for solution for injection vials | 1 vial [PoM] £172.80
Alteplase 20 mg Actilyse 20mg powder and solvent for solution for injection vials | 1 vial [PoM] £259.20

Powder and solvent for solution for infusion

▸ Actilyse (Boehringer Ingelheim Ltd)
Alteplase 50 mg Actilyse 50mg powder and solvent for solution for infusion vials | 1 vial [PoM] £432.00

⬛ **231**

Streptokinase

29-Jul-2020

● INDICATIONS AND DOSE

Acute myocardial infarction

▸ BY INTRAVENOUS INFUSION
▸ Adult: 1 500 000 units, to be initiated within 12 hours of symptom onset, dose to be given over 60 minutes

Deep-vein thrombosis | Central retinal venous or arterial thrombosis

▸ BY INTRAVENOUS INFUSION
▸ Adult: 250 000 units, dose to be given over 30 minutes, then 100 000 units every 1 hour for 12 hours for central retinal venous or arterial thrombosis, or for 72 hours for deep-vein thrombosis

Pulmonary embolism

▸ BY INTRAVENOUS INFUSION
▸ Adult: 250 000 units, dose to be given over 30 minutes, then 100 000 units every 1 hour for 24 hours, alternatively 1 500 000 units, dose to be given over 1–2 hours

Occlusive peripheral arterial disease

▸ BY INTRAVENOUS INFUSION
▸ Adult: 250 000 units, dose to be given over 30 minutes, then 100 000 units every 1 hour for up to 5 days
▸ BY INTRA-ARTERIAL INFUSION
▸ Adult: (consult product literature)

● CAUTIONS Cavernous pulmonary disease · recent streptococcal infections

● INTERACTIONS → Appendix 1: streptokinase

● SIDE-EFFECTS
▸ **Common or very common** Arrhythmias · asthenia · diarrhoea · epigastric pain · headache · malaise · pain
▸ **Uncommon** Respiratory arrest · splenic rupture
▸ **Rare or very rare** Arthritis · eye inflammation · hypersensitivity · nephritis · nerve disorders · neurological effects · pulmonary oedema non-cardiogenic (caused by reperfusion) · shock · vasculitis

● ALLERGY AND CROSS-SENSITIVITY Contra-indicated if previous allergic reaction to either streptokinase or anistreplase (no longer available). Prolonged persistence of antibodies to streptokinase and anistreplase (no longer available) can reduce the effectiveness of subsequent treatment; therefore, streptokinase should not be used again beyond 4 days of first administration of either streptokinase or anistreplase.

● DIRECTIONS FOR ADMINISTRATION Manufacturer advises for *intravenous infusion*, give continuously or intermittently; reconstitute with sodium chloride 0.9%, then dilute further with Glucose 5% or Sodium Chloride 0.9% or Compound Sodium Lactate after reconstitution.

2

Cardiovascular system

- MEDICINAL FORMS There can be variation in the licensing of different medicines containing the same drug.

Powder for solution for infusion

‣ Streptokinase (Non-proprietary)

Streptokinase 1.5 mega unit Streptokinase 1.5million unit powder for solution for infusion vials | 1 vial [PoM] £195.00

Streptokinase 250000 unit Streptokinase 250,000unit powder for solution for infusion vials | 1 vial [PoM] £97.50

Streptokinase 750000 unit Streptokinase 750,000unit powder for solution for infusion vials | 1 vial [PoM] £49.35

F 231

Tenecteplase

- **INDICATIONS AND DOSE**

Acute myocardial infarction

‣ BY INTRAVENOUS INJECTION

‣ Adult: 30–50 mg (max. per dose 50 mg), dose to be given over 10 seconds and Initiated within 6 hours of symptom onset, dose varies according to body weight— consult product literature

- INTERACTIONS → Appendix 1: tenecteplase

- SIDE-EFFECTS

‣ **Uncommon** Drowsiness · hemiparesis · venous thrombosis

- BREAST FEEDING Manufacturer advises avoid breast-feeding for 24 hours after dose (express and discard milk during this time).

- MEDICINAL FORMS There can be variation in the licensing of different medicines containing the same drug.

Powder and solvent for solution for injection

‣ Metalyse (Boehringer Ingelheim Ltd)

Tenecteplase 10000 unit Metalyse 10,000unit powder and solvent for solution for injection vials | 1 vial [PoM] £602.70

NITRATES

Nitrates

Overview

Nitrates have a useful role in *angina*. Although they are potent coronary vasodilators, their principal benefit follows from a reduction in venous return which reduces left ventricular work. Unwanted effects such as flushing, headache, and postural hypotension may limit therapy, especially when angina is severe or when patients are unusually sensitive to the effects of nitrates.

Sublingual glyceryl trinitrate below is one of the most effective drugs for providing rapid symptomatic relief of angina, but its effect lasts only for 20 to 30 minutes; the 300-microgram tablet is often appropriate when glyceryl trinitrate is first used. The *aerosol* spray provides an alternative method of rapid relief of symptoms for those who find difficulty in dissolving sublingual preparations. Duration of action may be prolonged by *transdermal* preparations (but tolerance may develop).

Isosorbide dinitrate p. 235 is active *sublingually* and is a more stable preparation for those who only require nitrates infrequently. It is also effective by mouth for prophylaxis; although the effect is slower in onset, it may persist for several hours. Duration of action of up to 12 hours is claimed for *modified-release* preparations. The activity of isosorbide dinitrate may depend on the production of active metabolites, the most important of which is isosorbide mononitrate p. 236. Isosorbide mononitrate itself is also licensed for angina prophylaxis; modified-release formulations (for once daily administration) are available.

Glyceryl trinitrate or isosorbide dinitrate may be tried by *intravenous injection* when the sublingual form is ineffective in patients with chest pain due to myocardial infarction or severe ischaemia. Intravenous injections are also useful in the treatment of congestive heart failure.

Nitrates

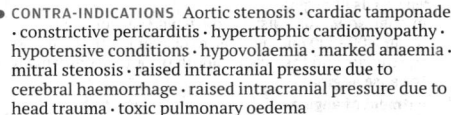

- CONTRA-INDICATIONS Aortic stenosis · cardiac tamponade · constrictive pericarditis · hypertrophic cardiomyopathy · hypotensive conditions · hypovolaemia · marked anaemia · mitral stenosis · raised intracranial pressure due to cerebral haemorrhage · raised intracranial pressure due to head trauma · toxic pulmonary oedema

- CAUTIONS Heart failure due to obstruction · hypothermia · hypothyroidism · hypoxaemia · malnutrition · metal-containing transdermal systems should be removed before magnetic resonance imaging procedures, cardioversion, or diathermy · recent history of myocardial infarction · susceptibility to angle-closure glaucoma · tolerance · ventilation and perfusion abnormalities

CAUTIONS, FURTHER INFORMATION

‣ Tolerance Many patients on long-acting or transdermal nitrates rapidly develop tolerance (with reduced therapeutic effects). Reduction of blood-nitrate concentrations to low levels for 4 to 12 hours each day usually maintains effectiveness in such patients. If tolerance is suspected during the use of transdermal patches they should be left off for 8–12 hours (usually overnight) in each 24 hours; in the case of modified-release tablets of isosorbide dinitrate (and conventional formulations of isosorbide mononitrate), the second of the two daily doses should be given after about 8 hours rather than after 12 hours. Conventional formulations of isosorbide mononitrate should not usually be given more than twice daily unless small doses are used; modified-release formulations of isosorbide mononitrate should only be given once daily, and used in this way do not produce tolerance.

‣ Elderly Prescription potentially inappropriate (STOPP criteria) if prescribed a **long-acting** nitrate with persistent postural hypotension i.e. recurrent drop in systolic blood pressure ≥ 20 mmHg (risk of syncope and falls).
See also Prescribing in the elderly p. 33.

- SIDE-EFFECTS

‣ **Common or very common** Arrhythmias · asthenia · cerebral ischaemia · dizziness · drowsiness · flushing · headache · hypotension · nausea · vomiting

‣ **Uncommon** Circulatory collapse · diarrhoea · skin reactions · syncope

- ALLERGY AND CROSS-SENSITIVITY [EvGr] Contra-indicated in nitrate hypersensitivity.

- BREAST FEEDING No information available— manufacturers advise use only if potential benefit outweighs risk.

- HEPATIC IMPAIRMENT In general, manufacturers advise caution in severe impairment.

- RENAL IMPAIRMENT Manufacturers advise use with caution in severe impairment.

- MONITORING REQUIREMENTS Monitor blood pressure and heart rate during intravenous infusion.

- TREATMENT CESSATION Avoid abrupt withdrawal.

F above

Glyceryl trinitrate

27-Jul-2018

- **INDICATIONS AND DOSE**

Prophylaxis of angina

‣ BY SUBLINGUAL ADMINISTRATION USING SUBLINGUAL TABLETS

‣ Adult: 1 tablet, to be administered prior to activity likely to cause angina

continued →

Treatment of angina
▸ BY SUBLINGUAL ADMINISTRATION USING SUBLINGUAL TABLETS
▸ Adult: 1 tablet, dose may be repeated at 5 minute intervals if required; if symptoms have not resolved after 3 doses, medical attention should be sought

Prophylaxis of angina
▸ BY SUBLINGUAL ADMINISTRATION USING AEROSOL SPRAY
▸ Adult: 400–800 micrograms, to be administered under the tongue and then close mouth prior to activity likely to cause angina

Treatment of angina
▸ BY SUBLINGUAL ADMINISTRATION USING AEROSOL SPRAY
▸ Adult: 400–800 micrograms, to be administered under the tongue and then close mouth, dose may be repeated at 5 minute intervals if required; if symptoms have not resolved after 3 doses, medical attention should be sought

Control of hypertension and myocardial ischaemia during and after cardiac surgery | Induction of controlled hypotension during surgery | Congestive heart failure | Unstable angina
▸ BY INTRAVENOUS INFUSION
▸ Adult: 10–200 micrograms/minute (max. per dose 400 micrograms/minute), adjusted according to response, consult product literature for recommended starting doses specific to indication

Anal fissure
▸ BY RECTUM USING OINTMENT
▸ Adult: Apply 2.5 centimetres every 12 hours until pain stops. Max. duration of use 8 weeks, apply to anal canal, 2.5 cm of ointment contains 1.5 mg of glyceryl trinitrate

DEPONIT ®

Prophylaxis of angina
▸ BY TRANSDERMAL APPLICATION
▸ Adult: One '5' or one '10' patch to be applied to lateral chest wall, upper arm, thigh, abdomen, or shoulder; increase to two '10' patches every 24 hours if necessary, to be replaced every 24 hours, siting replacement patch on different area

MINITRAN ®

Prophylaxis of angina
▸ BY TRANSDERMAL APPLICATION
▸ Adult: One '5' patch to be applied to chest or upper arm; replace every 24 hours, siting replacement patch on different area, dose to be adjusted according to response

Maintenance of venous patency ('5' patch only)
▸ BY TRANSDERMAL APPLICATION
▸ Adult: (consult product literature)

NITRO-DUR ®

Prophylaxis of angina
▸ BY TRANSDERMAL APPLICATION
▸ Adult: One '0.2mg/h' patch to be applied to chest or outer upper arm and replaced every 24 hours, siting replacement patch on different area, dose adjusted according to response; maximum 15 mg per day

PERCUTOL ®

Prophylaxis of angina
▸ TO THE SKIN
▸ Adult: Usual dose 1–2 inches every 3–4 hours as required, to be measured on to *Applirule*® and applied (usually to chest, arm, or thigh) without rubbing in and secured with surgical tape, approx. 800 micrograms/hour absorbed from 1 inch of ointment.

Prophylaxis of angina (to determine dose)
▸ TO THE SKIN
▸ Adult: ½ inch to be administered on first day then increased by ½ inch/day until headache occurs, then reduced by ½ inch, to be measured on to *Applirule*® and applied (usually to chest, arm, or thigh) without rubbing in and secured with surgical tape, approx. 800 micrograms/hour absorbed from 1 inch of ointment.

TRANSIDERM-NITRO ®

Prophylaxis of angina
▸ BY TRANSDERMAL APPLICATION
▸ Adult: One '5' or one '10' patch to be applied to lateral chest wall and replaced every 24 hours, siting replacement patch on different area, max. two '10' patches daily

Prophylaxis of phlebitis and extravasation ('5' patch only)
▸ BY TRANSDERMAL APPLICATION
▸ Adult: (consult product literature)

● INTERACTIONS → Appendix 1: nitrates
● SIDE-EFFECTS
▸ **Uncommon**
▸ With parenteral use Cardiac disorder · cyanosis
▸ With rectal use Anorectal disorder · anorectal haemorrhage · gastrointestinal discomfort
▸ With sublingual use Cyanosis
▸ **Rare or very rare**
▸ With parenteral or sublingual use Methaemoglobinaemia · respiratory disorder · restlessness
▸ With topical use Dyspepsia
▸ **Frequency not known**
▸ With parenteral use Hyperhidrosis
▸ With rectal use Vertigo
▸ With sublingual use Tongue blistering
▸ With transdermal use Palpitations
● PREGNANCY Not known to be harmful.
● DIRECTIONS FOR ADMINISTRATION
▸ With intravenous use For *intravenous infusion* (*Nitrocine*®, *Nitronal*®), give continuously in Glucose 5% or Sodium Chloride 0.9%. For *Nitrocine*®, suggested infusion concentration 100 micrograms/mL; incompatible with polyvinyl chloride infusion containers such as *Viaflex*® or *Steriflex*®; use glass or polyethylene containers or give via a syringe pump.
▸ With intravenous use Glass or polyethylene apparatus is preferable; loss of potency will occur if PVC is used. Glyceryl trinitrate 1 mg/ml to be diluted before use or given undiluted with syringe pump. Glyceryl trinitrate 5 mg/ml to be diluted before use.
● PRESCRIBING AND DISPENSING INFORMATION
▸ With sublingual use Glyceryl trinitrate tablets are available in strengths of 300-, 500- and 600-micrograms— manufacturer advises tablets should be supplied in glass containers of not more than 100 tablets, closed with a foil-lined cap, and containing no cotton wool wadding; they should be discarded after 8 weeks in use.
● PATIENT AND CARER ADVICE Rectal ointment should be discarded 8 weeks after first opening.

PERCUTOL ® Patients or carers should be given advice on how to administer glyceryl trinitrate ointment.
● NATIONAL FUNDING/ACCESS DECISIONS
For full details see funding body website

Scottish Medicines Consortium (SMC) decisions
▸ Glyceryl trinitrate 0.4% ointment (*Rectogesic*®) for relief of pain associated with chronic anal fissure (February 2008) SMC No. 200/05 Not recommended

● MEDICINAL FORMS There can be variation in the licensing of different medicines containing the same drug. Forms available from special-order manufacturers include: solution for infusion, ointment

Solution for infusion
EXCIPIENTS: May contain Ethanol, propylene glycol
▸ Glyceryl trinitrate (Non-proprietary)
    Glyceryl trinitrate 1 mg per 1 ml Glyceryl trinitrate 50mg/50ml solution for infusion vials | 1 vial [PoM] £15.90
    Glyceryl trinitrate 5 mg per 1 ml Glyceryl trinitrate 50mg/10ml solution for infusion ampoules | 5 ampoule [PoM] £64.90 (Hospital only)
    Glyceryl trinitrate 25mg/5ml solution for infusion ampoules | 5 ampoule [PoM] £32.45 (Hospital only)
▸ Nitrocine (Forum Health Products Ltd)
    Glyceryl trinitrate 1 mg per 1 ml Nitrocine 10mg/10ml solution for infusion ampoules | 10 ampoule [PoM] £58.75 (Hospital only)
▸ Nitronal (Intrapharm Laboratories Ltd)
    Glyceryl trinitrate 1 mg per 1 ml Nitronal 5mg/5ml solution for infusion ampoules | 10 ampoule [PoM] £18.04
    Nitronal 50mg/50ml solution for infusion vials | 1 vial [PoM] £14.76

Sublingual tablet
CAUTIONARY AND ADVISORY LABELS 16
▸ Glyceryl trinitrate (Non-proprietary)
    Glyceryl trinitrate 500 microgram Glyceryl trinitrate 500microgram sublingual tablets | 100 tablet [P] £2.43 DT = £2.07
    Glyceryl trinitrate 600 microgram Glyceryl trinitrate 600microgram sublingual tablets | 100 tablet [P] [⚠]

Transdermal patch
▸ Deponit (Forum Health Products Ltd)
    Glyceryl trinitrate 5 mg per 24 hour Deponit 5 transdermal patches | 28 patch [P] £12.77 DT = £12.77
    Glyceryl trinitrate 10 mg per 24 hour Deponit 10 transdermal patches | 28 patch [P] £14.06 DT = £14.06
▸ Minitran (Mylan)
    Glyceryl trinitrate 5 mg per 24 hour Minitran 5 transdermal patches | 30 patch [P] £11.62
    Glyceryl trinitrate 10 mg per 24 hour Minitran 10 transdermal patches | 30 patch [P] £12.87
    Glyceryl trinitrate 15 mg per 24 hour Minitran 15 transdermal patches | 30 patch [P] £14.19 DT = £14.19
▸ Transiderm-Nitro (Novartis Pharmaceuticals UK Ltd)
    Glyceryl trinitrate 5 mg per 24 hour Transiderm-Nitro 5 transdermal patches | 28 patch [P] £20.46 DT = £12.77
    Glyceryl trinitrate 10 mg per 24 hour Transiderm-Nitro 10 transdermal patches | 28 patch [P] £22.49 DT = £14.06

Rectal ointment
EXCIPIENTS: May contain Propylene glycol, woolfat and related substances (including lanolin)
▸ Rectogesic (Kyowa Kirin Ltd)
    Glyceryl trinitrate 4 mg per 1 gram Rectogesic 0.4% rectal ointment | 30 gram [P] £39.30 DT = £39.30

Sublingual spray
CAUTIONARY AND ADVISORY LABELS 15
▸ Glyceryl trinitrate (Non-proprietary)
    Glyceryl trinitrate 400 microgram per 1 dose Glyceryl trinitrate 400micrograms/dose pump sublingual spray | 180 dose [P] £3.10 DT = £2.71 | 200 dose [P] £3.44 DT = £2.91
    Glyceryl trinitrate 400micrograms/dose aerosol sublingual spray | 180 dose [P] £3.85 DT = £3.43 | 200 dose [P] £4.15 DT = £3.83
▸ Glytrin (Aspire Pharma Ltd)
    Glyceryl trinitrate 400 microgram per 1 dose Glytrin 400micrograms/dose aerosol sublingual spray | 200 dose [P] £3.44 DT = £3.83
▸ Nitrolingual (Intrapharm Laboratories Ltd)
    Glyceryl trinitrate 400 microgram per 1 dose Nitrolingual 400micrograms/dose pump sublingual spray | 75 dose [P] £2.50 (Hospital only) | 180 dose [P] £3.10 DT = £2.71 | 200 dose [P] £3.44 DT = £2.91

▰ 233

Isosorbide dinitrate
21-Jul-2020

● INDICATIONS AND DOSE

Prophylaxis and treatment of angina
▸ BY MOUTH USING IMMEDIATE-RELEASE MEDICINES
▸ Adult: 30–120 mg daily in divided doses

▸ BY INTRAVENOUS INFUSION
▸ Adult: 2–10 mg/hour, increased if necessary up to 20 mg/hour
▸ BY SUBLINGUAL ADMINISTRATION USING AEROSOL SPRAY
▸ Adult: 1–3 sprays, to be administered under tongue whilst holding breath, allow a 30 second interval between each dose

Left ventricular failure
▸ BY MOUTH USING IMMEDIATE-RELEASE MEDICINES
▸ Adult: 40–160 mg daily in divided doses, increased if necessary up to 240 mg daily in divided doses
▸ BY INTRAVENOUS INFUSION
▸ Adult: Initially 2–10 mg/hour, increased if necessary up to 20 mg/hour

Prophylaxis of angina
▸ BY MOUTH USING MODIFIED-RELEASE MEDICINES
▸ Adult: 40 mg daily in 1–2 divided doses, increased if necessary to 60–80 mg daily in 2–3 divided doses

● INTERACTIONS → Appendix 1: nitrates

● SIDE-EFFECTS
▸ **Common or very common**
▸ With oral use Peripheral oedema
▸ **Rare or very rare**
▸ With oral use Angioedema · angle closure glaucoma · hypoventilation · hypoxia · pituitary haemorrhage · Stevens-Johnson syndrome

● PREGNANCY May cross placenta—manufacturers advise avoid unless potential benefit outweighs risk.

● DIRECTIONS FOR ADMINISTRATION For *intravenous infusion*, manufacturer advises give continuously in Glucose 5% or Sodium chloride 0.9%. Absorbed to some extent by polyvinyl chloride infusion containers; preferably use glass or polyethylene containers or give via a syringe pump; 0.05% strength can alternatively be administered undiluted using a syringe pump with a glass or rigid plastic syringe. Glass or polyethylene infusion apparatus is preferable; loss of potency if PVC used.

● MEDICINAL FORMS There can be variation in the licensing of different medicines containing the same drug. Forms available from special-order manufacturers include: oral suspension, oral solution

Modified-release tablet
CAUTIONARY AND ADVISORY LABELS 25
▸ Isoket Retard (Forum Health Products Ltd)
    Isosorbide dinitrate 20 mg Isoket Retard 20 tablets | 56 tablet [P] £2.58 DT = £2.58
    Isosorbide dinitrate 40 mg Isoket Retard 40 tablets | 56 tablet [P] £6.36 DT = £6.36

Tablet
▸ Isosorbide dinitrate (Non-proprietary)
    Isosorbide dinitrate 10 mg Isosorbide dinitrate 10mg tablets | 56 tablet [P] £34.00 = £21.08
    Isosorbide dinitrate 20 mg Isosorbide dinitrate 20mg tablets | 56 tablet [PoM] [⚠] DT = £21.05

Solution for injection
▸ Isosorbide dinitrate (Non-proprietary)
    Isosorbide dinitrate 1 mg per 1 ml Isosorbide dinitrate 10mg/10ml concentrate for solution for injection ampoules | 10 ampoule [PoM] £29.60 (Hospital only)
▸ Isoket (Forum Health Products Ltd)
    Isosorbide dinitrate 1 mg per 1 ml Isoket 0.1% solution for injection 10ml ampoules | 10 ampoule [PoM] £26.93 (Hospital only)

Solution for infusion
▸ Isosorbide dinitrate (Non-proprietary)
    Isosorbide dinitrate 500 microgram per 1 ml Isosorbide dinitrate 25mg/50ml solution for infusion vials | 10 vial [PoM] £67.00
    Isosorbide dinitrate 1 mg per 1 ml Isosorbide dinitrate 50mg/50ml concentrate for solution for infusion vials | 10 vial [PoM] £86.70

2

Cardiovascular system

Isosorbide mononitrate

⊡ 233

● **INDICATIONS AND DOSE**

Prophylaxis of angina | Adjunct in congestive heart failure

▸ BY MOUTH USING IMMEDIATE-RELEASE MEDICINES
▸ Adult: Initially 20 mg 2–3 times a day, alternatively initially 40 mg twice daily, increased if necessary up to 120 mg daily in divided doses

Prophylaxis of angina (for patients who have not previously had a nitrate) | Adjunct in congestive heart failure (for patients who have not previously had a nitrate)

▸ BY MOUTH USING IMMEDIATE-RELEASE MEDICINES
▸ Adult: Initially 10 mg twice daily, increased if necessary up to 120 mg daily in divided doses

CHEMYDUR ® 60XL

Prophylaxis of angina

▸ BY MOUTH
▸ Adult: Initially 0.5 tablet daily for 2–4 days, to minimise possibility of headache, then 1 tablet daily, increased if necessary to 2 tablets daily, dose to be taken in the morning

ELANTAN ® LA

Prophylaxis of angina

▸ BY MOUTH
▸ Adult: 25–50 mg once daily, then increased if necessary to 50–100 mg once daily, dose to be taken in the morning, the lowest effective dose should be used

IMDUR ®

Prophylaxis of angina

▸ BY MOUTH
▸ Adult: Initially 0.5 tablet once daily, to minimise the occurrence of headache, then 1 tablet once daily, then increased if necessary to 2 tablets once daily, dose to be taken in the morning

ISIB ® 60XL

Prophylaxis of angina

▸ BY MOUTH
▸ Adult: Initially 0.5 tablet once daily for 2–4 days, to minimise the occurrence of headache, then 1 tablet once daily, increased if necessary to 2 tablets once daily, dose to be taken in the morning

ISMO RETARD ®

Prophylaxis of angina

▸ BY MOUTH
▸ Adult: 1 tablet once daily, dose to be taken in the morning

ISODUR ®

Prophylaxis of angina

▸ BY MOUTH
▸ Adult: 25–50 mg once daily, then increased if necessary to 50–100 mg once daily, dose to be taken in the morning

ISOTARD ®

Prophylaxis of angina

▸ BY MOUTH
▸ Adult: 25–60 mg once daily, if headaches occur with 60 mg tablet, half a 60 mg tablet may be given for 2–4 days, then increased if necessary to 50–120 mg once daily, dose to be taken in the morning

MODISAL ® XL

Prophylaxis of angina

▸ BY MOUTH
▸ Adult: Initially 0.5 tablet once daily for 2–4 days, to minimise the occurrence of headache, then 1 tablet

once daily, increased if necessary to 2 tablets once daily, dose to be taken in the morning

MONOMAX ® XL

Prophylaxis of angina

▸ BY MOUTH
▸ Adult: Initially 0.5 tablet once daily for 2–4 days, to minimise occurrence of headache, then 1 tablet once daily, increased if necessary to 2 tablets once daily, dose to be taken in the morning

MONOMIL ® XL

Prophylaxis of angina

▸ BY MOUTH
▸ Adult: Initially 0.5 tablet daily for 2–4 days, to minimise possibility of headache, then 1 tablet daily, increased if necessary to 2 tablets once daily, to be taken in the morning

MONOSORB ® XL60

Prophylaxis of angina

▸ BY MOUTH
▸ Adult: Initially 0.5 tablet once daily for the first 2–4 days, to minimise the occurrence of headache, then 1 tablet once daily, increased if necessary to 2 tablets once daily, dose to be taken in the morning

ZEMON ®

Prophylaxis of angina

▸ BY MOUTH
▸ Adult: Initially 30 mg once daily for 2–4 days, to minimise the occurrence of headache, then 40–60 mg once daily, increased if necessary to 80–120 mg once daily, dose to be taken in the morning

● **INTERACTIONS** → Appendix 1: nitrates
● **SIDE-EFFECTS**
▸ **Rare or very rare** Myalgia
● **PREGNANCY** Manufacturers advise avoid unless potential benefit outweighs risk.

● **MEDICINAL FORMS** There can be variation in the licensing of different medicines containing the same drug. Forms available from special-order manufacturers include: oral suspension, oral solution

Modified-release tablet

CAUTIONARY AND ADVISORY LABELS 25
▸ Carmil XL (Milpharm Ltd)
  Isosorbide mononitrate 60 mg Carmil XL 60mg tablets |
  28 tablet Ⓟ £5.75 DT = £10.50
▸ Chemydur 60XL (Advanz Pharma)
  Isosorbide mononitrate 60 mg Chemydur 60XL tablets |
  28 tablet Ⓟ £3.49 DT = £10.50
▸ Imdur (TopRidge Pharma (Ireland) Ltd)
  Isosorbide mononitrate 60 mg Imdur 60mg modified-release tablets | 28 tablet Ⓟ £10.50 DT = £10.50
▸ Isib XL (Alliance Pharmaceuticals Ltd)
  Isosorbide mononitrate 60 mg Isib 60XL tablets | 28 tablet Ⓟ £8.15 DT = £10.50
▸ Ismo Retard (Intrapharm Laboratories Ltd)
  Isosorbide mononitrate 40 mg Ismo Retard 40mg tablets |
  30 tablet Ⓟ £10.71
▸ Isotard XL (Kyowa Kirin Ltd)
  Isosorbide mononitrate 25 mg Isotard 25XL tablets | 28 tablet Ⓟ £6.75 DT = £6.75
  Isosorbide mononitrate 40 mg Isotard 40XL tablets | 28 tablet Ⓟ £6.75 DT = £6.75
  Isosorbide mononitrate 50 mg Isotard 50XL tablets | 28 tablet Ⓟ £6.75 DT = £6.75
  Isosorbide mononitrate 60 mg Isotard 60XL tablets | 28 tablet Ⓟ £5.75 DT = £10.50
▸ Modisal XL (Ennogen Pharma Ltd)
  Isosorbide mononitrate 40 mg Modisal XL 40mg tablets |
  28 tablet PoM £5.40 DT = £6.75
▸ Monomax XL (Chiesi Ltd)
  Isosorbide mononitrate 60 mg Monomax XL 60mg tablets |
  28 tablet Ⓟ £5.25 DT = £10.50

► Monomil XL (Teva UK Ltd)
Isosorbide mononitrate 60 mg Monomil XL 60mg tablets |
28 tablet P £3.49 DT = £10.50
► Monosorb XL (Dexcel-Pharma Ltd)
Isosorbide mononitrate 60 mg Monosorb XL 60 tablets |
28 tablet P £15.53 DT = £10.50
► Relosorb XL (Relonchem Ltd)
Isosorbide mononitrate 60 mg Relosorb XL 60mg tablets |
28 tablet PoM £22.45 DT = £10.50
► Tardisc XL (Dexcel-Pharma Ltd)
Isosorbide mononitrate 60 mg Tardisc XL 60 tablets | 28 tablet P
£3.49 DT = £10.50
► Trangina XL (Accord Healthcare Ltd)
Isosorbide mononitrate 60 mg Trangina XL 60mg tablets |
28 tablet PoM £4.55 DT = £10.50
► Xismox XL (Genus Pharmaceuticals Ltd)
Isosorbide mononitrate 60 mg Xismox XL 60 tablets |
28 tablet PoM £5.51 DT = £10.50
► Zemon XL (Kent Pharmaceuticals Ltd)
Isosorbide mononitrate 40 mg Zemon 40 XL tablets | 28 tablet P
£14.25 DT = £6.75

Tablet
CAUTIONARY AND ADVISORY LABELS 25
► Isosorbide mononitrate (Non-proprietary)
Isosorbide mononitrate 10 mg Isosorbide mononitrate 10mg
tablets | 56 tablet PoM £0.40–£13.10 DT = £1.21
Isosorbide mononitrate 20 mg Isosorbide mononitrate 20mg
tablets | 56 tablet PoM £0.41–£13.88 DT = £1.81
Isosorbide mononitrate 40 mg Isosorbide mononitrate 40mg
tablets | 56 tablet PoM £0.34–£20.55 DT = £2.10
► Ismo (Intrapharm Laboratories Ltd)
Isosorbide mononitrate 10 mg Ismo 10 tablets | 60 tablet P
£2.98
Isosorbide mononitrate 20 mg Ismo 20 tablets | 60 tablet P
£4.12

Modified-release capsule
CAUTIONARY AND ADVISORY LABELS 25
► Elantan LA (Forum Health Products Ltd)
Isosorbide mononitrate 25 mg Elantan LA25 capsules |
28 capsule P £3.40 DT = £3.40
Isosorbide mononitrate 50 mg Elantan LA50 capsules |
28 capsule P £3.69 DT = £3.69
► Isodur XL (Galen Ltd)
Isosorbide mononitrate 25 mg Isodur 25XL capsules |
28 capsule P £4.63 DT = £3.40
Isosorbide mononitrate 50 mg Isodur 50XL capsules |
28 capsule P £6.45 DT = £3.69
► Monomax SR (Ethypharm UK Ltd)
Isosorbide mononitrate 40 mg Nyzamac SR 40mg capsules |
28 capsule P £6.52 DT = £6.52
Isosorbide mononitrate 60 mg Nyzamac SR 60mg capsules |
28 capsule P £8.86 DT = £8.86

SYMPATHOMIMETICS > INOTROPIC

Dobutamine

11-Aug-2020

● DRUG ACTION Dobutamine is a cardiac stimulant which
acts on beta$_1$ receptors in cardiac muscle, and increases
contractility.

● **INDICATIONS AND DOSE**

**Inotropic support in infarction, cardiac surgery,
cardiomyopathies, septic shock, cardiogenic shock, and
during positive end expiratory pressure ventilation**
► BY INTRAVENOUS INFUSION
► Adult: Usual dose 2.5–10 micrograms/kg/minute,
adjusted according to response, alternatively
0.5–40 micrograms/kg/minute

Cardiac stress testing
► BY INTRAVENOUS INFUSION
► Adult: (consult product literature)

● CONTRA-INDICATIONS Phaeochromocytoma

● CAUTIONS Acute heart failure · acute myocardial infarction
· arrhythmias · correct hypercapnia before starting and
during treatment · correct hypovolaemia before starting

and during treatment · correct hypoxia before starting and
during treatment · correct metabolic acidosis before
starting and during treatment · diabetes mellitus · elderly ·
extravasation may cause tissue necrosis · extreme caution
or avoid in marked obstruction of cardiac ejection (such as
idiopathic hypertrophic subaortic stenosis) ·
hyperthyroidism · ischaemic heart disease · occlusive
vascular disease · severe hypotension · susceptibility to
angle-closure glaucoma · tachycardia · tolerance may
develop with continuous infusions longer than 72 hours

● INTERACTIONS → Appendix 1: sympathomimetics,
inotropic

● SIDE-EFFECTS
► **Common or very common** Arrhythmias · bronchospasm ·
chest pain · dyspnoea · eosinophilia · fever · headache ·
inflammation localised · ischaemic heart disease · nausea ·
palpitations · platelet aggregation inhibition (on
prolonged administration) · skin reactions · urinary
urgency · vasoconstriction
► **Uncommon** Myocardial infarction
► **Rare or very rare** Atrioventricular block · cardiac arrest ·
coronary vasospasm · hypertension exacerbated ·
hypokalaemia · hypotension exacerbated
► **Frequency not known** Anxiety · cardiomyopathy · feeling
hot · myoclonus · paraesthesia · tremor

● PREGNANCY No evidence of harm in *animal* studies—
manufacturers advise use only if potential benefit
outweighs risk.

● BREAST FEEDING Manufacturers advise avoid—no
information available.

● MONITORING REQUIREMENTS Monitor serum-potassium
concentration.

● DIRECTIONS FOR ADMINISTRATION Manufacturer advises
dobutamine *injection* should be diluted before use or given
undiluted with syringe pump. Dobutamine *concentrate* for
intravenous infusion should be diluted before use.
For *intravenous infusion*, manufacturer advises give
continuously in Glucose 5% or Sodium chloride 0.9%.
Dilute to a concentration of 0.5–1 mg/mL and give via an
infusion pump; give higher concentration (max. 5 mg/mL)
through central venous catheter; incompatible with
bicarbonate and other strong alkaline solutions.

● MEDICINAL FORMS There can be variation in the licensing of
different medicines containing the same drug. Forms available
from special-order manufacturers include: solution for infusion
Solution for infusion
EXCIPIENTS: May contain Sulfites
► Dobutamine (Non-proprietary)
**Dobutamine (as Dobutamine hydrochloride) 5 mg per
1 ml** Dobutamine 250mg/50ml solution for infusion vials |
1 vial PoM £7.50
**Dobutamine (as Dobutamine hydrochloride) 12.5 mg per
1 ml** Dobutamine 250mg/20ml concentrate for solution for infusion
ampoules | 5 ampoule PoM £12.00–£29.25 | 10 ampoule PoM
£52.50–£56.00

8.1a Cardiac arrest

Cardiopulmonary resuscitation

Overview
The algorithm for cardiopulmonary resuscitation (Life
support algorithm (image), see inside back pages) reflects the
most recent recommendations of the Resuscitation Council
(UK); this has been reproduced with the kind permission of
the Resuscitation Council (UK). The guidelines are available
at www.resus.org.uk.
Cardiac arrest can be associated with ventricular
fibrillation, pulseless ventricular tachycardia, asystole, and

2

Cardiovascular system

pulseless electrical activity (electromechanical dissociation). Adrenaline/epinephrine below 1 in 10000 (100 micrograms/mL) is recommended by intravenous injection repeated every 3–5 minutes if necessary. Administration through a central line results in a faster response than peripheral administration, however placement of a central line must not interfere with chest compressions; drugs administered peripherally must be followed by a flush of at least 20 mL Sodium Chloride 0.9% injection to aid entry into the central circulation. Intravenous injection of amiodarone hydrochloride p. 113 should be considered after adrenaline/epinephrine to treat ventricular fibrillation or pulseless ventricular tachycardia in cardiac arrest refractory to defibrillation. An additional dose of amiodarone hydrochloride can be given if necessary, followed by an amiodarone infusion of amiodarone hydrochloride. Lidocaine hydrochloride p. 111, is an alternative if amiodarone hydrochloride is not available. Atropine sulfate p. 1386 is no longer recommended in the treatment of asystole or pulseless electrical activity.

During cardiopulmonary arrest if intravenous access cannot be obtained, the intraosseous route can be used instead. Drug administration via the endotracheal route is no longer recommended.

For the management of acute anaphylaxis, see allergic emergencies under Antihistamines, allergen immunotherapy and allergic emergencies p. 292.

SYMPATHOMIMETICS ⟩ VASOCONSTRICTOR

I Adrenaline/epinephrine
21-May-2020

- **DRUG ACTION** Acts on both alpha and beta receptors and increases both heart rate and contractility (beta$_1$ effects); it can cause peripheral vasodilation (a beta$_2$ effect) or vasoconstriction (an alpha effect).

- **INDICATIONS AND DOSE**

Cardiopulmonary resuscitation
▸ BY INTRAVENOUS INJECTION
▸ Adult: 1 mg every 3–5 minutes as required, a 1 in 10 000 (100 micrograms/mL) solution is recommended

Acute hypotension
▸ BY CONTINUOUS INTRAVENOUS INFUSION
▸ Neonate: Initially 100 nanograms/kg/minute, adjusted according to response, higher doses up to 1.5 micrograms/kg/minute have been used in acute hypotension.
▸ Child: Initially 100 nanograms/kg/minute, adjusted according to response, higher doses up to 1.5 micrograms/kg/minute have been used in acute hypotension

Emergency treatment of acute anaphylaxis (under expert supervision) | Angioedema (if laryngeal oedema is present) (under expert supervision)
▸ BY INTRAMUSCULAR INJECTION
▸ Child 1 month-5 years: 150 micrograms, doses may be repeated several times if necessary at 5 minute intervals according to blood pressure, pulse, and respiratory function, suitable syringe to be used for measuring small volume; injected preferably into the anterolateral aspect of the middle third of the thigh
▸ Child 6-11 years: 300 micrograms, doses may be repeated several times if necessary at 5 minute intervals according to blood pressure, pulse, and respiratory function, to be injected preferably into the anterolateral aspect of the middle third of the thigh
▸ Child 12-17 years: 500 micrograms, to be injected preferably into the anterolateral aspect of the middle third of the thigh, doses may be repeated several times if necessary at 5 minute intervals according to blood

pressure, pulse, and respiratory function, 300 micrograms (0.3 mL) to be administered if child small or prepubertal
▸ Adult: 500 micrograms, to be injected preferably into the anterolateral aspect of the middle third of the thigh, doses may be repeated several times if necessary at 5 minute intervals according to blood pressure, pulse, and respiratory function

Acute anaphylaxis when there is doubt as to the adequacy of the circulation (specialist use only) | Angioedema (if laryngeal oedema is present) (specialist use only)
▸ BY SLOW INTRAVENOUS INJECTION
▸ Adult: 50 micrograms, using 0.5 mL of the dilute 1 in 10 000 adrenaline injection, dose to be repeated according to response, if multiple doses required, adrenaline should be given as a slow intravenous infusion stopping when a response has been obtained

Control of bradycardia in patients with arrhythmias after myocardial infarction, if there is a risk of asystole, or if the patient is unstable and has failed to respond to atropine
▸ BY INTRAVENOUS INFUSION
▸ Adult: 2–10 micrograms/minute, adjusted according to response

EMERADE ® 150 MICROGRAMS

Acute anaphylaxis (for self-administration)—product recalled, see Important Safety Information
▸ BY INTRAMUSCULAR INJECTION
▸ Child (body-weight up to 15 kg): 150 micrograms, then 150 micrograms after 5–15 minutes as required
▸ Child (body-weight 15-30 kg): 150 micrograms, then 150 micrograms after 5–15 minutes as required, on the basis of a dose of 10 micrograms/kg, 300 micrograms may be more appropriate for some children

EMERADE ® 300 MICROGRAMS

Acute anaphylaxis (for self-administration)—product recalled, see Important Safety Information
▸ BY INTRAMUSCULAR INJECTION
▸ Child (body-weight 30 kg and above): 300 micrograms, then 300 micrograms after 5–15 minutes as required
▸ Adult (body-weight 30 kg and above): 300 micrograms, then 300 micrograms after 5–15 minutes as required

EMERADE ® 500 MICROGRAMS

Acute anaphylaxis (for self-administration)—product recalled, see Important Safety Information
▸ BY INTRAMUSCULAR INJECTION
▸ Child 12-17 years: 500 micrograms, then 500 micrograms after 5–15 minutes as required
▸ Adult: 500 micrograms, then 500 micrograms after 5–15 minutes as required

EPIPEN ® AUTO-INJECTOR 0.3MG

Acute anaphylaxis (for self-administration)
▸ BY INTRAMUSCULAR INJECTION
▸ Child (body-weight 26 kg and above): 300 micrograms, then 300 micrograms after 5–15 minutes as required
▸ Adult: 300 micrograms, then 300 micrograms after 5–15 minutes as required

EPIPEN ® JR AUTO-INJECTOR 0.15MG

Acute anaphylaxis (for self-administration)
▸ BY INTRAMUSCULAR INJECTION
▸ Child (body-weight up to 15 kg): 150 micrograms, then 150 micrograms after 5–15 minutes as required
▸ Child (body-weight 15-25 kg): 150 micrograms, then 150 micrograms after 5–15 minutes as required, on the basis of a dose of 10 micrograms/kg, 300 micrograms may be more appropriate for some children

JEXT ® 150 MICROGRAMS

Acute anaphylaxis (for self-administration)
▸ BY INTRAMUSCULAR INJECTION
▸ Child (body-weight up to 15 kg): 150 micrograms, then 150 micrograms after 5–15 minutes as required
▸ Child (body-weight 15-30 kg): 150 micrograms, then 150 micrograms after 5–15 minutes as required, on the basis of a dose of 10 micrograms/kg, 300 micrograms may be more appropriate for some children

JEXT ® 300 MICROGRAMS

Acute anaphylaxis (for self-administration)
▸ BY INTRAMUSCULAR INJECTION
▸ Child (body-weight 31 kg and above): 300 micrograms, then 300 micrograms after 5–15 minutes as required
▸ Adult (body-weight 31 kg and above): 300 micrograms, then 300 micrograms after 5–15 minutes as required

● UNLICENSED USE
▸ With intramuscular use for acute anaphylaxis in children Auto-injectors delivering 150-microgram dose of adrenaline may not be licensed for use in children with body-weight under 15 kg.
▸ With intravenous use for acute hypotension in children Adrenaline 1 in 1000 (1 mg/mL) solution is not licensed for intravenous administration.

IMPORTANT SAFETY INFORMATION

SAFE PRACTICE
Intravenous route should be used with **extreme care** by specialists only.

MHRA/CHM ADVICE: ADRENALINE AUTO-INJECTORS: UPDATED ADVICE AFTER EUROPEAN REVIEW (AUGUST 2017)
Following a European review of all adrenaline auto-injectors approved in the EU, the MHRA recommend that 2 adrenaline auto-injectors are prescribed, which patients should carry at all times. This is particularly important for patients with allergic asthma, who are at increased risk of a severe anaphylactic reaction. Patients with allergies and their carers should be trained to use the particular auto-injector they have been prescribed and encouraged to practise using a trainer device. Patients are advised to check the expiry date of the adrenaline auto-injectors and obtain replacements before they expire.

MHRA/CHM ADVICE: CLASS 2 MEDICINES RECALL: *EMERADE*® 150 MICROGRAMS (MARCH 2020); *EMERADE*® 300 MICROGRAMS (APRIL 2020); *EMERADE*® 500 MICROGRAMS (MAY 2020) SOLUTION FOR INJECTION IN PRE-FILLED SYRINGES
The MHRA has advised that all unexpired batches of *Emerade*® 150 microgram, 300 microgram, and 500 microgram auto-injector pens are being recalled from patients due to an error in one component of the auto-injector believed to cause the failure of some pens to activate. Healthcare professionals are advised to identify these patients and review their adrenaline prescription. Patients and their carers should immediately be informed that a prescription for a suitable alternative brand of adrenaline auto-injector is required. They should be advised to return their current *Emerade*® pen(s) to a pharmacy once they have two pens of an alternative brand in their possession. Returned pens should be quarantined in pharmacies and returned to the supplier using the supplier's approved process. This advice also applies to *Emerade*® auto-injector pens that are kept in emergency anaphylaxis kits (e.g. in dental surgeries or schools). For patients who have been prescribed *Emerade*®**500 microgram** auto-injector pens, the MHRA advises that *EpiPen*® or *Jext*®**300 microgram** (maximum strength) pens will be a suitable replacement, based on results from a bioavailability study. The MHRA has produced a Patient Letter on the *Emerade*® recall for each strength of auto-injector which should be provided

to patients and their carers. Healthcare professionals are reminded to follow existing advice on the use of adrenaline auto-injectors—see *Prescribing and dispensing information*. For the latest safety alerts, see the MHRA website.

● CAUTIONS Arteriosclerosis (in adults) · arrhythmias · cerebrovascular disease · cor pulmonale · diabetes mellitus · elderly · hypercalcaemia · hyperreflexia · hypertension · hyperthyroidism · hypokalaemia · ischaemic heart disease · obstructive cardiomyopathy · occlusive vascular disease · organic brain damage · phaeochromocytoma · prostate disorders · psychoneurosis · severe angina · susceptibility to angle-closure glaucoma

CAUTIONS, FURTHER INFORMATION Cautions listed are only for non-life-threatening situations.

● INTERACTIONS → Appendix 1: sympathomimetics, vasoconstrictor

● SIDE-EFFECTS
GENERAL SIDE-EFFECTS
▸ **Rare or very rare** Cardiomyopathy
▸ **Frequency not known** Angina pectoris · angle closure glaucoma · anxiety · appetite decreased · arrhythmias · asthenia · CNS haemorrhage · confusion · dizziness · dry mouth · dyspnoea · headache · hepatic necrosis · hyperglycaemia · hyperhidrosis · hypersalivation · hypertension (increased risk of cerebral haemorrhage) · hypokalaemia · injection site necrosis · insomnia · intestinal necrosis · metabolic acidosis · mydriasis · myocardial infarction · nausea · pallor · palpitations · peripheral coldness · psychosis · pulmonary oedema (on excessive dosage or extreme sensitivity) · renal necrosis · soft tissue necrosis · tremor · urinary disorders · vomiting

SPECIFIC SIDE-EFFECTS
▸ With intramuscular use Muscle necrosis · necrotising fasciitis · peripheral ischaemia
▸ With intravenous use Hemiplegia · muscle rigidity

● PREGNANCY May reduce placental perfusion and cause tachycardia, cardiac irregularities, and extrasystoles in fetus. Can delay second stage of labour. Manufacturers advise use only if benefit outweighs risk.

● BREAST FEEDING Present in milk but unlikely to be harmful as poor oral bioavailability.

● RENAL IMPAIRMENT Manufacturers advise use with caution in severe impairment.

● MONITORING REQUIREMENTS Monitor blood pressure and ECG.

● DIRECTIONS FOR ADMINISTRATION
Acute hypotension
▸ With intravenous use in children For *continuous intravenous infusion*, dilute with Glucose 5% or Sodium Chloride 0.9% and give through a central venous catheter. Incompatible with bicarbonate and alkaline solutions. *Neonatal intensive care*, dilute 3 mg/kg body-weight to a final volume of 50 mL with infusion fluid; an intravenous infusion rate of 0.1 mL/hour provides a dose of 100 nanograms/kg/minute; infuse through a central venous catheter. Incompatible with bicarbonate and alkaline solutions. These infusions are usually made up with adrenaline 1 in 1000 (1 mg/mL) solution.
Cardiopulmonary resuscitation
▸ With intravenous use in adults Administration through a central line results in a faster response than peripheral administration, however placement of a central line must not interfere with chest compressions; drugs administered peripherally must be followed by a flush of at least 20 mL Sodium Chloride 0.9% injection to aid entry into the central circulation.

2

Cardiovascular system

- **PRESCRIBING AND DISPENSING INFORMATION**
  - ▶ With intramuscular use It is important, in acute anaphylaxis where intramuscular injection might still succeed, time should not be wasted seeking intravenous access. Great vigilance is needed to ensure that the *correct strength* of adrenaline injection is used; anaphylactic shock kits need to make a *very clear distinction* between the 1 in 10 000 strength and the 1 in 1000 strength. Patients with severe allergy should be instructed in the self-administration of adrenaline by intramuscular injection. Packs for self-administration need to be **clearly labelled with instructions** on how to administer adrenaline (intramuscularly, preferably at the midpoint of the outer thigh, through light clothing if necessary) so that in the case of rapid collapse someone else is able to give it. It is important to ensure individuals at risk and their carers understand that:
    - two injection devices should be carried at all times to treat symptoms until medical assistance is available; if, after the first injection, the individual does not start to feel better, the second injection should be given 5 to 15 minutes after the first;
    - an ambulance should be called after every administration, even if symptoms improve;
    - the individual should lie down with their legs raised (unless they have breathing difficulties, in which case they should sit up) and should not be left alone.

    Adrenaline for administration by intramuscular injection is available in 'auto-injectors' (e.g. *Emerade*®—product recalled, see *Important Safety Information, EpiPen*®, or *Jext*®), pre-assembled syringes fitted with a needle suitable for very rapid administration (if necessary by a bystander or a healthcare provider if it is the only preparation available); injection technique is device specific.

    To ensure patients receive the auto-injector device that they have been trained to use, prescribers should specify the brand to be dispensed. If switching between brands, patients should receive full training in use of the new auto-injector device.

    Licensed doses differ between brands of adrenaline auto-injectors. Adrenaline bioavailability has the potential to be influenced by a number of factors including formulation, propulsive force of the device and needle length—consult product literature for further information.

- **PATIENT AND CARER ADVICE**
  - ▶ With intramuscular use Individuals at considerable risk of anaphylaxis need to carry (or have available) adrenaline at all times and the patient, or their carers, need to be *instructed in advance* when and how to inject it.
  - ▶ With intramuscular use The MHRA has produced an advice sheet on the use of adrenaline auto-injectors, which should be provided to patients and their carers.
    Medicines for Children leaflet: Adrenaline auto-injector for anaphylaxis www.medicinesforchildren.org.uk/adrenaline-auto-injector-anaphylaxis-0

  JEXT® 300 MICROGRAMS 1.1 mL of the solution remains in the auto-injector device after use.

  JEXT® 150 MICROGRAMS 1.25 mL of the solution remains in the auto-injector device after use.

  EPIPEN® JR AUTO-INJECTOR 0.15MG 1.7 mL of the solution remains in the auto-injector device after use.

  EMERADE® 150 MICROGRAMS 0.35 mL of the solution remains in the auto-injector device after use.

  EPIPEN® AUTO-INJECTOR 0.3MG 1.7 mL of the solution remains in the auto-injector device after use.

  EMERADE® 500 MICROGRAMS No solution remains in the auto-injector device after use.

  EMERADE® 300 MICROGRAMS 0.2 mL of the solution remains in the auto-injector device after use.

- **EXCEPTIONS TO LEGAL CATEGORY**
  - ▶ With intramuscular use POM restriction does not apply to the intramuscular administration of up to 1 mg of adrenaline injection 1 in 1000 (1 mg/mL) for the emergency treatment of anaphylaxis.

- **MEDICINAL FORMS** There can be variation in the licensing of different medicines containing the same drug. Forms available from special-order manufacturers include: solution for injection

Solution for injection
EXCIPIENTS: May contain Sulfites
  - ▶ Adrenaline/epinephrine (Non-proprietary)
    Adrenaline 100 microgram per 1 ml Adrenaline (base) 100micrograms/1ml (1 in 10,000) dilute solution for injection ampoules | 10 ampoule [PoM] £92.59
    Adrenaline (base) 1mg/10ml (1 in 10,000) dilute solution for injection pre-filled syringes | 1 pre-filled disposable injection [PoM] £7.21 | 1 pre-filled disposable injection [PoM] £6.87–£18.00 (Hospital only) | 10 pre-filled disposable injection [PoM] £180.00 (Hospital only)
    Adrenaline (as Adrenaline acid tartrate) 100 microgram per 1 ml Adrenaline (base) 1mg/10ml (1 in 10,000) dilute solution for injection ampoules | 10 ampoule [PoM] £107.30
    Adrenaline (base) 500micrograms/5ml (1 in 10,000) dilute solution for injection ampoules | 10 ampoule [PoM] £98.64
    Adrenaline 1 mg per 1 ml Adrenaline (base) 10mg/10ml (1 in 1,000) solution for injection ampoules | 10 ampoule [PoM] £111.32 DT = £111.32
    Adrenaline (base) for anaphylaxis 1mg/1ml (1 in 1,000) solution for injection pre-filled syringes | 1 pre-filled disposable injection [PoM] £12.47 DT = £16.68
    Adrenaline (base) 1mg/1ml (1 in 1,000) solution for injection pre-filled syringes | 1 pre-filled disposable injection [PoM] £11.88–£14.47 DT = £16.68
    Adrenaline (as Adrenaline acid tartrate) 1 mg per 1 ml Adrenaline (base) 5mg/5ml (1 in 1,000) solution for injection ampoules | 10 ampoule [PoM] £113.49 DT = £113.49
    Adrenaline (base) 500micrograms/0.5ml (1 in 1,000) solution for injection ampoules | 10 ampoule [PoM] £90.85–£93.06 DT = £90.85
    Adrenaline (base) 1mg/1ml (1 in 1,000) solution for injection ampoules | 10 ampoule [PoM] £6.00–£10.50 DT = £10.34
  - ▶ Emerade (Bausch & Lomb UK Ltd)
    Adrenaline 1 mg per 1 ml Emerade 300micrograms/0.3ml (1 in 1,000) solution for injection auto-injectors | 1 pre-filled disposable injection [PoM] £25.99 DT = £34.30
    Adrenaline (as Adrenaline acid tartrate) 1 mg per 1 ml Emerade 150micrograms/0.15ml (1 in 1,000) solution for injection auto-injectors | 1 pre-filled disposable injection [PoM] £25.99 DT = £34.30
    Emerade 500micrograms/0.5ml (1 in 1,000) solution for injection auto-injectors | 1 pre-filled disposable injection [PoM] £26.99 DT = £26.99
  - ▶ EpiPen (Mylan)
    Adrenaline 500 microgram per 1 ml EpiPen Jr. 150micrograms/0.3ml (1 in 2,000) solution for injection auto-injectors | 1 pre-filled disposable injection [PoM] £34.30 DT = £34.30 | 2 pre-filled disposable injection [PoM] £68.60 DT = £68.60
    Adrenaline 1 mg per 1 ml EpiPen 300micrograms/0.3ml (1 in 1,000) solution for injection auto-injectors | 1 pre-filled disposable injection [PoM] £34.30 DT = £34.30 | 2 pre-filled disposable injection [PoM] £68.60
  - ▶ Jext (ALK-Abello Ltd)
    Adrenaline 1 mg per 1 ml Jext 300micrograms/0.3ml (1 in 1,000) solution for injection auto-injectors | 1 pre-filled disposable injection [PoM] £34.30 DT = £34.30
    Adrenaline (as Adrenaline acid tartrate) 1 mg per 1 ml Jext 150micrograms/0.15ml (1 in 1,000) solution for injection auto-injectors | 1 pre-filled disposable injection [PoM] £34.30 DT = £34.30

9 Oedema

Diuretics

14-Sep-2020

Overview

Thiazides are used to relieve oedema due to chronic heart failure and, in lower doses, to reduce blood pressure.

Loop diuretics are used in pulmonary oedema due to left ventricular failure and in patients with chronic heart failure.

Combination diuretic therapy may be effective in patients with oedema resistant to treatment with one diuretic. Vigorous diuresis, particularly with loop diuretics, may induce acute hypotension; rapid reduction of plasma volume should be avoided.

Thiazides and related diuretics

Thiazides and related compounds are moderately potent diuretics; they inhibit sodium reabsorption at the beginning of the distal convoluted tubule. They act within 1 to 2 hours of oral administration and most have a duration of action of 12 to 24 hours; they are usually administered early in the day so that the diuresis does not interfere with sleep.

In the management of *hypertension* a low dose of a thiazide produces a maximal or near-maximal blood pressure lowering effect, with very little biochemical disturbance. Higher doses cause more marked changes in plasma potassium, sodium, uric acid, glucose, and lipids, with little advantage in blood pressure control. Chlortalidone p. 246 and indapamide p. 181 are the preferred diuretics in the management of hypertension. Thiazides also have a role in chronic heart failure.

Bendroflumethiazide p. 180 can be used for mild or moderate heart failure; it is licensed for the treatment of hypertension but is no longer considered the first-line diuretic for this indication, although patients with stable and controlled blood pressure currently taking bendroflumethiazide can continue treatment.

Chlortalidone, a thiazide-related compound, has a longer duration of action than the thiazides and may be given on alternate days to control oedema. It is also useful if acute retention is liable to be precipitated by a more rapid diuresis or if patients dislike the altered pattern of micturition caused by other diuretics. Chlortalidone can also be used under close supervision for the treatment of ascites due to cirrhosis in stable patients.

Xipamide p. 247 and indapamide are chemically related to chlortalidone. Indapamide is claimed to lower blood pressure with less metabolic disturbance, particularly less aggravation of diabetes mellitus.

Metolazone p. 247 is particularly effective when combined with a loop diuretic (even in renal failure); profound diuresis can occur and the patient should therefore be monitored carefully.

The thiazide diuretics benzthiazide, clopamide, hydrochlorothiazide, and hydroflumethiazide do not offer any significant advantage over other thiazides and related diuretics.

Loop diuretics

Loop diuretics are used in pulmonary oedema due to left ventricular failure; intravenous administration produces relief of breathlessness and reduces pre-load sooner than would be expected from the time of onset of diuresis. Loop diuretics are also used in patients with chronic heart failure. Diuretic-resistant oedema (except lymphoedema and oedema due to peripheral venous stasis or calcium-channel blockers) can be treated with a loop diuretic combined with a thiazide or related diuretic (e.g. bendroflumethiazide or metolazone).

If necessary, a loop diuretic can be added to antihypertensive treatment to achieve better control of blood pressure in those with resistant hypertension, or in patients with impaired renal function or heart failure.

Loop diuretics can exacerbate diabetes (but hyperglycaemia is less likely than with thiazides) and gout. If there is an enlarged prostate, urinary retention can occur, although this is less likely if small doses and less potent diuretics are used initially.

Furosemide p. 243 and bumetanide p. 242 are similar in activity; both act within 1 hour of oral administration and diuresis is complete within 6 hours so that, if necessary, they can be given twice in one day without interfering with sleep. Following intravenous administration furosemide has a peak effect within 30 minutes. The diuresis associated with these drugs is dose related.

Torasemide p. 244 has properties similar to those of furosemide and bumetanide, and is indicated for oedema and for hypertension.

Potassium-sparing diuretics and aldosterone antagonists

Amiloride hydrochloride p. 245 and triamterene p. 246 on their own are weak diuretics. They cause retention of potassium and are therefore given with thiazide or loop diuretics as a more effective alternative to potassium supplements. See compound preparations with thiazides or loop diuretics.

Potassium supplements must **not** be given with potassium- sparing diuretics. Administration of a potassium sparing diuretic to a patient receiving an ACE inhibitor or an angiotensin-II receptor antagonist can also cause severe hyperkalaemia.

Aldosterone antagonists

Spironolactone p. 208 potentiates thiazide or loop diuretics by antagonising aldosterone; it is a potassium-sparing diuretic. Spironolactone is of value in the treatment of oedema and ascites caused by cirrhosis of the liver; furosemide can be used as an adjunct. Low doses of spironolactone are beneficial in moderate to severe heart failure and when used in resistant hypertension [unlicensed indication].

Spironolactone is also used in primary hyperaldosteronism (Conn's syndrome). It is given before surgery or if surgery is not appropriate, in the lowest effective dose for maintenance.

Eplerenone p. 208 is licensed for use as an adjunct in left ventricular dysfunction with evidence of heart failure after a myocardial infarction; it is also licensed as an adjunct in chronic mild heart failure with left ventricular systolic dysfunction.

Potassium supplements must **not** be given with aldosterone antagonists.

Potassium-sparing diuretics with other diuretics

Although it is preferable to prescribe thiazides and potassium-sparing diuretics separately, the use of fixed combinations may be justified if compliance is a problem. Potassium-sparing diuretics are not usually necessary in the routine treatment of hypertension, unless hypokalaemia develops.

Other diuretics

Mannitol p. 244 is an osmotic diuretic that can be used to treat cerebral oedema and raised intra-ocular pressure.

Mercurial diuretics are effective but are now almost never used because of their nephrotoxicity.

The carbonic anhydrase inhibitor acetazolamide p. 1225 is a weak diuretic and is little used for its diuretic effect. It is used for prophylaxis against mountain sickness [unlicensed indication] but is not a substitute for acclimatisation.

Eye drops of dorzolamide p. 1227 and brinzolamide p. 1226 inhibit the formation of aqueous humour and are used in glaucoma.

Diuretics with potassium

Many patients on diuretics do not need potassium supplements. For many of those who do, the amount of potassium in combined preparations may not be enough, and for this reason their use is to be discouraged.

Diuretics with potassium and potassium-sparing diuretics should **not** usually be given together. Diuretics and potassium supplements should be prescribed separately for children.

2

Cardiovascular system

Advanced Pharmacy Services

Patients taking diuretics may be eligible for the New Medicines Service / Medicines Use Review service provided by a community pharmacist. For further information, see *Advanced Pharmacy Services* in Medicines optimisation p. 18.

> **Other drugs used for Oedema** Diamorphine hydrochloride, p. 476

DIURETICS > LOOP DIURETICS

Loop diuretics

- **DRUG ACTION** Loop diuretics inhibit reabsorption from the ascending limb of the loop of Henlé in the renal tubule and are powerful diuretics.
- **CONTRA-INDICATIONS** Anuria · comatose and precomatose states associated with liver cirrhosis · renal failure due to nephrotoxic or hepatotoxic drugs · severe hypokalaemia · severe hyponatraemia
- **CAUTIONS** Can exacerbate diabetes (but hyperglycaemia less likely than with thiazides) · can excacerbate gout · hypotension should be corrected before initiation of treatment · hypovolaemia should be corrected before initiation of treatment · urinary retention can occur in prostatic hyperplasia

  CAUTIONS, FURTHER INFORMATION
- Elderly Manufacturer advises lower initial doses of diuretics may be necessary in the elderly because they are particularly susceptible to the side-effects. The dose should then be adjusted according to renal function. Prescription potentially inappropriate (STOPP criteria):
  - as a first-line treatment for hypertension (safer, more effective alternatives available)
  - for treatment of hypertension with concurrent urinary incontinence (may exacerbate incontinence)
  - for dependent ankle oedema without evidence of heart failure, liver failure, nephrotic syndrome or renal failure (leg elevation and/or compression hosiery usually more appropriate)

  See also Prescribing in the elderly p. 33.
- Potassium loss Hypokalaemia can occur with loop diuretics. Hypokalaemia is dangerous in severe cardiovascular disease and in patients also being treated with cardiac glycosides. Often the use of potassium-sparing diuretics avoids the need to take potassium supplements.

  In hepatic impairment, hypokalaemia caused by diuretics can precipitate encephalopathy.
- Urinary retention If there is an enlarged prostate, urinary retention can occur, although this is less likely if small doses and less potent diuretics are used initially; manufacturer advises adequate urinary output should be established before initiating treatment.
- **SIDE-EFFECTS**
- **Common or very common** Dizziness · electrolyte imbalance · fatigue · headache · metabolic alkalosis · muscle spasms · nausea
- **Uncommon** Diarrhoea
- **Rare or very rare** Bone marrow depression · photosensitivity reaction
- **Frequency not known** Deafness (more common in renal impairment) · leucopenia · paraesthesia · rash · severe cutaneous adverse reactions (SCARs) · thrombocytopenia · tinnitus (more common with rapid intravenous administration, and in renal impairment) · vomiting
- **HEPATIC IMPAIRMENT** Hypokalaemia induced by loop diuretics may precipitate hepatic encephalopathy and coma—potassium-sparing diuretics can be used to prevent this. Diuretics can increase the risk of hypomagnesaemia in alcoholic cirrhosis, leading to arrhythmias.

- **RENAL IMPAIRMENT** High doses or rapid intravenous administration can cause tinnitus and deafness. **Dose adjustments** High doses of loop diuretics may occasionally be needed in renal impairment.
- **MONITORING REQUIREMENTS** Monitor electrolytes during treatment.

▶ above

Bumetanide

- **INDICATIONS AND DOSE**

Oedema
- ▶ BY MOUTH
  - ▶ Adult: 1 mg, dose to be taken in the morning, then 1 mg after 6–8 hours if required
  - ▶ Elderly: 500 micrograms daily, this lower dose may be sufficient in elderly patients

Oedema, severe cases
- ▶ BY MOUTH
  - ▶ Adult: Initially 5 mg daily, increased in steps of 5 mg every 12–24 hours, adjusted according to response

- **INTERACTIONS** → Appendix 1: loop diuretics
- **SIDE-EFFECTS**
- **Common or very common** Dehydration · hypotension · skin reactions
- **Uncommon** Breast pain · chest discomfort · ear pain · vertigo
- **Rare or very rare** Hearing impairment
- **Frequency not known** Arthralgia · encephalopathy · gastrointestinal discomfort · gynaecomastia · hyperglycaemia · hyperuricaemia · muscle cramps · musculoskeletal pain (with high doses in renal failure)
- **PREGNANCY** Bumetanide should not be used to treat gestational hypertension because of the maternal hypovolaemia associated with this condition.
- **BREAST FEEDING** No information available. May inhibit lactation.

- **MEDICINAL FORMS** There can be variation in the licensing of different medicines containing the same drug. Forms available from special-order manufacturers include: oral suspension

Oral solution
- ▶ Bumetanide (Non-proprietary)
  Bumetanide 200 microgram per 1 ml Bumetanide 1mg/5ml oral solution sugar free sugar-free | 150 ml [PoM] £198.00 DT = £198.00

Tablet
- ▶ Bumetanide (Non-proprietary)
  Bumetanide 1 mg Bumetanide 1mg tablets | 28 tablet [PoM] £7.35 DT = £2.22
  Bumetanide 5 mg Bumetanide 5mg tablets | 28 tablet [PoM] £9.81 DT = £9.81

Combinations available: *Amiloride with bumetanide*, p. 246

Co-amilofruse

24-Sep-2020

- **INDICATIONS AND DOSE**

Oedema
- ▶ BY MOUTH
  - ▶ Adult: 2.5/20–10/80 mg daily, dose to be taken in the morning

  DOSE EQUIVALENCE AND CONVERSION
  - ▶ A mixture of amiloride hydrochloride and furosemide (frusemide) in the mass proportions of 1 part amiloride hydrochloride to 8 parts furosemide (frusemide).

- **CONTRA-INDICATIONS** Addison's disease · anuria · comatose or precomatose states associated with liver cirrhosis · dehydration · hyperkalaemia · hypovolaemia · renal failure · severe hypokalaemia · severe hyponatraemia

- CAUTIONS Correct hypovolaemia · diabetes mellitus · elderly · gout · hepatorenal syndrome · hypoproteinaemia · hypotension · impaired micturition · prostatic enlargement
- INTERACTIONS → Appendix 1: loop diuretics · potassium-sparing diuretics
- SIDE-EFFECTS
- ▶ **Uncommon** Hearing impairment
- ▶ **Frequency not known** Acute urinary retention · agranulocytosis · aplastic anaemia · cholestasis · constipation · diarrhoea · dizziness · electrolyte imbalance · eosinophilia · epigastric discomfort · gout · haemolytic anaemia · headache · leucopenia · loss of consciousness · lupus erythematosus · malaise · nausea · nephritis tubulointerstitial · pancreatitis acute · paraesthesia · psychiatric disorder · renal failure · severe cutaneous adverse reactions (SCARs) · skin eruption · syncope · tetany · thrombocytopenia · tinnitus · vasculitis · vomiting
- PREGNANCY Not used to treat hypertension in pregnancy.
- BREAST FEEDING Manufacturers advise avoid—no information regarding amiloride component available. Amount of furosemide in milk too small to be harmful. Furosemide may inhibit lactation.
- HEPATIC IMPAIRMENT Manufacturer advises caution in hepatic cirrhosis with renal impairment.
- RENAL IMPAIRMENT Risk of hyperkalaemia in renal impairment but may need higher doses. Avoid if eGFR less than 30 mL/minute/1.73 m^2.
  Monitoring Monitor plasma-potassium concentration.
- MONITORING REQUIREMENTS Monitor electrolytes.

- MEDICINAL FORMS There can be variation in the licensing of different medicines containing the same drug. Forms available from special-order manufacturers include: oral suspension, oral solution
  Tablet
  ▶ Co-amilofruse (Non-proprietary)
    Amiloride hydrochloride 2.5 mg, Furosemide 20 mg Co-amilofruse 2.5mg/20mg tablets | 28 tablet P̲o̲M̲ £12.86 DT = £8.58 | 56 tablet P̲o̲M̲ £17.16-£25.72
    Amiloride hydrochloride 5 mg, Furosemide 40 mg Co-amilofruse 5mg/40mg tablets | 28 tablet P̲o̲M̲ £7.94 DT = £5.29 | 56 tablet P̲o̲M̲ £15.88
    Amiloride hydrochloride 10 mg, Furosemide 80 mg Co-amilofruse 10mg/80mg tablets | 28 tablet P̲o̲M̲ £23.38 DT = £15.52
  ▶ Frumil (Sanofi)
    Amiloride hydrochloride 2.5 mg, Furosemide 20 mg Frumil LS 20mg/2.5mg tablets | 28 tablet P̲o̲M̲ £4.32 DT = £8.58
    Amiloride hydrochloride 5 mg, Furosemide 40 mg Frumil 40mg/5mg tablets | 28 tablet P̲o̲M̲ £5.29 DT = £5.29

F 242

Furosemide
(Frusemide)   24-Sep-2020

- **INDICATIONS AND DOSE**
Oedema
- ▶ BY MOUTH
- ▶ Adult: Initially 40 mg daily, dose to be taken in the morning, then maintenance 20–40 mg daily
- ▶ INITIALLY BY INTRAMUSCULAR INJECTION, OR BY SLOW INTRAVENOUS INJECTION, OR BY INTRAVENOUS INFUSION
- ▶ Adult: Initially 20–50 mg, then (by intramuscular injection or by intravenous injection or by intravenous infusion) increased in steps of 20 mg every 2 hours if required, doses greater than 50 mg given by intravenous infusion only; maximum 1.5 g per day

Resistant oedema
- ▶ BY MOUTH
- ▶ Adult: 80–120 mg daily

- ▶ INITIALLY BY INTRAMUSCULAR INJECTION, OR BY SLOW INTRAVENOUS INJECTION, OR BY INTRAVENOUS INFUSION
- ▶ Adult: Initially 20–50 mg, then (by intramuscular injection or by intravenous injection or by intravenous infusion) increased in steps of 20 mg every 2 hours if required, doses greater than 50 mg given by intravenous infusion only; maximum 1.5 g per day

Resistant hypertension
- ▶ BY MOUTH
- ▶ Adult: 40–80 mg daily
- ▶ INITIALLY BY INTRAMUSCULAR INJECTION, OR BY SLOW INTRAVENOUS INJECTION, OR BY INTRAVENOUS INFUSION
- ▶ Adult: Initially 20–50 mg, then (by intramuscular injection or by intravenous injection or by intravenous infusion) increased in steps of 20 mg every 2 hours if required, doses greater than 50 mg given by intravenous infusion only; maximum 1.5 g per day

- CAUTIONS Hepatorenal syndrome · hypoproteinaemia may reduce diuretic effect and increase risk of side-effects
- INTERACTIONS → Appendix 1: loop diuretics
- SIDE-EFFECTS
  GENERAL SIDE-EFFECTS
  Agranulocytosis · aplastic anaemia · auditory disorder (more common with rapid intravenous administration, and in renal impairment) · diabetes mellitus · eosinophilia · fever · gout · haemolytic anaemia · malaise · mucosal reaction · nephritis tubulointerstitial · pancreatitis acute · shock · skin eruption · tetany · vasculitis
  SPECIFIC SIDE-EFFECTS
- ▶ With oral use Acute kidney injury · hepatic disorders · metabolic acidosis · psychiatric disorder · urinary disorders
- ▶ With parenteral use Acute urinary retention · cholestasis
- PREGNANCY Furosemide should not be used to treat gestational hypertension because of the maternal hypovolaemia associated with this condition.
- BREAST FEEDING Amount too small to be harmful. May inhibit lactation.
- DIRECTIONS FOR ADMINISTRATION Intravenous administration rate should not usually exceed 4 mg/minute however single doses of up to 80 mg may be administered more rapidly; a lower rate of infusion may be necessary in renal impairment. For *intravenous infusion* (*Lasix*®), give continuously in Sodium chloride 0.9%; infusion pH must be above 5.5; glucose solutions are unsuitable.

- MEDICINAL FORMS There can be variation in the licensing of different medicines containing the same drug. Forms available from special-order manufacturers include: oral suspension, oral solution
  Tablet
  ▶ Furosemide (Non-proprietary)
    Furosemide 20 mg Furosemide 20mg tablets | 28 tablet P̲o̲M̲ £5.69 DT = £0.82 | 250 tablet P̲o̲M̲ £5.08-£7.32
    Furosemide 40 mg Furosemide 40mg tablets | 28 tablet P̲o̲M̲ £7.55 DT = £0.87 | 250 tablet P̲o̲M̲ £4.73-£7.77 | 1000 tablet P̲o̲M̲ £28.21-£45.00
    Furosemide 500 mg Furosemide 500mg tablets | 28 tablet P̲o̲M̲ £39.02 DT = £39.02
  ▶ Diuresal (Ennogen Pharma Ltd)
    Furosemide 500 mg Diuresal 500mg tablets | 28 tablet P̲o̲M̲ £39.02 DT = £39.02
  Solution for injection
  ▶ Furosemide (Non-proprietary)
    Furosemide 10 mg per 1 ml Furosemide 250mg/25ml solution for injection ampoules | 10 ampoule P̲o̲M̲ £30.00-£40.00
    Furosemide 40mg/4ml solution for injection ampoules | 10 ampoule P̲o̲M̲ £12.19 (Hospital only)
    Furosemide 50mg/5ml solution for injection ampoules | 10 ampoule P̲o̲M̲ £2.86-£17.00 | 10 ampoule P̲o̲M̲ £2.86-£4.20 (Hospital only)

Furosemide 20mg/2ml solution for injection ampoules | 10 ampoule [PoM] £7.00–£40.00 DT = £12.19 | 10 ampoule [PoM] £3.80–£12.19 DT = £12.19 (Hospital only)

Oral solution

EXCIPIENTS: May contain Alcohol

▸ Furosemide (Non-proprietary)

Furosemide 4 mg per 1 ml Furosemide 20mg/5ml oral solution sugar free sugar-free | 150 ml [PoM] £14.81 DT = £14.81
Furosemide 8 mg per 1 ml Furosemide 40mg/5ml oral solution sugar free sugar-free | 150 ml [PoM] £19.53 DT = £19.53
Furosemide 10 mg per 1 ml Furosemide 50mg/5ml oral solution sugar free sugar-free | 150 ml [PoM] £20.21 DT = £20.21

▸ Frusol (Rosemont Pharmaceuticals Ltd)

Furosemide 4 mg per 1 ml Frusol 20mg/5ml oral solution sugar-free | 150 ml [PoM] £12.07 DT = £14.81
Furosemide 8 mg per 1 ml Frusol 40mg/5ml oral solution sugar-free | 150 ml [PoM] £15.58 DT = £19.53
Furosemide 10 mg per 1 ml Frusol 50mg/5ml oral solution sugar-free | 150 ml [PoM] £16.84 DT = £20.21

Combinations available: *Spironolactone with furosemide,* p. 245

Furosemide with triamterene   24-Sep-2020

The properties listed below are those particular to the combination only. For the properties of the components please consider, furosemide p. 243, triamterene p. 246.

● **INDICATIONS AND DOSE**

Oedema

▸ BY MOUTH

▸ Adult: 0.5–2 tablets daily, dose to be taken in the morning

● CONTRA-INDICATIONS Anuria · dehydration · hyperkalaemia · hypovolaemia · renal failure · severe hypokalaemia · severe hyponatraemia

● CAUTIONS Diabetes mellitus · elderly · gout · hepatorenal syndrome · hypotension · impaired micturition · may cause blue fluorescence of urine · prostatic enlargement

● INTERACTIONS → Appendix 1: loop diuretics · potassium-sparing diuretics

● BREAST FEEDING Triamterene present in milk—manufacturer advises avoid. Furosemide may inhibit lactation.

● HEPATIC IMPAIRMENT Manufacturer advises caution; avoid in severe hepatic failure or hepatic coma.
Dose adjustments Manufacturer advises initial dose reduction.

● RENAL IMPAIRMENT Avoid in severe impairment.
Dose adjustments May need high doses.
Monitoring Monitor plasma-potassium concentration in renal impairment (high risk of hyperkalaemia).

● MONITORING REQUIREMENTS Monitor electrolytes.

● PATIENT AND CARER ADVICE Urine may look slightly blue in some lights.

● MEDICINAL FORMS There can be variation in the licensing of different medicines containing the same drug.
Tablet
CAUTIONARY AND ADVISORY LABELS 14
▸ Frusene (Orion Pharma (UK) Ltd)
Furosemide 40 mg, Triamterene 50 mg Frusene 50mg/40mg tablets | 56 tablet [PoM] £4.34 DT = £4.34

Torasemide   ▶ 242   05-Jun-2020

● **INDICATIONS AND DOSE**

Oedema

▸ BY MOUTH

▸ Adult: 5 mg once daily, to be taken preferably in the morning, then increased if necessary to 20 mg once daily; maximum 40 mg per day

Hypertension

▸ BY MOUTH

▸ Adult: 2.5 mg daily, then increased if necessary to 5 mg once daily

● INTERACTIONS → Appendix 1: loop diuretics

● SIDE-EFFECTS

▸ **Common or very common** Asthenia · gastrointestinal disorder

▸ **Uncommon** Bladder dilation · urinary retention

▸ **Rare or very rare** Allergic dermatitis

▸ **Frequency not known** Anaemia · cerebral ischaemia · confusion · dry mouth · embolism · ischaemic heart disease · myocardial infarction · pancreatitis · syncope · visual impairment

● PREGNANCY Manufacturer advises avoid—toxicity in *animal* studies.

● BREAST FEEDING Manufacturer advises avoid—no information available.

● MEDICINAL FORMS There can be variation in the licensing of different medicines containing the same drug.
Tablet
▸ Torasemide (Non-proprietary)
Torasemide 5 mg Torasemide 5mg tablets | 28 tablet [PoM] £14.50 DT = £5.53
Torasemide 10 mg Torasemide 10mg tablets | 28 tablet [PoM] £18.50 DT = £8.14
▸ Torem (Mylan)
Torasemide 2.5 mg Torem 2.5mg tablets | 28 tablet [PoM] £3.78 DT = £3.78
Torasemide 5 mg Torem 5mg tablets | 28 tablet [PoM] £5.53 DT = £5.53
Torasemide 10 mg Torem 10mg tablets | 28 tablet [PoM] £8.14 DT = £8.14

DIURETICS > OSMOTIC DIURETICS

Mannitol   09-Dec-2020

● **INDICATIONS AND DOSE**

Cerebral oedema

▸ BY INTRAVENOUS INFUSION

▸ Adult: 0.25–2 g/kg, repeated if necessary, to be administered over 30–60 minutes, dose may be repeated 1–2 times after 4–8 hours

Raised intra-ocular pressure

▸ BY INTRAVENOUS INFUSION

▸ Adult: 0.25–2 g/kg, repeated if necessary, to be administered over 30–60 minutes, dose may be repeated 1–2 times after 4–8 hours

● CONTRA-INDICATIONS Anuria · intracranial bleeding (except during craniotomy) · severe cardiac failure · severe dehydration · severe pulmonary oedema

● CAUTIONS Extravasation causes inflammation and thrombophlebitis

● SIDE-EFFECTS

▸ **Common or very common** Cough · headache · vomiting

▸ **Uncommon** Dizziness · fever · malaise · nausea · pain · skin reactions

▸ **Frequency not known** Arrhythmia · asthenia · azotaemia · chest pain · chills · coma · compartment syndrome ·

confusion · congestive heart failure · dry mouth · electrolyte imbalance · fluid imbalance · hyperhidrosis · hypersensitivity · hypertension · lethargy · metabolic acidosis · muscle complaints · musculoskeletal stiffness · nephrotic syndrome · neurotoxicity · peripheral oedema · pulmonary oedema · rebound intracranial pressure increase · renal impairment · rhinitis · seizure · thirst · urinary disorders · vision blurred

- PREGNANCY Manufacturer advises avoid unless essential— no information available.
- BREAST FEEDING Manufacturer advises avoid unless essential—no information available.
- RENAL IMPAIRMENT Use with caution in severe impairment.
- PRE-TREATMENT SCREENING Assess cardiac function before treatment.
- MONITORING REQUIREMENTS Monitor fluid and electrolyte balance, serum osmolality, and cardiac, pulmonary and renal function.
- DIRECTIONS FOR ADMINISTRATION For mannitol 20%, an in-line filter is recommended (15-micron filters have been used).

- MEDICINAL FORMS There can be variation in the licensing of different medicines containing the same drug. Forms available from special-order manufacturers include: infusion, solution for infusion

Infusion
▸ Mannitol (Non-proprietary)
   Mannitol 100 mg per 1 ml Mannitol 50g/500ml (10%) infusion Viaflo bags | 1 bag PoM 💲
   Polyfusor K mannitol 10% infusion 500ml bottles | 1 bottle PoM £5.43
   Mannitol 150 mg per 1 ml Mannitol 75g/500ml (15%) infusion Viaflo bags | 20 bag PoM 💲
   Mannitol 200 mg per 1 ml Mannitol 50g/250ml (20%) infusion Viaflex bags | 1 bag PoM 💲
   Polyfusor M mannitol 20% infusion 500ml bottles | 1 bottle PoM £7.12
   Mannitol 100g/500ml (20%) infusion Viaflex bags | 1 bag PoM 💲

DIURETICS > POTASSIUM-SPARING DIURETICS > ALDOSTERONE ANTAGONISTS

Spironolactone with furosemide

The properties listed below are those particular to the combination only. For the properties of the components please consider, spironolactone p. 208, furosemide p. 243.

- INDICATIONS AND DOSE
Resistant oedema
▸ BY MOUTH
  ▸ Adult: 20/50–80/200 mg daily

- INTERACTIONS → Appendix 1: aldosterone antagonists · loop diuretics

- MEDICINAL FORMS There can be variation in the licensing of different medicines containing the same drug.
Capsule
▸ Lasilactone (Sanofi)
  Furosemide 20 mg, Spironolactone 50 mg Lasilactone 20mg/50mg capsules | 28 capsule PoM £7.97 DT = £7.97

DIURETICS > POTASSIUM-SPARING DIURETICS > OTHER

Amiloride hydrochloride

11-Dec-2020

- INDICATIONS AND DOSE
Oedema (monotherapy)
▸ BY MOUTH
  ▸ Adult: Initially 10 mg daily, alternatively initially 5 mg twice daily, adjusted according to response; maximum 20 mg per day
Potassium conservation when used as an adjunct to thiazide or loop diuretics for hypertension or congestive heart failure
▸ BY MOUTH
  ▸ Adult: Initially 5–10 mg daily
Potassium conservation when used as an adjunct to thiazide or loop diuretics for hepatic cirrhosis with ascites
▸ BY MOUTH
  ▸ Adult: Initially 5 mg daily

- CONTRA-INDICATIONS Addison's disease · anuria · hyperkalaemia
- CAUTIONS Diabetes mellitus · elderly
- INTERACTIONS → Appendix 1: potassium-sparing diuretics
- SIDE-EFFECTS Alopecia · angina pectoris · aplastic anaemia · appetite decreased · arrhythmia · arthralgia · asthenia · atrioventricular block exacerbated · bladder spasm · chest pain · confusion · constipation · cough · depression · diarrhoea · dizziness · drowsiness · dry mouth · dyspnoea · dysuria · electrolyte imbalance · encephalopathy · gastrointestinal discomfort · gastrointestinal disorders · gastrointestinal haemorrhage · gout · headache · insomnia · jaundice · muscle cramps · nasal congestion · nausea · nervousness · neutropenia · pain · palpitations · paraesthesia · postural hypotension · sexual dysfunction · skin reactions · tinnitus · tremor · vertigo · visual impairment · vomiting
- PREGNANCY Not to be used to treat gestational hypertension.
- BREAST FEEDING Manufacturer advises avoid—no information available.
- RENAL IMPAIRMENT Manufacturers advise avoid in severe impairment.
  Monitoring Monitor plasma-potassium concentration (high risk of hyperkalaemia in renal impairment).
- MONITORING REQUIREMENTS Monitor electrolytes.

- MEDICINAL FORMS There can be variation in the licensing of different medicines containing the same drug. Forms available from special-order manufacturers include: oral suspension, oral solution
Oral solution
EXCIPIENTS: May contain Propylene glycol
▸ Amiloride hydrochloride (Non-proprietary)
  Amiloride hydrochloride 1 mg per 1 ml Amiloride 5mg/5ml oral solution sugar free sugar-free | 150 ml PoM £46.45 DT = £46.42
Tablet
▸ Amiloride hydrochloride (Non-proprietary)
  Amiloride hydrochloride 5 mg Amiloride 5mg tablets | 28 tablet PoM £39.82 DT = £33.09

Combinations available: *Co-amilofruse*, p. 242

Amiloride with bumetanide

The properties listed below are those particular to the combination only. For the properties of the components please consider, amiloride hydrochloride p. 245, bumetanide p. 242.

- ● **INDICATIONS AND DOSE**

Oedema
- ▸ BY MOUTH
- ▸ Adult: 1–2 tablets daily

- ● INTERACTIONS → Appendix 1: loop diuretics · potassium-sparing diuretics

- ● MEDICINAL FORMS There can be variation in the licensing of different medicines containing the same drug.
  Tablet
  - ▸ Amiloride with bumetanide (Non-proprietary)
    Bumetanide 1 mg, Amiloride hydrochloride 5 mg Amiloride 5mg / Bumetanide 1mg tablets | 28 tablet PoM £56.00 DT = £56.00

Triamterene

03-Sep-2020

- ● **INDICATIONS AND DOSE**

Oedema | Potassium conservation with thiazide and loop diuretics
- ▸ BY MOUTH
- ▸ Adult: Initially 150–250 mg daily for 1 week, lower initial dose when given with other diuretics, then reduced to 150–250 mg daily on alternate days, to be taken in divided doses after breakfast and lunch

- ● CONTRA-INDICATIONS Addison's disease · anuria · hyperkalaemia
- ● CAUTIONS Diabetes mellitus · elderly · gout · may cause blue fluorescence of urine
- ● INTERACTIONS → Appendix 1: potassium-sparing diuretics
- ● SIDE-EFFECTS
  - ▸ **Common or very common** Diarrhoea · hyperkalaemia · nausea · vomiting
  - ▸ **Uncommon** Dry mouth · headache · hyperuricaemia · renal failure (reversible on discontinuation) · skin reactions
  - ▸ **Rare or very rare** Megaloblastic anaemia · nephritis tubulointerstitial · pancytopenia · photosensitivity reaction · serum sickness · urolithiasis
  - ▸ **Frequency not known** Asthenia · jaundice · metabolic acidosis
- ● PREGNANCY Not used to treat gestational hypertension. Avoid unless essential.
- ● BREAST FEEDING Present in milk—manufacturer advises avoid.
- ● HEPATIC IMPAIRMENT Manufacturer advises caution; avoid in progressive impairment.
- ● RENAL IMPAIRMENT Avoid in progressive impairment.
  Monitoring Monitor plasma-potassium concentration (high risk of hyperkalaemia in renal impairment).
- ● MONITORING REQUIREMENTS Monitor electrolytes.
- ● PATIENT AND CARER ADVICE Urine may look slightly blue in some lights.

- ● MEDICINAL FORMS There can be variation in the licensing of different medicines containing the same drug.
  Capsule
  CAUTIONARY AND ADVISORY LABELS 14, 21
  - ▸ Triamterene (Non-proprietary)
    Triamterene 50 mg Triamterene 50mg capsules | 30 capsule PoM £41.90 DT = £41.90

  Combinations available: *Co-triamterzide,* p. 247 · *Furosemide with triamterene,* p. 244

Triamterene with chlortalidone

The properties listed below are those particular to the combination only. For the properties of the components please consider, triamterene above, chlortalidone below.

- ● **INDICATIONS AND DOSE**

Hypertension | Oedema
- ▸ BY MOUTH
- ▸ Adult: 50/50–100/100 mg once daily, dose to be taken in the morning
  DOSE EQUIVALENCE AND CONVERSION
  - ▸ Dose expressed as *x*/*y* mg of triamterene/chlortalidone.

- ● INTERACTIONS → Appendix 1: potassium-sparing diuretics · thiazide diuretics

- ● MEDICINAL FORMS There can be variation in the licensing of different medicines containing the same drug.
  Tablet
  CAUTIONARY AND ADVISORY LABELS 14, 21
  - ▸ Triamterene with chlortalidone (Non-proprietary)
    Chlortalidone 50 mg, Triamterene 50 mg Triamterene 50mg / Chlortalidone 50mg tablets | 28 tablet PoM £117.00 DT = £117.00

DIURETICS 〉 THIAZIDES AND RELATED DIURETICS

F 179

Chlortalidone

(Chlorthalidone)

- ● **INDICATIONS AND DOSE**

Ascites due to cirrhosis in stable patients (under close supervision) | Oedema due to nephrotic syndrome
- ▸ BY MOUTH
- ▸ Adult: Up to 50 mg daily

Hypertension
- ▸ BY MOUTH
- ▸ Adult: 25 mg daily, dose to be taken in the morning, then increased if necessary to 50 mg daily

Mild to moderate chronic heart failure
- ▸ BY MOUTH
- ▸ Adult: 25–50 mg daily, dose to be taken in the morning, then increased if necessary to 100–200 mg daily, reduce to lowest effective dose for maintenance

Nephrogenic diabetes insipidus | Partial pituitary diabetes insipidus
- ▸ BY MOUTH
- ▸ Adult: Initially 100 mg twice daily, then reduced to 50 mg daily

- ● INTERACTIONS → Appendix 1: thiazide diuretics
- ● SIDE-EFFECTS
  - ▸ **Common or very common** Appetite decreased · gastrointestinal discomfort
  - ▸ **Uncommon** Gout
  - ▸ **Rare or very rare** Arrhythmia · diabetes mellitus exacerbated · eosinophilia · glycosuria · hepatic disorders · nephritis tubulointerstitial · pulmonary oedema · respiratory disorder
- ● BREAST FEEDING The amount present in milk is too small to be harmful. Large doses may suppress lactation.

- ● MEDICINAL FORMS There can be variation in the licensing of different medicines containing the same drug. Forms available from special-order manufacturers include: oral suspension
  Tablet
  - ▸ Chlortalidone (Non-proprietary)
    Chlortalidone 25 mg Chlortalidone 25mg tablets | 100 tablet PoM Ⓢ

Chlortalidone 50 mg Chlortalidone 50mg tablets | 30 tablet PoM
£90.55 DT = £88.04

Combinations available: *Triamterene with chlortalidone,*
p. 246

Co-triamterzide
09-Oct-2020

The properties listed below are those particular to the
combination only. For the properties of the components
please consider, triamterene p. 246, hydrochlorothiazide
p. 180.

● **INDICATIONS AND DOSE**

Hypertension
▸ BY MOUTH
▸ Adult: 50/25 mg daily, increased if necessary up to
200/100 mg daily, dose to be taken after breakfast

Oedema
▸ BY MOUTH
▸ Adult: 50/25 mg twice daily, to be taken after breakfast
and after midday meal, increased if necessary to
150/75 mg daily, to be taken as 100/50 mg after
breakfast and 50/25 mg after midday meal;
maintenance 50/25 mg daily, alternatively
maintenance 100/50 mg once daily on alternate days;
maximum 200/100 mg per day

DOSE EQUIVALENCE AND CONVERSION
▸ Dose expressed as *x*/*y* mg of
triamterene/hydrochlorothiazide.

● INTERACTIONS → Appendix 1: potassium-sparing diuretics
· thiazide diuretics

● PATIENT AND CARER ADVICE Urine may look slightly blue
in some lights.

● MEDICINAL FORMS There can be variation in the licensing of
different medicines containing the same drug.

Tablet
CAUTIONARY AND ADVISORY LABELS 14, 21
▸ Dyazide (Advanz Pharma)
Hydrochlorothiazide 25 mg, Triamterene 50 mg Dyazide
50mg/25mg tablets | 30 tablet PoM £0.95 DT = £0.95

◀ 179

Metolazone
23-Sep-2020

● **INDICATIONS AND DOSE**

Oedema
▸ BY MOUTH
▸ Adult: 5–10 mg daily, dose to be taken in the morning;
increased if necessary to 20 mg daily, dose increased in
resistant oedema; maximum 80 mg per day

Hypertension
▸ BY MOUTH
▸ Adult: Initially 5 mg daily, dose to be taken in the
morning; maintenance 5 mg once daily on alternate
days

● CAUTIONS Acute porphyrias p. 1107

● INTERACTIONS → Appendix 1: thiazide diuretics

● SIDE-EFFECTS Appetite decreased · arthralgia · asthenia ·
chest discomfort · chills · drowsiness · gastrointestinal
discomfort · glycosuria · gout aggravated ·
haemoconcentration · hepatic disorders · hypoplastic
anaemia · hypovolaemia · muscle complaints · palpitations
· peripheral neuropathy · psychotic depression · severe
cutaneous adverse reactions (SCARs) · syncope · vasculitis ·
venous thrombosis · vertigo · vision blurred

● BREAST FEEDING The amount present in milk is too small
to be harmful. Large doses may suppress lactation.

● DIRECTIONS FOR ADMINISTRATION Expert sources advise
tablets may be crushed and mixed with water immediately
before use.

● MEDICINAL FORMS There can be variation in the licensing of
different medicines containing the same drug. Forms available
from special-order manufacturers include: tablet, oral
suspension, oral solution
Tablet
▸ Zaroxolyn (Imported (Canada))
Metolazone 2.5 mg Zaroxolyn 2.5mg tablets | 100 tablet PoM ⓧ
Metolazone 5 mg Zaroxolyn 5mg tablets | 50 tablet PoM ⓧ

◀ 179

Xipamide
23-Sep-2020

● **INDICATIONS AND DOSE**

Oedema
▸ BY MOUTH
▸ Adult: Initially 40 mg daily, dose to be taken in the
morning, increased if necessary to 80 mg daily, higher
dose to be used in resistant cases; maintenance 20 mg
daily, dose to be taken in the morning

Hypertension
▸ BY MOUTH
▸ Adult: 20 mg daily, dose to be taken in the morning

● CAUTIONS Acute porphyrias p. 1107

● INTERACTIONS → Appendix 1: thiazide diuretics

● SIDE-EFFECTS
▸ **Common or very common** Anxiety · gastrointestinal
discomfort · gouty arthritis · hyperhidrosis · lethargy ·
muscle complaints · palpitations
▸ **Rare or very rare** Cholecystitis acute · hyperlipidaemia ·
jaundice · nephritis acute interstitial · pancreatitis
haemorrhagic · vision disorders

● BREAST FEEDING No information available.

● MEDICINAL FORMS There can be variation in the licensing of
different medicines containing the same drug.
Tablet
▸ Diurexan (Mylan)
Xipamide 20 mg Diurexan 20mg tablets | 140 tablet PoM £19.46
DT = £19.46

10 Vascular disease

Peripheral vascular disease

Classification and management

Peripheral vascular disease can be either occlusive (e.g.
intermittent claudication) in which occlusion of the peripheral
arteries is caused by atherosclerosis, or vasospastic (e.g.
Raynaud's syndrome). Peripheral arterial occlusive disease is
associated with an increased risk of cardiovascular events;
this risk is reduced by measures such as Smoking cessation
p. 519, effective control of blood pressure, regulating blood
lipids, optimising glycaemic control in diabetes, taking
aspirin p. 132 in a dose of 75 mg daily, and possibly weight
reduction in obesity. Exercise training can improve
symptoms of intermittent claudication; revascularisation
procedures may be appropriate.

Naftidrofuryl oxalate p. 249 can alleviate symptoms of
intermittent claudication and improve pain-free walking
distance in moderate disease. Patients taking naftidrofuryl
oxalate should be assessed for improvement after
3–6 months.

Cilostazol p. 248 is licensed for use in intermittent
claudication to improve walking distance in patients without
peripheral tissue necrosis who do not have pain at rest; use is

restricted to second-line treatment where lifestyle modifications and other appropriate interventions have failed to improve symptoms. Cilostazol should be initiated by those experienced in the management of intermittent claudication. Patients receiving cilostazol should be assessed for improvement after 3 months; consider discontinuation of treatment if there is no clinically relevant improvement in walking distance.

Inositol nicotinate below and pentoxifylline p. 249 are not established as being effective for the treatment of intermittent claudication.

Intravenous iloprost p. 199 is a treatment option for critical limb ischaemia in patients unsuitable for surgery.

Management of *Raynaud's syndrome* includes avoidance of exposure to cold and Smoking cessation p. 519. More severe symptoms may require vasodilator treatment, which is most often successful in primary Raynaud's syndrome. Nifedipine p. 176 is useful for reducing the frequency and severity of vasospastic attacks. Alternatively, naftidrofuryl oxalate may produce symptomatic improvement; inositol nicotinate (a nicotinic acid derivative) may also be considered. Pentoxifylline, prazosin p. 829, and moxisylyte p. 249 are not established as being effective for the treatment of Raynaud's syndrome.

Vasodilator therapy is not established as being effective for *chilblains*.

Advanced Pharmacy Services

Patients with peripheral vascular disease may be eligible for the Medicines Use Review service provided by a community pharmacist. For further information, see *Advanced Pharmacy Services* in Medicines optimisation p. 18.

ANTITHROMBOTIC DRUGS > ANTIPLATELET DRUGS

Cilostazol

01-Sep-2020

● **INDICATIONS AND DOSE**

Intermittent claudication in patients without rest pain and no peripheral tissue necrosis

▸ BY MOUTH
▸ **Adult:** 100 mg twice daily, to be taken 30 minutes before food, cilostazol should be initiated by those experienced in the management of intermittent claudication, patients receiving cilostazol should be assessed for improvement after 3 months; consider discontinuation of treatment if there is no clinically relevant improvement in walking distance

DOSE ADJUSTMENTS DUE TO INTERACTIONS
▸ Manufacturer advises reduce dose to 50 mg twice daily with concurrent use of potent inhibitors of CYP3A4, potent inhibitors of CYP2C19, omeprazole and erythromycin.

● CONTRA-INDICATIONS Active peptic ulcer · congestive heart failure · coronary intervention in previous 6 months · haemorrhagic stroke in previous 6 months · history of severe tachyarrhythmia · myocardial infarction in previous 6 months · poorly controlled hypertension · predisposition to bleeding · proliferative diabetic retinopathy · prolongation of QT interval · unstable angina · ventricular arrhythmia

● CAUTIONS Atrial fibrillation · atrial flutter · atrial or ventricular ectopy · diabetes mellitus (higher risk of intraocular bleeding) · stable coronary disease · surgery

● INTERACTIONS → Appendix 1: cilostazol

● SIDE-EFFECTS
▸ **Common or very common** Appetite decreased · arrhythmias · diarrhoea · dizziness · gastrointestinal discomfort · gastrointestinal disorders · headache · increased risk of

infection · nausea · oedema · palpitations · skin reactions · vomiting
▸ **Uncommon** Anaemia · anxiety · congestive heart failure · cough · dyspnoea · haemorrhage · hyperglycaemia · hypotension · sleep disorders · syncope
▸ **Rare or very rare** Renal impairment · thrombocytosis
▸ **Frequency not known** Agranulocytosis · bone marrow disorders · conjunctivitis · fever · granulocytopenia · hepatic disorders · hot flush · hypertension · intracranial haemorrhage · leucopenia · paresis · severe cutaneous adverse reactions (SCARs) · thrombocytopenia · tinnitus · urinary frequency increased

● PREGNANCY Avoid—toxicity in *animal* studies.

● BREAST FEEDING Present in milk in *animal* studies—manufacturer advises avoid.

● HEPATIC IMPAIRMENT Manufacturer advises avoid in moderate-to-severe impairment—no information available.

● RENAL IMPAIRMENT Avoid if eGFR less than $25 \text{ mL/minute/1.73 m}^2$.

● PATIENT AND CARER ADVICE
Blood disorders Patients should be advised to report any unexplained bleeding, bruising, sore throat, or fever.

● NATIONAL FUNDING/ACCESS DECISIONS
For full details see funding body website
NICE decisions
▸ Cilostazol, naftidrofuryl oxalate, pentoxifylline and inositol nicotinate for the treatment of intermittent claudication in people with peripheral arterial disease (May 2011) NICE TA223 Not recommended

● MEDICINAL FORMS There can be variation in the licensing of different medicines containing the same drug.
Tablet
▸ Cilostazol (Non-proprietary)
Cilostazol 50 mg Cilostazol 50mg tablets | 56 tablet [PoM] £40.08 DT = £40.08
Cilostazol 100 mg Cilostazol 100mg tablets | 56 tablet [PoM] £33.37 DT = £5.96
▸ Pletal (Otsuka Pharmaceuticals (U.K.) Ltd)
Cilostazol 50 mg Pletal 50mg tablets | 56 tablet [PoM] £35.31 DT = £40.08
Cilostazol 100 mg Pletal 100mg tablets | 56 tablet [PoM] £33.37 DT = £5.96

LIPID MODIFYING DRUGS > NICOTINIC ACID DERIVATIVES

Inositol nicotinate

17-Jan-2020

● **INDICATIONS AND DOSE**

Peripheral vascular disease

▸ BY MOUTH
▸ **Adult:** 3 g daily in 2–3 divided doses; maximum 4 g per day

● CONTRA-INDICATIONS Acute phase of a cerebrovascular accident · recent myocardial infarction

● CAUTIONS Cerebrovascular insufficiency · unstable angina

● SIDE-EFFECTS
▸ **Uncommon** Dizziness · flushing · headache · nausea · oedema · paraesthesia · postural hypotension · rash · syncope · vomiting
▸ **Frequency not known** Myalgia

● PREGNANCY No information available—manufacturer advises avoid unless potential benefit outweighs risk.

● NATIONAL FUNDING/ACCESS DECISIONS
For full details see funding body website
NICE decisions
▸ Cilostazol, naftidrofuryl oxalate, pentoxifylline and inositol nicotinate for the treatment of intermittent claudication in

people with peripheral arterial disease (May 2011) NICE TA223
Not recommended

● LESS SUITABLE FOR PRESCRIBING Less suitable for
prescribing.

● MEDICINAL FORMS There can be variation in the licensing of
different medicines containing the same drug. Forms available
from special-order manufacturers include: oral suspension
Capsule
▸ Solgar No-Flush Niacin (Solgar Vitamin and Herb)
  Inositol nicotinate 500 mg Solgar No-Flush Niacin 500mg capsules
  | 50 capsule Ⓢ

VASODILATORS ⟩ FLAVONOIDS

Oxerutins

● INDICATIONS AND DOSE
**Relief of symptoms of oedema associated with chronic
venous insufficiency**
▸ BY MOUTH
▸ Adult: 500 mg twice daily

● SIDE-EFFECTS
▸ **Rare or very rare** Alopecia · arthralgia · diarrhoea ·
dizziness · fatigue · flushing · gastrointestinal discomfort ·
gastrointestinal disorders · headache · photosensitivity
reaction · skin reactions

● LESS SUITABLE FOR PRESCRIBING Oxerutins (rutosides)
are not vasodilators and are not generally regarded as
effective preparations as capillary sealants or for the
treatment of cramps; they are less suitable for prescribing.

● MEDICINAL FORMS There can be variation in the licensing of
different medicines containing the same drug.
Capsule
▸ Paroven (GlaxoSmithKline Consumer Healthcare)
  Oxerutins 250 mg Paroven 250mg capsules | 120 capsule Ⓟ
  £27.07 DT = £27.07

VASODILATORS ⟩ PERIPHERAL VASODILATORS

Moxisylyte
06-Feb-2020

(Thymoxamine)

● INDICATIONS AND DOSE
Primary Raynaud's syndrome (short-term treatment)
▸ BY MOUTH
▸ Adult: Initially 40 mg 4 times a day, increased if
necessary to 80 mg 4 times a day, increase dose if poor
initial response, discontinue after 2 weeks if no
response

● CAUTIONS Diabetes mellitus

● INTERACTIONS → Appendix 1: moxisylyte

● SIDE-EFFECTS
▸ **Rare or very rare** Hepatic disorders · rash
▸ **Frequency not known** Diarrhoea · flushing · headache ·
nausea · vertigo

● PREGNANCY Manufacturer advises avoid.

● HEPATIC IMPAIRMENT Manufacturer advises avoid in
active liver disease.

● LESS SUITABLE FOR PRESCRIBING Less suitable for
prescribing.

● MEDICINAL FORMS There can be variation in the licensing of
different medicines containing the same drug.
Tablet
CAUTIONARY AND ADVISORY LABELS 21
▸ Opilon (Kyowa Kirin Ltd)
  Moxisylyte (as Moxisylyte hydrochloride) 40 mg Opilon 40mg
  tablets | 112 tablet PoM £90.22 DT = £90.22

Naftidrofuryl oxalate

● INDICATIONS AND DOSE
Peripheral vascular disease
▸ BY MOUTH
▸ Adult: 100–200 mg 3 times a day, patients taking
naftidrofuryl should be assessed for improvement after
3–6 months
Cerebral vascular disease
▸ BY MOUTH
▸ Adult: 100 mg 3 times a day, patients taking
naftidrofuryl should be assessed for improvement after
3–6 months

● SIDE-EFFECTS
▸ **Uncommon** Diarrhoea · epigastric pain · nausea · rash ·
vomiting
▸ **Rare or very rare** Liver injury · oxalate nephrolithiasis
▸ **Frequency not known** Oesophagitis

● NATIONAL FUNDING/ACCESS DECISIONS
For full details see funding body website

NICE decisions
▸ **Cilostazol, naftidrofuryl oxalate, pentoxifylline and inositol
nicotinate for the treatment of intermittent claudication in
people with peripheral arterial disease (May 2011) NICE TA223**
Recommended

● MEDICINAL FORMS There can be variation in the licensing of
different medicines containing the same drug. Forms available
from special-order manufacturers include: oral solution
Capsule
CAUTIONARY AND ADVISORY LABELS 25, 27
▸ Naftidrofuryl oxalate (Non-proprietary)
  Naftidrofuryl oxalate 100 mg Naftidrofuryl 100mg capsules |
  84 capsule PoM £7.57 DT = £6.25
▸ Praxilene (Merck Serono Ltd)
  Naftidrofuryl oxalate 100 mg Praxilene 100mg capsules |
  84 capsule PoM £8.10 DT = £6.25

Pentoxifylline
06-Feb-2020

(Oxpentifylline)

● INDICATIONS AND DOSE
Peripheral vascular disease | Venous leg ulcer (adjunct)
▸ BY MOUTH
▸ Adult: 400 mg 2–3 times a day

● UNLICENSED USE Use of pentoxifylline as adjunct therapy
for venous leg ulcers is an unlicensed indication.

● CONTRA-INDICATIONS Acute myocardial infarction ·
cerebral haemorrhage · extensive retinal haemorrhage ·
severe cardiac arrhythmias

● CAUTIONS Avoid in Acute porphyrias p. 1107 · coronary
artery disease · hypotension

● INTERACTIONS → Appendix 1: pentoxifylline

● SIDE-EFFECTS Agitation · angina pectoris · angioedema ·
arrhythmias · bronchospasm · cholestasis · constipation ·
diarrhoea · dizziness · gastrointestinal discomfort ·
gastrointestinal disorder · haemorrhage · headache · hot
flush · hypersalivation · hypotension · leucopenia ·
meningitis aseptic · nausea · neutropenia · skin reactions ·
sleep disorder · thrombocytopenia · vomiting

● PREGNANCY Manufacturer advises avoid—no information
available.

● BREAST FEEDING Present in milk—manufacturer advises
use only if potential benefit outweighs risk.

● HEPATIC IMPAIRMENT Manufacturer advises caution in
severe impairment.
Dose adjustments Manufacturer advises consider dose
reduction in severe impairment.

2

Cardiovascular system

2

Cardiovascular system

• RENAL IMPAIRMENT
Dose adjustments Reduce dose by 30–50% if eGFR less than 30 mL/minute/1.73 m^2.

• NATIONAL FUNDING/ACCESS DECISIONS
For full details see funding body website
NICE decisions
▸ Cilostazol, naftidrofuryl oxalate, pentoxifylline and inositol nicotinate for the treatment of intermittent claudication in people with peripheral arterial disease (May 2011) NICE TA223 Not recommended

• LESS SUITABLE FOR PRESCRIBING Less suitable for prescribing.

• MEDICINAL FORMS There can be variation in the licensing of different medicines containing the same drug. Forms available from special-order manufacturers include: oral solution
Modified-release tablet
CAUTIONARY AND ADVISORY LABELS 21, 25
▸ Trental (Sanofi)
Pentoxifylline 400 mg Trental 400 modified-release tablets | 90 tablet [PoM] £19.39 DT = £19.39

10.1 Vein malformations

SCLEROSANTS

Sodium tetradecyl sulfate   24-Aug-2020

• **INDICATIONS AND DOSE**
Sclerotherapy of reticular veins and spider veins in legs and varicose veins
▸ BY INTRAVENOUS INJECTION
▸ Adult: Test dose recommended before each treatment (consult product literature)

• CONTRA-INDICATIONS Acute infection · asthma · blood disorders · deep vein thrombosis · high risk of thromboembolism · hyperthyroidism · inability to walk · neoplasm · occlusive arterial disease · phlebitis · pulmonary embolism · recent acute superficial thrombophlebitis · recent surgery · respiratory disease · significant valvular incompetence in deep veins · skin disease · symptomatic patent foramen ovale (if administered as foam) · uncontrolled diabetes mellitus · varicose veins caused by tumours (unless tumour removed)

• CAUTIONS Arterial disease · asymptomatic patent foramen ovale (use smaller volumes and avoid Valsalva manoeuvre immediately after administration) · extravasation may cause necrosis of tissues · history of migraine (use smaller volumes) · resuscitation facilities must be available · venous insufficiency with lymphoedema (pain and inflammation may worsen)

• SIDE-EFFECTS
▸ **Common or very common** Embolism and thrombosis · pain · paraesthesia
▸ **Uncommon** Skin reactions · telangiectasia
▸ **Rare or very rare** Arterial spasm · asthenia · asthma · cerebrovascular insufficiency · chest pressure · circulatory collapse · confusion · cough · diarrhoea · dry mouth · dyspnoea · fever · headaches · hot flush · hypersensitivity · local exfoliation · nausea · nerve damage · palpitations · presyncope · soft tissue necrosis · tongue swelling · vasculitis · vision disorders · vomiting

• PREGNANCY Avoid unless benefits outweigh risks—no information available.

• BREAST FEEDING Use with caution—no information available.

• MEDICINAL FORMS There can be variation in the licensing of different medicines containing the same drug.
Solution for injection
EXCIPIENTS: May contain Benzyl alcohol
▸ Fibro-Vein (STD Pharmaceutical Products Ltd)
Sodium tetradecyl sulfate 2 mg per 1 ml Fibrovein 0.2% solution for injection 5ml vials | 10 vial [PoM] £73.61
Sodium tetradecyl sulfate 5 mg per 1 ml Fibrovein 0.5% solution for injection 2ml ampoules | 5 ampoule [PoM] £18.93
Sodium tetradecyl sulfate 10 mg per 1 ml Fibrovein 1% solution for injection 2ml ampoules | 5 ampoule [PoM] £22.61
Sodium tetradecyl sulfate 30 mg per 1 ml Fibrovein 3% solution for injection 2ml ampoules | 5 ampoule [PoM] £33.65
Fibrovein 3% solution for injection 5ml vials | 10 vial [PoM] £166.66

Chapter 3
Respiratory system

CONTENTS

Respiratory system, drug delivery

30-Nov-2020

Inhalation

This route delivers the drug directly to the airways; the dose required is smaller than when given by mouth and side-effects are reduced.

Inhaler devices

These include *pressurised metered-dose inhalers*, *breath-actuated inhalers*, and *dry powder inhalers*. Many patients can be taught to use a pressurised metered-dose inhaler effectively but some patients, particularly the elderly and children, find them difficult to use. *Spacer devices* can help such patients because they remove the need to co-ordinate actuation with inhalation. Dry powder inhalers may be useful in adults and children over 5 years who are unwilling or unable to use a pressurised metered-dose inhaler. Alternatively, breath-actuated inhalers are suitable for adults and older children provided they can use the device effectively. EvGr Consider the patient's preference when testing alternative devices to a pressurised metered-dose inhaler; there is no evidence to dictate an order in which devices should be tested.

In adults with stable asthma, a pressurised metered-dose inhaler with or without a spacer is as effective as any other hand-held inhaler; a dry-powder inhaler may still be preferred. A spacer should always be used if the patient is on a high dose of inhaled corticosteroid.

In adults with mild or moderate acute asthma attacks, a pressurised metered-dose inhaler with a spacer is at least as effective as nebulisation. ⟨A⟩

On changing from a pressurised metered-dose inhaler to a dry powder inhaler, patients may notice a lack of sensation in the mouth and throat previously associated with each actuation. Coughing may also occur.

EvGr The patient should be instructed carefully on the use of the inhaler. It is important to check that the inhaler continues to be used correctly because inadequate inhalation technique may be mistaken for a lack of response to the drug. The number and different types of inhalers given to a patient should be minimised. To help reduce confusion and ensure patients receive inhalers they have been given training for, specify brand and inhaler when prescribing. ⟨A⟩

For more information on delivery systems used in the management of COPD, see Chronic obstructive pulmonary disease p. 258.

MHRA/CHM advice: Pressurised metered dose inhalers (pMDI): risk of airway obstruction from aspiration of loose objects (July 2018)
The MHRA have received reports of patients who have inhaled objects into the back of the throat—in some cases objects were aspirated, causing airway obstruction. Patients should be reminded to remove the mouthpiece cover fully,

shake the device and check that both the outside and inside of the mouthpiece are clear and undamaged before inhaling a dose, and to store the inhaler with the mouthpiece cover on.

Spacer devices

Spacer devices remove the need for coordination between actuation of a pressurised metered-dose inhaler and inhalation. The spacer device reduces the velocity of the aerosol and subsequent impaction on the oropharynx and allows more time for evaporation of the propellant so that a larger proportion of the particles can be inhaled and deposited in the lungs. Spacer devices are particularly useful for patients with poor inhalation technique, for children, for patients requiring high doses of inhaled corticosteroids, for nocturnal asthma, and for patients prone to candidiasis with inhaled corticosteroids. It is important to prescribe a spacer device that is compatible with the metered-dose inhaler, see devices below. Spacer devices should not be regarded as interchangeable; patients should be advised not to switch between spacer devices.

Use and care of spacer devices

Patients should inhale from the spacer device as soon as possible after actuation because the drug aerosol is very short-lived; single-dose actuation is recommended. Tidal breathing is as effective as single breaths. The device should be cleaned once a month by washing in mild detergent and then allowed to dry in air without rinsing; the mouthpiece should be wiped clean of detergent before use. Some manufacturers recommend more frequent cleaning, but this should be avoided since any electrostatic charge may affect drug delivery. Spacer devices should be replaced every 6–12 months.

Respiratory drug delivery, nebulisers

Solutions for nebulisation used in severe or life-threatening asthma attacks are administered over 5–10 minutes from a nebuliser, usually driven by oxygen.

EvGr Patients with a severe attack of asthma should preferably have oxygen during nebulisation since beta$_2$ agonists can increase arterial hypoxaemia. However, the absence of supplemental oxygen should not delay treatment. ⟨A⟩

A nebuliser converts a solution of a drug into an aerosol for inhalation. It is used to deliver higher doses of drug to the airways than is usual with standard inhalers. The main indications for use of a nebuliser are to deliver:

- a beta$_2$ agonist or ipratropium bromide p. 262 to a patient with an *acute exacerbation* of asthma or of chronic obstructive pulmonary disease;
- a beta$_2$ agonist, corticosteroid, or ipratropium bromide on a *regular basis* to a patient with severe asthma or reversible airways obstruction when the patient is unable to use other inhalational devices;

3

Respiratory system

- an antibiotic (such as colistimethate sodium p. 591) or a mucolytic to a patient with cystic fibrosis;
- Budesonide p. 275 or adrenaline/epinephrine p. 238 to a child with severe croup;
- Pentamidine isetionate p. 641 for the prophylaxis and treatment of pneumocystis pneumonia.

Before prescribing a nebuliser, a home trial should preferably be undertaken to monitor response for up to 2 weeks on standard treatment and up to 2 weeks on nebulised treatment. If prescribed, patients must:

- have clear instructions from a doctor, specialist nurse, physiotherapist, or pharmacist on the use of the nebuliser (including maintenance and cleaning) and on peak-flow monitoring;
- be instructed not to treat acute attacks at home without also seeking help;
- have regular follow up by a doctor, specialist nurse or physiotherapist after about 1 month and annually thereafter.

The proportion of a nebuliser solution that reaches the lungs depends on the type of nebuliser and although it can be as high as 30%, it is more frequently close to 10% and sometimes below 10%. The remaining solution is left in the nebuliser as residual volume or is deposited in the mouthpiece and tubing. The extent to which the nebulised solution is deposited in the airways or alveoli depends on the droplet size, pattern of breath inhalation, and condition of the lung. Droplets with a mass median diameter of 1–5 microns are deposited in the airways and are therefore appropriate for asthma, whereas a particle size of 1–2 microns is needed for alveolar deposition of pentamidine isetionate p. 641 to combat pneumocystis infection. The type of nebuliser is therefore chosen according to the deposition required and according to the viscosity of the solution.

Jet nebulisers
Jet nebulisers are more widely used than ultrasonic nebulisers. Most jet nebulisers require an optimum gas flow rate of 6–8 litres/minute and in hospital can be driven by piped air or oxygen; in acute asthma the nebuliser should be driven by oxygen. Domiciliary oxygen cylinders do not provide an adequate flow rate therefore an electrical compressor is required for domiciliary use.

For patients at risk of hypercapnia, such as those with chronic obstructive pulmonary disease, oxygen can be dangerous and the nebuliser should be driven by air. If oxygen is required, it should be given simultaneously by nasal cannula.

Tubing
The Department of Health has reminded users of the need to use the correct grade of tubing when connecting a nebuliser to a medical gas supply or compressor.

Ultrasonic nebulisers
Ultrasonic nebulisers produce an aerosol by ultrasonic vibration of the drug solution and therefore do not require a gas flow; they are not suitable for the nebulisation of some drugs, such as dornase alfa p. 309 and nebulised suspensions.

Nebuliser diluent
Nebulisation may be carried out using an undiluted nebuliser solution or it may require dilution beforehand. The usual diluent is sterile sodium chloride 0.9% (physiological saline).

In England and Wales nebulisers and compressors are not available on the NHS (but they are free of VAT); some nebulisers (but not compressors) are available on form GP10A in Scotland (for details consult Scottish Drug Tariff).

Oral

The oral route is used when administration by inhalation is not possible. Systemic side-effects occur more frequently when a drug is given orally rather than by inhalation. Drugs given by mouth for the treatment of asthma include corticosteroids, theophylline p. 289, and leukotriene receptor antagonists.

Parenteral

EvGr Drugs such as beta₂ agonists, corticosteroids, and aminophylline p. 288 can be given by injection in severe acute and life-threatening asthma when administration by nebulisation is inadequate or inappropriate. If the patient is being treated in the community, urgent transfer to hospital should be arranged. Ⓐ

Peak flow meters

When used in addition to symptom-based monitoring, peak flow monitoring has not been proven to improve asthma control in either adults or children, however measurement of peak flow may be of benefit in adult patients who are 'poor perceivers' and hence slow to detect deterioration in their asthma, and for those with more severe asthma.

When peak flow meters are used, patients must be given clear guidelines as to the action they should take if their peak flow falls below a certain level. Patients can be encouraged to adjust some of their own treatment (within specified limits) according to changes in peak flow rate.

Peak flow charts should be issued to patients where appropriate, and are available to purchase from:

3M Security Print and Systems Limited. Gorse Street, Chadderton, Oldham, OL9 9QH. Tel: 0845 610 1112

GP practices can obtain supplies through their Area Team stores.

NHS Hospitals can order supplies from www.nhsforms.co.uk/ or by emailing nhsforms@mmm.com.

In Scotland, peak flow charts can be obtained by emailing stockorders.dppas@apsgroup.co.uk.

1 Airways disease, obstructive

Asthma, chronic

06-May-2020

Description of condition

Asthma is a common chronic inflammatory condition of the airways, associated with airway hyperresponsiveness and variable airflow obstruction. The most frequent symptoms of asthma are cough, wheeze, chest tightness, and breathlessness. Asthma symptoms vary over time and in intensity and can gradually or suddenly worsen, provoking an acute asthma attack that, if severe, may require hospitalisation.

Asthma-COPD overlap syndrome (ACOS) is characterised by persistent airflow limitation displaying features of both asthma and COPD.

Aims of treatment

The aim of treatment is to achieve control of asthma. Complete control of asthma is defined as no daytime symptoms, no night-time awakening due to asthma, no asthma attacks, no need for rescue medication, no limitations on activity including exercise, normal lung function (in practical terms forced expiratory volume in 1 second (FEV₁) and/or peak expiratory flow (PEF) > 80% predicted or best), and minimal side-effects from treatment. In clinical practice, patients may choose to balance the aims of asthma management against the potential side-effects or inconvenience of taking medication necessary to achieve perfect control.

Lifestyle changes

EvGr Weight loss in overweight patients may lead to an improvement in asthma symptoms. Patients with asthma and parents of children with asthma should be advised about the dangers of smoking, to themselves and to their children, and be offered appropriate support to stop smoking. ⒶFor further information, see Smoking cessation p. 519.

EvGr Breathing exercise programmes (including physiotherapist-taught methods and audiovisual programmes), can be offered to adults as an adjuvant to drug treatment to improve quality of life and reduce symptoms. Ⓐ

Management

EvGr A stepwise approach aims to stop symptoms quickly and to improve peak flow. Treatment should be started at the level most appropriate to initial severity of asthma. The aim is to achieve early control and to maintain it by stepping up treatment as necessary and decreasing treatment when control is good. Before initiating a new drug or adjusting treatment, consider whether the diagnosis is correct, check adherence and inhaler technique, and eliminate trigger factors for acute attacks.

A self-management programme comprising of a written personalised action plan and education should be offered to all patients with asthma (and/or their family or carers), and should be supported with regular review by a healthcare professional. Ⓐ

For information on devices used in the management of asthma, see Respiratory system, drug delivery p. 251.

Recommendations on the management of chronic asthma from the *National Institute for Health and Care Excellence (NICE)—Asthma: diagnosis, monitoring and chronic asthma management guidelines (NG80, November 2017)*, and *British Thoracic Society (BTS) and Scottish Intercollegiate Guidelines Network (SIGN)—British guideline on the management of asthma (SIGN 158, July 2019)* differ significantly. Recommendations in BNF publications are based on NICE guidelines, and differences with BTS/SIGN (2019) have been highlighted.

For information on the management of patients during the COVID-19 pandemic, see COVID-19 p. 660.

Adult

NICE (2017) treatment recommendations for adults apply to patients aged 17 years and over. BTS/SIGN (2019) treatment recommendations for adults apply to patients over 12 years.

Intermittent reliever therapy

EvGr Start an inhaled short-acting beta$_2$ agonist (such as salbutamol p. 269 or terbutaline sulfate p. 271), to be used as required in all patients with asthma. For those with infrequent short-lived wheeze, occasional use of reliever therapy may be the only treatment required. Patients using more than one short-acting beta$_2$ agonist inhaler device a month should have their asthma urgently assessed and action taken to improve poorly controlled asthma. Ⓐ

Regular preventer (maintenance) therapy

NICE (2017) define inhaled corticosteroid (ICS) doses for adults as low, moderate, or high. BTS/SIGN (2019) instead define ICS doses for adults as low, medium or high (refer to individual guidelines for ICS dosing information).

EvGr A low-dose of ICS should be started as maintenance therapy in patients who present with any one of the following features: using an inhaled short-acting beta$_2$ agonist three times a week or more, symptomatic three times a week or more, or waking at night due to asthma symptoms at least once a week. BTS/SIGN (2019) also recommend initiation in patients who have had an asthma attack in the last 2 years, and starting an ICS at a dose appropriate to the severity of asthma.

BTS/SIGN (2019) recommend that inhaled corticosteroids (except ciclesonide p. 278) should initially be taken twice daily, however the same total daily dose taken once a day, can be considered in patients with milder disease if good or complete control of asthma is established. The dose of ICS should be adjusted over time to the lowest effective dose at which control of asthma is maintained.

BTS/SIGN (2019) recommend the prescribing of inhalers by brand. Ⓐ

Initial add-on therapy

EvGr If asthma is uncontrolled on a low-dose of ICS as maintenance therapy, a leukotriene receptor antagonist (LTRA—such as montelukast p. 285) should be offered in addition to the ICS, and the response to treatment reviewed in 4 to 8 weeks.

BTS/SIGN (2019) instead recommend a long-acting beta$_2$ agonist (LABA—such as salmeterol p. 268 or formoterol fumarate p. 266) as initial add-on therapy to low-dose ICS if asthma is uncontrolled. This can be given as either a fixed-dose ICS and LABA regimen, or a MART regimen (Maintenance And Reliever Therapy—a combination of an ICS and a fast-acting LABA such as formoterol in a single inhaler, see beclometasone with formoterol p. 274 and budesonide with formoterol p. 276). Combination inhalers containing both a LABA and an ICS are recommended to improve adherence, and ensure that the LABA is not taken alone without the ICS.

BTS/SIGN (2019) also recommend that a MART regimen should be considered in patients with a history of asthma attacks on a medium-dose ICS alone, or on a fixed-dose ICS and LABA regimen. Ⓐ

Additional controller therapies

EvGr If asthma is uncontrolled on a low-dose of ICS and a LTRA as maintenance therapy, a LABA in combination with the ICS should be offered with or without continued LTRA treatment, depending on the response achieved from the LTRA.

If asthma remains uncontrolled, offer to change the ICS and LABA maintenance therapy to a MART regimen, with a low-dose of ICS as maintenance. See beclometasone with formoterol p. 274 and budesonide with formoterol p. 276.

If asthma remains uncontrolled on a MART regimen with a low-dose of ICS as maintenance with or without a LTRA, consider increasing to a moderate-dose of ICS (either continuing a MART regimen, or changing to a fixed-dose regimen of an ICS and a LABA with a short-acting beta$_2$ agonist as reliever therapy).

If asthma is still uncontrolled in patients on a moderate-dose of ICS as maintenance with a LABA (either as a MART or a fixed-dose regimen), with or without a LTRA, consider the following options:

- Increasing the ICS dose to a high-dose as maintenance (this should only be offered as part of a fixed-dose regimen with a short-acting beta$_2$ agonist used as reliever therapy), or
- A trial of an additional drug, for example, a long-acting muscarinic receptor antagonist (such as tiotropium p. 263) or modified-release theophylline p. 289, or
- Seeking advice from an asthma specialist.

BTS/SIGN (2019) instead recommend that if the patient is gaining some benefit from addition of a LABA but control remains inadequate, the LABA should be continued and *either* the dose of ICS be increased to a medium-dose (if not already on this dose), or a LTRA be added.

If there is no response to the LABA, consider discontinuing it and *either* increasing the dose of the ICS to a medium-dose (if not already on this dose), or adding in a LTRA.

BTS/SIGN (2019) recommend that all patients whose asthma is not adequately controlled on recommended initial add-on therapy or additional controller therapies, should be referred for specialist asthma care. Ⓐ

High-dose ICS and further add-on treatment (specialist therapies)

[EvGr] Under specialist care, BTS/SIGN (2019) recommend that if asthma control remains inadequate on a medium-dose of ICS, plus a LABA or LTRA, the following interventions can be considered:

- Increasing the ICS to a high-dose—with high doses of ICS via a pressurised metered dose inhaler (pMDI) a spacer should be used, or
- Adding a LTRA (if not already tried), or modified-release theophylline p. 289, or tiotropium p. 263.

If a trial of a further add-on treatment is ineffective, stop the drug (or in the case of increased dose of ICS, reduce to the original dose). ⟨Ⓐ⟩

Continuous or frequent use of oral corticosteroids (specialist therapies)

[EvGr] Under specialist care, BTS/SIGN (2019) recommend adding a regular oral corticosteroid (prednisolone p. 718) at the lowest dose to provide adequate control in patients with very severe asthma uncontrolled on a high-dose ICS, and who have also tried (or are still receiving) a LABA, LTRA, tiotropium p. 263, or modified-release theophylline p. 289. ⟨Ⓐ⟩

For information on the general use and side effects of corticosteroids, see Corticosteroids, general use p. 709. For information on the cessation of oral corticosteroid treatment, see Treatment cessation for systemic corticosteroids (such as prednisolone).

Monoclonal antibodies and immunosuppressants (specialist therapies)

[EvGr] Under specialist initiation, BTS/SIGN (2019) recommend that monoclonal antibodies such as omalizumab p. 284 (for severe persistent allergic asthma), mepolizumab p. 284, benralizumab p. 283 and reslizumab p. 285 (in adults for severe eosinophilic asthma), and immunosuppressants such as methotrexate p. 957 [unlicensed], may be considered in patients with severe asthma to achieve control and reduce the use of oral corticosteroids. ⟨Ⓐ⟩ See National funding/access decisions for omalizumab p. 284, mepolizumab p. 284, reslizumab p. 285, and benralizumab.

Child aged over 5 years

For children aged over 5 years, NICE (2017) treatment recommendations for children apply to children aged 5–16 years, and adult treatment recommendations apply to those aged 17 years and over. Whereas, for children aged over 5 years, BTS/SIGN (2019) treatment recommendations for children apply to children aged 5–12 years, and adult treatment recommendations apply to those aged over 12 years.

Intermittent reliever therapy

[EvGr] Start an inhaled short-acting beta$_2$ agonist (such as salbutamol p. 269 or terbutaline sulfate p. 271), to be used as required in all children with asthma. For those with infrequent short-lived wheeze, occasional use of reliever therapy may be the only treatment required. Children using more than one short-acting beta$_2$ agonist inhaler device a month should have their asthma urgently assessed and action taken to improve poorly controlled asthma. ⟨Ⓐ⟩

Regular preventer (maintenance) therapy

NICE (2017) define inhaled corticosteroid (ICS) doses for children (aged 5–16 years) as paediatric low, moderate, or high. BTS/SIGN (2019) instead define ICS doses for children (aged 5–12 years) as very low, low, or medium, and for children aged over 12 years as low, medium or high (refer to individual guidelines for ICS dosing information).

[EvGr] A paediatric low-dose of ICS should be started as maintenance therapy in children who present with any one of the following features: using an inhaled short-acting beta$_2$ agonist three times a week or more, symptomatic three times a week or more, or waking at night due to asthma symptoms at least once a week.

BTS/SIGN (2019) instead recommend starting a very low-dose (child aged 5–12 years) or a low-dose (child aged over 12 years) of ICS in children presenting with any one of the following features: using an inhaled short-acting beta$_2$ agonist three times a week or more, symptomatic three times a week or more, waking at night due to asthma symptoms at least once a week, or have had an asthma attack in the last 2 years, and starting an ICS at a dose appropriate to the severity of asthma.

BTS/SIGN (2019) recommend that inhaled corticosteroids (except ciclesonide p. 278) should initially be taken twice daily, however the same total daily dose taken once a day, can be considered in patients with milder disease if good or complete control of asthma is established. The dose of ICS should be adjusted over time to the lowest effective dose at which control of asthma is maintained.

BTS/SIGN (2019) recommend the prescribing of inhalers by brand. ⟨Ⓐ⟩

Initial add-on therapy

[EvGr] If asthma is uncontrolled on a paediatric low-dose of ICS as maintenance therapy, consider a leukotriene receptor antagonist (LTRA—such as montelukast p. 285) in addition to the ICS, and review the response to treatment in 4 to 8 weeks.

BTS/SIGN (2019) instead recommend a long-acting beta$_2$ agonist (LABA—such as salmeterol p. 268 or formoterol fumarate p. 266) as initial add-on therapy to low-dose ICS if asthma is uncontrolled in children aged over 12 years. This can be given as either a fixed-dose ICS and LABA regimen, or a MART regimen (Maintenance And Reliever Therapy—a combination of an ICS and a fast-acting LABA such as formoterol in a single inhaler, see budesonide with formoterol p. 276). Combination inhalers containing both a LABA and an ICS are recommended to improve adherence, and ensure that the LABA is not taken alone without the ICS.

BTS/SIGN (2019) also recommend that a MART regimen should be considered in children aged over 12 years with a history of asthma attacks on a medium-dose ICS alone, or on a fixed-dose ICS and LABA regimen.

In children aged 5–12 years, BTS/SIGN (2019) recommend the addition of either a LABA or a LTRA, as initial add-on therapy to very low-dose ICS if asthma is uncontrolled. ⟨Ⓐ⟩

Additional controller therapies

[EvGr] If asthma is uncontrolled on a paediatric low-dose of ICS and a LTRA as maintenance therapy, consider discontinuation of the LTRA and initiation of a LABA in combination with the ICS.

If asthma remains uncontrolled on a paediatric low-dose of ICS and a LABA as maintenance therapy, consider changing to a MART regimen (Maintenance And Reliever Therapy—a combination of an ICS and fast-acting LABA such as formoterol in a single inhaler) with a paediatric low-dose of ICS as maintenance. See budesonide with formoterol p. 276 [not licensed in all age groups].

If asthma remains uncontrolled on a MART regimen with a paediatric low-dose of ICS as maintenance, consider increasing to a paediatric moderate-dose of ICS (either continuing a MART regimen, or changing to a fixed-dose regimen of an ICS and a LABA with a short-acting beta$_2$ agonist as reliever therapy).

If asthma is still uncontrolled on a paediatric moderate-dose of ICS as maintenance with a LABA (either as a MART or a fixed-dose regimen), consider seeking advice from an asthma specialist and the following options:

- Increasing the ICS dose to a paediatric high-dose as maintenance (this should only be offered as part of a fixed-dose regimen with a short-acting beta$_2$ agonist as reliever therapy), or
- A trial of an additional drug, such as modified-release theophylline p. 289.

BTS/SIGN (2019) instead recommend that in children aged 5–12 years who are gaining some benefit from the addition of a LABA or a LTRA but control remains inadequate, continue the LABA or LTRA and *either* increase the dose of the ICS to a low-dose (if not already on this dose), or add a LTRA or LABA (whichever is not being used).

In children aged over 12 years, BTS/SIGN (2019) recommend continuing the LABA and *either* increasing the ICS dose to a medium-dose (if not already on this dose), or adding a LTRA.

If there is no response to the LABA, consider discontinuing it and *either* increasing the dose of ICS to a low-dose (child aged 5–12 years) or medium-dose (child aged over 12 years) if not already on this dose, or adding a LTRA.

BTS/SIGN (2019) recommend that all patients whose asthma is not adequately controlled on recommended initial add-on therapy or additional controller therapies, should be referred for specialist asthma care. ⒶA

High-dose ICS and further add-on treatment (specialist therapies)

EvGr Under specialist care, BTS/SIGN (2019) recommend that if control remains inadequate on a low-dose (child aged 5–12 years) or medium-dose (child aged over 12 years) of ICS, plus a LABA or LTRA, the following interventions should be considered:

- Increasing the ICS to a medium-dose (child aged 5–12 years) or high-dose (child aged over 12 years)—with ICS via a pressurised metered dose inhaler (pMDI) a spacer should be used, or
- Adding a LTRA (if not already tried), or modified-release theophylline p. 289, or tiotropium p. 263 (in children over 12 years).

If a trial of a further add-on treatment is ineffective, stop the drug (or in the case of increased dose of ICS, reduce to the original dose). ⒶA

Continuous or frequent use of oral corticosteroids (specialist therapies)

EvGr Under specialist care, BTS/SIGN (2019) recommend adding a regular oral corticosteroid (prednisolone p. 718) at the lowest dose to provide adequate control in children with very severe asthma uncontrolled on a high-dose ICS, and who have also tried (or are still receiving) a LABA, LTRA, tiotropium p. 263 (child over 12 years), or modified-release theophylline p. 289. ⒶA

For information on the general use and side effects of corticosteroids, see Corticosteroids, general use p. 709. For information on the cessation of oral corticosteroid treatment, see *Treatment cessation* for systemic corticosteroids (such as prednisolone).

Monoclonal antibodies and immunosuppressants (specialist therapies)

EvGr Under specialist initiation, BTS/SIGN (2019) recommend that monoclonal antibodies such as omalizumab p. 284 (child over 6 years for severe persistent allergic asthma), and immunosuppressants such as methotrexate p. 957 [unlicensed] can be considered in children with severe asthma to achieve control and reduce the use of oral corticosteroids. ⒶA See *National funding/access decisions* for omalizumab p. 284.

Child aged under 5 years

Intermittent reliever therapy

EvGr A short-acting beta$_2$ agonist (such as salbutamol p. 269) as reliever therapy should be offered to children aged under 5 years with suspected asthma. A short-acting beta$_2$ agonist should be used for symptom relief alongside maintenance treatment.

Children using more than one short-acting beta$_2$ agonist inhaler device a month should have their asthma urgently assessed and action taken to improve poorly controlled asthma. ⒶA

Regular preventer (maintenance) therapy

NICE (2017) define inhaled corticosteroid (ICS) doses for children aged under 5 years as paediatric low or moderate. BTS/SIGN (2019) instead define ICS doses for

children aged under 5 years as very low (refer to individual guidelines for ICS dosing information).

EvGr Consider an 8-week trial of a paediatric moderate-dose of ICS in children presenting with any of the following features: asthma-related symptoms three times a week or more, experiencing night-time awakening at least once a week, or suspected asthma that is uncontrolled with a short-acting beta$_2$ agonist alone.

After 8 weeks, stop ICS treatment and continue to monitor the child's symptoms:

- If symptoms did not resolve during the trial period, review whether an alternative diagnosis is likely;
- If symptoms resolved then reoccurred within 4 weeks of stopping ICS treatment, restart the ICS at a paediatric low-dose as first-line maintenance therapy;
- If symptoms resolved but reoccurred beyond 4 weeks after stopping ICS treatment, repeat the 8-week trial of a paediatric moderate-dose of ICS.

BTS/SIGN (2019) instead recommend starting a very low-dose of ICS as initial regular preventer therapy in children presenting with any one of the following features: using an inhaled short-acting beta$_2$ agonist three times a week or more, symptomatic three times a week or more, or waking at night due to asthma symptoms at least once a week. In children unable to take an ICS, a leukotriene receptor antagonist (LRTA— such as montelukast p. 285) may be used as an alternative.

BTS/SIGN (2019) recommend the prescribing of inhalers by brand. ⒶA

Initial add-on therapy

EvGr If suspected asthma is uncontrolled in children aged under 5 years on a paediatric low-dose of ICS as maintenance therapy, consider a leukotriene receptor antagonist (LTRA—such as montelukast p. 285) in addition to the ICS.

If suspected asthma is uncontrolled in children aged under 5 years on a paediatric low-dose of ICS and a LTRA as maintenance therapy, stop the LTRA and refer the child to an asthma specialist. ⒶA

Decreasing treatment

EvGr Consider decreasing maintenance therapy when a patient's asthma has been controlled with their current maintenance therapy for at least three months. When deciding which drug to decrease first and at what rate, the severity of asthma, the side-effects of treatment, duration of current dose, the beneficial effect achieved, and the patient's preference should be considered. Patients should be regularly reviewed when decreasing treatment.

Patients should be maintained at the lowest possible dose of ICS. Reductions should be considered every three months, decreasing the dose by approximately 25–50% each time. Reduce the dose slowly as patients deteriorate at different rates. Only consider stopping ICS treatment completely for people who are using a paediatric or adult low-dose ICS alone as maintenance therapy and are symptom-free. ⒶA

Exercise-induced asthma

EvGr For most patients, exercise-induced asthma is an illustration of poorly controlled asthma and regular treatment including an ICS should therefore be reviewed. If exercise is a specific problem in patients already taking an ICS who are otherwise well controlled, consider adding either a LTRA, a long-acting beta$_2$ agonist, sodium cromoglicate p. 286 or nedocromil sodium, or theophylline p. 289. An inhaled short-acting beta$_2$ agonist used immediately before exercise is the drug of choice. ⒶA

Pregnancy

EvGr Women with asthma should be closely monitored during pregnancy. It is particularly important that asthma is well controlled during pregnancy; when this is achieved there is little or no increased risk of adverse maternal or fetal complications.

Women should be counselled about the importance and safety of taking their asthma medication during pregnancy to maintain good control. Women who smoke should be advised about the dangers to themselves and to their baby and be offered appropriate support to stop smoking. ⒶFor further information, see Smoking cessation p. 519.

EvGr Short-acting beta$_2$ agonists, LABAs, oral and inhaled corticosteroids, sodium cromoglicate p. 286 and nedocromil sodium, and oral and intravenous theophylline p. 289 (with appropriate monitoring) can be used as normal during pregnancy. There is limited information on use of a LTRA during pregnancy, however, where indicated to achieve adequate control, they should not be withheld. Ⓐ

Advanced Pharmacy Services

Patients with asthma may be eligible for the New Medicines Service / Medicines Use Review service provided by a community pharmacist. For further information, see *Advanced Pharmacy Services* in Medicines optimisation p. 18.

Useful Resources

Asthma: diagnosis, monitoring and chronic asthma management. National Institute for Health and Care Excellence. November 2017.
www.nice.org.uk/guidance/ng80

British guideline on the management of asthma. British Thoracic Society and Scottish Intercollegiate Guidelines Network. Full guidance - A national clinical guideline 158. July 2019.
www.sign.ac.uk/sign-158-british-guideline-on-the-management-of-asthma

Patient decision aid: Inhalers for asthma for use by people aged 17 years and over. National Institute for Health and Care Excellence. May 2019.
www.nice.org.uk/about/what-we-do/our-programmes/nice-guidance/nice-guidelines/shared-decision-making

---

Asthma, acute

07-Oct-2019

Description of condition

Acute asthma is the progressive worsening of asthma symptoms, including breathlessness, wheeze, cough, and chest tightness. An acute exacerbation is marked by a reduction in baseline objective measures of pulmonary function, such as peak expiratory flow rate and FEV$_1$.

Most asthma attacks severe enough to require hospitalisation develop relatively slowly over a period of six hours or more. In children, intermittent wheezing attacks are usually triggered by viral infections and response to asthma medication may be inconsistent. Low birth weight and/or prematurity may be risk factors for recurrent wheeze.

Aims of treatment

The aim of treatment is to relieve airflow obstruction and prevent future relapses. Early treatment is most advantageous.

Levels of severity

Adults

EvGr An acute exacerbation of asthma should be correctly differentiated from poor asthma control and its severity categorised in order to be appropriately treated. The categories are described as follows: Ⓐ

Moderate acute asthma

- Increasing symptoms;
- Peak flow > 50-75% best or predicted;
- No features of acute severe asthma.

Severe acute asthma

Any one of the following:

- Peak flow 33-50% best or predicted;
- Respiratory rate ≥ 25/min;
- Heart rate ≥ 110/min;
- Inability to complete sentences in one breath.

Life-threatening acute asthma

Any one of the following, in a patient with severe asthma:

- Peak flow < 33% best or predicted;
- Arterial oxygen saturation (SpO$_2$) < 92%;
- Partial arterial pressure of oxygen (PaO$_2$) < 8 kPa;
- Normal partial arterial pressure of carbon dioxide (PaCO$_2$) (4.6–6.0 kPa);
- Silent chest;
- Cyanosis;
- Poor respiratory effort;
- Arrhythmia;
- Exhaustion;
- Altered conscious level;
- Hypotension.

Near-fatal acute asthma

- Raised PaCO$_2$ and/or the need for mechanical ventilation with raised inflation pressures.

Children

EvGr An acute exacerbation of asthma should be correctly differentiated from poor asthma control and its severity categorised in order to be appropriately treated. The categories are described as follows: Ⓐ

Moderate acute asthma

- Able to talk in sentences;
- Arterial oxygen saturation (SpO$_2$) ≥ 92%;
- Peak flow ≥ 50% best or predicted;
- Heart rate ≤ 140/minute in children aged 1–5 years; heart rate ≤ 125/minute in children aged over 5 years;
- Respiratory rate ≤ 40/minute in children aged 1–5 years; respiratory rate ≤ 30/minute in children aged over 5 years.

Severe acute asthma

- Can't complete sentences in one breath or too breathless to talk or feed;
- SpO$_2$ < 92%;
- Peak flow 33–50% best or predicted;
- Heart rate > 140/minute in children aged 1–5 years; heart rate > 125/minute in children aged over 5 years;
- Respiratory rate > 40/minute in children aged 1–5 years; respiratory rate > 30/minute in children aged over 5 years.

Life-threatening acute asthma

Any one of the following in a child with severe asthma:

- SpO$_2$ < 92%;
- Peak flow < 33% best or predicted;
- Silent chest;
- Cyanosis;
- Poor respiratory effort;
- Hypotension;
- Exhaustion;
- Confusion.

Management in adults

EvGr Patients with moderate acute asthma should be treated at home or in primary care according to response to treatment, while patients with **severe** or **life-threatening** acute asthma should start treatment as soon as possible and be referred to hospital immediately following initial assessment. Hospital referral may also be warranted in other cases, such as failure to respond to initial treatment, social circumstances, or concomitant disease.

Supplementary oxygen should be given to all hypoxaemic patients with severe acute asthma to maintain an SpO$_2$ level between 94–98%. Do not delay if pulse oximetry is unavailable.

First-line treatment for acute asthma is a high-dose inhaled short-acting beta$_2$ agonist (salbutamol p. 269 or terbutaline sulfate p. 271) given as soon as possible. If the response to an initial dose of short-acting beta$_2$ agonist is poor, consider continuous nebulisation with an appropriate nebuliser. Intravenous beta$_2$ agonists are reserved for those patients in whom inhaled therapy cannot be used reliably.

In all cases of acute asthma, patients should be prescribed an adequate dose of oral prednisolone p. 718. Continue usual inhaled corticosteroid use during oral corticosteroid treatment. Parenteral hydrocortisone p. 716 or intramuscular methylprednisolone p. 717 are alternatives in patients who are unable to take oral prednisolone. ⟨A⟩

For information on the general use and side effects of corticosteroids, see Corticosteroids, general use p. 709. For information on the cessation of oral corticosteroid treatment, see *Treatment cessation* for systemic corticosteroids (such as prednisolone).

[EvGr] Nebulised ipratropium bromide p. 262 may be combined with a nebulised beta$_2$ agonist in patients with severe or life-threatening acute asthma, or in those with a poor initial response to beta$_2$ agonist therapy to provide greater bronchodilation. ⟨A⟩

There is some evidence that magnesium sulfate p. 1099 has bronchodilator effects. [EvGr] A single intravenous dose of magnesium sulfate may be considered in patients with severe acute asthma (peak flow < 50% best or predicted) who have not had a good initial response to inhaled bronchodilator therapy [unlicensed use]. ⟨A⟩ In an acute asthma attack, intravenous aminophylline p. 288 is not likely to produce any additional bronchodilation compared to standard therapy with inhaled bronchodilators and corticosteroids. However, in some patients with near-fatal or life-threatening acute asthma with a poor response to initial therapy, intravenous aminophylline may provide some benefit. [EvGr] Magnesium sulfate by intravenous infusion or aminophylline should only be used after consultation with senior medical staff. ⟨A⟩

Management in children aged 2 years and over

[EvGr] Children with **severe** or **life-threatening** acute asthma should start treatment as soon as possible and be referred to hospital immediately following initial assessment. Supplementary high flow oxygen (via a tight-fitting face mask or nasal cannula) should be given to all children with life-threatening acute asthma or SpO$_2$< 94% to achieve normal saturations of 94–98%.

First-line treatment for acute asthma is an inhaled short-acting beta$_2$ agonist (salbutamol or terbutaline sulfate) given as soon as possible. The dose given should be individualised according to severity and adjusted based on response. Discontinue long-acting beta$_2$ agonist use if a short-acting beta$_2$ agonist is given more than 4 hourly. Seek medical attention if symptoms are not controlled with 10 puffs of salbutamol via a spacer; give additional bronchodilator doses whilst awaiting medical attention if symptoms are severe.

In all cases of acute asthma, children should be prescribed an adequate dose of oral prednisolone. Treatment for up to 3 days is usually sufficient, but the length of the course should be tailored to the number of days necessary to bring about recovery. Repeat the dose in children who vomit and consider the intravenous route in those who are unable to retain oral medication. It is considered good practice that inhaled corticosteroids are continued at their usual maintenance dose whilst receiving additional treatment for the attack, but they should not be used as a replacement for the oral corticosteroid. ⟨A⟩

For information on the general use and side effects of corticosteroids, see Corticosteroids, general use p. 709. For information on the cessation of oral corticosteroid treatment, see *Treatment cessation* for systemic corticosteroids (such as prednisolone p. 718).

[EvGr] Nebulised ipratropium bromide p. 262 can be combined with beta$_2$ agonist treatment for children with a poor initial response to beta$_2$ agonist therapy to provide greater bronchodilation. Consider adding magnesium sulfate p. 1099 [unlicensed use] to each nebulised salbutamol p. 269 and ipratropium bromide in the first hour in children with a short duration of severe acute asthma symptoms presenting with an oxygen saturation less than 92%.

Children with continuing severe acute asthma despite frequent nebulised beta$_2$ agonists and ipratropium bromide plus oral corticosteroids, and those with life-threatening features, need urgent review by a specialist with a view to transfer to a high dependency unit or paediatric intensive care unit (PICU) to receive second-line intravenous therapies.

In children who respond poorly to first-line treatments, intravenous magnesium sulfate [unlicensed use] may be considered as first-line intravenous treatment. In a severe asthma attack where the child has not responded to initial inhaled therapy, early addition of a single bolus dose of intravenous salbutamol may be an option. Continuous intravenous infusion of salbutamol, administered under specialist supervision with continuous ECG and electrolyte monitoring, should be considered in children with unreliable inhalation or severe refractory asthma. Aminophylline p. 288 may be considered in children with severe or life-threatening acute asthma unresponsive to maximal doses of bronchodilators and corticosteroids. ⟨A⟩

Management in children aged under 2 years

[EvGr] Acute asthma treatment for all children aged under 2 years should be given in the hospital setting. Treatment of children aged under 1 year should be under the direct guidance of a respiratory paediatrician.

For moderate and severe acute asthma attacks, immediate treatment with oxygen via a tight-fitting face mask or nasal prongs should be given to achieve normal SpO$_2$ saturations of 94-98%. Trial an inhaled short-acting beta$_2$ agonist and if response is poor, combine nebulised ipratropium bromide to each nebulised beta$_2$ agonist dose. Consider oral prednisolone daily for up to 3 days, early in the management of severe asthma attacks.

In children not responsive to first-line treatments or have life-threatening features, discuss management with a senior paediatrician or the PICU team. ⟨A⟩

Follow up in all cases

[EvGr] Episodes of acute asthma may be a failure of preventative therapy, review is required to prevent further episodes. A careful history should be taken to establish the reason for the asthma attack. Inhaler technique should be checked and regular treatment should be reviewed. Patients should be given a written asthma action plan aimed at preventing relapse, optimising treatment, and preventing delay in seeking assistance in future attacks. It is essential that the patient's GP practice is informed within 24 hours of discharge from the emergency department or hospital following an asthma attack, and the patient be reviewed by their GP within 2 working days. Patients who have had a near-fatal asthma attack should be kept under specialist supervision indefinitely. A respiratory specialist should follow up all patients admitted with a severe asthma attack for at least one year after the admission. ⟨A⟩

Advanced Pharmacy Services

Patients with asthma may be eligible for the New Medicines Service / Medicines Use Review service provided by a community pharmacist. For further information, see *Advanced Pharmacy Services* in Medicines optimisation p. 18.

Useful Resources

British guideline on the management of asthma. British Thoracic Society and Scottish Intercollegiate Guidelines Network. Full guidance - A national clinical guideline 158. July 2019.
www.sign.ac.uk/sign-158-british-guideline-on-the-management-of-asthma

Chronic obstructive pulmonary disease

02-Oct-2020

Description of condition

Chronic obstructive pulmonary disease (COPD) is a common, largely preventable and treatable disease, characterised by persistent respiratory symptoms and airflow limitation that is usually progressive and not fully reversible. Airflow limitation is due to a combination of small airways disease (obstructive bronchiolitis) and parenchymal destruction (emphysema). Symptoms of COPD include dyspnoea, wheeze, chronic cough, and regular sputum production.

The main risk factor for development and exacerbations of COPD is tobacco smoking. Other risk factors include environmental pollution and occupational exposures, genetic factors (such as hereditary alpha-1 antitrypsin deficiency), and poor lung growth during childhood. Complications of COPD include cor pulmonale, depression, anxiety, type 2 respiratory failure, and secondary polycythaemia.

Asthma-COPD overlap syndrome (ACOS) is characterised by persistent airflow limitation that displays features of both asthma and COPD.

Aims of treatment

The primary aim of treatment is to reduce symptoms and exacerbations and improve quality of life.

Management of stable COPD:

For information on the management of patients during the COVID-19 pandemic, see COVID-19 p. 660.

Non-drug treatment

EvGr Patients who are smokers should be encouraged to stop smoking and be offered help to do so. For further information, see Smoking cessation p. 519.

All patients should receive care delivered by a multidisciplinary team. Pulmonary rehabilitation should be offered to appropriate patients, including those who view themselves as being functionally disabled by COPD. Pulmonary rehabilitation programmes should be tailored to the patient's individual needs, and include physical training, disease education, and nutritional, psychological and behavioural intervention.

Patients with excessive sputum production should be taught active cycle of breathing techniques, and how to use positive expiratory pressure devices by a physiotherapist.

Refer patients with a BMI that is abnormal or changing over time for dietetic input, and be attentive to changes in weight in the elderly.

Interventional procedures including surgery may be deemed appropriate following a respiratory review and input from the multidisciplinary team. A

Vaccinations

EvGr All patients should be offered the pneumococcal vaccine and annual influenza vaccine p. 1373. A

Inhaled treatment

EvGr The choice of inhaler device should be based on the patient's preference and ability to use the inhaler. When prescribing an inhaler, patients should be trained on how to use the device and be able to demonstrate satisfactory inhaler technique, and continue to have their inhaler technique regularly assessed. Where appropriate a spacer can be provided. Nebulised treatment should be considered for patients with distressing or disabling breathlessness despite maximal use of inhalers, and continued if an improvement is seen in symptoms, ability to undertake activities of daily living, exercise capacity, or lung function. A For information on devices used in the management of COPD, see Respiratory system, drug delivery p. 251.

Initial management for all patients

EvGr For initial empirical treatment, offer a short-acting bronchodilator as required to relieve breathlessness and exercise limitation. This can either be a short-acting beta$_2$ agonist (SABA) or a short-acting muscarinic antagonist (SAMA).

Before considering step-up treatment options, ensure that COPD is confirmed spirometrically, relevant vaccinations are given, non-drug treatment options have been optimised including smoking cessation, and that a short-acting bronchodilator is being used. A

Step-up treatment for patients without asthmatic features or features suggesting steroid responsiveness

EvGr In patients who continue to be breathless or have exacerbations, offer a long-acting beta$_2$ agonist (LABA) and a long-acting muscarinic antagonist (LAMA). Discontinue SAMA treatment if a LAMA is given. Treatment with a SABA as required may be continued in all stages of COPD.

In patients on a LAMA and LABA who have a severe exacerbation (requiring hospitalisation) or at least two moderate exacerbations (requiring systemic corticosteroids and/or antibacterial treatment) within a year, consider the addition of an inhaled corticosteroid (ICS)—triple therapy. If an ICS is given, review at least annually and document the reason for continuation.

In patients on a LAMA and LABA whose day-to-day symptoms continue to adversely impact their quality of life, consider trialling the addition of an ICS for 3 months. If symptoms have improved, continue triple therapy and review at least annually. If there has been no improvement, step back down to a LAMA and LABA combination. A

Step-up treatment for patients with asthmatic features or features suggesting steroid responsiveness

EvGr In patients who continue to be breathless or have exacerbations, consider treatment with a long-acting beta$_2$ agonist (LABA) and an inhaled corticosteroid (ICS). If an ICS is given, review annually documenting the reason for continuation.

In patients on a LABA and ICS who have a severe exacerbation (requiring hospitalisation) or at least two moderate exacerbations (requiring systemic corticosteroids and/or antibacterial treatment) within a year, or who continue to have day-to-day symptoms adversely impacting their quality of life, add a long-acting muscarinic antagonist (LAMA)—triple therapy. Discontinue SAMA treatment if a LAMA is given. Treatment with a SABA as required may be continued in all stages of COPD. A

Prophylactic antibiotics

EvGr After considering if respiratory specialist input is required, consider azithromycin p. 568 [unlicensed] prophylaxis to reduce the risk of exacerbations in patients who are non-smokers, have had all other treatment options optimised, and who continue to either have prolonged or frequent (4 or more per year) exacerbations with sputum production, or exacerbations resulting in hospitalisation. Ensure sputum culture and sensitivity testing, a CT scan of the thorax (to rule out other lung pathologies), a baseline ECG (to rule out QT prolongation), and LFTs are performed before offering prophylaxis. Review treatment after the first 3 months, then at least 6 monthly thereafter; only continue if benefits outweigh risks. A

Other treatments

EvGr Roflumilast p. 287 is recommended as add-on treatment to bronchodilator therapy in patients with severe COPD with chronic bronchitis (respiratory specialist initiation only), see *National funding/access decisions* for roflumilast. For guidance and the national funding access decision for roflumilast in Scotland, refer to the *Scottish Medicines Consortium*.

Consider mucolytic treatment in patients with chronic cough productive of sputum; only continue if symptomatic improvement is seen. Antitussive treatment should not be used in the management of stable COPD.

Modified-release theophylline p. 289 should only be used after a trial of short-acting and long-acting bronchodilators, or if the patient is unable to use inhaled treatment.

Be alert to the presence of anxiety or depression in patients, and manage accordingly. Ⓐ

For information on oxygen therapy in COPD patients, see Oxygen below.

For guidance on the management of COPD patients with cor pulmonale and/or pulmonary hypertension, see NICE guideline: **Chronic obstructive pulmonary disease in over 16s** (see *Useful resources*).

Management of exacerbations of COPD:

For information on the management of patients during the COVID-19 pandemic, see COVID-19 p. 660.

EvGr Together with the patient, action plans should be created for those at risk of exacerbations. In patients who have had an exacerbation within the last year, a short course of antibacterials (non-macrolide if on prophylactic azithromycin) and oral corticosteroids should be kept at home. Patients should understand and be confident with when and how to take these medicines, and to report having taken them to their healthcare professional. Patients may continue prophylactic azithromycin during an acute exacerbation.

Action plans may also include information on adjusting the short-acting bronchodilator dose, and a cognitive behavioural plan to manage symptoms of anxiety and associated breathlessness. Ⓐ

For guidance on assessing the need for hospital referral, see NICE guideline: **Chronic obstructive pulmonary disease in over 16s** (see *Useful resources*).

For guidance on antibacterial treatment in acute exacerbations of COPD, see *Chronic obstructive pulmonary disease, acute exacerbations* in Respiratory system infections, antibacterial therapy p. 538.

Non-drug treatment:

EvGr Where appropriate consider physiotherapy using positive expiratory pressure devices to help with sputum clearance. Ⓐ

Drug treatment

EvGr Give short-acting inhaled bronchodilators, usually at higher doses than the patient's maintenance treatment through a nebuliser or hand-held device to manage breathlessness. The choice should be dependant on the dose required, the patient's ability to use the device, and resources available to supervise administration. Withhold LAMA treatment if a SAMA is given.

In the absence of significant contra-indications in patients that present to hospital with an exacerbation, use a short course of prednisolone p. 718 along with other therapies. Consider a short course for patients in the community experiencing an exacerbation with a significant increase in breathlessness that interferes with daily activities. Consider osteoporosis prophylaxis for patients who require frequent courses of oral corticosteroids.

Long-term oral corticosteroid treatment is not usually recommended, however in some patients this may need to be continued when withdrawal following an exacerbation is not possible; the lowest dose possible should be used. Monitor patients for osteoporosis and give them appropriate prophylaxis. Start prophylaxis without monitoring for osteoporosis in patients aged over 65 years; for guidance on choice of therapy, see Osteoporosis p. 765. Ⓐ

For information on the general use and side effects of corticosteroids, see Corticosteroids, general use p. 709. For information on the cessation of oral corticosteroid treatment, see *Treatment cessation* for systemic corticosteroids (such as prednisolone).

EvGr Aminophylline p. 288 should only be used as add-on treatment when there is an inadequate response to nebulised bronchodilators; ensure therapeutic drug monitoring is performed and that previous oral theophylline use is considered to avoid toxicity.

If necessary, oxygen should be given to ensure oxygen saturation of arterial blood levels are kept within the target range for the patient. For further information, see Oxygen below.

For patients with persistant hypercapnic ventilatory failure, use non-invasive ventilation (NIV) if patients experience exacerbations despite the optimisation of medical treatment. If deemed necessary, invasive ventilation for COPD exacerbations should be given in an intensive care unit. Doxapram should only be given when NIV is inappropriate or unavailable in the clinical setting. Ⓐ

Advanced Pharmacy Services

Patients with chronic obstructive pulmonary disease may be eligible for the New Medicines Service / Medicines Use Review service provided by a community pharmacist. For further information, see *Advanced Pharmacy Services* in Medicines optimisation p. 18.

Useful Resources

Chronic obstructive pulmonary disease in over 16s: diagnosis and management. National Institute for Health and Care Excellence. NICE guideline 115; December 2018, updated July 2019.
www.nice.org.uk/guidance/ng115

Chronic obstructive pulmonary disease (acute exacerbation): antimicrobial prescribing. National Institute for Health and Care Excellence. NICE guideline 114; December 2018.
www.nice.org.uk/guidance/ng114

Oxygen

29-Sep-2019

Overview

Oxygen should be regarded as a drug. It is prescribed for hypoxaemic patients to increase alveolar oxygen tension and decrease the work of breathing. The concentration of oxygen required depends on the condition being treated; the administration of an inappropriate concentration of oxygen can have serious or even fatal consequences.

Oxygen is probably the most common drug used in medical emergencies. It should be prescribed initially to achieve a normal or near–normal oxygen saturation; in most acutely ill patients with a normal or low arterial carbon dioxide ($P_a CO_2$), oxygen saturation should be 94–98% oxygen saturation. However, in some clinical situations such as cardiac arrest and carbon monoxide poisoning it is more appropriate to aim for the highest possible oxygen saturation until the patient is stable. A lower target of 88–92% oxygen saturation is indicated for patients at risk of hypercapnic respiratory failure.

High concentration oxygen therapy is safe in uncomplicated cases of conditions such as pneumonia, pulmonary thromboembolism, pulmonary fibrosis, shock, severe trauma, sepsis, or anaphylaxis. In such conditions low arterial oxygen ($P_a O_2$) is usually associated with low or

3

Respiratory system

normal arterial carbon dioxide ($P_a CO_2$), and therefore there is little risk of hypoventilation and carbon dioxide retention.

In acute severe asthma, the arterial carbon dioxide ($P_a CO_2$) is usually subnormal but as asthma deteriorates it may rise steeply (particularly in children). These patients usually require high concentrations of oxygen and if the arterial carbon dioxide ($P_a CO_2$) remains high despite other treatment, intermittent positive-pressure ventilation needs to be considered urgently.

Low concentration oxygen therapy (controlled oxygen therapy) is reserved for patients at risk of hypercapnic respiratory failure, which is more likely in those with:

- chronic obstructive pulmonary disease (COPD);
- advanced cystic fibrosis;
- severe non-cystic fibrosis bronchiectasis;
- severe kyphoscoliosis or severe ankylosing spondylitis;
- severe lung scarring caused by tuberculosis;
- musculoskeletal disorders with respiratory weakness, especially if on home ventilation;
- an overdose of opioids, benzodiazepines, or other drugs causing respiratory depression.

[EvGr] Until blood gases can be measured, initial oxygen should be given using a controlled concentration of 24% or 28%, titrated towards a target oxygen saturation of 88–92% or the level specified on the patient's *oxygen alert card* if available. ⓐ The aim is to provide the patient with enough oxygen to achieve an acceptable arterial oxygen tension without worsening carbon dioxide retention and respiratory acidosis.

[EvGr] Patients with COPD and other at-risk conditions who have had an episode of hypercapnic respiratory failure, should be given a 24% or 28% Venturi mask and an oxygen alert card endorsed with the oxygen saturations required during previous exacerbations. Patients and their carers should be instructed to show the card to emergency healthcare providers in the event of an exacerbation. ⓐ

The oxygen alert card template is available at www.brit-thoracic.org.uk.

Domiciliary oxygen

Oxygen should only be prescribed for use in the home after careful evaluation in hospital by respiratory experts. Patients should be advised of the risks of continuing to smoke when receiving oxygen therapy, including the risk of fire. Smoking cessation p. 519 therapy should be recommended before home oxygen prescription. [EvGr] In patients with COPD, it should only be provided if the patient has stopped smoking. ⓐ

Air travel

Some patients with arterial hypoxaemia require supplementary oxygen for air travel. The patient's requirement should be discussed with the airline before travel.

Long-term oxygen therapy

Long-term administration of oxygen (usually at least 15 hours daily) improves survival in COPD patients with more severe hypoxaemia. [EvGr] The need for oxygen should be assessed in COPD patients with an FEV_1 less than 30% predicted (consider assessment if FEV_1 is 30-49%), cyanosis, polycythaemia, peripheral oedema, raised JVP, and when oxygen saturation levels are 92% or less breathing air. ⓐ

Assessment for long-term oxygen therapy requires measurement of arterial blood gas tensions. Measurements should be taken on 2 occasions at least 3 weeks apart to demonstrate clinical stability. Long-term oxygen therapy should be considered for patients with:

- [EvGr] COPD with $P_a O_2 < 7.3$ kPa when stable and who do not smoke (minimum of 15 hours per day);
- COPD with $P_a O_2$ 7.3–8 kPa when stable and do not smoke, and also have either secondary polycythaemia, peripheral

oedema, or evidence of pulmonary hypertension (minimum of 15 hours per day); ⓐ
- severe chronic asthma with $P_a O_2 < 7.3$ kPa or persistent disabling breathlessness;
- interstitial lung disease with $P_a O_2 < 8$ kPa and in patients with $P_a O_2 > 8$ kPa with disabling dyspnoea;
- cystic fibrosis when $P_a O_2 < 7.3$ kPa or if $P_a O_2$ 7.3–8 kPa in the presence of secondary polycythaemia, nocturnal hypoxaemia, pulmonary hypertension, or peripheral oedema;
- pulmonary hypertension, without parenchymal lung involvement when $P_a O_2 < 8$ kPa;
- neuromuscular or skeletal disorders, after specialist assessment;
- obstructive sleep apnoea despite continuous positive airways pressure therapy, after specialist assessment;
- pulmonary malignancy or other terminal disease with disabling dyspnoea;
- heart failure with daytime $P_a O_2 < 7.3$ kPa when breathing air or with nocturnal hypoxaemia;
- paediatric respiratory disease, after specialist assessment.

Increased respiratory depression is seldom a problem in patients with stable respiratory failure treated with low concentrations of oxygen although it may occur during exacerbations; patients and relatives should be warned to call for medical help if drowsiness or confusion occur.

[EvGr] A risk assessment should be carried out for all COPD patients being considered for long-term oxygen therapy and if treatment is given, should be reviewed at least annually. Offer smoking cessation advice, treatment and specialist referral for people who smoke or smokers living with the patient with COPD. Do not offer long-term oxygen therapy to patients who continue to smoke despite being offered smoking cessation interventions. ⓐ

Short-burst oxygen therapy

Oxygen is occasionally prescribed for short-burst (intermittent) use for episodes of breathlessness not relieved by other treatment in patients with interstitial lung disease, heart failure, and in palliative care. It is important, however, that the patient does not rely on oxygen instead of obtaining medical help or taking more specific treatment. Short-burst oxygen therapy can be used to improve exercise capacity and recovery; it should only be continued if there is proven improvement in breathlessness or exercise tolerance. [EvGr] It is not recommended for COPD patients who have mild or no hypoxaemia at rest. ⓐ

Ambulatory oxygen therapy

Ambulatory oxygen is prescribed for patients on long-term oxygen therapy who need to be away from home on a regular basis. Patients who are not on long-term oxygen therapy can be considered for ambulatory oxygen therapy if there is evidence of exercise-induced oxygen desaturation and of improvement in blood oxygen saturation and exercise capacity with oxygen. Ambulatory oxygen therapy is not recommended for patients with heart failure, COPD with mild or no hypoxaemia at rest, or those who smoke.

Oxygen therapy equipment

Under the NHS oxygen may be supplied as **oxygen cylinders**. Oxygen flow can be adjusted as the cylinders are equipped with an oxygen flow meter with 'medium' (2 litres/minute) and 'high' (4 litres/minute) settings. Oxygen delivered from a cylinder should be passed through a humidifier if used for long periods.

Oxygen concentrators are more economical for patients who require oxygen for long periods, and in England and Wales can be ordered on the NHS on a regional tendering basis. A concentrator is recommended for a patient who requires oxygen for more than 8 hours a day (or 21 cylinders per month). Exceptionally, if a higher concentration of oxygen is required the output of 2 oxygen concentrators can be combined using a 'Y' connection.

A nasal cannula is usually preferred for long-term oxygen therapy from an oxygen concentrator. It can, however, produce dermatitis and mucosal drying in sensitive individuals.

Giving oxygen by nasal cannula allows the patient to talk, eat, and drink, but the concentration of oxygen is not controlled; this may not be appropriate for acute respiratory failure. When oxygen is given through a nasal cannula at a rate of 1–2 litres/minute the inspiratory oxygen concentration is usually low, but it varies with ventilation and can be high if the patient is underventilating.

Arrangements for supplying oxygen

The following oxygen services may be ordered in England and Wales:

- emergency oxygen;
- short-burst (intermittent) oxygen therapy;
- long-term oxygen therapy;
- ambulatory oxygen.

The type of oxygen service (or combination of services) should be ordered on a Home Oxygen Order Form (HOOF); the amount of oxygen required (hours per day) and flow rate should be specified. The clinician will determine the appropriate equipment to be provided. Special needs or preferences should be specified on the HOOF.

The clinician should obtain the patient or carers consent, to pass on the patient's details to the supplier, the fire brigade, and other relevant organisations. The supplier will contact the patient to make arrangements for delivery, installation, and maintenance of the equipment. The supplier will also train the patient or carer to use the equipment.

The clinician should send the HOOF to the supplier who will continue to provide the service until a revised HOOF is received, or until notified that the patient no longer requires the home oxygen service.

- East of England, North East: BOC Medical: Tel: 0800 136 603 Fax: 0800 169 9989
- South West: Air Liquide: Tel: 0808 202 2229 Fax: 0191 497 4340
- London, East Midlands, North West: Air Liquide: Tel: 0500 823 773 Fax: 0800 781 4610
- Yorkshire and Humberside, West Midlands, Wales: Air Products: Tel: 0800 373 580 Fax: 0800 214 709
- South East Coast, South Central: Dolby Vivisol: Tel: 08443 814 402 Fax: 0800 781 4610

In **Scotland** refer the patient for assessment by a respiratory consultant. If the need for a concentrator is confirmed the consultant will arrange for the provision of a concentrator through the Common Services Agency. Prescribers should complete a Scottish Home Oxygen Order Form (SHOOF) and email it to Health Facilities Scotland. Health Facilities Scotland will then liaise with their contractor to arrange the supply of oxygen. Further information can be obtained at: www.dolbyvivisol.com/services/healthcare-professionals/.

In **Northern Ireland** oxygen concentrators and cylinders should be prescribed on form HS21; oxygen concentrators are supplied by a local contractor. Prescriptions for oxygen cylinders and accessories can be dispensed by pharmacists contracted to provide domiciliary oxygen services.

Croup

21-Oct-2020

Management

EvGr Mild croup is largely self-limiting, but treatment with a single dose of a corticosteroid (e.g. dexamethasone p. 714) by mouth may be of benefit.

Moderate to severe croup (or mild croup that might cause complications such as in those with chronic lung disease, immunodeficiency, impending respiratory failure, or in children aged under 3 months) calls for hospital admission; a single dose of a corticosteroid (e.g. dexamethasone or prednisolone p. 718 by mouth) should be administered while awaiting hospital admission. If the child is too unwell to receive oral medication, dexamethasone (by intramuscular injection) or budesonide p. 275 (by nebulisation) are suitable alternatives while awaiting hospital admission.

For severe croup not effectively controlled with corticosteroid treatment, nebulised adrenaline/epinephrine solution 1 in 1000 (1 mg/mL) p. 238 should be given with close clinical monitoring; ⟨A⟩ the clinical effects of nebulised adrenaline/epinephrine last at least 1 hour, but usually subside 2 hours after administration. EvGr The child needs to be monitored carefully for recurrence of severe respiratory distress. ⟨A⟩

> **Other drugs used for Airways disease, obstructive**
> Dupilumab, p. 1301

ANTIMUSCARINICS

Antimuscarinics (inhaled)

09-Feb-2016

- CAUTIONS Bladder outflow obstruction · paradoxical bronchospasm · prostatic hyperplasia · susceptibility to angle-closure glaucoma

  CAUTIONS, FURTHER INFORMATION
- ▸ Elderly Prescription potentially inappropriate (STOPP criteria) with a history of narrow-angle glaucoma (may exacerbate glaucoma) or bladder outflow obstruction (may cause urinary retention). See also Prescribing in the elderly p. 33.
- SIDE-EFFECTS
- ▸ **Common or very common** Arrhythmias · constipation · cough · dizziness · dry mouth · headache · nausea
- ▸ **Uncommon** Dysphonia · glaucoma · palpitations · skin reactions · stomatitis · urinary disorders · vision blurred

▰ **above**

▌Aclidinium bromide

17-Mar-2020

- ● INDICATIONS AND DOSE

Maintenance treatment of chronic obstructive pulmonary disease
- ▸ BY INHALATION OF POWDER
- ▸ Adult: 375 micrograms twice daily

  DOSE EQUIVALENCE AND CONVERSION
- ▸ Each 375 microgram inhalation of aclidinium bromide delivers 322 micrograms of aclidinium.

- CAUTIONS Arrhythmia (when newly diagnosed within last 3 months) · heart failure (hospitalisation with moderate or severe heart failure within last 12 months) · myocardial infarction within last 6 months · unstable angina
- INTERACTIONS → Appendix 1: aclidinium
- SIDE-EFFECTS
- ▸ **Common or very common** Diarrhoea · nasopharyngitis
- ▸ **Uncommon** Angioedema
- ▸ **Rare or very rare** Hypersensitivity
- PREGNANCY Manufacturer advises use only if potential benefit outweighs risk.
- BREAST FEEDING Manufacturer advises only use if potential benefits outweigh risks.
- PATIENT AND CARER ADVICE Patients or carers should be given advice on appropriate inhaler technique.

● MEDICINAL FORMS There can be variation in the licensing of different medicines containing the same drug.
Inhalation powder
▸ Eklira (AstraZeneca UK Ltd) ▼
 Aclidinium bromide 375 microgram per 1 dose Eklira 322micrograms/dose Genuair | 60 dose [PoM] £32.50 DT = £32.50

Aclidinium bromide with formoterol
16-Mar-2020

The properties listed below are those particular to the combination only. For the properties of the components please consider, aclidinium bromide p. 261, formoterol fumarate p. 266.

● **INDICATIONS AND DOSE**
Maintenance treatment of chronic obstructive pulmonary disease
▸ BY INHALATION OF POWDER
▸ Adult: 1 inhalation twice daily

● CAUTIONS Convulsive disorders · phaeochromocytoma
● INTERACTIONS → Appendix 1: aclidinium · beta₂ agonists
● PATIENT AND CARER ADVICE Patients or carers should be given advice on appropriate inhaler technique.

● MEDICINAL FORMS There can be variation in the licensing of different medicines containing the same drug.
Inhalation powder
▸ Duaklir (AstraZeneca UK Ltd) ▼
 Formoterol fumarate dihydrate 11.8 microgram per 1 dose, Aclidinium bromide 396 microgram per 1 dose Duaklir 340micrograms/dose / 12micrograms/dose Genuair | 60 dose [PoM] £32.50 DT = £32.50

⚑ 261
Glycopyrronium bromide
06-Nov-2020

(Glycopyrrolate)

● **INDICATIONS AND DOSE**
Maintenance treatment of chronic obstructive pulmonary disease
▸ BY INHALATION OF POWDER
▸ Adult: 1 capsule once daily, each capsule delivers 55 micrograms of glycopyrronium bromide (equivalent to 44 micrograms of glycopyrronium)

● CAUTIONS Arrhythmia (excluding chronic stable atrial fibrillation) · history of myocardial infarction · history of QT-interval prolongation · left ventricular failure · unstable ischaemic heart disease
● INTERACTIONS → Appendix 1: glycopyrronium
● SIDE-EFFECTS
▸ **Common or very common** Increased risk of infection · insomnia · pain
▸ **Uncommon** Asthenia · cystitis · dental caries · dyspepsia · epistaxis · hyperglycaemia · hypersensitivity · numbness · respiratory disorders · throat irritation
● PREGNANCY Manufacturer advises use only if potential benefit outweighs risk.
● BREAST FEEDING Manufacturer advises use only if potential benefit outweighs risk.
● RENAL IMPAIRMENT Manufacturer advises use only if potential benefit outweighs risk if eGFR less than 30 mL/minute/1.73 m².
● PATIENT AND CARER ADVICE Patients or carers should be given advice on appropriate inhaler technique.

● MEDICINAL FORMS There can be variation in the licensing of different medicines containing the same drug.
Inhalation powder
▸ Seebri Breezhaler (Novartis Pharmaceuticals UK Ltd)
 Glycopyrronium bromide 55 microgram Seebri Breezhaler 44microgram inhalation powder capsules with device | 10 capsule [PoM] £9.17 | 30 capsule [PoM] £27.50 DT = £27.50

Combinations available: *Beclometasone with formoterol and glycopyrronium,* p. 275 · *Mometasone furoate with glycopyrronium bromide and indacaterol,* p. 282

Glycopyrronium with indacaterol
16-Mar-2020

The properties listed below are those particular to the combination only. For the properties of the components please consider, glycopyrronium bromide above, indacaterol p. 267.

● **INDICATIONS AND DOSE**
Maintenance treatment of chronic obstructive pulmonary disease
▸ BY INHALATION OF POWDER
▸ Adult: 1 inhalation daily

● CAUTIONS Convulsive disorders
● INTERACTIONS → Appendix 1: beta₂ agonists · glycopyrronium
● PATIENT AND CARER ADVICE Patients or carers should be given advice on appropriate inhaler technique and reminded that the capsules are not for oral administration.

● MEDICINAL FORMS There can be variation in the licensing of different medicines containing the same drug.
Inhalation powder
▸ Ultibro Breezhaler (Novartis Pharmaceuticals UK Ltd)
 Glycopyrronium bromide 54 microgram per 1 dose, Indacaterol (as Indacaterol maleate) 85 microgram per 1 dose Ultibro Breezhaler 85microgram/43microgram inhalation powder capsules with device | 10 capsule [PoM] £10.83 | 30 capsule [PoM] £32.50 DT = £32.50

⚑ 261
Ipratropium bromide
20-Jul-2020

● **INDICATIONS AND DOSE**
Reversible airways obstruction
▸ BY INHALATION OF AEROSOL
▸ Child 1 month–5 years: 20 micrograms 3 times a day
▸ Child 6–11 years: 20–40 micrograms 3 times a day
▸ Child 12–17 years: 20–40 micrograms 3–4 times a day
Reversible airways obstruction, particularly in chronic obstructive pulmonary disease
▸ BY INHALATION OF AEROSOL
▸ Adult: 20–40 micrograms 3–4 times a day
▸ BY INHALATION OF NEBULISED SOLUTION
▸ Adult: 250–500 micrograms 3–4 times a day
Acute bronchospasm
▸ BY INHALATION OF NEBULISED SOLUTION
▸ Child 1 month–5 years: 125–250 micrograms as required; maximum 1 mg per day
▸ Child 6–11 years: 250 micrograms as required; maximum 1 mg per day
▸ Child 12–17 years: 500 micrograms as required, doses higher than max. can be given under medical supervision; maximum 2 mg per day
▸ Adult: 500 micrograms as required, doses higher than max. can be given under medical supervision; maximum 2 mg per day

Severe or life-threatening acute asthma
▶ BY INHALATION OF NEBULISED SOLUTION
▶ Child 1 month–11 years: 250 micrograms every 20–30 minutes for the first 2 hours, then 250 micrograms every 4–6 hours as required
▶ Child 12–17 years: 500 micrograms every 4–6 hours as required
▶ Adult: 500 micrograms every 4–6 hours as required

PHARMACOKINETICS
▶ The maximal effect of inhaled ipratropium occurs 30–60 minutes after use; its duration of action is 3 to 6 hours and bronchodilation can usually be maintained with treatment 3 times a day.

● UNLICENSED USE ⟨EvGr⟩ The dose of ipratropium for severe or life-threatening acute asthma is unlicensed. ⟨A⟩ *Inhalvent*® not licensed for use in children under 6 years.

> IMPORTANT SAFETY INFORMATION
> MHRA/CHM ADVICE: PRESSURISED METERED DOSE INHALERS (PMDI): RISK OF AIRWAY OBSTRUCTION FROM ASPIRATION OF LOOSE OBJECTS (JULY 2018)
> See Respiratory system, drug delivery p. 251.

● CAUTIONS Avoid spraying near eyes · cystic fibrosis
CAUTIONS, FURTHER INFORMATION
▶ Glaucoma *Acute angle-closure glaucoma* has been reported with nebulised ipratropium, particularly when given with nebulised salbutamol (and possibly other beta₂ agonists); care needed to protect the patient's eyes from nebulised drug or from drug powder.

● INTERACTIONS → Appendix 1: ipratropium

● SIDE-EFFECTS
▶ **Common or very common** Gastrointestinal motility disorder · throat complaints
▶ **Uncommon** Corneal oedema · diarrhoea · eye disorders · eye pain · respiratory disorders · vision disorders · vomiting

● ALLERGY AND CROSS-SENSITIVITY Contra-indicated in patients with hypersensitivity to atropine or its derivatives.

● PREGNANCY Manufacturer advises only use if potential benefit outweighs the risk.

● BREAST FEEDING No information available—manufacturer advises only use if potential benefit outweighs risk.

● DIRECTIONS FOR ADMINISTRATION Manufacturer advises if dilution of ipratropium bromide nebuliser solution is necessary use only sterile sodium chloride 0.9%.

● PATIENT AND CARER ADVICE Patients or carers should be counselled on appropriate administration technique and warned against accidental contact with the eye (due to risk of ocular complications).
Driving and skilled tasks Manufacturer advises patients and carers should be counselled on the effects on driving and performance of skilled tasks—increased risk of dizziness and vision disorders.

● MEDICINAL FORMS There can be variation in the licensing of different medicines containing the same drug.
Nebuliser liquid
▶ Ipratropium bromide (Non-proprietary)
Ipratropium bromide 250 microgram per 1 ml Ipratropium bromide 500micrograms/2ml nebuliser liquid unit dose vials | 20 unit dose [PoM] £3.69 DT = £3.21
Ipratropium bromide 250micrograms/1ml nebuliser liquid unit dose vials | 20 unit dose [PoM] £5.66 DT = £5.66
Ipratropium 250micrograms/1ml nebuliser liquid Steri-Neb unit dose vials | 20 unit dose [PoM] £6.99 DT = £5.66
Ipratropium 500micrograms/2ml nebuliser liquid Steri-Neb unit dose vials | 20 unit dose [PoM] £15.99 DT = £3.21
▶ Atrovent UDV (Boehringer Ingelheim Ltd)
Ipratropium bromide 250 microgram per 1 ml Atrovent 500micrograms/2ml nebuliser liquid UDVs | 20 unit dose [PoM] £4.87 DT = £3.21

Atrovent 250micrograms/1ml nebuliser liquid UDVs | 20 unit dose [PoM] £4.14 DT = £5.66
Pressurised inhalation
▶ Atrovent (Boehringer Ingelheim Ltd)
Ipratropium bromide 20 microgram per 1 dose Atrovent 20micrograms/dose inhaler CFC free | 200 dose [PoM] £5.56 DT = £5.56
▶ Inhalvent (Alissa Healthcare Research Ltd)
Ipratropium bromide 20 microgram per 1 dose Inhalvent 20micrograms/dose inhaler | 200 dose [PoM] £5.56 DT = £5.56

Ipratropium with salbutamol   16-Mar-2020

The properties listed below are those particular to the combination only. For the properties of the components please consider, ipratropium bromide p. 262, salbutamol p. 269.

● INDICATIONS AND DOSE
Bronchospasm in chronic obstructive pulmonary disease
▶ BY INHALATION OF NEBULISED SOLUTION
▶ Adult: 0.5/2.5 mg 3–4 times a day

● INTERACTIONS → Appendix 1: beta₂ agonists · ipratropium

● PRESCRIBING AND DISPENSING INFORMATION A mixture of ipratropium bromide and salbutamol (as sulfate); the proportions are expressed in the form x/y where x and y are the strengths in milligrams of ipratropium and salbutamol respectively.

● MEDICINAL FORMS There can be variation in the licensing of different medicines containing the same drug.
Nebuliser liquid
▶ Combivent (Boehringer Ingelheim Ltd)
Ipratropium bromide 200 microgram per 1 ml, Salbutamol (as Salbutamol sulfate) 1 mg per 1 ml Combivent nebuliser liquid 2.5ml UDVs | 60 unit dose [PoM] £24.10 DT = £24.10
▶ Ipramol (Teva UK Ltd)
Ipratropium bromide 200 microgram per 1 ml, Salbutamol (as Salbutamol sulfate) 1 mg per 1 ml Ipramol nebuliser solution 2.5ml Steri-Neb unit dose vials | 60 unit dose [PoM] £23.83 DT = £24.10

⧫ 261

Tiotropium   23-Oct-2020

● INDICATIONS AND DOSE
Maintenance treatment of chronic obstructive pulmonary disease
▶ BY INHALATION OF POWDER
▶ Adult: 1 capsule once daily

DOSE EQUIVALENCE AND CONVERSION
▶ For *Spiriva*® inhalation powder, 1 capsule contains a metered dose of 18 micrograms tiotropium; for *Braltus*® inhalation powder, 1 capsule contains a metered dose of 13 micrograms tiotropium.
▶ The delivered dose of *Spiriva*® and *Braltus*® inhalation powder products are the same (10 micrograms); no dose adjustment is necessary when switching between brands.

SPIRIVA RESPIMAT®
Maintenance treatment of chronic obstructive pulmonary disease | Severe asthma [add-on to inhaled corticosteroid (at least 800 micrograms budesonide daily or equivalent) and at least 1 controller in patients who have suffered one or more severe exacerbations in the last year]
▶ BY INHALATION
▶ Adult: 5 micrograms once daily   continued →

3

Respiratory system

Severe asthma [add-on to inhaled corticosteroid (over 400 micrograms budesonide daily or equivalent) and 1 controller, or inhaled corticosteroid (200–400 micrograms budesonide daily or equivalent) and 2 controllers, in patients who have suffered one or more severe exacerbations in the last year]
▸ BY INHALATION
▸ Child 6–11 years: 5 micrograms once daily

Severe asthma [add-on to inhaled corticosteroid (over 800 micrograms budesonide daily or equivalent) and 1 controller, or inhaled corticosteroid (400–800 micrograms budesonide daily or equivalent) and 2 controllers, in patients who have suffered one or more severe exacerbations in the last year]
▸ BY INHALATION
▸ Child 12–17 years: 5 micrograms once daily

DOSE EQUIVALENCE AND CONVERSION
▸ For *Spiriva Respimat*®: 2 puffs of inhalation solution is equivalent to 5 micrograms tiotropium.

IMPORTANT SAFETY INFORMATION
MHRA/CHM ADVICE: *BRALTUS*® (TIOTROPIUM): RISK OF INHALATION OF CAPSULE IF PLACED IN THE MOUTHPIECE OF THE INHALER (MAY 2018)
The MHRA have received reports of patients who have inhaled a *Braltus*® capsule from the mouthpiece into the back of the throat, resulting in coughing and risking aspiration or airway obstruction. Patients should be trained in the correct use of their inhaler and told to store capsules in the screw-top bottle provided (never in the inhaler) and to always check the mouthpiece is clear before inhaling. Pharmacists dispensing *Braltus*® capsules should remind patients always to read the instructions for use in the package leaflet and that they must never place a capsule directly into the mouthpiece.

MHRA/CHM ADVICE: PRESSURISED METERED DOSE INHALERS (PMDI): RISK OF AIRWAY OBSTRUCTION FROM ASPIRATION OF LOOSE OBJECTS (JULY 2018)
See Respiratory system, drug delivery p. 251.

● CAUTIONS Arrhythmia (unstable, life-threatening or requiring intervention in the previous 12 months) · heart failure (hospitalisation for moderate to severe heart failure in the previous 12 months) · myocardial infarction in the previous 6 months
● INTERACTIONS → Appendix 1: tiotropium
● SIDE-EFFECTS
▸ **Uncommon** Gastrointestinal disorders · increased risk of infection · taste altered
▸ **Rare or very rare** Bronchospasm · dysphagia · epistaxis · insomnia · oral disorders
▸ **Frequency not known** Dehydration · joint swelling · skin ulcer
● PREGNANCY Manufacturer advises avoid—limited data available.
● BREAST FEEDING Manufacturer advises avoid—no information available.
● RENAL IMPAIRMENT Manufacturer advises use only if potential benefit outweighs risk if creatinine clearance less than or equal to 50 mL/minute—plasma-tiotropium concentration raised.
● PATIENT AND CARER ADVICE Patients or carers should be advised that the *Respimat*® inhaler device is re-usable and can be used with a total of 6 cartridges before it needs to be replaced. Refer patients or carers to the Instructions for Use for information on how and when to replace the cartridge.
▸ In adults Patients or carers should be given advice on appropriate inhaler technique and reminded that the powder inhalation capsules are not for oral

administration; for *Braltus*®, see also *Important safety Information*.
▸ In children Patients or carers should be given advice on appropriate inhaler technique.
● NATIONAL FUNDING/ACCESS DECISIONS
For full details see funding body website
Scottish Medicines Consortium (SMC) decisions
▸ Tiotropium (*Spiriva Respimat*®) as add-on maintenance bronchodilator treatment in adults with asthma who are currently treated with the maintenance combination of inhaled corticosteroids (at least 800 micrograms budesonide/day or equivalent) and long-acting beta$_2$ agonists and who experienced one or more severe exacerbations in the previous year (August 2015) SMC No. 1028/15 Recommended
▸ Tiotropium (*Spiriva Respimat*®) as a maintenance bronchodilator treatment to relieve symptoms of patients with chronic obstructive pulmonary disease (COPD) (December 2017) SMC No. 411/07 Recommended
▸ Tiotropium (*Spiriva Respimat*®) as add-on maintenance bronchodilator treatment in patients aged 6 years and older with severe asthma who experienced one or more severe asthma exacerbations in the preceding year (January 2019) SMC No. SMC2118 Recommended
All Wales Medicines Strategy Group (AWMSG) decisions
▸ Tiotropium (*Spiriva Respimat*®) as add-on maintenance bronchodilator treatment in patients aged 6 years and older with severe asthma who experienced one or more severe asthma exacerbations in the preceding year (December 2018) AWMSG No. 1882 Recommended

● MEDICINAL FORMS There can be variation in the licensing of different medicines containing the same drug.
Inhalation powder
▸ Braltus (Teva UK Ltd)
Tiotropium (as Tiotropium bromide) 10 microgram Braltus 10microgram inhalation powder capsules with Zonda inhaler | 30 capsule [PoM] £25.80 DT = £25.80
▸ Spiriva (Boehringer Ingelheim Ltd)
Tiotropium (as Tiotropium bromide) 18 microgram Spiriva 18microgram inhalation powder capsules with HandiHaler | 30 capsule [PoM] £34.87 DT = £34.87
Spiriva 18microgram inhalation powder capsules | 30 capsule [PoM] £33.50 DT = £33.50 | 60 capsule [PoM] £67.00
Inhalation solution
▸ Spiriva Respimat (Boehringer Ingelheim Ltd)
Tiotropium (as Tiotropium bromide) 2.5 microgram per 1 dose Spiriva Respimat 2.5micrograms/dose inhalation solution cartridge with device | 60 dose [PoM] £23.00 DT = £23.00
Spiriva Respimat 2.5micrograms/dose inhalation solution refill cartridge | 60 dose [PoM] £23.00 DT = £23.00

Tiotropium with olodaterol   03-Sep-2020

The properties listed below are those particular to the combination only. For the properties of the components please consider, tiotropium p. 263, olodaterol p. 268.

● INDICATIONS AND DOSE
Maintenance treatment of chronic obstructive pulmonary disease
▸ BY INHALATION
▸ Adult: 2 puffs once daily
DOSE EQUIVALENCE AND CONVERSION
▸ 2 puffs of inhalation solution is equivalent to 5 micrograms tiotropium and 5 micrograms olodaterol.

● INTERACTIONS → Appendix 1: beta$_2$ agonists · tiotropium
● PATIENT AND CARER ADVICE Patient or carers should be given advice on appropriate inhaler technique. Patients or carers should be advised that the *Respimat*® inhaler device is re-usable and can be used with a total of 6 cartridges before it needs to be replaced. Refer patients or carers to

the Instructions for Use for information on how and when to replace the cartridge.

- MEDICINAL FORMS There can be variation in the licensing of different medicines containing the same drug.

Inhalation solution

- Spiolto Respimat (Boehringer Ingelheim Ltd)
  Olodaterol (as Olodaterol hydrochloride) 2.5 microgram per 1 dose, Tiotropium (as Tiotropium bromide) 2.5 microgram per 1 dose Spiolto Respimat 2.5micrograms/dose / 2.5micrograms/dose inhalation solution cartridge with device | 60 dose [PoM] £32.50 DT = £32.50
  Spiolto Respimat 2.5micrograms/dose / 2.5micrograms/dose inhalation solution refill cartridge | 60 dose [PoM] £32.50 DT = £32.50
- Yanimo Respimat (Boehringer Ingelheim Ltd)
  Yanimo Respimat 2.5micrograms/dose / 2.5micrograms/dose inhalation solution cartridge with device | 60 dose [PoM] £32.50 DT = £32.50

⧼ 261

Umeclidinium
02-Sep-2020

- **INDICATIONS AND DOSE**
Maintenance treatment of chronic obstructive pulmonary disease
- BY INHALATION OF POWDER
- Adult: 55 micrograms once daily
DOSE EQUIVALENCE AND CONVERSION
- Each 65 microgram inhalation of umeclidinium bromide delivers 55 micrograms of umeclidinium.

- CAUTIONS Cardiac disorders (particularly cardiac rhythm disorders)
- INTERACTIONS → Appendix 1: umeclidinium
- SIDE-EFFECTS
- **Uncommon** Taste altered
- **Rare or very rare** Eye pain
- PREGNANCY Manufacturer advises use only if potential benefit outweighs risk.
- BREAST FEEDING Manufacturer advises avoid—no information available.
- HEPATIC IMPAIRMENT Manufacturer advises caution in severe impairment (no information available).
- PATIENT AND CARER ADVICE Patient or carers should be given advice on appropriate inhaler technique.

- MEDICINAL FORMS There can be variation in the licensing of different medicines containing the same drug.

Inhalation powder
- Incruse Ellipta (GlaxoSmithKline UK Ltd) ▼
  Umeclidinium bromide 65 microgram per 1 dose Incruse Ellipta 55micrograms/dose dry powder inhaler | 30 dose [PoM] £27.50 DT = £27.50

Combinations available: *Fluticasone with umeclidinium and vilanterol,* p. 281

Umeclidinium with vilanterol
02-Sep-2020

The properties listed below are those particular to the combination only. For the properties of the components please consider, umeclidinium above.

- **INDICATIONS AND DOSE**
Maintenance treatment of chronic obstructive pulmonary disease
- BY INHALATION OF POWDER
- Adult: 1 inhalation once daily

- CAUTIONS Arrhythmias · cardiovascular disease · diabetes (risk of hyperglycaemia and ketoacidosis) · hypertension · hyperthyroidism · hypokalaemia · susceptibility to QT-interval prolongation

CAUTIONS, FURTHER INFORMATION
- Hypokalaemia Potentially serious hypokalaemia may result from beta$_2$ agonist therapy. Particular caution is required in severe asthma, because this effect may be potentiated by concomitant treatment with theophylline and its derivatives, corticosteroids, diuretics, and by hypoxia.
- INTERACTIONS → Appendix 1: beta$_2$ agonists · umeclidinium
- SIDE-EFFECTS
- **Common or very common** Constipation · dry mouth · headache · oropharyngeal pain · sinusitis
- **Uncommon** Arrhythmias · dysphonia · palpitations · taste altered · tremor
- **Rare or very rare** Bronchospasm paradoxical · glaucoma · urinary disorders · vision blurred
- **Frequency not known** Dizziness
- MONITORING REQUIREMENTS
- In severe asthma, plasma-potassium concentration should be monitored (risk of hypokalaemia).
- In patients with diabetes, monitor blood glucose (risk of hyperglycaemia and ketoacidosis, especially when beta$_2$ agonist given intravenously).
- PATIENT AND CARER ADVICE Patient or carers should be given advice on appropriate inhaler technique.

- MEDICINAL FORMS There can be variation in the licensing of different medicines containing the same drug.

Inhalation powder
- Umeclidinium with vilanterol (non-proprietary) ▼
  Vilanterol (as Vilanterol trifenatate) 22 microgram per 1 dose, Umeclidinium bromide 65 microgram per 1 dose Umeclidinium bromide 65micrograms/dose / Vilanterol 22micrograms/dose dry powder inhaler | 30 dose [PoM] 🅢 DT = £32.50
- Anoro Ellipta (GlaxoSmithKline UK Ltd) ▼
  Vilanterol (as Vilanterol trifenatate) 22 microgram per 1 dose, Umeclidinium bromide 65 microgram per 1 dose Anoro Ellipta 55micrograms/dose / 22micrograms/dose dry powder inhaler | 30 dose [PoM] £32.50 DT = £32.50

BETA$_2$-ADRENOCEPTOR AGONISTS, SELECTIVE

Beta$_2$ adrenoceptor agonists, selective
12-Feb-2016

- CAUTIONS Arrhythmias · cardiovascular disease · diabetes (risk of hyperglycaemia and ketoacidosis, especially with intravenous use) · hypertension · hyperthyroidism · hypokalaemia · susceptibility to QT-interval prolongation

CAUTIONS, FURTHER INFORMATION
- Hypokalaemia Potentially serious hypokalaemia may result from beta$_2$ agonist therapy. Particular caution is required in severe asthma, because this effect may be potentiated by concomitant treatment with theophylline and its derivatives, corticosteroids, diuretics, and by hypoxia.

- SIDE-EFFECTS
- **Common or very common** Arrhythmias · headache · hypokalaemia (with high doses) · muscle spasms · nasopharyngitis · nausea · palpitations · rash · tremor
- **Uncommon** Hyperglycaemia
- **Rare or very rare** Bronchospasm paradoxical (sometimes severe)
- PREGNANCY Women planning to become pregnant should be counselled about the importance of taking their asthma medication regularly to maintain good control.
- MONITORING REQUIREMENTS
- In severe asthma, plasma-potassium concentration should be monitored (risk of hypokalaemia).
- In patients with diabetes, monitor blood glucose (risk of hyperglycaemia and ketoacidosis, especially when beta$_2$ agonist given intravenously).

● PATIENT AND CARER ADVICE
▸ When used by inhalation The **dose**, the frequency, and the maximum number of inhalations in 24 hours of the beta$_2$ agonist should be **stated explicitly** to the patient or their carer. The patient or their carer should be advised to seek medical advice when the prescribed dose of beta$_2$ agonist fails to provide the usual degree of symptomatic relief because this usually indicates a worsening of the asthma and the patient may require a prophylactic drug. Patients or their carers should be advised to follow manufacturers' instructions on the care and cleansing of inhaler devices.

BETA$_2$-ADRENOCEPTOR AGONISTS, SELECTIVE > LONG-ACTING

⌐ 265

Bambuterol hydrochloride

05-Jun-2018

● DRUG ACTION Bambuterol is a pro-drug of terbutaline.

● INDICATIONS AND DOSE

Asthma (patients who have previously tolerated beta$_2$-agonists) | Other conditions associated with reversible airways obstruction (patients who have previously tolerated beta$_2$-agonists)
▸ BY MOUTH
▸ Adult: 20 mg once daily, dose to be taken at bedtime

Asthma (patients who have not previously tolerated beta$_2$-agonists) | Other conditions associated with reversible airways obstruction (patients who have not previously tolerated beta$_2$-agonists)
▸ BY MOUTH
▸ Adult: Initially 10 mg once daily for 1–2 weeks, then increased if necessary to 20 mg once daily, dose to be taken at bedtime

● INTERACTIONS → Appendix 1: beta$_2$ agonists

● SIDE-EFFECTS
▸ **Common or very common** Anxiety · behaviour abnormal · muscle cramps · sleep disorder
▸ **Frequency not known** Akathisia · angioedema · bronchospasm · circulatory collapse · dizziness · hypersensitivity · hypotension · myocardial ischaemia · urticaria

● PREGNANCY Manufacturer advises avoid—no information available.

● BREAST FEEDING Manufacturer advises avoid—no information available.

● HEPATIC IMPAIRMENT Manufacturer advises avoid in severe impairment or cirrhosis (risk of unpredictable conversion to terbutaline; direct terbutaline use preferred).

● RENAL IMPAIRMENT
Dose adjustments Reduce initial dose by half if eGFR less than 50 mL/minute/1.73 m^2.

● MEDICINAL FORMS There can be variation in the licensing of different medicines containing the same drug.
Tablet
▸ Bambec (AstraZeneca UK Ltd)
Bambuterol hydrochloride 10 mg Bambec 10mg tablets | 30 tablet [PoM] £30.99 DT = £30.99

⌐ 265

Formoterol fumarate

25-Nov-2019

(Eformoterol fumarate)

● INDICATIONS AND DOSE

Reversible airways obstruction in patients requiring long-term regular bronchodilator therapy | Nocturnal asthma in patients requiring long-term regular bronchodilator therapy | Prophylaxis of exercise-induced bronchospasm in patients requiring long-term regular bronchodilator therapy | Chronic asthma in patients who regularly use an inhaled corticosteroid
▸ BY INHALATION OF POWDER
▸ Child 6–11 years: 12 micrograms twice daily, a daily dose of 24 micrograms of formoterol should be sufficient for the majority of children, particularly for younger age-groups; higher doses should be used rarely, and only when control is not maintained on the lower dose
▸ Child 12–17 years: 12 micrograms twice daily, dose may be increased in more severe airway obstruction; increased to 24 micrograms twice daily, a daily dose of 24 micrograms of formoterol should be sufficient for the majority of children, particularly for younger age-groups; higher doses should be used rarely, and only when control is not maintained on the lower dose
▸ Adult: 12 micrograms twice daily, dose may be increased in more severe airway obstruction; increased to 24 micrograms twice daily
▸ BY INHALATION OF AEROSOL
▸ Child 12–17 years: 12 micrograms twice daily, dose may be increased in more severe airway obstruction; increased to 24 micrograms twice daily, a daily dose of 24 micrograms of formoterol should be sufficient for the majority of children, particularly for younger age-groups; higher doses should be used rarely, and only when control is not maintained on the lower dose
▸ Adult: 12 micrograms twice daily, dose may be increased in more severe airway obstruction; increased to 24 micrograms twice daily

Chronic obstructive pulmonary disease
▸ BY INHALATION OF POWDER
▸ Adult: 12 micrograms twice daily
▸ BY INHALATION OF AEROSOL
▸ Adult: 12 micrograms twice daily (max. per dose 24 micrograms), for symptom relief additional doses may be taken to maximum daily dose; maximum 48 micrograms per day

PHARMACOKINETICS
▸ At recommended inhaled doses, the duration of action of formoterol is about 12 hours.

OXIS ®

Chronic asthma
▸ BY INHALATION OF POWDER
▸ Child 6–17 years: 6–12 micrograms 1–2 times a day (max. per dose 12 micrograms), occasionally doses up to the maximum daily may be needed, reassess treatment if additional doses required on more than 2 days a week; maximum 48 micrograms per day
▸ Adult: 6–12 micrograms 1–2 times a day, increased if necessary up to 24 micrograms twice daily (max. per dose 36 micrograms), occasionally doses up to the maximum daily may be needed, reassess treatment if additional doses required on more than 2 days a week; maximum 72 micrograms per day

Relief of bronchospasm
▸ BY INHALATION OF POWDER
▸ Child 6–17 years: 6–12 micrograms
▸ Adult: 6–12 micrograms

Prophylaxis of exercise-induced bronchospasm
▸ BY INHALATION OF POWDER
▸ Child 6-17 years: 6–12 micrograms, dose to be taken before exercise
▸ Adult: 12 micrograms, dose to be taken before exercise

Chronic obstructive pulmonary disease
▸ BY INHALATION OF POWDER
▸ Adult: 12 micrograms 1–2 times a day (max. per dose 24 micrograms), for symptom relief additional doses up to maximum daily dose can be taken; maximum 48 micrograms per day

---

IMPORTANT SAFETY INFORMATION

CHM ADVICE

To ensure safe use, the CHM has advised that for the management of chronic asthma, long-acting beta$_2$ agonist (formoterol) should:
- be added only if regular use of standard-dose inhaled corticosteroids has failed to control asthma adequately;
- not be initiated in patients with rapidly deteriorating asthma;
- be introduced at a low dose and the effect properly monitored before considering dose increase;
- be discontinued in the absence of benefit;
- not be used for the relief of exercise-induced asthma symptoms unless regular inhaled corticosteroids are also used;
- be reviewed as clinically appropriate: stepping down therapy should be considered when good long-term asthma control has been achieved.

MHRA/CHM ADVICE: PRESSURISED METERED DOSE INHALERS (PMDI): RISK OF AIRWAY OBSTRUCTION FROM ASPIRATION OF LOOSE OBJECTS (JULY 2018)
See Respiratory system, drug delivery p. 251.

● CAUTIONS High doses of beta$_2$ agonists can be dangerous in some children
● INTERACTIONS → Appendix 1: beta$_2$ agonists
● SIDE-EFFECTS
▸ **Common or very common** Dizziness · muscle cramps
▸ **Uncommon** Angina pectoris · bronchospasm · skin reactions · sleep disorder · taste altered
▸ **Rare or very rare** Anxiety · QT interval prolongation
● PREGNANCY Inhaled drugs for asthma can be taken as normal during pregnancy.
● BREAST FEEDING Inhaled drugs for asthma can be taken as normal during breast-feeding.
● PATIENT AND CARER ADVICE Advise patients not to exceed prescribed dose, and to follow manufacturer's directions; if a previously effective dose of inhaled formoterol fails to provide adequate relief, a doctor's advice should be obtained as soon as possible. Patients should be advised to report any deterioration in symptoms following initiation of treatment with a long-acting beta$_2$ agonist. Patient or carer should be given advice on how to administer formoterol fumarate inhalers.

● MEDICINAL FORMS There can be variation in the licensing of different medicines containing the same drug.
Inhalation powder
▸ Easyhaler (formoterol) (Orion Pharma (UK) Ltd)
Formoterol fumarate dihydrate 12 microgram per 1 dose Formoterol Easyhaler 12micrograms/dose dry powder inhaler | 120 dose [PoM] £23.75 DT = £23.75
▸ Foradil (Novartis Pharmaceuticals UK Ltd)
Formoterol fumarate dihydrate 12 microgram Foradil 12microgram inhalation powder capsules with device | 60 capsule [PoM] £28.06 DT = £28.06

▸ Oxis Turbohaler (AstraZeneca UK Ltd)
Formoterol fumarate dihydrate 6 microgram per 1 dose Oxis 6 Turbohaler | 60 dose [PoM] £24.80 DT = £24.80
Formoterol fumarate dihydrate 12 microgram per 1 dose Oxis 12 Turbohaler | 60 dose [PoM] £24.80 DT = £24.80

Pressurised inhalation
EXCIPIENTS: May contain Alcohol
▸ Atimos Modulite (Chiesi Ltd)
Formoterol fumarate dihydrate 12 microgram per 1 dose Atimos Modulite 12micrograms/dose inhaler | 100 dose [PoM] £30.06 DT = £30.06

Combinations available: *Aclidinium bromide with formoterol,* p. 262 · *Beclometasone with formoterol,* p. 274 · *Beclometasone with formoterol and glycopyrronium,* p. 275 · *Budesonide with formoterol,* p. 276 · *Fluticasone with formoterol,* p. 279

F 265

Indacaterol

● INDICATIONS AND DOSE
Maintenance treatment of chronic obstructive pulmonary disease
▸ BY INHALATION OF POWDER
▸ Adult: 150 micrograms once daily, then increased to 300 micrograms once daily

● CAUTIONS Convulsive disorders
● INTERACTIONS → Appendix 1: beta$_2$ agonists
● SIDE-EFFECTS
▸ **Common or very common** Chest pain · cough · dizziness · increased risk of infection · oropharyngeal pain · peripheral oedema · rhinorrhoea · throat irritation
▸ **Uncommon** Diabetes mellitus · hypersensitivity · musculoskeletal pain · myalgia · myocardial ischaemia · paraesthesia · pruritus
● PREGNANCY Manufacturer advises use only if potential benefit outweighs risk.
● BREAST FEEDING Manufacturer advises avoid—present in milk in *animal* studies.
● HEPATIC IMPAIRMENT Manufacturer advises caution in severe impairment (no information available).
● PATIENT AND CARER ADVICE Patients or carers should be given advice on how to administer indacaterol inhalation powder.

● MEDICINAL FORMS There can be variation in the licensing of different medicines containing the same drug.
Inhalation powder
▸ Onbrez Breezhaler (Novartis Pharmaceuticals UK Ltd)
Indacaterol (as Indacaterol maleate) 150 microgram Onbrez Breezhaler 150microgram inhalation powder capsules with device | 30 capsule [PoM] £32.19 DT = £32.19
Indacaterol (as Indacaterol maleate) 300 microgram Onbrez Breezhaler 300microgram inhalation powder capsules with device | 30 capsule [PoM] £32.19 DT = £32.19

Combinations available: *Glycopyrronium with indacaterol,* p. 262 · *Indacaterol with mometasone furoate,* p. 282 · *Mometasone furoate with glycopyrronium bromide and indacaterol,* p. 282

3

Respiratory system

3

Respiratory system

⬅ 265

Olodaterol

03-Aug-2020

● **INDICATIONS AND DOSE**

Maintenance treatment of chronic obstructive pulmonary disease
▸ BY INHALATION
▸ **Adult:** 5 micrograms once daily

DOSE EQUIVALENCE AND CONVERSION
▸ 2 puffs is equivalent to 5 micrograms.

IMPORTANT SAFETY INFORMATION
MHRA/CHM ADVICE: PRESSURISED METERED DOSE INHALERS (PMDI): RISK OF AIRWAY OBSTRUCTION FROM ASPIRATION OF LOOSE OBJECTS (JULY 2018)
See Respiratory system, drug delivery p. 251.

● CAUTIONS Aneurysm · convulsive disorders
● INTERACTIONS → Appendix 1: beta₂ agonists
● **SIDE-EFFECTS**
▸ **Uncommon** Dizziness
▸ **Rare or very rare** Arthralgia · hypertension
▸ **Frequency not known** Dry mouth · fatigue · hypotension · insomnia · ischaemic heart disease · malaise · metabolic acidosis · nervousness
● PREGNANCY Manufacturer advises avoid—no information available.
● BREAST FEEDING Manufacturer advises avoid— present in milk in *animal* studies.
● HEPATIC IMPAIRMENT Manufacturer advises caution in severe hepatic impairment (no information available).
● PATIENT AND CARER ADVICE Patients or carers should be given advice on how to administer olodaterol solution for inhalation. Patients or carers should be advised that the *Respimat*® inhaler device is re-usable and can be used with a total of 6 cartridges before it needs to be replaced. Refer patients or carers to the Instructions for Use for information on how and when to replace the cartridge.

● MEDICINAL FORMS There can be variation in the licensing of different medicines containing the same drug.
Inhalation solution
▸ Striverdi Respimat (Boehringer Ingelheim Ltd) ▼
Olodaterol (as Olodaterol hydrochloride) 2.5 microgram per 1 dose Striverdi Respimat 2.5micrograms/dose inhalation solution cartridge with device | 60 dose [PoM] £26.35 DT = £26.35
Striverdi Respimat 2.5micrograms/dose inhalation solution refill cartridge | 60 dose [PoM] £26.35 DT = £26.35

Combinations available: *Tiotropium with olodaterol,* p. 264

⬅ 265

Salmeterol

25-Nov-2019

● **INDICATIONS AND DOSE**

Reversible airways obstruction in patients requiring long-term regular bronchodilator therapy | Nocturnal asthma in patients requiring long-term regular bronchodilator therapy | Prevention of exercise-induced bronchospasm in patients requiring long-term regular bronchodilator therapy | Chronic asthma only in patients who regularly use an inhaled corticosteroid (not for immediate relief of acute asthma)
▸ BY INHALATION OF AEROSOL, OR BY INHALATION OF POWDER
▸ **Child 5–11 years:** 50 micrograms twice daily
▸ **Child 12–17 years:** 50 micrograms twice daily, dose may be increased in more severe airway obstruction; increased to 100 micrograms twice daily
▸ **Adult:** 50 micrograms twice daily, dose may be increased in more severe airway obstruction; increased to 100 micrograms twice daily

Chronic obstructive pulmonary disease
▸ BY INHALATION OF AEROSOL, OR BY INHALATION OF POWDER
▸ **Adult:** 50 micrograms twice daily

PHARMACOKINETICS
▸ At recommended inhaled doses, the duration of action of salmeterol is about 12 hours.

● UNLICENSED USE *Neovent*® not licensed for use in children under 12 years.

IMPORTANT SAFETY INFORMATION
CHM ADVICE
To ensure safe use, the CHM has advised that for the management of chronic asthma, long-acting beta₂ agonist (salmeterol) should:
● be added only if regular use of standard-dose inhaled corticosteroids has failed to control asthma adequately;
● not be initiated in patients with rapidly deteriorating asthma;
● be introduced at a low dose and the effect properly monitored before considering dose increase;
● be discontinued in the absence of benefit;
● not be used for the relief of exercise-induced asthma symptoms unless regular inhaled corticosteroids are also used;
● be reviewed as clinically appropriate: stepping down therapy should be considered when good long-term asthma control has been achieved.

MHRA/CHM ADVICE: PRESSURISED METERED DOSE INHALERS (PMDI): RISK OF AIRWAY OBSTRUCTION FROM ASPIRATION OF LOOSE OBJECTS (JULY 2018)
See Respiratory system, drug delivery p. 251.

● CAUTIONS High doses of beta₂ agonists can be dangerous in some children
● INTERACTIONS → Appendix 1: beta₂ agonists
● **SIDE-EFFECTS**
▸ **Common or very common** Muscle cramps
▸ **Uncommon** Nervousness · skin reactions
▸ **Rare or very rare** Arthralgia · bronchospasm · chest pain · dizziness · insomnia · oedema · oropharyngeal irritation
● PREGNANCY Inhaled drugs for asthma can be taken as normal during pregnancy.
● BREAST FEEDING Inhaled drugs for asthma can be taken as normal during breast-feeding.
● PATIENT AND CARER ADVICE Advise patients that salmeterol should **not** be used for relief of acute attacks, not to exceed prescribed dose, and to follow manufacturer's directions; if a previously effective dose of inhaled salmeterol fails to provide adequate relief, a doctor's advice should be obtained as soon as possible. Patients should be advised to report any deterioration in symptoms following initiation of treatment with a long-acting beta₂ agonist.
Medicines for Children leaflet: Salmeterol inhaler for asthma
www.medicinesforchildren.org.uk/salmeterol-inhaler-asthma

● MEDICINAL FORMS There can be variation in the licensing of different medicines containing the same drug.
Inhalation powder
▸ Serevent Accuhaler (GlaxoSmithKline UK Ltd)
Salmeterol (as Salmeterol xinafoate) 50 microgram per 1 dose Serevent 50micrograms/dose Accuhaler | 60 dose [PoM] £35.11 DT = £35.11
Pressurised inhalation
▸ Neovent (Kent Pharmaceuticals Ltd)
Salmeterol (as Salmeterol xinafoate) 25 microgram per 1 dose Neovent 25micrograms/dose inhaler CFC free | 120 dose [PoM] £29.26 DT = £29.26

► Serevent Evohaler (GlaxoSmithKline UK Ltd)
Salmeterol (as Salmeterol xinafoate) 25 microgram per 1 dose Serevent 25micrograms/dose Evohaler | 120 dose PoM
£29.26 DT = £29.26
► Soltel (Cipla EU Ltd)
Salmeterol (as Salmeterol xinafoate) 25 microgram per 1 dose Soltel 25micrograms/dose inhaler CFC free | 120 dose PoM
£19.95 DT = £29.26

Combinations available: *Fluticasone with salmeterol*, p. 279

BETA$_2$-ADRENOCEPTOR AGONISTS, SELECTIVE > SHORT-ACTING

> F 265

Salbutamol

(Albuterol)

17-Nov-2020

● **INDICATIONS AND DOSE**

Asthma | Other conditions associated with reversible airways obstruction

► BY MOUTH USING IMMEDIATE-RELEASE MEDICINES
► Adult: 4 mg 3–4 times a day, maximum single dose 8 mg (but unlikely to provide much extra benefit or to be tolerated), inhalation route preferred over oral route, use elderly dose for sensitive patients
► Elderly: Initially 2 mg 3–4 times a day, maximum single dose 8 mg (but unlikely to provide much extra benefit or to be tolerated), inhalation route preferred over oral route
► BY SUBCUTANEOUS INJECTION, OR BY INTRAMUSCULAR INJECTION
► Adult: 500 micrograms every 4 hours if required
► BY SLOW INTRAVENOUS INJECTION
► Adult: 250 micrograms, repeated if necessary, injection to be diluted to a concentration of 50 micrograms/mL, reserve intravenous beta$_2$ agonists for those in whom inhaled therapy cannot be used reliably
► BY INTRAVENOUS INFUSION
► Adult: Initially 5 micrograms/minute, adjusted according to response and heart rate, usual dose 3–20 micrograms/minute, higher doses may be required, reserve intravenous beta$_2$ agonists for those in whom inhaled therapy cannot be used reliably
► BY INHALATION OF AEROSOL
► Adult: 100–200 micrograms, up to 4 times a day for persistent symptoms
► BY INHALATION OF NEBULISED SOLUTION
► Adult: 2.5–5 mg, repeated up to 4 times daily or more frequently in severe cases

Prophylaxis of allergen- or exercise-induced bronchospasm

► BY INHALATION OF AEROSOL
► Adult: 200 micrograms

Acute asthma

► BY INTRAVENOUS INJECTION
► Child 1–23 months: 5 micrograms/kg for 1 dose, dose to be administered over 5 minutes, reserve intravenous beta$_2$ agonists for those in whom inhaled therapy cannot be used reliably or there is no current effect
► Child 2–17 years: 15 micrograms/kg (max. per dose 250 micrograms) for 1 dose, dose to be administered over 5 minutes, reserve intravenous beta$_2$ agonists for those in whom inhaled therapy cannot be used reliably or there is no current effect

Moderate, severe, or life-threatening acute asthma

► BY INHALATION OF NEBULISED SOLUTION
► Child 1 month–4 years: 2.5 mg, repeat every 20–30 minutes or when required, give via oxygen-driven nebuliser if available

► Child 5–11 years: 2.5–5 mg, repeat every 20–30 minutes or when required, give via oxygen-driven nebuliser if available
► Child 12–17 years: 5 mg, repeat every 20–30 minutes or when required, give via oxygen-driven nebuliser if available
► Adult: 5 mg, repeat every 20–30 minutes or when required, give via oxygen-driven nebuliser if available

Moderate and severe acute asthma

► BY INHALATION OF AEROSOL
► Child: 2–10 puffs, each puff is to be inhaled separately, repeat every 10–20 minutes or when required, give via large volume spacer (and a close-fitting face mask in children under 3 years), each puff is equivalent to 100 micrograms
► Adult: 2–10 puffs, each puff is to be inhaled separately, repeat every 10–20 minutes or when required, give via large volume spacer, each puff is equivalent to 100 micrograms

Exacerbation of reversible airways obstruction (including nocturnal asthma) | Prophylaxis of allergen- or exercise-induced bronchospasm

► BY INHALATION OF AEROSOL
► Child: 100–200 micrograms, up to 4 times a day for persistent symptoms
► BY MOUTH USING IMMEDIATE-RELEASE MEDICINES
► Child 1 month–1 year: 100 micrograms/kg 3–4 times a day (max. per dose 2 mg), inhalation route preferred over oral route
► Child 2–5 years: 1–2 mg 3–4 times a day, inhalation route preferred over oral route
► Child 6–11 years: 2 mg 3–4 times a day, inhalation route preferred over oral route
► Child 12–17 years: 2–4 mg 3–4 times a day, inhalation route preferred over oral route

Uncomplicated premature labour (between 22 and 37 weeks of gestation) (specialist supervision in hospital)

► BY INTRAVENOUS INFUSION
► Adult: Initially 10 micrograms/minute, rate increased gradually according to response at 10-minute intervals until contractions diminish then increase rate slowly until contractions cease (maximum rate 45 micrograms/minute), maintain rate for 1 hour after contractions have stopped, then gradually reduce by 50% every 6 hours, maximum duration 48 hours

PHARMACOKINETICS
► At recommended inhaled doses, the duration of action of salbutamol is about 3 to 5 hours.

EASYHALER ® SALBUTAMOL

Acute bronchospasm

► BY INHALATION OF POWDER
► Adult: Initially 100–200 micrograms, increased if necessary to 400 micrograms; maximum 800 micrograms per day

Prophylaxis of allergen- or exercise-induced bronchospasm

► BY INHALATION OF POWDER
► Adult: 200 micrograms

SALBULIN NOVOLIZER ®

Acute bronchospasm

► BY INHALATION OF POWDER
► Adult: Initially 100–200 micrograms, up to 800 micrograms daily for persistent symptoms

Prophylaxis of allergen- or exercise-induced bronchospasm

► BY INHALATION OF POWDER
► Adult: 200 micrograms

continued →

3

Respiratory system

VENTOLIN ACCUHALER ®

Acute bronchospasm
▸ BY INHALATION OF POWDER
▸ Adult: Initially 200 micrograms, up to 4 times daily for persistent symptoms

Prophylaxis of allergen- or exercise-induced bronchospasm
▸ BY INHALATION OF POWDER
▸ Adult: 200 micrograms

● UNLICENSED USE Syrup and tablets not licensed for use in children under 2 years. Injection and solution for intravenous infusion not licensed for use in children under 12 years.
▸ With intravenous use in children Administration of undiluted salbutamol injection through a central venous catheter is not licensed.

IMPORTANT SAFETY INFORMATION

MHRA/CHM ADVICE: PRESSURISED METERED DOSE INHALERS (PMDI): RISK OF AIRWAY OBSTRUCTION FROM ASPIRATION OF LOOSE OBJECTS (JULY 2018)

See Respiratory system, drug delivery p. 251.

● CONTRA-INDICATIONS
▸ When used for uncomplicated premature labour under specialist supervision abruptio placenta · antepartum haemorrhage · cord compression · eclampsia · history of cardiac disease · intra-uterine fetal death · intra-uterine infection · placenta praevia · pulmonary hypertension · severe pre-eclampsia · significant risk factors for myocardial ischaemia · threatened miscarriage

● CAUTIONS
GENERAL CAUTIONS High doses of beta$_2$ agonists can be dangerous in some children
SPECIFIC CAUTIONS
▸ With intravenous use mild to moderate pre-eclampsia (when used for uncomplicated premature labour) · suspected cardiovascular disease (should be assessed by a cardiologist before initiating therapy for uncomplicated premature labour)

● INTERACTIONS → Appendix 1: beta$_2$ agonists

● SIDE-EFFECTS
GENERAL SIDE-EFFECTS
▸ **Common or very common** Muscle cramps
▸ **Rare or very rare** Akathisia · vasodilation
▸ **Frequency not known** Metabolic change · myocardial ischaemia
SPECIFIC SIDE-EFFECTS
▸ **Uncommon**
▸ When used by inhalation Oral irritation · throat irritation
▸ With parenteral use Pulmonary oedema
▸ **Frequency not known**
▸ With parenteral use Lactic acidosis (with high doses) · vomiting

● BREAST FEEDING Inhaled drugs for asthma can be taken as normal during breast-feeding.

● MONITORING REQUIREMENTS In uncomplicated premature labour it is important to monitor blood pressure, pulse rate (should not exceed 120 beats per minute), ECG (discontinue treatment if signs of myocardial ischaemia develop), blood glucose and lactate concentrations, and the patient's fluid and electrolyte status (avoid over-hydration—discontinue drug immediately and initiate diuretic therapy if pulmonary oedema occurs).

● DIRECTIONS FOR ADMINISTRATION
▸ With intravenous use in children For *continuous intravenous infusion*, dilute to a concentration of 200 micrograms/mL with Glucose 5% *or* Sodium Chloride 0.9%. If fluid-restricted, can be given undiluted through central venous

catheter [unlicensed]. For *intravenous injection*, dilute to a concentration of 50 micrograms/mL with Glucose 5%, Sodium Chloride 0.9%, *or* Water for injections.
▸ When used by inhalation For *nebulisation*, dilute nebuliser solution with a suitable volume of sterile Sodium Chloride 0.9% solution according to nebuliser type and duration of administration; salbutamol and ipratropium bromide solutions are compatible and can be mixed for nebulisation.
▸ With intravenous use in adults For *bronchodilation* by *continuous intravenous infusion*, dilute to a concentration of 200 micrograms/mL with glucose 5% or sodium chloride 0.9%. For *premature labour* by *continuous intravenous infusion*, dilute with glucose 5% to a concentration of 200 micrograms/mL for use in a syringe pump *or* for other infusion methods (preferably *via* controlled infusion device), dilute to a concentration of 20 micrograms/mL; close attention to patient's fluid and electrolyte status essential.

● PRESCRIBING AND DISPENSING INFORMATION For choice of therapy, see Asthma, acute p. 256 and Asthma, chronic p. 252.

● PATIENT AND CARER ADVICE *For inhalation by aerosol or dry powder*, advise patients and carers not to exceed prescribed dose and to follow manufacturer's directions; if a previously effective dose of inhaled salbutamol fails to provide at least 3 hours relief, a doctor's advice should be obtained as soon as possible. *For inhalation by nebuliser*, the dose given by nebuliser is substantially higher than that given by inhaler. Patients should therefore be warned that it is dangerous to exceed the prescribed dose and they should seek medical advice if they fail to respond to the usual dose of the respirator solution.
Medicines for Children leaflet: Salbutamol inhaler for asthma and wheeze www.medicinesforchildren.org.uk/salbutamol-inhaler-asthma-and-wheeze

● MEDICINAL FORMS There can be variation in the licensing of different medicines containing the same drug.
Tablet
▸ Salbutamol (Non-proprietary)
Salbutamol (as Salbutamol sulfate) 2 mg Salbutamol 2mg tablets | 28 tablet [PoM] £111.21 DT = £105.03
Salbutamol (as Salbutamol sulfate) 4 mg Salbutamol 4mg tablets | 28 tablet [PoM] £113.85 DT = £107.52
Inhalation powder
▸ Easyhaler (salbutamol) (Orion Pharma (UK) Ltd)
Salbutamol 100 microgram per 1 dose Easyhaler Salbutamol sulfate 100micrograms/dose dry powder inhaler | 200 dose [PoM] £3.31 DT = £3.31
Salbutamol 200 microgram per 1 dose Easyhaler Salbutamol sulfate 200micrograms/dose dry powder inhaler | 200 dose [PoM] £6.63 DT = £6.63
▸ Salbulin Novolizer (Mylan)
Salbutamol (as Salbutamol sulfate) 100 microgram per 1 dose Salbulin Novolizer 100micrograms/dose inhalation powder | 200 dose [PoM] £4.95 DT = £4.95
Salbulin Novolizer 100micrograms/dose inhalation powder refill | 200 dose [PoM] £2.75
▸ Ventolin Accuhaler (GlaxoSmithKline UK Ltd)
Salbutamol 200 microgram per 1 dose Ventolin 200micrograms/dose Accuhaler | 60 dose [PoM] £3.60 DT = £3.60
Solution for injection
▸ Ventolin (GlaxoSmithKline UK Ltd)
Salbutamol (as Salbutamol sulfate) 500 microgram per 1 ml Ventolin 500micrograms/1ml solution for injection ampoules | 5 ampoule [PoM] £1.91
Solution for infusion
▸ Ventolin (GlaxoSmithKline UK Ltd)
Salbutamol (as Salbutamol sulfate) 1 mg per 1 ml Ventolin 5mg/5ml solution for infusion ampoules | 10 ampoule [PoM] £24.81 DT = £24.81

Oral solution

▸ Salbutamol (Non-proprietary)

Salbutamol (as Salbutamol sulfate) 400 microgram per 1 ml Salbutamol 2mg/5ml oral solution sugar free sugar-free | 150 ml [PoM] Ⓢ DT = £1.50

▸ Ventolin (GlaxoSmithKline UK Ltd)

Salbutamol (as Salbutamol sulfate) 400 microgram per 1 ml Ventolin 2mg/5ml syrup sugar-free | 150 ml [PoM] £1.50 DT = £1.50

Pressurised inhalation

▸ Airomir (Teva UK Ltd)

Salbutamol (as Salbutamol sulfate) 100 microgram per 1 dose Airomir 100micrograms/dose inhaler | 200 dose [PoM] £1.97 DT = £1.50

▸ Airomir Autohaler (Teva UK Ltd)

Salbutamol (as Salbutamol sulfate) 100 microgram per 1 dose Airomir 100micrograms/dose Autohaler | 200 dose [PoM] £6.02 DT = £6.30

▸ Salamol (Teva UK Ltd)

Salbutamol (as Salbutamol sulfate) 100 microgram per 1 dose Salamol 100micrograms/dose inhaler CFC free | 200 dose [PoM] £1.46 DT = £1.50

▸ Salamol Easi-Breathe (Teva UK Ltd)

Salbutamol (as Salbutamol sulfate) 100 microgram per 1 dose Salamol 100micrograms/dose Easi-Breathe inhaler | 200 dose [PoM] £6.30 DT = £6.30

▸ Ventolin Evohaler (GlaxoSmithKline UK Ltd)

Salbutamol (as Salbutamol sulfate) 100 microgram per 1 dose Ventolin 100micrograms/dose Evohaler | 200 dose [PoM] £1.50 DT = £1.50

Nebuliser liquid

▸ Salbutamol (Non-proprietary)

Salbutamol (as Salbutamol sulfate) 1 mg per 1 ml Salbutamol 2.5mg/2.5ml nebuliser liquid unit dose vials | 20 unit dose [PoM] £3.98 DT = £3.96

Salbutamol (as Salbutamol sulfate) 2 mg per 1 ml Salbutamol 5mg/2.5ml nebuliser liquid unit dose vials | 20 unit dose [PoM] £6.31 DT = £6.30

▸ Ventolin (GlaxoSmithKline UK Ltd)

Salbutamol (as Salbutamol sulfate) 5 mg per 1 ml Ventolin 5mg/ml respirator solution | 20 ml [PoM] £2.18 DT = £2.18

▸ Ventolin Nebules (GlaxoSmithKline UK Ltd)

Salbutamol (as Salbutamol sulfate) 1 mg per 1 ml Ventolin 2.5mg Nebules | 20 unit dose [PoM] £1.98 DT = £3.96

Salbutamol (as Salbutamol sulfate) 2 mg per 1 ml Ventolin 5mg Nebules | 20 unit dose [PoM] £2.78 DT = £6.30

Combinations available: *Ipratropium with salbutamol*, p. 263

☞ 265

Terbutaline sulfate

● **INDICATIONS AND DOSE**

Asthma | Other conditions associated with reversible airways obstruction

▸ BY MOUTH

▸ **Adult:** Initially 2.5 mg 3 times a day for 1–2 weeks, then increased to up to 5 mg 3 times a day, use by inhalation preferred over by mouth

▸ BY SUBCUTANEOUS INJECTION, OR BY SLOW INTRAVENOUS INJECTION

▸ **Adult:** 250–500 micrograms up to 4 times a day, reserve intravenous beta$_2$ agonists for those in whom inhaled therapy cannot be used reliably or there is no current effect

▸ BY CONTINUOUS INTRAVENOUS INFUSION

▸ **Adult:** 90–300 micrograms/hour for 8-10 hours, to be administered as a solution containing 3–5 micrograms/mL, high doses require close monitoring, reserve intravenous beta$_2$ agonists for those in whom inhaled therapy cannot be used reliably or there is no current effect

▸ BY INHALATION OF POWDER

▸ **Adult:** 500 micrograms up to 4 times a day, for persistent symptoms

▸ BY INHALATION OF NEBULISED SOLUTION

▸ **Adult:** 5–10 mg 2–4 times a day, additional doses may be necessary in severe acute asthma

Acute asthma

▸ BY SUBCUTANEOUS INJECTION, OR BY SLOW INTRAVENOUS INJECTION

▸ **Child 2-14 years:** 10 micrograms/kg up to 4 times a day (max. per dose 300 micrograms), reserve intravenous beta$_2$ agonists for those in whom inhaled therapy cannot be used reliably or there is no current effect

▸ **Child 15-17 years:** 250–500 micrograms up to 4 times a day, reserve intravenous beta$_2$ agonists for those in whom inhaled therapy cannot be used reliably or there is no current effect

▸ BY CONTINUOUS INTRAVENOUS INFUSION

▸ **Child:** Loading dose 2–4 micrograms/kg, then 1–10 micrograms/kg/hour, dose to be adjusted according to response and heart rate, close monitoring is required for doses above 10 micrograms/kg/hour, reserve intravenous beta$_2$ agonists for those in whom inhaled therapy cannot be used reliably or there is no current effect

Moderate, severe, or life-threatening acute asthma

▸ BY INHALATION OF NEBULISED SOLUTION

▸ **Child 1 month-4 years:** 5 mg, repeat every 20–30 minutes or when required, give via oxygen-driven nebuliser if available

▸ **Child 5-11 years:** 5–10 mg, repeat every 20–30 minutes or when required, give via oxygen-driven nebuliser if available

▸ **Child 12-17 years:** 10 mg, repeat every 20–30 minutes or when required, give via oxygen-driven nebuliser if available

▸ **Adult:** 10 mg, repeat every 20–30 minutes or when required, give via oxygen-driven nebuliser if available

Exacerbation of reversible airways obstruction (including nocturnal asthma) | Prevention of exercise-induced bronchospasm

▸ BY INHALATION OF POWDER

▸ **Child 5-17 years:** 500 micrograms up to 4 times a day, for occasional use only

▸ BY MOUTH

▸ **Child 1 month-6 years:** 75 micrograms/kg 3 times a day (max. per dose 2.5 mg), administration by mouth is not recommended

▸ **Child 7-14 years:** 2.5 mg 2–3 times a day, administration by mouth is not recommended

▸ **Child 15-17 years:** Initially 2.5 mg 3 times a day, then increased if necessary to 5 mg 3 times a day, administration by mouth is not recommended

Uncomplicated premature labour (between 22 and 37 weeks of gestation) (specialist supervision in hospital)

▸ BY INTRAVENOUS INFUSION

▸ **Adult:** Initially 5 micrograms/minute for 20 minutes, then increased in steps of 2.5 micrograms/minute every 20 minutes until contractions have ceased (more than 10 micrograms/minute should **seldom** be given— 20 micrograms/minute should **not** be exceeded), continue for 1 hour, then reduced in steps of 2.5 micrograms/minute every 20 minutes to lowest dose that maintains suppression (maximum total duration 48 hours)

PHARMACOKINETICS

▸ At recommended inhaled doses, the duration of action of terbutaline is about 3 to 5 hours.

● UNLICENSED USE Tablets not licensed for use in children under 7 years. Injection not licensed for use in children under 2 years.

Respiratory system

3

- CONTRA-INDICATIONS
  ‣ When used for uncomplicated premature labour abruptio placenta · antepartum haemorrhage · cord compression · eclampsia · history of cardiac disease · intra-uterine fetal death · intra-uterine infection · placenta praevia · pulmonary hypertension · severe pre-eclampsia · significant risk factors for myocardial ischaemia · threatened miscarriage
- CAUTIONS High doses of beta$_2$ agonists can be dangerous in some children · mild to moderate pre-eclampsia (when used for uncomplicated premature labour) · suspected cardiovascular disease (should be assessed by a cardiologist before initiating therapy for uncomplicated premature labour))
- INTERACTIONS → Appendix 1: beta$_2$ agonists
- SIDE-EFFECTS
  GENERAL SIDE-EFFECTS
  ‣ **Common or very common** Hypotension
  ‣ **Rare or very rare** Myocardial ischaemia · vasodilation
  ‣ **Frequency not known** Angioedema · anxiety · behaviour abnormal · bronchospasm · circulatory collapse · oral irritation · sleep disorder · throat irritation · urticaria
  SPECIFIC SIDE-EFFECTS
  ‣ **Uncommon**
  ‣ With parenteral use Pulmonary oedema
  ‣ **Rare or very rare**
  ‣ With parenteral use Lactic acidosis
  ‣ **Frequency not known**
  ‣ With parenteral use Akathisia · bleeding tendency
- PREGNANCY Inhaled drugs for asthma can be taken as normal during pregnancy.
- BREAST FEEDING Inhaled drugs for asthma can be taken as normal during breast-feeding.
- MONITORING REQUIREMENTS In uncomplicated premature labour it is important to monitor blood pressure, pulse rate (should not exceed 120 beats per minute), ECG (discontinue treatment if signs of myocardial ischaemia develop), blood glucose and lactate concentrations, and the patient's fluid and electrolyte status (avoid over-hydration—discontinue drug immediately and initiate diuretic therapy if pulmonary oedema occurs).
- DIRECTIONS FOR ADMINISTRATION
  ‣ With intravenous use in children For *continuous intravenous infusion*, dilute to a concentration of 5 micrograms/mL with Glucose 5% *or* Sodium Chloride 0.9%; if fluid-restricted, dilute to a concentration of 100 micrograms/mL.
  ‣ When used by inhalation For *nebulisation*, dilute nebuliser solution with sterile Sodium Chloride 0.9% solution according to nebuliser type and duration of administration; terbutaline and ipratropium bromide solutions are compatible and may be mixed for nebulisation.
  ‣ With intravenous use in adults For *bronchodilation* by *continuous intravenous infusion*, dilute 1.5–2.5 mg with 500 mL glucose 5% or sodium chloride 0.9% and give over 8–10 hours. For *premature labour* by *continuous intravenous infusion*, dilute in glucose 5% and give *via* controlled infusion device preferably a syringe pump; if syringe pump available dilute to a concentration of 100 micrograms/mL; if syringe pump not available dilute to a concentration of 10 micrograms/mL; close attention to patient's fluid and electrolyte status essential.
- PATIENT AND CARER ADVICE
  ‣ When used by inhalation For *inhalation by dry powder*, advise patients and carers not to exceed prescribed dose and to follow manufacturer's directions; if a previously effective dose of inhaled terbutaline fails to provide at least 3 hours relief, a doctor's advice should be obtained as soon as possible. *For inhalation by nebuliser*, the dose given by nebuliser is substantially higher than that given by inhaler. Patients should therefore be warned that it is dangerous to exceed the prescribed dose and they should seek medical advice if they fail to respond to the usual dose of the respirator solution.

- MEDICINAL FORMS There can be variation in the licensing of different medicines containing the same drug.
  Tablet
  ‣ Bricanyl (AstraZeneca UK Ltd)
    Terbutaline sulfate 5 mg Bricanyl 5mg tablets | 100 tablet PoM £14.73 DT = £14.73
  Inhalation powder
  ‣ Bricanyl Turbohaler (AstraZeneca UK Ltd)
    Terbutaline sulfate 500 microgram per 1 dose Bricanyl 500micrograms/dose Turbohaler | 120 dose PoM £8.30 DT = £8.30
  Solution for injection
  ‣ Bricanyl (AstraZeneca UK Ltd)
    Terbutaline sulfate 500 microgram per 1 ml Bricanyl 2.5mg/5ml solution for injection ampoules | 10 ampoule PoM £20.09 DT = £20.09
    Bricanyl 500micrograms/1ml solution for injection ampoules | 5 ampoule PoM £6.48 DT = £6.48
  Nebuliser liquid
  ‣ Terbutaline sulfate (Non-proprietary)
    Terbutaline sulfate 2.5 mg per 1 ml Terbutaline 5mg/2ml nebuliser liquid unit dose vials | 20 unit dose PoM £4.82–£5.35 DT = £5.35
  ‣ Bricanyl Respules (AstraZeneca UK Ltd)
    Terbutaline sulfate 2.5 mg per 1 ml Bricanyl 5mg/2ml Respules | 20 unit dose PoM £11.64 DT = £5.35

CORTICOSTEROIDS

Corticosteroids (inhaled)

IMPORTANT SAFETY INFORMATION

MHRA/CHM ADVICE: CORTICOSTEROIDS: RARE RISK OF CENTRAL SEROUS CHORIORETINOPATHY WITH LOCAL AS WELL AS SYSTEMIC ADMINISTRATION (AUGUST 2017)

Central serous chorioretinopathy is a retinal disorder that has been linked to the systemic use of corticosteroids. Recently, it has also been reported after local administration of corticosteroids via inhaled and intranasal, epidural, intra-articular, topical dermal, and periocular routes. The MHRA recommends that patients should be advised to report any blurred vision or other visual disturbances with corticosteroid treatment given by any route; consider referral to an ophthalmologist for evaluation of possible causes if a patient presents with vision problems.

NHS IMPROVEMENT PATIENT SAFETY ALERT: STEROID EMERGENCY CARD TO SUPPORT EARLY RECOGNITION AND TREATMENT OF ADRENAL CRISIS IN ADULTS (AUGUST 2020)

A patient-held **Steroid Emergency Card** has been developed for patients with adrenal insufficiency and steroid dependence who are at risk of adrenal crisis. It aims to support healthcare staff with the early recognition of patients at risk of adrenal crisis and the emergency treatment of adrenal crisis. All eligible patients should be issued a Steroid Emergency Card. Providers that treat patients with acute physical illness or trauma, or who may require emergency treatment, elective surgery, or other invasive procedures, should establish processes to check for risk of adrenal crisis and confirm if the patient has a Steroid Emergency Card.

- SIDE-EFFECTS
  ‣ **Common or very common** Headache · oral candidiasis · pneumonia (in patients with COPD) · taste altered · voice alteration
  ‣ **Uncommon** Anxiety · bronchospasm paradoxical · cataract · vision blurred

- **Rare or very rare** Adrenal suppression · behaviour abnormal · glaucoma · growth retardation (in children) · sleep disorder

SIDE-EFFECTS, FURTHER INFORMATION Systemic absorption may follow inhaled administration particularly if high doses are used or if treatment is prolonged. Therefore also consider the side-effects of systemic corticosteroids.

    Candidiasis The risk of oral candidiasis can be reduced by using a spacer device with the corticosteroid inhaler; rinsing the mouth with water after inhalation of a dose may also be helpful. An anti-fungal oral suspension or oral gel can be used to treat oral candidiasis without discontinuing corticosteroid therapy.

    Paradoxical bronchospasm The potential for paradoxical bronchospasm (calling for discontinuation and alternative therapy) should be borne in mind. Mild bronchospasm may be prevented by inhalation of a short-acting beta$_2$ agonist beforehand (or by transfer from an aerosol inhalation to a dry powder inhalation).

- PREGNANCY Inhaled drugs for asthma can be taken as normal during pregnancy.
- BREAST FEEDING Inhaled corticosteroids for asthma can be taken as normal during breast-feeding.
- MONITORING REQUIREMENTS
▸ In children The height and weight of children receiving prolonged treatment with inhaled corticosteroids should be monitored annually; if growth is slowed, referral to a paediatrician should be considered.
- NATIONAL FUNDING/ACCESS DECISIONS
For full details see funding body website

NICE decisions
▸ **Inhaled corticosteroids for the treatment of chronic asthma in children under 12 years (November 2007)** NICE TA131 Recommended
▸ **Inhaled corticosteroids for the treatment of chronic asthma in adults and children over 12 years (March 2008)** NICE TA138 Recommended

◀ 272

Beclometasone dipropionate   16-Nov-2020

(Beclomethasone dipropionate)

- ● **INDICATIONS AND DOSE**
Prophylaxis of asthma
▸ BY INHALATION OF POWDER
▸ Child 5–11 years: 100–200 micrograms twice daily, dose to be adjusted as necessary
▸ Child 12–17 years: 200–400 micrograms twice daily; increased if necessary up to 800 micrograms twice daily, dose to be adjusted as necessary
▸ Adult: 200–400 micrograms twice daily; increased if necessary up to 800 micrograms twice daily, dose to be adjusted as necessary

DOSE EQUIVALENCE AND CONVERSION
▸ Dose adjustments may be required for some inhaler devices, see under individual preparations.

CLENIL MODULITE ®
Prophylaxis of asthma
▸ BY INHALATION OF AEROSOL
▸ Child 2–11 years: 100–200 micrograms twice daily
▸ Child 12–17 years: 200–400 micrograms twice daily, adjusted according to response; increased if necessary up to 1 mg twice daily
▸ Adult: 200–400 micrograms twice daily, adjusted according to response; increased if necessary up to 1 mg twice daily

KELHALE ®
Prophylaxis of asthma
▸ BY INHALATION OF AEROSOL
▸ Adult: 50–200 micrograms twice daily; increased if necessary up to 400 micrograms twice daily
POTENCY
▸ *Kelhale*® has extra-fine particles and is more potent than traditional beclometasone dipropionate CFC-containing inhalers.

QVAR ® PREPARATIONS
Prophylaxis of asthma
▸ BY INHALATION OF AEROSOL
▸ Child 5–11 years: 50–100 micrograms twice daily, using Autohaler or MDI device
▸ Child 12–17 years: 50–200 micrograms twice daily; increased if necessary up to 400 micrograms twice daily, using Autohaler, MDI, or Easi-Breathe device
▸ Adult: 50–200 micrograms twice daily; increased if necessary up to 400 micrograms twice daily, using Autohaler, MDI, or Easi-Breathe device
POTENCY
▸ *Qvar*® has extra-fine particles, is more potent than traditional beclometasone dipropionate CFC-containing inhalers and is approximately twice as potent as *Clenil Modulite*®.

SOPROBEC ®
Prophylaxis of asthma
▸ BY INHALATION OF AEROSOL
▸ Child: 100 micrograms twice daily; increased if necessary up to 400 micrograms daily in 2–4 divided doses
▸ Adult: 200 micrograms twice daily, adjusted according to response; increased if necessary up to 2 mg daily in 2–4 divided doses

- UNLICENSED USE *Easyhaler*® *Beclometasone Dipropionate* is not licensed for use in children. *Clenil Modulite*® 200 and 250 are not licensed for use in children.

> IMPORTANT SAFETY INFORMATION
> MHRA/CHM ADVICE (JULY 2008)
> Beclometasone dipropionate CFC-free pressurised metered-dose inhalers (*Qvar*® and *Clenil Modulite*®) are **not** interchangeable and should be prescribed by brand name; *Qvar*® has extra-fine particles, is more potent than traditional beclometasone dipropionate CFC-containing inhalers, and is approximately twice as potent as *Clenil Modulite*®.
>
> MHRA ADVICE: PRESSURISED METERED DOSE INHALERS (PMDI): RISK OF AIRWAY OBSTRUCTION FROM ASPIRATION OF LOOSE OBJECTS (JULY 2018)
> See Respiratory system, drug delivery p. 251.

- ● INTERACTIONS → Appendix 1: corticosteroids
- ● SIDE-EFFECTS
▸ **Common or very common** Throat irritation
▸ **Rare or very rare** Wheezing
- ● PRESCRIBING AND DISPENSING INFORMATION The MHRA has advised (July 2008) that beclometasone dipropionate CFC-free inhalers should be prescribed by brand name. Pressurised metered-doses inhalers with extra-fine particles (*Qvar*® and *Kelhale*®) are more potent than, and not interchangeable with, traditional CFC-containing and CFC-free inhalers (*Clenil Modulite*® and *Soprobec*®).

KELHALE ® Manufacturer advises when switching a patient with well-controlled asthma from another corticosteroid inhaler, initially a 100-microgram metered dose of *Kelhale*® should be prescribed for 200–250 micrograms of budesonide and for 100 micrograms of fluticasone propionate; the dose of *Kelhale*® should be adjusted according to response, up to a maximum of 800 micrograms daily. Manufacturer advises when switching a patient with poorly-controlled asthma from another corticosteroid inhaler, initially a 100-microgram metered dose of *Kelhale* ® should be prescribed for 100 micrograms of budesonide or fluticasone propionate; the dose of *Kelhale* ® should be adjusted according to response, up to a maximum of 800 micrograms daily.

QVAR ® PREPARATIONS When switching a patient with well-controlled asthma from another corticosteroid inhaler, initially a 100-microgram metered dose of *Qvar* ® should be prescribed for 200–250 micrograms of beclometasone dipropionate or budesonide and for 100 micrograms of fluticasone propionate. When switching a patient with poorly controlled asthma from another corticosteroid inhaler, initially a 100-microgram metered dose of *Qvar* ® should be prescribed for 100 micrograms of beclometasone dipropionate, budesonide, or fluticasone propionate; the dose of *Qvar* ® should be adjusted according to response.

- PATIENT AND CARER ADVICE Steroid card should be issued with high doses of inhaled beclometasone dipropionate. Medicines for Children leaflet: Beclometasone inhaler for asthma prevention (prophylaxis) www.medicinesforchildren.org.uk/beclometasone-inhaler-asthma-prevention-prophylaxis-0

- PROFESSION SPECIFIC INFORMATION
Dental practitioners' formulary
Clenil Modulite ® 50 micrograms/metered inhalation may be prescribed.

- MEDICINAL FORMS There can be variation in the licensing of different medicines containing the same drug.
Inhalation powder
CAUTIONARY AND ADVISORY LABELS 8, 10
  ▸ Easyhaler (beclometasone) (Orion Pharma (UK) Ltd)
  Beclometasone dipropionate 200 microgram per 1 dose Easyhaler Beclometasone 200micrograms/dose dry powder inhaler | 200 dose [PoM] £14.93 DT = £14.93

Pressurised inhalation
CAUTIONARY AND ADVISORY LABELS 8, 10
  ▸ Clenil Modulite (Chiesi Ltd)
  Beclometasone dipropionate 50 microgram per 1 dose Clenil Modulite 50micrograms/dose inhaler | 200 dose [PoM] £3.70 DT = £3.70
  Beclometasone dipropionate 100 microgram per 1 dose Clenil Modulite 100micrograms/dose inhaler | 200 dose [PoM] £7.42 DT = £7.42
  Beclometasone dipropionate 200 microgram per 1 dose Clenil Modulite 200micrograms/dose inhaler | 200 dose [PoM] £16.17 DT = £16.17
  Beclometasone dipropionate 250 microgram per 1 dose Clenil Modulite 250micrograms/dose inhaler | 200 dose [PoM] £16.29 DT = £16.29
  ▸ Kelhale (Cipla EU Ltd)
  Beclometasone dipropionate 50 microgram per 1 dose Kelhale 50micrograms/dose inhaler | 200 dose [PoM] £5.20 DT = £3.70
  Beclometasone dipropionate 100 microgram per 1 dose Kelhale 100micrograms/dose inhaler | 200 dose [PoM] £5.20 DT = £7.42
  ▸ Qvar (Teva UK Ltd)
  Beclometasone dipropionate 50 microgram per 1 dose Qvar 50 inhaler | 200 dose [PoM] £7.87 DT = £3.70
  Beclometasone dipropionate 100 microgram per 1 dose Qvar 100 inhaler | 200 dose [PoM] £17.21 DT = £7.42
  ▸ Qvar Autohaler (Teva UK Ltd)
  Beclometasone dipropionate 50 microgram per 1 dose Qvar 50 Autohaler | 200 dose [PoM] £7.87 DT = £7.87
  Beclometasone dipropionate 100 microgram per 1 dose Qvar 100 Autohaler | 200 dose [PoM] £17.21 DT = £17.21
  ▸ Qvar Easi-Breathe (Teva UK Ltd)
  Beclometasone dipropionate 50 microgram per 1 dose Qvar 50micrograms/dose Easi-Breathe inhaler | 200 dose [PoM] £7.74 DT = £7.87
  Beclometasone dipropionate 100 microgram per 1 dose Qvar 100micrograms/dose Easi-Breathe inhaler | 200 dose [PoM] £16.95 DT = £17.21

  ▸ Soprobec (Glenmark Pharmaceuticals Europe Ltd)
  Beclometasone dipropionate 50 microgram per 1 dose Soprobec 50micrograms/dose inhaler | 200 dose [PoM] £2.78 DT = £3.70
  Beclometasone dipropionate 100 microgram per 1 dose Soprobec 100micrograms/dose inhaler | 200 dose [PoM] £5.57 DT = £7.42
  Beclometasone dipropionate 200 microgram per 1 dose Soprobec 200micrograms/dose inhaler | 200 dose [PoM] £12.13 DT = £16.17
  Beclometasone dipropionate 250 microgram per 1 dose Soprobec 250micrograms/dose inhaler | 200 dose [PoM] £12.22 DT = £16.29

Beclometasone with formoterol

11-Nov-2020

The properties listed below are those particular to the combination only. For the properties of the components please consider, beclometasone dipropionate p. 273, formoterol fumarate p. 266.

- **INDICATIONS AND DOSE**

FOSTAIR NEXTHALER ® 100/6

Asthma maintenance therapy
  ▸ BY INHALATION OF POWDER
  ▸ Adult: 1–2 inhalations twice daily; maximum 4 inhalations per day

Asthma, maintenance and reliever therapy
  ▸ BY INHALATION OF POWDER
  ▸ Adult: Maintenance 1 inhalation twice daily; 1 inhalation as required, for relief of symptoms; maximum 8 inhalations per day

Chronic obstructive pulmonary disease with forced expiratory volume in 1 second < 50% of predicted
  ▸ BY INHALATION OF POWDER
  ▸ Adult: 2 inhalations twice daily

DOSE EQUIVALENCE AND CONVERSION
  ▸ For inhalation of powder, when switching patients from other beclometasone dipropionate formulations with non-extrafine particle size distribution to *Fostair NEXThaler* ®, the dose should be adjusted according to response.
  ▸ 1 inhalation is equivalent to 100 micrograms beclometasone dipropionate and 6 micrograms formoterol fumarate.

FOSTAIR NEXTHALER ® 200/6

Asthma maintenance therapy
  ▸ BY INHALATION OF POWDER
  ▸ Adult: 2 inhalations twice daily; maximum 4 inhalations per day

DOSE EQUIVALENCE AND CONVERSION
  ▸ For inhalation of powder, when switching patients from other beclometasone dipropionate formulations with non-extrafine particle size distribution to *Fostair NEXThaler* ®, the dose should be adjusted according to response.
  ▸ 1 inhalation is equivalent to 200 micrograms beclometasone dipropionate and 6 micrograms formoterol fumarate.

FOSTAIR ® 100/6

Asthma maintenance therapy
  ▸ BY INHALATION OF AEROSOL
  ▸ Adult: 1–2 inhalations twice daily; maximum 4 inhalations per day

Asthma, maintenance and reliever therapy
  ▸ BY INHALATION OF AEROSOL
  ▸ Adult: Maintenance 1 inhalation twice daily; 1 inhalation as required, for relief of symptoms; maximum 8 inhalations per day

Chronic obstructive pulmonary disease with forced expiratory volume in 1 second < 50% of predicted
▸ BY INHALATION OF AEROSOL
▸ Adult: 2 inhalations twice daily
DOSE EQUIVALENCE AND CONVERSION
▸ For inhalation of aerosol, when switching patients from other beclometasone dipropionate and formoterol fumarate inhalers, dose should be adjusted according to response—100 micrograms of beclometasone dipropionate extrafine in *Fostair*® is equivalent to 250 micrograms of beclometasone dipropionate in a non-extrafine formulation.
▸ 1 inhalation is equivalent to 100 micrograms beclometasone dipropionate and 6 micrograms formoterol fumarate.

FOSTAIR® 200/6

Asthma maintenance therapy
▸ BY INHALATION OF AEROSOL
▸ Adult: 2 inhalations twice daily; maximum 4 inhalations per day
DOSE EQUIVALENCE AND CONVERSION
▸ For inhalation of aerosol, when switching patients from other beclometasone dipropionate and formoterol fumarate inhalers, dose should be adjusted according to response—100 micrograms of beclometasone dipropionate extrafine in *Fostair*® is equivalent to 250 micrograms of beclometasone dipropionate in a non-extra-fine formulation.
▸ 1 inhalation is equivalent to 200 micrograms beclometasone dipropionate and 6 micrograms formoterol fumarate.

IMPORTANT SAFETY INFORMATION
MHRA/CHM ADVICE (JULY 2008)
Fostair® contains extra-fine particles of beclometasone dipropionate and is more potent than traditional beclometasone dipropionate CFC-free inhalers. The dose of beclometasone dipropionate in *Fostair*® should be lower than non-extra-fine formulations of beclometasone dipropionate and will need to be adjusted to the individual needs of the patient.

● INTERACTIONS → Appendix 1: beta₂ agonists · corticosteroids
● PATIENT AND CARER ADVICE Patients or carers should be given advice on how to administer beclometasone with formoterol aerosol for inhalation.
 With high doses, a steroid card should be supplied.

● MEDICINAL FORMS There can be variation in the licensing of different medicines containing the same drug.
Inhalation powder
CAUTIONARY AND ADVISORY LABELS 8, 10
▸ Fostair NEXThaler (Chiesi Ltd)
 Formoterol fumarate dihydrate 6 microgram per 1 dose, Beclometasone dipropionate 100 microgram per 1 dose Fostair NEXThaler 100micrograms/dose / 6micrograms/dose dry powder inhaler | 120 dose [PoM] £29.32 DT = £29.32
 Formoterol fumarate dihydrate 6 microgram per 1 dose, Beclometasone dipropionate 200 microgram per 1 dose Fostair NEXThaler 200micrograms/dose / 6micrograms/dose dry powder inhaler | 120 dose [PoM] £29.32 DT = £29.32
Pressurised inhalation
CAUTIONARY AND ADVISORY LABELS 8, 10
▸ Fostair (Chiesi Ltd)
 Formoterol fumarate dihydrate 6 microgram, Beclometasone dipropionate 200 microgram Fostair 200micrograms/dose / 6micrograms/dose inhaler | 120 dose [PoM] £29.32 DT = £29.32
 Formoterol fumarate dihydrate 6 microgram per 1 dose, Beclometasone dipropionate 100 microgram per 1 dose Fostair 100micrograms/dose / 6micrograms/dose inhaler | 120 dose [PoM] £29.32 DT = £29.32

Beclometasone with formoterol and glycopyrronium
03-Nov-2020

The properties listed below are those particular to the combination only. For the properties of the components please consider, beclometasone dipropionate p. 273, formoterol fumarate p. 266, glycopyrronium bromide p. 262.

● INDICATIONS AND DOSE
Moderate-to-severe chronic obstructive pulmonary disease
▸ BY INHALATION OF AEROSOL
▸ Adult: 2 inhalations twice daily

● INTERACTIONS → Appendix 1: beta₂ agonists · corticosteroids · glycopyrronium
● BREAST FEEDING Manufacturer advises avoid—no information available.
● HEPATIC IMPAIRMENT Manufacturer advises caution in severe impairment (no information available).
● NATIONAL FUNDING/ACCESS DECISIONS
 For full details see funding body website
Scottish Medicines Consortium (SMC) decisions
▸ Beclometasone with formoterol and glycopyrronium (*Trimbow*®) for maintenance treatment in adult patients with moderate to severe chronic obstructive pulmonary disease (COPD) who are not adequately treated by a combination of an inhaled corticosteroid and a long-acting beta₂-agonist (October 2017) SMC No. 1274/17 Recommended with restrictions

● MEDICINAL FORMS There can be variation in the licensing of different medicines containing the same drug.
Pressurised inhalation
CAUTIONARY AND ADVISORY LABELS 8, 10
▸ Trimbow (Chiesi Ltd)
 Formoterol fumarate dihydrate 5 microgram per 1 dose, Glycopyrronium (as Glycopyrronium bromide) 9 microgram per 1 dose, Beclometasone dipropionate 87 microgram per 1 dose Trimbow 87micrograms/dose / 5micrograms/dose / 9micrograms/dose inhaler | 120 dose [PoM] £44.50

F 272

Budesonide
12-Nov-2020

● DRUG ACTION Budesonide is a glucocorticoid, which exerts significant local anti-inflammatory effects.

● INDICATIONS AND DOSE
Prophylaxis of mild to moderate asthma (in patients stabilised on twice daily dose)
▸ BY INHALATION OF POWDER
▸ Child 6–11 years: 200–400 micrograms once daily, dose to be given in the evening
▸ Child 12–17 years: 200–400 micrograms once daily (max. per dose 800 micrograms), dose to be given in the evening
▸ Adult: 200–400 micrograms once daily (max. per dose 800 micrograms), dose to be given in the evening
Prophylaxis of asthma
▸ BY INHALATION OF POWDER
▸ Child 6–11 years: 100–400 micrograms twice daily, dose to be adjusted as necessary
▸ Child 12–17 years: 100–800 micrograms twice daily, dose to be adjusted as necessary
▸ Adult: 100–800 micrograms twice daily, dose to be adjusted as necessary
▸ BY INHALATION OF NEBULISED SUSPENSION
▸ Child 6 months–11 years: 125–500 micrograms twice daily, adjusted according to response; maximum 2 mg per day continued →

3

Respiratory system

▸ **Child 12-17 years:** Initially 0.25–1 mg twice daily, adjusted according to response, doses higher than recommended max. may be used in severe disease; maximum 2 mg per day

▸ **Adult:** Initially 0.25–1 mg twice daily, adjusted according to response, doses higher than recommended max. may be used in severe disease; maximum 2 mg per day

POTENCY

▸ Dose adjustments may be required for some inhaler devices, see under individual preparations.

BUDELIN NOVOLIZER ®

Prophylaxis of asthma

▸ BY INHALATION OF POWDER

▸ **Adult:** 200–800 micrograms twice daily, dose is adjusted as necessary

Alternative in mild to moderate asthma, for patients previously stabilised on a twice daily dose

▸ BY INHALATION OF POWDER

▸ **Adult:** 200–400 micrograms once daily (max. per dose 800 micrograms), to be taken in the evening

PULMICORT ® RESPULES

Prophylaxis of asthma

▸ BY INHALATION OF NEBULISED SUSPENSION

▸ **Child 3 months–11 years:** Initially 0.5–1 mg twice daily, reduced to 250–500 micrograms twice daily

▸ **Child 12-17 years:** Initially 1–2 mg twice daily, reduced to 0.5–1 mg twice daily

▸ **Adult:** Initially 1–2 mg twice daily, reduced to 0.5–1 mg twice daily

PULMICORT ® TURBOHALER

Prophylaxis of asthma

▸ BY INHALATION OF POWDER

▸ **Adult:** 100–800 micrograms twice daily, dose to be adjusted as necessary

Alternative in mild to moderate asthma, for patients previously stabilised on a twice daily dose

▸ BY INHALATION OF POWDER

▸ **Adult:** 200–400 micrograms once daily (max. per dose 800 micrograms), to be taken in the evening

● INTERACTIONS → Appendix 1: corticosteroids

● DIRECTIONS FOR ADMINISTRATION Budesonide nebuliser suspension is not suitable for use in ultrasonic nebulisers.

● PATIENT AND CARER ADVICE With high doses, a steroid card should be supplied. Patients or carers should be given advice on how to administer budesonide dry powder inhaler and nebuliser suspension.
Medicines for Children leaflet: Budesonide inhaler for asthma prevention (prophylaxis) www.medicinesforchildren.org.uk/budesonide-inhaler-asthma-prevention-prophylaxis

BUDELIN NOVOLIZER ® Patients or carers should be given advice on administration of *Budelin Novolizer®*.

● MEDICINAL FORMS There can be variation in the licensing of different medicines containing the same drug.

Inhalation powder

CAUTIONARY AND ADVISORY LABELS 8, 10

▸ Budelin Novolizer (Mylan)

Budesonide 200 microgram per 1 dose Budelin Novolizer 200micrograms/dose inhalation powder | 100 dose PoM £14.86 = £14.86
Budelin Novolizer 200micrograms/dose inhalation powder refill | 100 dose PoM £9.59 DT = £9.59

▸ Easyhaler (budesonide) (Orion Pharma (UK) Ltd)

Budesonide 100 microgram per 1 dose Easyhaler Budesonide 100micrograms/dose dry powder inhaler | 200 dose PoM £8.86 DT = £14.25

Budesonide 200 microgram per 1 dose Easyhaler Budesonide 200micrograms/dose dry powder inhaler | 200 dose PoM £17.71

Budesonide 400 microgram per 1 dose Easyhaler Budesonide 400micrograms/dose dry powder inhaler | 100 dose PoM £17.71

▸ Pulmicort Turbohaler (AstraZeneca UK Ltd)

Budesonide 100 microgram per 1 dose Pulmicort 100 Turbohaler | 200 dose PoM £14.25 DT = £14.25

Budesonide 200 microgram per 1 dose Pulmicort 200 Turbohaler | 100 dose PoM £14.25 DT = £14.25

Budesonide 400 microgram per 1 dose Pulmicort 400 Turbohaler | 50 dose PoM £14.25 DT = £14.25

Nebuliser liquid

CAUTIONARY AND ADVISORY LABELS 8, 10

▸ Budesonide (Non-proprietary)

Budesonide 250 microgram per 1 ml Budesonide 500micrograms/2ml nebuliser liquid unit dose vials | 20 unit dose PoM £25.68 DT = £25.65

Budesonide 500 microgram per 1 ml Budesonide 1mg/2ml nebuliser liquid unit dose vials | 20 unit dose PoM £39.45 DT = £39.45

▸ Pulmicort Respules (AstraZeneca UK Ltd)

Budesonide 250 microgram per 1 ml Pulmicort 0.5mg Respules | 20 unit dose PoM £31.70 DT = £25.65

Budesonide 500 microgram per 1 ml Pulmicort 1mg Respules | 20 unit dose PoM £48.00 DT = £39.45

Budesonide with formoterol
09-Dec-2020

The properties listed below are those particular to the combination only. For the properties of the components please consider, budesonide p. 275, formoterol fumarate p. 266.

● INDICATIONS AND DOSE

DUORESP SPIROMAX ® 160MICROGRAMS/4.5MICROGRAMS

Asthma, maintenance therapy

▸ BY INHALATION OF POWDER

▸ **Adult:** 1–2 inhalations twice daily, increased if necessary up to 4 inhalations twice daily

Asthma, maintenance and reliever therapy

▸ BY INHALATION OF POWDER

▸ **Adult:** Maintenance 2 inhalations daily in 1–2 divided doses, increased if necessary to 2 inhalations twice daily. 1 inhalation as required, for relief of symptoms, increased if necessary up to 6 inhalations as required, max. 8 inhalations per day; up to 12 inhalations daily can be used for a limited time but medical assessment is recommended

Chronic obstructive pulmonary disease with forced expiratory volume in 1 second <70% of predicted

▸ BY INHALATION OF POWDER

▸ **Adult:** 2 inhalations twice daily

DUORESP SPIROMAX ® 320MICROGRAMS/9MICROGRAMS

Asthma, maintenance therapy

▸ BY INHALATION OF POWDER

▸ **Adult:** 1 inhalation twice daily, increased if necessary up to 2 inhalations twice daily

Chronic obstructive pulmonary disease with forced expiratory volume in 1 second < 70% of predicted

▸ BY INHALATION OF POWDER

▸ **Adult:** 1 inhalation twice daily

FOBUMIX ® 160/4.5 EASYHALER

Asthma, maintenance therapy

▸ BY INHALATION OF POWDER

▸ **Adult:** 1–2 inhalations twice daily, increased if necessary up to 4 inhalations twice daily

Asthma, maintenance and reliever therapy

▸ BY INHALATION OF POWDER

▸ **Adult:** Maintenance 2 inhalations daily in 1–2 divided doses, increased if necessary to 2 inhalations twice daily. 1 inhalation as required for relief of symptoms, increased if necessary up to 6 inhalations as required, max. 8 inhalations per day; up to 12 inhalations daily can be used for a limited time but medical assessment is recommended

Chronic obstructive pulmonary disease with forced expiratory volume in 1 second < 70% of predicted (post-bronchodilator)
▸ BY INHALATION OF POWDER
▸ Adult: 2 inhalations twice daily

FOBUMIX ® 320/9 EASYHALER

Asthma, maintenance therapy
▸ BY INHALATION OF POWDER
▸ Adult: 1 inhalation twice daily; increased if necessary up to 2 inhalations twice daily

Chronic obstructive pulmonary disease with forced expiratory volume in 1 second < 70% of predicted (post-bronchodilator)
▸ BY INHALATION OF POWDER
▸ Adult: 1 inhalation twice daily

FOBUMIX ® 80/4.5 EASYHALER

Asthma, maintenance therapy
▸ BY INHALATION OF POWDER
▸ Adult: 1–2 inhalations twice daily, increased if necessary up to 4 inhalations twice daily

Asthma, maintenance and reliever therapy
▸ BY INHALATION OF POWDER
▸ Adult: Maintenance 2 inhalations daily in 1–2 divided doses. 1 inhalation as required for relief of symptoms, increased if necessary up to 6 inhalations as required, max. 8 inhalations per day; up to 12 inhalations daily can be used for a limited time but medical assessment is recommended

SYMBICORT 100/6 TURBOHALER ®

Asthma, maintenance therapy
▸ BY INHALATION OF POWDER
▸ Child 6-17 years: Initially 1–2 puffs twice daily; reduced to 1 puff daily, dose reduced only if control is maintained
▸ Adult: Initially 1–2 puffs twice daily, increased if necessary up to 4 puffs twice daily; reduced to 1 puff daily, dose reduced only if control is maintained

Asthma, maintenance and reliever therapy
▸ BY INHALATION OF POWDER
▸ Child 12-17 years: Maintenance 2 puffs daily in 1–2 divided doses; 1 puff as required for relief of symptoms, increased if necessary up to 6 puffs as required, max. 8 puffs per day; up to 12 puffs daily can be used for a limited time but medical assessment is recommended
▸ Adult: Maintenance 2 puffs daily in 1–2 divided doses; 1 puff as required for relief of symptoms, increased if necessary up to 6 puffs as required, max. 8 puffs per day; up to 12 puffs daily can be used for a limited time but medical assessment is recommended

SYMBICORT 200/6 TURBOHALER ®

Asthma, maintenance therapy
▸ BY INHALATION OF POWDER
▸ Child 12-17 years: Initially 1–2 puffs twice daily; reduced to 1 puff daily, dose reduced only if control is maintained
▸ Adult: Initially 1–2 puffs twice daily, increased if necessary up to 4 puffs twice daily; reduced to 1 puff daily, dose reduced only if control is maintained

Asthma, maintenance and reliever therapy
▸ BY INHALATION OF POWDER
▸ Child 12-17 years: Maintenance 2 puffs daily in 1–2 divided doses, increased if necessary to 2 puffs twice daily; 1 puff as required for relief of symptoms, increased if necessary up to 6 puffs as required, max. 8 puffs per day; up to 12 puffs daily can be used for a limited time but medical assessment is recommended

▸ Adult: Maintenance 2 puffs daily in 1–2 divided doses, increased if necessary to 2 puffs twice daily; 1 puff as required for relief of symptoms, increased if necessary up to 6 puffs as required, max. 8 puffs per day; up to 12 puffs daily can be used for a limited time but medical assessment is recommended

Chronic obstructive pulmonary disease with forced expiratory volume in 1 second < 70% of predicted (post bronchodilator)
▸ BY INHALATION OF POWDER
▸ Adult: 2 puffs twice daily

SYMBICORT 400/12 TURBOHALER ®

Asthma, maintenance therapy
▸ BY INHALATION OF POWDER
▸ Child 12-17 years: Initially 1 puff twice daily; reduced to 1 puff daily, dose reduced only if control is maintained
▸ Adult: Initially 1 puff twice daily, increased if necessary up to 2 puffs twice daily; reduced to 1 puff daily, dose reduced only if control is maintained

Chronic obstructive pulmonary disease with forced expiratory volume in 1 second < 70% of predicted (post bronchodilator)
▸ BY INHALATION OF POWDER
▸ Adult: 1 puff twice daily

SYMBICORT ® 100/3 PRESSURISED INHALER

Asthma, maintenance therapy
▸ BY INHALATION OF AEROSOL
▸ Child 12-17 years: Initially 2–4 inhalations twice daily; reduced to 1 inhalation daily, dose reduced only if control is maintained
▸ Adult: Initially 2–4 inhalations twice daily, increased if necessary up to 8 inhalations twice daily; reduced to 1 inhalation daily, dose reduced only if control is maintained

Asthma, maintenance and reliever therapy
▸ BY INHALATION OF AEROSOL
▸ Child 12-17 years: Maintenance 4 inhalations daily in 1–2 divided doses, increased if necessary up to 4 inhalations twice daily; 2 inhalations as required for relief of symptoms, increased if necessary up to 12 inhalations as required, usual max. 16 inhalations per day; up to 24 inhalations daily can be used for a limited time but medical assessment is recommended
▸ Adult: Maintenance 4 inhalations daily in 1–2 divided doses, increased if necessary up to 4 inhalations twice daily; 2 inhalations as required for relief of symptoms, increased if necessary up to 12 inhalations as required, usual max. 16 inhalations per day; up to 24 inhalations daily can be used for a limited time but medical assessment is recommended

SYMBICORT ® 200/6 PRESSURISED INHALER

Chronic obstructive pulmonary disease with forced expiratory volume in 1 second <70% of predicted (post bronchodilator)
▸ BY INHALATION OF AEROSOL
▸ Adult: 2 inhalations twice daily

● INTERACTIONS → Appendix 1: beta₂ agonists · corticosteroids

● PATIENT AND CARER ADVICE Patient counselling is advised for budesonide with formoterol inhalation (administration).
With high doses, a steroid card should be supplied.

● NATIONAL FUNDING/ACCESS DECISIONS
For full details see funding body website

Scottish Medicines Consortium (SMC) decisions
▸ Budesonide/formoterol 100/6, 200/6 inhalation powder turbohaler (*Symbicort* ® SMART ®) for asthma in adults (June 2007) SMC No. 362/07 Recommended

Respiratory system

3

▶ Budesonide/formoterol 100/6, 200/6 inhalation powder turbohaler (*Symbicort®* SMART®) for asthma in adolescents aged 12 years and over (June 2017) SMC No. 1244/17 Recommended

● MEDICINAL FORMS There can be variation in the licensing of different medicines containing the same drug.
Inhalation powder
CAUTIONARY AND ADVISORY LABELS 8, 10 (high doses)
▶ DuoResp Spiromax (Teva UK Ltd)
Formoterol fumarate dihydrate 6 microgram per 1 dose, Budesonide 200 microgram per 1 dose DuoResp Spiromax 160micrograms/dose / 4.5micrograms/dose dry powder inhaler | 120 dose [PoM] £27.97 DT = £28.00
Formoterol fumarate dihydrate 12 microgram per 1 dose, Budesonide 400 microgram per 1 dose DuoResp Spiromax 320micrograms/dose / 9micrograms/dose dry powder inhaler | 60 dose [PoM] £27.97 DT = £28.00
▶ Fobumix Easyhaler (Orion Pharma (UK) Ltd)
Formoterol fumarate dihydrate 6 microgram per 1 dose, Budesonide 100 microgram per 1 dose Fobumix Easyhaler 80micrograms/dose / 4.5micrograms/dose dry powder inhaler | 120 dose [PoM] £21.50 DT = £28.00
Formoterol fumarate dihydrate 6 microgram per 1 dose, Budesonide 200 microgram per 1 dose Fobumix Easyhaler 160micrograms/dose / 4.5micrograms/dose dry powder inhaler | 60 dose [PoM] £10.75 | 120 dose [PoM] £21.50 DT = £28.00
Formoterol fumarate dihydrate 12 microgram per 1 dose, Budesonide 400 microgram per 1 dose Fobumix Easyhaler 320micrograms/dose / 9micrograms/dose dry powder inhaler | 60 dose [PoM] £21.50 DT = £28.00
▶ Symbicort Turbohaler (AstraZeneca UK Ltd)
Formoterol fumarate dihydrate 6 microgram per 1 dose, Budesonide 100 microgram per 1 dose Symbicort 100/6 Turbohaler | 120 dose [PoM] £28.00 DT = £28.00
Formoterol fumarate dihydrate 6 microgram per 1 dose, Budesonide 200 microgram per 1 dose Symbicort 200/6 Turbohaler | 120 dose [PoM] £28.00 DT = £28.00
Formoterol fumarate dihydrate 12 microgram per 1 dose, Budesonide 400 microgram per 1 dose Symbicort 400/12 Turbohaler | 60 dose [PoM] £28.00 DT = £28.00
Pressurised inhalation
CAUTIONARY AND ADVISORY LABELS 8, 10 (high doses)
▶ Budesonide with formoterol (Non-proprietary)
Formoterol fumarate dihydrate 3 microgram per 1 dose, Budesonide 100 microgram per 1 dose Symbicort 100micrograms/dose / 3micrograms/dose pressurised inhaler | 120 dose [PoM] £14.00
▶ Symbicort (AstraZeneca UK Ltd)
Formoterol fumarate dihydrate 6 microgram per 1 dose, Budesonide 200 microgram per 1 dose Symbicort 200micrograms/dose / 6micrograms/dose pressurised inhaler | 120 dose [PoM] £28.00 DT = £28.00

F 272

Ciclesonide

25-Sep-2020

● INDICATIONS AND DOSE
Prophylaxis of asthma
▶ BY INHALATION OF AEROSOL
▶ Child 12-17 years: 160 micrograms once daily; reduced to 80 micrograms once daily, if control maintained; increased if necessary up to 320 micrograms twice daily, in severe asthma
▶ Adult: 160 micrograms once daily; reduced to 80 micrograms once daily, if control maintained; increased if necessary up to 320 micrograms twice daily, in severe asthma

IMPORTANT SAFETY INFORMATION
MHRA/CHM ADVICE: PRESSURISED METERED DOSE INHALERS (PMDI): RISK OF AIRWAY OBSTRUCTION FROM ASPIRATION OF LOOSE OBJECTS (JULY 2018)
See Respiratory system, drug delivery p. 251.

● INTERACTIONS → Appendix 1: corticosteroids

● SIDE-EFFECTS Cushing's syndrome

● HEPATIC IMPAIRMENT Manufacturer advises caution in severe impairment (risk of increased exposure, no information available).

● PATIENT AND CARER ADVICE Patients or carers should be given advice on how to administer ciclesonide aerosol inhaler.

● MEDICINAL FORMS There can be variation in the licensing of different medicines containing the same drug.
Pressurised inhalation
CAUTIONARY AND ADVISORY LABELS 8
▶ Alvesco (AstraZeneca UK Ltd)
Ciclesonide 80 microgram per 1 dose Alvesco 80 inhaler | 120 dose [PoM] £32.83 DT = £32.83
Ciclesonide 160 microgram per 1 dose Alvesco 160 inhaler | 60 dose [PoM] £19.31 DT = £19.31 | 120 dose [PoM] £38.62 DT = £38.62

F 272

Fluticasone

25-Sep-2020

● INDICATIONS AND DOSE
Prophylaxis of asthma
▶ BY INHALATION OF POWDER
▶ Child 5-15 years: Initially 50–100 micrograms twice daily (max. per dose 200 micrograms twice daily), dose to be adjusted as necessary
▶ Child 16-17 years: Initially 100–500 micrograms twice daily (max. per dose 1 mg twice daily), dose may be increased according to severity of asthma. Doses above 500 micrograms twice daily initiated by a specialist
▶ Adult: Initially 100–500 micrograms twice daily (max. per dose 1 mg twice daily), dose may be increased according to severity of asthma. Doses above 500 micrograms twice daily initiated by a specialist
▶ BY INHALATION OF AEROSOL
▶ Child 4-15 years: Initially 50–100 micrograms twice daily (max. per dose 200 micrograms twice daily), dose to be adjusted as necessary
▶ Child 16-17 years: Initially 100–500 micrograms twice daily (max. per dose 1 mg twice daily), dose may be increased according to severity of asthma. Doses above 500 micrograms twice daily initiated by a specialist
▶ Adult: Initially 100–500 micrograms twice daily (max. per dose 1 mg twice daily), dose may be increased according to severity of asthma. Doses above 500 micrograms twice daily initiated by a specialist
▶ BY INHALATION OF NEBULISED SUSPENSION
▶ Child 4-15 years: 1 mg twice daily
▶ Child 16-17 years: 0.5–2 mg twice daily
▶ Adult: 0.5–2 mg twice daily

IMPORTANT SAFETY INFORMATION
MHRA/CHM ADVICE: PRESSURISED METERED DOSE INHALERS (PMDI): RISK OF AIRWAY OBSTRUCTION FROM ASPIRATION OF LOOSE OBJECTS (JULY 2018)
See Respiratory system, drug delivery p. 251.

● INTERACTIONS → Appendix 1: corticosteroids

● SIDE-EFFECTS
▶ Rare or very rare Dyspepsia

● DIRECTIONS FOR ADMINISTRATION [EvGr] Fluticasone nebuliser liquid may be diluted with sterile sodium chloride 0.9%. It is not suitable for use in ultrasonic nebulisers. ⟨M⟩

● PATIENT AND CARER ADVICE Patients or carers should be given advice on how to administer all fluticasone inhalation preparations.
With high doses, a steroid card should be supplied.

Medicines for Children leaflet: Fluticasone inhaler for asthma prevention (prophylaxis) www.medicinesforchildren.org.uk/fluticasone-inhaler-asthma-prevention-prophylaxis

● MEDICINAL FORMS There can be variation in the licensing of different medicines containing the same drug.

Inhalation powder
CAUTIONARY AND ADVISORY LABELS 8, 10
▸ Flixotide Accuhaler (GlaxoSmithKline UK Ltd)
Fluticasone propionate 50 microgram per 1 dose Flixotide 50micrograms/dose Accuhaler | 60 dose [PoM] £4.00 DT = £4.00
Fluticasone propionate 100 microgram per 1 dose Flixotide 100micrograms/dose Accuhaler | 60 dose [PoM] £8.00 DT = £8.00
Fluticasone propionate 250 microgram per 1 dose Flixotide 250micrograms/dose Accuhaler | 60 dose [PoM] £25.51 DT = £25.51
Fluticasone propionate 500 microgram per 1 dose Flixotide 500micrograms/dose Accuhaler | 60 dose [PoM] £43.37 DT = £43.37

Pressurised inhalation
CAUTIONARY AND ADVISORY LABELS 8, 10
▸ Flixotide Evohaler (GlaxoSmithKline UK Ltd)
Fluticasone propionate 50 microgram per 1 dose Flixotide 50micrograms/dose Evohaler | 120 dose [PoM] £6.53 DT = £6.53
Fluticasone propionate 125 microgram per 1 dose Flixotide 125micrograms/dose Evohaler | 120 dose [PoM] £21.26 DT = £21.26
Fluticasone propionate 250 microgram per 1 dose Flixotide 250micrograms/dose Evohaler | 120 dose [PoM] £36.14 DT = £36.14

Nebuliser liquid
CAUTIONARY AND ADVISORY LABELS 8, 10
▸ Flixotide Nebule (GlaxoSmithKline UK Ltd)
Fluticasone propionate 250 microgram per 1 ml Flixotide 0.5mg/2ml Nebules | 10 unit dose [PoM] £9.34 DT = £9.34
Fluticasone propionate 1 mg per 1 ml Flixotide 2mg/2ml Nebules | 10 unit dose [PoM] £37.35 DT = £37.35

Fluticasone with formoterol 10-Nov-2020

The properties listed below are those particular to the combination only. For the properties of the components please consider, fluticasone p. 278, formoterol fumarate p. 266.

● INDICATIONS AND DOSE
FLUTIFORM ® 125
Prophylaxis of asthma
▸ BY INHALATION OF AEROSOL
▸ Child 12–17 years: 2 puffs twice daily
▸ Adult: 2 puffs twice daily

FLUTIFORM ® 250
Prophylaxis of asthma
▸ BY INHALATION OF AEROSOL
▸ Adult: 2 puffs twice daily

FLUTIFORM ® 50
Prophylaxis of asthma
▸ BY INHALATION OF AEROSOL
▸ Child 5–17 years: 2 puffs twice daily
▸ Adult: 2 puffs twice daily

FLUTIFORM ® K-HALER 125
Prophylaxis of asthma
▸ BY INHALATION OF AEROSOL
▸ Child 12–17 years: 2 puffs twice daily
▸ Adult: 2 puffs twice daily

FLUTIFORM ® K-HALER 50
Prophylaxis of asthma
▸ BY INHALATION OF AEROSOL
▸ Child 12–17 years: 2 puffs twice daily
▸ Adult: 2 puffs twice daily

● INTERACTIONS → Appendix 1: beta₂ agonists · corticosteroids

● SIDE-EFFECTS
▸ **Uncommon** Dry mouth · rash · sleep disorders

▸ **Rare or very rare** Asthenia · cough · diarrhoea · dyspepsia · hypertension · muscle spasms · oral fungal infection · peripheral oedema · vertigo

● PATIENT AND CARER ADVICE Patients or carers should be given advice on how to administer fluticasone with formoterol aerosol inhalation.
With high doses, a steroid card should be provided.

● NATIONAL FUNDING/ACCESS DECISIONS
For full details see funding body website
Scottish Medicines Consortium (SMC) decisions
▸ **Fluticasone propionate with formoterol fumarate (***Flutiform*®**) for the regular treatment of asthma (October 2012)** SMC No. 736/11 Recommended
▸ **Fluticasone propionate with formoterol fumarate (***Flutiform*® **50/5 metered dose inhaler) for the regular treatment of asthma in children aged 5 to 12 years (June 2019)** SMC No. SMC2178 Recommended

● MEDICINAL FORMS There can be variation in the licensing of different medicines containing the same drug.
Pressurised inhalation
CAUTIONARY AND ADVISORY LABELS 8, 10 (high doses)
▸ Flutiform (Napp Pharmaceuticals Ltd)
Formoterol fumarate dihydrate 5 microgram per 1 dose, Fluticasone propionate 50 microgram per 1 dose Flutiform 50micrograms/dose / 5micrograms/dose inhaler | 120 dose [PoM] £14.40 DT = £14.40
Formoterol fumarate dihydrate 5 microgram per 1 dose, Fluticasone propionate 125 microgram per 1 dose Flutiform 125micrograms/dose / 5micrograms/dose inhaler | 120 dose [PoM] £28.00 DT = £28.00
Formoterol fumarate dihydrate 10 microgram per 1 dose, Fluticasone propionate 250 microgram per 1 dose Flutiform 250micrograms/dose / 10micrograms/dose inhaler | 120 dose [PoM] £45.56 DT = £45.56
▸ Flutiform K-haler (Napp Pharmaceuticals Ltd)
Formoterol fumarate dihydrate 5 microgram per 1 dose, Fluticasone propionate 50 microgram per 1 dose Flutiform K-haler 50micrograms/dose / 5micrograms/dose breath actuated inhaler | 120 dose [PoM] £14.40 DT = £14.40
Formoterol fumarate dihydrate 5 microgram per 1 dose, Fluticasone propionate 125 microgram per 1 dose Flutiform K-haler 125micrograms/dose / 5micrograms/dose breath actuated inhaler | 120 dose [PoM] £28.00 DT = £28.00

Fluticasone with salmeterol 05-May-2020

The properties listed below are those particular to the combination only. For the properties of the components please consider, fluticasone p. 278, salmeterol p. 268.

● INDICATIONS AND DOSE
AIRFLUSAL FORSPIRO ®
Chronic obstructive pulmonary disease with forced expiratory volume in 1 second <60% of predicted | Prophylaxis of asthma
▸ BY INHALATION OF POWDER
▸ Adult: 1 inhalation twice daily

AIRFLUSAL ® 125
Prophylaxis of moderate-to-severe asthma
▸ BY INHALATION OF AEROSOL
▸ Adult: 2 inhalations twice daily

AIRFLUSAL ® 250
Prophylaxis of moderate-to-severe asthma
▸ BY INHALATION OF AEROSOL
▸ Adult: 2 inhalations twice daily

COMBISAL ® 25/125
Prophylaxis of asthma
▸ BY INHALATION OF AEROSOL
▸ Child 12–17 years: 2 inhalations twice daily
▸ Adult: 2 inhalations twice daily

continued →

COMBISAL® 25/250

Prophylaxis of asthma
‣ BY INHALATION OF AEROSOL
‣ Child 12-17 years: 2 inhalations twice daily
‣ Adult: 2 inhalations twice daily

COMBISAL® 25/50

Prophylaxis of asthma
‣ BY INHALATION OF AEROSOL
‣ Child 4-17 years: 2 inhalations twice daily, reduced to 2 inhalations once daily, use reduced dose only if control maintained
‣ Adult: 2 inhalations twice daily, reduced to 2 inhalations once daily, use reduced dose only if control maintained

FUSACOMB 50/250 EASYHALER®

Prophylaxis of asthma
‣ BY INHALATION OF POWDER
‣ Child 12-17 years: 1 inhalation twice daily, reduced to 1 inhalation once daily, use reduced dose only if control maintained
‣ Adult: 1 inhalation twice daily, reduced to 1 inhalation once daily, use reduced dose only if control maintained

FUSACOMB 50/500 EASYHALER®

Prophylaxis of asthma
‣ BY INHALATION OF POWDER
‣ Child 12-17 years: 1 inhalation twice daily
‣ Adult: 1 inhalation twice daily

Chronic obstructive pulmonary disease [with forced expiratory volume in 1 second <60% of predicted]
‣ BY INHALATION OF POWDER
‣ Adult: 1 inhalation twice daily

SEREFLO® 125

Moderate-to-severe asthma
‣ BY INHALATION OF AEROSOL
‣ Adult: 2 inhalations twice daily

SEREFLO® 250

Moderate-to-severe asthma
‣ BY INHALATION OF AEROSOL
‣ Adult: 2 inhalations twice daily

SERETIDE 100 ACCUHALER®

Prophylaxis of asthma
‣ BY INHALATION OF POWDER
‣ Child 4-17 years: 1 inhalation twice daily, reduced to 1 inhalation once daily, use reduced dose only if control maintained
‣ Adult: 1 inhalation twice daily, reduced to 1 inhalation once daily, use reduced dose only if control maintained

SERETIDE 125 EVOHALER®

Prophylaxis of asthma
‣ BY INHALATION OF AEROSOL
‣ Child 12-17 years: 2 puffs twice daily
‣ Adult: 2 puffs twice daily

SERETIDE 250 ACCUHALER®

Prophylaxis of asthma
‣ BY INHALATION OF POWDER
‣ Child 12-17 years: 1 inhalation twice daily
‣ Adult: 1 inhalation twice daily

SERETIDE 250 EVOHALER®

Prophylaxis of asthma
‣ BY INHALATION OF AEROSOL
‣ Child 12-17 years: 2 puffs twice daily
‣ Adult: 2 puffs twice daily

SERETIDE 50 EVOHALER®

Prophylaxis of asthma
‣ BY INHALATION OF AEROSOL
‣ Child 4-17 years: 2 puffs twice daily, reduced to 2 puffs once daily, use reduced dose only if control maintained
‣ Adult: 2 puffs twice daily, reduced to 2 puffs once daily, use reduced dose only if control maintained

SERETIDE 500 ACCUHALER®

Prophylaxis of asthma
‣ BY INHALATION OF POWDER
‣ Child 12-17 years: 1 inhalation twice daily
‣ Adult: 1 inhalation twice daily

Chronic obstructive pulmonary disease with forced expiratory volume in 1 second <60% of predicted
‣ BY INHALATION OF POWDER
‣ Adult: 1 inhalation twice daily

● INTERACTIONS → Appendix 1: beta$_2$ agonists · corticosteroids

● PRESCRIBING AND DISPENSING INFORMATION

SEREFLO® 125 Manufacturer advises spacer devices are not compatible—if spacer device required, switch to alternative fixed-dose combination preparation.

COMBISAL® 25/50 Manufacturer advises only AeroChamber Plus® spacer devices are compatible.

COMBISAL® 25/125 Manufacturer advises only AeroChamber Plus® spacer devices are compatible.

COMBISAL® 25/250 Manufacturer advises only AeroChamber Plus® spacer devices are compatible.

● PATIENT AND CARER ADVICE Patients or carers should be given advice on how to administer fluticasone with salmeterol dry powder inhalation and aerosol inhalation.
　With preparations containing greater than 100 micrograms fluticasone, a steroid card should be provided.

● NATIONAL FUNDING/ACCESS DECISIONS
For full details see funding body website

Scottish Medicines Consortium (SMC) decisions
‣ Fluticasone with salmeterol combination inhaler (*Seretide 500 Accuhaler*®) for symptomatic treatment of patients with chronic obstructive pulmonary disease (January 2009) SMC No. 450/08 Not recommended

● MEDICINAL FORMS There can be variation in the licensing of different medicines containing the same drug.

Inhalation powder
CAUTIONARY AND ADVISORY LABELS 8, 10 (excluding Seretide 100 Accuhaler®)
‣ AirFluSal Forspiro (Sandoz Ltd)
　Salmeterol (as Salmeterol xinafoate) 50 microgram per 1 dose, Fluticasone propionate 500 microgram per 1 dose AirFluSal Forspiro 50micrograms/dose / 500micrograms/dose dry powder inhaler | 60 dose PoM £29.97 DT = £32.74
‣ Fusacomb Easyhaler (Orion Pharma (UK) Ltd)
　Salmeterol (as Salmeterol xinafoate) 50 microgram per 1 dose, Fluticasone propionate 250 microgram per 1 dose Fusacomb Easyhaler 50micrograms/dose / 250micrograms/dose dry powder inhaler | 60 dose PoM £21.50 DT = £33.95
　Salmeterol (as Salmeterol xinafoate) 50 microgram per 1 dose, Fluticasone propionate 500 microgram per 1 dose Fusacomb Easyhaler 50micrograms/dose / 500micrograms/dose dry powder inhaler | 60 dose PoM £26.99 DT = £32.74
‣ Seretide Accuhaler (GlaxoSmithKline UK Ltd)
　Salmeterol (as Salmeterol xinafoate) 50 microgram per 1 dose, Fluticasone propionate 100 microgram per 1 dose Seretide 100 Accuhaler | 60 dose PoM £17.46 DT = £17.46
　Salmeterol (as Salmeterol xinafoate) 50 microgram per 1 dose, Fluticasone propionate 250 microgram per 1 dose Seretide 250 Accuhaler | 60 dose PoM £33.95 DT = £33.95
　Salmeterol (as Salmeterol xinafoate) 50 microgram per 1 dose, Fluticasone propionate 500 microgram per 1 dose Seretide 500 Accuhaler | 60 dose PoM £32.74 DT = £32.74

Pressurised inhalation

CAUTIONARY AND ADVISORY LABELS 8, 10 (excluding Seretide 50 Evohaler ®)

▸ AirFluSal (Sandoz Ltd)

Salmeterol (as Salmeterol xinafoate) 25 microgram per 1 dose, Fluticasone propionate 125 microgram per 1 dose AirFluSal 25micrograms/dose / 125micrograms/dose inhaler | 120 dose [PoM] £16.42 DT = £23.45

Salmeterol (as Salmeterol xinafoate) 25 microgram per 1 dose, Fluticasone propionate 250 microgram per 1 dose AirFluSal 25micrograms/dose / 250micrograms/dose inhaler | 120 dose [PoM] £20.52 DT = £29.32

▸ Combisal (Aspire Pharma Ltd)

Salmeterol (as Salmeterol xinafoate) 25 microgram per 1 dose, Fluticasone propionate 50 microgram per 1 dose Combisal 25micrograms/dose / 50micrograms/dose inhaler | 120 dose [PoM] £13.50 DT = £17.46

Salmeterol (as Salmeterol xinafoate) 25 microgram per 1 dose, Fluticasone propionate 125 microgram per 1 dose Combisal 25micrograms/dose / 125micrograms/dose inhaler | 120 dose [PoM] £17.59 DT = £23.45

Salmeterol (as Salmeterol xinafoate) 25 microgram per 1 dose, Fluticasone propionate 250 microgram per 1 dose Combisal 25micrograms/dose / 250micrograms/dose inhaler | 120 dose [PoM] £27.99 DT = £29.32

▸ Sereflo (Cipla EU Ltd)

Salmeterol (as Salmeterol xinafoate) 25 microgram per 1 dose, Fluticasone propionate 125 microgram per 1 dose Sereflo 25micrograms/dose / 125micrograms/dose inhaler | 120 dose [PoM] £14.99 DT = £23.45

Salmeterol (as Salmeterol xinafoate) 25 microgram per 1 dose, Fluticasone propionate 250 microgram per 1 dose Sereflo 25micrograms/dose / 250micrograms/dose inhaler | 120 dose [PoM] £19.99 DT = £29.32

▸ Seretide Evohaler (GlaxoSmithKline UK Ltd)

Salmeterol (as Salmeterol xinafoate) 25 microgram per 1 dose, Fluticasone propionate 50 microgram per 1 dose Seretide 50 Evohaler | 120 dose [PoM] £17.46 DT = £17.46

Salmeterol (as Salmeterol xinafoate) 25 microgram per 1 dose, Fluticasone propionate 125 microgram per 1 dose Seretide 125 Evohaler | 120 dose [PoM] £23.45 DT = £23.45

Salmeterol (as Salmeterol xinafoate) 25 microgram per 1 dose, Fluticasone propionate 250 microgram per 1 dose Seretide 250 Evohaler | 120 dose [PoM] £29.32 DT = £29.32

F 265

Fluticasone with umeclidinium and vilanterol
06-Nov-2020

The properties listed below are those particular to the combination only. For the properties of the components please consider, fluticasone p. 278, umeclidinium p. 265.

● **INDICATIONS AND DOSE**

Maintenance of moderate-to-severe chronic obstructive pulmonary disease

▸ BY INHALATION OF POWDER

▸ Adult: 1 inhalation once daily, dose should be taken at the same time each day

● CAUTIONS Convulsive disorders · pulmonary tuberculosis · thyrotoxicosis

● INTERACTIONS → Appendix 1: beta₂ agonists · corticosteroids · umeclidinium

● SIDE-EFFECTS

▸ **Common or very common** Arthralgia · back pain · constipation · cough · increased risk of infection · oropharyngeal pain

▸ **Uncommon** Bone fracture · dry mouth · dysphonia

▸ **Frequency not known** Vision disorders

● HEPATIC IMPAIRMENT Manufacturer advises caution in moderate to severe impairment.

● PATIENT AND CARER ADVICE Patients or carers should be given advice on appropriate inhaler technique.

● NATIONAL FUNDING/ACCESS DECISIONS
For full details see funding body website

Scottish Medicines Consortium (SMC) decisions

▸ Fluticasone furoate with umeclidinium and vilanterol (*Trelegy® Ellipta®*) for maintenance treatment in adult patients with moderate to severe chronic obstructive pulmonary disease who are not adequately treated by a combination of an inhaled corticosteroid and a long-acting beta₂-agonist (February 2018) SMC No. 1303/18 Recommended with restrictions

● MEDICINAL FORMS There can be variation in the licensing of different medicines containing the same drug.

Inhalation powder

▸ Trelegy Ellipta (GlaxoSmithKline UK Ltd) ▼

Vilanterol (as Vilanterol trifenatate) 22 microgram per 1 dose, Umeclidinium bromide 65 microgram per 1 dose, Fluticasone furoate 92 microgram per 1 dose Trelegy Ellipta 92micrograms/dose / 55micrograms/dose / 22micrograms/dose dry powder inhaler | 30 dose [PoM] £44.50

F 265

Fluticasone with vilanterol
27-Jul-2018

The properties listed below are those particular to the combination only. For the properties of the components please consider, fluticasone p. 278.

● **INDICATIONS AND DOSE**

RELVAR ELLIPTA® 184 MICROGRAMS/22 MICROGRAMS

Prophylaxis of asthma

▸ BY INHALATION OF POWDER

▸ Child 12–17 years: 1 inhalation once daily

▸ Adult: 1 inhalation once daily

RELVAR ELLIPTA® 92 MICROGRAMS/22 MICROGRAMS

Prophylaxis of asthma

▸ BY INHALATION OF POWDER

▸ Child 12–17 years: 1 inhalation once daily

▸ Adult: 1 inhalation once daily

Chronic obstructive pulmonary disease with forced expiratory volume in 1 second < 70% of predicted

▸ BY INHALATION OF POWDER

▸ Adult: 1 inhalation once daily

● INTERACTIONS → Appendix 1: beta₂ agonists · corticosteroids

● SIDE-EFFECTS

▸ **Common or very common** Abdominal pain · arthralgia · back pain · bone fracture · cough · dysphonia · fever · increased risk of infection · oropharyngeal pain

▸ **Uncommon** Vision blurred

▸ **Rare or very rare** Angioedema · anxiety

● PREGNANCY Manufacturer advises use only if potential benefit outweighs risk.

● BREAST FEEDING Manufacturer advises avoid—no information available.

● HEPATIC IMPAIRMENT Manufacturer advises caution.

Dose adjustments Manufacturer advises maximum dose of 92 microgram/22 microgram once daily in moderate to severe impairment.

● PATIENT AND CARER ADVICE Patients or carers should be given advice on how to administer fluticasone with vilanterol powder for inhalation.

A steroid card should be provided.

● NATIONAL FUNDING/ACCESS DECISIONS
For full details see funding body website

Scottish Medicines Consortium (SMC) decisions

▸ Fluticasone furoate with vilanterol (*Relvar® Ellipta®*) for symptomatic treatment of adults with chronic obstructive pulmonary disease with a forced expiratory volume in 1 second (FEV₁) less than 70% predicted normal (post-bronchodilator) with an exacerbation history despite regular bronchodilator therapy (April 2014) SMC No. 953/14 Recommended with restrictions

● MEDICINAL FORMS There can be variation in the licensing of different medicines containing the same drug.

Inhalation powder

CAUTIONARY AND ADVISORY LABELS 8, 10
▸ Relvar Ellipta (GlaxoSmithKline UK Ltd)
Vilanterol 22 microgram per 1 dose, Fluticasone furoate 92 microgram per 1 dose Relvar Ellipta 92micrograms/dose / 22micrograms/dose dry powder inhaler | 30 dose [PoM] £22.00 DT = £22.00
Vilanterol 22 microgram per 1 dose, Fluticasone furoate 184 microgram per 1 dose Relvar Ellipta 184micrograms/dose / 22micrograms/dose dry powder inhaler | 30 dose [PoM] £29.50 DT = £29.50

F 265

Indacaterol with mometasone furoate

19-Nov-2020

The properties listed below are those particular to the combination only. For the properties of the components please consider, mometasone furoate below.

● **INDICATIONS AND DOSE**

ATECTURA BREEZHALER ® 125/127.5
Prophylaxis of asthma
▸ BY INHALATION OF POWDER
▸ **Adult:** 1 inhalation once daily

ATECTURA BREEZHALER ® 125/260
Prophylaxis of asthma
▸ BY INHALATION OF POWDER
▸ **Adult:** 1 inhalation once daily

ATECTURA BREEZHALER ® 125/62.5
Prophylaxis of asthma
▸ BY INHALATION OF POWDER
▸ **Adult:** 1 inhalation once daily

● INTERACTIONS → Appendix 1: beta$_2$ agonists · corticosteroids

● SIDE-EFFECTS
▸ **Common or very common** Asthma exacerbated · dysphonia · hypersensitivity · increased risk of infection · myalgia · odynophagia · oral pain · oropharyngeal complaints · pain · skin reactions · tension headache · throat irritation
▸ **Uncommon** Anal pruritus · angioedema · cataract · eye inflammation · eye pruritus · genital pruritus · nasal pruritus · vision blurred

● PREGNANCY [EvGr] Use only if potential benefit outweighs risk. ◈

● BREAST FEEDING [EvGr] Avoid—present in milk in *animal* studies. ◈

● HEPATIC IMPAIRMENT [EvGr] Avoid in severe impairment unless potential benefit outweighs risk (no information available). ◈

● PATIENT AND CARER ADVICE [EvGr] Patients and carers should be given advice on appropriate inhaler technique and reminded that the capsules are not for oral administration. ◈

● MEDICINAL FORMS There can be variation in the licensing of different medicines containing the same drug.

Inhalation powder
▸ Atectura Breezhaler (Sandoz Ltd)
Mometasone furoate 62.5 microgram per 1 dose, Indacaterol (as Indacaterol acetate) 125 microgram per 1 dose Atectura Breezhaler 125micrograms/62.5micrograms inhalation powder capsules with device | 30 capsule [PoM] £17.49
Indacaterol (as Indacaterol acetate) 125 microgram per 1 dose, Mometasone furoate 127.5 microgram per 1 dose Atectura

Breezhaler 125micrograms/127.5micrograms inhalation powder capsules with device | 30 capsule [PoM] £21.50
Indacaterol (as Indacaterol acetate) 125 microgram per 1 dose, Mometasone furoate 260 microgram per 1 dose Atectura Breezhaler 125micrograms/260micrograms inhalation powder capsules with device | 30 capsule [PoM] £27.97

F 272

Mometasone furoate

10-Nov-2020

● **INDICATIONS AND DOSE**

Prophylaxis of asthma
▸ BY INHALATION OF POWDER
▸ **Child 12–17 years:** Initially 400 micrograms daily in 1–2 divided doses, single dose to be inhaled in the evening, reduced to 200 micrograms once daily, if control maintained
▸ **Adult:** Initially 400 micrograms daily in 1–2 divided doses, single dose to be inhaled in the evening, reduced to 200 micrograms once daily, if control maintained

Prophylaxis of severe asthma
▸ BY INHALATION OF POWDER
▸ **Child 12–17 years:** Increased if necessary up to 400 micrograms twice daily
▸ **Adult:** Increased if necessary up to 400 micrograms twice daily

● INTERACTIONS → Appendix 1: corticosteroids

● SIDE-EFFECTS
▸ **Common or very common** Candida infection

● PATIENT AND CARER ADVICE
Medicines for Children leaflet: Mometasone furoate inhaler for asthma prevention (prophylaxis) www.medicinesforchildren.org. uk/mometasone-furoate-inhaler-asthma-prevention-prophylaxis
Patients or carers should be given advice on how to administer mometasone by inhaler. With high doses, a steroid card should be supplied.

● NATIONAL FUNDING/ACCESS DECISIONS
For full details see funding body website

Scottish Medicines Consortium (SMC) decisions
▸ Mometasone furoate (*Asmanex® Twisthaler®*) for asthma (November 2003) SMC No. 79/03 Recommended with restrictions

● MEDICINAL FORMS There can be variation in the licensing of different medicines containing the same drug.

Inhalation powder
CAUTIONARY AND ADVISORY LABELS 8, 10
▸ Asmanex Twisthaler (Merck Sharp & Dohme Ltd)
Mometasone furoate 200 microgram per 1 dose Asmanex 200micrograms/dose Twisthaler | 30 dose [PoM] £15.70 DT = £15.70 | 60 dose [PoM] £23.54 DT = £23.54
Mometasone furoate 400 microgram per 1 dose Asmanex 400micrograms/dose Twisthaler | 30 dose [PoM] £21.78 DT = £21.78 | 60 dose [PoM] £36.05 DT = £36.05

F 265

Mometasone furoate with glycopyrronium bromide and indacaterol

27-Nov-2020

The properties listed below are those particular to the combination only. For the properties of the components please consider, mometasone furoate above, glycopyrronium bromide p. 262.

● **INDICATIONS AND DOSE**

Prophylaxis of asthma
▸ BY INHALATION OF POWDER
▸ **Adult:** 1 inhalation once daily

- INTERACTIONS → Appendix 1: beta$_2$ agonists · corticosteroids · glycopyrronium
- SIDE-EFFECTS
- ► **Common or very common** Asthma exacerbated · cough · cystitis · dysphonia · fever · gastrointestinal disorders · hypersensitivity · increased risk of infection · myalgia · odynophagia · oropharyngeal complaints · pain · skin reactions · tension headache · throat complaints
- ► **Uncommon** Cataract · dry mouth · dysuria · eye pruritus · genital pruritus
- PREGNANCY [EvGr] Use only if potential benefit outweighs risk—limited information available. ◁M▷
- BREAST FEEDING [EvGr] Avoid—present in milk in *animal* studies. ◁M▷
- HEPATIC IMPAIRMENT [EvGr] Avoid in severe impairment unless potential benefit outweighs risk (limited information available). ◁M▷
- RENAL IMPAIRMENT [EvGr] Use with caution in severe impairment or end-stage renal disease—limited information available. ◁M▷
- PATIENT AND CARER ADVICE [EvGr] Patients and carers should be given advice on appropriate inhaler technique and reminded that the capsules are not for oral administration. ◁M▷

- MEDICINAL FORMS There can be variation in the licensing of different medicines containing the same drug.
  Inhalation powder
  ► Enerzair Breezhaler (Sandoz Ltd)
    Glycopyrronium (as Glycopyrronium bromide) 46 microgram per 1 dose, Indacaterol (as Indacaterol acetate) 114 microgram per 1 dose, Mometasone furoate 136 microgram per 1 dose Enerzair Breezhaler 114micrograms/dose / 46micrograms/dose / 136micrograms/dose inhalation powder capsules with device | 30 capsule [PoM] £44.50

ENZYME INHIBITORS

Human alpha$_1$-proteinase inhibitor

20-Aug-2020

- DRUG ACTION Human alpha$_1$-proteinase inhibitor is a normal plasma constituent; it inhibits neutrophil elastase (an enzyme released in response to inflammation) in the lungs.

- INDICATIONS AND DOSE
  Progression of emphysema in patients with severe alpha$_1$-proteinase inhibitor deficiency, despite optimal treatment with other standard therapies (specialist use only)
  ► BY INTRAVENOUS INFUSION
  ► Adult: 60 mg/kg once weekly

- CONTRA-INDICATIONS IgA deficiency with confirmed antibodies against IgA—increased risk of severe hypersensitivity reactions
- CAUTIONS Consider vaccination against hepatitis A and hepatitis B · hypersensitivity reactions · IgA deficiency (without known antibodies to IgA)—increased risk of hypersensitivity reactions
  CAUTIONS, FURTHER INFORMATION
- ► **Hypersensitivity reactions** Hypersensitivity reactions may occur, even in patients who have previously tolerated treatment. Manufacturer advises close monitoring, including vital signs, during the first infusions. If a reaction occurs, manufacturer advises to decrease the rate of infusion or discontinue treatment; if symptoms improve promptly after stopping, the infusion may be resumed at a slower infusion rate.
- SIDE-EFFECTS
- ► **Common or very common** Dizziness · headache · nausea

- ► **Uncommon** Asthenia · confusion · flushing · hypersensitivity · hypotension · sensation abnormal · skin reactions · syncope · tachycardia · throat oedema
- ► **Rare or very rare** Chest pain · chills · fever · hyperhidrosis
- ► **Frequency not known** Eye swelling · facial swelling · lip swelling · lymph node pain
- PREGNANCY Manufacturer advises caution—no information available.
- BREAST FEEDING Manufacturer advises avoid—no information available.
- PRESCRIBING AND DISPENSING INFORMATION Manufacturer advises to record the brand name and batch number after each administration (in case of transmission of infective agents).
- PATIENT AND CARER ADVICE Manufacturer advises patients receiving treatment at home should receive appropriate training regarding self-administration, and be informed of the signs of hypersensitivity reactions.
  Driving and skilled tasks Manufacturer advises patients and carers should be counselled on the effects on driving and performance of skilled tasks—increased risk of dizziness.
- NATIONAL FUNDING/ACCESS DECISIONS
  For full details see funding body website
  Scottish Medicines Consortium (SMC) decisions
- ► Human alpha1-proteinase inhibitor (*Respreeza*®) for maintenance treatment, to slow the progression of emphysema in adults with documented severe alpha1-proteinase inhibitor (A1-PI) deficiency (August 2016) SMC No. 1157/16 Not recommended
  All Wales Medicines Strategy Group (AWMSG) decisions
- ► Human alpha1-proteinase inhibitor (*Respreeza*®) for maintenance treatment, to slow the progression of emphysema in adults with documented severe alpha1-proteinase inhibitor deficiency (March 2017) AWMSG No. 47 Not recommended

- MEDICINAL FORMS There can be variation in the licensing of different medicines containing the same drug.
  Powder and solvent for solution for infusion
  ELECTROLYTES: May contain Sodium
  ► Respreeza (CSL Behring UK Ltd)
    Human alpha1-proteinase inhibitor 1 gram Respreeza 1000mg powder and solvent for solution for infusion vials | 1 vial [PoM] £220.00

IMMUNOSUPPRESSANTS ⟩ MONOCLONAL ANTIBODIES

Benralizumab

03-Nov-2020

- DRUG ACTION Benralizumab is a humanised monoclonal antibody that interferes with interleukin-5 receptor binding, thereby reducing the survival of eosinophils and basophils.

- INDICATIONS AND DOSE
  Severe eosinophilic asthma (specialist use only)
  ► BY SUBCUTANEOUS INJECTION
  ► Adult: Initially 30 mg every 4 weeks for the first 3 doses, then maintenance 30 mg every 8 weeks, to be administered into the thigh, abdomen or upper arm
  PHARMACOKINETICS
  ► The half-life of benralizumab is approx. 15 days.

- CAUTIONS Pre-existing helminth infection
  CAUTIONS, FURTHER INFORMATION
- ► **Helminth infection** Manufacturer advises to treat pre-existing helminth infections before starting benralizumab—if patient becomes infected during therapy and does not respond to anti-helminth treatment, discontinue benralizumab until infection is resolved.

- SIDE-EFFECTS
  ▶ **Common or very common** Fever · headache · hypersensitivity (may be delayed) · increased risk of infection · skin reactions
  ▶ **Frequency not known** Anaphylactic reaction
- PREGNANCY Manufacturer advises avoid unless potential benefit outweighs risk—limited data available.
- BREAST FEEDING Manufacturer advises avoid—no information available.
- DIRECTIONS FOR ADMINISTRATION Manufacturer advises to take the syringe out of the refrigerator at least 30 minutes before administration, and to avoid injecting into areas of the skin that are tender, bruised, erythematous, or hardened—consult product literature for further information.
- HANDLING AND STORAGE Manufacturer advises store in a refrigerator (2–8°C) and protect from light.
- PATIENT AND CARER ADVICE Manufacturer advises patients and their carers should be instructed to seek medical advice if their asthma remains uncontrolled or if symptoms worsen after initiation of treatment.
- NATIONAL FUNDING/ACCESS DECISIONS
  For full details see funding body website
  NICE decisions
  ▶ Benralizumab for treating severe eosinophilic asthma (updated September 2019) NICE TA565 Recommended with restrictions
  Scottish Medicines Consortium (SMC) decisions
  ▶ Benralizumab (*Fasenra*®) as add-on maintenance treatment in adult patients with severe eosinophilic asthma inadequately controlled despite high-dose inhaled corticosteroids plus long-acting beta-agonists (June 2019) SMC No. SMC2155 Recommended with restrictions
- MEDICINAL FORMS There can be variation in the licensing of different medicines containing the same drug.
  Solution for injection
  ▶ Fasenra (AstraZeneca UK Ltd) ▼
    Benralizumab 30 mg per 1 ml Fasenra 30mg/1ml solution for injection pre-filled syringes | 1 pre-filled disposable injection PoM £1,955.00
    Fasenra 30mg/1ml solution for injection pre-filled pens | 1 pre-filled disposable injection PoM £1,955.00

| Mepolizumab

23-Oct-2020

- DRUG ACTION Mepolizumab is a humanised anti-interleukin-5 (anti-IL-5) monoclonal antibody; it reduces the production and survival of eosinophils.

- INDICATIONS AND DOSE
  Add on treatment for severe refractory eosinophilic asthma (under expert supervision)
  ▶ BY SUBCUTANEOUS INJECTION
  ▶ Adult: 100 mg every 4 weeks

- CAUTIONS Helminth infection
  CAUTIONS, FURTHER INFORMATION
  ▶ Helminth infections Manufacturer advises pre-existing helminth infections should be treated before initiation of therapy; if patients become infected during treatment and do not respond to anti-helminth treatment, consider treatment interruption.

- SIDE-EFFECTS
  ▶ **Common or very common** Abdominal pain upper · administration related reaction · back pain · eczema · fever · headache · hypersensitivity · increased risk of infection · nasal congestion

- PREGNANCY Manufacturer advises avoid unless potential benefit outweighs risk—limited data available.

- BREAST FEEDING Manufacturer advises avoid—present in milk in *animal* studies.
- DIRECTIONS FOR ADMINISTRATION Manufacturer advises injection is given into the thigh, abdomen, or upper arm. Patients may self-administer *Nucala*® pre-filled devices into the thigh or abdomen after appropriate training in preparation and administration.
- PRESCRIBING AND DISPENSING INFORMATION Mepolizumab is a biological medicine. Biological medicines must be prescribed and dispensed by brand name, see *Biological medicines* and *Biosimilar medicines*, under Guidance on prescribing p. 1; manufacturer advises to record the brand name and batch number after each administration.
- PATIENT AND CARER ADVICE
  Asthma Patients and their carers should be advised to seek medical advice if their asthma remains uncontrolled or worsens after initiation of treatment.
- NATIONAL FUNDING/ACCESS DECISIONS
  For full details see funding body website
  NICE decisions
  ▶ Mepolizumab for treating severe refractory eosinophilic asthma (January 2017) NICE TA431 Recommended with restrictions
  Scottish Medicines Consortium (SMC) decisions
  ▶ Mepolizumab (*Nucala*®) as an add-on treatment for severe refractory eosinophilic asthma in adult patients (June 2016) SMC No. 1149/16 Recommended with restrictions
- MEDICINAL FORMS There can be variation in the licensing of different medicines containing the same drug.
  Solution for injection
  EXCIPIENTS: May contain Edetic acid (edta), polysorbates
  ▶ Nucala (GlaxoSmithKline UK Ltd)
    Mepolizumab 100 mg per 1 ml Nucala 100mg/1ml solution for injection pre-filled pens | 1 pre-filled disposable injection PoM £840.00
    Nucala 100mg/1ml solution for injection pre-filled syringes | 1 pre-filled disposable injection PoM £840.00
  Powder for solution for injection
  EXCIPIENTS: May contain Polysorbates
  ▶ Nucala (GlaxoSmithKline UK Ltd)
    Mepolizumab 100 mg Nucala 100mg powder for solution for injection vials | 1 vial PoM £840.00 (Hospital only)

| Omalizumab

27-Mar-2020

- INDICATIONS AND DOSE
  Prophylaxis of severe persistent allergic asthma
  ▶ BY SUBCUTANEOUS INJECTION
  ▶ Adult: Dose according to immunoglobulin E concentration and body-weight (consult product literature)
  Add-on therapy for chronic spontaneous urticaria in patients who have had an inadequate response to H$_1$ antihistamine treatment
  ▶ BY SUBCUTANEOUS INJECTION
  ▶ Adult: 300 mg every 4 weeks

- CAUTIONS Autoimmune disease · susceptibility to helminth infection—discontinue if infection does not respond to anthelmintic

- SIDE-EFFECTS
  ▶ **Common or very common** Headache · skin reactions
  ▶ **Uncommon** Cough · diarrhoea · dizziness · drowsiness · dyspepsia · fatigue · flushing · increased risk of infection · influenza like illness · limb swelling · nausea · paraesthesia · photosensitivity reaction · postural hypotension · respiratory disorders · syncope · weight increased
  ▶ **Rare or very rare** Angioedema · hypersensitivity · systemic lupus erythematosus (SLE)

▶ **Frequency not known** Alopecia · eosinophilic granulomatosis with polyangiitis · immune thrombocytopenic purpura · joint disorders · lymphadenopathy · myalgia

SIDE-EFFECTS, FURTHER INFORMATION **Eosinophilic granulomatosis with polyangiitis (Churg-Strauss syndrome)** Churg-Strauss syndrome has occurred rarely in patients given omalizumab; the reaction is usually associated with the reduction of oral corticosteroid therapy. Churg-Strauss syndrome can present as eosinophilia, vasculitic rash, cardiac complications, worsening pulmonary symptoms, or peripheral neuropathy.

Hypersensitivity reactions Hypersensitivity reactions can also occur immediately following treatment with omalizumab or sometimes more than 24 hours after the first injection.

● PREGNANCY Manufacturer advises avoid unless essential—crosses the placenta.

● BREAST FEEDING Manufacturer advises avoid—present in milk in *animal* studies.

● HEPATIC IMPAIRMENT Manufacturer advises caution (no information available).

● RENAL IMPAIRMENT Manufacturer advises caution—no information available.

● NATIONAL FUNDING/ACCESS DECISIONS
For full details see funding body website
NICE decisions
▶ **Omalizumab for severe persistent allergic asthma (April 2013)** NICE TA278 Recommended
▶ **Omalizumab for previously treated chronic spontaneous urticaria (June 2015)** NICE TA339 Recommended with restrictions
Scottish Medicines Consortium (SMC) decisions
▶ **Omalizumab (*Xolair*®) as add-on therapy for the treatment of chronic spontaneous urticaria in adult and adolescent (12 years and above) patients with inadequate response to H$_1$-antihistamine treatment (January 2015)** SMC No. 1017/14 Recommended with restrictions

● MEDICINAL FORMS There can be variation in the licensing of different medicines containing the same drug.
Solution for injection
▶ Xolair (Novartis Pharmaceuticals UK Ltd)
Omalizumab 150 mg per 1 ml Xolair 150mg/1ml solution for injection pre-filled syringes | 1 pre-filled disposable injection PoM £256.17 DT = £256.17
Xolair 75mg/0.5ml solution for injection pre-filled syringes | 1 pre-filled disposable injection PoM £128.07 DT = £128.07

Reslizumab   25-Aug-2020

● DRUG ACTION Reslizumab is a humanised monoclonal antibody that interferes with interleukin-5 receptor binding, thereby reducing the survival and activity of eosinophils.

● INDICATIONS AND DOSE

Severe eosinophilic asthma (adjunctive therapy when inadequately controlled by high-dose corticosteroids plus another standard treatment) (specialist use only)
▶ BY INTRAVENOUS INFUSION
▶ Adult: (consult product literature)
PHARMACOKINETICS
▶ The half-life of reslizumab is approx. 24 days.

● CAUTIONS Hypersensitivity reactions · pre-existing helminth infection
CAUTIONS, FURTHER INFORMATION
▶ Helminth infection Manufacturer advises to treat pre-existing helminth infections before starting reslizumab—

consider temporarily discontinuing reslizumab if patient becomes infected during therapy and does not respond to anti-helminth treatment.
▶ Hypersensitivity reactions Serious hypersensitivity reactions, including life-threatening anaphylaxis, can occur and manufacturer advises to monitor closely during treatment and for at least 20 minutes after completion of infusion; in the event of a hypersensitivity reaction, treatment should be permanently discontinued.

● SIDE-EFFECTS
▶ **Uncommon** Anaphylactic reaction · myalgia
▶ **Frequency not known** Secondary malignancy

● PREGNANCY Manufacturer advises avoid—limited information available.

● BREAST FEEDING Manufacturer advises avoid during first few days after birth—risk of transfer of antibodies to infant cannot be excluded; present in milk in *animal* studies.

● DIRECTIONS FOR ADMINISTRATION For *intravenous infusion*, manufacturer advises give intermittently in Sodium chloride 0.9%; administer over 20–50 minutes through an in-line 0.2 micron filter.

● HANDLING AND STORAGE Manufacturer advises store in a refrigerator (2–8°C); consult product literature for storage conditions after preparation of infusion.

● PATIENT AND CARER ADVICE Manufacturer advises patients and their carers should be instructed to seek medical advice if their asthma remains uncontrolled or if symptoms worsen after initiation of treatment.

● NATIONAL FUNDING/ACCESS DECISIONS
For full details see funding body website
NICE decisions
▶ **Reslizumab for treating severe eosinophilic asthma (October 2017)** NICE TA479 Recommended with restrictions
Scottish Medicines Consortium (SMC) decisions
▶ **Reslizumab (*Cinqaero*®) as add-on therapy in adult patients with severe eosinophilic asthma inadequately controlled despite high-dose inhaled corticosteroids plus another medicinal product for maintenance treatment (December 2017)** SMC No. 1233/17 Not recommended

● MEDICINAL FORMS There can be variation in the licensing of different medicines containing the same drug.
Solution for infusion
EXCIPIENTS: May contain Sucrose
▶ Cinqaero (Teva UK Ltd) ▼
Reslizumab 10 mg per 1 ml Cinqaero 100mg/10ml concentrate for solution for infusion vials | 1 vial PoM £499.99
Cinqaero 25mg/2.5ml concentrate for solution for infusion vials | 1 vial PoM £124.99

LEUKOTRIENE RECEPTOR ANTAGONISTS

Montelukast   10-Nov-2020

● INDICATIONS AND DOSE

Prophylaxis of asthma
▶ BY MOUTH
▶ Child 6 months–5 years: 4 mg once daily, dose to be taken in the evening
▶ Child 6–14 years: 5 mg once daily, dose to be taken in the evening
▶ Child 15–17 years: 10 mg once daily, dose to be taken in the evening
▶ Adult: 10 mg once daily, dose to be taken in the evening

Symptomatic relief of seasonal allergic rhinitis in patients with asthma
▶ BY MOUTH
▶ Child 15–17 years: 10 mg once daily, dose to be taken in the evening continued →

3

Respiratory system

▸ **Adult:** 10 mg once daily, dose to be taken in the evening

> **IMPORTANT SAFETY INFORMATION**
>
> MHRA/CHM ADVICE: MONTELUKAST (*SINGULAIR*®): REMINDER OF THE RISK OF NEUROPSYCHIATRIC REACTIONS (SEPTEMBER 2019)
>
> Healthcare professionals are advised to be alert for neuropsychiatric reactions, including speech impairment and obsessive-compulsive symptoms, in adults, adolescents, and children taking montelukast. The risks and benefits of continuing treatment should be evaluated if these reactions occur. Patients should be advised to read the list of neuropsychiatric reactions in the information leaflet and seek immediate medical attention if they occur.

● INTERACTIONS → Appendix 1: montelukast

● SIDE-EFFECTS

▸ **Common or very common** Diarrhoea · fever · gastrointestinal discomfort · headache · nausea · skin reactions · upper respiratory tract infection · vomiting
▸ **Uncommon** Akathisia · anxiety · arthralgia · asthenia · behaviour abnormal · depression · dizziness · drowsiness · dry mouth · haemorrhage · irritability · malaise · muscle complaints · oedema · seizure · sensation abnormal · sleep disorders
▸ **Rare or very rare** Angioedema · concentration impaired · disorientation · eosinophilic granulomatosis with polyangiitis · erythema nodosum · hallucination · hepatic disorders · memory loss · palpitations · psychiatric disorders · pulmonary eosinophilia · speech disorder · suicidal behaviours · tremor

SIDE-EFFECTS, FURTHER INFORMATION Eosinophilic granulomatosis with polyangiitis (Churg-Strauss syndrome) has occurred very rarely in association with the use of montelukast; in many of the reported cases the reaction followed the reduction or withdrawal of oral corticosteroid therapy. Prescribers should be alert to the development of eosinophilia, vasculitic rash, worsening pulmonary symptoms, cardiac complications, or peripheral neuropathy.

● PREGNANCY Manufacturer advises avoid unless essential. There is limited evidence for the safe use of montelukast during pregnancy; however, it can be taken as normal in women who have shown a significant improvement in asthma not achievable with other drugs before becoming pregnant.

● BREAST FEEDING Manufacturer advises avoid unless essential.

● DIRECTIONS FOR ADMINISTRATION Manufacturer advises granules may be swallowed or mixed with cold, soft food (not liquid) and taken immediately.

● PRESCRIBING AND DISPENSING INFORMATION Flavours of chewable tablet formulations may include cherry.

● PATIENT AND CARER ADVICE

Administration Patients or carers should be given advice on how to administer montelukast granules.

Risk of neuropsychiatric reactions The MHRA advises patients and carers to seek medical attention if changes in speech or behaviour occur—see also *Important safety information*.

Medicines for Children leaflet: Montelukast for asthma www.medicinesforchildren.org.uk/montelukast-asthma

● MEDICINAL FORMS There can be variation in the licensing of different medicines containing the same drug.

Granules

▸ Montelukast (Non-proprietary)

Montelukast (as Montelukast sodium) **4 mg** Montelukast 4mg granules sachets sugar free sugar-free | 28 sachet PoM £19.99 DT = £5.28

▸ Singulair (Merck Sharp & Dohme Ltd)

Montelukast (as Montelukast sodium) **4 mg** Singulair Paediatric 4mg granules sachets sugar-free | 28 sachet PoM £25.69 DT = £5.28

Tablet

▸ Montelukast (Non-proprietary)

Montelukast (as Montelukast sodium) **10 mg** Montelukast 10mg tablets | 28 tablet PoM £26.97 DT = £2.88

▸ Singulair (Merck Sharp & Dohme Ltd)

Montelukast (as Montelukast sodium) **10 mg** Singulair 10mg tablets | 28 tablet PoM £26.97 DT = £2.88

Chewable tablet

CAUTIONARY AND ADVISORY LABELS 23, 24
EXCIPIENTS: May contain Aspartame

▸ Montelukast (Non-proprietary)

Montelukast (as Montelukast sodium) **4 mg** Montelukast 4mg chewable tablets sugar free sugar-free | 28 tablet PoM £25.69 DT = £2.04

Montelukast (as Montelukast sodium) **5 mg** Montelukast 5mg chewable tablets sugar free sugar-free | 28 tablet PoM £25.69 DT = £2.25

▸ Singulair (Merck Sharp & Dohme Ltd)

Montelukast (as Montelukast sodium) **4 mg** Singulair Paediatric 4mg chewable tablets sugar-free | 28 tablet PoM £25.69 DT = £2.04

Montelukast (as Montelukast sodium) **5 mg** Singulair Paediatric 5mg chewable tablets sugar-free | 28 tablet PoM £25.69 DT = £2.25

MAST-CELL STABILISERS

Sodium cromoglicate

23-Nov-2020

(Sodium cromoglycate)

● INDICATIONS AND DOSE

Prophylaxis of asthma

▸ BY INHALATION OF AEROSOL

▸ **Child 5–17 years:** Initially 10 mg 4 times a day, additional dose may also be taken before exercise, increased if necessary to 10 mg 6–8 times a day; maintenance 5 mg 4 times a day, 5 mg is equivalent to 1 puff

▸ **Adult:** Initially 10 mg 4 times a day, additional dose may also be taken before exercise, increased if necessary to 10 mg 6–8 times a day; maintenance 5 mg 4 times a day, 5 mg is equivalent to 1 puff

Food allergy (in conjunction with dietary restriction)

▸ BY MOUTH

▸ **Child 2–13 years:** Initially 100 mg 4 times a day for 2–3 weeks, then increased if necessary up to 40 mg/kg daily, then reduced according to response, to be taken before meals

▸ **Child 14–17 years:** Initially 200 mg 4 times a day for 2–3 weeks, then increased if necessary up to 40 mg/kg daily, then reduced according to response, to be taken before meals

▸ **Adult:** Initially 200 mg 4 times a day for 2–3 weeks, then increased if necessary up to 40 mg/kg daily, then reduced according to response, to be taken before meals

> **IMPORTANT SAFETY INFORMATION**
>
> MHRA/CHM ADVICE: PRESSURISED METERED DOSE INHALERS (PMDI): RISK OF AIRWAY OBSTRUCTION FROM ASPIRATION OF LOOSE OBJECTS (JULY 2018)
>
> See Respiratory system, drug delivery p. 251.

● CAUTIONS

▸ When used by inhalation Discontinue if eosinophilic pneumonia occurs

● SIDE-EFFECTS

▸ When used by inhalation Cough · headache · pneumonia eosinophilic · rhinitis · throat irritation
▸ With oral use Arthralgia · nausea · rash

SIDE-EFFECTS, FURTHER INFORMATION When used by inhalation, if paradoxical bronchospasm occurs, a short-acting beta$_2$-agonist should be used to control symptoms; treatment with sodium cromoglicate should be discontinued.

- PREGNANCY Not known to be harmful.
  - When used by inhalation Can be taken as normal during pregnancy.
- BREAST FEEDING Unlikely to be present in milk.
  - When used by inhalation Can be taken as normal during breast-feeding.
- TREATMENT CESSATION
  - When used by inhalation Withdrawal of sodium cromoglicate should be done gradually over a period of one week—symptoms of asthma may recur.
- DIRECTIONS FOR ADMINISTRATION
  - With oral use Expert sources advise capsules may be swallowed whole or the contents dissolved in hot water and diluted with cold water before taking.
- PATIENT AND CARER ADVICE
  - With oral use Patient counselling is advised for sodium cromoglicate capsules (administration).
  - When used by inhalation Patient counselling is advised for sodium cromoglicate pressurised inhalation (administration).

- MEDICINAL FORMS There can be variation in the licensing of different medicines containing the same drug. Forms available from special-order manufacturers include: oral solution

Capsule
CAUTIONARY AND ADVISORY LABELS 22
  - Nalcrom (Sanofi)
    Sodium cromoglicate 100 mg Nalcrom 100mg capsules | 100 capsule [PoM] £41.14 DT = £41.14

Pressurised inhalation
CAUTIONARY AND ADVISORY LABELS 8
  - Intal (Sanofi)
    Sodium cromoglicate 5 mg per 1 dose Intal 5mg/dose inhaler CFC free | 112 dose [PoM] £18.33 DT = £18.33

PHOSPHODIESTERASE TYPE-4 INHIBITORS

Roflumilast
02-Sep-2020

- DRUG ACTION Roflumilast is a phosphodiesterase type-4 inhibitor with anti-inflammatory properties.

- INDICATIONS AND DOSE
  Adjunct to bronchodilators for the maintenance treatment of patients with severe chronic obstructive pulmonary disease associated with chronic bronchitis and a history of frequent exacerbations
  - BY MOUTH
  - Adult: Initially 250 micrograms once daily for 28 days, then maintenance 500 micrograms once daily

- CONTRA-INDICATIONS Cancer (except basal cell carcinoma) · concomitant treatment with immunosuppressive drugs (except short-term systemic corticosteroids) · history of depression associated with suicidal ideation or behaviour · moderate to severe cardiac failure · severe acute infectious disease · severe immunological disease
- CAUTIONS History of psychiatric illness (discontinue if new or worsening psychiatric symptoms occur) · latent infection (such as tuberculosis, viral hepatitis, herpes infection)
- INTERACTIONS → Appendix 1: phosphodiesterase type-4 inhibitors
- SIDE-EFFECTS
  - **Common or very common** Appetite decreased · diarrhoea · gastrointestinal discomfort · headache · insomnia · nausea · weight decreased
  - **Uncommon** Anxiety · asthenia · back pain · dizziness · gastrointestinal disorders · malaise · muscle complaints ·

muscle weakness · palpitations · skin reactions · tremor · vertigo · vomiting
  - **Rare or very rare** Angioedema · constipation · depression · gynaecomastia · haematochezia · respiratory tract infection · suicidal behaviours · taste altered
- CONCEPTION AND CONTRACEPTION Women of child-bearing age should use effective contraception.
- PREGNANCY Manufacturer advises avoid—toxicity in *animal* studies.
- BREAST FEEDING Manufacturer advises avoid—present in milk in *animal* studies.
- HEPATIC IMPAIRMENT Manufacturer advises caution in mild impairment; avoid in moderate to severe impairment.
- MONITORING REQUIREMENTS Monitor body-weight.
- PATIENT AND CARER ADVICE Manufacturer advises patients and carers should be instructed to report changes in behaviour or mood and any suicidal ideation.
  Patient card Patients should be given a patient card before starting treatment and advised to record body-weight at regular intervals.
- NATIONAL FUNDING/ACCESS DECISIONS
  For full details see funding body website
  NICE decisions
  - Roflumilast for treating chronic obstructive pulmonary disease (July 2017) NICE TA461 Recommended with restrictions
  Scottish Medicines Consortium (SMC) decisions
  - Roflumilast (*Daxas*®) for the maintenance treatment of severe chronic obstructive pulmonary disease (COPD) (forced expiratory volume in one second [FEV1]) post-bronchodilator less than 50% predicted) associated with chronic bronchitis in adult patients with a history of frequent exacerbations as add on to bronchodilator treatment (September 2017) SMC No. 635/10 Not recommended

- MEDICINAL FORMS There can be variation in the licensing of different medicines containing the same drug.
Tablet
  - Daxas (AstraZeneca UK Ltd) ▼
    Roflumilast 250 microgram Daxas 250microgram tablets | 28 tablet [PoM] £35.20 DT = £35.20
    Roflumilast 500 microgram Daxas 500microgram tablets | 30 tablet [PoM] £37.71 DT = £37.71

SYMPATHOMIMETICS > VASOCONSTRICTOR

Ephedrine hydrochloride
04-Dec-2019

- INDICATIONS AND DOSE
  Reversal of hypotension from spinal or epidural anaesthesia
  - BY SLOW INTRAVENOUS INJECTION
  - Adult: 3–6 mg every 3–4 minutes (max. per dose 9 mg), adjusted according to response, injection solution to contain ephedrine hydrochloride 3 mg/ml; maximum 30 mg per course
  Reversible airways obstruction
  - BY MOUTH
  - Adult: 15–60 mg 3 times a day
  Neuropathic oedema
  - BY MOUTH
  - Adult: 30–60 mg 3 times a day

- UNLICENSED USE
  - With oral use Not licensed for neuropathic oedema.
- CAUTIONS
  GENERAL CAUTIONS Diabetes mellitus · elderly · hypertension · hyperthyroidism · ischaemic heart disease · prostatic hypertrophy (risk of acute urinary retention)

3

Respiratory system

SPECIFIC CAUTIONS
▸ With intravenous use Susceptibility to angle-closure glaucoma

● INTERACTIONS → Appendix 1: sympathomimetics, vasoconstrictor

● SIDE-EFFECTS
GENERAL SIDE-EFFECTS
▸ **Common or very common** Anxiety · headache · insomnia · nausea
▸ **Frequency not known** Tremor
SPECIFIC SIDE-EFFECTS
▸ **Common or very common**
▸ With intravenous use Arrhythmias · asthenia · confusion · depression · dyspnoea · hyperhidrosis · irritability · palpitations · vomiting
▸ **Rare or very rare**
▸ With intravenous use Acute urinary retention
▸ With oral use Myocardial infarction
▸ **Frequency not known**
▸ With intravenous use Acute angle closure glaucoma · angina pectoris · appetite decreased · cardiac arrest · dizziness · hypokalaemia · intracranial haemorrhage · psychotic disorder · pulmonary oedema
▸ With oral use Arrhythmias · circulation impaired · dry mouth · enuresis · hypertension · sedation

● PREGNANCY
▸ With oral use Manufacturer advises avoid.
▸ With intravenous use Increased fetal heart rate reported with parenteral ephedrine.

● BREAST FEEDING Present in milk; manufacturer advises avoid—irritability and disturbed sleep reported.

● RENAL IMPAIRMENT Use with caution.

● LESS SUITABLE FOR PRESCRIBING
▸ With oral use Ephedrine tablets are less suitable and less safe for use as a bronchodilator than the selective beta₂ agonists.

● EXCEPTIONS TO LEGAL CATEGORY
▸ With oral use For exceptions relating to ephedrine tablets see *Medicines, Ethics and Practice*, London, Pharmaceutical Press (always consult latest edition).

● MEDICINAL FORMS There can be variation in the licensing of different medicines containing the same drug. Forms available from special-order manufacturers include: oral suspension, oral solution, solution for injection

Tablet
▸ Ephedrine hydrochloride (Non-proprietary)
  Ephedrine hydrochloride 15 mg Ephedrine hydrochloride 15mg tablets | 28 tablet [PoM] £114.24 DT = £76.34
  Ephedrine hydrochloride 30 mg Ephedrine hydrochloride 30mg tablets | 28 tablet [PoM] £172.94 DT = £115.71

Solution for injection
▸ Ephedrine hydrochloride (Non-proprietary)
  Ephedrine hydrochloride 3 mg per 1 ml Ephedrine 30mg/10ml solution for injection ampoules | 10 ampoule [PoM] £112.81
  Ephedrine 30mg/10ml solution for injection pre-filled syringes | 1 pre-filled disposable injection [PoM] £9.50 | 12 pre-filled disposable injection [PoM] £114.00
  Ephedrine hydrochloride 30 mg per 1 ml Ephedrine 30mg/1ml solution for injection ampoules | 10 ampoule [PoM] £52.50-£69.62 DT = £69.62

XANTHINES

Aminophylline

16-Dec-2020

● INDICATIONS AND DOSE
Severe acute asthma in patients not previously treated with theophylline
▸ BY SLOW INTRAVENOUS INJECTION
▸ Child: 5 mg/kg (max. per dose 500 mg), to be followed by intravenous infusion

▸ Adult: 250–500 mg (max. per dose 5 mg/kg), to be followed by intravenous infusion
Severe acute asthma
▸ BY INTRAVENOUS INFUSION
▸ Child 1 month-11 years: 1 mg/kg/hour, adjusted according to plasma-theophylline concentration
▸ Child 12-17 years: 500–700 micrograms/kg/hour, adjusted according to plasma-theophylline concentration
▸ Adult: 500–700 micrograms/kg/hour, adjusted according to plasma-theophylline concentration
▸ Elderly: 300 micrograms/kg/hour, adjusted according to plasma-theophylline concentration
Severe acute exacerbation of chronic obstructive pulmonary disease in patients not previously treated with theophylline
▸ BY SLOW INTRAVENOUS INJECTION
▸ Adult: 250–500 mg (max. per dose 5 mg/kg), to be followed by intravenous infusion
Severe acute exacerbation of chronic obstructive pulmonary disease
▸ BY INTRAVENOUS INFUSION
▸ Adult: 500–700 micrograms/kg/hour, adjusted according to plasma-theophylline concentration
▸ Elderly: 300 micrograms/kg/hour, adjusted according to plasma-theophylline concentration
Chronic asthma
▸ BY MOUTH USING MODIFIED-RELEASE MEDICINES
▸ Child (body-weight 40 kg and above): Initially 225 mg twice daily for 1 week, then increased if necessary to 450 mg twice daily, adjusted according to plasma-theophylline concentration
Reversible airway obstruction
▸ BY MOUTH USING MODIFIED-RELEASE MEDICINES
▸ Adult (body-weight 40 kg and above): Initially 225 mg twice daily for 1 week, then increased if necessary to 450 mg twice daily, adjusted according to plasma-theophylline concentration
DOSE ADJUSTMENTS DUE TO INTERACTIONS
▸ Dose adjustment may be necessary if smoking started or stopped during treatment.
DOSES AT EXTREMES OF BODY-WEIGHT
▸ To avoid excessive dosage in obese patients, dose should be calculated on the basis of ideal weight for height.
PHARMACOKINETICS
▸ Aminophylline is a stable mixture or combination of theophylline and ethylenediamine; the ethylenediamine confers greater solubility in water.
▸ Theophylline is metabolised in the liver. The plasma-theophylline concentration is increased in heart failure, hepatic impairment, and in viral infections. The plasma-theophylline concentration is decreased in smokers, and by alcohol consumption. Differences in the half-life of aminophylline are important because the toxic dose is close to the therapeutic dose.

PHYLLOCONTIN CONTINUS ® FORTE
Reversible airways obstruction
▸ BY MOUTH USING MODIFIED-RELEASE MEDICINES
▸ Adult: Initially 350 mg twice daily for 1 week, then increased if necessary to 700 mg twice daily, increase dose according to plasma-theophylline concentration

● UNLICENSED USE Aminophylline injection not licensed for use in children under 6 months.

● CAUTIONS Arrhythmias following rapid intravenous injection · cardiac arrhythmias or other cardiac disease · elderly (increased plasma-theophylline concentration) · epilepsy · fever · hypertension · peptic ulcer · risk of hypokalaemia · thyroid disorder

- INTERACTIONS → Appendix 1: aminophylline
- SIDE-EFFECTS
  GENERAL SIDE-EFFECTS
  Headache · nausea · palpitations · seizure (more common when given too rapidly by intravenous injection)
  SPECIFIC SIDE-EFFECTS
  ▸ With intravenous use Abdominal pain · anxiety · arrhythmia (more common when given too rapidly by intravenous injection) · confusion · delirium · diarrhoea · dizziness · electrolyte imbalance · gastrointestinal haemorrhage · gastro-oesophageal reflux disease · hyperthermia · hyperventilation · hypotension (more common when given too rapidly by intravenous injection) · insomnia · mania · metabolic disorder · pain · skin reactions · tachycardia (more common when given too rapidly by intravenous injection) · thirst · tremor · vertigo · visual impairment · vomiting
  ▸ With oral use Arrhythmias · central nervous system stimulation · epigastric discomfort
  SIDE-EFFECTS, FURTHER INFORMATION Potentially serious hypokalaemia may result from beta$_2$-agonist therapy. Particular caution is required in severe asthma, because this effect may be potentiated by concomitant treatment with theophylline and its derivatives, corticosteroids, and diuretics, and by hypoxia. Plasma-potassium concentration should therefore be monitored in severe asthma.

  Overdose Theophylline and related drugs are often prescribed as modified-release formulations and toxicity can therefore be delayed. They cause vomiting (which may be severe and intractable), agitation, restlessness, dilated pupils, sinus tachycardia, and hyperglycaemia. More serious effects are haematemesis, convulsions, and supraventricular and ventricular arrhythmias. Severe hypokalaemia may develop rapidly.
  For specific details on the management of poisoning, see *Theophylline*, under **Emergency treatment of poisoning p. 1413**.

- ALLERGY AND CROSS-SENSITIVITY Allergy to ethylenediamine can cause urticaria, erythema, and exfoliative dermatitis.
- PREGNANCY Neonatal irritability and apnoea have been reported. Theophylline can be taken as normal during pregnancy as it is particularly important that asthma should be well controlled during pregnancy.
- BREAST FEEDING Present in milk—irritability in infant reported; modified-release preparations preferable. Theophylline can be taken as normal during breast-feeding.
- HEPATIC IMPAIRMENT Manufacturer advises caution (risk of reduced clearance).
  Dose adjustments ▸ With oral use Manufacturer advises consider dose reduction.
  ▸ With intravenous use Manufacturer advises maintenance dose reduction—consult product literature.
- MONITORING REQUIREMENTS
  ▸ Aminophylline is monitored therapeutically in terms of plasma-theophylline concentrations.
  ▸ Measurement of plasma-theophylline concentration may be helpful and is **essential** if a loading dose of intravenous aminophylline is to be given to patients who are already taking theophylline, because serious side-effects such as convulsions and arrhythmias can occasionally precede other symptoms of toxicity.
  ▸ In most individuals, a plasma-theophylline concentration of 10–20 mg/litre (55–110 micromol/litre) is required for satisfactory bronchodilation, although a lower plasma-theophylline concentration of 5–15 mg/litre may be effective. Adverse effects can occur within the range

10–20 mg/litre and both the frequency and severity increase at concentrations above 20 mg/litre.
  ▸ If aminophylline is given intravenously, a blood sample should be taken 4–6 hours after starting treatment.
  ▸ With oral use Plasma-theophylline concentration is measured 5 days after starting oral treatment and at least 3 days after any dose adjustment. A blood sample should usually be taken 4–6 hours after an oral dose of a modified-release preparation (sampling times may vary—consult local guidelines).
- DIRECTIONS FOR ADMINISTRATION
  ▸ With intravenous use For *intravenous injection*, manufacturer advises give **very slowly** over at least 20 minutes (with close monitoring).
  ▸ With intravenous use in children For *intravenous infusion*, expert sources advise dilute to a concentration of 1 mg/mL with Glucose 5% *or* Sodium Chloride 0.9%.
  ▸ With intravenous use in adults For *intravenous infusion*, manufacturer advises give continuously in Glucose 5% *or* Sodium Chloride 0.9%.
- PRESCRIBING AND DISPENSING INFORMATION Patients taking oral theophylline or aminophylline should not normally receive a loading dose of intravenous aminophylline.
  Consider intravenous aminophylline for treatment of severe and life-threatening acute asthma only after consultation with senior medical staff.
  Modified release The rate of absorption from modified-release preparations can vary between brands. If a prescription for a modified-release oral aminophylline preparation does not specify a brand name, the pharmacist should contact the prescriber and agree the brand to be dispensed. Additionally, it is essential that a patient discharged from hospital should be maintained on the brand on which that patient was stabilised as an in-patient.
  PHYLLOCONTIN CONTINUS ® FORTE
  Phyllocontin Continus ® Forte tablets are for smokers and other patients where theophylline half-life is shorter.

- MEDICINAL FORMS There can be variation in the licensing of different medicines containing the same drug. Forms available from special-order manufacturers include: solution for infusion
  Solution for injection
  ▸ Aminophylline (Non-proprietary)
    Aminophylline 25 mg per 1 ml Aminophylline 250mg/10ml solution for injection ampoules | 10 ampoule [PoM] £8.50 DT = £8.50
  Modified-release tablet
  CAUTIONARY AND ADVISORY LABELS 25
  ▸ Phyllocontin Continus (Napp Pharmaceuticals Ltd)
    Aminophylline hydrate 225 mg Phyllocontin Continus 225mg tablets | 56 tablet [P] £2.40 DT = £2.40
    Aminophylline hydrate 350 mg Phyllocontin Forte Continus 350mg tablets | 56 tablet [P] £4.22 DT = £4.22

Theophylline   27-Apr-2020

- INDICATIONS AND DOSE
  UNIPHYLLIN CONTINUS ®
  Chronic asthma
  ▸ BY MOUTH USING MODIFIED-RELEASE MEDICINES
  ▸ Child 2-11 years: 9 mg/kg every 12 hours (max. per dose 200 mg), dose may be increased in some children with chronic asthma; increased to 10–16 mg/kg every 12 hours (max. per dose 400 mg), may be appropriate to give larger evening or morning dose to achieve optimum therapeutic effect when symptoms most severe; in patients whose night or daytime symptoms persist despite other therapy, who are not currently receiving theophylline, total daily requirement may be added as single evening or morning dose continued →

▸ Child 12–17 years: 200 mg every 12 hours, adjusted according to response to 400 mg every 12 hours, may be appropriate to give larger evening or morning dose to achieve optimum therapeutic effect when symptoms most severe; in patients whose night or daytime symptoms persist despite other therapy, who are not currently receiving theophylline, total daily requirement may be added as single evening or morning dose

Reversible airways obstruction | Severe acute asthma | Chronic asthma

▸ BY MOUTH USING MODIFIED-RELEASE MEDICINES
▸ Adult: 200 mg every 12 hours, adjusted according to response to 400 mg every 12 hours, may be appropriate to give larger evening or morning dose to achieve optimum therapeutic effect when symptoms most severe; in patients whose night or daytime symptoms persist despite other therapy, who are not currently receiving theophylline, total daily requirement may be added as single evening or morning dose

DOSE ADJUSTMENTS DUE TO INTERACTIONS
▸ Dose adjustment may be necessary if smoking started or stopped during treatment.

PHARMACOKINETICS
▸ Theophylline is metabolised in the liver. The plasma-theophylline concentration is increased in heart failure, hepatic impairment, and in viral infections. The plasma-theophylline concentration is decreased in smokers, and by alcohol consumption. Differences in the half-life of theophylline are important because the toxic dose is close to the therapeutic dose.

● CAUTIONS Cardiac arrhythmias or other cardiac disease · elderly (increased plasma-theophylline concentration) · epilepsy · fever · hypertension · peptic ulcer · risk of hypokalaemia · thyroid disorder

CAUTIONS, FURTHER INFORMATION
▸ Elderly Prescription potentially inappropriate (STOPP criteria) as monotherapy for COPD (safer and more effective alternatives available; risk of adverse effects due to narrow therapeutic index). See also Prescribing in the elderly p. 33.

● INTERACTIONS → Appendix 1: theophylline

● SIDE-EFFECTS Anxiety · arrhythmias · diarrhoea · dizziness · gastrointestinal discomfort · gastrooesophageal reflux disease · headache · hyperuricaemia · nausea · palpitations · seizure · skin reactions · sleep disorders · tremor · urinary disorders · vomiting

SIDE-EFFECTS, FURTHER INFORMATION Potentially serious hypokalaemia may result from beta$_2$-agonist therapy. Particular caution is required in severe asthma, because this effect may be potentiated by concomitant treatment with theophylline and its derivatives, corticosteroids, and diuretics, and by hypoxia. Plasma-potassium concentration should therefore be monitored in severe asthma.

Overdose Theophylline in overdose can cause vomiting (which may be severe and intractable), agitation, restlessness, dilated pupils, sinus tachycardia, and hyperglycaemia. More serious effects are haematemesis, convulsions, and supraventricular and ventricular arrhythmias. Severe hypokalaemia may develop rapidly.
For details on the management of poisoning, see Theophylline, under Emergency treatment of poisoning p. 1413.

● PREGNANCY Neonatal irritability and apnoea have been reported. Theophylline can be taken as normal during pregnancy as it is particularly important that asthma should be well controlled during pregnancy.

● BREAST FEEDING Present in milk—irritability in infant reported; modified-release preparations preferable. Theophylline can be taken as normal during breast-feeding.

● HEPATIC IMPAIRMENT Manufacturer advises caution (risk of increased exposure).
Dose adjustments Manufacturer advises consider dose reduction.

● MONITORING REQUIREMENTS
▸ In most individuals, a plasma-theophylline concentration of 10–20 mg/litre (55–110 micromol/litre) is required for satisfactory bronchodilation, although a lower plasma-theophylline concentration of 5–15 mg/litre may be effective. Adverse effects can occur within the range 10–20 mg/litre and both the frequency and severity increase at concentrations above 20 mg/litre.
▸ Plasma-theophylline concentration is measured 5 days after starting oral treatment and at least 3 days after any dose adjustment. A blood sample should usually be taken 4–6 hours after an oral dose of a modified-release preparation (sampling times may vary—consult local guidelines).

● PRESCRIBING AND DISPENSING INFORMATION The rate of absorption from modified-release preparations can vary between brands. If a prescription for a modified-release oral theophylline preparation does not specify a brand name, the pharmacist should contact the prescriber and agree the brand to be dispensed. Additionally, it is essential that a patient discharged from hospital should be maintained on the brand on which that patient was stabilised as an in-patient.

● MEDICINAL FORMS There can be variation in the licensing of different medicines containing the same drug.
Modified-release tablet
CAUTIONARY AND ADVISORY LABELS 21, 25
▸ Uniphyllin Continus (Napp Pharmaceuticals Ltd)
Theophylline 200 mg Uniphyllin Continus 200mg tablets | 56 tablet [P] £2.96 DT = £2.96
Theophylline 300 mg Uniphyllin Continus 300mg tablets | 56 tablet [P] £4.77 DT = £4.77
Theophylline 400 mg Uniphyllin Continus 400mg tablets | 56 tablet [P] £5.65 DT = £5.65

Nebuliser solutions

● HYPERTONIC SODIUM CHLORIDE SOLUTIONS

● INDICATIONS AND DOSE
MUCOCLEAR ® 3%
Mobilise lower respiratory tract secretions in mucous consolidation (e.g. cystic fibrosis) | Mild to moderate acute viral bronchiolitis in infants
▸ BY INHALATION OF NEBULISED SOLUTION
▸ Adult: 4 mL 2–4 times a day, temporary irritation, such as coughing, hoarseness, or reversible bronchoconstriction may occur; an inhaled bronchodilator can be used before treatment with hypertonic sodium chloride to reduce the risk of these adverse effects

MucoClear 3% inhalation solution 4ml ampoules (Pari Medical Ltd) Sodium chloride 30 mg per 1 ml 20 ampoule · NHS indicative price = £12.98 · Drug Tariff (Part IXa)60 ampoule · NHS indicative price = £27.00 · Drug Tariff (Part IXa)

● INDICATIONS AND DOSE
MUCOCLEAR ® 6%
Mobilise lower respiratory tract secretions in mucous consolidation (e.g. cystic fibrosis)
▸ BY INHALATION OF NEBULISED SOLUTION
▸ Adult: 4 mL twice daily, temporary irritation, such as

coughing, hoarseness, or reversible bronchoconstriction may occur; an inhaled bronchodilator can be used before treatment with hypertonic sodium chloride to reduce the risk of these adverse effects

MucoClear 6% inhalation solution 4ml ampoules (Pari Medical Ltd) **Sodium chloride** 60 mg per 1 ml 20 ampoule · NHS indicative price = £12.98 · Drug Tariff (Part IXa)60 ampoule · NHS indicative price = £27.00 · Drug Tariff (Part IXa)

● INDICATIONS AND DOSE

NEBUSAL®

Mobilise lower respiratory tract secretions in mucous consolidation (e.g. cystic fibrosis)

▸ BY INHALATION OF NEBULISED SOLUTION

▸ Adult: 4 mL up to twice daily, temporary irritation, such as coughing, hoarseness, or reversible bronchoconstriction may occur; an inhaled bronchodilator can be used before treatment with hypertonic sodium chloride to reduce the risk of these adverse effects

Nebusal 7% inhalation solution 4ml vials (Forest Laboratories UK Ltd) **Sodium chloride** 70 mg per 1 ml 60 vial · NHS indicative price = £27.00 · Drug Tariff (Part IXa)

● INDICATIONS AND DOSE

PULMOCLEAR®

Mobilise lower respiratory tract secretions and prevent drying of bronchial mucous.

▸ BY INHALATION OF NEBULISED SOLUTION

▸ Adult: (consult product literature)

PulmoClear 6% inhalation solution 4ml vials (TriOn Pharma Ltd) 60 vial · NHS indicative price = £18.94 · Drug Tariff (Part IXa)

PulmoClear 3% inhalation solution 4ml vials (TriOn Pharma Ltd) **Sodium chloride** 30 mg per 1 ml 60 vial · NHS indicative price = £18.94 · Drug Tariff (Part IXa)

PulmoClear 7% inhalation solution 4ml vials (TriOn Pharma Ltd) **Sodium chloride** 70 mg per 1 ml 60 vial · NHS indicative price = £18.94 · Drug Tariff (Part IXa)

● INDICATIONS AND DOSE

RESP-EASE

Mobilise lower respiratory tract secretions and prevent drying of bronchial mucous.

▸ BY INHALATION OF NEBULISED SOLUTION

▸ Adult: (consult product literature)

Resp-Ease 7% inhalation solution 4ml vials (Venture Healthcare Ltd) **Sodium chloride** 70 mg per 1 ml 60 vial · NHS indicative price = £21.60 · Drug Tariff (Part IXa)

Peak flow meters: low range

● LOW RANGE PEAK FLOW METERS

MEDI® LOW RANGE

Range 40–420 litres/minute.

Compliant to standard EN ISO 23747:2007 except for scale range.

Medi peak flow meter low range (Medicareplus International Ltd) 1 device · NHS indicative price = £6.50 · Drug Tariff (Part IXa) price = £6.50

MINI-WRIGHT® LOW RANGE

Range 30–400 litres/minute.

Compliant to standard EN ISO 23747:2007 except for scale range.

Mini-Wright peak flow meter low range (Clement Clarke International Ltd) 1 device · NHS indicative price = £7.23 · Drug Tariff (Part IXa) price = £6.50

POCKETPEAK® LOW RANGE

Range 50–400 litres/minute.

Compliant to standard EN ISO 23747:2007 except for scale range.

nSpire Pocket Peak peak flow meter low range (nSpire Health Ltd) 1 device · NHS indicative price = £6.53 · Drug Tariff (Part IXa) price = £6.50

Peak flow meters: standard range

● STANDARD RANGE PEAK FLOW METERS

AIRZONE®

Range 60–720 litres/minute.

Conforms to standard EN ISO 23747:2007.

AirZone peak flow meter standard range (Clement Clarke International Ltd) 1 device · NHS indicative price = £4.76 · Drug Tariff (Part IXa) price = £4.50

MEDI® STANDARD RANGE

Range 60–800 litres/minute.

Conforms to standard EN ISO 23747:2007.

Medi peak flow meter standard range (Medicareplus International Ltd) 1 device · NHS indicative price = £4.50 · Drug Tariff (Part IXa) price = £4.50

MICROPEAK®

Range 60–900 litres/minute.

Conforms to standard EN ISO 23747:2007.

MicroPeak peak flow meter standard range (Micro Medical Ltd) 1 device · NHS indicative price = £6.50 · Drug Tariff (Part IXa) price = £4.50

MINI-WRIGHT® STANDARD RANGE

Range 60–800 litres/minute.

Conforms to standard EN ISO 23747:2007.

Mini-Wright peak flow meter standard range (Clement Clarke International Ltd) 1 device · NHS indicative price = £7.18 · Drug Tariff (Part IXa) price = £4.50

PIKO-1®

Range 15–999 litres/minute.

Conforms to standard EN ISO 23747:2007.

nSpire PiKo-1 peak flow meter standard range (nSpire Health Ltd) 1 device · NHS indicative price = £9.50 · Drug Tariff (Part IXa) price = £4.50

PINNACLE®

Range 60–900 litres/minute.

Conforms to standard EN ISO 23747:2007.

Fyne Dynamics Pinnacle peak flow meter standard range (Fyne Dynamics Ltd) 1 device · NHS indicative price = £6.50 · Drug Tariff (Part IXa) price = £4.50

POCKETPEAK® STANDARD RANGE

Range 60–800 litres/minute.

Conforms to standard EN ISO 23747:2007.

nSpire Pocket Peak peak flow meter standard range (nSpire Health Ltd) 1 device · NHS indicative price = £6.53 · Drug Tariff (Part IXa) price = £4.50

VITALOGRAPH®

Range 50–800 litres/minute.

Conforms to standard EN ISO 23747:2007.

Vitalograph peak flow meter standard range (Vitalograph Ltd) 1 device · NHS indicative price = £4.83 · Drug Tariff (Part IXa) price = £4.50

Spacers

● SPACERS

A2A SPACER®

For use with all pressurised (aerosol) inhalers.

A2A Spacer (Clement Clarke International Ltd) 1 device · NHS indicative price = £4.15 · Drug Tariff (Part IXa)

Respiratory system

3

Respiratory system

3

A2A Spacer with medium mask (Clement Clarke International Ltd)
1 device · NHS indicative price = £6.68 · Drug Tariff (Part IXa)

A2A Spacer with small mask (Clement Clarke International Ltd)
1 device · NHS indicative price = £6.68 · Drug Tariff (Part IXa)

ABLE SPACER ®

Small-volume device. For use with all pressurised (aerosol) inhalers.

Able Spacer (Clement Clarke International Ltd)
1 device · NHS indicative price = £4.39 · Drug Tariff (Part IXa)

Able Spacer with medium mask (Clement Clarke International Ltd)
1 device · NHS indicative price = £7.16 · Drug Tariff (Part IXa)

Able Spacer with small mask (Clement Clarke International Ltd)
1 device · NHS indicative price = £7.16 · Drug Tariff (Part IXa)

AEROCHAMBER PLUS ®

Medium-volume device. For use with all pressurised (aerosol) inhalers.

AeroChamber Plus (Trudell Medical UK Ltd)
1 device · NHS indicative price = £5.06 · Drug Tariff (Part IXa)

AeroChamber Plus with adult mask (Trudell Medical UK Ltd)
1 device · NHS indicative price = £8.44 · Drug Tariff (Part IXa)

AeroChamber Plus with child mask (Trudell Medical UK Ltd)
1 device · NHS indicative price = £8.44 · Drug Tariff (Part IXa)

AeroChamber Plus with infant mask (Trudell Medical UK Ltd)
1 device · NHS indicative price = £8.44 · Drug Tariff (Part IXa)

BABYHALER ®

For paediatric use with *Flixotide* ®, and *Ventolin* ® inhalers.

● PRESCRIBING AND DISPENSING INFORMATION
Not available for NHS prescription.

Babyhaler (GlaxoSmithKline UK Ltd)
1 device · No NHS indicative price available · Drug Tariff (Part IXa)

EASYCHAMBER ® SPACER

For use with all pressurised (aerosol) inhalers.

EasyChamber Spacer (TriOn Pharma Ltd)
1 device · NHS indicative price = £3.98 · Drug Tariff (Part IXa)

EasyChamber Spacer with adult mask (TriOn Pharma Ltd)
1 device · NHS indicative price = £6.59 · Drug Tariff (Part IXa)

EasyChamber Spacer with child mask (TriOn Pharma Ltd)
1 device · NHS indicative price = £6.55 · Drug Tariff (Part IXa)

EasyChamber Spacer with infant mask (TriOn Pharma Ltd)
1 device · NHS indicative price = £6.53 · Drug Tariff (Part IXa)

HALERAID ®

Device to place over pressurised (aerosol) inhalers to aid when strength in hands is impaired (e.g. in arthritis). For use with *Flixotide* ®, *Seretide* ®, *Serevent* ®, and *Ventolin* ® inhalers.

● PRESCRIBING AND DISPENSING INFORMATION
Not available for NHS prescription.

OPTICHAMBER ®

For use with all pressurised (aerosol) inhalers.

OptiChamber (Respironics (UK) Ltd)
1 device · NHS indicative price = £4.28 · Drug Tariff (Part IXa)

OPTICHAMBER ® DIAMOND

For use with all pressurised (aerosol) inhalers.

OptiChamber Diamond (Respironics (UK) Ltd)
1 device · NHS indicative price = £4.49 · Drug Tariff (Part IXa)

OptiChamber Diamond with large LiteTouch mask 5 years-adult (Respironics (UK) Ltd)
1 device · NHS indicative price = £7.49 · Drug Tariff (Part IXa)

OptiChamber Diamond with medium LiteTouch mask 1-5 years (Respironics (UK) Ltd)
1 device · NHS indicative price = £7.49 · Drug Tariff (Part IXa)

OptiChamber Diamond with small LiteTouch mask 0-18 months (Respironics (UK) Ltd)
1 device · NHS indicative price = £7.49 · Drug Tariff (Part IXa)

POCKET CHAMBER ®

Small volume device. For use with all pressurised (aerosol) inhalers.

Pocket Chamber (nSpire Health Ltd)
1 device · NHS indicative price = £4.18 · Drug Tariff (Part IXa)

Pocket Chamber with adult mask (nSpire Health Ltd)
1 device · NHS indicative price = £9.75 · Drug Tariff (Part IXa)

Pocket Chamber with child mask (nSpire Health Ltd)
1 device · NHS indicative price = £9.75 · Drug Tariff (Part IXa)

Pocket Chamber with infant mask (nSpire Health Ltd)
1 device · NHS indicative price = £9.75 · Drug Tariff (Part IXa)

Pocket Chamber with teenager mask (nSpire Health Ltd)
1 device · NHS indicative price = £9.75 · Drug Tariff (Part IXa)

SPACE CHAMBER PLUS ®

For use with all pressurised (aerosol) inhalers.

Space Chamber Plus (Medical Developments International Ltd)
1 device · NHS indicative price = £4.26 · Drug Tariff (Part IXa)

Space Chamber Plus with large mask (Medical Developments International Ltd)
1 device · NHS indicative price = £6.98 · Drug Tariff (Part IXa)

Space Chamber Plus with medium mask (Medical Developments International Ltd)
1 device · NHS indicative price = £6.98 · Drug Tariff (Part IXa)

Space Chamber Plus with small mask (Medical Developments International Ltd)
1 device · NHS indicative price = £6.98 · Drug Tariff (Part IXa)

VOLUMATIC ®

Large-volume device. For use with *Clenil Modulite* ®, *Flixotide* ®, *Seretide* ®, *Serevent* ®, and *Ventolin* ® inhalers.

Volumatic (GlaxoSmithKline UK Ltd)
1 device · NHS indicative price = £3.88 · Drug Tariff (Part IXa)

Volumatic with paediatric mask (GlaxoSmithKline UK Ltd)
1 device · NHS indicative price = £6.83 · Drug Tariff (Part IXa)

VORTEX ®

Medium-volume device. For use with all pressurised (aerosol) inhalers.

2   Allergic conditions

Antihistamines, allergen immunotherapy and allergic emergencies

28-Feb-2020

Antihistamines

All antihistamines are of potential value in the treatment of nasal allergies, particularly seasonal allergic rhinitis (hayfever), and they may be of some value in vasomotor rhinitis. They reduce rhinorrhoea and sneezing but are usually less effective for nasal congestion. Antihistamines are used topically in the eye, in the nose, and on the skin.

Oral antihistamines are also of some value in preventing urticaria and are used to treat urticarial rashes, pruritus, and insect bites and stings; they are also used in drug allergies. Injections of chlorphenamine maleate p. 299 or promethazine hydrochloride p. 302 are used as an adjunct to adrenaline/epinephrine p. 238 in the emergency treatment of anaphylaxis and angioedema. Antihistamines (including cinnarizine p. 456, cyclizine p. 449, and promethazine teoclate p. 457) may also have a role in nausea and vomiting. Buclizine is included as an anti-emetic in a preparation for migraine. Antihistamines may also have a role in occasional insomnia.

All older antihistamines cause sedation but alimemazine tartrate p. 298 and **promethazine** may be more sedating whereas chlorphenamine maleate and cyclizine may be less so. This sedating activity is sometimes used to manage the pruritus associated with some allergies. There is little evidence that any one of the older, 'sedating' antihistamines is superior to another and patients vary widely in their response.

Non-sedating antihistamines such as acrivastine p. 294, bilastine p. 294, cetirizine hydrochloride p. 295, desloratadine p. 295 (an active metabolite of loratadine

p. 297), fexofenadine hydrochloride p. 296 (an active metabolite of terfenadine), levocetirizine hydrochloride p. 296 (an isomer of cetirizine hydrochloride), loratadine and mizolastine p. 297 cause less sedation and psychomotor impairment than the older antihistamines because they penetrate the blood brain barrier only to a slight extent.

Considerations in the elderly

The use of first-generation antihistamines in elderly patients is potentially inappropriate (STOPP criteria) as safer, less toxic antihistamines are widely available.

For further information, see *STOPP/START criteria* in Prescribing in the elderly p. 33.

Allergen immunotherapy

Immunotherapy using allergen vaccines containing house dust mite, animal dander (cat or dog), or extracts of grass and tree pollen can reduce symptoms of asthma and allergic rhinoconjunctivitis. A vaccine containing extracts of wasp and bee venom is used to reduce the risk of severe anaphylaxis and systemic reactions in individuals with hypersensitivity to wasp and bee stings. An oral preparation of grass pollen extract (*Grazax*®) is also licensed for disease-modifying treatment of grass pollen-induced rhinitis and conjunctivitis. Those requiring immunotherapy must be referred to a hospital specialist for accurate diagnosis, assessment, and treatment.

Omalizumab p. 284 is a monoclonal antibody that binds to immunoglobulin E (IgE). It is used as additional therapy in individuals with proven IgE-mediated sensitivity to inhaled allergens, whose severe persistent allergic asthma cannot be controlled adequately with high dose inhaled corticosteroid together with a long-acting beta₂ agonist. Omalizumab should be initiated by physicians in specialist centres experienced in the treatment of severe persistent asthma. Omalizumab is also indicated as add-on therapy for the treatment of chronic spontaneous urticaria in patients who have had an inadequate response to H₁ antihistamine treatment.

Anaphylaxis and allergic emergencies

Anaphylaxis

Anaphylaxis is a severe, life-threatening, generalised or systemic hypersensitivity reaction. It is characterised by the rapid onset of respiratory and/or circulatory problems and is usually associated with skin and mucosal changes; prompt treatment is required. Patients with pre-existing asthma, especially poorly controlled asthma, are at particular risk of life-threatening reactions. Insect stings are a recognised risk (in particular wasp and bee stings). Latex and certain foods, including eggs, fish, cow's milk protein, peanuts, sesame, shellfish, soy, and tree nuts may also precipitate anaphylaxis (see Food allergy p. 92). Medicinal products particularly associated with anaphylaxis include blood products, vaccines, hyposensitising (allergen) preparations, antibacterials, aspirin and other NSAIDs, and neuromuscular blocking drugs. In the case of drugs, anaphylaxis is more likely after parenteral administration; resuscitation facilities must always be available for injections associated with special risk. Anaphylactic reactions may also be associated with *additives and excipients* in foods and medicines. Refined arachis (peanut) oil, which may be present in some medicinal products, is unlikely to cause an allergic reaction—nevertheless it is wise to check the full formula of preparations which may contain allergens.

Treatment of anaphylaxis

Adrenaline/epinephrine provides physiological reversal of the immediate symptoms associated with hypersensitivity reactions such as *anaphylaxis* and *angioedema*.

First-line treatment includes:

- securing the airway, restoration of blood pressure (laying the patient flat and raising the legs, or in the recovery position if unconscious or nauseous and at risk of vomiting);
- administering adrenaline/epinephrine (by **intramuscular** injection in a dose of 500 micrograms (a dose of 300 micrograms may be appropriate for *immediate self-administration*); the dose should be repeated if necessary at 5-minute intervals according to blood pressure, pulse, and respiratory function. Patients receiving beta-blockers require special consideration;
- administering high-flow **oxygen** and **intravenous fluids** is also of primary importance;
- administering an antihistamine, such as chlorphenamine maleate, by slow intravenous injection or intramuscular injection is a useful adjunctive treatment, given after adrenaline.
- Administering an intravenous corticosteroid such as hydrocortisone p. 716 (preferably as sodium succinate) is of secondary value in the initial management of anaphylaxis because the onset of action is delayed for several hours, but should be given to prevent further deterioration in severely affected patients.

Continuing respiratory deterioration requires further treatment with **bronchodilators** including inhaled or intravenous salbutamol p. 269, inhaled ipratropium bromide p. 262, intravenous aminophylline p. 288, or intravenous magnesium sulfate p. 1099 [unlicensed indication] (as for acute severe asthma); in addition to oxygen, assisted respiration and possibly emergency tracheotomy may be necessary.

When a patient is so ill that there is doubt about the adequacy of the circulation, the initial injection of adrenaline/epinephrine may need to be given as a *dilute solution by the intravenous route.*

Cardiopulmonary arrest may follow an anaphylactic reaction; resuscitation should be started immediately.

On discharge, patients should be considered for further treatment with an oral antihistamine and an oral corticosteroid for up to 3 days to reduce the risk of further reaction. Patients should be instructed to return to hospital if symptoms recur and to contact their general practitioner for follow-up.

Patients who are suspected of having had an anaphylactic reaction should be referred to a specialist for specific allergy diagnosis. Avoidance of the allergen is the principal treatment; if appropriate, an adrenaline/epinephrine auto-injector should be given for self-administration or a replacement supplied.

Intramuscular adrenaline (epinephrine)

The *intramuscular route* is the *first choice route* for the administration of adrenaline/epinephrine p. 238 in the management of anaphylaxis. Adrenaline/epinephrine is best given as an intramuscular injection into the anterolateral aspect of the middle third of the thigh; it has a rapid onset of action after intramuscular administration and in the shocked patient its absorption from the intramuscular site is faster and more reliable than from the subcutaneous site.

Patients with severe allergy should be instructed in the self-administration of adrenaline/epinephrine by intramuscular injection.

Prompt injection of adrenaline/epinephrine is of paramount importance. The adrenaline/epinephrine doses recommended for the emergency treatment of anaphylaxis by appropriately trained healthcare professionals are based on the revised recommendations of the Working Group of the Resuscitation Council (UK).

The MHRA/CHM have released important safety information regarding the use of adrenaline auto-injectors. For further information, see *Important safety information* for adrenaline/epinephrine.

3

Respiratory system

Intravenous adrenaline (epinephrine)

Intravenous adrenaline/epinephrine should be given only by those experienced in its use, in a setting where patients can be carefully monitored.

When the patient is severely ill and there is real doubt about the adequacy of the circulation and absorption after intramuscular injection, adrenaline/epinephrine can be given by **slow** *intravenous injection* repeated according to response; if multiple doses are required, adrenaline/epinephrine should be given as a **slow** intravenous infusion *stopping when a response has been obtained*.

It is important that, where intramuscular injection might still succeed, time should not be wasted seeking intravenous access.

The intravenous route is also used for *cardiac resuscitation*.

Angioedema

Angioedema is dangerous if *laryngeal oedema* is present. In this circumstance adrenaline/epinephrine injection and **oxygen** should be given as described under **Anaphylaxis**; antihistamines and corticosteroids should also be given. Tracheal intubation may be necessary.

Hereditary angioedema

The treatment of hereditary angioedema should be under specialist supervision. Unlike allergic angioedema, adrenaline/epinephrine, corticosteroids, and antihistamines should not be used for the treatment of acute attacks, including attacks involving laryngeal oedema, as they are ineffective and may delay appropriate treatment—intubation may be necessary. The administration of C1-esterase inhibitor p. 305, an endogenous complement blocker derived from human plasma, (in fresh frozen plasma or in partially purified form) can terminate acute attacks of *hereditary angioedema*; it can also be used for short-term prophylaxis before dental, medical or surgical procedures. Conestat alfa p. 305 and icatibant p. 306 are licensed for the treatment of acute attacks of hereditary angioedema in adults with C1-esterase inhibitor deficiency.

Tranexamic acid p. 118 and danazol p. 783 [unlicensed indication] are used for short-term and long-term prophylaxis of hereditary angioedema. Short-term prophylaxis with tranexamic acid or danazol is started several days before planned procedures (e.g. dental work) and continued for 2–5 days afterwards. Danazol should be avoided in children because of its androgenic effects.

Dose of intramuscular injection of adrenaline (epinephrine) for the emergency treatment of anaphylaxis by healthcare professionals

Age	Dose	Volume of adrenaline
▶ Child 1 month–5 years	150 micrograms	0.15 mL 1 in 1000 (1 mg/mL) adrenaline[1]
▶ Child 6–11 years	300 micrograms	0.3 mL 1 in 1000 (1 mg/mL) adrenaline
▶ Child 12–17 years	500 micrograms	0.5 mL 1 in 1000 (1 mg/mL) adrenaline[2]
▶ Adult	500 micrograms	0.5 mL 1 in 1000 (1 mg/mL) adrenaline

These doses may be repeated several times if necessary at 5-minute intervals according to blood pressure, pulse and respiratory function.

1. Use suitable syringe for measuring small volume
2. 300 micrograms (0.3 mL) if child is small or prepubertal

ANTIHISTAMINES ⟩ NON-SEDATING

Acrivastine
14-Dec-2020

● **INDICATIONS AND DOSE**

Symptomatic relief of allergy such as hayfever, chronic idiopathic urticaria
▶ BY MOUTH
▸ Child 12–17 years: 8 mg 3 times a day
▸ Adult: 8 mg 3 times a day

● CONTRA-INDICATIONS Avoid in Acute porphyrias p. 1107 · elderly

● INTERACTIONS → Appendix 1: antihistamines, non-sedating

● SIDE-EFFECTS
▸ **Common or very common** Drowsiness · dry mouth
▸ **Frequency not known** Dizziness · rash

SIDE-EFFECTS, FURTHER INFORMATION Non-sedating antihistamines such as acrivastine cause less sedation and psychomotor impairment than the older antihistamines, but can still occur; sedation is generally minimal. This is because non-sedating antihistamines penetrate the blood brain barrier to a much lesser extent.

● ALLERGY AND CROSS-SENSITIVITY EvGr Contra-indicated if history of hypersensitivity to triprolidine. Ⓜ

● PREGNANCY Most manufacturers of antihistamines advise avoiding their use during pregnancy; however, there is no evidence of teratogenicity.

● BREAST FEEDING Most antihistamines are present in breast milk in varying amounts; although not known to be harmful, most manufacturers advise avoiding their use in mothers who are breast-feeding.

● RENAL IMPAIRMENT Avoid in severe impairment.

● PATIENT AND CARER ADVICE
Driving and skilled tasks Patients and their carers should be advised that drowsiness can occur and may affect performance of skilled tasks (e.g. cycling or driving).

● MEDICINAL FORMS There can be variation in the licensing of different medicines containing the same drug.

Capsule
▸ Benadryl Allergy Relief (McNeil Products Ltd)
  Acrivastine 8 mg Benadryl Allergy Relief 8mg capsules | 24 capsule Ⓟ £5.45 | 48 capsule Ⓟ £9.91

Bilastine
14-Dec-2020

● **INDICATIONS AND DOSE**

Symptomatic relief of allergic rhinoconjunctivitis and urticaria
▶ BY MOUTH
▸ Child 12–17 years: 20 mg once daily
▸ Adult: 20 mg once daily

● CONTRA-INDICATIONS Avoid in Acute porphyrias p. 1107

● INTERACTIONS → Appendix 1: antihistamines, non-sedating

● SIDE-EFFECTS
▸ **Common or very common** Drowsiness · headache
▸ **Uncommon** Anxiety · appetite increased · asthenia · bundle branch block · diarrhoea · dry mouth · dyspnoea · fever · gastritis · gastrointestinal discomfort · insomnia · nasal complaints · nausea · oral herpes · pre-existing condition improved · pruritus · QT interval prolongation · sinus arrhythmia · thirst · tinnitus · vertigo · weight increased

SIDE-EFFECTS, FURTHER INFORMATION Non-sedating antihistamines such as bilastine cause less sedation and psychomotor impairment than the older antihistamines, but can still occur; sedation is generally minimal. This is because non-sedating antihistamines penetrate the blood brain barrier to a much lesser extent.

- PREGNANCY Avoid—limited information available. Most manufacturers of antihistamines advise avoiding their use during pregnancy; however, there is no evidence of teratogenicity.
- BREAST FEEDING Avoid—no information available. Most antihistamines are present in breast milk in varying amounts; although not known to be harmful, most manufacturers advise avoiding their use in mothers who are breast-feeding.
- DIRECTIONS FOR ADMINISTRATION Manufacturer advises tablet should be taken 1 hour before or 2 hours after food or fruit juice.
- PATIENT AND CARER ADVICE Patients or carers should be given advice on how to administer bilastine tablets.
  Driving and skilled tasks Patients and their carers should be advised that drowsiness can occur and may affect performance of skilled tasks (e.g. cycling or driving).

- MEDICINAL FORMS There can be variation in the licensing of different medicines containing the same drug.
  Tablet
  CAUTIONARY AND ADVISORY LABELS 23
  ▸ Ilaxten (A. Menarini Farmaceutica Internazionale SRL)
    Bilastine 20 mg Ilaxten 20mg tablets | 30 tablet [PoM] £6.00 DT = £6.00

Cetirizine hydrochloride
14-Dec-2020

- **INDICATIONS AND DOSE**
  Symptomatic relief of allergy such as hay fever, chronic idiopathic urticaria, atopic dermatitis
  ▸ BY MOUTH
  ▸ Child 2-5 years: 2.5 mg twice daily
  ▸ Child 6-11 years: 5 mg twice daily
  ▸ Child 12-17 years: 10 mg once daily
  ▸ Adult: 10 mg once daily

- CAUTIONS Epilepsy
- INTERACTIONS → Appendix 1: antihistamines, non-sedating
- SIDE-EFFECTS
  ▸ **Uncommon** Agitation · asthenia · diarrhoea · malaise · paraesthesia · skin reactions
  ▸ **Rare or very rare** Aggression · angioedema · confusion · depression · hallucination · hepatic function abnormal · insomnia · movement disorders · oculogyration · oedema · seizure · syncope · tachycardia · taste altered · thrombocytopenia · tic · tremor · urinary disorders · vision disorders · weight increased
  ▸ **Frequency not known** Abdominal pain · appetite increased · dizziness · drowsiness · dry mouth · headache · memory loss · nausea · pharyngitis · suicidal ideation · vertigo
  SIDE-EFFECTS, FURTHER INFORMATION Non-sedating antihistamines such as cetirizine hydrochloride cause less sedation and psychomotor impairment than the older antihistamines, but can still occur; sedation is generally minimal. This is because non-sedating antihistamines penetrate the blood brain barrier to a much lesser extent.
- PREGNANCY Most manufacturers of antihistamines advise avoiding their use during pregnancy; however, there is no evidence of teratogenicity.
- BREAST FEEDING Most antihistamines are present in breast milk in varying amounts; although not known to be harmful, most manufacturers advise avoiding their use in mothers who are breast-feeding.
- RENAL IMPAIRMENT
  ▸ In adults Avoid if eGFR less than 10 mL/minute/1.73 m^2.

▸ In children Avoid if estimated glomerular filtration rate less than 10 mL/minute/1.73 m^2.
  Dose adjustments ▸ In adults Use half normal dose if eGFR 30–50 mL/minute/1.73 m^2. Use half normal dose and reduce dose frequency to alternate days if eGFR 10–30 mL/minute/1.73 m^2.
  ▸ In children Use half normal dose if estimated glomerular filtration rate 30–50 mL/minute/1.73 m^2. Use half normal dose and reduce dose frequency to alternate days if estimated glomerular filtration rate 10–30 mL/minute/1.73 m^2.
- PATIENT AND CARER ADVICE
  Medicines for Children leaflet: Cetirizine for hay fever
  www.medicinesforchildren.org.uk/cetirizine-hay-fever-0
  Driving and skilled tasks Patients and their carers should be advised that drowsiness can occur and may affect performance of skilled tasks (e.g. cycling or driving).
- PROFESSION SPECIFIC INFORMATION
  Dental practitioners' formulary
  Cetirizine Tablets 10 mg may be prescribed.
    Cetirizine Oral Solution 5 mg/5 mL may be prescribed.

- MEDICINAL FORMS There can be variation in the licensing of different medicines containing the same drug.
  Oral solution
  EXCIPIENTS: May contain Propylene glycol
  ▸ Cetirizine hydrochloride (Non-proprietary)
    Cetirizine hydrochloride 1 mg per 1 ml Cetirizine 1mg/ml oral solution sugar free sugar-free | 200 ml [PoM] £1.55 DT = £1.55
  Tablet
  ▸ Cetirizine hydrochloride (Non-proprietary)
    Cetirizine hydrochloride 10 mg Cetirizine 10mg tablets | 30 tablet [PoM] £1.06 DT = £1.06
  Capsule
  ▸ Benadryl Allergy (McNeil Products Ltd)
    Cetirizine hydrochloride 10 mg Benadryl Allergy Liquid Release 10mg capsules | 7 capsule [GSL] £3.09 DT = £3.09

Desloratadine
14-Dec-2020

- **INDICATIONS AND DOSE**
  Symptomatic relief of allergy such as allergic rhinitis, urticaria, chronic idiopathic urticaria
  ▸ BY MOUTH
  ▸ Child 1-5 years: 1.25 mg once daily
  ▸ Child 6-11 years: 2.5 mg once daily
  ▸ Child 12-17 years: 5 mg once daily
  ▸ Adult: 5 mg once daily
  PHARMACOKINETICS
  ▸ Desloratadine is a metabolite of loratadine.

- INTERACTIONS → Appendix 1: antihistamines, non-sedating
- SIDE-EFFECTS
  ▸ **Common or very common** Asthenia · dry mouth · headache
  ▸ **Rare or very rare** Akathisia · arrhythmias · diarrhoea · dizziness · drowsiness · gastrointestinal discomfort · hallucination · hepatic disorders · insomnia · myalgia · nausea · palpitations · seizure · vomiting
  ▸ **Frequency not known** Behaviour abnormal · photosensitivity reaction · QT interval prolongation
  SIDE-EFFECTS, FURTHER INFORMATION Non-sedating antihistamines such as desloratadine cause less sedation and psychomotor impairment than the older antihistamines, but can still occur; sedation is generally minimal. This is because non-sedating antihistamines penetrate the blood brain barrier to a much lesser extent.
- ALLERGY AND CROSS-SENSITIVITY [EvGr] Contra-indicated if history of hypersensitivity to loratadine. Ⓜ

- PREGNANCY Most manufacturers of antihistamines advise avoiding their use during pregnancy; however, there is no evidence of teratogenicity.
- BREAST FEEDING Most antihistamines are present in breast milk in varying amounts; although not known to be harmful, most manufacturers advise avoiding their use in mothers who are breast-feeding.
- RENAL IMPAIRMENT Use with caution in severe impairment.
- PRESCRIBING AND DISPENSING INFORMATION Flavours of oral liquid formulations may include bubblegum.
- PATIENT AND CARER ADVICE
  Driving and skilled tasks Patients and their carers should be advised that drowsiness can occur and may affect performance of skilled tasks (e.g. cycling or driving).
- MEDICINAL FORMS There can be variation in the licensing of different medicines containing the same drug.
  Oral solution
  EXCIPIENTS: May contain Propylene glycol, sorbitol
  ▸ Desloratadine (Non-proprietary)
  Desloratadine 500 microgram per 1 ml Desloratadine 2.5mg/5ml oral solution sugar free sugar-free | 100 ml [PoM] £6.56 sugar-free | 150 ml [PoM] £8.12–£9.85 DT = £9.85
  ▸ Neoclarityn (Merck Sharp & Dohme Ltd)
  Desloratadine 500 microgram per 1 ml Neoclarityn 2.5mg/5ml oral solution sugar-free | 100 ml [PoM] £6.77 sugar-free | 150 ml [PoM] £10.15 DT = £9.85

  Tablet
  ▸ Desloratadine (Non-proprietary)
  Desloratadine 5 mg Desloratadine 5mg tablets | 30 tablet [PoM] £6.77 DT = £1.62
  ▸ Neoclarityn (Merck Sharp & Dohme Ltd)
  Desloratadine 5 mg Neoclarityn 5mg tablets | 30 tablet [PoM] £6.77 DT = £1.62

Fexofenadine hydrochloride
14-Dec-2020

- **INDICATIONS AND DOSE**
Symptomatic relief of seasonal allergic rhinitis
▸ BY MOUTH
▸ Child 6–11 years: 30 mg twice daily
▸ Child 12–17 years: 120 mg once daily
▸ Adult: 120 mg once daily
Symptomatic relief of chronic idiopathic urticaria
▸ BY MOUTH
▸ Child 12–17 years: 180 mg once daily
▸ Adult: 180 mg once daily
PHARMACOKINETICS
▸ Fexofenadine is a metabolite of terfenadine.

- INTERACTIONS → Appendix 1: antihistamines, non-sedating
- SIDE-EFFECTS
▸ **Common or very common** Dizziness · drowsiness · headache · nausea
▸ **Uncommon** Fatigue
▸ **Frequency not known** Diarrhoea · nervousness · palpitations · skin reactions · sleep disorders · tachycardia
  SIDE-EFFECTS, FURTHER INFORMATION Non-sedating antihistamines such as fexofenadine cause less sedation and psychomotor impairment than the older antihistamines, but can still occur; sedation is generally minimal. This is because non-sedating antihistamines penetrate the blood brain barrier to a much lesser extent.
- PREGNANCY Most manufacturers of antihistamines advise avoiding their use during pregnancy; however, there is no evidence of teratogenicity.
- BREAST FEEDING Most antihistamines are present in breast milk in varying amounts; although not known to be

harmful, most manufacturers advise avoiding their use in mothers who are breast-feeding.
- PATIENT AND CARER ADVICE
  Driving and skilled tasks Patients and their carers should be advised that drowsiness can occur and may affect performance of skilled tasks (e.g. cycling or driving).
- MEDICINAL FORMS There can be variation in the licensing of different medicines containing the same drug. Forms available from special-order manufacturers include: oral suspension, oral solution
  Tablet
  CAUTIONARY AND ADVISORY LABELS 5
  ▸ Fexofenadine hydrochloride (Non-proprietary)
  Fexofenadine hydrochloride 120 mg Fexofenadine 120mg tablets | 30 tablet [PoM] £6.23 DT = £2.16
  Fexofenadine hydrochloride 180 mg Fexofenadine 180mg tablets | 30 tablet [PoM] £7.89 DT = £3.04
  ▸ Telfast (Sanofi)
  Fexofenadine hydrochloride 30 mg Telfast 30mg tablets | 60 tablet [PoM] £5.46 DT = £5.46
  Fexofenadine hydrochloride 120 mg Telfast 120mg tablets | 30 tablet [PoM] £5.99 DT = £2.16
  Fexofenadine hydrochloride 180 mg Telfast 180mg tablets | 30 tablet [PoM] £7.58 DT = £3.04

Levocetirizine hydrochloride
14-Dec-2020

- **INDICATIONS AND DOSE**
Symptomatic relief of allergy such as hay fever, urticaria
▸ BY MOUTH
▸ Child 6–17 years: 5 mg once daily
▸ Adult: 5 mg once daily
PHARMACOKINETICS
▸ Levocetirizine is an isomer of cetirizine.

- CONTRA-INDICATIONS Avoid in Acute porphyrias p. 1107
- INTERACTIONS → Appendix 1: antihistamines, non-sedating
- SIDE-EFFECTS
▸ **Common or very common** Asthenia · constipation (in children) · drowsiness · dry mouth
▸ **Uncommon** Abdominal pain
▸ **Frequency not known** Aggression · agitation · angioedema · appetite increased · arthralgia · depression · diarrhoea (very common in children) · dizziness · dyspnoea · hallucination · hepatitis · myalgia · nausea · oedema · palpitations · paraesthesia · seizure · skin reactions · sleep disorders (very common in children) · suicidal ideation · syncope · tachycardia · taste altered · tremor · urinary disorders · vertigo · vision disorders · vomiting · weight increased
  SIDE-EFFECTS, FURTHER INFORMATION Non-sedating antihistamines such as levocetirizine cause less sedation and psychomotor impairment than the older antihistamines, but can still occur; sedation is generally minimal. This is because non-sedating antihistamines penetrate the blood brain barrier to a much lesser extent.
- PREGNANCY Most manufacturers of antihistamines advise avoiding their use during pregnancy; however, there is no evidence of teratogenicity.
- BREAST FEEDING Most antihistamines are present in breast milk in varying amounts; although not known to be harmful, most manufacturers advise avoiding their use in mothers who are breast-feeding.
- RENAL IMPAIRMENT
▸ In adults Avoid if eGFR less than 10 mL/minute/1.73 m^2.
▸ In children Avoid if estimated glomerular filtration rate less than 10 mL/minute/1.73 m^2.
  Dose adjustments ▸ In adults 5 mg on alternate days if eGFR 30–50 mL/minute/1.73 m^2. 5 mg every 3 days if eGFR 10–30 mL/minute/1.73 m^2.

▶ **In children** Reduce dose frequency to alternate days if estimated glomerular filtration rate 30–50 mL/minute/1.73 m². Reduce dose frequency to every 3 days if estimated glomerular filtration rate 10–30 mL/minute/1.73 m².

● PATIENT AND CARER ADVICE

Driving and skilled tasks Patients and their carers should be advised that drowsiness can occur and may affect performance of skilled tasks (e.g. cycling or driving).

● MEDICINAL FORMS There can be variation in the licensing of different medicines containing the same drug.

Oral solution

▶ Xyzal (UCB Pharma Ltd)
Levocetirizine dihydrochloride 500 microgram per 1 ml Xyzal 0.5mg/ml oral solution sugar-free | 200 ml PoM £6.00 DT = £6.00

Tablet

▶ Levocetirizine hydrochloride (Non-proprietary)
Levocetirizine dihydrochloride 5 mg Levocetirizine 5mg tablets | 30 tablet PoM £4.39 DT = £4.32
▶ Xyzal (UCB Pharma Ltd)
Levocetirizine dihydrochloride 5 mg Xyzal 5mg tablets | 30 tablet PoM £4.39 DT = £4.32

Loratadine

14-Dec-2020

● INDICATIONS AND DOSE

Symptomatic relief of allergy such as hay fever, chronic idiopathic urticaria

▶ BY MOUTH
▶ **Child 2–11 years (body-weight up to 31 kg):** 5 mg once daily
▶ **Child 2–11 years (body-weight 31 kg and above):** 10 mg once daily
▶ **Child 12–17 years:** 10 mg once daily
▶ **Adult:** 10 mg once daily

● INTERACTIONS → Appendix 1: antihistamines, non-sedating

● SIDE-EFFECTS

▶ **Common or very common** Drowsiness · nervousness (in children)
▶ **Uncommon** Appetite increased · headache (very common in children) · insomnia
▶ **Rare or very rare** Alopecia · angioedema · dizziness · dry mouth · fatigue (very common in children) · gastritis · hepatic function abnormal · nausea · palpitations · rash · seizure · tachycardia

SIDE-EFFECTS, FURTHER INFORMATION Non-sedating antihistamines such as loratadine cause less sedation and psychomotor impairment than the older antihistamines, but can still occur; sedation is generally minimal. This is because non-sedating antihistamines penetrate the blood brain barrier to a much lesser extent.

● PREGNANCY Most manufacturers of antihistamines advise avoiding their use during pregnancy; however, there is no evidence of teratogenicity.

● BREAST FEEDING Most antihistamines are present in breast milk in varying amounts; although not known to be harmful, most manufacturers advise avoiding their use in mothers who are breast-feeding.

● HEPATIC IMPAIRMENT Manufacturer advises caution in severe impairment (risk of increased exposure).
Dose adjustments Manufacturer advises initial dose reduction to alternate days in severe impairment.

● PATIENT AND CARER ADVICE

Medicines for Children leaflet: Loratadine for allergy symptoms www.medicinesforchildren.org.uk/loratadine-allergy-symptoms
Driving and skilled tasks Patients and their carers should be advised that drowsiness can occur and may affect performance of skilled tasks (e.g. cycling or driving).

● PROFESSION SPECIFIC INFORMATION

Dental practitioners' formulary
Loratadine 10 mg tablets may be prescribed.
Loratadine syrup 5 mg/5 mL may be prescribed.

● MEDICINAL FORMS There can be variation in the licensing of different medicines containing the same drug.

Oral solution
EXCIPIENTS: May contain Propylene glycol
▶ Loratadine (Non-proprietary)
Loratadine 1 mg per 1 ml Loratadine 5mg/5ml oral solution | 100 ml PoM £1.94 DT = £1.94

Tablet
▶ Loratadine (Non-proprietary)
Loratadine 10 mg Loratadine 10mg tablets | 30 tablet PoM X DT = £1.05

Mizolastine

14-Dec-2020

● INDICATIONS AND DOSE

Symptomatic relief of allergy such as hay fever, urticaria

▶ BY MOUTH
▶ **Child 12–17 years:** 10 mg once daily
▶ **Adult:** 10 mg once daily

● CONTRA-INDICATIONS Cardiac disease · susceptibility to QT-interval prolongation

● INTERACTIONS → Appendix 1: antihistamines, non-sedating

● SIDE-EFFECTS

▶ **Common or very common** Appetite increased · asthenia · diarrhoea · dizziness · drowsiness · dry mouth · gastrointestinal discomfort · headache · nausea · weight increased
▶ **Uncommon** Anxiety · arrhythmias · arthralgia · depression · myalgia · palpitations
▶ **Rare or very rare** Hypersensitivity
▶ **Frequency not known** Asthma exacerbated · bronchospasm · QT interval prolongation

SIDE-EFFECTS, FURTHER INFORMATION Non-sedating antihistamines such as mizolastine cause less sedation and psychomotor impairment than the older antihistamines, but can still occur; sedation is generally minimal. This is because non-sedating antihistamines penetrate the blood brain barrier to a much lesser extent.

● PREGNANCY Most manufacturers of antihistamines advise avoiding their use during pregnancy; however, there is no evidence of teratogenicity.

● BREAST FEEDING Most antihistamines are present in breast milk in varying amounts; although not known to be harmful, most manufacturers advise avoiding their use in mothers who are breast-feeding.

● HEPATIC IMPAIRMENT Manufacturer advises avoid in significant impairment.

● PATIENT AND CARER ADVICE

Driving and skilled tasks Patients and their carers should be advised that drowsiness can occur and may affect performance of skilled tasks (e.g. cycling or driving).

● MEDICINAL FORMS There can be variation in the licensing of different medicines containing the same drug.

Modified-release tablet
CAUTIONARY AND ADVISORY LABELS 25
▶ Mizollen (Sanofi)
Mizolastine 10 mg Mizollen 10mg modified-release tablets | 30 tablet PoM £6.92 DT = £6.92

3

Respiratory system

Rupatadine

29-Apr-2019

- **DRUG ACTION** Rupatadine is a second generation non-sedating antihistamine.

  - **INDICATIONS AND DOSE**

  Symptomatic relief of allergic rhinitis and urticaria
  - ▸ BY MOUTH USING TABLETS
  - ▸ Child 12–17 years: 10 mg once daily
  - ▸ Adult: 10 mg once daily

- **CAUTIONS** Elderly—limited information available · history of QT-interval prolongation · predisposition to arrhythmia · uncorrected hypokalaemia

- **INTERACTIONS** → Appendix 1: antihistamines, non-sedating

- **SIDE-EFFECTS**
  - ▸ **Common or very common** Asthenia · dizziness · drowsiness · dry mouth · headache
  - ▸ **Uncommon** Appetite increased · arthralgia · back pain · concentration impaired · constipation · cough · diarrhoea · dry throat · eosinophilia (in children) · epistaxis · fever · gastrointestinal discomfort · increased risk of infection · irritability · malaise · myalgia · nasal dryness · nausea · neutropenia (in children) · night sweats (in children) · oropharyngeal pain · skin reactions · thirst · vomiting · weight increased
  - ▸ **Rare or very rare** Palpitations · tachycardia

  SIDE-EFFECTS, FURTHER INFORMATION Non-sedating antihistamines such as rupatadine cause less sedation and psychomotor impairment than the older antihistamines, but can still occur; sedation is generally minimal. This is because non-sedating antihistamines penetrate the blood brain barrier to a much lesser extent.

- **PREGNANCY** Most manufacturers of antihistamines advise avoiding their use during pregnancy; however, there is no evidence of teratogenicity.

- **BREAST FEEDING** Most antihistamines are present in breast milk in varying amounts; although not known to be harmful, most manufacturers advise avoiding their use in mothers who are breast-feeding.

- **HEPATIC IMPAIRMENT** Manufacturer advises avoid (no information available).

- **RENAL IMPAIRMENT** Manufacturer advises avoid—no information available.

- **MEDICINAL FORMS** There can be variation in the licensing of different medicines containing the same drug.
  Tablet
  - ▸ Rupatadine (Non-proprietary)
    Rupatadine (as Rupatadine fumarate) 10 mg Rupatadine 10mg tablets | 30 tablet [PoM] £36.00 DT = £36.00

ANTIHISTAMINES > SEDATING

Alimemazine tartrate

28-Aug-2020

(Trimeprazine tartrate)

- **INDICATIONS AND DOSE**

  Urticaria | Pruritus
  - ▸ BY MOUTH
  - ▸ Child 2–4 years: 2.5 mg 3–4 times a day
  - ▸ Child 5–11 years: 5 mg 3–4 times a day
  - ▸ Child 12–17 years: 10 mg 2–3 times a day, in severe cases up to maximum daily dose has been used; maximum 100 mg per day
  - ▸ Adult: 10 mg 2–3 times a day, in severe cases up to maximum daily dose has been used; maximum 100 mg per day
  - ▸ Elderly: 10 mg 1–2 times a day

- **CONTRA-INDICATIONS** Epilepsy · hepatic dysfunction · history of narrow angle glaucoma · hypothyroidism · myasthenia gravis · Parkinson's disease · phaeochromocytoma · prostatic hypertrophy (in adults) · renal dysfunction

- **CAUTIONS** Cardiovascular diseases (due to tachycardia-inducing and hypotensive effects of phenothiazines) · elderly · exposure to sunlight should be avoided during treatment with high doses · pyloroduodenal obstruction · urinary retention · volume depleted patients who are more susceptible to orthostatic hypotension

- **INTERACTIONS** → Appendix 1: antihistamines, sedating

- **SIDE-EFFECTS** Agitation · agranulocytosis · amenorrhoea · atrioventricular block · autonomic dysfunction · bile thrombus · consciousness impaired · drug fever · dry mouth · eosinophilia · erectile dysfunction · eye disorder · galactorrhoea · gynaecomastia · hepatic disorders · hyperprolactinaemia · hyperthermia · hypotension · insomnia · leucopenia (on prolonged high dose) · movement disorders · muscle rigidity · nasal congestion · neuroleptic malignant syndrome · pallor · parkinsonism · photosensitivity reaction · postural hypotension (more common in the elderly or in volume depletion) · QT interval prolongation · respiratory depression · seizure · skin reactions · tardive dyskinesia (more common after long term high doses) · tremor · ventricular fibrillation (increased risk with hypokalamia and cardiac disease) · ventricular tachycardia (increased risk with hypokalamia and cardiac disease)

  SIDE-EFFECTS, FURTHER INFORMATION Drowsiness may diminish after a few days.

  Patients on high dosage may develop photosensitivity and should avoid exposure to direct sunlight.

  Children and elderly patients are more susceptible to side-effects.

- **PREGNANCY** Most manufacturers of antihistamines advise avoiding their use during pregnancy; however, there is no evidence of teratogenicity. Use in the latter part of the third trimester may cause adverse effects in neonates such as irritability, paradoxical excitability, and tremor.

- **BREAST FEEDING** Most antihistamines are present in breast milk in varying amounts; although not known to be harmful, most manufacturers advise avoiding their use in mothers who are breast-feeding.

- **HEPATIC IMPAIRMENT** Manufacturer advises avoid—no information available.

- **RENAL IMPAIRMENT** Avoid.

- **PATIENT AND CARER ADVICE**
  Driving and skilled tasks Drowsiness may affect performance of skilled tasks (e.g. cycling or driving); sedating effects enhanced by alcohol.

- **MEDICINAL FORMS** There can be variation in the licensing of different medicines containing the same drug. Forms available from special-order manufacturers include: oral solution
  Oral solution
  CAUTIONARY AND ADVISORY LABELS 2
  - ▸ Alimemazine tartrate (Non-proprietary)
    Alimemazine tartrate 1.5 mg per 1 ml Alfresed 7.5mg/5ml syrup | 100 ml [PoM] £179.58 DT = £179.58
    Alimemazine 7.5mg/5ml oral solution | 100 ml [PoM] £179.58 DT = £179.58
    Alimemazine tartrate 6 mg per 1 ml Alimemazine 30mg/5ml oral solution | 100 ml [PoM] £243.51 DT = £243.51
    Alfresed 30mg/5ml syrup | 100 ml [PoM] £243.51 DT = £243.51
  Tablet
  CAUTIONARY AND ADVISORY LABELS 2
  - ▸ Alimemazine tartrate (Non-proprietary)
    Alimemazine tartrate 10 mg Alimemazine 10mg tablets | 28 tablet [PoM] £112.88 DT = £112.88

Chlorphenamine maleate

14-Dec-2020

(Chlorpheniramine maleate)

● **INDICATIONS AND DOSE**

Symptomatic relief of allergy such as hay fever, urticaria, food allergy, drug reactions | Relief of itch associated with chickenpox

▸ BY MOUTH

▸ Child 1-23 months: 1 mg twice daily
▸ Child 2-5 years: 1 mg every 4–6 hours; maximum 6 mg per day
▸ Child 6-11 years: 2 mg every 4–6 hours; maximum 12 mg per day
▸ Child 12-17 years: 4 mg every 4–6 hours; maximum 24 mg per day
▸ Adult: 4 mg every 4–6 hours; maximum 24 mg per day
▸ Elderly: 4 mg every 4–6 hours; maximum 12 mg per day

Symptomatic relief of allergy such as hay fever, urticaria, food allergy, drug reactions

▸ BY INTRAMUSCULAR INJECTION, OR BY INTRAVENOUS INJECTION

▸ Child 1-5 months: 250 micrograms/kg (max. per dose 2.5 mg), repeated if necessary; maximum 4 doses per day
▸ Child 6 months-5 years: 2.5 mg, repeated if necessary; maximum 4 doses per day
▸ Child 6-11 years: 5 mg, repeated if necessary; maximum 4 doses per day
▸ Child 12-17 years: 10 mg, repeated if necessary; maximum 4 doses per day
▸ Adult: 10 mg, repeated if necessary; maximum 4 doses per day

Emergency treatment of anaphylactic reactions

▸ BY INTRAMUSCULAR INJECTION, OR BY INTRAVENOUS INJECTION

▸ Child 1-5 months: 250 micrograms/kg (max. per dose 2.5 mg), repeated if necessary; maximum 4 doses per day
▸ Child 6 months-5 years: 2.5 mg, repeated if necessary; maximum 4 doses per day
▸ Child 6-11 years: 5 mg, repeated if necessary; maximum 4 doses per day
▸ Child 12-17 years: 10 mg, repeated if necessary; maximum 4 doses per day
▸ Adult: 10 mg, repeated if necessary; maximum 4 doses per day

---

IMPORTANT SAFETY INFORMATION

MHRA/CHM ADVICE: OVER-THE-COUNTER COUGH AND COLD MEDICINES FOR CHILDREN (APRIL 2009)

Children under 6 years should not be given over-the-counter cough and cold medicines containing chlorphenamine.

● CAUTIONS Epilepsy · prostatic hypertrophy (in adults) · pyloroduodenal obstruction · susceptibility to angle-closure glaucoma · urinary retention

● INTERACTIONS → Appendix 1: antihistamines, sedating

● SIDE-EFFECTS

GENERAL SIDE-EFFECTS

▸ **Common or very common** Concentration impaired · coordination abnormal · dizziness · dry mouth · fatigue · headache · nausea · vision blurred

▸ **Frequency not known** Agitation · appetite decreased · blood disorder · bronchial secretion viscosity increased · depression · diarrhoea · haemolytic anaemia · hypotension · irritability · muscle twitching · muscle weakness · nightmare · palpitations · photosensitivity reaction · skin reactions · tinnitus · urinary retention · vomiting

SPECIFIC SIDE-EFFECTS

▸ **Common or very common**
▸ With oral use Drowsiness
▸ **Frequency not known**
▸ With oral use Angioedema · arrhythmias · chest tightness · confusion · gastrointestinal discomfort · hepatic disorders
▸ With parenteral use Central nervous system stimulation · confusional psychosis (in adults) · dyspepsia · gastrointestinal disorder · hepatitis · sedation

SIDE-EFFECTS, FURTHER INFORMATION Children and elderly patients are more susceptible to side-effects.

● PREGNANCY Most manufacturers of antihistamines advise avoiding their use during pregnancy; however, there is no evidence of teratogenicity. Use in the latter part of the third trimester may cause adverse effects in neonates such as irritability, paradoxical excitability, and tremor.

● BREAST FEEDING Most antihistamines are present in breast milk in varying amounts; although not known to be harmful, most manufacturers advise avoiding their use in mothers who are breast-feeding.

● HEPATIC IMPAIRMENT Manufacturer advises caution.

● DIRECTIONS FOR ADMINISTRATION For *intravenous injection*, manufacturer advises give over 1 minute; if small dose required, dilute with Sodium Chloride 0.9%.

● PATIENT AND CARER ADVICE

Medicines for Children leaflet: Chlorphenamine maleate for allergy symptoms www.medicinesforchildren.org.uk/chlorphenamine-maleate-allergy-symptoms-0

Driving and skilled tasks Drowsiness may affect performance of skilled tasks (e.g. cycling or driving); sedating effects enhanced by alcohol.

● PROFESSION SPECIFIC INFORMATION

Dental practitioners' formulary Chlorphenamine tablets may be prescribed. Chlorphenamine oral solution may be prescribed.

● EXCEPTIONS TO LEGAL CATEGORY

▸ With intramuscular use or intravenous use Prescription only medicine restriction does not apply to chlorphenamine injection where administration is for saving life in emergency.

● MEDICINAL FORMS There can be variation in the licensing of different medicines containing the same drug. Forms available from special-order manufacturers include: oral solution

Solution for injection

▸ Chlorphenamine maleate (Non-proprietary)
Chlorphenamine maleate 10 mg per 1 ml Chlorphenamine 10mg/1ml solution for injection ampoules | 5 ampoule [PoM] £22.50 DT = £22.50 | 5 ampoule [PoM] [⚠] DT = £22.50 (Hospital only)

Oral solution

CAUTIONARY AND ADVISORY LABELS 2

▸ Chlorphenamine maleate (Non-proprietary)
Chlorphenamine maleate 400 microgram per 1 ml Chlorphenamine 2mg/5ml oral solution sugar free sugar-free | 150 ml [P] £2.78 DT = £2.21

▸ Allerief (Crescent Pharma Ltd)
Chlorphenamine maleate 400 microgram per 1 ml Allerief 2mg/5ml oral solution sugar-free | 150 ml [P] £2.21 DT = £2.21

▸ Piriton (GlaxoSmithKline Consumer Healthcare)
Chlorphenamine maleate 400 microgram per 1 ml Piriton 2mg/5ml syrup | 150 ml [P] £2.78 DT = £2.78

Tablet

CAUTIONARY AND ADVISORY LABELS 2

▸ Chlorphenamine maleate (Non-proprietary)
Chlorphenamine maleate 4 mg Chlorphenamine 4mg tablets | 28 tablet [P] £3.23 DT = £1.91

▸ Allerief (Crescent Pharma Ltd)
Chlorphenamine maleate 4 mg Allerief 4mg tablets | 28 tablet [P] £1.74 DT = £1.91

▸ Hayleve (Genesis Pharmaceuticals Ltd)
Chlorphenamine maleate 4 mg Hayleve 4mg tablets | 28 tablet [P] £1.91 DT = £1.91

3

Respiratory system

▸ Piriton (GlaxoSmithKline Consumer Healthcare)
Chlorphenamine maleate 4 mg Piriton 4mg tablets | 500 tablet P
£6.96
Piriton Allergy 4mg tablets | 30 tablet P £2.23 | 60 tablet P £3.90
▸ Pollenase (chlorphenamine) (East Midlands Pharma Ltd)
Chlorphenamine maleate 4 mg Pollenase Antihistamine 4mg
tablets | 30 tablet P £1.00

Clemastine

04-Sep-2020

● **INDICATIONS AND DOSE**

Symptomatic relief of allergy such as hay fever, urticaria
▸ BY MOUTH
▸ Adult: 1 mg twice daily, increased if necessary up to
6 mg daily

● CONTRA-INDICATIONS Avoid in Acute porphyrias p. 1107
● CAUTIONS Elderly · epilepsy · prostatic hypertrophy ·
pyloroduodenal obstruction · stenosing peptic ulcer ·
susceptibility to angle-closure glaucoma · urinary
retention
● INTERACTIONS → Appendix 1: antihistamines, sedating
● SIDE-EFFECTS
▸ **Common or very common** Asthenia · sedation
▸ **Uncommon** Dizziness
▸ **Rare or very rare** Abdominal pain · agitation · constipation
· dry mouth · dyspnoea · headache · nausea · palpitations ·
rash · tachycardia
● PREGNANCY Most manufacturers of antihistamines advise
avoiding their use during pregnancy; however, there is no
evidence of teratogenicity. Use in the latter part of the
third trimester may cause adverse effects in neonates such
as irritability, paradoxical excitability, and tremor.
● BREAST FEEDING Most antihistamines are present in
breast milk in varying amounts; although not known to be
harmful, most manufacturers advise avoiding their use in
mothers who are breast-feeding.
● PATIENT AND CARER ADVICE
Driving and skilled tasks Drowsiness may affect
performance of skilled tasks (e.g. driving); sedating effects
enhanced by alcohol.
● MEDICINAL FORMS There can be variation in the licensing of
different medicines containing the same drug.
Tablet
CAUTIONARY AND ADVISORY LABELS 2
▸ Tavegil (GlaxoSmithKline Consumer Healthcare)
Clemastine (as Clemastine hydrogen fumarate) 1 mg Tavegil 1mg
tablets | 60 tablet P £7.33 DT = £7.33

Cyproheptadine hydrochloride

04-Sep-2020

● **INDICATIONS AND DOSE**

**Symptomatic relief of allergy such as hay fever, urticaria |
Pruritus**
▸ BY MOUTH
▸ Adult: 4 mg 3 times a day, usual dose 4–20 mg daily;
maximum 32 mg per day

● CONTRA-INDICATIONS Avoid in Acute porphyrias p. 1107
● CAUTIONS Epilepsy · prostatic hypertrophy ·
pyloroduodenal obstruction · susceptibility to angle-
closure glaucoma · urinary retention
● INTERACTIONS → Appendix 1: antihistamines, sedating
● SIDE-EFFECTS Aggression · agranulocytosis · anxiety ·
appetite abnormal · arrhythmias · bronchial secretion
viscosity increased · chest tightness · chills · confusion ·
constipation · coordination abnormal · diarrhoea ·
dizziness · drowsiness · dry mouth · dry throat · epigastric
distress · epistaxis · fatigue · haemolytic anaemia ·

hallucination · headache · hepatic disorders · hyperhidrosis
· hypotension · insomnia · labyrinthitis · leucopenia ·
menstruation irregular · mood altered · nasal complaints ·
nausea · neuritis · oedema · palpitations · paraesthesia ·
photosensitivity reaction · seizure · skin reactions ·
thrombocytopenia · tinnitus · tremor · urinary disorders ·
vertigo · vision disorders · vomiting · weight increased ·
wheezing
● PREGNANCY Most manufacturers of antihistamines advise
avoiding their use during pregnancy; however, there is no
evidence of teratogenicity. Use in the latter part of the
third trimester may cause adverse effects in neonates such
as irritability, paradoxical excitability, and tremor.
● BREAST FEEDING Most antihistamines are present in
breast milk in varying amounts; although not known to be
harmful, most manufacturers advise avoiding their use in
mothers who are breast-feeding.
● PATIENT AND CARER ADVICE
Driving and skilled tasks Drowsiness may affect
performance of skilled tasks (e.g. driving); sedating effects
enhanced by alcohol.
● MEDICINAL FORMS There can be variation in the licensing of
different medicines containing the same drug. Forms available
from special-order manufacturers include: oral suspension, oral
solution
Tablet
CAUTIONARY AND ADVISORY LABELS 2
▸ Periactin (Teva UK Ltd)
Cyproheptadine hydrochloride 4 mg Periactin 4mg tablets |
30 tablet P £5.99 DT = £5.99

Hydroxyzine hydrochloride

14-Dec-2020

● DRUG ACTION Hydroxyzine is a sedating antihistamine
which exerts its actions by antagonising the effects of
histamine.

● **INDICATIONS AND DOSE**

Pruritus
▸ BY MOUTH
▸ Child 6 months-5 years: 5–15 mg daily in divided doses,
dose adjusted according to weight; maximum 2 mg/kg
per day
▸ Child 6-17 years (body-weight up to 40 kg): Initially
15–25 mg daily in divided doses, dose increased as
necessary, adjusted according to weight; maximum
2 mg/kg per day
▸ Child 6-17 years (body-weight 40 kg and above): Initially
15–25 mg daily in divided doses, increased if necessary
to 50–100 mg daily in divided doses, dose adjusted
according to weight
▸ Adult: Initially 25 mg daily, dose to be taken at night;
increased if necessary to 25 mg 3–4 times a day
▸ Elderly: Initially 25 mg daily, dose to be taken at night;
increased if necessary to 25 mg twice daily

IMPORTANT SAFETY INFORMATION

MHRA/CHM ADVICE: RISK OF QT-INTERVAL PROLONGATION AND
TORSADE DE POINTES (APRIL 2015)

Following concerns of heart rhythm abnormalities, the
safety and efficacy of hydroxyzine has been reviewed by the
European Medicines Agency. The review concludes
that hydroxyzine is associated with a small risk of QT-
interval prolongation and torsade de pointes; these
events are most likely to occur in patients who have risk
factors for QT prolongation, e.g. concomitant use of
drugs that prolong the QT-interval, cardiovascular
disease, family history of sudden cardiac death,
significant electrolyte imbalance (low plasma-potassium
or plasma-magnesium concentrations), or significant
bradycardia. To minimise the risk of such adverse effects,

the following dose restrictions have been made and new cautions and contra-indications added:

- Hydroxyzine is contra-indicated in patients with prolonged QT-interval or who have risk factors for QT-interval prolongation;
- Avoid use in the elderly due to increased susceptibility to the side-effects of hydroxyzine;
- Consider the risks of QT-interval prolongation and torsade de pointes before prescribing to patients taking drugs that lower heart rate or plasma-potassium concentration;
- In children with body-weight up to 40 kg, the maximum daily dose is 2 mg/kg;
- In adults, the maximum daily dose is 100 mg;
- In the elderly, the maximum daily dose is 50 mg (if use of hydroxyzine cannot be avoided);
- The lowest effective dose for the shortest period of time should be prescribed.

- CONTRA-INDICATIONS Acquired or congenital QT interval prolongation · predisposition to QT interval prolongation
  CONTRA-INDICATIONS, FURTHER INFORMATION
  ‣ QT interval prolongation Risk factors for QT interval prolongation include significant electrolyte imbalance, bradycardia, cardiovascular disease, and family history of sudden cardiac death.
- CAUTIONS Bladder outflow obstruction · breathing problems · cardiovascular disease · children · decreased gastrointestinal motility · dementia · elderly · epilepsy · hypertension · hyperthyroidism · myasthenia gravis · prostatic hypertrophy (in adults) · pyloroduodenal obstruction · stenosing peptic ulcer · susceptibility to angle-closure glaucoma · urinary retention
  CAUTIONS, FURTHER INFORMATION Elderly patients are particularly susceptible to side-effects; manufacturers advise avoid or reduce dose. Children have an increased susceptibility to side-effects, particularly CNS effects.
- INTERACTIONS → Appendix 1: antihistamines, sedating
- SIDE-EFFECTS
  ‣ **Rare or very rare** Severe cutaneous adverse reactions (SCARs) · skin reactions
  ‣ **Frequency not known** Agranulocytosis · alopecia · anticholinergic syndrome · anxiety · appetite decreased · arrhythmias · asthenia · blood disorder · bronchial secretion viscosity increased · chest tightness · chills · coma · concentration impaired · confusion · constipation · depression · diarrhoea · dizziness · drowsiness · dry mouth · dry throat · dyskinesia (on discontinuation) · epigastric pain · fever · flushing · gastrointestinal disorders · haemolytic anaemia · hallucination · headache · hepatic function abnormal · hyperhidrosis · hypotension · irritability · labyrinthitis · leucopenia · malaise · menstruation irregular · movement disorders · myalgia · nasal congestion · nausea · palpitations · paraesthesia · QT interval prolongation · respiratory disorders · respiratory tract dryness · seizure (with high doses) · sexual dysfunction · sleep disorders · speech slurred · taste bitter · thrombocytopenia · tinnitus · tremor (with high doses) · urinary disorders · vertigo · vision disorders · vomiting
  SIDE-EFFECTS, FURTHER INFORMATION Paradoxical stimulation may occur rarely, especially with high doses or in the elderly. Drowsiness may diminish after a few days of treatment.
- ALLERGY AND CROSS-SENSITIVITY Manufacturer advises hydroxyzine should be avoided in patients with previous hypersensitivity to cetirizine or other piperazine derivatives, and aminophylline.
- PREGNANCY Manufacturers advise avoid—toxicity in *animal* studies with higher doses. Use in the latter part of the third trimester may cause irritability, paradoxical excitability, and tremor in the neonate.

- BREAST FEEDING Manufacturer advises avoid—expected to be present in milk but effect unknown.
- HEPATIC IMPAIRMENT Manufacturer advises caution in mild to moderate impairment (increased risk of accumulation); avoid in severe impairment.
  Dose adjustments Manufacturer advises dose reduction of 33% in mild to moderate impairment.
- RENAL IMPAIRMENT
  Dose adjustments Manufacturers advise reduce daily dose by half in moderate to severe renal impairment.
- EFFECT ON LABORATORY TESTS May interfere with methacholine test—manufacturer advises stop treatment 96 hours prior to test. May interfere with skin testing for allergy—manufacturer advises stop treatment one week prior to test.
- PATIENT AND CARER ADVICE
  Driving and skilled tasks Drowsiness may affect performance of skilled tasks (e.g. cycling or driving); sedating effects enhanced by alcohol.

- MEDICINAL FORMS There can be variation in the licensing of different medicines containing the same drug. Forms available from special-order manufacturers include: oral suspension, oral solution
  Tablet
  CAUTIONARY AND ADVISORY LABELS 2
  ‣ Hydroxyzine hydrochloride (Non-proprietary)
    Hydroxyzine hydrochloride 10 mg Hydroxyzine 10mg tablets | 84 tablet [PoM] £4.50 DT = £2.10
    Hydroxyzine hydrochloride 25 mg Hydroxyzine 25mg tablets | 28 tablet [PoM] £4.00 DT = £1.88

Ketotifen
14-Dec-2020

- **INDICATIONS AND DOSE**
  Allergic rhinitis
  ‣ BY MOUTH
  ‣ Child 3–17 years: 1 mg twice daily
  ‣ Adult: 1 mg twice daily, increased if necessary to 2 mg twice daily, to be taken with food
  Allergic rhinitis in readily sedated patients
  ‣ BY MOUTH
  ‣ Adult: Initially 0.5–1 mg once daily, dose to be taken at night

- CONTRA-INDICATIONS Avoid in Acute porphyrias p. 1107
- CAUTIONS Epilepsy · prostatic hypertrophy (in adults) · pyloroduodenal obstruction · susceptibility to angle-closure glaucoma · urinary retention
- INTERACTIONS → Appendix 1: antihistamines, sedating
- SIDE-EFFECTS
  ‣ **Common or very common** Anxiety · insomnia · irritability
  ‣ **Uncommon** Cystitis · dizziness · dry mouth · skin reactions
  ‣ **Rare or very rare** Hepatitis · sedation · seizure · Stevens-Johnson syndrome · weight increased
  SIDE-EFFECTS, FURTHER INFORMATION Drowsiness is a significant side-effect with most of the older antihistamines although paradoxical stimulation may occur rarely, especially with high doses or in children and the elderly. Drowsiness may diminish after a few days of treatment and is considerably less of a problem with the newer antihistamines.
- PREGNANCY Most manufacturers of antihistamines advise avoiding their use during pregnancy; however, there is no evidence of teratogenicity. Use in the latter part of the third trimester may cause adverse effects in neonates such as irritability, paradoxical excitability, and tremor.
- BREAST FEEDING Most antihistamines are present in breast milk in varying amounts; although not known to be

3

Respiratory system

harmful, most manufacturers advise avoiding their use in mothers who are breast-feeding.

● PATIENT AND CARER ADVICE
Driving and skilled tasks Drowsiness may affect performance of skilled tasks (e.g. driving or cycling); sedating effects enhanced by alcohol.

● MEDICINAL FORMS There can be variation in the licensing of different medicines containing the same drug. Forms available from special-order manufacturers include: oral solution

Oral solution
CAUTIONARY AND ADVISORY LABELS 2, 21
▸ Zaditen (CD Pharma Srl)
Ketotifen (as Ketotifen fumarate) 200 microgram per 1 ml Zaditen 1mg/5ml elixir sugar-free | 300 ml [PoM] £8.91 DT = £8.91

Tablet
CAUTIONARY AND ADVISORY LABELS 2, 21
▸ Zaditen (CD Pharma Srl)
Ketotifen (as Ketotifen fumarate) 1 mg Zaditen 1mg tablets | 60 tablet [PoM] £7.53 DT = £7.53

Promethazine hydrochloride   14-Dec-2020

● INDICATIONS AND DOSE

Symptomatic relief of allergy such as hay fever and urticaria | Insomnia associated with urticaria and pruritus
▸ BY MOUTH
▸ **Child 2-4 years:** 5 mg twice daily, alternatively 5–15 mg once daily, dose to be taken at night
▸ **Child 5-9 years:** 5–10 mg twice daily, alternatively 10–25 mg once daily, dose to be taken at night
▸ **Child 10-17 years:** 10–20 mg 2–3 times a day, alternatively 25 mg once daily, dose to be taken at night, increased if necessary to 25 mg twice daily
▸ **Adult:** 10–20 mg 2–3 times a day
▸ BY DEEP INTRAMUSCULAR INJECTION
▸ **Adult:** 25–50 mg (max. per dose 100 mg)

Emergency treatment of anaphylactic reactions
▸ BY SLOW INTRAVENOUS INJECTION
▸ **Adult:** 25–50 mg, to be administered as a solution containing 2.5 mg/mL in water for injections; maximum 100 mg per course

Sedation (short-term use)
▸ BY MOUTH
▸ **Child 2-4 years:** 15–20 mg
▸ **Child 5-9 years:** 20–25 mg
▸ **Child 10-17 years:** 25–50 mg
▸ **Adult:** 25–50 mg
▸ BY DEEP INTRAMUSCULAR INJECTION
▸ **Adult:** 25–50 mg

Nausea | Vomiting | Vertigo | Labyrinthine disorders | Motion sickness
▸ BY MOUTH
▸ **Child 2-4 years:** 5 mg, to be taken at bedtime on night before travel, repeat following morning if necessary
▸ **Child 5-9 years:** 10 mg, to be taken at bedtime on night before travel, repeat following morning if necessary
▸ **Child 10-17 years:** 20–25 mg, to be taken at bedtime on night before travel, repeat following morning if necessary

▸ **Adult:** 20–25 mg, to be taken at bedtime on night before travel, repeat following morning if necessary

┌───┐
IMPORTANT SAFETY INFORMATION
MHRA/CHM ADVICE: OVER-THE-COUNTER COUGH AND COLD MEDICINES FOR CHILDREN (APRIL 2009)
Children under 6 years should not be given over-the-counter cough and cold medicines containing promethazine.
└───┘

● CAUTIONS
GENERAL CAUTIONS Epilepsy · prostatic hypertrophy (in adults) · pyloroduodenal obstruction · severe coronary artery disease · susceptibility to angle-closure glaucoma · urinary retention
SPECIFIC CAUTIONS
▸ With intravenous use Avoid extravasation with intravenous injection

● INTERACTIONS → Appendix 1: antihistamines, sedating

● SIDE-EFFECTS
GENERAL SIDE-EFFECTS Arrhythmia · blood disorder · confusion · dizziness · drowsiness · dry mouth · headache · hypotension · jaundice · movement disorders · palpitations · photosensitivity reaction · urinary retention · vision blurred
SPECIFIC SIDE-EFFECTS
▸ With oral use Agranulocytosis · angle closure glaucoma · anticholinergic syndrome · anxiety · insomnia · leucopenia · nasal congestion · nausea · rash · seizure · thrombocytopenia · tinnitus · vomiting
▸ With parenteral use Appetite decreased · epigastric discomfort · fatigue · haemolytic anaemia · hypersensitivity · muscle spasms · nightmare · restlessness · skin reactions
SIDE-EFFECTS, FURTHER INFORMATION Elderly patients are more susceptible to anticholinergic side-effects.

● PREGNANCY Most manufacturers of antihistamines advise avoiding their use during pregnancy; however, there is no evidence of teratogenicity. Use in the latter part of the third trimester may cause adverse effects in neonates such as irritability, paradoxical excitability, and tremor.

● BREAST FEEDING Most antihistamines are present in breast milk in varying amounts; although not known to be harmful, most manufacturers advise avoiding their use in mothers who are breast-feeding.

● HEPATIC IMPAIRMENT Manufacturer advises caution.

● RENAL IMPAIRMENT Use with caution.

● PATIENT AND CARER ADVICE
Driving and skilled tasks Drowsiness may affect the performance of skilled tasks (e.g. cycling or driving); sedating effects enhanced by alcohol.

● PROFESSION SPECIFIC INFORMATION
Dental practitioners' formulary
Promethazine Hydrochloride Tablets 10 mg or 25 mg may be prescribed.
Promethazine Hydrochloride Oral Solution (elixir) 5 mg/5 mL may be prescribed.

● LESS SUITABLE FOR PRESCRIBING Promethazine is less suitable for prescribing for sedation.

● EXCEPTIONS TO LEGAL CATEGORY Prescription only medicine restriction does not apply to promethazine hydrochloride injection where administration is for saving life in emergency.

- MEDICINAL FORMS There can be variation in the licensing of different medicines containing the same drug. Forms available from special-order manufacturers include: oral suspension, oral solution

Solution for injection

EXCIPIENTS: May contain Sulfites

▶ Phenergan (Sanofi)

Promethazine hydrochloride 25 mg per 1 ml Phenergan 25mg/1ml solution for injection ampoules | 10 ampoule [PoM] £6.74 DT = £6.74

Oral solution

CAUTIONARY AND ADVISORY LABELS 2
EXCIPIENTS: May contain Sulfites
ELECTROLYTES: May contain Sodium

▶ Phenergan (Sanofi)

Promethazine hydrochloride 1 mg per 1 ml Phenergan 5mg/5ml elixir sugar-free | 100 ml [P] £2.85 DT = £2.85

Tablet

CAUTIONARY AND ADVISORY LABELS 2

▶ Promethazine hydrochloride (Non-proprietary)

Promethazine hydrochloride 10 mg Promethazine hydrochloride 10mg tablets | 56 tablet [PoM] £3.67 DT = £3.67

Promethazine hydrochloride 25 mg Promethazine hydrochloride 25mg tablets | 56 tablet [P] £4.51-£4.65 DT = £4.51

▶ Phenergan (Sanofi)

Promethazine hydrochloride 10 mg Phenergan 10mg tablets | 56 tablet [P] £2.96 DT = £3.67

Promethazine hydrochloride 25 mg Phenergan Nightime 25mg tablets | 14 tablet [P] £2.79

Phenergan 25mg tablets | 56 tablet [P] £4.65 DT = £4.51

▶ Sominex (Teva UK Ltd)

Promethazine hydrochloride 20 mg Sominex 20mg tablets | 8 tablet [P] £1.89 DT = £1.89 | 16 tablet [P] £2.69 DT = £2.69

VACCINES > ALLERGEN-TYPE VACCINES

Bee venom extract   28-Apr-2020

- **INDICATIONS AND DOSE**

Hypersensitivity to bee venom

▶ BY SUBCUTANEOUS INJECTION

▶ Adult: (consult product literature)

> IMPORTANT SAFETY INFORMATION
> DESENSITISING VACCINES
> In view of concerns about the safety of desensitising vaccines, it is recommended that they are used by specialists and only for the following indications:
> - seasonal allergic hay fever (caused by pollen) that has not responded to anti-allergic drugs;
> - hypersensitivity to wasp and bee venoms.
> Manufacturer advises desensitising vaccines should generally be avoided or used with particular care in patients with asthma.

- CONTRA-INDICATIONS Consult product literature
- CAUTIONS Consult product literature
- INTERACTIONS → Appendix 1: bee venom extract
- SIDE-EFFECTS

SIDE-EFFECTS, FURTHER INFORMATION Life-threatening hypersensitivity reactions can occur. Cardiopulmonary resuscitation must be immediately available. Manufacturer advises monitoring for at least 1 hour after injection.

- PREGNANCY Avoid.
- PRESCRIBING AND DISPENSING INFORMATION Each set of allergen extracts usually contains vials for the administration of graded amounts of allergen to patients undergoing hyposensitisation. Maintenance sets containing vials at the highest strength are also available. Product literature must be consulted for details of allergens, vial strengths, and administration.
- NATIONAL FUNDING/ACCESS DECISIONS For full details see funding body website

NICE decisions

▶ *Pharmalgen®* for the treatment of bee and wasp venom allergy (February 2012) NICE TA246 Recommended with restrictions

- MEDICINAL FORMS There can be variation in the licensing of different medicines containing the same drug.

Powder and solvent for solution for injection

▶ Bee Venom (ALK-Abello Ltd)

Bee venom 120 nanogram Pharmalgen Bee Venom 120nanogram powder and solvent for solution for injection vials | 1 vial [PoM] ⓢ

Bee venom 1.2 microgram Pharmalgen Bee Venom 1.2microgram powder and solvent for solution for injection vials | 1 vial [PoM] ⓢ

Bee venom 12 microgram Pharmalgen Bee Venom 12microgram powder and solvent for solution for injection vials | 1 vial [PoM] ⓢ

Bee venom 120 microgram Pharmalgen Bee Venom maintenance set 120microgram powder and solvent for solution for injection vials | 4 vial [PoM] £150.00

Grass pollen extract   27-Jul-2020

- **INDICATIONS AND DOSE**

Treatment of seasonal allergic hay fever due to grass pollen in patients who have failed to respond to anti-allergy drugs

▶ BY SUBCUTANEOUS INJECTION

▶ Adult: (consult product literature)

Treatment of seasonal allergic hay fever due to grass pollen in patients who have failed to respond to anti-allergy drugs (initiated under specialist supervision)

▶ BY MOUTH

▶ Adult: 1 tablet daily, treatment to be started at least 4 months before start of pollen season and continue for up to 3 years

> IMPORTANT SAFETY INFORMATION
> DESENSITISING VACCINES
> In view of concerns about the safety of desensitising vaccines, it is recommended that they are used by specialists and only for the following indications:
> - seasonal allergic hay fever (caused by pollen) that has not responded to anti-allergic drugs;
> - hypersensitivity to wasp and bee venoms.
> Manufacturer advises desensitising vaccines should generally be avoided or used with particular care in patients with asthma.

- CONTRA-INDICATIONS Consult product literature
- CAUTIONS Consult product literature
- INTERACTIONS → Appendix 1: grass pollen extract
- SIDE-EFFECTS

SIDE-EFFECTS, FURTHER INFORMATION Hypersensitivity reactions to immunotherapy can be life-threatening; bronchospasm usually develops within 1 hour and anaphylaxis within 30 minutes of injection. Therefore, cardiopulmonary resuscitation must be immediately available and patients need to be monitored for at least 1 hour after injection. If symptoms or signs of hypersensitivity develop (e.g. rash, urticaria, bronchospasm, faintness), **even when mild,** the patient should be observed until these have resolved completely.

- PREGNANCY Should be avoided in pregnant women— consult product literature.
- MONITORING REQUIREMENTS The first dose of grass pollen extract (*Grazax®*) should be taken under medical supervision and the patient should be monitored for 20–30 minutes.
- DIRECTIONS FOR ADMINISTRATION Manufacturer advises oral lyophilisates should be placed under the tongue and allowed to disperse. Advise patient not to swallow for

1 minute, or eat or drink for 5 minutes after taking the tablet. The first should be taken under medical supervision and the patient should be monitored for 20–30 minutes.

- PRESCRIBING AND DISPENSING INFORMATION Each set of allergen extracts usually contains vials for the administration of graded amounts of allergen to patients undergoing hyposensitisation. Maintenance sets containing vials at the highest strength are also available. Product literature must be consulted for details of allergens, vial strengths, and administration.

- PATIENT AND CARER ADVICE
  ▸ With oral use Patients or carers should be given advice on how to administer oral lyophilisates.

- MEDICINAL FORMS There can be variation in the licensing of different medicines containing the same drug.
  Suspension for injection
  ▸ Pollinex Grasses + Rye (Allergy Therapeutics (UK) Ltd)
    Pollinex Grasses + Rye suspension for injection treatment and extension course vials | 4 vial [PoM] £450.00
  Oral lyophilisate
  ▸ Grazax (ALK-Abello Ltd)
    Phleum pratense 75000 SQ-T Grazax 75,000 SQ-T oral lyophilisates sugar-free | 30 tablet [PoM] £80.12 DT = £80.12

Tree pollen extract

28-Apr-2020

- INDICATIONS AND DOSE
  Treatment of seasonal allergic hay fever due to tree pollen in patients who have failed to respond to anti-allergy drugs
  ▸ BY SUBCUTANEOUS INJECTION
  ▸ Adult: (consult product literature)

IMPORTANT SAFETY INFORMATION
DESENSITISING VACCINES
In view of concerns about the safety of desensitising vaccines, it is recommended that they are used by specialists and only for the following indications:
- seasonal allergic hay fever (caused by pollen) that has not responded to anti-allergic drugs;
- hypersensitivity to wasp and bee venoms.
Manufacturer advises desensitising vaccines should generally be avoided or used with particular care in patients with asthma.

- CONTRA-INDICATIONS Consult product literature
- CAUTIONS Consult product literature
- INTERACTIONS → Appendix 1: tree pollen extract
- SIDE-EFFECTS

SIDE-EFFECTS, FURTHER INFORMATION Hypersensitivity reactions to immunotherapy can be life-threatening. Cardiopulmonary resuscitation must be immediately available and patients need to be monitored for at least 1 hour after injection. If symptoms or signs of hypersensitivity develop (e.g. rash, urticaria, bronchospasm, faintness), **even when mild**, the patient should be observed until these have resolved completely.

- PREGNANCY Should be avoided in pregnant women— consult product literature.

- PRESCRIBING AND DISPENSING INFORMATION Each set of allergen extracts usually contains vials for the administration of graded amounts of allergen to patients undergoing hyposensitisation. Maintenance sets containing vials at the highest strength are also available. Product literature must be consulted for details of allergens, vial strengths, and administration.

- MEDICINAL FORMS There can be variation in the licensing of different medicines containing the same drug.
  Form unstated
  ▸ Pollinex Trees (Allergy Therapeutics (UK) Ltd)
    Pollinex Trees suspension for injection treatment and extension course vials | 4 vial [PoM] £450.00
  Suspension for injection
  ▸ Pollinex Trees (Allergy Therapeutics (UK) Ltd)
    Pollinex Trees No 3 suspension for injection 1ml vials | 1 vial [PoM] [X]
    Pollinex Trees No 2 suspension for injection 1ml vials | 1 vial [PoM] [X]
    Pollinex Trees No 1 suspension for injection 1ml vials | 1 vial [PoM] [X]

Wasp venom extract

28-Apr-2020

- INDICATIONS AND DOSE
  Hypersensitivity to wasp venom
  ▸ BY SUBCUTANEOUS INJECTION
  ▸ Adult: (consult product literature)

IMPORTANT SAFETY INFORMATION
DESENSITISING VACCINES
In view of concerns about the safety of desensitising vaccines, it is recommended that they are used by specialists and only for the following indications:
- seasonal allergic hay fever (caused by pollen) that has not responded to anti-allergic drugs;
- hypersensitivity to wasp and bee venoms.
Manufacturer advises desensitising vaccines should generally be avoided or used with particular care in patients with asthma.

- CONTRA-INDICATIONS Consult product literature
- CAUTIONS Consult product literature
- INTERACTIONS → Appendix 1: wasp venom extract
- SIDE-EFFECTS

SIDE-EFFECTS, FURTHER INFORMATION Hypersensitivity reactions to wasp venom extracts can be life-threatening; cardiopulmonary resuscitation must be immediately available and patients need to be monitored for at least 1 hour after injection. If symptoms or signs of hypersensitivity develop (e.g. rash, urticaria, bronchospasm, faintness), **even when mild,** the patient should be observed until these have resolved completely.

- PREGNANCY Avoid.

- PRESCRIBING AND DISPENSING INFORMATION Each set of allergen extracts usually contains vials for the administration of graded amounts of allergen to patients undergoing hyposensitisation. Maintenance sets containing vials at the highest strength are also available. Product literature must be consulted for details of allergens, vial strengths, and administration.

- NATIONAL FUNDING/ACCESS DECISIONS
  For full details see funding body website

  NICE decisions
  ▸ *Pharmalgen*® for bee and wasp venom allergy (February 2012) NICE TA246 Recommended with restrictions

- MEDICINAL FORMS There can be variation in the licensing of different medicines containing the same drug.
  Powder and solvent for solution for injection
  ▸ Pharmalgen Wasp Venom (ALK-Abello Ltd)
    Wasp venom 120 nanogram Pharmalgen Wasp Venom 120nanogram powder and solvent for solution for injection vials | 1 vial [PoM] [X]
    Wasp venom 1.2 microgram Pharmalgen Wasp Venom 1.2microgram powder and solvent for solution for injection vials | 1 vial [PoM] [X]
    Wasp venom 12 microgram Pharmalgen Wasp Venom 12microgram powder and solvent for solution for injection vials | 1 vial [PoM] [X]

Wasp venom 120 microgram Pharmalgen Wasp Venom maintenance set 120microgram vaccine powder and solvent for solution for injection vials | 4 vial [PoM] £150.00

2.1 Angioedema

Other drugs used for Angioedema Adrenaline/epinephrine, p. 238

DRUGS USED IN HEREDITARY ANGIOEDEMA >
COMPLEMENT REGULATORY PROTEINS

C1-esterase inhibitor

30-Oct-2020

● **INDICATIONS AND DOSE**

BERINERT ®

Acute attacks of hereditary angioedema (under expert supervision)
▸ BY SLOW INTRAVENOUS INJECTION, OR BY INTRAVENOUS INFUSION
▸ Adult: 20 units/kg

Short-term prophylaxis of hereditary angioedema before dental, medical, or surgical procedures (under expert supervision)
▸ BY SLOW INTRAVENOUS INJECTION, OR BY INTRAVENOUS INFUSION
▸ Adult: 1000 units for 1 dose, to be administered less than 6 hours before procedure

CINRYZE ®

Acute attacks of hereditary angioedema (under expert supervision)
▸ BY SLOW INTRAVENOUS INJECTION
▸ Adult: 1000 units for 1 dose, dose may be repeated if necessary after 60 minutes (or sooner for patients experiencing laryngeal attacks or if treatment initiation is delayed)

Short-term prophylaxis of hereditary angioedema before dental, medical, or surgical procedures (under expert supervision)
▸ BY SLOW INTRAVENOUS INJECTION
▸ Adult: 1000 units for 1 dose, to be administered up to 24 hours before procedure

Long-term prophylaxis of severe, recurrent attacks of hereditary angioedema where acute treatment is inadequate, or when oral prophylaxis is inadequate or not tolerated (under expert supervision)
▸ BY SLOW INTRAVENOUS INJECTION
▸ Adult: 1000 units every 3–4 days, interval between doses to be adjusted according to response

● CAUTIONS Vaccination against hepatitis A and hepatitis B may be required
● SIDE-EFFECTS
▸ Rare or very rare Dizziness · dyspnoea · flushing · headache · hypersensitivity · hypertension · hypotension · nausea · tachycardia · thrombosis (with high doses) · urticaria
● PREGNANCY Manufacturer advises avoid unless essential.
● PRESCRIBING AND DISPENSING INFORMATION C1-esterase inhibitor is prepared from human plasma.
● NATIONAL FUNDING/ACCESS DECISIONS
For full details see funding body website

All Wales Medicines Strategy Group (AWMSG) decisions
▸ C1 inhibitor (human) (Cinryze ®) for the treatment and pre-procedure prevention of attacks of hereditary angioedema (HAE) in adults; routine prevention of angioedema attacks in adults with severe and recurrent attacks of HAE, where acute treatment is inadequate, or when oral prophylaxis is

inadequate or not tolerated (October 2017) AWMSG No. 3295 Recommended

● MEDICINAL FORMS There can be variation in the licensing of different medicines containing the same drug.
Powder and solvent for solution for injection
ELECTROLYTES: May contain Sodium
▸ Berinert P (CSL Behring UK Ltd)
C1-esterase inhibitor 500 unit Berinert 500unit powder and solvent for solution for injection vials | 1 vial [PoM] £550.00 DT = £550.00
C1-esterase inhibitor 1500 unit Berinert 1,500unit powder and solvent for solution for injection vials | 1 vial [PoM] £1,650.00 DT = £1,650.00
▸ Cinryze (Shire Pharmaceuticals Ltd) ▼
C1-esterase inhibitor 500 unit Cinryze 500unit powder and solvent for solution for injection vials | 2 vial [PoM] £1,336.00

Conestat alfa

23-Oct-2020

● **INDICATIONS AND DOSE**
Acute attacks of hereditary angioedema in patients with C1-esterase inhibitor deficiency
▸ BY SLOW INTRAVENOUS INJECTION
▸ Adult (body-weight up to 84 kg): 50 units/kg for 1 dose, to be administered over 5 minutes, dose may be repeated if necessary; maximum 2 doses per day
▸ Adult (body-weight 84 kg and above): 4200 units for 1 dose, to be administered over 5 minutes, dose may be repeated if necessary; maximum 2 doses per day

● CONTRA-INDICATIONS Rabbit allergy
● SIDE-EFFECTS
▸ Common or very common Headache
▸ Uncommon Abdominal discomfort · diarrhoea · nausea · oral paraesthesia · paraesthesia · throat irritation · urticaria · vertigo
● PREGNANCY Use only if potential benefit outweighs risk—toxicity in *animal* studies.
● BREAST FEEDING Use only if potential benefit outweighs risk—no information available.
● NATIONAL FUNDING/ACCESS DECISIONS
For full details see funding body website

Scottish Medicines Consortium (SMC) decisions
▸ Conestat alfa (Ruconest ®) for the treatment of acute angioedema attacks in adults and adolescents with hereditary angioedema (HAE) due to C1 esterase inhibitor deficiency (August 2018) SMC No. 745/11 Recommended

All Wales Medicines Strategy Group (AWMSG) decisions
▸ Conestat alfa (Ruconest ®) for the treatment of acute angioedema attacks in adults and adolescents with hereditary angioedema due to C1 esterase inhibitor deficiency (November 2018) AWMSG No. 786 Recommended

● MEDICINAL FORMS There can be variation in the licensing of different medicines containing the same drug.
Powder for solution for injection
▸ Ruconest (Pharming Group N.V.)
Conestat alfa 2100 unit Ruconest 2,100unit powder for solution for injection vials | 1 vial [PoM] £750.00

3

Respiratory system

DRUGS USED IN HEREDITARY ANGIOEDEMA ›
KALLIKREIN INHIBITORS

Lanadelumab
09-Nov-2020

- **DRUG ACTION** Lanadelumab is a humanised monoclonal antibody which inhibits plasma kallikrein activity, thereby limiting the production of bradykinin, a potent vasodilator associated with angioedema attacks in patients with hereditary angioedema.

- **INDICATIONS AND DOSE**

Prevention of recurrent attacks of hereditary angioedema (initiated under specialist supervision)
  ▸ BY SUBCUTANEOUS INJECTION
  ▸ Adult: 300 mg every 2 weeks, reduced to 300 mg every 4 weeks, in those stable and attack free—consult product literature

- **CONTRA-INDICATIONS** Not a treatment for acute attacks of angioedema—initiate individualised treatment for breakthrough attacks
- **SIDE-EFFECTS**
▸ **Common or very common** Dizziness · hypersensitivity · myalgia · oral disorders · skin reactions
- **PREGNANCY** Manufacturer advises preferable to avoid—limited or no information available; *animal* studies do not indicate toxicity.
- **BREAST FEEDING** Manufacturer advises avoid during first few days after birth—possible risk from transfer of antibodies to infant. After this time, use during breast-feeding only if clinically needed.
- **EFFECT ON LABORATORY TESTS** Manufacturer advises may increase activated partial thromboplastin time (aPTT) due to an interaction with the aPTT assay—consult product literature.
- **DIRECTIONS FOR ADMINISTRATION** Manufacturer advises to withdraw dose from the vial into a syringe with an 18 gauge needle and inject, using a suitable gauge needle, into the abdomen, thigh, or upper outer arm within 2 hours—consult product literature for further information. *Takhzyro®* may be self-administered or administered by a carer after appropriate training in subcutaneous injection technique.
- **PRESCRIBING AND DISPENSING INFORMATION** Lanadelumab is a biological medicine. Biological medicines must be prescribed and dispensed by brand name, see *Biological medicines* and *Biosimilar medicines*, under Guidance on prescribing p. 1; manufacturer advises to record the brand name and batch number after each administration.
- **HANDLING AND STORAGE** Manufacturer advises store in a refrigerator (2–8°C) and protect from light—consult product literature for further information regarding storage outside refrigerator.
- **PATIENT AND CARER ADVICE**
Self-administration Manufacturer advises patients and their carers should be given training in subcutaneous injection technique if appropriate.
Missed doses Manufacturer advises if a dose is missed, it should be taken as soon as possible ensuring at least 10 days between doses.
- **NATIONAL FUNDING/ACCESS DECISIONS**
For full details see funding body website
NICE decisions
▸ Lanadelumab for preventing recurrent attacks of hereditary angioedema (October 2019) NICE TA606 Recommended with restrictions

Scottish Medicines Consortium (SMC) decisions
▸ Lanadelumab (*Takhzyro®*) for routine prevention of recurrent attacks of hereditary angioedema (HAE) in patients aged 12 years and older (December 2019) SMC No. SMC2206 Recommended with restrictions

- **MEDICINAL FORMS** There can be variation in the licensing of different medicines containing the same drug.
Solution for injection
EXCIPIENTS: May contain Polysorbates
▸ Lanadelumab (non-proprietary) ▼
Lanadelumab 150 mg per 1 ml Takhzyro 300mg/2ml solution for injection vials | 1 vial PoM £12,420.00 (Hospital only)

DRUGS USED IN HEREDITARY ANGIOEDEMA ›
SELECTIVE BRADYKININ B₂ ANTAGONISTS

Icatibant
22-Oct-2020

- **INDICATIONS AND DOSE**

Acute attacks of hereditary angioedema in patients with C1-esterase inhibitor deficiency
  ▸ BY SUBCUTANEOUS INJECTION
  ▸ Adult: 30 mg for 1 dose, then 30 mg after 6 hours if required, then 30 mg after 6 hours if required; maximum 3 doses per day

- **CAUTIONS** Ischaemic heart disease · stroke
- **INTERACTIONS** → Appendix 1: icatibant
- **SIDE-EFFECTS**
▸ **Common or very common** Dizziness · fever · headache · nausea · skin reactions
- **PREGNANCY** Manufacturer advises use only if potential benefit outweighs risk—toxicity in *animal* studies.
- **BREAST FEEDING** Manufacturer advises avoid for 12 hours after administration.
- **NATIONAL FUNDING/ACCESS DECISIONS**
For full details see funding body website
Scottish Medicines Consortium (SMC) decisions
▸ Icatibant (*Firazyr®*) for the symptomatic treatment of acute attacks of hereditary angioedema (HAE) in adults (type I and II HAE) (March 2012) SMC No. 476/08 Recommended
All Wales Medicines Strategy Group (AWMSG) decisions
▸ Icatibant acetate (*Firazyr®*) for the symptomatic treatment of acute attacks of hereditary angioedema (HAE) in adults, adolescents and children aged 2 years and older, with C1 esterase-inhibitor deficiency (June 2018) AWMSG No. 3293 Recommended

- **MEDICINAL FORMS** There can be variation in the licensing of different medicines containing the same drug.
Solution for injection
▸ Firazyr (Shire Pharmaceuticals Ltd)
Icatibant (as Icatibant acetate) 10 mg per 1 ml Firazyr 30mg/3ml solution for injection pre-filled syringes | 1 pre-filled disposable injection PoM £1,395.00

3 Conditions affecting sputum viscosity

MUCOLYTICS

Acetylcysteine
05-Oct-2020

- **INDICATIONS AND DOSE**
NACSYS® EFFERVESCENT TABLETS
Reduction of sputum viscosity
  ▸ BY MOUTH
  ▸ Adult: 600 mg once daily

- CAUTIONS History of peptic ulceration
- SIDE-EFFECTS
  - **Uncommon** Diarrhoea · fever · gastrointestinal discomfort · headache · hypotension · nausea · stomatitis · tinnitus · vomiting
  - **Rare or very rare** Haemorrhage
  - **Frequency not known** Face oedema

- MEDICINAL FORMS There can be variation in the licensing of different medicines containing the same drug. Forms available from special-order manufacturers include: effervescent tablet

Effervescent tablet
CAUTIONARY AND ADVISORY LABELS 13
ELECTROLYTES: May contain Sodium
- NACSYS (Alturix Ltd)
  Acetylcysteine 600 mg NACSYS 600mg effervescent tablets sugar-free | 30 tablet [PoM] £5.50 DT = £5.50

Carbocisteine

18-Mar-2020

- INDICATIONS AND DOSE
Reduction of sputum viscosity
- BY MOUTH
- Adult: Initially 2.25 g daily in divided doses, then reduced to 1.5 g daily in divided doses, as condition improves

- CONTRA-INDICATIONS Active peptic ulceration
- CAUTIONS History of peptic ulceration (may disrupt the gastric mucosal barrier)
- SIDE-EFFECTS Gastrointestinal haemorrhage · skin reactions · Stevens-Johnson syndrome · vomiting
- PREGNANCY Manufacturer advises avoid in first trimester.
- BREAST FEEDING No information available.
- PRESCRIBING AND DISPENSING INFORMATION Flavours of oral liquid formulations may include cherry, raspberry, cinnamon, or rum.

- MEDICINAL FORMS There can be variation in the licensing of different medicines containing the same drug.

Oral solution
- Carbocisteine (Non-proprietary)
  Carbocisteine 50 mg per 1 ml Carbocisteine 250mg/5ml oral solution sugar free sugar-free | 300 ml [PoM] £8.39-£9.49
  Carbocisteine 250mg/5ml oral solution | 300 ml [PoM] £8.99 DT = £7.29
  Carbocisteine 75 mg per 1 ml Carbocisteine 750mg/10ml oral solution 10ml sachets sugar free sugar-free | 15 sachet [PoM] £3.85 DT = £3.85
  Carbocisteine 150 mg per 1 ml Carbocisteine 750mg/5ml oral solution sugar free sugar-free | 200 ml [PoM] £18.98
- Mucodyne (Sanofi)
  Carbocisteine 50 mg per 1 ml Mucodyne Paediatric 250mg/5ml syrup | 125 ml [PoM] £12.60
  Mucodyne 250mg/5ml syrup | 300 ml [PoM] £8.39 DT = £7.29

Capsule
- Carbocisteine (Non-proprietary)
  Carbocisteine 375 mg Carbocisteine 375mg capsules | 120 capsule [PoM] £18.98 DT = £5.23
- Mucodyne (Sanofi)
  Carbocisteine 375 mg Mucodyne 375mg capsules | 120 capsule [PoM] £18.98 DT = £5.23

Erdosteine

05-Nov-2020

- INDICATIONS AND DOSE
Symptomatic treatment of acute exacerbations of chronic bronchitis
- BY MOUTH
- Adult: 300 mg twice daily for up to 10 days

- CAUTIONS History of peptic ulceration (may disrupt the gastric mucosal barrier)
- SIDE-EFFECTS
  - **Common or very common** Epigastric pain · taste altered
  - **Uncommon** Allergic dermatitis · angioedema · common cold · diarrhoea · dyspnoea · headache · nausea · vomiting
- PREGNANCY Manufacturer advises avoid—no information available.
- BREAST FEEDING Manufacturer advises avoid—no information available.
- HEPATIC IMPAIRMENT Manufacturer advises caution in mild to moderate hepatic failure; avoid in severe hepatic failure.
  Dose adjustments Manufacturer advises max. 300 mg daily in mild to moderate hepatic failure.
- RENAL IMPAIRMENT Avoid if eGFR less than 25 mL/minute/1.73 m^2—no information available.
- NATIONAL FUNDING/ACCESS DECISIONS
  For full details see funding body website
  Scottish Medicines Consortium (SMC) decisions
  - Erdosteine (*Erdotin*®) for chronic bronchitis in adults (November 2007) SMC No. 415/07 Not recommended

- MEDICINAL FORMS There can be variation in the licensing of different medicines containing the same drug.

Capsule
- Erdotin (Galen Ltd)
  Erdosteine 300 mg Erdotin 300mg capsules | 20 capsule [PoM] £5.00 DT = £5.00

3.1 Cystic fibrosis

Cystic fibrosis

06-May-2020

Description of condition

Cystic fibrosis is a genetic disorder affecting the lungs, pancreas, liver, intestine, and reproductive organs. The main clinical signs are pulmonary disease, with recurrent infections and the production of copious viscous sputum, and malabsorption due to pancreatic insufficiency. Other complications include hepatobiliary disease, osteoporosis, cystic fibrosis-related diabetes, and distal intestinal obstruction syndrome.

Aims of treatment

The aim of treatment includes preventing and managing lung infections, loosening and removing thick, sticky mucus from the lungs, preventing or treating intestinal obstruction, and providing sufficient nutrition and hydration.

Lung function is a key predictor of life expectancy in people with cystic fibrosis and optimising lung function is a major aim of care.

Non-drug treatment

Specialist physiotherapists should assess patients with cystic fibrosis and provide advice on airway clearance, nebuliser use, musculoskeletal disorders, physical activity, and urinary incontinence. The importance of airway clearance techniques should be discussed with patients and their parents or carers and appropriate training provided. Patients should be advised that regular exercise improves both lung function and overall fitness.

Drug treatment

Treatment for cystic fibrosis lung disease is based on the prevention of lung infection and the maintenance of lung function. [EvGr] In patients with cystic fibrosis, who have clinical evidence of lung disease, the frequency of routine review should be based on their clinical condition, but adults should be reviewed at least every 3 months. More frequent review is required immediately after diagnosis. ⒜

For information on the management of patients during the COVID-19 pandemic, see COVID-19 p. 660.

Mucolytics

ᴇᵥᴳʳ Patients with cystic fibrosis who have evidence of lung disease should be offered a mucolytic. Dornase alfa p. 309 is the first choice mucolytic. If there is an inadequate response, dornase alfa and hypertonic sodium chloride p. 290, or hypertonic sodium chloride alone should be considered.

Mannitol dry powder for inhalation p. 309 is recommended as an option when dornase alfa p. 309 is unsuitable (because of ineligibility, intolerance, or inadequate response), when lung function is rapidly declining, and if other osmotic drugs are not considered appropriate (see mannitol National funding/access decisions p. 310). ⒜

Lumacaftor with ivacaftor p. 310 is not recommended for treating cystic fibrosis within its marketing authorisation (see lumacaftor with ivacaftor National funding/access decisions p. 310).

Pulmonary infection

Staphylococcus aureus

ᴇᵥᴳʳ Patients who are not taking prophylaxis and have a new *Staphylococcus aureus* infection can be given an oral anti-*Staph. aureus* antibacterial, if they are clinically well. If they are clinically unwell and have pulmonary disease, oral or intravenous (depending on infection severity) broad-spectrum antibacterials with activity against *Staph. aureus* should be given (consult local protocol).

A long-term antibacterial should be considered to suppress **chronic***Staph. aureus* respiratory infections in patients whose pulmonary disease is stable. In patients with chronic *Staph. aureus* respiratory infections who become clinically unwell with pulmonary disease, oral or intravenous (depending on infection severity) broad-spectrum antibacterials with activity against *Staph. aureus* should be given. In those patients with new evidence of **meticillin-resistant***Staphylococcus aureus***(MRSA)** respiratory infection (with or without pulmonary exacerbation), specialist microbiological advice should be sought.

Antibacterials should not be routinely used to suppress chronic MRSA in patients with stable pulmonary disease.

If a patient with cystic fibrosis and chronic MRSA respiratory infection becomes unwell with a pulmonary exacerbation or shows a decline in pulmonary function, specialist microbiological advice should be sought. ⒜

Pseudomonas aeruginosa

ᴇᵥᴳʳ If a patient with cystic fibrosis develops a new *Pseudomonas aeruginosa* infection, eradication therapy with a course of oral antibacterial should be started (by intravenous injection, if they are clinically unwell), in combination with an inhaled antibacterial. An extended course of oral and inhaled antibacterial should follow (consult local protocol).

If eradication therapy is not successful, sustained treatment with an inhaled antibacterial should be offered. Nebulised colistimethate sodium p. 591 should be considered as first-line treatment (but see also colistimethate sodium by dry powder inhalation National funding/access decisions p. 591).

In patients with **chronic***Ps. aeruginosa* infection (when treatment has not eradicated the infection) who become clinically unwell with pulmonary exacerbations, an oral antibacterial or a combination of two intravenous antibacterial drugs of different classes (depending on infection severity) should be used. Changing antibacterial regimens should be considered to treat exacerbations (consult local protocol).

Nebulised aztreonam p. 574, nebulised tobramycin p. 547, or tobramycin dry powder for inhalation p. 547 (see tobramycin National funding/access decisions p. 547) should

be considered for those who are deteriorating despite regular inhaled colistimethate sodium p. 591. ⒜

Burkholderia cepacia **complex**

ᴇᵥᴳʳ Patients who develop a new *Burkholderia cepacia* complex infection, should be given eradication therapy with a combination of intravenous antibacterial drugs (specialist microbiological advice should be sought on the choice of antibacterials). ⒜ There is no evidence to support using antibacterials to suppress **chronic***Burkholderia cepacia* complex infection in patients with cystic fibrosis who have stable pulmonary status.

ᴇᵥᴳʳ Specialist microbiological advice should be sought for patients with chronic *Burkholderia cepacia* complex infection (when treatment has not eradicated the infection) and who become clinically unwell with a pulmonary disease exacerbation.

An inhaled antibacterial should be considered for those who have chronic *Burkholderia cepacia* complex infection and declining pulmonary status; treatment should be stopped if there is no observed benefit. ⒜

Haemophilus influenzae

ᴇᵥᴳʳ *Haemophilus influenzae* infection in the absence of clinical evidence of pulmonary infection should be treated with an appropriate oral antibacterial drug. In those who are unwell with clinical evidence of pulmonary infection, an appropriate antibacterial should be given by mouth or intravenously depending on the severity of the illness (consult local protocol). ⒜

Non-tuberculous mycobacteria

ᴇᵥᴳʳ Non-tuberculous mycobacterial eradication therapy should be considered for patients with cystic fibrosis who are clinically unwell and whose pulmonary disease has not responded to other recommended treatments. Specialist microbiological advice should be sought on the choice of antibacterial and on the duration of treatment. ⒜

Aspergillus fumigatus **complex**

ᴇᵥᴳʳ Treatment with an antifungal drug should only be considered to suppress **chronic***Aspergillus fumigatus* complex respiratory infection in patients with declining pulmonary status. Specialist microbiological advice should be sought on the choice of antifungal drug. ⒜

Unidentified infections

ᴇᵥᴳʳ An oral or intravenous (depending on the exacerbation severity) broad-spectrum antibacterial should be used for patients who have a pulmonary disease exacerbation and no clear cause. If a causative pathogen is identified, an appropriate treatment should be selected (consult local protocol). ⒜

Immunomodulatory drugs

ᴇᵥᴳʳ Long-term treatment with azithromycin p. 568 [unlicensed indication], at an immunomodulatory dose, should be offered to patients with deteriorating lung function or repeated pulmonary exacerbations. In those patients with continued deterioration in lung function or continuing pulmonary exacerbations, long-term azithromycin should be discontinued and the use of an oral corticosteroid considered. ⒜

Nutrition and exocrine pancreatic insufficiency

ᴇᵥᴳʳ The cystic fibrosis specialist dietitian should offer advice on optimal nutrition.

Pancreatin p. 104 should be offered to patients with exocrine pancreatic insufficiency. Dose should be adjusted as needed to minimise any symptoms or signs of malabsorption (see Exocrine pancreatic insufficiency p. 103). An acid-suppressing drug, such as an H_2 receptor antagonist or a proton pump inhibitor [unlicensed indications] can be considered for patients who have persistent symptoms or signs of malabsorption.

A short-term trial of an appetite stimulant (for example up to 3 months) [unlicensed indication] can be considered in adult patients if attempts to increase calorie intake are not effective. ⓐ

Distal intestinal obstruction syndrome

EvGr Oral or intravenous fluids should be offered to ensure adequate hydration for patients with distal intestinal obstruction syndrome. Meglumine amidotrizoate with sodium amidotrizoate solution (orally or via an enteral tube) should be considered as first-line treatment for distal intestinal obstruction syndrome. An iso-osmotic polyethylene glycol and electrolyte solution (macrogols) (orally or via an enteral tube) can be considered as a second-line treatment. Surgery is a last resort, if prolonged treatment with a polyethylene glycol solution is not effective. Suspected distal intestinal obstruction syndrome should be managed in a specialist cystic fibrosis centre. ⓐ

Liver disease

EvGr If liver function blood tests are abnormal in patients with cystic fibrosis, ursodeoxycholic acid p. 97 [unlicensed indication] can be given until liver function is restored. ⓐ

Bone mineral density

EvGr Patients should be monitored for cystic fibrosis-related low bone mineral density. ⓐ

Cystic fibrosis-related diabetes

EvGr Patients should be monitored for cystic fibrosis-related diabetes. ⓐ

Useful Resources

Cystic fibrosis: diagnosis and management. National Institute for Health and Care Excellence. NICE guideline 78. October 2017
www.nice.org.uk/guidance/NG78

MUCOLYTICS

▌Dornase alfa   17-Aug-2020

(Phosphorylated glycosylated recombinant human deoxyribonuclease 1 (rhDNase))

- DRUG ACTION Dornase alfa is a genetically engineered version of a naturally occurring human enzyme which cleaves extracellular deoxyribonucleic acid (DNA).

- ● INDICATIONS AND DOSE

Management of cystic fibrosis patients with a forced vital capacity (FVC) of greater than 40% of predicted to improve pulmonary function
▸ BY INHALATION OF NEBULISED SOLUTION
▸ Adult: 2500 units once daily, administered by jet nebuliser, patients over 21 years may benefit from twice daily dosage

DOSE EQUIVALENCE AND CONVERSION
▸ Dornase alfa 1000 units is equivalent to 1 mg

- ● SIDE-EFFECTS Chest pain · conjunctivitis · dyspepsia · dysphonia · dyspnoea · fever · increased risk of infection · skin reactions

- ● PREGNANCY No evidence of teratogenicity; manufacturer advises use only if potential benefit outweighs risk.

- ● BREAST FEEDING Amount probably too small to be harmful—manufacturer advises caution.

- ● DIRECTIONS FOR ADMINISTRATION Dornase alfa is administered undiluted by inhalation using a jet nebuliser; ultrasonic nebulisers are unsuitable. Expert sources advise usually once daily at least 1 hour before physiotherapy.

- ● MEDICINAL FORMS There can be variation in the licensing of different medicines containing the same drug.

Nebuliser liquid
▸ Pulmozyme (Roche Products Ltd)
  Dornase alfa 1 mg per 1 ml Pulmozyme 2.5mg nebuliser liquid 2.5ml ampoules | 30 ampoule PoM £496.43 DT = £496.43

▌Ivacaftor   20-Nov-2020

- DRUG ACTION Ivacaftor is a cystic fibrosis transmembrane conductance regulator (CFTR) protein potentiator that increases chloride transport in the abnormal CFTR protein.

- ● INDICATIONS AND DOSE

Cystic fibrosis (specialist use only)
▸ BY MOUTH
▸ Adult: 150 mg every 12 hours
DOSE ADJUSTMENTS DUE TO INTERACTIONS
▸ Manufacturer advises reduce dose to 150 mg twice a week with concurrent use of potent inhibitors of CYP3A4.
▸ Manufacturer advises reduce dose to 150 mg once daily with concurrent use of moderate inhibitors of CYP3A4.

- ● CONTRA-INDICATIONS Organ transplantation (no information available)

- ● INTERACTIONS → Appendix 1: ivacaftor

- ● SIDE-EFFECTS
▸ **Common or very common** Breast abnormalities · diarrhoea · dizziness · ear discomfort · headache · ototoxicity · rash · tympanic membrane hyperaemia
▸ **Uncommon** Gynaecomastia
▸ **Frequency not known** Hepatic function abnormal

SIDE-EFFECTS, FURTHER INFORMATION Manufacturer advises interrupt treatment if transaminase levels more than 5 times the upper limit of normal or transaminase levels more than 3 times the upper limit of normal **and** blood bilirubin more than twice the upper limit of normal—consult product literature.

- ● PREGNANCY Manufacturer advises avoid—limited information available.

- ● BREAST FEEDING Manufacturer advises avoid—present in milk in *animal* studies.

- ● HEPATIC IMPAIRMENT Manufacturer advises caution in moderate to severe impairment (limited information available).
Dose adjustments Manufacturer advises reduce dose to 150 mg once daily in moderate impairment; in severe impairment reduce starting dose to 150 mg on alternate days, adjust dosing interval according to clinical response and tolerability.

- ● RENAL IMPAIRMENT Manufacturer advises caution in severe impairment or end-stage renal disease—limited information available.

- ● MONITORING REQUIREMENTS Manufacturer advises monitor liver function before treatment, every 3 months during the first year of treatment, then annually thereafter (more frequent monitoring should be considered in patients with a history of transaminase elevations).

- ● DIRECTIONS FOR ADMINISTRATION Manufacturer advises tablets should be taken with fat-containing food.

- ● PRESCRIBING AND DISPENSING INFORMATION Ivacaftor should be prescribed by a physician experienced in the treatment of cystic fibrosis.

- ● PATIENT AND CARER ADVICE Patients or carers should be given advice on how to administer ivacaftor tablets.
Driving and skilled tasks Manufacturer advises that patients and their carers should be counselled on the effects on driving and skilled tasks—increased risk of dizziness.

3

Respiratory system

- NATIONAL FUNDING/ACCESS DECISIONS
  For full details see funding body website
  Scottish Medicines Consortium (SMC) decisions
  ▸ Ivacaftor (*Kalydeco*®) for the treatment of patients with cystic fibrosis (CF) aged 18 years and older who have an R117H mutation in the CF transmembrane conductance regulator (CFTR) gene (December 2016) SMC No. 1193/16 Not recommended

- MEDICINAL FORMS There can be variation in the licensing of different medicines containing the same drug.
  Tablet
  CAUTIONARY AND ADVISORY LABELS 25
  ▸ Kalydeco (Vertex Pharmaceuticals (UK) Ltd)
  Ivacaftor 150 mg Kalydeco 150mg tablets | 28 tablet [PoM]
  £7,000.00 | 56 tablet [PoM] £14,000.00

Lumacaftor with ivacaftor

20-Nov-2020

The properties listed below are those particular to the combination only. For the properties of the components please consider, ivacaftor p. 309.

- INDICATIONS AND DOSE
  Cystic fibrosis (specialist use only)
  ▸ BY MOUTH USING TABLETS
  ▸ Adult: 400/250 mg every 12 hours
  DOSE ADJUSTMENTS DUE TO INTERACTIONS
  ▸ Manufacturer advises reduce initial dose to 200/125 mg daily for the first week in those also taking a potent inhibitor of CYP3A4.
  DOSE EQUIVALENCE AND CONVERSION
  ▸ Dose expressed as x/y mg of lumacaftor/ivacaftor.

- CAUTIONS Forced expiratory volume in 1 second (FEV₁) less than 40% of the predicted normal value—additional monitoring recommended at initiation of treatment · pulmonary exacerbation—no information available
- INTERACTIONS → Appendix 1: ivacaftor · lumacaftor
- SIDE-EFFECTS
  ▸ **Common or very common** Breast abnormalities · diarrhoea · dizziness · ear discomfort · flatulence · gastrointestinal discomfort · headache · menstrual cycle irregularities · nausea · ototoxicity · rash · tympanic membrane hyperaemia · vomiting
  ▸ **Uncommon** Gynaecomastia · hepatic encephalopathy · hepatitis cholestatic · hypertension
  SIDE-EFFECTS, FURTHER INFORMATION Manufacturer advises interrupt treatment if transaminase levels more than 5 times the upper limit of normal *or* transaminase levels more than 3 times the upper limit of normal **and** blood bilirubin more than twice the upper limit of normal—consult product literature.
- HEPATIC IMPAIRMENT Manufacturer advises caution in moderate to severe impairment (risk of increased exposure).
  Dose adjustments Manufacturer advises dose reduction of evening dose to 200/125 mg in moderate impairment; in severe impairment, dose reduction to 200/125 mg every 12 hours is advised.
- PRE-TREATMENT SCREENING If the patient's genotype is unknown, a validated genotyping method should be performed to confirm the presence of the F508del mutation on both alleles of the CFTR gene before starting treatment.
- MONITORING REQUIREMENTS Manufacturer advises monitor blood pressure periodically during treatment.
- EFFECT ON LABORATORY TESTS False positive urine screening tests for tetrahydrocannabinol have been reported—manufacturer advises consider alternative confirmatory method.

- DIRECTIONS FOR ADMINISTRATION Manufacturer advises *tablets* should be taken with fat-containing food.
- PATIENT AND CARER ADVICE Patients or carers should be given advice on how to administer tablets.
  Missed doses Manufacturer advises if a dose is more than 6 hours late, the missed dose should not be taken and the next dose should be taken at the normal time.
- NATIONAL FUNDING/ACCESS DECISIONS
  For full details see funding body website
  NICE decisions
  ▸ Lumacaftor with ivacaftor for treating cystic fibrosis homozygous for the F508del mutation (July 2016) NICE TA398 Not recommended
  Scottish Medicines Consortium (SMC) decisions
  ▸ Lumacaftor with ivacaftor film-coated tablet (*Orkambi*®) for the treatment of cystic fibrosis (CF) in patients aged 12 years and older who are homozygous for the F508del mutation in the CF transmembrane conductance regulator (CFTR) gene (May 2016) SMC No. 1136/16 Not recommended

- MEDICINAL FORMS There can be variation in the licensing of different medicines containing the same drug.
  Tablet
  CAUTIONARY AND ADVISORY LABELS 25
  EXCIPIENTS: May contain Propylene glycol
  ▸ Orkambi (Vertex Pharmaceuticals (UK) Ltd) ▼
  Lumacaftor 100 mg, Ivacaftor 125 mg Orkambi 100mg/125mg tablets | 112 tablet [PoM] £8,000.00 (Hospital only)
  Ivacaftor 125 mg, Lumacaftor 200 mg Orkambi 200mg/125mg tablets | 112 tablet [PoM] £8,000.00 (Hospital only)

Mannitol

09-Dec-2020

- INDICATIONS AND DOSE
  Treatment of cystic fibrosis as an add-on therapy to standard care
  ▸ BY INHALATION OF POWDER
  ▸ Adult: Maintenance 400 mg twice daily, an initiation dose assessment must be carried out under medical supervision, for details of the initiation dose regimen, consult product literature

- CONTRA-INDICATIONS Bronchial hyperresponsiveness to inhaled mannitol · impaired lung function (forced expiratory volume in 1 second < 30% of predicted) · non-CF bronchiectasis
- CAUTIONS Asthma · haemoptysis
- SIDE-EFFECTS
  ▸ **Common or very common** Chest discomfort · condition aggravated · cough · haemoptysis · headache · respiratory disorders · throat complaints · vomiting
  ▸ **Uncommon** Abdominal pain upper · appetite decreased · asthma · burping · cold sweat · cystic fibrosis related diabetes · dehydration · diarrhoea · dizziness · dysphonia · dyspnoea · ear pain · fatigue · fever · gastrointestinal disorders · hypoxia · increased risk of infection · influenza like illness · insomnia · joint disorders · malaise · morbid thoughts · nausea · odynophagia · oral disorders · pain · rhinorrhoea · skin reactions · sputum discolouration · urinary incontinence
- PREGNANCY Manufacturer advises avoid.
- BREAST FEEDING Manufacturer advises avoid.
- PRE-TREATMENT SCREENING Patients must be assessed for bronchial hyperresponsiveness to inhaled mannitol before starting the therapeutic dose regimen; an initiation dose assessment must be carried out under medical supervision—for details of the initiation dose regimen, consult product literature.
- DIRECTIONS FOR ADMINISTRATION The dose should be administered 5–15 minutes after a bronchodilator and

before physiotherapy; the second daily dose should be taken 2–3 hours before bedtime.

- PATIENT AND CARER ADVICE Patients or carers should be given advice on how to administer mannitol inhalation powder.
- NATIONAL FUNDING/ACCESS DECISIONS For full details see funding body website

NICE decisions

▶ Mannitol dry powder for inhalation for treating cystic fibrosis (November 2012) NICE TA266 Recommended

Scottish Medicines Consortium (SMC) decisions

▶ Mannitol (*Bronchitol*®) for the treatment of cystic fibrosis (CF) in adults aged 18 years and above as an add-on therapy to best standard of care (December 2013) SMC No. 837/13 Recommended with restrictions

- MEDICINAL FORMS There can be variation in the licensing of different medicines containing the same drug. Forms available from special-order manufacturers include: infusion, solution for infusion

Inhalation powder

▶ Osmohale (Mawdsley-Brooks & Company Ltd)
Mannitol 5 mg Osmohale 5mg inhalation powder capsules | 1 capsule [PoM] 🔏
Mannitol 10 mg Osmohale 10mg inhalation powder capsules | 1 capsule [PoM] 🔏
Mannitol 20 mg Osmohale 20mg inhalation powder capsules | 1 capsule [PoM] 🔏
Mannitol 40 mg Osmohale 40mg inhalation powder capsules | 15 capsule [PoM] 🔏

▶ Bronchitol (Chiesi Ltd)
Mannitol 40 mg Bronchitol 40mg inhalation powder capsules with two devices | 280 capsule [PoM] £231.66 DT = £231.66
Bronchitol 40mg inhalation powder capsules with device | 10 capsule [PoM] £8.27

Tezacaftor with ivacaftor

16-Nov-2020

The properties listed below are those particular to the combination only. For the properties of the components please consider, ivacaftor p. 309.

- **INDICATIONS AND DOSE**

Cystic fibrosis (in combination with ivacaftor) (specialist use only)

▶ BY MOUTH
▶ Adult: 100/150 mg, to be taken in the morning and, *Ivacaftor* 150 mg to be taken in the evening

DOSE ADJUSTMENTS DUE TO INTERACTIONS

▶ With concurrent use of potent CYP3A4 inhibitors, manufacturer advises reduce dose to 100/150 mg tezacaftor/ivacaftor twice a week, taken approximately 3–4 days apart; the evening dose of ivacaftor should not be taken.
▶ With concurrent use of moderate CYP3A4 inhibitors, manufacturer advises reduce dose to 100/150 mg tezacaftor/ivacaftor every other morning, with ivacaftor 150 mg taken in the mornings alternate to tezacaftor/ivacaftor; the evening dose of ivacaftor should not be taken.

DOSE EQUIVALENCE AND CONVERSION

▶ Combination dose expressed as x/y mg of tezacaftor/ivacaftor.

- INTERACTIONS → Appendix 1: ivacaftor · tezacaftor
- SIDE-EFFECTS
▶ **Common or very common** Abdominal pain · breast abnormalities · diarrhoea · dizziness · ear discomfort · headache · nausea · ototoxicity · rash · tympanic membrane hyperaemia
▶ **Uncommon** Gynaecomastia
▶ **Frequency not known** Hepatic function abnormal

SIDE-EFFECTS, FURTHER INFORMATION Manufacturer advises interrupt treatment if transaminase levels more than 5 times the upper limit of normal *or* transaminase levels more than 3 times the upper limit of normal **and** blood bilirubin more than twice the upper limit of normal—consult product literature.

- HEPATIC IMPAIRMENT Manufacturer advises caution in moderate to severe impairment (risk of increased exposure).
Dose adjustments Manufacturer advises omit evening dose of ivacaftor in moderate to severe impairment; in severe impairment, adjust dosing interval according to clinical response and tolerability.
- PATIENT AND CARER ADVICE
Missed doses Manufacturer advises if a dose is more than 6 hours late, the missed dose should not be taken and the next dose should be taken at the normal time.
- NATIONAL FUNDING/ACCESS DECISIONS For full details see funding body website

Scottish Medicines Consortium (SMC) decisions

▶ Tezacaftor with ivacaftor (*Symkevi*®) for the treatment of patients with cystic fibrosis aged 12 years and older who are homozygous for the F508del mutation or who are heterozygous for the F508del mutation and have one of the following mutations in the cystic fibrosis transmembrane conductance regulator (CFTR) gene P67L, R117C, L206W, R352Q, A455E, D579G, 711+3A→G, S945L, S977F, R1070W, D1152H, 2789+5G→A, 3272-26A→G, and 3849+10kbC→T (August 2019) SMC No. SMC2183 Not recommended

- MEDICINAL FORMS There can be variation in the licensing of different medicines containing the same drug.
Tablet
CAUTIONARY AND ADVISORY LABELS 25
▶ Symkevi (Vertex Pharmaceuticals (UK) Ltd) ▼
Tezacaftor 100 mg, Ivacaftor 150 mg Symkevi 100mg/150mg tablets | 28 tablet [PoM] £6,293.91 (Hospital only)

Tezacaftor with ivacaftor and elexacaftor

22-Oct-2020

The properties listed below are those particular to the combination only. For the properties of the components please consider, ivacaftor p. 309, tezacaftor with ivacaftor above.

- **INDICATIONS AND DOSE**

Cystic fibrosis (in combination with ivacaftor) (specialist use only)

▶ BY MOUTH
▶ Adult: 2 tablets, to be taken in the morning and, *Ivacaftor* 150 mg to be taken in the evening (about 12 hours apart)

DOSE ADJUSTMENTS DUE TO INTERACTIONS

▶ With concurrent use of potent CYP3A4 inhibitors, manufacturer advises reduce dose to 2 tablets twice a week, taken approximately 3–4 days apart; the evening dose of ivacaftor should not be taken.
▶ With concurrent use of moderate CYP3A4 inhibitors, manufacturer advises reduce dose to 2 tablets every other morning, with ivacaftor 150 mg taken in the mornings alternate to tezacaftor/ivacaftor/elexacaftor; the evening dose of ivacaftor should not be taken.

DOSE EQUIVALENCE AND CONVERSION

▶ Tablet quantities refer to the number of *Kaftrio*® Tablets which should be taken. Each *Kaftrio*® Tablet contains tezacaftor 50 mg, ivacaftor 75 mg, and elexacaftor 100 mg.

- INTERACTIONS → Appendix 1: elexacaftor · ivacaftor · tezacaftor

- HEPATIC IMPAIRMENT Manufacturer advises avoid in severe impairment; use only if potential benefit outweighs risk in moderate impairment (risk of increased exposure). **Dose adjustments** Manufacturer advises alternate dose between 1 and 2 tablets in the mornings, and omit evening dose of ivacaftor in moderate impairment.
- PATIENT AND CARER ADVICE
  Missed doses Manufacturer advises if the morning dose is more than 6 hours late, the missed dose should be taken and the evening dose of ivacaftor omitted; the next morning dose should be taken at the normal time. If the evening dose of ivacaftor is more than 6 hours late, the missed dose should **not** be taken and the next morning dose should be taken at the normal time.

- MEDICINAL FORMS There can be variation in the licensing of different medicines containing the same drug.
  Tablet
  CAUTIONARY AND ADVISORY LABELS 25
  ‣ Kaftrio (Vertex Pharmaceuticals (UK) Ltd) ▼
  Tezacaftor 50 mg, Ivacaftor 75 mg, Elexacaftor 100 mg Kaftrio 75mg/50mg/100mg tablets | 56 tablet [PoM] £8,346.30 (Hospital only)

4   Cough and congestion

Aromatic inhalations, cough preparations and systemic nasal decongestants

Aromatic inhalations in adults

Inhalations containing volatile substances such as eucalyptus oil are traditionally used and although the vapour may contain little of the additive it encourages deliberate inspiration of warm moist air which is often comforting in bronchitis; boiling water should not be used owing to the risk of scalding. In practice, inhalations are also used for the relief of nasal obstruction in acute rhinitis or sinusitis.

Cough preparations in adults

Cough suppressants

Cough may be a symptom of an underlying disorder, such as asthma, gastro-oesophageal reflux disease, or rhinitis, which should be addressed before prescribing cough suppressants. Cough may be a side-effect of another drug, such as an ACE inhibitor, or it can be associated with smoking or environmental pollutants. Cough can also have a significant habit component. When there is no identifiable cause, cough suppressants may be useful, for example if sleep is disturbed. They may cause sputum retention and this may be harmful in patients with chronic bronchitis and bronchiectasis.

There is some evidence to suggest that codeine phosphate p. 475 provides no benefit for symptoms of acute cough. Codeine phosphate is also constipating and can cause dependence; **dextromethorphan** and pholcodine p. 313 have fewer side-effects.

Sedating antihistamines are used as the cough suppressant component of many compound cough preparations on sale to the public; all tend to cause drowsiness which may reflect their main mode of action.

Palliative care

Diamorphine hydrochloride p. 476 and methadone hydrochloride p. 524 have been used to control distressing cough in terminal lung cancer although morphine p. 483 is now preferred. In other circumstances they are contra-indicated because they induce sputum retention and ventilatory failure as well as causing opioid dependence.

Methadone hydrochloride linctus should be avoided because it has a long duration of action and tends to accumulate.

Demulcent and expectorant cough preparations

Demulcent cough preparations contain soothing substances such as syrup or glycerol and some patients believe that such preparations relieve a dry irritating cough. Preparations such as **simple linctus** have the advantage of being harmless and inexpensive; **paediatric simple linctus** is particularly useful in children.

Expectorants are claimed to promote expulsion of bronchial secretions, but there is no evidence that any drug can specifically facilitate expectoration.

[EvGr] An over-the-counter cough medicine containing the expectorant guaifenesin may be used for acute cough; there is some evidence to suggest it may reduce symptoms. ◇

Compound preparations are on sale to the public for the treatment of cough and colds but should not be used in children under 6 years; the rationale for some is dubious. Care should be taken to give the correct dose and to not use more than one preparation at a time.

Nasal decongestants, systemic

Nasal decongestants for administration by mouth may not be as effective as preparations for local application but they do not give rise to rebound nasal congestion on withdrawal. Pseudoephedrine hydrochloride p. 1246 is available over the counter; it has few sympathomimetic effects.

Aromatic inhalations in children

The use of strong aromatic decongestants (applied as rubs or to pillows) is not advised for infants under the age of 3 months. Carers of young infants in whom nasal obstruction with mucus is a problem can readily be taught appropriate techniques of suction aspiration but sodium chloride 0.9% p. 1089 given as nasal drops is preferred; administration before feeds may ease feeding difficulties caused by nasal congestion.

Cough preparations in children

The use of over-the-counter cough suppressants containing codeine phosphate should be avoided in children under 12 years and in children of any age known to be CYP2D6 ultra-rapid metabolisers. Cough suppressants containing similar opioid analgesics such as dextromethorphan and pholcodine are not generally recommended in children and should be avoided in children under 6 years; dextromethorphan should be avoided in children under 12 years.

MHRA/CHM advice (March 2008 and February 2009)
Children under 6 years should not be given over-the-counter cough and cold medicines containing the following ingredients:

- brompheniramine, chlorphenamine maleate p. 299, diphenhydramine, doxylamine, promethazine, or triprolidine (antihistamines);
- dextromethorphan or pholcodine (cough suppressants);
- guaifenesin or ipecacuanha (expectorants);
- Phenylephrine hydrochloride p. 203, pseudoephedrine hydrochloride, ephedrine hydrochloride p. 287, oxymetazoline, or xylometazoline hydrochloride p. 1247 (decongestants).

Over-the-counter cough and cold medicines can be considered for children aged 6–12 years after basic principles of best care have been tried, but treatment should be restricted to five days or less. Children should not be given more than 1 cough or cold preparation at a time because different brands may contain the same active ingredient; care should be taken to give the correct dose.

COUGH AND COLD PREPARATIONS 〉 COUGH SUPPRESSANTS

Pholcodine
21-Nov-2020

● **INDICATIONS AND DOSE**

Dry cough

▶ BY MOUTH USING LINCTUS
▶ Child 6-11 years: 2–5 mg 3–4 times a day
▶ Child 12-17 years: 5–10 mg 3–4 times a day
▶ Adult: 5–10 mg 3–4 times a day

IMPORTANT SAFETY INFORMATION

MHRA/CHM ADVICE (MARCH 2008 AND FEBRUARY 2009) OVER-THE-COUNTER COUGH AND COLD MEDICINES FOR CHILDREN
Children under 6 years should not be given over-the-counter cough and cold medicines containing pholcodine (cough suppressant).

Over-the-counter cough and cold medicines can be considered for children aged 6–12 years after basic principles of best care have been tried, but treatment should be restricted to 5 days or less. Children should not be given more than 1 cough or cold preparation at a time because different brands may contain the same active ingredient; care should be taken to give the correct dose.

● CONTRA-INDICATIONS Bronchiectasis · bronchiolitis (in children) · chronic bronchitis · chronic obstructive pulmonary disease (in adults) · patients at risk of respiratory failure
● CAUTIONS Asthma · chronic cough · history of drug abuse · persistent cough · productive cough
● INTERACTIONS → Appendix 1: pholcodine
● SIDE-EFFECTS Agitation · confusion · constipation · dizziness · drowsiness · gastrointestinal disorder · nausea · skin reactions · sputum retention · vomiting
● PREGNANCY Manufacturer advises avoid unless potential benefit outweighs risk.
● BREAST FEEDING Manufacturer advises avoid unless potential benefit outweighs risk—no information available.
● HEPATIC IMPAIRMENT Manufacturer advises caution; avoid in hepatic failure.
● RENAL IMPAIRMENT Use with caution in renal impairment. Avoid in severe renal impairment.
● PRESCRIBING AND DISPENSING INFORMATION Pholcodine is not generally recommended for children.
Flavours of oral liquid formulations may include orange.
When prepared extemporaneously, the BP states Pholcodine Linctus, BP consists of pholcodine 5 mg/5 mL in a suitable flavoured vehicle, containing citric acid monohydrate 1% and Pholcodine Linctus, Strong, BP consists of pholcodine 10 mg/5 mL in a suitable flavoured vehicle, containing citric acid monohydrate 2%

● MEDICINAL FORMS There can be variation in the licensing of different medicines containing the same drug.

Oral solution

▶ Pholcodine (Non-proprietary)
　Pholcodine 1 mg per 1 ml Pholcodine 5mg/5ml linctus | 200 ml [P] £1.23–£1.32 DT = £1.32 [CD5]
　Pholcodine 5mg/5ml linctus sugar free sugar-free | 200 ml £1.34 DT = £1.34 [CD5] sugar-free | 2000 ml [P] £13.40 [CD5]
　Pholcodine 2 mg per 1 ml Pholcodine 10mg/5ml linctus strong sugar free sugar-free | 2000 ml [P] £11.25 DT = £9.88 [CD5]
　Pholcodine 10mg/5ml linctus strong | 200 ml [P] £1.67 DT = £1.67 [CD5]
▶ Covonia Dry Cough (Thornton & Ross Ltd)
　Pholcodine 1 mg per 1 ml Covonia Dry Cough Sugar Free Formula 5mg/5ml oral solution sugar-free | 150 ml [P] £3.30 [CD5]

▶ Galenphol (Thornton & Ross Ltd)
　Pholcodine 1 mg per 1 ml Galenphol 5mg/5ml linctus sugar-free | 2000 ml [P] £8.50 [CD5]
　Pholcodine 2 mg per 1 ml Galenphol Strong 10mg/5ml linctus sugar-free | 2000 ml [P] £9.88 DT = £9.88 [CD5]

COUGH AND COLD PREPARATIONS 〉 OTHER

Citric acid
18-Mar-2020

(Formulated as Simple Linctus)

● **INDICATIONS AND DOSE**

Cough

▶ BY MOUTH
▶ Adult: 5 mL 3–4 times a day, this dose is for Simple Linctus, BP (2.5%)

● PRESCRIBING AND DISPENSING INFORMATION Flavours of oral liquid formulations may include anise.
When prepared extemporaneously, the BP states Simple Linctus, BP consists of citric acid monohydrate 2.5%, in a suitable vehicle with an anise flavour.

● MEDICINAL FORMS There can be variation in the licensing of different medicines containing the same drug.

Oral solution

▶ Citric acid (Non-proprietary)
　Citric acid monohydrate 25 mg per 1 ml Simple linctus sugar free sugar-free | 200 ml [GSL] £1.25 DT = £0.92 sugar-free | 2000 ml [GSL] £9.20
　Simple linctus | 200 ml [GSL] £0.93–£1.06 DT = £0.93

MENTHOL AND DERIVATIVES

Eucalyptus with menthol
18-Mar-2020

● **INDICATIONS AND DOSE**

Aromatic inhalation for relief of nasal congestion

▶ BY INHALATION
▶ Adult: Add one teaspoonful to a pint of hot, **not** boiling, water and inhale the vapour; repeat after 4 hours if necessary

● PRESCRIBING AND DISPENSING INFORMATION When prepared extemporaneously, the BP states Menthol and Eucalyptus Inhalation, BP 1980 consists of racementhol or levomenthol 2 g, eucalyptus oil 10 mL, light magnesium carbonate 7 g, water to 100 mL.

● PROFESSION SPECIFIC INFORMATION

Dental practitioners' formulary
Menthol and Eucalyptus Inhalation BP, 1980 may be prescribed.

● MEDICINAL FORMS There can be variation in the licensing of different medicines containing the same drug.

Inhalation vapour

▶ Eucalyptus with menthol (Non-proprietary)
　Menthol 20 mg per 1 ml, Magnesium carbonate light 70 mg per 1 ml, Eucalyptus oil 100 microlitre per 1 ml Menthol and Eucalyptus inhalation | 100 ml [GSL] £2.40

3

Respiratory system

Respiratory system

3

RESINS

Benzoin tincture, compound

18-Mar-2020

(Friars' Balsam)

- **INDICATIONS AND DOSE**

Aromatic inhalation for relief of nasal congestion

▸ BY INHALATION

▹ Child 3 months-17 years: Add 5 mL to a pint of hot, **not** boiling, water and inhale the vapour; repeat after 4 hours if necessary

▹ Adult: Add 5 mL to a pint of hot, **not** boiling, water and inhale the vapour; repeat after 4 hours if necessary

- SIDE-EFFECTS Skin sensitisation

- PRESCRIBING AND DISPENSING INFORMATION Not recommended (applied as a rub or to pillows) for infants under 3 months.
  When prepared extemporaneously, the BP states Benzoin Tincture, Compound, BP consists of balsamic acids approx. 4.5%.

- MEDICINAL FORMS There can be variation in the licensing of different medicines containing the same drug.
  Liquid
  CAUTIONARY AND ADVISORY LABELS 15
  ▸ Benzoin tincture, compound (Non-proprietary)
    Benzoin sumatra 100 mg per 1 ml, Storax prepared 100 mg per 1 ml Benzoin compound tincture | 500 ml £12.35 DT = £12.35
    Friars' Balsam | 50 ml GSL £2.11

5   Idiopathic pulmonary fibrosis

Other drugs used for Idiopathic pulmonary fibrosis
Nintedanib, p. 1036

ANTIFIBROTICS

Pirfenidone

03-Dec-2020

- DRUG ACTION The exact mechanism of action of pirfenidone is not yet understood, but it is believed to slow down the progression of idiopathic pulmonary fibrosis by exerting both antifibrotic and anti-inflammatory properties.

- **INDICATIONS AND DOSE**

Treatment of mild to moderate idiopathic pulmonary fibrosis (initiated under specialist supervision)

▸ BY MOUTH

▹ Adult: Initially 267 mg 3 times a day for 7 days, then increased to 534 mg 3 times a day for 7 days, then increased to 801 mg 3 times a day

DOSE ADJUSTMENTS DUE TO INTERACTIONS

▸ Caution with concomitant use with ciprofloxacin—reduce dose of pirfenidone to 534 mg three times daily with high-dose ciprofloxacin (750 mg twice daily).

IMPORTANT SAFETY INFORMATION

MHRA/CHM ADVICE: PIRFENIDONE (*ESBRIET* ®): RISK OF SERIOUS LIVER INJURY; UPDATED ADVICE ON LIVER FUNCTION TESTING (NOVEMBER 2020)

A European review of safety data identified severe, sometimes fatal, cases of drug-induced liver injury (including liver failure) associated with pirfenidone therapy. Healthcare professionals are advised to monitor liver function and counsel patients to seek immediate medical attention if they experience signs and symptoms

of liver injury; prompt clinical evaluation and measurement of liver function should be performed in those affected—see *Monitoring requirements*. Patients also taking inhibitors of cytochrome P450 isoenzymes involved in the metabolism of pirfenidone should be closely monitored for toxicity.

- CAUTIONS

  CAUTIONS, FURTHER INFORMATION

  ▸ Photosensitivity Manufacturer advises avoid exposure to direct sunlight—if photosensitivity reaction or rash occurs, dose adjustment or treatment interruption may be required (consult product literature).

  ▸ Treatment interruption If treatment is interrupted for 14 consecutive days or more, the initial 2 week titration regimen should be repeated; if treatment is interrupted for less than 14 consecutive days, the dose can be resumed at the previous daily dose without titration.

- INTERACTIONS → Appendix 1: pirfenidone

- SIDE-EFFECTS

  ▸ **Common or very common** Appetite decreased · arthralgia · asthenia · constipation · cough · diarrhoea · dizziness · drowsiness · dyspnoea · gastrointestinal discomfort · gastrointestinal disorders · headache · hot flush · increased risk of infection · insomnia · musculoskeletal chest pain · myalgia · nausea · photosensitivity reaction · skin reactions · sunburn · taste altered · vomiting · weight decreased

  ▸ **Uncommon** Angioedema · hepatic disorders

  ▸ **Rare or very rare** Agranulocytosis

  SIDE-EFFECTS, FURTHER INFORMATION Gastrointestinal side-effects may require dose reduction or treatment interruption—consult product literature.

- PREGNANCY Manufacturer advises avoid—no information available.

- BREAST FEEDING Manufacturer advises avoid—no information available.

- HEPATIC IMPAIRMENT Manufacturer advises caution in mild to moderate impairment (risk of increased exposure); avoid in severe impairment (no information available).

- RENAL IMPAIRMENT Avoid use if eGFR less than 30 mL/minute/1.73 m^2.

- MONITORING REQUIREMENTS

  ▸ Manufacturer advises monitor for weight loss.

  ▸ Manufacturer advises monitor liver function (ALT, AST, and bilirubin) before starting treatment, then at monthly intervals for the first 6 months, and then every 3 months thereafter; review if abnormal liver function tests—dose reduction, treatment interruption or discontinuation may be required (consult product literature).

- PATIENT AND CARER ADVICE

  Driving and skilled tasks Dizziness or malaise may affect performance of skilled tasks (e.g. driving).

- NATIONAL FUNDING/ACCESS DECISIONS
  For full details see funding body website

  NICE decisions

  ▸ Pirfenidone for treating idiopathic pulmonary fibrosis (February 2018) NICE TA504 Recommended with restrictions

  Scottish Medicines Consortium (SMC) decisions

  ▸ Pirfenidone (*Esbriet* ®) in adults for the treatment of mild to moderate idiopathic pulmonary fibrosis (IPF) (August 2013) SMC No. 835/13 Recommended with restrictions

- MEDICINAL FORMS There can be variation in the licensing of different medicines containing the same drug.
  Tablet
  CAUTIONARY AND ADVISORY LABELS 11, 21, 25
  ▸ Esbriet (Roche Products Ltd)
    Pirfenidone 267 mg Esbriet 267mg tablets | 63 tablet PoM
    £501.92 | 252 tablet PoM £2,007.70
    Pirfenidone 801 mg Esbriet 801mg tablets | 84 tablet PoM
    £2,007.70

Capsule

CAUTIONARY AND ADVISORY LABELS 21, 25, 11

▸ Esbriet (Roche Products Ltd)

Pirfenidone 267 mg Esbriet 267mg capsules | 252 capsule [PoM] £2,007.70 | 270 capsule [PoM] £2,151.10

6   Respiratory depression, respiratory distress syndrome and apnoea

Respiratory stimulants

Overview

Respiratory stimulants (analeptic drugs) have a limited place in the treatment of ventilatory failure in patients with chronic obstructive pulmonary disease. They are effective only when given by intravenous injection or infusion and have a short duration of action. Their use has largely been replaced by ventilatory support including nasal intermittent positive pressure ventilation. However, occasionally when ventilatory support is contra-indicated and in patients with hypercapnic respiratory failure who are becoming drowsy or comatose, respiratory stimulants in the short term may arouse patients sufficiently to co-operate and clear their secretions.

Respiratory stimulants can also be harmful in respiratory failure since they stimulate non-respiratory as well as respiratory muscles. They should only be given under **expert supervision** in hospital and must be combined with active physiotherapy. There is at present no oral respiratory stimulant available for long-term use in chronic respiratory failure.

RESPIRATORY STIMULANTS

Doxapram hydrochloride   28-Jun-2018

● **INDICATIONS AND DOSE**

Postoperative respiratory depression

▸ INITIALLY BY INTRAVENOUS INJECTION

▸ Adult: Initially 1–1.5 mg/kg, to be administered over at least 30 seconds, repeated if necessary after intervals of one hour, alternatively (by intravenous infusion) 2–3 mg/minute, adjusted according to response

Acute respiratory failure

▸ BY INTRAVENOUS INFUSION

▸ Adult: 1.5–4 mg/minute, adjusted according to response, to be given concurrently with oxygen and whenever possible monitor with frequent measurement of blood gas tensions

● CONTRA-INDICATIONS Cerebral oedema · cerebrovascular accident · coronary artery disease · epilepsy and other convulsive disorders · hyperthyroidism · physical obstruction of respiratory tract · severe hypertension · status asthmaticus

● CAUTIONS Give with beta$_2$ agonist in bronchoconstriction · give with oxygen in severe irreversible airways obstruction or severely decreased lung compliance (because of increased work load of breathing) · hypertension · impaired cardiac reserve · phaeochromocytoma

● INTERACTIONS → Appendix 1: doxapram

● SIDE-EFFECTS Arrhythmias · chest discomfort · confusion · cough · dizziness · dyspnoea · fever · flushing · hallucination · headache · hyperhidrosis · movement disorders · nausea · neuromuscular dysfunction · oral

disorders · perineal warmth · reflexes abnormal · respiratory disorders · seizure · urinary disorders · vomiting

● PREGNANCY No evidence of harm, but manufacturer advises avoid unless benefit outweighs risk.

● HEPATIC IMPAIRMENT Manufacturer advises use with caution.

● MONITORING REQUIREMENTS Frequent arterial blood gas and pH measurements are necessary during treatment to ensure correct dosage.

● MEDICINAL FORMS There can be variation in the licensing of different medicines containing the same drug.

Solution for injection

▸ Doxapram hydrochloride (Non-proprietary)

Doxapram hydrochloride 20 mg per 1 ml Doxapram 100mg/5ml solution for injection ampoules | 5 ampoule [PoM] £126.50

Chapter 4
Nervous system

1   Dementia

Dementia
14-Sep-2018

Description of condition

Dementia is a progressive clinical syndrome characterised by a range of cognitive and behavioural symptoms that can include memory loss, problems with reasoning and communication, a change in personality, and a reduced ability to carry out daily activities such as washing or dressing. Alzheimer's disease is the most common type of dementia; other common types of dementia include vascular dementia (due to cerebrovascular disease), dementia with Lewy bodies, mixed dementia, and frontotemporal dementia.

Aims of treatment

The aim of treatment is to promote independence, maintain function, and manage symptoms of dementia.

Non-drug treatment

EvGr Patients with all types of *mild-to-moderate* dementia presenting with **cognitive symptoms** should be given the opportunity to participate in a structured group cognitive stimulation programme. Group reminiscence therapy (use of life stories to improve psychological well-being), and cognitive rehabilitation or occupational therapy to support daily functional ability, should also be considered. ◁A▷

Management of cognitive symptoms

EvGr Some commonly prescribed drugs are associated with increased antimuscarinic (anticholinergic) burden, and therefore cognitive impairment; their use should be minimised. ◁A▷ Drugs with antimuscarinic effects include some antidepressants (e.g. amitriptyline hydrochloride p. 392, paroxetine p. 386), antihistamines (e.g. chlorphenamine maleate p. 299, promethazine hydrochloride p. 302), antipsychotics (e.g. olanzapine p. 419, quetiapine p. 422), and urinary antispasmodics (e.g. solifenacin succinate p. 824, tolterodine tartrate p. 824).

Alzheimer's disease

EvGr In newly diagnosed patients, drug treatment should only be initiated under the advice of a specialist clinician experienced in the management of Alzheimer's disease.

In patients with *mild-to-moderate* Alzheimer's disease, monotherapy with donepezil hydrochloride p. 317, galantamine p. 318, or rivastigmine p. 319 (acetylcholinesterase inhibitors) are first-line treatment options. If acetylcholinesterase inhibitors are not tolerated or contra-indicated, memantine hydrochloride p. 320 is a suitable alternative in patients with *moderate* Alzheimer's disease. Memantine hydrochloride is the drug of choice in patients with *severe* Alzheimer's disease.

In patients already receiving an acetylcholinesterase inhibitor to treat Alzheimer's disease, the addition of memantine hydrochloride should be considered if they develop *moderate* or *severe* disease; in this case, memantine hydrochloride can be initiated in primary care without advice from a specialist clinician. ◁A▷

In patients with moderate Alzheimer's disease, discontinuing acetylcholinesterase inhibitor treatment can cause a substantial worsening in cognitive function; EvGr treatment discontinuation should not be based on disease severity alone. ◁A▷

Non-Alzheimer's dementia

EvGr Donepezil hydrochloride [unlicensed indication] or rivastigmine [unlicensed indication] should be given to patients with *mild-to-moderate* dementia with Lewy bodies; galantamine [unlicensed indication] can be considered only if treatment with both donepezil hydrochloride or rivastigmine is not tolerated. Donepezil hydrochloride [unlicensed indication] or rivastigmine [unlicensed indication] can also be considered in patients with *severe* dementia with Lewy bodies. Memantine hydrochloride [unlicensed indication] can be considered as an alternative in patients with dementia with Lewy bodies in whom acetylcholinesterase inhibitors are contra-indicated or not tolerated.

Acetylcholinesterase inhibitors [unlicensed indication] or memantine hydrochloride [unlicensed indication] should only be considered in patients with vascular dementia if they have suspected co-morbid Alzheimer's disease, Parkinson's disease dementia, or dementia with Lewy bodies.

Acetylcholinesterase inhibitors and memantine hydrochloride are **not** recommended in patients with frontotemporal dementia or cognitive impairment caused by multiple sclerosis. Ⓐ

For management of Parkinson's disease dementia see Parkinson's disease p. 430.

Management of non-cognitive symptoms

Agitation, aggression, distress and psychosis

EvGr Patients with dementia should be offered psychosocial and environmental interventions such as counselling and management of pain and delirium to reduce distress.

Antipsychotic drugs should only be offered to patients with dementia if they are either at risk of harming themselves or others, or experiencing agitation, hallucinations or delusions that are causing them severe distress. ⒶThe CHM/MHRA has reported (2009) an increased risk of stroke and a small increased risk of death when antipsychotic drugs are used in elderly patients with dementia. The balance of risks and benefits should be carefully assessed, including any previous history of stroke or transient ischaemic attack and any risk factors for cerebrovascular disease such as hypertension, diabetes, smoking, and atrial fibrillation.

EvGr Antipsychotic drugs should be used at the lowest effective dose and for the shortest time possible, with a regular review at least every 6 weeks. Ⓐ

In patients who have dementia with Lewy bodies or Parkinson's disease dementia, antipsychotic drugs can worsen the motor features of the condition, and in some cases cause severe antipsychotic sensitivity reactions. See also management of psychotic symptoms in Parkinson's disease p. 430.

Depression and anxiety

EvGr Psychological treatments (e.g. cognitive behavioural therapy (CBT), multisensory stimulation, relaxation, or animal-assisted therapies) should be considered for patients with *mild-to-moderate* dementia who have mild to moderate depression or anxiety; antidepressants should be reserved for pre-existing severe mental health problems. Ⓐ

Sleep disturbances

EvGr Patients should be offered non-drug treatment approaches to manage sleep problems and insomnia, including sleep hygiene education, exposure to daylight, and increasing exercise and activity. Ⓐ

Useful Resources

Dementia: assessment, management and support for people living with dementia and their carers. National Institute for Health and Care Excellence. NICE guideline 97. June 2018.
www.nice.org.uk/guidance/ng97

> **Other drugs used for Dementia** Risperidone, p. 423

ANTICHOLINESTERASES ⟩ CENTRALLY ACTING

▌Donepezil hydrochloride   02-Sep-2020

- **DRUG ACTION** Donepezil is a reversible inhibitor of acetylcholinesterase.

  - **INDICATIONS AND DOSE**
  ### Mild to moderate dementia in Alzheimer's disease
  ▸ BY MOUTH
  ▸ Adult: Initially 5 mg once daily for one month, then increased if necessary up to 10 mg daily, doses to be given at bedtime

- **CAUTIONS** Asthma · chronic obstructive pulmonary disease · sick sinus syndrome · supraventricular conduction abnormalities · susceptibility to peptic ulcers

CAUTIONS, FURTHER INFORMATION
▸ Elderly For acetylcholinesterase inhibitors, prescription potentially inappropriate (STOPP criteria) in patients with a known history of persistent bradycardia (heart rate less than 60 beats per minute), heart block, recurrent unexplained syncope, or concurrent treatment with drugs that reduce heart rate (risk of cardiac conduction failure, syncope and injury).
See also Prescribing in the elderly p. 33.

- **INTERACTIONS** → Appendix 1: anticholinesterases, centrally acting

- **SIDE-EFFECTS**
▸ **Common or very common** Aggression · agitation · appetite decreased · common cold · diarrhoea · dizziness · fatigue · gastrointestinal disorders · hallucination · headache · injury · muscle cramps · nausea · pain · skin reactions · sleep disorders · syncope · urinary incontinence · vomiting
▸ **Uncommon** Bradycardia · gastrointestinal haemorrhage · hypersalivation · seizure
▸ **Rare or very rare** Cardiac conduction disorders · extrapyramidal symptoms · hepatic disorders · neuroleptic malignant syndrome · rhabdomyolysis

SIDE-EFFECTS, FURTHER INFORMATION Dose should be started low and increased if tolerated and necessary.

- **HEPATIC IMPAIRMENT** Manufacturer advises caution (risk of increased exposure in mild to moderate impairment; no information available in severe impairment).
Dose adjustments Manufacturer advises dose escalation should be performed according to individual tolerability in mild to moderate impairment.

- **DIRECTIONS FOR ADMINISTRATION** Manufacturer advises donepezil orodispersible tablet should be placed on the tongue, allowed to disperse, and swallowed.

- **PATIENT AND CARER ADVICE** Patient or carers should be given advice on how to administer donepezil hydrochloride orodispersible tablets.

- **NATIONAL FUNDING/ACCESS DECISIONS**
For full details see funding body website
NICE decisions
▸ **Donepezil, galantamine, rivastigmine, and memantine for the treatment of Alzheimer's disease (updated June 2018)**
NICE TA217 Recommended with restrictions

- **MEDICINAL FORMS** There can be variation in the licensing of different medicines containing the same drug. Forms available from special-order manufacturers include: oral suspension
Oral solution
▸ Donepezil hydrochloride (Non-proprietary)
   Donepezil hydrochloride 1 mg per 1 ml Donepezil 1mg/ml oral solution sugar free sugar-free | 150 ml [PoM] £53.73 DT = £53.71
Orodispersible tablet
▸ Donepezil hydrochloride (Non-proprietary)
   Donepezil hydrochloride 5 mg Donepezil 5mg orodispersible tablets sugar free sugar-free | 28 tablet [PoM] £9.38–£50.87 DT = £9.38
   Donepezil hydrochloride 10 mg Donepezil 10mg orodispersible tablets sugar free sugar-free | 28 tablet [PoM] £10.43–£71.31 DT = £10.43
▸ Aricept Evess (Eisai Ltd)
   Donepezil hydrochloride 5 mg Aricept Evess 5mg orodispersible tablets sugar-free | 28 tablet [PoM] £59.85 DT = £9.38
   Donepezil hydrochloride 10 mg Aricept Evess 10mg orodispersible tablets sugar-free | 28 tablet [PoM] £83.89 DT = £10.43
Tablet
▸ Donepezil hydrochloride (Non-proprietary)
   Donepezil hydrochloride 5 mg Donepezil 5mg tablets | 28 tablet [PoM] £59.85 DT = £1.34
   Donepezil hydrochloride 10 mg Donepezil 10mg tablets | 28 tablet [PoM] £83.89 DT = £1.52
▸ Aricept (Eisai Ltd)
   Donepezil hydrochloride 5 mg Aricept 5mg tablets | 28 tablet [PoM] £59.85 DT = £1.34
   Donepezil hydrochloride 10 mg Aricept 10mg tablets | 28 tablet [PoM] £83.89 DT = £1.52

4

Nervous system

Galantamine

25-Jul-2018

- DRUG ACTION Galantamine is a reversible inhibitor of acetylcholinesterase and it also has nicotinic receptor agonist properties.

- ● **INDICATIONS AND DOSE**

Mild to moderately severe dementia in Alzheimer's disease
- ▶ BY MOUTH USING IMMEDIATE-RELEASE MEDICINES
  - ▶ Adult: Initially 4 mg twice daily for 4 weeks, increased to 8 mg twice daily for at least 4 weeks; maintenance 8–12 mg twice daily
- ▶ BY MOUTH USING MODIFIED-RELEASE CAPSULES
  - ▶ Adult: Initially 8 mg once daily for 4 weeks, increased to 16 mg once daily for at least 4 weeks; maintenance 16–24 mg daily

- CAUTIONS Avoid in gastro-intestinal obstruction · avoid in urinary outflow obstruction · avoid whilst recovering from bladder surgery · avoid whilst recovering from gastro-intestinal surgery · cardiac disease · chronic obstructive pulmonary disease · congestive heart failure · electrolyte disturbances · history of seizures · history of severe asthma · pulmonary infection · sick sinus syndrome · supraventricular conduction abnormalities · susceptibility to peptic ulcers · unstable angina

  CAUTIONS, FURTHER INFORMATION
  - ▶ Elderly For acetylcholinesterase inhibitors, prescription potentially inappropriate (STOPP criteria) in patients with a known history of persistent bradycardia (heart rate less than 60 beats per minute), heart block, recurrent unexplained syncope or concurrent treatment with drugs that reduce heart rate (risk of cardiac conduction failure, syncope and injury).
    See also Prescribing in the elderly p. 33.

- INTERACTIONS → Appendix 1: anticholinesterases, centrally acting

- SIDE-EFFECTS
  - ▶ **Common or very common** Appetite decreased · arrhythmias · asthenia · depression · diarrhoea · dizziness · drowsiness · fall · gastrointestinal discomfort · hallucinations · headache · hypertension · malaise · muscle spasms · nausea · skin reactions · syncope · tremor · vomiting · weight decreased
  - ▶ **Uncommon** Atrioventricular block · dehydration · flushing · hyperhidrosis · hypersomnia · hypotension · muscle weakness · palpitations · paraesthesia · seizure · taste altered · tinnitus · vision blurred
  - ▶ **Rare or very rare** Hepatitis · severe cutaneous adverse reactions (SCARs)

- PREGNANCY Use with caution—toxicity in *animal* studies.

- BREAST FEEDING Avoid—no information available.

- HEPATIC IMPAIRMENT Manufacturer advises caution in moderate impairment (risk of increased plasma concentrations); avoid in severe impairment (no information available).
  Dose adjustments Manufacturer advises for *immediate-release* preparations in moderate impairment, initially 4 mg once daily (preferably in the morning) for at least 7 days, then 4 mg twice daily for at least 4 weeks; maximum 8 mg twice daily.
  Manufacturer advises for *modified-release* preparations in moderate impairment, initially 8 mg on alternate days (preferably in the morning) for 7 days, then 8 mg once daily for 4 weeks; maximum 16 mg daily.

- RENAL IMPAIRMENT Avoid if eGFR less than 9 mL/minute/1.73 m².

- PATIENT AND CARER ADVICE Manufacturer recommends that patients are warned of the signs of serious skin reactions; they should be advised to stop taking galantamine immediately and seek medical advice if symptoms occur.

- NATIONAL FUNDING/ACCESS DECISIONS
  For full details see funding body website
  NICE decisions
  - ▶ **Donepezil, galantamine, rivastigmine, and memantine for the treatment of Alzheimer's disease** (updated June 2018)
    NICE TA217 Recommended with restrictions

- MEDICINAL FORMS There can be variation in the licensing of different medicines containing the same drug. Forms available from special-order manufacturers include: tablet

Oral solution
CAUTIONARY AND ADVISORY LABELS 3, 21
- ▶ Galantamine (Non-proprietary)
  Galantamine (as Galantamine hydrobromide) 4 mg per 1 ml Galantamine 20mg/5ml oral solution sugar free sugar-free | 100 ml PoM £120.00 DT = £120.00
- ▶ Galzemic (Creo Pharma Ltd)
  Galantamine (as Galantamine hydrobromide) 4 mg per 1 ml Galzemic 4mg/ml oral solution sugar-free | 100 ml £90.00 DT = £120.00
- ▶ Reminyl (Shire Pharmaceuticals Ltd)
  Galantamine (as Galantamine hydrobromide) 4 mg per 1 ml Reminyl 4mg/ml oral solution sugar-free | 100 ml PoM £120.00 DT = £120.00

Modified-release capsule
CAUTIONARY AND ADVISORY LABELS 3, 21, 25
- ▶ Acumor XL (Mylan)
  Galantamine (as Galantamine hydrobromide) 8 mg Acumor XL 8mg capsules | 28 capsule PoM £49.26 DT = £51.88
  Galantamine (as Galantamine hydrobromide) 24 mg Acumor XL 24mg capsules | 28 capsule PoM £75.81 DT = £79.80
- ▶ Consion XL (Dr Reddy's Laboratories (UK) Ltd)
  Galantamine (as Galantamine hydrobromide) 8 mg Consion XL 8mg capsules | 28 capsule PoM £25.94 DT = £51.88
  Galantamine (as Galantamine hydrobromide) 16 mg Consion XL 16mg capsules | 28 capsule PoM £32.45 DT = £64.90
  Galantamine (as Galantamine hydrobromide) 24 mg Consion XL 24mg capsules | 28 capsule PoM £39.90 DT = £79.80
- ▶ Elmino (Zentiva)
  Galantamine (as Galantamine hydrobromide) 8 mg Elmino XL 8mg capsules | 28 capsule PoM £51.88 DT = £51.88
  Galantamine (as Galantamine hydrobromide) 16 mg Elmino XL 16mg capsules | 28 capsule PoM £64.90 DT = £64.90
  Galantamine (as Galantamine hydrobromide) 24 mg Elmino XL 24mg capsules | 28 capsule PoM £79.80 DT = £79.80
- ▶ Gaalin (Milpharm Ltd)
  Galantamine (as Galantamine hydrobromide) 8 mg Gaalin 8mg modified-release capsules | 28 capsule PoM £51.88 DT = £51.88
  Galantamine (as Galantamine hydrobromide) 16 mg Gaalin 16mg modified-release capsules | 28 capsule PoM £64.90 DT = £64.90
  Galantamine (as Galantamine hydrobromide) 24 mg Gaalin 24mg modified-release capsules | 28 capsule PoM £79.80 DT = £79.80
- ▶ Galantex XL (Creo Pharma Ltd)
  Galantamine (as Galantamine hydrobromide) 8 mg Galzemic XL 8mg capsules | 28 capsule PoM £19.03 DT = £51.88
  Galantamine (as Galantamine hydrobromide) 16 mg Galzemic XL 16mg capsules | 28 capsule PoM £23.82 DT = £64.90
  Galantamine (as Galantamine hydrobromide) 24 mg Galzemic XL 24mg capsules | 28 capsule PoM £29.30 DT = £79.80
- ▶ Galsya XL (Consilient Health Ltd)
  Galantamine (as Galantamine hydrobromide) 8 mg Galsya XL 8mg capsules | 28 capsule PoM £44.09 DT = £51.88
  Galantamine (as Galantamine hydrobromide) 16 mg Galsya XL 16mg capsules | 28 capsule PoM £55.16 DT = £64.90
  Galantamine (as Galantamine hydrobromide) 24 mg Galsya XL 24mg capsules | 28 capsule PoM £67.83 DT = £79.80
- ▶ Gatalin XL (Aspire Pharma Ltd)
  Galantamine (as Galantamine hydrobromide) 8 mg Gatalin XL 8mg capsules | 28 capsule PoM £25.94 DT = £51.88
  Galantamine (as Galantamine hydrobromide) 16 mg Gatalin XL 16mg capsules | 28 capsule PoM £32.45 DT = £64.90
  Galantamine (as Galantamine hydrobromide) 24 mg Gatalin XL 24mg capsules | 28 capsule PoM £39.90 DT = £79.80
- ▶ Gazylan XL (Teva UK Ltd)
  Galantamine (as Galantamine hydrobromide) 8 mg Gazylan XL 8mg capsules | 28 capsule PoM £19.04 DT = £51.88

Galantamine (as Galantamine hydrobromide) 16 mg   Gazylan XL
16mg capsules | 28 capsule PoM £23.83 DT = £64.90
Galantamine (as Galantamine hydrobromide) 24 mg   Gazylan XL
24mg capsules | 28 capsule PoM £29.31 DT = £79.80
▸ Lotprosin XL (Accord Healthcare Ltd)
Galantamine (as Galantamine hydrobromide) 8 mg   Lotprosin XL
8mg capsules | 28 capsule PoM £51.88 DT = £51.88
Galantamine (as Galantamine hydrobromide) 16 mg   Lotprosin XL
16mg capsules | 28 capsule PoM £64.90 DT = £64.90
Galantamine (as Galantamine hydrobromide) 24 mg   Lotprosin XL
24mg capsules | 28 capsule PoM £79.80 DT = £79.80
▸ Luventa XL (Fontus Health Ltd)
Galantamine (as Galantamine hydrobromide) 8 mg   Luventa XL
8mg capsules | 28 capsule PoM £25.42 DT = £51.88
Galantamine (as Galantamine hydrobromide) 16 mg   Luventa XL
16mg capsules | 28 capsule PoM £31.80 DT = £64.90
Galantamine (as Galantamine hydrobromide) 24 mg   Luventa XL
24mg capsules | 28 capsule PoM £39.10 DT = £79.80
▸ Reminyl XL (Shire Pharmaceuticals Ltd)
Galantamine (as Galantamine hydrobromide) 8 mg   Reminyl XL
8mg capsules | 28 capsule PoM £51.88 DT = £51.88
Galantamine (as Galantamine hydrobromide) 16 mg   Reminyl XL
16mg capsules | 28 capsule PoM £64.90 DT = £64.90
Galantamine (as Galantamine hydrobromide) 24 mg   Reminyl XL
24mg capsules | 28 capsule PoM £79.80 DT = £79.80

Rivastigmine

12-Nov-2020

● **DRUG ACTION** Rivastigmine is a reversible non-competitive inhibitor of acetylcholinesterases.

● **INDICATIONS AND DOSE**

Mild to moderate dementia in Alzheimer's disease
▸ BY MOUTH
▸ **Adult:** Initially 1.5 mg twice daily, increased in steps of 1.5 mg twice daily, dose to be increased at intervals of at least 2 weeks according to response and tolerance; usual dose 3–6 mg twice daily (max. per dose 6 mg twice daily), if treatment interrupted for more than several days, retitrate from 1.5 mg twice daily
▸ BY TRANSDERMAL APPLICATION USING PATCHES
▸ **Adult:** Apply 4.6 mg/24 hours daily for at least 4 weeks, increased if tolerated to 9.5 mg/24 hours daily for a further 6 months, then increased if necessary to 13.3 mg/24 hours daily, increase to 13.3 mg/24 hours patch if well tolerated and cognitive deterioration or functional decline demonstrated; use caution in patients with body-weight less than 50 kg, if treatment interrupted for more than 3 days, retitrate from 4.6 mg/24 hours patch

Mild to moderate dementia in Parkinson's disease
▸ BY MOUTH
▸ **Adult:** Initially 1.5 mg twice daily, increased in steps of 1.5 mg twice daily, dose to be increased at intervals of at least 2 weeks according to response and tolerance; usual dose 3–6 mg twice daily (max. per dose 6 mg twice daily), if treatment interrupted for more than several days, retitrate from 1.5 mg twice daily

DOSE EQUIVALENCE AND CONVERSION
▸ When switching from oral to transdermal therapy, patients taking 3–6 mg by mouth daily should initially switch to 4.6 mg/24 hours patch, then titrate as above. Patients taking 9 mg by mouth daily should switch to 9.5 mg/24 hours patch if oral dose stable and well tolerated; if oral dose not stable or well tolerated patients should switch to 4.6 mg/24 hours patch, then titrate as above. Patients taking 12 mg by mouth daily should switch to 9.5 mg/24 hours patch. The first patch should be applied on the day following the last oral dose

● CAUTIONS Bladder outflow obstruction · conduction abnormalities · duodenal ulcers · gastric ulcers · history of asthma · history of chronic obstructive pulmonary disease ·

history of seizures · risk of fatal overdose with patch administration errors · sick sinus syndrome · susceptibility to ulcers

CAUTIONS, FURTHER INFORMATION
▸ **Elderly** For acetylcholinesterase inhibitors, prescription potentially inappropriate (STOPP criteria) in patients with a known history of persistent bradycardia (heart rate less than 60 beats per minute), heart block, recurrent unexplained syncope or concurrent treatment with drugs that reduce heart rate (risk of cardiac conduction failure, syncope and injury).
  See also Prescribing in the elderly p. 33.

● INTERACTIONS → Appendix 1: anticholinesterases, centrally acting

● SIDE-EFFECTS

GENERAL SIDE-EFFECTS
▸ **Common or very common** Anxiety · appetite decreased · arrhythmias · asthenia · dehydration · depression · diarrhoea · dizziness · drowsiness · fall · gastrointestinal discomfort · headache · hyperhidrosis · hypersalivation · hypertension · movement disorders · nausea · skin reactions · syncope · tremor · urinary incontinence · urinary tract infection · vomiting · weight decreased
▸ **Uncommon** Aggression · atrioventricular block
▸ **Rare or very rare** Pancreatitis · seizure
▸ **Frequency not known** Hepatitis

SPECIFIC SIDE-EFFECTS
▸ **Common or very common**
▸ With oral use Confusion · gait abnormal · hallucinations · malaise · parkinsonism · sleep disorders
▸ **Uncommon**
▸ With oral use Hypotension
▸ With transdermal use Gastric ulcer
▸ **Rare or very rare**
▸ With oral use Angina pectoris · gastrointestinal disorders · gastrointestinal haemorrhage
▸ **Frequency not known**
▸ With transdermal use Hallucination · nightmare

SIDE-EFFECTS, FURTHER INFORMATION Dose should be started low and increased according to response if tolerated.
  Treatment should be interrupted if dehydration resulting from prolonged vomiting or diarrhoea occurs and withheld until resolution—retitrate dose if necessary.
  Transdermal administration is less likely to cause side-effects.

● HEPATIC IMPAIRMENT Manufacturer advises caution (risk of increased exposure; no information available in severe impairment).
Dose adjustments Manufacturer advises cautious dose titration according to individual tolerability.

● RENAL IMPAIRMENT
Dose adjustments Titrate according to individual tolerability.

● MONITORING REQUIREMENTS Monitor body-weight.

● DIRECTIONS FOR ADMINISTRATION
▸ With transdermal use Manufacturer advises apply patches to clean, dry, non-hairy, non-irritated skin on back, upper arm, or chest, removing after 24 hours and siting a replacement patch on a different area (avoid using the same area for 14 days).

● PATIENT AND CARER ADVICE
EXELON ® PATCHES Advise patients and carers of patch administration instructions, particularly to remove the previous day's patch before applying the new patch—consult product literature.

● NATIONAL FUNDING/ACCESS DECISIONS
For full details see funding body website

4

Nervous system

NICE decisions
▶ Donepezil, galantamine, rivastigmine, and memantine for the treatment of Alzheimer's disease (updated June 2018)
NICE TA217 Recommended with restrictions

● MEDICINAL FORMS There can be variation in the licensing of different medicines containing the same drug.

Oral solution
CAUTIONARY AND ADVISORY LABELS 21
▶ Rivastigmine (Non-proprietary)
Rivastigmine (as Rivastigmine hydrogen tartrate) 2 mg per 1 ml Rivastigmine 2mg/ml oral solution sugar free sugar-free | 120 ml PoM £96.82 DT = £96.82

Capsule
CAUTIONARY AND ADVISORY LABELS 21, 25
▶ Rivastigmine (Non-proprietary)
Rivastigmine (as Rivastigmine hydrogen tartrate)
1.5 mg Rivastigmine 1.5mg capsules | 28 capsule PoM £28.26 DT = £3.71 | 56 capsule PoM £3.82
Rivastigmine (as Rivastigmine hydrogen tartrate)
3 mg Rivastigmine 3mg capsules | 28 capsule PoM £33.25 DT = £5.30 | 56 capsule PoM £4.88-£66.51
Rivastigmine (as Rivastigmine hydrogen tartrate)
4.5 mg Rivastigmine 4.5mg capsules | 28 capsule PoM £33.25 DT = £32.56 | 56 capsule PoM £47.02-£66.51
Rivastigmine (as Rivastigmine hydrogen tartrate)
6 mg Rivastigmine 6mg capsules | 28 capsule PoM £33.15 DT = £33.15 | 56 capsule PoM £54.34-£66.51
▶ Nimvastid (Consilient Health Ltd)
Rivastigmine (as Rivastigmine hydrogen tartrate)
1.5 mg Nimvastid 1.5mg capsules | 28 capsule PoM £28.26 DT = £3.71
Rivastigmine (as Rivastigmine hydrogen tartrate) 3 mg Nimvastid 3mg capsules | 28 capsule PoM £28.26 DT = £5.30
Rivastigmine (as Rivastigmine hydrogen tartrate)
4.5 mg Nimvastid 4.5mg capsules | 28 capsule PoM £28.26 DT = £32.56
Rivastigmine (as Rivastigmine hydrogen tartrate)
6 mg Nimvastid 6mg capsules | 28 capsule PoM £28.26 DT = £33.15

Transdermal patch
▶ Almuriva (Sandoz Ltd)
Rivastigmine 4.6 mg per 24 hour Almuriva 4.6mg/24hours transdermal patches | 30 patch PoM £77.97 DT = £77.97
Rivastigmine 9.5 mg per 24 hour Almuriva 9.5mg/24hours transdermal patches | 30 patch PoM £77.97 DT = £19.97
▶ Alzest (Dr Reddy's Laboratories (UK) Ltd)
Rivastigmine 4.6 mg per 24 hour Alzest 4.6mg/24hours transdermal patches | 30 patch PoM £35.10 DT = £77.97
Rivastigmine 9.5 mg per 24 hour Alzest 9.5mg/24hours transdermal patches | 30 patch PoM £19.97 DT = £19.97
▶ Exelon (Novartis Pharmaceuticals UK Ltd)
Rivastigmine 4.6 mg per 24 hour Exelon 4.6mg/24hours transdermal patches | 30 patch PoM £77.97 DT = £77.97
Rivastigmine 9.5 mg per 24 hour Exelon 9.5mg/24hours transdermal patches | 30 patch PoM £77.97 DT = £19.97
Rivastigmine 13.3 mg per 24 hour Exelon 13.3mg/24hours transdermal patches | 30 patch PoM £77.97 DT = £77.97
▶ Prometax (Sandoz Ltd)
Rivastigmine 4.6 mg per 24 hour Prometax 4.6mg/24hours transdermal patches | 30 patch PoM £77.97 DT = £77.97
Rivastigmine 9.5 mg per 24 hour Prometax 9.5mg/24hours transdermal patches | 30 patch PoM £77.97 DT = £19.97
▶ Rivatev (Teva UK Ltd)
Rivastigmine 13.3 mg per 24 hour Erastig 13.3mg/24hours transdermal patches | 30 patch PoM £73.90 DT = £77.97
▶ Voleze (Advanz Pharma)
Rivastigmine 4.6 mg per 24 hour Voleze 4.6mg/24hours transdermal patches | 30 patch PoM £77.97 DT = £77.97
Rivastigmine 13.3 mg per 24 hour Voleze 13.3mg/24hours transdermal patches | 30 patch PoM £77.97 DT = £77.97

DOPAMINERGIC DRUGS ❭ NMDA RECEPTOR ANTAGONISTS

Memantine hydrochloride
03-Aug-2020

● DRUG ACTION Memantine is a glutamate receptor antagonist.

● **INDICATIONS AND DOSE**
Moderate to severe dementia in Alzheimer's disease
▶ BY MOUTH
▶ Adult: Initially 5 mg once daily, then increased in steps of 5 mg every week; usual maintenance 20 mg daily; maximum 20 mg per day
Oscillopsia in multiple sclerosis
▶ BY MOUTH
▶ Adult: Initially 10 mg daily, then increased to 40 mg daily, over 1 week; increased if necessary to 60 mg daily, over 1 week, on specialist advice only

● UNLICENSED USE EvGr Memantine hydrochloride is used for oscillopsia in multiple sclerosis, Ⓔbut is not licensed for this indication.

● CAUTIONS Epilepsy · history of convulsions · risk factors for epilepsy

● INTERACTIONS → Appendix 1: memantine

● SIDE-EFFECTS
▶ **Common or very common** Balance impaired · constipation · dizziness · drowsiness · dyspnoea · headache · hypersensitivity · hypertension
▶ **Uncommon** Confusion · embolism and thrombosis · fatigue · fungal infection · hallucination · heart failure · vomiting
▶ **Rare or very rare** Seizure
▶ **Frequency not known** Hepatitis · pancreatitis · psychotic disorder

● PREGNANCY Manufacturer advises avoid unless essential—no information available.

● BREAST FEEDING Manufacturer advises avoid—no information available.

● HEPATIC IMPAIRMENT Manufacturer advises avoid in severe impairment—no information available.

● RENAL IMPAIRMENT Avoid if eGFR less than 5 mL/minute/1.73 m^2.
Dose adjustments Reduce dose to 10 mg daily if eGFR 30–49 mL/minute/1.73 m^2, if well tolerated after at least 7 days dose can be increased in steps to 20 mg daily; reduce dose to 10 mg daily if eGFR 5–29 mL/minute/1.73 m^2.

● DIRECTIONS FOR ADMINISTRATION For *oral solution*, manufacturer advises solution should be dosed onto a spoon or into a glass of water.

● NATIONAL FUNDING/ACCESS DECISIONS
For full details see funding body website
NICE decisions
▶ Donepezil, galantamine, rivastigmine, and memantine for the treatment of Alzheimer's disease (updated June 2018)
NICE TA217 Recommended with restrictions

● MEDICINAL FORMS There can be variation in the licensing of different medicines containing the same drug.

Oral solution
▶ Memantine hydrochloride (Non-proprietary)
Memantine hydrochloride 10 mg per 1 ml Memantine 10mg/ml oral solution sugar free sugar-free | 50 ml PoM £61.61 DT = £55.15 sugar-free | 100 ml PoM £97.98-£123.23
▶ Ebixa (Lundbeck Ltd)
Memantine hydrochloride 10 mg per 1 ml Ebixa 5mg/0.5ml pump actuation oral solution sugar-free | 50 ml PoM £61.61 DT = £55.15 sugar-free | 100 ml PoM £123.23

Orodispersible tablet
EXCIPIENTS: May contain Aspartame
▸ Valios (Dr Reddy's Laboratories (UK) Ltd)
Memantine hydrochloride 5 mg Valios 5mg orodispersible tablets sugar free sugar-free | 7 tablet [PoM] [⚕]
Memantine hydrochloride 10 mg Valios 10mg orodispersible tablets sugar free sugar-free | 28 tablet [PoM] £24.99 DT = £24.99
Memantine hydrochloride 15 mg Valios 15mg orodispersible tablets sugar free sugar-free | 7 tablet [PoM] [⚕]
Memantine hydrochloride 20 mg Valios 20mg orodispersible tablets sugar free sugar-free | 28 tablet [PoM] £49.98 DT = £49.98
Valios 5mg/10mg/15mg/20mg orodispersible tablets initiation pack sugar-free | 28 tablet [PoM] £31.24 DT = £31.24

Tablet
▸ Memantine hydrochloride (Non-proprietary)
Memantine hydrochloride 5 mg Memantine 5mg tablets | 7 tablet [PoM] [⚕]
Memantine hydrochloride 10 mg Memantine 10mg tablets | 28 tablet [PoM] £34.50 DT = £3.54 | 56 tablet [PoM] £10.10
Memantine hydrochloride 15 mg Memantine 15mg tablets | 7 tablet [PoM] [⚕]
Memantine hydrochloride 20 mg Memantine 20mg tablets | 28 tablet [PoM] £69.01 DT = £8.46
Memantine 5mg/10mg/15mg/20mg tablets treatment initiation pack | 28 tablet [PoM] £43.13 DT = £43.13
▸ Ebixa (Lundbeck Ltd)
Memantine hydrochloride 5 mg Ebixa 5mg tablets | 7 tablet [PoM] [⚕]
Memantine hydrochloride 10 mg Ebixa 10mg tablets | 28 tablet [PoM] £34.50 DT = £3.54
Memantine hydrochloride 15 mg Ebixa 15mg tablets | 7 tablet [PoM] [⚕]
Memantine hydrochloride 20 mg Ebixa 20mg tablets | 28 tablet [PoM] £69.01 DT = £8.46
Ebixa tablets treatment initiation pack | 28 tablet [PoM] £43.13 DT = £43.13
▸ Maruxa (Consilient Health Ltd)
Memantine hydrochloride 10 mg Marixino 10mg tablets | 28 tablet [PoM] £29.32 DT = £3.54
Memantine hydrochloride 20 mg Marixino 20mg tablets | 28 tablet [PoM] £58.65 DT = £8.46
▸ Nemdatine (Actavis UK Ltd)
Memantine hydrochloride 5 mg Nemdatine 5mg tablets | 7 tablet [PoM] [⚕]
Memantine hydrochloride 15 mg Nemdatine 15mg tablets | 7 tablet [PoM] [⚕]

2 Epilepsy and other seizure disorders

Epilepsy

14-Sep-2020

Epilepsy control

The object of treatment is to prevent the occurrence of seizures by maintaining an effective dose of one or more antiepileptic drugs. Careful adjustment of doses is necessary, starting with low doses and increasing gradually until seizures are controlled or there are significant adverse effects.

When choosing an antiepileptic drug, the presenting epilepsy syndrome should first be considered. If the syndrome is not clear, the seizure type should determine the choice of treatment. Concomitant medication, co-morbidity, age, and sex should also be taken into account.

The dosage frequency is often determined by the plasma-drug half-life, and should be kept as low as possible to encourage adherence with the prescribed regimen. Most antiepileptics, when used in the usual dosage, can be given twice daily. Lamotrigine p. 335, perampanel p. 339, phenobarbital p. 353, and phenytoin p. 340, which have long half-lives, can be given once daily at bedtime. However, with large doses, some antiepileptics may need to be given more frequently to avoid adverse effects associated with high peak plasma-drug concentration.

Management

When monotherapy with a first-line antiepileptic drug has failed, monotherapy with a second drug should be tried; the diagnosis should be checked before starting an alternative drug if the first drug showed lack of efficacy. The change from one antiepileptic drug to another should be cautious, slowly withdrawing the first drug only when the new regimen has been established. Combination therapy with two or more antiepileptic drugs may be necessary, but the concurrent use of antiepileptic drugs increases the risk of adverse effects and drug interactions. If combination therapy does not bring about worthwhile benefits, revert to the regimen (monotherapy or combination therapy) that provided the best balance between tolerability and efficacy. A single antiepileptic drug should be prescribed wherever possible.

MHRA/CHM advice: Antiepileptic drugs: updated advice on switching between different manufacturers' products (November 2017)
The CHM has reviewed spontaneous adverse reactions received by the MHRA and publications that reported potential harm arising from switching of antiepileptic drugs in patients previously stabilised on a branded product to a generic. The CHM concluded that reports of loss of seizure control and/or worsening of side-effects around the time of switching between products could be explained as chance associations, but that a causal role of switching could not be ruled out in all cases. The following guidance has been issued to help minimise risk:

● Different antiepileptic drugs vary considerably in their characteristics, which influences the risk of whether switching between different manufacturers' products of a particular drug may cause adverse effects or loss of seizure control;
● Antiepileptic drugs have been divided into three risk-based categories to help healthcare professionals decide whether it is necessary to maintain continuity of supply of a specific manufacturer's product. These categories are listed below;
● If it is felt desirable for a patient to be maintained on a specific manufacturer's product this should be prescribed either by specifying a brand name, or by using the generic drug name and name of the manufacturer (otherwise known as the Marketing Authorisation Holder);
● This advice relates only to antiepileptic drug use for treatment of epilepsy; it does not apply to their use in other indications (e.g. mood stabilisation, neuropathic pain);
● Please report on a Yellow Card any suspected adverse reactions to antiepileptic drugs;
● Dispensing pharmacists should ensure the continuity of supply of a particular product when the prescription specifies it. If the prescribed product is unavailable, it may be necessary to dispense a product from a different manufacturer to maintain continuity of treatment of that antiepileptic drug. Such cases should be discussed and agreed with both the prescriber and patient (or carer);
● Usual dispensing practice can be followed when a specific product is not stated.

Category 1
Carbamazepine p. 327, phenobarbital, phenytoin, primidone p. 354. For these drugs, doctors are advised to ensure that their patient is maintained on a specific manufacturer's product.

Category 2
Clobazam p. 355, clonazepam p. 355, eslicarbazepine acetate p. 329, lamotrigine, oxcarbazepine p. 338, perampanel, rufinamide p. 343, topiramate p. 349, valproate, zonisamide p. 352. For these drugs, the need for continued supply of a particular manufacturer's product

should be based on clinical judgement and consultation with the patient and/or carer taking into account factors such as seizure frequency, treatment history, and potential implications to the patient of having a breakthrough seizure. Non-clinical factors as for Category 3 drugs should also be considered.

Category 3

Brivaracetam p. 326, **ethosuximide p. 330**, **gabapentin p. 332**, **lacosamide p. 333**, **levetiracetam p. 337**, **pregabalin p. 342**, **tiagabine p. 348**, **vigabatrin p. 351**. For these drugs, it is usually unnecessary to ensure that patients are maintained on a specific manufacturer's product as therapeutic equivalence can be assumed, however, other factors are important when considering whether switching is appropriate. Differences between alternative products (e.g. product name, packaging, appearance, and taste) may be perceived negatively by patients and/or carers, and may lead to dissatisfaction, anxiety, confusion, dosing errors, and reduced adherence. In addition, difficulties for patients with co-morbid autism, mental health problems, or learning disability should also be considered.

MHRA/CHM advice: Antiepileptics: risk of suicidal thoughts and behaviour (August 2008)

A Europe-wide review concluded that all antiepileptic drugs may be associated with a small increased risk of suicidal thoughts and behaviour; symptoms may occur as early as 1 week after starting treatment. The MHRA has recommended that patients and their carers should be advised to seek medical advice if any mood changes, distressing thoughts, or feelings about suicide or self-harming develop, and that the patient should be referred for appropriate treatment if necessary. Patients should also be advised not to stop or switch antiepileptic treatment and to seek advice from a healthcare professional if concerned.

Antiepileptic hypersensitivity syndrome

Antiepileptic hypersensitivity syndrome is a rare but potentially fatal syndrome associated with some antiepileptic drugs (**carbamazepine**, **lacosamide**, **lamotrigine**, **oxcarbazepine**, **phenobarbital**, **phenytoin**, **primidone**, and **rufinamide**); rarely cross-sensitivity occurs between some of these antiepileptic drugs. Some other antiepileptics (**eslicarbazepine**, **stiripentol**, and **zonisamide**) have a theoretical risk. The symptoms usually start between 1 and 8 weeks of exposure; fever, rash, and lymphadenopathy are most commonly seen. Other systemic signs include liver dysfunction, haematological, renal, and pulmonary abnormalities, vasculitis, and multi-organ failure. If signs or symptoms of hypersensitivity syndrome occur, the drug should be withdrawn immediately, the patient must not be re-exposed, and expert advice should be sought.

Interactions

Interactions between antiepileptics are complex and may increase toxicity without a corresponding increase in antiepileptic effect. Interactions are usually caused by hepatic enzyme induction or inhibition; displacement from protein binding sites is not usually a problem. These interactions are highly variable and unpredictable.

Withdrawal

Antiepileptic drugs should be withdrawn under specialist supervision. Avoid abrupt withdrawal, particularly of barbiturates and benzodiazepines, because this can precipitate severe rebound seizures. Reduction in dosage should be gradual and, in the case of barbiturates, withdrawal of the drug may take months.

The decision to withdraw antiepileptic drugs from a seizure-free patient, and its timing, is often difficult and depends on individual circumstances. Even in patients who have been seizure-free for several years, there is a significant risk of seizure recurrence on drug withdrawal. In patients receiving several antiepileptic drugs, only one drug should be withdrawn at a time.

Driving

If a driver has a seizure (of any type) they must stop driving immediately and inform the Driver and Vehicle Licensing Agency (DVLA)

Patients who have had a first unprovoked epileptic seizure or a single isolated seizure must not drive for 6 months; driving may then be resumed, provided the patient has been assessed by a specialist as fit to drive and investigations do not suggest a risk of further seizures.

Patients with established epilepsy may drive a motor vehicle provided they are not a danger to the public and are compliant with treatment and follow up. To continue driving, these patients must be seizure-free for at least one year (or have a pattern of seizures established for one year where there is no influence on their level of consciousness or the ability to act); also, they must not have a history of unprovoked seizures.

Note: additional criteria apply for drivers of large goods or passenger carrying vehicles—consult DVLA guidance.

Patients who have had a *seizure while asleep* are not permitted to drive for one year from the date of each seizure, unless:

- a history or pattern of sleep seizures occurring **only** ever while asleep has been established over the course of at least one year from the date of the first sleep seizure; or
- an established pattern of purely asleep seizures can be demonstrated over the course of three years if the patient has previously had seizures whilst awake (or awake and asleep).

The DVLA recommends that patients should not drive during medication changes or withdrawal of antiepileptic drugs, and for 6 months after their last dose. If a seizure occurs due to a prescribed change or withdrawal of epilepsy treatment, the patient will have their driving license revoked for 1 year; relicensing may be considered earlier if treatment has been reinstated for 6 months and no further seizures have occurred.

Pregnancy

Women of child-bearing potential should discuss with a specialist the impact of both epilepsy, and its treatment, on the outcome of pregnancy.

There is an increased risk of teratogenicity associated with the use of antiepileptic drugs (especially if used during the first trimester and particularly if the patient takes two or more antiepileptic drugs). Valproate is associated with the highest risk of serious developmental disorders (up to 30–40% risk) and congenital malformations (approx. 10% risk). Valproate must **not** be used in females of childbearing potential unless the conditions of the Pregnancy Prevention Programme are met and alternative treatments are ineffective or not tolerated; during pregnancy, it must not be used for epilepsy, unless it is the only possible treatment. There is also an increased risk of teratogenicity with phenytoin, primidone, phenobarbital, lamotrigine, and carbamazepine. Topiramate carries an increased risk of congenital malformations (including cleft palate, hypospadias, and anomalies involving various body systems) if taken in the first trimester of pregnancy. There is not enough evidence to establish the risk of teratogenicity with other antiepileptic drugs.

Prescribers should also consider carefully the choice of antiepileptic therapy in pre-pubescent girls who may later become pregnant. Women of child-bearing potential who take antiepileptic drugs should be given advice about the need for an effective contraception method to avoid unplanned pregnancy—for further information, see *Conception and contraception* in the individual drug monographs. Some antiepileptic drugs can reduce the efficacy of hormonal contraceptives, and the efficacy of some antiepileptics may be affected by hormonal contraceptives.

Women who want to become pregnant should be referred to a specialist for advice in advance of conception. For some women, the severity of seizure or the seizure type may not pose a serious threat, and drug withdrawal may be considered; therapy may be resumed after the first trimester. If treatment with antiepileptic drugs must continue throughout pregnancy, then monotherapy is preferable at the lowest effective dose.

Once an unplanned pregnancy is discovered it is usually too late for changes to be made to the treatment regimen; the risk of harm to the mother and fetus from convulsive seizures outweighs the risk of continued therapy. The likelihood of a woman who is taking antiepileptic drugs having a baby with no malformations is at least 90%, and it is important that women do not stop taking essential treatment because of concern over harm to the fetus. To reduce the risk of neural tube defects, folate supplementation is advised before conception and throughout the first trimester. In the case of sodium valproate p. 345 and valproic acid p. 373 an urgent consultation is required to reconsider the benefits and risks of valproate therapy.

The concentration of antiepileptic drugs in the plasma can change during pregnancy. Doses of phenytoin, carbamazepine, and lamotrigine should be adjusted on the basis of plasma-drug concentration monitoring; the dose of other antiepileptic drugs should be monitored carefully during pregnancy and after birth, and adjustments made on a clinical basis. Plasma-drug concentration monitoring during pregnancy is also useful to check compliance. Additionally, in patients taking topiramate or levetiracetam, it is recommended that fetal growth should be monitored. Women who have seizures in the second half of pregnancy should be assessed for eclampsia before any change is made to antiepileptic treatment. Status epilepticus should be treated according to the standard protocol.

Routine injection of vitamin K at birth minimises the risk of neonatal haemorrhage associated with antiepileptics. Withdrawal effects in the newborn may occur with some antiepileptic drugs, in particular benzodiazepines and phenobarbital.

Epilepsy and Pregnancy Register

All pregnant women with epilepsy, whether taking medication or not, should be encouraged to notify the UK Epilepsy and Pregnancy Register (Tel: 0800 389 1248).

Breast-feeding

Women taking antiepileptic monotherapy should generally be encouraged to breast-feed; if a woman is on combination therapy or if there are other risk factors, such as premature birth, specialist advice should be sought.

All infants should be monitored for sedation, feeding difficulties, adequate weight gain, and developmental milestones. Infants should also be monitored for adverse effects associated with the antiepileptic drug particularly with newer antiepileptics, if the antiepileptic is readily transferred into breast-milk causing high infant serum-drug concentrations (e.g. ethosuximide, lamotrigine, primidone, and zonisamide), or if slower metabolism in the infant causes drugs to accumulate (e.g. phenobarbital and lamotrigine). Serum-drug concentration monitoring should be undertaken in breast-fed infants if suspected adverse reactions develop; if toxicity develops it may be necessary to introduce formula feeds to limit the infant's drug exposure, or to wean the infant off breast-milk altogether.

Primidone, phenobarbital, and the benzodiazepines are associated with an established risk of drowsiness in breast-fed babies and caution is required.

Withdrawal effects may occur in infants if a mother suddenly stops breast-feeding, particularly if she is taking phenobarbital, primidone, or lamotrigine.

Focal seizures with or without secondary generalisation

Carbamazepine p. 327 and lamotrigine p. 335 are first-line options for treating newly diagnosed focal seizures; oxcarbazepine p. 338, sodium valproate p. 345 and levetiracetam p. 337 may be used if carbamazepine or lamotrigine are unsuitable or not tolerated. If monotherapy is unsuccessful with two of these first-line antiepileptic drugs, adjunctive treatment may be considered. Options for adjunctive treatment include carbamazepine, clobazam p. 355, gabapentin p. 332, lamotrigine, levetiracetam, oxcarbazepine, sodium valproate, or topiramate p. 349. If adjunctive treatment is ineffective or not tolerated, a tertiary epilepsy specialist should be consulted who may consider eslicarbazepine acetate p. 329, lacosamide p. 333, phenobarbital p. 353, phenytoin p. 340, pregabalin p. 342, tiagabine p. 348, vigabatrin p. 351 and zonisamide p. 352.

Generalised seizures

Tonic-clonic seizures

Sodium valproate is the first-line treatment for newly diagnosed generalised tonic-clonic seizures (except in female patients who are premenopausal, see *Valproate* below). Lamotrigine is the alternative choice if sodium valproate is not suitable, but may exacerbate myoclonic seizures. In those with established epilepsy with generalised tonic-clonic seizures only, lamotrigine or sodium valproate may be prescribed as the first-line treatment.

Carbamazepine and oxcarbazepine may also be considered in newly diagnosed and established tonic-clonic seizures, but may exacerbate myoclonic and absence seizures. Clobazam, lamotrigine, levetiracetam, sodium valproate or topiramate may be used as adjunctive treatment if monotherapy is ineffective or not tolerated.

Absence seizures

Ethosuximide p. 330, or sodium valproate (except in female patients who are premenopausal, see *Valproate* below), are the drugs of choice in absence seizures and syndromes; lamotrigine is a suitable alternative when ethosuximide and sodium valproate are unsuitable, ineffective or not tolerated. Sodium valproate should be used as the first choice if there is a high risk of generalised tonic-clonic seizures. A combination of any two of these drugs may be used if monotherapy is ineffective. Clobazam, clonazepam p. 355, levetiracetam, topiramate or zonisamide may be considered by a tertiary epilepsy specialist if adjunctive treatment fails. Carbamazepine, gabapentin, oxcarbazepine, phenytoin, pregabalin, tiagabine and vigabatrin are not recommended in absence seizures or syndromes.

Myoclonic seizures

Myoclonic seizures (myoclonic jerks) occur in a variety of syndromes, and response to treatment varies considerably. Sodium valproate is the drug of choice in newly diagnosed myoclonic seizures (except in female patients who are premenopausal, see *Valproate* below); topiramate and levetiracetam are alternative options if sodium valproate is unsuitable but consideration should be given to the less favourable side-effect profile of topiramate. A combination of two of these drugs may be used if monotherapy is ineffective or not tolerated. If adjunctive treatment fails, a tertiary epilepsy specialist should be consulted and may consider clobazam, clonazepam, zonisamide or piracetam p. 427. Carbamazepine, gabapentin, oxcarbazepine, phenytoin, pregabalin, tiagabine and vigabatrin are not recommended for the treatment of myoclonic seizures.

Sodium valproate and levetiracetam are effective in treating the generalised tonic-clonic seizures that coexist with myoclonic seizures in idiopathic generalised epilepsy.

4

Nervous system

Atonic and tonic seizures

Atonic and tonic seizures are usually seen in childhood, in specific epilepsy syndromes, or associated with cerebral damage or mental retardation. They may respond poorly to the traditional drugs. Sodium valproate is the drug of choice (except in female patients who are premenopausal, see *Valproate* below); lamotrigine can be added as adjunctive treatment. If adjunctive treatment is ineffective or not tolerated, a tertiary epilepsy specialist should be consulted, and may consider rufinamide p. 343 or topiramate. Carbamazepine, gabapentin, oxcarbazepine, pregabalin, tiagabine or vigabatrin are not recommended in atonic and tonic seizures.

Epilepsy syndromes

Some drugs are licensed for use in particular epilepsy syndromes. The epilepsy syndromes are specific types of epilepsy that are characterised according to a number of features including seizure type, age of onset, and EEG characteristics. For more information on epilepsy syndromes in children see BNF *for children*.

Dravet syndrome

A tertiary specialist should be involved in decisions regarding treatment of Dravet syndrome. Sodium valproate (except in pregnancy or females of childbearing potential, see *Valproate* below) or topiramate are first-line treatment options in children with Dravet syndrome. Clobazam or stiripentol p. 348 may be considered as adjunctive treatment in children and adults if first-line treatments are ineffective or not tolerated. Carbamazepine, gabapentin, lamotrigine, oxcarbazepine, phenytoin, pregabalin, tiagabine, and vigabatrin should not be used as they may exacerbate myoclonic seizures.

Lennox-Gastaut syndrome

A tertiary specialist should be involved in decisions regarding treatment of Lennox-Gastaut syndrome. Sodium valproate is the first-line drug for treating children with Lennox-Gastaut syndrome (except in pregnancy or females of childbearing potential, see *Valproate* below); lamotrigine can be used as adjunctive treatment in children and adults if sodium valproate is unsuitable, ineffective or not tolerated. If adjunctive treatment is ineffective or not tolerated, rufinamide may be considered by tertiary specialists. Carbamazepine, gabapentin, oxcarbazepine, pregabalin, tiagabine, and vigabatrin should not be used. Felbamate [unlicensed] may be used in tertiary specialist centres when all other treatment options have failed.

Antiepileptic drugs

Carbamazepine and related antiepileptics

Carbamazepine is a drug of choice for simple and complex focal seizures and is a first-line treatment option for generalised tonic-clonic seizures. It can be used as adjunctive treatment for focal seizures when monotherapy has been ineffective. It is essential to initiate carbamazepine therapy at a low dose and build this up slowly. Carbamazepine p. 327 may exacerbate tonic, atonic, myoclonic and absence seizures and is therefore not recommended if these seizures are present.

Oxcarbazepine p. 338 is licensed as monotherapy or adjunctive therapy for the treatment of focal seizures with or without secondary generalised tonic-clonic seizures. It can also be considered for the treatment of primary generalised tonic-clonic seizures [unlicensed]. Oxcarbazepine is not recommended in tonic, atonic, absence or myoclonic seizures due to the risk of seizure exacerbation.

Eslicarbazepine acetate p. 329 is licensed for adjunctive treatment in adults with focal seizures with or without secondary generalisation.

Ethosuximide

Ethosuximide p. 330 is a first-line treatment option for absence seizures. It may also be prescribed as adjunctive treatment for absence seizures when monotherapy is ineffective. Ethosuximide is also licensed for myoclonic seizures.

Gabapentin and pregabalin

Gabapentin p. 332 and pregabalin p. 342 are used for the treatment of focal seizures with or without secondary generalisation. They are not recommended if tonic, atonic, absence or myoclonic seizures are present. Both are also licensed for the treatment of neuropathic pain. Pregabalin is licensed for the treatment of generalised anxiety disorder.

Lamotrigine

Lamotrigine p. 335 is an antiepileptic drug recommended as a first-line treatment for focal seizures and primary and secondary generalised tonic-clonic seizures. It is also licensed for typical absence seizures in children (but efficacy may not be maintained in all children) and is an unlicensed treatment option in adults if first-line treatments have been unsuccessful. Lamotrigine can also be used as adjunctive treatment in atonic or tonic seizures if first-line treatment has failed [unlicensed]. Myoclonic seizures may be exacerbated by lamotrigine and it can cause serious rashes especially in children; dose recommendations should be adhered to closely.

Lamotrigine is used either as sole treatment or as an adjunct to treatment with other antiepileptic drugs. Valproate increases plasma-lamotrigine concentration, whereas the enzyme-inducing antiepileptics reduce it; care is therefore required in choosing the appropriate initial dose and subsequent titration. When the potential for interaction is not known, treatment should be initiated with lower doses, such as those used with valproate.

Levetiracetam and brivaracetam

Levetiracetam p. 337 is used for monotherapy and adjunctive treatment of focal seizures with or without secondary generalisation, and for adjunctive treatment of myoclonic seizures in patients with juvenile myoclonic epilepsy and primary generalised tonic-clonic seizures. Levetiracetam may be prescribed alone and in combination for the treatment of myoclonic seizures, and under specialist supervision for absence seizures [both unlicensed].

Brivaracetam p. 326 is used as adjunctive therapy in the treatment of partial-onset seizures with or without secondary generalisation.

Phenobarbital and primidone

Phenobarbital p. 353 is effective for tonic-clonic and focal seizures but may be sedative in adults. It may be tried for atypical absence, atonic, and tonic seizures. Rebound seizures may be a problem on withdrawal.

Primidone p. 354 is largely converted to phenobarbital and this is probably responsible for its antiepileptic action. A low initial dose of primidone is essential.

Phenytoin

Phenytoin p. 340 is licensed for tonic-clonic and focal seizures but may exacerbate absence or myoclonic seizures and should be avoided if these seizures are present. It has a narrow therapeutic index and the relationship between dose and plasma-drug concentration is non-linear; small dosage increases in some patients may produce large increases in plasma concentration with acute toxic side-effects. Similarly, a few missed doses or a small change in drug absorption may result in a marked change in plasma-drug concentration. Monitoring of plasma-drug concentration improves dosage adjustment.

When only parenteral administration is possible, fosphenytoin sodium p. 331, a pro-drug of phenytoin, may be convenient to give. Unlike phenytoin (which should only be given intravenously), fosphenytoin sodium may also be given by intramuscular injection.

Rufinamide

Rufinamide p. 343 is licensed for the adjunctive treatment of seizures in Lennox-Gastaut syndrome. It may be considered by a tertiary specialist for the treatment of refractory tonic or atonic seizures [unlicensed].

Topiramate

Topiramate p. 349 can be given alone or as adjunctive treatment in generalised tonic-clonic seizures or focal seizures with or without secondary generalisation. It can be used as adjunctive treatment for seizures associated with Lennox-Gastaut syndrome and for absence, tonic and atonic seizures under specialist supervision [unlicensed]. It can also be considered as an option in myoclonic seizures [unlicensed]. Female patients should be fully informed of the risks related to the use of topiramate during pregnancy and the need to use effective contraception—for further information, see *Conception and contraception* and *Pregnancy* in the topiramate drug monograph.

Valproate

Sodium valproate p. 345 is effective in controlling tonic-clonic seizures, particularly in primary generalised epilepsy. It is a drug of choice in primary generalised tonic-clonic seizures, focal seizures, generalised absences and myoclonic seizures, and can be tried in atypical absence seizures. It is recommended as a first-line option in atonic and tonic seizures. Sodium valproate has widespread metabolic effects and monitoring of liver function tests and full blood count is essential. Because of its high teratogenic potential, valproate must not be used in females of childbearing potential unless the conditions of the Pregnancy Prevention Programme are met and alternative treatments are ineffective or not tolerated. During pregnancy, it must not be used for epilepsy unless it is the only possible treatment. For further information see *Important safety information*, *Conception and contraception*, and *Pregnancy* in the sodium valproate and valproic acid p. 373 drug monographs.

Valproic acid (as semisodium valproate) is licensed for acute mania associated with bipolar disorder.

Zonisamide

Zonisamide p. 352 can be used alone for the treatment of focal seizures with or without secondary generalisation in adults with newly diagnosed epilepsy, and as adjunctive treatment for refractory focal seizures with or without secondary generalisation in adults and children aged 6 years and above. It can also be used under the supervision of a specialist for refractory absence and myoclonic seizures [unlicensed indications].

Benzodiazepines

Clobazam p. 355 may be used as adjunctive therapy in the treatment of generalised tonic-clonic and refractory focal seizures. It may be prescribed under the care of a specialist for refractory absence and myoclonic seizures. Clonazepam p. 355 may be prescribed by a specialist for refractory absence and myoclonic seizures, but its sedative side-effects may be prominent.

Other drugs

Acetazolamide p. 1225, a carbonic anhydrase inhibitor, has a specific role in treating epilepsy associated with menstruation. Piracetam p. 427 is used as adjunctive treatment for cortical myoclonus.

Status epilepticus

Convulsive status epilepticus

Immediate measures to manage status epilepticus include positioning the patient to avoid injury, supporting respiration including the provision of oxygen, maintaining blood pressure, and the correction of any hypoglycaemia. Parenteral thiamine p. 1130 should be considered if alcohol abuse is suspected; pyridoxine hydrochloride p. 1130 should be given if the status epilepticus is caused by pyridoxine hydrochloride deficiency.

Seizures lasting longer than 5 minutes should be treated urgently with intravenous lorazepam p. 357 (repeated once after 10 minutes if seizures recur or fail to respond). Intravenous diazepam p. 362 is effective but it carries a high risk of thrombophlebitis (reduced by using an emulsion formulation). Absorption of diazepam from intramuscular injection or from suppositories is too slow for treatment of status epilepticus. Patients should be monitored for respiratory depression and hypotension.

Where facilities for resuscitation are not immediately available, diazepam can be administered as a rectal solution or midazolam oromucosal solution p. 358 can be given into the buccal cavity.

Important

If, after initial treatment with benzodiazepines, seizures recur or fail to respond 25 minutes after onset, phenytoin sodium, fosphenytoin sodium p. 331, or phenobarbital sodium should be used; contact intensive care unit if seizures continue. If these measures fail to control seizures 45 minutes after onset, anaesthesia with thiopental sodium p. 356, midazolam, or a non-barbiturate anaesthetic such as propofol p. 1382 [unlicensed indication], should be instituted with full intensive care support.

Phenytoin sodium can be given by slow intravenous injection, followed by the maintenance dosage if appropriate.

Alternatively, fosphenytoin sodium (a pro-drug of phenytoin), can be given more rapidly and when given intravenously causes fewer injection-site reactions than phenytoin sodium. Although it can also be given intramuscularly, absorption is too slow by this route for treatment of status epilepticus. Doses of fosphenytoin sodium should be expressed in terms of phenytoin sodium.

Non-convulsive status epilepticus

The urgency to treat non-convulsive status epilepticus depends on the severity of the patient's condition. If there is incomplete loss of awareness, usual oral antiepileptic therapy should be continued or restarted. Patients who fail to respond to oral antiepileptic therapy or have complete lack of awareness can be treated in the same way as for convulsive status epilepticus, although anaesthesia is rarely needed.

Febrile convulsions

Brief febrile convulsions need no specific treatment; antipyretic medication (e.g. paracetamol p. 464), is commonly used to reduce fever and prevent further convulsions but evidence to support this practice is lacking. *Prolonged febrile convulsions* (those lasting 5 minutes or longer), or *recurrent febrile convulsions* without recovery must be treated actively (as for convulsive status epilepticus). Long-term anticonvulsant prophylaxis for febrile convulsions is rarely indicated.

> **Other drugs used for Epilepsy and other seizure disorders** Magnesium sulfate, p. 1099

4

Nervous system

ANTIEPILEPTICS

Brivaracetam

13-Nov-2020

● **INDICATIONS AND DOSE**

Adjunctive therapy of focal seizures with or without secondary generalisation

▸ BY MOUTH, OR BY INTRAVENOUS INJECTION, OR BY INTRAVENOUS INFUSION

▸ Adult: Initially 25–50 mg twice daily, adjusted according to response; usual maintenance 25–100 mg twice daily (max. per dose 100 mg twice daily)

IMPORTANT SAFETY INFORMATION

MHRA/CHM ADVICE: ANTIEPILEPTICS: RISK OF SUICIDAL THOUGHTS AND BEHAVIOUR (AUGUST 2008)
See Epilepsy p. 321.

MHRA/CHM ADVICE: ANTIEPILEPTIC DRUGS: UPDATED ADVICE ON SWITCHING BETWEEN DIFFERENT MANUFACTURERS' PRODUCTS (NOVEMBER 2017)
See Epilepsy p. 321.

● INTERACTIONS → Appendix 1: antiepileptics

● SIDE-EFFECTS

▸ **Common or very common** Anxiety · appetite decreased · constipation · cough · depression · dizziness · drowsiness · fatigue · increased risk of infection · insomnia · irritability · nausea · vertigo · vomiting

▸ **Uncommon** Aggression · psychotic disorder

▸ **Frequency not known** Suicidal behaviours

● PREGNANCY Manufacturer advises avoid unless potential benefit outweighs risk—limited information available. See also *Pregnancy* in Epilepsy p. 321.

● BREAST FEEDING Manufacturer advises avoid—present in milk in *animal* studies.

● HEPATIC IMPAIRMENT Manufacturer advises caution (risk of increased exposure).
Dose adjustments Manufacturer advises consider initial dose of 25 mg twice daily; max. maintenance dose of 75 mg twice daily (limited information available).

● TREATMENT CESSATION Manufacturer advises avoid abrupt withdrawal—reduce daily dose in steps of 50 mg at weekly intervals, then reduce to 20 mg daily for a final week.

● DIRECTIONS FOR ADMINISTRATION

▸ With intravenous use For intermittent *intravenous infusion*, manufacturer advises dilute in Glucose 5% *or* Sodium Chloride 0.9% *or* Lactated Ringer's solution; give over 15 minutes.

▸ With oral use Manufacturer advises oral solution can be diluted in water or juice shortly before swallowing.

● PRESCRIBING AND DISPENSING INFORMATION
Manufacturer advises if switching between oral therapy and intravenous therapy (for those temporarily unable to take oral medication), the total daily dose and the frequency of administration should be maintained.

● PATIENT AND CARER ADVICE
Missed doses Manufacturer advises if one or more doses are missed, a single dose should be taken as soon as possible and the next dose should be taken at the usual time.
Driving and skilled tasks Manufacturer advises patients and carers should be cautioned on the effects on driving and performance of skilled tasks—increased risk of dizziness.

● NATIONAL FUNDING/ACCESS DECISIONS
For full details see funding body website
Scottish Medicines Consortium (SMC) decisions

▸ Brivaracetam (*Briviact*®) as adjunctive therapy in the treatment of partial-onset seizures with or without secondary generalisation in adult and adolescent patients from 16 years of age with epilepsy (July 2016) SMC No. 1160/16 Recommended with restrictions

All Wales Medicines Strategy Group (AWMSG) decisions

▸ Brivaracetam (*Briviact*®) as adjunctive therapy in the treatment of partial-onset seizures with or without secondary generalisation in patients from 4 years of age with epilepsy (December 2018) AWMSG No. 3387 Recommended with restrictions

● MEDICINAL FORMS There can be variation in the licensing of different medicines containing the same drug.

Solution for injection
CAUTIONARY AND ADVISORY LABELS 2
ELECTROLYTES: May contain Sodium

▸ Briviact (UCB Pharma Ltd)
Brivaracetam 10 mg per 1 ml Briviact 50mg/5ml solution for injection vials | 10 vial (PoM) £222.75

Oral solution
CAUTIONARY AND ADVISORY LABELS 2, 8
EXCIPIENTS: May contain Sorbitol
ELECTROLYTES: May contain Sodium

▸ Briviact (UCB Pharma Ltd)
Brivaracetam 10 mg per 1 ml Briviact 10mg/ml oral solution sugar-free | 300 ml (PoM) £115.83 DT = £115.83

Tablet
CAUTIONARY AND ADVISORY LABELS 2, 8, 25

▸ Briviact (UCB Pharma Ltd)
Brivaracetam 10 mg Briviact 10mg tablets | 14 tablet (PoM) £34.64 DT = £34.64
Brivaracetam 25 mg Briviact 25mg tablets | 56 tablet (PoM) £129.64 DT = £129.64
Brivaracetam 50 mg Briviact 50mg tablets | 56 tablet (PoM) £129.64 DT = £129.64
Brivaracetam 75 mg Briviact 75mg tablets | 56 tablet (PoM) £129.64 DT = £129.64
Brivaracetam 100 mg Briviact 100mg tablets | 56 tablet (PoM) £129.64 DT = £129.64

Cannabidiol

03-Nov-2020

● **INDICATIONS AND DOSE**

Seizures associated with Lennox-Gastaut syndrome [adjunctive treatment with clobazam] (specialist use only)

▸ BY MOUTH

▸ Adult: Initially 2.5 mg/kg twice daily for 1 week, then increased to 5 mg/kg twice daily, then increased in steps of 2.5 mg/kg twice daily, adjusted according to response, dose to be increased at weekly intervals, food may affect absorption (take at the same time with respect to food); maximum 20 mg/kg per day

Seizures associated with Dravet syndrome [adjunctive treatment with clobazam] (specialist use only)

▸ BY MOUTH

▸ Adult: Initially 2.5 mg/kg twice daily for 1 week, then increased to 5 mg/kg twice daily, then increased in steps of 2.5 mg/kg twice daily, adjusted according to response, dose to be increased at weekly intervals, food may affect absorption (take at the same time with respect to food); maximum 20 mg/kg per day

---

IMPORTANT SAFETY INFORMATION

MHRA/CHM ADVICE: ANTIEPILEPTICS: RISK OF SUICIDAL THOUGHTS AND BEHAVIOUR (AUGUST 2008)
See Epilepsy p. 321.

MHRA/CHM ADVICE: ANTIEPILEPTIC DRUGS: UPDATED ADVICE ON SWITCHING BETWEEN DIFFERENT MANUFACTURERS' PRODUCTS (NOVEMBER 2017)
See Epilepsy p. 321.

● CAUTIONS Elderly

● INTERACTIONS → Appendix 1: cannabidiol

- SIDE-EFFECTS
▶ **Common or very common** Agitation · appetite abnormal · behaviour abnormal · cough · diarrhoea · drooling · drowsiness · fatigue · fever · increased risk of infection · insomnia · irritability · rash · tremor · vomiting · weight decreased
▶ **Frequency not known** Anaemia · seizure · suicidal behaviours

- PREGNANCY Manufacturer advises avoid unless potential benefit outweighs risk—toxicity in *animal* studies.

- BREAST FEEDING Manufacturer advises avoid—limited information available.

- HEPATIC IMPAIRMENT Manufacturer advises caution in moderate to severe impairment (risk of increased exposure).
Dose adjustments Manufacturer advises dose reduction in moderate to severe impairment—consult product literature.

- MONITORING REQUIREMENTS Manufacturer advises monitor liver function at baseline, at 1 month, 3 months, and 6 months of treatment, then periodically thereafter; more frequent monitoring is recommended in patients with raised baseline ALT or AST or taking valproate. Restart monitoring schedule if dose increased above 10 mg/kg/day. If transaminase or bilirubin levels increase significantly or symptoms of hepatic dysfunction occur, treatment should be withheld or permanently discontinued based on severity—consult product literature.

- TREATMENT CESSATION Manufacturer advises avoid abrupt withdrawal—withdraw treatment gradually.

- PATIENT AND CARER ADVICE
Missed doses Manufacturer advises if more than 7 doses are missed, dose titration should be re-started.
Driving and skilled tasks Manufacturer advises patients and carers should be counselled on the effects on driving and performance of skilled tasks—increased risk of somnolence and sedation. Effects of alcohol increased.
   For information on 2015 legislation regarding driving whilst taking certain controlled drugs, including cannabis, see Drugs and driving under Guidance on prescribing p. 1.

- NATIONAL FUNDING/ACCESS DECISIONS
For full details see funding body website
NICE decisions
▶ Cannabidiol with clobazam for treating seizures associated with Dravet syndrome (December 2019) NICE TA614 Recommended with restrictions
▶ Cannabidiol with clobazam for treating seizures associated with Lennox–Gastaut syndrome (December 2019) NICE TA615 Recommended with restrictions
Scottish Medicines Consortium (SMC) decisions
▶ Cannabidiol (*Epidyolex*®) as adjunctive therapy of seizures associated with Dravet syndrome (DS) in conjunction with clobazam, for patients 2 years of age and older (September 2020) SMC No. SMC2262 Recommended
▶ Cannabidiol (*Epidyolex*®) as adjunctive therapy of seizures associated with Lennox-Gastaut syndrome (LGS) in conjunction with clobazam, for patients 2 years of age and older (September 2020) SMC No. SMC2263 Recommended

- MEDICINAL FORMS There can be variation in the licensing of different medicines containing the same drug. Forms available from special-order manufacturers include: oral solution
Oral solution
CAUTIONARY AND ADVISORY LABELS 2, 8
EXCIPIENTS: May contain Ethanol, sesame oil
▶ Epidyolex (GW Pharma Ltd)
   Cannabidiol 100 mg per 1 ml Epidyolex 100mg/ml oral solution sugar-free | 100 ml PoM ▣ CD5

Carbamazepine   07-Dec-2020

- INDICATIONS AND DOSE
Focal and secondary generalised tonic-clonic seizures |
Primary generalised tonic-clonic seizures
▶ BY MOUTH USING IMMEDIATE-RELEASE MEDICINES
▶ Adult: Initially 100–200 mg 1–2 times a day, increased in steps of 100–200 mg every 2 weeks; usual dose 0.8–1.2 g daily in divided doses; increased if necessary up to 1.6–2 g daily in divided doses
▶ Elderly: Reduce initial dose
▶ BY RECTUM
▶ Adult: Up to 1 g daily in 4 divided doses for up to 7 days, for short-term use when oral therapy temporarily not possible

Trigeminal neuralgia
▶ BY MOUTH USING IMMEDIATE-RELEASE MEDICINES
▶ Adult: Initially 100 mg 1–2 times a day, some patients may require higher initial dose, increase gradually according to response; usual dose 200 mg 3–4 times a day, increased if necessary up to 1.6 g daily

Prophylaxis of bipolar disorder unresponsive to lithium
▶ BY MOUTH USING IMMEDIATE-RELEASE MEDICINES
▶ Adult: Initially 400 mg daily in divided doses, increased until symptoms controlled; usual dose 400–600 mg daily; maximum 1.6 g per day

Adjunct in acute alcohol withdrawal
▶ BY MOUTH USING IMMEDIATE-RELEASE MEDICINES
▶ Adult: Initially 800 mg daily in divided doses, then reduced to 200 mg daily for usual treatment duration of 7–10 days, dose to be reduced gradually over 5 days

Diabetic neuropathy
▶ BY MOUTH USING IMMEDIATE-RELEASE MEDICINES
▶ Adult: Initially 100 mg 1–2 times a day, increased gradually according to response; usual dose 200 mg 3–4 times a day, increased if necessary up to 1.6 g daily

Focal and generalised tonic-clonic seizures
▶ BY MOUTH USING IMMEDIATE-RELEASE MEDICINES
▶ Child 1 month-11 years: Initially 5 mg/kg once daily, dose to be taken at night, alternatively initially 2.5 mg/kg twice daily, then increased in steps of 2.5–5 mg/kg every 3–7 days as required; maintenance 5 mg/kg 2–3 times a day, increased if necessary up to 20 mg/kg daily
▶ Child 12–17 years: Initially 100–200 mg 1–2 times a day, then increased to 200–400 mg 2–3 times a day, increased if necessary up to 1.8 g daily, dose should be increased slowly

DOSE EQUIVALENCE AND CONVERSION
▶ Suppositories of 125 mg may be considered to be approximately equivalent in therapeutic effect to tablets of 100 mg but final adjustment should always depend on clinical response (plasma concentration monitoring recommended).

CARBAGEN ® SR
Focal and secondary generalised tonic-clonic seizures |
Primary generalised tonic-clonic seizures
▶ BY MOUTH
▶ Adult: Initially 100–400 mg daily in 1–2 divided doses, increased in steps of 100–200 mg every 2 weeks, dose should be increased slowly; usual dose 0.8–1.2 g daily in 1–2 divided doses, increased if necessary up to 1.6–2 g daily in 1–2 divided doses
▶ Elderly: Reduce initial dose

Trigeminal neuralgia
▶ BY MOUTH
▶ Adult: Initially 100–200 mg daily in 1–2 divided doses, some patients may require higher initial dose, increase gradually according to response; usual dose   continued →

4

Nervous system

600–800 mg daily in 1–2 divided doses, increased if necessary up to 1.6 g daily in 1–2 divided doses

Prophylaxis of bipolar disorder unresponsive to lithium
▶ BY MOUTH
▸ Adult: Initially 400 mg daily in 1–2 divided doses, increased until symptoms controlled; usual dose 400–600 mg daily in 1–2 divided doses; maximum 1.6 g per day

Focal and generalised tonic-clonic seizures | Prophylaxis of bipolar disorder
▶ BY MOUTH
▸ Child 5–11 years: Initially 5 mg/kg daily in 1–2 divided doses, then increased in steps of 2.5–5 mg/kg every 3–7 days as required, dose should be increased slowly; maintenance 10–15 mg/kg daily in 1–2 divided doses, increased if necessary up to 20 mg/kg daily in 1–2 divided doses
▸ Child 12–17 years: Initially 100–400 mg daily in 1–2 divided doses, then increased to 400–1200 mg daily in 1–2 divided doses, increased if necessary up to 1.8 g daily in 1–2 divided doses, dose should be increased slowly

TEGRETOL ® PROLONGED RELEASE

Focal and secondary generalised tonic-clonic seizures | Primary generalised tonic-clonic seizures
▶ BY MOUTH
▸ Adult: Initially 100–400 mg daily in 2 divided doses, increased in steps of 100–200 mg every 2 weeks, dose should be increased slowly; usual dose 0.8–1.2 g daily in 2 divided doses, increased if necessary up to 1.6–2 g daily in 2 divided doses
▸ Elderly: Reduce initial dose

Focal and generalised tonic-clonic seizures | Prophylaxis of bipolar disorder
▶ BY MOUTH
▸ Child 5–11 years: Initially 5 mg/kg daily in 2 divided doses, then increased in steps of 2.5–5 mg/kg every 3–7 days as required; maintenance 10–15 mg/kg daily in 2 divided doses, increased if necessary up to 20 mg/kg daily in 2 divided doses
▸ Child 12–17 years: Initially 100–400 mg daily in 2 divided doses, dose should be increased slowly; maintenance 400–1200 mg daily in 2 divided doses, increased if necessary up to 1.8 g daily in 2 divided doses

Trigeminal neuralgia
▶ BY MOUTH
▸ Adult: Initially 100–200 mg daily in 2 divided doses, some patients may require higher initial dose. After initial dose, increase according to response; usual dose 600–800 mg daily in 2 divided doses, increased if necessary up to 1.6 g daily in 2 divided doses, dose should be increased slowly

Prophylaxis of bipolar disorder unresponsive to lithium
▶ BY MOUTH
▸ Adult: Initially 400 mg daily in 2 divided doses, increased until symptoms controlled; usual dose 400–600 mg daily in 2 divided doses; maximum 1.6 g per day

● UNLICENSED USE
▸ In children Not licensed for use in trigeminal neuralgia or prophylaxis of bipolar disorder.
▸ In adults Not licensed for use in acute alcohol withdrawal. Use in diabetic neuropathy is an unlicensed indication.

⎡ **IMPORTANT SAFETY INFORMATION**
MHRA/CHM ADVICE: ANTIEPILEPTICS: RISK OF SUICIDAL THOUGHTS AND BEHAVIOUR (AUGUST 2008)
See Epilepsy p. 321.

MHRA/CHM ADVICE: ANTIEPILEPTIC DRUGS: UPDATED ADVICE ON SWITCHING BETWEEN DIFFERENT MANUFACTURERS' PRODUCTS (NOVEMBER 2017)
See Epilepsy p. 321 and see also *Prescribing and dispensing information.*

● CONTRA-INDICATIONS Acute porphyrias p. 1107 · AV conduction abnormalities (unless paced) · history of bone-marrow depression
● CAUTIONS Cardiac disease · history of haematological reactions to other drugs · may exacerbate absence and myoclonic seizures · skin reactions · susceptibility to angle-closure glaucoma
CAUTIONS, FURTHER INFORMATION Consider vitamin D supplementation in patients who are immobilised for long periods or who have inadequate sun exposure or dietary intake of calcium.
▸ Blood, hepatic, or skin disorders Carbamazepine should be withdrawn immediately in cases of aggravated liver dysfunction or acute liver disease. Leucopenia that is severe, progressive, or associated with clinical symptoms requires withdrawal (if necessary under cover of a suitable alternative).
● INTERACTIONS → Appendix 1: antiepileptics
● SIDE-EFFECTS
▸ **Common or very common** Dizziness · drowsiness · dry mouth · eosinophilia · fatigue · fluid imbalance · gastrointestinal discomfort · headache · hyponatraemia · leucopenia · movement disorders · nausea · oedema · skin reactions · thrombocytopenia · vision disorders · vomiting · weight increased
▸ **Uncommon** Constipation · diarrhoea · eye disorders · tic · tremor
▸ **Rare or very rare** Aggression · agranulocytosis · albuminuria · alopecia · anaemia · angioedema · anxiety · appetite decreased · arrhythmias · arthralgia · azotaemia · bone disorders · bone marrow disorders · cardiac conduction disorders · circulatory collapse · confusion · congestive heart failure · conjunctivitis · coronary artery disease aggravated · depression · dyspnoea · embolism and thrombosis · erythema nodosum · fever · folate deficiency · galactorrhoea · gynaecomastia · haematuria · haemolytic anaemia · hallucinations · hearing impairment · hepatic disorders · hirsutism · hyperacusia · hyperhidrosis · hypersensitivity · hypertension · hypogammaglobulinaemia · hypotension · lens opacity · leucocytosis · lymphadenopathy · meningitis aseptic · muscle complaints · muscle weakness · nephritis tubulointerstitial · nervous system disorder · neuroleptic malignant syndrome · oral disorders · pancreatitis · paraesthesia · paresis · peripheral neuropathy · photosensitivity reaction · pneumonia · pneumonitis · pseudolymphoma · psychosis · red blood cell abnormalities · renal impairment · severe cutaneous adverse reactions (SCARs) · sexual dysfunction · speech impairment · spermatogenesis abnormal · syncope · systemic lupus erythematosus (SLE) · taste altered · tinnitus · urinary disorders · vanishing bile duct syndrome · vasculitis
▸ **Frequency not known** Bone fracture · colitis · human herpesvirus 6 infection reactivation · memory loss · nail loss · suicidal behaviours
SIDE-EFFECTS, FURTHER INFORMATION Some side-effects (such as headache, ataxia, drowsiness, nausea, vomiting, blurring of vision, dizziness and allergic skin reactions) are dose-related, and may be dose-limiting. These side-effects are more common at the start of treatment and in the elderly.
Overdose For details on the management of poisoning, see Active elimination techniques, under Emergency treatment of poisoning p. 1413.

- **ALLERGY AND CROSS-SENSITIVITY** Antiepileptic hypersensitivity syndrome associated with carbamazepine. See under Epilepsy p. 321 for more information. EvGr Caution—cross-sensitivity reported with oxcarbazepine, phenytoin, primidone, and phenobarbital. ⟨M⟩
- **PREGNANCY** See *Pregnancy* in Epilepsy p. 321.
  Monitoring Doses should be adjusted on the basis of plasma-drug concentration monitoring.
- **BREAST FEEDING** Amount probably too small to be harmful.
  Monitoring Monitor infant for possible adverse reactions.
- **HEPATIC IMPAIRMENT** Manufacturer advises caution and close monitoring—no information available.
- **RENAL IMPAIRMENT** Use with caution.
- **PRE-TREATMENT SCREENING** Test for HLA-B*1502 allele in individuals of Han Chinese or Thai origin (avoid unless no alternative—risk of Stevens-Johnson syndrome in presence of HLA-B*1502 allele).
- **MONITORING REQUIREMENTS**
- ▸ Plasma concentration for optimum response 4–12 mg/litre (20–50 micromol/litre) measured after 1–2 weeks.
- ▸ Manufacturer recommends blood counts and hepatic and renal function tests (but evidence of practical value uncertain).
- **TREATMENT CESSATION** When stopping treatment with carbamazepine for bipolar disorder, reduce the dose gradually over a period of at least 4 weeks.
- **DIRECTIONS FOR ADMINISTRATION**
- ▸ In children Expert sources advise oral liquid has been used rectally—should be retained for at least 2 hours (but may have laxative effect).
  TEGRETOL® PROLONGED RELEASE Manufacturer advises *Tegretol® Prolonged Release* tablets can be halved but should not be chewed.
- **PRESCRIBING AND DISPENSING INFORMATION** Switching between formulations Different formulations of oral preparations may vary in bioavailability. Patients being treated for epilepsy should be maintained on a specific manufacturer's product.
- **PATIENT AND CARER ADVICE** Blood, hepatic, or skin disorders Patients or their carers should be told how to recognise signs of blood, liver, or skin disorders, and advised to seek immediate medical attention if symptoms such as fever, rash, mouth ulcers, bruising, or bleeding develop.
  Medicines for Children leaflet: Carbamazepine (oral) for preventing seizures www.medicinesforchildren.org.uk/carbamazepine-oral-preventing-seizures-0
- **PROFESSION SPECIFIC INFORMATION**
  Dental practitioners' formulary
  Carbamazepine Tablets may be prescribed.
- **MEDICINAL FORMS** There can be variation in the licensing of different medicines containing the same drug. Forms available from special-order manufacturers include: oral suspension, oral solution

Modified-release tablet
CAUTIONARY AND ADVISORY LABELS 3, 8, 25
- ▸ Tegretol Retard (Novartis Pharmaceuticals UK Ltd)
  Carbamazepine 200 mg Tegretol Prolonged Release 200mg tablets | 56 tablet [PoM] £5.20 DT = £5.20
  Carbamazepine 400 mg Tegretol Prolonged Release 400mg tablets | 56 tablet [PoM] £10.24 DT = £10.24

Tablet
CAUTIONARY AND ADVISORY LABELS 3, 8
- ▸ Carbamazepine (Non-proprietary)
  Carbamazepine 100 mg Carbamazepine 100mg tablets | 84 tablet [PoM] £2.07 DT = £2.07
  Carbamazepine 200 mg Carbamazepine 200mg tablets | 84 tablet [PoM] £3.83 DT = £3.83

Carbamazepine 400 mg Carbamazepine 400mg tablets | 56 tablet [PoM] £5.02 DT = £5.02
- ▸ Tegretol (Novartis Pharmaceuticals UK Ltd)
  Carbamazepine 100 mg Tegretol 100mg tablets | 84 tablet [PoM] £2.07 DT = £2.07
  Carbamazepine 200 mg Tegretol 200mg tablets | 84 tablet [PoM] £3.83 DT = £3.83
  Carbamazepine 400 mg Tegretol 400mg tablets | 56 tablet [PoM] £5.02 DT = £5.02

Suppository
CAUTIONARY AND ADVISORY LABELS 3, 8
- ▸ Carbamazepine (Non-proprietary)
  Carbamazepine 125 mg Carbamazepine 125mg suppositories | 5 suppository [PoM] £120.00 DT = £120.00
  Carbamazepine 250 mg Carbamazepine 250mg suppositories | 5 suppository [PoM] £140.00 DT = £140.00

Oral suspension
CAUTIONARY AND ADVISORY LABELS 3, 8
- ▸ Carbamazepine (Non-proprietary)
  Carbamazepine 20 mg per 1 ml Carbamazepine 100mg/5ml oral suspension sugar free sugar-free | 300 ml [PoM] £9.30 DT = £9.06
- ▸ Tegretol (Novartis Pharmaceuticals UK Ltd)
  Carbamazepine 20 mg per 1 ml Tegretol 100mg/5ml liquid sugar-free | 300 ml [PoM] £6.12 DT = £9.06

Eslicarbazepine acetate
10-Dec-2020

- **INDICATIONS AND DOSE**

Monotherapy of focal seizures with or without secondary generalisation
- ▸ BY MOUTH
- ▸ Adult: Initially 400 mg once daily for 1–2 weeks, then increased to 800 mg once daily, then increased if necessary to 1.2 g once daily (max. per dose 1.6 g)
- ▸ Elderly: Initially 400 mg once daily for 1–2 weeks, then increased to 800 mg once daily (max. per dose 1.2 g)

Adjunctive therapy of focal seizures with or without secondary generalisation
- ▸ BY MOUTH
- ▸ Adult: Initially 400 mg once daily for 1–2 weeks, then increased to 800 mg once daily (max. per dose 1.2 g)

IMPORTANT SAFETY INFORMATION

MHRA/CHM ADVICE: ANTIEPILEPTICS: RISK OF SUICIDAL THOUGHTS AND BEHAVIOUR (AUGUST 2008)
See Epilepsy p. 321.

MHRA/CHM ADVICE: ANTIEPILEPTIC DRUGS: UPDATED ADVICE ON SWITCHING BETWEEN DIFFERENT MANUFACTURERS' PRODUCTS (NOVEMBER 2017)
See Epilepsy p. 321 and see also *Prescribing and dispensing information.*

- **CONTRA-INDICATIONS** Second- or third-degree AV block
- **CAUTIONS** Hyponatraemia · PR-interval prolongation
- **INTERACTIONS** → Appendix 1: antiepileptics
- **SIDE-EFFECTS**
- ▸ **Common or very common** Appetite decreased · asthenia · concentration impaired · diarrhoea · dizziness · drowsiness · electrolyte imbalance · gait abnormal · headaches · movement disorders · nausea · skin reactions · sleep disorders · vertigo · vision disorders · vomiting
- ▸ **Uncommon** Alopecia · anaemia · anxiety · bradycardia · chest pain · chills · confusion · constipation · depression · dry mouth · eye disorders · flushing · gastritis · gastrointestinal discomfort · haemorrhage · hearing impairment · hyperhidrosis · hypertension · hypotension · hypothyroidism · increased risk of infection · liver disorder · malaise · mood altered · muscle weakness · myalgia · pain in extremity · palpitations · peripheral coldness · peripheral neuropathy · peripheral oedema · psychomotor retardation · psychotic disorder · sensation abnormal · speech impairment · tinnitus · toothache · weight decreased

4

Nervous system

▸ **Frequency not known** Angioedema · leucopenia · pancreatitis · severe cutaneous adverse reactions (SCARs) · suicidal behaviours · thrombocytopenia

● ALLERGY AND CROSS-SENSITIVITY Antiepileptic hypersensitivity syndrome theoretically associated with eslicarbazepine. See under Epilepsy p. 321 for more information.

● PREGNANCY Manufacturer advises minimum effective doses and monotherapy if possible—reproductive toxicity in *animal* studies.
Monitoring The dose should be monitored carefully during pregnancy and after birth, and adjustments made on a clinical basis.

● BREAST FEEDING Manufacturer advises avoid—present in milk in *animal* studies.

● HEPATIC IMPAIRMENT Manufacturer advises caution in mild to moderate impairment—limited information; avoid in severe impairment—no information available.

● RENAL IMPAIRMENT Manufacturer advises avoid if creatinine creatinine clearance less than 30 mL/minute.
Dose adjustments Manufacturer advises reduce initial dose to 200 mg once daily or 400 mg every other day for 2 weeks, then increase to 400 mg once daily if creatinine clearance 30–60 mL/minute. The dose may be further increased based on individual response.

● PRE-TREATMENT SCREENING Test for HLA-B*1502 allele in individuals of Han Chinese or Thai origin (avoid unless no alternative— risk of Stevens-Johnson syndrome in presence of HLA-B*1502 allele).

● MONITORING REQUIREMENTS Monitor plasma-sodium concentration in patients at risk of hyponatraemia and discontinue treatment if hyponatraemia occurs.

● PRESCRIBING AND DISPENSING INFORMATION
Switching between formulations Care should be taken when switching between oral formulations. The need for continued supply of a particular manufacturer's product should be based on clinical judgement and consultation with the patient or their carer, taking into account factors such as seizure frequency and treatment history.

● PATIENT AND CARER ADVICE
Driving and skilled tasks Manufacturer advises patients and carers should be cautioned on the effects on driving and performance of skilled tasks—increased risk of dizziness, somnolence and visual disorders.

● NATIONAL FUNDING/ACCESS DECISIONS
For full details see funding body website
Scottish Medicines Consortium (SMC) decisions
▸ Eslicarbazepine acetate (*Zebinix*®) for the treatment of adjunctive therapy in adults with partial-onset seizures with or without secondary generalisation (November 2010) SMC No. 592/09 Recommended with restrictions
All Wales Medicines Strategy Group (AWMSG) decisions
▸ Eslicarbazepine acetate (*Zebinix*®) as adjunctive therapy in adults, adolescents and children aged above six years, with partial-onset seizures with or without secondary generalisation (June 2019) AWMSG No. 1214 Recommended with restrictions

● MEDICINAL FORMS There can be variation in the licensing of different medicines containing the same drug.
Oral suspension
CAUTIONARY AND ADVISORY LABELS 8
▸ Zebinix (Eisai Ltd)
Eslicarbazepine acetate 50 mg per 1 ml Zebinix 50mg/1ml oral suspension sugar-free | 200 ml PoM £56.67 DT = £56.67
Tablet
CAUTIONARY AND ADVISORY LABELS 8
▸ Zebinix (Eisai Ltd)
Eslicarbazepine acetate 200 mg Zebinix 200mg tablets | 60 tablet PoM £68.00 DT = £68.00

Eslicarbazepine acetate 800 mg Zebinix 800mg tablets | 30 tablet PoM £136.00 DT = £136.00

Ethosuximide

10-Dec-2020

● **INDICATIONS AND DOSE**

Absence seizures | Atypical absence seizures (adjunct) | Myoclonic seizures

▸ BY MOUTH

▸ **Child 1 month-5 years:** Initially 5 mg/kg twice daily (max. per dose 125 mg), dose to be increased every 5–7 days; maintenance 10–20 mg/kg twice daily (max. per dose 500 mg), total daily dose may rarely be given in 3 divided doses

▸ **Child 6-17 years:** Initially 250 mg twice daily, then increased in steps of 250 mg every 5–7 days; usual dose 500–750 mg twice daily, increased if necessary up to 1 g twice daily

▸ **Adult:** Initially 500 mg daily in 2 divided doses, then increased in steps of 250 mg every 5–7 days; usual dose 1–1.5 g daily in 2 divided doses, increased if necessary up to 2 g daily

---

IMPORTANT SAFETY INFORMATION

MHRA/CHM ADVICE: ANTIEPILEPTICS: RISK OF SUICIDAL THOUGHTS AND BEHAVIOUR (AUGUST 2008)
See Epilepsy p. 321.

MHRA/CHM ADVICE: ANTIEPILEPTIC DRUGS: UPDATED ADVICE ON SWITCHING BETWEEN DIFFERENT MANUFACTURERS' PRODUCTS (NOVEMBER 2017)
See Epilepsy p. 321.

● CAUTIONS Avoid in Acute porphyrias p. 1107

● INTERACTIONS → Appendix 1: antiepileptics

● SIDE-EFFECTS Aggression · agranulocytosis · appetite decreased · blood disorder · bone marrow disorders · concentration impaired · depression · diarrhoea · dizziness · drowsiness · erythema nodosum · fatigue · gastrointestinal discomfort · generalised tonic-clonic seizure · headache · hiccups · leucopenia · libido increased · lupus-like syndrome · mood altered · movement disorders · nausea · nephrotic syndrome · oral disorders · psychosis · rash · sleep disorders · Stevens-Johnson syndrome · suicidal behaviours · vaginal haemorrhage · vision disorders · vomiting · weight decreased

SIDE-EFFECTS, FURTHER INFORMATION Blood counts required if features of fever, sore throat, mouth ulcers, bruising or bleeding.

● PREGNANCY See also *Pregnancy* in Epilepsy p. 321.
Monitoring The dose should be monitored carefully during pregnancy and after birth, and adjustments made on a clinical basis.

● BREAST FEEDING Present in milk. Hyperexcitability and sedation reported.

● HEPATIC IMPAIRMENT Use with caution.

● RENAL IMPAIRMENT Use with caution.

● PATIENT AND CARER ADVICE
Blood disorders Patients or their carers should be told how to recognise signs of blood disorders, and advised to seek immediate medical attention if symptoms such as fever, mouth ulcers, bruising, or bleeding develop.
Medicines for Children leaflet: Ethosuximide for preventing seizures www.medicinesforchildren.org.uk/ethosuximide-preventing-seizures

- MEDICINAL FORMS There can be variation in the licensing of different medicines containing the same drug.

Oral solution
CAUTIONARY AND ADVISORY LABELS 8
- ▸ Ethosuximide (Non-proprietary)
 Ethosuximide 50 mg per 1 ml Ethosuximide 250mg/5ml syrup | 200 ml [PoM] £173.00 DT = £173.00
 Ethosuximide 250mg/5ml oral solution sugar free sugar-free | 125 ml [PoM] £86.50–£108.13 sugar-free | 200 ml [PoM] £173.00–£212.36 sugar-free | 250 ml [PoM] £216.25 DT = £216.25

Capsule
CAUTIONARY AND ADVISORY LABELS 8
- ▸ Ethosuximide (Non-proprietary)
 Ethosuximide 250 mg Ethosuximide 250mg capsules | 56 capsule [PoM] £191.00 DT = £190.97

Fosphenytoin sodium   10-Dec-2020

- DRUG ACTION Fosphenytoin is a pro-drug of phenytoin.

● INDICATIONS AND DOSE

Status epilepticus
- ▸ BY INTRAVENOUS INFUSION
- ▸ Adult: Initially 20 mg(PE)/kg, dose to be administered at a rate of 100–150 mg(PE)/minute, then 4–5 mg (PE)/kg daily in 1–2 divided doses, dose to be administered at a rate of 50–100 mg(PE)/minute, dose to be adjusted according to response and trough plasma-phenytoin concentration
- ▸ Elderly: Consider 10–25% reduction in dose or infusion rate

Prophylaxis or treatment of seizures associated with neurosurgery or head injury
- ▸ BY INTRAMUSCULAR INJECTION, OR BY INTRAVENOUS INFUSION
- ▸ Adult: Initially 10–15 mg(PE)/kg, intravenous infusion to be administered at a rate of 50–100 mg(PE)/minute, then 4–5 mg(PE)/kg daily in 1–2 divided doses, intravenous infusion to be administered at a rate of 50–100 mg(PE)/minute, dose to be adjusted according to response and trough plasma-phenytoin concentration
- ▸ Elderly: Consider 10–25% reduction in dose or infusion rate

Temporary substitution for oral phenytoin
- ▸ BY INTRAMUSCULAR INJECTION, OR BY INTRAVENOUS INFUSION
- ▸ Adult: Same dose and same dosing frequency as oral phenytoin therapy, intravenous infusion to be administered at a rate of 50–100 mg(PE)/minute
- ▸ Elderly: Consider 10–25% reduction in dose or infusion rate

DOSE EQUIVALENCE AND CONVERSION
- ▸ Doses are expressed as phenytoin sodium equivalent (PE); fosphenytoin sodium 1.5 mg ≡ phenytoin sodium 1 mg.

- UNLICENSED USE Fosphenytoin sodium doses in BNF may differ from those in product literature.

> IMPORTANT SAFETY INFORMATION
> MHRA/CHM ADVICE: ANTIEPILEPTICS: RISK OF SUICIDAL THOUGHTS AND BEHAVIOUR (AUGUST 2008)
> **See Epilepsy p. 321.**
> MHRA/CHM ADVICE: ANTIEPILEPTIC DRUGS: UPDATED ADVICE ON SWITCHING BETWEEN DIFFERENT MANUFACTURERS' PRODUCTS (NOVEMBER 2017)
> **See Epilepsy p. 321.**

- CONTRA-INDICATIONS Acute porphyrias p. 1107 · second-degree heart block · sino-atrial block · sinus bradycardia · Stokes-Adams syndrome · third-degree heart block

- CAUTIONS Heart failure · hypotension · injection solutions alkaline (irritant to tissues) · respiratory depression · resuscitation facilities must be available

- INTERACTIONS → Appendix 1: antiepileptics

- SIDE-EFFECTS
- ▸ **Common or very common** Asthenia · chills · dizziness · drowsiness · dry mouth · dysarthria · euphoric mood · headache · hypotension · movement disorders · nausea · nystagmus · sensation abnormal · skin reactions · stupor · taste altered · tinnitus · tremor · vasodilation · vertigo · vision disorders · vomiting
- ▸ **Uncommon** Cardiac arrest · confusion · hearing impairment · muscle complaints · muscle weakness · nervousness · oral disorders · reflexes abnormal · severe cutaneous adverse reactions (SCARs) · systemic lupus erythematosus (SLE) · thinking abnormal
- ▸ **Frequency not known** Acute psychosis · agranulocytosis · appetite disorder · atrial conduction depression (more common if injection too rapid) · atrioventricular block · bone disorders · bone fracture · bone marrow disorders · bradycardia · cardiotoxicity · cerebrovascular insufficiency · circulatory collapse (more common if injection too rapid) · coarsening of the facial features · constipation · delirium · Dupuytren's contracture · encephalopathy · granulocytopenia · groin tingling · hair changes · hepatic disorders · hyperglycaemia · hypersensitivity · insomnia · leucopenia · lymphadenopathy · nephritis tubulointerstitial · Peyronie's disease · polyarteritis nodosa · polyarthritis · purple glove syndrome · respiratory disorders · sensory peripheral polyneuropathy · suicidal behaviours · thrombocytopenia · tonic seizure · ventricular conduction depression (more common if injection too rapid) · ventricular fibrillation (more common if injection too rapid)

 SIDE-EFFECTS, FURTHER INFORMATION Fosphenytoin has been associated with severe cardiovascular reactions including asystole, ventricular fibrillation, and cardiac arrest. Hypotension, bradycardia, and heart block have also been reported. The following are recommended: monitor heart rate, blood pressure, and respiratory function for duration of infusion; observe patient for at least 30 minutes after infusion; if hypotension occurs, reduce infusion rate or discontinue; reduce dose or infusion rate in elderly, and in renal or hepatic impairment.

- ALLERGY AND CROSS-SENSITIVITY Cross-sensitivity reported with carbamazepine.

- PREGNANCY See also *Pregnancy* in Epilepsy p. 321.
 Monitoring Changes in plasma-protein binding make interpretation of plasma-phenytoin concentrations difficult—monitor unbound fraction.
 The dose should be monitored carefully during pregnancy and after birth, and adjustments made on a clinical basis.

- BREAST FEEDING Small amounts present in milk, but not known to be harmful.

- HEPATIC IMPAIRMENT Manufacturer advises caution—monitor free plasma-phenytoin concentration (rather than total plasma-phenytoin concentration) in hepatic impairment or hypoalbuminaemia and in hyperbilirubinaemia.
 Dose adjustments Manufacturer advises consider a 10–25% reduction in dose or infusion rate (except in the treatment of status epilepticus) in hepatic impairment or hypoalbuminaemia.

- RENAL IMPAIRMENT
 Dose adjustments Consider 10–25% reduction in dose or infusion rate (except initial dose for status epilepticus).

- PRE-TREATMENT SCREENING HLA-B* 1502 allele in individuals of Han Chinese or Thai origin—avoid unless essential (increased risk of Stevens-Johnson syndrome).

4

Nervous system

4

Nervous system

- MONITORING REQUIREMENTS
- ▶ Manufacturer recommends blood counts (but evidence of practical value uncertain).
- ▶ With intravenous use Monitor heart rate, blood pressure, ECG, and respiratory function for during infusion.
- DIRECTIONS FOR ADMINISTRATION For *intermittent intravenous infusion* (*Pro-Epanutin®*), manufacturer advises give *in* Glucose 5% *or* Sodium chloride 0.9%; dilute to a concentration of 1.5–25 mg (phenytoin sodium equivalent (PE))/mL.
- PRESCRIBING AND DISPENSING INFORMATION
  Prescriptions for fosphenytoin sodium should state the dose in terms of phenytoin sodium equivalent (PE); fosphenytoin sodium 1.5 mg ≡ phenytoin sodium 1 mg.

- MEDICINAL FORMS There can be variation in the licensing of different medicines containing the same drug.
  Solution for injection
  ELECTROLYTES: May contain Phosphate
  - ▶ Pro-Epanutin (Pfizer Ltd)
    Fosphenytoin sodium 75 mg per 1 ml Pro-Epanutin 750mg/10ml concentrate for solution for injection vials | 10 vial [PoM] £400.00 (Hospital only)

Gabapentin

07-Oct-2020

- INDICATIONS AND DOSE

Adjunctive treatment of focal seizures with or without secondary generalisation
- ▶ BY MOUTH
  - ▶ Child 6–11 years: 10 mg/kg once daily (max. per dose 300 mg) on day 1, then 10 mg/kg twice daily (max. per dose 300 mg) on day 2, then 10 mg/kg 3 times a day (max. per dose 300 mg) on day 3; usual dose 25–35 mg/kg daily in 3 divided doses, some children may not tolerate daily increments; longer intervals (up to weekly) may be more appropriate, daily dose maximum to be given in 3 divided doses; maximum 70 mg/kg per day
  - ▶ Child 12–17 years: Initially 300 mg once daily on day 1, then 300 mg twice daily on day 2, then 300 mg 3 times a day on day 3, alternatively initially 300 mg 3 times a day on day 1, then increased in steps of 300 mg every 2–3 days in 3 divided doses, adjusted according to response; usual dose 0.9–3.6 g daily in 3 divided doses (max. per dose 1.6 g 3 times a day), some children may not tolerate daily increments; longer intervals (up to weekly) may be more appropriate
  - ▶ Adult: Initially 300 mg once daily on day 1, then 300 mg twice daily on day 2, then 300 mg 3 times a day on day 3, alternatively initially 300 mg 3 times a day on day 1, then increased in steps of 300 mg every 2–3 days in 3 divided doses, adjusted according to response; usual dose 0.9–3.6 g daily in 3 divided doses (max. per dose 1.6 g 3 times a day)

Monotherapy for focal seizures with or without secondary generalisation
- ▶ BY MOUTH
  - ▶ Child 12–17 years: Initially 300 mg once daily on day 1, then 300 mg twice daily on day 2, then 300 mg 3 times a day on day 3, alternatively initially 300 mg 3 times a day on day 1, then increased in steps of 300 mg every 2–3 days in 3 divided doses, adjusted according to response; usual dose 0.9–3.6 g daily in 3 divided doses (max. per dose 1.6 g 3 times a day), some children may not tolerate daily increments; longer intervals (up to weekly) may be more appropriate
  - ▶ Adult: Initially 300 mg once daily on day 1, then 300 mg twice daily on day 2, then 300 mg 3 times a day on day 3, alternatively initially 300 mg 3 times a day on day 1, then increased in steps of 300 mg every

2–3 days in 3 divided doses, adjusted according to response; usual dose 0.9–3.6 g daily in 3 divided doses (max. per dose 1.6 g 3 times a day)

Peripheral neuropathic pain
- ▶ BY MOUTH
  - ▶ Adult: Initially 300 mg once daily on day 1, then 300 mg twice daily on day 2, then 300 mg 3 times a day on day 3, alternatively initially 300 mg 3 times a day on day 1, then increased in steps of 300 mg every 2–3 days in 3 divided doses, adjusted according to response; maximum 3.6 g per day

Menopausal symptoms, particularly hot flushes, in women with breast cancer
- ▶ BY MOUTH
  - ▶ Adult: 300 mg 3 times a day, initial dose should be lower and titrated up over three days

Oscillopsia in multiple sclerosis
- ▶ BY MOUTH
  - ▶ Adult: Initially 300 mg once daily, then increased in steps of 300 mg, every 4–7 days, adjusted according to response; usual maximum 900 mg 3 times a day

Spasticity in multiple sclerosis
- ▶ BY MOUTH
  - ▶ Adult: Initially 300 mg once daily for 1–2 weeks, then 300 mg twice daily for 1–2 weeks, then 300 mg 3 times a day for 1–2 weeks, alternatively initially 100 mg 3 times a day, then increased in steps of 100 mg 3 times a day, every 1–2 weeks, adjusted according to response; usual maximum 900 mg 3 times a day

- UNLICENSED USE
- ▶ In children Not licensed at doses over 50 mg/kg daily in children under 12 years.
- ▶ In adults [EvGr] Gabapentin is used for the treatment of menopausal symptoms, Ⓐ but is not licensed for this indication. [EvGr] Gabapentin is used for oscillopsia in multiple sclerosis, Ⓔ but is not licensed for this indication. [EvGr] Gabapentin is used for spasticity in multiple sclerosis, Ⓔ but is not licensed for this indication.

> IMPORTANT SAFETY INFORMATION
> The levels of propylene glycol, acesulfame K and saccharin sodium may exceed the recommended WHO daily intake limits if high doses of gabapentin oral solution (Rosemont brand) are given to adolescents or adults with low body-weight (39–50 kg)—consult product literature.
>
> MHRA/CHM ADVICE: ANTIEPILEPTICS: RISK OF SUICIDAL THOUGHTS AND BEHAVIOUR (AUGUST 2008)
> See Epilepsy p. 321.
>
> MHRA/CHM ADVICE: GABAPENTIN (*NEURONTIN®*): RISK OF SEVERE RESPIRATORY DEPRESSION (OCTOBER 2017)
> Gabapentin has been associated with a rare risk of severe respiratory depression even without concomitant opioid medicines. Patients with compromised respiratory function, respiratory or neurological disease, renal impairment, concomitant use of central nervous system (CNS) depressants, and elderly people might be at higher risk of experiencing severe respiratory depression and dose adjustments may be necessary in these patients.
>
> MHRA/CHM ADVICE: ANTIEPILEPTIC DRUGS: UPDATED ADVICE ON SWITCHING BETWEEN DIFFERENT MANUFACTURERS' PRODUCTS (NOVEMBER 2017)
> See Epilepsy p. 321.
>
> MHRA/CHM ADVICE: GABAPENTIN (*NEURONTIN®*) AND RISK OF ABUSE AND DEPENDENCE: NEW SCHEDULING REQUIREMENTS FROM 1 APRIL (APRIL 2019)
> Following concerns about abuse, gabapentin has been reclassified as a Class C controlled substance and is now a Schedule 3 drug, but is exempt from safe custody

requirements. Healthcare professionals should evaluate patients carefully for a history of drug abuse before prescribing gabapentin, and observe patients for signs of abuse and dependence. Patients should be informed of the potentially fatal risks of interactions between gabapentin and alcohol, and with other medicines that cause CNS depression, particularly opioids.

- CAUTIONS Diabetes mellitus · elderly · high doses of oral solution in adolescents and adults with low body-weight · history of psychotic illness · history of substance abuse · mixed seizures (including absences)
- INTERACTIONS → Appendix 1: antiepileptics
- SIDE-EFFECTS
- ► **Common or very common** Anxiety · appetite abnormal · arthralgia · asthenia · behaviour abnormal · confusion · constipation · cough · depression · diarrhoea · dizziness · drowsiness · dry mouth · dysarthria · dyspnoea · emotional lability · flatulence · gait abnormal · gastrointestinal discomfort · headache · hypertension · increased risk of infection · insomnia · leucopenia · malaise · movement disorders · muscle complaints · nausea · nystagmus · oedema · pain · reflexes abnormal · seizure (in children) · sensation abnormal · sexual dysfunction · skin reactions · thinking abnormal · tooth disorder · tremor · vasodilation · vertigo · visual impairment · vomiting
- ► **Uncommon** Cognitive impairment · palpitations
- ► **Frequency not known** Acute kidney injury · alopecia · angioedema · breast enlargement · drug use disorders · gynaecomastia · hallucination · hepatic disorders · hyponatraemia · pancreatitis · rhabdomyolysis · severe cutaneous adverse reactions (SCARs) · suicidal behaviours · thrombocytopenia · tinnitus · urinary incontinence
- PREGNANCY Manufacturer advises avoid unless benefit outweighs risk — toxicity reported. See also *Pregnancy* in Epilepsy p. 321.
- BREAST FEEDING Present in milk—manufacturer advises use only if potential benefit outweighs risk. See also *Breast-feeding* in Epilepsy p. 321.
- RENAL IMPAIRMENT

   Dose adjustments ► In adults Manufacturer advises reduce dose to 600–1800 mg daily in 3 divided doses if creatinine clearance 50–79 mL/minute. Manufacturer advises reduce dose to 300–900 mg daily in 3 divided doses if creatinine clearance 30–49 mL/minute. Manufacturer advises reduce dose to 150–600 mg daily in 3 divided doses if creatinine clearance 15–29 mL/minute (150 mg daily dose to be given as 300 mg in 3 divided doses on alternate days). Manufacturer advises reduce dose to 150–300 mg daily in 3 divided doses if creatinine clearance is less than 15 mL/minute (150 mg daily dose to be given as 300 mg in 3 divided doses on alternate days)—further dose reductions may be required in proportion to creatinine clearance, consult product literature.
   ► In children Reduce dose if estimated glomerular filtration rate less than 80 mL/minute/1.73 m^2; consult product literature.
- MONITORING REQUIREMENTS Monitor for signs of gabapentin abuse.
- EFFECT ON LABORATORY TESTS False positive readings with some urinary protein tests.
- DIRECTIONS FOR ADMINISTRATION Expert sources advise capsules can be opened but the bitter taste is difficult to mask.
- PATIENT AND CARER ADVICE

   Medicines for Children leaflet: Gabapentin for neuropathic pain www.medicinesforchildren.org.uk/gabapentin-neuropathic-pain
   Medicines for Children leaflet: Gabapentin for preventing seizures www.medicinesforchildren.org.uk/gabapentin-preventing-seizures

Patient leaflet NHS England has produced a patient leaflet with information on the reclassification of gabapentin.

- MEDICINAL FORMS There can be variation in the licensing of different medicines containing the same drug. Forms available from special-order manufacturers include: oral suspension, oral solution

Tablet
CAUTIONARY AND ADVISORY LABELS 3, 5, 8, 25
► Gabapentin (Non-proprietary)
   Gabapentin 600 mg Gabapentin 600mg tablets | 100 tablet [PoM] £106.00 DT = £11.29 [CD3]
   Gabapentin 800 mg Gabapentin 800mg tablets | 100 tablet [PoM] £78.00 DT = £27.45 [CD3]
► Neurontin (Upjohn UK Ltd)
   Gabapentin 600 mg Neurontin 600mg tablets | 100 tablet [PoM] £84.80 DT = £11.29 [CD3]
   Gabapentin 800 mg Neurontin 800mg tablets | 100 tablet [PoM] £98.13 DT = £27.45 [CD3]

Oral solution
CAUTIONARY AND ADVISORY LABELS 3, 5, 8
EXCIPIENTS: May contain Propylene glycol
ELECTROLYTES: May contain Potassium, sodium
► Gabapentin (Non-proprietary)
   Gabapentin 50mg/ml oral solution sugar free sugar-free | 150 ml [PoM] £67.29 DT = £66.07 [CD3]

Capsule
CAUTIONARY AND ADVISORY LABELS 3, 5, 8, 25
► Gabapentin (Non-proprietary)
   Gabapentin 100 mg Gabapentin 100mg capsules | 100 capsule [PoM] £18.29 DT = £2.42 [CD3]
   Gabapentin 300 mg Gabapentin 300mg capsules | 100 capsule [PoM] £42.40 DT = £3.64 [CD3]
   Gabapentin 400 mg Gabapentin 400mg capsules | 100 capsule [PoM] £49.06 DT = £4.07 [CD3]
► Neurontin (Upjohn UK Ltd)
   Gabapentin 100 mg Neurontin 100mg capsules | 100 capsule [PoM] £18.29 DT = £2.42 [CD3]
   Gabapentin 300 mg Neurontin 300mg capsules | 100 capsule [PoM] £42.40 DT = £3.64 [CD3]
   Gabapentin 400 mg Neurontin 400mg capsules | 100 capsule [PoM] £49.06 DT = £4.07 [CD3]

Lacosamide   10-Dec-2020

- INDICATIONS AND DOSE

Monotherapy of focal seizures with or without secondary generalisation
► BY MOUTH, OR BY INTRAVENOUS INFUSION
► Child (body-weight 50 kg and above): Initially 50 mg twice daily, then increased to 100 mg twice daily, after one week, alternatively initially 100 mg twice daily; increased in steps of 50 mg twice daily (max. per dose 300 mg twice daily) if necessary and if tolerated, dose to be increased at weekly intervals
► Child 4-17 years (body-weight up to 50 kg): (consult product literature)
► Adult: Initially 50 mg twice daily, then increased to 100 mg twice daily, after one week, alternatively initially 100 mg twice daily; increased in steps of 50 mg twice daily (max. per dose 300 mg twice daily) if necessary and if tolerated, dose to be increased at weekly intervals

Monotherapy of focal seizures with or without secondary generalisation (alternative loading dose regimen when it is necessary to rapidly attain therapeutic plasma concentrations) (under close medical supervision)
► BY MOUTH, OR BY INTRAVENOUS INFUSION
► Child (body-weight 50 kg and above): Loading dose 200 mg, followed by 100 mg twice daily, to be given 12 hours after initial dose; increased in steps of 50 mg twice daily (max. per dose 300 mg twice daily) if necessary and if tolerated, dose to be increased at weekly intervals continued →

► Adult: Loading dose 200 mg, followed by 100 mg twice daily, to be given 12 hours after initial dose; increased in steps of 50 mg twice daily (max. per dose 300 mg twice daily) if necessary and if tolerated, dose to be increased at weekly intervals

Adjunctive treatment of focal seizures with or without secondary generalisation

▶ BY MOUTH, OR BY INTRAVENOUS INFUSION

► Child (body-weight 50 kg and above): Initially 50 mg twice daily, then increased to 100 mg twice daily, after one week; increased in steps of 50 mg twice daily (max. per dose 200 mg twice daily) if necessary and if tolerated, dose to be increased at weekly intervals

► Child 4-17 years (body-weight up to 50 kg): (consult product literature)

► Adult: Initially 50 mg twice daily, then increased to 100 mg twice daily, after one week; increased in steps of 50 mg twice daily (max. per dose 200 mg twice daily) if necessary and if tolerated, dose to be increased at weekly intervals

Adjunctive treatment of focal seizures with or without secondary generalisation (alternative loading dose regimen when it is necessary to rapidly attain therapeutic plasma concentrations) (under close medical supervision)

▶ BY MOUTH, OR BY INTRAVENOUS INFUSION

► Child (body-weight 50 kg and above): Loading dose 200 mg, followed by 100 mg twice daily, to be given 12 hours after initial dose; increased in steps of 50 mg twice daily (max. per dose 200 mg twice daily) if necessary and if tolerated, dose to be increased at weekly intervals

► Adult: Loading dose 200 mg, followed by 100 mg twice daily, to be given 12 hours after initial dose; increased in steps of 50 mg twice daily (max. per dose 200 mg twice daily) if necessary and if tolerated, dose to be increased at weekly intervals

---

IMPORTANT SAFETY INFORMATION

MHRA/CHM ADVICE: ANTIEPILEPTICS: RISK OF SUICIDAL THOUGHTS AND BEHAVIOUR (AUGUST 2008)
See Epilepsy p. 321.

MHRA/CHM ADVICE: ANTIEPILEPTIC DRUGS: UPDATED ADVICE ON SWITCHING BETWEEN DIFFERENT MANUFACTURERS' PRODUCTS (NOVEMBER 2017)
See Epilepsy p. 321.

● CONTRA-INDICATIONS Second- or third-degree AV block
● CAUTIONS Conduction problems · elderly · risk of PR-interval prolongation · severe cardiac disease
● INTERACTIONS → Appendix 1: antiepileptics
● SIDE-EFFECTS
▶ Common or very common Asthenia · concentration impaired · confusion · constipation · depression · diarrhoea · dizziness · drowsiness · dry mouth · dysarthria · dyspepsia · flatulence · gait abnormal · headache · insomnia · mood altered · movement disorders · muscle spasms · nausea · nystagmus · sensation abnormal · skin reactions · tinnitus · vertigo · vision disorders · vomiting
▶ Uncommon Aggression · agitation · angioedema · arrhythmias · atrioventricular block · hallucination · psychotic disorder · suicidal behaviours · syncope
▶ Frequency not known Agranulocytosis
● ALLERGY AND CROSS-SENSITIVITY Antiepileptic hypersensitivity syndrome associated with lacosamide. See under Epilepsy p. 321 for more information.
● PREGNANCY See also *Pregnancy* in Epilepsy p. 321.
Monitoring The dose should be monitored carefully during pregnancy and after birth, and adjustments made on a clinical basis.

● BREAST FEEDING Manufacturer advises avoid—present in milk in *animal* studies.
● HEPATIC IMPAIRMENT Manufacturer advises caution (risk of increased exposure), particularly in severe impairment (no information available).
Dose adjustments Manufacturer advises consider dose reduction—consult product literature.
● RENAL IMPAIRMENT Consult product literature.
● DIRECTIONS FOR ADMINISTRATION
▶ With intravenous use For *intermittent intravenous infusion*, manufacturer advises give undiluted or dilute with Glucose 5% *or* Sodium Chloride 0.9% *or* Lactated Ringer's Solution; give over 15–60 minutes—give doses greater than 200 mg over at least 30 minutes.
● PRESCRIBING AND DISPENSING INFORMATION Flavours of syrup may include strawberry.
● PATIENT AND CARER ADVICE
Medicines for Children leaflet: Lacosamide for preventing seizures www.medicinesforchildren.org.uk/lacosamide-preventing-seizures
● NATIONAL FUNDING/ACCESS DECISIONS
For full details see funding body website

Scottish Medicines Consortium (SMC) decisions

► Lacosamide (*Vimpat*®) as adjunctive therapy in the treatment of partial-onset seizures with or without secondary generalisation in patients with epilepsy aged 16 years or older (February 2009) SMC No. 532/09 Recommended with restrictions

► Lacosamide (*Vimpat*®) as adjunctive therapy in the treatment of partial-onset seizures with or without secondary generalisation in adolescents and children from 4 years of age with epilepsy (February 2018) SMC No. 1301/18 Recommended with restrictions

All Wales Medicines Strategy Group (AWMSG) decisions

► Lacosamide (*Vimpat*®) as adjunctive treatment of partial-onset seizures with or without secondary generalisation in children from 4 years of age up to 15 years of age with epilepsy (March 2018) AWMSG No. 3343 Recommended

---

● MEDICINAL FORMS There can be variation in the licensing of different medicines containing the same drug.

Solution for infusion

ELECTROLYTES: May contain Sodium
► Vimpat (UCB Pharma Ltd)
Lacosamide 10 mg per 1 ml Vimpat 200mg/20ml solution for infusion vials | 1 vial [PoM] £29.70

Oral solution

CAUTIONARY AND ADVISORY LABELS 8
EXCIPIENTS: May contain Aspartame, propylene glycol
ELECTROLYTES: May contain Sodium
► Vimpat (UCB Pharma Ltd)
Lacosamide 10 mg per 1 ml Vimpat 10mg/ml syrup sugar-free | 200 ml [PoM] £25.74 DT = £25.74

Tablet

CAUTIONARY AND ADVISORY LABELS 8
► Vimpat (UCB Pharma Ltd)
Lacosamide 50 mg Vimpat 50mg tablets | 14 tablet [PoM] £10.81 DT = £10.81
Lacosamide 100 mg Vimpat 100mg tablets | 14 tablet [PoM] £21.62 | 56 tablet [PoM] £86.50 DT = £86.50
Lacosamide 150 mg Vimpat 150mg tablets | 14 tablet [PoM] £32.44 | 56 tablet [PoM] £129.74 DT = £129.74
Lacosamide 200 mg Vimpat 200mg tablets | 56 tablet [PoM] £144.16 DT = £144.16

Lamotrigine
10-Dec-2020

● **INDICATIONS AND DOSE**

Monotherapy of focal seizures | Monotherapy of primary and secondary generalised tonic-clonic seizures | Monotherapy of seizures associated with Lennox-Gastaut syndrome

▸ BY MOUTH

▸ **Child 12-17 years:** Initially 25 mg once daily for 14 days, then increased to 50 mg once daily for further 14 days, then increased in steps of up to 100 mg every 7–14 days; maintenance 100–200 mg daily in 1–2 divided doses; increased if necessary up to 500 mg daily, dose titration should be repeated if restarting after interval of more than 5 days

▸ **Adult:** Initially 25 mg once daily for 14 days, then increased to 50 mg once daily for further 14 days, then increased in steps of up to 100 mg every 7–14 days; maintenance 100–200 mg daily in 1–2 divided doses; increased if necessary up to 500 mg daily, dose titration should be repeated if restarting after interval of more than 5 days

Adjunctive therapy of focal seizures with valproate | Adjunctive therapy of primary and secondary generalised tonic-clonic seizures with valproate | Adjunctive therapy of seizures associated with Lennox-Gastaut syndrome with valproate

▸ BY MOUTH

▸ **Child 2-11 years (body-weight up to 13 kg):** Initially 2 mg once daily on alternate days for first 14 days, then 300 micrograms/kg once daily for further 14 days, then increased in steps of up to 300 micrograms/kg every 7–14 days; maintenance 1–5 mg/kg daily in 1–2 divided doses, dose titration should be repeated if restarting after interval of more than 5 days; maximum 200 mg per day

▸ **Child 2-11 years (body-weight 13 kg and above):** Initially 150 micrograms/kg once daily for 14 days, then 300 micrograms/kg once daily for further 14 days, then increased in steps of up to 300 micrograms/kg every 7–14 days; maintenance 1–5 mg/kg daily in 1–2 divided doses, dose titration should be repeated if restarting after interval of more than 5 days; maximum 200 mg per day

▸ **Child 12-17 years:** Initially 25 mg once daily on alternate days for 14 days, then 25 mg once daily for further 14 days, then increased in steps of up to 50 mg every 7–14 days; maintenance 100–200 mg daily in 1–2 divided doses, dose titration should be repeated if restarting after interval of more than 5 days

▸ **Adult:** Initially 25 mg once daily on alternate days for 14 days, then 25 mg once daily for further 14 days, then increased in steps of up to 50 mg every 7–14 days; maintenance 100–200 mg daily in 1–2 divided doses, dose titration should be repeated if restarting after interval of more than 5 days

Adjunctive therapy of focal seizures (with enzyme inducing drugs) without valproate | Adjunctive therapy of primary and secondary generalised tonic-clonic seizures (with enzyme inducing drugs) without valproate | Adjunctive therapy of seizures associated with Lennox-Gastaut syndromes (with enzyme inducing drugs) without valproate

▸ BY MOUTH

▸ **Child 2-11 years:** Initially 300 micrograms/kg twice daily for 14 days, then 600 micrograms/kg twice daily for further 14 days, then increased in steps of up to 1.2 mg/kg every 7–14 days; maintenance 5–15 mg/kg daily in 1–2 divided doses, dose titration should be repeated if restarting after interval of more than 5 days; maximum 400 mg per day

▸ **Child 12-17 years:** Initially 50 mg once daily for 14 days, then 50 mg twice daily for further 14 days, then increased in steps of up to 100 mg every 7–14 days; maintenance 200–400 mg daily in 2 divided doses, increased if necessary up to 700 mg daily, dose titration should be repeated if restarting after interval of more than 5 days

▸ **Adult:** Initially 50 mg once daily for 14 days, then 50 mg twice daily for further 14 days, then increased in steps of up to 100 mg every 7–14 days; maintenance 200–400 mg daily in 2 divided doses, increased if necessary up to 700 mg daily, dose titration should be repeated if restarting after interval of more than 5 days

Adjunctive therapy of focal seizures (without enzyme inducing drugs) without valproate | Adjunctive therapy of primary and secondary generalised tonic-clonic seizures (without enzyme inducing drugs) without valproate | Adjunctive therapy of seizures associated with Lennox-Gastaut syndromes (without enzyme inducing drugs) without valproate

▸ BY MOUTH

▸ **Child 2-11 years:** Initially 300 micrograms/kg daily in 1–2 divided doses for 14 days, then 600 micrograms/kg daily in 1–2 divided doses for further 14 days, then increased in steps of up to 600 micrograms/kg every 7–14 days; maintenance 1–10 mg/kg daily in 1–2 divided doses, dose titration should be repeated if restarting after interval of more than 5 days; maximum 200 mg per day

▸ **Child 12-17 years:** Initially 25 mg once daily for 14 days, then increased to 50 mg once daily for further 14 days, then increased in steps of up to 100 mg every 7–14 days; maintenance 100–200 mg daily in 1–2 divided doses, dose titration should be repeated if restarting after interval of more than 5 days

▸ **Adult:** Initially 25 mg once daily for 14 days, then increased to 50 mg once daily for further 14 days, then increased in steps of up to 100 mg every 7–14 days; maintenance 100–200 mg daily in 1–2 divided doses, dose titration should be repeated if restarting after interval of more than 5 days

Monotherapy or adjunctive therapy of bipolar disorder (without enzyme inducing drugs) without valproate

▸ BY MOUTH

▸ **Adult:** Initially 25 mg once daily for 14 days, then 50 mg daily in 1–2 divided doses for further 14 days, then 100 mg daily in 1–2 divided doses for further 7 days; maintenance 200 mg daily in 1–2 divided doses, patients stabilised on lamotrigine for bipolar disorder may require dose adjustments if other drugs are added to or withdrawn from their treatment regimens— consult product literature, dose titration should be repeated if restarting after interval of more than 5 days; maximum 400 mg per day

Adjunctive therapy of bipolar disorder with valproate

▸ BY MOUTH

▸ **Adult:** Initially 25 mg once daily on alternate days for 14 days, then 25 mg once daily for further 14 days, then 50 mg daily in 1–2 divided doses for further 7 days; maintenance 100 mg daily in 1–2 divided doses, patients stabilised on lamotrigine for bipolar disorder may require dose adjustments if other drugs are added to or withdrawn from their treatment regimens— consult product literature, dose titration should be repeated if restarting after interval of more than 5 days; maximum 200 mg per day

Adjunctive therapy of bipolar disorder (with enzyme inducing drugs) without valproate

▸ BY MOUTH

▸ **Adult:** Initially 50 mg once daily for 14 days, then 50 mg twice daily for further 14 days, then continued →

4

Nervous system

increased to 100 mg twice daily for further 7 days, then increased to 150 mg twice daily for further 7 days; maintenance 200 mg twice daily, patients stabilised on lamotrigine for bipolar disorder may require dose adjustments if other drugs are added to or withdrawn from their treatment regimens—consult product literature, dose titration should be repeated if restarting after interval of more than 5 days

> **IMPORTANT SAFETY INFORMATION**
>
> MHRA/CHM ADVICE: ANTIEPILEPTICS: RISK OF SUICIDAL THOUGHTS AND BEHAVIOUR (AUGUST 2008)
> See Epilepsy p. 321.
>
> MHRA/CHM ADVICE: ANTIEPILEPTIC DRUGS: UPDATED ADVICE ON SWITCHING BETWEEN DIFFERENT MANUFACTURERS' PRODUCTS (NOVEMBER 2017)
> See Epilepsy p. 321 and see also *Prescribing and dispensing information.*

* CAUTIONS Brugada syndrome · myoclonic seizures (may be exacerbated) · Parkinson's disease (may be exacerbated) (in adults)
* INTERACTIONS → Appendix 1: antiepileptics
* SIDE-EFFECTS
  ▸ **Common or very common** Aggression · agitation · arthralgia · diarrhoea · dizziness · drowsiness · dry mouth · fatigue · headache · irritability · nausea · pain · rash · sleep disorders · tremor · vomiting
  ▸ **Uncommon** Alopecia · movement disorders · vision disorders
  ▸ **Rare or very rare** Confusion · conjunctivitis · disseminated intravascular coagulation · face oedema · fever · haemophagocytic lymphohistiocytosis · hallucination · hepatic disorders · lupus-like syndrome · lymphadenopathy · meningitis aseptic · multi organ failure · nystagmus · seizure · severe cutaneous adverse reactions (SCARs) · tic
  ▸ **Frequency not known** Suicidal behaviours
  SIDE-EFFECTS, FURTHER INFORMATION Serious skin reactions including Stevens-Johnson syndrome and toxic epidermal necrolysis have developed (especially in children); most rashes occur in the first 8 weeks. Rash is sometimes associated with hypersensitivity syndrome and is more common in patients with history of allergy or rash from other antiepileptic drugs. Consider withdrawal if rash or signs of hypersensitivity syndrome develop. Factors associated with increased risk of serious skin reactions include concomitant use of valproate, initial lamotrigine dosing higher than recommended, and more rapid dose escalation than recommended.
* ALLERGY AND CROSS-SENSITIVITY Antiepileptic hypersensitivity syndrome associated with lamotrigine. See under Epilepsy p. 321 for more information.
* PREGNANCY See also *Pregnancy* in Epilepsy p. 321. **Monitoring** Doses should be adjusted on the basis of plasma-drug concentration monitoring.
* BREAST FEEDING Present in milk, but limited data suggest no harmful effect on infant.
* HEPATIC IMPAIRMENT Manufacturer advises caution in moderate to severe impairment.
  Dose adjustments Manufacturer advises dose reduction of approx. 50% in moderate impairment, and approx. 75% in severe impairment; adjust according to response.
* RENAL IMPAIRMENT Caution in renal failure; metabolite may accumulate.
  Dose adjustments Consider reducing maintenance dose in significant impairment.
* TREATMENT CESSATION Avoid abrupt withdrawal (taper off over 2 weeks or longer) unless serious skin reaction occurs.

* PRESCRIBING AND DISPENSING INFORMATION Patients being treated for epilepsy may need to be maintained on a specific manufacturer's branded or generic lamotrigine product.
  Switching between formulations Care should be taken when switching between oral formulations in the treatment of epilepsy. The need for continued supply of a particular manufacturer's product should be based on clinical judgement and consultation with the patient or their carer, taking into account factors such as seizure frequency and treatment history.
* PATIENT AND CARER ADVICE
  Skin reactions Warn patients and carers to see their doctor immediately if rash or signs or symptoms of hypersensitivity syndrome develop.
  Blood disorders Patients and their carers should be alert for symptoms and signs suggestive of bone-marrow failure, such as anaemia, bruising, or infection. Aplastic anaemia, bone-marrow depression, and pancytopenia have been associated rarely with lamotrigine.
  Medicines for Children leaflet: Lamotrigine for preventing seizures www.medicinesforchildren.org.uk/lamotrigine-preventing-seizures

* MEDICINAL FORMS There can be variation in the licensing of different medicines containing the same drug. Forms available from special-order manufacturers include: oral suspension, oral solution

Dispersible tablet

CAUTIONARY AND ADVISORY LABELS 8, 13
▸ Lamotrigine (Non-proprietary)
  Lamotrigine 5 mg Lamotrigine 5mg dispersible tablets sugar free sugar-free | 28 tablet [PoM] £15.00 DT = £6.82
  Lamotrigine 25 mg Lamotrigine 25mg dispersible tablets sugar free sugar-free | 56 tablet [PoM] £20.00 DT = £7.39
  Lamotrigine 100 mg Lamotrigine 100mg dispersible tablets sugar free sugar-free | 56 tablet [PoM] £58.68 DT = £13.30
▸ Lamictal (GlaxoSmithKline UK Ltd)
  Lamotrigine 2 mg Lamictal 2mg dispersible tablets sugar-free | 30 tablet [PoM] £18.81 DT = £18.81
  Lamotrigine 5 mg Lamictal 5mg dispersible tablets sugar-free | 28 tablet [PoM] £9.38 DT = £6.82
  Lamotrigine 25 mg Lamictal 25mg dispersible tablets sugar-free | 56 tablet [PoM] £23.53 DT = £7.39
  Lamotrigine 100 mg Lamictal 100mg dispersible tablets sugar-free | 56 tablet [PoM] £69.04 DT = £13.30

Tablet

CAUTIONARY AND ADVISORY LABELS 8
▸ Lamotrigine (Non-proprietary)
  Lamotrigine 25 mg Lamotrigine 25mg tablets | 56 tablet [PoM] £23.53 DT = £1.66
  Lamotrigine 50 mg Lamotrigine 50mg tablets | 56 tablet [PoM] £40.02 DT = £1.92
  Lamotrigine 100 mg Lamotrigine 100mg tablets | 56 tablet [PoM] £69.04 DT = £2.98
  Lamotrigine 200 mg Lamotrigine 200mg tablets | 56 tablet [PoM] £117.35 DT = £3.07
▸ Lamictal (GlaxoSmithKline UK Ltd)
  Lamotrigine 25 mg Lamictal 25mg tablets | 56 tablet [PoM] £23.53 DT = £1.66
  Lamotrigine 50 mg Lamictal 50mg tablets | 56 tablet [PoM] £40.02 DT = £1.92
  Lamotrigine 100 mg Lamictal 100mg tablets | 56 tablet [PoM] £69.04 DT = £2.98
  Lamotrigine 200 mg Lamictal 200mg tablets | 56 tablet [PoM] £117.35 DT = £3.07

Levetiracetam

07-Oct-2020

● **INDICATIONS AND DOSE**

Monotherapy of focal seizures with or without secondary generalisation

▶ **BY MOUTH, OR BY INTRAVENOUS INFUSION**

▶ **Child 16-17 years:** Initially 250 mg once daily for 1 week, then increased to 250 mg twice daily, then increased in steps of 250 mg twice daily (max. per dose 1.5 g twice daily), adjusted according to response, dose to be increased every 2 weeks

▶ **Adult:** Initially 250 mg once daily for 1–2 weeks, then increased to 250 mg twice daily, then increased in steps of 250 mg twice daily (max. per dose 1.5 g twice daily), adjusted according to response, dose to be increased every 2 weeks

Adjunctive therapy of focal seizures with or without secondary generalisation

▶ **BY MOUTH**

▶ **Child 1-5 months:** Initially 7 mg/kg once daily, then increased in steps of up to 7 mg/kg twice daily (max. per dose 21 mg/kg twice daily), dose to be increased every 2 weeks

▶ **Child 6 months-17 years (body-weight up to 50 kg):** Initially 10 mg/kg once daily, then increased in steps of up to 10 mg/kg twice daily (max. per dose 30 mg/kg twice daily), dose to be increased every 2 weeks

▶ **Child 12-17 years (body-weight 50 kg and above):** Initially 250 mg twice daily, then increased in steps of 500 mg twice daily (max. per dose 1.5 g twice daily), dose to be increased every 2–4 weeks

▶ **Adult:** Initially 250 mg twice daily, then increased in steps of 500 mg twice daily (max. per dose 1.5 g twice daily), dose to be increased every 2–4 weeks

▶ **BY INTRAVENOUS INFUSION**

▶ **Child 4-17 years (body-weight up to 50 kg):** Initially 10 mg/kg once daily, then increased in steps of up to 10 mg/kg twice daily (max. per dose 30 mg/kg twice daily), dose to be increased every 2 weeks

▶ **Child 12-17 years (body-weight 50 kg and above):** Initially 250 mg twice daily, then increased in steps of 500 mg twice daily (max. per dose 1.5 g twice daily), dose to be increased every 2 weeks

▶ **Adult:** Initially 250 mg twice daily, then increased in steps of 500 mg twice daily (max. per dose 1.5 g twice daily), dose to be increased every 2–4 weeks

Adjunctive therapy of myoclonic seizures and tonic-clonic seizures

▶ **BY MOUTH, OR BY INTRAVENOUS INFUSION**

▶ **Child 12-17 years (body-weight up to 50 kg):** Initially 10 mg/kg once daily, then increased in steps of up to 10 mg/kg twice daily (max. per dose 30 mg/kg twice daily), dose to be increased every 2 weeks

▶ **Child 12-17 years (body-weight 50 kg and above):** Initially 250 mg twice daily, then increased in steps of 500 mg twice daily (max. per dose 1.5 g twice daily), dose to be increased every 2 weeks

▶ **Adult:** Initially 250 mg twice daily, then increased in steps of 500 mg twice daily (max. per dose 1.5 g twice daily), dose to be increased every 2–4 weeks

● **UNLICENSED USE** EvGr Initial dosing recommendations for levetiracetam ⓔ in BNF Publications differ from product licence.

▶ With oral use in children Manufacturer advises *granules* not licensed for use in children under 6 years, for initial treatment in children with body-weight less than 25 kg, or

for the administration of doses below 250 mg—oral solution should be used.

IMPORTANT SAFETY INFORMATION

MHRA/CHM ADVICE: ANTIEPILEPTICS: RISK OF SUICIDAL THOUGHTS AND BEHAVIOUR (AUGUST 2008)
See Epilepsy p. 321.

MHRA/CHM ADVICE: ANTIEPILEPTIC DRUGS: UPDATED ADVICE ON SWITCHING BETWEEN DIFFERENT MANUFACTURERS' PRODUCTS (NOVEMBER 2017)
See Epilepsy p. 321.

● **INTERACTIONS** → Appendix 1: antiepileptics

● **SIDE-EFFECTS**

▶ **Common or very common** Anxiety · appetite decreased · asthenia · behaviour abnormal · cough · depression · diarrhoea · dizziness · drowsiness · gastrointestinal discomfort · headache · increased risk of infection · insomnia · mood altered · movement disorders · nausea · skin reactions · vertigo · vomiting

▶ **Uncommon** Alopecia · concentration impaired · confusion · hallucination · leucopenia · muscle weakness · myalgia · paraesthesia · psychotic disorder · suicidal behaviours · thrombocytopenia · vision disorders · weight changes

▶ **Rare or very rare** Acute kidney injury · agranulocytosis · hepatic disorders · hyponatraemia · neutropenia · pancreatitis · pancytopenia · personality disorder · rhabdomyolysis · severe cutaneous adverse reactions (SCARs) · thinking abnormal

● **PREGNANCY** See also *Pregnancy* in Epilepsy p. 321.
Monitoring The dose should be monitored carefully during pregnancy and after birth, and adjustments made on a clinical basis.
It is recommended that the fetal growth should be monitored.

● **BREAST FEEDING** Present in milk—manufacturer advises avoid.

● **HEPATIC IMPAIRMENT** Manufacturer advises caution in severe impairment.
Dose adjustments Manufacturer advises maintenance dose reduction of 50% in severe impairment if creatinine clearance is less than 60 mL/minute/1.73 m^2—consult product literature.

● **RENAL IMPAIRMENT**
Dose adjustments ▶ In children Reduce dose if estimated glomerular filtration rate less than 80 mL/minute/1.73 m^2 (consult product literature).
▶ In adults Maximum 2 g daily if eGFR 50–80 mL/minute/1.73 m^2. Maximum 1.5 g daily if eGFR 30–50 mL/minute/1.73 m^2. Maximum 1 g daily if eGFR less than 30 mL/minute/1.73 m^2.

● **DIRECTIONS FOR ADMINISTRATION**

▶ With intravenous use For *intravenous infusion* (Keppra®), manufacturer advises dilute requisite dose with at least 100 mL Glucose 5% or Sodium Chloride 0.9%; give over 15 minutes.

▶ With oral use For administration of *oral solution*, manufacturer advises requisite dose may be diluted in a glass of water.

● **PRESCRIBING AND DISPENSING INFORMATION** If switching between oral therapy and intravenous therapy (for those temporarily unable to take oral medication), the intravenous dose should be the same as the established oral dose.

● **PATIENT AND CARER ADVICE**
Medicines for Children leaflet: Levetiracetam for preventing seizures www.medicinesforchildren.org.uk/levetiracetam-preventing-seizures

- MEDICINAL FORMS There can be variation in the licensing of different medicines containing the same drug. Forms available from special-order manufacturers include: oral suspension, oral solution

Granules
CAUTIONARY AND ADVISORY LABELS 8
- Desitrend (Desitin Pharma Ltd)
  Levetiracetam 250 mg Desitrend 250mg granules sachets sugar-free | 60 sachet [PoM] £22.41 DT = £22.41
  Levetiracetam 500 mg Desitrend 500mg granules sachets sugar-free | 60 sachet [PoM] £39.46 DT = £39.46
  Levetiracetam 1 gram Desitrend 1000mg granules sachets sugar-free | 60 sachet [PoM] £76.27 DT = £76.27

Tablet
CAUTIONARY AND ADVISORY LABELS 8
- Levetiracetam (Non-proprietary)
  Levetiracetam 250 mg Levetiracetam 250mg tablets | 60 tablet [PoM] £28.01 DT = £3.15
  Levetiracetam 500 mg Levetiracetam 500mg tablets | 60 tablet [PoM] £49.32 DT = £5.25
  Levetiracetam 750 mg Levetiracetam 750mg tablets | 60 tablet [PoM] £84.02 DT = £5.40
  Levetiracetam 1 gram Levetiracetam 1g tablets | 60 tablet [PoM] £95.34 DT = £7.32
- Keppra (UCB Pharma Ltd)
  Levetiracetam 250 mg Keppra 250mg tablets | 60 tablet [PoM] £28.01 DT = £3.15
  Levetiracetam 500 mg Keppra 500mg tablets | 60 tablet [PoM] £49.32 DT = £5.25
  Levetiracetam 750 mg Keppra 750mg tablets | 60 tablet [PoM] £84.02 DT = £5.40
  Levetiracetam 1 gram Keppra 1g tablets | 60 tablet [PoM] £95.34 DT = £7.32

Solution for infusion
ELECTROLYTES: May contain Sodium
- Levetiracetam (Non-proprietary)
  Levetiracetam 100 mg per 1 ml Levetiracetam 500mg/5ml concentrate for solution for infusion vials | 10 vial [PoM] £127.31 DT = £127.31 (Hospital only)
- Desitrend (Desitin Pharma Ltd)
  Levetiracetam 100 mg per 1 ml Desitrend 500mg/5ml concentrate for solution for infusion ampoules | 10 ampoule [PoM] £127.31 DT = £127.31
- Keppra (UCB Pharma Ltd)
  Levetiracetam 100 mg per 1 ml Keppra 500mg/5ml concentrate for solution for infusion vials | 10 vial [PoM] £127.31 DT = £127.31 (Hospital only)

Oral solution
CAUTIONARY AND ADVISORY LABELS 8
- Levetiracetam (Non-proprietary)
  Levetiracetam 100 mg per 1 ml Levetiracetam 100mg/ml oral solution sugar free sugar-free | 150 ml [PoM] £27.00 sugar-free | 300 ml [PoM] £66.95 DT = £6.73
- Keppra (UCB Pharma Ltd)
  Levetiracetam 100 mg per 1 ml Keppra 100mg/ml oral solution sugar-free | 150 ml [PoM] £33.48 sugar-free | 300 ml [PoM] £66.95 DT = £6.73

Oxcarbazepine

10-Dec-2020

- **INDICATIONS AND DOSE**

Monotherapy for the treatment of focal seizures with or without secondary generalised tonic-clonic seizures
- BY MOUTH
  - Child 6–17 years: Initially 4–5 mg/kg twice daily (max. per dose 300 mg), then increased in steps of up to 5 mg/kg twice daily, adjusted according to response, dose to be adjusted at weekly intervals; maximum 46 mg/kg per day
  - Adult: Initially 300 mg twice daily, then increased in steps of up to 600 mg daily, adjusted according to response, dose to be adjusted at weekly intervals; usual dose 0.6–2.4 g daily in divided doses

Adjunctive therapy for the treatment of focal seizures with or without secondary generalised tonic-clonic seizures
- BY MOUTH
  - Child 6–17 years: Initially 4–5 mg/kg twice daily (max. per dose 300 mg), then increased in steps of up to 5 mg/kg twice daily, adjusted according to response, dose to be adjusted at weekly intervals; maintenance 15 mg/kg twice daily; maximum 46 mg/kg per day
  - Adult: Initially 300 mg twice daily, then increased in steps of up to 600 mg daily, adjusted according to response, dose to be adjusted at weekly intervals; usual dose 0.6–2.4 g daily in divided doses

Treatment of primary generalised tonic-clonic seizures
- BY MOUTH
  - Adult: Initially 300 mg twice daily, then increased in steps of up to 600 mg daily, adjusted according to response, dose to be increased at weekly intervals; usual dose 0.6–2.4 g daily in divided doses

DOSE ADJUSTMENTS DUE TO INTERACTIONS
- In adjunctive therapy, the dose of concomitant antiepileptics may need to be reduced when using high doses of oxcarbazepine.

- UNLICENSED USE Not licensed for the treatment of primary generalised tonic-clonic seizures.

IMPORTANT SAFETY INFORMATION

MHRA/CHM ADVICE: ANTIEPILEPTICS: RISK OF SUICIDAL THOUGHTS AND BEHAVIOUR (AUGUST 2008)
See Epilepsy p. 321.

MHRA/CHM ADVICE: ANTIEPILEPTIC DRUGS: UPDATED ADVICE ON SWITCHING BETWEEN DIFFERENT MANUFACTURERS' PRODUCTS (NOVEMBER 2017)
See Epilepsy p. 321 and see also *Prescribing and dispensing information.*

- CAUTIONS Avoid in Acute porphyrias p. 1107 · cardiac conduction disorders · heart failure · hyponatraemia · may exacerbate absence and myoclonic seizures
- INTERACTIONS → Appendix 1: antiepileptics
- SIDE-EFFECTS
  - **Common or very common** Abdominal pain · agitation · alopecia · asthenia · ataxia · concentration impaired · constipation · depression · diarrhoea · dizziness · drowsiness · emotional lability · headache · hyponatraemia · nausea · nystagmus · skin reactions · vertigo · vision disorders · vomiting
  - **Uncommon** Leucopenia
  - **Rare or very rare** Angioedema · arrhythmia · atrioventricular block · hepatitis · hypothyroidism · pancreatitis · severe cutaneous adverse reactions (SCARs) · systemic lupus erythematosus (SLE) · thrombocytopenia
  - **Frequency not known** Agranulocytosis · bone disorders · bone marrow disorders · hypertension · inappropriate antidiuretic hormone secretion like-syndrome · neutropenia · speech impairment · suicidal behaviours
- ALLERGY AND CROSS-SENSITIVITY Caution in patients with hypersensitivity to carbamazepine. Antiepileptic hypersensitivity syndrome associated with oxcarbazepine. See under Epilepsy p. 321 for more information.
- PREGNANCY See also *Pregnancy* in Epilepsy p. 321.
  Monitoring The dose should be monitored carefully during pregnancy and after birth, and adjustments made on a clinical basis.
- BREAST FEEDING Amount probably too small to be harmful but manufacturer advises avoid.
- HEPATIC IMPAIRMENT Manufacturer advises caution in severe impairment (no information available).

- **RENAL IMPAIRMENT**
  Dose adjustments ▸ In adults Halve initial dose if eGFR less than 30 mL/minute/1.73 m²; increase according to response at intervals of at least 1 week.
  ▸ In children Halve initial dose if estimated glomerular filtration rate less than 30 mL/minute/1.73 m², increase according to response at intervals of at least 1 week.
- **PRE-TREATMENT SCREENING** Test for HLA-B*1502 allele in individuals of Han Chinese or Thai origin (avoid unless no alternative—risk of Stevens-Johnson syndrome in presence of HLA-B*1502 allele).
- **MONITORING REQUIREMENTS**
  ▸ Monitor plasma-sodium concentration in patients at risk of hyponatraemia.
  ▸ Monitor body-weight in patients with heart failure.
- **PRESCRIBING AND DISPENSING INFORMATION** Patients may need to be maintained on a specific manufacturer's branded or generic oxcarbazepine product.
  Switching between formulations Care should be taken when switching between oral formulations. The need for continued supply of a particular manufacturer's product should be based on clinical judgement and consultation with the patient or their carer, taking into account factors such as seizure frequency and treatment history.
- **PATIENT AND CARER ADVICE**
  Blood, hepatic, or skin disorders Patients or their carers should be told how to recognise signs of blood, liver, or skin disorders, and advised to seek immediate medical attention if symptoms such as lethargy, confusion, muscular twitching, fever, rash, blistering, mouth ulcers, bruising, or bleeding develop.
  Medicines for Children: Oxcarbazepine for preventing seizures www.medicinesforchildren.org.uk/oxcarbazepine-preventing-seizures

- **MEDICINAL FORMS** There can be variation in the licensing of different medicines containing the same drug. Forms available from special-order manufacturers include: oral suspension
  Oral suspension
  CAUTIONARY AND ADVISORY LABELS 3, 8
  EXCIPIENTS: May contain Propylene glycol
  ▸ Trileptal (Novartis Pharmaceuticals UK Ltd)
  Oxcarbazepine 60 mg per 1 mL Trileptal 60mg/ml oral suspension sugar-free | 250 ml [PoM] £48.96 DT = £48.96
  Tablet
  CAUTIONARY AND ADVISORY LABELS 3, 8
  ▸ Oxcarbazepine (Non-proprietary)
  Oxcarbazepine 150 mg Oxcarbazepine 150mg tablets | 50 tablet [PoM] £11.14 DT = £8.37
  Oxcarbazepine 300 mg Oxcarbazepine 300mg tablets | 50 tablet [PoM] £22.61 DT = £7.42
  Oxcarbazepine 600 mg Oxcarbazepine 600mg tablets | 50 tablet [PoM] £45.19 DT = £38.71
  ▸ Trileptal (Novartis Pharmaceuticals UK Ltd)
  Oxcarbazepine 150 mg Trileptal 150mg tablets | 50 tablet [PoM] £12.24 DT = £8.37
  Oxcarbazepine 300 mg Trileptal 300mg tablets | 50 tablet [PoM] £24.48 DT = £7.42
  Oxcarbazepine 600 mg Trileptal 600mg tablets | 50 tablet [PoM] £48.96 DT = £38.71

Perampanel
11-Nov-2020

- **INDICATIONS AND DOSE**
  Adjunctive treatment of focal seizures with or without secondary generalised seizures
  ▸ BY MOUTH
  ▸ Child 12–17 years: Initially 2 mg once daily, dose to be taken before bedtime, then increased, if tolerated, in steps of 2 mg at intervals of at least every 2 weeks, adjusted according to response; maintenance 4–8 mg once daily; maximum 12 mg per day

▸ Adult: Initially 2 mg once daily, dose to be taken before bedtime, then increased, if tolerated, in steps of 2 mg at intervals of at least every 2 weeks, adjusted according to response; maintenance 4–8 mg once daily; maximum 12 mg per day

Adjunctive treatment of primary generalised tonic-clonic seizures
▸ BY MOUTH
▸ Child 12–17 years: Initially 2 mg once daily, dose to be taken before bedtime, then increased, if tolerated, in steps of 2 mg at intervals of at least every 2 weeks, adjusted according to response, maintenance up to 8 mg once daily; maximum 12 mg per day
▸ Adult: Initially 2 mg once daily, dose to be taken before bedtime, then increased, if tolerated, in steps of 2 mg at intervals of at least every 2 weeks, adjusted according to response, maintenance up to 8 mg once daily; maximum 12 mg per day

DOSE ADJUSTMENTS DUE TO INTERACTIONS
▸ Titrate at intervals of at least 1 week with concomitant carbamazepine, fosphenytoin, oxcarbazepine, or phenytoin.

IMPORTANT SAFETY INFORMATION
MHRA/CHM ADVICE: ANTIEPILEPTICS: RISK OF SUICIDAL THOUGHTS AND BEHAVIOUR (AUGUST 2008)
See Epilepsy p. 321.

MHRA/CHM ADVICE: ANTIEPILEPTIC DRUGS: UPDATED ADVICE ON SWITCHING BETWEEN DIFFERENT MANUFACTURERS' PRODUCTS (NOVEMBER 2017)
See Epilepsy p. 321 and see also *Prescribing and dispensing information*.

- **INTERACTIONS** → Appendix 1: antiepileptics
- **SIDE-EFFECTS**
  ▸ **Common or very common** Anxiety · appetite abnormal · back pain · behaviour abnormal · confusion · dizziness · drowsiness · dysarthria · fatigue · gait abnormal · irritability · movement disorders · nausea · vertigo · vision disorders · weight increased
  ▸ **Frequency not known** Severe cutaneous adverse reactions (SCARs) · suicidal behaviours
- **PREGNANCY** Manufacturer advises avoid. See also *Pregnancy* in Epilepsy p. 321.
  Monitoring The dose should be monitored carefully during pregnancy and after birth, and adjustments made on a clinical basis.
- **BREAST FEEDING** Avoid—present in milk in *animal* studies.
- **HEPATIC IMPAIRMENT** Manufacturer advises caution in mild to moderate impairment; avoid in severe impairment.
  Dose adjustments Manufacturer advises maximum 8 mg per day in mild to moderate impairment.
- **RENAL IMPAIRMENT** Avoid in moderate or severe impairment.
- **PRESCRIBING AND DISPENSING INFORMATION**
  Switching between formulations Care should be taken when switching between oral formulations. The need for continued supply of a particular manufacturer's product should be based on clinical judgement and consultation with the patient or their carer, taking into account factors such as seizure frequency and treatment history.
  Patients may need to be maintained on a specific manufacturer's branded or generic perampanel product.
- **PATIENT AND CARER ADVICE**
  Driving and skilled tasks Manufacturer advises patients and carers should be cautioned on the effects on driving and performance of skilled tasks—increased risk of dizziness and drowsiness.
- **NATIONAL FUNDING/ACCESS DECISIONS**
  For full details see funding body website

4

Nervous system

▶ Perampanel (*Fycompa*®) for the adjunctive treatment of partial-onset seizures with or without secondary generalised seizures in patients with epilepsy aged 12 years and older (December 2012) SMC No. 819/12 Recommended with restrictions

▶ Perampanel oral suspension (*Fycompa*®) for the adjunctive treatment of partial-onset seizures with or without secondary generalised seizures in patients with epilepsy aged 12 years and older (August 2019) SMC No. SMC2172 Recommended with restrictions

● MEDICINAL FORMS There can be variation in the licensing of different medicines containing the same drug. Forms available from special-order manufacturers include: oral suspension

Oral suspension

CAUTIONARY AND ADVISORY LABELS 3, 8

EXCIPIENTS: May contain Sorbitol

▶ Fycompa (Eisai Ltd)

Perampanel 500 microgram per 1 ml Fycompa 0.5mg/ml oral suspension sugar-free | 340 ml [PoM] £127.50 DT = £127.50

Tablet

CAUTIONARY AND ADVISORY LABELS 3, 8, 25

▶ Fycompa (Eisai Ltd)

Perampanel 2 mg Fycompa 2mg tablets | 7 tablet [PoM] £35.00 DT = £35.00 | 28 tablet [PoM] £140.00 DT = £140.00

Perampanel 4 mg Fycompa 4mg tablets | 28 tablet [PoM] £140.00 DT = £140.00

Perampanel 6 mg Fycompa 6mg tablets | 28 tablet [PoM] £140.00 DT = £140.00

Perampanel 8 mg Fycompa 8mg tablets | 28 tablet [PoM] £140.00 DT = £140.00

Perampanel 10 mg Fycompa 10mg tablets | 28 tablet [PoM] £140.00 DT = £140.00

Perampanel 12 mg Fycompa 12mg tablets | 28 tablet [PoM] £140.00 DT = £140.00

Phenytoin

07-Dec-2020

● INDICATIONS AND DOSE

Tonic-clonic seizures | Focal seizures

▶ BY MOUTH

▶ Child 1 month–11 years: Initially 1.5–2.5 mg/kg twice daily, then adjusted according to response to 2.5–5 mg/kg twice daily (max. per dose 7.5 mg/kg twice daily), dose also adjusted according to plasma-phenytoin concentration; maximum 300 mg per day

▶ Child 12–17 years: Initially 75–150 mg twice daily, then adjusted according to response to 150–200 mg twice daily (max. per dose 300 mg twice daily), dose also adjusted according to plasma-phenytoin concentration

Tonic-clonic seizures | Focal seizures | Prevention and treatment of seizures during or following neurosurgery or severe head injury

▶ BY MOUTH

▶ Adult: Initially 3–4 mg/kg daily, alternatively 150–300 mg once daily, alternatively 150–300 mg daily in 2 divided doses; usual maintenance 200–500 mg daily, to be taken preferably with or after food, dose to be increased gradually as necessary (with plasma-phenytoin concentration monitoring), exceptionally, higher doses may be used

Prevention and treatment of seizures during or following neurosurgery or severe head injury

▶ BY MOUTH

▶ Child: Initially 2.5 mg/kg twice daily, then adjusted according to response to 4–8 mg/kg daily, dose also adjusted according to plasma-phenytoin concentration; maximum 300 mg per day

Status epilepticus | Acute symptomatic seizures associated with head trauma or neurosurgery

▶ INITIALLY BY SLOW INTRAVENOUS INJECTION, OR BY INTRAVENOUS INFUSION

▶ Child 1 month–11 years: Loading dose 20 mg/kg, then (by slow intravenous injection or by intravenous infusion) 2.5–5 mg/kg twice daily

▶ Child 12–17 years: Loading dose 20 mg/kg, then (by intravenous infusion or by slow intravenous injection) up to 100 mg 3–4 times a day

▶ Adult: Loading dose 20 mg/kg (max. per dose 2 g), then (by intravenous infusion or by slow intravenous injection or by mouth) maintenance 100 mg every 6–8 hours adjusted according to plasma-concentration monitoring

DOSE EQUIVALENCE AND CONVERSION

▶ Preparations containing phenytoin sodium are **not** bioequivalent to those containing phenytoin base (such as *Epanutin Infatabs*® and *Epanutin*® suspension); 100 mg of phenytoin sodium is approximately equivalent in therapeutic effect to 92 mg phenytoin base. The dose is the same for all phenytoin products when initiating therapy. However, if switching between these products the difference in phenytoin content may be clinically significant. Care is needed when making changes between formulations and plasma-phenytoin concentration monitoring is recommended.

● UNLICENSED USE

▶ With oral use in children Licensed for use in children (age range not specified by manufacturer).

▶ With intravenous use Phenytoin doses in BNF publications may differ from those in product literature.

> IMPORTANT SAFETY INFORMATION
>
> MHRA/CHM ADVICE: ANTIEPILEPTICS: RISK OF SUICIDAL THOUGHTS AND BEHAVIOUR (AUGUST 2008)
> See Epilepsy p. 321.
>
> NHS IMPROVEMENT PATIENT SAFETY ALERT: RISK OF DEATH AND SEVERE HARM FROM ERROR WITH INJECTABLE PHENYTOIN (NOVEMBER 2016)
> Use of injectable phenytoin is error-prone throughout the prescribing, preparation, administration and monitoring processes; all relevant staff should be made aware of appropriate guidance on the safe use of injectable phenytoin to reduce the risk of error.
>
> MHRA/CHM ADVICE: ANTIEPILEPTIC DRUGS: UPDATED ADVICE ON SWITCHING BETWEEN DIFFERENT MANUFACTURERS' PRODUCTS (NOVEMBER 2017)
> See Epilepsy p. 321 and see also *Prescribing and dispensing information*.

● CONTRA-INDICATIONS

GENERAL CONTRA-INDICATIONS Acute porphyrias p. 1107

SPECIFIC CONTRA-INDICATIONS

▶ With intravenous use Second- and third-degree heart block · sino-atrial block · sinus bradycardia · Stokes-Adams syndrome

● CAUTIONS

GENERAL CAUTIONS Enteral feeding (interrupt feeding for 2 hours before and after dose; more frequent monitoring may be necessary)

SPECIFIC CAUTIONS

▶ With intravenous use Heart failure · hypotension · injection solutions alkaline (irritant to tissues) · respiratory depression · resuscitation facilities must be available

CAUTIONS, FURTHER INFORMATION Consider vitamin D supplementation in patients who are immobilised for long periods or who have inadequate sun exposure or dietary intake of calcium.

Intramuscular phenytoin should not be used (absorption is slow and erratic).

● INTERACTIONS → Appendix 1: antiepileptics

● SIDE-EFFECTS

GENERAL SIDE-EFFECTS

Agranulocytosis · bone disorders · bone fracture · bone marrow disorders · cerebrovascular insufficiency · coarsening of the facial features · confusion · constipation · dizziness · drowsiness · Dupuytren's contracture · dysarthria · eosinophilia · fever · gingival hyperplasia (maintain good oral hygiene) · granulocytopenia · hair changes · headache · hepatic disorders · hypersensitivity · insomnia · joint disorders · leucopenia · lip swelling · lymphatic abnormalities · macrocytosis · megaloblastic anaemia · movement disorders · muscle twitching · nausea · neoplasms · nephritis tubulointerstitial · nervousness · nystagmus · paraesthesia · Peyronie's disease · polyarteritis nodosa · pseudolymphoma · sensory peripheral polyneuropathy · severe cutaneous adverse reactions (SCARs) · skin reactions · suicidal behaviours · systemic lupus erythematosus (SLE) · taste altered · thrombocytopenia · tremor · vertigo · vomiting

SPECIFIC SIDE-EFFECTS

▸ With oral use Electrolyte imbalance · pneumonitis · vitamin D deficiency

▸ With parenteral use Arrhythmias · atrial conduction depression (more common if injection too rapid) · cardiac arrest · extravasation necrosis · hypotension · injection site necrosis · purple glove syndrome · respiratory arrest (more common if injection too rapid) · respiratory disorders · tonic seizure (more common if injection too rapid) · ventricular conduction depression (more common if injection too rapid) · ventricular fibrillation (more common if injection too rapid)

SIDE-EFFECTS, FURTHER INFORMATION **Rash** Discontinue; if mild re-introduce cautiously but discontinue immediately if recurrence.

Bradycardia and hypotension With intravenous use; reduce rate of administration if bradycardia or hypotension occurs.

Overdose Symptoms of phenytoin toxicity include nystagmus, diplopia, slurred speech, ataxia, confusion, and hyperglycaemia.

● ALLERGY AND CROSS-SENSITIVITY Cross-sensitivity reported with carbamazepine. Antiepileptic hypersensitivity syndrome associated with phenytoin. See under Epilepsy p. 321 for more information.

● PREGNANCY See also *Pregnancy* in Epilepsy p. 321. **Monitoring** Changes in plasma-protein binding make interpretation of plasma-phenytoin concentrations difficult—monitor unbound fraction.
Doses should be adjusted on the basis of plasma-drug concentration monitoring.

● BREAST FEEDING Small amounts present in milk, but not known to be harmful.

● HEPATIC IMPAIRMENT Manufacturer advises caution (increased risk of accumulation and toxicity due to decreased protein binding in hepatic impairment, hypoalbuminaemia, or hyperbilirubinaemia).
Dose adjustments ▸ With oral use Manufacturer advises consider dose reduction.
▸ With intravenous use Manufacturer advises consider maintenance dose reduction.

● PRE-TREATMENT SCREENING HLAB* 1502 allele in individuals of Han Chinese or Thai origin—avoid unless essential (increased risk of Stevens- Johnson syndrome).

● MONITORING REQUIREMENTS

▸ **Blood counts** Manufacturer recommends blood counts (but evidence of practical value uncertain).

▸ In adults The usual total plasma-phenytoin concentration for optimum response is 10–20 mg/litre (or 40–80 micromol/litre). In pregnancy, the elderly, and certain disease states where protein binding may be reduced, careful interpretation of total plasma-phenytoin concentration is necessary; it may be more appropriate to measure free plasma-phenytoin concentration.

▸ In children Therapeutic plasma-phenytoin concentrations reduced in first 3 months of life because of reduced protein binding. Trough plasma concentration for optimum response: neonate–3 months, 6–15 mg/litre (25–60 micromol/litre); child 3 months–18 years, 10–20 mg/litre (40–80 micromol/litre).

▸ With intravenous use Monitor ECG and blood pressure.

● DIRECTIONS FOR ADMINISTRATION Manufacturer advises each injection or infusion should be preceded and followed by an injection of Sodium Chloride 0.9% through the same needle or catheter to avoid local venous irritation.

▸ With intravenous use in children [EvGr] For *intravenous injection*, give into a large vein at a rate not exceeding 1 mg/kg/minute (max. 50 mg/minute). ⒹManufacturer advises for *intravenous infusion*, dilute to a concentration not exceeding 10 mg/mL with Sodium Chloride 0.9% and give into a large vein through an in-line filter (0.22–0.50 micron). [EvGr] Give at a rate not exceeding 1 mg/kg/minute (max. 50 mg/minute). ⒹComplete administration within 1 hour of preparation.

▸ With intravenous use in adults Manufacturer advises for *intravenous injection*, give into a large vein at a rate not exceeding 50 mg/minute; rate of 25 mg/minute or lower may be more appropriate in some patients (including the elderly and those with heart disease). Manufacturer advises for *intravenous infusion*, dilute in 50–100 mL Sodium Chloride 0.9% (final concentration not to exceed 10 mg/mL) and give into a large vein through an in-line filter (0.22–0.50 micron) at a rate not exceeding 50 mg/minute; rate of 25 mg/minute or lower may be more appropriate in some patients (including the elderly and those with heart disease). Complete administration within 1 hour of preparation.

● PRESCRIBING AND DISPENSING INFORMATION
Switching between formulations Different formulations of oral preparations may vary in bioavailability. Patients being treated for epilepsy should be maintained on a specific manufacturer's product.

● PATIENT AND CARER ADVICE
Blood or skin disorders Patients or their carers should be told how to recognise signs of blood or skin disorders, and advised to seek immediate medical attention if symptoms such as fever, rash, mouth ulcers, bruising, or bleeding develop. Leucopenia that is severe, progressive, or associated with clinical symptoms requires withdrawal (if necessary under cover of a suitable alternative).
Medicines for Children leaflet: Phenytoin for preventing seizures
www.medicinesforchildren.org.uk/phenytoin-preventing-seizures

● MEDICINAL FORMS There can be variation in the licensing of different medicines containing the same drug. Forms available from special-order manufacturers include: chewable tablet, oral suspension, oral solution

Tablet
CAUTIONARY AND ADVISORY LABELS 8
▸ Phenytoin (Non-proprietary)
Phenytoin sodium 100 mg Phenytoin sodium 100mg tablets | 28 tablet [PoM] £30.00 DT = £10.45

4

Nervous system

Solution for injection

EXCIPIENTS: May contain Alcohol, propylene glycol
ELECTROLYTES: May contain Sodium

▸ Phenytoin (Non-proprietary)

Phenytoin sodium 50 mg per 1 ml Phenytoin sodium 250mg/5ml solution for injection ampoules | 5 ampoule [PoM] £24.40 (Hospital only)

▸ Epanutin (Upjohn UK Ltd)

Phenytoin sodium 50 mg per 1 ml Epanutin Ready-Mixed Parenteral 250mg/5ml solution for injection ampoules | 10 ampoule [PoM] £48.79 (Hospital only)

Oral suspension

CAUTIONARY AND ADVISORY LABELS 8

▸ Epanutin (Upjohn UK Ltd)

Phenytoin 6 mg per 1 ml Epanutin 30mg/5ml oral suspension | 500 ml [PoM] £4.27 DT = £4.27

Chewable tablet

CAUTIONARY AND ADVISORY LABELS 8, 24

▸ Epanutin (Upjohn UK Ltd)

Phenytoin 50 mg Epanutin Infatabs 50mg chewable tablets | 200 tablet [PoM] £13.18 DT = £13.18

Capsule

CAUTIONARY AND ADVISORY LABELS 8

▸ Phenytoin (Non-proprietary)

Phenytoin sodium 25 mg Phenytoin sodium 25mg capsules | 28 capsule [PoM] £7.24 DT = £7.24

Phenytoin sodium 50 mg Phenytoin sodium 50mg capsules | 28 capsule [PoM] £7.07 DT = £7.07

Phenytoin sodium 100 mg Phenytoin sodium 100mg capsules | 84 capsule [PoM] £67.50 DT = £12.78

Phenytoin sodium 300 mg Phenytoin sodium 300mg capsules | 28 capsule [PoM] £9.11 DT = £9.11

Pregabalin

18-Nov-2020

● INDICATIONS AND DOSE

Peripheral and central neuropathic pain

▸ BY MOUTH

▸ **Adult:** Initially 150 mg daily in 2–3 divided doses, then increased if necessary to 300 mg daily in 2–3 divided doses, dose to be increased after 3–7 days, then increased if necessary up to 600 mg daily in 2–3 divided doses, dose to be increased after 7 days

Adjunctive therapy for focal seizures with or without secondary generalisation

▸ BY MOUTH

▸ **Adult:** Initially 25 mg twice daily, then increased in steps of 50 mg daily, dose to be increased at 7 day intervals, increased to 300 mg daily in 2–3 divided doses for 7 days, then increased if necessary up to 600 mg daily in 2–3 divided doses

Generalised anxiety disorder

▸ BY MOUTH

▸ **Adult:** Initially 150 mg daily in 2–3 divided doses, then increased in steps of 150 mg daily if required, dose to be increased at 7 day intervals, increased if necessary up to 600 mg daily in 2–3 divided doses

● UNLICENSED USE Pregabalin doses in BNF may differ from those in product literature.

IMPORTANT SAFETY INFORMATION

MHRA/CHM ADVICE: ANTIEPILEPTICS: RISK OF SUICIDAL THOUGHTS AND BEHAVIOUR (AUGUST 2008)
See Epilepsy p. 321.

MHRA/CHM ADVICE: ANTIEPILEPTIC DRUGS: UPDATED ADVICE ON SWITCHING BETWEEN DIFFERENT MANUFACTURERS' PRODUCTS (NOVEMBER 2017)
See Epilepsy p. 321.

MHRA/CHM ADVICE: PREGABALIN (*LYRICA*®) AND RISK OF ABUSE AND DEPENDENCE: NEW SCHEDULING REQUIREMENTS FROM 1 APRIL (APRIL 2019)
Following concerns about abuse, pregabalin has been reclassified as a Class C controlled substance and is now

---

a Schedule 3 drug, but is exempt from safe custody requirements. Healthcare professionals should evaluate patients carefully for a history of drug abuse before prescribing pregabalin, and observe patients for signs of abuse and dependence. Patients should be informed of the potentially fatal risks of interactions between pregabalin and alcohol, and with other medicines that cause CNS depression, particularly opioids.

● CAUTIONS Conditions that may precipitate encephalopathy · history of substance abuse · severe congestive heart failure

● INTERACTIONS → Appendix 1: antiepileptics

● SIDE-EFFECTS

▸ **Common or very common** Abdominal distension · appetite abnormal · asthenia · cervical spasm · concentration impaired · confusion · constipation · diarrhoea · dizziness · drowsiness · dry mouth · feeling abnormal · gait abnormal · gastrointestinal disorders · headache · increased risk of infection · joint disorders · memory loss · mood altered · movement disorders · muscle complaints · nausea · oedema · pain · sensation abnormal · sexual dysfunction · sleep disorders · speech impairment · vertigo · vision disorders · vomiting · weight changes

▸ **Uncommon** Aggression · anxiety · arrhythmias · atrioventricular block · breast abnormalities · chest tightness · chills · consciousness impaired · cough · depression · dry eye · dyspnoea · epistaxis · eye discomfort · eye disorders · eye inflammation · fever · hallucination · hyperacusia · hypertension · hypoglycaemia · hypotension · malaise · menstrual cycle irregularities · nasal complaints · neutropenia · oral disorders · peripheral coldness · psychiatric disorders · reflexes decreased · skin reactions · snoring · sweat changes · syncope · taste loss · thirst · urinary disorders · vasodilation

▸ **Rare or very rare** Altered smell sensation · ascites · dysgraphia · dysphagia · gynaecomastia · hepatic disorders · pancreatitis · QT interval prolongation · renal impairment · rhabdomyolysis · Stevens-Johnson syndrome · throat tightness

▸ **Frequency not known** Drug use disorders · suicidal behaviours

● PREGNANCY Manufacturer advises avoid unless potential benefit outweighs risk — toxicity in animal studies. See also *Pregnancy* in Epilepsy p. 321.

● BREAST FEEDING See *Breast-feeding* in Epilepsy p. 321.

● RENAL IMPAIRMENT
Dose adjustments Initially 75 mg daily and maximum 300 mg daily if eGFR 30–60 mL/minute/1.73 m^2.
Initially 25–50 mg daily and maximum 150 mg daily in 1–2 divided doses if eGFR 15–30 mL/minute/1.73 m^2.
Initially 25 mg once daily and maximum 75 mg once daily if eGFR less than 15 mL/minute/1.73 m^2.

● MONITORING REQUIREMENTS Monitor for signs of pregabalin abuse.

● TREATMENT CESSATION Avoid abrupt withdrawal (taper over at least 1 week).

● PRESCRIBING AND DISPENSING INFORMATION Flavours of oral liquid formulations may include strawberry.

● PATIENT AND CARER ADVICE
Patient leaflet NHS England has produced a patient leaflet with information on the reclassification of pregabalin.

● NATIONAL FUNDING/ACCESS DECISIONS
For full details see funding body website
Scottish Medicines Consortium (SMC) decisions

▸ Pregabalin (*Lyrica*®) for central neuropathic pain in adults (August 2007) SMC No. 389/07 Not recommended

▸ Pregabalin oral solution (*Lyrica*®) for the treatment of peripheral and central neuropathic pain in adults, and as adjunctive therapy in adults with partial seizures with or

without secondary generalization (June 2012) SMC No. 765/12
Recommended with restrictions

● MEDICINAL FORMS There can be variation in the licensing of different medicines containing the same drug. Forms available from special-order manufacturers include: oral suspension, oral solution

Oral solution
CAUTIONARY AND ADVISORY LABELS 3, 8
▶ Pregabalin (Non-proprietary)
  Pregabalin 20 mg per 1 ml Pregabalin 20mg/ml oral solution sugar free sugar-free | 473 ml [PoM] £99.48 DT = £99.48 Schedule 3 (CD No Register Exempt Exempt Safe Custody) sugar-free | 500 ml [PoM] £75.00–£105.16 [CD3]
▶ Lyrica (Upjohn UK Ltd)
  Lyrica 20 mg per 1 ml Lyrica 20mg/ml oral solution sugar-free | 473 ml [PoM] £99.48 DT = £99.48 [CD3]

Capsule
CAUTIONARY AND ADVISORY LABELS 3, 8
▶ Pregabalin (Non-proprietary)
  Pregabalin 25 mg Pregabalin 25mg capsules | 56 capsule [PoM] £64.40 DT = £2.06 [CD3] | 84 capsule [PoM] £2.76–£96.60 [CD3]
  Pregabalin 50 mg Pregabalin 50mg capsules | 56 capsule [PoM] £8.96 [CD3] | 84 capsule [PoM] £96.60 DT = £2.80 [CD3]
  Pregabalin 75 mg Pregabalin 75mg capsules | 14 capsule [PoM] £3.21 [CD3] | 56 capsule [PoM] £64.40 DT = £2.17 [CD3]
  Pregabalin 100 mg Pregabalin 100mg capsules | 84 capsule [PoM] £96.60 DT = £3.60 [CD3]
  Pregabalin 150 mg Pregabalin 150mg capsules | 56 capsule [PoM] £64.40 DT = £3.01 [CD3]
  Pregabalin 200 mg Pregabalin 200mg capsules | 84 capsule [PoM] £96.60 DT = £4.68 [CD3]
  Pregabalin 225 mg Pregabalin 225mg capsules | 56 capsule [PoM] £64.40 DT = £3.54 [CD3]
  Pregabalin 300 mg Pregabalin 300mg capsules | 56 capsule [PoM] £64.40 DT = £4.73 [CD3]
▶ Alzain (Dr Reddy's Laboratories (UK) Ltd)
  Pregabalin 25 mg Alzain 25mg capsules | 56 capsule [PoM] £4.99 DT = £2.06 [CD3]
  Pregabalin 50 mg Alzain 50mg capsules | 56 capsule [PoM] £5.99 [CD3] | 84 capsule [PoM] £6.99 DT = £2.80 [CD3]
  Pregabalin 75 mg Alzain 75mg capsules | 56 capsule [PoM] £5.99 DT = £2.17 [CD3]
  Pregabalin 100 mg Alzain 100mg capsules | 84 capsule [PoM] £6.99 DT = £3.60 [CD3]
  Pregabalin 150 mg Alzain 150mg capsules | 56 capsule [PoM] £6.99 DT = £3.01 [CD3]
  Pregabalin 200 mg Alzain 200mg capsules | 84 capsule [PoM] £8.99 DT = £4.68 [CD3]
  Pregabalin 225 mg Alzain 225mg capsules | 56 capsule [PoM] £7.99 DT = £3.54 [CD3]
  Pregabalin 300 mg Alzain 300mg capsules | 56 capsule [PoM] £8.99 DT = £4.73 [CD3]
▶ Axalid (Kent Pharmaceuticals Ltd)
  Pregabalin 25 mg Axalid 25mg capsules | 56 capsule [PoM] £19.95 DT = £2.06 [CD3]
  Pregabalin 50 mg Axalid 50mg capsules | 56 capsule [PoM] £19.95 [CD3]
  Pregabalin 75 mg Axalid 75mg capsules | 56 capsule [PoM] £19.95 DT = £2.17 [CD3]
  Pregabalin 100 mg Axalid 100mg capsules | 56 capsule [PoM] £19.95 [CD3]
  Pregabalin 150 mg Axalid 150mg capsules | 56 capsule [PoM] £19.95 DT = £3.01 [CD3]
  Pregabalin 200 mg Axalid 200mg capsules | 56 capsule [PoM] £19.95 [CD3]
  Pregabalin 225 mg Axalid 225mg capsules | 56 capsule [PoM] £19.95 DT = £3.54 [CD3]
  Pregabalin 300 mg Axalid 300mg capsules | 56 capsule [PoM] £19.95 DT = £4.73 [CD3]
▶ Lecaent (Accord Healthcare Ltd)
  Pregabalin 25 mg Lecaent 25mg capsules | 56 capsule [PoM] £64.39 DT = £2.06 [CD3]
  Pregabalin 50 mg Lecaent 50mg capsules | 84 capsule [PoM] £96.59 DT = £2.80 [CD3]
  Pregabalin 100 mg Lecaent 100mg capsules | 84 capsule [PoM] £96.59 DT = £3.60 [CD3]
  Pregabalin 150 mg Lecaent 150mg capsules | 56 capsule [PoM] £64.39 DT = £3.01 [CD3]

▶ Lyrica (Upjohn UK Ltd)
  Pregabalin 25 mg Lyrica 25mg capsules | 56 capsule [PoM] £64.40 DT = £2.06 [CD3] | 84 capsule [PoM] £96.60 [CD3]
  Pregabalin 50 mg Lyrica 50mg capsules | 84 capsule [PoM] £96.60 DT = £2.80 [CD3]
  Pregabalin 75 mg Lyrica 75mg capsules | 56 capsule [PoM] £64.40 DT = £2.17 [CD3]
  Pregabalin 100 mg Lyrica 100mg capsules | 84 capsule [PoM] £96.60 DT = £3.60 [CD3]
  Pregabalin 150 mg Lyrica 150mg capsules | 56 capsule [PoM] £64.40 DT = £3.01 [CD3]
  Pregabalin 200 mg Lyrica 200mg capsules | 84 capsule [PoM] £96.60 DT = £4.68 [CD3]
  Pregabalin 225 mg Lyrica 225mg capsules | 56 capsule [PoM] £64.40 DT = £3.54 [CD3]
  Pregabalin 300 mg Lyrica 300mg capsules | 56 capsule [PoM] £64.40 DT = £4.73 [CD3]

Rufinamide
02-Dec-2020

● **INDICATIONS AND DOSE**
Adjunctive treatment of seizures in Lennox-Gastaut syndrome without valproate (initiated by a specialist)
▶ BY MOUTH
▶ **Child 1–3 years:** Initially 5 mg/kg twice daily, then increased in steps of up to 5 mg/kg twice daily (max. per dose 22.5 mg/kg twice daily), adjusted according to response, dose to be increased at intervals of not less than 3 days to the target dose (maximum dose), each dose should be given to the nearest 0.5 mL
▶ **Child 4–17 years (body-weight up to 30 kg):** Initially 100 mg twice daily, then increased in steps of 100 mg twice daily (max. per dose 500 mg twice daily), adjusted according to response, dose to be increased at intervals of not less than 3 days
▶ **Child 4–17 years (body-weight 30–50 kg):** Initially 200 mg twice daily, then increased in steps of 200 mg twice daily (max. per dose 900 mg twice daily), adjusted according to response, dose to be increased at intervals of not less than 2 days
▶ **Child 4–17 years (body-weight 50.1–70 kg):** Initially 200 mg twice daily, then increased in steps of 200 mg twice daily (max. per dose 1.2 g twice daily), adjusted according to response, dose to be increased at intervals of not less than 2 days
▶ **Child 4–17 years (body-weight 70.1 kg and above):** Initially 200 mg twice daily, then increased in steps of 200 mg twice daily (max. per dose 1.6 g twice daily), adjusted according to response, dose to be increased at intervals of not less than 2 days
▶ **Adult (body-weight 30–50 kg):** Initially 200 mg twice daily, then increased in steps of 200 mg twice daily (max. per dose 900 mg twice daily), adjusted according to response, dose to be increased at intervals of not less than 2 days
▶ **Adult (body-weight 50.1–70 kg):** Initially 200 mg twice daily, then increased in steps of 200 mg twice daily (max. per dose 1.2 g twice daily), adjusted according to response, dose to be increased at intervals of not less than 2 days
▶ **Adult (body-weight 70.1 kg and above):** Initially 200 mg twice daily, then increased in steps of 200 mg twice daily (max. per dose 1.6 g twice daily), adjusted according to response, dose to be increased at intervals of not less than 2 days

Adjunctive treatment of seizures in Lennox-Gastaut syndrome with valproate (initiated by a specialist)
▶ BY MOUTH
▶ **Child 1–3 years:** Initially 5 mg/kg twice daily, then increased in steps of up to 5 mg/kg twice daily (max. per dose 15 mg/kg twice daily), adjusted according to response, dose to be increased at intervals continued →

of not less than 3 days to the target dose (maximum dose), each dose should be given to the nearest 0.5 mL
‣ Child 4-17 years (body-weight up to 30 kg): Initially 100 mg twice daily, then increased in steps of 100 mg twice daily (max. per dose 300 mg twice daily), adjusted according to response, dose to be increased at intervals of not less than 2 days
‣ Child 4-17 years (body-weight 30-50 kg): Initially 200 mg twice daily, then increased in steps of 200 mg twice daily (max. per dose 600 mg twice daily), adjusted according to response, dose to be increased at intervals of not less than 2 days
‣ Child 4-17 years (body-weight 50.1-70 kg): Initially 200 mg twice daily, then increased in steps of 200 mg twice daily (max. per dose 800 mg twice daily), adjusted according to response, dose to be increased at intervals of not less than 2 days
‣ Child 4-17 years (body-weight 70.1 kg and above): Initially 200 mg twice daily, then increased in steps of 200 mg twice daily (max. per dose 1.1 g twice daily), adjusted according to response, dose to be increased at intervals of not less than 2 days
‣ Adult (body-weight 30-50 kg): Initially 200 mg twice daily, then increased in steps of 200 mg twice daily (max. per dose 600 mg twice daily), adjusted according to response, dose to be increased at intervals of not less than 2 days
‣ Adult (body-weight 50.1-70 kg): Initially 200 mg twice daily, then increased in steps of 200 mg twice daily (max. per dose 800 mg twice daily), adjusted according to response, dose to be increased at intervals of not less than 2 days
‣ Adult (body-weight 70.1 kg and above): Initially 200 mg twice daily, then increased in steps of 200 mg twice daily (max. per dose 1.1 g twice daily), adjusted according to response, dose to be increased at intervals of not less than 2 days

---

IMPORTANT SAFETY INFORMATION

MHRA/CHM ADVICE: ANTIEPILEPTICS: RISK OF SUICIDAL THOUGHTS AND BEHAVIOUR (AUGUST 2008)
See Epilepsy p. 321.

MHRA/CHM ADVICE: ANTIEPILEPTIC DRUGS: UPDATED ADVICE ON SWITCHING BETWEEN DIFFERENT MANUFACTURERS' PRODUCTS (NOVEMBER 2017)
See Epilepsy p. 321 and see also *Prescribing and dispensing information.*

● CAUTIONS Patients at risk of further shortening of QTc interval
● INTERACTIONS → Appendix 1: antiepileptics
● SIDE-EFFECTS
‣ **Common or very common** Anxiety · appetite decreased · back pain · constipation · diarrhoea · dizziness · drowsiness · eating disorder · epistaxis · fatigue · gait abnormal · gastrointestinal discomfort · headache · increased risk of infection · insomnia · movement disorders · nausea · nystagmus · oligomenorrhoea · seizures · skin reactions · tremor · vertigo · vision disorders · vomiting · weight decreased
‣ **Uncommon** Hypersensitivity
‣ **Frequency not known** Suicidal behaviours
● ALLERGY AND CROSS-SENSITIVITY Antiepileptic hypersensitivity syndrome associated with rufinamide. See under Epilepsy p. 321 for more information.
● PREGNANCY Manufacturer advises avoid unless essential—toxicity in *animal* studies. See also *Pregnancy* in Epilepsy p. 321.
● BREAST FEEDING Manufacturer advises avoid—no information available.

● HEPATIC IMPAIRMENT Manufacturer advises caution in mild to moderate impairment; avoid in severe impairment (no information available).
Dose adjustments Manufacturer advises cautious dose titration in mild to moderate impairment.
● DIRECTIONS FOR ADMINISTRATION Manufacturer advises tablets may be crushed and given in half a glass of water.
● PRESCRIBING AND DISPENSING INFORMATION
Switching between formulations Care should be taken when switching between oral formulations. The need for continued supply of a particular manufacturer's product should be based on clinical judgement and consultation with the patient or their carer, taking into account factors such as seizure frequency and treatment history.
Patients may need to be maintained on a specific manufacturer's branded or generic rufinamide product.
● PATIENT AND CARER ADVICE Counselling on antiepileptic hypersensitivity syndrome is advised.
Medicines for Children leaflet: Rufinamide for preventing seizures www.medicinesforchildren.org.uk/rufinamide-preventing-seizures
Driving and skilled tasks Manufacturer advises patients and carers should be cautioned on the effects on driving and performance of skilled tasks—increased risk of dizziness, somnolence and blurred vision.
● NATIONAL FUNDING/ACCESS DECISIONS
For full details see funding body website
Scottish Medicines Consortium (SMC) decisions
‣ Rufinamide (*Inovelon*®) as adjunctive therapy in the treatment of seizures associated with Lennox-Gastaut syndrome in patients four years and older (November 2008) SMC No. 416/07 Recommended with restrictions
‣ Rufinamide 40 mg/mL oral suspension (*Inovelon*®) as adjunctive therapy in the treatment of seizures associated with Lennox-Gastaut syndrome (LGS) in patients 4 years of age or older (July 2012) SMC No. 795/12 Recommended with restrictions
‣ Rufinamide (*Inovelon*®) as adjunctive therapy in the treatment of seizures associated with Lennox-Gastaut syndrome in patients aged 1 year up to 4 years (April 2019) SMC No. SMC2146 Recommended with restrictions
All Wales Medicines Strategy Group (AWMSG) decisions
‣ Rufinamide 40 mg/mL oral suspension (*Inovelon*®) as adjunctive therapy in the treatment of seizures associated with Lennox-Gastaut syndrome in patients 1 year of age and older (June 2019) AWMSG No. 991 Recommended with restrictions

● MEDICINAL FORMS There can be variation in the licensing of different medicines containing the same drug.
Oral suspension
CAUTIONARY AND ADVISORY LABELS 8, 21
EXCIPIENTS: May contain Propylene glycol
‣ Inovelon (Eisai Ltd)
Rufinamide 40 mg per 1 ml Inovelon 40mg/ml oral suspension sugar-free | 460 ml [PoM] £94.71 DT = £94.71
Tablet
CAUTIONARY AND ADVISORY LABELS 8, 21
‣ Inovelon (Eisai Ltd)
Rufinamide 100 mg Inovelon 100mg tablets | 10 tablet [PoM] £5.15 DT = £5.15
Rufinamide 200 mg Inovelon 200mg tablets | 60 tablet [PoM] £61.77 DT = £61.77
Rufinamide 400 mg Inovelon 400mg tablets | 60 tablet [PoM] £102.96 DT = £102.96

Sodium valproate

24-Nov-2020

● **INDICATIONS AND DOSE**

All forms of epilepsy

▶ BY MOUTH USING IMMEDIATE-RELEASE MEDICINES
▶ Child 1 month–11 years: Initially 10–15 mg/kg daily in 1–2 divided doses (max. per dose 600 mg); maintenance 25–30 mg/kg daily in 2 divided doses, doses up to 60 mg/kg daily in 2 divided doses may be used in infantile spasms; monitor clinical chemistry and haematological parameters if dose exceeds 40 mg/kg daily
▶ Child 12–17 years: Initially 600 mg daily in 1–2 divided doses, increased in steps of 150–300 mg every 3 days; maintenance 1–2 g daily in 2 divided doses; maximum 2.5 g per day
▶ Adult: Initially 600 mg daily in 1–2 divided doses, then increased in steps of 150–300 mg every 3 days; maintenance 1–2 g daily, alternatively maintenance 20–30 mg/kg daily; maximum 2.5 g per day

Initiation of valproate treatment

▶ INITIALLY BY INTRAVENOUS INJECTION
▶ Adult: Initially 10 mg/kg, (usually 400–800 mg), followed by (by intravenous infusion or by intravenous injection) up to 2.5 g daily in 2–4 divided doses, alternatively (by continuous intravenous infusion) up to 2.5 g daily; (by intravenous injection or by intravenous infusion or by continuous intravenous infusion) usual dose 1–2 g daily, alternatively (by intravenous injection or by intravenous infusion or by continuous intravenous infusion) usual dose 20–30 mg/kg daily, intravenous injection to be administered over 3–5 minutes

Continuation of valproate treatment

▶ BY INTRAVENOUS INJECTION, OR BY INTRAVENOUS INFUSION, OR BY CONTINUOUS INTRAVENOUS INFUSION
▶ Adult: If switching from oral therapy to intravenous therapy give the same dose as current oral daily dose, give over 3–5 minutes by intravenous injection *or* in 2–4 divided doses by intravenous infusion

Migraine prophylaxis

▶ BY MOUTH USING IMMEDIATE-RELEASE MEDICINES
▶ Adult: Initially 200 mg twice daily, then increased if necessary to 1.2–1.5 g daily in divided doses

EPILIM CHRONOSPHERE ®

All forms of epilepsy

▶ BY MOUTH
▶ Adult: Total daily dose to be given in 1–2 divided doses (consult product literature)

EPILIM CHRONO ®

All forms of epilepsy

▶ BY MOUTH
▶ Adult: Total daily dose to be given in 1–2 divided doses (consult product literature)

EPISENTA ® CAPSULES

All forms of epilepsy

▶ BY MOUTH
▶ Adult: Total daily dose to be given in 1–2 divided doses (consult product literature)

Mania

▶ BY MOUTH
▶ Adult: Initially 750 mg daily in 1–2 divided doses, adjusted according to response, usual dose 1–2 g daily in 1–2 divided doses, doses greater than 45 mg/kg daily require careful monitoring

EPISENTA ® GRANULES

All forms of epilepsy

▶ BY MOUTH
▶ Adult: Total daily dose to be given in 1–2 divided doses (consult product literature)

Mania

▶ BY MOUTH
▶ Adult: Initially 750 mg daily in 1–2 divided doses, adjusted according to response, usual dose 1–2 g daily in 1–2 divided doses, doses greater than 45 mg/kg daily require careful monitoring

EPIVAL ®

All forms of epilepsy

▶ BY MOUTH
▶ Adult: Total daily dose to be given in 1–2 divided doses (consult product literature)

● **UNLICENSED USE** Not licensed for migraine prophylaxis.

IMPORTANT SAFETY INFORMATION

MHRA/CHM ADVICE: ANTIEPILEPTICS: RISK OF SUICIDAL THOUGHTS AND BEHAVIOUR (AUGUST 2008)
See Epilepsy p. 321.

MHRA/CHM ADVICE: ANTIEPILEPTIC DRUGS: UPDATED ADVICE ON SWITCHING BETWEEN DIFFERENT MANUFACTURERS' PRODUCTS (NOVEMBER 2017)
See Epilepsy p. 321 and see also *Prescribing and dispensing information.*

MHRA/CHM ADVICE: VALPROATE MEDICINES: CONTRA-INDICATED IN WOMEN AND GIRLS OF CHILDBEARING POTENTIAL UNLESS CONDITIONS OF PREGNANCY PREVENTION PROGRAMME ARE MET (APRIL 2018)
Valproate is highly teratogenic and evidence supports that use in pregnancy leads to neurodevelopmental disorders (approx. 30–40% risk) and congenital malformations (approx. 10% risk).

Valproate must not be used in women and girls of childbearing potential unless the conditions of the Pregnancy Prevention Programme are met (see *Conception and contraception*) and only if other treatments are ineffective or not tolerated, as judged by an experienced specialist.

Use of valproate in pregnancy is contra-indicated for migraine prophylaxis [unlicensed] and bipolar disorder; it must only be considered for epilepsy if there is no suitable alternative treatment (see *Pregnancy*).

Women and girls (and their carers) must be fully informed of the risks and the need to avoid exposure to valproate medicines in pregnancy; supporting materials have been provided to use in the implementation of the Pregnancy Prevention Programme (see *Prescribing and dispensing Information*). The MHRA advises that:

● GPs must recall all women and girls who may be of childbearing potential, provide the Patient Guide, check they have been reviewed by a specialist in the last year and are on highly effective contraception;
● Specialists must book in review appointments at least annually with women and girls under the Pregnancy Prevention Programme, re-evaluate treatment as necessary, explain clearly the conditions as outlined in the supporting materials and complete and sign the Risk Acknowledgement Form—copies of the form must be given to the patient or carer and sent to their GP;
● Pharmacists must ensure valproate medicines are dispensed in whole packs whenever possible—all packs dispensed to women and girls of childbearing potential should have a warning label either on the carton or via a sticker. They must also discuss risks in pregnancy with female patients each time valproate medicines are dispensed, ensure they have the Patient Guide and have seen their GP or specialist to discuss their treatment and the need for contraception.

4

Nervous system

MHRA/CHM ADVICE: VALPROATE MEDICINES: ARE YOU ACTING IN COMPLIANCE WITH THE PREGNANCY PREVENTION MEASURES? (DECEMBER 2018)

The MHRA advises that all healthcare professionals must continue to identify and review all female patients on valproate, including when used outside licensed indications (off-label use) and provide them with the patient information materials every time they attend appointments or receive their medicines.

Guidance for psychiatrists on the withdrawal of, and alternatives to, valproate in women of childbearing potential who have a psychiatric illness is available from the Royal College of Psychiatrists.

MHRA/CHM ADVICE: VALPROATE MEDICINES AND SERIOUS HARMS IN PREGNANCY: NEW ANNUAL RISK ACKNOWLEDGEMENT FORM AND CLINICAL GUIDANCE FROM PROFESSIONAL BODIES TO SUPPORT COMPLIANCE WITH THE PREGNANCY PREVENTION PROGRAMME (APRIL 2019)

The Annual Risk Acknowledgement Form has been updated and should be used for all future reviews of female patients on valproate. Specialists should comply with guidance given on the form if they consider the patient is not at risk of pregnancy, including the need for review in case her risk status changes.

Guidance has been published to support healthcare professionals with the use of valproate. These include a summary by NICE of their guidance and safety advice, pan-college guidance by national healthcare bodies, and paediatric guidance by the British Paediatric Neurology Association and the Royal College of Paediatrics and Child Health.

MHRA/CHM ADVICE (UPDATED JANUARY 2020): VALPROATE PREGNANCY PREVENTION PROGRAMME

The Guide for Healthcare Professionals has been updated and should be used for all future reviews of female patients on valproate medicines, in conjunction with other supporting materials (see *Prescribing and dispensing Information*).

MHRA/CHM ADVICE (UPDATED MAY 2020): VALPROATE PREGNANCY PREVENTION PROGRAMME: TEMPORARY ADVICE FOR MANAGEMENT DURING CORONAVIRUS (COVID-19)

The MHRA has issued temporary guidance for female patients on valproate during the coronavirus (COVID-19) pandemic to support adherence to the Pregnancy Prevention Programme, particularly for those who are shielding due to other health conditions, and should be followed until further notice.

- CONTRA-INDICATIONS Acute porphyrias p. 1107 · known or suspected mitochondrial disorders (higher rate of acute liver failure and liver-related deaths) · personal or family history of severe hepatic dysfunction · urea cycle disorders (risk of hyperammonaemia)

- CAUTIONS Systemic lupus erythematosus

CAUTIONS, FURTHER INFORMATION Consider vitamin D supplementation in patients that are immobilised for long periods or who have inadequate sun exposure or dietary intake of calcium.

▸ Liver toxicity Liver dysfunction (including fatal hepatic failure) has occurred in association with valproate (especially in children under 3 years and in those with metabolic or degenerative disorders, organic brain disease or severe seizure disorders associated with mental retardation) usually in first 6 months and usually involving multiple antiepileptic therapy. Raised liver enzymes during valproate treatment are usually transient but patients should be reassessed clinically and liver function (including prothrombin time) monitored until return to normal—discontinue if abnormally prolonged prothrombin time (particularly in association with other relevant abnormalities).

- INTERACTIONS → Appendix 1: antiepileptics

- SIDE-EFFECTS

GENERAL SIDE-EFFECTS

- ▸ **Common or very common** Abdominal pain · agitation · alopecia (regrowth may be curly) · anaemia · behaviour abnormal · concentration impaired · confusion · deafness · diarrhoea · drowsiness · haemorrhage · hallucination · headache · hepatic disorders · hypersensitivity · hyponatraemia · memory loss · menstrual cycle irregularities · movement disorders · nail disorder · nausea · nystagmus · oral disorders · seizures · stupor · thrombocytopenia · tremor · urinary disorders · vomiting · weight increased

- ▸ **Uncommon** Androgenetic alopecia · angioedema · bone disorders · bone fracture · bone marrow disorders · coma · encephalopathy · hair changes · hypothermia · leucopenia · pancreatitis · paraesthesia · parkinsonism · peripheral oedema · pleural effusion · renal failure · SIADH · skin reactions · vasculitis · virilism

- ▸ **Rare or very rare** Agranulocytosis · cerebral atrophy · cognitive disorder · dementia · diplopia · gynaecomastia · hyperammonaemia · hypothyroidism · infertility male · learning disability · myelodysplastic syndrome · nephritis tubulointerstitial · obesity · polycystic ovaries · red blood cell abnormalities · rhabdomyolysis · severe cutaneous adverse reactions (SCARs) · systemic lupus erythematosus (SLE) · urine abnormalities

- ▸ **Frequency not known** Alertness increased · suicidal behaviours

SPECIFIC SIDE-EFFECTS

- ▸ **Common or very common**

- ▸ With intravenous use Dizziness

SIDE-EFFECTS, FURTHER INFORMATION **Hepatic dysfunction** Withdraw treatment immediately if persistent vomiting and abdominal pain, anorexia, jaundice, oedema, malaise, drowsiness, or loss of seizure control.

Pancreatitis Discontinue treatment if symptoms of pancreatitis develop.

- CONCEPTION AND CONTRACEPTION The MHRA advises that all women and girls of childbearing potential being treated with valproate medicines must be supported on a Pregnancy Prevention Programme—pregnancy should be excluded before treatment initiation and highly effective contraception must be used during treatment.

- PREGNANCY For *migraine prophylaxis*[unlicensed] and *bipolar disorder*, the MHRA advises that valproate must not be used. For *epilepsy*, the MHRA advises valproate must not be used unless there is no suitable alternative treatment; in such cases, access to counselling about the risks should be provided (see Healthcare Professional Guide for more information) and a Risk Acknowledgement Form signed by both specialist and patient. If valproate is to be used during pregnancy, the lowest effective dose should be prescribed in divided doses or as modified-release tablets to avoid peaks in plasma-valproate concentrations; doses greater than 1 g daily are associated with an increased risk of teratogenicity. Neonatal bleeding (related to hypofibrinaemia) reported. Neonatal hepatotoxicity also reported. See also *Pregnancy* in Epilepsy p. 321.

Monitoring Specialist prenatal monitoring should be instigated when valproate has been taken in pregnancy.

The dose should be monitored carefully during pregnancy and after birth, and adjustments made on a clinical basis.

- BREAST FEEDING Present in milk—risk of haematological disorders in breast-fed newborns and infants.

- HEPATIC IMPAIRMENT Manufacturer advises avoid.

● **RENAL IMPAIRMENT**
Dose adjustments Reduce dose.

● **MONITORING REQUIREMENTS**
▶ Plasma-valproate concentrations are not a useful index of efficacy, therefore routine monitoring is unhelpful.
▶ Monitor liver function before therapy and during first 6 months especially in patients most at risk.
▶ Measure full blood count and ensure no undue potential for bleeding before starting and before surgery.

● **EFFECT ON LABORATORY TESTS** False-positive urine tests for ketones.

● **TREATMENT CESSATION** [EvGr] Avoid abrupt withdrawal; if treatment with valproate is stopped, reduce the dose gradually over at least 4 weeks. ⟨A⟩

● **DIRECTIONS FOR ADMINISTRATION**
▶ With intravenous use Manufacturer advises for *intravenous injection*, give over 3–5 minutes. For *intravenous infusion*, dilute with Glucose 5% or Sodium Chloride 0.9%. Reconstitute *Epilim* ® with solvent provided then dilute with infusion fluid if required. Displacement value may be significant, consult local guidelines.
EPIVAL ® Manufacturer advises tablets may be halved but not crushed or chewed.
EPISENTA ® CAPSULES Manufacturer advises contents of capsule may be mixed with soft food or drink that is cold or at room temperature and swallowed immediately without chewing.
EPILIM ® SYRUP Manufacturer advises may be diluted, preferably in Syrup BP; use within 14 days.
EPISENTA ® GRANULES, EPILIM CHRONOSPHERE ® Manufacturer advises granules may be mixed with soft food or drink that is cold or at room temperature and swallowed immediately without chewing.

● **PRESCRIBING AND DISPENSING INFORMATION** The Pregnancy Prevention Programme is supported by the following materials provided by the manufacturer: *Patient Guide, Guide for Healthcare Professionals, Risk Acknowledgement Form*, and for pharmacists, *Patient Cards* and *Stickers with warning symbols*; the MHRA has also produced a patient information sheet providing advice for women and girls taking valproate medicines.
   The Royal Pharmaceutical Society has also produced a safe supply algorithm, available at: www.rpharms.com/safesupplyvalproate
Switching between formulations Care should be taken when switching between oral formulations in the treatment of epilepsy. The need for continued supply of a particular manufacturer's product should be based on clinical judgement and consultation with the patient or their carer, taking into account factors such as seizure frequency and treatment history.
   Patients being treated for epilepsy may need to be maintained on a specific manufacturer's branded or generic oral sodium valproate product.
EPILIM CHRONOSPHERE ® Prescribe dose to the nearest whole 50-mg sachet.

● **PATIENT AND CARER ADVICE**
Valproate use by women and girls The MHRA advises women and girls should **not** stop taking valproate without first discussing it with their doctor.
Blood or hepatic disorders Patients or their carers should be told how to recognise signs and symptoms of blood or liver disorders and advised to seek immediate medical attention if symptoms develop.
Pancreatitis Patients or their carers should be told how to recognise signs and symptoms of pancreatitis and advised to seek immediate medical attention if symptoms such as abdominal pain, nausea, or vomiting develop.

Pregnancy Prevention Programme Pharmacists must ensure that female patients have a patient card—see also *Important safety information.*
Medicines for Children leaflet: Sodium valproate for preventing seizures www.medicinesforchildren.org.uk/sodium-valproate-preventing-seizures
Medicines for Children leaflet: Sodium valproate and pregnancy - information for girls and young women
www.medicinesforchildren.org.uk/sodium-valproate-and-pregnancy-information-girls-and-young-women
Medicines for Children leaflet: Sodium valproate and pregnancy - information for parents and carers www.medicinesforchildren.org.uk/sodium-valproate-and-pregnancy-information-parents-and-carers

EPISENTA ® CAPSULES Patients and carers should be counselled on the administration of capsules.

EPISENTA ® GRANULES Patients and carers should be counselled on the administration of granules.

EPILIM CHRONOSPHERE ® Patients and carers should be counselled on the administration of granules.

● **MEDICINAL FORMS** There can be variation in the licensing of different medicines containing the same drug. Forms available from special-order manufacturers include: oral suspension, oral solution, suppository

Modified-release tablet
CAUTIONARY AND ADVISORY LABELS 8, 10, 21, 25
▶ Sodium valproate (Non-proprietary)
Sodium valproate 200 mg Dyzantil 200mg modified-release tablets | 30 tablet [PoM] £2.45 DT = £3.50
Sodium valproate 300 mg Dyzantil 300mg modified-release tablets | 30 tablet [PoM] £3.67 DT = £5.24
Sodium valproate 500 mg Dyzantil 500mg modified-release tablets | 30 tablet [PoM] £6.11 DT = £8.73
▶ Epilim Chrono (Sanofi) ▼
Sodium valproate 200 mg Epilim Chrono 200 tablets | 30 tablet [PoM] £3.50 DT = £3.50
Sodium valproate 300 mg Epilim Chrono 300 tablets | 30 tablet [PoM] £5.24 DT = £5.24
Sodium valproate 500 mg Epilim Chrono 500 tablets | 30 tablet [PoM] £8.73 DT = £8.73
▶ Epival CR (Healthcare Pharma Ltd) ▼
Sodium valproate 300 mg Epival CR 300mg tablets | 30 tablet [PoM] £5.24 DT = £5.24 | 100 tablet [PoM] £17.47
Sodium valproate 500 mg Epival CR 500mg tablets | 30 tablet [PoM] £8.73 DT = £8.73

Gastro-resistant tablet
CAUTIONARY AND ADVISORY LABELS 5, 8, 10, 25
▶ Sodium valproate (non-proprietary) ▼
Sodium valproate 200 mg Sodium valproate 200mg gastro-resistant tablets | 30 tablet [PoM] £2.77 DT = £2.85 | 100 tablet [PoM] £9.51–£14.51 DT = £9.51
Sodium valproate 500 mg Sodium valproate 500mg gastro-resistant tablets | 30 tablet [PoM] £6.93 DT = £6.79 | 100 tablet [PoM] £22.62–£34.95 DT = £22.62
▶ Epilim (Sanofi) ▼
Sodium valproate 200 mg Epilim 200 gastro-resistant tablets | 30 tablet [PoM] £2.31 DT = £2.85
Sodium valproate 500 mg Epilim 500 gastro-resistant tablets | 30 tablet [PoM] £5.78 DT = £6.79

Tablet
CAUTIONARY AND ADVISORY LABELS 8, 10, 21
▶ Epilim (Sanofi) ▼
Sodium valproate 100 mg Epilim 100mg crushable tablets | 30 tablet [PoM] £1.68 DT = £1.68

Powder and solvent for solution for injection
▶ Sodium valproate (non-proprietary) ▼
Sodium valproate 400 mg Sodium valproate 400mg powder and solvent for solution for injection vials | 4 vial [PoM] £49.00
▶ Epilim (Sanofi) ▼
Sodium valproate 400 mg Epilim Intravenous 400mg powder and solvent for solution for injection vials | 1 vial [PoM] £13.32 DT = £13.32

Solution for injection

‣ Sodium valproate (non-proprietary) ▼
Sodium valproate 100 mg per 1 ml Sodium valproate 400mg/4ml solution for injection ampoules | 5 ampoule [PoM] £57.90 DT = £57.90

‣ Episenta (Desitin Pharma Ltd) ▼
Sodium valproate 100 mg per 1 ml Episenta 300mg/3ml solution for injection ampoules | 5 ampoule [PoM] £35.00 DT = £35.00

Modified-release capsule

CAUTIONARY AND ADVISORY LABELS 8, 10, 21, 25

‣ Episenta (Desitin Pharma Ltd) ▼
Sodium valproate 150 mg Episenta 150mg modified-release capsules | 100 capsule [PoM] £7.00 DT = £7.00
Sodium valproate 300 mg Episenta 300mg modified-release capsules | 100 capsule [PoM] £13.00 DT = £13.00

Oral solution

CAUTIONARY AND ADVISORY LABELS 8, 10, 21

‣ Sodium valproate (non-proprietary) ▼
Sodium valproate 40 mg per 1 ml Sodium valproate 200mg/5ml oral solution sugar free sugar-free | 300 ml [PoM] £14.66 DT = £9.61
Sodium valproate 200 mg per 1 ml Depakin 200mg/ml oral solution | 40 ml [PoM] ⬛

‣ Epilim (Sanofi) ▼
Sodium valproate 40 mg per 1 ml Epilim 200mg/5ml liquid sugar-free | 300 ml [PoM] £7.78 DT = £9.61
Epilim 200mg/5ml syrup | 300 ml [PoM] £9.33 DT = £9.33

Modified-release granules

CAUTIONARY AND ADVISORY LABELS 8, 10, 21, 25

‣ Epilim Chronosphere MR (Sanofi) ▼
Sodium valproate 50 mg Epilim Chronosphere MR 50mg granules sachets sugar-free | 30 sachet [PoM] £30.00 DT = £30.00
Sodium valproate 100 mg Epilim Chronosphere MR 100mg granules sachets sugar-free | 30 sachet [PoM] £30.00 DT = £30.00
Sodium valproate 250 mg Epilim Chronosphere MR 250mg granules sachets sugar-free | 30 sachet [PoM] £30.00 DT = £30.00
Sodium valproate 500 mg Epilim Chronosphere MR 500mg granules sachets sugar-free | 30 sachet [PoM] £30.00 DT = £30.00
Sodium valproate 750 mg Epilim Chronosphere MR 750mg granules sachets sugar-free | 30 sachet [PoM] £30.00 DT = £30.00
Sodium valproate 1 gram Epilim Chronosphere MR 1000mg granules sachets sugar-free | 30 sachet [PoM] £30.00 DT = £30.00

‣ Episenta (Desitin Pharma Ltd) ▼
Sodium valproate 500 mg Episenta 500mg modified-release granules sachets sugar-free | 100 sachet [PoM] £21.00 DT = £21.00
Sodium valproate 1 gram Episenta 1000mg modified-release granules sachets sugar-free | 100 sachet [PoM] £41.00 DT = £41.00

Stiripentol

04-Nov-2020

● INDICATIONS AND DOSE

Adjunctive therapy of refractory generalised tonic-clonic seizures in patients with severe myoclonic epilepsy in infancy (Dravet syndrome) in combination with clobazam and valproate (under expert supervision)

‣ BY MOUTH

‣ Adult: Doses of up to 50 mg/kg daily in 2–3 divided doses should be continued for as long as efficacy is observed

DOSE EQUIVALENCE AND CONVERSION

‣ Stiripentol capsules and oral powder sachets are **not** bioequivalent. If a switch of formulation is required, manufacturer advises this is done under clinical supervision in case of intolerance.

IMPORTANT SAFETY INFORMATION

MHRA/CHM ADVICE: ANTIEPILEPTICS: RISK OF SUICIDAL THOUGHTS AND BEHAVIOUR (AUGUST 2008)
See Epilepsy p. 321.

MHRA/CHM ADVICE: ANTIEPILEPTIC DRUGS: UPDATED ADVICE ON SWITCHING BETWEEN DIFFERENT MANUFACTURERS' PRODUCTS (NOVEMBER 2017)
See Epilepsy p. 321.

● CONTRA-INDICATIONS History of psychosis in the form of episodes of delirium

● INTERACTIONS → Appendix 1: antiepileptics

● SIDE-EFFECTS

‣ **Common or very common** Agitation · appetite decreased · behaviour abnormal · drowsiness · irritability · movement disorders · muscle tone decreased · nausea · neutropenia · sleep disorders · vomiting · weight decreased

‣ **Uncommon** Diplopia · fatigue · photosensitivity reaction · skin reactions

‣ **Rare or very rare** Thrombocytopenia

‣ **Frequency not known** Suicidal behaviours

● ALLERGY AND CROSS-SENSITIVITY Antiepileptic hypersensitivity syndrome theoretically associated with stiripentol. See under Epilepsy p. 321 for more information.

● PREGNANCY See also *Pregnancy* in Epilepsy p. 321.
Monitoring The dose should be monitored carefully during pregnancy and after birth, and adjustments made on a clinical basis.

● BREAST FEEDING Present in milk in *animal* studies.

● HEPATIC IMPAIRMENT Manufacturer advises avoid (no information available).

● RENAL IMPAIRMENT Avoid—no information available.

● MONITORING REQUIREMENTS Perform full blood count and liver function tests prior to initiating treatment and every 6 months thereafter.

● NATIONAL FUNDING/ACCESS DECISIONS
For full details see funding body website

Scottish Medicines Consortium (SMC) decisions

‣ Stiripentol (*Diacomit*®) for use in conjunction with clobazam and valproate as adjunctive therapy of refractory generalised tonic-clonic seizures in patients with severe myoclonic epilepsy in infancy (SMEI; Dravet' s syndrome) whose seizures are not adequately controlled with clobazam and valproate (September 2017) SMC No. 524/08 Recommended

All Wales Medicines Strategy Group (AWMSG) decisions

‣ Stiripentol (*Diacomit*®) for use in conjunction with clobazam and valproate as adjunctive therapy of refractory generalized tonic-clonic seizures in patients with severe myoclonic epilepsy in infancy (SMEI; Dravet syndrome) whose seizures are not adequately controlled with clobazam and valproate (November 2017) AWMSG No. 3468 Recommended

● MEDICINAL FORMS There can be variation in the licensing of different medicines containing the same drug.

Powder

CAUTIONARY AND ADVISORY LABELS 1, 8, 13, 21
EXCIPIENTS: May contain Aspartame

‣ Diacomit (Alan Pharmaceuticals)
Stiripentol 250 mg Diacomit 250mg oral powder sachets | 60 sachet [PoM] £284.00 DT = £284.00
Stiripentol 500 mg Diacomit 500mg oral powder sachets | 60 sachet [PoM] £493.00 DT = £493.00

Capsule

CAUTIONARY AND ADVISORY LABELS 1, 8, 21

‣ Diacomit (Alan Pharmaceuticals)
Stiripentol 250 mg Diacomit 250mg capsules | 60 capsule [PoM] £284.00 DT = £284.00
Stiripentol 500 mg Diacomit 500mg capsules | 60 capsule [PoM] £493.00 DT = £493.00

Tiagabine

13-Dec-2020

● INDICATIONS AND DOSE

Adjunctive treatment for focal seizures with or without secondary generalisation that are not satisfactorily controlled by other antiepileptics (with enzyme-inducing drugs)

‣ BY MOUTH

‣ Child 12–17 years: Initially 5–10 mg daily in 1–2 divided doses, then increased in steps of 5–10 mg/24 hours every week; maintenance 30–45 mg daily in 2–3 divided doses

▸ **Adult:** Initially 5–10 mg daily in 1–2 divided doses, then increased in steps of 5–10 mg/24 hours every week; maintenance 30–45 mg daily in 2–3 divided doses

Adjunctive treatment for focal seizures with or without secondary generalisation that are not satisfactorily controlled by other antiepileptics (without enzyme-inducing drugs)

▸ BY MOUTH
▸ **Child 12–17 years:** Initially 5–10 mg daily in 1–2 divided doses, then increased in steps of 5–10 mg/24 hours every week; maintenance 15–30 mg daily in 2–3 divided doses
▸ **Adult:** Initially 5–10 mg daily in 1–2 divided doses, then increased in steps of 5–10 mg/24 hours every week; maintenance 15–30 mg daily in 2–3 divided doses

---

IMPORTANT SAFETY INFORMATION

MHRA/CHM ADVICE: ANTIEPILEPTICS: RISK OF SUICIDAL THOUGHTS AND BEHAVIOUR (AUGUST 2008)
See Epilepsy p. 321.

MHRA/CHM ADVICE: ANTIEPILEPTIC DRUGS: UPDATED ADVICE ON SWITCHING BETWEEN DIFFERENT MANUFACTURERS' PRODUCTS (NOVEMBER 2017)
See Epilepsy p. 321.

● CAUTIONS Avoid in Acute porphyrias p. 1107
  CAUTIONS, FURTHER INFORMATION Tiagabine may worsen seizures. [EvGr] It should be avoided in absence, myoclonic, tonic and atonic seizures. Ⓐ
● INTERACTIONS → Appendix 1: antiepileptics
● SIDE-EFFECTS
▸ **Common or very common** Abdominal pain · behaviour abnormal · concentration impaired · depression · diarrhoea · dizziness · emotional lability · fatigue · gait abnormal · insomnia · nausea · nervousness · speech disorder · tremor · vision disorders · vomiting
▸ **Uncommon** Drowsiness · psychosis · skin reactions
▸ **Rare or very rare** Delusions · hallucination
▸ **Frequency not known** Suicidal behaviours
● PREGNANCY See also *Pregnancy* in Epilepsy p. 321.
  Monitoring The dose should be monitored carefully during pregnancy and after birth, and adjustments made on a clinical basis.
● HEPATIC IMPAIRMENT Manufacturer advises caution in mild to moderate impairment (risk of increased exposure); avoid in severe impairment.
  Dose adjustments Manufacturer advises dose reduction and/or longer dose interval with careful titration in mild to moderate impairment.
● PATIENT AND CARER ADVICE
  Medicines for Children leaflet: Tiagabine for preventing seizures www.medicinesforchildren.org.uk/tiagabine-preventing-seizures
  Driving and skilled tasks May impair performance of skilled tasks (e.g. driving).

● MEDICINAL FORMS There can be variation in the licensing of different medicines containing the same drug. Forms available from special-order manufacturers include: oral suspension

Tablet
CAUTIONARY AND ADVISORY LABELS 21
▸ Gabitril (Teva UK Ltd)
  Tiagabine (as Tiagabine hydrochloride monohydrate)
  5 mg Gabitril 5mg tablets | 100 tablet [PoM] £52.04 DT = £52.04
  Tiagabine (as Tiagabine hydrochloride monohydrate)
  10 mg Gabitril 10mg tablets | 100 tablet [PoM] £104.09 DT = £104.09
  Tiagabine (as Tiagabine hydrochloride monohydrate)
  15 mg Gabitril 15mg tablets | 100 tablet [PoM] £156.13 DT = £156.13

Topiramate

10-Dec-2020

● **INDICATIONS AND DOSE**

Monotherapy of generalised tonic-clonic seizures or focal seizures with or without secondary generalisation

▸ BY MOUTH
▸ **Child 6–17 years:** Initially 0.5–1 mg/kg once daily (max. per dose 25 mg) for 1 week, dose to be taken at night, then increased in steps of 250–500 micrograms/kg twice daily, dose to be increased by a maximum of 25 mg twice daily at intervals of 1–2 weeks; usual dose 50 mg twice daily (max. per dose 7.5 mg/kg twice daily), if child cannot tolerate titration regimens recommended above then smaller steps or longer interval between steps may be used; maximum 500 mg per day
▸ **Adult:** Initially 25 mg once daily for 1 week, dose to be taken at night, then increased in steps of 25–50 mg every 1–2 weeks, dose to be taken in 2 divided doses; usual dose 100–200 mg daily in 2 divided doses, adjusted according to response, doses of 1 g daily have been used in refractory epilepsy; maximum 500 mg per day

Adjunctive treatment of generalised tonic-clonic seizures or focal seizures with or without secondary generalisation | Adjunctive treatment for seizures associated with Lennox-Gastaut syndrome

▸ BY MOUTH
▸ **Child 2–17 years:** Initially 1–3 mg/kg once daily (max. per dose 25 mg) for 1 week, dose to be taken at night, then increased in steps of 0.5–1.5 mg/kg twice daily, dose to be increased by a maximum of 25 mg twice daily at intervals of 1–2 weeks; usual dose 2.5–4.5 mg/kg twice daily (max. per dose 7.5 mg/kg twice daily), if child cannot tolerate recommended titration regimen then smaller steps or longer interval between steps may be used; maximum 400 mg per day
▸ **Adult:** Initially 25–50 mg once daily for 1 week, dose to be taken at night, then increased in steps of 25–50 mg every 1–2 weeks, dose to be taken in 2 divided doses; usual dose 200–400 mg daily in 2 divided doses; maximum 400 mg per day

Migraine prophylaxis
▸ BY MOUTH
▸ **Adult:** Initially 25 mg once daily for 1 week, dose to be taken at night, then increased in steps of 25 mg every week; usual dose 50–100 mg daily in 2 divided doses; maximum 200 mg per day

---

IMPORTANT SAFETY INFORMATION

MHRA/CHM ADVICE: ANTIEPILEPTICS: RISK OF SUICIDAL THOUGHTS AND BEHAVIOUR (AUGUST 2008)
See Epilepsy p. 321.

MHRA/CHM ADVICE: ANTIEPILEPTIC DRUGS: UPDATED ADVICE ON SWITCHING BETWEEN DIFFERENT MANUFACTURERS' PRODUCTS (NOVEMBER 2017)
See Epilepsy p. 321 and see also *Prescribing and dispensing information.*

● CAUTIONS Avoid in Acute porphyrias p. 1107 · risk of metabolic acidosis · risk of nephrolithiasis—ensure adequate hydration (especially in strenuous activity or warm environment)
● INTERACTIONS → Appendix 1: antiepileptics
● SIDE-EFFECTS
▸ **Common or very common** Alopecia · anaemia · anxiety · appetite abnormal · asthenia · behaviour abnormal · cognitive impairment · concentration impaired · confusion · constipation · cough · depression · diarrhoea · dizziness ·

drowsiness · dry mouth · dyspnoea · ear discomfort · eye disorders · feeling abnormal · fever (in children) · gait abnormal · gastrointestinal discomfort · gastrointestinal disorders · haemorrhage · hypersensitivity · joint disorders · malaise · memory loss · mood altered · movement disorders · muscle complaints · muscle weakness · nasal complaints · nasopharyngitis · nausea · oral disorders · pain · seizures · sensation abnormal · skin reactions · sleep disorders · speech impairment · taste altered · tinnitus · tremor · urinary disorders · urolithiases · vertigo (in children) · vision disorders · vomiting (in children) · weight changes

▸ **Uncommon** Abnormal sensation in eye · anhidrosis · arrhythmias · aura · cerebellar syndrome · consciousness impaired · crying · drooling · dry eye · dysgraphia · dysphonia · eosinophilia (in children) · facial swelling · hallucinations · hearing impairment · hyperthermia (in children) · hypokalaemia · hypotension · influenza like illness · learning disability (in children) · leucopenia · lymphadenopathy · metabolic acidosis · musculoskeletal stiffness · palpitations · pancreatitis · paranasal sinus hypersecretion · peripheral coldness · peripheral neuropathy · polydipsia · psychotic disorder · renal pain · sexual dysfunction · smell altered · suicidal behaviours · syncope · thinking abnormal · thirst · thrombocytopenia · vasodilation

▸ **Rare or very rare** Eye inflammation · face oedema · glaucoma · hepatic disorders · limb discomfort · neutropenia · Raynaud's phenomenon · renal tubular acidosis · severe cutaneous adverse reactions (SCARs) · unresponsive to stimuli

SIDE-EFFECTS, FURTHER INFORMATION Topiramate has been associated with acute myopia with secondary angle-closure glaucoma, typically occurring within 1 month of starting treatment. Choroidal effusions resulting in anterior displacement of the lens and iris have also been reported. If raised intra-ocular pressure occurs: seek specialist ophthalmological advice; use appropriate measures to reduce intra-ocular pressure and stop topiramate as rapidly as feasible.

● CONCEPTION AND CONTRACEPTION Manufacturer advises perform pregnancy test before the initiation of treatment—a highly effective contraceptive method is advised in women of child-bearing potential; patients should be fully informed of the risks related to the use of topiramate during pregnancy.

● PREGNANCY Increased risk of major congenital malformations following exposure during the first trimester. *For migraine prophylaxis* manufacturer advises avoid. *For epilepsy* manufacturer advises consider alternative treatment options. See also *Pregnancy* in Epilepsy p. 321.

Monitoring Manufacturer advises in case of administration during first trimester, careful prenatal monitoring should be performed.

It is recommended that the fetal growth should be monitored.

The dose should be monitored carefully during pregnancy and after birth, and adjustments made on a clinical basis.

● BREAST FEEDING Manufacturer advises avoid—present in milk.

● HEPATIC IMPAIRMENT Manufacturer advises caution (risk of decreased clearance).

● RENAL IMPAIRMENT Use with caution.

Dose adjustments ▸ In adults Half usual starting and maintenance dose if eGFR less than 70 mL/minute/1.73 m^2—reduced clearance and longer time to steady-state plasma concentration.

▸ In children Half usual starting and maintenance dose if estimated glomerular filtration less than 70 mL/minute/1.73 m^2—reduced clearance and longer time to steady-state plasma concentration.

● DIRECTIONS FOR ADMINISTRATION

TOPAMAX ® CAPSULES Manufacturer advises swallow whole or sprinkle contents of capsule on soft food and swallow immediately without chewing.

● PRESCRIBING AND DISPENSING INFORMATION

Switching between formulations Care should be taken when switching between oral formulations in the treatment of epilepsy. The need for continued supply of a particular manufacturer's product should be based on clinical judgement and consultation with the patient or their carer, taking into account factors such as seizure frequency and treatment history.

Patients being treated for epilepsy may need to be maintained on a specific manufacturer's branded or generic topiramate product.

● PATIENT AND CARER ADVICE

Medicines for Children leaflet: Topiramate for preventing seizures www.medicinesforchildren.org.uk/topiramate-preventing-seizures

TOPAMAX ® CAPSULES Patients or carers should be given advice on how to administer *Topamax* ® *Sprinkle* capsules.

● MEDICINAL FORMS There can be variation in the licensing of different medicines containing the same drug. Forms available from special-order manufacturers include: oral suspension, oral solution

Oral suspension

▸ Topiramate (Non-proprietary)

Topiramate 10 mg per 1 ml Topiramate 50mg/5ml oral suspension sugar free sugar-free | 150 ml [PoM] £186.00 DT = £186.00

Topiramate 20 mg per 1 ml Topiramate 100mg/5ml oral suspension sugar free sugar-free | 280 ml [PoM] £263.70 DT = £263.70

Tablet

CAUTIONARY AND ADVISORY LABELS 3, 8

▸ Topiramate (Non-proprietary)

Topiramate 25 mg Topiramate 25mg tablets | 60 tablet [PoM] £19.29 DT = £3.46

Topiramate 50 mg Topiramate 50mg tablets | 60 tablet [PoM] £36.75 DT = £5.15

Topiramate 100 mg Topiramate 100mg tablets | 60 tablet [PoM] £56.76 DT = £8.58

Topiramate 200 mg Topiramate 200mg tablets | 60 tablet [PoM] £110.23 DT = £41.31

▸ Topamax (Janssen-Cilag Ltd)

Topiramate 25 mg Topamax 25mg tablets | 60 tablet [PoM] £19.29 DT = £3.46

Topiramate 50 mg Topamax 50mg tablets | 60 tablet [PoM] £31.69 DT = £5.15

Topiramate 100 mg Topamax 100mg tablets | 60 tablet [PoM] £56.76 DT = £8.58

Topiramate 200 mg Topamax 200mg tablets | 60 tablet [PoM] £110.23 DT = £41.31

Capsule

CAUTIONARY AND ADVISORY LABELS 3, 8

▸ Topamax (Janssen-Cilag Ltd)

Topiramate 15 mg Topamax 15mg sprinkle capsules | 60 capsule [PoM] £14.79 DT = £14.79

Topiramate 25 mg Topamax 25mg sprinkle capsules | 60 capsule [PoM] £22.18 DT = £13.94

Topiramate 50 mg Topamax 50mg sprinkle capsules | 60 capsule [PoM] £36.45 DT = £36.45

Vigabatrin

13-Dec-2020

● **INDICATIONS AND DOSE**

Adjunctive treatment of focal seizures with or without secondary generalisation not satisfactorily controlled with other antiepileptics (under expert supervision)

▸ BY MOUTH

▸ Child 1-23 months: Initially 15–20 mg/kg twice daily (max. per dose 250 mg), to be increased over 2–3 weeks to usual maintenance dose, usual maintenance 30–40 mg/kg twice daily (max. per dose 75 mg/kg)

▸ Child 2-11 years: Initially 15–20 mg/kg twice daily (max. per dose 250 mg), to be increased over 2–3 weeks to usual maintenance dose, usual maintenance 30–40 mg/kg twice daily (max. per dose 1.5 g)

▸ Child 12-17 years: Initially 250 mg twice daily, to be increased over 2–3 weeks to usual maintenance dose, usual maintenance 1–1.5 g twice daily

▸ Adult: Initially 1 g once daily, alternatively initially 1 g daily in 2 divided doses, then increased in steps of 500 mg every week, adjusted according to response; usual dose 2–3 g daily; maximum 3 g per day

▸ BY RECTUM

▸ Child 1-23 months: Initially 15–20 mg/kg twice daily (max. per dose 250 mg), to be increased over 2–3 weeks to usual maintenance dose, usual maintenance 30–40 mg/kg twice daily (max. per dose 75 mg/kg)

▸ Child 2-11 years: Initially 15–20 mg/kg twice daily (max. per dose 250 mg), to be increased over 2–3 weeks to usual maintenance dose, usual maintenance 30–40 mg/kg twice daily (max. per dose 1.5 g)

▸ Child 12-17 years: Initially 250 mg twice daily, to be increased over 2–3 weeks to usual maintenance dose, usual maintenance 1–1.5 g twice daily

● UNLICENSED USE Granules not licensed for rectal use. Tablets not licensed to be crushed and dispersed in liquid. Vigabatrin doses in BNF publications may differ from those in product literature.

IMPORTANT SAFETY INFORMATION

MHRA/CHM ADVICE: ANTIEPILEPTICS: RISK OF SUICIDAL THOUGHTS AND BEHAVIOUR (AUGUST 2008)
See Epilepsy p. 321.

MHRA/CHM ADVICE: ANTIEPILEPTIC DRUGS: UPDATED ADVICE ON SWITCHING BETWEEN DIFFERENT MANUFACTURERS' PRODUCTS (NOVEMBER 2017)
See Epilepsy p. 321.

● CONTRA-INDICATIONS Visual field defects

● CAUTIONS Elderly · history of behavioural problems · history of depression · history of psychosis

CAUTIONS, FURTHER INFORMATION Vigabatrin may worsen seizures. EvGr It should be avoided in absence, myoclonic, tonic and atonic seizures. Ⓐ

▸ Visual field defects Vigabatrin is associated with visual field defects. The onset of symptoms varies from 1 month to several years after starting. In most cases, visual field defects have persisted despite discontinuation, and further deterioration after discontinuation cannot be excluded. EvGr Visual field testing should be carried out before treatment and at 6-month intervals. Patients and their carers should be warned to report any new visual symptoms that develop and those with symptoms should be referred for an urgent ophthalmological opinion. Gradual withdrawal of vigabatrin should be considered. Ⓜ

● INTERACTIONS → Appendix 1: antiepileptics

● SIDE-EFFECTS

GENERAL SIDE-EFFECTS

▸ **Rare or very rare** Suicidal behaviours

SPECIFIC SIDE-EFFECTS

▸ **Common or very common**

▹ With oral use Abdominal pain · anaemia · anxiety · arthralgia · behaviour abnormal · concentration impaired · depression · dizziness · drowsiness · eye disorders · fatigue · headache · memory loss · mood altered · nausea · oedema · paraesthesia · speech disorder · thinking abnormal · tremor · vision disorders · vomiting · weight increased

▸ **Uncommon**

▹ With oral use Movement disorders · psychotic disorder · seizure (patients with myoclonic seizures at greater risk) · skin reactions

▸ **Rare or very rare**

▹ With oral use Angioedema · encephalopathy · hallucination · hepatitis · optic neuritis

▸ **Frequency not known**

▹ With oral use Muscle tone increased

SIDE-EFFECTS, FURTHER INFORMATION **Encephalopathic symptoms** Encephalopathic symptoms including marked sedation, stupor, and confusion with non-specific slow wave EEG can occur rarely -reduce dose or withdraw.

Visual field defects About one-third of patients treated with vigabatrin have suffered visual field defects; counselling and careful monitoring for this side-effect are required.

● PREGNANCY See also *Pregnancy* in Epilepsy p. 321.
Monitoring The dose should be monitored carefully during pregnancy and after birth, and adjustments made on a clinical basis.

● BREAST FEEDING Present in milk—manufacturer advises avoid.

● RENAL IMPAIRMENT

Dose adjustments ▸ In adults Consider reduced dose or increased dose interval if eGFR less than 60 mL/minute/1.73 m^2.

▸ In children Consider reduced dose or increased dose interval if estimated glomerular filtration rate less than 60 mL/minute/1.73 m^2.

● MONITORING REQUIREMENTS Closely monitor neurological function.

● DIRECTIONS FOR ADMINISTRATION

▸ With oral use Manufacturer advises contents of a sachet should be dissolved in water, fruit juice or milk immediately before taking. Expert sources advise tablets may be crushed and dispersed in liquid.

▸ With rectal use Expert sources advise contents of a sachet should be dissolved in a small amount of water and administered rectally.

● PATIENT AND CARER ADVICE Patients and their carers should be warned to report any new visual symptoms that develop.
Medicines for Children leaflet: Vigabatrin for preventing seizures www.medicinesforchildren.org.uk/vigabatrin-preventing-seizures

● MEDICINAL FORMS There can be variation in the licensing of different medicines containing the same drug. Forms available from special-order manufacturers include: oral solution

Powder

CAUTIONARY AND ADVISORY LABELS 3, 8, 13

▸ Sabril (Sanofi)
Vigabatrin 500 mg Sabril 500mg oral powder sachets sugar-free | 50 sachet PoM £24.60 DT = £24.60

Tablet

CAUTIONARY AND ADVISORY LABELS 3, 8

▸ Sabril (Sanofi)
Vigabatrin 500 mg Sabril 500mg tablets | 100 tablet PoM £44.41 DT = £44.41

4

Nervous system

4

Nervous system

Zonisamide

10-Dec-2020

● INDICATIONS AND DOSE

Monotherapy for treatment of focal seizures with or without secondary generalisation in adults with newly diagnosed epilepsy

▶ BY MOUTH

▸ **Adult:** Initially 100 mg once daily for 2 weeks, then increased in steps of 100 mg every 2 weeks, usual maintenance dose 300 mg once daily; maximum 500 mg per day

Adjunctive treatment for refractory focal seizures with or without secondary generalisation

▶ BY MOUTH

▸ **Child 6–17 years (body-weight 20–54 kg):** Initially 1 mg/kg once daily for 7 days, then increased in steps of 1 mg/kg every 7 days, usual maintenance 6–8 mg/kg once daily (max. per dose 500 mg once daily), dose to be increased at 2-week intervals in patients who are **not** receiving concomitant carbamazepine, phenytoin, phenobarbital or other potent inducers of cytochrome P450 enzyme CYP3A4

▸ **Child 6–17 years (body-weight 55 kg and above):** Initially 1 mg/kg once daily for 7 days, then increased in steps of 1 mg/kg every 7 days, usual maintenance 300–500 mg once daily, dose to be increased at 2-week intervals in patients who are **not** receiving concomitant carbamazepine, phenytoin, phenobarbital or other potent inducers of cytochrome P450 enzyme CYP3A4

▸ **Adult:** Initially 50 mg daily in 2 divided doses for 7 days, then increased to 100 mg daily in 2 divided doses, then increased in steps of 100 mg every 7 days, usual maintenance 300–500 mg daily in 1–2 divided doses, dose to be increased at 2-week intervals in patients who are **not** receiving concomitant carbamazepine, phenytoin, phenobarbital or other potent inducers of cytochrome P450 enzyme CYP3A4

IMPORTANT SAFETY INFORMATION

MHRA/CHM ADVICE: ANTIEPILEPTICS: RISK OF SUICIDAL THOUGHTS AND BEHAVIOUR (AUGUST 2008)

See Epilepsy p. 321.

MHRA/CHM ADVICE: ANTIEPILEPTIC DRUGS: UPDATED ADVICE ON SWITCHING BETWEEN DIFFERENT MANUFACTURERS' PRODUCTS (NOVEMBER 2017)

See Epilepsy p. 321 and see also *Prescribing and dispensing information.*

● CAUTIONS Elderly · history of eye disorders · low body-weight or poor appetite—monitor weight throughout treatment (fatal cases of weight loss reported in children) · metabolic acidosis—monitor serum bicarbonate concentration in children and those with other risk factors (consider dose reduction or discontinuation if metabolic acidosis develops) · risk factors for renal stone formation (particularly predisposition to nephrolithiasis)

CAUTIONS, FURTHER INFORMATION [EvGr] Avoid overheating and ensure adequate hydration especially in children, during strenuous activity or if in warm environment (fatal cases of heat stroke reported in children). [M]

● INTERACTIONS → Appendix 1: antiepileptics

● SIDE-EFFECTS

▶ **Common or very common** Alopecia · anxiety · appetite decreased · ataxia · bradyphrenia · concentration impaired · confusion · constipation · depression · diarrhoea · dizziness · drowsiness · fatigue · fever · gastrointestinal discomfort · hypersensitivity · influenza like illness · insomnia · memory loss · mood altered · nausea · nystagmus · paraesthesia · peripheral oedema · psychosis · rash (consider

discontinuation) · skin reactions · speech disorder · tremor · urolithiases · vision disorders · vomiting · weight decreased

▶ **Uncommon** Behaviour abnormal · gallbladder disorders · hallucination · hypokalaemia · increased risk of infection · leucopenia · respiratory disorders · seizures · suicidal behaviours · thrombocytopenia

▶ **Rare or very rare** Agranulocytosis · angle closure glaucoma · anhidrosis · bone marrow disorders · coma · dyspnoea · eye pain · heat stroke · hepatocellular injury · hydronephrosis · leucocytosis · lymphadenopathy · metabolic acidosis · myasthenic syndrome · neuroleptic malignant syndrome · pancreatitis · renal failure · renal tubular acidosis · rhabdomyolysis · severe cutaneous adverse reactions (SCARs) · urine abnormal

▶ **Frequency not known** Sudden unexplained death in epilepsy

● ALLERGY AND CROSS-SENSITIVITY Contra-indicated in sulfonamide hypersensitivity.

Antiepileptic hypersensitivity syndrome theoretically associated with zonisamide. See under Epilepsy p. 321 for more information.

● CONCEPTION AND CONTRACEPTION Manufacturer advises women of childbearing potential should use effective contraception during treatment and for one month after last dose—avoid in women of childbearing potential not using effective contraception unless clearly necessary and the potential benefit outweighs risk; patients should be fully informed of the risks related to the use of zonisamide during pregnancy.

● PREGNANCY Manufacturer advises use only if clearly necessary and the potential benefit outweighs risk—toxicity in *animal* studies; patients should be fully informed of the risks related to the use of zonisamide during pregnancy. See also *Pregnancy* in Epilepsy p. 321. **Monitoring** The dose should be monitored carefully during pregnancy and after birth, and adjustments made on a clinical basis.

● BREAST FEEDING Manufacturer advises avoid for 4 weeks after last dose.

● HEPATIC IMPAIRMENT Avoid in severe impairment. **Dose adjustments** Initially increase dose at 2-week intervals if mild or moderate impairment.

● RENAL IMPAIRMENT **Dose adjustments** Initially increase dose at 2-week intervals; discontinue if renal function deteriorates.

● TREATMENT CESSATION Avoid abrupt withdrawal (consult product literature for recommended withdrawal regimens in children).

● PRESCRIBING AND DISPENSING INFORMATION Switching between formulations Care should be taken when switching between oral formulations. The need for continued supply of a particular manufacturer's product should be based on clinical judgement and consultation with the patient or their carer, taking into account factors such as seizure frequency and treatment history.

Patients may need to be maintained on a specific manufacturer's branded or generic zonisamide product.

● PATIENT AND CARER ADVICE Children and their carers should be made aware of how to prevent and recognise overheating and dehydration.

Medicines for Children leaflet: Zonisamide for preventing seizures www.medicinesforchildren.org.uk/zonisamide-preventing-seizures

● NATIONAL FUNDING/ACCESS DECISIONS For full details see funding body website

Scottish Medicines Consortium (SMC) decisions

▶ Zonisamide (*Zonegran*®) as adjunctive therapy in the treatment of partial seizures, with or without secondary generalisation, in adolescents, and children aged 6 years and

above (March 2014) SMC No. 949/14 Recommended with restrictions

- ● MEDICINAL FORMS There can be variation in the licensing of different medicines containing the same drug. Forms available from special-order manufacturers include: oral suspension, oral solution

Capsule

CAUTIONARY AND ADVISORY LABELS 3, 8, 10

- ▸ Zonisamide (Non-proprietary)
  Zonisamide 25 mg Zonisamide 25mg capsules | 14 capsule [PoM]
  £10.70 DT = £8.50
  Zonisamide 50 mg Zonisamide 50mg capsules | 56 capsule [PoM]
  £54.00 DT = £44.87
  Zonisamide 100 mg Zonisamide 100mg capsules | 56 capsule [PoM]
  £75.48 DT = £6.94
- ▸ Zonegran (Eisai Ltd)
  Zonisamide 25 mg Zonegran 25mg capsules | 14 capsule [PoM]
  £8.82 DT = £8.50
  Zonisamide 50 mg Zonegran 50mg capsules | 56 capsule [PoM]
  £47.04 DT = £44.87
  Zonisamide 100 mg Zonegran 100mg capsules | 56 capsule [PoM]
  £62.72 DT = £6.94

ANTIEPILEPTICS › BARBITURATES

Phenobarbital
10-Dec-2020

(Phenobarbitone)

- ● INDICATIONS AND DOSE

All forms of epilepsy except typical absence seizures
- ▸ BY MOUTH
- ▸ Child 1 month–11 years: Initially 1–1.5 mg/kg twice daily, then increased in steps of 2 mg/kg daily as required; maintenance 2.5–4 mg/kg 1–2 times a day
- ▸ Child 12–17 years: 60–180 mg once daily
- ▸ Adult: 60–180 mg once daily, dose to be taken at night

Status epilepticus
- ▸ BY INTRAVENOUS INJECTION
- ▸ Adult: 10 mg/kg (max. per dose 1 g), dose to be administered at a rate not more than 100 mg/minute, injection to be diluted 1 in 10 with water for injections
- ▸ BY SLOW INTRAVENOUS INJECTION

- ▸ Neonate: Initially 20 mg/kg, dose to be administered at a rate no faster than 1 mg/kg/minute, then 2.5–5 mg/kg 1–2 times a day.

- ▸ Child 1 month–11 years: Initially 20 mg/kg, dose to be administered at a rate no faster than 1 mg/kg/minute, then 2.5–5 mg/kg 1–2 times a day
- ▸ Child 12–17 years: Initially 20 mg/kg (max. per dose 1 g), dose to be administered at a rate no faster than 1 mg/kg/minute, then 300 mg twice daily

DOSE EQUIVALENCE AND CONVERSION
- ▸ For therapeutic purposes phenobarbital and phenobarbital sodium may be considered equivalent in effect.

IMPORTANT SAFETY INFORMATION

MHRA/CHM ADVICE: ANTIEPILEPTICS: RISK OF SUICIDAL THOUGHTS AND BEHAVIOUR (AUGUST 2008)
See Epilepsy p. 321.

MHRA/CHM ADVICE: ANTIEPILEPTIC DRUGS: UPDATED ADVICE ON SWITCHING BETWEEN DIFFERENT MANUFACTURERS' PRODUCTS (NOVEMBER 2017)
See Epilepsy p. 321 and see also *Prescribing and dispensing information.*

- ● CAUTIONS Avoid in Acute porphyrias p. 1107 · children · debilitated · elderly · history of alcohol abuse · history of drug abuse · respiratory depression (avoid if severe)

CAUTIONS, FURTHER INFORMATION MHRA advises consider vitamin D supplementation in patients who are immobilised for long periods or who have inadequate sun exposure or dietary intake of calcium.

- ● INTERACTIONS → Appendix 1: antiepileptics
- ● SIDE-EFFECTS

GENERAL SIDE-EFFECTS
Agranulocytosis · anticonvulsant hypersensitivity syndrome · behaviour abnormal · bone disorders · bone fracture · cognitive impairment · confusion · depression · drowsiness · folate deficiency · hepatic disorders · memory loss · movement disorders · nystagmus · respiratory depression · skin reactions · suicidal behaviours

SPECIFIC SIDE-EFFECTS
- ▸ With oral use Anxiety · hallucination · hypotension · megaloblastic anaemia · severe cutaneous adverse reactions (SCARs) · thrombocytopenia
- ▸ With parenteral use Agitation · anaemia · aplastic anaemia · Dupuytren's contracture · hypocalcaemia · irritability · toxic epidermal necrolysis

Overdose For details on the management of poisoning, see Active elimination techniques, under Emergency treatment of poisoning p. 1413.

- ● ALLERGY AND CROSS-SENSITIVITY Cross-sensitivity reported with carbamazepine. Antiepileptic hypersensitivity syndrome associated with phenobarbital. See under Epilepsy p. 321 for more information.

- ● PREGNANCY
Monitoring The dose should be monitored carefully during pregnancy and after birth, and adjustments made on a clinical basis.

- ● BREAST FEEDING Avoid if possible; drowsiness may occur.

- ● HEPATIC IMPAIRMENT Manufacturer advises caution in mild to moderate impairment; avoid in severe impairment.

- ● RENAL IMPAIRMENT Use with caution.

- ● MONITORING REQUIREMENTS
- ▸ Plasma-phenobarbital concentration for optimum response is 15–40 mg/litre (60–180 micromol/litre); however, monitoring the plasma-drug concentration is less useful than with other drugs because tolerance occurs.

- ● TREATMENT CESSATION Avoid abrupt withdrawal (dependence with prolonged use).

- ● DIRECTIONS FOR ADMINISTRATION
- ▸ With oral use For administration by *mouth*, tablets may be crushed.
- ▸ With intravenous use in adults Solution for injection must be diluted before intravenous administration.
- ▸ With intravenous use in children For *intravenous injection*, dilute to a concentration of 20 mg/mL with Water for Injections; give over 20 minutes (no faster than 1 mg/kg/minute).

- ● PRESCRIBING AND DISPENSING INFORMATION
- ▸ In children The RCPCH and NPPG recommend that, when a liquid special of phenobarbital is required, it is alcohol-free and the following strength is used: 50 mg/5 mL. Switching between formulations Different formulations of oral preparations may vary in bioavailability. Patients should be maintained on a specific manufacturer's product.

- ● PATIENT AND CARER ADVICE
Medicines for Children leaflet: Phenobarbital for preventing seizures www.medicinesforchildren.org.uk/phenobarbital-preventing-seizures

4

● MEDICINAL FORMS There can be variation in the licensing of different medicines containing the same drug. Forms available from special-order manufacturers include: tablet, capsule, oral suspension, oral solution

Tablet

CAUTIONARY AND ADVISORY LABELS 2, 8
▸ Phenobarbital (Non-proprietary)
Phenobarbital 15 mg Phenobarbital 15mg tablets | 28 tablet PoM £24.95 DT = £22.69 CD3
Phenobarbital 30 mg Phenobarbital 30mg tablets | 28 tablet PoM £5.99 DT = £1.06 CD3
Phenobarbital 60 mg Phenobarbital 60mg tablets | 28 tablet PoM £7.99 DT = £7.61 CD3

Solution for injection

EXCIPIENTS: May contain Propylene glycol
▸ Phenobarbital (Non-proprietary)
Phenobarbital sodium 30 mg per 1 ml Phenobarbital 30mg/1ml solution for injection ampoules | 10 ampoule PoM £116.51-£119.35 DT = £116.51 CD3
Phenobarbital sodium 60 mg per 1 ml Phenobarbital 60mg/1ml solution for injection ampoules | 10 ampoule PoM £125.93 DT = £125.93 CD3
Phenobarbital sodium 200 mg per 1 ml Phenobarbital 200mg/1ml solution for injection ampoules | 10 ampoule PoM £100.23-£102.67 DT = £100.23 CD3

Oral solution

CAUTIONARY AND ADVISORY LABELS 2, 8
EXCIPIENTS: May contain Alcohol
▸ Phenobarbital (Non-proprietary)
Phenobarbital 3 mg per 1 ml Phenobarbital 15mg/5ml elixir | 500 ml PoM £83.00-£83.01 DT = £83.01 CD3

Primidone

07-Dec-2020

● INDICATIONS AND DOSE

All forms of epilepsy except typical absence seizures
▸ BY MOUTH
▸ Child 1 month-1 year: Initially 125 mg daily, dose to be taken at bedtime, then increased in steps of 125 mg every 3 days, adjusted according to response; maintenance 125-250 mg twice daily
▸ Child 2-4 years: Initially 125 mg once daily, dose to be taken at bedtime, then increased in steps of 125 mg every 3 days, adjusted according to response; maintenance 250-375 mg twice daily
▸ Child 5-8 years: Initially 125 mg once daily, dose to be taken at bedtime, then increased in steps of 125 mg every 3 days, adjusted according to response; maintenance 375-500 mg twice daily
▸ Child 9-17 years: Initially 125 mg once daily, dose to be taken at bedtime, then increased in steps of 125 mg every 3 days, increased to 250 mg twice daily, then increased in steps of 250 mg every 3 days (max. per dose 750 mg twice daily), adjusted according to response
▸ Adult: Initially 125 mg once daily, dose to be taken at bedtime, then increased in steps of 125 mg every 3 days, increased to 500 mg daily in 2 divided doses, then increased in steps of 250 mg every 3 days, adjusted according to response; maintenance 0.75-1.5 g daily in 2 divided doses

Essential tremor
▸ BY MOUTH
▸ Adult: Initially 50 mg daily, then adjusted according to response to up to 750 mg daily, dose to be increased over 2-3 weeks

IMPORTANT SAFETY INFORMATION
MHRA/CHM ADVICE: ANTIEPILEPTICS: RISK OF SUICIDAL THOUGHTS AND BEHAVIOUR (AUGUST 2008)
See Epilepsy p. 321.

MHRA/CHM ADVICE: ANTIEPILEPTIC DRUGS: UPDATED ADVICE ON SWITCHING BETWEEN DIFFERENT MANUFACTURERS' PRODUCTS (NOVEMBER 2017)
See Epilepsy p. 321 and see also *Prescribing and dispensing information.*

● CAUTIONS Avoid in Acute porphyrias p. 1107 · children · debilitated · elderly · history of alcohol abuse · history of drug abuse · respiratory depression (avoid if severe)
CAUTIONS, FURTHER INFORMATION Consider vitamin D supplementation in patients who are immobilised for long periods or who have inadequate sun exposure or dietary intake of calcium.

● INTERACTIONS → Appendix 1: antiepileptics

● SIDE-EFFECTS
▸ **Common or very common** Apathy · ataxia · drowsiness · nausea · nystagmus · visual impairment
▸ **Uncommon** Dizziness · headache · hypersensitivity · skin reactions · vomiting
▸ **Rare or very rare** Arthralgia · blood disorder · bone disorders · Dupuytren's contracture · megaloblastic anaemia (may be treated with folic acid) · personality change · psychotic disorder · severe cutaneous adverse reactions (SCARs) · systemic lupus erythematosus (SLE)
▸ **Frequency not known** Bone fracture · suicidal behaviours
● ALLERGY AND CROSS-SENSITIVITY Cross-sensitivity reported with carbamazepine. Antiepileptic hypersensitivity syndrome associated with primidone. See under Epilepsy p. 321 for more information.

● PREGNANCY
Monitoring The dose should be monitored carefully during pregnancy and after birth, and adjustments made on a clinical basis.

● HEPATIC IMPAIRMENT Manufacturer advises caution.
Dose adjustments Manufacturer advises consider dose reduction.

● RENAL IMPAIRMENT Use with caution.

● MONITORING REQUIREMENTS
▸ Monitor plasma concentrations of derived phenobarbital; plasma concentration for optimum response is 15-40 mg/litre (60-180 micromol/litre).

● TREATMENT CESSATION Avoid abrupt withdrawal (dependence with prolonged use).

● PRESCRIBING AND DISPENSING INFORMATION
Switching between formulations Different formulations of oral preparations may vary in bioavailability. Patients being treated for epilepsy should be maintained on a specific manufacturer's product.

● MEDICINAL FORMS There can be variation in the licensing of different medicines containing the same drug. Forms available from special-order manufacturers include: capsule, oral suspension

Oral suspension
▸ Liskantin Saft (Imported (Germany))
Primidone 25 mg per 1 ml Liskantin Saft 125mg/5ml oral suspension | 250 ml PoM ⊠

Tablet
CAUTIONARY AND ADVISORY LABELS 2, 8
▸ Primidone (Non-proprietary)
Primidone 50 mg Primidone 50mg tablets | 100 tablet PoM £112.50 DT = £111.66
Primidone 250 mg Primidone 250mg tablets | 100 tablet PoM £99.65-£123.00 DT = £116.48

HYPNOTICS, SEDATIVES AND ANXIOLYTICS > BENZODIAZEPINES

F 361

Clobazam

07-Oct-2020

● **INDICATIONS AND DOSE**

Adjunct in epilepsy
▶ BY MOUTH
▶ Child 6-17 years: Initially 5 mg daily, dose to be increased if necessary at intervals of 5 days, maintenance 0.3–1 mg/kg daily, daily doses of up to 30 mg may be given as a single dose at bedtime, higher doses should be divided; maximum 60 mg per day
▶ Adult: 20–30 mg daily, then increased if necessary up to 60 mg daily

Anxiety (short-term use)
▶ BY MOUTH
▶ Adult: 20–30 mg daily in divided doses, alternatively 20–30 mg once daily, dose to be taken at bedtime; increased if necessary up to 60 mg daily in divided doses, dose only increased in severe anxiety (in hospital patients), for debilitated patients, use elderly dose
▶ Elderly: 10–20 mg daily

● **UNLICENSED USE**
▶ In children Not licensed as monotherapy.

IMPORTANT SAFETY INFORMATION

SAFE PRACTICE
Clobazam has been confused with clonazepam; care must be taken to ensure the correct drug is prescribed and dispensed.

MHRA/CHM ADVICE: ANTIEPILEPTICS: RISK OF SUICIDAL THOUGHTS AND BEHAVIOUR (AUGUST 2008)
See Epilepsy p. 321.

MHRA/CHM ADVICE: ANTIEPILEPTIC DRUGS: UPDATED ADVICE ON SWITCHING BETWEEN DIFFERENT MANUFACTURERS' PRODUCTS (NOVEMBER 2017)
See Epilepsy p. 321 and see also *Prescribing and dispensing information.*

● **CONTRA-INDICATIONS** Respiratory depression
● **CAUTIONS** Muscle weakness · organic brain changes
CAUTIONS, FURTHER INFORMATION The effectiveness of clobazam may decrease significantly after weeks or months of continuous therapy.
● **INTERACTIONS** → Appendix 1: benzodiazepines
● **SIDE-EFFECTS** Appetite decreased · consciousness impaired · constipation · drug abuse · dry mouth · fall · gait unsteady · libido loss · movement disorders · muscle spasms · nystagmus · respiratory disorder · severe cutaneous adverse reactions (SCARs) · skin reactions · speech impairment · suicidal behaviours · weight increased
● **BREAST FEEDING** Benzodiazepines are present in milk, and should be avoided if possible during breast-feeding.
Monitoring All infants should be monitored for sedation, feeding difficulties, adequate weight gain, and developmental milestones.
● **RENAL IMPAIRMENT**
Dose adjustments Start with small doses in severe impairment.
● **MONITORING REQUIREMENTS**
▶ In children Routine measurement of plasma concentrations of antiepileptic drugs is not usually justified, because the target concentration ranges are arbitrary and often vary between individuals. However, plasma drug concentrations may be measured in children with worsening seizures, status epilepticus, suspected noncompliance, or suspected toxicity. Similarly,

haematological and biochemical monitoring should not be undertaken unless clinically indicated.
● **PRESCRIBING AND DISPENSING INFORMATION**
Switching between formulations Care should be taken when switching between oral formulations in the treatment of epilepsy. The need for continued supply of a particular manufacturer's product should be based on clinical judgement and consultation with the patient or their carer, taking into account factors such as seizure frequency and treatment history.

Patients being treated for epilepsy may need to be maintained on a specific manufacturer's branded or generic clobazam product.
● **PATIENT AND CARER ADVICE**
Medicines for Children leaflet: Clobazam for preventing seizures www.medicinesforchildren.org.uk/clobazam-preventing-seizures-0
● **NATIONAL FUNDING/ACCESS DECISIONS**
NHS restrictions Clobazam is not prescribable in NHS primary care except for the treatment of epilepsy; endorse prescription 'SLS'.
● **MEDICINAL FORMS** There can be variation in the licensing of different medicines containing the same drug. Forms available from special-order manufacturers include: capsule, oral suspension

Oral suspension
CAUTIONARY AND ADVISORY LABELS 2, 8, 19
▶ Clobazam (Non-proprietary)
Clobazam 1 mg per 1 ml Clobazam 5mg/5ml oral suspension sugar free sugar-free | 150 ml [PoM] £90.00 DT = £90.00 [CD4-1] sugar-free | 250 ml [PoM] £150.00 [CD4-1]
Clobazam 2 mg per 1 ml Clobazam 10mg/5ml oral suspension sugar free sugar-free | 150 ml [PoM] £95.00 DT = £95.00 [CD4-1] sugar-free | 250 ml [PoM] £158.33 [CD4-1]
▶ Perizam (Rosemont Pharmaceuticals Ltd)
Clobazam 1 mg per 1 ml Perizam 1mg/ml oral suspension sugar-free | 150 ml [PoM] £90.00 DT = £90.00 [CD4-1]
Clobazam 2 mg per 1 ml Perizam 2mg/ml oral suspension sugar-free | 150 ml [PoM] £95.00 DT = £95.00 [CD4-1]
▶ Tapclob (Martindale Pharmaceuticals Ltd)
Clobazam 1 mg per 1 ml Tapclob 5mg/5ml oral suspension sugar-free | 150 ml [PoM] £90.00 DT = £90.00 [CD4-1] sugar-free | 250 ml [PoM] £150.00 [CD4-1]
Clobazam 2 mg per 1 ml Tapclob 10mg/5ml oral suspension sugar-free | 150 ml [PoM] £95.00 DT = £95.00 [CD4-1] sugar-free | 250 ml [PoM] £158.34 [CD4-1]
▶ Zacco (Thame Laboratories Ltd)
Clobazam 1 mg per 1 ml Zacco 5mg/5ml oral suspension sugar-free | 150 ml [PoM] £82.00 DT = £90.00 [CD4-1]
Clobazam 2 mg per 1 ml Zacco 10mg/5ml oral suspension sugar-free | 150 ml [PoM] £87.00 DT = £95.00 [CD4-1]

Tablet
CAUTIONARY AND ADVISORY LABELS 2, 8, 19
▶ Clobazam (Non-proprietary)
Clobazam 10 mg Clobazam 10mg tablets | 30 tablet [PoM] £3.75 DT = £3.75 [CD4-1]
▶ Frisium (Sanofi)
Clobazam 10 mg Frisium 10mg tablets | 30 tablet [PoM] £2.51 DT = £3.75 [CD4-1]

F 361

Clonazepam

01-Oct-2020

● **INDICATIONS AND DOSE**

All forms of epilepsy
▶ BY MOUTH
▶ Child 1-11 months: Initially 250 micrograms once daily for 4 nights, dose to be increased over 2–4 weeks, usual dose 0.5–1 mg daily, dose to be taken at night; may be given in 3 divided doses if necessary
▶ Child 1-4 years: Initially 250 micrograms once daily for 4 nights, dose to be increased over 2–4 weeks, usual dose 1–3 mg daily, dose to be taken at night; may be given in 3 divided doses if necessary continued →

4

Nervous system

▸ **Child 5–11 years:** Initially 500 micrograms once daily for 4 nights, dose to be increased over 2–4 weeks, usual dose 3–6 mg daily, dose to be taken at night; may be given in 3 divided doses if necessary
▸ **Child 12–17 years:** Initially 1 mg once daily for 4 nights, dose to be increased over 2–4 weeks, usual dose 4–8 mg daily, dose usually taken at night; may be given in 3–4 divided doses if necessary

All forms of epilepsy | Myoclonus
▸ BY MOUTH
▸ **Adult:** Initially 1 mg once daily for 4 nights, dose to be increased over 2–4 weeks, usual dose 4–8 mg daily, adjusted according to response, dose usually taken at night; may be given in 3–4 divided doses if necessary
▸ **Elderly:** Initially 500 micrograms once daily for 4 nights, dose to be increased over 2–4 weeks, usual dose 4–8 mg daily, adjusted according to response, dose usually taken at night; may be given in 3–4 divided doses if necessary

Panic disorders (with or without agoraphobia) resistant to antidepressant therapy
▸ BY MOUTH
▸ **Adult:** 1–2 mg daily

● **UNLICENSED USE** Clonazepam doses in BNF may differ from those in product literature. Use for panic disorders (with or without agoraphobia) resistant to antidepressant therapy is an unlicensed indication.

> **IMPORTANT SAFETY INFORMATION**
>
> SAFE PRACTICE
> Clonazepam has been confused with clobazam; care must be taken to ensure the correct drug is prescribed and dispensed.
>
> MHRA/CHM ADVICE: ANTIEPILEPTICS: RISK OF SUICIDAL THOUGHTS AND BEHAVIOUR (AUGUST 2008)
> See Epilepsy p. 321.
>
> MHRA/CHM ADVICE: ANTIEPILEPTIC DRUGS: UPDATED ADVICE ON SWITCHING BETWEEN DIFFERENT MANUFACTURERS' PRODUCTS (NOVEMBER 2017)
> See Epilepsy p. 321 and see also *Prescribing and dispensing information.*

● **CONTRA-INDICATIONS** Coma · current alcohol abuse · current drug abuse · respiratory depression
● **CAUTIONS** Acute porphyrias p. 1107 · airways obstruction · brain damage · cerebellar ataxia · depression · spinal ataxia · suicidal ideation
CAUTIONS, FURTHER INFORMATION The effectiveness of clonazepam may decrease significantly after weeks or months of continuous therapy.
● **INTERACTIONS** → Appendix 1: benzodiazepines
● **SIDE-EFFECTS** Alopecia · bronchial secretion increased (in children) · concentration impaired · coordination abnormal · drooling (in children) · hypersalivation (in children) · incomplete precocious puberty (in children) · increased risk of fall (in adults) · increased risk of fracture (in adults) · muscle tone decreased · nystagmus · seizures · sexual dysfunction · skin reactions · speech impairment · suicidal behaviours
● **BREAST FEEDING** Present in milk, and should be avoided if possible during breast-feeding.
Monitoring All infants should be monitored for sedation, feeding difficulties, adequate weight gain, and developmental milestones.
● **RENAL IMPAIRMENT**
Dose adjustments Start with small doses in severe impairment.
● **MONITORING REQUIREMENTS**
▸ In children Routine measurement of plasma concentrations of antiepileptic drugs is not usually justified, because the

target concentration ranges are arbitrary and often vary between individuals. However, plasma drug concentrations may be measured in children with worsening seizures, status epilepticus, suspected noncompliance, or suspected toxicity. Similarly, haematological and biochemical monitoring should not be undertaken unless clinically indicated.
● **PRESCRIBING AND DISPENSING INFORMATION** The RCPCH and NPPG recommend that, when a liquid special of clonazepam is required, the following strength is used: 2 mg/5 mL.
Switching between formulations Care should be taken when switching between oral formulations in the treatment of epilepsy. The need for continued supply of a particular manufacturer's product should be based on clinical judgement and consultation with the patient or their carer, taking into account factors such as seizure frequency and treatment history.
  Patients being treated for epilepsy may need to be maintained on a specific manufacturer's branded or generic oral clonazepam product.
● **PATIENT AND CARER ADVICE**
Medicines for Children leaflet: Clonazepam for preventing seizures www.medicinesforchildren.org.uk/clonazepam-preventing-seizures-0

● **MEDICINAL FORMS** There can be variation in the licensing of different medicines containing the same drug. Forms available from special-order manufacturers include: orodispersible tablet, oral suspension, oral solution

Tablet
CAUTIONARY AND ADVISORY LABELS 2, 8
▸ Clonazepam (Non-proprietary)
  Clonazepam 500 microgram Clonazepam 500microgram tablets | 100 tablet [PoM] £31.82 DT = £31.82 [CD4-1]
  Clonazepam 2 mg Clonazepam 2mg tablets | 100 tablet [PoM] £34.50 DT = £34.50 [CD4-1]

Oral solution
CAUTIONARY AND ADVISORY LABELS 2, 8
EXCIPIENTS: May contain Ethanol
▸ Clonazepam (Non-proprietary)
  Clonazepam 100 microgram per 1 ml Clonazepam 500micrograms/5ml oral solution sugar free sugar-free | 150 ml [PoM] £77.09 DT = £77.09 [CD4-1]
  Clonazepam 400 microgram per 1 ml Clonazepam 2mg/5ml oral solution sugar free sugar-free | 150 ml [PoM] £108.38 DT = £108.38 [CD4-1]

2.1   Status epilepticus

> **Other drugs used for Status epilepticus** Diazepam, p. 362 · Fosphenytoin sodium, p. 331 · Phenobarbital, p. 353 · Phenytoin, p. 340

ANTIEPILEPTICS ⟩ BARBITURATES

Thiopental sodium
10-Dec-2020

(Thiopentone sodium)

● **INDICATIONS AND DOSE**
Status epilepticus (only if other measures fail)
▸ BY SLOW INTRAVENOUS INJECTION
▸ **Adult:** 75–125 mg for 1 dose, to be administered as a 2.5% (25 mg/mL) solution
Induction of anaesthesia
▸ BY SLOW INTRAVENOUS INJECTION
▸ **Adult:** Initially 100–150 mg, to be administered over 10–15 seconds usually as a 2.5% (25 mg/mL) solution, followed by 100–150 mg after 0.5–1 minute if required, dose to be given in fit and premedicated adults;

debilitated patients or adults over 65 years may require a lower dose or increased administration time, alternatively initially up to 4 mg/kg (max. per dose 500 mg)

Anaesthesia of short duration
▶ BY SLOW INTRAVENOUS INJECTION
▶ Adult: Initially 100–150 mg, to be administered over 10–15 seconds usually as a 2.5% (25 mg/mL) solution, followed by 100–150 mg after 0.5–1 minute if required, dose to be given in fit and premedicated adults; debilitated patients or adults over 65 years may require a lower dose or increased administration time, alternatively initially up to 4 mg/kg (max. per dose 500 mg)

Reduction of raised intracranial pressure if ventilation controlled
▶ BY SLOW INTRAVENOUS INJECTION
▶ Adult: 1.5–3 mg/kg, repeated if necessary

> **IMPORTANT SAFETY INFORMATION**
> Thiopental sodium should only be administered by, or under the direct supervision of, personnel experienced in its use, with adequate training in anaesthesia and airway management, and when resuscitation equipment is available.

● CONTRA-INDICATIONS Acute porphyrias p. 1107 · myotonic dystrophy
● CAUTIONS Acute circulatory failure (shock) · avoid intra-arterial injection · cardiovascular disease · elderly · hypovolaemia · reconstituted solution is highly alkaline (extravasation causes tissue necrosis and severe pain) · respiratory diseases (avoid in acute asthma)
● INTERACTIONS → Appendix 1: thiopental
● SIDE-EFFECTS
▶ **Common or very common** Arrhythmia · myocardial contractility decreased
▶ **Frequency not known** Appetite decreased · circulatory collapse · cough · electrolyte imbalance · extravasation necrosis · hypotension · respiratory disorders · skin eruption · sneezing
● PREGNANCY May depress neonatal respiration when used during delivery.
● BREAST FEEDING Breast-feeding can be resumed as soon as mother has recovered sufficiently from anaesthesia.
● HEPATIC IMPAIRMENT Manufacturer advises caution.
  Dose adjustments Manufacturer advises dose reduction.
● RENAL IMPAIRMENT Caution in severe impairment.
● PATIENT AND CARER ADVICE
  Driving and skilled tasks Patients given sedatives and analgesics during minor outpatient procedures should be very carefully warned about the risk of driving or undertaking skilled tasks afterwards. For a short general anaesthetic the risk extends to **at least 24 hours** after administration. Responsible persons should be available to take patients home. The dangers of taking **alcohol** should also be emphasised.

● MEDICINAL FORMS There can be variation in the licensing of different medicines containing the same drug. Forms available from special-order manufacturers include: solution for injection

Powder for solution for injection
▶ Thiopental sodium (Non-proprietary)
  Thiopental sodium 500 mg Thiopental 500mg powder for solution for injection vials | 10 vial [PoM] £57.60–£69.00

HYPNOTICS, SEDATIVES AND
ANXIOLYTICS > BENZODIAZEPINES

F 361

Lorazepam

21-Oct-2019

● INDICATIONS AND DOSE
Short-term use in anxiety
▶ BY MOUTH
▶ Adult: 1–4 mg daily in divided doses, for debilitated patients, use elderly dose
▶ Elderly: 0.5–2 mg daily in divided doses

Short-term use in insomnia associated with anxiety
▶ BY MOUTH
▶ Adult: 1–2 mg daily, to be taken at bedtime

Acute panic attacks
▶ BY INTRAMUSCULAR INJECTION, OR BY SLOW INTRAVENOUS INJECTION
▶ Adult: 25–30 micrograms/kg every 6 hours if required; usual dose 1.5–2.5 mg every 6 hours if required, intravenous injection to be administered into a large vein, only use intramuscular route when oral and intravenous routes not possible

Conscious sedation for procedures
▶ BY MOUTH
▶ Adult: 2–3 mg, to be taken the night before operation; 2–4 mg, to be taken 1–2 hours before operation
▶ BY SLOW INTRAVENOUS INJECTION
▶ Adult: 50 micrograms/kg, to be administered 30–45 minutes before operation
▶ BY INTRAMUSCULAR INJECTION
▶ Adult: 50 micrograms/kg, to be administered 60–90 minutes before operation

Premedication
▶ BY MOUTH
▶ Adult: 2–3 mg, to be taken the night before operation; 2–4 mg, to be taken 1–2 hours before operation
▶ BY SLOW INTRAVENOUS INJECTION
▶ Adult: 50 micrograms/kg, to be administered 30–45 minutes before operation
▶ BY INTRAMUSCULAR INJECTION
▶ Adult: 50 micrograms/kg, to be administered 60–90 minutes before operation

Status epilepticus | Febrile convulsions | Convulsions caused by poisoning
▶ BY SLOW INTRAVENOUS INJECTION
▶ Child 1 month–11 years: 100 micrograms/kg (max. per dose 4 mg) for 1 dose, then 100 micrograms/kg after 10 minutes (max. per dose 4 mg) if required for 1 dose, to be administered into a large vein
▶ Child 12–17 years: 4 mg for 1 dose, then 4 mg after 10 minutes if required for 1 dose, to be administered into a large vein
▶ Adult: 4 mg for 1 dose, then 4 mg after 10 minutes if required for 1 dose, to be administered into a large vein

● UNLICENSED USE
▶ In children Not licensed for use in febrile convulsions. Not licensed for use in convulsions caused by poisoning.

> **IMPORTANT SAFETY INFORMATION**
> ANAESTHESIA
> Benzodiazepines should only be administered for anaesthesia by, or under the direct supervision of, personnel experienced in their use, with adequate training in anaesthesia and airway management.

● CONTRA-INDICATIONS Avoid injections containing benzyl alcohol in neonates · CNS depression · compromised airway · respiratory depression

- CAUTIONS Muscle weakness · organic brain changes · parenteral administration
  CAUTIONS, FURTHER INFORMATION
  ▸ Paradoxical effects A paradoxical increase in hostility and aggression may be reported by patients taking benzodiazepines. The effects range from talkativeness and excitement to aggressive and antisocial acts. Adjustment of the dose (up or down) sometimes attenuates the impulses. Increased anxiety and perceptual disorders are other paradoxical effects.
  ▸ Special precautions for parenteral administration When given parenterally, facilities for managing respiratory depression with mechanical ventilation must be available. Close observation required until full recovery from sedation.
- INTERACTIONS → Appendix 1: benzodiazepines
- SIDE-EFFECTS
  GENERAL SIDE-EFFECTS
  ▸ **Common or very common** Apnoea · asthenia · coma · disinhibition · extrapyramidal symptoms · hypothermia · memory loss · speech slurred · suicide attempt
  ▸ **Uncommon** Allergic dermatitis · constipation · sexual dysfunction
  ▸ **Rare or very rare** Agranulocytosis · hyponatraemia · pancytopenia · SIADH · thrombocytopenia
  SPECIFIC SIDE-EFFECTS
  ▸ **Rare or very rare**
  ▸ With oral use Saliva altered
  ▸ **Frequency not known**
  ▸ With parenteral use Leucopenia
- BREAST FEEDING Benzodiazepines are present in milk, and should be avoided if possible during breast-feeding.
- RENAL IMPAIRMENT
  Dose adjustments Start with small doses in severe impairment.
- DIRECTIONS FOR ADMINISTRATION
  ▸ With intravenous use in children For *intravenous injection*, dilute with an equal volume of Sodium Chloride 0.9% (for neonates, dilute injection solution to a concentration of 100 micrograms/mL). Give over 3–5 minutes; max. rate 50 micrograms/kg over 3 minutes.
  ▸ With intramuscular use in adults For intramuscular injection, solution for injection should be diluted with an equal volume of water for injections or sodium chloride 0.9% (but only use when oral and intravenous routes not possible).
  ▸ With intravenous use in adults For slow intravenous injection, solution for injection should preferably be diluted with an equal volume of water for injections or sodium chloride 0.9%.
- PATIENT AND CARER ADVICE
  Driving and skilled tasks Patients given sedatives and analgesics during minor outpatient procedures should be very carefully warned about the risks of undertaking skilled tasks (e.g. driving) afterwards. For intravenous benzodiazepines the risk extends to at least 24 hours after administration. Responsible persons should be available to take patients home afterwards. The dangers of taking **alcohol** should be emphasised.

- MEDICINAL FORMS There can be variation in the licensing of different medicines containing the same drug. Forms available from special-order manufacturers include: oral suspension, oral solution, solution for injection
  Solution for injection
  EXCIPIENTS: May contain Benzyl alcohol, propylene glycol
  ▸ Lorazepam (Non-proprietary)
  Lorazepam 2 mg per 1 ml Lorazepam 2mg/1ml solution for injection Carpuject cartridges | 10 cartridge [PoM] 🅢 (Hospital only) [CD4-1]
  Lorazepam 2mg/1ml solution for injection vials | 10 vial [PoM] 🅢 [CD4-1]

  ▸ Ativan (Pfizer Ltd)
  Lorazepam 4 mg per 1 ml Ativan 4mg/1ml solution for injection ampoules | 10 ampoule [PoM] £3.54 [CD4-1]

  Oral solution
  CAUTIONARY AND ADVISORY LABELS 2, 19
  EXCIPIENTS: May contain Ethanol
  ▸ Lorazepam (Non-proprietary)
  Lorazepam 1 mg per 1 ml Lorazepam 1mg/ml oral solution sugar free sugar-free | 150 ml [PoM] £103.62 DT = £103.62 [CD4-1]

  Tablet
  CAUTIONARY AND ADVISORY LABELS 2, 19
  ▸ Lorazepam (Non-proprietary)
  Lorazepam 500 microgram Lorazepam 500microgram tablets | 28 tablet [PoM] £14.04–£16.50 DT = £14.04 [CD4-1]
  Lorazepam 1 mg Lorazepam 1mg tablets | 28 tablet [PoM] £6.59 DT = £3.46 [CD4-1]
  Lorazepam 2.5 mg Lorazepam 2.5mg tablets | 28 tablet [PoM] £11.43 DT = £6.67 [CD4-1]

🏴 361

Midazolam

10-Nov-2020

- INDICATIONS AND DOSE
  Status epilepticus | Febrile convulsions
  ▸ BY BUCCAL ADMINISTRATION
  ▸ Child 1-2 months: 300 micrograms/kg (max. per dose 2.5 mg), then 300 micrograms/kg after 10 minutes (max. per dose 2.5 mg) if required
  ▸ Child 3-11 months: 2.5 mg, then 2.5 mg after 10 minutes if required
  ▸ Child 1-4 years: 5 mg, then 5 mg after 10 minutes if required
  ▸ Child 5-9 years: 7.5 mg, then 7.5 mg after 10 minutes if required
  ▸ Child 10-17 years: 10 mg, then 10 mg after 10 minutes if required
  ▸ Adult: 10 mg, then 10 mg after 10 minutes if required

  Conscious sedation for procedures
  ▸ BY SLOW INTRAVENOUS INJECTION
  ▸ Adult: Initially 2–2.5 mg, to be administered 5–10 minutes before procedure at a rate of approximately 2 mg/minute, increased in steps of 1 mg if required, usual total dose is 3.5–5 mg; maximum 7.5 mg per course
  ▸ Elderly: Initially 0.5–1 mg, to be administered 5–10 minutes before procedure at a rate of approximately 2 mg/minute, increased in steps of 0.5–1 mg if required; maximum 3.5 mg per course

  Sedative in combined anaesthesia
  ▸ INITIALLY BY INTRAVENOUS INJECTION
  ▸ Adult: 30–100 micrograms/kg, repeated if necessary, alternatively (by continuous intravenous infusion) 30–100 micrograms/kg/hour
  ▸ Elderly: Lower doses needed

  Premedication
  ▸ BY DEEP INTRAMUSCULAR INJECTION
  ▸ Adult: 70–100 micrograms/kg, to be administered 20–60 minutes before induction, for debilitated patients, use elderly dose
  ▸ Elderly: 25–50 micrograms/kg, to be administered 20–60 minutes before induction
  ▸ BY INTRAVENOUS INJECTION
  ▸ Adult: 1–2 mg, repeated if necessary, to be administered 5–30 minutes before procedure, for debilitated patients, use elderly dose
  ▸ Elderly: 0.5 mg, repeated if necessary, initial dose to be administered 5–30 minutes before procedure, repeat dose slowly as required

  Induction of anaesthesia (but rarely used)
  ▸ BY SLOW INTRAVENOUS INJECTION
  ▸ Adult: 150–200 micrograms/kg daily in divided doses (max. per dose 5 mg), dose to be given at intervals of

2 minutes, maximum total dose 600 micrograms/kg, for debilitated patients, use elderly dose
▸ **Elderly:** 50–150 micrograms/kg daily in divided doses (max. per dose 5 mg), dose to be given at intervals of 2 minutes, maximum total dose 600 micrograms/kg

Sedation of patient receiving intensive care
▸ **INITIALLY BY SLOW INTRAVENOUS INJECTION**
▸ **Adult:** Initially 30–300 micrograms/kg, dose to be given in steps of 1–2.5 mg every 2 minutes, then (by slow intravenous injection or by continuous intravenous infusion) 30–200 micrograms/kg/hour, reduce dose (or reduce or omit initial dose) in hypovolaemia, vasoconstriction, or hypothermia, lower doses may be adequate if opioid analgesic also used

Adjunct to antipsychotic for confusion and restlessness in palliative care
▸ **BY SUBCUTANEOUS INFUSION**
▸ **Adult:** Initially 10–20 mg/24 hours, adjusted according to response; usual dose 20–60 mg/24 hours

Convulsions in palliative care
▸ **BY CONTINUOUS SUBCUTANEOUS INFUSION**
▸ **Adult:** Initially 20–40 mg/24 hours

● **UNLICENSED USE** Unlicensed oromucosal formulations are also available and may have different doses—refer to product literature.
▸ In adults Oromucosal solution not licensed for use in adults over 18 years.
▸ In children Oromucosal solution not licensed for use in children under 3 months. Injection not licensed for use in status epilepticus or febrile convulsions. Not licensed for use in children under 6 months for premedication and conscious sedation. Not licensed for use by mouth. Not licensed for use by buccal administration for conscious sedation.

IMPORTANT SAFETY INFORMATION

ANAESTHESIA
Benzodiazepines should only be administered for anaesthesia by, or under the direct supervision of, personnel experienced in their use, with adequate training in anaesthesia and airway management.

NHS NEVER EVENT: MIS-SELECTION OF HIGH-STRENGTH MIDAZOLAM DURING CONSCIOUS SEDATION (JANUARY 2018).
In clinical areas performing conscious sedation, high-strength preparations (5 mg/mL in 2 mL and 10 mL ampoules, or 2 mg/mL in 5 mL ampoules) should **not** be selected in place of the 1 mg/mL preparation.
    The areas where high-strength midazolam is used should be restricted to those performing general anaesthesia, intensive care, palliative care, or areas where its use has been formally risk-assessed in the organisation. In these situations the higher strength may be more appropriate to administer the prescribed dose.
    It is advised that flumazenil is available when midazolam is used, to reverse the effects if necessary.

● **CONTRA-INDICATIONS** CNS depression · compromised airway · severe respiratory depression
● **CAUTIONS** Cardiac disease · children (particularly if cardiovascular impairment) · concentration of midazolam in children under 15 kg not to exceed 1 mg/mL · debilitated patients (reduce dose) (in children) · hypothermia · hypovolaemia (risk of severe hypotension) · neonates · risk of airways obstruction and hypoventilation in children under 6 months (monitor respiratory rate and oxygen saturation) · vasoconstriction

CAUTIONS, FURTHER INFORMATION
▸ Recovery when used for sedation Midazolam has a fast onset of action, recovery is faster than for other benzodiazepines such as diazepam, but may be significantly longer in the

elderly, in patients with a low cardiac output, or after repeated dosing.
● **INTERACTIONS** → Appendix 1: benzodiazepines
● **SIDE-EFFECTS**
    GENERAL SIDE-EFFECTS
▸ **Common or very common** Vomiting
▸ **Uncommon** Skin reactions
▸ **Rare or very rare** Dry mouth · dyspnoea · hiccups · movement disorders · respiratory disorders
▸ **Frequency not known** Disinhibition (severe; with sedative and peri-operative use) (in children)
    SPECIFIC SIDE-EFFECTS
▸ **Common or very common**
▸ With buccal use Level of consciousness decreased
▸ **Rare or very rare**
▸ With buccal use Apnoea · bradycardia · cardiac arrest · constipation · physical assault · vasodilation
▸ **Frequency not known**
▸ With buccal use Appetite increased · fall · saliva altered · thrombosis
▸ With parenteral use Angioedema · apnoea · appetite increased · bradycardia · cardiac arrest · constipation · drug abuse · drug withdrawal seizure · embolism and thrombosis · fall · level of consciousness decreased · physical assault · saliva altered · vasodilation

SIDE-EFFECTS, FURTHER INFORMATION Higher doses are associated with prolonged sedation and risk of hypoventilation. The co-administration of midazolam with other sedative, hypnotic, or CNS-depressant drugs results in increased sedation. Midazolam accumulates in adipose tissue, which can significantly prolong sedation, especially in patients with obesity, hepatic impairment or renal impairment.

Overdose There have been reports of overdosage when high strength midazolam has been used for conscious sedation. The use of high-strength midazolam (5mg/mL in 2mL and 10mL ampoules, or 2mg/mL in 5mL ampoules) should be restricted to general anaesthesia, intensive care, palliative care, or other situations where the risk has been assessed. It is advised that flumazenil is available when midazolam is used, to reverse the effects if necessary.

● **BREAST FEEDING** Small amount present in milk—avoid breast-feeding for 24 hours after administration (although amount probably too small to be harmful after single doses).
● **HEPATIC IMPAIRMENT** For *parenteral preparations* manufacturer advises caution in all degrees of impairment. **Dose adjustments** For *parenteral preparations* manufacturer advises consider dose reduction in all degrees of impairment.
● **RENAL IMPAIRMENT** Use with caution in chronic renal failure.
● **DIRECTIONS FOR ADMINISTRATION**
▸ With intravenous use in adults For *intravenous infusion* (*Hypnovel®*), give continuously in Glucose 5% or Sodium chloride 0.9%.
● **PRESCRIBING AND DISPENSING INFORMATION**
Palliative care For further information on the use of midazolam in palliative care, see www.medicinescomplete. com/#/content/palliative/benzodiazepines-and-z-drugs.
● **PATIENT AND CARER ADVICE** Patients or carers should be given advice on how and when to administer midazolam oromucosal solution.
    Patients given sedatives and analgesics during minor outpatient procedures should be very carefully warned about the risks of undertaking skilled tasks (e.g. driving) afterwards. For intravenous benzodiazepines the risk extends to **at least 24 hours** after administration. Responsible persons should be available to take patients

home afterwards. The dangers of taking **alcohol** should be emphasised.

Medicines for Children leaflet: Midazolam for stopping seizures www.medicinesforchildren.org.uk/midazolam-stopping-seizures

● NATIONAL FUNDING/ACCESS DECISIONS

EPISTATUS OROMUCOSAL SOLUTION For full details see funding body website

Scottish Medicines Consortium (SMC) decisions

▶ **Midazolam oromucosal solution (*Epistatus* ®) for the treatment of prolonged, acute, convulsive seizures in children and adolescents aged 10 to less than 18 years (November 2017)** SMC No. 1279/17 Recommended

● MEDICINAL FORMS There can be variation in the licensing of different medicines containing the same drug. Forms available from special-order manufacturers include: oromucosal solution, solution for injection, infusion, solution for infusion

Solution for injection

▶ Midazolam (Non-proprietary)
  Midazolam (as Midazolam hydrochloride) 1 mg per 1 ml Midazolam 5mg/5ml solution for injection ampoules | 10 ampoule [PoM] £16.89 DT = £10.29 [CD3]
  Midazolam 2mg/2ml solution for injection ampoules | 10 ampoule [PoM] £4.50–£6.00 DT = £6.00 [CD3]
  Midazolam (as Midazolam hydrochloride) 2 mg per 1 ml Midazolam 10mg/5ml solution for injection ampoules | 10 ampoule [PoM] £7.51 DT = £7.26 [CD3]
  Midazolam (as Midazolam hydrochloride) 5 mg per 1 ml Midazolam 50mg/10ml solution for injection ampoules | 10 ampoule [PoM] £7.26 DT = £29.25 (Hospital only) [CD3] | 10 ampoule [PoM] £33.77 DT = £29.25 [CD3]
  Midazolam 15mg/3ml solution for injection ampoules | 10 ampoule [PoM] £7.26 (Hospital only) [CD3]
  Midazolam 10mg/2ml solution for injection ampoules | 10 ampoule [PoM] £7.65 DT = £7.13 [CD3]

▶ Hypnovel (Cheplapharm Arzneimittel GmbH)
  Midazolam (as Midazolam hydrochloride) 5 mg per 1 ml Hypnovel 10mg/2ml solution for injection ampoules | 10 ampoule [PoM] £7.11 DT = £7.13 [CD3]

Solution for infusion

▶ Midazolam (Non-proprietary)
  Midazolam (as Midazolam hydrochloride) 1 mg per 1 ml Midazolam 50mg/50ml solution for infusion pre-filled syringes | 1 pre-filled disposable injection [PoM] ▣ (Hospital only) [CD3]
  Midazolam 50mg/50ml solution for infusion vials | 1 vial [PoM] £9.56–£12.00 [CD3]
  Midazolam (as Midazolam hydrochloride) 2 mg per 1 ml Midazolam 100mg/50ml solution for infusion vials | 1 vial [PoM] £9.96–£13.50 [CD3]
  Midazolam 100mg/50ml solution for infusion pre-filled syringes | 1 pre-filled disposable injection [PoM] ▣ (Hospital only) [CD3]

Oromucosal solution

CAUTIONARY AND ADVISORY LABELS 2
EXCIPIENTS: May contain Ethanol

▶ Buccolam (Shire Pharmaceuticals Ltd)
  Midazolam (as Midazolam hydrochloride) 5 mg per 1 ml Buccolam 10mg/2ml oromucosal solution pre-filled oral syringes sugar-free | 4 unit dose [PoM] £91.50 DT = £91.50 [CD3]
  Buccolam 7.5mg/1.5ml oromucosal solution pre-filled oral syringes sugar-free | 4 unit dose [PoM] £89.00 DT = £89.00 [CD3]
  Buccolam 5mg/1ml oromucosal solution pre-filled oral syringes sugar-free | 4 unit dose [PoM] £85.50 DT = £85.50 [CD3]
  Buccolam 2.5mg/0.5ml oromucosal solution pre-filled oral syringes sugar-free | 4 unit dose [PoM] £82.00 DT = £82.00 [CD3]

▶ Epistatus (Veriton Pharma Ltd)
  Midazolam (as Midazolam maleate) 10 mg per 1 ml Epistatus 10mg/1ml oromucosal solution pre-filled oral syringes sugar-free | 1 unit dose [PoM] £45.76 DT = £45.76 [CD3]

3 Mental health disorders

3.1 Anxiety

Other drugs used for Anxiety Duloxetine, p. 387 · Escitalopram, p. 384 · Lorazepam, p. 357 · Moclobemide, p. 382 · Paroxetine, p. 386 · Pericyazine, p. 408 · Pregabalin, p. 342 · Trazodone hydrochloride, p. 390 · Trifluoperazine, p. 410 · Venlafaxine, p. 388

ANTIDEPRESSANTS ⟩ SEROTONIN RECEPTOR AGONISTS

▌Buspirone hydrochloride

20-Oct-2020

● INDICATIONS AND DOSE

Anxiety (short-term use)

▶ BY MOUTH
▶ Adult: 5 mg 2–3 times a day, increased if necessary up to 45 mg daily, dose to be increased at intervals of 2–3 days; usual dose 15–30 mg daily in divided doses

DOSE ADJUSTMENTS DUE TO INTERACTIONS
▶ Manufacturer advises reduce dose to 2.5 mg twice daily with concurrent use of potent inhibitors of CYP3A4.

● CONTRA-INDICATIONS Epilepsy

● CAUTIONS Angle-closure glaucoma · does not alleviate symptoms of benzodiazepine withdrawal · myasthenia gravis

CAUTIONS, FURTHER INFORMATION Manufacturer advises a patient taking a benzodiazepine still needs to have the benzodiazepine withdrawn gradually; it is advisable to do this before starting buspirone.

● INTERACTIONS → Appendix 1: buspirone

● SIDE-EFFECTS
▶ Common or very common Abdominal pain · anger · anxiety · chest pain · cold sweat · concentration impaired · confusion · constipation · depression · diarrhoea · dizziness · drowsiness · dry mouth · fatigue · headache · laryngeal pain · movement disorders · musculoskeletal pain · nasal congestion · nausea · paraesthesia · skin reactions · sleep disorders · tachycardia · tinnitus · tremor · vision disorders · vomiting
▶ Rare or very rare Depersonalisation · emotional lability · galactorrhoea · hallucination · memory loss · parkinsonism · psychotic disorder · seizure · serotonin syndrome · syncope · urinary retention

● PREGNANCY Avoid.

● BREAST FEEDING Avoid.

● HEPATIC IMPAIRMENT Manufacturer advises caution; avoid in severe hepatic failure.
Dose adjustments Manufacturer advises titrate individual dose carefully in cirrhosis—consult product literature.

● RENAL IMPAIRMENT Avoid if eGFR less than 20 mL/minute/1.73 m².
Dose adjustments Reduce dose.

● PATIENT AND CARER ADVICE
Driving and skilled tasks May affect performance of skilled tasks (e.g. driving); effects of alcohol may be enhanced.

● MEDICINAL FORMS There can be variation in the licensing of different medicines containing the same drug. Forms available from special-order manufacturers include: oral suspension, oral solution

Tablet

▶ Buspirone hydrochloride (Non-proprietary)
  Buspirone hydrochloride 5 mg Buspirone 5mg tablets | 30 tablet [PoM] £14.36 DT = £14.36

Buspirone hydrochloride **7.5 mg** Buspirone 7.5mg tablets |
30 tablet [PoM] £15.00 DT = £25.99
Buspirone hydrochloride **10 mg** Buspirone 10mg tablets |
30 tablet [PoM] £15.62 DT = £15.47

HYPNOTICS, SEDATIVES AND ANXIOLYTICS >
BENZODIAZEPINES

Benzodiazepines

IMPORTANT SAFETY INFORMATION

MHRA/CHM ADVICE: BENZODIAZEPINES AND OPIOIDS: REMINDER OF RISK OF POTENTIALLY FATAL RESPIRATORY DEPRESSION (MARCH 2020)
The MHRA reminds healthcare professionals that benzodiazepines and benzodiazepine-like drugs co-prescribed with opioids can produce additive CNS depressant effects, thereby increasing the risk of sedation, respiratory depression, coma, and death. Healthcare professionals are advised to only co-prescribe if there is no alternative and, if necessary, the lowest possible doses should be given for the shortest duration. Patients should be closely monitored for signs of respiratory depression at initiation of treatment and when there is any change in prescribing, such as dose adjustments or new interactions. If methadone is co-prescribed with a benzodiazepine or benzodiazepine-like drug, the respiratory depressant effect of methadone may be delayed; patients should be monitored for at least 2 weeks after initiation or changes in prescribing. Patients should be informed of the signs and symptoms of respiratory depression and sedation, and advised to seek urgent medical attention should these occur.

● CONTRA-INDICATIONS Acute pulmonary insufficiency · marked neuromuscular respiratory weakness · not for use alone to treat chronic psychosis (in adults) · not for use alone to treat depression (or anxiety associated with depression) (in adults) · obsessional states · phobic states · sleep apnoea syndrome · unstable myasthenia gravis

● CAUTIONS Avoid prolonged use (and abrupt withdrawal thereafter) · debilitated patients (reduce dose) (in adults) · elderly (reduce dose) · history of alcohol dependence or abuse · history of drug dependence or abuse · myasthenia gravis · personality disorder (within the fearful group—dependent, avoidant, obsessive-compulsive) may increase risk of dependence · respiratory disease

CAUTIONS, FURTHER INFORMATION
▸ **Paradoxical effects** A paradoxical increase in hostility and aggression may be reported by patients taking benzodiazepines. The effects range from talkativeness and excitement to aggressive and antisocial acts. Adjustment of the dose (up or down) sometimes attenuates the impulses. Increased anxiety and perceptual disorders are other paradoxical effects.
▸ **Elderly** Prescription potentially inappropriate (STOPP criteria):
 ● for a duration of 4 weeks or longer (no indication for longer treatment; risk of adverse events; all benzodiazepines should be withdrawn gradually if taken for more than 2 weeks as there is a risk of causing a benzodiazepine withdrawal syndrome if stopped abruptly)
 ● with acute or chronic respiratory failure i.e. $PaO_2 < 8$ kPa with or without $PaCO_2 > 6.5$ kPa (risk of exacerbation of respiratory failure)
 ● in patients prone to falls (sedative, may cause reduced sensorium and impair balance)
 See also Prescribing in the elderly p. 33.

● SIDE-EFFECTS
▸ **Common or very common** Alertness decreased · anxiety · ataxia (more common in elderly) · confusion (more common in elderly) · depression · dizziness · drowsiness · dysarthria · fatigue · gastrointestinal disorder · headache · hypotension · mood altered · muscle weakness · nausea · respiratory depression (particularly with high dose and intravenous use—facilities for its treatment are essential) · sleep disorders · suicidal ideation · tremor · vertigo · vision disorders · withdrawal syndrome
▸ **Uncommon** Agitation (more common in children and elderly) · anterograde amnesia · behaviour abnormal · hallucination · libido disorder · rash · urinary disorders
▸ **Rare or very rare** Aggression (more common in children and elderly) · blood disorder · delusions · jaundice · paradoxical drug reaction · psychosis · restlessness (with sedative and peri-operative use)
▸ **Frequency not known** Drug dependence
 Overdose Benzodiazepines taken alone cause drowsiness, ataxia, dysarthria, nystagmus, and occasionally respiratory depression, and coma. For details on the management of poisoning, see Benzodiazepines, under Emergency treatment of poisoning p. 1413.

● PREGNANCY Risk of neonatal withdrawal symptoms when used during pregnancy. Avoid regular use and use only if there is a clear indication such as seizure control. High doses administered during late pregnancy or labour may cause neonatal hypothermia, hypotonia, and respiratory depression.

● HEPATIC IMPAIRMENT In general, manufacturers advise caution in mild to moderate impairment; avoid in severe impairment. Benzodiazepines with a shorter half-life are considered safer.
 Dose adjustments In general, manufacturers advise dose reduction in mild to moderate impairment, adjust dose according to response.

● RENAL IMPAIRMENT Increased cerebral sensitivity to benzodiazepines.

● PATIENT AND CARER ADVICE
 Driving and skilled tasks May cause drowsiness, impair judgement and increase reaction time, and so affect ability to drive or perform skilled tasks; effects of alcohol increased. Moreover the hangover effects of a night dose may impair performance on the following day.
 For information on 2015 legislation regarding driving whilst taking certain controlled drugs, including benzodiazepines, see *Drugs and driving* under Guidance on prescribing p. 1.

◤ above

Alprazolam

21-Oct-2019

● INDICATIONS AND DOSE

Short-term use in anxiety
▸ BY MOUTH
▸ Adult: 250–500 micrograms 3 times a day, increased if necessary up to 3 mg daily, for debilitated patients, use elderly dose
▸ Elderly: 250 micrograms 2–3 times a day, increased if necessary up to 3 mg daily

● CONTRA-INDICATIONS Respiratory depression
● CAUTIONS Muscle weakness · organic brain changes
● INTERACTIONS → Appendix 1: benzodiazepines
● SIDE-EFFECTS
▸ **Common or very common** Appetite decreased · concentration impaired · constipation · dermatitis · dry mouth · memory loss · movement disorders · sexual dysfunction · weight changes
▸ **Uncommon** Menstruation irregular

▶ **Frequency not known** Angioedema · autonomic dysfunction · hepatic disorders · hyperprolactinaemia · peripheral oedema · photosensitivity reaction · suicide · thinking abnormal

● BREAST-FEEDING Benzodiazepines are present in milk, and should be avoided if possible during breast-feeding.

● RENAL IMPAIRMENT
Dose adjustments Start with small doses in severe impairment.

● NATIONAL FUNDING/ACCESS DECISIONS
NHS restrictions Alprazolam tablets are not prescribable in NHS primary care.

● MEDICINAL FORMS There can be variation in the licensing of different medicines containing the same drug.
Tablet
CAUTIONARY AND ADVISORY LABELS 2
▶ Xanax (Upjohn UK Ltd)
Alprazolam 250 microgram Xanax 250microgram tablets | 60 tablet PoM £3.18 CD4-1
Alprazolam 500 microgram Xanax 500microgram tablets | 60 tablet PoM £6.09 CD4-1

▶ 361

Chlordiazepoxide hydrochloride

21-Oct-2019

● **INDICATIONS AND DOSE**
Short-term use in anxiety
▶ BY MOUTH
▶ Adult: 10 mg 3 times a day, increased if necessary to 60–100 mg daily in divided doses, for debilitated patients, use elderly dose
▶ Elderly: 5 mg 3 times a day, increased if necessary to 30–50 mg daily in divided doses

Treatment of alcohol withdrawal in moderate dependence
▶ BY MOUTH
▶ Adult: 10–30 mg 4 times a day, dose to be gradually reduced over 5–7 days, consult local protocols for titration regimens

Treatment of alcohol withdrawal in severe dependence
▶ BY MOUTH
▶ Adult: 10–50 mg 4 times a day and 10–40 mg as required for the first 2 days, dose to be gradually reduced over 7–10 days, consult local protocols for titration regimens; maximum 250 mg per day

● CONTRA-INDICATIONS Chronic psychosis · respiratory depression

● CAUTIONS Muscle weakness · organic brain changes

● INTERACTIONS → Appendix 1: benzodiazepines

● SIDE-EFFECTS
▶ **Common or very common** Movement disorders
▶ **Rare or very rare** Abdominal distress · agranulocytosis · bone marrow disorders · erectile dysfunction · leucopenia · menstrual disorder · skin eruption · thrombocytopenia
▶ **Frequency not known** Appetite increased · gait abnormal · increased risk of fall · level of consciousness decreased · memory loss · saliva altered · suicide attempt

● BREAST FEEDING Benzodiazepines are present in milk, and should be avoided if possible during breast-feeding.

● HEPATIC IMPAIRMENT
Dose adjustments Manufacturer advises dose reduction to max. 50% of the usual dose in mild to moderate impairment.

● RENAL IMPAIRMENT
Dose adjustments Start with small doses in severe impairment.

● NATIONAL FUNDING/ACCESS DECISIONS
NHS restrictions *Librium* ® is not prescribable in NHS primary care.

● MEDICINAL FORMS There can be variation in the licensing of different medicines containing the same drug. Forms available from special-order manufacturers include: oral suspension, oral solution
Capsule
CAUTIONARY AND ADVISORY LABELS 2
▶ Chlordiazepoxide hydrochloride (Non-proprietary)
Chlordiazepoxide hydrochloride 5 mg Chlordiazepoxide 5mg capsules | 100 capsule PoM £15.16 DT = £15.16 CD4-1
Chlordiazepoxide hydrochloride 10 mg Chlordiazepoxide 10mg capsules | 100 capsule PoM £18.00 DT = £18.00 CD4-1
▶ Librium (Mylan)
Chlordiazepoxide hydrochloride 5 mg Librium 5mg capsules | 100 capsule PoM £5.38 DT = £15.16 CD4-1
Chlordiazepoxide hydrochloride 10 mg Librium 10mg capsules | 100 capsule PoM £7.46 DT = £18.00 CD4-1

▶ 361

Diazepam

12-Oct-2020

● **INDICATIONS AND DOSE**
Muscle spasm of varied aetiology
▶ BY MOUTH
▶ Adult: 2–15 mg daily in divided doses, then increased if necessary to 60 mg daily, adjusted according to response, dose only increased in spastic conditions

Acute muscle spasm
▶ BY INTRAMUSCULAR INJECTION, OR BY SLOW INTRAVENOUS INJECTION
▶ Adult: 10 mg, then 10 mg after 4 hours if required, intravenous injection to be administered into a large vein at a rate of no more than 5 mg/minute

Tetanus
▶ BY INTRAVENOUS INJECTION
▶ Child: 100–300 micrograms/kg every 1–4 hours
▶ Adult: 100–300 micrograms/kg every 1–4 hours
▶ BY INTRAVENOUS INFUSION, OR BY NASODUODENAL TUBE
▶ Child: 3–10 mg/kg, adjusted according to response, to be given over 24 hours
▶ Adult: 3–10 mg/kg, adjusted according to response, to be given over 24 hours

Muscle spasm in cerebral spasticity or in postoperative skeletal muscle spasm
▶ BY MOUTH
▶ Child 1-11 months: Initially 250 micrograms/kg twice daily
▶ Child 1-4 years: Initially 2.5 mg twice daily
▶ Child 5-11 years: Initially 5 mg twice daily
▶ Child 12-17 years: Initially 10 mg twice daily; maximum 40 mg per day

Anxiety
▶ BY MOUTH
▶ Adult: 2 mg 3 times a day, then increased if necessary to 15–30 mg daily in divided doses, for debilitated patients, use elderly dose
▶ Elderly: 1 mg 3 times a day, then increased if necessary to 7.5–15 mg daily in divided doses

Insomnia associated with anxiety
▶ BY MOUTH
▶ Adult: 5–15 mg daily, to be taken at bedtime

Severe acute anxiety | Control of acute panic attacks | Acute alcohol withdrawal
▶ BY INTRAMUSCULAR INJECTION, OR BY SLOW INTRAVENOUS INJECTION
▶ Adult: 10 mg, then 10 mg after at least 4 hours if required, intravenous injection to be administered into a large vein, at a rate of not more than 5 mg/minute

Acute drug-induced dystonic reactions
▸ BY INTRAVENOUS INJECTION
▸ Adult: 5–10 mg, then 5–10 mg after at least 10 minutes as required, to be administered into a large vein, at a rate of not more than 5 mg/minute

Acute anxiety and agitation
▸ BY RECTUM
▸ Adult: 500 micrograms/kg, then 500 micrograms/kg after 12 hours as required
▸ Elderly: 250 micrograms/kg, then 250 micrograms/kg after 12 hours as required

Premedication
▸ BY MOUTH
▸ Adult: 5–10 mg, to be given 1–2 hours before procedure, for debilitated patients, use elderly dose
▸ Elderly: 2.5–5 mg, to be given 1–2 hours before procedure
▸ BY INTRAVENOUS INJECTION
▸ Adult: 100–200 micrograms/kg, to be administered into a large vein at a rate of not more than 5 mg/minute, immediately before procedure

Sedation in dental procedures carried out in hospital
▸ BY MOUTH
▸ Adult: Up to 20 mg, to be given 1–2 hours before procedure

Conscious sedation for procedures, and in conjunction with local anaesthesia
▸ BY MOUTH
▸ Adult: 5–10 mg, to be given 1–2 hours before procedure, for debilitated patients, use elderly dose
▸ Elderly: 2.5–5 mg, to be given 1–2 hours before procedure

Sedative cover for minor surgical and medical procedures
▸ BY INTRAVENOUS INJECTION
▸ Adult: 10–20 mg, to be administered into a large vein over 2–4 minutes, immediately before procedure

Status epilepticus | Febrile convulsions | Convulsions due to poisoning
▸ BY INTRAVENOUS INJECTION
▸ Neonate: 300–400 micrograms/kg, then 300–400 micrograms/kg after 10 minutes if required, to be given over 3–5 minutes.

▸ Child 1 month-11 years: 300–400 micrograms/kg (max. per dose 10 mg), then 300–400 micrograms/kg after 10 minutes if required, to be given over 3–5 minutes
▸ Child 12-17 years: 10 mg, then 10 mg after 10 minutes if required, to be given over 3–5 minutes
▸ Adult: 10 mg, then 10 mg after 10 minutes if required, administered at a rate of 1 mL (5 mg) per minute
▸ BY RECTUM
▸ Neonate: 1.25–2.5 mg, then 1.25–2.5 mg after 10 minutes if required.

▸ Child 1 month-1 year: 5 mg, then 5 mg after 10 minutes if required
▸ Child 2-11 years: 5–10 mg, then 5–10 mg after 10 minutes if required
▸ Child 12-17 years: 10–20 mg, then 10–20 mg after 10 minutes if required
▸ Adult: 10–20 mg, then 10–20 mg after 10–15 minutes if required
▸ Elderly: 10 mg, then 10 mg after 10–15 minutes if required

Life-threatening acute drug-induced dystonic reactions
▸ BY INTRAVENOUS INJECTION
▸ Child 1 month-11 years: 100 micrograms/kg, repeated if necessary, to be given over 3–5 minutes
▸ Child 12-17 years: 5–10 mg, repeated if necessary, to be given over 3–5 minutes

Dyspnoea associated with anxiety in palliative care
▸ BY MOUTH
▸ Adult: 5–10 mg daily
Pain of muscle spasm in palliative care
▸ BY MOUTH
▸ Adult: 5–10 mg daily

● UNLICENSED USE
▸ With rectal use in children *Diazepam Desitin* ®, *Diazepam Rectubes* ®, and *Stesolid Rectal Tubes* ® not licensed for use in children under 1 year.

IMPORTANT SAFETY INFORMATION
ANAESTHESIA
Benzodiazepines should only be administered for anaesthesia by, or under the direct supervision of, personnel experienced in their use, with adequate training in anaesthesia and airway management.

● CONTRA-INDICATIONS Avoid injections containing benzyl alcohol in neonates · chronic psychosis (in adults) · CNS depression · compromised airway · hyperkinesis · respiratory depression

● CAUTIONS
GENERAL CAUTIONS Muscle weakness · organic brain changes · parenteral administration (close observation required until full recovery from sedation)
SPECIFIC CAUTIONS
▸ With intravenous use high risk of venous thrombophlebitis with intravenous use (reduced by using an emulsion formulation)
CAUTIONS, FURTHER INFORMATION
▸ Special precautions for intravenous injection
▸ With intravenous use When given intravenously facilities for reversing respiratory depression with mechanical ventilation must be immediately available.

● INTERACTIONS → Appendix 1: benzodiazepines

● SIDE-EFFECTS
GENERAL SIDE-EFFECTS
▸ **Common or very common** Appetite abnormal · concentration impaired · movement disorders · muscle spasms · palpitations · sensory disorder · vomiting
▸ **Uncommon** Constipation · diarrhoea · hypersalivation · speech slurred
▸ **Rare or very rare** Bradycardia · bronchial secretion increased · cardiac arrest · dry mouth · gynaecomastia · heart failure · leucopenia · loss of consciousness · memory loss · respiratory arrest · sexual dysfunction · syncope
▸ **Frequency not known** Apnoea · nystagmus
SPECIFIC SIDE-EFFECTS
▸ **Uncommon**
▸ With intravenous use Skin reactions
▸ With oral use Skin reactions
▸ With rectal use Skin reactions
▸ **Rare or very rare**
▸ With intravenous use Psychiatric disorder
▸ With oral use Psychiatric disorder
▸ **Frequency not known**
▸ With intramuscular use Chest pain · embolism and thrombosis · fall · increased risk of dementia · psychiatric disorders · soft tissue necrosis · urticaria

● PREGNANCY Women who have seizures in the second half of pregnancy should be assessed for eclampsia before any change is made to antiepileptic treatment. Status epilepticus should be treated according to the standard protocol.
Epilepsy and Pregnancy Register All pregnant women with epilepsy, whether taking medication or not, should be encouraged to notify the UK Epilepsy and Pregnancy Register (Tel: 0800 389 1248).

4

Nervous system

4

Nervous system

- BREAST FEEDING Present in milk, and should be avoided if possible during breast-feeding.
- RENAL IMPAIRMENT
  Dose adjustments Start with small doses in severe impairment.
- DIRECTIONS FOR ADMINISTRATION
  ‣ With intravenous use Diazepam is adsorbed by plastics of infusion bags and giving sets. Expert sources advise emulsion formulation preferred for intravenous use.
  ‣ With intravenous use in children EvGr For *continuous intravenous infusion* (emulsion) (*Diazemuls®*), dilute to a concentration of max. 400 micrograms/mL with Glucose 5% or 10%; max. 6 hours between addition and completion of infusion. For *continuous intravenous infusion* (solution) (*Diazepam*, Hameln), dilute to a concentration of max. 80 micrograms/mL with Glucose 5% or Sodium Chloride 0.9%. ⟨M⟩
  ‣ With intravenous use in adults EvGr For *intravenous infusion* (solution) (*Diazepam*, Hameln), give continuously *in* Glucose 5% or Sodium Chloride 0.9%. Dilute to a concentration of not more than 40 mg in 500 mL. For *intravenous infusion* (emulsion) (*Diazemuls®*), give continuously *in* Glucose 5% or 10%. May be diluted to a max. concentration of 200 mg in 500 mL; max. 6 hours between addition and completion of administration. May be given *via* drip tubing *in* Glucose 5% or 10% or Sodium Chloride 0.9%. ⟨M⟩
  ‣ With intramuscular use or intravenous use in adults EvGr Solution for injection should not be diluted, except for intravenous infusion. ⟨M⟩
  ‣ With intramuscular use EvGr Only use intramuscular route when oral and intravenous routes not possible. ⟨M⟩
- PRESCRIBING AND DISPENSING INFORMATION
  Palliative care For further information on the use of diazepam in palliative care, see www.medicinescomplete.com/#/content/palliative/benzodiazepines-and-z-drugs.
- PATIENT AND CARER ADVICE Patients or carers should be given advice on how and when to administer rectal diazepam. Patients given sedatives and analgesics during minor outpatient procedures should be very carefully warned about the risks of undertaking skilled tasks (e.g. driving) afterwards. For intravenous benzodiazepines, the risk extends to **at least 24 hours** after administration. Responsible persons should be available to take patients home afterwards. The dangers of taking **alcohol** should be emphasised.
  Medicines for Children leaflet: Diazepam (rectal) for stopping seizures www.medicinesforchildren.org.uk/diazepam-rectal-stopping-seizures-0
  Medicines for Children leaflet: Diazepam for muscle spasm www.medicinesforchildren.org.uk/diazepam-muscle-spasm-0
- PROFESSION SPECIFIC INFORMATION
  Dental practitioners' formulary
  Diazepam Tablets may be prescribed.
  Diazepam Oral Solution 2 mg/5 mL may be prescribed.
- MEDICINAL FORMS There can be variation in the licensing of different medicines containing the same drug. Forms available from special-order manufacturers include: oral suspension, oral solution, suppository

Tablet
CAUTIONARY AND ADVISORY LABELS 2, 19
‣ Diazepam (Non-proprietary)
  Diazepam 2 mg Diazepam 2mg tablets | 28 tablet PoM £1.10 DT = £0.85 CD4-1
  Diazepam 5 mg Diazepam 5mg tablets | 28 tablet PoM £1.12 DT = £0.89 CD4-1
  Diazepam 10 mg Diazepam 10mg tablets | 28 tablet PoM £4.99 DT = £0.98 CD4-1

Emulsion for injection
‣ Diazemuls (Accord Healthcare Ltd)
  Diazepam 5 mg per 1 ml Diazemuls 10mg/2ml emulsion for injection ampoules | 10 ampoule PoM £9.05 CD4-1
Solution for injection
EXCIPIENTS: May contain Benzyl alcohol, ethanol, propylene glycol
‣ Diazepam (Non-proprietary)
  Diazepam 5 mg per 1 ml Diazepam 10mg/2ml solution for injection ampoules | 10 ampoule PoM £6.44–£6.50 DT = £6.44 CD4-1
Oral suspension
CAUTIONARY AND ADVISORY LABELS 2, 19
‣ Diazepam (Non-proprietary)
  Diazepam 400 microgram per 1 ml Diazepam 2mg/5ml oral suspension | 100 ml PoM £31.75–£55.56 DT = £55.07 CD4-1
Oral solution
CAUTIONARY AND ADVISORY LABELS 2, 19
‣ Diazepam (Non-proprietary)
  Diazepam 400 microgram per 1 ml Diazepam 2mg/5ml oral solution sugar free sugar-free | 100 ml PoM £58.35 DT = £56.02 CD4-1
Enema
CAUTIONARY AND ADVISORY LABELS 2, 19
‣ Diazepam (Non-proprietary)
  Diazepam 2 mg per 1 ml Diazepam 5mg RecTubes | 5 tube PoM £5.85 DT = £6.55 CD4-1
  Diazepam 2.5mg RecTubes | 5 tube PoM £5.65 DT = £5.65 CD4-1
  Diazepam 5mg/2.5ml rectal solution tube | 5 tube PoM £5.85–£6.49 DT = £6.55 CD4-1
  Diazepam 4 mg per 1 ml Diazepam 10mg RecTubes | 5 tube PoM £7.35 DT = £7.40 CD4-1
  Diazepam 10mg/2.5ml rectal solution tube | 5 tube PoM £7.40 DT = £7.40 CD4-1
‣ Stesolid (Accord Healthcare Ltd)
  Diazepam 2 mg per 1 ml Stesolid 5mg rectal tube | 5 tube PoM £6.89 DT = £6.55 CD4-1
  Diazepam 4 mg per 1 ml Stesolid 10mg rectal tube | 5 tube PoM £8.78 DT = £7.40 CD4-1

F 361

Oxazepam
21-Oct-2019

- INDICATIONS AND DOSE
Anxiety (short-term use)
‣ BY MOUTH
‣ Adult: 15–30 mg 3–4 times a day, for debilitated patients, use elderly dose
‣ Elderly: 10–20 mg 3–4 times a day
Insomnia associated with anxiety
‣ BY MOUTH
‣ Adult: 15–25 mg once daily (max. per dose 50 mg), dose to be taken at bedtime

- CONTRA-INDICATIONS Chronic psychosis · respiratory depression
- CAUTIONS Muscle weakness · organic brain changes
  CAUTIONS, FURTHER INFORMATION
  ‣ Paradoxical effects A paradoxical increase in hostility and aggression may be reported by patients taking benzodiazepines. The effects range from talkativeness and excitement to aggressive and antisocial acts. Adjustment of the dose (up or down) sometimes attenuates the impulses. Increased anxiety and perceptual disorders are other paradoxical effects.
- INTERACTIONS → Appendix 1: benzodiazepines
- SIDE-EFFECTS Fever · leucopenia · memory loss · oedema · saliva altered · speech slurred · syncope · urticaria
- BREAST FEEDING Benzodiazepines are present in milk, and should be avoided if possible during breast-feeding.
- RENAL IMPAIRMENT
  Dose adjustments Start with small doses in severe impairment.

- **MEDICINAL FORMS** There can be variation in the licensing of different medicines containing the same drug. Forms available from special-order manufacturers include: oral suspension

Tablet

CAUTIONARY AND ADVISORY LABELS 2

▸ Oxazepam (Non-proprietary)

Oxazepam 10 mg Oxazepam 10mg tablets | 28 tablet [PoM] £13.73
DT = £6.32 [CD4-1]

Oxazepam 15 mg Oxazepam 15mg tablets | 28 tablet [PoM] £13.44
DT = £6.23 [CD4-1]

HYPNOTICS, SEDATIVES AND ANXIOLYTICS ⟩

NON-BENZODIAZEPINE HYPNOTICS AND SEDATIVES

Meprobamate

26-May-2020

- ● **INDICATIONS AND DOSE**

Short-term use in anxiety—not recommended

▸ BY MOUTH

▸ Adult: 400 mg 3–4 times a day

▸ Elderly: Up to 200 mg 3–4 times a day

IMPORTANT SAFETY INFORMATION

MHRA/CHM ADVICE: MEPROBAMATE: LICENCE TO BE CANCELLED (APRIL 2016)

Following an EU-wide review of meprobamate, the UK licence holder has ceased manufacturing and the licence is due to be cancelled by December 2016. No new stock will be released into the normal distribution chain after 31 December 2016, although existing stock placed on the market before that date is likely to be dispensed until the products approach their expiry date.

Prescribers should review the treatment of any patient who is currently receiving a meprobamate-containing medicine with a view to switching them to an alternative treatment, and not start any new patients on medicines that contain meprobamate.

- **CONTRA-INDICATIONS** Acute porphyrias p. 1107 · acute pulmonary insufficiency · respiratory depression
- **CAUTIONS** Abrupt withdrawal (may precipitate convulsions) · avoid prolonged use · elderly · emotionally unstable personality (if taken over long periods)—increased risk of dependence · epilepsy (may induce seizures) · history of alcohol dependence · history of drug dependence · muscle weakness · respiratory disease
- **INTERACTIONS** → Appendix 1: meprobamate
- **SIDE-EFFECTS** Agitation · agranulocytosis · anal inflammation · ataxia · blood disorder · bone marrow disorders · dizziness · drowsiness · hypersensitivity · hypotension · nausea · paraesthesia · purpura non-thrombocytopenic · skin reactions · Stevens-Johnson syndrome · stomatitis · thrombocytopenia · vomiting · withdrawal syndrome
- **PREGNANCY** Avoid if possible.
- **BREAST FEEDING** Avoid. Concentration in milk may exceed maternal plasma concentrations fourfold and may cause drowsiness in infant.
- **HEPATIC IMPAIRMENT** Elimination may be prolonged in chronic impairment.
- **RENAL IMPAIRMENT** Increased cerebral sensitivity.
  Dose adjustments Start with small doses in severe impairment.
- **PATIENT AND CARER ADVICE**
  Driving and skilled tasks Drowsiness may affect performance of skilled tasks (e.g. driving); effects of alcohol enhanced.
- **LESS SUITABLE FOR PRESCRIBING** Meprobamate is less suitable for prescribing.

- **MEDICINAL FORMS** Forms available from special-order manufacturers include: oral suspension, oral solution

3.2   Attention deficit hyperactivity disorder

Attention deficit hyperactivity disorder

04-Aug-2018

Description of condition

Attention deficit hyperactivity disorder (ADHD) is a behavioural disorder characterised by hyperactivity, impulsivity and inattention, which can lead to functional impairment such as psychological, social, educational or occupational difficulties. While these symptoms tend to co-exist, some patients are predominantly hyperactive and impulsive, while others are principally inattentive. Symptoms typically appear in children aged 3–7 years, but may not be recognised until after 7 years of age, especially if hyperactivity is not present. ADHD is more commonly diagnosed in males than in females.

ADHD is usually a persisting disorder and some children continue to have symptoms throughout adolescence and into adulthood, where inattentive symptoms tend to persist, and hyperactive-impulsive symptoms tend to recede over time. ADHD is also associated with an increased risk of disorders such as oppositional defiant disorder (ODD), conduct disorder, and possibly mood disorders such as depression, mania, and anxiety, as well as substance misuse.

Aims of treatment

The aims of treatment are to reduce functional impairment, severity of symptoms, and to improve quality of life.

Non-drug treatment

[EvGr] Patients should be advised about the importance of a balanced diet, good nutrition and regular exercise. ⟨A⟩

Environmental modifications are changes made to the physical environment that can help reduce the impact of ADHD symptoms on a person's day-to-day life. [EvGr] The modifications should be specific to the person's circumstances, and may involve changes to seating arrangements, lighting and noise, reducing distractions, optimising work or education by having shorter periods of focus with movement breaks, and reinforcing verbal requests with written instructions. These changes should form part of the discussion at the time of diagnosis of ADHD and be trialled and reviewed for effectiveness before drug treatment is started.

ADHD focused psychological interventions which may involve elements of, or a complete course of cognitive behavioural therapy (CBT) may be effective in patients who have refused drug treatment, have difficulty with adherence, are intolerant of, or unresponsive to drug treatment. In patients who have benefited from drug treatment, but whose symptoms are still causing significant impairment in at least one area of function (such as interpersonal relationships, education and occupational attainment, and risk awareness), consider a combination of non-drug treatment with drug treatment. ⟨A⟩

Drug treatment

[EvGr] Drug treatment should be initiated by a specialist trained in the diagnosis and management of ADHD. Following dose stabilisation, continuation and monitoring of drug treatment can be undertaken by the patient's general practitioner under a shared care arrangement. Treatment should be started in patients with ADHD whose symptoms

4

Nervous system

4

Nervous system

are still causing significant impairment in at least one area of function, despite environmental modifications. Patients with ADHD and anxiety disorder, tic disorder, or autism spectrum disorder should be offered the same treatment options as other patients with ADHD.

Lisdexamfetamine mesilate p. 370 or methylphenidate hydrochloride p. 367 are recommended as first-line treatment. If symptoms have not improved following a 6-week trial of either drug, switching to the alternative first-line treatment should be considered. Dexamfetamine sulfate p. 369 [unlicensed] can be tried if the patient is having a beneficial response to lisdexamfetamine mesilate but cannot tolerate its longer duration of effect.

Modified-release preparations of stimulants are preferred because of their pharmacokinetic profile, convenience, improved adherence, reduced risk of drug diversion (drugs being forwarded to others for non-prescription use or misuse), and the lack of need to be taken to work. Immediate-release preparations can be given when more flexible dosing regimens are required, or during initial dose titration. A combination of modified-release and immediate-release preparations taken at different times of the day can be used to extend the duration of effect. The magnitude, duration of effect, and side-effects of stimulants vary between patients.

In patients who are intolerant to both methylphenidate hydrochloride p. 367 and lisdexamfetamine mesilate, or who have not responded to separate 6-week trials of both drugs, treatment with the non-stimulant atomoxetine below can be considered.

Advice from, or referral to a tertiary specialist ADHD service should be considered if the patient is unresponsive to one or more stimulant drugs (e.g. methylphenidate hydrochloride p. 367 and lisdexamfetamine mesilate) and atomoxetine below. A specialist service should also be consulted for advice before starting treatment with guanfacine p. 372 [unlicensed], or an atypical antipsychotic in addition to stimulants in patients with ADHD and co-existing pervasive aggression, rages or irritability. If sustained orthostatic hypotension or fainting episodes occur with guanfacine p. 372 treatment, the dose should be reduced or an alternative treatment offered. ⟨A⟩

Other treatment options such as bupropion hydrochloride p. 520, modafinil p. 513, tricyclic antidepressants, and venlafaxine p. 388 [all unlicensed] have been used in the management of ADHD, but due to limited evidence their use is not recommended without specialist advice.

EvGr Patients should be monitored for effectiveness of medication and side-effects, as well as changes in sleep pattern, sexual dysfunction (associated with atomoxetine below), and stimulant diversion or misuse. If the patient develops new, or has worsening of existing seizures, review drug treatment and stop any drug that might be contributing to the seizures; treatment can be cautiously reintroduced if it is unlikely to be the cause. Monitor patients for the development of tics associated with stimulant use. If tics are stimulant related, consider a dose reduction, stopping treatment, or changing to a non-stimulant drug. If there is worsening of behaviour, consider adjusting drug treatment and reviewing the diagnosis.

Treatment should be reviewed by a specialist at least once a year and trials of treatment-free periods, or dose reductions considered where appropriate. ⟨A⟩

Useful Resources

Attention deficit hyperactivity disorder: diagnosis and management. National Institute for Health and Care Excellence. Clinical guideline 87. March 2018.
www.nice.org.uk/guidance/ng87

CNS STIMULANTS ⟩ CENTRALLY ACTING SYMPATHOMIMETICS

Atomoxetine

16-Nov-2020

● **INDICATIONS AND DOSE**

Attention deficit hyperactivity disorder (initiated by a specialist)

▸ BY MOUTH

⟩ **Child 6–17 years (body-weight up to 70 kg):** Initially 500 micrograms/kg daily for 7 days, dose is increased according to response; maintenance 1.2 mg/kg daily, total daily dose may be given either as a single dose in the morning or in 2 divided doses with last dose no later than early evening, high daily doses to be given under the direction of a specialist; maximum 1.8 mg/kg per day; maximum 120 mg per day

⟩ **Child 6–17 years (body-weight 70 kg and above):** Initially 40 mg daily for 7 days, dose is increased according to response; maintenance 80 mg daily, total daily dose may be given either as a single dose in the morning or in 2 divided doses with last dose no later than early evening, high daily doses to be given under the direction of a specialist; maximum 120 mg per day

⟩ **Adult (body-weight up to 70 kg):** Initially 500 micrograms/kg daily for 7 days, dose is increased according to response; maintenance 1.2 mg/kg daily, total daily dose may be given either as a single dose in the morning or in 2 divided doses with last dose no later than early evening, high daily doses to be given under the direction of a specialist; maximum 1.8 mg/kg per day; maximum 120 mg per day

⟩ **Adult (body-weight 70 kg and above):** Initially 40 mg daily for 7 days, dose is increased according to response; maintenance 80–100 mg daily, total daily dose may be given either as a single dose in the morning or in 2 divided doses with last dose no later than early evening, high daily doses to be given under the direction of a specialist; maximum 120 mg per day

● UNLICENSED USE Atomoxetine doses in BNF may differ from those in product literature.
▸ In children Doses above 100 mg daily not licensed.
▸ In adults Dose maximum of 120 mg not licensed.

● CONTRA-INDICATIONS Phaeochromocytoma · severe cardiovascular disease · severe cerebrovascular disease

● CAUTIONS Aggressive behaviour · cardiovascular disease · cerebrovascular disease · emotional lability · history of seizures · hostility · hypertension · mania · psychosis · QT-interval prolongation · structural cardiac abnormalities · susceptibility to angle-closure glaucoma · tachycardia

● INTERACTIONS → Appendix 1: atomoxetine

● SIDE-EFFECTS
▸ **Common or very common** Anxiety · appetite decreased · arrhythmias (uncommon in children) · asthenia · chills (in adults) · constipation · depression · dizziness · drowsiness · dry mouth (in adults) · feeling jittery (in adults) · flatulence (in adults) · gastrointestinal discomfort · genital pain (rare in children) · headaches · hyperhidrosis (uncommon in children) · menstrual cycle irregularities (in adults) · mood altered · mydriasis (in children) · nausea · palpitations (uncommon in children) · prostatitis (in adults) · sensation abnormal (uncommon in children) · sexual dysfunction (rare in children) · skin reactions · sleep disorders · taste altered (in adults) · thirst (in adults) · tremor (uncommon in children) · urinary disorders (rare in children) · vasodilation (in adults) · vomiting · weight decreased
▸ **Uncommon** Behaviour abnormal · chest pain (very common in children) · dyspnoea · feeling cold (in adults) · hypersensitivity · muscle spasms (in adults) · peripheral coldness (in adults) · QT interval prolongation · suicidal

behaviour · syncope · tic (very common in children) · vision blurred
▶ **Rare or very rare** Hallucination (uncommon in children) · hepatic disorders · psychosis (uncommon in children) · Raynaud's phenomenon · seizure (uncommon in children)
▶ **Frequency not known** Sudden cardiac death
● PREGNANCY Manufacturer advises avoid unless potential benefit outweighs risk.
● BREAST FEEDING Avoid-present in milk in *animal* studies.
● HEPATIC IMPAIRMENT
Dose adjustments Manufacturer advises halve dose in moderate impairment and quarter dose in severe impairment.
● MONITORING REQUIREMENTS
▶ Monitor for appearance or worsening of anxiety, depression or tics.
▶ Pulse, blood pressure, psychiatric symptoms, appetite, weight and height should be recorded at initiation of therapy, following each dose adjustment, and at least every 6 months thereafter.
● PATIENT AND CARER ADVICE
Suicidal ideation Following reports of suicidal thoughts and behaviour, patients and their carers should be informed about the risk and told to report clinical worsening, suicidal thoughts or behaviour, irritability, agitation, or depression.
Hepatic impairment Following rare reports of hepatic disorders, patients and carers should be advised of the risk and be told how to recognise symptoms; prompt medical attention should be sought in case of abdominal pain, unexplained nausea, malaise, darkening of the urine, or jaundice.
Medicines for Children leaflet: Atomoxetine for attention deficit hyperactivity disorder (ADHD) www.medicinesforchildren.org.uk/atomoxetine-attention-deficit-hyperactivity-disorder-adhd
● NATIONAL FUNDING/ACCESS DECISIONS
For full details see funding body website
Scottish Medicines Consortium (SMC) decisions
▶ Atomoxetine oral solution (*Strattera®*) for treatment of **attention-deficit/hyperactivity disorder (ADHD) in children of 6 years and older, in adolescents and in adults as part of a comprehensive treatment programme (December 2015)** SMC No. 1107/15 Recommended with restrictions

● MEDICINAL FORMS There can be variation in the licensing of different medicines containing the same drug. Forms available from special-order manufacturers include: oral suspension, oral solution

Oral solution
CAUTIONARY AND ADVISORY LABELS 3
▶ Strattera (Eli Lilly and Company Ltd)
Atomoxetine (as Atomoxetine hydrochloride) 4 mg per 1 ml Strattera 4mg/1ml oral solution sugar-free | 300 ml PoM £85.00 DT = £85.00

Capsule
CAUTIONARY AND ADVISORY LABELS 3
▶ Atomoxetine (Non-proprietary)
Atomoxetine (as Atomoxetine hydrochloride) 10 mg Atomoxetine 10mg capsules | 7 capsule PoM £11.94–£13.28 | 28 capsule PoM £53.09 DT = £48.52
Atomoxetine (as Atomoxetine hydrochloride) 18 mg Atomoxetine 18mg capsules | 7 capsule PoM £11.94–£13.28 | 28 capsule PoM £53.09 DT = £48.52
Atomoxetine (as Atomoxetine hydrochloride) 25 mg Atomoxetine 25mg capsules | 7 capsule PoM £11.94–£13.28 | 28 capsule PoM £53.09 DT = £48.01
Atomoxetine (as Atomoxetine hydrochloride) 40 mg Atomoxetine 40mg capsules | 7 capsule PoM £11.94–£13.28 | 28 capsule PoM £53.09 DT = £48.01
Atomoxetine (as Atomoxetine hydrochloride) 60 mg Atomoxetine 60mg capsules | 28 capsule PoM £53.09 DT = £48.44
Atomoxetine (as Atomoxetine hydrochloride) 80 mg Atomoxetine 80mg capsules | 28 capsule PoM £70.79 DT = £64.59

Atomoxetine (as Atomoxetine hydrochloride)
100 mg Atomoxetine 100mg capsules | 28 capsule PoM £70.79 DT = £64.59
▶ Strattera (Eli Lilly and Company Ltd)
Atomoxetine (as Atomoxetine hydrochloride) 10 mg Strattera 10mg capsules | 7 capsule PoM £13.28 | 28 capsule PoM £53.09 DT = £48.52
Atomoxetine (as Atomoxetine hydrochloride) 18 mg Strattera 18mg capsules | 7 capsule PoM £13.28 | 28 capsule PoM £53.09 DT = £48.52
Atomoxetine (as Atomoxetine hydrochloride) 25 mg Strattera 25mg capsules | 7 capsule PoM £13.28 | 28 capsule PoM £53.09 DT = £48.01
Atomoxetine (as Atomoxetine hydrochloride) 40 mg Strattera 40mg capsules | 7 capsule PoM £13.28 | 28 capsule PoM £53.09 DT = £48.01
Atomoxetine (as Atomoxetine hydrochloride) 60 mg Strattera 60mg capsules | 28 capsule PoM £53.09 DT = £48.44
Atomoxetine (as Atomoxetine hydrochloride) 80 mg Strattera 80mg capsules | 28 capsule PoM £70.79 DT = £64.59
Atomoxetine (as Atomoxetine hydrochloride) 100 mg Strattera 100mg capsules | 28 capsule PoM £70.79 DT = £64.59

Methylphenidate hydrochloride
04-Sep-2020

● INDICATIONS AND DOSE
Attention deficit hyperactivity disorder (initiated under specialist supervision)
▶ BY MOUTH USING IMMEDIATE-RELEASE MEDICINES
▶ Child 6-17 years: Initially 5 mg 1–2 times a day, increased in steps of 5–10 mg daily if required, at weekly intervals, increased if necessary up to 60 mg daily in 2–3 divided doses, increased if necessary up to 2.1 mg/kg daily in 2–3 divided doses, the licensed maximum dose is 60 mg daily in 2–3 doses, higher dose (up to a maximum of 90 mg daily) under the direction of a specialist, discontinue if no response after 1 month, if effect wears off in evening (with rebound hyperactivity) a dose at bedtime may be appropriate (establish need with trial bedtime dose). Treatment may be started using a modified-release preparation
▶ Adult: Initially 5 mg 2–3 times a day, dose is increased if necessary at weekly intervals according to response, increased if necessary up to 100 mg daily in 2–3 divided doses, if effect wears off in evening (with rebound hyperactivity) a dose at bedtime may be appropriate (establish need with trial bedtime dose). Treatment may be started using a modified-release preparation

Narcolepsy
▶ BY MOUTH USING IMMEDIATE-RELEASE MEDICINES
▶ Adult: 10–60 mg daily in divided doses; usual dose 20–30 mg daily in divided doses, dose to be taken before meals

DOSE EQUIVALENCE AND CONVERSION
▶ When switching from *immediate-release* preparations to *modified-release* preparations—consult product literature.

CONCERTA® XL
Attention deficit hyperactivity disorder
▶ BY MOUTH
▶ Child 6-17 years: Initially 18 mg once daily, dose to be taken in the morning, increased in steps of 18 mg every week, adjusted according to response; increased if necessary up to 2.1 mg/kg daily, licensed max. dose is 54 mg once daily, to be increased to higher dose only under direction of specialist; discontinue if no response after 1 month; maximum 108 mg per day
▶ Adult: Initially 18 mg once daily, dose to be taken in the morning; adjusted at weekly intervals according to response; maximum 108 mg per day continued →

Nervous system

4

DOSE EQUIVALENCE AND CONVERSION
▸ Total daily dose of 15 mg of standard-release formulation is considered equivalent to *Concerta*® XL 18 mg once daily.

DELMOSART® PROLONGED-RELEASE TABLET

Attention deficit hyperactivity disorder (under expert supervision)
▸ BY MOUTH
▸ Child 6-17 years: Initially 18 mg once daily, dose to be taken in the morning, then increased in steps of 18 mg every week if required, discontinue if no response after 1 month; maximum 54 mg per day
▸ Adult: Initially 18 mg once daily, dose to be taken in the morning, then increased in steps of 18 mg every week if required, discontinue if no response after 1 month; maximum 54 mg per day

DOSE EQUIVALENCE AND CONVERSION
▸ Total daily dose of 15 mg of standard-release formulation is considered equivalent to *Delmosart*® 18 mg once daily.

EQUASYM® XL

Attention deficit hyperactivity disorder
▸ BY MOUTH
▸ Child 6-17 years: Initially 10 mg once daily, dose to be taken in the morning before breakfast; increased gradually at weekly intervals if necessary; increased if necessary up to 2.1 mg/kg daily, licensed max. dose is 60 mg daily, to be increased to higher dose only under direction of specialist; discontinue if no response after 1 month; maximum 90 mg per day
▸ Adult: Initially 10 mg once daily, dose to be taken in the morning before breakfast; increased gradually at weekly intervals if necessary; maximum 100 mg per day

MEDIKINET® XL

Attention deficit hyperactivity disorder
▸ BY MOUTH
▸ Child 6-17 years: Initially 10 mg once daily, dose to be taken in the morning with breakfast; adjusted at weekly intervals according to response; increased if necessary up to 2.1 mg/kg daily, licensed max. dose is 60 mg daily, to be increased to higher dose only under direction of specialist; discontinue if no response after 1 month; maximum 90 mg per day
▸ Adult: Initially 10 mg once daily, dose to be taken in the morning with breakfast; adjusted at weekly intervals according to response; maximum 100 mg per day

XAGGITIN® XL

Attention deficit hyperactivity disorder (under expert supervision)
▸ BY MOUTH
▸ Child 6-17 years: Initially 18 mg once daily, dose to be taken in the morning, increased in steps of 18 mg every week, adjusted according to response, discontinue if no response after 1 month; maximum 54 mg per day
▸ Adult: Initially 18 mg once daily, dose to be taken in the morning, increased in steps of 18 mg every week, adjusted according to response, discontinue if no response after 1 month; maximum 54 mg per day

DOSE EQUIVALENCE AND CONVERSION
▸ Total daily dose of 15 mg of standard-release formulation is considered equivalent to *Xaggitin*® XL 18 mg once daily.

● UNLICENSED USE Doses over 60 mg daily not licensed; doses of *Concerta XL* over 54 mg daily not licensed.
▸ In adults Not licensed for use in narcolepsy. Not licensed for use in adults for attention deficit hyperactivity disorder.

● CONTRA-INDICATIONS Anorexia nervosa · arrhythmias · cardiomyopathy · cardiovascular disease · cerebrovascular disorders · heart failure · hyperthyroidism · mania · phaeochromocytoma · psychosis · severe depression · severe hypertension · structural cardiac abnormalities · suicidal tendencies · uncontrolled bipolar disorder · vasculitis

● CAUTIONS Agitation · alcohol dependence · anxiety · drug dependence · epilepsy (discontinue if increased seizure frequency) · family history of Tourette syndrome · susceptibility to angle-closure glaucoma · tics
CONCERTA® XL, DELMOSART® PROLONGED-RELEASE TABLET Dysphagia (dose form not appropriate) · restricted gastro-intestinal lumen (dose form not appropriate)
XAGGITIN® XL Dysphagia (dose form not appropriate)

● INTERACTIONS → Appendix 1: methylphenidate

● SIDE-EFFECTS
▸ **Common or very common** Aggression (or hostility) · alopecia · anxiety · appetite decreased · arrhythmias · arthralgia · behaviour abnormal · cough · depression · diarrhoea · dizziness · drowsiness · dry mouth · fever · gastrointestinal discomfort · growth retardation (in children) · headaches · hypertension · laryngeal pain · mood altered · movement disorders · nasopharyngitis · nausea · palpitations · sleep disorders · vomiting · weight decreased
▸ **Uncommon** Chest discomfort · constipation · dyspnoea · fatigue · haematuria · hallucinations · muscle complaints · psychotic disorder · suicidal behaviours · tic · tremor · vision disorders
▸ **Rare or very rare** Anaemia · angina pectoris · cardiac arrest · cerebrovascular insufficiency · confusion · gynaecomastia · hepatic coma · hyperfocus · hyperhidrosis · leucopenia · mydriasis · myocardial infarction · neuroleptic malignant syndrome · peripheral coldness · Raynaud's phenomenon · seizures · sexual dysfunction · skin reactions · sudden cardiac death · thinking abnormal · thrombocytopenia
▸ **Frequency not known** Delusions · drug dependence · hyperpyrexia · intracranial haemorrhage · logorrhea · pancytopenia · vasculitis

● PREGNANCY Limited experience—avoid unless potential benefit outweighs risk.

● BREAST FEEDING Limited information available—avoid.

● MONITORING REQUIREMENTS
▸ Monitor for psychiatric disorders.
▸ Pulse, blood pressure, psychiatric symptoms, appetite, weight and height should be recorded at initiation of therapy, following each dose adjustment, and at least every 6 months thereafter.

● TREATMENT CESSATION Avoid abrupt withdrawal.

● DIRECTIONS FOR ADMINISTRATION
MEDIKINET® XL Manufacturer advises contents of capsule can be sprinkled on a tablespoon of apple sauce or yoghurt (then swallowed immediately without chewing).
EQUASYM® XL Manufacturer advises contents of capsule can be sprinkled on a tablespoon of apple sauce (then swallowed immediately without chewing).

● PRESCRIBING AND DISPENSING INFORMATION Different versions of modified-release preparations may not have the same clinical effect. To avoid confusion between these different formulations of methylphenidate, prescribers should specify the brand to be dispensed.
CONCERTA® XL Consists of an immediate-release component (22% of the dose) and a modified-release component (78% of the dose).
MEDIKINET® XL Consists of an immediate-release component (50% of the dose) and a modified-release component (50% of the dose).

EQUASYM ® XL Consists of an immediate-release component (30% of the dose) and a modified-release component (70% of the dose).

● PATIENT AND CARER ADVICE

Medicines for Children leaflet: Methylphenidate for attention deficit hyperactivity disorder (ADHD) www.medicinesforchildren. org.uk/methylphenidate-attention-deficit-hyperactivity-disorder-adhd

Driving and skilled tasks   **Drugs and Driving** Prescribers and other healthcare professionals should advise patients if treatment is likely to affect their ability to perform skilled tasks (e.g. driving). This applies especially to drugs with sedative effects; patients should be warned that these effects are increased by alcohol. General information about a patient's fitness to drive is available from the Driver and Vehicle Licensing Agency at www.gov.uk/ government/organisations/driver-and-vehicle-licensing-agency.

2015 legislation regarding driving whilst taking certain drugs, may also apply to methylphenidate, see *Drugs and driving* under Guidance on prescribing p. 1.

CONCERTA ® XL Tablet membrane may pass through gastro-intestinal tract unchanged.

DELMOSART ® PROLONGED-RELEASE TABLET Manufacturer advises tablet membrane may pass through gastro-intestinal tract unchanged.

● MEDICINAL FORMS There can be variation in the licensing of different medicines containing the same drug. Forms available from special-order manufacturers include: modified-release tablet, oral suspension, oral solution

Modified-release tablet

CAUTIONARY AND ADVISORY LABELS 25

▸ Concerta XL (Janssen-Cilag Ltd)
Methylphenidate hydrochloride 18 mg Concerta 18mg tablets | 30 tablet [PoM] £31.19 DT = £31.19 [CD2]
Methylphenidate hydrochloride 27 mg Concerta 27mg tablets | 30 tablet [PoM] £36.81 DT = £36.81 [CD2]
Methylphenidate hydrochloride 36 mg Concerta 36mg tablets | 30 tablet [PoM] £42.45 DT = £42.45 [CD2]
Methylphenidate hydrochloride 54 mg Concerta XL 54mg tablets | 30 tablet [PoM] £73.62 DT = £36.80 [CD2]

▸ Delmosart (Accord Healthcare Ltd)
Methylphenidate hydrochloride 18 mg Delmosart 18mg modified-release tablets | 30 tablet [PoM] £15.57 DT = £31.19 [CD2]
Methylphenidate hydrochloride 27 mg Delmosart 27mg modified-release tablets | 30 tablet [PoM] £18.39 DT = £36.81 [CD2]
Methylphenidate hydrochloride 36 mg Delmosart 36mg modified-release tablets | 30 tablet [PoM] £21.21 DT = £42.45 [CD2]
Methylphenidate hydrochloride 54 mg Delmosart 54mg modified-release tablets | 30 tablet [PoM] £36.79 DT = £36.80 [CD2]

▸ Matoride XL (Sandoz Ltd)
Methylphenidate hydrochloride 18 mg Matoride XL 18mg tablets | 30 tablet [PoM] £15.58 DT = £31.19 [CD2]
Methylphenidate hydrochloride 36 mg Matoride XL 36mg tablets | 30 tablet [PoM] £21.22 DT = £42.45 [CD2]
Methylphenidate hydrochloride 54 mg Matoride XL 54mg tablets | 30 tablet [PoM] £36.80 DT = £36.80 [CD2]

▸ Ritalin-SR (Imported (United States))
Methylphenidate hydrochloride 20 mg Ritalin-SR 20mg tablets | 100 tablet [PoM] [Ⓢ][CD2]

▸ Xaggitin XL (Ethypharm UK Ltd)
Methylphenidate hydrochloride 18 mg Xaggitin XL 18mg tablets | 30 tablet [PoM] £15.58 DT = £31.19 [CD2]
Methylphenidate hydrochloride 27 mg Xaggitin XL 27mg tablets | 30 tablet [PoM] £18.40 DT = £36.81 [CD2]
Methylphenidate hydrochloride 36 mg Xaggitin XL 36mg tablets | 30 tablet [PoM] £21.22 DT = £42.45 [CD2]
Methylphenidate hydrochloride 54 mg Xaggitin XL 54mg tablets | 30 tablet [PoM] £36.80 DT = £36.80 [CD2]

▸ Xenidate XL (Mylan)
Methylphenidate hydrochloride 18 mg Xenidate XL 18mg tablets | 30 tablet [PoM] £15.57 DT = £31.19 [CD2]
Methylphenidate hydrochloride 27 mg Xenidate XL 27mg tablets | 30 tablet [PoM] £18.39 DT = £36.81 [CD2]
Methylphenidate hydrochloride 36 mg Xenidate XL 36mg tablets | 30 tablet [PoM] £21.21 DT = £42.45 [CD2]

Methylphenidate hydrochloride 54 mg Xenidate XL 54mg tablets | 30 tablet [PoM] £36.79 DT = £36.80 [CD2]

Tablet

▸ Methylphenidate hydrochloride (Non-proprietary)
Methylphenidate hydrochloride 5 mg Methylphenidate 5mg tablets | 30 tablet [PoM] £3.95 DT = £3.03 [CD2]
Methylphenidate hydrochloride 10 mg Methylphenidate 10mg tablets | 30 tablet [PoM] £5.29 DT = £3.77 [CD2]
Methylphenidate hydrochloride 20 mg Methylphenidate 20mg tablets | 30 tablet [PoM] £12.71 DT = £10.92 [CD2]

▸ Medikinet (Flynn Pharma Ltd)
Methylphenidate hydrochloride 5 mg Medikinet 5mg tablets | 30 tablet [PoM] £3.03 DT = £3.03 [CD2]
Methylphenidate hydrochloride 10 mg Medikinet 10mg tablets | 30 tablet [PoM] £5.49 DT = £3.77 [CD2]
Methylphenidate hydrochloride 20 mg Medikinet 20mg tablets | 30 tablet [PoM] £10.92 DT = £10.92 [CD2]

▸ Ritalin (Novartis Pharmaceuticals UK Ltd)
Methylphenidate hydrochloride 10 mg Ritalin 10mg tablets | 30 tablet [PoM] £6.68 DT = £3.77 [CD2]

▸ Tranquilyn (Genesis Pharmaceuticals Ltd)
Methylphenidate hydrochloride 5 mg Tranquilyn 5mg tablets | 30 tablet [PoM] £3.03 DT = £3.03 [CD2]
Methylphenidate hydrochloride 10 mg Tranquilyn 10mg tablets | 30 tablet [PoM] £3.77 DT = £3.77 [CD2]
Methylphenidate hydrochloride 20 mg Tranquilyn 20mg tablets | 30 tablet [PoM] £10.92 DT = £10.92 [CD2]

Modified-release capsule

CAUTIONARY AND ADVISORY LABELS 25

▸ Methylphenidate hydrochloride (Non-proprietary)
Methylphenidate hydrochloride 10 mg Ritalin XL 10mg capsules | 30 capsule [PoM] £23.92 DT = £25.00 [CD2]
Methylphenidate hydrochloride 20 mg Ritalin XL 20mg capsules | 30 capsule [PoM] £28.72 DT = £30.00 [CD2]
Methylphenidate hydrochloride 30 mg Ritalin XL 30mg capsules | 30 capsule [PoM] £33.49 DT = £35.00 [CD2]
Methylphenidate hydrochloride 40 mg Ritalin XL 40mg capsules | 30 capsule [PoM] £57.43 DT = £57.72 [CD2]
Methylphenidate hydrochloride 60 mg Ritalin XL 60mg capsules | 30 capsule [PoM] £66.98 DT = £67.32 [CD2]

▸ Equasym XL (Shire Pharmaceuticals Ltd)
Methylphenidate hydrochloride 10 mg Equasym XL 10mg capsules | 30 capsule [PoM] £25.00 DT = £25.00 [CD2]
Methylphenidate hydrochloride 20 mg Equasym XL 20mg capsules | 30 capsule [PoM] £30.00 DT = £30.00 [CD2]
Methylphenidate hydrochloride 30 mg Equasym XL 30mg capsules | 30 capsule [PoM] £35.00 DT = £35.00 [CD2]

▸ Medikinet XL (Flynn Pharma Ltd) ▼
Methylphenidate hydrochloride 5 mg Medikinet XL 5mg capsules | 30 capsule [PoM] £24.04 DT = £24.04 [CD2]
Methylphenidate hydrochloride 10 mg Medikinet XL 10mg capsules | 30 capsule [PoM] £24.04 DT = £25.00 [CD2]
Methylphenidate hydrochloride 20 mg Medikinet XL 20mg capsules | 30 capsule [PoM] £28.86 DT = £30.00 [CD2]
Methylphenidate hydrochloride 30 mg Medikinet XL 30mg capsules | 30 capsule [PoM] £33.66 DT = £35.00 [CD2]
Methylphenidate hydrochloride 40 mg Medikinet XL 40mg capsules | 30 capsule [PoM] £57.72 DT = £57.72 [CD2]
Methylphenidate hydrochloride 50 mg Medikinet XL 50mg capsules | 30 capsule [PoM] £62.52 DT = £62.52 [CD2]
Methylphenidate hydrochloride 60 mg Medikinet XL 60mg capsules | 30 capsule [PoM] £67.32 DT = £67.32 [CD2]

CNS STIMULANTS ❯ CENTRALLY ACTING SYMPATHOMIMETICS ❯ AMFETAMINES

Dexamfetamine sulfate

24-Nov-2020

(Dexamphetamine sulfate)

● INDICATIONS AND DOSE

Narcolepsy

▸ BY MOUTH
▸ **Adult:** Initially 10 mg daily in divided doses, increased in steps of 10 mg every week, maintenance dose to be given in 2–4 divided doses; maximum 60 mg per day continued →

4

Nervous system

▸ **Elderly:** Initially 5 mg daily in divided doses, increased in steps of 5 mg every week, maintenance dose to be given in 2–4 divided doses; maximum 60 mg per day

Refractory attention deficit hyperactivity disorder (initiated under specialist supervision)
▸ BY MOUTH
▸ **Child 6-17 years:** Initially 2.5 mg 2–3 times a day, increased in steps of 5 mg once weekly if required;, usual maximum 1 mg/kg daily, up to 20 mg daily (40 mg daily has been required in some children); maintenance dose to be given in 2–4 divided doses
▸ **Adult:** Initially 5 mg twice daily, dose is increased at weekly intervals according to response, maintenance dose to be given in 2–4 divided doses; maximum 60 mg per day

● UNLICENSED USE Not licensed for use in adults for refractory attention deficit hyperactivity disorder.
● CONTRA-INDICATIONS Advanced arteriosclerosis · anorexia · arrhythmias (life-threatening) · cardiomyopathies · cardiovascular disease · cerebrovascular disorders · heart failure · history of alcohol abuse · history of drug abuse · hyperexcitability · hyperthyroidism · moderate hypertension · psychiatric disorders · psychosis · severe hypertension · structural cardiac abnormalities · suicidal tendencies
  CONTRA-INDICATIONS, FURTHER INFORMATION
▸ Psychiatric disorders Psychiatric disorders include severe depression, schizophrenia, borderline personality disorder and uncontrolled bipolar disorder. Co-morbidity with psychiatric disorders is common in attention deficit hyperactivity disorder. Manufacturer advises if new psychiatric symptoms develop or exacerbation of psychiatric disorders occurs, continue use only if benefits outweigh risks.
● CAUTIONS History of epilepsy (discontinue if seizures occur) · mild hypertension · susceptibility to angle-closure glaucoma · tics · Tourette syndrome
  CAUTIONS, FURTHER INFORMATION
▸ Tics and Tourette syndrome Discontinue use if tics occur.
▸ Growth restriction in children Monitor height and weight as growth restriction may occur during prolonged therapy (drug-free periods may allow catch-up in growth but withdraw slowly to avoid inducing depression or renewed hyperactivity).
● INTERACTIONS → Appendix 1: amfetamines
● SIDE-EFFECTS
▸ **Common or very common** Abdominal pain · anxiety · appetite decreased · arrhythmias · arthralgia · behaviour abnormal · depression · dry mouth · headache · mood altered · movement disorders · muscle cramps · nausea · palpitations · poor weight gain · sleep disorders · vertigo · vomiting · weight decreased
▸ **Rare or very rare** Anaemia · angina pectoris · cardiac arrest · cerebrovascular insufficiency · fatigue · growth retardation · hallucination · hepatic coma · hepatic function abnormal · intracranial haemorrhage · leucopenia · mydriasis · psychosis · seizure · skin reactions · suicidal behaviours · thrombocytopenia · tic (in those at risk) · vasculitis cerebral · vision disorders
▸ **Frequency not known** Acidosis · alopecia · cardiomyopathy · chest pain · circulatory collapse · colitis ischaemic · concentration impaired · confusion · diarrhoea · dizziness · drug dependence · hyperhidrosis · hypermetabolism · hyperpyrexia · kidney injury · myocardial infarction · neuroleptic malignant syndrome · obsessive-compulsive disorder · reflexes increased · rhabdomyolysis · sexual dysfunction · sudden death · taste altered · tremor
  Overdose Amfetamines cause wakefulness, excessive activity, paranoia, hallucinations, and hypertension followed by exhaustion, convulsions, hyperthermia, and

coma. See Stimulants under **Emergency treatment of poisoning p. 1413**.
● PREGNANCY Avoid (retrospective evidence of uncertain significance suggesting possible embryotoxicity).
● BREAST FEEDING Significant amount in milk—avoid.
● RENAL IMPAIRMENT Use with caution.
● MONITORING REQUIREMENTS
▸ Monitor growth in children.
▸ Monitor for aggressive behaviour or hostility during initial treatment.
▸ Pulse, blood pressure, psychiatric symptoms, appetite, weight and height should be recorded at initiation of therapy, following each dose adjustment, and at least every 6 months thereafter.
● TREATMENT CESSATION Avoid abrupt withdrawal.
● DIRECTIONS FOR ADMINISTRATION
▸ In children Manufacturer advises tablets can be halved.
● PRESCRIBING AND DISPENSING INFORMATION Data on safety and efficacy of long-term use not complete.
● PATIENT AND CARER ADVICE
  Driving and skilled tasks   **Drugs and Driving** Prescribers and other healthcare professionals should advise patients if treatment is likely to affect their ability to perform skilled tasks (e.g. driving). This applies especially to drugs with sedative effects; patients should be warned that these effects are increased by alcohol.
  For information on 2015 legislation regarding driving whilst taking certain controlled drugs, including amfetamines, see *Drugs and driving* under Guidance on prescribing p. 1.

● MEDICINAL FORMS There can be variation in the licensing of different medicines containing the same drug. Forms available from special-order manufacturers include: modified-release capsule, oral suspension, oral solution

Oral solution
▸ Dexamfetamine sulfate (Non-proprietary)
  Dexamfetamine sulfate 1 mg per 1 ml Dexamfetamine 5mg/5ml oral solution sugar free sugar-free | 150 ml [PoM] £114.49 DT = £114.49 [CD2]

Modified-release capsule
▸ Dexedrine Spansules (Imported (United States))
  Dexamfetamine sulfate 5 mg Dexedrine 5mg Spansules | 100 capsule [PoM] [℞] [CD2]
  Dexamfetamine sulfate 10 mg Dexedrine 10mg Spansules | 100 capsule [PoM] [℞] [CD2]
  Dexamfetamine sulfate 15 mg Dexedrine 15mg Spansules | 100 capsule [PoM] [℞] [CD2]

Tablet
▸ Dexamfetamine sulfate (Non-proprietary)
  Dexamfetamine sulfate 5 mg Dexamfetamine 5mg tablets | 28 tablet [PoM] £24.75 DT = £24.73 [CD2]
▸ Amfexa (Flynn Pharma Ltd)
  Dexamfetamine sulfate 5 mg Amfexa 5mg tablets | 30 tablet [PoM] £19.89 [CD2]
  Dexamfetamine sulfate 10 mg Amfexa 10mg tablets | 30 tablet [PoM] £39.78 DT = £39.78 [CD2]
  Dexamfetamine sulfate 20 mg Amfexa 20mg tablets | 30 tablet [PoM] £79.56 DT = £79.56 [CD2]

Lisdexamfetamine mesilate   29-Oct-2020

● DRUG ACTION Lisdexamfetamine is a prodrug of dexamfetamine.

● INDICATIONS AND DOSE

Attention deficit hyperactivity disorder (initiated by a specialist)
▸ BY MOUTH
▸ **Child 6-17 years:** Initially 30 mg once daily, alternatively initially 20 mg once daily, increased in steps of 10–20 mg every week if required, dose to be taken in

the morning, discontinue if response insufficient after 1 month; maximum 70 mg per day
► **Adult:** Initially 30 mg once daily, increased in steps of 20 mg every week if required, dose to be taken in the morning, discontinue if response insufficient after 1 month; maximum 70 mg per day

● CONTRA-INDICATIONS Advanced arteriosclerosis · agitated states · hyperthyroidism · moderate hypertension · severe hypertension · symptomatic cardiovascular disease

● CAUTIONS Bipolar disorder · history of cardiovascular disease · history of substance abuse · may lower seizure threshold (discontinue if seizures occur) · psychotic disorders · susceptibility to angle-closure glaucoma · tics · Tourette syndrome

CAUTIONS, FURTHER INFORMATION
► **Cardiovascular disease** Manufacturer advises caution in patients with underlying conditions that might be compromised by increases in blood pressure or heart rate; see also *Contra-indications*.

● INTERACTIONS → Appendix 1: amfetamines

● SIDE-EFFECTS
► **Common or very common** Abdominal pain upper · anxiety · appetite decreased · behaviour abnormal · constipation · diarrhoea · dizziness · dry mouth · dyspnoea · fatigue · feeling jittery · headache · hyperhidrosis (uncommon in children) · insomnia · mood altered · movement disorders (uncommon in children) · nausea · palpitations · sexual dysfunction (uncommon in children) · tachycardia · tremor · weight decreased
► **Uncommon** Depression (very common in children) · drowsiness (very common in children) · fever (very common in children) · logorrhea · psychiatric disorders (very common in children) · skin reactions (very common in children) · taste altered · vision blurred · vomiting (very common in children)
► **Frequency not known** Angioedema · cardiomyopathy (uncommon in children) · drug dependence · hallucination (uncommon in children) · hepatitis allergic · mydriasis (uncommon in children) · psychotic disorder · Raynaud's phenomenon (uncommon in children) · seizure · Stevens-Johnson syndrome

Overdose Amfetamines cause wakefulness, excessive activity, paranoia, hallucinations, and hypertension followed by exhaustion, convulsions, hyperthermia, and coma. See Stimulants under Emergency treatment of poisoning p. 1413.

● PREGNANCY Manufacturer advises use only if potential benefit outweighs risk.

● BREAST FEEDING Manufacturer advises avoid—present in human milk.

● RENAL IMPAIRMENT
Dose adjustments Manufacturer advises max. dose 50 mg daily in severe impairment.

● MONITORING REQUIREMENTS
► Manufacturer advises monitor for aggressive behaviour or hostility during initial treatment.
► Manufacturer advises monitor pulse, blood pressure, and for psychiatric symptoms before treatment initiation, following each dose adjustment, and at least every 6 months thereafter. Monitor weight in adults before treatment initiation and during treatment; in children, height and weight should be recorded before treatment initiation, and height, weight and appetite monitored at least every 6 months during treatment.

● TREATMENT CESSATION Avoid abrupt withdrawal.

● DIRECTIONS FOR ADMINISTRATION Manufacturer advises swallow whole or mix contents of capsule with soft food such as yoghurt or in a glass of water or orange juice;

contents should be dispersed completely and consumed immediately.

● PATIENT AND CARER ADVICE Patients and carers should be counselled on the administration of capsules.
Driving and skilled tasks   **Drugs and Driving** Prescribers and other healthcare professionals should advise patients if treatment is likely to affect their ability to perform skilled tasks (e.g. driving). This applies especially to drugs with sedative effects; patients should be warned that these effects are increased by alcohol. General information about a patient's fitness to drive is available from the Driver and Vehicle Licensing Agency at www.gov.uk/government/organisations/driver-and-vehicle-licensing-agency.
For information on 2015 legislation regarding driving whilst taking certain controlled drugs, including amfetamines, see *Drugs and driving* under Guidance on prescribing p. 1.

● NATIONAL FUNDING/ACCESS DECISIONS
For full details see funding body website
Scottish Medicines Consortium (SMC) decisions
► **Lisdexamfetamine dimesylate (*Elvanse*®)** for use as part of a comprehensive treatment programme for attention deficit/hyperactivity disorder (ADHD) in children aged 6 years of age and over when response to previous methylphenidate treatment is considered clinically inadequate **(May 2013)** SMC No. 863/13 Recommended
► **Lisdexamfetamine dimesylate (*Elvanse Adult*®)** for use as part of a comprehensive treatment programme for attention deficit/hyperactivity disorder (ADHD) in adults **(September 2015)** SMC No. 1079/15 Recommended
All Wales Medicines Strategy Group (AWMSG) decisions
► **Lisdexamfetamine dimesylate (*Elvanse*®)** for use as part of a treatment programme for attention deficit/hyperactivity disorder (ADHD) in children aged 6 years and over when response to previous methylphenidate treatment is considered clinically inadequate **(December 2013)** AWMSG No. 188 Recommended
► **Lisdexamfetamine dimesylate (*Elvanse Adult*®)** for use as part of a comprehensive treatment programme for attention deficit/hyperactivity disorder (ADHD) in adults **(October 2015)** AWMSG No. 2534 Recommended

● MEDICINAL FORMS There can be variation in the licensing of different medicines containing the same drug.
Capsule
CAUTIONARY AND ADVISORY LABELS 3, 25
► Elvanse (Shire Pharmaceuticals Ltd)
Lisdexamfetamine dimesylate 20 mg Elvanse 20mg capsules | 28 capsule PoM £54.62 DT = £54.62 CD2
Lisdexamfetamine dimesylate 30 mg Elvanse Adult 30mg capsules | 28 capsule PoM £58.24 DT = £58.24 CD2
Elvanse 30mg capsules | 28 capsule PoM £58.24 DT = £58.24 CD2
Lisdexamfetamine dimesylate 40 mg Elvanse 40mg capsules | 28 capsule PoM £62.82 DT = £62.82 CD2
Lisdexamfetamine dimesylate 50 mg Elvanse Adult 50mg capsules | 28 capsule PoM £68.60 DT = £68.60 CD2
Elvanse 50mg capsules | 28 capsule PoM £68.60 DT = £68.60 CD2
Lisdexamfetamine dimesylate 60 mg Elvanse 60mg capsules | 28 capsule PoM £75.18 DT = £75.18 CD2
Lisdexamfetamine dimesylate 70 mg Elvanse 70mg capsules | 28 capsule PoM £83.16 DT = £83.16 CD2
Elvanse Adult 70mg capsules | 28 capsule PoM £83.16 DT = £83.16 CD2

4

Nervous system

4

Nervous system

Guanfacine

27-Jul-2020

● **INDICATIONS AND DOSE**

Attention deficit hyperactivity disorder in children for whom stimulants are not suitable, not tolerated or ineffective (initiated under specialist supervision)

▸ BY MOUTH

▸ **Child 6-12 years (body-weight 25 kg and above):** Initially 1 mg once daily; adjusted in steps of 1 mg every week if necessary and if tolerated; maintenance 0.05–0.12 mg/kg once daily (max. per dose 4 mg), for optimal weight-adjusted dose titrations, consult product literature

▸ **Child 13-17 years (body-weight 34–41.4 kg):** Initially 1 mg once daily; adjusted in steps of 1 mg every week if necessary and if tolerated; maintenance 0.05–0.12 mg/kg once daily (max. per dose 4 mg), for optimal weight-adjusted dose titrations, consult product literature

▸ **Child 13-17 years (body-weight 41.5-49.4 kg):** Initially 1 mg once daily; adjusted in steps of 1 mg every week if necessary and if tolerated; maintenance 0.05–0.12 mg/kg once daily (max. per dose 5 mg), for optimal weight-adjusted dose titrations, consult product literature

▸ **Child 13-17 years (body-weight 49.5-58.4 kg):** Initially 1 mg once daily; adjusted in steps of 1 mg every week if necessary and if tolerated; maintenance 0.05–0.12 mg/kg once daily (max. per dose 6 mg), for optimal weight-adjusted dose titrations, consult product literature

▸ **Child 13-17 years (body-weight 58.5 kg and above):** Initially 1 mg once daily; adjusted in steps of 1 mg every week if necessary and if tolerated; maintenance 0.05–0.12 mg/kg once daily (max. per dose 7 mg), for optimal weight-adjusted dose titrations, consult product literature

DOSE ADJUSTMENTS DUE TO INTERACTIONS

▸ Manufacturer advises reduce dose by half with concurrent use of moderate and potent inhibitors of CYP3A4.

▸ Manufacturer advises increase dose up to max. 7 mg daily with concurrent use of potent inducers of CYP3A4—no specific recommendation made for children.

● CAUTIONS Bradycardia (risk of torsade de pointes) · heart block (risk of torsade de pointes) · history of cardiovascular disease · history of QT-interval prolongation · hypokalaemia (risk of torsade de pointes)

CAUTIONS, FURTHER INFORMATION

▸ **Elderly** For centrally-acting antihypertensives, prescription potentially inappropriate (STOPP criteria), unless clear intolerance of, or lack of efficacy with, other classes of antihypertensives (generally less well tolerated by older people). See also Prescribing in the elderly p. 33.

● INTERACTIONS → Appendix 1: guanfacine

● SIDE-EFFECTS

▸ **Common or very common** Anxiety · appetite decreased · arrhythmias · asthenia · constipation · depression · diarrhoea · dizziness · drowsiness · dry mouth · gastrointestinal discomfort · headache · hypotension · mood altered · nausea · skin reactions · sleep disorders · urinary disorders · vomiting · weight increased

▸ **Uncommon** Asthma · atrioventricular block · chest pain · hallucination · loss of consciousness · pallor · seizure · syncope

▸ **Rare or very rare** Hypertension · hypertensive encephalopathy · malaise

▸ **Frequency not known** Erectile dysfunction

SIDE-EFFECTS, FURTHER INFORMATION Somnolence and sedation may occur, predominantly during the first 2-3 weeks of treatment and with dose increases; manufacturer advises to consider dose reduction or discontinuation of treatment if symptoms are clinically significant or persistent.

Overdose Features may include hypotension, initial hypertension, bradycardia, lethargy, and respiratory depression. Manufacturer advises that patients who develop lethargy should be observed for development of more serious toxicity for up to 24 hours.

● CONCEPTION AND CONTRACEPTION Manufacturer recommends effective contraception in females of childbearing potential.

● PREGNANCY Manufacturer advises avoid—toxicity in *animal* studies.

● BREAST FEEDING Manufacturer advises avoid—present in milk in *animal* studies.

● HEPATIC IMPAIRMENT Manufacturer advises caution (pharmacokinetics have not been assessed in paediatric patients with hepatic impairment).
Dose adjustments Manufacturer advises consider dose reduction.

● RENAL IMPAIRMENT
Dose adjustments Manufacturer advises consider dose reduction in severe impairment and end-stage renal disease.

● MONITORING REQUIREMENTS

▸ Manufacturer advises to conduct a baseline evaluation to identify patients at risk of somnolence, sedation, hypotension, bradycardia, QT-prolongation, and arrhythmia; this should include assessment of cardiovascular status. Monitor for signs of these adverse effects weekly during dose titration and then every 3 months during the first year of treatment, and every 6 months thereafter. Monitor BMI prior to treatment and then every 3 months for the first year of treatment, and every 6 months thereafter. More frequent monitoring is advised following dose adjustments.

▸ Monitor blood pressure and pulse during dose downward titration and following discontinuation of treatment.

● TREATMENT CESSATION Manufacturer advises avoid abrupt withdrawal; consider dose tapering to minimise potential withdrawal effects.

● DIRECTIONS FOR ADMINISTRATION Manufacturer advises avoid administration with high fat meals (may increase absorption).

● PATIENT AND CARER ADVICE Patients or carers should be counselled on administration of guanfacine modified-release tablets.
Missed doses Manufacturer advises that patients and carers should inform their prescriber if more than one dose is missed; consider dose re-titration.
Driving and skilled tasks Manufacturer advises patients and carers should be counselled about the effects on driving and performance of skilled tasks—increased risk of dizziness and syncope.

● MEDICINAL FORMS There can be variation in the licensing of different medicines containing the same drug.
Modified-release tablet
CAUTIONARY AND ADVISORY LABELS 2, 25
▸ Intuniv (Shire Pharmaceuticals Ltd) ▼
Guanfacine (as Guanfacine hydrochloride) 1 mg Intuniv 1mg modified-release tablets | 28 tablet PoM £56.00 DT = £56.00
Guanfacine (as Guanfacine hydrochloride) 2 mg Intuniv 2mg modified-release tablets | 28 tablet PoM £58.52 DT = £58.52

Guanfacine (as Guanfacine hydrochloride) 3 mg Intuniv 3mg
modified-release tablets | 28 tablet [PoM] £65.52 DT = £65.52
Guanfacine (as Guanfacine hydrochloride) 4 mg Intuniv 4mg
modified-release tablets | 28 tablet [PoM] £76.16 DT = £76.16

3.3　Bipolar disorder and mania

Mania and hypomania   14-Sep-2020

Overview

Antimanic drugs are used to control acute attacks and to prevent recurrence of episodes of mania or hypomania.

An antidepressant drug may also be required for the treatment of co-existing depression, but should be avoided in patients with rapid-cycling bipolar disorder, a recent history of hypomania, or with rapid mood fluctuations.

MHRA/CHM important safety information

When using antiepileptics for the management of mania and hypomania, see Epilepsy p. 321 for information on the use of antiepileptic drugs and the risk of suicidal thoughts and behaviour.

Benzodiazepines

Use of benzodiazepines (such as lorazepam p. 357) may be helpful in the initial stages of treatment for behavioural disturbance or agitation; they should not be used for long periods because of the risk of dependence.

Antipsychotic drugs

Antipsychotic drugs (normally olanzapine p. 419, quetiapine p. 422, or risperidone p. 423) are useful in acute episodes of mania and hypomania; if the response to antipsychotic drugs is inadequate, lithium or valproate may be added. An antipsychotic drug may be used concomitantly with lithium or valproate in the initial treatment of severe acute mania. See *Important safety information, Conception and contraception*, and *Pregnancy* in the valproic acid below and sodium valproate p. 345 monographs.

Olanzapine can be used for the long-term management of bipolar disorder in patients whose manic episode responded to olanzapine therapy. It can be given either as monotherapy, or in combination with lithium or valproate if the patient has frequent relapses or continuing functional impairment.

Asenapine p. 375, a second-generation antipsychotic, is licensed for the treatment of moderate to severe manic episodes associated with bipolar disorder.

When discontinuing antipsychotics, the dose should be reduced gradually over at least 4 weeks if the patient is continuing with other antimanic drugs; if the patient is not continuing with other antimanic drugs or if there is a history of manic relapse, a withdrawal period of up to 3 months should be considered.

Carbamazepine

Carbamazepine p. 327 may be used under specialist supervision for the prophylaxis of bipolar disorder (manic-depressive disorder) in patients unresponsive to a combination of other prophylactic drugs; it is used in patients with rapid-cycling manic-depressive illness (4 or more affective episodes per year). The dose of carbamazepine should not normally be increased if an acute episode of mania occurs.

Valproate

Valproate (valproic acid (as the semisodium salt) and sodium valproate) is used for the treatment of manic episodes associated with bipolar disorder. It must be started and supervised by a specialist experienced in managing bipolar disorder. Valproate (valproic acid and sodium valproate) is also used for the prophylaxis of bipolar disorder. Because of its high teratogenic risk, valproate must not be used in females of childbearing potential unless the conditions of the Pregnancy Prevention Programme are met and alternative treatments are ineffective or not tolerated. Valproic acid and sodium valproate must not be used during pregnancy in bipolar disorder. The benefit and risk of valproate therapy should be carefully reconsidered at regular treatment reviews. For further information, see *Important safety information, Conception and contraception*, and *Pregnancy* in the valproic acid and sodium valproate monographs.

In patients with frequent relapse or continuing functional impairment, consider switching therapy to lithium or olanzapine, or adding lithium or olanzapine to valproate. If a patient taking valproate experiences an acute episode of mania that is not ameliorated by increasing the valproate dose, consider concomitant therapy with olanzapine, quetiapine, or risperidone.

Lithium

Lithium salts are used in the prophylaxis and treatment of mania, hypomania and depression in bipolar disorder (manic-depressive disorder), and in the prophylaxis and treatment of recurrent unipolar depression. Lithium is also used as concomitant therapy with antidepressant medication in patients who have had an incomplete response to treatment for acute bipolar depression and to augment other antidepressants in patients with treatment-resistant depression [unlicensed indication]. It is also licensed for the treatment of aggressive or self-harming behaviour.

The decision to give prophylactic lithium requires specialist advice, and must be based on careful consideration of the likelihood of recurrence in the individual patient, and the benefit of treatment weighed against the risks. The full prophylactic effect of lithium may not occur for six to twelve months after the initiation of therapy. Olanzapine or valproate (given alone or as adjunctive therapy with lithium) are alternative prophylactic treatments in patients who experience frequent relapses or continued functional impairment.

> **Other drugs used for Bipolar disorder and mania**
> Aripiprazole, p. 415 · Chlorpromazine hydrochloride, p. 404 · Haloperidol, p. 405 · Lamotrigine, p. 335 · Paliperidone, p. 420 · Prochlorperazine, p. 408 · Zuclopenthixol acetate, p. 411

ANTIEPILEPTICS

▌Valproic acid   24-Nov-2020

● **INDICATIONS AND DOSE**

Treatment of manic episodes associated with bipolar disorder
▸ BY MOUTH
  ▸ Adult: Initially 750 mg daily in 2–3 divided doses, then increased to 1–2 g daily, adjusted according to response, doses greater than 45 mg/kg daily require careful monitoring

Migraine prophylaxis
▸ BY MOUTH
  ▸ Adult: Initially 250 mg twice daily, then increased if necessary to 1 g daily in divided doses

DOSE EQUIVALENCE AND CONVERSION
▸ Semisodium valproate comprises equimolar amounts of sodium valproate and valproic acid.

CONVULEX®

Epilepsy
▸ BY MOUTH
  ▸ Adult: Initially 600 mg daily in 2–4 divided doses, increased in steps of 150–300 mg every 3 days;

continued →

4

Nervous system

usual maintenance 1–2 g daily in 2–4 divided doses, max. 2.5 g daily in 2–4 divided doses

DOSE EQUIVALENCE AND CONVERSION
▸ *Convulex*® has a 1:1 dose relationship with products containing sodium valproate, but nevertheless care is needed if switching or making changes.

● UNLICENSED USE Not licensed for migraine prophylaxis.

IMPORTANT SAFETY INFORMATION

MHRA/CHM ADVICE: ANTIEPILEPTICS: RISK OF SUICIDAL THOUGHTS AND BEHAVIOUR (AUGUST 2008)
See Epilepsy p. 321.

MHRA/CHM ADVICE: ANTIEPILEPTIC DRUGS: UPDATED ADVICE ON SWITCHING BETWEEN DIFFERENT MANUFACTURERS' PRODUCTS (NOVEMBER 2017)
See Epilepsy p. 321 and see also *Prescribing and dispensing information*.

MHRA/CHM ADVICE: VALPROATE MEDICINES: CONTRA-INDICATED IN WOMEN AND GIRLS OF CHILDBEARING POTENTIAL UNLESS CONDITIONS OF PREGNANCY PREVENTION PROGRAMME ARE MET (APRIL 2018)
Valproate is highly teratogenic and evidence supports that use in pregnancy leads to neurodevelopmental disorders (approx. 30–40% risk) and congenital malformations (approx. 10% risk).

Valproate must not be used in women and girls of childbearing potential unless the conditions of the Pregnancy Prevention Programme are met (see *Conception and contraception*) and only if other treatments are ineffective or not tolerated, as judged by an experienced specialist.

Use of valproate in pregnancy is contra-indicated for migraine prophylaxis [unlicensed] and bipolar disorder; it must only be considered for epilepsy if there is no suitable alternative treatment (see *Pregnancy*).

Women and girls (and their carers) must be fully informed of the risks and the need to avoid exposure to valproate medicines in pregnancy; supporting materials have been provided to use in the implementation of the Pregnancy Prevention Programme (see *Prescribing and dispensing information*). The MHRA advises that:
● GPs must recall all women and girls who may be of childbearing potential, provide the Patient Guide, check they have been reviewed by a specialist in the last year and are on highly effective contraception;
● Specialists must book in review appointments at least annually with women and girls under the Pregnancy Prevention Programme, re-evaluate treatment as necessary, explain clearly the conditions as outlined in the supporting materials and complete and sign the Risk Acknowledgement Form—copies of the form must be given to the patient or carer and sent to their GP;
● Pharmacists must ensure valproate medicines are dispensed in whole packs whenever possible—all packs dispensed to women and girls of childbearing potential should have a warning label either on the carton or via a sticker. They must also discuss risks in pregnancy with female patients each time valproate medicines are dispensed, ensure they have the Patient Guide and have seen their GP or specialist to discuss their treatment and the need for contraception.

MHRA/CHM ADVICE: VALPROATE MEDICINES: ARE YOU ACTING IN COMPLIANCE WITH THE PREGNANCY PREVENTION MEASURES? (DECEMBER 2018)
The MHRA advises that all healthcare professionals must continue to identify and review all female patients on valproate, including when used outside licensed indications (off-label use) and provide them with the patient information materials every time they attend appointments or receive their medicines.

Guidance for psychiatrists on the withdrawal of, and alternatives to, valproate in women of childbearing

potential who have a psychiatric illness is available from the Royal College of Psychiatrists.

MHRA/CHM ADVICE: VALPROATE MEDICINES AND SERIOUS HARMS IN PREGNANCY: NEW ANNUAL RISK ACKNOWLEDGEMENT FORM AND CLINICAL GUIDANCE FROM PROFESSIONAL BODIES TO SUPPORT COMPLIANCE WITH THE PREGNANCY PREVENTION PROGRAMME (APRIL 2019)
The Annual Risk Acknowledgement Form has been updated and should be used for all future reviews of female patients on valproate. Specialists should comply with guidance given on the form if they consider the patient is not at risk of pregnancy, including the need for review in case her risk status changes.

Guidance has been published to support healthcare professionals with the use of valproate. These include a summary by NICE of their guidance and safety advice, pan-college guidance by national healthcare bodies, and paediatric guidance by the British Paediatric Neurology Association and the Royal College of Paediatrics and Child Health.

MHRA/CHM ADVICE (UPDATED JANUARY 2020): VALPROATE PREGNANCY PREVENTION PROGRAMME
The Guide for Healthcare Professionals has been updated and should be used for all future reviews of female patients on valproate medicines, in conjunction with other supporting materials (see *Prescribing and dispensing Information*).

MHRA/CHM ADVICE (UPDATED MAY 2020): VALPROATE PREGNANCY PREVENTION PROGRAMME: TEMPORARY ADVICE FOR MANAGEMENT DURING CORONAVIRUS (COVID-19)
The MHRA has issued temporary guidance for female patients on valproate during the coronavirus (COVID-19) pandemic to support adherence to the Pregnancy Prevention Programme, particularly for those who are shielding due to other health conditions, and should be followed until further notice.

● CONTRA-INDICATIONS Acute porphyrias p. 1107 · known or suspected mitochondrial disorders (higher rate of acute liver failure and liver-related deaths) · personal or family history of severe hepatic dysfunction

● CAUTIONS Systemic lupus erythematosus

CAUTIONS, FURTHER INFORMATION
▸ Liver toxicity Liver dysfunction (including fatal hepatic failure) has occurred in association with valproate (especially in children under 3 years and in those with metabolic or degenerative disorders, organic brain disease or severe seizure disorders associated with mental retardation) usually in first 6 months and usually involving multiple antiepileptic therapy. Raised liver enzymes during valproate treatment are usually transient but patients should be reassessed clinically and liver function (including prothrombin time) monitored until return to normal—discontinue if abnormally prolonged prothrombin time (particularly in association with other relevant abnormalities).

Consider vitamin D supplementation in patients who are immobilised for long periods or who have inadequate sun exposure or dietary intake of calcium.

● INTERACTIONS → Appendix 1: antiepileptics

● SIDE-EFFECTS Abdominal pain · alertness increased · alopecia (regrowth may be curly) · anaemia · behaviour abnormal · bone disorders · bone fracture · cerebral atrophy · coma · confusion · consciousness impaired · dementia · diarrhoea · diplopia · drowsiness · encephalopathy · fine postural tremor · gastrointestinal disorder · gynaecomastia · haemorrhage · hallucination · hearing loss · hepatic disorders · hirsutism · hyperammonaemia · leucopenia · menstrual cycle irregularities · movement disorders · nail disorder · nausea · obesity · pancreatitis · pancytopenia · parkinsonism · peripheral oedema · seizure · severe cutaneous adverse reactions (SCARs) · skin reactions ·

suicidal behaviours · thrombocytopenia · urine abnormalities · vasculitis · vomiting · weight increased

SIDE-EFFECTS, FURTHER INFORMATION **Hepatic dysfunction** Withdraw treatment immediately if persistent vomiting and abdominal pain, anorexia, jaundice, oedema, malaise, drowsiness, or loss of seizure control.

Pancreatitis Discontinue treatment if symptoms of pancreatitis develop.

● CONCEPTION AND CONTRACEPTION The MHRA advises that all women and girls of childbearing potential being treated with valproate medicines must be supported on a Pregnancy Prevention Programme—pregnancy should be excluded before treatment initiation and highly effective contraception must be used during treatment.

● PREGNANCY For *migraine prophylaxis*[unlicensed] and *bipolar disorder*, the MHRA advises that valproate must not be used. For *epilepsy*, the MHRA advises valproate must not be used unless there is no suitable alternative treatment; in such cases, access to counselling about the risks should be provided (see Healthcare Professional Guide for more information) and a Risk Acknowledgement Form signed by both specialist and patient. If valproate is to be used during pregnancy, the lowest effective dose should be prescribed in divided doses to avoid peaks in plasma-valproate concentrations; doses greater than 1 g daily are associated with an increased risk of teratogenicity. Neonatal bleeding (related to hypofibrinaemia). Neonatal hepatotoxicity also reported. See also *Pregnancy* in Epilepsy p. 321.
Monitoring Specialist prenatal monitoring should be instigated when valproate has been taken in pregnancy.

The dose should be monitored carefully during pregnancy and after birth, and adjustments made on a clinical basis.

● BREAST FEEDING Present in milk—risk of haematological disorders in breast-fed newborns and infants.

● HEPATIC IMPAIRMENT Manufacturer advises avoid.

● RENAL IMPAIRMENT
Dose adjustments Reduce dose.

● MONITORING REQUIREMENTS
▸ Monitor closely if dose greater than 45 mg/kg daily.
▸ Monitor liver function before therapy and during first 6 months especially in patients most at risk.
▸ Measure full blood count and ensure no undue potential for bleeding before starting and before surgery.

● EFFECT ON LABORATORY TESTS False-positive urine tests for ketones.

● TREATMENT CESSATION [EvGr] In bipolar disorder, avoid abrupt withdrawal; if treatment with valproate is stopped, reduce the dose gradually over at least 4 weeks. Ⓐ

● PRESCRIBING AND DISPENSING INFORMATION The Pregnancy Prevention Programme is supported by the following materials provided by the manufacturer: *Patient Guide, Guide for Healthcare Professionals, Risk Acknowledgement Form*, and for pharmacists, *Patient Cards* and *Stickers with warning symbols*; the MHRA has also produced a patient information sheet providing advice for women and girls taking valproate medicines.

The Royal Pharmaceutical Society has also produced a safe supply algorithm, available at: www.rpharms.com/safesupplyvalproate

CONVULEX ® Patients being treated for epilepsy may need to be maintained on a specific manufacturer's branded or generic oral valproic acid product.

● PATIENT AND CARER ADVICE
Valproate use by women and girls The MHRA advises women and girls should **not** stop taking valproate without first discussing it with their doctor.

Blood or hepatic disorders Patients or their carers should be told how to recognise signs and symptoms of blood or liver disorders and advised to seek immediate medical attention if symptoms develop.
Pancreatitis Patients or their carers should be told how to recognise signs and symptoms of pancreatitis and advised to seek immediate medical attention if symptoms such as abdominal pain, nausea, or vomiting develop.
Pregnancy Prevention Programme Pharmacists must ensure that female patients have a patient card—see also *Important safety information*.

● MEDICINAL FORMS There can be variation in the licensing of different medicines containing the same drug. Forms available from special-order manufacturers include: oral suspension, oral solution

Gastro-resistant capsule
CAUTIONARY AND ADVISORY LABELS 8, 10, 21, 25
▸ Depakote (Imported (United States))
Valproic acid (as Valproate semisodium) 125 mg Depakote 125mg sprinkle gastro-resistant capsules | 100 capsule [PoM] ⓢ
▸ Convulex (G.L. Pharma UK Ltd) ▼
Valproic acid 150 mg Convulex 150mg gastro-resistant capsules | 30 capsule [PoM] £3.41
Valproic acid 300 mg Convulex 300mg gastro-resistant capsules | 30 capsule [PoM] £6.83
Valproic acid 500 mg Convulex 500mg gastro-resistant capsules | 30 capsule [PoM] £9.00

Gastro-resistant tablet
CAUTIONARY AND ADVISORY LABELS 10, 21, 25
▸ Depakote (Sanofi) ▼
Valproic acid (as Valproate semisodium) 250 mg Depakote 250mg gastro-resistant tablets | 30 tablet [PoM] £5.69 DT = £5.69
Valproic acid (as Valproate semisodium) 500 mg Depakote 500mg gastro-resistant tablets | 30 tablet [PoM] £11.37 DT = £11.37

ANTIPSYCHOTICS ⟩ SECOND-GENERATION

▮ Asenapine   10-Aug-2020

● INDICATIONS AND DOSE
Moderate to severe manic episodes associated with bipolar disorder, as monotherapy or combination therapy
▸ BY SUBLINGUAL ADMINISTRATION
▸ Adult: 5 mg twice daily, increased if necessary to 10 mg twice daily, adjusted according to response

● CAUTIONS Dementia with Lewy bodies

● INTERACTIONS → Appendix 1: antipsychotics, second generation

● SIDE-EFFECTS
▸ **Common or very common** Anxiety · appetite increased · fatigue · muscle rigidity · nausea · oral disorders · taste altered
▸ **Uncommon** Bundle branch block · dysarthria · dysphagia · hyperglycaemia · sexual dysfunction · syncope
▸ **Rare or very rare** Accommodation disorder · rhabdomyolysis

● PREGNANCY Use only if potential benefit outweighs risk—toxicity in *animal* studies.

● BREAST FEEDING Manufacturer advises discontinue breast-feeding—present in milk in *animal* studies.

● HEPATIC IMPAIRMENT Manufacturer advises caution in moderate impairment; avoid in severe impairment (risk of increased exposure).

● RENAL IMPAIRMENT Use with caution if eGFR less than 15 mL/minute/1.73 m² —no information available.

● DIRECTIONS FOR ADMINISTRATION Manufacturer advises *sublingual tablets* should be placed under the tongue and allowed to dissolve completely. Patients should be advised not to consume food or drink for at least 10 minutes after administration. When used as combination therapy, asenapine sublingual tablets should be administered last.

● PATIENT AND CARER ADVICE Patient or carer should be given advice on how to administer asenapine sublingual tablets.

● MEDICINAL FORMS There can be variation in the licensing of different medicines containing the same drug.

Sublingual tablet
CAUTIONARY AND ADVISORY LABELS 2, 26
▸ Sycrest (Merck Sharp & Dohme Ltd)
Asenapine (as Asenapine maleate) 5 mg Sycrest 5mg sublingual tablets sugar-free | 60 tablet [PoM] £102.60 DT = £102.60
Asenapine (as Asenapine maleate) 10 mg Sycrest 10mg sublingual tablets sugar-free | 60 tablet [PoM] £102.60 DT = £102.60

ANTIPSYCHOTICS > LITHIUM SALTS

Lithium salts

● CONTRA-INDICATIONS Addison's disease · cardiac disease associated with rhythm disorder · cardiac insufficiency · dehydration · family history of Brugada syndrome · low sodium diets · personal history of Brugada syndrome · untreated hypothyroidism

● CAUTIONS Avoid abrupt withdrawal · cardiac disease · concurrent ECT (may lower seizure threshold) · diuretic treatment (risk of toxicity) · elderly (reduce dose) · epilepsy (may lower seizure threshold) · myasthenia gravis · psoriasis (risk of exacerbation) · QT interval prolongation · review dose as necessary in diarrhoea · review dose as necessary in intercurrent infection (especially if sweating profusely) · review dose as necessary in vomiting · surgery
CAUTIONS, FURTHER INFORMATION
▸ Long-term use Long-term use of lithium has been associated with thyroid disorders and mild cognitive and memory impairment. Long-term treatment should therefore be undertaken only with careful assessment of risk and benefit, and with monitoring of thyroid function every 6 months (more often if there is evidence of deterioration).
  The need for continued therapy should be assessed regularly and patients should be maintained on lithium after 3–5 years only if benefit persists.

● SIDE-EFFECTS
▸ **Rare or very rare** Nephropathy
▸ **Frequency not known** Abdominal discomfort · alopecia · angioedema · appetite decreased · arrhythmias · atrioventricular block · cardiomyopathy · cerebellar syndrome · circulatory collapse · coma · delirium · diarrhoea · dizziness · dry mouth · electrolyte imbalance · encephalopathy · folliculitis · gastritis · goitre · hyperglycaemia · hyperparathyroidism · hypersalivation · hypotension · hypothyroidism · idiopathic intracranial hypertension · leucocytosis · memory loss · movement disorders · muscle weakness · myasthenia gravis · nausea · neoplasms · nystagmus · peripheral neuropathy · peripheral oedema · polyuria · QT interval prolongation · reflexes abnormal · renal disorders · renal impairment · rhabdomyolysis · seizure · sexual dysfunction · skin reactions · skin ulcer · speech impairment · taste altered · thyrotoxicosis · tremor · vertigo · vision disorders · vomiting · weight increased

SIDE-EFFECTS, FURTHER INFORMATION **Overdose** Signs of intoxication require withdrawal of treatment and include increasing gastro-intestinal disturbances (vomiting, diarrhoea), visual disturbances, polyuria, muscle weakness, fine tremor increasing to coarse tremor, CNS disturbances (confusion and drowsiness increasing to lack of coordination, restlessness, stupor); abnormal reflexes, myoclonus, incontinence, hypernatraemia. With severe

overdosage seizures, cardiac arrhythmias (including sino-atrial block, bradycardia and first-degree heart block), blood pressure changes, circulatory failure, renal failure, coma and sudden death reported.
  For details on the management of poisoning, see Lithium, under Emergency treatment of poisoning p. 1413.

● CONCEPTION AND CONTRACEPTION Manufacturer advises effective contraception during treatment for women of child bearing potential.

● PREGNANCY Avoid if possible, particularly in the first trimester (risk of teratogenicity, including cardiac abnormalities).
Dose adjustments Dose requirements increased during the second and third trimesters (but on delivery return abruptly to normal).
Monitoring Close monitoring of serum-lithium concentration advised in pregnancy (risk of toxicity in neonate).

● BREAST FEEDING Present in milk and risk of toxicity in infant—avoid.

● RENAL IMPAIRMENT Caution in mild to moderate impairment. Avoid in severe impairment.
Monitoring In renal impairment monitor serum-lithium concentration closely and adjust dose accordingly.

● MONITORING REQUIREMENTS
▸ Serum concentrations Lithium salts have a narrow therapeutic/toxic ratio and should therefore not be prescribed unless facilities for monitoring serum-lithium concentrations are available.
Samples should be taken 12 hours after the dose to achieve a serum-lithium concentration of 0.4–1 mmol/litre (lower end of the range for maintenance therapy and elderly patients).
A target serum-lithium concentration of 0.8–1 mmol/litre is recommended for acute episodes of mania, and for patients who have previously relapsed or have sub-syndromal symptoms. It is important to determine the optimum range for each individual patient.
[EvGr] Routine serum-lithium monitoring should be performed weekly after initiation and after each dose change until concentrations are stable, then every 3 months for the first year, and every 6 months thereafter. Patients who are 65 years and older, taking drugs that interact with lithium, at risk of impaired renal or thyroid function, raised calcium levels or other complications, have poor symptom control or poor adherence, or whose last serum-lithium concentration was 0.8 mmol/litre or higher, should be monitored every 3 months. ⒶAdditional serum-lithium measurements should be made if a patient develops significant intercurrent disease or if there is a significant change in a patient's sodium or fluid intake.
▸ Manufacturer advises to assess renal, cardiac, and thyroid function before treatment initiation. [EvGr] An ECG is recommended in patients with cardiovascular disease or risk factors for it. Body-weight or BMI, serum electrolytes, and a full blood count should also be measured before treatment initiation.
▸ Monitor body-weight or BMI, serum electrolytes, eGFR, and thyroid function every 6 months during treatment, and more often if there is evidence of impaired renal or thyroid function, or raised calcium levels. Ⓐ
Manufacturer also advises to monitor cardiac function regularly.

● TREATMENT CESSATION While there is no clear evidence of withdrawal or rebound psychosis, abrupt discontinuation of lithium increases the risk of relapse. If lithium is to be discontinued, the dose should be reduced gradually over a period of at least 4 weeks (preferably over a period of up to 3 months). Patients and their carers should be warned of the risk of relapse if lithium is discontinued abruptly. If lithium is stopped or is to be discontinued abruptly, consider changing therapy to an atypical antipsychotic or valproate.

● PATIENT AND CARER ADVICE Patients should be advised to report signs and symptoms of lithium toxicity, hypothyroidism, renal dysfunction (including polyuria and polydipsia), and benign intracranial hypertension (persistent headache and visual disturbance). Maintain adequate fluid intake and avoid dietary changes which reduce or increase sodium intake.

Lithium treatment packs A lithium treatment pack should be given to patients on initiation of treatment with lithium. The pack consists of a patient information booklet, lithium alert card, and a record book for tracking serum-lithium concentration. Packs may be purchased from

3M
0845 610 1112
nhsforms@mmm.uk.com

Driving and skilled tasks May impair performance of skilled tasks (e.g. driving, operating machinery).

◤ 376

Lithium carbonate

● INDICATIONS AND DOSE

Treatment and prophylaxis of mania | Treatment and prophylaxis of bipolar disorder | Treatment and prophylaxis of recurrent depression | Treatment and prophylaxis of aggressive or self-harming behaviour
▸ BY MOUTH
▸ Adult: Dose adjusted according to serum-lithium concentration, doses are initially divided throughout the day, but once daily administration is preferred when serum-lithium concentration stabilised

DOSE EQUIVALENCE AND CONVERSION
▸ **Preparations vary widely in bioavailability**; changing the preparation requires the same precautions as initiation of treatment.

CAMCOLIT ® IMMEDIATE-RELEASE TABLET

Treatment of mania | Treatment of bipolar disorder | Treatment of recurrent depression | Treatment of aggressive or self-harming behaviour
▸ BY MOUTH
▸ Adult: Initially 1–1.5 g daily, dose adjusted according to serum-lithium concentration, doses are initially divided throughout the day, but once daily administration is preferred when serum-lithium concentration stabilised
▸ Elderly: Reduce initial dose, dose adjusted according to serum-lithium concentration, doses are initially divided throughout the day, but once daily administration is preferred when serum-lithium concentration stabilised

Prophylaxis of mania | Prophylaxis of bipolar disorder | Prophylaxis of recurrent depression | Prophylaxis of aggressive or self-harming behaviour
▸ BY MOUTH
▸ Adult: Initially 300–400 mg daily, dose adjusted according to serum-lithium concentration, doses are initially divided throughout the day, but once daily administration is preferred when serum-lithium concentration stabilised

CAMCOLIT ® MODIFIED-RELEASE TABLET

Treatment of mania | Treatment of bipolar disorder | Treatment of recurrent depression | Treatment of aggressive or self-harming behaviour
▸ BY MOUTH
▸ Adult: Initially 1–1.5 g daily, dose adjusted according to serum-lithium concentration, doses are initially divided throughout the day, but once daily

administration is preferred when serum-lithium concentration stabilised
▸ Elderly: Reduce initial dose, dose adjusted according to serum-lithium concentration, doses are initially divided throughout the day, but once daily administration is preferred when serum-lithium concentration stabilised

Prophylaxis of mania | Prophylaxis of bipolar disorder | Prophylaxis of recurrent depression | Prophylaxis of aggressive or self-harming behaviour
▸ BY MOUTH
▸ Adult: Initially 300–400 mg daily, dose adjusted according to serum-lithium concentration, doses are initially divided throughout the day, but once daily administration is preferred when serum-lithium concentration stabilised

LISKONUM ®

Treatment of mania | Treatment of bipolar disorder | Treatment of recurrent depression | Treatment of aggressive or self-harming behaviour
▸ BY MOUTH
▸ Adult: Initially 450–675 mg twice daily, dose adjusted according to serum-lithium concentration, doses are initially divided throughout the day, but once daily administration is preferred when serum-lithium concentration stabilised
▸ Elderly: Initially 225 mg twice daily, dose adjusted according to serum-lithium concentration, doses are initially divided throughout the day, but once daily administration is preferred when serum-lithium concentration stabilised

Prophylaxis of mania | Prophylaxis of bipolar disorder | Prophylaxis of recurrent depression | Prophylaxis of aggressive or self-harming behaviour
▸ BY MOUTH
▸ Adult: Initially 450 mg twice daily, dose adjusted according serum-lithium concentration, doses are initially divided throughout the day, but once daily administration is preferred when serum-lithium concentration stabilised
▸ Elderly: Initially 225 mg twice daily, dose adjusted according to serum-lithium concentration, doses are initially divided throughout the day, but once daily administration is preferred when serum-lithium concentration stabilised

PRIADEL ® TABLETS

Treatment and prophylaxis of mania | Treatment and prophylaxis of bipolar disorder | Treatment and prophylaxis of recurrent depression | Treatment and prophylaxis of aggressive or self-harming behaviour
▸ BY MOUTH
▸ Adult (body-weight up to 50 kg): Initially 200–400 mg daily, dose adjusted according to serum-lithium concentration, doses are initially divided throughout the day, but once daily administration is preferred when serum-lithium concentration stabilised
▸ Adult (body-weight 50 kg and above): Initially 0.4–1.2 g once daily, alternatively initially 0.4–1.2 g daily in 2 divided doses, dose adjusted according to serum-lithium concentration, doses are initially divided throughout the day, but once daily administration is preferred when serum-lithium concentration stabilised
▸ Elderly: Initially 200–400 mg daily, dose adjusted according to serum-lithium concentration, doses are initially divided throughout the day, but once daily administration is preferred when serum-lithium concentration stabilised

● INTERACTIONS → Appendix 1: lithium

- **MEDICINAL FORMS** There can be variation in the licensing of different medicines containing the same drug. Forms available from special-order manufacturers include: oral suspension

Modified-release tablet

CAUTIONARY AND ADVISORY LABELS 10, 25
  ▸ Camcolit (Essential Pharma Ltd)
    Lithium carbonate 400 mg Camcolit 400 modified-release tablets | 100 tablet [PoM] £48.18 DT = £4.02
  ▸ Liskonum (Teofarma)
    Lithium carbonate 450 mg Liskonum 450mg modified-release tablets | 60 tablet [PoM] £11.84 DT = £11.84
  ▸ Priadel (lithium carbonate) (Essential Pharma M)
    Lithium carbonate 200 mg Priadel 200mg modified-release tablets | 100 tablet [PoM] £7.50 DT = £2.76
    Lithium carbonate 400 mg Priadel 400mg modified-release tablets | 100 tablet [PoM] £8.50 DT = £4.02

Tablet

CAUTIONARY AND ADVISORY LABELS 10
  ▸ Lithium carbonate (Non-proprietary)
    Lithium carbonate 250 mg Lithium carbonate 250mg tablets | 100 tablet [PoM] £87.00 DT = £87.00

F 376

Lithium citrate

- **INDICATIONS AND DOSE**

Treatment and prophylaxis of mania | Treatment and prophylaxis of bipolar disorder | Treatment and prophylaxis of recurrent depression | Treatment and prophylaxis of aggressive or self-harming behaviour
  ▸ BY MOUTH
  ▸ Adult: Dose adjusted according to serum-lithium concentration; doses are initially divided throughout the day, but once daily administration is preferred when serum-lithium concentration stabilised

DOSE EQUIVALENCE AND CONVERSION
  ▸ Preparations vary widely in bioavailability; changing the preparation requires the same precautions as initiation of treatment.

LI-LIQUID ®

Treatment and prophylaxis of mania | Treatment and prophylaxis of bipolar disorder | Treatment and prophylaxis of recurrent depression | Treatment and prophylaxis of aggressive or self-harming behaviour
  ▸ BY MOUTH
  ▸ Adult (body-weight up to 50 kg): Initially 509 mg daily in 2 divided doses, dose adjusted according to serum-lithium concentration
  ▸ Adult (body-weight 50 kg and above): Initially 1.018–3.054 g daily in 2 divided doses, dose adjusted according to serum-lithium concentration
  ▸ Elderly: Initially 509 mg daily in 2 divided doses, dose adjusted according to serum-lithium concentration

DOSE EQUIVALENCE AND CONVERSION
  ▸ For Li-Liquid®: Lithium citrate tetrahydrate 509 mg is equivalent to lithium carbonate 200 mg.

PRIADEL ® LIQUID

Treatment and prophylaxis of mania | Treatment and prophylaxis of bipolar disorder | Treatment and prophylaxis of recurrent depression | Treatment and prophylaxis of aggressive or self-harming behaviour
  ▸ BY MOUTH
  ▸ Adult (body-weight up to 50 kg): Initially 520 mg twice daily, dose adjusted according to serum-lithium concentration, doses are initially divided throughout the day, but once daily administration is preferred when serum-lithium concentration stabilised
  ▸ Adult (body-weight 50 kg and above): Initially 1.04–3.12 g daily in 2 divided doses, dose adjusted according to serum-lithium concentration, doses are initially divided throughout the day, but once daily administration is preferred when serum-lithium concentration stabilised
  ▸ Elderly: Initially 520 mg twice daily, dose adjusted according to serum-lithium concentration, doses are initially divided throughout the day, but once daily administration is preferred when serum-lithium concentration stabilised

DOSE EQUIVALENCE AND CONVERSION
  ▸ For Priadel ® liquid : Lithium citrate tetrahydrate 520 mg is equivalent to lithium carbonate 204 mg.

- **INTERACTIONS** → Appendix 1: lithium
- **SIDE-EFFECTS** Polydipsia

- **MEDICINAL FORMS** There can be variation in the licensing of different medicines containing the same drug.

Oral solution

CAUTIONARY AND ADVISORY LABELS 10
  ▸ Li-Liquid (Rosemont Pharmaceuticals Ltd)
    Lithium citrate 101.8 mg per 1 ml Li-Liquid 509mg/5ml oral solution | 150 ml [PoM] £5.79 DT = £5.79
    Lithium citrate 203.6 mg per 1 ml Li-Liquid 1.018g/5ml oral solution | 150 ml [PoM] £17.49 DT = £17.49
  ▸ Priadel (lithium citrate) (Essential Pharma M)
    Lithium citrate 104 mg per 1 ml Priadel 520mg/5ml liquid sugar-free | 150 ml [PoM] £6.73 DT = £6.73

3.4 Depression

Antidepressant drugs

14-Sep-2020

Overview

Antidepressant drugs are effective for treating moderate to severe depression associated with psychomotor and physiological changes such as loss of appetite and sleep disturbance; improvement in sleep is usually the first benefit of therapy. Ideally, patients with moderate to severe depression should be treated with psychological therapy in addition to drug therapy. Antidepressant drugs are also effective for dysthymia (lower grade chronic depression (typically of at least 2 years duration)).

Antidepressant drugs should not be used routinely in mild depression, and psychological therapy should be considered initially; however, a trial of antidepressant therapy may be considered in cases refractory to psychological treatments or in those associated with psychosocial or medical problems. Drug treatment of mild depression may also be considered in patients with a history of moderate or severe depression.

Choice

The major classes of antidepressant drugs include the tricyclic and related antidepressants, the selective serotonin re-uptake inhibitors (SSRIs), and the monoamine oxidase inhibitors (MAOIs). A number of antidepressant drugs cannot be accommodated easily into this classification.

There is little to choose between the different classes of antidepressant drugs in terms of efficacy, so choice should be based on the individual patient's requirements, including the presence of concomitant disease, existing therapy, suicide risk, and previous response to antidepressant therapy. Since there may be an interval of 2 weeks before the antidepressant action takes place, electroconvulsive treatment may be required in severe depression when delay is hazardous or intolerable. During the first few weeks of treatment, there is an increased potential for agitation, anxiety, and suicidal ideation.

SSRIs are better tolerated and are safer in overdose than other classes of antidepressants and should be considered first-line for treating depression. In patients with unstable angina or who have had a recent myocardial infarction, sertraline p. 387 has been shown to be safe.

Tricyclic antidepressants have similar efficacy to SSRIs but are more likely to be discontinued because of side-effects; toxicity in overdosage is also a problem. SSRIs are less sedating and have fewer antimuscarinic and cardiotoxic effects than tricyclic antidepressants.

MAOIs have dangerous interactions with some foods and drugs, and should be reserved for use by specialists.

Although anxiety is often present in depressive illness (and may be the presenting symptom), the use of an antipsychotic or an anxiolytic may mask the true diagnosis. Anxiolytics or antipsychotic drugs should therefore be used with caution in depression but they are useful adjuncts in agitated patients. Augmenting antidepressants with antipsychotics under specialist supervision may also be necessary in patients who have depression with psychotic symptoms.

St John's wort (*Hypericum perforatum*) is a popular herbal remedy on sale to the public for treating mild depression. It should not be prescribed or recommended for depression because St John's wort can induce drug metabolising enzymes and a number of important interactions with conventional drugs, including conventional antidepressants, have been identified. Furthermore, the amount of active ingredient varies between different preparations of St John's wort and switching from one to another can change the degree of enzyme induction. If a patient stops taking St John's wort, the concentration of interacting drugs may increase, leading to toxicity.

Management
Patients should be reviewed every 1–2 weeks at the start of antidepressant treatment. Treatment should be continued for at least 4 weeks (6 weeks in the elderly) before considering whether to switch antidepressant due to lack of efficacy. In cases of partial response, continue for a further 2–4 weeks (elderly patients may take longer to respond).

Following remission, antidepressant treatment should be continued at the same dose for at least 6 months (about 12 months in the elderly), or for at least 12 months in patients receiving treatment for generalised anxiety disorder (as the likelihood of relapse is high). Patients with a history of recurrent depression should receive maintenance treatment for at least 2 years.

Hyponatraemia and antidepressant therapy
Hyponatraemia (usually in the elderly and possibly due to inappropriate secretion of antidiuretic hormone) has been associated with all types of antidepressants; however, it has been reported more frequently with SSRIs than with other antidepressants. Hyponatraemia should be considered in all patients who develop drowsiness, confusion, or convulsions while taking an antidepressant.

Suicidal behaviour and antidepressant therapy
The use of antidepressants has been linked with suicidal thoughts and behaviour; children, young adults, and patients with a history of suicidal behaviour are particularly at risk. Where necessary patients should be monitored for suicidal behaviour, self-harm, or hostility, particularly at the beginning of treatment or if the dose is changed.

Serotonin syndrome
Serotonin syndrome or serotonin toxicity is a relatively uncommon adverse drug reaction caused by excessive central and peripheral serotonergic activity. Onset of symptoms, which range from mild to lifethreatening, can occur within hours or days following the initiation, dose escalation, or overdose of a serotonergic drug, the addition of a new serotonergic drug, or the replacement of one serotonergic drug by another without allowing a long enough washout period in-between, particularly when the first drug is an irreversible MAOI or a drug with a long half-life. Severe toxicity, which is a medical emergency, usually occurs with a combination of serotonergic drugs, one of which is generally an MAOI.

The characteristic symptoms of serotonin syndrome fall into 3 main areas, although features from each group may not be seen in all patients—neuromuscular hyperactivity (such as tremor, hyperreflexia, clonus, myoclonus, rigidity), autonomic dysfunction (tachycardia, blood pressure changes, hyperthermia, diaphoresis, shivering, diarrhoea), and altered mental state (agitation, confusion, mania).

Treatment consists of withdrawal of the serotonergic medication and supportive care; specialist advice should be sought.

Failure to respond
Failure to respond to initial treatment with an SSRI may require an increase in the dose, or switching to a different SSRI or mirtazapine p. 391. Other second-line choices include lofepramine p. 397, moclobemide p. 382, and reboxetine p. 383. Other tricyclic antidepressants and venlafaxine p. 388 should be considered for more severe forms of depression; irreversible MAOIs should only be prescribed by specialists. Failure to respond to a second antidepressant may require the addition of another antidepressant of a different class, or use of an augmenting agent (such as lithium, aripiprazole p. 415 [unlicensed], olanzapine p. 419 [unlicensed], quetiapine p. 422, or risperidone p. 423 [unlicensed]), but such adjunctive treatment should be initiated only by doctors with special experience of these combinations. Electroconvulsive therapy may be initiated in severe refractory depression.

Anxiety disorders and obsessive-compulsive disorder
Management of acute anxiety generally involves the use of a benzodiazepine or buspirone hydrochloride p. 360. For chronic anxiety (of longer than 4 weeks' duration) it may be appropriate to use an antidepressant. Combined therapy with a benzodiazepine may be required until the antidepressant takes effect. Patients with *generalised anxiety disorder*, a form of chronic anxiety, should be offered psychological treatment before initiating an antidepressant. If drug treatment is needed, an SSRI such as escitalopram p. 384, paroxetine p. 386, or sertraline p. 387 [unlicensed], can be used. Duloxetine p. 387 and venlafaxine p. 388 (serotonin and noradrenaline reuptake inhibitors) are also recommended for the treatment of generalised anxiety disorder; if the patient cannot tolerate SSRIs or serotonin and noradrenaline reuptake inhibitors (or if treatment has failed to control symptoms), pregabalin p. 342 can be considered. The MHRA/CHM have released important safety information on the use of antiepileptic drugs and the risk of suicidal thoughts and behaviour. For further information, see Epilepsy p. 321.

Panic disorder, obsessive-compulsive disorder, post-traumatic stress disorder, and phobic states such as *social anxiety disorder* are treated with SSRIs. Clomipramine hydrochloride p. 393 or imipramine hydrochloride p. 396 can be used second-line in panic disorder [unlicensed]; clomipramine hydrochloride can also be used second-line for obsessive-compulsive disorder. Moclobemide p. 382 is licensed for the treatment of social anxiety disorder.

Tricyclic and related antidepressant drugs
Choice
Tricyclic and related antidepressants block the re-uptake of both serotonin and noradrenaline, although to different extents. For example, clomipramine hydrochloride is more selective for serotonergic transmission, and imipramine hydrochloride is more selective for noradrenergic transmission. Tricyclic and related antidepressant drugs can be roughly divided into those with additional sedative properties and those that are less sedating. Agitated and anxious patients tend to respond best to the sedative compounds, whereas withdrawn and apathetic patients will often obtain most benefit from the less sedating ones. Those with **sedative** properties include amitriptyline hydrochloride p. 392, clomipramine hydrochloride, dosulepin

4

Nervous system

hydrochloride p. 394, doxepin p. 395, mianserin hydrochloride p. 391, trazodone hydrochloride p. 390, and trimipramine p. 398. Those with **less sedative** properties include imipramine hydrochloride, lofepramine p. 397, and nortriptyline p. 397.

Tricyclic and related antidepressants also have varying degrees of antimuscarinic side-effects and cardiotoxicity in overdosage, which may be important in individual patients. Lofepramine has a lower incidence of side-effects and is less dangerous in overdosage but is infrequently associated with hepatic toxicity. Imipramine hydrochloride is also well established, but has more marked antimuscarinic side-effects than other tricyclic and related antidepressants. Amitriptyline hydrochloride and dosulepin hydrochloride are effective but they are particularly dangerous in overdosage and are not recommended for the treatment of depression; dosulepin hydrochloride should be initiated by a specialist.

Dosage

About 10 to 20% of patients fail to respond to tricyclic and related antidepressant drugs and inadequate dosage may account for some of these failures. It is important to use doses that are sufficiently high for effective treatment but not so high as to cause toxic effects. Low doses should be used for initial treatment in the **elderly**. In most patients the long half-life of tricyclic antidepressant drugs allows **once-daily** administration, usually at night; the use of modified-release preparations is therefore unnecessary.

Some tricyclic antidepressants are used in the management of *panic* and other *anxiety disorders*. Some tricyclic antidepressants may also have a role in some forms of *neuralgia* and in *nocturnal enuresis* in children.

Children and adolescents

Studies have shown that tricyclic antidepressants are not effective for treating depression in children.

Considerations in the elderly

The use of tricyclic antidepressants in elderly patients is potentially inappropriate (STOPP criteria):

- if prescribed in those with dementia, narrow angle glaucoma, cardiac conduction abnormalities, prostatism, or history of urinary retention (risk of worsening these conditions);
- if initiated as first-line antidepressant treatment (higher risk of adverse drug reactions than with SSRIs or SNRIs).

For further information, see *STOPP/START criteria* in Prescribing in the elderly p. 33.

Monoamine-oxidase inhibitors

Monoamine-oxidase inhibitors are used much less frequently than tricyclic and related antidepressants, or SSRIs and related antidepressants because of the dangers of dietary and drug interactions and the fact that it is easier to prescribe MAOIs when tricyclic antidepressants have been unsuccessful than vice versa.

Tranylcypromine p. 382 has a greater stimulant action than phenelzine p. 382 or isocarboxazid p. 381 and is more likely to cause a hypertensive crisis. Isocarboxazid and phenelzine are more likely to cause hepatotoxicity than tranylcypromine.

Moclobemide should be reserved as a second line treatment.

Phobic patients and depressed patients with atypical, hypochondriacal, or hysterical features are said to respond best to MAOIs. However, MAOIs should be tried in any patients who are refractory to treatment with other antidepressants as there is occasionally a dramatic response. Response to treatment may be delayed for 3 weeks or more and may take an additional 1 or 2 weeks to become maximal.

Interactions

Other antidepressants should not be started for 2 weeks after treatment with MAOIs has been stopped (3 weeks if starting clomipramine or imipramine). Conversely, an MAOI should not be started until:

- at least 2 weeks after a previous MAOI has been stopped (then started at a reduced dose)
- at least 7–14 days after a tricyclic or related antidepressant (3 weeks in the case of clomipramine or imipramine) has been stopped
- at least a week after an SSRI or related antidepressant (at least 5 weeks in the case of fluoxetine) has been stopped

Other antidepressant drugs

The thioxanthene flupentixol (Fluanxol ®) p. 405 has antidepressant properties when given by mouth in low doses. Flupentixol is also used for the treatment of psychoses.

Vortioxetine p. 399, an antidepressant thought to directly modulate serotonergic receptor activity and inhibit the re-uptake of serotonin, is recommended in patients whose condition has responded inadequately to 2 antidepressants within the current episode.

Tryptophan is licensed for use in treatment-resistant depression, used as monotherapy and as an adjunct to other antidepressant drugs; it should be initiated by hospital specialists.

> **Other drugs used for Depression** Lithium carbonate, p. 377
> · Lithium citrate, p. 378

ANTIDEPRESSANTS 〉 MELATONIN RECEPTOR AGONISTS

Agomelatine

11-Nov-2020

- **DRUG ACTION** A melatonin receptor agonist and a selective serotonin-receptor antagonist; it does not affect the uptake of serotonin, noradrenaline, or dopamine.

- **INDICATIONS AND DOSE**

Major depression

  ▶ BY MOUTH

  ▸ Adult: 25 mg daily, dose to be taken at bedtime, dose to be increased if necessary after 2 weeks, increased if necessary to 50 mg daily, dose to be taken at bedtime

- **CAUTIONS** Alcoholism · bipolar disorder · diabetes · elderly with dementia (safety and efficacy not established) · excessive alcohol consumption · hypomania · mania · non-alcoholic fatty liver disease · obesity · patients 75 years of age or older (safety and efficacy not established)

- **INTERACTIONS** → Appendix 1: agomelatine

- **SIDE-EFFECTS**

  ▶ **Common or very common** Abdominal pain · anxiety · back pain · constipation · diarrhoea · dizziness · drowsiness · fatigue · headaches · nausea · sleep disorders · vomiting · weight changes

  ▶ **Uncommon** Aggression · confusion · hyperhidrosis · mood altered · movement disorders · paraesthesia · skin reactions · suicidal behaviours · tinnitus · vision blurred

  ▶ **Rare or very rare** Angioedema · face oedema · hallucination · hepatic disorders · urinary retention

  SIDE-EFFECTS, FURTHER INFORMATION The use of antidepressants has been linked with suicidal thoughts and behaviour; children, young adults, and patients with a history of suicidal behaviour are particularly at risk. Where necessary patients should be monitored for suicidal behaviour, self-harm, or hostility, particularly at the beginning of treatment or if the dose is changed.

- **PREGNANCY** Manufacturer advises avoid.

- BREAST FEEDING Avoid—present in milk in *animal* studies.
- HEPATIC IMPAIRMENT Manufacturer advises caution if transaminases are elevated; avoid in hepatic impairment or if transaminases exceed 3 times the upper limit of normal.
- RENAL IMPAIRMENT Caution in moderate to severe impairment.
- MONITORING REQUIREMENTS Test liver function before treatment and after 3, 6, 12 and 24 weeks of treatment, and then regularly thereafter when clinically indicated (restart monitoring schedule if dose increased); discontinue if serum transaminases exceed 3 times the upper limit of reference range or symptoms of liver disorder.
- PATIENT AND CARER ADVICE
Hepatotoxicity Patients should be told how to recognise signs of liver disorder, and advised to seek immediate medical attention if symptoms such as dark urine, light coloured stools, jaundice, bruising, fatigue, abdominal pain, or pruritus develop.
Patients should be given a booklet with more information on the risk of hepatic side-effects.

- MEDICINAL FORMS There can be variation in the licensing of different medicines containing the same drug.
Tablet
  ▸ Agomelatine (Non-proprietary)
    Agomelatine 25 mg Agomelatine 25mg tablets | 28 tablet PoM £30.91 DT = £30.29
  ▸ Valdoxan (Servier Laboratories Ltd)
    Agomelatine 25 mg Valdoxan 25mg tablets | 28 tablet PoM £30.00 DT = £30.29

ANTIDEPRESSANTS › MONOAMINE-OXIDASE INHIBITORS

Monoamine-oxidase inhibitors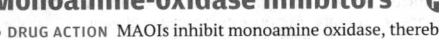

- DRUG ACTION MAOIs inhibit monoamine oxidase, thereby causing an accumulation of amine neurotransmitters.
- CONTRA-INDICATIONS Cerebrovascular disease · not indicated in manic phase · phaeochromocytoma · severe cardiovascular disease
- CAUTIONS Acute porphyrias p. 1107 · avoid in agitated patients · blood disorders · cardiovascular disease · concurrent electroconvulsive therapy · diabetes mellitus · elderly (great caution) · epilepsy · severe hypertensive reactions to certain drugs and foods · surgery
- SIDE-EFFECTS Akathisia · anxiety · appetite increased · arrhythmia · asthenia · behaviour abnormal · blood disorder · confusion · constipation · dizziness · drowsiness · dry mouth · dysuria · hallucination · headache · hyperhidrosis · insomnia · jaundice · nausea · paraesthesia · peripheral neuritis · postural hypotension (more common in elderly) · reflexes increased · skin reactions · suicidal behaviours · tremor · vision blurred · vomiting · weight increased

  SIDE-EFFECTS, FURTHER INFORMATION Risk of postural hypotension and hypertensive responses. Discontinue if palpitations or frequent headaches occur.

- PREGNANCY Increased risk of neonatal malformations—manufacturer advise avoid unless there are compelling reasons.
- HEPATIC IMPAIRMENT In general, manufacturers advise avoid.
- MONITORING REQUIREMENTS Monitor blood pressure (risk of postural hypotension and hypertensive responses).
- TREATMENT CESSATION
Withdrawal If possible avoid abrupt withdrawal.

MAOIs are associated with withdrawal symptoms on cessation of therapy. Symptoms include agitation, irritability, ataxia, movement disorders, insomnia, drowsiness, vivid dreams, cognitive impairment, and slowed speech. Withdrawal symptoms occasionally experienced when discontinuing MAOIs include hallucinations and paranoid delusions. If possible MAOIs should be withdrawn slowly.

Withdrawal effects may occur within 5 days of stopping treatment with antidepressant drugs; they are usually mild and self-limiting, but in some cases may be severe. The risk of withdrawal symptoms is increased if the antidepressant is stopped suddenly after regular administration for 8 weeks or more. The dose should preferably be reduced gradually over about 4 weeks, or longer if withdrawal symptoms emerge (6 months in patients who have been on long-term maintenance treatment).

- PATIENT AND CARER ADVICE Patients should be advised to eat only fresh foods and avoid food that is suspected of being stale or 'going off'. This is especially important with meat, fish, poultry or offal; game should be avoided. The danger of interaction persists for up to 2 weeks after treatment with MAOIs is discontinued. Patients should also be advised to avoid alcoholic drinks or de-alcoholised (low alcohol) drinks.
Driving and skilled tasks Drowsiness may affect performance of skilled tasks (e.g. driving).

ANTIDEPRESSANTS › MONOAMINE-OXIDASE A AND B INHIBITORS, IRREVERSIBLE

◀ above

Isocarboxazid
21-May-2020

- INDICATIONS AND DOSE
Depressive illness
  ▸ BY MOUTH
  ▸ Adult: Initially 30 mg daily until improvement occurs, initial dose may be given in single or divided doses, dose may be increased if necessary after 4 weeks, increased if necessary up to 60 mg daily for 4–6 weeks, dose to be increased under close supervision only, then reduced to 10–20 mg daily, usual maintenance dose, but up to 40 mg daily may be required
  ▸ Elderly: 5–10 mg daily

- INTERACTIONS → Appendix 1: MAOIs, irreversible
- SIDE-EFFECTS Granulocytopenia · peripheral oedema · sexual dysfunction
- BREAST FEEDING Avoid.
- RENAL IMPAIRMENT Use with caution.
- LESS SUITABLE FOR PRESCRIBING Less suitable for prescribing.

- MEDICINAL FORMS There can be variation in the licensing of different medicines containing the same drug. Forms available from special-order manufacturers include: oral suspension
Tablet
CAUTIONARY AND ADVISORY LABELS 3, 10
  ▸ Isocarboxazid (Non-proprietary)
    Isocarboxazid 10 mg Isocarboxazid 10mg tablets | 56 tablet PoM £249.10 DT = £233.43

Phenelzine

21-May-2020

● **INDICATIONS AND DOSE**

Depressive illness

▸ BY MOUTH

▸ Adult: Initially 15 mg 3 times a day, response is usually seen within first week; dose may be increased if necessary after 2 weeks if response is not evident, increased if necessary to 15 mg 4 times a day, doses up to 30 mg three times a day may be used in hospital patients; response may not become apparent for up to 4 weeks; once satisfactory response has been achieved, reduce dose gradually to lowest suitable maintenance dose (15 mg on alternate days may be adequate)

● INTERACTIONS → Appendix 1: MAOIs, irreversible

● SIDE-EFFECTS Cardiovascular insufficiency · delirium · electrolyte imbalance · fatal progressive hepatocellular necrosis · feeling jittery · fever · gastrointestinal disorder · glaucoma · hypermetabolism · hypertensive crisis · impaired driving ability · intracranial haemorrhage · lupus-like syndrome · malaise · mood altered · movement disorders · muscle tone increased · muscle twitching · neuroleptic malignant syndrome · nystagmus · oedema · respiratory disorders · schizophrenia · seizure · sexual dysfunction · shock-like coma · speech repetitive

● BREAST FEEDING Avoid—no information available.

● LESS SUITABLE FOR PRESCRIBING Less suitable for prescribing.

● MEDICINAL FORMS Forms available from special-order manufacturers include: tablet

Tranylcypromine

22-May-2020

● **INDICATIONS AND DOSE**

Depressive illness

▸ BY MOUTH

▸ Adult: Initially 10 mg twice daily, dose to be taken at a time no later than 3 p.m., dose may be increased if necessary after 1 week, increased if necessary to 30 mg daily in divided doses, 10 mg to be taken in the morning and 20 mg to be taken in the afternoon, doses above 30 mg daily under close supervision only; maintenance 10 mg daily

● CONTRA-INDICATIONS History of hepatic disease · hyperthyroidism

● INTERACTIONS → Appendix 1: MAOIs, irreversible

● SIDE-EFFECTS

▸ Rare or very rare Hepatocellular injury

▸ Frequency not known Chest pain · diarrhoea · drug dependence · extrasystole · flushing · hypertension · hypomania · mydriasis · pain · pallor · photophobia · sleep disorder · throbbing headache

● BREAST FEEDING Present in milk in *animal* studies.

● LESS SUITABLE FOR PRESCRIBING Less suitable for prescribing.

● MEDICINAL FORMS There can be variation in the licensing of different medicines containing the same drug.

Tablet

CAUTIONARY AND ADVISORY LABELS 3, 10

▸ Tranylcypromine (Non-proprietary)

Tranylcypromine (as Tranylcypromine sulfate)

10 mg Tranylcypromine 10mg tablets | 28 tablet PoM £367.65 DT = £367.65

Moclobemide

08-Nov-2020

● DRUG ACTION Moclobemide is reported to act by reversible inhibition of monoamine oxidase type A (it is therefore termed a RIMA).

● **INDICATIONS AND DOSE**

Depressive illness

▸ BY MOUTH

▸ Adult: Initially 300 mg daily in divided doses, adjusted according to response; usual dose 150–600 mg daily, dose to be taken after food

Social anxiety disorder

▸ BY MOUTH

▸ Adult: Initially 300 mg daily for 3 days, then increased to 600 mg daily in 2 divided doses continued for 8–12 weeks to assess efficacy

DOSE ADJUSTMENTS DUE TO INTERACTIONS

▸ Manufacturer advises reduce dose to half or one-third of the usual dose with concurrent use of cimetidine.

● CONTRA-INDICATIONS Acute confusional states · phaeochromocytoma

● CAUTIONS Avoid in agitated or excited patients (or give with sedative for up to 2–3 weeks) · may provoke manic episodes in bipolar disorders · thyrotoxicosis

● INTERACTIONS → Appendix 1: moclobemide

● SIDE-EFFECTS

▸ Common or very common Anxiety · constipation · diarrhoea · dizziness · dry mouth · headache · hypotension · irritability · nausea · paraesthesia · skin reactions · sleep disorder · vomiting

▸ Uncommon Asthenia · confusion · flushing · oedema · suicidal behaviours · taste altered · visual impairment

▸ Rare or very rare Appetite decreased · delusions · hyponatraemia · serotonin syndrome

● PREGNANCY Safety in pregnancy has not been established—manufacturer advises avoid unless there are compelling reasons.

● BREAST FEEDING Amount too small to be harmful, but patient information leaflet advises avoid.

● HEPATIC IMPAIRMENT Manufacturer advises caution in severe impairment (risk of decreased metabolism). **Dose adjustments** Manufacturer advises dose reduction to half or one-third of the daily dose in severe impairment,

● TREATMENT CESSATION Withdrawal effects may occur within 5 days of stopping treatment with antidepressant drugs; they are usually mild and self-limiting, but in some cases may be severe. The risk of withdrawal symptoms is increased if the antidepressant is stopped suddenly after regular administration for 8 weeks or more. The dose should preferably be reduced gradually over about 4 weeks, or longer if withdrawal symptoms emerge (6 months in patients who have been on long-term maintenance treatment).

● PATIENT AND CARER ADVICE Moclobemide is claimed to cause less potentiation of the pressor effect of tyramine than the traditional (irreversible) MAOIs, but patients should avoid consuming large amounts of tyramine-rich food (such as mature cheese, yeast extracts and fermented soya bean products).

- MEDICINAL FORMS There can be variation in the licensing of different medicines containing the same drug. Forms available from special-order manufacturers include: oral suspension

Tablet

CAUTIONARY AND ADVISORY LABELS 10, 21

▸ Moclobemide (Non-proprietary)

Moclobemide 150 mg Moclobemide 150mg tablets | 30 tablet PoM £22.10 DT = £28.25

Moclobemide 300 mg Moclobemide 300mg tablets | 30 tablet PoM £15.00 DT = £13.99

▸ Manerix (Mylan)

Moclobemide 150 mg Manerix 150mg tablets | 30 tablet PoM £9.33 DT = £28.25

Moclobemide 300 mg Manerix 300mg tablets | 30 tablet PoM £13.99 DT = £13.99

ANTIDEPRESSANTS > NORADRENALINE REUPTAKE INHIBITORS

Reboxetine
19-Oct-2020

- DRUG ACTION Reboxetine is a selective inhibitor of noradrenaline re-uptake.

- ● INDICATIONS AND DOSE

Major depression

▸ BY MOUTH

▸ Adult 18–65 years: 4 mg twice daily for 3–4 weeks, then increased if necessary to 10 mg daily in divided doses; maximum 12 mg per day

- CAUTIONS Bipolar disorder · history of cardiovascular disease · history of epilepsy · prostatic hypertrophy · susceptibility to angle-closure glaucoma · urinary retention

- INTERACTIONS → Appendix 1: reboxetine

- SIDE-EFFECTS

▸ **Common or very common** Accommodation disorder · akathisia · anxiety · appetite decreased · chills · constipation · dizziness · dry mouth · headache · hyperhidrosis · hypertension · hypotension · insomnia · nausea · palpitations · paraesthesia · sexual dysfunction · skin reactions · tachycardia · taste altered · urinary disorders · urinary tract infection · vasodilation · vomiting

▸ **Uncommon** Mydriasis · vertigo

▸ **Rare or very rare** Glaucoma

▸ **Frequency not known** Aggression · hallucination · hyponatraemia · irritability · peripheral coldness · potassium depletion (long term use) · Raynaud's phenomenon · suicidal behaviours · testicular pain

- PREGNANCY Use only if potential benefit outweighs risk— limited information available.

- BREAST FEEDING Small amount present in milk—use only if potential benefit outweighs risk.

- HEPATIC IMPAIRMENT Manufacturer advises caution (risk of increased exposure).
Dose adjustments Manufacturer advises initial dose reduction to 2 mg twice daily, increased according to tolerance.

- RENAL IMPAIRMENT
Dose adjustments Initial dose 2 mg twice daily, increased according to tolerance.

- TREATMENT CESSATION Caution— avoid abrupt withdrawal.

- PATIENT AND CARER ADVICE
Driving and skilled tasks Counselling advised.

- MEDICINAL FORMS There can be variation in the licensing of different medicines containing the same drug.

Tablet

▸ Edronax (Pfizer Ltd)

Reboxetine (as Reboxetine mesilate) 4 mg Edronax 4mg tablets | 60 tablet PoM £18.91 DT = £18.91

Selective serotonin re-uptake inhibitors
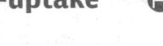

- DRUG ACTION Selectively inhibit the re-uptake of serotonin (5-hydroxytryptamine, 5-HT).

- CONTRA-INDICATIONS Poorly controlled epilepsy · SSRIs should not be used if the patient enters a manic phase

- CAUTIONS Cardiac disease · concurrent electroconvulsive therapy · diabetes mellitus · epilepsy (discontinue if convulsions develop) · history of bleeding disorders (especially gastro-intestinal bleeding) · history of mania · susceptibility to angle-closure glaucoma

CAUTIONS, FURTHER INFORMATION

▸ Elderly Prescription potentially inappropriate (STOPP criteria) with current or recent significant hyponatraemia i.e. serum sodium less than 130 mmol/L (risk of exacerbating or precipitating hyponatraemia).
See also Prescribing in the elderly p. 33.

- SIDE-EFFECTS

▸ **Common or very common** Anxiety · appetite abnormal · arrhythmias · arthralgia · asthenia · concentration impaired · confusion · constipation · depersonalisation · diarrhoea · dizziness · drowsiness · dry mouth · fever · gastrointestinal discomfort · haemorrhage · headache · hyperhidrosis · malaise · memory loss · menstrual cycle irregularities · myalgia · mydriasis · nausea (dose-related) · palpitations · paraesthesia · QT interval prolongation · sexual dysfunction · skin reactions · sleep disorders · taste altered · tinnitus · tremor · urinary disorders · visual impairment · vomiting · weight changes · yawning

▸ **Uncommon** Alopecia · angioedema · behaviour abnormal · hallucination · mania · movement disorders · photosensitivity reaction · postural hypotension · seizure · suicidal behaviours · syncope

▸ **Rare or very rare** Galactorrhoea · hepatitis · hyperprolactinaemia · hyponatraemia · serotonin syndrome · severe cutaneous adverse reactions (SCARs) · SIADH · thrombocytopenia

▸ **Frequency not known** Withdrawal syndrome

SIDE-EFFECTS, FURTHER INFORMATION Symptoms of sexual dysfunction may persist after treatment has stopped.

Overdose Symptoms of poisoning by selective serotonin re-uptake inhibitors include nausea, vomiting, agitation, tremor, nystagmus, drowsiness, and sinus tachycardia; convulsions may occur. Rarely, severe poisoning results in the serotonin syndrome, with marked neuropsychiatric effects, neuromuscular hyperactivity, and autonomic instability; hyperthermia, rhabdomyolysis, renal failure, and coagulopathies may develop.
For details on the management of poisoning, see Selective serotonin re-uptake inhibitors, under Emergency treatment of poisoning p. 1413.

- PREGNANCY Manufacturers advise avoid during pregnancy unless the potential benefit outweighs the risk. There is a small increased risk of congenital heart defects when taken during early pregnancy. If used during the third trimester there is a risk of neonatal withdrawal symptoms, and persistent pulmonary hypertension in the newborn has been reported.

- HEPATIC IMPAIRMENT In general, manufacturers advise caution (prolonged half-life).

- TREATMENT CESSATION Gastro-intestinal disturbances, headache, anxiety, dizziness, paraesthesia, electric shock sensation in the head, neck, and spine, tinnitus, sleep disturbances, fatigue, influenza-like symptoms, and sweating are the most common features of abrupt

Nervous system   **4**

withdrawal of an SSRI or marked reduction of the dose; palpitation and visual disturbances can occur less commonly. The dose should be tapered over at least a few weeks to avoid these effects. For some patients, it may be necessary to withdraw treatment over a longer period; consider obtaining specialist advice if symptoms persist.

Withdrawal effects may occur within 5 days of stopping treatment with antidepressant drugs; they are usually mild and self-limiting, but in some cases may be severe. The risk of withdrawal symptoms is increased if the antidepressant is stopped suddenly after regular administration for 8 weeks or more.

● PATIENT AND CARER ADVICE
Driving and skilled tasks May also impair performance of skilled tasks (e.g. driving, operating machinery).

F 383

Citalopram

30-Jul-2020

● **INDICATIONS AND DOSE**

Depressive illness

▶ BY MOUTH USING TABLETS
▶ Adult: 20 mg once daily, increased in steps of 20 mg daily if required, dose to be increased at intervals of 3–4 weeks; maximum 40 mg per day
▶ Elderly: 10–20 mg once daily; maximum 20 mg per day
▶ BY MOUTH USING ORAL DROPS
▶ Adult: 16 mg once daily, increased in steps of 16 mg daily if required, dose to be increased at intervals of 3–4 weeks; maximum 32 mg per day
▶ Elderly: 8–16 mg daily; maximum 16 mg per day

Panic disorder

▶ BY MOUTH USING TABLETS
▶ Adult: Initially 10 mg daily, increased in steps of 10 mg daily if required, dose to be increased gradually; usual dose 20–30 mg daily; maximum 40 mg per day
▶ Elderly: Initially 10 mg daily, increased in steps of 10 mg daily if required, dose to be increased gradually; maximum 20 mg per day
▶ BY MOUTH USING ORAL DROPS
▶ Adult: Initially 8 mg once daily, increased in steps of 8 mg if required, dose to be increased gradually; usual dose 16–24 mg daily; maximum 32 mg per day
▶ Elderly: Initially 8 mg once daily, increased in steps of 8 mg if required, dose to be increased gradually; maximum 16 mg per day

DOSE EQUIVALENCE AND CONVERSION
▶ 4 oral drops (8 mg) is equivalent in therapeutic effect to 10 mg tablet.

● CONTRA-INDICATIONS QT-interval prolongation
● CAUTIONS Susceptibility to QT-interval prolongation
● INTERACTIONS → Appendix 1: SSRIs
● SIDE-EFFECTS
▶ **Common or very common** Acute angle closure glaucoma · apathy · flatulence · hypersalivation · migraine · rhinitis
▶ **Uncommon** Oedema
▶ **Rare or very rare** Cough · generalised tonic-clonic seizure
▶ **Frequency not known** Hypokalaemia
● BREAST FEEDING Present in milk—use with caution.
● HEPATIC IMPAIRMENT
Dose adjustments For *tablets* manufacturer advises initial dose of 10 mg daily for the first two weeks in mild to moderate impairment—dose may be increased to max. 20 mg daily; use with extra caution and careful dose titration in severe impairment.
For *oral drops* manufacturer advises initial dose of 8 mg daily for the first two weeks in mild to moderate impairment—dose may be increased to max. 16 mg daily; use with extra caution and careful dose titration in severe impairment.

● RENAL IMPAIRMENT No information available for eGFR less than 20 mL/minute/1.73 m^2.
● TREATMENT CESSATION The dose should preferably be reduced gradually over about 4 weeks, or longer if withdrawal symptoms emerge (6 months in patients who have been on long-term maintenance treatment).
● DIRECTIONS FOR ADMINISTRATION Manufacturer advises *Cipramil*® oral drops should be mixed with water, orange juice, or apple juice before taking.
● PATIENT AND CARER ADVICE Counselling on administration of oral drops is advised.
Driving and skilled tasks Patients should be advised of the effects of citalopram on driving and skilled tasks.

● MEDICINAL FORMS There can be variation in the licensing of different medicines containing the same drug.
Oral drops
EXCIPIENTS: May contain Alcohol
▶ Citalopram (Non-proprietary)
Citalopram (as Citalopram hydrochloride) 40 mg per 1 ml Citalopram 40mg/ml oral drops sugar free sugar-free | 15 ml PoM £17.98 DT = £12.84
▶ Cipramil (Lundbeck Ltd)
Citalopram (as Citalopram hydrochloride) 40 mg per 1 ml Cipramil 40mg/ml drops sugar-free | 15 ml PoM £10.08 DT = £12.84
Tablet
▶ Citalopram (Non-proprietary)
Citalopram (as Citalopram hydrobromide) 10 mg Citalopram 10mg tablets | 28 tablet PoM £12.36 DT = £1.00 | 250 tablet PoM £13.25
Citalopram (as Citalopram hydrobromide) 20 mg Citalopram 20mg tablets | 28 tablet PoM £14.66 DT = £1.05 | 250 tablet PoM £8.50
Citalopram (as Citalopram hydrobromide) 40 mg Citalopram 40mg tablets | 28 tablet PoM £16.47 DT = £1.46
▶ Cipramil (Lundbeck Ltd)
Citalopram (as Citalopram hydrobromide) 20 mg Cipramil 20mg tablets | 28 tablet PoM £8.95 DT = £1.05

F 383

Escitalopram

29-Oct-2020

● DRUG ACTION Escitalopram is the active enantiomer of citalopram.

● **INDICATIONS AND DOSE**

Depressive illness | Generalised anxiety disorder | Obsessive-compulsive disorder

▶ BY MOUTH
▶ Adult: 10 mg once daily; increased if necessary up to 20 mg daily
▶ Elderly: Initially 5 mg once daily; maximum 10 mg per day

Panic disorder

▶ BY MOUTH
▶ Adult: Initially 5 mg once daily for 7 days, then increased to 10 mg daily; maximum 20 mg per day
▶ Elderly: Initially 5 mg once daily; maximum 10 mg per day

Social anxiety disorder

▶ BY MOUTH
▶ Adult: Initially 10 mg once daily for 2–4 weeks, dose to be adjusted after 2-4 weeks of treatment; usual dose 5–20 mg daily

DOSE EQUIVALENCE AND CONVERSION
▶ 1 drop of oral solution contains 1 mg of escitalopram.

● CONTRA-INDICATIONS QT-interval prolongation
● CAUTIONS Susceptibility to QT-interval prolongation
● INTERACTIONS → Appendix 1: SSRIs
● SIDE-EFFECTS
▶ **Common or very common** Sinusitis

- **Uncommon** Oedema
- **BREAST FEEDING** Present in breast milk; avoid.
- **HEPATIC IMPAIRMENT**
  Dose adjustments Manufacturer advises initially 5 mg once daily for 2 weeks in mild to moderate impairment; thereafter increased to 10 mg once daily according to response; titrate dose with extra caution in severe impairment.
- **RENAL IMPAIRMENT** Caution if eGFR less than 30 mL/minute/1.73m².
- **TREATMENT CESSATION** The dose should preferably be reduced gradually over about 4 weeks, or longer if withdrawal symptoms emerge (6 months in patients who have been on long-term maintenance treatment).
- **DIRECTIONS FOR ADMINISTRATION** Manufacturer advises oral drops can be mixed with water, orange juice, or apple juice before taking.
- **PATIENT AND CARER ADVICE** Counselling on administration of oral drops advised.
  Driving and skilled tasks Patients should be counselled about the effects on driving.

- **MEDICINAL FORMS** There can be variation in the licensing of different medicines containing the same drug.
  Oral drops
  ▸ Cipralex (Lundbeck Ltd)
  Escitalopram (as Escitalopram oxalate) 20 mg per 1 ml Cipralex 20mg/ml oral drops sugar-free | 15 ml [PoM] £20.16 DT = £20.16
  Tablet
  ▸ Escitalopram (Non-proprietary)
  Escitalopram (as Escitalopram oxalate) 5 mg Escitalopram 5mg tablets | 28 tablet [PoM] £8.97 DT = £1.97
  Escitalopram (as Escitalopram oxalate) 10 mg Escitalopram 10mg tablets | 28 tablet [PoM] £14.91 DT = £1.92
  Escitalopram (as Escitalopram oxalate) 20 mg Escitalopram 20mg tablets | 28 tablet [PoM] £25.20 DT = £2.16
  ▸ Cipralex (Lundbeck Ltd)
  Escitalopram (as Escitalopram oxalate) 5 mg Cipralex 5mg tablets | 28 tablet [PoM] £8.97 DT = £1.97
  Escitalopram (as Escitalopram oxalate) 10 mg Cipralex 10mg tablets | 28 tablet [PoM] £14.91 DT = £1.92
  Escitalopram (as Escitalopram oxalate) 20 mg Cipralex 20mg tablets | 28 tablet [PoM] £25.20 DT = £2.16

F 383

Fluoxetine
10-Sep-2020

- **INDICATIONS AND DOSE**
  Major depression
  ▸ BY MOUTH
  ▸ Adult: Initially 20 mg daily, dose is increased after 3–4 weeks if necessary, and at appropriate intervals thereafter, daily dose may be administered as a single or divided dose; maximum 60 mg per day
  ▸ Elderly: Initially 20 mg daily, dose is increased after 3–4 weeks if necessary, and at appropriate intervals thereafter, daily dose may be administered as a single or divided dose, usual maximum dose is 40 mg daily but doses up to 60 mg daily can be used

  Bulimia nervosa
  ▸ BY MOUTH
  ▸ Adult: 60 mg daily, daily dose may be administered as a single or divided dose
  ▸ Elderly: Up to 40 mg daily, daily dose may be administered as a single or divided dose, usual maximum dose is 40 mg daily but doses up to 60 mg daily can be used

  Obsessive-compulsive disorder
  ▸ BY MOUTH
  ▸ Adult: 20 mg daily, increased if necessary up to 60 mg daily, daily dose may be administered as a single or divided dose, dose to be increased gradually, review

treatment if inadequate response after 10 weeks; maximum 60 mg per day
  ▸ Elderly: 20 mg daily, increased if necessary up to 40 mg daily, daily dose may be administered as a single or divided dose, dose to be increased gradually, review treatment if inadequate response after 10 weeks, usual maximum dose is 40 mg daily but doses up to 60 mg daily can be used

Menopausal symptoms, particularly hot flushes, in women with breast cancer (except those taking tamoxifen)
  ▸ BY MOUTH
  ▸ Adult: 20 mg once daily
  PHARMACOKINETICS
  ▸ Consider the long half-life of fluoxetine when adjusting dosage (or in overdosage).

- **UNLICENSED USE** [EvGr] Fluoxetine is used for menopausal symptoms, Ⓑ but it is not licensed for this indication.
- **INTERACTIONS** → Appendix 1: SSRIs
- **SIDE-EFFECTS**
  ▸ **Common or very common** Chills · feeling abnormal · postmenopausal haemorrhage · uterine disorder · vasodilation · vision blurred
  ▸ **Uncommon** Cold sweat · dysphagia · dyspnoea · hypotension · mood altered · muscle twitching · self-injurious behaviour · temperature sensation altered · thinking abnormal
  ▸ **Rare or very rare** Buccoglossal syndrome · leucopenia · neutropenia · oesophageal pain · pharyngitis · respiratory disorders · serum sickness · speech disorder · vasculitis
  ▸ **Frequency not known** Bone fracture
- **BREAST FEEDING** Present in milk—avoid.
- **HEPATIC IMPAIRMENT**
  Dose adjustments Manufacturer advises dose reduction or increasing dose interval.
- **DIRECTIONS FOR ADMINISTRATION** Manufacturer advises dispersible tablets can be dispersed in water for administration or swallowed whole with plenty of water.
- **PATIENT AND CARER ADVICE** Patients and carers should be counselled on the administration of dispersible tablets.
  Driving and skilled tasks Patients should be counselled about the effects on driving and skilled tasks.

- **MEDICINAL FORMS** There can be variation in the licensing of different medicines containing the same drug. Forms available from special-order manufacturers include: capsule, oral suspension, oral solution
  Tablet
  ▸ Fluoxetine (Non-proprietary)
  Fluoxetine (as Fluoxetine hydrochloride) 10 mg Fluoxetine 10mg tablets | 30 tablet [PoM] £61.73 DT = £61.73
  Dispersible tablet
  CAUTIONARY AND ADVISORY LABELS 10
  ▸ Olena (Advanz Pharma)
  Fluoxetine (as Fluoxetine hydrochloride) 20 mg Olena 20mg dispersible tablets sugar-free | 28 tablet [PoM] £3.44 DT = £3.44
  Oral solution
  ▸ Fluoxetine (Non-proprietary)
  Fluoxetine (as Fluoxetine hydrochloride) 4 mg per 1 ml Fluoxetine 20mg/5ml oral solution | 70 ml [PoM] £12.75 DT = £4.22
  Fluoxetine 20mg/5ml oral solution sugar free sugar-free | 70 ml [PoM] £12.95 DT = £12.95
  ▸ Prozep (Chemidex Pharma Ltd)
  Fluoxetine (as Fluoxetine hydrochloride) 4 mg per 1 ml Prozep 20mg/5ml oral solution sugar-free | 70 ml [PoM] £12.95 DT = £12.95
  Capsule
  ▸ Fluoxetine (Non-proprietary)
  Fluoxetine (as Fluoxetine hydrochloride) 10 mg Fluoxetine 10mg capsules | 30 capsule [PoM] £61.43 DT = £61.43
  Fluoxetine (as Fluoxetine hydrochloride) 20 mg Fluoxetine 20mg capsules | 30 capsule [PoM] £5.00 DT = £1.12 | 100 capsule [PoM] £4.70

Fluoxetine (as Fluoxetine hydrochloride) 30 mg Fluoxetine 30mg capsules | 30 capsule [PoM] £2.43 DT = £1.80
Fluoxetine (as Fluoxetine hydrochloride) 40 mg Fluoxetine 40mg capsules | 30 capsule [PoM] £2.41 DT = £1.80
Fluoxetine (as Fluoxetine hydrochloride) 60 mg Fluoxetine 60mg capsules | 30 capsule [PoM] £54.36 DT = £7.46

Fluvoxamine maleate

⚑ 383

02-Sep-2020

● **INDICATIONS AND DOSE**

Depressive illness
▶ BY MOUTH
▶ Adult: Initially 50–100 mg daily, dose to be taken in the evening, dose to be increased gradually, increased if necessary up to 300 mg daily, doses over 150 mg daily are given in divided doses; maintenance 100 mg daily

Obsessive-compulsive disorder
▶ BY MOUTH
▶ Adult: Initially 50 mg daily, dose to be taken in the evening, dose is increased gradually if necessary after several weeks, increased if necessary up to 300 mg daily; maintenance 100–300 mg daily, doses over 150 mg daily are given in divided doses, if no improvement in obsessive-compulsive disorder within 10 weeks, treatment should be reconsidered

● INTERACTIONS → Appendix 1: SSRIs

● SIDE-EFFECTS
▶ **Rare or very rare** Hepatic function abnormal (discontinue)
▶ **Frequency not known** Bone fracture · glaucoma · neuroleptic malignant-like syndrome · withdrawal syndrome neonatal

● BREAST FEEDING Present in milk—avoid.

● HEPATIC IMPAIRMENT
Dose adjustments Manufacturer advises low initial dose.

● RENAL IMPAIRMENT
Dose adjustments Start with low dose.

● TREATMENT CESSATION The dose should preferably be reduced gradually over about 4 weeks, or longer if withdrawal symptoms emerge (6 months in patients who have been on long-term maintenance treatment).

● PATIENT AND CARER ADVICE
Driving and skilled tasks Patients should be counselled about the effects on driving and skilled tasks.

● MEDICINAL FORMS There can be variation in the licensing of different medicines containing the same drug. Forms available from special-order manufacturers include: oral suspension
Tablet
▶ Fluvoxamine maleate (Non-proprietary)
Fluvoxamine maleate 50 mg Fluvoxamine 50mg tablets | 60 tablet [PoM] £18.90 DT = £17.53
Fluvoxamine maleate 100 mg Fluvoxamine 100mg tablets | 30 tablet [PoM] £20.98 DT = £17.70
▶ Faverin (Mylan)
Fluvoxamine maleate 50 mg Faverin 50mg tablets | 60 tablet [PoM] £17.10 DT = £17.53
Fluvoxamine maleate 100 mg Faverin 100mg tablets | 30 tablet [PoM] £17.10 DT = £17.70

Paroxetine

⚑ 383

02-Sep-2020

● **INDICATIONS AND DOSE**

Major depression | Social anxiety disorder | Post-traumatic stress disorder | Generalised anxiety disorder
▶ BY MOUTH
▶ Adult: 20 mg daily, dose to be taken in the morning, no evidence of greater efficacy at higher doses; maximum 50 mg per day

▶ Elderly: 20 mg daily, dose to be taken in the morning, no evidence of greater efficacy at higher doses; maximum 40 mg per day

Obsessive-compulsive disorder
▶ BY MOUTH
▶ Adult: Initially 20 mg daily, dose to be taken in the morning, increased in steps of 10 mg, dose to be increased gradually, increased to 40 mg daily, no evidence of greater efficacy at higher doses; maximum 60 mg per day
▶ Elderly: Initially 20 mg daily, dose to be taken in the morning, increased in steps of 10 mg, dose to be increased gradually; maximum 40 mg per day

Panic disorder
▶ BY MOUTH
▶ Adult: Initially 10 mg daily, dose to be taken in the morning, increased in steps of 10 mg, dose to be increased gradually, increased to 40 mg daily, no evidence of greater efficacy at higher doses; maximum 60 mg per day
▶ Elderly: Initially 10 mg daily, dose to be taken in the morning, increased in steps of 10 mg, dose to be increased gradually; maximum 40 mg per day

Menopausal symptoms, particularly hot flushes, in women with breast cancer (except those taking tamoxifen).
▶ BY MOUTH
▶ Adult: 10 mg once daily

● UNLICENSED USE [EvGr] Paroxetine is used for menopausal symptoms, Ⓑ but it is not licensed for this indication.

● CAUTIONS Achlorhydria · high gastric pH
CAUTIONS, FURTHER INFORMATION
▶ Achlorhydria or high gastric pH Causes reduced absorption of the oral suspension.

● INTERACTIONS → Appendix 1: SSRIs

● SIDE-EFFECTS
▶ **Common or very common** Vision blurred
▶ **Uncommon** Diabetic control impaired
▶ **Rare or very rare** Acute glaucoma · hepatic disorders · peripheral oedema

● PREGNANCY Increased risk of congenital malformations, especially if used in the first trimester.

● BREAST FEEDING Present in milk but amount too small to be harmful.

● HEPATIC IMPAIRMENT
Dose adjustments Manufacturer advises dose at the lower end of the range.

● RENAL IMPAIRMENT
Dose adjustments Reduce dose if eGFR less than 30 mL/minute/1.73 m^2.

● TREATMENT CESSATION Associated with a higher risk of withdrawal reactions. The dose should preferably be reduced gradually over about 4 weeks, or longer if withdrawal symptoms emerge (6 months in patients who have been on long-term maintenance treatment).

● PATIENT AND CARER ADVICE
Driving and skilled tasks Patients should be counselled about the effect on driving.

● MEDICINAL FORMS There can be variation in the licensing of different medicines containing the same drug. Forms available from special-order manufacturers include: oral suspension, oral solution
Oral suspension
CAUTIONARY AND ADVISORY LABELS 5, 21
▶ Seroxat (GlaxoSmithKline UK Ltd)
Paroxetine (as Paroxetine hydrochloride) 2 mg per 1 ml Seroxat 20mg/10ml liquid sugar-free | 150 ml [PoM] £9.12 DT = £9.12

Tablet

CAUTIONARY AND ADVISORY LABELS 21

▸ Paroxetine (Non-proprietary)
Paroxetine (as Paroxetine hydrochloride) 10 mg Paroxetine 10mg tablets | 28 tablet [PoM] £17.03 DT = £4.27
Paroxetine (as Paroxetine hydrochloride) 20 mg Paroxetine 20mg tablets | 30 tablet [PoM] £12.18 DT = £1.67
Paroxetine (as Paroxetine hydrochloride) 30 mg Paroxetine 30mg tablets | 30 tablet [PoM] £2.65 DT = £2.04
Paroxetine (as Paroxetine hydrochloride) 40 mg Paroxetine 40mg tablets | 28 tablet [PoM] £17.03 DT = £16.91 | 30 tablet [PoM] £18.12–£25.07

▸ Seroxat (GlaxoSmithKline UK Ltd)
Paroxetine (as Paroxetine hydrochloride) 10 mg Seroxat 10mg tablets | 28 tablet [PoM] £14.21 DT = £4.27
Paroxetine (as Paroxetine hydrochloride) 20 mg Seroxat 20mg tablets | 30 tablet [PoM] £15.23 DT = £1.67
Paroxetine (as Paroxetine hydrochloride) 30 mg Seroxat 30mg tablets | 30 tablet [PoM] £26.74 DT = £2.04

⚑ 383

Sertraline
19-Mar-2018

● **INDICATIONS AND DOSE**

Depressive illness
▸ BY MOUTH
▸ **Adult:** Initially 50 mg daily, then increased in steps of 50 mg at intervals of at least 1 week if required; maintenance 50 mg daily; maximum 200 mg per day

Obsessive-compulsive disorder
▸ BY MOUTH
▸ **Adult:** Initially 50 mg daily, then increased in steps of 50 mg at intervals of at least 1 week if required; maximum 200 mg per day

Panic disorder | Post-traumatic stress disorder | Social anxiety disorder
▸ BY MOUTH
▸ **Adult:** Initially 25 mg daily for 1 week, then increased to 50 mg daily, then increased in steps of 50 mg at intervals of at least 1 week if required, increase only if response is partial and if drug is tolerated; maximum 200 mg per day

● INTERACTIONS → Appendix 1: SSRIs

● SIDE-EFFECTS
▸ **Common or very common** Chest pain · depression · gastrointestinal disorders · increased risk of infection · neuromuscular dysfunction · vasodilation
▸ **Uncommon** Back pain · burping · chills · cold sweat · dysphagia · dyspnoea · ear pain · euphoric mood · hypertension · hypothyroidism · migraine · muscle complaints · muscle weakness · oedema · oral disorders · osteoarthritis · periorbital oedema · respiratory disorders · sensation abnormal · speech disorder · thinking abnormal · thirst
▸ **Rare or very rare** Balanoposthitis · bone disorder · cardiac disorder · coma · conversion disorder · diabetes mellitus · drug dependence · dysphonia · eye disorders · gait abnormal · genital discharge · glaucoma · hair texture abnormal · hepatic disorders · hiccups · hypercholesterolaemia · hypoglycaemia · injury · lymphadenopathy · myocardial infarction · neoplasms · oliguria · peripheral ischaemia · psychotic disorder · vasodilation procedure · vision disorders · vulvovaginal atrophy
▸ **Frequency not known** Cerebrovascular insufficiency · gynaecomastia · hyperglycaemia · leucopenia · neuroleptic malignant syndrome · pancreatitis

● BREAST FEEDING Not known to be harmful but consider discontinuing breast-feeding.

● HEPATIC IMPAIRMENT Manufacturer advises avoid in severe impairment (no information available).

Dose adjustments Manufacturer advises dose reduction or increasing dose interval in mild to moderate impairment.

● RENAL IMPAIRMENT Use with caution.

● TREATMENT CESSATION The dose should preferably be reduced gradually over about 4 weeks, or longer if withdrawal symptoms emerge (6 months in patients who have been on long-term maintenance treatment).

● PATIENT AND CARER ADVICE
Driving and skilled tasks Patients should be counselled on the effects on driving and skilled tasks.

● MEDICINAL FORMS There can be variation in the licensing of different medicines containing the same drug. Forms available from special-order manufacturers include: tablet, oral suspension

Tablet

▸ Sertraline (Non-proprietary)
Sertraline (as Sertraline hydrochloride) 25 mg Sertraline 25mg tablets | 28 tablet [PoM] £12.20
Sertraline (as Sertraline hydrochloride) 50 mg Sertraline 50mg tablets | 28 tablet [PoM] £17.00 DT = £4.22 | 500 tablet [PoM] £12.45
Sertraline (as Sertraline hydrochloride) 100 mg Sertraline 100mg tablets | 28 tablet [PoM] £28.00 DT = £5.89 | 500 tablet [PoM] £16.39

▸ Lustral (Upjohn UK Ltd)
Sertraline (as Sertraline hydrochloride) 50 mg Lustral 50mg tablets | 28 tablet [PoM] £17.82 DT = £4.22
Sertraline (as Sertraline hydrochloride) 100 mg Lustral 100mg tablets | 28 tablet [PoM] £29.16 = £5.89

ANTIDEPRESSANTS ❭ SEROTONIN AND NORADRENALINE RE-UPTAKE INHIBITORS

Duloxetine
19-Oct-2020

● DRUG ACTION Inhibits the re-uptake of serotonin and noradrenaline.

● **INDICATIONS AND DOSE**

Major depressive disorder
▸ BY MOUTH
▸ **Adult:** 60 mg once daily

Generalised anxiety disorder
▸ BY MOUTH
▸ **Adult:** Initially 30 mg once daily, increased if necessary to 60 mg once daily; maximum 120 mg per day

Diabetic neuropathy
▸ BY MOUTH
▸ **Adult:** 60 mg once daily, discontinue if inadequate response after 2 months; review treatment at least every 3 months, maximum dose to be given in divided doses; maximum 120 mg per day

Moderate to severe stress urinary incontinence
▸ BY MOUTH
▸ **Adult (female):** 40 mg twice daily, patient should be assessed for benefit and tolerability after 2–4 weeks, alternatively initially 20 mg twice daily for 2 weeks, this can minimise side effects, then increased to 40 mg twice daily, the patient should be assessed for benefit and tolerability after 2–4 weeks.

● CAUTIONS Bleeding disorders · cardiac disease · elderly · history of mania · history of seizures · hypertension (avoid if uncontrolled) · raised intra-ocular pressure · susceptibility to angle-closure glaucoma

● INTERACTIONS → Appendix 1: duloxetine

● SIDE-EFFECTS
▸ **Common or very common** Anxiety · appetite decreased · constipation · diarrhoea · dizziness · drowsiness · dry mouth · fall · fatigue · flushing · gastrointestinal discomfort · gastrointestinal disorders · headache · muscle complaints · nausea · pain · palpitations · paraesthesia · sexual dysfunction · skin reactions · sleep disorders · sweat

4

Nervous system

4

Nervous system

changes · tinnitus · tremor · urinary disorders · vision disorders · vomiting · weight changes · yawning
▸ **Uncommon** Apathy · arrhythmias · behaviour abnormal · burping · chills · concentration impaired · disorientation · dysphagia · ear pain · feeling abnormal · gait abnormal · haemorrhage · hepatic disorders · hyperglycaemia · increased risk of infection · malaise · menstrual disorder · movement disorders · mydriasis · peripheral coldness · photosensitivity reaction · postural hypotension · suicidal behaviours · syncope · taste altered · temperature sensation altered · testicular pain · thirst · throat tightness · vertigo
▸ **Rare or very rare** Angioedema · cutaneous vasculitis · dehydration · galactorrhoea · glaucoma · hallucination · hyperprolactinaemia · hypertensive crisis · hyponatraemia · hypothyroidism · mania · menopausal symptoms · oral disorders · seizure · serotonin syndrome · SIADH · Stevens-Johnson syndrome · urine odour abnormal

SIDE-EFFECTS, FURTHER INFORMATION Symptoms of sexual dysfunction may persist after treatment has stopped.

● PREGNANCY Toxicity in *animal* studies—avoid in patients with stress urinary incontinence; in other conditions use only if potential benefit outweighs risk. Risk of neonatal withdrawal symptoms if used near term.

● BREAST FEEDING Present in milk—manufacturer advises avoid.

● HEPATIC IMPAIRMENT Manufacturer advises avoid.

● RENAL IMPAIRMENT Avoid if eGFR less than 30 mL/minute/1.73 m².

● TREATMENT CESSATION Nausea, vomiting, headache, anxiety, dizziness, paraesthesia, sleep disturbances, and tremor are the most common features of abrupt withdrawal or marked reduction of the dose; dose should be reduced over at least 1–2 weeks.

● NATIONAL FUNDING/ACCESS DECISIONS
CYMBALTA® For full details see funding body website
Scottish Medicines Consortium (SMC) decisions
▸ Duloxetine (*Cymbalta*®) for diabetic peripheral neuropathic pain in adults (September 2006) SMC No. 285/06
Recommended with restrictions

● MEDICINAL FORMS There can be variation in the licensing of different medicines containing the same drug.

Gastro-resistant capsule
CAUTIONARY AND ADVISORY LABELS 2
▸ Duloxetine (Non-proprietary)
Duloxetine (as Duloxetine hydrochloride) 20 mg Duloxetine 20mg gastro-resistant capsules | 28 capsule [PoM] £18.48 DT = £5.25
Duloxetine (as Duloxetine hydrochloride) 30 mg Duloxetine 30mg gastro-resistant capsules | 28 capsule [PoM] £22.40 DT = £1.67
Duloxetine (as Duloxetine hydrochloride) 40 mg Duloxetine 40mg gastro-resistant capsules | 56 capsule [PoM] £36.96 DT = £11.12
Duloxetine (as Duloxetine hydrochloride) 60 mg Duloxetine 60mg gastro-resistant capsules | 28 capsule [PoM] £27.72 DT = £2.30
▸ Cymbalta (Eli Lilly and Company Ltd)
Duloxetine (as Duloxetine hydrochloride) 30 mg Cymbalta 30mg gastro-resistant capsules | 28 capsule [PoM] £22.40 DT = £1.67
Duloxetine (as Duloxetine hydrochloride) 60 mg Cymbalta 60mg gastro-resistant capsules | 28 capsule [PoM] £27.72 DT = £2.30
▸ Depalta (Disposable Medical Equipment Ltd)
Duloxetine (as Duloxetine hydrochloride) 30 mg Depalta 30mg gastro-resistant capsules | 28 capsule [PoM] £2.95 DT = £1.67
Duloxetine (as Duloxetine hydrochloride) 60 mg Depalta 60mg gastro-resistant capsules | 28 capsule [PoM] £4.25 DT = £2.30
▸ Duciltia (Aristo Pharma Ltd)
Duloxetine (as Duloxetine hydrochloride) 30 mg Duciltia 30mg gastro-resistant capsules | 28 capsule [PoM] £22.40 DT = £1.67
Duloxetine (as Duloxetine hydrochloride) 60 mg Duciltia 60mg gastro-resistant capsules | 28 capsule [PoM] £27.72 DT = £2.30
▸ Yentreve (Eli Lilly and Company Ltd)
Duloxetine (as Duloxetine hydrochloride) 20 mg Yentreve 20mg gastro-resistant capsules | 28 capsule [PoM] £18.48 DT = £5.25
Duloxetine (as Duloxetine hydrochloride) 40 mg Yentreve 40mg gastro-resistant capsules | 56 capsule [PoM] £36.96 DT = £11.12

Venlafaxine

19-Oct-2020

● DRUG ACTION A serotonin and noradrenaline re-uptake inhibitor.

● INDICATIONS AND DOSE
Major depression
▸ BY MOUTH USING IMMEDIATE-RELEASE MEDICINES
▸ Adult: Initially 75 mg daily in 2 divided doses, then increased if necessary up to 375 mg daily, dose to be increased if necessary at intervals of at least 2 weeks, faster dose titration may be necessary in some patients; maximum 375 mg per day
▸ BY MOUTH USING MODIFIED-RELEASE MEDICINES
▸ Adult: Initially 75 mg once daily, increased if necessary up to 375 mg once daily, dose to be increased if necessary at intervals of at least 2 weeks, faster dose titration may be necessary in some patients; maximum 375 mg per day

Generalised anxiety disorder
▸ BY MOUTH USING MODIFIED-RELEASE MEDICINES
▸ Adult: 75 mg once daily, increased if necessary up to 225 mg once daily, dose to be increased at intervals of at least 2 weeks; maximum 225 mg per day

Social anxiety disorder
▸ BY MOUTH USING MODIFIED-RELEASE MEDICINES
▸ Adult: 75 mg once daily, there is no evidence of greater efficacy at higher doses, increased if necessary up to 225 mg once daily, dose to be increased if necessary at intervals of at least 2 weeks; maximum 225 mg per day

Panic disorder
▸ BY MOUTH USING MODIFIED-RELEASE MEDICINES
▸ Adult: Initially 37.5 mg once daily for 7 days, increased to 75 mg once daily, increased if necessary up to 225 mg once daily, dose to be increased at intervals of at least 2 weeks; maximum 225 mg per day

Menopausal symptoms, particularly hot flushes, in women with breast cancer
▸ BY MOUTH USING MODIFIED-RELEASE MEDICINES
▸ Adult: 37.5 mg once daily for one week, then increased if necessary to 75 mg once daily

● UNLICENSED USE [EvGr] Venlafaxine is used for menopausal symptoms, ⒶbutⒶ it is not licensed for this indication.

● CONTRA-INDICATIONS Uncontrolled hypertension

● CAUTIONS Conditions associated with high risk of cardiac arrhythmia · diabetes · heart disease (monitor blood pressure) · history of bleeding disorders · history of epilepsy · history or family history of mania · susceptibility to angle-closure glaucoma

● INTERACTIONS → Appendix 1: venlafaxine

● SIDE-EFFECTS
▸ **Common or very common** Anxiety · appetite decreased · arrhythmias · asthenia · chills · confusion · constipation · depersonalisation · diarrhoea · dizziness · dry mouth · dyspnoea · headache · hot flush · hypertension · menstrual cycle irregularities · movement disorders · muscle tone increased · mydriasis · nausea · palpitations · paraesthesia · sedation · sexual dysfunction · skin reactions · sleep disorders · sweat changes · taste altered · tinnitus · tremor · urinary disorders · vision disorders · vomiting · weight changes · yawning
▸ **Uncommon** Alopecia · angioedema · apathy · behaviour abnormal · derealisation · haemorrhage · hallucination · hypotension · mood altered · photosensitivity reaction · syncope
▸ **Rare or very rare** Agranulocytosis · angle closure glaucoma · bone marrow disorders · delirium · hepatitis · hyponatraemia · neuroleptic malignant syndrome · neutropenia · pancreatitis · QT interval prolongation · respiratory disorders · rhabdomyolysis · seizure · serotonin

syndrome · severe cutaneous adverse reactions (SCARs) · SIADH · thrombocytopenia

▸ **Frequency not known** Suicidal behaviours · vertigo · withdrawal syndrome

SIDE-EFFECTS, FURTHER INFORMATION Symptoms of sexual dysfunction may persist after treatment has stopped.

● PREGNANCY Avoid unless potential benefit outweighs risk—toxicity in *animal* studies. Risk of withdrawal effects in neonate.

● BREAST FEEDING Present in milk—avoid.

● HEPATIC IMPAIRMENT Manufacturer advises caution (inter-individual variability in clearance; limited information available in severe impairment).
Dose adjustments Manufacturer advises consider dose reduction of 50% in mild to moderate impairment and of more than 50% in severe impairment.

● RENAL IMPAIRMENT Use with caution.
Dose adjustments Use half normal dose (immediate-release tablets may be given once daily) if eGFR less than 30 mL/minute/1.73 m^2.

● TREATMENT CESSATION Associated with a higher risk of withdrawal effects compared with other antidepressants.
Gastro-intestinal disturbances, headache, anxiety, dizziness, paraesthesia, tremor, sleep disturbances, and sweating are most common features of withdrawal if treatment stopped abruptly or if dose reduced markedly; dose should be reduced over several weeks.

● PATIENT AND CARER ADVICE
Driving and skilled tasks May affect performance of skilled tasks (e.g. driving).

● MEDICINAL FORMS There can be variation in the licensing of different medicines containing the same drug. Forms available from special-order manufacturers include: oral suspension, oral solution

Modified-release tablet
CAUTIONARY AND ADVISORY LABELS 3, 21, 25
▸ Venlafaxine (Non-proprietary)
Venlafaxine (as Venlafaxine hydrochloride) 150 mg Venlafaxine 150mg modified-release tablets | 28 tablet [PoM] £18.70
▸ Sunveniz XL (Sun Pharmaceutical Industries Europe B.V.)
Venlafaxine (as Venlafaxine hydrochloride) 75 mg Sunveniz XL 75mg tablets | 30 tablet [PoM] £11.14 DT = £2.60
Venlafaxine (as Venlafaxine hydrochloride) 150 mg Sunveniz XL 150mg tablets | 30 tablet [PoM] £18.64 DT = £3.90
▸ Venladex XL (Dexcel-Pharma Ltd)
Venlafaxine (as Venlafaxine hydrochloride) 75 mg Venladex XL 75mg tablets | 28 tablet [PoM] £11.20
Venlafaxine (as Venlafaxine hydrochloride) 150 mg Venladex XL 150mg tablets | 28 tablet [PoM] £18.70
Venlafaxine (as Venlafaxine hydrochloride) 225 mg Venladex XL 225mg tablets | 28 tablet [PoM] £31.36
▸ Venlalic XL (Ethypharm UK Ltd)
Venlafaxine (as Venlafaxine hydrochloride) 37.5 mg Venlalic XL 37.5mg tablets | 30 tablet [PoM] £6.60 DT = £6.60
Venlafaxine (as Venlafaxine hydrochloride) 75 mg Venlalic XL 75mg tablets | 30 tablet [PoM] £2.60 DT = £2.60
Venlafaxine (as Venlafaxine hydrochloride) 150 mg Venlalic XL 150mg tablets | 30 tablet [PoM] £3.90 DT = £3.90
Venlafaxine (as Venlafaxine hydrochloride) 225 mg Venlalic XL 225mg tablets | 30 tablet [PoM] £33.60 DT = £33.60
Venlafaxine (as Venlafaxine hydrochloride) 300 mg Venlalic XL 300mg tablets | 30 tablet [PoM] £35.00
▸ ViePax XL (Dexcel-Pharma Ltd)
Venlafaxine (as Venlafaxine hydrochloride) 75 mg ViePax XL 75mg tablets | 28 tablet [PoM] £2.60
Venlafaxine (as Venlafaxine hydrochloride) 150 mg ViePax XL 150mg tablets | 28 tablet [PoM] £3.90
Venlafaxine (as Venlafaxine hydrochloride) 225 mg ViePax XL 225mg tablets | 28 tablet [PoM] £31.36

Tablet
CAUTIONARY AND ADVISORY LABELS 3
▸ Venlafaxine (Non-proprietary)
Venlafaxine (as Venlafaxine hydrochloride) 37.5 mg Venlafaxine 37.5mg tablets | 56 tablet [PoM] £7.95 DT = £4.86

Venlafaxine (as Venlafaxine hydrochloride) 75 mg Venlafaxine 75mg tablets | 56 tablet [PoM] £15.95 DT = £9.56

Modified-release capsule
CAUTIONARY AND ADVISORY LABELS 3, 21, 25
▸ Venlafaxine (Non-proprietary)
Venlafaxine (as Venlafaxine hydrochloride) 225 mg Venlafaxine 225mg modified-release capsules | 28 capsule [PoM] ⚠ DT = £47.11 | 30 capsule [PoM] £44.75
▸ Alventa XL (Consilient Health Ltd)
Venlafaxine (as Venlafaxine hydrochloride) 75 mg Alventa XL 75mg capsules | 28 capsule [PoM] £19.12 DT = £2.60
Venlafaxine (as Venlafaxine hydrochloride) 150 mg Alventa XL 150mg capsules | 28 capsule [PoM] £31.88 DT = £3.90
▸ Depefex XL (Chiesi Ltd)
Venlafaxine (as Venlafaxine hydrochloride) 75 mg Depefex XL 75mg capsules | 28 capsule [PoM] £10.40 DT = £2.60
Venlafaxine (as Venlafaxine hydrochloride) 150 mg Depefex XL 150mg capsules | 28 capsule [PoM] £17.40 DT = £3.90
▸ Efexor XL (Upjohn UK Ltd)
Venlafaxine (as Venlafaxine hydrochloride) 75 mg Efexor XL 75mg capsules | 28 capsule [PoM] £22.08 DT = £2.60
Venlafaxine (as Venlafaxine hydrochloride) 150 mg Efexor XL 150mg capsules | 28 capsule [PoM] £36.81 DT = £3.90
Venlafaxine (as Venlafaxine hydrochloride) 225 mg Efexor XL 225mg capsules | 28 capsule [PoM] £47.11 DT = £47.11
▸ Majoven XL (Bristol Laboratories Ltd)
Venlafaxine (as Venlafaxine hydrochloride) 37.5 mg Majoven XL 37.5mg capsules | 28 capsule [PoM] £5.25 DT = £5.25
Venlafaxine (as Venlafaxine hydrochloride) 75 mg Majoven XL 75mg capsules | 28 capsule [PoM] £22.08 DT = £2.60
Venlafaxine (as Venlafaxine hydrochloride) 150 mg Majoven XL 150mg capsules | 28 capsule [PoM] £36.81 DT = £3.90
▸ Politid XL (Accord Healthcare Ltd)
Venlafaxine (as Venlafaxine hydrochloride) 75 mg Politid XL 75mg capsules | 28 capsule [PoM] £23.41 DT = £2.60
Venlafaxine (as Venlafaxine hydrochloride) 150 mg Politid XL 150mg capsules | 28 capsule [PoM] £39.03 DT = £3.90
▸ Venaxx XL (Advanz Pharma)
Venlafaxine (as Venlafaxine hydrochloride) 75 mg Venaxx XL 75mg capsules | 28 capsule [PoM] £10.40 DT = £2.60
Venlafaxine (as Venlafaxine hydrochloride) 150 mg Venaxx XL 150mg capsules | 28 capsule [PoM] £17.40 DT = £3.90
▸ Vencarm XL (Aspire Pharma Ltd)
Venlafaxine (as Venlafaxine hydrochloride) 37.5 mg Vencarm XL 37.5mg capsules | 28 capsule [PoM] £3.30 DT = £5.25
Venlafaxine (as Venlafaxine hydrochloride) 75 mg Vencarm XL 75mg capsules | 28 capsule [PoM] £2.59 DT = £2.60
Venlafaxine (as Venlafaxine hydrochloride) 150 mg Vencarm XL 150mg capsules | 28 capsule [PoM] £3.89 DT = £3.90
Venlafaxine (as Venlafaxine hydrochloride) 225 mg Vencarm XL 225mg capsules | 28 capsule [PoM] £9.90 DT = £47.11
▸ Venablue XL (Zentiva)
Venlafaxine (as Venlafaxine hydrochloride) 37.5 mg Venablue XL 37.5mg capsules | 28 capsule [PoM] £5.25 DT = £5.25
Venlafaxine (as Venlafaxine hydrochloride) 75 mg Venablue XL 75mg capsules | 28 capsule [PoM] £6.95 DT = £2.60
Venlafaxine (as Venlafaxine hydrochloride) 150 mg Venablue XL 150mg capsules | 28 capsule [PoM] £9.95 DT = £3.90
▸ Venlasov XL (Sovereign Medical Ltd)
Venlafaxine (as Venlafaxine hydrochloride) 75 mg Venlasov XL 75mg capsules | 28 capsule [PoM] £2.98 DT = £2.60
Venlafaxine (as Venlafaxine hydrochloride) 150 mg Venlasov XL 150mg capsules | 28 capsule [PoM] £3.97 DT = £3.90
▸ Vensir XL (Morningside Healthcare Ltd)
Venlafaxine (as Venlafaxine hydrochloride) 75 mg Vensir XL 75mg capsules | 28 capsule [PoM] £2.60 DT = £2.60
Venlafaxine (as Venlafaxine hydrochloride) 150 mg Vensir XL 150mg capsules | 28 capsule [PoM] £3.90 DT = £3.90
Venlafaxine (as Venlafaxine hydrochloride) 225 mg Vensir XL 225mg capsules | 28 capsule [PoM] £21.90 DT = £47.11
▸ Venzip XL (Milpharm Ltd)
Venlafaxine (as Venlafaxine hydrochloride) 75 mg Venzip XL 75mg capsules | 28 capsule [PoM] £22.08 DT = £2.60
Venlafaxine (as Venlafaxine hydrochloride) 150 mg Venzip XL 150mg capsules | 28 capsule [PoM] £36.81 DT = £3.90

4

Nervous system

4

Nervous system

Trazodone hydrochloride

21-Oct-2020

- **INDICATIONS AND DOSE**

Depressive illness (particularly where sedation is required)

▶ BY MOUTH

▶ Adult: Initially 150 mg daily in divided doses, dose to be taken after food, alternatively initially 150 mg once daily, dose to be taken at bedtime, increased if necessary to 300 mg daily; increased if necessary to 600 mg daily in divided doses, higher dose for use in hospital patients only

▶ Elderly: Initially 100 mg daily in divided doses, dose to be taken after food, alternatively initially 100 mg once daily, dose to be taken at bedtime, increased if necessary to 300 mg daily; increased if necessary to 600 mg daily in divided doses, higher dose for use in hospital patients only

Anxiety

▶ BY MOUTH

▶ Adult: 75 mg daily, increased if necessary to 300 mg daily

- **CONTRA-INDICATIONS** During the manic phase of bipolar disorder · immediate recovery period after myocardial infarction

- **CAUTIONS** Arrhythmias · cardiovascular disease · chronic constipation · epilepsy · history of bipolar disorder · history of psychosis · hyperthyroidism (risk of arrhythmias) · increased intra-ocular pressure · patients with a significant risk of suicide · prostatic hypertrophy · susceptibility to angle-closure glaucoma · urinary retention

CAUTIONS, FURTHER INFORMATION Manufacturer advises treatment should be stopped if the patient enters a manic phase.

Elderly patients are particularly susceptible to many of the side-effects of tricyclic antidepressants; manufacturer advises low initial doses should be used, with close monitoring, particularly for psychiatric and cardiac side-effects.

- **INTERACTIONS** → Appendix 1: trazodone

- **SIDE-EFFECTS** Aggression · agranulocytosis · alertness decreased · anaemia · anxiety · aphasia · appetite abnormal · arrhythmias · arthralgia · asthenia · blood disorder · chest pain · confusion · constipation · delirium · delusions · diarrhoea · dizziness · drowsiness · dry mouth · dyspnoea · eosinophilia · fever · gastroenteritis · gastrointestinal discomfort · hallucination · headache · hepatic disorders · hyperhidrosis · hypersalivation · hypertension · hyponatraemia · influenza like illness · jaundice (discontinue) · leucopenia · libido decreased · mania · memory loss · movement disorders · myalgia · nasal congestion · nausea · neuroleptic malignant syndrome · oedema · pain · palpitations · paraesthesia · paralytic ileus · postural hypotension · priapism (discontinue) · QT interval prolongation · seizure · serotonin syndrome · SIADH · skin reactions · sleep disorders · suicidal behaviours · syncope · taste altered · thrombocytopenia · tremor · urinary disorder · vertigo · vision blurred · vomiting · weight decreased · withdrawal syndrome

SIDE-EFFECTS, FURTHER INFORMATION The risk of side-effects is reduced by titrating slowly to the minimum effective dose (every 2–3 days). Consider using a lower starting dose in elderly patients.

Overdose The tricyclic-related antidepressant drugs may be associated with a lower risk of cardiotoxicity in overdosage.

Tricyclic and related antidepressants cause dry mouth, coma of varying degree, hypotension, hypothermia, hyperreflexia, extensor plantar responses, convulsions, respiratory failure, cardiac conduction defects, and arrhythmias. Dilated pupils and urinary retention also occur. For details on the management of poisoning see Tricyclic and related antidepressants under Emergency treatment of poisoning p. 1413.

- **PREGNANCY** Avoid during first trimester—limited information available. Monitor infant for signs of withdrawal if used until delivery.

- **BREAST FEEDING** The amount secreted into breast milk is too small to be harmful.

- **HEPATIC IMPAIRMENT** Manufacturer advises caution, particularly in severe impairment (increased risk of side-effects).

- **RENAL IMPAIRMENT** Use with caution in severe impairment.

- **TREATMENT CESSATION** Withdrawal effects may occur within 5 days of stopping treatment with antidepressant drugs; they are usually mild and self-limiting, but in some cases may be severe. The risk of withdrawal symptoms is increased if the antidepressant is stopped suddenly after regular administration for 8 weeks or more. The dose should preferably be reduced gradually over about 4 weeks, or longer if withdrawal symptoms emerge (6 months in patients who have been on long-term maintenance treatment). If possible tricyclic and related antidepressants should be withdrawn slowly.

- **PRESCRIBING AND DISPENSING INFORMATION** Limited quantities of tricyclic antidepressants should be prescribed at any one time because their cardiovascular and epileptogenic effects are dangerous in overdosage.

- **PATIENT AND CARER ADVICE**

Driving and skilled tasks Drowsiness may affect the performance of skilled tasks (e.g. driving). Effects of alcohol enhanced.

- **MEDICINAL FORMS** There can be variation in the licensing of different medicines containing the same drug. Forms available from special-order manufacturers include: oral suspension, oral solution

Oral solution

CAUTIONARY AND ADVISORY LABELS 2, 21

▶ Trazodone hydrochloride (Non-proprietary)

Trazodone hydrochloride **10 mg per 1 ml** Trazodone 50mg/5ml oral solution sugar free sugar-free | 120 ml PoM £180.00 DT = £24.40

Trazodone hydrochloride **20 mg per 1 ml** Trazodone 100mg/5ml oral solution sugar free sugar-free | 120 ml PoM £232.50 DT = £232.50

Tablet

CAUTIONARY AND ADVISORY LABELS 2, 21

▶ Trazodone hydrochloride (Non-proprietary)

Trazodone hydrochloride **50 mg** Trazodone 50mg tablets | 84 tablet PoM £20.00

Trazodone hydrochloride **100 mg** Trazodone 100mg tablets | 56 tablet PoM £25.00

Trazodone hydrochloride **150 mg** Trazodone 150mg tablets | 28 tablet PoM £34.00 DT = £2.90

▶ Molipaxin (Zentiva)

Trazodone hydrochloride **150 mg** Molipaxin 150mg tablets | 28 tablet PoM £16.08 DT = £2.90

Capsule

CAUTIONARY AND ADVISORY LABELS 2, 21

▶ Trazodone hydrochloride (Non-proprietary)

Trazodone hydrochloride **50 mg** Trazodone 50mg capsules | 84 capsule PoM £35.00 DT = £3.57

Trazodone hydrochloride **100 mg** Trazodone 100mg capsules | 56 capsule PoM £41.00 DT = £3.74

▶ Molipaxin (Zentiva)

Trazodone hydrochloride **50 mg** Molipaxin 50mg capsules | 84 capsule PoM £23.92 DT = £3.57

Trazodone hydrochloride 100 mg Molipaxin 100mg capsules |
56 capsule PoM £28.14 DT = £3.74

ANTIDEPRESSANTS > TETRACYCLIC ANTIDEPRESSANTS

Mianserin hydrochloride   21-Oct-2020

● **INDICATIONS AND DOSE**

Depressive illness (particularly where sedation is required)

▸ BY MOUTH

▸ Adult: Initially 30–40 mg daily in divided doses, alternatively initially 30–40 mg once daily, dose to be taken at bedtime, increase dose gradually as necessary; usual dose 30–90 mg

▸ Elderly: Initially 30 mg daily in divided doses, alternatively initially 30 mg once daily, dose to be taken at bedtime, increase dose gradually as necessary; usual dose 30–90 mg

● CONTRA-INDICATIONS Acute porphyrias p. 1107 · during the manic phase of bipolar disorder

● CAUTIONS Arrhythmias · cardiovascular disease · diabetes · elderly · epilepsy · heart block · history of bipolar disorder · history of psychosis · immediate recovery period after myocardial infarction · increased intra-ocular pressure · patients with a significant risk of suicide · phaeochromocytoma (risk of arrhythmias) · prostatic hypertrophy · susceptibility to angle-closure glaucoma

CAUTIONS, FURTHER INFORMATION Manufacturer advises treatment should be stopped if the patient enters a manic phase.

● INTERACTIONS → Appendix 1: mianserin

● SIDE-EFFECTS Agranulocytosis · arthritis · bone marrow disorders · breast abnormalities · dizziness · granulocytopenia · gynaecomastia · hepatic disorders · hyperhidrosis · hyponatraemia · joint disorders · lactation in absence of pregnancy · leucopenia · mood altered · neuromuscular irritability · oedema · paranoid delusions · postural hypotension · psychosis · rash · seizure · sexual dysfunction · suicidal behaviours · tremor · withdrawal syndrome

SIDE-EFFECTS, FURTHER INFORMATION The risk of side-effects is reduced by titrating slowly to the minimum effective dose (every 2–3 days). Consider using a lower starting dose in elderly patients.

Overdose The tricyclic-related antidepressant drugs may be associated with a lower risk of cardiotoxicity in overdosage.

Tricyclic and related antidepressants cause dry mouth, coma of varying degree, hypotension, hypothermia, hyperreflexia, extensor plantar responses, convulsions, respiratory failure, cardiac conduction defects, and arrhythmias. Dilated pupils and urinary retention also occur. For details on the management of poisoning see Tricyclic and related antidepressants under Emergency treatment of poisoning p. 1413.

● PREGNANCY Avoid.

● BREAST FEEDING The amount secreted into breast milk is too small to be harmful.

● HEPATIC IMPAIRMENT Manufacturer advises caution; avoid in severe impairment.

● RENAL IMPAIRMENT

Dose adjustments Caution in renal impairment.

● MONITORING REQUIREMENTS A full **blood count** is recommended every 4 weeks during the first 3 months of treatment; clinical monitoring should continue subsequently and treatment should be stopped and a full

blood count obtained if *fever, sore throat, stomatitis,* or other signs of infection develop.

● TREATMENT CESSATION Withdrawal effects may occur within 5 days of stopping treatment with antidepressant drugs; they are usually mild and self-limiting, but in some cases may be severe. The risk of withdrawal symptoms is increased if the antidepressant is stopped suddenly after regular administration for 8 weeks or more. The dose should preferably be reduced gradually over about 4 weeks, or longer if withdrawal symptoms emerge (6 months in patients who have been on long-term maintenance treatment). If possible tricyclic and related antidepressants should be withdrawn slowly.

● PRESCRIBING AND DISPENSING INFORMATION Limited quantities of tricyclic antidepressants should be prescribed at any one time because their cardiovascular and epileptogenic effects are dangerous in overdosage.

● PATIENT AND CARER ADVICE
Driving and skilled tasks Drowsiness may affect the performance of skilled tasks (e.g. driving). Effects of alcohol enhanced.

● MEDICINAL FORMS There can be variation in the licensing of different medicines containing the same drug. Forms available from special-order manufacturers include: oral suspension, oral solution

Tablet
CAUTIONARY AND ADVISORY LABELS 2, 25
▸ Mianserin hydrochloride (Non-proprietary)
   Mianserin hydrochloride 10 mg Mianserin 10mg tablets |
   28 tablet PoM £14.10 DT = £14.10
   Mianserin hydrochloride 30 mg Mianserin 30mg tablets |
   28 tablet PoM £34.44 DT = £34.44

Mirtazapine   21-Oct-2020

● DRUG ACTION Mirtazapine is a presynaptic alpha$_2$-adrenoreceptor antagonist which increases central noradrenergic and serotonergic neurotransmission.

● **INDICATIONS AND DOSE**

Major depression
▸ BY MOUTH
▸ Adult: Initially 15–30 mg daily for 2–4 weeks, dose to be taken at bedtime, then adjusted according to response to up to 45 mg once daily, alternatively up to 45 mg daily in 2 divided doses

● CAUTIONS Cardiac disorders · diabetes mellitus · elderly · history of mania (discontinue if patient entering manic phase) · history of seizures · history of urinary retention · hypotension · psychoses (may aggravate psychotic symptoms) · susceptibility to angle-closure glaucoma

● INTERACTIONS → Appendix 1: mirtazapine

● SIDE-EFFECTS
▸ **Common or very common** Anxiety · appetite increased · arthralgia · back pain · confusion · constipation · diarrhoea · dizziness · drowsiness · dry mouth · fatigue · headache (on discontinuation) · myalgia · nausea · oedema · postural hypotension · sleep disorders · tremor · vomiting · weight increased
▸ **Uncommon** Hallucination · mania · movement disorders · oral disorders · syncope
▸ **Rare or very rare** Aggression · pancreatitis
▸ **Frequency not known** Agranulocytosis · arrhythmias · bone marrow disorders · dysarthria · eosinophilia · granulocytopenia · hyponatraemia · jaundice (discontinue) · QT interval prolongation · rhabdomyolysis · seizure · serotonin syndrome · severe cutaneous adverse reactions (SCARs) · SIADH · skin reactions · sudden death · suicidal behaviours · thrombocytopenia · urinary retention · withdrawal syndrome

4

Nervous system

- PREGNANCY Use with caution—limited experience; monitor neonate for withdrawal effects.
- BREAST FEEDING Present in milk; use only if potential benefit outweighs risk.
- HEPATIC IMPAIRMENT Manufacturer advises caution (risk of increased plasma concentration, no information available in severe impairment).
- RENAL IMPAIRMENT Clearance reduced by 30% if eGFR less than 40 mL/minute/1.73 m^2; clearance reduced by 50% if eGFR less than 10 mL/minute/1.73 m^2.
- TREATMENT CESSATION Nausea, vomiting, dizziness, agitation, anxiety, and headache are most common features of withdrawal if treatment stopped abruptly or if dose reduced markedly; dose should be reduced over several weeks.
- DIRECTIONS FOR ADMINISTRATION Orodispersible tablet should be placed on the tongue, allowed to disperse and swallowed.
- PATIENT AND CARER ADVICE Counselling on administration of orodispersible tablet advised. Blood Disorders Patients should be advised to report any fever, sore throat, stomatitis or other signs of infection during treatment. Blood count should be performed and the drug stopped immediately if blood dyscrasia suspected.

- MEDICINAL FORMS There can be variation in the licensing of different medicines containing the same drug. Forms available from special-order manufacturers include: capsule, oral suspension, oral solution

Tablet
CAUTIONARY AND ADVISORY LABELS 2, 25
▸ Mirtazapine (Non-proprietary)
  Mirtazapine 15 mg Mirtazapine 15mg tablets | 28 tablet [PoM]
  £4.60 DT = £2.74
  Mirtazapine 30 mg Mirtazapine 30mg tablets | 28 tablet [PoM]
  £4.50 DT = £2.83
  Mirtazapine 45 mg Mirtazapine 45mg tablets | 28 tablet [PoM]
  £6.00 DT = £3.09

Oral solution
CAUTIONARY AND ADVISORY LABELS 2
▸ Mirtazapine (Non-proprietary)
  Mirtazapine 15 mg per 1 ml Mirtazapine 15mg/ml oral solution
  sugar free sugar-free | 66 ml [PoM] £80.55 DT = £68.98

Orodispersible tablet
CAUTIONARY AND ADVISORY LABELS 2
EXCIPIENTS: May contain Aspartame
▸ Mirtazapine (Non-proprietary)
  Mirtazapine 15 mg Mirtazapine 15mg orodispersible tablets |
  30 tablet [PoM] £3.95 DT = £2.16
  Mirtazapine 30 mg Mirtazapine 30mg orodispersible tablets |
  30 tablet [PoM] £19.19 DT = £2.42
  Mirtazapine 45 mg Mirtazapine 45mg orodispersible tablets |
  30 tablet [PoM] £4.95 DT = £2.62

ANTIDEPRESSANTS ❯ TRICYCLIC ANTIDEPRESSANTS

| Amitriptyline hydrochloride
20-Oct-2020

● **INDICATIONS AND DOSE**

Abdominal pain or discomfort (in patients who have not responded to laxatives, loperamide, or antispasmodics)
▸ BY MOUTH
▸ Adult: Initially 5–10 mg daily, to be taken at night; increased in steps of 10 mg at least every 2 weeks as required; maximum 30 mg per day

Major depressive disorder [not recommended—increased risk of fatality in overdose]
▸ BY MOUTH
▸ Adult: Initially 50 mg daily in 2 divided doses, then increased in steps of 25 mg once daily on alternate days if required, maximum 150 mg daily in 2 divided doses

▸ Elderly: Initially 10–25 mg daily, increased if necessary up to 100–150 mg daily in 2 divided doses, dose increases dependent on individual patient response and tolerability—doses above 100 mg should be used with caution

Major depressive disorder in patients with cardiovascular disease [not recommended—increased risk of fatality in overdose]
▸ BY MOUTH
▸ Adult: Initially 10–25 mg daily, increased if necessary up to 100–150 mg daily in 2 divided doses, dose increases dependent on individual patient response and tolerability—doses above 100 mg should be used with caution

Neuropathic pain | Migraine prophylaxis | Chronic tension-type headache prophylaxis
▸ BY MOUTH
▸ Adult: Initially 10–25 mg daily, dose to be taken in the evening, then increased, if tolerated, in steps of 10–25 mg every 3–7 days in 1–2 divided doses; usual dose 25–75 mg daily, dose to be taken in the evening, doses above 100 mg should be used with caution (doses above 75 mg should be used with caution in the elderly and in patients with cardiovascular disease); maximum per dose 75 mg

Emotional lability in multiple sclerosis
▸ BY MOUTH
▸ Adult: Initially 10–25 mg daily; increased, if tolerated, in steps of 10–25 mg every 1–7 days; maximum 75 mg per day

- UNLICENSED USE Not licensed for use in abdominal pain or discomfort in patients who have not responded to laxatives, loperamide, or antispasmodics. [EvGr] Amitriptyline hydrochloride is used for emotional lability in multiple sclerosis, ⟨Ε⟩ but is not licensed for this indication.
- CONTRA-INDICATIONS Arrhythmias · during manic phase of bipolar disorder · heart block · immediate recovery period after myocardial infarction
- CAUTIONS Cardiovascular disease · chronic constipation · diabetes · epilepsy · history of bipolar disorder · history of psychosis · hyperthyroidism (risk of arrhythmias) · increased intra-ocular pressure · patients with a significant risk of suicide · phaeochromocytoma (risk of arrhythmias) · prostatic hypertrophy · pyloric stenosis · susceptibility to angle-closure glaucoma · urinary retention
  CAUTIONS, FURTHER INFORMATION [EvGr] Treatment should be stopped if the patient enters a manic phase. ⟨Μ⟩
    Elderly patients are particularly susceptible to many of the side-effects of tricyclic antidepressants; [EvGr] low initial doses should be used, with close monitoring, particularly for psychiatric and cardiac side-effects. ⟨Μ⟩
- INTERACTIONS → Appendix 1: tricyclic antidepressants
- SIDE-EFFECTS
▸ Common or very common Anticholinergic syndrome · drowsiness · QT interval prolongation
▸ Frequency not known Agranulocytosis · alopecia · anxiety · appetite abnormal · arrhythmias · asthenia · bone marrow depression · breast enlargement · cardiac conduction disorders · coma · concentration impaired · confusion · constipation · delirium · delusions · diarrhoea · dizziness · dry mouth · dysarthria · eosinophilia · epigastric distress · face oedema · galactorrhoea · gynaecomastia · hallucination · headache · hepatic disorders · hyperhidrosis · hyperpyrexia · hypertension · hyponatraemia · hypotension · leucopenia · mood altered · movement disorders · mydriasis · myocardial infarction · nausea · neuroleptic malignant syndrome · oral disorders · palpitations · paralytic ileus · peripheral neuropathy · photosensitivity reaction · seizure · sensation abnormal ·

4

sexual dysfunction · SIADH · skin reactions · sleep disorders · stroke · sudden cardiac death · suicidal behaviours · syncope · taste altered · testicular swelling · thrombocytopenia · tinnitus · tremor · urinary disorders · urinary tract dilation · vision disorders · vomiting · weight changes · withdrawal syndrome

SIDE-EFFECTS, FURTHER INFORMATION The risk of side-effects is reduced by titrating slowly to the minimum effective dose (every 2–3 days). Consider using a lower starting dose in elderly patients.

Overdose Overdosage with amitriptyline is associated with a relatively high rate of fatality. Symptoms of overdosage may include dry mouth, coma of varying degree, hypotension, hypothermia, hyperreflexia, extensor plantar responses, convulsions, respiratory failure, cardiac conduction defects, and arrhythmias. Dilated pupils and urinary retention also occur. For details on the management of poisoning, see Tricyclic and related antidepressants, under Emergency treatment of poisoning p. 1413.

● PREGNANCY Use only if potential benefit outweighs risk.

● BREAST FEEDING The amount secreted into breast milk is too small to be harmful.

● HEPATIC IMPAIRMENT Manufacturer advises use with caution in mild-to-moderate impairment; avoid in severe impairment.

● TREATMENT CESSATION Withdrawal effects may occur within 5 days of stopping treatment with antidepressant drugs; they are usually mild and self-limiting, but in some cases may be severe. The risk of withdrawal symptoms is increased if the antidepressant is stopped suddenly after regular administration for 8 weeks or more. The dose should preferably be reduced gradually over about 4 weeks, or longer if withdrawal symptoms emerge (6 months in patients who have been on long-term maintenance treatment). If possible tricyclic and related antidepressants should be withdrawn slowly.

● PRESCRIBING AND DISPENSING INFORMATION Limited quantities of tricyclic antidepressants should be prescribed at any one time because their cardiovascular and epileptogenic effects are dangerous in overdosage.

● PATIENT AND CARER ADVICE

Driving and skilled tasks Drowsiness may affect the performance of skilled tasks (e.g. driving). Effects of alcohol enhanced.

● LESS SUITABLE FOR PRESCRIBING Amitriptyline hydrochloride is less suitable for prescribing, see Tricyclic and related antidepressant drugs in Antidepressant drugs p. 378.

● MEDICINAL FORMS There can be variation in the licensing of different medicines containing the same drug. Forms available from special-order manufacturers include: oral suspension, oral solution

Oral solution
CAUTIONARY AND ADVISORY LABELS 2
▸ Amitriptyline hydrochloride (Non-proprietary)
  Amitriptyline hydrochloride 2 mg per 1 ml Amitriptyline 10mg/5ml oral solution sugar free sugar-free | 150 ml PoM £136.47 DT = £136.47
  Amitriptyline hydrochloride 5 mg per 1 ml Amitriptyline 25mg/5ml oral solution sugar free sugar-free | 150 ml PoM £18.00 DT = £18.00
  Amitriptyline hydrochloride 10 mg per 1 ml Amitriptyline 50mg/5ml oral solution sugar free sugar-free | 150 ml PoM £24.00 DT = £19.20

Tablet
CAUTIONARY AND ADVISORY LABELS 2
▸ Amitriptyline hydrochloride (Non-proprietary)
  Amitriptyline hydrochloride 10 mg Amitriptyline 10mg tablets | 28 tablet PoM £1.50 DT = £1.02
  Amitriptyline hydrochloride 25 mg Amitriptyline 25mg tablets | 28 tablet PoM £1.75 DT = £0.94

  Amitriptyline hydrochloride 50 mg Amitriptyline 50mg tablets | 28 tablet PoM £5.99 DT = £1.72

Clomipramine hydrochloride
24-Nov-2020

● **INDICATIONS AND DOSE**

Depressive illness
▸ BY MOUTH
▸ Adult: Initially 10 mg daily, then increased if necessary to 30–150 mg daily in divided doses, dose to be increased gradually, alternatively increased if necessary to 30–150 mg once daily, dose to be taken at bedtime; maximum 250 mg per day
▸ Elderly: Initially 10 mg daily, then increased to 30–75 mg daily, dose to be increased carefully over approximately 10 days

Phobic and obsessional states
▸ BY MOUTH
▸ Adult: Initially 25 mg daily, then increased to 100–150 mg daily, dose to be increased gradually over 2 weeks; maximum 250 mg per day
▸ Elderly: Initially 10 mg daily, then increased to 100–150 mg daily, dose to be increased gradually over 2 weeks; maximum 250 mg per day

Adjunctive treatment of cataplexy associated with narcolepsy
▸ BY MOUTH
▸ Adult: Initially 10 mg daily, dose to be gradually increased until satisfactory response; increased if necessary to 10–75 mg daily

● CONTRA-INDICATIONS Acute porphyrias p. 1107 · arrhythmias · during the manic phase of bipolar disorder · heart block · immediate recovery period after myocardial infarction

● CAUTIONS Cardiovascular disease · chronic constipation · epilepsy · history of bipolar disorder · history of psychosis · hyperthyroidism (risk of arrhythmias) · increased intra-ocular pressure · patients with a significant risk of suicide · phaeochromocytoma (risk of arrhythmias) · prostatic hypertrophy · risk factors for QT interval prolongation—correct hypokalaemia before initiating treatment · susceptibility to angle-closure glaucoma · urinary retention

CAUTIONS, FURTHER INFORMATION EvGr Treatment should be stopped or dose reduced if the patient enters a manic phase. ⓜ
  Elderly patients are particularly susceptible to many of the side-effects of tricyclic antidepressants; EvGr low initial doses should be used, with close monitoring, particularly for psychiatric and cardiac side-effects. ⓜ

● INTERACTIONS → Appendix 1: tricyclic antidepressants

● SIDE-EFFECTS
▸ **Common or very common** Aggression · anxiety · arrhythmias · breast enlargement · concentration impaired · confusion · constipation · delirium · depersonalisation · depression exacerbated · diarrhoea · dizziness · drowsiness · dry mouth · fatigue · galactorrhoea · gastrointestinal disorder · hallucination · headache · hot flush · hyperhidrosis · hypotension · memory loss · mood altered · movement disorders · muscle tone increased · muscle weakness · mydriasis · nausea · palpitations · paraesthesia · photosensitivity reaction · sexual dysfunction · skin reactions · sleep disorders · speech disorder · taste altered · tinnitus · tremor · urinary disorders · vision disorders · vomiting · weight increased · yawning
▸ **Uncommon** Psychosis · seizure
▸ **Rare or very rare** Agranulocytosis · alopecia · cardiac conduction disorders · eosinophilia · glaucoma · hepatic disorders · hyperpyrexia · leucopenia · neuroleptic

malignant syndrome · oedema · QT interval prolongation · respiratory disorders · thrombocytopenia · vaginal haemorrhage
▸ **Frequency not known** Rhabdomyolysis · serotonin syndrome · suicidal behaviours · withdrawal syndrome
SIDE-EFFECTS, FURTHER INFORMATION The patient should be encouraged to persist with treatment as some tolerance to these side-effects seems to develop.

The risk of side-effects is reduced by titrating slowly to the minimum effective dose (every 2–3 days). Consider using a lower starting dose in elderly patients.

Overdose Tricyclic and related antidepressants cause dry mouth, coma of varying degree, hypotension, hypothermia, hyperreflexia, extensor plantar responses, convulsions, respiratory failure, cardiac conduction defects, and arrhythmias. Dilated pupils and urinary retention also occur. For details on the management of poisoning see Tricyclic and related antidepressants under Emergency treatment of poisoning p. 1413.

● PREGNANCY Neonatal withdrawal symptoms reported if used during third trimester.

● BREAST FEEDING The amount secreted into breast milk is too small to be harmful.

● HEPATIC IMPAIRMENT Manufacturer advises caution; avoid in severe impairment (risk of hypertensive crisis).

● MONITORING REQUIREMENTS Manufacturer advises monitor cardiac and hepatic function during long-term use.

● TREATMENT CESSATION Withdrawal effects may occur within 5 days of stopping treatment with antidepressant drugs; they are usually mild and self-limiting, but in some cases may be severe. The risk of withdrawal symptoms is increased if the antidepressant is stopped suddenly after regular administration for 8 weeks or more. The dose should preferably be reduced gradually over about 4 weeks, or longer if withdrawal symptoms emerge (6 months in patients who have been on long-term maintenance treatment). If possible tricyclic and related antidepressants should be withdrawn slowly.

● PRESCRIBING AND DISPENSING INFORMATION Limited quantities of tricyclic antidepressants should be prescribed at any one time because their cardiovascular and epileptogenic effects are dangerous in overdosage.

● PATIENT AND CARER ADVICE
Driving and skilled tasks Drowsiness may affect the performance of skilled tasks (e.g. driving).
Effects of alcohol enhanced.

● MEDICINAL FORMS There can be variation in the licensing of different medicines containing the same drug. Forms available from special-order manufacturers include: modified-release tablet, oral suspension, oral solution

Capsule
CAUTIONARY AND ADVISORY LABELS 2
▸ Clomipramine hydrochloride (Non-proprietary)
  Clomipramine hydrochloride 10 mg Clomipramine 10mg capsules | 28 capsule [PoM] £6.72 DT = £2.65
  Clomipramine hydrochloride 25 mg Clomipramine 25mg capsules | 28 capsule [PoM] £9.36 DT = £2.85
  Clomipramine hydrochloride 50 mg Clomipramine 50mg capsules | 28 capsule [PoM] £11.76 DT = £5.30

Dosulepin hydrochloride
03-Nov-2020
(Dothiepin hydrochloride)

● INDICATIONS AND DOSE
Depressive illness, particularly where sedation is required (not recommended—increased risk of fatality in overdose) (initiated by a specialist)
▸ BY MOUTH
▸ Adult: Initially 75 mg daily in divided doses, alternatively initially 75 mg once daily, dose to be taken at bedtime, increased if necessary to 150 mg daily, doses to be increased gradually; up to 225 mg daily in some circumstances (e.g. hospital use)
▸ Elderly: Initially 50–75 mg daily in divided doses, alternatively initially 50–75 mg once daily, dose to be taken at bedtime, increased if necessary to 75–150 mg daily, doses to be increased gradually; up to 225 mg daily in some circumstances (e.g. hospital use)

● CONTRA-INDICATIONS Acute porphyrias p. 1107 · arrhythmias · during the manic phase of bipolar disorder · heart block · immediate recovery period after myocardial infarction

● CAUTIONS Cardiovascular disease · chronic constipation · diabetes · epilepsy · history of bipolar disorder · history of psychosis · hyperthyroidism (risk of arrhythmias) · increased intra-ocular pressure · patients with a significant risk of suicide · phaeochromocytoma (risk of arrhythmias) · prostatic hypertrophy · susceptibility to angle-closure glaucoma · urinary retention
CAUTIONS, FURTHER INFORMATION [EvGr] Treatment should be stopped if the patient enters a manic phase. ◁Ⓜ▷

Elderly patients are particularly susceptible to many of the side-effects of tricyclic antidepressants; [EvGr] low initial doses should be used, with close monitoring, particularly for psychiatric and cardiac side-effects. ◁Ⓜ▷

● INTERACTIONS → Appendix 1: tricyclic antidepressants

● SIDE-EFFECTS Accommodation disorder · agranulocytosis · alveolitis · anticholinergic syndrome · appetite abnormal · arrhythmias · asthenia · bone marrow depression · cardiac conduction disorder · confusion · constipation · dizziness · drowsiness · dry mouth · endocrine disorder · eosinophilia · epigastric discomfort · galactorrhoea · gynaecomastia · hepatic disorders · hyperhidrosis · hypertension · hyponatraemia · hypotension · increased risk of fracture · leucopenia · mood altered · movement disorders · nausea · nervousness · paranoid delusions · photosensitivity reaction · psychosis · seizures · sexual dysfunction · SIADH · skin reactions · speech disorder · suicidal behaviours · testicular hypertrophy · thrombocytopenia · tremor · urinary hesitation · vomiting · weight changes · withdrawal syndrome
SIDE-EFFECTS, FURTHER INFORMATION The risk of side-effects are reduced by titrating slowly to the minimum effective dose (every 2–3 days). Consider using a lower starting dose in elderly patients.

Overdose Overdosage with dosulepin is associated with a relatively high rate of fatality.

Tricyclic and related antidepressants cause dry mouth, coma of varying degree, hypotension, hypothermia, hyperreflexia, extensor plantar responses, convulsions, respiratory failure, cardiac conduction defects, and arrhythmias. Dilated pupils and urinary retention also occur. For details on the management of poisoning see Tricyclic and related antidepressants under Emergency treatment of poisoning.

● PREGNANCY Use only if potential benefit outweighs risk.

● BREAST FEEDING The amount secreted into breast milk is too small to be harmful.

- HEPATIC IMPAIRMENT Manufacturer advises caution in mild to moderate impairment; avoid in severe impairment.
- TREATMENT CESSATION Withdrawal effects may occur within 5 days of stopping treatment with antidepressant drugs; they are usually mild and self-limiting, but in some cases may be severe. The risk of withdrawal symptoms is increased if the antidepressant is stopped suddenly after regular administration for 8 weeks or more. The dose should preferably be reduced gradually over about 4 weeks, or longer if withdrawal symptoms emerge. (6 months in patients who have been on long-term maintenance treatment). If possible tricyclic and related antidepressants should be withdrawn slowly.
- PRESCRIBING AND DISPENSING INFORMATION Limited quantities of tricyclic antidepressants should be prescribed at any one time because their cardiovascular and epileptogenic effects are dangerous in overdosage.

  A maximum prescription equivalent to 2 weeks' supply of 75 mg daily should be considered in patients with increased risk factors for suicide at initiation of treatment, during any dose adjustment, and until improvement occurs.
- PATIENT AND CARER ADVICE
  Driving and skilled tasks Drowsiness may affect the performance of skilled tasks (e.g. driving).
  Effects of alcohol enhanced.
- LESS SUITABLE FOR PRESCRIBING Dosulepin hydrochloride is less suitable for prescribing, see Tricyclic and related antidepressant drugs in Antidepressant drugs p. 378.

- MEDICINAL FORMS There can be variation in the licensing of different medicines containing the same drug. Forms available from special-order manufacturers include: oral suspension, oral solution

Tablet
CAUTIONARY AND ADVISORY LABELS 2
▸ Dosulepin hydrochloride (Non-proprietary)
  Dosulepin hydrochloride 75 mg Dosulepin 75mg tablets |
  28 tablet [PoM] £17.48 DT = £16.50
▸ Prothiaden (Teofarma)
  Dosulepin hydrochloride 75 mg Prothiaden 75mg tablets |
  28 tablet [PoM] £2.97 DT = £16.50

Capsule
CAUTIONARY AND ADVISORY LABELS 2
▸ Dosulepin hydrochloride (Non-proprietary)
  Dosulepin hydrochloride 25 mg Dosulepin 25mg capsules |
  28 capsule [PoM] £3.50 DT = £1.53
▸ Prothiaden (Teofarma)
  Dosulepin hydrochloride 25 mg Prothiaden 25mg capsules |
  28 capsule [PoM] £1.70 DT = £1.53

Doxepin
02-Sep-2020

- INDICATIONS AND DOSE
Depressive illness (particularly where sedation is required)
▸ BY MOUTH
▸ Adult: Initially 75 mg daily in divided doses, alternatively 75 mg once daily, adjusted according to response, dose to taken at bedtime; maintenance 25–300 mg daily, doses above 100 mg given in 3 divided doses
▸ Elderly: Start with lower doses and adjust according to response

- CONTRA-INDICATIONS Acute porphyrias p. 1107 · during manic phase of bipolar disorder
- CAUTIONS Arrhythmias · cardiovascular disease · chronic constipation · diabetes · epilepsy · heart block · history of bipolar disorder · history of psychosis · hyperthyroidism (risk of arrhythmias) · immediate recovery period after

myocardial infarction · increased intra-ocular pressure · patients with significant risk of suicide · phaeochromocytoma (risk of arrhythmias) · prostatic hypertrophy · susceptibility to angle-closure glaucoma · urinary retention
  CAUTIONS, FURTHER INFORMATION Treatment should be stopped if the patient enters a manic phase.
  ▸ Elderly Elderly patients are particularly susceptible to many of the side-effects of tricyclic antidepressants; low initial doses should be used, with close monitoring, particularly for psychiatric and cardiac side-effects.
- INTERACTIONS → Appendix 1: tricyclic antidepressants
- SIDE-EFFECTS Agitation · agranulocytosis · alopecia · anticholinergic syndrome · appetite decreased · asthenia · asthma exacerbated · bone marrow depression · breast enlargement · cardiovascular effects · chills · confusion · constipation · diarrhoea · dizziness · drowsiness · dry mouth · dyspepsia · eosinophilia · face oedema · flushing · galactorrhoea · gynaecomastia · haemolytic anaemia · hallucination · headache · hyperhidrosis · hyperpyrexia · increased risk of fracture · jaundice · leucopenia · mania · movement disorders · nausea · oral ulceration · paranoid delusions · photosensitivity reaction · postural hypotension · psychosis · seizure · sensation abnormal · sexual dysfunction · SIADH · skin reactions · sleep disorders · suicidal behaviours · tachycardia · taste altered · testicular swelling · thrombocytopenia · tinnitus · tremor · urinary retention · vision blurred · vomiting · weight increased
  SIDE-EFFECTS, FURTHER INFORMATION The risk of side-effects is reduced by titrating slowly to the minimum effective dose (every 2–3 days). Consider using a lower starting dose in elderly patients.

  Overdose Tricyclic and related antidepressants cause dry mouth, coma of varying degree, hypotension, hypothermia, hyperreflexia, extensor plantar responses, convulsions, respiratory failure, cardiac conduction defects, and arrhythmias. Dilated pupils and urinary retention also occur. For details on the management of poisoning see Tricyclic and related antidepressants under Emergency treatment of poisoning p. 1413.
- PREGNANCY Use with caution—limited information available.
- BREAST FEEDING The amount secreted into breast milk is too small to be harmful. Accumulation of metabolite may cause sedation and respiratory depression in neonate.
- HEPATIC IMPAIRMENT Manufacturer advises caution in mild to moderate impairment; avoid in severe impairment.
  Dose adjustments Manufacturer advises consider dose reduction in mild to moderate impairment.
- RENAL IMPAIRMENT Use with caution.
- TREATMENT CESSATION Withdrawal effects may occur within 5 days of stopping treatment with antidepressant drugs; they are usually mild and self-limiting, but in some cases may be severe. The risk of withdrawal symptoms is increased if the antidepressant is stopped suddenly after regular administration for 8 weeks or more. The dose should preferably be reduced gradually over about 4 weeks, or longer if withdrawal symptoms emerge (6 months in patients who have been on long-term maintenance treatment). If possible tricyclic and related antidepressants should be withdrawn slowly.
- PRESCRIBING AND DISPENSING INFORMATION Limited quantities of tricyclic antidepressants should be prescribed at any one time because their cardiovascular and epileptogenic effects are dangerous in overdosage.
- PATIENT AND CARER ADVICE
  Driving and skilled tasks Drowsiness may affect performance of skilled tasks (e.g. driving).
  Effects of alcohol enhanced.

• MEDICINAL FORMS There can be variation in the licensing of different medicines containing the same drug. Forms available from special-order manufacturers include: capsule, oral suspension, oral solution

Capsule

CAUTIONARY AND ADVISORY LABELS 2

▸ Doxepin (Non-proprietary)
   Doxepin (as Doxepin hydrochloride) 25 mg Doxepin 25mg capsules
   | 28 capsule [PoM] £97.00 DT = £97.00
   Doxepin (as Doxepin hydrochloride) 50 mg Doxepin 50mg capsules
   | 28 capsule [PoM] £154.00 DT = £154.00

Imipramine hydrochloride   04-Nov-2020

• INDICATIONS AND DOSE

Depressive illness

▸ BY MOUTH
▸ **Adult:** Initially up to 75 mg daily in divided doses, then increased to 150–200 mg daily, up to 150 mg may be given as a single dose at bedtime, dose to be increased gradually
▸ **Elderly:** Initially 10 mg daily, increased to 30–50 mg daily, dose to be increased gradually

Depressive illness in hospital patients

▸ BY MOUTH
▸ **Adult:** Initially up to 75 mg daily in divided doses, dose to be increased gradually, increased to up to 300 mg daily in divided doses

Nocturnal enuresis

▸ BY MOUTH
▸ **Child 6-7 years:** 25 mg once daily, to be taken at bedtime, initial period of treatment (including gradual withdrawal) 3 months—full physical examination before further course
▸ **Child 8-10 years:** 25–50 mg once daily, to be taken at bedtime, initial period of treatment (including gradual withdrawal) 3 months—full physical examination before further course
▸ **Child 11-17 years:** 50–75 mg once daily, to be taken at bedtime, initial period of treatment (including gradual withdrawal) 3 months—full physical examination before further course

• CONTRA-INDICATIONS Immediate recovery period after myocardial infarction · Acute porphyrias p. 1107 · arrhythmia · during the manic phase of bipolar disorder · heart block

• CAUTIONS Cardiovascular disease · chronic constipation · diabetes · epilepsy · history of bipolar disorder · history of psychosis · hyperthyroidism (risk of arrhythmias) · increased intra-ocular pressure · patients with a significant risk of suicide · phaeochromocytoma (risk of arrhythmias) · prostatic hypertrophy (in adults) · susceptibility to angle-closure glaucoma · urinary retention

   CAUTIONS, FURTHER INFORMATION [EvGr] Treatment should be stopped if the patient enters a manic phase. ⟨M⟩
   Elderly patients are particularly susceptible to many of the side-effects of tricyclic antidepressants; [EvGr] low initial doses should be used, with close monitoring, particularly for psychiatric and cardiac side-effects. ⟨M⟩

• INTERACTIONS → Appendix 1: tricyclic antidepressants

• SIDE-EFFECTS

▸ **Common or very common** Anxiety · appetite decreased · arrhythmias · asthenia · cardiac conduction disorders · confusion · delirium · depression · dizziness · drowsiness · epilepsy · hallucination · headache · hepatic disorders · hypotension · mood altered · nausea · palpitations · paraesthesia · sexual dysfunction · skin reactions · sleep disorder · tremor · vomiting · weight changes
▸ **Uncommon** Psychosis

▸ **Rare or very rare** Aggression · agranulocytosis · alopecia · bone marrow depression · enlarged mammary gland · eosinophilia · fever · galactorrhoea · gastrointestinal disorders · glaucoma · heart failure · leucopenia · movement disorders · mydriasis · oedema · oral disorders · peripheral vasospastic reaction · photosensitivity reaction · respiratory disorders · SIADH · speech disorder · thrombocytopenia
▸ **Frequency not known** Anticholinergic syndrome · cardiovascular effects · drug fever · hyponatraemia · increased risk of fracture · neurological effects · paranoid delusions exacerbated · psychiatric disorder · suicidal behaviours · tinnitus · urinary disorder · withdrawal syndrome

   SIDE-EFFECTS, FURTHER INFORMATION The risk of side-effects is reduced by titrating slowly to the minimum effective dose (every 2–3 days). Consider using a lower starting dose in elderly patients.

   Overdose Tricyclic and related antidepressants cause dry mouth, coma of varying degree, hypotension, hypothermia, hyperreflexia, extensor plantar responses, convulsions, respiratory failure, cardiac conduction defects, and arrhythmias. Dilated pupils and urinary retention also occur. For details on the management of poisoning see Tricyclic and related antidepressants under Emergency treatment of poisoning p. 1413.

• PREGNANCY Colic, tachycardia, dyspnoea, irritability, muscle spasms, respiratory depression and withdrawal symptoms reported in neonates when used in the third trimester.

• BREAST FEEDING The amount secreted into breast milk is too small to be harmful.

• HEPATIC IMPAIRMENT Manufacturer advises caution in mild to moderate impairment; avoid in severe impairment.

• RENAL IMPAIRMENT Use with caution in severe impairment.

• TREATMENT CESSATION Withdrawal effects may occur within 5 days of stopping treatment with antidepressant drugs; they are usually mild and self-limiting, but in some cases may be severe. The risk of withdrawal symptoms is increased if the antidepressant is stopped suddenly after regular administration for 8 weeks or more. The dose should preferably be reduced gradually over about 4 weeks, or longer if withdrawal symptoms emerge (6 months in patients who have been on long-term maintenance treatment). If possible tricyclic antidepressants should be withdrawn slowly.

• PRESCRIBING AND DISPENSING INFORMATION Limited quantities of tricyclic antidepressants should be prescribed at any one time because their cardiovascular and epileptogenic effects are dangerous in overdosage.

• PATIENT AND CARER ADVICE
   Medicines for Children leaflet: Imipramine for various conditions
   www.medicinesforchildren.org.uk/imipramine-various-conditions
   Driving and skilled tasks Drowsiness may affect the performance of skilled tasks (e.g. driving).
   Effects of alcohol enhanced.

• MEDICINAL FORMS There can be variation in the licensing of different medicines containing the same drug. Forms available from special-order manufacturers include: oral suspension, oral solution

Oral solution

CAUTIONARY AND ADVISORY LABELS 2

▸ Imipramine hydrochloride (Non-proprietary)
   Imipramine hydrochloride 5 mg per 1 ml Imipramine 25mg/5ml
   oral solution sugar free sugar-free | 150 ml [PoM] £49.09 DT = £49.09

Tablet

CAUTIONARY AND ADVISORY LABELS 2

▸ Imipramine hydrochloride (Non-proprietary)

Imipramine hydrochloride 10 mg Imipramine 10mg tablets |
28 tablet PoM £1.93 DT = £1.93

Imipramine hydrochloride 25 mg Imipramine 25mg tablets |
28 tablet PoM £9.99 DT = £6.63

Lofepramine
15-Nov-2020

● **INDICATIONS AND DOSE**

Depressive illness

▸ BY MOUTH

▸ Adult: 140–210 mg daily in divided doses

▸ Elderly: May respond to lower doses

● CONTRA-INDICATIONS Acute porphyrias p. 1107 ·
arrhythmias · during the manic phase of bipolar disorder ·
heart block · immediate recovery period after myocardial
infarction

● CAUTIONS Cardiovascular disease · chronic constipation ·
diabetes · epilepsy · history of bipolar disorder · history of
psychosis · hyperthyroidism (risk of arrhythmias) ·
increased intra-ocular pressure · patients with a significant
risk of suicide · phaeochromocytoma (risk of arrhythmias) ·
prostatic hypertrophy · susceptibility to angle-closure
glaucoma · urinary retention

CAUTIONS, FURTHER INFORMATION EvGr Treatment should
be stopped if the patient enters a manic phase. Ⓜ

Elderly patients are particularly susceptible to many of
the side-effects of tricyclic antidepressants; EvGr low
initial doses should be used, with close monitoring,
particularly for psychiatric and cardiac side-effects Ⓜ.

● INTERACTIONS → Appendix 1: tricyclic antidepressants

● SIDE-EFFECTS Accommodation disorder · agitation ·
agranulocytosis · arrhythmias · bone marrow disorders ·
cardiac conduction disorder · confusion · constipation ·
coordination abnormal · dizziness · drowsiness · dry mouth
· eosinophilia · face oedema · galactorrhoea · glaucoma ·
granulocytopenia · gynaecomastia · hallucination ·
headache · heart failure aggravated · hepatic disorders ·
hyperhidrosis (on discontinuation) · hyponatraemia ·
hypotension · increased risk of fracture · leucopenia ·
malaise · mood altered · mucositis · nausea · paraesthesia ·
paranoid delusions · photosensitivity reaction · psychosis ·
respiratory depression · seizure · sexual dysfunction ·
SIADH · skin haemorrhage · skin reactions · sleep disorder ·
suicidal behaviours · taste altered · testicular disorders ·
thrombocytopenia · tinnitus · tremor · urinary disorders ·
vomiting · withdrawal syndrome

SIDE-EFFECTS, FURTHER INFORMATION The risk of side-
effects is reduced by titrating slowly to the minimum
effective dose (every 2–3 days). Consider using a lower
starting dose in elderly patients.

Overdose Tricyclic and related antidepressants cause dry
mouth, coma of varying degree, hypotension,
hypothermia, hyperreflexia, extensor plantar responses,
convulsions, respiratory failure, cardiac conduction
defects, and arrhythmias. Dilated pupils and urinary
retention also occur. Lofepramine is associated with the
lowest risk of fatality in overdosage, in comparison with
other tricyclic antidepressant drugs. For details on the
management of poisoning see Tricyclic and related
antidepressants under Emergency treatment of poisoning
p. 1413.

● PREGNANCY Neonatal withdrawal symptoms and
respiratory depression reported if used during third
trimester.

● BREAST FEEDING The amount secreted into breast milk is
too small to be harmful.

● HEPATIC IMPAIRMENT Manufacturer advises caution in
mild to moderate impairment; avoid in severe impairment.

● RENAL IMPAIRMENT Avoid in severe impairment.

● TREATMENT CESSATION Withdrawal effects may occur
within 5 days of stopping treatment with antidepressant
drugs; they are usually mild and self-limiting, but in some
cases may be severe. The risk of withdrawal symptoms is
increased if the antidepressant is stopped suddenly after
regular administration for 8 weeks or more. The dose
should preferably be reduced gradually over about 4 weeks,
or longer if withdrawal symptoms emerge (6 months in
patients who have been on long-term maintenance
treatment). If possible tricyclic and related antidepressants
should be withdrawn slowly.

● PRESCRIBING AND DISPENSING INFORMATION Limited
quantities of tricyclic antidepressants should be prescribed
at any one time because their cardiovascular and
epileptogenic effects are dangerous in overdosage.

● PATIENT AND CARER ADVICE
Driving and skilled tasks Drowsiness may affect the
performance of skilled tasks (e.g. driving). Effects of
alcohol enhanced.

● MEDICINAL FORMS There can be variation in the licensing of
different medicines containing the same drug. Forms available
from special-order manufacturers include: oral suspension, oral
solution

Oral suspension

CAUTIONARY AND ADVISORY LABELS 2

▸ Lofepramine (Non-proprietary)

**Lofepramine (as Lofepramine hydrochloride) 14 mg per
1 ml** Lofepramine 70mg/5ml oral suspension sugar free sugar-free |
150 ml PoM £33.87 DT = £33.87

Tablet

CAUTIONARY AND ADVISORY LABELS 2

▸ Lofepramine (Non-proprietary)

Lofepramine (as Lofepramine hydrochloride) 70 mg Lofepramine
70mg tablets | 56 tablet PoM £29.00 DT = £19.71

Nortriptyline
07-Nov-2020

● **INDICATIONS AND DOSE**

Depressive illness

▸ BY MOUTH

▸ Adult: To be initiated at a low dose, then increased if
necessary to 75–100 mg daily in divided doses,
alternatively increased if necessary to 75–100 mg once
daily; maximum 150 mg per day

▸ Elderly: To be initiated at a low dose, then increased if
necessary to 30–50 mg daily in divided doses

Neuropathic pain

▸ BY MOUTH

▸ Adult: Initially 10 mg once daily, to be taken at night,
increased if necessary to 75 mg daily, dose to be
increased gradually; higher doses to be given under
specialist supervision

● UNLICENSED USE Not licensed for use in neuropathic pain.

● CONTRA-INDICATIONS Arrhythmias · during the manic
phase of bipolar disorder · heart block · immediate recovery
period after myocardial infarction

● CAUTIONS Cardiovascular disease · chronic constipation ·
diabetes · epilepsy · history of bipolar disorder · history of
psychosis · hyperthyroidism (risk of arrhythmias) ·
increased intra-ocular pressure · patients with a significant
risk of suicide · phaeochromocytoma (risk of arrhythmias) ·
prostatic hypertrophy · susceptibility to angle-closure
glaucoma · urinary retention

CAUTIONS, FURTHER INFORMATION EvGr Treatment should
be stopped if the patient enters a manic phase. Ⓜ

4

Nervous system

Elderly patients are particularly susceptible to many of the side-effects of tricyclic antidepressants; EvGr low initial doses should be used, with close monitoring, particularly for psychiatric and cardiac side-effects. ⟨M⟩

● INTERACTIONS → Appendix 1: tricyclic antidepressants

● SIDE-EFFECTS Agranulocytosis · alopecia · anxiety · appetite decreased · arrhythmias · asthenia · atrioventricular block · bone marrow disorders · breast enlargement · confusion · constipation · delusions · diarrhoea · dizziness · drowsiness · drug cross-reactivity · drug fever · dry mouth · eosinophilia · fever · flushing · galactorrhoea · gastrointestinal discomfort · gynaecomastia · hallucination · headache · hepatic disorders · hyperhidrosis · hypertension · hypomania · hypotension · increased risk of fracture · increased risk of infection · malaise · movement disorders · mydriasis · myocardial infarction · nausea · oedema · oral disorders · palpitations · paralytic ileus · peripheral neuropathy · photosensitivity reaction · psychosis exacerbated · seizure · sensation abnormal · sexual dysfunction · SIADH · skin reactions · sleep disorders · stroke · suicidal behaviours · taste altered · testicular swelling · thrombocytopenia · tinnitus · tremor · urinary disorders · urinary tract dilation · vision disorders · vomiting · weight changes

SIDE-EFFECTS, FURTHER INFORMATION The risk of side-effects is reduced by titrating slowly to the minimum effective dose (every 2–3 days). Consider using a lower starting dose in elderly patients.

Overdose Tricyclic and related antidepressants cause dry mouth, coma of varying degree, hypotension, hypothermia, hyperreflexia, extensor plantar responses, convulsions, respiratory failure, cardiac conduction defects, and arrhythmias. Dilated pupils and urinary retention also occur. For details on the management of poisoning see Tricyclic and related antidepressants under Emergency treatment of poisoning p. 1413.

● PREGNANCY Use only if potential benefit outweighs risk.

● BREAST FEEDING The amount secreted into breast milk is too small to be harmful.

● HEPATIC IMPAIRMENT Manufacture advises avoid in severe impairment.

● MONITORING REQUIREMENTS
▶ Manufacturer advises plasma-nortriptyline concentration monitoring if dose above 100 mg daily, but evidence of practical value uncertain.

● TREATMENT CESSATION Withdrawal effects may occur within 5 days of stopping treatment with antidepressant drugs; they are usually mild and self-limiting, but in some cases may be severe. The risk of withdrawal symptoms is increased if the antidepressant is stopped suddenly after regular administration for 8 weeks or more. The dose should preferably be reduced gradually over about 4 weeks, or longer if withdrawal symptoms emerge (6 months in patients who have been on long-term maintenance treatment). If possible tricyclic and related antidepressants should be withdrawn slowly.

● PRESCRIBING AND DISPENSING INFORMATION Limited quantities of tricyclic antidepressants should be prescribed at any one time because their cardiovascular and epileptogenic effects are dangerous in overdosage.

● PATIENT AND CARER ADVICE Drowsiness may affect the performance of skilled tasks (e.g. driving). Effects of alcohol enhanced.

● MEDICINAL FORMS There can be variation in the licensing of different medicines containing the same drug. Forms available from special-order manufacturers include: oral suspension, oral solution

Oral solution
▶ Nortriptyline (Non-proprietary)
Nortriptyline (as Nortriptyline hydrochloride) 2 mg per 1 ml Nortriptyline 10mg/5ml oral solution sugar free sugar-free | 250 ml PoM £246.00 DT = £246.00
Nortriptyline (as Nortriptyline hydrochloride) 5 mg per 1 ml Nortriptyline 25mg/5ml oral solution sugar free sugar-free | 250 ml PoM £324.00

Tablet
CAUTIONARY AND ADVISORY LABELS 2
▶ Nortriptyline (Non-proprietary)
Nortriptyline (as Nortriptyline hydrochloride) 10 mg Nortriptyline 10mg tablets | 28 tablet PoM £1.48-£2.14 | 30 tablet PoM £10.02-£11.79 | 84 tablet PoM £3.39-£6.42 | 100 tablet PoM £39.30 DT = £4.04
Nortriptyline (as Nortriptyline hydrochloride) 25 mg Nortriptyline 25mg tablets | 28 tablet PoM £1.85-£2.46 | 30 tablet PoM £6.81-£12.43 | 84 tablet PoM £5.56-£7.38 | 100 tablet PoM £41.44 DT = £5.30
Nortriptyline (as Nortriptyline hydrochloride) 50 mg Nortriptyline 50mg tablets | 30 tablet PoM £42.00 DT = £41.81

Trimipramine
15-Nov-2020

● INDICATIONS AND DOSE

Depressive illness (particularly where sedation required)
▶ BY MOUTH
▶ Adult: Initially 50–75 mg daily in divided doses, alternatively initially 50–75 mg once daily, dose to be taken at bedtime, increased if necessary to 150–300 mg daily
▶ Elderly: Initially 10–25 mg 3 times a day, maintenance 75–150 mg daily

● CONTRA-INDICATIONS Acute porphyrias p. 1107 · arrhythmias · during the manic phase of bipolar disorder · heart block · immediate recovery period after myocardial infarction

● CAUTIONS Cardiovascular disease · chronic constipation · diabetes · epilepsy · history of bipolar disorder · history of psychosis · hyperthyroidism (risk of arrhythmias) · increased intra-ocular pressure · patients with a significant risk of suicide · phaeochromocytoma (risk of arrhythmias) · prostatic hypertrophy · susceptibility to angle-closure glaucoma · urinary retention

CAUTIONS, FURTHER INFORMATION EvGr Treatment should be stopped if the patient enters a manic phase. ⟨M⟩

Elderly patients are particularly susceptible to many of the side-effects of tricyclic antidepressants; EvGr low initial doses should be used, with close monitoring, particularly for psychiatric and cardiac side-effects. ⟨M⟩

● INTERACTIONS → Appendix 1: tricyclic antidepressants

● SIDE-EFFECTS Accommodation disorder · agitation · agranulocytosis · anticholinergic syndrome · arrhythmias · bone fracture · bone marrow depression · constipation · drowsiness · dry mouth · hyperglycaemia · hyperhidrosis · hypotension · jaundice cholestatic · mood altered · paranoid delusions · peripheral neuropathy · rash · respiratory depression · seizure · sexual dysfunction · suicidal behaviours · tremor · urinary hesitation · withdrawal syndrome

SIDE-EFFECTS, FURTHER INFORMATION The risk of side-effects is reduced by titrating slowly to the minimum effective dose (every 2–3 days). Consider using a lower starting dose in elderly patients.

Overdose Tricyclic and related antidepressants cause dry mouth, coma of varying degree, hypotension, hypothermia, hyperreflexia, extensor plantar responses, convulsions, respiratory failure, cardiac conduction defects, and arrhythmias. Dilated pupils and urinary retention also occur. For details on the management of poisoning see Tricyclic and related antidepressants under Emergency treatment of poisoning p. 1413.

- PREGNANCY Use only if potential benefit outweighs risk.
- BREAST FEEDING The amount secreted into breast milk is too small to be harmful.
- HEPATIC IMPAIRMENT Manufacturer advises avoid in severe impairment.
- TREATMENT CESSATION Withdrawal effects may occur within 5 days of stopping treatment with antidepressant drugs; they are usually mild and self-limiting, but in some cases may be severe. The risk of withdrawal symptoms is increased if the antidepressant is stopped suddenly after regular administration for 8 weeks or more. The dose should preferably be reduced gradually over about 4 weeks, or longer if withdrawal symptoms emerge (6 months in patients who have been on long-term maintenance treatment). If possible tricyclic and related antidepressants should be withdrawn slowly.
- PRESCRIBING AND DISPENSING INFORMATION Limited quantities of tricyclic antidepressants should be prescribed at any one time because their cardiovascular and epileptogenic effects are dangerous in overdosage.
- PATIENT AND CARER ADVICE
  Driving and skilled tasks Drowsiness may affect the performance of skilled tasks (e.g. driving).
  Effects of alcohol enhanced.
- MEDICINAL FORMS There can be variation in the licensing of different medicines containing the same drug. Forms available from special-order manufacturers include: oral suspension, oral solution

Tablet
CAUTIONARY AND ADVISORY LABELS 2
‣ Trimipramine (Non-proprietary)
   Trimipramine (as Trimipramine maleate) 10 mg Trimipramine 10mg tablets | 28 tablet PoM £197.18 DT = £179.18
   Trimipramine (as Trimipramine maleate) 25 mg Trimipramine 25mg tablets | 28 tablet PoM £205.44 DT = £200.50

Capsule
CAUTIONARY AND ADVISORY LABELS 2
‣ Trimipramine (Non-proprietary)
   Trimipramine (as Trimipramine maleate) 50 mg Trimipramine 50mg capsules | 28 capsule PoM £217.50 DT = £217.50

OTHER ANTIDEPRESSANTS

| Tryptophan
04-Oct-2017

(L-Tryptophan)

- DRUG ACTION Tryptophan is an essential dietary amino acid, and is a precursor of serotonin; it re-establishes the inhibitory action of serotonin on the amygdaloid nuclei, thereby reducing feelings of anxiety and depression.

- INDICATIONS AND DOSE
  Treatment-resistant depression (used alone or as adjunct to other antidepressant drugs) (initiated under direction of hospital consultant)
  ‣ BY MOUTH
  ‣ Adult: 1 g 3 times a day; maximum 6 g per day

- CONTRA-INDICATIONS History of eosinophilia myalgia syndrome following use of tryptophan
- INTERACTIONS → Appendix 1: tryptophan
- SIDE-EFFECTS Asthenia · dizziness · drowsiness · eosinophilia myalgia syndrome · headache · myalgia · myopathy · nausea · oedema · suicidal behaviours
  SIDE-EFFECTS, FURTHER INFORMATION If patients experience any symptoms of eosinophilia myalgia

syndrome (EMS), manufacturer advises to withhold treatment until possibility of EMS is excluded.

- PREGNANCY Manufacturer advises caution—no information available.
- BREAST FEEDING Manufacturer advises avoid—no information available.
- MONITORING REQUIREMENTS Manufacturer advises close monitoring for signs of suicidal thoughts, particularly in patients at high risk and during early treatment and dose changes.
- PATIENT AND CARER ADVICE Manufacturer advises patients and carers should be advised to seek medical advice immediately if any clinical worsening, suicidal thoughts, or unusual behaviour develops.
  Driving and skilled tasks Manufacturer advises patients should be counselled on the effects on driving and performance of skilled tasks—increased risk of drowsiness.

- MEDICINAL FORMS There can be variation in the licensing of different medicines containing the same drug. Forms available from special-order manufacturers include: capsule

Capsule
‣ Optimax (Special Order)
   Tryptophan 500 mg Optimax 500mg capsules | 84 capsule PoM ⓢ

| Vortioxetine
20-Oct-2020

- DRUG ACTION Vortioxetine inhibits the re-uptake of serotonin (5-HT) and is an antagonist at 5-HT_3 and an agonist at 5-HT_{1A} receptors. This multimodal activity appears to be associated with antidepressant and anxiolytic-like effects.

- INDICATIONS AND DOSE
  Major depression
  ‣ BY MOUTH
  ‣ Adult: Initially 10 mg once daily; adjusted according to response to 5–20 mg once daily
  ‣ Elderly: Initially 5 mg once daily; increased if necessary up to 20 mg once daily

- CAUTIONS Bleeding disorders · cirrhosis of the liver (risk of hyponatraemia) · elderly (risk of hyponatraemia) · history of mania (discontinue if patient entering manic phase) · history of seizures · susceptibility to angle-closure glaucoma · unstable epilepsy
  CAUTIONS, FURTHER INFORMATION
  ‣ Seizures Manufacturer advises discontinue treatment in patients who develop seizures or if there is an increase in seizure frequency.
  ‣ Elderly Manufacturer advises caution when treating elderly patients with doses over 10 mg daily—limited information.
- INTERACTIONS → Appendix 1: vortioxetine
- SIDE-EFFECTS
  ‣ **Common or very common** Abnormal dreams · constipation · diarrhoea · dizziness · nausea · skin reactions · vomiting
  ‣ **Uncommon** Flushing · night sweats
  ‣ **Frequency not known** Angioedema · haemorrhage · hyponatraemia · neuroleptic malignant syndrome (discontinue immediately) · serotonin syndrome (discontinue immediately)
- PREGNANCY Manufacturer advises avoid unless potential benefit outweighs risk—toxicity in *animal* studies. If used during the later stages of pregnancy, there is a risk of neonatal withdrawal symptoms and persistent pulmonary hypertension in the newborn.
- BREAST FEEDING Manufacturer advises avoid—present in milk in *animal* studies.
- HEPATIC IMPAIRMENT Manufacturer advises caution in severe impairment (no information available).

- RENAL IMPAIRMENT Manufacturer advises caution in severe impairment—limited information available.
- TREATMENT CESSATION Manufacturer advises treatment can be stopped abruptly, without need for gradual dose reduction.
- PATIENT AND CARER ADVICE
  Driving and skilled tasks Manufacturer advises patients and carers should be counselled on the effects on driving and performance of skilled tasks, especially when starting treatment or changing the dose.
- NATIONAL FUNDING/ACCESS DECISIONS
  For full details see funding body website
  NICE decisions
  ▸ Vortioxetine for treating major depressive episodes (November 2015) NICE TA367 Recommended with restrictions
- MEDICINAL FORMS There can be variation in the licensing of different medicines containing the same drug.
  Tablet
  ▸ Brintellix (Lundbeck Ltd)
  Vortioxetine (as Vortioxetine hydrobromide) 5 mg Brintellix 5mg tablets | 28 tablet [PoM] £27.72 DT = £27.72
  Vortioxetine (as Vortioxetine hydrobromide) 10 mg Brintellix 10mg tablets | 28 tablet [PoM] £27.72 DT = £27.72
  Vortioxetine (as Vortioxetine hydrobromide) 20 mg Brintellix 20mg tablets | 28 tablet [PoM] £27.72 DT = £27.72

3.5 Inappropriate sexual behaviour

ANTIPSYCHOTICS ⟩ FIRST-GENERATION

F 403

Benperidol

07-Jun-2018

- **INDICATIONS AND DOSE**
  Control of deviant antisocial sexual behaviour
  ▸ BY MOUTH
  ▸ Adult: 0.25–1.5 mg daily in divided doses, adjusted according to response, for debilitated patients, use elderly dose
  ▸ Elderly: Initially 0.125–0.75 mg daily in divided doses, adjusted according to response

- CONTRA-INDICATIONS CNS depression · comatose states · phaeochromocytoma
- CAUTIONS Risk factors for stroke
- INTERACTIONS → Appendix 1: benperidol
- SIDE-EFFECTS Appetite decreased · blood disorder · cardiac arrest · confusion · depression · dyspepsia · headache · hepatic disorders · hyperhidrosis · hypersalivation · hypertension · muscle rigidity · nausea · oculogyric crisis · oedema · oligomenorrhoea · paradoxical drug reaction · pruritus · psychiatric disorder · temperature regulation disorders · weight change
- PREGNANCY Extrapyramidal effects and withdrawal syndrome have been reported occasionally in the neonate when antipsychotic drugs are taken during the third trimester of pregnancy. Following maternal use of antipsychotic drugs in the third trimester, neonates should be monitored for symptoms including agitation, hypertonia, hypotonia, tremor, drowsiness, feeding problems, and respiratory distress.
- BREAST FEEDING There is limited information available on the short- and long-term effects of antipsychotic drugs on the breast-fed infant. *Animal* studies indicate possible adverse effects of antipsychotic medicines on the developing nervous system. Chronic treatment with antipsychotic drugs whilst breast-feeding should be avoided unless absolutely necessary.

- HEPATIC IMPAIRMENT Manufacturer advises caution.
- RENAL IMPAIRMENT
  Dose adjustments Start with small doses in severe renal impairment because of increased cerebral sensitivity.
- MONITORING REQUIREMENTS Manufacturer advises regular blood counts and liver function tests during long-term treatment.
- PRESCRIBING AND DISPENSING INFORMATION The proprietary name *Benquil*® has been used for benperidol tablets.

- MEDICINAL FORMS There can be variation in the licensing of different medicines containing the same drug. Forms available from special-order manufacturers include: oral suspension
  Tablet
  CAUTIONARY AND ADVISORY LABELS 2
  ▸ Anquil (Neon Healthcare Ltd)
  Benperidol 250 microgram Anquil 250microgram tablets | 112 tablet [PoM] £200.32 DT = £200.32

3.6 Psychoses and schizophrenia

Psychoses and related disorders

10-Sep-2020

Advice of Royal College of Psychiatrists on doses of antipsychotic drugs above BNF upper limit

Unless otherwise stated, doses in the BNF are licensed doses—any higher dose is therefore **unlicensed**

- Consider alternative approaches including adjuvant therapy and newer or second-generation antipsychotic drugs such as clozapine.
- Bear in mind risk factors, including obesity; particular caution is indicated in older patients, especially those over 70.
- Consider potential for drug interactions—see interactions: Appendix 1 (antipsychotics).
- Carry out ECG to exclude untoward abnormalities such as prolonged QT interval; repeat ECG periodically and reduce dose if prolonged QT interval or other adverse cardiac abnormality develops.
- Increase dose slowly and not more often than once weekly.
- Carry out regular pulse, blood pressure, and temperature checks; ensure that patient maintains adequate fluid intake.
- Consider high-dose therapy to be for limited period and review regularly; abandon if no improvement after 3 months (return to standard dosage).

Important: When prescribing an antipsychotic for administration on an emergency basis, the intramuscular dose should be **lower** than the corresponding oral dose (owing to absence of first-pass effect), particularly if the patient is very active (increased blood flow to muscle considerably increases the rate of absorption). The prescription should specify the dose for **each route** and should **not** imply that the same dose can be given by mouth or by intramuscular injection. The dose of antipsychotic for emergency use should be reviewed at least **daily**.

MHRA/CHM advice: Clozapine and other antipsychotics

The MHRA/CHM have released important safety information regarding antipsychotics and monitoring blood concentrations for toxicity. For further information, see *Important safety information* in the amisulpride p. 414, aripiprazole p. 415, clozapine p. 417, olanzapine p. 419, olanzapine embonate p. 425, quetiapine p. 422, risperidone p. 423, and sulpiride p. 409 monographs.

Antipsychotic drugs

Antipsychotic drugs are also known as 'neuroleptics' and (misleadingly) as 'major tranquillisers'.

In the short term they are used to calm disturbed patients whatever the underlying psychopathology, which may be schizophrenia, brain damage, mania, toxic delirium, or agitated depression. Antipsychotic drugs are used to alleviate severe anxiety but this too should be a short-term measure.

Schizophrenia

The aim of treatment is to alleviate the suffering of the patient (and carer) and to improve social and cognitive functioning. Many patients require life-long treatment with antipsychotic medication. Antipsychotic drugs relieve positive psychotic symptoms such as thought disorder, hallucinations, and delusions, and prevent relapse; they are usually less effective on negative symptoms such as apathy and social withdrawal. In many patients, negative symptoms persist between episodes of treated positive symptoms, but earlier treatment of psychotic illness may protect against the development of negative symptoms over time. Patients with acute schizophrenia generally respond better than those with chronic symptoms.

Long-term treatment of a patient with a definitive diagnosis of schizophrenia is usually required after the first episode of illness in order to prevent relapses. Doses that are effective in acute episodes should generally be continued as prophylaxis.

First-generation antipsychotic drugs

The first-generation antipsychotic drugs act predominantly by blocking dopamine D_2 receptors in the brain. First-generation antipsychotic drugs are not selective for any of the four dopamine pathways in the brain and so can cause a range of side-effects, particularly extrapyramidal symptoms and elevated prolactin. The **phenothiazine** derivatives can be divided into 3 main groups:

- **Group 1**: chlorpromazine hydrochloride p. 404, levomepromazine p. 459, and promazine hydrochloride p. 427, generally characterised by pronounced sedative effects and moderate antimuscarinic and extrapyramidal side-effects.
- **Group 2**: pericyazine p. 408, generally characterised by moderate sedative effects, but fewer extrapyramidal side-effects than groups 1 or 3.
- **Group 3**: fluphenazine decanoate p. 412, perphenazine, prochlorperazine p. 408, and trifluoperazine p. 410, generally characterised by fewer sedative and antimuscarinic effects, but more pronounced extrapyramidal side-effects than groups 1 and 2.

Butyrophenones (benperidol p. 400 and haloperidol p. 405) resemble the group 3 phenothiazines in their clinical properties. **Thioxanthenes** (flupentixol p. 405 and zuclopenthixol p. 410) have moderate sedative, antimuscarinic effects, and extrapyramidal effects. **Diphenylbutylpiperidines** (pimozide p. 408) and the **substituted benzamides** (sulpiride) have reduced sedative, antimuscarinic, and extrapyramidal effects.

Second-generation antipsychotic drugs

The second-generation antipsychotic drugs (sometimes referred to as atypical antipsychotic drugs) act on a range of receptors in comparison to first-generation antipsychotic drugs and have more distinct clinical profiles, particularly with regard to side-effects.

Prescribing for the elderly

The balance of risks and benefit should be considered before prescribing antipsychotic drugs for elderly patients. In elderly patients with dementia, antipsychotic drugs are associated with a small increased risk of mortality and an increased risk of stroke or transient ischaemic attack (see Dementia p. 316). Furthermore, elderly patients are particularly susceptible to postural hypotension and to hyper- and hypothermia in hot or cold weather.

It is recommended that:

- Antipsychotic drugs should not be used in elderly patients to treat mild to moderate psychotic symptoms.
- Initial doses of antipsychotic drugs in elderly patients should be reduced (to half the adult dose or less), taking into account factors such as the patient's weight, co-morbidity, and concomitant medication.
- Treatment should be reviewed regularly.

Prescribing of antipsychotic drugs in patients with learning disabilities

EvGr When prescribing for patients with learning disabilities who are prescribed antipsychotic drugs and who are not experiencing psychotic symptoms, the following considerations should be taken into account:

- a reduction in dose or the discontinuation of long-term antipsychotic treatment;
- review of the patient's condition after dose reduction or discontinuation of an antipsychotic drug;
- referral to a psychiatrist experienced in working with patients who have learning disabilities and mental health problems;
- annual documentation of the reasons for continuing a prescription if the antipsychotic is not reduced in dose or discontinued ⟨A⟩.

Side effects of antipsychotic drugs

Side-effects caused by antipsychotic drugs are common and contribute significantly to non-adherence to therapy.

Extrapyramidal symptoms

Extrapyramidal symptoms occur most frequently with the piperazine phenothiazines (fluphenazine, perphenazine, prochlorperazine, and trifluoperazine), the butyrophenones (benperidol and haloperidol), and the first-generation depot preparations. They are easy to recognise but cannot be predicted accurately because they depend on the dose, the type of drug, and on individual susceptibility.

Extrapyramidal symptoms consist of:

- *parkinsonian symptoms* (including tremor), which may occur more commonly in adults or the elderly and may appear gradually;
- *dystonia* (abnormal face and body movements) and *dyskinesia*, which occur more commonly in children or young adults and appear after only a few doses;
- *akathisia* (restlessness), which characteristically occurs after large initial doses and may resemble an exacerbation of the condition being treated;
- *tardive dyskinesia* (rhythmic, involuntary movements of tongue, face, and jaw), which usually develops on long-term therapy or with high dosage, but it may develop on short-term treatment with low doses—short-lived tardive dyskinesia may occur after withdrawal of the drug.

Parkinsonian symptoms remit if the drug is withdrawn and may be suppressed by the administration of antimuscarinic drugs. However, routine administration of such drugs is not justified because not all patients are affected and they may unmask or worsen tardive dyskinesia.

Tardive dyskinesia is the most serious manifestation of extrapyramidal symptoms; it is of particular concern because it may be irreversible on withdrawing therapy and treatment is usually ineffective. In children, tardive dyskinesia is more likely to occur when the antipsychotic drug is withdrawn. However, some manufacturers suggest that drug withdrawal at the earliest signs of tardive dyskinesia (fine vermicular movements of the tongue) may halt its full development. Tardive dyskinesia occurs fairly frequently, especially in the elderly, and treatment must be carefully and regularly reviewed.

Hyperprolactinaemia

Most antipsychotic drugs, both first- and second-generation, increase prolactin concentration to some extent because dopamine inhibits prolactin release. Aripiprazole reduces prolactin because it is a dopamine-receptor partial agonist. Risperidone, amisulpride, and first-generation antipsychotic drugs are most likely to cause symptomatic hyperprolactinaemia. The clinical symptoms of hyperprolactinaemia include sexual dysfunction, reduced bone mineral density, menstrual disturbances, breast enlargement, and galactorrhoea.

Sexual dysfunction

Sexual dysfunction is one of the main causes of non-adherence to antipsychotic medication; physical illness, psychiatric illness, and substance misuse are contributing factors. Antipsychotic-induced sexual dysfunction is caused by more than one mechanism. Reduced dopamine transmission and hyperprolactinaemia decrease libido; antimuscarinic effects can cause disorders of arousal; and alpha₁-adrenoceptor antagonists are associated with erection and ejaculation problems in men. Risperidone and haloperidol commonly cause sexual dysfunction. If sexual dysfunction is thought to be antipsychotic-induced, dose reduction or switching medication should be considered.

Cardiovascular side-effects

Antipsychotic drugs have been associated with cardiovascular side-effects such as tachycardia, arrhythmias, and hypotension. QT-interval prolongation is a particular concern with pimozide and haloperidol. There is also a higher probability of QT-interval prolongation in patients using any intravenous antipsychotic drug, or any antipsychotic drug or combination of antipsychotic drugs with doses exceeding the recommended maximum. Cases of sudden death have occurred.

Hyperglycaemia and weight gain

Hyperglycaemia, and sometimes diabetes, can occur with antipsychotic drugs, particularly clozapine, olanzapine, quetiapine, and risperidone. All antipsychotic drugs may cause weight gain, but the risk and extent varies. Clozapine and olanzapine commonly cause weight gain.

Hypotension and interference with temperature regulation

Hypotension and interference with temperature regulation are dose-related side-effects that are liable to cause dangerous falls and hypothermia or hyperthermia in the elderly. Clozapine, chlorpromazine, lurasidone, and quetiapine can cause postural hypotension (especially during initial dose titration) which may be associated with syncope or reflex tachycardia in some patients.

Neuroleptic malignant syndrome

Neuroleptic malignant syndrome (hyperthermia, fluctuating level of consciousness, muscle rigidity, and autonomic dysfunction with pallor, tachycardia, labile blood pressure, sweating, and urinary incontinence) is a rare but potentially fatal side-effect of all antipsychotic drugs. Discontinuation of the antipsychotic drug is essential because there is no proven effective treatment, but bromocriptine and dantrolene have been used. The syndrome, which usually lasts for 5–7 days after drug discontinuation, may be unduly prolonged if depot preparations have been used.

Blood dyscrasias

Perform blood counts if unexplained infection or fever develops.

Choice

There is little meaningful difference in efficacy between each of the antipsychotic drugs (other than clozapine p. 417), and response and tolerability to each antipsychotic drug varies. There is no first-line antipsychotic drug which is suitable for all patients. Choice of antipsychotic medication is influenced by the patient's medication history, the degree of sedation required (although tolerance to this usually develops), and consideration of individual patient factors such as risk of extrapyramidal side-effects, weight gain, impaired glucose tolerance, QT-interval prolongation, or the presence of negative symptoms.

Negative symptoms

Second generation antipsychotic drugs may be better at treating the negative symptoms of schizophrenia.

Extrapyramidal side-effects

Second-generation antipsychotic drugs should be prescribed if extrapyramidal side-effects are a particular concern. Of these, aripiprazole p. 415, clozapine, olanzapine p. 419, and quetiapine p. 422 are least likely to cause extrapyramidal side-effects. Although amisulpride p. 414 is a dopamine-receptor antagonist, extrapyramidal side-effects are less common than with the first-generation antipsychotic drugs because amisulpride selectively blocks mesolimbic dopamine receptors, and extrapyramidal symptoms are caused by blockade of the striatal dopamine pathway.

QT interval

Aripiprazole has negligible effect on the QT interval. Other antipsychotic drugs with a reduced tendency to prolong QT interval include amisulpride, clozapine, flupentixol p. 405, fluphenazine decanoate p. 412, olanzapine, perphenazine, prochlorperazine p. 408, risperidone p. 423, and sulpiride p. 409.

Diabetes

Schizophrenia is associated with insulin resistance and diabetes; the risk of diabetes is increased in patients with schizophrenia who take antipsychotic drugs. First-generation antipsychotic drugs are less likely to cause diabetes than second-generation antipsychotic drugs, and of the first-generation antipsychotic drugs, fluphenazine decanoate and haloperidol p. 405 are lowest risk. Amisulpride and aripiprazole have the lowest risk of diabetes of the second-generation antipsychotic drugs. Amisulpride, aripiprazole, haloperidol, sulpiride, and trifluoperazine p. 410 are least likely to cause weight gain.

Sexual dysfunction and prolactin

The antipsychotic drugs with the lowest risk of sexual dysfunction are aripiprazole and quetiapine. Olanzapine may be considered if sexual dysfunction is judged to be secondary to hyperprolactinaemia. Hyperprolactinaemia is usually not clinically significant with aripiprazole, clozapine, olanzapine, and quetiapine treatment. When changing from other antipsychotic drugs, a reduction in prolactin concentration may increase fertility.

Patients should receive an antipsychotic drug for 4–6 weeks before it is deemed ineffective. Prescribing more than one antipsychotic drug at a time should be avoided except in exceptional circumstances (e.g. clozapine augmentation or when changing medication during titration) because of the increased risk of adverse effects such as extrapyramidal symptoms, QT-interval prolongation, and sudden cardiac death.

Clozapine is licensed for the treatment of schizophrenia in patients unresponsive to, or intolerant of, other antipsychotic drugs. Clozapine should be introduced if schizophrenia is not controlled despite the sequential use of two or more antipsychotic drugs (one of which should be a second-generation antipsychotic drug), each for at least 6–8 weeks. If symptoms do not respond adequately to an optimised dose of clozapine p. 417, plasma-clozapine concentration should be checked before adding a second antipsychotic drug to augment clozapine; allow 8–10 weeks' treatment to assess response. Patients must be registered with a clozapine patient monitoring service.

Monitoring

Full blood count, urea and electrolytes, and liver function test monitoring is required at the start of therapy with antipsychotic drugs, and then annually thereafter.

Blood lipids and weight should be measured at baseline, at 3 months (weight should be measured at frequent intervals during the first 3 months), and then yearly.

Fasting blood glucose should be measured at baseline, at 4–6 months, and then yearly.

Before initiating antipsychotic drugs, an ECG may be required, particularly if physical examination identifies cardiovascular risk factors, if there is a personal history of cardiovascular disease, or if the patient is being admitted as an inpatient.

Blood pressure monitoring is advised before starting therapy and frequently during dose titration of antipsychotic drugs.

Other uses
Some antipsychotic drugs can be used for the treatment of nausea and vomiting, choreas, and motor tics. Chlorpromazine hydrochloride p. 404 and haloperidol p. 405 can be used for intractable hiccup. Benperidol p. 400 is used in deviant antisocial sexual behaviour but its value is not established.

Psychomotor agitation should be investigated for an underlying cause; it can be managed with low doses of chlorpromazine hydrochloride or haloperidol used for short periods. Antipsychotic drugs can be used with caution for the short-term treatment of severe agitation and restlessness in the elderly.

Dosage
After an initial period of stabilisation, in most patients, the total daily oral dose can be given as a single dose. The Royal College of Psychiatrists has published advice on doses of antipsychotic drugs above BNF upper limit.

Antipsychotic depot injections
Long-acting depot injections are used for maintenance therapy especially when compliance with oral treatment is unreliable. However, depot injections of conventional antipsychotics may give rise to a higher incidence of extrapyramidal reactions than oral preparations; extrapyramidal reactions occur less frequently with second-generation antipsychotic depot preparations, such as risperidone p. 423 and olanzapine embonate p. 425.

Choice
There is no clear-cut division in the use of the conventional antipsychotics, but zuclopenthixol p. 410 may be suitable for the treatment of agitated or aggressive patients whereas flupentixol decanoate p. 411 can cause over-excitement in such patients. Zuclopenthixol decanoate p. 413 may be more effective in preventing relapses than other conventional antipsychotic depot preparations. The incidence of extrapyramidal reactions is similar for the conventional antipsychotics.

Dosage
Individual responses to neuroleptic drugs are variable and to achieve optimum effect, dosage and dosage interval must be titrated according to the patient's response.

ANTIPSYCHOTICS

Antipsychotic drugs

● CAUTIONS Blood dyscrasias · cardiovascular disease · conditions predisposing to seizures · depression · diabetes (may raise blood glucose) · epilepsy · history of jaundice · myasthenia gravis · Parkinson's disease (may be exacerbated) (in adults) · photosensitisation (may occur with higher dosages) · prostatic hypertrophy (in adults) · severe respiratory disease · susceptibility to angle-closure glaucoma

CAUTIONS, FURTHER INFORMATION
▶ **Cardiovascular disease** An ECG may be required, particularly if physical examination identifies cardiovascular risk factors, personal history of cardiovascular disease, or if the patient is being admitted as an inpatient.
▶ **Elderly** Prescription potentially inappropriate (STOPP criteria):
 ● for all antipsychotics (other than quetiapine and clozapine) in patients with parkinsonism or Lewy Body Disease (risk of severe extrapyramidal symptoms)
 ● in behavioural and psychological symptoms of dementia (BPSD), unless symptoms are severe and other non-pharmacological treatments have failed (increased risk of stroke)
 ● for use as a hypnotic, unless sleep disorder is due to psychosis or dementia (risk of confusion, hypotension, extrapyramidal side-effects and falls)
 ● in patients prone to falls (may cause gait dyspraxia, parkinsonism)
 ● if prescribed a **phenothiazine** (other than prochlorperazine for nausea, vomiting or vertigo; chlorpromazine for relief of persistent hiccups; levomepromazine as an antiemetic in palliative care) as first-line treatment (sedative, significant antimuscarinic (anticholinergic) toxicity in older people, and safer and more efficacious alternatives exist)—
 ● if prescribed an antipsychotic drug with **moderate or marked antimuscarinic effects** (e.g. chlorpromazine, clozapine, flupenthixol, fluphenazine, pipothiazine, promazine and zuclopenthixol) in patients with a history of prostatism or urinary retention (high risk of urinary retention).
See also Prescribing in the elderly p. 33.

● SIDE-EFFECTS
▶ **Common or very common** Agitation · amenorrhoea · arrhythmias · constipation · dizziness · drowsiness · dry mouth · erectile dysfunction · galactorrhoea · gynaecomastia · hyperprolactinaemia · hypotension (dose-related) · insomnia · leucopenia · movement disorders · neutropenia · parkinsonism · QT interval prolongation · rash · seizure · tremor · urinary retention · vomiting · weight increased
▶ **Uncommon** Agranulocytosis · embolism and thrombosis · neuroleptic malignant syndrome (discontinue—potentially fatal)
▶ **Rare or very rare** Sudden death · withdrawal syndrome neonatal

SIDE-EFFECTS, FURTHER INFORMATION For depot antipsychotics—side-effects may persist until the drug has been cleared from its depot site.

Overdose Phenothiazines cause less depression of consciousness and respiration than other sedatives. Hypotension, hypothermia, sinus tachycardia, and arrhythmias may complicate poisoning. For details on the management of poisoning see Antipsychotics under Emergency treatment of poisoning p. 1413.

● PREGNANCY Extrapyramidal effects and withdrawal syndrome have been reported occasionally in the neonate when antipsychotic drugs are taken during the third trimester of pregnancy. Following maternal use of antipsychotic drugs in the third trimester, neonates should be monitored for symptoms including agitation, hypertonia, hypotonia, tremor, drowsiness, feeding problems, and respiratory distress.

● BREAST FEEDING There is limited information available on the short- and long-term effects of antipsychotic drugs on the breast-fed infant. *Animal studies* indicate possible adverse effects of antipsychotic medicines on the developing nervous system. Chronic treatment with antipsychotic drugs whilst breast-feeding should be avoided unless absolutely necessary. Phenothiazine

4

Nervous system

derivatives are sometimes used in breast-feeding women for short-term treatment of nausea and vomiting.

- MONITORING REQUIREMENTS
- It is advisable to monitor prolactin concentration at the start of therapy, at 6 months, and then yearly. Patients taking antipsychotic drugs not normally associated with symptomatic hyperprolactinaemia should be considered for prolactin monitoring if they show symptoms of hyperprolactinaemia (such as breast enlargement and galactorrhoea).
- Patients with schizophrenia should have physical health monitoring (including cardiovascular disease risk assessment) at least once per year.
- In children Regular clinical monitoring of endocrine function should be considered when children are taking an antipsychotic drug known to increase prolactin levels; this includes measuring weight and height, assessing sexual maturation, and monitoring menstrual function.
- TREATMENT CESSATION There is a high risk of relapse if medication is stopped after 1–2 years. Withdrawal of antipsychotic drugs after long-term therapy should always be gradual and closely monitored to avoid the risk of acute withdrawal syndromes or rapid relapse. Patients should be monitored for 2 years after withdrawal of antipsychotic medication for signs and symptoms of relapse.
- PRESCRIBING AND DISPENSING INFORMATION
Patient decision aid
- In adults Antipsychotic medicines for treating agitation, aggression and distress in people living with dementia. National Institute for Health and Care Excellence. June 2018. www.nice.org.uk/about/what-we-do/our-programmes/nice-guidance/nice-guidelines/shared-decision-making
- PATIENT AND CARER ADVICE As photosensitisation may occur with higher dosages, patients should avoid direct sunlight.
Driving and skilled tasks Drowsiness may affect performance of skilled tasks (e.g. driving or operating machinery), especially at start of treatment; effects of alcohol are enhanced.

ANTIPSYCHOTICS › FIRST-GENERATION

F 403

Chlorpromazine hydrochloride   13-Mar-2020

- INDICATIONS AND DOSE

Schizophrenia and other psychoses | Mania | Short-term adjunctive management of severe anxiety | Psychomotor agitation, excitement, and violent or dangerously impulsive behaviour
- BY MOUTH
- Adult: Initially 25 mg 3 times a day, adjusted according to response, alternatively initially 75 mg once daily, adjusted according to response, dose to be taken at night; maintenance 75–300 mg daily, increased if necessary up to 1 g daily, this dose may be required in psychoses; use a third to half adult dose in the elderly or debilitated patients
- BY RECTUM
- Adult: 100 mg every 6–8 hours, dose expressed as chlorpromazine base

Intractable hiccup
- BY MOUTH
- Adult: 25–50 mg 3–4 times a day

Relief of acute symptoms of psychoses (under expert supervision)
- BY DEEP INTRAMUSCULAR INJECTION
- Adult: 25–50 mg every 6–8 hours

Nausea and vomiting in palliative care (where other drugs have failed or are not available)
- BY MOUTH
- Child 1–5 years: 500 micrograms/kg every 4–6 hours; maximum 40 mg per day
- Child 6–11 years: 500 micrograms/kg every 4–6 hours; maximum 75 mg per day
- Child 12–17 years: 10–25 mg every 4–6 hours
- Adult: 10–25 mg every 4–6 hours
- BY DEEP INTRAMUSCULAR INJECTION
- Child 1–5 years: 500 micrograms/kg every 6–8 hours; maximum 40 mg per day
- Child 6–11 years: 500 micrograms/kg every 6–8 hours; maximum 75 mg per day
- Child 12–17 years: Initially 25 mg, then 25–50 mg every 3–4 hours until vomiting stops
- Adult: Initially 25 mg, then 25–50 mg every 3–4 hours until vomiting stops
- BY RECTUM
- Adult: 100 mg every 6–8 hours

DOSE EQUIVALENCE AND CONVERSION
- For equivalent therapeutic effect 100 mg chlorpromazine base given *rectally* as a suppository ≡ 20–25 mg chlorpromazine hydrochloride *by intramuscular injection* ≡ 40–50 mg of chlorpromazine base or hydrochloride given *by mouth*.

- UNLICENSED USE Rectal route is not licensed.
- CONTRA-INDICATIONS CNS depression · comatose states · hypothyroidism · phaeochromocytoma
- INTERACTIONS → Appendix 1: phenothiazines
- SIDE-EFFECTS
GENERAL SIDE-EFFECTS
- **Common or very common** Anxiety · glucose tolerance impaired · mood altered · muscle tone increased
- **Frequency not known** Accommodation disorder · angioedema · atrioventricular block · cardiac arrest · eye deposit · eye disorders · gastrointestinal disorders · hepatic disorders · hyperglycaemia · hypertriglyceridaemia · hyponatraemia · photosensitivity reaction · respiratory disorders · sexual dysfunction · SIADH · skin reactions · systemic lupus erythematosus (SLE) · temperature regulation disorder · trismus
SPECIFIC SIDE-EFFECTS
- With intramuscular use Muscle rigidity · nasal congestion
SIDE-EFFECTS, FURTHER INFORMATION Acute dystonic reactions may occur; children are particularly susceptible.
- HEPATIC IMPAIRMENT Manufacturer advises caution in severe hepatic failure (increased risk of accumulation).
- RENAL IMPAIRMENT
Dose adjustments Start with small doses in severe renal impairment because of increased cerebral sensitivity.
- MONITORING REQUIREMENTS
- With intramuscular use Patients should remain supine, with blood pressure monitoring for 30 minutes after intramuscular injection.
- PRESCRIBING AND DISPENSING INFORMATION
Palliative care For further information on the use of chlorpromazine hydrochloride in palliative care, see www.medicinescomplete.com/#/content/palliative/antipsychotics.
- HANDLING AND STORAGE Owing to the risk of contact sensitisation, pharmacists, nurses, and other health workers should avoid direct contact with chlorpromazine; tablets should not be crushed and solutions should be handled with care.

● MEDICINAL FORMS There can be variation in the licensing of different medicines containing the same drug. Forms available from special-order manufacturers include: tablet, capsule, oral suspension, oral solution, suppository

Tablet
CAUTIONARY AND ADVISORY LABELS 2, 11
▸ Chlorpromazine hydrochloride (Non-proprietary)
   Chlorpromazine hydrochloride 25 mg Chlorpromazine 25mg tablets | 28 tablet PoM £37.13 DT = £17.55
   Chlorpromazine hydrochloride 50 mg Chlorpromazine 50mg tablets | 28 tablet PoM £37.50 DT = £17.77
   Chlorpromazine hydrochloride 100 mg Chlorpromazine 100mg tablets | 28 tablet PoM £39.99 DT = £17.71

Solution for injection
▸ Largactil (Sanofi)
   Chlorpromazine hydrochloride 25 mg per 1 ml Largactil 50mg/2ml solution for injection ampoules | 10 ampoule PoM £7.51

Oral solution
CAUTIONARY AND ADVISORY LABELS 2, 11
▸ Chlorpromazine hydrochloride (Non-proprietary)
   Chlorpromazine hydrochloride 5 mg per 1 ml Chlorpromazine 25mg/5ml syrup | 150 ml PoM £2.35 DT = £2.35
   Chlorpromazine 25mg/5ml oral solution sugar free sugar-free | 150 ml PoM £2.54 DT = £2.66
   Chlorpromazine 25mg/5ml oral solution | 150 ml PoM £2.35 DT = £2.35
   Chlorpromazine hydrochloride 20 mg per 1 ml Chlorpromazine 100mg/5ml oral solution | 150 ml PoM £5.50 DT = £5.50

Flupentixol
(Flupenthixol)

09-Aug-2019

◤ 403

● INDICATIONS AND DOSE

Schizophrenia and other psychoses, particularly with apathy and withdrawal but not mania or psychomotor hyperactivity
▸ BY MOUTH
▸ Adult: Initially 3–9 mg twice daily, adjusted according to response, for debilitated patients, use elderly dose; maximum 18 mg per day
▸ Elderly: Initially 0.75–4.5 mg twice daily, adjusted according to response

Depressive illness
▸ BY MOUTH
▸ Adult: Initially 1 mg once daily, dose to be taken in the morning, increased if necessary to 2 mg after 1 week, doses above 2 mg to be given in divided doses, last dose to be taken before 4 pm; discontinue if no response after 1 week at maximum dosage; maximum 3 mg per day
▸ Elderly: Initially 500 micrograms daily, dose to be taken in the morning, then increased if necessary to 1 mg after 1 week, doses above 1 mg to be given in divided doses, last dose to be taken before 4 pm; discontinue if no response after 1 week at maximum dosage; maximum 1.5 mg per day

● CONTRA-INDICATIONS Circulatory collapse · CNS depression · comatose states · excitable patients · impaired consciousness · overactive patients

● CAUTIONS Cardiac disorders · cardiovascular disease · cerebral arteriosclerosis · elderly · hyperthyroidism · hypothyroidism · parkinsonism · phaeochromocytoma · QT-interval prolongation · senile confusional states

● INTERACTIONS → Appendix 1: flupentixol

● SIDE-EFFECTS
▸ **Common or very common** Appetite abnormal · asthenia · concentration impaired · depression · diarrhoea · dyspnoea · gastrointestinal discomfort · headache · hyperhidrosis · hypersalivation · muscle complaints · nervousness · palpitations · sexual dysfunction · skin reactions · urinary disorder · vision disorders

▸ **Uncommon** Confusion · flatulence · hot flush · nausea · oculogyration · photosensitivity reaction · speech disorder
▸ **Rare or very rare** Glucose tolerance impaired · hyperglycaemia · jaundice · thrombocytopenia
▸ **Frequency not known** Suicidal behaviours

● PREGNANCY Avoid unless potential benefit outweighs risk.

● BREAST FEEDING Present in breast milk—avoid.

● HEPATIC IMPAIRMENT Manufacturer advises caution—monitor serum drug concentration.

● RENAL IMPAIRMENT Manufacturer advises caution in renal failure.
   Dose adjustments Start with small doses of antipsychotic drugs in severe renal impairment because of increased cerebral sensitivity.

● PATIENT AND CARER ADVICE Although drowsiness may occur, can also have an alerting effect so should not be taken in the evening.

● MEDICINAL FORMS There can be variation in the licensing of different medicines containing the same drug. Forms available from special-order manufacturers include: oral suspension, oral solution

Tablet
CAUTIONARY AND ADVISORY LABELS 2
▸ Depixol (Lundbeck Ltd)
   Flupentixol (as Flupentixol dihydrochloride) 3 mg Depixol 3mg tablets | 100 tablet PoM £13.92 DT = £13.92
▸ Fluanxol (Lundbeck Ltd)
   Flupentixol (as Flupentixol dihydrochloride)
   500 microgram Fluanxol 500microgram tablets | 60 tablet PoM £2.88 DT = £2.88
   Flupentixol (as Flupentixol dihydrochloride) 1 mg Fluanxol 1mg tablets | 60 tablet PoM £4.86 DT = £4.86

◤ 403

Haloperidol

20-Nov-2019

● INDICATIONS AND DOSE

Prophylaxis of postoperative nausea and vomiting [in patients at moderate to high risk and when alternatives ineffective or not tolerated]
▸ BY INTRAMUSCULAR INJECTION
▸ Adult: 1–2 mg, to be given at induction or 30 minutes before the end of anaesthesia
▸ Elderly: 500 micrograms, to be given at induction or 30 minutes before the end of anaesthesia

Combination treatment of postoperative nausea and vomiting [when alternatives ineffective or not tolerated]
▸ BY INTRAMUSCULAR INJECTION
▸ Adult: 1–2 mg
▸ Elderly: 500 micrograms

Nausea and vomiting in palliative care
▸ BY MOUTH
▸ Adult: Initially 1.5 mg 1–2 times a day, increased if necessary to 5–10 mg daily in divided doses
▸ BY SUBCUTANEOUS INFUSION
▸ Adult: 2.5–10 mg/24 hours

Schizophrenia and schizoaffective disorder
▸ BY MOUTH
▸ Adult: 2–10 mg daily in 1–2 divided doses; usual dose 2–4 mg daily, in first-episode schizophrenia, up to 10 mg daily, in multiple-episode schizophrenia, dose adjusted according to response at intervals of 1–7 days. Individual benefit-risk should be assessed when considering doses above 10 mg daily; maximum 20 mg per day
▸ Elderly: Initially, use half the lowest adult dose, then adjust gradually according to response up to maximum 5 mg daily, doses above 5 mg daily should only be considered in patients who have tolerated higher doses and after reassessment of the individual benefit-risk

continued →

Acute delirium [when non-pharmacological treatments ineffective]
▸ BY MOUTH
▸ Adult: 1–10 mg daily in 1–3 divided doses, treatment should be started at the lowest possible dose and adjusted in increments at 2–4 hourly intervals if required; maximum 10 mg per day
▸ Elderly: Initially, use half the lowest adult dose, then adjust gradually according to response up to maximum 5 mg daily, doses above 5 mg daily should only be considered in patients who have tolerated higher doses and after reassessment of the individual benefit-risk
▸ BY INTRAMUSCULAR INJECTION
▸ Adult: 1–10 mg, treatment should be started at the lowest possible dose and adjusted in increments at 2–4 hourly intervals if required; maximum 10 mg per day
▸ Elderly: Initially 500 micrograms, dose adjusted gradually according to response up to maximum 5 mg daily, doses above 5 mg daily should only be considered in patients who have tolerated higher doses and after reassessment of the individual benefit-risk

Moderate to severe manic episodes associated with bipolar I disorder
▸ BY MOUTH
▸ Adult: 2–10 mg daily in 1–2 divided doses, dose adjusted according to response at intervals of 1–3 days. Individual benefit-risk should be assessed when considering doses above 10 mg daily; continued use should be evaluated early in treatment; maximum 15 mg per day
▸ Elderly: Initially, use half the lowest adult dose, then adjust gradually according to response up to maximum 5 mg daily, doses above 5 mg daily should only be considered in patients who have tolerated higher doses and after reassessment of the individual benefit-risk; continued use should be evaluated early in treatment

Acute psychomotor agitation associated with psychotic disorder or manic episodes of bipolar I disorder
▸ BY MOUTH
▸ Adult: 5–10 mg, dose may be repeated after 12 hours if necessary; continued use should be evaluated early in treatment; maximum 20 mg per day
▸ Elderly: Initially 2.5 mg, dose may be repeated after 12 hours if necessary up to maximum 5 mg daily, doses above 5 mg daily should only be considered in patients who have tolerated higher doses and after reassessment of the individual benefit-risk; continued use should be evaluated early in treatment

Rapid control of severe acute psychomotor agitation associated with psychotic disorder or manic episodes of bipolar I disorder [when oral therapy is not appropriate]
▸ BY INTRAMUSCULAR INJECTION
▸ Adult: 5 mg, dose may be repeated hourly if required—up to 15 mg daily is usually sufficient; continued use should be evaluated early in treatment; maximum 20 mg per day
▸ Elderly: 2.5 mg, dose may be repeated hourly if required up to maximum 5 mg daily, doses above 5 mg daily should only be considered in patients who have tolerated higher doses and after reassessment of the individual benefit-risk; continued use should be evaluated early in treatment

Persistent aggression and psychotic symptoms in moderate to severe Alzheimer's dementia and vascular dementia [when non-pharmacological treatments ineffective and there is a risk of harm to self or others]
▸ BY MOUTH
▸ Adult: 0.5–5 mg daily in 1–2 divided doses, dose adjusted according to response at intervals of 1–3 days. Reassess treatment after no more than 6 weeks

▸ Elderly: 500 micrograms daily, reassess treatment after no more than 6 weeks

Severe tic disorders, including Tourette's syndrome [when educational, psychological and other pharmacological treatments ineffective]
▸ BY MOUTH
▸ Adult: 0.5–5 mg daily in 1–2 divided doses, dose adjusted according to response at intervals of 1–7 days. Reassess treatment every 6–12 months
▸ Elderly: Initially, use half the lowest adult dose, then adjust gradually according to response up to maximum 5 mg daily. Reassess treatment every 6–12 months

Mild to moderate chorea in Huntington's disease [when alternatives ineffective or not tolerated]
▸ BY MOUTH
▸ Adult: 2–10 mg daily in 1–2 divided doses, dose adjusted according to response at intervals of 1–3 days
▸ Elderly: Initially, use half the lowest adult dose, then adjust gradually according to response up to maximum 5 mg daily, doses above 5 mg daily should only be considered in patients who have tolerated higher doses and after reassessment of the individual benefit-risk

Mild to moderate chorea in Huntington's disease [when alternatives ineffective or not tolerated and oral therapy inappropriate]
▸ BY INTRAMUSCULAR INJECTION
▸ Adult: 2–5 mg, dose may be repeated hourly if required; maximum 10 mg per day
▸ Elderly: Initially 1 mg, dose may be repeated hourly if required up to maximum 5 mg daily, doses above 5 mg daily should only be considered in patients who have tolerated higher doses and after reassessment of the individual benefit-risk

Restlessness and confusion in palliative care
▸ BY MOUTH
▸ Adult: 2 mg, then 2 mg every 2 hours if required
▸ BY SUBCUTANEOUS INJECTION
▸ Adult: 2.5 mg, then 2.5 mg every 2 hours if required
▸ BY SUBCUTANEOUS INFUSION
▸ Adult: 5–15 mg/24 hours

● UNLICENSED USE Not licensed for use in palliative care.

> IMPORTANT SAFETY INFORMATION
> When prescribing, dispensing or administering, check that this injection is the correct preparation—this preparation is usually used in hospital for the rapid control of an *acute episode* and should **not** be confused with depot preparations which are usually used in the community or clinics for *maintenance* treatment.

● CONTRA-INDICATIONS CNS depression · comatose states · congenital long QT syndrome · dementia with Lewy bodies · history of torsade de pointes · history of ventricular arrhythmia · Parkinson's disease · progressive supranuclear palsy · QTc-interval prolongation · recent acute myocardial infarction · uncompensated heart failure · uncorrected hypokalaemia

● CAUTIONS Bradycardia · electrolyte disturbances (correct before treatment initiation) · family history of QTc-interval prolongation · history of heavy alcohol exposure · hyperthyroidism · hypotension (including orthostatic hypotension) · prolactin-dependent tumours · prolactinaemia · risk factors for stroke

● INTERACTIONS → Appendix 1: haloperidol

● SIDE-EFFECTS
GENERAL SIDE-EFFECTS
▸ **Common or very common** Depression · eye disorders · headache · hypersalivation · nausea · neuromuscular dysfunction · psychotic disorder · vision disorders · weight decreased

▶ **Uncommon** Breast abnormalities · confusion · dyspnoea · gait abnormal · hepatic disorders · hyperhidrosis · menstrual cycle irregularities · muscle complaints · musculoskeletal stiffness · oedema · photosensitivity reaction · restlessness · sexual dysfunction · skin reactions · temperature regulation disorders

▶ **Rare or very rare** Hypoglycaemia · respiratory disorders · SIADH · trismus

▶ **Frequency not known** Hypersensitivity vasculitis · pancytopenia · rhabdomyolysis · thrombocytopenia

SPECIFIC SIDE-EFFECTS

▶ With oral use Angioedema

▶ With parenteral use Hypertension · severe cutaneous adverse reactions (SCARs)

SIDE-EFFECTS, FURTHER INFORMATION Haloperidol is a less sedating antipsychotic.

● PREGNANCY Manufacturer advises it is preferable to avoid—moderate amount of data indicate no malformative or fetal/neonatal toxicity, however there are isolated case reports of birth defects following fetal exposure, mostly in combination with other drugs; reproductive toxicity shown in *animal* studies.

● HEPATIC IMPAIRMENT Manufacturer advises caution.
Dose adjustments Manufacturer advises halve initial dose and then adjust if necessary with smaller increments and at longer intervals.

● RENAL IMPAIRMENT Manufacturer advises use with caution.
Dose adjustments Manufacturer advises consider lower initial dose in severe impairment and then adjust if necessary with smaller increments and at longer intervals.

● MONITORING REQUIREMENTS

▶ Manufacturer advises monitor electrolytes before treatment initiation and periodically during treatment.

▶ Manufacturer advises perform ECG before treatment initiation and assess need for further ECGs during treatment on an individual basis; continuous ECG monitoring is recommended for repeated *intramuscular* doses, and for up to 6 hours after administration of *intramuscular* doses for prophylaxis or treatment of postoperative nausea and vomiting.

● PRESCRIBING AND DISPENSING INFORMATION
Palliative care For further information on the use of haloperidol in palliative care, see www.medicinescomplete. com/#/content/palliative/haloperidol.

● MEDICINAL FORMS There can be variation in the licensing of different medicines containing the same drug. Forms available from special-order manufacturers include: oral suspension, oral solution

Solution for injection

▶ Haloperidol (Non-proprietary)
Haloperidol 5 mg per 1 ml Haloperidol 5mg/1ml solution for injection ampoules | 10 ampoule [PoM] £42.00 DT = £35.00

Oral solution

CAUTIONARY AND ADVISORY LABELS 2

▶ Haloperidol (Non-proprietary)
Haloperidol 1 mg per 1 ml Haloperidol 5mg/5ml oral solution sugar free sugar-free | 100 ml [PoM] £6.48 DT = £6.48 sugar-free | 500 ml [PoM] £32.40
Haloperidol 2 mg per 1 ml Haloperidol 10mg/5ml oral solution sugar free sugar-free | 100 ml [PoM] £46.75 DT = £7.10

▶ Haldol (Janssen-Cilag Ltd)
Haloperidol 2 mg per 1 ml Haldol 2mg/ml oral solution sugar-free | 100 ml [PoM] £4.45 DT = £7.10

▶ Halkid (Thame Laboratories Ltd)
Haloperidol 200 microgram per 1 ml Halkid 200micrograms/ml oral solution sugar-free | 100 ml [PoM] £89.90 DT = £89.90

Tablet

CAUTIONARY AND ADVISORY LABELS 2

▶ Haloperidol (Non-proprietary)
Haloperidol 500 microgram Haloperidol 500microgram tablets | 28 tablet [PoM] £117.00 DT = £104.59

Haloperidol 1.5 mg Haloperidol 1.5mg tablets | 28 tablet [PoM] £14.00 DT = £4.97
Haloperidol 5 mg Haloperidol 5mg tablets | 28 tablet [PoM] £16.00 DT = £5.35
Haloperidol 10 mg Haloperidol 10mg tablets | 28 tablet [PoM] £18.97 DT = £17.55

▶ F 403

Loxapine
25-Apr-2017

● DRUG ACTION Loxapine is a dopamine D_2 and serotonin 5-HT_{2A} receptor antagonist. It also binds to noradrenergic, histaminergic, and cholinergic receptors.

● INDICATIONS AND DOSE
Rapid control of mild-to-moderate agitation in patients with schizophrenia or bipolar disorder (specialist supervision in hospital)

▶ BY INHALATION

▶ Adult: 9.1 mg as a single dose, followed by 9.1 mg after 2 hours if required, alternatively 4.5 mg as a single dose, followed by 4.5 mg after 2 hours if required, lower dose may be given if more appropriate or if the higher dose not previously tolerated

● CONTRA-INDICATIONS Acute respiratory symptoms · asthma · cardiovascular disease · cerebrovascular disease · chronic obstructive pulmonary disease · dehydration—risk of hypotension · elderly patients (especially those with dementia-related psychosis) · hypovolaemia—risk of hypotension

● CAUTIONS Bronchodilator treatment should be available for treatment of possible severe respiratory side-effects (bronchospasm) · history of extrapyramidal symptoms · risk factors for hypoventilation

● INTERACTIONS → Appendix 1: loxapine

● SIDE-EFFECTS

▶ **Common or very common** Fatigue · taste altered · throat irritation

▶ **Uncommon** Bronchospasm · oculogyration · restlessness

▶ **Frequency not known** Dry eye · hypertension · syncope · vision blurred

● PREGNANCY Manufacturer advises use only if potential benefit outweighs risk.

● BREAST FEEDING Manufacturer advises to avoid for 48 hours after dose (express and discard milk produced during this time)—present in milk in *animal* studies.

● MONITORING REQUIREMENTS Manufacturer advises to observe patient during the first hour after each dose for signs and symptoms of bronchospasm.

● DIRECTIONS FOR ADMINISTRATION Manufacturer advises remove pull-tab and wait for green light to turn on (product must be used within 15 minutes of pulling tab); instruct patient to inhale through mouthpiece and then hold breath briefly. When green light turns off, this indicates the dose has been delivered.

● PRESCRIBING AND DISPENSING INFORMATION Educational risk minimisation materials are available for health care professionals.
Adasuve® 4.5 mg inhalation powder may be difficult to obtain.

● MEDICINAL FORMS There can be variation in the licensing of different medicines containing the same drug.
Inhalation powder

▶ Adasuve (Galen Ltd)
Loxapine 9.1 mg Adasuve 9.1mg/dose inhalation powder | 1 dose [PoM] £58.30 (Hospital only)

F 403

Pericyazine

(Periciazine)

● INDICATIONS AND DOSE

Schizophrenia | Psychoses
▸ BY MOUTH
▸ Adult: Initially 75 mg daily in divided doses, then increased in steps of 25 mg every week, adjusted according to response; maximum 300 mg per day
▸ Elderly: Initially 15–30 mg daily in divided doses, then increased in steps of 25 mg every week, adjusted according to response; maximum 300 mg per day

Short-term adjunctive management of severe anxiety, psychomotor agitation, and violent or dangerously impulsive behaviour
▸ BY MOUTH
▸ Adult: Initially 15–30 mg daily in 2 divided doses, adjusted according to response, larger dose to be taken at bedtime
▸ Elderly: Initially 5–10 mg daily in 2 divided doses, adjusted according to response, larger dose to be taken at bedtime

● CONTRA-INDICATIONS CNS depression · comatose states · phaeochromocytoma
● CAUTIONS Hypothyroidism
● INTERACTIONS → Appendix 1: phenothiazines
● SIDE-EFFECTS Atrioventricular block · cardiac arrest · consciousness impaired · contact dermatitis · glucose tolerance impaired · hepatic disorders · hyperglycaemia · hyperthermia · nasal congestion · priapism · respiratory depression
● HEPATIC IMPAIRMENT Can precipitate coma; phenothiazines are hepatotoxic.
● RENAL IMPAIRMENT Avoid in renal impairment.

● MEDICINAL FORMS There can be variation in the licensing of different medicines containing the same drug. Forms available from special-order manufacturers include: oral suspension, oral solution
Oral solution
CAUTIONARY AND ADVISORY LABELS 2
▸ Pericyazine (Non-proprietary)
Pericyazine 2 mg per 1 ml Pericyazine 10mg/5ml oral solution | 100 ml [PoM] £82.80 DT = £82.80
Tablet
CAUTIONARY AND ADVISORY LABELS 2
▸ Pericyazine (Non-proprietary)
Pericyazine 2.5 mg Pericyazine 2.5mg tablets | 84 tablet [PoM] £27.90 DT = £27.90
Pericyazine 10 mg Pericyazine 10mg tablets | 84 tablet [PoM] £72.00 DT = £72.00

F 403

Pimozide

● INDICATIONS AND DOSE

Schizophrenia
▸ BY MOUTH
▸ Adult: Initially 2 mg daily, adjusted according to response, then increased in steps of 2–4 mg at intervals of not less than 1 week; usual dose 2–20 mg daily
▸ Elderly: Initially 1 mg daily, adjusted according to response, increased in steps of 2–4 mg at intervals of not less than 1 week; usual dose 2–20 mg daily

Monosymptomatic hypochondriacal psychosis | Paranoid psychosis
▸ BY MOUTH
▸ Adult: Initially 4 mg daily, adjusted according to response, then increased in steps of 2–4 mg at intervals of not less than 1 week; maximum 16 mg per day
▸ Elderly: Initially 2 mg daily, adjusted according to response, increased in steps of 2–4 mg at intervals of not less than 1 week; maximum 16 mg per day

● CONTRA-INDICATIONS CNS depression · comatose states · history of arrhythmias · history or family history of congenital QT prolongation · phaeochromocytoma
● INTERACTIONS → Appendix 1: pimozide
● SIDE-EFFECTS
▸ Common or very common Appetite decreased · depression · fatigue · headache · hyperhidrosis · hypersalivation · muscle complaints · restlessness · sebaceous gland overactivity · urinary disorders · vision blurred
▸ Uncommon Dysarthria · face oedema · oculogyric crisis · skin reactions
▸ Frequency not known Cardiac arrest · generalised tonic-clonic seizure · glycosuria · hyperglycaemia · hyponatraemia · libido decreased · neck stiffness · temperature regulation disorders
● HEPATIC IMPAIRMENT Manufacturer advises caution.
● RENAL IMPAIRMENT
Dose adjustments Start with small doses in severe renal impairment because of increased cerebral sensitivity.
● MONITORING REQUIREMENTS
▸ ECG monitoring Following reports of sudden unexplained death, an ECG is recommended before treatment. It is also recommended that patients taking pimozide should have an annual ECG (if the QT interval is prolonged, treatment should be reviewed and either withdrawn or dose reduced under close supervision) and that pimozide should not be given with other antipsychotic drugs (including depot preparations), tricyclic antidepressants or other drugs which prolong the QT interval, such as certain antimalarials, antiarrhythmic drugs and certain antihistamines and should not be given with drugs which cause electrolyte disturbances (especially diuretics).

● MEDICINAL FORMS There can be variation in the licensing of different medicines containing the same drug. Forms available from special-order manufacturers include: oral suspension
Tablet
CAUTIONARY AND ADVISORY LABELS 2
▸ Orap (Eumedica Pharmaceuticals)
Pimozide 1 mg Orap 1mg tablets | 100 tablet [PoM] [℥]
Pimozide 4 mg Orap 4mg tablets | 100 tablet [PoM] £40.31 DT = £40.31

F 403

Prochlorperazine

04-Aug-2020

● INDICATIONS AND DOSE

Schizophrenia and other psychoses | Mania
▸ BY MOUTH
▸ Adult: 12.5 mg twice daily for 7 days, dose to be adjusted at intervals of 4–7 days according to response; usual dose 75–100 mg daily
▸ BY DEEP INTRAMUSCULAR INJECTION
▸ Adult: 12.5–25 mg 2–3 times a day

Short-term adjunctive management of severe anxiety
▸ BY MOUTH
▸ Adult: 15–20 mg daily in divided doses; maximum 40 mg per day

Nausea and vomiting, acute attack
▸ BY MOUTH
▸ Adult: Initially 20 mg, then 10 mg after 2 hours

▸ BY DEEP INTRAMUSCULAR INJECTION
▸ Adult: 12.5 mg as required, to be followed if necessary after 6 hours by an oral dose

Nausea and vomiting, prevention
▸ BY MOUTH
▸ Adult: 5–10 mg 2–3 times a day
▸ BY DEEP INTRAMUSCULAR INJECTION
▸ Adult: 12.5 mg as required, to be followed if necessary after 6 hours by an oral dose

Prevention and treatment of nausea and vomiting
▸ BY MOUTH
▸ Child 1–11 years (body-weight 10 kg and above): 250 micrograms/kg 2–3 times a day
▸ Child 12–17 years: 5–10 mg up to 3 times a day if required
▸ BY INTRAMUSCULAR INJECTION
▸ Child 2–4 years: 1.25–2.5 mg up to 3 times a day if required
▸ Child 5–11 years: 5–6.25 mg up to 3 times a day if required
▸ Child 12–17 years: 12.5 mg up to 3 times a day if required

Labyrinthine disorders
▸ BY MOUTH
▸ Adult: 5 mg 3 times a day, increased if necessary to 30 mg daily in divided doses, dose to be increased gradually, then reduced to 5–10 mg daily, dose is reduced after several weeks

Nausea and vomiting in previously diagnosed migraine
▸ BY MOUTH USING BUCCAL TABLET
▸ Child 12–17 years: 3–6 mg twice daily, tablets to be placed high between upper lip and gum and left to dissolve
▸ Adult: 3–6 mg twice daily, tablets to be placed high between upper lip and gum and left to dissolve

Acute migraine
▸ BY MOUTH
▸ Adult: 10 mg for 1 dose, to be taken as soon as migraine symptoms develop

DOSE EQUIVALENCE AND CONVERSION
▸ Doses are expressed as prochlorperazine maleate or mesilate; 1 mg prochlorperazine maleate ≡ 1 mg prochlorperazine mesilate.

● UNLICENSED USE [EvGr] Prochlorperazine is used for the treatment of acute migraine, ⓐ but is not licensed for this indication.
    Injection not licensed for use in children. *Buccastem M*® tablets not licensed for use in children.

● CONTRA-INDICATIONS Avoid oral route in child under 10 kg · CNS depression · comatose states · phaeochromocytoma

● CAUTIONS
GENERAL CAUTIONS Elderly · hypotension (more likely after intramuscular injection)
SPECIFIC CAUTIONS
▸ With systemic use Hypothyroidism (in adults)
CAUTIONS, FURTHER INFORMATION
▸ Elderly Prescription potentially inappropriate (STOPP criteria) in patients with parkinsonism (risk of exacerbating parkinsonian symptoms). See also Prescribing in the elderly p. 33.

● INTERACTIONS → Appendix 1: phenothiazines

● SIDE-EFFECTS
GENERAL SIDE-EFFECTS
▸ **Rare or very rare** Glucose tolerance impaired · hyperglycaemia · hyponatraemia · SIADH
▸ **Frequency not known** Photosensitivity reaction
SPECIFIC SIDE-EFFECTS
▸ **Rare or very rare**
▸ With buccal use Blood disorder · hepatic disorders

▸ **Frequency not known**
▸ With buccal use Oral disorders · skin eruption
▸ With intramuscular use Atrioventricular block · cardiac arrest · eye disorders · jaundice · muscle rigidity · nasal congestion · respiratory depression · skin reactions
▸ With oral use Atrioventricular block · autonomic dysfunction · cardiac arrest · consciousness impaired · hyperthermia · jaundice · muscle rigidity · nasal congestion · oculogyric crisis · respiratory depression · skin reactions
SIDE-EFFECTS, FURTHER INFORMATION Acute dytonias are more common with potent first-generation antipsychotics. The risk is increased in men, young adults, children, antipsychotic-naïve patients, rapid dose escalation, and abrupt treatment discontinuation.

● HEPATIC IMPAIRMENT Manufacturer advises avoid.

● RENAL IMPAIRMENT
Dose adjustments Start with small doses in severe renal impairment because of increased cerebral sensitivity.

● DIRECTIONS FOR ADMINISTRATION
▸ With buccal use Manufacturer advises buccal tablets are placed high between upper lip and gum and left to dissolve.

● PATIENT AND CARER ADVICE
▸ With buccal use Patients or carers should be given advice on how to administer prochlorperazine buccal tablets.

● MEDICINAL FORMS There can be variation in the licensing of different medicines containing the same drug.
Tablet
CAUTIONARY AND ADVISORY LABELS 2
▸ Prochlorperazine (Non-proprietary)
    Prochlorperazine maleate 5 mg Prochlorperazine 5mg tablets | 28 tablet [PoM] £1.98 DT = £1.16 | 84 tablet [PoM] £2.58–£3.68
▸ Stemetil (Sanofi)
    Prochlorperazine maleate 5 mg Stemetil 5mg tablets 28 tablet [PoM] £1.98 DT = £1.16 | 84 tablet [PoM] £5.94
Solution for injection
▸ Stemetil (Sanofi)
    Prochlorperazine mesilate 12.5 mg per 1 ml Stemetil 12.5mg/1ml solution for injection ampoules | 10 ampoule [PoM] £5.23 DT = £5.23
Buccal tablet
CAUTIONARY AND ADVISORY LABELS 2
▸ Prochlorperazine (Non-proprietary)
    Prochlorperazine maleate 3 mg Prochlorperazine 3mg buccal tablets | 8 tablet [PoM] £3.85 | 50 tablet [PoM] £50.27 DT = £28.05
Oral solution
CAUTIONARY AND ADVISORY LABELS 2
▸ Stemetil (Sanofi)
    Prochlorperazine mesilate 1 mg per 1 ml Stemetil 5mg/5ml syrup | 100 ml [PoM] £3.34 DT = £3.34

F 403

Sulpiride
04-Sep-2020

● INDICATIONS AND DOSE
Schizophrenia with predominantly negative symptoms
▸ BY MOUTH
▸ Adult: 200–400 mg twice daily; maximum 800 mg per day
▸ Elderly: Lower initial dose to be given, increased gradually according to response

Schizophrenia with mainly positive symptoms
▸ BY MOUTH
▸ Adult: 200–400 mg twice daily; maximum 2.4 g per day
continued →

4   Nervous system

‣ **Elderly:** Lower initial dose to be given, increased gradually according to response

---

IMPORTANT SAFETY INFORMATION

MHRA/CHM ADVICE: CLOZAPINE AND OTHER ANTIPSYCHOTICS: MONITORING BLOOD CONCENTRATIONS FOR TOXICITY (AUGUST 2020)

Following fatal cases involving toxicity of clozapine and other antipsychotic medicines, the MHRA advises that monitoring blood concentration of sulpiride may be helpful in certain circumstances, such as patients presenting symptoms suggestive of toxicity, or when concomitant medicines may interact to increase blood concentration of sulpiride.

● CONTRA-INDICATIONS CNS depression · comatose states · phaeochromocytoma

● CAUTIONS Aggressive patients (even low doses may aggravate symptoms) · agitated patients (even low doses may aggravate symptoms) · excited patients (even low doses may aggravate symptoms)

● INTERACTIONS → Appendix 1: sulpiride

● SIDE-EFFECTS
  ‣ **Common or very common** Breast abnormalities
  ‣ **Uncommon** Hypersalivation · muscle tone increased · orgasm abnormal
  ‣ **Rare or very rare** Oculogyric crisis
  ‣ **Frequency not known** Cardiac arrest · confusion · dyspnoea · hyponatraemia · SIADH · trismus · urticaria

● RENAL IMPAIRMENT
  Dose adjustments Start with small doses in severe renal impairment because of increased cerebral sensitivity.

● MONITORING REQUIREMENTS Sulpiride does not affect blood pressure to the same extent as other antipsychotic drugs and so blood pressure monitoring is not mandatory for this drug.

● PRESCRIBING AND DISPENSING INFORMATION Flavours of oral liquid formulations may include lemon and aniseed.

● MEDICINAL FORMS There can be variation in the licensing of different medicines containing the same drug. Forms available from special-order manufacturers include: oral suspension, oral solution

Oral solution
CAUTIONARY AND ADVISORY LABELS 2
  ‣ Sulpiride (Non-proprietary)
    Sulpiride 40 mg per 1 ml Sulpiride 200mg/5ml oral solution sugar free sugar-free | 150 ml [PoM] £50.89 DT = £43.61

Tablet
CAUTIONARY AND ADVISORY LABELS 2
  ‣ Sulpiride (Non-proprietary)
    Sulpiride 200 mg Sulpiride 200mg tablets | 30 tablet [PoM] £12.20 DT = £9.26
    Sulpiride 400 mg Sulpiride 400mg tablets | 30 tablet [PoM] £23.50 DT = £22.49

F 403

Trifluoperazine

● INDICATIONS AND DOSE

Schizophrenia and other psychoses | Short-term adjunctive management of psychomotor agitation, excitement, and violent or dangerously impulsive behaviour
  ‣ BY MOUTH
  ‣ **Adult:** Initially 5 mg twice daily, daily dose may be increased by 5 mg after 1 week. If necessary, dose may be further increased in steps of 5 mg at intervals of 3 days. When satisfactory control has been achieved, reduce gradually until an effective maintenance level has been established

‣ **Elderly:** Initially up to 2.5 mg twice daily, daily dose may be increased by 5 mg after 1 week. If necessary, dose may be further increased in steps of 5 mg at intervals of 3 days. When satisfactory control has been achieved, reduce gradually until an effective maintenance level has been established

Short-term adjunctive management of severe anxiety
  ‣ BY MOUTH
  ‣ **Adult:** 2–4 mg daily in divided doses, increased if necessary to 6 mg daily
  ‣ **Elderly:** Up to 2 mg daily in divided doses, increased if necessary to 6 mg daily

Severe nausea and vomiting
  ‣ BY MOUTH
  ‣ **Adult:** 2–4 mg daily in divided doses; maximum 6 mg per day

● CONTRA-INDICATIONS CNS depression · comatose states · phaeochromocytoma

● INTERACTIONS → Appendix 1: phenothiazines

● SIDE-EFFECTS Alertness decreased · anxiety · appetite decreased · blood disorder · cardiac arrest · confusion · fatigue · hyperpyrexia · jaundice cholestatic · lens opacity · muscle weakness · oedema · pancytopenia · photosensitivity reaction · postural hypotension (dose-related) · skin reactions · thrombocytopenia · urinary hesitation · vision blurred · withdrawal syndrome

SIDE-EFFECTS, FURTHER INFORMATION Extrapyramidal symptoms are more frequent at doses exceeding 6mg daily. Acute dystonias are more common with potent first generation antipsychotics. The risk is increased in men, young adults, children, antipsychotic-naïve patients, rapid dose escalation, and abrupt treatment discontinuation.

● HEPATIC IMPAIRMENT Manufacturer advises avoid.

● RENAL IMPAIRMENT
  Dose adjustments Start with small doses in severe renal impairment because of increased cerebral sensitivity.

● MONITORING REQUIREMENTS Trifluoperazine does not affect blood pressure to the same extent as other antipsychotic drugs and so blood pressure monitoring is not mandatory for this drug.

● MEDICINAL FORMS There can be variation in the licensing of different medicines containing the same drug.

Oral solution
CAUTIONARY AND ADVISORY LABELS 2
  ‣ Trifluoperazine (Non-proprietary)
    Trifluoperazine (as Trifluoperazine hydrochloride) 200 microgram per 1 ml Trifluoperazine 1mg/5ml oral solution sugar free sugar-free | 200 ml [PoM] £125.00 DT = £125.00
    Trifluoperazine (as Trifluoperazine hydrochloride) 1 mg per 1 ml Trifluoperazine 5mg/5ml oral solution sugar free sugar-free | 150 ml [PoM] £30.00 DT = £30.00

Tablet
CAUTIONARY AND ADVISORY LABELS 2
  ‣ Trifluoperazine (Non-proprietary)
    Trifluoperazine (as Trifluoperazine hydrochloride) 1 mg Trifluoperazine 1mg tablets | 112 tablet [PoM] £59.12–£99.80 DT = £59.12
    Trifluoperazine (as Trifluoperazine hydrochloride) 5 mg Trifluoperazine 5mg tablets | 112 tablet [PoM] £134.89–£165.00 DT = £134.89

F 403

Zuclopenthixol

● INDICATIONS AND DOSE

Schizophrenia and other psychoses
  ‣ BY MOUTH
  ‣ **Adult:** Initially 20–30 mg daily in divided doses, increased if necessary up to 150 mg daily; usual

maintenance 20–50 mg daily (max. per dose 40 mg), for debilitated patients, use elderly dose
▸ **Elderly:** Initially 5–15 mg daily in divided doses, increased if necessary up to 150 mg daily; usual maintenance 20–50 mg daily (max. per dose 40 mg)

● CONTRA-INDICATIONS Apathetic states · CNS depression · comatose states · phaeochromocytoma · withdrawn states

● CAUTIONS Hyperthyroidism · hypothyroidism

● INTERACTIONS → Appendix 1: zuclopenthixol

● SIDE-EFFECTS Anxiety · appetite abnormal · asthenia · concentration impaired · confusion · depression · diarrhoea · dyspnoea · eye disorders · fever · flatulence · gait abnormal · gastrointestinal discomfort · glucose tolerance impaired · headaches · hepatic disorders · hot flush · hyperacusia · hyperglycaemia · hyperhidrosis · hyperlipidaemia · hypersalivation · hypothermia · malaise · memory loss · muscle complaints · nasal congestion · nausea · neuromuscular dysfunction · pain · palpitations · paraesthesia · photosensitivity reaction · reflexes increased · seborrhoea · sexual dysfunction · skin reactions · sleep disorders · speech disorder · syncope · thirst · thrombocytopenia · tinnitus · urinary disorders · vertigo · vision disorders · vulvovaginal dryness · weight decreased · withdrawal syndrome

● HEPATIC IMPAIRMENT Manufacturer advises caution—monitor serum drug concentration.
Dose adjustments Manufacturer advises dose reduction of half the recommended dose.

● RENAL IMPAIRMENT
Dose adjustments Halve dose in renal failure; smaller starting doses used in severe renal impairment because of increased cerebral sensitivity.

● MEDICINAL FORMS There can be variation in the licensing of different medicines containing the same drug.
Oral drops
▸ Ciatyl-Z (Imported (Germany))
Zuclopenthixol (as Zuclopenthixol dihydrochloride) 20 mg per 1 ml Ciatyl-Z 20mg/ml oral drops | 30 ml [PoM] Ⓢ
Tablet
CAUTIONARY AND ADVISORY LABELS 2
▸ Clopixol (Lundbeck Ltd)
Zuclopenthixol (as Zuclopenthixol dihydrochloride) 2 mg Clopixol 2mg tablets | 100 tablet [PoM] £3.14 DT = £3.14
Zuclopenthixol (as Zuclopenthixol dihydrochloride) 10 mg Clopixol 10mg tablets | 100 tablet [PoM] £8.06 DT = £8.06
Zuclopenthixol (as Zuclopenthixol dihydrochloride) 25 mg Clopixol 25mg tablets | 100 tablet [PoM] £16.13 DT = £16.13

⚑ 403

Zuclopenthixol acetate
20-Nov-2019

● **INDICATIONS AND DOSE**

Short-term management of acute psychosis | Short-term management of mania | Short-term management of exacerbation of chronic psychosis
▸ BY DEEP INTRAMUSCULAR INJECTION
▸ **Adult:** 50–150 mg, then 50–150 mg after 2–3 days if required, (1 additional dose may be needed 1–2 days after the first injection); maximum cumulative dose 400 mg in 2 weeks and maximum 4 injections; maximum duration of treatment 2 weeks—if maintenance treatment necessary change to an oral antipsychotic 2–3 days after last injection, or to a longer acting antipsychotic depot injection given concomitantly with last injection of zuclopenthixol acetate; to be administered into the gluteal muscle or lateral thigh
▸ **Elderly:** 50–100 mg, then 50–100 mg after 2–3 days if required, (1 additional dose may be needed 1–2 days after the first injection); maximum cumulative dose

400 mg in 2 weeks and maximum 4 injections; maximum duration of treatment 2 weeks—if maintenance treatment necessary change to an oral antipsychotic 2–3 days after last injection, or to a longer acting antipsychotic depot injection given concomitantly with last injection of zuclopenthixol acetate; to be administered into the gluteal muscle or lateral thigh

---

IMPORTANT SAFETY INFORMATION
When prescribing, dispensing, or administering, check that this is the correct preparation—this preparation is usually used in hospital for an *acute episode* and should **not** be confused with depot preparations which are usually used in the community or clinics for *maintenance* treatment.

SAFE PRACTICE
Zuclopenthixol acetate has been confused with zuclopenthixol decanoate; care must be taken to ensure the correct drug is prescribed and dispensed.

● CONTRA-INDICATIONS CNS depression · comatose states · phaeochromocytoma

● CAUTIONS Hyperthyroidism · hypothyroidism

● INTERACTIONS → Appendix 1: zuclopenthixol

● SIDE-EFFECTS Anxiety · appetite abnormal · asthenia · concentration impaired · confusion · depression · diarrhoea · dyspnoea · eye disorders · fever · flatulence · gait abnormal · gastrointestinal discomfort · glucose tolerance impaired · headaches · hepatic disorders · hot flush · hyperacusia · hyperglycaemia · hyperhidrosis · hyperlipidaemia · hypersalivation · hypothermia (dose-related) · malaise · memory loss · muscle complaints · nasal congestion · nausea · neuromuscular dysfunction · pain · palpitations · paraesthesia · photosensitivity reaction · reflexes increased · seborrhoea · sexual dysfunction · skin reactions · sleep disorders · speech disorder · syncope · thirst · thrombocytopenia · tinnitus · urinary disorders · vertigo · vision disorders · vulvovaginal dryness · weight decreased · withdrawal syndrome

● HEPATIC IMPAIRMENT Manufacturer advises caution—monitor serum drug concentration.
Dose adjustments Manufacturer advises dose reduction to half the recommended dose.

● RENAL IMPAIRMENT
Dose adjustments Start with small doses in severe renal impairment because of increased cerebral sensitivity.

● MEDICINAL FORMS There can be variation in the licensing of different medicines containing the same drug.
Solution for injection
▸ Clopixol Acuphase (Lundbeck Ltd)
Zuclopenthixol acetate 50 mg per 1 ml Clopixol Acuphase 50mg/1ml solution for injection ampoules | 5 ampoule [PoM] £24.21 DT = £24.21 (Hospital only)

ANTIPSYCHOTICS ⟩ FIRST-GENERATION (DEPOT INJECTIONS)

⚑ 403

Flupentixol decanoate
22-Oct-2020

(Flupenthixol Decanoate)

● **INDICATIONS AND DOSE**

Maintenance in schizophrenia and other psychoses
▸ BY DEEP INTRAMUSCULAR INJECTION
▸ **Adult:** Test dose 20 mg, dose to be injected into the upper outer buttock or lateral thigh, then 20–40 mg after at least 7 days, then 20–40 mg every 2–4 weeks, adjusted according to response, usual continued →

maintenance dose 50 mg every 4 weeks to 300 mg every 2 weeks; maximum 400 mg per week
- Elderly: Dose is initially quarter to half adult dose

- CONTRA-INDICATIONS Children · CNS depression · comatose states · excitable patients · overactive patients
- CAUTIONS An alternative antipsychotic may be necessary if symptoms such as aggression or agitation appear · hyperthyroidism · hypothyroidism · phaeochromocytoma · when transferring from oral to depot therapy, the dose by mouth should be reduced gradually
- INTERACTIONS → Appendix 1: flupentixol
- SIDE-EFFECTS
- **Common or very common** Appetite abnormal · asthenia · concentration impaired · depression · diarrhoea · dyspnoea · gastrointestinal discomfort · headache · hyperhidrosis · hypersalivation · muscle complaints · nervousness · palpitations · sexual dysfunction · skin reactions · urinary disorder · vision disorders
- **Uncommon** Confusion · flatulence · hot flush · nausea · oculogyration · photosensitivity reaction · speech disorder
- **Rare or very rare** Glucose tolerance impaired · hyperglycaemia · jaundice · thrombocytopenia
- **Frequency not known** Suicidal behaviours

  SIDE-EFFECTS, FURTHER INFORMATION Side-effects may persist until the drug has been cleared from its depot site.
- HEPATIC IMPAIRMENT Manufacturer advises caution—monitor serum drug concentration.

  Dose adjustments Manufacturer advises initiate at low dose orally to check for tolerability before switching to depot formulation.
- RENAL IMPAIRMENT

  Dose adjustments Start with small doses in severe renal impairment because of increased cerebral sensitivity.
- MONITORING REQUIREMENTS Treatment requires careful monitoring for optimum effect.
- DIRECTIONS FOR ADMINISTRATION In general, manufacturers advise not more than 2–3 mL of oily injection should be administered at any one site (consult product literature). Use correct injection technique (including use of z-track technique) and rotate injection sites. When initiating therapy with sustained-release preparations of conventional antipsychotics, expert sources advise patients should first be given a small test-dose as undesirable side-effects are prolonged.

- MEDICINAL FORMS There can be variation in the licensing of different medicines containing the same drug.

  Solution for injection
  - Depixol (Lundbeck Ltd)

    Flupentixol decanoate 20 mg per 1 ml Depixol 40mg/2ml solution for injection ampoules | 10 ampoule [PoM] £25.39 DT = £25.39
    Depixol 20mg/1ml solution for injection ampoules | 10 ampoule [PoM] £15.17 DT = £15.17
    Flupentixol decanoate 100 mg per 1 ml Depixol Conc 100mg/1ml solution for injection ampoules | 10 ampoule [PoM] £62.51 DT = £62.51
    Flupentixol decanoate 200 mg per 1 ml Depixol Low Volume 200mg/1ml solution for injection ampoules | 5 ampoule [PoM] £97.59 DT = £97.59
  - Psytixol (Mylan)

    Flupentixol decanoate 20 mg per 1 ml Psytixol 40mg/2ml solution for injection ampoules | 10 ampoule [PoM] £25.38 DT = £25.39
    Psytixol 20mg/1ml solution for injection ampoules | 10 ampoule [PoM] £15.16 DT = £15.17
    Flupentixol decanoate 100 mg per 1 ml Psytixol 50mg/0.5ml solution for injection ampoules | 10 ampoule [PoM] £34.12 DT = £34.12
    Psytixol 100mg/1ml solution for injection ampoules | 10 ampoule [PoM] £62.50 DT = £62.51
    Flupentixol decanoate 200 mg per 1 ml Psytixol 200mg/1ml solution for injection ampoules | 5 ampoule [PoM] £97.58 DT = £97.59

Fluphenazine decanoate

403 | 22-Oct-2020

- **INDICATIONS AND DOSE**

  Maintenance in schizophrenia and other psychoses
  - BY DEEP INTRAMUSCULAR INJECTION
  - Adult: Test dose 12.5 mg, dose to be administered into the gluteal muscle, then 12.5–100 mg after 4–7 days, then 12.5–100 mg every 14–35 days, adjusted according to response
  - Elderly: Test dose 6.25 mg, dose to be administered into the gluteal muscle, then 12.5–100 mg after 4–7 days, then 12.5–100 mg every 14–35 days, adjusted according to response

- CONTRA-INDICATIONS Children · CNS depression · comatose states · marked cerebral atherosclerosis · phaeochromocytoma
- CAUTIONS Hypothyroidism · QT-interval prolongation · when transferring from oral to depot therapy, the dose by mouth should be reduced gradually
- INTERACTIONS → Appendix 1: phenothiazines
- SIDE-EFFECTS Acute kidney injury · blood disorder · cognitive impairment · epileptiform seizure · headache · hepatic disorders · hyponatraemia · lens opacity · leucocytosis · nasal congestion · oculogyric crisis · oedema · oligomenorrhoea · sexual dysfunction · SIADH · skin pigmentation change · systemic lupus erythematosus (SLE) · temperature regulation disorder · thrombocytopenia · urinary disorders · vision blurred

  SIDE-EFFECTS, FURTHER INFORMATION Side-effects may persist until the drug has been cleared from its depot site
- HEPATIC IMPAIRMENT Manufacturer advises caution; avoid in hepatic failure.
- RENAL IMPAIRMENT Manufacturer advises caution. Avoid in renal failure.

  Dose adjustments Start with small doses of antipsychotic drugs in severe renal impairment because of increased cerebral sensitivity.
- MONITORING REQUIREMENTS Treatment requires careful monitoring for optimum effect.
- DIRECTIONS FOR ADMINISTRATION In general, manufacturers advise not more than 2–3 mL of oily injection should be administered at any one site (consult product literature). Use correct injection technique (including use of z-track technique) and rotate injection sites. When initiating therapy with sustained-release preparations of conventional antipsychotics, expert sources advise patients should first be given a small test-dose as undesirable side-effects are prolonged.

- MEDICINAL FORMS There can be variation in the licensing of different medicines containing the same drug.

  Solution for injection
  EXCIPIENTS: May contain Sesame oil
  - Modecate (Imported (Germany))

    Fluphenazine decanoate 25 mg per 1 ml Modecate 25mg/1ml solution for injection ampoules | 5 ampoule [PoM] [S]
    Fluphenazine decanoate 100 mg per 1 ml Modecate Concentrate 100mg/1ml solution for injection ampoules | 5 ampoule [PoM] [S] DT = £43.73

F 403

Haloperidol decanoate

22-Oct-2020

- ● **INDICATIONS AND DOSE**

Maintenance in schizophrenia and schizoaffective disorder [in patients currently stabilised on oral haloperidol]

- ▶ BY DEEP INTRAMUSCULAR INJECTION
- ▶ Adult: Initially 25–150 mg every 4 weeks, initial dose should be based on previous daily dose of oral haloperidol (10–15 times the daily dose of oral haloperidol is recommended), adjusted in steps of up to 50 mg every 4 weeks if required, adjustment of the dosing interval may be required, depending on individual patient response; usual maintenance 50–200 mg every 4 weeks (max. per dose 300 mg every 4 weeks), dose to be administered into gluteal muscle, the individual benefit-risk should be assessed when considering doses above 200 mg every 4 weeks, if supplementation with oral haloperidol is required, the combined total dose of haloperidol from both formulations must not exceed the corresponding maximum oral haloperidol dose of 20 mg per day
- ▶ Elderly: Initially 12.5–25 mg every 4 weeks, increased if necessary to 25–75 mg every 4 weeks, adjustment of the dosing interval may be required, depending on individual patient response, dose to be administered into gluteal muscle, doses above 75 mg every 4 weeks should only be considered in patients who have tolerated higher doses and after reassessment of the individual benefit-risk, if supplementation with oral haloperidol is required, the combined total dose of haloperidol from both formulations must not exceed the corresponding maximum oral haloperidol dose of 5 mg per day, or the previously administered oral haloperidol dose in patients who have received long-term treatment with oral haloperidol

DOSE EQUIVALENCE AND CONVERSION

- ▶ A range of equivalent doses is quoted in the literature; the consensus is that 2 mg per day of *oral* haloperidol is approximately equivalent to 15 mg per week of haloperidol decanoate *depot injection.*

IMPORTANT SAFETY INFORMATION
When prescribing, dispensing or administering, check that this is the correct preparation—this preparation is used for *maintenance* treatment and should **not** be used for the rapid control of an *acute episode.*

- ● CONTRA-INDICATIONS CNS depression · comatose states · congenital long QT syndrome · dementia with Lewy bodies · history of torsade de pointes · history of ventricular arrhythmia · Parkinson's disease · progressive supranuclear palsy · QT-interval prolongation · recent acute myocardial infarction · uncompensated heart failure · uncorrected hypokalaemia
- ● CAUTIONS Bradycardia · electrolyte disturbances (correct before treatment initiation) · family history of QTc-interval prolongation · history of heavy alcohol exposure · hyperthyroidism · hypotension (including orthostatic hypotension) · prolactin-dependent tumours · prolactinaemia · risk factors for stroke · when transferring from oral to depot therapy, the dose by mouth should be reduced gradually
- ● INTERACTIONS → Appendix 1: haloperidol
- ● SIDE-EFFECTS
- ▶ **Common or very common** Depression · hypersalivation · muscle complaints · sexual dysfunction
- ▶ **Uncommon** Eye disorders · headache · neuromuscular dysfunction · vision disorders

- ▶ **Frequency not known** Angioedema · breast abnormalities · cardiac arrest · confusion · dyspnoea · gait abnormal · hepatic disorders · hyperhidrosis · hypersensitivity vasculitis · hypoglycaemia · menstrual cycle irregularities · musculoskeletal stiffness · nausea · oedema · pancytopenia · photosensitivity reaction · psychotic disorder · respiratory disorders · restlessness · rhabdomyolysis · SIADH · skin reactions · temperature regulation disorders · thrombocytopenia · trismus · weight decreased

SIDE-EFFECTS, FURTHER INFORMATION Haloperidol is a less sedating antipsychotic.

- ● PREGNANCY Manufacturer advises it is preferable to avoid—moderate amount of data indicate no malformative or fetal/neonatal toxicity, however there are isolated case reports of birth defects following fetal exposure, mostly in combination with other drugs; reproductive toxicity shown in *animal* studies.
- ● HEPATIC IMPAIRMENT Manufacturer advises caution. **Dose adjustments** Manufacturer advises halve initial dose and then adjust if necessary with smaller increments and at longer intervals.
- ● RENAL IMPAIRMENT Manufacturer advises use with caution. **Dose adjustments** Manufacturer advises consider lower initial dose in severe impairment and then adjust if necessary with smaller increments and at longer intervals.
- ● MONITORING REQUIREMENTS
- ▶ Manufacturer advises perform ECG before treatment initiation and assess need for further ECGs during treatment on an individual basis.
- ▶ Manufacturer advises monitor electrolytes before treatment initiation and periodically during treatment.
- ● DIRECTIONS FOR ADMINISTRATION In general, manufacturers advise not more than 2–3 mL of oily injection should be administered at any one site. Use correct injection technique (including use of z-track technique) and rotate injection sites. When initiating therapy with sustained-release preparations of conventional antipsychotics, expert sources advise patients should first be given a small test-dose as undesirable side-effects are prolonged.

- ● MEDICINAL FORMS There can be variation in the licensing of different medicines containing the same drug.
Solution for injection
EXCIPIENTS: May contain Benzyl alcohol, sesame oil
- ▶ Haldol decanoate (Janssen-Cilag Ltd)
Haloperidol (as Haloperidol decanoate) 50 mg per 1 ml Haldol Decanoate 50mg/1ml solution for injection ampoules | 5 ampoule [PoM] £19.06 DT = £19.06
Haloperidol (as Haloperidol decanoate) 100 mg per 1 ml Haldol Decanoate 100mg/1ml solution for injection ampoules | 5 ampoule [PoM] £25.26 DT = £25.26

F 403

Zuclopenthixol decanoate

22-Oct-2020

- ● **INDICATIONS AND DOSE**

Maintenance in schizophrenia and paranoid psychoses

- ▶ BY DEEP INTRAMUSCULAR INJECTION
- ▶ Adult: Test dose 100 mg, dose to be administered into the upper outer buttock or lateral thigh, followed by 200–500 mg after at least 7 days, then 200–500 mg every 1–4 weeks, adjusted according to response, higher doses of more than 500mg can be used: do not exceed 600 mg weekly
- ▶ Elderly: A quarter to half usual starting dose to be used

IMPORTANT SAFETY INFORMATION
When prescribing, dispensing, or administering, check that this is the correct preparation—this preparation is

4

Nervous system

used for *maintenance* treatment and should **not** be used for the short-term management of an *acute episode*.

SAFE PRACTICE
Zuclopenthixol decanoate has been confused with zuclopenthixol acetate; care must be taken to ensure the correct drug is prescribed and dispensed.

- CONTRA-INDICATIONS CNS depression · comatose states · phaeochromocytoma
- CAUTIONS Hyperthyroidism · hypothyroidism · QT interval prolongation · when transferring from oral to depot therapy, the dose by mouth should be reduced gradually
- INTERACTIONS → Appendix 1: zuclopenthixol
- SIDE-EFFECTS Anxiety · appetite abnormal · asthenia · concentration impaired · confusion · depression · diarrhoea · dyspnoea · eye disorders · fever · flatulence · gait abnormal · gastrointestinal discomfort · glucose tolerance impaired · headaches · hepatic disorders · hot flush · hyperacusia · hyperglycaemia · hyperhidrosis · hyperlipidaemia · hypersalivation · hypothermia · malaise · memory loss · muscle complaints · nasal congestion · nausea · neuromuscular dysfunction · pain · palpitations · paraesthesia · photosensitivity reaction · reflexes increased · seborrhoea · sexual dysfunction · skin reactions · sleep disorders · speech disorder · syncope · thirst · thrombocytopenia · tinnitus · urinary disorders · vertigo · vision disorders · vulvovaginal dryness · weight decreased · withdrawal syndrome

SIDE-EFFECTS, FURTHER INFORMATION Side-effects may persist until the drug has been cleared from its depot site.
- HEPATIC IMPAIRMENT Manufacturer advises caution—monitor serum drug concentration.
Dose adjustments Manufacturer advises dose reduction to half the recommended dose.
- RENAL IMPAIRMENT
Dose adjustments Start with small doses in severe renal impairment because of increased cerebral sensitivity.
- MONITORING REQUIREMENTS Treatment requires careful monitoring for optimum effect.
- DIRECTIONS FOR ADMINISTRATION In general, manufacturers advise not more than 2–3 mL of oily injection should be administered at any one site (consult product literature). Use correct injection technique (including use of z-track technique) and rotate injection sites. When initiating therapy with sustained-release preparations of conventional antipsychotics, expert sources advise patients should first be given a small test-dose as undesirable side-effects are prolonged.

- MEDICINAL FORMS There can be variation in the licensing of different medicines containing the same drug.
Solution for injection
- Clopixol (Lundbeck Ltd)
  Zuclopenthixol decanoate 200 mg per 1 ml Clopixol 200mg/1ml solution for injection ampoules | 10 ampoule PoM £31.51 DT = £31.51
  Zuclopenthixol decanoate 500 mg per 1 ml Clopixol Conc 500mg/1ml solution for injection ampoules | 5 ampoule PoM £37.18 DT = £37.18

ANTIPSYCHOTICS ⟩ SECOND-GENERATION
F 403

Amisulpride

09-Sep-2020

- DRUG ACTION Amisulpride is a selective dopamine receptor antagonist with high affinity for mesolimbic D_2 and D_3 receptors.

- INDICATIONS AND DOSE
Acute psychotic episode in schizophrenia
▸ BY MOUTH
  ▸ Adult: 400–800 mg daily in 2 divided doses, adjusted according to response; maximum 1.2 g per day
Schizophrenia with predominantly negative symptoms
▸ BY MOUTH
  ▸ Adult: 50–300 mg daily

IMPORTANT SAFETY INFORMATION
MHRA/CHM ADVICE: CLOZAPINE AND OTHER ANTIPSYCHOTICS: MONITORING BLOOD CONCENTRATIONS FOR TOXICITY (AUGUST 2020)
Following fatal cases involving toxicity of clozapine and other antipsychotic medicines, the MHRA advises that monitoring blood concentration of amisulpride may be helpful in certain circumstances, such as patients presenting symptoms suggestive of toxicity, or when concomitant medicines may interact to increase blood concentration of amisulpride.

- CONTRA-INDICATIONS CNS depression · comatose states · phaeochromocytoma · prolactin-dependent tumours
- INTERACTIONS → Appendix 1: antipsychotics, second generation
- SIDE-EFFECTS
  ▸ **Common or very common** Anxiety · breast pain · hypersalivation · muscle rigidity · nausea · oculogyric crisis · orgasm abnormal · trismus
  ▸ **Uncommon** Hyperglycaemia
  ▸ **Frequency not known** Angioedema · bone disorders · cardiac arrest · confusion · dyslipidaemia · hyponatraemia · nasal congestion · neoplasms · SIADH · urticaria · vision blurred
- PREGNANCY Avoid.
- BREAST FEEDING Avoid—no information available.
- RENAL IMPAIRMENT No information available if eGFR less than 10 mL/minute/1.73 m².
Dose adjustments Halve dose if eGFR 30–60 mL/minute/1.73 m². Use one-third dose if eGFR 10–30 mL/minute/1.73 m².
- MONITORING REQUIREMENTS Amisulpride does not affect blood pressure to the same extent as other antipsychotic drugs and so blood pressure monitoring is not mandatory for this drug.
- PRESCRIBING AND DISPENSING INFORMATION Flavours of oral liquid formulations may include caramel.

- MEDICINAL FORMS There can be variation in the licensing of different medicines containing the same drug. Forms available from special-order manufacturers include: oral suspension, oral solution
Oral solution
CAUTIONARY AND ADVISORY LABELS 2
- Amisulpride (Non-proprietary)
  Amisulpride 100 mg per 1 ml Amisulpride 100mg/ml oral solution sugar free sugar-free | 60 ml PoM £88.50 DT = £88.42
- Solian (Sanofi)
  Amisulpride 100 mg per 1 ml Solian 100mg/ml oral solution sugar-free | 60 ml PoM £33.76 DT = £88.42

Tablet

CAUTIONARY AND ADVISORY LABELS 2

▶ Amisulpride (Non-proprietary)

Amisulpride 50 mg Amisulpride 50mg tablets | 60 tablet [PoM] £19.74 DT = £4.51

Amisulpride 100 mg Amisulpride 100mg tablets | 60 tablet [PoM] £39.48 DT = £7.11

Amisulpride 200 mg Amisulpride 200mg tablets | 60 tablet [PoM] £66.00 DT = £10.49

Amisulpride 400 mg Amisulpride 400mg tablets | 60 tablet [PoM] £132.00 DT = £42.08

▶ Solian (Sanofi)

Amisulpride 50 mg Solian 50 tablets | 60 tablet [PoM] £22.76 DT = £4.51

Amisulpride 100 mg Solian 100 tablets | 60 tablet [PoM] £35.29 DT = £7.11

Amisulpride 200 mg Solian 200 tablets | 60 tablet [PoM] £58.99 DT = £10.49

Amisulpride 400 mg Solian 400 tablets | 60 tablet [PoM] £117.97 DT = £42.08

☞ 403

Aripiprazole
22-Oct-2020

● DRUG ACTION Aripiprazole is a dopamine D_2 partial agonist with weak $5\text{-}HT_{1a}$ partial agonism and $5\text{-}HT_{2A}$ receptor antagonism.

● **INDICATIONS AND DOSE**

Maintenance of schizophrenia in patients stabilised with oral aripiprazole (CYP2D6 poor metabolisers)

▶ BY INTRAMUSCULAR INJECTION

▶ Adult: 300 mg every month, to be injected into the gluteal or deltoid muscle, minimum of 26 days between injections, treatment with 10–20 mg oral aripiprazole daily should be continued for 14 consecutive days after the first injection, for dose adjustment due to side-effects and for advice on missed doses, consult product literature

Maintenance of schizophrenia in patients stabilised with oral aripiprazole

▶ BY INTRAMUSCULAR INJECTION

▶ Adult: 400 mg every month, to be injected into the gluteal or deltoid muscle, minimum of 26 days between injections, treatment with 10–20 mg oral aripiprazole daily should be continued for 14 consecutive days after the first injection, for dose adjustment due to side-effects and for advice on missed doses, consult product literature

Schizophrenia

▶ BY MOUTH

▶ Adult: 10–15 mg once daily; usual dose 15 mg once daily (max. per dose 30 mg once daily)

Treatment and recurrence prevention of mania

▶ BY MOUTH

▶ Adult: 15 mg once daily, increased if necessary up to 30 mg once daily

Control of agitation and disturbed behaviour in schizophrenia

▶ BY INTRAMUSCULAR INJECTION

▶ Adult: Initially 5.25–15 mg for 1 dose, alternatively usual dose 9.75 mg for 1 dose, followed by 5.25–15 mg after 2 hours if required, maximum 3 injections daily; maximum daily combined oral and parenteral dose 30 mg

DOSE ADJUSTMENTS DUE TO INTERACTIONS

▶ With oral use Manufacturer advises double the dose with concurrent use of potent inducers of CYP3A4. Manufacturer advises reduce dose by half with concurrent use of potent inhibitors of CYP3A4 or CYP2D6.

▶ With intramuscular use For dose adjustments due to concurrent use of interacting drugs—consult product literature.

IMPORTANT SAFETY INFORMATION

When prescribing, dispensing, or administering, check that the correct preparation is used—the preparation usually used in hospital for the rapid control of an *acute episode* (solution for injection containing aripiprazole 7.5 mg/mL) should **not** be confused with depot preparations (aripiprazole 400-mg vial with solvent), which are usually used in the community or clinics for *maintenance treatment.*

MHRA/CHM ADVICE: CLOZAPINE AND OTHER ANTIPSYCHOTICS: MONITORING BLOOD CONCENTRATIONS FOR TOXICITY (AUGUST 2020)

Following fatal cases involving toxicity of clozapine and other antipsychotic medicines, the MHRA advises that monitoring blood concentration of aripiprazole may be helpful in certain circumstances, such as patients presenting symptoms suggestive of toxicity, or when concomitant medicines may interact to increase blood concentration of aripiprazole.

● CONTRA-INDICATIONS CNS depression · comatose state · phaeochromocytoma

● CAUTIONS

GENERAL CAUTIONS Cerebrovascular disease · elderly (reduce initial dose)

SPECIFIC CAUTIONS

▶ With intramuscular use when transferring from oral to depot therapy, the dose by mouth should be reduced gradually

● INTERACTIONS → Appendix 1: antipsychotics, second generation

● SIDE-EFFECTS

▶ **Common or very common** Anxiety · appetite abnormal · diabetes mellitus · fatigue · gastrointestinal discomfort · headache · hypersalivation · nausea · vision disorders

▶ **Uncommon** Depression · hiccups · hyperglycaemia · sexual dysfunction

▶ **Frequency not known** Aggression · alopecia · cardiac arrest · chest pain · diabetic hyperosmolar coma · diabetic ketoacidosis · diarrhoea · dysphagia · generalised tonic-clonic seizure · hepatic disorders · hyperhidrosis · hypertension · hyponatraemia · laryngospasm · musculoskeletal stiffness · myalgia · oropharyngeal spasm · pancreatitis · pathological gambling · peripheral oedema · photosensitivity reaction · pneumonia aspiration · rhabdomyolysis · serotonin syndrome · speech disorder · suicidal behaviours · syncope · temperature regulation disorder · thrombocytopenia · urinary incontinence · weight decreased

● PREGNANCY Use only if potential benefit outweighs risk.

● BREAST FEEDING Manufacturer advises avoid—present in milk.

● HEPATIC IMPAIRMENT Manufacturer advises caution in severe impairment (oral treatment preferred to intramuscular administration; limited information available).

● MONITORING REQUIREMENTS

▶ Aripiprazole does not affect blood pressure to the same extent as other antipsychotic drugs and so blood pressure monitoring is not mandatory for this drug.

▶ With intramuscular use Treatment requires careful monitoring for optimum effect.

● DIRECTIONS FOR ADMINISTRATION

▶ With oral use Orodispersible tablets should be placed on the tongue and allowed to dissolve, or be dispersed in water and swallowed.

4

Nervous system

‣ With intramuscular use Use correct injection technique (including the use of z-track technique) and rotate injection sites.

● PATIENT AND CARER ADVICE

‣ With oral use Patients or carers should be given advice on how to administer aripiprazole orodispersible tablets.

● NATIONAL FUNDING/ACCESS DECISIONS

For full details see funding body website

Scottish Medicines Consortium (SMC) decisions

‣ Aripiprazole prolonged-release suspension for injection (*Abilify Maintena*®) for maintenance treatment of schizophrenia in adult patients stabilised with oral aripiprazole (May 2014) SMC No. 962/14 Recommended

● MEDICINAL FORMS There can be variation in the licensing of different medicines containing the same drug. Forms available from special-order manufacturers include: oral solution

Tablet

CAUTIONARY AND ADVISORY LABELS 2

‣ Aripiprazole (Non-proprietary)

Aripiprazole 5 mg Aripiprazole 5mg tablets | 28 tablet [PoM] £96.04 DT = £1.34

Aripiprazole 10 mg Aripiprazole 10mg tablets | 28 tablet [PoM] £96.04 DT = £1.40

Aripiprazole 15 mg Aripiprazole 15mg tablets | 28 tablet [PoM] £96.04 DT = £1.55

Aripiprazole 30 mg Aripiprazole 30mg tablets | 28 tablet [PoM] £192.08 DT = £13.74

‣ Abilify (Otsuka Pharmaceuticals (U.K.) Ltd)

Aripiprazole 5 mg Abilify 5mg tablets | 28 tablet [PoM] £96.04 DT = £1.34

Aripiprazole 10 mg Abilify 10mg tablets | 28 tablet [PoM] £96.04 DT = £1.40

Aripiprazole 15 mg Abilify 15mg tablets | 28 tablet [PoM] £96.04 DT = £1.55

Aripiprazole 30 mg Abilify 30mg tablets | 28 tablet [PoM] £192.08 DT = £13.74

‣ Arpoya (Torrent Pharma (UK) Ltd)

Aripiprazole 5 mg Arpoya 5mg tablets | 28 tablet [PoM] £96.04 DT = £1.34

Aripiprazole 10 mg Arpoya 10mg tablets | 28 tablet [PoM] £96.04 DT = £1.40

Aripiprazole 15 mg Arpoya 15mg tablets | 28 tablet [PoM] £96.04 DT = £1.55

Aripiprazole 30 mg Arpoya 30mg tablets | 28 tablet [PoM] £192.08 DT = £13.74

Solution for injection

‣ Abilify (Otsuka Pharmaceuticals (U.K.) Ltd)

Aripiprazole 7.5 mg per 1 ml Abilify 9.75mg/1.3ml solution for injection vials | 1 vial [PoM] £3.43

Oral solution

CAUTIONARY AND ADVISORY LABELS 2

‣ Aripiprazole (Non-proprietary)

Aripiprazole 1 mg per 1 ml Aripiprazole 1mg/ml oral solution sugar free sugar-free | 150 ml [PoM] £101.20
Aripiprazole 1mg/ml oral solution | 150 ml [PoM] £102.90 DT = £99.82

‣ Abilify (Otsuka Pharmaceuticals (U.K.) Ltd)

Aripiprazole 1 mg per 1 ml Abilify 1mg/ml oral solution | 150 ml [PoM] £102.90 DT = £99.82

Powder and solvent for suspension for injection

‣ Abilify Maintena (Otsuka Pharmaceuticals (U.K.) Ltd)

Aripiprazole 400 mg Abilify Maintena 400mg powder and solvent for prolonged-release suspension for injection pre-filled syringes | 1 pre-filled disposable injection [PoM] £220.41 DT = £220.41
Abilify Maintena 400mg powder and solvent for prolonged-release suspension for injection vials | 1 vial [PoM] £220.41 DT = £220.41

Orodispersible tablet

CAUTIONARY AND ADVISORY LABELS 2

EXCIPIENTS: May contain Aspartame

‣ Aripiprazole (Non-proprietary)

Aripiprazole 10 mg Aripiprazole 10mg orodispersible tablets sugar free sugar-free | 28 tablet [PoM] £96.04 DT = £59.38

Aripiprazole 15 mg Aripiprazole 15mg orodispersible tablets sugar free sugar-free | 28 tablet [PoM] £96.04 DT = £59.38

‣ Abilify (Otsuka Pharmaceuticals (U.K.) Ltd)

Aripiprazole 10 mg Abilify 10mg orodispersible tablets sugar-free | 28 tablet [PoM] £96.04 DT = £59.38

Aripiprazole 15 mg Abilify 15mg orodispersible tablets sugar-free | 28 tablet [PoM] £96.04 DT = £59.38

⚑ 403

Cariprazine

29-Oct-2020

● INDICATIONS AND DOSE

Schizophrenia

‣ BY MOUTH

‣ Adult: 1.5 mg once daily, increased in steps of 1.5 mg if required; maximum 6 mg per day

● INTERACTIONS → Appendix 1: antipsychotics, second generation

● SIDE-EFFECTS

‣ **Common or very common** Anxiety · appetite abnormal · bradyphrenia · drooling · dyslipidaemia · eye disorders · fatigue · gait abnormal · hypertension · joint stiffness · muscle complaints · musculoskeletal stiffness · nausea · oral disorders · pain · reflexes abnormal · sleep disorders · speech impairment · teeth grinding · vision disorders

‣ **Uncommon** Anaemia · cardiac conduction disorder · delirium · depression · diabetes mellitus · dysaesthesia · eosinophilia · eye irritation · gastrooesophageal reflux disease · grimacing · hiccups · pruritus · sexual dysfunction · suicidal behaviour · thirst · urinary disorders · vertigo

‣ **Rare or very rare** Cataract · dysphagia · hypothyroidism · memory loss · rhabdomyolysis

‣ **Frequency not known** Hepatitis toxic

● CONCEPTION AND CONTRACEPTION Manufacturer advises highly effective contraception in women of childbearing potential during treatment and for at least 10 weeks after the last dose; addition of barrier method recommended in women using systemically-acting hormonal contraceptives.

● PREGNANCY Manufacturer advises avoid—toxicity in *animal* studies.

● BREAST FEEDING Manufacturer advises avoid—present in milk in *animal* studies.

● HEPATIC IMPAIRMENT Manufacturer advises avoid in severe impairment (no information available).

● RENAL IMPAIRMENT Manufacturer advises avoid in severe impairment (no information available).

● NATIONAL FUNDING/ACCESS DECISIONS

For full details see funding body website

Scottish Medicines Consortium (SMC) decisions

‣ Cariprazine (*Reagila*®) for the treatment of schizophrenia in adult patients (May 2019) SMC No. SMC2137 Recommended with restrictions

All Wales Medicines Strategy Group (AWMSG) decisions

‣ Cariprazine (*Reagila*®) for the treatment of schizophrenia in adult patients (August 2020) AWMSG No. 731 Not recommended

● MEDICINAL FORMS There can be variation in the licensing of different medicines containing the same drug.

Capsule

‣ Reagila (Recordati Pharmaceuticals Ltd) ▼

Cariprazine (as Cariprazine hydrochloride) 1.5 mg Reagila 1.5mg capsules | 28 capsule [PoM] £80.36 DT = £80.36

Cariprazine (as Cariprazine hydrochloride) 3 mg Reagila 3mg capsules | 28 capsule [PoM] £80.36 DT = £80.36

Cariprazine (as Cariprazine hydrochloride) 4.5 mg Reagila 4.5mg capsules | 28 capsule [PoM] £80.36 DT = £80.36

Cariprazine (as Cariprazine hydrochloride) 6 mg Reagila 6mg capsules | 28 capsule [PoM] £80.36 DT = £80.36

Clozapine

403

15-Sep-2020

- DRUG ACTION Clozapine is a dopamine D_1, dopamine D_2, 5-HT$_{2A}$, alpha$_1$-adrenoceptor, and muscarinic-receptor antagonist.

- INDICATIONS AND DOSE

Schizophrenia in patients unresponsive to, or intolerant of, conventional antipsychotic drugs
▶ BY MOUTH
▶ Adult 18–59 years: 12.5 mg 1–2 times a day for day 1, then 25–50 mg for day 2, then increased, if tolerated, in steps of 25–50 mg daily, dose to be increased gradually over 14–21 days, increased to up to 300 mg daily in divided doses, larger dose to be taken at night, up to 200 mg daily may be taken as a single dose at bedtime; increased in steps of 50–100 mg 1–2 times a week if required, it is preferable to increase once a week; usual dose 200–450 mg daily, max. 900 mg per day, if restarting after interval of more than 48 hours, 12.5 mg once or twice on first day (but may be feasible to increase more quickly than on initiation)—extreme caution if previous respiratory or cardiac arrest with initial dosing
▶ Adult 60 years and over: 12.5 mg once daily for day 1, then increased to 25–37.5 mg for day 2, then increased, if tolerated, in steps of up to 25 mg daily, dose to be increased gradually over 14–21 days, increased to up to 300 mg daily in divided doses, larger dose at to be taken night, up to 200 mg daily may be taken as a single dose at bedtime; increased in steps of 50–100 mg 1–2 times a week if required, it is preferable to increase once a week; usual dose 200–450 mg daily, max. 900 mg per day, if restarting after interval of more than 48 hours, 12.5 mg once or twice on first day (but may be feasible to increase more quickly than on initiation)—extreme caution if previous respiratory or cardiac arrest with initial dosing

Psychosis in Parkinson's disease
▶ BY MOUTH
▶ Adult: 12.5 mg once daily, dose to be taken at bedtime, then increased in steps of 12.5 mg up to twice weekly, adjusted according to response; usual dose 25–37.5 mg once daily, dose to be taken at bedtime; increased in steps of 12.5 mg once weekly, this applies only in exceptional cases, increased if necessary up to 100 mg daily in 1–2 divided doses; Usual maximum 50 mg/24 hours

IMPORTANT SAFETY INFORMATION
MHRA/CHM ADVICE: CLOZAPINE: REMINDER OF POTENTIALLY FATAL RISK OF INTESTINAL OBSTRUCTION, FAECAL IMPACTION, AND PARALYTIC ILEUS (OCTOBER 2017)
Clozapine has been associated with varying degrees of impairment of intestinal peristalsis—see Cautions and Contra-indications for further information. Patients and their carers should be advised to seek immediate medical advice before taking the next dose of clozapine if constipation develops.

MHRA/CHM ADVICE: CLOZAPINE AND OTHER ANTIPSYCHOTICS: MONITORING BLOOD CONCENTRATIONS FOR TOXICITY (AUGUST 2020)
Following fatal cases involving toxicity of clozapine and other antipsychotic medicines, the MHRA recommends monitoring blood concentration of clozapine for toxicity in certain clinical situations such as when:
- a patient stops smoking or switches to an e-cigarette;
- concomitant medicines may interact to increase blood clozapine levels;
- a patient has pneumonia or other serious infection;
- reduced clozapine metabolism is suspected;

- toxicity is suspected.
Clozapine blood concentration monitoring should be carried out in addition to the required blood tests to manage the risk of agranulocytosis.

- CONTRA-INDICATIONS Alcoholic and toxic psychoses · bone-marrow disorders · coma · drug intoxication · history of agranulocytosis · history of circulatory collapse · history of neutropenia · paralytic ileus · severe cardiac disorders (e.g. myocarditis) · severe CNS depression · uncontrolled epilepsy

- CAUTIONS Age over 60 years · prostatic hypertrophy · susceptibility to angle-closure glaucoma · taper off other antipsychotics before starting

CAUTIONS, FURTHER INFORMATION
▶ Agranulocytosis Neutropenia and potentially fatal agranulocytosis reported. Leucocyte and differential blood counts must be normal before starting; minor counts every week for 18 weeks then at least every 2 weeks and if clozapine continued and blood count stable after 1 year at least every 4 weeks (and 4 weeks after discontinuation); if leucocyte count below 3000 /mm^3 or if absolute neutrophil count below 1500 /mm^3 discontinue permanently and refer to haematologist. Patients who have a low white blood cell count because of benign ethnic neutropenia may be started on clozapine with the agreement of a haematologist. Avoid drugs which depress leucopoiesis; patients should report immediately symptoms of infection, especially influenza-like illness.
▶ Myocarditis and cardiomyopathy Fatal myocarditis (most commonly in first 2 months) and cardiomyopathy reported.
  - Perform physical examination and take full medical history before starting
  - Specialist examination required if cardiac abnormalities or history of heart disease found—clozapine initiated only in absence of severe heart disease and if benefit outweighs risk
  - Persistent tachycardia especially in first 2 months should prompt observation for other indicators for myocarditis or cardiomyopathy
  - If myocarditis or cardiomyopathy suspected clozapine should be stopped and patient evaluated urgently by cardiologist
  - Discontinue permanently in clozapine-induced myocarditis or cardiomyopathy
▶ Intestinal obstruction Impairment of intestinal peristalsis, including constipation, intestinal obstruction, faecal impaction, and paralytic ileus, (including fatal cases) reported. Clozapine should be used with caution in patients receiving drugs that may cause constipation (e.g. antimuscarinic drugs) or in those with a history of colonic disease or lower abdominal surgery. It is essential that constipation is recognised and actively treated.

- INTERACTIONS → Appendix 1: antipsychotics, second generation

- SIDE-EFFECTS
▶ **Common or very common** Appetite decreased · eosinophilia · fatigue · fever · headache · hypertension · leucocytosis · muscle complaints · nausea · oral disorders · postural hypotension (dose-related) · speech impairment · sweating abnormal · syncope · temperature regulation disorders · urinary disorders · vision blurred
▶ **Uncommon** Fall
▶ **Rare or very rare** Anaemia · cardiac arrest · cardiac inflammation · cardiomyopathy · circulatory collapse · confusion · delirium · diabetes mellitus · dyslipidaemia · dysphagia · gastrointestinal disorders · glucose tolerance impaired · hepatic disorders · hyperglycaemia · increased risk of infection · intestinal obstruction (including fatal cases) · ketoacidosis · nephritis tubulointerstitial ·

obsessive-compulsive disorder · pancreatitis · pericardial effusion · respiratory disorders · restlessness · sexual dysfunction · skin reactions · sleep apnoea · thrombocytopenia · thrombocytosis

▶ **Frequency not known** Angina pectoris · angioedema · chest pain · cholinergic syndrome · diarrhoea · gastrointestinal discomfort · hypersensitivity vasculitis · mitral valve incompetence · muscle weakness · myocardial infarction · nasal congestion · palpitations · polyserositis · pseudophaeochromocytoma · renal failure · rhabdomyolysis · sepsis · systemic lupus erythematosus (SLE)

SIDE-EFFECTS, FURTHER INFORMATION Hypersalivation associated with clozapine therapy can be treated with hyoscine hydrobromide [unlicensed indication], provided that the patient is not at particular risk from the additive antimuscarinic side-effects of hyoscine and clozapine.

● **PREGNANCY** Use with caution.

● **BREAST FEEDING** Avoid.

● **HEPATIC IMPAIRMENT** Manufacturer advises caution—monitor liver function (discontinue if liver enzymes are greater than 3 times the upper limit of normal or jaundice occurs); avoid in symptomatic or progressive impairment and in hepatic failure.

● **RENAL IMPAIRMENT** Avoid in severe impairment.

● **MONITORING REQUIREMENTS**
▶ Monitor leucocyte and differential blood counts. Clozapine requires differential white blood cell monitoring weekly for 18 weeks, then fortnightly for up to one year, and then monthly as part of the clozapine patient monitoring service.
▶ Blood clozapine concentration should be monitored in certain clinical situations—consult product literature.
▶ Close medical supervision during initiation (risk of collapse because of hypotension and convulsions).
▶ Blood lipids and weight should be measured at baseline, at 3 months (weight should be measured at frequent intervals during the first 3 months), and then yearly with antipsychotics. Patients taking clozapine require more frequent monitoring of these parameters: every 3 months for the first year, then yearly.
▶ Fasting blood glucose should be measured at baseline, at 4–6 months, and then yearly. Patients taking clozapine should have fasting blood glucose tested at baseline, after one months' treatment, then every 4–6 months.
▶ Patient, prescriber, and supplying pharmacist must be registered with the appropriate Patient Monitoring Service—it takes several days to do this.

● **TREATMENT CESSATION** On planned withdrawal reduce dose over 1–2 weeks to avoid risk of rebound psychosis. If abrupt withdrawal necessary observe patient carefully.

● **DIRECTIONS FOR ADMINISTRATION** Manufacturer advises shake oral suspension well for 90 seconds when dispensing or if visibly settled and stand for 24 hours before use; otherwise shake well for 10 seconds before use. May be diluted with water. Orodispersible tablets should be placed on the tongue, allowed to dissolve and swallowed.

● **PRESCRIBING AND DISPENSING INFORMATION** Clozapine has been used for psychosis in Parkinson's disease in children aged 16 years and over.

● **PATIENT AND CARER ADVICE** Patients or carers should be given advice on how to administer clozapine oral suspension and orodispersible tablets.

● **MEDICINAL FORMS** There can be variation in the licensing of different medicines containing the same drug. Forms available from special-order manufacturers include: oral suspension, oral solution

Tablet
CAUTIONARY AND ADVISORY LABELS 2, 10
▶ Clozaril (Mylan)
Clozapine 25 mg Clozaril 25mg tablets | 28 tablet [PoM] £3.02 (Hospital only) | 84 tablet [PoM] £8.40 DT = £16.64 (Hospital only) | 100 tablet [PoM] £10.00 (Hospital only)
Clozapine 100 mg Clozaril 100mg tablets | 28 tablet [PoM] £12.07 (Hospital only) | 84 tablet [PoM] £33.60 DT = £66.53 (Hospital only) | 100 tablet [PoM] £39.00 (Hospital only)

▶ Denzapine (Britannia Pharmaceuticals Ltd)
Clozapine 25 mg Denzapine 25mg tablets | 84 tablet [PoM] £16.64 DT = £16.64 | 100 tablet [PoM] £19.80
Clozapine 50 mg Denzapine 50mg tablets | 100 tablet [PoM] £39.60 DT = £39.60
Clozapine 100 mg Denzapine 100mg tablets | 84 tablet [PoM] £66.53 DT = £66.53 | 100 tablet [PoM] £79.20
Clozapine 200 mg Denzapine 200mg tablets | 100 tablet [PoM] £158.40 DT = £158.40

▶ Zaponex (Leyden Delta B.V.)
Clozapine 25 mg Zaponex 25mg tablets | 84 tablet [PoM] £8.28 DT = £16.64 | 500 tablet [PoM] £48.39
Clozapine 100 mg Zaponex 100mg tablets | 84 tablet [PoM] £33.88 DT = £66.53 | 500 tablet [PoM] £196.43

Oral suspension
CAUTIONARY AND ADVISORY LABELS 2, 10
▶ Denzapine (Britannia Pharmaceuticals Ltd)
Clozapine 50 mg per 1 ml Denzapine 50mg/ml oral suspension sugar-free | 100 ml [PoM] £39.60 DT = £39.60

Orodispersible tablet
CAUTIONARY AND ADVISORY LABELS 2, 10
EXCIPIENTS: May contain Aspartame
▶ Zaponex (Leyden Delta B.V.)
Clozapine 12.5 mg Zaponex 12.5mg orodispersible tablets sugar-free | 28 tablet [PoM] £2.77
Clozapine 25 mg Zaponex 25mg orodispersible tablets sugar-free | 28 tablet [PoM] £5.55
Clozapine 50 mg Zaponex 50mg orodispersible tablets sugar-free | 28 tablet [PoM] £11.09
Clozapine 100 mg Zaponex 100mg orodispersible tablets sugar-free | 28 tablet [PoM] £22.18
Clozapine 200 mg Zaponex 200mg orodispersible tablets sugar-free | 28 tablet [PoM] £44.35

F 403

Lurasidone hydrochloride
23-Jul-2020

● **DRUG ACTION** Lurasidone is a dopamine D_2, 5-HT_{2A}, 5-HT_7, alpha$_{2A}$- and alpha$_{2C}$- adrenoceptor antagonist, and is a partial agonist at 5-HT_{1a} receptors.

● **INDICATIONS AND DOSE**

Schizophrenia
▶ BY MOUTH
▶ Adult: Initially 37 mg once daily, increased if necessary up to 148 mg once daily

Schizophrenia when given with concomitant moderate CYP3A4 inhibitors (e.g. diltiazem, erythromycin, fluconazole, and verapamil)
▶ BY MOUTH
▶ Adult: Initially 18.5 mg once daily (max. per dose 74 mg once daily)

● **CAUTIONS** High doses in elderly · susceptibility to QT-interval prolongation

● **INTERACTIONS** → Appendix 1: antipsychotics, second generation

● **SIDE-EFFECTS**
▶ **Common or very common** Anxiety · drooling · fatigue · gastrointestinal discomfort · muscle complaints · musculoskeletal stiffness · nausea · oculogyric crisis · oral disorders · pain · psychiatric disorders · sleep disorders

▶ **Uncommon** Appetite decreased · dysarthria · dysuria · gait abnormal · gastrointestinal disorders · hot flush · hyperhidrosis · hypertension · joint stiffness · nasopharyngitis · vision blurred

▶ **Rare or very rare** Eosinophilia · rhabdomyolysis

▶ **Frequency not known** Anaemia · angina pectoris · angioedema · atrioventricular block · breast abnormalities · diarrhoea · dysmenorrhoea · dysphagia · pruritus · renal failure · Stevens-Johnson syndrome · suicidal behaviour · vertigo

● PREGNANCY Use only if potential benefit outweighs risk—limited information available.

● HEPATIC IMPAIRMENT Manufacturer advises caution in moderate to severe impairment (risk of increased exposure).
Dose adjustments Manufacturer advises initially 18.5 mg once daily in moderate to severe impairment, increased if necessary up to 74 mg once daily in moderate impairment, or up to max. 37 mg once daily in severe impairment.

● RENAL IMPAIRMENT Manufacturer advises use only if potential benefit outweighs risk if eGFR less than 15 mL/minute/1.73 m².
Dose adjustments Initially 18.5 mg once daily, up to max. 74 mg once daily if eGFR less than 50 mL/minute/1.73 m².

● DIRECTIONS FOR ADMINISTRATION Manufacturer advises patients on doses higher than 111 mg once daily whose treatment is interrupted for longer than 3 days should restart on 111 mg once daily and titrate to usual dose; for all other doses, restart on usual dose.

● MEDICINAL FORMS There can be variation in the licensing of different medicines containing the same drug.

Tablet
CAUTIONARY AND ADVISORY LABELS 2, 21, 25
▶ Latuda (Sunovion Pharmaceuticals Europe Ltd)
Lurasidone (as Lurasidone hydrochloride) **18.5 mg** Latuda 18.5mg tablets | 28 tablet PoM £90.72 DT = £90.72
Lurasidone (as Lurasidone hydrochloride) **37 mg** Latuda 37mg tablets | 28 tablet PoM £90.72 DT = £90.72
Lurasidone (as Lurasidone hydrochloride) **74 mg** Latuda 74mg tablets | 28 tablet PoM £90.72 DT = £90.72

▶ 403

Olanzapine
04-Sep-2020

● DRUG ACTION Olanzapine is a dopamine D_1, D_2, D_4, 5-HT_2, histamine- 1-, and muscarinic-receptor antagonist.

● INDICATIONS AND DOSE
Schizophrenia | Combination therapy for mania
▶ BY MOUTH
▶ Adult: 10 mg daily, adjusted according to response, usual dose 5–20 mg daily, doses greater than 10 mg daily only after reassessment, when one or more factors present that might result in slower metabolism (e.g. female gender, elderly, non-smoker) consider lower initial dose and more gradual dose increase; maximum 20 mg per day

Preventing recurrence in bipolar disorder
▶ BY MOUTH
▶ Adult: 10 mg daily, adjusted according to response, usual dose 5–20 mg daily, doses greater than 10 mg daily only after reassessment, when one or more factors present that might result in slower metabolism (e.g. female gender, elderly, non-smoker) consider lower initial dose and more gradual dose increase; maximum 20 mg per day

Monotherapy for mania
▶ BY MOUTH
▶ Adult: 15 mg daily, adjusted according to response, usual dose 5–20 mg daily, doses greater than 15 mg daily only after reassessment, when one or more

factors present that might result in slower metabolism (e.g. female gender, elderly, non-smoker) consider lower initial dose and more gradual dose increase; maximum 20 mg per day

Control of agitation and disturbed behaviour in schizophrenia or mania
▶ BY INTRAMUSCULAR INJECTION
▶ Adult: Initially 5–10 mg for 1 dose; usual dose 10 mg for 1 dose, followed by 5–10 mg after 2 hours if required, maximum 3 injections daily for 3 days; maximum daily combined oral and parenteral dose 20 mg, when one or more factors present that might result in slower metabolism (e.g. female gender, elderly, non-smoker) consider lower initial dose and more gradual dose increase
▶ Elderly: Initially 2.5–5 mg, followed by 2.5–5 mg after 2 hours if required, maximum 3 injections daily for 3 days; maximum daily combined oral and parenteral dose 20 mg, when one or more factors present that might result in slower metabolism (e.g. female gender, elderly, non-smoker) consider lower initial dose and more gradual dose increase

---

IMPORTANT SAFETY INFORMATION

MHRA/CHM ADVICE: CLOZAPINE AND OTHER ANTIPSYCHOTICS: MONITORING BLOOD CONCENTRATIONS FOR TOXICITY (AUGUST 2020)
Following fatal cases involving toxicity of clozapine and other antipsychotic medicines, the MHRA advises that monitoring blood concentration of olanzapine may be helpful in certain circumstances, such as patients presenting symptoms suggestive of toxicity, or when concomitant medicines may interact to increase blood concentration of olanzapine.

● CONTRA-INDICATIONS
▶ With intramuscular use Acute myocardial infarction · bradycardia · recent heart surgery · severe hypotension · sick sinus syndrome · unstable angina

● CAUTIONS Bone-marrow depression · hypereosinophilic disorders · low leucocyte count · low neutrophil count · myeloproliferative disease · paralytic ileus
CAUTIONS, FURTHER INFORMATION
▶ CNS and respiratory depression
▶ With intramuscular use Blood pressure, pulse and respiratory rate should be monitored for at least 4 hours after intramuscular injection, particularly in those also receiving a benzodiazepine or another antipsychotic (leave at least one hour between administration of olanzapine intramuscular injection and parenteral benzodiazepines).

● INTERACTIONS → Appendix 1: antipsychotics, second generation

● SIDE-EFFECTS
GENERAL SIDE-EFFECTS
▶ **Common or very common** Anticholinergic syndrome · appetite increased · arthralgia · asthenia · eosinophilia · fever · glycosuria · oedema · sexual dysfunction
▶ **Uncommon** Abdominal distension · alopecia · breast enlargement · diabetes mellitus · dysarthria · epistaxis · memory loss · photosensitivity reaction · urinary disorders
▶ **Rare or very rare** Hepatic disorders · hypothermia · pancreatitis · rhabdomyolysis · thrombocytopenia
SPECIFIC SIDE-EFFECTS
▶ **Common or very common**
▶ With intramuscular use Dyslipidaemia
▶ With oral use Hypersomnia
▶ **Uncommon**
▶ With intramuscular use Hypoventilation
▶ With oral use Diabetic coma · ketoacidosis · oculogyration
▶ **Rare or very rare**
▶ With intramuscular use Withdrawal syndrome

► **Frequency not known**

► **With intramuscular use** Cardiovascular event · erythema · fall · gait abnormal · hallucinations · pneumonia

● PREGNANCY Use only if potential benefit outweighs risk; neonatal lethargy, tremor, and hypertonia reported when used in third trimester.

● BREAST FEEDING Avoid—present in milk.

● HEPATIC IMPAIRMENT Manufacturer advises caution.
Dose adjustments Manufacturer advises consider initial dose of 5 mg daily and cautious titration.

● RENAL IMPAIRMENT
Dose adjustments Consider initial dose of 5 mg daily.

● MONITORING REQUIREMENTS

► Blood lipids and weight should be measured at baseline, at 3 months (weight should be measured at frequent intervals during the first 3 months), and then yearly with antipsychotic drugs. Patients taking olanzapine require more frequent monitoring of these parameters: every 3 months for the first year, then yearly.

► Fasting blood glucose should be measured at baseline, at 4–6 months, and then yearly. Patients taking olanzapine should have fasting blood glucose tested at baseline, after one months' treatment, and then every 4–6 months.

● DIRECTIONS FOR ADMINISTRATION Manufacturer advises olanzapine orodispersible tablet may be placed on the tongue and allowed to dissolve, or dispersed in water, orange juice, apple juice, milk, or coffee.

● PRESCRIBING AND DISPENSING INFORMATION

► **With intramuscular use** When prescribing, dispensing, or administering, check that this injection is the correct preparation—this preparation is usually used in hospital for the rapid control of an *acute episode* and should **not** be confused with depot preparations which are usually used in the community or clinics for *maintenance* treatment. Available from specialist importing companies.

● PATIENT AND CARER ADVICE Patients or carers should be given advice on how to administer orodispersible tablets.

● MEDICINAL FORMS There can be variation in the licensing of different medicines containing the same drug. Forms available from special-order manufacturers include: oral suspension, oral solution

Tablet
CAUTIONARY AND ADVISORY LABELS 2

► Olanzapine (Non-proprietary)
Olanzapine 2.5 mg Olanzapine 2.5mg tablets | 28 tablet [PoM] £21.85 DT = £1.48
Olanzapine 5 mg Olanzapine 5mg tablets | 28 tablet [PoM] £43.70 DT = £1.78
Olanzapine 7.5 mg Olanzapine 7.5mg tablets | 28 tablet [PoM] £62.27 DT = £1.86 | 56 tablet [PoM] £3.72–£131.10
Olanzapine 10 mg Olanzapine 10mg tablets | 28 tablet [PoM] £87.40 DT = £2.10
Olanzapine 15 mg Olanzapine 15mg tablets | 28 tablet [PoM] £119.18 DT = £2.25
Olanzapine 20 mg Olanzapine 20mg tablets | 28 tablet [PoM] £158.90 DT = £3.09

► Zalasta (Consilient Health Ltd)
Olanzapine 2.5 mg Zalasta 2.5mg tablets | 28 tablet [PoM] £18.57 DT = £1.48
Olanzapine 5 mg Zalasta 5mg tablets | 28 tablet [PoM] £37.14 DT = £1.78
Olanzapine 7.5 mg Zalasta 7.5mg tablets | 56 tablet [PoM] £111.43
Olanzapine 10 mg Zalasta 10mg tablets | 28 tablet [PoM] £74.29 DT = £2.10
Olanzapine 15 mg Zalasta 15mg tablets | 28 tablet [PoM] £101.30 DT = £2.25
Olanzapine 20 mg Zalasta 20mg tablets | 28 tablet [PoM] £135.06 DT = £3.09

► Zyprexa (Eli Lilly and Company Ltd)
Olanzapine 2.5 mg Zyprexa 2.5mg tablets | 28 tablet [PoM] £21.85 DT = £1.48
Olanzapine 5 mg Zyprexa 5mg tablets | 28 tablet [PoM] £43.70 DT = £1.78

Olanzapine 7.5 mg Zyprexa 7.5mg tablets | 56 tablet [PoM] £131.10
Olanzapine 10 mg Zyprexa 10mg tablets | 28 tablet [PoM] £87.40 DT = £2.10
Olanzapine 15 mg Zyprexa 15mg tablets | 28 tablet [PoM] £119.18 DT = £2.25
Olanzapine 20 mg Zyprexa 20mg tablets | 28 tablet [PoM] £158.90 DT = £3.09

Oral lyophilisate

► Zyprexa (Eli Lilly and Company Ltd)
Olanzapine 5 mg Zyprexa 5mg Velotabs sugar-free | 28 tablet [PoM] £48.07 DT = £48.07
Olanzapine 10 mg Zyprexa 10mg Velotabs sugar-free | 28 tablet [PoM] £87.40 DT = £87.40
Olanzapine 15 mg Zyprexa 15mg Velotabs sugar-free | 28 tablet [PoM] £131.10 DT = £131.10
Olanzapine 20 mg Zyprexa 20mg Velotabs sugar-free | 28 tablet [PoM] £174.79 DT = £174.79

Orodispersible tablet
CAUTIONARY AND ADVISORY LABELS 2
EXCIPIENTS: May contain Aspartame

► Olanzapine (Non-proprietary)
Olanzapine 5 mg Olanzapine 5mg orodispersible tablets sugar free sugar-free | 28 tablet [PoM] £6.86–£40.85 DT = £7.97
Olanzapine 5mg orodispersible tablets | 28 tablet [PoM] £30.00 DT = £29.77
Olanzapine 10 mg Olanzapine 10mg orodispersible tablets | 28 tablet [PoM] £50.00 DT = £49.64
Olanzapine 10mg orodispersible tablets sugar free sugar-free | 28 tablet [PoM] £11.50–£74.29 DT = £13.30
Olanzapine 15 mg Olanzapine 15mg orodispersible tablets sugar free sugar-free | 28 tablet [PoM] £11.65–£111.44 DT = £25.98
Olanzapine 15mg orodispersible tablets | 28 tablet [PoM] £48.80 DT = £48.79
Olanzapine 20 mg Olanzapine 20mg orodispersible tablets sugar free sugar-free | 28 tablet [PoM] £18.93–£148.57 DT = £18.93
Olanzapine 20mg orodispersible tablets | 28 tablet [PoM] £80.00 DT = £79.61

► Zalasta (Consilient Health Ltd)
Olanzapine 5 mg Zalasta 5mg orodispersible tablets sugar-free | 28 tablet [PoM] £40.85 DT = £7.97
Olanzapine 10 mg Zalasta 10mg orodispersible tablets sugar-free | 28 tablet [PoM] £74.20 DT = £13.30
Olanzapine 15 mg Zalasta 15mg orodispersible tablets sugar-free | 28 tablet [PoM] £111.43 DT = £25.98
Olanzapine 20 mg Zalasta 20mg orodispersible tablets sugar-free | 28 tablet [PoM] £148.57 DT = £18.93

F 403

Paliperidone

12-Nov-2020

● DRUG ACTION Paliperidone is a metabolite of risperidone.

● **INDICATIONS AND DOSE**

Schizophrenia | Psychotic or manic symptoms of schizoaffective disorder
► BY MOUTH
► **Adult:** 6 mg once daily, dose to be taken in the morning, then adjusted in steps of 3 mg if required, dose to be adjusted over at least 5 days; usual dose 3–12 mg daily

TREVICTA ® PRE-FILLED SYRINGES

Maintenance of schizophrenia in patients who are clinically stable on once-monthly intramuscular paliperidone
► BY DEEP INTRAMUSCULAR INJECTION
► **Adult:** Initially 175–525 mg every 3 months, adjusted according to response, to be administered into the deltoid or gluteal muscle, dose is based on previous once-monthly intramuscular paliperidone and should be initiated in place of the next scheduled dose—consult product literature

XEPLION ® PRE-FILLED SYRINGES
Maintenance in schizophrenia in patients previously responsive to paliperidone or risperidone
▶ BY DEEP INTRAMUSCULAR INJECTION
▶ **Adult:** 150 mg for 1 dose on day 1, then 100 mg for 1 dose on day 8, to be injected into the deltoid muscle, dose subsequently adjusted at monthly intervals according to response; maintenance 75 mg once a month, alternatively maintenance 25–150 mg once a month, following the second dose, monthly maintenance doses can be administered into either the deltoid or gluteal muscle

● CAUTIONS

GENERAL CAUTIONS Cataract surgery (risk of intraoperative floppy iris syndrome) · dementia with Lewy bodies · elderly patients with dementia · elderly patients with risk factors for stroke · predisposition to gastro-intestinal obstruction · prolactin-dependent tumours
SPECIFIC CAUTIONS
▶ With intramuscular use when transferring from oral to depot therapy, the dose by mouth should be reduced gradually
● INTERACTIONS → Appendix 1: antipsychotics, second generation
● SIDE-EFFECTS
GENERAL SIDE-EFFECTS
▶ **Common or very common** Anxiety · appetite abnormal · asthenia · cardiac conduction disorders · cough · depression · diarrhoea · fever · gastrointestinal discomfort · headache · hyperglycaemia · hypertension · increased risk of infection · joint disorders · laryngeal pain · mood altered · nasal congestion · nausea · oral disorders · pain · skin reactions · vision disorders
▶ **Uncommon** Alopecia · anaemia · breast abnormalities · chest discomfort · chills · conjunctivitis · cystitis · dry eye · dysarthria · dysphagia · dyspnoea · ear pain · epistaxis · fall · gait abnormal · gastrointestinal disorders · generalised tonic-clonic seizure · hypoglycaemia · induration · malaise · menstrual cycle irregularities · muscle spasms · muscle weakness · oedema · palpitations · respiratory disorders · sensation abnormal · sexual dysfunction · sleep disorders · syncope · taste altered · thirst · thrombocytopenia · tinnitus · urinary disorders · vertigo
▶ **Rare or very rare** Angioedema · cerebrovascular insufficiency · coma · consciousness impaired · dandruff · diabetic ketoacidosis · dysphonia · eye disorders · flushing · glaucoma · hypothermia · ischaemia · jaundice · pancreatitis · polydipsia · posture abnormal · rhabdomyolysis · SIADH · sleep apnoea · vaginal discharge · water intoxication · withdrawal syndrome
SPECIFIC SIDE-EFFECTS
▶ **Common or very common**
▶ With oral use Weight decreased
▶ **Uncommon**
▶ With oral use Concentration impaired · confusion · diabetes mellitus
▶ **Frequency not known**
▶ With intramuscular use Injection site necrosis
● PREGNANCY Use only if potential benefit outweighs risk—toxicity in *animal* studies; if discontinuation during pregnancy is necessary, withdraw gradually.
TREVICTA ® PRE-FILLED SYRINGES Manufacturer advises to consider long-acting nature of formulation—paliperidone detected in plasma up to 18 months after single dose.
● BREAST FEEDING Manufacturer advises avoid—present in milk.
TREVICTA ® PRE-FILLED SYRINGES Manufacturer advises to consider long-acting nature of formulation—paliperidone detected in plasma up to 18 months after single dose.

● HEPATIC IMPAIRMENT Manufacturer advises caution in severe impairment (no information available).
● RENAL IMPAIRMENT
▶ With oral use Manufacturer advises avoid if creatinine clearance less than 10 mL/minute.
▶ With intramuscular use Manufacturer advises avoid if creatinine clearance less than 50 mL/minute.
Dose adjustments ▶ With oral use Manufacturer advises reduce initial dose to 3 mg once daily if creatinine clearance 50–80 mL/minute (max. 6 mg once daily). Manufacturer advises reduce initial dose to 1.5 mg once daily if creatinine clearance 10–50 mL/minute (max. 3 mg once daily).
TREVICTA ® PRE-FILLED SYRINGES **Dose adjustments** Manufacturer advises dose should be adjusted and stabilised using once-monthly injectable paliperidone before switching to three-monthly injectable paliperidone, if creatinine clearance 50–80 mL/minute.
XEPLION ® PRE-FILLED SYRINGES **Dose adjustments** Manufacturer advises initial dose 100 mg on day 1 and then 75 mg on day 8 if creatinine clearance 50–80 mL/minute; recommended maintenance dose 50 mg (range 25–100 mg) monthly if creatinine clearance 50–80 mL/minute.
● MONITORING REQUIREMENTS
▶ With intramuscular use Treatment requires careful monitoring for optimum effect.
● DIRECTIONS FOR ADMINISTRATION
▶ With intramuscular use Use correct injection technique (including the use of z-track technique) and rotate injection sites.
▶ With oral use Manufacturer advises always take with breakfast or always take on an empty stomach.
● PRESCRIBING AND DISPENSING INFORMATION
XEPLION ® PRE-FILLED SYRINGES *Xeplion* ® 25 mg pre-filled syringes may be difficult to obtain.
● PATIENT AND CARER ADVICE
▶ With oral use Patients or carers should be given advice on how to administer paliperidone tablets.
Missed doses ▶ With intramuscular use For missed doses see product literature.
● NATIONAL FUNDING/ACCESS DECISIONS
TREVICTA ® PRE-FILLED SYRINGES For full details see funding body website
Scottish Medicines Consortium (SMC) decisions
▶ **Paliperidone palmitate (*Trevicta* ®), a three-monthly injection, is indicated for the maintenance treatment of schizophrenia in adult patients who are clinically stable on one-monthly paliperidone palmitate injectable product (September 2016)** SMC No. 1181/16 Recommended

● MEDICINAL FORMS There can be variation in the licensing of different medicines containing the same drug.
Prolonged-release suspension for injection
▶ Trevicta (Janssen-Cilag Ltd)
Paliperidone (as Paliperidone palmitate) 200 mg per 1 ml Trevicta 175mg/0.875ml prolonged-release suspension for injection pre-filled syringes | 1 pre-filled disposable injection PoM £551.76 DT = £551.76
Trevicta 263mg/1.315ml prolonged-release suspension for injection pre-filled syringes | 1 pre-filled disposable injection PoM £734.70 DT = £734.70
Trevicta 350mg/1.75ml prolonged-release suspension for injection pre-filled syringes | 1 pre-filled disposable injection PoM £942.21 DT = £942.21
Trevicta 525mg/2.625ml prolonged-release suspension for injection pre-filled syringes | 1 pre-filled disposable injection PoM £1,177.77 DT = £1,177.77

Nervous system

Modified-release tablet
CAUTIONARY AND ADVISORY LABELS 2, 25
▶ Invega (Janssen-Cilag Ltd)
  Paliperidone 3 mg Invega 3mg modified-release tablets |
  28 tablet [PoM] £97.28 DT = £97.28
  Paliperidone 6 mg Invega 6mg modified-release tablets |
  28 tablet [PoM] £97.28 DT = £97.28
  Paliperidone 9 mg Invega 9mg modified-release tablets |
  28 tablet [PoM] £145.92 DT = £145.92

Suspension for injection
▶ Xeplion (Janssen-Cilag Ltd)
  Paliperidone (as Paliperidone palmitate) 100 mg per 1 ml Xeplion
  150mg/1.5ml suspension for injection pre-filled syringes | 1 pre-filled
  disposable injection [PoM] £392.59 DT = £392.59
  Xeplion 75mg/0.75ml suspension for injection pre-filled syringes |
  1 pre-filled disposable injection [PoM] £244.90 DT = £244.90
  Xeplion 100mg/1ml suspension for injection pre-filled syringes |
  1 pre-filled disposable injection [PoM] £314.07 DT = £314.07
  Xeplion 50mg/0.5ml suspension for injection pre-filled syringes |
  1 pre-filled disposable injection [PoM] £183.92 DT = £183.92

F 403

Quetiapine
09-Sep-2020

● DRUG ACTION Quetiapine is a dopamine D_1, dopamine D_2,
5-HT_2, alpha$_1$-adrenoceptor, and histamine-1 receptor
antagonist.

● INDICATIONS AND DOSE
Schizophrenia
▶ BY MOUTH USING IMMEDIATE-RELEASE MEDICINES
▶ Adult: 25 mg twice daily for day 1, then 50 mg twice
  daily for day 2, then 100 mg twice daily for day 3, then
  150 mg twice daily for day 4, then, adjusted according
  to response, usual dose 300–450 mg daily in 2 divided
  doses, the rate of dose titration may need to be slower
  and the daily dose lower in elderly patients; maximum
  750 mg per day
▶ BY MOUTH USING MODIFIED-RELEASE MEDICINES
▶ Adult: 300 mg once daily for day 1, then 600 mg once
  daily for day 2, then, adjusted according to response,
  usual dose 600 mg once daily, maximum dose under
  specialist supervision; maximum 800 mg per day
▶ Elderly: Initially 50 mg once daily, adjusted according
  to response. adjusted in steps of 50 mg daily

Treatment of mania in bipolar disorder
▶ BY MOUTH USING IMMEDIATE-RELEASE MEDICINES
▶ Adult: 50 mg twice daily for day 1, then 100 mg twice
  daily for day 2, then 150 mg twice daily for day 3, then
  200 mg twice daily for day 4, then adjusted in steps of
  up to 200 mg daily, adjusted according to response,
  usual dose 400–800 mg daily in 2 divided doses, the
  rate of dose titration may need to be slower and the
  daily dose lower in elderly patients; maximum 800 mg
  per day
▶ BY MOUTH USING MODIFIED-RELEASE MEDICINES
▶ Adult: 300 mg once daily for day 1, then 600 mg once
  daily for day 2, then, adjusted according to response,
  usual dose 400–800 mg once daily
▶ Elderly: Initially 50 mg once daily, adjusted according
  to response. adjusted in steps of 50 mg daily

Treatment of depression in bipolar disorder
▶ BY MOUTH USING IMMEDIATE-RELEASE MEDICINES
▶ Adult: 50 mg once daily for day 1, dose to be taken at
  bedtime, then 100 mg once daily for day 2, then 200 mg
  once daily for day 3, then 300 mg once daily for day 4,
  then, adjusted according to response; usual dose
  300 mg once daily, the rate of dose titration may need
  to be slower and the daily dose lower in elderly
  patients; maximum 600 mg per day
▶ BY MOUTH USING MODIFIED-RELEASE MEDICINES
▶ Adult: 50 mg once daily for day 1, dose to be taken at
  bedtime, then 100 mg once daily for day 2, then 200 mg
  once daily for day 3, then 300 mg once daily for day 4,

then, adjusted according to response; usual dose
300 mg once daily; maximum 600 mg per day

Prevention of mania and depression in bipolar disorder
▶ BY MOUTH USING IMMEDIATE-RELEASE MEDICINES
▶ Adult: Continue at the dose effective for treatment of
  bipolar disorder and adjust to lowest effective dose;
  usual dose 300–800 mg daily in 2 divided doses
▶ BY MOUTH USING MODIFIED-RELEASE MEDICINES
▶ Adult: Continue at the dose effective for treatment of
  bipolar disorder and adjust to lowest effective dose;
  usual dose 300–800 mg once daily

Adjunctive treatment of major depression
▶ BY MOUTH USING MODIFIED-RELEASE MEDICINES
▶ Adult: 50 mg once daily for 2 days, dose to be taken at
  bedtime, then 150 mg once daily for 2 days, then,
  adjusted according to response, usual dose
  150–300 mg once daily
▶ Elderly: Initially 50 mg once daily for 3 days, then
  increased if necessary to 100 mg once daily for 4 days,
  then adjusted in steps of 50 mg, adjusted according to
  response, usual dose 50–300 mg once daily, dose of
  300 mg should not be reached before day 22 of
  treatment

DOSE EQUIVALENCE AND CONVERSION
▶ Patients can be switched from immediate-release to
  modified-release tablets at the equivalent daily dose;
  to maintain clinical response, dose titration may be
  required.

IMPORTANT SAFETY INFORMATION
MHRA/CHM ADVICE: CLOZAPINE AND OTHER ANTIPSYCHOTICS:
MONITORING BLOOD CONCENTRATIONS FOR TOXICITY (AUGUST
2020)
Following fatal cases involving toxicity of clozapine and
other antipsychotic medicines, the MHRA advises that
monitoring blood concentration of quetiapine may be
helpful in certain circumstances, such as patients
presenting symptoms suggestive of toxicity, or when
concomitant medicines may interact to increase blood
concentration of quetiapine.

● CAUTIONS Cerebrovascular disease · elderly · patients at
  risk of aspiration pneumonia · treatment of depression in
  patients under 25 years (increased risk of suicide)
● INTERACTIONS → Appendix 1: antipsychotics, second
  generation
● SIDE-EFFECTS
▶ **Common or very common** Appetite increased · asthenia ·
  dysarthria · dyspepsia · dyspnoea · fever · headache ·
  hyperglycaemia · irritability · palpitations · peripheral
  oedema · rhinitis · sleep disorders · suicidal behaviour
  (particularly on initiation) · suicidal ideation (particularly
  on initiation) · syncope · vision blurred · withdrawal
  syndrome
▶ **Uncommon** Anaemia · diabetes mellitus · dysphagia ·
  hyponatraemia · hypothyroidism · sexual dysfunction · skin
  reactions · thrombocytopenia
▶ **Rare or very rare** Angioedema · breast swelling ·
  gastrointestinal disorders · hepatic disorders · hypothermia
  · menstrual disorder · metabolic syndrome · pancreatitis ·
  rhabdomyolysis · severe cutaneous adverse reactions
  (SCARs) · SIADH
● PREGNANCY Use only if potential benefit outweighs risk.
● BREAST FEEDING Manufacturer advises avoid.
● HEPATIC IMPAIRMENT Manufacturer advises caution (risk
  of increased plasma concentrations).
  Dose adjustments Manufacturer advises for *immediate-
  release tablets*, initially 25 mg daily, increased daily in steps
  of 25–50 mg.
  Manufacturer advises for *modified-release tablets*,
  initially 50 mg daily, increased daily in steps of 50 mg.

● MEDICINAL FORMS There can be variation in the licensing of different medicines containing the same drug. Forms available from special-order manufacturers include: oral suspension, oral solution, powder

Modified-release tablet

CAUTIONARY AND ADVISORY LABELS 2, 23, 25

▸ Atrolak XL (Accord Healthcare Ltd)
Quetiapine (as Quetiapine fumarate) **50 mg** Atrolak XL 50mg tablets | 60 tablet [PoM] £67.65 DT = £67.66
Quetiapine (as Quetiapine fumarate) **150 mg** Atrolak XL 150mg tablets | 60 tablet [PoM] £107.45 DT = £113.10
Quetiapine (as Quetiapine fumarate) **200 mg** Atrolak XL 200mg tablets | 60 tablet [PoM] £113.09 DT = £113.10
Quetiapine (as Quetiapine fumarate) **300 mg** Atrolak XL 300mg tablets | 60 tablet [PoM] £169.99 DT = £170.00
Quetiapine (as Quetiapine fumarate) **400 mg** Atrolak XL 400mg tablets | 60 tablet [PoM] £226.19 DT = £226.20

▸ Biquelle XL (Aspire Pharma Ltd)
Quetiapine (as Quetiapine fumarate) **50 mg** Biquelle XL 50mg tablets | 60 tablet [PoM] £29.45 DT = £67.66
Quetiapine (as Quetiapine fumarate) **150 mg** Biquelle XL 150mg tablets | 60 tablet [PoM] £49.45 DT = £113.10
Quetiapine (as Quetiapine fumarate) **200 mg** Biquelle XL 200mg tablets | 60 tablet [PoM] £49.45 DT = £113.10
Quetiapine (as Quetiapine fumarate) **300 mg** Biquelle XL 300mg tablets | 60 tablet [PoM] £74.45 DT = £170.00
Quetiapine (as Quetiapine fumarate) **400 mg** Biquelle XL 400mg tablets | 60 tablet [PoM] £98.95 DT = £226.20
Quetiapine (as Quetiapine fumarate) **600 mg** Biquelle XL 600mg tablets | 30 tablet [PoM] £70.73

▸ Brancico XL (Zentiva)
Quetiapine (as Quetiapine fumarate) **50 mg** Brancico XL 50mg tablets | 60 tablet [PoM] £8.99 DT = £67.66
Quetiapine (as Quetiapine fumarate) **150 mg** Brancico XL 150mg tablets | 60 tablet [PoM] £19.49 DT = £113.10
Quetiapine (as Quetiapine fumarate) **200 mg** Brancico XL 200mg tablets | 60 tablet [PoM] £19.49 DT = £113.10
Quetiapine (as Quetiapine fumarate) **300 mg** Brancico XL 300mg tablets | 60 tablet [PoM] £33.74 DT = £170.00
Quetiapine (as Quetiapine fumarate) **400 mg** Brancico XL 400mg tablets | 60 tablet [PoM] £44.99 DT = £226.20

▸ Mintreleq XL (Aristo Pharma Ltd)
Quetiapine (as Quetiapine fumarate) **50 mg** Mintreleq XL 50mg tablets | 60 tablet [PoM] £14.99 DT = £67.66
Quetiapine (as Quetiapine fumarate) **150 mg** Mintreleq XL 150mg tablets | 60 tablet [PoM] £29.99 DT = £113.10
Quetiapine (as Quetiapine fumarate) **200 mg** Mintreleq XL 200mg tablets | 60 tablet [PoM] £29.99 DT = £113.10
Quetiapine (as Quetiapine fumarate) **300 mg** Mintreleq XL 300mg tablets | 60 tablet [PoM] £49.99 DT = £170.00
Quetiapine (as Quetiapine fumarate) **400 mg** Mintreleq XL 400mg tablets | 60 tablet [PoM] £64.99 DT = £226.20

▸ Seroquel XL (Luye Pharma Ltd)
Quetiapine (as Quetiapine fumarate) **50 mg** Seroquel XL 50mg tablets | 60 tablet [PoM] £67.66 DT = £67.66
Quetiapine (as Quetiapine fumarate) **150 mg** Seroquel XL 150mg tablets | 60 tablet [PoM] £113.10 DT = £113.10
Quetiapine (as Quetiapine fumarate) **200 mg** Seroquel XL 200mg tablets | 60 tablet [PoM] £113.10 DT = £113.10
Quetiapine (as Quetiapine fumarate) **300 mg** Seroquel XL 300mg tablets | 60 tablet [PoM] £170.00 DT = £170.00
Quetiapine (as Quetiapine fumarate) **400 mg** Seroquel XL 400mg tablets | 60 tablet [PoM] £226.20 DT = £226.20

▸ Sondate XL (Teva UK Ltd)
Quetiapine (as Quetiapine fumarate) **50 mg** Sondate XL 50mg tablets | 60 tablet [PoM] £11.99 DT = £67.66
Quetiapine (as Quetiapine fumarate) **150 mg** Sondate XL 150mg tablets | 60 tablet [PoM] £25.99 DT = £113.10
Quetiapine (as Quetiapine fumarate) **200 mg** Sondate XL 200mg tablets | 60 tablet [PoM] £25.99 DT = £113.10
Quetiapine (as Quetiapine fumarate) **300 mg** Sondate XL 300mg tablets | 60 tablet [PoM] £44.99 DT = £170.00
Quetiapine (as Quetiapine fumarate) **400 mg** Sondate XL 400mg tablets | 60 tablet [PoM] £59.99 DT = £226.20

▸ Zaluron XL (Fontus Health Ltd)
Quetiapine (as Quetiapine fumarate) **50 mg** Zaluron XL 50mg tablets | 60 tablet [PoM] £27.96 DT = £67.66

Quetiapine (as Quetiapine fumarate) **150 mg** Zaluron XL 150mg tablets | 60 tablet [PoM] £46.96 DT = £113.10
Quetiapine (as Quetiapine fumarate) **200 mg** Zaluron XL 200mg tablets | 60 tablet [PoM] £46.96 DT = £113.10
Quetiapine (as Quetiapine fumarate) **300 mg** Zaluron XL 300mg tablets | 60 tablet [PoM] £70.71 DT = £170.00
Quetiapine (as Quetiapine fumarate) **400 mg** Zaluron XL 400mg tablets | 60 tablet [PoM] £93.98 DT = £226.20

Tablet

CAUTIONARY AND ADVISORY LABELS 2

▸ Quetiapine (Non-proprietary)
Quetiapine (as Quetiapine fumarate) **25 mg** Quetiapine 25mg tablets | 60 tablet [PoM] £38.05 DT = £2.11
Quetiapine (as Quetiapine fumarate) **100 mg** Quetiapine 100mg tablets | 60 tablet [PoM] £113.10 DT = £4.75
Quetiapine (as Quetiapine fumarate) **150 mg** Quetiapine 150mg tablets | 60 tablet [PoM] £113.10 DT = £4.34
Quetiapine (as Quetiapine fumarate) **200 mg** Quetiapine 200mg tablets | 60 tablet [PoM] £133.10 DT = £5.26
Quetiapine (as Quetiapine fumarate) **300 mg** Quetiapine 300mg tablets | 60 tablet [PoM] £170.00 DT = £6.44

▸ Seroquel (Luye Pharma Ltd)
Quetiapine (as Quetiapine fumarate) **25 mg** Seroquel 25mg tablets | 60 tablet [PoM] £48.60 DT = £2.11
Quetiapine (as Quetiapine fumarate) **100 mg** Seroquel 100mg tablets | 60 tablet [PoM] £135.72 DT = £4.75
Quetiapine (as Quetiapine fumarate) **200 mg** Seroquel 200mg tablets | 60 tablet [PoM] £135.72 DT = £5.26
Quetiapine (as Quetiapine fumarate) **300 mg** Seroquel 300mg tablets | 60 tablet [PoM] £204.00 DT = £6.44

Oral suspension

CAUTIONARY AND ADVISORY LABELS 2

▸ Quetiapine (Non-proprietary)
Quetiapine (as Quetiapine fumarate) **20 mg per 1 ml** Quetiapine 20mg/ml oral suspension sugar free sugar-free | 150 ml [PoM] £99.28–£132.00 DT = £132.00

◼ 403

Risperidone

22-Oct-2020

● DRUG ACTION Risperidone is a dopamine D_2, 5-HT_{2A}, alpha$_1$-adrenoceptor, and histamine-1 receptor antagonist.

● INDICATIONS AND DOSE

Schizophrenia and other psychoses in patients tolerant to risperidone by mouth and taking oral risperidone up to 4 mg daily

▸ BY DEEP INTRAMUSCULAR INJECTION

▸ Adult: Initially 25 mg every 2 weeks, to be administered into the deltoid or gluteal muscle, adjusted in steps of 12.5 mg (max. per dose 50 mg every 2 weeks) at intervals of at least 4 weeks, during initiation risperidone by mouth may need to be continued for 4–6 weeks; risperidone by mouth may also be used during dose adjustment of depot injection

Schizophrenia and other psychoses in patients tolerant to risperidone by mouth and taking oral risperidone over 4 mg daily

▸ BY DEEP INTRAMUSCULAR INJECTION

▸ Adult: Initially 37.5 mg every 2 weeks, adjusted in steps of 12.5 mg (max. per dose 50 mg every 2 weeks) at intervals of at least 4 weeks, during initiation risperidone by mouth may need to be continued for 4–6 weeks; risperidone by mouth may also be used during dose adjustment of depot injection

Acute and chronic psychosis

▸ BY MOUTH

▸ Adult: 2 mg daily in 1–2 divided doses for day 1, then 4 mg daily in 1–2 divided doses for day 2, slower titration is appropriate in some patients, usual dose 4–6 mg daily, doses above 10 mg daily only if benefit considered to outweigh risk; maximum 16 mg per day

continued →

▸ **Elderly:** Initially 500 micrograms twice daily, then increased in steps of 500 micrograms twice daily, increased to 1–2 mg twice daily

Mania

▸ BY MOUTH
▸ **Adult:** Initially 2 mg once daily, then increased in steps of 1 mg daily if required; usual dose 1–6 mg daily
▸ **Elderly:** Initially 500 micrograms twice daily, then increased in steps of 500 micrograms twice daily, increased to 1–2 mg twice daily

Short-term treatment (up to 6 weeks) of persistent aggression in patients with moderate to severe Alzheimer's dementia unresponsive to non-pharmacological interventions and when there is a risk of harm to self or others

▸ BY MOUTH
▸ **Adult:** Initially 250 micrograms twice daily, then increased in steps of 250 micrograms twice a day on alternate days, adjusted according to response; usual dose 500 micrograms twice daily (max. per dose 1 mg twice daily)

IMPORTANT SAFETY INFORMATION

SAFE PRACTICE
Risperidone has been confused with ropinirole; care must be taken to ensure the correct drug is prescribed and dispensed.

MHRA/CHM ADVICE: CLOZAPINE AND OTHER ANTIPSYCHOTICS: MONITORING BLOOD CONCENTRATIONS FOR TOXICITY (AUGUST 2020)
Following fatal cases involving toxicity of clozapine and other antipsychotic medicines, the MHRA advises that monitoring blood concentration of risperidone may be helpful in certain circumstances, such as patients presenting symptoms suggestive of toxicity, or when concomitant medicines may interact to increase blood concentration of risperidone.

● CAUTIONS
GENERAL CAUTIONS Avoid in Acute porphyrias p. 1107 · cataract surgery (risk of intra-operative floppy iris syndrome) · dehydration · dementia with Lewy bodies · prolactin-dependent tumours

SPECIFIC CAUTIONS
▸ **With intramuscular use** When transferring from oral to depot therapy, the dose by mouth should be reduced gradually

● INTERACTIONS → Appendix 1: antipsychotics, second generation

● SIDE-EFFECTS
▸ **Common or very common** Anaemia · anxiety · appetite abnormal · asthenia · chest discomfort · conjunctivitis · cough · depression · diarrhoea · dyspnoea · epistaxis · fall · fever · gastrointestinal discomfort · headache · hyperglycaemia · hypertension · increased risk of infection · joint disorders · laryngeal pain · muscle spasms · nasal congestion · nausea · oedema · oral disorders · pain · sexual dysfunction · skin reactions · sleep disorders · urinary disorders · vision disorders · weight decreased
▸ **Uncommon** Alopecia · breast abnormalities · cardiac conduction disorders · cerebrovascular insufficiency · chills · coma · concentration impaired · confusion · consciousness impaired · cystitis · diabetes mellitus · dry eye · dysarthria · dysphagia · dysphonia · ear pain · eye disorders · feeling abnormal · flushing · gait abnormal · gastrointestinal disorders · induration · malaise · menstrual cycle irregularities · mood altered · muscle weakness · palpitations · polydipsia · posture abnormal · procedural pain · respiratory disorders · sensation abnormal · syncope · taste altered · thirst · thrombocytopenia · tinnitus · vaginal discharge · vertigo

▸ **Rare or very rare** Angioedema · dandruff · diabetic ketoacidosis · eyelid crusting · glaucoma · hypoglycaemia · hypothermia · jaundice · pancreatitis · peripheral coldness · rhabdomyolysis · SIADH · sleep apnoea · water intoxication · withdrawal syndrome
▸ **Frequency not known** Cardiac arrest

● PREGNANCY Use only if potential benefit outweighs risk.

● BREAST FEEDING Use only if potential benefit outweighs risk—small amount present in milk.

● HEPATIC IMPAIRMENT Manufacturer advises caution.
Dose adjustments ▸ With intramuscular use Manufacturer advises if an oral dose of at least 2 mg daily tolerated, 25 mg as a depot injection can be given every 2 weeks (no information available).
▸ With oral use Manufacturer advises dose reduction to half the usual dose, and slower dose titration.

● RENAL IMPAIRMENT
Dose adjustments Initial and subsequent oral doses should be halved.

● MONITORING REQUIREMENTS
▸ With intramuscular use Treatment requires careful monitoring for optimum effect.

● DIRECTIONS FOR ADMINISTRATION
▸ With oral use Orodispersible tablets should be placed on the tongue, allowed to dissolve and swallowed. Manufacturer advises oral liquid may be diluted with any non-alcoholic drink, except tea.
▸ With intramuscular use Use correct injection technique (including the use of z-track technique) and rotate injection sites.

● PATIENT AND CARER ADVICE
▸ With oral use Patients or carers should be given advice on how to administer risperidone orodispersible tablets and oral liquid (counselling on use of dose syringe advised).

● MEDICINAL FORMS There can be variation in the licensing of different medicines containing the same drug. Forms available from special-order manufacturers include: oral solution

Tablet
CAUTIONARY AND ADVISORY LABELS 2
▸ Risperidone (Non-proprietary)
Risperidone 250 microgram Risperidone 250microgram tablets | 20 tablet [PoM] £12.00–£14.40
Risperidone 500 microgram Risperidone 500microgram tablets | 20 tablet [PoM] £6.95 DT = £1.45
Risperidone 1 mg Risperidone 1mg tablets | 20 tablet [PoM] £10.16 DT = £1.67 | 60 tablet [PoM] £5.00–£17.56
Risperidone 2 mg Risperidone 2mg tablets | 60 tablet [PoM] £60.10 DT = £4.53
Risperidone 3 mg Risperidone 3mg tablets | 60 tablet [PoM] £88.38 DT = £5.46
Risperidone 4 mg Risperidone 4mg tablets | 60 tablet [PoM] £116.67 DT = £6.04
Risperidone 6 mg Risperidone 6mg tablets | 28 tablet [PoM] £82.50 DT = £49.21
▸ Risperdal (Janssen-Cilag Ltd)
Risperidone 500 microgram Risperdal 500microgram tablets | 20 tablet [PoM] £5.08 DT = £1.45
Risperidone 1 mg Risperdal 1mg tablets | 20 tablet [PoM] £8.36 DT = £1.67
Risperidone 2 mg Risperdal 2mg tablets | 60 tablet [PoM] £34.62 DT = £4.53
Risperidone 3 mg Risperdal 3mg tablets | 60 tablet [PoM] £50.91 DT = £5.46
Risperidone 4 mg Risperdal 4mg tablets | 60 tablet [PoM] £67.20 DT = £6.04
Risperidone 6 mg Risperdal 6mg tablets | 28 tablet [PoM] £67.88 DT = £49.21

Oral solution
CAUTIONARY AND ADVISORY LABELS 2
▸ Risperidone (Non-proprietary)
Risperidone 1 mg per 1 ml Risperidone 1mg/ml oral solution sugar free sugar-free | 100 ml [PoM] £58.22 DT = £3.88

▶ Risperdal (Janssen-Cilag Ltd)
  Risperidone 1 mg per 1 ml Risperdal 1mg/ml oral solution sugar-free | 100 ml [PoM] £37.01 DT = £3.88

Powder and solvent for suspension for injection

▶ Risperdal Consta (Janssen-Cilag Ltd)
  Risperidone 25 mg Risperdal Consta 25mg powder and solvent for suspension for injection vials | 1 vial [PoM] £79.69 DT = £79.69
  Risperidone 37.5 mg Risperdal Consta 37.5mg powder and solvent for injection for injection vials | 1 vial [PoM] £111.32 DT = £111.32
  Risperidone 50 mg Risperdal Consta 50mg powder and solvent for suspension for injection vials | 1 vial [PoM] £142.76 DT = £142.76

Orodispersible tablet
CAUTIONARY AND ADVISORY LABELS 2
EXCIPIENTS: May contain Aspartame

▶ Risperidone (Non-proprietary)
  Risperidone 500 microgram Risperidone 500microgram orodispersible tablets sugar free sugar-free | 28 tablet [PoM] £18.64 DT = £18.28
  Risperidone 1 mg Risperidone 1mg orodispersible tablets sugar free sugar-free | 28 tablet [PoM] £22.50 DT = £22.50
  Risperidone 2 mg Risperidone 2mg orodispersible tablets sugar free sugar-free | 28 tablet [PoM] £38.18 DT = £29.26
  Risperidone 3 mg Risperidone 3mg orodispersible tablets sugar free sugar-free | 28 tablet [PoM] £43.50 DT = £43.50
  Risperidone 4 mg Risperidone 4mg orodispersible tablets sugar free sugar-free | 28 tablet [PoM] £50.29 DT = £50.29

ANTIPSYCHOTICS ⟩ SECOND-GENERATION (DEPOT INJECTIONS)

🏳 403

Olanzapine embonate

22-Oct-2020

(Olanzapine pamoate)

● **INDICATIONS AND DOSE**

Maintenance in schizophrenia in patients tolerant to olanzapine by mouth (patients taking 10 mg oral olanzapine daily)

▶ BY DEEP INTRAMUSCULAR INJECTION
▶ Adult 18–75 years: Initially 210 mg every 2 weeks, alternatively initially 405 mg every 4 weeks, then maintenance 150 mg every 2 weeks, alternatively maintenance 300 mg every 4 weeks, maintenance dose to be started after 2 months of initial treatment, dose to be administered into the gluteal muscle, consult product literature if supplementation with oral olanzapine required

Maintenance in schizophrenia in patients tolerant to olanzapine by mouth (patients taking 15 mg oral olanzapine daily)

▶ BY DEEP INTRAMUSCULAR INJECTION
▶ Adult 18–75 years: Initially 300 mg every 2 weeks, then maintenance 210 mg every 2 weeks, alternatively maintenance 405 mg every 4 weeks, maintenance dose to be started after 2 months of initial treatment, dose to be administered into the gluteal muscle, consult product literature if supplementation with oral olanzapine required

Maintenance in schizophrenia in patients tolerant to olanzapine by mouth (patients taking 20 mg oral olanzapine daily)

▶ BY DEEP INTRAMUSCULAR INJECTION
▶ Adult: Initially 300 mg every 2 weeks, then maintenance 300 mg every 2 weeks (max. per dose 300 mg every 2 weeks), adjusted according to response, dose to be administered into the gluteal muscle, consult product literature if supplementation with oral olanzapine required

IMPORTANT SAFETY INFORMATION
When prescribing, dispensing or administering, check that this is the correct preparation—this preparation is

used for *maintenance* treatment and should **not** be used for the rapid control of an *acute* episode.

MHRA/CHM ADVICE: CLOZAPINE AND OTHER ANTIPSYCHOTICS: MONITORING BLOOD CONCENTRATIONS FOR TOXICITY (AUGUST 2020)
Following fatal cases involving toxicity of clozapine and other antipsychotic medicines, the MHRA advises that monitoring blood concentration of olanzapine may be helpful in certain circumstances, such as patients presenting symptoms suggestive of toxicity, or when concomitant medicines may interact to increase blood concentration of olanzapine.

● CAUTIONS Bone-marrow depression · hypereosinophilic disorders · low leucocyte count · low neutrophil count · myeloproliferative disease · paralytic ileus · when transferring from oral to depot therapy, the dose by mouth should be reduced gradually

● INTERACTIONS → Appendix 1: antipsychotics, second generation

● SIDE-EFFECTS

▶ **Common or very common** Anticholinergic syndrome · appetite increased · arthralgia · asthenia · eosinophilia · fever · glycosuria · oedema · sexual dysfunction

▶ **Uncommon** Abdominal distension · alopecia · breast enlargement · diabetes mellitus · diabetic coma · dysarthria · epistaxis · ketoacidosis · memory loss · oculogyration · photosensitivity reaction · urinary disorders

▶ **Rare or very rare** Drug reaction with eosinophilia and systemic symptoms (DRESS) · hepatic disorders · hypothermia · pancreatitis · rhabdomyolysis · thrombocytopenia

▶ **Frequency not known** Erythema · gait abnormal · increased risk of fall · pneumonia · visual hallucinations

SIDE-EFFECTS, FURTHER INFORMATION Side-effects may persist until the drug has been cleared from its depot site.
Overdose Post-injection reactions have been reported leading to signs and symptoms of overdose.

● PREGNANCY Use only if potential benefit outweighs risk; neonatal lethargy, tremor, and hypertonia reported when used in third trimester.

● BREAST FEEDING Avoid—present in milk.

● HEPATIC IMPAIRMENT Manufacturer advises caution.
Dose adjustments Manufacturer advises consider initial dose of 150 mg every 4 weeks.

● RENAL IMPAIRMENT
Dose adjustments Initially 150 mg every 4 weeks.

● MONITORING REQUIREMENTS

▶ Observe patient for at least 3 hours after injection.
▶ Treatment requires careful monitoring for optimum effect.
▶ Blood lipids and weight should be measured at baseline, at 3 months (weight should be measured at frequent intervals during the first 3 months), and then yearly with antipsychotic drugs. Patients taking olanzapine require more frequent monitoring of these parameters: every 3 months for the first year, then yearly.
▶ Fasting blood glucose should be measured at baseline, at 4–6 months, and then yearly. Patients taking olanzapine should have fasting blood glucose tested at baseline, after one months' treatment, then every 4–6 months.

● DIRECTIONS FOR ADMINISTRATION Use correct injection technique (including use of z-track technique) and rotate injection sites.

● MEDICINAL FORMS There can be variation in the licensing of different medicines containing the same drug.
Powder and solvent for suspension for injection

▶ Zypadhera (Eli Lilly and Company Ltd)
  Olanzapine (as Olanzapine embonate monohydrate)
  210 mg Zypadhera 210mg powder and solvent for suspension for injection vials | 1 vial [PoM] £142.76 DT = £142.76

Olanzapine (as Olanzapine embonate monohydrate)
300 mg Zypadhera 300mg powder and solvent for suspension for injection vials | 1 vial PoM £222.64 DT = £222.64
Olanzapine (as Olanzapine embonate monohydrate)
405 mg Zypadhera 405mg powder and solvent for suspension for injection vials | 1 vial PoM £285.52 DT = £285.52

4 Movement disorders

Cerebral palsy and spasticity
05-Apr-2019

Overview

Cerebral palsy is a group of permanent, non-progressive abnormalities of the developing fetal or neonatal brain that lead to movement and posture disorders, causing activity limitation and functional impact. There can be accompanying clinical and developmental comorbidities. These include disturbances of sensation, perception, cognition, communication and behaviour, epilepsy, and secondary musculoskeletal problems (such as muscle contracture and abnormal torsion). Cerebral palsy is not curable and the comorbidities can impact on many areas of participation and quality of life, particularly eating, drinking, comfort, and sleep.

There are an increasing number of adults now living with cerebral palsy. These patients have a wide range of abilities — from full independence in everyday life to requiring 24 hour care and attention. It is therefore important that patients and their family and carers are provided with information about the network of general and specialised adult services available, to ensure their changing needs are met. The management of adults with cerebral palsy is a continuation from childhood under the care of specialists. For guidance on the management of patients with cerebral palsy, see *Cerebral Palsy and Spasticity* in BNF for Children.

Useful Resources

Cerebral palsy in under 25s: assessment and management. National Institute for Health and Care Excellence. Clinical guideline 62. January 2017.
www.nice.org.uk/guidance/ng62

Spasticity in under 19s: management. National Institute for Health and Care Excellence. Clinical guideline 145. July 2012 (updated November 2016).
www.nice.org.uk/guidance/cg145

Cerebral Palsy in adults. National Institute for Health and Care Excellence. Clinical guideline 119. January 2019.
www.nice.org.uk/guidance/ng119

Motor neurone disease
13-Nov-2020

Description of condition

Motor neurone disease is a neurodegenerative condition affecting the brain and spinal cord. Degeneration of motor neurones leads to progressive muscle weakness; resulting symptoms include muscle cramps, wasting and stiffness, loss of dexterity, reduced respiratory function and cognitive dysfunction. The most common form is amyotrophic lateral sclerosis.

EvGr Patients suspected of having developed motor neurone disease should be referred to a neurologist without delay. ◁A▷

Aims of treatment

As there is no cure, treatment focuses on maintaining functional ability and managing symptoms.

Non-drug treatment

Non-drug treatment includes nutrition, psychosocial support, physiotherapy, exercise programmes and use of special equipment or mobility aids.

Management of symptoms

Muscular symptoms

EvGr Quinine p. 658 [unlicensed indication] is recommended as first line treatment for muscle cramps. If quinine is ineffective, not tolerated or contra-indicated, baclofen p. 1173 [unlicensed indication] should be considered as second line treatment. Subsequent treatment options include tizanidine p. 1175 [unlicensed indication], dantrolene sodium p. 1400 [unlicensed indication] or gabapentin p. 332 [unlicensed indication].

Symptoms of muscle stiffness, spasticity or increased tone can be managed with baclofen, tizanidine, dantrolene sodium or gabapentin [unlicensed indication]. Treatment of severe spasticity may require specialist referral. ◁A▷

The MHRA/CHM have released important safety information on the use of antiepileptic drugs and the risk of suicidal thoughts and behaviour. For further information, see Epilepsy p. 321.

Saliva problems

EvGr A trial of an antimuscarinic drug [unlicensed indication] can be considered for excessive drooling of saliva. Glycopyrronium bromide p. 1387 is recommended in patients who have cognitive impairment as it has fewer central nervous system side-effects. If initial treatment is ineffective, not tolerated or contra-indicated, referral for specialist administration of botulinum toxin type A p. 428 may be required.

Humidification, nebulisers and carbocisteine p. 307 can be used to treat patients with thick, tenacious saliva. ◁A▷

Respiratory symptoms

EvGr Reversible causes of worsening respiratory impairment (such as respiratory tract infections or secretion problems) should be treated before considering other options.

Patients experiencing breathlessness can be treated with opioids [unlicensed indication], or benzodiazepines [unlicensed indication] if the patient's symptoms are exacerbated by anxiety. Non-invasive ventilation should be considered in patients with respiratory impairment. ◁A▷

Amyotrophic lateral sclerosis

Riluzole p. 1169 is licensed for use in patients with amyotrophic lateral sclerosis to extend life or to extend the time to mechanical ventilation—see *National funding/access decisions* under riluzole.

Useful Resources

Motor neurone disease: assessment and management. National Institute for Health and Care Excellence. Clinical guideline NG42. February 2016.
www.nice.org.uk/guidance/ng42

4.1 Dystonias and other involuntary movements

Essential tremor, chorea, tics, and related disorders
14-Sep-2020

Drugs used in essential tremor, chorea, tics, and related disorders

Tetrabenazine p. 428 is mainly used to control movement disorders in Huntington's chorea and related disorders. Tetrabenazine can also be prescribed for the treatment of tardive dyskinesia if switching or withdrawing the causative antipsychotic drug is not effective. It acts by depleting nerve endings of dopamine. It is effective in only a proportion of patients and its use may be limited by the development of depression.

Haloperidol p. 405 [unlicensed indication], olanzapine p. 419 [unlicensed indication], risperidone p. 423 [unlicensed indication], and quetiapine p. 422 [unlicensed indication], can also be used to suppress chorea in Huntington's disease.

Haloperidol can also improve motor tics and symptoms of Tourette syndrome and related choreas. Other treatments for Tourette syndrome include pimozide p. 408 [unlicensed indication] (**important**: ECG monitoring required), clonidine hydrochloride p. 159 [unlicensed indication], and sulpiride p. 409 [unlicensed indication]. Trihexyphenidyl hydrochloride p. 432 in high dosage can also improve some movement disorders; it is sometimes necessary to build the dose up over many weeks. Chlorpromazine hydrochloride p. 404 and haloperidol are used to relieve intractable hiccup.

Propranolol hydrochloride p. 164 or another beta-adrenoceptor blocking drug may be useful in treating essential tremor or tremors associated with anxiety or thyrotoxicosis.

Primidone p. 354 in some cases provides relief from benign essential tremor; the dose is increased slowly to reduce side-effects. The MHRA/CHM have released important safety information on the use of antiepileptic drugs and the risk of suicidal thoughts and behaviour. For further information, see Epilepsy p. 321.

Piracetam below is used as an adjunctive treatment for myoclonus of cortical origin. After an acute episode, attempts should be made every 6 months to decrease or discontinue treatment.

Riluzole p. 1169 is used to extend life in patients with motor neurone disease who have amyotrophic lateral sclerosis.

Torsion dystonia and other involuntary movements
Treatment with botulinum toxin type A p. 428 can be considered after an acquired non-progressive brain injury if rapid-onset spasticity causes postural or functional difficulties.

Other drugs used for Dystonias and other involuntary movements Clozapine, p. 417 · Diazepam, p. 362 · Orphenadrine hydrochloride, p. 431 · Pericyazine, p. 408 · Pramipexole, p. 442 · Prochlorperazine, p. 408 · Procyclidine hydrochloride, p. 432 · Ropinirole, p. 444 · Rotigotine, p. 445 · Trifluoperazine, p. 410

ANTIPSYCHOTICS > FIRST-GENERATION

◄ 403

Promazine hydrochloride

- **INDICATIONS AND DOSE**

Short-term adjunctive management of psychomotor agitation
▸ BY MOUTH
▸ Adult: 100–200 mg 4 times a day

Agitation and restlessness in elderly
▸ BY MOUTH
▸ Elderly: 25–50 mg 4 times a day

- CONTRA-INDICATIONS CNS depression · comatose states · phaeochromocytoma
- CAUTIONS Cerebral arteriosclerosis
- INTERACTIONS → Appendix 1: phenothiazines
- SIDE-EFFECTS Apathy · autonomic dysfunction · cardiac arrest · cardiovascular effects · confusion · consciousness impaired · corneal opacity · epilepsy · eye discolouration · gastrointestinal disorder · glaucoma · haemolytic anaemia ·

headache · hepatic disorders · hyperpyrexia · hypersensitivity · hyperthermia (dose-related) · hypothermia (dose-related) · lens opacity · menstrual disorder · muscle rigidity · nasal congestion · photosensitivity reaction · skin reactions · urinary hesitation · vision blurred · withdrawal syndrome
- HEPATIC IMPAIRMENT Manufacturer advises caution.
- RENAL IMPAIRMENT
  Dose adjustments Start with small doses in severe renal impairment because of increased cerebral sensitivity.
- LESS SUITABLE FOR PRESCRIBING Promazine hydrochloride is less suitable for prescribing.

- MEDICINAL FORMS There can be variation in the licensing of different medicines containing the same drug. Forms available from special-order manufacturers include: oral suspension, oral solution

Oral solution
CAUTIONARY AND ADVISORY LABELS 2
▸ Promazine hydrochloride (Non-proprietary)
  Promazine hydrochloride 5 mg per 1 ml Promazine 25mg/5ml syrup | 150 ml [PoM] £40.78 DT = £33.87
  Promazine 25mg/5ml oral solution | 150 ml [PoM] £40.78 DT = £33.87
  Promazine hydrochloride 10 mg per 1 ml Promazine 50mg/5ml syrup | 150 ml [PoM] £51.10 DT = £42.13
  Promazine 50mg/5ml oral solution | 150 ml [PoM] £51.10 DT = £42.13

Tablet
CAUTIONARY AND ADVISORY LABELS 2
▸ Promazine hydrochloride (Non-proprietary)
  Promazine hydrochloride 25 mg Promazine 25mg tablets | 100 tablet [PoM] £49.99 DT = £45.34
  Promazine hydrochloride 50 mg Promazine 50mg tablets | 100 tablet [PoM] £76.49 DT = £76.18

CNS STIMULANTS

Piracetam

04-Aug-2020

- **INDICATIONS AND DOSE**

Adjunctive treatment of cortical myoclonus
▸ BY MOUTH
▸ Adult: Initially 7.2 g daily in 2–3 divided doses, then increased in steps of 4.8 g every 3–4 days, adjusted according to response, subsequently, attempts should be made to reduce dose of concurrent therapy; maximum 24 g per day

- CONTRA-INDICATIONS Cerebral haemorrhage · Huntington's chorea
- CAUTIONS Gastric ulcer · history of haemorrhagic stroke · increased risk of bleeding · major surgery · underlying disorders of haemostasis
- SIDE-EFFECTS
- **Common or very common** Anxiety · movement disorders · weight increased
- **Uncommon** Asthenia · depression · drowsiness
- **Frequency not known** Angioedema · confusion · diarrhoea · epilepsy exacerbated · gastrointestinal discomfort · haemorrhagic disorder · hallucination · headache · insomnia · nausea · skin reactions · vertigo · vomiting
- PREGNANCY Avoid.
- BREAST FEEDING Avoid.
- HEPATIC IMPAIRMENT Manufacturer advises caution in combined hepatic and renal impairment.
  Dose adjustments Manufacturer advises dose reduction in combined hepatic and renal impairment.
- RENAL IMPAIRMENT Avoid if eGFR less than 20 mL/minute/1.73 m^2.
  Dose adjustments Use two-thirds of normal dose if eGFR 50–80 mL/minute/1.73 m^2; use one-third of normal dose in 2 divided doses if eGFR 30–50 mL/minute/1.73 m^2; use one-sixth of normal dose as a single dose if eGFR 20–30 mL/minute/1.73 m^2.

4

Nervous system

- TREATMENT CESSATION Avoid abrupt withdrawal.
- DIRECTIONS FOR ADMINISTRATION Manufacturer advises follow the oral solution with a glass of water (or soft drink) to reduce bitter taste.
- PRESCRIBING AND DISPENSING INFORMATION Piracetam has been used in children 16 years and over as adjunctive treatment for cortical myoclonus.
- MEDICINAL FORMS There can be variation in the licensing of different medicines containing the same drug.

Oral solution
CAUTIONARY AND ADVISORY LABELS 3
▸ Nootropil (UCB Pharma Ltd)
  Piracetam 333.3 mg per 1 ml Nootropil 33% oral solution sugar-free | 300 ml [PoM] £16.31 DT = £16.31

Tablet
CAUTIONARY AND ADVISORY LABELS 3
▸ Nootropil (UCB Pharma Ltd)
  Piracetam 800 mg Nootropil 800mg tablets | 90 tablet [PoM] £11.75 DT = £11.75
  Piracetam 1.2 gram Nootropil 1200mg tablets | 60 tablet [PoM] £10.97 DT = £10.97

MONOAMINE DEPLETING DRUGS

Tetrabenazine

21-Nov-2020

- INDICATIONS AND DOSE
Movement disorders due to Huntington's chorea, hemiballismus, senile chorea, and related neurological conditions
▸ BY MOUTH
▸ Adult: Initially 25 mg 3 times a day, then increased, if tolerated, in steps of 25 mg every 3–4 days; maximum 200 mg per day
▸ Elderly: Lower initial dose may be necessary
Moderate to severe tardive dyskinesia
▸ BY MOUTH
▸ Adult: Initially 12.5 mg daily, dose to be gradually increased according to response

- CONTRA-INDICATIONS Depression · parkinsonism · phaeochromocytoma · prolactin-dependent tumours
- CAUTIONS Susceptibility to QT-interval prolongation
- INTERACTIONS → Appendix 1: tetrabenazine
- SIDE-EFFECTS
▸ **Common or very common** Anxiety · confusion · constipation · depression · diarrhoea · drowsiness · hypotension · insomnia · nausea · parkinsonism · vomiting
▸ **Uncommon** Consciousness impaired · hyperthermia
▸ **Rare or very rare** Neuroleptic malignant syndrome · skeletal muscle damage
▸ **Frequency not known** Bradycardia · dizziness · dry mouth · epigastric pain · suicidal ideation
- PREGNANCY Avoid unless essential—toxicity in *animal* studies.
- BREAST FEEDING Avoid.
- HEPATIC IMPAIRMENT Manufacturer advises caution (increased risk of exposure), particularly in severe impairment (no information available).
  Dose adjustments Manufacturer advises initial dose reduction of 50% and slower dose titration in mild to moderate impairment.
- RENAL IMPAIRMENT Use with caution.
- TREATMENT CESSATION Avoid abrupt withdrawal.
- PATIENT AND CARER ADVICE
  Driving and skilled tasks May affect performance of skilled tasks (e.g. driving).

- MEDICINAL FORMS There can be variation in the licensing of different medicines containing the same drug. Forms available from special-order manufacturers include: oral suspension
Tablet
CAUTIONARY AND ADVISORY LABELS 2
▸ Tetrabenazine (Non-proprietary)
  Tetrabenazine 25 mg Tetrabenazine 25mg tablets | 112 tablet [PoM] £107.69 DT = £107.69
▸ Tardiben (AOP Orphan Ltd)
  Tetrabenazine 25 mg Tardiben 25mg tablets | 112 tablet [PoM] £100.00 DT = £107.69
▸ Xenazine (Alliance Pharmaceuticals Ltd)
  Tetrabenazine 25 mg Xenazine 25 tablets | 112 tablet [PoM] £100.00 DT = £107.69

MUSCLE RELAXANTS ❯ PERIPHERALLY ACTING ❯ NEUROTOXINS (BOTULINUM TOXINS)

Botulinum toxin type A

03-Nov-2020

- INDICATIONS AND DOSE
Hand and wrist disability due to upper limb spasticity associated with stroke (specialist use only) | Foot and ankle disability due to lower limb spasticity associated with stroke (specialist use only) | Blepharospasm (specialist use only) | Hemifacial spasm (specialist use only) | Spasmodic torticollis (specialist use only) | Severe hyperhidrosis of the axillae (specialist use only) | Prophylaxis of headaches in chronic migraine (specialist use only) | Temporary improvement of moderate to severe upper facial lines in adults under 65 years (specialist use only) | Management of bladder dysfunctions (specialist use only) | Chronic sialorrhoea [due to neurological disorders] (specialist use only)
▸ BY SUBCUTANEOUS INJECTION, OR BY INTRADERMAL INJECTION, OR BY INTRAMUSCULAR INJECTION, OR BY LOCAL INFILTRATION
▸ Adult: (consult product literature)
DOSE EQUIVALENCE AND CONVERSION
▸ **Important**: information is specific to each individual preparation.

- CONTRA-INDICATIONS Acute urinary retention (specific to use in bladder disorders only) · catheterisation difficulties (specific to use in bladder disorders only) · infection at injection site · presence of bladder calculi (specific to use in bladder disorders only) · urinary tract infection (specific to use in bladder disorders only)
- CAUTIONS
GENERAL CAUTIONS Atrophy in target muscle · chronic respiratory disorder · elderly · excessive weakness in target muscle · history of aspiration · history of dysphagia · inflammation in target muscle · neurological disorders · neuromuscular disorders · off-label use (fatal adverse events reported)
SPECIFIC CAUTIONS
▸ When used for Blepharospasm or Hemifacial spasm Risk of angle-closure glaucoma
CAUTIONS, FURTHER INFORMATION Neuromuscular or neurological disorders can lead to increased sensitivity and exaggerated muscle weakness including dysphagia and respiratory compromise.
▸ Blepharospasm or hemifacial spasm When used for blepharospasm and hemifacial spasm, reduced blinking can lead to corneal exposure, persistent epithelial defect and corneal ulceration (especially in those with VIIth nerve disorders)—careful testing of corneal sensation in previously operated eyes, avoidance of injection in lower lid area to avoid ectropion, and vigorous treatment of epithelial defect needed.
- INTERACTIONS → Appendix 1: botulinum toxins

- SIDE-EFFECTS
- **Common or very common** Alopecia · asthenia · autonomic dysreflexia · bladder diverticulum · constipation · dizziness · drowsiness · dry eye · dry mouth · dysphagia (most common after injection into sternocleidomastoid muscle and salivary gland) · ecchymosis (minimised by applying gentle pressure at injection site immediately after injection) · eye discomfort · eye disorders · eye inflammation · fall · fever · gait abnormal · haematuria · headaches · hot flush · increased risk of infection · influenza like illness · insomnia · joint disorders · leukocyturia · malaise · muscle complaints · muscle weakness · musculoskeletal stiffness · nausea · neuromuscular dysfunction · oedema · pain · paresis · sensation abnormal · skin reactions · subcutaneous nodule · urinary disorders · vision disorders
- **Uncommon** Anxiety · coordination abnormal · depression · dysphonia · dyspnoea · facial paralysis · memory loss · oral paraesthesia · photosensitivity reaction · postural hypotension · speech impairment · taste altered · vertigo
- **Frequency not known** Abdominal pain · angioedema · angle closure glaucoma · appetite decreased · arrhythmia · diarrhoea · hearing impairment · hypersensitivity · myocardial infarction · myopathy · nerve disorders · respiratory disorders · seizure · syncope · tinnitus · vomiting
- CONCEPTION AND CONTRACEPTION Avoid in women of child-bearing age unless using effective contraception.
- PREGNANCY Avoid unless essential—toxicity in *animal* studies (manufacturer of *Botox®* advise avoid).
- BREAST FEEDING Low risk of systemic absorption but avoid unless essential.
- PRESCRIBING AND DISPENSING INFORMATION Preparations are not interchangeable.
- PATIENT AND CARER ADVICE Patients and carers should be warned of the signs and symptoms of toxin spread, such as muscle weakness and breathing difficulties; they should be advised to seek immediate medical attention if swallowing, speech or breathing difficulties occur.
- NATIONAL FUNDING/ACCESS DECISIONS For full details see funding body website

NICE decisions
- Botulinum toxin type A for the prevention of headaches in adults with chronic migraine (June 2012) NICE TA260 Recommended with restrictions
- Xeomin ® (botulinum neurotoxin type A) for treating chronic sialorrhoea (October 2019) NICE TA605 Recommended

Scottish Medicines Consortium (SMC) decisions
- Botulinum toxin type A (*Botox®*) for the management of bladder dysfunctions in adult patients who are not adequately managed with anticholinergics: overactive bladder with symptoms of urinary incontinence, urgency and frequency (July 2014) SMC No. 931/13 Recommended with restrictions
- Botulinum toxin A (*Botox®*) for the prophylaxis of headaches in adults with chronic migraine (headaches on at least 15 days per month of which at least 8 days are with migraine) (February 2017) SMC No. 692/11 Recommended with restrictions
- Clostridium botulinum neurotoxin type A (*Xeomin®*) for adult patients with chronic sialorrhoea due to neurological conditions (November 2019) SMC No. SMC2212 Recommended

- MEDICINAL FORMS There can be variation in the licensing of different medicines containing the same drug.

Powder for solution for injection
- Azzalure (Galderma (UK) Ltd)
  Botulinum toxin type A 125 unit Azzalure 125unit powder for solution for injection vials | 1 vial PoM £64.00 | 2 vial PoM £128.00
- Bocouture (Merz Pharma UK Ltd)
  Botulinum toxin type A 50 unit Bocouture 50unit powder for solution for injection vials | 1 vial PoM £72.00

Botulinum toxin type A 100 unit Bocouture 100unit powder for solution for injection vials | 1 vial PoM £229.90
- Botox (Allergan Ltd)
  Botulinum toxin type A 50 unit Botox 50unit powder for solution for injection vials | 1 vial PoM £77.50 (Hospital only)
  Botulinum toxin type A 100 unit Botox 100unit powder for solution for injection vials | 1 vial PoM £138.20 (Hospital only)
  Botulinum toxin type A 200 unit Botox 200unit powder for solution for injection vials | 1 vial PoM £276.40 (Hospital only)
- Dysport (Ipsen Ltd)
  Botulinum toxin type A 300 unit Dysport 300unit powder for solution for injection vials | 1 vial PoM £92.40
  Botulinum toxin type A 500 unit Dysport 500unit powder for solution for injection vials | 2 vial PoM £308.00
- Xeomin (Merz Pharma UK Ltd)
  Botulinum toxin type A 50 unit Xeomin 50unit powder for solution for injection vials | 1 vial PoM £72.00
  Botulinum toxin type A 100 unit Xeomin 100unit powder for solution for injection vials | 1 vial PoM £129.90
  Botulinum toxin type A 200 unit Xeomin 200unit powder for solution for injection vials | 1 vial PoM £259.80 (Hospital only)

Botulinum toxin type B
02-Sep-2020

- **INDICATIONS AND DOSE**
Spasmodic torticollis (cervical dystonia) (specialist use only)
- BY INTRAMUSCULAR INJECTION
- Adult: Initially 5000–10 000 units, adjusted according to response, dose to be divided between 2–4 most affected muscles

DOSE EQUIVALENCE AND CONVERSION
- **Important**: information specific to each individual preparation.

- CONTRA-INDICATIONS Neuromuscular disorders · neuromuscular junctional disorders
- CAUTIONS History of dysphagia or aspiration · off-label use (risk of toxin spread) · tolerance may occur
- INTERACTIONS → Appendix 1: botulinum toxins
- SIDE-EFFECTS
- **Common or very common** Dry mouth · dysphagia · dysphonia · headache · influenza like illness · muscle weakness · neck pain · taste altered · vision disorders
- **Frequency not known** Angioedema · asthenia · constipation · dyspnoea · pneumonia aspiration · ptosis · skin reactions · vomiting
- PREGNANCY Low risk of systemic absorption but avoid unless essential.
- BREAST FEEDING Low risk of systemic absorption but avoid unless essential.
- DIRECTIONS FOR ADMINISTRATION Manufacturer advises injection may be diluted with sodium chloride 0.9%.
- PRESCRIBING AND DISPENSING INFORMATION **Important: not** interchangeable with other botulinum toxin preparations.
- PATIENT AND CARER ADVICE Patients should be warned of the signs and symptoms of toxin spread, such as muscle weakness and breathing difficulties; they should be advised to seek immediate medical attention if swallowing, speech or breathing difficulties occur.

- MEDICINAL FORMS There can be variation in the licensing of different medicines containing the same drug.

Solution for injection
- NeuroBloc (Sloan Pharma Sarl)
  Botulinum toxin type B 5000 unit per 1 ml NeuroBloc 5,000units/1ml solution for injection vials | 1 vial PoM £148.27 (Hospital only)
  NeuroBloc 10,000units/2ml solution for injection vials | 1 vial PoM £197.69 (Hospital only)
  NeuroBloc 2,500units/0.5ml solution for injection vials | 1 vial PoM £111.20 (Hospital only)

4

Nervous system

4.2 Parkinson's disease

Parkinson's disease

13-Nov-2020

Description of condition

Parkinson's disease is a progressive neurodegenerative condition resulting from the death of dopaminergic cells of the substantia nigra in the brain.

Patients with Parkinson's disease classically present with motor-symptoms including hypokinesia, bradykinesia, rigidity, rest tremor, and postural instability.

Non-motor symptoms include dementia, depression, sleep disturbances, bladder and bowel dysfunction, speech and language changes, swallowing problems and weight loss.

EvGr Patients with suspected Parkinson's disease should be referred to a specialist and reviewed every 6 to 12 months. When Parkinson's disease diagnosis is confirmed, patients should be advised to inform the DVLA and their car insurer. Ⓐ

Aims of treatment

Parkinson's disease is an incurable progressive condition, and the aim of treatment is to control the symptoms and to improve the patient's quality of life.

Non-drug treatment

EvGr Parkinson's disease patients should be offered physiotherapy if balance or motor function problems are present, speech and language therapy if they develop communication, swallowing or saliva problems, and occupational therapy if they experience difficulties with their daily activities. Dietitian referral should be considered. Ⓐ

Drug treatment

Drug management of motor symptoms in Parkinson's disease
First-line treatment
EvGr In early stages of Parkinson's disease, patients whose motor symptoms decrease their quality of life should be offered *levodopa* combined with *carbidopa* (co-careldopa p. 435) or *benserazide* (co-beneldopa p. 434).

Parkinson's disease patients whose motor symptoms *do not* affect their quality of life, could be prescribed a choice of *levodopa, non-ergot-derived dopamine-receptor agonists* (pramipexole p. 442, ropinirole p. 444 or rotigotine p. 445) or *monoamine-oxidase-B inhibitors* (rasagiline p. 446 or selegiline hydrochloride p. 447).

Before starting antiparkinsonian treatment, the patient's individual circumstances, including symptoms, comorbidities and preferences, should be discussed together with the potential benefits and harms from the different drugs available.

Patients and their carers should be informed about the risk of adverse reactions from antiparkinsonian drugs, including psychotic symptoms, excessive sleepiness and sudden onset of sleep with dopamine-receptor agonists, and impulse control disorders with all dopaminergic therapy (especially *dopamine-receptor agonists*). For further information *see Impulse control disorders*. Ⓐ

Levodopa treatment is associated with motor complications, including response fluctuations and dyskinesias. Response fluctuations are characterised by large variations in motor performance, with normal function during the 'on' period, and weakness and restricted mobility during the 'off' period. 'End-of-dose' deterioration with progressively shorter duration of benefit can also occur. Modified-release preparations may help with 'end-of-dose' deterioration or nocturnal immobility.

The overall improvement in motor performance is more noticeable with *levodopa* than with *dopamine-receptor agonists*, and motor complications are less likely to occur with *dopamine-receptor agonists* when used alone long-term. Conversely, excessive sleepiness, hallucinations, and impulse control disorders are more likely to occur with *dopamine-receptor agonists* than with *levodopa*.

EvGr To avoid the potential for acute akinesia or neuroleptic malignant syndrome, antiparkinsonian drug concentrations should not be allowed to fall suddenly due to poor absorption or abrupt withdrawal. Ⓐ

Adjuvant therapy
EvGr If a patient with Parkinson's disease develops dyskinesia or motor fluctuations, specialist advice should be sought before modifying antiparkinsonian drug therapy.

Patients who develop dyskinesia or motor fluctuations despite optimal *levodopa* therapy should be offered a choice of *non-ergotic dopamine-receptor agonists* (pramipexole, ropinirole, rotigotine), *monoamine oxidase B inhibitors* (rasagiline or selegiline hydrochloride) or COMT inhibitors (entacapone p. 433 or tolcapone p. 433) as an adjunct to *levodopa*.

An *ergot-derived dopamine-receptor agonist* (bromocriptine p. 440, cabergoline p. 441 or pergolide) should **only** be considered as an adjunct to *levodopa* if symptoms are not adequately controlled with a *non-ergot-derived dopamine-receptor agonist*.

If dyskinesia is not adequately managed by modifying existing therapy, amantadine hydrochloride p. 438 should be considered. Ⓐ

Drug management of non-motor symptoms in Parkinson's disease
Daytime sleepiness and sudden onset of sleep
EvGr Patients who experience daytime sleepiness or sudden onset of sleep, should have their Parkinson's drug treatment adjusted under specialist medical guidance. If reversible pharmacological and physical causes have been excluded, modafinil p. 513 should be considered to treat excessive daytime sleepiness, and treatment should be reviewed at least every 12 months.

Patients with Parkinson's disease who have daytime sleepiness or sudden onset of sleep should be advised not to drive, to inform the DVLA about their symptoms, and to think about any occupational hazards. Ⓐ

Nocturnal akinesia
EvGr When treating nocturnal akinesia in patients with Parkinson's disease, *levodopa* or oral *dopamine-receptor agonists* should be considered as first-line options and rotigotine p. 445 as second-line (if both *levodopa* or oral *dopamine-receptor agonists* are ineffective). Ⓐ

Postural hypotension
EvGr Patients with Parkinson's disease who develop postural hypotension should have their drug treatment reviewed to address any pharmacological cause. If drug therapy is required, midodrine hydrochloride p. 202 should be considered as the first option and fludrocortisone acetate p. 715 [unlicensed indication] as an alternative. Ⓐ

Depression
See Antidepressant drugs p. 378.

Psychotic symptoms
EvGr Hallucinations and delusions need not be treated if they are well tolerated. Otherwise, the dosage of any antiparkinsonism drugs that might have triggered hallucinations or delusions should be reduced, taking into account the severity of symptoms and possible withdrawal effects. Specialist advice should be sought before modifying drug treatment.

In Parkinson's disease patients with no cognitive impairment, quetiapine p. 422 [unlicensed indication] can be considered to treat hallucinations and delusions. If standard treatment is not effective, clozapine p. 417 should be offered to treat hallucinations and delusions in patients with Parkinson's disease. Ⓐ It is important to acknowledge that other antipsychotic medicines (such as phenothiazines and butyrophenones) can worsen the motor features of Parkinson's disease.

Rapid eye movement sleep behaviour disorder

EvGr Clonazepam p. 355 [unlicensed indication] or melatonin p. 510 [unlicensed indication] should be used to treat rapid eye movement sleep behaviour disorder in Parkinson's patients once possible pharmacological causes have been addressed. Ⓐ The MHRA/CHM have released important safety information on the use of antiepileptic drugs and the risk of suicidal thoughts and behaviour. For further information, see Epilepsy p. 321.

Drooling of saliva

EvGr Drug treatment for drooling of saliva in patients with Parkinson's disease should only be considered if non-drug treatment such as speech and language therapy is not available or is ineffective.

Glycopyrronium bromide p. 1387 [unlicensed indication] should be considered as first-line treatment and botulinum toxin type A p. 428 as second-line.

Other antimuscarinic drugs, should only be considered if the risk of cognitive adverse effects is thought to be minimal; topical preparations, such as *atropine* [unlicensed indication], should be used if possible to reduce the risk of adverse events. Ⓐ

Parkinson's disease dementia

EvGr An acetylcholinesterase inhibitor should be offered to patients with mild-to-moderate Parkinson's disease dementia and considered for patients with severe Parkinson's disease dementia [unlicensed indications apart from rivastigmine capsules and oral solution p. 319 for the treatment of mild-to-moderate dementia in patients with Parkinson's disease]. If acetylcholinesterase inhibitors are not tolerated or contra-indicated, memantine hydrochloride p. 320 [unlicensed indication] should be considered. Ⓐ For further information *see* Dementia p. 316

Advanced Parkinson's disease

EvGr Patients with advanced Parkinson's disease can be offered apomorphine hydrochloride p. 438 as intermittent injections or continuous subcutaneous infusions. Ⓐ To control nausea and vomiting associated with *apomorphine*, the manufacturers recommend that administration of domperidone p. 451 [unlicensed in those weighing less than 35 kg] will usually need to be started two days before *apomorphine* therapy, and then discontinued as soon as possible. To reduce the risk of serious arrhythmia due to QT prolongation associated to the concomitant use of domperidone p. 451 and apomorphine hydrochloride p. 438, the MHRA/CHM recommend an assessment of cardiac risk factors and ECG monitoring and to ensure that the benefits outweighs the risks when initiating treatment. In addition, the MHRA/CHM have released important safety information and restrictions regarding the use of domperidone for nausea and vomiting in those weighing less than 35 kg, and a reminder of contra-indications. For further information, see *Important safety information* for domperidone p. 451.

Levodopa-carbidopa intestinal gel is used for the treatment of advanced levodopa-responsive Parkinson's disease with severe motor fluctuations and hyperkinesia or dyskinesia. The gel is administered with a portable pump directly into the duodenum or upper jejunum.

EvGr Deep brain stimulation should *only* be considered for patients with advanced Parkinson's disease whose symptoms are *not* adequately controlled by best drug therapy. Ⓐ

Impulse control disorders

Impulse control disorders (compulsive gambling, hypersexuality, binge eating, or obsessive shopping) can develop in a person with Parkinson's disease who is on any dopaminergic therapy at any stage in the disease course particularly if the patient has a history of previous impulsive behaviours, alcohol consumption, or smoking. EvGr Patients should be informed about the different types of impulse control disorders and that dopamine-receptor agonist therapy may be reduced or stopped if problematic impulse control disorders develop.

When managing impulse control disorders, dopamine-receptor agonist doses should be reduced gradually and patients should be monitored for symptoms of dopamine agonist withdrawal. Specialist cognitive behavioural therapy should be offered if modifying dopaminergic therapy is not effective. Ⓐ

Useful Resources

Parkinson's disease in adults. National Institute for Health and Care Excellence. NICE guideline 71. July 2017. www.nice.org.uk/guidance/NG71

ANTIMUSCARINICS

Orphenadrine hydrochloride
20-Dec-2019

- **DRUG ACTION** Orphenadrine exerts its antiparkinsonian action by reducing the effects of the relative central cholinergic excess that occurs as a result of dopamine deficiency.

- **INDICATIONS AND DOSE**

Parkinsonism | Drug-induced extrapyramidal symptoms (but not tardive dyskinesia)
▶ BY MOUTH
  ▸ Adult: Initially 150 mg daily in divided doses, then increased in steps of 50 mg every 2–3 days, adjusted according to response; usual dose 150–300 mg daily in divided doses; maximum 400 mg per day
  ▸ Elderly: Preferably dose at lower end of range

- **CONTRA-INDICATIONS** Acute porphyrias p. 1107 · gastro-intestinal obstruction

- **CAUTIONS** Cardiovascular disease · elderly · hypertension · in patients susceptible to angle-closure glaucoma · liable to abuse · prostatic hypertrophy · psychotic disorders · pyrexia

- **INTERACTIONS** → Appendix 1: orphenadrine

- **SIDE-EFFECTS**
▶ **Common or very common** Accommodation disorder · anxiety · dizziness · dry mouth · gastrointestinal disorder · nausea
▶ **Uncommon** Confusion · constipation · coordination abnormal · euphoric mood · hallucination · insomnia · sedation · seizure · tachycardia · urinary retention
▶ **Rare or very rare** Memory loss

- **PREGNANCY** Caution.

- **BREAST FEEDING** Caution.

- **HEPATIC IMPAIRMENT** Manufacturer advises caution.

- **RENAL IMPAIRMENT** Use with caution.

- **TREATMENT CESSATION** Avoid abrupt withdrawal in patients taking long-term treatment.

- **PATIENT AND CARER ADVICE**
  Driving and skilled tasks May affect performance of skilled tasks (e.g. driving).

- **MEDICINAL FORMS** There can be variation in the licensing of different medicines containing the same drug. Forms available from special-order manufacturers include: oral solution
  Oral solution
  ▸ Orphenadrine hydrochloride (Non-proprietary)
    Orphenadrine hydrochloride 10 mg per 1 ml Orphenadrine 50mg/5ml oral solution sugar free sugar-free | 150 ml PoM £67.00 DT = £56.14

Procyclidine hydrochloride
31-Oct-2019

- **DRUG ACTION** Procyclidine exerts its antiparkinsonian action by reducing the effects of the relative central cholinergic excess that occurs as a result of dopamine deficiency.

- **INDICATIONS AND DOSE**

Parkinsonism | Extrapyramidal symptoms (but not tardive dyskinesia)
- ▶ BY MOUTH
- ▶ Adult: 2.5 mg 3 times a day, then increased in steps of 2.5–5 mg daily if required; increased if necessary up to 30 mg daily in 2–4 divided doses, to be increased at 2–3 day intervals. Maximum daily dose only to be used in exceptional circumstances; maximum 60 mg per day
- ▶ Elderly: Lower end of range preferable

Acute dystonia
- ▶ BY INTRAMUSCULAR INJECTION, OR BY INTRAVENOUS INJECTION
- ▶ Adult: 5–10 mg, occasionally, more than 10 mg, dose usually effective in 5–10 minutes but may need 30 minutes for relief
- ▶ Elderly: Lower end of range preferable

- **CONTRA-INDICATIONS** Gastro-intestinal obstruction
- **CAUTIONS** Cardiovascular disease · elderly · hypertension · liable to abuse · prostatic hypertrophy · psychotic disorders · pyrexia · those susceptible to angle-closure glaucoma
- **INTERACTIONS** → Appendix 1: procyclidine
- **SIDE-EFFECTS**
- ▶ **Common or very common** Constipation · dry mouth · urinary retention · vision blurred
- ▶ **Uncommon** Anxiety · cognitive impairment · confusion · dizziness · gingivitis · hallucination · memory loss · nausea · rash · vomiting
- ▶ **Rare or very rare** Psychotic disorder
- **PREGNANCY** Use only if potential benefit outweighs risk.
- **BREAST FEEDING** No information available.
- **HEPATIC IMPAIRMENT** Manufacturer advises caution.
- **RENAL IMPAIRMENT** Use with caution.
- **TREATMENT CESSATION** Avoid abrupt withdrawal in patients taking long-term treatment.
- **PATIENT AND CARER ADVICE**
Driving and skilled tasks May affect performance of skilled tasks (e.g. driving).

- **MEDICINAL FORMS** There can be variation in the licensing of different medicines containing the same drug. Forms available from special-order manufacturers include: oral suspension, oral solution

Solution for injection
- ▶ Procyclidine hydrochloride (Non-proprietary)
Procyclidine hydrochloride 5 mg per 1 ml Procyclidine 10mg/2ml solution for injection ampoules | 5 ampoule [PoM] £72.50–£86.89 DT = £79.54

Oral solution
- ▶ Procyclidine hydrochloride (Non-proprietary)
Procyclidine hydrochloride 500 microgram per 1 ml Procyclidine 2.5mg/5ml oral solution sugar free sugar-free | 150 ml [PoM] £23.09 DT = £20.00
Procyclidine hydrochloride 1 mg per 1 ml Procyclidine 5mg/5ml oral solution sugar free sugar-free | 150 ml [PoM] £33.25 DT = £28.85

Tablet
- ▶ Procyclidine hydrochloride (Non-proprietary)
Procyclidine hydrochloride 5 mg Procyclidine 5mg tablets | 28 tablet [PoM] £12.65 DT = £1.97 | 100 tablet [PoM] £7.04–£8.94 | 500 tablet [PoM] £35.18–£44.63
- ▶ Kemadrin (Aspen Pharma Trading Ltd)
Procyclidine hydrochloride 5 mg Kemadrin 5mg tablets | 100 tablet [PoM] £4.72 | 500 tablet [PoM] £23.62

Trihexyphenidyl hydrochloride
03-Sep-2020

(Benzhexol hydrochloride)

- **DRUG ACTION** Trihexyphenidyl exerts its effects by reducing the effects of the relative central cholinergic excess that occurs as a result of dopamine deficiency.

- **INDICATIONS AND DOSE**

Parkinson's disease (if used in combination with co-careldopa or co-beneldopa)
- ▶ BY MOUTH
- ▶ Adult: Maintenance 2–6 mg daily in divided doses, use not recommended because of toxicity in the elderly and the risk of aggravating dementia

Parkinsonism | Drug-induced extrapyramidal symptoms (but not tardive dyskinesia)
- ▶ BY MOUTH
- ▶ Adult: 1 mg daily, then increased in steps of 2 mg every 3–5 days, adjusted according to response; maintenance 5–15 mg daily in 3–4 divided doses, not recommended for use in Parkinson's disease because of toxicity in the elderly and the risk of aggravating dementia; maximum 20 mg per day
- ▶ Elderly: Lower end of range preferable, not recommended for use in Parkinson's disease because of toxicity in the elderly and the risk of aggravating dementia

- **CONTRA-INDICATIONS** Myasthenia gravis
- **CAUTIONS** Cardiovascular disease · elderly · gastro-intestinal obstruction · hypertension · liable to abuse · prostatic hypertrophy · psychotic disorders · pyrexia · those susceptible to angle-closure glaucoma
- **INTERACTIONS** → Appendix 1: trihexyphenidyl
- **SIDE-EFFECTS** Anxiety · bronchial secretion decreased · confusion · constipation · delusions · dizziness · dry mouth · dysphagia · euphoric mood · fever · flushing · hallucination · insomnia · memory loss · myasthenia gravis aggravated · mydriasis · nausea · skin reactions · tachycardia · thirst · urinary disorders · vision disorders · vomiting
- **PREGNANCY** Use only if potential benefit outweighs risk.
- **BREAST FEEDING** Avoid.
- **HEPATIC IMPAIRMENT** Manufacturer advises caution.
- **RENAL IMPAIRMENT** Use with caution.
- **TREATMENT CESSATION** Avoid abrupt withdrawal in patients taking long-term treatment.
- **DIRECTIONS FOR ADMINISTRATION** Manufacturer advises tablets should be taken with or after food.
- **PATIENT AND CARER ADVICE**
Driving and skilled tasks May affect performance of skilled tasks (e.g. driving).

- **MEDICINAL FORMS** There can be variation in the licensing of different medicines containing the same drug. Forms available from special-order manufacturers include: oral suspension, oral solution

Oral solution
EXCIPIENTS: May contain Propylene glycol
- ▶ Trihexyphenidyl hydrochloride (Non-proprietary)
Trihexyphenidyl hydrochloride 1 mg per 1 ml Trihexyphenidyl 5mg/5ml oral solution | 200 ml [PoM] £53.41 DT = £42.51
Trihexyphenidyl 5mg/5ml syrup | 200 ml [PoM] £53.41 DT = £42.51

Tablet
- ▶ Trihexyphenidyl hydrochloride (Non-proprietary)
Trihexyphenidyl hydrochloride 2 mg Trihexyphenidyl 2mg tablets | 84 tablet [PoM] £8.53 DT = £8.53
Trihexyphenidyl hydrochloride 5 mg Trihexyphenidyl 5mg tablets | 84 tablet [PoM] £20.62 DT = £20.62

DOPAMINERGIC DRUGS > CATECHOL-O-METHYLTRANSFERASE INHIBITORS

Entacapone

04-Sep-2020

- **DRUG ACTION** Entacapone prevents the peripheral breakdown of levodopa, by inhibiting catechol- *O*-methyltransferase, allowing more levodopa to reach the brain.

- **INDICATIONS AND DOSE**

Adjunct to co-beneldopa or co-careldopa in Parkinson's disease with 'end-of-dose' motor fluctuations (under expert supervision)
  - ▸ BY MOUTH
    - ▸ Adult: 200 mg, dose to be given with each dose of levodopa with dopa-decarboxylase inhibitor; maximum 2 g per day

- **CONTRA-INDICATIONS** History of neuroleptic malignant syndrome · history of non-traumatic rhabdomyolysis · phaeochromocytoma
- **CAUTIONS** Concurrent levodopa dose may need to be reduced by about 10–30% · ischaemic heart disease
- **INTERACTIONS** → Appendix 1: entacapone
- **SIDE-EFFECTS**
  - ▸ **Common or very common** Abdominal pain · confusion · constipation · diarrhoea · dizziness · dry mouth · fall · fatigue · hallucination · hyperhidrosis · ischaemic heart disease · movement disorders · nausea · sleep disorders · urine discolouration · vomiting
  - ▸ **Uncommon** Myocardial infarction
  - ▸ **Rare or very rare** Agitation · appetite decreased · skin reactions · weight decreased
  - ▸ **Frequency not known** Colitis · drowsiness · hair colour changes · hepatic disorders · impulse-control disorder · nail discolouration · neuroleptic malignant syndrome · rhabdomyolysis
- **PREGNANCY** Avoid—no information available.
- **BREAST FEEDING** Avoid—present in milk in *animal* studies.
- **HEPATIC IMPAIRMENT** Manufacturer advises avoid.
- **TREATMENT CESSATION** Avoid abrupt withdrawal.
- **PATIENT AND CARER ADVICE** Patient counselling is advised (may colour urine reddish-brown, concomitant iron containing products).

- **MEDICINAL FORMS** There can be variation in the licensing of different medicines containing the same drug. Forms available from special-order manufacturers include: oral suspension, oral solution

Tablet
CAUTIONARY AND ADVISORY LABELS 14
  - ▸ Entacapone (Non-proprietary)
    Entacapone 200 mg Entacapone 200mg tablets | 30 tablet [PoM] £16.38 DT = £3.87 | 100 tablet [PoM] £16.01–£54.58
  - ▸ Comtess (Orion Pharma (UK) Ltd)
    Entacapone 200 mg Comtess 200mg tablets | 30 tablet [PoM] £17.24 DT = £3.87 | 100 tablet [PoM] £57.45

Combinations available: *Levodopa with carbidopa and entacapone*, p. 437

Opicapone

11-Apr-2017

- **DRUG ACTION** Opicapone prevents the peripheral breakdown of levodopa, by inhibiting catechol- *O*-methyltransferase, allowing more levodopa to reach the brain.

- **INDICATIONS AND DOSE**

Adjunct to co-beneldopa or co-careldopa in Parkinson's disease with 'end-of-dose' motor fluctuations (under expert supervision)
  - ▸ BY MOUTH
    - ▸ Adult: 50 mg once daily, dose to be taken at bedtime, at least one hour before or after levodopa combinations

- **CONTRA-INDICATIONS** Catecholamine-secreting neoplasms · history of neuroleptic malignant syndrome · history of non-traumatic rhabdomyolysis · paraganglioma · phaeochromocytoma
- **CAUTIONS** Concurrent levodopa dose may need to be reduced · elderly over 85 years (limited information available)
- **INTERACTIONS** → Appendix 1: opicapone
- **SIDE-EFFECTS**
  - ▸ **Common or very common** Constipation · dizziness · drowsiness · dry mouth · hallucinations · headache · hypotension · movement disorders · muscle complaints · sleep disorders · vomiting
  - ▸ **Uncommon** Anxiety · appetite decreased · depression · dry eye · dyspnoea · ear congestion · gastrointestinal discomfort · hypertension · hypertriglyceridaemia · musculoskeletal stiffness · nocturia · pain in extremity · palpitations · syncope · taste altered · urine discolouration · weight decreased

  SIDE-EFFECTS, FURTHER INFORMATION Manufacturer advises consider liver function tests in patients who experience progressive anorexia, asthenia and weight decrease within a relatively short period of time.

- **PREGNANCY** Manufacturer advises avoid—limited information available.
- **BREAST FEEDING** Manufacturer advises avoid—no information available.
- **HEPATIC IMPAIRMENT** Manufacturer advises caution in moderate impairment (risk of increased exposure); avoid in severe impairment (no information available).
  Dose adjustments Manufacturer advises consider dose reduction in moderate impairment.

- **MEDICINAL FORMS** There can be variation in the licensing of different medicines containing the same drug.
Capsule
  - ▸ Ongentys (BIAL Pharma UK Ltd) ▼
    Opicapone 50 mg Ongentys 50mg capsules | 30 capsule [PoM] £93.90 DT = £93.90

Tolcapone

03-Sep-2020

- **DRUG ACTION** Tolcapone prevents the peripheral breakdown of levodopa, by inhibiting catechol- O-methyltransferase, allowing more levodopa to reach the brain.

- **INDICATIONS AND DOSE**

Adjunct to co-beneldopa or co-careldopa in Parkinson's disease with 'end-of-dose' motor fluctuations if another inhibitor of peripheral catechol-O-methyltransferase inappropriate (under expert supervision)
  - ▸ BY MOUTH
    - ▸ Adult: 100 mg 3 times a day (max. per dose 200 mg 3 times a day) continuing beyond 3 weeks **only** if substantial improvement, leave 6 hours continued →

4

Nervous system

4

Nervous system

between each dose; first daily dose should be taken at the same time as levodopa with dopa-decarboxylase inhibitor, dose maximum only in exceptional circumstances

- CONTRA-INDICATIONS Phaeochromocytoma · previous history of hyperthermia · previous history of neuroleptic malignant syndrome · previous history of rhabdomyolysis · severe dyskinesia
- CAUTIONS Most patients receiving more than 600 mg levodopa daily require reduction of levodopa dose by about 30%

  CAUTIONS, FURTHER INFORMATION
  ▸ Hepatotoxicity Potentially life-threatening hepatotoxicity including fulminant hepatitis reported rarely, usually in women and during the first 6 months, but late-onset liver injury also reported; discontinue if abnormal liver function tests or symptoms of liver disorder; do not re-introduce tolcapone once discontinued.
- INTERACTIONS → Appendix 1: tolcapone
- SIDE-EFFECTS
  ▸ Common or very common Appetite decreased · chest pain · confusion · constipation · diarrhoea · dizziness · drowsiness · dry mouth · gastrointestinal discomfort · hallucination · headache · hyperhidrosis · influenza like illness · movement disorders · nausea · postural hypotension · sleep disorders · syncope · upper respiratory tract infection · urine discolouration · vomiting
  ▸ Uncommon Hepatocellular injury
  ▸ Rare or very rare Eating disorders · neuroleptic malignant syndrome (reported on dose reduction or withdrawal) · pathological gambling · psychiatric disorders · sexual dysfunction
- PREGNANCY Toxicity in *animal* studies—use only if potential benefit outweighs risk.
- BREAST FEEDING Avoid—present in milk in *animal* studies.
- HEPATIC IMPAIRMENT Manufacturer advises avoid.
- RENAL IMPAIRMENT Caution if eGFR less than 30 mL/minute/1.73 m^2.
- MONITORING REQUIREMENTS Test liver function before treatment, and monitor every 2 weeks for first year, every 4 weeks for next 6 months and then every 8 weeks thereafter (restart monitoring schedule if dose increased).
- TREATMENT CESSATION Avoid abrupt withdrawal.
- PATIENT AND CARER ADVICE Patients should be told how to recognise signs of liver disorder and advised to seek immediate medical attention if symptoms such as anorexia, nausea, vomiting, fatigue, abdominal pain, dark urine, or pruritus develop.

- MEDICINAL FORMS There can be variation in the licensing of different medicines containing the same drug.
  Tablet
  CAUTIONARY AND ADVISORY LABELS 14, 25
  ▸ Tasmar (Mylan)
  Tolcapone 100 mg Tasmar 100mg tablets | 100 tablet [PoM] £95.20 DT = £95.20

DOPAMINERGIC DRUGS > DOPAMINE PRECURSORS

Co-beneldopa

27-Jul-2020

- INDICATIONS AND DOSE
  Parkinson's disease
  ▸ BY MOUTH USING IMMEDIATE-RELEASE MEDICINES
  ▸ Adult: Initially 50 mg 3–4 times a day, then increased in steps of 100 mg daily, dose to be increased once or twice weekly according to response; maintenance 400–800 mg daily in divided doses

- ▸ Elderly: Initially 50 mg 1–2 times a day, then increased in steps of 50 mg daily, dose to be increased every 3–4 days according to response

Parkinson's disease (in advanced disease)
▸ BY MOUTH USING IMMEDIATE-RELEASE MEDICINES
▸ Adult: Initially 100 mg 3 times a day, then increased in steps of 100 mg daily, dose to be increased once or twice weekly according to response; maintenance 400–800 mg daily in divided doses

Parkinson's disease (patients not taking levodopa/dopa-decarboxylase inhibitor therapy)
▸ BY MOUTH USING MODIFIED-RELEASE MEDICINES
▸ Adult: Initially 1 capsule 3 times a day; maximum 6 capsules per day

Parkinson's disease (patients transferring from immediate-release levodopa/dopa-decarboxylase inhibitor preparations)
▸ BY MOUTH USING MODIFIED-RELEASE MEDICINES
▸ Adult: Initially 1 capsule substituted for every 100 mg of levodopa and given at same dosage frequency, increased every 2–3 days according to response; average increase of 50% needed over previous levodopa dose and titration may take up to 4 weeks, supplementary dose of immediate-release *Madopar*® may be needed with first morning dose; if response still poor to total daily dose of *Madopar*® CR plus *Madopar*® corresponding to 1.2 g levodopa—consider alternative therapy.

DOSE EQUIVALENCE AND CONVERSION
▸ Dose is expressed as levodopa.

IMPORTANT SAFETY INFORMATION
IMPULSE CONTROL DISORDERS
Treatment with levodopa is associated with impulse control disorders, including pathological gambling, binge eating, and hypersexuality. Patients and their carers should be informed about the risk of impulse control disorders. See Parkinson's disease p. 430.

- CAUTIONS Cushing's syndrome · diabetes mellitus · endocrine disorders · history of convulsions · history of myocardial infarction with residual arrhythmia · history of peptic ulcer · hyperthyroidism · osteomalacia · phaeochromocytoma · psychiatric illness (avoid if severe and discontinue if deterioration) · severe cardiovascular disease · severe pulmonary disease · susceptibility to angle-closure glaucoma
- INTERACTIONS → Appendix 1: levodopa
- SIDE-EFFECTS
  ▸ Common or very common Anxiety · appetite decreased · arrhythmia · depression · diarrhoea · hallucination · movement disorders · nausea · parkinsonism · postural hypotension · sleep disorders · taste altered · vomiting
  ▸ Rare or very rare Leucopenia
  ▸ Frequency not known Aggression · compulsions · confusion · delusions · dopamine dysregulation syndrome · drowsiness · eating disorders · euphoric mood · flushing · gastrointestinal haemorrhage · haemolytic anaemia · hyperhidrosis · oral disorders · pathological gambling · psychosis · sexual dysfunction · skin reactions · thrombocytopenia · tongue discolouration · tooth discolouration · urine discolouration
- PREGNANCY Caution in pregnancy—toxicity has occurred in *animal* studies.
- BREAST FEEDING May suppress lactation; present in milk—avoid.
- HEPATIC IMPAIRMENT Manufacturer advises caution in mild to moderate impairment; avoid in decompensated hepatic function.
- RENAL IMPAIRMENT Use with caution.

- EFFECT ON LABORATORY TESTS False positive tests for urinary ketones have been reported.
- TREATMENT CESSATION Avoid abrupt withdrawal (risk of neuroleptic malignant syndrome and rhabdomyolysis).
- DIRECTIONS FOR ADMINISTRATION Manufacturer advises the dispersible tablets can be dispersed in water or orange squash (not orange juice).
- PRESCRIBING AND DISPENSING INFORMATION Co-beneldopa is a mixture of benserazide hydrochloride and levodopa in mass proportions corresponding to 1 part of benserazide and 4 parts of levodopa.

  When transferring patients from another levodopa/dopa-decarboxylase inhibitor preparation, the previous preparation should be discontinued 12 hours before (although interval can be shorter).

  When switching from modified-release levodopa to dispersible co-beneldopa, reduce dose by approximately 30%.

  When administered as an adjunct to other antiparkinsonian drugs, once therapeutic effect apparent, the other drugs may be reduced or withdrawn.
- PATIENT AND CARER ADVICE Patients or carers should be given advice on how to administer co-beneldopa dispersible tablets.

  Dopamine dysregulation syndrome Manufacturer advises patients and their carers should be informed of the risk of developing dopamine dysregulation syndrome; addiction-like symptoms should be reported.

  Driving and skilled tasks   **Sudden onset of sleep** Excessive daytime sleepiness and sudden onset of sleep can occur with co-beneldopa.

  Patients starting treatment with these drugs should be warned of the risk and of the need to exercise caution when driving or operating machinery. Those who have experienced excessive sedation or sudden onset of sleep should refrain from driving or operating machines until these effects have stopped occurring.

  Management of excessive daytime sleepiness should focus on the identification of an underlying cause, such as depression or concomitant medication. Patients should be counselled on improving sleep behaviour.

- MEDICINAL FORMS There can be variation in the licensing of different medicines containing the same drug. Forms available from special-order manufacturers include: oral suspension, oral solution

Dispersible tablet

CAUTIONARY AND ADVISORY LABELS 10, 14, 21
- Madopar (Roche Products Ltd)

  Benserazide (as Benserazide hydrochloride) 12.5 mg, Levodopa 50 mg Madopar 50mg/12.5mg dispersible tablets sugar-free | 100 tablet PoM DT = £5.90

  Benserazide (as Benserazide hydrochloride) 25 mg, Levodopa 100 mg Madopar 100mg/25mg dispersible tablets sugar-free | 100 tablet PoM £10.45 DT = £10.45

Modified-release capsule

CAUTIONARY AND ADVISORY LABELS 5, 10, 14, 25
- Madopar CR (Roche Products Ltd)

  Benserazide (as Benserazide hydrochloride) 25 mg, Levodopa 100 mg Madopar CR capsules | 100 capsule PoM £12.77 DT = £12.77

Capsule

CAUTIONARY AND ADVISORY LABELS 10, 14, 21
- Co-beneldopa (Non-proprietary)

  Benserazide (as Benserazide hydrochloride) 12.5 mg, Levodopa 50 mg Co-beneldopa 12.5mg/50mg capsules | 100 capsule PoM £4.96 DT = £4.96

  Benserazide (as Benserazide hydrochloride) 50 mg, Levodopa 200 mg Co-beneldopa 50mg/200mg capsules | 100 capsule PoM ⓧ DT = £11.78
- Madopar (Roche Products Ltd)

  Benserazide (as Benserazide hydrochloride) 12.5 mg, Levodopa 50 mg Madopar 50mg/12.5mg capsules | 100 capsule PoM £4.96 DT = £4.96

Benserazide (as Benserazide hydrochloride) 25 mg, Levodopa 100 mg Madopar 100mg/25mg capsules | 100 capsule PoM £6.91 DT = £6.91

Benserazide (as Benserazide hydrochloride) 50 mg, Levodopa 200 mg Madopar 200mg/50mg capsules | 100 capsule PoM £11.78 DT = £11.78

Co-careldopa
29-Oct-2020

- INDICATIONS AND DOSE

Parkinson's disease
▶ BY MOUTH
- Adult: Initially 25/100 mg 3 times a day, then increased in steps of 12.5/50 mg once daily or on alternate days, alternatively increased in steps of 25/100 mg once daily or on alternate days, dose to be adjusted according to response; dose increased until 800 mg levodopa (with 200 mg carbidopa) daily in divided doses is reached, then maintenance up to 200/2000 mg daily in divided doses, adjusted according to response, when co-careldopa is used, the total daily dose of carbidopa should be at least 70 mg. A lower dose may not achieve full inhibition of extracerebral dopa-decarboxylase, with a resultant increase in side-effects

Parkinson's disease—alternative regimen
▶ BY MOUTH
- Adult: Initially 12.5/50 mg 3–4 times a day, alternatively initially 10/100 mg 3–4 times a day, then increased in steps of 12.5/50 mg once daily or on alternate days, adjusted according to response, alternatively increased in steps of 10/100 mg once daily or on alternate days, adjusted according to response, dose increased until 800 mg levodopa (with up to 200 mg carbidopa) daily in divided doses is reached, then maintenance up to 200/2000 mg daily in divided doses, adjusted according to response, when co-careldopa is used, the total daily dose of carbidopa should be at least 70 mg. A lower dose may not achieve full inhibition of extracerebral dopa-decarboxylase, with a resultant increase in side-effects

DOSE EQUIVALENCE AND CONVERSION
- The proportions are expressed in the form x/y where x and y are the strengths in milligrams of carbidopa and levodopa respectively.
- 2 tablets *Sinemet*® 12.5 mg/50 mg is equivalent to 1 tablet *Sinemet*® Plus 25 mg/100 mg.

CARAMET® CR

Parkinson's disease (patients not receiving levodopa/dopa-decarboxylase inhibitor preparations, expressed as levodopa)
▶ BY MOUTH USING MODIFIED-RELEASE TABLETS
- Adult: Initially 100–200 mg twice daily, dose to be given at least 6 hours apart; dose adjusted according to response at intervals of at least 2 days

Parkinson's disease (patients transferring from immediate-release levodopa/dopa-decarboxylase inhibitor preparations)
▶ BY MOUTH USING MODIFIED-RELEASE TABLETS
- Adult: Discontinue previous preparation at least 12 hours before first dose of *Caramet*® CR; substitute *Caramet*® CR to provide a similar amount of levodopa daily and extend dosing interval by 30–50%; dose then adjusted according to response at intervals of at least 2 days.

DUODOPA®

Severe Parkinson's disease inadequately controlled by other preparations
- Adult: Administered as intestinal gel, for use with enteral tube (consult product literature)   continued →

4

Nervous system

HALF SINEMET ® CR

Parkinson's disease (for fine adjustment of Sinemet ® CR dose)
▸ BY MOUTH
▸ Adult: (consult product literature)

SINEMET ® CR

Parkinson's disease (patients not receiving levodopa/dopa-decarboxylase inhibitor therapy)
▸ BY MOUTH
▸ Adult: Initially 1 tablet twice daily, both dose and interval then adjusted according to response at intervals of not less than 3 days

Parkinson's disease (patients transferring from immediate-release levodopa/dopa-decarboxylase inhibitor preparations)
▸ BY MOUTH
▸ Adult: 1 tablet twice daily, dose can be substituted for a daily dose of levodopa 300–400 mg in immediate-release *Sinemet* ® tablets (substitute *Sinemet* ® CR to provide approximately 10% more levodopa per day and extend dosing interval by 30–50%); dose and interval then adjusted according to response at intervals of not less than 3 days.

IMPORTANT SAFETY INFORMATION
IMPULSE CONTROL DISORDERS
Treatment with levodopa is associated with impulse control disorders, including pathological gambling, binge eating, and hypersexuality. Patients and their carers should be informed about the risk of impulse control disorders. See Parkinson's disease p. 430.

● CAUTIONS Cushing's syndrome · diabetes mellitus · endocrine disorders · history of convulsions · history of myocardial infarction with residual arrhythmia · history of peptic ulcer · hyperthyroidism · osteomalacia · phaeochromocytoma · psychiatric illness (avoid if severe and discontinue if deterioration) · severe cardiovascular disease · severe pulmonary disease · susceptibility to angle-closure glaucoma
● INTERACTIONS → Appendix 1: carbidopa · levodopa
● SIDE-EFFECTS
▸ Rare or very rare Drowsiness · seizure · sleep disorders
▸ Frequency not known Agranulocytosis · alertness decreased · alopecia · anaemia · angioedema · anxiety · appetite decreased · asthenia · cardiac disorder · chest pain · compulsions · confusion · constipation · delusions · dementia · depression · diarrhoea · dizziness · dopamine dysregulation syndrome · dry mouth · dyskinesia (may be dose-limiting) · dysphagia · dyspnoea · eating disorders · euphoric mood · eye disorders · fall · focal tremor · gait abnormal · gastrointestinal discomfort · gastrointestinal disorders · gastrointestinal haemorrhage · haemolytic anaemia · hallucination · headache · Henoch-Schönlein purpura · hiccups · hoarseness · Horner's syndrome exacerbated · hypertension · hypotension · leucopenia · malaise · malignant melanoma · movement disorders · muscle complaints · nausea · neuroleptic malignant syndrome (on abrupt discontinuation) · oedema · on and off phenomenon · oral disorders · palpitations · pathological gambling · postural disorders · psychotic disorder · respiration abnormal · sensation abnormal · sexual dysfunction · skin reactions · suicidal ideation · sweat changes · syncope · taste bitter · teeth grinding · thrombocytopenia · trismus · urinary disorders · urine dark · vasodilation · vision disorders · vomiting · weight changes
● PREGNANCY Use with caution—toxicity has occurred in *animal* studies.
● BREAST FEEDING May suppress lactation; present in milk—avoid.

● HEPATIC IMPAIRMENT Manufacturer advises use with caution in hepatic disease.
DUODOPA ® **Dose adjustments** Manufacturer advises titrate dose with caution in severe impairment.
● RENAL IMPAIRMENT Use with caution.
● EFFECT ON LABORATORY TESTS False positive tests for urinary ketones have been reported.
● TREATMENT CESSATION Avoid abrupt withdrawal (risk of neuroleptic malignant syndrome and rhabdomyolysis).
● PRESCRIBING AND DISPENSING INFORMATION Co-careldopa is a mixture of carbidopa and levodopa; the proportions are expressed in the form x/y where x and y are the strengths in milligrams of carbidopa and levodopa respectively.
    When transferring patients from another levodopa/dopa-decarboxylase inhibitor preparation, the previous preparation should be discontinued at least 12 hours before.
    Co-careldopa 25/100 provides an adequate dose of carbidopa when low doses of levodopa are needed.
● PATIENT AND CARER ADVICE Manufacturer advises patients and their carers should be informed of the risk of developing dopamine dysregulation syndrome; addiction-like symptoms should be reported.
Driving and skilled tasks   Sudden onset of sleep Excessive daytime sleepiness and sudden onset of sleep can occur with co-careldopa.
    Patients starting treatment with these drugs should be warned of the risk and of the need to exercise caution when driving or operating machinery. Those who have experienced excessive sedation or sudden onset of sleep should refrain from driving or operating machines until these effects have stopped occurring.
    Management of excessive daytime sleepiness should focus on the identification of an underlying cause, such as depression or concomitant medication. Patients should be counselled on improving sleep behaviour.
● NATIONAL FUNDING/ACCESS DECISIONS
DUODOPA ® For full details see funding body website
Scottish Medicines Consortium (SMC) decisions
▸ Co-careldopa (*Duodopa* ®) for the treatment of advanced levodopa-responsive Parkinson's disease with severe motor fluctuations and hyper-/dyskinesia when available combinations of Parkinson medicinal products have not given satisfactory results (June 2016) SMC No. 316/06 Recommended with restrictions
All Wales Medicines Strategy Group (AWMSG) decisions
▸ Levodopa-carbidopa intestinal gel (*Duodopa* ®) for the treatment of advanced levodopa-responsive Parkinson's disease with severe motor fluctuations and hyper-/dyskinesia when available combinations of Parkinson medicinal products have not given satisfactory results and patients are not eligible for deep brain stimulation (March 2018) AWMSG No. 3397 Recommended with restrictions

● MEDICINAL FORMS There can be variation in the licensing of different medicines containing the same drug. Forms available from special-order manufacturers include: oral suspension, oral solution
Modified-release tablet
CAUTIONARY AND ADVISORY LABELS 10, 14, 25
▸ Caramet CR (Teva UK Ltd)
    Carbidopa (as Carbidopa monohydrate) 25 mg, Levodopa 100 mg Caramet 25mg/100mg CR tablets | 60 tablet PoM £11.47 DT = £11.60
▸ Half Sinemet CR (Merck Sharp & Dohme Ltd)
    Carbidopa (as Carbidopa monohydrate) 25 mg, Levodopa 100 mg Half Sinemet CR 25mg/100mg tablets | 60 tablet PoM £11.60 DT = £11.60

▸ Lecado (Sandoz Ltd)
 Carbidopa (as Carbidopa monohydrate) 25 mg, Levodopa
 100 mg Lecado 100mg/25mg modified-release tablets |
 60 tablet [PoM] £9.86 DT = £11.60
 Carbidopa (as Carbidopa monohydrate) 50 mg, Levodopa
 200 mg Lecado 200mg/50mg modified-release tablets |
 60 tablet [PoM] £9.86 DT = £11.60
▸ Sinemet CR (Merck Sharp & Dohme Ltd)
 Carbidopa (as Carbidopa monohydrate) 50 mg, Levodopa
 200 mg Sinemet CR 50mg/200mg tablets | 60 tablet [PoM] £11.60
 DT = £11.60

Tablet

CAUTIONARY AND ADVISORY LABELS 10, 14
▸ Co-careldopa (Non-proprietary)
 Carbidopa (as Carbidopa monohydrate) 12.5 mg, Levodopa
 50 mg Co-careldopa 12.5mg/50mg tablets | 90 tablet [PoM] £21.67
 DT = £21.67
 Carbidopa (as Carbidopa monohydrate) 25 mg, Levodopa
 100 mg Co-careldopa 25mg/100mg tablets | 100 tablet [PoM]
 £26.99 DT = £21.45
 Carbidopa (as Carbidopa monohydrate) 10 mg, Levodopa
 100 mg Co-careldopa 10mg/100mg tablets | 100 tablet [PoM]
 £14.00 DT = £13.96
 Carbidopa (as Carbidopa monohydrate) 25 mg, Levodopa
 250 mg Co-careldopa 25mg/250mg tablets | 100 tablet [PoM]
 £35.00 DT = £34.99
▸ Sinemet 110 (Merck Sharp & Dohme Ltd)
 Carbidopa (as Carbidopa monohydrate) 10 mg, Levodopa
 100 mg Sinemet 10mg/100mg tablets | 100 tablet [PoM] £7.30 DT =
 £13.96
▸ Sinemet 275 (Merck Sharp & Dohme Ltd)
 Carbidopa (as Carbidopa monohydrate) 25 mg, Levodopa
 250 mg Sinemet 25mg/250mg tablets | 100 tablet [PoM] £18.29 DT =
 £34.99
▸ Sinemet 62.5 (Merck Sharp & Dohme Ltd)
 Carbidopa (as Carbidopa monohydrate) 12.5 mg, Levodopa
 50 mg Sinemet 12.5mg/50mg tablets | 90 tablet [PoM] £6.28 DT =
 £21.67
▸ Sinemet Plus (Merck Sharp & Dohme Ltd)
 Carbidopa (as Carbidopa monohydrate) 25 mg, Levodopa
 100 mg Sinemet Plus 25mg/100mg tablets | 100 tablet [PoM] £12.88
 DT = £21.45

Gel

CAUTIONARY AND ADVISORY LABELS 10, 14
▸ Duodopa (AbbVie Ltd)
 Carbidopa (as Carbidopa monohydrate) 5 mg per 1 ml, Levodopa
 20 mg per 1 ml Duodopa intestinal gel 100ml cassette | 7 bag [PoM]
 £539.00

Levodopa with carbidopa and entacapone

The properties listed below are those particular to the
combination only. For the properties of the components
please consider, co-careldopa p. 435, entacapone p. 433.

● INDICATIONS AND DOSE
STALEVO ® 100/25/200

**Parkinson's disease and end-of-dose motor fluctuations
not adequately controlled with levodopa and dopa-
decarboxylase inhibitor treatment**
▸ BY MOUTH
▸ Adult: 1 tablet for each dose; maximum 10 tablets per
 day

STALEVO ® 125/31.25/200

**Parkinson's disease and end-of-dose motor fluctuations
not adequately controlled with levodopa and dopa-
decarboxylase inhibitor treatment**
▸ BY MOUTH
▸ Adult: 1 tablet for each dose; maximum 10 tablets per
 day

STALEVO ® 150/37.5/200

**Parkinson's disease and end-of-dose motor fluctuations
not adequately controlled with levodopa and dopa-
decarboxylase inhibitor treatment**
▸ BY MOUTH
▸ Adult: 1 tablet for each dose; maximum 10 tablets per
 day

STALEVO ® 175/43.75/200

**Parkinson's disease and end-of-dose motor fluctuations
not adequately controlled with levodopa and dopa-
decarboxylase inhibitor treatment**
▸ BY MOUTH
▸ Adult: 1 tablet for each dose; maximum 8 tablets per
 day

STALEVO ® 200/50/200

**Parkinson's disease and end-of-dose motor fluctuations
not adequately controlled with levodopa and dopa-
decarboxylase inhibitor treatment**
▸ BY MOUTH
▸ Adult: 1 tablet for each dose; maximum 7 tablets per
 day

STALEVO ® 50/12.5/200

**Parkinson's disease and end-of-dose motor fluctuations
not adequately controlled with levodopa and dopa-
decarboxylase inhibitor treatment**
▸ BY MOUTH
▸ Adult: 1 tablet for each dose; maximum 10 tablets per
 day

STALEVO ® 75/18.75/200

**Parkinson's disease and end-of-dose motor fluctuations
not adequately controlled with levodopa and dopa-
decarboxylase inhibitor treatment**
▸ BY MOUTH
▸ Adult: 1 tablet for each dose; maximum 10 tablets per
 day

● INTERACTIONS → Appendix 1: carbidopa · entacapone ·
 levodopa

● PRESCRIBING AND DISPENSING INFORMATION Patients
 receiving standard-release co-careldopa or co-beneldopa
 alone, initiate *Stalevo* ® at a dose that provides similar (or
 slightly lower) amount of levodopa.
  Patients with dyskinesia or receiving more than 800 mg
 levodopa daily, introduce entacapone before transferring
 to *Stalevo* ® (levodopa dose may need to be reduced by
 10–30% initially).
  Patients receiving entacapone and standard-release co-
 careldopa or co-beneldopa, initiate *Stalevo* ® at a dose that
 provides similar (or slightly higher) amount of levodopa.

● PATIENT AND CARER ADVICE
 Driving and skilled tasks **Sudden onset of sleep** Excessive
 daytime sleepiness and sudden onset of sleep can occur
 with carbidopa with entacapone and levodopa.
  Patients starting treatment with these drugs should be
 warned of the risk and of the need to exercise caution
 when driving or operating machinery. Those who have
 experienced excessive sedation or sudden onset of sleep
 should refrain from driving or operating machines until
 these effects have stopped occurring.
  Management of excessive daytime sleepiness should
 focus on the identification of an underlying cause, such as
 depression or concomitant medication. Patients should be
 counselled on improving sleep behaviour.

4

Nervous system

- MEDICINAL FORMS There can be variation in the licensing of different medicines containing the same drug.

Tablet

CAUTIONARY AND ADVISORY LABELS 10, 14(urine reddish-brown), 25

▸ Stalevo (Orion Pharma (UK) Ltd)

Carbidopa 25 mg, Levodopa 100 mg, Entacapone 200 mg Stalevo 100mg/25mg/200mg tablets | 30 tablet [PoM] £20.79 DT = £20.79 | 100 tablet [PoM] £69.31 DT = £69.31

Carbidopa 18.75 mg, Levodopa 75 mg, Entacapone 200 mg Stalevo 75mg/18.75mg/200mg tablets | 30 tablet [PoM] £20.79 DT = £20.79 | 100 tablet [PoM] £69.31 DT = £69.31

Carbidopa 37.5 mg, Levodopa 150 mg, Entacapone 200 mg Stalevo 150mg/37.5mg/200mg tablets | 30 tablet [PoM] £20.79 DT = £20.79 | 100 tablet [PoM] £69.31 DT = £69.31

Carbidopa 12.5 mg, Levodopa 50 mg, Entacapone 200 mg Stalevo 50mg/12.5mg/200mg tablets | 30 tablet [PoM] £20.79 DT = £20.79 | 100 tablet [PoM] £69.31 DT = £69.31

Carbidopa 31.25 mg, Levodopa 125 mg, Entacapone 200 mg Stalevo 125mg/31.25mg/200mg tablets | 30 tablet [PoM] £20.79 DT = £20.79 | 100 tablet [PoM] £69.31 DT = £69.31

Carbidopa 43.75 mg, Levodopa 175 mg, Entacapone 200 mg Stalevo 175mg/43.75mg/200mg tablets | 30 tablet [PoM] £20.79 DT = £20.79 | 100 tablet [PoM] £69.31 DT = £69.31

Carbidopa 50 mg, Entacapone 200 mg, Levodopa 200 mg Stalevo 200mg/50mg/200mg tablets | 30 tablet [PoM] £20.79 DT = £20.79 | 100 tablet [PoM] £69.31 DT = £69.31

DOPAMINERGIC DRUGS › DOPAMINE RECEPTOR AGONISTS

Amantadine hydrochloride

28-Aug-2020

- DRUG ACTION Amantadine is a weak dopamine agonist with modest antiparkinsonian effects.

- **INDICATIONS AND DOSE**

Parkinson's disease

▸ BY MOUTH

▸ Adult: 100 mg daily for 1 week, then increased to 100 mg twice daily, usually administered in conjunction with other treatment. Some patients may require higher doses; maximum 400 mg per day

▸ Elderly: 100 mg daily, adjusted according to response

Post-herpetic neuralgia

▸ BY MOUTH

▸ Adult: 100 mg twice daily for 14 days (continued for another 14 days if necessary)

Treatment of influenza A (but not recommended)

▸ BY MOUTH

▸ Adult: 100 mg daily 4–5 days

Prophylaxis of influenza A (but not recommended)

▸ BY MOUTH

▸ Adult: 100 mg daily usually for 6 weeks or with influenza vaccination for 2–3 weeks after vaccination

Fatigue in multiple sclerosis (initiated by a specialist)

▸ BY MOUTH

▸ Adult: 100 mg daily for 1 week, dose to be taken in the morning, then increased to 100 mg twice daily; maximum 400 mg per day

- UNLICENSED USE [EvGr] Amantadine is used for fatigue in multiple sclerosis, ⟨€⟩ but is not licensed for this indication.

- CONTRA-INDICATIONS Epilepsy · history of gastric ulceration

- CAUTIONS Confused or hallucinatory states · congestive heart disease (may exacerbate oedema) · elderly · tolerance to the effects of amantadine may develop in Parkinson's disease

- INTERACTIONS → Appendix 1: dopamine receptor agonists

- SIDE-EFFECTS

▸ **Common or very common** Anxiety · appetite decreased · concentration impaired · confusion · constipation · depression · dizziness · dry mouth · hallucination · headache · hyperhidrosis · lethargy · mood altered · movement disorders · myalgia · nausea · palpitations · peripheral oedema · postural hypotension · skin reactions · sleep disorders · speech slurred · vision disorders · vomiting

▸ **Uncommon** Neuroleptic malignant-like syndrome · psychosis · seizure · tremor

▸ **Rare or very rare** Cardiovascular insufficiency · diarrhoea · eye disorders · eye inflammation · heart failure · leucopenia · photosensitivity reaction · urinary disorders

▸ **Frequency not known** Delirium

- PREGNANCY Avoid; toxicity in *animal* studies.

- BREAST FEEDING Avoid; present in milk; toxicity in infant reported.

- HEPATIC IMPAIRMENT Manufacturer advises use with caution in liver disorders.

- RENAL IMPAIRMENT Avoid if eGFR less than 15 mL/minute/1.73 m^2.

Dose adjustments Reduce dose.

- TREATMENT CESSATION Avoid abrupt withdrawal in Parkinson's disease.

- PATIENT AND CARER ADVICE

Driving and skilled tasks May affect performance of skilled tasks (e.g. driving).

- NATIONAL FUNDING/ACCESS DECISIONS

For full details see funding body website

NICE decisions

▸ Oseltamivir, amantadine (review) and zanamivir for the prophylaxis of influenza (September 2008) NICE TA158 Not recommended

▸ Amantadine, oseltamivir and zanamivir for the treatment of influenza (February 2009) NICE TA168 Not recommended

- MEDICINAL FORMS There can be variation in the licensing of different medicines containing the same drug. Forms available from special-order manufacturers include: tablet

Oral solution

▸ Amantadine hydrochloride (Non-proprietary)

Amantadine hydrochloride 10 mg per 1 ml Amantadine 50mg/5ml oral solution sugar free sugar-free | 150 ml [PoM] £140.00 DT = £129.04

Capsule

▸ Amantadine hydrochloride (Non-proprietary)

Amantadine hydrochloride 100 mg Amantadine 100mg capsules | 14 capsule [PoM] £9.44–£10.25 | 56 capsule [PoM] £41.00 DT = £26.87

Apomorphine hydrochloride

20-Dec-2019

- **INDICATIONS AND DOSE**

Refractory motor fluctuations in Parkinson's disease ('off' episodes) inadequately controlled by co-beneldopa or co-careldopa or other dopaminergics (for capable and motivated patients) (under expert supervision)

▸ BY SUBCUTANEOUS INJECTION

▸ Adult: Initially 1 mg, dose to be administered at the first sign of 'off' episode, then 2 mg after 30 minutes, dose to be given if inadequate or no response following initial dose, thereafter increase dose at minimum 40-minute intervals until satisfactory response obtained, this determines threshold dose; usual dose 3–30 mg daily in divided doses (max. per dose 10 mg), subcutaneous infusion may be preferable in those requiring division of injections into more than 10 doses; maximum 100 mg per day

Refractory motor fluctuations in Parkinson's disease ('off' episodes) inadequately controlled by co-beneldopa or co-careldopa or other dopaminergics (in patients requiring division into more than 10 injections daily) (under expert supervision)

▶ BY CONTINUOUS SUBCUTANEOUS INFUSION

▶ Adult: Initially 1 mg/hour, adjusted according to response, then increased in steps of up to 500 micrograms/hour, dose to be increased at intervals not more often than every 4 hours; usual dose 1–4 mg/hour, alternatively usual dose 15–60 micrograms/kg/hour, change infusion site every 12 hours and give during waking hours only (tolerance may occur unless there is a 4-hour treatment-free period at night—24-hour infusions not recommended unless severe night time symptoms); intermittent bolus doses may be needed; maximum 100 mg per day

---

IMPORTANT SAFETY INFORMATION

IMPULSE CONTROL DISORDERS

Treatment with dopamine-receptor agonists are associated with impulse control disorders, including pathological gambling, binge eating, and hypersexuality. Patients and their carers should be informed about the risk of impulse control disorders. Ergot- and non-ergot-derived dopamine-receptor agonists do not differ in their propensity to cause impulse control disorders, so switching between dopamine-receptor agonists will not control these side-effects. See Parkinson's disease p. 430.

● CONTRA-INDICATIONS Avoid if 'on' response to levodopa marred by severe dyskinesia or dystonia · dementia · psychosis · respiratory depression

● CAUTIONS Cardiovascular disease · history of postural hypotension (special care on initiation) · neuropsychiatric conditions · pulmonary disease · susceptibility to QT-interval prolongation

● INTERACTIONS → Appendix 1: dopamine receptor agonists

● SIDE-EFFECTS

▶ Common or very common Confusion · dizziness · drowsiness · hallucinations · nausea · psychiatric disorders · subcutaneous nodule · vomiting · yawning

▶ Uncommon Dyskinesia (may require discontinuation) · dyspnoea · haemolytic anaemia · injection site necrosis · postural hypotension · skin reactions · sudden onset of sleep · thrombocytopenia

▶ Rare or very rare Bronchospasm · eosinophilia · hypersensitivity

▶ Frequency not known Aggression · agitation · dopamine dysregulation syndrome · eating disorders · pathological gambling · peripheral oedema · sexual dysfunction · syncope

● ALLERGY AND CROSS-SENSITIVITY Contra-indicated if history of hypersensitivity to opioids.

● PREGNANCY Avoid unless clearly necessary.

● BREAST FEEDING No information available; may suppress lactation.

● HEPATIC IMPAIRMENT Manufacturer advises avoid in hepatic insufficiency.

● RENAL IMPAIRMENT Use with caution.

● MONITORING REQUIREMENTS

▶ Monitor hepatic, haemopoietic, renal, and cardiovascular function.

▶ *With concomitant levodopa* test initially and every 6 months for haemolytic anaemia and thrombocytopenia (development calls for specialist haematological care with dose reduction and possible discontinuation).

● TREATMENT CESSATION Antiparkinsonian drug therapy should never be stopped abruptly as this carries a small risk of neuroleptic malignant syndrome.

● PATIENT AND CARER ADVICE Manufacturer advises patients and their carers should be informed of the risk of developing dopamine dysregulation syndrome; addiction-like symptoms should be reported.

Driving and skilled tasks   Sudden onset of sleep Excessive daytime sleepiness and sudden onset of sleep can occur with dopamine-receptor agonists.

Patients starting treatment with these drugs should be warned of the risk and of the need to exercise caution when driving or operating machinery. Those who have experienced excessive sedation or sudden onset of sleep should refrain from driving or operating machines until these effects have stopped occurring.

Management of excessive daytime sleepiness should focus on the identification of an underlying cause, such as depression or concomitant medication. Patients should be counselled on improving sleep behaviour.

Drugs and driving Prescribers and other healthcare professionals should advise patients if treatment is likely to affect their ability to perform skilled tasks (e.g. driving). This applies especially to drugs with sedative effects; patients should be warned that these effects are increased by alcohol. General information about a patient's fitness to drive is available from the Driver and Vehicle Licensing Agency at www.gov.uk/government/organisations/driver-and-vehicle-licensing-agency.

2015 legislation regarding driving whilst taking certain drugs, may also apply to apomorphine, see *Drugs and driving* under Guidance on prescribing p. 1.

Hypotensive reactions Hypotensive reactions can occur in some patients taking dopamine-receptor agonists; these can be particularly problematic during the first few days of treatment and care should be exercised when driving or operating machinery.

● MEDICINAL FORMS There can be variation in the licensing of different medicines containing the same drug. Forms available from special-order manufacturers include: solution for injection, solution for infusion

Solution for injection

CAUTIONARY AND ADVISORY LABELS 10

EXCIPIENTS: May contain Sulfites

▶ APO-go (Britannia Pharmaceuticals Ltd)

Apomorphine hydrochloride 10 mg per 1 ml APO-go 50mg/5ml solution for injection ampoules | 5 ampoule `PoM` £73.11 DT = £73.11

▶ APO-go Pen (Britannia Pharmaceuticals Ltd)

Apomorphine hydrochloride 10 mg per 1 ml APO-go PEN 30mg/3ml solution for injection | 5 pre-filled disposable injection `PoM` £123.91 DT = £123.91

▶ Dacepton (Ever Pharma UK Ltd)

Apomorphine hydrochloride hemihydrate 10 mg per 1 ml Dacepton 30mg/3ml solution for injection cartridges | 5 cartridge `PoM` £123.00 DT = £123.00

Solution for infusion

CAUTIONARY AND ADVISORY LABELS 10

EXCIPIENTS: May contain Sulfites

▶ APO-go PFS (Britannia Pharmaceuticals Ltd)

Apomorphine hydrochloride 5 mg per 1 ml APO-go PFS 50mg/10ml solution for infusion pre-filled syringes | 5 pre-filled disposable injection `PoM` £73.11 DT = £73.11

▶ Dacepton (Ever Pharma UK Ltd)

Apomorphine hydrochloride hemihydrate 5 mg per 1 ml Dacepton 100mg/20ml solution for infusion vials | 5 vial `PoM` £145.00 DT = £145.00

4

Nervous system

Bromocriptine

20-Nov-2020

- **DRUG ACTION** Bromocriptine is a stimulant of dopamine receptors in the brain; it also inhibits release of prolactin by the pituitary.

- **INDICATIONS AND DOSE**

Prevention of lactation
▸ BY MOUTH
  ▹ Adult: Initially 2.5 mg daily for 1 day, then 2.5 mg twice daily for 14 days

Suppression of lactation
▸ BY MOUTH
  ▹ Adult: Initially 2.5 mg daily for 2–3 days, then 2.5 mg twice daily for 14 days

Hypogonadism | Galactorrhoea | Infertility
▸ BY MOUTH
  ▹ Adult: Initially 1–1.25 mg daily, dose to be taken at bedtime, increase dose gradually; usual dose 7.5 mg daily in divided doses, increased if necessary up to 30 mg daily, usual dose in infertility without hyperprolactinaemia is 2.5 mg twice daily

Acromegaly
▸ BY MOUTH
  ▹ Adult: Initially 1–1.25 mg daily, dose to be taken at bedtime, then increased to 5 mg every 6 hours, increase dose gradually

Prolactinoma
▸ BY MOUTH
  ▹ Adult: Initially 1–1.25 mg daily, dose to be taken at bedtime, then increased to 5 mg every 6 hours, increase dose gradually. Occasionally patients may require up to 30 mg daily

Parkinson's disease
▸ BY MOUTH
  ▹ Adult: Initially 1–1.25 mg daily for 1 week, dose to be taken at night, then 2–2.5 mg daily for 1 week, dose to be taken at night, then 2.5 mg twice daily for 1 week, then 2.5 mg 3 times a day for 1 week, then increased in steps of 2.5 mg every 3–14 days, adjusted according to response; maintenance 10–30 mg daily

---

IMPORTANT SAFETY INFORMATION

FIBROTIC REACTIONS

Bromocriptine has been associated with pulmonary, retroperitoneal, and pericardial fibrotic reactions.

Manufacturer advises exclude cardiac valvulopathy with echocardiography before starting treatment with these ergot derivatives for Parkinson's disease or chronic endocrine disorders (excludes suppression of lactation); it may also be appropriate to measure the erythrocyte sedimentation rate and serum creatinine and to obtain a chest X-ray. Patients should be monitored for dyspnoea, persistent cough, chest pain, cardiac failure, and abdominal pain or tenderness. If long-term treatment is expected, then lung-function tests may also be helpful.

IMPULSE CONTROL DISORDERS

Treatment with dopamine-receptor agonists are associated with impulse control disorders, including pathological gambling, binge eating, and hypersexuality. Patients and their carers should be informed about the risk of impulse control disorders. Ergot- and non-ergot-derived dopamine-receptor agonists do not differ in their propensity to cause impulse control disorders, so switching between dopamine-receptor agonists will not control these side-effects. See Parkinson's disease p. 430.

- **CONTRA-INDICATIONS** Cardiac valvulopathy (exclude before treatment) · hypertension in postpartum women or in puerperium · hypertensive disorders of pregnancy (e.g.

pre-eclampsia, eclampsia or pregnancy-induced hypertension)

CONTRA-INDICATIONS, FURTHER INFORMATION
▸ Use in Suppression of lactation or other non-life threatening indications Manufacturer advises avoid in these indications for patients with a history of severe cardiovascular conditions, including coronary artery disease, or symptoms (or history) of serious mental disorder. Very rarely hypertension, myocardial infarction, seizures or stroke (both sometimes preceded by severe headache or visual disturbances), and mental disorders have been reported in postpartum women given bromocriptine for lactation suppression—caution with antihypertensive therapy and avoid other ergot alkaloids. Discontinue immediately if hypertension, unremitting headache, or signs of CNS toxicity develop.

- **CAUTIONS** Cardiovascular disease · history of peptic ulcer (particularly in acromegalic patients) · history of serious mental disorders (especially psychotic disorders) · Raynaud's syndrome

CAUTIONS, FURTHER INFORMATION
▸ Hyperprolactinemic patients In hyperprolactinaemic patients, the source of the hyperprolactinaemia should be established (i.e. exclude pituitary tumour before treatment).

- **INTERACTIONS** → Appendix 1: dopamine receptor agonists

- **SIDE-EFFECTS**
▸ **Common or very common** Constipation · drowsiness · headache · nasal congestion · nausea
▸ **Uncommon** Allergic dermatitis · alopecia · confusion · dizziness · dry mouth · fatigue · hallucination · hypotension · leg cramps · movement disorders · vomiting
▸ **Rare or very rare** Abdominal pain · arrhythmias · cardiac valvulopathy · diarrhoea · dyspnoea · gastrointestinal disorders · gastrointestinal haemorrhage · neuroleptic malignant-like syndrome · pallor · paraesthesia · pericardial effusion · pericarditis · peripheral oedema · psychotic disorder · respiratory disorders · sleep disorders · tinnitus · vision disorders
▸ **Frequency not known** Eating disorders · hypertension · myocardial infarction · pathological gambling · psychiatric disorders · seizure · sexual dysfunction · stroke

SIDE-EFFECTS, FURTHER INFORMATION Treatment should be withdrawn if gastro-intestinal bleeding occurs.

- **ALLERGY AND CROSS-SENSITIVITY** [EvGr] Bromocriptine should not be used in patients with hypersensitivity to ergot alkaloids. ⓜ

- **CONCEPTION AND CONTRACEPTION** Caution—provide contraceptive advice if appropriate (oral contraceptives may increase prolactin concentration).

- **BREAST FEEDING** Suppresses lactation; avoid breast feeding for about 5 days if lactation prevention fails.

- **HEPATIC IMPAIRMENT**
Dose adjustments Manufacturer advises dose adjustment may be necessary—risk of increased plasma concentration.

- **MONITORING REQUIREMENTS**
▸ Specialist evaluation—monitor for pituitary enlargement, particularly during pregnancy; monitor visual field to detect secondary field loss in macroprolactinoma.
▸ Monitor for fibrotic disease.
▸ Monitor blood pressure for a few days after starting treatment and following dosage increase.

- **TREATMENT CESSATION** Antiparkinsonian drug therapy should never be stopped abruptly as this carries a small risk of neuroleptic malignant syndrome.

- **PATIENT AND CARER ADVICE**
Driving and skilled tasks **Sudden onset of sleep** Excessive daytime sleepiness and sudden onset of sleep can occur with dopamine-receptor agonists.

Patients starting treatment with these drugs should be warned of the risk and of the need to exercise caution when driving or operating machinery. Those who have experienced excessive sedation or sudden onset of sleep should refrain from driving or operating machines until these effects have stopped occurring.

Management of excessive daytime sleepiness should focus on the identification of an underlying cause, such as depression or concomitant medication. Patients should be counselled on improving sleep behaviour.

Hypotensive reactions Hypotensive reactions can occur in some patients taking dopamine-receptor agonists; these can be particularly problematic during the first few days of treatment and care should be exercised when driving or operating machinery.

- MEDICINAL FORMS There can be variation in the licensing of different medicines containing the same drug. Forms available from special-order manufacturers include: oral suspension

Tablet

CAUTIONARY AND ADVISORY LABELS 10, 21
▸ Bromocriptine (Non-proprietary)
  Bromocriptine (as Bromocriptine mesilate) 2.5 mg Bromocriptine 2.5mg tablets | 30 tablet [PoM] £74.99 DT = £74.99

Cabergoline   20-Nov-2020

- DRUG ACTION Cabergoline is a stimulant of dopamine receptors in the brain and it also inhibits release of prolactin by the pituitary.

- INDICATIONS AND DOSE

Prevention of lactation
▸ BY MOUTH
▸ Adult: 1 mg, to be taken as a single dose on the first day postpartum

Suppression of established lactation
▸ BY MOUTH
▸ Adult: 250 micrograms every 12 hours for 2 days

Hyperprolactinaemic disorders
▸ BY MOUTH
▸ Adult: Initially 500 micrograms once weekly, dose may be taken as a single dose or as 2 divided doses on separate days, then increased in steps of 500 micrograms every month until optimal therapeutic response reached, increase dose following monthly monitoring of serum prolactin levels; usual dose 0.25–2 mg once weekly, usually 1 mg weekly; reduce initial dose and increase more gradually if patient intolerant, doses over 1 mg weekly to be given as divided dose; maximum 4.5 mg per week

Alone or as adjunct to co-beneldopa or co-careldopa in Parkinson's disease where dopamine-receptor agonists other than ergot derivative not appropriate
▸ BY MOUTH
▸ Adult: Initially 1 mg daily, then increased in steps of 0.5–1 mg every 7–14 days, concurrent dose of levodopa may be decreased gradually while dose of cabergoline is increased; maximum 3 mg per day

---

IMPORTANT SAFETY INFORMATION

FIBROTIC REACTIONS

Cabergoline has been associated with pulmonary, retroperitoneal, and pericardial fibrotic reactions.

Manufacturer advises exclude cardiac valvulopathy with echocardiography before starting treatment with these ergot derivatives for Parkinson's disease or chronic endocrine disorders (excludes suppression of lactation); it may also be appropriate to measure the erythrocyte sedimentation rate and serum creatinine and to obtain a chest X-ray. Patients should be monitored for dyspnoea,

---

persistent cough, chest pain, cardiac failure, and abdominal pain or tenderness. If long-term treatment is expected, then lung-function tests may also be helpful. Patients taking cabergoline should be regularly monitored for cardiac fibrosis by echocardiography (within 3–6 months of initiating treatment and subsequently at 6–12 month intervals).

IMPULSE CONTROL DISORDERS

Treatment with dopamine-receptor agonists are associated with impulse control disorders, including pathological gambling, binge eating, and hypersexuality. Patients and their carers should be informed about the risk of impulse control disorders. Ergot- and non-ergot-derived dopamine-receptor agonists do not differ in their propensity to cause impulse control disorders, so switching between dopamine-receptor agonists will not control these side-effects. See Parkinson's disease p. 430.

- CONTRA-INDICATIONS Avoid in pre-eclampsia · cardiac valvulopathy—exclude before treatment (does not apply to suppression of lactation) · history of pericardial fibrotic disorders · history of puerperal psychosis · history of pulmonary fibrotic disorders · history of retroperitoneal fibrotic disorders

- CAUTIONS Cardiovascular disease · history of peptic ulcer (particularly in acromegalic patients) · history of serious mental disorders (especially psychotic disorders) · Raynaud's syndrome

  CAUTIONS, FURTHER INFORMATION
  ▸ Hyperprolactinemic patients In hyperprolactinaemic patients, the source of the hyperprolactinaemia should be established (i.e. exclude pituitary tumour before treatment).

- INTERACTIONS → Appendix 1: dopamine receptor agonists

- SIDE-EFFECTS
  ▸ **Common or very common** Angina pectoris · asthenia · cardiac valvulopathy · confusion · constipation · dizziness · drowsiness · dyspepsia · dyspnoea · gastritis · hallucination · headache · hypotension · movement disorders · nausea · oedema · pericardial effusion · pericarditis · sexual dysfunction · sleep disorders · vertigo · vomiting
  ▸ **Uncommon** Delusions · erythromelalgia · hepatic function abnormal · psychotic disorder · rash · respiratory disorders
  ▸ **Rare or very rare** Fibrosis
  ▸ **Frequency not known** Aggression · alopecia · chest pain · digital vasospasm · leg cramps · pathological gambling · syncope · tremor · visual impairment

- ALLERGY AND CROSS-SENSITIVITY [EvGr] Cabergoline should not be used in patients with hypersensitivity to ergot alkaloids. ⓂⓌ

- CONCEPTION AND CONTRACEPTION Exclude pregnancy before starting and perform monthly pregnancy tests during the amenorrhoeic period. Caution—advise non-hormonal contraception if pregnancy not desired. Discontinue 1 month before intended conception (ovulatory cycles persist for 6 months).

- PREGNANCY Discontinue if pregnancy occurs during treatment (specialist advice needed).

- BREAST FEEDING Suppresses lactation; avoid breast-feeding if lactation prevention fails.

- HEPATIC IMPAIRMENT Manufacturer advises caution in severe impairment (risk of increased of exposure).
  Dose adjustments Manufacturer advises consider dose reduction in severe impairment.

- MONITORING REQUIREMENTS
  ▸ Monitor for fibrotic disease.
  ▸ Monitor blood pressure for a few days after starting treatment and following dosage increase.

- **TREATMENT CESSATION** Antiparkinsonian drug therapy should never be stopped abruptly as this carries a small risk of neuroleptic malignant syndrome.
- **PRESCRIBING AND DISPENSING INFORMATION** Dispense in original container (contains desiccant).
- **PATIENT AND CARER ADVICE**
  Driving and skilled tasks **Sudden onset of sleep** Excessive daytime sleepiness and sudden onset of sleep can occur with dopamine-receptor agonists.
  Patients starting treatment with these drugs should be warned of the risk and of the need to exercise caution when driving or operating machinery. Those who have experienced excessive sedation or sudden onset of sleep should refrain from driving or operating machines until these effects have stopped occurring.
  Management of excessive daytime sleepiness should focus on the identification of an underlying cause, such as depression or concomitant medication. Patients should be counselled on improving sleep behaviour.
  Hypotensive reactions Hypotensive reactions can occur in some patients taking dopamine-receptor agonists; these can be particularly problematic during the first few days of treatment and care should be exercised when driving or operating machinery.

- **MEDICINAL FORMS** There can be variation in the licensing of different medicines containing the same drug.
  Tablet
  CAUTIONARY AND ADVISORY LABELS 10, 21
  ▸ Cabergoline (Non-proprietary)
  Cabergoline 500 microgram Cabergoline 500microgram tablets | 8 tablet PoM £35.95 DT = £35.93
  Cabergoline 1 mg Cabergoline 1mg tablets | 20 tablet PoM £66.00 DT = £64.25
  Cabergoline 2 mg Cabergoline 2mg tablets | 20 tablet PoM £73.14 DT = £73.12
  ▸ Cabaser (Pfizer Ltd)
  Cabergoline 1 mg Cabaser 1mg tablets | 20 tablet PoM £83.00 DT = £64.25
  Cabergoline 2 mg Cabaser 2mg tablets | 20 tablet PoM £83.00 DT = £73.12
  ▸ Dostinex (Pfizer Ltd)
  Cabergoline 500 microgram Dostinex 500microgram tablets | 8 tablet PoM £30.04 DT = £35.93

Pramipexole

20-Dec-2019

- **INDICATIONS AND DOSE**

Parkinson's disease, used alone or as an adjunct to co-beneldopa or co-careldopa
▸ BY MOUTH USING IMMEDIATE-RELEASE MEDICINES
▸ Adult: Initially 88 micrograms 3 times a day, if tolerated dose to be increased by doubling dose every 5–7 days, increased to 350 micrograms 3 times a day, then increased in steps of 180 micrograms 3 times a day if required, dose to be increased at weekly intervals, during dose titration and maintenance, levodopa dose may be reduced, maximum daily dose to be given in 3 divided doses; maximum 3.3 mg per day
▸ BY MOUTH USING MODIFIED-RELEASE MEDICINES
▸ Adult: Initially 260 micrograms once daily, dose to be increased by doubling dose every 5–7 days, increased to 1.05 mg once daily, then increased in steps of 520 micrograms every week if required, during dose titration and maintenance, levodopa dose may be reduced according to response; maximum 3.15 mg per day

Moderate to severe restless legs syndrome
▸ BY MOUTH USING IMMEDIATE-RELEASE MEDICINES
▸ Adult: Initially 88 micrograms once daily, dose to be taken 2–3 hours before bedtime, dose to be increased by doubling dose every 4–7 days if necessary, repeat

dose titration if restarting treatment after an interval of more than a few days; maximum 540 micrograms per day

DOSE EQUIVALENCE AND CONVERSION
▸ Doses and strengths are stated in terms of pramipexole (base).
▸ Equivalent strengths of pramipexole (base) in terms of pramipexole dihydrochloride monohydrate (salt) for immediate-release preparations are as follows:
▸ 88 micrograms base ≡ 125 micrograms salt;
▸ 180 micrograms base ≡ 250 micrograms salt;
▸ 350 micrograms base ≡ 500 micrograms salt;
▸ 700 micrograms base ≡ 1 mg salt.
▸ Equivalent strengths of pramipexole (base) in terms of pramipexole dihydrochloride monohydrate (salt) for modified-release preparations are as follows:
▸ 260 micrograms base ≡ 375 micrograms salt;
▸ 520 micrograms base ≡ 750 micrograms salt;
▸ 1.05 mg base ≡ 1.5 mg salt;
▸ 1.57 mg base ≡ 2.25 mg salt;
▸ 2.1 mg base ≡ 3 mg salt;
▸ 2.62 mg base ≡ 3.75 mg salt;
▸ 3.15 mg base ≡ 4.5 mg salt.

IMPORTANT SAFETY INFORMATION

IMPULSE CONTROL DISORDERS
Treatment with dopamine-receptor agonists is associated with impulse control disorders, including pathological gambling, binge eating, and hypersexuality. Patients and their carers should be informed about the risk of impulse control disorders. Ergot- and non-ergot-derived dopamine-receptor agonists do not differ in their propensity to cause impulse control disorders, so switching between dopamine-receptor agonists will not control these side-effects. See Parkinson's disease p. 430

- **CAUTIONS** Psychotic disorders · risk of visual disorders (ophthalmological testing recommended) · severe cardiovascular disease
- **INTERACTIONS** → Appendix 1: dopamine receptor agonists
- **SIDE-EFFECTS**
  ▸ **Common or very common** Appetite abnormal · behaviour abnormal · confusion · constipation · dizziness · drowsiness · fatigue · hallucination · headache · hypotension · movement disorders · nausea · peripheral oedema · psychiatric disorders · sleep disorders · vision disorders · vomiting · weight changes
  ▸ **Uncommon** Anxiety · binge eating · delirium · delusions · dyspnoea · heart failure · hiccups · mania · memory loss · pathological gambling · pneumonia · sexual dysfunction · SIADH · skin reactions · syncope
  ▸ **Frequency not known** Depression · dopamine agonist withdrawal syndrome · generalised pain · sweating abnormal
- **PREGNANCY** Use only if potential benefit outweighs risk—no information available.
- **BREAST FEEDING** May suppress lactation; avoid—present in milk in *animal* studies.
- **RENAL IMPAIRMENT** For *modified-release* tablets, avoid if eGFR less than 30 mL/minute/1.73 m^2.
  Dose adjustments For *immediate-release* tablets in Parkinson's disease, initially 88 micrograms twice daily (max. 1.57 mg daily in 2 divided doses) if eGFR 20–50 mL/minute/1.73 m^2; initially 88 micrograms once daily (max. 1.1 mg once daily) if eGFR less than 20 mL/minute/1.73 m^2. If renal function declines during treatment, reduce dose by the same percentage as the decline in eGFR.
  For *immediate-release* tablets in restless legs syndrome, reduce dose if eGFR less than 20 mL/minute/1.73 m^2.

For *modified-release* tablets, initially 260 micrograms on alternate days if eGFR 30–50 mL/minute/1.73 m², increased to 260 micrograms once daily after 1 week, further increased if necessary by 260 micrograms daily at weekly intervals to max. 1.57 mg daily.

- MONITORING REQUIREMENTS Risk of postural hypotension (especially on initiation)—monitor blood pressure.
- TREATMENT CESSATION Antiparkinsonian drug therapy should never be stopped abruptly as this carries a small risk of neuroleptic malignant syndrome.
- PATIENT AND CARER ADVICE

Driving and skilled tasks   Sudden onset of sleep Excessive daytime sleepiness and sudden onset of sleep can occur with dopamine-receptor agonists.

Patients starting treatment with these drugs should be warned of the risk and of the need to exercise caution when driving or operating machinery. Those who have experienced excessive sedation or sudden onset of sleep should refrain from driving or operating machines until these effects have stopped occurring.

Management of excessive daytime sleepiness should focus on the identification of an underlying cause, such as depression or concomitant medication. Patients should be counselled on improving sleep behaviour.

Hypotensive reactions Hypotensive reactions can occur in some patients taking dopamine-receptor agonists; these can be particularly problematic during the first few days of treatment and care should be exercised when driving or operating machinery.

- MEDICINAL FORMS There can be variation in the licensing of different medicines containing the same drug.

Modified-release tablet
CAUTIONARY AND ADVISORY LABELS 10, 25
▸ Pramipexole (Non-proprietary)
Pramipexole (as Pramipexole dihydrochloride monohydrate)
260 microgram Pramipexole 260microgram modified-release tablets | 30 tablet [PoM] £30.87 DT = £29.29
Pramipexole (as Pramipexole dihydrochloride monohydrate)
520 microgram Pramipexole 520microgram modified-release tablets | 30 tablet [PoM] £61.73 DT = £29.24
Pramipexole (as Pramipexole dihydrochloride monohydrate)
1.05 mg Pramipexole 1.05mg modified-release tablets | 30 tablet [PoM] £123.46 DT = £49.15
Pramipexole (as Pramipexole dihydrochloride monohydrate)
1.57 mg Pramipexole 1.57mg modified-release tablets | 30 tablet [PoM] £192.24 DT = £182.50
Pramipexole (as Pramipexole dihydrochloride monohydrate)
2.1 mg Pramipexole 2.1mg modified-release tablets | 30 tablet [PoM] £246.91 DT = £234.22
Pramipexole (as Pramipexole dihydrochloride monohydrate)
2.62 mg Pramipexole 2.62mg modified-release tablets | 30 tablet [PoM] £320.41 DT = £153.46
Pramipexole (as Pramipexole dihydrochloride monohydrate)
3.15 mg Pramipexole 3.15mg modified-release tablets | 30 tablet [PoM] £370.38 DT = £351.49
▸ Mirapexin (Boehringer Ingelheim Ltd)
Pramipexole (as Pramipexole dihydrochloride monohydrate)
260 microgram Mirapexin 0.26mg modified-release tablets | 30 tablet [PoM] £32.49 DT = £29.29
Pramipexole (as Pramipexole dihydrochloride monohydrate)
520 microgram Mirapexin 0.52mg modified-release tablets | 30 tablet [PoM] £64.98 DT = £29.24
Pramipexole (as Pramipexole dihydrochloride monohydrate)
1.05 mg Mirapexin 1.05mg modified-release tablets | 30 tablet [PoM] £129.96 DT = £49.15
Pramipexole (as Pramipexole dihydrochloride monohydrate)
1.57 mg Mirapexin 1.57mg modified-release tablets | 30 tablet [PoM] £202.36 DT = £182.50
Pramipexole (as Pramipexole dihydrochloride monohydrate)
2.1 mg Mirapexin 2.1mg modified-release tablets | 30 tablet [PoM] £259.91 DT = £234.22
Pramipexole (as Pramipexole dihydrochloride monohydrate)
2.62 mg Mirapexin 2.62mg modified-release tablets | 30 tablet [PoM] £337.27 DT = £153.46

Pramipexole (as Pramipexole dihydrochloride monohydrate)
3.15 mg Mirapexin 3.15mg modified-release tablets | 30 tablet [PoM] £389.87 DT = £351.49
▸ Oprymea (Consilient Health Ltd)
Pramipexole (as Pramipexole dihydrochloride monohydrate)
260 microgram Oprymea 0.26mg modified-release tablets | 30 tablet [PoM] £25.56 DT = £29.29
Pramipexole (as Pramipexole dihydrochloride monohydrate)
520 microgram Oprymea 0.52mg modified-release tablets | 30 tablet [PoM] £51.14 DT = £29.24
Pramipexole (as Pramipexole dihydrochloride monohydrate)
1.05 mg Oprymea 1.05mg modified-release tablets | 30 tablet [PoM] £102.28 DT = £49.15
Pramipexole (as Pramipexole dihydrochloride monohydrate)
1.57 mg Oprymea 1.57mg modified-release tablets | 30 tablet [PoM] £159.26 DT = £182.50
Pramipexole (as Pramipexole dihydrochloride monohydrate)
2.1 mg Oprymea 2.1mg modified-release tablets | 30 tablet [PoM] £204.56 DT = £234.22
Pramipexole (as Pramipexole dihydrochloride monohydrate)
2.62 mg Oprymea 2.62mg modified-release tablets | 30 tablet [PoM] £337.27 DT = £153.46
Pramipexole (as Pramipexole dihydrochloride monohydrate)
3.15 mg Oprymea 3.15mg modified-release tablets | 30 tablet [PoM] £389.87 DT = £351.49
▸ Pipexus (Ethypharm UK Ltd)
Pramipexole (as Pramipexole dihydrochloride monohydrate)
260 microgram Pipexus 0.26mg modified-release tablets | 30 tablet [PoM] £16.25 DT = £29.29
Pramipexole (as Pramipexole dihydrochloride monohydrate)
520 microgram Pipexus 0.52mg modified-release tablets | 30 tablet [PoM] £32.49 DT = £29.24
Pramipexole (as Pramipexole dihydrochloride monohydrate)
1.05 mg Pipexus 1.05mg modified-release tablets | 30 tablet [PoM] £64.98 DT = £49.15
Pramipexole (as Pramipexole dihydrochloride monohydrate)
1.57 mg Pipexus 1.57mg modified-release tablets | 30 tablet [PoM] £101.18 DT = £182.50
Pramipexole (as Pramipexole dihydrochloride monohydrate)
2.1 mg Pipexus 2.1mg modified-release tablets | 30 tablet [PoM] £129.96 DT = £234.22
Pramipexole (as Pramipexole dihydrochloride monohydrate)
2.62 mg Pipexus 2.62mg modified-release tablets | 30 tablet [PoM] £168.64 DT = £153.46
Pramipexole (as Pramipexole dihydrochloride monohydrate)
3.15 mg Pipexus 3.15mg modified-release tablets | 30 tablet [PoM] £194.94 DT = £351.49

Tablet
CAUTIONARY AND ADVISORY LABELS 10
▸ Pramipexole (Non-proprietary)
Pramipexole (as Pramipexole dihydrochloride monohydrate)
88 microgram Pramipexole 88microgram tablets | 30 tablet [PoM] £9.55 DT = £4.17
Pramipexole (as Pramipexole dihydrochloride monohydrate)
180 microgram Pramipexole 180microgram tablets | 30 tablet [PoM] £19.12 DT = £2.20 | 100 tablet [PoM] £7.32–£7.33
Pramipexole (as Pramipexole dihydrochloride monohydrate)
350 microgram Pramipexole 350microgram tablets | 30 tablet [PoM] £38.22 DT = £13.90 | 100 tablet [PoM] £46.33–£46.50
Pramipexole (as Pramipexole dihydrochloride monohydrate)
700 microgram Pramipexole 700microgram tablets | 30 tablet [PoM] £68.76 DT = £1.97 | 100 tablet [PoM] £6.57–£254.85
▸ Mirapexin (Boehringer Ingelheim Ltd)
Pramipexole (as Pramipexole dihydrochloride monohydrate)
88 microgram Mirapexin 0.088mg tablets | 30 tablet [PoM] £11.24 DT = £4.17
Pramipexole (as Pramipexole dihydrochloride monohydrate)
180 microgram Mirapexin 0.18mg tablets | 30 tablet [PoM] £22.49 DT = £2.20 | 100 tablet [PoM] £74.95
Pramipexole (as Pramipexole dihydrochloride monohydrate)
350 microgram Mirapexin 0.35mg tablets | 30 tablet [PoM] £44.97 DT = £13.90 | 100 tablet [PoM] £149.90
Pramipexole (as Pramipexole dihydrochloride monohydrate)
700 microgram Mirapexin 0.7mg tablets | 30 tablet [PoM] £89.94 DT = £1.97 | 100 tablet [PoM] £299.82
▸ Oprymea (Consilient Health Ltd)
Pramipexole (as Pramipexole dihydrochloride monohydrate)
88 microgram Oprymea 0.088mg tablets | 30 tablet [PoM] £3.23 DT = £4.17

Pramipexole (as Pramipexole dihydrochloride monohydrate)
180 microgram Oprymea 0.18mg tablets | 30 tablet [PoM] £6.09 DT
= £2.20 | 100 tablet [PoM] £15.46

Pramipexole (as Pramipexole dihydrochloride monohydrate)
350 microgram Oprymea 0.35mg tablets | 30 tablet [PoM] £32.47
DT = £13.90 | 100 tablet [PoM] £108.23

Pramipexole (as Pramipexole dihydrochloride monohydrate)
700 microgram Oprymea 0.7mg tablets | 30 tablet [PoM] £18.26 DT
= £1.97 | 100 tablet [PoM] £117.63

Ropinirole

10-Nov-2020

● **INDICATIONS AND DOSE**

Parkinson's disease, either used alone or as adjunct to co-beneldopa or co-careldopa
▶ BY MOUTH USING IMMEDIATE-RELEASE MEDICINES
▶ **Adult:** Initially 750 micrograms daily in 3 divided doses, then increased in steps of 750 micrograms daily, dose to be increased at weekly intervals, increased to 3 mg daily in 3 divided doses, then increased in steps of 1.5–3 mg daily, adjusted according to response, dose to be increased at weekly intervals; usual dose 9–16 mg daily in 3 divided doses, higher doses may be required if used with levodopa, when administered as adjunct to levodopa, concurrent dose of levodopa may be reduced by approx. 20%; daily maximum dose to be given in 3 divided doses; maximum 24 mg per day
▶ BY MOUTH USING MODIFIED-RELEASE MEDICINES
▶ **Adult:** Initially 2 mg once daily for 1 week, then 4 mg once daily, increased in steps of 2 mg at intervals of at least 1 week, adjusted according to response, increased to up to 8 mg once daily, dose to be increased further if still no response; increased in steps of 2–4 mg at intervals of at least 2 weeks if required, consider slower titration in patients over 75 years, when administered as adjunct to levodopa, concurrent dose of levodopa may gradually be reduced by approx. 30%; maximum 24 mg per day

Parkinson's disease in patients transferring from ropinirole immediate-release tablets
▶ BY MOUTH USING MODIFIED-RELEASE MEDICINES
▶ **Adult:** Initially ropinirole modified-release once daily substituted for total daily dose equivalent of ropinirole immediate-release tablets; if control not maintained after switching, titrate dose as above

Moderate to severe restless legs syndrome
▶ BY MOUTH USING IMMEDIATE-RELEASE MEDICINES
▶ **Adult:** Initially 250 micrograms once daily for 2 days, increased if tolerated to 500 micrograms once daily for 5 days, then increased if tolerated to 1 mg once daily for 7 days, then increased in steps of 500 micrograms daily, adjusted according to response, dose to be increased at weekly intervals; usual dose 2 mg once daily, doses to be taken at night; maximum 4 mg per day

● **UNLICENSED USE** Doses in the BNF may differ from those in product literature.

IMPORTANT SAFETY INFORMATION

SAFE PRACTICE
Ropinirole has been confused with risperidone; care must be taken to ensure the correct drug is prescribed and dispensed.

IMPULSE CONTROL DISORDERS
Treatment with dopamine-receptor agonists is associated with impulse control disorders, including pathological gambling, binge eating, and hypersexuality. Patients and their carers should be informed about the risk of impulse control disorders. Ergot- and non-ergot-derived dopamine-receptor agonists do not differ in their propensity to cause impulse control disorders, so

switching between dopamine-receptor agonists will not control these side-effects. See Parkinson's disease p. 430

● **CAUTIONS** Elderly · major psychotic disorders · severe cardiovascular disease (risk of hypotension—monitor blood pressure)

● **INTERACTIONS** → Appendix 1: dopamine receptor agonists

● **SIDE-EFFECTS**
▶ **Common or very common** Confusion · dizziness · drowsiness · fatigue · gastrointestinal discomfort · hallucination · movement disorders · nausea · nervousness · peripheral oedema · sleep disorders · syncope · vertigo · vomiting
▶ **Uncommon** Hypotension · sexual dysfunction
▶ **Rare or very rare** Hepatic reaction
▶ **Frequency not known** Behaviour abnormal · compulsions · delirium · delusions · dopamine dysregulation syndrome · eating disorders · pathological gambling · psychotic disorder

● **PREGNANCY** Avoid unless potential benefit outweighs risk—toxicity in *animal* studies.

● **BREAST FEEDING** May suppress lactation—avoid.

● **HEPATIC IMPAIRMENT**
▶ When used for Parkinson's disease Manufacturer advises avoid (no information available).
▶ When used for Restless legs syndrome Manufacturer advises caution in moderate impairment; avoid in severe impairment.

● **RENAL IMPAIRMENT** Avoid if eGFR less than 30 mL/minute/1.73 m^2.

● **TREATMENT CESSATION** Antiparkinsonian drug therapy should never be stopped abruptly as this carries a small risk of neuroleptic malignant syndrome.

● **PATIENT AND CARER ADVICE** Manufacturer advises patients and their carers should be informed of the risk of developing dopamine dysregulation syndrome; addiction-like symptoms should be reported.

Missed doses
▶ When used for Parkinson's disease Manufacturer advises if treatment is interrupted for one day or more, re-initiation by dose titration should be considered—consult product literature.
▶ When used for Moderate to severe restless legs syndrome Manufacturer advises if treatment is interrupted for more than a few days, re-initiation by dose titration is recommended.

Driving and skilled tasks   Sudden onset of sleep Excessive daytime sleepiness and sudden onset of sleep can occur with dopamine-receptor agonists.

Patients starting treatment with these drugs should be warned of the risk and of the need to exercise caution when driving or operating machinery. Those who have experienced excessive sedation or sudden onset of sleep should refrain from driving or operating machines until these effects have stopped occurring.

Management of excessive daytime sleepiness should focus on the identification of an underlying cause, such as depression or concomitant medication. Patients should be counselled on improving sleep behaviour.

Hypotensive reactions Hypotensive reactions can occur in some patients taking dopamine-receptor agonists; these can be particularly problematic during the first few days of treatment and care should be exercised when driving or operating machinery.

● **NATIONAL FUNDING/ACCESS DECISIONS**
For full details see funding body website

Scottish Medicines Consortium (SMC) decisions
▶ Ropinirole tablets (*Adartrel*®) for the treatment of moderate to severe idiopathic restless legs syndrome (July 2006) SMC No. 165/05 Recommended with restrictions

▶ Ropinirole (*Requip XL*®) for the treatment of idiopathic Parkinson's Disease (September 2008) SMC No. 491/08 Recommended

● MEDICINAL FORMS There can be variation in the licensing of different medicines containing the same drug. Forms available from special-order manufacturers include: oral suspension, oral solution

Modified-release tablet
CAUTIONARY AND ADVISORY LABELS 10, 25
▶ Ropinirole (Non-proprietary)
Ropinirole (as Ropinirole hydrochloride) 2 mg Ropinirole 2mg modified-release tablets | 28 tablet [PoM] £10.66 DT = £12.54
Ropinirole (as Ropinirole hydrochloride) 4 mg Ropinirole 4mg modified-release tablets | 28 tablet [PoM] £21.33 DT = £25.09
Ropinirole (as Ropinirole hydrochloride) 8 mg Ropinirole 8mg modified-release tablets | 28 tablet [PoM] £35.79 DT = £42.11

▶ Eppinix XL (Ethypharm UK Ltd)
Ropinirole (as Ropinirole hydrochloride) 2 mg Ipinnia XL 2mg tablets | 28 tablet [PoM] £5.64 DT = £12.54
Ropinirole (as Ropinirole hydrochloride) 3 mg Ipinnia XL 3mg tablets | 28 tablet [PoM] £8.46 DT = £8.46
Ropinirole (as Ropinirole hydrochloride) 4 mg Ipinnia XL 4mg tablets | 28 tablet [PoM] £11.29 DT = £25.09
Ropinirole (as Ropinirole hydrochloride) 6 mg Ipinnia XL 6mg tablets | 28 tablet [PoM] £15.32 DT = £15.32
Ropinirole (as Ropinirole hydrochloride) 8 mg Ipinnia XL 8mg tablets | 28 tablet [PoM] £18.95 DT = £42.11

▶ Ralnea XL (Consilient Health Ltd)
Ropinirole (as Ropinirole hydrochloride) 2 mg Ralnea XL 2mg tablets | 28 tablet [PoM] £10.65 DT = £12.54
Ropinirole (as Ropinirole hydrochloride) 4 mg Ralnea XL 4mg tablets | 28 tablet [PoM] £21.32 DT = £25.09
Ropinirole (as Ropinirole hydrochloride) 8 mg Ralnea XL 8mg tablets | 28 tablet [PoM] £35.79 DT = £42.11

▶ Raponer XL (Accord Healthcare Ltd)
Ropinirole (as Ropinirole hydrochloride) 2 mg Raponer XL 2mg tablets | 28 tablet [PoM] £12.54 DT = £12.54
Ropinirole (as Ropinirole hydrochloride) 4 mg Raponer XL 4mg tablets | 28 tablet [PoM] £25.09 DT = £25.09
Ropinirole (as Ropinirole hydrochloride) 8 mg Raponer XL 8mg tablets | 28 tablet [PoM] £42.11 DT = £42.11

▶ ReQuip XL (GlaxoSmithKline UK Ltd)
Ropinirole (as Ropinirole hydrochloride) 2 mg ReQuip XL 2mg tablets | 28 tablet [PoM] £12.54 DT = £12.54
Ropinirole (as Ropinirole hydrochloride) 4 mg ReQuip XL 4mg tablets | 28 tablet [PoM] £25.09 DT = £25.09
Ropinirole (as Ropinirole hydrochloride) 8 mg ReQuip XL 8mg tablets | 28 tablet [PoM] £42.11 DT = £42.11

▶ Repinex XL (Aspire Pharma Ltd)
Ropinirole (as Ropinirole hydrochloride) 2 mg Repinex XL 2mg tablets | 28 tablet [PoM] £6.20 DT = £12.54
Ropinirole (as Ropinirole hydrochloride) 4 mg Repinex XL 4mg tablets | 28 tablet [PoM] £12.50 DT = £25.09
Ropinirole (as Ropinirole hydrochloride) 8 mg Repinex XL 8mg tablets | 28 tablet [PoM] £21.00 DT = £42.11

▶ Ropiqual XL (Milpharm Ltd)
Ropinirole (as Ropinirole hydrochloride) 2 mg Ropiqual XL 2mg tablets | 28 tablet [PoM] £12.54 DT = £12.54
Ropinirole (as Ropinirole hydrochloride) 4 mg Ropiqual XL 4mg tablets | 28 tablet [PoM] £25.09 DT = £25.09
Ropinirole (as Ropinirole hydrochloride) 8 mg Ropiqual XL 8mg tablets | 28 tablet [PoM] £42.11 DT = £42.11

▶ Spiroco XL (Teva UK Ltd)
Ropinirole (as Ropinirole hydrochloride) 2 mg Spiroco XL 2mg tablets | 28 tablet [PoM] £5.63 DT = £12.54
Ropinirole (as Ropinirole hydrochloride) 4 mg Spiroco XL 4mg tablets | 28 tablet [PoM] £11.28 DT = £25.09
Ropinirole (as Ropinirole hydrochloride) 8 mg Spiroco XL 8mg tablets | 28 tablet [PoM] £18.94 DT = £42.11

Tablet
CAUTIONARY AND ADVISORY LABELS 10, 21
▶ Ropinirole (Non-proprietary)
Ropinirole (as Ropinirole hydrochloride) 250 microgram Ropinirole 250microgram tablets | 12 tablet [PoM] £15.00 DT = £2.76
Ropinirole (as Ropinirole hydrochloride) 500 microgram Ropinirole 500microgram tablets | 28 tablet [PoM] £25.00 DT = £5.43

Ropinirole (as Ropinirole hydrochloride) 1 mg Ropinirole 1mg tablets | 84 tablet [PoM] £57.10 DT = £57.10
Ropinirole (as Ropinirole hydrochloride) 2 mg Ropinirole 2mg tablets | 28 tablet [PoM] £49.99 DT = £9.50 | 84 tablet [PoM] £28.50-£37.94
Ropinirole (as Ropinirole hydrochloride) 5 mg Ropinirole 5mg tablets | 84 tablet [PoM] £185.63 DT = £185.63

▶ Adartrel (GlaxoSmithKline UK Ltd)
Ropinirole (as Ropinirole hydrochloride) 250 microgram Adartrel 250microgram tablets | 12 tablet [PoM] £3.94 DT = £2.76
Ropinirole (as Ropinirole hydrochloride) 500 microgram Adartrel 500microgram tablets | 28 tablet [PoM] £15.75 DT = £5.43
Ropinirole (as Ropinirole hydrochloride) 2 mg Adartrel 2mg tablets | 28 tablet [PoM] £31.51 DT = £9.50

▶ ReQuip (GlaxoSmithKline UK Ltd)
Ropinirole (as Ropinirole hydrochloride) 250 microgram ReQuip 250microgram tablets | 21 tablet [PoM] £5.70
Ropinirole (as Ropinirole hydrochloride) 1 mg ReQuip 1mg tablets | 84 tablet [PoM] £56.71 DT = £57.10
Ropinirole (as Ropinirole hydrochloride) 2 mg ReQuip 2mg tablets | 84 tablet [PoM] £113.44
Ropinirole (as Ropinirole hydrochloride) 5 mg ReQuip 5mg tablets | 84 tablet [PoM] £195.92 DT = £185.63

Rotigotine
20-Jul-2020

● INDICATIONS AND DOSE
Monotherapy in Parkinson's disease
▶ BY TRANSDERMAL APPLICATION USING PATCHES
▶ Adult: Initially 2 mg/24 hours, then increased in steps of 2 mg/24 hours every week if required; maximum 8 mg/24 hours per day

Adjunctive therapy with co-beneldopa or co-careldopa in Parkinson's disease
▶ BY TRANSDERMAL APPLICATION USING PATCHES
▶ Adult: Initially 4 mg/24 hours, then increased in steps of 2 mg/24 hours every week if required; maximum 16 mg/24 hours per day

Moderate to severe restless legs syndrome
▶ BY TRANSDERMAL APPLICATION USING PATCHES
▶ Adult: Initially 1 mg/24 hours, then increased in steps of 1 mg/24 hours every week if required; maximum 3 mg/24 hours per day

---

IMPORTANT SAFETY INFORMATION

IMPULSE CONTROL DISORDERS
Treatment with dopamine-receptor agonists is associated with impulse control disorders, including pathological gambling, binge eating, and hypersexuality. Patients and their carers should be informed about the risk of impulse control disorders. Ergot- and non-ergot-derived dopamine-receptor agonists do not differ in their propensity to cause impulse control disorders, so switching between dopamine-receptor agonists will not control these side-effects. See Parkinson's disease p. 430

● CAUTIONS Avoid exposure of patch to heat · remove patch (aluminium-containing) before magnetic resonance imaging or cardioversion

● INTERACTIONS → Appendix 1: dopamine receptor agonists

● SIDE-EFFECTS
▶ **Common or very common** Asthenia · behaviour abnormal · constipation · dizziness · drowsiness · dry mouth · dyskinesia · eating disorders · fall · gastrointestinal discomfort · hallucinations · headache · hiccups · hyperhidrosis · hypertension · hypotension · loss of consciousness · malaise · nausea · palpitations · pathological gambling · perception altered · peripheral oedema · psychiatric disorders · skin reactions · sleep disorders · syncope · vertigo · vomiting · weight changes
▶ **Uncommon** Agitation · angioedema · arrhythmias · confusion · sexual dysfunction · vision disorders

▶ **Rare or very rare** Delirium · delusions · irritability · psychotic disorder · seizure
▶ **Frequency not known** Dopamine dysregulation syndrome
● PREGNANCY Avoid—no information available.
● BREAST FEEDING May suppress lactation; avoid—present in milk in *animal* studies.
● HEPATIC IMPAIRMENT Manufacturer advises caution in severe impairment (no information available).
Dose adjustments Manufacturer advises consider dose reduction in severe impairment.
● MONITORING REQUIREMENTS Ophthalmic testing recommended.
● TREATMENT CESSATION Antiparkinsonian drug therapy should never be stopped abruptly as this carries a small risk of neuroleptic malignant syndrome.
● DIRECTIONS FOR ADMINISTRATION Manufacturer advises apply patch to clean, dry, intact, healthy and non-irritated skin on torso, thigh, hip, shoulder or upper arm by pressing the patch firmly against the skin for about 30 seconds. Patches should be removed after 24 hours and the replacement patch applied on a different area (avoid using the same area for 14 days)—consult product literature for further information.
● PATIENT AND CARER ADVICE Manufacturer advises patients and their carers should be informed of the risk of developing dopamine dysregulation syndrome; addiction-like symptoms should be reported.
Driving and skilled tasks **Sudden onset of sleep** Excessive daytime sleepiness and sudden onset of sleep can occur with dopamine-receptor agonists.
Patients starting treatment with these drugs should be warned of the risk and of the need to exercise caution when driving or operating machinery. Those who have experienced excessive sedation or sudden onset of sleep should refrain from driving or operating machines until these effects have stopped occurring.
Management of excessive daytime sleepiness should focus on the identification of an underlying cause, such as depression or concomitant medication. Patients should be counselled on improving sleep behaviour.
Hypotensive reactions Hypotensive reactions can occur in some patients taking dopamine-receptor agonists; these can be particularly problematic during the first few days of treatment and care should be exercised when driving or operating machinery.
● NATIONAL FUNDING/ACCESS DECISIONS
For full details see funding body website
Scottish Medicines Consortium (SMC) decisions
▶ Rotigotine (*Neupro*®) for advanced-stage idiopathic Parkinson's disease (August 2007) SMC No. 392/07 Recommended with restrictions
▶ Rotigotine (*Neupro*®) for early-stage Parkinson's disease (July 2007) SMC No. 289/06 Recommended
▶ Rotigotine (*Neupro*®) for Restless Legs Syndrome (RLS) (August 2009) SMC No. 548/09 Recommended with restrictions
● MEDICINAL FORMS There can be variation in the licensing of different medicines containing the same drug.
Transdermal patch
CAUTIONARY AND ADVISORY LABELS 10
▶ Neupro (UCB Pharma Ltd)
Rotigotine 1 mg per 24 hour Neupro 1mg/24hours transdermal patches | 28 patch [PoM] £77.24 DT = £77.24
Rotigotine 2 mg per 24 hour Neupro 2mg/24hours transdermal patches | 28 patch [PoM] £81.10 DT = £81.10
Rotigotine 3 mg per 24 hour Neupro 3mg/24hours transdermal patches | 28 patch [PoM] £102.35 DT = £102.35
Rotigotine 4 mg per 24 hour Neupro 4mg/24hours transdermal patches | 28 patch [PoM] £123.60 DT = £123.60
Rotigotine 6 mg per 24 hour Neupro 6mg/24hours transdermal patches | 28 patch [PoM] £149.93 DT = £149.93

Rotigotine 8 mg per 24 hour Neupro 8mg/24hours transdermal patches | 28 patch [PoM] £149.93 DT = £149.93

DOPAMINERGIC DRUGS > MONOAMINE-OXIDASE B INHIBITORS

Rasagiline
26-May-2020

● DRUG ACTION Rasagiline is a monoamine-oxidase B inhibitor.

● **INDICATIONS AND DOSE**

Parkinson's disease, used alone or as adjunct to co-beneldopa or co-careldopa for 'end-of-dose' fluctuations
▶ BY MOUTH
▶ Adult: 1 mg daily

● INTERACTIONS → Appendix 1: MAO-B inhibitors
● SIDE-EFFECTS
▶ **Common or very common** Abdominal pain · angina pectoris · arthralgia · arthritis · conjunctivitis · depression · dermatitis · dry mouth · fall · fever · flatulence · hallucination · headache · increased risk of infection · leucopenia · malaise · nausea · neoplasms · pain · postural hypotension · sleep disorders · urinary urgency · vertigo · vomiting · weight decreased
▶ **Uncommon** Appetite decreased · confusion
▶ **Frequency not known** Dopamine dysregulation syndrome · drowsiness · eating disorders · pathological gambling · psychiatric disorders · sexual dysfunction
● PREGNANCY Manufacturer advises avoid—no information available.
● BREAST FEEDING Use with caution—may suppress lactation.
● HEPATIC IMPAIRMENT Manufacturer advises caution in mild impairment; avoid in moderate to severe impairment (risk of increased exposure).
● TREATMENT CESSATION Avoid abrupt withdrawal.

● MEDICINAL FORMS There can be variation in the licensing of different medicines containing the same drug. Forms available from special-order manufacturers include: oral suspension, oral solution
Tablet
▶ Rasagiline (Non-proprietary)
Rasagiline 1 mg Rasagiline 1mg tablets | 28 tablet [PoM] £70.72 DT = £3.16
▶ Azilect (Teva UK Ltd)
Rasagiline 1 mg Azilect 1mg tablets | 28 tablet [PoM] £70.72 DT = £3.16

Safinamide
18-Jul-2017

● DRUG ACTION Safinamide is a monoamine-oxidase-B inhibitor.

● **INDICATIONS AND DOSE**

Parkinson's disease, as an adjunct to levodopa alone or in combination with other antiparkinsonian drugs, for mid- to late-stage fluctuations
▶ BY MOUTH
▶ Adult: 50 mg once daily, increased if necessary to 100 mg once daily

● CONTRA-INDICATIONS Active retinopathy · albinism · family history of hereditary retinal disease · retinal degeneration · uveitis
● CAUTIONS Hypertension (may raise blood pressure) · may exacerbate pre-existing dyskinesia (requiring levodopa dose reduction)
● INTERACTIONS → Appendix 1: MAO-B inhibitors

- SIDE-EFFECTS
▶ **Common or very common** Cataract · dizziness · drowsiness · headache · hypotension · injury · nausea · sleep disorders
▶ **Uncommon** Anaemia · anxiety · appetite abnormal · arrhythmias · asthenia · cognitive disorder · confusion · constipation · cough · decreased leucocytes · depression · diarrhoea · dry mouth · dysarthria · dyslipidaemia · dyspnoea · emotional lability · eye disorders · eye inflammation · gastrointestinal discomfort · gastrointestinal disorders · glaucoma · hallucination · hyperglycaemia · hypertension · increased risk of infection · joint disorders · movement disorders · muscle complaints · muscle weakness · neoplasms · oral disorders · pain · palpitations · peripheral oedema · photosensitivity reaction · psychotic disorder · QT interval prolongation · red blood cell abnormality · rhinorrhoea · sensation abnormal · sensation of pressure · sexual dysfunction · skin reactions · sweat changes · syncope · temperature sensation altered · urinary disorders · varicose veins · vertigo · vision disorders · vomiting · weight changes
▶ **Rare or very rare** Alopecia · arterial spasm · atherosclerosis · benign prostatic hyperplasia · breast abnormalities · bronchospasm · cachexia · concentration impaired · delirium · diabetic retinopathy · dysphonia · eosinophilia · eye pain · fat embolism · fever · gambling · haemorrhage · hyperbilirubinaemia · hyperkalaemia · illusion · malaise · myocardial infarction · oropharyngeal complaints · osteoarthritis · paranoia · psychiatric disorders · pyuria · reflexes decreased · suicidal ideation · taste altered
- PREGNANCY Manufacturer advises avoid—toxicity in *animal* studies.
- BREAST FEEDING Manufacturer advises avoid—present in milk in *animal* studies.
- HEPATIC IMPAIRMENT Manufacturer advises caution in moderate impairment (risk of increased exposure); avoid in severe impairment.
  Dose adjustments Manufacturer advises max. daily dose should not exceed 50 mg daily in moderate impairment.
- MEDICINAL FORMS There can be variation in the licensing of different medicines containing the same drug.
  Tablet
  ▶ Xadago (Profile Pharma Ltd)
  Safinamide (as Safinamide methansulfonate) 50 mg Xadago 50mg tablets | 30 tablet [PoM] £69.00 DT = £69.00
  Safinamide (as Safinamide methansulfonate) 100 mg Xadago 100mg tablets | 30 tablet [PoM] £69.00 DT = £69.00

Selegiline hydrochloride

- DRUG ACTION Selegiline is a monoamine-oxidase-B inhibitor.

- INDICATIONS AND DOSE
  Parkinson's disease, used alone or as adjunct to co-beneldopa or co-careldopa to reduce 'end of dose' deterioration | Symptomatic parkinsonism
  ▶ BY MOUTH USING IMMEDIATE-RELEASE MEDICINES
  ▶ Adult: Initially 5 mg once daily for 2–4 weeks, then increased if tolerated to 10 mg daily, dose to be taken in the morning
  ▶ BY MOUTH USING ORAL LYOPHILISATE
  ▶ Adult: 1.25 mg once daily, dose to be taken before breakfast

  DOSE EQUIVALENCE AND CONVERSION
  ▶ 1.25-mg oral lyophilisate is equivalent to 10-mg tablet.
  ▶ Patients receiving 10 mg conventional selegiline hydrochloride tablets can be switched to oral lyophilisates (*Zelapar®*) 1.25 mg.

- CONTRA-INDICATIONS Active duodenal ulceration · active gastric ulceration · avoid or use with great caution in

postural hypotension (when used in combination with levodopa)
- CAUTIONS Angina · arrhythmias · duodenal ulceration · gastric ulceration · history of hepatic dysfunction · patients predisposed to confusion and psychosis · psychosis · uncontrolled hypertension
- INTERACTIONS → Appendix 1: MAO-B inhibitors
- SIDE-EFFECTS
▶ **Common or very common** Arrhythmias · arthralgia · back pain · confusion · constipation · depression · diarrhoea · dizziness · dry mouth · fall · fatigue · hallucination · headache · hyperhidrosis · hypertension · hypotension · movement disorders · muscle cramps · nasal congestion · nausea · oral disorders · sleep disorders · throat pain · tremor · vertigo
▶ **Uncommon** Alopecia · angina pectoris · anxiety · appetite decreased · chest pain · dyspnoea · leucopenia · mood altered · myopathy · palpitations · peripheral oedema · pharyngitis · psychosis · skin eruption · thrombocytopenia · urinary disorders · vision blurred
▶ **Frequency not known** Hypersexuality
  SIDE-EFFECTS, FURTHER INFORMATION Side-effects of levodopa may be increased—concurrent levodopa dosage can be reduced by 10–30% in steps of 10% every 3–4 days.
- PREGNANCY Avoid—no information available.
- BREAST FEEDING Avoid—no information available.
- HEPATIC IMPAIRMENT Manufacturer advises caution in severe impairment.
- RENAL IMPAIRMENT Use with caution in severe impairment.
- TREATMENT CESSATION Avoid abrupt withdrawal.
- DIRECTIONS FOR ADMINISTRATION Oral lyophilisates should be placed on the tongue and allowed to dissolve. Advise patient not to drink, rinse, or wash mouth out for 5 minutes after taking the tablet.
- PATIENT AND CARER ADVICE Patients or carers should be advised on how to administer selegiline hydrochloride oral lyophilisates.
  Driving and skilled tasks   **Drugs and driving** Prescribers and other healthcare professionals should advise patients if treatment is likely to affect their ability to perform skilled tasks (e.g. driving). This applies especially to drugs with sedative effects; patients should be warned that these effects are increased by alcohol. General information about a patient's fitness to drive is available from the Driver and Vehicle Licensing Agency at www.dvla.gov.uk.
  2015 legislation regarding driving whilst taking certain drugs, may also apply to selegiline, see *Drugs and driving* under Guidance on prescribing p. 1.

- MEDICINAL FORMS There can be variation in the licensing of different medicines containing the same drug. Forms available from special-order manufacturers include: oral solution
  Tablet
  ▶ Eldepryl (Orion Pharma (UK) Ltd)
  Selegiline hydrochloride 5 mg Eldepryl 5mg tablets | 100 tablet [PoM] £16.52 DT = £16.52
  Selegiline hydrochloride 10 mg Eldepryl 10mg tablets | 100 tablet [PoM] £32.23 DT = £32.23

5 Nausea and labyrinth disorders

Nausea and labyrinth disorders

19-Feb-2020

Drug treatment

Antiemetics should be prescribed only when the cause of vomiting is known because otherwise they may delay diagnosis, particularly in children. Antiemetics are unnecessary and sometimes harmful when the cause can be treated, such as in diabetic ketoacidosis, or in digoxin p. 117 or antiepileptic overdose.

If antiemetic drug treatment is indicated, the drug is chosen according to the aetiology of vomiting.

Antihistamines are effective against nausea and vomiting resulting from many underlying conditions. There is no evidence that any one antihistamine is superior to another but their duration of action and incidence of adverse effects (drowsiness and antimuscarinic effects) differ.

The **phenothiazines** are dopamine antagonists and act centrally by blocking the chemoreceptor trigger zone. They are of considerable value for the prophylaxis and treatment of nausea and vomiting associated with diffuse neoplastic disease, radiation sickness, and the emesis caused by drugs such as opioids, general anaesthetics, and cytotoxics. Prochlorperazine p. 408, perphenazine, and trifluoperazine p. 410 are less sedating than chlorpromazine hydrochloride p. 404; severe dystonic reactions sometimes occur with phenothiazines, especially in children. Some phenothiazines are available as rectal suppositories, which can be useful in patients with persistent vomiting or with severe nausea; prochlorperazine can also be administered as a buccal tablet which is placed between the upper lip and the gum.

Other antipsychotic drugs including haloperidol p. 405 and levomepromazine p. 459 are used for the relief of nausea and vomiting in terminal illness.

Metoclopramide hydrochloride p. 451 is an effective antiemetic and its activity closely resembles that of the phenothiazines. Metoclopramide hydrochloride also acts directly on the gastro-intestinal tract and it may be superior to the phenothiazines for emesis associated with gastroduodenal, hepatic, and biliary disease.

Domperidone p. 451 acts at the chemoreceptor trigger zone. It has the advantage over metoclopramide hydrochloride and the phenothiazines of being less likely to cause central effects such as sedation and dystonic reactions because it does not readily cross the blood-brain barrier. In Parkinson's disease, domperidone [unlicensed in those weighing less than 35 kg] can be used to treat nausea caused by dopaminergic drugs. The MHRA and CHM have released important safety information and restrictions regarding the use of domperidone for nausea and vomiting in those weighing less than 35 kg, and a reminder of contra-indications. For further information, see *Important safety information* for domperidone.

Granisetron p. 453 and ondansetron p. 454 are of value in the management of nausea and vomiting in patients receiving cytotoxics and in postoperative nausea and vomiting. Palonosetron p. 456 is licensed for prevention of nausea and vomiting associated with moderately or highly emetogenic cytotoxic chemotherapy. Palonosetron is also available in combination with netupitant, a neurokinin 1-receptor antagonist, for the prevention of acute and delayed nausea and vomiting associated with moderately emetogenic chemotherapy and highly emetogenic cisplatin-based chemotherapy.

Dexamethasone p. 714 has antiemetic effects and it is used in vomiting associated with cancer chemotherapy. It can be used alone or with metoclopramide hydrochloride, prochlorperazine, lorazepam p. 357, or a 5HT$_3$-receptor antagonist.

Aprepitant p. 452, fosaprepitant p. 453, and rolapitant are neurokinin 1-receptor antagonists. Aprepitant is licensed for the prevention of nausea and vomiting associated with highly and moderately emetogenic chemotherapy; fosaprepitant is licensed for the prevention of acute and delayed nausea and vomiting associated with highly emetogenic cisplatin-based chemotherapy and the prevention of nausea and vomiting associated with moderately emetogenic chemotherapy; rolapitant is licensed for the prevention of delayed nausea and vomiting associated with highly and moderately emetogenic chemotherapy. These drugs are given with dexamethasone and a 5HT$_3$-receptor antagonist. For further information on the prevention of nausea and vomiting caused by chemotherapy, see Cytotoxic drugs p. 932.

Nabilone p. 450 is a synthetic cannabinoid. EvGr It can be considered as an add-on treatment for chemotherapy-induced nausea and vomiting unresponsive to optimised conventional antiemetics. ⒶÏ

Vomiting during pregnancy

Nausea in the first trimester of pregnancy is generally mild and does not require drug therapy. On rare occasions if vomiting is severe, short-term treatment with an antihistamine, such as **promethazine**, may be required. Prochlorperazine or metoclopramide hydrochloride are alternatives. If symptoms do not settle in 24 to 48 hours then specialist opinion should be sought. Hyperemesis gravidarum is a more serious condition, which requires regular antiemetic therapy, intravenous fluid and electrolyte replacement and sometimes nutritional support. Supplementation with thiamine p. 1130 must be considered in order to reduce the risk of Wernicke's encephalopathy.

Postoperative nausea and vomiting

The incidence of postoperative nausea and vomiting depends on many factors including the anaesthetic used, and the type and duration of surgery. Other risk factors include female sex, non-smokers, a history of postoperative nausea and vomiting or motion sickness, and intraoperative and postoperative use of opioids. Therapy to prevent postoperative nausea and vomiting should be based on the assessed risk of postoperative nausea and vomiting in each patient. Drugs used include **5HT$_3$-receptor antagonists**, droperidol p. 459, dexamethasone, some **phenothiazines** (e.g. prochlorperazine), and **antihistamines** (e.g. cyclizine p. 449). A combination of two or more antiemetic drugs that have different mechanisms of action is often indicated in those at high risk of postoperative nausea and vomiting or where postoperative vomiting presents a particular danger (e.g. in some types of surgery). When a prophylactic antiemetic drug has failed, postoperative nausea and vomiting should be treated with one or more drugs from a different class.

Motion sickness

Antiemetics should be given to prevent motion sickness rather than after nausea or vomiting develop. The most effective drug for the prevention of motion sickness is hyoscine hydrobromide p. 458. The sedating antihistamines are slightly less effective against motion sickness, but are generally better tolerated than hyoscine. If a sedative effect is desired **promethazine** is useful, but generally a slightly less sedating antihistamine such as cyclizine or cinnarizine p. 456 is preferred. Domperidone, metoclopramide hydrochloride, 5HT$_3$-receptor antagonists, and the phenothiazines (except the antihistamine phenothiazine promethazine) are **ineffective** in motion sickness.

Other vestibular disorders

Management of vestibular diseases is aimed at treating the underlying cause as well as treating symptoms of the balance disturbance and associated nausea and vomiting. Vertigo and nausea associated with Ménière's disease and middle-ear surgery can be difficult to treat.

Betahistine dihydrochloride p. 460 is an analogue of histamine and is claimed to reduce endolymphatic pressure by improving the microcirculation. Betahistine dihydrochloride is licensed for vertigo, tinnitus, and hearing loss associated with Ménière's disease.

A **diuretic** alone or combined with salt restriction may provide some benefit in vertigo associated with Ménière's disease; **antihistamines** (such as cinnarizine p. 456), and **phenothiazines** (such as prochlorperazine p. 408) are also used. Where possible, prochlorperazine should be reserved for the treatment of acute symptoms.

Nausea and vomiting associated with migraine

For information on the use of antiemetics in migraine attacks, see Migraine p. 494.

> **Other drugs used for Nausea and labyrinth disorders**
> Paracetamol with metoclopramide, p. 496 · Promethazine hydrochloride, p. 302

ANTIEMETICS AND ANTINAUSEANTS ›
ANTIHISTAMINES

Cyclizine   04-Sep-2020

● **INDICATIONS AND DOSE**

Nausea | Vomiting | Vertigo | Motion sickness | Labyrinthine disorders
▸ BY MOUTH
▸ Adult: 50 mg up to 3 times a day, for motion sickness, take 1–2 hours before departure
▸ BY INTRAVENOUS INJECTION, OR BY INTRAMUSCULAR INJECTION
▸ Adult: 50 mg 3 times a day

Nausea and vomiting of known cause | Nausea and vomiting associated with vestibular disorders
▸ BY MOUTH, OR BY INTRAVENOUS INJECTION
▸ Child 1 month–5 years: 0.5–1 mg/kg up to 3 times a day (max. per dose 25 mg), intravenous injection to be given over 3–5 minutes, for motion sickness, take 1–2 hours before departure
▸ Child 6–11 years: 25 mg up to 3 times a day, intravenous injection to be given over 3–5 minutes, for motion sickness, take 1–2 hours before departure
▸ Child 12–17 years: 50 mg up to 3 times a day, intravenous injection to be given over 3–5 minutes, for motion sickness, take 1–2 hours before departure
▸ BY RECTUM
▸ Child 2–5 years: 12.5 mg up to 3 times a day
▸ Child 6–11 years: 25 mg up to 3 times a day
▸ Child 12–17 years: 50 mg up to 3 times a day
▸ BY CONTINUOUS INTRAVENOUS INFUSION, OR BY SUBCUTANEOUS INFUSION
▸ Child 1–23 months: 3 mg/kg, dose to be given over 24 hours
▸ Child 2–5 years: 50 mg, dose to be given over 24 hours
▸ Child 6–11 years: 75 mg, dose to be given over 24 hours
▸ Child 12–17 years: 150 mg, dose to be given over 24 hours

Nausea and vomiting in palliative care
▸ BY SUBCUTANEOUS INFUSION
▸ Child 1–23 months: 3 mg/kg, dose to be given over 24 hours
▸ Child 2–5 years: 50 mg, dose to be given over 24 hours
▸ Child 6–11 years: 75 mg, dose to be given over 24 hours
▸ Child 12–17 years: 150 mg, dose to be given over 24 hours
▸ Adult: 150 mg, dose to be given over 24 hours
▸ BY MOUTH
▸ Child 1 month–5 years: 0.5–1 mg/kg up to 3 times a day (max. per dose 25 mg)
▸ Child 6–11 years: 25 mg up to 3 times a day
▸ Child 12–17 years: 50 mg up to 3 times a day
▸ Adult: 50 mg up to 3 times a day
▸ BY INTRAVENOUS INJECTION
▸ Child 1 month–5 years: 0.5–1 mg/kg up to 3 times a day (max. per dose 25 mg), intravenous injection to be given over 3–5 minutes
▸ Child 6–11 years: 25 mg up to 3 times a day, intravenous injection to be given over 3–5 minutes
▸ Child 12–17 years: 50 mg up to 3 times a day, intravenous injection to be given over 3–5 minutes
▸ BY CONTINUOUS INTRAVENOUS INFUSION
▸ Child 1–23 months: 3 mg/kg, dose to be given over 24 hours
▸ Child 2–5 years: 50 mg, dose to be given over 24 hours
▸ Child 6–11 years: 75 mg, dose to be given over 24 hours
▸ Child 12–17 years: 150 mg, dose to be given over 24 hours
▸ BY RECTUM
▸ Child 2–5 years: 12.5 mg up to 3 times a day
▸ Child 6–11 years: 25 mg up to 3 times a day
▸ Child 12–17 years: 50 mg up to 3 times a day

● UNLICENSED USE
▸ In children Tablets not licensed for use in children under 6 years. Injection not licensed for use in children.

● CAUTIONS Epilepsy · glaucoma (in children) · may counteract haemodynamic benefits of opioids · neuromuscular disorders—increased risk of transient paralysis with intravenous use · prostatic hypertrophy (in adults) · pyloroduodenal obstruction · severe heart failure—may cause fall in cardiac output and associated increase in heart rate, mean arterial pressure and pulmonary wedge pressure · susceptibility to angle-closure glaucoma (in adults) · urinary retention

● INTERACTIONS → Appendix 1: antihistamines, sedating

● SIDE-EFFECTS

GENERAL SIDE-EFFECTS
▸ **Rare or very rare** Agitation (more common at high doses) · angle closure glaucoma · depression
▸ **Frequency not known** Abdominal pain · agranulocytosis · angioedema · anxiety · apnoea · appetite decreased · arrhythmias · asthenia · bronchospasm · constipation · diarrhoea · disorientation · dizziness · drowsiness · dry mouth · dry throat · euphoric mood · haemolytic anaemia · hallucinations · headache · hepatic disorders · hypertension · hypotension · increased gastric reflux · insomnia · leucopenia · movement disorders · muscle complaints · nasal dryness · nausea · oculogyric crisis · palpitations · paraesthesia · photosensitivity reaction · seizure · skin reactions · speech disorder · thrombocytopenia · tinnitus · tremor · urinary retention · vision blurred · vomiting

SPECIFIC SIDE-EFFECTS
▸ With oral use Level of consciousness decreased
▸ With parenteral use Chills · consciousness impaired · injection site necrosis · pain · paralysis · sensation of pressure · thrombophlebitis

4

Nervous system

4

Nervous system

- PREGNANCY Manufacturer advises avoid; however, there is no evidence of teratogenicity. The use of sedating antihistamines in the latter part of the third trimester may cause adverse effects in neonates such as irritability, paradoxical excitability, and tremor.
- BREAST FEEDING No information available. Most antihistamines are present in breast milk in varying amounts; although not known to be harmful, most manufacturers advise avoiding their use in mothers who are breast-feeding.
- HEPATIC IMPAIRMENT Manufacturer advises caution.
- DIRECTIONS FOR ADMINISTRATION For administration *by mouth*, tablets may be crushed.
  Mixing and compatibility for the use of syringe drivers in palliative care Cyclizine may precipitate at concentrations above 10 mg/mL or in the presence of sodium chloride 0.9% *or* as the concentration of diamorphine relative to cyclizine increases; mixtures of diamorphine and cyclizine are also likely to precipitate after 24 hours.
- PRESCRIBING AND DISPENSING INFORMATION
  Palliative care For further information on the use of cyclizine in palliative care, see www.medicinescomplete. com/#/content/palliative/antihistaminic-antimuscarinic-anti-emetics.
- PATIENT AND CARER ADVICE
  Driving and skilled tasks Drowsiness may affect performance of skilled tasks (e.g. cycling, driving); effects of alcohol enhanced.

- MEDICINAL FORMS There can be variation in the licensing of different medicines containing the same drug. Forms available from special-order manufacturers include: oral suspension, oral solution, suppository
  Tablet
  CAUTIONARY AND ADVISORY LABELS 2
  ▸ Cyclizine (Non-proprietary)
  Cyclizine hydrochloride 50 mg Cyclizine 50mg tablets | 30 tablet P £2.24–£5.00 | 100 tablet P £9.27 DT = £7.46
  Solution for injection
  ▸ Cyclizine (Non-proprietary)
  Cyclizine lactate 50 mg per 1 ml Cyclizine 50mg/1ml solution for injection ampoules | 5 ampoule PoM £18.75 DT = £18.75 | 10 ampoule PoM £25.00–£37.50

Doxylamine with pyridoxine

13-Aug-2020

- DRUG ACTION Doxylamine is a first-generation antihistamine which selectively binds H_1 receptors in the brain; pyridoxine (vitamin B_6) is a water-soluble vitamin.

- INDICATIONS AND DOSE
  Nausea and vomiting in pregnancy
  ▸ BY MOUTH
  ▸ Adult: 20/20 mg once daily for 2 days, to be taken at bedtime; increased if necessary to 10/10 mg, to be taken in the morning and 20/20 mg, to be taken at bedtime; increased if necessary to 10/10 mg, to be taken in the morning, 10/10 mg, to be taken mid-afternoon and 20/20 mg, to be taken at bedtime; maximum 40/40 mg per day
  DOSE EQUIVALENCE AND CONVERSION
  ▸ Dose expressed as *x/y* mg of doxylamine/pyridoxine.

- CAUTIONS Asthma · bladder neck obstruction · increased intra-ocular pressure · narrow angle glaucoma · pyloroduodenal obstruction · stenosing peptic ulcer
- INTERACTIONS → Appendix 1: antihistamines, sedating
- SIDE-EFFECTS
  ▸ **Common or very common** Dizziness · drowsiness · dry mouth · fatigue

- ▸ **Frequency not known** Akathisia · anxiety · chest discomfort · constipation · diarrhoea · disorientation · dyspnoea · gastrointestinal discomfort · headaches · hyperhidrosis · irritability · malaise · palpitations · paraesthesia · skin reactions · sleep disorders · tachycardia · urinary disorders · vertigo · vision disorders
- PATIENT AND CARER ADVICE
  Driving and skilled tasks Manufacturer advises patients and carers should be counselled on the effects on driving and performance of skilled tasks—increased risk of somnolence and dizziness.
- NATIONAL FUNDING/ACCESS DECISIONS
  For full details see funding body website
  Scottish Medicines Consortium (SMC) decisions
  ▸ Doxylamine succinate and pyridoxine hydrochloride (*Xonvea*®) for the treatment of nausea and vomiting of pregnancy in women who do not respond to conservative management (May 2019) SMC No. SMC2140 Not recommended
  All Wales Medicines Strategy Group (AWMSG) decisions
  ▸ Doxylamine succinate/pyridoxine hydrochloride (*Xonvea*®) for the treatment of nausea and vomiting of pregnancy in those patients who do not respond to conservative management (June 2019) AWMSG No. 2170 Not recommended

- MEDICINAL FORMS There can be variation in the licensing of different medicines containing the same drug.
  Gastro-resistant tablet
  CAUTIONARY AND ADVISORY LABELS 2, 23, 25
  ▸ Xonvea (Alliance Pharmaceuticals Ltd)
  Doxylamine succinate 10 mg, Pyridoxine hydrochloride 10 mg Xonvea 10mg/10mg gastro-resistant tablets | 20 tablet PoM £28.50 DT = £28.50

ANTIEMETICS AND ANTINAUSEANTS ›
CANNABINOIDS

Nabilone

21-Jan-2020

- INDICATIONS AND DOSE
  Nausea and vomiting caused by cytotoxic chemotherapy, unresponsive to conventional antiemetics (preferably in hospital setting) (under close medical supervision)
  ▸ BY MOUTH
  ▸ Adult: Initially 1 mg twice daily, increased if necessary to 2 mg twice daily throughout each cycle of cytotoxic therapy and, if necessary, for 48 hours after the last dose of each cycle, the first dose should be taken the night before initiation of cytotoxic treatment and the second dose 1–3 hours before the first dose of cytotoxic drug, daily dose maximum should be given in 3 divided doses; maximum 6 mg per day

- CAUTIONS Adverse effects on mental state can persist for 48–72 hours after stopping · elderly · heart disease · history of psychiatric disorder · hypertension
- INTERACTIONS → Appendix 1: nabilone
- SIDE-EFFECTS Abdominal pain · appetite decreased · concentration impaired · confusion · depression · dizziness · drowsiness · drug use disorders · dry mouth · euphoric mood · feeling of relaxation · hallucination · headache · hypotension · movement disorders · nausea · psychosis · sleep disorder · tachycardia · tremor · vertigo · visual impairment
  SIDE-EFFECTS, FURTHER INFORMATION Drowsiness and dizziness occur frequently with standard doses.
- PREGNANCY Avoid unless essential.
- BREAST FEEDING Avoid—no information available.
- HEPATIC IMPAIRMENT Manufacturer advises avoid in severe impairment (primarily biliary excretion).

● PATIENT AND CARER ADVICE
Behavioural effects Patients should be made aware of possible changes of mood and other adverse behavioural effects.
Driving and skilled tasks Drowsiness may affect performance of skilled tasks (e.g. driving).
　Effects of alcohol enhanced.
For information on 2015 legislation regarding driving whilst taking certain controlled drugs, including nabilone, see *Drugs and driving* under Guidance on prescribing p. 1.

● MEDICINAL FORMS There can be variation in the licensing of different medicines containing the same drug. Forms available from special-order manufacturers include: capsule
Capsule
CAUTIONARY AND ADVISORY LABELS 2
▸ Nabilone (Non-proprietary)
　Nabilone 250 microgram Nabilone 250microgram capsules |
　20 capsule PoM £150.00 DT = £150.00 CD2
　Nabilone 1 mg Nabilone 1mg capsules | 20 capsule PoM £196.00
　DT = £196.00 CD2

ANTIEMETICS AND ANTINAUSEANTS 〉
DOPAMINE RECEPTOR ANTAGONISTS

Domperidone
06-Nov-2020

● INDICATIONS AND DOSE
Relief of nausea and vomiting
▸ BY MOUTH
▸ Child 12–17 years (body-weight 35 kg and above): 10 mg up to 3 times a day for a usual maximum of 1 week; maximum 30 mg per day
▸ Adult (body-weight 35 kg and above): 10 mg up to 3 times a day for a usual maximum of 1 week; maximum 30 mg per day

Gastro-intestinal pain in palliative care
▸ BY MOUTH
▸ Adult: 10 mg 3 times a day, before meals

IMPORTANT SAFETY INFORMATION
MHRA/CHM ADVICE (UPDATED DECEMBER 2019): DOMPERIDONE FOR NAUSEA AND VOMITING: LACK OF EFFICACY IN CHILDREN; REMINDER OF CONTRA-INDICATIONS IN ADULTS AND ADOLESCENTS
Domperidone is no longer indicated for the relief of nausea and vomiting in children aged under 12 years or those weighing less than 35 kg. A European review concluded that domperidone is not as effective in this population as previously thought and alternative treatments should be considered. Healthcare professionals are advised to adhere to the licensed dose and to use the lowest effective dose for the shortest possible duration (max. treatment duration should not usually exceed 1 week).
　Healthcare professionals are also reminded of the existing contra-indications for use of domperidone (see *Contra-indications, Hepatic impairment,* and *Interactions*).

● CONTRA-INDICATIONS Cardiac disease · conditions where cardiac conduction is, or could be, impaired · gastro-intestinal haemorrhage · gastro-intestinal mechanical obstruction · gastro-intestinal mechanical perforation · if increased gastro-intestinal motility harmful · prolactinoma
● CAUTIONS Patients over 60 years—increased risk of ventricular arrhythmia
● INTERACTIONS → Appendix 1: domperidone
● SIDE-EFFECTS
▸ **Common or very common** Dry mouth
▸ **Uncommon** Anxiety · asthenia · breast abnormalities · diarrhoea · drowsiness · headache · lactation disorders · libido loss

▸ **Frequency not known** Arrhythmias · depression · gynaecomastia · menstrual cycle irregularities · movement disorders · oculogyric crisis · QT interval prolongation · seizure · sudden cardiac death · urinary retention
● PREGNANCY Use only if potential benefit outweighs risk.
● BREAST FEEDING Amount too small to be harmful.
● HEPATIC IMPAIRMENT Manufacturer advises avoid in moderate to severe impairment.
● RENAL IMPAIRMENT
Dose adjustments Reduce frequency.
● PRESCRIBING AND DISPENSING INFORMATION
Palliative care For further information on the use of domperidone in palliative care, see www.medicinescomplete.com/#/content/palliative/domperidone.
● PATIENT AND CARER ADVICE
Arrhythmia Patients and their carers should be told how to recognise signs of arrhythmia and advised to seek medical attention if symptoms such as palpitation or syncope develop.

● MEDICINAL FORMS There can be variation in the licensing of different medicines containing the same drug. Forms available from special-order manufacturers include: oral suspension
Oral suspension
CAUTIONARY AND ADVISORY LABELS 22
▸ Domperidone (Non-proprietary)
　Domperidone 1 mg per 1 ml Domperidone 1mg/ml oral suspension sugar free sugar-free | 200 ml PoM £24.85 DT = £24.85
Tablet
CAUTIONARY AND ADVISORY LABELS 22
▸ Domperidone (Non-proprietary)
　Domperidone (as Domperidone maleate) 10 mg Domperidone 10mg tablets | 30 tablet PoM £2.71 DT = £0.95 | 100 tablet PoM £9.04 DT = £3.17
▸ Motilium (Zentiva)
　Domperidone (as Domperidone maleate) 10 mg Motilium 10mg tablets | 30 tablet PoM £2.71 DT = £0.95 | 100 tablet PoM £9.04 DT = £3.17

Metoclopramide hydrochloride
12-Aug-2020

● INDICATIONS AND DOSE
Symptomatic treatment of nausea and vomiting including that associated with acute migraine | Delayed (but not acute) chemotherapy-induced nausea and vomiting | Radiotherapy-induced nausea and vomiting | Prevention of postoperative nausea and vomiting
▸ BY MOUTH, OR BY INTRAMUSCULAR INJECTION, OR BY SLOW INTRAVENOUS INJECTION
▸ Adult (body-weight up to 60 kg): Up to 500 micrograms/kg daily in 3 divided doses, when administered by slow intravenous injection, to be given over at least 3 minutes
▸ Adult (body-weight 60 kg and above): 10 mg up to 3 times a day, when administered by slow intravenous injection, to be given over at least 3 minutes
Hiccup in palliative care
▸ BY MOUTH, OR BY INTRAMUSCULAR INJECTION, OR BY SUBCUTANEOUS INJECTION
▸ Adult: 10 mg every 6–8 hours
Nausea and vomiting in palliative care
▸ BY MOUTH
▸ Adult: 10 mg 3 times a day
▸ BY SUBCUTANEOUS INFUSION
▸ Adult: 30–100 mg/24 hours
Acute migraine
▸ BY MOUTH, OR BY SLOW INTRAVENOUS INJECTION, OR BY INTRAMUSCULAR INJECTION
▸ Adult: 10 mg for 1 dose, to be administered as soon as migraine symptoms develop; intravenous injection to be given over at least 3 minutes

- UNLICENSED USE EvGr Metoclopramide is used for the treatment of acute migraine, Ⓐ but is not licensed for this indication.

IMPORTANT SAFETY INFORMATION

MHRA/CHM ADVICE—METOCLOPRAMIDE: RISK OF NEUROLOGICAL ADVERSE EFFECTS—RESTRICTED DOSE AND DURATION OF USE (AUGUST 2013)

The benefits and risks of metoclopramide have been reviewed by the European Medicines Agency's Committee on Medicinal Products for Human Use, which concluded that the risk of neurological effects such as extrapyramidal disorders and tardive dyskinesia outweigh the benefits in long-term or high-dose treatment. To help minimise the risk of potentially serious neurological adverse effects, the following restrictions to indications, dose, and duration of use have been made:

- In adults over 18 years, metoclopramide should only be used for prevention of postoperative nausea and vomiting, radiotherapy-induced nausea and vomiting, delayed (but not acute) chemotherapy-induced nausea and vomiting, and symptomatic treatment of nausea and vomiting, including that associated with acute migraine (where it may also be used to improve absorption of oral analgesics);
- Metoclopramide should only be prescribed for short-term use (up to 5 days);
- Usual dose is 10 mg, repeated up to 3 times daily; max. daily dose is 500 micrograms/kg;
- Intravenous doses should be administered as a slow bolus over at least 3 minutes;
- Oral liquid formulations should be given via an appropriately designed, graduated oral syringe to ensure dose accuracy.

This advice does not apply to unlicensed uses of metoclopramide (e.g. palliative care).

- CONTRA-INDICATIONS 3–4 days after gastrointestinal surgery · epilepsy · gastro-intestinal haemorrhage · gastro-intestinal obstruction · gastro-intestinal perforation · phaeochromocytoma
- CAUTIONS Asthma · atopic allergy · bradycardia · cardiac conduction disturbances · children · elderly · may mask underlying disorders such as cerebral irritation · Parkinson's disease · uncorrected electrolyte imbalance · young adults

  CAUTIONS, FURTHER INFORMATION
  ▸ Elderly Prescription potentially inappropriate (STOPP criteria) in patients with parkinsonism (risk of exacerbating parkinsonian symptoms). See also Prescribing in the elderly p. 33.

- INTERACTIONS → Appendix 1: metoclopramide
- SIDE-EFFECTS

  GENERAL SIDE-EFFECTS
  ▸ **Common or very common** Asthenia · depression · diarrhoea · drowsiness · hypotension · menstrual cycle irregularities · movement disorders · parkinsonism
  ▸ **Uncommon** Arrhythmias · hallucination · hyperprolactinaemia · level of consciousness decreased
  ▸ **Rare or very rare** Confusion · galactorrhoea · seizure
  ▸ **Frequency not known** Atrioventricular block · blood disorders · cardiac arrest · gynaecomastia · hypertension · neuroleptic malignant syndrome · QT interval prolongation · shock · syncope · tremor

  SPECIFIC SIDE-EFFECTS
  ▸ With parenteral use Anxiety · dizziness · dyspnoea · oedema · skin reactions · visual impairment

  SIDE-EFFECTS, FURTHER INFORMATION Metoclopramide can induce acute dystonic reactions involving facial and skeletal muscle spasms and oculogyric crises. These

dystonic effects are more common in the young (especially girls and young women) and the very old; they usually occur shortly after starting treatment with metoclopramide and subside within 24 hours of stopping it. Injection of an antiparkinsonian drug such as procyclidine will abort dystonic attacks.

- PREGNANCY Not known to be harmful.
- BREAST FEEDING Small amount present in milk; avoid.
- HEPATIC IMPAIRMENT Manufacturer advises caution in severe impairment (risk of accumulation).

  Dose adjustments Manufacturer advises dose reduction of 50% in severe impairment.

- RENAL IMPAIRMENT

  Dose adjustments Avoid or use small dose in severe impairment; increased risk of extrapyramidal reactions.

- DIRECTIONS FOR ADMINISTRATION Manufacturer advises oral liquid preparation to be given via a graduated oral dosing syringe.
- PRESCRIBING AND DISPENSING INFORMATION

  Palliative care For further information on the use of metoclopramide hydrochloride in palliative care, see www.medicinescomplete.com/#/content/palliative/metoclopramide.

- PATIENT AND CARER ADVICE Counselling on use of pipette advised with oral solution.

- MEDICINAL FORMS There can be variation in the licensing of different medicines containing the same drug. Forms available from special-order manufacturers include: oral solution

  Solution for injection
  ▸ Metoclopramide hydrochloride (Non-proprietary)
  Metoclopramide hydrochloride 5 mg per 1 ml Metoclopramide 10mg/2ml solution for injection ampoules | 5 ampoule PoM £1.31–£15.00 | 10 ampoule PoM £25.00 DT = £2.88 | 10 ampoule PoM £3.80 DT = £2.88 (Hospital only)
  ▸ Maxolon (Advanz Pharma)
  Metoclopramide hydrochloride 5 mg per 1 ml Maxolon High Dose 100mg/20ml solution for injection ampoules | 10 ampoule PoM £26.68

  Oral solution
  ▸ Metoclopramide hydrochloride (Non-proprietary)
  Metoclopramide hydrochloride 1 mg per 1 ml Metoclopramide 5mg/5ml oral solution sugar free sugar-free | 150 ml PoM £19.79 DT = £19.79

  Tablet
  ▸ Metoclopramide hydrochloride (Non-proprietary)
  Metoclopramide hydrochloride 10 mg Metoclopramide 10mg tablets | 28 tablet PoM £2.04 DT = £1.33
  ▸ Maxolon (Advanz Pharma)
  Metoclopramide hydrochloride 10 mg Maxolon 10mg tablets | 84 tablet PoM £5.24

  Combinations available: *Paracetamol with metoclopramide,* p. 496

ANTIEMETICS AND ANTINAUSEANTS >
NEUROKININ RECEPTOR ANTAGONISTS

Aprepitant

11-Sep-2018

- INDICATIONS AND DOSE

  Adjunct treatment to prevent nausea and vomiting associated with moderately and highly emetogenic chemotherapy
  ▸ BY MOUTH
  ▸ Adult: Initially 125 mg, dose to be taken 1 hour before chemotherapy, then 80 mg once daily for 2 days, consult product literature for dose of concomitant dexamethasone and 5HT$_3$-antagonist

- CONTRA-INDICATIONS Acute porphyrias p. 1107
- INTERACTIONS → Appendix 1: neurokinin-1 receptor antagonists

- SIDE-EFFECTS
- ▶ **Common or very common** Appetite decreased · asthenia · constipation · gastrointestinal discomfort · headache · hiccups
- ▶ **Uncommon** Anaemia · anxiety · burping · dizziness · drowsiness · dry mouth · febrile neutropenia · gastrointestinal disorders · hot flush · malaise · nausea · palpitations · skin reactions · urinary disorders · vomiting
- ▶ **Rare or very rare** Bradycardia · cardiovascular disorder · chest discomfort · cognitive disorder · conjunctivitis · cough · disorientation · euphoric mood · gait abnormal · hyperhidrosis · increased risk of infection · muscle spasms · muscle weakness · oedema · oropharyngeal pain · photosensitivity reaction · polydipsia · seborrhoea · severe cutaneous adverse reactions (SCARs) · sneezing · stomatitis · taste altered · throat irritation · tinnitus · weight decreased
- ▶ **Frequency not known** Dysarthria · dyspnoea · insomnia · miosis · sensation abnormal · visual acuity decreased · wheezing
- CONCEPTION AND CONTRACEPTION Manufacturer advises effectiveness of hormonal contraceptives may be reduced—alternative non-hormonal methods of contraception necessary during treatment and for 2 months after stopping aprepitant.
- PREGNANCY Manufacturer advises avoid unless clearly necessary—no information available.
- BREAST FEEDING Manufacturer advises avoid—present in milk in *animal* studies.
- HEPATIC IMPAIRMENT Manufacturer advises caution in moderate to severe impairment—limited information available.

- MEDICINAL FORMS There can be variation in the licensing of different medicines containing the same drug. Forms available from special-order manufacturers include: oral suspension

Capsule
- ▶ Aprepitant (Non-proprietary)
  Aprepitant 80 mg Aprepitant 80mg capsules | 2 capsule `PoM` £26.87-£31.61 DT = £31.61 | 2 capsule `PoM` £31.61 DT = £31.61 (Hospital only)
  Aprepitant 125 mg Aprepitant 125mg capsules | 5 capsule `PoM` £67.18-£79.03 DT = £79.03 | 5 capsule `PoM` £79.03 DT = £79.03 (Hospital only)
- ▶ Emend (Merck Sharp & Dohme Ltd)
  Aprepitant 80 mg Emend 80mg capsules | 2 capsule `PoM` £31.61 DT = £31.61
  Aprepitant 125 mg Emend 125mg capsules | 5 capsule `PoM` £79.03 DT = £79.03

Fosaprepitant
02-Nov-2020

- DRUG ACTION Fosaprepitant is a prodrug of aprepitant.

- INDICATIONS AND DOSE

Adjunct to dexamethasone and a 5HT$_3$-receptor antagonist in preventing nausea and vomiting associated with moderately and highly emetogenic chemotherapy
- ▶ BY INTRAVENOUS INFUSION
- ▶ Adult: 150 mg, dose to be administered over 20–30 minutes and given 30 minutes before chemotherapy on day 1 of cycle only, consult product literature for dose of concomitant corticosteroid and 5HT$_3$-receptor antagonist

- CONTRA-INDICATIONS Acute porphyrias p. 1107
- INTERACTIONS → Appendix 1: neurokinin-1 receptor antagonists
- SIDE-EFFECTS
- ▶ **Common or very common** Appetite decreased · asthenia · constipation · gastrointestinal discomfort · headache · hiccups

- ▶ **Uncommon** Anaemia · anxiety · burping · dizziness · drowsiness · dry mouth · febrile neutropenia · flushing · gastrointestinal disorders · malaise · nausea · palpitations · skin reactions · thrombophlebitis · urinary disorders · vomiting
- ▶ **Rare or very rare** Bradycardia · cardiovascular disorder · chest discomfort · cognitive disorder · conjunctivitis · cough · disorientation · euphoric mood · gait abnormal · hyperhidrosis · increased risk of infection · muscle spasms · muscle weakness · oedema · oropharyngeal pain · photosensitivity reaction · polydipsia · seborrhoea · severe cutaneous adverse reactions (SCARs) · sneezing · stomatitis · taste altered · throat irritation · tinnitus · weight decreased
- ▶ **Frequency not known** Dysarthria · dyspnoea · insomnia · miosis · sensation abnormal · visual acuity decreased · wheezing
- CONCEPTION AND CONTRACEPTION Effectiveness of hormonal contraceptives reduced—effective non-hormonal methods of contraception necessary during treatment and for 2 months after stopping fosaprepitant.
- PREGNANCY Avoid unless potential benefit outweighs risk—no information available.
- BREAST FEEDING Avoid—present in milk in *animal* studies.
- HEPATIC IMPAIRMENT Manufacturer advises caution in moderate to severe impairment—limited information available.
- DIRECTIONS FOR ADMINISTRATION For *intravenous infusion* (*Ivemend®*), manufacturer advises give intermittently *in* Sodium chloride 0.9%; reconstitute each 150 mg vial with 5 mL sodium chloride 0.9% gently without shaking to avoid foaming, then dilute in 145 mL infusion fluid; give over 20–30 minutes.
- NATIONAL FUNDING/ACCESS DECISIONS
  For full details see funding body website
  Scottish Medicines Consortium (SMC) decisions
- ▶ **Fosaprepitant (*Ivemend®*) for the prevention of acute and delayed nausea and vomiting associated with highly emetogenic cisplatin based cancer chemotherapy in adults (March 2011) SMC No. 678/11 Recommended**

- MEDICINAL FORMS There can be variation in the licensing of different medicines containing the same drug.
  Powder for solution for infusion
- ▶ Ivemend (Merck Sharp & Dohme Ltd)
  Fosaprepitant (as Fosaprepitant dimeglumine) 150 mg Ivemend 150mg powder for solution for infusion vials | 1 vial `PoM` £47.42

ANTIEMETICS AND ANTINAUSEANTS ⟩
SEROTONIN (5HT3) RECEPTOR ANTAGONISTS

Granisetron
16-Jul-2020

- DRUG ACTION Granisetron is a specific 5HT$_3$-receptor antagonist which blocks 5HT$_3$ receptors in the gastro-intestinal tract and in the CNS.

- INDICATIONS AND DOSE

Nausea and vomiting induced by cytotoxic chemotherapy for planned duration of 3–5 days where oral antiemetics cannot be used
- ▶ BY TRANSDERMAL APPLICATION USING PATCHES
- ▶ Adult: Apply 3.1 mg/24 hours, apply patch to clean, dry, non-irritated, non-hairy skin on upper arm (or abdomen if upper arm cannot be used) 24–48 hours before treatment, patch may be worn for up to 7 days; remove at least 24 hours after completing chemotherapy

continued →

Prevention of postoperative nausea and vomiting
▸ BY INTRAVENOUS INJECTION
▸ Adult: 1 mg, to be administered before induction of anaesthesia, dose to be diluted to 5 mL and given over 30 seconds

Treatment of postoperative nausea and vomiting
▸ BY INTRAVENOUS INJECTION
▸ Adult: 1 mg, dose to be diluted to 5 mL and given over 30 seconds; maximum 3 mg per day

Management of nausea and vomiting induced by cytotoxic chemotherapy or radiotherapy
▸ BY MOUTH
▸ Adult: 1–2 mg, to be taken within 1 hour before start of treatment, then 2 mg daily in 1–2 divided doses for up to 1 week following treatment, when intravenous route also used, maximum combined total dose 9 mg in 24 hours
▸ BY INTRAVENOUS INJECTION, OR BY INTRAVENOUS INFUSION
▸ Adult: 10–40 micrograms/kg (max. per dose 3 mg), to be given 5 minutes before start of treatment, dose may be repeated if necessary, further maintenance doses must not be given less than 10 minutes apart, for intravenous injection, each 1 mg granisetron diluted to 5 mL and given over not less than 30 seconds, for intravenous infusion, to be given over 5 minutes; maximum 9 mg per day

● CAUTIONS Subacute intestinal obstruction · susceptibility to QT-interval prolongation (including electrolyte disturbances)

● INTERACTIONS → Appendix 1: 5-HT3-receptor antagonists

● SIDE-EFFECTS
GENERAL SIDE-EFFECTS
▸ **Common or very common** Constipation · headache
SPECIFIC SIDE-EFFECTS
▸ **Common or very common**
▸ With intravenous or oral use Diarrhoea · insomnia
▸ **Uncommon**
▸ With intravenous or oral use Extrapyramidal symptoms · QT interval prolongation · serotonin syndrome
▸ With transdermal use Appetite decreased · arthralgia · dry mouth · flushing · generalised oedema · vertigo
▸ **Rare or very rare**
▸ With transdermal use Dystonia

● PREGNANCY Manufacturer advises avoid.

● BREAST FEEDING Avoid—no information available.

● HEPATIC IMPAIRMENT Manufacturer advises caution.

● DIRECTIONS FOR ADMINISTRATION
▸ With intravenous use For *intravenous infusion*, manufacturer advises give intermittently in Glucose 5% or Sodium Chloride 0.9%; dilute up to 3 mL in 20–50 mL infusion fluid; give over 5 minutes.

● PATIENT AND CARER ADVICE
▸ With transdermal use Patients should be advised not to expose the site of the patch to sunlight during use and for 10 days after removal.

● MEDICINAL FORMS There can be variation in the licensing of different medicines containing the same drug.
Solution for injection
▸ Granisetron (Non-proprietary)
Granisetron (as Granisetron hydrochloride) 1 mg per 1 ml Granisetron 3mg/3ml concentrate for solution for injection ampoules | 10 ampoule [PoM] £60.00
Granisetron 1mg/1ml concentrate for solution for injection ampoules | 5 ampoule [PoM] £10.00 | 10 ampoule [PoM] £20.00
Tablet
▸ Granisetron (Non-proprietary)
Granisetron (as Granisetron hydrochloride) 1 mg Granisetron 1mg tablets | 10 tablet [PoM] £52.39 DT = £40.80

Granisetron (as Granisetron hydrochloride) 2 mg Granisetron 2mg tablets | 5 tablet [PoM] [℥] DT = £52.39
▸ Kytril (Atnahs Pharma UK Ltd)
Granisetron (as Granisetron hydrochloride) 1 mg Kytril 1mg tablets | 10 tablet [PoM] £52.39 DT = £40.80
Granisetron (as Granisetron hydrochloride) 2 mg Kytril 2mg tablets | 5 tablet [PoM] £52.39 DT = £52.39
Transdermal patch
▸ Sancuso (Kyowa Kirin Ltd)
Granisetron 3.1 mg per 24 hour Sancuso 3.1mg/24hours transdermal patches | 1 patch [PoM] £56.00 DT = £56.00

Ondansetron

04-Dec-2020

● DRUG ACTION Ondansetron is a specific 5HT$_3$-receptor antagonist which blocks 5HT$_3$ receptors in the gastro-intestinal tract and in the CNS.

● INDICATIONS AND DOSE
Moderately emetogenic chemotherapy or radiotherapy
▸ BY MOUTH
▸ Adult: Initially 8 mg, dose to be taken 1–2 hours before treatment, then 8 mg every 12 hours for up to 5 days
▸ BY RECTUM
▸ Adult: Initially 16 mg, dose to be taken 1–2 hours before treatment, then 16 mg daily for up to 5 days
▸ INITIALLY BY INTRAMUSCULAR INJECTION, OR BY SLOW INTRAVENOUS INJECTION
▸ Adult: Initially 8 mg, dose to be administered immediately before treatment, then (by mouth) 8 mg every 12 hours for up to 5 days, alternatively (by rectum) 16 mg daily for up to 5 days
▸ INITIALLY BY INTRAMUSCULAR INJECTION, OR BY INTRAVENOUS INFUSION
▸ Elderly: Initially 8 mg, dose to be administered immediately before treatment, intravenous infusion to be given over at least 15 minutes, then (by mouth) 8 mg every 12 hours for up to 5 days, alternatively (by rectum) 16 mg daily for up to 5 days

Severely emetogenic chemotherapy (consult product literature for dose of concomitant corticosteroid)
▸ BY MOUTH
▸ Adult: 24 mg, dose to be taken 1–2 hours before treatment, then 8 mg every 12 hours for up to 5 days
▸ BY RECTUM
▸ Adult: 16 mg, dose to be administered 1–2 hours before treatment, then 16 mg daily for up to 5 days
▸ INITIALLY BY INTRAMUSCULAR INJECTION, OR BY SLOW INTRAVENOUS INJECTION
▸ Adult: Initially 8 mg, dose to be administered immediately before treatment, followed by (by intramuscular injection or by slow intravenous injection) 8 mg every 4 hours if required for 2 doses, alternatively, followed by (by continuous intravenous infusion) 1 mg/hour for up to 24 hours, then (by mouth) 8 mg every 12 hours for up to 5 days, alternatively (by rectum) 16 mg daily for up to 5 days
▸ INITIALLY BY INTRAMUSCULAR INJECTION
▸ Adult 65-74 years: Initially 8 mg, to be given immediately before treatment, followed by (by intramuscular injection) 8 mg every 4 hours if required for 2 doses, alternatively, followed by (by continuous intravenous infusion) 1 mg/hour for up to 24 hours, then (by mouth) 8 mg every 12 hours for up to 5 days, alternatively (by rectum) 16 mg daily for up to 5 days
▸ INITIALLY BY INTRAVENOUS INFUSION
▸ Adult: Initially 16 mg, immediately before treatment (over at least 15 minutes), followed by (by intramuscular injection or by slow intravenous injection) 8 mg every 4 hours if required for 2 doses, then (by mouth) 8 mg every 12 hours for up to 5 days, alternatively (by rectum) 16 mg daily for up to 5 days

▸ **Adult 65-74 years:** Initially 8–16 mg, immediately before treatment (over at least 15 minutes), followed by (by intramuscular injection or by intravenous infusion) 8 mg every 4 hours if required for 2 doses, then (by mouth) 8 mg every 12 hours for up to 5 days, alternatively (by rectum) 16 mg daily for up to 5 days

▸ **Adult 75 years and over:** Initially 8 mg, immediately before treatment (over at least 15 minutes), followed by (by intravenous infusion) 8 mg every 4 hours if required for 2 doses, then (by mouth) 8 mg every 12 hours for up to 5 days, alternatively (by rectum) 16 mg daily for up to 5 days

Prevention of postoperative nausea and vomiting
▸ INITIALLY BY MOUTH
▸ **Adult:** 16 mg, dose to be taken 1 hour before anaesthesia, alternatively (by intramuscular injection or by slow intravenous injection) 4 mg, dose to be administered at induction of anaesthesia

Treatment of postoperative nausea and vomiting
▸ BY INTRAMUSCULAR INJECTION, OR BY SLOW INTRAVENOUS INJECTION
▸ **Adult:** 4 mg for 1 dose

IMPORTANT SAFETY INFORMATION

MHRA/CHM ADVICE: ONDANSETRON: SMALL INCREASED RISK OF ORAL CLEFTS FOLLOWING USE IN THE FIRST 12 WEEKS OF PREGNANCY (JANUARY 2020)

Epidemiological studies have identified a small increased risk of cleft lip and/or cleft palate in babies born to women who used oral ondansetron during the first trimester of pregnancy. Healthcare professionals are advised that if there is a clinical need for ondansetron in pregnancy, patients should be counselled on the potential benefits and risks, and the final decision made jointly.

● CONTRA-INDICATIONS Congenital long QT syndrome
● CAUTIONS Adenotonsillar surgery · subacute intestinal obstruction · susceptibility to QT-interval prolongation (including electrolyte disturbances)
● INTERACTIONS → Appendix 1: 5-HT3-receptor antagonists
● SIDE-EFFECTS
▸ **Common or very common** Constipation · feeling hot · headache · sensation abnormal
▸ **Uncommon** Arrhythmias · chest pain · hiccups · hypotension · movement disorders · oculogyric crisis · seizure
▸ **Rare or very rare** Dizziness · QT interval prolongation · vision disorders
● PREGNANCY Manufacturer advises avoid in first trimester—small increased risk of congenital abnormalities such as orofacial clefts, see *Important safety information*.
● BREAST FEEDING Present in milk in *animal* studies—avoid.
● HEPATIC IMPAIRMENT Manufacturer advises caution in moderate to severe impairment (decreased clearance). **Dose adjustments** Manufacturer advises maximum 8 mg daily in moderate to severe impairment.
● DIRECTIONS FOR ADMINISTRATION
▸ With intravenous use For *intravenous infusion (Zofran®)*, give continuously or intermittently in Glucose 5% or Glucose 5% with Potassium chloride 0.3% or Sodium chloride 0.9% or Sodium chloride 0.9% with Potassium chloride 0.3% or Mannitol 10% or Ringers solution; for intermittent infusion, dilute the required dose in 50–100 mL of infusion fluid and give over at least 15 minutes.
▸ With oral use Orodispersible films and lyophylisates should be placed on the tongue, allowed to disperse and swallowed.

● PRESCRIBING AND DISPENSING INFORMATION Flavours of oral liquid formulations may include strawberry.
● PATIENT AND CARER ADVICE Patients or carers should be given advice on how to administer orodispersible films and lyophilisates.

● MEDICINAL FORMS There can be variation in the licensing of different medicines containing the same drug. Forms available from special-order manufacturers include: oral suspension, oral solution

Tablet
▸ Ondansetron (Non-proprietary)
  Ondansetron (as Ondansetron hydrochloride) 4 mg Ondansetron 4mg tablets | 10 tablet PoM £30.57 DT = £1.24 | 30 tablet PoM £3.72–£107.91
  Ondansetron (as Ondansetron hydrochloride) 8 mg Ondansetron 8mg tablets | 10 tablet PoM £71.94 DT = £1.56
▸ Zofran (Novartis Pharmaceuticals UK Ltd)
  Ondansetron (as Ondansetron hydrochloride) 4 mg Zofran 4mg tablets | 30 tablet PoM £107.91
  Ondansetron (as Ondansetron hydrochloride) 8 mg Zofran 8mg tablets | 10 tablet PoM £71.94 DT = £1.56

Suppository
▸ Zofran (Novartis Pharmaceuticals UK Ltd)
  Ondansetron 16 mg Zofran 16mg suppositories | 1 suppository PoM £14.39 DT = £14.39

Solution for injection
▸ Ondansetron (Non-proprietary)
  Ondansetron (as Ondansetron hydrochloride) 2 mg per 1 ml Ondansetron 8mg/4ml solution for injection ampoules | 5 ampoule PoM £11.20–£56.95 DT = £59.95 (Hospital only) | 5 ampoule PoM £8.97–£58.45 DT = £59.95
  Ondansetron 4mg/2ml solution for injection ampoules | 5 ampoule PoM £5.40–£28.47 DT = £29.97 (Hospital only) | 5 ampoule PoM £5.80–£35.47 DT = £29.97 | 10 ampoule PoM £10.00–£15.00 DT = £15.00
▸ Zofran Flexi-amp (Novartis Pharmaceuticals UK Ltd)
  Ondansetron (as Ondansetron hydrochloride) 2 mg per 1 ml Zofran Flexi-amp 4mg/2ml solution for injection ampoules | 5 ampoule PoM £29.97 DT = £29.97
  Zofran Flexi-amp 8mg/4ml solution for injection ampoules | 5 ampoule PoM £59.95 DT = £59.95

Oral solution
▸ Ondansetron (Non-proprietary)
  Ondansetron (as Ondansetron hydrochloride) 800 microgram per 1 ml Ondansetron 4mg/5ml oral solution sugar free sugar-free | 50 ml PoM £39.88 DT = £39.62
▸ Zofran (Novartis Pharmaceuticals UK Ltd)
  Ondansetron (as Ondansetron hydrochloride) 800 microgram per 1 ml Zofran 4mg/5ml syrup sugar-free | 50 ml PoM £35.97 DT = £39.62

Orodispersible film
▸ Setofilm (Norgine Pharmaceuticals Ltd)
  Ondansetron 4 mg Setofilm 4mg orodispersible films sugar-free | 10 film PoM £28.50 DT = £28.50
  Ondansetron 8 mg Setofilm 8mg orodispersible films sugar-free | 10 film PoM £57.00 DT = £57.00

Oral lyophilisate
EXCIPIENTS: May contain Aspartame
▸ Zofran Melt (Novartis Pharmaceuticals UK Ltd)
  Ondansetron 4 mg Zofran Melt 4mg oral lyophilisates sugar-free | 10 tablet PoM £35.97 DT = £35.97
  Ondansetron 8 mg Zofran Melt 8mg oral lyophilisates sugar-free | 10 tablet PoM £71.94 DT = £71.94

Orodispersible tablet
▸ Ondansetron (Non-proprietary)
  Ondansetron 4 mg Ondansetron 4mg orodispersible tablets | 10 tablet PoM £43.48 DT = £43.48
  Ondansetron 8 mg Ondansetron 8mg orodispersible tablets | 10 tablet PoM £85.43 DT = £85.43

4

Nervous system

Palonosetron

22-Jan-2020

- DRUG ACTION Palonosetron is a specific 5HT$_3$-receptor antagonist which blocks 5HT$_3$ receptors in the gastro-intestinal tract and in the CNS.

  - ● INDICATIONS AND DOSE
  Moderately emetogenic chemotherapy
    ▸ INITIALLY BY MOUTH
    ▸ Adult: 500 micrograms, dose to be taken 1 hour before treatment, alternatively (by intravenous injection) 250 micrograms for 1 dose, to be administered over 30 seconds, 30 minutes before treatment
  Severely emetogenic chemotherapy
    ▸ BY INTRAVENOUS INJECTION
    ▸ Adult: 250 micrograms for 1 dose, dose to be administered over 30 seconds, 30 minutes before treatment

- ● CAUTIONS History of constipation · intestinal obstruction · susceptibility to QT-interval prolongation (including electrolyte disturbances)
- ● INTERACTIONS → Appendix 1: 5-HT3-receptor antagonists
- ● SIDE-EFFECTS
  GENERAL SIDE-EFFECTS
  ▸ **Common or very common** Constipation · headache
  SPECIFIC SIDE-EFFECTS
  ▸ **Common or very common**
  ▸ With intravenous use Diarrhoea · dizziness · electrolyte imbalance · metabolic disorder
  ▸ **Uncommon**
  ▸ With intravenous use Amblyopia · anxiety · appetite decreased · arrhythmias · arthralgia · asthenia · drowsiness · dry mouth · dyspepsia · euphoric mood · eye irritation · feeling hot · fever · flatulence · glycosuria · hiccups · hyperbilirubinaemia · hyperglycaemia · hypertension · hypotension · influenza like illness · motion sickness · myocardial ischaemia · paraesthesia · peripheral neuropathy · QT interval prolongation · skin reactions · sleep disorders · tinnitus · urinary retention · vasodilation · vein discolouration
  ▸ With oral use Atrioventricular block · dyspnoea · eye swelling · insomnia · myalgia
  ▸ **Rare or very rare**
  ▸ With intravenous use Shock
- ● PREGNANCY Avoid—no information available.
- ● BREAST FEEDING Avoid—no information available.
- ● PATIENT AND CARER ADVICE
  Driving and skilled tasks Dizziness or drowsiness may affect performance of skilled tasks (e.g. driving).

- ● MEDICINAL FORMS There can be variation in the licensing of different medicines containing the same drug.
  Solution for injection
    ▸ Palonosetron (Non-proprietary)
    Palonosetron (as Palonosetron hydrochloride) 50 microgram per 1 ml Palonosetron 250micrograms/5ml solution for injection vials | 1 vial [PoM] £53.10 (Hospital only) | 10 vial [PoM] £646.90
    ▸ Aloxi (Chugai Pharma UK Ltd)
    Palonosetron (as Palonosetron hydrochloride) 50 microgram per 1 ml Aloxi 250micrograms/5ml solution for injection vials | 1 vial [PoM] £55.89
  Capsule
    ▸ Aloxi (Chugai Pharma UK Ltd)
    Palonosetron (as Palonosetron hydrochloride) 500 microgram Aloxi 500microgram capsules | 1 capsule [PoM] £55.89

Palonosetron with netuptitant

12-Nov-2020

The properties listed below are those particular to the combination only. For the properties of the components please consider, palonosetron above.

- ● INDICATIONS AND DOSE
  Moderately emetogenic chemotherapy | Highly emetogenic cisplatin-based chemotherapy
    ▸ BY MOUTH
    ▸ Adult: 1 capsule, to be taken approximately 1 hour before the start of each chemotherapy cycle

- ● CAUTIONS Patients over 75 years
- ● INTERACTIONS → Appendix 1: 5-HT3-receptor antagonists · neurokinin-1 receptor antagonists
- ● SIDE-EFFECTS
  ▸ **Common or very common** Asthenia · constipation · headache
  ▸ **Uncommon** Alopecia · cardiac conduction disorders · cardiomyopathy · diarrhoea · dizziness · flatulence · gastrointestinal discomfort · hiccups · hypertension · increased leucocytes · neutropenia · QT interval prolongation · sleep disorders · urticaria · vertigo
  ▸ **Rare or very rare** Acute psychosis · arrhythmias · conjunctivitis · cystitis · dysphagia · feeling hot · hypokalaemia · hypotension · leucopenia · mitral valve incompetence · mood altered · myocardial ischaemia · numbness · pain · tongue coated · vision blurred
- ● CONCEPTION AND CONTRACEPTION Manufacturer recommends exclude pregnancy before treatment in females of childbearing age; ensure effective contraception during treatment and for one month after treatment.
- ● PREGNANCY Manufacturer advises avoid—toxicity in *animal* studies.
- ● BREAST FEEDING Manufacturer advises avoid during treatment and for 1 month after last dose—no information available.
- ● HEPATIC IMPAIRMENT Manufacturer advises caution in severe impairment (risk of increased exposure, limited information available).
- ● NATIONAL FUNDING/ACCESS DECISIONS
  For full details see funding body website
  Scottish Medicines Consortium (SMC) decisions
    ▸ Palonosetron with netupitant (*Akynzeo*®) in adults for the prevention of acute and delayed nausea and vomiting associated with highly emetogenic cisplatin-based cancer chemotherapy and moderately emetogenic cancer chemotherapy (January 2016) SMC No. 1109/15 Recommended with restrictions

- ● MEDICINAL FORMS There can be variation in the licensing of different medicines containing the same drug.
  Capsule
  CAUTIONARY AND ADVISORY LABELS 25
    ▸ Akynzeo (Chugai Pharma UK Ltd)
    Palonosetron (as Palonosetron hydrochloride) 500 microgram, Netupitant 300 mg Akynzeo 300mg/0.5mg capsules | 1 capsule [PoM] £69.00 (Hospital only)

ANTIHISTAMINES ❭ SEDATING ANTIHISTAMINES

Cinnarizine

04-Sep-2020

- ● INDICATIONS AND DOSE
  Relief of symptoms of vestibular disorders, such as vertigo, tinnitus, nausea, and vomiting in Ménière's disease
    ▸ BY MOUTH
    ▸ Child 5–11 years: 15 mg 3 times a day

▸ Child 12-17 years: 30 mg 3 times a day
▸ Adult: 30 mg 3 times a day

Motion sickness
▸ BY MOUTH
▸ Child 5-11 years: Initially 15 mg, dose to be taken 2 hours before travel, then 7.5 mg every 8 hours if required, dose to be taken during journey
▸ Child 12-17 years: Initially 30 mg, dose to be taken 2 hours before travel, then 15 mg every 8 hours if required, dose to be taken during journey
▸ Adult: Initially 30 mg, dose to be taken 2 hours before travel, then 15 mg every 8 hours if required, dose to be taken during journey

● CONTRA-INDICATIONS Avoid in Acute porphyrias p. 1107
● CAUTIONS Epilepsy · glaucoma (in children) · Parkinson's disease (in adults) · prostatic hypertrophy (in adults) · pyloroduodenal obstruction · susceptibility to angle-closure glaucoma (in adults) · urinary retention
● INTERACTIONS → Appendix 1: antihistamines, sedating
● SIDE-EFFECTS
▸ **Common or very common** Drowsiness · gastrointestinal discomfort · nausea · weight increased
▸ **Uncommon** Fatigue · hyperhidrosis · vomiting
▸ **Frequency not known** Dry mouth · gastrointestinal disorder · headache · jaundice cholestatic · movement disorders · muscle rigidity · parkinsonism · skin reactions · subacute cutaneous lupus erythematosus · tremor
● PREGNANCY Manufacturer advises avoid; however, there is no evidence of teratogenicity. The use of sedating antihistamines in the latter part of the third trimester may cause adverse effects in neonates such as irritability, paradoxical excitability, and tremor.
● BREAST FEEDING Most antihistamines are present in breast milk in varying amounts; although not known to be harmful, most manufacturers advise avoiding their use in mothers who are breast-feeding.
● HEPATIC IMPAIRMENT Manufacturer advises caution in hepatic insufficiency—no information available.
● RENAL IMPAIRMENT Use with caution—no information available.
● PATIENT AND CARER ADVICE
Driving and skilled tasks Drowsiness may affect performance of skilled tasks (e.g. cycling, driving); sedating effects enhanced by alcohol.

● MEDICINAL FORMS There can be variation in the licensing of different medicines containing the same drug. Forms available from special-order manufacturers include: oral suspension
Tablet
CAUTIONARY AND ADVISORY LABELS 2
▸ Cinnarizine (Non-proprietary)
Cinnarizine 15 mg Cinnarizine 15mg tablets | 84 tablet [PoM] £6.88 DT = £4.65

Cinnarizine with dimenhydrinate
10-Sep-2020

The properties listed below are those particular to the combination only. For the properties of the components please consider, cinnarizine p. 456.

● INDICATIONS AND DOSE
Vertigo
▸ BY MOUTH
▸ Adult: 1 tablet 3 times a day

● INTERACTIONS → Appendix 1: antihistamines, sedating · dimenhydrinate

● MEDICINAL FORMS There can be variation in the licensing of different medicines containing the same drug.
Tablet
CAUTIONARY AND ADVISORY LABELS 2, 21
▸ Arlevert (Hennig Arzneimittel GmbH & Co. KG)
Cinnarizine 20 mg, Dimenhydrinate 40 mg Arlevert tablets | 100 tablet [PoM] £24.00 DT = £24.00

Promethazine teoclate
14-Dec-2020

● INDICATIONS AND DOSE
Nausea | Vomiting | Labyrinthine disorders
▸ BY MOUTH
▸ Child 5-9 years: 12.5–37.5 mg daily
▸ Child 10-17 years: 25–75 mg daily; maximum 100 mg per day
▸ Adult: 25–75 mg daily; maximum 100 mg per day
Motion sickness prevention (acts longer than promethazine hydrochloride)
▸ BY MOUTH
▸ Child 5-9 years: 12.5 mg once daily, dose to be taken at bedtime on night before travel or 1–2 hours before travel
▸ Child 10-17 years: 25 mg once daily, dose to be taken at bedtime on night before travel or 1–2 hours before travel
▸ Adult: 25 mg once daily, dose to be taken at bedtime on night before travel or 1–2 hours before travel
Motion sickness treatment (acts longer than promethazine hydrochloride)
▸ BY MOUTH
▸ Child 5-9 years: 12.5 mg, dose to be taken at onset of motion sickness, then 12.5 mg daily for 2 days, dose to be taken at bedtime
▸ Child 10-17 years: 25 mg, dose to be taken at onset of motion sickness, then 25 mg once daily for 2 days, dose to be taken at bedtime
▸ Adult: 25 mg, dose to be taken at onset of motion sickness, then 25 mg once daily for 2 days, dose to be taken at bedtime

---

IMPORTANT SAFETY INFORMATION

MHRA/CHM ADVICE: OVER-THE-COUNTER COUGH AND COLD MEDICINES FOR CHILDREN (APRIL 2009)
Children under 6 years should not be given over-the-counter cough and cold medicines containing promethazine.

● CAUTIONS Asthma · bronchiectasis · bronchitis · epilepsy · prostatic hypertrophy (in adults) · pyloroduodenal obstruction · Reye's syndrome · severe coronary artery disease · susceptibility to angle-closure glaucoma · urinary retention
● INTERACTIONS → Appendix 1: antihistamines, sedating
● SIDE-EFFECTS Anticholinergic syndrome · anxiety · appetite decreased · arrhythmia · blood disorder · bronchial secretion viscosity increased · confusion · dizziness · drowsiness · dry mouth · epigastric discomfort · fatigue · haemolytic anaemia · headache · hypotension · jaundice · movement disorders · muscle spasms · nightmare · palpitations · photosensitivity reaction · urinary retention · vision blurred
SIDE-EFFECTS, FURTHER INFORMATION Elderly patients are more susceptible to anticholinergic side-effects. In children paradoxical stimulation may occur, especially with high doses.
● PREGNANCY Most manufacturers of antihistamines advise avoiding their use during pregnancy; however, there is no evidence of teratogenicity. Use in the latter part of the

Nervous system

4

third trimester may cause adverse effects in neonates such as irritability, paradoxical excitability, and tremor.

- **BREAST FEEDING** Most antihistamines are present in breast milk in varying amounts; although not known to be harmful, most manufacturers advise avoiding their use in mothers who are breast-feeding.
- **HEPATIC IMPAIRMENT** Manufacturer advises caution.
- **RENAL IMPAIRMENT** Use with caution.
- **PATIENT AND CARER ADVICE**
  Driving and skilled tasks Drowsiness may affect performance of skilled tasks (e.g. cycling or driving); sedating effects enhanced by alcohol.

- **MEDICINAL FORMS** There can be variation in the licensing of different medicines containing the same drug.
  Tablet
  CAUTIONARY AND ADVISORY LABELS 2
  ▸ Avomine (Manx Healthcare Ltd)
  Promethazine teoclate 25 mg Avomine 25mg tablets |
  10 tablet Ⓟ £1.13 | 28 tablet Ⓟ £3.13 DT = £3.13
  ▸ Vertigon (Manx Healthcare Ltd)
  Promethazine teoclate 25 mg Vertigon 25mg tablets |
  28 tablet Ⓟ Ⓝ DT = £3.13

ANTIMUSCARINICS

Ⓕ 821

Hyoscine hydrobromide

03-Aug-2020

(Scopolamine hydrobromide)

- ● **INDICATIONS AND DOSE**

Motion sickness
▸ BY MOUTH
▸ Child 4-9 years: 75–150 micrograms, dose to be taken up to 30 minutes before the start of journey, then 75–150 micrograms every 6 hours if required; maximum 450 micrograms per day
▸ Child 10-17 years: 150–300 micrograms, dose to be taken up to 30 minutes before the start of journey, then 150–300 micrograms every 6 hours if required; maximum 900 micrograms per day
▸ Adult: 150–300 micrograms, dose to be taken up to 30 minutes before the start of journey, then 150–300 micrograms every 6 hours if required; maximum 900 micrograms per day
▸ BY TRANSDERMAL APPLICATION
▸ Child 10-17 years: Apply 1 patch, apply behind ear 5–6 hours before journey, then apply 1 patch after 72 hours if required, remove old patch and site replacement patch behind the other ear
▸ Adult: Apply 1 patch, apply behind ear 5–6 hours before journey, then apply 1 patch after 72 hours if required, remove old patch and site replacement patch behind the other ear

Hypersalivation associated with clozapine therapy
▸ BY MOUTH
▸ Adult: 300 micrograms up to 3 times a day; maximum 900 micrograms per day

Excessive respiratory secretion in palliative care
▸ BY SUBCUTANEOUS INJECTION
▸ Adult: 400 micrograms every 4 hours as required, hourly use is occasionally necessary, particularly in excessive respiratory secretions
▸ BY CONTINUOUS SUBCUTANEOUS INFUSION
▸ Adult: 1.2–2 mg/24 hours

Bowel colic in palliative care
▸ BY SUBCUTANEOUS INJECTION
▸ Adult: 400 micrograms every 4 hours as required, hourly use is occasionally necessary
▸ BY SUBCUTANEOUS INFUSION
▸ Adult: 1.2–2 mg/24 hours

Bowel colic pain in palliative care
▸ BY MOUTH USING SUBLINGUAL TABLETS
▸ Adult: 300 micrograms 3 times a day, as *Kwells ®*.

Premedication
▸ BY SUBCUTANEOUS INJECTION, OR BY INTRAMUSCULAR INJECTION
▸ Adult: 200–600 micrograms, to be administered 30–60 minutes before induction of anaesthesia

- ● **UNLICENSED USE** Not licensed for hypersalivation associated with clozapine therapy.

> **IMPORTANT SAFETY INFORMATION**
> Antimuscarinic drugs used for premedication to general anaesthesia should only be administered by, or under the direct supervision of, personnel experienced in their use.

- ● **CAUTIONS** Epilepsy
  CAUTIONS, FURTHER INFORMATION
  ▸ Anticholinergic syndrome
  ▸ With systemic use in adults In some patients, especially the elderly, hyoscine may cause the central anticholinergic syndrome (excitement, ataxia, hallucinations, behavioural abnormalities, and drowsiness).
  ▸ With systemic use in children In some children hyoscine may cause the central anticholinergic syndrome (excitement, ataxia, hallucinations, behavioural abnormalities, and drowsiness).

- ● **INTERACTIONS** → Appendix 1: hyoscine

- ● **SIDE-EFFECTS**
  ▸ **Common or very common**
  ▸ With transdermal use Eye disorders · eyelid irritation
  ▸ **Rare or very rare**
  ▸ With transdermal use Concentration impaired · glaucoma · hallucinations · memory loss · restlessness
  ▸ **Frequency not known**
  ▸ With oral use Asthma · cardiovascular disorders · central nervous system stimulation · gastrointestinal disorder · hallucination · hypersensitivity · hyperthermia · hypohidrosis · mydriasis · oedema · respiratory tract reaction · restlessness · seizure
  ▸ With parenteral use Agitation · angle closure glaucoma · arrhythmias · delirium · dysphagia · dyspnoea · epilepsy exacerbated · hallucination · hypersensitivity · idiosyncratic drug reaction · loss of consciousness · mydriasis · neuroleptic malignant syndrome · psychotic disorder · thirst
  ▸ With transdermal use Balance impaired

- ● **PREGNANCY** Use only if potential benefit outweighs risk. Injection may depress neonatal respiration.
- ● **BREAST FEEDING** Amount too small to be harmful.
- ● **HEPATIC IMPAIRMENT** Manufacturer advises caution.
- ● **RENAL IMPAIRMENT** Use with caution.
- ● **DIRECTIONS FOR ADMINISTRATION**
  ▸ With transdermal use in children Expert sources advise *patch* applied to hairless area of skin behind ear; if less than whole patch required **either** cut with scissors along full thickness ensuring membrane is not peeled away **or** cover portion to prevent contact with skin.
  ▸ With oral use in children For administration by *mouth*, expert sources advise injection solution may be given orally.
- ● **PRESCRIBING AND DISPENSING INFORMATION** Flavours of chewable tablet formulations may include raspberry.
  Palliative care For further information on the use of hyoscine hydrobromide in palliative care, see www.medicinescomplete.com/#/content/palliative/hyoscine-hydrobromide.

- PATIENT AND CARER ADVICE
▸ With transdermal use Explain accompanying instructions to patient and in particular emphasise advice to wash hands after handling and to wash application site after removing, and to use one patch at a time.
  Driving and skilled tasks ▸ With transdermal use Drowsiness may persist for up to 24 hours or longer after removal of patch; effects of alcohol enhanced.

- MEDICINAL FORMS There can be variation in the licensing of different medicines containing the same drug. Forms available from special-order manufacturers include: oral suspension, oral solution, eye drops

Tablet
CAUTIONARY AND ADVISORY LABELS 2
▸ Kwells (Dexcel-Pharma Ltd)
  Hyoscine hydrobromide 150 microgram Kwells Kids 150microgram tablets | 12 tablet ℗ £1.84 DT = £1.84
  Hyoscine hydrobromide 300 microgram Kwells 300microgram tablets | 12 tablet ℗ £1.84 DT = £1.84
▸ Travel Calm (The Boots Company Plc)
  Hyoscine hydrobromide 300 microgram Travel Calm 300microgram tablets | 12 tablet ℗ Ⓢ DT = £1.84

Solution for injection
▸ Hyoscine hydrobromide (Non-proprietary)
  Hyoscine hydrobromide 400 microgram per 1 ml Hyoscine hydrobromide 400micrograms/1ml solution for injection ampoules | 10 ampoule PoM £47.21 DT = £47.21
  Hyoscine hydrobromide 600 microgram per 1 ml Hyoscine hydrobromide 600micrograms/1ml solution for injection ampoules | 10 ampoule £59.32 DT = £59.32

Transdermal patch
CAUTIONARY AND ADVISORY LABELS 19
▸ Scopoderm (GlaxoSmithKline Consumer Healthcare)
  Hyoscine 1 mg per 72 hour Scopoderm 1.5mg patches | 2 patch ℗ £12.87 DT = £12.87

Chewable tablet
CAUTIONARY AND ADVISORY LABELS 2, 24
▸ Joy-Rides (Teva UK Ltd)
  Hyoscine hydrobromide 150 microgram Joy-rides 150microgram chewable tablets sugar-free | 12 tablet ℗ £1.99 DT = £1.99

ANTIPSYCHOTICS 〉 FIRST-GENERATION

⚑ 403

Droperidol
06-Aug-2019

- DRUG ACTION Droperidol is a butyrophenone, structurally related to haloperidol, which blocks dopamine receptors in the chemoreceptor trigger zone.

- INDICATIONS AND DOSE

Prevention and treatment of postoperative nausea and vomiting
▸ BY INTRAVENOUS INJECTION
▸ Adult: 0.625–1.25 mg, dose to be given 30 minutes before end of surgery, then 0.625–1.25 mg every 6 hours as required
▸ Elderly: 625 micrograms, dose to be given 30 minutes before end of surgery, then 625 micrograms every 6 hours as required

Prevention of nausea and vomiting caused by opioid analgesics in postoperative patient-controlled analgesia (PCA)
▸ BY INTRAVENOUS INJECTION
▸ Adult: 15–50 micrograms of droperidol for every 1 mg of morphine in PCA, reduce dose in elderly; maximum 5 mg per day

- CONTRA-INDICATIONS Bradycardia · comatose states · hypokalaemia · hypomagnesaemia · phaeochromocytoma · QT-interval prolongation

- CAUTIONS Chronic obstructive pulmonary disease · CNS depression · electrolyte disturbances · history of alcohol abuse · respiratory failure

- INTERACTIONS → Appendix 1: droperidol
- SIDE-EFFECTS
▸ **Uncommon** Anxiety · oculogyration
▸ **Rare or very rare** Blood disorder · cardiac arrest · confusion · dysphoria
▸ **Frequency not known** Coma · epilepsy · hallucination · oligomenorrhoea · respiratory disorders · SIADH · syncope
- BREAST FEEDING Limited information available—avoid repeated administration.
- HEPATIC IMPAIRMENT Manufacturer advises caution.
  Dose adjustments
  ▸ When used for Prevention and treatment of postoperative nausea and vomiting Manufacturer advises maximum 625 micrograms repeated every 6 hours as required.
  ▸ When used for Prevention of nausea and vomiting caused by opioid analgesics in postoperative patient-controlled analgesia Manufacturer advises dose reduction (no information available).
- RENAL IMPAIRMENT
  Dose adjustments In postoperative nausea and vomiting, max. 625 micrograms repeated every 6 hours as required.
  For nausea and vomiting caused by opioid analgesics in postoperative patient-controlled analgesia, reduce dose.
- MONITORING REQUIREMENTS Continuous pulse oximetry required if risk of ventricular arrhythmia—continue for 30 minutes following administration.

- MEDICINAL FORMS There can be variation in the licensing of different medicines containing the same drug.
Solution for injection
▸ Droperidol (Non-proprietary)
  Droperidol 2.5 mg per 1 ml Droperidol 2.5mg/1ml solution for injection ampoules | 10 ampoule PoM £39.40
▸ Xomolix (Kyowa Kirin Ltd)
  Droperidol 2.5 mg per 1 ml Xomolix 2.5mg/1ml solution for injection ampoules | 10 ampoule PoM £39.40

⚑ 403

Levomepromazine
12-Aug-2020
(Methotrimeprazine)

- INDICATIONS AND DOSE

Pain in palliative care (reserved for distressed patients with severe pain unresponsive to other measures)
▸ BY CONTINUOUS SUBCUTANEOUS INFUSION, OR BY INTRAMUSCULAR INJECTION, OR BY INTRAVENOUS INJECTION
▸ Adult: Seek specialist advice

Restlessness and confusion in palliative care
▸ BY CONTINUOUS SUBCUTANEOUS INFUSION
▸ Child 1–11 years: 0.35–3 mg/kg, to be administered over 24 hours
▸ Child 12–17 years: 12.5–200 mg, to be administered over 24 hours
▸ BY MOUTH
▸ Adult: 6 mg every 2 hours as required
▸ BY SUBCUTANEOUS INJECTION
▸ Adult: 6.25 mg every 2 hours as required
▸ BY SUBCUTANEOUS INFUSION
▸ Adult: Initially 12.5–50 mg/24 hours, titrated according to response (doses greater than 100 mg/24 hours should be given under specialist supervision)

Nausea and vomiting in palliative care
▸ BY CONTINUOUS INTRAVENOUS INFUSION, OR BY SUBCUTANEOUS INFUSION
▸ Child 1 month–11 years: 100–400 micrograms/kg, to be administered over 24 hours
▸ Child 12–17 years: 5–25 mg, to be administered over 24 hours

continued →

4 Nervous system

Nervous system

4

▸ BY MOUTH
▸ Adult: 6 mg once daily, dose to be taken at bedtime, increased if necessary to 12.5–25 mg twice daily
▸ BY SUBCUTANEOUS INJECTION
▸ Adult: 6.25 mg once daily, dose to be given at bedtime, increased if necessary to 12.5–25 mg twice daily
▸ BY SUBCUTANEOUS INFUSION
▸ Adult: 5–25 mg/24 hours, sedation can limit the dose

Schizophrenia (bed patients)
▸ BY MOUTH
▸ Adult: Initially 100–200 mg daily in 3 divided doses, increased if necessary to 1 g daily

Schizophrenia
▸ BY MOUTH
▸ Adult: Initially 25–50 mg daily in divided doses, dose can be increased as necessary

● CONTRA-INDICATIONS CNS depression · comatose states · phaeochromocytoma
● CAUTIONS Patients receiving large initial doses should remain supine
  CAUTIONS, FURTHER INFORMATION
▸ In adults Risk of postural hypotension; not recommended for ambulant patients over 50 years unless risk of hypotensive reaction assessed.
● INTERACTIONS → Appendix 1: phenothiazines
● SIDE-EFFECTS
▸ **Common or very common** Asthenia · heat stroke
▸ **Rare or very rare** Cardiac arrest · hepatic disorders
▸ **Frequency not known** Allergic dermatitis · confusion · delirium · gastrointestinal disorders · glucose tolerance impaired · hyperglycaemia · hyponatraemia · photosensitivity reaction · priapism · SIADH
● HEPATIC IMPAIRMENT Manufacturer advises consider avoiding.
● RENAL IMPAIRMENT
  Dose adjustments Start with small doses in severe renal impairment because of increased cerebral sensitivity.
● DIRECTIONS FOR ADMINISTRATION
▸ With subcutaneous use in children For administration by *subcutaneous infusion*, manufacturer advises dilute with a suitable volume of Sodium Chloride 0.9%.
● PRESCRIBING AND DISPENSING INFORMATION
  Palliative care For further information on the use of levomepromazine in palliative care, see www.medicinescomplete.com/#/content/palliative/levomepromazine.

● MEDICINAL FORMS There can be variation in the licensing of different medicines containing the same drug. Forms available from special-order manufacturers include: oral suspension, oral solution
  Tablet
  CAUTIONARY AND ADVISORY LABELS 2
▸ Levomepromazine (Non-proprietary)
  Levomepromazine maleate 6 mg Levomepromazine 6mg tablets | 28 tablet [PoM] £240.00
  Levomepromazine maleate 25 mg Levomepromazine 25mg tablets | 84 tablet [PoM] [Ⓢ] DT = £20.26
  Levomepromazine maleate 50 mg Levomepromazine 50mg tablets | 28 tablet [PoM] [Ⓢ]
  Levomepromazine maleate 100 mg Levomepromazine 100mg tablets | 28 tablet [PoM] [Ⓢ] (Hospital only)
▸ Nozinan (Sanofi)
  Levomepromazine maleate 25 mg Nozinan 25mg tablets | 84 tablet [PoM] £20.26 DT = £20.26
  Levomepromazine maleate 100 mg Nozinan 100mg tablets | 100 tablet [PoM] [Ⓢ] (Hospital only)

Solution for injection
▸ Levomepromazine (Non-proprietary)
  Levomepromazine hydrochloride 25 mg per 1 ml Levomepromazine 25mg/1ml solution for injection ampoules | 10 ampoule [PoM] £20.13 DT = £20.13
▸ Nozinan (Sanofi)
  Levomepromazine hydrochloride 25 mg per 1 ml Nozinan 25mg/1ml solution for injection ampoules | 10 ampoule [PoM] £20.13 DT = £20.13

5.1 Ménière's disease

HISTAMINE ANALOGUES

Betahistine dihydrochloride
23-Nov-2020

● **INDICATIONS AND DOSE**

  Vertigo, tinnitus and hearing loss associated with Ménière's disease
▸ BY MOUTH
▸ Adult: Initially 16 mg 3 times a day, dose preferably taken with food; maintenance 24–48 mg daily

● CONTRA-INDICATIONS Phaeochromocytoma
● CAUTIONS Asthma · history of peptic ulcer
● INTERACTIONS → Appendix 1: betahistine
● SIDE-EFFECTS
▸ **Common or very common** Gastrointestinal discomfort · headache · nausea
▸ **Frequency not known** Allergic dermatitis · vomiting
● PREGNANCY Avoid unless clearly necessary—no information available.
● BREAST FEEDING Use only if potential benefit outweighs risk—no information available.

● MEDICINAL FORMS There can be variation in the licensing of different medicines containing the same drug. Forms available from special-order manufacturers include: oral suspension, oral solution
  Tablet
  CAUTIONARY AND ADVISORY LABELS 21
▸ Betahistine dihydrochloride (Non-proprietary)
  Betahistine dihydrochloride 8 mg Betahistine 8mg tablets | 84 tablet [PoM] £10.50 DT = £2.07 | 120 tablet [PoM] £2.95
  Betahistine dihydrochloride 16 mg Betahistine 16mg tablets | 84 tablet [PoM] £17.19 DT = £3.71
▸ Serc (Mylan)
  Betahistine dihydrochloride 8 mg Serc 8mg tablets | 120 tablet [PoM] £9.04
  Betahistine dihydrochloride 16 mg Serc 16mg tablets | 84 tablet [PoM] £12.65 DT = £3.71

---

6 Pain

Pain, Chronic
01-Oct-2019

Overview

Pain is described as an unpleasant sensory and emotional experience associated with actual or potential tissue damage. Physiologically, it can be described as **neuropathic** or **nociceptive**, and classified as either **acute** or **chronic** in nature. Nociceptive pain generally responds to treatment with conventional analgesics whereas neuropathic pain responds poorly to conventional analgesics and can be difficult to treat.

  Chronic pain is defined as pain that has been present for more than 12 weeks; beyond the expected time of wound healing. It is a complex phenomenon and can have a considerable impact on quality of life, resulting in significant suffering and disability.

Aims of treatment

Treatment aims to reduce the impact of chronic pain on quality of life, mood and function.

Management of chronic pain

A wide range of both pharmacological and non-pharmacological management strategies are available for chronic pain. For guidance on the management of chronic pain in osteoarthritis, see Osteoarthritis and soft-tissue disorders p. 1140, for musculoskeletal conditions, see Soft-tissue disorders p. 1201, and for neuropathic pain, see Neuropathic pain p. 504.

EvGr Consider specialist referral when non-specialist management is failing, the pain is poorly controlled, the patient is experiencing significant distress, and/or where a specialist intervention is being considered. ◇A◇

Non-drug treatment

EvGr Exercise and exercise therapies, regardless of their form, are recommended in the management of chronic pain; strategies to improve adherence (such as supervised exercise sessions) should be implemented.

Transcutaneous electrical nerve stimulation (either high or low frequency) should be considered for the relief of chronic pain.

Referral to a pain management programme and psychologically based interventions such as cognitive behavioural therapy, biofeedback, and progressive relaxation should be considered for patients with chronic pain; brief education should be given to all patients.

The use of self-management resources (safe, low-technology, community-based, and affordable programmes) should be considered to complement other therapies in the treatment of chronic pain. For information on self-management resources, see SIGN clinical guideline: **Management of chronic pain** (see *Useful resources*). ◇A◇

Drug treatment

A variety of analgesics are used in the treatment of chronic pain and can be divided into **non-opioid** and **opioid** analgesics. Although developed and validated for cancer pain, the World Health Organisation (WHO) analgesic ladder is widely used to guide the basic treatment of acute and chronic pain; whilst there is little evidence to support its use in chronic pain it may provide an analgesic strategy for non-specialists. The WHO analgesic ladder is available at: www.who.int/cancer/palliative/painladder/en/.

Individual responses to analgesia vary considerably, both in terms of efficacy and side effects; even with the same chronic pain syndrome, the underlying pain mechanisms may differ between individuals. This provides challenges with assessment and management in routine clinical practice. EvGr If an individual either fails to tolerate, or has an inadequate response to a drug, then it is worthwhile considering a different agent from the same class.

Individuals using analgesics to manage chronic pain should be reviewed at least annually, with review frequency increased if there are any changes to their medication, underlying pain syndrome or comorbidities. ◇A◇

For comparative information on analgesic options, see Analgesics p. 462.

EvGr **Depression** is a common comorbidity in those with chronic pain; individuals should be monitored and treated for depression when necessary. Optimising antidepressant therapy should be considered in individuals with moderate depression and chronic pain. ◇A◇ For information on the treatment of depression in adults, see Antidepressant drugs p. 378.

Non-opioid analgesics

Non-opioid analgesics include paracetamol p. 464 and non-steroidal anti-inflammatory drugs (NSAIDs). For information on the use of NSAIDs, see Non-steroidal anti-inflammatory drugs p. 1176.

EvGr Cannabis-based medicinal products (nabilone, dronabinol, delta-9-tetrahydrocannabinol (THC), and combination cannabidiol (CBD) with THC) are not recommended for managing chronic pain. The use of CBD is not recommended unless as part of a clinical trial. If the patient is already using cannabis-based treatment for chronic pain, it may be continued until they and the appropriate clinician deem it suitable to stop. ◇A◇

Topical analgesic preparations may be useful for the management of chronic pain in different disorders. Preparations include capsaicin or lidocaine (see Neuropathic pain p. 504), NSAIDs (see Osteoarthritis and soft-tissue disorders p. 1140), and rubefacients (see Soft-tissue disorders p. 1201).

Compound preparations

EvGr The use of single-ingredient analgesics is preferred to allow for independent titration of each drug; however, fixed dose combination analgesics (except those with low-dose opioids) may be considered for those with stable chronic pain. ◇A◇

Opioids

Opioid analgesics can be divided into those used for mild-to-moderate pain (such as codeine phosphate p. 475) and those used for moderate-to-severe pain (such as morphine p. 483 or oxycodone hydrochloride p. 486).

EvGr Opioids should only be considered in carefully selected individuals for the short- to medium-term treatment of chronic non-malignant pain, when other therapies have been insufficient; the benefits should outweigh the risks of serious harms (such as addiction, overdose and death). With continuous longer-term use of opioids, tolerance and dependence compromise both safety and efficacy. Prescribers should have knowledge of opioid pharmacology, and be competent and experienced in the use of strong opioids.

When starting treatment with an opioid there should be an agreement between the prescriber and patient about the expected outcomes—with advanced agreement on the reduction and cessation of the opioid if these are not met. Opioids should be reviewed at least annually but more frequently if required; consideration should be given to a gradual reduction of the opioid to the lowest effective dose or complete cessation. Pain specialist advice or review should be sought for individuals taking doses >90 mg/day morphine equivalent. ◇A◇

There is a rationale for switching between opioids if the initial choice is ineffective or if side effects are unacceptable. EvGr Caution should be used with dose comparisons and switching due to limited evidence for the accuracy of dose equivalence tables and considerable variation between individuals. ◇A◇ For more information on opioid dose conversions or equivalents, see Prescribing in palliative care p. 28. Resources for the prescribing of opioids have been produced by the *Faculty of Pain Medicine* in partnership with *Public Health England*, and are available at: fpm.ac.uk/opioids-aware.

Useful Resources

Management of chronic pain. Scottish Intercollegiate Guidelines Network. SIGN guideline 136. August 2019. www.sign.ac.uk/sign-136-management-of-chronic-pain.html

4

Nervous system

Analgesics

06-Oct-2020

Pain relief

The non-opioid drugs, paracetamol p. 464 and aspirin p. 132 (and other NSAIDs), are particularly suitable for pain in musculoskeletal conditions, whereas the opioid analgesics are more suitable for moderate to severe pain, particularly of visceral origin. The MHRA/CHM have issued important safety information on the use of opioids and risk of dependence and addiction. For further information, see *Important safety information* in individual drug monographs.

Pain in sickle-cell disease

The pain of mild sickle-cell crises is managed with paracetamol, a NSAID, codeine phosphate p. 475, or dihydrocodeine tartrate p. 477. Severe crises may require the use of morphine p. 483 or diamorphine hydrochloride p. 476; concomitant use of a NSAID may potentiate analgesia and allow lower doses of the opioid to be used. Pethidine hydrochloride p. 489 should be avoided if possible because accumulation of a neurotoxic metabolite can precipitate seizures; the relatively short half-life of pethidine hydrochloride necessitates frequent injections.

Dental and orofacial pain

Analgesics should be used judiciously in dental care as a **temporary** measure until the cause of the pain has been dealt with.

Dental pain of inflammatory origin, such as that associated with pulpitis, apical infection, localised osteitis or pericoronitis is usually best managed by treating the infection, providing drainage, restorative procedures, and other local measures. Analgesics provide temporary relief of pain (usually for about 1 to 7 days) until the causative factors have been brought under control. In the case of pulpitis, intra-osseous infection or abscess, reliance on analgesics alone is usually inappropriate.

Similarly the pain and discomfort associated with acute problems of the oral mucosa (e.g. acute herpetic gingivostomatitis, erythema multiforme) may be relieved by benzydamine hydrochloride mouthwash or spray p. 1259 until the cause of the mucosal disorder has been dealt with. However, where a patient is febrile, the antipyretic action of paracetamol or ibuprofen p. 1186 is often helpful.

The *choice* of an analgesic for dental purposes should be based on its suitability for the patient. Most dental pain is relieved effectively by non-steroidal anti-inflammatory drugs (NSAIDs). NSAIDs that are used for dental pain include ibuprofen, diclofenac sodium p. 1181, and aspirin. Paracetamol has analgesic and antipyretic effects but no anti-inflammatory effect.

Opioid analgesics such as dihydrocodeine tartrate act on the central nervous system and are traditionally used for *moderate to severe pain*. However, opioid analgesics are relatively ineffective in dental pain and their side-effects can be unpleasant. Paracetamol, ibuprofen, or aspirin are adequate for most cases of dental pain and an opioid is rarely required.

Combining a non-opioid with an opioid analgesic can provide greater relief of pain than either analgesic given alone. However, this applies only when an adequate dose of each analgesic is used. Most combination analgesic preparations have not been shown to provide greater relief of pain than an adequate dose of the non-opioid component given alone. Moreover, combination preparations have the disadvantage of an increased number of side-effects.

Any analgesic given before a dental procedure should have a low risk of increasing postoperative bleeding. In the case of pain after the dental procedure, taking an analgesic before the effect of the local anaesthetic has worn off can improve control. Postoperative analgesia with ibuprofen or aspirin is usually continued for about 24 to 72 hours.

Temporomandibular dysfunction can be related to anxiety in some patients who may clench or grind their teeth (bruxism) during the day or night. The muscle spasm (which appears to be the main source of pain) may be treated empirically with an overlay appliance which provides a free sliding occlusion and may also interfere with grinding. In addition, diazepam p. 362, which has muscle relaxant as well as anxiolytic properties, may be helpful but it should only be prescribed on a short-term basis during the acute phase. Analgesics such as aspirin or ibuprofen may also be required.

Dysmenorrhoea

Use of an oral contraceptive prevents the pain of dysmenorrhoea which is generally associated with ovulatory cycles. If treatment is necessary paracetamol or a NSAID will generally provide adequate relief of pain. The vomiting and severe pain associated with dysmenorrhoea in women with endometriosis may call for an antiemetic (in addition to an analgesic). Antispasmodics (such as alverine citrate p. 94) have been advocated for dysmenorrhoea but the antispasmodic action does not generally provide significant relief.

Non-opioid analgesics and compound analgesic preparations

Aspirin is indicated for headache, transient musculoskeletal pain, dysmenorrhoea, and pyrexia. In inflammatory conditions, most physicians prefer anti-inflammatory treatment with another NSAID which may be better tolerated and more convenient for the patient. Aspirin is used increasingly for its antiplatelet properties. Aspirin tablets or dispersible aspirin tablets are adequate for most purposes as they act rapidly.

Gastric irritation may be a problem; it is minimised by taking the dose after food. Enteric-coated preparations are available, but have a slow onset of action and are therefore unsuitable for single-dose analgesic use (though their prolonged action may be useful for night pain).

Aspirin interacts significantly with a number of other drugs and its interaction with warfarin sodium p. 153 is a **special hazard**.

Paracetamol is similar in efficacy to aspirin, but has no demonstrable anti-inflammatory activity; it is less irritant to the stomach and for that reason is now generally preferred to aspirin, particularly in the elderly. **Overdosage** with paracetamol is particularly dangerous as it may cause hepatic damage which is sometimes not apparent for 4 to 6 days.

Nefopam hydrochloride p. 466 may have a place in the relief of persistent pain unresponsive to other non-opioid analgesics. It causes little or no respiratory depression, but sympathomimetic and antimuscarinic side-effects may be troublesome.

Non-steroidal anti-inflammatory analgesics (NSAIDs) are particularly useful for the treatment of patients with chronic disease accompanied by pain and inflammation. Some of them are also used in the short-term treatment of mild to moderate pain including transient musculoskeletal pain but paracetamol is now often preferred, particularly in the elderly. They are also suitable for the relief of pain in *dysmenorrhoea* and to treat pain caused by *secondary bone tumours*, many of which produce lysis of bone and release prostaglandins. Selective inhibitors of cyclo-oxygenase-2 may be used in preference to non-selective NSAIDs for patients at high risk of developing serious gastro-intestinal side-effects. Several NSAIDs are also used for postoperative analgesia.

A non-opioid analgesic administered by intrathecal infusion (**ziconotide** (*Prialt®*), available from Eisai) is licensed for the treatment of chronic severe pain; ziconotide can be used by a hospital specialist as an adjunct to opioid analgesics.

Compound analgesic preparations

Compound analgesic preparations that contain a simple analgesic (such as aspirin p. 132 or paracetamol p. 464) with an opioid component reduce the scope for effective titration of the individual components in the management of pain of varying intensity.

Compound analgesic preparations containing paracetamol or aspirin with a *low dose* of an opioid analgesic (e.g. 8 mg of codeine phosphate p. 475 per compound tablet) are commonly used, but the advantages have not been substantiated. The low dose of the opioid may be enough to cause opioid side-effects (in particular, constipation) and can complicate the treatment of **overdosage** yet may not provide significant additional relief of pain.

A *full dose* of the opioid component (e.g. 60 mg codeine phosphate) in compound analgesic preparations effectively augments the analgesic activity but is associated with the full range of opioid side-effects (including nausea, vomiting, severe constipation, drowsiness, respiratory depression, and risk of dependence on long-term administration).

Important: the elderly are particularly susceptible to opioid side-effects and should receive lower doses.

In general, when assessing pain, it is necessary to weigh up carefully whether there is a need for a non-opioid and an opioid analgesic to be taken simultaneously.

Caffeine is a weak stimulant that is often included, in small doses, in analgesic preparations. It is claimed that the addition of caffeine may enhance the analgesic effect, but the alerting effect, mild habit-forming effect and possible provocation of headache may not always be desirable. Moreover, in excessive dosage or on withdrawal caffeine may itself induce headache.

Co-proxamol tablets (dextropropoxyphene in combination with paracetamol) are no longer licensed because of safety concerns, particularly toxicity in overdose. Co-proxamol tablets [unlicensed] may still be prescribed for patients who find it difficult to change, because alternatives are not effective or suitable.

Opioid analgesics and dependence

Opioid analgesics are usually used to relieve moderate to severe pain particularly of visceral origin. Repeated administration may cause dependence and tolerance, but this is no deterrent in the control of pain in terminal illness. Regular use of a potent opioid may be appropriate for certain cases of chronic non-malignant pain.

For general guidance on the use of opioid analgesics in chronic pain, see Pain, Chronic p. 460.

Strong opioids

Morphine p. 483 remains the most valuable opioid analgesic for severe pain although it frequently causes nausea and vomiting. It is the standard against which other opioid analgesics are compared. In addition to relief of pain, morphine also confers a state of euphoria and mental detachment.

Morphine is the opioid of choice for the oral treatment of *severe pain in palliative care*. It is given regularly every 4 hours (or every 12 or 24 hours as modified-release preparations).

Buprenorphine p. 468 has both opioid agonist and antagonist properties and may precipitate withdrawal symptoms, including pain, in patients dependent on other opioids. It has abuse potential and may itself cause dependence. It has a much longer duration of action than morphine and sublingually is an effective analgesic for 6 to 8 hours. Unlike most opioid analgesics, the effects of buprenorphine are only partially reversed by naloxone hydrochloride p. 1424.

Dipipanone hydrochloride used alone is less sedating than morphine but the only preparation available contains an antiemetic and is therefore not suitable for regular regimens in palliative care.

Diamorphine hydrochloride (heroin) p. 476 is a powerful opioid analgesic. It may cause less nausea and hypotension than morphine. In *palliative care* the greater solubility of diamorphine hydrochloride allows effective doses to be injected in smaller volumes and this is important in the emaciated patient.

Alfentanil p. 1397, fentanyl p. 478 and remifentanil p. 1398 are used by injection for intra-operative analgesia; fentanyl is available in a transdermal drug delivery system as a self-adhesive patch which is changed every 72 hours.

Methadone hydrochloride p. 524 is less sedating than morphine and acts for longer periods. In prolonged use, methadone hydrochloride should not be administered more often than twice daily to avoid the risk of accumulation and opioid overdosage. Methadone hydrochloride may be used instead of morphine in the occasional patient who experiences excitation (or exacerbation of pain) with morphine.

Oxycodone hydrochloride p. 486 has an efficacy and side-effect profile similar to that of morphine. It is commonly used as a second-line drug if morphine is not tolerated or does not control the pain.

Papaveretum is rarely used; morphine is easier to prescribe and less prone to error with regard to the strength and dose.

Pentazocine p. 489 has both agonist and antagonist properties and precipitates withdrawal symptoms, including pain in patients dependent on other opioids. By injection it is more potent than dihydrocodeine tartrate p. 477 or codeine phosphate, but hallucinations and thought disturbances may occur. It is not recommended and, in particular, should be avoided after myocardial infarction as it may increase pulmonary and aortic blood pressure as well as cardiac work.

Pethidine hydrochloride p. 489 produces prompt but short-lasting analgesia; it is less constipating than morphine, but even in high doses is a less potent analgesic. It is not suitable for severe continuing pain. It is used for analgesia in labour; however, other opioids, such as morphine or diamorphine hydrochloride, are often preferred for obstetric pain.

Tapentadol p. 490 produces analgesia by two mechanisms. It is an opioid-receptor agonist and it also inhibits noradrenaline reuptake. Nausea, vomiting, and constipation are less likely to occur with tapentadol than with other strong opioid analgesics.

Tramadol hydrochloride p. 491 produces analgesia by two mechanisms: an opioid effect and an enhancement of serotonergic and adrenergic pathways. It has fewer of the typical opioid side-effects (notably, less respiratory depression, less constipation and less addiction potential); psychiatric reactions have been reported.

Weak opioids

Codeine phosphate can be used for the relief of mild to moderate pain where other painkillers such as paracetamol or ibuprofen p. 1186 have proved ineffective.

Dihydrocodeine tartrate has an analgesic efficacy similar to that of codeine phosphate. Higher doses may provide some additional pain relief but this may be at the cost of more nausea and vomiting.

Meptazinol p. 483 is claimed to have a low incidence of repiratory depression. It has a reported length of action of 2 to 7 hours with onset within 15 minutes.

Postoperative analgesia

[EvGr] Offer a multimodal approach using a combination of analgesics from different classes to manage postoperative pain. ⓐ For further information on postoperative analgesia, see Peri-operative analgesia p. 1392. The use of intra-operative opioids affects the prescribing of postoperative analgesics. A postoperative opioid analgesic should be given with care since it may potentiate any residual respiratory depression.

Morphine p. 483 is used most widely. Tramadol hydrochloride p. 491 is not as effective in severe pain as other opioid analgesics. Buprenorphine p. 468 may antagonise the analgesic effect of previously administered opioids and is generally not recommended. Pethidine hydrochloride p. 489 is generally not recommended for postoperative pain because it is metabolised to norpethidine which may accumulate, particularly in renal impairment; norpethidine stimulates the central nervous system and may cause convulsions.

Opioids are also given epidurally [unlicensed route] in the postoperative period but are associated with side-effects such as pruritus, urinary retention, nausea and vomiting; respiratory depression can be delayed, particularly with morphine.

Patient-controlled analgesia (PCA) can be used to relieve postoperative pain—consult individual hospital protocols.

Pain management and opioid dependence
Although caution is necessary, patients who are dependent on opioids or have a history of drug dependence may be treated with opioid analgesics when there is a clinical need. Treatment with opioid analgesics in this patient group should normally be carried out with the advice of specialists. However, doctors do not require a special licence to prescribe opioid analgesics to patients with opioid dependence for relief of pain due to organic disease or injury.

> **Other drugs used for Pain** Dexibuprofen, p. 1179 ·
> Diclofenac potassium, p. 1180 · Levomepromazine, p. 459 ·
> Mefenamic acid, p. 1191

ANAESTHETICS, GENERAL ❭ VOLATILE LIQUID ANAESTHETICS

▌Methoxyflurane

30-Jan-2018

● **INDICATIONS AND DOSE**

Moderate-to-severe pain associated with trauma (under close medical supervision)
▶ BY INHALATION
▶ Adult: 3–6 mL as required, avoid administration on consecutive days; administer using inhaler device; maximum 15 mL per week

> **IMPORTANT SAFETY INFORMATION**
> Manufacturer advises methoxyflurane should only be self-administered under the supervision of personnel experienced in its use, using a hand-held *Penthrox*® inhaler device.

● CONTRA-INDICATIONS Cardiovascular disease · history of liver damage associated with use of methoxyflurane or other halogenated anaesthetics · impaired consciousness · respiratory depression · susceptibility to malignant hyperthermia
● CAUTIONS Elderly—increased risk of hypotension · repeated administration more than once every 3 months—increased risk of hepatic injury · risk factors for hepatic impairment · risk factors for renal impairment
● INTERACTIONS → Appendix 1: volatile halogenated anaesthetics
● SIDE-EFFECTS
▶ **Common or very common** Cough · dizziness · drowsiness · dry mouth · dysarthria · feeling abnormal · headache · hypotension · memory loss · mood altered · nausea · taste altered
▶ **Uncommon** Anxiety · appetite increased · chills · depression · fatigue · flushing · hyperhidrosis · oral discomfort · paraesthesia · peripheral neuropathy · vision disorders

▶ **Frequency not known** Choking · confusion · consciousness impaired · dissociation · hepatic disorders · hypoxia · nystagmus · renal failure · vomiting
● ALLERGY AND CROSS-SENSITIVITY Contra-indicated in patients with hypersensitivity to fluorinated anaesthetics.
● PREGNANCY Manufacturer advises use with caution—limited information available.
● BREAST FEEDING Manufacturer advises use with caution—limited information available.
● HEPATIC IMPAIRMENT Manufacturer advises caution (risk of increased exposure).
● RENAL IMPAIRMENT Manufacturer advises avoid.
● PRESCRIBING AND DISPENSING INFORMATION The manufacturer of *Penthrox*® has provided an *Administration Checklist* and an *Administration Guide* for healthcare professionals.
● HANDLING AND STORAGE Manufacturer advises exposure of healthcare professionals to methoxyflurane should be minimised—risk of serious side-effects.
● PATIENT AND CARER ADVICE Manufacturer advises patients should be given advice on appropriate inhaler technique.
  A patient alert card should be provided.
  Driving and skilled tasks Manufacturer advises patients and carers should be counselled on the effects on driving and performance of skilled tasks—increased risk of dizziness and drowsiness.

● MEDICINAL FORMS There can be variation in the licensing of different medicines containing the same drug.
  Inhalation vapour
  EXCIPIENTS: May contain Butylated hydroxytoluene
  ▶ Penthrox (Galen Ltd) ▼
    Methoxyflurane 999 mg per 1 gram Penthrox inhalation vapour 3ml bottles with device | 1 bottle [PoM] £17.89 (Hospital only)

ANALGESICS ❭ NON-OPIOID

▌Paracetamol

16-Nov-2020

(Acetaminophen)

● **INDICATIONS AND DOSE**

Mild to moderate pain | Pyrexia
▶ BY MOUTH
▶ Adult: 0.5–1 g every 4–6 hours; maximum 4 g per day
▶ BY INTRAVENOUS INFUSION
▶ Adult (body-weight up to 50 kg): 15 mg/kg every 4–6 hours, dose to be administered over 15 minutes; maximum 60 mg/kg per day
▶ Adult (body-weight 50 kg and above): 1 g every 4–6 hours, dose to be administered over 15 minutes; maximum 4 g per day
▶ BY RECTUM
▶ Adult: 0.5–1 g every 4–6 hours; maximum 4 g per day

Mild to moderate pain in patients with risk factors for hepatotoxicity | Pyrexia in patients with risk factors for hepatotoxicity
▶ BY INTRAVENOUS INFUSION
▶ Adult (body-weight up to 50 kg): 15 mg/kg every 4–6 hours, dose to be administered over 15 minutes; maximum 60 mg/kg per day
▶ Adult (body-weight 50 kg and above): 1 g every 4–6 hours, dose to be administered over 15 minutes; maximum 3 g per day

Pain | Pyrexia with discomfort
▶ BY MOUTH
▶ Child 3-5 months: 60 mg every 4–6 hours; maximum 4 doses per day

▸ Child 6–23 months: 120 mg every 4–6 hours; maximum 4 doses per day
▸ Child 2–3 years: 180 mg every 4–6 hours; maximum 4 doses per day
▸ Child 4–5 years: 240 mg every 4–6 hours; maximum 4 doses per day
▸ Child 6–7 years: 240–250 mg every 4–6 hours; maximum 4 doses per day
▸ Child 8–9 years: 360–375 mg every 4–6 hours; maximum 4 doses per day
▸ Child 10–11 years: 480–500 mg every 4–6 hours; maximum 4 doses per day
▸ Child 12–15 years: 480–750 mg every 4–6 hours; maximum 4 doses per day
▸ Child 16–17 years: 0.5–1 g every 4–6 hours; maximum 4 doses per day
▸ BY RECTUM
▸ Child 3–11 months: 60–125 mg every 4–6 hours as required; maximum 4 doses per day
▸ Child 1–4 years: 125–250 mg every 4–6 hours as required; maximum 4 doses per day
▸ Child 5–11 years: 250–500 mg every 4–6 hours as required; maximum 4 doses per day
▸ Child 12–17 years: 500 mg every 4–6 hours

Post-immunisation pyrexia in infants
▸ BY MOUTH
▸ Child 2–3 months: 60 mg for 1 dose, then 60 mg after 4–6 hours if required
▸ Child 4 months: 60 mg for 1 dose, then 60 mg after 4–6 hours; maximum 4 doses per day

Acute migraine
▸ BY MOUTH
▸ Adult: 1 g for 1 dose, to be taken as soon as migraine symptoms develop

● UNLICENSED USE
▸ In children Paracetamol oral suspension 500 mg/5 mL not licensed for use in children under 16 years. [EvGr] Not licensed for use as prophylaxis of post-immunisation pyrexia following immunisation with meningococcal group B vaccine. ◁Ⓔ
● CAUTIONS Before administering, check when paracetamol last administered and cumulative paracetamol dose over previous 24 hours · body-weight under 50 kg · chronic alcohol consumption · chronic dehydration · chronic malnutrition · long-term use (especially in those who are malnourished)
CAUTIONS, FURTHER INFORMATION [EvGr] Some patients may be at increased risk of experiencing toxicity at therapeutic doses, particularly those with a body-weight under 50 kg and those with risk factors for hepatotoxicity. Clinical judgement should be used to adjust the dose of oral and intravenous paracetamol in these patients.
Co-administration of enzyme-inducing antiepileptic medications may increase toxicity; doses should be reduced. ◁Ⓔ
● INTERACTIONS → Appendix 1: paracetamol
● SIDE-EFFECTS
GENERAL SIDE-EFFECTS
▸ Rare or very rare Thrombocytopenia
SPECIFIC SIDE-EFFECTS
▸ Common or very common
▸ With rectal use Anorectal erythema
▸ Rare or very rare
▸ With intravenous use Hypersensitivity · hypotension · leucopenia · malaise · neutropenia
▸ With rectal use Angioedema · liver injury · skin reactions
▸ Frequency not known
▸ With intravenous use Flushing · skin reactions · tachycardia

▸ With oral use Agranulocytosis · bronchospasm · hepatic function abnormal · rash · severe cutaneous adverse reactions (SCARs)
▸ With rectal use Agranulocytosis · blood disorder · severe cutaneous adverse reactions (SCARs)
Overdose Liver damage and less frequently renal damage can occur following overdose.
Nausea and vomiting, the only early features of poisoning, usually settle within 24 hours. Persistence beyond this time, often associated with the onset of right subcostal pain and tenderness, usually indicates development of hepatic necrosis.
For specific details on the management of poisoning, see Paracetamol, under Emergency treatment of poisoning p. 1413.
● PREGNANCY Not known to be harmful.
● BREAST FEEDING Amount too small to be harmful.
● HEPATIC IMPAIRMENT Manufacturer advises caution (increased risk of toxicity).
● RENAL IMPAIRMENT
Dose adjustments ▸ In adults Increase infusion dose interval to every 6 hours if eGFR less than 30 mL/minute/1.73 m^2.
▸ In children Increase infusion dose interval to every 6 hours if estimated glomerular filtration rate less than 30 mL/minute/1.73 m^2.
● DIRECTIONS FOR ADMINISTRATION
▸ With intravenous infusion (Perfalgan®), manufacturer advises give in Glucose 5% or Sodium Chloride 0.9%; dilute to a concentration of not less than 1 mg/mL and use within an hour; may also be given undiluted.
● PRESCRIBING AND DISPENSING INFORMATION BP directs that when Paediatric Paracetamol Oral Suspension or Paediatric Paracetamol Mixture is prescribed Paracetamol Oral Suspension 120 mg/5 mL should be dispensed.
● PATIENT AND CARER ADVICE
Medicines for Children leaflet: Paracetamol for mild-to-moderate pain www.medicinesforchildren.org.uk/paracetamol-mild-moderate-pain
● PROFESSION SPECIFIC INFORMATION
Dental practitioners' formulary
Paracetamol Tablets may be prescribed.
Paracetamol Soluble Tablets 500 mg may be prescribed.
Paracetamol Oral Suspension may be prescribed.
● EXCEPTIONS TO LEGAL CATEGORY Paracetamol capsules or tablets can be sold to the public provided packs contain no more than 32 capsules or tablets; pharmacists can sell multiple packs up to a total quantity of 100 capsules or tablets in justifiable circumstances.
● MEDICINAL FORMS There can be variation in the licensing of different medicines containing the same drug. Forms available from special-order manufacturers include: oral suspension, oral solution, suppository, powder

Tablet
CAUTIONARY AND ADVISORY LABELS 29 (500 mg tablets in adults), 30
▸ Paracetamol (Non-proprietary)
Paracetamol 500 mg Paracetamol 500mg caplets | 100 tablet [PoM] £3.53 DT = £3.53
Paracetamol 500mg tablets | 100 tablet [PoM] £3.53 DT = £3.53 | 1000 tablet [PoM] £35.30
Paracetamol 1 gram Paracetamol 1g tablets | 100 tablet [PoM] £3.50 DT = £3.50
▸ Mandanol (M & A Pharmachem Ltd)
Paracetamol 500 mg Mandanol 500mg caplets | 100 tablet [PoM] £1.34 DT = £3.53
Mandanol 500mg tablets | 100 tablet [PoM] £1.34 DT = £3.53
▸ Paravict (Ecogen Europe Ltd)
Paracetamol 500 mg Paravict 500mg tablets | 100 tablet [PoM] £1.62 DT = £3.53

Nervous system

4

Suppository

CAUTIONARY AND ADVISORY LABELS 30

▸ Paracetamol (Non-proprietary)

Paracetamol 80 mg Paracetamol 80mg suppositories |
10 suppository [P] £10.00 DT = £10.00

Paracetamol 120 mg Paracetamol 120mg suppositories |
10 suppository [P] £12.39 DT = £12.39

Paracetamol 125 mg Paracetamol 125mg suppositories |
10 suppository [P] £15.00 DT = £13.80

Paracetamol 240 mg Paracetamol 240mg suppositories |
10 suppository [P] £22.01 DT = £22.01

Paracetamol 250 mg Paracetamol 250mg suppositories |
10 suppository [P] £35.07 DT = £27.60

Paracetamol 500 mg Paracetamol 500mg suppositories |
10 suppository [P] £41.50 DT = £41.15

Paracetamol 1 gram Paracetamol 1g suppositories |
10 suppository [P] £60.00 DT = £59.50

▸ Alvedon (Intrapharm Laboratories Ltd)

Paracetamol 60 mg Alvedon 60mg suppositories |
10 suppository [P] £11.95 DT = £11.95

Paracetamol 125 mg Alvedon 125mg suppositories |
10 suppository [P] £13.80 DT = £13.80

Paracetamol 250 mg Alvedon 250mg suppositories |
10 suppository [P] £27.60 DT = £27.60

Oral suspension

CAUTIONARY AND ADVISORY LABELS 30

▸ Paracetamol (Non-proprietary)

Paracetamol 24 mg per 1 ml Paracetamol 120mg/5ml oral
suspension paediatric | 100 ml [P] £1.25–£1.76 | 500 ml [P] [⊠] DT =
£7.93

Paracetamol 120mg/5ml oral suspension paediatric sugar free sugar-
free | 100 ml [P] £1.85 DT = £1.58 sugar-free | 200 ml [P] £3.16–
£3.18 sugar-free | 500 ml [P] £7.23–£7.90 sugar-free | 1000 ml [P]
£15.90

Paracetamol 50 mg per 1 ml Paracetamol 250mg/5ml oral
suspension | 100 ml [P] £2.72 DT = £2.72 | 500 ml [P] £10.00–£13.60
Paracetamol 250mg/5ml oral suspension sugar free sugar-free |
100 ml [P] £1.43–£1.63 sugar-free | 200 ml [P] £2.85 DT = £2.85
sugar-free | 500 ml [P] £7.10–£7.13 sugar-free | 1000 ml [P] £12.38

Paracetamol 100 mg per 1 ml Paracetamol 500mg/5ml oral
suspension sugar free sugar-free | 150 ml [PoM] £24.00 DT = £24.00

▸ Calpol (McNeil Products Ltd)

Paracetamol 24 mg per 1 ml Calpol Infant 120mg/5ml oral
suspension | 200 ml [P] £3.78

Calpol Infant 120mg/5ml oral suspension sugar free sugar-free |
200 ml [P] £3.78

Paracetamol 50 mg per 1 ml Calpol Six Plus 250mg/5ml oral
suspension | 200 ml [P] £4.40

Calpol Six Plus 250mg/5ml oral suspension sugar free sugar-free |
100 ml [P] £2.64 sugar-free | 200 ml [P] £4.40 DT = £2.85

Effervescent tablet

CAUTIONARY AND ADVISORY LABELS 13, 29(500 mg tablets in
adults), 30

▸ Paracetamol (Non-proprietary)

Paracetamol 500 mg Paracetamol 500mg soluble tablets |
100 tablet [PoM] [⊠] DT = £8.79

Paracetamol 500mg effervescent tablets | 24 tablet [PoM] £1.57–
£2.19 | 60 tablet [PoM] £4.10–£5.27 | 100 tablet [PoM] £8.79 DT =
£8.79

▸ Altridexamol (TriOn Pharma Ltd)

Paracetamol 1 gram Altridexamol 1000mg effervescent tablets
sugar-free | 50 tablet [PoM] £6.59 DT = £6.59

Solution for infusion

▸ Paracetamol (Non-proprietary)

Paracetamol 10 mg per 1 ml Paracetamol 500mg/50ml solution for
infusion bottles | 10 bottle [PoM] £11.00 (Hospital only)

Paracetamol 500mg/50ml solution for infusion vials | 10 vial [PoM]
£15.10

Paracetamol 1g/100ml solution for infusion bottles |
10 bottle [PoM] [⊠]

Paracetamol 1g/100ml solution for infusion vials | 10 vial [PoM]
£12.00 DT = £12.00 (Hospital only) | 10 vial [PoM] £16.40 DT = £12.00
| 12 vial [PoM] £14.40 (Hospital only) | 20 vial [PoM] £24.00 (Hospital
only)

Paracetamol 100mg/10ml solution for infusion ampoules |
20 ampoule [PoM] £12.00

▸ Perfalgan (Bristol-Myers Squibb Pharmaceuticals Ltd)

Paracetamol 10 mg per 1 ml Perfalgan 1g/100ml solution for
infusion vials | 12 vial [PoM] £14.96

Perfalgan 500mg/50ml solution for infusion vials | 12 vial [PoM]
£13.60

Oral solution

CAUTIONARY AND ADVISORY LABELS 30

▸ Paracetamol (Non-proprietary)

Paracetamol 24 mg per 1 ml Paracetamol 120mg/5ml oral solution
paediatric sugar free sugar-free | 2000 ml [P] £23.80 DT = £23.80

Paracetamol 100 mg per 1 ml Paracetamol 500mg/5ml oral
solution sugar free sugar-free | 200 ml [PoM] £18.00 DT = £18.00

Powder

▸ Paracetamol (Non-proprietary)

Paracetamol 650 mg Boots Cold & Flu Relief 650mg oral powder
sachets | 10 sachet [GSL] [⊠]

Value Health Cold Relief Powders Lemon Flavour | 5 sachet [GSL] [⊠]

Capsule

CAUTIONARY AND ADVISORY LABELS 29 (500 mg capsules in adults),
30

▸ Paracetamol (Non-proprietary)

Paracetamol 500 mg Paracetamol 500mg capsules | 100 capsule
[PoM] £5.06 DT = £5.06

Orodispersible tablet

CAUTIONARY AND ADVISORY LABELS 30

▸ Calpol Fastmelts (McNeil Products Ltd)

Paracetamol 250 mg Calpol Six Plus Fastmelts 250mg tablets sugar-
free | 24 tablet [P] £4.12 DT = £4.12

Combinations available: Co-codamol, p. 474 · *Dihydrocodeine
with paracetamol,* p. 477 · *Tramadol with paracetamol,* p. 493

ANALGESICS › NON-OPIOID, CENTRALLY ACTING

Nefopam hydrochloride

09-Nov-2020

● INDICATIONS AND DOSE

Moderate pain

▸ BY MOUTH

▸ **Adult:** Initially 60 mg 3 times a day, adjusted according
to response; usual dose 30–90 mg 3 times a day

▸ **Elderly:** Initially 30 mg 3 times a day, adjusted
according to response; usual dose 30–90 mg 3 times a
day

● CONTRA-INDICATIONS Convulsive disorders · not indicated
for myocardial infarction

● CAUTIONS Angle-closure glaucoma · elderly · urinary
retention

● INTERACTIONS → Appendix 1: nefopam

● SIDE-EFFECTS

▸ **Uncommon** Coma · drowsiness · headache · hyperhidrosis ·
insomnia · tachycardia · vision blurred · vomiting

▸ **Rare or very rare** Urine red

▸ **Frequency not known** Abdominal pain · angioedema ·
confusion · diarrhoea · dizziness · dry mouth ·
gastrointestinal disorder · hallucination · hypotension ·
nausea · nervousness · palpitations · paraesthesia · seizure ·
syncope · tremor · urinary retention

● PREGNANCY No information available—avoid unless no
safer treatment.

● HEPATIC IMPAIRMENT Manufacturer advises caution.

● RENAL IMPAIRMENT Caution.

● MEDICINAL FORMS There can be variation in the licensing of
different medicines containing the same drug. Forms available
from special-order manufacturers include: oral suspension

Tablet

CAUTIONARY AND ADVISORY LABELS 2, 14

▸ Nefopam hydrochloride (Non-proprietary)

Nefopam hydrochloride 30 mg Nefopam 30mg tablets |
30 tablet [PoM] £2.95–£3.97 | 90 tablet [PoM] £68.39 DT = £11.91

ANALGESICS > NON-STEROIDAL ANTI-INFLAMMATORY DRUGS

Aspirin with codeine

14-Jul-2020

The properties listed below are those particular to the combination only. For the properties of the components please consider, aspirin p. 132, codeine phosphate p. 475.

- **INDICATIONS AND DOSE**

  Mild to moderate pain | Pyrexia
  - ▶ BY MOUTH
  - ▶ Adult: 1–2 tablets every 4–6 hours as required; maximum 8 tablets per day

- **INTERACTIONS** → Appendix 1: aspirin · opioids
- **PRESCRIBING AND DISPENSING INFORMATION** When co-codaprin tablets or dispersible tablets are prescribed and no strength is stated, tablets or dispersible tablets, respectively, containing codeine phosphate 8 mg and aspirin 400 mg should be dispensed.
- **LESS SUITABLE FOR PRESCRIBING** Aspirin with codeine is less suitable for prescribing.
- **EXCEPTIONS TO LEGAL CATEGORY** Aspirin with codeine can be sold to the public provided packs contain no more than 32 capsules or tablets; pharmacists can sell multiple packs up to a total quantity of 100 capsules or tablets in justifiable circumstances.

- **MEDICINAL FORMS** There can be variation in the licensing of different medicines containing the same drug.

  Dispersible tablet
  CAUTIONARY AND ADVISORY LABELS 13, 21, 32
  - ▶ Codis (Reckitt Benckiser Healthcare (UK) Ltd)
    Codeine phosphate 8 mg, Aspirin 500 mg Codis 500 dispersible tablets sugar-free | 32 tablet Ⓟ £3.23 CD5

  Tablet
  - ▶ Boots Aspirin and Codeine (The Boots Company Plc)
    Codeine phosphate 8 mg, Aspirin 400 mg Boots Aspirin and Codeine tablets | 32 tablet Ⓟ Ⓢ CD5

ANALGESICS > OPIOIDS

Opioids

IMPORTANT SAFETY INFORMATION

MHRA/CHM ADVICE: BENZODIAZEPINES AND OPIOIDS: REMINDER OF RISK OF POTENTIALLY FATAL RESPIRATORY DEPRESSION (MARCH 2020)

The MHRA reminds healthcare professionals that opioids co-prescribed with benzodiazepines and benzodiazepine-like drugs can produce additive CNS depressant effects, thereby increasing the risk of sedation, respiratory depression, coma, and death. Healthcare professionals are advised to only co-prescribe if there is no alternative and, if necessary, the lowest possible doses should be given for the shortest duration. Patients should be closely monitored for signs of respiratory depression at initiation of treatment and when there is any change in prescribing, such as dose adjustments or new interactions. If methadone is co-prescribed with a benzodiazepine or benzodiazepine-like drug, the respiratory depressant effect of methadone may be delayed; patients should be monitored for at least 2 weeks after initiation or changes in prescribing. Patients should be informed of the signs and symptoms of respiratory depression and sedation, and advised to seek urgent medical attention should these occur.

MHRA/CHM ADVICE: OPIOIDS: RISK OF DEPENDENCE AND ADDICTION (SEPTEMBER 2020)

New safety recommendations have been issued following a review of the risks of dependence and addiction associated with prolonged use (longer than 3 months) of opioids for non-malignant pain.

Healthcare professionals are advised to:
- discuss with patients that prolonged use of opioids, even at therapeutic doses, may lead to dependence and addiction;
- agree a treatment strategy and plan for end of treatment with the patient before starting opioids;
- counsel patients and their carers on the risks of tolerance and potentially fatal unintentional overdose, as well as signs and symptoms of overdose;
- provide regular monitoring and support to patients at increased risk, such as those with current or history of substance use disorder (including alcohol misuse) or mental health disorders;
- taper dosage slowly at the end of treatment to reduce the risk of withdrawal effects associated with abrupt discontinuation (tapering high doses may take weeks or months);
- consider hyperalgesia in patients on long-term opioid treatment who present with increased pain sensitivity;
- consult product literature for the latest advice and warnings for opioid use during pregnancy (see also *Pregnancy*).

The MHRA has also issued a safety leaflet for patients—see *Patient and carer advice*.

- **CONTRA-INDICATIONS** Acute respiratory depression · comatose patients · head injury (opioid analgesics interfere with pupillary responses vital for neurological assessment) · raised intracranial pressure (opioid analgesics interfere with pupillary responses vital for neurological assessment) · risk of paralytic ileus

- **CAUTIONS** Adrenocortical insufficiency (reduced dose is recommended) · asthma (avoid during an acute attack) · central sleep apnoea · convulsive disorders · current or history of mental health disorder · current or history of substance use disorder · debilitated patients (reduced dose is recommended) (in adults) · diseases of the biliary tract · elderly (reduced dose is recommended) · hypotension · hypothyroidism (reduced dose is recommended) · impaired respiratory function (avoid in chronic obstructive pulmonary disease) · inflammatory bowel disorders · myasthenia gravis · obstructive bowel disorders · prostatic hypertrophy (in adults) · shock · urethral stenosis

  CAUTIONS, FURTHER INFORMATION
  - ▶ Dependence and addiction Prolonged use of opioid analgesics may lead to drug dependence and addiction, even at therapeutic doses. There is an increased risk in individuals with current or history of substance use disorder or mental health disorders. See also *Important safety information*.
  - ▶ Central sleep apnoea Opioids cause a dose-dependent increased risk of central sleep apnoea, EvGr consider total opioid dose reduction. ◆
  - ▶ Palliative care EvGr In the control of pain in terminal illness, the cautions listed should not necessarily be a deterrent to the use of opioid analgesics. ◆
  - ▶ Elderly Prescription potentially inappropriate (STOPP criteria):
    - if prescribed a **strong**, **oral** or **transdermal** opioid (i.e. morphine, oxycodone, fentanyl, buprenorphine, diamorphine, methadone, tramadol, pethidine, pentazocine) as first-line therapy for mild pain (WHO analgesic ladder not observed)
    - if used regularly without concomitant laxative (risk of severe constipation)
    - if prescribed a **long-acting (modified-release)** opioid without a **short-acting (immediate-release)** opioid for breakthrough pain (risk of persistence of severe pain)

    See also Prescribing in the elderly p. 33.

● SIDE-EFFECTS

▶ **Common or very common** Arrhythmias · confusion · constipation · dizziness · drowsiness · dry mouth · euphoric mood · flushing · hallucination · headache · hyperhidrosis · hypotension (with high doses) · miosis · nausea (more common on initiation) · palpitations · respiratory depression (with high doses) · skin reactions · urinary retention · vertigo · visual impairment · vomiting (more common on initiation) · withdrawal syndrome

▶ **Uncommon** Drug dependence · dysphoria

SIDE-EFFECTS, FURTHER INFORMATION **Respiratory depression** Respiratory depression is a major concern with opioid analgesics and it may be treated by artificial ventilation or be reversed by naloxone.

Dependence, addiction, and withdrawal Long term use of opioids in non-malignant pain (longer than 3 months) carries an increased risk of dependence and addiction, even at therapeutic doses. At the end of treatment the dosage should be tapered slowly to reduce the risk of withdrawal effects; tapering from a high dose may take weeks or months. See also *Important safety information*.

Overdose Opioids (narcotic analgesics) cause coma, respiratory depression, and pinpoint pupils. For details on the management of poisoning, see Opioids, under Emergency treatment of poisoning p. 1413 and consider the specific antidote, naloxone hydrochloride.

● PREGNANCY Respiratory depression and withdrawal symptoms can occur in the neonate if opioid analgesics are used during delivery; also gastric stasis and inhalation pneumonia has been reported in the mother if opioid analgesics are used during labour.

● TREATMENT CESSATION Avoid abrupt withdrawal after long-term treatment; they should be withdrawn gradually to avoid abstinence symptoms.

● PRESCRIBING AND DISPENSING INFORMATION The *Faculty of Pain Medicine* has produced resources for healthcare professionals around opioid prescribing: www.fpm.ac.uk/faculty-of-pain-medicine/opioids-aware

● PATIENT AND CARER ADVICE

MHRA safety leaflet: Opioid medicines and the risk of addiction www.gov.uk/guidance/opioid-medicines-and-the-risk-of-addiction

Driving and skilled tasks Drowsiness may affect performance of skilled tasks (e.g. driving); effects of alcohol enhanced. Driving at the start of therapy with opioid analgesics, and following dose changes, should be avoided.

For information on 2015 legislation regarding driving whilst taking certain controlled drugs, including opioids, see *Drugs and driving* under Guidance on prescribing p. 1.

Ｆ 467

Buprenorphine
29-Oct-2020

● DRUG ACTION Buprenorphine is an opioid-receptor partial agonist (it has opioid agonist and antagonist properties).

● INDICATIONS AND DOSE

Moderate to severe pain

▶ BY SUBLINGUAL ADMINISTRATION

▶ Child (body-weight 16-25 kg): 100 micrograms every 6–8 hours

▶ Child (body-weight 25-37.5 kg): 100–200 micrograms every 6–8 hours

▶ Child (body-weight 37.5-50 kg): 200–300 micrograms every 6–8 hours

▶ Child (body-weight 50 kg and above): 200–400 micrograms every 6–8 hours

▶ Adult: 200–400 micrograms every 6–8 hours

▶ BY INTRAMUSCULAR INJECTION, OR BY SLOW INTRAVENOUS INJECTION

▶ Child 6 months-11 years: 3–6 micrograms/kg every 6–8 hours (max. per dose 9 micrograms/kg)

▶ Child 12-17 years: 300–600 micrograms every 6–8 hours

▶ Adult: 300–600 micrograms every 6–8 hours

Premedication

▶ BY SUBLINGUAL ADMINISTRATION

▶ Adult: 400 micrograms

▶ BY INTRAMUSCULAR INJECTION

▶ Adult: 300 micrograms

Intra-operative analgesia

▶ BY SLOW INTRAVENOUS INJECTION

▶ Adult: 300–450 micrograms

Adjunct in the treatment of opioid dependence

▶ BY SUBLINGUAL ADMINISTRATION USING SUBLINGUAL TABLETS

▶ Adult: Initially 0.8–4 mg for 1 dose on the first day, adjusted in steps of 2–4 mg daily if required; usual dose 12–24 mg daily; maximum 32 mg per day

▶ BY MOUTH USING ORAL LYOPHILISATE

▶ Adult: Initially 2 mg daily, followed by 2–4 mg if required on day one, adjusted in steps of 2–6 mg daily if required, for adjustment of dosing interval following stabilisation, consult product literature; maximum 18 mg per day

DOSE EQUIVALENCE AND CONVERSION

▶ For opioid substitution therapy, in patients taking methadone who want to switch to buprenorphine, the dose of methadone should be reduced to a maximum of 30 mg daily before starting buprenorphine treatment—consult product literature. For *sublingual tablets*, if the dose of methadone is over 10 mg daily, buprenorphine can be started at a dose of 4 mg daily and titrated according to requirements; if the methadone dose is below 10 mg daily, buprenorphine can be started at a dose of 2 mg daily.

BUTRANS ®

Moderate, non-malignant pain unresponsive to non-opioid analgesics

▶ BY TRANSDERMAL APPLICATION USING PATCHES

▶ Adult: Initially 5 micrograms/hour up to every 7 days, dose adjustments—when starting, analgesic effect should not be evaluated until the system has been worn for 72 hours (to allow for gradual increase in plasma-buprenorphine concentration)—if necessary, dose should be adjusted at intervals of at least 3 days using a patch of the next strength or a combination of 2 patches applied in different places (applied at *same time* to avoid confusion). Maximum 2 patches can be used at any one time

BUPEAZE ®

Moderate to severe chronic cancer pain in patients who have not previously received strong opioid analgesic | Severe pain unresponsive to non-opioid analgesics in patients who have not previously received strong opioid analgesic

▶ BY TRANSDERMAL APPLICATION USING PATCHES

▶ Adult: Initially 35 micrograms/hour up to every 96 hours, dose adjustment—when starting, analgesic effect should not be evaluated until the system has been worn for 24 hours (to allow for gradual increase in plasma-buprenorphine concentration)—if necessary, dose should be adjusted at intervals of no longer than 96 hours using a patch of the next strength or using 2 patches of the same strength (applied at *same time* to avoid confusion). Maximum 2 patches can be used at any one time

Moderate to severe chronic cancer pain in patients who have previously received strong opioid analgesic | Severe pain unresponsive to non-opioid analgesics in patients who have previously received strong opioid analgesic
▶ BY TRANSDERMAL APPLICATION USING PATCHES
▶ Adult: The initial dose should be based on previous 24-hour opioid requirement, consult product literature, dose adjustment—when starting, analgesic effect should not be evaluated until the system has been worn for 24 hours (to allow for gradual increase in plasma-buprenorphine concentration)—if necessary, dose should be adjusted at intervals of no longer than 96 hours using a patch of the next strength or using 2 patches of the same strength (applied at *same time* to avoid confusion). Maximum 2 patches can be used at any one time

PHARMACOKINETICS
▶ For *Bupeaze*®: It may take approximately 30 hours for the plasma-buprenorphine concentration to decrease by 50% after patch is removed.

BUPLAST ®

Moderate to severe chronic cancer pain in patients who have not previously received strong opioid analgesic | Severe pain unresponsive to non-opioid analgesics in patients who have not previously received strong opioid analgesic
▶ BY TRANSDERMAL APPLICATION USING PATCHES
▶ Adult: Initially 35 micrograms/hour up to every 96 hours, dose adjustment—when starting, analgesic effect should not be evaluated until the system has been worn for 24 hours (to allow for gradual increase in plasma-buprenorphine concentration)—if necessary, dose should be adjusted at intervals of no longer than 96 hours using a patch of the next strength or using 2 patches of the same strength (applied at *same time* to avoid confusion). Maximum 2 patches can be used at any one time

Moderate to severe chronic cancer pain in patients who have previously received strong opioid analgesic | Severe pain unresponsive to non-opioid analgesics in patients who have previously received strong opioid analgesic
▶ BY TRANSDERMAL APPLICATION USING PATCHES
▶ Adult: The initial dose should be based on previous 24-hour opioid requirement, consult product literature, dose adjustment—when starting, analgesic effect should not be evaluated until the system has been worn for 24 hours (to allow for gradual increase in plasma-buprenorphine concentration)—if necessary, dose should be adjusted at intervals of no longer than 96 hours using a patch of the next strength or using 2 patches of the same strength (applied at *same time* to avoid confusion). Maximum 2 patches can be used at any one time

PHARMACOKINETICS
▶ For *Buplast*®: It may take approximately 30 hours for the plasma-buprenorphine concentration to decrease by 50% after patch is removed.

BUPRAMYL ®

Moderate, non-malignant pain unresponsive to non-opioid analgesics
▶ BY TRANSDERMAL APPLICATION USING PATCHES
▶ Adult: Initially 5 micrograms/hour up to every 7 days, dose adjustments—when starting, analgesic effect should not be evaluated until the system has been worn for 72 hours (to allow for gradual increase in plasma-buprenorphine concentration)—if necessary, dose should be adjusted at intervals of at least 3 days using a patch of the next strength or a combination of 2 patches applied in different places (applied at

same time to avoid confusion). Maximum 2 patches can be used at any one time

PHARMACOKINETICS
▶ For *Bupramyl*®: It may take approximately 12 hours for the plasma-buprenorphine concentration to decrease by 50% after patch is removed.

BUTEC ®

Moderate, non-malignant pain unresponsive to non-opioid analgesics
▶ BY TRANSDERMAL APPLICATION USING PATCHES
▶ Adult: Initially 5 micrograms/hour up to every 7 days, dose adjustments—when starting, analgesic effect should not be evaluated until the system has been worn for 72 hours (to allow for gradual increase in plasma-buprenorphine concentration)—if necessary, dose should be adjusted at intervals of at least 3 days using a patch of the next strength or a combination of 2 patches applied in different places (applied at *same time* to avoid confusion). Maximum 2 patches can be used at any one time

PHARMACOKINETICS
▶ For *Butec*®: It may take approximately 12 hours for the plasma-buprenorphine concentration to decrease by 50% after patch is removed.

BUVIDAL ®

Adjunct in the treatment of opioid dependence
▶ BY SUBCUTANEOUS INJECTION
▶ Adult: (consult product literature)

PHARMACOKINETICS
▶ Weekly *Buvidal*® has a terminal half-life ranging from 3 to 5 days.
▶ Monthly *Buvidal*® has a terminal half-life ranging from 19 to 25 days.

HAPOCTASIN ®

Moderate to severe chronic cancer pain in patients who have not previously received strong opioid analgesic | Severe pain unresponsive to non-opioid analgesics in patients who have not previously received strong opioid analgesic
▶ BY TRANSDERMAL APPLICATION USING PATCHES
▶ Adult: Initially 35 micrograms/hour up to every 72 hours, dose adjustment—when starting, analgesic effect should not be evaluated until the system has been worn for 24 hours (to allow for gradual increase in plasma-buprenorphine concentration)—if necessary, dose should be adjusted at intervals of no longer than 72 hours using a patch of the next strength or using 2 patches of the same strength (applied at *same time* to avoid confusion). Maximum 2 patches can be used at any one time, for breakthrough pain, consider 200–400 micrograms buprenorphine sublingually

Moderate to severe chronic cancer pain in patients who have previously received strong opioid analgesic | Severe pain unresponsive to non-opioid analgesics in patients who have previously received strong opioid analgesic
▶ BY TRANSDERMAL APPLICATION USING PATCHES
▶ Adult: The initial dose should be based on previous 24-hour opioid requirement, consult product literature, dose adjustment—when starting, analgesic effect should not be evaluated until the system has been worn for 24 hours (to allow for gradual increase in plasma-buprenorphine concentration)—if necessary, dose should be adjusted at intervals of no longer than 72 hours using a patch of the next strength or using 2 patches of the same strength (applied at *same time* to avoid confusion). Maximum 2 patches can be used at any one time, for breakthrough pain, consider 200–400 micrograms buprenorphine sublingually

continued →

4

Nervous system

PHARMACOKINETICS
▶ For *Hapoctasin*®: It may take approximately 25 hours for the plasma-buprenorphine concentration to decrease by 50% after patch is removed.

PANITAZ ®

Moderate, non-malignant pain unresponsive to non-opioid analgesics
▶ BY TRANSDERMAL APPLICATION USING PATCHES
▶ Adult: Initially 5 micrograms/hour up to every 7 days, dose adjustments—when starting, analgesic effect should not be evaluated until the system has been worn for 72 hours (to allow for gradual increase in plasma-buprenorphine concentration)—if necessary, dose should be adjusted at intervals of at least 3 days using a patch of the next strength or a combination of 2 patches applied in different places (applied at *same time* to avoid confusion). Maximum 2 patches can be used at any one time

PHARMACOKINETICS
▶ For *Panitaz*®: It may take approximately 12 hours for the plasma-buprenorphine concentration to decrease by 50% after patch is removed.

PRENOTRIX ®

Moderate to severe chronic cancer pain in patients who have not previously received strong opioid analgesic | Severe pain unresponsive to non-opioid analgesics in patients who have not previously received strong opioid analgesic
▶ BY TRANSDERMAL APPLICATION USING PATCHES
▶ Adult: Initially 35 micrograms/hour up to every 72 hours, dose adjustment—when starting, analgesic effect should not be evaluated until the system has been worn for 24 hours (to allow for gradual increase in plasma-buprenorphine concentration)—if necessary, dose should be adjusted at intervals of no longer than 72 hours using a patch of the next strength or using 2 patches of the same strength (applied at *same time* to avoid confusion). Maximum 2 patches can be used at any one time

Moderate to severe chronic cancer pain in patients who have previously received strong opioid analgesic | Severe pain unresponsive to non-opioid analgesics in patients who have previously received strong opioid analgesic
▶ BY TRANSDERMAL APPLICATION USING PATCHES
▶ Adult: The initial dose should be based on previous 24-hour opioid requirement, consult product literature, dose adjustment—when starting, analgesic effect should not be evaluated until the system has been worn for 24 hours (to allow for gradual increase in plasma-buprenorphine concentration)—if necessary, dose should be adjusted at intervals of no longer than 72 hours using a patch of the next strength or using 2 patches of the same strength (applied at *same time* to avoid confusion). Maximum 2 patches can be used at any one time

PHARMACOKINETICS
▶ For *Prenotrix*®: It may take approximately 25 hours for the plasma-buprenorphine concentration to decrease by 50% after patch is removed.

RELETRANS ®

Moderate, non-malignant pain unresponsive to non-opioid analgesics
▶ BY TRANSDERMAL APPLICATION USING PATCHES
▶ Adult: Initially 5 micrograms/hour up to every 7 days, dose adjustments—when starting, analgesic effect should not be evaluated until the system has been worn for 72 hours (to allow for gradual increase in plasma-buprenorphine concentration)—if necessary, dose should be adjusted at intervals of at least

3 days using a patch of the next strength or a combination of 2 patches applied in different places (applied at *same time* to avoid confusion). Maximum 2 patches can be used at any one time

PHARMACOKINETICS
▶ For *Reletrans*®: It may take approximately 12 hours for the plasma-buprenorphine concentration to decrease by 50% after patch is removed.

RELEVTEC ®

Moderate to severe chronic cancer pain in patients who have not previously received strong opioid analgesic | Severe pain unresponsive to non-opioid analgesics in patients who have not previously received strong opioid analgesic
▶ BY TRANSDERMAL APPLICATION USING PATCHES
▶ Adult: Initially 35 micrograms/hour up to every 96 hours, dose adjustment—when starting, analgesic effect should not be evaluated until the system has been worn for 24 hours (to allow for gradual increase in plasma-buprenorphine concentration)—if necessary, dose should be adjusted at intervals of no longer than 96 hours using a patch of the next strength or using 2 patches of the same strength (applied at *same time* to avoid confusion). Maximum 2 patches can be used at any one time

Moderate to severe chronic cancer pain in patients who have previously received strong opioid analgesic | Severe pain unresponsive to non-opioid analgesics in patients who have previously received strong opioid analgesic
▶ BY TRANSDERMAL APPLICATION USING PATCHES
▶ Adult: The initial dose should be based on previous 24-hour opioid requirement, consult product literature, dose adjustment—when starting, analgesic effect should not be evaluated until the system has been worn for 24 hours (to allow for gradual increase in plasma-buprenorphine concentration)—if necessary, dose should be adjusted at intervals of no longer than 96 hours using a patch of the next strength or using 2 patches of the same strength (applied at *same time* to avoid confusion). Maximum 2 patches can be used at any one time

PHARMACOKINETICS
▶ For *Relevtec*®: It may take approximately 30 hours for the plasma-buprenorphine concentration to decrease by 50% after patch is removed.

SEVODYNE ®

Moderate, non-malignant pain unresponsive to non-opioid analgesics
▶ BY TRANSDERMAL APPLICATION USING PATCHES
▶ Adult: Initially 5 micrograms/hour up to every 7 days, dose adjustments—when starting, analgesic effect should not be evaluated until the system has been worn for 72 hours (to allow for gradual increase in plasma-buprenorphine concentration)—if necessary, dose should be adjusted at intervals of at least 3 days using a patch of the next strength or a combination of 2 patches applied in different places (applied at *same time* to avoid confusion). Maximum 2 patches can be used at any one time

PHARMACOKINETICS
▶ For *Sevodyne*®: It may take approximately 12 hours for the plasma-buprenorphine concentration to decrease by 50% after patch is removed.

TRANSTEC ®

Moderate to severe chronic cancer pain in patients who have not previously received strong opioid analgesic | Severe pain unresponsive to non-opioid analgesics in patients who have not previously received strong opioid analgesic

▶ BY TRANSDERMAL APPLICATION USING PATCHES

▶ Adult: Initially 35 micrograms/hour up to every 96 hours, dose adjustment—when starting, analgesic effect should not be evaluated until the system has been worn for 24 hours (to allow for gradual increase in plasma-buprenorphine concentration)—if necessary, dose should be adjusted at intervals of no longer than 96 hours using a patch of the next strength or using 2 patches of the same strength (applied at *same time* to avoid confusion). Maximum 2 patches can be used at any one time, for breakthrough pain, consider 200–400 micrograms buprenorphine sublingually

Moderate to severe chronic cancer pain in patients who have previously received strong opioid analgesic | Severe pain unresponsive to non-opioid analgesics in patients who have previously received strong opioid analgesic

▶ BY TRANSDERMAL APPLICATION USING PATCHES

▶ Adult: The initial dose should be based on previous 24-hour opioid requirement, consult product literature, dose adjustment—when starting, analgesic effect should not be evaluated until the system has been worn for 24 hours (to allow for gradual increase in plasma-buprenorphine concentration)—if necessary, dose should be adjusted at intervals of no longer than 96 hours using a patch of the next strength or using 2 patches of the same strength (applied at *same time* to avoid confusion). Maximum 2 patches can be used at any one time, for breakthrough pain, consider 200–400 micrograms buprenorphine sublingually

PHARMACOKINETICS

▶ For *Transtec* ®: It may take approximately 30 hours for the plasma-buprenorphine concentration to decrease by 50% after patch is removed.

● UNLICENSED USE

▶ With oral use in children Sublingual tablets not licensed for use in children under 6 years.

> IMPORTANT SAFETY INFORMATION
> ▶ With transdermal use
> Do not confuse the formulations of transdermal patches which are available as 72-hourly, 96-hourly and 7-day patches, see *Prescribing and dispensing information*.

● CAUTIONS

GENERAL CAUTIONS Impaired consciousness

SPECIFIC CAUTIONS

▶ With transdermal use Fever or external heat · other opioids should not be administered within 24 hours of patch removal (long duration of action)

▶ When used for adjunct in the treatment of opioid dependence Hepatitis B infection · hepatitis C infection · pre-existing liver enzyme abnormalities

CAUTIONS, FURTHER INFORMATION

▶ Fever or external heat

▶ With transdermal use Manufacturer advises monitor patients using patches for increased side-effects if fever present (increased absorption possible); avoid exposing application site to external heat (may also increase absorption).

BUVIDAL ® Susceptibility to QT-interval prolongation

● INTERACTIONS → Appendix 1: opioids

● SIDE-EFFECTS

GENERAL SIDE-EFFECTS

▶ **Common or very common** Anxiety · appetite decreased · depression · diarrhoea · dyspnoea · syncope · tremor

SPECIFIC SIDE-EFFECTS

▶ **Common or very common**

▶ With parenteral use Arthralgia (in adults) · asthenia (in adults) · asthma (in adults) · behaviour abnormal (in adults) · chest pain (in adults) · chills (in adults) · cough (in adults) · dysmenorrhoea (in adults) · eye disorders (in adults) · fever (in adults) · gastrointestinal discomfort (in adults) · gastrointestinal disorders (in adults) · hypersensitivity · increased risk of infection (in adults) · insomnia (in adults) · lymphadenopathy (in adults) · malaise (in adults) · migraine (in adults) · muscle complaints (in adults) · muscle tone increased (in adults) · pain (in adults) · paraesthesia (in adults) · peripheral oedema (in adults) · speech disorder (in adults) · thinking abnormal (in adults) · vasodilation (in adults) · withdrawal syndrome neonatal · yawning (in adults)

▶ With sublingual use Fatigue · sleep disorders

▶ With transdermal use Asthenia · gastrointestinal discomfort · muscle weakness · oedema · sleep disorders

▶ **Uncommon**

▶ With parenteral use Procedural dizziness (in adults)

▶ With sublingual use Apnoea · atrioventricular block · coma · conjunctivitis · coordination abnormal · cyanosis · depersonalisation · diplopia · dyspepsia · hypertension · pallor · paraesthesia · psychosis · seizure · speech slurred · tinnitus · urinary disorder

▶ With transdermal use Aggression · chest pain · chills · circulatory collapse · concentration impaired · cough · dry eye · fever · gastrointestinal disorders · hiccups · hypertension · injury · memory loss · migraine · mood altered · movement disorders · muscle complaints · respiratory disorders · sensation abnormal · sexual dysfunction · speech impairment · taste altered · tinnitus · urinary disorders · vision blurred · weight decreased

▶ **Rare or very rare**

▶ With sublingual use Angioedema · bronchospasm

▶ With transdermal use Angina pectoris · asthma exacerbated · dehydration · dysphagia · ear pain · eyelid oedema · increased risk of infection · influenza like illness · muscle contractions involuntary · psychotic disorder · vasodilation

▶ **Frequency not known**

▶ With parenteral use Angioedema · bronchospasm · death (in adults) · hepatic disorders · hepatic encephalopathy (in adults) · psychotic disorder · vision blurred

▶ With sublingual use Cerebrospinal fluid pressure increased · circulation impaired · haemorrhagic diathesis · hepatic disorders · oral disorders

▶ With transdermal use Biliary colic · depersonalisation · seizure · withdrawal syndrome neonatal

Overdose The effects of buprenorphine are only partially reversed by naloxone.

● BREAST FEEDING Present in low levels in breast milk. **Monitoring** Neonates should be monitored for drowsiness, adequate weight gain, and developmental milestones.

● HEPATIC IMPAIRMENT Manufacturer advises caution; avoid in severe impairment (limited information available).

▶ In adults For *transdermal patch*, manufacturer advises consider avoiding in severe impairment. **Dose adjustments** ▶ In adults For *oral lyophilisate*, manufacturer advises initial dose reduction in mild to moderate impairment.

● RENAL IMPAIRMENT Avoid use or reduce dose; opioid effects increased and prolonged; increased cerebral sensitivity.

● PRE-TREATMENT SCREENING Documentation of viral hepatitis status is recommended before commencing therapy for opioid dependence.

- MONITORING REQUIREMENTS Monitor liver function; when used in opioid dependence baseline liver function test is recommended before commencing therapy, and regular liver function tests should be performed throughout treatment.
- DIRECTIONS FOR ADMINISTRATION
  - In children Manufacturer advises *sublingual tablets* may be halved.
  - In adults Manufacturer advises *oral lyophilisates* should be placed on the tongue and allowed to dissolve. Patients should be advised not to swallow for 2 minutes and not to consume food or drink for at least 5 minutes after administration.

    BUTRANS ® Manufacturer advises apply patch to dry, non-irritated, non-hairy skin on upper torso, removing after 7 days and siting replacement patch on a different area (avoid same area for at least 3 weeks).

    HAPOCTASIN ®, PRENOTRIX ® Manufacturer advises apply patch to dry, non-irritated, non-hairy skin on upper torso, removing after no longer than 72 hours and siting replacement patch on a different area (avoid same area for at least 7 days).

    BUPRAMYL ®, BUTEC ®, PANITAZ ®, RELETRANS ®, SEVODYNE ® Manufacturer advises apply patch to dry, non-irritated, non-hairy skin on upper torso or upper outer arm, removing after 7 days and siting replacement patch on a different area (avoid same area for at least 3 weeks).

    BUPEAZE ®, BUPLAST ®, RELEVTEC ®, TRANSTEC ® Manufacturer advises apply patch to dry, non-irritated, non-hairy skin on upper torso, removing after no longer than 96 hours and siting replacement patch on a different area (avoid same area for at least 7 days).

- PRESCRIBING AND DISPENSING INFORMATION
  - In adults Transdermal buprenorphine patches are not suitable for acute pain or in those patients whose analgesic requirements are changing rapidly because the long time to steady state prevents rapid titration of the dose. Transdermal patches are available as 72-hourly, 96-hourly and 7-day formulations; prescribers and dispensers must ensure that the correct preparation is prescribed and dispensed. Preparations that should be applied up to every 72 hours include *Hapoctasin* ® and *Prenotrix* ®. Preparations that should be applied up to every 96 hours include *Bupeaze* ®, *Buplast* ®, *Relevtec* ®, and *Transtec* ®. Preparations that should be applied up to every 7 days include *Bupramyl* ®, *Butec* ®, *BuTrans* ®, *Panitaz* ®, *Reletrans* ®, and *Sevodyne* ®. *Espranor* ® oral lyophilisate has different bioavailability to other buprenorphine products and is not interchangeable with them—consult product literature before switching between products.
- PATIENT AND CARER ADVICE Patients or carers should be given advice on how to administer buprenorphine products.
- NATIONAL FUNDING/ACCESS DECISIONS
  For full details see funding body website

NICE decisions
- Methadone and buprenorphine for the management of opioid dependence (January 2007) NICE TA114 Recommended

Scottish Medicines Consortium (SMC) decisions
- Buprenorphine transdermal patches (*Butec* ®) for the treatment of chronic non-malignant pain of moderate intensity when an opioid is necessary for obtaining adequate analgesia in adults (January 2017) SMC No. 1213/17 Recommended with restrictions
- Buprenorphine oral lyophilisate (*Espranor* ®) as substitution treatment for opioid drug dependence, within a framework of medical, social and psychological treatment (June 2017) SMC No. 1245/17 Recommended with restrictions

- Buprenorphine (*Buvidal* ®) for the treatment of opioid dependence within a framework of medical, social and psychological treatment (August 2019) SMC No. SMC2169 Recommended with restrictions

All Wales Medicines Strategy Group (AWMSG) decisions
- Buprenorphine (*Buvidal* ®) for the treatment of opioid dependence within a framework of medical, social and psychological treatment (September 2019) AWMSG No. 3977 Recommended

- MEDICINAL FORMS There can be variation in the licensing of different medicines containing the same drug.

Solution for injection
- Temgesic (Indivior UK Ltd)
  Buprenorphine (as Buprenorphine hydrochloride)
  300 microgram per 1 ml Temgesic 300micrograms/1ml solution for injection ampoules | 5 ampoule [PoM] £2.46 [CD3]

Sublingual tablet
CAUTIONARY AND ADVISORY LABELS 2, 26
- Buprenorphine (Non-proprietary)
  Buprenorphine (as Buprenorphine hydrochloride)
  400 microgram Buprenorphine 400microgram sublingual tablets sugar free sugar-free | 7 tablet [PoM] £1.67 DT = £1.36 [CD3] sugar-free | 50 tablet [PoM] £13.87 DT = £10.07 [CD3]
  Buprenorphine (as Buprenorphine hydrochloride)
  2 mg Buprenorphine 2mg sublingual tablets sugar free sugar-free | 7 tablet [PoM] £8.35 DT = £4.29 [CD3]
  Buprenorphine (as Buprenorphine hydrochloride)
  8 mg Buprenorphine 8mg sublingual tablets sugar free sugar-free | 7 tablet [PoM] £22.50 DT = £8.98 [CD3]
- Natzon (Morningside Healthcare Ltd)
  Buprenorphine (as Buprenorphine hydrochloride)
  400 microgram Natzon 0.4mg sublingual tablets sugar-free | 7 tablet [PoM] £1.60 DT = £1.36 [CD3]
  Buprenorphine (as Buprenorphine hydrochloride) 2 mg Natzon 2mg sublingual tablets sugar-free | 7 tablet [PoM] £6.35 DT = £4.29 [CD3]
  Buprenorphine (as Buprenorphine hydrochloride) 8 mg Natzon 8mg sublingual tablets sugar-free | 7 tablet [PoM] £19.05 DT = £8.98 [CD3]
- Prefibin (Sandoz Ltd)
  Buprenorphine (as Buprenorphine hydrochloride)
  400 microgram Prefibin 0.4mg sublingual tablets sugar-free | 7 tablet [PoM] £1.60 DT = £1.36 [CD3]
  Buprenorphine (as Buprenorphine hydrochloride) 2 mg Prefibin 2mg sublingual tablets sugar-free | 7 tablet [PoM] £5.38 DT = £4.29 [CD3]
  Buprenorphine (as Buprenorphine hydrochloride) 8 mg Prefibin 8mg sublingual tablets sugar-free | 7 tablet [PoM] £16.15 DT = £8.98 [CD3]
- Subutex (Indivior UK Ltd)
  Buprenorphine (as Buprenorphine hydrochloride)
  400 microgram Subutex 0.4mg sublingual tablets sugar-free | 7 tablet [PoM] £1.36 DT = £1.36 [CD3]
  Buprenorphine (as Buprenorphine hydrochloride) 2 mg Subutex 2mg sublingual tablets sugar-free | 7 tablet [PoM] £4.45 DT = £4.29 [CD3]
  Buprenorphine (as Buprenorphine hydrochloride) 8 mg Subutex 8mg sublingual tablets sugar-free | 7 tablet [PoM] £13.34 DT = £8.98 [CD3]
- Temgesic (Indivior UK Ltd)
  Buprenorphine (as Buprenorphine hydrochloride)
  200 microgram Temgesic 200microgram sublingual tablets sugar-free | 50 tablet [PoM] £5.04 DT = £5.04 [CD3]
  Buprenorphine (as Buprenorphine hydrochloride)
  400 microgram Temgesic 400microgram sublingual tablets sugar-free | 50 tablet [PoM] £10.07 DT = £10.07 [CD3]
- Tephine (Sandoz Ltd)
  Buprenorphine (as Buprenorphine hydrochloride)
  200 microgram Tephine 200microgram sublingual tablets sugar-free | 50 tablet [PoM] £4.27 DT = £5.04 [CD3]
  Buprenorphine (as Buprenorphine hydrochloride)
  400 microgram Tephine 400microgram sublingual tablets sugar-free | 50 tablet [PoM] £8.54 DT = £10.07 [CD3]

Transdermal patch

CAUTIONARY AND ADVISORY LABELS 2

▶ Rebrikel (Zentiva)

Buprenorphine 5 microgram per 1 hour Rebrikel
5micrograms/hour transdermal patches | 4 patch [PoM] £5.53 DT =
£17.60 [CD3]

Buprenorphine 10 microgram per 1 hour Rebrikel
10micrograms/hour transdermal patches | 4 patch [PoM] £9.93 DT =
£31.55 [CD3]

Buprenorphine 20 microgram per 1 hour Rebrikel
20micrograms/hour transdermal patches | 4 patch [PoM] £18.09 DT =
£57.46 [CD3]

▶ BuTrans (Napp Pharmaceuticals Ltd)

Buprenorphine 5 microgram per 1 hour BuTrans
5micrograms/hour transdermal patches | 4 patch [PoM] £17.60 DT =
£17.60 [CD3]

Buprenorphine 10 microgram per 1 hour BuTrans
10micrograms/hour transdermal patches | 4 patch [PoM] £31.55 DT =
£31.55 [CD3]

Buprenorphine 15 microgram per 1 hour BuTrans
15micrograms/hour transdermal patches | 4 patch [PoM] £49.15 DT =
£49.15 [CD3]

Buprenorphine 20 microgram per 1 hour BuTrans
20micrograms/hour transdermal patches | 4 patch [PoM] £57.46 DT =
£57.46 [CD3]

▶ Bunov (Glenmark Pharmaceuticals Europe Ltd)

Buprenorphine 5 microgram per 1 hour Bunov 5micrograms/hour
transdermal patches | 4 patch [PoM] £5.54 DT = £17.60 [CD3]

Buprenorphine 10 microgram per 1 hour Bunov
10micrograms/hour transdermal patches | 4 patch [PoM] £9.94 DT =
£31.55 [CD3]

Buprenorphine 20 microgram per 1 hour Bunov
20micrograms/hour transdermal patches | 4 patch [PoM] £18.10 DT =
£57.46 [CD3]

▶ Bupeaze (Dr Reddy's Laboratories (UK) Ltd)

Buprenorphine 35 microgram per 1 hour Bupeaze
35micrograms/hour transdermal patches | 4 patch [PoM] £9.47 DT =
£15.80 [CD3]

Buprenorphine 52.5 microgram per 1 hour Bupeaze
52.5micrograms/hour transdermal patches | 4 patch [PoM] £13.99 DT
= £23.71 [CD3]

Buprenorphine 70 microgram per 1 hour Bupeaze
70micrograms/hour transdermal patches | 4 patch [PoM] £17.99 DT =
£31.60 [CD3]

▶ Buplast (Mylan)

Buprenorphine 70 microgram per 1 hour Buplast
70micrograms/hour transdermal patches | 4 patch [PoM] £31.60 DT =
£31.60 [CD3]

▶ Bupramyl (Mylan)

Buprenorphine 5 microgram per 1 hour Bupramyl
5micrograms/hour transdermal patches | 4 patch [PoM] £7.04 DT =
£17.60 [CD3]

Buprenorphine 10 microgram per 1 hour Bupramyl
10micrograms/hour transdermal patches | 4 patch [PoM] £12.62 DT =
£31.55 [CD3]

Buprenorphine 20 microgram per 1 hour Bupramyl
20micrograms/hour transdermal patches | 4 patch [PoM] £22.98 DT =
£57.46 [CD3]

▶ Butec (Qdem Pharmaceuticals Ltd)

Buprenorphine 5 microgram per 1 hour Butec 5micrograms/hour
transdermal patches | 4 patch [PoM] £7.92 DT = £17.60 [CD3]

Buprenorphine 10 microgram per 1 hour Butec
10micrograms/hour transdermal patches | 4 patch [PoM] £14.20 DT =
£31.55 [CD3]

Buprenorphine 15 microgram per 1 hour Butec
15micrograms/hour transdermal patches | 4 patch [PoM] £22.12 DT =
£49.15 [CD3]

Buprenorphine 20 microgram per 1 hour Butec
20micrograms/hour transdermal patches | 4 patch [PoM] £25.86 DT =
£57.46 [CD3]

▶ Carlosafine (Glenmark Pharmaceuticals Europe Ltd)

Buprenorphine 35 microgram per 1 hour Carlosafine
35micrograms/hour transdermal patches | 4 patch [PoM] £9.48 DT =
£15.80 [CD3]

Buprenorphine 52.5 microgram per 1 hour Carlosafine
52.5micrograms/hour transdermal patches | 4 patch [PoM] £14.23 DT
= £23.71 [CD3]

Buprenorphine 70 microgram per 1 hour Carlosafine
70micrograms/hour transdermal patches | 4 patch [PoM] £18.96 DT =
£31.60 [CD3]

▶ Hapoctasin (Accord Healthcare Ltd)

Buprenorphine 35 microgram per 1 hour Hapoctasin
35micrograms/hour transdermal patches | 4 patch [PoM] £9.48 DT =
£15.80 [CD3]

Buprenorphine 52.5 microgram per 1 hour Hapoctasin
52.5micrograms/hour transdermal patches | 4 patch [PoM] £14.23 DT
= £23.71 [CD3]

Buprenorphine 70 microgram per 1 hour Hapoctasin
70micrograms/hour transdermal patches | 4 patch [PoM] £18.96 DT =
£31.60 [CD3]

▶ Panitaz (Dr Reddy's Laboratories (UK) Ltd)

Buprenorphine 5 microgram per 1 hour Panitaz 5micrograms/hour
transdermal patches | 4 patch [PoM] £7.04 DT = £17.60 [CD3]

Buprenorphine 10 microgram per 1 hour Panitaz
10micrograms/hour transdermal patches | 4 patch [PoM] £12.62 DT =
£31.55 [CD3]

Buprenorphine 20 microgram per 1 hour Panitaz
20micrograms/hour transdermal patches | 4 patch [PoM] £22.98 DT =
£57.46 [CD3]

▶ Reletrans (Sandoz Ltd)

Buprenorphine 5 microgram per 1 hour Reletrans
5micrograms/hour transdermal patches | 4 patch [PoM] £6.34 DT =
£17.60 [CD3]

Buprenorphine 10 microgram per 1 hour Reletrans
10micrograms/hour transdermal patches | 4 patch [PoM] £11.36 DT =
£31.55 [CD3]

Buprenorphine 15 microgram per 1 hour Reletrans
15micrograms/hour transdermal patches | 4 patch [PoM] £17.70 DT =
£49.15 [CD3]

Buprenorphine 20 microgram per 1 hour Reletrans
20micrograms/hour transdermal patches | 4 patch [PoM] £20.06 DT =
£57.46 [CD3]

▶ Relevtec (Sandoz Ltd)

Buprenorphine 35 microgram per 1 hour Relevtec
35micrograms/hour transdermal patches | 4 patch [PoM] £11.06 DT =
£15.80 [CD3]

Buprenorphine 52.5 microgram per 1 hour Relevtec
52.5micrograms/hour transdermal patches | 4 patch [PoM] £16.60 DT
= £23.71 [CD3]

Buprenorphine 70 microgram per 1 hour Relevtec
70micrograms/hour transdermal patches | 4 patch [PoM] £22.12 DT =
£31.60 [CD3]

▶ Sevodyne (Aspire Pharma Ltd)

Buprenorphine 5 microgram per 1 hour Sevodyne
5micrograms/hour transdermal patches | 4 patch [PoM] £5.53 DT =
£17.60 [CD3]

Buprenorphine 10 microgram per 1 hour Sevodyne
10micrograms/hour transdermal patches | 4 patch [PoM] £9.93 DT =
£31.55 [CD3]

Buprenorphine 15 microgram per 1 hour Sevodyne
15micrograms/hour transdermal patches | 4 patch [PoM] £15.48 DT =
£49.15 [CD3]

Buprenorphine 20 microgram per 1 hour Sevodyne
20micrograms/hour transdermal patches | 4 patch [PoM] £18.09 DT =
£57.46 [CD3]

▶ Transtec (Napp Pharmaceuticals Ltd)

Buprenorphine 35 microgram per 1 hour Transtec
35micrograms/hour transdermal patches | 4 patch [PoM] £15.80 DT =
£15.80 [CD3]

Buprenorphine 52.5 microgram per 1 hour Transtec
52.5micrograms/hour transdermal patches | 4 patch [PoM] £23.71 DT
= £23.71 [CD3]

Buprenorphine 70 microgram per 1 hour Transtec
70micrograms/hour transdermal patches | 4 patch [PoM] £31.60 DT =
£31.60 [CD3]

Oral lyophilisate

CAUTIONARY AND ADVISORY LABELS 2
EXCIPIENTS: May contain Aspartame, gelatin

▶ Espranor (Martindale Pharmaceuticals Ltd)

Buprenorphine (as Buprenorphine hydrochloride) 2 mg Espranor
2mg oral lyophilisates sugar-free | 28 tablet [PoM] £25.40 [CD3]

Buprenorphine (as Buprenorphine hydrochloride) 8 mg Espranor
8mg oral lyophilisates sugar-free | 28 tablet [PoM] £76.20 [CD3]

Prolonged-release solution for injection

▶ Buvidal (Camurus AB)

Buprenorphine 50 mg per 1 ml Buvidal 16mg/0.32ml prolonged-
release solution for injection pre-filled syringes | 1 pre-filled
disposable injection [PoM] £55.93 DT = £55.93 [CD3]
Buvidal 8mg/0.16ml prolonged-release solution for injection pre-filled
syringes | 1 pre-filled disposable injection [PoM] £55.93 DT =
£55.93 [CD3]

Buvidal 24mg/0.48ml prolonged-release solution for injection pre-filled syringes | 1 pre-filled disposable injection [PoM] £55.93 DT = £55.93 [CD3]

Buvidal 32mg/0.64ml prolonged-release solution for injection pre-filled syringes | 1 pre-filled disposable injection [PoM] £55.93 DT = £55.93 [CD3]

Buprenorphine 355.56 mg per 1 ml Buvidal 96mg/0.27ml prolonged-release solution for injection pre-filled syringes | 1 pre-filled disposable injection [PoM] £239.70 DT = £239.70 [CD3]

Buvidal 64mg/0.18ml prolonged-release solution for injection pre-filled syringes | 1 pre-filled disposable injection [PoM] £239.70 DT = £239.70 [CD3]

Buvidal 128mg/0.36ml prolonged-release solution for injection pre-filled syringes | 1 pre-filled disposable injection [PoM] £239.70 DT = £239.70 [CD3]

Co-codamol

F 467

13-Nov-2020

The properties listed below are those particular to the combination only. For the properties of the components please consider, paracetamol p. 464.

● **INDICATIONS AND DOSE**

Moderate pain (using co-codamol 8/500 preparations only)
▸ BY MOUTH
▸ Adult: 8/500–16/1000 mg every 4–6 hours as required; maximum 64/4000 mg per day

Moderate pain (using co-codamol 15/500 preparations only)
▸ BY MOUTH
▸ Adult: 15/500–30/1000 mg every 4–6 hours as required; maximum 120/4000 mg per day

Moderate to severe pain (using co-codamol 30/500 preparations only)
▸ BY MOUTH
▸ Adult: 30/500–60/1000 mg every 4–6 hours as required; maximum 240/4000 mg per day

KAPAKE ® 15/500

Mild to moderate pain
▸ BY MOUTH
▸ Adult: 2 tablets every 4–6 hours as required; maximum 8 tablets per day

SOLPADOL ® CAPLETS

Severe pain
▸ BY MOUTH
▸ Adult: 2 tablets every 4–6 hours as required; maximum 8 tablets per day

SOLPADOL ® CAPSULES

Severe pain
▸ BY MOUTH
▸ Adult: 2 capsules every 4–6 hours as required; maximum 8 capsules per day

SOLPADOL ® EFFERVESCENT TABLETS

Severe pain
▸ BY MOUTH USING EFFERVESCENT TABLETS
▸ Adult: 2 tablets every 4–6 hours as required, tablets to be dispersed in water; maximum 8 tablets per day

● CONTRA-INDICATIONS Acute ulcerative colitis · antibiotic-associated colitis · conditions where abdominal distention develops · conditions where inhibition of peristalsis should be avoided · known ultra-rapid codeine metabolisers

● CAUTIONS Acute abdomen · alcohol dependence · avoid abrupt withdrawal after long-term treatment · cardiac arrhythmias · chronic alcoholism · chronic dehydration · chronic malnutrition · not recommended for adolescents aged 12–18 years with breathing problems

CAUTIONS, FURTHER INFORMATION
▸ Variation in metabolism The capacity to metabolise codeine to morphine can vary considerably between individuals;

there is a marked increase in morphine toxicity in patients who are ultra-rapid codeine metabolisers (CYP2D6 ultra-rapid metabolisers) and a reduced therapeutic effect in poor codeine metabolisers.

● INTERACTIONS → Appendix 1: opioids · paracetamol

● SIDE-EFFECTS Abdominal pain · addiction · agranulocytosis · blood disorder · irritability · pancreatitis · restlessness · severe cutaneous adverse reactions (SCARs) · thrombocytopenia

Overdose Liver damage (and less frequently renal damage) following overdosage with paracetamol.

● BREAST FEEDING Manufacturer advises avoid (recommendation also supported by MHRA and specialist sources). Present in milk and mothers vary considerably in their capacity to metabolise codeine; risk of opioid toxicity in infant.

● HEPATIC IMPAIRMENT Manufacturer advises caution in mild to moderate impairment; avoid in severe impairment. **Dose adjustments** Manufacturer advises consider dose reduction in mild to moderate impairment.

● RENAL IMPAIRMENT Reduce dose or avoid codeine; increased and prolonged effect; increased cerebral sensitivity.

● PRESCRIBING AND DISPENSING INFORMATION Co-codamol is a mixture of codeine phosphate and paracetamol; the proportions are expressed in the form x/y, where x and y are the strengths in milligrams of codeine phosphate and paracetamol respectively.

When co-codamol tablets, dispersible (or effervescent) tablets, or capsules are prescribed and **no strength is stated**, tablets, dispersible (or effervescent) tablets, or capsules, respectively, containing codeine phosphate 8 mg and paracetamol 500 mg should be dispensed.

The Drug Tariff allows tablets of co-codamol labelled 'dispersible' to be dispensed against an order for 'effervescent' and *vice versa*.

● LESS SUITABLE FOR PRESCRIBING Co-codamol is less suitable for prescribing.

● EXCEPTIONS TO LEGAL CATEGORY Co-codamol 8/500 can be sold to the public in certain circumstances; for exemptions see *Medicines, Ethics and Practice*, London, Pharmaceutical Press (always consult latest edition).

● MEDICINAL FORMS There can be variation in the licensing of different medicines containing the same drug. Forms available from special-order manufacturers include: oral suspension, oral solution

Tablet
CAUTIONARY AND ADVISORY LABELS 2(does not apply to the 8/500 tablet), 29, 30
▸ Co-codamol (Non-proprietary)
Codeine phosphate 8 mg, Paracetamol 500 mg Co-codamol 8mg/500mg tablets | 100 tablet [PoM] £5.75 DT = £4.50 [CD5] | 500 tablet [PoM] £22.50 [CD5] | 1000 tablet [PoM] £45.00 [CD5]
Codeine phosphate 15 mg, Paracetamol 500 mg Co-codamol 15mg/500mg tablets | 100 tablet [PoM] £15.00 DT = £3.70 [CD5]
Codeine phosphate 30 mg, Paracetamol 500 mg Co-codamol 30mg/500mg caplets | 100 tablet [PoM] £5.70 DT = £5.70 [CD5] | Co-codamol 30mg/500mg tablets | 30 tablet [PoM] £1.71 DT = £1.71 [CD5] | 100 tablet [PoM] £7.53 DT = £5.70 [CD5]
▸ Codipar (Advanz Pharma)
Codeine phosphate 15 mg, Paracetamol 500 mg Codipar 15mg/500mg tablets | 100 tablet [PoM] £8.25 DT = £3.70 [CD5]
▸ Emcozin (M & A Pharmachem Ltd)
Codeine phosphate 30 mg, Paracetamol 500 mg Emcozin 30mg/500mg tablets | 100 tablet [PoM] £2.94 DT = £5.70 [CD5]
▸ Kapake (Galen Ltd)
Codeine phosphate 30 mg, Paracetamol 500 mg Kapake 30mg/500mg tablets | 100 tablet [PoM] £7.10 DT = £5.70 [CD5]
▸ Migraleve Yellow (McNeil Products Ltd)
Codeine phosphate 8 mg, Paracetamol 500 mg Migraleve Yellow tablets | 16 tablet [PoM] [℞] [CD5]

▸ Panadol Ultra (GlaxoSmithKline Consumer Healthcare)
Codeine phosphate 12.8 mg, Paracetamol 500 mg Panadol Ultra 12.8mg/500mg tablets | 20 tablet P £2.61 DT = £3.81 CD5
▸ Solpadeine Max (Omega Pharma Ltd)
Codeine phosphate 12.8 mg, Paracetamol 500 mg Solpadeine Max 12.8mg/500mg tablets | 20 tablet P £3.81 DT = £3.81 CD5 | 30 tablet P £4.91 DT = £4.91 CD5
▸ Solpadol (Sanofi)
Codeine phosphate 30 mg, Paracetamol 500 mg Solpadol 30mg/500mg caplets | 30 tablet PoM £2.02 DT = £1.71 CD5 | 100 tablet PoM £6.74 DT = £5.70 CD5
▸ Zapain (Advanz Pharma)
Codeine phosphate 30 mg, Paracetamol 500 mg Zapain 30mg/500mg tablets | 100 tablet PoM £3.11 DT = £5.70 CD5

Effervescent tablet
CAUTIONARY AND ADVISORY LABELS 2(does not apply to the 8/500 tablet), 13, 29, 30
EXCIPIENTS: May contain Aspartame
ELECTROLYTES: May contain Sodium
▸ Co-codamol (Non-proprietary)
Codeine phosphate 8 mg, Paracetamol 500 mg Co-codamol 8mg/500mg effervescent tablets sugar free sugar-free | 100 tablet PoM £5.00 CD5
Co-codamol 8mg/500mg effervescent tablets | 100 tablet PoM £8.75 DT = £8.38 CD5
Codeine phosphate 30 mg, Paracetamol 500 mg Co-codamol 30mg/500mg effervescent tablets | 32 tablet PoM £5.40 DT = £2.59 CD5 | 100 tablet PoM £19.20 DT = £8.09 CD5
▸ Codipar (Advanz Pharma)
Codeine phosphate 15 mg, Paracetamol 500 mg Codipar 15mg/500mg effervescent tablets sugar-free | 100 tablet PoM £8.25 DT = £8.25 CD5
▸ Solpadol (Sanofi)
Codeine phosphate 30 mg, Paracetamol 500 mg Solpadol 30mg/500mg effervescent tablets | 32 tablet PoM £2.59 DT = £2.59 CD5 | 100 tablet PoM £8.90 DT = £8.09 CD5

Oral solution
▸ Co-codamol (Non-proprietary)
Codeine phosphate 6 mg per 1 ml, Paracetamol 100 mg per 1 ml Co-codamol 30mg/500mg/5ml oral solution sugar free sugar-free | 150 ml PoM £11.99 CD5 sugar-free | 150 ml PoM £1.99 (Hospital only) CD5

Capsule
CAUTIONARY AND ADVISORY LABELS 2(does not apply to the 8/500 capsule), 29, 30
EXCIPIENTS: May contain Sulfites
▸ Co-codamol (Non-proprietary)
Codeine phosphate 8 mg, Paracetamol 500 mg Co-codamol 8mg/500mg capsules | 32 capsule PoM ℞ DT = £7.16 CD5 | 100 capsule PoM £23.63 DT = £22.36 CD5
Codeine phosphate 15 mg, Paracetamol 500 mg Co-codamol 15mg/500mg capsules | 100 capsule PoM £9.05 DT = £9.05 CD5
Codeine phosphate 30 mg, Paracetamol 500 mg Co-codamol 30mg/500mg capsules | 100 capsule PoM £7.01 DT = £5.70 CD5
▸ Codipar (Advanz Pharma)
Codeine phosphate 15 mg, Paracetamol 500 mg Codipar 15mg/500mg capsules | 100 capsule PoM £7.25 DT = £9.05 CD5
▸ Kapake (Galen Ltd)
Codeine phosphate 30 mg, Paracetamol 500 mg Kapake 30mg/500mg capsules | 100 capsule PoM £7.10 DT = £5.70 CD5
▸ Solpadol (Sanofi)
Codeine phosphate 30 mg, Paracetamol 500 mg Solpadol 30mg/500mg capsules | 100 capsule PoM £6.74 DT = £5.70 CD5
▸ Tylex (UCB Pharma Ltd)
Codeine phosphate 30 mg, Paracetamol 500 mg Tylex 30mg/500mg capsules | 100 capsule PoM £7.93 DT = £5.70 CD5
▸ Zapain (Advanz Pharma)
Codeine phosphate 30 mg, Paracetamol 500 mg Zapain 30mg/500mg capsules | 100 capsule PoM £3.85 DT = £5.70 CD5

◤ 467

Codeine phosphate
13-Nov-2020

● **INDICATIONS AND DOSE**

Acute diarrhoea
▸ BY MOUTH
▸ Child 12–17 years: 30 mg 3–4 times a day; usual dose 15–60 mg 3–4 times a day

▸ Adult: 30 mg 3–4 times a day; usual dose 15–60 mg 3–4 times a day

Mild to moderate pain
▸ BY MOUTH
▸ Adult: 30–60 mg every 4 hours if required; maximum 240 mg per day
▸ BY INTRAMUSCULAR INJECTION
▸ Adult: 30–60 mg every 4 hours if required

Short-term treatment of acute moderate pain
▸ BY MOUTH, OR BY INTRAMUSCULAR INJECTION
▸ Child 12–17 years: 30–60 mg every 6 hours if required for maximum 3 days; maximum 240 mg per day

Dry or painful cough
▸ BY MOUTH USING LINCTUS
▸ Adult: 15–30 mg 3–4 times a day

IMPORTANT SAFETY INFORMATION

MHRA/CHM ADVICE (JULY 2013) CODEINE FOR ANALGESIA: RESTRICTED USE IN CHILDREN DUE TO REPORTS OF MORPHINE TOXICITY

Codeine should only be used to relieve acute moderate pain in children older than 12 years and only if it cannot be relieved by other painkillers such as paracetamol or ibuprofen alone. A significant risk of serious and life-threatening adverse reactions has been identified in children with obstructive sleep apnoea who received codeine after tonsillectomy or adenoidectomy:
- in children aged 12–18 years, the maximum daily dose of codeine should not exceed 240 mg. Doses may be taken up to four times a day at intervals of no less than 6 hours. The lowest effective dose should be used and duration of treatment should be limited to 3 days
- codeine is contra-indicated in all children (under 18 years) who undergo the removal of tonsils or adenoids for the treatment of obstructive sleep apnoea
- codeine is not recommended for use in children whose breathing may be compromised, including those with neuromuscular disorders, severe cardiac or respiratory conditions, respiratory infections, multiple trauma or extensive surgical procedures
- codeine is contra-indicated in patients of any age who are known to be ultra-rapid metabolisers of codeine (CYP2D6 ultra-rapid metabolisers)
- codeine should not be used in breast-feeding mothers because it can pass to the baby through breast milk
- parents and carers should be advised on how to recognise signs and symptoms of morphine toxicity, and to stop treatment and seek medical attention if signs or symptoms of toxicity occur (including reduced consciousness, lack of appetite, somnolence, constipation, respiratory depression, 'pin-point' pupils, nausea, vomiting)

MHRA/CHM ADVICE (APRIL 2015) CODEINE FOR COUGH AND COLD: RESTRICTED USE IN CHILDREN
Do not use codeine in children under 12 years as it is associated with a risk of respiratory side effects. Codeine is not recommended for adolescents (12–18 years) who have problems with breathing. When prescribing or dispensing codeine-containing medicines for cough and cold, consider that codeine is contra-indicated in:
- children younger than 12 years old
- patients of any age known to be CYP2D6 ultra-rapid metabolisers
- breastfeeding mothers

● **CONTRA-INDICATIONS** Acute ulcerative colitis · antibiotic-associated colitis · children under 18 years who undergo the removal of tonsils or adenoids for the treatment of obstructive sleep apnoea · conditions where abdominal distension develops · conditions where inhibition of peristalsis should be avoided · known ultra-rapid codeine metabolisers

- CAUTIONS Acute abdomen · cardiac arrhythmias · gallstones · not recommended for adolescents aged 12–18 years with breathing problems
  CAUTIONS, FURTHER INFORMATION
  ‣ Variation in metabolism The capacity to metabolise codeine to morphine can vary considerably between individuals; there is a marked increase in morphine toxicity in patients who are ultra-rapid codeine metabolisers (CYP2D6 ultra-rapid metabolisers) and a reduced therapeutic effect in poor codeine metabolisers.
- INTERACTIONS → Appendix 1: opioids
- SIDE-EFFECTS
  GENERAL SIDE-EFFECTS
  Biliary spasm · hypothermia · mood altered · sexual dysfunction · ureteral spasm
  SPECIFIC SIDE-EFFECTS
  ‣ With oral use Abdominal cramps · addiction · appetite decreased · depression · drug reaction with eosinophilia and systemic symptoms (DRESS) · dyskinesia · dyspnoea · face oedema · fatigue · fever · hyperglycaemia · hypersensitivity · intracranial pressure increased · lymphadenopathy · malaise · muscle rigidity (with high doses) · nightmare · pancreatitis · restlessness · seizure · splenomegaly · urinary disorders · vision disorders
  ‣ With parenteral use Dysuria
- BREAST FEEDING Manufacturer advises avoid (recommendation also supported by MHRA and specialist sources). Present in milk and mothers vary considerably in their capacity to metabolise codeine; risk of opioid toxicity in infant.
- HEPATIC IMPAIRMENT
  ‣ With oral use Manufacturer advises caution in mild to moderate impairment; avoid in severe impairment.
  ‣ With intramuscular use Manufacturer advises avoid.
  Dose adjustments ‣ With oral use Manufacturer advises dose reduction in mild to moderate impairment.
- RENAL IMPAIRMENT Avoid use or reduce dose; opioid effects increased and prolonged and increased cerebral sensitivity occurs.
- PRESCRIBING AND DISPENSING INFORMATION BP directs that when Diabetic Codeine Linctus is prescribed, Codeine Linctus formulated with a vehicle appropriate for administration to diabetics, whether or not labelled 'Diabetic Codeine Linctus', shall be dispensed or supplied.
- PATIENT AND CARER ADVICE
  Medicines for Children leaflet: Codeine phosphate for pain
  www.medicinesforchildren.org.uk/codeine-phosphate-pain-0

- MEDICINAL FORMS There can be variation in the licensing of different medicines containing the same drug. Forms available from special-order manufacturers include: oral suspension, oral solution, solution for injection

Tablet
CAUTIONARY AND ADVISORY LABELS 2
‣ Codeine phosphate (Non-proprietary)
Codeine phosphate 15 mg Codeine 15mg tablets | 28 tablet [PoM] £1.40 DT = £1.06 [CD5] | 100 tablet [PoM] £3.79 DT = £3.79 [CD5]
Codeine phosphate 30 mg Codeine 30mg tablets | 28 tablet [PoM] £1.59 DT = £1.23 [CD5] | 100 tablet [PoM] £5.68 DT = £4.39 [CD5] | 500 tablet [PoM] £21.95 [CD5]
Codeine phosphate 60 mg Codeine 60mg tablets | 28 tablet [PoM] £2.50 DT = £2.50 [CD5]

Solution for injection
‣ Codeine phosphate (Non-proprietary)
Codeine phosphate 60 mg per 1 ml Codeine 60mg/1ml solution for injection ampoules | 10 ampoule [PoM] £27.20 DT = £24.19 [CD2]

Oral solution
CAUTIONARY AND ADVISORY LABELS 2
‣ Codeine phosphate (Non-proprietary)
Codeine phosphate 3 mg per 1 ml Codeine 15mg/5ml linctus sugar free sugar-free | 200 ml [P] £1.90 DT = £1.63 [CD5] sugar-free | 2000 ml [P] £16.30 [CD5]
Codeine 15mg/5ml linctus | 200 ml [P] £1.73–£1.90 DT = £1.90 [CD5]
Codeine phosphate 5 mg per 1 ml Codeine 25mg/5ml oral solution | 500 ml [PoM] £6.64 DT = £6.64 [CD5]
‣ Galcodine (Thornton & Ross Ltd)
Codeine phosphate 3 mg per 1 ml Galcodine 15mg/5ml linctus sugar-free | 2000 ml [P] £9.90 [CD5]

Combinations available: **Aspirin with codeine**, p. 467

⌐ 467

Diamorphine hydrochloride

13-Nov-2020

(Heroin hydrochloride)

- INDICATIONS AND DOSE
Acute pain
▸ BY INTRAMUSCULAR INJECTION, OR BY SUBCUTANEOUS INJECTION
‣ Adult: 5 mg every 4 hours if required
▸ BY SLOW INTRAVENOUS INJECTION
‣ Adult: 1.25–2.5 mg every 4 hours if required
Acute pain (heavier, well-muscled patients)
▸ BY INTRAMUSCULAR INJECTION, OR BY SUBCUTANEOUS INJECTION
‣ Adult: Up to 10 mg every 4 hours if required
▸ BY SLOW INTRAVENOUS INJECTION
‣ Adult: 2.5–5 mg every 4 hours if required
Chronic pain not currently treated with a strong opioid analgesic
▸ BY SUBCUTANEOUS INJECTION, OR BY INTRAMUSCULAR INJECTION
‣ Adult: Initially 2.5–5 mg every 4 hours, adjusted according to response
▸ BY SUBCUTANEOUS INFUSION
‣ Adult: Initially 5–10 mg, adjusted according to response, dose to be administered over 24 hours
Acute pulmonary oedema
▸ BY SLOW INTRAVENOUS INJECTION
‣ Adult: 2.5–5 mg, dose to be administered at a rate of 1 mg/minute
Myocardial infarction
▸ BY SLOW INTRAVENOUS INJECTION
‣ Adult: 5 mg, followed by 2.5–5 mg if required, dose to be administered at a rate of 1–2 mg/minute
‣ Elderly: 2.5 mg, followed by 1.25–2.5 mg if required, dose to be administered at a rate of 1–2 mg/minute
Myocardial infarction (frail patients)
▸ BY SLOW INTRAVENOUS INJECTION
‣ Adult: 2.5 mg, followed by 1.25–2.5 mg if required, dose to be administered at a rate of 1–2 mg/minute

- CONTRA-INDICATIONS Delayed gastric emptying · phaeochromocytoma
- CAUTIONS CNS depression · severe cor pulmonale · severe diarrhoea · toxic psychosis
- INTERACTIONS → Appendix 1: opioids
- SIDE-EFFECTS Biliary spasm · circulatory depression · intracranial pressure increased · mood altered
- BREAST FEEDING Therapeutic doses unlikely to affect infant; withdrawal symptoms in infants of dependent mothers; breast-feeding not best method of treating dependence in offspring.
- HEPATIC IMPAIRMENT Manufacturer advises caution.
  Dose adjustments Manufacturer advises dose reduction.

● RENAL IMPAIRMENT Avoid use or reduce dose; opioid effects increased and prolonged; increased cerebral sensitivity.

● MEDICINAL FORMS There can be variation in the licensing of different medicines containing the same drug. Forms available from special-order manufacturers include: capsule, oral solution, solution for injection, powder for solution for injection

Powder for solution for injection
▸ Diamorphine hydrochloride (Non-proprietary)
Diamorphine hydrochloride 5 mg Diamorphine 5mg powder for solution for injection ampoules | 5 ampoule [PoM] £12.81 DT = £12.81 [CD2]
Diamorphine hydrochloride 10 mg Diamorphine 10mg powder for solution for injection ampoules | 5 ampoule [PoM] £15.97-£16.56 [CD2]
Diamorphine hydrochloride 30 mg Diamorphine 30mg powder for solution for injection ampoules | 5 ampoule [PoM] £16.72 DT = £15.33 [CD2]
Diamorphine hydrochloride 100 mg Diamorphine 100mg powder for solution for injection ampoules | 5 ampoule [PoM] £42.44 DT = £42.44 [CD2]
Diamorphine hydrochloride 500 mg Diamorphine 500mg powder for solution for injection ampoules | 5 ampoule [PoM] £187.80 DT = £187.80 [CD2]

F 467

Dihydrocodeine tartrate
12-Nov-2020

● INDICATIONS AND DOSE

Moderate to severe pain
▸ BY MOUTH USING IMMEDIATE-RELEASE MEDICINES
▸ Child 4-11 years: 0.5-1 mg/kg every 4-6 hours (max. per dose 30 mg)
▸ Child 12-17 years: 30 mg every 4-6 hours
▸ Adult: 30 mg every 4-6 hours as required
▸ BY DEEP SUBCUTANEOUS INJECTION, OR BY INTRAMUSCULAR INJECTION
▸ Adult: Up to 50 mg every 4-6 hours if required

Chronic severe pain
▸ BY MOUTH USING MODIFIED-RELEASE MEDICINES
▸ Child 12-17 years: 60-120 mg every 12 hours
▸ Adult: 60-120 mg every 12 hours

DF118 FORTE®

Severe pain
▸ BY MOUTH
▸ Child 12-17 years: 40-80 mg 3 times a day; maximum 240 mg per day
▸ Adult: 40-80 mg 3 times a day; maximum 240 mg per day

● CAUTIONS Pancreatitis · severe cor pulmonale

● INTERACTIONS → Appendix 1: opioids

● SIDE-EFFECTS

GENERAL SIDE-EFFECTS
Dysuria · mood altered
SPECIFIC SIDE-EFFECTS
▸ With oral use Biliary spasm · bronchospasm · hypothermia · sexual dysfunction · ureteral spasm

● BREAST FEEDING Use only if potential benefit outweighs risk.

● HEPATIC IMPAIRMENT Manufacturer advises caution; consider avoiding.
Dose adjustments Manufacturer advises dose reduction, if used.

● RENAL IMPAIRMENT Avoid use or reduce dose; opioid effects increased and prolonged and increased cerebral sensitivity occurs.

● PROFESSION SPECIFIC INFORMATION
Dental practitioners' formulary
Dihydrocodeine tablets 30 mg may be prescribed.

● MEDICINAL FORMS There can be variation in the licensing of different medicines containing the same drug. Forms available from special-order manufacturers include: oral suspension, oral solution

Modified-release tablet
CAUTIONARY AND ADVISORY LABELS 2, 25
▸ DHC Continus (Napp Pharmaceuticals Ltd)
Dihydrocodeine tartrate 60 mg DHC Continus 60mg tablets | 56 tablet [PoM] £5.20 DT = £5.20 [CD5]
Dihydrocodeine tartrate 90 mg DHC Continus 90mg tablets | 56 tablet [PoM] £8.66 DT = £8.66 [CD5]
Dihydrocodeine tartrate 120 mg DHC Continus 120mg tablets | 56 tablet [PoM] £10.95 DT = £10.95 [CD5]

Tablet
CAUTIONARY AND ADVISORY LABELS 2
▸ Dihydrocodeine tartrate (Non-proprietary)
Dihydrocodeine tartrate 30 mg Dihydrocodeine 30mg tablets | 28 tablet [PoM] £1.26 DT = £1.26 [CD5] | 30 tablet [PoM] £1.34-£1.63 [CD5] | 100 tablet [PoM] £4.50 DT = £4.50 [CD5]

Solution for injection
▸ Dihydrocodeine tartrate (Non-proprietary)
Dihydrocodeine tartrate 50 mg per 1 ml Dihydrocodeine 50mg/1ml solution for injection ampoules | 10 ampoule [PoM] £133.75 DT = £133.75 [CD2]

F 467

Dihydrocodeine with paracetamol
13-Nov-2020

The properties listed below are those particular to the combination only. For the properties of the components please consider, paracetamol p. 464.

● INDICATIONS AND DOSE

Mild to moderate pain (using 10/500 preparations only)
▸ BY MOUTH
▸ Adult: 10/500-20/1000 mg every 4-6 hours as required; maximum 80/4000 mg per day

Severe pain (using 20/500 preparations only)
▸ BY MOUTH
▸ Adult: 20/500-40/1000 mg every 4-6 hours as required; maximum 160/4000 mg per day

Severe pain (using 30/500 preparations only)
▸ BY MOUTH
▸ Adult: 30/500-60/1000 mg every 4-6 hours as required; maximum 240/4000 mg per day

DOSE EQUIVALENCE AND CONVERSION
▸ A mixture of dihydrocodeine tartrate and paracetamol; the proportions are expressed in the form x/y, where x and y are the strengths in milligrams of dihydrocodeine and paracetamol respectively.

IMPORTANT SAFETY INFORMATION
MHRA/CHM ADVICE: DIHYDROCODEINE WITH PARACETAMOL (CO-DYDRAMOL): PRESCRIBE AND DISPENSE BY STRENGTH TO MINIMISE RISK OF MEDICATION ERROR (JANUARY 2018)
The MHRA has advised that dihydrocodeine with paracetamol preparations are prescribed and dispensed by strength to minimise dispensing errors and the risk of accidental opioid overdose—see Prescribing and dispensing information.

● CAUTIONS Alcohol dependence · before administering, check when paracetamol last administered and cumulative paracetamol dose over previous 24 hours · chronic alcoholism · chronic dehydration · chronic malnutrition · pancreatitis · severe cor pulmonale

● INTERACTIONS → Appendix 1: opioids · paracetamol

4

Nervous system

- SIDE-EFFECTS Abdominal pain · blood disorder · leucopenia · malaise · neutropenia · pancreatitis · paraesthesia · paralytic ileus · severe cutaneous adverse reactions (SCARs) · thrombocytopenia

  Overdose Liver damage (and less frequently renal damage) following overdosage with paracetamol.
- BREAST FEEDING Amount of dihydrocodeine too small to be harmful but use only if potential benefit outweighs risk.
- HEPATIC IMPAIRMENT Manufacturer advises consider avoiding in mild to moderate impairment; avoid in severe impairment.

  Dose adjustments Manufacturer advises dose reduction in mild to moderate impairment, if used.
- RENAL IMPAIRMENT Reduce dose or avoid dihydrocodeine; increased and prolonged effect; increased cerebral sensitivity.
- PRESCRIBING AND DISPENSING INFORMATION The MHRA advises when prescribing dihydrocodeine with paracetamol, the tablet strength and dose must be clearly indicated; when dispensing dihydrocodeine with paracetamol, ensure the prescribed strength is supplied—contact the prescriber if in doubt.

  The BP defines *Co-dydramol* Tablets as containing dihydrocodeine tartrate 10 mg and paracetamol 500 mg.
- LESS SUITABLE FOR PRESCRIBING Dihydrocodeine with paracetamol is less suitable for prescribing.

- MEDICINAL FORMS There can be variation in the licensing of different medicines containing the same drug. Forms available from special-order manufacturers include: oral suspension, oral solution

  Tablet

  CAUTIONARY AND ADVISORY LABELS 2, 29, 30
  - Dihydrocodeine with paracetamol (Non-proprietary)
  Dihydrocodeine tartrate 10 mg, Paracetamol 500 mg Co-dydramol 10mg/500mg tablets | 30 tablet [PoM] £2.49 DT = £1.69 [CD5] | 100 tablet [PoM] £8.30 DT = £5.63 [CD5] | 500 tablet [PoM] £28.15 [CD5]
  Dihydrocodeine tartrate 20 mg, Paracetamol 500 mg Co-dydramol 20mg/500mg tablets | 56 tablet [PoM] £5.87–£7.01 [CD5] | 112 tablet [PoM] £14.01 DT = £14.01 [CD5]
  Dihydrocodeine tartrate 30 mg, Paracetamol 500 mg Co-dydramol 30mg/500mg tablets | 56 tablet [PoM] £10.51 DT = £10.51 [CD5]
  - Paramol (SSL International Plc)
  Dihydrocodeine tartrate 7.46 mg, Paracetamol 500 mg Paramol tablets | 12 tablet [P] £2.45 [CD5] | 24 tablet [P] £4.20 [CD5] | 32 tablet [P] £4.85 [CD5]
  - Remedeine (Crescent Pharma Ltd)
  Dihydrocodeine tartrate 20 mg, Paracetamol 500 mg Remedeine tablets | 56 tablet [PoM] £5.87 [CD5] | 112 tablet [PoM] £11.13 DT = £14.01 [CD5]
  Dihydrocodeine tartrate 30 mg, Paracetamol 500 mg Remedeine Forte tablets | 56 tablet [PoM] £6.82 DT = £10.51 [CD5]

F 467

Dipipanone hydrochloride with cyclizine

- INDICATIONS AND DOSE

  Acute pain
  - BY MOUTH
  - Adult: Initially 1 tablet every 6 hours, then increased if necessary up to 3 tablets every 6 hours, dose to be increased gradually

- CAUTIONS Diabetes mellitus · palliative care (not recommended) · phaeochromocytoma
- INTERACTIONS → Appendix 1: antihistamines, sedating · opioids
- SIDE-EFFECTS Agranulocytosis · anxiety · biliary spasm · consciousness impaired · dry throat · dysuria · hallucinations · hepatic disorders · insomnia · intracranial

pressure increased · mood altered · movement disorders · muscle complaints · nasal dryness · psychosis · renal spasm · seizure · speech disorder · tremor · vision blurred

- BREAST FEEDING No information available.
- HEPATIC IMPAIRMENT Manufacturer advises caution in mild to moderate impairment; avoid in severe impairment. **Dose adjustments** Manufacturer advises dose reduction in mild to moderate impairment; adjust according to response.
- RENAL IMPAIRMENT Avoid use or reduce dose; opioid effects increased and prolonged and increased cerebral sensitivity occurs.

- MEDICINAL FORMS There can be variation in the licensing of different medicines containing the same drug.

  Tablet
  - Dipipanone hydrochloride with cyclizine (Non-proprietary)
  Dipipanone hydrochloride 10 mg, Cyclizine hydrochloride 30 mg Dipipanone 10mg / Cyclizine 30mg tablets | 50 tablet [PoM] £440.65 DT = £440.65 [CD2]

F 467

Fentanyl

03-Dec-2020

- INDICATIONS AND DOSE

  Chronic intractable pain not currently treated with a strong opioid analgesic (not opioid-naive patients)
  - BY TRANSDERMAL APPLICATION
  - Child 16-17 years: Initially 12 micrograms/hour every 72 hours, alternatively initially 25 micrograms/hour every 72 hours, when starting, evaluation of the analgesic effect should not be made before the system has been worn for 24 hours (to allow for the gradual increase in plasma-fentanyl concentration)—previous analgesic therapy should be phased out gradually from time of first patch application, dose should be adjusted at 72 hour intervals in steps of 12–25 micrograms/hour if necessary. After a dose increase, the system should be worn through two 72-hour applications before any further increase in dose, more than one patch may be used at a time (but applied at the same time to avoid confusion)—consider additional or alternative analgesic therapy if dose required exceeds 300 micrograms/hour (important: it takes 20 hours or more for the plasma-fentanyl concentration to decrease by 50%—replacement opioid therapy should be initiated at a low dose and increased gradually)
  - Adult: Initially 12 micrograms/hour every 72 hours, alternatively initially 25 micrograms/hour every 72 hours, when starting, evaluation of the analgesic effect should not be made before the system has been worn for 24 hours (to allow for the gradual increase in plasma-fentanyl concentration)—previous analgesic therapy should be phased out gradually from time of first patch application, dose should be adjusted at 72 hour intervals in steps of 12–25 micrograms/hour if necessary. After a dose increase, the system should be worn through two 72-hour applications before any further increase in dose, more than one patch may be used at a time (but applied at the same time to avoid confusion)—consider additional or alternative analgesic therapy if dose required exceeds 300 micrograms/hour (important: it takes 20 hours or more for the plasma-fentanyl concentration to decrease by 50%—replacement opioid therapy should be initiated at a low dose and increased gradually)

  Chronic intractable pain currently treated with a strong opioid analgesic
  - BY TRANSDERMAL APPLICATION
  - Child 2-17 years: Initial dose based on previous 24-hour opioid requirement—consult product literature, for

evaluating analgesic efficacy and dose increments—consult product literature, for conversion from long term oral morphine to transdermal fentanyl, see *Pain management with opioids* under Prescribing in palliative care p. 28.

▸ Adult: Initial dose based on previous 24-hour opioid requirement—consult product literature, for evaluating analgesic efficacy and dose increments, see under *Chronic intractable pain not currently treated with a strong opioid analgesic (not opioid-naive patients)*, for conversion from long term oral morphine to transdermal fentanyl, see *Pain management with opioids* under Prescribing in palliative care p. 28.

Spontaneous respiration: analgesia and enhancement of anaesthesia, during operation
▸ BY SLOW INTRAVENOUS INJECTION
▸ Adult: Initially 50–100 micrograms (max. per dose 200 micrograms), dose maximum on specialist advice, then 25–50 micrograms as required
▸ BY INTRAVENOUS INFUSION
▸ Adult: 3–4.8 micrograms/kg/hour, adjusted according to response

Assisted ventilation: analgesia and enhancement of anaesthesia during operation
▸ BY SLOW INTRAVENOUS INJECTION
▸ Adult: Initially 300–3500 micrograms, then 100–200 micrograms as required
▸ BY INTRAVENOUS INFUSION
▸ Adult: Initially 10 micrograms/kg, dose to be given over 10 minutes, then 6 micrograms/kg/hour, adjusted according to response, may require up to 180 micrograms/kg/hour during cardiac surgery

Assisted ventilation: analgesia and respiratory depression in intensive care
▸ BY SLOW INTRAVENOUS INJECTION
▸ Adult: Initially 300–3500 micrograms, then 100–200 micrograms as required
▸ BY INTRAVENOUS INFUSION
▸ Adult: Initially 10 micrograms/kg, dose to be given over 10 minutes, then 6 micrograms/kg/hour, adjusted according to response, may require up to 180 micrograms/kg/hour during cardiac surgery

Breakthrough pain in patients receiving opioid therapy for chronic cancer pain
▸ BY BUCCAL ADMINISTRATION USING LOZENGES
▸ Child 16–17 years: Initially 200 micrograms, dose to be given over 15 minutes, then 200 micrograms after 15 minutes if required, no more than 2 dose units for each pain episode; if adequate pain relief not achieved with 1 dose unit for consecutive breakthrough pain episodes, increase the strength of the dose unit until adequate pain relief achieved with 4 lozenges or less daily, if more than 4 episodes of breakthrough pain each day, adjust background analgesia
▸ Adult: Initially 200 micrograms, dose to be given over 15 minutes, then 200 micrograms after 15 minutes if required, no more than 2 dose units for each pain episode; if adequate pain relief not achieved with 1 dose unit for consecutive breakthrough pain episodes, increase the strength of the dose unit until adequate pain relief achieved with 4 lozenges or less daily, if more than 4 episodes of breakthrough pain each day, adjust background analgesia
▸ BY BUCCAL ADMINISTRATION USIOG BUCCAL FILMS
▸ Adult: Initially 200 micrograms, adjusted according to response, consult product literature for information on dose adjustments, maximum 1.2 mg per episode of breakthrough pain; leave at least 4 hours between treatment of episodes of breakthrough pain, if more than 4 episodes of breakthrough pain each day occur

on more than 4 consecutive days, adjust background analgesia

DOSE EQUIVALENCE AND CONVERSION
▸ Fentanyl films are **not bioequivalent** to other fentanyl preparations.
▸ Fentanyl preparations for the treatment of breakthrough pain are not interchangeable; if patients are switched from another fentanyl-containing preparation, a new dose titration is required.

DOSES AT EXTREMES OF BODY-WEIGHT
▸ To avoid excessive dosage in obese patients, weight-based doses may need to be calculated on the basis of ideal bodyweight.

ABSTRAL ®
Breakthrough pain in patients receiving opioid therapy for chronic cancer pain
▸ BY MOUTH USING SUBLINGUAL TABLETS
▸ Adult: Initially 100 micrograms, then 100 micrograms after 15–30 minutes if required, dose to be adjusted according to response—consult product literature, no more than 2 dose units 15–30 minutes apart, for each pain episode; max. 800 micrograms per episode of breakthrough pain; leave at least 2 hours between treatment of episodes of breakthrough pain, if more than 4 episodes of breakthrough pain each day, adjust background analgesia

EFFENTORA ®
Breakthrough pain in patients receiving opioid therapy for chronic cancer pain
▸ BY MOUTH USING BUCCAL TABLET
▸ Adult: Initially 100 micrograms, then 100 micrograms after 30 minutes if required, dose to be adjusted according to response—consult product literature, no more than 2 dose units for each pain episode; max. 800 micrograms per episode of breakthrough pain; leave at least 4 hours between treatment of episodes of breakthrough pain during titration

INSTANYL ®
Breakthrough pain in patients receiving opioid therapy for chronic cancer pain
▸ BY INTRANASAL ADMINISTRATION
▸ Adult: Initially 50 micrograms, dose to be administered into one nostril, then 50 micrograms after 10 minutes if required, dose to be adjusted according to response, maximum 2 sprays for each pain episode and minimum 4 hours between treatment of each pain episode, if more than 4 breakthrough pain episodes daily, adjust background analgesia

PECFENT ®
Breakthrough pain in patients receiving opioid therapy for chronic cancer pain
▸ BY INTRANASAL ADMINISTRATION
▸ Adult: Initially 100 micrograms, adjusted according to response, dose to be administered into one nostril only, maximum 2 sprays for each pain episode and minimum 4 hours between treatment of each pain episode, if more than 4 breakthrough pain episodes daily, adjust background analgesia

---

IMPORTANT SAFETY INFORMATION
MHRA/CHM ADVICE: TRANSDERMAL FENTANYL PATCHES: LIFE-THREATENING AND FATAL OPIOID TOXICITY FROM ACCIDENTAL EXPOSURE, PARTICULARLY IN CHILDREN (OCTOBER 2018)
Accidental exposure to transdermal fentanyl can occur if a patch is swallowed or transferred to another individual. Always fully inform patients and their carers about directions for safe use of fentanyl patches, including the importance of:
● not exceeding the prescribed dose;

4

Nervous system

- following the correct frequency of patch application, avoiding touching the adhesive side of patches, and washing hands after application;
- not cutting patches and avoiding exposure of patches to heat including via hot water;
- ensuring that old patches are removed before applying a new one;
- following instructions for safe storage and properly disposing of used patches or those which are not needed.

Patients and carers should be advised to seek immediate medical attention if overdose is suspected—see *Side-effects* and *Patient and carer advice* for further information.

MHRA/CHM ADVICE: TRANSDERMAL FENTANYL PATCHES FOR NON-CANCER PAIN: DO NOT USE IN OPIOID-NAIVE PATIENTS (SEPTEMBER 2020)

A review noted that serious harm, including fatalities, has been reported with the use of fentanyl patches in both opioid-naive and opioid-tolerant patients. There is considerable risk of respiratory depression with the use of fentanyl, especially in opioid-naive patients, and significant risk with too rapid an escalation of dose, even in long-term opioid-tolerant patients.

The MHRA advises healthcare professionals that the use of fentanyl transdermal patches is contra-indicated in opioid-naive patients; other analgesics and other opioids for non-malignant pain should be used before prescribing fentanyl patches. Patients and their carers should be reminded about the directions for safe use of fentanyl patches (see above).

- CONTRA-INDICATIONS
▸ With transdermal use Opioid-naive patients

- CAUTIONS
  GENERAL CAUTIONS Bradyarrhythmias · cerebral tumour · diabetes mellitus (with *Actiq*® and *Cynril*® lozenges) · impaired consciousness

  SPECIFIC CAUTIONS
▸ With buccal use mucositis—absorption from oral preparations may be increased, caution during dose titration

  CAUTIONS, FURTHER INFORMATION
▸ With transdermal use [EvGr] Transdermal fentanyl patches are not suitable for acute pain or in those patients whose analgesic requirements are changing rapidly because the long time to steady state prevents rapid titration of the dose. ⟨M⟩
▸ With intravenous use [EvGr] Repeated intra-operative doses should be given with care since the resulting respiratory depression can persist postoperatively and occasionally it may become apparent for the first time postoperatively when monitoring of the patient might be less intensive. ⟨M⟩

- INTERACTIONS → Appendix 1: opioids

- SIDE-EFFECTS
▸ **Common or very common**
▸ With parenteral use Apnoea · hypertension · movement disorders · muscle rigidity · post procedural complications · respiratory disorders · vascular pain
▸ With sublingual use Asthenia · dyspnoea · oral disorders
▸ With transdermal use Anxiety · appetite decreased · asthenia · depression · diarrhoea · dyspnoea · gastrointestinal discomfort · hypertension · insomnia · malaise · muscle complaints · peripheral oedema · sensation abnormal · temperature sensation altered · tremor
▸ **Uncommon**
▸ With parenteral use Airway complication of anaesthesia · chills · hiccups · hypothermia
▸ With sublingual use Altered smell sensation · anxiety · appetite decreased · bruising tendency · concentration

impaired · depression · emotional lability · erectile dysfunction · gastrointestinal discomfort · impaired gastric emptying · joint disorders · malaise · memory loss · musculoskeletal stiffness · night sweats · numbness · oropharyngeal pain · overdose · paranoia · psychiatric disorder · sleep disorders · taste altered · throat tightness · tremor · vision blurred
▸ With transdermal use Consciousness impaired · cyanosis · fever · gastrointestinal disorders · influenza like illness · memory loss · respiratory disorders · seizures · sexual dysfunction · vision blurred
▸ **Rare or very rare**
▸ With transdermal use Apnoea
▸ **Frequency not known**
▸ With buccal use Adrenal insufficiency · androgen deficiency · anxiety · appetite decreased · asthenia · coma · depersonalisation · depression · diarrhoea · dyspnoea · emotional lability · fever · gait abnormal · gastrointestinal discomfort · gastrointestinal disorders · gingival haemorrhage · gingivitis · injury · loss of consciousness · malaise · myoclonus · oral disorders · peripheral oedema · seizure · sensation abnormal · sleep disorders · speech slurred · taste altered · thinking abnormal · throat oedema · vasodilation · vision disorders · weight decreased · withdrawal syndrome neonatal
▸ With intranasal use Diarrhoea · epistaxis · fatigue · fever · hot flush · insomnia · malaise · motion sickness · myoclonus · nasal complaints · peripheral oedema · seizure · sensation abnormal · stomatitis · taste altered · throat irritation
▸ With parenteral use Biliary spasm · cardiac arrest · cough · hyperalgesia · loss of consciousness · seizure
▸ With sublingual use Addiction · consciousness impaired · diarrhoea · fall · fever · hot flush · peripheral oedema · seizure · withdrawal syndrome neonatal
▸ With transdermal use Myoclonus · withdrawal syndrome neonatal

SIDE-EFFECTS, FURTHER INFORMATION **Muscle rigidity** Intravenous administration of fentanyl can cause muscle rigidity, which may involve the thoracic muscles. Manufacturer advises administration by slow intravenous injection to avoid; higher doses may require premedication with benzodiazepines and muscle relaxants.

Transdermal use Monitor patients using patches for increased side-effects if fever is present (increased absorption possible); avoid exposing application site to external heat, for example a hot bath or sauna (may also increase absorption).

- BREAST FEEDING
▸ With buccal use or intranasal use or sublingual use Manufacturer advises avoid during treatment and for 5 days after last administration—present in milk.
▸ With intravenous use Manufacturer advises avoid during treatment and for 24 hours after last administration—present in milk.
▸ With transdermal use Manufacturer advises avoid during treatment and for 72 hours after removal of patch—present in milk.

- HEPATIC IMPAIRMENT Manufacturer advises caution (risk of accumulation).
  Dose adjustments Manufacturer advises cautious dose titration.

- RENAL IMPAIRMENT Avoid use or reduce dose; opioid effects increased and prolonged and increased cerebral sensitivity occurs.

- DIRECTIONS FOR ADMINISTRATION
▸ With transdermal use [EvGr] For *patches*, apply to dry, non-irritated, non-irradiated, non-hairy skin on torso or upper arm, removing after 72 hours and siting replacement patch on a different area (avoid using the same area for several days). ⟨M⟩

With intravenous use [EvGr] For *intravenous infusion*, give continuously or intermittently in Glucose 5% or Sodium Chloride 0.9%. ◁M▷

With buccal use in adults [EvGr] For buccal films, moisten mouth, place film on inner lining of cheek (pink side to cheek), hold for at least 5 seconds until it sticks, and leave to dissolve (15–30 minutes); if more than 1 film required do not overlap, but use another area of the mouth. Avoid liquids for 5 minutes after application; avoid food until the film has dissolved. ◁M▷

With buccal use [EvGr] Patients should be advised to place the lozenge in the mouth against the cheek and move it around the mouth using the applicator; each lozenge should be sucked over a 15 minute period. In patients with a dry mouth, water may be used to moisten the buccal mucosa. Patients with diabetes should be advised each lozenge contains approximately 2 g glucose. ◁M▷

INSTANYL ® Patient should sit or stand during administration.

EFFENTORA ® Place tablet between cheek and gum and leave to dissolve; if more than 1 tablet required, place second tablet on the other side of the mouth; tablet may alternatively be placed under the tongue (sublingually).

● **PRESCRIBING AND DISPENSING INFORMATION**

With transdermal use Prescriptions for fentanyl patches can be written to show the strength in terms of the release rate and it is acceptable to write *'Fentanyl 25 patches'* to prescribe patches that release fentanyl 25 micrograms per hour. The dosage should be expressed in terms of the interval between applying a patch and replacing it with a new one, e.g. *'one patch to be applied every 72 hours'*. The total quantity of patches to be supplied should be written in words and figures.

● **PATIENT AND CARER ADVICE**

With transdermal use Patients and carers should be informed about safe use, including correct administration and disposal, strict adherence to dosage instructions, and the symptoms and signs of opioid overdose. Patches should be removed immediately in case of breathing difficulties, marked drowsiness, confusion, dizziness, or impaired speech, and patients and carers should seek prompt medical attention.

Patients or carers should be given advice on how to administer fentanyl buccal films or fentanyl lozenges. Patients or carers should be given advice on how to administer fentanyl nasal spray.

Medicines for Children leaflet: Fentanyl lozenges for pain www.medicinesforchildren.org.uk/fentanyl-lozenges-pain

Medicines for Children leaflet: Fentanyl patches for pain www.medicinesforchildren.org.uk/fentanyl-patches-pain

PECFENT ® Avoid concomitant use of other nasal preparations.

Patients or carers should be given advice on how to administer *PecFent®* spray.

INSTANYL ® Avoid concomitant use of other nasal preparations.

Patients or carers should be given advice on how to administer *Instanyl®* spray.

EFFENTORA ® Patients or carers should be given advice on how to administer *Effentora®* buccal tablets.

Tablet should be advised not to eat or drink until the tablet is completely dissolved; after 30 minutes, if any remnants remain, they may be swallowed with a glass of water. Patients with a dry mouth should be advised to drink water to moisten the buccal mucosa before administration of the tablets; if appropriate effervescence does not occur, a switch of therapy may be advised.

ABSTRAL ® Patients should be advised not to eat or drink until the tablet is completely dissolved.

In patients with a dry mouth, the buccal mucosa may be moistened with water before administration of tablet.

● **NATIONAL FUNDING/ACCESS DECISIONS**

PECFENT ® For full details see funding body website

Scottish Medicines Consortium (SMC) decisions

▸ Fentanyl pectin nasal spray (*PecFent®*) for the management of breakthrough pain in adults who are already receiving maintenance opioid therapy for chronic cancer pain (January 2011) SMC No. 663/10 Recommended with restrictions

INSTANYL ® For full details see funding body website

Scottish Medicines Consortium (SMC) decisions

▸ Fentanyl nasal spray (*Instanyl®*) for the management of breakthrough pain in adults already receiving maintenance opioid therapy for chronic cancer pain (November 2009) SMC No. 579/09 Recommended with restrictions

EFFENTORA ® For full details see funding body website

Scottish Medicines Consortium (SMC) decisions

▸ Fentanyl buccal tablets (*Effentora®*) for breakthrough pain in adults with cancer (February 2009) SMC No. 510/08 Recommended with restrictions

ABSTRAL ® For full details see funding body website

Scottish Medicines Consortium (SMC) decisions

▸ Fentanyl sublingual tablets (*Abstral®*) for the management of breakthrough pain in adult patients using opioid therapy for chronic cancer pain (February 2009) SMC No. 534/09 Recommended with restrictions

● **MEDICINAL FORMS** There can be variation in the licensing of different medicines containing the same drug. Forms available from special-order manufacturers include: solution for injection, infusion, solution for infusion

Solution for injection

▸ Fentanyl (Non-proprietary)

Fentanyl (as Fentanyl citrate) 50 microgram per 1 ml Fentanyl 100micrograms/2ml solution for injection ampoules | 10 ampoule [PoM] £11.50–£14.33 DT = £14.33 [CD2] Fentanyl 500micrograms/10ml solution for injection ampoules | 10 ampoule [PoM] £14.50–£16.15 [CD2]

▸ Sublimaze (Piramal Critical Care Ltd)

Fentanyl (as Fentanyl citrate) 50 microgram per 1 ml Sublimaze 500micrograms/10ml solution for injection ampoules | 5 ampoule [PoM] £6.53 [CD2]

Spray

CAUTIONARY AND ADVISORY LABELS 2

▸ Instanyl (Takeda UK Ltd)

Fentanyl (as Fentanyl citrate) 50 microgram per 1 dose Instanyl 50micrograms/dose nasal spray | 6 dose [PoM] £35.70 [CD2]

Fentanyl (as Fentanyl citrate) 100 microgram per 1 dose Instanyl 100micrograms/dose nasal spray | 6 dose [PoM] £35.70 DT = £35.70 [CD2]

Fentanyl (as Fentanyl citrate) 200 microgram per 1 dose Instanyl 200micrograms/dose nasal spray | 6 dose [PoM] £35.70 [CD2]

▸ PecFent (Kyowa Kirin Ltd)

Fentanyl (as Fentanyl citrate) 100 microgram per 1 dose PecFent 100micrograms/dose nasal spray | 8 dose [PoM] £36.48 DT = £36.48 [CD2] | 32 dose [PoM] £145.92 DT = £145.92 [CD2]

Fentanyl (as Fentanyl citrate) 400 microgram per 1 dose PecFent 400micrograms/dose nasal spray | 8 dose [PoM] £36.48 DT = £36.48 [CD2] | 32 dose [PoM] £145.92 DT = £145.92 [CD2]

Buccal tablet

CAUTIONARY AND ADVISORY LABELS 2

ELECTROLYTES: May contain Sodium

▸ Effentora (Teva UK Ltd)

Fentanyl (as Fentanyl citrate) 100 microgram Effentora 100microgram buccal tablets sugar-free | 4 tablet [PoM] £19.96 [CD2] sugar-free | 28 tablet [PoM] £139.72 DT = £139.72 [CD2]

Fentanyl (as Fentanyl citrate) 200 microgram Effentora 200microgram buccal tablets sugar-free | 4 tablet [PoM] £19.96 [CD2] sugar-free | 28 tablet [PoM] £139.72 DT = £139.72 [CD2]

Fentanyl (as Fentanyl citrate) 400 microgram Effentora 400microgram buccal tablets sugar-free | 4 tablet [PoM] £19.96 [CD2] sugar-free | 28 tablet [PoM] £139.72 DT = £139.72 [CD2]

Fentanyl (as Fentanyl citrate) 600 microgram Effentora 600microgram buccal tablets sugar-free | 4 tablet [PoM] £19.96 [CD2] sugar-free | 28 tablet [PoM] £139.72 DT = £139.72 [CD2]

Fentanyl (as Fentanyl citrate) 800 microgram Effentora 800microgram buccal tablets sugar-free | 4 tablet [PoM] £19.96 [CD2] sugar-free | 28 tablet [PoM] £139.72 DT = £139.72 [CD2]

4

Nervous system

4

Nervous system

Solution for infusion

▶ Fentanyl (Non-proprietary)

Fentanyl (as Fentanyl citrate) 50 microgram per 1 ml Fentanyl 2.5mg/50ml solution for infusion vials | 1 vial [PoM] £5.50 [CD2]

Sublingual tablet

CAUTIONARY AND ADVISORY LABELS 2, 26

▶ Abstral (Kyowa Kirin Ltd)

Fentanyl (as Fentanyl citrate) 100 microgram Abstral 100microgram sublingual tablets sugar-free | 10 tablet [PoM] £49.99 DT = £49.99 [CD2] sugar-free | 30 tablet [PoM] £149.70 [CD2]

Fentanyl (as Fentanyl citrate) 200 microgram Abstral 200microgram sublingual tablets sugar-free | 10 tablet [PoM] £49.99 DT = £49.99 [CD2] sugar-free | 30 tablet [PoM] £149.70 [CD2]

Fentanyl (as Fentanyl citrate) 300 microgram Abstral 300microgram sublingual tablets sugar-free | 10 tablet [PoM] £49.99 DT = £49.99 [CD2] sugar-free | 30 tablet [PoM] £149.70 [CD2]

Fentanyl (as Fentanyl citrate) 400 microgram Abstral 400microgram sublingual tablets sugar-free | 10 tablet [PoM] £49.99 DT = £49.99 [CD2] sugar-free | 30 tablet [PoM] £149.70 [CD2]

Fentanyl (as Fentanyl citrate) 600 microgram Abstral 600microgram sublingual tablets sugar-free | 30 tablet [PoM] £149.70 DT = £149.70 [CD2]

Fentanyl (as Fentanyl citrate) 800 microgram Abstral 800microgram sublingual tablets sugar-free | 30 tablet [PoM] £149.70 DT = £149.70 [CD2]

Transdermal patch

CAUTIONARY AND ADVISORY LABELS 2

▶ Durogesic DTrans (Janssen-Cilag Ltd)

Fentanyl 12 microgram per 1 hour Durogesic DTrans 12micrograms/hour transdermal patches | 5 patch [PoM] £12.59 DT = £12.59 [CD2]

Fentanyl 25 microgram per 1 hour Durogesic DTrans 25micrograms/hour transdermal patches | 5 patch [PoM] £17.99 DT = £17.99 [CD2]

Fentanyl 50 microgram per 1 hour Durogesic DTrans 50micrograms/hour transdermal patches | 5 patch [PoM] £33.66 DT = £33.66 [CD2]

Fentanyl 75 microgram per 1 hour Durogesic DTrans 75micrograms/hour transdermal patches | 5 patch [PoM] £46.99 DT = £46.99 [CD2]

Fentanyl 100 microgram per 1 hour Durogesic DTrans 100micrograms/hour transdermal patches | 5 patch [PoM] £57.86 DT = £57.86 [CD2]

▶ Fencino (Ethypharm UK Ltd)

Fentanyl 12 microgram per 1 hour Fencino 12micrograms/hour transdermal patches | 5 patch [PoM] £8.46 DT = £12.59 [CD2]

Fentanyl 25 microgram per 1 hour Fencino 25micrograms/hour transdermal patches | 5 patch [PoM] £12.10 DT = £17.99 [CD2]

Fentanyl 50 microgram per 1 hour Fencino 50micrograms/hour transdermal patches | 5 patch [PoM] £22.62 DT = £33.66 [CD2]

Fentanyl 75 microgram per 1 hour Fencino 75micrograms/hour transdermal patches | 5 patch [PoM] £31.54 DT = £46.99 [CD2]

Fentanyl 100 microgram per 1 hour Fencino 100micrograms/hour transdermal patches | 5 patch [PoM] £38.88 DT = £57.86 [CD2]

▶ Fentalis (Sandoz Ltd)

Fentanyl 25 microgram per 1 hour Fentalis Reservoir 25micrograms/hour transdermal patches | 5 patch [PoM] £22.89 DT = £17.99 [CD2]

Fentanyl 50 microgram per 1 hour Fentalis Reservoir 50micrograms/hour transdermal patches | 5 patch [PoM] £42.77 DT = £33.66 [CD2]

Fentanyl 75 microgram per 1 hour Fentalis Reservoir 75micrograms/hour transdermal patches | 5 patch [PoM] £59.62 DT = £46.99 [CD2]

Fentanyl 100 microgram per 1 hour Fentalis Reservoir 100micrograms/hour transdermal patches | 5 patch [PoM] £73.49 DT = £57.86 [CD2]

▶ Matrifen (Teva UK Ltd)

Fentanyl 12 microgram per 1 hour Matrifen 12micrograms/hour transdermal patches | 5 patch [PoM] £7.52 DT = £12.59 [CD2]

Fentanyl 25 microgram per 1 hour Matrifen 25micrograms/hour transdermal patches | 5 patch [PoM] £10.76 DT = £17.99 [CD2]

Fentanyl 50 microgram per 1 hour Matrifen 50micrograms/hour transdermal patches | 5 patch [PoM] £20.12 DT = £33.66 [CD2]

Fentanyl 75 microgram per 1 hour Matrifen 75micrograms/hour transdermal patches | 5 patch [PoM] £28.06 DT = £46.99 [CD2]

Fentanyl 100 microgram per 1 hour Matrifen 100micrograms/hour transdermal patches | 5 patch [PoM] £34.59 DT = £57.86 [CD2]

▶ Mezolar Matrix (Sandoz Ltd)

Fentanyl 12 microgram per 1 hour Mezolar Matrix 12micrograms/hour transdermal patches | 5 patch [PoM] £7.53 DT = £12.59 [CD2]

Fentanyl 25 microgram per 1 hour Mezolar Matrix 25micrograms/hour transdermal patches | 5 patch [PoM] £10.77 DT = £17.99 [CD2]

Fentanyl 37.5 microgram per 1 hour Mezolar Matrix 37.5micrograms/hour transdermal patches | 5 patch [PoM] £15.46 = £15.46 [CD2]

Fentanyl 50 microgram per 1 hour Mezolar Matrix 50micrograms/hour transdermal patches | 5 patch [PoM] £20.13 DT = £33.66 [CD2]

Fentanyl 75 microgram per 1 hour Mezolar Matrix 75micrograms/hour transdermal patches | 5 patch [PoM] £28.07 DT = £46.99 [CD2]

Fentanyl 100 microgram per 1 hour Mezolar Matrix 100micrograms/hour transdermal patches | 5 patch [PoM] £34.60 DT = £57.86 [CD2]

▶ Victanyl (Accord Healthcare Ltd)

Fentanyl 12 microgram per 1 hour Victanyl 12micrograms/hour transdermal patches | 5 patch [PoM] £12.58 DT = £12.59 [CD2]

Fentanyl 25 microgram per 1 hour Victanyl 25micrograms/hour transdermal patches | 5 patch [PoM] £25.89 DT = £17.99 [CD2]

Fentanyl 50 microgram per 1 hour Victanyl 50micrograms/hour transdermal patches | 5 patch [PoM] £48.36 DT = £33.66 [CD2]

Fentanyl 75 microgram per 1 hour Victanyl 75micrograms/hour transdermal patches | 5 patch [PoM] £67.41 DT = £46.99 [CD2]

Fentanyl 100 microgram per 1 hour Victanyl 100micrograms/hour transdermal patches | 5 patch [PoM] £83.09 DT = £57.86 [CD2]

▶ Yemex (Sandoz Ltd)

Fentanyl 12 microgram per 1 hour Yemex 12micrograms/hour transdermal patches | 5 patch [PoM] £12.59 DT = £12.59 [CD2]

Fentanyl 25 microgram per 1 hour Yemex 25micrograms/hour transdermal patches | 5 patch [PoM] £17.99 DT = £17.99 [CD2]

Fentanyl 50 microgram per 1 hour Yemex 50micrograms/hour transdermal patches | 5 patch [PoM] £33.66 DT = £33.66 [CD2]

Fentanyl 75 microgram per 1 hour Yemex 75micrograms/hour transdermal patches | 5 patch [PoM] £46.99 DT = £46.99 [CD2]

Fentanyl 100 microgram per 1 hour Yemex 100micrograms/hour transdermal patches | 5 patch [PoM] £57.86 DT = £57.86 [CD2]

Lozenge

CAUTIONARY AND ADVISORY LABELS 2
EXCIPIENTS: May contain Propylene glycol

▶ Actiq (Teva UK Ltd)

Fentanyl (as Fentanyl citrate) 200 microgram Actiq 200microgram lozenges with integral oromucosal applicator | 3 lozenge [PoM] £21.05 DT = £21.05 [CD2] | 30 lozenge [PoM] £210.41 DT = £210.41 [CD2]

Fentanyl (as Fentanyl citrate) 400 microgram Actiq 400microgram lozenges with integral oromucosal applicator | 3 lozenge [PoM] £21.05 DT = £21.05 [CD2] | 30 lozenge [PoM] £210.41 DT = £210.41 [CD2]

Fentanyl (as Fentanyl citrate) 600 microgram Actiq 600microgram lozenges with integral oromucosal applicator | 3 lozenge [PoM] £21.05 DT = £21.05 [CD2] | 30 lozenge [PoM] £210.41 DT = £210.41 [CD2]

Fentanyl (as Fentanyl citrate) 800 microgram Actiq 800microgram lozenges with integral oromucosal applicator | 3 lozenge [PoM] £21.05 DT = £21.05 [CD2] | 30 lozenge [PoM] £210.41 DT = £210.41 [CD2]

Fentanyl (as Fentanyl citrate) 1.2 mg Actiq 1.2mg lozenges with integral oromucosal applicator | 3 lozenge [PoM] £21.05 DT = £21.05 [CD2] | 30 lozenge [PoM] £210.41 DT = £210.41 [CD2]

Fentanyl (as Fentanyl citrate) 1.6 mg Actiq 1.6mg lozenges with integral oromucosal applicator | 3 lozenge [PoM] £21.05 DT = £21.05 [CD2] | 30 lozenge [PoM] £210.41 DT = £210.41 [CD2]

F 467

Hydromorphone hydrochloride 13-Nov-2020

● INDICATIONS AND DOSE

Severe pain in cancer

▶ **BY MOUTH USING IMMEDIATE-RELEASE MEDICINES**

▸ Child 12–17 years: 1.3 mg every 4 hours, dose to be increased if necessary according to severity of pain

▸ Adult: 1.3 mg every 4 hours, dose to be increased if necessary according to severity of pain

▸ BY MOUTH USING MODIFIED-RELEASE MEDICINES
▸ Child 12–17 years: 4 mg every 12 hours, dose to be increased if necessary according to severity of pain
▸ Adult: 4 mg every 12 hours, dose to be increased if necessary according to severity of pain

● CONTRA-INDICATIONS Acute abdomen
● CAUTIONS Pancreatitis · toxic psychosis
● INTERACTIONS → Appendix 1: opioids
● SIDE-EFFECTS
▸ **Common or very common** Abdominal pain · anxiety · appetite decreased · asthenia · sleep disorders
▸ **Uncommon** Depression · diarrhoea · dyspnoea · erectile dysfunction · malaise · movement disorders · paraesthesia · peripheral oedema · taste altered · tremor
▸ **Frequency not known** Hyperalgesia · paralytic ileus · seizure · withdrawal syndrome neonatal
● BREAST FEEDING Avoid—no information available.
● HEPATIC IMPAIRMENT Manufacturer advises avoid.
● RENAL IMPAIRMENT Avoid use or reduce dose; opioid effects increased and prolonged and increased cerebral sensitivity occurs.
● DIRECTIONS FOR ADMINISTRATION For *immediate-release* capsules, manufacturer advises swallow whole capsule or sprinkle contents on soft food. For *modified-release* capsules, manufacturer advises swallow whole or open capsule and sprinkle contents on soft cold food (swallow the pellets within the capsule whole; do not crush or chew).
● PATIENT AND CARER ADVICE Patients or carers should be given advice on how to administer hydromorphone hydrochloride capsules and modified-release capsules.

● MEDICINAL FORMS There can be variation in the licensing of different medicines containing the same drug. Forms available from special-order manufacturers include: oral solution
Modified-release capsule
CAUTIONARY AND ADVISORY LABELS 2
▸ Palladone SR (Napp Pharmaceuticals Ltd)
Hydromorphone hydrochloride 2 mg Palladone SR 2mg capsules | 56 capsule PoM £20.98 DT = £20.98 CD2
Hydromorphone hydrochloride 4 mg Palladone SR 4mg capsules | 56 capsule PoM £28.75 DT = £28.75 CD2
Hydromorphone hydrochloride 8 mg Palladone SR 8mg capsules | 56 capsule PoM £56.08 DT = £56.08 CD2
Hydromorphone hydrochloride 16 mg Palladone SR 16mg capsules | 56 capsule PoM £106.53 DT = £106.53 CD2
Hydromorphone hydrochloride 24 mg Palladone SR 24mg capsules | 56 capsule PoM £159.82 DT = £159.82 CD2
Capsule
CAUTIONARY AND ADVISORY LABELS 2
▸ Palladone (Napp Pharmaceuticals Ltd)
Hydromorphone hydrochloride 1.3 mg Palladone 1.3mg capsules | 56 capsule PoM £8.82 DT = £8.82 CD2
Hydromorphone hydrochloride 2.6 mg Palladone 2.6mg capsules | 56 capsule PoM £17.64 DT = £17.64 CD2

⚑ 467

Meptazinol

● INDICATIONS AND DOSE
Moderate to severe pain, including post-operative pain and renal colic
▸ BY MOUTH
▸ Adult: 200 mg every 3–6 hours as required
▸ BY INTRAMUSCULAR INJECTION
▸ Adult: 75–100 mg every 2–4 hours if required
▸ BY SLOW INTRAVENOUS INJECTION
▸ Adult: 50–100 mg every 2–4 hours if required
Obstetric analgesia
▸ BY INTRAMUSCULAR INJECTION
▸ Adult: 2 mg/kg, usual dose 100–150 mg

● CONTRA-INDICATIONS Myocardial infarction · phaeochromocytoma
● INTERACTIONS → Appendix 1: opioids
● SIDE-EFFECTS
▸ **Common or very common** Diarrhoea · gastrointestinal discomfort
Overdose Effects only partially reversed by naloxone.
● BREAST FEEDING Use only if potential benefit outweighs risk.
● HEPATIC IMPAIRMENT Manufacturer advises caution.
Dose adjustments Manufacturer advises dose reduction.
● RENAL IMPAIRMENT Avoid use or reduce dose; opioid effects increased and prolonged and increased cerebral sensitivity occurs.

● MEDICINAL FORMS There can be variation in the licensing of different medicines containing the same drug.
Solution for injection
▸ Meptid (Almirall Ltd)
Meptazinol (as Meptazinol hydrochloride) 100 mg per 1 ml Meptid 100mg/1ml solution for injection ampoules | 10 ampoule PoM £19.21
Tablet
CAUTIONARY AND ADVISORY LABELS 2
▸ Meptid (Almirall Ltd)
Meptazinol (as Meptazinol hydrochloride) 200 mg Meptid 200mg tablets | 112 tablet PoM £22.11 DT = £22.11

⚑ 467

Morphine

13-Nov-2020

● INDICATIONS AND DOSE
Pain
▸ BY SUBCUTANEOUS INJECTION
▸ Child 1–5 months: Initially 100–200 micrograms/kg every 6 hours, adjusted according to response
▸ Child 6 months-1 year: Initially 100–200 micrograms/kg every 4 hours, adjusted according to response
▸ Child 2–11 years: Initially 200 micrograms/kg every 4 hours, adjusted according to response
▸ Child 12–17 years: Initially 2.5–10 mg every 4 hours, adjusted according to response
▸ INITIALLY BY INTRAVENOUS INJECTION
▸ Child 1–5 months: 100 micrograms/kg every 6 hours, adjusted according to response, dose to be administered over at least 5 minutes, alternatively (by intravenous injection) initially 100 micrograms/kg, dose to be administered over at least 5 minutes, followed by (by continuous intravenous infusion) 10–30 micrograms/kg/hour, adjusted according to response
▸ Child 6 months–11 years: 100 micrograms/kg every 4 hours, adjusted according to response, dose to be administered over at least 5 minutes, alternatively (by intravenous injection) initially 100 micrograms/kg, dose to be administered over at least 5 minutes, followed by (by continuous intravenous infusion) 20–30 micrograms/kg/hour, adjusted according to response
▸ Child 12–17 years: 5 mg every 4 hours, adjusted according to response, dose to be administered over at least 5 minutes, alternatively (by intravenous injection) initially 5 mg, dose to be administered over at least 5 minutes, followed by (by continuous intravenous infusion) 20–30 micrograms/kg/hour, adjusted according to response
▸ BY MOUTH, OR BY RECTUM
▸ Child 1–2 months: Initially 50–100 micrograms/kg every 4 hours, adjusted according to response
▸ Child 3–5 months: 100–150 micrograms/kg every 4 hours, adjusted according to response continued →

▸ **Child 6-11 months:** 200 micrograms/kg every 4 hours, adjusted according to response
▸ **Child 1 year:** Initially 200–300 micrograms/kg every 4 hours, adjusted according to response
▸ **Child 2-11 years:** Initially 200–300 micrograms/kg every 4 hours (max. per dose 10 mg), adjusted according to response
▸ **Child 12-17 years:** Initially 5–10 mg every 4 hours, adjusted according to response

Acute pain
▶ BY MOUTH, OR BY SUBCUTANEOUS INJECTION, OR BY INTRAMUSCULAR INJECTION
▸ **Adult:** Initially 10 mg every 4 hours, adjusted according to response, subcutaneous injection not suitable for oedematous patients, dose can be given more frequently during titration, use dose for elderly in frail patients
▸ **Elderly:** Initially 5 mg every 4 hours, adjusted according to response, subcutaneous injection not suitable for oedematous patients, dose can be given more frequently during titration
▶ BY SLOW INTRAVENOUS INJECTION
▸ **Adult:** Initially 5 mg every 4 hours, adjusted according to response, dose can be adjusted more frequently during titration, reduced dose recommended in frail and elderly patients

Chronic pain
▶ BY MOUTH, OR BY SUBCUTANEOUS INJECTION, OR BY INTRAMUSCULAR INJECTION
▸ **Adult:** Initially 5–10 mg every 4 hours, adjusted according to response, subcutaneous injection not suitable for oedematous patients
▶ BY RECTUM
▸ **Adult:** Initially 15–30 mg every 4 hours, adjusted according to response

Pain (with modified-release 12-hourly preparations)
▶ BY MOUTH USING MODIFIED-RELEASE MEDICINES
▸ **Adult:** Every 12 hours, dose adjusted according to daily morphine requirements, dosage requirements should be reviewed if the brand is altered

Pain (with modified-release 24-hourly preparations)
▶ BY MOUTH USING MODIFIED-RELEASE MEDICINES
▸ **Adult:** Every 24 hours, dose adjusted according to daily morphine requirements, dosage requirements should be reviewed if the brand is altered

Pain management in palliative care (starting dose for opioid-naïve patients)
▶ BY MOUTH
▸ **Adult:** 20–30 mg daily in divided doses, using immediate-release preparation 4-hourly or a 12-hourly modified-release preparation, for management of breakthrough pain and other general advice, see *Pain management with opioids* under Prescribing in palliative care p. 28.

Pain management in palliative care (starting dose for patients being switched from a regular weak opioid)
▶ BY MOUTH
▸ **Adult:** 40–60 mg daily in divided doses, using immediate-release preparation 4-hourly or 12-hourly modified-release preparation, for management of breakthrough pain and other general advice, see *Pain management with opioids* under Prescribing in palliative care p. 28.

Pain in palliative care (following initial titration)
▶ BY MOUTH USING IMMEDIATE-RELEASE MEDICINES
▸ **Adult:** Usual dose 30 mg every 4 hours; up to 200 mg every 4 hours, higher dose may be required for some patients (occasionally more is needed); for management of breakthrough pain and other general

advice, see *Pain management with opioids* under Prescribing in palliative care p. 28.
▶ BY MOUTH USING MODIFIED-RELEASE MEDICINES
▸ **Adult:** Usual dose 100 mg every 12 hours; up to 600 mg every 12 hours, higher dose may be required for some patients (occasionally more is needed); for management of breakthrough pain and other general advice, see *Pain management with opioids* under Prescribing in palliative care p. 28.

Cough in palliative care
▶ BY MOUTH
▸ **Adult:** Initially 5 mg every 4 hours

Premedication
▶ BY SUBCUTANEOUS INJECTION, OR BY INTRAMUSCULAR INJECTION
▸ **Adult:** Up to 10 mg, dose to be administered 60–90 minutes before operation

Patient controlled analgesia (PCA)
▶ BY INTRAVENOUS INFUSION
▸ **Adult:** (consult local protocol)

Myocardial infarction
▶ BY SLOW INTRAVENOUS INJECTION
▸ **Adult:** 5–10 mg, followed by 5–10 mg if required, dose to be administered at a rate of 1–2 mg/minute, use dose for elderly in frail patients
▸ **Elderly:** 2.5–5 mg, followed by 2.5–5 mg if required, dose to be administered at a rate of 1–2 mg/minute

Acute pulmonary oedema
▶ BY SLOW INTRAVENOUS INJECTION
▸ **Adult:** 5–10 mg, dose to be administered at a rate of 2 mg/minute, use dose for elderly in frail patients
▸ **Elderly:** 2.5–5 mg, dose to be administered at a rate of 2 mg/minute

Dyspnoea at rest in palliative care
▶ BY MOUTH
▸ **Adult:** Initially 5 mg every 4 hours, to be given in carefully titrated doses

DOSE EQUIVALENCE AND CONVERSION
▸ The doses stated refer equally to morphine hydrochloride and sulfate.

● UNLICENSED USE
▸ With oral use in children *Oramorph* ® solution and *MXL* ® capsules not licensed for use in children under 1 year. *Sevredol* ® tablets not licensed for use in children under 3 years. *Oramorph* ® unit dose vials and *Filnarine* ® SR tablets not licensed for use in children under 6 years. *MST Continus* ® preparations licensed to treat children with cancer pain (age-range not specified by manufacturer).
▸ With rectal use in children Suppositories are not licensed for use in children.

> IMPORTANT SAFETY INFORMATION
> Do not confuse modified-release 12-hourly preparations with 24-hourly preparations, see *Prescribing and dispensing information.*

● CONTRA-INDICATIONS Acute abdomen · delayed gastric emptying · heart failure secondary to chronic lung disease · phaeochromocytoma
● CAUTIONS Cardiac arrhythmias · pancreatitis · severe cor pulmonale
● INTERACTIONS → Appendix 1: opioids
● SIDE-EFFECTS
▶ **Common or very common**
▸ With oral use Appetite decreased · asthenic conditions · gastrointestinal discomfort · insomnia · neuromuscular dysfunction
▶ **Uncommon**
▸ With oral use Agitation · bronchospasm · ileus · mood altered · myoclonus · peripheral oedema · pulmonary

oedema · seizure · sensation abnormal · syncope · taste altered
▶ **Frequency not known**
▶ With oral use Amenorrhoea · biliary pain · cough decreased · hyperalgesia · hypertension · pancreatitis exacerbated · sexual dysfunction · thinking abnormal · ureteral spasm
▶ With parenteral use Alertness decreased · bile duct disorders · mood altered · myoclonus · sexual dysfunction · ureteral spasm · urinary disorders · vision disorders
● BREAST FEEDING Therapeutic doses unlikely to affect infant.
● HEPATIC IMPAIRMENT Manufacturer advises caution. Avoid *oral preparations* in acute impairment; for *injectable preparations*—consult product literature.
Dose adjustments Manufacturer advises consider dose reduction—consult product literature.
● RENAL IMPAIRMENT Avoid use or reduce dose; opioid effects increased and prolonged; increased cerebral sensitivity.
● MONITORING REQUIREMENTS Possible association between acute chest syndrome in patients with sickle cell disease treated with morphine during a vaso-occlusive crisis—manufacturer advises close monitoring for acute chest syndrome symptoms during treatment.
● DIRECTIONS FOR ADMINISTRATION
▶ With intravenous use in children For *continuous intravenous infusion*, dilute with Glucose 5% or 10% or Sodium Chloride 0.9%.
▶ With oral use For *modified release capsules*—swallow whole or open capsule and sprinkle contents on soft food.
● PRESCRIBING AND DISPENSING INFORMATION Modified-release preparations are available as 12-hourly or 24-hourly formulations; prescribers must ensure that the correct preparation is prescribed. Preparations that should be given 12-hourly include *Filnarine® SR, MST Continus®, Morphgesic® SR* and *Zomorph®*. Preparations that should be given 24-hourly include *MXL®*.
  Prescriptions must specify the 'form'.
▶ With rectal use Both the strength of the suppositories and the morphine salt contained in them must be specified by the prescriber.
Palliative care For further information on the use of morphine in palliative care, see www.medicinescomplete.com/#/content/palliative/morphine.
● PATIENT AND CARER ADVICE
▶ With oral use Patients or carers should be given advice on how to administer morphine modified-release capsules.
Medicines for Children leaflet: Morphine for pain www.medicinesforchildren.org.uk/morphine-pain
● EXCEPTIONS TO LEGAL CATEGORY
Morphine Oral Solutions Prescription-only medicines or schedule 2 controlled drug. The proportion of morphine hydrochloride can be altered when specified by the prescriber; if above 13 mg per 5 mL the solution becomes a schedule 2 controlled drug. It is usual to adjust the strength so that the dose volume is 5 or 10 mL.
  Oral solutions of morphine can be prescribed by writing the formula:
  Morphine hydrochloride 5 mg
  Chloroform water to 5 mL

● MEDICINAL FORMS There can be variation in the licensing of different medicines containing the same drug. Forms available from special-order manufacturers include: capsule, oral solution, solution for injection, infusion, solution for infusion, suppository
Modified-release tablet
CAUTIONARY AND ADVISORY LABELS 2, 25
▶ MST Continus (Napp Pharmaceuticals Ltd)
  Morphine sulfate 5 mg MST Continus 5mg tablets | 60 tablet [PoM] £3.29 DT = £3.29 [CD2]

Morphine sulfate 10 mg MST Continus 10mg tablets | 60 tablet [PoM] £5.20 DT = £5.20 [CD2]
Morphine sulfate 15 mg MST Continus 15mg tablets | 60 tablet [PoM] £9.10 DT = £9.10 [CD2]
Morphine sulfate 30 mg MST Continus 30mg tablets | 60 tablet [PoM] £12.47 DT = £12.47 [CD2]
Morphine sulfate 60 mg MST Continus 60mg tablets | 60 tablet [PoM] £24.32 DT = £24.32 [CD2]
Morphine sulfate 100 mg MST Continus 100mg tablets | 60 tablet [PoM] £38.50 DT = £38.50 [CD2]
Morphine sulfate 200 mg MST Continus 200mg tablets | 60 tablet [PoM] £81.34 DT = £81.34 [CD2]
▶ Morphgesic SR (Advanz Pharma)
Morphine sulfate 10 mg Morphgesic SR 10mg tablets | 60 tablet [PoM] £3.85 DT = £5.20 [CD2]
Morphine sulfate 30 mg Morphgesic SR 30mg tablets | 60 tablet [PoM] £9.24 DT = £12.47 [CD2]
Morphine sulfate 60 mg Morphgesic SR 60mg tablets | 60 tablet [PoM] £18.04 DT = £24.32 [CD2]
Morphine sulfate 100 mg Morphgesic SR 100mg tablets | 60 tablet [PoM] £28.54 DT = £38.50 [CD2]
Tablet
CAUTIONARY AND ADVISORY LABELS 2
▶ Sevredol (Napp Pharmaceuticals Ltd)
Morphine sulfate 10 mg Sevredol 10mg tablets | 56 tablet [PoM] £5.31 = £5.31 [CD2]
Morphine sulfate 20 mg Sevredol 20mg tablets | 56 tablet [PoM] £10.61 DT = £10.61 [CD2]
Morphine sulfate 50 mg Sevredol 50mg tablets | 56 tablet [PoM] £28.02 DT = £28.02 [CD2]
Solution for injection
▶ Morphine (Non-proprietary)
Morphine sulfate 1 mg per 1 ml Morphine sulfate 5mg/5ml solution for injection ampoules | 10 ampoule [PoM] £48.30 DT = £48.30 [CD2] Morphine sulfate 1mg/1ml solution for injection ampoules | 10 ampoule [PoM] £38.20 [CD2]
Morphine sulfate 10mg/10ml solution for injection ampoules | 10 ampoule [PoM] £15.00–£50.60 [CD2]
Morphine sulfate 10 mg per 1 ml Morphine sulfate 10mg/1ml solution for injection ampoules | 10 ampoule [PoM] [S] DT = £11.45 (Hospital only) [CD2] | 10 ampoule [PoM] £11.87 DT = £11.45 [CD2]
Morphine sulfate 15 mg per 1 ml Morphine sulfate 15mg/1ml solution for injection ampoules | 10 ampoule [PoM] [S] DT = £10.74 (Hospital only) [CD2] | 10 ampoule [PoM] £10.74–£13.10 = £10.74 [CD2]
Morphine sulfate 20 mg per 1 ml Morphine sulfate 20mg/1ml solution for injection ampoules | 10 ampoule [PoM] £77.75–£79.64 DT = £77.75 [CD2]
Morphine sulfate 30 mg per 1 ml Morphine sulfate 30mg/1ml solution for injection ampoules | 10 ampoule [PoM] [S] DT = £11.49 (Hospital only) [CD2] | 10 ampoule [PoM] £14.02 DT = £11.49 [CD2] Morphine sulfate 60mg/2ml solution for injection ampoules | 5 ampoule [PoM] £10.07 DT = £10.07 [CD2]
Modified-release capsule
CAUTIONARY AND ADVISORY LABELS 2
▶ MXL (Napp Pharmaceuticals Ltd)
Morphine sulfate 30 mg MXL 30mg capsules | 28 capsule [PoM] £10.91 [CD2]
Morphine sulfate 60 mg MXL 60mg capsules | 28 capsule [PoM] £14.95 [CD2]
Morphine sulfate 90 mg MXL 90mg capsules | 28 capsule [PoM] £22.04 DT = £22.04 [CD2]
Morphine sulfate 120 mg MXL 120mg capsules | 28 capsule [PoM] £29.15 DT = £29.15 [CD2]
Morphine sulfate 150 mg MXL 150mg capsules | 28 capsule [PoM] £36.43 DT = £36.43 [CD2]
Morphine sulfate 200 mg MXL 200mg capsules | 28 capsule [PoM] £46.15 [CD2]
▶ Zomorph (Ethypharm UK Ltd)
Morphine sulfate 10 mg Zomorph 10mg modified-release capsules | 60 capsule [PoM] £3.47 DT = £3.47 [CD2]
Morphine sulfate 30 mg Zomorph 30mg modified-release capsules | 60 capsule [PoM] £8.30 DT = £8.30 [CD2]
Morphine sulfate 60 mg Zomorph 60mg modified-release capsules | 60 capsule [PoM] £16.20 DT = £16.20 [CD2]
Morphine sulfate 100 mg Zomorph 100mg modified-release capsules | 60 capsule [PoM] £21.80 DT = £21.80 [CD2]
Morphine sulfate 200 mg Zomorph 200mg modified-release capsules | 60 capsule [PoM] £43.60 DT = £43.60 [CD2]

4

Nervous system

4

Nervous system

Solution for infusion

▸ Morphine (Non-proprietary)

Morphine sulfate 1 mg per 1 ml Morphine sulfate 50mg/50ml solution for infusion vials | 1 vial [PoM] £4.48–£5.78 DT = £5.78 [CD2] | 10 vial [PoM] £44.80 [CD2]

Morphine sulfate 2 mg per 1 ml Morphine sulfate 100mg/50ml solution for infusion vials | 1 vial [PoM] £6.48 [CD2] | 10 vial [PoM] £73.20 [CD2]

Oral solution

CAUTIONARY AND ADVISORY LABELS 2

▸ Morphine (Non-proprietary)

Morphine sulfate 2 mg per 1 ml Morphine sulfate 10mg/5ml oral solution | 100 ml [PoM] £2.00–£3.00 [CD5] | 300 ml [PoM] £9.00 DT = £6.01 [CD5] | 500 ml [PoM] £10.01–£15.00 [CD5]

▸ Oramorph (Boehringer Ingelheim Ltd)

Morphine sulfate 2 mg per 1 ml Oramorph 10mg/5ml oral solution | 100 ml [PoM] £1.89 [CD5] | 300 ml [PoM] £5.45 DT = £6.01 [CD5] | 500 ml [PoM] £8.50 [CD5]

Morphine sulfate 20 mg per 1 ml Oramorph 20mg/ml concentrated oral solution sugar-free | 120 ml [PoM] £19.50 DT = £19.50 [CD2]

Modified-release granules

CAUTIONARY AND ADVISORY LABELS 2, 13

▸ MST Continus (Napp Pharmaceuticals Ltd)

Morphine sulfate 20 mg MST Continus suspension 20mg granules sachets sugar-free | 30 sachet [PoM] £24.58 DT = £24.58 [CD2]

Morphine sulfate 30 mg MST Continus suspension 30mg granules sachets sugar-free | 30 sachet [PoM] £25.54 DT = £25.54 [CD2]

Morphine sulfate 60 mg MST Continus suspension 60mg granules sachets sugar-free | 30 sachet [PoM] £51.09 DT = £51.09 [CD2]

Morphine sulfate 100 mg MST Continus suspension 100mg granules sachets sugar-free | 30 sachet [PoM] £85.15 DT = £85.15 [CD2]

Morphine sulfate 200 mg MST Continus suspension 200mg granules sachets sugar-free | 30 sachet [PoM] £170.30 DT = £170.30 [CD2]

Morphine with cyclizine

The properties listed below are those particular to the combination only. For the properties of the components please consider, morphine p. 483, cyclizine p. 449.

● INDICATIONS AND DOSE

CYCLIMORPH-10 ®

Moderate to severe pain (short-term use only)

▸ BY SUBCUTANEOUS INJECTION, OR BY INTRAMUSCULAR INJECTION, OR BY INTRAVENOUS INJECTION

▸ **Adult:** 1 mL, do not repeat dose more often than every 4 hours; maximum 3 doses per day

CYCLIMORPH-15 ®

Moderate to severe pain (short-term use only)

▸ BY SUBCUTANEOUS INJECTION, OR BY INTRAMUSCULAR INJECTION, OR BY INTRAVENOUS INJECTION

▸ **Adult:** 1 mL, do not repeat dose more often than every 4 hours; maximum 3 doses per day

● CAUTIONS Myocardial infarction (cyclizine may aggravate severe heart failure and counteract the haemodynamic benefits of opioids) · not recommended in palliative care

● INTERACTIONS → Appendix 1: antihistamines, sedating · opioids

● MEDICINAL FORMS There can be variation in the licensing of different medicines containing the same drug.

Solution for injection

▸ Cyclimorph (Advanz Pharma)

Morphine tartrate 15 mg per 1 ml, Cyclizine tartrate 50 mg per 1 ml Cyclimorph 15 solution for injection 1ml ampoules | 5 ampoule [PoM] £9.12 DT = £9.12 [CD2]

Morphine tartrate 10 mg per 1 ml, Cyclizine tartrate 50 mg per 1 ml Cyclimorph 10 solution for injection 1ml ampoules | 5 ampoule [PoM] £8.77 DT = £8.77 [CD2]

▶ 467

Oxycodone hydrochloride

13-Nov-2020

● INDICATIONS AND DOSE

Postoperative pain | Severe pain

▸ BY MOUTH USING IMMEDIATE-RELEASE MEDICINES

▸ **Adult:** Initially 5 mg every 4–6 hours, dose to be increased if necessary according to severity of pain, some patients may require higher doses than the maximum daily dose; maximum 400 mg per day

▸ BY MOUTH USING MODIFIED-RELEASE MEDICINES

▸ **Adult:** Initially 10 mg every 12 hours (max. per dose 200 mg every 12 hours), dose to be increased if necessary according to severity of pain, some patients might require higher doses than the maximum daily dose, use 12-hourly modified-release preparations for this dose; see *Prescribing and dispensing information*

▸ BY SLOW INTRAVENOUS INJECTION

▸ **Adult:** 1–10 mg every 4 hours as required

▸ BY INTRAVENOUS INFUSION

▸ **Adult:** Initially 2 mg/hour, adjusted according to response

▸ BY SUBCUTANEOUS INJECTION

▸ **Adult:** Initially 5 mg every 4 hours as required

▸ BY SUBCUTANEOUS INFUSION

▸ **Adult:** Initially 7.5 mg/24 hours, adjusted according to response

Patient controlled analgesia (PCA)

▸ BY INTRAVENOUS INFUSION

▸ **Adult:** (consult local protocol)

Moderate to severe pain in palliative care

▸ BY MOUTH USING IMMEDIATE-RELEASE MEDICINES

▸ **Adult:** Initially 5 mg every 4–6 hours, dose to be increased if necessary according to severity of pain, some patients may require higher doses than the maximum daily dose; maximum 400 mg per day

▸ BY MOUTH USING MODIFIED-RELEASE MEDICINES

▸ **Adult:** Initially 10 mg every 12 hours (max. per dose 200 mg every 12 hours), dose to be increased if necessary according to severity of pain, some patients might require higher doses than the maximum daily dose, use 12-hourly modified-release preparations for this dose; see *Prescribing and dispensing information*

▸ BY SLOW INTRAVENOUS INJECTION

▸ **Adult:** 1–10 mg every 4 hours as required

▸ BY INTRAVENOUS INFUSION

▸ **Adult:** Initially 2 mg/hour, adjusted according to response

▸ BY SUBCUTANEOUS INJECTION

▸ **Adult:** Initially 5 mg every 4 hours as required

▸ BY SUBCUTANEOUS INFUSION

▸ **Adult:** Initially 7.5 mg/24 hours, adjusted according to response

DOSE EQUIVALENCE AND CONVERSION

▸ When switching between formulations in patients already receiving oxycodone, 2 mg oral oxycodone is approximately equivalent to 1 mg parenteral oxycodone.

ONEXILA XL®

Severe pain

▸ BY MOUTH

▸ **Adult:** Initially 10 mg every 24 hours, dose to be increased if necessary according to severity of pain, some patients may require higher doses than the maximum daily dose; maximum 400 mg per day

IMPORTANT SAFETY INFORMATION

Do not confuse modified-release 12-hourly preparations with 24-hourly preparations, see *Prescribing and dispensing information*.

- CONTRA-INDICATIONS Acute abdomen · chronic constipation · cor pulmonale · delayed gastric emptying
- CAUTIONS Pancreatitis · toxic psychosis
- INTERACTIONS → Appendix 1: opioids
- SIDE-EFFECTS

GENERAL SIDE-EFFECTS

▸ **Common or very common** Anxiety · bronchospasm · depression · diarrhoea · dyspnoea · gastrointestinal discomfort · hiccups · mood altered · tremor

▸ **Uncommon** Biliary colic · burping · chills · dehydration · dysphagia · gastrointestinal disorders · malaise · memory loss · neuromuscular dysfunction · oedema · seizure · sensation abnormal · sexual dysfunction · speech disorder · syncope · taste altered · thirst · vasodilation

▸ **Frequency not known** Aggression · amenorrhoea · cholestasis

SPECIFIC SIDE-EFFECTS

▸ **Common or very common**

▸ With oral use Appetite abnormal · asthenic conditions · cognitive impairment · insomnia · movement disorders · perception altered · psychiatric disorders · urinary frequency increased

▸ With parenteral use Appetite decreased · asthenia · cough decreased · sleep disorders · thinking abnormal

▸ **Uncommon**

▸ With oral use Chest pain · cough · hyperacusia · increased risk of infection · injury · lacrimation disorder · migraine · oral disorders · pain · SIADH · voice alteration

▸ With parenteral use Fever · hypogonadism · ureteral spasm

▸ **Rare or very rare**

▸ With oral use Haemorrhage · lymphadenopathy · muscle spasms · photosensitivity reaction · tooth discolouration · weight changes

▸ **Frequency not known**

▸ With parenteral use Dental caries · hyperalgesia · withdrawal syndrome neonatal

- BREAST FEEDING Present in milk—avoid.
- HEPATIC IMPAIRMENT Manufacturer advises caution in mild impairment; avoid in moderate to severe impairment.
Dose adjustments Manufacturer advises initial dose reduction of 50% in mild impairment; adjust according to response.
- RENAL IMPAIRMENT Opioid effects increased and prolonged and increased cerebral sensitivity occurs. Avoid if eGFR less than 10 mL/minute/1.73 m².
Dose adjustments Max. initial dose 2.5 mg every 6 hours in patients not currently treated with an opioid with mild to moderate impairment.
- DIRECTIONS FOR ADMINISTRATION
▸ With intravenous use For intravenous infusion (*Oxynorm*®), manufacturer advises give continuously *or* intermittently in Glucose 5% or Sodium chloride 0.9%; dilute to a concentration of 1 mg/mL.
- PRESCRIBING AND DISPENSING INFORMATION Modified-release preparations are available as 12-hourly or 24-hourly formulations. Preparations that should be given 12-hourly include *Abtard*®, *Carexil*®, *Ixyldone*®, *Leveraxo*®, *Longtec*®, *Oxeltra*®, *OxyContin*®, *Oxypro*®, *Oxylan*®, *Reltebon*®, and *Renocontin*®. Preparations that should be given 24-hourly include *Onexila*® XL.

Palliative care For further information on the use of oxycodone in palliative care, see www.medicinescomplete. com/#/content/palliative/oxycodone.

- NATIONAL FUNDING/ACCESS DECISIONS
For full details see funding body website
Scottish Medicines Consortium (SMC) decisions
▸ Oxycodone injection (*OxyNorm*®) for the treatment of moderate to severe pain in patients with cancer (October 2004) SMC No. 125/04 Recommended with restrictions

▸ Oxycodone 5 mg, 10 mg, 20 mg, 40 mg and 80 mg prolonged release tablets (*OxyContin*®) for the treatment of severe non-malignant pain requiring a strong opioid (September 2005) SMC No. 197/05 Recommended

▸ Oxycodone hydrochloride 50 mg/mL injection (*OxyNorm*®) for the treatment of moderate to severe pain in patients with cancer (November 2010) SMC No. 648/10 Recommended with restrictions

- MEDICINAL FORMS There can be variation in the licensing of different medicines containing the same drug. Forms available from special-order manufacturers include: oral solution, solution for infusion

Modified-release tablet

CAUTIONARY AND ADVISORY LABELS 2, 25

▸ Abtard (Ethypharm UK Ltd)
Oxycodone hydrochloride 15 mg Abtard 15mg modified-release tablets | 56 tablet [PoM] £19.06 DT = £38.12 [CD2]
Oxycodone hydrochloride 30 mg Abtard 30mg modified-release tablets | 56 tablet [PoM] £38.11 DT = £76.23 [CD2]
Oxycodone hydrochloride 40 mg Abtard 40mg modified-release tablets | 56 tablet [PoM] £50.09 DT = £100.19 [CD2]
Oxycodone hydrochloride 60 mg Abtard 60mg modified-release tablets | 56 tablet [PoM] £76.24 DT = £152.49 [CD2]
Oxycodone hydrochloride 80 mg Abtard 80mg modified-release tablets | 56 tablet [PoM] £100.19 DT = £200.39 [CD2]

▸ Carexil (Sandoz Ltd)
Oxycodone hydrochloride 5 mg Carexil 5mg modified-release tablets | 28 tablet [PoM] £6.26 DT = £12.52 [CD2]
Oxycodone hydrochloride 20 mg Carexil 20mg modified-release tablets | 56 tablet [PoM] £25.04 DT = £50.08 [CD2]
Oxycodone hydrochloride 40 mg Carexil 40mg modified-release tablets | 56 tablet [PoM] £60.11 DT = £100.19 [CD2]
Oxycodone hydrochloride 80 mg Carexil 80mg modified-release tablets | 56 tablet [PoM] £120.23 DT = £200.39 [CD2]

▸ Ixyldone (Morningside Healthcare Ltd)
Oxycodone hydrochloride 5 mg Ixyldone 5mg modified-release tablets | 28 tablet [PoM] £2.96 DT = £12.52 [CD2]
Oxycodone hydrochloride 10 mg Ixyldone 10mg modified-release tablets | 56 tablet [PoM] £5.94 DT = £25.04 [CD2]
Oxycodone hydrochloride 15 mg Ixyldone 15mg modified-release tablets | 56 tablet [PoM] £9.05 DT = £38.12 [CD2]
Oxycodone hydrochloride 20 mg Ixyldone 20mg modified-release tablets | 56 tablet [PoM] £11.88 DT = £50.08 [CD2]
Oxycodone hydrochloride 30 mg Ixyldone 30mg modified-release tablets | 56 tablet [PoM] £18.10 DT = £76.23 [CD2]
Oxycodone hydrochloride 40 mg Ixyldone 40mg modified-release tablets | 56 tablet [PoM] £23.79 DT = £100.19 [CD2]
Oxycodone hydrochloride 60 mg Ixyldone 60mg modified-release tablets | 56 tablet [PoM] £36.19 DT = £152.49 [CD2]
Oxycodone hydrochloride 80 mg Ixyldone 80mg modified-release tablets | 56 tablet [PoM] £47.58 DT = £200.39 [CD2]

▸ Leveraxo (Mylan)
Oxycodone hydrochloride 30 mg Leveraxo 30mg modified-release tablets | 56 tablet [PoM] £75.47 DT = £76.23 [CD2]
Oxycodone hydrochloride 60 mg Leveraxo 60mg modified-release tablets | 56 tablet [PoM] £150.97 DT = £152.49 [CD2]

▸ Longtec (Qdem Pharmaceuticals Ltd)
Oxycodone hydrochloride 5 mg Longtec 5mg modified-release tablets | 28 tablet [PoM] £6.26 DT = £12.52 [CD2]
Oxycodone hydrochloride 10 mg Longtec 10mg modified-release tablets | 56 tablet [PoM] £12.52 DT = £25.04 [CD2]
Oxycodone hydrochloride 15 mg Longtec 15mg modified-release tablets | 56 tablet [PoM] £19.06 DT = £38.12 [CD2]
Oxycodone hydrochloride 20 mg Longtec 20mg modified-release tablets | 56 tablet [PoM] £25.04 DT = £50.08 [CD2]
Oxycodone hydrochloride 30 mg Longtec 30mg modified-release tablets | 56 tablet [PoM] £38.11 DT = £76.23 [CD2]
Oxycodone hydrochloride 40 mg Longtec 40mg modified-release tablets | 56 tablet [PoM] £50.09 DT = £100.19 [CD2]
Oxycodone hydrochloride 60 mg Longtec 60mg modified-release tablets | 56 tablet [PoM] £76.24 DT = £152.49 [CD2]
Oxycodone hydrochloride 80 mg Longtec 80mg modified-release tablets | 56 tablet [PoM] £100.19 DT = £200.39 [CD2]
Oxycodone hydrochloride 120 mg Longtec 120mg modified-release tablets | 56 tablet [PoM] £152.51 DT = £305.02 [CD2]

▸ Onexila XL (Aspire Pharma Ltd)
Oxycodone hydrochloride 10 mg Onexila XL 10mg tablets | 28 tablet [PoM] £12.52 [CD2]

Oxycodone hydrochloride 20 mg Onexila XL 20mg tablets | 28 tablet PoM £12.52 CD2

Oxycodone hydrochloride 40 mg Onexila XL 40mg tablets | 28 tablet PoM £25.04 CD2

Oxycodone hydrochloride 80 mg Onexila XL 80mg tablets | 28 tablet PoM £50.09 CD2

‣ Oxeltra (Wockhardt UK Ltd)

Oxycodone hydrochloride 5 mg Oxeltra 5mg modified-release tablets | 28 tablet PoM £3.13 DT = £12.52 CD2

Oxycodone hydrochloride 10 mg Oxeltra 10mg modified-release tablets | 56 tablet PoM £6.26 DT = £25.04 CD2

Oxycodone hydrochloride 15 mg Oxeltra 15mg modified-release tablets | 56 tablet PoM £9.53 DT = £38.12 CD2

Oxycodone hydrochloride 20 mg Oxeltra 20mg modified-release tablets | 56 tablet PoM £12.52 DT = £50.08 CD2

Oxycodone hydrochloride 30 mg Oxeltra 30mg modified-release tablets | 56 tablet PoM £19.06 DT = £76.23 CD2

Oxycodone hydrochloride 40 mg Oxeltra 40mg modified-release tablets | 56 tablet PoM £25.05 DT = £100.19 CD2

Oxycodone hydrochloride 60 mg Oxeltra 60mg modified-release tablets | 56 tablet PoM £38.12 DT = £152.49 CD2

Oxycodone hydrochloride 80 mg Oxeltra 80mg modified-release tablets | 56 tablet PoM £50.10 DT = £200.39 CD2

‣ OxyContin (Napp Pharmaceuticals Ltd)

Oxycodone hydrochloride 5 mg OxyContin 5mg modified-release tablets | 28 tablet PoM £12.52 DT = £12.52 CD2

Oxycodone hydrochloride 10 mg OxyContin 10mg modified-release tablets | 56 tablet PoM £25.04 DT = £25.04 CD2

Oxycodone hydrochloride 15 mg OxyContin 15mg modified-release tablets | 56 tablet PoM £38.12 DT = £38.12 CD2

Oxycodone hydrochloride 20 mg OxyContin 20mg modified-release tablets | 56 tablet PoM £50.08 DT = £50.08 CD2

Oxycodone hydrochloride 30 mg OxyContin 30mg modified-release tablets | 56 tablet PoM £76.23 DT = £76.23 CD2

Oxycodone hydrochloride 40 mg OxyContin 40mg modified-release tablets | 56 tablet PoM £100.19 DT = £100.19 CD2

Oxycodone hydrochloride 60 mg OxyContin 60mg modified-release tablets | 56 tablet PoM £152.49 DT = £152.49 CD2

Oxycodone hydrochloride 80 mg OxyContin 80mg modified-release tablets | 56 tablet PoM £200.39 DT = £200.39 CD2

Oxycodone hydrochloride 120 mg OxyContin 120mg modified-release tablets | 56 tablet PoM £305.02 DT = £305.02 CD2

‣ Oxylan (Healthcare Pharma Ltd)

Oxycodone hydrochloride 5 mg Oxylan 5mg modified-release tablets | 28 tablet PoM £12.50 DT = £12.52 CD2

Oxycodone hydrochloride 10 mg Oxylan 10mg modified-release tablets | 56 tablet PoM £24.99 DT = £25.04 CD2

Oxycodone hydrochloride 20 mg Oxylan 20mg modified-release tablets | 56 tablet PoM £49.98 DT = £50.08 CD2

Oxycodone hydrochloride 40 mg Oxylan 40mg modified-release tablets | 56 tablet PoM £99.98 DT = £100.19 CD2

Oxycodone hydrochloride 80 mg Oxylan 80mg modified-release tablets | 56 tablet PoM £199.97 DT = £200.39 CD2

‣ Oxypro (Ridge Pharma Ltd)

Oxycodone hydrochloride 5 mg Oxypro 5mg modified-release tablets | 28 tablet PoM £3.13 DT = £12.52 CD2

Oxycodone hydrochloride 10 mg Oxypro 10mg modified-release tablets | 56 tablet PoM £6.26 DT = £25.04 CD2

Oxycodone hydrochloride 15 mg Oxypro 15mg modified-release tablets | 56 tablet PoM £9.53 DT = £38.12 CD2

Oxycodone hydrochloride 20 mg Oxypro 20mg modified-release tablets | 56 tablet PoM £12.52 DT = £50.08 CD2

Oxycodone hydrochloride 30 mg Oxypro 30mg modified-release tablets | 56 tablet PoM £19.06 DT = £76.23 CD2

Oxycodone hydrochloride 40 mg Oxypro 40mg modified-release tablets | 56 tablet PoM £25.05 DT = £100.19 CD2

Oxycodone hydrochloride 60 mg Oxypro 60mg modified-release tablets | 56 tablet PoM £38.12 DT = £152.49 CD2

Oxycodone hydrochloride 80 mg Oxypro 80mg modified-release tablets | 56 tablet PoM £50.10 DT = £200.39 CD2

‣ Reltebon (Accord Healthcare Ltd)

Oxycodone hydrochloride 5 mg Reltebon 5mg modified-release tablets | 28 tablet PoM £6.26 DT = £12.52 CD2

Oxycodone hydrochloride 10 mg Reltebon 10mg modified-release tablets | 56 tablet PoM £12.52 DT = £25.04 CD2

Oxycodone hydrochloride 15 mg Reltebon 15mg modified-release tablets | 56 tablet PoM £19.06 DT = £38.12 CD2

Oxycodone hydrochloride 20 mg Reltebon 20mg modified-release tablets | 56 tablet PoM £25.04 DT = £50.08 CD2

Oxycodone hydrochloride 30 mg Reltebon 30mg modified-release tablets | 56 tablet PoM £38.11 DT = £76.23 CD2

Oxycodone hydrochloride 40 mg Reltebon 40mg modified-release tablets | 56 tablet PoM £50.09 DT = £100.19 CD2

Oxycodone hydrochloride 60 mg Reltebon 60mg modified-release tablets | 56 tablet PoM £76.24 DT = £152.49 CD2

Oxycodone hydrochloride 80 mg Reltebon 80mg modified-release tablets | 56 tablet PoM £100.19 DT = £200.39 CD2

‣ Renocontin (Glenmark Pharmaceuticals Europe Ltd)

Oxycodone hydrochloride 5 mg Renocontin 5mg modified-release tablets | 28 tablet PoM £2.75 DT = £12.52 CD2

Oxycodone hydrochloride 10 mg Renocontin 10mg modified-release tablets | 56 tablet PoM £5.50 DT = £25.04 CD2

Oxycodone hydrochloride 15 mg Renocontin 15mg modified-release tablets | 56 tablet PoM £8.00 DT = £38.12 CD2

Oxycodone hydrochloride 20 mg Renocontin 20mg modified-release tablets | 56 tablet PoM £9.90 DT = £50.08 CD2

Oxycodone hydrochloride 30 mg Renocontin 30mg modified-release tablets | 56 tablet PoM £16.50 DT = £76.23 CD2

Oxycodone hydrochloride 40 mg Renocontin 40mg modified-release tablets | 56 tablet PoM £21.50 DT = £100.19 CD2

Oxycodone hydrochloride 60 mg Renocontin 60mg modified-release tablets | 56 tablet PoM £33.50 DT = £152.49 CD2

Solution for injection

‣ Oxycodone hydrochloride (Non-proprietary)

Oxycodone hydrochloride 10 mg per 1 ml Oxycodone 20mg/2ml solution for injection ampoules | 5 ampoule PoM £16.00 DT = £16.00 CD2 | 10 ampoule PoM £30.00 CD2

Oxycodone 10mg/1ml solution for injection ampoules | 5 ampoule PoM £8.00 DT = £8.00 CD2 | 10 ampoule PoM £15.00 CD2

Oxycodone hydrochloride 50 mg per 1 ml Oxycodone 50mg/1ml solution for injection ampoules | 5 ampoule PoM £70.10 DT = £70.10 CD2 | 10 ampoule PoM £135.00 CD2

‣ OxyNorm (Napp Pharmaceuticals Ltd)

Oxycodone hydrochloride 10 mg per 1 ml OxyNorm 10mg/1ml solution for injection ampoules | 5 ampoule PoM £8.00 DT = £8.00 CD2

OxyNorm 20mg/2ml solution for injection ampoules | 5 ampoule PoM £16.00 DT = £16.00 CD2

Oxycodone hydrochloride 50 mg per 1 ml OxyNorm 50mg/1ml solution for injection ampoules | 5 ampoule PoM £70.10 DT = £70.10 CD2

‣ Shortec (Qdem Pharmaceuticals Ltd)

Oxycodone hydrochloride 10 mg per 1 ml Shortec 20mg/2ml solution for injection ampoules | 5 ampoule PoM £13.60 DT = £16.00 CD2

Shortec 10mg/1ml solution for injection ampoules | 5 ampoule PoM £6.80 DT = £8.00 CD2

Oxycodone hydrochloride 50 mg per 1 ml Shortec 50mg/1ml solution for injection ampoules | 5 ampoule PoM £59.59 DT = £70.10 CD2

Oral solution

CAUTIONARY AND ADVISORY LABELS 2

‣ Oxycodone hydrochloride (Non-proprietary)

Oxycodone hydrochloride 1 mg per 1 ml Oxycodone 5mg/5ml oral solution sugar free sugar-free | 250 ml PoM £11.63 DT = £9.71 CD2

Oxycodone hydrochloride 10 mg per 1 ml Oxycodone 10mg/ml oral solution sugar free sugar-free | 120 ml PoM £55.95 DT = £46.63 CD2

‣ OxyNorm (Napp Pharmaceuticals Ltd)

Oxycodone hydrochloride 1 mg per 1 ml OxyNorm liquid 1mg/ml oral solution sugar-free | 250 ml PoM £9.71 DT = £9.71 CD2

Oxycodone hydrochloride 10 mg per 1 ml OxyNorm 10mg/ml concentrate oral solution sugar-free | 120 ml PoM £46.63 CD2

‣ Shortec (Qdem Pharmaceuticals Ltd)

Oxycodone hydrochloride 1 mg per 1 ml Shortec liquid 1mg/ml oral solution sugar-free | 250 ml PoM £8.25 DT = £9.71 CD2

Oxycodone hydrochloride 10 mg per 1 ml Shortec 10mg/ml concentrate oral solution sugar-free | 120 ml PoM £39.64 DT = £46.63 CD2

Capsule

CAUTIONARY AND ADVISORY LABELS 2

‣ Lynlor (Accord Healthcare Ltd)

Oxycodone hydrochloride 5 mg Lynlor 5mg capsules | 56 capsule PoM £6.86 DT = £11.43 CD2

Oxycodone hydrochloride 10 mg Lynlor 10mg capsules | 56 capsule PoM £13.72 DT = £22.86 CD2

Oxycodone hydrochloride 20 mg Lynlor 20mg capsules | 56 capsule PoM £27.43 DT = £45.71 CD2

► OxyNorm (Napp Pharmaceuticals Ltd)
Oxycodone hydrochloride 5 mg OxyNorm 5mg capsules |
56 capsule PoM £11.43 DT = £11.43 CD2
Oxycodone hydrochloride 10 mg OxyNorm 10mg capsules |
56 capsule PoM £22.86 DT = £22.86 CD2
Oxycodone hydrochloride 20 mg OxyNorm 20mg capsules |
56 capsule PoM £45.71 DT = £45.71 CD2
► Shortec (Qdem Pharmaceuticals Ltd)
Oxycodone hydrochloride 5 mg Shortec 5mg capsules |
56 capsule PoM £6.86 DT = £11.43 CD2
Oxycodone hydrochloride 10 mg Shortec 10mg capsules |
56 capsule PoM £13.72 DT = £22.86 CD2
Oxycodone hydrochloride 20 mg Shortec 20mg capsules |
56 capsule PoM £27.43 DT = £45.71 CD2

Oxycodone with naloxone

The properties listed below are those particular to the
combination only. For the properties of the components
please consider, oxycodone hydrochloride p. 486, naloxone
hydrochloride p. 1424.

● **INDICATIONS AND DOSE**

**Severe pain requiring opioid analgesia in patients not
currently treated with opioid analgesics**
► BY MOUTH
► Adult: Initially 10/5 mg every 12 hours (max. per dose
40/20 mg every 12 hours), dose to be increased
according to response; patients already receiving
opioid analgesics can start with a higher dose

**Second-line treatment of symptomatic severe to very
severe idiopathic restless legs syndrome after failure of
dopaminergic therapy**
► BY MOUTH
► Adult: Initially 5/2.5 mg every 12 hours, adjusted
weekly according to response, usual dose 10/5 mg
every 12 hours; maximum 60/30 mg per day

DOSE EQUIVALENCE AND CONVERSION
► Dose quantities are expressed in the form x/y where x
and y are the strengths in milligrams of oxycodone and
naloxone respectively.

● INTERACTIONS → Appendix 1: opioids

● MEDICINAL FORMS There can be variation in the licensing of
different medicines containing the same drug. Forms available
from special-order manufacturers include: oral suspension
Modified-release tablet
CAUTIONARY AND ADVISORY LABELS 2, 25
► Targinact (Napp Pharmaceuticals Ltd)
**Naloxone hydrochloride 2.5 mg, Oxycodone hydrochloride
5 mg** Targinact 5mg/2.5mg modified-release tablets |
28 tablet PoM £21.16 DT = £21.16 CD2
**Naloxone hydrochloride 5 mg, Oxycodone hydrochloride
10 mg** Targinact 10mg/5mg modified-release tablets |
56 tablet PoM £42.32 DT = £42.32 CD2
**Naloxone hydrochloride 10 mg, Oxycodone hydrochloride
20 mg** Targinact 20mg/10mg modified-release tablets |
56 tablet PoM £84.62 DT = £84.62 CD2
**Naloxone hydrochloride 20 mg, Oxycodone hydrochloride
40 mg** Targinact 40mg/20mg modified-release tablets |
56 tablet PoM £169.28 DT = £169.28 CD2

F 467

Pentazocine

13-Nov-2020

● **INDICATIONS AND DOSE**
Moderate to severe pain
► BY MOUTH
► Adult: 50 mg every 3–4 hours, dose to be taken
preferably after food, usual dose 25–100 mg every
3–4 hours; maximum 600 mg per day

Moderate pain
► BY SUBCUTANEOUS INJECTION, OR BY INTRAMUSCULAR
INJECTION, OR BY INTRAVENOUS INJECTION
► Adult: 30 mg every 3–4 hours as required; maximum
360 mg per day
Severe pain
► BY SUBCUTANEOUS INJECTION, OR BY INTRAMUSCULAR
INJECTION, OR BY INTRAVENOUS INJECTION
► Adult: 45–60 mg every 3–4 hours as required;
maximum 360 mg per day

● CONTRA-INDICATIONS Acute porphyrias p. 1107 · heart
failure secondary to chronic lung disease · patients
dependent on opioids (can precipitate withdrawal)
● CAUTIONS Arterial hypertension · cardiac arrhythmias ·
myocardial infarction · pancreatitis · phaeochromocytoma ·
pulmonary hypertension
● INTERACTIONS → Appendix 1: opioids
● SIDE-EFFECTS Biliary spasm · blood disorder · chills ·
circulatory depression · face oedema · facial plethora ·
generalised tonic-clonic seizure · hypertension ·
hypothermia · intracranial pressure increased · mood
altered · myalgia · paraesthesia · sexual dysfunction · sleep
disorders · syncope · toxic epidermal necrolysis · tremor ·
ureteral spasm
Overdose Effects only partially reversed by naloxone.
● BREAST FEEDING Use with caution—limited information
available.
● HEPATIC IMPAIRMENT Manufacturer advises caution in
severe impairment (risk of increased bioavailability).
Dose adjustments Manufacturer advises consider dose
reduction in severe impairment.
● RENAL IMPAIRMENT Avoid use or reduce dose; opioid
effects increased and prolonged and increased cerebral
sensitivity occurs.
● LESS SUITABLE FOR PRESCRIBING Pentazocine is less
suitable for prescribing.

● MEDICINAL FORMS There can be variation in the licensing of
different medicines containing the same drug.
Tablet
CAUTIONARY AND ADVISORY LABELS 2, 21
► Pentazocine (Non-proprietary)
Pentazocine hydrochloride 25 mg Pentazocine 25mg tablets |
28 tablet PoM £25.04 DT = £25.04 CD3
Capsule
CAUTIONARY AND ADVISORY LABELS 2, 21
► Pentazocine (Non-proprietary)
Pentazocine hydrochloride 50 mg Pentazocine 50mg capsules |
28 capsule PoM £28.50 DT = £28.50 CD3

F 467

Pethidine hydrochloride

13-Nov-2020

(Meperidine)

● **INDICATIONS AND DOSE**
Acute pain
► BY MOUTH
► Adult: 50–150 mg every 4 hours
► BY SUBCUTANEOUS INJECTION, OR BY INTRAMUSCULAR
INJECTION
► Adult: 25–100 mg, then 25–100 mg after 4 hours, for
debilitated patients use dose described for elderly
patients
► Elderly: Initially 25 mg, then 25–100 mg after 4 hours
► BY SLOW INTRAVENOUS INJECTION
► Adult: 25–50 mg, then 25–50 mg after 4 hours, for
debilitated patients use dose described for elderly
patients
► Elderly: Initially 25 mg, then 25–50 mg after 4 hours

continued →

4

Nervous system

Obstetric analgesia
▸ BY SUBCUTANEOUS INJECTION, OR BY INTRAMUSCULAR INJECTION
▸ Adult: 50–100 mg, then 50–100 mg after 1–3 hours if required; maximum 400 mg per day

Premedication
▸ BY INTRAMUSCULAR INJECTION
▸ Adult: 25–100 mg, dose to be given 1 hour before operation, for debilitated patients use dose described for elderly patients
▸ Elderly: 25 mg, dose to be given 1 hour before operation

Postoperative pain
▸ BY SUBCUTANEOUS INJECTION, OR BY INTRAMUSCULAR INJECTION
▸ Adult: 25–100 mg every 2–3 hours if required, for debilitated patients use dose described for elderly patients
▸ Elderly: Initially 25 mg every 2–3 hours if required

● CONTRA-INDICATIONS Phaeochromocytoma
● CAUTIONS Accumulation of metabolites may result in toxicity · cardiac arrhythmias · not suitable for severe continuing pain · severe cor pulmonale
● INTERACTIONS → Appendix 1: opioids
● SIDE-EFFECTS
GENERAL SIDE-EFFECTS
Biliary spasm · dysuria · hypothermia
SPECIFIC SIDE-EFFECTS
▸ With oral use Agitation · mood altered · muscle rigidity · sexual dysfunction · ureteral spasm
▸ With parenteral use Anxiety · asthenia · coordination abnormal · delirium · seizure · syncope · tremor
Overdose Convulsions reported in overdosage.
● BREAST FEEDING Present in milk but not known to be harmful.
● HEPATIC IMPAIRMENT Manufacturer advises caution in mild to moderate impairment; avoid in severe impairment.
Dose adjustments Manufacturer advises dose reduction in mild to moderate impairment.
● RENAL IMPAIRMENT Avoid use or reduce dose; opioid effects increased and prolonged and increased cerebral sensitivity occurs.

● MEDICINAL FORMS There can be variation in the licensing of different medicines containing the same drug. Forms available from special-order manufacturers include: capsule, oral solution, solution for injection
Tablet
CAUTIONARY AND ADVISORY LABELS 2
▸ Pethidine hydrochloride (Non-proprietary)
Pethidine hydrochloride 50 mg Pethidine 50mg tablets | 50 tablet PoM £49.92 DT = £49.92 CD2
Solution for injection
▸ Pethidine hydrochloride (Non-proprietary)
Pethidine hydrochloride 50 mg per 1 ml Pethidine 50mg/1ml solution for injection ampoules | 10 ampoule PoM £5.11 DT = £5.11 CD2
Pethidine 100mg/2ml solution for injection ampoules | 10 ampoule PoM £4.66 DT = £4.66 CD2

F 467

Tapentadol
16-Nov-2020

● INDICATIONS AND DOSE
Moderate to severe acute pain which can be managed only with opioid analgesics
▸ BY MOUTH USING IMMEDIATE-RELEASE MEDICINES
▸ Adult: Initially 50 mg every 4–6 hours, adjusted according to response, on the first day of treatment, an additional dose of 50 mg may be taken 1 hour after the initial dose; maximum 700 mg in the first 24 hours; maximum 600 mg per day

Severe chronic pain
▸ BY MOUTH USING MODIFIED-RELEASE MEDICINES
▸ Adult: Initially 50 mg every 12 hours, adjusted according to response; maximum 500 mg per day

---

IMPORTANT SAFETY INFORMATION

MHRA/CHM ADVICE: TAPENTADOL (*PALEXIA* ®): RISK OF SEIZURES AND REPORTS OF SEROTONIN SYNDROME WHEN CO-ADMINISTERED WITH OTHER MEDICINES (JANUARY 2019)
Tapentadol can induce seizures and should be prescribed with caution in patients with a history of seizure disorders or epilepsy. Seizure risk may be increased in patients taking other medicines that lower seizure threshold, for example, antidepressants such as selective serotonin reuptake inhibitors (SSRIs), serotonin-noradrenaline reuptake inhibitors (SNRIs), tricyclic antidepressants, and antipsychotics.

Serotonin syndrome has been reported when tapentadol is used in combination with serotonergic antidepressants—withdrawal of the serotonergic medicine, together with supportive symptomatic care, usually brings about a rapid improvement in serotonin syndrome.

● INTERACTIONS → Appendix 1: opioids
● SIDE-EFFECTS
▸ **Common or very common** Anxiety · appetite decreased · asthenia · diarrhoea · feeling of body temperature change · gastrointestinal discomfort · muscle spasms · sleep disorders · tremor
▸ **Uncommon** Concentration impaired · depressed mood · dysarthria · dyspnoea · feeling abnormal · irritability · memory loss · movement disorders · muscle contractions involuntary · oedema · sensation abnormal · urinary disorders
▸ **Rare or very rare** Angioedema · impaired gastric emptying · level of consciousness decreased · seizure · thinking abnormal
● BREAST FEEDING Avoid—no information available.
● HEPATIC IMPAIRMENT Manufacturer advises caution in moderate impairment; avoid in severe impairment (no information available).
Dose adjustments Manufacturer advises reduce initial daily dose in moderate impairment. For *immediate-release tablets*, initiate at 50 mg up to every 8 hours; for *oral solution*, initiate at 25 mg up to every 8 hours; for *modified-release tablets*, initiate at 50 mg up to every 24 hours.
● RENAL IMPAIRMENT Manufacturer advises avoid in severe impairment (no information available).
● NATIONAL FUNDING/ACCESS DECISIONS
For full details see funding body website
Scottish Medicines Consortium (SMC) decisions
▸ Tapentadol (*Palexia SR* ®) for the management of severe chronic pain in adults (June 2011) SMC No. 654/10 Recommended with restrictions

---

● MEDICINAL FORMS There can be variation in the licensing of different medicines containing the same drug.
Oral solution
CAUTIONARY AND ADVISORY LABELS 2
EXCIPIENTS: May contain Propylene glycol
▸ Palexia (Grunenthal Ltd)
Tapentadol (as Tapentadol hydrochloride) 20 mg per 1 ml Palexia 20mg/ml oral solution sugar-free | 100 ml PoM £17.80 DT = £17.80 CD2

Modified-release tablet
CAUTIONARY AND ADVISORY LABELS 2, 25
▸ Palexia SR (Grunenthal Ltd)
  Tapentadol (as Tapentadol hydrochloride) 50 mg Palexia SR 50mg
  tablets | 28 tablet PoM £12.46 DT = £12.46 CD2 | 56 tablet PoM
  £24.91 DT = £24.91 CD2
  Tapentadol (as Tapentadol hydrochloride) 100 mg Palexia SR
  100mg tablets | 56 tablet PoM £49.82 DT = £49.82 CD2
  Tapentadol (as Tapentadol hydrochloride) 150 mg Palexia SR
  150mg tablets | 56 tablet PoM £74.73 DT = £74.73 CD2
  Tapentadol (as Tapentadol hydrochloride) 200 mg Palexia SR
  200mg tablets | 56 tablet PoM £99.64 DT = £99.64 CD2
  Tapentadol (as Tapentadol hydrochloride) 250 mg Palexia SR
  250mg tablets | 56 tablet PoM £124.55 DT = £124.55 CD2

Tablet
CAUTIONARY AND ADVISORY LABELS 2
▸ Palexia (Grunenthal Ltd)
  Tapentadol (as Tapentadol hydrochloride) 50 mg Palexia 50mg
  tablets | 28 tablet PoM £12.46 DT = £12.46 CD2 | 56 tablet PoM
  £24.91 CD2
  Tapentadol (as Tapentadol hydrochloride) 75 mg Palexia 75mg
  tablets | 28 tablet PoM £18.68 DT = £18.68 CD2 | 56 tablet PoM
  £37.37 DT = £37.37 CD2

▰ 467

Tramadol hydrochloride

13-Nov-2020

● **INDICATIONS AND DOSE**
Moderate to severe pain
▸ BY INTRAMUSCULAR INJECTION, OR BY INTRAVENOUS
  INJECTION, OR BY INTRAVENOUS INFUSION, OR BY
  SUBCUTANEOUS INJECTION
▸ Adult: 50–100 mg every 4–6 hours, intravenous
  injection to be given over 2–3 minutes; Usual
  maximum 400 mg/24 hours
Moderate to severe acute pain
▸ BY MOUTH USING IMMEDIATE-RELEASE MEDICINES
▸ Child 12-17 years: Initially 100 mg, then 50–100 mg
  every 4–6 hours; Usual maximum 400 mg/24 hours
▸ Adult: Initially 100 mg, then 50–100 mg every
  4–6 hours; Usual maximum 400 mg/24 hours
Moderate to severe chronic pain
▸ BY MOUTH USING IMMEDIATE-RELEASE MEDICINES
▸ Child 12-17 years: Initially 50 mg, then, adjusted
  according to response; Usual maximum
  400 mg/24 hours
▸ Adult: Initially 50 mg, then, adjusted according to
  response; Usual maximum 400 mg/24 hours
Postoperative pain
▸ BY INTRAVENOUS INJECTION, OR BY INTRAMUSCULAR
  INJECTION, OR BY INTRAVENOUS INFUSION, OR BY
  SUBCUTANEOUS INJECTION
▸ Adult: Initially 100 mg, then 50 mg every
  10–20 minutes if required up to total maximum 250 mg
  (including initial dose) in first hour, then 50–100 mg
  every 4–6 hours, intravenous injection to be given over
  2–3 minutes; Usual maximum 400 mg/24 hours
**Moderate to severe pain (with modified-release 12-hourly
preparations)**
▸ BY MOUTH USING MODIFIED-RELEASE MEDICINES
▸ Child 12-17 years: 50–100 mg twice daily, increased if
  necessary to 150–200 mg twice daily, doses exceeding
  the usual maximum not generally required; Usual
  maximum 400 mg/24 hours
▸ Adult: 50–100 mg twice daily, increased if necessary to
  150–200 mg twice daily, doses exceeding the usual
  maximum not generally required; Usual maximum
  400 mg/24 hours

**Moderate to severe pain (with modified-release 24-hourly
preparations)**
▸ BY MOUTH USING MODIFIED-RELEASE MEDICINES
▸ Child 12-17 years: Initially 100–150 mg once daily,
  increased if necessary up to 400 mg once daily; Usual
  maximum 400 mg/24 hours
▸ Adult: Initially 100–150 mg once daily, increased if
  necessary up to 400 mg once daily; Usual maximum
  400 mg/24 hours
ZYDOL® XL
Moderate to severe pain
▸ BY MOUTH USING MODIFIED-RELEASE TABLETS
▸ Child 12-17 years: Initially 150 mg once daily, increased
  if necessary up to 400 mg once daily
▸ Adult: Initially 150 mg once daily, increased if
  necessary up to 400 mg once daily

┌───┐
│ IMPORTANT SAFETY INFORMATION   │
│ Do not confuse modified-release 12-hourly   │
│ preparations with 24-hourly preparations, see   │
│ *Prescribing and dispensing information*.   │
└───┘

● CONTRA-INDICATIONS Acute intoxication with alcohol ·
  acute intoxication with analgesics · acute intoxication with
  hypnotics · acute intoxication with opioids · compromised
  respiratory function (in children) · not suitable for narcotic
  withdrawal treatment · uncontrolled epilepsy
● CAUTIONS Excessive bronchial secretions · history of
  epilepsy—use tramadol only if compelling reasons ·
  impaired consciousness · not suitable as a substitute in
  opioid-dependent patients · postoperative use (in
  children) · susceptibility to seizures—use tramadol only if
  compelling reasons · variation in metabolism
  CAUTIONS, FURTHER INFORMATION
▸ Variation in metabolism The capacity to metabolise tramadol
  can vary considerably between individuals; there is a risk
  of developing side-effects of opioid toxicity in patients
  who are ultra-rapid tramadol metabolisers (CYP2D6 ultra-
  rapid metabolisers) and the therapeutic effect may be
  reduced in poor tramadol metabolisers.
▸ Postoperative use Manufacturer advises extreme caution
  when used for postoperative pain relief in children—
  reports of rare, but life threatening adverse events after
  tonsillectomy and/or adenoidectomy for obstructive sleep
  apnoea; if used, monitor closely for symptoms of opioid
  toxicity.
● INTERACTIONS → Appendix 1: opioids
● SIDE-EFFECTS
  GENERAL SIDE-EFFECTS
▸ **Common or very common** Fatigue
▸ **Rare or very rare** Dyspnoea · epileptiform seizure ·
  respiratory disorders · sleep disorders · vision blurred
▸ **Frequency not known** Asthma exacerbated · hypoglycaemia
  SPECIFIC SIDE-EFFECTS
▸ **Uncommon**
▸ With parenteral use Circulatory collapse · gastrointestinal
  discomfort
▸ **Rare or very rare**
▸ With parenteral use Angioedema · appetite change ·
  behaviour abnormal · cognitive disorder · dysuria ·
  hypersensitivity · mood altered · movement disorders ·
  muscle weakness · perception disorders · psychiatric
  disorder · sensation abnormal
▸ **Frequency not known**
▸ With oral use Anxiety · blood disorder · gastrointestinal
  disorder · hyperkinesia · hypertension · paraesthesia ·
  syncope · tremor · urinary disorder
● PREGNANCY Embryotoxic in *animal* studies—
  manufacturers advise avoid.

4

Nervous system

4

Nervous system

- **BREAST FEEDING** Amount probably too small to be harmful, but manufacturer advises avoid.
- **HEPATIC IMPAIRMENT** Manufacturers advise caution (risk of delayed elimination); some *oral preparations* should be avoided in severe impairment—consult product literature. **Dose adjustments** Manufacturers advise consider increasing dosage interval.
- **RENAL IMPAIRMENT** Avoid use or reduce dose; opioid effects increased and prolonged and increased cerebral sensitivity occurs. Caution (avoid for *oral drops*) in severe impairment.
- **TREATMENT CESSATION** Manufacturer advises consider tapering the dose gradually to prevent withdrawal symptoms.
- **DIRECTIONS FOR ADMINISTRATION** Manufacturer advises tramadol hydrochloride *orodispersible tablets* should be sucked and then swallowed. May also be dispersed in water. Manufacturers advise some tramadol hydrochloride modified-release capsule preparations may be opened and the contents swallowed immediately without chewing— check individual preparations.

  For *intravenous infusion*, manufacturer advises dilute in Glucose 5% or Sodium Chloride 0.9%.
- **PRESCRIBING AND DISPENSING INFORMATION** Modified-release preparations are available as 12-hourly or 24-hourly formulations. Non-proprietary preparations of modified-release tramadol may be available as either 12-hourly or 24-hourly formulations; prescribers and dispensers must ensure that the correct formulation is prescribed and dispensed. Branded preparations that should be given 12-hourly include *Invodol*® SR, *Mabron*®, *Maneo*®, *Marol*®, *Maxitram*® SR, *Oldaram*®, *Tilodol*® SR, *Tramquel*® SR, *Tramulief*® SR, *Zamadol*® SR, *Zeridame*® SR and *Zydol SR*®. Preparations that should be given 24-hourly include *Tradorec XL*®, *Zamadol*® 24hr, and *Zydol XL*®.
- **PATIENT AND CARER ADVICE** Patients or carers should be given advice on how to administer tramadol hydrochloride orodispersible tablets.

  Medicines for Children leaflet: Tramadol for pain
  www.medicinesforchildren.org.uk/tramadol-pain

- **MEDICINAL FORMS** There can be variation in the licensing of different medicines containing the same drug. Forms available from special-order manufacturers include: oral suspension

Modified-release tablet
CAUTIONARY AND ADVISORY LABELS 2, 25
▸ Brimisol PR (Bristol Laboratories Ltd)
Tramadol hydrochloride 100 mg Brimisol PR 100mg tablets | 60 tablet [PoM] [🔬] [CD3]
Tramadol hydrochloride 200 mg Brimisol PR 200mg tablets | 60 tablet [PoM] £36.00 [CD3]
▸ Invodol SR (Ennogen Healthcare Ltd)
Tramadol hydrochloride 100 mg Invodol SR 100mg tablets | 60 tablet [PoM] £5.55 [CD3]
Tramadol hydrochloride 150 mg Invodol SR 150mg tablets | 60 tablet [PoM] £8.31 [CD3]
Tramadol hydrochloride 200 mg Invodol SR 200mg tablets | 60 tablet [PoM] £11.35 [CD3]
▸ Mabron (Teva UK Ltd)
Tramadol hydrochloride 100 mg Mabron 100mg modified-release tablets | 60 tablet [PoM] £15.52 [CD3]
Tramadol hydrochloride 150 mg Mabron 150mg modified-release tablets | 60 tablet [PoM] £23.28 [CD3]
▸ Marol (Teva UK Ltd)
Tramadol hydrochloride 100 mg Marol 100mg modified-release tablets | 60 tablet [PoM] £6.94 [CD3]
Tramadol hydrochloride 150 mg Marol 150mg modified-release tablets | 60 tablet [PoM] £10.39 [CD3]
Tramadol hydrochloride 200 mg Marol 200mg modified-release tablets | 60 tablet [PoM] £14.19 [CD3]
▸ Tilodol SR (Sandoz Ltd)
Tramadol hydrochloride 100 mg Tilodol SR 100mg tablets | 60 tablet [PoM] £15.52 [CD3]

Tramadol hydrochloride 150 mg Tilodol SR 150mg tablets | 60 tablet [PoM] £23.28 [CD3]
Tramadol hydrochloride 200 mg Tilodol SR 200mg tablets | 60 tablet [PoM] £31.04 [CD3]
▸ Tradorec XL (Endo Ventures Ltd)
Tramadol hydrochloride 100 mg Tradorec XL 100mg tablets | 30 tablet [PoM] £14.10 [CD3]
Tramadol hydrochloride 200 mg Tradorec XL 200mg tablets | 30 tablet [PoM] £14.98 [CD3]
Tramadol hydrochloride 300 mg Tradorec XL 300mg tablets | 30 tablet [PoM] £22.47 [CD3]
▸ Tramulief SR (Advanz Pharma)
Tramadol hydrochloride 100 mg Tramulief SR 100mg tablets | 60 tablet [PoM] £6.98 [CD3]
Tramadol hydrochloride 150 mg Tramulief SR 150mg tablets | 60 tablet [PoM] £10.48 [CD3]
Tramadol hydrochloride 200 mg Tramulief SR 200mg tablets | 60 tablet [PoM] £14.28 [CD3]
▸ Zamadol 24hr (Mylan)
Tramadol hydrochloride 150 mg Zamadol 24hr 150mg modified-release tablets | 28 tablet [PoM] £10.70 [CD3]
Tramadol hydrochloride 200 mg Zamadol 24hr 200mg modified-release tablets | 28 tablet [PoM] £14.26 [CD3]
Tramadol hydrochloride 300 mg Zamadol 24hr 300mg modified-release tablets | 28 tablet [PoM] £21.39 [CD3]
Tramadol hydrochloride 400 mg Zamadol 24hr 400mg modified-release tablets | 28 tablet [PoM] £28.51 DT = £28.51 [CD3]
▸ Zydol SR (Grunenthal Ltd)
Tramadol hydrochloride 50 mg Zydol SR 50mg tablets | 60 tablet [PoM] £4.60 DT = £4.60 [CD3]
Tramadol hydrochloride 100 mg Zydol SR 100mg tablets | 60 tablet [PoM] £17.22 [CD3]
Tramadol hydrochloride 150 mg Zydol SR 150mg tablets | 60 tablet [PoM] £25.83 [CD3]
Tramadol hydrochloride 200 mg Zydol SR 200mg tablets | 60 tablet [PoM] £34.40 [CD3]
▸ Zydol XL (Grunenthal Ltd)
Tramadol hydrochloride 150 mg Zydol XL 150mg tablets | 30 tablet [PoM] £12.18 [CD3]
Tramadol hydrochloride 200 mg Zydol XL 200mg tablets | 30 tablet [PoM] £17.98 [CD3]
Tramadol hydrochloride 300 mg Zydol XL 300mg tablets | 30 tablet [PoM] £24.94 [CD3]
Tramadol hydrochloride 400 mg Zydol XL 400mg tablets | 30 tablet [PoM] £32.47 [CD3]

Soluble tablet
CAUTIONARY AND ADVISORY LABELS 2, 13
▸ Zydol (Grunenthal Ltd)
Tramadol hydrochloride 50 mg Zydol 50mg soluble tablets sugar-free | 20 tablet [PoM] £2.79 Schedule 3 (CD No Register Exempt Safe Custody) sugar-free | 100 tablet [PoM] £13.33 DT = £13.33 [CD3]

Solution for injection
▸ Tramadol hydrochloride (Non-proprietary)
Tramadol hydrochloride 50 mg per 1 ml Tramadol 100mg/2ml solution for injection ampoules | 5 ampoule [PoM] £4.00 DT = £4.00 (Hospital only) [CD3] | 5 ampoule [PoM] £4.90 DT = £4.00 [CD3] | 10 ampoule [PoM] £10.00 [CD3]
▸ Zamadol (Mylan)
Tramadol hydrochloride 50 mg per 1 ml Zamadol 100mg/2ml solution for injection ampoules | 5 ampoule [PoM] £5.49 DT = £4.00 [CD3]
▸ Zydol (Grunenthal Ltd)
Tramadol hydrochloride 50 mg per 1 ml Zydol 100mg/2ml solution for injection ampoules | 5 ampoule [PoM] £4.00 DT = £4.00 [CD3]

Modified-release capsule
CAUTIONARY AND ADVISORY LABELS 2, 25
▸ Maxitram SR (Chiesi Ltd)
Tramadol hydrochloride 50 mg Maxitram SR 50mg capsules | 60 capsule [PoM] £4.55 DT = £7.24 [CD3]
Tramadol hydrochloride 100 mg Maxitram SR 100mg capsules | 60 capsule [PoM] £12.14 DT = £14.47 [CD3]
Tramadol hydrochloride 150 mg Maxitram SR 150mg capsules | 60 capsule [PoM] £18.21 DT = £21.71 [CD3]
Tramadol hydrochloride 200 mg Maxitram SR 200mg capsules | 60 capsule [PoM] £24.28 DT = £28.93 [CD3]
▸ Tramquel SR (Mylan)
Tramadol hydrochloride 100 mg Tramquel SR 100mg capsules | 60 capsule [PoM] £14.47 DT = £14.47 [CD3]
Tramadol hydrochloride 150 mg Tramquel SR 150mg capsules | 60 capsule [PoM] £21.71 DT = £21.71 [CD3]

Tramadol hydrochloride 200 mg Tramquel SR 200mg capsules |
60 capsule [PoM] £28.93 DT = £28.93 [CD3]
▸ Zamadol SR (Mylan)
Tramadol hydrochloride 50 mg Zamadol SR 50mg capsules |
60 capsule [PoM] £7.24 DT = £7.24 [CD3]
Tramadol hydrochloride 100 mg Zamadol SR 100mg capsules |
60 capsule [PoM] £14.47 DT = £14.47 [CD3]
Tramadol hydrochloride 150 mg Zamadol SR 150mg capsules |
60 capsule [PoM] £21.71 DT = £21.71 [CD3]
Tramadol hydrochloride 200 mg Zamadol SR 200mg capsules |
60 capsule [PoM] £28.93 DT = £28.93 [CD3]

Oral drops
CAUTIONARY AND ADVISORY LABELS 2, 13
▸ Tramadol hydrochloride (Non-proprietary)
Tramadol (as Tramadol hydrochloride) 100 mg per 1 ml Tramadol
100mg/ml oral drops | 10 ml [PoM] £25.00 DT = £25.00 [CD3]

Capsule
CAUTIONARY AND ADVISORY LABELS 2
▸ Tramadol hydrochloride (Non-proprietary)
Tramadol hydrochloride 50 mg Tramadol 50mg capsules |
30 capsule [PoM] £1.20 DT = £0.93 [CD3] | 100 capsule [PoM] £14.40
DT = £3.10 [CD3]
▸ Zamadol (Mylan)
Tramadol hydrochloride 50 mg Zamadol 50mg capsules |
100 capsule [PoM] £8.00 DT = £3.10 [CD3]
▸ Zydol (Grunenthal Ltd)
Tramadol hydrochloride 50 mg Zydol 50mg capsules |
30 capsule [PoM] £2.29 DT = £0.93 [CD3] | 100 capsule [PoM] £7.63 DT
= £3.10 [CD3]

Orodispersible tablet
CAUTIONARY AND ADVISORY LABELS 2
▸ Zamadol Melt (Mylan)
Tramadol hydrochloride 50 mg Zamadol Melt 50mg tablets sugar-
free | 60 tablet [PoM] £7.12 DT = £7.12 [CD3]

Tramadol with dexketoprofen 24-Apr-2018

The properties listed below are those particular to the
combination only. For the properties of the components
please consider, tramadol hydrochloride p. 491,
dexketoprofen p. 1180.

● **INDICATIONS AND DOSE**

Moderate to severe acute pain
▸ BY MOUTH
▸ Adult: 75/25 mg every 8 hours as required for up to
5 days
▸ Elderly: 75/25 mg every 8 hours as required for up to
5 days; Usual maximum 150/50 mg/24 hours

DOSE EQUIVALENCE AND CONVERSION
▸ Dose expressed as x/y mg of tramadol/dexketoprofen.

● INTERACTIONS → Appendix 1: NSAIDs · opioids

● MEDICINAL FORMS There can be variation in the licensing of
different medicines containing the same drug.

Tablet
CAUTIONARY AND ADVISORY LABELS 2, 22
▸ Skudexa (A. Menarini Farmaceutica Internazionale SRL) ▼
Dexketoprofen 25 mg, Tramadol hydrochloride 75 mg Skudexa
75mg/25mg tablets | 10 tablet [PoM] £3.68 [CD3] | 20 tablet [PoM]
£5.52 DT = £5.52 [CD3]

Tramadol with paracetamol 22-Feb-2018

The properties listed below are those particular to the
combination only. For the properties of the components
please consider, paracetamol p. 464, tramadol hydrochloride
p. 491.

● **INDICATIONS AND DOSE**

Moderate to severe pain
▸ BY MOUTH
▸ Child 12–17 years: 75/650 mg every 6 hours as required

▸ Adult: 75/650 mg every 6 hours as required

DOSE EQUIVALENCE AND CONVERSION
▸ The proportions are expressed in the form x/y, where x
and y are the strengths in milligrams of tramadol and
paracetamol respectively.

● INTERACTIONS → Appendix 1: opioids · paracetamol

● MEDICINAL FORMS There can be variation in the licensing of
different medicines containing the same drug.

Effervescent tablet
CAUTIONARY AND ADVISORY LABELS 2, 13, 29, 30
ELECTROLYTES: May contain Sodium
▸ Tramacet (Grunenthal Ltd)
Tramadol hydrochloride 37.5 mg, Paracetamol 325 mg Tramacet
37.5mg/325mg effervescent tablets sugar-free | 60 tablet [PoM] £9.68
DT = £9.68 [CD3]

Tablet
CAUTIONARY AND ADVISORY LABELS 2, 25, 29, 30
▸ Tramadol with paracetamol (Non-proprietary)
Tramadol hydrochloride 37.5 mg, Paracetamol 325 mg Tramadol
37.5mg / Paracetamol 325mg tablets | 60 tablet [PoM] £9.68 DT =
£2.29 [CD3]
Tramadol hydrochloride 75 mg, Paracetamol 650 mg Tramadol
75mg / Paracetamol 650mg tablets | 30 tablet [PoM] £19.50 [CD3]
▸ Tramacet (Grunenthal Ltd)
Tramadol hydrochloride 37.5 mg, Paracetamol 325 mg Tramacet
37.5mg/325mg tablets | 60 tablet [PoM] £9.68 DT = £2.29 [CD3]

6.1 Headache

Cluster headache and other trigeminal autonomic cephalalgias

Management

Cluster headache rarely responds to standard analgesics.
Sumatriptan p. 502 given by subcutaneous injection is the
drug of choice for the *treatment* of cluster headache. If an
injection is unsuitable, sumatriptan nasal spray or
zolmitriptan nasal spray p. 503 [both unlicensed use] may be
used. Alternatively, 100% oxygen at a rate of
10–15 litres/minute for 10–20 minutes is useful in aborting
an attack.

Prophylaxis of cluster headache is considered if the attacks
are frequent, last over 3 weeks, or if they cannot be treated
effectively. Verapamil hydrochloride p. 178 or lithium [both
unlicensed use] are used for prophylaxis.

Prednisolone p. 718 can be used for short-term
prophylaxis of episodic cluster headache [unlicensed use]
either as monotherapy, or in combination with verapamil
hydrochloride during verapamil titration.

Ergotamine tartrate p. 499, used on an intermittent basis is
an alternative for patients with short bouts, but it should not
be used for prolonged periods.

The other trigeminal autonomic cephalalgias, paroxysmal
hemicrania (sensitive to indometacin p. 1189), and short-
lasting unilateral neuralgiform headache attacks with
conjunctival injection and tearing, are seen rarely and are
best managed by a specialist.

> **Other drugs used for Headache** Clonidine hydrochloride,
> p. 159

4

Nervous system

ANTIHISTAMINES > SEDATING ANTIHISTAMINES

Pizotifen
14-Dec-2020

- **INDICATIONS AND DOSE**

Prevention of vascular headache | Prevention of classical migraine | Prevention of common migraine | Prevention of cluster headache

▶ BY MOUTH

▶ Adult: Initially 500 micrograms once daily, then increased to 1.5 mg once daily, dose to be increased gradually and taken at night, alternatively increased to 1.5 mg daily in 3 divided doses, doses to be increased gradually; increased if necessary up to 4.5 mg daily (max. per dose 3 mg)

Prophylaxis of migraine

▶ BY MOUTH

▶ Child 5–17 years: Initially 500 micrograms once daily, dose to be taken at night, then increased if necessary up to 1.5 mg daily in divided doses, dose to be increased gradually, max. single dose (at night) 1 mg

- **CONTRA-INDICATIONS** Acute porphyrias p. 1107
- **CAUTIONS** Avoid abrupt withdrawal · history of epilepsy · susceptibility to angle-closure glaucoma · urinary retention
- **INTERACTIONS** → Appendix 1: antihistamines, sedating
- **SIDE-EFFECTS**
▶ **Common or very common** Appetite increased · dizziness · drowsiness · dry mouth · fatigue · nausea · weight increased
▶ **Uncommon** Constipation
▶ **Rare or very rare** Aggression · anxiety · arthralgia · central nervous system stimulation · depression · hallucination · muscle complaints · paraesthesia · seizure · skin reactions · sleep disorders
▶ **Frequency not known** Hepatic disorders
- **PREGNANCY** Avoid unless potential benefit outweighs risk.
- **BREAST FEEDING** Amount probably too small to be harmful, but manufacturer advises avoid.
- **HEPATIC IMPAIRMENT** Manufacturer advises caution. **Dose adjustments** Manufacturer advises consider dose reduction.
- **RENAL IMPAIRMENT** Use with caution.
- **PATIENT AND CARER ADVICE** Medicines for Children leaflet: Pizotifen to prevent migraine headaches www.medicinesforchildren.org.uk/pizotifen-prevent-migraine-headaches **Driving and skilled tasks** Drowsiness may affect performance of skilled tasks (e.g. driving); effects of alcohol enhanced.
- **MEDICINAL FORMS** There can be variation in the licensing of different medicines containing the same drug. Forms available from special-order manufacturers include: oral solution

Tablet

CAUTIONARY AND ADVISORY LABELS 2

▶ Pizotifen (Non-proprietary)
  Pizotifen (as Pizotifen hydrogen malate)
  500 microgram Pizotifen 500microgram tablets | 28 tablet [PoM] £16.25 DT = £2.70
  Pizotifen (as Pizotifen hydrogen malate) 1.5 mg Pizotifen 1.5mg tablets | 28 tablet [PoM] £16.25 DT = £7.18

6.1a Migraine

Migraine
14-Sep-2020

Description of condition

Migraine is a common type of primary headache disorder. It occurs more commonly in women than in men, and is characterised by recurrent attacks of typically moderate to severe headaches that usually last between 4–72 hours. The headache is usually unilateral, pulsating, aggravated by routine physical activity, and may be severe enough to impact or prevent daily activities. It is frequently accompanied by nausea and vomiting, photophobia and phonophobia, or both. Migraine is subdivided into migraine *with* or *without* aura, and is defined as either episodic or chronic.

Migraine *with* aura consists of visual symptoms (zigzag or flickering lights, spots, lines, or loss of vision), sensory symptoms (pins and needles, or numbness), or dysphasia, which usually precede the onset of headache. Symptoms usually develop gradually and resolve within 1 hour.

Episodic migraine is defined as headache which occurs on less than 15 days per month, and can be further subdivided into low frequency (1–9 days per month) and high frequency (10–14 days per month). Chronic migraine is defined as headache which occurs on at least 15 days per month and has the characteristics of a migraine headache on at least 8 days per month for greater than 3 months.

In some women, the drop in oestrogen levels just before menstruation is a trigger for migraine, with symptoms generally occurring from two days before the start of bleeding up until three days after.

Medication-overuse headache is a complication of migraine; the frequent use of acute treatment for migraine increases the frequency and intensity of headache, and can become the cause of the headache.

Aims of treatment

Treatment of acute migraine aims to stop the attack, or to significantly reduce the severity of the headache and other associated symptoms. Preventative treatment aims to reduce the frequency, severity and duration of migraine attacks, and development of medication-overuse headache.

Lifestyle advice

[EvGr] Patients should be encouraged to eat regular meals, and to maintain adequate hydration, sleep and exercise. [A] Other potential triggers include stress, relaxation after stress, some foods and drinks, and bright lights. [EvGr] Known triggers should be avoided; keeping a headache diary may be useful to identify potential triggers and should be continued for a minimum of 8 weeks. [A]

Acute migraine treatment

[EvGr] The choice of treatment for acute migraine should be guided by the patient's preference, response to previous treatment, the severity and frequency of headache attacks, other associated symptoms, and co-morbidities. Treatment should ideally be restricted to 2 days per week and patients should be advised of the risk of developing medication-overuse headache.

Monotherapy, with either aspirin p. 132, ibuprofen p. 1186, or a $5HT_1$-receptor agonist ('triptan') is recommended as first-line treatment and should be taken as soon as the patient knows that they are developing a migraine (start of headache phase).

In patients who experience aura with their migraine, it is recommended that $5HT_1$-receptor agonists are taken at the start of the headache and not at the start of the aura (unless the aura and headache start at the same time). Treatment with a 5HT$_1$-receptor agonist can be repeated after 2 hours with the same or different drug if there has been an inadequate response to the initial dose.

Based on its clinical efficacy and safety profile, sumatriptan p. 502 is the 5HT$_1$-receptor agonist of choice. ⒶAlternative 5HT$_1$-receptor agonists include almotriptan p. 499, eletriptan p. 500, frovatriptan p. 500, naratriptan p. 501, rizatriptan p. 501, and zolmitriptan p. 503. [EvGr] In patients who do not respond to one 5HT$_1$-receptor agonist, a different 5HT$_1$-receptor agonist should be tried as response can be variable between patients. Subcutaneous sumatriptan p. 502 or nasal zolmitriptan p. 503 can be given to patients who present with early vomiting or who have severe migraine attacks. Ⓐ

[EvGr] Other NSAIDs that may be used for the treatment of acute migraine include, naproxen p. 1194 [unlicensed indication], tolfenamic acid p. 496, and diclofenac potassium p. 1180. In patients presenting with severe nausea and vomiting, diclofenac sodium suppositories p. 1181 [unlicensed indication] may be an option. Mefenamic acid p. 1191 [unlicensed indication] can also be used for menstrual migraine in women already using it for other indications such as dysmenorrhea, or menorrhagia. Ⓔ [EvGr] Treatment with paracetamol p. 464 can be considered in patients who are unable to take other acute treatment options.

In patients who fail to respond to monotherapy, combination therapy with sumatriptan p. 502 and naproxen p. 1194 can be given.

In addition to their use as antiemetics, metoclopramide hydrochloride p. 451 [unlicensed indication] or prochlorperazine p. 408 [unlicensed indication] can also be given as a single dose at the onset of migraine symptoms for the treatment of headache. They can be given orally or by injection, depending on the severity of the patients' symptoms and the setting. Ⓐ

Antiemetics

[EvGr] Metoclopramide hydrochloride p. 451 or prochlorperazine p. 408 can be given orally or by injection to relieve nausea or vomiting. Metoclopramide hydrochloride p. 451 should not be used regularly due to the risk of extrapyramidal side effects. Ⓐ The MHRA/CHM have released important safety information regarding the use of metoclopramide and risk of neurological adverse effects. See *Important safety information* for metoclopramide hydrochloride p. 451.

[EvGr] Domperidone p. 451 [unlicensed in those weighing less than 35 kg] may be used as an alternative antiemetic. Ⓔ The MHRA/CHM have released important safety information and restrictions regarding the use of domperidone for nausea and vomiting in those weighing less than 35 kg, and a reminder of contra-indications. For further information, see *Important safety information* for domperidone.

Preventative migraine treatment

[EvGr] The decision to start prophylactic treatment should be based on the impact of the migraine on the patient's quality of life. The choice of treatment depends on factors such as patient preference, drug interactions, and other co-morbidities. Treatment should be started at a low dose and gradually increased to the maximum effective and tolerated dose.

Propranolol hydrochloride p. 164 is recommended as first-line preventative treatment in patients with episodic or chronic migraine. Ⓐ[EvGr] For patients in whom propranolol is unsuitable, other beta-blockers that can be considered are metoprolol tartrate p. 169, atenolol p. 166 [unlicensed indication], nadolol p. 164, and timolol maleate p. 165. Bisoprolol fumarate p. 167 [unlicensed indication] may also be considered, especially in patients already taking it for cardiac reasons under the advice of their cardiologist.

Ⓔ[EvGr] Topiramate p. 349 can be given if a beta-blocker is unsuitable, however in women of childbearing potential, advice should be given on the associated risks during pregnancy, the need to use highly effective contraception and to seek further information if pregnant or planning a pregnancy. Ⓐ See *Conception and contraception,* and *Pregnancy* in the topiramate p. 349 drug monograph for further information. The MHRA/CHM have released important safety information on the use of antiepileptic drugs and the risk of suicidal thoughts and behaviour. For further information, see Epilepsy p. 321.

[EvGr] Amitriptyline hydrochloride p. 392 is effective for migraine prophylaxis and should be considered for patients with episodic or chronic migraine. A less sedative tricyclic antidepressant can be used if amitriptyline hydrochloride p. 392 is not tolerated.

Candesartan cilexetil p. 189 [unlicensed indication] can be considered in patients with episodic or chronic migraine, although there is limited evidence to support its use.

Sodium valproate p. 345 [unlicensed indication] can also be considered in patients with episodic or chronic migraine. Ⓐ The MHRA/CHM have released important safety information on the use of antiepileptic drugs and the risk of suicidal thoughts and behaviour. For further information, see Epilepsy p. 321. In addition, the MHRA has advised that sodium valproate must not be used in women of childbearing potential unless the conditions of the Pregnancy Prevention Programme are met and alternative treatments are ineffective or not tolerated; it must not be used during pregnancy for migraine prophylaxis. For further information, see *Important safety information,Conception and contraception,* and *Pregnancy* in the sodium valproate p. 345 drug monograph.

[EvGr] Flunarizine [unlicensed] can also be considered in patients with episodic or chronic migraine (specialist use only). Pizotifen p. 494 is used but evidence to recommend its use is limited.

Preventative treatment should be tried for at least 3 months at the maximum tolerated dose, before deciding whether or not it is effective. Ⓐ A good response to treatment is defined as a 50% reduction in the severity and frequency of migraine attacks. [EvGr] A review of ongoing prophylaxis should be considered after 6–12 months; treatment can be gradually withdrawn in many patients. Patients should be referred to a neurology or specialist headache clinic if trials with 3 or more drugs have been unsuccessful.

Botulinum toxin type A p. 428 (specialist use only) is recommended for prophylaxis of chronic migraine where medication-overuse has been addressed and where 3 or more oral prophylactic treatments have failed. Ⓐ

Menstrual migraine prophylaxis

[EvGr] Frovatriptan p. 500 [unlicensed indication] can be given instead of, or in addition to, standard prophylactic treatment in women with perimenstrual migraine. It is given from 2 days before until 3 days after menstruation starts. Zolmitriptan p. 503 [unlicensed indication] or naratriptan p. 501 [unlicensed indication] are suitable alternatives to frovatriptan p. 500. In order for treatment to be effective, the patient's menstrual cycle must be regular.

Women with menstrual-related migraine who are using 5HT$_1$-receptor agonists for both perimenstrual prophylaxis and at other times in the month should be advised of the increased risk of developing medication-overuse headache. Ⓐ

Medication-overuse headache

[EvGr] Medication overuse should be addressed in patients overusing acute treatments such as 5HT$_1$-receptor agonists, combination analgesics, ergots, or opioids for migraine. Ⓐ Withdrawing the overused medication can reduce the frequency and intensity of headaches but is often associated

Nervous system

4

with transient worsening. Not all patients overusing acute treatment will develop medication-overuse headache; in some patients, continued headaches may be a sign of poorly treated migraine.

Useful Resources

Pharmacological management of migraine. Scottish Intercollegiate Guidelines Network. A national clinical guideline 155. February 2018.
www.sign.ac.uk/assets/sign155.pdf

> **Other drugs used for Migraine** Clonidine hydrochloride, p. 159 · Cyclizine, p. 449 · Trifluoperazine, p. 410 · Valproic acid, p. 373

ANALGESICS > NON-OPIOID

Paracetamol with isometheptene

11-Nov-2019

The properties listed below are those particular to the combination only. For the properties of the components please consider, paracetamol p. 464.

- **INDICATIONS AND DOSE**
  Treatment of acute attacks of migraine
  ▸ BY MOUTH
  ▸ Adult: 2 capsules, dose to be taken at onset of attack, followed by 1 capsule every 1 hour if required, maximum of 5 capsules in 12 hours

- CONTRA-INDICATIONS Acute porphyrias p. 1107 · glaucoma · severe cardiovascular disease · severe hypertension
- INTERACTIONS → Appendix 1: paracetamol · sympathomimetics, vasoconstrictor
- PATIENT AND CARER ADVICE Patient counselling is advised (dosage).
- LESS SUITABLE FOR PRESCRIBING Isometheptene with paracetamol is less suitable for prescribing (more effective treatments available).

- MEDICINAL FORMS There can be variation in the licensing of different medicines containing the same drug.
  Capsule
  CAUTIONARY AND ADVISORY LABELS 30
  ▸ Midrid (DHP Healthcare Ltd)
    Isometheptene mucate 65 mg, Paracetamol 325 mg Midrid 325mg/65mg capsules | 30 capsule PoM £7.50 DT = £7.50

Paracetamol with metoclopramide

22-Jan-2020

The properties listed below are those particular to the combination only. For the properties of the components please consider, paracetamol p. 464, metoclopramide hydrochloride p. 451.

- **INDICATIONS AND DOSE**
  Acute migraine
  ▸ BY MOUTH USING TABLETS
  ▸ Adult: 2 tablets, to be taken at the onset of attack, followed by 2 tablets every 4 hours if required; maximum 6 tablets per day
  ▸ BY MOUTH USING EFFERVESCENT POWDER SACHETS
  ▸ Adult: 2 sachets, to be taken at the onset of attack, followed by 2 sachets every 4 hours if required, sachets

to be dissolved in a quarter tumblerful of water; maximum 6 sachets per day

> IMPORTANT SAFETY INFORMATION
> Metoclopramide can cause **severe extrapyramidal effects**, particularly in young adults.

- CAUTIONS Treatment should not exceed 3 months due to risk of tardive dyskinesia
- INTERACTIONS → Appendix 1: metoclopramide · paracetamol

- MEDICINAL FORMS No licensed medicines listed.

ANALGESICS > NON-STEROIDAL ANTI-INFLAMMATORY DRUGS

Aspirin with metoclopramide

14-Jul-2020

The properties listed below are those particular to the combination only. For the properties of the components please consider, aspirin p. 132, metoclopramide hydrochloride p. 451.

- **INDICATIONS AND DOSE**
  Acute migraine
  ▸ BY MOUTH
  ▸ Adult: 1 sachet, sachet to be mixed in water, and dose to be taken at the start of the attack, then 1 sachet after 2 hours if required; maximum 3 sachets per day

> IMPORTANT SAFETY INFORMATION
> Metoclopramide can cause **severe extrapyramidal effects**, particularly in children and young adults.

- CAUTIONS Treatment should not exceed 3 months due to risk of tardive dyskinesia
- INTERACTIONS → Appendix 1: aspirin · metoclopramide
- PRESCRIBING AND DISPENSING INFORMATION Flavours of oral powder formulations may include lemon.

- MEDICINAL FORMS There can be variation in the licensing of different medicines containing the same drug.
  Powder
  CAUTIONARY AND ADVISORY LABELS 13, 21, 32
  EXCIPIENTS: May contain Aspartame
  ▸ MigraMax (Zentiva)
    Metoclopramide hydrochloride 10 mg, Aspirin DL-Lysine 900 mg MigraMax oral powder sachets sugar-free | 6 sachet PoM £6.61 DT = £6.61

Tolfenamic acid

17-Nov-2020

- **INDICATIONS AND DOSE**
  Treatment of acute migraine
  ▸ BY MOUTH
  ▸ Adult: 200 mg, dose to be taken at onset, then 200 mg after 1–2 hours if required

- CONTRA-INDICATIONS Active gastro-intestinal bleeding · active gastro-intestinal ulceration · history of gastro-intestinal bleeding related to previous NSAID therapy · history of gastro-intestinal haemorrhage (two or more distinct episodes) · history of gastro-intestinal perforation related to previous NSAID therapy · history of recurrent gastro-intestinal ulceration (two or more distinct episodes) · severe heart failure
- CAUTIONS Allergic disorders · cardiac impairment (NSAIDs may impair renal function) · cerebrovascular disease · coagulation defects · connective-tissue disorders · dehydration (risk of renal impairment) · elderly (risk of

serious side-effects and fatalities) · heart failure · history of gastro-intestinal disorders (e.g. ulcerative colitis, Crohn's disease) · ischaemic heart disease · may mask symptoms of infection · peripheral arterial disease · risk factors for cardiovascular events · uncontrolled hypertension

- INTERACTIONS → Appendix 1: NSAIDs
- SIDE-EFFECTS Agranulocytosis · angioedema · aplastic anaemia · asthma · confusion · constipation · Crohn's disease aggravated · depression · diarrhoea · dizziness · drowsiness · dyspnoea · dysuria (most common in men) · euphoric mood · fatigue · fertility decreased female · gastrointestinal discomfort · gastrointestinal disorders · haemolytic anaemia · haemorrhage · hallucination · headache · heart failure · hepatic disorders · hypersensitivity · hypertension · increased risk of arterial thromboembolism · malaise · meningitis aseptic (patients with connective-tissue disorders such as systemic lupus erythematosus may be especially susceptible) · nausea · nephritis tubulointerstitial · nephropathy · neutropenia · oedema · optic neuritis · oral ulceration · pancreatitis · paraesthesia · photosensitivity reaction · renal failure (more common in patients with pre-existing renal impairment) · respiratory disorders · severe cutaneous adverse reactions (SCARs) · skin reactions · thrombocytopenia · tinnitus · tremor · vertigo · visual impairment · vomiting

SIDE-EFFECTS, FURTHER INFORMATION For information about cardiovascular and gastrointestinal side-effects, and a possible exacerbation of symptoms in asthma, see Non-steroidal anti-inflammatory drugs. p. 1176

- ALLERGY AND CROSS-SENSITIVITY EvGr Contra-indicated in patients with a history of hypersensitivity to aspirin or any other NSAID—which includes those in whom attacks of asthma, angioedema, urticaria or rhinitis have been precipitated by aspirin or any other NSAID. ◁M▷
- CONCEPTION AND CONTRACEPTION Caution—long-term use of some NSAIDs is associated with reduced female fertility, which is reversible on stopping treatment.
- PREGNANCY Avoid unless the potential benefit outweighs the risk. Avoid during the third trimester (risk of closure of fetal ductus arteriosus *in utero* and possibly persistent pulmonary hypertension of the newborn); onset of labour may be delayed and duration may be increased.
- BREAST FEEDING Amount too small to be harmful. Use with caution during breast-feeding.
- HEPATIC IMPAIRMENT Manufacturer advises caution in mild to moderate impairment; avoid in severe impairment.
- RENAL IMPAIRMENT Avoid if possible or use with caution.
  Dose adjustments The lowest effective dose should be used for the shortest possible duration.
  Monitoring In renal impairment monitor renal function; sodium and water retention may occur and renal function may deteriorate, possibly leading to renal failure.
- MEDICINAL FORMS There can be variation in the licensing of different medicines containing the same drug.
  Tablet
  CAUTIONARY AND ADVISORY LABELS 21
  ▸ Tolfenamic acid (Non-proprietary)
    Tolfenamic acid 200 mg Tolfenamic acid 200mg tablets | 10 tablet PoM £24.63 DT = £24.63
  ▸ Clotam Rapid (Galen Ltd)
    Tolfenamic acid 200 mg Clotam Rapid 200mg tablets | 10 tablet PoM £12.75 DT = £24.63

Paracetamol with buclizine hydrochloride and codeine phosphate

22-Nov-2019

The properties listed below are those particular to the combination only. For the properties of the components please consider, paracetamol p. 464, codeine phosphate p. 475.

- **INDICATIONS AND DOSE**
  MIGRALEVE®
  Acute migraine
  ▸ BY MOUTH
    ▸ Child 12–15 years: Initially 1 tablet, (pink tablet) to be taken at onset of attack, or if it is imminent, followed by 1 tablet every 4 hours if required, (yellow tablet) to be taken following initial dose; maximum 1 pink and 3 yellow tablets in 24 hours
    ▸ Child 16–17 years: Initially 2 tablets, (pink tablets) to be taken at onset of attack or if it is imminent, followed by 2 tablets every 4 hours if required, (yellow tablets) to be taken following initial dose; maximum 2 pink and 6 yellow tablets in 24 hours
    ▸ Adult: Initially 2 tablets, (pink tablets) to be taken at onset of attack or if it is imminent, followed by 2 tablets every 4 hours if required, (yellow tablets) to be taken following initial dose; maximum 2 pink and 6 yellow tablets in 24 hours

- INTERACTIONS → Appendix 1: antihistamines, sedating · opioids · paracetamol
- PRESCRIBING AND DISPENSING INFORMATION See co-codamol p. 474 for Migraleve Yellow preparations.
- LESS SUITABLE FOR PRESCRIBING
  MIGRALEVE® *Migraleve®* is less suitable for prescribing.

- MEDICINAL FORMS There can be variation in the licensing of different medicines containing the same drug.
  Tablet
  CAUTIONARY AND ADVISORY LABELS 2, 17, 30
  ▸ Migraleve Pink (McNeil Products Ltd)
    Buclizine hydrochloride 6.25 mg, Codeine phosphate 8 mg, Paracetamol 500 mg Migraleve Pink tablets | 12 tablet P £3.97 CD5 | 24 tablet P £6.37 CD5 | 48 tablet PoM £3.97 CD5

CALCITONIN GENE-RELATED PEPTIDE INHIBITORS

Erenumab

05-Nov-2020

- DRUG ACTION Erenumab is a human monoclonal antibody that binds to the calcitonin gene-related peptide (CGRP) receptor, inhibiting the function of CGRP, and thereby preventing migraine attacks.

- **INDICATIONS AND DOSE**
  Prophylaxis of migraine (in patients who have at least 4 migraine days per month) (initiated by a specialist)
  ▸ BY SUBCUTANEOUS INJECTION
    ▸ Adult: 70 mg every 4 weeks; increased if necessary to 140 mg every 4 weeks, consider discontinuing if no response after 3 months of treatment

- SIDE-EFFECTS
  ▸ **Common or very common** Constipation · muscle spasms · skin reactions
  ▸ **Frequency not known** Oedema · swelling
- PREGNANCY Manufacturer advises avoid—limited information available.

4

Nervous system

- BREAST FEEDING Manufacturer advises avoid during first few days after birth—possible risk from transfer of antibodies to infant. After this time, use during breast-feeding only if clinically needed.
- DIRECTIONS FOR ADMINISTRATION Manufacturer advises injection into the abdomen, thigh, or upper arm (if not self-administered). Patients may self-administer Aimovig® after appropriate training in subcutaneous injection technique.
- PRESCRIBING AND DISPENSING INFORMATION Erenumab is a biological medicine. Biological medicines must be prescribed and dispensed by brand name, see *Biological medicines* and *Biosimilar medicines*, under Guidance on prescribing p. 1; manufacturer advises to record the brand name and batch number after each administration.
- HANDLING AND STORAGE Manufacturer advises store in a refrigerator (2-8°C) and protect from light—consult product literature for further information regarding storage outside refrigerator.
- PATIENT AND CARER ADVICE
  Self-administration Manufacturer advises that patients and their carers should be given training in subcutaneous injection technique if appropriate.
- NATIONAL FUNDING/ACCESS DECISIONS
  For full details see funding body website
  Scottish Medicines Consortium (SMC) decisions
  ‣ Erenumab (*Aimovig*®) for the prophylaxis of migraine in adults who have at least 4 migraine days per month (April 2019) SMC No. SMC2134 Recommended with restrictions

- MEDICINAL FORMS There can be variation in the licensing of different medicines containing the same drug.
  Solution for injection
  EXCIPIENTS: May contain Polysorbates, sucrose
  ‣ Aimovig (Novartis Pharmaceuticals UK Ltd) ▼
    Erenumab 70 mg per 1 ml Aimovig 70mg/1ml solution for injection pre-filled pens | 1 pre-filled disposable injection [PoM] £386.50
    Erenumab 140 mg per 1 ml Aimovig 140mg/1ml solution for injection pre-filled pens | 1 pre-filled disposable injection [PoM] £386.50 (Hospital only)

Fremanezumab

06-Nov-2020

- DRUG ACTION Fremanezumab is a humanised monoclonal antibody that binds to the calcitonin gene-related peptide (CGRP) ligand, inhibiting the function of CGRP at its receptor, and thereby preventing migraine attacks.

- INDICATIONS AND DOSE
  Prophylaxis of migraine [in patients who have at least 4 migraine days per month] (initiated by a specialist)
  ▶ BY SUBCUTANEOUS INJECTION
  ‣ Adult: 225 mg once a month, alternatively 675 mg every 3 months, review treatment within first 3 months and regularly thereafter

- CAUTIONS Major cardiovascular disease (no information available)
- SIDE-EFFECTS Hypersensitivity
- PREGNANCY Manufacturer advises avoid—limited information available.
- BREAST FEEDING Manufacturer advises avoid during first few days after birth—possible risk from transfer of antibodies to infant. After this time, use during breast-feeding only if clinically needed.
- DIRECTIONS FOR ADMINISTRATION Manufacturer advises injection into the abdomen, thigh or upper arm. Patients may self-administer *Ajovy*® after appropriate training in subcutaneous injection technique.
- PRESCRIBING AND DISPENSING INFORMATION
  Fremanezumab is a biological medicine. Biological

medicines must be prescribed and dispensed by brand name, see *Biological medicines* and *Biosimilar medicines*, under Guidance on prescribing p. 1; manufacturer advises to record the brand name and batch number after each administration.
- HANDLING AND STORAGE Manufacturer advises store in a refrigerator (2-8°C) and protect from light—consult product literature for further information regarding storage outside refrigerator.
- PATIENT AND CARER ADVICE
  Self-administration Manufacturer advises patients and their carers should be given training in subcutaneous injection technique if appropriate.
- NATIONAL FUNDING/ACCESS DECISIONS
  For full details see funding body website
  NICE decisions
  ‣ Fremanezumab for preventing migraine (June 2020)
  NICE TA631 Recommended with restrictions
  Scottish Medicines Consortium (SMC) decisions
  ‣ Fremanezumab (*Ajovy*®) for the prophylaxis of migraine in adults who have at least four migraine days per month (January 2020) SMC No. SMC2226 Recommended with restrictions

- MEDICINAL FORMS There can be variation in the licensing of different medicines containing the same drug.
  Solution for injection
  EXCIPIENTS: May contain Edetic acid (edta), polysorbates, sucrose
  ‣ Ajovy (Teva UK Ltd) ▼
    Fremanezumab 150 mg per 1 ml Ajovy 225mg/1.5ml solution for injection pre-filled syringes | 1 pre-filled disposable injection [PoM] £450.00
    Ajovy 225mg/1.5ml solution for injection pre-filled pens | 1 pre-filled disposable injection [PoM] £450.00

Galcanezumab

03-Dec-2020

- DRUG ACTION Galcanezumab is a humanised monoclonal antibody that binds to the calcitonin gene-related peptide (CGRP) ligand, inhibiting the function of CGRP at its receptor, and thereby preventing migraine attacks.

- INDICATIONS AND DOSE
  Prophylaxis of migraine [in patients who have at least 4 migraine days per month] (initiated by a specialist)
  ▶ BY SUBCUTANEOUS INJECTION
  ‣ Adult: Loading dose 240 mg for 1 dose, then maintenance 120 mg once a month, maintenance dosing to start 1 month after loading dose. Review treatment 3 months after initiation

- SIDE-EFFECTS
- Common or very common Constipation · skin reactions · vertigo
- PREGNANCY Manufacturer advises avoid—limited information available.
- BREAST FEEDING Manufacturer advises avoid during first few days after birth—possible risk from transfer of antibodies to infant. After this time, use during breast-feeding only if clinically needed.
- DIRECTIONS FOR ADMINISTRATION Manufacturer advises injection into the abdomen, thigh, back of the upper arm, or the gluteal region. Patients may self-administer *Emgality*® after appropriate training in subcutaneous injection technique.
- PRESCRIBING AND DISPENSING INFORMATION
  Galcanezumab is a biological medicine. Biological medicines must be prescribed and dispensed by brand name, see *Biological medicines* and *Biosimilar medicines*, under Guidance on prescribing p. 1; manufacturer advises

to record the brand name and batch number after each administration.

- **HANDLING AND STORAGE** Manufacturer advises store in a refrigerator (2-8°C) and protect from light—consult product literature for further information regarding storage outside refrigerator.
- **PATIENT AND CARER ADVICE**
  Self-administration Manufacturer advises patients and their carers should be given training in subcutaneous injection technique if appropriate.
  Driving and skilled tasks Manufacturer advises patients and their carers should be counselled on the effects on driving and performance of skilled tasks—increased risk of vertigo.
- **NATIONAL FUNDING/ACCESS DECISIONS**
  For full details see funding body website
  NICE decisions
  ▸ Galcanezumab for preventing migraine (November 2020) NICE TA659 Recommended with restrictions
- **MEDICINAL FORMS** There can be variation in the licensing of different medicines containing the same drug.
  Solution for injection
  EXCIPIENTS: May contain Polysorbates
  ▸ Emgality (Eli Lilly and Company Ltd) ▼
     Galcanezumab 120 mg per 1 ml Emgality 120mg/1ml solution for injection pre-filled pens | 1 pre-filled disposable injection [PoM] £450.00

ERGOT ALKALOIDS

Ergotamine tartrate

- **INDICATIONS AND DOSE**
  Management of cluster headache
  ▸ BY MOUTH USING TABLETS
  ▸ Adult: 1 mg once daily for 6 nights in 7; occasionally given for 1–2 weeks, dose to be taken at night

- **UNLICENSED USE** Not licensed for the management of cluster headache.
- **CONTRA-INDICATIONS** Acute porphyrias p. 1107 · coronary heart disease · hyperthyroidism · inadequately controlled hypertension · obliterative vascular disease · peripheral vascular disease · Raynaud's syndrome · sepsis · severe hypertension · temporal arteritis
- **CAUTIONS** Anaemia · cardiac disease · dependence · elderly · risk of peripheral vasospasm
- **INTERACTIONS** → Appendix 1: ergotamine
- **SIDE-EFFECTS**
  ▸ **Common or very common** Abdominal pain · dizziness · nausea · vomiting
  ▸ **Uncommon** Cyanosis · diarrhoea · muscle weakness · pain in extremity · sensation abnormal · vasoconstriction
  ▸ **Rare or very rare** Arrhythmias · cardiac valve fibrosis · dyspnoea · ergot poisoning (including absence of pulse and numbness in extremities) · gangrene · intestinal ischaemia · myalgia · myocardial infarction · myocardial ischaemia · skin reactions
  ▸ **Frequency not known** Anxiety · arthralgia · blood disorder · cerebral ischaemia · confusion · constipation · depression · drowsiness · dry mouth · extrapyramidal symptoms · hallucination · renal artery spasm · seizure · sleep disorder · thrombosis · tremor · urinary retention · vision blurred
- **PREGNANCY** Avoid; oxytocic effect on the uterus.
- **BREAST FEEDING** Avoid; ergotism may occur in infant; repeated doses may inhibit lactation.
- **HEPATIC IMPAIRMENT** Avoid in severe impairment—risk of toxicity increased.
- **RENAL IMPAIRMENT** Avoid; risk of renal vasoconstriction.

- **PATIENT AND CARER ADVICE**
  Peripheral vasospasm Warn patient to stop treatment immediately if numbness or tingling of extremities develops and to contact doctor.
- **LESS SUITABLE FOR PRESCRIBING** Ergotamine tartrate is less suitable for prescribing.

- **MEDICINAL FORMS** No licensed medicines listed.

Ergotamine tartrate with caffeine hydrate and cyclizine hydrochloride

22-Nov-2019

The properties listed below are those particular to the combination only. For the properties of the components please consider, ergotamine tartrate above, cyclizine p. 449.

- **INDICATIONS AND DOSE**
  Treatment of acute migraine
  ▸ BY MOUTH
  ▸ Adult: 1 tablet, to be taken at onset, then 0.5–1 tablet every 30 minutes if required, max. 3 tablets in 24 hours, max. 4 tablets per attack, max. 6 tablets in one week, max. 2 courses of treatment in one month

- **INTERACTIONS** → Appendix 1: antihistamines, sedating · ergotamine
- **PATIENT AND CARER ADVICE** Patient counselling is advised for cyclizine hydrochloride with caffeine hydrate and ergotamine tartrate tablets (dosage).
- **LESS SUITABLE FOR PRESCRIBING** Cyclizine hydrochloride with caffeine hydrate and ergotamine tartrate (*Migril*®) is less suitable for prescribing.

- **MEDICINAL FORMS** No licensed medicines listed.

TRIPTANS

Almotriptan

17-Nov-2020

- **INDICATIONS AND DOSE**
  Treatment of acute migraine
  ▸ BY MOUTH
  ▸ Adult: 12.5 mg, dose to be taken as soon as possible after onset, followed by 12.5 mg after 2 hours if required, dose to be taken only if migraine recurs (patient not responding to initial dose should not take second dose for same attack); maximum 25 mg per day

- **UNLICENSED USE** Not licensed for use in elderly.
- **CONTRA-INDICATIONS** Coronary vasospasm · ischaemic heart disease · peripheral vascular disease · previous cerebrovascular accident · previous myocardial infarction · previous transient ischaemic attack · Prinzmetal's angina · severe hypertension · uncontrolled hypertension
- **CAUTIONS** Conditions which predispose to coronary artery disease · elderly
- **INTERACTIONS** → Appendix 1: triptans
- **SIDE-EFFECTS**
  ▸ **Common or very common** Asthenia · dizziness · drowsiness · nausea · vomiting
  ▸ **Uncommon** Bone pain · chest pain · diarrhoea · dry mouth · dyspepsia · headache · myalgia · palpitations · paraesthesia · throat tightness · tinnitus
  ▸ **Rare or very rare** Coronary vasospasm · myocardial infarction · tachycardia
  ▸ **Frequency not known** Intestinal ischaemia · seizure · vision disorders

4

Nervous system

SIDE-EFFECTS, FURTHER INFORMATION Discontinue if symptoms of heat, heaviness, pressure or tightness (including throat and chest) occur.

● ALLERGY AND CROSS-SENSITIVITY EvGr Caution in patients with sensitivity to sulfonamides. ⊛

● PREGNANCY There is limited experience of using 5HT$_1$-receptor agonists during pregnancy; manufacturers advise that they should be avoided unless the potential benefit outweighs the risk.

● BREAST FEEDING Present in milk in *animal* studies—withhold breast-feeding for 24 hours.

● HEPATIC IMPAIRMENT Manufacturer advises caution in mild to moderate impairment; avoid in severe impairment—no information available.

● RENAL IMPAIRMENT
Dose adjustments Max. 12.5 mg in 24 hours if eGFR less than 30 mL/minute/1.73 m^2.

● MEDICINAL FORMS There can be variation in the licensing of different medicines containing the same drug.
Tablet
CAUTIONARY AND ADVISORY LABELS 3
▸ Almotriptan (Non-proprietary)
Almotriptan (as Almotriptan hydrogen malate)
12.5 mg Almotriptan 12.5mg tablets | 3 tablet [PoM] £9.58 DT = £8.34 | 6 tablet [PoM] £18.14 DT = £16.68 | 9 tablet [PoM] £27.20 DT = £25.53

Eletriptan

05-Mar-2020

● INDICATIONS AND DOSE
Treatment of acute migraine
▸ BY MOUTH
▸ Adult: 40 mg, followed by 40 mg after 2 hours if required, dose to be taken only if migraine recurs (patient not responding to initial dose should not take second dose for same attack); increased if necessary to 80 mg, dose to be taken for subsequent attacks if 40 mg dose inadequate; maximum 80 mg per day

● UNLICENSED USE Not licensed for use in elderly.

● CONTRA-INDICATIONS Arrhythmias · coronary vasospasm · heart failure · ischaemic heart disease · peripheral vascular disease · previous cerebrovascular accident · previous myocardial infarction · previous transient ischaemic attack · Prinzmetal's angina · severe hypertension · uncontrolled hypertension

● CAUTIONS Conditions which predispose to coronary artery disease · elderly

● INTERACTIONS → Appendix 1: triptans

● SIDE-EFFECTS
▸ **Common or very common** Arrhythmias · asthenia · chest discomfort · chills · dizziness · drowsiness · dry mouth · feeling hot · flushing · gastrointestinal discomfort · headache · hyperhidrosis · increased risk of infection · muscle complaints · muscle tone increased · muscle weakness · nausea · pain · palpitations · sensation abnormal · throat tightness · vertigo
▸ **Uncommon** Agitation · appetite decreased · arthralgia · arthritis · confusion · depersonalisation · depression · diarrhoea · dyspnoea · ear pain · eye pain · insomnia · lacrimation disorder · malaise · mood altered · movement disorders · oedema · oral disorders · peripheral vascular disease · respiratory disorder · skin reactions · speech disorder · stupor · taste altered · thinking abnormal · thirst · tinnitus · tremor · urinary disorders · urinary tract disorder · vision disorders · yawning
▸ **Rare or very rare** Asthma · breast pain · burping · conjunctivitis · constipation · gastrointestinal disorders ·

hyperbilirubinaemia · lymphadenopathy · menorrhagia · myopathy · shock · voice alteration
▸ **Frequency not known** Coronary vasospasm · hypertension · myocardial infarction · myocardial ischaemia · serotonin syndrome · stroke · syncope · vomiting

SIDE-EFFECTS, FURTHER INFORMATION Discontinue if symptoms of heat, heaviness, pressure or tightness (including throat and chest) occur.

● PREGNANCY There is limited experience of using 5HT$_1$-receptor agonists during pregnancy; manufacturers advise that they should be avoided unless the potential benefit outweighs the risk.

● BREAST FEEDING Present in milk—avoid breast-feeding for 24 hours.

● HEPATIC IMPAIRMENT Manufacturer advises avoid in severe impairment.

● RENAL IMPAIRMENT Avoid if eGFR less than 30 mL/minute/1.73 m^2.
Dose adjustments Reduce initial dose to 20 mg; maximum 40 mg in 24 hours.

● MEDICINAL FORMS There can be variation in the licensing of different medicines containing the same drug.
Tablet
CAUTIONARY AND ADVISORY LABELS 3
▸ Relpax (Upjohn UK Ltd)
Eletriptan (as Eletriptan hydrobromide) 20 mg Relpax 20mg tablets | 6 tablet [PoM] £22.50 DT = £22.50
Eletriptan (as Eletriptan hydrobromide) 40 mg Relpax 40mg tablets | 6 tablet [PoM] £22.50 DT = £22.50

Frovatriptan

04-Mar-2020

● INDICATIONS AND DOSE
Treatment of acute migraine
▸ BY MOUTH
▸ Adult: 2.5 mg, dose to be taken as soon as possible after onset, followed by 2.5 mg after 2 hours if required, dose to be taken only if migraine recurs (patient not responding to initial dose should not take second dose for same attack); maximum 5 mg per day
Menstrual migraine prophylaxis
▸ BY MOUTH
▸ Adult: 2.5 mg twice daily, to be taken from 2 days before until 3 days after bleeding starts

● UNLICENSED USE Not licensed for use in elderly.
EvGr Frovatriptan may be used for menstrual migraine prophylaxis, ⚠ but it is not licensed for this indication.

● CONTRA-INDICATIONS Coronary vasospasm · ischaemic heart disease · peripheral vascular disease · previous cerebrovascular accident · previous myocardial infarction · previous transient ischaemic attack · Prinzmetal's angina · severe hypertension · uncontrolled hypertension

● CAUTIONS Conditions which predispose to coronary artery disease · elderly

● INTERACTIONS → Appendix 1: triptans

● SIDE-EFFECTS
▸ **Common or very common** Asthenia · chest discomfort · dizziness · drowsiness · dry mouth · flushing · gastrointestinal discomfort · headache · hyperhidrosis · nausea · sensation abnormal · throat complaints · vision disorders
▸ **Uncommon** Anxiety · arrhythmias · arthralgia · concentration impaired · confusion · dehydration · depression · diarrhoea · dysphagia · ear discomfort · eye discomfort · gastrointestinal disorders · hypertension · increased risk of infection · malaise · musculoskeletal stiffness · neuromuscular dysfunction · pain · palpitations · peripheral coldness · psychiatric disorders · skin reactions ·

sleep disorders · taste altered · temperature sensation altered · thirst · tinnitus · tremor · urinary disorders · vertigo

▸ **Rare or very rare** Breast tenderness · burping · constipation · ear disorder · epistaxis · fever · hiccups · hyperacusia · hypoglycaemia · irritable bowel syndrome · lymphadenopathy · memory loss · movement disorder · oesophageal spasm · oral disorders · piloerection · reflexes decreased · renal pain · respiratory disorders · self mutilation

▸ **Frequency not known** Angioedema · coronary vasospasm · hypersensitivity · myocardial infarction

SIDE-EFFECTS, FURTHER INFORMATION Discontinue if symptoms of heat, heaviness, pressure or tightness (including throat and chest) occur.

● PREGNANCY There is limited experience of using 5HT$_1$-receptor agonists during pregnancy; manufacturers advise that they should be avoided unless the potential benefit outweighs the risk.

● BREAST FEEDING Present in milk in *animal* studies—withhold breast-feeding for 24 hours.

● HEPATIC IMPAIRMENT Manufacturer advises avoid in severe impairment—no information available.

● MEDICINAL FORMS There can be variation in the licensing of different medicines containing the same drug.

Tablet
CAUTIONARY AND ADVISORY LABELS 3
▸ Frovatriptan (Non-proprietary)
Frovatriptan (as Frovatriptan succinate monohydrate)
2.5 mg Frovatriptan 2.5mg tablets | 6 tablet [PoM] £16.67 DT = £6.14
▸ Migard (A. Menarini Farmaceutica Internazionale SRL)
Frovatriptan (as Frovatriptan succinate monohydrate)
2.5 mg Migard 2.5mg tablets | 6 tablet [PoM] £16.67 DT = £6.14
▸ Mylatrip (Mylan)
Frovatriptan (as Frovatriptan succinate monohydrate)
2.5 mg Mylatrip 2.5mg tablets | 6 tablet [PoM] £16.50 DT = £6.14

▎Naratriptan   02-Dec-2020

● **INDICATIONS AND DOSE**
Treatment of acute migraine
▸ BY MOUTH
▸ Adult: 2.5 mg, followed by 2.5 mg after at least 4 hours if required, to be taken only if migraine recurs (patient not responding to initial dose should not take second dose for same attack); maximum 5 mg per day

Menstrual migraine prophylaxis
▸ BY MOUTH
▸ Adult: 2.5 mg twice daily, to be taken from 2 days before until 3 days after bleeding starts

● UNLICENSED USE [EvGr] Naratriptan is used for menstrual migraine prophylaxis, ⟨A⟩ but is not licensed for this indication. Not licensed for use in elderly.

● CONTRA-INDICATIONS Coronary vasospasm · ischaemic heart disease · moderate or severe hypertension · peripheral vascular disease · previous cerebrovascular accident · previous myocardial infarction · previous transient ischaemic attack · Prinzmetal's angina · uncontrolled hypertension

● CAUTIONS Conditions which predispose to coronary artery disease · elderly

● INTERACTIONS → Appendix 1: triptans

● SIDE-EFFECTS
▸ **Common or very common** Dizziness · drowsiness · fatigue · feeling hot · malaise · nausea · paraesthesia · vomiting
▸ **Uncommon** Arrhythmias · feeling abnormal · pain · palpitations · visual impairment

---

▸ **Rare or very rare** Angina pectoris · colitis ischaemic · coronary vasospasm · face oedema · myocardial infarction · peripheral vascular disease · skin reactions

SIDE-EFFECTS, FURTHER INFORMATION Discontinue if symptoms of heat, heaviness, pressure or tightness (including throat and chest) occur.

● ALLERGY AND CROSS-SENSITIVITY [EvGr] Caution in patients with sensitivity to sulfonamides. ⟨M⟩

● PREGNANCY There is limited experience of using 5HT$_1$-receptor agonists during pregnancy; manufacturers advise that they should be avoided unless the potential benefit outweighs the risk.

● BREAST FEEDING Withhold breast-feeding for 24 hours.

● HEPATIC IMPAIRMENT Manufacturer advises caution in mild to moderate impairment (risk of decreased clearance); avoid in severe impairment.
Dose adjustments Manufacturer advises maximum 2.5 mg in 24 hours in mild to moderate impairment.

● RENAL IMPAIRMENT Avoid if eGFR less than 15 mL/minute/1.73 m^2.
Dose adjustments Max. 2.5 mg in 24 hours.

● PATIENT AND CARER ADVICE
Driving and skilled tasks Drowsiness may affect performance of skilled tasks (e.g. driving).

● MEDICINAL FORMS There can be variation in the licensing of different medicines containing the same drug.

Tablet
CAUTIONARY AND ADVISORY LABELS 3
▸ Naratriptan (Non-proprietary)
Naratriptan (as Naratriptan hydrochloride) 2.5 mg Naratriptan 2.5mg tablets | 6 tablet [PoM] £24.55 DT = £2.96 | 12 tablet [PoM] £8.68–£46.00 DT = £5.92
▸ Naramig (GlaxoSmithKline UK Ltd)
Naratriptan (as Naratriptan hydrochloride) 2.5 mg Naramig 2.5mg tablets | 6 tablet [PoM] £24.55 DT = £2.96

▎Rizatriptan   13-Oct-2020

● **INDICATIONS AND DOSE**
Treatment of acute migraine
▸ BY MOUTH
▸ Adult: 10 mg, dose to be taken as soon as possible after onset, followed by 10 mg after 2 hours if required, dose to be taken only if migraine recurs (patient not responding to initial dose should not take second dose for same attack); maximum 20 mg per day

DOSE ADJUSTMENTS DUE TO INTERACTIONS
▸ Manufacturer advises reduce dose to 5 mg with concurrent use of propranolol.

● UNLICENSED USE Not licensed for use in elderly.

● CONTRA-INDICATIONS Coronary vasospasm · ischaemic heart disease · peripheral vascular disease · previous cerebrovascular accident · previous myocardial infarction · previous transient ischaemic attack · Prinzmetal's angina · severe hypertension · uncontrolled hypertension

● CAUTIONS Conditions which predispose to coronary artery disease · elderly

● INTERACTIONS → Appendix 1: triptans

● SIDE-EFFECTS
▸ **Common or very common** Alertness decreased · asthenia · diarrhoea · dizziness · drowsiness · dry mouth · dyspepsia · feeling abnormal · headache · insomnia · musculoskeletal stiffness · nausea · pain · palpitations · sensation abnormal · throat complaints · vasodilation · vomiting
▸ **Uncommon** Angioedema · arrhythmias · ataxia · disorientation · dyspnoea · face oedema · hyperhidrosis · hypertension · muscle weakness · myalgia · nervousness ·

4

Nervous system

skin reactions · syncope · taste altered · thirst · tongue swelling · tremor · vertigo · vision blurred
▶ **Rare or very rare** Hypersensitivity · stroke · wheezing
▶ **Frequency not known** Colitis ischaemic · myocardial infarction · myocardial ischaemia · peripheral vascular disease · seizure · serotonin syndrome · toxic epidermal necrolysis
SIDE-EFFECTS, FURTHER INFORMATION Discontinue if symptoms of heat, heaviness, pressure or tightness (including throat and chest) occur.
● PREGNANCY There is limited experience of using 5HT$_1$-receptor agonists during pregnancy; manufacturers advise that they should be avoided unless the potential benefit outweighs the risk.
● BREAST FEEDING Present in milk in *animal* studies— withhold breast-feeding for 24 hours.
● HEPATIC IMPAIRMENT Manufacturer advises caution in mild to moderate impairment; avoid in severe impairment (no information available).
Dose adjustments Manufacturer advises dose reduction to 5 mg in mild to moderate impairment.
● RENAL IMPAIRMENT Avoid in severe impairment.
Dose adjustments Reduce dose to 5 mg in mild to moderate impairment.
● DIRECTIONS FOR ADMINISTRATION Rizatriptan orodispersible tablets should be placed on the tongue, allowed to disperse and swallowed. Rizatriptan oral lyophilisates should be placed on the tongue and allowed to dissolve.
● PATIENT AND CARER ADVICE Patients or carers should be given advice on how to administer rizatriptan orodispersible tablets and oral lyophilisates.
Driving and skilled tasks Drowsiness may affect performance of skilled tasks (e.g. driving).

● MEDICINAL FORMS There can be variation in the licensing of different medicines containing the same drug.
Orodispersible tablet
CAUTIONARY AND ADVISORY LABELS 3
EXCIPIENTS: May contain Aspartame
▶ Rizatriptan (Non-proprietary)
Rizatriptan (as Rizatriptan benzoate) 10 mg Rizatriptan 10mg orodispersible tablets sugar free sugar-free | 3 tablet [PoM] £13.37 DT = £3.05 sugar-free | 6 tablet [PoM] £6.10–£26.74
Tablet
CAUTIONARY AND ADVISORY LABELS 3
▶ Rizatriptan (Non-proprietary)
Rizatriptan (as Rizatriptan benzoate) 5 mg Rizatriptan 5mg tablets | 3 tablet [PoM] £13.37 | 6 tablet [PoM] £26.74 DT = £26.73
Rizatriptan (as Rizatriptan benzoate) 10 mg Rizatriptan 10mg tablets | 3 tablet [PoM] £13.37 DT = £2.87 | 6 tablet [PoM] £5.74–£26.74
▶ Maxalt (Merck Sharp & Dohme Ltd)
Rizatriptan (as Rizatriptan benzoate) 5 mg Maxalt 5mg tablets | 6 tablet [PoM] £26.74 DT = £26.73
Rizatriptan (as Rizatriptan benzoate) 10 mg Maxalt 10mg tablets | 3 tablet [PoM] £13.37 DT = £2.87 | 6 tablet [PoM] £26.74
Oral lyophilisate
CAUTIONARY AND ADVISORY LABELS 3
EXCIPIENTS: May contain Aspartame
▶ Maxalt Melt (Merck Sharp & Dohme Ltd)
Rizatriptan (as Rizatriptan benzoate) 10 mg Maxalt Melt 10mg oral lyophilisates sugar-free | 3 tablet [PoM] £13.37 DT = £13.37 sugar-free | 6 tablet [PoM] £26.74 DT = £26.74 sugar-free | 12 tablet [PoM] £53.48 DT = £53.48

Sumatriptan

09-Dec-2020

● INDICATIONS AND DOSE
Treatment of acute migraine
▶ BY MOUTH
▶ **Adult:** Initially 50–100 mg for 1 dose, followed by 50–100 mg after at least 2 hours if required, to be taken only if migraine recurs (patient not responding to initial dose should not take second dose for same attack); maximum 300 mg per day
▶ BY SUBCUTANEOUS INJECTION
▶ **Adult 18–65 years:** Initially 3–6 mg for 1 dose, followed by 3–6 mg after at least 1 hour if required, to be taken only if migraine recurs (patient not responding to initial dose should not take second dose for same attack), dose to be administered using an auto-injector; not for intravenous injection which may cause coronary vasospasm and angina; maximum 12 mg per day
▶ BY INTRANASAL ADMINISTRATION
▶ **Adult 18–65 years:** Initially 10–20 mg, to be administered into one nostril, followed by 10–20 mg after at least 2 hours if required, to be taken only if migraine recurs (patient not responding to initial dose should not take second dose for same attack); maximum 40 mg per day
Treatment of acute cluster headache
▶ BY SUBCUTANEOUS INJECTION
▶ **Adult:** Initially 6 mg for 1 dose, followed by 6 mg after at least 1 hour if required, to be taken only if headache recurs (patient not responding to initial dose should not take second dose for same attack), dose to be administered using an auto-injector; not for intravenous injection which may cause coronary vasospasm and angina; maximum 12 mg per day
▶ BY INTRANASAL ADMINISTRATION
▶ **Adult 18–65 years:** Initially 10–20 mg, dose to be administered into one nostril, followed by 10–20 mg after at least 2 hours if required, to be taken only if headache recurs (patient not responding to initial dose should not take second dose for same attack); maximum 40 mg per day

● UNLICENSED USE Not licensed for use in elderly.
● CONTRA-INDICATIONS Coronary vasospasm · ischaemic heart disease · mild uncontrolled hypertension · moderate and severe hypertension · peripheral vascular disease · previous cerebrovascular accident · previous myocardial infarction · previous transient ischaemic attack · Prinzmetal's angina
● CAUTIONS Conditions which predispose to coronary artery disease · elderly · history of seizures · mild, controlled hypertension · risk factors for seizures
● INTERACTIONS → Appendix 1: triptans
● SIDE-EFFECTS
GENERAL SIDE-EFFECTS
▶ **Common or very common** Asthenia · dizziness · drowsiness · dyspnoea · feeling abnormal · flushing · myalgia · nausea · pain · sensation abnormal · skin reactions · temperature sensation altered · vomiting
▶ **Rare or very rare** Hypersensitivity
▶ **Frequency not known** Angina pectoris · anxiety · arrhythmias · arthralgia · colitis ischaemic · coronary vasospasm · diarrhoea · dystonia · hyperhidrosis · hypotension · myocardial infarction · nystagmus · palpitations · Raynaud's phenomenon · seizure · tremor · vision disorders
SPECIFIC SIDE-EFFECTS
▶ **Common or very common**
▶ With intranasal use Epistaxis · nasal irritation · taste altered · throat irritation

▸ With subcutaneous use Haemorrhage · swelling

SIDE-EFFECTS, FURTHER INFORMATION Discontinue if symptoms of heat, heaviness, pressure or tightness (including throat and chest) occur.

● ALLERGY AND CROSS-SENSITIVITY EvGr Caution in patients with sensitivity to sulfonamides. Ⓜ

● PREGNANCY There is limited experience of using 5HT$_1$-receptor agonists during pregnancy; manufacturers advise that they should be avoided unless the potential benefit outweighs the risk.

● BREAST FEEDING Present in milk but amount probably too small to be harmful; withhold breast-feeding for 12 hours after treatment.

● HEPATIC IMPAIRMENT Manufacturer advises caution (reduced pre-systemic clearance increases exposure); avoid in severe impairment (no information available).
Dose adjustments ▸ With oral use Manufacturer advises consider dose reduction to 25–50 mg in mild to moderate impairment.

● RENAL IMPAIRMENT Use with caution.

● PATIENT AND CARER ADVICE
Driving and skilled tasks Drowsiness may affect performance of skilled tasks (e.g. driving).

● EXCEPTIONS TO LEGAL CATEGORY
▸ With oral use Sumatriptan 50 mg tablets can be sold to the public to treat previously diagnosed migraine; max. daily dose 100 mg.

● MEDICINAL FORMS There can be variation in the licensing of different medicines containing the same drug.
Solution for injection
CAUTIONARY AND ADVISORY LABELS 3, 10
▸ Sumatriptan (Non-proprietary)
Sumatriptan (as Sumatriptan succinate) 6 mg per 1 ml Sumatriptan 3mg/0.5ml solution for injection pre-filled pens | 2 pre-filled disposable injection [PoM] £39.50-£54.00
Sumatriptan (as Sumatriptan succinate) 12 mg per 1 ml Sumatriptan 6mg/0.5ml solution for injection pre-filled pens | 2 pre-filled disposable injection [PoM] £45.00 DT = £45.00
▸ Imigran Subject (GlaxoSmithKline UK Ltd)
Sumatriptan (as Sumatriptan succinate) 12 mg per 1 ml Imigran Subject 6mg/0.5ml solution for injection syringe refill pack | 2 pre-filled disposable injection [PoM] £48.49 DT = £48.49
Imigran Subject 6mg/0.5ml solution for injection pre-filled syringes with device | 2 pre-filled disposable injection [PoM] £50.96 DT = £50.96
Spray
CAUTIONARY AND ADVISORY LABELS 3, 10
▸ Imigran (GlaxoSmithKline UK Ltd)
Sumatriptan 100 mg per 1 ml Imigran 10mg nasal spray | 2 unit dose [PoM] £14.16 DT = £14.16
Sumatriptan 200 mg per 1 ml Imigran 20mg nasal spray | 2 unit dose [PoM] £14.16 | 6 unit dose [PoM] £42.47 DT = £42.47
Tablet
CAUTIONARY AND ADVISORY LABELS 3, 10
▸ Sumatriptan (Non-proprietary)
Sumatriptan (as Sumatriptan succinate) 50 mg Sumatriptan 50mg tablets | 6 tablet [PoM] £31.85 DT = £1.29
Sumatriptan (as Sumatriptan succinate) 100 mg Sumatriptan 100mg tablets | 6 tablet [PoM] £51.48 DT = £1.50
▸ Imigran (GlaxoSmithKline UK Ltd)
Sumatriptan (as Sumatriptan succinate) 50 mg Imigran Radis 50mg tablets | 6 tablet [PoM] £23.90 DT = £1.29
Imigran 50mg tablets | 6 tablet [PoM] £31.85 DT = £1.29
Sumatriptan (as Sumatriptan succinate) 100 mg Imigran 100mg tablets | 6 tablet [PoM] £51.48 DT = £1.50
Imigran Radis 100mg tablets | 6 tablet [PoM] £42.90 DT = £1.50
▸ Migraitan (Bristol Laboratories Ltd)
Sumatriptan (as Sumatriptan succinate) 50 mg Migraitan 50mg tablets | 2 tablet [P] £4.44

▌Zolmitriptan
03-Sep-2020

● INDICATIONS AND DOSE
Treatment of acute migraine
▸ BY MOUTH
▸ Adult: 2.5 mg, followed by 2.5 mg after at least 2 hours if required, dose to be taken only if migraine recurs, then increased if necessary to 5 mg, dose to be taken only for subsequent attacks in patients not achieving satisfactory relief with 2.5 mg dose; maximum 10 mg per day
▸ BY INTRANASAL ADMINISTRATION
▸ Adult: 5 mg, dose to be administered as soon as possible after onset into one nostril only, followed by 5 mg after at least 2 hours if required, dose to be administered only if migraine recurs; maximum 10 mg per day

Treatment of acute cluster headache
▸ BY INTRANASAL ADMINISTRATION
▸ Adult: 5 mg, dose to be administered as soon as possible after onset into one nostril only, followed by 5 mg after at least 2 hours if required, dose to be administered only if migraine recurs; maximum 10 mg per day

Menstrual migraine prophylaxis
▸ BY MOUTH
▸ Adult: 2.5 mg 3 times a day, to be taken from 2 days before until 3 days after bleeding starts

DOSE ADJUSTMENTS DUE TO INTERACTIONS
▸ Manufacturer advises max. dose 5 mg in 24 hours with concurrent use of moderate and potent inhibitors of CYP1A2, cimetidine and moclobemide.

DOSE EQUIVALENCE AND CONVERSION
▸ 1 spray of Zomig® nasal spray = 5 mg zolmitriptan.

● UNLICENSED USE EvGr Zolmitriptan is used for menstrual migraine prophylaxis, Ⓐ but is not licensed for this indication. Not licensed for use in elderly. Not licensed for treatment of cluster headaches.

● CONTRA-INDICATIONS Arrhythmias associated with accessory cardiac conduction pathways · coronary vasospasm · ischaemic heart disease · moderate to severe hypertension · peripheral vascular disease · previous cerebrovascular accident · previous myocardial infarction · Prinzmetal's angina · transient ischaemic attack · uncontrolled hypertension · Wolff-Parkinson-White syndrome

● CAUTIONS Conditions which predispose to coronary artery disease · elderly

● INTERACTIONS → Appendix 1: triptans

● SIDE-EFFECTS
GENERAL SIDE-EFFECTS
▸ **Common or very common** Abdominal pain · asthenia · chest discomfort · dizziness · drowsiness · dry mouth · dysphagia · feeling hot · headache · limb discomfort · muscle weakness · nausea · pain · palpitations · sensation abnormal · vomiting
▸ **Uncommon** Tachycardia · urinary disorders
▸ **Rare or very rare** Angina pectoris · angioedema · coronary vasospasm · gastrointestinal disorders · gastrointestinal infarction · hypersensitivity · myocardial infarction · splenic infarction · urticaria
SPECIFIC SIDE-EFFECTS
▸ **Common or very common**
▸ With intranasal use Feeling abnormal · haemorrhage · myalgia · nasal discomfort · taste altered · throat pain
▸ With oral use Muscle complaints · sensation of pressure · throat complaints
▸ **Rare or very rare**
▸ With oral use Diarrhoea

SIDE-EFFECTS, FURTHER INFORMATION Discontinue if symptoms of heat, heaviness, pressure or tightness (including throat and chest) occur.

- **PREGNANCY** There is limited experience of using 5HT$_1$-receptor agonists during pregnancy; manufacturers advise that they should be avoided unless the potential benefit outweighs the risk.
- **BREAST FEEDING** Use with caution—present in milk in *animal* studies.
- **HEPATIC IMPAIRMENT** Manufacturer advises caution in moderate to severe impairment (risk of increased exposure).
  Dose adjustments Manufacturer advises maximum 5 mg in 24 hours in moderate to severe impairment.
- **DIRECTIONS FOR ADMINISTRATION** Zolmitriptan orodispersible tablets should be placed on the tongue, allowed to disperse and swallowed.
- **PATIENT AND CARER ADVICE** Patients or carers should be given advice on how to administer zolmitriptan orodispersible tablets.

- **MEDICINAL FORMS** There can be variation in the licensing of different medicines containing the same drug.
  Spray
  ▸ Zomig (Grunenthal Ltd)
  Zolmitriptan 50 mg per 1 ml Zomig 5mg/0.1ml nasal spray 0.1ml unit dose | 6 unit dose [PoM] £36.50 DT = £36.50
  Orodispersible tablet
  EXCIPIENTS: May contain Aspartame
  ▸ Zolmitriptan (Non-proprietary)
  Zolmitriptan 2.5 mg Zolmitriptan 2.5mg orodispersible tablets sugar free sugar-free | 6 tablet [PoM] £20.35 DT = £9.92
  Zolmitriptan 5 mg Zolmitriptan 5mg orodispersible tablets sugar free sugar-free | 6 tablet [PoM] £20.35 DT = £13.41
  ▸ Zomig Rapimelt (Grunenthal Ltd)
  Zolmitriptan 2.5 mg Zomig Rapimelt 2.5mg orodispersible tablets sugar-free | 6 tablet [PoM] £23.99 DT = £9.92
  Zolmitriptan 5 mg Zomig Rapimelt 5mg orodispersible tablets sugar-free | 6 tablet [PoM] £23.94 DT = £13.41
  Tablet
  ▸ Zolmitriptan (Non-proprietary)
  Zolmitriptan 2.5 mg Zolmitriptan 2.5mg tablets | 6 tablet [PoM] £23.94 DT = £3.18 | 12 tablet [PoM] £21.00 DT = £6.36
  Zolmitriptan 5 mg Zolmitriptan 5mg tablets | 6 tablet [PoM] £43.20 DT = £36.00
  ▸ Zomig (Grunenthal Ltd)
  Zolmitriptan 2.5 mg Zomig 2.5mg tablets | 6 tablet [PoM] £23.94 DT = £3.18

6.2 Neuropathic pain

Neuropathic pain

06-Oct-2020

MHRA/CHM important safety information

When using antiepileptics for the management of neuropathic pain, see Epilepsy p. 321 for information on the use of antiepileptic drugs and the risk of suicidal thoughts and behaviour.

For information on the use of opioids and risk of dependence and addiction, see *Important safety information* in individual drug monographs.

Overview and management

Neuropathic pain, which occurs as a result of damage to neural tissue, includes *phantom limb pain*, *compression neuropathies*, *peripheral neuropathies* (e.g. due to Diabetic complications p. 728, chronic excessive alcohol intake, HIV infection p. 679, chemotherapy, idiopathic neuropathy), *trauma*, *central pain* (e.g. pain following stroke, spinal cord injury, and syringomyelia), and *postherpetic neuralgia* (peripheral nerve damage following acute herpes zoster infection (shingles)). The pain may occur in an area of sensory deficit and is sometimes accompanied by pain that is evoked by a non-noxious stimulus (allodynia).

Trigeminal neuralgia is also caused by dysfunction of neural tissue, but its management is distinct from other forms of neuropathic pain.

Neuropathic pain is generally managed with a **tricyclic antidepressant** or with certain **antiepileptic drugs**. Amitriptyline hydrochloride p. 392 and pregabalin p. 342 are effective treatments for neuropathic pain. Amitriptyline hydrochloride and pregabalin can be used in combination if the patient has an inadequate response to either drug at the maximum tolerated dose.

Nortriptyline p. 397 [unlicensed indication] may be better tolerated than amitriptyline hydrochloride.

Gabapentin p. 332 is also effective for the treatment of neuropathic pain.

Neuropathic pain may respond to **opioid analgesics**. There is evidence of efficacy for tramadol hydrochloride p. 491, morphine p. 483, and oxycodone hydrochloride p. 486; however, treatment with morphine or oxycodone hydrochloride should be initiated only under specialist supervision. Tramadol hydrochloride can be prescribed when other treatments have been unsuccessful, while the patient is waiting for assessment by a specialist.

Patients with localised superficial pain who are unable to take oral medicines may benefit from **topical local anaesthetic preparations**, such as lidocaine hydrochloride medicated plasters p. 1406, while awaiting specialist review.

Capsaicin p. 505 is licensed for neuropathic pain (but the intense burning sensation during initial treatment may limit use). Capsaicin 0.075% cream is licensed for the symptomatic relief of *postherpetic neuralgia*. A self-adhesive patch containing capsaicin 8% is licensed for the treatment of peripheral neuropathic pain. It should be used under specialist supervision.

A corticosteroid may help to relieve pressure in compression neuropathy and thereby reduce pain.

Neuromodulation by spinal cord stimulation may be of benefit in some patients. Many patients with chronic neuropathic pain require multidisciplinary management, including physiotherapy and psychological support.

Trigeminal neuralgia

Surgery may be the treatment of choice in many patients; a neurological assessment will identify those who stand to benefit. Carbamazepine p. 327 taken during the acute stages of trigeminal neuralgia, reduces the frequency and severity of attacks. It is very effective for the severe pain associated with trigeminal neuralgia and (less commonly) glossopharyngeal neuralgia. Blood counts and electrolytes should be monitored when high doses are given. Small doses should be used initially to reduce the incidence of side-effects e.g. dizziness. Some cases respond to phenytoin p. 340; the drug may be given by intravenous infusion (possibly as fosphenytoin sodium p. 331) in a crisis (specialist use only).

Chronic facial pain

Chronic oral and facial pain including *persistent idiopathic facial pain* (also termed 'atypical facial pain') and *temporomandibular dysfunction* (previously termed temporomandibular joint pain dysfunction syndrome) may call for prolonged use of analgesics or for other drugs. **Tricyclic antidepressants** may be useful for facial pain [unlicensed indication], but are not on the Dental Practitioners' List. Disorders of this type require specialist referral and psychological support to accompany drug treatment. Patients on long-term therapy need to be monitored both for progress and for side-effects.

Other drugs used for Neuropathic pain Amantadine hydrochloride, p. 438

4

Nervous system

ANALGESICS > PLANT ALKALOIDS

Capsaicin
09-Nov-2020

- **INDICATIONS AND DOSE**

Localised neuropathic pain
▶ TO THE SKIN USING CREAM
▶ Adult: Apply 3–4 times a day, using 0.075% strength; apply sparingly, not more often than every 4 hours

AXSAIN ®

Post-herpetic neuralgia
▶ TO THE SKIN
▶ Adult: Apply 3–4 times a day, apply sparingly; **important; after** lesions have healed, not more often than every 4 hours

Painful diabetic neuropathy (under expert supervision)
▶ TO THE SKIN
▶ Adult: Apply 3–4 times a day for 8 weeks then review, apply sparingly, not more often than every 4 hours

QUTENZA ®

Peripheral neuropathic pain (under the supervision of a physician)
▶ BY TRANSDERMAL APPLICATION USING PATCHES
▶ Adult: (consult product literature)

ZACIN ®

Symptomatic relief in osteoarthritis
▶ TO THE SKIN
▶ Adult: Apply 4 times a day, apply sparingly, not more often than every 4 hours

- UNLICENSED USE [EvGr] Capsaicin is used in the treatment of localised neuropathic pain, ⟨E⟩ but is not licensed for this indication.

- **CAUTIONS**
GENERAL CAUTIONS Avoid contact with broken skin · avoid contact with inflamed skin
SPECIFIC CAUTIONS
▶ With topical use Avoid contact with eyes · avoid hot shower or bath just before or after application (burning sensation enhanced) · avoid inhalation of vapours · not to be used under tight bandages
▶ With transdermal use Avoid contact with the face, scalp or in proximity to mucous membranes · avoid holding near eyes or mucous membranes · diabetes · history of cardiovascular disease · uncontrolled hypertension
CAUTIONS, FURTHER INFORMATION
▶ Diabetes
▶ With transdermal use [EvGr] Particular attention should be given to diabetic patients with coronary artery disease, hypertension, or cardiovascular autonomic neuropathy. ⟨M⟩

- **SIDE-EFFECTS**
GENERAL SIDE-EFFECTS
▶ **Uncommon** Cough
SPECIFIC SIDE-EFFECTS
▶ **Common or very common**
▶ With transdermal use Sensation abnormal
▶ **Uncommon**
▶ With transdermal use Atrioventricular block · eye irritation · muscle spasms · nausea · palpitations · peripheral oedema · skin reactions · tachycardia · taste altered · throat irritation
▶ **Rare or very rare**
▶ With topical use Sneezing · watering eye
▶ **Frequency not known**
▶ With topical use Asthma exacerbated · dyspnoea · skin burning sensation (particularly if too much used or if administered more than 4 times daily) · skin irritation

- MONITORING REQUIREMENTS
▶ With transdermal use Monitor blood pressure during treatment procedure.

- HANDLING AND STORAGE
▶ With topical use Wash hands immediately after use (or wash hands 30 minutes after application if hands treated).
▶ With transdermal use Nitrile gloves to be worn while handling patches and cleaning treatment areas (latex gloves do not provide adequate protection).

- NATIONAL FUNDING/ACCESS DECISIONS
For full details see funding body website
Scottish Medicines Consortium (SMC) decisions
▶ Capsaicin (*Qutenza*®) for the treatment of peripheral neuropathic pain in non-diabetic adults either alone or in combination with other medicinal products for pain (October 2014) SMC No. 673/11 Recommended with restrictions

- MEDICINAL FORMS There can be variation in the licensing of different medicines containing the same drug. Forms available from special-order manufacturers include: cream
Cutaneous patch
EXCIPIENTS: May contain Butylated hydroxyanisole
▶ Qutenza (Grunenthal Ltd)
   Capsaicin 179 mg Qutenza 179mg cutaneous patches | 1 patch [PoM] £210.00 DT = £210.00
Cream
EXCIPIENTS: May contain Benzyl alcohol, cetostearyl alcohol (including cetyl and stearyl alcohol)
▶ Axsain (Teva UK Ltd)
   Capsaicin 750 microgram per 1 gram Axsain 0.075% cream | 45 gram [PoM] £14.58 DT = £14.58
▶ Zacin (Teva UK Ltd)
   Capsaicin 250 microgram per 1 gram Zacin 0.025% cream | 45 gram [PoM] £17.71 DT = £17.71

7 Sleep disorders

7.1 Insomnia

Hypnotics and anxiolytics

Overview

Most anxiolytics ('sedatives') will induce sleep when given at night and most hypnotics will sedate when given during the day. Prescribing of these drugs is widespread but dependence (both physical and psychological) and tolerance occur. This may lead to difficulty in withdrawing the drug after the patient has been taking it regularly for more than a few weeks. Hypnotics and anxiolytics should therefore be reserved for short courses to alleviate acute conditions after causal factors have been established.

Benzodiazepines are the most commonly used anxiolytics and hypnotics; they act at benzodiazepine receptors which are associated with gamma-aminobutyric acid (GABA) receptors. Older drugs such as meprobamate p. 365 and barbiturates are **not** recommended—they have more side-effects and interactions than benzodiazepines and are much more dangerous in overdosage.

Benzodiazepine indications

- Benzodiazepines are indicated for the short-term relief (two to four weeks only) of anxiety that is severe, disabling, or causing the patient unacceptable distress, occurring alone or in association with insomnia or short-term psychosomatic, organic, or psychotic illness.
- The use of benzodiazepines to treat short-term 'mild' anxiety is inappropriate.
- Benzodiazepines should be used to treat insomnia only when it is severe, disabling, or causing the patient extreme distress.

4

Nervous system

Dependence and withdrawal

Withdrawal of a benzodiazepine should be gradual because abrupt withdrawal may produce confusion, toxic psychosis, convulsions, or a condition resembling delirium tremens. The benzodiazepine withdrawal syndrome may develop at any time up to 3 weeks after stopping a long-acting benzodiazepine, but may occur within a day in the case of a short-acting one. It is characterised by insomnia, anxiety, loss of appetite and of body-weight, tremor, perspiration, tinnitus, and perceptual disturbances. Some symptoms may be similar to the original complaint and encourage further prescribing; some symptoms may continue for weeks or months after stopping benzodiazepines.

Benzodiazepine withdrawal should be flexible and carried out at a reduction rate that is tolerable for the patient. The rate should depend on the initial dose of benzodiazepine, duration of use, and the patient's clinical response. Short-term users of benzodiazepines (2–4 weeks only) can usually taper off within 2–4 weeks. However, long-term users should be withdrawn over a much longer period of several months or more.

A suggested protocol for withdrawal for prescribed long-term benzodiazepine patients is as follows:

- Transfer patient stepwise, one dose at a time over about a week, to an equivalent daily dose of diazepam preferably taken at night.
- Reduce diazepam dose, usually by 1–2 mg every 2–4 weeks (in patients taking high doses of benzodiazepines, initially it may be appropriate to reduce the dose by up to one-tenth every 1–2 weeks). If uncomfortable withdrawal symptoms occur, maintain this dose until symptoms lessen.
- Reduce diazepam dose further, if necessary in smaller steps; steps of 500 micrograms may be appropriate towards the end of withdrawal. Then stop completely.
- For long-term patients, the period needed for complete withdrawal may vary from several months to a year or more.

Approximate equivalent doses, diazepam 5 mg

≡ alprazolam 250 micrograms
≡ clobazam 10 mg
≡ clonazepam 250 micrograms
≡ flurazepam 7.5–15 mg
≡ chlordiazepoxide 12.5 mg
≡ loprazolam 0.5–1 mg
≡ lorazepam 500 micrograms
≡ lormetazepam 0.5–1 mg
≡ nitrazepam 5 mg
≡ oxazepam 10 mg
≡ temazepam 10 mg

Withdrawal symptoms for long-term users usually resolve within 6–18 months of the last dose. Some patients will recover more quickly, others may take longer. The addition of beta-blockers, antidepressants and antipsychotics should be **avoided** where possible.

Counselling can be of considerable help both during and after the taper.

Hypnotics

Before a hypnotic is prescribed the cause of the insomnia should be established and, where possible, underlying factors should be treated. However, it should be noted that some patients have unrealistic sleep expectations, and others understate their alcohol consumption which is often the cause of the insomnia. Short-acting hypnotics are preferable in patients with sleep onset insomnia, when sedation the following day is undesirable, or when prescribing for elderly patients. Long-acting hypnotics are indicated in patients with poor sleep maintenance (e.g. early morning waking) that causes daytime effects, when an anxiolytic effect is needed during the day, or when sedation the following day is acceptable.

Transient insomnia may occur in those who normally sleep well and may be due to extraneous factors such as noise, shift work, and jet lag. If a hypnotic is indicated one that is rapidly eliminated should be chosen, and only one or two doses should be given.

Short-term insomnia is usually related to an emotional problem or serious medical illness. It may last for a few weeks and may recur; a hypnotic can be useful but should not be given for more than three weeks (preferably only one week). Intermittent use is desirable with omission of some doses. A short-acting drug is usually appropriate.

Chronic insomnia is rarely benefited by hypnotics and is sometimes due to mild dependence caused by injudicious prescribing of hypnotics. Psychiatric disorders such as anxiety, depression, and abuse of drugs and alcohol are common causes. Sleep disturbance is very common in depressive illness and early wakening is often a useful pointer. The underlying psychiatric complaint should be treated, adapting the drug regimen to alleviate insomnia. For example, clomipramine hydrochloride p. 393 or mirtazapine p. 391 prescribed for depression will also help to promote sleep if taken at night. Other causes of insomnia include daytime cat-napping and physical causes such as pain, pruritus, and dyspnoea.

Hypnotics should **not** be prescribed indiscriminately and routine prescribing is undesirable. They should be reserved for short courses in the acutely distressed. Tolerance to their effects develops within 3 to 14 days of continuous use and long-term efficacy cannot be assured. A major drawback of long-term use is that withdrawal can cause rebound insomnia and a withdrawal syndrome.

Where prolonged administration is unavoidable hypnotics should be discontinued as soon as feasible and the patient warned that sleep may be disturbed for a few days before normal rhythm is re-established; broken sleep with vivid dreams may persist for several weeks.

Elderly

Benzodiazepines and the Z–drugs should be avoided in the elderly, because the elderly are at greater risk of becoming ataxic and confused, leading to falls and injury.

Dental patients

Some anxious patients may benefit from the use of hypnotics during dental procedures such as temazepam p. 509 or diazepam p. 362. Temazepam is preferred when it is important to minimise any residual effect the following day.

Benzodiazepines

Benzodiazepines used as hypnotics include nitrazepam p. 508 and flurazepam p. 507 which have a prolonged action and may give rise to residual effects on the following day; repeated doses tend to be cumulative.

Loprazolam p. 508, lormetazepam p. 508, and temazepam act for a shorter time and they have little or no hangover effect. Withdrawal phenomena are more common with the short-acting benzodiazepines.

If insomnia is associated with daytime anxiety then the use of a long-acting benzodiazepine anxiolytic such as diazepam given as a single dose at night may effectively treat both symptoms.

Zolpidem, and zopiclone

Zolpidem tartrate p. 511 and zopiclone p. 512 are non-benzodiazepine hypnotics (sometimes referred to as Z-drugs), but they act at the benzodiazepine receptor. They are not licensed for long-term use; dependence has been reported in a small number of patients. Both zolpidem tartrate and zopiclone have a short duration of action.

Chloral and derivatives

There is no convincing evidence that they are particularly useful in the elderly and their role as hypnotics is now very limited.

Clomethiazole

Clomethiazole p. 510 may be a useful hypnotic for elderly patients because of its freedom from hangover but, as with all hypnotics, routine administration is undesirable and dependence occurs.

Antihistamines

Some **antihistamines** such as promethazine hydrochloride p. 302 are on sale to the public for occasional insomnia; their prolonged duration of action can often cause drowsiness the following day. The sedative effect of antihistamines may diminish after a few days of continued treatment; antihistamines are associated with headache, psychomotor impairment and antimuscarinic effects.

Alcohol

Alcohol is a poor hypnotic because the diuretic action interferes with sleep during the latter part of the night. Alcohol also disturbs sleep patterns, and so can worsen sleep disorders.

Melatonin

Melatonin p. 510 is a pineal hormone; it is licensed for the short-term treatment of insomnia in adults over 55 years; and for the short-term treatment of jet-lag in adults.

Anxiolytics

Benzodiazepine anxiolytics can be effective in alleviating anxiety states. Although these drugs are sometimes prescribed for stress-related symptoms, unhappiness, or minor physical disease, their use in such conditions is inappropriate. Benzodiazepine anxiolytics should not be used as sole treatment for chronic anxiety, and they are not appropriate for treating depression or chronic psychosis. In bereavement, psychological adjustment may be inhibited by benzodiazepines.

Anxiolytic benzodiazepine treatment should be limited to the lowest possible dose for the shortest possible time. Dependence is particularly likely in patients with a history of alcohol or drug abuse and in patients with marked personality disorders.

Some antidepressant drugs are licensed for use in anxiety and related disorders. Some antipsychotic drugs, in low doses, are also sometimes used in severe anxiety for their sedative action, but long-term use should be avoided because of the risk of adverse effects. The use of antihistamines (e.g. hydroxyzine hydrochloride p. 300) for their sedative effect in anxiety is not appropriate.

Beta-adrenoceptor blocking drugs do not affect psychological symptoms of anxiety, such as worry, tension, and fear, but they do reduce autonomic symptoms, such as palpitation and tremor; they do not reduce non-autonomic symptoms, such as muscle tension. Beta-blockers are therefore indicated for patients with predominantly somatic symptoms; this, in turn, may prevent the onset of worry and fear.

Benzodiazepines

Benzodiazepines are indicated for the *short-term relief of severe anxiety*; long-term use should be avoided. Diazepam, alprazolam p. 361, chlordiazepoxide hydrochloride p. 362, and clobazam p. 355 have a sustained action. Shorter-acting compounds such as lorazepam p. 357 and oxazepam p. 364 may be preferred in patients with hepatic impairment but they carry a greater risk of withdrawal symptoms.

In *panic disorders* (with or without agoraphobia) resistant to antidepressant therapy, a benzodiazepine may be used; alternatively, a benzodiazepine may be used as short-term adjunctive therapy at the start of antidepressant treatment to prevent the initial worsening of symptoms.

Diazepam or lorazepam are very occasionally administered intravenously for the *control of panic attacks*. This route is the most rapid but the procedure is not without risk and should be used only when alternative measures have failed. The intramuscular route has no advantage over the oral route.

Buspirone

Buspirone hydrochloride p. 360 is thought to act at specific serotonin (5HT$_{1A}$) receptors. Response to treatment may take up to 2 weeks. It does not alleviate the symptoms of benzodiazepine withdrawal. Therefore a patient taking a benzodiazepine still needs to have the benzodiazepine withdrawn gradually; it is advisable to do this before starting buspirone hydrochloride. The dependence and abuse potential of buspirone hydrochloride is low; it is, however, licensed for short-term use only (but specialists occasionally use it for several months).

Meprobamate

Meprobamate p. 365 is **less effective** than the benzodiazepines, more hazardous in overdosage, and can also induce dependence. It is **not** recommended.

Barbiturates

The intermediate-acting **barbiturates** have a place only in the treatment of severe intractable insomnia in patients **already taking** barbiturates; they should be **avoided** in the elderly. Intermediate-acting barbiturate preparations containing amobarbital sodium, butobarbital, and secobarbital sodium are available on a named patient basis.

The long-acting barbiturate phenobarbital is still sometimes of value in epilepsy but its use as a sedative is unjustified.

The very short-acting barbiturate thiopental sodium p. 356 is used in anaesthesia.

Increased hostility and aggression after barbiturates and alcohol usually indicates intoxication.

HYPNOTICS, SEDATIVES AND ANXIOLYTICS > BENZODIAZEPINES

↑361

Flurazepam

21-Oct-2019

● **INDICATIONS AND DOSE**

Insomnia (short-term use)

▸ BY MOUTH
  ▹ Adult: 15–30 mg once daily, dose to be taken at bedtime, for debilitated patients, use elderly dose
  ▹ Elderly: 15 mg once daily, dose to be taken at bedtime

● CONTRA-INDICATIONS Respiratory depression

● CAUTIONS Acute porphyrias p. 1107 · hypoalbuminaemia · muscle weakness

CAUTIONS, FURTHER INFORMATION
▸ Paradoxical effects A paradoxical increase in hostility and aggression may be reported by patients taking benzodiazepines. The effects range from talkativeness and excitement to aggressive and antisocial acts. Adjustment of the dose (up or down) sometimes attenuates the impulses. Increased anxiety and perceptual disorders are other paradoxical effects.

● INTERACTIONS → Appendix 1: benzodiazepines

● SIDE-EFFECTS
▸ **Common or very common** Taste altered
▸ **Rare or very rare** Abdominal discomfort · skin eruption
▸ **Frequency not known** Agranulocytosis · extrapyramidal symptoms · leucopenia · pancytopenia · suicide attempt · thrombocytopenia

● BREAST FEEDING Benzodiazepines are present in milk, and should be avoided if possible during breast-feeding.

4

Nervous system

- **HEPATIC IMPAIRMENT**
  Dose adjustments Manufacturer advises dose of 15 mg in mild to moderate impairment.
- **RENAL IMPAIRMENT**
  Dose adjustments Start with small doses in severe impairment.
- **NATIONAL FUNDING/ACCESS DECISIONS**
  NHS restrictions Flurazepam capsules are not prescribable in NHS primary care.
- **MEDICINAL FORMS** There can be variation in the licensing of different medicines containing the same drug.
  Capsule
  CAUTIONARY AND ADVISORY LABELS 19
  ▸ Dalmane (Mylan)
  Flurazepam (as Flurazepam hydrochloride) 15 mg Dalmane 15mg capsules | 30 capsule [PoM] £6.73 [CD4-1]
  Flurazepam (as Flurazepam hydrochloride) 30 mg Dalmane 30mg capsules | 30 capsule [PoM] £8.63 [CD4-1]

F 361

Loprazolam

05-Nov-2019

- **INDICATIONS AND DOSE**

Insomnia (short-term use)
▸ BY MOUTH
▸ Adult: 1 mg once daily, then increased to 1.5–2 mg once daily if required, dose to be taken at bedtime, for debilitated patients, use elderly dose
▸ Elderly: 0.5–1 mg once daily, dose to be taken at bedtime

- **CONTRA-INDICATIONS** Respiratory depression
- **CAUTIONS** Acute porphyrias p. 1107 · hypoalbuminaemia · muscle weakness
  CAUTIONS, FURTHER INFORMATION
  ▸ Paradoxical effects A paradoxical increase in hostility and aggression may be reported by patients taking benzodiazepines. The effects range from talkativeness and excitement to aggressive and antisocial acts. Adjustment of the dose (up or down) sometimes attenuates the impulses. Increased anxiety and perceptual disorders are other paradoxical effects.
- **INTERACTIONS** → Appendix 1: benzodiazepines
- **SIDE-EFFECTS** Adjustment disorder · cognitive disorder · muscle tone decreased · speech disorder
- **BREAST FEEDING** Benzodiazepines are present in milk, and should be avoided if possible during breast-feeding.
- **RENAL IMPAIRMENT**
  Dose adjustments Start with small doses in severe impairment.
- **MEDICINAL FORMS** There can be variation in the licensing of different medicines containing the same drug.
  Tablet
  CAUTIONARY AND ADVISORY LABELS 19
  ▸ Loprazolam (Non-proprietary)
  Loprazolam (as Loprazolam mesilate) 1 mg Loprazolam 1mg tablets | 28 tablet [PoM] £27.00 DT = £22.50 [CD4-1]

F 361

Lormetazepam

21-Oct-2019

- **INDICATIONS AND DOSE**

Insomnia (short-term use)
▸ BY MOUTH
▸ Adult: 0.5–1.5 mg once daily, dose to be taken at bedtime, for debilitated patients, use elderly dose
▸ Elderly: 500 micrograms once daily, dose to be taken at bedtime

- **CONTRA-INDICATIONS** Not for use alone to treat insomnia associated with depression · respiratory depression
- **CAUTIONS** Acute porphyrias p. 1107 · hypoalbuminaemia · muscle weakness
  CAUTIONS, FURTHER INFORMATION
  ▸ Paradoxical effects A paradoxical increase in hostility and aggression may be reported by patients taking benzodiazepines. The effects range from talkativeness and excitement to aggressive and antisocial acts. Adjustment of the dose (up or down) sometimes attenuates the impulses. Increased anxiety and perceptual disorders are other paradoxical effects.
- **INTERACTIONS** → Appendix 1: benzodiazepines
- **SIDE-EFFECTS**
  ▸ **Common or very common** Asthenia
  ▸ **Rare or very rare** Agranulocytosis · allergic dermatitis · apnoea · appetite change · coma · constipation · disinhibition · extrapyramidal symptoms · hyponatraemia · hypothermia · leucopenia · memory loss · obstructive pulmonary disease exacerbated · pancytopenia · saliva altered · sexual dysfunction · SIADH · speech slurred · thrombocytopenia
  ▸ **Frequency not known** Suicide attempt
- **BREAST FEEDING** Benzodiazepines are present in milk, and should be avoided if possible during breast-feeding.
- **RENAL IMPAIRMENT**
  Dose adjustments Start with small doses in severe impairment.
- **MEDICINAL FORMS** There can be variation in the licensing of different medicines containing the same drug. Forms available from special-order manufacturers include: oral suspension
  Tablet
  CAUTIONARY AND ADVISORY LABELS 19
  ▸ Lormetazepam (Non-proprietary)
  Lormetazepam 500 microgram Lormetazepam 500microgram tablets | 30 tablet [PoM] £64.17 DT = £18.94 [CD4-1]
  Lormetazepam 1 mg Lormetazepam 1mg tablets | 30 tablet [PoM] £17.77 DT = £17.77 [CD4-1]

F 361

Nitrazepam

05-Nov-2019

- **INDICATIONS AND DOSE**

Insomnia (short-term use)
▸ BY MOUTH
▸ Adult: 5–10 mg daily, dose to be taken at bedtime, for debilitated patients, use elderly dose
▸ Elderly: 2.5–5 mg daily, dose to be taken at bedtime

- **CONTRA-INDICATIONS** Chronic psychosis · respiratory depression
- **CAUTIONS** Acute porphyrias p. 1107 · hypoalbuminaemia · muscle weakness
  CAUTIONS, FURTHER INFORMATION
  ▸ Paradoxical effects A paradoxical increase in hostility and aggression may be reported by patients taking benzodiazepines. The effects range from talkativeness and excitement to aggressive and antisocial acts. Adjustment of the dose (up or down) sometimes attenuates the impulses. Increased anxiety and perceptual disorders are other paradoxical effects.
- **INTERACTIONS** → Appendix 1: benzodiazepines
- **SIDE-EFFECTS**
  ▸ **Common or very common** Movement disorders
  ▸ **Uncommon** Concentration impaired
  ▸ **Rare or very rare** Abdominal distress · muscle cramps · psychiatric disorder · skin reactions · Stevens-Johnson syndrome
  ▸ **Frequency not known** Drug abuse

- **BREAST FEEDING** Benzodiazepines are present in milk, and should be avoided if possible during breast-feeding.
- **RENAL IMPAIRMENT**
  Dose adjustments Start with small doses in severe impairment.

- **MEDICINAL FORMS** There can be variation in the licensing of different medicines containing the same drug. Forms available from special-order manufacturers include: oral suspension

Oral suspension
CAUTIONARY AND ADVISORY LABELS 19
▸ Nitrazepam (Non-proprietary)
  Nitrazepam 500 microgram per 1 ml Nitrazepam 2.5mg/5ml oral suspension | 70 ml [PoM] £114.00 DT = £114.00 [CD4-1]

Tablet
CAUTIONARY AND ADVISORY LABELS 19
▸ Nitrazepam (Non-proprietary)
  Nitrazepam 5 mg Nitrazepam 5mg tablets | 28 tablet [PoM] £7.22 DT = £3.43 [CD4-1]
▸ Mogadon (Mylan)
  Nitrazepam 5 mg Mogadon 5mg tablets | 30 tablet [PoM] £5.76 [CD4-1]

━━━━━━━━━━━━━━━━━━━━━━━━ ⚑ 361

Temazepam
21-Oct-2019

- **INDICATIONS AND DOSE**

Insomnia (short-term use)
▸ BY MOUTH
  ▸ Adult: 10–20 mg once daily, alternatively 30–40 mg once daily, higher dose range only to be administered in exceptional circumstances, dose to be taken at bedtime, for debilitated patients, use elderly dose
  ▸ Elderly: 10 mg once daily, alternatively 20 mg once daily, higher dose only to be administered in exceptional circumstances, dose to be taken at bedtime

Conscious sedation for dental procedures
▸ BY MOUTH
  ▸ Adult: 15–30 mg, to be administered 30–60 minutes before procedure

Premedication before surgery or investigatory procedures
▸ BY MOUTH
  ▸ Adult: 10–20 mg, to be taken 1–2 hours before procedure, alternatively 30 mg, to be taken 1–2 hours before procedure, higher alternate dose only administered in exceptional circumstances
  ▸ Elderly: 10 mg, to be taken 1–2 hours before procedure, alternatively 20 mg, to be taken 1–2 hours before procedure, higher alternate dose only administered in exceptional circumstances

- **UNLICENSED USE** Temazepam doses in BNF may differ from those in product literature.
  Not licensed for conscious sedation for dental procedures.
- **CONTRA-INDICATIONS** Chronic psychosis · CNS depression · compromised airway · respiratory depression
- **CAUTIONS** Hypoalbuminaemia · muscle weakness · organic brain changes
  CAUTIONS, FURTHER INFORMATION
  ▸ Paradoxical effects A paradoxical increase in hostility and aggression may be reported by patients taking benzodiazepines. The effects range from talkativeness and excitement to aggressive and antisocial acts. Adjustment of the dose (up or down) sometimes attenuates the impulses. Increased anxiety and perceptual disorders are other paradoxical effects.
- **INTERACTIONS** → Appendix 1: benzodiazepines
- **SIDE-EFFECTS** Drug abuse · dry mouth · hypersalivation · speech slurred
- **BREAST FEEDING** Benzodiazepines are present in milk, and should be avoided if possible during breast-feeding.

- **HEPATIC IMPAIRMENT**
  Dose adjustments
  ▸ When used for insomnia Manufacturer advises initiate at 5 mg once daily, increase to 10 mg or 20 mg once daily in extreme cases. Dose to be taken at bedtime.
- **RENAL IMPAIRMENT**
  Dose adjustments Start with small doses in severe impairment.
- **PATIENT AND CARER ADVICE**
  Driving and skilled tasks Patients given sedatives and analgesics during minor outpatient procedures should be very carefully warned about the risks of undertaking skilled tasks (e.g. driving) afterwards. Responsible persons should be available to take patients home afterwards. The dangers of taking **alcohol** should be emphasised.
- **PROFESSION SPECIFIC INFORMATION**
  Dental practitioners' formulary
  Temazepam Tablets and Oral Solution may be prescribed.
- **MEDICINAL FORMS** There can be variation in the licensing of different medicines containing the same drug. Forms available from special-order manufacturers include: oral suspension, oral solution

Oral solution
CAUTIONARY AND ADVISORY LABELS 19
▸ Temazepam (Non-proprietary)
  Temazepam 2 mg per 1 ml Temazepam 10mg/5ml oral solution sugar free sugar-free | 300 ml [PoM] £183.28 DT = £183.28 [CD3]

Tablet
CAUTIONARY AND ADVISORY LABELS 19
▸ Temazepam (Non-proprietary)
  Temazepam 10 mg Temazepam 10mg tablets | 28 tablet [PoM] £35.00 DT = £1.69 [CD3] | 500 tablet [PoM] £30.18 [CD3]
  Temazepam 20 mg Temazepam 20mg tablets | 28 tablet [PoM] £35.00 DT = £1.65 [CD3] | 250 tablet [PoM] £14.73–£307.94 [CD3]

HYPNOTICS, SEDATIVES AND ANXIOLYTICS ›
NON-BENZODIAZEPINE HYPNOTICS AND SEDATIVES

Chloral hydrate
23-Jul-2020

- **INDICATIONS AND DOSE**

Insomnia (short-term use), using chloral hydrate 143.3 mg/5 mL oral solution
▸ BY MOUTH USING ORAL SOLUTION
  ▸ Adult: 430–860 mg once daily (max. per dose 2 g), dose to be taken with water or milk at bedtime

Insomnia (short-term use), using chloral betaine 707 mg (≡ 414 mg chloral hydrate) tablets
▸ BY MOUTH USING TABLETS
  ▸ Adult: 1–2 tablets, alternatively 414–828 mg once daily, dose to be taken with water or milk at bedtime; maximum 4 tablets per day; maximum 2 g per day

- **CONTRA-INDICATIONS** Acute porphyrias p. 1107 · gastritis · severe cardiac disease
- **CAUTIONS** Avoid contact with mucous membranes · avoid contact with skin · avoid prolonged use (and abrupt withdrawal thereafter) · reduce dose in frail elderly
- **INTERACTIONS** → Appendix 1: chloral hydrate
- **SIDE-EFFECTS** Agitation · allergic dermatitis · ataxia · confusion · delirium (more common on abrupt discontinuation) · drug use disorders · gastrointestinal discomfort · gastrointestinal disorders · headache · injury · ketonuria · kidney injury
- **PREGNANCY** Avoid.
- **BREAST FEEDING** Risk of sedation in infant—avoid.
- **HEPATIC IMPAIRMENT** Manufacturer advises avoid in marked impairment.
  Dose adjustments Manufacturer advises consider dose reduction in the elderly with hepatic impairment.

4

Nervous system

- RENAL IMPAIRMENT Avoid in severe impairment.
- DIRECTIONS FOR ADMINISTRATION For administration *by mouth*, expert sources advise dilute liquid with plenty of water or juice to mask unpleasant taste.
- PRESCRIBING AND DISPENSING INFORMATION Flavours of oral liquid formulations may include black currant.
- PATIENT AND CARER ADVICE
  Driving and skilled tasks Drowsiness may persist the next day and affect performance of skilled tasks (e.g. driving); effects of alcohol enhanced.
- LESS SUITABLE FOR PRESCRIBING Chloral hydrate is less suitable for prescribing in insomnia.

- MEDICINAL FORMS There can be variation in the licensing of different medicines containing the same drug. Forms available from special-order manufacturers include: oral suspension, oral solution, suppository, enema

  Tablet
  CAUTIONARY AND ADVISORY LABELS 19, 27
  ▸ Chloral hydrate (Non-proprietary)
    Cloral betaine 707 mg Cloral betaine 707mg tablets | 30 tablet [PoM] [⚠] DT = £138.59

  Oral solution
  CAUTIONARY AND ADVISORY LABELS 1(paediatric solution only), 19 (solution other than paediatric only), 27
  ▸ Chloral hydrate (Non-proprietary)
    Chloral hydrate 28.66 mg per 1 ml Chloral hydrate 143.3mg/5ml oral solution BP | 150 ml [PoM] £244.25 DT = £244.25

Clomethiazole

04-Sep-2020

(Chlormethiazole)

- INDICATIONS AND DOSE

Severe insomnia (short-term use)
▸ BY MOUTH USING CAPSULES
▸ Elderly: 192–384 mg once daily, dose to be taken at bedtime
▸ BY MOUTH USING ORAL SOLUTION
▸ Elderly: 5–10 mL once daily, dose to be taken at bedtime

Restlessness and agitation
▸ BY MOUTH USING CAPSULES
▸ Elderly: 192 mg 3 times a day
▸ BY MOUTH USING ORAL SOLUTION
▸ Elderly: 5 mL 3 times a day

Alcohol withdrawal
▸ BY MOUTH USING CAPSULES
▸ Adult: Initially 2–4 capsules, to be repeated if necessary after some hours. 9–12 capsules daily in 3–4 divided doses on day 1 (first 24 hours), then 6–8 capsules daily in 3–4 divided doses on day 2, then 4–6 capsules daily in 3–4 divided doses on day 3, dose then to be gradually reduced over days 4–6, total duration of treatment for no more than 9 days
▸ BY MOUTH USING ORAL SOLUTION
▸ Adult: Initially 10–20 mL, to be repeated if necessary after some hours, then 45–60 mL daily in 3–4 divided doses on day 1 (first 24 hours), then 30–40 mL daily in 3–4 divided doses on day 2, then 20–30 mL daily in 3–4 divided doses on day 3, dose then to be gradually reduced over days 4–6, total duration of treatment for no more than 9 days

- CONTRA-INDICATIONS Acute pulmonary insufficiency · alcohol-dependent patients who continue to drink
- CAUTIONS Avoid prolonged use (and abrupt withdrawal thereafter) · cardiac disease (confusional state may indicate hypoxia) · chronic pulmonary insufficiency · elderly · excessive sedation may occur (particularly with higher doses) · history of drug abuse · marked personality

disorder · respiratory disease (confusional state may indicate hypoxia) · sleep apnoea syndrome
- INTERACTIONS → Appendix 1: clomethiazole
- SIDE-EFFECTS Agitation · bronchial secretion increased · confusion · conjunctival irritation · drug dependence · excessive sedation · gastrointestinal disorder · hangover · nasal complaints · skin reactions · upper airway secretion increased
- PREGNANCY Avoid if possible—especially during the first and third trimesters.
- BREAST FEEDING Use only if benefit outweighs risk—present in breast milk but effects unknown.
- HEPATIC IMPAIRMENT Manufacturer advises caution in moderate to severe impairment (risk of increased exposure).
  Dose adjustments Manufacturer advises consider dose reduction in moderate hepatic disorders associated with alcoholism.
- RENAL IMPAIRMENT Increased cerebral sensitivity.
  Dose adjustments Start with small doses in severe impairment.
- PATIENT AND CARER ADVICE
  Driving and skilled tasks Drowsiness may persist the next day and affect performance of skilled tasks (e.g. driving); effects of alcohol enhanced.

- MEDICINAL FORMS There can be variation in the licensing of different medicines containing the same drug.

  Oral solution
  CAUTIONARY AND ADVISORY LABELS 19
  EXCIPIENTS: May contain Alcohol
  ▸ Clomethiazole (Non-proprietary)
    Clomethiazole (as Clomethiazole edisilate) 50 mg per 1 ml Clomethiazole 31.5mg/ml oral solution sugar free sugar-free | 300 ml [PoM] £30.00 DT = £30.00

  Capsule
  CAUTIONARY AND ADVISORY LABELS 19
  ▸ Clomethiazole (Non-proprietary)
    Clomethiazole 192 mg Clomethiazole 192mg capsules | 60 capsule [PoM] £32.80 DT = £32.80

Melatonin

02-Nov-2020

- INDICATIONS AND DOSE

Insomnia [short-term use]
▸ BY MOUTH USING MODIFIED-RELEASE TABLETS
▸ Adult 55 years and over: 2 mg once daily for up to 13 weeks, dose to be taken 1–2 hours before bedtime

Jet lag [short-term use]
▸ BY MOUTH USING IMMEDIATE-RELEASE MEDICINES
▸ Adult: 3 mg once daily, increased if necessary to 6 mg once daily for up to 5 days, the first dose should be taken at the habitual bedtime after arrival at destination. Doses should not be taken before 8pm or after 4am. Maximum of 16 treatment courses per year

Insomnia in patients with learning disabilities [where sleep hygiene measures have been insufficient] (initiated under specialist supervision)
▸ BY MOUTH USING MODIFIED-RELEASE TABLETS
▸ Adult: Initially 2 mg once daily, increased if necessary to 4–6 mg once daily, dose to be taken 30–60 minutes before bedtime; maximum 10 mg per day

PHARMACOKINETICS
▸ The intake of food with *immediate-release* melatonin may increase the bioavailability of melatonin

- UNLICENSED USE [EvGr] Melatonin is used for insomnia in patients with learning disabilities, [Ⓔ] but is not licensed for this indication.

- CAUTIONS Autoimmune disease (manufacturer advises avoid—no information available)
- INTERACTIONS → Appendix 1: melatonin
- SIDE-EFFECTS
- ▶ **Common or very common** Arthralgia · headaches · increased risk of infection · pain
- ▶ **Uncommon** Anxiety · asthenia · chest pain · dizziness · drowsiness · dry mouth · gastrointestinal discomfort · hyperbilirubinaemia · hypertension · menopausal symptoms · mood altered · movement disorders · nausea · night sweats · oral disorders · skin reactions · sleep disorders · urine abnormalities · weight increased
- ▶ **Rare or very rare** Aggression · angina pectoris · arthritis · concentration impaired · crying · depression · disorientation · electrolyte imbalance · excessive tearing · gastrointestinal disorders · haematuria · hot flush · hypertriglyceridaemia · leucopenia · memory loss · muscle complaints · nail disorder · palpitations · paraesthesia · partial complex seizure · prostatitis · sexual dysfunction · syncope · thirst · thrombocytopenia · urinary disorders · vertigo · vision disorders · vomiting
- ▶ **Frequency not known** Angioedema · galactorrhoea · hyperglycaemia
- PREGNANCY No information available—avoid.
- BREAST FEEDING Present in milk—avoid.
- HEPATIC IMPAIRMENT Manufacturer advises avoid (risk of decreased clearance; limited information available).
- RENAL IMPAIRMENT No information available—use with caution.
- DIRECTIONS FOR ADMINISTRATION Manufacturers advise that modified-release tablets should be taken with or after food. Licensed immediate-release formulations should be taken on an empty stomach, 2 hours before or 2 hours after food—intake with carbohydrate-rich meals may impair blood glucose control.

- MEDICINAL FORMS There can be variation in the licensing of different medicines containing the same drug. Forms available from special-order manufacturers include: tablet, modified-release tablet, oral solution

Modified-release tablet
CAUTIONARY AND ADVISORY LABELS 2, 21, 25
▶ Melatonin (Non-proprietary)
  Melatonin 2 mg Melatonin 2mg modified-release tablets | 30 tablet PoM £15.39 DT = £15.39
  Melatonin 3 mg Melatonin 3mg modified-release tablets | 120 tablet PoM ⓢ
▶ Circadin (Flynn Pharma Ltd)
  Melatonin 2 mg Circadin 2mg modified-release tablets | 30 tablet PoM £15.39 DT = £15.39
▶ Slenyto (Flynn Pharma Ltd)
  Melatonin 1 mg Slenyto 1mg modified-release tablets | 60 tablet PoM £41.20 DT = £41.20
  Melatonin 5 mg Slenyto 5mg modified-release tablets | 30 tablet PoM £103.00 DT = £103.00

Tablet
CAUTIONARY AND ADVISORY LABELS 2, 25
▶ Melatonin (Non-proprietary)
  Melatonin 1 mg Melatonin 1mg tablets | 90 tablet PoM ⓢ
  Melatonin 3 mg Melatonin 3mg tablets | 30 tablet PoM £65.00 DT = £29.75
  Melatonin 5 mg Melatonin Extra Strength 5mg tablets | 60 tablet PoM ⓢ
▶ VesPro Melatonin (Imported (United States))
  Melatonin 500 microgram VesPro Melatonin 500microgram tablets | 1000 tablet PoM ⓢ

Oral solution
CAUTIONARY AND ADVISORY LABELS 2
EXCIPIENTS: May contain Ethanol, propylene glycol, sorbitol
▶ Melatonin (Non-proprietary)
  Melatonin 1 mg per 1 ml Melatonin 1mg/ml oral solution sugar free sugar-free | 150 ml PoM £130.00 DT = £130.00

Zolpidem tartrate
03-Sep-2020

- INDICATIONS AND DOSE
Insomnia (short-term use)
▶ BY MOUTH
  ▶ Adult: 10 mg daily for up to 4 weeks, dose to be taken at bedtime, for debilitated patients, use elderly dose
  ▶ Elderly: 5 mg daily for up to 4 weeks, dose to be taken at bedtime

- CONTRA-INDICATIONS Acute respiratory depression · marked neuromuscular respiratory weakness · myasthenia gravis · obstructive sleep apnoea · psychotic illness · severe respiratory depression
- CAUTIONS Avoid prolonged use (and abrupt withdrawal thereafter) · depression · elderly · history of alcohol abuse · history of drug abuse · muscle weakness
  CAUTIONS, FURTHER INFORMATION
  ▶ Elderly For hypnotic Z-drugs, prescription potentially inappropriate (STOPP criteria) in elderly (may cause protracted daytime sedation and/or ataxia).
    See also Prescribing in the elderly p. 33.
- INTERACTIONS → Appendix 1: zolpidem
- SIDE-EFFECTS
- ▶ **Common or very common** Abdominal pain · anterograde amnesia · anxiety · back pain · diarrhoea · dizziness · fatigue · hallucination · headache · increased risk of infection · nausea · sleep disorders · vomiting
- ▶ **Uncommon** Confusion · diplopia · irritability
- ▶ **Frequency not known** Angioedema · behaviour abnormal · concentration impaired · delusions · depression · drug dependence · fall · gait abnormal · hepatic disorders · hyperhidrosis · level of consciousness decreased · libido disorder · muscle weakness · psychosis · respiratory depression · skin reactions · speech disorder · withdrawal syndrome
- PREGNANCY Avoid regular use (risk of neonatal withdrawal symptoms); high doses during late pregnancy or labour may cause neonatal hypothermia, hypotonia, and respiratory depression.
- BREAST FEEDING Small amounts present in milk—avoid.
- HEPATIC IMPAIRMENT Manufacturer advises caution in mild to moderate impairment (risk of decreased clearance); avoid in severe impairment.
  Dose adjustments Manufacturer advises initial dose reduction to 5 mg daily in mild to moderate impairment.
- RENAL IMPAIRMENT Use with caution.
- PATIENT AND CARER ADVICE
  Driving and skilled tasks Drowsiness may persist the next day—leave at least 8 hours between taking zolpidem and performing skilled tasks (e.g. driving, or operating machinery); effects of alcohol and other CNS depressants enhanced.
- NATIONAL FUNDING/ACCESS DECISIONS
  For full details see funding body website
  NICE decisions
  ▶ Guidance on the use of zaleplon, zolpidem, and zopiclone for the short-term management of insomnia (April 2004)
  NICE TA77 Recommended

- MEDICINAL FORMS There can be variation in the licensing of different medicines containing the same drug.
  Tablet
  CAUTIONARY AND ADVISORY LABELS 19
  ▶ Zolpidem tartrate (Non-proprietary)
    Zolpidem tartrate 5 mg Zolpidem 5mg tablets | 28 tablet PoM £3.08 DT = £1.95 CD4-1
    Zolpidem tartrate 10 mg Zolpidem 10mg tablets | 28 tablet PoM £4.48 DT = £1.52 CD4-1

4

Nervous system

4

Nervous system

▸ Stilnoct (Sanofi)
Zolpidem tartrate 10 mg Stilnoct 10mg tablets | 28 tablet [PoM]
£1.00 DT = £1.52 [CD4-1]

Zopiclone

03-Sep-2020

● **INDICATIONS AND DOSE**

Insomnia (short-term use)
▸ BY MOUTH
▸ **Adult:** 7.5 mg once daily for up to 4 weeks, dose to be taken at bedtime
▸ **Elderly:** Initially 3.75 mg once daily for up to 4 weeks, dose to be taken at bedtime, increased if necessary to 7.5 mg daily

Insomnia (short-term use) in patients with chronic pulmonary insufficiency
▸ BY MOUTH
▸ **Adult:** Initially 3.75 mg once daily for up to 4 weeks, dose to be taken at bedtime, increased if necessary to 7.5 mg daily

● **CONTRA-INDICATIONS** Marked neuromuscular respiratory weakness · myasthenia gravis · respiratory failure · severe sleep apnoea syndrome

● **CAUTIONS** Avoid prolonged use (risk of tolerance and withdrawal symptoms) · chronic pulmonary insufficiency (increased risk of respiratory depression) · depression · elderly · history of alcohol abuse · history of drug abuse · muscle weakness · psychiatric illness

CAUTIONS, FURTHER INFORMATION
▸ **Elderly** For hypnotic Z-drugs, prescription potentially inappropriate (STOPP criteria) in elderly (may cause protracted daytime sedation and /or ataxia).
See also Prescribing in the elderly p. 33.

● **INTERACTIONS** → Appendix 1: zopiclone

● **SIDE-EFFECTS**
▸ **Common or very common** Dry mouth · taste bitter
▸ **Uncommon** Anxiety · dizziness · fatigue · headache · nausea · sleep disorders · vomiting
▸ **Rare or very rare** Behaviour abnormal · confusion · dyspnoea · fall · hallucination · irritability · libido disorder · memory impairment · skin reactions
▸ **Frequency not known** Cognitive disorder · concentration impaired · delusions · depressed mood · diplopia · drug dependence · dyspepsia · movement disorders · muscle weakness · paraesthesia · respiratory depression · speech disorder · withdrawal syndrome

● **PREGNANCY** Not recommended (risk of neonatal withdrawal symptoms). Use during late pregnancy or labour may cause neonatal hypothermia, hypotonia, and respiratory depression.

● **BREAST FEEDING** Present in milk—avoid.

● **HEPATIC IMPAIRMENT** Manufacturer advises caution in mild to moderate impairment; avoid in severe impairment (risk of decreased elimination).
Dose adjustments Manufacturer advises dose reduction to 3.75 mg in mild to moderate impairment, dose can be increased with caution if necessary.

● **RENAL IMPAIRMENT** Increased cerebral sensitivity.
Dose adjustments Start with reduced dose of 3.75 mg.

● **PATIENT AND CARER ADVICE**
Driving and skilled tasks Drowsiness may persist the next day and affect performance of skilled tasks (e.g. driving); effects of alcohol enhanced.

● **NATIONAL FUNDING/ACCESS DECISIONS**
For full details see funding body website

NICE decisions
▸ **Guidance on the use of zaleplon, zolpidem and zopiclone for the short-term management of insomnia (April 2004)**
NICE TA77 Recommended

● **MEDICINAL FORMS** There can be variation in the licensing of different medicines containing the same drug. Forms available from special-order manufacturers include: oral suspension, oral solution

Tablet
CAUTIONARY AND ADVISORY LABELS 19, 25
▸ Zopiclone (Non-proprietary)
Zopiclone 3.75 mg Zopiclone 3.75mg tablets | 28 tablet [PoM] £2.49 DT = £1.20 [CD4-1]
Zopiclone 7.5 mg Zopiclone 7.5mg tablets | 28 tablet [PoM] £3.75 DT = £1.19 [CD4-1]
▸ Zimovane (Sanofi)
Zopiclone 3.75 mg Zimovane LS 3.75mg tablets | 28 tablet [PoM] £2.24 DT = £1.20 [CD4-1]
Zopiclone 7.5 mg Zimovane 7.5mg tablets | 28 tablet [PoM] £3.26 DT = £1.19 [CD4-1]

7.2 Narcolepsy

Other drugs used for Narcolepsy Dexamfetamine sulfate, p. 369 · Methylphenidate hydrochloride, p. 367

CENTRAL NERVOUS SYSTEM DEPRESSANTS

Sodium oxybate

23-Nov-2020

● **DRUG ACTION** A central nervous system depressant.

● **INDICATIONS AND DOSE**

Narcolepsy with cataplexy (under expert supervision)
▸ BY MOUTH
▸ **Adult:** Initially 2.25 g daily, dose to be taken on retiring and 2.25 g after 2.5–4 hours, then increased in steps of 1.5 g daily in 2 divided doses, dose adjusted according to response at intervals of 1–2 weeks; dose titration should be repeated if restarting after interval of more than 14 days, maximum 9 g daily in 2 divided doses

DOSE ADJUSTMENTS DUE TO INTERACTIONS
▸ Manufacturer advises reduce dose by 20 % with concurrent use of sodium valproate or valproic acid.

● **CONTRA-INDICATIONS** Major depression · succinic semi-aldehyde dehydrogenase deficiency

● **CAUTIONS** Body mass index of 40 kg/m^2 or greater (higher risk of sleep apnoea) · elderly · epilepsy · heart failure (high sodium content) · history of depression · history of drug abuse · hypertension (high sodium content) · respiratory disorders · risk of discontinuation effects including rebound cataplexy and withdrawal symptoms

● **INTERACTIONS** → Appendix 1: sodium oxybate

● **SIDE-EFFECTS**
▸ **Common or very common** Abdominal pain upper · anxiety · appetite abnormal · arthralgia · asthenia · back pain · concentration impaired · confusion · depression · diarrhoea · dizziness · dyspnoea · fall · feeling drunk · headache · hyperhidrosis · hypertension · increased risk of infection · movement disorders · muscle spasms · nasal congestion · nausea · palpitations · peripheral oedema · sedation · sensation abnormal · skin reactions · sleep disorders · sleep paralysis · snoring · taste altered · tremor · urinary disorders · vertigo · vision blurred · vomiting · weight decreased
▸ **Uncommon** Behaviour abnormal · faecal incontinence · hallucination · memory loss · psychosis · suicidal behaviours · thinking abnormal

▸ **Frequency not known** Angioedema · dehydration · delusions · dry mouth · homicidal ideation · loss of consciousness · mood altered · respiratory depression · seizure · sleep apnoea
● PREGNANCY Avoid.
● HEPATIC IMPAIRMENT Manufacturer advises caution (risk of increased exposure).
Dose adjustments Manufacturer advises initial dose reduction of 50%.
● RENAL IMPAIRMENT Caution—contains 3.96 mmol Na$^+$ per mL.
● DIRECTIONS FOR ADMINISTRATION Manufacturer advises dilute each dose with 60 mL water; prepare both doses before retiring. Observe the same time interval (2–3 hours) each night between the last meal and the first dose.
● PATIENT AND CARER ADVICE Patients or carers should be given advice on how to administer sodium oxybate oral solution.
Driving and skilled tasks Leave at least 6 hours between taking sodium oxybate and performing skilled tasks (e.g. driving or operating machinery); effects of alcohol and other CNS depressants enhanced.

● MEDICINAL FORMS There can be variation in the licensing of different medicines containing the same drug.
Oral solution
CAUTIONARY AND ADVISORY LABELS 13, 19
ELECTROLYTES: May contain Sodium
▸ Sodium oxybate (Non-proprietary)
Sodium oxybate 500 mg per 1 ml Sodium oxybate 500mg/ml oral solution sugar free sugar-free | 180 ml [PoM] £360.00 DT = £360.00 (Hospital only) [CD2]
▸ Xyrem (UCB Pharma Ltd)
Sodium oxybate 500 mg per 1 ml Xyrem 500mg/ml oral solution sugar-free | 180 ml [PoM] £360.00 DT = £360.00 (Hospital only) [CD2]

CNS STIMULANTS

Pitolisant
11-Apr-2017

● DRUG ACTION Pitolisant is a histamine H$_3$-receptor antagonist which enhances the activity of brain histaminergic neurons.

● INDICATIONS AND DOSE
Narcolepsy with or without cataplexy (initiated by a specialist)
▸ BY MOUTH
▸ Adult: Initially 9 mg once daily for 1 week, then increased if necessary to 18 mg once daily for 1 week, then increased if necessary to 36 mg once daily, dose to be taken in the morning with breakfast, dose can be decreased (down to 4.5 mg per day) or increased (up to 36 mg per day) according to response and tolerance

● CAUTIONS Acid-related gastric disorders · epilepsy · history of psychiatric disorders · severe anorexia · severe obesity
● INTERACTIONS → Appendix 1: pitolisant
● SIDE-EFFECTS
▸ **Common or very common** Anxiety · asthenia · depression · dizziness · gastrointestinal discomfort · headaches · mood altered · nausea · sleep disorders · tremor · vertigo · vomiting
▸ **Uncommon** Appetite abnormal · arrhythmias · arthralgia · blepharospasm · chest pain · concentration impaired · constipation · diarrhoea · drowsiness · dry mouth · epilepsy · feeling abnormal · fluid retention · gastrointestinal disorders · hallucinations · hot flush · hypertension · hypotension · malaise · metrorrhagia · movement disorders · muscle complaints · muscle weakness · oedema · on and off phenomenon · oral paraesthesia · pain · paraesthesia · QT interval prolongation · sexual dysfunction · skin

reactions · sweat changes · tinnitus · urinary frequency increased · visual acuity decreased · weight decreased (review treatment if significant) · weight increased (review treatment if significant) · yawning
▸ **Rare or very rare** Behaviour abnormal · cognitive impairment · confusion · loss of consciousness · memory loss · obsessive thoughts · photosensitivity reaction · sense of oppression · swallowing difficulty
● CONCEPTION AND CONTRACEPTION Manufacturer advises effective contraception in women of childbearing potential for at least 21 days after treatment discontinuation—pitolisant may reduce the effectiveness of hormonal contraceptives.
● PREGNANCY Manufacturer advises avoid unless potential benefit outweighs risk—toxicity in *animal* studies.
● BREAST FEEDING Manufacturer advises avoid—present in milk in *animal* studies.
● HEPATIC IMPAIRMENT Manufacturer advises caution in moderate impairment; avoid in severe impairment.
Dose adjustments Manufacturer advises consider dose increase two weeks after initiation in moderate impairment; maximum daily dose of 18 mg.
● RENAL IMPAIRMENT
Dose adjustments Manufacturer advises use with caution; maximum daily dose should not exceed 18 mg.

● MEDICINAL FORMS There can be variation in the licensing of different medicines containing the same drug.
Tablet
▸ Wakix (Lincoln Medical Ltd) ▼
Pitolisant (as Pitolisant hydrochloride) 4.5 mg Wakix 4.5mg tablets | 30 tablet [PoM] £310.00 DT = £310.00
Pitolisant (as Pitolisant hydrochloride) 18 mg Wakix 18mg tablets | 30 tablet [PoM] £310.00 DT = £310.00

CNS STIMULANTS 〉 CENTRALLY ACTING SYMPATHOMIMETICS

Modafinil
03-Dec-2020

● INDICATIONS AND DOSE
Excessive sleepiness associated with narcolepsy with or without cataplexy
▸ BY MOUTH
▸ Adult: Initially 200 mg daily in 2 divided doses, dose to be taken in the morning and at noon, alternatively initially 200 mg once daily, dose to be taken in the morning, adjusted according to response to 200–400 mg daily in 2 divided doses, alternatively adjusted according to response to 200–400 mg once daily
▸ Elderly: Initially 100 mg daily

IMPORTANT SAFETY INFORMATION
MHRA/CHM ADVICE (UPDATED NOVEMBER 2020): MODAFINIL (*PROVIGIL*®): INCREASED RISK OF CONGENITAL MALFORMATIONS IF USED DURING PREGNANCY
A European review and other safety data found that use of modafinil during pregnancy potentially increases the risk of congenital malformations such as heart defects, hypospadias, and orofacial clefts. Healthcare professionals are advised that modafinil should not be used during pregnancy; alternative treatment options should be considered, including behaviour modifying measures, sleep hygiene, and scheduled daytime naps. Modafinil may also reduce the effectiveness of some hormonal contraceptives, including oral contraceptives, therefore alternative or additional methods of contraception are required—see also *Interactions*. Females of childbearing potential should be advised on the use of contraception (see *Conception and*

Nervous system

4

contraception) and informed of the risk of congenital malformations.

- CONTRA-INDICATIONS Arrhythmia · history of clinically significant signs of CNS stimulant-induced mitral valve prolapse (including ischaemic ECG changes, chest pain and arrhythmias) · history of cor pulmonale · history of left ventricular hypertrophy · moderate to severe uncontrolled hypertension
- CAUTIONS History of alcohol abuse · history of depression · history of drug abuse · history of mania · history of psychosis · possibility of dependence
- INTERACTIONS → Appendix 1: modafinil
- SIDE-EFFECTS
  ▸ **Common or very common** Anxiety · appetite abnormal · arrhythmias · asthenia · chest pain · confusion · constipation · depression · diarrhoea · dizziness · drowsiness · dry mouth · gastrointestinal discomfort · headaches · mood altered · nausea · palpitations · sensation abnormal · sleep disorders · thinking abnormal · vasodilation · vision disorders
  ▸ **Uncommon** Allergic rhinitis · arthralgia · asthma · behaviour abnormal · central nervous system stimulation · cough aggravated · diabetes mellitus · dry eye · dysphagia · dyspnoea · eosinophilia · epistaxis · gastrointestinal disorders · hypercholesterolaemia · hyperglycaemia · hyperhidrosis · hypertension · hypotension · increased risk of infection · leucopenia · libido decreased · memory loss · menstrual disorder · movement disorders · muscle complaints · muscle tone increased · muscle weakness · oral disorders · pain · peripheral oedema · psychiatric disorders · skin reactions · speech disorder · suicidal ideation · taste altered · thirst · tremor · urinary frequency increased · urine abnormal · vertigo · vomiting · weight changes
  ▸ **Rare or very rare** Hallucination · psychosis
  ▸ **Frequency not known** Angioedema · delusions · fever · hypersensitivity · lymphadenopathy · severe cutaneous adverse reactions (SCARs)
  SIDE-EFFECTS, FURTHER INFORMATION Discontinue treatment if rash develops. Discontinue treatment if psychiatric symptoms develop.
- CONCEPTION AND CONTRACEPTION The MHRA advises females of childbearing potential should use effective contraception during treatment and for 2 months after last treatment—see also *Important safety information*.
- PREGNANCY Manufacturer advises avoid—increased risk of congenital malformations (see also *Important safety information*).
- BREAST FEEDING Avoid—present in milk in *animal* studies.
- HEPATIC IMPAIRMENT Manufacturer advises caution in severe impairment (risk of increased plasma concentrations).
  Dose adjustments Manufacturer advises dose reduction of 50% in severe impairment.
- RENAL IMPAIRMENT Use with caution—limited information available.
- PRE-TREATMENT SCREENING ECG required before initiation.
- MONITORING REQUIREMENTS Monitor blood pressure and heart rate in hypertensive patients.

- MEDICINAL FORMS There can be variation in the licensing of different medicines containing the same drug. Forms available from special-order manufacturers include: oral suspension, oral solution
  Tablet
  ▸ Modafinil (Non-proprietary)
  Modafinil 100 mg Modafinil 100mg tablets | 30 tablet [PoM] £105.21 DT = £3.31

Modafinil 200 mg Modafinil 200mg tablets | 30 tablet [PoM] £105.21 DT = £6.45
▸ Provigil (Teva UK Ltd)
Modafinil 100 mg Provigil 100mg tablets | 30 tablet [PoM] £52.60 DT = £3.31

Solriamfetol
09-Oct-2020

- DRUG ACTION Solriamfetol increases the levels of dopamine and noradrenaline in the brain by inhibiting re-uptake, thereby improving wakefulness.

● INDICATIONS AND DOSE

Excessive sleepiness associated with narcolepsy [with or without cataplexy] (initiated by a specialist)
▸ BY MOUTH
  ▸ Adult: 75 mg once daily, increased if necessary up to 150 mg once daily, dose to be taken upon awakening and not within 9 hours of bedtime, dose to be increased by doubling the dose after at least 3 days, according to response, in patients with severe symptoms, a starting dose of 150 mg once daily may be considered; maximum 150 mg per day

Excessive sleepiness associated with obstructive sleep apnoea (initiated by a specialist)
▸ BY MOUTH
  ▸ Adult: 37.5 mg once daily, increased if necessary up to 150 mg once daily, dose to be taken upon awakening and not within 9 hours of bedtime, dose to be increased by doubling the dose at intervals of at least 3 days, according to response; maximum 150 mg per day

- CONTRA-INDICATIONS Cardiac arrhythmias · hypertension (uncontrolled) · myocardial infarction (within the past year) · unstable angina pectoris
- CAUTIONS Elderly (limited information available—consider lower doses and close monitoring) · history of alcohol abuse · history of stimulant abuse · history of, or concurrent, psychosis or bipolar disorder (risk of exacerbation of psychiatric symptoms) · increased intra-ocular pressure (risk of mydriasis) · patients at risk of angle-closure glaucoma (risk of mydriasis) · patients at risk of major cardiovascular events
- INTERACTIONS → Appendix 1: solriamfetol
- SIDE-EFFECTS
  ▸ **Common or very common** Abdominal pain · anxiety · appetite decreased · chest discomfort · constipation · cough · diarrhoea · dizziness · dry mouth · feeling jittery · headache · hyperhidrosis · insomnia · irritability · nausea · palpitations · teeth grinding · vomiting
  ▸ **Uncommon** Concentration impaired · dyspnoea · hypertension · tachycardia · thirst · tremor · weight decreased
  ▸ **Frequency not known** Mydriasis
- CONCEPTION AND CONTRACEPTION Manufacturer advises females of childbearing potential or their male partners should use effective contraception during treatment.
- PREGNANCY Manufacturer advises avoid—toxicity in *animal* studies.
- BREAST FEEDING Specialist sources indicate use with caution—limited information available. Monitor breast-fed infants for adverse reactions such as agitation, insomnia, poor feeding, and reduced weight gain.
- RENAL IMPAIRMENT Manufacturer advises caution in moderate to severe impairment—increased risk of elevations in blood pressure and heart rate; avoid in end-stage renal disease.
  Dose adjustments Manufacturer advises a starting dose of 37.5 mg once daily, increased if necessary after 5 days to a maximum of 75 mg once daily, in moderate impairment; a

dose of 37.5 mg once daily should not be exceeded in severe impairment.

- MONITORING REQUIREMENTS Manufacturer advises assess blood pressure and heart rate before initiation and monitor periodically during treatment, including after dose increases; pre-existing hypertension should be controlled before starting treatment.

- PATIENT AND CARER ADVICE
Driving and skilled tasks Manufacturer advises patients and carers should be counselled on the effects on driving and performance of skilled tasks—increased risk of dizziness and attention disturbances.

    Patients should be frequently reassessed, and if appropriate, advised to avoid driving or any other potentially dangerous activity, especially at the start of treatment or when a dose is changed. Patients with abnormal levels of sleepiness should be advised that their level of wakefulness may not return to normal.

- MEDICINAL FORMS There can be variation in the licensing of different medicines containing the same drug.

Tablet
- Solriamfetol (non-proprietary) ▼
    Solriamfetol (as Solriamfetol hydrochloride) 75 mg Sunosi 75mg tablets | 28 tablet [PoM] £177.52 (Hospital only)
    Solriamfetol (as Solriamfetol hydrochloride) 150 mg Sunosi 150mg tablets | 28 tablet [PoM] £248.64 (Hospital only)

8   Substance dependence

Substance dependence   08-Apr-2018

Guidance on treatment of drug misuse

The UK health departments have produced guidance on the treatment of drug misuse in the UK. *Drug Misuse and Dependence: UK Guidelines on Clinical Management* (2017) is available at www.gov.uk/government/publications/drug-misuse-and-dependence-uk-guidelines-on-clinical-management.

Alcohol dependence

See Alcohol dependence p. 516.

Nicotine dependence

See Smoking cessation p. 519.

Opioid dependence

The management of opioid dependence requires medical, social, and psychological treatment; access to a multidisciplinary team is recommended. Treatment for opioid dependence should be initiated under the supervision of an appropriately qualified prescriber.

    Untreated heroin dependence shows early withdrawal symptoms within 8 hours, with peak symptoms at 36–72 hours; symptoms subside substantially after 5 days. Methadone hydrochloride p. 524 or buprenorphine p. 468 withdrawal occurs later, with longer-lasting symptoms.

Opioid substitution therapy

Methadone hydrochloride and buprenorphine are used as substitution therapy in opioid dependence. Substitute medication should be commenced with a short period of stabilisation, followed by either a withdrawal regimen or by maintenance treatment. Maintenance treatment enables patients to achieve stability, reduces drug use and crime, and improves health; it should be regularly reviewed to ensure the patient continues to derive benefit. The prescriber should monitor for signs of toxicity, and the patient should be told to be aware of warning signs of toxicity on initiation and during titration.

A withdrawal regimen after stabilisation with methadone hydrochloride or buprenorphine should be attempted only after careful consideration. Enforced withdrawal is ineffective for sustained abstinence, and it increases the risk of patients relapsing and subsequently overdosing because of loss of tolerance. Complete withdrawal from opioids usually takes up to 4 weeks in an inpatient or residential setting, and up to 12 weeks in a community setting. If abstinence is not achieved, illicit drug use is resumed, or the patient cannot tolerate withdrawal, the withdrawal regimen should be stopped and maintenance therapy should be resumed at the optimal dose. Following successful withdrawal treatment, further support and monitoring to maintain abstinence should be provided for a period of at least 6 months.

Missed doses
Patients who miss 3 days or more of their regular prescribed dose of opioid maintenance therapy are at risk of overdose because of loss of tolerance. Consider reducing the dose in these patients.

    If the patient misses 5 or more days of treatment, an assessment of illicit drug use is also recommended before restarting substitution therapy; this is particularly important for patients taking buprenorphine because of the risk of precipitated withdrawal.

Buprenorphine
Buprenorphine is preferred by some patients because it is less sedating than methadone hydrochloride; for this reason it may be more suitable for employed patients or those undertaking other skilled tasks such as driving. Buprenorphine is safer than methadone hydrochloride when used in conjunction with other sedating drugs, and has fewer drug interactions. Dose reductions may be easier than with methadone hydrochloride because the withdrawal symptoms are milder, and patients generally require fewer adjunctive medications; there is also a lower risk of overdose. Buprenorphine can be given on alternate days in higher doses and it requires a shorter drug-free period than methadone hydrochloride before induction with naltrexone hydrochloride p. 519 for prevention of relapse.

    Patients dependent on high doses of opioids may be at increased risk of precipitated withdrawal. Precipitated withdrawal can occur in any patient if buprenorphine is administered when other opioid agonist drugs are in circulation. Precipitated opioid withdrawal, if it occurs, starts within 1–3 hours of the first buprenorphine dose and peaks at around 6 hours. Non-opioid adjunctive therapy, such as lofexidine hydrochloride p. 526, may be required if symptoms are severe.

    To reduce the risk of precipitated withdrawal, the first dose of buprenorphine should be given when the patient is exhibiting signs of withdrawal, or 6–12 hours after the last use of heroin (or other short-acting opioid), or 24–48 hours after the last dose of methadone hydrochloride. It is possible to titrate the dose of buprenorphine within one week—more rapidly than with methadone hydrochloride therapy—but care is still needed to avoid toxicity or precipitated withdrawal; dividing the dose on the first day may be useful.

    A combination preparation containing buprenorphine with naloxone (*Suboxone®*) p. 525 can be prescribed for patients when there is a risk of dose diversion for parenteral administration; the naloxone hydrochloride p. 1424 component precipitates withdrawal if the preparation is injected, but it has little effect when the preparation is taken sublingually.

    Where there is a risk of diversion of opioid substitution medicines, or difficulties with adherence to daily supervised opioid substitution medication, buprenorphine prolonged-release injection may be an option.

Methadone
Methadone hydrochloride, a long-acting opioid agonist, is usually administered in a single daily dose as

methadone hydrochloride oral solution 1 mg/mL. Patients with a long history of opioid misuse, those who typically abuse a variety of sedative drugs and alcohol, and those who experience increased anxiety during withdrawal of opioids may prefer methadone hydrochloride to buprenorphine because it has a more pronounced sedative effect.

Methadone hydrochloride is initiated at least 8 hours after the last heroin dose, provided that there is objective evidence of withdrawal symptoms. A supplementary dose on the first day may be considered if there is evidence of persistent opioid withdrawal symptoms. Because of the long half-life, plasma concentrations progressively rise during initial treatment even if the patient remains on the same daily dose (it takes 3–10 days for plasma concentrations to reach steady-state in patients on a stable dose); a dose tolerated on the first day of treatment may become a toxic dose on the third day as cumulative toxicity develops. Thus, titration to the optimal dose in methadone hydrochloride maintenance treatment may take several weeks.

Opioid substitution during pregnancy
Acute withdrawal of opioids should be avoided in pregnancy because it can cause fetal death. Opioid substitution therapy is recommended during pregnancy because it carries a lower risk to the fetus than continued use of illicit drugs. If a woman who is stabilised on methadone hydrochloride or buprenorphine for treatment of opioid dependence becomes pregnant, therapy should be continued [buprenorphine is not licensed for use in pregnancy]. Many pregnant patients choose a withdrawal regimen, but withdrawal during the first trimester should be avoided because it is associated with an increased risk of spontaneous miscarriage. Withdrawal of methadone hydrochloride or buprenorphine should be undertaken gradually during the second trimester, with dose reductions made every 3–5 days. If illicit drug use occurs, the patient should be re-stabilised at the optimal maintenance dose and consideration should be given to stopping the withdrawal regimen.

Further withdrawal of methadone hydrochloride p. 524 or buprenorphine p. 468 in the third trimester is not recommended because maternal withdrawal, even if mild, is associated with fetal distress, stillbirth, and the risk of neonatal mortality. Drug metabolism can be increased in the third trimester; it may be necessary to either increase the dose of methadone hydrochloride or change to twice-daily consumption (or a combination of both strategies) to prevent withdrawal symptoms from developing.

The neonate should be monitored for respiratory depression and signs of withdrawal if the mother is prescribed high doses of opioid substitute.

Signs of neonatal withdrawal from opioids usually develop 24–72 hours after delivery but symptoms may be delayed for up to 14 days, so monitoring may be required for several weeks. Symptoms include a high-pitched cry, rapid breathing, hungry but ineffective suckling, and excessive wakefulness; severe, but rare symptoms include hypertonicity and convulsions.

Opioid substitution during breastfeeding
Doses of methadone and buprenorphine should be kept as low as possible in breast-feeding mothers. Increased sleepiness, breathing difficulties, or limpness in breast-fed babies of mothers taking opioid substitutes should be reported urgently to a healthcare professional.

Adjunctive therapy and symptomatic treatment
Adjunctive therapy may be required for the management of opioid withdrawal symptoms. Loperamide hydrochloride p. 72 may be used for the control of diarrhoea; mebeverine hydrochloride p. 94 for controlling stomach cramps; paracetamol p. 464 and **non-steroidal anti-inflammatory drugs** for muscular pains and headaches; metoclopramide hydrochloride p. 451 or prochlorperazine p. 408 may be useful for nausea or vomiting. Topical **rubefacients** can be helpful for relieving muscle pain associated with

methadone hydrochloride withdrawal. If a patient is suffering from insomnia, short-acting **benzodiazepines** or zopiclone p. 512 may be prescribed, but because of the potential for abuse, prescriptions should be limited to a short course of a few days only. If anxiety or agitation is severe, specialist advice should be sought.

Lofexidine
Lofexidine hydrochloride p. 526 may alleviate some of the physical symptoms of opioid withdrawal by attenuating the increase in adrenergic neurotransmission that occurs during opioid withdrawal. Lofexidine hydrochloride can be prescribed as an adjuvant to opioid substitution therapy, initiated either at the same time as the opioid substitute or during withdrawal of the opioid substitute. Alternatively, lofexidine hydrochloride may be prescribed instead of an opioid substitute in patients who have mild or uncertain dependence (including young people), and those with a short history of illicit drug use.

Opioid-receptor antagonists
Patients dependant on opioids can be given a supply of naloxone hydrochloride p. 1424 to be used in case of accidental overdose.

Naltrexone hydrochloride p. 519 precipitates withdrawal symptoms in opioid-dependent subjects. Because the effects of opioid-receptor agonists are blocked by naltrexone hydrochloride, it is prescribed as an aid to prevent relapse in formerly opioid-dependent patients.

Opioid dependence in children

In younger patients (under 18 years), the harmful effects of drug misuse are more often related to acute intoxication than to dependence, so substitution therapy is usually inappropriate. Maintenance treatment with opioid substitution therapy is therefore controversial in young people; however, it may be useful for the older adolescent who has a history of opioid use to undergo a period of stabilisation with buprenorphine or methadone hydrochloride before starting a withdrawal regimen.

8.1 Alcohol dependence

Alcohol dependence

14-Sep-2020

Description of condition

Alcohol dependence is a cluster of behavioural, cognitive and physiological factors that typically include a strong desire to drink alcohol, tolerance to its effects, and difficulties controlling its use. Someone who is alcohol-dependent may persist in drinking, despite harmful consequences, such as physical or mental health problems.

In severely dependent patients who have been drinking excessively for a prolonged period of time, an abrupt reduction in alcohol intake may result in the development of an alcohol withdrawal syndrome, which, in the absence of medical management, can lead to seizures, delirium tremens, and death.

Assisted alcohol withdrawal

EvGr Patients with mild alcohol dependence usually do not need assisted alcohol withdrawal. Patients with moderate dependence can generally be treated in a community setting unless they are at high risk of developing alcohol withdrawal seizures or delirium tremens; individuals with severe dependence should undergo withdrawal in an inpatient setting. Patients with decompensated liver disease should be treated under specialist supervision.

A long-acting benzodiazepine, such as chlordiazepoxide hydrochloride p. 362 or diazepam p. 362, is recommended to attenuate alcohol withdrawal symptoms; local clinical protocols should be followed.

In primary care, *fixed-dose reducing regimens* are used. This involves using a *standard, initial dose* (determined by the severity of alcohol dependence or level of alcohol consumption), followed by dose reduction to zero, usually over 7–10 days. In inpatient or residential settings, a *fixed-dose regimen* or a *symptom-triggered regimen* can be used. A symptom-triggered approach involves tailoring the drug regimen according to the severity of withdrawal and any complications in an individual patient; adequate monitoring facilities should be available. The patient should be monitored on a regular basis and treatment only continued as long as there are withdrawal symptoms.

Carbamazepine p. 327 [unlicensed indication] can be used as an alternative treatment in acute alcohol withdrawal. ⒶThe MHRA/CHM have released important safety information on the use of antiepileptic drugs and the risk of suicidal thoughts and behaviour. For further information, see Epilepsy p. 321.

EvGr Clomethiazole p. 510 may be considered as an alternative to a benzodiazepine or carbamazepine p. 327. It should only be used in an inpatient setting and should not be prescribed if the patient is liable to continue drinking alcohol. ⒶNote: Alcohol combined with clomethiazole p. 510, particularly in patients with cirrhosis, can lead to fatal respiratory depression even with short-term use.

EvGr When managing withdrawal from **co-existing** benzodiazepine and alcohol dependence, the dose of benzodiazepine used for withdrawal should be increased. The initial daily dose is calculated, based on the requirements for alcohol withdrawal plus the equivalent regularly used daily dose of benzodiazepine. A single benzodiazepine (chlordiazepoxide hydrochloride p. 362 or diazepam p. 362) should be used rather than multiple benzodiazepines. Inpatient withdrawal regimens should last for 2–3 weeks or longer, depending on the severity of benzodiazepine dependence. When withdrawal is managed in the community, or where there is a high level of benzodiazepine dependence, or both, the regimen should last for a minimum of 3 weeks (according to the patient's symptoms).

If alcohol withdrawal seizures occur, a fast-acting benzodiazepine (such as lorazepam p. 357 [unlicensed indication]) should be prescribed to reduce the likelihood of further seizures. If alcohol withdrawal seizures develop in a person during treatment for acute alcohol withdrawal, review their withdrawal drug regimen. Ⓐ

Delirium tremens

EvGr Delirium tremens is a medical emergency that requires specialist inpatient care. In patients with delirium tremens (characterised by agitation, confusion, paranoia, and visual and auditory hallucinations), oral lorazepam p. 357 should be used as first-line treatment. If symptoms persist or oral medication is declined, parenteral lorazepam p. 357 [unlicensed], or haloperidol p. 405 [unlicensed] can be given as adjunctive therapy. If delirium tremens develops during treatment for acute alcohol withdrawal, the withdrawal drug regimen should also be reviewed. Ⓐ

Alcohol dependence

EvGr In harmful drinkers or patients with mild alcohol dependence, a psychological intervention (such as cognitive behavioural therapy) should be offered. In those who have not responded to psychological interventions alone or who have specifically requested a pharmacological treatment, acamprosate calcium p. 518 or oral naltrexone hydrochloride p. 519 can be used in combination with a psychological intervention.

Acamprosate calcium p. 518 or oral naltrexone hydrochloride p. 519 in combination with a psychological intervention are recommended for relapse prevention in patients with moderate and severe alcohol dependence, to start after successful assisted withdrawal. Disulfiram below is an alternative for patients in whom acamprosate calcium p. 518 and oral naltrexone hydrochloride p. 519 are not suitable, or if the patient prefers disulfiram below and understands the risks of taking the drug.

Nalmefene p. 518 is recommended for the reduction of alcohol consumption in patients with alcohol dependence who have a high drinking risk level, without physical withdrawal symptoms, and who do not require immediate detoxification (see *National funding/access decisions* for nalmefene p. 518).

Patients with severe alcohol-related hepatitis with a discriminant function of 32 or more can be given corticosteroids but only after any active infection or gastro-intestinal bleeding is treated, any renal impairment is controlled, and following discussion of the potential benefits and risks of treatment. Corticosteroid treatment has been shown to improve survival in the short term (1 month) but not over a longer term (3 months to 1 year). It has also been shown to increase the risk of serious infections within the first 3 months of starting treatment.

Patients with chronic alcohol-related pancreatitis should be offered nutritional support; those who have symptoms of steatorrhoea or who have poor nutritional status due to Exocrine pancreatic insufficiency p. 103 should be prescribed pancreatic enzyme supplements; supplements are not indicated when pain is the only symptom. Ⓐ

Wernicke's encephalopathy

EvGr Patients with alcohol dependence are at risk of developing Wernicke's encephalopathy; patients at high risk are those who are malnourished, at risk of malnourishment, or have decompensated liver disease. Parenteral thiamine p. 1130, followed by oral thiamine p. 1130, should be given to patients with suspected Wernicke's encephalopathy, those who are malnourished or at risk of malnourishment, those who have decompensated liver disease or who are attending hospital for acute treatment. Prophylactic oral thiamine p. 1130 should also be given to harmful or dependent drinkers if they are in acute withdrawal, or before and during assisted alcohol withdrawal. Ⓐ Parenteral thiamine is available as part of a vitamin B substances with ascorbic acid p. 1131 preparation.

Useful Resources

Alcohol-use disorders: diagnosis, assessment and management of harmful drinking and alcohol dependence. National Institute for Health and Care Excellence. Clinical guideline 115. February 2011.
www.nice.org.uk/guidance/cg115

Alcohol-use disorders: diagnosis and management of physical complications. National Institute for Health and Care Excellence. Clinical guideline 100. June 2010 (updated April 2017).
www.nice.org.uk/guidance/cg100

ALDEHYDE DEHYDROGENASE INHIBITORS

Disulfiram
02-Sep-2020

● **INDICATIONS AND DOSE**

Adjunct in the treatment of alcohol dependence (under expert supervision)

▶ BY MOUTH
  ▶ Adult: 200 mg daily, increased if necessary up to 500 mg daily

● UNLICENSED USE Disulfiram doses in BNF may differ from those in product literature.

● CONTRA-INDICATIONS Cardiac failure · coronary artery disease · history of cerebrovascular accident · hypertension · psychosis · severe personality disorder · suicide risk

- CAUTIONS Alcohol challenge **not** recommended on routine basis (if considered essential—specialist units only with resuscitation facilities) · avoid in Acute porphyrias p. 1107 · diabetes mellitus · epilepsy · respiratory disease
- INTERACTIONS → Appendix 1: disulfiram
- SIDE-EFFECTS Allergic dermatitis · breath odour · depression · drowsiness · encephalopathy · fatigue · hepatocellular injury · libido decreased · mania · nausea · nerve disorders · paranoia · psychotic disorder · vomiting
- PREGNANCY High concentrations of acetaldehyde which occur in presence of alcohol may be teratogenic; avoid in first trimester.
- BREAST FEEDING Avoid—no information available.
- HEPATIC IMPAIRMENT Manufacturer advises caution.
- RENAL IMPAIRMENT Use with caution.
- PRE-TREATMENT SCREENING Before initiating disulfiram, prescribers should evaluate the patient's suitability for treatment, because some patient factors, for example memory impairment or social circumstances, make compliance to treatment or abstinence from alcohol difficult.
- MONITORING REQUIREMENTS During treatment with disulfiram, patients should be monitored at least every 2 weeks for the first 2 months, then each month for the following 4 months, and at least every 6 months thereafter.
- PATIENT AND CARER ADVICE Manufacturer advises patients and their carers should be counselled on the disulfiram-alcohol reaction—reactions may occur following exposure to small amounts of alcohol found in perfume, aerosol sprays, or low alcohol and "non-alcohol" beers and wines; symptoms may be severe and life-threatening and can include nausea, flushing, palpitations, arrhythmias, hypotension, respiratory depression, and coma. EvGr Patients and their carers should be counselled on the signs of hepatotoxicity—patients should discontinue treatment and seek immediate medical attention if they feel unwell or symptoms such as fever or jaundice develop. ⟨A⟩
- MEDICINAL FORMS There can be variation in the licensing of different medicines containing the same drug.
  Tablet
  CAUTIONARY AND ADVISORY LABELS 2
  ▸ Disulfiram (Non-proprietary)
    Disulfiram 200 mg Disulfiram 200mg tablets | 50 tablet [PoM] £127.22 DT = £111.54
  ▸ Antabuse (Imported (United States))
    Disulfiram 250 mg Antabuse 250mg tablets | 100 tablet [PoM] Ⓢ
  ▸ Esperal (Imported (France))
    Disulfiram 500 mg Esperal 500mg tablets | 20 tablet [PoM] Ⓢ

GAMMA-AMINOBUTYRIC ACID ANALOGUES AND DERIVATIVES

Acamprosate calcium
10-Sep-2018

- **INDICATIONS AND DOSE**
  Maintenance of abstinence in alcohol-dependent patients
  ▸ BY MOUTH
  ▸ Adult 18–65 years (body-weight up to 60 kg): 666 mg once daily at breakfast and 333 mg twice daily at midday and at night
  ▸ Adult 18–65 years (body-weight 60 kg and above): 666 mg 3 times a day

- CAUTIONS Continued alcohol abuse (risk of treatment failure)

- SIDE-EFFECTS
  ▸ Common or very common Abdominal pain · diarrhoea · flatulence · nausea · sexual dysfunction · skin reactions · vomiting
- PREGNANCY Manufacturer advises avoid unless potential benefit outweighs risk.
- BREAST FEEDING Avoid.
- HEPATIC IMPAIRMENT Manufacturer advises caution in severe hepatic failure—no information available.
- RENAL IMPAIRMENT Avoid if serum-creatinine greater than 120 micromol/litre.
- PRESCRIBING AND DISPENSING INFORMATION Acamprosate calcium has been used for the maintenance of abstinence in alcohol dependence in children aged 16 years and over.

- MEDICINAL FORMS There can be variation in the licensing of different medicines containing the same drug.
  Gastro-resistant tablet
  CAUTIONARY AND ADVISORY LABELS 5, 21, 25
  ELECTROLYTES: May contain Calcium
  ▸ Acamprosate calcium (Non-proprietary)
    Acamprosate calcium 333 mg Acamprosate 333mg gastro-resistant tablets | 168 tablet [PoM] £38.25 DT = £38.25
  ▸ Campral EC (Merck Serono Ltd)
    Acamprosate calcium 333 mg Campral EC 333mg tablets | 168 tablet [PoM] £28.80 DT = £38.25

OPIOID RECEPTOR ANTAGONISTS

Nalmefene

- **INDICATIONS AND DOSE**
  Reduction of alcohol consumption in patients with alcohol dependence who have a high drinking risk level without physical withdrawal symptoms, and who do not require immediate detoxification
  ▸ BY MOUTH
  ▸ Adult: 18 mg daily if required, taken on each day there is a risk of drinking alcohol, preferably taken 1–2 hours before the anticipated time of drinking, if a dose has not been taken before drinking alcohol, 1 dose should be taken as soon as possible; maximum 18 mg per day

- CONTRA-INDICATIONS Recent history of acute alcohol withdrawal syndrome · recent or current opioid use
- CAUTIONS Continued treatment for more than 1 year · history of seizure disorders (including alcohol withdrawal seizures) · psychiatric illness
- INTERACTIONS → Appendix 1: nalmefene
- SIDE-EFFECTS
  ▸ Common or very common Appetite decreased · asthenia · concentration impaired · confusion · diarrhoea · dizziness · drowsiness · dry mouth · feeling abnormal · headache · hyperhidrosis · libido decreased · malaise · muscle spasms · nausea · palpitations · restlessness · sensation abnormal · sleep disorders · tachycardia · tremor · vomiting · weight decreased
  ▸ Frequency not known Dissociation · hallucinations
- PREGNANCY Manufacturer advises avoid—toxicity in *animal* studies.
- BREAST FEEDING Manufacturer advises avoid—present in milk in *animal* studies.
- HEPATIC IMPAIRMENT Manufacturer advises caution in mild to moderate impairment (risk of increased exposure); avoid in severe impairment (no information available).
- RENAL IMPAIRMENT Use with caution—avoid in severe impairment.
- PRE-TREATMENT SCREENING Before initiating treatment, prescribers should evaluate the patient's clinical status, alcohol dependence, and level of alcohol consumption.

4

Nervous system

Nalmefene should only be prescribed for patients who continue to have a high drinking risk level two weeks after the initial assessment.

- MONITORING REQUIREMENTS During treatment, patients should be monitored regularly and the need for continued treatment assessed.
- NATIONAL FUNDING/ACCESS DECISIONS For full details see funding body website

NICE decisions
▶ **Nalmefene for reducing alcohol consumption in people with alcohol dependence (November 2014)** NICE TA325 Recommended with restrictions

- MEDICINAL FORMS There can be variation in the licensing of different medicines containing the same drug.
Tablet
CAUTIONARY AND ADVISORY LABELS 25
▶ Selincro (Lundbeck Ltd)
Nalmefene (as Nalmefene hydrochloride) 18 mg Selincro 18mg tablets | 14 tablet [PoM] £42.42 DT = £42.42 | 28 tablet [PoM] £84.84

Naltrexone hydrochloride
17-Aug-2017

- DRUG ACTION Naltrexone is an opioid-receptor antagonist.

● **INDICATIONS AND DOSE**

Adjunct to prevent relapse in formerly opioid-dependent patients (who have remained opioid-free for at least 7–10 days) (initiated under specialist supervision)
▶ BY MOUTH
▶ Adult: Initially 25 mg daily, then increased to 50 mg daily, total weekly dose may be divided and given on 3 days of the week for improved compliance (e.g. 100 mg on Monday and Wednesday, and 150 mg on Friday); maximum 350 mg per week

Adjunct to prevent relapse in formerly alcohol-dependent patients (initiated under specialist supervision)
▶ BY MOUTH
▶ Adult: 25 mg once daily on the first day, then increased if tolerated to 50 mg daily

- UNLICENSED USE 25 mg dose for adjunct to prevent relapse in formerly alcohol-dependent patients is an unlicensed dose.
- CONTRA-INDICATIONS Patients currently dependent on opioids
- CAUTIONS Concomitant use of opioids
CAUTIONS, FURTHER INFORMATION
▶ Concomitant use of opioids Concomitant use of opioids should be avoided but increased dose of opioid analgesic may be required for pain—manufacturer advises to monitor for opioid intoxication.
- INTERACTIONS → Appendix 1: naltrexone
- SIDE-EFFECTS
▶ **Common or very common** Abdominal pain · anxiety · appetite abnormal · arthralgia · asthenia · chest pain · chills · constipation · diarrhoea · dizziness · eye disorders · headache · hyperhidrosis · mood altered · myalgia · nausea · palpitations · sexual dysfunction · skin reactions · sleep disorders · tachycardia · thirst · vomiting
▶ **Uncommon** Alopecia · confusion · cough · depression · drowsiness · dry mouth · dysphonia · dyspnoea · ear discomfort · eye discomfort · eye swelling · feeling hot · fever · flatulence · flushing · hallucination · hepatic disorders · lymphadenopathy · nasal complaints · oropharyngeal pain · pain · paranoia · peripheral coldness · seborrhoea · sinus disorder · sputum increased · tinnitus · tremor · ulcer · urinary disorders · vertigo · vision disorders · weight changes · yawning

▶ **Rare or very rare** Immune thrombocytopenic purpura · rhabdomyolysis · suicidal behaviours
▶ **Frequency not known** Withdrawal syndrome
- PREGNANCY Use only if benefit outweighs risk.
- BREAST FEEDING Avoid—potential toxicity.
- HEPATIC IMPAIRMENT Manufacturer advises caution in mild to moderate impairment; avoid in severe or acute impairment, acute hepatitis, or hepatic failure.
Dose adjustments Manufacturer advises consider dose adjustment in mild to moderate impairment.
- RENAL IMPAIRMENT Avoid in severe impairment.
- PRE-TREATMENT SCREENING Test for opioid dependence with naloxone before treatment.
- MONITORING REQUIREMENTS Liver function tests needed before and during treatment.
- PATIENT AND CARER ADVICE Patients should be warned that an attempt to overcome the blockade of opioid receptors by overdosing could result in acute opioid intoxication.
- NATIONAL FUNDING/ACCESS DECISIONS For full details see funding body website

NICE decisions
▶ **Naltrexone for the management of opioid dependence (January 2007)** NICE TA115 Recommended

- MEDICINAL FORMS There can be variation in the licensing of different medicines containing the same drug. Forms available from special-order manufacturers include: capsule, oral suspension, oral solution
Tablet
▶ Naltrexone hydrochloride (Non-proprietary)
Naltrexone hydrochloride 50 mg Naltrexone 50mg tablets | 28 tablet [PoM] £70.11 DT = £68.74
▶ Adepend (AOP Orphan Ltd)
Naltrexone hydrochloride 50 mg Adepend 50mg tablets | 28 tablet [PoM] £47.43 DT = £68.74

8.2 Nicotine dependence

Smoking cessation
14-Aug-2018

Overview

Smoking tobacco is the main cause of preventable illness and premature death in the UK. It is linked to a number of diseases such as cancer (primarily lung cancer), chronic obstructive pulmonary disease, and cardiovascular disease, and can lead to complications during pregnancy. Smoking cessation reduces the risk of developing or worsening of smoking-related illnesses, and the benefits begin as soon as a person stops smoking.

Smoking cessation may be associated with temporary withdrawal symptoms caused by nicotine dependence, making it difficult for people to stop. These symptoms include nicotine cravings, irritability, depression, restlessness, poor concentration, light-headedness, sleep disturbances, and increased appetite. Weight gain is a concern for many people who stop smoking, however it is less likely to occur when drug treatment is used to aid smoking cessation.

Non-drug treatment

[EvGr] All smokers, including those who smoke e-cigarettes, should be advised to stop smoking and be offered support to facilitate smoking cessation. They should also be advised that stopping in one step ('abrupt quitting') offers the best chance of lasting success, and that a combination of drug treatment and behavioural support is likely to be the most effective approach Ⓐ 'Abrupt quitting' is when a smoker makes a commitment to stop smoking on or before a particular date (the quit date), rather than by gradually reducing their smoking.

EvGr Smokers who wish to stop smoking should be referred to their local NHS Stop Smoking Services, where they will be provided with advice, drug treatment, and behavioural support options such as individual counselling or group meetings. Smokers who decline to attend their local NHS Stop Smoking Services should be referred to a suitable healthcare professional who can also offer drug treatment and practical advice. ◁A▷

Drug treatment

Nicotine replacement therapy (NRT), varenicline p. 524, and bupropion hydrochloride below, are effective drug treatments to aid smoking cessation. EvGr The choice of drug treatment should take into consideration the smoker's likely adherence, preferences, and previous experience of smoking-cessation aids, as well as contra-indications and side-effects of each preparation. Varenicline, or a combination of long-acting NRT (transdermal patch) and short-acting NRT (lozenges, gum, sublingual tablets, inhalator, nasal spray and oral spray), are the most effective treatment options and thus the preferred choices. If these options are not appropriate, bupropion hydrochloride or single therapy NRT should be considered instead. ◁A▷

Nicotine transdermal patches are generally applied for 16 hours, with the patch removed overnight; if smokers experience strong nicotine cravings upon waking, a 24-hour patch can be used instead. Short-acting nicotine preparations are used whenever the urge to smoke occurs or to prevent cravings; there is no evidence that one form of NRT is more effective than another. EvGr The use of NRT combined with varenicline or bupropion hydrochloride is not recommended, and both varenicline and bupropion hydrochloride should not be prescribed together.

A quit date should be agreed when drug treatment is prescribed for smoking cessation, and treatment should be available before the person stops smoking. Smokers should be prescribed enough treatment to last 2 weeks after their agreed quit date and be re-assessed shortly before their supply finishes.

Smokers who are unwilling or not ready to stop smoking may also benefit from the use of NRT as part of a 'harm reduction approach', because the amount of nicotine in NRT is much lower and less addictive than in smoking tobacco. Harm reduction approaches include stopping smoking whilst using NRT to prevent relapse, and smoking reduction or temporary abstinence with or without the use of NRT. These smokers should be advised that NRT will make it easier to reduce how much they smoke and improve their chance of stopping smoking in the long-term. ◁A▷

E-cigarettes

E-cigarettes deliver nicotine without the toxins found in tobacco smoke. Evidence suggests that e-cigarettes are substantially less harmful to health than tobacco smoking, but long-term effects are still largely unknown. Some smokers have found e-cigarettes useful for smoking cessation, however they cannot be prescribed or supplied by smoking cessation services. EvGr People who wish to use e-cigarettes should be advised that although these products are not licensed drugs, they are regulated by the Tobacco and Related Products Regulations 2016. ◁A▷ In the UK, sale of e-cigarettes is prohibited in children under 18 years of age.

Pregnancy

EvGr Pregnant females should be advised to stop smoking completely, and be informed about the risks to the unborn child of smoking during pregnancy, and the harmful effects of exposure to second-hand smoke for both mother and baby. All pregnant females who smoke or have stopped smoking in the last 2 weeks should be referred to their local NHS Stop Smoking Services, and ongoing support should be offered during and following pregnancy. Smoking cessation should also be encouraged for all members of the household. Pregnant females who smoke should be advised to contact the NHS Pregnancy Smoking Helpline for further information (Tel: 0800 169 9169).

NRT should only be used in pregnant females if non-drug treatment options have failed. Clinical judgement should be used when deciding whether to prescribe NRT following a discussion about its risks and benefits. Subsequent prescriptions should only be given to pregnant females who have demonstrated they are still not smoking. ◁A▷

Concomitant drugs

Polycyclic aromatic hydrocarbons found in tobacco smoke increase the metabolism of some drugs by inducing hepatic enzymes, often requiring an increase in dose. Information about drugs interacting with tobacco smoke can be found under *Interactions* of the relevant drug monograph.

Useful Resources

Stop smoking interventions and services. National Institute for Health and Care Excellence. NICE guideline 92. March 2018.
www.nice.org.uk/guidance/ng92

Smoking: harm reduction. National Institute for Health and Care Excellence. Public health guidance 45. June 2013.
www.nice.org.uk/guidance/ph45

National Centre for Smoking Cessation and Training.
www.ncsct.co.uk

ANTIDEPRESSANTS > SEROTONIN AND NORADRENALINE RE-UPTAKE INHIBITORS

Bupropion hydrochloride
(Amfebutamone hydrochloride)

27-Nov-2020

● **INDICATIONS AND DOSE**

To aid smoking cessation in combination with motivational support in nicotine-dependent patients

▸ BY MOUTH

▸ **Adult:** Initially 150 mg daily for 6 days, then 150 mg twice daily (max. per dose 150 mg), minimum 8 hours between doses; period of treatment 7–9 weeks, start treatment 1–2 weeks before target stop date, discontinue if abstinence not achieved at 7 weeks, consider maximum 150 mg daily in patients with risk factors for seizures; maximum 300 mg per day

▸ **Elderly:** 150 mg daily for 7–9 weeks, start treatment 1–2 weeks before target stop date, discontinue if abstinence not achieved at 7 weeks; maximum 150 mg per day

---

IMPORTANT SAFETY INFORMATION

MHRA/CHM ADVICE: BUPROPION (*ZYBAN*®): RISK OF SEROTONIN SYNDROME WITH USE WITH OTHER SEROTONERGIC DRUGS (NOVEMBER 2020)

Cases of serotonin syndrome have been reported in patients taking bupropion with other serotonergic drugs, such as selective serotonin re-uptake inhibitors (SSRIs) and serotonin and noradrenaline re-uptake inhibitors (SNRIs); some cases were associated with an overdose of bupropion.

The MHRA reminds healthcare professionals not to exceed the recommended dose when prescribing bupropion with other serotonergic drugs; patients should be counselled on the milder symptoms of serotonin syndrome and advised to seek medical attention should these occur, particularly during treatment initiation and dose increases. They should also be advised to never exceed the prescribed dose of bupropion, and encouraged to read the patient information leaflet for information on side-effects. If serotonin syndrome is suspected, a dose reduction or discontinuation of bupropion, depending on the severity of the symptoms, should be considered.

- CONTRA-INDICATIONS Acute alcohol withdrawal · acute benzodiazepine withdrawal · bipolar disorder · CNS tumour · eating disorders · history of seizures · severe hepatic cirrhosis
- CAUTIONS Alcohol abuse · diabetes · elderly · history of head trauma · predisposition to seizures (prescribe only if benefit clearly outweighs risk)
- INTERACTIONS → Appendix 1: bupropion
- SIDE-EFFECTS
- ► **Common or very common** Abdominal pain · anxiety · concentration impaired · constipation · dizziness · dry mouth · fever · gastrointestinal disorder · headache · hyperhidrosis · hypersensitivity · insomnia (reduced by avoiding dose at bedtime) · nausea · skin reactions · taste altered · tremor · vomiting
- ► **Uncommon** Appetite decreased · asthenia · chest pain · confusion · tachycardia · tinnitus · vasodilation · visual impairment
- ► **Rare or very rare** Angioedema · arthralgia · behaviour abnormal · bronchospasm · delusions · depersonalisation · dyspnoea · hallucination · hepatic disorders · irritability · memory loss · movement disorders · muscle complaints · palpitations · paraesthesia · parkinsonism · postural hypotension · seizure · sleep disorders · Stevens-Johnson syndrome · syncope · urinary disorders
- ► **Frequency not known** Anaemia · hyponatraemia · leucopenia · psychosis · suicidal behaviours · thrombocytopenia
- PREGNANCY Avoid—no information available.
- BREAST FEEDING Present in milk—avoid.
- HEPATIC IMPAIRMENT Manufacturer advises use with caution—monitor closely for adverse effects; avoid in severe cirrhosis.
  Dose adjustments Manufacturer advises reduce dose to 150 mg daily in mild to moderate impairment
- RENAL IMPAIRMENT
  Dose adjustments Reduce dose to 150 mg daily.
- MONITORING REQUIREMENTS Manufacturer advises monitor blood pressure before and during treatment.
- PATIENT AND CARER ADVICE Manufacturer advises patients and carers should be instructed to report any clinical worsening of depression, suicidal behaviour or thoughts and unusual changes in behaviour.
  Driving and skilled tasks Manufacturer advises patients and carers should be counselled on the effects on driving and performance of skilled tasks—increased risk of dizziness and light-headedness.

- MEDICINAL FORMS There can be variation in the licensing of different medicines containing the same drug.
  Modified-release tablet
  CAUTIONARY AND ADVISORY LABELS 25
  ► Bupropion hydrochloride (Non-proprietary)
    Bupropion hydrochloride 150 mg Bupropion 150mg modified-release tablets | 60 tablet [PoM] 🛇 DT = £41.76
  ► Zyban (GlaxoSmithKline UK Ltd)
    Bupropion hydrochloride 150 mg Zyban 150mg modified-release tablets | 60 tablet [PoM] £41.76 DT = £41.76

NICOTINIC RECEPTOR AGONISTS

▌Nicotine

- ● INDICATIONS AND DOSE
Nicotine replacement therapy in individuals who smoke fewer than 20 cigarettes each day
- ► BY MOUTH USING CHEWING GUM
- ► Adult: 2 mg as required, chew 1 piece of gum when the urge to smoke occurs or to prevent cravings, if attempting smoking cessation, treatment should continue for 3 months before reducing the dose
- ► BY SUBLINGUAL ADMINISTRATION USING SUBLINGUAL TABLETS
- ► Adult: 1 tablet every 1 hour, increased to 2 tablets every 1 hour if required, if attempting smoking cessation, treatment should continue for up to 3 months before reducing the dose; maximum 40 tablets per day

Nicotine replacement therapy in individuals who smoke more than 20 cigarettes each day or who require more than 15 pieces of 2-mg strength gum each day
- ► BY MOUTH USING CHEWING GUM
- ► Adult: 4 mg as required, chew 1 piece of gum when the urge to smoke occurs or to prevent cravings, individuals should not exceed 15 pieces of 4-mg strength gum daily, if attempting smoking cessation, treatment should continue for 3 months before reducing the dose

Nicotine replacement therapy in individuals who smoke more than 20 cigarettes each day
- ► BY SUBLINGUAL ADMINISTRATION USING SUBLINGUAL TABLETS
- ► Adult: 2 tablets every 1 hour, if attempting smoking cessation, treatment should continue for up to 3 months before reducing the dose; maximum 40 tablets per day

Nicotine replacement therapy
- ► BY INHALATION USING INHALATOR
- ► Adult: As required, the cartridges can be used when the urge to smoke occurs or to prevent cravings, individuals should not exceed 12 cartridges of the 10-mg strength daily, or 6 cartridges of the 15-mg strength daily
- ► BY MOUTH USING LOZENGES
- ► Adult: 1 lozenge every 1–2 hours as required, one lozenge should be used when the urge to smoke occurs, individuals who smoke less than 20 cigarettes each day should usually use the lower-strength lozenges; individuals who smoke more than 20 cigarettes each day and those who fail to stop smoking with the low-strength lozenges should use the higher-strength lozenges; If attempting smoking cessation, treatment should continue for 6–12 weeks before attempting a reduction in dose; maximum 15 lozenges per day
- ► BY MOUTH USING OROMUCOSAL SPRAY
- ► Adult: 1–2 sprays as required, individuals can spray in the mouth when the urge to smoke occurs or to prevent cravings, individuals should not exceed 2 sprays per episode (up to 4 sprays every hour); maximum 64 sprays per day
- ► BY INTRANASAL ADMINISTRATION USING NASAL SPRAY
- ► Adult: 1 spray as required, individuals can spray into each nostril when the urge to smoke occurs, up to twice every hour for 16 hours daily, if attempting smoking cessation, treatment should continue for 8 weeks before reducing the dose; maximum 64 sprays per day
- ► BY TRANSDERMAL APPLICATION USING PATCHES
- ► Adult: Individuals who smoke more than 10 cigarettes daily should apply a high-strength patch daily for 6–8 weeks, followed by the medium-strength patch for 2 weeks, and then the low-strength patch for the final 2 weeks; individuals who smoke fewer than 10 cigarettes daily can usually start with the continued →

4

Nervous system

medium-strength patch for 6–8 weeks, followed by the low-strength patch for 2–4 weeks; a slower titration schedule can be used in individuals who are not ready to quit but want to reduce cigarette consumption before a quit attempt; if abstinence is not achieved, or if withdrawal symptoms are experienced, the strength of the patch used should be maintained or increased until the patient is stabilised; individuals using the high-strength patch who experience excessive side-effects, that do not resolve within a few days, should change to a medium-strength patch for the remainder of the initial period and then use the low-strength patch for 2–4 weeks

● CAUTIONS

GENERAL CAUTIONS Diabetes mellitus—blood-glucose concentration should be monitored closely when initiating treatment · haemodynamically unstable patients hospitalised with cerebrovascular accident · haemodynamically unstable patients hospitalised with myocardial infarction · haemodynamically unstable patients hospitalised with severe arrhythmias · phaeochromocytoma · uncontrolled hyperthyroidism

SPECIFIC CAUTIONS
▸ When used by inhalation Bronchospastic disease · chronic throat disease · obstructive lung disease
▸ With intranasal use Bronchial asthma (may exacerbate)
▸ With oral use gastritis (can be aggravated by swallowed nicotine) · gum may also stick to and damage dentures · oesophagitis (can be aggravated by swallowed nicotine) · peptic ulcers (can be aggravated by swallowed nicotine)
▸ With transdermal use patches should not be placed on broken skin · patients with skin disorders

CAUTIONS, FURTHER INFORMATION Most warnings for nicotine replacement therapy also apply to continued cigarette smoking, but the risk of continued smoking outweighs any risks of using nicotine preparations.

Specific cautions for individual preparations are usually related to the local effect of nicotine.

● SIDE-EFFECTS
GENERAL SIDE-EFFECTS
▸ **Common or very common** Dizziness · headache · hyperhidrosis · nausea · palpitations · skin reactions · vomiting
▸ **Uncommon** Flushing
SPECIFIC SIDE-EFFECTS
▸ **Common or very common**
▸ When used by inhalation Asthenia · cough · dry mouth · flatulence · gastrointestinal discomfort · hiccups · hypersensitivity · nasal complaints · oral disorders · taste altered · throat complaints
▸ With intranasal use Chest discomfort · cough · dyspnoea · epistaxis · nasal complaints · paraesthesia · throat irritation
▸ With oral use Anxiety · appetite abnormal · burping · diarrhoea · dyspepsia (may be caused by swallowed nicotine) · gastrointestinal disorders · hiccups · increased risk of infection · mood altered · oral disorders · sleep disorders
▸ With sublingual use Asthenia · cough · dry mouth · flatulence · gastrointestinal discomfort · hiccups · hypersensitivity · oral disorders · rhinitis · taste altered · throat complaints
▸ **Uncommon**
▸ When used by inhalation Abnormal dreams · arrhythmias · bronchospasm · burping · chest discomfort · dysphonia · dyspnoea · hypertension · malaise
▸ With intranasal use Abnormal dreams · asthenia · hypertension · malaise
▸ With oral use Anger · asthma exacerbated · cough · dyspepsia aggravated · dysphagia · haemorrhage · laryngospasm · nasal complaints · nocturia · numbness · overdose · pain · palpitations exacerbated · peripheral

oedema · tachycardia · taste altered · throat complaints · vascular disorders
▸ With sublingual use Abnormal dreams · arrhythmias · bronchospasm · burping · chest discomfort · dysphonia · dyspnoea · hypertension · malaise · nasal complaints
▸ With transdermal use Arrhythmias · asthenia · chest discomfort · dyspnoea · hypertension · malaise · myalgia · paraesthesia
▸ **Rare or very rare**
▸ When used by inhalation Dysphagia
▸ With intranasal use Arrhythmias
▸ With oral use Coagulation disorder · platelet disorder
▸ With sublingual use Dysphagia
▸ With transdermal use Abdominal discomfort · angioedema · pain in extremity
▸ **Frequency not known**
▸ When used by inhalation Angioedema · excessive tearing · vision blurred
▸ With intranasal use Abdominal discomfort · angioedema · excessive tearing · oropharyngeal complaints
▸ With sublingual use Excessive tearing · muscle tightness · vision blurred

SIDE-EFFECTS, FURTHER INFORMATION Some systemic effects occur on initiation of therapy, particularly if the patient is using high-strength preparations; however, the patient may confuse side-effects of the nicotine-replacement preparation with nicotine withdrawal symptoms. Common symptoms of nicotine withdrawal include malaise, headache, dizziness, sleep disturbance, coughing, influenza–like symptoms, depression, irritability, increased appetite, weight gain, restlessness, anxiety, drowsiness, aphthous ulcers, decreased heart rate, and impaired concentration.

● PREGNANCY The use of nicotine replacement therapy in pregnancy is preferable to the continuation of smoking, but should be used only if smoking cessation without nicotine replacement fails. Intermittent therapy is preferable to patches but avoid liquorice-flavoured nicotine products. Patches are useful, however, if the patient is experiencing pregnancy-related nausea and vomiting. If patches are used, they should be removed before bed.

● BREAST FEEDING Nicotine is present in milk; however, the amount to which the infant is exposed is small and less hazardous than second-hand smoke. Intermittent therapy is preferred.

● HEPATIC IMPAIRMENT Manufacturer advises caution in moderate to severe impairment (risk of decreased clearance).

● RENAL IMPAIRMENT Use with caution in severe renal impairment.

● DIRECTIONS FOR ADMINISTRATION Acidic beverages, such as coffee or fruit juice, may decrease the absorption of nicotine through the buccal mucosa and should be avoided for 15 minutes before the use of oral nicotine replacement therapy.
Administration by transdermal patch Patches should be applied on waking to dry, non-hairy skin on the hip, trunk, or upper arm and held in position for 10–20 seconds to ensure adhesion; place next patch on a different area and avoid using the same site for several days.
Administration by nasal spray Initially 1 spray should be used in both nostrils but when withdrawing from therapy, the dose can be gradually reduced to 1 spray in 1 nostril.
Administration by oral spray The oral spray should be released into the mouth, holding the spray as close to the mouth as possible and avoiding the lips. The patient should not inhale while spraying and avoid swallowing for a few seconds after use. If using the oral spray for the first time, or if unit not used for 2 or more days, prime the unit before administration.

Administration by sublingual tablet Each tablet should be placed under the tongue and allowed to dissolve.

Administration by lozenge Slowly allow each lozenge to dissolve in the mouth; periodically move the lozenge from one side of the mouth to the other. Lozenges last for 10–30 minutes, depending on their size.

Administration by inhalation Insert the cartridge into the device and draw in air through the mouthpiece; each session can last for approximately 5 minutes. The amount of nicotine from 1 puff of the cartridge is less than that from a cigarette, therefore it is necessary to inhale more often than when smoking a cigarette. A single 10 mg cartridge lasts for approximately 20 minutes of intense use; a single 15 mg cartridge lasts for approximately 40 minutes of intense use.

Administration by medicated chewing gum Chew the gum until the taste becomes strong, then rest it between the cheek and gum; when the taste starts to fade, repeat this process. One piece of gum lasts for approximately 30 minutes.

● PRESCRIBING AND DISPENSING INFORMATION Flavours of chewing gum and lozenges may include mint, freshfruit, freshmint, icy white, or cherry.

● PATIENT AND CARER ADVICE Patient or carers should be given advice on how to administer nicotine chewing gum, inhalators, lozenges, sublingual tablets, oral spray, nasal spray and patches.

● MEDICINAL FORMS There can be variation in the licensing of different medicines containing the same drug.

Spray
EXCIPIENTS: May contain Ethanol
▸ Nicorette QuickMist SmartTrack (McNeil Products Ltd)
Nicotine 1 mg per 1 actuation Nicorette QuickMist SmartTrack 1mg/dose mouthspray sugar-free | 13.2 ml (GSL) £14.30 DT = £13.66 sugar-free | 26.4 ml (GSL) £23.12

Sublingual tablet
CAUTIONARY AND ADVISORY LABELS 26
▸ Nicorette Microtab (McNeil Products Ltd)
Nicotine (as Nicotine cyclodextrin complex) 2 mg Nicorette Microtab 2mg sublingual tablets sugar-free | 100 tablet (GSL) £15.95 DT = £15.95

Transdermal patch
▸ NiQuitin (Omega Pharma Ltd)
Nicotine 7 mg per 24 hour NiQuitin 7mg patches | 7 patch (GSL) £11.48 DT = £9.12
Nicotine 14 mg per 24 hour NiQuitin 14mg patches | 7 patch (GSL) £11.48 DT = £9.40
Nicotine 21 mg per 24 hour NiQuitin 21mg patches | 7 patch (GSL) £11.48 DT = £9.97 | 14 patch (GSL) £18.79
▸ NiQuitin Clear (Omega Pharma Ltd)
Nicotine 7 mg per 24 hour NiQuitin Clear 7mg patches | 7 patch (GSL) £11.48 DT = £9.12
Nicotine 14 mg per 24 hour NiQuitin Clear 14mg patches | 7 patch (GSL) £11.48 DT = £9.40 | 14 patch (GSL) £18.79
Nicotine 21 mg per 24 hour NiQuitin Clear 21mg patches | 7 patch (GSL) £11.48 DT = £9.97 | 14 patch (GSL) £18.79
NiQuitin Pre-Quit Clear 21mg patches | 7 patch (GSL) £11.48 DT = £9.97
▸ Nicorette invisi (McNeil Products Ltd)
Nicotine 10 mg per 16 hour Nicorette invisi 10mg/16hours patches | 7 patch (GSL) £11.43 = £11.43
Nicotine 15 mg per 16 hour Nicorette invisi 15mg/16hours patches | 7 patch (GSL) £11.43 = £11.43
Nicotine 25 mg per 16 hour Nicorette invisi 25mg/16hours patches | 7 patch (GSL) £11.43 = £11.43 | 14 patch (GSL) £18.72
▸ Nicotinell TTS (GlaxoSmithKline Consumer Healthcare)
Nicotine 7 mg per 24 hour Nicotinell TTS 10 patches | 7 patch (GSL) £9.12 DT = £9.12
Nicotine 14 mg per 24 hour Nicotinell TTS 20 patches | 7 patch (GSL) £9.40 DT = £9.40
Nicotine 21 mg per 24 hour Nicotinell TTS 30 patches | 7 patch (GSL) £9.97 DT = £9.97 | 21 patch (GSL) £24.51

Medicated chewing-gum
▸ Nicorette (McNeil Products Ltd)
Nicotine 2 mg Nicorette Freshmint 2mg medicated chewing gum sugar-free | 25 piece (GSL) £3.69 sugar-free | 105 piece (GSL) £10.55 sugar-free | 210 piece (GSL) £17.04
Nicorette Fruitfusion 2mg medicated chewing gum sugar-free | 75 piece (GSL) £5.58 sugar-free | 105 piece (GSL) £10.55
Nicorette Original 2mg medicated chewing gum sugar-free | 75 piece (GSL) £5.58 sugar-free | 105 piece (GSL) £10.55 sugar-free | 165 piece (GSL) £11.49 sugar-free | 210 piece (GSL) £17.04
Nicotine 4 mg Nicorette Fruitfusion 4mg medicated chewing gum sugar-free | 75 piece (GSL) £5.58 sugar-free | 105 piece (GSL) £12.91
Nicorette Original 4mg medicated chewing gum sugar-free | 105 piece (GSL) £12.90 sugar-free | 210 piece (GSL) £21.05
Nicorette Freshmint 4mg medicated chewing gum sugar-free | 25 piece (GSL) £3.70 sugar-free | 105 piece (GSL) £12.90
▸ Nicorette Icy White (McNeil Products Ltd)
Nicotine 2 mg Nicorette Icy White 2mg medicated chewing gum sugar-free | 25 piece (GSL) £3.69 sugar-free | 75 piece (GSL) £5.58 sugar-free | 105 piece (GSL) £10.54 sugar-free | 165 piece (GSL) £11.49 sugar-free | 210 piece (GSL) £17.03
Nicotine 4 mg Nicorette Icy White 4mg medicated chewing gum sugar-free | 75 piece (GSL) £5.58 sugar-free | 105 piece (GSL) £12.89 sugar-free | 165 piece (GSL) £11.49
▸ Nicotinell (GlaxoSmithKline Consumer Healthcare)
Nicotine 2 mg Nicotinell Mint 2mg medicated chewing gum sugar-free | 96 piece (GSL) £8.26 DT = £8.26 sugar-free | 204 piece (GSL) £14.23
Nicotinell Fruit 2mg medicated chewing gum sugar-free | 96 piece (GSL) £8.26 DT = £8.26 sugar-free | 204 piece (GSL) £14.23
Nicotine 4 mg Nicotinell Mint 4mg medicated chewing gum sugar-free | 96 piece (GSL) £10.26 DT = £10.26
Nicotinell Fruit 4mg medicated chewing gum sugar-free | 96 piece (GSL) £10.26 DT = £10.26

Lozenge
EXCIPIENTS: May contain Aspartame
ELECTROLYTES: May contain Sodium
▸ NiQuitin (Omega Pharma Ltd)
Nicotine 1.5 mg NiQuitin Minis Mint 1.5mg lozenges sugar-free | 20 lozenge (GSL) £4.14 sugar-free | 60 lozenge (GSL) £10.85 DT = £10.85 sugar-free | 100 lozenge (GSL) £14.04
Nicotine 2 mg NiQuitin Mint 2mg lozenges sugar-free | 72 lozenge (GSL) £7.40 DT = £7.40
Nicotine 4 mg NiQuitin Mint 4mg lozenges sugar-free | 36 lozenge (GSL) £5.91 sugar-free | 72 lozenge (GSL) £7.40 DT = £7.40
NiQuitin Minis Mint 4mg lozenges sugar-free | 60 lozenge (GSL) £10.85 DT = £10.85 sugar-free | 100 lozenge (GSL) £14.04
▸ Nicorette (McNeil Products Ltd)
Nicotine 2 mg Nicorette Fruit 2mg lozenges sugar-free | 80 lozenge (GSL) £12.05 DT = £12.05
Nicorette Cools 2mg lozenges sugar-free | 20 lozenge (GSL) £3.34 DT = £3.34 sugar-free | 80 lozenge (GSL) £12.05 DT = £12.05
Nicotine 4 mg Nicorette Cools 4mg lozenges sugar-free | 80 lozenge (GSL) £12.17 DT = £12.17
▸ Nicotinell (GlaxoSmithKline Consumer Healthcare)
Nicotine (as Nicotine bitartrate) 1 mg Nicotinell 1mg lozenges sugar-free | 12 lozenge (GSL) £1.59 sugar-free | 96 lozenge (GSL) £9.12 DT = £9.12 sugar-free | 144 lozenge (GSL) £11.48 sugar-free | 204 lozenge (GSL) £12.77
Nicotine (as Nicotine bitartrate) 2 mg Nicotinell 2mg lozenges sugar-free | 96 lozenge (GSL) £10.60 DT = £10.60 sugar-free | 144 lozenge (GSL) £13.50 DT = £13.50 sugar-free | 204 lozenge (GSL) £14.94 DT = £14.94

Inhalation vapour
▸ Nicorette (McNeil Products Ltd)
Nicotine 15 mg Nicorette 15mg Inhalator | 4 cartridge (GSL) £5.21 DT = £5.21 | 20 cartridge (GSL) £19.02 DT = £19.02 | 36 cartridge (GSL) £30.26 DT = £30.26

4

Nervous system

Varenicline

03-Sep-2020

- DRUG ACTION Varenicline is a selective nicotine-receptor partial agonist.

- **INDICATIONS AND DOSE**

To aid smoking cessation

▸ BY MOUTH

▸ Adult: Initially 500 micrograms once daily for 3 days, increased to 500 micrograms twice daily for 4 days, then 1 mg twice daily for 11 weeks; reduced if not tolerated to 500 micrograms twice daily, usually to be started 1–2 weeks before target stop date but can be started up to a maximum of 5 weeks before target stop date, 12-week course can be repeated in abstinent individuals to reduce risk of relapse

- CAUTIONS Conditions that may lower seizure threshold · history of cardiovascular disease · history of psychiatric illness (may exacerbate underlying illness including depression) · predisposition to seizures

- SIDE-EFFECTS

▸ **Common or very common** Appetite abnormal · asthenia · chest discomfort · constipation · diarrhoea · dizziness · drowsiness · dry mouth · gastrointestinal discomfort · gastrointestinal disorders · headache · joint disorders · muscle complaints · nausea · oral disorders · pain · skin reactions · sleep disorders · vomiting · weight increased

▸ **Uncommon** Allergic rhinitis · anxiety · arrhythmias · behaviour abnormal · burping · conjunctivitis · depression · eye pain · fever · fungal infection · haemorrhage · hallucination · hot flush · hyperglycaemia · influenza like illness · malaise · menorrhagia · mood swings · numbness · palpitations · seizure · sexual dysfunction · suicidal ideation · sweat changes · thinking abnormal · tinnitus · tremor · urinary disorders

▸ **Rare or very rare** Angioedema · bradyphrenia · coordination abnormal · costochondritis · cyst · diabetes mellitus · dysarthria · eye disorders · feeling cold · glycosuria · muscle tone increased · polydipsia · psychosis · scleral discolouration · severe cutaneous adverse reactions (SCARs) · snoring · vaginal discharge · vision disorders

▸ **Frequency not known** Loss of consciousness

- PREGNANCY Avoid—toxicity in *animal* studies.

- BREAST FEEDING Avoid—present in milk in *animal* studies.

- RENAL IMPAIRMENT

Dose adjustments If eGFR less than 30 mL/minute/1.73 m^2, initial dose 500 micrograms once daily, increased after 3 days to 1 mg once daily.

- TREATMENT CESSATION Risk of relapse, irritability, depression, and insomnia on discontinuation; consider dose tapering on completion of 12-week course.

- PATIENT AND CARER ADVICE

Driving and skilled tasks Manufacturer advises patients and carers should be cautioned on the effects on driving and performance of skilled tasks—increased risk of dizziness, somnolence, and transient loss of consciousness.

- NATIONAL FUNDING/ACCESS DECISIONS

For full details see funding body website

NICE decisions

▸ Varenicline for smoking cessation (July 2007) NICE TA123 Recommended

- MEDICINAL FORMS There can be variation in the licensing of different medicines containing the same drug.

Tablet

CAUTIONARY AND ADVISORY LABELS 3

▸ Champix (Pfizer Ltd)

Varenicline (as Varenicline tartrate) 500 microgram Champix 0.5mg tablets | 56 tablet [PoM] £54.60 DT = £54.60
Varenicline (as Varenicline tartrate) 1 mg Champix 1mg tablets | 28 tablet [PoM] £27.30 DT = £27.30 | 56 tablet [PoM] £54.60

Varenicline (as Varenicline tartrate) 500 microgram/1 mg Champix 0.5mg/1mg 2 week treatment initiation pack | 25 tablet [PoM] £27.30 DT = £27.30
Champix 0.5mg/1mg 4 week treatment initiation pack | 53 tablet [PoM] £54.60

8.3 Opioid dependence

Other drugs used for Opioid dependence Buprenorphine, p. 468 · Naltrexone hydrochloride, p. 519

ANALGESICS ❭ OPIOIDS

◤467

Methadone hydrochloride

13-Nov-2020

- **INDICATIONS AND DOSE**

Severe pain

▸ BY MOUTH, OR BY SUBCUTANEOUS INJECTION, OR BY INTRAMUSCULAR INJECTION

▸ Adult: 5–10 mg every 6–8 hours, adjusted according to response, on prolonged use not to be given more frequently than every 12 hours

Adjunct in treatment of opioid dependence

▸ BY MOUTH USING ORAL SOLUTION

▸ Adult: Initially 10–30 mg daily, increased in steps of 5–10 mg daily if required until no signs of withdrawal nor evidence of intoxication, dose to be increased in the first week, then increased every few days as necessary up to usual dose, maximum weekly dose increase of 30 mg; usual dose 60–120 mg daily

Adjunct in treatment of opioid dependence if tolerance low or not known

▸ BY MOUTH USING ORAL SOLUTION

▸ Adult: Initially 10–20 mg daily, increased in steps of 5–10 mg daily if required until no signs of withdrawal nor evidence of intoxication, dose to be increased in the first week, then increased every few days as necessary up to usual dose, maximum weekly dose increase of 30 mg; usual dose 60–120 mg daily

Adjunct in treatment of opioid dependence if tolerance high (under expert supervision)

▸ BY MOUTH USING ORAL SOLUTION

▸ Adult: Initially up to 40 mg daily, increased in steps of 5–10 mg daily if required until no signs of withdrawal nor evidence of intoxication, dose to be increased in the first week, then increased every few days as necessary up to usual dose, maximum weekly dose increase of 30 mg; usual dose 60–120 mg daily

Cough in palliative care

▸ INITIALLY BY MOUTH USING LINCTUS

▸ Adult: 1–2 mg every 4–6 hours, (by mouth) reduced to 1–2 mg twice daily, use twice daily frequency if prolonged use

DOSE EQUIVALENCE AND CONVERSION

▸ See buprenorphine p. 468 for dose adjustments in opioid substitution therapy, for patients taking methadone who want to switch to buprenorphine.

- UNLICENSED USE Methadone hydrochloride doses for opioid dependence in the BNF may differ from those in the product literature.

IMPORTANT SAFETY INFORMATION

Many preparations of Methadone oral solution are licensed for opioid drug addiction only but some are also licensed for analgesia in severe pain.

- CONTRA-INDICATIONS Phaeochromocytoma

- CAUTIONS Risk factors for QT-interval prolongation

CAUTIONS, FURTHER INFORMATION
▸ QT-interval prolongation EvGr ECG monitoring recommended in patients with the following risk factors for QT-interval prolongation while taking methadone: history of cardiac conduction abnormalities, family history of sudden death, heart or liver disease, electrolyte abnormalities, or concomitant treatment with drugs that can prolong QT interval; patients requiring more than 100 mg daily should also be monitored. ⟨M⟩

● INTERACTIONS → Appendix 1: opioids

● SIDE-EFFECTS

GENERAL SIDE-EFFECTS
Asthma exacerbated · dry eye · dysuria · hyperprolactinaemia · hypothermia · menstrual cycle irregularities · mood altered · nasal dryness · QT interval prolongation

SPECIFIC SIDE-EFFECTS
▸ With oral use Galactorrhoea · intracranial pressure increased
▸ With parenteral use Biliary spasm · muscle rigidity · oedema · restlessness · sexual dysfunction · sleep disorder · ureteral spasm · withdrawal syndrome neonatal

SIDE-EFFECTS, FURTHER INFORMATION Methadone is a long-acting opioid therefore effects may be cumulative.
Methadone, even in low doses is a special hazard for children; non-dependent adults are also at risk of toxicity; dependent adults are at risk if tolerance is incorrectly assessed during induction.

Overdose Methadone has a very long duration of action; patients may need to be monitored for long periods following large overdoses.

● BREAST FEEDING Withdrawal symptoms in infant; breast-feeding permissible during maintenance but dose should be as low as possible and infant monitored to avoid sedation (high doses of methadone carry an increased risk of sedation and respiratory depression in the neonate).

● HEPATIC IMPAIRMENT Manufacturer advises caution; consider avoiding in severe impairment (risk of increased exposure).
Dose adjustments Manufacturer advises consider dose reduction.

● RENAL IMPAIRMENT Avoid use or reduce dose; opioid effects increased and prolonged and increased cerebral sensitivity occurs.

● TREATMENT CESSATION Avoid abrupt withdrawal.

● PRESCRIBING AND DISPENSING INFORMATION Flavours of oral liquid formulations may include tolu.

Palliative care For further information on the use of methadone in palliative care, see www.medicinescomplete.com/#/content/palliative/methadone

METHADOSE ® The final strength of the methadone mixture to be dispensed to the patient must be specified on the prescription.
Important—care is required in prescribing and dispensing the **correct strength** since any confusion could lead to an overdose; this preparation should be dispensed only **after dilution** as appropriate with *Methadose* ® Diluent (life of diluted solution 3 months) and is for drug dependent persons.

● NATIONAL FUNDING/ACCESS DECISIONS
For full details see funding body website

NICE decisions
▸ Methadone and buprenorphine for the management of opioid dependence (January 2007) NICE TA114 Recommended

● LESS SUITABLE FOR PRESCRIBING Methadone linctus is less suitable for prescribing for cough in terminal disease (has a tendency to accumulate).

● MEDICINAL FORMS There can be variation in the licensing of different medicines containing the same drug. Forms available from special-order manufacturers include: tablet, capsule, oral suspension, oral solution, solution for injection, suppository

Tablet
CAUTIONARY AND ADVISORY LABELS 2
▸ Physeptone (Martindale Pharmaceuticals Ltd)
Methadone hydrochloride 5 mg Physeptone 5mg tablets | 50 tablet PoM £2.84 DT = £2.84 CD2

Solution for injection
▸ Physeptone (Martindale Pharmaceuticals Ltd)
Methadone hydrochloride 10 mg per 1 ml Physeptone 10mg/1ml solution for injection ampoules | 10 ampoule PoM £7.63 DT = £7.63 CD2
Methadone hydrochloride 50 mg per 1 ml Physeptone 50mg/1ml solution for injection ampoules | 10 ampoule PoM £17.72 DT = £17.72 CD2

Oral solution
CAUTIONARY AND ADVISORY LABELS 2
▸ Methadone hydrochloride (Non-proprietary)
Methadone hydrochloride 1 mg per 1 ml Methadone 1mg/ml oral solution | 100 ml PoM £1.15–£1.20 DT = £1.15 CD2 | 500 ml PoM £4.30–£5.75 DT = £5.75 CD2 | 2500 ml PoM £28.75–£32.10 CD2
Methadone 1mg/ml oral solution sugar free-free | 50 ml PoM £1.00 CD2 sugar-free | 100 ml PoM £1.20 DT = £1.16 CD2 sugar-free | 500 ml PoM £4.30–£6.00 DT = £5.80 CD2 sugar-free | 2500 ml PoM £29.00–£32.10 CD2
▸ Methadose (Rosemont Pharmaceuticals Ltd)
Methadone hydrochloride 10 mg per 1 ml Methadose 10mg/ml oral solution concentrate sugar-free | 150 ml PoM £12.01 DT = £12.01 CD2 sugar-free | 500 ml PoM £30.75 CD2
Methadone hydrochloride 20 mg per 1 ml Methadose 20mg/ml oral solution concentrate sugar-free | 150 ml PoM £24.02 DT = £24.02 CD2
▸ Metharose (Rosemont Pharmaceuticals Ltd)
Methadone hydrochloride 1 mg per 1 ml Metharose 1mg/ml oral solution sugar free-free | 500 ml PoM £6.82 DT = £5.80 CD2
▸ Physeptone (Martindale Pharmaceuticals Ltd)
Methadone hydrochloride 1 mg per 1 ml Physeptone 1mg/ml mixture | 100 ml PoM £1.27 DT = £1.15 CD2 | 500 ml PoM £6.42 DT = £5.75 CD2 | 2500 ml PoM £32.10 CD2
Physeptone 1mg/ml oral solution sugar free sugar-free | 100 ml PoM £1.27 DT = £1.16 CD2 sugar-free | 500 ml PoM £6.42 DT = £5.80 CD2 sugar-free | 2500 ml PoM £32.10 CD2

OPIOID RECEPTOR ANTAGONISTS

Buprenorphine with naloxone   03-Nov-2020

The properties listed below are those particular to the combination only. For the properties of the components please consider, buprenorphine p. 468, naloxone hydrochloride p. 1424.

● INDICATIONS AND DOSE

Adjunct in the treatment of opioid dependence (dose expressed as buprenorphine)
▸ BY SUBLINGUAL ADMINISTRATION
▸ Adult: Initially 2–4 mg once daily, an additional dose of 2–4 mg may be administered on day 1 depending on the individual patient's requirement, increased in steps of 2–8 mg, adjusted according to response, total weekly dose may be divided and given on alternate days or 3 times weekly; maximum 24 mg per day

● INTERACTIONS → Appendix 1: opioids

● NATIONAL FUNDING/ACCESS DECISIONS
For full details see funding body website

Scottish Medicines Consortium (SMC) decisions
▸ Buprenorphine/naloxone (*Suboxone* ®) as substitution treatment for opioid drug dependence (March 2007) SMC No. 355/07 Recommended with restrictions

- MEDICINAL FORMS There can be variation in the licensing of different medicines containing the same drug.

Sublingual tablet

CAUTIONARY AND ADVISORY LABELS 2, 26

▶ Buprenorphine with naloxone (Non-proprietary)

Naloxone (as Naloxone hydrochloride dihydrate) 500 microgram, Buprenorphine (as Buprenorphine hydrochloride)

2 mg Buprenorphine 2mg / Naloxone 500microgram sublingual tablets sugar free sugar-free | 28 tablet (PoM) £25.60 DT = £25.60 (CD3)

Naloxone (as Naloxone hydrochloride dihydrate) 2 mg, Buprenorphine (as Buprenorphine hydrochloride)

8 mg Buprenorphine 8mg / Naloxone 2mg sublingual tablets sugar free sugar-free | 28 tablet (PoM) £76.73 DT = £76.73 (CD3)

▶ Suboxone (Indivior UK Ltd)

Naloxone (as Naloxone hydrochloride dihydrate) 500 microgram, Buprenorphine (as Buprenorphine hydrochloride) Suboxone 2mg/500microgram sublingual tablets sugar-free | 28 tablet (PoM) £25.40 DT = £25.60 (CD3)

Naloxone (as Naloxone hydrochloride dihydrate) 2 mg, Buprenorphine (as Buprenorphine hydrochloride)

8 mg Suboxone 8mg/2mg sublingual tablets sugar-free | 28 tablet (PoM) £76.19 DT = £76.73 (CD3)

Naloxone (as Naloxone hydrochloride dihydrate) 4 mg, Buprenorphine (as Buprenorphine hydrochloride)

16 mg Suboxone 16mg/4mg sublingual tablets sugar-free | 28 tablet (PoM) £152.38 DT = £152.38 (CD3)

SYMPATHOMIMETICS › ALPHA₂-ADRENOCEPTOR AGONISTS

▌Lofexidine hydrochloride

03-Apr-2020

- DRUG ACTION Lofexidine is an alpha₂-adrenergic agonist.

- **INDICATIONS AND DOSE**

Management of symptoms of opioid withdrawal

▶ BY MOUTH

▶ Adult: Initially 800 micrograms daily in divided doses, increased in steps of 400–800 micrograms daily (max. per dose 800 micrograms) as required recommended duration of treatment 7–10 days if no opioid use (but longer may be required); maximum 2.4 mg per day

- CAUTIONS Bradycardia · cerebrovascular disease · depression · hypotension (monitor pulse rate and blood pressure) · metabolic disturbances · recent myocardial infarction · risk factors for QT interval prolongation · severe coronary insufficiency

- INTERACTIONS → Appendix 1: lofexidine

- SIDE-EFFECTS

▶ **Common or very common** Bradycardia · dizziness · drowsiness · hypotension · mucosal dryness

▶ **Frequency not known** QT interval prolongation

- PREGNANCY Use only if benefit outweighs risk—no information available.

- BREAST FEEDING Use only if benefit outweighs risk—no information available.

- RENAL IMPAIRMENT Caution in chronic impairment.

- MONITORING REQUIREMENTS Monitoring of blood pressure and pulse rate is recommended on initiation, for at least 72 hours or until a stable dose is achieved, and on discontinuation.

- TREATMENT CESSATION Treatment should be withdrawn gradually over 2–4 days (or longer) to reduce the risk of rebound hypertension and associated symptoms.

- PRESCRIBING AND DISPENSING INFORMATION Lofexidine has been used in children over 12 years in the management of symptoms of opioid withdrawal. Available from specialist importing companies.

- PATIENT AND CARER ADVICE The patient should take part of the dose at bedtime to offset insomnia associated with opioid withdrawal.

- MEDICINAL FORMS No licensed medicines listed.

Chapter 5
Infection

CONTENTS

1 Amoebic infection

Other drugs used for Amoebic infection Metronidazole, p. 575 · Tinidazole, p. 577

ANTIPROTOZOALS

Mepacrine hydrochloride
01-Jul-2020

- **INDICATIONS AND DOSE**

Giardiasis
▸ BY MOUTH
▸ Adult: 100 mg every 8 hours for 5–7 days

- **UNLICENSED USE** Not licensed for use in giardiasis.
- **CAUTIONS** Avoid in psoriasis · elderly · history of psychosis
- **INTERACTIONS** → Appendix 1: mepacrine
- **SIDE-EFFECTS** Aplastic anaemia (long term use) · central nervous system stimulation (with high doses) · corneal deposits · dermatosis (long term use) · dizziness · exfoliative dermatitis (severe; long term use) · gastrointestinal disorder · headache · hepatitis (long term use) · nail discolouration · nausea (with high doses) · oral discolouration · skin discolouration (long term use) · toxic psychosis (transient; with high doses) · urine discolouration (long term use) · visual impairment · vomiting (with high doses)
- **HEPATIC IMPAIRMENT** Use with caution.

- **MEDICINAL FORMS** Forms available from special-order manufacturers include: tablet

2 Bacterial infection

Antibacterials, principles of therapy

15-Sep-2020

Antibacterial drug choice

Before selecting an antibacterial the clinician must first consider three factors— the patient, the known or likely causative organism, and the risk of bacterial resistance with repeated courses.

Factors related to the patient which must be considered include history of allergy, renal and hepatic function, susceptibility to infection (i.e. whether immunocompromised), ability to tolerate drugs by mouth, severity of illness, risk of complications, ethnic origin, age, whether taking other medication and, if female, whether pregnant, breast-feeding or taking an oral contraceptive.

The known or likely organism and its antibacterial sensitivity, in association with the factors above, will provide one or more antibacterial option. EvGr In patients receiving antibacterial prophylaxis, an antibacterial from a different class should be used. ⬦

Some patients may be at higher risk of treatment failure. They include those who have had repeated antibacterial courses, a previous or current culture with resistant bacteria, or those at higher risk of developing complications.

Antibacterials, considerations before starting therapy

The following precepts should be considered before starting:
- Viral infections should not be treated with antibacterials. However, antibacterials may be used to treat secondary bacterial infection (e.g. bacterial pneumonia secondary to influenza);
- Samples should be taken for culture and sensitivity testing as appropriate; '**blind**' antibacterial prescribing for unexplained pyrexia usually leads to further difficulty in establishing the diagnosis;
- Knowledge of **prevalent organisms** and their current sensitivity is of great help in choosing an antibacterial

before bacteriological confirmation is available. Generally, narrow-spectrum antibacterials are preferred to broad-spectrum antibacterials unless there is a clear clinical indication (e.g. life-threatening sepsis);

- The **dose** of an antibacterial varies according to a number of factors including age, weight, hepatic function, renal function, and severity of infection. The prescribing of the so-called 'standard' dose in serious infections may result in failure of treatment or even death of the patient; therefore it is important to prescribe a dose appropriate to the condition. An inadequate dose may also increase the likelihood of antibacterial resistance. On the other hand, for an antibacterial with a narrow margin between the toxic and therapeutic dose (e.g. an aminoglycoside) it is also important to avoid an excessive dose and the concentration of the drug in the plasma may need to be monitored;

- The **route** of administration of an antibacterial often depends on the severity of the infection. Life-threatening infections require intravenous therapy. Antibacterials that are well absorbed may be given by mouth even for some serious infections. Parenteral administration is also appropriate when the oral route cannot be used (e.g. because of vomiting) or if absorption is inadequate. Whenever possible, painful intramuscular injections should be avoided in children;

- **Duration** of therapy depends on the nature of the infection and the response to treatment. Courses should not be unduly prolonged because they encourage resistance, they may lead to side-effects and they are costly. However, in certain infections such as tuberculosis or osteomyelitis it may be necessary to treat for prolonged periods. The prescription for an antibacterial should specify the duration of treatment or the date when treatment is to be reviewed.

For further guidance on the appropriate and effective use of antibacterials, see Antimicrobial stewardship p. 20

Advice to be given to patients and their family and/or carers

If an antibacterial is given, advise patients about directions for correct use and possible side-effects using verbal and written information.

If an antibacterial is **not** given, advise patients about an antibacterial not being needed currently—discuss alternative options as appropriate, such as self-care with over-the-counter preparations, back-up (delayed) prescribing, or other non-pharmacological interventions.

Patients should be advised to seek medical help if symptoms worsen rapidly or significantly at any time, if symptoms do not start to improve within an agreed time, if problems arise as a result of treatment, or if the patient becomes systemically very unwell.

For further information on advice for patients and their family and/or carers when deciding if antibacterial treatment is necessary, see *Advice for patients and their family and/or carers* in Antimicrobial stewardship p. 20.

Antibacterials, considerations during therapy

EvGr Review choice of antibacterial if susceptibility results indicate bacterial resistance and symptoms are not improving—consult local microbiologist as needed. ⒶIf no bacterium is cultured, the antibacterial can be continued or stopped on clinical grounds.

EvGr Review intravenous antibacterials within 48 hours and consider stepping down to oral antibacterials where possible. Ⓐ

Superinfection

In general, broad-spectrum antibacterial drugs such as the cephalosporins are more likely to be associated with adverse reactions related to the selection of resistant organisms e.g.

fungal infections or antibiotic-associated colitis (pseudomembranous colitis); other problems associated with superinfection include vaginitis and pruritus ani.

Notifiable diseases

In England and Wales, registered medical practitioners must notify the proper officer at their local council or local health protection team of any patient(s) suspected of suffering from any of the diseases listed below; a notification form should be completed immediately. For further information on reporting notifiable diseases, see **Public Health England** collection at: www.gov.uk/government/collections/notifications-of-infectious-diseases-noids.

Anthrax	Mumps
Botulism	Paratyphoid fever
Brucellosis	Plague
Cholera	Poliomyelitis (acute)
COVID-19	Rabies
Diarrhoea (infectious bloody)	Rubella
Diphtheria	Severe acute respiratory
Encephalitis, acute	syndrome (SARS)
Food poisoning	Scarlet fever
Haemolytic uraemic syndrome	Smallpox
(HUS)	Streptococcal disease (Group A,
Haemorrhagic fever (viral)	invasive)
Hepatitis (acute infectious)	Tetanus
Legionnaires' disease	Tuberculosis
Leprosy	Typhoid fever
Malaria	Typhus
Measles	Whooping cough
Meningitis (acute)	Yellow fever
Meningococcal septicaemia	

Note It is good practice for registered medical practitioners to report other diseases that may present a significant risk to human health. These should be done under the category 'other significant disease'.

In Northern Ireland, information on notifiable diseases is available from the **Department of Health** (www.health-ni.gov. uk/articles/public-health-act-northern-ireland-1967).

In Scotland, information on notifiable diseases is available from **Health Protection Scotland** (www.hps.scot.nhs.uk/web-resources-container/notification-of-infectious-disease-or-health-risk-state-form/).

Sepsis, early management

EvGr Patients identified as being at high risk of severe illness or death due to suspected sepsis should be given a broad-spectrum antibacterial at the maximum recommended dose without delay (ideally within one hour). Microbiological samples and blood cultures must be taken prior to administration of antibiotics; the prescription should be adjusted subsequently according to susceptibility results.

A thorough clinical examination should be carried out to identify sources of infection. If the source of infection is identified, treat in line with local antibacterial guidance or susceptibility results.

Patients who require empirical intravenous treatment for a suspected infection, but who have no confirmed diagnosis, should be treated with an intravenous antibiotic from the local formulary and in line with national guidelines.

The need for intravenous fluids, inotropes, vasopressors and oxygen should also be assessed without delay, taking into consideration the patient's lactate concentration, systolic blood pressure, and their risk of severe illness or death. Patients at high risk should be monitored continuously if possible, and no less than every 30 minutes.

Patients with suspected sepsis who are not immediately deemed to be at high risk of severe illness or death, should be re-assessed regularly for the need for empirical treatment, taking into consideration all risk factors including lactate concentration and evidence of acute kidney injury. ⟨A⟩

Antibacterials, use for prophylaxis

17-Aug-2020

Rheumatic fever: prevention of recurrence

- Phenoxymethylpenicillin p. 581 or sulfadiazine p. 599.

Invasive group A streptococcal infection: prevention of secondary cases

- Phenoxymethylpenicillin.
- Patients who are penicillin allergic, either erythromycin p. 572 or azithromycin p. 568 [unlicensed indication].

For details of those who should receive chemoprophylaxis contact a consultant in communicable disease control (or a consultant in infectious diseases or the local Public Health England Laboratory).

Meningococcal meningitis: prevention of secondary cases

- Ciprofloxacin p. 593 or rifampicin p. 619 or i/m ceftriaxone p. 558 [unlicensed indication].

For details of those who should receive chemoprophylaxis contact a consultant in communicable disease control (or a consultant in infectious diseases or the local Public Health England laboratory). Unless there has been direct exposure of the mouth or nose to infectious droplets from a patient with meningococcal disease who has received less than 24 hours of antibacterial treatment, healthcare workers do not generally require chemoprophylaxis.

Haemophilus influenzae type b infection: prevention of secondary disease

Haemophilus influenzae type b (Hib) can cause severe life-threatening disease in healthy individuals. With invasive Hib disease, the index case has a small, but significant risk of secondary Hib infection, particularly within 6 months of the first episode. Close contacts of the index case (mainly in a household, or a pre-school or primary school setting) are also at increased risk of developing invasive Hib disease, especially within the first week of the index case becoming ill. Antibacterial prophylaxis aims to reduce the risk of secondary disease in the index case and among close contacts by eliminating asymptomatic pharyngeal carriage of Hib.

The following recommendations on antibacterial prophylaxis reflect advice from Public Health England's (PHE) guidance: **Revised recommendations for the prevention of secondary Haemophilus influenzae type b (Hib) disease** (see Useful resources).

For confirmed or probable cases of invasive Hib disease in all children aged under 10 years, and in individuals of any age who have a vulnerable individual (any individual who is immunosuppressed or has asplenia, or any child aged under 10 years old) in their household, antibacterial prophylaxis should be given prior to hospital discharge.

All household contacts of a confirmed or probable index case should be given antibacterial prophylaxis if there is a vulnerable individual in the household.

For a pre-school or primary school setting that has an outbreak (2 or more cases of invasive Hib disease within 120 days), antibacterial prophylaxis is recommended for all room contacts, including staff.

For a pre-school or primary school setting where the levels of contact are similar to those in a household (e.g. a small number of children attending the same child-minder for several hours each day), antibacterial prophylaxis for the close contact group should be considered.

For all eligible contacts, antibacterial prophylaxis should be offered up to 4 weeks after illness onset in the index case.

In addition to antibacterial prophylaxis, vaccination with a Hib-containing vaccine should be considered following a case of invasive Hib disease. For information on vaccination, see Post-exposure management of invasive Haemophilus influenzae type b disease in Haemophilus influenzae type b conjugate vaccine p. 1344.

Choice of antibacterial prophylaxis

- First line:
  ‣ Rifampicin;
  ‣ Alternative if rifampicin unsuitable: ceftriaxone [unlicensed] (based on limited evidence), or oral ciprofloxacin [unlicensed] or azithromycin [unlicensed] (however effectiveness in healthy individuals has not been determined).

Diphtheria in non-immune patients: prevention of secondary cases

- Erythromycin (or another macrolide e.g. azithromycin or clarithromycin p. 569).

Treat for further 10 days if nasopharyngeal swabs positive after first 7 days treatment.

Pertussis, antibacterial prophylaxis

- Clarithromycin (or azithromycin or erythromycin).

Within 3 weeks of onset of cough in the index case, give antibacterial prophylaxis to all close contacts if amongst them there is at least one unimmunised or partially immunised child under 1 year of age, or if there is at least one individual who has not received a pertussis-containing vaccine more than 1 week and less than 5 years ago (so long as that individual lives or works with children under 4 months of age, is pregnant at over 32 weeks gestation, or is a healthcare worker who works with children under 1 year of age or with pregnant women).

Pneumococcal infection in asplenia or in patients with sickle-cell disease, antibacterial prophylaxis

- Phenoxymethylpenicillin.
- If penicillin-allergic, erythromycin.

Antibacterial prophylaxis is not fully reliable. Antibacterial prophylaxis may be discontinued in children over 5 years of age with sickle-cell disease who have received pneumococcal immunisation and who do not have a history of severe pneumococcal infection.

Tuberculosis antibacterial prophylaxis in susceptible close contacts or those who have become tuberculin positive

See Close contacts and Treatment of latent tuberculosis under Tuberculosis p. 616.

Animal and human bites, antibacterial prophylaxis

- Co-amoxiclav p. 585 alone (or doxycycline p. 601+ metronidazole p. 575 if penicillin-allergic).

Cleanse wound thoroughly. For tetanus-prone wound, give human tetanus immunoglobulin p. 1337 (with a tetanus-containing vaccine if necessary, according to immunisation history and risk of infection).

Consider rabies prophylaxis for bites from animals in endemic countries. Assess risk of blood-borne viruses (including HIV, hepatitis B and C) and give appropriate prophylaxis to prevent viral spread.

Antibacterial prophylaxis recommended for wounds less than 48–72 hours old when the risk of infection is high (e.g. bites from humans or cats; bites to the hand, foot, face, or genital area; bites involving oedema, crush or puncture injury, or other moderate to severe injury; wounds that cannot be debrided adequately; patients with diabetes mellitus, cirrhosis, asplenia, prosthetic joints or valves, or those who are immunocompromised). Give antibacterial prophylaxis for up to 5 days.

Early-onset neonatal infection, antibacterial prophylaxis

- i/v benzylpenicillin sodium p. 580 (or i/v clindamycin p. 566 if history of allergy to penicillins).

Give intrapartum prophylaxis to women with group B streptococcal colonisation, bacteriuria, or infection in the current pregnancy, or to women who had a previous baby with an invasive group B streptococcal infection. Consider prophylaxis for women in preterm labour if there is prelabour rupture of membranes or if intrapartum rupture of membranes lasting more than 18 hours is suspected.

Gastro-intestinal procedures, antibacterial prophylaxis

Operations on stomach or oesophagus

- Single dose of i/v gentamicin p. 545 or i/v cefuroxime p. 555 or i/v co-amoxiclav (additional intra-operative or postoperative doses may be given for prolonged procedures or if there is major blood loss).

Intravenous antibacterial prophylaxis should be given up to 30 minutes before the procedure.

Add i/v teicoplanin p. 563 (or vancomycin p. 565) if high risk of meticillin-resistant *Staphylococcus aureus*.

Open biliary surgery

- Single dose of i/v cefuroxime p. 555+ i/v metronidazole p. 575 or i/v gentamicin p. 545+ i/v metronidazole or i/v co-amoxiclav p. 585 alone (additional intra-operative or postoperative doses may be given for prolonged procedures or if there is major blood loss).

Intravenous antibacterial prophylaxis should be given up to 30 minutes before the procedure.

Where i/v metronidazole is suggested, it may alternatively be given by suppository but to allow adequate absorption, it should be given 2 hours before surgery.

Add i/v teicoplanin p. 563 (or vancomycin p. 565) if high risk of meticillin-resistant *Staphylococcus aureus*.

Resections of colon and rectum for carcinoma, and resections in inflammatory bowel disease, and appendicectomy

- Single dose of i/v gentamicin + i/v metronidazole or i/v cefuroxime + i/v metronidazole or i/v co-amoxiclav alone (additional intra-operative or postoperative doses may be given for prolonged procedures or if there is major blood loss).

Intravenous antibacterial prophylaxis should be given up to 30 minutes before the procedure.

Where i/v metronidazole is suggested, it may alternatively be given by suppository but to allow adequate absorption, it should be given 2 hours before surgery.

Add i/v teicoplanin (or vancomycin) if high risk of meticillin-resistant *Staphylococcus aureus*.

Endoscopic retrograde cholangiopancreatography

- Single dose of i/v gentamicin or oral or i/v ciprofloxacin p. 593.

Intravenous antibacterial prophylaxis should be given up to 30 minutes before the procedure.

Prophylaxis recommended if pancreatic pseudocyst, immunocompromised, history of liver transplantation, or risk of incomplete biliary drainage. For biliary complications following liver transplantation, add i/v amoxicillin p. 582 or i/v teicoplanin (or vancomycin).

Percutaneous endoscopic gastrostomy or jejunostomy

- Single dose of i/v co-amoxiclav or i/v cefuroxime.

Intravenous antibacterial prophylaxis should be given up to 30 minutes before the procedure.

Use single dose of i/v clindamycin (or vancomycin) if history of allergy to penicillins or cephalosporins, or if high risk of meticillin-resistant *Staphylococcus aureus*.

Orthopaedic surgery, antibacterial prophylaxis

Joint replacement including hip and knee

- Single dose of i/v cefuroxime alone or i/v flucloxacillin p. 589+ i/v gentamicin (additional intra-operative or postoperative doses may be given for prolonged procedures or if there is major blood loss).

Intravenous antibacterial prophylaxis should be given up to 30 minutes before the procedure.

If history of allergy to penicillins or to cephalosporins or if high risk of meticillin-resistant *Staphylococcus aureus*, use single dose of i/v teicoplanin (or vancomycin) + i/v gentamicin (additional intra-operative or postoperative doses may be given for prolonged procedures or if there is major blood loss).

Closed fractures

- Single dose of i/v cefuroxime or i/v flucloxacillin (additional intra-operative or postoperative doses may be given for prolonged procedures or if there is major blood loss).

Intravenous antibacterial prophylaxis should be given up to 30 minutes before the procedure.

If history of allergy to penicillins or to cephalosporins or if high risk of meticillin-resistant *Staphylococcus aureus*, use single dose of i/v teicoplanin (or vancomycin) (additional intra-operative or postoperative doses may be given for prolonged procedures or if there is major blood loss).

Open fractures

- Use i/v co-amoxiclav alone or i/v cefuroxime + i/v metronidazole (or i/v clindamycin p. 566 alone if history of allergy to penicillins or to cephalosporins).

Add i/v teicoplanin (or vancomycin) if high risk of meticillin-resistant *Staphylococcus aureus*. Start prophylaxis within 3 hours of injury and continue until soft tissue closure (max. 72 hours).

At first debridement also use a single dose of i/v cefuroxime + i/v metronidazole + i/v gentamicin or i/v co-amoxiclav + i/v gentamicin (or i/v clindamycin + i/v gentamicin if history of allergy to penicillins or to cephalosporins).

At time of skeletal stabilisation and definitive soft tissue closure use a single dose of i/v gentamicin + i/v teicoplanin (or vancomycin) (intravenous antibacterial prophylaxis should be given up to 30 minutes before the procedure).

High lower-limb amputation

- Use i/v co-amoxiclav alone or i/v cefuroxime + i/v metronidazole.

Intravenous antibacterial prophylaxis should be given up to 30 minutes before the procedure.

Continue antibacterial prophylaxis for at least 2 doses after procedure (max. duration of prophylaxis 5 days). If history of allergy to penicillin or to cephalosporins or if high risk of meticillin-resistant *Staphylococcus aureus*, use i/v teicoplanin (or vancomycin) + i/v gentamicin + i/v metronidazole.

Where i/v metronidazole is suggested, it may alternatively be given by suppository but to allow adequate absorption, it should be given 2 hours before surgery.

Urological procedures, antibacterial prophylaxis

Transrectal prostate biopsy

- Single dose of oral ciprofloxacin + oral metronidazole or i/v gentamicin + i/v metronidazole (additional intra-operative or postoperative doses may be given for prolonged procedures or if there is major blood loss).

Intravenous antibacterial prophylaxis should be given up to 30 minutes before the procedure.

Use single dose of i/v gentamicin + i/v metronidazole if high risk of meticillin-resistant *Staphylococcus aureus* (additional intra-operative or postoperative doses of antibacterial may be given for prolonged procedures or if there is major blood loss).

Where i/v metronidazole is suggested, it may alternatively be given by suppository but to allow adequate absorption, it should be given 2 hours before surgery.

Transurethral resection of prostate

- Single dose of oral ciprofloxacin *or* i/v gentamicin *or* i/v cefuroxime (additional intra-operative or postoperative doses may be given for prolonged procedures or if there is major blood loss).

Intravenous antibacterial prophylaxis should be given up to 30 minutes before the procedure.

Use single dose of i/v gentamicin if high risk of meticillin-resistant *Staphylococcus aureus* (additional intra-operative or postoperative doses may be given for prolonged procedures or if there is major blood loss).

Obstetric and gynaecological surgery, antibacterial prophylaxis

Caesarean section

- Single dose of i/v cefuroxime (additional intra-operative or postoperative doses may be given for prolonged procedures or if there is major blood loss).

Intravenous antibacterial prophylaxis should be given up to 30 minutes before the procedure.

Substitute i/v clindamycin if history of allergy to penicillins or cephalosporins. Add i/v teicoplanin (*or* vancomycin) if high risk of meticillin-resistant *Staphylococcus aureus*.

Hysterectomy

- Single dose of i/v cefuroxime + i/v metronidazole *or* i/v gentamicin + i/v metronidazole *or* i/v co-amoxiclav alone (additional intra-operative or postoperative doses may be given for prolonged procedures or if there is major blood loss).

Intravenous antibacterial prophylaxis should be given up to 30 minutes before the procedure.

Use single dose of i/v gentamicin + i/v metronidazole or add i/v teicoplanin (*or* vancomycin) to other regimens if high risk of meticillin-resistant *Staphylococcus aureus* (additional intra-operative or postoperative doses may be given for prolonged procedures or if there is major blood loss).

Where i/v metronidazole p. 575 is suggested, it may alternatively be given by suppository but to allow adequate absorption, it should be given 2 hours before surgery.

Termination of pregnancy

- Single dose of oral metronidazole (additional intra-operative or postoperative doses may be given for prolonged procedures or if there is major blood loss).

If genital chlamydial infection cannot be ruled out, give doxycycline p. 601 postoperatively.

Cardiology procedures, antibacterial prophylaxis

Cardiac pacemaker insertion

- Single dose of i/v cefuroxime p. 555 alone *or* i/v flucloxacillin p. 589+ i/v gentamicin p. 545 *or* i/v teicoplanin p. 563 (*or* vancomycin p. 565) + i/v gentamicin (additional intra-operative or postoperative doses may be given for prolonged procedures or if there is major blood loss).

Intravenous antibacterial prophylaxis should be given up to 30 minutes before the procedure.

Use single dose of i/v teicoplanin (*or* vancomycin) + i/v cefuroxime *or* i/v teicoplanin (*or* vancomycin) + i/v gentamicin if high risk of meticillin-resistant *Staphylococcus aureus* (additional intra-operative or postoperative doses may be given for prolonged procedures or if there is major blood loss).

Vascular surgery, antibacterial prophylaxis

Reconstructive arterial surgery of abdomen, pelvis or legs

- Single dose of i/v cefuroxime alone *or* i/v flucloxacillin + i/v gentamicin (additional intra-operative or postoperative doses may be given for prolonged procedures or if there is major blood loss).

Intravenous antibacterial prophylaxis should be given up to 30 minutes before the procedure.

Add i/v metronidazole for patients at risk from anaerobic infections including those with diabetes, gangrene, or undergoing amputation. Use single dose of i/v teicoplanin (*or* vancomycin) + i/v gentamicin if history of allergy to penicillins or cephalosporins, or if high risk of meticillin-resistant *Staphylococcus aureus* (additional intra-operative or postoperative doses may be given for prolonged procedures or if there is major blood loss).

Infective endocarditis, antibacterial prophylaxis

NICE guidance: Antimicrobial prophylaxis against infective endocarditis in adults and children undergoing interventional procedures (March 2008, updated 2016)

- Chlorhexidine mouthwash is **not** recommended for the prevention of infective endocarditis in at risk patients undergoing dental procedures.

Antibacterial prophylaxis is **not** *routinely* recommended for the prevention of infective endocarditis in patients undergoing the following procedures:

- dental;
- upper and lower respiratory tract (including ear, nose, and throat procedures and bronchoscopy);
- genito-urinary tract (including urological, gynaecological, and obstetric procedures);
- upper and lower gastro-intestinal tract.

Whilst these procedures can cause bacteraemia, there is no clear association with the development of infective endocarditis. Prophylaxis may expose patients to the adverse effects of antimicrobials when the evidence of benefit has not been proven.

Any infection in patients at risk of endocarditis should be investigated promptly and treated appropriately to reduce the risk of endocarditis.

If patients at risk of endocarditis are undergoing a gastro-intestinal or genito-urinary tract procedure at a site where infection is suspected, they should receive appropriate antibacterial therapy that includes cover against organisms that cause infective endocarditis.

Patients at risk of infective endocarditis should be:

- advised to maintain good oral hygiene;
- told how to recognise signs of infective endocarditis, and advised when to seek expert advice.

Patients at risk of infective endocarditis include those with valve replacement, acquired valvular heart disease with stenosis or regurgitation, structural congenital heart disease (including surgically corrected or palliated structural conditions, but excluding isolated atrial septal defect, fully repaired ventricular septal defect, fully repaired patent ductus arteriosus, and closure devices considered to be endothelialised), hypertrophic cardiomyopathy, or a previous episode of infective endocarditis.

Dermatological procedures

Advice of a Working Party of the British Society for Antimicrobial Chemotherapy is that patients who undergo dermatological procedures do not require antibacterial prophylaxis against endocarditis.

The British Association of Dermatologists Therapy Guidelines and Audit Subcommittee advise that such dermatological procedures include skin biopsies and excision of moles or of malignant lesions.

Joint prostheses and dental treatment, antibacterial prophylaxis

Advice of a Working Party of the British Society for Antimicrobial Chemotherapy is that patients with prosthetic joint implants (including total hip replacements) do not require antibiotic prophylaxis for dental treatment. The Working Party considers that it is unacceptable to expose patients to the adverse effects of antibiotics when there is no evidence that such prophylaxis is of any benefit, but that those who develop any intercurrent infection require prompt treatment with antibiotics to which the infecting organisms are sensitive.

The Working Party has commented that joint infections have rarely been shown to follow dental procedures and are even more rarely caused by oral streptococci.

Immunosuppression and indwelling intraperitoneal catheters

Advice of a Working Party of the British Society for Antimicrobial Chemotherapy is that patients who are immunosuppressed (including transplant patients) and patients with indwelling intraperitoneal catheters do not require antibiotic prophylaxis for dental treatment provided there is no other indication for prophylaxis.

The Working Party has commented that there is little evidence that dental treatment is followed by infection in immunosuppressed and immunodeficient patients nor is there evidence that dental treatment is followed by infection in patients with indwelling intraperitoneal catheters.

Useful Resources

Revised recommendations for the prevention of secondary *Haemophilus influenzae* type b (Hib) disease. Public Health England. 2009, updated July 2013. www.gov.uk/government/publications/haemophilus-influenzae-type-b-hib-revised-recommendations-for-the-prevention-of-secondary-cases

Blood infections, antibacterial therapy

Septicaemia (community-acquired)

- A broad-spectrum antipseudomonal penicillin (e.g. piperacillin with tazobactam p. 579, ticarcillin with clavulanic acid) *or* a broad-spectrum cephalosporin (e.g. cefuroxime p. 555)
- If meticillin-resistant *Staphylococcus aureus* suspected, add vancomycin p. 565 (*or* teicoplanin p. 563).
- If anaerobic infection suspected, add metronidazole p. 575 to broad-spectrum cephalosporin.
- If other resistant micro-organisms suspected, use a more broad-spectrum beta-lactam antibacterial (e.g. meropenem p. 550).

Septicaemia (hospital-acquired)

- A broad-spectrum antipseudomonal beta-lactam antibacterial (e.g. piperacillin with tazobactam, ticarcillin with clavulanic acid, ceftazidime p. 557, imipenem with cilastatin p. 549, *or* meropenem)
- If meticillin-resistant *Staphylococcus aureus* suspected, add vancomycin (*or* teicoplanin).

- If anaerobic infection suspected, add metronidazole to broad-spectrum cephalosporin

Septicaemia related to vascular catheter

- Vancomycin (*or* teicoplanin)
- If Gram-negative sepsis suspected, especially in the immunocompromised, add a broad-spectrum antipseudomonal beta-lactam.
- Consider removing vascular catheter, particularly if infection caused by *Staphylococcus aureus*, pseudomonas, or *Candida* species.

Meningococcal septicaemia

If meningococcal disease suspected, a single dose of benzylpenicillin sodium p. 580 should be given before urgent transfer to hospital, so long as this does not delay the transfer; cefotaxime p. 557 may be an alternative in penicillin allergy; chloramphenicol p. 605 may be used if history of immediate hypersensitivity reaction to penicillin or to cephalosporins.

- Benzylpenicillin sodium or cefotaxime (*or* ceftriaxone p. 558)
- *If history of immediate hypersensitivity reaction to penicillin or to cephalosporins*, chloramphenicol

To eliminate nasopharyngeal carriage, ciprofloxacin p. 593, or rifampicin p. 619, or ceftriaxone may be used.

Cardiovascular system infections, antibacterial therapy

Endocarditis: initial 'blind' therapy

- *Native valve endocarditis*, amoxicillin p. 582 (*or* ampicillin p. 584)
- Consider adding low-dose gentamicin p. 545
- If penicillin-allergic, or if meticillin-resistant *Staphylococcus aureus* suspected, or if severe sepsis, use vancomycin p. 565+ low-dose gentamicin
- If severe sepsis with risk factors for Gram-negative infection, use vancomycin + meropenem p. 550
- *If prosthetic valve endocarditis*, vancomycin + rifampicin p. 619+ low-dose gentamicin

Endocarditis (native valve) caused by staphylococci

- Flucloxacillin p. 589
- *Suggested duration of treatment* 4 weeks (at least 6 weeks if secondary lung abscess or osteomyelitis also present)
- *If penicillin-allergic or if meticillin-resistant Staphylococcus aureus*, vancomycin + rifampicin
- *Suggested duration of treatment* 4 weeks (at least 6 weeks if secondary lung absecess or osteomyelitis also present)

Endocarditis (prosthetic valve) caused by staphylococci

- Flucloxacillin + rifampicin + low-dose gentamicin
- *Suggested duration of treatment* at least 6 weeks; review need to continue gentamicin at 2 weeks—seek specialist advice if gentamicin considered necessary beyond 2 weeks
- *If penicillin-allergic or if meticillin-resistant Staphylococcus aureus*, vancomycin + rifampicin + low-dose gentamicin
- *Suggested duration of treatment* at least 6 weeks; review need to continue gentamicin at 2 weeks—seek specialist advice if gentamicin considered necessary beyond 2 weeks

Endocarditis caused by fully-sensitive streptococci

- Benzylpenicillin sodium p. 580
- ▸ *Suggested duration of treatment* 4–6 weeks (6 weeks for prosthetic valve endocarditis)
- *If penicillin-allergic*, vancomycin (*or* teicoplanin p. 563) + low-dose gentamicin
- ▸ *Suggested duration of treatment* 4–6 weeks (stop gentamicin after 2 weeks)

Endocarditis caused by less-sensitive streptococci

- Benzylpenicillin sodium + low-dose gentamicin
- ▸ *Suggested duration of treatment* 4–6 weeks (6 weeks for prosthetic valve endocarditis); review need to continue gentamicin at 2 weeks—seek specialist advice if gentamicin considered necessary beyond 2 weeks; stop gentamicin at 2 weeks if micro-organisms moderately sensitive to penicillin
- *If penicillin-allergic or highly penicillin-resistant*, vancomycin (*or* teicoplanin) + low-dose gentamicin
- ▸ *Suggested duration of treatment* 4–6 weeks (6 weeks for prosthetic valve endocarditis); review need to continue gentamicin at 2 weeks—seek specialist advice if gentamicin considered necessary beyond 2 weeks; stop gentamicin at 2 weeks if micro-organisms moderately sensitive to penicillin

Endocarditis caused by enterococci

- Amoxicillin (*or* ampicillin) + low dose gentamicin *or* benzylpenicillin sodium + low-dose gentamicin
- ▸ *Suggested duration of treatment* 4–6 weeks (6 weeks for prosthetic valve endocarditis); review need to continue gentamicin at 2 weeks—seek specialist advice if gentamicin considered necessary beyond 2 weeks
- *If penicillin-allergic or penicillin-resistant*, vancomycin (*or* teicoplanin) + low-dose gentamicin
- ▸ *Suggested duration of treatment* 4–6 weeks (6 weeks for prosthetic valve endocarditis); review need to continue gentamicin at 2 weeks—seek specialist advice if gentamicin considered necessary beyond 2 weeks
- If gentamicin resistant, amoxicillin (*or* ampicillin)
- ▸ Add streptomycin p. 547 (if susceptible) for 2 weeks
- ▸ *Suggested duration of treatment* at least 6 weeks

Endocarditis caused by *Haemophilus, Actinobacillus, Cardiobacterium, Eikenella,* and *Kingella* species ('HACEK' micro-organisms)

- Amoxicillin (*or* ampicillin) + low-dose gentamicin
- ▸ *Suggested duration of treatment* 4 weeks (6 weeks for prosthetic valve endocarditis); stop gentamicin after 2 weeks
- *If* amoxicillin *-resistant*, ceftriaxone p. 558 (*or* cefotaxime p. 557) + low-dose gentamicin
- ▸ *Suggested duration of treatment* 4 weeks (6 weeks for prosthetic valve endocarditis); stop gentamicin after 2 weeks

Central nervous system infections, antibacterial therapy

Meningitis: initial empirical therapy

- Transfer patient to hospital urgently.
- If *meningococcal disease* (meningitis with non-blanching rash or meningococcal septicaemia) suspected, benzylpenicillin sodium p. 580 should be given before transfer to hospital, so long as this does not delay the transfer. If a patient with suspected bacterial meningitis

without non-blanching rash cannot be transferred to hospital urgently, benzylpenicillin sodium should be given before the transfer. Cefotaxime p. 557 may be an alternative in penicillin allergy; chloramphenicol p. 605 may be used if history of immediate hypersensitivity reaction to penicillin or to cephalosporins.
- In hospital, consider adjunctive treatment with dexamethasone p. 714 (particularly if pneumococcal meningitis suspected in adults), preferably starting before or with first dose of antibacterial, but no later than 12 hours after starting antibacterial; avoid dexamethasone in septic shock, meningococcal septicaemia, or if immunocompromised, or in meningitis following surgery.

In hospital, if aetiology unknown:

- *Adult and child* 3 *months–50 years*, cefotaxime (*or* ceftriaxone p. 558)
- ▸ Consider adding vancomycin p. 565 if prolonged or multiple use of other antibacterials in the last 3 months, or if travelled, in the last 3 months, to areas outside the UK with highly penicillin- and cephalosporin-resistant pneumococci.
- ▸ *Suggested duration of treatment* at least 10 days
- *Adult over* 50 *years* cefotaxime (*or* ceftriaxone) + amoxicillin p. 582 (*or* ampicillin p. 584)
- ▸ Consider adding vancomycin if prolonged or multiple use of other antibacterials in the last 3 months, or if travelled, in the last 3 months, to areas outside the UK with highly penicillin- and cephalosporin-resistant pneumococci.
- ▸ *Suggested duration of treatment* at least 10 days

Meningitis caused by meningococci

- Benzylpenicillin sodium *or* cefotaxime (*or* ceftriaxone)
- ▸ *Suggested duration of treatment* 7 days.
- *If history of immediate hypersensitivity reaction to penicillin or to cephalosporins*, chloramphenicol
- ▸ *Suggested duration of treatment* 7 days.

Meningitis caused by pneumococci

- Cefotaxime (*or* ceftriaxone)
- ▸ Consider adjunctive treatment with dexamethasone, preferably starting before or with first dose of antibacterial, but no later than 12 hours after starting antibacterial (may reduce penetration of vancomycin into cerebrospinal fluid).
- ▸ If micro-organism penicillin-sensitive, replace cefotaxime with benzylpenicillin sodium.
- ▸ If micro-organism highly penicillin- and cephalosporin-resistant, add vancomycin and if necessary rifampicin p. 619.
- ▸ *Suggested duration of antibacterial treatment* 14 days

Meningitis caused by *Haemophilus influenzae*

- Cefotaxime (*or* ceftriaxone)
- ▸ Consider adjunctive treatment with dexamethasone, preferably starting before or with first dose of antibacterial, but no later than 12 hours after starting antibacterial.
- ▸ *Suggested duration of antibacterial treatment* 10 days.
- ▸ For *H. influenzae* type b give rifampicin for 4 days before hospital discharge to those under 10 years of age or to those in contact with vulnerable household contacts
- *If history of immediate hypersensitivity reaction to penicillin or to cephalosporins, or if micro-organism resistant to* cefotaxime , chloramphenicol
- ▸ Consider adjunctive treatment with dexamethasone, preferably starting before or with first dose of antibacterial, but no later than 12 hours after starting antibacterial.
- ▸ *Suggested duration of antibacterial treatment* 10 days.
- ▸ For *H. influenzae* type b give rifampicin for 4 days before

5

Infection

hospital discharge to those under 10 years of age or to those in contact with vulnerable household contacts

Meningitis caused by Listeria

- Amoxicillin (*or* ampicillin) + gentamicin p. 545
  - ▸ *Suggested duration of treatment* 21 days.
  - ▸ Consider stopping gentamicin after 7 days.
- *If history of immediate hypersensitivity reaction to penicillin,* co-trimoxazole p. 598
  - ▸ *Suggested duration of treatment* 21 days.

Diabetic foot infections, antibacterial therapy

13-Nov-2019

Diabetic foot infection

Diabetic foot infection is defined as any type of skin, soft tissue or bone infection below the ankle in patients with diabetes. It includes cellulitis, paronychia, abscesses, myositis, tendonitis, necrotising fasciitis, osteomyelitis, and septic arthritis. It is defined clinically by the presence of at least 2 of the following: local swelling or induration, erythema, local tenderness or pain, local warmth, or purulent discharge.

For guidance on classification of infection severity, see NICE guideline: **Diabetic foot problems** (see *Useful resources*).

Treatment

EvGr Refer patients immediately to acute services and inform the multidisciplinary foot care service if they have a limb-threatening or life-threatening problem, such as ulceration with fever or any signs of sepsis, ulceration with limb ischaemia, or gangrene.

Antibacterial treatment should be started as soon as possible if diabetic foot infection is suspected. Samples (such as soft tissue, bone sample, or deep swab) should be taken for microbiological testing before, or as close as possible to, the start of antibacterial treatment.

Offer an antibacterial taking into account the severity of infection, risk of complications, previous microbiological results, recent antibacterial use, and patient preferences. ⒶEvGr

For other considerations such as switching from intravenous to oral antibacterials, and for advice to be given to patients, see Antibacterials, principles of therapy p. 527.

Reassessment

EvGr Reassess if symptoms worsen rapidly or significantly at any time, do not start to improve within 1–2 days of starting antibacterial treatment, or the patient becomes systemically very unwell or has severe pain out of proportion to the infection. Take into account other diagnoses (such as pressure sores, gout, or non-infected ulcers), signs and symptoms of a more serious illness (such as limb ischaemia, osteomyelitis, necrotising fasciitis, or sepsis), and previous antibacterial use.

Review the choice of antibacterial when microbiological results are available and change according to the results, using a narrower-spectrum antibacterial if appropriate. ⒶEvGr

Choice of antibacterial therapy

EvGr Treatment should be based on clinical assessment, infection severity, suspected micro-organism, and be guided by microbiological results when available. Treatment duration should be based on the severity of infection, and clinical assessment of response to treatment. Review the need for continued antibacterials regularly.

Offer oral antibacterials to patients who are able to take oral treatment and the severity of their condition does not require intravenous treatment. ⒶEvGr

Mild infection
- ***Oral** first line* :
  - ▸ EvGr Flucloxacillin p. 589.
  - ▸ Alternative in penicillin allergy or flucloxacillin unsuitable: clarithromycin p. 569, doxycycline p. 601, or erythromycin p. 572 (in pregnancy). Ⓐ

Moderate or severe infection
Treatment duration is based on clinical assessment; minimum of 7 days and up to 6 weeks for osteomyelitis (use oral antibacterials for prolonged treatment). In severe infection, intravenous antibacterials should be given for at least 48 hours (until stabilised).

- ***Oral** or **Intravenous** first line* :
  - ▸ EvGr Flucloxacillin **with** or **without** intravenous gentamicin p. 545 **and/or** metronidazole p. 575, *or* co-amoxiclav p. 585 **with** or **without** intravenous gentamicin p. 545, *or* intravenous ceftriaxone p. 558 **with** metronidazole p. 575.
  - ▸ Alternative in penicillin allergy: co-trimoxazole p. 598 [unlicensed] **with** or **without** intravenous gentamicin p. 545 **and/or** metronidazole p. 575.
  - ▸ Additional antibacterial choices if *Pseudomonas aeruginosa* suspected or confirmed: intravenous piperacillin with tazobactam p. 579, *or* clindamycin p. 566 **with** ciprofloxacin p. 593 **and/or** intravenous gentamicin p. 545.
  - ▸ If meticillin-resistant *Staphylococcus aureus* (MRSA) confirmed or suspected **add** intravenous vancomycin p. 565, *or* intravenous teicoplanin p. 563, or linezolid p. 609 (specialist use only if vancomycin or teicoplanin cannot be used).
  - ▸ Other antibacterials may be appropriate based on microbiological results and specialist advice. Ⓐ

Useful Resources

Diabetic foot problems: prevention and management. National Institute for Health and Care Excellence. NICE guideline 19. August 2015, updated October 2019. www.nice.org.uk/guidance/ng19

Ear infections, antibacterial therapy

03-Sep-2018

Otitis externa

Otitis externa can be triggered by a bacterial infection caused by *Pseudomonas aeruginosa* or *Staphylococcus aureus*. Consider systemic antibacterial if spreading cellulitis or patient systemically unwell.

Choice of antibacterial therapy
No penicillin allergy
- Flucloxacillin p. 589

Penicillin allergy or intolerance
- Clarithromycin p. 569 (*or* azithromycin p. 568 *or* erythromycin p. 572)

If pseudomonas suspected
- Ciprofloxacin p. 593 (*or* an aminoglycoside)

For topical treatments, see *Otitis externa*, under Ear p. 1238.

Otitis media

Acute otitis media is an inflammation in the middle ear associated with effusion and accompanied by an ear infection. Acute otitis media is commonly seen in children and is generally caused by viruses (respiratory syncytial virus and rhinovirus) or bacteria (*Haemophilus influenzae, Streptococcus pneumoniae, Streptococcus pyogenes,* and *Moraxella catarrhalis*); both virus and bacteria often co-exist. For further information see *Acute otitis media* in Ear p. 1238.

EvGr Antibacterial therapy should be offered to children with acute otitis media who are systemically very unwell, have signs and symptoms of a more serious illness, or those who are at high-risk of serious complications due to pre-existing comorbidities. Antibacterial therapy should also be considered if otorrhoea (discharge following perforation of the eardrum) is present, or in children under 2 years of age with bilateral otitis media. Ⓐ

Choice of antibacterial therapy in children

No penicillin allergy

- *First line*: EvGr amoxicillin p. 582. Ⓐ
- *Second line* (worsening symptoms despite 2 to 3 days of antibacterial treatment): EvGr co-amoxiclav p. 585. Ⓐ

Penicillin allergy or intolerance

- *First line*: EvGr clarithromycin p. 569 or erythromycin p. 572 (preferred in pregnancy). Ⓐ
- *Second line* (worsening symptoms despite 2 to 3 days of antibacterial treatment): EvGr Consult local microbiologist. Ⓐ

Eye infections, antibacterial therapy

Conjunctivitis (purulent)

- Chloramphenicol eye drops p. 1217.

Gastro-intestinal system infections, antibacterial therapy

20-Feb-2020

Gastro-enteritis

Frequently self-limiting and may not be bacterial.

- Antibacterial not usually indicated

Campylobacter enteritis

Frequently self-limiting; treat if immunocompromised or if severe infection.

- Clarithromycin p. 569 (*or* azithromycin p. 568 *or* erythromycin p. 572)
- *Alternative*, ciprofloxacin p. 593
  - ▸ Strains with decreased sensitivity to ciprofloxacin isolated frequently

Diverticulitis, acute

Acute diverticulitis is a condition where diverticula (small pouches protruding from the walls of the large intestine) suddenly become inflamed or infected. Complicated acute diverticulitis refers to diverticulitis associated with complications such as abscess, bowel perforation and peritonitis, fistula, intestinal obstruction, haemorrhage, or sepsis. For further information on acute diverticulitis including the non-antibacterial management, see Diverticular disease and diverticulitis p. 40.

Treatment

EvGr For patients with acute diverticulitis who are systemically well, consider a watchful waiting and a no antibacterial prescribing strategy. Advise patients to re-present if symptoms persist or worsen.

For patients who are systemically unwell, immunosuppressed, or have significant comorbidities, an antibacterial prescribing strategy should be offered.

Oral antibacterials should be offered to patients who are systemically unwell but do not meet the referral criteria for suspected complicated acute diverticulitis.

Patients with persistent or worsening symptoms should be reassessed in primary care and considered for referral to hospital for further assessment.

Patients with suspected complicated acute diverticulitis and uncontrolled abdominal pain should be referred for same-day hospital assessment.

Patients admitted to hospital with suspected or confirmed complicated acute diverticulitis should be treated with intravenous antibacterials. Ⓐ For guidance on the management of suspected sepsis, see NICE guideline **Sepsis** at: www.nice.org.uk/guidance/ng51.

For other considerations such as switching from intravenous to oral antibacterials, and for advice to be given to patients, see Antibacterials, principles of therapy p. 527.

EvGr Antibacterial prophylaxis is not recommended to prevent recurrent acute diverticulitis. Ⓐ

Choice of antibacterial therapy

EvGr Patients unable to take oral treatment should be referred to hospital. Ⓐ

Suspected or confirmed **uncomplicated** acute diverticulitis

- *Oral* first line :
  - ▸ EvGr Co-amoxiclav p. 585.
  - ▸ Alternative in penicillin allergy or co-amoxiclav unsuitable: cefalexin p. 552 (caution in penicillin allergy) **with** metronidazole p. 575, *or* trimethoprim p. 610 **with** metronidazole p. 575, *or* ciprofloxacin p. 593 (only if switching from intravenous route with specialist advice) **with** metronidazole p. 575. Ⓐ

Suspected or confirmed **complicated** acute diverticulitis

- *Intravenous* first line :
  - ▸ EvGr Co-amoxiclav, *or* cefuroxime p. 555 **with** metronidazole p. 575, *or* amoxicillin p. 582 **with** gentamicin p. 545 **and** metronidazole p. 575.
  - ▸ Alternative in penicillin and cephalosporins allergy: ciprofloxacin p. 593 **with** metronidazole p. 575.
  - ▸ For alternative antibacterials consult local microbiologist. Ⓐ

Salmonella (non-typhoid)

Treat invasive or severe infection. Do not treat less severe infection unless there is a risk of developing invasive infection (e.g. immunocompromised patients, those with haemoglobinopathy, or children under 6 months of age).

- Ciprofloxacin *or* cefotaxime p. 557

Shigellosis

Antibacterial not indicated for mild cases.

- Ciprofloxacin *or* azithromycin
- *Alternatives if micro-organism sensitive*, amoxicillin p. 582 *or* trimethoprim p. 610

Typhoid fever

Infections from Middle-East, South Asia, and South-East Asia may be multiple-antibacterial-resistant and sensitivity should be tested.

- Cefotaxime (*or* ceftriaxone p. 558)
  - ▸ azithromycin may be an alternative in mild or moderate disease caused by multiple-antibacterial-resistant organisms.
- *Alternative if micro-organism sensitive*, ciprofloxacin

Clostridioides difficile infection

Clostridioides difficile infection is caused by colonisation of the colon with *Clostridioides difficile* and production of toxin. It often follows antibiotic therapy and is usually of acute onset, but may become chronic. It is a particular hazard of ampicillin p. 584, amoxicillin, co-amoxiclav, second- and third-generation cephalosporins, clindamycin p. 566, and quinolones, but few antibiotics are free of this side-effect. Treatment options include metronidazole p. 575, vancomycin p. 565, and fidaxomicin p. 606.

- *For first episode of mild to moderate infection*, oral metronidazole
  - ▸ *Suggested duration of treatment* 10–14 days

- *For second or subsequent episode of infection, for severe infection, for infection not responding to* metronidazole , *or in patients intolerant of* metronidazole, oral vancomycin
▸ For severe infection in patients with multiple co-morbidities who are receiving treatment with other antibacterials, or for second or subsequent episode of infection, fidaxomicin can replace vancomycin
- *Suggested duration of treatment* 10–14 days
- *For infection not responding to* vancomycin *or* fidaxomicin , *for life-threatening infection, or in patients with ileus*, oral vancomycin + i/v metronidazole
▸ For infection not responding to vancomycin in patients without life-threatening infection or ileus, fidaxomicin can be used instead of vancomycin + metronidazole
- *Suggested duration of treatment* 10–14 days

Biliary-tract infection

- Ciprofloxacin *or* gentamicin p. 545 *or* a cephalosporin

Peritonitis

- A cephalosporin + metronidazole *or* gentamicin + metronidazole *or* gentamicin + clindamycin *or* piperacillin with tazobactam p. 579 alone

Peritonitis: peritoneal dialysis-associated

- Vancomycin (*or* teicoplanin p. 563) + ceftazidime p. 557 added to dialysis fluid *or* vancomycin added to dialysis fluid + ciprofloxacin by mouth
▸ *Suggested duration of treatment* 14 days or longer

Genital system infections, antibacterial therapy

07-Feb-2020

Bacterial vaginosis

- Oral metronidazole p. 575
▸ *Suggested duration of treatment* 5–7 days (or high-dose metronidazole as a single dose)
- *Alternatively*, topical metronidazole for 5 days *or* topical clindamycin p. 566 for 7 days

Uncomplicated genital chlamydial infection, non-gonococcal urethritis, and non-specific genital infection

Contact tracing recommended.

- Azithromycin p. 568 *or* doxycycline p. 601
▸ *Suggested duration of treatment* azithromycin as a single dose or doxycycline for 7 days
- *Alternatively*, erythromycin p. 572.
▸ *Suggested duration of treatment* 14 days

Gonorrhoea: uncomplicated

EvGr Contact tracing and test of cure following treatment are recommended. Consider chlamydia co-infection. Treatment is only recommended for those presenting within 14 days of exposure, or those presenting 14 days after exposure with a positive test. Sexual intercourse should be avoided until 7 days after patients and their partner(s) have completed treatment. Choice of alternative antibacterial regimen depends on locality where infection is acquired. Ⓐ

- *First line*:
▸ EvGr If antimicrobial susceptibility unknown: intramuscular ceftriaxone p. 558.
▸ If micro-organism is sensitive to ciprofloxacin: oral ciprofloxacin p. 593. Ⓐ
- *Alternatives due to allergy, needle phobia or contra-indications*:

▸ EvGr Intramuscular gentamicin p. 545 **plus** oral azithromycin.
▸ If parenteral administration is not possible: oral cefixime p. 556 [unlicensed] **plus** oral azithromycin.
▸ In non-pharyngeal infections: intramuscular spectinomycin [unlicensed] **plus** oral azithromycin.
▸ If unable to take standard therapy: oral azithromycin. Ⓐ

For information on the management of other types of gonorrhoeal infections, see the British Association for Sexual Health and HIV guideline: **Management of infection with *Neisseria gonorrhoeae*** (see *Useful resources*). For other considerations such as in patients receiving prophylactic antibacterial therapy and for advice to be given to patients, see Antibacterials, principles of therapy p. 527.

Pelvic inflammatory disease

Contact tracing recommended.

- Doxycycline + metronidazole + single-dose of i/m ceftriaxone *or* ofloxacin p. 597+ metronidazole
▸ *Suggested duration of treatment* 14 days (except i/m ceftriaxone).
▸ In severely ill patients initial treatment with doxycycline + i/v ceftriaxone + i/v metronidazole, then switch to oral treatment with doxycycline + metronidazole to complete 14 days' treatment

Early syphilis (infection of less than 2 years)

Contact tracing recommended.

- Benzathine benzylpenicillin p. 579
▸ *Suggested duration of treatment* single-dose (repeat dose after 7 days for women in the third trimester of pregnancy)
- *Alternatively*, doxycycline or erythromycin
▸ *Suggested duration of treatment* 14 days

Late latent syphilis (asymptomatic infection of more than 2 years)

Contact tracing recommended.

- Benzathine benzylpenicillin
▸ *Suggested duration of treatment* once weekly for 2 weeks
- *Alternatively*, doxycycline
▸ *Suggested duration of treatment* 28 days

Asymptomatic contacts of patients with infectious syphilis

- Doxycycline
▸ *Suggested duration of treatment* 14 days

Useful Resources

British Association for Sexual Health and HIV national guideline for the management of infection with *Neisseria gonorrhoeae*. British Association for Sexual Health and HIV. 2011, updated 2019.
www.bashhguidelines.org/media/1208/gc-2019.pdf

Musculoskeletal system infections, antibacterial therapy

Osteomyelitis

For management of osteomyelitis below the ankle in individuals with diabetes mellitus, see Diabetic foot infections, antibacterial therapy p. 534.

Seek specialist advice if chronic infection or prostheses present.

- Flucloxacillin p. 589
▸ Consider adding fusidic acid p. 608 or rifampicin p. 619 for initial 2 weeks.
▸ *Suggested duration of treatment* 6 weeks for acute infection

- *If penicillin-allergic*, clindamycin p. 566
▶ Consider adding fusidic acid or rifampicin for initial 2 weeks.
▶ *Suggested duration of treatment* 6 weeks for acute infection
- *If meticillin-resistant Staphylococcus aureus suspected*, vancomycin p. 565 (*or* teicoplanin p. 563)
▶ Consider adding fusidic acid or rifampicin for initial 2 weeks.
▶ *Suggested duration of treatment* 6 weeks for acute infection

Septic arthritis

For management of septic arthritis below the ankle in individuals with diabetes mellitus, see Diabetic foot infections, antibacterial therapy p. 534.
    Seek specialist advice if prostheses present.
- Flucloxacillin
▶ *Suggested duration of treatment* 4–6 weeks (longer if infection complicated).
- *If penicillin-allergic*, clindamycin
▶ *Suggested duration of treatment* 4–6 weeks (longer if infection complicated).
- *If meticillin-resistant Staphylococcus aureus suspected*, vancomycin (*or* teicoplanin)
▶ *Suggested duration of treatment* 4–6 weeks (longer if infection complicated).
- *If gonococcal arthritis or Gram-negative infection suspected*, cefotaxime p. 557 (*or* ceftriaxone p. 558)
▶ *Suggested duration of treatment* 4–6 weeks (longer if infection complicated; treat gonococcal infection for 2 weeks).

Nose infections, antibacterial therapy

31-Oct-2017

Sinusitis (acute)

Acute sinusitis is generally triggered by a viral infection, although occasionally it may become complicated by a bacterial infection caused by *Streptococcus pneumoniae*, *Haemophilus influenzae*, *Moraxella catharrhalis*, or *Staphylococcus aureus*. For further information *see* Sinusitis (acute) p. 1247.

Treatment

EvGr Antibacterial therapy should *only* be offered to patients with acute sinusitis who are systemically very unwell, have signs and symptoms of a more serious illness, those who are at high-risk of complications due to pre-existing comorbidities, or whenever bacterial sinusitis is suspected.
    Patients presenting with symptoms for around 10 days or more with no improvement may be prescribed a back-up antibiotic prescription, which can be used if symptoms do not improve within 7 days or if they worsen significantly at any time. Ⓐ For further information *see*, Sinusitis (acute) p. 1247.

Choice of antibacterial therapy
No penicillin allergy
- *First line*:
▶ EvGr Non-life threatening symptoms: phenoxymethylpenicillin p. 581.
▶ Systemically very unwell, signs and symptoms of a more serious illness, or at high-risk of complications: co-amoxiclav p. 585. Ⓐ
- *Second line* (worsening symptoms despite 2 or 3 days of antibiotic treatment):
▶ EvGr Non-life threatening symptoms: co-amoxiclav.

▶ Systemically very unwell, signs and symptoms of a more serious illness or at high-risk of complications: consult local microbiologist. Ⓐ

Penicillin allergy or intolerance
- *First line*: EvGr doxycycline p. 601 or clarithromycin p. 569 (erythromycin p. 572 in pregnancy). Ⓐ
- *Second line* (worsening symptoms despite 2 or 3 days of antibiotic treatment): EvGr Consult local microbiologist. Ⓐ

Useful Resources

Sinusitis (acute): antimicrobial prescribing. National Institute for Health and Care Excellence. NICE guideline 79. October 2017.
www.nice.org.uk/guidance/ng79

Oral bacterial infections

Antibacterial drugs

Antibacterial drugs should only be prescribed for the *treatment* of oral infections on the basis of defined need. They may be used in conjunction with (but not as an alternative to) other appropriate measures, such as providing drainage or extracting a tooth.
    The 'blind' prescribing of an antibacterial for unexplained pyrexia, cervical lymphadenopathy, or facial swelling can lead to difficulty in establishing the diagnosis. In severe oral infections, a sample should always be taken for bacteriology.
    Oral infections which may require antibacterial treatment include acute periapical or periodontal abscess, cellulitis, acutely created oral-antral communication (and acute sinusitis), severe pericoronitis, localised osteitis, acute necrotising ulcerative gingivitis, and destructive forms of chronic periodontal disease. Most of these infections are readily resolved by the early establishment of drainage and removal of the cause (typically an infected necrotic pulp). Antibacterials may be required if treatment has to be delayed, in immunocompromised patients, or in those with conditions such as diabetes or Paget's disease. Certain rarer infections including bacterial sialadenitis, osteomyelitis, actinomycosis, and infections involving fascial spaces such as Ludwig's angina, require antibiotics and specialist hospital care.
    Antibacterial drugs may also be useful after dental surgery in some cases of spreading infection. Infection may spread to involve local lymph nodes, to fascial spaces (where it can cause airway obstruction), or into the bloodstream (where it can lead to cavernous sinus thrombosis and other serious complications). Extension of an infection can also lead to maxillary sinusitis; osteomyelitis is a complication, which usually arises when host resistance is reduced.
    If the oral infection fails to respond to antibacterial treatment within 48 hours the antibacterial should be changed, preferably on the basis of bacteriological investigation. Failure to respond may also suggest an incorrect diagnosis, lack of essential additional measures (such as drainage), poor host resistance, or poor patient compliance.
    Combination of a penicillin (or a macrolide) with metronidazole p. 575 may sometimes be helpful for the treatment of severe oral infections or oral infections that have not responded to initial antibacterial treatment.

Penicillins

Phenoxymethylpenicillin p. 581 is effective for dentoalveolar abscess.

Broad-spectrum penicillins
Amoxicillin p. 582 is as effective as phenoxymethylpenicillin but is better absorbed; however, it may encourage emergence of resistant organisms.

5

Infection

Like phenoxymethylpenicillin, amoxicillin is ineffective against bacteria that produce beta-lactamases.

Amoxicillin may be useful for short course oral regimens. Co-amoxiclav p. 585 is active against beta-lactamase-producing bacteria that are resistant to amoxicillin. Co-amoxiclav may be used for severe dental infection with spreading cellulitis or dental infection not responding to first-line antibacterial treatment.

Cephalosporins

The cephalosporins offer little advantage over the penicillins in dental infections, often being less active against anaerobes. Infections due to oral streptococci (often termed viridans streptococci) which become resistant to penicillin are usually also resistant to cephalosporins. This is of importance in the case of patients who have had rheumatic fever and are on long-term penicillin therapy. Cefalexin p. 552 and cefradine p. 554 have been used in the treatment of oral infections.

Tetracyclines

In adults, tetracyclines can be effective against oral anaerobes but the development of resistance (especially by oral streptococci) has reduced their usefulness for the treatment of acute oral infections; they may still have a role in the treatment of destructive (refractory) forms of periodontal disease. Doxycycline p. 601 has a longer duration of action than tetracycline p. 604 or oxytetracycline p. 603 and need only be given once daily; it is reported to be more active against anaerobes than some other tetracyclines.

Doxycycline may have a role in the treatment of recurrent aphthous ulceration, or as an adjunct to gingival scaling and root planing for periodontitis.

Macrolides

The macrolides are an alternative for oral infections in penicillin-allergic patients or where a beta-lactamase producing organism is involved. However, many organisms are now resistant to macrolides or rapidly develop resistance; their use should therefore be limited to short courses.

Clindamycin

Clindamycin p. 566 should not be used routinely for the treatment of oral infections because it may be no more effective than penicillins against anaerobes and there may be cross-resistance with erythromycin p. 572-resistant bacteria. Clindamycin can be used for the treatment of dentoalveolar abscess that has not responded to penicillin or to metronidazole.

Metronidazole and tinidazole

Metronidazole is an alternative to a penicillin for the treatment of many oral infections where the patient is allergic to penicillin or the infection is due to beta-lactamase-producing anaerobes. It is the drug of first choice for the treatment of acute necrotising ulcerative gingivitis (Vincent's infection) and pericoronitis; amoxicillin is a suitable alternative. For these purposes metronidazole for 3 days is sufficient, but the duration of treatment may need to be longer in pericoronitis. Tinidazole p. 577 is licensed for the treatment of acute ulcerative gingivitis.

Respiratory system infections, antibacterial therapy
06-May-2020

Epiglottitis (*Haemophilus influenzae*)

- Cefotaxime p. 557 (*or* ceftriaxone p. 558)

- *If history of immediate hypersensitivity reaction to penicillin or to cephalosporins*, chloramphenicol p. 605

Bronchiectasis (non-cystic fibrosis), acute exacerbation

Bronchiectasis is a persistent or progressive condition, caused by chronic inflammatory damage to the airways and is characterised by thick-walled, dilated bronchi. Signs and symptoms may range from intermittent expectoration and infection, to chronic cough, persistent daily production of sputum, bacterial colonisation, and recurrent infections. An acute exacerbation is defined as sustained deterioration of the patient's signs and symptoms from their baseline, and presents with worsening local symptoms, with or without increased wheeze, breathlessness or haemoptysis and may be accompanied by fever or pleurisy.

Treatment

[EvGr] Obtain a sputum sample and send for culture and susceptibility testing. Antibacterial therapy should be given to all patients with an acute exacerbation. [A]

For patients receiving prophylactic antibacterial therapy, switching from intravenous to oral antibacterials, and for advice to be given to patients, see Antibacterials, principles of therapy p. 527.

[EvGr] Refer patients to hospital if they have signs or symptoms suggestive of a more serious illness such as cardiorespiratory failure or sepsis. [A]

Reassessment

[EvGr] Reassess if symptoms worsen rapidly or significantly at any time and consider:

- Other diagnoses such as pneumonia, or signs and symptoms of a more serious illness such as cardiorespiratory failure, or sepsis;
- Previous antibacterial use that may have led to resistance.

Review choice of antibacterial if susceptibility results indicate bacterial resistance and symptoms are not improving—consult local microbiologist as needed. [A]

Choice of antibacterial therapy

[EvGr] The recommended total duration of treatment is 7–14 days.

Treatment should be guided by the most recent sputum culture and susceptibility results when available.

Seek specialist advice for patients whose symptoms are not improving with repeated courses, or who are resistant to, or cannot take oral antibacterials. [A]

- *Oral first line* :
  - [EvGr] Amoxicillin p. 582, clarithromycin p. 569, or doxycycline p. 601.
  - Alternative if at high risk of treatment failure (repeated courses of antibacterials, previous culture with resistant or atypical bacteria, or high risk of complications): co-amoxiclav p. 585, or levofloxacin p. 595. [A]
- *Intravenous first line* (severely unwell or unable to take oral treatment):
  - [EvGr] Co-amoxiclav, piperacillin with tazobactam p. 579, or levofloxacin. [A]

Antibacterial prophylaxis

[EvGr] For patients with repeated acute exacerbations, a trial of antibacterial prophylaxis may be given on specialist advice only. [A]

Chronic obstructive pulmonary disease, acute exacerbation

An acute exacerbation of chronic obstructive pulmonary disease (COPD) is a sustained worsening of symptoms from the patient's usual stable state, that is beyond the usual day to day variations. Many exacerbations are not caused by bacterial infections, but instead can be triggered by other factors such as smoking or viral infections.

For the non-antibacterial management of acute exacerbations of COPD, see Chronic obstructive pulmonary disease p. 258.

Treatment

EvGr Consider antibacterial treatment taking into account:

- The severity of symptoms, sputum colour changes and increases in volume and thickness;
- The need for hospital admission;
- Previous exacerbations and hospital admission history, and risk of developing complications. (A)

For other considerations such as in patients receiving prophylactic antibacterial therapy, switching from intravenous to oral antibacterials, and for advice to be given to patients, see Antibacterials, principles of therapy p. 527.

EvGr Refer patients to hospital if they have signs or symptoms suggestive of a more serious illness such as cardiorespiratory failure or sepsis. (A)

Reassessment

EvGr Reassess if symptoms worsen rapidly or significantly at any time and consider:

- Other diagnoses such as pneumonia, or signs and symptoms of a more serious illness such as cardiorespiratory failure, or sepsis;
- Previous antibacterial use that may have led to resistance.

Send a sputum sample for testing if there is no improvement after antibacterial therapy and this has not already been done.

Review choice of antibacterial if susceptibility results indicate bacterial resistance and symptoms are not improving—consult local microbiologist as needed. (A)

Choice of antibacterial therapy

EvGr The recommended total duration of treatment is 5 days.

Treatment should be guided by the most recent sputum culture and susceptibility results when available.

Seek specialist advice for patients whose symptoms are not improving with repeated courses, or who are resistant to, or cannot take oral antibacterials. (A)

- **Oral** *first line* :
  ▸ EvGr Amoxicillin, clarithromycin, or doxycycline.
  ▸ Alternative if at high risk of treatment failure (repeated courses of antibacterials, previous culture with resistant or atypical bacteria, or high risk of complications): co-amoxiclav, or levofloxacin. (A)
- **Oral** *second line* (if no improvement after at least 2 to 3 days):
  ▸ EvGr Use a first line antibacterial from a different class to the antibacterial used previously.
  ▸ Alternative if at high risk of treatment failure: co-amoxiclav, levofloxacin, or co-trimoxazole p. 598 (only when sensitivities are available and there is good reason to use co-trimoxazole over single antibacterials). (A)
- **Intravenous** *first line* (severely unwell or unable to take oral treatment):
  ▸ EvGr Amoxicillin, co-amoxiclav, clarithromycin, co-trimoxazole, or piperacillin with tazobactam. (A)
- **Intravenous** *second line* : EvGr Choice should be made in consultation with a local microbiologist. (A)

Cough, acute

Acute cough is usually self-limiting and often resolves within 3–4 weeks without antibacterials. It is most commonly caused by a viral upper respiratory tract infection, but can have other infective causes such as acute bronchitis or pneumonia, or non-infective causes such as interstitial lung disease or gastro-oesophageal reflux disease.

Treatment

EvGr Patients should be advised that an acute cough is usually self-limiting and to manage their symptoms using

self-care treatments. These include honey and over-the-counter cough medicines containing expectorants or cough suppressants, however there is limited evidence to support the use of such products. For more information, see Aromatic inhalations, cough preparations and systemic nasal decongestants p. 312.

Patients with an acute cough who are systemically very unwell should be offered immediate antibacterial treatment.

Do not routinely offer an antibacterial to treat an acute cough associated with an upper respiratory tract infection or acute bronchitis in patients who are not systemically very unwell or at higher risk of complications. (A)

Patients with a pre-existing co-morbidity, young children who were born prematurely, and patients aged over 65 years of age and the presence of certain criteria (hospitalisation in the previous year, type 1 or 2 diabetes, history of congestive heart failure, or currently taking oral corticosteroids) are considered to be at a higher risk of complications if they present with an acute cough. EvGr Immediate or back-up antibacterial treatment should be considered in these patients based on the face-to-face clinical examination. If back-up treatment is given, advise patients to start treatment if symptoms worsen rapidly or significantly at any time. (A)

For general advice to give to patients, see Antibacterials, principles of therapy p. 527.

EvGr Seek specialist advice, or refer patients with an acute cough to hospital if they have signs or symptoms of a more serious illness or condition. (A)

Reassessment

EvGr Reassess if symptoms worsen rapidly or significantly taking into account alternative diagnoses, signs or symptoms suggestive of a more serious condition, and previous antibacterial use which may have led to resistant bacteria. (A)

Choice of antibacterial therapy

EvGr The recommended duration of oral treatment is 5 days. (A)

- *First line*
  ▸ EvGr Doxycycline p. 601.
  ▸ Alternative *first line* choices: amoxicillin p. 582, clarithromycin p. 569, or erythromycin p. 572. (A)
- Choice during pregnancy:
  ▸ EvGr Amoxicillin or erythromycin. (A)

Pneumonia, community-acquired

Pneumonia is an acute infection of the lung parenchyma that presents with symptoms such as cough, chest pain, dyspnoea, and fever. It is classified as community-acquired if acquired outside of hospital or in a nursing home.

For recommendations on the management of pneumonia during the COVID-19 pandemic, see NICE rapid guidelines: **Managing suspected or confirmed pneumonia in adults in the community** (available at: www.nice.org.uk/guidance/ng165), and **Antibiotics for pneumonia in adults in hospital** for patients presenting to hospital with community acquired pneumonia (available at: www.nice.org.uk/guidance/ng173). Where the new recommendations cover existing recommendations discussed below, follow the rapid guideline recommendations during the pandemic. For further information on COVID-19, see COVID-19 p. 660.

Treatment

EvGr Offer an antibacterial taking into account the severity assessment, risk of complications, local antimicrobial resistance and surveillance data, recent antibacterial use, and recent microbiological results. (A) For severity assessment and guidance on monitoring, see NICE guideline on pneumonia in adults (see *Useful resources*).

EvGr Antibacterial treatment should be started as soon as possible and within 4 hours of establishing a diagnosis (within 1 hour if the patient has suspected sepsis and meets any of the high risk criteria for this — see NICE guideline on sepsis at: www.nice.org.uk/guidance/ng51).

Refer patients to hospital as recommended in the NICE guideline on pneumonia in adults, or if they have signs or symptoms suggestive of a more serious illness (such as cardiorespiratory failure or sepsis).

In patients with moderate or high-severity community-acquired pneumonia, obtain blood and sputum cultures and consider performing pneumococcal and legionella urinary antigen tests.

Do not routinely offer a glucocorticoid to patients with community-acquired pneumonia unless they have other conditions for which glucocorticoid treatment is indicated. Ⓐ

For other considerations such as switching from intravenous to oral antibacterials, and for advice to be given to patients, see Antibacterials, principles of therapy p. 527.

Reassessment

EvGr Reassess if signs or symptoms do not improve or worsen rapidly or significantly, and consider other possible non-bacterial causes such as influenza.

If a sample has been sent for microbiological testing, review the choice of antibacterial and consider changing according to the results, using a narrower-spectrum antibacterial if appropriate.

Send a sample (such as sputum sample) for testing if there is no improvement after antibacterial therapy and this has not already been done.

Refer patients to hospital if symptoms do not improve as expected with antibacterial treatment. ⒶEv

Choice of antibacterial therapy

EvGr Treatment should be based on severity assessment using clinical judgement and CRB65 or CURB65, suspected micro-organism, and in moderate and high-severity community-acquired pneumonia microbiological results when available.

Offer oral antibacterials to patients who are able to take oral treatment and the severity of their condition does not require intravenous treatment.

Consider referral to hospital or seeking specialist advice if bacteria are resistant to oral antibacterials or patients cannot take oral treatment. ⒶEv

Low severity

• **Oral** *first line* :
  ▸ EvGr Amoxicillin.
  ▸ Alternative in penicillin allergy or amoxicillin unsuitable (e.g. atypical pathogens suspected): clarithromycin, doxycycline, or erythromycin (in pregnancy). ⒶEv

Moderate severity

• **Oral** *first line* :
  ▸ EvGr Amoxicillin.
  ▸ If atypical pathogens suspected: amoxicillin **with** clarithromycin **or** erythromycin (in pregnancy).
  ▸ Alternative in penicillin allergy: clarithromycin, or doxycycline. ⒶEv

High severity

• **Oral** *or* **Intravenous** *first line* :
  ▸ EvGr Co-amoxiclav p. 585 **with** clarithromycin **or** oral erythromycin (in pregnancy).
  ▸ Alternative in penicillin allergy: levofloxacin p. 595 (consult local microbiologist if fluoroquinolone not appropriate). ⒶEv

Pneumonia, hospital-acquired

Pneumonia is an acute infection of the lung parenchyma that presents with symptoms such as cough, chest pain, dyspnoea, and fever. It is classified as hospital-acquired when it develops 48 hours or more after hospital admission.

For recommendations on the management of suspected or confirmed pneumonia during the COVID-19 pandemic, see NICE rapid guideline: **Antibiotics for pneumonia in adults**

in hospital (available at: www.nice.org.uk/guidance/ng173). Where the new recommendations cover existing recommendations discussed below, follow the rapid guideline recommendations during the pandemic. For further information on COVID-19, see COVID-19 p. 660.

Treatment

EvGr In patients with signs or symptoms of pneumonia starting within 48 hours of hospital admission, follow recommendations for patients with community-acquired pneumonia.

Offer an antibacterial taking into account:

• The severity of signs or symptoms;
• The number of days in hospital before onset of symptoms;
• The risk of complications;
• Local hospital and ward-based antimicrobial resistance data;
• Recent antibacterial use;
• Recent microbiological test results;
• Recent contact with health or social care settings;
• Risk of adverse effects such as *Clostridioides difficile* infection.

Antibacterial treatment should be started as soon as possible and within 4 hours of establishing a diagnosis (within 1 hour if the patient has suspected sepsis and meets any of the high risk criteria for this — see NICE guideline on sepsis at: www.nice.org.uk/guidance/ng51).

A sample (for example, sputum sample, nasopharyngeal swab, or tracheal aspirate) should be taken for microbiological testing. ⒶEv

For other considerations such as switching from intravenous to oral antibacterials, and for advice to be given to patients, see Antibacterials, principles of therapy p. 527.

Reassessment

EvGr Reassess if symptoms do not improve or worsen rapidly or significantly.

When microbiological results are available, review choice of antibacterial and change treatment according to the results, using a narrower-spectrum antibacterial if appropriate.

Seek advice from a microbiologist if symptoms do not improve as expected with treatment, or multidrug-resistant bacteria are present. ⒶEv

Choice of antibacterial therapy

EvGr For patients with non-severe signs or symptoms and not at higher risk of resistance, treatment should be guided by microbiological results when available. For patients with severe signs or symptoms or at higher risk of resistance, treatment should be based on specialist microbiological advice and local resistance data.

Higher risk of resistance includes signs or symptoms starting more than 5 days after hospital admission, relevant comorbidity, recent use of broad-spectrum antibacterials, colonisation with multidrug-resistant bacteria, and recent contact with a health or social care setting before the current admission.

In patients with signs or symptoms of pneumonia starting within 3 to 5 days of hospital admission who are not at higher risk of resistance, consider following the recommendations for community-acquired pneumonia for choice of antibacterial treatment. ⒶEv

Non-severe signs or symptoms and not at higher risk of resistance

• **Oral** *first line* :
  ▸ EvGr Co-amoxiclav p. 585.
  ▸ Alternative in penicillin allergy or co-amoxiclav unsuitable (based on specialist microbiological advice and local resistance data): doxycycline p. 601, cefalexin p. 552 (caution in penicillin allergy), co-trimoxazole p. 598 [unlicensed], or levofloxacin p. 595 [unlicensed] (only if switching from intravenous levofloxacin under specialist advice). ⒶEv

Severe signs or symptoms or at higher risk of resistance

● **Intravenous** *first line* :

▸ EvGr Piperacillin with tazobactam p. 579, ceftazidime p. 557, ceftazidime with avibactam p. 560, ceftriaxone p. 558, cefuroxime p. 555, levofloxacin [unlicensed], or meropenem p. 550.

▸ If meticillin-resistant *Staphylococcus aureus* confirmed or suspected **add** vancomycin p. 565, or teicoplanin p. 563, or linezolid p. 609 (under specialist advice only if vancomycin cannot be used). Ⓐ

Useful resources

Bronchiectasis (non-cystic fibrosis), acute exacerbation: antimicrobial prescribing. National Institute for Health and Care Excellence. NICE guideline 117. December 2018.
www.nice.org.uk/guidance/ng117

Chronic obstructive pulmonary disease (acute exacerbation): antimicrobial prescribing. National Institute for Health and Care Excellence. NICE guideline 114. December 2018.
www.nice.org.uk/guidance/ng114

Cough (acute): antimicrobial prescribing. National Institute for Health and Care Excellence. NICE guideline 120. February 2019.
www.nice.org.uk/guidance/ng120

Pneumonia in adults: diagnosis and management. National Institute for Health and Care Excellence. Clinical guideline 191. December 2014, updated September 2019.
www.nice.org.uk/guidance/cg191

Pneumonia (community-acquired): antimicrobial prescribing. National Institute for Health and Care Excellence. NICE guideline 138. September 2019.
www.nice.org.uk/guidance/ng138

Pneumonia (hospital-acquired): antimicrobial prescribing. National Institute for Health and Care Excellence. NICE guideline 139. September 2019.
www.nice.org.uk/guidance/ng139

Skin infections, antibacterial therapy

28-Sep-2020

Impetigo

Impetigo is a contagious, superficial bacterial infection of the skin that affects all age groups, but it is more common in young children. Transmission occurs directly through close contact with an infected individual or indirectly via contaminated objects such as toys, clothing, or towels.

Impetigo can develop as a primary infection or as a secondary complication of pre-existing skin conditions such as eczema, scabies, or chickenpox. The two main clinical forms are non-bullous impetigo (most common form) and bullous impetigo. Non-bullous impetigo is characterised by thin-walled vesicles or pustules that rupture quickly, forming a golden-brown crust, while bullous impetigo is characterised by the presence of fluid-filled vesicles and blisters that rupture, leaving a thin, flat, yellow-brown crust.

Initial treatment

EvGr Patients, and if appropriate their family or carers, should be advised on good hygiene measures to reduce the spread of impetigo to other body areas and to other people.

In patients with **localised non-bullous impetigo** who are not systemically unwell or at high risk of complications, consider hydrogen peroxide 1% cream p. 1322; if unsuitable (e.g. if impetigo is around the eyes), offer a topical antibacterial.

In patients with **widespread non-bullous impetigo** who are not systemically unwell or at high risk of complications, offer a topical **or** oral antibacterial. Take into account that both routes of administration are effective; any previous use of topical antibacterials that could have led to resistance;

and the preferences of the patient and, their family or carers (if appropriate), including the practicalities of administration (particularly to large areas).

In patients with **non-bullous impetigo** who are systemically unwell or at high risk of complications and in all patients with **bullous impetigo**, offer an oral antibacterial. Combination treatment with a topical and oral antibacterial is not recommended. Ⓐ

For other considerations such as advice to be given to patients, and if appropriate their family or carers, see Antibacterials, principles of therapy p. 527.

EvGr Refer patients to hospital if they have any signs or symptoms suggestive of a more serious condition or illness, or if they have widespread impetigo and are immunocompromised.

Consider referral to hospital or seeking specialist advice for patients who are systemically unwell, have a higher risk of complications, or if impetigo is difficult to treat (such as bullous impetigo (particularly in children aged under 1 year) or frequently recurrent impetigo). Ⓐ

Reassessment and further treatment

EvGr Reassess if symptoms worsen rapidly or significantly at any time, or do not improve after completion of the treatment course. Take into consideration other possible diagnoses (such as herpes simplex infection), signs or symptoms suggesting a more serious illness or condition (such as cellulitis), and previous antibacterial use that might have led to resistance.

For patients whose impetigo is worsening or has not improved after treatment with hydrogen peroxide 1% cream, offer a topical antibacterial if the infection remains localised, or a topical **or** oral antibacterial if infection has become widespread.

Offer an oral antibacterial to patients whose impetigo is worsening or has not improved after completing a course of topical antibacterial.

For patients whose impetigo is worsening or has not improved after completing a course of topical or oral antibacterials, consider sending a skin swab for microbiological testing.

For patients with impetigo that recurs frequently, send a skin swab for microbiological testing and consider taking a nasal swab and starting treatment for decolonisation (using topical treatments and personal hygiene measures).

If a skin swab has been sent for microbiological testing, review the choice of antibacterial and change according to the results if symptoms are not improving, using a narrower-spectrum antibacterial if possible. Ⓐ

Choice of antibacterial therapy

EvGr Treatment should be based on infection severity and number of lesions, suspected micro-organism, local antibacterial resistance data, and be guided by microbiological results if available. Ⓐ

● **Topical** *first line* if hydrogen peroxide unsuitable or ineffective:

▸ EvGr fusidic acid p. 608.

▸ Alternative if fusidic acid resistance suspected or confirmed: mupirocin p. 1276. Ⓐ

● **Oral** *first line* :

▸ EvGr Flucloxacillin p. 589.

▸ Alternative if penicillin allergy or flucloxacillin unsuitable: clarithromycin p. 569 or erythromycin p. 572 (in pregnancy). Ⓐ

● If meticillin-resistant *Staphylococcus aureus* (MRSA) infection suspected or confirmed: EvGr Consult local microbiologist. Ⓐ

Cellulitis and erysipelas

Cellulitis and erysipelas are infections of the subcutaneous tissues, which usually result from contamination of a break in the skin. Both conditions are characterised by acute

5

Infection

localised inflammation and oedema. Lesions are more superficial in erysipelas and have a well-defined, raised margin.

For management of an infected leg ulcer, see *Leg Ulcer*, and for infection below the ankle in patients with diabetes, see Diabetic foot infections, antibacterial therapy p. 534.

Treatment

EvGr Consider taking a swab for microbiological testing **only** if the skin is broken and there is risk of infection by an uncommon pathogen (for example, after a penetrating injury, exposure to water-born organisms, or an infection acquired outside the UK).

Drawing around the extent of the infection to monitor progress before initiating antibacterial treatment can also be considered, taking into account that redness may be less visible on darker skin tones.

Offer an antibacterial taking into account the severity of symptoms, site of infection, risk of uncommon pathogens, previous microbiological results from a swab, and the patient's meticillin-resistant *Staphylococcus aureus* (MRSA) status if known. A

For other considerations such as in patients receiving prophylactic antibacterial therapy, switching from intravenous to oral antibacterials, and for advice to be given to patients, see Antibacterials, principles of therapy p. 527.

EvGr Manage any underlying condition that may predispose to cellulitis or erysipelas, such as diabetes mellitus, venous insufficiency, eczema, and oedema.

Refer patients to hospital if they have signs or symptoms suggestive of a more serious illness, such as orbital cellulitis, osteomyelitis, septic arthritis, necrotising fasciitis, or sepsis.

Consider referral to hospital or seeking specialist advice for patients who have lymphangitis, are severely unwell, are unable to take oral antibacterials, have infection near the eyes or nose, or that could be caused by an uncommon pathogen. A

Reassessment

EvGr Reassess if symptoms worsen rapidly or significantly at any time, do not improve within 2–3 days of starting an antibacterial, or the patient becomes systemically very unwell, has severe pain out of proportion to the infection, or has redness or swelling spreading beyond the initial presentation (taking into account that some initial spreading may occur). Take into consideration other possible diagnoses (such as an inflammatory reaction to an insect bite or deep vein thrombosis), any underlying condition that may predispose to cellulitis or erysipelas, signs or symptoms suggesting a more serious illness, results from microbiological tests, and previous antibacterial use that might have led to resistance.

Consider taking a swab for testing if the skin is broken and this has not already been done.

If a swab has been sent for microbiological testing, review the choice of antibacterial and change according to the results if signs or symptoms are not improving, using a narrower-spectrum antibacterial if possible.

Consider referral to hospital or seeking specialist advice if the infection has spread and is not responding to oral antibacterials. A

Choice of antibacterial therapy

EvGr Treatment should be based on clinical assessment, infection severity, suspected micro-organism, and site of infection.

Offer oral antibacterials to patients who are able to take oral treatment and the severity of their condition does not require intravenous treatment.

Consider referral to hospital or seeking specialist advice if bacteria are resistant to oral antibacterials, patients cannot take oral treatment, or have infection near the eyes or nose. A

First choice antibacterials

- **Oral** *or* **Intravenous** *first line* :
  ‣ EvGr Flucloxacillin p. 589.
  ‣ Alternative in penicillin allergy or flucloxacillin unsuitable: clarithromycin p. 572, oral erythromycin p. 569 (in pregnancy), or oral doxycycline p. 601. A

- **Oral** *or* **Intravenous** *first line if infection near the eyes or nose* :
  ‣ EvGr Co-amoxiclav p. 585.
  ‣ Alternative in penicillin allergy or co-amoxiclav unsuitable: clarithromycin **with** metronidazole p. 575. A

Alternative choice antibacterials for severe infection

- **Oral** *or* **Intravenous**:
  ‣ EvGr Co-amoxiclav, clindamycin p. 566, intravenous cefuroxime p. 555, or intravenous ceftriaxone p. 558 (ambulatory care only).
  ‣ If meticillin-resistant *Staphylococcus aureus* confirmed or suspected, **add** intravenous vancomycin p. 565, intravenous teicoplanin p. 563, or linezolid p. 609 (specialist use only if vancomycin or teicoplanin cannot be used).
  ‣ For ambulatory care, and in MRSA confirmed or suspected infections, other antibacterials may be appropriate based on microbiological results and specialist advice. A

Antibacterial prophylaxis

EvGr For patients who have been treated in hospital, or under specialist advice, for at least 2 separate episodes of cellulitis or erysipelas in the previous 12 months, a trial of antibacterial prophylaxis may be considered by a specialist.

If cellulitis or erysipelas recurs, stop or change the prophylactic antibacterial to an alternative once the acute infection has been treated.

Review antibacterial prophylaxis at least every 6 months, assessing the success of therapy and discussing continuing, stopping or changing prophylaxis taking into account the patient's preference for antibacterial use and the risk of antibacterial resistance. A

Insect bites and stings

Redness, itchiness, or pain and swelling after an insect sting or bite (including bites from spiders and ticks) is often caused by a localised inflammatory or allergic reaction rather than an infection, especially when there is a rapid onset. Rarely, symptoms may last for up to 10 days.

For the management of patients with a known or suspected tick bite, see Lyme disease p. 614. EvGr Consider referral or seeking specialist advice for patients with fever or persistent lesions after an insect bite or sting from outside the UK, as this may indicate a more serious illness such as rickettsial infection or malaria.

Antibacterials are not recommended for an insect bite or sting unless the patient has signs or symptoms of an infection. For the management of patients with a suspected infection, see *Cellulitis and erysipelas*. A

Leg Ulcer

Leg ulcers usually develop on the lower leg, between the shin and the ankle, and take more than 4–6 weeks to heal. Although the majority of leg ulcers may be colonised with bacteria, this does not necessarily mean that the wound is infected. Signs and symptoms of an infected leg ulcer include redness (may be less visible on darker skin tones) or swelling spreading beyond the ulcer, localised warmth, increased pain, or fever.

Treatment

EvGr Any underlying condition that may cause a leg ulcer, such as venous insufficiency and oedema should be managed to promote healing.

Taking a sample for microbiological testing at initial presentation with a leg ulcer is not recommended, even if the ulcer may be infected.

Offer an antibacterial to patients who have signs or symptoms of infection taking into account the severity of signs or symptoms, risk of developing complications, and previous antibacterial use. ⒶEvGr

For other considerations such as switching from intravenous to oral antibacterials and for advice to be given to patients, see Antibacterials, principles of therapy p. 527.

EvGr Refer patients to hospital if they have signs or symptoms suggestive of a more serious condition or illness, such as sepsis, necrotising fasciitis, or osteomyelitis.

Consider referral to hospital or seeking specialist advice for patients with an infected leg ulcer who have lymphangitis or a higher risk of complications due to comorbidities, such as diabetes or immunosuppression. Ⓐ

Reassessment

EvGr Reassess if signs or symptoms worsen rapidly or significantly at any time, do not improve within 2–3 days, or the patient becomes systemically unwell or has severe pain out of proportion to the infection. Take into consideration previous antibacterial use that might have led to resistance, and be aware that full resolution of an infected leg ulcer is not expected until after the antibacterial course is completed.

Consider taking a sample from the leg ulcer (after cleaning) for microbiological testing if signs or symptoms of infection are worsening or have not improved as expected. Review the choice of antibacterial(s) and change according to the results if signs or symptoms are not improving, using a narrower-spectrum antibacterial if possible.

Consider referral to hospital or seeking specialist advice if patients have a spreading infection that is not responding to oral antibacterials. Ⓐ

Choice of antibacterial therapy

EvGr Treatment should be based on clinical assessment, infection severity, suspected micro-organism, and be guided by microbiological results if available.

Offer oral antibacterials to patients who are able to take oral treatment and the severity of their condition does not require intravenous treatment. For patients unable to take oral treatment, consider referring or seeking specialist advice and where appropriate, explore options for administration of intravenous or intramuscular antibiotics at home or in the community. Ⓐ

Non-severely unwell patients

● *Oral* first line :
  ▸ EvGr Flucloxacillin.
  ▸ Alternative in penicillin allergy or flucloxacillin unsuitable: doxycycline, clarithromycin, or erythromycin (in pregnancy). Ⓐ
● *Oral* second line (guided by microbiological results when available):
  ▸ EvGr Co-amoxiclav.
  ▸ Alternative in penicillin allergy: co-trimoxazole p. 598 [unlicensed]. Ⓐ

Severely unwell patients

● *Oral* or *Intravenous* first line (guided by microbiological results if available):
  ▸ EvGr Intravenous flucloxacillin **with** or **without** intravenous gentamicin p. 545 **and/or** metronidazole, *or* intravenous co-amoxiclav **with** or **without** intravenous gentamicin.
  ▸ Alternative in penicillin allergy: intravenous co-trimoxazole [unlicensed] **with** or **without** intravenous gentamicin p. 545 **and/or** metronidazole p. 575. Ⓐ
● *Oral* or *Intravenous* second line (guided by microbiological results when available or following specialist advice):
  ▸ EvGr Intravenous piperacillin with tazobactam p. 579, *or* intravenous ceftriaxone p. 558 **with** or **without** metronidazole. Ⓐ

Antibacterials to be added if meticillin-resistant Staphylococcus aureus (MRSA) infection suspected or confirmed

● *Oral* or *Intravenous* (in addition to antibacterials listed above):
  ▸ EvGr Intravenous vancomycin p. 565, intravenous teicoplanin p. 563, or linezolid p. 609 (specialist use only if vancomycin or teicoplanin cannot be used). Ⓐ

Animal and human bites

Cleanse wound thoroughly. For tetanus-prone wound, give human tetanus immunoglobulin p. 1337 (with a tetanus-containing vaccine if necessary, according to immunisation history and risk of infection). Consider rabies prophylaxis for bites from animals in endemic countries. Assess risk of blood-borne viruses (including HIV, hepatitis B and C) and give appropriate prophylaxis to prevent viral spread.

● Co-amoxiclav p. 585
● *If penicillin-allergic*, doxycycline p. 601+ metronidazole

Mastitis during breast-feeding

Treat if severe, if systemically unwell, if nipple fissure present, if symptoms do not improve after 12–24 hours of effective milk removal, or if culture indicates infection. Continue breast-feeding or expressing milk during treatment.

● Flucloxacillin p. 589
  ▸ *Suggested duration of treatment* 10–14 days.
● *If penicillin-allergic*, erythromycin p. 572
  ▸ *Suggested duration of treatment* 10–14 days.

Useful Resources

Cellulitis and erysipelas: antimicrobial prescribing. National Institute for Health and Care Excellence. NICE guideline 141. September 2019.
www.nice.org.uk/guidance/ng141

Impetigo: antimicrobial prescribing. National Institute for Health and Care Excellence. NICE guideline 153. February 2020.
www.nice.org.uk/guidance/ng153

Insect bites and stings: antimicrobial prescribing. National Institute for Health and Care Excellence. NICE guideline 182. September 2020.
www.nice.org.uk/guidance/ng182

Leg ulcer infection: antimicrobial prescribing. National Institute for Health and Care Excellence. NICE guideline 152. February 2020.
www.nice.org.uk/guidance/ng152

ANTIBACTERIALS ❯ AMINOGLYCOSIDES

Aminoglycosides

Overview

These include amikacin p. 545, gentamicin p. 545, neomycin sulfate p. 546, streptomycin p. 546, and tobramycin p. 547. All are bactericidal and active against some Gram-positive and many Gram-negative organisms. Amikacin, gentamicin, and tobramycin are also active against *Pseudomonas aeruginosa*; streptomycin is active against *Mycobacterium tuberculosis* and is now almost entirely reserved for tuberculosis.

The aminoglycosides are not absorbed from the gut (although there is a risk of absorption in inflammatory bowel disease and liver failure) and must therefore be given by injection for systemic infections.

Gentamicin is the aminoglycoside of choice in the UK and is used widely for the treatment of serious infections. It has a broad spectrum but is inactive against anaerobes and has poor activity against haemolytic streptococci and pneumococci. When used for the 'blind' therapy of undiagnosed serious infections it is usually given in

5

Infection

Infection

5

conjunction with a penicillin or metronidazole p. 575 (or both). Gentamicin is used together with another antibiotic for the treatment of endocarditis. Streptomycin may be used as an alternative in gentamicin-resistant enterococcal endocarditis.

Loading and maintenance doses of gentamicin may be calculated on the basis of the patient's weight and renal function (e.g. using a nomogram); adjustments are then made according to serum-gentamicin concentrations. High doses are occasionally indicated for serious infections, especially in the neonate, in the patient with cystic fibrosis, or in the immunocompromised patient. Whenever possible treatment should not exceed 7 days.

Amikacin is more stable than gentamicin to enzyme inactivation. Amikacin is used in the treatment of serious infections caused by gentamicin-resistant Gram-negative bacilli.

Tobramycin has similar activity to gentamicin. It is slightly more active against *Ps. aeruginosa* but shows less activity against certain other Gram-negative bacteria. Tobramycin can be administered by nebuliser or by inhalation of powder on a cyclical basis (28 days of tobramycin followed by a 28-day tobramycin-free interval) for the treatment of chronic pulmonary *Ps. aeruginosa* infection in cystic fibrosis; however, resistance may develop and some patients do not respond to treatment.

Neomycin sulfate is too toxic for parenteral administration and can only be used for infections of the skin or mucous membranes or to reduce the bacterial population of the colon prior to bowel surgery or in hepatic failure. Oral administration may lead to malabsorption. Small amounts of neomycin sulfate may be absorbed from the gut in patients with hepatic failure and, as these patients may also be uraemic, cumulation may occur with resultant ototoxicity.

Once daily dosage

Once daily administration of aminoglycosides is more convenient, provides adequate serum concentrations, and in many cases has largely superseded *multiple-daily dose regimens* (given in 2–3 divided doses during the 24 hours). Local guidelines on dosage and serum concentrations should be consulted. A once-daily, high-dose regimen of an aminoglycoside should be avoided in patients with endocarditis due to Gram-positive bacteria, HACEK endocarditis, burns of more than 20% of the total body surface area, or creatinine clearance less than 20 mL/minute. There is insufficient evidence to recommend a once daily, high-dose regimen of an aminoglycoside in pregnancy.

Serum concentrations

Serum concentration monitoring avoids both excessive and subtherapeutic concentrations thus preventing toxicity and ensuring efficacy. Serum-aminoglycoside concentrations should be monitored in patients receiving parenteral aminoglycosides and **must** be determined in the elderly, in obesity, and in cystic fibrosis, or if high doses are being given, or if there is renal impairment.

Aminoglycosides (by injection) 🅟

- CONTRA-INDICATIONS Myasthenia gravis (aminoglycosides may impair neuromuscular transmission)
- CAUTIONS Auditory disorder · care must be taken with dosage (the main side-effects of the aminoglycosides are dose-related) · conditions characterised by muscular weakness (aminoglycosides may impair neuromuscular transmission) · if possible, dehydration should be corrected before starting an aminoglycoside · vestibular disorder · whenever possible, parenteral treatment should not exceed 7 days

- SIDE-EFFECTS
  ▸ **Common or very common** Skin reactions · tinnitus
  ▸ **Uncommon** Nausea · vomiting
  ▸ **Rare or very rare** Anaemia · azotaemia · bronchospasm · eosinophilia · fever · headache · hearing impairment · hypomagnesaemia · paraesthesia · renal impairment
  ▸ **Frequency not known** Confusion · lethargy · leucopenia · nephrotoxicity · thrombocytopenia · vertigo

  SIDE-EFFECTS, FURTHER INFORMATION Ototoxicity and nephrotoxicity are important side-effects to consider with aminoglycoside therapy. Nephrotoxicity occurs most commonly in patients with renal impairment, who may require reduced doses; monitoring is particularly important in the elderly.

- PREGNANCY There is a risk of auditory or vestibular nerve damage in the infant when aminoglycosides are used in the second and third trimesters of pregnancy. The risk is greatest with streptomycin. The risk is probably very small with gentamicin and tobramycin, but their use should be avoided unless essential.
  Monitoring If given during pregnancy, serum-aminoglycoside concentration monitoring is essential.

- RENAL IMPAIRMENT Excretion of aminoglycosides is principally via the kidney and accumulation occurs in renal impairment. Ototoxicity and nephrotoxicity occur commonly in patients with renal failure.
  ▸ In adults A once-daily, high-dose regimen of an aminoglycoside should be avoided in patients with a creatinine clearance less than 20 mL/minute.
  ▸ In children A once-daily, high-dose regimen of an aminoglycoside should be avoided in children over 1 month of age with a creatinine clearance less than 20 mL/minute/1.73 m^2.
  Dose adjustments If there is impairment of renal function, the interval between doses must be increased; if the renal impairment is severe, the dose itself should be reduced as well.
  Monitoring Serum-aminoglycoside concentrations **must** be monitored in patients with renal impairment; earlier and more frequent measurement of aminoglycoside concentration may be required.

- MONITORING REQUIREMENTS
  ▸ Serum concentrations Serum concentration monitoring avoids both excessive and subtherapeutic concentrations thus preventing toxicity and ensuring efficacy. Serum-aminoglycoside concentrations should be measured in all patients receiving parenteral aminoglycosides and **must** be determined in obesity, if high doses are being given and in cystic fibrosis.
  ▸ In adults Serum aminoglycoside concentrations **must** be determined in the elderly. In patients with normal renal function, aminoglycoside concentrations should be measured after 3 or 4 doses of a multiple daily dose regimen and after a dose change. For multiple daily dose regimens, blood samples should be taken approximately 1 hour after intramuscular or intravenous administration ('peak' concentration) and also just before the next dose ('trough') concentration). If the pre-dose ('trough') concentration is high, the interval between doses must be increased. If the post-dose ('peak') concentration is high, the dose must be decreased. For once daily dose regimens, consult local guidelines on serum concentration monitoring.
  ▸ In children In children with normal renal function, aminoglycoside concentrations should be measured after 3 or 4 doses of a multiple daily dose regimen. Blood samples should be taken just before the next dose is administered ('trough' concentration). If the pre-dose ('trough') concentration is high, the interval between doses must be increased. For multiple daily dose regimens, blood samples should also be taken approximately 1 hour after intramuscular or intravenous administration ('peak'

concentration). If the post-dose ('peak') concentration is high, the dose must be decreased.

▸ Renal function should be assessed before starting an aminoglycoside and during treatment.

▸ Auditory and vestibular function should also be monitored during treatment.

F 544

Amikacin

12-Aug-2020

● INDICATIONS AND DOSE

Serious Gram-negative infections resistant to gentamicin (multiple daily dose regimen)
▸ BY INTRAMUSCULAR INJECTION, OR BY SLOW INTRAVENOUS INJECTION, OR BY INTRAVENOUS INFUSION
▸ Adult: 15 mg/kg daily in 2 divided doses, increased to 22.5 mg/kg daily in 3 divided doses for up to 10 days, higher dose to be used in severe infections; maximum 1.5 g per day; maximum 15 g per course

Serious Gram-negative infections resistant to gentamicin (once daily dose regimen)
▸ BY INTRAVENOUS INFUSION
▸ Adult: Initially 15 mg/kg once daily (max. per dose 1.5 g once daily), dose to be adjusted according to serum-amikacin concentration; maximum 15 g per course

Acute prostatitis (once daily dose regimen)
▸ BY INTRAVENOUS INFUSION, OR BY SLOW INTRAVENOUS INJECTION
▸ Adult: Initially 15 mg/kg once daily (max. per dose 1.5 g once daily), dose to be adjusted according to serum-amikacin concentration; maximum 15 g per course

Acute pyelonephritis (once daily dose regimen) | Urinary tract infection (catheter-associated, once daily dose regimen)
▸ BY INTRAVENOUS INFUSION, OR BY SLOW INTRAVENOUS INJECTION
▸ Adult: Initially 15 mg/kg once daily (max. per dose 1.5 g once daily), dose to be adjusted according to serum-amikacin concentration; maximum 15 g per course

DOSES AT EXTREMES OF BODY-WEIGHT
▸ To avoid excessive dosage in obese patients, use ideal weight for height to calculate dose and monitor serum-amikacin concentration closely

● INTERACTIONS → Appendix 1: aminoglycosides

● SIDE-EFFECTS
▸ **Uncommon** Superinfection
▸ **Rare or very rare** Albuminuria · arthralgia · balance impaired · hypotension · muscle twitching · tremor
▸ **Frequency not known** Apnoea · neuromuscular blockade · paralysis

● MONITORING REQUIREMENTS
▸ With intravenous use *Multiple daily dose regimen*: one-hour ('peak') serum concentration should not exceed 30 mg/litre; pre-dose ('trough') concentration should be less than 10 mg/litre. *Once daily dose regimen*: pre-dose ('trough') concentration should be less than 5 mg/litre.

● DIRECTIONS FOR ADMINISTRATION
▸ With intravenous use For *intravenous infusion (Amikin ®)*; manufacturer advises dilute in Glucose 5% *or* Sodium Chloride 0.9%. To be given over 30–60 minutes.

● PRESCRIBING AND DISPENSING INFORMATION Once daily dose regimen not to be used for endocarditis, febrile neutropenia, or meningitis. Consult local guidelines.

● MEDICINAL FORMS There can be variation in the licensing of different medicines containing the same drug. Forms available from special-order manufacturers include: solution for injection

Solution for injection
▸ Amikacin (Non-proprietary)
  Amikacin (as Amikacin sulfate) 250 mg per 1 ml Amikacin 500mg/2ml solution for injection vials | 5 vial [PoM] £60.00 (Hospital only)
▸ Amikin (Vianex S.A.)
  Amikacin (as Amikacin sulfate) 50 mg per 1 ml Amikin 100mg/2ml solution for injection vials | 5 vial [PoM] £10.33

F 544

Gentamicin

04-Dec-2020

● INDICATIONS AND DOSE

Moderate diabetic foot infection | Severe diabetic foot infection | Acute diverticulitis [in combination with amoxicillin and metronidazole]
▸ BY INTRAVENOUS INFUSION
▸ Adult: Initially 5–7 mg/kg once daily, subsequent doses adjusted according to serum-gentamicin concentration

Leg ulcer infection [in combination with other drugs]
▸ BY INTRAVENOUS INFUSION
▸ Adult: Initially 5–7 mg/kg, subsequent dosing adjusted according to serum-gentamicin concentration

Gram-positive bacterial endocarditis or HACEK endocarditis (in combination with other antibacterials)
▸ BY INTRAMUSCULAR INJECTION, OR BY SLOW INTRAVENOUS INJECTION, OR BY INTRAVENOUS INFUSION
▸ Adult: 1 mg/kg every 12 hours, intravenous injection to be administered over at least 3 minutes, to be given in a multiple daily dose regimen

Septicaemia | Meningitis and other CNS infections | Biliary-tract infection | Endocarditis | Pneumonia in hospital patients | Adjunct in listerial meningitis | Prostatitis
▸ BY INTRAVENOUS INFUSION, OR BY SLOW INTRAVENOUS INJECTION, OR BY INTRAMUSCULAR INJECTION
▸ Adult: 3–5 mg/kg daily in 3 divided doses, to be given in a multiple daily dose regimen, divided doses to be given every 8 hours, intravenous injection to be administered over at least 3 minutes
▸ BY INTRAVENOUS INFUSION
▸ Adult: Initially 5–7 mg/kg, subsequent doses adjusted according to serum-gentamicin concentration, to be given in a once daily dose regimen

CNS infections (administered on expert advice)
▸ BY INTRATHECAL INJECTION
▸ Adult: 1 mg daily, increased if necessary to 5 mg daily, seek specialist advice

Surgical prophylaxis
▸ BY SLOW INTRAVENOUS INJECTION
▸ Adult: 1.5 mg/kg, intravenous injection to be administered over at least 3 minutes, administer dose up to 30 minutes before the procedure, dose may be repeated every 8 hours for high-risk procedures; up to 3 further doses may be given

Surgical prophylaxis in joint replacement surgery
▸ BY INTRAVENOUS INFUSION
▸ Adult: 5 mg/kg for 1 dose, administer dose up to 30 minutes before the procedure

Acute pyelonephritis (once daily dose regimen) | Urinary tract infection (catheter-associated, once daily dose regimen)
▸ BY INTRAVENOUS INFUSION
▸ Adult: Initially 5–7 mg/kg once daily, subsequent doses adjusted according to serum-gentamicin concentration

continued →

5

Infection

Uncomplicated gonorrhoea [anogenital and pharyngeal infection—in combination with azithromycin]

▸ BY INTRAMUSCULAR INJECTION
▸ Adult: 240 mg for 1 dose

DOSES AT EXTREMES OF BODY-WEIGHT
▸ With intramuscular use or intravenous use To avoid excessive dosage in obese patients, use ideal weight for height to calculate parenteral dose and monitor serum-gentamicin concentration closely.

● UNLICENSED USE Gentamicin doses in BNF publications may differ from those in product literature.

⟨EvGr⟩ Gentamicin is used in the doses provided in the BNF for the treatment of uncomplicated gonorrhoea, ⟨Ⓐ⟩ but these are not licensed.

IMPORTANT SAFETY INFORMATION

MHRA/CHM ADVICE: POTENTIAL FOR HISTAMINE-RELATED ADVERSE DRUG REACTIONS WITH SOME BATCHES (NOVEMBER 2017)

Following reports that some batches of gentamicin sulphate active pharmaceutical ingredient (API) used to manufacture gentamicin may contain higher than expected levels of histamine, which is a residual from the manufacturing process, the MHRA advise to monitor patients for signs of histamine-related adverse reactions; particular caution is required in patients taking concomitant drugs known to cause histamine release, in children, and in patients with severe renal impairment.

● INTERACTIONS → Appendix 1: aminoglycosides
● SIDE-EFFECTS Antibiotic associated colitis · blood disorder · depression · encephalopathy · hallucination · hepatic reaction · neurotoxicity · peripheral neuropathy · seizure · stomatitis · vestibular damage
● MONITORING REQUIREMENTS
▸ With intramuscular use or intravenous use For multiple daily dose regimen, one-hour ('peak') serum concentration should be 5–10 mg/litre; pre-dose ('trough') concentration should be less than 2 mg/litre. For multiple daily dose regimen in endocarditis, one-hour ('peak') serum concentration should be 3–5 mg/litre; pre-dose ('trough') concentration should be less than 1 mg/litre. Serum-gentamicin concentration should be measured after 3 or 4 doses, then at least every 3 days and after a dose change (more frequently in renal impairment).
▸ With intravenous use For once-daily dose regimen, consult local guidelines on monitoring serum-gentamicin concentration.
● DIRECTIONS FOR ADMINISTRATION
▸ With intrathecal use For *intrathecal* injection, use preservative-free intrathecal preparations only.
▸ With intravenous use ⟨EvGr⟩ For *intravenous infusion*, give intermittently *or* via drip tubing in Glucose 5% or Sodium Chloride 0.9%. Suggested volume for intermittent infusion 50–100 mL given over 20–30 minutes (given over 60 minutes for once daily dose regimen). ⟨Ⓜ⟩
● PRESCRIBING AND DISPENSING INFORMATION For choice of antibacterial therapy, see Antibacterials, use for prophylaxis p. 529, Blood infections, antibacterial therapy p. 532, Cardiovascular system infections, antibacterial therapy p. 532, Central nervous system infections, antibacterial therapy p. 533, Diabetic foot infections, antibacterial therapy p. 534, Gastro-intestinal system infections, antibacterial therapy p. 535, Respiratory system infections, antibacterial therapy p. 538, Skin infections, antibacterial therapy p. 541, Urinary-tract infections p. 626.
▸ With intravenous use Local guidelines may vary in the dosing advice provided for once daily administration.
▸ With intrathecal use Only preservative-free intrathecal preparation should be used.

● MEDICINAL FORMS There can be variation in the licensing of different medicines containing the same drug. Forms available from special-order manufacturers include: infusion, eye drops

Solution for injection
▸ Gentamicin (Non-proprietary)
  Gentamicin (as Gentamicin sulfate) 5 mg per 1 ml Gentamicin Intrathecal 5mg/1ml solution for injection ampoules | 5 ampoule [PoM] £36.28 DT = £36.28 (Hospital only)
  Gentamicin (as Gentamicin sulfate) 10 mg per 1 ml Gentamicin 20mg/2ml solution for injection ampoules | 5 ampoule [PoM] £11.25 DT = £11.25
  Gentamicin Paediatric 20mg/2ml solution for injection vials | 5 vial [PoM] £11.25 DT = £11.25
  Gentamicin (as Gentamicin sulfate) 40 mg per 1 ml Gentamicin 80mg/2ml solution for injection vials | 5 vial [PoM] £20.00 DT = £6.88 (Hospital only)
  Gentamicin 80mg/2ml solution for injection ampoules | 5 ampoule [PoM] £6.88 DT = £6.88 | 10 ampoule [PoM] £12.00
▸ Cidomycin (Sanofi)
  Gentamicin (as Gentamicin sulfate) 40 mg per 1 ml Cidomycin 80mg/2ml solution for injection vials | 5 vial [PoM] £6.88 DT = £6.88 (Hospital only)
  Cidomycin 80mg/2ml solution for injection ampoules | 5 ampoule [PoM] £6.88 DT = £6.88

Infusion
▸ Gentamicin (Non-proprietary)
  Gentamicin (as Gentamicin sulfate) 1 mg per 1 ml Gentamicin 80mg/80ml infusion bags | 20 bag [PoM] £40.17–£44.19
  Gentamicin (as Gentamicin sulfate) 3 mg per 1 ml Gentamicin 240mg/80ml infusion bags | 20 bag [PoM] £122.58–£134.83
  Gentamicin 360mg/120ml infusion bags | 20 bag [PoM] £174.07–£191.48

Neomycin sulfate

● INDICATIONS AND DOSE
Bowel sterilisation before surgery
▸ BY MOUTH
▸ Adult: 1 g every 1 hour for 4 hours, then 1 g every 4 hours for 2–3 days

Hepatic coma
▸ BY MOUTH
▸ Adult: Up to 4 g daily in divided doses usually for 5–7 days

● CONTRA-INDICATIONS Intestinal obstruction · myasthenia gravis (aminoglycosides may impair neuromuscular transmission)
● CAUTIONS Avoid prolonged use

CAUTIONS, FURTHER INFORMATION Although neomycin is associated with the same cautions as other aminoglycosides it is generally considered too toxic for systemic use.

● INTERACTIONS → Appendix 1: neomycin
● SIDE-EFFECTS Blood disorder · confusion · diarrhoea · drug cross-reactivity · electrolyte imbalance · gastrointestinal disorders · haemolytic anaemia · nausea · nephrotoxicity · nystagmus · oral disorders · ototoxicity · paraesthesia · superinfection · vomiting

SIDE-EFFECTS, FURTHER INFORMATION Although neomycin is associated with the same side effects as other aminoglycosides, it is poorly absorbed after oral administration.

● PREGNANCY There is a risk of auditory or vestibular nerve damage in the infant when aminoglycosides are used in the second and third trimesters of pregnancy.
● HEPATIC IMPAIRMENT Manufacturer advises caution (increased risk of ototoxicity and nephrotoxicity).
● RENAL IMPAIRMENT Avoid–risk of ototoxicity and nephrotoxicity.

● MONITORING REQUIREMENTS
▶ Renal function should be assessed before starting an aminoglycoside and during treatment.
▶ Auditory and vestibular function should also be monitored during treatment.

● MEDICINAL FORMS There can be variation in the licensing of different medicines containing the same drug. Forms available from special-order manufacturers include: oral solution

Oral solution
▶ Neo-Fradin (Imported (United States))
Neomycin sulfate 25 mg per 1 ml Neo-Fradin 125mg/5ml oral solution | 480 ml [PoM] ⓈⓁ

Tablet
▶ Neomycin sulfate (Non-proprietary)
Neomycin sulfate 500 mg Neomycin 500mg tablets | 100 tablet [PoM] £34.69 DT = £34.69

`▶ 544`

Streptomycin

● INDICATIONS AND DOSE

Tuberculosis, resistant to other treatment, in combination with other drugs
▶ BY DEEP INTRAMUSCULAR INJECTION
▶ Adult: 15 mg/kg daily (max. per dose 1 g), reduce dose in those under 50 kg and those over 40 years

Adjunct to doxycycline in brucellosis (administered on expert advice)
▶ BY DEEP INTRAMUSCULAR INJECTION
▶ Adult: (consult local protocol)

Enterococcal endocarditis
▶ Adult: (consult local protocol)

● UNLICENSED USE Use in tuberculosis is an unlicensed indication.

IMPORTANT SAFETY INFORMATION
Side-effects increase after a cumulative dose of 100 g, which should only be exceeded in exceptional circumstances.

● INTERACTIONS → Appendix 1: aminoglycosides
● SIDE-EFFECTS Amblyopia · angioedema · Clostridioides difficile colitis · haemolytic anaemia · muscle weakness · ototoxicity · pancytopenia
● RENAL IMPAIRMENT
Dose adjustments Should preferably be avoided. If essential, use with great care and consider dose reduction.
● MONITORING REQUIREMENTS
▶ One-hour ('peak') concentration should be 15–40 mg/litre; pre-dose ('trough') concentration should be less than 5 mg/litre (less than 1 mg/litre in renal impairment or in those over 50 years).

● MEDICINAL FORMS Forms available from special-order manufacturers include: powder for solution for injection

`▶ 544`

Tobramycin

03-Sep-2020

● INDICATIONS AND DOSE

Septicaemia | Meningitis and other CNS infections | Biliary-tract infection | Acute pyelonephritis or prostatitis | Pneumonia in hospital patients
▶ BY INTRAMUSCULAR INJECTION, OR BY SLOW INTRAVENOUS INJECTION, OR BY INTRAVENOUS INFUSION
▶ Adult: 3 mg/kg daily in 3 divided doses; increased if necessary up to 5 mg/kg daily in 3–4 divided doses, increased dose used in severe infection; dose to be reduced back to 3 mg/kg daily as soon as clinically indicated

Urinary-tract infection
▶ BY INTRAMUSCULAR INJECTION
▶ Adult: 2–3 mg/kg for 1 dose

Chronic *Pseudomonas aeruginosa* infection in patients with cystic fibrosis
▶ BY INHALATION OF NEBULISED SOLUTION
▶ Adult: 300 mg every 12 hours for 28 days, subsequent courses repeated after 28-day interval without tobramycin nebuliser solution
▶ BY INHALATION OF POWDER
▶ Adult: 112 mg every 12 hours for 28 days, subsequent courses repeated after 28-day interval without tobramycin inhalation powder

DOSES AT EXTREMES OF BODY-WEIGHT
▶ With intramuscular use or intravenous use To avoid excessive dosage in obese patients, use ideal weight for height to calculate parenteral dose and monitor serum-tobramycin concentration closely.

VANTOBRA® NEBULISER SOLUTION
Chronic pulmonary *Pseudomonas aeruginosa* infection in patients with cystic fibrosis
▶ BY INHALATION OF NEBULISED SOLUTION
▶ Adult: 170 mg every 12 hours for 28 days, subsequent courses repeated after 28-day interval without tobramycin nebuliser solution

● CAUTIONS
▶ When used by inhalation Auditory disorder · conditions characterised by muscular weakness (may impair neuromuscular transmission) · history of prolonged previous or concomitant intravenous aminoglycosides (increased risk of ototoxicity) · renal impairment (limited information available) · severe haemoptysis (risk of further haemorrhage) · vestibular disorder

● INTERACTIONS → Appendix 1: aminoglycosides

● SIDE-EFFECTS
GENERAL SIDE-EFFECTS
▶ **Rare or very rare** Diarrhoea · dizziness
SPECIFIC SIDE-EFFECTS
▶ **Common or very common**
▶ When used by inhalation Dysphonia · malaise · respiratory disorder · sputum discolouration
▶ **Uncommon**
▶ When used by inhalation Cough
▶ **Rare or very rare**
▶ When used by inhalation Abdominal pain · aphonia · appetite decreased · asthenia · asthma · chest discomfort · drowsiness · ear disorder · ear pain · haemorrhage · hypoxia · increased risk of infection · lymphadenopathy · oral ulceration · pain · taste altered
▶ **Frequency not known**
▶ When used by inhalation Oropharyngeal pain
▶ With parenteral use Granulocytopenia · leucocytosis · nerve disorders · urine abnormalities

SIDE-EFFECTS, FURTHER INFORMATION Manufacturer advises to monitor serum-tobramycin concentration in patients with known or suspected signs of auditory dysfunction; if ototoxicity develops — discontinue treatment until serum concentration falls below 2 mg/litre.

● RENAL IMPAIRMENT
▶ When used by inhalation Manufacturer advises monitor serum-tobramycin concentration; if nephrotoxicity develops—discontinue treatment until serum concentration falls below 2 mg/litre.

● MONITORING REQUIREMENTS
▶ With intramuscular use or intravenous use One-hour ('peak') serum concentration should not exceed 10 mg/litre; pre-dose ('trough') concentration should be less than 2 mg/litre.

5

Infection

▸ **When used by inhalation** Measure lung function before and after initial dose of tobramycin and monitor for bronchospasm; if bronchospasm occurs in a patient not using a bronchodilator, repeat test using bronchodilator. Manufacturer advises monitor renal function before treatment and then annually.

● DIRECTIONS FOR ADMINISTRATION

▸ **With intravenous use** For *intravenous infusion (Nebcin ®)*; manufacturer advises give intermittently or via drip tubing in Glucose 5% or Sodium chloride 0.9%. For adult intermittent infusion suggested volume 50–100 mL given over 20–60 minutes.

▸ **When used by inhalation** Manufacturer advises other inhaled drugs should be administered before tobramycin.

● PATIENT AND CARER ADVICE

▸ **When used by inhalation** Patient counselling is advised for Tobramycin dry powder for inhalation (administration).

VANTOBRA ® NEBULISER SOLUTION

Missed doses ▸ **When used by inhalation** Manufacturer advises if a dose is more than 6 hours late, the missed dose should not be taken and the next dose should be taken at the normal time.

● NATIONAL FUNDING/ACCESS DECISIONS
For full details see funding body website

NICE decisions

▸ **Tobramycin by dry powder inhalation for pseudomonal lung infection in cystic fibrosis (March 2013)** NICE TA276 Recommended with restrictions

● MEDICINAL FORMS There can be variation in the licensing of different medicines containing the same drug.

Solution for injection
▸ Tobramycin (Non-proprietary)
Tobramycin 40 mg per 1 ml Tobramycin 80mg/2ml solution for injection vials | 1 vial PoM £5.37 DT = £5.37 | 5 vial PoM £20.80 DT = £20.80
Tobramycin 240mg/6ml solution for injection vials | 1 vial PoM £19.20 DT = £19.20

Inhalation powder
▸ Tobi Podhaler (Mylan)
Tobramycin 28 mg Tobi Podhaler 28mg inhalation powder capsules with device | 224 capsule PoM £1,790.00 DT = £1,790.00

Nebuliser liquid
▸ Tobramycin (Non-proprietary)
Tobramycin 60 mg per 1 ml Tobramycin 300mg/5ml nebuliser liquid ampoules | 56 ampoule PoM £719.00-£1,187.00 DT = £780.00
▸ Bramitob (Chiesi Ltd)
Tobramycin 75 mg per 1 ml Bramitob 300mg/4ml nebuliser solution 4ml ampoules | 56 ampoule PoM £1,187.00 DT = £1,187.00
▸ TOBI (Mylan)
Tobramycin 60 mg per 1 ml Tobi 300mg/5ml nebuliser solution 5ml ampoules | 56 ampoule PoM £1,305.92 DT = £780.00
▸ Tymbrineb (Teva UK Ltd)
Tobramycin 60 mg per 1 ml Tymbrineb 300mg/5ml nebuliser solution 5ml ampoules | 56 ampoule PoM £780.00 DT = £780.00
▸ Vantobra (Pari Medical Ltd)
Tobramycin 100 mg per 1 ml Vantobra 170mg/1.7ml nebuliser solution 1.7ml ampoules | 56 ampoule PoM £1,305.00

ANTIBACTERIALS > CARBAPENEMS

Carbapenems

Overview

The carbapenems are beta-lactam antibacterials with a broad-spectrum of activity which includes many Gram-positive and Gram-negative bacteria, and anaerobes; **imipenem** (imipenem with cilastatin p. 549) and meropenem p. 550 have good activity against *Pseudomonas aeruginosa*. The carbapenems are not active against meticillin-resistant *Staphylococcus aureus* and *Enterococcus faecium*.

Imipenem (imipenem with cilastatin) and meropenem are used for the treatment of severe hospital-acquired infections and polymicrobial infections including septicaemia, hospital-acquired pneumonia, intra-abdominal infections, skin and soft-tissue infections, and complicated urinary-tract infections.

Ertapenem below is licensed for treating abdominal and gynaecological infections and for community-acquired pneumonia, but it is not active against atypical respiratory pathogens and it has limited activity against penicillin-resistant pneumococci. It is also licensed for treating foot infections of the skin and soft tissue in patients with diabetes. Unlike the other carbapenems, ertapenem is not active against *Pseudomonas* or against *Acinetobacter spp.*

Imipenem is partially inactivated in the kidney by enzymatic activity and is therefore administered in combination with **cilastatin** (imipenem with cilastatin), a specific enzyme inhibitor, which blocks its renal metabolism. Meropenem and ertapenem are stable to the renal enzyme which inactivates imipenem and therefore can be given without cilastatin.

Side-effects of imipenem with cilastatin are similar to those of other beta-lactam antibiotics. Meropenem has less seizure-inducing potential and can be used to treat central nervous system infection.

Ertapenem

24-Nov-2020

● INDICATIONS AND DOSE

Abdominal infections | Acute gynaecological infections | Community-acquired pneumonia
▸ BY INTRAVENOUS INFUSION
▸ **Adult:** 1 g once daily

Diabetic foot infections of the skin and soft-tissue
▸ BY INTRAVENOUS INFUSION
▸ **Adult:** 1 g once daily

Surgical prophylaxis, colorectal surgery
▸ BY INTRAVENOUS INFUSION
▸ **Adult:** 1 g for 1 dose, dose to be completed within 1 hour before surgery

● CAUTIONS CNS disorders—risk of seizures · elderly

● INTERACTIONS → Appendix 1: carbapenems

● SIDE-EFFECTS

▸ **Common or very common** Diarrhoea · headache · nausea · skin reactions · thrombophlebitis · vomiting

▸ **Uncommon** Appetite decreased · arrhythmias · asthenia · confusion · constipation · dizziness · drowsiness · dry mouth · gastrointestinal discomfort · gastrointestinal disorders · hypotension · increased risk of infection · insomnia · oedema · pseudomembranous enterocolitis · seizure · swelling · taste altered · throat discomfort

▸ **Rare or very rare** Anxiety · cholecystitis · depression · dysphagia · eye disorder · haemorrhage · hepatic disorders · hypersensitivity · hypoglycaemia · malaise · muscle cramps · nasal congestion · neutropenia · renal impairment · shoulder pain · syncope · thrombocytopenia · tremor

▸ **Frequency not known** Aggression · delirium · drug reaction with eosinophilia and systemic symptoms (DRESS) · gait abnormal · hallucination · level of consciousness decreased · movement disorders · muscle weakness · psychiatric disorder · tooth discolouration

● ALLERGY AND CROSS-SENSITIVITY EvG Avoid if history of **immediate hypersensitivity** reaction to beta-lactam antibacterials.
Use with caution in patients with sensitivity to beta-lactam antibacterials. ⓜ

● PREGNANCY Manufacturer advises avoid unless potential benefit outweighs risk.

- **BREAST FEEDING** Present in milk—manufacturer advises avoid.
- **RENAL IMPAIRMENT**
  Dose adjustments Risk of seizures; max. 500 mg daily if eGFR less than 30 mL/minute/1.73 m².
- **DIRECTIONS FOR ADMINISTRATION** For *intravenous infusion* (*Invanz®*), manufacturer advises give intermittently in Sodium chloride 0.9%. Reconstitute 1 g with 10 mL Water for injections *or* Sodium chloride 0.9%; dilute requisite dose in infusion fluid to a final concentration not exceeding 20 mg/mL; give over 30 minutes; incompatible with glucose solutions.
- **PRESCRIBING AND DISPENSING INFORMATION** For choice of antibacterial therapy, see Antibacterials, use for prophylaxis p. 529, Diabetic foot infections, antibacterial therapy p. 534, Gastro-intestinal system infections, antibacterial therapy p. 535, Respiratory system infections, antibacterial therapy p. 538.

- **MEDICINAL FORMS** There can be variation in the licensing of different medicines containing the same drug.
  Powder for solution for infusion
  ELECTROLYTES: May contain Sodium
  ▸ Ertapenem (Non-proprietary)
    Ertapenem (as Ertapenem sodium) 1 gram Ertapenem 1g powder for concentrate for solution for infusion vials | 10 vial P̲o̲M̲ £316.50
  ▸ Invanz (Merck Sharp & Dohme Ltd)
    Ertapenem (as Ertapenem sodium) 1 gram Invanz 1g powder for solution for infusion vials | 1 vial P̲o̲M̲ £31.65 DT = £31.65 (Hospital only)

Imipenem with cilastatin
24-Nov-2020

- **INDICATIONS AND DOSE**

Aerobic and anaerobic Gram-positive and Gram-negative infections (not indicated for CNS infections) | Hospital-acquired septicaemia
  ▸ BY INTRAVENOUS INFUSION
  ▸ Adult: 500 mg every 6 hours, alternatively 1 g every 8 hours

Infection caused by *Pseudomonas* or other less sensitive organisms | Empirical treatment of infection in febrile patients with neutropenia | Life-threatening infection
  ▸ BY INTRAVENOUS INFUSION
  ▸ Adult: 1 g every 6 hours

DOSE EQUIVALENCE AND CONVERSION
  ▸ Dose expressed in terms of imipenem.

- **CAUTIONS** CNS disorders · epilepsy
- **INTERACTIONS** → Appendix 1: carbapenems
- **SIDE-EFFECTS**
  ▸ **Common or very common** Diarrhoea · eosinophilia · nausea · skin reactions · thrombophlebitis · vomiting
  ▸ **Uncommon** Bone marrow disorders · confusion · dizziness · drowsiness · hallucination · hypotension · leucopenia · movement disorders · psychiatric disorder · seizure · thrombocytopenia · thrombocytosis
  ▸ **Rare or very rare** Agranulocytosis · anaphylactic reaction · angioedema · antibiotic associated colitis · chest discomfort · colitis haemorrhagic · cyanosis · dyspnoea · encephalopathy · flushing · focal tremor · gastrointestinal discomfort · haemolytic anaemia · headache · hearing loss · hepatic disorders · hyperhidrosis · hyperventilation · increased risk of infection · myasthenia gravis aggravated · oral disorders · palpitations · paraesthesia · polyarthralgia · polyuria · renal impairment · severe cutaneous adverse reactions (SCARs) · spinal pain · tachycardia · taste altered · tinnitus · tongue discolouration · tooth discolouration · urine discolouration · vertigo
  ▸ **Frequency not known** Agitation

- **ALLERGY AND CROSS-SENSITIVITY** E̲v̲G̲r̲ Avoid if history of **immediate hypersensitivity** reaction to beta-lactam antibacterials.
  Use with caution in patients with sensitivity to beta-lactam antibacterials. Ⓜ
- **PREGNANCY** Manufacturer advises avoid unless potential benefit outweighs risk (toxicity in *animal* studies).
- **BREAST FEEDING** E̲v̲G̲r̲ Specialist sources indicate suitable for use in breast-feeding. Ⓓ
- **RENAL IMPAIRMENT** Manufacturer advises caution if creatinine clearance less than 90 mL/minute.
  Dose adjustments Manufacturer advises reduce dose if creatinine clearance less than 90 mL/minute (risk of CNS side-effects)—consult product literature.
- **EFFECT ON LABORATORY TESTS** Positive Coombs' test.
- **DIRECTIONS FOR ADMINISTRATION** For *intravenous infusion*, manufacturer advises dilute to a concentration of 5 mg (as imipenem)/mL in Sodium chloride 0.9%; give up to 500 mg (as imipenem) over 20–30 minutes, give dose greater than 500 mg (as imipenem) over 40–60 minutes.

- **MEDICINAL FORMS** There can be variation in the licensing of different medicines containing the same drug.
  Powder for solution for infusion
  ELECTROLYTES: May contain Sodium
  ▸ Imipenem with cilastatin (Non-proprietary)
    Cilastatin (as Cilastatin sodium) 500 mg, Imipenem (as Imipenem monohydrate) 500 mg Imipenem 500mg / Cilastatin 500mg powder for solution for infusion vials | 10 vial P̲o̲M̲ £130.30
  ▸ Primaxin I.V. (Merck Sharp & Dohme Ltd)
    Cilastatin (as Cilastatin sodium) 500 mg, Imipenem (as Imipenem monohydrate) 500 mg Primaxin IV 500mg powder for solution for infusion vials | 1 vial P̲o̲M̲ £12.00

Imipenem with cilastatin and relebactam
21-Sep-2020

The properties listed below are those particular to the combination only. For the properties of the components please consider, imipenem with cilastatin above.

- **INDICATIONS AND DOSE**

Aerobic Gram-negative infections [in patients with limited treatment options] (administered on expert advice)
  ▸ BY INTRAVENOUS INFUSION
  ▸ Adult: 500 mg every 6 hours, duration should be tailored to site of infection—consult product literature

DOSE EQUIVALENCE AND CONVERSION
  ▸ Dose expressed in terms of imipenem.

- **CAUTIONS** Neutropenia (consider alternative treatment options) · severe infections (consider alternative treatment options) · supra-normal creatinine clearance
  CAUTIONS, FURTHER INFORMATION
  ▸ Supra-normal creatinine clearance Manufacturer advises the usual dose may not be sufficient to treat patients with creatinine clearance 150 mL/minute or more, and alternative treatment options should be considered.
- **INTERACTIONS** → Appendix 1: carbapenems
- **RENAL IMPAIRMENT** Manufacturer advises caution if creatinine clearance less than 90 mL/minute.
  Dose adjustments Manufacturer advises reduce dose if creatinine clearance less than 90 mL/minute—consult product literature.
- **DIRECTIONS FOR ADMINISTRATION** Manufacturer advises for *intravenous infusion*, dilute to a concentration of 5 mg (as imipenem)/mL with Sodium Chloride 0.9% (preferably) *or* Glucose 5%; give intermittently over 30 minutes. For a list of compatible infusion bags and infusion sets—consult product literature.

5

Infection

● MEDICINAL FORMS There can be variation in the licensing of different medicines containing the same drug.
Powder for solution for infusion
ELECTROLYTES: May contain Sodium
▸ Recarbrio (Merck Sharp & Dohme Ltd) ▼
Relebactam (as Relebactam monohydrate) 250 mg, Cilastatin (as Cilastatin sodium) 500 mg, Imipenem (as Imipenem monohydrate) 500 mg Recarbrio 500mg/500mg/250mg powder for solution for infusion vials | 25 vial PoM £3,838.75

Meropenem

17-Nov-2020

● INDICATIONS AND DOSE

Aerobic and anaerobic Gram-positive and Gram-negative infections | Hospital-acquired septicaemia
▸ BY INTRAVENOUS INFUSION, OR BY INTRAVENOUS INJECTION
▸ Adult: 0.5–1 g every 8 hours

Exacerbations of chronic lower respiratory-tract infection in cystic fibrosis
▸ BY INTRAVENOUS INFUSION, OR BY INTRAVENOUS INJECTION
▸ Adult: 2 g every 8 hours

Meningitis
▸ BY INTRAVENOUS INFUSION, OR BY INTRAVENOUS INJECTION
▸ Adult: 2 g every 8 hours

Endocarditis (in combination with another antibacterial)
▸ BY INTRAVENOUS INFUSION, OR BY INTRAVENOUS INJECTION
▸ Adult: 2 g every 8 hours

● UNLICENSED USE Not licensed for use in endocarditis.
● INTERACTIONS → Appendix 1: carbapenems
● SIDE-EFFECTS
▸ **Common or very common** Abdominal pain · diarrhoea · headache · inflammation · nausea · pain · skin reactions · thrombocytosis · vomiting
▸ **Uncommon** Agranulocytosis · antibiotic associated colitis · eosinophilia · haemolytic anaemia · increased risk of infection · leucopenia · neutropenia · paraesthesia · severe cutaneous adverse reactions (SCARs) · thrombocytopenia · thrombophlebitis
▸ **Rare or very rare** Seizure
● ALLERGY AND CROSS-SENSITIVITY EvGr Avoid if history of **immediate hypersensitivity** reaction to beta-lactam antibacterials.
Use with caution in patients with sensitivity to beta-lactam antibacterials. ⓜ
● PREGNANCY Use only if potential benefit outweighs risk—no information available.
● BREAST FEEDING Unlikely to be absorbed (however, manufacturer advises avoid).
● RENAL IMPAIRMENT
Dose adjustments Use normal dose every 12 hours if eGFR 26–50 mL/minute/1.73 m².
Use half normal dose every 12 hours if eGFR 10–25 mL/minute/1.73 m².
Use half normal dose every 24 hours if eGFR less than 10 mL/minute/1.73 m².
● MONITORING REQUIREMENTS Manufacturer advises monitor liver function—risk of hepatotoxicity.
● EFFECT ON LABORATORY TESTS Positive Coombs' test.
● DIRECTIONS FOR ADMINISTRATION Manufacturer advises *intravenous injection* to be administered over 5 minutes.
For *intravenous infusion* (*Meronem*®), manufacturer advises give intermittently in Glucose 5% *or* Sodium chloride 0.9%. Dilute dose in infusion fluid to a final concentration of 1–20 mg/mL; give over 15–30 minutes.

● MEDICINAL FORMS There can be variation in the licensing of different medicines containing the same drug.
Powder for solution for injection
ELECTROLYTES: May contain Sodium
▸ Meropenem (Non-proprietary)
Meropenem (as Meropenem trihydrate) 500 mg Meropenem 500mg powder for solution for injection vials | 10 vial PoM £103.14 DT = £93.30 (Hospital only)
Meropenem (as Meropenem trihydrate) 1 gram Meropenem 1g powder for solution for injection vials | 10 vial PoM £206.30 DT = £186.70 (Hospital only)
▸ Meronem (Pfizer Ltd)
Meropenem (as Meropenem trihydrate) 500 mg Meronem 500mg powder for solution for injection vials | 10 vial PoM £103.14 DT = £93.30 (Hospital only)
Meropenem (as Meropenem trihydrate) 1 gram Meronem 1g powder for solution for injection vials | 10 vial PoM £206.28 DT = £186.70 (Hospital only)

Meropenem with vaborbactam

11-Nov-2020

The properties listed below are those particular to the combination only. For the properties of the components please consider, meropenem above.

● INDICATIONS AND DOSE

Complicated urinary-tract infection [including pyelonephritis] | Complicated intra-abdominal infection
▸ BY INTRAVENOUS INFUSION
▸ Adult: 2 g every 8 hours for 5–10 days; may be continued for up to 14 days

Hospital-acquired pneumonia | Ventilator-associated pneumonia
▸ BY INTRAVENOUS INFUSION
▸ Adult: 2 g every 8 hours for 7–14 days

Bacteraemia [occurring in association with or suspected to be associated with the licensed indications]
▸ BY INTRAVENOUS INFUSION
▸ Adult: 2 g every 8 hours, duration should be tailored to site of infection

Aerobic Gram-negative infections [in patients with limited treatment options] (administered on expert advice)
▸ BY INTRAVENOUS INFUSION
▸ Adult: 2 g every 8 hours, duration should be tailored to site of infection

DOSE EQUIVALENCE AND CONVERSION
▸ Dose expressed in terms of meropenem.

● INTERACTIONS → Appendix 1: carbapenems · vaborbactam
● SIDE-EFFECTS
▸ **Common or very common** Diarrhoea · electrolyte imbalance · headache · hypoglycaemia · hypotension · nausea · thrombocytosis · vomiting
▸ **Uncommon** Appetite decreased · bronchospasm · chest discomfort · Clostridioides difficile colitis · dizziness · eosinophilia · gastrointestinal discomfort · hallucination · hyperglycaemia · increased risk of infection · infusion related reaction · insomnia · lethargy · leucopenia · neutropenia · pain · paraesthesia · renal impairment · skin reactions · thrombocytopenia · tremor · urinary incontinence · vascular pain
▸ **Rare or very rare** Seizure
▸ **Frequency not known** Agranulocytosis · angioedema · haemolytic anaemia · severe cutaneous adverse reactions (SCARs)
● PREGNANCY Manufacturer advises avoid—no or limited information available.
● BREAST FEEDING Manufacturer advises discontinue breast-feeding.
● RENAL IMPAIRMENT
Dose adjustments Manufacturer advises reduce dose to 1 g every 8 hours if creatinine clearance 20–39 mL/minute.

Manufacturer advises reduce dose to 1 g every 12 hours if creatinine clearance 10–19 mL/minute.

Manufacturer advises reduce dose to 0.5 g every 12 hours if creatinine clearance less than 10 mL/minute.

- DIRECTIONS FOR ADMINISTRATION For *continuous intravenous infusion*, manufacturer advises reconstitute each 1 g (as meropenem) vial to produce a 0.05 g (as meropenem)/mL solution with 20 mL Sodium Chloride 0.9%. Dilute reconstituted solution to a final volume of 250 mL with Sodium Chloride 0.9%; give over 3 hours.

- PATIENT AND CARER ADVICE
Driving and skilled tasks Manufacturer advises patients and carers should be counselled on the effects on driving and performance of skilled tasks—increased risk of dizziness, lethargy, and paraesthesia.

- NATIONAL FUNDING/ACCESS DECISIONS
For full details see funding body website
Scottish Medicines Consortium (SMC) decisions
▸ Meropenem/vaborbactam (*Vaborem*®) for the treatment of: complicated urinary tract infection; complicated intra-abdominal infection; hospital-acquired pneumonia; bacteraemia that occurs in association with, or is suspected to be associated with any of these infections; infections due to aerobic Gram-negative organisms in adults with limited treatment options (October 2020) SMC No. SMC2278
Recommended with restrictions

All Wales Medicines Strategy Group (AWMSG) decisions
▸ Meropenem/vaborbactam (*Vaborem*®) for the treatment of: complicated urinary tract infection; complicated intra-abdominal infection; hospital-acquired pneumonia; bacteraemia that occurs in association with, or is suspected to be associated with any of these infections; infections due to aerobic Gram-negative organisms in adults with limited treatment options (October 2020) AWMSG No. 2760
Recommended with restrictions

- MEDICINAL FORMS There can be variation in the licensing of different medicines containing the same drug.
Powder for solution for infusion
ELECTROLYTES: May contain Sodium
▸ Vaborem (A. Menarini Farmaceutica Internazionale SRL) ▼
Meropenem (as Meropenem trihydrate) 1 gram, Vaborbactam 1 gram Vaborem 1g/1g powder for concentrate for solution for infusion vials | 6 vial [PoM] £334.00 (Hospital only)

ANTIBACTERIALS › CEPHALOSPORINS

Cephalosporins

Overview
The cephalosporins are broad-spectrum antibiotics which are used for the treatment of septicaemia, pneumonia, meningitis, biliary-tract infections, peritonitis, and urinary-tract infections. The pharmacology of the cephalosporins is similar to that of the penicillins, excretion being principally renal. Cephalosporins penetrate the cerebrospinal fluid poorly unless the meninges are inflamed; cefotaxime p. 557 and ceftriaxone p. 558 are suitable cephalosporins for infections of the CNS (e.g meningitis).

The principal side-effect of the cephalosporins is hypersensitivity and about 0.5–6.5% of penicillin-sensitive patients will also be allergic to the cephalosporins. If a cephalosporin is essential in patients with a history of immediate hypersensitivity to penicillin, because a suitable alternative antibacterial is not available, then cefixime p. 556, cefotaxime, ceftazidime p. 557, ceftriaxone, or cefuroxime p. 555 can be used with caution; cefaclor p. 554, cefadroxil p. 552, cefalexin p. 552, cefradine p. 554, and ceftaroline fosamil p. 562 should be avoided.

The orally active 'first generation' cephalosporins, cefalexin, cefradine, and cefadroxil and the 'second generation' cephalosporin, cefaclor, have a similar antimicrobial spectrum. They are useful for urinary-tract infections, respiratory-tract infections, otitis media, and skin and soft-tissue infections. Cefaclor has good activity against *H. influenzae*. Cefadroxil has a long duration of action and can be given twice daily; it has poor activity against *H. influenzae*. **Cefuroxime axetil**, an ester of the 'second generation' cephalosporin cefuroxime, has the same antibacterial spectrum as the parent compound; it is poorly absorbed and needs to be given with food to maximise absorption.

Cefixime is an orally active 'third generation' cephalosporin. It has a longer duration of action than the other cephalosporins that are active by mouth. It is only licensed for acute infections.

Cefuroxime is a 'second generation' cephalosporin that is less susceptible than the earlier cephalosporins to inactivation by beta-lactamases. It is, therefore, active against certain bacteria which are resistant to the other drugs and has greater activity against *Haemophilus influenzae*.

Cefotaxime, ceftazidime and ceftriaxone are 'third generation' cephalosporins with greater activity than the 'second generation' cephalosporins against certain Gram-negative bacteria. However, they are less active than cefuroxime against Gram-positive bacteria, most notably *Staphylococcus aureus*. Their broad antibacterial spectrum may encourage superinfection with resistant bacteria or fungi.

Ceftazidime has good activity against pseudomonas. It is also active against other Gram-negative bacteria.

Ceftriaxone has a longer half-life and therefore needs to be given only once daily. Indications include serious infections such as septicaemia, pneumonia, and meningitis. The calcium salt of ceftriaxone forms a precipitate in the gall bladder which may rarely cause symptoms but these usually resolve when the antibiotic is stopped.

Ceftaroline fosamil is a 'fifth generation' cephalosporin with bactericidal activity similar to cefotaxime; however, ceftaroline fosamil has an extended spectrum of activity against Gram-positive bacteria that includes meticillin-resistant *Staphylococcus aureus* and multi-drug resistant *Streptococcus pneumoniae*. Ceftaroline fosamil is licensed for the treatment of community-acquired pneumonia and complicated skin and soft-tissue infections, but there is no experience of its use in pneumonia caused by meticillin-resistant *S. aureus*.

Cephalosporins

- DRUG ACTION Cephalosporins are antibacterials that attach to penicillin binding proteins to interrupt cell wall biosynthesis, leading to bacterial cell lysis and death.

- SIDE-EFFECTS
▸ **Common or very common** Abdominal pain · diarrhoea · dizziness · eosinophilia · headache · leucopenia · nausea · neutropenia · pseudomembranous enterocolitis · skin reactions · thrombocytopenia · vomiting · vulvovaginal candidiasis
▸ **Uncommon** Anaphylactic reaction · angioedema
▸ **Rare or very rare** Agranulocytosis · haemolytic anaemia · nephritis tubulointerstitial (reversible) · severe cutaneous adverse reactions (SCARs)

- ALLERGY AND CROSS-SENSITIVITY Contra-indicated in patients with cephalosporin hypersensitivity.
▸ Cross-sensitivity with other beta-lactam antibacterials About 0.5–6.5% of penicillin-sensitive patients will also be allergic to the cephalosporins. Patients with a history of **immediate hypersensitivity** to penicillin and other beta-lactams should not receive a cephalosporin.

Cephalosporins should be used with caution in patients with sensitivity to penicillin and other beta-lactams.

- EFFECT ON LABORATORY TESTS False positive urinary glucose (if tested for reducing substances). False positive Coombs' test.

ANTIBACTERIALS > CEPHALOSPORINS, FIRST-GENERATION

F 551

Cefadroxil

- INDICATIONS AND DOSE

Susceptible infections due to sensitive Gram-positive and Gram-negative bacteria
▸ BY MOUTH
  - Child 6–17 years (body-weight up to 40 kg): 0.5 g twice daily
  - Child 6–17 years (body-weight 40 kg and above): 0.5–1 g twice daily
  - Adult: 0.5–1 g twice daily

Skin infections | Soft-tissue infections | Uncomplicated urinary-tract infections
▸ BY MOUTH
  - Child 6–17 years (body-weight 40 kg and above): 1 g once daily
  - Adult: 1 g daily

- INTERACTIONS → Appendix 1: cephalosporins
- SIDE-EFFECTS
▸ **Common or very common** Dyspepsia · glossitis
▸ **Uncommon** Fungal infection
▸ **Rare or very rare** Arthralgia · drug fever · fatigue · hepatic disorders · insomnia · nervousness · serum sickness-like reaction
- PREGNANCY Not known to be harmful.
- BREAST FEEDING Present in milk in low concentration, but appropriate to use.
- RENAL IMPAIRMENT

Dose adjustments ▸ In adults 1 g initially, then 500 mg every 12 hours if eGFR 26–50 mL/minute/1.73 m². 1 g initially, then 500 mg every 24 hours if eGFR 11–26 mL/minute/1.73 m². 1 g initially, then 500 mg every 36 hours if eGFR less than 11 mL/minute/1.73 m².
  ▸ In children Reduce dose if estimated glomerular filtration rate less than 50 mL/minute/1.73 m².

- MEDICINAL FORMS There can be variation in the licensing of different medicines containing the same drug.

Capsule
CAUTIONARY AND ADVISORY LABELS 9
▸ Cefadroxil (Non-proprietary)
  Cefadroxil (as Cefadroxil monohydrate) 500 mg Cefadroxil 500mg capsules | 20 capsule PoM £22.38 DT = £22.38

F 551

Cefalexin

26-Mar-2020

(Cephalexin)

- INDICATIONS AND DOSE

Susceptible infections due to sensitive Gram-positive and Gram-negative bacteria
▸ BY MOUTH
  - Child 1–11 months: 12.5 mg/kg twice daily, alternatively 125 mg twice daily
  - Child 1–4 years: 12.5 mg/kg twice daily, alternatively 125 mg 3 times a day
  - Child 5–11 years: 12.5 mg/kg twice daily, alternatively 250 mg 3 times a day
  - Child 12–17 years: 500 mg 2–3 times a day

- Adult: 250 mg every 6 hours, alternatively 500 mg every 8–12 hours; increased to 1–1.5 g every 6–8 hours, increased dose to be used for severe infections

Serious susceptible infections due to sensitive Gram-positive and Gram-negative bacteria
▸ BY MOUTH
  - Child 1 month–11 years: 25 mg/kg 2–4 times a day (max. per dose 1 g 4 times a day)
  - Child 12–17 years: 1–1.5 g 3–4 times a day

Hospital-acquired pneumonia | Acute diverticulitis [in combination with metronidazole]
▸ BY MOUTH
  - Adult: 500 mg 2–3 times a day; increased if necessary to 1–1.5 g 3–4 times a day for 5 days then review, use increased dose in severe infection

Prophylaxis of recurrent urinary-tract infection
▸ BY MOUTH
  - Child 3 months–15 years: 12.5 mg/kg once daily (max. per dose 125 mg), dose to be taken at night
  - Child 16–17 years: 125 mg once daily, dose to be taken at night, alternatively 500 mg for 1 dose, following exposure to a trigger
  - Adult: 125 mg once daily, dose to be taken at night, alternatively 500 mg for 1 dose, following exposure to a trigger

Acute pyelonephritis | Urinary-tract infection (catheter-associated)
▸ BY MOUTH
  - Child 3–11 months: 12.5 mg/kg twice daily for 7 to 10 days, alternatively 125 mg twice daily; increased if necessary to 25 mg/kg 2–4 times a day (max. per dose 1 g 4 times a day), increased dose used in severe infections
  - Child 1–4 years: 12.5 mg/kg twice daily, alternatively 125 mg 3 times a day for 7 to 10 days; increased if necessary to 25 mg/kg 2–4 times a day (max. per dose 1 g 4 times a day), increased dose used in severe infections
  - Child 5–11 years: 12.5 mg/kg twice daily, alternatively 250 mg 3 times a day for 7 to 10 days; increased if necessary to 25 mg/kg 2–4 times a day (max. per dose 1 g 4 times a day), increased dose used in severe infections
  - Child 12–17 years: 500 mg 2–3 times a day for 7 to 10 days; increased to 1–1.5 g 3–4 times a day, increased dose used in severe infections
  - Adult: 500 mg 2–3 times a day for 7 to 10 days; increased if necessary to 1–1.5 g 3–4 times a day, increased dose used in severe infections

Lower urinary-tract infection in pregnancy
▸ BY MOUTH
  - Child 12–17 years: 500 mg twice daily for 7 days
  - Adult: 500 mg twice daily for 7 days

Lower urinary-tract infection
▸ BY MOUTH
  - Child 3–11 months: 12.5 mg/kg twice daily, alternatively 125 mg twice daily for 3 days
  - Child 1–4 years: 12.5 mg/kg twice daily, alternatively 125 mg 3 times a day for 3 days
  - Child 5–11 years: 12.5 mg/kg twice daily, alternatively 250 mg 3 times a day for 3 days
  - Child 12–15 years: 500 mg twice daily for 3 days

- UNLICENSED USE EvGr Cefalexin is used for prophylaxis of recurrent urinary-tract infection, ⒶEvGr but is not licensed for this indication.
- INTERACTIONS → Appendix 1: cephalosporins
- SIDE-EFFECTS Agitation · arthritis · confusion · fatigue · fungal infection · gastrointestinal discomfort · genital pruritus · hallucination · hepatitis (transient) ·

hypersensitivity · jaundice cholestatic (transient) · joint disorders · vaginal discharge
● **PREGNANCY** Not known to be harmful.
● **BREAST FEEDING** Present in milk in low concentration, but appropriate to use.
● **RENAL IMPAIRMENT**
Dose adjustments ▸ In adults Max. 3 g daily if eGFR 40–50 mL/minute/1.73 m². Max. 1.5 g daily if eGFR 10–40 mL/minute/1.73 m². Max. 750 mg daily if eGFR less than 10 mL/minute/1.73 m².
  ▸ In children Reduce dose in moderate impairment.
● **PRESCRIBING AND DISPENSING INFORMATION** For choice of antibacterial therapy, see Gastro-intestinal system infections, antibacterial therapy p. 535, Respiratory system infections, antibacterial therapy p. 538, Urinary-tract infections p. 626.
● **PATIENT AND CARER ADVICE**
Medicines for Children leaflet: Cefalexin for bacterial infections www.medicinesforchildren.org.uk/cefalexin-bacterial-infections-0
● **PROFESSION SPECIFIC INFORMATION**
Dental practitioners' formulary
Cefalexin Capsules may be prescribed.
Cefalexin Tablets may be prescribed.
Cefalexin Oral Suspension may be prescribed.

● **MEDICINAL FORMS** There can be variation in the licensing of different medicines containing the same drug.
Oral suspension
CAUTIONARY AND ADVISORY LABELS 9
▸ Cefalexin (Non-proprietary)
Cefalexin 25 mg per 1 ml Cefalexin 125mg/5ml oral suspension sugar free sugar-free | 100 ml [PoM] £0.84 DT = £2.92
Cefalexin 125mg/5ml oral suspension | 100 ml [PoM] £3.27 DT = £2.87
Cefalexin 50 mg per 1 ml Cefalexin 250mg/5ml oral suspension sugar free sugar-free | 100 ml [PoM] £1.72 DT = £3.38
Cefalexin 250mg/5ml oral suspension | 100 ml [PoM] £3.41 DT = £2.95
Tablet
CAUTIONARY AND ADVISORY LABELS 9
▸ Cefalexin (Non-proprietary)
Cefalexin 250 mg Cefalexin 250mg tablets | 28 tablet [PoM] £2.69 DT = £2.69
Cefalexin 500 mg Cefalexin 500mg tablets | 21 tablet [PoM] £5.35 DT = £2.77
Capsule
CAUTIONARY AND ADVISORY LABELS 9
▸ Cefalexin (Non-proprietary)
Cefalexin 250 mg Cefalexin 250mg capsules | 28 capsule [PoM] £2.20 DT = £2.20
Cefalexin 500 mg Cefalexin 500mg capsules | 21 capsule [PoM] £2.46 DT = £2.46

F 551

Cefazolin
25-Aug-2020

● **INDICATIONS AND DOSE**
Surgical prophylaxis
▸ BY SLOW INTRAVENOUS INJECTION, OR BY INTRAVENOUS INFUSION, OR BY DEEP INTRAMUSCULAR INJECTION
▸ Adult: 1 g, to be administered 30–60 minutes before surgery, then 0.5–1 g if required, during surgery (in procedures lasting 2 hours or more)
Skin infection | Soft tissue infection | Bone infection | Joint infection
▸ BY SLOW INTRAVENOUS INJECTION, OR BY INTRAVENOUS INFUSION, OR BY DEEP INTRAMUSCULAR INJECTION
▸ Adult: 1–2 g daily in 2–3 divided doses, for sensitive bacteria; increased to 3–4 g daily in 3–4 divided doses, for moderately-sensitive bacteria; increased if necessary up to 6 g daily in 3–4 divided doses, for severe infections, single doses greater than 1 g should be given by intravenous infusion

● INTERACTIONS → Appendix 1: cephalosporins
● SIDE-EFFECTS
▸ **Common or very common** Appetite decreased
▸ **Uncommon** Drug fever · oral candidiasis (particularly in long term use) · respiratory disorders · seizure (in renal impairment) · thrombophlebitis
▸ **Rare or very rare** Akathisia · anaemia · anal pruritus · anxiety · asthenia · bone marrow disorders · chest pain · coagulation disorder · colour vision change · confusion · cough · drowsiness · dyspnoea · epileptogenic activity · face oedema · genital pruritus · hepatitis (transient) · hot flush · hyperglycaemia · hypersensitivity · hypoglycaemia · increased leucocytes · increased risk of infection · jaundice cholestatic (transient) · lymphopenia · malaise · nephropathy · proteinuria · sleep disorders · tongue swelling · vertigo
SIDE-EFFECTS, FURTHER INFORMATION Blood disorders including: leucopenia, granulocytopenia, thrombocytopenia, lymphopenia, eosinophillia and increased leucocytes are reversible.
● **PREGNANCY** Manufacturer advises avoid unless essential—limited data available but not known to be harmful in *animal* studies. [EvGr] Specialist sources indicate suitable for use in pregnancy. ⟨D⟩
● **BREAST FEEDING** Present in milk in low concentration, but appropriate to use.
● **RENAL IMPAIRMENT** Manufacturer advises caution if creatinine clearance 54 mL/minute or less, or serum creatinine 1.6 mg/dL or above (increased risk of convulsions).
Dose adjustments Manufacturer advises dose reduction in impairment—consult product literature.
● **DIRECTIONS FOR ADMINISTRATION** Displacement value may be significant when reconstituting injection, consult local guidelines or product literature.
For *intravenous injection*, manufacturer advises reconstitute with Water for Injection *or* Glucose 5 or 10% *or* Sodium Chloride 0.9%; give over 3 to 5 minutes—consult product literature.
For intermittent *intravenous infusion*, manufacturer advises dilute reconstituted solution with Water for Injection *or* Glucose 5% *or* Sodium Chloride 0.9% *or* Compound Sodium Lactate *or* Ringer's Solution; give over 30 to 60 minutes—consult product literature.
For *intramuscular injection*, manufacturer advises reconstitute with Water for Injection *or* Glucose 10% *or* Sodium Chloride 0.9% *or* Lidocaine Hydrochloride 0.5%; give as a deep *intramuscular injection*—consult product literature.
● **PRESCRIBING AND DISPENSING INFORMATION** For choice of antibacterial therapy, see Antibacterials, use for prophylaxis p. 529, Skin infections, antibacterial therapy p. 541, Musculoskeletal system infections, antibacterial therapy p. 536.

● **MEDICINAL FORMS** There can be variation in the licensing of different medicines containing the same drug.
Powder for solution for injection
ELECTROLYTES: May contain Sodium
▸ Cefazolin (Non-proprietary)
Cefazolin (as Cefazolin sodium) 1 gram Cefazolin 1g powder for solution for injection vials | 10 vial [PoM] £161.83
Cefazolin (as Cefazolin sodium) 2 gram Cefazolin 2g powder for solution for injection vials | 10 vial [PoM] £183.90

5

Infection

Cefradine
F 551

(Cephradine)

● **INDICATIONS AND DOSE**

Susceptible infections due to sensitive Gram-positive and Gram-negative bacteria | Surgical prophylaxis

▸ BY MOUTH
▸ Child 7-11 years: 25–50 mg/kg daily in 2–4 divided doses
▸ Child 12-17 years: 250–500 mg 4 times a day, alternatively 0.5–1 g twice daily; increased if necessary up to 1 g 4 times a day, increased dose may be used in severe infections
▸ Adult: 250–500 mg 4 times a day, alternatively 0.5–1 g twice daily; increased if necessary up to 1 g 4 times a day, increased dose may be used in severe infections

● **UNLICENSED USE**
▸ In children Not licensed for use in children for prevention of *Staphylococcus aureus* lung infection in cystic fibrosis.

● **INTERACTIONS** → Appendix 1: cephalosporins

● **SIDE-EFFECTS** Akathisia · antibiotic associated colitis · aplastic anaemia · arthralgia · blood disorder · chest tightness · confusion · gastrointestinal discomfort · glossitis · hepatitis (transient) · hypersensitivity · increased risk of infection · jaundice cholestatic · muscle tone increased · nervousness · oedema · sleep disorder

● **PREGNANCY** Not known to be harmful.

● **BREAST FEEDING** Present in milk in low concentration, but appropriate to use.

● **RENAL IMPAIRMENT**
Dose adjustments ▸ In adults Use half normal dose if eGFR 5–20 mL/minute/1.73 m^2. Use one-quarter normal dose if eGFR less than 5 mL/minute/1.73 m^2.
▸ In children Reduce dose if estimated glomerular filtration rate less than 20 mL/minute/1.73 m^2.

● **PROFESSION SPECIFIC INFORMATION**
Dental practitioners' formulary
Cefradine Capsules may be prescribed.

● **MEDICINAL FORMS** There can be variation in the licensing of different medicines containing the same drug.
Capsule
CAUTIONARY AND ADVISORY LABELS 9
▸ Cefradine (Non-proprietary)
Cefradine 250 mg Cefradine 250mg capsules | 20 capsule PoM £6.00 DT = £4.61
Cefradine 500 mg Cefradine 500mg capsules | 20 capsule PoM £8.75 DT = £6.06

ANTIBACTERIALS > CEPHALOSPORINS, SECOND-GENERATION
F 551

Cefaclor

● **INDICATIONS AND DOSE**

Susceptible infections due to sensitive Gram-positive and Gram-negative bacteria

▸ BY MOUTH USING IMMEDIATE-RELEASE MEDICINES
▸ Child 1-11 months: 20 mg/kg daily in 3 divided doses, alternatively 62.5 mg 3 times a day
▸ Child 1-4 years: 20 mg/kg daily in 3 divided doses, alternatively 125 mg 3 times a day
▸ Child 5-11 years: 20 mg/kg daily in 3 divided doses, usual max. 1 g daily, alternatively 250 mg 3 times a day
▸ Child 12-17 years: 250 mg 3 times a day; maximum 4 g per day
▸ Adult: 250 mg 3 times a day; maximum 4 g per day

▸ BY MOUTH USING MODIFIED-RELEASE MEDICINES
▸ Child 12-17 years: 375 mg every 12 hours, dose to be taken with food
▸ Adult: 375 mg every 12 hours, dose to be taken with food

Severe susceptible infections due to sensitive Gram-positive and Gram-negative bacteria

▸ BY MOUTH USING IMMEDIATE-RELEASE MEDICINES
▸ Child 1-11 months: 40 mg/kg daily in 3 divided doses, usual max. 1 g daily, alternatively 125 mg 3 times a day
▸ Child 1-4 years: 40 mg/kg daily in 3 divided doses, usual max. 1 g daily, alternatively 250 mg 3 times a day
▸ Child 5-11 years: 40 mg/kg daily in 3 divided doses, usual max. 1 g daily
▸ Child 12-17 years: 500 mg 3 times a day; maximum 4 g per day
▸ Adult: 500 mg 3 times a day; maximum 4 g per day

Pneumonia

▸ BY MOUTH USING MODIFIED-RELEASE TABLETS
▸ Child 12-17 years: 750 mg every 12 hours, dose to be taken with food
▸ Adult: 750 mg every 12 hours, dose to be taken with food

Lower urinary-tract infections

▸ BY MOUTH USING MODIFIED-RELEASE MEDICINES
▸ Child 12-17 years: 375 mg every 12 hours, dose to be taken with food
▸ Adult: 375 mg every 12 hours, dose to be taken with food

Asymptomatic carriage of *Haemophilus influenzae* or mild exacerbations in cystic fibrosis

▸ BY MOUTH USING IMMEDIATE-RELEASE MEDICINES
▸ Child 1-11 months: 125 mg every 8 hours
▸ Child 1-6 years: 250 mg 3 times a day
▸ Child 7-17 years: 500 mg 3 times a day

● **INTERACTIONS** → Appendix 1: cephalosporins

● **SIDE-EFFECTS** Akathisia · anxiety · aplastic anaemia · arthralgia · arthritis · asthenia · colitis · confusion · drowsiness · dyspnoea · fever · fungal infection · genital pruritus · hallucination · hepatitis (transient) · hypersensitivity · insomnia · jaundice cholestatic (transient) · lymphadenopathy · lymphocytosis · muscle tone increased · oedema · paraesthesia · proteinuria · syncope · vasodilation

SIDE-EFFECTS, FURTHER INFORMATION Cefaclor is associated with protracted skin reactions, especially in children.

● **PREGNANCY** Not known to be harmful.

● **BREAST FEEDING** Present in milk in low concentration, but appropriate to use.

● **RENAL IMPAIRMENT** Manufacturer advises caution.
Dose adjustments No dose adjustment required.

● **MEDICINAL FORMS** There can be variation in the licensing of different medicines containing the same drug.
Oral suspension
CAUTIONARY AND ADVISORY LABELS 9
▸ Distaclor (Flynn Pharma Ltd)
Cefaclor (as Cefaclor monohydrate) 25 mg per 1 ml Distaclor 125mg/5ml oral suspension | 100 ml PoM £4.13 DT = £4.13
Cefaclor (as Cefaclor monohydrate) 50 mg per 1 ml Distaclor 250mg/5ml oral suspension | 100 ml PoM £8.26 DT = £8.26
Modified-release tablet
CAUTIONARY AND ADVISORY LABELS 9, 21, 25
▸ Distaclor MR (Flynn Pharma Ltd)
Cefaclor (as Cefaclor monohydrate) 375 mg Distaclor MR 375mg tablets | 14 tablet PoM £9.10 DT = £9.10

Capsule

CAUTIONARY AND ADVISORY LABELS 9

▶ Distaclor (Flynn Pharma Ltd)
Cefaclor (as Cefaclor monohydrate) 500 mg Distaclor 500mg capsules | 21 capsule [PoM] £7.50 DT = £7.50

🏳 551

Cefoxitin

21-Aug-2019

● **INDICATIONS AND DOSE**

Complicated urinary tract infection | Pyelonephritis

▶ BY SLOW INTRAVENOUS INJECTION
▶ Adult: 2 g every 4–6 hours; maximum 12 g per day

● INTERACTIONS → Appendix 1: cephalosporins

● SIDE-EFFECTS Anaemia · bone marrow failure · encephalopathy · fever · hypersensitivity · local reaction · myasthenia gravis aggravated · overgrowth of nonsusceptible organisms · renal impairment · thrombophlebitis

● PREGNANCY Manufacturer advises not known to be harmful.

● BREAST FEEDING [EvGr] Specialist sources indicate present in milk in low concentrations, but appropriate to use. Ⓓ

● RENAL IMPAIRMENT
Dose adjustments Manufacturer advises increase dosing interval to every 8-12 hours if creatinine clearance 30-50 mL/minute, or every 12-24 hours if creatinine clearance 10-29 mL/minute. Consult product literature if creatinine clearance less than 10 mL/minute.

● DIRECTIONS FOR ADMINISTRATION For *slow intravenous injection*, reconstitute with 10 mL water for injections; give over 3 to 5 minutes.

● MEDICINAL FORMS There can be variation in the licensing of different medicines containing the same drug. Forms available from special-order manufacturers include: powder for solution for injection
Powder for solution for injection
ELECTROLYTES: May contain Sodium
▶ Renoxitin (Renascience Pharma Ltd)
Cefoxitin (as Cefoxitin sodium) 1 gram Renoxitin 1g powder for solution for injection vials | 10 vial [PoM] £163.80 (Hospital only)
Cefoxitin (as Cefoxitin sodium) 2 gram Renoxitin 2g powder for solution for injection vials | 10 vial [PoM] £282.45 (Hospital only)

🏳 551

Cefuroxime

10-Nov-2020

● **INDICATIONS AND DOSE**

Susceptible infections due to Gram-positive and Gram-negative bacteria

▶ BY MOUTH
▶ Child 3 months-1 year: 10 mg/kg twice daily (max. per dose 125 mg)
▶ Child 2-11 years: 15 mg/kg twice daily (max. per dose 250 mg)
▶ Child 12-17 years: 250 mg twice daily, dose may be doubled in severe lower respiratory-tract infections or if pneumonia is suspected
▶ Adult: 250 mg twice daily, dose may be doubled in severe lower respiratory-tract infections or if pneumonia is suspected
▶ BY INTRAVENOUS INFUSION, OR BY INTRAVENOUS INJECTION, OR BY INTRAMUSCULAR INJECTION
▶ Child: 20 mg/kg every 8 hours (max. per dose 750 mg); increased to 50–60 mg/kg every 6–8 hours (max. per dose 1.5 g), increased dose used for severe infection and cystic fibrosis
▶ Adult: 750 mg every 6–8 hours; increased if necessary up to 1.5 g every 6–8 hours, increased dose used for severe infections

Hospital-acquired pneumonia

▶ BY INTRAVENOUS INJECTION, OR BY INTRAVENOUS INFUSION
▶ Adult: 750 mg every 8 hours; increased if necessary to 750 mg every 6 hours, alternatively 1.5 g every 6–8 hours, increased dose used for severe infections

Cellulitis | Erysipelas

▶ BY INTRAVENOUS INJECTION, OR BY INTRAVENOUS INFUSION
▶ Child: 20 mg/kg every 8 hours (max. per dose 750 mg); increased if necessary up to 50–60 mg/kg every 6–8 hours (max. per dose 1.5 g)
▶ Adult: 750 mg every 6–8 hours; increased if necessary up to 1.5 g every 6–8 hours

Acute diverticulitis [in combination with metronidazole]

▶ BY INTRAVENOUS INJECTION, OR BY INTRAVENOUS INFUSION
▶ Adult: 750 mg every 6–8 hours; increased if necessary up to 1.5 g every 6–8 hours, use increased dose in severe infection

Lyme disease

▶ BY MOUTH
▶ Child 3 months-11 years: 15 mg/kg twice daily (max. per dose 500 mg) for 14–21 days (for 28 days in Lyme arthritis)
▶ Child 12-17 years: 500 mg twice daily for 14–21 days (for 28 days in Lyme arthritis)
▶ Adult: 500 mg twice daily for 14–21 days (for 28 days in Lyme arthritis)

Surgical prophylaxis

▶ INITIALLY BY INTRAVENOUS INJECTION
▶ Adult: 1.5 g, to be administered up to 30 minutes before the procedure, then (by intravenous injection or by intramuscular injection) 750 mg every 8 hours if required for up to 3 doses (in high risk procedures)

Open fractures, prophylaxis

▶ BY INTRAVENOUS INFUSION, OR BY INTRAVENOUS INJECTION
▶ Adult: 1.5 g every 8 hours until soft tissue closure (maximum duration 72 hours)

Acute prostatitis

▶ BY INTRAVENOUS INFUSION, OR BY INTRAVENOUS INJECTION
▶ Adult: 1.5 g every 6–8 hours

Urinary-tract infection (lower)

▶ BY MOUTH
▶ Child (body-weight up to 40 kg): 15 mg/kg twice daily (max. per dose 250 mg)
▶ Child (body-weight 40 kg and above): 250 mg twice daily
▶ Adult: 250 mg twice daily

Urinary tract infection (catheter-associated)

▶ BY INTRAVENOUS INFUSION, OR BY INTRAVENOUS INJECTION
▶ Child 3 months-15 years: 20 mg/kg every 8 hours (max. per dose 750 mg); increased to 50–60 mg/kg every 6–8 hours (max. per dose 1.5 g), increased dose used for severe infection
▶ Child 16-17 years: 0.75–1.5 g every 6–8 hours
▶ Adult: 0.75–1.5 g every 6–8 hours

Acute pyelonephritis

▶ BY MOUTH
▶ Child (body-weight up to 40 kg): 15 mg/kg twice daily (max. per dose 250 mg)
▶ Child (body-weight 40 kg and above): 250 mg twice daily
▶ Adult: 250 mg twice daily
▶ BY INTRAVENOUS INFUSION, OR BY INTRAVENOUS INJECTION
▶ Child 3 months-15 years: 20 mg/kg every 8 hours (max. per dose 750 mg); increased to 50–60 mg/kg every 6–8 hours (max. per dose 1.5 g), increased dose used for severe infection
▶ Child 16-17 years: 0.75–1.5 g every 6–8 hours
▶ Adult: 0.75–1.5 g every 6–8 hours

- UNLICENSED USE
  - In adults EvGr Cefuroxime is used for the treatment of hospital-acquired pneumonia, ⒶＷ but is not licensed for this indication.
  - In children EvGr Cefuroxime is used for the treatment of cellulitis, ⒶＷ but the dose increase is not licensed for this indication. EvGr Cefuroxime is used for the treatment of erysipelas, ⒶＷ but the dose increase is not licensed for this indication.
  - With oral use in children Not licensed for treatment of Lyme disease in children under 12 years.
  - With oral use Duration of treatment in Lyme disease is unlicensed.
- INTERACTIONS → Appendix 1: cephalosporins
- SIDE-EFFECTS
  - Common or very common
  - With oral use Increased risk of infection
  - Uncommon
  - With parenteral use Gastrointestinal disorder
  - Frequency not known
  - With oral use Drug fever · hepatic disorders · Jarisch-Herxheimer reaction · serum sickness
  - With parenteral use Cutaneous vasculitis · drug fever · increased risk of infection
- PREGNANCY Not known to be harmful.
- BREAST FEEDING Present in milk in low concentration, but appropriate to use.
- RENAL IMPAIRMENT
  Dose adjustments ► With intravenous use in adults Use parenteral dose of 750 mg twice daily if eGFR 10–20 mL/minute/1.73 m². Use parenteral dose of 750 mg once daily if eGFR less than 10 mL/minute/1.73 m².
  ► In children Reduce parenteral dose if estimated glomerular filtration rate less than 20 mL/minute/1.73 m².
- DIRECTIONS FOR ADMINISTRATION
  - With intramuscular use or intravenous use Manufacturer advises single doses over 750 mg should be administered by the intravenous route only.
  - With intravenous use in children Displacement value may be significant when reconstituting injection, consult local guidelines. For intermittent intravenous infusion, manufacturer advises dilute reconstituted solution further in Glucose 5% or Sodium Chloride 0.9%; give over 30–60 minutes.
  - With intravenous use in adults For *intravenous infusion* (*Zinacef*®), manufacturer advises give intermittently or via drip tubing in Glucose 5% or Sodium Chloride 0.9%. Dissolve initially in water for injections (at least 2 mL for each 250 mg, 15 mL for 1.5 g); suggested volume 50–100 mL given over 30–60 minutes.
- PRESCRIBING AND DISPENSING INFORMATION For choice of antibacterial therapy, see Antibacterials, use for prophylaxis p. 529, Gastro-intestinal system infections, antibacterial therapy p. 535, Lyme disease p. 614, Skin infections, antibacterial therapy p. 541, Respiratory system infections, antibacterial therapy p. 538, Urinary-tract infections p. 626.

- MEDICINAL FORMS There can be variation in the licensing of different medicines containing the same drug. Forms available from special-order manufacturers include: solution for injection, infusion

Tablet
CAUTIONARY AND ADVISORY LABELS 9, 21, 25
  ► Cefuroxime (Non-proprietary)
    Cefuroxime (as Cefuroxime axetil) 250 mg Cefuroxime 250mg tablets | 14 tablet PoM £17.72 DT = £17.72
  ► Zinnat (GlaxoSmithKline UK Ltd)
    Cefuroxime (as Cefuroxime axetil) 125 mg Zinnat 125mg tablets | 14 tablet PoM £4.56 DT = £4.56
    Cefuroxime (as Cefuroxime axetil) 250 mg Zinnat 250mg tablets | 14 tablet PoM £9.11 DT = £17.72

Powder for injection
ELECTROLYTES: May contain Sodium
  ► Cefuroxime (Non-proprietary)
    Cefuroxime (as Cefuroxime sodium) 250 mg Cefuroxime 250mg powder for injection vials | 10 vial PoM £9.25 (Hospital only)
    Cefuroxime (as Cefuroxime sodium) 750 mg Cefuroxime 750mg powder for injection vials | 1 vial PoM £2.52 (Hospital only) | 10 vial PoM £25.20 | 10 vial PoM £25.20-£26.10 (Hospital only)
    Cefuroxime (as Cefuroxime sodium) 1.5 gram Cefuroxime 1.5g powder for injection vials | 1 vial PoM £5.05 (Hospital only) | 10 vial PoM £50.50 | 10 vial PoM £50.50-£53.00 (Hospital only)
  ► Zinacef (GlaxoSmithKline UK Ltd)
    Cefuroxime (as Cefuroxime sodium) 250 mg Zinacef 250mg powder for injection vials | 5 vial PoM £4.70 (Hospital only)
    Cefuroxime (as Cefuroxime sodium) 750 mg Zinacef 750mg powder for injection vials | 5 vial PoM £11.72 (Hospital only)
    Cefuroxime (as Cefuroxime sodium) 1.5 gram Zinacef 1.5g powder for injection vials | 1 vial PoM £4.70 (Hospital only)

Oral suspension
CAUTIONARY AND ADVISORY LABELS 9, 21
EXCIPIENTS: May contain Aspartame, sucrose
  ► Zinnat (GlaxoSmithKline UK Ltd)
    Cefuroxime (as Cefuroxime axetil) 25 mg per 1 ml Zinnat 125mg/5ml oral suspension | 70 ml PoM £5.20 DT = £5.20

ANTIBACTERIALS 〉 CEPHALOSPORINS, THIRD-GENERATION

▐ Cefixime   25-Aug-2020

⊩ 551

- INDICATIONS AND DOSE
Acute infections due to sensitive Gram-positive and Gram-negative bacteria
  ► BY MOUTH
  - Child 6-11 months: 75 mg daily
  - Child 1-4 years: 100 mg daily
  - Child 5-9 years: 200 mg daily
  - Child 10-17 years: 200–400 mg daily, alternatively 100–200 mg twice daily
  - Adult: 200–400 mg daily in 1–2 divided doses

Uncomplicated gonorrhoea [anogenital and pharyngeal infection—in combination with azithromycin]
  ► BY MOUTH
  - Adult: 400 mg for 1 dose

Disseminated gonococcal infection [when sensitivity confirmed]
  ► BY MOUTH
  - Adult: 400 mg twice daily, following intravenous antibacterial treatment, starting 24–48 hours after symptoms improve, to give 7 days treatment in total

- UNLICENSED USE EvGr Cefixime is used for the treatment of uncomplicated gonorrhoea and disseminated gonococcal infection, ⒶＷ but is not licensed for these indications.
- INTERACTIONS → Appendix 1: cephalosporins
- SIDE-EFFECTS Acute kidney injury · arthralgia · drug fever · dyspepsia · dyspnoea · face oedema · flatulence · genital pruritus · hypereosinophilia · jaundice · serum sickness-like reaction · thrombocytosis
- PREGNANCY Not known to be harmful.
- BREAST FEEDING Manufacturer advises avoid unless essential—no information available.
- RENAL IMPAIRMENT
  Dose adjustments ► In adults Reduce dose if eGFR less than 20 mL/minute/1.73 m² (max. 200 mg once daily).
  ► In children Reduce dose if estimated glomerular filtration rate less than 20 mL/minute/1.73 m².
- PRESCRIBING AND DISPENSING INFORMATION For choice of antibacterial therapy, see Genital system infections, antibacterial therapy p. 536.

● MEDICINAL FORMS There can be variation in the licensing of different medicines containing the same drug.

Tablet

CAUTIONARY AND ADVISORY LABELS 9

▸ Suprax (Sanofi)
  Cefixime 200 mg Suprax 200mg tablets | 7 tablet PoM £13.23 DT = £13.23

⚑ 551

Cefotaxime
12-Aug-2020

● **INDICATIONS AND DOSE**

Uncomplicated gonorrhoea
▸ BY INTRAMUSCULAR INJECTION
▸ Adult: 500 mg for 1 dose

Disseminated gonococcal infection
▸ BY INTRAMUSCULAR INJECTION, OR BY INTRAVENOUS INFUSION
▸ Adult: 1 g every 8 hours for 7 days, may be switched 24–48 hours after symptoms improve to a suitable oral antibacterial

Infections due to sensitive Gram-positive and Gram-negative bacteria | Surgical prophylaxis | Haemophilus epiglottitis
▸ BY INTRAMUSCULAR INJECTION, OR BY INTRAVENOUS INJECTION, OR BY INTRAVENOUS INFUSION
▸ Adult: 1 g every 12 hours

Severe susceptible infections due to sensitive Gram-positive and Gram-negative bacteria | Meningitis
▸ BY INTRAMUSCULAR INJECTION, OR BY INTRAVENOUS INJECTION, OR BY INTRAVENOUS INFUSION
▸ Adult: 8 g daily in 4 divided doses, increased if necessary to 12 g daily in 3–4 divided doses, intramuscular doses over 1 g should be divided between more than one site

Emergency treatment of suspected bacterial meningitis or meningococcal disease, before urgent transfer to hospital, in patients who cannot be given benzylpenicillin (e.g. because of an allergy)
▸ BY INTRAVENOUS INJECTION, OR BY INTRAMUSCULAR INJECTION
▸ Child 1 month–11 years: 50 mg/kg for 1 dose
▸ Child 12–17 years: 1 g for 1 dose
▸ Adult: 1 g for 1 dose

● INTERACTIONS → Appendix 1: cephalosporins

● SIDE-EFFECTS
▸ **Uncommon** Drug fever · Jarisch-Herxheimer reaction · renal impairment · seizure
▸ **Frequency not known** Arrhythmia (following rapid injection) · bronchospasm · encephalopathy · fungal infection · hepatic disorders

● PREGNANCY Not known to be harmful.

● BREAST FEEDING Present in milk in low concentration, but appropriate to use.

● RENAL IMPAIRMENT
  Dose adjustments ▸ In adults If eGFR less than 5 mL/minute/1.73 m^2, initial dose of 1 g then use half normal dose.
  ▸ In children Usual initial dose, then use half normal dose if estimated glomerular filtration rate less than 5 mL/minute/1.73 m^2.

● DIRECTIONS FOR ADMINISTRATION
▸ With intravenous use in children Displacement value may be significant, consult local guidelines. For intermittent *intravenous infusion*, manufacturer advises dilute reconstituted solution in Glucose 5% *or* Sodium Chloride 0.9%; administer over 20–60 minutes; incompatible with alkaline solutions.
▸ With intravenous use in adults For *intravenous infusion*, manufacturer advises give reconstituted solution intermittently *in* Glucose 5% *or* Sodium Chloride 0.9%.

Suggested volume 40–100 mL given over 20–60 minutes; incompatible with alkaline solutions.

● PRESCRIBING AND DISPENSING INFORMATION For choice of antibacterial therapy, see Antibacterials, use for prophylaxis p. 529, Central nervous system infections, antibacterial therapy p. 533, Genital system infections, antibacterial therapy p. 536, Respiratory system infections, antibacterial therapy p. 538.

● MEDICINAL FORMS There can be variation in the licensing of different medicines containing the same drug.

Powder for solution for injection
▸ Cefotaxime (Non-proprietary)
  Cefotaxime (as Cefotaxime sodium) 500 mg Cefotaxime 500mg powder for solution for injection vials | 10 vial PoM £21.00-£30.00 (Hospital only)
  Cefotaxime (as Cefotaxime sodium) 1 gram Cefotaxime 1g powder for solution for injection vials | 10 vial PoM £35.00-£42.00 (Hospital only)
  Cefotaxime (as Cefotaxime sodium) 2 gram Cefotaxime 2g powder for solution for injection vials | 10 vial PoM £37.50

⚑ 551

Ceftazidime
06-Nov-2020

● **INDICATIONS AND DOSE**

Prophylaxis for transurethral resection of prostate
▸ BY INTRAVENOUS INJECTION, OR BY INTRAVENOUS INFUSION, OR BY DEEP INTRAMUSCULAR INJECTION
▸ Adult: 1 g, single dose to be administered up to 30 minutes before procedure and may be repeated if necessary when catheter removed

Pseudomonal lung infection in cystic fibrosis
▸ BY INTRAVENOUS INFUSION, OR BY INTRAVENOUS INJECTION, OR BY DEEP INTRAMUSCULAR INJECTION
▸ Adult: 100–150 mg/kg daily in 3 divided doses; maximum 9 g per day

Complicated urinary-tract infection
▸ BY INTRAVENOUS INJECTION, OR BY INTRAVENOUS INFUSION, OR BY DEEP INTRAMUSCULAR INJECTION
▸ Adult: 1–2 g every 8–12 hours

Septicaemia | Hospital-acquired pneumonia
▸ BY INTRAVENOUS INFUSION, OR BY INTRAVENOUS INJECTION
▸ Adult: 2 g every 8 hours

Febrile neutropenia
▸ BY INTRAVENOUS INFUSION, OR BY INTRAVENOUS INJECTION
▸ Adult: 2 g every 8 hours

Meningitis
▸ BY INTRAVENOUS INFUSION, OR BY INTRAVENOUS INJECTION
▸ Adult: 2 g every 8 hours

Susceptible infections due to sensitive Gram-positive and Gram-negative bacteria
▸ BY INTRAVENOUS INFUSION, OR BY INTRAVENOUS INJECTION, OR BY DEEP INTRAMUSCULAR INJECTION
▸ Adult: 1–2 g every 8 hours

● INTERACTIONS → Appendix 1: cephalosporins

● SIDE-EFFECTS
▸ **Common or very common** Thrombocytosis · thrombophlebitis
▸ **Uncommon** Antibiotic associated colitis · fungal infection
▸ **Rare or very rare** Acute kidney injury
▸ **Frequency not known** Coma · encephalopathy · jaundice · lymphocytosis · myoclonus · neurological effects · paraesthesia · seizure · taste altered · tremor

● PREGNANCY Not known to be harmful.

● BREAST FEEDING Present in milk in low concentration, but appropriate to use.

● HEPATIC IMPAIRMENT Manufacturer advises caution in severe impairment (no information available).

5

Infection

- RENAL IMPAIRMENT [EvGr] Use with caution. ⟨M⟩
  Dose adjustments [EvGr] Reduce dose if creatinine clearance 50 mL/minute or less—consult product literature. ⟨M⟩
- DIRECTIONS FOR ADMINISTRATION Intramuscular administration used when intravenous administration not possible; single doses over 1 g by intravenous route only.
- With intravenous use For *intravenous infusion* give intermittently *or via* drip tubing in Glucose 5% or 10% *or* Sodium chloride 0.9%. Dissolve 2 g initially in 10 mL (3 g in 15 mL) infusion fluid. For *Fortum*® dilute further to a concentration of 40 mg/mL. For *Kefadim*® dilute further to a concentration of 20 mg/mL. Give over up to 30 minutes.

- MEDICINAL FORMS There can be variation in the licensing of different medicines containing the same drug. Forms available from special-order manufacturers include: infusion, solution for infusion

Powder for solution for injection
ELECTROLYTES: May contain Sodium
- Ceftazidime (Non-proprietary)
  Ceftazidime (as Ceftazidime pentahydrate) 500 mg Ceftazidime 500mg powder for solution for injection vials | 1 vial [PoM] £4.25–£4.91 (Hospital only)
  Ceftazidime (as Ceftazidime pentahydrate) 1 gram Ceftazidime 1g powder for solution for injection vials | 1 vial [PoM] £9.51 (Hospital only) | 10 vial [PoM] £13.90–£79.10 (Hospital only)
  Ceftazidime (as Ceftazidime pentahydrate) 2 gram Ceftazidime 2g powder for solution for injection vials | 1 vial [PoM] £20.04 (Hospital only) | 5 vial [PoM] £79.15 (Hospital only) | 10 vial [PoM] £27.70–£176.00 (Hospital only)
  Ceftazidime (as Ceftazidime pentahydrate) 3 gram Ceftazidime 3g powder for solution for injection vials | 10 vial [PoM] £257.60 (Hospital only)
- Fortum (GlaxoSmithKline UK Ltd)
  Ceftazidime (as Ceftazidime pentahydrate) 500 mg Fortum 500mg powder for solution for injection vials | 1 vial [PoM] £4.40 (Hospital only)
  Ceftazidime (as Ceftazidime pentahydrate) 1 gram Fortum 1g powder for solution for injection vials | 1 vial [PoM] £8.79 (Hospital only)
  Ceftazidime (as Ceftazidime pentahydrate) 2 gram Fortum 2g powder for solution for injection vials | 1 vial [PoM] £17.59 (Hospital only)

Combinations available: **Ceftazidime with avibactam**, p. 560

⟨F 551⟩

Ceftazidime

28-Jul-2020

- INDICATIONS AND DOSE

Community-acquired pneumonia | Hospital-acquired pneumonia | Intra-abdominal infections | Complicated urinary-tract infections | Acute exacerbations of chronic obstructive pulmonary disease
- BY INTRAVENOUS INFUSION, OR BY INTRAVENOUS INJECTION, OR BY DEEP INTRAMUSCULAR INJECTION
- Adult: 1–2 g once daily, 2 g dose to be used for hospital-acquired pneumonia and severe cases

Cellulitis | Erysipelas | Moderate diabetic foot infection | Severe diabetic foot infection | Leg ulcer infection
- BY INTRAVENOUS INJECTION, OR BY INTRAVENOUS INFUSION
- Adult: 2 g once daily

Complicated skin and soft tissue infections | Infections of bones and joints
- BY INTRAVENOUS INFUSION, OR BY INTRAVENOUS INJECTION, OR BY DEEP INTRAMUSCULAR INJECTION
- Adult: 2 g once daily

Suspected bacterial infection in neutropenic patients
- BY INTRAVENOUS INFUSION, OR BY INTRAVENOUS INJECTION, OR BY DEEP INTRAMUSCULAR INJECTION
- Adult: 2–4 g daily, doses at the higher end of the recommended range used in severe cases

Bacterial meningitis | Bacterial endocarditis
- BY INTRAVENOUS INFUSION, OR BY INTRAVENOUS INJECTION, OR BY DEEP INTRAMUSCULAR INJECTION
- Adult: 2–4 g daily, doses at the higher end of the recommended range used in severe cases
- BY INTRAVENOUS INFUSION
- Child 1 month–11 years (body-weight up to 50 kg): 80–100 mg/kg once daily, 100 mg/kg once daily dose should be used for bacterial endocarditis; maximum 4 g per day
- Child 9–11 years (body-weight 50 kg and above): 2–4 g once daily, doses at the higher end of the recommended range used in severe cases
- Child 12–17 years: 2–4 g once daily, doses at the higher end of the recommended range used in severe cases
- BY INTRAVENOUS INJECTION
- Child 9–11 years (body-weight 50 kg and above): 2–4 g once daily, doses at the higher end of the recommended range used in severe cases; doses of 50 mg/kg or more should be given by infusion
- Child 12–17 years: 2–4 g once daily, doses at the higher end of the recommended range used in severe cases
- BY DEEP INTRAMUSCULAR INJECTION
- Child 1 month–11 years (body-weight up to 50 kg): 80–100 mg/kg daily, 100 mg/kg daily dose should be used for bacterial endocarditis; maximum 4 g per day
- Child 9–11 years (body-weight 50 kg and above): 2–4 g daily, doses at the higher end of the recommended range used in severe cases
- Child 12–17 years: 2–4 g daily, doses at the higher end of the recommended range used in severe cases

Surgical prophylaxis
- BY INTRAVENOUS INFUSION, OR BY INTRAVENOUS INJECTION, OR BY DEEP INTRAMUSCULAR INJECTION
- Adult: 2 g for 1 dose, dose to be administered 30–90 minutes before procedure

Pelvic inflammatory disease
- BY DEEP INTRAMUSCULAR INJECTION
- Adult: 500 mg for 1 dose

Gonococcal conjunctivitis | Uncomplicated gonorrhoea [anogenital and pharyngeal infection, when sensitivity unknown]
- BY DEEP INTRAMUSCULAR INJECTION
- Adult: 1 g for 1 dose

Gonococcal epididymo-orchitis
- BY DEEP INTRAMUSCULAR INJECTION
- Adult: 1 g for 1 dose, to be followed by an additional antibacterial course to treat epididymo-orchitis

Disseminated gonococcal infection
- BY DEEP INTRAMUSCULAR INJECTION, OR BY INTRAVENOUS INFUSION, OR BY INTRAVENOUS INJECTION
- Adult: 1 g every 24 hours for 7 days, may be switched 24–48 hours after symptoms improve to a suitable oral antibacterial

Syphilis
- BY INTRAVENOUS INFUSION, OR BY INTRAVENOUS INJECTION, OR BY DEEP INTRAMUSCULAR INJECTION
- Adult: 0.5–1 g once daily for 10–14 days, dose increased to 2 g once daily for neurosyphilis

Lyme disease [affecting central nervous system]
- BY INTRAVENOUS INFUSION, OR BY INTRAVENOUS INJECTION
- Adult: 2 g twice daily for 21 days, alternatively 4 g once daily for 21 days

Lyme arthritis | Acrodermatitis chronica atrophicans
- BY INTRAVENOUS INFUSION, OR BY INTRAVENOUS INJECTION
- Adult: 2 g once daily for 28 days

Lyme carditis
- BY INTRAVENOUS INFUSION, OR BY INTRAVENOUS INJECTION
- Adult: 2 g once daily for 21 days

Prevention of secondary case of meningococcal meningitis
▸ BY INTRAMUSCULAR INJECTION
▸ Adult: 250 mg for 1 dose

Prevention of secondary case of *Haemophilus influenzae* type b disease
▸ BY INTRAMUSCULAR INJECTION, OR BY INTRAVENOUS INJECTION, OR BY INTRAVENOUS INFUSION
▸ Adult: 1 g daily for 2 days

Acute otitis media
▸ BY DEEP INTRAMUSCULAR INJECTION
▸ Adult: 1–2 g for 1 dose, dose can be given for 3 days if severely ill or previous therapy failed

Acute prostatitis
▸ BY SLOW INTRAVENOUS INJECTION, OR BY INTRAVENOUS INFUSION
▸ Adult: 2 g once daily

● UNLICENSED USE EvGr Not licensed for prophylaxis of *Haemophilus influenzae* type b disease. Ⓔ Not licensed for prophylaxis of meningococcal meningitis.
▸ In adults EvGr Dose not licensed for treatment of pelvic inflammatory disease in adults over 18 years. Ceftriaxone is used for Lyme disease affecting the central nervous system, Ⓐ but the dose is not licensed for this indication.

● CAUTIONS
GENERAL CAUTIONS History of hypercalciuria · history of kidney stones
SPECIFIC CAUTIONS
▸ With intravenous use concomitant treatment with intravenous calcium (including total parenteral nutrition containing calcium)

● INTERACTIONS → Appendix 1: cephalosporins

● SIDE-EFFECTS
▸ **Uncommon** Anaemia · coagulation disorder · fungal infection
▸ **Rare or very rare** Bronchospasm · glycosuria · haematuria · oedema
▸ **Frequency not known** Antibiotic associated colitis · cholelithiasis · hypersensitivity · nephrolithiasis · oral disorders · pancreatitis · seizure · vertigo
SIDE-EFFECTS, FURTHER INFORMATION Precipitates of calcium ceftriaxone can occur in the gall bladder and urine (particularly in very young, dehydrated or those who are immobilised)—consider discontinuation if symptomatic.

● PREGNANCY Manufacturer advises use only if benefit outweighs risk—limited data available but not known to be harmful in *animal* studies. EvGr Specialist sources indicate suitable for use in pregnancy. Ⓓ

● BREAST FEEDING EvGr Specialist sources advise ceftriaxone is compatible with breastfeeding—present in milk in low concentration but limited effects to breast-fed infant. Ⓓ

● HEPATIC IMPAIRMENT Manufacturer advises caution in severe impairment (no information available).

● RENAL IMPAIRMENT
Dose adjustments Manufacturer advises reduce dose and monitor efficacy in patients with severe renal impairment in combination with hepatic impairment—no information available.
▸ In adults Manufacturer advises reduce dose if eGFR less than 10 mL/minute/1.73 m^2 (max. 2 g daily).
▸ In children Manufacturer advises reduce dose if estimated glomeruler filtration rate less than 10 mL/minute/1.73 m^2 max. 50 mg/kg daily or max. 2 g daily).

● MONITORING REQUIREMENTS Manufacturer advises to monitor full blood count regularly during prolonged treatment.

● DIRECTIONS FOR ADMINISTRATION
▸ With intramuscular use or intravenous use Twice daily dosing may be considered for doses greater than 2 g daily.
▸ With intravenous use in children For *intravenous infusion* (preferred route), dilute reconstituted solution with Glucose 5% (or 10% in neonates) *or* Sodium Chloride 0.9%; give over at least 30 minutes (60 minutes in neonates— may displace bilirubin from serum albumin). Not to be given simultaneously with parenteral nutrition or infusion fluids containing calcium, even by different infusion lines; in children, may be infused sequentially with infusion fluids containing calcium if infusion lines at different sites are used, or if the infusion lines are replaced or thoroughly flushed between infusions with Sodium Chloride 0.9% to avoid precipitation—consult product literature. Displacement value may be significant, consult local guidelines. For *intravenous injection*, give over 5 minutes.
▸ With intramuscular use in children For *intramuscular injection*, may be mixed with 1% Lidocaine Hydrochloride Injection to reduce pain at intramuscular injection site. Intramuscular injection should only be considered when the intravenous route is not possible or less appropriate. If administered by intramuscular injection, the lower end of the dose range should be used for the shortest time possible; volume depends on the age and size of the child, but doses over 1 g must be divided between more than one site. Displacement value may be significant, consult local guidelines. The maximum single intramuscular dose is 2 g, doses greater than 2 g must be given in divided doses *or* by intravenous administration (see above).
▸ With intravenous use in adults For *intravenous infusion* (preferred route) (*Rocephin*®; *Ceftriaxone Injection*, Genus), give intermittently *or via* drip tubing *in* Glucose 5% or 10% *or* Sodium Chloride 0.9%. Reconstitute 2-g vial with 40 mL infusion fluid. Give by intermittent infusion over at least 30 minutes. Not to be given simultaneously with total parenteral nutrition or infusion fluids containing calcium, even by different infusion lines. May be infused sequentially with infusion fluids containing calcium if infusion lines at different sites are used, or if the infusion lines are replaced or thoroughly flushed between infusions with Sodium Chloride 0.9% to avoid precipitation—consult product literature. For *intravenous injection*, give over 5 minutes.
▸ With intramuscular use in adults For *intramuscular injection*, doses over 1 g must be divided between more than one site. Displacement value may be significant, consult local guidelines. The maximum single intramuscular dose is 2 g, doses greater than 2 g must be given in divided doses *or* by intravenous administration.

● PRESCRIBING AND DISPENSING INFORMATION For choice of antibacterial therapy, see Antibacterials, use for prophylaxis p. 529, Cardiovascular system infections, antibacterial therapy p. 532, Central nervous system infections, antibacterial therapy p. 533, Diabetic foot infections, antibacterial therapy p. 534, Ear infections, antibacterial therapy p. 534, Gastro-intestinal system infections, antibacterial therapy p. 535, Genital system infections, antibacterial therapy p. 536, Lyme disease p. 614, Musculoskeletal system infections, antibacterial therapy p. 536, Respiratory system infections, antibacterial therapy p. 538, Skin infections, antibacterial therapy p. 541, Urinary-tract infections p. 626.

● MEDICINAL FORMS There can be variation in the licensing of different medicines containing the same drug. Forms available from special-order manufacturers include: infusion
Powder for solution for injection
ELECTROLYTES: May contain Sodium
▸ Ceftriaxone (Non-proprietary)
Ceftriaxone (as Ceftriaxone sodium) 250 mg Ceftriaxone 250mg powder for solution for injection vials | 1 vial PoM £2.30 DT = £2.40 (Hospital only)

Ceftriaxone (as Ceftriaxone sodium) 1 gram Ceftriaxone 1g powder for solution for injection vials | 1 vial [PoM] £3.62 DT = £9.58 (Hospital only) | 10 vial [PoM] £95.80 | 10 vial [PoM] £36.00–£95.80 (Hospital only)

Ceftriaxone (as Ceftriaxone sodium) 2 gram Ceftriaxone 2g powder for solution for injection vials | 1 vial [PoM] £18.30 DT = £19.18 (Hospital only) | 10 vial [PoM] £122.00–£191.80 (Hospital only) Ceftriaxone 2g powder for solution for infusion vials | 1 vial [PoM] £19.18 DT = £19.18 (Hospital only) | 10 vial [PoM] £191.80 (Hospital only)

▸ Rocephin (Roche Products Ltd)

Ceftriaxone (as Ceftriaxone sodium) 250 mg Rocephin 250mg powder for solution for injection vials | 1 vial [PoM] £2.40 DT = £2.40 (Hospital only)

Ceftriaxone (as Ceftriaxone sodium) 1 gram Rocephin 1g powder for solution for injection vials | 1 vial [PoM] £9.58 DT = £9.58 (Hospital only)

Ceftriaxone (as Ceftriaxone sodium) 2 gram Rocephin 2g powder for solution for injection vials | 1 vial [PoM] £19.18 DT = £19.18 (Hospital only)

ANTIBACTERIALS> ❭ CEPHALOSPORINS, THIRD-GENERATION WITH BETA-LACTAMASE INHIBITOR

F 551

Ceftazidime with avibactam

06-Nov-2020

The properties listed below are those particular to the combination only. For the properties of the components please consider, ceftazidime p. 557.

● **INDICATIONS AND DOSE**

Complicated intra-abdominal infection
▸ BY INTRAVENOUS INFUSION
▸ Adult: 2/0.5 g every 8 hours for 5–14 days

Complicated urinary tract infection, including pyelonephritis
▸ BY INTRAVENOUS INFUSION
▸ Adult: 2/0.5 g every 8 hours for 5–10 days

Hospital-acquired pneumonia, including ventilator-associated pneumonia
▸ BY INTRAVENOUS INFUSION
▸ Adult: 2/0.5 g every 8 hours for 7–14 days

Infections due to Gram-negative bacteria with limited treatment options
▸ BY INTRAVENOUS INFUSION
▸ Adult: 2/0.5 g every 8 hours, duration of treatment guided by infection severity, pathogen, and response

DOSE EQUIVALENCE AND CONVERSION
▸ Dose expressed as x/y g ceftazidime/avibactam

● INTERACTIONS → Appendix 1: cephalosporins
● SIDE-EFFECTS
▸ **Common or very common** Increased risk of infection · thrombocytosis
▸ **Uncommon** Acute kidney injury · antibiotic associated colitis · lymphocytosis · paraesthesia · taste altered
▸ **Frequency not known** Coma · encephalopathy · jaundice · myoclonus · neurological effects · seizures · tremor
● PREGNANCY Manufacturer advises avoid unless potential benefit outweighs risk—toxicity in *animal* studies.
● BREAST FEEDING Manufacturer advises avoid—presence of avibactam in milk unknown.
● RENAL IMPAIRMENT [EvGr] Use with caution. ⬙
Dose adjustments [EvGr] Reduce dose if creatinine clearance 50 mL/minute or less—consult product literature. ⬙
● DIRECTIONS FOR ADMINISTRATION Manufacturer advises for *intravenous infusion* (Zavicefta ®) give in Glucose 5%, *or* Sodium Chloride 0.9%, *or* Sodium Chloride 0.45% with Glucose 2.5% combination *or* Lactated Ringer's solution. Reconstitute each 2 g/0.5 g vial with 10 mL water for injections; dilute requisite dose in an appropriate infusion bag and give over 120 minutes.

● PATIENT AND CARER ADVICE
Driving and skilled tasks Manufacturer advises patients and carers should be counselled on the effects on driving and performance of skilled tasks—risk of dizziness.

● MEDICINAL FORMS There can be variation in the licensing of different medicines containing the same drug.
Powder for solution for infusion
ELECTROLYTES: May contain Sodium
▸ Zavicefta (Pfizer Ltd) ▼
Avibactam (as Avibactam sodium) 500 mg, Ceftazidime (as Ceftazidime pentahydrate) 2 gram Zavicefta 2g/0.5g powder for concentrate for solution for infusion vials | 10 vial [PoM] £857.00 (Hospital only)

F 551

Ceftolozane with tazobactam

31-Aug-2020

● **INDICATIONS AND DOSE**

Complicated intra-abdominal infection
▸ BY INTRAVENOUS INFUSION
▸ Adult: 1/0.5 g every 8 hours for 4–14 days

Complicated urinary tract infection | Acute pyelonephritis
▸ BY INTRAVENOUS INFUSION
▸ Adult: 1/0.5 g every 8 hours for 7 days

Hospital-acquired pneumonia | Ventilator-associated pneumonia
▸ BY INTRAVENOUS INFUSION
▸ Adult: 2/1 g every 8 hours for 8–14 days

DOSE EQUIVALENCE AND CONVERSION
▸ Dose expressed as x/y g where x and y are ceftolozane and tazobactam respectively.

● INTERACTIONS → Appendix 1: cephalosporins
● SIDE-EFFECTS
▸ **Common or very common** Antibiotic associated colitis · anxiety · constipation · electrolyte imbalance · hypotension · insomnia · thrombocytosis
▸ **Uncommon** Anaemia · angina pectoris · arrhythmias · dyspnoea · gastrointestinal discomfort · gastrointestinal disorders · hyperglycaemia · increased risk of infection · ischaemic stroke · renal impairment · venous thrombosis
● PREGNANCY Manufacturer advises to use only if potential benefit outweighs risk—toxicity in *animal* studies with tazobactam.
● BREAST FEEDING Manufacturer advises avoid—no information available.
● RENAL IMPAIRMENT Manufacturer advises monitor for changes in renal function.
Dose adjustments
▸ When used for Complicated intra-abdominal infection or Complicated urinary tract infection or Acute pyelonephritis Manufacturer advises reduce dose to 500/250 mg every 8 hours if creatinine clearance 30–50 mL/minute and 250/125 mg every 8 hours if creatinine clearance 15–29 mL/minute.
▸ When used for Hospital-acquired pneumonia or Ventilator-associated pneumonia Manufacturer advises reduce dose to 1/0.5 g every 8 hours if creatinine clearance 30–50 mL/minute and 500/250 mg every 8 hours if creatinine clearance 15–29 mL/minute.
● DIRECTIONS FOR ADMINISTRATION For *intravenous infusion* (Zerbaxa ®), give intermittently in Glucose 5% or Sodium chloride 0.9%; reconstitute initially each vial with 10 mL Water for Injections or Sodium chloride 0.9% to give a final volume of 11.4 mL; dilute requisite dose in 100 mL of Glucose 5% or Sodium chloride 0.9%; give over 1 hour.
● HANDLING AND STORAGE Manufacturer advises store in a refrigerator at 2°C–8°C.

● PATIENT AND CARER ADVICE
Driving and skilled tasks Manufacturer advises ceftolozane with tazobactam may influence driving and performance of skilled tasks—increased risk of dizziness.

● NATIONAL FUNDING/ACCESS DECISIONS
For full details see funding body website
Scottish Medicines Consortium (SMC) decisions
▶ Ceftolozane with tazobactam (*Zerbaxa*®) for the treatment of the following infections in adults: complicated intra-abdominal infections, acute pyelonephritis, and complicated urinary tract infections (May 2016) SMC No. 1146/16 Not recommended

● MEDICINAL FORMS There can be variation in the licensing of different medicines containing the same drug.
Powder for solution for infusion
ELECTROLYTES: May contain Sodium
▶ Zerbaxa (Merck Sharp & Dohme Ltd)
Tazobactam (as Tazobactam sodium) 500 mg, Ceftolozane (as Ceftolozane sulfate) 1 gram Zerbaxa 1g/0.5g powder for concentrate for solution for infusion vials | 10 vial PoM £670.30 (Hospital only)

ANTIBACTERIALS > CEPHALOSPORINS, OTHER

�F 551

Cefepime
19-Aug-2020

● INDICATIONS AND DOSE
Infections due to sensitive Gram-positive and Gram-negative bacteria
▶ BY INTRAVENOUS INJECTION, OR BY INTRAVENOUS INFUSION, OR BY INTRAMUSCULAR INJECTION
▶ Adult (body-weight up to 41 kg): 50 mg/kg every 12 hours (max. per dose 2 g), increased if necessary to 50 mg/kg every 8 hours (max. per dose 2 g), increased dose used for severe infections, intravenous route preferred in severe infections

Mild to moderate urinary tract infections
▶ BY INTRAVENOUS INJECTION, OR BY INTRAVENOUS INFUSION, OR BY INTRAMUSCULAR INJECTION
▶ Adult (body-weight 41 kg and above): 0.5–1 g every 12 hours

Mild to moderate infections due to sensitive Gram-positive and Gram-negative bacteria
▶ BY INTRAVENOUS INJECTION, OR BY INTRAVENOUS INFUSION, OR BY INTRAMUSCULAR INJECTION
▶ Adult (body-weight 41 kg and above): 1 g every 12 hours

Severe infections due to sensitive Gram-positive and Gram-negative bacteria
▶ BY INTRAVENOUS INJECTION, OR BY INTRAVENOUS INFUSION
▶ Adult (body-weight 41 kg and above): 2 g every 12 hours, increased if necessary to 2 g every 8 hours, increased dose used for very severe infections

● INTERACTIONS → Appendix 1: cephalosporins

● SIDE-EFFECTS
▶ **Common or very common** Anaemia
▶ **Uncommon** Gastrointestinal disorders · increased risk of infection
▶ **Rare or very rare** Constipation · dyspnoea · genital pruritus · paraesthesia · seizure · taste altered · vasodilation
▶ **Frequency not known** Anaphylactic shock · aplastic anaemia · coma · confusion · consciousness impaired · encephalopathy · haemorrhage · hallucination · myoclonus · nephrotoxicity · renal failure

● PREGNANCY Manufacturer advises caution—no data available but not known to be harmful in *animal* studies.

● BREAST FEEDING Manufacturer advises caution—present in milk in very low quantities.

● RENAL IMPAIRMENT Manufacturer advises use with caution.
Dose adjustments Manufacturer advises reduce dose—consult product literature.

● DIRECTIONS FOR ADMINISTRATION After reconstitution the solution is yellow to yellow-brown. Displacement value may be significant when reconstituting injection, consult local guidelines. For *intravenous infusion*, manufacturer advises reconstitute with 50 mL Glucose 5% or 10% or Sodium Chloride 0.9%; give over 30 minutes. For *intravenous injection*, manufacturer advises reconstitute with 10 mL Glucose 5% or 10% or Sodium Chloride 0.9%. For *intramuscular injection*, manufacturer advises reconstitute with 3 mL Water for Injection.

● NATIONAL FUNDING/ACCESS DECISIONS
For full details see funding body website
All Wales Medicines Strategy Group (AWMSG) decisions
▶ Cefepime (*Renapime*®) for resistant pseudomonas infections (November 2019) AWMSG No. 4129 Recommended with restrictions

● MEDICINAL FORMS There can be variation in the licensing of different medicines containing the same drug.
Powder for solution for injection
▶ Renapime (Renascience Pharma Ltd)
Cefepime (as Cefepime dihydrochloride monohydrate) 1 gram Renapime 1g powder for solution for injection vials | 10 vial PoM £70.00
Cefepime (as Cefepime dihydrochloride monohydrate) 2 gram Renapime 2g powder for solution for injection vials | 10 vial PoM £110.00

�F 551

Cefiderocol
02-Oct-2020

● INDICATIONS AND DOSE
Aerobic Gram-negative infections [in patients with limited treatment options] (administered on expert advice)
▶ BY INTRAVENOUS INFUSION
▶ Adult: 2 g every 8 hours, duration should be tailored to site of infection—consult product literature

● CAUTIONS Seizure disorders · supra-normal creatinine clearance
CAUTIONS, FURTHER INFORMATION
▶ **Supra-normal creatinine clearance** Manufacturer advises to increase frequency of infusion to 2 g every 6 hours in patients with creatinine clearance of 120 mL/minute or more.

● INTERACTIONS → Appendix 1: cephalosporins

● SIDE-EFFECTS
▶ **Common or very common** Clostridioides difficile colitis · cough · hepatic function abnormal · increased risk of infection

● PREGNANCY Manufacturer advises avoid—limited data available but not known to be harmful in *animal* studies.

● BREAST FEEDING Manufacturer advises avoid—not known if present in human milk. A specialist source confirms lack of information in human lactation, but states acceptable to use (cephalosporins generally not expected to cause adverse effects in breastfed infants).

● RENAL IMPAIRMENT Manufacturer advises use with caution if creatinine clearance less than 60 mL/minute.
Dose adjustments Manufacturer advises reduce dose if creatinine clearance less than 60 mL/minute—consult product literature.

● MONITORING REQUIREMENTS Manufacturer advises monitor renal function regularly—dose adjustment may be required.

- EFFECT ON LABORATORY TESTS Manufacturer advises may cause false-positive urine tests for protein, ketones, or occult blood.
- DIRECTIONS FOR ADMINISTRATION Manufacturer advises for *intravenous infusion*, give intermittently in Glucose 5% or Sodium Chloride 0.9%. Dilute reconstituted solution to 100 mL with infusion fluid; give over 3 hours.
- HANDLING AND STORAGE Store in a refrigerator (2–8°C)—consult product literature for storage after reconstitution and dilution. Protect from light.

- MEDICINAL FORMS There can be variation in the licensing of different medicines containing the same drug.
  Powder for solution for infusion
  ELECTROLYTES: May contain Sodium
  ‣ Fetcroja (Shionogi BV) ▼
    Cefiderocol (as Cefiderocol sulfate tosylate) 1 gram Fetcroja 1g powder for concentrate for solution for infusion vials | 10 vial [PoM] £1,319.00 (Hospital only)

Ceftaroline fosamil

F 551
04-Nov-2020

- INDICATIONS AND DOSE

Community-acquired pneumonia
  ‣ BY INTRAVENOUS INFUSION
  ‣ Adult: 600 mg every 12 hours for 5–7 days

Complicated skin infections | Complicated soft-tissue infections
  ‣ BY INTRAVENOUS INFUSION
  ‣ Adult: 600 mg every 12 hours for 5–14 days, for high dose regimen consult product literature

- CAUTIONS Seizure disorders
- INTERACTIONS → Appendix 1: cephalosporins
- SIDE-EFFECTS
‣ **Uncommon** Anaemia · antibiotic associated colitis · hypersensitivity
- PREGNANCY Manufacturer advises avoid unless essential—limited information; *animal* studies do not indicate toxicity.
- BREAST FEEDING Manufacturer advises avoid—no information available.
- RENAL IMPAIRMENT
  Dose adjustments Manufacturer advises reduce dose if creatinine clearance less than 51 mL/minute—consult product literature.
- DIRECTIONS FOR ADMINISTRATION For *intravenous infusion*, give intermittently in Glucose 5% or Sodium chloride 0.9%. Dilute reconstituted solution to 50, 100, or 250 mL with infusion fluid; give over 5 to 60 minutes. Consult product literature for administration of high-dose regimen.
- NATIONAL FUNDING/ACCESS DECISIONS
  For full details see funding body website
  Scottish Medicines Consortium (SMC) decisions
  ‣ Ceftaroline fosamil (*Zinforo*®) for the treatment of complicated skin and soft tissue infections (cSSTIs) (January 2013) SMC No. 830/12 Recommended with restrictions

- MEDICINAL FORMS There can be variation in the licensing of different medicines containing the same drug.
  Powder for solution for infusion
  ‣ Zinforo (Pfizer Ltd)
    Ceftaroline fosamil (as Ceftaroline fosamil acetic acid solvate monohydrate) 600 mg Zinforo 600mg powder for concentrate for solution for infusion vials | 10 vial [PoM] £375.00 (Hospital only)

Ceftobiprole

F 551
07-Aug-2020

- INDICATIONS AND DOSE

Hospital-acquired pneumonia (excluding ventilator-associated pneumonia) | Community-acquired pneumonia
  ‣ BY INTRAVENOUS INFUSION
  ‣ Adult: 500 mg every 8 hours

- CAUTIONS Pre-existing seizure disorder—increased risk of seizures · supra-normal creatinine clearance
  CAUTIONS, FURTHER INFORMATION
  ‣ Supra-normal creatinine clearance Manufacturer advises to measure baseline renal function and increase duration of infusion if creatinine clearance greater than 150 mL/minute.
- INTERACTIONS → Appendix 1: cephalosporins
- SIDE-EFFECTS
‣ **Common or very common** Drowsiness · dyspepsia · electrolyte imbalance · fungal infection · hypersensitivity · taste altered
‣ **Uncommon** Anaemia · antibiotic associated colitis · anxiety · asthma · dyspnoea · laryngeal pain · muscle spasms · peripheral oedema · renal failure · sleep disorders · thrombocytosis
‣ **Frequency not known** Seizure
- PREGNANCY Manufacturer advises avoid unless essential—no information available.
- BREAST FEEDING Manufacturer advises avoid—present in milk in *animal* studies.
- RENAL IMPAIRMENT Manufacturer advises use with caution in severe impairment—limited information available.
  Dose adjustments Reduce dose to 500 mg every 12 hours in moderate impairment and 250 mg every 12 hours in severe impairment.
- DIRECTIONS FOR ADMINISTRATION Manufacturer advises for *intravenous infusion* (*Zevtera*®), give intermittently in Glucose 5%, or Sodium Chloride 0.9%, or Lactated Ringer's solution; reconstitute each 500 mg with 10 mL Water for injections or Glucose 5%; dilute in 250 mL infusion fluid and give over 2 hours (increased to 4 hours if creatinine clearance greater than 150 mL/minute). Do not mix with calcium-containing solutions (except Lactated Ringer's solution) in the same intravenous line—precipitation may occur.
- HANDLING AND STORAGE Manufacturer advises store in a refrigerator (2–8°C)—consult product literature for storage after reconstitution and dilution.
- PATIENT AND CARER ADVICE
  Driving and skilled tasks Manufacturer advises patients and carers should be counselled on the effects on driving and performance of skilled tasks—increased risk of dizziness.

- MEDICINAL FORMS There can be variation in the licensing of different medicines containing the same drug.
  Powder for solution for infusion
  ELECTROLYTES: May contain Sodium
  ‣ Zevtera (Correvio UK Ltd)
    Ceftobiprole (as Ceftobiprole medocaril sodium) 500 mg Zevtera 500mg powder for concentrate for solution for infusion vials | 10 vial [PoM] £396.30 (Hospital only)

ANTIBACTERIALS > GLYCOPEPTIDE
ANTIBACTERIALS

Dalbavancin

20-Oct-2020

- DRUG ACTION Dalbavancin is a glycopeptide antibacterial; it has bactericidal activity against Gram-positive bacteria including various staphylococci. However, there are reports of *Staphylococcus aureus* with reduced susceptibility to glycopeptides and increasing reports of glycopeptide-resistant enterococci.

- INDICATIONS AND DOSE

Acute bacterial skin and skin structure infections
▸ BY INTRAVENOUS INFUSION
▸ Adult: 1500 mg for 1 dose, alternatively 1000 mg, then 500 mg after 1 week

- SIDE-EFFECTS
▸ **Common or very common** Diarrhoea · headache · nausea
▸ **Uncommon** Anaemia · antibiotic associated colitis · appetite decreased · constipation · cough · dizziness · eosinophilia · flushing · gastrointestinal discomfort · increased risk of infection · infusion related reaction · insomnia · leucopenia · neutropenia · skin reactions · taste altered · thrombocytosis · vomiting · vulvovaginal pruritus
▸ **Rare or very rare** Bronchospasm
▸ **Frequency not known** Ototoxicity

- ALLERGY AND CROSS-SENSITIVITY Manufacturer advises use with caution in patients with other glycopeptide sensitivity.

- PREGNANCY
Dose adjustments Manufacturer advises avoid unless essential—toxicity in *animal* studies.

- BREAST FEEDING
Dose adjustments Manufacturer advises avoid—present in milk in *animal* studies.

- HEPATIC IMPAIRMENT Manufacturer advises caution in moderate to severe impairment (no information available).

- RENAL IMPAIRMENT
Dose adjustments Manufacturer advises reduce dose to 1000 mg as a single infusion *or* reduce dose to 750 mg followed one week later by 375 mg if creatinine clearance <30 mL/minute.

- DIRECTIONS FOR ADMINISTRATION Manufacturer advises for *intravenous infusion (Xydalba®)*, reconstitute each 500 mg vial to produce a 20 mg/mL solution with 25 mL water for injections. Dilute reconstituted solution to a concentration of 1–5 mg/mL with Glucose 5%; give intermittently over 30 minutes (avoid rapid infusion—risk of 'red man' syndrome).

- NATIONAL FUNDING/ACCESS DECISIONS
For full details see funding body website
Scottish Medicines Consortium (SMC) decisions
▸ Dalbavancin (*Xydalba®*) for the treatment of acute bacterial skin and skin structure infections (ABSSSI) in adults (January 2017) SMC No. 1105/15 Recommended with restrictions
All Wales Medicines Strategy Group (AWMSG) decisions
▸ Dalbavancin (*Xydalba®*) for the treatment of acute bacterial skin and skin structure infections (ABSSSI) in adults (July 2018) AWMSG No. 2001 Recommended with restrictions

- MEDICINAL FORMS There can be variation in the licensing of different medicines containing the same drug.
Powder for solution for infusion
▸ Xydalba (Correvio UK Ltd)
Dalbavancin (as Dalbavancin hydrochloride) 500 mg Xydalba 500mg powder for concentrate for solution for infusion vials | 1 vial PoM £558.70 (Hospital only)

Teicoplanin

17-Nov-2020

- DRUG ACTION The glycopeptide antibiotic teicoplanin has bactericidal activity against aerobic and anaerobic Gram-positive bacteria including multi-resistant staphylococci. However, there are reports of *Staphylococcus aureus* with reduced susceptibility to glycopeptides and increasing reports of glycopeptide-resistant enterococci. Teicoplanin is similar to vancomycin, but has a significantly longer duration of action, allowing once daily administration after the loading dose.

- INDICATIONS AND DOSE

***Clostridioides difficile* infection**
▸ BY MOUTH
▸ Adult: 100–200 mg twice daily for 7–14 days
Moderate diabetic foot infection | Severe diabetic foot infection | Leg ulcer infection
▸ BY INTRAVENOUS INJECTION, OR BY INTRAVENOUS INFUSION
▸ Adult: Initially 6 mg/kg every 12 hours for 3 doses, then 6 mg/kg once daily
Cellulitis | Erysipelas
▸ BY INTRAVENOUS INJECTION, OR BY INTRAVENOUS INFUSION
▸ Adult: Initially 6 mg/kg every 12 hours for 3 doses, then 6 mg/kg once daily
Serious infections caused by Gram-positive bacteria (e.g. complicated skin and soft-tissue infections, pneumonia, complicated urinary tract infections)
▸ BY INTRAVENOUS INJECTION, OR BY INTRAVENOUS INFUSION, OR BY INTRAMUSCULAR INJECTION
▸ Adult: Initially 6 mg/kg every 12 hours for 3 doses, then 6 mg/kg once daily
Streptococcal or enterococcal endocarditis (in combination with another antibacterial) | Bone and joint infections
▸ INITIALLY BY INTRAVENOUS INJECTION, OR BY INTRAVENOUS INFUSION
▸ Adult: 12 mg/kg every 12 hours for 3–5 doses, then (by intravenous injection or by intravenous infusion or by intramuscular injection) 12 mg/kg once daily
Surgical prophylaxis
▸ BY INTRAVENOUS INJECTION
▸ Adult: 400 mg, to be administered up to 30 minutes before the procedure
Surgical prophylaxis in open fractures
▸ BY INTRAVENOUS INFUSION
▸ Adult: 800 mg, to be administered up to 30 minutes before skeletal stabilisation and definitive soft-tissue closure
Peritonitis associated with peritoneal dialysis (added to dialysis fluid)
▸ BY INTRAPERITONEAL INFUSION
▸ Adult: (consult local protocol)
PHARMACOKINETICS
▸ Teicoplanin should **not** be given by mouth for systemic infections because it is not absorbed significantly.

- UNLICENSED USE Not licensed for surgical prophylaxis.
- INTERACTIONS → Appendix 1: teicoplanin
- SIDE-EFFECTS
▸ **Common or very common** Fever · pain · skin reactions
▸ **Uncommon** Bronchospasm · diarrhoea · dizziness · eosinophilia · headache · hearing impairment · hypersensitivity · leucopenia · nausea · ototoxicity · thrombocytopenia · vomiting
▸ **Rare or very rare** Abscess · red man syndrome
▸ **Frequency not known** Agranulocytosis · angioedema · chills · neutropenia · overgrowth of nonsusceptible organisms · renal impairment · seizure · severe cutaneous adverse reactions (SCARs) · thrombophlebitis

5

Infection

SIDE-EFFECTS, FURTHER INFORMATION Teicoplanin is associated with a lower incidence of nephrotoxicity than vancomycin.

● ALLERGY AND CROSS-SENSITIVITY [EvGr] Caution if history of vancomycin sensitivity. ◈

● PREGNANCY Manufacturer advises use only if potential benefit outweighs risk.

● BREAST FEEDING No information available.

● RENAL IMPAIRMENT
Dose adjustments Use normal dose regimen on days 1–4, then use normal maintenance dose every 48 hours if eGFR 30–80 mL/minute/1.73 m² and use normal maintenance dose every 72 hours if eGFR less than 30 mL/minute/1.73 m².
Monitoring Monitor renal and auditory function during prolonged treatment in renal impairment.

● MONITORING REQUIREMENTS
▸ With intramuscular use or intravenous use Manufacturer advises monitor serum-teicoplanin trough concentration at steady state after completion of loading dose and during maintenance treatment—consult product literature.
▸ Blood counts and liver and kidney function tests required.
▸ Manufacturer advises monitoring for adverse reactions when doses of 12 mg/kg twice daily are administered.

● DIRECTIONS FOR ADMINISTRATION
▸ With intravenous use For intravenous infusion (*Targocid*®), manufacturer advises give intermittently in Glucose 5% or Sodium chloride 0.9%; reconstitute initially with water for injections provided; infuse over 30 minutes. Continuous infusion not usually recommended.
▸ With oral use Manufacturer advises injection can be used to prepare solution for oral administration.

● PRESCRIBING AND DISPENSING INFORMATION For choice of antibacterial therapy, see Antibacterials, use for prophylaxis p. 529, Cardiovascular system infections, antibacterial therapy p. 532, Diabetic foot infections, antibacterial therapy p. 534, Gastro-intestinal system infections, antibacterial therapy p. 535, Musculoskeletal system infections, antibacterial therapy p. 536, Respiratory system infections, antibacterial therapy p. 538, Skin infections, antibacterial therapy p. 541, Urinary-tract infections p. 626.

● MEDICINAL FORMS There can be variation in the licensing of different medicines containing the same drug. Forms available from special-order manufacturers include: solution for injection

Powder and solvent for solution for injection
ELECTROLYTES: May contain Sodium
▸ Teicoplanin (non-proprietary) ▼
  Teicoplanin 200 mg Teicoplanin 200mg powder and solvent for solution for injection vials | 1 vial [PoM] £4.45 DT = £3.93
  Teicoplanin 400 mg Teicoplanin 400mg powder and solvent for solution for injection vials | 1 vial [PoM] £7.57 DT = £7.32
▸ Targocid (Sanofi) ▼
  Teicoplanin 200 mg Targocid 200mg powder and solvent for solution for injection vials | 1 vial [PoM] £3.93 DT = £3.93
  Teicoplanin 400 mg Targocid 400mg powder and solvent for solution for injection vials | 1 vial [PoM] £7.32 DT = £7.32

Telavancin

● DRUG ACTION Telavancin is a glycopeptide antibacterial; it has bactericidal activity against aerobic and anaerobic Gram-positive bacteria including multi-resistant staphylococci. However, there are reports of *Staphylococcus aureus* with reduced susceptibility to glycopeptides. There are increasing reports of glycopeptide-resistant enterococci.

● INDICATIONS AND DOSE

Hospital-acquired pneumonia, known or suspected to be caused by meticillin-resistant *Staphylococcus aureus* when other antibacterials cannot be used
▸ BY INTRAVENOUS INFUSION
▸ Adult: 10 mg/kg once daily for 7–21 days

● CAUTIONS Conditions that predispose to renal impairment · predisposition to QT interval prolongation (including electrolyte disturbances, congenital long QT syndrome, uncompensated heart failure, severe left ventricular hypertrophy)

● INTERACTIONS → Appendix 1: telavancin

● SIDE-EFFECTS
▸ **Common or very common** Asthenia · constipation · diarrhoea · dizziness · headaches · increased risk of infection · insomnia · nausea · renal impairment · skin reactions · taste altered · urine abnormalities · vomiting
▸ **Uncommon** Altered smell sensation · anaemia · angina pectoris · anxiety · appetite decreased · arrhythmias · arthralgia · Clostridium colitis · confusion · congestive heart failure · depression · drowsiness · dry mouth · dyspnoea · electrolyte imbalance · eye irritation · flatulence · flushing · gastrointestinal discomfort · haematuria · hepatitis · hiccups · hyperglycaemia · hyperhidrosis · hypertension · hypoglycaemia · hypotension · laryngeal pain · leucopenia · muscle complaints · nasal congestion · oedema · oral hypoaesthesia · pain · palpitations · paraesthesia · QT interval prolongation · red man syndrome · thrombocytopenia · thrombocytosis · tinnitus · tremor · urinary disorders · vision blurred
▸ **Rare or very rare** Deafness

● ALLERGY AND CROSS-SENSITIVITY Use with caution in patients with vancomycin or teicoplanin sensitivity.

● CONCEPTION AND CONTRACEPTION Effective contraception required during treatment.

● PREGNANCY Avoid (teratogenic in *animal* studies).

● BREAST FEEDING Manufacturer advises avoid unless potential benefit outweighs risk—no information available.

● HEPATIC IMPAIRMENT Manufacturer advises caution in severe impairment (no information available).

● RENAL IMPAIRMENT Avoid in acute renal failure—risk of mortality increased. In chronic renal failure, avoid if eGFR less than 30 mL/minute/1.73 m².
Dose adjustments In chronic renal failure, use 7.5 mg/kg once daily if eGFR 30–50 mL/minute/1.73 m².

● MONITORING REQUIREMENTS Monitor renal function daily for at least the first 3–5 days, then every 2–3 days thereafter.

● DIRECTIONS FOR ADMINISTRATION For *intravenous infusion* (*Vibativ*®). Avoid rapid infusion (can cause 'red man' syndrome). Give intermittently *in* Glucose 5% or Sodium chloride 0.9%; reconstitute each 750 mg with 45 mL glucose 5%, sodium chloride 0.9%, or water for injections to produce a 15 mg/mL solution; for doses of 150–800 mg, dilute requisite dose in 100 to 250 mL infusion fluid; for doses outside this range, dilute to a final concentration of 0.6–8 mg/mL; give over at least 60 minutes.

● MEDICINAL FORMS There can be variation in the licensing of
different medicines containing the same drug.

Powder for solution for infusion
▸ Vibativ (Clinigen Healthcare Ltd)
    Telavancin (as Telavancin hydrochloride) 750 mg Vibativ 750mg
    powder for solution for infusion vials | 1 vial [PoM] £645.00 (Hospital
    only)

Vancomycin   02-Dec-2020

● DRUG ACTION The glycopeptide antibiotic vancomycin has
bactericidal activity against aerobic and anaerobic Gram-
positive bacteria including multi-resistant staphylococci.
However, there are reports of *Staphylococcus aureus* with
reduced susceptibility to glycopeptides. There are
increasing reports of glycopeptide-resistant enterococci.
Penetration into cerebrospinal fluid is poor.

● **INDICATIONS AND DOSE**

Clostridioides difficile infection [first episode]
▸ BY MOUTH
▸ Adult: 125 mg every 6 hours for 10 days; increased if
    necessary to 500 mg every 6 hours for 10 days,
    increased dose if severe or complicated infection

Clostridioides difficile infection [multiple recurrences]
▸ BY MOUTH
▸ Adult: 125 mg every 6 hours for 10 days, followed by,
    either tapering the dose (gradually reducing until
    125 mg daily) or a pulse regimen (125–500 mg every
    2–3 days for at least 3 weeks)

Moderate diabetic foot infection | Severe diabetic foot infection | Leg ulcer infection
▸ BY INTRAVENOUS INFUSION
▸ Adult: 15–20 mg/kg every 8–12 hours (max. per dose
    2 g) adjusted according to plasma-concentration
    monitoring

Cellulitis | Erysipelas
▸ BY INTRAVENOUS INFUSION
▸ Adult: 15–20 mg/kg every 8–12 hours (max. per dose
    2 g) adjusted according to plasma-concentration
    monitoring

Complicated skin and soft tissue infections | Bone infections | Joint infections | Community-acquired pneumonia | Hospital-acquired pneumonia [including ventilator-associated pneumonia] | Infective endocarditis | Acute bacterial meningitis | Bacteraemia [occurring in association with or suspected to be associated with the licensed indications]
▸ BY INTRAVENOUS INFUSION
▸ Adult: 15–20 mg/kg every 8–12 hours (max. per dose
    2 g) adjusted according to plasma-concentration
    monitoring, duration should be tailored to type and
    severity of infection and the individual clinical
    response—consult product literature for further
    information, in seriously ill patients, a loading dose of
    25–30 mg/kg (usual max. 2 g) can be used to facilitate
    rapid attainment of the target trough serum-
    vancomycin concentration

Perioperative prophylaxis of bacterial endocarditis [in patients at high risk of developing bacterial endocarditis when undergoing major surgical procedures]
▸ BY INTRAVENOUS INFUSION
▸ Adult: 15 mg/kg, to be given prior to induction of
    anaesthesia, a second dose may be required depending
    on duration of surgery

Surgical prophylaxis (when high risk of MRSA)
▸ BY INTRAVENOUS INFUSION
▸ Adult: 1 g for 1 dose

Peritonitis associated with peritoneal dialysis
▸ BY INTRAPERITONEAL ADMINISTRATION
▸ Adult: (consult local protocol)

PHARMACOKINETICS
▸ Vancomycin should **not** be given by mouth for systemic
    infections because it is not absorbed significantly.

● UNLICENSED USE Vancomycin doses in BNF publications
may differ from those in product literature. Use of
vancomycin (added to dialysis fluid) for the treatment of
peritonitis associated with peritoneal dialysis is an
unlicensed route.

● CONTRA-INDICATIONS
▸ With intravenous use Previous hearing loss

● CAUTIONS
▸ With oral use Systemic absorption may be enhanced in
patients with inflammatory disorders of the intestinal
mucosa or with *Clostridioides difficile*-induced
pseudomembranous colitis (increased risk of adverse
reactions)

● INTERACTIONS → Appendix 1: vancomycin

● SIDE-EFFECTS

GENERAL SIDE-EFFECTS
Agranulocytosis · dizziness · drug fever · eosinophilia ·
hypersensitivity · nausea · nephritis tubulointerstitial ·
neutropenia (more common after 1 week or cumulative
dose of 25 g) · renal failure · severe cutaneous adverse
reactions (SCARs) · skin reactions · thrombocytopenia ·
tinnitus (discontinue) · vasculitis · vertigo

SPECIFIC SIDE-EFFECTS
▸ With intravenous use Back pain · bradycardia · cardiac arrest
(on rapid intravenous injection) · cardiogenic shock (on
rapid intravenous injection) · chest pain · dyspnoea ·
hearing loss · hypotension · muscle complaints ·
pseudomembranous enterocolitis · red man syndrome ·
wheezing

SIDE-EFFECTS, FURTHER INFORMATION Vancomycin is
associated with a higher incidence of nephrotoxicity than
teicoplanin.

● ALLERGY AND CROSS-SENSITIVITY [EvGr] Caution if
teicoplanin sensitivity. ◁

● PREGNANCY Manufacturer advises use only if potential
benefit outweighs risk.
Monitoring Plasma-vancomycin concentration monitoring
essential to reduce risk of fetal toxicity.

● BREAST FEEDING Present in milk—significant absorption
following oral administration unlikely.

● RENAL IMPAIRMENT Manufacturer advises serial
monitoring of renal function.
▸ With intravenous use Manufacturer advises use with
caution—increased risk of toxic effects with prolonged
high blood concentration.
Dose adjustments ▸ With oral use Manufacturer advises
dose adjustment is unlikely to be required unless
substantial oral absorption occurs in inflammatory
disorders of the intestinal mucosa or with *Clostridioides
difficile*-induced pseudomembranous colitis, see
Monitoring.
    ▸ With intravenous use Manufacturer advises initial dose
    must not be reduced—consult product literature.

● MONITORING REQUIREMENTS
▸ With intravenous use Manufacturer advises initial doses
should be based on body-weight; subsequent dose
adjustments should be based on serum-vancomycin
concentrations to achieve targeted therapeutic
concentrations. All patients require serum-vancomycin
measurement (on the second day of treatment,
immediately before the next dose if renal function normal,
earlier if renal impairment—consult product literature).
Frequency of monitoring depends on the clinical situation

and response to treatment; regular monitoring indicated in high-dose therapy and longer-term use, particularly in patients with impaired renal function, impaired hearing, or concurrent use of nephrotoxic or ototoxic drugs. Manufacturer advises pre-dose ('trough') concentration should normally be 10–20 mg/litre depending on the site of infection and the susceptibility of the pathogen; trough concentration of 15–20 mg/litre is usually recommended to cover susceptible pathogens with MIC greater than or equal to 1 mg/litre—consult product literature.

▶ With intravenous use Manufacturer advises periodic testing of auditory function. Manufacturer advises monitor blood counts, urinalysis, hepatic and renal function periodically in all patients; monitor leucocyte count regularly in patients receiving long-term vancomycin or if given concurrently with other drugs that may cause neutropenia or agranulocytosis.

▶ With intravenous use Manufacturer advises monitor vestibular and auditory function during and after treatment in the elderly; avoid concurrent or sequential use of other ototoxic drugs.

▶ With oral use Manufacturer advises monitoring serum-vancomycin concentration in inflammatory intestinal disorders.

▶ With oral use Manufacturer advises serial tests of auditory function may be helpful to minimise the risk of ototoxicity in patients with an underlying hearing loss, or who are receiving concomitant therapy with other ototoxic drugs.

● DIRECTIONS FOR ADMINISTRATION

▶ With intravenous use Avoid rapid infusion (risk of anaphylactoid reactions) and rotate infusion sites.
  For intravenous infusion, give intermittently in Glucose 5% or Sodium chloride 0.9%; reconstitute each 500 mg with 10 mL water for injections and dilute with infusion fluid to a concentration of up to 5 mg/mL (10 mg/mL in fluid restriction but increased risk of infusion-related effects); give over at least 60 minutes (rate not to exceed 10 mg/minute for doses over 500 mg); use continuous infusion only if intermittent not feasible.

▶ With oral use Injection can be used to prepare solution for oral administration—consult product literature.

● PRESCRIBING AND DISPENSING INFORMATION For choice of antibacterial therapy, see Antibacterials, use for prophylaxis p. 529, Blood infections, antibacterial therapy p. 532, Cardiovascular system infections, antibacterial therapy p. 532, Central nervous system infections, antibacterial therapy p. 533, Diabetic foot infections, antibacterial therapy p. 534, Gastro-intestinal system infections, antibacterial therapy p. 535, Musculoskeletal system infections, antibacterial therapy p. 536, Respiratory system infections, antibacterial therapy p. 538, Skin infections, antibacterial therapy p. 541.

● MEDICINAL FORMS There can be variation in the licensing of different medicines containing the same drug. Forms available from special-order manufacturers include: oral suspension, oral solution, solution for injection, infusion

Powder for solution for infusion

▶ Vancomycin (Non-proprietary)
  Vancomycin (as Vancomycin hydrochloride) 500 mg Vancomycin 500mg powder for solution for infusion vials | 1 vial [PoM] £7.25 DT = £5.49 (Hospital only) | 10 vial [PoM] £62.50 DT = £62.50 (Hospital only)
  Vancomycin 500mg powder for concentrate for solution for infusion vials | 1 vial [PoM] £5.49–£8.50 DT = £5.49 (Hospital only) | 10 vial [PoM] £62.50–£72.50 DT = £62.50 (Hospital only)
  Vancomycin (as Vancomycin hydrochloride) 1 gram Vancomycin 1g powder for solution for infusion vials | 1 vial [PoM] £14.50 DT = £11.25 (Hospital only) | 10 vial [PoM] £125.00 DT = £125.00 (Hospital only)
  Vancomycin 1g powder for concentrate for solution for infusion vials | 1 vial [PoM] £11.25–£17.25 DT = £11.25 (Hospital only) | 10 vial [PoM] £125.00 DT = £125.00 (Hospital only)

▶ Vancocin (Flynn Pharma Ltd)
  Vancomycin (as Vancomycin hydrochloride) 500 mg Vancocin 500mg powder for solution for infusion vials | 1 vial [PoM] £6.25 DT = £5.49 (Hospital only)
  Vancomycin (as Vancomycin hydrochloride) 1 gram Vancocin 1g powder for solution for infusion vials | 1 vial [PoM] £12.50 DT = £11.25 (Hospital only)

Capsule

CAUTIONARY AND ADVISORY LABELS 9

▶ Vancomycin (Non-proprietary)
  Vancomycin (as Vancomycin hydrochloride) 125 mg Vancomycin 125mg capsules | 28 capsule [PoM] £132.49 DT = £132.49
  Vancomycin (as Vancomycin hydrochloride) 250 mg Vancomycin 250mg capsules | 28 capsule [PoM] £135.40 DT = £135.40

▶ Vancocin Matrigel (Flynn Pharma Ltd)
  Vancomycin (as Vancomycin hydrochloride) 125 mg Vancocin Matrigel 125mg capsules | 28 capsule [PoM] £88.31 DT = £132.49

ANTIBACTERIALS ⟩ LINCOSAMIDES

Clindamycin

25-Nov-2020

● DRUG ACTION
Clindamycin is active against Gram-positive cocci, including streptococci and penicillin-resistant staphylococci, and also against many anaerobes, especially *Bacteroides fragilis*. It is well concentrated in bone and excreted in bile and urine.

● INDICATIONS AND DOSE

Staphylococcal bone and joint infections such as osteomyelitis | Peritonitis | Intra-abdominal sepsis | Meticillin-resistant *Staphylococcus aureus* (MRSA) in bronchiectasis, bone and joint infections, and skin and soft-tissue infections

▶ BY MOUTH
▶ Child: 3–6 mg/kg 4 times a day (max. per dose 450 mg)
▶ Adult: 150–300 mg every 6 hours; increased if necessary up to 450 mg every 6 hours if required, increased dose used in severe infection
▶ BY DEEP INTRAMUSCULAR INJECTION, OR BY INTRAVENOUS INFUSION
▶ Adult: 0.6–2.7 g daily in 2–4 divided doses; increased if necessary up to 4.8 g daily, increased dose used in life-threatening infection, single doses above 600 mg to be administered by intravenous infusion only, single doses by intravenous infusion not to exceed 1.2 g, doses administered using **solution for injection ampoules**

Staphylococcal bone and joint infections | Chronic sinusitis | Lower respiratory-tract infections | Complicated intra-abdominal infections | Pelvic and female genital infections | Skin and soft-tissue infections

▶ BY INTRAVENOUS INFUSION
▶ Adult: 1.2–1.8 g daily in 2–4 divided doses, for less complicated infections; increased to 1.8–2.7 g daily in 2–3 divided doses, for severe infections; increased if necessary up to 4.8 g daily, for life-threatening infections, doses administered using **solution for infusion bags**

Moderate diabetic foot infection | Severe diabetic foot infection

▶ BY MOUTH
▶ Adult: 150–300 mg every 6 hours; increased if necessary up to 450 mg every 6 hours
▶ BY INTRAVENOUS INFUSION
▶ Adult: 0.6–2.7 g daily in 2–4 divided doses; increased if necessary up to 4.8 g daily, increased dose used in life-threatening infection, single doses not to exceed 1.2 g

Cellulitis | Erysipelas

▶ BY MOUTH
▶ Child: 3–6 mg/kg 4 times a day (max. per dose 450 mg) for 7 days then review

▸ Adult: 150–300 mg every 6 hours; increased if necessary up to 450 mg every 6 hours for 7 days then review
▸ BY INTRAVENOUS INFUSION
▸ Adult: 0.6–2.7 g daily in 2–4 divided doses; increased if necessary to 1.2 g 4 times a day, increased dose used in life-threatening infection

Treatment of mild to moderate pneumocystis pneumonia (in combination with primaquine)
▸ BY MOUTH
▸ Adult: 600 mg every 8 hours

Treatment of falciparum malaria (to be given with or following quinine)
▸ BY MOUTH
▸ Child: 7–13 mg/kg every 8 hours (max. per dose 450 mg) for 7 days
▸ Adult: 450 mg every 8 hours for 7 days

● UNLICENSED USE Not licensed for treatment of mild to moderate pneumocystis infection. Not licensed for treatment of falciparum malaria.
▸ With intravenous use in adults [EvGr] Clindamycin is used in the doses provided in the BNF for the treatment of diabetic foot infections, cellulitis and erysipelas, ◈Ⓜ but licensed dosing for intravenous infusion bags may differ.
▸ With intravenous use in children [EvGr] Clindamycin is used in the doses provided in the BNF for the treatment of cellulitis and erysipelas, ◈Ⓜ but licensed dosing for intravenous infusion bags may differ. Intravenous infusion bags are not licensed in children under 12 years.
● CONTRA-INDICATIONS Diarrhoeal states
● CAUTIONS Avoid in Acute porphyrias p. 1107
● INTERACTIONS → Appendix 1: clindamycin
● SIDE-EFFECTS
GENERAL SIDE-EFFECTS
▸ **Common or very common** Skin reactions
SPECIFIC SIDE-EFFECTS
▸ **Common or very common**
▸ With oral use Abdominal pain · antibiotic associated colitis · diarrhoea (discontinue)
▸ **Uncommon**
▸ With oral use Nausea · vomiting
▸ **Frequency not known**
▸ With oral use Agranulocytosis · angioedema · eosinophilia · gastrointestinal disorders · jaundice · leucopenia · neutropenia · severe cutaneous adverse reactions (SCARs) · taste altered · thrombocytopenia · vulvovaginal infection
▸ With parenteral use Abdominal pain · agranulocytosis · antibiotic associated colitis · cardiac arrest · diarrhoea (discontinue) · eosinophilia · hypotension · jaundice · leucopenia · nausea · neutropenia · severe cutaneous adverse reactions (SCARs) · taste altered · thrombocytopenia · thrombophlebitis · vomiting · vulvovaginal infection

SIDE-EFFECTS, FURTHER INFORMATION Clindamycin has been associated with antibiotic-associated colitis, which may be fatal. Although antibiotic-associated colitis can occur with most antibacterials, it occurs more frequently with clindamycin. If *C difficile* infection is suspected or confirmed, discontinue the antibiotic if appropriate. Seek specialist advice if the antibiotic cannot be stopped and the diarrhoea is severe.
● PREGNANCY Manufacturer advises not known to be harmful in the second and third trimesters; use with caution in the first trimester—limited data.
● BREAST FEEDING [EvGr] Specialist sources indicate use with caution—present in milk. Monitor infant for effects on the gastrointestinal flora such as diarrhoea, candidiasis, or rarely, blood in the stool indicating possible antibiotic-associated colitis. ◈Ⓓ

● MONITORING REQUIREMENTS Monitor liver and renal function if treatment exceeds 10 days.
▸ In children Monitor liver and renal function in neonates and infants.
● DIRECTIONS FOR ADMINISTRATION
▸ With intravenous use Avoid rapid intravenous administration. For *intravenous infusion bags*, manufacturer advises give over 10–60 minutes without further dilution. For *intravenous infusion (Dalacin® C Phosphate)*, manufacturer advises give continuously or intermittently in Glucose 5% or Sodium Chloride 0.9%; dilute to not more than 18 mg/mL and give over 10–60 minutes at a rate not exceeding 30 mg/minute (1.2 g over at least 60 minutes; higher doses by continuous infusion).
● PRESCRIBING AND DISPENSING INFORMATION For choice of antibacterial therapy, see Diabetic foot infections, antibacterial therapy p. 534, Gastro-intestinal system infections, antibacterial therapy p. 535, Genital system infections, antibacterial therapy p. 536, Malaria, treatment p. 652, MRSA p. 615, Musculoskeletal system infections, antibacterial therapy p. 536, Pneumocystis pneumonia p. 640, Respiratory system infections, antibacterial therapy p. 538, Skin infections, antibacterial therapy p. 541.
● PATIENT AND CARER ADVICE Patients and their carers should be advised to discontinue and contact a doctor immediately if severe, prolonged or bloody diarrhoea develops.
▸ With oral use Capsules should be swallowed with a glass of water.
● PROFESSION SPECIFIC INFORMATION
Dental practitioners' formulary
▸ With oral use Clindamycin capsules may be prescribed.

● MEDICINAL FORMS There can be variation in the licensing of different medicines containing the same drug. Forms available from special-order manufacturers include: oral suspension, oral solution

Solution for injection
EXCIPIENTS: May contain Benzyl alcohol
▸ Clindamycin (Non-proprietary)
Clindamycin (as Clindamycin phosphate) 150 mg per 1 ml Clindamycin 600mg/4ml solution for injection ampoules | 5 ampoule [PoM] £59.00–£61.75 (Hospital only)
Clindamycin 300mg/2ml solution for injection ampoules | 5 ampoule [PoM] £29.50–£31.01 (Hospital only)
▸ Dalacin C (Pfizer Ltd)
Clindamycin (as Clindamycin phosphate) 150 mg per 1 ml Dalacin C Phosphate 300mg/2ml solution for injection ampoules | 5 ampoule [PoM] £31.01 (Hospital only)
Dalacin C Phosphate 600mg/4ml solution for injection ampoules | 5 ampoule [PoM] £61.75 (Hospital only)

Capsule
CAUTIONARY AND ADVISORY LABELS 9, 27
▸ Clindamycin (Non-proprietary)
Clindamycin (as Clindamycin hydrochloride) 75 mg Clindamycin 75mg capsules | 24 capsule [PoM] £7.45 DT = £7.45
Clindamycin (as Clindamycin hydrochloride) 150 mg Clindamycin 150mg capsules | 24 capsule [PoM] £13.72 DT = £2.46 | 100 capsule [PoM] £4.26–£55.08
Clindamycin (as Clindamycin hydrochloride) 300 mg Clindamycin 300mg capsules | 30 capsule [PoM] £42.00 DT = £38.23
▸ Dalacin C (Pfizer Ltd)
Clindamycin (as Clindamycin hydrochloride) 75 mg Dalacin C 75mg capsules | 24 capsule [PoM] £7.45 DT = £7.45
Clindamycin (as Clindamycin hydrochloride) 150 mg Dalacin C 150mg capsules | 24 capsule [PoM] £13.72 DT = £2.46 | 100 capsule [PoM] £55.08

Infusion
EXCIPIENTS: May contain Disodium edetate, glucose
▸ Clindamycin (Non-proprietary)
Clindamycin (as Clindamycin phosphate) 6 mg per 1 ml Clindamycin 300mg/50ml infusion bags | 10 bag [PoM] £49.50 (Hospital only)

Clindamycin (as Clindamycin phosphate) 12 mg per 1 ml Clindamycin 600mg/50ml infusion bags | 10 bag [PoM] £99.00 (Hospital only)

ANTIBACTERIALS > MACROLIDES

Macrolides

18-Jun-2018

Overview

The macrolides have an antibacterial spectrum that is similar but not identical to that of penicillin; they are thus an alternative in penicillin-allergic patients. They are active against many-penicillin-resistant staphylococci, but some are now also resistant to the macrolides.

Indications for the macrolides include campylobacter enteritis, respiratory infections (including pneumonia, whooping cough, Legionella, chlamydia, and mycoplasma infection), and skin infections.

Erythromycin p. 572 is also used in the treatment of early syphilis, uncomplicated genital chlamydial infection, and non-gonococcal urethritis. Erythromycin has poor activity against *Haemophilus influenzae*. Erythromycin causes nausea, vomiting, and diarrhoea in some patients; in mild to moderate infections this can be avoided by giving a lower dose, but if a more serious infection, such as Legionella pneumonia, is suspected higher doses are needed.

Azithromycin below is a macrolide with slightly less activity than erythromycin against Gram-positive bacteria, but enhanced activity against some Gram-negative organisms including *H. influenzae*. Plasma concentrations are very low, but tissue concentrations are much higher. It has a long tissue half-life and once daily dosage is recommended. Azithromycin is also used in the treatment of uncomplicated genital chlamydial infection, non-gonococcal urethritis, uncomplicated gonorrhoea, typhoid [unlicensed indication], trachoma [unlicensed indication], and Lyme disease [unlicensed indication].

Clarithromycin p. 569 is an erythromycin derivative with slightly greater activity than the parent compound. Tissue concentrations are higher than with erythromycin. Clarithromycin is also used in regimens for *Helicobacter pylori* eradication.

Spiramycin is also a macrolide which is used for the treatment of toxoplasmosis.

Macrolides

- CAUTIONS
▶ With intravenous use or oral use electrolyte disturbances (predisposition to QT interval prolongation) · may aggravate myasthenia gravis · predisposition to QT interval prolongation

- SIDE-EFFECTS
▶ **Common or very common** Appetite decreased · diarrhoea · dizziness · gastrointestinal discomfort · gastrointestinal disorders · headache · hearing impairment · insomnia · nausea · pancreatitis · paraesthesia · skin reactions · taste altered · vasodilation · vision disorders · vomiting
▶ **Uncommon** Angioedema · anxiety · arrhythmias · candida infection · chest pain · constipation · drowsiness · eosinophilia · hepatic disorders · leucopenia · neutropenia · palpitations · QT interval prolongation · severe cutaneous adverse reactions (SCARs) · tinnitus · vertigo
▶ **Rare or very rare** Antibiotic associated colitis · myasthenia gravis · nephritis tubulointerstitial
▶ **Frequency not known** Hallucination · hypotension · seizure · smell altered · thrombocytopenia · tongue discolouration

F above

Azithromycin

29-Jul-2020

- INDICATIONS AND DOSE

Prevention of secondary case of invasive group A streptococcal infection in patients who are allergic to penicillin
▶ BY MOUTH
  ▹ Child 6 months-11 years: 12 mg/kg once daily (max. per dose 500 mg) for 5 days
  ▹ Child 12-17 years: 500 mg once daily for 5 days
  ▹ Adult: 500 mg once daily for 5 days

Respiratory-tract infections, otitis media, skin and soft-tissue infections
▶ BY MOUTH
  ▹ Child 6 months-17 years: 10 mg/kg once daily (max. per dose 500 mg) for 3 days
  ▹ Child 6 months-17 years (body-weight 15-25 kg): 200 mg once daily for 3 days
  ▹ Child 6 months-17 years (body-weight 26-35 kg): 300 mg once daily for 3 days
  ▹ Child 6 months-17 years (body-weight 36-45 kg): 400 mg once daily for 3 days
  ▹ Child 6 months-17 years (body-weight 46 kg and above): 500 mg once daily for 3 days
  ▹ Adult: 500 mg once daily for 3 days, alternatively initially 500 mg once daily for 1 day, then 250 mg once daily for 4 days

Uncomplicated genital chlamydial infections | Non-gonococcal urethritis
▶ BY MOUTH
  ▹ Child 12-17 years: 1 g for 1 dose
  ▹ Adult: 1 g for 1 dose

Uncomplicated gonorrhoea [anogenital and pharyngeal infection]
▶ BY MOUTH
  ▹ Adult: 2 g for 1 dose

Lyme disease [erythema migrans and/or non-focal symptoms]
▶ BY MOUTH
  ▹ Adult: 500 mg daily for 17 days

Mild to moderate typhoid due to multiple-antibacterial resistant organisms
▶ BY MOUTH
  ▹ Adult: 500 mg once daily for 7 days

Community-acquired pneumonia, low to moderate severity
▶ BY MOUTH
  ▹ Adult: 500 mg once daily for 3 days, alternatively initially 500 mg once daily for 1 day, then 250 mg once daily for 4 days

Community-acquired pneumonia, high severity
▶ INITIALLY BY INTRAVENOUS INFUSION
  ▹ Adult: Initially 500 mg once daily for at least 2 days, then (by mouth) 500 mg once daily for a total duration of 7–10 days

Antibacterial prophylaxis for insertion of intra-uterine device
▶ BY MOUTH
  ▹ Adult: 1 g for 1 dose

- UNLICENSED USE
▶ In children Azithromycin may be used as detailed below, although this situation is considered outside the scope of its licence:
  • prevention of group A streptococcal infection
▶ With oral use in adults Azithromycin may be used as detailed below, although these situations are considered outside the scope of its licence:
  • prevention of group A streptococcal infection;

- EvGr Lyme disease ⟨A⟩;
- mild to moderate typhoid due to multiple-antibacterial resistant organisms;
- community-acquired pneumonia (high severity) when oral treatment continues for more than 3 days.

● INTERACTIONS → Appendix 1: macrolides

● SIDE-EFFECTS
▸ **Common or very common**
▸ With oral use Arthralgia
▸ **Uncommon** Numbness · oedema · photosensitivity reaction
▸ **Frequency not known** Acute kidney injury · aggression · akathisia · haemolytic anaemia · syncope

● PREGNANCY Manufacturers advise use only if adequate alternatives not available.

● BREAST FEEDING Present in milk; use only if no suitable alternatives.

● HEPATIC IMPAIRMENT Manufacturer advises caution; consider avoiding in severe impairment (no information available).

● RENAL IMPAIRMENT
▸ In adults Use with caution if eGFR less than 10 mL/minute/1.73 m².
▸ In children Use with caution if estimated glomerular filtration rate less than 10 mL/minute/1.73 m².

● DIRECTIONS FOR ADMINISTRATION
▸ With intravenous use in adults For *intravenous infusion* (*Zedbac®*), manufacturer advises give intermittently *in* Glucose 5% *or* Sodium Chloride 0.9%. Reconstitute 500 mg with 4.8 mL water for injections to produce a 100 mg/mL solution, then dilute 5 mL of solution with infusion fluid to a final concentration of 1 or 2 mg/mL; give the 1 mg/mL solution over 3 hours *or* give the 2 mg/mL solution over 1 hour.

● PRESCRIBING AND DISPENSING INFORMATION For choice of antibacterial therapy, see Antibacterials, use for prophylaxis p. 529, Ear infections, antibacterial therapy p. 534, Genital system infections, antibacterial therapy p. 536, Lyme disease p. 614, Respiratory system infections, antibacterial therapy p. 538, Skin infections, antibacterial therapy p. 541.

● PATIENT AND CARER ADVICE
Medicines for Children leaflet: Azithromycin for bacterial infections www.medicinesforchildren.org.uk/azithromycin-bacterial-infections-0

● PROFESSION SPECIFIC INFORMATION
Dental practitioners' formulary
▸ With oral use Azithromycin Capsules may be prescribed. Azithromycin Tablets may be prescribed. Azithromycin Oral Suspension 200 mg/5 mL may be prescribed.

● EXCEPTIONS TO LEGAL CATEGORY Azithromycin tablets can be sold to the public for the treatment of confirmed, asymptomatic *Chlamydia trachomatis* genital infection in those over 16 years of age, and for the epidemiological treatment of their sexual partners, subject to maximum single dose of 1 g, maximum daily dose 1 g, and a pack size of 1 g.

● MEDICINAL FORMS There can be variation in the licensing of different medicines containing the same drug. Forms available from special-order manufacturers include: oral suspension

Tablet
CAUTIONARY AND ADVISORY LABELS 5, 9
▸ Azithromycin (Non-proprietary)
Azithromycin 250 mg Azithromycin 250mg tablets | 4 tablet PoM £10.11 DT = £1.54 | 6 tablet PoM £2.24–£2.59
Azithromycin 500 mg Azithromycin 500mg tablets | 3 tablet PoM £7.45 DT = £1.54

Oral suspension
CAUTIONARY AND ADVISORY LABELS 5, 9
▸ Azithromycin (Non-proprietary)
Azithromycin 40 mg per 1 ml Azithromycin 200mg/5ml oral suspension | 15 ml PoM £6.18 DT = £4.06 | 30 ml PoM £11.04 DT = £11.04
▸ Zithromax (Pfizer Ltd)
Azithromycin 40 mg per 1 ml Zithromax 200mg/5ml oral suspension | 15 ml PoM £4.06 DT = £4.06 | 22.5 ml PoM £6.10 DT = £6.10 | 30 ml PoM £11.04 DT = £11.04

Powder for solution for infusion
ELECTROLYTES: May contain Sodium
▸ Zedbac (Aspire Pharma Ltd)
Azithromycin (as Azithromycin dihydrate) 500 mg Zedbac 500mg powder for solution for infusion vials | 1 vial PoM £9.50 (Hospital only)

Capsule
CAUTIONARY AND ADVISORY LABELS 5, 9, 23
▸ Azithromycin (Non-proprietary)
Azithromycin (as Azithromycin dihydrate) 250 mg Azithromycin 250mg capsules | 4 capsule PoM £1.73–£10.10 | 6 capsule PoM £15.15 DT = £2.60
▸ Zithromax (Pfizer Ltd)
Azithromycin (as Azithromycin dihydrate) 250 mg Zithromax 250mg capsules | 4 capsule PoM £7.16 | 6 capsule PoM £10.74 DT = £2.60

⟁ 568

Clarithromycin

14-Dec-2020

● INDICATIONS AND DOSE
Mild diabetic foot infection
▸ BY MOUTH USING IMMEDIATE-RELEASE MEDICINES
▸ Adult: 500 mg twice daily for 7 days then review

Leg ulcer infection
▸ BY MOUTH USING IMMEDIATE-RELEASE MEDICINES
▸ Adult: 500 mg twice daily for 7 days

Cellulitis | Erysipelas
▸ BY MOUTH USING IMMEDIATE-RELEASE MEDICINES
▸ Child 1 month–11 years (body-weight up to 8 kg): 7.5 mg/kg twice daily for 5–7 days then review (review after 7 days if infection near the eyes or nose)
▸ Child 1 month–11 years (body-weight 8–11 kg): 62.5 mg twice daily for 5–7 days then review (review after 7 days if infection near the eyes or nose)
▸ Child 1 month–11 years (body-weight 12–19 kg): 125 mg twice daily for 5–7 days then review (review after 7 days if infection near the eyes or nose)
▸ Child 1 month–11 years (body-weight 20–29 kg): 187.5 mg twice daily for 5–7 days then review (review after 7 days if infection near the eyes or nose)
▸ Child 1 month–11 years (body-weight 30–40 kg): 250 mg twice daily for 5–7 days then review (review after 7 days if infection near the eyes or nose)
▸ Child 12–17 years: 250–500 mg twice daily for 5–7 days then review (review after 7 days if infection near the eyes or nose)
▸ Adult: 500 mg twice daily for 5–7 days then review (review after 7 days if infection near the eyes or nose)
▸ BY INTRAVENOUS INFUSION
▸ Adult: 500 mg every 12 hours

Impetigo
▸ BY MOUTH USING IMMEDIATE-RELEASE MEDICINES
▸ Child 1 month–11 years (body-weight up to 8 kg): 7.5 mg/kg twice daily for 5–7 days
▸ Child 1 month–11 years (body-weight 8–11 kg): 62.5 mg twice daily for 5–7 days
▸ Child 1 month–11 years (body-weight 12–19 kg): 125 mg twice daily for 5–7 days
▸ Child 1 month–11 years (body-weight 20–29 kg): 187.5 mg twice daily for 5–7 days
▸ Child 1 month–11 years (body-weight 30–40 kg): 250 mg twice daily for 5–7 days

continued →

5

Infection

Child 12-17 years: 250 mg twice daily for 5–7 days, increased if necessary to 500 mg twice daily, increased dose used in severe infections
- Adult: 250 mg twice daily for 5–7 days, increased if necessary to 500 mg twice daily, increased dose used in severe infections

Community-acquired pneumonia
▸ BY MOUTH USING IMMEDIATE-RELEASE MEDICINES
- Child 1 month-11 years (body-weight up to 8 kg): 7.5 mg/kg twice daily for 5 days
- Child 1 month-11 years (body-weight 8-11 kg): 62.5 mg twice daily for 5 days
- Child 1 month-11 years (body-weight 12-19 kg): 125 mg twice daily for 5 days
- Child 1 month-11 years (body-weight 20-29 kg): 187.5 mg twice daily for 5 days
- Child 1 month-11 years (body-weight 30-40 kg): 250 mg twice daily for 5 days
- Child 12-17 years: 250–500 mg twice daily for 5 days
- Adult: 500 mg twice daily for 5 days
▸ BY INTRAVENOUS INFUSION
- Adult: 500 mg every 12 hours

Hospital-acquired pneumonia
▸ BY MOUTH USING IMMEDIATE-RELEASE MEDICINES
- Child 1 month-11 years (body-weight up to 8 kg): 7.5 mg/kg twice daily for 5 days then review
- Child 1 month-11 years (body-weight 8-11 kg): 62.5 mg twice daily for 5 days then review
- Child 1 month-11 years (body-weight 12-19 kg): 125 mg twice daily for 5 days then review
- Child 1 month-11 years (body-weight 20-29 kg): 187.5 mg twice daily for 5 days then review
- Child 1 month-11 years (body-weight 30-40 kg): 250 mg twice daily for 5 days then review
- Child 12-17 years: 500 mg twice daily for 5 days then review

Respiratory-tract infections | Mild to moderate skin and soft-tissue infections
▸ BY MOUTH USING IMMEDIATE-RELEASE MEDICINES
- Child 1 month-11 years (body-weight up to 8 kg): 7.5 mg/kg twice daily
- Child 1 month-11 years (body-weight 8-11 kg): 62.5 mg twice daily
- Child 1 month-11 years (body-weight 12-19 kg): 125 mg twice daily
- Child 1 month-11 years (body-weight 20-29 kg): 187.5 mg twice daily
- Child 1 month-11 years (body-weight 30-40 kg): 250 mg twice daily
- Child 12-17 years: 250 mg twice daily usually for 7–14 days, increased to 500 mg twice daily, if required in severe infections
- Adult: 250 mg twice daily usually for 7–14 days, increased to 500 mg twice daily, if required in severe infections
▸ BY MOUTH USING MODIFIED-RELEASE MEDICINES
- Child 12-17 years: 500 mg once daily usually for 7–14 days, increased to 1 g once daily, if required in severe infections
- Adult: 500 mg once daily usually for 7–14 days, increased to 1 g once daily, if required in severe infections
▸ BY INTRAVENOUS INFUSION
- Adult: 500 mg every 12 hours maximum duration 5 days, switch to oral route when appropriate, to be administered into a large proximal vein

Acute exacerbation of chronic obstructive pulmonary disease
▸ BY MOUTH USING IMMEDIATE-RELEASE MEDICINES
- Adult: 500 mg twice daily for 5 days

▸ BY INTRAVENOUS INFUSION
- Adult: 500 mg every 12 hours, to be administered into a large proximal vein

Acute exacerbation of bronchiectasis
▸ BY MOUTH USING IMMEDIATE-RELEASE MEDICINES
- Child 1 month-11 years (body-weight up to 8 kg): 7.5 mg/kg twice daily for 7–14 days
- Child 1 month-11 years (body-weight 8-11 kg): 62.5 mg twice daily for 7–14 days
- Child 1 month-11 years (body-weight 12-19 kg): 125 mg twice daily for 7–14 days
- Child 1 month-11 years (body-weight 20-29 kg): 187.5 mg twice daily for 7–14 days
- Child 1 month-11 years (body-weight 30-40 kg): 250 mg twice daily for 7–14 days
- Child 12-17 years: 250–500 mg twice daily for 7–14 days
- Adult: 500 mg twice daily for 7–14 days

Acute cough [if systemically very unwell or at higher risk of complications] | Acute sore throat
▸ BY MOUTH USING IMMEDIATE-RELEASE MEDICINES
- Child 1 month-11 years (body-weight up to 8 kg): 7.5 mg/kg twice daily for 5 days
- Child 1 month-11 years (body-weight 8-11 kg): 62.5 mg twice daily for 5 days
- Child 1 month-11 years (body-weight 12-19 kg): 125 mg twice daily for 5 days
- Child 1 month-11 years (body-weight 20-29 kg): 187.5 mg twice daily for 5 days
- Child 1 month-11 years (body-weight 30-40 kg): 250 mg twice daily for 5 days
- Child 12-17 years: 250–500 mg twice daily for 5 days
- Adult: 250–500 mg twice daily for 5 days

Acute otitis media
▸ BY MOUTH USING IMMEDIATE-RELEASE MEDICINES
- Child 1 month-11 years (body-weight up to 8 kg): 7.5 mg/kg twice daily for 5–7 days
- Child 1 month-11 years (body-weight 8-11 kg): 62.5 mg twice daily for 5–7 days
- Child 1 month-11 years (body-weight 12-19 kg): 125 mg twice daily for 5–7 days
- Child 1 month-11 years (body-weight 20-29 kg): 187.5 mg twice daily for 5–7 days
- Child 1 month-11 years (body-weight 30-40 kg): 250 mg twice daily for 5–7 days
- Child 12-17 years: 250–500 mg twice daily for 5–7 days
- Adult: 250 mg twice daily usually for 7–14 days, increased to 500 mg twice daily, if required in severe infections
▸ BY INTRAVENOUS INFUSION
- Adult: 500 mg every 12 hours maximum duration 5 days, switch to oral route when appropriate, to be administered into a large proximal vein

Prevention of pertussis
▸ BY MOUTH USING IMMEDIATE-RELEASE MEDICINES
- Child 1 month-11 years (body-weight up to 8 kg): 7.5 mg/kg twice daily for 7 days
- Child 1 month-11 years (body-weight 8-11 kg): 62.5 mg twice daily for 7 days
- Child 1 month-11 years (body-weight 12-19 kg): 125 mg twice daily for 7 days
- Child 1 month-11 years (body-weight 20-29 kg): 187.5 mg twice daily for 7 days
- Child 1 month-11 years (body-weight 30-40 kg): 250 mg twice daily for 7 days
- Child 12-17 years: 500 mg twice daily for 7 days
- Adult: 500 mg twice daily for 7 days

Helicobacter pylori eradication [in combination with other drugs (see Helicobacter pylori infection p. 90)]
▶ BY MOUTH
▶ Adult: 500 mg twice daily for 7 days for first- and second-line eradication therapy; 10 days for third-line eradication therapy

Acute sinusitis
▶ BY MOUTH USING IMMEDIATE-RELEASE MEDICINES
▶ Child 1 month–11 years (body-weight up to 8 kg): 7.5 mg/kg twice daily for 5 days
▶ Child 1 month–11 years (body-weight 8–11 kg): 62.5 mg twice daily for 5 days
▶ Child 1 month–11 years (body-weight 12–19 kg): 125 mg twice daily for 5 days
▶ Child 1 month–11 years (body-weight 20–29 kg): 187.5 mg twice daily for 5 days
▶ Child 1 month–11 years (body-weight 30–40 kg): 250 mg twice daily for 5 days
▶ Child 12–17 years: 250 mg twice daily for 5 days, alternatively 500 mg twice daily for 5 days
▶ Adult: 500 mg twice daily for 5 days

● UNLICENSED USE EvGr Duration of treatment for acute sinusitis differs from product literature and adheres to national guidelines. ⒶA
▶ With oral use in children EvGr Duration of treatment for acute otitis media differs from product literature and adheres to national guidelines. ⒶA Tablets not licensed for use in children under 12 years; oral suspension not licensed for use in infants under 6 months.
▶ In adults EvGr Combination regimens and durations for *Helicobacter pylori* eradication may differ from product literature but adhere to national guidelines. ⒶA
● INTERACTIONS → Appendix 1: macrolides
● SIDE-EFFECTS
  GENERAL SIDE-EFFECTS
▶ **Uncommon** Burping · dry mouth · muscle complaints · oral disorders · thrombocytosis · tremor
▶ **Frequency not known** Abnormal dreams · agranulocytosis · depersonalisation · depression · mania · myopathy · psychotic disorder · renal failure · tooth discolouration · urine discolouration
  SPECIFIC SIDE-EFFECTS
▶ **Uncommon**
▶ With oral use Epistaxis
▶ With parenteral use Cardiac arrest · dyskinesia · haemorrhage · loss of consciousness · pulmonary embolism
● PREGNANCY Manufacturer advises avoid, particularly in the first trimester, unless potential benefit outweighs risk.
● BREAST FEEDING Manufacturer advises avoid unless potential benefit outweighs risk—present in milk.
● HEPATIC IMPAIRMENT Manufacturer advises caution; avoid in severe failure if renal impairment also present.
● RENAL IMPAIRMENT Avoid if severe hepatic impairment also present.
▶ With oral use in adults Avoid *Klaricid XL*® or clarithromycin m/r preparations if eGFR less than 30 mL/minute/1.73 m².
▶ With oral use in children Avoid *Klaricid XL*® or clarithromyin m/r preparations if estimated glomerular filtration rate less than 30 mL/minute/1.73 m².
  Dose adjustments ▶ In adults Use half normal dose if eGFR less than 30 mL/minute/1.73 m², max. duration 14 days.
  ▶ In children Use half normal dose if estimated glomerular filtration rate less than 30 mL/minute/1.73 m², max. duration 14 days.
● DIRECTIONS FOR ADMINISTRATION
▶ With intravenous use For *intravenous infusion (Klaricid*® *I.V.)*, manufacturer advises give intermittently in Glucose 5% or Sodium Chloride 0.9%; dissolve initially in

water for injections (500 mg in 10 mL) then dilute to a concentration of 2 mg/mL; give over 60 minutes.
● PRESCRIBING AND DISPENSING INFORMATION For choice of antibacterial therapy, see Antibacterials, use for prophylaxis p. 529, Diabetic foot infections, antibacterial therapy p. 534, Ear infections, antibacterial therapy p. 534, Helicobacter pylori infection p. 90, Nose infections, antibacterial therapy p. 537, Oropharyngeal infections, antibacterial therapy p. 1261, Respiratory system infections, antibacterial therapy p. 538, Skin infections, antibacterial therapy p. 541.
● PATIENT AND CARER ADVICE
  Medicines for Children leaflet: Clarithromycin for bacterial infections www.medicinesforchildren.org.uk/clarithromycin-bacterial-infections
● PROFESSION SPECIFIC INFORMATION
  Dental practitioners' formulary
  Clarithromycin Tablets may be prescribed.
    Clarithromycin Oral Suspension may be prescribed.

● MEDICINAL FORMS There can be variation in the licensing of different medicines containing the same drug. Forms available from special-order manufacturers include: infusion
  Modified-release tablet
  CAUTIONARY AND ADVISORY LABELS 9, 21, 25
  ▶ Klaricid XL (Mylan)
    Clarithromycin 500 mg Klaricid XL 500mg tablets | 7 tablet PoM £6.72 DT = £6.72 | 14 tablet PoM £13.23
  ▶ Xetinin XL (Morningside Healthcare Ltd)
    Clarithromycin 500 mg Xetinin XL 500mg tablets | 7 tablet PoM £6.72 DT = £6.72 | 14 tablet PoM £13.23
  Granules
  CAUTIONARY AND ADVISORY LABELS 9, 13
  ▶ Klaricid (Mylan)
    Clarithromycin 250 mg Klaricid Adult 250mg granules sachets | 14 sachet PoM £11.68 DT = £11.68
  Tablet
  CAUTIONARY AND ADVISORY LABELS 9
  ▶ Clarithromycin (Non-proprietary)
    Clarithromycin 250 mg Clarithromycin 250mg tablets | 14 tablet PoM £10.50 DT = £1.59
    Clarithromycin 500 mg Clarithromycin 500mg tablets | 14 tablet PoM £21.50 DT = £2.80
  Oral suspension
  CAUTIONARY AND ADVISORY LABELS 9
  ▶ Clarithromycin (Non-proprietary)
    Clarithromycin 25 mg per 1 ml Clarithromycin 125mg/5ml oral suspension | 70 ml PoM £4.62 DT = £4.62
    Clarithromycin 50 mg per 1 ml Clarithromycin 250mg/5ml oral suspension | 70 ml PoM £7.59 DT = £7.59
  ▶ Klaricid (Mylan)
    Clarithromycin 25 mg per 1 ml Klaricid Paediatric 125mg/5ml oral suspension | 70 ml PoM £5.26 DT = £4.62 | 100 ml PoM £9.04
    Clarithromycin 50 mg per 1 ml Klaricid Paediatric 250mg/5ml oral suspension | 70 ml PoM £10.51 DT = £7.59
  Powder for solution for infusion
  ELECTROLYTES: May contain Sodium
  ▶ Clarithromycin (Non-proprietary)
    Clarithromycin 500 mg Clarithromycin 500mg powder for solution for infusion vials | 1 vial PoM £9.45–£11.25 DT = £9.45 (Hospital only) | 10 vial PoM £111.50 (Hospital only)
    Clarithromycin 500mg powder for concentrate for solution for infusion vials | 1 vial PoM £11.15 DT = £9.45 (Hospital only) | 10 vial PoM £111.50 (Hospital only)
  ▶ Klaricid (Mylan)
    Clarithromycin 500 mg Klaricid IV 500mg powder for solution for infusion vials | 1 vial PoM £9.45 DT = £9.45 (Hospital only)

Erythromycin

F 568

28-Jul-2020

● **INDICATIONS AND DOSE**

Susceptible infections in patients with penicillin hypersensitivity (e.g. respiratory-tract infections (including Legionella infection), skin and oral infections, and campylobacter enteritis)
▸ BY MOUTH
▸ Child 1-23 months: 125 mg 4 times a day, total daily dose may alternatively be given in two divided doses, increased to 250 mg 4 times a day, dose increase may be used in severe infections
▸ Child 2-7 years: 250 mg 4 times a day, total daily dose may alternatively be given in two divided doses, increased to 500 mg 4 times a day, dose increase may be used in severe infections
▸ Child 8-17 years: 250–500 mg 4 times a day, total daily dose may alternatively be given in two divided doses, increased to 500–1000 mg 4 times a day, dose increase may be used in severe infections
▸ Adult: 250–500 mg 4 times a day, total daily dose may alternatively be given in two divided doses, increased to 500–1000 mg 4 times a day, dose increase may be used in severe infections
▸ BY INTRAVENOUS INFUSION
▸ Child: 12.5 mg/kg every 6 hours (max. per dose 1 g)
▸ Adult: 6.25 mg/kg every 6 hours, for mild infections when oral treatment not possible, increased to 12.5 mg/kg every 6 hours, dose increase may be used in severe infections

Impetigo
▸ BY MOUTH
▸ Child 8-17 years: 250–500 mg 4 times a day for 5–7 days
▸ Adult: 250–500 mg 4 times a day for 5–7 days

Cellulitis | Erysipelas
▸ BY MOUTH
▸ Child 8-17 years: 250–500 mg 4 times a day for 5–7 days then review
▸ Adult: 500 mg 4 times a day for 5–7 days then review

Prevention of recurrent cellulitis (specialist use only) | Prevention of recurrent erysipelas (specialist use only)
▸ BY MOUTH
▸ Adult: 250 mg twice daily

Mild diabetic foot infection
▸ BY MOUTH
▸ Adult: 500 mg 4 times a day for 7 days then review

Leg ulcer infection
▸ BY MOUTH
▸ Adult: 500 mg 4 times a day for 7 days

Community-acquired pneumonia
▸ BY MOUTH
▸ Child 8-17 years: 250–500 mg 4 times a day for 5 days
▸ Adult: 500 mg 4 times a day for 5 days

Acute cough [if systemically very unwell or at higher risk of complications] | Acute sore throat
▸ BY MOUTH
▸ Child 1-23 months: 125 mg 4 times a day for 5 days, alternatively 250 mg twice daily for 5 days
▸ Child 2-7 years: 250 mg 4 times a day for 5 days, alternatively 500 mg twice daily for 5 days
▸ Child 8-17 years: 250–500 mg 4 times a day for 5 days, alternatively 500–1000 mg twice daily for 5 days
▸ Adult: 250–500 mg 4 times a day for 5 days, alternatively 500–1000 mg twice daily for 5 days

Acute otitis media
▸ BY MOUTH
▸ Child 1-23 months: 125 mg 4 times a day for 5–7 days, alternatively 250 mg twice daily for 5–7 days

▸ Child 2-7 years: 250 mg 4 times a day for 5–7 days, alternatively 500 mg twice daily for 5–7 days
▸ Child 8-17 years: 250–500 mg 4 times a day for 5–7 days, alternatively 500–1000 mg twice daily for 5–7 days

Early syphilis
▸ BY MOUTH
▸ Adult: 500 mg 4 times a day for 14 days

Uncomplicated genital chlamydia | Non-gonococcal urethritis
▸ BY MOUTH
▸ Adult: 500 mg twice daily for 14 days

Chronic prostatitis
▸ BY MOUTH
▸ Adult: 250–500 mg 4 times a day, total daily dose may alternatively be given in two divided doses, increased to 4 g daily in divided doses, dose increase may be used in severe infections
▸ BY INTRAVENOUS INFUSION
▸ Adult: 6.25 mg/kg every 6 hours, for mild infections when oral treatment is not possible, increased to 12.5 mg/kg every 6 hours, dose increase may be used in severe infections

Prevention and treatment of pertussis
▸ BY MOUTH
▸ Child 1-23 months: 125 mg 4 times a day, total daily dose may alternatively be given in two divided doses, increased to 250 mg 4 times a day, dose increase may be used in severe infections
▸ Child 2-7 years: 250 mg 4 times a day, total daily dose may alternatively be given in two divided doses, increased to 500 mg 4 times a day, dose increase may be used in severe infections
▸ Child 8-17 years: 250–500 mg 4 times a day, total daily dose may alternatively be given in two divided doses, increased to 500–1000 mg 4 times a day, dose increase may be used in severe infections
▸ Adult: (consult local protocol)

Prevention of secondary case of diphtheria in non-immune patient
▸ BY MOUTH
▸ Adult: 500 mg every 6 hours for 7 days, treat for further 10 days if nasopharyngeal swabs positive after first 7 days' treatment

Prevention of secondary case of invasive group A streptococcal infection in penicillin allergic patients
▸ BY MOUTH
▸ Adult: 250–500 mg every 6 hours for 10 days

Prevention of pneumococcal infection in asplenia or in patients with sickle-cell disease (if penicillin-allergic)
▸ BY MOUTH
▸ Adult: 500 mg twice daily, antibiotic prophylaxis is not fully reliable. It may be discontinued in those with sickle-cell disease who have received pneumococcal immunisation and who do not have a history of severe pneumococcal infection

Rosacea
▸ BY MOUTH
▸ Adult: 500 mg twice daily courses usually last 6–12 weeks and are repeated intermittently

Acne
▸ BY MOUTH
▸ Adult: 500 mg twice daily

Gastro-intestinal stasis
▸ BY MOUTH
▸ Adult: 250–500 mg 3 times a day for up to 4 weeks, to be taken before food
▸ BY INTRAVENOUS INFUSION
▸ Adult: 3 mg/kg 3 times a day

● UNLICENSED USE [EvGr] Duration of treatment for acute otitis media differs from product literature and adheres to national guidelines. ⟨A⟩
▸ In adults [EvGr] Erythromycin is used for the prevention of recurrent cellulitis, ⟨A⟩ but the dose is not licensed for this indication. [EvGr] Erythromycin is used for the prevention of recurrent erysipelas, ⟨A⟩ but the dose is not licensed for this indication. [EvGr] Erythromycin may be used for gastro-intestinal stasis, ⟨E⟩ but it is not licensed for this indication.

● CAUTIONS Avoid in Acute porphyrias p. 1107

● INTERACTIONS → Appendix 1: macrolides

● SIDE-EFFECTS
GENERAL SIDE-EFFECTS
▸ **Rare or very rare** Hearing loss (can occur after large doses)
SPECIFIC SIDE-EFFECTS
▸ With oral use Cerebral impairment
▸ With parenteral use Atrioventricular block

● PREGNANCY Not known to be harmful.

● BREAST FEEDING Only small amounts in milk—not known to be harmful.

● HEPATIC IMPAIRMENT Manufacturer advises caution.

● RENAL IMPAIRMENT
Dose adjustments ▸ In adults Max. 1.5 g daily in severe renal impairment (ototoxicity).
▸ In children Reduce dose in severe renal impairment (ototoxicity).

● DIRECTIONS FOR ADMINISTRATION
▸ With intravenous use in children Dilute reconstituted solution further in glucose 5% (neutralised with Sodium bicarbonate) or sodium chloride 0.9% to a concentration of 1–5 mg/mL; give over 20–60 minutes. Concentration of up to 10 mg/mL may be used in fluid-restriction if administered via a central venous catheter.
▸ With intravenous use in adults For *intravenous infusion* (as lactobionate), give intermittently *in* Glucose 5% (neutralised with sodium bicarbonate) *or* Sodium chloride 0.9%; dissolve initially in water for injections (1 g in 20 mL) then dilute to a concentration of 1–5 mg/mL; give over 20–60 minutes.

● PRESCRIBING AND DISPENSING INFORMATION For choice of antibacterial therapy, see Antibacterials, use for prophylaxis p. 529, Ear infections, antibacterial therapy p. 534, Diabetic foot infections, antibacterial therapy p. 534, Gastro-intestinal system infections, antibacterial therapy p. 535, Genital system infections, antibacterial therapy p. 536, Oropharyngeal infections, antibacterial therapy p. 1261, Respiratory system infections, antibacterial therapy p. 538, Skin infections, antibacterial therapy p. 541.

● PATIENT AND CARER ADVICE
Medicines for Children leaflet: Erythromycin for bacterial infections www.medicinesforchildren.org.uk/erythromycin-bacterial-infections

● PROFESSION SPECIFIC INFORMATION
Dental practitioners' formulary
▸ With oral use Erythromycin tablets e/c may be prescribed. Erythromycin ethyl succinate oral suspension may be prescribed. Erythromycin stearate tablets may be prescribed. Erythromycin ethyl succinate tablets may be prescribed.

● MEDICINAL FORMS There can be variation in the licensing of different medicines containing the same drug.
Gastro-resistant tablet
CAUTIONARY AND ADVISORY LABELS 5, 9, 25
▸ Erythromycin (Non-proprietary)
Erythromycin 250 mg Erythromycin 250mg gastro-resistant tablets | 28 tablet [PoM] £12.31 DT = £4.28 | 500 tablet [PoM] £76.43

Tablet
CAUTIONARY AND ADVISORY LABELS 9
▸ Erythromycin (Non-proprietary)
Erythromycin (as Erythromycin stearate) 250 mg Erythromycin stearate 250mg tablets | 28 tablet [PoM] £5.10
Erythromycin (as Erythromycin ethyl succinate) 500 mg Erythromycin ethyl succinate 500mg tablets | 28 tablet [PoM] £15.95 DT = £10.78
Erythromycin (as Erythromycin stearate) 500 mg Erythromycin stearate 500mg tablets | 28 tablet [PoM] £10.19
▸ Erythrocin (Advanz Pharma)
Erythromycin (as Erythromycin stearate) 250 mg Erythrocin 250 tablets | 100 tablet [PoM] £18.20 DT = £18.20
Erythromycin (as Erythromycin stearate) 500 mg Erythrocin 500 tablets | 100 tablet [PoM] £36.40 DT = £36.40
▸ Erythrolar (Ennogen Pharma Ltd)
Erythromycin (as Erythromycin stearate) 250 mg Erythrolar 250mg tablets | 100 tablet [PoM] £22.80 DT = £18.20
Erythromycin (as Erythromycin stearate) 500 mg Erythrolar 500mg tablets | 100 tablet [PoM] £45.60 DT = £36.40
▸ Erythroped A (Advanz Pharma)
Erythromycin (as Erythromycin ethyl succinate) 500 mg Erythroped A 500mg tablets | 28 tablet [PoM] £10.78 DT = £10.78

Oral suspension
CAUTIONARY AND ADVISORY LABELS 9
▸ Erythromycin (Non-proprietary)
Erythromycin (as Erythromycin ethyl succinate) 25 mg per 1 ml Erythromycin ethyl succinate 125mg/5ml oral suspension | 100 ml [PoM] £5.86 DT = £5.86
Erythromycin ethyl succinate 125mg/5ml oral suspension sugar free sugar-free | 100 ml [PoM] £5.35 DT = £5.35
Erythromycin (as Erythromycin ethyl succinate) 50 mg per 1 ml Erythromycin ethyl succinate 250mg/5ml oral suspension | 100 ml [PoM] £8.89 DT = £8.89
Erythromycin ethyl succinate 250mg/5ml oral suspension sugar free sugar-free | 100 ml [PoM] £8.87 DT = £8.87
Erythromycin (as Erythromycin ethyl succinate) 100 mg per 1 ml Erythromycin ethyl succinate 500mg/5ml oral suspension | 100 ml [PoM] £15.73 DT = £15.73
Erythromycin ethyl succinate 500mg/5ml oral suspension sugar free sugar-free | 100 ml [PoM] ⓢ
▸ Erythroped (Advanz Pharma)
Erythromycin (as Erythromycin ethyl succinate) 25 mg per 1 ml Erythroped PI SF 125mg/5ml oral suspension sugar-free | 140 ml [PoM] £61.13
Erythromycin (as Erythromycin ethyl succinate) 50 mg per 1 ml Erythroped SF 250mg/5ml oral suspension sugar-free | 140 ml [PoM] £5.95
Erythromycin (as Erythromycin ethyl succinate) 100 mg per 1 ml Erythroped Forte SF 500mg/5ml oral suspension sugar-free | 140 ml [PoM] £10.56 DT = £10.56

Powder for solution for infusion
▸ Erythromycin (Non-proprietary)
Erythromycin (as Erythromycin lactobionate)
1 gram Erythromycin 1g powder for solution for infusion vials | 1 vial [PoM] £22.00–£22.92 (Hospital only)

5

Infection

5

Infection

ANTIBACTERIALS > MONOBACTAMS

Aztreonam

14-Dec-2020

- **DRUG ACTION** Aztreonam is a monocyclic beta-lactam ('monobactam') antibiotic with an antibacterial spectrum limited to Gram-negative aerobic bacteria including *Pseudomonas aeruginosa*, *Neisseria meningitidis*, and *Haemophilus influenzae*; it should not be used alone for 'blind' treatment since it is not active against Gram-positive organisms. Aztreonam is also effective against *Neisseria gonorrhoeae* (but not against concurrent chlamydial infection).

- **INDICATIONS AND DOSE**

Gram-negative infections including *Pseudomonas aeruginosa*, *Haemophilus influenzae*, and *Neisseria meningitidis*
- ▸ BY DEEP INTRAMUSCULAR INJECTION, OR BY INTRAVENOUS INFUSION, OR BY INTRAVENOUS INJECTION
- ▸ Adult: 1 g every 8 hours, alternatively 2 g every 12 hours, single doses over 1 g intravenous route only

Severe gram-negative infections including *Pseudomonas aeruginosa*, *Haemophilus influenzae*, *Neisseria meningitidis*, and lung infections in cystic fibrosis
- ▸ BY INTRAVENOUS INFUSION, OR BY INTRAVENOUS INJECTION
- ▸ Adult: 2 g every 6–8 hours

Gonorrhoea | Cystitis
- ▸ BY INTRAMUSCULAR INJECTION
- ▸ Adult: 1 g for 1 single dose

Urinary-tract infections
- ▸ BY DEEP INTRAMUSCULAR INJECTION, OR BY INTRAVENOUS INFUSION, OR BY INTRAVENOUS INJECTION
- ▸ Adult: 0.5–1 g every 8–12 hours

Chronic pulmonary *Pseudomonas aeruginosa* infection in patients with cystic fibrosis
- ▸ BY INHALATION OF NEBULISED SOLUTION
- ▸ Adult: 75 mg 3 times a day for 28 days, doses to be administered at least 4 hours apart, subsequent courses repeated after 28-day interval without aztreonam nebuliser solution

- **CAUTIONS**
- ▸ When used by inhalation Haemoptysis— risk of further haemorrhage
- **SIDE-EFFECTS**
  GENERAL SIDE-EFFECTS
- **Common or very common** Dyspnoea · respiratory disorders
  SPECIFIC SIDE-EFFECTS
- **Common or very common**
- ▸ When used by inhalation Cough · haemoptysis · joint disorders · laryngeal pain · nasal complaints · rash
- ▸ **Rare or very rare**
- ▸ With parenteral use Anaemia · asthenia · breast tenderness · chest pain · confusion · diplopia · dizziness · eosinophilia · haemorrhage · headache · hepatic disorders · hypotension · insomnia · leucocytosis · myalgia · nasal congestion · neutropenia · oral disorders · pancytopenia · paraesthesia · pseudomembranous enterocolitis · seizure · thrombocytopenia · thrombocytosis · tinnitus · vertigo · vulvovaginal candidiasis
- ▸ **Frequency not known**
- ▸ With parenteral use Abdominal pain · angioedema · diarrhoea · nausea · skin reactions · taste altered · toxic epidermal necrolysis · vomiting
- **ALLERGY AND CROSS-SENSITIVITY** EvGr Contra-indicated in aztreonam hypersensitivity.
  Use with caution in patients with hypersensitivity to other beta-lactam antibiotics (although aztreonam may be less likely than other beta-lactams to cause hypersensitivity in penicillin-sensitive patients). ⓜ

- **PREGNANCY**
- ▸ With systemic use No information available; manufacturer of injection advises avoid.
- ▸ When used by inhalation No information available; manufacturer of powder for nebuliser solution advises avoid unless essential.
- **BREAST FEEDING** Amount in milk probably too small to be harmful.
- **HEPATIC IMPAIRMENT**
- ▸ With systemic use Manufacturer advises caution in chronic impairment with cirrhosis.
  Dose adjustments ▸ With systemic use Manufacturer advises dose reduction of 20—25% for long term treatment of patients with chronic impairment with cirrhosis, especially in alcoholic cirrhosis and concomitant renal impairment.
- **RENAL IMPAIRMENT**
  Dose adjustments ▸ With systemic use If eGFR 10–30 mL/minute/1.73 m^2, usual initial dose of injection, then half normal dose. If eGFR less than 10 mL/minute/1.73 m^2, usual initial dose of injection, then one-quarter normal dose.
- **MONITORING REQUIREMENTS**
- ▸ When used by inhalation Measure lung function before and after initial dose of aztreonam and monitor for bronchospasm.
- **DIRECTIONS FOR ADMINISTRATION**
- ▸ With intravenous use For *intravenous injection*, manufacturer advises give over 3–5 minutes. For *intravenous infusion* (*Azactam*®), manufacturer advises give intermittently *in* Glucose 5% *or* Sodium chloride 0.9%. Dissolve initially in water for injections (1 g per 3 mL) then dilute to a concentration of less than 20 mg/mL; to be given over 20–60 minutes.
- ▸ When used by inhalation Manufacturer advises other inhaled drugs should be administered before aztreonam; a bronchodilator should be administered before each dose.
- **NATIONAL FUNDING/ACCESS DECISIONS**
  For full details see funding body website
  Scottish Medicines Consortium (SMC) decisions
- ▸ Aztreonam lysine (*Cayston*®) for suppressive therapy of chronic pulmonary infections due to *Pseudomonas aeruginosa* in patients with cystic fibrosis aged six years and older (January 2015) SMC No. 753/12 Recommended with restrictions

- **MEDICINAL FORMS** There can be variation in the licensing of different medicines containing the same drug.
  Powder and solvent for nebuliser solution
- ▸ Cayston (Gilead Sciences Ireland UC)
  Aztreonam (as Aztreonam lysine) 75 mg Cayston 75mg powder and solvent for nebuliser solution vials with Altera Nebuliser Handset | 84 vial PoM £2,181.53 DT = £2,181.53
  Powder for solution for injection
- ▸ Azactam (Bristol-Myers Squibb Pharmaceuticals Ltd)
  Aztreonam 1 gram Azactam 1g powder for solution for injection vials | 1 vial PoM £9.40 (Hospital only)
  Aztreonam 2 gram Azactam 2g powder for solution for injection vials | 1 vial PoM £18.82 (Hospital only)

Metronidazole

24-Nov-2020

- **DRUG ACTION** Metronidazole is an antimicrobial drug with high activity against anaerobic bacteria and protozoa.

- **INDICATIONS AND DOSE**

Anaerobic infections
▶ BY MOUTH
▷ Child 1 month: 7.5 mg/kg every 12 hours usually treated for 7 days (for 10–14 days in *Clostridioides difficile* infection)
▷ Child 2 months-11 years: 7.5 mg/kg every 8 hours (max. per dose 400 mg) usually treated for 7 days (for 10–14 days in *Clostridioides difficile* infection)
▷ Child 12-17 years: 400 mg every 8 hours usually treated for 7 days (for 10–14 days in *Clostridioides difficile* infection)
▷ Adult: 400 mg every 8 hours, alternatively 500 mg every 8 hours usually treated for 7 days (for 10–14 days in *Clostridioides difficile* infection)
▶ BY RECTUM
▷ Child 1-11 months: 125 mg 3 times a day for 3 days, then 125 mg twice daily, for usual total treatment duration of 7 days
▷ Child 1-4 years: 250 mg 3 times a day for 3 days, then 250 mg twice daily, for usual total treatment duration of 7 days
▷ Child 5-9 years: 500 mg 3 times a day for 3 days, then 500 mg twice daily, for usual total treatment duration of 7 days
▷ Child 10-17 years: 1 g 3 times a day for 3 days, then 1 g twice daily, for usual total treatment duration of 7 days
▷ Adult: 1 g 3 times a day for 3 days, then 1 g twice daily, for usual total treatment duration of 7 days
▶ BY INTRAVENOUS INFUSION
▷ Adult: 500 mg every 8 hours usually treated for 7 days (for 10–14 days in *Clostridioides difficile* infection), to be given over 20 minutes

Moderate diabetic foot infection | Severe diabetic foot infection | Leg ulcer infection [in combination with other drugs]
▶ BY MOUTH
▷ Adult: 400 mg every 8 hours
▶ BY INTRAVENOUS INFUSION
▷ Adult: 500 mg every 8 hours

Cellulitis | Erysipelas
▶ BY MOUTH
▷ Child 1 month: 7.5 mg/kg every 12 hours for 7 days then review
▷ Child 2 months-11 years: 7.5 mg/kg every 8 hours (max. per dose 400 mg) for 7 days then review
▷ Child 12-17 years: 400 mg every 8 hours for 7 days then review
▷ Adult: 400 mg every 8 hours for 7 days then review
▶ BY INTRAVENOUS INFUSION
▷ Adult: 500 mg every 8 hours

Helicobacter pylori eradication [in combination with other drugs (see Helicobacter pylori infection p. 90)]
▶ BY MOUTH
▷ Adult: 400 mg twice daily for 7 days for first- and second-line eradication therapy; 10 days for third-line eradication therapy

Fistulating Crohn's disease
▶ BY MOUTH
▷ Adult: 10–20 mg/kg daily in divided doses, usual dose 400–500 mg 3 times a day usually given for 1 month but no longer than 3 months because of concerns about peripheral neuropathy

Acute diverticulitis [in combination with other drugs (see Diverticular disease and diverticulitis p. 40)]
▶ BY MOUTH
▷ Adult: 400 mg 3 times a day for 5 days then review
▶ BY INTRAVENOUS INFUSION
▷ Adult: 500 mg every 8 hours
Pressure sores
▶ BY MOUTH
▷ Adult: 400 mg every 8 hours for 7 days
Bacterial vaginosis (notably *Gardnerella vaginalis* infection)
▶ BY MOUTH
▷ Adult: 400–500 mg twice daily for 5–7 days, alternatively 2 g for 1 dose
Bacterial vaginosis
▶ BY VAGINA USING VAGINAL GEL
▷ Adult: 1 applicatorful daily for 5 days, dose to be administered at night

DOSE EQUIVALENCE AND CONVERSION
▷ 1 applicatorful of vaginal gel delivers a 5 g dose of metronidazole 0.75%.
Pelvic inflammatory disease
▶ BY MOUTH
▷ Adult: 400 mg twice daily for 14 days
Acute ulcerative gingivitis
▶ BY MOUTH
▷ Child 1-2 years: 50 mg every 8 hours for 3 days
▷ Child 3-6 years: 100 mg every 12 hours for 3 days
▷ Child 7-9 years: 100 mg every 8 hours for 3 days
▷ Child 10-17 years: 200–250 mg every 8 hours for 3 days
▷ Adult: 400 mg every 8 hours for 3 days
Acute oral infections
▶ BY MOUTH
▷ Child 1-2 years: 50 mg every 8 hours for 3–7 days
▷ Child 3-6 years: 100 mg every 12 hours for 3–7 days
▷ Child 7-9 years: 100 mg every 8 hours for 3–7 days
▷ Child 10-17 years: 200–250 mg every 8 hours for 3–7 days
▷ Adult: 400 mg every 8 hours for 3–7 days
Surgical prophylaxis
▶ BY MOUTH
▷ Adult: 400–500 mg, to be administered 2 hours before surgery, then 400–500 mg every 8 hours if required for up to 3 doses (in high-risk procedures)
▶ BY RECTUM
▷ Adult: 1 g, to be administered 2 hours before surgery, then 1 g every 8 hours if required for up to 3 doses (in high-risk procedures)
▶ BY INTRAVENOUS INFUSION
▷ Adult: 500 mg, to be administered up to 30 minutes before the procedure (if rectal administration inappropriate), then 500 mg every 8 hours if required for up to 3 further doses (in high-risk procedures)
Invasive intestinal amoebiasis | Extra-intestinal amoebiasis (including liver abscess)
▶ BY MOUTH
▷ Child 1-2 years: 200 mg 3 times a day for 5 days in intestinal infection (for 5–10 days in extra-intestinal infection)
▷ Child 3-6 years: 200 mg 4 times a day for 5 days in intestinal infection (for 5–10 days in extra-intestinal infection)
▷ Child 7-9 years: 400 mg 3 times a day for 5 days in intestinal infection (for 5–10 days in extra-intestinal infection)
▷ Child 10-17 years: 800 mg 3 times a day for 5 days in intestinal infection (for 5–10 days in extra-intestinal infection)
▷ Adult: 800 mg 3 times a day for 5 days in intestinal infection (for 5–10 days in extra-intestinal infection)

continued →

Urogenital trichomoniasis
▶ BY MOUTH
▸ Child 1-2 years: 50 mg 3 times a day for 7 days
▸ Child 3-6 years: 100 mg twice daily for 7 days
▸ Child 7-9 years: 100 mg 3 times a day for 7 days
▸ Child 10-17 years: 200 mg 3 times a day for 7 days, alternatively 400–500 mg twice daily for 5–7 days, alternatively 2 g for 1 dose
▸ Adult: 200 mg 3 times a day for 7 days, alternatively 400–500 mg twice daily for 5–7 days, alternatively 2 g for 1 dose

Giardiasis
▶ BY MOUTH
▸ Child 1-2 years: 500 mg once daily for 3 days
▸ Child 3-6 years: 600–800 mg once daily for 3 days
▸ Child 7-9 years: 1 g once daily for 3 days
▸ Child 10-17 years: 2 g once daily for 3 days, alternatively 400 mg 3 times a day for 5 days, alternatively 500 mg twice daily for 7–10 days
▸ Adult: 2 g once daily for 3 days, alternatively 400 mg 3 times a day for 5 days, alternatively 500 mg twice daily for 7–10 days

Established case of tetanus
▶ BY INTRAVENOUS INFUSION
▸ Adult: (consult product literature)

● UNLICENSED USE [EvGr] Metronidazole is used for the treatment of cellulitis, ⟨Å⟩ but is not licensed for this indication.
[EvGr] Metronidazole is used for the treatment of erysipelas, ⟨Å⟩ but is not licensed for this indication.
▸ With systemic use in adults Metronidazole doses in the BNF may differ from those in product literature.
[EvGr] Combination regimens and durations for *Helicobacter pylori* eradication may differ from product literature but adhere to national guidelines. ⟨Å⟩

● CAUTIONS
▸ With vaginal use Not recommended during menstruation · some systemic absorption may occur with vaginal gel

● INTERACTIONS → Appendix 1: metronidazole

● SIDE-EFFECTS
▸ **Common or very common**
▸ With systemic use Dry mouth · myalgia · nausea · oral disorders · taste metallic · vomiting
▸ With vaginal use Pelvic discomfort · vulvovaginal candidiasis · vulvovaginal disorders
▸ **Uncommon**
▸ With systemic use Asthenia · headache · leucopenia (with long term or intensive therapy)
▸ With vaginal use Menstrual cycle irregularities · vaginal haemorrhage
▸ **Rare or very rare**
▸ With systemic use Agranulocytosis · angioedema · appetite decreased · ataxia · cerebellar syndrome · confusion · diarrhoea · dizziness · drowsiness · encephalopathy · epigastric pain · epileptiform seizure (with long term or intensive therapy) · flushing · hallucination · hepatic disorders · meningitis aseptic · mucositis · nerve disorders · neutropenia · pancreatitis · pancytopenia · peripheral neuropathy (with long term or intensive therapy) · psychotic disorder · seizure · severe cutaneous adverse reactions (SCARs) · skin reactions · thrombocytopenia · urine dark · vision disorders
▸ **Frequency not known**
▸ With systemic use Depressed mood · gastrointestinal disorder · hearing impairment · taste altered · tinnitus

● PREGNANCY
▸ With systemic use Manufacturer advises avoidance of high-dose regimens; use only if potential benefit outweighs risk.

● BREAST FEEDING
▸ With systemic use Significant amount in milk; manufacturer advises avoid large single doses though otherwise compatible; may give milk a bitter taste.

● HEPATIC IMPAIRMENT
▸ With oral use or rectal use Manufacturer advises caution in hepatic encephalopathy (risk of decreased clearance).
▸ With intravenous use Manufacturer advises caution in severe impairment (risk of decreased clearance).
Dose adjustments ▸ With oral use or rectal use Manufacturer advises dose reduction to one-third of the daily dose in hepatic encephalopathy (dose may be given once daily).
▸ With intravenous use Manufacturer advises consider dose reduction in severe impairment.

● MONITORING REQUIREMENTS
▸ With systemic use Clinical and laboratory monitoring advised if treatment exceeds 10 days.

● DIRECTIONS FOR ADMINISTRATION
▸ With intravenous use [EvGr] For *intravenous infusion*, give over 20–60 minutes. ⟨M⟩

● PRESCRIBING AND DISPENSING INFORMATION For choice of antibacterial therapy, see Antibacterials, use for prophylaxis p. 529, Antiprotozoal drugs p. 645, Diabetic foot infections, antibacterial therapy p. 534, Gastro-intestinal system infections, antibacterial therapy p. 535, Genital system infections, antibacterial therapy p. 536, Helicobacter pylori infection p. 90, Oropharyngeal infections, antibacterial therapy p. 1261, Skin infections, antibacterial therapy p. 541.
▸ With systemic use Metronidazole is well absorbed orally and the intravenous route is normally reserved for severe infections. Metronidazole by the rectal route is an effective alternative to the intravenous route when oral administration is not possible.

● PATIENT AND CARER ADVICE
Medicines for Children leaflet: Metronidazole for bacterial infections www.medicinesforchildren.org.uk/metronidazole-bacterial-infections

● PROFESSION SPECIFIC INFORMATION
Dental practitioners' formulary
▸ With oral use Metronidazole Tablets may be prescribed. Metronidazole Oral Suspension may be prescribed.

● MEDICINAL FORMS There can be variation in the licensing of different medicines containing the same drug. Forms available from special-order manufacturers include: oral suspension, oral solution, suppository, cream, gel
Tablet
CAUTIONARY AND ADVISORY LABELS 4, 9, 21, 25, 27
▸ Metronidazole (Non-proprietary)
Metronidazole 200 mg Metronidazole 200mg tablets | 21 tablet [PoM] £4.03 DT = £4.03
Metronidazole 400 mg Metronidazole 400mg tablets | 21 tablet [PoM] £5.64 DT = £3.38
Metronidazole 500 mg Metronidazole 500mg tablets | 21 tablet [PoM] £39.29 DT = £39.29
▸ Flagyl (Sanofi)
Metronidazole 200 mg Flagyl 200mg tablets | 21 tablet [PoM] £4.49 DT = £4.03
Metronidazole 400 mg Flagyl 400mg tablets | 14 tablet [PoM] £6.34
Suppository
CAUTIONARY AND ADVISORY LABELS 4, 9
▸ Flagyl (Sanofi)
Metronidazole 500 mg Flagyl 500mg suppositories | 10 suppository [PoM] £15.18 DT = £15.18
Metronidazole 1 gram Flagyl 1g suppositories | 10 suppository [PoM] £23.06 DT = £23.06

Oral suspension
CAUTIONARY AND ADVISORY LABELS 4, 9
▸ Metronidazole (Non-proprietary)
Metronidazole (as Metronidazole benzoate) 40 mg per 1 ml Metronidazole 200mg/5ml oral suspension | 100 ml [PoM] £37.29 DT = £37.29

Vaginal gel
EXCIPIENTS: May contain Disodium edetate, hydroxybenzoates (parabens), propylene glycol
▸ Zidoval (Mylan)
Metronidazole 7.5 mg per 1 gram Zidoval 0.75% vaginal gel | 40 gram [PoM] £4.31 DT = £4.31

Infusion
ELECTROLYTES: May contain Sodium
▸ Metronidazole (Non-proprietary)
Metronidazole 5 mg per 1 ml Metronidazole 500mg/100ml infusion 100ml bags | 20 bag [PoM] £67.05 DT = £67.05

Tinidazole
07-Aug-2020

● DRUG ACTION Tinidazole is an antimicrobial drug with high activity against anaerobic bacteria and protozoa; it has a longer duration of action than metronidazole.

● INDICATIONS AND DOSE
Anaerobic infections
▸ BY MOUTH
▸ Adult: Initially 2 g, followed by 1 g daily usually for 5–6 days, alternatively 500 mg twice daily usually for 5–6 days

Bacterial vaginosis | Acute ulcerative gingivitis
▸ BY MOUTH
▸ Adult: 2 g for 1 single dose

Abdominal surgery prophylaxis
▸ BY MOUTH
▸ Adult: 2 g for 1 single dose, to be administered approximately 12 hours before surgery

Intestinal amoebiasis
▸ BY MOUTH
▸ Child 1 month–11 years: 50–60 mg/kg once daily (max. per dose 2 g) for 3 days
▸ Child 12–17 years: 2 g once daily for 2–3 days
▸ Adult: 2 g once daily for 2–3 days

Amoebic involvement of liver
▸ BY MOUTH
▸ Child 1 month–11 years: 50–60 mg/kg once daily (max. per dose 2 g) for 5 days
▸ Child 12–17 years: 1.5–2 g once daily for 3–6 days
▸ Adult: 1.5–2 g once daily for 3–6 days

Urogenital trichomoniasis | Giardiasis
▸ BY MOUTH
▸ Child 1 month–11 years: 50–75 mg/kg (max. per dose 2 g) for 1 single dose, dose may be repeated once if necessary
▸ Child 12–17 years: 2 g for 1 single dose, dose may be repeated once if necessary
▸ Adult: 2 g for 1 single dose

***Helicobacter pylori* eradication**
▸ BY MOUTH
▸ Adult: (consult local protocol)

● INTERACTIONS → Appendix 1: tinidazole
● SIDE-EFFECTS
▸ **Common or very common** Abdominal pain · appetite decreased · diarrhoea · headache · nausea · skin reactions · vertigo · vomiting
▸ **Frequency not known** Angioedema · ataxia · dizziness · fatigue · flushing · leucopenia · oral disorders · peripheral neuropathy · seizure · sensation abnormal · taste altered · tongue discolouration · urine discolouration
● PREGNANCY Manufacturer advises avoid in first trimester.

● BREAST FEEDING Present in milk—manufacturer advises avoid breast-feeding during and for 3 days after stopping treatment.

● MONITORING REQUIREMENTS Clinical and laboratory monitoring advised if treatment exceeds 10 days.

● MEDICINAL FORMS There can be variation in the licensing of different medicines containing the same drug.

Tablet
CAUTIONARY AND ADVISORY LABELS 4, 9, 21, 25
▸ Fasigyn (Pfizer Ltd)
Tinidazole 500 mg Fasigyn 500mg tablets | 16 tablet [PoM] £11.04 DT = £11.04

ANTIBACTERIALS ⟩ PENICILLINS

Penicillins

Benzylpenicillin and phenoxymethylpenicillin

Benzylpenicillin sodium p. 580 (Penicillin G) remains an important and useful antibiotic but is inactivated by bacterial beta-lactamases. It is effective for many streptococcal (including pneumococcal), gonococcal, and meningococcal infections and also for anthrax, diphtheria, gas-gangrene, and leptospirosis. Pneumococci, meningococci, and gonococci which have decreased sensitivity to penicillin have been isolated; benzylpenicillin sodium is no longer the drug of first choice for pneumococcal meningitis. Although benzylpenicillin sodium is effective in the treatment of tetanus, metronidazole p. 575 is preferred. Benzylpenicillin is inactivated by gastric acid and absorption from the gastro-intestinal tract is low; therefore it must be given by injection.

Benzathine benzylpenicillin p. 579 is used for the treatment of early syphilis and late latent syphilis; it is given by intramuscular injection.

Phenoxymethylpenicillin p. 581 (Penicillin V) has a similar antibacterial spectrum to benzylpenicillin sodium, but is less active. It is gastric acid-stable, so is suitable for oral administration. It should not be used for serious infections because absorption can be unpredictable and plasma concentrations variable. It is indicated principally for respiratory-tract infections in children, for streptococcal tonsillitis, and for continuing treatment after one or more injections of benzylpenicillin sodium when clinical response has begun. It should not be used for meningococcal or gonococcal infections. Phenoxymethylpenicillin is used for prophylaxis against streptococcal infections following rheumatic fever and against pneumococcal infections following splenectomy or in sickle-cell disease.

Penicillinase-resistant penicillins

Most staphylococci are now resistant to benzylpenicillin because they produce penicillinases. Flucloxacillin p. 589, however, is not inactivated by these enzymes and is thus effective in infections caused by penicillin-resistant staphylococci, which is the sole indication for its use. Flucloxacillin is acid-stable and can, therefore, be given by mouth as well as by injection. Flucloxacillin is well absorbed from the gut.

Temocillin p. 590 is active against Gram-negative bacteria and is stable against a wide range of beta-lactamases. It should be reserved for the treatment of infections caused by beta-lactamase-producing strains of Gram-negative bacteria, including those resistant to third-generation cephalosporins. Temocillin is not active against *Pseudomonas aeruginosa* or *Acinetobacter* spp.

Broad-spectrum penicillins

Ampicillin p. 584 is active against certain Gram-positive and Gram-negative organisms but is inactivated by penicillinases including those produced by *Staphylococcus aureus* and by

5

Infection

common Gram-negative bacilli such as *Escherichia coli*. Almost all staphylococci, approx. 60% of *E. coli* strains and approx. 20% of *Haemophilus influenzae* strains are now resistant. The likelihood of resistance should therefore be considered before using ampicillin for the 'blind' treatment of infections; in particular, it should not be used for hospital patients without checking sensitivity.

Ampicillin is well excreted in the bile and urine. It is principally indicated for the treatment of exacerbations of chronic bronchitis and middle ear infections, both of which may be due to *Streptococcus pneumoniae* and *H. influenzae*, and for urinary-tract infections.

Ampicillin can be given by mouth but less than half the dose is absorbed, and absorption is further decreased by the presence of food in the gut.

Maculopapular rashes commonly occur with ampicillin (and amoxicillin p. 582) but are not usually related to true penicillin allergy. They almost always occur in patients with glandular fever; broad-spectrum penicillins should not therefore be used for 'blind' treatment of a sore throat. The risk of rash is also increased in patients with acute or chronic lymphocytic leukaemia or in cytomegalovirus infection.

Amoxicillin is a derivative of ampicillin and has a similar antibacterial spectrum. It is better absorbed than ampicillin when given by mouth, producing higher plasma and tissue concentrations; unlike ampicillin, absorption is not affected by the presence of food in the stomach. Amoxicillin is also used for the treatment of Lyme disease.

Co-amoxiclav p. 585 consists of amoxicillin with the betalactamase inhibitor clavulanic acid. Clavulanic acid itself has no significant antibacterial activity but, by inactivating beta-lactamases, it makes the combination active against beta-lactamase-producing bacteria that are resistant to amoxicillin. These include resistant strains of *Staph. aureus*, *E. coli*, and *H. influenzae*, as well as many *Bacteroides* and *Klebsiella* spp. Co-amoxiclav should be reserved for infections likely, or known, to be caused by amoxicillin-resistant beta-lactamase-producing strains.

A combination of ampicillin with flucloxacillin (as co-fluampicil p. 585 is available to treat infections involving either streptococci or staphylococci.

Antipseudomonal penicillins

Piperacillin, a ureidopenicillin, is only available in combination with the beta-lactamase inhibitor tazobactam. **Ticarcillin**, a carboxypenicillin, is only available in combination with the beta-lactamase inhibitor clavulanic acid. Both preparations have a broad spectrum of activity against a range of Gram-positive and Gram-negative bacteria, and anaerobes. Piperacillin with tazobactam p. 579 has activity against a wider range of Gram-negative organisms than ticarcillin with clavulanic acid and it is more active against *Pseudomonas aeruginosa*. These antibacterials are not active against MRSA. They are used in the treatment of septicaemia, hospital-acquired pneumonia, and complicated infections involving the urinary tract, skin and soft tissues, or intra-abdomen. For severe pseudomonas infections these antipseudomonal penicillins can be given with an aminoglycoside (e.g. gentamicin p. 545) since they have a synergistic effect.

Mecillinams

Pivmecillinam hydrochloride p. 588 has significant activity against many Gram-negative bacteria including *Escherichia coli*, klebsiella, enterobacter, and salmonellae. It is not active against *Pseudomonas aeruginosa* or enterococci.

Pivmecillinam hydrochloride is hydrolysed to mecillinam, which is the active drug.

Penicillins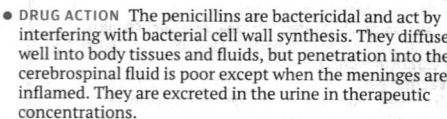

- **DRUG ACTION** The penicillins are bactericidal and act by interfering with bacterial cell wall synthesis. They diffuse well into body tissues and fluids, but penetration into the cerebrospinal fluid is poor except when the meninges are inflamed. They are excreted in the urine in therapeutic concentrations.

- **CAUTIONS** History of allergy

- **SIDE-EFFECTS**
  ▸ **Common or very common** Diarrhoea · hypersensitivity · nausea · skin reactions · thrombocytopenia · vomiting
  ▸ **Uncommon** Antibiotic associated colitis · arthralgia · leucopenia
  ▸ **Rare or very rare** Agranulocytosis · angioedema · haemolytic anaemia · hepatic disorders · nephritis tubulointerstitial · neutropenia · seizure · severe cutaneous adverse reactions (SCARs)

  SIDE-EFFECTS, FURTHER INFORMATION Diarrhoea frequently occurs during oral penicillin therapy. It is most common with broad-spectrum penicillins, which can cause antibiotic-associated colitis.

- **ALLERGY AND CROSS-SENSITIVITY** The most important side-effect of the penicillins is hypersensitivity which causes rashes and anaphylaxis and can be fatal. Allergic reactions to penicillins occur in 1–10% of exposed individuals; anaphylactic reactions occur in fewer than 0.05% of treated patients. Patients with a history of atopic allergy (e.g. asthma, eczema, hay fever) are at a higher risk of anaphylactic reactions to penicillins. Individuals with a history of anaphylaxis, urticaria, or rash immediately after penicillin administration are at risk of immediate hypersensitivity to a penicillin; these individuals should not receive a penicillin. Individuals with a history of a minor rash (i.e. non-confluent, non-pruritic rash restricted to a small area of the body) or a rash that occurs more than 72 hours after penicillin administration are probably not allergic to penicillin and in these individuals a penicillin should not be withheld unnecessarily for serious infections; the possibility of an allergic reaction should, however, be borne in mind. Other beta-lactam antibiotics (including cephalosporins) can be used in these patients.

  Patients who are allergic to one penicillin will be allergic to all because the hypersensitivity is related to the basic penicillin structure. Patients with a history of immediate hypersensitivity to penicillins may also react to the cephalosporins and other beta-lactam antibiotics, they should not receive these antibiotics. If a penicillin (or another beta-lactam antibiotic) is essential in an individual with immediate hypersensitivity to penicillin then specialist advice should be sought on hypersensitivity testing or using a beta-lactam antibiotic with a different structure to the penicillin that caused the hypersensitivity.

ANTIBACTERIALS > PENICILLINS,
ANTIPSEUDOMONAL WITH BETA-
LACTAMASE INHIBITOR

F 578

Piperacillin with tazobactam   22-May-2020

● **INDICATIONS AND DOSE**

Hospital-acquired pneumonia | Septicaemia | Complicated infections involving the urinary-tract | Complicated infections involving the skin | Complicated infections involving the soft-tissues | Acute exacerbation of chronic obstructive pulmonary disease | Acute exacerbation of bronchiectasis | Moderate diabetic foot infection | Severe diabetic foot infection | Leg ulcer infection

▸ BY INTRAVENOUS INFUSION
▸ Adult: 4.5 g every 8 hours; increased if necessary to 4.5 g every 6 hours, increased frequency may be used for severe infections

Infections in neutropenic patients

▸ BY INTRAVENOUS INFUSION
▸ Adult: 4.5 g every 6 hours

● UNLICENSED USE [EvGr] Piperacillin with tazobactam is used for the treatment of acute exacerbation of chronic obstructive pulmonary disease, <A> but is not licensed for this indication.
    [EvGr] Piperacillin with tazobactam is used for the treatment of acute exacerbation of bronchiectasis, <A> but is not licensed for this indication.

● CAUTIONS High doses may lead to hypernatraemia (owing to sodium content of preparations)

● INTERACTIONS → Appendix 1: penicillins

● SIDE-EFFECTS
▸ **Common or very common** Anaemia · candida infection · constipation · gastrointestinal discomfort · headache · insomnia
▸ **Uncommon** Flushing · hypokalaemia · hypotension · myalgia · thrombophlebitis
▸ **Rare or very rare** Epistaxis · stomatitis
▸ **Frequency not known** Eosinophilia · pancytopenia · pneumonia eosinophilic · renal failure · thrombocytosis

● PREGNANCY Manufacturers advise use only if potential benefit outweighs risk.

● BREAST FEEDING Trace amount in milk, but appropriate to use.

● RENAL IMPAIRMENT
Dose adjustments Max. 4.5 g every 8 hours if eGFR 20–40 mL/minute/1.73 m^2.
    Max. 4.5 g every 12 hours if eGFR less than 20 mL/minute/1.73 m^2.

● EFFECT ON LABORATORY TESTS False-positive urinary glucose (if tested for reducing substances).

● DIRECTIONS FOR ADMINISTRATION For *intravenous infusion*, give intermittently in Glucose 5% or Sodium chloride 0.9%. Reconstitute initially (2.25 g in 10 mL, 4.5 g in 20 mL) with water for injections, or glucose 5% (*Tazocin*® brand only), or sodium chloride 0.9%, then dilute to 50–150 mL with infusion fluid; give over 30 minutes.

● PRESCRIBING AND DISPENSING INFORMATION Dose expressed as a combination of piperacillin and tazobactam (both as sodium salts) in a ratio of 8:1.
    For choice of antibacterial therapy, see Blood infections, antibacterial therapy p. 532, Diabetic foot infections, antibacterial therapy p. 534, Respiratory system infections, antibacterial therapy p. 538, Skin infections, antibacterial therapy p. 541, Urinary-tract infections p. 626.

● MEDICINAL FORMS There can be variation in the licensing of different medicines containing the same drug. Forms available from special-order manufacturers include: infusion, powder for solution for infusion

Powder for solution for infusion
ELECTROLYTES: May contain Sodium
▸ Piperacillin with tazobactam (Non-proprietary)
    Tazobactam (as Tazobactam sodium) 250 mg, Piperacillin (as Piperacillin sodium) 2 gram Piperacillin 2g / Tazobactam 250mg powder for solution for infusion vials | 1 vial [PoM] £9.55 DT = £7.65 (Hospital only) | 10 vial [PoM] £7.65–£86.40 (Hospital only)
    Tazobactam (as Tazobactam sodium) 500 mg, Piperacillin (as Piperacillin sodium) 4 gram Piperacillin 4g / Tazobactam 500mg powder for solution for infusion vials | 1 vial [PoM] £12.90–£19.97 (Hospital only) | 10 vial [PoM] £48.00–£99.00 (Hospital only)
▸ Tazocin (Pfizer Ltd)
    Tazobactam (as Tazobactam sodium) 250 mg, Piperacillin (as Piperacillin sodium) 2 gram Tazocin 2g/0.25g powder for solution for infusion vials | 1 vial [PoM] £7.65 DT = £7.65 (Hospital only)
    Tazobactam (as Tazobactam sodium) 500 mg, Piperacillin (as Piperacillin sodium) 4 gram Tazocin 4g/0.5g powder for solution for infusion vials | 1 vial [PoM] £15.17 (Hospital only)

ANTIBACTERIALS > PENICILLINS, BETA-
LACTAMASE SENSITIVE

F 578

Benzathine benzylpenicillin   24-Apr-2020

(Benzathine penicillin G)

● **INDICATIONS AND DOSE**

Erysipelas | Yaws | Pinta
▸ BY DEEP INTRAMUSCULAR INJECTION
▸ Adult: 1.2 million units as a single dose, outer quadrant of the gluteus maximus or Hochstetter's ventrogluteal field is the preferred site of injection

Syphilis [primary and secondary stage]
▸ BY DEEP INTRAMUSCULAR INJECTION
▸ Adult: 2.4 million units as a single dose, outer quadrant of the gluteus maximus or Hochstetter's ventrogluteal field is the preferred site of injection, if clinical symptoms recur or laboratory findings remain positive—repeat treatment

Syphilis [late-stage (latent seropositive)]
▸ BY DEEP INTRAMUSCULAR INJECTION
▸ Adult: 2.4 million units once weekly for 3 weeks, outer quadrant of the gluteus maximus or Hochstetter's ventrogluteal field is the preferred site of injection

Prophylaxis of rheumatic fever [without cardiac involvement] | Prophylaxis of poststreptococcal glomerulonephritis [without cardiac involvement] | Prophylaxis of erysipelas [without cardiac involvement]
▸ BY DEEP INTRAMUSCULAR INJECTION
▸ Adult: 1.2 million units every 3–4 weeks for at least 5 years or up to 21 years of age (whichever is longer), outer quadrant of the gluteus maximus or Hochstetter's ventrogluteal field is the preferred site of injection

Prophylaxis of rheumatic fever [transient cardiac involvement] | Prophylaxis of poststreptococcal glomerulonephritis [transient cardiac involvement] | Prophylaxis of erysipelas [transient cardiac involvement]
▸ BY DEEP INTRAMUSCULAR INJECTION
▸ Adult: 1.2 million units every 3–4 weeks for at least 10 years or up to 21 years of age (whichever is longer), outer quadrant of the gluteus maximus or Hochstetter's ventrogluteal field is the preferred site of injection   continued →

5

Infection

Prophylaxis of rheumatic fever [persistent cardiac involvement] | Prophylaxis of poststreptococcal glomerulonephritis [persistent cardiac involvement] | Prophylaxis of erysipelas [persistent cardiac involvement]

▸ BY DEEP INTRAMUSCULAR INJECTION

▸ Adult: 1.2 million units every 3–4 weeks for at least 10 years or up to 40 years of age (whichever is longer); life-long prophylaxis may be necessary, outer quadrant of the gluteus maximus or Hochstetter's ventrogluteal field is the preferred site of injection

● INTERACTIONS → Appendix 1: penicillins

● SIDE-EFFECTS

▸ **Common or very common** Increased risk of infection

▸ **Uncommon** Oral disorders

▸ **Rare or very rare** Nephropathy

▸ **Frequency not known** Encephalopathy · Hoigne's syndrome · Jarisch-Herxheimer reaction

● ALLERGY AND CROSS-SENSITIVITY Contra-indicated in patients allergic to peanuts or soya (contains phospholipids from soya lecithin).

● PREGNANCY Manufacturer advises not known to be harmful.

● BREAST FEEDING Manufacturer advises present in milk in small amounts but not known to be harmful. Monitor infant for effects on the gastrointestinal flora; discontinue breast feeding if diarrhoea, candidiasis or rash in the infant occur.

● HEPATIC IMPAIRMENT Manufacturer advises caution in impairment (possible risk of delayed metabolism and excretion in severe impairment).

● RENAL IMPAIRMENT Manufacturer advises caution in impairment (possible risk of delayed metabolism and excretion in severe impairment).

Dose adjustments Manufacturer advises reduce daily dose by 25% and give as a single dose if creatinine clearance 15–59 mL/minute; reduce daily dose by 50–80% and give in 2–3 divided doses if creatinine clearance less than 15 mL/minute (maximum 1–3 million units per day).

● MONITORING REQUIREMENTS

▸ Manufacturer advises observe the patient for hypersensitivity reactions for at least 30 minutes after the injection.

▸ Manufacturer advises monitor renal, hepatic and haematopoietic function periodically in patients on long-term treatment.

● EFFECT ON LABORATORY TESTS False-positive direct Coombs' test. False-positive urinary glucose. False-positive urobilinogen. False-positive urinary protein using precipitation techniques, the Folin-Ciocalteu-Lowry method, or the biuret method. False-positive urinary amino acids using the ninhydrin method. Increased levels of urinary 17-ketosteriods using the Zimmermann reaction.

● DIRECTIONS FOR ADMINISTRATION For *deep intramuscular injection*, manufacturer advises reconstitute with water for injection and inject slowly with low pressure. No more than 5 mL should be administered per injection site and do not administer into tissues with reduced perfusion. Avoid rubbing the injection site after the injection.

● MEDICINAL FORMS There can be variation in the licensing of different medicines containing the same drug.

Powder and solvent for suspension for injection

EXCIPIENTS: May contain Lecithin, polysorbates

▸ Benzathine benzylpenicillin (Non-proprietary)

Benzathine benzylpenicillin 1.2 mega unit Benzathine benzylpenicillin 1.2million unit powder and solvent for suspension for injection vials | 1 vial PoM £9.50

Benzathine benzylpenicillin 2.4 mega unit Benzathine benzylpenicillin 2.4million unit powder and solvent for suspension for injection vials | 1 vial PoM £9.50

▸ Extencilline (Imported (France))

Benzathine benzylpenicillin 600000 unit Extencilline 600,000units powder and solvent for suspension for injection vials | 50 vial PoM ⓢ

Benzathine benzylpenicillin 1.2 mega unit Extencilline 1.2million unit powder and solvent for suspension for injection vials | 50 vial PoM ⓢ

F 578

Benzylpenicillin sodium

21-May-2020

(Penicillin G)

● INDICATIONS AND DOSE

Mild to moderate susceptible infections | Throat infections | Otitis media | Pneumonia | Cellulitis

▸ BY INTRAMUSCULAR INJECTION, OR BY SLOW INTRAVENOUS INJECTION, OR BY INTRAVENOUS INFUSION

▸ Adult: 0.6–1.2 g every 6 hours, dose may be increased if necessary in more serious infections (consult product literature), single doses over 1.2 g to be given by intravenous route only

Endocarditis (in combination with other antibacterial if necessary)

▸ BY SLOW INTRAVENOUS INJECTION, OR BY INTRAVENOUS INFUSION

▸ Adult: 1.2 g every 4 hours, increased if necessary to 2.4 g every 4 hours, dose may be increased in infections such as enterococcal endocarditis

Anthrax (in combination with other antibacterials)

▸ BY SLOW INTRAVENOUS INJECTION, OR BY INTRAVENOUS INFUSION

▸ Adult: 2.4 g every 4 hours

Intrapartum prophylaxis against group B streptococcal infection

▸ BY SLOW INTRAVENOUS INJECTION, OR BY INTRAVENOUS INFUSION

▸ Adult: Initially 3 g for 1 dose, then 1.5 g every 4 hours until delivery

Meningitis | Meningococcal disease

▸ BY SLOW INTRAVENOUS INJECTION, OR BY INTRAVENOUS INFUSION

▸ Adult: 2.4 g every 4 hours

▸ BY INTRAVENOUS INFUSION

▸ Neonate up to 7 days: 50 mg/kg every 12 hours.

▸ Neonate 7 days to 28 days: 50 mg/kg every 8 hours.

▸ Child: 50 mg/kg every 4–6 hours (max. per dose 2.4 g every 4 hours)

Suspected meningococcal disease (meningitis with non-blanching rash or meningococcal septicaemia) prior to urgent transfer to hospital

▸ BY INTRAVENOUS INJECTION, OR BY INTRAMUSCULAR INJECTION

▸ Child 1-11 months: 300 mg, administer as single dose prior to urgent transfer to hospital so long as does not delay transfer

▸ Child 1-9 years: 600 mg, administer as single dose prior to urgent transfer to hospital so long as does not delay transfer

▸ Child 10-17 years: 1.2 g, administer as single dose prior to urgent transfer to hospital so long as does not delay transfer

▸ Adult: 1.2 g, administer as single dose prior to urgent transfer to hospital so long as does not delay transfer

Suspected bacterial meningitis without non-blanching rash where patient cannot be transferred to hospital urgently

▶ BY INTRAVENOUS INJECTION, OR BY INTRAMUSCULAR INJECTION

▹ Child 1-11 months: 300 mg, administer as single dose prior to transfer to hospital

▹ Child 1-9 years: 600 mg, administer as single dose prior to transfer to hospital

▹ Child 10-17 years: 1.2 g, administer as single dose prior to transfer to hospital

▹ Adult: 1.2 g, administer as single dose prior to transfer to hospital

● UNLICENSED USE

▶ In adults Benzylpenicillin doses in the BNF may differ from those in product literature.

> IMPORTANT SAFETY INFORMATION
> Intrathecal injection of benzylpenicillin is **not** recommended.

● CAUTIONS Accumulation of sodium from injection can occur with high doses

● INTERACTIONS → Appendix 1: penicillins

● SIDE-EFFECTS

▶ **Common or very common** Fever · Jarisch-Herxheimer reaction

▶ **Rare or very rare** Neurotoxicity

▶ **Frequency not known** Coma

● PREGNANCY Not known to be harmful.

● BREAST FEEDING Trace amounts in milk, but appropriate to use.

● RENAL IMPAIRMENT Accumulation of sodium from injection can occur in renal failure. High doses may cause neurotoxicity, including cerebral irritation, convulsions, or coma.

Dose adjustments ▶ In adults Reduce dose—consult product literature.

▶ In children Estimated glomerular filtration rate 10–50 mL/minute/1.73 m^2, use normal dose every 8–12 hours. Estimated glomerular filtration rate less than 10 mL/minute/1.73 m^2 use normal dose every 12 hours.

● EFFECT ON LABORATORY TESTS False-positive urinary glucose (if tested for reducing substances).

● DIRECTIONS FOR ADMINISTRATION

▶ With intravenous use in children Intravenous route recommended in neonates and infants. For *intravenous infusion*, dilute with Glucose 5% or Sodium Chloride 0.9%; give over 15–30 minutes. Longer administration time is particularly important when using doses of 50 mg/kg (or greater) to avoid CNS toxicity.

▶ With intravenous use in adults For *intravenous infusion* (Crystapen®), give intermittently in Glucose 5% or Sodium chloride 0.9%; suggested volume 100 mL given over 30–60 minutes. Continuous infusion not usually recommended.

● PRESCRIBING AND DISPENSING INFORMATION For choice of antibacterial therapy, see Anthrax p. 613, Antibacterials, use for prophylaxis p. 529, Blood infections, antibacterial therapy p. 532, Cardiovascular system infections, antibacterial therapy p. 532, Central nervous system infections, antibacterial therapy p. 533, Ear infections, antibacterial therapy p. 534, Oropharyngeal infections, antibacterial therapy p. 1261, Respiratory system infections, antibacterial therapy p. 538, Skin infections, antibacterial therapy p. 541.

● MEDICINAL FORMS There can be variation in the licensing of different medicines containing the same drug. Forms available from special-order manufacturers include: infusion

Powder for solution for injection

ELECTROLYTES: May contain Sodium

▶ Benzylpenicillin sodium (Non-proprietary)

Benzylpenicillin sodium 600 mg Benzylpenicillin 600mg powder for solution for injection vials | 2 vial PoM £6.01-£6.02 DT = £6.02 | 25 vial PoM £75.12-£75.25

Benzylpenicillin sodium 1.2 gram Benzylpenicillin 1.2g powder for solution for injection vials | 25 vial PoM £109.49-£109.51 DT = £109.50

▶ 578

Phenoxymethylpenicillin

18-May-2020

(Penicillin V)

● INDICATIONS AND DOSE

Oral infections | Otitis media

▶ BY MOUTH

▹ Child 1-11 months: 62.5 mg 4 times a day; increased if necessary up to 12.5 mg/kg 4 times a day

▹ Child 1-5 years: 125 mg 4 times a day; increased if necessary up to 12.5 mg/kg 4 times a day

▹ Child 6-11 years: 250 mg 4 times a day; increased if necessary up to 12.5 mg/kg 4 times a day

▹ Child 12-17 years: 500 mg 4 times a day; increased if necessary up to 1 g 4 times a day

▹ Adult: 500 mg every 6 hours, increased if necessary up to 1 g every 6 hours

Acute sore throat

▶ BY MOUTH

▹ Child 1-11 months: 62.5 mg 4 times a day, alternatively 125 mg twice daily for 5–10 days

▹ Child 1-5 years: 125 mg 4 times a day, alternatively 250 mg twice daily for 5–10 days

▹ Child 6-11 years: 250 mg 4 times a day, alternatively 500 mg twice daily for 5–10 days

▹ Child 12-17 years: 500 mg 4 times a day, alternatively 1000 mg twice daily for 5–10 days

▹ Adult: 500 mg 4 times a day, alternatively 1000 mg twice daily for 5–10 days

Prevention of recurrent cellulitis (specialist use only) | Prevention of recurrent erysipelas (specialist use only)

▶ BY MOUTH

▹ Adult: 250 mg twice daily

Prevention of recurrence of rheumatic fever

▶ BY MOUTH

▹ Child 1 month-5 years: 125 mg twice daily

▹ Child 6-17 years: 250 mg twice daily

▹ Adult: 250 mg twice daily

Prevention of secondary case of invasive group A streptococcal infection

▶ BY MOUTH

▹ Child 1-11 months: 62.5 mg every 6 hours for 10 days

▹ Child 1-5 years: 125 mg every 6 hours for 10 days

▹ Child 6-11 years: 250 mg every 6 hours for 10 days

▹ Child 12-17 years: 250–500 mg every 6 hours for 10 days

▹ Adult: 250–500 mg every 6 hours for 10 days

Prevention of pneumococcal infection in asplenia or in patients with sickle-cell disease

▶ BY MOUTH

▹ Child 1-11 months: 62.5 mg twice daily

▹ Child 1-4 years: 125 mg twice daily

▹ Child 5-17 years: 250 mg twice daily

▹ Adult: 250 mg twice daily

Acute sinusitis

▶ BY MOUTH

▹ Child 1-11 months: 62.5 mg 4 times a day for 5 days

▹ Child 1-5 years: 125 mg 4 times a day for 5 days

▹ Child 6-11 years: 250 mg 4 times a day for 5 days

continued →

5

Infection

> ▸ Child 12–17 years: 500 mg 4 times a day for 5 days
> ▸ Adult: 500 mg 4 times a day for 5 days

- **UNLICENSED USE** EvGr Duration of treatment for acute sinusitis adheres to national guidelines. Ⓐ See Sinusitis (acute) p. 1247 for further information.
  ▸ In adults EvGr Phenoxymethylpenicillin is used for the prevention of recurrent cellulitis, Ⓐ but is not licensed for this indication. EvGr Phenoxymethylpenicillin is used for the prevention of recurrent erysipelas, Ⓐ but is not licensed for this indication.
    Phenoxymethylpenicillin doses in the BNF may differ from product literature.
- **INTERACTIONS** → Appendix 1: penicillins
- **SIDE-EFFECTS** Circulatory collapse · coagulation disorder · eosinophilia · faeces soft · fever · increased risk of infection · neurotoxicity · oral disorders · paraesthesia
- **PREGNANCY** Not known to be harmful.
- **BREAST FEEDING** Trace amounts in milk, but appropriate to use.
- **EFFECT ON LABORATORY TESTS** False-positive urinary glucose (if tested for reducing substances).
- **PRESCRIBING AND DISPENSING INFORMATION** For choice of antibacterial therapy, see Antibacterials, use for prophylaxis p. 529, Ear infections, antibacterial therapy p. 534, Nose infections, antibacterial therapy p. 537, Oral bacterial infections p. 537, Oropharyngeal infections, antibacterial therapy p. 1261, Skin infections, antibacterial therapy p. 541.
- **PATIENT AND CARER ADVICE**
  Medicines for Children leaflet: Penicillin V for bacterial infections www.medicinesforchildren.org.uk/penicillin-v-bacterial-infections
  Medicines for Children leaflet: Penicillin V for prevention of pneumococcal infection www.medicinesforchildren.org.uk/penicillin-v-prevention-pneumococcal-infection
- **PROFESSION SPECIFIC INFORMATION**
  Dental practitioners' formulary
  Phenoxymethylpenicillin Tablets may be prescribed.
    Phenoxymethylpenicillin Oral Solution may be prescribed.

- **MEDICINAL FORMS** There can be variation in the licensing of different medicines containing the same drug.
  Oral solution
  CAUTIONARY AND ADVISORY LABELS 9, 23
  ▸ Phenoxymethylpenicillin (Non-proprietary)
    Phenoxymethylpenicillin (as Phenoxymethylpenicillin potassium) 25 mg per 1 ml Phenoxymethylpenicillin 125mg/5ml oral solution | 100 ml PoM £34.00 DT = £2.27
    Phenoxymethylpenicillin 125mg/5ml oral solution sugar free sugar-free | 100 ml PoM £25.00 DT = £7.04
    Phenoxymethylpenicillin (as Phenoxymethylpenicillin potassium) 50 mg per 1 ml Phenoxymethylpenicillin 250mg/5ml oral solution | 100 ml PoM £35.00 DT = £3.91
    Phenoxymethylpenicillin 250mg/5ml oral solution sugar free sugar-free | 100 ml PoM £35.00 DT = £8.46
  Tablet
  CAUTIONARY AND ADVISORY LABELS 9, 23
  ▸ Phenoxymethylpenicillin (Non-proprietary)
    Phenoxymethylpenicillin (as Phenoxymethylpenicillin potassium) 250 mg Phenoxymethylpenicillin 250mg tablets | 28 tablet PoM £5.00 DT = £1.25

ANTIBACTERIALS ⟩ PENICILLINS, BROAD-SPECTRUM

F 578

Amoxicillin
(Amoxycillin)

24-Nov-2020

- **INDICATIONS AND DOSE**
Susceptible infections (e.g. sinusitis, salmonellosis, oral infections)
▸ BY MOUTH
▸ Child 1–11 months: 125 mg 3 times a day; increased if necessary up to 30 mg/kg 3 times a day
▸ Child 1–4 years: 250 mg 3 times a day; increased if necessary up to 30 mg/kg 3 times a day
▸ Child 5–11 years: 500 mg 3 times a day; increased if necessary up to 30 mg/kg 3 times a day (max. per dose 1 g)
▸ Child 12–17 years: 500 mg 3 times a day; increased if necessary up to 1 g 3 times a day, use increased dose in severe infections
▸ Adult: 500 mg every 8 hours, increased if necessary to 1 g every 8 hours, increased dose used in severe infections
▸ BY INTRAMUSCULAR INJECTION
▸ Adult: 500 mg every 8 hours
▸ BY INTRAVENOUS INJECTION, OR BY INTRAVENOUS INFUSION
▸ Adult: 500 mg every 8 hours, increased to 1 g every 6 hours, use increased dose in severe infections

Community-acquired pneumonia
▸ BY MOUTH
▸ Child 1–11 months: 125 mg 3 times a day for 5 days; increased if necessary up to 30 mg/kg 3 times a day
▸ Child 1–4 years: 250 mg 3 times a day for 5 days; increased if necessary up to 30 mg/kg 3 times a day
▸ Child 5–11 years: 500 mg 3 times a day for 5 days; increased if necessary up to 30 mg/kg 3 times a day (max. per dose 1 g 3 times a day)
▸ Child 12–17 years: 500 mg 3 times a day for 5 days; increased if necessary up to 1 g 3 times a day
▸ Adult: 500 mg 3 times a day for 5 days; increased if necessary to 1 g 3 times a day

Acute exacerbation of bronchiectasis
▸ BY MOUTH
▸ Child 1–11 months: 125 mg 3 times a day for 7–14 days
▸ Child 1–4 years: 250 mg 3 times a day for 7–14 days
▸ Child 5–17 years: 500 mg 3 times a day for 7–14 days
▸ Adult: 500 mg 3 times a day for 7–14 days

Acute exacerbation of chronic obstructive pulmonary disease
▸ BY MOUTH
▸ Adult: 500 mg 3 times a day for 5 days, increased if necessary to 1 g 3 times a day, increased dose used in severe infections
▸ BY INTRAVENOUS INJECTION, OR BY INTRAVENOUS INFUSION
▸ Adult: 500 mg every 8 hours, increased to 1 g every 6 hours, increased dose used in severe infections

Acute cough [if systemically very unwell or at higher risk of complications]
▸ BY MOUTH
▸ Child 1–11 months: 125 mg 3 times a day for 5 days
▸ Child 1–4 years: 250 mg 3 times a day for 5 days
▸ Child 5–17 years: 500 mg 3 times a day for 5 days
▸ Adult: 500 mg 3 times a day for 5 days

Acute otitis media
▸ BY MOUTH
▸ Child 1–11 months: 125 mg 3 times a day for 5–7 days
▸ Child 1–4 years: 250 mg 3 times a day for 5–7 days
▸ Child 5–17 years: 500 mg 3 times a day for 5–7 days

Lyme disease [erythema migrans and/or non-focal symptoms] | Lyme disease [affecting cranial nerves or peripheral nervous system]
▸ BY MOUTH
 ▸ Adult: 1 g 3 times a day for 21 days

Lyme arthritis | Acrodermatitis chronica atrophicans
▸ BY MOUTH
 ▸ Adult: 1 g 3 times a day for 28 days

Anthrax (treatment and post-exposure prophylaxis)
▸ BY MOUTH
 ▸ Adult: 500 mg 3 times a day

Dental abscess (short course)
▸ BY MOUTH
 ▸ Adult: 3 g, then 3 g after 8 hours

Listerial meningitis (in combination with another antibiotic)
▸ BY INTRAVENOUS INFUSION
 ▸ Adult: 2 g every 4 hours

Endocarditis (in combination with another antibiotic if necessary)
▸ BY INTRAVENOUS INFUSION
 ▸ Adult: 2 g every 4 hours

***Helicobacter pylori* eradication [in combination with other drugs (see Helicobacter pylori infection p. 90)]**
▸ BY MOUTH
 ▸ Adult: 1 g twice daily for 7 days for first- and second-line eradication therapy; 10 days for third-line eradication therapy

Acute diverticulitis [in combination with gentamicin and metronidazole]
▸ BY INTRAVENOUS INJECTION, OR BY INTRAVENOUS INFUSION
 ▸ Adult: 500 mg every 8 hours; increased if necessary to 1 g every 6 hours, increased dose used in severe infections

Prophylaxis of recurrent urinary-tract infection
▸ BY MOUTH
 ▸ Adult: 250 mg once daily, dose to be taken at night, alternatively 500 mg for 1 dose, following exposure to a trigger

Lower urinary-tract infection in pregnancy
▸ BY MOUTH
 ▸ Adult: 500 mg 3 times a day for 7 days

Lower urinary-tract infection
▸ BY MOUTH
 ▸ Child 3-11 months: 125 mg 3 times a day for 3 days
 ▸ Child 1-4 years: 250 mg 3 times a day for 3 days
 ▸ Child 5-15 years: 500 mg 3 times a day for 3 days

Urinary-tract infections (short course)
▸ BY MOUTH
 ▸ Adult: 3 g, then 3 g after 10–12 hours

Asymptomatic bacteriuria in pregnancy
▸ BY MOUTH
 ▸ Adult: 250–500 mg 3 times a day, alternatively 750–1000 mg twice daily

Urinary-tract infection (catheter-associated)
▸ BY MOUTH
 ▸ Child 16-17 years: 500 mg 3 times a day for 7 days
 ▸ Adult: 500 mg 3 times a day for 7 days

● UNLICENSED USE Amoxicillin doses in BNF Publications may differ from those in product literature.
   EvGr Duration of treatment for acute otitis media differs from product literature and adheres to national guidelines. Amoxicillin is used for the treatment of acute exacerbation of bronchiectasis, ⟨A⟩ but is not licensed for this indication.
   EvGr Amoxicillin is used for prophylaxis of recurrent urinary-tract infection, ⟨A⟩ but is not licensed for this indication.

EvGr Combination regimens and durations for *Helicobacter pylori* eradication may differ from product literature but adhere to national guidelines. ⟨A⟩

● CAUTIONS
   GENERAL CAUTIONS Acute lymphocytic leukaemia (increased risk of erythematous rashes) · chronic lymphocytic leukaemia (increased risk of erythematous rashes) · cytomegalovirus infection (increased risk of erythematous rashes) · glandular fever (erythematous rashes common) · maintain adequate hydration with high doses (particularly during parenteral therapy)
   SPECIFIC CAUTIONS
 ▸ With intravenous use accumulation of sodium can occur with high parenteral doses

● INTERACTIONS → Appendix 1: penicillins

● SIDE-EFFECTS
   GENERAL SIDE-EFFECTS
 ▸ **Rare or very rare** Colitis haemorrhagic · crystalluria · dizziness · hyperkinesia · hypersensitivity vasculitis · mucocutaneous candidiasis
 ▸ **Frequency not known** Jarisch-Herxheimer reaction
   SPECIFIC SIDE-EFFECTS
 ▸ **Rare or very rare**
 ▸ With oral use Black hairy tongue

● PREGNANCY Not known to be harmful.

● BREAST FEEDING Trace amount in milk, but appropriate to use.

● HEPATIC IMPAIRMENT Manufacturer advises caution.

● RENAL IMPAIRMENT Risk of crystalluria with high doses (particularly during parenteral therapy).
 ▸ With intravenous use Accumulation of sodium from injection can occur in patients with renal failure.
   Dose adjustments Reduce dose in severe impairment; rashes more common.

● DIRECTIONS FOR ADMINISTRATION
 ▸ With intravenous use in adults For *intravenous infusion* (*Amoxil*®), give intermittently *in* Glucose 5% *or* Sodium chloride 0.9%. Reconstituted solutions diluted and given without delay; suggested volume 100 mL given over 30–60 minutes or *give via* drip tubing in Glucose 5% *or* Sodium chloride 0.9%; continuous infusion not usually recommended.

● PRESCRIBING AND DISPENSING INFORMATION For choice of antibacterial therapy, see Anthrax p. 613, Cardiovascular system infections, antibacterial therapy p. 532, Central nervous system infections, antibacterial therapy p. 533, Ear infections, antibacterial therapy p. 534, Gastro-intestinal system infections, antibacterial therapy p. 535, Helicobacter pylori infection p. 90, Lyme disease p. 614, Nose infections, antibacterial therapy p. 537, Oral bacterial infections p. 537, Respiratory system infections, antibacterial therapy p. 538, Urinary-tract infections p. 626.
 ▸ In children For choice of antibacterial therapy, see Antibacterials, use for prophylaxis p. 529.

● PATIENT AND CARER ADVICE Patient counselling is advised for amoxicillin oral suspension (use of oral dosing syringe).
   Medicines for Children leaflet: Amoxicillin for bacterial infections www.medicinesforchildren.org.uk/amoxicillin-bacterial-infections-0

● PROFESSION SPECIFIC INFORMATION
   Dental practitioners' formulary
   Amoxicillin capsules may be prescribed.
     Amoxicillin sachets may be prescribed as Amoxicillin Oral Powder.
     Amoxicillin Oral Suspension may be prescribed.

● MEDICINAL FORMS There can be variation in the licensing of different medicines containing the same drug.

Powder for solution for injection
ELECTROLYTES: May contain Sodium
▸ Amoxicillin (Non-proprietary)
Amoxicillin (as Amoxicillin sodium) 250 mg Amoxicillin 250mg powder for solution for injection vials | 10 vial [PoM] £4.80 | 10 vial [PoM] £4.50 (Hospital only)
Amoxicillin (as Amoxicillin sodium) 500 mg Amoxicillin 500mg powder for solution for injection vials | 10 vial [PoM] £9.60 DT = £5.48 | 10 vial [PoM] £12.00 DT = £5.48 (Hospital only)
Amoxicillin (as Amoxicillin sodium) 1 gram Amoxicillin 1g powder for solution for injection vials | 1 vial [PoM] £1.92 | 10 vial [PoM] £16.50 DT = £10.96 (Hospital only)
▸ Amoxil (GlaxoSmithKline UK Ltd)
Amoxicillin (as Amoxicillin sodium) 500 mg Amoxil 500mg powder for solution for injection vials | 10 vial [PoM] £5.48 DT = £5.48
Amoxicillin (as Amoxicillin sodium) 1 gram Amoxil 1g powder for solution for injection vials | 10 vial [PoM] £10.96 DT = £10.96

Oral suspension
CAUTIONARY AND ADVISORY LABELS 9
EXCIPIENTS: May contain Sucrose
▸ Amoxicillin (Non-proprietary)
Amoxicillin (as Amoxicillin trihydrate) 25 mg per 1 ml Amoxicillin 125mg/5ml oral suspension sugar free sugar-free | 100 ml [PoM] £25.00 DT = £1.48
Amoxicillin 125mg/5ml oral suspension | 100 ml [PoM] £25.00 DT = £1.97
Amoxicillin (as Amoxicillin trihydrate) 50 mg per 1 ml Amoxicillin 250mg/5ml oral suspension sugar free sugar-free | 100 ml [PoM] £35.00 DT = £1.76
Amoxicillin 250mg/5ml oral suspension | 100 ml [PoM] £35.00 DT = £2.12

Powder
CAUTIONARY AND ADVISORY LABELS 9, 13
▸ Amoxicillin (Non-proprietary)
Amoxicillin (as Amoxicillin trihydrate) 3 gram Amoxicillin 3g oral powder sachets sugar free sugar-free | 2 sachet [PoM] £15.00 DT = £10.48

Capsule
CAUTIONARY AND ADVISORY LABELS 9
▸ Amoxicillin (Non-proprietary)
Amoxicillin (as Amoxicillin trihydrate) 250 mg Amoxicillin 250mg capsules | 15 capsule [PoM] £5.00 DT = £1.14 | 21 capsule [PoM] £8.99 DT = £1.60 | 500 capsule [PoM] £38.00–£120.00
Amoxicillin (as Amoxicillin trihydrate) 500 mg Amoxicillin 500mg capsules | 15 capsule [PoM] £7.50 DT = £1.23 | 21 capsule [PoM] £15.00 DT = £1.72 | 100 capsule [PoM] £8.19–£75.00

Combinations available: *Co-amoxiclav*, p. 585

▌Ampicillin   ⚑ 578

21-May-2020

● INDICATIONS AND DOSE

Susceptible infections (including bronchitis, urinary-tract infections, otitis media, sinusitis, uncomplicated community-acquired pneumonia, salmonellosis)
▸ BY MOUTH
▸ Child 1–11 months: 125 mg 4 times a day; increased if necessary up to 30 mg/kg 4 times a day
▸ Child 1–4 years: 250 mg 4 times a day; increased if necessary up to 30 mg/kg 4 times a day
▸ Child 5–11 years: 500 mg 4 times a day; increased if necessary up to 30 mg/kg 4 times a day (max. per dose 1 g)
▸ Child 12–17 years: 500 mg 4 times a day; increased if necessary to 1 g 4 times a day, use increased dose in severe infection
▸ Adult: 0.5–1 g every 6 hours
▸ BY INTRAVENOUS INJECTION, OR BY INTRAVENOUS INFUSION
▸ Adult: 500 mg every 4–6 hours
▸ BY INTRAMUSCULAR INJECTION
▸ Adult: 500 mg every 4–6 hours

Endocarditis (in combination with another antibiotic if necessary) | Listerial meningitis (in combination with another antibiotic)
▸ BY INTRAVENOUS INFUSION
▸ Adult: 2 g every 4 hours

● UNLICENSED USE
▸ In adults Ampicillin doses in BNF may differ from those in product literature.

● CAUTIONS
GENERAL CAUTIONS Acute lymphocytic leukaemia (increased risk of erythematous rashes) · chronic lymphocytic leukaemia (increased risk of erythematous rashes) · cytomegalovirus infection (increased risk of erythematous rashes) · glandular fever (erythematous rashes common)
SPECIFIC CAUTIONS
▸ With intravenous use Accumulation of electrolytes contained in parenteral preparations can occur with high doses

● INTERACTIONS → Appendix 1: penicillins
● SIDE-EFFECTS Colitis haemorrhagic
● PREGNANCY Not known to be harmful.
● BREAST FEEDING Trace amounts in milk, but appropriate to use.
● RENAL IMPAIRMENT
▸ With intravenous use Accumulation of electrolytes contained in parenteral preparations can occur in patients with renal failure.
Dose adjustments ▸ In adults Reduce dose if eGFR less than 10 mL/minute/1.73 m²; rashes more common.
▸ In children If estimated glomerular filtration rate less than 10 mL/minute/1.73 m² reduce dose or frequency; rashes more common.

● DIRECTIONS FOR ADMINISTRATION
▸ With oral use Administer at least 30 minutes before food.
▸ With intravenous use in adults For *intravenous infusion* (*Penbritin*®), give intermittently in Glucose 5% or Sodium chloride 0.9%. Reconstituted solutions diluted and given without delay; suggested volume 100 mL given over 30–60 minutes *via* drip tubing in Glucose 5% or Sodium chloride 0.9%. Continuous infusion not usually recommended.

● PATIENT AND CARER ADVICE
Medicines for Children leaflet: Ampicillin for bacterial infection
www.medicinesforchildren.org.uk/ampicillin-bacterial-infection

● MEDICINAL FORMS There can be variation in the licensing of different medicines containing the same drug.
Oral suspension
CAUTIONARY AND ADVISORY LABELS 9, 23
▸ Ampicillin (Non-proprietary)
Ampicillin 25 mg per 1 ml Ampicillin 125mg/5ml oral suspension | 100 ml [PoM] £29.86 DT = £29.86
Ampicillin 50 mg per 1 ml Ampicillin 250mg/5ml oral suspension | 100 ml [PoM] £38.86 DT = £38.86

Capsule
CAUTIONARY AND ADVISORY LABELS 9, 23
▸ Ampicillin (Non-proprietary)
Ampicillin 250 mg Ampicillin 250mg capsules | 28 capsule [PoM] £25.03 DT = £23.98
Ampicillin 500 mg Ampicillin 500mg capsules | 28 capsule [PoM] £49.51 DT = £46.28

Powder for solution for injection
▸ Ampicillin (Non-proprietary)
Ampicillin (as Ampicillin sodium) 500 mg Ampicillin 500mg powder for solution for injection vials | 10 vial [PoM] £78.30 DT = £78.30

Co-fluampicil

☞ 578

26-May-2020

● INDICATIONS AND DOSE

Mixed infections involving beta-lactamase-producing staphylococci

▶ BY MOUTH
- Child 10–17 years: 250/250 mg every 6 hours
- Adult: 250/250 mg every 6 hours

Severe mixed infections involving beta-lactamase-producing staphylococci

▶ BY MOUTH
- Child 10–17 years: 500/500 mg every 6 hours
- Adult: 500/500 mg every 6 hours

IMPORTANT SAFETY INFORMATION

HEPATIC DISORDERS

Cholestatic jaundice and hepatitis may occur very rarely, up to two months after treatment with flucloxacillin has been stopped. Administration for more than 2 weeks and increasing age are risk factors. Manufacturer advises:
- flucloxacillin should not be used in patients with a history of hepatic dysfunction associated with flucloxacillin;
- flucloxacillin should be used with caution in patients with hepatic impairment;
- careful enquiry should be made about hypersensitivity reactions to beta-lactam antibacterials.

- CAUTIONS Acute lymphocytic leukaemia (increased risk of erythematous rashes) · chronic lymphocytic leukaemia (increased risk of erythematous rashes) · cytomegalovirus infection (increased risk of erythematous rashes) · glandular fever (erythematous rashes common)
- INTERACTIONS → Appendix 1: penicillins
- SIDE-EFFECTS Bronchospasm · coma · dyspnoea · electrolyte imbalance · eosinophilia · erythema nodosum · gastrointestinal disorder · hallucination · Jarisch-Herxheimer reaction · myalgia · purpura non-thrombocytopenic · vasculitis
- PREGNANCY Not known to be harmful.
- BREAST FEEDING Trace amount in milk, but appropriate to use.
- HEPATIC IMPAIRMENT Manufacturer advises caution.
- RENAL IMPAIRMENT
  Dose adjustments ▶ In adults Reduce dose if eGFR less than 10 mL/minute/1.73 m^2; rashes more common.
  ▶ In children Reduce dose or frequency if estimated glomerular filtration rate less than 10 mL/minute/1.73 m^2; rashes more common.
- EFFECT ON LABORATORY TESTS False-positive urinary glucose (if tested for reducing substances).
- PRESCRIBING AND DISPENSING INFORMATION Dose expressed as a combination of equal parts by mass of flucloxacillin and ampicillin.

- MEDICINAL FORMS There can be variation in the licensing of different medicines containing the same drug.

Capsule

CAUTIONARY AND ADVISORY LABELS 9, 22
▶ Co-fluampicil (Non-proprietary)
  Ampicillin (as Ampicillin trihydrate) 250 mg, Flucloxacillin (as Flucloxacillin sodium) 250 mg Co-fluampicil 250mg/250mg capsules | 28 capsule [PoM] £28.71 DT = £18.18 | 100 capsule [PoM] £64.93

ANTIBACTERIALS ⟩ PENICILLINS, BROAD-SPECTRUM WITH BETA-LACTAMASE INHIBITOR

☞ 578

Co-amoxiclav

04-Dec-2020

● INDICATIONS AND DOSE

Infections due to beta-lactamase-producing strains (where amoxicillin alone not appropriate), including respiratory tract infections, bone and joint infections, genito-urinary and abdominal infections, and animal bites

▶ BY MOUTH USING TABLETS
- Child 12–17 years: 250/125 mg every 8 hours; increased to 500/125 mg every 8 hours, increased dose used for severe infection
- Adult: 250/125 mg every 8 hours; increased to 500/125 mg every 8 hours, increased dose used for severe infection
▶ BY INTRAVENOUS INJECTION, OR BY INTRAVENOUS INFUSION
- Adult: 1.2 g every 8 hours

Infections due to beta-lactamase-producing strains (where amoxicillin alone not appropriate) including respiratory-tract infections, bone and joint infections, genito-urinary and abdominal infections, and animal bites (doses for 125/31 suspension)

▶ BY MOUTH USING ORAL SUSPENSION
- Child 1–11 months: 0.25 mL/kilogram 3 times a day, dose doubled in severe infection
- Child 1–5 years: 0.25 mL/kilogram 3 times a day, alternatively 5 mL 3 times a day, dose doubled in severe infection

Infections due to beta-lactamase-producing strains (where amoxicillin alone not appropriate) including respiratory-tract infections, bone and joint infections, genito-urinary and abdominal infections, and animal bites (doses for 250/62 suspension)

▶ BY MOUTH USING ORAL SUSPENSION
- Child 6–11 years: 0.15 mL/kilogram 3 times a day, alternatively 5 mL 3 times a day, dose doubled in severe infection

Infections due to beta-lactamase-producing strains (where amoxicillin alone not appropriate) including respiratory-tract infections, bone and joint infections, genito-urinary and abdominal infections, and animal bites (doses for 400/57 suspension)

▶ BY MOUTH USING ORAL SUSPENSION
- Child 2–23 months: 0.15 mL/kilogram twice daily, doubled in severe infection
- Child 2–6 years (body-weight 13–21 kg): 2.5 mL twice daily, doubled in severe infection
- Child 7–12 years (body-weight 22–40 kg): 5 mL twice daily, doubled in severe infection
- Child 12–17 years (body-weight 41 kg and above): 10 mL twice daily; increased if necessary to 10 mL 3 times a day, increased frequency to be used in severe infection
- Adult: 10 mL twice daily; increased if necessary to 10 mL 3 times a day, increased frequency to be used in severe infection

Acute diverticulitis

▶ BY MOUTH
- Adult: 500/125 mg 3 times a day for 5 days then review
▶ BY INTRAVENOUS INFUSION, OR BY INTRAVENOUS INJECTION
- Adult: 1.2 g every 8 hours

Moderate diabetic foot infection | Severe diabetic foot infection

▶ BY MOUTH USING TABLETS
- Adult: 500/125 mg every 8 hours
▶ BY INTRAVENOUS INJECTION, OR BY INTRAVENOUS INFUSION
- Adult: 1.2 g every 8 hours

continued →

5

Infection

Leg ulcer infection
▸ BY MOUTH USING TABLETS
- Adult: 500/125 mg every 8 hours for 7 days
▸ BY INTRAVENOUS INJECTION, OR BY INTRAVENOUS INFUSION
- Adult: 1.2 g every 8 hours

Cellulitis | Erysipelas
▸ BY MOUTH USING TABLETS
- Child 12–17 years: 250/125 mg every 8 hours, alternatively 500/125 mg every 8 hours for 5–7 days then review (review after 7 days in severe infection or if infection near the eyes or nose)
- Adult: 500/125 mg every 8 hours for 7 days then review
▸ BY INTRAVENOUS INJECTION, OR BY INTRAVENOUS INFUSION
- Adult: 1.2 g every 8 hours

Cellulitis (doses for 125/31 suspension) | Erysipelas (doses for 125/31 suspension)
▸ BY MOUTH USING ORAL SUSPENSION
- Child 1–11 months: 0.25 mL/kilogram 3 times a day for 5–7 days then review (review after 7 days in severe infection or if infection near the eyes or nose), dose doubled in severe infection
- Child 1–5 years: 0.25 mL/kilogram 3 times a day, alternatively 5 mL 3 times a day for 5–7 days then review (review after 7 days in severe infection or if infection near the eyes or nose), dose doubled in severe infection

Cellulitis (doses for 250/62 suspension) | Erysipelas (doses for 250/62 suspension)
▸ BY MOUTH USING ORAL SUSPENSION
- Child 6–11 years: 0.15 mL/kilogram 3 times a day, alternatively 5 mL 3 times a day for 5–7 days then review (review after 7 days in severe infection or if infection near the eyes or nose), dose doubled in severe infection

Severe dental infection with spreading cellulitis | Dental infection not responding to first-line antibacterial
▸ BY MOUTH USING TABLETS
- Child 12–17 years: 250/125 mg every 8 hours for 5 days
- Adult: 250/125 mg every 8 hours for 5 days

Surgical prophylaxis
▸ BY INTRAVENOUS INJECTION, OR BY INTRAVENOUS INFUSION
- Adult: 1.2 g, to be administered up to 30 minutes before the procedure, then 1.2 g every 8 hours for up to 2–3 further doses in high risk procedures

Community-acquired pneumonia (doses for 125/31 suspension)
▸ BY MOUTH USING ORAL SUSPENSION
- Child 1–11 months: 0.5 mL/kilogram 3 times a day for 5 days
- Child 1–5 years: 0.5 mL/kilogram 3 times a day for 5 days, alternatively 10 mL 3 times a day for 5 days

Community-acquired pneumonia (doses for 250/62 suspension)
▸ BY MOUTH USING ORAL SUSPENSION
- Child 6–11 years: 0.3 mL/kilogram 3 times a day for 5 days, alternatively 10 mL 3 times a day for 5 days

Community-acquired pneumonia
▸ BY MOUTH USING TABLETS
- Child 12–17 years: 500/125 mg 3 times a day for 5 days
- Adult: 500/125 mg 3 times a day for 5 days
▸ BY INTRAVENOUS INJECTION, OR BY INTRAVENOUS INFUSION
- Adult: 1.2 g every 8 hours

Hospital-acquired pneumonia (doses for 125/31 suspension)
▸ BY MOUTH USING ORAL SUSPENSION
- Child 1–11 months: 0.5 mL/kilogram 3 times a day for 5 days then review
- Child 1–5 years: 0.5 mL/kilogram 3 times a day for 5 days then review, alternatively 10 mL 3 times a day for 5 days then review

Hospital-acquired pneumonia (doses for 250/62 suspension)
▸ BY MOUTH USING ORAL SUSPENSION
- Child 6–11 years: 0.3 mL/kilogram 3 times a day for 5 days then review, alternatively 10 mL 3 times a day for 5 days then review

Hospital-acquired pneumonia
▸ BY MOUTH USING TABLETS
- Child 12–17 years: 500/125 mg 3 times a day for 5 days then review
- Adult: 500/125 mg 3 times a day for 5 days then review

Acute exacerbation of bronchiectasis (doses for 125/31 suspension)
▸ BY MOUTH USING ORAL SUSPENSION
- Child 1–11 months: 0.25 mL/kilogram 3 times a day for 7–14 days
- Child 1–5 years: 5 mL 3 times a day for 7–14 days, alternatively 0.25 mL/kilogram 3 times a day for 7–14 days

Acute exacerbation of bronchiectasis (doses for 250/62 suspension)
▸ BY MOUTH USING ORAL SUSPENSION
- Child 6–11 years: 5 mL 3 times a day for 7–14 days, alternatively 0.15 mL/kilogram 3 times a day for 7–14 days

Acute exacerbation of bronchiectasis
▸ BY MOUTH USING TABLETS
- Child 12–17 years: 250/125 mg 3 times a day for 7–14 days, alternatively 500/125 mg 3 times a day for 7–14 days
- Adult: 500/125 mg 3 times a day for 7–14 days
▸ BY INTRAVENOUS INFUSION, OR BY INTRAVENOUS INJECTION
- Adult: 1.2 g every 8 hours

Acute exacerbation of chronic obstructive pulmonary disease
▸ BY MOUTH USING TABLETS
- Adult: 500/125 mg 3 times a day for 5 days
▸ BY INTRAVENOUS INJECTION, OR BY INTRAVENOUS INFUSION
- Adult: 1.2 g every 8 hours

Acute sinusitis (doses for 125/31 suspension)
▸ BY MOUTH USING ORAL SUSPENSION
- Child 1–11 months: 0.25 mL/kilogram 3 times a day for 5 days
- Child 1–5 years: 5 mL 3 times a day for 5 days, alternatively 0.25 mL/kilogram 3 times a day for 5 days

Acute sinusitis (doses for 250/62 suspension)
▸ BY MOUTH USING ORAL SUSPENSION
- Child 6–11 years: 5 mL 3 times a day for 5 days, alternatively 0.15 mL/kilogram 3 times a day for 5 days

Acute sinusitis
▸ BY MOUTH USING TABLETS
- Child 12–17 years: 250/125 mg 3 times a day for 5 days, alternatively 500/125 mg 3 times a day for 5 days
- Adult: 500/125 mg 3 times a day for 5 days

Acute otitis media (doses for 125/31 suspension)
▸ BY MOUTH USING ORAL SUSPENSION
- Child 1–11 months: 0.25 mL/kilogram 3 times a day for 5–7 days
- Child 1–5 years: 5 mL 3 times a day for 5–7 days, alternatively 0.25 mL/kilogram 3 times a day for 5–7 days

Acute otitis media (doses for 250/62 suspension)
▸ BY MOUTH USING ORAL SUSPENSION
- Child 6–11 years: 5 mL 3 times a day for 5–7 days, alternatively 0.15 mL/kilogram 3 times a day for 5–7 days

Acute otitis media
▶ BY MOUTH USING TABLETS
▪ Child 12–17 years: 250/125 mg 3 times a day for
5–7 days, alternatively 500/125 mg 3 times a day for
5–7 days

**Acute pyelonephritis (doses for 125/31 suspension) |
Urinary-tract infection (catheter-associated) (doses for
125/31 suspension)**
▶ BY MOUTH USING ORAL SUSPENSION
▪ Child 3–11 months: 0.25 mL/kilogram 3 times a day for
7 to 10 days, dose doubled in severe infection
▪ Child 1–5 years: 0.25 mL/kilogram 3 times a day,
alternatively 5 mL 3 times a day for 7 to 10 days, dose
doubled in severe infection

**Acute pyelonephritis (doses for 250/62 suspension) |
Urinary-tract infection (catheter-associated) (doses for
250/62 suspension)**
▶ BY MOUTH USING ORAL SUSPENSION
▪ Child 6–11 years: 0.15 mL/kilogram 3 times a day,
alternatively 5 mL 3 times a day for 7 to 10 days, dose
doubled in severe infection

**Acute pyelonephritis | Urinary-tract infection (catheter-
associated)**
▶ BY MOUTH USING TABLETS
▪ Child 12–15 years: 250/125 mg 3 times a day for
7–10 days, alternatively 500/125 mg 3 times a day for
7–10 days
▪ Child 16–17 years: 500/125 mg 3 times a day for
7–10 days
▪ Adult: 500/125 mg 3 times a day for 7–10 days
▶ BY SLOW INTRAVENOUS INJECTION, OR BY INTRAVENOUS
INFUSION
▪ Adult: 1.2 g every 8 hours

DOSE EQUIVALENCE AND CONVERSION
▶ Doses are expressed as co-amoxiclav.
▶ A mixture of amoxicillin (as the trihydrate or as the
sodium salt) and clavulanic acid (as potassium
clavulanate); the proportions are expressed in the form
x/y where x and y are the strengths in milligrams of
amoxicillin and clavulanic acid respectively.

● UNLICENSED USE Co-amoxiclav may be used as detailed
below, although these situations are considered
unlicensed:
  ● EvGr treatment of acute exacerbation of bronchiectasis
  ● treatment of hospital-acquired pneumonia
  ● duration of treatment for acute sinusitis
  ● duration of treatment for acute otitis media
  Co-amoxiclav is used for the treatment of acute
diverticulitis ⟨A⟩, but is not licensed orally for this
indication.
● CONTRA-INDICATIONS History of co-amoxiclav-associated
jaundice or hepatic dysfunction · history of penicillin-
associated jaundice or hepatic dysfunction
● CAUTIONS
GENERAL CAUTIONS Acute lymphocytic leukaemia
(increased risk of erythematous rashes) · chronic
lymphocytic leukaemia (increased risk of erythematous
rashes) · cytomegalovirus infection (increased risk of
erythematous rashes) · glandular fever (erythematous
rashes common) · maintain adequate hydration with high
doses (particularly during parental therapy)
SPECIFIC CAUTIONS
▶ With intravenous use accumulation of electrolytes contained
in parenteral preparations can occur with high doses
● INTERACTIONS → Appendix 1: clavulanate · penicillins
● SIDE-EFFECTS
GENERAL SIDE-EFFECTS
▶ **Common or very common** Increased risk of infection
▶ **Uncommon** Dizziness · dyspepsia · headache

▶ **Frequency not known** Colitis haemorrhagic · crystalluria ·
hypersensitivity vasculitis · meningitis aseptic
SPECIFIC SIDE-EFFECTS
▶ With oral use Akathisia · black hairy tongue · cholangitis ·
Kounis syndrome

SIDE-EFFECTS, FURTHER INFORMATION Hepatic events
have been reported mostly in males and elderly patients
and may be associated with prolonged treatment.
    Signs and symptoms usually occur during or shortly after
treatment but in some cases may occur several weeks after
discontinuation.
● PREGNANCY Specialist sources indicate not known to be
harmful. Avoid in preterm prelabour rupture of the
membranes (PPROM)—possible increased risk of
necrotising enterocolitis in the neonate.
● BREAST FEEDING Trace amount in milk, but appropriate to
use.
● HEPATIC IMPAIRMENT Manufacturer advises caution.
Monitoring Monitor liver function in liver disease.
● RENAL IMPAIRMENT Risk of crystalluria with high doses
(particularly during parenteral therapy).
▶ With intravenous use Accumulation of electrolytes
contained in parenteral preparations can occur in patients
with renal failure.
Dose adjustments ▶ With oral use in adults *Co-amoxiclav
250/125 tablets or 500/125 tablets*: if eGFR
10–30 mL/minute/1.73 m^2, one 250/125 strength tablet
every 12 hours or one 500/125 strength tablet every
12 hours; if eGFR less than 10 mL/minute/1.73 m^2, one
250/125 strength tablet every 24 hours or one 500/125
strength tablet every 24 hours.
  ▶ With oral use in adults *Co-amoxiclav 400/57 suspension*:
avoid if eGFR less than 30 mL/minute/1.73 m^2.
  ▶ With intravenous use in adults *Co-amoxiclav injection*
(expressed as co-amoxiclav): if eGFR
10–30 mL/minute/1.73 m^2, 1.2 g initially, then 600 mg
every 12 hours; if eGFR less than 10 mL/minute/1.73 m^2,
1.2 g initially, then 600 mg every 24 hours.
  ▶ With oral use in children *Co-amoxiclav 125/31 suspension,
250/62 suspension, 250/125 tablets, or 500/125 tablets*: use
normal dose every 12 hours if estimated glomerular
filtration rate 10–30 mL/minute/1.73 m^2. Use the normal
dose recommended for mild or moderate infections every
12 hours if estimated glomerular filtration rate less than
10 mL/minute/1.73 m^2.
  ▶ With oral use in children *Co-amoxiclav 400/57 suspension*:
avoid if estimated glomerular filtration rate less than
30 mL/minute/1.73 m^2.
● DIRECTIONS FOR ADMINISTRATION For *intravenous infusion*
(*Augmentin*®), manufacturer advises give intermittently *in*
Sodium chloride 0.9%. Reconstitute 600 mg initially with
10 mL water for injections, then dilute with 50 mL infusion
fluid; reconstitute 1.2 g initially with 20 mL water for
injections, then dilute with 100 mL infusion fluid; give
over 30–40 minutes. For *intravenous injection*, administer
over 3–4 minutes. *Via* drip tubing *in* Sodium chloride 0.9%.
● PRESCRIBING AND DISPENSING INFORMATION Doses are
expressed as co-amoxiclav: a mixture of amoxicillin (as the
trihydrate or as the sodium salt) and clavulanic acid (as
potassium clavulanate); the proportions are expressed in
the form x/y where x and y are the strengths in milligrams
of amoxicillin and clavulanic acid respectively.
    For choice of antibacterial therapy, see Antibacterials,
use for prophylaxis p. 529, Diabetic foot infections,
antibacterial therapy p. 534, Ear infections, antibacterial
therapy p. 534, Gastro-intestinal system infections,
antibacterial therapy p. 535, Musculoskeletal system
infections, antibacterial therapy p. 536, Nose infections,
antibacterial therapy p. 537, Oropharyngeal infections,
antibacterial therapy p. 1261, Respiratory system
infections, antibacterial therapy p. 538, Skin infections,

5

Infection

antibacterial therapy p. 541, Urinary-tract infections p. 626.

● PATIENT AND CARER ADVICE
Medicines for Children leaflet: Co-amoxiclav for bacterial infections
www.medicinesforchildren.org.uk/co-amoxiclav-bacterial-infections-0

● PROFESSION SPECIFIC INFORMATION

Dental practitioners' formulary
Co-amoxiclav 250/125 Tablets may be prescribed.
 Co-amoxiclav 125/31 Suspension may be prescribed.
 Co-amoxiclav 250/62 Suspension may be prescribed.

● MEDICINAL FORMS There can be variation in the licensing of different medicines containing the same drug. Forms available from special-order manufacturers include: infusion

Oral suspension
CAUTIONARY AND ADVISORY LABELS 9
EXCIPIENTS: May contain Aspartame
▸ Co-amoxiclav (Non-proprietary)
Clavulanic acid (as Potassium clavulanate) 6.25 mg per 1 ml, Amoxicillin (as Amoxicillin trihydrate) 25 mg per 1 ml Co-amoxiclav 125mg/31mg/5ml oral suspension | 100 ml [PoM] £5.00 DT = £5.00
Co-amoxiclav 125mg/31mg/5ml oral suspension sugar free sugar-free | 100 ml [PoM] £2.33 DT = £2.33
Clavulanic acid (as Potassium clavulanate) 12.5 mg per 1 ml, Amoxicillin (as Amoxicillin trihydrate) 50 mg per 1 ml Co-amoxiclav 250mg/62mg/5ml oral suspension | 100 ml [PoM] £5.00 DT = £5.00
Co-amoxiclav 250mg/62mg/5ml oral suspension sugar free sugar-free | 70 ml [PoM] £2.05 sugar-free | 100 ml [PoM] £2.06 DT = £1.87
Clavulanic acid (as Potassium clavulanate) 11.4 mg per 1 ml, Amoxicillin (as Amoxicillin trihydrate) 80 mg per 1 ml Co-amoxiclav 400mg/57mg/5ml oral suspension sugar free sugar-free | 35 ml [PoM] £4.13 DT = £4.13 sugar-free | 70 ml [PoM] £6.97 DT = £5.79
▸ Augmentin (GlaxoSmithKline UK Ltd)
Clavulanic acid (as Potassium clavulanate) 6.25 mg per 1 ml, Amoxicillin (as Amoxicillin trihydrate) 25 mg per 1 ml Augmentin 125/31 SF oral suspension sugar-free | 100 ml [PoM] £3.54 DT = £2.33
Clavulanic acid (as Potassium clavulanate) 12.5 mg per 1 ml, Amoxicillin (as Amoxicillin trihydrate) 50 mg per 1 ml Augmentin 250/62 SF oral suspension sugar-free | 100 ml [PoM] £3.60 DT = £1.87
▸ Augmentin-Duo (GlaxoSmithKline UK Ltd)
Clavulanic acid (as Potassium clavulanate) 11.4 mg per 1 ml, Amoxicillin (as Amoxicillin trihydrate) 80 mg per 1 ml Augmentin-Duo 400/57 oral suspension sugar-free | 35 ml [PoM] £4.13 DT = £4.13 sugar-free | 70 ml [PoM] £5.79 DT = £5.79

Tablet
CAUTIONARY AND ADVISORY LABELS 9
▸ Co-amoxiclav (Non-proprietary)
Clavulanic acid (as Potassium clavulanate) 125 mg, Amoxicillin (as Amoxicillin trihydrate) 250 mg Co-amoxiclav 250mg/125mg tablets | 21 tablet [PoM] £6.00 DT = £1.69
Clavulanic acid (as Potassium clavulanate) 125 mg, Amoxicillin (as Amoxicillin trihydrate) 500 mg Co-amoxiclav 500mg/125mg tablets | 21 tablet [PoM] £15.00 DT = £2.72
Clavulanic acid (as Potassium clavulanate) 125 mg, Amoxicillin (as Amoxicillin trihydrate) 875 mg Co-amoxiclav 875mg/125mg tablets | 14 tablet [PoM] £18.00 DT = £18.00
▸ Augmentin (GlaxoSmithKline UK Ltd)
Clavulanic acid (as Potassium clavulanate) 125 mg, Amoxicillin (as Amoxicillin trihydrate) 250 mg Augmentin 375mg tablets | 21 tablet [PoM] £5.03 DT = £1.69
Clavulanic acid (as Potassium clavulanate) 125 mg, Amoxicillin (as Amoxicillin trihydrate) 500 mg Augmentin 625mg tablets | 21 tablet [PoM] £9.60 DT = £2.72

Powder for solution for injection
ELECTROLYTES: May contain Potassium, sodium
▸ Co-amoxiclav (Non-proprietary)
Clavulanic acid (as Potassium clavulanate) 100 mg, Amoxicillin (as Amoxicillin sodium) 500 mg Co-amoxiclav 500mg/100mg powder for solution for injection vials | 10 vial [PoM] £10.60–£14.90 (Hospital only)
Clavulanic acid (as Potassium clavulanate) 200 mg, Amoxicillin (as Amoxicillin sodium) 1000 mg Co-amoxiclav 1000mg/200mg powder for solution for injection vials | 10 vial [PoM] £10.60–£39.70 (Hospital only)

▸ Augmentin Intravenous (GlaxoSmithKline UK Ltd)
Clavulanic acid (as Potassium clavulanate) 100 mg, Amoxicillin (as Amoxicillin sodium) 500 mg Augmentin Intravenous 600mg powder for solution for injection vials | 10 vial [PoM] £10.60 (Hospital only)
Clavulanic acid (as Potassium clavulanate) 200 mg, Amoxicillin (as Amoxicillin sodium) 1000 mg Augmentin Intravenous 1.2g powder for solution for injection vials | 10 vial [PoM] £10.60 (Hospital only)

ANTIBACTERIALS › PENICILLINS, MECILLINAM-TYPE

⚑ 578

Pivmecillinam hydrochloride
04-Aug-2020

● INDICATIONS AND DOSE

Acute uncomplicated cystitis
▸ BY MOUTH
▸ Child (body-weight 40 kg and above): Initially 400 mg for 1 dose, then 200 mg every 8 hours to a total of 10 tablets
▸ Adult (body-weight 40 kg and above): Initially 400 mg for 1 dose, then 200 mg every 8 hours to a total of 10 tablets

Chronic or recurrent bacteriuria
▸ BY MOUTH
▸ Child (body-weight 40 kg and above): 400 mg every 6–8 hours
▸ Adult (body-weight 40 kg and above): 400 mg every 6–8 hours

Urinary-tract infections
▸ BY MOUTH
▸ Child (body-weight up to 40 kg): 5–10 mg/kg every 6 hours, alternatively 20–40 mg/kg daily in 3 divided doses

● UNLICENSED USE
▸ In children Not licensed for use in children under 3 months.

● CONTRA-INDICATIONS Carnitine deficiency · gastro-intestinal obstruction · oesophageal strictures

● CAUTIONS Avoid in Acute porphyrias p. 1107

● INTERACTIONS → Appendix 1: penicillins

● SIDE-EFFECTS
▸ Common or very common Vulvovaginal fungal infection
▸ Uncommon Dizziness · fatigue · gastrointestinal discomfort · gastrointestinal disorders · headache · oral ulceration · vertigo

● PREGNANCY Not known to be harmful, but manufacturer advises avoid.

● BREAST FEEDING Trace amount in milk, but appropriate to use.

● MONITORING REQUIREMENTS Liver and renal function tests required in long-term use.

● EFFECT ON LABORATORY TESTS False positive urinary glucose (if tested for reducing substances). False positive newborn screening results for isovaleric acidaemia may occur in neonates born to mothers receiving pivmecillinam during late pregnancy.

● DIRECTIONS FOR ADMINISTRATION Manufacturer advises tablets should be swallowed whole with plenty of fluid during meals while sitting or standing.

● PATIENT AND CARER ADVICE Patient counselling is advised on administration of pivmecillinam hydrochloride tablets (posture).

● MEDICINAL FORMS There can be variation in the licensing of different medicines containing the same drug.

Tablet

CAUTIONARY AND ADVISORY LABELS 9, 21, 27

▸ Pivmecillinam hydrochloride (Non-proprietary)

Pivmecillinam hydrochloride 200 mg Pivmecillinam 200mg tablets | 10 tablet [PoM] £6.95 DT = £5.40

▸ Selexid (Karo Pharma)

Pivmecillinam hydrochloride 200 mg Selexid 200mg tablets | 10 tablet [PoM] £5.40 DT = £5.40 | 18 tablet [PoM] £9.72

ANTIBACTERIALS › PENICILLINS, PENICILLINASE-RESISTANT

▶ 578

Flucloxacillin

21-May-2020

● INDICATIONS AND DOSE

Infections due to beta-lactamase-producing staphylococci including otitis externa | Adjunct in pneumonia

▸ BY MOUTH
▹ Child 1 month-1 year: 62.5–125 mg 4 times a day
▹ Child 2-9 years: 125–250 mg 4 times a day
▹ Child 10-17 years: 250–500 mg 4 times a day
▹ Adult: 250–500 mg 4 times a day
▸ BY INTRAMUSCULAR INJECTION
▹ Adult: 250–500 mg every 6 hours
▸ BY SLOW INTRAVENOUS INJECTION, OR BY INTRAVENOUS INFUSION
▹ Adult: 0.25–2 g every 6 hours

Impetigo

▸ BY MOUTH
▹ Child 1 month-1 year: 62.5–125 mg 4 times a day for 5–7 days
▹ Child 2-9 years: 125–250 mg 4 times a day for 5–7 days
▹ Child 10-17 years: 250–500 mg 4 times a day for 5–7 days
▹ Adult: 500 mg 4 times a day for 5–7 days
▸ BY INTRAMUSCULAR INJECTION
▹ Adult: 250–500 mg every 6 hours
▸ BY SLOW INTRAVENOUS INJECTION, OR BY INTRAVENOUS INFUSION
▹ Adult: 0.25–2 g every 6 hours

Cellulitis | Erysipelas

▸ BY MOUTH
▹ Child 1 month-1 year: 62.5–125 mg 4 times a day for 5–7 days then review
▹ Child 2-9 years: 125–250 mg 4 times a day for 5–7 days then review
▹ Child 10-17 years: 250–500 mg 4 times a day for 5–7 days then review
▹ Adult: 0.5–1 g 4 times a day for 5–7 days then review
▸ BY SLOW INTRAVENOUS INJECTION, OR BY INTRAVENOUS INFUSION
▹ Adult: 1–2 g every 6 hours

Mild diabetic foot infection

▸ BY MOUTH
▹ Adult: 0.5–1 g 4 times a day for 7 days then review

Moderate diabetic foot infection | Severe diabetic foot infection

▸ BY MOUTH
▹ Adult: 1 g 4 times a day
▸ BY SLOW INTRAVENOUS INJECTION, OR BY INTRAVENOUS INFUSION
▹ Adult: 1–2 g every 6 hours

Leg ulcer infection

▸ BY MOUTH
▹ Adult: 0.5–1 g 4 times a day for 7 days
▸ BY SLOW INTRAVENOUS INJECTION, OR BY INTRAVENOUS INFUSION
▹ Adult: 1–2 g every 6 hours

Endocarditis (in combination with other antibacterial if necessary)

▸ BY SLOW INTRAVENOUS INJECTION, OR BY INTRAVENOUS INFUSION
▹ Adult (body-weight up to 85 kg): 8 g daily in 4 divided doses
▹ Adult (body-weight 85 kg and above): 12 g daily in 6 divided doses

Osteomyelitis

▸ BY SLOW INTRAVENOUS INJECTION, OR BY INTRAVENOUS INFUSION
▹ Adult: Up to 8 g daily in 3–4 divided doses

Surgical prophylaxis

▸ INITIALLY BY SLOW INTRAVENOUS INJECTION, OR BY INTRAVENOUS INFUSION
▹ Adult: 1–2 g, to be administered up to 30 minutes before the procedure, then (by mouth or by intramuscular injection or by slow intravenous injection or by intravenous infusion) 500 mg every 6 hours if required for up to 4 further doses in high risk procedures

Staphylococcal lung infection in cystic fibrosis

▸ BY MOUTH
▹ Child: 25 mg/kg 4 times a day (max. per dose 1 g), alternatively 100 mg/kg daily in 3 divided doses; maximum 4 g per day

Prevention of *Staphylococcus aureus* lung infection in cystic fibrosis—primary prevention

▸ BY MOUTH
▹ Child 1 month-3 years: 125 mg twice daily

Prevention of *Staphylococcus aureus* lung infection in cystic fibrosis—secondary prevention

▸ BY MOUTH
▹ Child: 50 mg/kg twice daily (max. per dose 1 g twice daily)

● UNLICENSED USE Flucloxacillin doses in the BNF may differ from those in product literature.

IMPORTANT SAFETY INFORMATION

HEPATIC DISORDERS

Cholestatic jaundice and hepatitis may occur very rarely, up to two months after treatment with flucloxacillin has been stopped. Administration for more than 2 weeks and increasing age are risk factors. Manufacturer advises:

● flucloxacillin should not be used in patients with a history of hepatic dysfunction associated with flucloxacillin
● flucloxacillin should be used with caution in patients with hepatic impairment
● careful enquiry should be made about hypersensitivity reactions to beta-lactam antibacterials

---

● CAUTIONS
» With intravenous use accumulation of electrolytes can occur with high doses

● INTERACTIONS → Appendix 1: penicillins

● SIDE-EFFECTS

GENERAL SIDE-EFFECTS

▶ Rare or very rare Fever

SPECIFIC SIDE-EFFECTS

▶ Common or very common
» With oral use Gastrointestinal disorder
▶ Rare or very rare
» With oral use Eosinophilia · myalgia
▶ Frequency not known
» With parenteral use Bronchospasm · coma · dyspnoea · electrolyte imbalance · erythema nodosum · hallucination · Jarisch-Herxheimer reaction · nephropathy · neurotoxicity

5

Infection

· oral candidiasis · platelet dysfunction · purpura non-thrombocytopenic · vasculitis
- PREGNANCY Not known to be harmful.
- BREAST FEEDING Trace amounts in milk, but appropriate to use.
- HEPATIC IMPAIRMENT Manufacturer advises caution; including in those with risk factors for hepatic reactions.
- RENAL IMPAIRMENT
▸ With intravenous use Accumulation of electrolytes can occur in patients with renal failure.
  Dose adjustments ▸ In adults Reduce dose if eGFR less than 10 mL/minute/1.73 m².
  ▸ In children Use normal dose every 8 hours if estimated glomerular filtration rate less than 10 mL/minute/1.73 m².
- EFFECT ON LABORATORY TESTS False-positive urinary glucose (if tested for reducing substances).
- DIRECTIONS FOR ADMINISTRATION For *intravenous infusion* (*Floxapen*®), give intermittently *in* Glucose 5% *or* Sodium chloride 0.9%; suggested volume 100 mL given over 30–60 minutes. *Via* drip tubing *in* Glucose 5% *or* Sodium chloride 0.9%; continuous infusion not usually recommended.
- PRESCRIBING AND DISPENSING INFORMATION For choice of antibacterial therapy, see Antibacterials, use for prophylaxis p. 529, Cardiovascular system infections, antibacterial therapy p. 532, Diabetic foot infections, antibacterial therapy p. 534, Ear infections, antibacterial therapy p. 534, Musculoskeletal system infections, antibacterial therapy p. 536, Respiratory system infections, antibacterial therapy p. 538, Skin infections, antibacterial therapy p. 541.
- PATIENT AND CARER ADVICE
Medicines for Children leaflet: Flucloxacillin for bacterial infections
www.medicinesforchildren.org.uk/flucloxacillin-bacterial-infections

- MEDICINAL FORMS There can be variation in the licensing of different medicines containing the same drug. Forms available from special-order manufacturers include: infusion

Oral solution
CAUTIONARY AND ADVISORY LABELS 9, 23
▸ Flucloxacillin (Non-proprietary)
  Flucloxacillin (as Flucloxacillin sodium) 25 mg per 1 ml Flucloxacillin 125mg/5ml oral solution | 100 ml [PoM] £20.99 DT = £2.17
  Flucloxacillin 125mg/5ml oral solution sugar free sugar-free | 100 ml [PoM] £18.79 DT = £16.55
  Flucloxacillin (as Flucloxacillin sodium) 50 mg per 1 ml Flucloxacillin 250mg/5ml oral solution sugar free sugar-free | 100 ml [PoM] £19.04 DT = £17.08
  Flucloxacillin 250mg/5ml oral solution | 100 ml [PoM] £47.10 DT = £6.39

Capsule
CAUTIONARY AND ADVISORY LABELS 9, 23
▸ Flucloxacillin (Non-proprietary)
  Flucloxacillin (as Flucloxacillin sodium) 250 mg Flucloxacillin 250mg capsules | 28 capsule [PoM] £1.80 DT = £1.80 | 100 capsule [PoM] £6.43–£17.80
  Flucloxacillin (as Flucloxacillin sodium) 500 mg Flucloxacillin 500mg capsules | 28 capsule [PoM] £10.50 DT = £2.45 | 100 capsule [PoM] £8.75–£37.50

Powder for solution for injection
▸ Flucloxacillin (Non-proprietary)
  Flucloxacillin (as Flucloxacillin sodium) 250 mg Flucloxacillin 250mg powder for solution for injection vials | 10 vial [PoM] £8.60–£12.25 DT = £8.60 (Hospital only)
  Flucloxacillin (as Flucloxacillin sodium) 500 mg Flucloxacillin 500mg powder for solution for injection vials | 10 vial [PoM] £17.20–£35.00 DT = £17.20 (Hospital only)
  Flucloxacillin (as Flucloxacillin sodium) 1 gram Flucloxacillin 1g powder for solution for injection vials | 10 vial [PoM] £34.50–£49.00 DT = £34.50 (Hospital only)

Flucloxacillin (as Flucloxacillin sodium) 2 gram Flucloxacillin 2g powder for solution for injection vials | 1 vial [PoM] £6.00 DT = £6.00 (Hospital only)

Combinations available: *Co-fluampicil*, p. 585

F 578

Temocillin

22-May-2020

- INDICATIONS AND DOSE

Septicaemia | Urinary-tract infections | Lower respiratory-tract infections caused by susceptible Gram-negative bacteria
▸ BY INTRAMUSCULAR INJECTION, OR BY SLOW INTRAVENOUS INJECTION, OR BY INTRAVENOUS INFUSION
▸ Adult: 2 g every 12 hours, alternatively 2 g every 8 hours, higher daily dose to be used in critically ill patients
▸ BY CONTINUOUS INTRAVENOUS INFUSION
▸ Adult: (consult product literature)

- CAUTIONS Accumulation of sodium from injection can occur with high doses
- INTERACTIONS → Appendix 1: penicillins
- SIDE-EFFECTS Fever · myalgia · nervous system disorder · thrombophlebitis
- PREGNANCY Not known to be harmful.
- BREAST FEEDING Trace amounts in milk.
- RENAL IMPAIRMENT Accumulation of sodium from injection can occur in patients with renal failure.
  Dose adjustments Manufacturer advises reduce usual dose to 1 g every 12 hours if creatinine clearance 30–60 mL/minute; reduce usual dose to 1 g every 24 hours if creatinine clearance 10–30 mL/minute; reduce usual dose to 1 g every 48 hours *or* 500 mg every 24 hours if creatinine clearance less than 10 mL/minute; no information available to recommend dose adjustments with higher daily dose for use in critically ill patients.
- EFFECT ON LABORATORY TESTS False-positive urinary glucose (if tested for reducing substances).
- DIRECTIONS FOR ADMINISTRATION Manufacturer advises for *intramuscular injection*, reconstitute 1 g with 2 mL water for injections *or* Sodium chloride 0.9% *(or* 0.5 or 1% lidocaine solution, if pain is experienced at injection site). Manufacturer advises for *slow intravenous injection*, reconstitute 1 g with 10 mL water for injections *or* Sodium chloride 0.9%; give over 3–4 minutes. Manufacturer advises for *intermittent intravenous infusion*, give in Glucose 5% or 10% *or* Sodium chloride 0.9% *or* Ringer's solution *or* Lactated Ringer's solution. Reconstitute 1 g with 10 mL water for injections *or* infusion fluid, then dilute in up to 150 mL infusion fluid; give over 30–40 minutes. For *continuous intravenous infusion*, consult product literature.

- MEDICINAL FORMS There can be variation in the licensing of different medicines containing the same drug.
Powder for solution for injection
ELECTROLYTES: May contain Sodium
▸ Negaban (Eumedica Pharmaceuticals)
  Temocillin (as Temocillin sodium) 1 gram Negaban 1g powder for solution for injection vials | 1 vial [PoM] £25.45 DT = £25.45 (Hospital only)

Colistimethate sodium

13-Nov-2020

(Colistin sulfomethate sodium)

- **DRUG ACTION** The polymyxin antibiotic, colistimethate sodium (colistin sulfomethate sodium), is active against Gram-negative organisms including *Pseudomonas aeruginosa*, *Acinetobacter baumanii*, and *Klebsiella pneumoniae*. It is not absorbed by mouth and thus needs to be given by injection for a systemic effect.

- **INDICATIONS AND DOSE**

Serious infections due to selected aerobic Gram-negative bacteria in patients with limited treatment options

▸ BY INTRAVENOUS INFUSION

▸ Adult: 9 million units daily in 2–3 divided doses, an initial loading dose of 9 million units should be used in those who are critically ill, loading and maintenance doses of up to 12 million units may be required in some cases, however clinical experience is limited and safety has not been established—consult product literature for details

Management of chronic pulmonary infections due to *Pseudomonas aeruginosa* in patients with cystic fibrosis

▸ BY INHALATION OF NEBULISED SOLUTION

▸ Child 2-17 years: 1–2 million units 2–3 times a day, for specific advice on administration using nebulisers—consult product literature; maximum 6 million units per day

▸ Adult: 1–2 million units 2–3 times a day, for specific advice on administration using nebulisers—consult product literature; maximum 6 million units per day

▸ BY INHALATION OF POWDER

▸ Adult: 1.66 million units twice daily

- **CONTRA-INDICATIONS** Myasthenia gravis

- **CAUTIONS**

▸ When used by inhalation Severe haemoptysis—risk of further haemorrhage

- **INTERACTIONS** → Appendix 1: colistimethate

- **SIDE-EFFECTS**

▸ **Common or very common**

▸ When used by inhalation Arthralgia · asthenia · asthma · balance impaired · chest discomfort · cough · dysphonia · dyspnoea · fever · haemorrhage · headache · lower respiratory tract infection · nausea · respiratory disorders · taste altered · throat complaints · tinnitus · vomiting

▸ **Uncommon**

▸ When used by inhalation Anxiety · appetite decreased · diarrhoea · drowsiness · ear congestion · flatulence · oral disorders · proteinuria · seizure · sputum purulent · thirst · weight change

▸ **Rare or very rare**

▸ With parenteral use Confusion · nephrotoxicity · presyncope · psychosis · speech slurred · visual impairment

▸ **Frequency not known**

▸ With parenteral use Apnoea · neurological effects · neurotoxicity · renal disorder · sensory disorder

SIDE-EFFECTS, FURTHER INFORMATION Neurotoxicity and nephrotoxicity are dose-related.

- **PREGNANCY**

▸ When used by inhalation Clinical use suggests probably safe.

▸ With intravenous use Manufacturer advises use only if potential benefit outweighs risk.

- **BREAST FEEDING** Present in milk but poorly absorbed from gut; manufacturers advise avoid (or use only if potential benefit outweighs risk).

- **HEPATIC IMPAIRMENT**

▸ With intravenous use Manufacturer advises caution (no information available).

- **RENAL IMPAIRMENT**

▸ When used by inhalation Manufacturer advises caution.

Dose adjustments ▸ With intravenous use in adults Manufacturer advises reduce maintenance dose if creatinine clearance less than 50 mL/minute—consult product literature.

Monitoring ▸ With intravenous use In renal impairment, monitor plasma colistimethate sodium concentration during parenteral treatment—consult product literature. Recommended 'peak' plasma colistimethate sodium concentration (approx. 1 hour after intravenous injection or infusion) 5–15 mg/litre; pre-dose ('trough') concentration 2–6 mg/litre.

- **MONITORING REQUIREMENTS**

▸ With intravenous use Monitor renal function.

▸ When used by inhalation Measure lung function before and after initial dose of colistimethate sodium and monitor for bronchospasm; if bronchospasm occurs in a patient not using a bronchodilator, repeat test using a bronchodilator before the dose of colistimethate sodium.

- **DIRECTIONS FOR ADMINISTRATION**

▸ When used by inhalation Manufacturer advises if other treatments are being administered, they should be taken in the order recommended by the physician. For *nebulisation*, consult product literature for information on reconstitution and dilution.

▸ With intravenous use in adults For *intravenous infusion*, manufacturer advises following reconstitution, dilute requisite dose, usually with 50 mL Sodium Chloride 0.9%; give over 30–60 minutes. Patients fitted with a totally implantable venous access device may tolerate an injection. For *slow intravenous injection* into a totally implantable venous access device, dilute to a concentration of 200 000 units/mL with Sodium Chloride 0.9%; give over at least 5 minutes.

- **PRESCRIBING AND DISPENSING INFORMATION** Colistimethate sodium is included in some preparations for topical application.

- **PATIENT AND CARER ADVICE**

▸ When used by inhalation Patient should be advised to rinse mouth with water after each dose of dry powder inhalation. Patients or carers should be given advice on how to administer colistimethate sodium; first dose should be given under medical supervision.

Driving and skilled tasks Manufacturer advises patients and carers should be counselled on the effects on driving and performance of skilled tasks—increased risk of dizziness, confusion and visual disturbances.

- **NATIONAL FUNDING/ACCESS DECISIONS** For full details see funding body website

NICE decisions

▸ **Colistimethate sodium and tobramycin dry powders for inhalation for treating pseudomonas lung infection in cystic fibrosis (March 2013)** NICE TA276 Recommended with restrictions

- **MEDICINAL FORMS** There can be variation in the licensing of different medicines containing the same drug.

Powder for solution for injection

ELECTROLYTES: May contain Sodium

▸ Colistimethate sodium (Non-proprietary)

Colistimethate sodium 1000000 unit Colistimethate 1million unit powder for solution for injection vials | 10 vial [PoM] £30.00 DT = £18.00 (Hospital only)

▸ Colomycin (Teva UK Ltd)

Colistimethate sodium 1000000 unit Colomycin 1million unit powder for solution for injection vials | 10 vial [PoM] £18.00 DT = £18.00 (Hospital only)

5

Infection

5

Infection

Colistimethate sodium 2000000 unit Colomycin 2million unit powder for solution for injection vials | 10 vial [PoM] £32.40 DT = £32.40

▸ Promixin (Profile Pharma Ltd)
Colistimethate sodium 1000000 unit Promixin 1million unit powder for solution for injection vials | 10 vial [PoM] £37.50 DT = £18.00 (Hospital only)

Inhalation powder

▸ Colobreathe (Teva UK Ltd)
Colistimethate sodium 1662500 unit Colobreathe 1,662,500unit inhalation powder capsules | 56 capsule [PoM] £968.80 DT = £968.80

Powder for nebuliser solution

▸ Promixin (Profile Pharma Ltd)
Colistimethate sodium 1000000 unit Promixin 1million unit powder for nebuliser solution unit dose vials | 30 unit dose [PoM] £204.00 DT = £204.00

ANTIBACTERIALS > QUINOLONES

Quinolones

31-Oct-2017

MHRA/CHM advice: Systemic and inhaled fluoroquinolones (November 2018, and March 2019)

The MHRA and CHM have released important safety information regarding the use of systemic and inhaled fluoroquinolones. For restrictions and precautions, see *Important safety information* for all quinolones: ciprofloxacin p. 593, levofloxacin p. 595, moxifloxacin p. 596, and ofloxacin p. 597.

Overview

In the UK, only fluoroquinolones are available; the recommendations below therefore refer to the use of fluoroquinolones.

Ciprofloxacin is active against both Gram-positive and Gram-negative bacteria. It is particularly active against Gram-negative bacteria, including *Salmonella*, *Shigella*, *Campylobacter*, *Neisseria*, and *Pseudomonas*. Ciprofloxacin has only moderate activity against Gram-positive bacteria such as *Streptococcus pneumoniae* and *Enterococcus faecalis*; it should not be used for pneumococcal pneumonia. It is active against *Chlamydia* and some mycobacteria. Most anaerobic organisms are not susceptible. Ciprofloxacin can be used for respiratory tract infections (but not for pneumococcal pneumonia), infections of the gastro-intestinal system (including typhoid fever), bone and joint infections, gonorrhoea and septicaemia caused by sensitive organisms.

Ofloxacin is licensed for urinary-tract infections, lower respiratory-tract infections, gonorrhoea, and non-gonococcal urethritis and cervicitis.

Levofloxacin is active against Gram-positive and Gram-negative organisms. It has greater activity against *Pneumococci* than ciprofloxacin.

Many *Staphylococci* are resistant to quinolones and their use should be avoided in MRSA infections.

Moxifloxacin is active against Gram-positive and Gram-negative organisms. It has greater activity against Gram-positive organisms, including *Pneumococci*, than ciprofloxacin. Moxifloxacin is not active against *Pseudomonas aeruginosa* or meticillin-resistant *Staphylococcus aureus* (MRSA).

Quinolones

IMPORTANT SAFETY INFORMATION

▸ With intravenous use or oral use or when used by inhalation
The CSM has warned that quinolones may induce **convulsions** in patients with or without a history of convulsions; taking NSAIDs at the same time may also induce them.

TENDON DAMAGE

▸ With intravenous use or oral use or when used by inhalation
Tendon damage (including rupture) has been reported rarely in patients receiving quinolones. Tendon rupture may occur within 48 hours of starting treatment; cases have also been reported several months after stopping a quinolone. Healthcare professionals are reminded that:

● quinolones are contra-indicated in patients with a history of tendon disorders related to quinolone use;
● patients over 60 years of age are more prone to tendon damage;
● the risk of tendon damage is increased by the concomitant use of corticosteroids;
● if tendinitis is suspected, the quinolone should be discontinued immediately.

MHRA/CHM ADVICE: SYSTEMIC AND INHALED FLUOROQUINOLONES: SMALL INCREASED RISK OF AORTIC ANEURYSM AND DISSECTION; ADVICE FOR PRESCRIBING IN HIGH-RISK PATIENTS (NOVEMBER 2018)

▸ With intravenous use or oral use or when used by inhalation
The MHRA advises that benefit-risk should be assessed and other therapeutic options considered before using fluoroquinolones in patients at risk of aortic aneurysm and dissection. Patients (particularly the elderly and those at risk) and their carers should be informed about rare events of aortic aneurysm and dissection, and advised to seek immediate medical attention if sudden-onset severe abdominal, chest, or back pain develops.

MHRA/CHM ADVICE: FLUOROQUINOLONE ANTIBIOTICS: NEW RESTRICTIONS AND PRECAUTIONS FOR USE DUE TO VERY RARE REPORTS OF DISABLING AND POTENTIALLY LONG-LASTING OR IRREVERSIBLE SIDE EFFECTS (MARCH 2019)

▸ With intravenous use or oral use or when used by inhalation in adults

Disabling, long-lasting or potentially irreversible adverse reactions affecting musculoskeletal and nervous systems have been reported very rarely with fluoroquinolone antibiotics. Healthcare professionals are advised to inform patients to stop treatment at the first signs of a serious adverse reaction, such as tendinitis or tendon rupture, muscle pain, muscle weakness, joint pain, joint swelling, peripheral neuropathy, and CNS effects, and to contact their doctor immediately. Fluoroquinolones should not be prescribed for non-severe or self-limiting infections, or non-bacterial conditions. Unless other commonly recommended antibiotics are inappropriate, fluoroquinolones should not be prescribed for some mild to moderate infections, such as acute exacerbation of chronic bronchitis and chronic obstructive pulmonary disease, and ciprofloxacin or levofloxacin should not be prescribed for uncomplicated cystitis. Fluoroquinolones should be avoided in patients who have previously had serious adverse reactions. Use of fluoroquinolones with corticosteroids should also be avoided as it may exacerbate fluoroquinolone-induced tendinitis and tendon rupture. Fluoroquinolones should be prescribed with caution in patients older than 60 years and in patients with renal impairment or solid-organ transplants as they are at a higher risk of tendon injury.

MHRA/CHM ADVICE: FLUOROQUINOLONE ANTIBIOTICS: NEW RESTRICTIONS AND PRECAUTIONS FOR USE DUE TO VERY RARE REPORTS OF DISABLING AND POTENTIALLY LONG-LASTING OR IRREVERSIBLE SIDE EFFECTS (MARCH 2019)

▸ With intravenous use or oral use in children
Disabling, long-lasting or potentially irreversible adverse reactions affecting musculoskeletal and nervous systems have been reported very rarely with fluoroquinolone antibiotics. Healthcare professionals are advised to inform patients to stop treatment at the first signs of a serious adverse reaction, such as tendinitis or tendon rupture, muscle pain, muscle weakness, joint pain, joint swelling, peripheral neuropathy, and CNS effects, and to

5

Infection

contact their doctor immediately. Fluoroquinolones should not be prescribed for non-severe or self-limiting infections, or non-bacterial infections. Unless other commonly recommended antibiotics are inappropriate, fluoroquinolones should not be prescribed for mild to moderate infections. Fluoroquinolones should be avoided in patients who have previously had serious adverse reactions. Use of fluoroquinolones with corticosteroids should also be avoided as it may exacerbate fluoroquinolone-induced tendinitis and tendon rupture. Fluoroquinolones should be prescribed with caution in patients with renal impairment or solid-organ transplants as they are at a higher risk of tendon injury.

● CONTRA-INDICATIONS
▸ With intravenous use or oral use or when used by inhalation History of tendon disorders related to quinolone use
● CAUTIONS
▸ With intravenous use or oral use or when used by inhalation Can prolong the QT interval · conditions that predispose to seizures · diabetes (may affect blood glucose) · exposure to excessive sunlight and UV radiation should be avoided during treatment and for 48 hours after stopping treatment · G6PD deficiency · history of epilepsy · myasthenia gravis (risk of exacerbation) · psychiatric disorders
▸ With intravenous use or oral use Children or adolescents (arthropathy has developed in weight-bearing joints in young *animals*)
  CAUTIONS, FURTHER INFORMATION
▸ With intravenous use or oral use in children Quinolones cause arthropathy in the weight-bearing joints of immature *animals* and are therefore generally not recommended in children and growing adolescents. However, the significance of this effect in humans is uncertain and in some specific circumstances use of ciprofloxacin may be justified in children.
● SIDE-EFFECTS
▸ **Common or very common** Appetite decreased · arthralgia · asthenia · constipation · diarrhoea · dizziness · dyspnoea · eye discomfort · eye disorders · fever · fungal infection · gastrointestinal discomfort · headache · myalgia · nausea · QT interval prolongation · skin reactions · sleep disorders · taste altered · tinnitus · vision disorders · vomiting
▸ **Uncommon** Altered smell sensation · anaemia · anxiety · arrhythmias · chest pain · confusion · cough · depression · drowsiness · dry eye · eosinophilia · eye inflammation · flatulence · hallucination · hearing impairment · hepatic disorders · hyperglycaemia · hyperhidrosis · hypersensitivity · hypoglycaemia · hypotension · leucopenia · muscle weakness · neutropenia · pain · palpitations · peripheral neuropathy (sometimes irreversible) · pseudomembranous enterocolitis (in adults) · renal impairment · seizure · sensation abnormal · stomatitis · tendon disorders · thrombocytopenia · tremor · vertigo
▸ **Rare or very rare** Agranulocytosis · angioedema · arthritis · coordination abnormal · gait abnormal · haemolytic anaemia · idiopathic intracranial hypertension · myasthenia gravis aggravated · pancreatitis · photosensitivity reaction · polyneuropathy · psychotic disorder · severe cutaneous adverse reactions (SCARs) · suicidal behaviours · syncope · vasculitis
▸ **Frequency not known** Hypoglycaemic coma · increased risk of aortic aneurysm (more common in elderly) · increased risk of aortic dissection (more common in elderly)
  SIDE-EFFECTS, FURTHER INFORMATION The drug should be discontinued if neurological, psychiatric, tendon disorders or hypersensitivity reactions (including severe rash) occur.

For more information regarding the safety of fluoroquinolones, please see Important Safety Information.
● ALLERGY AND CROSS-SENSITIVITY EvGr Use of quinolones contra-indicated in quinolone hypersensitivity. ◈
● PREGNANCY
▸ With intravenous use or oral use or when used by inhalation Avoid in pregnancy—shown to cause arthropathy in *animal* studies; safer alternatives are available.
● PATIENT AND CARER ADVICE
▸ With intravenous use or oral use or when used by inhalation The MHRA has produced an advice sheet on serious adverse reactions affecting musculoskeletal and nervous systems associated with fluoroquinolone use, which should be provided to patients and their carers.

F 592

Ciprofloxacin

18-Nov-2020

● INDICATIONS AND DOSE

Moderate diabetic foot infection | Severe diabetic foot infection
▸ BY MOUTH
▸ Adult: 500 mg twice daily
▸ BY INTRAVENOUS INFUSION
▸ Adult: 400 mg every 8–12 hours, to be given over 60 minutes

Fistulating Crohn's disease
▸ BY MOUTH
▸ Adult: 500 mg twice daily

Acute diverticulitis [in combination with metronidazole] (administered on expert advice)
▸ BY MOUTH
▸ Adult: 500 mg twice daily for 5 days then review
▸ BY INTRAVENOUS INFUSION
▸ Adult: 400 mg every 8–12 hours, to be given over 60 minutes

Respiratory-tract infections
▸ BY MOUTH
▸ Adult: 500–750 mg twice daily
▸ BY INTRAVENOUS INFUSION
▸ Adult: 400 mg every 8–12 hours, to be given over 60 minutes

Pseudomonal lower respiratory-tract infection in cystic fibrosis
▸ BY MOUTH
▸ Adult: 750 mg twice daily

Urinary-tract infections
▸ BY MOUTH
▸ Adult: 250–750 mg twice daily
▸ BY INTRAVENOUS INFUSION
▸ Adult: 400 mg every 8–12 hours, to be given over 60 minutes

Acute prostatitis
▸ BY MOUTH
▸ Adult: 500 mg twice daily for 14 days then carry out a clinical assessment to decide whether to continue for a further 14 days
▸ BY INTRAVENOUS INFUSION
▸ Adult: 400 mg every 8–12 hours

Uncomplicated gonorrhoea [anogenital and pharyngeal infection, when sensitivity confirmed]
▸ BY MOUTH
▸ Adult: 500 mg for 1 dose

continued →

Disseminated gonococcal infection [when sensitivity confirmed]
▶ BY INTRAVENOUS INFUSION
▸ Adult: 500 mg every 12 hours for 7 days, may be switched 24–48 hours after symptoms improve to a suitable oral antibacterial
▶ BY MOUTH
▸ Adult: 500 mg twice daily, following intravenous antibacterial treatment, starting 24–48 hours after symptoms improve, to give 7 days treatment in total

Most other infections
▶ BY MOUTH
▸ Adult: Initially 500 mg twice daily; increased to 750 mg twice daily, in severe or deep-seated infection
▶ BY INTRAVENOUS INFUSION
▸ Adult: 400 mg every 8–12 hours, to be given over 60 minutes

Surgical prophylaxis
▶ BY MOUTH
▸ Adult: 750 mg, to be taken 60 minutes before procedure

Anthrax (treatment and post-exposure prophylaxis)
▶ BY MOUTH
▸ Adult: 500 mg twice daily
▶ BY INTRAVENOUS INFUSION
▸ Adult: 400 mg every 12 hours, to be given over 60 minutes

Prevention of secondary case of meningococcal meningitis
▶ BY MOUTH
▸ Child 1 month-4 years: 30 mg/kg (max. per dose 125 mg) for 1 dose
▸ Child 5-11 years: 250 mg for 1 dose
▸ Child 12-17 years: 500 mg for 1 dose
▸ Adult: 500 mg for 1 dose

Acute pyelonephritis | Urinary tract infection (catheter-associated)
▶ BY MOUTH
▸ Adult: 500 mg twice daily for 7 days
▶ BY INTRAVENOUS INFUSION
▸ Adult: 400 mg every 8–12 hours

● UNLICENSED USE [EvGr] Ciprofloxacin is used for the treatment of disseminated gonococcal infection, ⚠ but is not licensed for this indication.
   Not licensed for use in children under 1 year of age. Not licensed for use in children for prophylaxis of meningococcal meningitis.

● CAUTIONS Acute myocardial infarction (risk factor for QT interval prolongation) · avoid excessive alkalinity of urine (risk of crystalluria) · bradycardia (risk factor for QT interval prolongation) · congenital long QT syndrome (risk factor for QT interval prolongation) · electrolyte disturbances (risk factor for QT interval prolongation) · ensure adequate fluid intake (risk of crystalluria) · heart failure with reduced left ventricular ejection fraction (risk factor for QT interval prolongation) · history of symptomatic arrhythmias (risk factor for QT interval prolongation)

● INTERACTIONS → Appendix 1: quinolones

● SIDE-EFFECTS
▶ **Common or very common** Arthropathy (in children)
▶ **Uncommon** Akathisia · fungal superinfection · oedema · thrombocytosis · vasodilation
▶ **Rare or very rare** Antibiotic associated colitis · asthma · bone marrow disorders · crystalluria · erythema nodosum · haematuria · intracranial pressure increased · leucocytosis · migraine · muscle cramps · muscle tone increased · nephritis tubulointerstitial · oedema · olfactory nerve disorder · status epilepticus · thrombocytosis · vasodilation
▶ **Frequency not known** Mood altered · self-injurious behaviour

● PREGNANCY A single dose of ciprofloxacin may be used for the prevention of a secondary case of meningococcal meningitis.

● BREAST FEEDING Amount too small to be harmful but manufacturer advises avoid.

● RENAL IMPAIRMENT
Dose adjustments ▸ With oral use in adults Give 250–500 mg every 12 hours if eGFR 30–60 mL/minute/1.73 m² (every 24 hours if eGFR less than 30 mL/minute/1.73 m²).
▸ With intravenous use in adults Give (200 mg over 30 minutes), 200–400 mg every 12 hours if eGFR 30–60 mL/minute/1.73m² (every 24 hours if eGFR less than 30 mL/minute/1.73 m²).
▸ In children Reduce dose if estimated glomerular filtration rate less than 30 mL/minute/1.73 m²—consult product literature.

● PRESCRIBING AND DISPENSING INFORMATION For choice of antibacterial therapy, see Antibacterials, use for prophylaxis p. 529, Anthrax p. 613, Diabetic foot infections, antibacterial therapy p. 534, Ear infections, antibacterial therapy p. 534, Gastro-intestinal system infections, antibacterial therapy p. 535, Genital system infections, antibacterial therapy p. 536, Respiratory system infections, antibacterial therapy p. 538, Urinary-tract infections p. 626.

● PATIENT AND CARER ADVICE
Medicines for Children leaflet: Ciprofloxacin for bacterial infections www.medicinesforchildren.org.uk/ciprofloxacin-bacterial-infection

Driving and skilled tasks May impair performance of skilled tasks (e.g. driving); effects enhanced by alcohol.

● MEDICINAL FORMS There can be variation in the licensing of different medicines containing the same drug. Forms available from special-order manufacturers include: oral suspension

Tablet
CAUTIONARY AND ADVISORY LABELS 7, 9, 25
▸ Ciprofloxacin (Non-proprietary)
   Ciprofloxacin (as Ciprofloxacin hydrochloride)
   100 mg Ciprofloxacin 100mg tablets | 6 tablet [PoM] £4.50 DT = £2.11
   Ciprofloxacin (as Ciprofloxacin hydrochloride)
   250 mg Ciprofloxacin 250mg tablets | 10 tablet [PoM] £7.21 DT = £0.82 | 20 tablet [PoM] £1.64-£14.42 | 100 tablet [PoM] £7.90
   Ciprofloxacin (as Ciprofloxacin hydrochloride)
   500 mg Ciprofloxacin 500mg tablets | 10 tablet [PoM] £12.49 DT = £1.36 | 20 tablet [PoM] £1.84-£27.29 | 100 tablet [PoM] £9.10-£18.60
   Ciprofloxacin (as Ciprofloxacin hydrochloride)
   750 mg Ciprofloxacin 750mg tablets | 10 tablet [PoM] £17.78 DT = £8.00 | 20 tablet [PoM] £15.99
▸ Ciproxin (Bayer Plc)
   Ciprofloxacin (as Ciprofloxacin hydrochloride) 500 mg Ciproxin 500mg tablets | 10 tablet [PoM] £12.49 DT = £1.36

Oral suspension
CAUTIONARY AND ADVISORY LABELS 7, 9, 25
▸ Ciproxin (Bayer Plc)
   Ciprofloxacin 50 mg per 1 ml Ciproxin 250mg/5ml oral suspension | 100 ml [PoM] £21.29 DT = £21.29

Solution for infusion
ELECTROLYTES: May contain Sodium
▸ Ciprofloxacin (Non-proprietary)
   Ciprofloxacin (as Ciprofloxacin lactate) 2 mg per 1 ml Ciprofloxacin 200mg/100ml solution for infusion vials | 1 vial [PoM] £10.00
   Ciprofloxacin 200mg/100ml solution for infusion bottles | 10 bottle [PoM] £131.00-£144.50 (Hospital only)
   Ciprofloxacin 100mg/50ml solution for infusion vials | 1 vial [PoM] £10.00
   Ciprofloxacin 400mg/200ml solution for infusion bottles | 1 bottle [PoM] £10.00 (Hospital only) | 10 bottle [PoM] £195.90-£199.20 (Hospital only)
   Ciprofloxacin 400mg/200ml solution for infusion vials | 1 vial [PoM] £10.00

▸ Ciproxin (Bayer Plc)

Ciprofloxacin (as Ciprofloxacin lactate) 2 mg per 1 ml Ciproxin 100mg/50ml solution for infusion bottles | 1 bottle PoM £7.61 (Hospital only)

Ciproxin 200mg/100ml solution for infusion bottles | 1 bottle PoM £15.01 (Hospital only)

Ciproxin 400mg/200ml solution for infusion bottles | 1 bottle PoM £22.85 (Hospital only) | 5 bottle PoM £114.23 (Hospital only)

Infusion

▸ Ciprofloxacin (Non-proprietary)

Ciprofloxacin (as Ciprofloxacin lactate) 2 mg per 1 ml Ciprofloxacin 200mg/100ml infusion bags | 5 bag PoM £60.00 (Hospital only) | 10 bag PoM £120.00 (Hospital only)

Ciprofloxacin 400mg/200ml infusion bags | 5 bag PoM £85.00 (Hospital only) | 10 bag PoM £170.00-£228.46 (Hospital only)

⚑ 592

Delafloxacin

18-Aug-2020

● **INDICATIONS AND DOSE**

Acute bacterial skin and skin structure infections

▸ BY INTRAVENOUS INFUSION
▸ Adult: 300 mg every 12 hours for 5–14 days, to be given over 60 minutes, switch from intravenous to oral route when clinically appropriate

▸ BY MOUTH
▸ Adult: 450 mg twice daily for 5–14 days

● INTERACTIONS → Appendix 1: quinolones

● SIDE-EFFECTS
▸ **Common or very common** Hypertransaminasaemia
▸ **Uncommon** Alopecia · auditory hallucinations · chills · dry mouth · dry throat · flushing · gastrointestinal disorders · haematuria · hypertension · increased risk of infection · local swelling · muscle spasms · myositis · oral disorders · peripheral oedema · seasonal allergy · sweat changes · wound complications
▸ **Rare or very rare** Paranoia
▸ **Frequency not known** Intracranial pressure increased · memory impairment · toxic psychosis

● CONCEPTION AND CONTRACEPTION Manufacturer advises females of childbearing potential should use effective contraception during treatment.

● BREAST FEEDING Manufacturer advises avoid—present in milk in *animal* studies.

● RENAL IMPAIRMENT Avoid in end-stage renal disease.
▸ With intravenous use Manufacturer advises monitor serum creatinine in patients with moderate to severe renal impairment as intravenous vehicle may accumulate—if serum creatinine increases, consider switching to oral formulation (no dose adjustment required).
▸ With oral use Manufacturer advises caution in severe renal impairment—monitor renal function.
Dose adjustments ▸ With intravenous use Manufacturer advises reduce dose to 200 mg every 12 hours if creatinine clearance is less than 30 mL/min; alternatively, consider switching to oral formulation (no dose adjustment required).

● DIRECTIONS FOR ADMINISTRATION
▸ With intravenous use For *continuous intravenous infusion*, manufacturer advises reconstitute each 300 mg vial to produce a 25 mg/mL solution with 10.5 mL Glucose 5% *or* Sodium Chloride 0.9%, then dilute required dose in 250 mL Glucose 5% *or* Sodium Chloride 0.9%; give over 60 minutes.

● PRESCRIBING AND DISPENSING INFORMATION For choice of antibacterial therapy, see Skin infections, antibacterial therapy p. 541.

● HANDLING AND STORAGE
▸ With intravenous use Consult product literature for storage after reconstitution or dilution.
▸ With oral use Manufacturer advises protect from light.

● PATIENT AND CARER ADVICE
Driving and skilled tasks May impair performance of skilled tasks (e.g. driving).

● MEDICINAL FORMS There can be variation in the licensing of different medicines containing the same drug.
Powder for solution for infusion
EXCIPIENTS: May contain Disodium edetate, sulfobutylether beta cyclodextrin sodium
ELECTROLYTES: May contain Sodium
▸ Quofenix (A. Menarini Farmaceutica Internazionale SRL) ▼
Delafloxacin (as Delafloxacin meglumine) 300 mg Quofenix 300mg powder for concentrate for solution for infusion vials | 10 vial PoM £615.00
Tablet
ELECTROLYTES: May contain Sodium
▸ Quofenix (A. Menarini Farmaceutica Internazionale SRL) ▼
Delafloxacin (as Delafloxacin meglumine) 450 mg Quofenix 450mg tablets | 10 tablet PoM £615.00

⚑ 592

Levofloxacin

26-Nov-2020

● **INDICATIONS AND DOSE**

Acute sinusitis
▸ BY MOUTH
▸ Adult: 500 mg once daily for 10–14 days

Acute exacerbation of chronic obstructive pulmonary disease
▸ BY MOUTH
▸ Adult: 500 mg once daily for 5 days

Acute exacerbation of bronchiectasis
▸ BY MOUTH
▸ Adult: 500 mg 1–2 times a day for 7–14 days
▸ BY INTRAVENOUS INFUSION
▸ Adult: 500 mg 1–2 times a day, to be given over at least 60 minutes

Community-acquired pneumonia
▸ BY MOUTH
▸ Adult: 500 mg twice daily for 5 days
▸ BY INTRAVENOUS INFUSION
▸ Adult: 500 mg twice daily for 5 days, to be given over at least 60 minutes

Hospital-acquired pneumonia (administered on expert advice)
▸ BY MOUTH
▸ Adult: 500 mg 1–2 times a day for 5 days then review
▸ BY INTRAVENOUS INFUSION
▸ Adult: 500 mg 1–2 times a day, to be given over at least 60 minutes, use twice daily if severe infection

Urinary-tract infections
▸ BY MOUTH
▸ Adult: 500 mg once daily for 7–14 days

Complicated urinary-tract infections
▸ BY INTRAVENOUS INFUSION
▸ Adult: 500 mg once daily, to be given over at least 60 minutes

Prostatitis (initiated under specialist supervision)
▸ BY MOUTH
▸ Adult: 500 mg once daily for 14 or 28 days based on clinical assessment
▸ BY INTRAVENOUS INFUSION
▸ Adult: 500 mg once daily, to be given over at least 60 minutes

Complicated skin infections | Complicated soft-tissue infections
▸ BY MOUTH
▸ Adult: 500 mg 1–2 times a day for 7–14 days
▸ BY INTRAVENOUS INFUSION
▸ Adult: 500 mg 1–2 times a day, to be given over at least 60 minutes   continued →

5

Infection

Inhalation of anthrax (treatment and post-exposure prophylaxis)
▸ BY MOUTH
▸ Adult: 500 mg once daily for 8 weeks
▸ BY INTRAVENOUS INFUSION
▸ Adult: 500 mg once daily, to be given over at least 60 minutes

Chronic pulmonary infections due to *Pseudomonas aeruginosa* in cystic fibrosis
▸ BY INHALATION OF NEBULISED SOLUTION
▸ Adult: 240 mg twice daily for 28 days, subsequent courses repeated after 28-day interval without levofloxacin nebuliser solution

Helicobacter pylori eradication [in combination with other drugs (see Helicobacter pylori infection p. 90)]
▸ BY MOUTH
▸ Adult: 250 mg twice daily for 7 days for second-line eradication therapy; 10 days for third-line eradication therapy

● UNLICENSED USE Levofloxacin may be used as detailed below, although these situations are considered unlicensed:
  ● EvGr treatment of acute exacerbation of bronchiectasis
  ● treatment of hospital-acquired pneumonia
  ● duration of treatment for acute exacerbation of chronic obstructive pulmonary disease
  ● duration of treatment for community-acquired pneumonia
  ● eradication of *Helicobacter pylori* Ⓐ

● CAUTIONS Risk factors for QT interval prolongation (e.g. electrolyte disturbances, acute myocardial infarction, heart failure with reduced left ventricular ejection fraction, bradycardia, congenital long QT syndrome, history of symptomatic arrhythmias)

● INTERACTIONS → Appendix 1: quinolones

● SIDE-EFFECTS
▸ **Common or very common**
▸ When used by inhalation Bronchial secretion changes · dysphonia · haemoptysis · increased risk of infection · respiratory disorders · weight decreased
▸ **Uncommon**
▸ When used by inhalation Costochondritis · hyperbilirubinaemia · joint stiffness
▸ With intravenous or oral use Increased risk of infection
▸ **Rare or very rare**
▸ With intravenous or oral use Nephritis tubulointerstitial · paranoia · SIADH
▸ **Frequency not known**
▸ When used by inhalation Memory impairment
▸ With intravenous or oral use Anosmia · cardiac arrest · Clostridioides difficile colitis · diarrhoea haemorrhagic · ligament rupture · memory impairment · movement disorders · muscle rupture · pancytopenia · respiratory disorders · rhabdomyolysis · self-endangering behaviour

SIDE-EFFECTS, FURTHER INFORMATION Systemic side-effects may occur with nebulised levofloxacin.
  Bronchospasm Manufacturer advises if acute symptomatic bronchospasm occurs after receiving nebulised levofloxacin, patients may benefit from the use of a short-acting inhaled bronchodilator at least 15 minutes to 4 hours prior to subsequent doses.

● BREAST FEEDING Manufacturer advises avoid.

● RENAL IMPAIRMENT
  Dose adjustments ▸ With intravenous use or oral use Usual initial dose, then use half normal dose if eGFR 20–50 mL/minute/1.73 m^2; consult product literature if eGFR less than 20 mL/minute/1.73 m^2.
  ▸ When used by inhalation Manufacturer advises avoid if creatinine clearance less than 20 mL/minute.

● PATIENT AND CARER ADVICE
▸ When used by inhalation Manufacturer advises patients and carers should be given advice on how to administer levofloxacin.
  Missed doses ▸ When used by inhalation Manufacturer advises if a dose is more than 4 hours late, the missed dose should not be taken and the next dose should be taken at the normal time.
  Driving and skilled tasks May impair performance of skilled tasks (e.g. driving).

● NATIONAL FUNDING/ACCESS DECISIONS
  For full details see funding body website
  Scottish Medicines Consortium (SMC) decisions
▸ Levofloxacin (*Quinsair*®) for the management of chronic pulmonary infections due to *Pseudomonas aeruginosa* in adult patients with cystic fibrosis (August 2016)
  SMC No. 1162/16 Recommended with restrictions
  All Wales Medicines Strategy Group (AWMSG) decisions
▸ Levofloxacin (*Quinsair*®) for use as third-line therapy in patients who do not respond to, or are intolerant of, second-line treatment with tobramycin for the management of chronic pulmonary infections due to *Pseudomonas aeruginosa* in adult patients with cystic fibrosis (November 2016)
  AWMSG No. 1012 Recommended with restrictions

● MEDICINAL FORMS There can be variation in the licensing of different medicines containing the same drug.
  Tablet
  CAUTIONARY AND ADVISORY LABELS 6, 9, 25
▸ Levofloxacin (Non-proprietary)
    Levofloxacin (as Levofloxacin hemihydrate) 250 mg Levofloxacin 250mg tablets | 5 tablet PoM £5.54 DT = £5.55 | 10 tablet PoM £11.09 DT = £11.09
    Levofloxacin (as Levofloxacin hemihydrate) 500 mg Levofloxacin 500mg tablets | 5 tablet PoM £12.93 DT = £12.30 | 10 tablet PoM £25.85 DT = £24.60
  Solution for infusion
  ELECTROLYTES: May contain Sodium
▸ Levofloxacin (Non-proprietary)
    Levofloxacin (as Levofloxacin hemihydrate) 5 mg per 1 ml Levofloxacin 500mg/100ml solution for infusion vials | 1 vial PoM £25.00 (Hospital only)
    Levofloxacin 500mg/100ml solution for infusion bottles | 1 bottle PoM £24.40 (Hospital only) | 1 bottle PoM £12.00 | 10 bottle PoM £273.00
  Nebuliser liquid
▸ Quinsair (Chiesi Ltd) ▼
    Levofloxacin (as Levofloxacin hemihydrate) 100 mg per 1 ml Quinsair 240mg nebuliser solution ampoules | 56 ampoule PoM £2,181.53 DT = £2,181.53
  Infusion
▸ Levofloxacin (Non-proprietary)
    Levofloxacin (as Levofloxacin hemihydrate) 5 mg per 1 ml Levofloxacin 500mg/100ml infusion bags | 1 bag PoM £4.00 | 10 bag PoM £250.00 (Hospital only) | 20 bag PoM £502.00 (Hospital only)

🏴 592

Moxifloxacin

17-Apr-2020

● INDICATIONS AND DOSE
Sinusitis
▸ BY MOUTH
▸ Adult: 400 mg once daily for 7 days
Community-acquired pneumonia
▸ BY MOUTH
▸ Adult: 400 mg once daily for 7–14 days
▸ BY INTRAVENOUS INFUSION
▸ Adult: 400 mg once daily for 7–14 days, to be given over 60 minutes
Exacerbations of chronic bronchitis
▸ BY MOUTH
▸ Adult: 400 mg once daily for 5–10 days

Mild to moderate pelvic inflammatory disease
▶ BY MOUTH
▶ Adult: 400 mg once daily for 14 days

Complicated skin and soft-tissue infections which have failed to respond to other antibacterials or for patients who cannot be treated with other antibacterials
▶ BY MOUTH
▶ Adult: 400 mg once daily for 7–21 days
▶ BY INTRAVENOUS INFUSION
▶ Adult: 400 mg once daily for 7–21 days, to be given over 60 minutes

● CONTRA-INDICATIONS Acute myocardial infarction (risk factor for QT interval prolongation) · bradycardia (risk factor for QT interval prolongation) · congenital long QT syndrome (risk factor for QT interval prolongation) · electrolyte disturbances (risk factor for QT interval prolongation) · heart failure with reduced left ventricular ejection fraction (risk factor for QT interval prolongation) · history of symptomatic arrhythmias (risk factor for QT interval prolongation)

● INTERACTIONS → Appendix 1: quinolones

● SIDE-EFFECTS
▶ **Common or very common**
▶ With systemic use Increased risk of infection
▶ **Uncommon**
▶ With systemic use Akathisia · angina pectoris · antibiotic associated colitis · asthma · dehydration · gastritis · hyperlipidaemia · malaise · oedema · pelvic pain · thrombocytosis · vasodilation
▶ **Rare or very rare**
▶ With systemic use Cardiac arrest · concentration impaired · depersonalisation · dysphagia · emotional lability · generalised tonic-clonic seizure · hypertension · hyperuricaemia · memory loss · muscle complaints · self-injurious behaviour · respiratory disorders · smell disorders · speech disorder
▶ With oral use Anosmia

● BREAST FEEDING Manufacturer advises avoid—present in milk in *animal* studies.

● HEPATIC IMPAIRMENT Manufacturer advises avoid in severe impairment or increased transaminases (5 times upper limit of normal).

● PATIENT AND CARER ADVICE
Driving and skilled tasks May impair performance of skilled tasks (e.g. driving).

● MEDICINAL FORMS There can be variation in the licensing of different medicines containing the same drug.
Tablet
CAUTIONARY AND ADVISORY LABELS 6, 9
▶ Moxifloxacin (Non-proprietary)
Moxifloxacin (as Moxifloxacin hydrochloride)
400 mg Moxifloxacin 400mg tablets | 5 tablet [PoM] £11.19 DT = £10.49
▶ Avelox (Bayer Plc)
Moxifloxacin (as Moxifloxacin hydrochloride) 400 mg Avelox 400mg tablets | 5 tablet [PoM] £12.43 DT = £10.49
Solution for infusion
ELECTROLYTES: May contain Sodium
▶ Moxifloxacin (Non-proprietary)
Moxifloxacin (as Moxifloxacin hydrochloride) 1.6 mg per 1 ml Moxifloxacin 400mg/250ml solution for infusion bottles | 10 bottle [PoM] £399.50–£535.40 (Hospital only)
▶ Avelox (Bayer Plc)
Moxifloxacin (as Moxifloxacin hydrochloride) 1.6 mg per 1 ml Avelox 400mg/250ml solution for infusion bottles | 1 bottle [PoM] £39.95 (Hospital only) | 5 bottle [PoM] £199.75 (Hospital only)
Infusion
▶ Avelox (Imported (United States))
Moxifloxacin (as Moxifloxacin hydrochloride) 1.6 mg per 1 ml Avelox I.V. 400mg/250ml infusion bags | 1 bag [PoM] [⚠]

▌**Ofloxacin**   ▶ 592
26-Aug-2020

● INDICATIONS AND DOSE
Urinary-tract infections
▶ BY MOUTH
▶ Adult: 200–400 mg daily for 3 days, preferably taken in the morning

Complicated urinary-tract infections | Acute pyelonephritis | Lower respiratory-tract infections
▶ BY MOUTH
▶ Adult: 400 mg daily, preferably taken in the morning, increased if necessary to 400 mg twice daily for 7–10 days, dose increased for severe or complicated infections
▶ BY INTRAVENOUS INFUSION
▶ Adult: 200 mg twice daily, increased if necessary to 400 mg twice daily, dose increased for severe or complicated infections, to be given over at least 30 minutes for each 200 mg

Prostatitis
▶ BY MOUTH
▶ Adult: 200 mg twice daily for 14 or 28 days based on clinical assessment

Complicated skin and soft-tissue infections
▶ BY MOUTH
▶ Adult: 400 mg twice daily for 7–10 days
▶ BY INTRAVENOUS INFUSION
▶ Adult: 400 mg twice daily, to be given over at least 30 minutes for each 200 mg

Uncomplicated gonorrhoea
▶ BY MOUTH
▶ Adult: 400 mg as a single dose

Disseminated gonococcal infection [when sensitivity confirmed]
▶ BY MOUTH
▶ Adult: 400 mg twice daily, following intravenous antibacterial treatment, starting 24–48 hours after symptoms improve, to give 7 days treatment in total

Uncomplicated genital chlamydial infection | Non-gonococcal urethritis and cervicitis
▶ BY MOUTH
▶ Adult: 400 mg daily for 7 days, dose may be taken as a single daily dose or in divided doses

Pelvic inflammatory disease
▶ BY MOUTH
▶ Adult: 400 mg twice daily for 14 days

● UNLICENSED USE [EvGr] Ofloxacin is used for the treatment of disseminated gonococcal infection, [Ⓐ] but is not licensed for this indication.

● CAUTIONS Acute myocardial infarction (risk factor for QT interval prolongation) · bradycardia (risk factor for QT interval prolongation) · congenital long QT syndrome (risk factor for QT interval prolongation) · electrolyte disturbances (risk factor for QT interval prolongation) · heart failure with reduced left ventricular ejection fraction (risk factor for QT interval prolongation) · history of symptomatic arrhythmias (risk factor for QT interval prolongation)

● INTERACTIONS → Appendix 1: quinolones

● SIDE-EFFECTS
▶ **Uncommon** Increased risk of infection
▶ **Rare or very rare** Enterocolitis · enterocolitis haemorrhagic · hot flush · movement disorders · respiratory disorders
▶ **Frequency not known** Bone marrow failure · ligament rupture · muscle rupture · myopathy · nephritis acute interstitial · self-endangering behaviour

● BREAST FEEDING Amount probably too small to be harmful but manufacturer advises avoid.

- HEPATIC IMPAIRMENT Manufacturer advises caution.
Dose adjustments Manufacturer advises maximum 400 mg
daily in hepatic failure (risk of decreased elimination).
- RENAL IMPAIRMENT
Dose adjustments Usual initial dose, then use half normal
dose if eGFR 20–50 mL/minute/1.73 m^2; 100 mg every
24 hours if eGFR less than 20 mL/minute/1.73 m^2
- PRESCRIBING AND DISPENSING INFORMATION For choice
of antibacterial therapy, see Genital system infections,
antibacterial therapy p. 536, Respiratory system
infections, antibacterial therapy p. 538, Skin infections,
antibacterial therapy p. 541, Urinary-tract infections
p. 626.
- PATIENT AND CARER ADVICE
Driving and skilled tasks May affect performance of skilled
tasks (e.g. driving); effects enhanced by alcohol.

- MEDICINAL FORMS There can be variation in the licensing of
different medicines containing the same drug. Forms available
from special-order manufacturers include: oral suspension, oral
solution

Tablet
CAUTIONARY AND ADVISORY LABELS 6, 9, 11
- Ofloxacin (Non-proprietary)
Ofloxacin 200 mg Ofloxacin 200mg tablets | 10 tablet [PoM] £9.00
DT = £8.78
Ofloxacin 400 mg Ofloxacin 400mg tablets | 5 tablet [PoM] £13.09
DT = £13.05 | 10 tablet [PoM] £4.59–£26.10
Solution for infusion
- Tarivid (Sanofi)
Ofloxacin (as Ofloxacin hydrochloride) 2 mg per 1 ml Tarivid
200mg/100ml solution for infusion bottles | 1 bottle [PoM] £16.16

ANTIBACTERIALS > SULFONAMIDES

Co-trimoxazole

16-Oct-2020

- DRUG ACTION Sulfamethoxazole and trimethoprim are
used in combination (as co-trimoxazole) because of their
synergistic activity (the importance of the sulfonamides
has decreased as a result of increasing bacterial resistance
and their replacement by antibacterials which are
generally more active and less toxic).

- INDICATIONS AND DOSE
Treatment of susceptible infections
▸ BY MOUTH
- Child 6 weeks–5 months: 120 mg twice daily,
alternatively 24 mg/kg twice daily
- Child 6 months–5 years: 240 mg twice daily, alternatively
24 mg/kg twice daily
- Child 6–11 years: 480 mg twice daily, alternatively
24 mg/kg twice daily
- Child 12–17 years: 960 mg twice daily
- Adult: 960 mg twice daily
▸ BY INTRAVENOUS INFUSION
- Adult: 960 mg every 12 hours, increased to 1.44 g every
12 hours, increased dose used in severe infection
**Moderate diabetic foot infection | Severe diabetic foot
infection**
▸ BY MOUTH
- Adult: 960 mg twice daily
▸ BY INTRAVENOUS INFUSION
- Adult: 960 mg every 12 hours, increased if necessary to
1.44 g every 12 hours
Leg ulcer infection
▸ BY MOUTH
- Adult: 960 mg twice daily for 7 days
▸ BY INTRAVENOUS INFUSION
- Adult: 960 mg every 12 hours, increased to 1.44 g every
12 hours, increased dose used in severe infection

Hospital-acquired pneumonia
▸ BY MOUTH
- Adult: 960 mg twice daily for 5 days then review
**Acute exacerbation of chronic obstructive pulmonary
disease**
▸ BY MOUTH
- Adult: 960 mg twice daily for 5 days
▸ BY INTRAVENOUS INFUSION
- Adult: 960 mg every 12 hours, increased if necessary to
1.44 g every 12 hours, increased dose used in severe
infection

**Treatment of *Pneumocystis jirovecii* (*Pneumocystis
carinii*) infections (undertaken where facilities for
appropriate monitoring available—consult
microbiologist and product literature)**
▸ BY MOUTH, OR BY INTRAVENOUS INFUSION
- Child: 120 mg/kg daily in 2–4 divided doses for
14–21 days, oral route preferred for children
- Adult: 120 mg/kg daily in 2–4 divided doses for
14–21 days
**Prophylaxis of *Pneumocystis jirovecii* (*Pneumocystis
carinii*) infections**
▸ BY MOUTH
- Child: 450 mg/m^2 twice daily (max. per dose 960 mg
twice daily) for 3 days of the week (either consecutively
or on alternate days), dose regimens may vary, consult
local guidelines
- Adult: 960 mg once daily, reduced if not tolerated to
480 mg once daily, alternatively 960 mg once daily on
alternate days, alternate day dose to be given 3 times
weekly, alternatively 960 mg twice a day on alternate
days, alternate day dose to be given 3 times weekly
Acute prostatitis (initiated under specialist supervision)
▸ BY MOUTH
- Adult: 960 mg twice daily for 14 or 28 days based on
clinical assessment

DOSE EQUIVALENCE AND CONVERSION
- 480 mg of co-trimoxazole consists of sulfamethoxazole
400 mg and trimethoprim 80 mg.

- UNLICENSED USE Co-trimoxazole may be used as detailed
below, although these situations are considered
unlicensed:
  - Treatment of *Burkholderia cepacia* infections in cystic
fibrosis;
  - Treatment of *Stenotrophomonas maltophilia* infections
  - [EvGr] treatment of hospital-acquired pneumonia
  - treatment of moderate diabetic foot infection
  - treatment of severe diabetic foot infection
  - treatment of leg ulcer infection Ⓐ
- In children Not licensed for use in children under 6 weeks.

> **IMPORTANT SAFETY INFORMATION**
> RESTRICTIONS ON THE USE OF CO-TRIMOXAZOLE
> Co-trimoxazole is licensed for the prophylaxis and
> treatment of *Pneumocystis jirovecii* (*Pneumocystis carinii*)
> pneumonia and toxoplasmosis; it is also licensed for the
> treatment of nocardiosis. *Stenotrophomonas maltophilia*
> has demonstrated susceptibility to co-trimoxazole. It
> should only be considered for use in acute exacerbations
> of chronic bronchitis and infections of the urinary tract
> when there is bacteriological evidence of sensitivity to
> co-trimoxazole and good reason to prefer this
> combination to a single antibacterial; similarly it should
> only be used in acute otitis media in children when there
> is good reason to prefer it.

- CONTRA-INDICATIONS Acute porphyrias p. 1107
- CAUTIONS Asthma · avoid in blood disorders (unless under
specialist supervision) · avoid in infants under 6 weeks
(except for treatment or prophylaxis of pneumocystis

pneumonia) because of the risk of kernicterus · elderly (increased risk of serious side-effects) · G6PD deficiency (risk of haemolytic anaemia) · maintain adequate fluid intake · predisposition to folate deficiency · predisposition to hyperkalaemia

- INTERACTIONS → Appendix 1: sulfonamides · trimethoprim
- SIDE-EFFECTS
  - ▶ **Common or very common** Diarrhoea · electrolyte imbalance · fungal overgrowth · headache · nausea · skin reactions
  - ▶ **Uncommon** Vomiting
  - ▶ **Rare or very rare** Agranulocytosis · angioedema · aplastic anaemia · appetite decreased · arthralgia · ataxia · cough · depression · dizziness · dyspnoea · eosinophilia · fever · haemolysis · haemolytic anaemia · hallucination · hepatic disorders · hypoglycaemia · leucopenia · lung infiltration · megaloblastic anaemia · meningitis aseptic · metabolic acidosis · methaemoglobinaemia · myalgia · myocarditis allergic · nephritis tubulointerstitial · neutropenia · oral disorders · pancreatitis · peripheral neuritis · photosensitivity reaction · pseudomembranous enterocolitis · renal impairment · renal tubular acidosis · seizure · serum sickness · severe cutaneous adverse reactions (SCARs) · systemic lupus erythematosus (SLE) · thrombocytopenia · tinnitus · uveitis · vasculitis · vertigo
  - SIDE-EFFECTS, FURTHER INFORMATION Co-trimoxazole is associated with rare but serious side effects. Discontinue immediately if blood disorders (including leucopenia, thrombocytopenia, megaloblastic anaemia, eosinophilia) or rash (including Stevens-Johnson syndrome or toxic epidermal necrolysis) develop.
- PREGNANCY Teratogenic risk in first trimester (trimethoprim a folate antagonist). Neonatal haemolysis and methaemoglobinaemia in third trimester; fear of increased risk of kernicterus in neonates appears to be unfounded.
- BREAST FEEDING Small risk of kernicterus in jaundiced infants and of haemolysis in G6PD-deficient infants (due to sulfamethoxazole).
- HEPATIC IMPAIRMENT Manufacturer advises avoid in severe liver disease.
- RENAL IMPAIRMENT
  - ▶ In adults Avoid if eGFR less than 15 mL/minute/1.73 m^2 and if plasma-sulfamethoxazole concentration cannot be monitored.
  - ▶ In children Avoid if estimated glomerular filtration rate less than 15 mL/minute/1.73 m^2 and if plasma-sulfamethoxazole concentration cannot be monitored.
  - **Dose adjustments** ▶ In adults Use half normal dose if eGFR 15–30 mL/minute/1.73 m^2.
  - ▶ In children Use half normal dose if estimated glomerular filtration rate 15–30 mL/minute/1.73 m^2.
- MONITORING REQUIREMENTS
  - ▶ Monitor blood counts on prolonged treatment.
  - ▶ In children Plasma concentration monitoring may be required with high doses; seek expert advice.
- DIRECTIONS FOR ADMINISTRATION
  - ▶ With intravenous use in children For intermittent *intravenous infusion*, manufacturer advises may be further diluted in glucose 5% and 10% or sodium chloride 0.9%. Dilute contents of 1 ampoule (5 mL) to 125 mL, 2 ampoules (10 mL) to 250 mL or 3 ampoules (15 mL) to 500 mL; suggested duration of infusion 60–90 minutes (but may be adjusted according to fluid requirements); if fluid restriction necessary, 1 ampoule (5 mL) may be diluted with 75 mL glucose 5% and the required dose infused over max. 60 minutes; check container for haze or precipitant during administration. Expert sources advise in severe fluid restriction may be given undiluted via a central venous line.
  - ▶ With intravenous use in adults For *intravenous infusion*, manufacturer advises give intermittently *in* Glucose 5% or

10% *or* Sodium chloride 0.9%. Dilute contents of 1 ampoule (5 mL) to 125 mL, 2 ampoules (10 mL) to 250 mL or 3 ampoules (15 mL) to 500 mL; suggested duration of infusion 60–90 minutes (but may be adjusted according to fluid requirements); if fluid restriction necessary, 1 ampoule (5 mL) may be diluted with 75 mL glucose 5% and infused over max. 60 minutes.

- PRESCRIBING AND DISPENSING INFORMATION Co-trimoxazole is a mixture of trimethoprim and sulfamethoxazole (sulphamethoxazole) in the proportions of 1 part to 5 parts.

  For choice of antibacterial therapy, see Diabetic foot infections, antibacterial therapy p. 534, Pneumocystis pneumonia p. 640, Respiratory system infections, antibacterial therapy p. 538, Skin infections, antibacterial therapy p. 541, Urinary-tract infections p. 626.

- MEDICINAL FORMS There can be variation in the licensing of different medicines containing the same drug.

  Solution for infusion
  EXCIPIENTS: May contain Alcohol, propylene glycol, sulfites
  ELECTROLYTES: May contain Sodium
  - ▶ Co-trimoxazole (Non-proprietary)
    Trimethoprim 80 mg, Sulfamethoxazole 80 mg per 1 ml Co-trimoxazole 80mg/400mg/5ml solution for infusion ampoules | 10 ampoule [PoM] £47.15 DT = £47.15

  Oral suspension
  CAUTIONARY AND ADVISORY LABELS 9
  - ▶ Co-trimoxazole (Non-proprietary)
    Trimethoprim 8 mg per 1 ml, Sulfamethoxazole 40 mg per 1 ml Co-trimoxazole 40mg/200mg/5ml oral suspension sugar free sugar-free | 100 ml [PoM] £9.96 DT = £9.96
    Trimethoprim 16 mg per 1 ml, Sulfamethoxazole 80 mg per 1 ml Co-trimoxazole 80mg/400mg/5ml oral suspension | 100 ml [PoM] £10.95–£10.96 DT = £10.96

  Tablet
  CAUTIONARY AND ADVISORY LABELS 9
  - ▶ Co-trimoxazole (Non-proprietary)
    Trimethoprim 80 mg, Sulfamethoxazole 400 mg Co-trimoxazole 80mg/400mg tablets | 28 tablet [PoM] £15.50 DT = £2.33 | 100 tablet [PoM] £8.32–£10.91
    Trimethoprim 160 mg, Sulfamethoxazole 800 mg Co-trimoxazole 160mg/800mg tablets | 100 tablet [PoM] £23.48 DT = £23.48

Sulfadiazine
26-May-2020

(Sulphadiazine)

- DRUG ACTION Sulfadiazine is a short-acting sulphonamide with bacteriostatic activity against a broad spectrum of organisms. The importance of the sulfonamides has decreased as a result of increasing bacterial resistance and their replacement by antibacterials which are generally more active and less toxic.

- INDICATIONS AND DOSE
  Prevention of rheumatic fever recurrence
  - ▶ BY MOUTH
    - ▶ Adult (body-weight up to 30 kg): 500 mg daily
    - ▶ Adult (body-weight 30 kg and above): 1 g daily

> IMPORTANT SAFETY INFORMATION
>
> SAFE PRACTICE
> Sulfadiazine has been confused with sulfasalazine; care must be taken to ensure the correct drug is prescribed and dispensed.

- CONTRA-INDICATIONS Acute porphyrias p. 1107
- CAUTIONS Asthma · avoid in blood disorders · elderly · G6PD deficiency (risk of haemolytic anaemia) · maintain adequate fluid intake · predisposition to folate deficiency
- INTERACTIONS → Appendix 1: sulfonamides

● SIDE-EFFECTS
▸ **Rare or very rare** Haemolytic anaemia
▸ **Frequency not known** Agranulocytosis · aplastic anaemia · appetite decreased · ataxia · back pain · blood disorders · cough · crystalluria · cyanosis · depression · diarrhoea · dizziness · drowsiness · dyspnoea · eosinophilia · erythema nodosum · fatigue · fever · haematuria · hallucination · headache · hepatic disorders · hypoglycaemia · hypoprothrombinaemia · hypothyroidism · idiopathic intracranial hypertension · insomnia · leucopenia · meningitis aseptic · myocarditis · nausea · nephritis tubulointerstitial · nephrotoxicity · nerve disorders · neurological effects · neutropenia · oral disorders · pancreatitis · photosensitivity reaction · pseudomembranous enterocolitis · psychosis · renal impairment · renal tubular necrosis · respiratory disorders · seizure · serum sickness-like reaction · severe cutaneous adverse reactions (SCARs) · skin reactions · systemic lupus erythematosus (SLE) · thrombocytopenia · tinnitus · vasculitis · vertigo · vomiting

SIDE-EFFECTS, FURTHER INFORMATION Discontinue immediately if blood disorders (including leucopenia, thrombocytopenia, megaloblastic anaemia, eosinophilia) or rash (including Stevens-Johnson syndrome, toxic epidermal necrolysis) develop.

● PREGNANCY Risk of neonatal haemolysis and methaemoglobinaemia in third trimester; fear of increased risk of kernicterus in neonates appears to be unfounded.

● BREAST FEEDING Small risk of kernicterus in jaundiced infants and of haemolysis in G6PD-deficient infants.

● HEPATIC IMPAIRMENT Manufacturer advises caution in mild to moderate impairment; avoid in severe impairment or jaundice.

● RENAL IMPAIRMENT Use with caution in mild to moderate impairment; avoid in severe impairment; high risk of crystalluria.

● MONITORING REQUIREMENTS Monitor blood counts on prolonged treatment.

● MEDICINAL FORMS There can be variation in the licensing of different medicines containing the same drug. Forms available from special-order manufacturers include: oral suspension

Tablet
CAUTIONARY AND ADVISORY LABELS 9, 27
▸ Sulfadiazine (Non-proprietary)
Sulfadiazine 500 mg Sulfadiazine 500mg tablets | 56 tablet PoM
£308.30 DT = £302.54

ANTIBACTERIALS 〉TETRACYCLINES AND RELATED DRUGS

Tetracyclines

Overview

The tetracyclines are broad-spectrum antibiotics whose value has decreased owing to increasing bacterial resistance. They remain, however, the treatment of choice for infections caused by chlamydia (trachoma, psittacosis, salpingitis, urethritis, and lymphogranuloma venereum), rickettsia (including Q-fever), brucella (doxycycline p. 601 with either streptomycin p. 547 or rifampicin p. 619), and the spirochaete, *Borrelia burgdorferi* (See Lyme disease). They are also used in respiratory and genital mycoplasma infections, in acne, in destructive (refractory) periodontal disease, in exacerbations of chronic bronchitis (because of their activity against *Haemophilus influenzae*), and for leptospirosis in penicillin hypersensitivity (as an alternative to erythromycin p. 572).

Tetracyclines have a role in the management of meticillin-resistant *Staphylococcus aureus* (MRSA) infection.

Microbiologically, there is little to choose between the various tetracyclines, the only exception being minocycline p. 603 which has a broader spectrum; it is active against *Neisseria meningitidis* and has been used for meningococcal prophylaxis but is no longer recommended because of side-effects including dizziness and vertigo. Compared to other tetracyclines, minocycline is associated with a greater risk of lupus-erythematosus-like syndrome. Minocycline sometimes causes irreversible pigmentation.

Tetracyclines

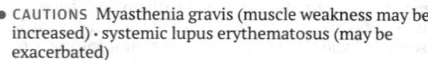

● CAUTIONS Myasthenia gravis (muscle weakness may be increased) · systemic lupus erythematosus (may be exacerbated)

● SIDE-EFFECTS
▸ **Common or very common** Angioedema · diarrhoea · headache · Henoch-Schönlein purpura · hypersensitivity · nausea · pericarditis · photosensitivity reaction · skin reactions · systemic lupus erythematosus exacerbated · vomiting
▸ **Rare or very rare** Appetite decreased · discolouration of thyroid gland · dysphagia · eosinophilia · fontanelle bulging (in infants) · gastrointestinal disorders · haemolytic anaemia · hepatic disorders · idiopathic intracranial hypertension · increased risk of infection · neutropenia · oral disorders · pancreatitis · pseudomembranous enterocolitis · Stevens-Johnson syndrome · thrombocytopenia
▸ **Frequency not known** Dizziness · tooth discolouration

SIDE-EFFECTS, FURTHER INFORMATION Headache and visual disturbances may indicate benign intracranial hypertension (discontinue treatment if raised intracranial pressure develops).

● PREGNANCY Should **not** be given to pregnant women; effects on skeletal development have been documented in the first trimester in *animal* studies. Administration during the second or third trimester may cause discolouration of the child's teeth, and maternal hepatotoxicity has been reported with large parenteral doses.

● BREAST FEEDING Should **not** be given to women who are breast-feeding (although absorption and therefore discolouration of teeth in the infant is probably usually prevented by chelation with calcium in milk).

● HEPATIC IMPAIRMENT In general, manufacturers advise caution.

◤ above

Demeclocycline hydrochloride 01-Sep-2020

● INDICATIONS AND DOSE
Susceptible infections (e.g. chlamydia, rickettsia and mycoplasma)
▸ BY MOUTH
▸ Adult: 150 mg 4 times a day, alternatively 300 mg twice daily

Treatment of hyponatraemia resulting from inappropriate secretion of antidiuretic hormone, if fluid restriction alone does not restore sodium concentration or is not tolerable
▸ BY MOUTH
▸ Adult: Initially 0.9–1.2 g daily in divided doses, maintenance 600–900 mg daily

● CAUTIONS Photosensitivity more common than with other tetracyclines

● INTERACTIONS → Appendix 1: tetracyclines

- SIDE-EFFECTS
- ▶ **Rare or very rare** Agranulocytosis · aplastic anaemia · hearing impairment · nephritis · severe cutaneous adverse reactions (SCARs)
- ▶ **Frequency not known** Intracranial pressure increased · muscle weakness · nephrogenic diabetes insipidus · vision disorders
- HEPATIC IMPAIRMENT

Dose adjustments Manufacturer advises maximum 1 g daily in divided doses.

- RENAL IMPAIRMENT May exacerbate renal failure and should **not** be given to patients with renal impairment.
- PATIENT AND CARER ADVICE Patients should be advised to avoid exposure to sunlight or sun lamps.

- MEDICINAL FORMS There can be variation in the licensing of different medicines containing the same drug. Forms available from special-order manufacturers include: tablet, oral suspension, oral solution

Tablet
- ▶ Demeclocycline hydrochloride (Non-proprietary)
  Demeclocycline hydrochloride 150 mg Demeclocycline 150mg tablets | 100 tablet PoM ⓧ

Capsule
CAUTIONARY AND ADVISORY LABELS 7, 9, 11, 23
- ▶ Demeclocycline hydrochloride (Non-proprietary)
  Demeclocycline hydrochloride 150 mg Demeclocycline 150mg capsules | 28 capsule PoM £217.73 DT = £217.73
- ▶ Ledermycin (Imported (Netherlands))
  Demeclocycline hydrochloride 300 mg Ledermycin 300mg capsules | 16 capsule PoM ⓧ

Ϝ 600

Doxycycline

02-Sep-2020

- INDICATIONS AND DOSE

Susceptible infections (e.g. chlamydia, rickettsia and mycoplasma)
- ▶ BY MOUTH USING IMMEDIATE-RELEASE MEDICINES
- ▶ Child 12-17 years: Initially 200 mg daily in 1–2 divided doses for 1 day, then maintenance 100 mg daily
- ▶ Adult: Initially 200 mg daily in 1–2 divided doses for 1 day, then maintenance 100 mg daily

Severe infections (including refractory urinary-tract infections)
- ▶ BY MOUTH USING IMMEDIATE-RELEASE MEDICINES
- ▶ Child 12-17 years: 200 mg daily
- ▶ Adult: 200 mg daily

Acute sinusitis | Acute cough [if systemically very unwell or at higher risk of complications] | Community-acquired pneumonia
- ▶ BY MOUTH USING IMMEDIATE-RELEASE MEDICINES
- ▶ Child 12-17 years: Initially 200 mg daily for 1 dose, then maintenance 100 mg once daily for 5 days in total
- ▶ Adult: Initially 200 mg daily for 1 dose, then maintenance 100 mg once daily for 5 days in total

Hospital-acquired pneumonia
- ▶ BY MOUTH USING IMMEDIATE-RELEASE MEDICINES
- ▶ Adult: Initially 200 mg daily for 1 dose, then maintenance 100 mg once daily for 5 days in total then review

Acute exacerbation of bronchiectasis
- ▶ BY MOUTH USING IMMEDIATE-RELEASE MEDICINES
- ▶ Child 12-17 years: Initially 200 mg daily for 1 dose, then maintenance 100 mg once daily for 7–14 days in total
- ▶ Adult: Initially 200 mg daily for 1 dose, then maintenance 100 mg once daily for 7–14 days in total

Acute exacerbation of chronic obstructive pulmonary disease
- ▶ BY MOUTH USING IMMEDIATE-RELEASE MEDICINES
- ▶ Adult: Initially 200 mg daily for 1 dose, then maintenance 100 mg once daily for 5 days in total, increased if necessary to 200 mg once daily, increased dose used in severe infections

Mild diabetic foot infection
- ▶ BY MOUTH USING IMMEDIATE-RELEASE MEDICINES
- ▶ Adult: Initially 200 mg daily for 1 dose, then maintenance 100 mg once daily for 7 days in total then review, increased if necessary to 200 mg once daily

Cellulitis | Erysipelas
- ▶ BY MOUTH USING IMMEDIATE-RELEASE MEDICINES
- ▶ Adult: Initially 200 mg daily for 1 dose, then maintenance 100 mg once daily for 5–7 days in total then review

Leg ulcer infection
- ▶ BY MOUTH USING IMMEDIATE-RELEASE MEDICINES
- ▶ Adult: Initially 200 mg daily for 1 dose, then maintenance 100 mg once daily for 7 days in total, increased if necessary to 200 mg once daily

Acne
- ▶ BY MOUTH USING IMMEDIATE-RELEASE MEDICINES
- ▶ Child 12-17 years: 100 mg once daily
- ▶ Adult: 100 mg once daily

Rosacea
- ▶ BY MOUTH USING IMMEDIATE-RELEASE MEDICINES
- ▶ Adult: 100 mg once daily

Papulopustular facial rosacea (without ocular involvement)
- ▶ BY MOUTH USING MODIFIED-RELEASE MEDICINES
- ▶ Adult: 40 mg once daily for 16 weeks, dose to be taken in the morning, consider discontinuing treatment if no response after 6 weeks

Early syphilis
- ▶ BY MOUTH USING IMMEDIATE-RELEASE MEDICINES
- ▶ Child 12-17 years: 100 mg twice daily for 14 days
- ▶ Adult: 100 mg twice daily for 14 days

Late latent syphilis
- ▶ BY MOUTH USING IMMEDIATE-RELEASE MEDICINES
- ▶ Child 12-17 years: 100 mg twice daily for 28 days
- ▶ Adult: 100 mg twice daily for 28 days

Neurosyphilis
- ▶ BY MOUTH USING IMMEDIATE-RELEASE MEDICINES
- ▶ Adult: 200 mg twice daily for 28 days

Uncomplicated genital chlamydia | Non-gonococcal urethritis
- ▶ BY MOUTH USING IMMEDIATE-RELEASE MEDICINES
- ▶ Child 12-17 years: 100 mg twice daily for 7 days
- ▶ Adult: 100 mg twice daily for 7 days

Pelvic inflammatory disease
- ▶ BY MOUTH USING IMMEDIATE-RELEASE MEDICINES
- ▶ Child 12-17 years: 100 mg twice daily for 14 days
- ▶ Adult: 100 mg twice daily for 14 days

Lyme disease [erythema migrans and/or non-focal symptoms] | Lyme disease [affecting cranial nerves or peripheral nervous system] | Lyme carditis
- ▶ BY MOUTH USING IMMEDIATE-RELEASE MEDICINES
- ▶ Adult: 200 mg daily in 1–2 divided doses for 21 days

Lyme disease [affecting central nervous system]
- ▶ BY MOUTH USING IMMEDIATE-RELEASE MEDICINES
- ▶ Adult: 400 mg daily in 1–2 divided doses for 21 days

Lyme arthritis | Acrodermatitis chronica atrophicans
- ▶ BY MOUTH USING IMMEDIATE-RELEASE MEDICINES
- ▶ Adult: 200 mg daily in 1–2 divided doses for 28 days

continued →

5

Infection

Anthrax (treatment or post-exposure prophylaxis)
▶ BY MOUTH USING IMMEDIATE-RELEASE MEDICINES
- Child 12–17 years: 100 mg twice daily
- Adult: 100 mg twice daily

Prophylaxis of malaria
▶ BY MOUTH USING IMMEDIATE-RELEASE MEDICINES
- Child 12–17 years (body-weight 25 kg and above): 100 mg once daily, to be started 1–2 days before entering endemic area and continued for 4 weeks after leaving
- Adult: 100 mg once daily, to be started 1–2 days before entering endemic area and continued for 4 weeks after leaving

Adjunct to quinine in treatment of *Plasmodium falciparum* malaria
▶ BY MOUTH USING IMMEDIATE-RELEASE MEDICINES
- Child 12–17 years: 200 mg daily for 7 days
- Adult: 200 mg daily for 7 days

Periodontitis (as an adjunct to gingival scaling and root planing)
▶ BY MOUTH USING IMMEDIATE-RELEASE MEDICINES
- Child 12–17 years: 20 mg twice daily for 3 months
- Adult: 20 mg twice daily for 3 months

Rocky Mountain spotted fever
▶ BY MOUTH USING DISPERSIBLE TABLETS
- Adult: 100 mg twice daily, continue treatment for at least 3 days after fever subsides, minimum treatment duration is 5–7 days

- **UNLICENSED USE** Doxycycline may be used as detailed below, although these situations are considered outside the scope of its licence:
  - EvGr Duration of treatment for acute sinusitis;
  - Lyme disease A ;
  - treatment or post-exposure prophylaxis of anthrax;
  - malaria prophylaxis during pregnancy;
  - recurrent aphthous ulceration.
  Immediate-release doxycycline may be used for the treatment of rosacea, but it is not licensed for this indication.
- **CAUTIONS** Alcohol dependence
- **INTERACTIONS** → Appendix 1: tetracyclines
- **SIDE-EFFECTS**
▶ **Common or very common** Dyspnoea · hypotension · peripheral oedema · tachycardia
▶ **Uncommon** Gastrointestinal discomfort
▶ **Rare or very rare** Antibiotic associated colitis · anxiety · arthralgia · flushing · intracranial pressure increased with papilloedema · Jarisch-Herxheimer reaction · myalgia · photoonycholysis · severe cutaneous adverse reactions (SCARs) · skin hyperpigmentation (long term use) · tinnitus · vision disorders
- **PREGNANCY** When travel to malarious areas is unavoidable during pregnancy, doxycycline can be used for malaria prophylaxis if other regimens are unsuitable, and if the entire course of doxycycline can be completed before 15 weeks' gestation.
- **RENAL IMPAIRMENT** Use with caution (avoid excessive doses).
- **MONITORING REQUIREMENTS** When used for periodontitis, monitor for superficial fungal infection, particularly if predisposition to oral candidiasis.
- **DIRECTIONS FOR ADMINISTRATION** Manufacturer advises capsules and tablets should be swallowed whole with plenty of fluid, while sitting or standing.
- **PRESCRIBING AND DISPENSING INFORMATION** For choice of antibacterial therapy, see Anthrax p. 613, Diabetic foot infections, antibacterial therapy p. 534, Genital system infections, antibacterial therapy p. 536, Lyme disease p. 614, Malaria, prophylaxis p. 646, Malaria, treatment p. 652, Nose infections, antibacterial therapy p. 537,

Oropharyngeal infections, antibacterial therapy p. 1261, Respiratory system infections, antibacterial therapy p. 538, Skin infections, antibacterial therapy p. 541, Urinary-tract infections p. 626.
- **PATIENT AND CARER ADVICE** Counselling on administration advised.
  Photosensitivity Patients should be advised to avoid exposure to sunlight or sun lamps.
- **PROFESSION SPECIFIC INFORMATION**
Dental practitioners' formulary
Doxycycline Capsules 100 mg may be prescribed.
  Dispersible tablets may be prescribed as Dispersible Doxycycline Tablets.
  Tablets may be prescribed as Doxycycline Tablets 20 mg.

- **MEDICINAL FORMS** There can be variation in the licensing of different medicines containing the same drug. Forms available from special-order manufacturers include: oral suspension, oral solution

Tablet
CAUTIONARY AND ADVISORY LABELS 6, 11, 27
▶ Doxycycline (Non-proprietary)
  Doxycycline (as Doxycycline hyclate) 100 mg Doxycycline 100mg tablets | 10 tablet [PoM] £1.64
▶ Periostat (Alliance Pharmaceuticals Ltd)
  Doxycycline (as Doxycycline hyclate) 20 mg Periostat 20mg tablets | 56 tablet [PoM] £17.30 DT = £17.30

Dispersible tablet
CAUTIONARY AND ADVISORY LABELS 6, 9, 11, 13
▶ Vibramycin-D (Pfizer Ltd)
  Doxycycline (as Doxycycline monohydrate) 100 mg Vibramycin-D 100mg dispersible tablets sugar-free | 8 tablet [PoM] £4.91 DT = £4.91

Modified-release capsule
CAUTIONARY AND ADVISORY LABELS 6, 11, 27
▶ Efracea (Galderma (UK) Ltd)
  Doxycycline (as Doxycycline monohydrate) 40 mg Efracea 40mg modified-release capsules | 14 capsule [PoM] £7.99 DT = £7.99 | 56 capsule [PoM] £21.71

Capsule
CAUTIONARY AND ADVISORY LABELS 6, 9, 11, 27
▶ Doxycycline (Non-proprietary)
  Doxycycline (as Doxycycline hyclate) 50 mg Doxycycline 50mg capsules | 28 capsule [PoM] £4.00 DT = £2.23
  Doxycycline (as Doxycycline hyclate) 100 mg Doxycycline 100mg capsules | 8 capsule [PoM] £3.00 DT = £1.34 | 14 capsule [PoM] £5.25 | 50 capsule [PoM] £8.37–£19.00

Ⅎ 600

Lymecycline

14-Nov-2018

- **INDICATIONS AND DOSE**
Susceptible infections (e.g. chlamydia, rickettsia and mycoplasma)
▶ BY MOUTH
- Child 12–17 years: 408 mg twice daily, increased to 1.224–1.632 g daily, (in severe infection)
- Adult: 408 mg twice daily, increased to 1.224–1.632 g daily, (in severe infection)

Acne
▶ BY MOUTH
- Child 12–17 years: 408 mg daily for at least 8 weeks
- Adult: 408 mg daily for at least 8 weeks

- **INTERACTIONS** → Appendix 1: tetracyclines
- **SIDE-EFFECTS**
▶ **Common or very common** Gastrointestinal discomfort
▶ **Frequency not known** Visual impairment
- **RENAL IMPAIRMENT** May exacerbate renal failure and should **not** be given to patients with renal impairment.

● MEDICINAL FORMS There can be variation in the licensing of different medicines containing the same drug.

Capsule

CAUTIONARY AND ADVISORY LABELS 6, 9

▸ Lymecycline (Non-proprietary)

Lymecycline 408 mg Lymecycline 408mg capsules | 28 capsule PoM £8.25 DT = £8.10 | 56 capsule PoM £16.20 DT = £16.20

▸ Tetralysal (Galderma (UK) Ltd)

Lymecycline 408 mg Tetralysal 300 capsules | 28 capsule PoM £6.95 DT = £8.10 | 56 capsule PoM £11.53 DT = £16.20

⚑ 600

Minocycline

13-Aug-2020

● INDICATIONS AND DOSE

Susceptible infections (e.g. chlamydia, rickettsia and mycoplasma)

▸ BY MOUTH USING IMMEDIATE-RELEASE MEDICINES
▸ Child 12–17 years: 100 mg twice daily
▸ Adult: 100 mg twice daily

Acne

▸ BY MOUTH USING IMMEDIATE-RELEASE MEDICINES
▸ Child 12–17 years: 100 mg once daily, alternatively 50 mg twice daily
▸ Adult: 100 mg once daily, alternatively 50 mg twice daily
▸ BY MOUTH USING MODIFIED-RELEASE MEDICINES
▸ Child 12–17 years: 100 mg daily
▸ Adult: 100 mg daily

Prophylaxis of asymptomatic meningococcal carrier state (but no longer recommended)

▸ BY MOUTH USING IMMEDIATE-RELEASE MEDICINES
▸ Adult: 100 mg twice daily for 5 days, minocycline treatment is usually followed by administration of rifampicin

● CAUTIONS Systemic lupus erythematosus

● INTERACTIONS → Appendix 1: tetracyclines

● SIDE-EFFECTS

▸ **Rare or very rare** Acute kidney injury · hearing impairment · respiratory disorders · tinnitus

▸ **Frequency not known** Alopecia · antibiotic associated colitis · arthralgia · ataxia · breast secretion · conjunctival discolouration · drug reaction with eosinophilia and systemic symptoms (DRESS) · dyspepsia · hyperbilirubinaemia · hyperhidrosis · polyarteritis nodosa · sensation abnormal · tear discolouration · tongue discolouration · vertigo

● RENAL IMPAIRMENT Use with caution (avoid excessive doses).

● MONITORING REQUIREMENTS If treatment continued for longer than 6 months, monitor every 3 months for hepatotoxicity, pigmentation and for systemic lupus erythematosus—discontinue if these develop or if pre-existing systemic lupus erythematosus worsens.

● DIRECTIONS FOR ADMINISTRATION Manufacturer advises tablets or capsules should be swallowed whole with plenty of fluid while sitting or standing.

● PATIENT AND CARER ADVICE Counselling on administration advised (posture).

● LESS SUITABLE FOR PRESCRIBING Less suitable for prescribing (compared with other tetracyclines, minocycline is associated with a greater risk of lupus-erythematosus-like syndrome; it sometimes causes irreversible pigmentation).

● MEDICINAL FORMS There can be variation in the licensing of different medicines containing the same drug. Forms available from special-order manufacturers include: oral suspension, oral solution

Tablet

CAUTIONARY AND ADVISORY LABELS 6, 9

▸ Minocycline (Non-proprietary)

Minocycline (as Minocycline hydrochloride) 50 mg Minocycline 50mg tablets | 28 tablet PoM £8.50 DT = £6.19

Minocycline (as Minocycline hydrochloride) 100 mg Minocycline 100mg tablets | 28 tablet PoM £14.50 DT = £14.18

Modified-release capsule

CAUTIONARY AND ADVISORY LABELS 6, 25

▸ Acnamino MR (Dexcel-Pharma Ltd)

Minocycline (as Minocycline hydrochloride) 100 mg Acnamino MR 100mg capsules | 56 capsule PoM £21.14 DT = £20.08

▸ Minocin MR (Mylan)

Minocycline (as Minocycline hydrochloride) 100 mg Minocin MR 100mg capsules | 56 capsule PoM £20.08 DT = £20.08

Capsule

CAUTIONARY AND ADVISORY LABELS 6, 9

▸ Aknemin (Almirall Ltd)

Minocycline (as Minocycline hydrochloride) 100 mg Aknemin 100mg capsules | 28 capsule PoM £13.09 DT = £13.09

⚑ 600

Oxytetracycline

14-Nov-2018

● INDICATIONS AND DOSE

Susceptible infections (e.g. chlamydia, rickettsia and mycoplasma)

▸ BY MOUTH
▸ Child 12–17 years: 250–500 mg 4 times a day
▸ Adult: 250–500 mg 4 times a day

Rosacea

▸ BY MOUTH
▸ Adult: 500 mg twice daily usually for 6–12 weeks (course may be repeated intermittently)

Acne

▸ BY MOUTH
▸ Child 12–17 years: 500 mg twice daily for at least 3 months, if there is no improvement after the first 3 months another oral antibacterial should be used, maximum improvement usually occurs after 4 to 6 months but in more severe cases treatment may need to be continued for 2 years or longer
▸ Adult: 500 mg twice daily for at least 3 months, if there is no improvement after the first 3 months another oral antibacterial should be used, maximum improvement usually occurs after 4 to 6 months but in more severe cases treatment may need to be continued for 2 years or longer

● INTERACTIONS → Appendix 1: tetracyclines

● SIDE-EFFECTS Gastrointestinal discomfort · renal impairment

● HEPATIC IMPAIRMENT

Dose adjustments Manufacturer advises avoid in high doses.

● RENAL IMPAIRMENT May exacerbate renal failure and should **not** be given to patients with renal impairment.

● PROFESSION SPECIFIC INFORMATION

Dental practitioners' formulary

Oxytetracycline Tablets may be prescribed.

● MEDICINAL FORMS There can be variation in the licensing of different medicines containing the same drug. Forms available from special-order manufacturers include: oral suspension

Tablet

CAUTIONARY AND ADVISORY LABELS 7, 9, 23

▸ Oxytetracycline (Non-proprietary)

Oxytetracycline (as Oxytetracycline dihydrate) 250 mg Oxytetracycline 250mg tablets | 28 tablet PoM £9.79 DT = £4.93

5

Infection

Tetracycline

F 600

03-Sep-2020

● INDICATIONS AND DOSE

Susceptible infections (e.g. chlamydia, rickettsia, mycoplasma)
▶ BY MOUTH
▷ Child 12-17 years: 250 mg 4 times a day, increased if necessary to 500 mg 3–4 times a day, increased dose used in severe infections
▷ Adult: 250 mg 4 times a day, increased if necessary to 500 mg 3–4 times a day, increased dose used in severe infections

Rosacea
▶ BY MOUTH
▷ Adult: 500 mg twice daily usually for 6–12 weeks (course may be repeated intermittently)

Acne
▶ BY MOUTH
▷ Child 12-17 years: 500 mg twice daily for at least 3 months, if there is no improvement after the first 3 months another oral antibacterial should be used, maximum improvement usually occurs after 4 to 6 months but in more severe cases treatment may need to be continued for 2 years or longer
▷ Adult: 500 mg twice daily for at least 3 months, if there is no improvement after the first 3 months another oral antibacterial should be used, maximum improvement usually occurs after 4 to 6 months but in more severe cases treatment may need to be continued for 2 years or longer

Diabetic diarrhoea in autonomic neuropathy
▶ BY MOUTH
▷ Adult: 250 mg for 2 or 3 doses

Non-gonococcal urethritis
▶ BY MOUTH
▷ Child 12-17 years: 500 mg 4 times a day for 7–14 days (21 days if failure or relapse after first course)
▷ Adult: 500 mg 4 times a day for 7–14 days (21 days if failure or relapse after first course)

Helicobacter pylori eradication [in combination with other drugs (see Helicobacter pylori infection p. 90)]
▶ BY MOUTH
▷ Adult: 500 mg 4 times a day for 7 days for first- and second-line eradication therapy; 10 days for third-line eradication therapy

● UNLICENSED USE Not licensed for treatment of diabetic diarrhoea in *autonomic neuropathy*. EvGr Tetracycline is used for the eradication of *Helicobacter pylori*, ⒶⒷ but is not licensed for this indication.

● INTERACTIONS → Appendix 1: tetracyclines

● SIDE-EFFECTS
▶ **Rare or very rare** Agranulocytosis · aplastic anaemia · nephritis · renal impairment
▶ **Frequency not known** Gastrointestinal discomfort · toxic epidermal necrolysis

● HEPATIC IMPAIRMENT
Dose adjustments Manufacturer advises avoid in high doses.

● RENAL IMPAIRMENT May exacerbate renal failure and should **not** be given to patients with renal impairment.

● DIRECTIONS FOR ADMINISTRATION Manufacturer advises tablets should be swallowed whole with plenty of fluid while sitting or standing.

● PATIENT AND CARER ADVICE Counselling on administration advised.

● PROFESSION SPECIFIC INFORMATION
Dental practitioners' formulary
Tetracycline Tablets may be prescribed.

● MEDICINAL FORMS There can be variation in the licensing of different medicines containing the same drug. Forms available from special-order manufacturers include: capsule, oral solution
Tablet
CAUTIONARY AND ADVISORY LABELS 7, 9, 23
▷ Tetracycline (Non-proprietary)
Tetracycline hydrochloride 250 mg Tetracycline 250mg tablets | 28 tablet PoM £7.46 DT = £5.75

Tigecycline

02-Dec-2020

● DRUG ACTION Tigecycline is a glycylcycline antibacterial structurally related to the tetracyclines. Tigecycline is active against Gram-positive and Gram-negative bacteria, including tetracycline-resistant organisms, and some anaerobes. It is also active against meticillin-resistant *Staphylococcus aureus* and vancomycin-resistant enterococci, but *Pseudomonas aeruginosa* and many strains of *Proteus spp* are resistant to tigecycline.

● INDICATIONS AND DOSE

Complicated skin and soft tissue infections (when other antibiotics are not suitable) | Complicated intra-abdominal infections (when other antibiotics are not suitable)
▶ BY INTRAVENOUS INFUSION
▷ Adult: Initially 100 mg, followed by 50 mg every 12 hours for 5–14 days

● CONTRA-INDICATIONS Diabetic foot infections

● CAUTIONS Cholestasis

● INTERACTIONS → Appendix 1: tigecycline

● SIDE-EFFECTS
▶ **Common or very common** Abscess · appetite decreased · diarrhoea · dizziness · gastrointestinal discomfort · headache · healing impaired · hyperbilirubinaemia · hypoglycaemia · hypoproteinaemia · increased risk of infection · nausea · sepsis · skin reactions · vomiting
▶ **Uncommon** Hepatic disorders · pancreatitis · thrombocytopenia · thrombophlebitis
▶ **Frequency not known** Acidosis · azotaemia · hyperphosphataemia · hypofibrinogenaemia · idiopathic intracranial hypertension · photosensitivity reaction · pseudomembranous enterocolitis · severe cutaneous adverse reactions (SCARs) · tooth discolouration

SIDE-EFFECTS, FURTHER INFORMATION Side-effects similar to those of the tetracyclines can potentially occur.

● ALLERGY AND CROSS-SENSITIVITY EvGr Contra-indicated in patients hypersensitive to tetracyclines. Ⓜ

● PREGNANCY Tetracyclines should **not** be given to pregnant women; effects on skeletal development have been documented in the first trimester in *animal* studies. Administration during the second or third trimester may cause discoloration of the child's teeth, and maternal hepatotoxicity has been reported with large parenteral doses.

● BREAST FEEDING Manufacturer advises avoid—present in milk in *animal* studies.

● HEPATIC IMPAIRMENT Manufacturer advises caution in severe impairment.
Dose adjustments Manufacturer advises dose reduction to 25 mg every 12 hours following the loading dose in severe impairment.

● DIRECTIONS FOR ADMINISTRATION For *intravenous infusion* (*Tygacil®*), give intermittently in Glucose 5% or Sodium Chloride 0.9%. Reconstitute each vial with 5.3 mL infusion fluid to produce a 10 mg/mL solution; dilute requisite dose in 100 mL infusion fluid; give over 30–60 minutes.

- PATIENT AND CARER ADVICE
Driving and skilled tasks Manufacturer advises patients and carers should be cautioned on the effects on driving and performance of skilled tasks—increased risk of dizziness.

- MEDICINAL FORMS There can be variation in the licensing of different medicines containing the same drug.
Powder for solution for infusion
  ▸ Tigecycline (Non-proprietary)
   Tigecycline 50 mg Tigecycline 50mg powder for solution for infusion vials | 10 vial [PoM] £290.79 (Hospital only)
  ▸ Tygacil (Pfizer Ltd)
   Tigecycline 50 mg Tygacil 50mg powder for solution for infusion vials | 10 vial [PoM] £323.10 (Hospital only)

ANTIBACTERIALS > OTHER

Chloramphenicol
09-Nov-2020

- DRUG ACTION Chloramphenicol is a potent broad-spectrum antibiotic.

- INDICATIONS AND DOSE

Life threatening infections particularly those caused by *Haemophilus influenzae* | Typhoid fever
  ▸ BY MOUTH, OR BY INTRAVENOUS INJECTION, OR BY INTRAVENOUS INFUSION
  ▸ Adult: 12.5 mg/kg every 6 hours, in exceptional cases dose can be doubled for severe infections such as septicaemia and meningitis, providing high doses reduced as soon as clinically indicated

- CONTRA-INDICATIONS Acute porphyrias p. 1107
- CAUTIONS Avoid repeated courses and prolonged treatment
- INTERACTIONS → Appendix 1: chloramphenicol
- SIDE-EFFECTS
▸ **Rare or very rare**
▸ With parenteral use Aplastic anaemia (reversible or irreversible, with reports of resulting leukaemia)
▸ **Frequency not known**
▸ With oral use Bone marrow disorders · circulatory collapse · diarrhoea · enterocolitis · nausea · optic neuritis · oral disorders · ototoxicity · vomiting
▸ With parenteral use Agranulocytosis · bone marrow disorders · depression · diarrhoea · dry mouth · fungal superinfection · headache · nausea · nerve disorders · thrombocytopenic purpura · urticaria · vision disorders · vomiting
  SIDE-EFFECTS, FURTHER INFORMATION Associated with serious haematological side-effects when given systemically and should therefore be reserved for the treatment of life-threatening infections.

- PREGNANCY Manufacturer advises avoid; neonatal 'grey-baby syndrome' if used in third trimester.

- BREAST FEEDING Manufacturer advises avoid; use another antibiotic; may cause bone-marrow toxicity in infant; concentration in milk usually insufficient to cause 'grey syndrome'.

- HEPATIC IMPAIRMENT Manufacturer advises caution (increased risk of bone-marrow depression)—monitor plasma-chloramphenicol concentration.
Dose adjustments Manufacturer advises consider dose reduction.
Monitoring Monitor plasma-chloramphenicol concentration in hepatic impairment.

- RENAL IMPAIRMENT Avoid in severe renal impairment unless no alternative; dose-related depression of haematopoiesis.

- MONITORING REQUIREMENTS
▸ Plasma concentration monitoring preferred in the elderly.
▸ Recommended peak plasma concentration (approx. 2 hours after administration by mouth, intravenous injection or infusion) 10–25 mg/litre; pre-dose ('trough') concentration should not exceed 15 mg/litre.
▸ Blood counts required before and periodically during treatment.

- DIRECTIONS FOR ADMINISTRATION
▸ With intravenous use [EvG] For *intravenous infusion*, give intermittently or via drip tubing in Glucose 5% *or* Sodium Chloride 0.9%. ⟨M⟩

- MEDICINAL FORMS There can be variation in the licensing of different medicines containing the same drug.
Powder for solution for injection
ELECTROLYTES: May contain Sodium
  ▸ Chloramphenicol (Non-proprietary)
   Chloramphenicol (as Chloramphenicol sodium succinate)
   1 gram Chloramphenicol 1g powder for solution for injection vials | 1 vial [PoM] £88.00 DT = £88.00
Capsule
  ▸ Chloramphenicol (Non-proprietary)
   Chloramphenicol 250 mg Chloramphenicol 250mg capsules | 60 capsule [PoM] £377.00 DT = £377.00

Daptomycin
04-Nov-2020

- DRUG ACTION Daptomycin is a lipopeptide antibacterial with a spectrum of activity similar to vancomycin but its efficacy against enterococci has not been established. It needs to be given with other antibacterials for mixed infections involving Gram-negative bacteria and some anaerobes.

- INDICATIONS AND DOSE

Complicated skin and soft-tissue infections caused by Gram-positive bacteria
  ▸ BY INTRAVENOUS INFUSION
  ▸ Child 12-23 months: 10 mg/kg once daily for up to 14 days, alternatively 12 mg/kg once daily, higher dose only if associated with *Staphylococcus aureus* bacteraemia—duration of treatment in accordance with risk of complications in individual patients
  ▸ Child 2-6 years: 9 mg/kg once daily for up to 14 days, alternatively 12 mg/kg once daily, higher dose only if associated with *Staphylococcus aureus* bacteraemia—duration of treatment in accordance with risk of complications in individual patients
  ▸ Child 7-11 years: 7 mg/kg once daily for up to 14 days, alternatively 9 mg/kg once daily, higher dose only if associated with *Staphylococcus aureus* bacteraemia—duration of treatment in accordance with risk of complications in individual patients
  ▸ Child 12-17 years: 5 mg/kg once daily for up to 14 days, alternatively 7 mg/kg once daily, higher dose only if associated with *Staphylococcus aureus* bacteraemia—duration of treatment in accordance with risk of complications in individual patients

Complicated skin and soft-tissue infections caused by Gram-positive bacteria
  ▸ BY SLOW INTRAVENOUS INJECTION, OR BY INTRAVENOUS INFUSION
  ▸ Adult: 4 mg/kg once daily for 7–14 days or longer if necessary, alternatively 6 mg/kg once daily, higher dose only if associated with *Staphylococcus aureus* bacteraemia—duration of treatment may need to be longer than 14 days in accordance with risk of complications in individual patients
continued →

5

Infection

Right-sided infective endocarditis caused by *Staphylococcus aureus* (administered on expert advice)

▶ BY SLOW INTRAVENOUS INJECTION, OR BY INTRAVENOUS INFUSION

▸ Adult: 6 mg/kg once daily, duration of treatment in accordance with official recommendations

● CAUTIONS Obesity (limited information on safety and efficacy)

● INTERACTIONS → Appendix 1: daptomycin

● SIDE-EFFECTS

▶ **Common or very common** Anaemia · anxiety · asthenia · constipation · diarrhoea · dizziness · fever · flatulence · gastrointestinal discomfort · headache · hypertension · hypotension · increased risk of infection · insomnia · nausea · pain · skin reactions · vomiting

▶ **Uncommon** Appetite decreased · arrhythmias · arthralgia · electrolyte imbalance · eosinophilia · flushing · gastritis · hyperglycaemia · muscle weakness · myalgia · myopathy · paraesthesia · renal impairment · taste altered · thrombocytosis · tremor · vertigo

▶ **Rare or very rare** Jaundice

▶ **Frequency not known** Acute generalised exanthematous pustulosis (AGEP) · antibiotic associated colitis · chills · cough · infusion related reaction · peripheral neuropathy · respiratory disorders · syncope

SIDE-EFFECTS, FURTHER INFORMATION If unexplained muscle pain, tenderness, weakness, or cramps develop during treatment, measure creatine kinase every 2 days; discontinue if unexplained muscular symptoms and creatine elevated markedly.

● PREGNANCY Manufacturer advises use only if potential benefit outweighs risk—no information available.

● BREAST FEEDING Present in milk in small amounts, but absorption from gastrointestinal tract negligible.

● HEPATIC IMPAIRMENT Manufacturer advises caution in severe impairment—no information available.

● RENAL IMPAIRMENT

▸ In children Manufacturer advises the dosage regimen has not been established—use with caution and monitor renal function regularly.

▸ In adults Manufacturer advises use only when potential benefit outweighs risk—higher risk of developing myopathy; monitor renal function regularly.

Dose adjustments ▸ In adults Use normal dose every 48 hours if eGFR less than 30 mL/minute/1.73 m^2.

● MONITORING REQUIREMENTS

▸ Manufacturer advises monitor plasma creatine phosphokinase (CPK) before treatment and then at least weekly during treatment; monitor CPK more frequently in patients at higher risk of developing myopathy, including those with renal impairment, taking other drugs associated with myopathy, or if CPK elevated more than 5 times upper limit of normal before treatment.

▸ Manufacturer advises monitor renal function regularly during concomitant administration of potentially nephrotoxic drugs.

● EFFECT ON LABORATORY TESTS Interference with assay for prothrombin time and INR—take blood sample immediately before daptomycin dose.

● DIRECTIONS FOR ADMINISTRATION

▸ In children For *intravenous infusion*, manufacturer advises give intermittently in Sodium Chloride 0.9%; reconstitute with Sodium Chloride 0.9% (350 mg in 7 mL, 500 mg in 10 mL); gently rotate vial without shaking; allow to stand for at least 10 minutes then rotate gently to dissolve; dilute requisite dose in 50 mL infusion fluid and give over 60 minutes for children aged 1–6 years and over 30 minutes for children aged 7–17 years.

▸ In adults For *intravenous infusion*, manufacturer advises give intermittently in Sodium Chloride 0.9%; reconstitute with Sodium Chloride 0.9% (350 mg in 7 mL, 500 mg in 10 mL); gently rotate vial without shaking; allow to stand for at least 10 minutes then rotate gently to dissolve; dilute requisite dose in 50 mL infusion fluid and give over 30 minutes. For *intravenous injection*, give over 2 minutes.

● HANDLING AND STORAGE Manufacturer advises store in a refrigerator (2–8 °C)—consult product literature for further information regarding storage after reconstitution and dilution.

● NATIONAL FUNDING/ACCESS DECISIONS For full details see funding body website

Scottish Medicines Consortium (SMC) decisions

▸ Daptomycin (*Cubicin*®) for complicated skin and soft tissue infections in adults (April 2006) SMC No. 248/06 Recommended with restrictions

▸ Daptomycin (*Cubicin*®) for the treatment of *Staphylococcus aureus* bacteraemia (SAB) when associated with right-sided infective endocarditis or with complicated skin and soft-tissue infection in adults (March 2008) SMC No. 449/08 Recommended with restrictions

● MEDICINAL FORMS There can be variation in the licensing of different medicines containing the same drug.

Powder for solution for infusion

▸ Daptomycin (Non-proprietary)

Daptomycin 350 mg Daptomycin 350mg powder for solution for infusion vials | 1 vial [PoM] £60.00–£62.00 (Hospital only)

Daptomycin 500 mg Daptomycin 500mg powder for solution for infusion vials | 1 vial [PoM] £88.00–£88.57 (Hospital only)

▸ Cubicin (Merck Sharp & Dohme Ltd)

Daptomycin 350 mg Cubicin 350mg powder for concentrate for solution for infusion vials | 1 vial [PoM] £62.00 (Hospital only)

Daptomycin 500 mg Cubicin 500mg powder for concentrate for solution for infusion vials | 1 vial [PoM] £88.57 (Hospital only)

| Fidaxomicin

24-Nov-2020

● DRUG ACTION Fidaxomicin is a macrocyclic antibacterial that is poorly absorbed from the gastro-intestinal tract, and, therefore, it should not be used to treat systemic infections.

● INDICATIONS AND DOSE

Clostridioides difficile infection

▶ BY MOUTH

▸ Adult: 200 mg every 12 hours for 10 days, limited clinical data is available on the use of fidaxomicin in severe or life-threatening *Clostridioides difficile* infection

● CAUTIONS Severe or life-threatening *C. difficile* infection

● INTERACTIONS → Appendix 1: fidaxomicin

● SIDE-EFFECTS

▶ **Common or very common** Constipation · nausea · vomiting

▶ **Uncommon** Abdominal distension · appetite decreased · dizziness · dry mouth · flatulence · headache · skin reactions · taste altered

▶ **Frequency not known** Angioedema · dyspnoea · hypersensitivity

● ALLERGY AND CROSS-SENSITIVITY [EvGr] Use with caution in macrolide hypersensitivity. ⓜ

● PREGNANCY Manufacturer advises avoid—no information available.

● BREAST FEEDING Manufacturer advises avoid—no information available.

● HEPATIC IMPAIRMENT Manufacturer advises caution in moderate to severe impairment—limited information available.

- RENAL IMPAIRMENT Manufacturer advises caution in severe impairment—no information available.
- NATIONAL FUNDING/ACCESS DECISIONS For full details see funding body website

Scottish Medicines Consortium (SMC) decisions
▸ Fidaxomicin (*Dificlir*®) for the treatment of *Clostridium difficile* infections (CDI) also known as *C. Difficile*-associated diarrhoea (CDAD) (July 2012) SMC No. 791/12 Recommended with restrictions

- MEDICINAL FORMS There can be variation in the licensing of different medicines containing the same drug.

Tablet
CAUTIONARY AND ADVISORY LABELS 9
▸ Dificlir (Astellas Pharma Ltd)
Fidaxomicin 200 mg Dificlir 200mg tablets | 20 tablet [PoM] £1,350.00 DT = £1,350.00

Fosfomycin

06-Nov-2020

- DRUG ACTION Fosfomycin, a phosphonic acid antibacterial, is active against a range of Gram-positive and Gram-negative bacteria including *Staphylococcus aureus* and Enterobacteriaceae.

- INDICATIONS AND DOSE

Acute uncomplicated lower urinary-tract infections
▸ BY MOUTH USING GRANULES
▸ Adult: 3 g for 1 dose

Prophylaxis of urinary-tract infections in transurethral surgical procedures
▸ BY MOUTH USING GRANULES
▸ Adult: 3 g, to be given 3 hours before surgery. Dose may be repeated once, 24 hours after surgery

Osteomyelitis when first-line treatments are inappropriate or ineffective | Hospital-acquired lower respiratory-tract infections when first-line treatments are inappropriate or ineffective
▸ BY INTRAVENOUS INFUSION
▸ Adult: 12–24 g daily in 2–3 divided doses (max. per dose 8 g), use the high-dose regimen in severe infection suspected or known to be caused by less sensitive organisms

Complicated urinary-tract infections when first-line treatment ineffective or inappropriate
▸ BY INTRAVENOUS INFUSION
▸ Adult: 12–16 g daily in 2–3 divided doses (max. per dose 8 g)

Bacterial meningitis when first-line treatment ineffective or inappropriate
▸ BY INTRAVENOUS INFUSION
▸ Adult: 16–24 g daily in 3–4 divided doses (max. per dose 8 g), use the high-dose regimen in severe infection suspected or known to be caused by less sensitive organisms

- CAUTIONS
▸ With intravenous use Cardiac insufficiency · elderly (high doses) · hyperaldosteronism · hypernatraemia · hypertension · pulmonary oedema

- SIDE-EFFECTS

GENERAL SIDE-EFFECTS
▸ **Common or very common** Abdominal pain · diarrhoea · headache · nausea · vomiting
▸ **Uncommon** Skin reactions
▸ **Frequency not known** Antibiotic associated colitis

SPECIFIC SIDE-EFFECTS
▸ **Common or very common**
▸ With oral use Dizziness · vulvovaginal infection

▸ **Uncommon**
▸ With parenteral use Appetite decreased · dyspnoea · electrolyte imbalance · fatigue · oedema · taste altered · vertigo
▸ **Rare or very rare**
▸ With parenteral use Bone marrow disorders · eosinophilia · hepatic disorders · visual impairment
▸ **Frequency not known**
▸ With parenteral use Agranulocytosis · asthmatic attack · confusion · leucopenia · neutropenia · tachycardia · thrombocytopenia

- PREGNANCY Manufacturer advises use only if potential benefit outweighs risk.
- BREAST FEEDING Manufacturer advises use only if potential benefit outweighs risk—present in milk.
- RENAL IMPAIRMENT
▸ With oral use Avoid *oral* treatment if eGFR less than 10 mL/minute/1.73 m^2.
▸ With intravenous use Use *intravenous* treatment with caution if eGFR 40–80 mL/minute/1.73 m^2 and consult product literature for dose if eGFR less than 40 mL/minute/1.73 m^2.
- MONITORING REQUIREMENTS
▸ With intravenous use Monitor electrolytes and fluid balance.
- DIRECTIONS FOR ADMINISTRATION
▸ With intravenous use For *intravenous infusion* (*Fomicyt*®), manufacturer advises give intermittently *in* Glucose 5% *or* 10% *or* Water for Injections; reconstitute each 2-g or 4-g vial with 20 mL and 8-g vial with 40 mL infusion fluid; dilute reconstituted solution to a concentration of 40 mg/mL; give 2 g over 15 minutes.
▸ With oral use Manufacturer advises granules should be taken on an empty stomach (about 2–3 hours before or after a meal), preferably before bedtime and after emptying the bladder. The granules should be dissolved into a glass of water and taken immediately.
- PRESCRIBING AND DISPENSING INFORMATION Doses expressed as fosfomycin base.
- NATIONAL FUNDING/ACCESS DECISIONS For full details see funding body website

Scottish Medicines Consortium (SMC) decisions
▸ Fosfomycin (*Fomicyt*®) for the treatment of the following infections in adults and children including neonates: acute osteomyelitis; complicated urinary tract infections; nosocomial lower respiratory tract infections; bacterial meningitis; bacteraemia that occurs in association with, or is suspected to be associated with, any of the infections listed above (March 2015) SMC No. 1033/15 Recommended with restrictions
▸ Fosfomycin trometamol (*Monuril*®) for the treatment of acute lower uncomplicated urinary tract infections, caused by pathogens sensitive to fosfomycin in adult and adolescent female, and for prophylaxis in diagnostic and surgical transurethral procedures (September 2016) SMC No. 1163/16 Recommended

- MEDICINAL FORMS There can be variation in the licensing of different medicines containing the same drug. Forms available from special-order manufacturers include: capsule

Oral suspension
▸ Fosfocina (Imported (Spain))
Fosfomycin calcium 50 mg per 1 ml Fosfocina 250mg/5ml oral suspension | 120 ml [PoM] [⅀]
Powder for solution for infusion
ELECTROLYTES: May contain Sodium
▸ Infectofos (Imported (Germany))
Fosfomycin (as Fosfomycin sodium) 5 gram Infectofos 5g powder for solution for infusion vials | 10 vial [PoM] [⅀]
▸ Fomicyt (Kent Pharmaceuticals Ltd)
Fosfomycin (as Fosfomycin sodium) 2 gram Fomicyt 2g powder for solution for infusion vials | 10 vial [PoM] £150.00
Fosfomycin (as Fosfomycin sodium) 4 gram Fomicyt 4g powder for solution for infusion vials | 10 vial [PoM] £300.00

Granules

CAUTIONARY AND ADVISORY LABELS 9, 13, 23
EXCIPIENTS: May contain Sucrose
▸ Fosfomycin (Non-proprietary)
Fosfomycin (as Fosfomycin trometamol) 3 gram Fosfomycin 3g
granules sachets | 1 sachet [PoM] £75.45 DT = £4.86
▸ Monuril (Profile Pharma Ltd)
Fosfomycin (as Fosfomycin trometamol) 3 gram Monuril 3g
granules sachets | 1 sachet [PoM] £4.86 DT = £4.86

Fusidic acid

30-Apr-2020

● DRUG ACTION Fusidic acid and its salts are narrow-spectrum antibiotics used for staphylococcal infections.

● INDICATIONS AND DOSE

Staphylococcal skin infection
▸ TO THE SKIN
▹ Child: Apply 3–4 times a day usually for 7 days
▹ Adult: Apply 3–4 times a day
▸ BY MOUTH USING TABLETS
▹ Child 12–17 years: 250 mg every 12 hours for 5-10 days, dose expressed as sodium fusidate
▹ Adult: 250 mg every 12 hours for 5-10 days, dose expressed as sodium fusidate

Non-bullous impetigo [in patients who are not systemically unwell or at high risk of complications]
▸ TO THE SKIN
▹ Child: Apply 3 times a day for 5–7 days
▹ Adult: Apply 3 times a day for 5–7 days

Penicillin-resistant staphylococcal infection including osteomyelitis | Staphylococcal endocarditis in combination with other antibacterials
▸ BY MOUTH USING ORAL SUSPENSION
▹ Child 1-11 months: 15 mg/kg 3 times a day
▹ Child 1-4 years: 250 mg 3 times a day
▹ Child 5-11 years: 500 mg 3 times a day
▹ Child 12-17 years: 750 mg 3 times a day
▹ Adult: 750 mg 3 times a day
▸ BY MOUTH USING TABLETS
▹ Child 12-17 years: 500 mg every 8 hours, increased to 1 g every 8 hours, increased dose can be used for severe infections, dose expressed as sodium fusidate
▹ Adult: 500 mg every 8 hours, increased to 1 g every 8 hours, increased dose can be used for severe infections, dose expressed as sodium fusidate

Staphylococcal infections due to susceptible organisms
▸ BY INTRAVENOUS INFUSION
▹ Child (body-weight up to 50 kg): 6–7 mg/kg 3 times a day, dose expressed as sodium fusidate
▹ Child (body-weight 50 kg and above): 500 mg 3 times a day, dose expressed as sodium fusidate
▹ Adult (body-weight up to 50 kg): 6–7 mg/kg 3 times a day, dose expressed as sodium fusidate
▹ Adult (body-weight 50 kg and above): 500 mg 3 times a day, dose expressed as sodium fusidate

DOSE EQUIVALENCE AND CONVERSION
▸ With oral use
▹ Fusidic acid is incompletely absorbed and doses recommended for suspension are proportionately higher than those for sodium fusidate tablets.

● CAUTIONS
▸ With systemic use Impaired transport and metabolism of bilirubin
▸ With topical use Avoid contact of cream or ointment with eyes

CAUTIONS, FURTHER INFORMATION
▸ Avoiding resistance
▸ With topical use To avoid the development of resistance, fusidic acid should not be used for longer than 10 days and

local microbiology advice should be sought before using it in hospital.

● INTERACTIONS → Appendix 1: fusidate

● SIDE-EFFECTS

GENERAL SIDE-EFFECTS
▸ **Uncommon** Skin reactions

SPECIFIC SIDE-EFFECTS
▸ **Common or very common**
▹ With intravenous use Dizziness · drowsiness · hepatic disorders · hyperbilirubinaemia · thrombophlebitis · vascular pain (reduced if given via central vein)
▹ With oral use Diarrhoea · dizziness · drowsiness · gastrointestinal discomfort · nausea · vomiting
▸ **Uncommon**
▹ With intravenous use Appetite decreased · asthenia · headache · malaise
▹ With oral use Appetite decreased · asthenia · headache · malaise · rash pustular
▸ **Rare or very rare**
▹ With topical use Angioedema · conjunctivitis
▸ **Frequency not known**
▹ With intravenous use Agranulocytosis · anaemia · leucopenia · neutropenia · pancytopenia · renal failure · rhabdomyolysis · thrombocytopenia
▹ With oral use Agranulocytosis · anaemia · hepatic disorders · hyperbilirubinaemia · leucopenia · neutropenia · pancytopenia · renal failure · rhabdomyolysis · thrombocytopenia

SIDE-EFFECTS, FURTHER INFORMATION Elevated liver enzymes, hyperbilirubinaemia and jaundice can occur with systemic use—these effects are usually reversible following withdrawal of therapy.

● PREGNANCY
▸ With systemic use Not known to be harmful; manufacturer advises use only if potential benefit outweighs risk.

● BREAST FEEDING
▸ With systemic use Present in milk—manufacturer advises caution.

● HEPATIC IMPAIRMENT
▸ With systemic use Manufacturer advises caution.

● MONITORING REQUIREMENTS
▸ With systemic use Manufacturer advises monitor liver function with high doses or on prolonged therapy; monitoring also advised for patients with biliary tract obstruction, those taking potentially hepatotoxic medication, or those taking concurrent medication with a similar excretion pathway.

● DIRECTIONS FOR ADMINISTRATION
▸ With intravenous use Manufacturer advises *for intravenous infusion*, give intermittently in Sodium chloride 0.9% or Glucose 5%; reconstitute each vial with 10 mL buffer solution, then add contents of vial to 500 mL infusion fluid to give a solution containing approximately 1 mg/mL. Give requisite dose via a central line over 2 hours (give over at least 6 hours if administered via a large peripheral vein).

● PRESCRIBING AND DISPENSING INFORMATION For choice of antibacterial therapy, see Cardiovascular system infections, antibacterial therapy p. 532, Musculoskeletal system infections, antibacterial therapy p. 536, Skin infections, antibacterial therapy p. 541.

● PROFESSION SPECIFIC INFORMATION

Dental practitioners' formulary
▸ With topical use May be prescribed as Sodium Fusidate ointment.

- MEDICINAL FORMS There can be variation in the licensing of different medicines containing the same drug.

Tablet
CAUTIONARY AND ADVISORY LABELS 9
▸ Fucidin (LEO Pharma)
Sodium fusidate 250 mg Fucidin 250mg tablets | 10 tablet [PoM] £6.02 DT = £6.02 | 100 tablet [PoM] £54.99 DT = £54.99

Oral suspension
CAUTIONARY AND ADVISORY LABELS 9
▸ Fucidin (LEO Pharma)
Fusidic acid 50 mg per 1 ml Fucidin 250mg/5ml oral suspension | 90 ml [PoM] £12.11 DT = £12.11

Cream
EXCIPIENTS: May contain Butylated hydroxyanisole, cetostearyl alcohol (including cetyl and stearyl alcohol)
▸ Fusidic acid (Non-proprietary)
Fusidic acid 20 mg per 1 gram Fusidic acid 2% cream | 15 gram [PoM] £3.08 DT = £3.08 | 30 gram [PoM] £6.16 DT = £6.16
▸ Fucidin (LEO Pharma)
Fusidic acid 20 mg per 1 gram Fucidin 20mg/g cream | 15 gram [PoM] £1.92 DT = £3.08 | 30 gram [PoM] £3.59 DT = £6.16

Ointment
EXCIPIENTS: May contain Cetostearyl alcohol (including cetyl and stearyl alcohol), woolfat and related substances (including lanolin)
▸ Fucidin (LEO Pharma)
Sodium fusidate 20 mg per 1 gram Fucidin 20mg/g ointment | 15 gram [PoM] £2.68 DT = £2.68 | 30 gram [PoM] £4.55 DT = £4.55

Powder and solvent for solution for infusion
ELECTROLYTES: May contain Sodium
▸ Fusidic acid (Non-proprietary)
Sodium fusidate 500 mg Sodium fusidate 500mg powder and solvent for solution for infusion vials | 1 vial [PoM] £20.50–£20.90 DT = £20.70

Linezolid
23-Jul-2020

- DRUG ACTION Linezolid, an oxazolidinone antibacterial, is active against Gram-positive bacteria including meticillin-resistant *Staphylococcus aureus* (MRSA), and glycopeptide-resistant enterococci. Resistance to linezolid can develop with prolonged treatment or if the dose is less than that recommended. Linezolid is **not** active against common Gram-negative organisms; it must be given in combination with other antibacterials for mixed infections that also involve Gram-negative organisms.

- INDICATIONS AND DOSE

Pneumonia (when other antibacterials e.g. a glycopeptide, such as vancomycin, cannot be used) (initiated under specialist supervision) | Complicated skin and soft-tissue infections caused by Gram-positive bacteria, when other antibacterials cannot be used (initiated under specialist supervision)
▸ BY MOUTH
▸ Adult: 600 mg every 12 hours usually for 10–14 days (maximum duration of treatment 28 days)
▸ BY INTRAVENOUS INFUSION
▸ Adult: 600 mg every 12 hours

Cellulitis (specialist use only) | Erysipelas (specialist use only)
▸ BY MOUTH, OR BY INTRAVENOUS INFUSION
▸ Adult: 600 mg every 12 hours

Moderate diabetic foot infection (specialist use only) | Severe diabetic foot infection (specialist use only) | Leg ulcer infection (specialist use only)
▸ BY MOUTH, OR BY INTRAVENOUS INFUSION
▸ Adult: 600 mg every 12 hours

IMPORTANT SAFETY INFORMATION
CHM ADVICE (OPTIC NEUROPATHY)
Severe optic neuropathy may occur rarely, particularly if linezolid is used for longer than 28 days. The CHM recommends that:

- patients should be warned to report symptoms of visual impairment (including blurred vision, visual field defect, changes in visual acuity and colour vision) immediately;
- patients experiencing new visual symptoms (regardless of treatment duration) should be evaluated promptly, and referred to an ophthalmologist if necessary;
- visual function should be monitored regularly if treatment is required for longer than 28 days.

BLOOD DISORDERS
Haematopoietic disorders (including thrombocytopenia, anaemia, leucopenia, and pancytopenia) have been reported in patients receiving linezolid. It is recommended that full blood counts are monitored weekly. Close monitoring is recommended in patients who:
- receive treatment for more than 10–14 days;
- have pre-existing myelosuppression;
- are receiving drugs that may have adverse effects on haemoglobin, blood counts, or platelet function;
- have severe renal impairment.
If significant myelosuppression occurs, treatment should be stopped unless it is considered essential, in which case intensive monitoring of blood counts and appropriate management should be implemented.

- CAUTIONS Acute confusional states · bipolar depression · carcinoid tumour · elderly (increased risk of blood disorders) · history of seizures · phaeochromocytoma · schizophrenia · thyrotoxicosis · uncontrolled hypertension
CAUTIONS, FURTHER INFORMATION
- Close observation Unless close observation and blood pressure monitoring possible, linezolid should be avoided in uncontrolled hypertension, phaeochromocytoma, carcinoid tumour, thyrotoxicosis, bipolar depression, schizophrenia, or acute confusional states.

- INTERACTIONS → Appendix 1: linezolid

- SIDE-EFFECTS
▸ **Common or very common** Anaemia · constipation · diarrhoea · dizziness · gastrointestinal discomfort · headache · hypertension · increased risk of infection · insomnia · localised pain · nausea · skin reactions · taste altered · vomiting
▸ **Uncommon** Arrhythmia · chills · dry mouth · eosinophilia · fatigue · gastritis · hyperhidrosis · hyponatraemia · leucopenia · neutropenia · oral disorders · pancreatitis · polyuria · renal failure · seizure · sensation abnormal · thirst · thrombocytopenia · thrombophlebitis · tinnitus · tongue discolouration · transient ischaemic attack · vision disorders · vulvovaginal disorder
▸ **Rare or very rare** Antibiotic associated colitis · bone marrow disorders · tooth discolouration
▸ **Frequency not known** Alopecia · angioedema · lactic acidosis · nerve disorders · serotonin syndrome · severe cutaneous adverse reactions (SCARs)

- PREGNANCY Manufacturer advises use only if potential benefit outweighs risk—no information available.

- BREAST FEEDING Manufacturer advises avoid—present in milk in *animal* studies.

- HEPATIC IMPAIRMENT Manufacturer advises caution in severe impairment (no information available).

- RENAL IMPAIRMENT Manufacturer advises metabolites may accumulate if eGFR less than 30 mL/minute/1.73 m^2.

- MONITORING REQUIREMENTS Monitor full blood count (including platelet count) weekly.

- DIRECTIONS FOR ADMINISTRATION
▸ With intravenous use Manufacturer advises infusion to be administered over 30–120 minutes.

- PRESCRIBING AND DISPENSING INFORMATION For choice of antibacterial therapy, see Diabetic foot infections, antibacterial therapy p. 534, Respiratory system infections, antibacterial therapy p. 538, Skin infections, antibacterial therapy p. 541.
- PATIENT AND CARER ADVICE Patients should be advised to read the patient information leaflet given with linezolid.
- MEDICINAL FORMS There can be variation in the licensing of different medicines containing the same drug.

Infusion

EXCIPIENTS: May contain Glucose

ELECTROLYTES: May contain Sodium

▸ Linezolid (Non-proprietary)

Linezolid 2 mg per 1 ml Linezolid 600mg/300ml infusion bags | 10 bag PoM £445.00-£541.00 (Hospital only)

▸ Zyvox (Pfizer Ltd)

Linezolid 2 mg per 1 ml Zyvox 600mg/300ml infusion bags | 10 bag PoM £445.00 (Hospital only)

Oral suspension

CAUTIONARY AND ADVISORY LABELS 9, 10

EXCIPIENTS: May contain Aspartame

▸ Zyvox (Pfizer Ltd)

Linezolid 20 mg per 1 ml Zyvox 100mg/5ml granules for oral suspension | 150 ml PoM £222.50 DT = £222.50

Tablet

CAUTIONARY AND ADVISORY LABELS 9, 10

▸ Linezolid (Non-proprietary)

Linezolid 600 mg Linezolid 600mg tablets | 10 tablet PoM £239.16 DT = £327.24 (Hospital only) | 10 tablet PoM £312.41-£445.00 DT = £327.24

▸ Zyvox (Pfizer Ltd)

Linezolid 600 mg Zyvox 600mg tablets | 10 tablet PoM £445.00 DT = £327.24

Tedizolid

16-Nov-2020

- DRUG ACTION Tedizolid is an oxazolidinone antibacterial, which inhibits bacterial protein synthesis.

● INDICATIONS AND DOSE

Treatment of acute bacterial skin and skin structure infections

▸ BY INTRAVENOUS INFUSION, OR BY MOUTH

▸ Adult: 200 mg once daily for 6 days, patients should be switched from the intravenous to the oral route when clinically appropriate

- CAUTIONS Neutropenia—limited clinical experience · patients aged 75 years and over—limited clinical experience
- INTERACTIONS → Appendix 1: tedizolid
- SIDE-EFFECTS

GENERAL SIDE-EFFECTS

▸ **Common or very common** Diarrhoea · dizziness · fatigue · headache · nausea · skin reactions · vomiting

▸ **Uncommon** Abscess · alopecia · antibiotic associated colitis · anxiety · arthralgia · bradycardia · chills · constipation · cough · dehydration · diabetic control impaired · drowsiness · dry mouth · fever · gastrointestinal discomfort · gastrointestinal disorders · haematochezia · hyperhidrosis · hyperkalaemia · increased risk of infection · irritability · limb discomfort · lymphadenopathy · muscle spasms · nasal dryness · pain · peripheral oedema · pulmonary congestion · sensation abnormal · sleep disorders · taste altered · tremor · urine odour abnormal · vasodilation · vision blurred · vitreous floater · vulvovaginal pruritus

SPECIFIC SIDE-EFFECTS

▸ **Uncommon**

▸ With intravenous use Infusion related reaction

- CONCEPTION AND CONTRACEPTION Manufacturer recommends effective contraception in women of childbearing potential; an additional method of

contraception is advised in women taking hormonal contraceptives—effectiveness may be reduced.

- PREGNANCY Manufacturer advises avoid—fetal developmental toxicity in *animal* studies.
- BREAST FEEDING Manufacturer advises avoid—present in milk in *animal* studies.
- DIRECTIONS FOR ADMINISTRATION For *intravenous infusion* (*Sivextro*®), manufacturer advises give intermittently in Sodium Chloride 0.9%; reconstitute each 200 mg vial with 4 mL Water for Injections, then dilute reconstituted solution in 250 mL sodium chloride 0.9%; give over approx. 1 hour.
- PATIENT AND CARER ADVICE

Optic neuropathy Although neuropathy (peripheral and optic) has not been reported in patients treated with tedizolid, manufacturer advises patients and carers are warned to report symptoms of visual impairment (including blurred vision, visual field defect, changes in visual acuity and colour vision) immediately; patients should be evaluated promptly, and referred to an ophthalmologist if necessary.

Missed doses Manufacturer advises that if a dose is more than 16 hours late, the missed dose should not be taken and the next dose should be taken at the normal time.

Driving and skilled tasks Patients and carers should be counselled on the effects on driving and skilled tasks—increased risk of dizziness and fatigue.

- NATIONAL FUNDING/ACCESS DECISIONS

For full details see funding body website

Scottish Medicines Consortium (SMC) decisions

▸ Tedizolid (*Sivextro*®) for the treatment of acute bacterial skin and skin structure infections in adults (August 2015) SMC No. 1080/15 Recommended with restrictions

- MEDICINAL FORMS There can be variation in the licensing of different medicines containing the same drug.

Powder for solution for infusion

▸ Sivextro (Merck Sharp & Dohme Ltd)

Tedizolid phosphate 200 mg Sivextro 200mg powder for concentrate for solution for infusion vials | 6 vial PoM £862.00

Tablet

▸ Sivextro (Merck Sharp & Dohme Ltd)

Tedizolid phosphate 200 mg Sivextro 200mg tablets | 6 tablet PoM £862.00

Trimethoprim

03-Sep-2020

● INDICATIONS AND DOSE

Respiratory-tract infections

▸ BY MOUTH

▸ Child 4-5 weeks: 4 mg/kg twice daily (max. per dose 200 mg)

▸ Child 6 weeks-5 months: 4 mg/kg twice daily (max. per dose 200 mg), alternatively 25 mg twice daily

▸ Child 6 months-5 years: 4 mg/kg twice daily (max. per dose 200 mg), alternatively 50 mg twice daily

▸ Child 6-11 years: 4 mg/kg twice daily (max. per dose 200 mg), alternatively 100 mg twice daily

▸ Child 12-17 years: 200 mg twice daily

▸ Adult: 200 mg twice daily

Prophylaxis of recurrent urinary-tract infection

▸ BY MOUTH

▸ Child 4-5 weeks: 2 mg/kg once daily, dose to be taken at night

▸ Child 6 weeks-5 months: 2 mg/kg once daily, alternatively 12.5 mg once daily, dose to be taken at night

▸ Child 6 months-5 years: 2 mg/kg once daily (max. per dose 100 mg), alternatively 25 mg once daily, dose to be taken at night

▸ Child 6–11 years: 2 mg/kg once daily (max. per dose 100 mg), alternatively 50 mg once daily, dose to be taken at night
▸ Child 12–15 years: 100 mg once daily, dose to be taken at night
▸ Child 16–17 years: 100 mg once daily, dose to be taken at night, alternatively 200 mg for 1 dose, following exposure to a trigger
▸ Adult: 100 mg once daily, dose to be taken at night, alternatively 200 mg for 1 dose, following exposure to a trigger

Treatment of mild to moderate *Pneumocystis jirovecii* (*Pneumocystis carinii*) pneumonia in patients who cannot tolerate co-trimoxazole (in combination with dapsone)
▸ BY MOUTH
▸ Child: 5 mg/kg every 6–8 hours
▸ Adult: 5 mg/kg every 6–8 hours

Acne resistant to other antibacterials
▸ BY MOUTH
▸ Adult: 300 mg twice daily

Shigellosis | Invasive salmonella infection
▸ BY MOUTH
▸ Adult: (consult product literature)

Acute diverticulitis [in combination with metronidazole]
▸ BY MOUTH
▸ Adult: 200 mg twice daily for 5 days then review

Acute prostatitis
▸ BY MOUTH
▸ Adult: 200 mg twice daily for 14 or 28 days based on clinical assessment

Acute pyelonephritis
▸ BY MOUTH
▸ Child 16–17 years: 200 mg twice daily for 14 days
▸ Adult: 200 mg twice daily for 14 days

Urinary-tract infection (catheter-associated)
▸ BY MOUTH
▸ Child 3–5 months: 4 mg/kg twice daily (max. per dose 200 mg) for 7–10 days, alternatively 25 mg twice daily for 7–10 days
▸ Child 6 months–5 years: 4 mg/kg twice daily (max. per dose 200 mg) for 7–10 days, alternatively 50 mg twice daily for 7–10 days
▸ Child 6–11 years: 4 mg/kg twice daily (max. per dose 200 mg) for 7–10 days, alternatively 100 mg twice daily for 7–10 days
▸ Child 12–15 years: 200 mg twice daily for 7–10 days
▸ Child 16–17 years: 200 mg twice daily for 7 days (14 days if upper urinary-tract symptoms are present)
▸ Adult: 200 mg twice daily for 7 days (14 days if upper urinary-tract symptoms are present)

Lower urinary-tract infection
▸ BY MOUTH
▸ Child 4–5 weeks: 4 mg/kg twice daily (max. per dose 200 mg)
▸ Child 6 weeks–2 months: 4 mg/kg twice daily (max. per dose 200 mg), alternatively 25 mg twice daily
▸ Child 3–5 months: 4 mg/kg twice daily (max. per dose 200 mg) for 3 days, alternatively 25 mg twice daily for 3 days
▸ Child 6 months–5 years: 4 mg/kg twice daily (max. per dose 200 mg) for 3 days, alternatively 50 mg twice daily for 3 days
▸ Child 6–11 years: 4 mg/kg twice daily (max. per dose 200 mg) for 3 days, alternatively 100 mg twice daily for 3 days
▸ Child 12–15 years: 200 mg twice daily for 3 days
▸ Child 16–17 years: 200 mg twice daily for 3 days (7 days in males)
▸ Adult: 200 mg twice daily for 3 days (7 days in males)

● UNLICENSED USE EvGr Trimethoprim can be given as a single dose for the prophylaxis of recurrent urinary-tract infection following exposure to a trigger, ⒶⒹ but this dosing regimen is not licensed. Not licensed for treatment of pneumocystis pneumonia. Not licensed for treatment of acne resistant to other antibacterials.
▸ In children Not licensed for use in children under 6 months for the prophylaxis of recurrent urinary-tract infection. Not licensed for use in children under 6 weeks.

● CONTRA-INDICATIONS Blood dyscrasias

● CAUTIONS Acute porphyrias p. 1107 · elderly · predisposition to folate deficiency

● INTERACTIONS → Appendix 1: trimethoprim

● SIDE-EFFECTS
▸ **Common or very common** Diarrhoea · electrolyte imbalance · fungal overgrowth · headache · nausea · skin reactions · vomiting
▸ **Rare or very rare** Agranulocytosis · angioedema · anxiety · appetite decreased · arthralgia · behaviour abnormal · bone marrow disorders · confusion · constipation · cough · depression · dizziness · dyspnoea · eosinophilia · erythema nodosum · fever · haemolysis · haemolytic anaemia · haemorrhage · hallucination · hepatic disorders · hypoglycaemia · lethargy · leucopenia · meningitis aseptic · movement disorders · myalgia · neutropenia · oral disorders · pancreatitis · paraesthesia · peripheral neuritis · photosensitivity reaction · pseudomembranous enterocolitis · renal impairment · seizure · severe cutaneous adverse reactions (SCARs) · sleep disorders · syncope · systemic lupus erythematosus (SLE) · thrombocytopenia · tinnitus · tremor · uveitis · vasculitis · vertigo · wheezing
▸ **Frequency not known** Gastrointestinal disorder · megaloblastic anaemia · methaemoglobinaemia

● PREGNANCY Teratogenic risk in first trimester (folate antagonist). Manufacturers advise avoid during pregnancy.

● BREAST FEEDING Present in milk—short-term use not known to be harmful.

● RENAL IMPAIRMENT Manufacturer advises caution in impairment.
Dose adjustments ▸ In adults Manufacturer advises dose reduction to half normal dose after 3 days if eGFR 15–30 mL/minute/1.73 m^2. Manufacturer advises dose reduction to half normal dose if eGFR less than 15 mL/minute/1.73 m^2.
▸ In children Manufacturer advises dose reduction to half normal dose after 3 days if estimated glomerular filtration rate 15–30 mL/minute/1.73 m^2. Manufacturer advises dose reduction to half normal dose if estimated glomerular filtration rate less than 15 mL/minute/1.73 m^2.

● MONITORING REQUIREMENTS
▸ Manufacturer advises monitor blood counts with long-term use and in those with, or at risk of, folate deficiency.
▸ Manufacturer advises monitor serum electrolytes in patients at risk of developing hyperkalaemia, and consider monitoring in other patients, particularly with long-term use.
▸ Manufacturer advises consider monitoring renal function, particularly with long-term use.
▸ Manufacturer advises monitoring of plasma-trimethoprim concentration may be considered with long-term use and under specialist advice.

● PRESCRIBING AND DISPENSING INFORMATION For choice of antibacterial therapy, see Gastro-intestinal system infections, antibacterial therapy p. 535, Pneumocystis pneumonia p. 640, Respiratory system infections, antibacterial therapy p. 538, Urinary-tract infections p. 626.

5

Infection

Infection

5

- **PATIENT AND CARER ADVICE**
Blood disorders On long-term treatment, patients and their carers should be told how to recognise signs of blood disorders and advised to seek immediate medical attention if symptoms such as fever, sore throat, rash, mouth ulcers, purpura, bruising or bleeding develop.
Medicines for Children leaflet: Trimethoprim for bacterial infections www.medicinesforchildren.org.uk/trimethoprim-bacterial-infections

- **MEDICINAL FORMS** There can be variation in the licensing of different medicines containing the same drug. Forms available from special-order manufacturers include: oral suspension, oral solution

Oral suspension
CAUTIONARY AND ADVISORY LABELS 9
▸ Trimethoprim (Non-proprietary)
Trimethoprim 10 mg per 1 ml Trimethoprim 50mg/5ml oral suspension sugar free sugar-free | 100 ml [PoM] £8.97 DT = £6.68
▸ Monotrim (Chemidex Pharma Ltd)
Trimethoprim 10 mg per 1 ml Monotrim 50mg/5ml oral suspension sugar-free | 100 ml [PoM] £1.77 DT = £6.68

Tablet
CAUTIONARY AND ADVISORY LABELS 9
▸ Trimethoprim (Non-proprietary)
Trimethoprim 100 mg Trimethoprim 100mg tablets | 28 tablet [PoM] £3.32 DT = £1.67
Trimethoprim 200 mg Trimogal 200mg tablets | 14 tablet [PoM] £0.91 DT = £1.27
Trimethoprim 200mg tablets | 6 tablet [PoM] £2.15 DT = £0.54 | 14 tablet [PoM] £5.00 DT = £1.27

Combinations available: *Co-trimoxazole*, p. 598

ANTIMYCOBACTERIALS ⟩ RIFAMYCINS

Rifabutin

02-Dec-2020

- **INDICATIONS AND DOSE**
Prophylaxis of *Mycobacterium avium* complex infections in immunosuppressed patients with low CD4 count
▸ BY MOUTH
▸ Adult: 300 mg once daily, also consult product literature
Treatment of non-tuberculous mycobacterial disease, in combination with other drugs
▸ BY MOUTH
▸ Adult: 450–600 mg once daily for up to 6 months after cultures negative
Treatment of pulmonary tuberculosis, in combination with other drugs
▸ BY MOUTH
▸ Adult: 150–450 mg once daily for at least 6 months
***Helicobacter pylori* eradication [in combination with other drugs (see Helicobacter pylori infection p. 90)]**
▸ BY MOUTH
▸ Adult: 150 mg twice daily for 10 days for third-line eradication therapy

- **UNLICENSED USE** [EvGr] Rifabutin is used for the eradication of *Helicobacter pylori*, ⟨Å⟩ but is not licensed for this indication.
- **CAUTIONS** Acute porphyrias p. 1107 · discolours soft contact lenses
- **INTERACTIONS** → Appendix 1: rifamycins
- **SIDE-EFFECTS** Agranulocytosis · anaemia · arthralgia · bronchospasm · chest pain · corneal deposits · decreased leucocytes · dyspnoea · eosinophilia · fever · haemolysis · hepatic disorders · influenza like illness · myalgia · nausea · neutropenia · pancytopenia · skin reactions · thrombocytopenia · urine discolouration · uveitis (more common following high doses or concomitant use with drugs that increase plasma concentration) · vomiting

- **ALLERGY AND CROSS-SENSITIVITY** [EvGr] Contra-indicated in patients with rifamycin hypersensitivity. ⟨M⟩
- **CONCEPTION AND CONTRACEPTION**
Important Rifabutin induces hepatic enzymes and the effectiveness of hormonal contraceptives is reduced; alternative family planning advice should be offered.
- **PREGNANCY** Manufacturer advises avoid—no information available.
- **BREAST FEEDING** Manufacturer advises avoid—no information available.
- **HEPATIC IMPAIRMENT** Manufacturer advises caution in severe impairment.
- **RENAL IMPAIRMENT**
Dose adjustments Use half normal dose if eGFR less than 30 mL/minute/1.73 m^2.
- **MONITORING REQUIREMENTS**
▸ *Renal function* should be checked before treatment.
▸ *Hepatic function* should be checked before treatment. If there is no evidence of liver disease (and pre-treatment liver function is normal), further checks are only necessary if the patient develops fever, malaise, vomiting, jaundice or unexplained deterioration during treatment. However, hepatic function should be monitored on prolonged therapy.
▸ Blood counts should be monitored on prolonged therapy.
▸ Those with alcohol dependence should have frequent checks of hepatic function, particularly in the first 2 months. Blood counts should also be monitored in these patients.
- **PRESCRIBING AND DISPENSING INFORMATION** If treatment interruption occurs, re-introduce with low dosage and increase gradually.
- **PATIENT AND CARER ADVICE**
Soft contact lenses Patients or their carers should be advised that rifabutin discolours soft contact lenses.
Hepatic disorders Patients or their carers should be told how to recognise signs of liver disorder, and advised to discontinue treatment and seek immediate medical attention if symptoms such as persistent nausea, vomiting, malaise or jaundice develop.

- **MEDICINAL FORMS** There can be variation in the licensing of different medicines containing the same drug. Forms available from special-order manufacturers include: oral suspension, oral solution

Capsule
CAUTIONARY AND ADVISORY LABELS 8, 14
▸ Mycobutin (Pfizer Ltd)
Rifabutin 150 mg Mycobutin 150mg capsules | 30 capsule [PoM] £90.38 DT = £90.38

Rifaximin

02-Dec-2020

- **DRUG ACTION** Rifaximin is a rifamycin that is poorly absorbed from the gastro-intestinal tract, and, therefore, should not be used to treat systemic infections.

- **INDICATIONS AND DOSE**
Travellers' diarrhoea that is not associated with fever, bloody diarrhoea, blood or leucocytes in the stool, or 8 or more unformed stools in the previous 24 hours
▸ BY MOUTH
▸ Adult: 200 mg every 8 hours for 3 days
Reduction in recurrence of hepatic encephalopathy
▸ BY MOUTH
▸ Adult: 550 mg twice daily

- **CONTRA-INDICATIONS** Intestinal obstruction
- **INTERACTIONS** → Appendix 1: rifaximin

SIDE-EFFECTS

▶ **Common or very common** Arthralgia · ascites · constipation · depression · dizziness · dyspnoea · gastrointestinal discomfort · gastrointestinal disorders · headaches · muscle complaints · nausea · oedema · skin reactions · vomiting

▶ **Uncommon** Anaemia · anxiety · appetite decreased · asthenia · balance impaired · concentration impaired · confusion · cough · diplopia · drowsiness · dry lips · dry mouth · dry throat · ear pain · fall · haematuria · hot flush · hyperhidrosis · hyperkalaemia · increased risk of infection · lymphocytosis · memory loss · muscle weakness · nasal complaints · neutropenia · oropharyngeal pain · pain · palpitations · polymenorrhoea · respiratory disorders · seizure · sensation abnormal · sleep disorders · sunburn · taste altered · urinary disorders · urine abnormalities · vertigo

▶ **Rare or very rare** Hypertension · hypotension

▶ **Frequency not known** Angioedema · syncope · thrombocytopenia · urine discolouration

● **ALLERGY AND CROSS-SENSITIVITY** EvGr Contra-indicated if history of rifamycin hypersensitivity. ⊛

● **PREGNANCY** Manufacturer advises avoid—toxicity in *animal* studies.

● **BREAST FEEDING** Unlikely to be present in milk in significant amounts, but manufacturer advises avoid.

● **HEPATIC IMPAIRMENT**

▶ **When used for hepatic encephalopathy** Manufacturer advises caution in severe impairment (risk of increased exposure).

● **PRESCRIBING AND DISPENSING INFORMATION** Not recommended for diarrhoea associated with invasive organisms such as *Campylobacter* and *Shigella*.

● **NATIONAL FUNDING/ACCESS DECISIONS** For full details see funding body website

NICE decisions

▶ **Rifaximin for preventing episodes of overt hepatic encephalopathy (March 2015)** NICE TA337 Recommended

● **MEDICINAL FORMS** There can be variation in the licensing of different medicines containing the same drug. Forms available from special-order manufacturers include: oral suspension

Oral suspension

▶ Normix (Imported (Italy))
Rifaximin 20 mg per 1 ml Normix 100mg/5ml granules for oral suspension | 100 ml PoM ⓢ

Tablet

CAUTIONARY AND ADVISORY LABELS 9(Xifaxantan ® brand only), 14

▶ Targaxan (Norgine Pharmaceuticals Ltd)
Rifaximin 550 mg Targaxan 550mg tablets | 56 tablet PoM £259.23 DT = £259.23

▶ Xifaxanta (Norgine Pharmaceuticals Ltd)
Rifaximin 200 mg Xifaxanta 200mg tablets | 9 tablet PoM £15.15 DT = £15.15

2.1 Anthrax

Anthrax

Treatment and post-exposure prophylaxis

Inhalation or *gastro-intestinal anthrax* should be treated initially with either ciprofloxacin p. 593 or, in patients over 12 years, doxycycline p. 601 [unlicensed indication] combined with one or two other antibacterials (such as amoxicillin p. 582, benzylpenicillin sodium p. 580, chloramphenicol p. 605, clarithromycin p. 569, clindamycin p. 566, imipenem with cilastatin p. 549, rifampicin p. 619 [unlicensed indication], and vancomycin p. 565). When the condition improves and the sensitivity of the *Bacillus anthracis* strain is known, treatment may be switched to a single antibacterial. Treatment should continue for 60 days because germination may be delayed.

Cutaneous anthrax should be treated with either ciprofloxacin [unlicensed indication] or doxycycline [unlicensed indication] for 7 days. Treatment may be switched to amoxicillin if the infecting strain is susceptible. Treatment may need to be extended to 60 days if exposure is due to aerosol. A combination of antibacterials for 14 days is recommended for cutaneous anthrax with systemic features, extensive oedema, or lesions of the head or neck.

Ciprofloxacin or doxycycline may be given for *post-exposure prophylaxis*. If exposure is confirmed, antibacterial prophylaxis should continue for 60 days. Antibacterial prophylaxis may be switched to amoxicillin after 10–14 days if the strain of *B. anthracis* is susceptible. Vaccination against anthrax may allow the duration of antibacterial prophylaxis to be shortened.

2.2 Leprosy

Leprosy

Management

Advice from a member of the Panel of Leprosy Opinion is essential for the treatment of leprosy (Hansen's disease). Details can be obtained from the Hospital for Tropical Diseases, London (telephone (020) 3456 7890).

The World Health Organization has made recommendations to overcome the problem of dapsone p. 614 resistance and to prevent the emergence of resistance to other antileprotic drugs. Drugs recommended are dapsone, rifampicin p. 619, and clofazimine p. 614. Other drugs with significant activity against *Mycobacterium leprae* include ofloxacin p. 597, minocycline p. 603 and clarithromycin p. 569, but none of these are as active as rifampicin; at present they should be reserved as second-line drugs for leprosy.

A three-drug regimen is recommended for *multibacillary leprosy* (lepromatous, borderline-lepromatous, and borderline leprosy) and a two-drug regimen for *paucibacillary leprosy* (borderline-tuberculoid, tuberculoid, and indeterminate).

Multibacillary leprosy should be treated with a combination of rifampicin, dapsone and clofazimine for at least 2 years. Treatment should be continued unchanged during both type I (reversal) or type II (erythema nodosum leprosum) reactions. During reversal reactions neuritic pain or weakness can herald the rapid onset of permanent nerve damage. Treatment with prednisolone p. 718 should be instituted at once. Mild type II reactions may respond to aspirin. Severe type II reactions may require corticosteroids; thalidomide p. 1004 [unlicensed] is also useful in patients who have become corticosteroid dependent, but it should be used only under **specialist supervision**. Thalidomide is teratogenic and, therefore, contra-indicated in pregnancy; it must **not** be given to women of child-bearing potential unless they comply with a pregnancy prevention programme. Increased doses of clofazimine are also useful.

Paucibacillary leprosy should be treated with rifampicin and dapsone for 6 months. If treatment is interrupted the regimen should be recommenced where it was left off to complete the full course.

Neither the multibacillary nor the paucibacillary antileprosy regimen is sufficient to treat tuberculosis.

5

Infection

ANTIMYCOBACTERIALS > OTHER

Clofazimine

07-May-2020

● INDICATIONS AND DOSE

Multibacillary leprosy in combination with rifampicin and dapsone (3-drug regimen) (administered on expert advice)

▸ BY MOUTH

▹ Adult: 300 mg once a month, to be administered under supervision and 50 mg daily, to be self-administered, alternatively 300 mg once a month, to be administered under supervision and 100 mg once daily on alternate days, to be self-administered

Lepromatous lepra reactions (administered on expert advice)

▸ BY MOUTH

▹ Adult: 300 mg daily for max. 3 months

Severe type II (erythema nodosum leprosum) reactions (administered on expert advice)

▸ BY MOUTH

▹ Adult: 100 mg 3 times a day for one month, subsequent dose reductions are required, may take 4–6 weeks to attain full effect

● CAUTIONS Avoid if persistent abdominal pain and diarrhoea · may discolour soft contact lenses

● INTERACTIONS → Appendix 1: clofazimine

● SIDE-EFFECTS Abdominal pain · appetite decreased · dry eye · eye discolouration · fatigue · gastrointestinal disorders · hair colour changes (reversible) · headache · lymphadenopathy · nausea · photosensitivity reaction · red discolouration of body fluids · skin discolouration (including areas exposed to light) · skin reactions · splenic infarction · urine red · visual impairment · vomiting (hospitalise if persistent) · weight decreased

● PREGNANCY Use with caution.

● BREAST FEEDING May alter colour of milk; skin discoloration of infant.

● HEPATIC IMPAIRMENT Use with caution.

● RENAL IMPAIRMENT Use with caution.

● MEDICINAL FORMS There can be variation in the licensing of different medicines containing the same drug. Forms available from special-order manufacturers include: capsule

Capsule

CAUTIONARY AND ADVISORY LABELS 8, 14, 21

▹ Lamprene (Imported (United States))

Clofazimine 50 mg Lamprene 50mg capsules | 100 capsule [PoM] ⓢ

Dapsone

05-May-2020

● INDICATIONS AND DOSE

Multibacillary leprosy in combination with rifampicin and clofazimine (3-drug regimen) | Paucibacillary leprosy in combination with rifampicin (2-drug regimen)

▸ BY MOUTH

▹ Adult (body-weight up to 35 kg): 50 mg daily, alternatively 1–2 mg/kg daily, may be self-administered

▹ Adult (body-weight 35 kg and above): 100 mg daily, may be self-administered

Dermatitis herpetiformis

▸ BY MOUTH

▹ Adult: (consult product literature or local protocols)

Treatment of mild to moderate *Pneumocystis jirovecii* (*Pneumocystis carinii*) pneumonia (in combination with trimethoprim)

▸ BY MOUTH

▹ Adult: 100 mg once daily

Prophylaxis of *Pneumocystis jirovecii* (*Pneumocystis carinii*) pneumonia

▸ BY MOUTH

▹ Adult: 100 mg daily

● UNLICENSED USE Not licensed for treatment of pneumocystis (*P. jirovecii*) pneumonia.

● CAUTIONS Anaemia (treat severe anaemia before starting) · avoid in Acute porphyrias p. 1107 · cardiac disease · G6PD deficiency · pulmonary disease · susceptibility to haemolysis

● INTERACTIONS → Appendix 1: dapsone

● SIDE-EFFECTS Agranulocytosis · appetite decreased · haemolysis · haemolytic anaemia · headache · hepatic disorders · hypoalbuminaemia · insomnia · lepra reaction · methaemoglobinaemia · motor loss · nausea · peripheral neuropathy · photosensitivity reaction · psychosis · severe cutaneous adverse reactions (SCARs) · skin reactions · tachycardia · vomiting

SIDE-EFFECTS, FURTHER INFORMATION Side-effects are dose-related. If dapsone syndrome occurs (rash with fever and eosinophilia)—discontinue immediately (may progress to exfoliative dermatitis, hepatitis, hypoalbuminaemia, psychosis and death).

● PREGNANCY Folic acid p. 1071 (higher dose) should be given to mother throughout pregnancy; neonatal haemolysis and methaemoglobinaemia reported in third trimester.

● BREAST FEEDING Haemolytic anaemia; although significant amount in milk, risk to infant very small unless infant is G6PD deficient.

● PATIENT AND CARER ADVICE

Blood disorders On long-term treatment, patients and their carers should be told how to recognise signs of blood disorders and advised to seek immediate medical attention if symptoms such as fever, sore throat, rash, mouth ulcers, purpura, bruising or bleeding develop.

● MEDICINAL FORMS There can be variation in the licensing of different medicines containing the same drug. Forms available from special-order manufacturers include: oral suspension, oral solution

Tablet

CAUTIONARY AND ADVISORY LABELS 8

▹ Dapsone (Non-proprietary)

Dapsone 50 mg Dapsone 50mg tablets | 28 tablet [PoM] £36.22 DT = £9.97

Dapsone 100 mg Dapsone 100mg tablets | 28 tablet [PoM] £97.39 DT = £40.68

2.3 Lyme disease

Lyme disease

14-Nov-2018

Description of condition

Lyme disease, also known as Lyme borreliosis, is an infection caused by bacteria called *Borrelia burgdorferi*. It is transmitted to humans by the bite of an infected tick. Ticks are mainly found in grassy and wooded areas including urban gardens and parks. Most tick bites do not cause Lyme disease, and the prompt and correct removal of the tick reduces the risk of infection.

Lyme disease usually presents with a characteristic erythema migrans rash. This usually becomes visible

1–4 weeks after a tick bite, but can appear from 3 days to 3 months, and last for several weeks. It may be accompanied by non-focal (non-organ related) symptoms, such as fever, swollen glands, malaise, fatigue, neck pain or stiffness, joint or muscle pain, headache, cognitive impairment, or paraesthesia.

Other signs and symptoms of Lyme disease may also appear months or years after the initial infection and are typically characterised by focal symptoms (relating to at least 1 organ system). These include neurological (affecting cranial nerves, peripheral and central nervous systems), joint (Lyme arthritis), cardiac (Lyme carditis), or skin (acrodermatitis chronica atrophicans) manifestations.

Drug treatment

EvGr Patients diagnosed with Lyme disease should be given treatment with an antibacterial drug; the choice of drug should be based on presenting symptoms. In patients who present with focal symptoms, a discussion with, or referral to, a specialist should be considered but should not delay treatment.

In patients presenting with *erythema migrans rash with or without non-focal symptoms*, oral doxycycline p. 601 [unlicensed indication] is recommended as first-line treatment. If doxycycline p. 601 cannot be given, oral amoxicillin p. 582 should be used as an alternative. Oral azithromycin p. 568 [unlicensed indication] should be given if both doxycycline p. 601 and amoxicillin p. 582 are unsuitable.

In patients presenting with focal symptoms of *cranial nerve or peripheral nervous system* involvement, oral doxycycline p. 601 [unlicensed indication] is recommended as first-line treatment. If doxycycline p. 601 cannot be given, oral amoxicillin p. 582 should be used as an alternative.

In patients presenting with symptoms of *central nervous system* involvement, intravenous ceftriaxone p. 558 is recommended as first-line treatment. Oral doxycycline p. 601 [unlicensed indication] should be used as an alternative if ceftriaxone p. 558 cannot be given, or when switching to oral antibacterial treatment.

In patients with symptoms of *Lyme arthritis or acrodermatitis chronica atrophicans*, oral doxycycline p. 601 [unlicensed indication] is recommended as first-line treatment. If doxycycline p. 601 cannot be given, oral amoxicillin p. 582 should be used as an alternative. Intravenous ceftriaxone p. 558 should be given if both doxycycline p. 601 and amoxicillin p. 582 are unsuitable.

In patients with symptoms of *Lyme carditis who are haemodynamically stable*, oral doxycycline p. 601 [unlicensed indication] is recommended as first-line treatment. If doxycycline p. 601 cannot be given, intravenous ceftriaxone p. 558 should be used as an alternative.

In patients with symptoms of *Lyme carditis who are haemodynamically unstable*, intravenous ceftriaxone p. 558 is recommended. Oral doxycycline p. 601 [unlicensed indication] should be given when switching to oral antibacterial treatment. (A)

Ongoing symptom management

EvGr If symptoms continue to persist or worsen after antibacterial treatment, patients should be assessed for possible alternative causes, re-infection with Lyme disease, treatment failure or non-adherence to previous antibacterial treatment, or progression to organ damage caused by Lyme disease (such as nerve palsy).

A second course of antibacterial treatment should be given to patients presenting with signs and symptoms of re-infection. In patients presenting with ongoing symptoms due to possible treatment failure, treatment with an alternative antibacterial drug should be considered. A third course of antibacterial treatment is not recommended, and further management should be discussed with a national

reference laboratory or suitable specialist depending on symptoms (for example, a rheumatologist or neurologist). (A)

Useful Resources

Lyme disease. National Institute for Health and Care Excellence. NICE guideline 95. April 2018.
www.nice.org.uk/guidance/ng95

'Be tick aware'–Toolkit for raising awareness of the potential risk posed by ticks and tick-borne disease in England. Public Health England. March 2018.
www.gov.uk/government/publications/tick-bite-risks-and-prevention-of-lyme-disease

2.4 Methicillin-resistant staphylococcus aureus

MRSA

Management

Infection from *Staphylococcus aureus* strains resistant to meticillin [now discontinued] (meticillin-resistant *Staph. aureus*, MRSA) and to flucloxacillin p. 589 can be difficult to manage. Treatment is guided by the sensitivity of the infecting strain.

Rifampicin p. 619 or fusidic acid p. 608 should **not** be used alone because resistance may develop rapidly. A **tetracycline** alone or a combination of rifampicin and fusidic acid can be used for *skin* and *soft-tissue infections* caused by MRSA; clindamycin p. 566 alone is an alternative. A **glycopeptide** (e.g. vancomycin p. 565) can be used for severe skin and soft-tissue infections associated with MRSA; if a glycopeptide is unsuitable, linezolid p. 609 can be used on expert advice. As linezolid is **not** active against Gram-negative organisms, it can be used for mixed skin and soft-tissue infections only when other treatments are not available; linezolid must be given with other antibacterials if the infection also involves Gram-negative organisms. A combination of a glycopeptide and fusidic acid *or* a glycopeptide and rifampicin can be considered for skin and soft-tissue infections that have failed to respond to a single antibacterial.

Tigecycline p. 604 and daptomycin p. 605 are licensed for the treatment of complicated skin and soft-tissue infections involving MRSA.

A **tetracycline** or clindamycin can be used for *bronchiectasis* caused by MRSA. A **glycopeptide** can be used for *pneumonia* associated with MRSA; if a glycopeptide is unsuitable, linezolid can be used on expert advice. Linezolid must be given with other antibacterials if the infection also involves Gram-negative organisms.

A **tetracycline** can be used for *urinary-tract infections* caused by MRSA; trimethoprim p. 610 or nitrofurantoin p. 628 are alternatives. A **glycopeptide** can be used for urinary-tract infections that are severe or resistant to other antibacterials.

A **glycopeptide** can be used for *septicaemia* associated with MRSA.

See the management of *endocarditis, osteomyelitis,* or *septic arthritis* associated with MRSA.

Prophylaxis with vancomycin or teicoplanin p. 563 (alone or in combination with another antibacterial active against other pathogens) is appropriate for patients undergoing surgery if:

- there is a history of MRSA colonisation or infection without documented eradication;
- there is a risk that the patient's MRSA carriage has recurred;

- the patient comes from an area with a high prevalence of MRSA.

See eradication of nasal carriage of MRSA in Nose p. 1245.

2.5 Tuberculosis

Tuberculosis

24-Oct-2019

Overview

Tuberculosis is a curable infectious disease caused by bacteria of the *Mycobacterium tuberculosis* complex (*M. tuberculosis*, *M. africanum*, *M. bovis* or *M. microti*) and is spread by breathing in infected respiratory droplets from a person with infectious tuberculosis. The most common form of tuberculosis infection is in the lungs (**pulmonary**) but infection can also spread and develop in other parts of the body (**extrapulmonary**).

The initial infection with tuberculosis clears in the majority of individuals. However, in some cases the bacteria may become dormant and remain in the body with no symptoms (**latent** tuberculosis) or progress to being symptomatic (**active** tuberculosis) over the following weeks or months. In individuals with latent tuberculosis only a small proportion will develop active tuberculosis.

Many cases of tuberculosis can be prevented by public health measures and when clinical disease does occur most individuals can be cured if treated properly with the correct dose, combination and duration of treatment. Drug-resistant strains of tuberculosis are much harder to treat and significantly increase an individual's risk of long-term complications or death.

Treatment phases, overview

The standard treatment of active tuberculosis is completed in two phases—an **initial phase** using four drugs and a **continuation phase** using two drugs, in fully sensitive cases. [EvGr] The management of tuberculosis should be under specialist care by clinicians with training in, and experience of, the specialised care of individuals with tuberculosis. This tuberculosis service should include specialised nurses and health visitors. (A)

Within the UK there are two regimens recommended for the treatment of tuberculosis: **unsupervised** or **supervised**. The choice of either regimen is dependent on a risk assessment to identify if an individual needs enhanced case management.

[EvGr] In all phases of treatment for tuberculosis, fixed-dose combination tablets should be used, and a daily dosing schedule should be considered in active tuberculosis. (A)

Initial phase

[EvGr] As standard treatment for individuals with active tuberculosis, offer rifampicin p. 619, ethambutol hydrochloride p. 623, pyrazinamide p. 625 and isoniazid p. 624 (with pyridoxine hydrochloride p. 1130) in the initial phase of therapy; modified according to drug susceptibility testing; and continued for 2 months.

Treatment should be started without waiting for culture results if clinical signs and symptoms are consistent with a tuberculosis diagnosis; consider completing the standard treatment even if subsequent culture results are negative. (A)

Continuation phase

[EvGr] After the initial phase, offer standard continuation treatment with rifampicin and isoniazid (with pyridoxine hydrochloride) for a further 4 months in individuals with active tuberculosis without central nervous system involvement. Longer treatment for 10 months should be offered in individuals with active tuberculosis of the central nervous system, with or without spinal involvement.

Treatment should be modified according to drug susceptibility testing. (A)

Unsupervised treatment

The unsupervised treatment regimen is for individuals who are likely to take antituberculosis drugs reliably and willingly without supervision.

Supervised treatment

For individuals requiring supervised treatment (directly observed therapy, DOT), this is offered as part of enhanced case management. [EvGr] A 3 times weekly dosing schedule can be considered in individuals with tuberculosis if they require enhanced case management and daily directly observed therapy is not available. Antituberculosis treatment dosing regimens of fewer than 3 times a week are not recommended.

Directly observed therapy should be offered to individuals who:

- have a current risk or history of non-adherence;
- have previously been treated for tuberculosis;
- have a history of homelessness, drug or alcohol misuse;
- are in prison or a young offender institution, or have been in the past 5 years;
- have a major psychiatric, memory or cognitive disorder;
- are in denial of the tuberculosis diagnosis;
- have multi-drug resistant tuberculosis;
- request directly observed therapy after discussion with the clinical team;
- are too ill to self-administer treatment. (A)

Individuals with comorbidities or coexisting conditions, including the immunocompromised

[EvGr] Individuals with comorbidities or coexisting conditions (such as HIV, severe liver disease, chronic kidney disease, diabetes, eye disease or vision impairment, a history of alcohol or substance misuse, or who are pregnant or breastfeeding) should be managed by a specialist multidisciplinary team with experience in managing tuberculosis and the comorbidity or coexisting condition.

For individuals who are HIV-positive with active TB, treatment with the standard regimen should not routinely exceed 6 months, unless the tuberculosis has central nervous system involvement, in which case treatment should not routinely extend beyond 12 months.

Care should be taken to avoid drug interactions when co-prescribing antiretroviral and antituberculosis drugs. (A) For further information on the management of tuberculosis in HIV infection, see British HIV Association guideline: **Management of tuberculosis in adults living with HIV** (available at www.bhiva.org/guidelines).

Extrapulmonary tuberculosis

Central nervous system tuberculosis

[EvGr] Individuals with central nervous system tuberculosis should be offered standard treatment with **initial phase** drugs for 2 months (see *Initial phase* for specific drugs). After completion of the initial treatment phase, standard treatment with **continuation phase** drugs should then be offered (see *Continuation phase* for specific drugs); and continued for a further 10 months. Treatment for tuberculous meningitis should be offered if clinical signs and other laboratory findings are consistent with the diagnosis, even if a rapid diagnostic test is negative.

An initial high dose of *dexamethasone* or *prednisolone* should be offered at the same time as antituberculosis treatment, then slowly withdrawn over 4–8 weeks. (A) For additional information on corticosteroid use, see NICE clinical guideline: **Tuberculosis** (see *Useful resources*).

[EvGr] Referral for surgery should only be considered in individuals who have raised intracranial pressure; or have spinal TB with spinal instability or evidence of spinal cord compression. (A)

Recommended dosage for standard unsupervised 6-month treatment

Rifampicin with isoniazid and pyrazinamide	Adult: ▸ body-weight up to 40 kg 3 tablets daily for 2 months (initial phase), use *Rifater*® Tablets, preferably taken before breakfast; ▸ body-weight 40–49 kg 4 tablets daily for 2 months (initial phase), use *Rifater*® Tablets, preferably taken before breakfast; ▸ body-weight 50–64 kg 5 tablets daily for 2 months (initial phase), use *Rifater*® Tablets, preferably taken before breakfast; ▸ body-weight 65 kg and above 6 tablets daily for 2 months (initial phase), use *Rifater*® Tablets, preferably taken before breakfast
Ethambutol hydrochloride	Adult: 15 mg/kg once daily for 2 months (initial phase)
Rifampicin with isoniazid	Adult: ▸ body-weight up to 50 kg 450/300 mg daily for 4 months (continuation phase after 2-month initial phase), use *Rifinah*® *150/100* Tablets, preferably taken before breakfast; ▸ body-weight 50 kg and above 600/300 mg daily for 4 months (continuation phase after 2-month initial phase), use *Rifinah*® *300/150* Tablets, preferably taken before breakfast
or (if combination preparations not appropriate):	
Isoniazid	Child: 10 mg/kg once daily (max. per dose 300 mg) for 6 months (initial and continuation phases) Adult: 300 mg daily for 6 months (initial and continuation phases)
Rifampicin	Child: ▸ body-weight up to 50 kg 15 mg/kg once daily for 6 months (initial and continuation phases); maximum 450 mg per day; ▸ body-weight 50 kg and above 15 mg/kg once daily for 6 months (initial and continuation phases); maximum 600 mg per day Adult: ▸ body-weight up to 50 kg 450 mg once daily for 6 months (initial and continuation phases); ▸ body-weight 50 kg and above 600 mg once daily for 6 months (initial and continuation phases)
Pyrazinamide	Child: ▸ body-weight up to 50 kg 35 mg/kg once daily for 2 months (initial phase); maximum 1.5 g per day; ▸ body-weight 50 kg and above 35 mg/kg once daily for 2 months (initial phase); maximum 2 g per day Adult: ▸ body-weight up to 50 kg 1.5 g once daily for 2 months (initial phase); ▸ body-weight 50 kg and above 2 g once daily for 2 months (initial phase)
Ethambutol hydrochloride	Child: 20 mg/kg once daily for 2 months (initial phase) Adult: 15 mg/kg once daily for 2 months (initial phase)

In general, doses should be rounded up to facilitate administration of suitable volumes of liquid or an appropriate strength of tablet. The exception is ethambutol hydrochloride p. 623 due to the risk of toxicity. Doses may also need to be recalculated to allow for weight gain in younger children. The fixed-dose combination preparations (*Rifater*®, *Rifinah*®) are unlicensed for use in children. Consideration may be given to use of these preparations in older children, provided the respective dose of each drug is appropriate for the weight of the child.

Recommended dosage for intermittent supervised 6-month treatment

Isoniazid	Child: 15 mg/kg 3 times a week (max. per dose 900 mg) for 6 months (initial and continuation phases) Adult: 15 mg/kg 3 times a week (max. per dose 900 mg) for 6 months (initial and continuation phases)
Rifampicin	Child: 15 mg/kg 3 times a week (max. per dose 900 mg) for 6 months (initial and continuation phases) Adult: 600–900 mg 3 times a week for 6 months (initial and continuation phases)
Pyrazinamide	Child: ▸ body-weight up to 50 kg 50 mg/kg 3 times a week (max. per dose 2 g 3 times a week) for 2 months (initial phase); ▸ body-weight 50 kg and above 50 mg/kg 3 times a week (max. per dose 2.5 g 3 times a week) for 2 months (initial phase) Adult: ▸ body-weight up to 50 kg 2 g 3 times a week for 2 months (initial phase); ▸ body-weight 50 kg and above 2.5 g 3 times a week for 2 months (initial phase)
Ethambutol hydrochloride	Child: 30 mg/kg 3 times a week for 2 months (initial phase) Adult: 30 mg/kg 3 times a week for 2 months (initial phase)

In general, doses should be rounded up to facilitate administration of suitable volumes of liquid or an appropriate strength of tablet. The exception is ethambutol hydrochloride due to the risk of toxicity. Doses may also need to be recalculated to allow for weight gain in younger children. The fixed-dose combination preparations (*Rifater*®, *Rifinah*®) are unlicensed for use in children. Consideration may be given to use of these preparations in older children, provided the respective dose of each drug is appropriate for the weight of the child.

5

Infection

Pericardial tuberculosis

EvGr An initial high dose of oral *prednisolone* should be offered to individuals with active pericardial tuberculosis, at the same time as antituberculosis treatment, then slowly withdrawn over 2–3 weeks. A For additional information on corticosteroid use, see NICE clinical guideline: **Tuberculosis** (see *Useful resources*).

Latent tuberculosis

Some individuals with latent tuberculosis are at increased risk of developing active tuberculosis (such as individuals who are HIV-positive, diabetic, injecting drug users, or receiving treatment with an anti-tumor necrosis factor alpha inhibitor). EvGr If for any reason these individuals do not have treatment for latent tuberculosis, they should be informed of the risks and symptoms of active tuberculosis. A

Close contacts

EvGr Anyone aged under 65 years who is a close contact (prolonged, frequent or intense contact, for example household contacts or partners) of a person with pulmonary or laryngeal tuberculosis should be tested for latent tuberculosis. Drug treatment should be offered to all individuals aged under 65 years with evidence of latent tuberculosis, if the close contact has *suspected infectious* or *confirmed active* pulmonary or laryngeal drug-sensitive tuberculosis. A

Immunocompromised

EvGr Individuals who are anticipated to be, or who are currently immunocompromised, should have a risk assessment carried out to establish whether tuberculosis testing should be offered. Take into account the severity and duration of their immunocompromise and any risk factors for tuberculosis (such as country of birth or recent contact with an index case with suspected infectious or confirmed pulmonary or laryngeal tuberculosis).

Individuals who are severely immunocompromised (such as those with HIV and a CD4 count of less than 200 cells/mm^3, or who have had a solid organ or allogeneic stem cell transplant) should be tested for latent tuberculosis using an appropriate method. Individuals who test positive should then be assessed for active disease, and if negative, offered treatment for latent tuberculosis. A For further information on tuberculosis testing methods, see NICE clinical guideline: **Tuberculosis** (see *Useful resources*).

Healthcare workers

EvGr Any new NHS employees who are new entrants from a high incidence country should be offered appropriate testing for latent tuberculosis. Those who are not new entrants from a high incidence country, but who will be in contact with patients or clinical materials should be offered appropriate testing for latent tuberculosis if prior BCG vaccination cannot be verified. A For further information on tuberculosis testing methods, see NICE clinical guideline: **Tuberculosis** (see *Useful resources*) and Bacillus Calmette-Guérin vaccine p. 1343.

EvGr Those who test positive should then be assessed for active disease, and if negative, offered treatment for latent tuberculosis.

For healthcare workers who are immunocompromised, follow standard advice for testing and treatment (see *Immunocompromised* above). A

Treatment of latent tuberculosis

EvGr For individuals aged below 65 years, including those with HIV where treatment for latent tuberculosis is indicated, offer drug treatment with either 3 months of isoniazid (with pyridoxine hydrochloride p. 1130) and rifampicin or 6 months of isoniazid (with pyridoxine hydrochloride). A

The choice of regimen is dependent on clinical factors, including age, risk of hepatotoxicity and possible drug

interactions. EvGr Testing for HIV, hepatitis B and hepatitis C should be offered before starting antituberculosis treatment as this may affect choice of therapy.

Individuals aged 35 to 65 years should only be offered treatment if hepatotoxicity is not a concern.

For individuals aged under 35 years offer treatment with 3 months of isoniazid (with pyridoxine hydrochloride) and rifampicin if hepatotoxicity is a concern after an assessment of both liver function (including transaminase levels) and risk factors.

For individuals where interactions with rifamycins are a concern (for example, in people with HIV or who those have had a transplant), offer treatment with 6 months of isoniazid (with pyridoxine hydrochloride).

Individuals with severe liver disease should be treated under the care of a specialist team. Careful monitoring of liver function is necessary in individuals with non-severe liver disease, abnormal liver function, or who misuse alcohol or drugs. A

For advice on immunisation against tuberculosis, see Bacillus Calmette-Guérin vaccine p. 1343.

Treatment failure

Major causes of treatment failure include incorrect prescribing by the clinician and inadequate compliance by the infected individual. EvGr All individuals diagnosed with tuberculosis should have an allocated case manager to help with the development of a health and social care plan, supervision of treatment, and support with the completion of treatment. Multidisciplinary tuberculosis teams should implement strategies (such as random urine tests, pill counts, home visits, health education counselling, and language appropriate reminder services) to help with adherence to, and successful completion of treatment. A

Treatment interruptions

A break in antituberculosis treatment of at least 2 weeks (during the initial phase) or missing more than 20% of prescribed doses is classified as treatment interruption. Re-establishing treatment appropriately following interruptions is key to ensuring treatment success without relapse, drug resistance or further adverse events. EvGr If an adverse reaction recurs upon re-introducing a particular drug, do not give that drug in future regimens and consider extending the total regimen accordingly. A

Treatment interruptions due to drug-induced hepatotoxicity

EvGr Following treatment interruption due to drug-induced hepatotoxicty, all potential causes of hepatotoxicity should be investigated. Once aspartate or alanine transaminase levels fall below twice the upper limit of normal, bilirubin levels have returned to the normal range, and hepatotoxic symptoms have resolved, antituberculosis therapy should be sequentially re-introduced at previous full doses over a period of no more than 10 days. Start with ethambutol hydrochloride p. 623 and either isoniazid p. 624 (with pyridoxine hydrochloride) or rifampicin p. 619.

In individuals with severe or highly infectious tuberculosis who need to interrupt the standard regimen, consider continuing treatment with at least 2 drugs with low risk of hepatotoxicity, such as ethambutol hydrochloride and streptomycin p. 547 (with or without a fluoroquinolone antibiotic, such as levofloxacin p. 595 or moxifloxacin p. 596), with ongoing monitoring by a liver specialist. A

Treatment interruptions due to cutaneous reactions

EvGr If an individual with severe or highly infectious tuberculosis has a cutaneous reaction, consider continuing treatment with a combination of at least 2 drugs with low risk for causing cutaneous reactions, such as ethambutol hydrochloride and streptomycin, with monitoring by a dermatologist. A

Drug-resistant tuberculosis

EvGr Treatment of drug-resistant tuberculosis should be managed by a multidisciplinary team with experience in such cases, and where appropriate facilities for infection-control exist. Ⓐ The risk of resistance is minimised by ensuring therapy is administered in the correct dose and combination for the prescribed duration.

Single drug-resistant tuberculosis

EvGr For single drug-resistance in individuals with tuberculosis with central nervous system involvement, refer to a specialist with experience in managing drug-resistant tuberculosis. Ⓐ For those without central nervous system involvement, the following treatment regimens are recommended:

Resistance to isoniazid:
● EvGr First 2 months (initial phase): rifampicin, pyrazinamide p. 625 and ethambutol hydrochloride;
● Continue with (continuation phase): rifampicin and ethambutol hydrochloride for 7 months (up to 10 months for extensive disease). Ⓐ

Resistance to pyrazinamide:
● EvGr First 2 months (initial phase): rifampicin, ethambutol hydrochloride and isoniazid (with pyridoxine hydrochloride);
● Continue with (continuation phase): rifampicin and isoniazid (with pyridoxine hydrochloride) for 7 months. Ⓐ

Resistance to ethambutol hydrochloride:
● EvGr First 2 months (initial phase): rifampicin, pyrazinamide and isoniazid (with pyridoxine hydrochloride);
● Continue with (continuation phase): rifampicin and isoniazid p. 624 (with pyridoxine hydrochloride p. 1130) for 4 months. Ⓐ

Resistance to rifampicin below:
● EvGr Offer treatment with at least 6 antituberculosis drugs to which the mycobacterium is likely to be sensitive. Ⓐ

Multi-drug resistant tuberculosis

EvGr In multidrug-resistant tuberculosis (*resistance to isoniazid and rifampicin, with or without any other resistance*), positive cases of rifampicin resistance require treatment with at least 6 antituberculosis drugs to which the mycobacterium is likely to be sensitive. Testing for resistance to second-line drugs is recommended and treatment should be modified according to susceptibility. Ⓐ

Useful Resources

Tuberculosis. National Institute for Health and Care Excellence. NICE guideline 33. September 2019. www.nice.org.uk/guidance/ng33

> **Other drugs used for Tuberculosis** Rifabutin, p. 612

ANTIMYCOBACTERIALS ⟩ RIFAMYCINS

Rifampicin
02-Dec-2020

● INDICATIONS AND DOSE

Brucellosis in combination with other antibacterials | Legionnaires disease in combination with other antibacterials | Serious staphylococcal infections in combination with other antibacterials
▸ BY MOUTH, OR BY INTRAVENOUS INFUSION
▸ Child 1–11 months: 5–10 mg/kg twice daily
▸ Child 1–17 years: 10 mg/kg twice daily (max. per dose 600 mg)

▸ Adult: 0.6–1.2 g daily in 2–4 divided doses

Endocarditis in combination with other drugs
▸ BY MOUTH, OR BY INTRAVENOUS INFUSION
▸ Adult: 0.6–1.2 g daily in 2–4 divided doses

Tuberculosis, in combination with other drugs (intermittent supervised 6-month treatment) (under expert supervision)
▸ BY MOUTH
▸ Child: 15 mg/kg 3 times a week (max. per dose 900 mg) for 6 months (initial and continuation phases)
▸ Adult: 600–900 mg 3 times a week for 6 months (initial and continuation phases)

Tuberculosis, in combination with other drugs (standard unsupervised 6-month treatment)
▸ BY MOUTH
▸ Child (body-weight up to 50 kg): 15 mg/kg once daily for 6 months (initial and continuation phases); maximum 450 mg per day
▸ Child (body-weight 50 kg and above): 15 mg/kg once daily for 6 months (initial and continuation phases); maximum 600 mg per day
▸ Adult (body-weight up to 50 kg): 450 mg once daily for 6 months (initial and continuation phases)
▸ Adult (body-weight 50 kg and above): 600 mg once daily for 6 months (initial and continuation phases)

Prevention of tuberculosis in susceptible close contacts or those who have become tuberculin positive, in combination with isoniazid
▸ BY MOUTH
▸ Child 1 month–11 years (body-weight up to 50 kg): 15 mg/kg daily for 3 months; maximum 450 mg per day
▸ Child 1 month–11 years (body-weight 50 kg and above): 15 mg/kg daily for 3 months; maximum 600 mg per day
▸ Child 12–17 years (body-weight up to 50 kg): 450 mg daily for 3 months
▸ Child 12–17 years (body-weight 50 kg and above): 600 mg daily for 3 months
▸ Adult (body-weight up to 50 kg): 450 mg daily for 3 months
▸ Adult (body-weight 50 kg and above): 600 mg daily for 3 months

Prevention of tuberculosis in susceptible close contacts or those who have become tuberculin positive, who are isoniazid-resistant
▸ BY MOUTH
▸ Child 1 month–11 years (body-weight up to 50 kg): 15 mg/kg daily for 6 months; maximum 450 mg per day
▸ Child 1 month–11 years (body-weight 50 kg and above): 15 mg/kg daily for 6 months; maximum 600 mg per day
▸ Child 12–17 years (body-weight up to 50 kg): 450 mg daily for 6 months
▸ Child 12–17 years (body-weight 50 kg and above): 600 mg daily for 6 months

Prevention of tuberculosis in susceptible close contacts or those who have become tuberculin positive, who are isoniazid-resistant and under 35 years
▸ BY MOUTH
▸ Adult 18–34 years (body-weight up to 50 kg): 450 mg daily for 6 months
▸ Adult 18–34 years (body-weight 50 kg and above): 600 mg daily for 6 months

Prevention of secondary case of *Haemophilus influenzae* type b disease
▸ BY MOUTH
▸ Child 1–2 months: 10 mg/kg once daily for 4 days
▸ Child 3 months–11 years: 20 mg/kg once daily (max. per dose 600 mg) for 4 days
▸ Child 12–17 years: 600 mg once daily for 4 days
▸ Adult: 600 mg once daily for 4 days continued →

Prevention of secondary case of meningococcal meningitis
▸ BY MOUTH
  ▸ Child 1–11 months: 5 mg/kg every 12 hours for 2 days
  ▸ Child 1–11 years: 10 mg/kg every 12 hours (max. per dose 600 mg), for 2 days
  ▸ Child 12–17 years: 600 mg every 12 hours for 2 days
  ▸ Adult: 600 mg every 12 hours for 2 days

Multibacillary leprosy in combination with dapsone and clofazimine (3-drug regimen) | Paucibacillary leprosy in combination with dapsone (2-drug regimen)
▸ BY MOUTH
  ▸ Adult (body-weight up to 35 kg): 450 mg once a month, supervised administration
  ▸ Adult (body-weight 35 kg and above): 600 mg once a month, supervised administration

● CONTRA-INDICATIONS Acute porphyrias p. 1107 · jaundice
● CAUTIONS Discolours soft contact lenses
● INTERACTIONS → Appendix 1: rifamycins
● SIDE-EFFECTS
  GENERAL SIDE-EFFECTS
  ▸ **Common or very common** Nausea · thrombocytopenia · vomiting
  ▸ **Uncommon** Diarrhoea · leucopenia
  ▸ **Frequency not known** Abdominal discomfort · acute kidney injury · adrenal insufficiency · agranulocytosis · appetite decreased · disseminated intravascular coagulation · dyspnoea · eosinophilia · flushing · haemolytic anaemia · hepatitis · hypersensitivity · influenza · intracranial haemorrhage · menstrual disorder · muscle weakness · myopathy · oedema · pseudomembranous enterocolitis · severe cutaneous adverse reactions (SCARs) · shock · skin reactions · sputum discolouration · sweat discolouration · tear discolouration · urine discolouration · vasculitis · wheezing
  SPECIFIC SIDE-EFFECTS
  ▸ With intravenous use Bone pain · gastrointestinal disorder · hyperbilirubinaemia · psychotic disorder
  ▸ With oral use Psychosis
  SIDE-EFFECTS, FURTHER INFORMATION Side-effects that mainly occur with intermittent therapy include influenza-like symptoms (with chills, fever, dizziness, bone pain), respiratory symptoms (including shortness of breath), collapse and shock, haemolytic anaemia, thrombocytopenic purpura, and acute renal failure. Discontinue if serious side-effects develop.
● ALLERGY AND CROSS-SENSITIVITY EvGr Contra-indicated in patients with rifamycin hypersensitivity. ◈
● CONCEPTION AND CONTRACEPTION
  Important Effectiveness of hormonal contraceptives is reduced and alternative family planning advice should be offered.
● PREGNANCY Manufacturers advise very high doses teratogenic in *animal* studies in first trimester; risk of neonatal bleeding may be increased in third trimester.
● BREAST FEEDING Amount too small to be harmful.
● HEPATIC IMPAIRMENT Manufacturer advises caution—monitor liver function weekly for two weeks, then every two weeks for the next six weeks.
  Dose adjustments Manufacturer advises maximum 8 mg/kg per day.
● RENAL IMPAIRMENT
  ▸ In children Use with caution if doses above 10 mg/kg daily.
  ▸ In adults Use with caution if dose above 600 mg daily.
● MONITORING REQUIREMENTS
  ▸ *Renal function* should be checked before treatment.
  ▸ *Hepatic function* should be checked before treatment. If there is no evidence of liver disease (and pre-treatment liver function is normal), further checks are only necessary

if the patient develops fever, malaise, vomiting, jaundice or unexplained deterioration during treatment. However, liver function should be monitored on prolonged therapy.
  ▸ Blood counts should be monitored in patients on prolonged therapy.
  ▸ In adults Those with alcohol dependence should have frequent checks of hepatic function, particularly in the first 2 months. Blood counts should also be monitored in these patients.
● DIRECTIONS FOR ADMINISTRATION
  ▸ With intravenous use in adults For *intravenous infusion* (*Rifadin ®*), give intermittently in Glucose 5% *or* Sodium chloride 0.9%; reconstitute with solvent provided then dilute with 500 mL infusion fluid; give over 2–3 hours.
  ▸ With intravenous use in children Displacement value may be significant, consult local reconstitution guidelines; reconstitute with solvent provided. May be further diluted with Glucose 5% *or* Sodium chloride 0.9% to a final concentration of 1.2 mg/mL. Infuse over 2–3 hours.
● PRESCRIBING AND DISPENSING INFORMATION If treatment interruption occurs, re-introduce with low dosage and increase gradually.
  Flavours of syrup may include raspberry.
  ▸ With oral use in children In general, doses should be rounded up to facilitate administration of suitable volumes of liquid or an appropriate strength of tablet. Doses may also need to be recalculated to allow for weight gain in younger children.
● PATIENT AND CARER ADVICE
  Soft contact lenses Patients or their carers should be advised that rifampicin discolours soft contact lenses.
  Hepatic disorders Patients or their carers should be told how to recognise signs of liver disorder, and advised to discontinue treatment and seek immediate medical attention if symptoms such as persistent nausea, vomiting, malaise or jaundice develop.
  Medicines for Children leaflet: Rifampicin for meningococcal prophylaxis www.medicinesforchildren.org.uk/rifampicin-meningococcal-prophylaxis
  Medicines for Children leaflet: Rifampicin for the treatment of tuberculosis www.medicinesforchildren.org.uk/rifampicin-treatment-tuberculosis

● MEDICINAL FORMS There can be variation in the licensing of different medicines containing the same drug. Forms available from special-order manufacturers include: oral suspension, oral solution

Powder and solvent for solution for injection
  ▸ RIFA (Imported (Germany))
    Rifampicin 300 mg RIFA parenteral 300mg powder and solvent for solution for injection vials | 1 vial PoM ⚠

Oral suspension
CAUTIONARY AND ADVISORY LABELS 8, 14, 23
EXCIPIENTS: May contain Sucrose
  ▸ Rifadin (Sanofi)
    Rifampicin 20 mg per 1 ml Rifadin 100mg/5ml syrup | 120 ml PoM £4.27 DT = £4.27

Capsule
CAUTIONARY AND ADVISORY LABELS 8, 14, 23
  ▸ Rifampicin (Non-proprietary)
    Rifampicin 150 mg Rifampicin 150mg capsules | 100 capsule PoM £54.67 DT = £54.66
    Rifampicin 300 mg Rifampicin 300mg capsules | 100 capsule PoM £123.90 DT = £123.90
  ▸ Rifadin (Sanofi)
    Rifampicin 150 mg Rifadin 150mg capsules | 100 capsule PoM £18.32 DT = £54.66
    Rifampicin 300 mg Rifadin 300mg capsules | 100 capsule PoM £36.63 DT = £123.90
  ▸ Rimactane (Sandoz Ltd)
    Rifampicin 300 mg Rimactane 300mg capsules | 60 capsule PoM £21.98

Powder and solvent for solution for infusion

ELECTROLYTES: May contain Sodium

▸ Rifadin (Sanofi)
Rifampicin 600 mg Rifadin 600mg powder and solvent for solution for infusion vials | 1 vial $\boxed{PoM}$ £9.20

Rifampicin with ethambutol, isoniazid and pyrazinamide

14-May-2020

The properties listed below are those particular to the combination only. For the properties of the components please consider, rifampicin p. 619, ethambutol hydrochloride p. 623, isoniazid p. 624, pyrazinamide p. 625.

● INDICATIONS AND DOSE

Initial treatment of tuberculosis

▸ BY MOUTH
▸ Adult (body-weight 30–39 kg): 2 tablets daily for 2 months (initial phase)
▸ Adult (body-weight 40–54 kg): 3 tablets daily for 2 months (initial phase)
▸ Adult (body-weight 55–69 kg): 4 tablets daily for 2 months (initial phase)
▸ Adult (body-weight 70 kg and above): 5 tablets daily for 2 months (initial phase)

DOSE EQUIVALENCE AND CONVERSION
▸ Tablet quantities refer to the number of *Voractiv*® Tablets which should be taken. Each *Voractiv*® Tablet contains ethambutol hydrochloride 275 mg, isoniazid 75 mg, pyrazinamide 400 mg and rifampicin 150 mg.

● INTERACTIONS → Appendix 1: ethambutol · isoniazid · pyrazinamide · rifamycins

● MEDICINAL FORMS There can be variation in the licensing of different medicines containing the same drug.

Tablet
CAUTIONARY AND ADVISORY LABELS 8, 14, 22
▸ Voractiv (Genus Pharmaceuticals Ltd)
Isoniazid 75 mg, Rifampicin 150 mg, Ethambutol hydrochloride 275 mg, Pyrazinamide 400 mg Voractiv tablets | 60 tablet $\boxed{PoM}$ £39.50

Rifampicin with isoniazid

10-Mar-2020

The properties listed below are those particular to the combination only. For the properties of the components please consider, rifampicin p. 619, isoniazid p. 624.

● INDICATIONS AND DOSE

Treatment of tuberculosis (continuation phase)

▸ BY MOUTH
▸ Adult (body-weight up to 50 kg): 450/300 mg daily for 4 months (continuation phase after 2-month initial phase), use *Rifinah*® 150/100 Tablets, preferably taken before breakfast.
▸ Adult (body-weight 50 kg and above): 600/300 mg daily for 4 months (continuation phase after 2-month initial phase), use *Rifinah*® 300/150 Tablets, preferably taken before breakfast.

DOSE EQUIVALENCE AND CONVERSION
▸ *Rifinah*® Tablets contain rifampicin and isoniazid; the proportions are expressed in the form x/y where x and y are the strengths in milligrams of rifampicin and isoniazid respectively.
▸ Each *Rifinah*® 150/100 Tablet contains rifampicin 150 mg and isoniazid 100 mg.
▸ Each *Rifinah*® 300/150 Tablet contains rifampicin 300 mg and isoniazid 150 mg.

● INTERACTIONS → Appendix 1: isoniazid · rifamycins

● MEDICINAL FORMS There can be variation in the licensing of different medicines containing the same drug.

Tablet
CAUTIONARY AND ADVISORY LABELS 8, 14, 23
▸ Rifinah (Sanofi)
Isoniazid 100 mg, Rifampicin 150 mg Rifinah 150mg/100mg tablets | 84 tablet $\boxed{PoM}$ £19.09 DT = £19.09
Isoniazid 150 mg, Rifampicin 300 mg Rifinah 300mg/150mg tablets | 56 tablet $\boxed{PoM}$ £25.22 DT = £25.22

Rifampicin with isoniazid and pyrazinamide

The properties listed below are those particular to the combination only. For the properties of the components please consider, rifampicin p. 619, isoniazid p. 624, pyrazinamide p. 625.

● INDICATIONS AND DOSE

Initial unsupervised treatment of tuberculosis (in combination with ethambutol)

▸ BY MOUTH
▸ Adult (body-weight up to 40 kg): 3 tablets daily for 2 months (initial phase), use *Rifater*® Tablets, preferably taken before breakfast.
▸ Adult (body-weight 40–49 kg): 4 tablets daily for 2 months (initial phase), use *Rifater*® Tablets, preferably taken before breakfast.
▸ Adult (body-weight 50–64 kg): 5 tablets daily for 2 months (initial phase), use *Rifater*® Tablets, preferably taken before breakfast.
▸ Adult (body-weight 65 kg and above): 6 tablets daily for 2 months (initial phase), use *Rifater*® Tablets, preferably taken before breakfast.

DOSE EQUIVALENCE AND CONVERSION
▸ Tablet quantities refer to the number of *Rifater*® Tablets which should be taken. Each *Rifater*® Tablet contains isoniazid 50 mg, pyrazinamide 300 mg and rifampicin 120 mg.

● INTERACTIONS → Appendix 1: isoniazid · pyrazinamide · rifamycins

● MEDICINAL FORMS There can be variation in the licensing of different medicines containing the same drug.

Tablet
CAUTIONARY AND ADVISORY LABELS 8, 14, 22
▸ Rifater (Sanofi)
Isoniazid 50 mg, Rifampicin 120 mg, Pyrazinamide 300 mg Rifater tablets | 100 tablet $\boxed{PoM}$ £26.34

ANTIMYCOBACTERIALS ⟩ OTHER

Aminosalicylic acid

03-Sep-2020

● INDICATIONS AND DOSE

Multiple-drug resistant tuberculosis, in combination with other drugs

▸ BY MOUTH
▸ Adult: 4 g every 8 hours for a usual treatment duration of 24 months; maximum 12 g per day

Desensitisation regimen

▸ BY MOUTH
▸ Adult: (consult product literature)

● CAUTIONS Peptic ulcer

● INTERACTIONS → Appendix 1: aminosalicylic acid

● SIDE-EFFECTS
▸ **Common or very common** Diarrhoea · dizziness · gastrointestinal discomfort · gastrointestinal disorders · hypersensitivity · nausea · skin reactions · vestibular syndrome · vomiting

▸ **Uncommon** Appetite decreased
▸ **Rare or very rare** Agranulocytosis · anaemia · crystalluria · gastrointestinal haemorrhage · headache · hepatic disorders · hypoglycaemia · hypothyroidism · leucopenia · methaemoglobinaemia · peripheral neuropathy · taste metallic · tendon pain · thrombocytopenia · visual impairment · weight decreased

● PREGNANCY Manufacturer advises avoid unless essential—toxicity in *animal* studies (highest risk during first trimester).

● BREAST FEEDING Present in milk—manufacturer advises avoid.

● HEPATIC IMPAIRMENT Manufacturer advises use with caution.

● RENAL IMPAIRMENT Use with caution in mild to moderate impairment. Avoid in severe impairment due to accumulation of inactive metabolites.

● MONITORING REQUIREMENTS
▸ Monitor for hypersensitivity reaction during the first 3 months of treatment—for desensitisation dosing regimen consult product literature.
▸ Monitor liver function—discontinue immediately if signs or symptoms of hepatic toxicity (including rash, fever and gastrointestinal disturbance).

● DIRECTIONS FOR ADMINISTRATION Manufacturer advises disperse granules in orange or tomato juice and take immediately (granules will not dissolve, ensure all granules are swallowed). Granules can be sprinkled on apple sauce or yoghurt for administration.

● PATIENT AND CARER ADVICE Patients should be advised that the skeletons of the granules may be seen in the stools. Counselling advised on administration.

● MEDICINAL FORMS There can be variation in the licensing of different medicines containing the same drug.
Gastro-resistant granules
CAUTIONARY AND ADVISORY LABELS 9, 25
▸ Granupas (Eurocept International bv)
Aminosalicylic acid 1 gram per 1 gram Granupas gastro-resistant granules 4g sachets sugar-free | 30 sachet [PoM] £331.00 DT = £331.00

Bedaquiline

28-Oct-2020

● INDICATIONS AND DOSE
Multiple-drug resistant pulmonary tuberculosis, in combination with other drugs
▸ BY MOUTH
▸ Adult: Initially 400 mg once daily for 2 weeks, then 200 mg 3 times a week for 22 weeks, intervals of at least 48 hours between each dose, continue appropriate combination therapy after bedaquiline

● CONTRA-INDICATIONS QTc interval more than 500 milliseconds (derived using Fridericia's formula) · ventricular arrhythmia

● CAUTIONS Hypothyroidism · QTc interval (derived using Fridericia's formula) 450–500 milliseconds · risk factors for QT interval prolongation (e.g. electrolyte disturbances, heart failure, history of symptomatic arrhythmias, bradycardia, congenital long QT syndrome)

● INTERACTIONS → Appendix 1: bedaquiline

● SIDE-EFFECTS
▸ **Common or very common** Arthralgia · diarrhoea · dizziness · headache · hepatic function abnormal · myalgia · nausea · QT interval prolongation · vomiting
SIDE-EFFECTS, FURTHER INFORMATION If syncope occurs, obtain ECG.

● PREGNANCY Manufacturer advises avoid unless potential benefit outweighs risk.

● BREAST FEEDING Manufacturer advises avoid—present in milk in *animal* studies.

● HEPATIC IMPAIRMENT Manufacturer advises caution in moderate impairment; avoid in severe impairment—no information available.

● RENAL IMPAIRMENT Manufacturer advises caution if eGFR less than 30 mL/minute/1.73 m^2.

● MONITORING REQUIREMENTS
▸ Determine serum potassium, calcium, and magnesium before starting treatment (correct if abnormal)—remeasure if QT prolongation occurs during treatment.
▸ Obtain ECG before starting treatment, and then at least monthly during treatment or more frequently if concomitant use with other drugs known to prolong the QT interval.
▸ Monitor liver function before starting treatment and then at least monthly during treatment—discontinue treatment if severe abnormalities in liver function tests.

● PATIENT AND CARER ADVICE
Missed doses If a dose is missed during the first two weeks of treatment, the missed dose should not be taken and the next dose should be taken at the usual time; if a dose is missed during weeks 3–24 of treatment, the missed dose should be taken as soon as possible and then the usual regimen resumed.
Driving and skilled tasks Dizziness may affect performance of skilled tasks (e.g. driving).

● NATIONAL FUNDING/ACCESS DECISIONS
For full details see funding body website

All Wales Medicines Strategy Group (AWMSG) decisions
▸ Bedaquiline (*Sirturo*®) for use as part of an appropriate combination regimen for pulmonary multidrug-resistant tuberculosis in adults and adolescent patients (12 years to less than 18 years of age and weighing at least 30 kg) when an effective treatment regimen cannot otherwise be composed for reasons of resistance or tolerability (September 2020) AWMSG No. 3726 Recommended

● MEDICINAL FORMS There can be variation in the licensing of different medicines containing the same drug.
Tablet
CAUTIONARY AND ADVISORY LABELS 4, 8, 21, 25
▸ Sirturo (Janssen-Cilag Ltd) ▼
Bedaquiline (as Bedaquiline fumarate) 100 mg Sirturo 100mg tablets | 24 tablet [PoM] £2,387.28

Capreomycin

05-May-2020

● INDICATIONS AND DOSE
Tuberculosis resistant to first-line drugs, in combination with other drugs
▸ BY DEEP INTRAMUSCULAR INJECTION
▸ Adult: 1 g daily (max. per dose 20 mg/kg) for 2–4 months, then reduced to 1 g 2–3 times a week

● CAUTIONS Auditory impairment

● INTERACTIONS → Appendix 1: capreomycin

● SIDE-EFFECTS Eosinophilia · febrile disorders · hearing impairment · leucocytosis · leucopenia · nephrotoxicity · pain · pseudo-Bartter syndrome · skin reactions · thrombocytopenia · tinnitus · vertigo

● PREGNANCY Manufacturer advises use only if potential benefit outweighs risk—teratogenic in *animal* studies.

● BREAST FEEDING Manufacturer advises caution—no information available.

● RENAL IMPAIRMENT Nephrotoxic; ototoxic.
Dose adjustments Reduce dose—consult product literature.

● MONITORING REQUIREMENTS Monitor renal, hepatic, auditory, and vestibular function and electrolytes.

● MEDICINAL FORMS There can be variation in the licensing of different medicines containing the same drug.
Powder for solution for injection
▸ Capreomycin (Non-proprietary)
Capreomycin (as Capreomycin sulfate) 1 gram Capreomycin 1g powder for solution for injection vials | 1 vial PoM £31.47

Cycloserine

● INDICATIONS AND DOSE
Tuberculosis resistant to first-line drugs, in combination with other drugs
▸ BY MOUTH
▸ Adult: Initially 250 mg every 12 hours for 2 weeks, then increased if necessary up to 500 mg every 12 hours, dose to be increased according to blood concentration and response
PHARMACOKINETICS
▸ Cycloserine penetrates the CNS.

● CONTRA-INDICATIONS Alcohol dependence · depression · epilepsy · psychotic states · severe anxiety
● INTERACTIONS → Appendix 1: cycloserine
● SIDE-EFFECTS Behaviour abnormal · coma · confusion · congestive heart failure · drowsiness · dysarthria · headache · hyperirritability · megaloblastic anaemia · memory loss · neurological effects · paraesthesia · paresis · psychosis · rash · reflexes increased · seizures · suicidal ideation · tremor · vertigo
SIDE-EFFECTS, FURTHER INFORMATION **CNS toxicity**
Discontinue or reduce dose if symptoms of CNS toxicity occur.
Rashes or allergic dermatitis Discontinue or reduce dose if rashes or allergic dermatitis develop.
● PREGNANCY Manufacturer advises use only if potential benefit outweighs risk—crosses the placenta.
● BREAST FEEDING Present in milk—amount too small to be harmful.
● RENAL IMPAIRMENT
Dose adjustments Increase interval between doses if creatinine clearance less than 50 mL/minute.
Monitoring Monitor blood-cycloserine concentration if creatinine clearance less than 50 mL/minute.
● MONITORING REQUIREMENTS
▸ Blood concentration monitoring required especially in renal impairment or if dose exceeds 500 mg daily or if signs of toxicity; blood concentration should not exceed 30 mg/litre.
▸ Monitor haematological, renal, and hepatic function.
● MEDICINAL FORMS There can be variation in the licensing of different medicines containing the same drug.
Capsule
CAUTIONARY AND ADVISORY LABELS 2, 8
▸ Cycloserine (Non-proprietary)
Cycloserine 250 mg Cycloserine 250mg capsules | 100 capsule PoM £442.89 DT = £442.89

Delamanid

11-May-2020

● INDICATIONS AND DOSE
Multiple-drug resistant pulmonary tuberculosis, in combination with other drugs
▸ BY MOUTH
▸ Adult: 100 mg twice daily for 24 weeks, continue appropriate combination therapy after delamanid
● CONTRA-INDICATIONS QTc interval more than 500 milliseconds (derived using Fridericia's formula) · serum albumin less than 28 g/litre

● CAUTIONS Risk factors for QT interval prolongation (e.g. electrolyte disturbances, acute myocardial infarction, heart failure with reduced left ventricular ejection fraction, severe hypertension, left ventricular hypertrophy, bradycardia, congenital long QT syndrome, history of symptomatic arrhythmias)
● INTERACTIONS → Appendix 1: delamanid
● SIDE-EFFECTS
▸ **Common or very common** Anxiety · appetite decreased · asthenia · chest pain · cough · depression · dyslipidaemia · dyspnoea · ear pain · electrolyte imbalance · gastrointestinal discomfort · haemoptysis · headache · hyperhidrosis · hypertension · hypotension · malaise · muscle weakness · nausea · oropharyngeal pain · osteochondrosis · pain · palpitations · peripheral neuropathy · photophobia · psychotic disorder · QT interval prolongation · reticulocytosis · sensation abnormal · skin reactions · sleep disorders · throat irritation · tinnitus · tremor · vomiting
▸ **Uncommon** Aggression · atrioventricular block · balance impaired · dehydration · delusional disorder, persecutory type · dysphagia · extrasystole · hepatic function abnormal · increased risk of infection · lethargy · leucopenia · oral paraesthesia · psychiatric disorders · thrombocytopenia · urinary disorders
● CONCEPTION AND CONTRACEPTION Effective contraception required during treatment.
● PREGNANCY Manufacturer advises avoid—toxicity in *animal* studies.
● BREAST FEEDING Manufacturer advises avoid—present in milk in *animal* studies.
● HEPATIC IMPAIRMENT Manufacturer advises avoid in moderate to severe impairment.
● RENAL IMPAIRMENT Manufacturer advises avoid in severe impairment—no information available.
● MONITORING REQUIREMENTS
▸ Monitor serum albumin and electrolytes before starting treatment and then during treatment—discontinue treatment if serum albumin less than 28 g/litre.
▸ Obtain ECG before starting treatment and then monthly during treatment (more frequently if serum albumin 28–34 g/litre, or if concomitant use of potent CYP3A4 inhibitors, or if risk factors for QT interval prolongation, or if QTc interval 450–500 milliseconds in men or 470–500 milliseconds in women)—discontinue treatment if QTc interval more than 500 milliseconds (derived using Fridericia's formula).
● HANDLING AND STORAGE Dispense in original container (contains desiccant).

● MEDICINAL FORMS There can be variation in the licensing of different medicines containing the same drug.
Tablet
CAUTIONARY AND ADVISORY LABELS 8, 21
▸ Deltyba (Otsuka Novel Products GmbH) ▼
Delamanid 50 mg Deltyba 50mg tablets | 48 tablet PoM £1,250.00

Ethambutol hydrochloride

04-Sep-2020

● INDICATIONS AND DOSE
Tuberculosis, in combination with other drugs (standard unsupervised 6-month treatment)
▸ BY MOUTH
▸ Child: 20 mg/kg once daily for 2 months (initial phase)
▸ Adult: 15 mg/kg once daily for 2 months (initial phase)
continued →

5

Infection

Tuberculosis, in combination with other drugs (intermittent supervised 6-month treatment) (under expert supervision)
▶ BY MOUTH
  ▶ Child: 30 mg/kg 3 times a week for 2 months (initial phase)
  ▶ Adult: 30 mg/kg 3 times a week for 2 months (initial phase)

● CONTRA-INDICATIONS Optic neuritis · poor vision
● CAUTIONS Elderly · young children
  CAUTIONS, FURTHER INFORMATION
  ▶ Understanding warnings Patients who cannot understand warnings about visual side-effects should, if possible, be given an alternative drug. In particular, ethambutol should be used with caution in children until they are at least 5 years old and capable of reporting symptomatic visual changes accurately.
● INTERACTIONS → Appendix 1: ethambutol
● SIDE-EFFECTS
  ▶ Common or very common Hyperuricaemia · nerve disorders · visual impairment
  ▶ Rare or very rare Nephritis tubulointerstitial
  ▶ Frequency not known Alveolitis allergic · appetite decreased · asthenia · confusion · dizziness · eosinophilia · fever · flatulence · gastrointestinal discomfort · gout · hallucination · headache · jaundice · leucopenia · nausea · nephrotoxicity · neutropenia · photosensitive lichenoid eruption · sensation abnormal · severe cutaneous adverse reactions (SCARs) · skin reactions · taste metallic · thrombocytopenia · tremor · vomiting
  SIDE-EFFECTS, FURTHER INFORMATION Ocular toxicity is more common where excessive dosage is used or if the patient's renal function is impaired. Early discontinuation of the drug is almost always followed by recovery of eyesight.
● PREGNANCY Not known to be harmful.
● BREAST FEEDING Amount too small to be harmful.
● RENAL IMPAIRMENT Risk of optic nerve damage. Should preferably be avoided in patients with renal impairment.
  Dose adjustments ▶ In adults If creatinine clearance less than 30 mL/minute, use 15–25 mg/kg (max. 2.5 g) 3 times a week.
  ▶ In children If creatinine clearance less than 30 mL/minute/1.73 m^2, use 15–25 mg/kg (max. 2.5 g) 3 times a week.
  Monitoring If creatinine clearance less than 30 mL/minute, monitor plasma-ethambutol concentration.
● MONITORING REQUIREMENTS
  ▶ 'Peak' concentration (2–2.5 hours after dose) should be 2–6 mg/litre (7–22 micromol/litre); 'trough' (pre-dose) concentration should be less than 1 mg/litre (4 micromol/litre).
  ▶ Renal function should be checked before treatment.
  ▶ Visual acuity should be tested by Snellen chart before treatment with ethambutol.
  ▶ In children In young children, routine ophthalmological monitoring recommended.
● PRESCRIBING AND DISPENSING INFORMATION The RCPCH and NPPG recommend that, when a liquid special of ethambutol is required, the following strength is used: 400 mg/5 mL.
● PATIENT AND CARER ADVICE
  Ocular toxicity The earliest features of ocular toxicity are subjective and patients should be advised to discontinue therapy immediately if they develop deterioration in vision and promptly seek further advice.
  Medicines for Children leaflet: Ethambutol for the treatment of tuberculosis www.medicinesforchildren.org.uk/ethambutol-treatment-tuberculosis

● MEDICINAL FORMS There can be variation in the licensing of different medicines containing the same drug. Forms available from special-order manufacturers include: oral suspension, oral solution

Tablet
CAUTIONARY AND ADVISORY LABELS 8
▶ Ethambutol hydrochloride (Non-proprietary)
  Ethambutol hydrochloride 100 mg Ethambutol 100mg tablets | 56 tablet [PoM] £17.00 DT = £11.51
  Ethambutol hydrochloride 400 mg Ethambutol 400mg tablets | 56 tablet [PoM] £42.74 DT = £42.74

Combinations available: *Rifampicin with ethambutol, isoniazid and pyrazinamide*, p. 621

Isoniazid

08-May-2020

● INDICATIONS AND DOSE

Tuberculosis, in combination with other drugs (standard unsupervised 6-month treatment)
▶ BY MOUTH, OR BY INTRAMUSCULAR INJECTION, OR BY INTRAVENOUS INJECTION
  ▶ Child: 10 mg/kg once daily (max. per dose 300 mg) for 6 months (initial and continuation phases)
  ▶ Adult: 300 mg daily for 6 months (initial and continuation phases)

Tuberculosis, in combination with other drugs (intermittent supervised 6-month treatment) (under expert supervision)
▶ BY MOUTH, OR BY INTRAMUSCULAR INJECTION, OR BY INTRAVENOUS INJECTION
  ▶ Child: 15 mg/kg 3 times a week (max. per dose 900 mg) for 6 months (initial and continuation phases)
  ▶ Adult: 15 mg/kg 3 times a week (max. per dose 900 mg) for 6 months (initial and continuation phases)

Prevention of tuberculosis in susceptible close contacts or those who have become tuberculin positive
▶ INITIALLY BY MOUTH, OR BY INTRAMUSCULAR INJECTION, OR BY INTRAVENOUS INJECTION
  ▶ Child 1 month–11 years: 10 mg/kg daily (max. per dose 300 mg) for 6 months, alternatively (by mouth) 10 mg/kg daily (max. per dose 300 mg) for 3 months, to be taken in combination with rifampicin
  ▶ Child 12–17 years: 300 mg daily for 6 months, alternatively (by mouth) 300 mg daily for 3 months, to be taken in combination with rifampicin
  ▶ Adult: 300 mg daily for 6 months, alternatively (by mouth) 300 mg daily for 3 months, to be taken in combination with rifampicin

● CONTRA-INDICATIONS Drug-induced liver disease
● CAUTIONS Acute porphyrias p. 1107 · alcohol dependence · diabetes mellitus · epilepsy · history of psychosis · HIV infection · malnutrition · slow acetylator status (increased risk of side-effects)
  CAUTIONS, FURTHER INFORMATION
  ▶ Peripheral neuropathy Pyridoxine hydrochloride p. 1130 should be given prophylactically in all patients from the start of treatment. Peripheral neuropathy is more likely to occur where there are pre-existing risk factors such as diabetes, alcohol dependence, chronic renal failure, pregnancy, malnutrition and HIV infection.
● INTERACTIONS → Appendix 1: isoniazid
● SIDE-EFFECTS
  ▶ Uncommon Hepatic disorders
  ▶ Rare or very rare Severe cutaneous adverse reactions (SCARs)
  ▶ Frequency not known Agranulocytosis · alopecia · anaemia · aplastic anaemia · eosinophilia · fever · gynaecomastia · haemolytic anaemia · hyperglycaemia · lupus-like syndrome · nerve disorders · optic atrophy · pancreatitis ·

pellagra · psychosis · seizure · skin reactions · thrombocytopenia · vasculitis

SIDE-EFFECTS, FURTHER INFORMATION Hepatitis more common in those aged over 35 years and those with a daily alcohol intake.

- PREGNANCY Not known to be harmful; prophylactic pyridoxine recommended.
- BREAST FEEDING Theoretical risk of convulsions and neuropathy; prophylactic pyridoxine advisable in mother. **Monitoring** In breast-feeding, monitor infant for possible toxicity.
- HEPATIC IMPAIRMENT Manufacturer advises caution (increased risk of hepatotoxicity).
  Monitoring In patients with pre-existing liver disease or hepatic impairment monitor liver function regularly and particularly frequently in the first 2 months.
- RENAL IMPAIRMENT Risk of ototoxicity and peripheral neuropathy; prophylactic pyridoxine hydrochloride p. 1130 recommended.
- MONITORING REQUIREMENTS
  ▸ *Renal function* should be checked before treatment.
  ▸ *Hepatic function* should be checked before treatment. If there is no evidence of liver disease (and pre-treatment liver function is normal), further checks are only necessary if the patient develops fever, malaise, vomiting, jaundice or unexplained deterioration during treatment.
  ▸ In adults Those with alcohol dependence should have frequent checks of hepatic function, particularly in the first 2 months.
- PRESCRIBING AND DISPENSING INFORMATION
  ▸ With oral use in children In general, doses should be rounded up to facilitate administration of suitable volumes of liquid or an appropriate strength of tablet. The RCPCH and NPPG recommend that, when a liquid special of isoniazid is required, the following strength is used: 50 mg/5 mL.
  ▸ In children Doses may need to be recalculated to allow for weight gain in younger children.
- PATIENT AND CARER ADVICE
  Hepatic disorders Patients or their carers should be told how to recognise signs of liver disorder, and advised to discontinue treatment and seek immediate medical attention if symptoms such as persistent nausea, vomiting, malaise or jaundice develop.
  Medicines for Children leaflet: Isoniazid for latent tuberculosis www.medicinesforchildren.org.uk/isoniazid-latent-tuberculosis
  Medicines for Children leaflet: Isoniazid for the treatment of tuberculosis www.medicinesforchildren.org.uk/isoniazid-treatment-tuberculosis

- MEDICINAL FORMS There can be variation in the licensing of different medicines containing the same drug. Forms available from special-order manufacturers include: oral suspension, oral solution

Solution for injection
▸ Cemidon (Imported (Spain))
  Isoniazid 60 mg per 1 ml Cemidon Intravenoso 300mg/5ml solution for injection ampoules | 5 ampoule [PoM] 🔣
▸ Isoniazid (Non-proprietary)
  Isoniazid 25 mg per 1 ml Isoniazid 50mg/2ml solution for injection ampoules | 10 ampoule [PoM] £387.32
▸ Tebesium-S (Imported (Germany))
  Isoniazid 20 mg per 1 ml Tebesium-S 100mg/5ml solution for injection ampoules | 12 ampoule [PoM] 🔣

Tablet
CAUTIONARY AND ADVISORY LABELS 8, 22
▸ Isoniazid (Non-proprietary)
  Isoniazid 50 mg Isoniazid 50mg tablets | 56 tablet [PoM] £19.25 DT = £19.25
  Isoniazid 100 mg Isoniazid 100mg tablets | 28 tablet [PoM] £25.13 DT = £25.13

▸ Isoniazid (Imported (United States))
  Isoniazid 300 mg Isoniazid 300mg tablets | 30 tablet [PoM] 🔣

Combinations available: *Rifampicin with ethambutol, isoniazid and pyrazinamide*, p. 621 · *Rifampicin with isoniazid*, p. 621 · *Rifampicin with isoniazid and pyrazinamide*, p. 621

Pyrazinamide

12-May-2020

- INDICATIONS AND DOSE
  Tuberculosis, in combination with other drugs (standard unsupervised 6-month treatment)
  ▸ BY MOUTH
  ▸ Child (body-weight up to 50 kg): 35 mg/kg once daily for 2 months (initial phase); maximum 1.5 g per day
  ▸ Child (body-weight 50 kg and above): 35 mg/kg once daily for 2 months (initial phase); maximum 2 g per day
  ▸ Adult (body-weight up to 50 kg): 1.5 g once daily for 2 months (initial phase)
  ▸ Adult (body-weight 50 kg and above): 2 g once daily for 2 months (initial phase)

  Tuberculosis, in combination with other drugs (intermittent supervised 6-month treatment) (under expert supervision)
  ▸ BY MOUTH
  ▸ Child (body-weight up to 50 kg): 50 mg/kg 3 times a week (max. per dose 2 g 3 times a week) for 2 months (initial phase)
  ▸ Child (body-weight 50 kg and above): 50 mg/kg 3 times a week (max. per dose 2.5 g 3 times a week) for 2 months (initial phase)
  ▸ Adult (body-weight up to 50 kg): 2 g 3 times a week for 2 months (initial phase)
  ▸ Adult (body-weight 50 kg and above): 2.5 g 3 times a week for 2 months (initial phase)

- CONTRA-INDICATIONS Acute attack of gout (in adults)
- CAUTIONS Diabetes · gout (in adults)
- INTERACTIONS → Appendix 1: pyrazinamide
- SIDE-EFFECTS Appetite decreased · arthralgia · dysuria · flushing · gout aggravated · hepatic disorders · malaise · nausea · peptic ulcer aggravated · photosensitivity reaction · sideroblastic anaemia · skin reactions · splenomegaly · vomiting
- PREGNANCY Manufacturer advises use only if potential benefit outweighs risk.
- BREAST FEEDING Amount too small to be harmful.
- HEPATIC IMPAIRMENT Manufacturer advises avoid in severe impairment, acute hepatic disease and for up to 6 months after occurrence of hepatitis (risk of increased exposure).
- RENAL IMPAIRMENT
  Dose adjustments ▸ In adults 25–30 mg/kg 3 times a week if eGFR less than 30 mL/minute/1.73 m^2.
  ▸ In children If estimated glomerular filtration rate less than 30 mL/minute/1.73 m^2, use 25–30 mg/kg 3 times a week.
  Monitoring Monitor for gout in renal impairment.
- MONITORING REQUIREMENTS
  ▸ *Renal function* should be checked before treatment.
  ▸ *Hepatic function* should be checked before treatment. If there is no evidence of liver disease (and pre-treatment liver function is normal), further checks are only necessary if the patient develops fever, malaise, vomiting, jaundice or unexplained deterioration during treatment.
  ▸ In adults Those with alcohol dependence should have frequent checks of hepatic function, particularly in the first 2 months.

5

Infection

- **PRESCRIBING AND DISPENSING INFORMATION**
  - ▸ In children In general, doses should be rounded up to facilitate administration of suitable volumes of liquid or an appropriate strength of tablet. Doses may also need to be recalculated to allow for weight gain in younger children. The RCPCH and NPPG recommend that, when a liquid special of pyrazinamide is required, the following strength is used: 500 mg/5 mL.

- **PATIENT AND CARER ADVICE**
  Hepatic disorders Patients or their carers should be told how to recognise signs of liver disorder, and advised to discontinue treatment and seek immediate medical attention if symptoms such as persistent nausea, vomiting, malaise or jaundice develop.
  Medicines for Children leaflet: Pyrazinamide for treatment of tuberculosis www.medicinesforchildren.org.uk/pyrazinamide-treatment-tuberculosis

- **MEDICINAL FORMS** There can be variation in the licensing of different medicines containing the same drug. Forms available from special-order manufacturers include: oral suspension, oral solution

  Tablet
  CAUTIONARY AND ADVISORY LABELS 8
  - ▸ Pyrazinamide (Non-proprietary)
    Pyrazinamide 500 mg Pyrazinamide 500mg tablets |
    30 tablet [PoM] £40.06 DT = £40.06
  - ▸ Zinamide (Genus Pharmaceuticals Ltd)
    Pyrazinamide 500 mg Zinamide 500mg tablets | 30 tablet [PoM]
    £31.35 DT = £40.06

  Combinations available: *Rifampicin with ethambutol, isoniazid and pyrazinamide,* p. 621 · *Rifampicin with isoniazid and pyrazinamide,* p. 621

2.6 Urinary tract infections

Urinary-tract infections

12-Feb-2019

Description of condition

Urinary-tract infections (UTIs) are common infections that can affect any part of the urinary tract. They occur more frequently in women, and are usually independent of any risk factor. UTIs are predominantly caused by bacteria from the gastrointestinal tract entering the urinary tract, with *Escherichia coli* being the most common cause. Infection due to *Candida albicans* is rare, but may occur in hospitalised patients who are immunocompromised or have an indwelling catheter.

Lower UTIs are associated with inflammation of the bladder (cystitis) and urethra (urethritis). In some patients infection can ascend the urinary tract and lead to an upper UTI. Upper UTIs affect the proximal part of the ureters (pyelitis) or the proximal part of the ureters and the kidneys (pyelonephritis), and can cause renal scarring, abscess or failure, and sepsis. The most common signs and symptoms of lower UTIs are dysuria, increased urinary frequency and urgency, urine that is strong smelling, cloudy or contains blood, and persistent lower abdominal pain. Upper UTIs usually present with accompanying loin pain and fever.

In pregnant women, asymptomatic bacteriuria is a risk factor for pyelonephritis and premature labour. UTIs in pregnancy have been associated with developmental delay and cerebral palsy in the infant, as well as fetal death.

Insertion of a catheter into the urinary tract increases the risk of developing a UTI, and the longer the catheter is in place for, further increases the risk of bacteriuria.

UTIs are considered recurrent after at least two episodes within 6 months, or three or more episodes within 12 months.

Acute prostatitis is an infection of the prostate gland and is usually caused by a UTI. It can occur spontaneously or after certain medical procedures and can last for several weeks. Common symptoms include sudden onset of fever, acute urinary retention or irritative voiding symptoms. Possible complications include prostatic abscess, bacteraemia, epididymitis, and pyelonephritis. Chronic prostatitis is a complication of acute prostatitis and is defined as at least 3 months of urogenital pain usually associated with lower urinary tract symptoms.

Aims of treatment

The aims of treatment are to relieve symptoms, treat the underlying infection, prevent systemic infection, and to reduce the risk of complications.

Non-drug treatment

[EvGr] Patients with a UTI should be advised to drink plenty of fluids to avoid dehydration, and to use self-care strategies to reduce the risk of recurrent infections. These include wiping from front to back after defaecation, not delaying urination, and not wearing occlusive underwear.

D-mannose, cranberry or urine alkalinising products may be used as self-care treatment strategies, however the benefit of these products for the prevention and treatment of UTIs has not been established. Patients should be advised to consider the sugar content of these products. ⟨A⟩

Drug treatment

[EvGr] When prescribing antibacterial therapy the severity of symptoms, risk of developing complications, previous urine culture and susceptibility results, and previous antibacterial use should be taken into consideration.

With the exception of pregnant women, asymptomatic bacteriuria is not routinely treated with antibacterials. ⟨A⟩

For other considerations such as for patients receiving prophylactic antibacterial therapy, switching from *intravenous* to *oral* antibacterials, and for advice to give to patients, see Antibacterials, principles of therapy p. 527.

[EvGr] Reassess patients if symptoms worsen at any time, or do not start to improve within 48 hours of starting treatment.

Refer patients to hospital if they have any symptoms or signs suggestive of a more serious illness or condition.

Review choice of antibacterial when microbiological results are available, and change treatment as appropriate if susceptibility results indicate bacterial resistance.

Advise patients that paracetamol or ibuprofen can be used for pain relief. Where appropriate codeine may be used in patients with acute pyelonephritis or prostatitis. ⟨A⟩

Lower urinary-tract infection

Non-pregnant women

[EvGr] Consider a back-up antibacterial prescription for use if symptoms worsen or do not improve within 48 hours **or** an immediate antibacterial prescription. ⟨A⟩

Choice of antibacterial therapy

- **Oral** *first line* :
  - ▸ [EvGr] Nitrofurantoin p. 628, or trimethoprim p. 610 (if low risk of resistance). ⟨A⟩

- **Oral** *second line* (if no improvement after at least 48 hours, **or** first line not suitable):
  - ▸ [EvGr] Nitrofurantoin (if not used first line), fosfomycin p. 607, or pivmecillinam hydrochloride p. 588. ⟨A⟩

Men

[EvGr] An immediate antibacterial prescription should be given and a midstream urine sample obtained before treatment is taken and sent for culture and susceptibility testing. ⟨A⟩

Choice of antibacterial therapy

- **Oral** *first line* :
  - ▸ [EvGr] Nitrofurantoin, or trimethoprim. ⟨A⟩

- **Oral** *second line* (if no improvement after at least 48 hours, or first line not suitable):
▶ Consider pyelonephritis or prostatitis. See *pyelonephritis, acute*, or *prostatitis, acute* below for guidance.

Pregnant women

EvGr An immediate antibacterial prescription should be given and a midstream urine sample obtained before treatment is taken and sent for culture and susceptibility testing. Ⓐ

Choice of antibacterial therapy

- **Oral** *first line* :
▶ EvGr Nitrofurantoin. Ⓐ
- **Oral** *second line* (if no improvement after at least 48 hours, or first line not suitable):
▶ EvGr Amoxicillin p. 582 (only if culture susceptible), or cefalexin p. 552. Ⓐ
- **Alternative** *second line* :
▶ EvGr Consult local microbiologist. Ⓐ
- **Asymptomatic bacteriuria**:
▶ EvGr Amoxicillin, cefalexin, or nitrofurantoin. Ⓐ

Prostatitis, acute

EvGr An immediate antibacterial prescription should be given and a midstream urine sample obtained before treatment is taken and sent for culture and susceptibility testing.

Refer patients to hospital if symptoms are not improving after 48 hours of treatment, or if they have any signs or symptoms suggestive of a more serious condition such as sepsis, acute urinary retention, or prostatic abscess. Ⓐ

Choice of antibacterial therapy

- **Oral** *first line* :
▶ EvGr Ciprofloxacin p. 593, or ofloxacin p. 597.
▶ Alternative first line (if unable to take fluoroquinolones): trimethoprim. Ⓐ
- **Oral** *second line* (on specialist advice):
▶ EvGr Levofloxacin p. 595, or co-trimoxazole p. 598. Ⓐ
- **Intravenous** *first line* (if severely unwell or unable to take oral treatment). EvGr Antibacterials may be combined if concerned about sepsis.
▶ Amikacin p. 545, ceftriaxone p. 558, cefuroxime p. 555, ciprofloxacin, gentamicin p. 545, or levofloxacin. Ⓐ
- **Intravenous** *second line* :
▶ EvGr Consult local microbiologist. Ⓐ

Pyelonephritis, acute

EvGr An immediate antibacterial prescription should be given and a midstream urine sample obtained before treatment is taken and sent for culture and susceptibility testing.

Consider referring or seeking specialist advice for patients with acute pyelonephritis who are significantly dehydrated or are unable to take oral fluids and medicines, are pregnant, or have a higher risk of developing complications. Ⓐ

Non-pregnant women and men
Choice of antibacterial therapy

- **Oral** *first line* :
▶ EvGr Cefalexin p. 552, or ciprofloxacin p. 593. If sensitivity known: co-amoxiclav p. 585, or trimethoprim p. 610. Ⓐ
- **Intravenous** *first line* (if severely unwell or unable to take oral treatment). EvGr Antibacterials may be combined if concerned about susceptibility or sepsis. Ⓐ
▶ EvGr Amikacin p. 545, ceftriaxone p. 558, cefuroxime p. 555, ciprofloxacin, or gentamicin p. 545. Co-amoxiclav may be used if given in combination or sensitivity known. Ⓐ

- **Intravenous** *second line* :
▶ EvGr Consult local microbiologist. Ⓐ

Pregnant women
Choice of antibacterial therapy

- **Oral** *first line* :
▶ EvGr Cefalexin. Ⓐ
- **Intravenous** *first line* (if severely unwell or unable to take oral treatment):
▶ EvGr Cefuroxime. Ⓐ
- **Second line** or combining antibacterials if concerned about susceptibility or sepsis:
▶ EvGr Consult local microbiologist. Ⓐ

Recurrent urinary-tract infection

EvGr For patients with recurrent UTIs, refer or seek specialist advice for men, pregnant women, patients with suspected cancer, those presenting with recurrent upper UTI, and those with recurrent lower UTI with an unknown cause.

For postmenopausal women experiencing recurrent UTIs, consider a vaginal oestrogen [unlicensed indication] at the lowest effective dose if behavioural and personal hygiene measures alone are not effective or appropriate. Treatment should be reviewed within 12 months. Oral oestrogens (hormone replacement therapy) should not be given to postmenopausal women specifically to reduce the risk of recurrent UTIs.

In non-pregnant women, consider a trial of antibacterial prophylaxis if behavioural and personal hygiene measures, and vaginal oestrogen (in postmenopausal women) are not effective or appropriate. Single-dose antibacterial prophylaxis [unlicensed indication] should be considered for use when exposed to an identifiable trigger. Daily antibacterial prophylaxis should be considered in non-pregnant women who have had no improvement after single-dose antibacterial prophylaxis, or who have no identifiable triggers.

With specialist advice, daily antibacterial prophylaxis should be considered for men and pregnant women if behavioural and personal hygiene measures alone are not effective or appropriate.

Advise patients about the risk of resistance with long-term antibacterial use, seeking medical help if symptoms of an acute UTI develop, and to return for review within 6 months.

Review the success and ongoing need of prophylaxis at least every 6 months. If antibacterial prophylaxis is stopped ensure the patient has rapid access to treatment if they develop an acute UTI. Ⓐ

Women and men
Choice of antibacterial therapy

- **Oral** *first line* :
▶ EvGr Trimethoprim, or nitrofurantoin p. 628. Ⓐ
- **Oral** *second line* :
▶ EvGr Amoxicillin p. 582 [unlicensed indication], or cefalexin. Ⓐ

Catheter-associated urinary-tract infection

EvGr For people with a catheter-associated urinary-tract infection, consider removing or changing the catheter as soon as possible if it has been in place for longer than 7 days, without delaying antibacterial treatment. An immediate antibacterial prescription should be given and a urine sample obtained before treatment is taken and sent for culture and susceptibility testing.

Consider referring or seeking specialist advice for patients with a catheter-associated UTI who are significantly dehydrated or unable to take oral fluids and medicines, are pregnant, have a higher risk of developing complications, have recurrent catheter-associated UTIs, or have bacteria resistant to oral antibacterials. Ⓐ

5

Infection

Infection

5

Non-pregnant women and men
Choice of antibacterial therapy

- *Oral first line* (if **no** upper UTI symptoms):
  ▸ EvGr Amoxicillin (only if culture susceptible), nitrofurantoin, or trimethoprim (if low risk of resistance). Ⓐ
- *Oral second line* (if **no** upper UTI symptoms and first-line not suitable):
  ▸ EvGr Pivmecillinam hydrochloride p. 588. Ⓐ
- *Oral first line* (upper UTI symptoms):
  ▸ EvGr Cefalexin, ciprofloxacin, co-amoxiclav (if culture susceptible), or trimethoprim (if culture susceptible). Ⓐ
- *Intravenous first line* (if severely unwell or unable to take oral treatment): EvGr Antibacterials may be combined if concerned about susceptibility or sepsis.
  ▸ Amikacin, ceftriaxone, cefuroxime, ciprofloxacin, gentamicin, or co-amoxiclav (only in combination, unless culture results confirm susceptibility). Ⓐ
- *Intravenous second line* :
  ▸ EvGr Consult local microbiologist. Ⓐ

Pregnant women
Choice of antibacterial therapy

- *Oral first line* :
  ▸ EvGr Cefalexin. Ⓐ
- *Intravenous first line* (if severely unwell or unable to take oral treatment):
  ▸ EvGr Cefuroxime. Ⓐ
- *Second line or combining if concerned about susceptibility or sepsis*:
  ▸ EvGr Consult local microbiologist. Ⓐ

Useful Resources

Urinary tract infection (lower): antimicrobial prescribing. National Institute for Health and Care Excellence. Clinical Guideline 109. October 2018.
www.nice.org.uk/guidance/ng109

Prostatitis (acute): antimicrobial prescribing. National Institute for Health and Care Excellence. Clinical Guideline 110. October 2018.
www.nice.org.uk/guidance/ng110

Pyelonephritis (acute): antimicrobial prescribing. National Institute for Health and Care Excellence. Clinical Guideline 111. October 2018.
www.nice.org.uk/guidance/ng111

Urinary tract infection (recurrent): antimicrobial prescribing. National Institute for Health and Care Excellence. Clinical Guideline 112. October 2018.
www.nice.org.uk/guidance/ng112

Urinary tract infection (catheter-associated): antimicrobial prescribing. National Institute for Health and Care Excellence. Clinical Guideline 113. November 2018.
www.nice.org.uk/guidance/ng113

Patient decision aids: Urinary tract infection (lower); Urinary tract infection (recurrent) National Institute for Health and Care Excellence. November 2018.
www.nice.org.uk/about/what-we-do/our-programmes/nice-guidance/nice-guidelines/shared-decision-making

ANTIBACTERIALS ⟩ OTHER

Methenamine hippurate

20-Aug-2020

(Hexamine hippurate)

● **INDICATIONS AND DOSE**

Prophylaxis and long-term treatment of chronic or recurrent uncomplicated lower urinary-tract infections
▸ BY MOUTH
▸ Adult: 1 g every 12 hours

Prophylaxis and long-term treatment of chronic or recurrent uncomplicated lower urinary-tract infections in patients with catheters
▸ BY MOUTH
▸ Adult: 1 g every 8–12 hours

● CONTRA-INDICATIONS Gout · metabolic acidosis · severe dehydration
● INTERACTIONS → Appendix 1: methenamine
● SIDE-EFFECTS
▸ **Uncommon** Epigastric discomfort · skin reactions
● PREGNANCY There is inadequate evidence of safety, but it has been in wide use for many years without apparent ill consequence, however, manufacturer advises it is preferable to avoid.
● BREAST FEEDING Amount too small to be harmful.
● HEPATIC IMPAIRMENT Manufacturer advises avoid.
● RENAL IMPAIRMENT Avoid if eGFR less than 10 mL/minute/1.73 m^2—risk of hippurate crystalluria.
● EFFECT ON LABORATORY TESTS False results for urinary steroids, catecholamines and 5-hydroxyindole acetic acid can occur.
● LESS SUITABLE FOR PRESCRIBING Methenamine (hexamine) hippurate should **not** generally be used because it requires an acidic urine for its antimicrobial activity and it is ineffective for upper urinary-tract infections; it may, however, have a role in the prophylaxis and treatment of chronic or recurrent uncomplicated lower urinary-tract infections. It is considered less suitable for prescribing.

● MEDICINAL FORMS There can be variation in the licensing of different medicines containing the same drug.
Tablet
CAUTIONARY AND ADVISORY LABELS 9
▸ Methenamine hippurate (Non-proprietary)
Methenamine hippurate 1 gram Methenamine hippurate 1g tablets | 60 tablet Ⓟ £19.74–£23.68 DT = £19.74
▸ Hiprex (Mylan)
Methenamine hippurate 1 gram Hiprex 1g tablets | 60 tablet Ⓟ £19.74 DT = £19.74

Nitrofurantoin

07-Aug-2020

● **INDICATIONS AND DOSE**

Lower urinary-tract infections
▸ BY MOUTH USING IMMEDIATE-RELEASE MEDICINES
▸ Child 3 months–11 years: 750 micrograms/kg 4 times a day for 3 days
▸ Child 12–15 years: 50 mg 4 times a day for 3 days (7 days in pregnant women)
▸ Child 16–17 years: 50 mg 4 times a day for 3 days (7 days in males and pregnant women)
▸ Adult: 50 mg 4 times a day for 3 days (7 days in males and pregnant women)
▸ BY MOUTH USING MODIFIED-RELEASE MEDICINES
▸ Child 12–15 years: 100 mg twice daily for 3 days (7 days in pregnant women)
▸ Child 16–17 years: 100 mg twice daily for 3 days (7 days in males and pregnant women)
▸ Adult: 100 mg twice daily for 3 days (7 days in males and pregnant women)

Urinary-tract infections (catheter-associated)
▸ BY MOUTH USING IMMEDIATE-RELEASE MEDICINES
▸ Child 16–17 years: 50 mg 4 times a day for 7 days, to be used if modified-release preparations are unavailable
▸ Adult: 50 mg 4 times a day for 7 days, to be used if modified-release preparations are unavailable
▸ BY MOUTH USING MODIFIED-RELEASE MEDICINES
▸ Child 16–17 years: 100 mg twice daily for 7 days

▸ **Adult:** 100 mg twice daily for 7 days

Severe chronic recurrent urinary-tract infections
▶ BY MOUTH USING IMMEDIATE-RELEASE MEDICINES
▸ **Child 12-17 years:** 100 mg 4 times a day for 3–7 days
▸ **Adult:** 100 mg 4 times a day for 7 days

Prophylaxis of recurrent urinary-tract infection
▶ BY MOUTH USING IMMEDIATE-RELEASE MEDICINES
▸ **Child 3 months-11 years:** 1 mg/kg once daily, dose to be taken at night
▸ **Child 12-15 years:** 50–100 mg once daily, dose to be taken at night
▸ **Child 16-17 years:** 50–100 mg once daily, dose to be taken at night, alternatively 100 mg for 1 dose, following exposure to a trigger
▸ **Adult:** 50–100 mg once daily, dose to be taken at night, alternatively 100 mg for 1 dose, following exposure to a trigger

Genito-urinary surgical prophylaxis
▶ BY MOUTH USING MODIFIED-RELEASE MEDICINES
▸ **Child 12-17 years:** 100 mg twice daily on day of procedure and for 3 days after
▸ **Adult:** 100 mg twice daily on day of procedure and for 3 days after

● UNLICENSED USE EvGr Duration of treatment for lower urinary-tract infection differs from product literature and adheres to national guidelines. Ⓐ See Urinary-tract infections p. 626 for further information. EvGr Nitrofurantoin can be given as a single dose for the prophylaxis of recurrent urinary tract infection following exposure to a trigger, Ⓐ but this dosing regimen is not licensed. See Urinary-tract infections p. 626 for further information.

● CONTRA-INDICATIONS Acute porphyrias p. 1107 · G6PD deficiency

● CAUTIONS Anaemia · diabetes mellitus · electrolyte imbalance · folate deficiency · pulmonary disease · susceptibility to peripheral neuropathy · urine may be coloured yellow or brown · vitamin B deficiency

● INTERACTIONS → Appendix 1: nitrofurantoin

● SIDE-EFFECTS Agranulocytosis · alopecia · anaemia · angioedema · aplastic anaemia · appetite decreased · arthralgia · asthenia · chest pain · chills · circulatory collapse · confusion · cough · cyanosis · depression · diarrhoea · dizziness · drowsiness · dyspnoea · eosinophilia · euphoric mood · fever · granulocytopenia · haemolytic anaemia · headache · hepatic disorders · idiopathic intracranial hypertension · increased risk of infection · leucopenia · lupus-like syndrome · nausea · nerve disorders · nystagmus · pancreatitis · psychotic disorder · pulmonary hypersensitivity · pulmonary reaction (possible association with lupus erythematosus-like syndrome) · respiratory disorders · skin reactions · Stevens-Johnson syndrome · thrombocytopenia · urine discolouration · vertigo · vomiting

● PREGNANCY Avoid at term—may produce neonatal haemolysis.

● BREAST FEEDING Avoid; only small amounts in milk but enough to produce haemolysis in G6PD-deficient infants.

● HEPATIC IMPAIRMENT Manufacturer advises caution.

● RENAL IMPAIRMENT Risk of peripheral neuropathy; antibacterial efficacy depends on renal secretion of the drug into urinary tract.
▸ In adults Avoid if eGFR less than 45 mL/minute/1.73 m²; may be used with caution if eGFR 30–44 mL/minute/1.73 m² as a short-course only (3 to 7 days), to treat uncomplicated lower urinary-tract infection caused by suspected or proven multidrug resistant bacteria and only if potential benefit outweighs risk.

▸ In children Avoid if estimated glomerular filtration rate less than 45 mL/minute/1.73 m²; may be used with caution if estimated glomerular filtration rate 30–44 mL/minute/1.73 m² as a short-course only (3 to 7 days), to treat uncomplicated lower urinary-tract infection caused by suspected or proven multidrug resistant bacteria and only if potential benefit outweighs risk.

● MONITORING REQUIREMENTS On long-term therapy, monitor liver function and monitor for pulmonary symptoms, especially in the elderly (discontinue if deterioration in lung function).

● EFFECT ON LABORATORY TESTS False positive urinary glucose (if tested for reducing substances).

● PATIENT AND CARER ADVICE
Medicines for Children leaflet: Nitrofurantoin for urinary tract infections www.medicinesforchildren.org.uk/nitrofurantoin-urinary-tract-infections

● MEDICINAL FORMS There can be variation in the licensing of different medicines containing the same drug. Forms available from special-order manufacturers include: oral suspension, oral solution

Tablet
CAUTIONARY AND ADVISORY LABELS 9, 14, 21
▶ Nitrofurantoin (Non-proprietary)
Nitrofurantoin 50 mg Nitrofurantoin 50mg tablets | 28 tablet PoM £31.33 DT = £9.48 | 100 tablet PoM £33.86-£111.89
Nitrofurantoin 100 mg Nitrofurantoin 100mg tablets | 28 tablet PoM £12.99 DT = £7.94 | 100 tablet PoM £22.14-£28.36

Oral suspension
CAUTIONARY AND ADVISORY LABELS 9, 14, 21
▶ Nitrofurantoin (Non-proprietary)
Nitrofurantoin 5 mg per 1 ml Nitrofurantoin 25mg/5ml oral suspension sugar free sugar-free | 300 ml PoM £588.16 DT = £529.09

Modified-release capsule
CAUTIONARY AND ADVISORY LABELS 9, 14, 21, 25
▶ Macrobid (Advanz Pharma)
Nitrofurantoin 100 mg Macrobid 100mg modified-release capsules | 14 capsule PoM £9.50 DT = £9.50

Capsule
CAUTIONARY AND ADVISORY LABELS 9, 14, 21
▶ Nitrofurantoin (Non-proprietary)
Nitrofurantoin 50 mg Nitrofurantoin 50mg capsules | 30 capsule PoM £15.42 DT = £8.72
Nitrofurantoin 100 mg Nitrofurantoin 100mg capsules | 30 capsule PoM £10.43 DT = £10.43

3   Fungal infection

Antifungals, systemic use

Fungal infections

The systemic treatment of common fungal infections is outlined below; specialist treatment is required in most forms of systemic or disseminated fungal infections. Local treatment is suitable for a number of fungal infections (genital, bladder, eye, ear, oropharynx, and skin).

Aspergillosis
Aspergillosis most commonly affects the respiratory tract but in severely immunocompromised patients, invasive forms can affect the heart, brain, and skin. Voriconazole p. 638 is the treatment of choice for aspergillosis; liposomal amphotericin B p. 632 is an alternative first-line treatment when voriconazole cannot be used. Caspofungin p. 631, or itraconazole p. 636, can be used in patients who are refractory to, or intolerant of voriconazole and liposomal amphotericin B. Itraconazole is also used for the treatment of chronic pulmonary aspergillosis or as an adjunct in the treatment of allergic bronchopulmonary aspergillosis [unlicensed indication]. Posaconazole p. 637 is licensed for

5

Infection

use in patients with invasive aspergillosis who are refractory to, or intolerant of itraconazole or amphotericin B.

Candidiasis

Many superficial candidal infections including infections of the skin are treated locally; widespread or intractable infection requires systemic antifungal treatment. Vaginal candidiasis may be treated with locally acting antifungals or with fluconazole p. 634 given by mouth; for resistant organisms in adults, itraconazole can be given by mouth.

Oropharyngeal candidiasis generally responds to topical therapy; fluconazole is given by mouth for unresponsive infections; it is effective and is reliably absorbed. Itraconazole may be used for infections that do not respond to fluconazole. Topical therapy may not be adequate in immunocompromised patients and an oral triazole antifungal is preferred.

For *invasive or disseminated candidiasis*, an **echinocandin** can be used. Fluconazole is an alternative for *Candida albicans* infection in clinically stable patients who have not received an azole antifungal recently. Amphotericin B is an alternative when an echinocandin or fluconazole cannot be used, however, amphotericin B should be considered for the initial treatment of CNS candidiasis. Voriconazole can be used for infections caused by fluconazole-resistant *Candida* spp. when oral therapy is required, or in patients intolerant of amphotericin B or an echinocandin. In refractory cases, flucytosine p. 639 can be used with intravenous amphotericin B.

Cryptococcosis

Cryptococcosis is uncommon but infection in the immunocompromised, especially in HIV-positive patients, can be life-threatening; cryptococcal meningitis is the most common form of fungal meningitis. The treatment of choice in cryptococcal meningitis is amphotericin B by intravenous infusion and flucytosine by intravenous infusion for 2 weeks, followed by fluconazole by mouth for 8 weeks or until cultures are negative. In cryptococcosis, fluconazole is sometimes given alone as an alternative in HIV-positive patients with mild, localised infections or in those who cannot tolerate amphotericin B. Following successful treatment, fluconazole can be used for prophylaxis against relapse until immunity recovers.

Histoplasmosis

Histoplasmosis is rare in temperate climates; it can be life-threatening, particularly in HIV-infected persons. Itraconazole can be used for the treatment of immunocompetent patients with indolent non-meningeal infection, including chronic pulmonary histoplasmosis. Amphotericin B by intravenous infusion is used for the initial treatment of fulminant or severe infections, followed by a course of itraconazole by mouth. Following successful treatment, itraconazole can be used for prophylaxis against relapse until immunity recovers.

Skin and nail infections

Mild localised fungal infections of the skin (including tinea corporis, tinea cruris, and tinea pedis) respond to topical therapy. Systemic therapy is appropriate if topical therapy fails, if many areas are affected, or if the site of infection is difficult to treat such as in infections of the nails (onychomycosis) and of the scalp (tinea capitis). Oral imidazole or triazole antifungals (particularly itraconazole) and terbinafine p. 1279 are used more frequently than griseofulvin p. 640 because they have a broader spectrum of activity and require a shorter duration of treatment.

Tinea capitis is treated systemically; additional topical application of an antifungal may reduce transmission. Griseofulvin is used for tinea capitis in adults and children; it is effective against infections caused by *Trichophyton tonsurans* and *Microsporum spp.* Terbinafine is used for tinea capitis caused by *T. tonsurans* [unlicensed indication]. The

role of terbinafine in the management of *Microsporum* infections is uncertain.

Pityriasis versicolor may be treated with itraconazole by mouth if topical therapy is ineffective; fluconazole by mouth is an alternative. Oral terbinafine is **not** effective for pityriasis versicolor.

Antifungal treatment may not be necessary in asymptomatic patients with tinea infection of the nails. If treatment is necessary, a systemic antifungal is more effective than topical therapy. Terbinafine and itraconazole have largely replaced griseofulvin for the systemic treatment of *onychomycosis*, particularly of the toenail; terbinafine is considered to be the drug of choice. Itraconazole can be administered as intermittent 'pulse' therapy. Topical antifungals also have a role in the treatment of onychomycosis.

Immunocompromised patients

Immunocompromised patients are at particular risk of fungal infections and may receive antifungal drugs prophylactically; oral triazole antifungals are the drugs of choice for prophylaxis. Fluconazole is more reliably absorbed than itraconazole, but fluconazole is not effective against *Aspergillus* spp. Itraconazole is preferred in patients at risk of invasive aspergillosis. Posaconazole can be used for prophylaxis in patients who are undergoing haematopoietic stem cell transplantation or receiving chemotherapy for acute myeloid leukaemia or myelodysplastic syndrome. Micafungin p. 632 can be used for prophylaxis of candidiasis in patients undergoing haematopoietic stem cell transplantation when fluconazole, itraconazole or posaconazole cannot be used.

Amphotericin B by intravenous infusion or caspofungin is used for the empirical *treatment* of serious fungal infections; caspofungin is not effective against fungal infections of the CNS.

Triazole antifungals

Triazole antifungal drugs have a role in the prevention and systemic treatment of fungal infections.

Fluconazole is very well absorbed after oral administration. It also achieves good penetration into the cerebrospinal fluid to treat fungal meningitis. Fluconazole is excreted largely unchanged in the urine and can be used to treat candiduria.

Itraconazole is active against a wide range of dermatophytes. Itraconazole capsules require an acid environment in the stomach for optimal absorption. Itraconazole has been associated with liver damage and should be avoided or used with caution in patients with liver disease; fluconazole is less frequently associated with hepatotoxicity.

Posaconazole is licensed for the treatment of invasive fungal infections unresponsive to conventional treatment.

Voriconazole is a broad-spectrum antifungal drug which is licensed for use in life-threatening infections.

Imidazole antifungals

The imidazole antifungals include clotrimazole p. 876, econazole nitrate p. 876, ketoconazole p. 876, and tioconazole p. 1278. They are used for the local treatment of vaginal candidiasis and for dermatophyte infections. Miconazole p. 877 can be used locally for oral infections; it is also effective in intestinal infections. Systemic absorption may follow use of miconazole oral gel p. 877 and may result in significant drug interactions.

Polyene antifungals

The polyene antifungals include amphotericin B p. 632 and nystatin p. 1263; neither drug is absorbed when given by mouth. Nystatin is used for oral, oropharyngeal, and perioral infections by local application in the mouth. Nystatin is also used for *Candida albicans* infection of the skin.

Amphotericin B by intravenous infusion is used for the treatment of systemic fungal infections and is active against most fungi and yeasts. It is highly protein bound and penetrates poorly into body fluids and tissues. When given parenterally amphotericin B is toxic and side-effects are common. Lipid formulations of amphotericin B (*Abelcet*® and *AmBisome*®) are significantly less toxic and are recommended when the conventional formulation of amphotericin B is contra-indicated because of toxicity, especially nephrotoxicity or when response to conventional amphotericin B is inadequate; lipid formulations are more expensive.

Echinocandin antifungals

The echinocandin antifungals include anidulafungin below, caspofungin below and micafungin p. 632. They are only active against *Aspergillus* spp. and *Candida* spp.; however, anidulafungin and micafungin are not used for the treatment of aspergillosis. Echinocandins are not effective against fungal infections of the CNS.

Other antifungals

Flucytosine p. 639 is used with amphotericin B in a synergistic combination. Bone marrow depression can occur which limits its use, particularly in HIV-positive patients; weekly blood counts are necessary during prolonged therapy. Resistance to flucytosine can develop during therapy and sensitivity testing is essential before and during treatment. Flucytosine has a role in the treatment of systemic candidiasis and cryptococcal meningitis.

Griseofulvin p. 640 is effective for widespread or intractable dermatophyte infections but has been superseded by newer antifungals, particularly for nail infections. It is the drug of choice for trichophyton infections in children. Duration of therapy is dependent on the site of the infection and may extend to a number of months.

Terbinafine p. 1279 is the drug of choice for fungal nail infections and is also used for ringworm infections where oral treatment is considered appropriate.

ANTIFUNGALS > ECHINOCANDIN ANTIFUNGALS

Anidulafungin   24-Nov-2020

● **INDICATIONS AND DOSE**

Invasive candidiasis
▸ BY INTRAVENOUS INFUSION
▸ Adult: Initially 200 mg once daily for 1 day, then 100 mg once daily

● SIDE-EFFECTS
▸ **Common or very common** Bronchospasm · cholestasis · diarrhoea · dyspnoea · headache · hyperglycaemia · hypertension · hypokalaemia · hypotension · nausea · seizure · skin reactions · vomiting
▸ **Uncommon** Abdominal pain upper · coagulation disorder · vasodilation

● PREGNANCY Manufacturer advises avoid unless potential benefit outweighs risk—toxicity in *animal* studies.

● BREAST FEEDING Manufacturer advises avoid unless potential benefit outweighs risk—present in milk in *animal* studies.

● DIRECTIONS FOR ADMINISTRATION For *intravenous infusion* (*Ecalta*®), give intermittently *in* Glucose 5% *or* Sodium chloride 0.9%. Reconstitute each 100 mg with 30 mL water for injections and allow up to 5 minutes for reconstitution; dilute dose in infusion fluid to a concentration of 770 micrograms/mL; give at a rate not exceeding 1.1 mg/minute.

● MEDICINAL FORMS There can be variation in the licensing of different medicines containing the same drug.
Powder for solution for infusion
▸ Anidulafungin (Non-proprietary)
  Anidulafungin 100 mg Anidulafungin 100mg powder for concentrate for solution for infusion vials | 1 vial POM £299.98 DT = £299.98 (Hospital only)
▸ Ecalta (Pfizer Ltd)
  Anidulafungin 100 mg Ecalta 100mg powder for concentrate for solution for infusion vials | 1 vial POM £299.99 DT = £299.98 (Hospital only)

Caspofungin   07-Aug-2020

● **INDICATIONS AND DOSE**

Invasive aspergillosis | Invasive candidiasis | Empirical treatment of systemic fungal infections in patients with neutropenia
▸ BY INTRAVENOUS INFUSION
▸ Adult (body-weight up to 81 kg): 70 mg once daily for 1 day, then 50 mg once daily
▸ Adult (body-weight 81 kg and above): 70 mg once daily

DOSE ADJUSTMENTS DUE TO INTERACTIONS
▸ Manufacturer advises increase dose to 70 mg daily with concurrent use of some enzyme inducers (such as carbamazepine, dexamethasone, phenytoin, and rifampicin); no dose adjustment required for patients already on 70 mg daily.

● INTERACTIONS → Appendix 1: caspofungin

● SIDE-EFFECTS
▸ **Common or very common** Arthralgia · diarrhoea · dyspnoea · electrolyte imbalance · fever · headache · hyperhidrosis · nausea · skin reactions · vomiting
▸ **Uncommon** Anaemia · anxiety · appetite decreased · arrhythmias · ascites · chest discomfort · coagulation disorder · congestive heart failure · constipation · cough · disorientation · dizziness · drowsiness · dry mouth · dysphagia · excessive tearing · eyelid oedema · fatigue · flatulence · fluid overload · flushing · gastrointestinal discomfort · haematuria · hepatic disorders · hyperbilirubinaemia · hyperglycaemia · hypertension · hypotension · hypoxia · induration · insomnia · laryngeal pain · leucopenia · malaise · metabolic acidosis · muscle weakness · myalgia · nasal congestion · oedema · pain · palpitations · renal impairment · respiratory disorders · sensation abnormal · taste altered · thrombocytopenia · thrombophlebitis · tremor · vision blurred
▸ **Frequency not known** Severe cutaneous adverse reactions (SCARs)

● PREGNANCY Manufacturer advises avoid unless essential—toxicity in *animal* studies.

● BREAST FEEDING Present in milk in *animal* studies—manufacturer advises avoid.

● HEPATIC IMPAIRMENT No information available for severe impairment.
Dose adjustments 70 mg on first day then 35 mg once daily in moderate impairment.

● DIRECTIONS FOR ADMINISTRATION For *intravenous infusion* (*Cancidas*®), manufacturer advises give intermittently *in* Sodium chloride 0.9%. Allow vial to reach room temperature; initially reconstitute each vial with 10.5 mL water for injections, mixing gently to dissolve then dilute requisite dose in 250 mL infusion fluid (35- or 50-mg doses may be diluted in 100 ml infusion fluid if necessary); give over 60 minutes; incompatible with glucose solutions.

5

Infection

- MEDICINAL FORMS There can be variation in the licensing of different medicines containing the same drug.

Powder for solution for infusion

▸ Caspofungin (Non-proprietary)

Caspofungin (as Caspofungin acetate) 50 mg Caspofungin 50mg powder for concentrate for solution for infusion vials | 1 vial PoM £42.90–£327.67

Caspofungin (as Caspofungin acetate) 70 mg Caspofungin 70mg powder for concentrate for solution for infusion vials | 1 vial PoM £52.91–£416.78

▸ Cancidas (Merck Sharp & Dohme Ltd)

Caspofungin (as Caspofungin acetate) 50 mg Cancidas 50mg powder for solution for infusion vials | 1 vial PoM £327.67

Micafungin

29-Jul-2020

- INDICATIONS AND DOSE

Invasive candidiasis

▸ BY INTRAVENOUS INFUSION

▸ Adult (body-weight up to 40 kg): 2 mg/kg once daily for at least 14 days; increased if necessary to 4 mg/kg once daily, increase dose if response inadequate

▸ Adult (body-weight 40 kg and above): 100 mg once daily for at least 14 days; increased if necessary to 200 mg once daily, increase dose if response inadequate

Oesophageal candidiasis

▸ BY INTRAVENOUS INFUSION

▸ Adult (body-weight up to 40 kg): 3 mg/kg once daily

▸ Adult (body-weight 40 kg and above): 150 mg once daily

Prophylaxis of candidiasis in patients undergoing bone-marrow transplantation or who are expected to become neutropenic for over 10 days

▸ BY INTRAVENOUS INFUSION

▸ Adult (body-weight up to 40 kg): 1 mg/kg once daily continue for at least 7 days after neutrophil count is in desirable range

▸ Adult (body-weight 40 kg and above): 50 mg once daily continue for at least 7 days after neutrophil count is in desirable range

- INTERACTIONS → Appendix 1: micafungin

- SIDE-EFFECTS Anaemia · anxiety · appetite decreased · arrhythmias · confusion · constipation · diarrhoea · disseminated intravascular coagulation · dizziness · drowsiness · dyspnoea · electrolyte imbalance · eosinophilia · flushing · gastrointestinal discomfort · haemolysis · haemolytic anaemia · headache · hepatic disorders · hepatic failure (potentially life-threatening) · hyperbilirubinaemia · hyperhidrosis · hypersensitivity · hypertension · hypoalbuminaemia · hypotension · insomnia · leucopenia · nausea · neutropenia · palpitations · pancytopenia · peripheral oedema · renal impairment · severe cutaneous adverse reactions (SCARs) · shock · skin reactions · taste altered · thrombocytopenia · tremor · vomiting

- PREGNANCY Manufacturer advises avoid unless essential—toxicity in *animal* studies.

- BREAST FEEDING Manufacturer advises use only if potential benefit outweighs risk—present in milk in *animal* studies.

- HEPATIC IMPAIRMENT Manufacturer advises caution in chronic impairment; avoid in severe impairment (limited information available).

- RENAL IMPAIRMENT Use with caution; renal function may deteriorate.

- MONITORING REQUIREMENTS

▸ Monitor renal function.

▸ Monitor liver function—discontinue if significant and persistent abnormalities in liver function tests develop.

- DIRECTIONS FOR ADMINISTRATION For *intravenous infusion* (*Mycamine*®), manufacturer advises give intermittently in

Glucose 5% or Sodium chloride 0.9%. Reconstitute each vial with 5 mL infusion fluid; gently rotate vial, without shaking, to dissolve; dilute requisite dose with infusion fluid to 100 mL (final concentration of 0.5–2 mg/mL); protect infusion from light; give over 60 minutes.

- MEDICINAL FORMS There can be variation in the licensing of different medicines containing the same drug.

Powder for solution for infusion

▸ Micafungin (Non-proprietary)

Micafungin (as Micafungin sodium) 50 mg Micafungin 50mg powder for concentrate for solution for infusion vials | 1 vial PoM £166.67–£196.08 (Hospital only)

Micafungin (as Micafungin sodium) 100 mg Micafungin 100mg powder for concentrate for solution for infusion vials | 1 vial PoM £289.85–£341.00 (Hospital only)

▸ Mycamine (Astellas Pharma Ltd)

Micafungin (as Micafungin sodium) 50 mg Mycamine 50mg powder for solution for infusion vials | 1 vial PoM £196.08

Micafungin (as Micafungin sodium) 100 mg Mycamine 100mg powder for solution for infusion vials | 1 vial PoM £341.00

ANTIFUNGALS ⟩ POLYENE ANTIFUNGALS

Amphotericin B

26-Aug-2020

(Amphotericin)

- INDICATIONS AND DOSE

ABELCET®

Severe invasive candidiasis | Severe systemic fungal infections in patients not responding to conventional amphotericin B or to other antifungal drugs or where toxicity or renal impairment precludes conventional amphotericin B, including invasive aspergillosis, cryptococcal meningitis and disseminated cryptococcosis in HIV patients

▸ BY INTRAVENOUS INFUSION

▸ Adult: Test dose 1 mg, to be given over 15 minutes, then 5 mg/kg once daily for at least 14 days

AMBISOME®

Severe systemic or deep mycoses where toxicity (particularly nephrotoxicity) precludes use of conventional amphotericin B | Suspected or proven infection in febrile neutropenic patients unresponsive to broad-spectrum antibacterials

▸ BY INTRAVENOUS INFUSION

▸ Adult: Test dose 1 mg, to be given over 10 minutes, then 3 mg/kg once daily; maximum 5 mg/kg per day

Aspergillosis

▸ BY INTRAVENOUS INFUSION

▸ Adult: Test dose 1 mg, to be given over 10 minutes, then 3 mg/kg once daily; maximum 5 mg/kg per day

Visceral leishmaniasis (unresponsive to the antimonial alone)

▸ BY INTRAVENOUS INFUSION

▸ Adult: 1–3 mg/kg daily for 10–21 days to a cumulative dose of 21–30 mg/kg, alternatively 3 mg/kg for 5 consecutive days, followed by 3 mg/kg after 6 days for 1 dose

FUNGIZONE®

Systemic fungal infections

▸ BY INTRAVENOUS INFUSION

▸ Adult: Test dose 1 mg, to be given over 20–30 minutes, then 250 micrograms/kg daily, gradually increased over 2–4 days, increased if tolerated to 1 mg/kg daily, max. (severe infection) 1.5 mg/kg daily or on alternate days. Prolonged treatment usually necessary; if interrupted for longer than 7 days recommence at 250 micrograms/kg daily and increase gradually

● UNLICENSED USE

AMBISOME ® Use at the maximum dose of 5 mg/kg once daily is an unlicensed dose.

IMPORTANT SAFETY INFORMATION

MHRA/CHM ADVICE: LIPOSOMAL AND LIPID-COMPLEX FORMULATIONS: NAME CHANGE TO REDUCE MEDICATION ERRORS (JULY 2020)

Serious harm and fatal overdoses have occurred following confusion between liposomal, pegylated-liposomal, lipid-complex, and conventional formulations of the same drug substance. Medicines with these formulations will explicitly include 'liposomal', 'pegylated-liposomal', or 'lipid-complex' within their name to reduce the risk of potentially fatal medication errors.

The MHRA reminds healthcare professionals that liposomal, pegylated-liposomal, lipid-complex, and conventional formulations containing the same drug substance are **not** interchangeable. Healthcare professionals are advised to make a clear distinction between formulations when prescribing, dispensing, administering, and communicating about amphotericin B. The product name and dose should be verified before administration and the maximum dose should not be exceeded.

● CAUTIONS Avoid rapid infusion (risk of arrhythmias) · when given parenterally, toxicity common (close supervision necessary and close observation required for at least 30 minutes after test dose)

CAUTIONS, FURTHER INFORMATION

▸ Anaphylaxis Anaphylaxis can occur with any intravenous amphotericin B product and a test dose is advisable before the first infusion in a new course; the patient should be carefully observed for at least 30 minutes after the test dose.

▸ Infusion-related reactions Manufacturer advises prophylactic antipyretics or hydrocortisone can be used in patients who have previously experienced infusion-related reactions (in whom continued treatment with amphotericin B is essential).

● INTERACTIONS → Appendix 1: amphotericin B

● SIDE-EFFECTS

▸ **Common or very common** Anaemia · appetite decreased · azotaemia · chills · diarrhoea · dyspnoea · electrolyte imbalance · fever · headache · hepatic function abnormal (discontinue) · hypothenuria · hypotension · nausea · nephrocalcinosis · renal impairment · renal tubular acidosis · skin reactions · vomiting

▸ **Uncommon** Agranulocytosis · arrhythmias · flushing · gastrointestinal discomfort · hepatic disorders · leucopenia · myalgia · peripheral neuropathy · respiratory disorders · thrombocytopenia

▸ **Rare or very rare** Arthralgia · cardiac arrest · coagulation disorder · deafness · encephalopathy · eosinophilia · haemorrhage · heart failure · hypersensitivity · hypertension · malaise · nephrogenic diabetes insipidus · pain · pulmonary oedema non-cardiogenic · seizure · severe cutaneous adverse reactions (SCARs) · shock · tinnitus · vertigo · vision disorders · weight decreased

● PREGNANCY Not known to be harmful but manufacturers advise avoid unless potential benefit outweighs risk.

● BREAST FEEDING No information available.

● RENAL IMPAIRMENT Use only if no alternative; nephrotoxicity may be reduced with use of lipid formulation.

● MONITORING REQUIREMENTS Hepatic and renal function tests, blood counts, and plasma electrolyte (including plasma-potassium and magnesium concentration) monitoring required.

● DIRECTIONS FOR ADMINISTRATION

ABELCET ® **Amphotericin B (lipid complex)**

For *intravenous infusion*, manufacturer advises give intermittently *in* Glucose 5%. Allow suspension to reach room temperature, shake gently to ensure no yellow settlement, withdraw requisite dose (using 17-19 gauge needle) into one or more 20-mL syringes; replace needle on syringe with a 5-micron filter needle provided (fresh needle for each syringe) and dilute in Glucose 5% to a concentration of 1 mg/mL (2 mg/mL can be used in fluid restriction); preferably give *via* an infusion pump at a rate of 2.5 mg/kg/hour (initial test dose of 1 mg over 15 minutes); an in-line filter (pore size no less than 15 micron) may be used; do not use sodium chloride or other electrolyte solutions, flush existing intravenous line with Glucose 5% or use separate line.

AMBISOME ® **Amphotericin B (liposomal)**

For *intravenous infusion*, manufacturer advises give intermittently *in* Glucose 5% or 10%. Reconstitute each vial with 12 mL Water for Injections and shake vigorously to produce a preparation containing 4 mg/mL; withdraw requisite dose from vial and introduce into Glucose 5% or 10% through the 5 micron filter provided, to produce a final concentration of 0.2–2 mg/mL; infuse over 30–60 minutes, or if non-anaphylactic infusion-related reactions occur infuse over 2 hours (initial test dose of 1 mg over 10 minutes); an in-line filter (pore size no less than 1 micron) may be used; incompatible with sodium chloride solutions, flush existing intravenous line with glucose 5% or 10%, or use separate line.

FUNGIZONE ® **Amphotericin B (as sodium deoxycholate complex)**

For *intravenous infusion*, manufacturer advises give intermittently *in* Glucose 5%. Reconstitute each vial with 10 mL Water for Injections and shake immediately to produce a 5 mg/mL colloidal solution; dilute further in Glucose 5% to a concentration of 100 micrograms/mL; pH of the glucose must not be below 4.2 (check each container—consult product literature for details of the buffer); infuse over 2–6 hours (initial test dose of 1 mg over 20–30 minutes); begin infusion immediately after dilution; protect from light; incompatible with sodium chloride solutions, flush existing intravenous line with glucose 5% or use separate line; an in-line filter (pore size no less than 1 micron) may be used.

● PRESCRIBING AND DISPENSING INFORMATION

Amphotericin B is available as *conventional*, *liposomal* and *lipid-complex* formulations. These different formulations vary in their licensed indications, pharmacokinetics, dosage and administration, and are **not** interchangeable.

● MEDICINAL FORMS There can be variation in the licensing of different medicines containing the same drug.

Suspension for infusion

ELECTROLYTES: May contain Sodium

▸ Abelcet (Teva UK Ltd)

Amphotericin B (as Amphotericin B phospholipid complex) 5 mg per 1 ml Abelcet 100mg/20ml concentrate for suspension for infusion vials | 10 vial [PoM] £775.04 (Hospital only)

Powder for dispersion for infusion

EXCIPIENTS: May contain Sucrose

ELECTROLYTES: May contain Sodium

▸ AmBisome (Gilead Sciences Ireland UC)

Amphotericin B liposomal 50 mg AmBisome Liposomal 50mg powder for dispersion for infusion vials | 10 vial [PoM] £821.87 (Hospital only)

Powder for solution for infusion

▸ Fungizone (Neon Healthcare Ltd)

Amphotericin B 50 mg Fungizone 50mg powder for concentrate for solution for infusion vials | 1 vial [PoM] £3.88 DT = £3.88

ANTIFUNGALS ＞ TRIAZOLE ANTIFUNGALS

Fluconazole

10-Mar-2020

● INDICATIONS AND DOSE

Candidal balanitis
▸ BY MOUTH
▸ Child 16-17 years: 150 mg for 1 dose
▸ Adult: 150 mg for 1 dose

Vaginal candidiasis
▸ BY MOUTH
▸ Adult: 150 mg for 1 dose

Vulvovaginal candidiasis (recurrent)
▸ BY MOUTH
▸ Adult: Initially 150 mg every 72 hours for 3 doses, then 150 mg once weekly for 6 months

Mucosal candidiasis (except genital)
▸ BY MOUTH, OR BY INTRAVENOUS INFUSION
▸ Child 1 month-11 years: 3–6 mg/kg, dose to be given on first day, then 3 mg/kg daily (max. per dose 100 mg) for 7–14 days in oropharyngeal candidiasis (max. 14 days except in severely immunocompromised patients); for 14–30 days in other mucosal infections (e.g. oesophagitis, candiduria, non-invasive bronchopulmonary infections)
▸ Child 12-17 years: 50 mg daily for 7–14 days in oropharyngeal candidiasis (max. 14 days except in severely immunocompromised patients); for 14–30 days in other mucosal infections (e.g. oesophagitis, candiduria, non-invasive bronchopulmonary infections); increased to 100 mg daily, increased dose only for unusually difficult infections
▸ BY MOUTH
▸ Adult: 50 mg daily given for 7–14 days in oropharyngeal candidiasis (max. 14 days except in severely immunocompromised patients); for 14 days in atrophic oral candidiasis associated with dentures; for 14–30 days in other mucosal infections (e.g. oesophagitis, candiduria, non-invasive bronchopulmonary infections; increased to 100 mg daily, increased dose only for unusually difficult infections

Tinea pedis, corporis, cruris, pityriasis versicolor | Dermal candidiasis
▸ BY MOUTH
▸ Adult: 50 mg daily for 2–4 weeks (for up to 6 weeks in tinea pedis); max. duration of treatment 6 weeks

Invasive candidal infections (including candidaemia and disseminated candidiasis) and cryptococcal infections (including meningitis)
▸ BY MOUTH, OR BY INTRAVENOUS INFUSION
▸ Child: 6–12 mg/kg daily (max. per dose 800 mg), treatment continued according to response (at least 8 weeks for cryptococcal meningitis)
▸ Adult: 400 mg, dose to be given on first day, then 200–400 mg daily (max. per dose 800 mg once daily), treatment continued according to response (at least 8 weeks for cryptococcal meningitis), maximum dose for use in severe infections

Prevention of fungal infections in immunocompromised patients
▸ BY MOUTH, OR BY INTRAVENOUS INFUSION
▸ Child: 3–12 mg/kg daily (max. per dose 400 mg), commence treatment before anticipated onset of neutropenia and continue for 7 days after neutrophil count in desirable range, dose given according to extent and duration of neutropenia
▸ Adult: 50–400 mg daily, commence treatment before anticipated onset of neutropenia and continue for 7 days after neutrophil count in desirable range, dose adjusted according to risk

Prevention of fungal infections in immunocompromised patients (for patients with high risk of systemic infections e.g. following bone-marrow transplantation)
▸ BY MOUTH, OR BY INTRAVENOUS INFUSION
▸ Adult: 400 mg daily, commence treatment before anticipated onset of neutropenia and continue for 7 days after neutrophil count in desirable range

Prevention of relapse of cryptococcal meningitis in HIV-infected patients after completion of primary therapy
▸ BY MOUTH, OR BY INTRAVENOUS INFUSION
▸ Adult: 200 mg daily

● CONTRA-INDICATIONS Acute porphyrias p. 1107
● CAUTIONS Susceptibility to QT interval prolongation
● INTERACTIONS → Appendix 1: antifungals, azoles
● SIDE-EFFECTS

GENERAL SIDE-EFFECTS
▸ **Common or very common** Diarrhoea · gastrointestinal discomfort · headache · nausea · skin reactions · vomiting
▸ **Uncommon** Dizziness · flatulence · hepatic disorders · seizure · taste altered
▸ **Rare or very rare** Agranulocytosis · alopecia · dyslipidaemia · hypokalaemia · leucopenia · neutropenia · QT interval prolongation · severe cutaneous adverse reactions (SCARs) · thrombocytopenia · torsade de pointes

SPECIFIC SIDE-EFFECTS
▸ **Uncommon**
▹ With parenteral use Anaemia · appetite decreased · asthenia · constipation · drowsiness · dry mouth · fever · hyperhidrosis · insomnia · malaise · myalgia · paraesthesia · vertigo
▸ **Rare or very rare**
▹ With parenteral use Angioedema · face oedema · tremor
▸ **Frequency not known**
▹ With oral use Cardio-respiratory distress · oedema

SIDE-EFFECTS, FURTHER INFORMATION If rash occurs, discontinue treatment (or monitor closely if infection invasive or systemic); severe cutaneous reactions are more likely in patients with AIDS.
● PREGNANCY Manufacturer advises avoid—multiple congenital abnormalities reported with long-term high doses.
● BREAST FEEDING Present in milk but amount probably too small to be harmful.
● HEPATIC IMPAIRMENT Manufacturer advises caution—limited information available.
● RENAL IMPAIRMENT
Dose adjustments ▸ In adults Usual initial dose then halve subsequent doses if eGFR less than 50 mL/minute/1.73 m^2.
▸ In children Usual initial dose then halve subsequent doses if estimated glomerular filtration rate less than 50 mL/minute/1.73 m^2.
● MONITORING REQUIREMENTS Monitor liver function with high doses or extended courses—discontinue if signs or symptoms of hepatic disease (risk of hepatic necrosis).
● DIRECTIONS FOR ADMINISTRATION
▸ With intravenous use in children For *intravenous infusion*, give over 10–30 minutes; do not exceed an infusion rate of 5–10 mL/minute.
● PRESCRIBING AND DISPENSING INFORMATION Flavours of oral liquid formulations may include orange.
● PATIENT AND CARER ADVICE
Medicines for Children leaflet: Fluconazole for yeast and fungal infections www.medicinesforchildren.org.uk/fluconazole-yeast-and-fungal-infections

- **PROFESSION SPECIFIC INFORMATION**

Dental practitioners' formulary
Fluconazole Capsules 50 mg may be prescribed.
Fluconazole Oral Suspension 50 mg/5 mL may be
prescribed.

- **EXCEPTIONS TO LEGAL CATEGORY** Fluconazole capsules
can be sold to the public for vaginal candidiasis and
associated candidal balanitis in those aged 16–60 years, in
a container or packaging containing not more than 150 mg
and labelled to show a max. dose of 150 mg.

- **MEDICINAL FORMS** There can be variation in the licensing of
different medicines containing the same drug.

Infusion
▶ Fluconazole (Non-proprietary)
  Fluconazole 2 mg per 1 ml Fluconazole 200mg/100ml infusion bags
  | 5 bag [PoM] £19.45 (Hospital only) | 10 bag [PoM] £65.00 (Hospital
  only)
  Fluconazole 400mg/200ml infusion bags | 5 bag [PoM] £72.50
  (Hospital only)

Solution for infusion
ELECTROLYTES: May contain Sodium
▶ Fluconazole (Non-proprietary)
  Fluconazole 2 mg per 1 ml Fluconazole 200mg/100ml solution for
  infusion vials | 1 vial [PoM] £28.80 DT = £29.28 (Hospital only) |
  1 vial [PoM] £15.00–£29.28 DT = £29.28
  Fluconazole 100mg/50ml solution for infusion vials | 5 vial [PoM]
  £12.60 (Hospital only)
  Fluconazole 50mg/25ml solution for infusion vials | 1 vial [PoM]
  £20.00
  Fluconazole 200mg/100ml solution for infusion bottles |
  10 bottle [PoM] £392.30 | 20 bottle [PoM] £603.17

Oral suspension
CAUTIONARY AND ADVISORY LABELS 9
▶ Fluconazole (Non-proprietary)
  Fluconazole 10 mg per 1 ml Fluconazole 50mg/5ml oral suspension
  | 35 ml [PoM] £25.85 DT = £25.85
▶ Diflucan (Pfizer Ltd)
  Fluconazole 10 mg per 1 ml Diflucan 50mg/5ml oral suspension |
  35 ml [PoM] £16.61 DT = £25.85
  Fluconazole 40 mg per 1 ml Diflucan 200mg/5ml oral suspension |
  35 ml [PoM] £66.42 DT = £66.42

Capsule
CAUTIONARY AND ADVISORY LABELS 9 (50 mg and 200 mg strengths
only)
▶ Canesten (fluconazole) (Bayer Plc)
  Fluconazole 150 mg Canesten Thrush Oral 150mg capsules |
  1 capsule [P] £6.33 DT = £0.93
▶ Diflucan (Pfizer Ltd)
  Fluconazole 50 mg Diflucan 50mg capsules | 7 capsule [PoM]
  £16.61 DT = £1.02
  Fluconazole 150 mg Diflucan 150mg capsules | 1 capsule [PoM]
  £7.12 DT = £0.93
  Fluconazole 200 mg Diflucan 200mg capsules | 7 capsule [PoM]
  £66.42 DT = £5.46
▶ Fluconazole (Non-proprietary)
  Fluconazole 50 mg Fluconazole 50mg capsules | 7 capsule [PoM]
  £1.02 DT = £1.02
  Fluconazole 150 mg Fluconazole 150mg capsules | 1 capsule [PoM]
  £8.50 DT = £0.93
  Fluconazole 200 mg Fluconazole 200mg capsules | 7 capsule [PoM]
  £6.38 DT = £5.46

Isavuconazole   18-Aug-2020

- **DRUG ACTION** Isavuconazole is a triazole antifungal that
blocks the synthesis of ergosterol, a key component of the
fungal cell membrane.

- **INDICATIONS AND DOSE**

**Invasive aspergillosis | Mucormycosis in patients for whom
amphotericin B is inappropriate**
▶ BY MOUTH, OR BY INTRAVENOUS INFUSION
▶ Adult: Loading dose 200 mg every 8 hours for 48 hours
  (6 administrations in total), then maintenance 200 mg
  once daily, maintenance dose to be started at least

12 hours after the last loading dose; long-term
treatment should be reviewed after 6-months

- **CONTRA-INDICATIONS** Acute porphyrias p. 1107 · short QT
syndrome
- **CAUTIONS** Elderly—limited information
- **INTERACTIONS** → Appendix 1: antifungals, azoles
- **SIDE-EFFECTS**

GENERAL SIDE-EFFECTS
▶ **Common or very common** Appetite decreased · asthenia ·
  chest pain · confusion · delirium · diarrhoea · drowsiness ·
  dyspnoea · electrolyte imbalance · gastrointestinal
  discomfort · headache · hepatic disorders ·
  hyperbilirubinaemia · nausea · renal failure · respiratory
  disorders · skin reactions · thrombophlebitis · vomiting
▶ **Uncommon** Alopecia · anaemia · arrhythmias · back pain ·
  circulatory collapse · constipation · depression · dizziness ·
  encephalopathy · haemorrhage · hypersensitivity ·
  hypoalbuminaemia · hypoglycaemia · hypotension ·
  insomnia · leucopenia · malaise · malnutrition ·
  neutropenia · palpitations · pancytopenia · paraesthesia ·
  peripheral neuropathy · peripheral oedema · seizures ·
  syncope · taste altered · thrombocytopenia · vertigo
▶ **Frequency not known** Severe cutaneous adverse reactions
  (SCARs)

SPECIFIC SIDE-EFFECTS
▶ With intravenous use Infusion related reaction
SIDE-EFFECTS, FURTHER INFORMATION Infusion-related
reactions have been reported, including hypotension,
dyspnoea, dizziness, paraesthesia, nausea, and headache—
manufacturer advises discontinue treatment if these
reactions occur.

- **PREGNANCY** Manufacturer advises avoid unless severe or
life-threatening infection—toxicity in *animal* studies.
- **BREAST FEEDING** Manufacturer advises avoid—present in
milk in *animal* studies.
- **HEPATIC IMPAIRMENT** Manufacturer advises caution in
severe impairment (no information available)—monitor
for drug toxicity.
- **DIRECTIONS FOR ADMINISTRATION**
▶ With intravenous use For *intravenous infusion*, manufacturer
  advises reconstitute each 200 mg with 5 mL Water for
  Injection; dilute dose to concentration of 0.8 mg/mL with
  Glucose 5% or Sodium Chloride 0.9% and give via a
  0.2–1.2 micron filter over at least 1 hour.
- **HANDLING AND STORAGE**
▶ With intravenous use Manufacturer advises store in a
  refrigerator (2–8°C)—consult product literature for storage
  after reconstitution or dilution.
- **PATIENT AND CARER ADVICE**
Driving and skilled tasks Manufacturer advises patients and
carers should be cautioned on the effects on driving and
performance of skilled tasks—increased risk of confusion,
syncope and dizziness.
- **NATIONAL FUNDING/ACCESS DECISIONS**
For full details see funding body website
All Wales Medicines Strategy Group (AWMSG) decisions
▶ Isavuconazole (*Cresemba*®) for the treatment of invasive
  aspergillosis in adults and the treatment of mucormycosis in
  adult patients for whom amphotericin B is inappropriate
  (January 2017) AWMSG No. 2433 Recommended

- **MEDICINAL FORMS** There can be variation in the licensing of
different medicines containing the same drug.
Powder for solution for infusion
CAUTIONARY AND ADVISORY LABELS 3
▶ Cresemba (Pfizer Ltd)
  Isavuconazole (as Isavuconazonium sulfate) 200 mg Cresemba
  200mg powder for concentrate for solution for infusion vials |
  1 vial [PoM] £297.84 (Hospital only)

5

Infection

Capsule

CAUTIONARY AND ADVISORY LABELS 3, 25
- Cresemba (Pfizer Ltd)

Isavuconazole (as Isavuconazonium sulfate) 100 mg Cresemba 100mg capsules | 14 capsule [PoM] £599.28 (Hospital only)

Itraconazole

11-Aug-2020

● **INDICATIONS AND DOSE**

Vulvovaginal candidiasis
- BY MOUTH
- Adult: 200 mg twice daily for 1 day

Vulvovaginal candidiasis (recurrent)
- BY MOUTH
- Adult: 50–100 mg daily for 6 months

Oral or oesophageal candidiasis that has not responded to fluconazole
- BY MOUTH USING ORAL SOLUTION
- Adult: 100–200 mg twice daily for 2 weeks (continue for another 2 weeks if no response; the higher dose should not be used for longer than 2 weeks if no signs of improvement)

Oral or oesophageal candidiasis in HIV-positive or other immunocompromised patients
- BY MOUTH USING ORAL SOLUTION
- Adult: 200 mg daily in 1–2 divided doses for 1 week (continue for another week if no response)

Systemic candidiasis where other antifungal drugs inappropriate or ineffective
- BY MOUTH
- Adult: 100–200 mg once daily
- BY INTRAVENOUS INFUSION
- Adult: 200 mg every 12 hours for 2 days, then 200 mg once daily for max. 12 days

Systemic candidiasis (invasive or disseminated) where other antifungal drugs inappropriate or ineffective
- BY MOUTH
- Adult: 200 mg twice daily

Pityriasis versicolor
- BY MOUTH
- Adult: 200 mg once daily for 7 days

Tinea pedis | Tinea manuum
- BY MOUTH
- Adult: 100 mg once daily for 30 days, alternatively 200 mg twice daily for 7 days

Tinea corporis | Tinea cruris
- BY MOUTH
- Adult: 100 mg once daily for 15 days, alternatively 200 mg once daily for 7 days

Onychomycosis
- BY MOUTH
- Adult: 200 mg once daily for 3 months, alternatively 200 mg twice daily for 7 days, subsequent courses repeated after 21-day intervals; fingernails 2 courses, toenails 3 courses

Aspergillosis
- BY MOUTH
- Adult: 200 mg twice daily

Systemic aspergillosis where other antifungal drugs inappropriate or ineffective
- BY INTRAVENOUS INFUSION
- Adult: 200 mg every 12 hours for 2 days, then 200 mg once daily for max. 12 days

Histoplasmosis
- BY MOUTH
- Adult: 200 mg 3 times a day for 3 days, then 200 mg 1–2 times a day

- BY INTRAVENOUS INFUSION
- Adult: 200 mg every 12 hours for 2 days, then 200 mg once daily for max. 12 days

Systemic cryptococcosis including cryptococcal meningitis where other antifungal drugs inappropriate or ineffective
- BY MOUTH
- Adult: 200 mg once daily, dose increased in invasive or disseminated disease and in cryptococcal meningitis, increased to 200 mg twice daily
- BY INTRAVENOUS INFUSION
- Adult: 200 mg every 12 hours for 2 days, then 200 mg once daily for max. 12 days

Maintenance in HIV-infected patients to prevent relapse of underlying fungal infection and prophylaxis in neutropenia when standard therapy inappropriate
- BY MOUTH
- Adult: 200 mg once daily, then increased to 200 mg twice daily, dose increased only if low plasma-itraconazole concentration

Prophylaxis of deep fungal infections (when standard therapy inappropriate) in patients with haematological malignancy or undergoing bone-marrow transplantation who are expected to become neutropenic
- BY MOUTH USING ORAL SOLUTION
- Adult: 5 mg/kg daily in 2 divided doses, to be started before transplantation or before chemotherapy (taking care to avoid interaction with cytotoxic drugs) and continued until neutrophil count recovers, safety and efficacy not established in elderly patients

DOSE ADJUSTMENTS DUE TO INTERACTIONS
- Manufacturer advises max. dose 200 mg daily with concurrent use of cobicistat.

● UNLICENSED USE Itraconazole doses in BNF may differ from those in product literature.

● CONTRA-INDICATIONS Acute porphyrias p. 1107

● CAUTIONS Active liver disease · elderly · history of hepatotoxicity with other drugs · susceptibility to congestive heart failure

CAUTIONS, FURTHER INFORMATION
- Susceptibility to congestive heart failure There have been reports of heart failure associated with itraconazole. Those at risk may include patients receiving higher daily doses and longer courses, patients with cardiac disease, patients with chronic lung disease, and patients receiving treatment with calcium channel blockers. Manufacturer advises avoid in patients with ventricular dysfunction, such as history of congestive heart failure, unless the infection is serious.

● INTERACTIONS → Appendix 1: antifungals, azoles

● SIDE-EFFECTS

GENERAL SIDE-EFFECTS
- **Common or very common** Alopecia · constipation · diarrhoea · dyspnoea · gastrointestinal discomfort · headache · heart failure · hepatic disorders · hyperbilirubinaemia · nausea · oedema · pulmonary oedema · skin reactions · vision disorders · vomiting
- **Uncommon** Hearing loss · taste altered
- **Rare or very rare** Angioedema · hypersensitivity vasculitis · hypertriglyceridaemia · pancreatitis · photosensitivity reaction · severe cutaneous adverse reactions (SCARs)
- **Frequency not known** Peripheral neuropathy (discontinue)

SPECIFIC SIDE-EFFECTS
- **Common or very common**
- With intravenous use Chest pain · confusion · cough · dizziness · drowsiness · electrolyte imbalance · fatigue · gastrointestinal disorder · granulocytopenia · hyperglycaemia · hyperhidrosis · hypersensitivity ·

hypertension · hypotension · myalgia · pain · renal impairment · tachycardia · tremor · urinary incontinence
▸ **Uncommon**
▸ With intravenous use Dysphonia · numbness · thrombocytopenia
▸ With oral use Flatulence · increased risk of infection · menstrual disorder
▸ **Rare or very rare**
▸ With oral use Erectile dysfunction · leucopenia · sensation abnormal · serum sickness · tinnitus · urinary frequency increased

SIDE-EFFECTS, FURTHER INFORMATION Potentially life-threatening hepatotoxicity reported very rarely — discontinue if signs of hepatitis develop.

● CONCEPTION AND CONTRACEPTION Ensure effective contraception during treatment and until the next menstrual period following end of treatment.

● PREGNANCY Manufacturer advises use only in life-threatening situations (toxicity at high doses in *animal* studies).

● BREAST FEEDING Small amounts present in milk—may accumulate; manufacturer advises avoid.

● HEPATIC IMPAIRMENT Manufacturer advises use only in serious or life-saving situations where potential benefit outweighs risk of hepatotoxicity.

● RENAL IMPAIRMENT Risk of congestive heart failure.
▸ With oral use Bioavailability of oral formulations possibly reduced.
▸ With intravenous use Use intravenous infusion with caution if eGFR 30–80 mL/minute/1.73 m^2; avoid intravenous infusion if eGFR less than 30 mL/minute/1.73 m^2.

● MONITORING REQUIREMENTS
▸ Absorption reduced in AIDS and neutropenia (monitor plasma-itraconazole concentration and increase dose if necessary).
▸ Monitor liver function if treatment continues for longer than one month, if receiving other hepatotoxic drugs, or if history of hepatotoxicity with other drugs.

● DIRECTIONS FOR ADMINISTRATION
▸ With intravenous use For *intravenous infusion (Sporanox®)*, manufacturer advises give intermittently in Sodium Chloride 0.9%; dilute 250 mg in 50 mL infusion fluid and infuse only 60 mL through an in-line filter (0.2 micron) over 60 minutes.
▸ With oral use For *oral liquid*, manufacturer advises do not take with food; swish around mouth and swallow, do not rinse afterwards.

● PRESCRIBING AND DISPENSING INFORMATION Flavours of oral liquid formulations may include cherry.

● PATIENT AND CARER ADVICE Patients should be told how to recognise signs of liver disorder and advised to seek prompt medical attention if symptoms such as anorexia, nausea, vomiting, fatigue, abdominal pain or dark urine develop.
▸ With oral use Patients or carers should be given advice on how to administer itraconazole oral liquid.

● MEDICINAL FORMS There can be variation in the licensing of different medicines containing the same drug. Forms available from special-order manufacturers include: oral suspension, oral solution

Solution for infusion
EXCIPIENTS: May contain Propylene glycol
▸ Sporanox (Janssen-Cilag Ltd)
Itraconazole 10 mg per 1 ml Sporanox I.V. 250mg/25ml solution for infusion ampoules and diluent | 1 ampoule PoM £79.71

Oral solution
CAUTIONARY AND ADVISORY LABELS 9, 23
▸ Itraconazole (Non-proprietary)
Itraconazole 10 mg per 1 ml Itraconazole 50mg/5ml oral solution sugar free sugar-free | 150 ml PoM £59.28 DT = £59.28

▸ Sporanox (Janssen-Cilag Ltd)
Itraconazole 10 mg per 1 ml Sporanox 50mg/5ml oral solution sugar-free | 150 ml PoM £58.34 DT = £59.28

Capsule
CAUTIONARY AND ADVISORY LABELS 5, 9, 21, 25
▸ Itraconazole (Non-proprietary)
Itraconazole 100 mg Itraconazole 100mg capsules | 15 capsule PoM £13.77 DT = £4.26 | 60 capsule PoM £17.03–£55.10
▸ Sporanox (Janssen-Cilag Ltd)
Itraconazole 100 mg Sporanox-Pulse 100mg capsules | 28 capsule PoM £25.72
Sporanox 100mg capsules | 4 capsule PoM £3.67 | 60 capsule PoM £55.10

Posaconazole

10-Nov-2017

● **INDICATIONS AND DOSE**
Invasive aspergillosis either refractory to, or in patients intolerant of, itraconazole or amphotericin B | Fusariosis either refractory to, or in patients intolerant of, amphotericin B | Chromoblastomycosis and mycetoma either refractory to, or in patients intolerant of, itraconazole | Coccidioidomycosis either refractory to, or in patients intolerant of, amphotericin B, itraconazole, or fluconazole
▸ BY MOUTH USING ORAL SUSPENSION
▸ Adult: 400 mg twice daily, to be taken with food, alternatively 200 mg 4 times a day, if unable to tolerate food
▸ BY MOUTH USING TABLETS, OR BY INTRAVENOUS INFUSION
▸ Adult: Loading dose 300 mg twice daily on first day, then 300 mg once daily, switch from intravenous to oral route when appropriate

Oropharyngeal candidiasis (severe infection or in immunocompromised patients only)
▸ BY MOUTH USING ORAL SUSPENSION
▸ Adult: Loading dose 200 mg on first day, then 100 mg once daily for 13 days, dose to be taken with food

Prophylaxis of invasive fungal infections in patients at high risk and undergoing high-dose immunosuppressive therapy for haematopoietic stem cell transplantation or receiving chemotherapy for acute myeloid leukaemia or myelodysplastic syndrome and expected to develop prolonged neutropenia
▸ BY MOUTH USING ORAL SUSPENSION
▸ Adult: 200 mg 3 times a day, dose to be taken with food, for chemotherapy patients, start several days before the expected onset of neutropenia and continue for 7 days after neutrophil count rises above 500 cells/mm^3
▸ BY MOUTH USING TABLETS, OR BY INTRAVENOUS INFUSION
▸ Adult: Loading dose 300 mg twice daily on first day, then 300 mg once daily, for chemotherapy patients, start several days before the expected onset of neutropenia and continue for 7 days after neutrophil count rises above 500 cells/mm^3, switch from intravenous to oral route when appropriate

DOSE EQUIVALENCE AND CONVERSION
▸ Posaconazole oral suspension is **not** interchangeable with tablets on a milligram-for-milligram basis.

PHARMACOKINETICS
▸ Posaconazole oral suspension should be taken with food (preferably a high fat meal) or nutritional supplement to ensure adequate exposure for systemic effects. Where possible, tablets should be used in preference to suspension because tablets have a higher bioavailability.

● CONTRA-INDICATIONS Acute porphyrias p. 1107
● CAUTIONS Administration by intravenous infusion, particularly by peripheral catheter—increased risk of QTc

5

Infection

interval prolongation · body-weight over 120 kg—risk of treatment failure possibly increased · body-weight under 60 kg—risk of side effects increased · bradycardia · cardiomyopathy · history of QTc interval prolongation · symptomatic arrhythmias

● INTERACTIONS → Appendix 1: antifungals, azoles

● SIDE-EFFECTS

▸ **Common or very common** Appetite decreased · asthenia · constipation · diarrhoea · dizziness · drowsiness · dry mouth · electrolyte imbalance · gastrointestinal discomfort · gastrointestinal disorders · headache · hypertension · nausea · neutropenia · sensation abnormal · skin reactions · taste altered · vomiting

▸ **Uncommon** Alopecia · anaemia · aphasia · arrhythmias · burping · chest discomfort · confusion · cough · embolism and thrombosis · eosinophilia · feeling jittery · haemorrhage · hepatic disorders · hiccups · hyperglycaemia · hypoglycaemia · hypotension · leucopenia · lymphadenopathy · malaise · menstrual disorder · mucositis · nasal congestion · oedema · oral disorders · pain · palpitations · pancreatitis · peripheral neuropathy · QT interval prolongation · renal impairment · respiratory disorders · seizure · sleep disorders · splenic infarction · thrombocytopenia · tremor · vasculitis · vision disorders

▸ **Rare or very rare** Adrenal insufficiency · breast pain · cardiac arrest · coagulation disorder · depression · encephalopathy · haemolytic uraemic syndrome · hearing impairment · heart failure · myocardial infarction · nephritis tubulointerstitial · pancytopenia · psychotic disorder · pulmonary hypertension · renal tubular acidosis · Stevens-Johnson syndrome · stroke · sudden cardiac death · syncope

● CONCEPTION AND CONTRACEPTION Manufacturer recommends effective contraception during treatment.

● PREGNANCY Manufacturer advises avoid unless potential benefit outweighs risk; toxicity in *animal* studies.

● BREAST FEEDING Manufacturer advises avoid—present in milk in *animal* studies.

● HEPATIC IMPAIRMENT Manufacturer advises caution (risk of increased exposure, limited information available).

● RENAL IMPAIRMENT Manufacturer advises monitor efficacy in severe impairment—variable exposure expected.

▸ With intravenous use Manufacturer advises caution if eGFR less than 50 mL/minute/1.73 m² —intravenous vehicle may accumulate.

● MONITORING REQUIREMENTS

▸ Monitor electrolytes (including potassium, magnesium, and calcium) before and during therapy.

▸ Monitor liver function before and during therapy.

● DIRECTIONS FOR ADMINISTRATION

▸ With intravenous use Manufacturer advises for *intravenous infusion* (Noxafil®), give continuously in Glucose 5% *or* Sodium Chloride 0.9%; dilute requisite dose in infusion fluid to produce a final concentration of 1–2 mg/mL; give via a central venous catheter or peripherally inserted central catheter over approx. 90 minutes (can give a single dose via peripheral venous catheter if central access not established—dilute to a final concentration of 2 mg/mL and give over approx. 30 minutes).

● PRESCRIBING AND DISPENSING INFORMATION Flavours of oral liquid formulations may include cherry.

● HANDLING AND STORAGE

▸ With intravenous use Manufacturer advises store in a refrigerator (2–8 °C).

● PATIENT AND CARER ADVICE

Driving and skilled tasks Manufacturer advises patients and carers should be counselled on the effects on driving and performance of skilled tasks—increased risk of dizziness and somnolence.

● MEDICINAL FORMS There can be variation in the licensing of different medicines containing the same drug.

Solution for infusion
ELECTROLYTES: May contain Sodium
▸ Noxafil (Merck Sharp & Dohme Ltd)
  Posaconazole 18 mg per 1 ml Noxafil 300mg/16.7ml concentrate for solution for infusion vials | 1 vial PoM £211.00 (Hospital only)

Oral suspension
CAUTIONARY AND ADVISORY LABELS 3, 9, 21
▸ Posaconazole (Non-proprietary)
  Posaconazole 40 mg per 1 ml Posaconazole 40mg/ml oral suspension | 105 ml PoM £491.20 DT = £491.20
▸ Noxafil (Merck Sharp & Dohme Ltd)
  Posaconazole 40 mg per 1 ml Noxafil 40mg/ml oral suspension | 105 ml PoM £491.20 DT = £491.20 (Hospital only)

Gastro-resistant tablet
CAUTIONARY AND ADVISORY LABELS 3, 9, 25
▸ Posaconazole (Non-proprietary)
  Posaconazole 100 mg Posaconazole 100mg gastro-resistant tablets | 24 tablet PoM £58.50–£596.96 DT = £596.96 | 24 tablet PoM £507.42 DT = £596.96 (Hospital only) | 96 tablet PoM £229.11–£2,387.85 | 96 tablet PoM £2,029.67–£2,387.85 (Hospital only)
▸ Noxafil (Merck Sharp & Dohme Ltd)
  Posaconazole 100 mg Noxafil 100mg gastro-resistant tablets | 24 tablet PoM £596.96 DT = £596.96 | 96 tablet PoM £2,387.85

Voriconazole

06-Nov-2020

● INDICATIONS AND DOSE

Invasive aspergillosis | Serious infections caused by *Scedosporium* spp., *Fusarium* spp., or invasive fluconazole-resistant *Candida* spp. (including *C. krusei*)

▸ BY MOUTH

▸ **Adult (body-weight up to 40 kg):** Initially 200 mg every 12 hours for 2 doses, then 100 mg every 12 hours, increased if necessary to 150 mg every 12 hours

▸ **Adult (body-weight 40 kg and above):** Initially 400 mg every 12 hours for 2 doses, then 200 mg every 12 hours, increased if necessary to 300 mg every 12 hours

▸ BY INTRAVENOUS INFUSION

▸ **Adult:** Initially 6 mg/kg every 12 hours for 2 doses, then 4 mg/kg every 12 hours; reduced if not tolerated to 3 mg/kg every 12 hours; for max. 6 months

DOSE ADJUSTMENTS DUE TO INTERACTIONS

▸ With intravenous use Manufacturer advises increase maintenance dose to 5 mg/kg every 12 hours with concurrent use of fosphenytoin, phenytoin or rifabutin.

▸ With oral use
Manufacturer advises increase maintenance dose with concurrent use of fosphenytoin or phenytoin; 400 mg every 12 hours for patients of body-weight 40 kg and above; 200 mg every 12 hours for patients of body-weight less than 40 kg. Manufacturer advises if concurrent use of rifabutin is unavoidable, increase maintenance dose to 350 mg every 12 hours for patients of body-weight 40 kg and above; 200 mg every 12 hours for patients of body-weight less than 40 kg.

● CONTRA-INDICATIONS Acute porphyrias p. 1107

● CAUTIONS Avoid exposure to sunlight · bradycardia · cardiomyopathy · electrolyte disturbances · history of QT interval prolongation · patients at risk of pancreatitis · symptomatic arrhythmias

● INTERACTIONS → Appendix 1: antifungals, azoles

● SIDE-EFFECTS

GENERAL SIDE-EFFECTS

▸ **Common or very common** Acute kidney injury · agranulocytosis · alopecia · anaemia · anxiety · arrhythmias · asthenia · bone marrow disorders · chest pain · chills · confusion · constipation · depression · diarrhoea · dizziness · drowsiness · dyspnoea · electrolyte imbalance · eye disorders · eye inflammation · fever · gastrointestinal discomfort · haemorrhage · hallucination · headache · hepatic disorders · hypoglycaemia · hypotension · increased risk of infection · insomnia · leucopenia · muscle tone increased · nausea · neutropenia · oedema · oral disorders · pain · pulmonary oedema · respiratory disorders · seizure · sensation abnormal · skin reactions · syncope · tetany · thrombocytopenia · tremor · vision disorders · vomiting

► **Uncommon** Adrenal insufficiency · arthritis · brain oedema · duodenitis · encephalopathy · eosinophilia · gallbladder disorders · hearing impairment · hypothyroidism · influenza like illness · lymphadenopathy · lymphangitis · movement disorders · nephritis · nerve disorders · pancreatitis · parkinsonism · phototoxicity · proteinuria · pseudomembranous enterocolitis · QT interval prolongation · renal tubular necrosis · severe cutaneous adverse reactions (SCARs) · taste altered · thrombophlebitis · tinnitus · vertigo

► **Rare or very rare** Angioedema · cardiac conduction disorders · disseminated intravascular coagulation · hyperthyroidism

► **Frequency not known** Cutaneous lupus erythematosus · periostitis (more common in transplant patients) · squamous cell carcinoma (more common in presence of phototoxicity)

SPECIFIC SIDE-EFFECTS

► With intravenous use Infusion related reaction

SIDE-EFFECTS, FURTHER INFORMATION **Hepatotoxicity** Hepatitis, cholestasis, and acute hepatic failure have been reported; risk of hepatotoxicity increased in patients with haematological malignancy. Consider treatment discontinuation if severe abnormalities in liver function tests.

Phototoxicity Phototoxicity occurs uncommonly. If phototoxicity occurs, consider treatment discontinuation; if treatment is continued, monitor for pre-malignant skin lesions and squamous cell carcinoma, and discontinue treatment if they occur.

● CONCEPTION AND CONTRACEPTION Effective contraception required during treatment.

● PREGNANCY Toxicity in *animal* studies—manufacturer advises avoid unless potential benefit outweighs risk.

● BREAST FEEDING Manufacturer advises avoid—no information available.

● HEPATIC IMPAIRMENT Manufacturer advises caution, particularly in severe impairment (no information available).
Dose adjustments Manufacturer advises use usual initial loading dose then halve maintenance dose in mild to moderate cirrhosis.

● RENAL IMPAIRMENT Intravenous vehicle may accumulate if eGFR less than 50 mL/minute/1.73 m^2—use intravenous infusion only if potential benefit outweighs risk, and monitor renal function; alternatively, use tablets or oral suspension (no dose adjustment required).

● MONITORING REQUIREMENTS
► Monitor renal function.
► Monitor liver function before starting treatment, then at least weekly for 1 month, and then monthly during treatment.

● DIRECTIONS FOR ADMINISTRATION
► With intravenous use For *intravenous infusion*, manufacturer advises reconstitute each 200 mg with 19 mL Water for Injections or Sodium Chloride 0.9% to produce a 10 mg/mL solution; dilute dose to concentration of 0.5–5 mg/mL with Glucose 5% or Sodium Chloride 0.9% and give intermittently at a rate not exceeding 3 mg/kg/hour.

● PRESCRIBING AND DISPENSING INFORMATION Flavours of oral liquid formulations may include orange.

● PATIENT AND CARER ADVICE Patients and their carers should be told how to recognise symptoms of liver disorder, and advised to seek immediate medical attention if symptoms such as persistent nausea, vomiting, malaise or jaundice develop.

Patients and their carers should be advised that patients should avoid exposure to direct sunlight, and to avoid the use of sunbeds. In sunlight, patients should cover sun-exposed areas of skin and use a sunscreen with a high sun protection factor. Patients should seek medical attention if they experience sunburn or a severe skin reaction following exposure to light or sun.

Patients and their carers should be advised to keep the alert card with them at all times.

● MEDICINAL FORMS There can be variation in the licensing of different medicines containing the same drug.

Powder for solution for infusion
EXCIPIENTS: May contain Sulfobutylether beta cyclodextrin sodium
ELECTROLYTES: May contain Sodium
► Voriconazole (Non-proprietary)
Voriconazole 200 mg Voriconazole 200mg powder for solution for infusion vials | 1 vial [PoM] £77.00–£77.14 (Hospital only)
► VFEND (Pfizer Ltd)
Voriconazole 200 mg VFEND 200mg powder for solution for infusion vials | 1 vial [PoM] £77.14 (Hospital only)

Oral suspension
CAUTIONARY AND ADVISORY LABELS 9, 11, 23
► VFEND (Pfizer Ltd)
Voriconazole 40 mg per 1 ml VFEND 40mg/ml oral suspension | 75 ml [PoM] £551.37 DT = £551.37

Tablet
CAUTIONARY AND ADVISORY LABELS 9, 11, 23
► Voriconazole (Non-proprietary)
Voriconazole 50 mg Voriconazole 50mg tablets | 28 tablet [PoM] £275.68 DT = £161.72 | 28 tablet [PoM] £47.47 DT = £161.72 (Hospital only)
Voriconazole 100 mg Voriconazole 100mg tablets | 28 tablet [PoM] £275.68 DT = £275.68
Voriconazole 200 mg Voriconazole 200mg tablets | 28 tablet [PoM] £164.58 DT = £633.87 (Hospital only) | 28 tablet [PoM] £160.00–£1,102.74 DT = £633.87
► VFEND (Pfizer Ltd)
Voriconazole 50 mg VFEND 50mg tablets | 28 tablet [PoM] £275.68 DT = £161.72
Voriconazole 200 mg VFEND 200mg tablets | 28 tablet [PoM] £1,102.74 DT = £633.87

ANTIFUNGALS > OTHER

Flucytosine

17-Nov-2020

● **INDICATIONS AND DOSE**

Systemic yeast and fungal infections | Adjunct to amphotericin B in severe systemic candidiasis and in other severe or long-standing infections
► BY INTRAVENOUS INFUSION
► Adult: Usual dose 200 mg/kg daily in 4 divided doses usually for not more than 7 days, alternatively 100–150 mg/kg daily in 4 divided doses, lower dose may be sufficient for extremely sensitive organisms

Cryptococcal meningitis (adjunct to amphotericin B)
► BY INTRAVENOUS INFUSION
► Adult: 100 mg/kg daily in 4 divided doses for 2 weeks

● UNLICENSED USE Use in cryptococcal meningitis for 2 weeks is an unlicensed duration.

IMPORTANT SAFETY INFORMATION

MHRA/CHM ADVICE: FLUCYTOSINE (*ANCOTIL*®): NEW CONTRA-INDICATION IN PATIENTS WITH DPD DEFICIENCY (OCTOBER 2020)
Patients with partial or complete dihydropyrimidine dehydrogenase (DPD) deficiency are at increased risk of severe and fatal toxicity during treatment with fluoropyrimidines. Healthcare professionals are advised

that pre-treatment testing for DPD deficiency is not required in order to avoid delay in antimycotic therapy with flucytosine. However, if drug toxicity is confirmed or suspected, testing of DPD activity and withdrawal of treatment should be considered. Flucytosine is contra-indicated in patients with known complete DPD deficiency.

- CONTRA-INDICATIONS Complete dihydropyrimidine dehydrogenase deficiency
- CAUTIONS Blood disorders · elderly · partial dihydropyrimidine dehydrogenase deficiency
- INTERACTIONS → Appendix 1: flucytosine
- SIDE-EFFECTS Agranulocytosis · aplastic anaemia · blood disorder · cardiotoxicity · confusion · diarrhoea · hallucination · headache · hepatic disorders · leucopenia · nausea · rash · sedation · seizure · thrombocytopenia · toxic epidermal necrolysis · ventricular dysfunction · vertigo · vomiting
- PREGNANCY Teratogenic in *animal* studies; manufacturer advises use only if potential benefit outweighs risk.
- BREAST FEEDING Manufacturer advises avoid.
- RENAL IMPAIRMENT
  Dose adjustments Use 50 mg/kg every 12 hours if creatinine clearance 20–40 mL/minute; use 50 mg/kg every 24 hours if creatinine clearance 10–20 mL/minute; use initial dose of 50 mg/kg if creatinine clearance less than 10 mL/minute and then adjust dose according to plasma-flucytosine concentration.
  Monitoring In renal impairment liver- and kidney-function tests and blood counts required weekly.
- MONITORING REQUIREMENTS
  ▸ For plasma concentration monitoring, blood should be taken shortly before starting the next infusion; plasma concentration for optimum response 25–50 mg/litre (200–400 micromol/litre)—should not be allowed to exceed 80 mg/litre (620 micromol/litre).
  ▸ Liver- and kidney-function tests and blood counts required (weekly in blood disorders).
- DIRECTIONS FOR ADMINISTRATION For *intravenous infusion*, manufacturer advises give over 20–40 minutes.
- MEDICINAL FORMS There can be variation in the licensing of different medicines containing the same drug.
  Solution for infusion
  ELECTROLYTES: May contain Sodium
  ▸ Ancotil (Mylan)
  Flucytosine 10 mg per 1 ml Ancotil 2.5g/250ml solution for infusion bottles | 5 bottle [PoM] £151.67 (Hospital only)

Griseofulvin

16-Jan-2020

- **INDICATIONS AND DOSE**
  Dermatophyte infections of the skin, scalp, hair and nails where topical therapy has failed or is inappropriate
  ▸ BY MOUTH
  ▸ Adult: 500 mg daily, increased if necessary to 1 g daily, for severe infections; reduce dose when response occurs, daily dose may be taken once daily or in divided doses
  Tinea capitis caused by *Trichophyton tonsurans*
  ▸ BY MOUTH
  ▸ Adult: 1 g once daily, alternatively 1 g daily in divided doses

- UNLICENSED USE Griseofulvin doses in BNF may differ from those in product literature.
- CONTRA-INDICATIONS Acute porphyrias p. 1107 · systemic lupus erythematosus (risk of exacerbation)
- INTERACTIONS → Appendix 1: griseofulvin

- SIDE-EFFECTS
  ▸ **Common or very common** Diarrhoea · epigastric discomfort · headache · nausea · vomiting
  ▸ **Uncommon** Appetite decreased · confusion · coordination abnormal · dizziness · drowsiness · insomnia · irritability · peripheral neuropathy · photosensitivity reaction · skin reactions · taste altered · toxic epidermal necrolysis
  ▸ **Rare or very rare** Anaemia · hepatic disorders · leucopenia · neutropenia · systemic lupus erythematosus (SLE)
- CONCEPTION AND CONTRACEPTION Effective contraception required during and for at least 1 month after administration to women (important: effectiveness of oral contraceptives may be reduced, additional contraceptive precautions e.g. barrier method, required). Men should avoid fathering a child during and for at least 6 months after administration
- PREGNANCY Avoid (fetotoxicity and teratogenicity in *animals*).
- BREAST FEEDING Avoid—no information available.
- HEPATIC IMPAIRMENT Manufacturer advises caution in mild to moderate impairment (risk of deterioration); avoid in severe impairment.
- PATIENT AND CARER ADVICE
  Driving and skilled tasks May impair performance of skilled tasks (e.g. driving); effects of alcohol enhanced.
- MEDICINAL FORMS There can be variation in the licensing of different medicines containing the same drug. Forms available from special-order manufacturers include: oral suspension
  Tablet
  CAUTIONARY AND ADVISORY LABELS 9, 21
  ▸ Griseofulvin (Non-proprietary)
  Griseofulvin 125 mg Griseofulvin 125mg tablets | 100 tablet [PoM] £96.67 DT = £96.67
  Griseofulvin 500 mg Griseofulvin 500mg tablets | 90 tablet [PoM] £81.32 | 100 tablet [PoM] £90.34 DT = £90.35

3.1 Pneumocystis pneumonia

Pneumocystis pneumonia

Overview

Pneumonia caused by *Pneumocystis jirovecii* (*Pneumocystis carinii*) occurs in immunosuppressed patients; it is a common cause of pneumonia in AIDS. Pneumocystis pneumonia should generally be treated by those experienced in its management. Blood gas measurement is used to assess disease severity.

Treatment

Mild to moderate disease
Co-trimoxazole p. 598 in high dosage is the drug of choice for the treatment of mild to moderate pneumocystis pneumonia.

Atovaquone p. 641 is licensed for the treatment of mild to moderate pneumocystis infection in patients who cannot tolerate co-trimoxazole. A combination of dapsone p. 614 with trimethoprim p. 610 is given by mouth for the treatment of mild to moderate disease [unlicensed indication].

A combination of clindamycin p. 566 and primaquine p. 657 by mouth is used in the treatment of mild to moderate disease [unlicensed indication]; this combination is associated with considerable toxicity.

Severe disease
Co-trimoxazole in high dosage, given by mouth or by intravenous infusion, is the drug of choice for the treatment of severe pneumocystis pneumonia. Pentamidine isetionate p. 641 given by intravenous infusion is an alternative for

patients who cannot tolerate co-trimoxazole, or who have not responded to it. Pentamidine isetionate is a potentially toxic drug that can cause severe hypotension during or immediately after infusion.

Corticosteroid treatment can be lifesaving in those with severe pneumocystis pneumonia.

Adjunctive therapy
In moderate to severe infections associated with HIV infection, prednisolone p. 718 is given by mouth for 5 days (alternatively, hydrocortisone p. 716 may be given parenterally); the dose is then reduced to complete 21 days of treatment. Corticosteroid treatment should ideally be started at the same time as the anti-pneumocystis therapy and certainly no later than 24–72 hours afterwards. The corticosteroid should be withdrawn before anti-pneumocystis treatment is complete.

Prophylaxis
Prophylaxis against pneumocystis pneumonia should be given to all patients with a history of the infection. Prophylaxis against pneumocystis pneumonia should also be considered for severely immunocompromised patients. Prophylaxis should continue until immunity recovers sufficiently. It should not be discontinued if the patient has oral candidiasis, continues to lose weight, or is receiving cytotoxic therapy or long-term immunosuppressant therapy.

Co-trimoxazole by mouth is the drug of choice for prophylaxis against pneumocystis pneumonia. It is given daily or on alternate days (3 times a week); the dose may be reduced to improve tolerance.

Inhaled pentamidine isetionate is better tolerated than parenteral pentamidine isetionate. Intermittent inhalation of pentamidine isetionate is used for prophylaxis against pneumocystis pneumonia in patients unable to tolerate co-trimoxazole. It is effective but patients may be prone to extrapulmonary infection. Alternatively, dapsone can be used. Atovaquone has also been used for prophylaxis [unlicensed indication].

ANTIPROTOZOALS > OTHER

Atovaquone

27-May-2020

● **INDICATIONS AND DOSE**

Treatment of mild to moderate *Pneumocystis jirovecii* (*Pneumocystis carinii*) pneumonia in patients intolerant of co-trimoxazole

▸ BY MOUTH

▸ Adult: 750 mg twice daily for 21 days, dose to be taken with food, particularly high fat food

Prophylaxis against pneumocystis pneumonia

▸ BY MOUTH

▸ Adult: 750 mg twice daily

● UNLICENSED USE Not licensed for prophylaxis against pneumocystis pneumonia.

● CAUTIONS Elderly · initial diarrhoea and difficulty in taking with food may reduce absorption (and require alternative therapy) · other causes of pulmonary disease should be sought and treated

● INTERACTIONS → Appendix 1: antimalarials

● SIDE-EFFECTS

▸ **Common or very common** Anaemia · angioedema · bronchospasm · diarrhoea · headache · hypersensitivity · hyponatraemia · insomnia · nausea · neutropenia · skin reactions · throat tightness · vomiting

▸ **Frequency not known** Stevens-Johnson syndrome

● PREGNANCY Manufacturer advises avoid unless potential benefit outweighs risk—no information available.

● BREAST FEEDING Manufacturer advises avoid.

● HEPATIC IMPAIRMENT Manufacturer advises use with caution in significant impairment and monitor closely—no information available.

● RENAL IMPAIRMENT Manufacturer advises caution.
Monitoring Monitor more closely in renal impairment.

● PRESCRIBING AND DISPENSING INFORMATION Flavours of oral liquid formulations may include tutti-frutti.

● MEDICINAL FORMS There can be variation in the licensing of different medicines containing the same drug.

Oral suspension
CAUTIONARY AND ADVISORY LABELS 21
▸ Atovaquone (Non-proprietary)
    Atovaquone 150 mg per 1 ml Atovaquone 750mg/5ml oral suspension sugar free sugar-free | 250 ml [PoM] £470.60–£543.00
▸ Wellvone (GlaxoSmithKline UK Ltd)
    Atovaquone 150 mg per 1 ml Wellvone 750mg/5ml oral suspension sugar-free | 226 ml [PoM] £486.37 DT = £486.37

Pentamidine isetionate

30-Jul-2020

● **INDICATIONS AND DOSE**

Treatment of *Pneumocystis jirovecii* (*Pneumocystis carinii*) pneumonia (specialist use only)

▸ BY INTRAVENOUS INFUSION

▸ Adult: 4 mg/kg once daily for at least 14 days

Prophylaxis of *Pneumocystis jirovecii* (*Pneumocystis carinii*) pneumonia (specialist use only)

▸ BY INHALATION OF NEBULISED SOLUTION

▸ Adult: 300 mg every 4 weeks, alternatively 150 mg every 2 weeks, using suitable equipment—consult product literature

Visceral leishmaniasis (specialist use only)

▸ BY DEEP INTRAMUSCULAR INJECTION

▸ Adult: 3–4 mg/kg once daily on alternate days, maximum total of 10 injections, course may be repeated if necessary

Cutaneous leishmaniasis (specialist use only)

▸ BY DEEP INTRAMUSCULAR INJECTION

▸ Adult: 3–4 mg/kg 1–2 times a week until condition resolves

Trypanosomiasis (specialist use only)

▸ BY DEEP INTRAMUSCULAR INJECTION, OR BY INTRAVENOUS INFUSION

▸ Adult: 4 mg/kg once daily or on alternate days for a total of 7–10 injections

● UNLICENSED USE Not licensed for primary prevention of *Pneumocystis jirovecii* (*Pneumocystis carinii*) pneumonia by inhalation of nebulised solution.

● CAUTIONS Anaemia · bradycardia · cardiac disease · history of ventricular arrhythmias · hyperglycaemia · hypertension · hypoglycaemia · hypokalaemia · hypomagnesaemia · hypotension · leucopenia · risk of severe hypotension following administration · thrombocytopenia

● INTERACTIONS → Appendix 1: pentamidine

● SIDE-EFFECTS

  GENERAL SIDE-EFFECTS

▸ **Common or very common** Dizziness · hypoglycaemia (can be severe and sometimes fatal) · hypotension (can be severe and sometimes fatal) · local reaction · nausea · rash · taste altered

▸ **Rare or very rare** QT interval prolongation

▸ **Frequency not known** Pancreatitis acute (can be severe and sometimes fatal)

  SPECIFIC SIDE-EFFECTS

▸ **Common or very common**

▸ When used by inhalation Cough · dyspnoea · respiratory disorders

5

Infection

5

Infection

▸ With parenteral use Acute kidney injury · anaemia · azotaemia · electrolyte imbalance · flushing · haematuria · hyperglycaemia · induration · leucopenia · localised pain · myopathy · syncope · thrombocytopenia · vomiting
▸ **Rare or very rare**
▸ With parenteral use Arrhythmia (can be severe and sometimes fatal) · pancreatitis (can be severe and sometimes fatal)
▸ **Frequency not known**
▸ When used by inhalation Angioedema · appetite decreased · bradycardia · fatigue · renal failure
▸ With parenteral use Arrhythmias · perioral hypoaesthesia · sensation abnormal · Stevens-Johnson syndrome

● PREGNANCY Manufacturer advises avoid unless essential.

● BREAST FEEDING Manufacturer advises avoid unless essential—no information available.

● HEPATIC IMPAIRMENT Manufacturer advises caution.

● RENAL IMPAIRMENT
Dose adjustments Reduce intravenous dose for pneumocystis pneumonia if creatinine clearance less than 10 mL/minute: in *life-threatening infection*, use 4 mg/kg once daily for 7–10 days, then 4 mg/kg on alternate days to complete course of at least 14 doses; in *less severe infection*, use 4 mg/kg on alternate days for at least 14 doses.

● MONITORING REQUIREMENTS
▸ Monitor blood pressure before starting treatment, during administration, and at regular intervals, until treatment concluded.
▸ Carry out laboratory monitoring according to product literature.

● DIRECTIONS FOR ADMINISTRATION Manufacturer advises patient should be lying down when receiving drug parenterally. Direct intravenous injection should be avoided whenever possible and **never** given rapidly; intramuscular injections should be deep and preferably given into the buttock. For *intravenous infusion*, manufacturer advises reconstitute 300 mg with 3–5 mL Water for Injections (displacement value may be significant), then dilute required dose with 50–250 mL Glucose 5% *or* Sodium Chloride 0.9%; give over at least 60 minutes.
Powder for injection (dissolved in water for injection) may be used for nebulisation.

● HANDLING AND STORAGE Pentamidine isetionate is toxic and personnel should be adequately protected during handling and administration—consult product literature.

● MEDICINAL FORMS There can be variation in the licensing of different medicines containing the same drug.
Powder for solution for injection
▸ Pentacarinat (Sanofi)
Pentamidine isetionate 300 mg Pentacarinat 300mg powder for solution for injection vials | 5 vial PoM £158.86

4   Helminth infection

Helminth infections

Specialist centres
Advice on prophylaxis and treatment of helminth infections is available from the following specialist centres:

Birmingham	(0121) 424 0357
Scotland	Contact local Infectious Diseases Unit
Liverpool	(0151) 705 3100
London	0845 155 5000 (treatment)

Threadworms
Anthelmintics are effective in threadworm (pinworms, *Enterobius vermicularis*) infections, but their use needs to be combined with hygienic measures to break the cycle of auto-infection. All members of the family require treatment.
Adult threadworms do not live for longer than 6 weeks and for development of fresh worms, ova must be swallowed and exposed to the action of digestive juices in the upper intestinal tract. Direct multiplication of worms does not take place in the large bowel. Adult female worms lay ova on the perianal skin which causes pruritus; scratching the area then leads to ova being transmitted on fingers to the mouth, often via food eaten with unwashed hands. Washing hands and scrubbing nails before each meal and after each visit to the toilet is essential. A bath taken immediately after rising will remove ova laid during the night.
Mebendazole p. 644 is the drug of choice for treating threadworm infection in patients of all ages over 6 months. It is given as a single dose; as reinfection is very common, a second dose may be given after 2 weeks.

Ascaricides (common roundworm infections)
Mebendazole is effective against *Ascaris lumbricoides* and is generally considered to be the drug of choice.
Levamisole p. 644 [unlicensed] (available from 'special-order' manufacturers or specialist importing companies) is an alternative when mebendazole cannot be used. It is very well tolerated.

Tapeworm infections
Taenicides
Niclosamide [unlicensed] (available from 'special-order' manufacturers or specialist importing companies) is the most widely used drug for tapeworm infections and side-effects are limited to occasional gastro-intestinal upset, lightheadedness, and pruritus; it is not effective against larval worms. Fears of developing cysticercosis in *Taenia solium* infections have proved unfounded. All the same, an antiemetic can be given before treatment and a laxative can be given 2 hours after niclosamide.
Praziquantel p. 644 [unlicensed] (available from 'special-order' manufacturers or specialist importing companies) is as effective as niclosamide.

Hydatid disease
Cysts caused by *Echinococcus granulosus* grow slowly and asymptomatic patients do not always require treatment. Surgical treatment remains the method of choice in many situations. Albendazole p. 643 [unlicensed] (available from 'special-order' manufacturers or specialist importing companies) is used in conjunction with surgery to reduce the risk of recurrence or as primary treatment in inoperable cases. Alveolar echinococcosis due to *E. multilocularis* is usually fatal if untreated. Surgical removal with albendazole cover is the treatment of choice, but where effective surgery is impossible, repeated cycles of albendazole (for a year or more) may help. Careful monitoring of liver function is particularly important during drug treatment.

Hookworms
Hookworms (ancylostomiasis, necatoriasis) live in the upper small intestine and draw blood from the point of their attachment to their host. An iron-deficiency anaemia may occur and, if present, effective treatment of the infection requires not only expulsion of the worms but treatment of the anaemia.
Mebendazole has a useful broad-spectrum activity, and is effective against hookworms. Albendazole [unlicensed] (available from 'special-order' manufacturers or specialist importing companies) is an alternative. Levamisole is also is also effective in children.

Schistosomicides (bilharziasis)

Adult *Schistosoma haematobium* worms live in the genito-urinary veins and adult *S. mansoni* in those of the colon and mesentery. *S. japonicum* is more widely distributed in veins of the alimentary tract and portal system.

Praziquantel [unlicensed] is available from Merck Serono (*Cysticide*®) and is effective against all human schistosomes. No serious adverse effects have been reported. Of all the available schistosomicides, it has the most attractive combination of effectiveness, broad-spectrum activity, and low toxicity.

Filaricides

Diethylcarbamazine [unlicensed] (available from 'special-order' manufacturers or specialist importing companies) is effective against microfilariae and adults of *Loa loa*, *Wuchereria bancrofti*, and *Brugia malayi*. To minimise reactions, treatment in adults and children over 1 month, is commenced with a dose of diethylcarbamazine citrate on the first day and increased gradually over 3 days. Length of treatment varies according to infection type, and usually gives a radical cure for these infections. Close medical supervision is necessary particularly in the early phase of treatment.

In heavy infections there may be a febrile reaction, and in heavy *Loa loa* infection there is a small risk of encephalopathy. In such cases specialist advice should be sought, and treatment must be given under careful in-patient supervision and stopped at the first sign of cerebral involvement.

Ivermectin below [unlicensed] (available from 'special-order' manufacturers or specialist importing companies) is very effective in *onchocerciasis* and it is now the drug of choice; reactions are usually slight. Diethylcarbamazine or suramin should no longer be used for *onchocerciasis* because of their toxicity.

Cutaneous larva migrans (creeping eruption)

Dog and cat hookworm larvae may enter human skin where they produce slowly extending itching tracks usually on the foot. Single tracks can be treated with topical tiabendazole (no commercial preparation available). Multiple infections respond to ivermectin, albendazole or **tiabendazole** (thiabendazole) by mouth [all unlicensed] (available from 'special-order' manufacturers or specialist importing companies).

Strongyloidiasis

Adult *Strongyloides stercoralis* live in the gut and produce larvae which penetrate the gut wall and invade the tissues, setting up a cycle of auto-infection. Ivermectin [unlicensed] (available from 'special-order' manufacturers or specialist importing companies) is the treatment of choice for chronic *Strongyloides* infection in adults and children over 5 years. Albendazole [unlicensed] (available from 'special order' manufacturers or specialist importing companies) is an alternative given to adults and children over 2 years.

ANTHELMINTICS

Albendazole

- **INDICATIONS AND DOSE**

Chronic *Strongyloides* infection
▸ BY MOUTH
▸ Adult: 400 mg twice daily for 3 days, dose may be repeated after 3 weeks if necessary

Hydatid disease, in conjunction with surgery to reduce the risk of recurrence or as primary treatment in inoperable cases
▸ BY MOUTH
▸ Adult: (consult product literature)

Hookworm infections
▸ BY MOUTH
▸ Adult: 400 mg for 1 dose

- UNLICENSED USE Albendazole is an unlicensed drug.

- INTERACTIONS → Appendix 1: albendazole

- MEDICINAL FORMS There can be variation in the licensing of different medicines containing the same drug. Forms available from special-order manufacturers include: tablet, chewable tablet, oral suspension

Tablet
CAUTIONARY AND ADVISORY LABELS 9
▸ Eskazole (Imported (France))
Albendazole 400 mg Eskazole 400mg tablets | 60 tablet [PoM] [✗]

Chewable tablet
CAUTIONARY AND ADVISORY LABELS 9
▸ Zentel (Imported)
Albendazole 200 mg Zentel 200mg chewable tablets | 6 tablet [PoM] [✗]
Albendazole 400 mg Zentel 400mg chewable tablets | 1 tablet [PoM] [✗]

Diethylcarbamazine

- **INDICATIONS AND DOSE**

***Wuchereria bancrofti* infections | *Brugia malayi* infections**
▸ BY MOUTH
▸ Adult: Initially 1 mg/kg daily on the first day, then increased to 6 mg/kg daily in divided doses, dose to be increased gradually over 3 days

***Loa loa* infections**
▸ BY MOUTH
▸ Adult: Initially 1 mg/kg daily on the first day, then increased to 6 mg/kg daily in divided doses, dose to be increased gradually over 3 days; maximum 9 mg/kg per day

- UNLICENSED USE Diethylcarbamazine is an unlicensed drug.

- MEDICINAL FORMS No licensed medicines listed.

Ivermectin   20-Aug-2020

- **INDICATIONS AND DOSE**

Chronic *Strongyloides* infection
▸ BY MOUTH
▸ Adult: 200 micrograms/kg daily for 2 days

Onchocerciasis
▸ BY MOUTH
▸ Adult: 150 micrograms/kg for 1 dose, retreatment at intervals of 6 to 12 months, depending on symptoms, must be given until the adult worms die out

Scabies, in combination with topical drugs, for the treatment of hyperkeratotic (crusted or 'Norwegian') scabies that does not respond to topical treatment alone
▸ BY MOUTH
▸ Adult: 200 micrograms/kg for 1 dose, further doses of 200 micrograms/kg may be required

- UNLICENSED USE Ivermectin is unlicensed.

- INTERACTIONS → Appendix 1: ivermectin

- SIDE-EFFECTS
▸ **Common or very common** Skin reactions

5

Infection

▶ **Frequency not known** Abnormal sensation in eye · anaemia · appetite decreased · asthenia · asthma exacerbated · chest discomfort · coma · confusion · conjunctival haemorrhage · constipation · diarrhoea · difficulty standing · difficulty walking · dizziness · drowsiness · dyspnoea · encephalopathy · eosinophilia · eye inflammation · faecal incontinence · fever · gastrointestinal discomfort · headache · hepatitis · hypotension · joint disorders · leucopenia · lymphatic abnormalities · Mazzotti reaction aggravated · myalgia · nausea · oedema · pain · psychiatric disorder · seizure · severe cutaneous adverse reactions (SCARs) · stupor · tachycardia · tremor · urinary incontinence · vertigo · vomiting

● MEDICINAL FORMS There can be variation in the licensing of different medicines containing the same drug. Forms available from special-order manufacturers include: tablet
Tablet
▶ Stromectol (Imported (France))
Ivermectin 3 mg Stromectol 3mg tablets | 4 tablet PoM ⓢ

Levamisole

10-Mar-2020

● **INDICATIONS AND DOSE**
Roundworm infections
▶ BY MOUTH
▶ Adult: 120–150 mg for 1 dose

● UNLICENSED USE Not licensed.
● CONTRA-INDICATIONS Blood disorders
● CAUTIONS Epilepsy · Sjögren's syndrome
● INTERACTIONS → Appendix 1: levamisole
● SIDE-EFFECTS Arthralgia (long term use) · blood disorder (long term use) · diarrhoea · dizziness · headache · influenza like illness (long term use) · insomnia (long term use) · myalgia (long term use) · nausea · rash (long term use) · seizure (long term use) · taste altered (long term use) · vasculitis (long term use) · vomiting
● PREGNANCY Embryotoxic in *animal* studies, avoid if possible.
● BREAST FEEDING No information available.
● HEPATIC IMPAIRMENT
Dose adjustments Use with caution—dose adjustment may be necessary.

● MEDICINAL FORMS There can be variation in the licensing of different medicines containing the same drug. Forms available from special-order manufacturers include: tablet
Tablet
CAUTIONARY AND ADVISORY LABELS 4
▶ Ergamisol (Imported (Belgium))
Levamisole (as Levamisole hydrochloride) 50 mg Ergamisol 50mg tablets | 20 tablet PoM ⓢ

Mebendazole

10-Mar-2020

● **INDICATIONS AND DOSE**
Threadworm infections
▶ BY MOUTH
▶ Child 6 months–17 years: 100 mg for 1 dose, if reinfection occurs, second dose may be needed after 2 weeks
▶ Adult: 100 mg for 1 dose, if reinfection occurs, second dose may be needed after 2 weeks
Whipworm infections | Hookworm infections
▶ BY MOUTH
▶ Child 1–17 years: 100 mg twice daily for 3 days
▶ Adult: 100 mg twice daily for 3 days

Roundworm infections
▶ BY MOUTH
▶ Child 1 year: 100 mg twice daily for 3 days
▶ Child 2–17 years: 100 mg twice daily for 3 days, alternatively 500 mg for 1 dose
▶ Adult: 100 mg twice daily for 3 days, alternatively 500 mg for 1 dose

Threadworm infections (dose approved for use by community practitioner nurse prescribers)
▶ BY MOUTH
▶ Child 2–17 years: 100 mg for 1 dose, if reinfection occurs, second dose may be needed after 2 weeks
▶ Adult: 100 mg for 1 dose, if reinfection occurs, second dose may be needed after 2 weeks

● UNLICENSED USE Not licensed for use as a single dose of 500 mg in roundworm infections.
▶ In children Not licensed for use in children under 2 years.
● INTERACTIONS → Appendix 1: mebendazole
● SIDE-EFFECTS
▶ **Common or very common** Gastrointestinal discomfort
▶ **Uncommon** Diarrhoea · flatulence
▶ **Rare or very rare** Alopecia · dizziness · hepatitis · neutropenia · seizure · severe cutaneous adverse reactions (SCARs) · skin reactions
● PREGNANCY Manufacturer advises avoid—toxicity in *animal* studies.
● BREAST FEEDING Amount present in milk too small to be harmful but manufacturer advises avoid.
● PRESCRIBING AND DISPENSING INFORMATION Flavours of oral liquid formulations may include banana.
● PATIENT AND CARER ADVICE
Medicines for Children leaflet: Mebendazole for worm infections www.medicinesforchildren.org.uk/mebendazole-worm-infections
● EXCEPTIONS TO LEGAL CATEGORY Mebendazole tablets can be sold to the public if supplied for oral use in the treatment of enterobiasis in adults and children over 2 years provided its container or package is labelled to show a max. single dose of 100 mg and it is supplied in a container or package containing not more than 800 mg.

● MEDICINAL FORMS There can be variation in the licensing of different medicines containing the same drug.
Oral suspension
▶ Vermox (Janssen-Cilag Ltd)
Mebendazole 20 mg per 1 ml Vermox 100mg/5ml oral suspension | 30 ml PoM £1.55 DT = £1.55
Chewable tablet
▶ Vermox (Janssen-Cilag Ltd)
Mebendazole 100 mg Vermox 100mg chewable tablets sugar-free | 6 tablet PoM £1.34 DT = £1.34

Praziquantel

● **INDICATIONS AND DOSE**
Tapeworm infections (*Taenia solium*)
▶ BY MOUTH
▶ Adult: 5–10 mg/kg for 1 dose, to be taken after a light breakfast
Tapeworm infections (*Hymenolepis nana*)
▶ BY MOUTH
▶ Adult: 25 mg/kg for 1 dose, to be taken after a light breakfast
***Schistosoma haematobium* worm infections | *Schistosoma mansoni* worm infections**
▶ BY MOUTH
▶ Adult: 20 mg/kg, followed by 20 mg/kg after 4–6 hours

***Schistosoma japonicum* worm infections**
▶ BY MOUTH
  ▶ Adult: 20 mg/kg 3 times a day for 1 day

● UNLICENSED USE Praziquantel is an unlicensed drug.
● INTERACTIONS → Appendix 1: praziquantel

● MEDICINAL FORMS There can be variation in the licensing of different medicines containing the same drug. Forms available from special-order manufacturers include: tablet

Tablet
▶ Biltricide (Imported (Germany))
  Praziquantel 600 mg Biltricide 600mg tablets | 6 tablet PoM Ⓢ
▶ Cesol (Imported (Germany))
  Praziquantel 150 mg Cesol 150mg tablets | 6 tablet PoM Ⓢ
▶ Cysticide (Imported (Germany))
  Praziquantel 500 mg Cysticide 500mg tablets | 90 tablet PoM Ⓢ

5　Protozoal infection

Antiprotozoal drugs

Amoebicides

Metronidazole p. 575 is the drug of choice for *acute invasive amoebic dysentery* since it is very effective against vegetative forms of *Entamoeba histolytica* in ulcers. Tinidazole p. 577 is also effective. Metronidazole and tinidazole are also active against amoebae which may have migrated to the liver. Treatment with metronidazole (or tinidazole) is followed by a 10-day course of diloxanide furoate.

Diloxanide furoate is the drug of choice for asymptomatic patients with *E. histolytica* cysts in the faeces; metronidazole and tinidazole are relatively ineffective. Diloxanide furoate is relatively free from toxic effects and the usual course is of 10 days, given alone for chronic infections or following metronidazole or tinidazole treatment.

For *amoebic abscesses* of the liver metronidazole is effective; tinidazole is an alternative. Aspiration of the abscess is indicated where it is suspected that it may rupture or where there is no improvement after 72 hours of metronidazole; the aspiration may need to be repeated. Aspiration aids penetration of metronidazole and, for abscesses with more than 100 mL of pus, if carried out in conjunction with drug therapy, may reduce the period of disability.

Diloxanide furoate is not effective against hepatic amoebiasis, but a 10-day course should be given at the completion of metronidazole or tinidazole treatment to destroy any amoebae in the gut.

Trichomonacides

Metronidazole is the treatment of choice for *Trichomonas vaginalis* infection. Contact tracing is recommended and sexual contacts should be treated simultaneously. If metronidazole is ineffective, tinidazole may be tried.

Antigiardial drugs

Metronidazole is the treatment of choice for *Giardia lamblia* infections. Alternative treatments are tinidazole or mepacrine hydrochloride p. 527.

Leishmaniacides

Cutaneous leishmaniasis frequently heals spontaneously but if skin lesions are extensive or unsightly, treatment is indicated, as it is in visceral leishmaniasis (kala-azar). Leishmaniasis should be treated under specialist supervision.

Sodium stibogluconate, an organic pentavalent antimony compound, is used for visceral leishmaniasis. The dosage varies with different geographical regions and expert advice

should be obtained. Some early non-inflamed lesions of cutaneous leishmaniasis can be treated with intralesional injections of sodium stibogluconate under specialist supervision.

Amphotericin B p. 632 is used with or after an antimony compound for visceral leishmaniasis unresponsive to the antimonial alone; side-effects may be reduced by using liposomal amphotericin B (*AmBisome®*). *Abelcet®*, a lipid formulation of amphotericin B, is also likely to be effective but less information is available.

Pentamidine isetionate p. 641 has been used in antimony-resistant visceral leishmaniasis, but although the initial response is often good, the relapse rate is high; it is associated with serious side-effects. Other treatments include paromomycin [unlicensed] (available from 'special-order' manufacturers or specialist importing companies).

Trypanocides

The prophylaxis and treatment of trypanosomiasis is difficult and differs according to the strain of organism. Expert advice should therefore be obtained.

Toxoplasmosis

Most infections caused by *Toxoplasma gondii* are self-limiting, and treatment is not necessary. Exceptions are patients with eye involvement (toxoplasma choroidoretinitis), and those who are immunosuppressed. Toxoplasmic encephalitis is a common complication of AIDS. The treatment of choice is a combination of pyrimethamine p. 659 and sulfadiazine p. 599, given for several weeks (expert advice **essential**). Pyrimethamine is a folate antagonist, and adverse reactions to this combination are relatively common (folinic acid supplements and weekly blood counts needed). Alternative regimens use combinations of pyrimethamine with clindamycin p. 566 or clarithromycin p. 569 or azithromycin p. 568. Long-term secondary prophylaxis is required after treatment of toxoplasmosis in immunocompromised patients; prophylaxis should continue until immunity recovers.

If toxoplasmosis is acquired in pregnancy, transplacental infection may lead to severe disease in the fetus; specialist advice should be sought on management. Spiramycin [unlicensed] (available from 'special-order' manufacturers or specialist importing companies) may reduce the risk of transmission of maternal infection to the fetus.

5.1　Malaria

Antimalarials　　　　　　　　　　　　　　20-Nov-2019

Artemether with lumefantrine

Artemether with lumefantrine p. 653 is licensed for the *treatment of acute uncomplicated falciparum malaria*.

Artenimol with piperaquine

Artenimol with piperaquine phosphate p. 654 is not recommended for the first-line treatment of *acute uncomplicated falciparum malaria* because there is limited experience of its use in travellers who usually reside in areas where malaria is not endemic. Piperaquine has a long half-life.

Atovaquone with proguanil

Atovaquone with proguanil hydrochloride p. 654 is licensed for the *prophylaxis of falciparum malaria* (for details, see Recommended regimens for prophylaxis against malaria p. 647) and for the treatment of *acute, uncomplicated falciparum malaria*.

Chloroquine

Chloroquine p. 655 is usually used with proguanil hydrochloride p. 658 for the *prophylaxis of malaria* in areas of the world where there is little chloroquine resistance (for details, see Recommended regimens for prophylaxis against malaria p. 647).

Guidelines for malaria prevention in travellers from the United Kingdom (2019) published by Public Health England state that patients already taking hydroxychloroquine sulfate p. 1144 for another indication, and for whom chloroquine would be an appropriate antimalarial, can remain on hydroxychloroquine sulfate.

Chloroquine is **no longer recommended** for the *treatment of falciparum malaria* owing to widespread resistance, nor is it recommended if the infective species is *not known* or if the infection is *mixed*; in these cases treatment should be with quinine p. 658, atovaquone with proguanil hydrochloride p. 654, or artemether with lumefantrine. It is still recommended for the *treatment of non-falciparum malaria*.

Doxycycline

Doxycycline p. 601 is used in adults and children over 12 years as an option for the *prophylaxis of malaria* in areas of *chloroquine resistance*. Doxycycline is also used as an alternative to mefloquine p. 656 or atovaquone with proguanil hydrochloride p. 654, (for details, see Recommended regimens for prophylaxis against malaria p. 647).

Mefloquine

Mefloquine is used for the *prophylaxis of malaria* in areas of *chloroquine resistance*. Mefloquine is also used as an alternative to doxycycline or atovaquone with proguanil hydrochloride p. 654, (for details, see Recommended regimens for prophylaxis against malaria p. 647).

Mefloquine is now rarely used for the *treatment of falciparum malaria* because of increased resistance. It is rarely used for the *treatment of non-falciparum malaria* because better tolerated alternatives are available. Mefloquine should not be used for treatment if it has been used for prophylaxis.

Primaquine

Primaquine p. 657 is used to eliminate the liver stages of *P. vivax* or *P. ovale* following chloroquine treatment.

Proguanil

Proguanil hydrochloride is usually used in combination with chloroquine or atovaquone for the *prophylaxis of malaria*, (for details, see Recommended regimens for prophylaxis against malaria p. 647).

Proguanil hydrochloride used alone is not suitable for the *treatment of malaria*; however, atovaquone with proguanil hydrochloride p. 654 is licensed for the treatment of acute uncomplicated falciparum malaria. Atovaquone with proguanil hydrochloride p. 654 is also used for the *prophylaxis of falciparum malaria* in areas of *chloroquine resistance*. Atovaquone with proguanil hydrochloride p. 654 is also used as an alternative to mefloquine or doxycycline. Atovaquone with proguanil hydrochloride p. 654 is particularly suitable for short trips to chloroquine-resistant areas because it needs to be taken only for 7 days after leaving an endemic area.

Pyrimethamine

Pyrimethamine p. 659 should not be used alone, but is used with sulfadoxine.

Pyrimethamine with sulfadoxine can be used in the *treatment of falciparum malaria with (or following) quinine*.

Quinine

Quinine is used for the *treatment of falciparum malaria*, if the infective species is *not known*, or if the infection is mixed (for details see Malaria, treatment p. 652).

Useful resources

Recommendations on prophylaxis against malaria reflect guidelines agreed by the Advisory Committee on Malaria Prevention (ACMP), published in the Public Health England (PHE) Guidelines for malaria prevention in travellers from the United Kingdom, 2019. The advice is aimed at residents of the UK who travel to endemic areas. www.gov.uk/government/publications/malaria-prevention-guidelines-for-travellers-from-the-uk

Malaria, prophylaxis

20-Nov-2019

Prophylaxis against malaria

The recommendations on prophylaxis reflect guidelines agreed by the Advisory Committee on Malaria Prevention (ACMP), published in the Public Health England (PHE) Guidelines for malaria prevention in travellers from the United Kingdom, 2019. The advice is aimed at residents of the UK who travel to endemic areas.

For specialist centres offering advice on specific malaria-related problems, see Malaria, treatment p. 652. The choice of drug for a particular individual should take into account:
- risk of exposure to malaria
- extent of drug resistance
- efficacy of the recommended drugs
- side-effects of the drugs
- patient-related factors (e.g. age, pregnancy, renal or hepatic impairment, compliance with prophylactic regimen)

For more information on choice of drug, see also Antimalarials p. 645.

Protection against bites

Prophylaxis is not absolute, and breakthrough infection can occur with any of the drugs recommended. Personal protection against being bitten is very important and is recommended even in malaria-free areas as a preventive measure against other insect vector-borne diseases. Mosquito nets impregnated with a pyrethroid insecticide, such as permethrin p. 1281, improves protection against insects and should be used if sleeping outdoors or in unscreened lodging; vaporised insecticides are also useful. Long sleeves and trousers worn after dusk also provide protection against bites.

Insect repellents give protection against bites, but attention to the correct application of product is required. Diethyltoluamide (DEET) 20–50% (available in various preparations including sprays and modified-release polymer formulations) is safe and effective when applied to the skin of adults and children over 2 months of age. It can also be used during pregnancy and breast-feeding. However, ingestion should be avoided, therefore breast-feeding mothers should wash their hands and breast tissue before handling infants. The duration of protection varies according to the concentration of DEET and is longest for DEET 50%. When sunscreen is also required, DEET should be applied after the sunscreen. DEET reduces the SPF of sunscreen, so a sunscreen of SPF 30–50 should be applied. If DEET is not tolerated or is unavailable, for alternative options, see Public Health England Guidelines for malaria prevention in travellers from the United Kingdom (see *Useful resources*).

Key to recommended regimens for prophylaxis against malaria

Codes for regimens	Details of regimens for prophylaxis against malaria
-	No risk
1	Chemoprophylaxis not recommended, but avoid mosquito bites and consider malaria if fever presents
2	Chloroquine only
3	Chloroquine with proguanil
4	Atovaquone with proguanil hydrochloride or doxycycline or mefloquine

Specific recommendations

Country	Comments on risk of malaria and regional or seasonal variation	Codes for regimens
Afghanistan	Low risk below 2000 m from May–November	1
	Very low risk below 2000 m from December–April	1
Algeria	No risk	1
Andaman and Nicobar Islands (India)	Low risk	1
Angola	High risk	4
Argentina	No risk	1
Armenia	No risk	1
Azerbaijan	Very low risk	1
Bangladesh	High risk in Chittagong Hill Tract districts (but not Chittagong city)	4
	Very low risk in Chittagong city and other areas, except Chittagong Hill Tract districts	1
Belize	Low risk in rural areas	1
	No risk in Belize district (including Belize city and islands)	-
Benin	High risk	4
Bhutan	Low risk in southern belt districts, along border with India: Chukha, Geyleg-phug, Samchi, Samdrup Jonkhar, and Shemgang	1
	No risk in areas other than those above	-
Bolivia	Low risk in Amazon basin	1
	Low risk in rural areas below 2500 m (other than above)	1
	No risk above 2500 m	-
Botswana	High risk from November–June in northern half, including Okavango Delta area	4
	Low risk from July–October in northern half, including Okavango Delta area	1
	Very low risk in southern half	1
Brazil	Low risk in Amazon basin, including city of Manaus	1
	Very low risk in areas other than those above	1
	No risk in Iguaçu Falls	-
Brunei Darussalam	Very low risk	1
Burkina Faso	High risk	4
Burundi	High risk	4
Cambodia	Low risk. Mefloquine resistance widespread in western provinces bordering Thailand	1
	Very low risk in Angkor Wat and Lake Tonle Sap, including Siem Reap	1
	No risk in Phnom Penh	-
Cameroon	High risk	4
Cape Verde	Individuals travelling to Praia who are at increased risk of malaria (such as long-term travellers and those at risk of severe complications from malaria including pregnant women, infants and young children, the elderly, and asplenic individuals) should consider taking antimalarials, seek advice from a travel health advisor. Very low risk on island of Santiago (Sao Tiago) and Boa Vista	1
Central African Republic	High risk	4
Chad	High risk	4

Country	Comments on risk of malaria and regional or seasonal variation	Codes for regimens
China	Low risk in Yunnan and Hainan provinces	1
	Very low risk in southern and some central provinces, including Anhui, Ghuizhou, Hena, Hubei, and Jiangsu below 1500 m	1
	Very low risk in areas other than those above and below	1
	No risk in Hong Kong	-
Colombia	Low risk in rural areas below 1600 m	1
	Very low risk above 1600 m and in Cartagena	1
Comoros	High risk	4
Congo	High risk	4
Costa Rica	Low risk in Limon province, but not city of Limon (Puerto Limon)	1
	Very low risk in areas other than those above	1
Cote d'Ivoire (Ivory Coast)	High risk	4
Democratic Republic of the Congo	High risk	4
Djibouti	High risk	4
Dominican Republic	Low risk	1
	No risk in cities of Santiago and Santo Domingo	-
East Timor (Timor-Leste)	Risk present	4
Ecuador	Low risk in areas below 1500 m including coastal provinces and Amazon basin	1
	No risk in Galapagos islands or city of Guayaquil	-
Egypt	No risk	1
El Salvador	Low risk in rural areas of Santa Ana, Ahuachapán, and La Unión provinces in western part of country	1
	Very low risk in areas other than those above	1
Equatorial Guinea	High risk	4
Eritrea	High risk below 2200 m	4
	No risk in Asmara or in areas above 2200 m	-
Ethiopia	High risk below 2000 m	4
	No risk in Addis Ababa or in areas above 2000 m	-
French Guiana	Risk present (particularly in border areas) except city of Cayenne or Devil's Island (Ile du Diable)	4
	Low risk in city of Cayenne or Devil's Island (Ile du Diable)	1
Gabon	High risk	4
Gambia	High risk	4
Georgia	Very low risk from June–October in rural south east	1
	No risk from November–May in rural south east	-
Ghana	High risk	4
Guatemala	Low risk below 1500 m	1
	No risk in Guatemala City, Antigua, or Lake Atitlan and above 1500 m	-
Guinea	High risk	4
Guinea-Bissau	High risk	4
Guyana	Risk present in all interior regions	4
	Very low risk in Georgetown and coastal region	1
Haiti	Risk present	3
Honduras	Low risk below 1000 m and in Roatán and other Bay Islands	1
	No risk in San Pedro Sula or Tegucigalpa and areas above 1000 m	-
India	Risk present in states of Assam and Orissa, districts of East Godavari, Srikakulam, Vishakhapatnam, and Vizianagaram in the state of Andhra Pradesh, and districts of Balaghat, Dindori, Mandla, and Seoni in the state of Madhya Pradesh	4
	Low risk in areas other than those above or below (including Goa, Andaman and Nicobar islands)	1
	Exceptional circumstances in low risk areas (dependent on individual risk assessment)	3
	No risk in Lakshadweep islands	-

Key to recommended regimens for prophylaxis against malaria

Codes for regimens	Details of regimens for prophylaxis against malaria
-	No risk
1	Chemoprophylaxis not recommended, but avoid mosquito bites and consider malaria if fever presents
2	Chloroquine only
3	Chloroquine with proguanil
4	Atovaquone with proguanil hydrochloride or doxycycline or mefloquine

Specific recommendations

Country	Comments on risk of malaria and regional or seasonal variation	Codes for regimens
Indonesia	High risk in Irian Jaya (Papua)	4
	Low risk in Bali, Lombok and islands of Java and Sumatra	1
	No risk in city of Jakarta	-
Indonesia (Borneo)	Low risk	1
Iran	Low risk from March–November in rural south eastern provinces and in north, along Azerbaijan border in Ardabil, and near Turkmenistan border in North Khorasan	1
	Very low risk in areas other than those above	1
Iraq	Very low risk from May–November in rural northern area below 1500 m	1
	No risk in areas other than those above	-
Kenya	High risk (except city of Nairobi)	4
	Very low risk in the highlands above 2500 m and in city of Nairobi	1
Kyrgyzstan	No risk	-
Lao People's Democratic Republic (Laos)	Low risk	1
	Very low risk in city of Vientiane	1
Liberia	High risk	4
Libya	No risk	1
Madagascar	High risk	4
Malawi	High risk	4
Malaysia	Low risk in mainland Malaysia	1
Malaysia (Borneo)	Low risk in inland areas of Sabah and in inland, forested areas of Sarawak	1
	Very low risk in areas other than those above, including coastal areas of Sabah and Sarawak	1
Mali	High risk	4
Mauritania	High risk all year in southern provinces, and from July–October in the northern provinces	4
	Low risk from November–June in the northern provinces	1
Mauritius	No risk	1
Mayotte	Risk present	4
Mexico	Very low risk	1
Mozambique	High risk	4
Myanmar	Low risk	1
Namibia	High risk all year in regions of Caprivi Strip, Kavango, and Kunene river, and from November–June in northern third of country	4
	Low risk from July–October in northern third of country, except as above in regions of Caprivi Strip, Kavango, and Kunene river	1
	Very low risk in areas other than those above	1
Nepal	Low risk below 1500 m, including the Terai district	1
	No risk in city of Kathmandu and on typical Himalayan treks	-
Nicaragua	Low risk (except Managua)	1
	Very low risk in Managua	1
Niger	High risk	4
Nigeria	High risk	4
North Korea	Very low risk in some southern areas	1

Country	Comments on risk of malaria and regional or seasonal variation	Codes for regimens
Pakistan	Low risk below 2000 m	1
	Very low risk above 2000 m	1
Panama	Low risk east of Canal Zone	1
	Very low risk west of Canal Zone	1
	No risk in Panama City or Canal Zone itself	-
Papua New Guinea	High risk below 1800 m	4
	Very low risk above 1800 m	1
Paraguay	No risk	1
Peru	Low risk in Amazon basin along border with Brazil, particularly in Loreto province and in rural areas below 2000 m including the Amazon basin bordering Bolivia	1
	No risk in city of Lima and coastal region south of Chiclayo	-
Philippines	Low risk in rural areas below 600 m and on islands of Luzon, Mindanao, Mindoro, and Palawan	1
	No risk in cities or on islands of Boracay, Bohol, Catanduanes, Cebu, or Leyte	-
Rwanda	High risk	4
São Tomé and Principe	High risk	4
Saudi Arabia	Low risk in south-western provinces along border with Yemen, including below 2000 m in Asir province	1
	No risk in cities of Jeddah, Makkah (Mecca), Medina, Riyadh, or Ta'if, or above 2000 m in Asir province	-
Senegal	High risk	4
Sierra Leone	High risk	4
Singapore	No risk	1
Solomon Islands	High risk	4
Somalia	High risk	4
South Africa	Risk from September–May in low altitude areas of Mpumalanga and Limpopo, particularly those bordering Mozambique, Swaziland (Estwatini), and Zimbabwe (including Kruger National Park)	4
	Low risk in north-east KwaZulu-Natal and in designated areas of Mpumalanga and Limpopo	1
	Very low risk in North West Province (adjacent to Molopo river) and Northern Cape Province (adjacent to Orange river)	1
South Korea	Very low risk in northern areas, in Gangwon-do and Gyeonggi-do provinces, and Incheon city (towards Demilitarized Zone)	1
South Sudan	High risk	4
Sri Lanka	No risk	1
Sudan	High risk in central and southern areas; risk also present in rest of country (except Khartoum)	4
	Very low risk in Khartoum	1
Suriname	Risk present on the French Guiana border	4
	Low risk in areas other than above and below	1
	No risk in city of Paramaribo	-
Swaziland	Risk in northern and eastern regions bordering Mozambique and South Africa, including all of Lubombo district and Big Bend, Mhlume, Simunye, and Tshaneni regions	4
	Very low risk in the areas other than those above	1
Syria	Very low risk in small, remote foci of El Hasakah	1
Tajikistan	Very low risk	1
	No risk above 2000 m	-
Tanzania	High risk below 1800 m; risk also in Zanzibar	4
	No risk above 1800 m	-
Thailand	Mefloquine resistance present. Low risk in rural forested borders with Cambodia, Laos, and Myanmar	1
	Very low risk in areas other than those above, including Kanchanaburi (Kwai Bridge)	1
	No risk in cities of Bangkok, Chiang Mai, Chiang Rai, Koh Phangan, Koh Samui, and Pattaya	-

Key to recommended regimens for prophylaxis against malaria

Codes for regimens	Details of regimens for prophylaxis against malaria
-	No risk
1	Chemoprophylaxis not recommended, but avoid mosquito bites and consider malaria if fever presents
2	Chloroquine only
3	Chloroquine with proguanil
4	Atovaquone with proguanil hydrochloride or doxycycline or mefloquine

Specific recommendations

Country	Comments on risk of malaria and regional or seasonal variation	Codes for regimens
Togo	High risk	4
Turkey	Very low risk	1
Uganda	High risk	4
Uzbekistan	No risk	1
Vanuatu	Risk present	4
Venezuela	Risk in all areas south of, and including, the Orinoco river and Angel Falls, rural areas of Apure, Monagas, Sucre, and Zulia states	1
	Increase in reported malaria cases between 2010 and 2017, mainly in the Bolivar state	1
	No risk in city of Caracas or on Margarita Island	-
Vietnam	Low risk in rural areas, and in southern provinces of Tay Ninh, Lam Dong, Dac Lac, Gia Lai, and Kon Tum	1
	No risk in large cities (including Ho Chi Minh City (Saigon) and Hanoi), the Red River delta, coastal areas north of Nha Trang and Phu Quoc Island	1
Western Sahara	No risk	1
Yemen	Risk below 2000 m	3
	Very low risk on Socrota Island	1
	No risk above 2000 m, including Sana'a city	1
Zambia	High risk	4
Zimbabwe	High risk all year in Zambezi valley, and from November-June in areas below 1200 m	4
	Low risk from July-October in areas below 1200 m	1
	Very low risk all year in Harare and Bulawayo	1

Length of prophylaxis

Prophylaxis should generally be started before travel into an endemic area; 1 week before travel for chloroquine p. 655 and proguanil hydrochloride p. 658; 2–3 weeks before travel for mefloquine p. 656; and 1–2 days before travel for atovaquone with proguanil hydrochloride p. 654 or doxycycline p. 601. Prophylaxis should be continued for **4 weeks after leaving the area** (except for atovaquone with proguanil hydrochloride prophylaxis which should be stopped 1 week after leaving). For extensive journeys across different regions, the traveller must be protected in all areas of risk.

In those requiring long-term prophylaxis, chloroquine and proguanil hydrochloride may be used. However, there is considerable concern over the protective efficacy of the combination of chloroquine and proguanil hydrochloride in certain areas where it was previously useful. Mefloquine is licensed for use up to 1 year (although, if it is tolerated in the short term, there is no evidence of harm when it is used for up to 3 years). Doxycycline can be used for up to 2 years, and atovaquone with proguanil hydrochloride for up to 1 year. Prophylaxis with mefloquine, doxycycline, or atovaquone with proguanil hydrochloride may be considered for longer durations if it is justified by the risk of exposure to malaria. Specialist advice may be sought for long-term prophylaxis.

Return from malarial region

It is important to consider that any illness that occurs within 1 year and **especially within 3 months of return might be malaria** even if all recommended precautions against malaria were taken. Travellers should be warned of this and told that if they develop any illness after their return they should see a doctor early, and specifically mention their risk of exposure to malaria.

Epilepsy

Both chloroquine and mefloquine are unsuitable for malaria prophylaxis in individuals with a history of epilepsy. In these patients, doxycycline or atovaquone with proguanil hydrochloride may be used. However doxycycline may interact with some antiepileptics and its dose may need to be adjusted, see *interactions* information for doxycycline.

Asplenia

Asplenic individuals (or those with severe splenic dysfunction) are at particular risk of severe malaria. If travel to malarious areas is unavoidable, rigorous precautions are required against contracting the disease.

Pregnancy

Travel to malarious areas should be avoided during pregnancy; if travel is unavoidable, pregnant individuals must be informed about the risks and benefits of effective prophylaxis. Chloroquine and proguanil hydrochloride can be given in the usual doses during pregnancy, but these

5

Infection

drugs are not appropriate for most areas because their effectiveness has declined. In the case of proguanil hydrochloride, folic acid p. 1071 (dosed as a pregnancy at 'high-risk' of neural tube defects) should be given for the length of time that it is used during pregnancy. If travelling to high risk areas or there is resistance to other drugs, mefloquine may be considered during the second or third trimester of pregnancy. Mefloquine can be used in the first trimester with caution if the benefits outweigh the risks. Doxycycline is contra-indicated during pregnancy; however, it can be used for malaria prophylaxis if other regimens are unsuitable, and if the entire course of doxycycline can be completed before 15 weeks' gestation [unlicensed]. Atovaquone with proguanil hydrochloride should be avoided during pregnancy, however, it can be considered during the second and third trimesters if there is no suitable alternative. Folic acid (dosed as a pregnancy at 'high-risk' of neural tube defects) should be given for the length of time that atovaquone with proguanil hydrochloride is used during pregnancy.

Breast-feeding

Some antimalarials should be avoided when breast feeding, see individual drugs for details.

Prophylaxis is required in **breast-fed infants**; although antimalarials are present in milk, the amounts are too variable to give reliable protection.

Anticoagulants

Travellers taking warfarin sodium p. 153 should begin chemoprophylaxis 2–3 weeks before departure and the INR should be stable before departure. The INR should be measured before starting chemoprophylaxis, 7 days after starting, and after completing the course. For prolonged stays, the INR should be checked at regular intervals.

There is relatively limited experience of chemoprophylaxis in those travellers taking direct oral anticoagulants (DOACs).

Other medical conditions

For additional information on malaria prophylaxis in patients with other medical conditions, see Public Health England Guidelines for malaria prevention in travellers from the United Kingdom (see *Useful resources*).

Emergency standby treatment

Travellers on prophylaxis and visiting remote, malarious areas should carry standby emergency treatment if they are likely to be more than 24 hours away from medical care. Standby emergency treatment should also be considered in long-term travellers living in or visiting remote, malarious areas that may be far from appropriate medical attention; this does not replace the need to consider prophylaxis. Self-medication should be **avoided** if medical help is accessible.

In order to use standby treatment appropriately, the traveller should be provided with **written instructions** which include seeking urgent medical attention if fever (38°C or more) develops 7 days (or more) after arriving in a malarious area and that self-treatment is indicated if medical help is not available within 24 hours of fever onset.

In view of the continuing emergence of resistant strains and of the different regimens required for different areas expert advice should be sought on the best treatment course for an individual traveller. A drug used for chemoprophylaxis should not be considered for standby treatment for the same traveller due to concerns over drug resistance and to minimise drug toxicity.

Malaria prophylaxis, specific recommendations

Travellers planning journeys across continents can travel into areas that have different malaria prophylaxis recommendations. The choice of prophylaxis medication must reflect overall risk to ensure protection in all areas; it may be possible to change from one regimen to another. Those travelling to remote or little-visited areas may require expert advice. For further information see *Recommended*

regimens for prophylaxis against malaria, and Public Health England Guidelines for malaria prevention in travellers from the United Kingdom (see *Useful resources*).

Important

Settled immigrants (or long-term visitors) to the UK may be unaware that **any immunity they may have acquired while living in malarious areas is lost rapidly** after migration to the UK, or that any non-malarious areas where they lived previously **may now be malarious.**

Useful resources

Public Health England guideline: Guidelines for malaria prevention in travellers from the United Kingdom. September 2019.
www.gov.uk/government/publications/malaria-prevention-guidelines-for-travellers-from-the-uk

Malaria, treatment

20-Jul-2020

Advice for healthcare professionals

A number of specialist centres are able to provide advice on specific problems.

Public Health England (PHE) Malaria Reference Laboratory (prophylaxis) www.gov.uk/government/collections/malaria-reference-laboratory-mrl

National Travel Health Network and Centre (NaTHNaC) 0845 602 6712 www.travelhealthpro.org

TRAVAX (Health Protection Scotland) 0141 300 1130 www.travax.nhs.uk (for registered users of the NHS Travax website only)

Hospital for Tropical Diseases (HTD) (treatment) www.thehtd.org/

Liverpool School of Tropical Medicine (LSTM) (treatment) 0151 705 3100 Monday to Friday: 9 a.m.–5 p.m. and via Royal Liverpool Hospital switchboard at all other times 0151 706 2000 www.lstmed.ac.uk/

Birmingham 0121 424 2358

Your local infectious diseases unit

Advice for travellers

Hospital for Tropical Diseases Travel Healthline 020 7950 7799 www.fitfortravel.nhs.uk/home

WHO advice on international travel and health www.who.int/ith/en/

National Travel Health Network and Centre (NaTHNaC) www.travelhealthpro.org.uk/

Treatment of malaria

Recommendations on the treatment of malaria reflect guidelines agreed by UK malaria specialists.

If the infective species is **not known**, or if the infection is **mixed**, initial treatment should be as for *falciparum malaria* with quinine p. 658, atovaquone with proguanil hydrochloride p. 654, or *Riamet®* (artemether with lumefantrine p. 653). Falciparum malaria can progress rapidly in unprotected individuals and antimalarial treatment should be considered in those with features of severe malaria and possible exposure, even if the initial blood tests for the organism are negative.

Falciparum malaria (treatment)

Falciparum malaria (malignant malaria) is caused by *Plasmodium falciparum.* In most parts of the world *P. falciparum* is now resistant to chloroquine p. 655 which should not therefore be given for treatment.

Quinine, atovaquone with proguanil hydrochloride, or *Riamet®* (artemether with lumefantrine) can be given *by mouth* if the patient can swallow and retain tablets and there are no serious manifestations (e.g. impaired consciousness); quinine should be given *by intravenous infusion* if the patient is seriously ill or unable to take tablets. Mefloquine p. 656 is now rarely used for treatment because of concerns about resistance.

Oral quinine is given by mouth for 5–7 days, together with or followed by either doxycycline p. 601 for 7 days or clindamycin p. 566 for 7 days [unlicensed].

If the parasite is likely to be sensitive, pyrimethamine with sulfadoxine as a single dose [unlicensed] may be given (instead of either clindamycin or doxycycline) together with, or after, a course of quinine.

Alternatively, atovaquone with proguanil hydrochloride or *Riamet*® may be given instead of quinine. It is not necessary to give clindamycin, doxycycline, or pyrimethamine with sulfadoxine after atovaquone with proguanil hydrochloride or *Riamet*® treatment.

If the patient is seriously ill or unable to take tablets, or if more than 2% of red blood cell are parasitized, quinine should be given by *intravenous infusion*[unlicensed] (until patient can swallow tablets to complete the 7-day course *together with* or *followed by either* doxycycline or clindamycin).

Specialist advice should be sought in difficult cases (e.g. very high parasite count, deterioration on optimal doses of quinine, infection acquired in quinine-resistant areas of south east Asia) because intravenous **artesunate** may be available for 'named-patient' use.

Pregnancy

Falciparum malaria is particularly dangerous in pregnancy, especially in the last trimester. The adult treatment doses or oral and intravenous quinine (including the loading dose) can safely be given to pregnant women. Clindamycin should be given after quinine [unlicensed indication]. Doxycycline should be avoided in pregnancy (affects teeth and skeletal development); pyrimethamine with sulfadoxine, atovaquone with proguanil hydrochloride, and *Riamet*® are also best avoided until more information is available. Specialist advice should be sought in difficult cases (e.g. very high parasite count, deterioration on optimal doses of quinine, infection acquired in quinine-resistant areas of south east Asia) because intravenous artesunate may be available for 'named patient' use.

Non-falciparum malaria (treatment)

Non-falciparum malaria is usually caused by *Plasmodium vivax* and less commonly by *P. ovale* and *P. malariae*.*P. knowlesi* is also present in the Asia-Pacific region. Chloroquine is the drug of choice for the treatment of non-falciparum malaria (but chloroquine-resistant *P. vivax* has been reported in the Indonesian archipelago, the Malay Peninsula, including Myanmar, and eastward to Southern Vietnam).

For the treatment of chloroquine-resistant non-falciparum malaria, atovaquone with proguanil hydrochloride [unlicensed indication], quinine, or *Riamet*®[unlicensed indication] can be used; as with chloroquine, primaquine p. 657 should be given for radical cure.

Chloroquine alone is adequate for *P. malariae* and *P. knowlesi* infections but in the case of *P. vivax* and *P. ovale*, a *radical cure* (to destroy parasites in the liver and thus prevent relapses) is required. This is achieved with primaquine [unlicensed] given after chloroquine, with the dose dependent on the infecting organism. For a radical cure, primaquine [unlicensed] is then given for 14 days, with the dose also dependent on the infecting organism.

Parenteral

Parenteral If the patient is unable to take oral therapy, quinine can be given by intravenous infusion [unlicensed], changed to oral chloroquine as soon as the patient's condition permits.

Pregnancy

The adult treatment doses of chloroquine can be given for non-falciparum malaria. In the case of *P. vivax* or *P. ovale*, however, the radical cure with primaquine should be

postponed until the pregnancy is over; instead chloroquine should be continued, given weekly during the pregnancy.

ANTIPROTOZOALS > ANTIMALARIALS

Artemether with lumefantrine　　03-Sep-2020

● **INDICATIONS AND DOSE**

Treatment of acute uncomplicated falciparum malaria | Treatment of chloroquine-resistant non-falciparum malaria

▶ BY MOUTH

▸ Adult (body-weight 35 kg and above): Initially 4 tablets, followed by 4 tablets for 5 doses each given at 8, 24, 36, 48 and 60 hours (total 24 tablets over 60 hours)

● UNLICENSED USE Use in treatment of non-falciparum malaria is an unlicensed indication.

● CONTRA-INDICATIONS Family history of congenital QT interval prolongation · family history of sudden death · history of arrhythmias · history of clinically relevant bradycardia · history of congestive heart failure accompanied by reduced left ventricular ejection fraction

● CAUTIONS Avoid in Acute porphyrias p. 1107 · electrolyte disturbances (correct before and during treatment)

● INTERACTIONS → Appendix 1: antimalarials

● SIDE-EFFECTS

▶ **Common or very common** Abdominal pain · appetite decreased · arthralgia · asthenia · cough · diarrhoea · dizziness · gait abnormal · headache · movement disorders · myalgia · nausea · palpitations · QT interval prolongation · sensation abnormal · skin reactions · sleep disorders · vomiting

▶ **Uncommon** Drowsiness

▶ **Frequency not known** Angioedema

● PREGNANCY Toxicity in *animal* studies with artemether. Manufacturer advises use only if potential benefit outweighs risk.

● BREAST FEEDING Manufacturer advises avoid breastfeeding for at least 1 week after last dose. Present in milk in *animal* studies.

● HEPATIC IMPAIRMENT Manufacturer advises caution in severe impairment (no information available)—monitor ECG and plasma potassium concentration.

● RENAL IMPAIRMENT Manufacturer advises caution in severe impairment.
Monitoring In severe renal impairment monitor ECG and plasma potassium concentration.

● MONITORING REQUIREMENTS Monitor patients unable to take food (greater risk of recrudescence).

● DIRECTIONS FOR ADMINISTRATION Manufacturer advises tablets may be crushed just before administration.

● PATIENT AND CARER ADVICE
Driving and skilled tasks Dizziness may affect performance of skilled tasks (e.g. driving).

● MEDICINAL FORMS There can be variation in the licensing of different medicines containing the same drug.
Tablet
CAUTIONARY AND ADVISORY LABELS 21
▸ Riamet (Novartis Pharmaceuticals UK Ltd)
Artemether 20 mg, Lumefantrine 120 mg Riamet tablets | 24 tablet [PoM] £22.50

5

Infection

5

Infection

Artenimol with piperaquine phosphate

03-Sep-2020

(Piperaquine tetraphosphate with dihydroartemisinin)

● INDICATIONS AND DOSE

Treatment of uncomplicated falciparum malaria
▸ BY MOUTH
▸ Child 6 months-17 years (body-weight 7-12 kg): 0.5 tablet once daily for 3 days, max. 2 courses in 12 months; second course given at least 2 months after first course
▸ Child 6 months-17 years (body-weight 13-23 kg): 1 tablet once daily for 3 days, max. 2 courses in 12 months; second course given at least 2 months after first course
▸ Child 6 months-17 years (body-weight 24-35 kg): 2 tablets once daily for 3 days, max. 2 courses in 12 months; second course given at least 2 months after first course
▸ Child 6 months-17 years (body-weight 36-74 kg): 3 tablets once daily for 3 days, max. 2 courses in 12 months; second course given at least 2 months after first course
▸ Child 6 months-17 years (body-weight 75-99 kg): 4 tablets once daily for 3 days, max. 2 courses in 12 months; second course given at least 2 months after first course
▸ Adult (body-weight 36-74 kg): 3 tablets once daily for 3 days, max. 2 courses in 12 months; second course given at least 2 months after first course
▸ Adult (body-weight 75-99 kg): 4 tablets once daily for 3 days, max. 2 courses in 12 months; second course given at least 2 months after first course

● CONTRA-INDICATIONS Acute myocardial infarction · bradycardia · congenital long QT syndrome · electrolyte disturbances · family history of sudden death · heart failure with reduced left ventricular ejection fraction · history of symptomatic arrhythmias · left ventricular hypertrophy · risk factors for QT interval prolongation · severe hypertension

● INTERACTIONS → Appendix 1: antimalarials

● SIDE-EFFECTS
▸ **Common or very common** Anaemia · arrhythmias (in adults) · asthenia · conjunctivitis (in children) · eosinophilia · fever · headache (uncommon in children) · leucocytosis (in children) · leucopenia (in children) · neutropenia (in children) · QT interval prolongation · thrombocytopenia (in children)
▸ **Uncommon** Abdominal pain (very common in children) · appetite decreased (very common in children) · arthralgia · cardiac conduction disorder · cough (very common in children) · diarrhoea (very common in children) · dizziness (in adults) · epistaxis (in children) · hepatic disorders · hypochromia (in children) · increased risk of infection (very common in children) · lymphadenopathy (in children) · myalgia (in adults) · nausea · rhinorrhoea (in children) · seizure · skin reactions (very common in children) · splenomegaly (in children) · stomatitis (in children) · thrombocytosis (in children) · vomiting (very common in children)
● PREGNANCY Teratogenic in *animal* studies—manufacturer advises use only if other antimalarials cannot be used.
● BREAST FEEDING Manufacturer advises avoid—present in milk in *animal* studies.
● HEPATIC IMPAIRMENT Manufacturer advises caution in jaundice or in moderate to severe hepatic failure (no information available)—monitor ECG and plasma potassium concentration.
Monitoring Manufacturer advises monitor ECG and plasma-potassium concentration in moderate to severe hepatic impairment.
● RENAL IMPAIRMENT No information available in moderate to severe impairment.

Monitoring Manufacturer advises monitor ECG and plasma-potassium concentration in moderate to severe renal impairment.

● MONITORING REQUIREMENTS
▸ Consider obtaining ECG in all patients before third dose and 4–6 hours after third dose. If QT_C interval more than 500 milliseconds, discontinue treatment and monitor ECG for a further 24–48 hours.
▸ Obtain ECG as soon as possible after starting treatment then continue monitoring in those taking medicines that increase plasma-piperaquine concentration, in children who are vomiting, in females, or in the elderly.
● DIRECTIONS FOR ADMINISTRATION Manufacturer advises tablets to be taken at least 3 hours before and at least 3 hours after food. Tablets may be crushed and mixed with water immediately before administration.
● PATIENT AND CARER ADVICE Patients or carers should be given advice on how to administer tablets containing piperaquine phosphate with artenimol.

● MEDICINAL FORMS There can be variation in the licensing of different medicines containing the same drug.
Tablet
▸ Eurartesim (Logixx Pharma Solutions Ltd)
  Artenimol 40 mg, Piperaquine phosphate 320 mg Eurartesim 320mg/40mg tablets | 12 tablet [PoM] £40.00

Atovaquone with proguanil hydrochloride

15-Jul-2020

● INDICATIONS AND DOSE

Prophylaxis of falciparum malaria, particularly where resistance to other antimalarial drugs suspected [using 250 mg/100 mg tablets]
▸ BY MOUTH
▸ Adult (body-weight 40 kg and above): 1 tablet once daily, to be started 1–2 days before entering endemic area and continued for 1 week after leaving

Prophylaxis of falciparum malaria, particularly where resistance to other antimalarial drugs suspected [using 62.5 mg/25 mg tablets]
▸ BY MOUTH
▸ Adult (body-weight 30-39 kg): 3 tablets once daily, to be started 1–2 days before entering endemic area and continued for 1 week after leaving

Treatment of acute uncomplicated falciparum malaria [using 250 mg/100 mg tablets] | Treatment of non-falciparum malaria [using 250 mg/100 mg tablets]
▸ BY MOUTH
▸ Adult: 4 tablets once daily for 3 days

DOSE EQUIVALENCE AND CONVERSION
▸ Each 250 mg/100 mg tablet contains 250 mg of atovaquone and 100 mg of proguanil hydrochloride.
▸ Each 62.5 mg/25 mg tablet contains 62.5 mg of atovaquone and 25 mg of proguanil hydrochloride.

● UNLICENSED USE Not licensed for treatment of non-falciparum malaria.
● CAUTIONS Diarrhoea or vomiting (reduced absorption of atovaquone) · efficacy not evaluated in cerebral or complicated malaria (including hyperparasitaemia, pulmonary oedema or renal failure)
● INTERACTIONS → Appendix 1: antimalarials
● SIDE-EFFECTS
▸ **Common or very common** Abdominal pain · appetite decreased · cough · depression · diarrhoea · dizziness · fever · headache · nausea · skin reactions · sleep disorders · vomiting
▸ **Uncommon** Alopecia · anxiety · blood disorder · hyponatraemia · oral disorders · palpitations

- **Frequency not known** Hallucination · hepatic disorders · photosensitivity reaction · seizure · Stevens-Johnson syndrome · tachycardia · vasculitis
- **PREGNANCY** Manufacturer advises use only if potential benefit outweighs risk. See also *Pregnancy* in Malaria, prophylaxis p. 646.
- **BREAST FEEDING** Use only if no suitable alternative available.
- **RENAL IMPAIRMENT** Avoid for malaria prophylaxis (and if possible for malaria treatment) if eGFR less than 30 mL/minute/1.73m^2.
- **PATIENT AND CARER ADVICE** Warn travellers about **importance** of avoiding mosquito bites, **importance** of taking prophylaxis regularly, and **importance** of immediate visit to doctor if ill within 1 year and **especially** within 3 months of return.
- **NATIONAL FUNDING/ACCESS DECISIONS**
  NHS restrictions Drugs for malaria prophylaxis are not prescribable in NHS primary care; health authorities may investigate circumstances under which antimalarials are prescribed.

- **MEDICINAL FORMS** There can be variation in the licensing of different medicines containing the same drug.

Tablet
CAUTIONARY AND ADVISORY LABELS 21
- Atovaquone with proguanil hydrochloride (Non-proprietary)
  Proguanil hydrochloride 100 mg, Atovaquone 250 mg Proguanil 100mg / Atovaquone 250mg tablets | 12 tablet [PoM] £31.78 DT = £31.78
- Malarone (GlaxoSmithKline UK Ltd)
  Proguanil hydrochloride 25 mg, Atovaquone 62.5 mg Malarone Paediatric 62.5mg/25mg tablets | 12 tablet [PoM] £6.26 DT = £6.26
  Proguanil hydrochloride 100 mg, Atovaquone 250 mg Malarone 250mg/100mg tablets | 12 tablet [PoM] £25.21 DT = £31.78

Chloroquine

13-May-2020

- **INDICATIONS AND DOSE**

Active rheumatoid arthritis (administered on expert advice) | Systemic and discoid lupus erythematosus (administered on expert advice)
- BY MOUTH USING TABLETS
- Adult: 155 mg daily; maximum 2.5 mg/kg per day

Prophylaxis of malaria
- BY MOUTH USING SYRUP
- Child (body-weight up to 4.5 kg): 25 mg once weekly, started 1 week before entering endemic area and continued for 4 weeks after leaving
- Child (body-weight 4.5-7 kg): 50 mg once weekly, started 1 week before entering endemic area and continued for 4 weeks after leaving
- Child (body-weight 8-10 kg): 75 mg once weekly, started 1 week before entering endemic area and continued for 4 weeks after leaving
- Child (body-weight 11-14 kg): 100 mg once weekly, started 1 week before entering endemic area and continued for 4 weeks after leaving
- Child (body-weight 15-16.4 kg): 125 mg once weekly, started 1 week before entering endemic area and continued for 4 weeks after leaving
- Child (body-weight 16.5-24 kg): 150 mg once weekly, started 1 week before entering endemic area and continued for 4 weeks after leaving
- Child (body-weight 25-44 kg): 225 mg once weekly, started 1 week before entering endemic area and continued for 4 weeks after leaving
- Child (body-weight 45 kg and above): 300 mg once weekly, started 1 week before entering endemic area and continued for 4 weeks after leaving

- Adult (body-weight 45 kg and above): 300 mg once weekly, started 1 week before entering endemic area and continued for 4 weeks after leaving
- BY MOUTH USING TABLETS
- Child (body-weight up to 6 kg): 38.75 mg once weekly, started 1 week before entering endemic area and continued for 4 weeks after leaving
- Child (body-weight 6-9 kg): 77.5 mg once weekly, started 1 week before entering endemic area and continued for 4 weeks after leaving
- Child (body-weight 10-15 kg): 116.25 mg once weekly, started 1 week before entering endemic area and continued for 4 weeks after leaving
- Child (body-weight 16-24 kg): 155 mg once weekly, started 1 week before entering endemic area and continued for 4 weeks after leaving
- Child (body-weight 25-44 kg): 232.5 mg once weekly, started 1 week before entering endemic area and continued for 4 weeks after leaving
- Child (body-weight 45 kg and above): 310 mg once weekly, started 1 week before entering endemic area and continued for 4 weeks after leaving
- Adult (body-weight 25-44 kg): 232.5 mg once weekly, started 1 week before entering endemic area and continued for 4 weeks after leaving
- Adult (body-weight 45 kg and above): 310 mg once weekly, started 1 week before entering endemic area and continued for 4 weeks after leaving

Treatment of non-falciparum malaria
- BY MOUTH
- Child: Initially 10 mg/kg (max. per dose 620 mg), then 5 mg/kg after 6-8 hours (max. per dose 310 mg), then 5 mg/kg daily (max. per dose 310 mg) for 2 days
- Adult: Initially 620 mg, then 310 mg after 6-8 hours, then 310 mg daily for 2 days, approximate total cumulative dose of 25 mg/kg of base

***P. vivax* or *P. ovale* infection during pregnancy while radical cure is postponed**
- BY MOUTH
- Adult: 310 mg once weekly

DOSE EQUIVALENCE AND CONVERSION
- Doses expressed as chloroquine base.
- Each tablet contains 155 mg of chloroquine base (equivalent to 250 mg of chloroquine phosphate). Syrup contains 50 mg/5 mL of chloroquine base (equivalent to 80 mg/5 mL of chloroquine phosphate).

DOSES AT EXTREMES OF BODY-WEIGHT
- With oral use in adults In active rheumatoid arthritis and systemic and discoid lupus erythematosus, to avoid excessive dosage in obese patients, the daily maximum dose should be calculated on the basis of ideal body weight.

- **UNLICENSED USE** Chloroquine doses for the treatment and prophylaxis of malaria in BNF publications may differ from those in product literature.

> IMPORTANT SAFETY INFORMATION
> - In adults
> Ocular toxicity is unlikely if the dose of chloroquine phosphate does not exceed 4 mg/kg daily (equivalent to chloroquine base approx. 2.5 mg/kg daily).

- **CAUTIONS** Acute porphyrias p. 1107 · diabetes (may lower blood glucose) · G6PD deficiency · long-term therapy (risk of retinopathy and cardiomyopathy) · may aggravate myasthenia gravis · may exacerbate psoriasis · neurological disorders, especially epilepsy (may lower seizure threshold)—avoid for prophylaxis of malaria if history of epilepsy · severe gastro-intestinal disorders

5

Infection

- Monitoring for retinopathy
- In adults A review group convened by the Royal College of Ophthalmologists has updated guidelines on monitoring for chloroquine and hydroxychloroquine retinopathy (*Hydroxychloroquine and Chloroquine Retinopathy: Recommendations on Monitoring* 2020). Chloroquine appears to be more retinotoxic than hydroxychloroquine. Monitoring recommendations for chloroquine:
  - All patients planning to be on long-term treatment should receive a baseline examination (including fundus photography and spectral domain optical coherence tomography) within 6-12 months of treatment initiation;
  - Annual monitoring is recommended in all patients who have taken chloroquine for greater than 1 year.
- INTERACTIONS → Appendix 1: antimalarials
- SIDE-EFFECTS
- **Rare or very rare** Cardiomyopathy · hallucination · hepatitis
- **Frequency not known** Abdominal pain · agranulocytosis · alopecia · anxiety · atrioventricular block · bone marrow disorders · confusion · corneal deposits · depression · diarrhoea · eye disorders · gastrointestinal disorder · headache · hearing impairment · hypoglycaemia · hypotension · insomnia · interstitial lung disease · movement disorders · myopathy · nausea · neuromyopathy · neutropenia · personality change · photosensitivity reaction · psychotic disorder · QT interval prolongation · seizure · severe cutaneous adverse reactions (SCARs) · skin reactions · thrombocytopenia · tinnitus · tongue protrusion · vision disorders · vomiting

SIDE-EFFECTS, FURTHER INFORMATION Side-effects which occur at doses used in the prophylaxis or treatment of malaria are generally not serious.

Overdose Chloroquine is very toxic in overdosage; overdosage is extremely hazardous and difficult to treat. Urgent advice from the National Poisons Information Service is essential. Life-threatening features include arrhythmias (which can have a very rapid onset) and convulsions (which can be intractable).

- PREGNANCY Benefit of use in prophylaxis and treatment in malaria outweighs risk. For rheumatoid disease, it is not necessary to withdraw an antimalarial drug during pregnancy if the disease is well controlled.
- BREAST FEEDING Present in breast milk and breast-feeding should be avoided when used to treat rheumatic disease. Amount in milk probably too small to be harmful when used for malaria.
- HEPATIC IMPAIRMENT Manufacturer advises caution, particularly in cirrhosis.
- RENAL IMPAIRMENT Manufacturers advise caution.
  Dose adjustments Only partially excreted by the kidneys and reduction of the dose is not required for prophylaxis of malaria except in severe impairment.
  For rheumatoid arthritis and lupus erythematosus, reduce dose.
- MONITORING REQUIREMENTS
- In adults Manufacturer advises regular ophthalmological examination but the evidence of practical value is unsatisfactory (see *Cautions, further information* for advice of the Royal College of Ophthalmologists).
- In children Expert sources advise ophthalmic examination with long-term therapy.
- PATIENT AND CARER ADVICE Warn travellers going to malarious areas about **importance** of avoiding mosquito bites, **importance** of taking prophylaxis regularly, and **importance** of immediate visit to doctor if ill within 1 year and **especially** within 3 months of return.

- NATIONAL FUNDING/ACCESS DECISIONS
  NHS restrictions Drugs for malaria prophylaxis are not prescribable in NHS primary care; health authorities may investigate circumstances under which antimalarials are prescribed.
- EXCEPTIONS TO LEGAL CATEGORY *Tablets* can be sold to the public provided it is licensed and labelled for the prophylaxis of malaria.
- MEDICINAL FORMS There can be variation in the licensing of different medicines containing the same drug. Forms available from special-order manufacturers include: oral solution

Oral solution
CAUTIONARY AND ADVISORY LABELS 5
- Malarivon (Wallace Manufacturing Chemists Ltd)
  Chloroquine phosphate 16 mg per 1 ml Malarivon 80mg/5ml syrup | 75 ml [PoM] £30.00 DT = £30.00

Tablet
CAUTIONARY AND ADVISORY LABELS 5
- Avloclor (Alliance Pharmaceuticals Ltd)
  Chloroquine phosphate 250 mg Avloclor 250mg tablets | 20 tablet [P] £8.59 DT = £8.59

Chloroquine with proguanil

The properties listed below are those particular to the combination only. For the properties of the components please consider, chloroquine p. 655, proguanil hydrochloride p. 658.

- INDICATIONS AND DOSE
  Prophylaxis of malaria
  - BY MOUTH
  - Adult: (consult product literature)

- INTERACTIONS → Appendix 1: antimalarials
- EXCEPTIONS TO LEGAL CATEGORY Can be sold to the public provided it is licensed and labelled for the prophylaxis of malaria.

- MEDICINAL FORMS There can be variation in the licensing of different medicines containing the same drug.
  Tablet
  - Paludrine/Avloclor (Alliance Pharmaceuticals Ltd)
    Paludrine/Avloclor tablets anti-malarial travel pack | 112 tablet [P] £13.50

Mefloquine

02-Dec-2020

- INDICATIONS AND DOSE
  Treatment of malaria
  - BY MOUTH
  - Adult: (consult product literature)
  Prophylaxis of malaria
  - BY MOUTH
  - Child (body-weight 5-15 kg): 62.5 mg once weekly, dose to be started 2-3 weeks before entering endemic area and continued for 4 weeks after leaving
  - Child (body-weight 16-24 kg): 125 mg once weekly, dose to be started 2-3 weeks before entering endemic area and continued for 4 weeks after leaving
  - Child (body-weight 25-44 kg): 187.5 mg once weekly, dose to be started 2-3 weeks before entering endemic area and continued for 4 weeks after leaving
  - Child (body-weight 45 kg and above): 250 mg once weekly, dose to be started 2-3 weeks before entering endemic area and continued for 4 weeks after leaving
  - Adult (body-weight 25-44 kg): 187.5 mg once weekly, dose to be started 2-3 weeks before entering endemic area and continued for 4 weeks after leaving

▸ **Adult (body-weight 45 kg and above):** 250 mg once weekly, dose to be started 2–3 weeks before entering endemic area and continued for 4 weeks after leaving

- **UNLICENSED USE** Mefloquine doses in BNF Publications may differ from those in product literature.
- ▸ **In children** Not licensed for use in children under 5 kg body-weight and under 3 months.
- **CONTRA-INDICATIONS** Avoid for prophylaxis if history of psychiatric disorders (including depression) or convulsions · avoid for standby treatment if history of convulsions · history of blackwater fever
- **CAUTIONS** Cardiac conduction disorders · epilepsy (avoid for prophylaxis) · infants less than 3 months (limited experience) · not recommended in infants under 5 kg · traumatic brain injury

  CAUTIONS, FURTHER INFORMATION
- ▸ **Neuropsychiatric reactions** Mefloquine is associated with potentially serious neuropsychiatric reactions. Abnormal dreams, insomnia, anxiety, and depression occur commonly. Psychosis, suicidal ideation, and suicide have also been reported. Psychiatric symptoms such as insomnia, nightmares, acute anxiety, depression, restlessness, or confusion should be regarded as potentially prodromal for a more serious event. Adverse reactions may occur and persist up to several months after discontinuation because mefloquine has a long half-life. For a prescribing checklist, and further information on side-effects, particularly neuropsychiatric side-effects, which may be associated with the use of mefloquine for malaria prophylaxis, see the *Guide for Healthcare Professionals* provided by the manufacturer.
- **INTERACTIONS** → Appendix 1: antimalarials
- **SIDE-EFFECTS**
- ▸ **Common or very common** Anxiety · depression · diarrhoea · dizziness · gastrointestinal discomfort · headache · nausea · skin reactions · sleep disorders · vision disorders · vomiting
- ▸ **Frequency not known** Acute kidney injury · agranulocytosis · alopecia · aplastic anaemia · appetite decreased · arrhythmias · arthralgia · asthenia · behaviour abnormal · cardiac conduction disorders · cataract · chest pain · chills · concentration impaired · confusion · cranial nerve paralysis · delusional disorder · depersonalisation · drowsiness · dyspnoea · encephalopathy · eye disorder · fever · flushing · gait abnormal · hallucination · hearing impairment · hepatic disorders · hyperacusia · hyperhidrosis · hypertension · hypotension · leucocytosis · leucopenia · malaise · memory loss · mood altered · movement disorders · muscle complaints · muscle weakness · nephritis · nerve disorders · oedema · palpitations · pancreatitis · paraesthesia · pneumonia · pneumonitis · psychosis · seizure · self-endangering behaviour · speech disorder · Stevens-Johnson syndrome · suicidal behaviours · syncope · thrombocytopenia · tinnitus · tremor · vertigo
- **ALLERGY AND CROSS-SENSITIVITY** [EvGr] Contra-indicated in patients with hypersensitivity to quinine. ⟨M⟩
- **CONCEPTION AND CONTRACEPTION** Manufacturer advises adequate contraception during prophylaxis and for 3 months after stopping (teratogenicity in *animal* studies).
- **PREGNANCY** Manufacturer advises avoid (particularly in the first trimester) unless the potential benefit outweighs the risk; however, studies of mefloquine in pregnancy (including use in the first trimester) indicate that it can be considered for travel to chloroquine-resistant areas.
- **BREAST FEEDING** Present in milk but risk to infant minimal.
- **HEPATIC IMPAIRMENT** Manufacturer advises avoid in severe impairment—elimination may be prolonged.
- **RENAL IMPAIRMENT** Manufacturer advises caution.

- **DIRECTIONS FOR ADMINISTRATION** Expert sources advise tablet may be crushed and mixed with food such as jam or honey just before administration.
- **PATIENT AND CARER ADVICE** Manufacturer advises that patients receiving mefloquine for malaria prophylaxis should be informed to discontinue its use if neuropsychiatric symptoms occur and seek immediate medical advice so that mefloquine can be replaced with an alternative antimalarial. Travellers should also be warned about **importance** of avoiding mosquito bites, **importance** of taking prophylaxis regularly, and **importance** of immediate visit to doctor if ill within 1 year and especially within 3 months of return.

  A patient alert card should be provided.

  Driving and skilled tasks Dizziness or a disturbed sense of balance may affect performance of skilled tasks (e.g. driving); effects may occur and persist up to several months after stopping mefloquine.
- **NATIONAL FUNDING/ACCESS DECISIONS**

  NHS restrictions Drugs for malaria prophylaxis are not prescribable in NHS primary care; health authorities may investigate circumstances under which antimalarials are prescribed.

- **MEDICINAL FORMS** There can be variation in the licensing of different medicines containing the same drug.

  Tablet

  CAUTIONARY AND ADVISORY LABELS 10, 21, 27
  - ▸ Lariam (Neon Healthcare Ltd)
    Mefloquine (as Mefloquine hydrochloride) 250 mg Lariam 250mg tablets | 8 tablet [PoM] £14.53 DT = £14.53

Primaquine

05-Aug-2020

- **INDICATIONS AND DOSE**

  Adjunct in the treatment of non-falciparum malaria caused by *Plasmodium vivax* infection
  - ▸ BY MOUTH
  - ▸ **Adult:** 30 mg daily for 14 days

  Adjunct in the treatment of non-falciparum malaria caused by *Plasmodium ovale* infection
  - ▸ BY MOUTH
  - ▸ **Adult:** 15 mg daily for 14 days

  Adjunct in the treatment of non-falciparum malaria caused by *Plasmodium vivax* infection in patients with mild G6PD deficiency (administered on expert advice) | **Adjunct in the treatment of non-falciparum malaria caused by *Plasmodium ovale* infection in patients with mild G6PD deficiency (administered on expert advice)**
  - ▸ BY MOUTH
  - ▸ **Adult:** 45 mg once weekly for 8 weeks

  Treatment of mild to moderate pneumocystis infection (in combination with clindamycin)
  - ▸ BY MOUTH
  - ▸ **Adult:** 30 mg daily, this combination is associated with considerable toxicity

- **UNLICENSED USE** Not licensed.
- **CAUTIONS** G6PD deficiency · systemic diseases associated with granulocytopenia (e.g. rheumatoid arthritis, lupus erythematosus)
- **INTERACTIONS** → Appendix 1: antimalarials
- **SIDE-EFFECTS** Arrhythmia · dizziness · gastrointestinal discomfort · haemolytic anaemia (in G6PD deficiency) · leucopenia · methaemoglobinaemia (in NADH methaemoglobin reductase deficiency) · nausea · QT interval prolongation · skin reactions · vomiting
- **PREGNANCY** Risk of neonatal haemolysis and methaemoglobinaemia in third trimester.

5

Infection

- BREAST FEEDING No information available; theoretical risk of haemolysis in G6PD-deficient infants.
- PRE-TREATMENT SCREENING Before starting primaquine, blood should be tested for glucose-6-phosphate dehydrogenase (G6PD) activity since the drug can cause haemolysis in G6PD-deficient patients. Specialist advice should be obtained in G6PD deficiency.

- MEDICINAL FORMS There can be variation in the licensing of different medicines containing the same drug. Forms available from special-order manufacturers include: oral suspension

Tablet
  ▸ Primaquine (Non-proprietary)
    Primaquine (as Primaquine phosphate) 7.5 mg Primaquine 7.5mg tablets | 100 tablet 🖳
  ▸ Primaquine (Imported (United States))
    Primaquine (as Primaquine phosphate) 15 mg Primaquine 15mg tablets | 100 tablet PoM 🖳

Proguanil hydrochloride
04-Aug-2020

- INDICATIONS AND DOSE
Prophylaxis of malaria
▸ BY MOUTH
  ▸ Child (body-weight up to 6 kg): 25 mg once daily, dose to be started 1 week before entering endemic area and continued for 4 weeks after leaving
  ▸ Child (body-weight 6–9 kg): 50 mg once daily, dose to be started 1 week before entering endemic area and continued for 4 weeks after leaving
  ▸ Child (body-weight 10–15 kg): 75 mg once daily, dose to be started 1 week before entering endemic area and continued for 4 weeks after leaving
  ▸ Child (body-weight 16–24 kg): 100 mg once daily, dose to be started 1 week before entering endemic area and continued for 4 weeks after leaving
  ▸ Child (body-weight 25–44 kg): 150 mg once daily, dose to be started 1 week before entering endemic area and continued for 4 weeks after leaving
  ▸ Child (body-weight 45 kg and above): 200 mg once daily, dose to be started 1 week before entering endemic area and continued for 4 weeks after leaving
  ▸ Adult (body-weight 25–44 kg): 150 mg once daily, dose to be started 1 week before entering endemic area and continued for 4 weeks after leaving
  ▸ Adult (body-weight 45 kg and above): 200 mg once daily, dose to be started 1 week before entering endemic area and continued for 4 weeks after leaving

- UNLICENSED USE Proguanil doses in BNF Publications may differ from those in product literature.
- INTERACTIONS → Appendix 1: antimalarials
- SIDE-EFFECTS Alopecia · angioedema · bone marrow disorders · cholestasis · constipation · diarrhoea · fever · gastric disorder · megaloblastic anaemia · oral disorders · skin reactions · vasculitis
- PREGNANCY Benefit of prophylaxis in malaria outweighs risk. Adequate folate supplements should be given to mother.
- BREAST FEEDING Amount in milk probably too small to be harmful when used for malaria prophylaxis.
- RENAL IMPAIRMENT
  Dose adjustments ▸ In children Use half normal dose if estimated glomerular filtration rate 20–60 mL/minute/1.73m². Use one-quarter normal dose on alternate days if estimated glomerular filtration rate 10–20 mL/minute/1.73m². Use one-quarter normal dose once weekly if estimated glomerular filtration rate less than 10 mL/minute/1.73m²; increased risk of haematological toxicity in severe impairment.

  ▸ In adults 100 mg once daily if eGFR 20–60 mL/minute/1.73m². 50 mg on alternate days if eGFR 10–20 mL/minute/1.73m². 50 mg once weekly if eGFR less than 10 mL/minute/1.73m²; increased risk of haematological toxicity in severe impairment.

- DIRECTIONS FOR ADMINISTRATION Manufacturer advises tablet may be crushed and mixed with food such as milk, jam, or honey just before administration.
- PATIENT AND CARER ADVICE Warn travellers about **importance** of avoiding mosquito bites, **importance** of taking prophylaxis regularly, and **importance** of immediate visit to doctor if ill within 1 year and **especially** within 3 months of return.
- NATIONAL FUNDING/ACCESS DECISIONS
  NHS restrictions Drugs for malaria prophylaxis are not prescribable in NHS primary care; health authorities may investigate circumstances under which antimalarials are prescribed.
- EXCEPTIONS TO LEGAL CATEGORY Can be sold to the public provided it is licensed and labelled for the prophylaxis of malaria.
- MEDICINAL FORMS There can be variation in the licensing of different medicines containing the same drug. Forms available from special-order manufacturers include: oral suspension, oral solution

Tablet
CAUTIONARY AND ADVISORY LABELS 21
  ▸ Paludrine (Alliance Pharmaceuticals Ltd)
    Proguanil hydrochloride 100 mg Paludrine 100mg tablets | 98 tablet P £11.95 DT = £11.95

Quinine
27-Jul-2020

- INDICATIONS AND DOSE
Nocturnal leg cramps
▸ BY MOUTH
  ▸ Adult: 200–300 mg once daily, to be taken at bedtime
Non-falciparum malaria
▸ BY INTRAVENOUS INFUSION
  ▸ Adult: 10 mg/kg every 8 hours (max. per dose 700 mg), infused over 4 hours, given if patient is unable to take oral therapy. Change to oral chloroquine as soon as the patient's condition permits, reduce dose to 5–7 mg/kg if parenteral treatment is required for more than 48 hours
Falciparum malaria
▸ BY MOUTH
  ▸ Child: 10 mg/kg every 8 hours (max. per dose 600 mg) for 7 days, to be given together with or followed by either doxycycline (in children over 12 years), or clindamycin
  ▸ Adult: 600 mg every 8 hours for 5–7 days, to be given together with or followed by either doxycycline or clindamycin
▸ BY INTRAVENOUS INFUSION
  ▸ Adult: Loading dose 20 mg/kg (max. per dose 1.4 g), infused over 4 hours, the loading dose of 20 mg/kg should **not** be used if the patient has received quinine or mefloquine during the previous 12 hours, then maintenance 10 mg/kg every 8 hours (max. per dose 700 mg) until patient can swallow tablets to complete the 7-day course, maintenance dose to be given 8 hours after the start of the loading dose and infused over 4 hours, to be given together with or followed by either doxycycline or clindamycin, reduce maintenance dose to 5–7 mg/kg if parenteral treatment is required for more than 48 hours

Falciparum malaria (in intensive care unit)

▶ BY INTRAVENOUS INFUSION

▶ **Adult:** Loading dose 7 mg/kg, infused over 30 minutes, followed immediately by 10 mg/kg, infused over 4 hours, then maintenance 10 mg/kg every 8 hours (max. per dose 700 mg) until patient can swallow tablets to complete the 7-day course, maintenance dose to be given 8 hours after the start of the loading dose and infused over 4 hours, to be given together with or followed by either doxycycline or clindamycin, reduce maintenance dose to 5–7 mg/kg if parenteral treatment is required for more than 48 hours

DOSE EQUIVALENCE AND CONVERSION

▶ When using quinine for malaria, doses are valid for quinine hydrochloride, dihydrochloride, and sulfate; they are **not valid** for quinine bisulfate which contains a correspondingly smaller amount of quinine.

▶ Quinine (anhydrous base) 100 mg = quinine bisulfate 169 mg; quinine dihydrochloride 122 mg; quinine hydrochloride 122 mg; and quinine sulfate 121 mg. Quinine bisulfate 300 mg tablets are available but provide less quinine than 300 mg of the dihydrochloride, hydrochloride, or sulfate.

● UNLICENSED USE Injection not licensed.

IMPORTANT SAFETY INFORMATION

MHRA/CHM ADVICE: REMINDER OF DOSE-DEPENDENT QT-PROLONGING EFFECTS (NOVEMBER 2017)

Quinine has been associated with dose-dependent QT-interval-prolonging effects and should be used with caution in patients with risk factors for QT prolongation or in those with atrioventricular block—see Cautions for further information.

● CONTRA-INDICATIONS Haemoglobinuria · myasthenia gravis · optic neuritis · tinnitus

● CAUTIONS Atrial fibrillation (monitor ECG during parenteral treatment) · cardiac disease (monitor ECG during parenteral treatment) · conduction defects (monitor ECG during parenteral treatment) · elderly (monitor ECG during parenteral treatment) · electrolyte disturbance · G6PD deficiency · heart block (monitor ECG during parenteral treatment)

● INTERACTIONS → Appendix 1: antimalarials

● SIDE-EFFECTS Abdominal pain · agitation · agranulocytosis · angioedema · asthma · atrioventricular conduction changes · bronchospasm · cardiotoxicity · cerebral impairment · coagulation disorders · coma · confusion · death · diarrhoea · dyspnoea · fever · flushing · gastrointestinal disorder · haemoglobinuria · haemolysis · haemolytic uraemic syndrome · headache · hearing impairment · hypersensitivity · loss of consciousness · muscle weakness · myasthenia gravis aggravated · nausea · ocular toxicity · oedema · pancytopenia · photosensitivity reaction · QT interval prolongation · renal impairment · skin reactions · thrombocytopenia · tinnitus · vertigo · vision disorders · vomiting

Overdose Quinine is very toxic in overdosage; life-threatening features include arrhythmias (which can have a very rapid onset) and convulsions (which can be intractable).
For details on the management of poisoning, see Emergency treatment of poisoning p. 1413.

● PREGNANCY High doses are teratogenic in *first trimester*, but in malaria benefit of treatment outweighs risk.

● BREAST FEEDING Present in milk but not known to be harmful.

● HEPATIC IMPAIRMENT
▶ With oral use Manufacturer advises caution (risk of prolonged half-life).

Dose adjustments ▶ With intravenous use For treatment of malaria in severe impairment, reduce parenteral maintenance dose to 5–7 mg/kg of quinine salt.
▶ With oral use Manufacturer advises dose reduction or increased dose interval.

● RENAL IMPAIRMENT

Dose adjustments ▶ With intravenous use For treatment of malaria in severe impairment, reduce parenteral maintenance dose to 5–7 mg/kg of quinine salt.

● MONITORING REQUIREMENTS
▶ With intravenous use Monitor blood glucose and electrolyte concentration during parenteral treatment.
▶ In adults Patients taking quinine for nocturnal leg cramps should be monitored closely during the early stages for adverse effects as well as for benefit.

● DIRECTIONS FOR ADMINISTRATION For *intravenous infusion*, expert sources advise give continuously in Glucose 5% or Sodium Chloride 0.9%. To be given over 4 hours.

● PRESCRIBING AND DISPENSING INFORMATION
▶ With intravenous use Intravenous injection of quinine is so hazardous that it has been superseded by infusion.

● MEDICINAL FORMS There can be variation in the licensing of different medicines containing the same drug. Forms available from special-order manufacturers include: capsule, oral suspension, oral solution, solution for infusion

Tablet
▶ Quinine (Non-proprietary)
Quinine sulfate 200 mg Quinine sulfate 200mg tablets |
28 tablet PoM £2.90 DT = £2.42
Quinine bisulfate 300 mg Quinine bisulfate 300mg tablets |
28 tablet PoM £9.75 DT = £8.97
Quinine sulfate 300 mg Quinine sulfate 300mg tablets |
28 tablet PoM £6.16 DT = £6.16

5.2 Toxoplasmosis

ANTIPROTOZOALS

Pyrimethamine   01-Jun-2020

● INDICATIONS AND DOSE

Toxoplasmosis in pregnancy (in combination with sulfadiazine and folinic acid)

▶ BY MOUTH
▶ **Adult:** 50 mg once daily until delivery

● CAUTIONS History of seizures—avoid large loading doses · predisposition to folate deficiency

● INTERACTIONS → Appendix 1: antimalarials

● SIDE-EFFECTS
▶ **Common or very common** Anaemia · diarrhoea · dizziness · headache · leucopenia · nausea · skin reactions · thrombocytopenia · vomiting
▶ **Uncommon** Fever
▶ **Rare or very rare** Abdominal pain · oral ulceration · pancytopenia · pneumonia eosinophilic · seizure

● PREGNANCY Theoretical teratogenic risk in *first trimester* (folate antagonist). Adequate folate supplements should be given to the mother.

● BREAST FEEDING Significant amount in milk—avoid administration of other folate antagonists to infant. Avoid breast-feeding during toxoplasmosis treatment.

● HEPATIC IMPAIRMENT Manufacturer advises caution.

● RENAL IMPAIRMENT Manufacturer advises caution.

● MONITORING REQUIREMENTS Blood counts required with prolonged treatment.

5

Infection

● MEDICINAL FORMS There can be variation in the licensing of different medicines containing the same drug. Forms available from special-order manufacturers include: oral suspension

Tablet

▸ Daraprim (GlaxoSmithKline UK Ltd)

Pyrimethamine 25 mg Daraprim 25mg tablets | 30 tablet PoM
£13.00 DT = £13.00

6 Viral infection

6.1 Coronavirus

COVID-19

21-Aug-2020

Description of condition

COVID-19 is the syndrome caused by a novel coronavirus, SARS-CoV-2, which was originally detected late 2019 in Wuhan, Hubei Province, China. Primary transmission between people is through respiratory droplets generated by coughing and sneezing, and through contact with contaminated surfaces.

COVID-19 is predominantly a respiratory illness with early non-specific symptoms that can last 2–10 days before more specific signs or symptoms develop. The most common symptoms are fever, cough, and shortness of breath. Other symptoms, such as anxiety, delirium, agitation, fatigue, muscle aches, headache, and a loss of sense of smell may also be present. The illness varies in severity from no symptoms present in some individuals to severe pneumonia in others. Older patients and/or those with co-morbidities (such as chronic obstructive pulmonary disease, cystic fibrosis, asthma, cardiovascular disease, and diabetes), frailty, impaired immunity, or a reduced ability to cough and clear secretions are more likely to develop severe pneumonia. Patients with severe symptoms of COVID-19 may deteriorate rapidly and older patients with co-morbidities may have a higher risk of deteriorating.

Management

Medical practitioners must notify the proper officer at their local council or local health protection team of all suspected cases of COVID-19. For further information, see *Notifiable diseases* in Antibacterials, principles of therapy p. 527.

The National Institute of Health and Care Excellence (NICE) have developed rapid guidelines to maximise patient safety, optimise treatment management, protect staff from infection, and make the best use of NHS resources. These guidelines provide recommendations around the provision of care during the pandemic (such as critical care in adults and systemic anticancer treatments), and for managing symptoms (including at the end of life) and suspected/confirmed pneumonia. They also include recommendations for patients with conditions that increase the risk of developing COVID-19 (such as in immunocompromised patients; those with severe asthma; cystic fibrosis; rheumatological autoimmune, inflammatory and metabolic bone disorders; or conditions treated with drugs that affect the immune response). NICE are also developing rapid evidence summaries focusing on whether certain medications (such as non-steroidal anti-inflammatory drugs) may increase the severity/length of the COVID-19 illness, and advice on the safety and efficacy of COVID-19 treatments (such as remdesivir p. 661). For further information, see NICE rapid guidelines and evidence summaries: **Coronavirus (COVID-19)**(see *Useful resources*).

NHS England and NHS Improvement have produced guidance for clinicians and NHS managers working in primary and secondary care, and community-based health, social care, mental health trusts and ambulance services. For further information, see NHS England: **Coronavirus guidance for clinicians and NHS managers** (see *Useful resources*).

Public Health England (PHE) have also produced guidance for health professionals, the public, and those in non-clinical settings; on infection prevention and control; and sampling and diagnostics. For further information, see the PHE collection: **Coronavirus (COVID-19): guidance** (see *Useful resources*).

The Medicines and Healthcare products Regulatory Agency (MHRA) have issued COVID-19 guidance for industry, information about medications and COVID-19, and guidance on medical devices (such as COVID-19 tests and testing kits). For further information, see the MHRA collection: **MHRA guidance on coronavirus (COVID-19)** (see *Useful resources*). In addition, information on the use of dexamethasone for the management of COVID-19 is available at: www.gov.uk/drug-safety-update/letters-and-drug-alerts-sent-to-healthcare-professionals-in-may-2020.

The UK Teratology Information Service (UKTIS) have produced an information page summarising the fetal and neonatal risks of exposure to COVID-19 treatments that have either been identified as possible options or listed as investigational medicinal products. For further information, see UKTIS: **Medications used to treat COVID-19 in pregnancy** (see *Useful resources*).

The UK Drugs in Lactation Advisory Service (UKDILAS) are updating breastfeeding advice for drugs that may be used for COVID-19 (such as remdesivir) on the Specialist Pharmacy Service website (available at: www.sps.nhs.uk/articles/ukdilas/).

The Joint Committee on Vaccination and Immunisation (JCVI) have issued statements on immunisation prioritisation and delivery of the routine human papillomavirus vaccination programme for children, during the COVID-19 pandemic (available at: tinyurl.com/yygw3ea4 and tinyurl.com/yyla flue).

The Scottish Intercollegiate Guidelines Network (SIGN) have issued position statements that provide guidance around the provision of care (such as maternal critical care), and management of patients with COVID-19 (such as presentation and management of older people in acute care, and prevention and management of thromboembolism in hospitalised patients). SIGN have also produced an evidence review with advice on assessment of patients with COVID-19 in primary care. For further information, see SIGN: **COVID-19 guidance** (see *Useful resources*).

Additional country-specific guidance is available for Northern Ireland, Scotland, and Wales (see *Useful resources*).

Useful Resources

Medicines and Healthcare products Regulatory Agency. MHRA guidance on coronavirus (COVID-19) collection. www.gov.uk/government/collections/mhra-guidance-on-coronavirus-covid-19

National Health Service England and National Health Service Improvement. Coronavirus guidance for clinicians and NHS managers. www.england.nhs.uk/coronavirus/

National Institute for Health and Care Excellence. Coronavirus (COVID-19) rapid guidelines and evidence summaries. www.nice.org.uk/covid-19

Public Health England. Coronavirus (COVID-19) collection. www.gov.uk/government/collections/coronavirus-covid-19-list-of-guidance

Scottish Intercollegiate Guidelines Network. COVID-19 guidance. www.sign.ac.uk/

UK Teratology Information Service. Medications used to treat COVID-19 in pregnancy. www.medicinesinpregnancy.org/bumps/monographs/MEDICATIONS-USED-TO-TREAT-COVID-19-IN-PREGNANCY/

Northern Ireland Government Services. Coronavirus (COVID-19).
www.nidirect.gov.uk/campaigns/coronavirus-covid-19
Public Health Agency in Northern Ireland. Coronavirus (COVID-19).
www.publichealth.hscni.net/covid-19-coronavirus
Scottish Government. Coronavirus in Scotland.
www.gov.scot/coronavirus-covid-19/
Health Protection Scotland. Coronavirus (COVID-19).
www.hps.scot.nhs.uk/a-to-z-of-topics/covid-19/
Welsh Government. Coronavirus (COVID-19).
gov.wales/coronavirus
Public Health Wales. Novel Coronavirus (COVID-19).
phw.nhs.wales/topics/latest-information-on-novel-coronavirus-covid-19/

ANTIVIRALS ⟩ OTHER

Remdesivir
09-Nov-2020

- **DRUG ACTION** Remdesivir (a prodrug), is an RNA polymerase inhibitor that disrupts the production of viral RNA, preventing multiplication of the virus.

- **INDICATIONS AND DOSE**

COVID-19 in patients with pneumonia requiring supplemental oxygen (under close medical supervision)
  ▶ BY INTRAVENOUS INFUSION
  ▹ Adult (body-weight 40 kg and above): Loading dose 200 mg daily for 1 dose, then maintenance 100 mg once daily for 5–10 days in total

- **INTERACTIONS** → Appendix 1: remdesivir

- **SIDE-EFFECTS**
- **Common or very common** Headache · nausea · rash
▶ **Rare or very rare** Hypersensitivity · infusion related reaction

  SIDE-EFFECTS, FURTHER INFORMATION Manufacturer advises slower infusion rates, with a maximum infusion time of up to 120 minutes, to prevent signs and symptoms of hypersensitivity. If significant hypersensitivity occurs, discontinue immediately.

- **CONCEPTION AND CONTRACEPTION** Manufacturer advises females of childbearing potential should use effective contraception during treatment.

- **PREGNANCY** Manufacturer advises avoid unless potential benefit outweighs risk—no information available.

- **BREAST FEEDING** Specialist sources indicate use with caution—limited information. Minimal oral absorption expected, but monitor breast-fed infants for adverse reactions such as diarrhoea, rash, hypotension, liver and renal impairment (increased risk of accumulation due to long half-life).

- **HEPATIC IMPAIRMENT** Manufacturer advises caution (no information available)—treatment should not be started if ALT is ≥5 times the upper limit of normal. If ALT increases during treatment, remdesivir may need to be withheld, consult product literature for further information.

- **RENAL IMPAIRMENT** Manufacturer advises avoid if eGFR less than 30 mL/minute/1.73 m^2— *Veklury*® formulation excipient (sulfobutylether beta cyclodextrin sodium) may accumulate.

- **MONITORING REQUIREMENTS**
▶ Manufacturer advises monitor liver function at baseline and periodically during treatment as indicated.
▶ Manufacturer advises monitor eGFR at baseline and periodically during treatment as indicated—severe renal toxicity in *animal* studies.

- **DIRECTIONS FOR ADMINISTRATION** EvGr For *intravenous infusion* (*Veklury*® concentrate for solution for infusion), dilute in Sodium Chloride 0.9%; give over 30–120 minutes.

For *intravenous infusion* (*Veklury*® powder for concentrate for solution for infusion), reconstitute each vial with 19 mL Water for Injections, then dilute in Sodium Chloride 0.9%; give over 30–120 minutes. ⓜ For further information on dilution and infusion rates—consult product literature.

- **HANDLING AND STORAGE** *Veklury*® concentrate for solution for infusion should be stored in a refrigerator (2–8°C)—consult product literature about storage after dilution. For *Veklury*® powder for concentrate for solution for infusion—consult product literature about storage after reconstitution and dilution.

- **MEDICINAL FORMS** There can be variation in the licensing of different medicines containing the same drug.
Solution for infusion
EXCIPIENTS: May contain Sulfobutylether beta cyclodextrin sodium
  ▶ Veklury (Gilead Sciences Ireland UC) ▼
  Remdesivir 5 mg per 1 ml Veklury 100mg/20ml concentrate for solution for infusion vials | 1 vial PoM £340.00 (Hospital only)
Powder for solution for infusion
EXCIPIENTS: May contain Sulfobutylether beta cyclodextrin sodium
  ▶ Veklury (Gilead Sciences Ireland UC) ▼
  Remdesivir 100 mg Veklury 100mg powder for concentrate for solution for infusion vials | 1 vial PoM £340.00 (Hospital only)

6.2 Hepatitis

Hepatitis

Overview

Treatment for viral hepatitis should be initiated by a specialist. The management of uncomplicated acute viral hepatitis is largely symptomatic. Early treatment of acute hepatitis C with interferon alfa [unlicensed indication] may reduce the risk of chronic infection. Hepatitis B and hepatitis C viruses are major causes of chronic hepatitis. Active or passive immunisation against hepatitis A and B infections can be given.

Chronic hepatitis B

Peginterferon alfa p. 664 is an option for the initial treatment of chronic hepatitis B and may be preferable to interferon alfa. The use of peginterferon alfa and interferon alfa is limited by a response rate of 30–40% and relapse is frequent. Treatment should be discontinued if no improvement occurs after 4 months. The manufacturers of peginterferon alfa-2a and interferon alfa contraindicate use in decompensated liver disease, but low doses can be used with great caution in these patients. Although interferon alfa is contra-indicated in patients receiving immunosuppressant treatment (or who have received it recently), cautious use of peginterferon alfa-2a may be justified in some cases.

Entecavir p. 662 or tenofovir disoproxil p. 692 are options for the initial treatment of chronic hepatitis B. If the response is inadequate after 6–9 months of treatment, a change in treatment should be considered.

Entecavir alone, tenofovir disoproxil alone, or a combination of lamivudine p. 691 with either adefovir dipivoxil p. 663 or tenofovir disoproxil can be used in patients with decompensated liver disease.

If drug-resistant hepatitis B virus emerges during treatment, another antiviral drug to which the virus is sensitive should be added. Hepatitis B viruses with reduced susceptibility to lamivudine have emerged following extended therapy. Adefovir dipivoxil or tenofovir disoproxil can be given with lamivudine in lamivudine-resistant chronic hepatitis B; telbivudine or entecavir should not be used because cross-resistance can occur.

If there is no toxicity or loss in efficacy, treatment with adefovir dipivoxil, entecavir, lamivudine, telbivudine, or tenofovir disoproxil is usually continued until 6 months after adequate seroconversion has occurred. Treatment is usually continued long-term in patients with decompensated liver disease.

Tenofovir disoproxil, or a combination of tenofovir disoproxil with either emtricitabine p. 689 or lamivudine may be used with other antiretrovirals, as part of 'highly active antiretroviral therapy' in patients who require treatment for both HIV and chronic hepatitis B. If patients infected with both HIV and chronic hepatitis B only require treatment for chronic hepatitis B, they should receive antivirals that are not active against HIV, such as peginterferon alfa or adefovir dipivoxil. Treatment may be continued long-term, even if adequate seroconversion occurs. Management of these patients should be coordinated between HIV and hepatology specialists.

Chronic hepatitis C

Before starting treatment, the genotype of the infecting hepatitis C virus should be determined and the viral load measured as this may affect the choice and duration of treatment. A combination of ribavirin p. 666 and peginterferon alfa is used for the treatment of chronic hepatitis C. The combination of ribavirin and interferon alfa is less effective than the combination of peginterferon alfa and ribavirin. Peginterferon alfa alone should be used if ribavirin is contra-indicated or not tolerated. Ribavirin monotherapy is ineffective.

Daclatasvir is licensed for use in combination with sofosbuvir p. 668 for the treatment of chronic hepatitis C infection of genotypes 1 or 4, with or without compensated cirrhosis; the addition of ribavirin should be considered for patients with advanced liver disease or with other negative prognostic factors, such as prior treatment experience. It is also licensed in combination with sofosbuvir and ribavirin for the treatment of chronic hepatitis C infection of genotype 3 in patients who are treatment experienced, with or without compensated cirrhosis, and in combination with peginterferon alfa and ribavirin for the treatment of chronic hepatitis C infection of genotype 4. Daclatasvir must not be given as monotherapy.

Ombitasvir with paritaprevir and ritonavir p. 665 (*Viekirax*®), is licensed for use in combination with dasabuvir p. 670, with or without ribavirin, for the treatment of chronic hepatitis C infection of genotype 1 in patients with or without compensated cirrhosis; it is also licensed for use in combination with ribavirin for the treatment of chronic hepatitis C infection of genotype 4 with or without compensated cirrhosis.

Ribavirin inhibits a wide range of DNA and RNA viruses. It is given by mouth for the treatment of chronic hepatitis C infection, in double therapy with peginterferon alfa, interferon alfa, or sofosbuvir, or in triple therapy with peginterferon alfa and one protease inhibitor or sofosbuvir. Ribavirin is also effective in Lassa fever [unlicensed indication].

Sofosbuvir is a pro-drug of a nucleoside inhibitor that is effective against hepatitis C virus polymerase NS5B. It is licensed for use in combination with ribavirin, with or without peginterferon alfa, for the treatment of chronic hepatitis C infection of genotypes 1, 2, 3, 4, 5, or 6 in patients with compensated liver disease. Sofosbuvir monotherapy is not recommended because it is less effective than combination therapy.

Ledipasvir is licensed for use in combination with sofosbuvir (ledipasvir with sofosbuvir p. 668), with or without ribavirin, for the treatment of chronic hepatitis C infections of genotypes 1, 3, 4, 5 or 6.

Sofosbuvir with velpatasvir and voxilaprevir p. 669 is licensed for the treatment of chronic hepatitis C of all genotypes.

6.3 Hepatitis infections

6.3a Chronic hepatitis B

> **Other drugs used for Chronic hepatitis B** Lamivudine, p. 691 · Tenofovir disoproxil, p. 692

ANTIVIRALS 〉 NUCLEOSIDE ANALOGUES

❘ Entecavir

03-Aug-2020

● **INDICATIONS AND DOSE**

Chronic hepatitis B in patients with compensated liver disease (with evidence of viral replication, and histologically documented active liver inflammation or fibrosis) not previously treated with nucleoside analogues

▸ BY MOUTH
  ▸ Adult: 500 micrograms once daily

Chronic hepatitis B in patients with compensated liver disease (with evidence of viral replication, and histologically documented active liver inflammation or fibrosis) and lamivudine-resistance

▸ BY MOUTH
  ▸ Adult: 1 mg once daily, consider other treatment if inadequate response after 6 months

Chronic hepatitis B in patients with decompensated liver disease

▸ BY MOUTH
  ▸ Adult: 1 mg once daily

● CAUTIONS HIV infection—risk of HIV resistance in patients not receiving 'highly active antiretroviral therapy' · lamivudine-resistant chronic hepatitis B—risk of entecavir resistance

CAUTIONS, FURTHER INFORMATION Manufacturer advises review treatment and consider discontinuation if deterioration in liver function occurs (risk of lactic acidosis)—consult product literature.

● SIDE-EFFECTS

▸ **Common or very common** Diarrhoea · dizziness · drowsiness · dyspepsia · fatigue · headache · insomnia · nausea · vomiting

▸ **Uncommon** Alopecia · rash

▸ **Frequency not known** Lactic acidosis

● CONCEPTION AND CONTRACEPTION Effective contraception required during treatment.

● PREGNANCY Toxicity in *animal* studies—manufacturer advises use only if potential benefit outweighs risk.

● BREAST FEEDING Manufacturer advises avoid—present in milk in *animal* studies.

● RENAL IMPAIRMENT Consult product literature.
  Dose adjustments Reduce dose if eGFR less than 50 mL/minute/1.73 m^2.

● MONITORING REQUIREMENTS Monitor liver function tests every 3 months, and viral markers for hepatitis B every 3–6 months during treatment (continue monitoring for at least 1 year after discontinuation—recurrent hepatitis may occur on discontinuation).

● DIRECTIONS FOR ADMINISTRATION Manufacturer advises to be taken at least 2 hours before or 2 hours after food.

● PRESCRIBING AND DISPENSING INFORMATION Flavours of oral liquid formulations may include orange.

● PATIENT AND CARER ADVICE Patients or carers should be counselled on the administration of entecavir tablets and oral solution.

5

Infection

- **NATIONAL FUNDING/ACCESS DECISIONS**
  For full details see funding body website
  NICE decisions
- ▶ Entecavir for the treatment of chronic hepatitis B (August 2008) NICE TA153 Recommended

- **MEDICINAL FORMS** There can be variation in the licensing of different medicines containing the same drug.
  Oral solution
  ▶ Baraclude (Bristol-Myers Squibb Pharmaceuticals Ltd)
  Entecavir (as Entecavir monohydrate) 50 microgram per 1 ml Baraclude 0.05mg/ml oral solution sugar-free | 210 ml [PoM]
  £423.80 DT = £423.80
  Tablet
  ▶ Entecavir (Non-proprietary)
  Entecavir (as Entecavir monohydrate) 500 microgram Entecavir 500microgram tablets | 30 tablet [PoM] £363.26 DT = £363.26 | 30 tablet [PoM] £363.26 DT = £363.26 (Hospital only)
  Entecavir (as Entecavir monohydrate) 1 mg Entecavir 1mg tablets | 30 tablet [PoM] £363.26 DT = £363.26 | 30 tablet [PoM] £363.26 DT = £363.26 (Hospital only)
  ▶ Baraclude (Bristol-Myers Squibb Pharmaceuticals Ltd)
  Entecavir (as Entecavir monohydrate) 500 microgram Baraclude 0.5mg tablets | 30 tablet [PoM] £363.26 DT = £363.26
  Entecavir (as Entecavir monohydrate) 1 mg Baraclude 1mg tablets | 30 tablet [PoM] £363.26 DT = £363.26

ANTIVIRALS > NUCLEOSIDE REVERSE TRANSCRIPTASE INHIBITORS

⚑ 685

Tenofovir alafenamide
26-Feb-2018

- **INDICATIONS AND DOSE**
  Chronic hepatitis B (initiated by a specialist)
  ▶ BY MOUTH
  ▶ Adult: 25 mg once daily (for duration of treatment consult product literature)

- **CAUTIONS** Decompensated liver disease · HIV co-infection
- **INTERACTIONS** → Appendix 1: tenofovir alafenamide
- **SIDE-EFFECTS**
- ▶ **Common or very common** Abdominal distension · arthralgia
- ▶ **Frequency not known** Hepatitis aggravated (during or following treatment) · nephrotoxicity

- **BREAST FEEDING** Manufacturer advises avoid—present in milk in *animal* studies.

- **HEPATIC IMPAIRMENT** Manufacturer advises caution in decompensated hepatic disease (no information available).

- **PRE-TREATMENT SCREENING** Manufacturer advises HIV antibody testing should be offered to those with unknown HIV-1 status before initiation of treatment.

- **MONITORING REQUIREMENTS** Manufacturer advises monitor liver function tests at repeated intervals during treatment and for at least 6 months after last dose— recurrent hepatitis may occur on discontinuation.

- **PATIENT AND CARER ADVICE**
  Missed doses Manufacturer advises if a dose is more than 18 hours late, the missed dose should not be taken and the next dose should be taken at the normal time.

- **MEDICINAL FORMS** There can be variation in the licensing of different medicines containing the same drug.
  Tablet
  CAUTIONARY AND ADVISORY LABELS 21
  ▶ Vemlidy (Gilead Sciences Ireland UC) ▼
  Tenofovir alafenamide (as Tenofovir alafenamide fumarate) 25 mg Vemlidy 25mg tablets | 30 tablet [PoM] £325.73

ANTIVIRALS > NUCLEOTIDE ANALOGUES

Adefovir dipivoxil
25-Jun-2020

- **INDICATIONS AND DOSE**
  Chronic hepatitis B infection with either compensated liver disease with evidence of viral replication, and histologically documented active liver inflammation and fibrosis, when other treatment not appropriate or decompensated liver disease in combination with another antiviral for chronic hepatitis B that has no cross-resistance to adefovir
  ▶ BY MOUTH
  ▶ Adult: 10 mg once daily

- **CAUTIONS** Elderly
  CAUTIONS, FURTHER INFORMATION Manufacturer advises review treatment and consider discontinuation if deterioration in liver function occurs (risk of lactic acidosis)—consult product literature.

- **INTERACTIONS** → Appendix 1: adefovir

- **SIDE-EFFECTS**
- ▶ **Common or very common** Asthenia · diarrhoea · flatulence · gastrointestinal discomfort · headache · nausea · renal impairment · skin reactions · vomiting
- ▶ **Frequency not known** Bone fracture · bone pain · hypophosphataemia · myopathy · nephrotoxicity · osteomalacia · pancreatitis · proximal renal tubulopathy

- **CONCEPTION AND CONTRACEPTION** Effective contraception required during treatment.

- **PREGNANCY** Toxicity in *animal* studies—manufacturer advises use only if potential benefit outweighs risk.

- **BREAST FEEDING** Manufacturer advises avoid—no information available.

- **RENAL IMPAIRMENT** No information available if eGFR less than 10 mL/minute/1.73 m^2.
  Dose adjustments 10 mg every 48 hours if eGFR 30–50 mL/minute/1.73 m^2; 10 mg every 72 hours if eGFR 10–30 mL/minute/1.73 m^2.
  Monitoring Monitor renal function more frequently in patients with renal impairment.

- **MONITORING REQUIREMENTS**
- ▶ Monitor liver function tests every 3 months, and viral markers for hepatitis B every 3–6 months during treatment (continue monitoring for at least 1 year after discontinuation—recurrent hepatitis may occur on discontinuation).
- ▶ Monitor renal function before treatment then every 3 months, more frequently in patients receiving nephrotoxic drugs.

- **MEDICINAL FORMS** There can be variation in the licensing of different medicines containing the same drug.
  Tablet
  ▶ Hepsera (Gilead Sciences Ireland UC)
  Adefovir dipivoxil 10 mg Hepsera 10mg tablets | 30 tablet [PoM] £252.22 DT = £252.22

IMMUNOSTIMULANTS 〉 INTERFERONS

Peginterferon alfa

20-Nov-2020

- DRUG ACTION Polyethylene glycol-conjugated ('pegylated') derivatives of interferon alfa (**peginterferon alfa-2a** and **peginterferon alfa-2b**) are available; pegylation increases the persistence of the interferon in the blood.

- INDICATIONS AND DOSE

  PEGASYS ®

  Combined with ribavirin for chronic hepatitis C | Monotherapy for chronic hepatitis C if ribavirin not tolerated or contra-indicated | Monotherapy for chronic hepatitis B
  - ▸ BY SUBCUTANEOUS INJECTION
  - ▸ Adult: (consult product literature)

- CONTRA-INDICATIONS For contra-indications consult product literature.
- CAUTIONS For cautions consult product literature.
- INTERACTIONS → Appendix 1: interferons
- SIDE-EFFECTS
  - ▸ **Common or very common** Alopecia · anaemia · anxiety · appetite abnormal · arrhythmias · arthralgia · arthritis · asthenia · ataxia · behaviour abnormal · breast pain · chest discomfort · chills · concentration impaired · confusion · constipation · cough · crying · dehydration · depression · diarrhoea · dizziness · drowsiness · dry eye · dry mouth · dysphagia · dysphonia · dyspnoea · ear pain · eye discomfort · eye disorders · eye inflammation · feeling abnormal · fever · gastrointestinal discomfort · gastrointestinal disorders · haemolytic anaemia · haemorrhage · hair texture abnormal · headaches · hearing impairment · hyperbilirubinaemia · hypertension · hyperthyroidism · hyperuricaemia · hypotension · hypothyroidism · increased risk of infection · influenza like illness · leucopenia · lymphadenopathy · malaise · memory loss · menstrual cycle irregularities · mood altered · muscle complaints · muscle tone increased · muscle weakness · nail disorder · nasal complaints · nausea · neutropenia · oedema · oral disorders · ovarian disorder · pain · palpitations · photosensitivity reaction · prostatitis · respiratory disorders · sensation abnormal · sepsis · sexual dysfunction · skin reactions · sleep disorders · sweat changes · syncope · taste altered · thirst · throat complaints · thrombocytopenia · tinnitus · tremor · urinary disorders · urine abnormal · vaginal disorder · vasodilation · vertigo · vision disorders · vomiting · weight decreased
  - ▸ **Uncommon** Diabetes mellitus · hallucination · hypersensitivity · hypertriglyceridaemia · myocardial infarction · nerve disorders · pancreatitis · psychosis · sarcoidosis · suicidal behaviours · thyroiditis
  - ▸ **Rare or very rare** Angioedema · bone marrow disorders · cardiac inflammation · cardiomyopathy · cerebral ischaemia · CNS haemorrhage · coma · congestive heart failure · diabetic ketoacidosis · embolism and thrombosis · encephalopathy · facial paralysis · injection site necrosis · ischaemic heart disease · myopathy · renal failure · retinopathy · seizure (more common with high doses in the elderly) · severe cutaneous adverse reactions (SCARs) · systemic lupus erythematosus (SLE) · ulcerative colitis · vasculitis
  - ▸ **Frequency not known** Homicidal ideation · pericardial effusion · peripheral ischaemia · pulmonary arterial hypertension · pure red cell aplasia · solid organ transplant rejection · tongue discolouration
- CONCEPTION AND CONTRACEPTION Effective contraception required during treatment—consult product literature.

- PREGNANCY Manufacturers recommend avoid unless potential benefit outweighs risk (toxicity in *animal* studies).
- BREAST FEEDING Manufacturers advise avoid—no information available.
- HEPATIC IMPAIRMENT Manufacturer advises avoid in severe impairment and decompensated cirrhosis.
- RENAL IMPAIRMENT For further information on peginterferon alfa use in renal impairment consult product literature.

  Dose adjustments Reduce dose in moderate to severe impairment.

  Monitoring Close monitoring required in renal impairment.
- MONITORING REQUIREMENTS Monitoring of lipid concentration is recommended.
- NATIONAL FUNDING/ACCESS DECISIONS For full details see funding body website

  NICE decisions
  - ▸ **Peginterferon alfa and ribavirin for the treatment of chronic hepatitis C (September 2010)** NICE TA200 Recommended with restrictions

- MEDICINAL FORMS There can be variation in the licensing of different medicines containing the same drug.

  Solution for injection

  EXCIPIENTS: May contain Benzyl alcohol
  - ▸ Pegasys (Roche Products Ltd)

    Interferon alfa-2a (as Peginterferon alfa-2a) 180 microgram per 1 ml Pegasys 90micrograms/0.5ml solution for injection pre-filled syringes | 1 pre-filled disposable injection [PoM] £76.51

    Interferon alfa-2a (as Peginterferon alfa-2a) 270 microgram per 1 ml Pegasys 135micrograms/0.5ml solution for injection pre-filled syringes | 1 pre-filled disposable injection [PoM] £107.76 DT = £107.76

    Interferon alfa-2a (as Peginterferon alfa-2a) 360 microgram per 1 ml Pegasys 180micrograms/0.5ml solution for injection pre-filled syringes | 4 pre-filled disposable injection [PoM] £497.60

6.3b Chronic hepatitis C

Other drugs used for Chronic hepatitis C Peginterferon alfa, above

ANTIVIRALS 〉 HCV INHIBITORS

Elbasvir with grazoprevir

31-Aug-2020

- DRUG ACTION Elbasvir is an HCV NS5A inhibitor and grazoprevir is an HCV NS3/4A protease inhibitor; they reduce viral load by inhibiting hepatitis C virus RNA replication.

- INDICATIONS AND DOSE

  Chronic hepatitis C infection of genotypes 1 or 4 (with or without ribavirin) (initiated by a specialist)
  - ▸ BY MOUTH
  - ▸ Adult: 50/100 mg once daily for 12 weeks (may extend to 16 weeks in some circumstances—consult product literature)

  DOSE EQUIVALENCE AND CONVERSION
  - ▸ Dose expressed as x/y mg elbasvir/grazoprevir.

  IMPORTANT SAFETY INFORMATION

  MHRA/CHM ADVICE: DIRECT-ACTING ANTIVIRALS TO TREAT CHRONIC HEPATITIS C: RISK OF INTERACTION WITH VITAMIN K ANTAGONISTS AND CHANGES IN INR (JANUARY 2017)

  An EU-wide review has identified that changes in liver function, secondary to hepatitis C treatment with direct-acting antivirals, may affect the efficacy of vitamin K antagonists; the MHRA has advised that INR should be monitored closely in patients receiving concomitant treatment.

MHRA/CHM ADVICE: DIRECT-ACTING ANTIVIRAL INTERFERON-FREE REGIMENS TO TREAT CHRONIC HEPATITIS C: RISK OF HEPATITIS B REACTIVATION (JANUARY 2017)

An EU-wide review has concluded that direct-acting antiviral interferon-free regimens for chronic hepatitis C can cause hepatitis B reactivation in patients co-infected with hepatitis B and C viruses; the MHRA recommends to screen patients for hepatitis B before starting treatment—patients infected with both hepatitis B and C viruses must be monitored and managed according to current clinical guidelines.

MHRA/CHM ADVICE: DIRECT-ACTING ANTIVIRALS FOR CHRONIC HEPATITIS C: RISK OF HYPOGLYCAEMIA IN PATIENTS WITH DIABETES (DECEMBER 2018)

Rapid reduction in hepatitis C viral load during direct-acting antiviral therapy for hepatitis C may improve glucose metabolism in patients with diabetes and result in symptomatic hypoglycaemia if diabetic treatment is continued at the same dose.

The MHRA advises healthcare professionals:
- to monitor glucose levels closely in patients with diabetes during direct-acting antiviral therapy for hepatitis C, especially within the first 3 months of treatment and modify diabetic medication or doses when necessary;
- to be vigilant for changes in glucose tolerance and advise patients of the risk of hypoglycaemia;
- to inform the healthcare professional in charge of the diabetic care of the patient when direct-acting antiviral therapy is initiated.

- CAUTIONS Hepatitis B co-infection · re-treatment following previous exposure to elbasvir with grazoprevir, or to drugs of the same classes (NS5A inhibitors or NS3/4A inhibitors other than telaprevir, simeprevir, boceprevir)—efficacy not demonstrated

- INTERACTIONS → Appendix 1: elbasvir · grazoprevir

- SIDE-EFFECTS
- **Common or very common** Alopecia · anxiety · appetite decreased · arthralgia · asthenia · constipation · depression · diarrhoea · dizziness · dry mouth · gastrointestinal discomfort · headache · insomnia · irritability · myalgia · nausea · pruritus · vomiting
- **Uncommon** Anaemia · transient ischaemic attack

- PREGNANCY Manufacturer advises use only if potential benefit outweighs risk.

- BREAST FEEDING Manufacturer advises avoid—present in milk in *animal* studies.

- HEPATIC IMPAIRMENT Manufacturer advises avoid in moderate to severe impairment.

- MONITORING REQUIREMENTS Manufacturer advises monitor liver function before treatment, at week 8 in all patients, at week 12 in patients receiving 16 weeks of treatment, and then as clinically indicated—consider discontinuing treatment if alanine aminotransferase (ALT) is greater than 10 times the upper limit of normal; discontinue treatment if ALT elevation is accompanied by signs or symptoms of hepatic impairment or inflammation.

- PATIENT AND CARER ADVICE
Hepatic effects Manufacturer advises that patients and their carers should consult a healthcare professional if signs and symptoms of hepatic dysfunction occur (including fatigue, weakness, lack of appetite, nausea and vomiting, jaundice or discoloured faeces).
Vomiting Manufacturer advises if vomiting occurs within 4 hours of a dose, an additional dose should be taken.
Missed doses Manufacturer advises if a dose is more than 16 hours late, the missed dose should not be taken and the next dose should be taken at the normal time.

- NATIONAL FUNDING/ACCESS DECISIONS
For full details see funding body website
NICE decisions
▸ Elbasvir–grazoprevir for treating chronic hepatitis C (October 2016) NICE TA413 Recommended
Scottish Medicines Consortium (SMC) decisions
▸ Elbasvir with grazoprevir (*Zepatier*®) for chronic hepatitis C (January 2017) SMC No. 1203/17 Recommended

- MEDICINAL FORMS There can be variation in the licensing of different medicines containing the same drug.
Tablet
CAUTIONARY AND ADVISORY LABELS 3
ELECTROLYTES: May contain Sodium
▸ Zepatier (Merck Sharp & Dohme Ltd) ▼
Elbasvir 50 mg, Grazoprevir 100 mg Zepatier 50mg/100mg tablets | 28 tablet PoM £12,166.67

ANTIVIRALS > NON-STRUCTURAL PROTEIN 5A INHIBITORS

Ombitasvir with paritaprevir and ritonavir

06-May-2020

The properties listed below are those particular to the combination only. For the properties of the components please consider, ritonavir p. 698.

- INDICATIONS AND DOSE
Chronic hepatitis C of genotype 1 (in combination with dasabuvir, with or without ribavirin) | Chronic hepatitis C of genotype 4 (in combination with ribavirin)
▸ BY MOUTH
▸ Adult: 2 tablets once daily for duration of treatment consult product literature, to be taken with food

IMPORTANT SAFETY INFORMATION
MHRA/CHM ADVICE: DIRECT-ACTING ANTIVIRALS TO TREAT CHRONIC HEPATITIS C: RISK OF INTERACTION WITH VITAMIN K ANTAGONISTS AND CHANGES IN INR (JANUARY 2017)

An EU-wide review has identified that changes in liver function, secondary to hepatitis C treatment with direct-acting antivirals, may affect the efficacy of vitamin K antagonists; the MHRA has advised that INR should be monitored closely in patients receiving concomitant treatment.

MHRA/CHM ADVICE: DIRECT-ACTING ANTIVIRAL INTERFERON-FREE REGIMENS TO TREAT CHRONIC HEPATITIS C: RISK OF HEPATITIS B REACTIVATION (JANUARY 2017)

An EU-wide review has concluded that direct-acting antiviral interferon-free regimens for chronic hepatitis C can cause hepatitis B reactivation in patients co-infected with hepatitis B and C viruses; the MHRA recommends to screen patients for hepatitis B before starting treatment—patients infected with both hepatitis B and C viruses must be monitored and managed according to current clinical guidelines.

MHRA/CHM ADVICE: DIRECT-ACTING ANTIVIRALS FOR CHRONIC HEPATITIS C: RISK OF HYPOGLYCAEMIA IN PATIENTS WITH DIABETES (DECEMBER 2018)

Rapid reduction in hepatitis C viral load during direct-acting antiviral therapy for hepatitis C may improve glucose metabolism in patients with diabetes and result in symptomatic hypoglycaemia if diabetic treatment is continued at the same dose.

The MHRA advises healthcare professionals:
- to monitor glucose levels closely in patients with diabetes during direct-acting antiviral therapy for hepatitis C, especially within the first 3 months of treatment and modify diabetic medication or doses when necessary;

5

Infection

- to be vigilant for changes in glucose tolerance and advise patients of the risk of hypoglycaemia;
- to inform the healthcare professional in charge of the diabetic care of the patient when direct-acting antiviral therapy is initiated.

- CONTRA-INDICATIONS HIV co-infection without suppressive antiretroviral therapy
- CAUTIONS Psychiatric disorders · retreatment—efficacy not established
- INTERACTIONS → Appendix 1: HIV-protease inhibitors · ombitasvir · paritaprevir
- SIDE-EFFECTS
- ▸ **Common or very common** Anaemia · asthenia · diarrhoea · insomnia · nausea · pruritus · vomiting
- ▸ **Uncommon** Dehydration
- ▸ **Rare or very rare** Angioedema
- ▸ **Frequency not known** Depression · hepatic failure · hepatitis B reactivation · suicidal behaviours

  SIDE-EFFECTS, FURTHER INFORMATION Side-effects listed are reported when ombitasvir with paritaprevir and ritonavir is used in combination with dasabuvir, with or without ribavirin.
- CONCEPTION AND CONTRACEPTION For women of child-bearing potential, exclude pregnancy before initiation of treatment; effective contraception should be used during treatment.
- PREGNANCY Manufacturer advises avoid—toxicity in *animal* studies.
- BREAST FEEDING Manufacturer advises avoid—present in milk in *animal* studies.
- HEPATIC IMPAIRMENT Manufacturer advises avoid in moderate to severe impairment.
- PATIENT AND CARER ADVICE
  Missed doses If a dose is more than 12 hours late, the missed dose should not be taken and the next dose should be taken at the normal time.
- NATIONAL FUNDING/ACCESS DECISIONS
  For full details see funding body website
  NICE decisions
- ▸ Ombitasvir with paritaprevir and ritonavir with or without dasabuvir for treating chronic hepatitis C (November 2015) NICE TA365 Recommended with restrictions

- MEDICINAL FORMS No licensed medicines listed.

ANTIVIRALS ⟩ NUCLEOSIDE ANALOGUES

▍Ribavirin

(Tribavirin)

20-Nov-2020

- INDICATIONS AND DOSE
  Bronchiolitis
- ▸ BY INHALATION OF AEROSOL, OR BY INHALATION OF NEBULISED SOLUTION
- ▸ **Child 1-23 months:** Inhale a solution containing 20 mg/mL for 12–18 hours for at least 3 days, maximum of 7 days, to be administered via small particle aerosol generator

  Life-threatening RSV, parainfluenza virus, and adenovirus infection in immunocompromised children (administered on expert advice)
- ▸ BY INTRAVENOUS INFUSION
- ▸ **Child:** 33 mg/kg for 1 dose, to be administered over 15 minutes, then 16 mg/kg every 6 hours for 4 days, then 8 mg/kg every 8 hours for 3 days

COPEGUS® TABLETS

Chronic hepatitis C (in combination with direct acting antivirals, or interferon alfa 2a, or peginterferon alfa 2a with or without direct acting antivirals)
- ▸ BY MOUTH
- ▸ **Adult (body-weight up to 75 kg):** 400 mg, dose to be taken in the morning and 600 mg, dose to be taken in the evening
- ▸ **Adult (body-weight 75 kg and above):** 600 mg twice daily

Chronic hepatitis C (in combination with peginterferon alfa 2b with or without direct acting antivirals)
- ▸ BY MOUTH
- ▸ **Adult (body-weight up to 65 kg):** 400 mg twice daily
- ▸ **Adult (body-weight 65-80 kg):** 400 mg, to be taken in the morning and 600 mg, to be taken in the evening
- ▸ **Adult (body-weight 81-105 kg):** 600 mg twice daily
- ▸ **Adult (body-weight 106 kg and above):** 600 mg, to be taken in the morning and 800 mg, to be taken in the evening

Chronic hepatitis C genotype 2 or 3 (not previously treated), or patients infected with HIV and hepatitis C (in combination with peginterferon alfa)
- ▸ BY MOUTH
- ▸ **Adult:** Usual dose 400 mg twice daily

REBETOL® CAPSULES

Chronic hepatitis C (in combination with interferon alfa 2b, or peginterferon alfa 2b with or without boceprevir)
- ▸ BY MOUTH
- ▸ **Adult (body-weight up to 65 kg):** 400 mg twice daily
- ▸ **Adult (body-weight 65-80 kg):** 400 mg, dose to be taken in the morning and 600 mg, dose to be taken in the evening
- ▸ **Adult (body-weight 81-104 kg):** 600 mg twice daily
- ▸ **Adult (body-weight 105 kg and above):** 600 mg, dose to be taken in the morning and 800 mg, dose to be taken in the evening

REBETOL® ORAL SOLUTION

Chronic hepatitis C (in combination with interferon alfa 2b, or peginterferon alfa 2b with or without boceprevir)
- ▸ BY MOUTH
- ▸ **Adult (body-weight up to 65 kg):** 400 mg twice daily
- ▸ **Adult (body-weight 65-80 kg):** 400 mg, dose to be taken in the morning and 600 mg, dose to be taken in the evening
- ▸ **Adult (body-weight 81-104 kg):** 600 mg twice daily
- ▸ **Adult (body-weight 105 kg and above):** 600 mg, dose to be taken in the morning and 800 mg, dose to be taken in the evening

- UNLICENSED USE
- ▸ When used by inhalation in children Inhalation licensed for use in children (age range not specified by manufacturer).
- ▸ With intravenous use in children Intravenous preparation not licensed.
- CONTRA-INDICATIONS
- ▸ With systemic use consult product literature for specific contra-indications when ribavirin used in combination with other medicinal products · haemoglobinopathies · severe cardiac disease (in adults) · severe, uncontrolled cardiac disease in children with chronic hepatitis C · unstable or uncontrolled cardiac disease in previous 6 months (in adults)
- CAUTIONS
- ▸ When used by inhalation maintain standard supportive respiratory and fluid management therapy
- ▸ With systemic use anaemia (haemoglobin concentration should be monitored during the treatment and corrective action taken) (in adults) · cardiac disease (assessment including ECG recommended before and during treatment—discontinue if deterioration) · consult product

literature for specific cautions when ribavirin used in combination with other medicinal products · gout (in adults) · haemolysis (haemoglobin concentration should be monitored during the treatment and corrective action taken) (in adults) · patients with a transplant—risk of rejection · risk of growth retardation in children, the reversibility of which is uncertain—if possible, consider starting treatment after pubertal growth spurt · severe dental disorders (in adults) · severe ocular disorders (in adults) · severe periodontal disorders (in adults) · severe psychiatric effects (in adults)

● INTERACTIONS → Appendix 1: ribavirin

● SIDE-EFFECTS
▸ **Common or very common** Alopecia · anaemia · anxiety · appetite decreased · arrhythmias · arthralgia · arthritis · asthenia · behaviour abnormal · chest pain · chills · concentration impaired · constipation · cough · depression · diarrhoea · dizziness · drowsiness · dry mouth · dysphagia · dyspnoea · ear pain · eye disorders · eye inflammation · eye pain · fever · gastrointestinal discomfort · gastrointestinal disorders · haemorrhage · headaches · hyperthyroidism · hypotension · hypothyroidism · increased risk of infection · influenza like illness · lymphadenopathy · malaise · memory loss · mood altered · muscle complaints · muscle weakness · nasal congestion · nausea · neutropenia · oral disorders · pain · palpitations · peripheral oedema · photosensitivity reaction · respiratory disorders · sensation abnormal · sexual dysfunction · skin reactions · sleep disorders · sweat changes · syncope · taste altered · thirst · throat pain · thrombocytopenia · tinnitus · tremor · vasodilation · vertigo · vision disorders · vomiting · weight decreased
▸ **Uncommon** Dehydration · diabetes mellitus · hallucination · hearing loss · hepatic disorders · hypertension · nerve disorders · sarcoidosis · suicidal behaviours · thyroiditis
▸ **Rare or very rare** Angina pectoris · angioedema · bone marrow disorders · cardiac inflammation · cerebral ischaemia · cholangitis · coma · congestive heart failure · facial paralysis · hepatic failure (discontinue) · hypersensitivity · intracranial haemorrhage · myocardial infarction · myopathy · pancreatitis · psychotic disorder · pulmonary embolism · retinopathy · seizure · severe cutaneous adverse reactions (SCARs) · systemic lupus erythematosus (SLE) · vasculitis
▸ **Frequency not known** Haemolytic anaemia · homicidal ideation · nephrotic syndrome · pure red cell aplasia · renal failure · solid organ transplant rejection · tongue discolouration · ulcerative colitis

SIDE-EFFECTS, FURTHER INFORMATION Side effects listed are reported when oral ribavirin is used in combination with peginterferon alfa or interferon alfa, consult product literature for details.

● CONCEPTION AND CONTRACEPTION
▸ With systemic use Exclude pregnancy before treatment in females of childbearing age. Effective contraception essential during treatment and for 4 months after treatment in females and for 7 months after treatment in males of childbearing age. Routine monthly pregnancy tests recommended. Condoms must be used if partner of male patient is pregnant (ribavirin excreted in semen).
▸ When used by inhalation Women planning pregnancy should avoid exposure to aerosol.

● PREGNANCY Avoid; teratogenicity in *animal* studies.
▸ When used by inhalation Pregnant women should avoid exposure to aerosol.

● BREAST FEEDING Avoid—no information available.

● RENAL IMPAIRMENT Plasma-ribavirin concentration increased.
▸ In adults Manufacturer advises avoid oral ribavirin unless essential if eGFR less than 50 mL/minute/1.73 m²— monitor haemoglobin concentration closely.

▸ In children Manufacturer advises avoid oral ribavirin if estimated glomerular filtration rate less than 50 mL/minute/1.73 m²—monitor haemoglobin concentration closely. Manufacturer advises use intravenous preparation with caution if estimated glomerular filtration rate less than 30 mL/minute/1.73 m².

● MONITORING REQUIREMENTS
▸ When used by inhalation Monitor electrolytes closely. Monitor equipment for precipitation.
▸ With systemic use in children Determine full blood count, platelets, electrolytes, serum creatinine, liver function tests and uric acid before starting treatment and then on weeks 2 and 4 of treatment, then as indicated clinically— adjust dose if adverse reactions or laboratory abnormalities develop (consult product literature). Test thyroid function before treatment and then every 3 months.
▸ With oral use in children Eye examination recommended before treatment. Eye examination also recommended during treatment if pre-existing ophthalmological disorder or if decrease in vision reported—discontinue treatment if ophthalmological disorder deteriorates or if new ophthalmological disorder develops.
▸ With systemic use in adults Determine full blood count, platelets, electrolytes, glucose, serum creatinine, liver function tests and uric acid before starting treatment and then on weeks 2 and 4 of treatment, then as indicated clinically—adjust dose if adverse reactions or laboratory abnormalities develop (consult product literature).

● PRESCRIBING AND DISPENSING INFORMATION Flavours of oral liquid formulations may include bubble-gum.

● NATIONAL FUNDING/ACCESS DECISIONS
For full details see funding body website
NICE decisions
▸ **Peginterferon alfa and ribavirin for the treatment of chronic hepatitis C (September 2010)** NICE TA200 Recommended with restrictions
▸ **Peginterferon alfa and ribavirin for treating chronic hepatitis C in children and young people (November 2013)** NICE TA300 Recommended

● LESS SUITABLE FOR PRESCRIBING Ribavirin inhalation is less suitable for prescribing.

● MEDICINAL FORMS There can be variation in the licensing of different medicines containing the same drug.

Oral solution
CAUTIONARY AND ADVISORY LABELS 21
▸ Rebetol (Merck Sharp & Dohme Ltd)
Ribavirin 40 mg per 1 ml Rebetol 40mg/ml oral solution | 100 ml PoM £67.08

Tablet
CAUTIONARY AND ADVISORY LABELS 21
▸ Ribavirin (Non-proprietary)
Ribavirin 200 mg Ribavirin 200mg tablets | 42 tablet PoM £92.50 | 112 tablet PoM £246.65 | 168 tablet PoM £369.98

Capsule
CAUTIONARY AND ADVISORY LABELS 21
▸ Ribavirin (Non-proprietary)
Ribavirin 200 mg Ribavirin 200mg capsules | 84 capsule PoM £160.69 | 140 capsule PoM £267.81 | 168 capsule PoM £321.38

5

Infection

ANTIVIRALS > NUCLEOTIDE ANALOGUES

Ledipasvir with sofosbuvir

09-Nov-2020

The properties listed below are those particular to the combination only. For the properties of the components please consider, sofosbuvir below.

- **DRUG ACTION** Sofosbuvir is a nucleotide analogue inhibitor and ledipasvir is an HCV inhibitor; they reduce viral load by inhibiting hepatitis C virus RNA replication.

- **INDICATIONS AND DOSE**

Chronic hepatitis C infection (initiated by a specialist)
- ▸ BY MOUTH
- ▸ Adult: 90/400 mg once daily, for duration of treatment consult product literature

DOSE ADJUSTMENTS DUE TO INTERACTIONS
- ▸ Manufacturer advises reduce dose of concurrent H₂-receptor antagonist if above a dose comparable to famotidine 40 mg twice daily.
- ▸ Manufacturer advises reduce dose of concurrent proton pump inhibitor if above a dose comparable to omeprazole 20 mg; take at the same time as sofosbuvir with ledipasvir.

DOSE EQUIVALENCE AND CONVERSION
- ▸ Dose expressed as x/y mg ledipasvir/sofosbuvir.

- **CAUTIONS** Retreatment following treatment failure—efficacy not established
- **INTERACTIONS** → Appendix 1: ledipasvir · sofosbuvir
- **SIDE-EFFECTS**
- ▸ **Common or very common** Fatigue · headache · rash
- ▸ **Frequency not known** Angioedema · arrhythmia · Stevens-Johnson syndrome
- **PRESCRIBING AND DISPENSING INFORMATION** Dispense in original container (contains desiccant).
- **PATIENT AND CARER ADVICE**
  Vomiting If vomiting occurs within 5 hours of administration, an additional dose should be taken.
  Missed doses If a dose is more than 18 hours late, the missed dose should not be taken and the next dose should be taken at the normal time.
- **NATIONAL FUNDING/ACCESS DECISIONS**
  For full details see funding body website
  NICE decisions
- ▸ Ledipasvir-sofosbuvir for treating chronic hepatitis C (November 2015) NICE TA363 Recommended with restrictions
  Scottish Medicines Consortium (SMC) decisions
- ▸ Ledipasvir with sofosbuvir (*Harvoni*®) for the treatment of chronic hepatitis C (CHC) in adults (March 2015) SMC No. 1030/15 Recommended with restrictions
- ▸ Ledipasvir with sofosbuvir (*Harvoni*®) for the treatment of genotype 3 chronic hepatitis C (CHC) in adults (September 2015) SMC No. 1084/15 Recommended with restrictions

- **MEDICINAL FORMS** There can be variation in the licensing of different medicines containing the same drug.
  Tablet
  CAUTIONARY AND ADVISORY LABELS 25
  - ▸ Harvoni (Gilead Sciences Ireland UC) ▼
    Ledipasvir 90 mg, Sofosbuvir 400 mg Harvoni 90mg/400mg tablets | 28 tablet [PoM] £12,993.33

Sofosbuvir

08-Dec-2020

- **INDICATIONS AND DOSE**

Chronic hepatitis C infection
- ▸ BY MOUTH
- ▸ Adult: 400 mg once daily, for duration of treatment consult product literature

---

IMPORTANT SAFETY INFORMATION

MHRA/CHM ADVICE: DIRECT-ACTING ANTIVIRALS TO TREAT CHRONIC HEPATITIS C: RISK OF INTERACTION WITH VITAMIN K ANTAGONISTS AND CHANGES IN INR (JANUARY 2017)
An EU-wide review has identified that changes in liver function, secondary to hepatitis C treatment with direct-acting antivirals, may affect the efficacy of vitamin K antagonists; the MHRA has advised that INR should be monitored closely in patients receiving concomitant treatment.

MHRA/CHM ADVICE: DIRECT-ACTING ANTIVIRAL INTERFERON-FREE REGIMENS TO TREAT CHRONIC HEPATITIS C: RISK OF HEPATITIS B REACTIVATION (JANUARY 2017)
An EU-wide review has concluded that direct-acting antiviral interferon-free regimens for chronic hepatitis C can cause hepatitis B reactivation in patients co-infected with hepatitis B and C viruses; the MHRA recommends to screen patients for hepatitis B before starting treatment—patients infected with both hepatitis B and C viruses must be monitored and managed according to current clinical guidelines.

MHRA/CHM ADVICE: DIRECT-ACTING ANTIVIRALS FOR CHRONIC HEPATITIS C: RISK OF HYPOGLYCAEMIA IN PATIENTS WITH DIABETES (DECEMBER 2018)
Rapid reduction in hepatitis C viral load during direct-acting antiviral therapy for hepatitis C may improve glucose metabolism in patients with diabetes and result in symptomatic hypoglycaemia if diabetic treatment is continued at the same dose.
The MHRA advises healthcare professionals:
- to monitor glucose levels closely in patients with diabetes during direct-acting antiviral therapy for hepatitis C, especially within the first 3 months of treatment and modify diabetic medication or doses when necessary;
- to be vigilant for changes in glucose tolerance and advise patients of the risk of hypoglycaemia;
- to inform the healthcare professional in charge of the diabetic care of the patient when direct-acting antiviral therapy is initiated.

- **CAUTIONS** Manufacturer advises in chronic hepatitis C of genotype 1, 4, 5, or 6, only use sofosbuvir with ribavirin dual therapy in those with intolerance or contra-indications to peginterferon alfa who require urgent treatment.
- **INTERACTIONS** → Appendix 1: sofosbuvir
- **SIDE-EFFECTS**
- ▸ **Common or very common** Alopecia · anaemia · anxiety · appetite decreased · arthralgia · asthenia · chest pain · chills · concentration impaired · constipation · cough · depression · diarrhoea · dizziness · dry mouth · dyspnoea · fever · gastrointestinal discomfort · gastrooesophageal reflux disease · headaches · influenza like illness · insomnia · irritability · memory loss · muscle complaints · nasopharyngitis · nausea · neutropenia · pain · skin reactions · vision blurred · vomiting · weight decreased
- ▸ **Frequency not known** Arrhythmia · hepatitis B reactivation · Stevens-Johnson syndrome

SIDE-EFFECTS, FURTHER INFORMATION Side-effects listed are reported when sofosbuvir is used in combination with ribavirin or with ribavirin and peginterferon alfa.

- PREGNANCY Manufacturer advises avoid—limited information available.
- BREAST FEEDING Manufacturer advises avoid—present in milk in *animal* studies.
- RENAL IMPAIRMENT Safety and efficacy not established if eGFR less than 30 mL/minute/1.73 m^2—accumulation may occur.
- PRESCRIBING AND DISPENSING INFORMATION Dispense in original container (contains desiccant).
- PATIENT AND CARER ADVICE
  Missed doses Manufacturer advises if a dose is more than 18 hours late, the missed dose should not be taken and the next dose should be taken at the normal time.
- NATIONAL FUNDING/ACCESS DECISIONS
  For full details see funding body website
  NICE decisions
  ‣ Sofosbuvir for treating chronic hepatitis C [with peginterferon alfa and ribavirin for adults with genotype 1, 3, 4, 5, or 6; with ribavirin for adults with genotype 2 or 3] (February 2015) NICE TA330 Recommended with restrictions
  ‣ Sofosbuvir for treating chronic hepatitis C [with ribavirin for adults with genotype 1, 4, 5, or 6] (February 2015) NICE TA330 Not recommended
  Scottish Medicines Consortium (SMC) decisions
  ‣ Sofosbuvir (*Sovaldi*®) in combination with other medicinal products for the treatment of chronic hepatitis C (CHC) in adults (June 2014) SMC No. 964/14 Recommended with restrictions
- MEDICINAL FORMS There can be variation in the licensing of different medicines containing the same drug.
  Tablet
  CAUTIONARY AND ADVISORY LABELS 21, 25
  ‣ Sovaldi (Gilead Sciences Ireland UC) ▼
  Sofosbuvir 400 mg Sovaldi 400mg tablets | 28 tablet [PoM] £11,660.98

Sofosbuvir with velpatasvir
04-Dec-2020

The properties listed below are those particular to the combination only. For the properties of the components please consider, sofosbuvir p. 668.

- DRUG ACTION Sofosbuvir is a nucleotide analogue inhibitor and velpatasvir is an HCV inhibitor; they reduce viral load by inhibiting hepatitis C virus RNA replication.

- INDICATIONS AND DOSE
  Chronic hepatitis C infection, with or without ribavirin (initiated by a specialist)
  ‣ BY MOUTH
  ‣ Adult: 400/100 mg once daily for 12 weeks (may extend to 24 weeks in some circumstances—consult product literature)
  DOSE ADJUSTMENTS DUE TO INTERACTIONS
  ‣ Manufacturer advises reduce dose of concurrent H$_2$-receptor antagonist if above a dose comparable to famotidine 40 mg twice daily.
  ‣ Manufacturer advises reduce dose of concurrent proton pump inhibitor if above a dose comparable to omeprazole 20 mg; take 4 hours after sofosbuvir with velpatasvir.
  DOSE EQUIVALENCE AND CONVERSION
  ‣ Dose expressed as x/y mg sofosbuvir/velpatasvir.

- CAUTIONS Hepatitis B co-infection
- INTERACTIONS → Appendix 1: sofosbuvir · velpatasvir
- SIDE-EFFECTS Atrioventricular block · bradycardia · fatigue · headache · nausea

- PATIENT AND CARER ADVICE
  Vomiting Manufacturer advises if vomiting occurs within 3 hours of administration, an additional dose should be taken.
- NATIONAL FUNDING/ACCESS DECISIONS
  For full details see funding body website
  NICE decisions
  ‣ Sofosbuvir-velpatasvir for treating chronic hepatitis C (January 2017) NICE TA430 Recommended
  Scottish Medicines Consortium (SMC) decisions
  ‣ Sofosbuvir with velpatasvir (*Epclusa*®) for the treatment of chronic hepatitis C virus (HCV) infection in adults [with genotype 3 chronic HCV infection] (November 2016) SMC No. 1195/16 Recommended with restrictions
  ‣ Sofosbuvir with velpatasvir (*Epclusa*®) for the treatment of chronic hepatitis C virus (HCV) infection in adults [with genotype 2, 5 or 6 chronic HCV infection, or decompensated cirrhosis, irrespective of chronic HCV genotype] (October 2017) SMC No. 1271/17 Recommended with restrictions
  ‣ Sofosbuvir with velpatasvir (*Epclusa*®) for the treatment of chronic hepatitis C virus (HCV) infection in adults [with genotype 1 or 4 chronic HCV infection] (April 2018) SMC No. 1271/17 Recommended with restrictions

- MEDICINAL FORMS There can be variation in the licensing of different medicines containing the same drug.
  Tablet
  CAUTIONARY AND ADVISORY LABELS 25
  ‣ Epclusa (Gilead Sciences Ireland UC) ▼
  Velpatasvir 100 mg, Sofosbuvir 400 mg Epclusa 400mg/100mg tablets | 28 tablet [PoM] £12,993.33

Sofosbuvir with velpatasvir and voxilaprevir
10-Nov-2020

The properties listed below are those particular to the combination only. For the properties of the components please consider, sofosbuvir p. 668.

- INDICATIONS AND DOSE
  Chronic hepatitis C infection (specialist use only)
  ‣ BY MOUTH
  ‣ Adult: 1 tablet once daily, for duration of treatment, consult product literature
  DOSE ADJUSTMENTS DUE TO INTERACTIONS
  ‣ Manufacturer advises reduce dose of concurrent H$_2$-receptor antagonist if above a dose comparable to famotidine 40 mg twice daily.
  ‣ Manufacturer advises reduce dose of concurrent proton pump inhibitor if above a dose comparable to omeprazole 20 mg.

- CAUTIONS Hepatitis B co-infection
- INTERACTIONS → Appendix 1: sofosbuvir · velpatasvir · voxilaprevir
- HEPATIC IMPAIRMENT Manufacturer advises avoid in moderate to severe impairment.
- PATIENT AND CARER ADVICE
  Vomiting Manufacturer advises if vomiting occurs within 4 hours of administration, an additional dose should be taken.
- NATIONAL FUNDING/ACCESS DECISIONS
  For full details see funding body website
  NICE decisions
  ‣ Sofosbuvir-velpatasvir-voxilaprevir for treating chronic hepatitis C (February 2018) NICE TA507 Recommended with restrictions

5

Infection

5

Infection

▶ Sofosbuvir with velpatasvir and voxilaprevir (*Vosevi*®) for the treatment of chronic hepatitis C virus (HCV) infection in adults (April 2018) SMC No. 1317/18 Recommended with restrictions

● MEDICINAL FORMS There can be variation in the licensing of different medicines containing the same drug.
Tablet
CAUTIONARY AND ADVISORY LABELS 21, 25
▶ Vosevi (Gilead Sciences Ireland UC) ▼
Velpatasvir 100 mg, Voxilaprevir 100 mg, Sofosbuvir 400 mg Vosevi 400mg/100mg/100mg tablets | 28 tablet [PoM] £14,942.33

ANTIVIRALS > PROTEASE INHIBITORS, HEPATITIS

Glecaprevir with pibrentasvir
02-Nov-2020

● INDICATIONS AND DOSE
Chronic hepatitis C (specialist use only)
▶ BY MOUTH
▶ Adult: 300/120 mg once daily, for duration of treatment, consult product literature
DOSE EQUIVALENCE AND CONVERSION
▶ Dose expressed as x/y mg glecaprevir/pibrentasvir.

IMPORTANT SAFETY INFORMATION
HEPATITIS B INFECTION
Cases of hepatitis B reactivation, sometimes fatal, have been reported in patients co-infected with hepatitis B and C viruses; manufacturer advises to assess patients for hepatitis B prior to initiation of therapy and manage according to current clinical guidelines.

MHRA/CHM ADVICE: DIRECT-ACTING ANTIVIRALS TO TREAT CHRONIC HEPATITIS C: RISK OF INTERACTION WITH VITAMIN K ANTAGONISTS AND CHANGES IN INR (JANUARY 2017)
An EU-wide review has identified that changes in liver function, secondary to hepatitis C treatment with direct-acting antivirals, may affect the efficacy of vitamin K antagonists; the MHRA has advised that INR should be monitored closely in patients receiving concomitant treatment.

MHRA/CHM ADVICE: DIRECT-ACTING ANTIVIRALS FOR CHRONIC HEPATITIS C: RISK OF HYPOGLYCAEMIA IN PATIENTS WITH DIABETES (DECEMBER 2018)
Rapid reduction in hepatitis C viral load during direct-acting antiviral therapy for hepatitis C may improve glucose metabolism in patients with diabetes and result in symptomatic hypoglycaemia if diabetic treatment is continued at the same dose.
The MHRA advises healthcare professionals:
● to monitor glucose levels closely in patients with diabetes during direct-acting antiviral therapy for hepatitis C, especially within the first 3 months of treatment and modify diabetic medication or doses when necessary;
● to be vigilant for changes in glucose tolerance and advise patients of the risk of hypoglycaemia;
● to inform the healthcare professional in charge of the diabetic care of the patient when direct-acting antiviral therapy is initiated.

● CAUTIONS Hepatitis B infection · post-liver transplant patients · re-treatment of patients with prior exposure to NS3/4A- or NS5A-inhibitors—efficacy not established
● INTERACTIONS → Appendix 1: glecaprevir · pibrentasvir
● SIDE-EFFECTS
▶ **Common or very common** Asthenia · diarrhoea · headache · nausea
▶ **Frequency not known** Pruritus · transient ischaemic attack

● PREGNANCY Manufacturer advises avoid—limited information available.
● BREAST FEEDING Manufacturer advises avoid—present in milk in *animal* studies.
● HEPATIC IMPAIRMENT Manufacturer advises avoid in moderate to severe impairment (risk of increased exposure).
● PATIENT AND CARER ADVICE
Missed doses Manufacturer advises if a dose is more than 18 hours late, the missed dose should not be taken and the next dose should be taken at the normal time.
● NATIONAL FUNDING/ACCESS DECISIONS
For full details see funding body website
NICE decisions
▶ Glecaprevir–pibrentasvir for treating chronic hepatitis C (January 2018) NICE TA499 Recommended with restrictions
Scottish Medicines Consortium (SMC) decisions
▶ Glecaprevir with pibrentasvir (*Maviret*®) for the treatment of chronic hepatitis C virus (HCV) infection in adults (November 2017) SMC No. 1278/17 Recommended

● MEDICINAL FORMS There can be variation in the licensing of different medicines containing the same drug.
Tablet
CAUTIONARY AND ADVISORY LABELS 21, 25
▶ Maviret (AbbVie Ltd) ▼
Pibrentasvir 40 mg, Glecaprevir 100 mg Maviret 100mg/40mg tablets | 84 tablet [PoM] £12,993.66

ANTIVIRALS > OTHER

Dasabuvir
27-May-2020

● DRUG ACTION Dasabuvir is a non-nucleoside inhibitor of hepatitis C virus polymerase NS5B, which is an essential component of the hepatitis C virus replication process.

● INDICATIONS AND DOSE
Chronic hepatitis C infection of genotype 1, in combination with other antiviral drugs (ombitasvir with paritaprevir and ritonavir, with or without ribavirin)
▶ BY MOUTH
▶ Adult: 250 mg twice daily for details of duration of treatment, consult product literature, dose to be taken in the morning and evening

IMPORTANT SAFETY INFORMATION
MHRA/CHM ADVICE: DIRECT-ACTING ANTIVIRALS TO TREAT CHRONIC HEPATITIS C: RISK OF INTERACTION WITH VITAMIN K ANTAGONISTS AND CHANGES IN INR (JANUARY 2017)
A EU-wide review has identified that changes in liver function, secondary to hepatitis C treatment with direct-acting antivirals, may affect the efficacy of vitamin K antagonists; the MHRA has advised that INR should be monitored closely in patients receiving concomitant treatment.

MHRA/CHM ADVICE: DIRECT-ACTING ANTIVIRAL INTERFERON-FREE REGIMENS TO TREAT CHRONIC HEPATITIS C: RISK OF HEPATITIS B REACTIVATION (JANUARY 2017)
An EU-wide review has concluded that direct-acting antiviral interferon-free regimens for chronic hepatitis C can cause hepatitis B reactivation in patients co-infected with hepatitis B and C viruses; the MHRA recommends to screen patients for hepatitis B before starting treatment—patients infected with both hepatitis B and C viruses must be monitored and managed according to current clinical guidelines.

MHRA/CHM ADVICE: DIRECT-ACTING ANTIVIRALS FOR CHRONIC HEPATITIS C: RISK OF HYPOGLYCAEMIA IN PATIENTS WITH DIABETES (DECEMBER 2018)
Rapid reduction in hepatitis C viral load during direct-acting antiviral therapy for hepatitis C may improve

glucose metabolism in patients with diabetes and result in symptomatic hypoglycaemia if diabetic treatment is continued at the same dose.

The MHRA advises healthcare professionals:
- to monitor glucose levels closely in patients with diabetes during direct-acting antiviral therapy for hepatitis C, especially within the first 3 months of treatment and modify diabetic medication or doses when necessary;
- to be vigilant for changes in glucose tolerance and advise patients of the risk of hypoglycaemia;
- to inform the healthcare professional in charge of the diabetic care of the patient when direct-acting antiviral therapy is initiated.

- **CONTRA-INDICATIONS** HIV co-infection without suppressive antiretroviral therapy
- **CAUTIONS** Psychiatric disorders · retreatment—efficacy not established
- **INTERACTIONS** → Appendix 1: dasabuvir
- **SIDE-EFFECTS**
  ▸ **Common or very common** Anaemia · asthenia · diarrhoea · insomnia · nausea · pruritus · vomiting
  ▸ **Uncommon** Dehydration
  ▸ **Rare or very rare** Angioedema
  ▸ **Frequency not known** Depression · hepatic failure · hepatitis B reactivation · suicidal behaviours

  SIDE-EFFECTS, FURTHER INFORMATION Side-effects listed are reported when dasabuvir is used in combination with Viekirax (ombitasvir with paritaprevir and ritonavir), with or without ribavirin.

- **PREGNANCY** Manufacturer advises avoid—no information available.
- **BREAST FEEDING** Manufacturer advises avoid—present in milk in *animal* studies.
- **HEPATIC IMPAIRMENT** Manufacturer advises caution in cirrhosis —monitor for signs and symptoms of hepatic decompensation and assess hepatic function (including direct bilirubin) at baseline, during the first 4 weeks of treatment and thereafter as clinically indicated, discontinue if hepatic decompensation develops; avoid in moderate to severe impairment.
- **PATIENT AND CARER ADVICE**
  Missed doses If a dose is more than 6 hours late, the missed dose should not be taken and the next dose should be taken at the normal time.
- **NATIONAL FUNDING/ACCESS DECISIONS**
  For full details see funding body website
  NICE decisions
  ▸ Ombitasvir with paritaprevir and ritonavir with or without dasabuvir for treating chronic hepatitis C (November 2015) NICE TA365 Recommended with restrictions

- **MEDICINAL FORMS** No licensed medicines listed.

6.4 Herpesvirus infections

Herpesvirus infections   07-Sep-2020

Herpes simplex infections

Herpes infection of the mouth and lips and in the eye is generally associated with herpes simplex virus serotype 1 (HSV-1); other areas of the skin may also be infected, especially in immunodeficiency. Genital infection is most often associated with HSV-2 and also HSV-1.

EvGr Topical antiviral treatment is not routinely recommended in immunocompetent individuals with uncomplicated infection of the lips (herpes labialis or cold sores) or herpetic gingivostomatitis. However, some patients may find application of a topical antiviral drug helpful when used from the onset of the prodromal phase. Oral paracetamol p. 464 and/or ibuprofen p. 1186 may be given to relieve pain and fever. Other preparations that may be considered for symptom relief include topical anaesthetics or analgesics, and mouthwashes. Oral antiviral treatment may be considered in patients with severe, frequent or persistent oral infection.

Primary or recurrent genital herpes simplex infection is treated with an antiviral drug given by mouth.

Individuals suspected of having ocular herpes simplex infection should be referred for urgent, same-day specialist referral; treatment should not be initiated whilst awaiting review. If same-day review is not possible, specialist advice should be sought, which may include topical antiviral treatment in primary care. Some optometrists with appropriate expertise and training can initiate topical antiviral treatment in certain suspected cases.

Refer or seek specialist advice for treatment of herpes simplex infection in pregnancy. Ⓐ

Varicella-zoster infections

Chickenpox is an acute disease caused by the varicella-zoster virus. EvGr Specialist advice on the management of chickenpox (varicella) in neonates should be sought due to the higher risk of severe disease and complications. Chickenpox in otherwise healthy children is usually self-limiting and complications are rare; antiviral treatment is not routinely recommended.

Chickenpox is more severe in adolescents (aged 14 years and over) and adults than in children; antiviral treatment started within 24 hours of the onset of rash may be considered, particularly for those with severe infection or at risk of complications. Specialist advice should be sought on the diagnosis and management of chickenpox in immunocompromised patients. Ⓐ

Pregnant women who develop severe chickenpox may be at risk of complications, especially varicella pneumonia. EvGr Immediate specialist advice should be sought for the treatment of chickenpox during pregnancy. Ⓐ

Public Health England advise that individuals at high risk of severe chickenpox (neonates, infants, pregnant women, or immunocompromised patients) who have been exposed to the varicella-zoster virus, may require post-exposure prophylaxis with varicella-zoster immunoglobulin p. 1337 or an antiviral [unlicensed] to reduce the impact of chickenpox infection, and risk of complications (such as pneumonitis). For further information, see *Varicella-zoster immunoglobulin* in Immunoglobulins p. 1331.

Shingles (herpes zoster) is a viral infection of an individual nerve and the skin surface affected by the nerve. The infection is caused by the reactivation of the varicella-zoster virus, the same virus that causes chickenpox. EvGr Oral antiviral treatment should be offered to patients with shingles who are immunocompromised, have non-truncal involvement (e.g. neck, limbs, perineum), or to those with moderate to severe pain or rash. Consider oral antiviral treatment for patients aged over 50 years to reduce the risk of post-herpetic neuralgia. Treatment with the antiviral should be started within 72 hours of the onset of rash. Immunocompromised patients with severe or widespread infection, or severely immunocompromised patients, or patients with shingles in the ophthalmic distribution of the trigeminal nerve, should be admitted to hospital or specialist advice should be sought. Ⓐ

Chronic pain which persists after the rash has healed (post-herpetic neuralgia) requires specific management. For further information, see Neuropathic pain p. 504.

The risk and incidence of varicella-zoster infections can be reduced through vaccination of selected individuals. For further information, see Varicella-zoster vaccine p. 1358.

5

Infection

Drug choice

Aciclovir below is active against herpesviruses but does not eradicate them. EvGr Uses of aciclovir include systemic treatment of varicella-zoster and the systemic and topical treatment of herpes simplex infections of the skin and mucous membranes. ◇A◇ Aciclovir eye ointment is licensed for herpes simplex infections of the eye.

EvGr Famciclovir p. 674, a prodrug of penciclovir, is similar to aciclovir and may be used in the treatment of herpes zoster and genital herpes.

Valaciclovir p. 675 is an ester of aciclovir, which may be used in the treatment of herpes zoster and herpes simplex infections of the skin and mucous membranes (including genital herpes); ◇A◇ it is also licensed for preventing cytomegalovirus disease following solid organ transplantation.

Intravenous foscarnet sodium p. 678 is licensed for mucocutaneous herpes simplex virus infection unresponsive to aciclovir in immunocompromised patients. Oral inosine pranobex below is also licensed for mucocutaneous infections due to the herpes simplex virus.

Cytomegalovirus infection

Cytomegalovirus (CMV) is a member of the herpesvirus group. In immunocompetent patients, CMV infection is often asymptomatic and self-limiting therefore treatment is not always required. In immunocompromised patients, such as those with AIDS and transplant recipients, the infection manifests more severely causing diseases associated with greater morbidity and mortality.

Drugs licensed for use in the management of CMV disease include ganciclovir p. 676 (related to aciclovir), cidofovir p. 676, foscarnet sodium, letermovir p. 678, valaciclovir, and valganciclovir p. 677 (an ester of ganciclovir). There is a possibility of ganciclovir resistance in those who repeatedly have a poor treatment response or when viral excretion continues despite treatment.

ANTIVIRALS > INOSINE COMPLEXES

Inosine pranobex

27-May-2020

(Inosine acedoben dimepranol)

● **INDICATIONS AND DOSE**

Mucocutaneous herpes simplex
▸ BY MOUTH
  ▸ Adult: 1 g 4 times a day for 7–14 days

Adjunctive treatment of genital warts
▸ BY MOUTH
  ▸ Adult: 1 g 3 times a day for 14–28 days

Subacute sclerosing panencephalitis
▸ BY MOUTH
  ▸ Adult: 50–100 mg/kg daily in 6 divided doses

● CAUTIONS History of gout · history of hyperuricaemia · history of urolithiasis
● SIDE-EFFECTS Arthralgia · constipation · diarrhoea · drowsiness · epigastric discomfort · fatigue · headache · insomnia · malaise · nausea · nervousness · polyuria · skin reactions · vertigo · vomiting
● PREGNANCY Manufacturer advises avoid.
● RENAL IMPAIRMENT Manufacturer advises caution; metabolised to uric acid.
● LESS SUITABLE FOR PRESCRIBING Inosine pranobex is less suitable for prescribing.

● MEDICINAL FORMS There can be variation in the licensing of different medicines containing the same drug.

Tablet
CAUTIONARY AND ADVISORY LABELS 9
▸ Imunovir (KoRa Healthcare)
   Inosine acedoben dimepranol 500 mg Imunovir 500mg tablets |
   100 tablet PoM £39.50 DT = £39.50

ANTIVIRALS > NUCLEOSIDE ANALOGUES

Aciclovir

09-Jun-2020

(Acyclovir)

● **INDICATIONS AND DOSE**

Herpes simplex, suppression
▸ BY MOUTH
  ▸ Child 12–17 years: 400 mg twice daily, alternatively 200 mg 4 times a day; increased to 400 mg 3 times a day, dose may be increased if recurrences occur on standard suppressive therapy or for suppression of genital herpes during late pregnancy (from 36 weeks gestation), therapy interrupted every 6–12 months to reassess recurrence frequency—consider restarting after two or more recurrences
  ▸ Adult: 400 mg twice daily, alternatively 200 mg 4 times a day; increased to 400 mg 3 times a day, dose may be increased if recurrences occur on standard suppressive therapy or for suppression of genital herpes during late pregnancy (from 36 weeks gestation), therapy interrupted every 6–12 months to reassess recurrence frequency—consider restarting after two or more recurrences

Herpes simplex, prophylaxis in the immunocompromised
▸ BY MOUTH
  ▸ Child 1–23 months: 100–200 mg 4 times a day
  ▸ Child 2–17 years: 200–400 mg 4 times a day
  ▸ Adult: 200–400 mg 4 times a day
▸ BY INTRAVENOUS INFUSION
  ▸ Adult: 5 mg/kg every 8 hours

Herpes simplex, treatment (non-genital)
▸ BY MOUTH
  ▸ Adult: 200 mg 5 times a day usually for 5 days (longer if new lesions appear during treatment or if healing incomplete)

Herpes simplex, treatment (non-genital) in immunocompromised or if absorption impaired
▸ BY MOUTH
  ▸ Adult: 400 mg 5 times a day usually for 5 days (longer if new lesions appear during treatment or if healing incomplete)

Herpes simplex, treatment
▸ BY MOUTH
  ▸ Child 1–23 months: 100 mg 5 times a day usually for 5 days (longer if new lesions appear during treatment or if healing incomplete)
  ▸ Child 2–17 years: 200 mg 5 times a day usually for 5 days (longer if new lesions appear during treatment or if healing incomplete)

Herpes simplex, treatment, in immunocompromised or if absorption impaired
▸ BY MOUTH
  ▸ Child 1–23 months: 200 mg 5 times a day usually for 5 days (longer if new lesions appear during treatment or if healing incomplete)
  ▸ Child 2–17 years: 400 mg 5 times a day usually for 5 days (longer if new lesions appear during treatment or if healing incomplete)

Genital herpes simplex, treatment of first episode
▶ BY MOUTH
▶ Adult: 200 mg 5 times a day, alternatively 400 mg 3 times a day both courses usually for 5 days (longer if new lesions appear during treatment or if healing incomplete)

Genital herpes simplex, treatment of first episode, in immunocompromised or HIV-positive
▶ BY MOUTH
▶ Adult: 400 mg 5 times a day for 7–10 days (longer if new lesions appear during treatment or if healing incomplete)

Severe genital herpes simplex, treatment, initial infection | Treatment of herpes simplex in the immunocompromised
▶ BY INTRAVENOUS INFUSION
▶ Adult: Initially 5 mg/kg every 8 hours usually for 5 days, alternatively 10 mg/kg every 8 hours for at least 14 days in encephalitis (at least 21 days if also immunocompromised)—confirm cerebrospinal fluid negative for herpes simplex virus before stopping treatment, higher dose to be used only if resistant organisms suspected or in simplex encephalitis

Genital herpes simplex, treatment of recurrent infection
▶ BY MOUTH
▶ Adult: 800 mg 3 times a day for 2 days, alternatively 200 mg 5 times a day for 5 days, alternatively 400 mg 3 times a day for 3–5 days

Genital herpes simplex, treatment of recurrent infection in immunocompromised or HIV-positive patients
▶ BY MOUTH
▶ Adult: 400 mg 3 times a day for 5–10 days

Varicella zoster (chickenpox), treatment | Herpes zoster (shingles), treatment
▶ BY MOUTH
▶ Child 1–23 months: 200 mg 4 times a day for 5 days
▶ Child 2–5 years: 400 mg 4 times a day for 5 days
▶ Child 6–11 years: 800 mg 4 times a day for 5 days
▶ Child 12–17 years: 800 mg 5 times a day for 7 days
▶ Adult: 800 mg 5 times a day for 7 days
▶ BY INTRAVENOUS INFUSION
▶ Adult: 5 mg/kg every 8 hours usually for 5 days

Varicella zoster (chickenpox), treatment in immunocompromised | Herpes zoster (shingles), treatment in immunocompromised
▶ BY INTRAVENOUS INFUSION
▶ Adult: 10 mg/kg every 8 hours usually for 5 days

Herpes zoster (shingles), treatment in immunocompromised
▶ BY MOUTH
▶ Child 1–23 months: 200 mg 4 times a day continued for 2 days after crusting of lesions
▶ Child 2–5 years: 400 mg 4 times a day continued for 2 days after crusting of lesions
▶ Child 6–11 years: 800 mg 4 times a day continued for 2 days after crusting of lesions
▶ Child 12–17 years: 800 mg 5 times a day continued for 2 days after crusting of lesions
▶ Adult: 800 mg 5 times a day continued for 2 days after crusting of lesions

Herpes zoster, treatment in encephalitis | Varicella zoster, treatment in encephalitis
▶ BY INTRAVENOUS INFUSION
▶ Adult: 10 mg/kg every 8 hours given for 10–14 days in encephalitis, possibly longer if also immunocompromised or if severe infection

Varicella zoster (chickenpox), attenuation of infection if varicella–zoster immunoglobulin not indicated
▶ BY MOUTH
▶ Child: 10 mg/kg 4 times a day for 7 days, to be started 1 week after exposure
▶ Adult: 10 mg/kg 4 times a day for 7 days, to be started 1 week after exposure

DOSES AT EXTREMES OF BODY-WEIGHT
▶ With intravenous use To avoid excessive dosage in obese patients parenteral dose should be calculated on the basis of ideal weight for height.

● UNLICENSED USE
▶ With oral use in children Tablets and suspension not licensed for suppression of herpes simplex or for treatment of herpes zoster in children (age range not specified by manufacturer).
▶ With oral use Aciclovir doses in BNF may differ from those in product literature. Attenuation of chickenpox is an unlicensed indication.

● CAUTIONS Elderly (risk of neurological reactions) · maintain adequate hydration (especially with infusion or high doses)

● INTERACTIONS → Appendix 1: aciclovir

● SIDE-EFFECTS
▶ Common or very common
▶ With intravenous use Nausea · photosensitivity reaction · skin reactions · vomiting
▶ With oral use Abdominal pain · diarrhoea · dizziness · fatigue · fever · headache · nausea · photosensitivity reaction · skin reactions · vomiting
▶ Uncommon
▶ With intravenous use Anaemia · leucopenia · thrombocytopenia
▶ Rare or very rare
▶ With intravenous use Abdominal pain · agitation · angioedema · ataxia · coma · confusion · diarrhoea · dizziness · drowsiness · dysarthria · dyspnoea · encephalopathy · fatigue · fever · hallucination · headache · hepatic disorders · inflammation localised · psychosis · renal impairment · renal pain · seizure · tremor
▶ With oral use Agitation · anaemia · angioedema · ataxia · coma · confusion · drowsiness · dysarthria · dyspnoea · encephalopathy · hallucination · hepatic disorders · leucopenia · psychosis · renal impairment · renal pain · seizure · thrombocytopenia · tremor
▶ Frequency not known
▶ With intravenous use Crystalluria
▶ With oral use Alopecia · crystalluria

● PREGNANCY Not known to be harmful—manufacturers advise use only when potential benefit outweighs risk.

● BREAST FEEDING Significant amount in milk after systemic administration—not known to be harmful but manufacturer advises caution.

● RENAL IMPAIRMENT Risk of neurological reactions increased. Maintain adequate hydration (especially during renal impairment).
Dose adjustments ▶ With intravenous use in adults Use normal intravenous dose every 12 hours if eGFR 25–50 mL/minute/1.73 m^2 (every 24 hours if eGFR 10–25 mL/minute/1.73 m^2). Consult product literature for intravenous dose if eGFR less than 10 mL/minute/1.73 m^2.
▶ With oral use in adults For *herpes zoster*, use normal oral dose every 8 hours if eGFR 10–25 mL/minute/1.73 m^2 (every 12 hours if eGFR less than 10 mL/minute/1.73 m^2). For *herpes simplex*, use normal oral dose every 12 hours if eGFR less than 10 mL/minute/1.73 m^2.
▶ With oral use in children For *herpes zoster*, use normal oral dose every 8 hours if estimated glomerular filtration rate 10–25 mL/minute/1.73 m^2 (every 12 hours if estimated glomerular filtration rate less than 10 mL/minute/1.73 m^2).

For *herpes simplex*, use normal dose every 12 hours if estimated glomerular filtration rate less than 10 mL/minute/1.73 m².

- **DIRECTIONS FOR ADMINISTRATION**
  ‣ With intravenous use in adults For *intravenous infusion Zovirax IV®*, *Aciclovir IV* (Genus), give intermittently *in* Sodium chloride 0.9% *or* Sodium chloride and glucose; initially reconstitute to 25 mg/mL in water for injection or sodium chloride 0.9% then dilute to not more than 5 mg/mL with the infusion fluid; to be given over 1 hour; alternatively, may be administered in a concentration of 25 mg/mL using a suitable infusion pump and given over 1 hour; for *Aciclovir IV* (Hospira) dilute to not more than 5 mg/mL with infusion fluid; give over 1 hour.
- **PRESCRIBING AND DISPENSING INFORMATION** Flavours of oral liquid preparations may include banana, or orange.
- **PATIENT AND CARER ADVICE**
  Medicines for Children leaflet: Aciclovir (oral) for viral infections
  www.medicinesforchildren.org.uk/aciclovir-oral-viral-infections-0
- **PROFESSION SPECIFIC INFORMATION**
  Dental practitioners' formulary
  ‣ With oral use Aciclovir Tablets 200 mg or 800 mg may be prescribed. Aciclovir Oral Suspension 200 mg/5mL may be prescribed.

- **MEDICINAL FORMS** There can be variation in the licensing of different medicines containing the same drug.

  Tablet
  CAUTIONARY AND ADVISORY LABELS 9
  ‣ Aciclovir (Non-proprietary)
  Aciclovir 200 mg Aciclovir 200mg tablets | 25 tablet PoM £2.03 DT = £1.67
  Aciclovir 400 mg Aciclovir 400mg tablets | 56 tablet PoM £4.62 DT = £3.40
  Aciclovir 800 mg Aciclovir 800mg tablets | 35 tablet PoM £6.41 DT = £4.52

  Dispersible tablet
  CAUTIONARY AND ADVISORY LABELS 9
  ‣ Aciclovir (Non-proprietary)
  Aciclovir 200 mg Aciclovir 200mg dispersible tablets | 25 tablet PoM £1.82 DT = £1.81
  Aciclovir 400 mg Aciclovir 400mg dispersible tablets | 56 tablet PoM £11.99 DT = £11.99
  Aciclovir 800 mg Aciclovir 800mg dispersible tablets | 35 tablet PoM £10.99 DT = £10.99
  ‣ Zovirax (GlaxoSmithKline UK Ltd)
  Aciclovir 200 mg Zovirax 200mg dispersible tablets | 25 tablet PoM £2.85 DT = £1.81
  Aciclovir 800 mg Zovirax 800mg dispersible tablets | 35 tablet PoM £10.50 DT = £10.99

  Oral suspension
  CAUTIONARY AND ADVISORY LABELS 9
  ‣ Aciclovir (Non-proprietary)
  Aciclovir 40 mg per 1 ml Aciclovir 200mg/5ml oral suspension sugar free sugar-free | 125 ml PoM £35.78 DT = £35.78
  Aciclovir 80 mg per 1 ml Aciclovir 400mg/5ml oral suspension sugar free sugar-free | 100 ml PoM £39.49 DT = £39.49
  ‣ Zovirax (GlaxoSmithKline UK Ltd)
  Aciclovir 40 mg per 1 ml Zovirax 200mg/5ml oral suspension sugar-free | 125 ml PoM £29.56 DT = £35.78
  Aciclovir 80 mg per 1 ml Zovirax Double Strength 400mg/5ml oral suspension sugar-free | 100 ml PoM £33.02 DT = £39.49

  Solution for infusion
  ELECTROLYTES: May contain Sodium
  ‣ Aciclovir (Non-proprietary)
  Aciclovir (as Aciclovir sodium) 25 mg per 1 ml Aciclovir 1g/40ml solution for infusion vials | 1 vial PoM £40.00 (Hospital only)
  Aciclovir 250mg/10ml concentrate for solution for infusion vials | 5 vial PoM £10.00–£50.00 (Hospital only)
  Aciclovir 500mg/20ml solution for infusion vials | 5 vial PoM £50.00–£100.00 (Hospital only)
  Aciclovir 500mg/20ml concentrate for solution for infusion vials | 5 vial PoM £20.00–£40.00 (Hospital only)

Powder for solution for infusion
ELECTROLYTES: May contain Sodium
‣ Aciclovir (Non-proprietary)
Aciclovir (as Aciclovir sodium) 250 mg Aciclovir 250mg powder for solution for Infusion vials | 5 vial PoM £16.50 (Hospital only)
Aciclovir 250mg powder for solution for infusion vials | 5 vial PoM £49.30 (Hospital only) | 10 vial PoM £91.30 (Hospital only)
Aciclovir (as Aciclovir sodium) 500 mg Aciclovir 500mg powder for solution for infusion vials | 10 vial PoM £182.00 (Hospital only)
‣ Zovirax I.V. (GlaxoSmithKline UK Ltd)
Aciclovir (as Aciclovir sodium) 250 mg Zovirax I.V. 250mg powder for solution for infusion vials | 5 vial PoM £16.70 (Hospital only)
Aciclovir (as Aciclovir sodium) 500 mg Zovirax I.V. 500mg powder for solution for infusion vials | 5 vial PoM £17.00 (Hospital only)

Famciclovir

23-Jul-2018

- **INDICATIONS AND DOSE**

Herpes zoster infection, treatment
‣ BY MOUTH
‣ **Adult:** 500 mg 3 times a day for 7 days, alternatively 750 mg 1–2 times a day for 7 days

Herpes zoster infection, treatment in immunocompromised patients
‣ BY MOUTH
‣ **Adult:** 500 mg 3 times a day for 10 days, continue for 2 days after crusting of lesions

Genital herpes, suppression
‣ BY MOUTH
‣ **Adult:** 250 mg twice daily, therapy to be interrupted every 6–12 months to reassess recurrence frequency—consider restarting after two or more recurrences

Genital herpes, suppression in immunocompromised or HIV-positive patients
‣ BY MOUTH
‣ **Adult:** 500 mg twice daily, therapy to be interrupted every 6–12 months to reassess recurrence frequency—consider restarting after two or more recurrences

Genital herpes infection, treatment of first episode
‣ BY MOUTH
‣ **Adult:** 250 mg 3 times a day for 5 days or longer if new lesions appear during treatment or if healing incomplete

Genital herpes infection, treatment of first episode in immunocompromised or HIV-positive patients
‣ BY MOUTH
‣ **Adult:** 500 mg twice daily for 10 days

Genital herpes infection, treatment of recurrent infection
‣ BY MOUTH
‣ **Adult:** 125 mg twice daily for 5 days, alternatively 1 g twice daily for 1 day

Genital herpes infection, treatment of recurrent infections in immunocompromised or HIV-positive patients
‣ BY MOUTH
‣ **Adult:** 500 mg twice daily for 5–10 days

Herpes simplex infection (non-genital), treatment in immunocompromised patients
‣ BY MOUTH
‣ **Adult:** 500 mg twice daily for 7 days

- **UNLICENSED USE** Famciclovir doses in BNF may differ from those in product literature.
- **SIDE-EFFECTS**
  ‣ **Common or very common** Abdominal pain · diarrhoea · dizziness · headache · nausea · skin reactions · vomiting
  ‣ **Uncommon** Angioedema · confusion · drowsiness
  ‣ **Rare or very rare** Hallucination · jaundice cholestatic · palpitations · thrombocytopenia
- **PREGNANCY** Manufacturers advise avoid unless potential benefit outweighs risk.

- **BREAST FEEDING** No information available—present in milk in *animal* studies.
- **HEPATIC IMPAIRMENT** Manufacturer advises efficacy may be decreased in severe impairment (risk of impaired conversion to active metabolite, no information available).
- **RENAL IMPAIRMENT**
  Dose adjustments Reduce dose; consult product literature.
- **PRESCRIBING AND DISPENSING INFORMATION** Famciclovir is a pro-drug of penciclovir.

- **MEDICINAL FORMS** There can be variation in the licensing of different medicines containing the same drug. Forms available from special-order manufacturers include: tablet

Tablet
CAUTIONARY AND ADVISORY LABELS 9
▸ Famciclovir (Non-proprietary)
  Famciclovir 125 mg Famciclovir 125mg tablets | 10 tablet PoM
  £65.42 DT = £65.42
  Famciclovir 250 mg Famciclovir 250mg tablets | 15 tablet
  £110.59-£187.81 | 21 tablet PoM £246.44 DT = £246.44 |
  56 tablet PoM £412.85-£701.14
  Famciclovir 500 mg Famciclovir 500mg tablets | 14 tablet PoM
  £302.56 DT = £276.90
▸ Famvir (Phoenix Labs Ltd)
  Famciclovir 125 mg Famvir 125mg tablets | 10 tablet PoM £53.45
  DT = £65.42
  Famciclovir 250 mg Famvir 250mg tablets | 15 tablet PoM
  £160.34 | 56 tablet PoM £598.56
  Famciclovir 500 mg Famvir 500mg tablets | 30 tablet PoM
  £641.21

Valaciclovir
09-Jun-2020

- **INDICATIONS AND DOSE**

Herpes zoster infection, treatment
▸ BY MOUTH
  ▹ Adult: 1 g 3 times a day for 7 days

Herpes zoster infection, treatment in immunocompromised patients
▸ BY MOUTH
  ▹ Adult: 1 g 3 times a day for at least 7 days and continued for 2 days after crusting of lesions

Herpes simplex, treatment of first infective episode
▸ BY MOUTH
  ▹ Adult: 500 mg twice daily for 5 days (longer if new lesions appear during treatment or healing is incomplete)

Herpes simplex infections treatment of first episode in immunocompromised or HIV-positive patients
▸ BY MOUTH
  ▹ Adult: 1 g twice daily for 10 days

Herpes simplex, treatment of recurrent infections
▸ BY MOUTH
  ▹ Adult: 500 mg twice daily for 3–5 days

Treatment of recurrent herpes simplex infections in immunocompromised or HIV-positive patients
▸ BY MOUTH
  ▹ Adult: 1 g twice daily for 5–10 days

Herpes labialis treatment
▸ BY MOUTH
  ▹ Child 12-17 years: Initially 2 g, then 2 g after 12 hours
  ▹ Adult: Initially 2 g, then 2 g after 12 hours

Herpes simplex, suppression of infections
▸ BY MOUTH
  ▹ Adult: 500 mg daily in 1–2 divided doses, therapy to be interrupted every 6–12 months to reassess recurrence frequency—consider restarting after two or more recurrences

Herpes simplex, suppression of infections in immunocompromised or HIV-positive patients
▸ BY MOUTH
  ▹ Adult: 500 mg twice daily, therapy to be interrupted every 6–12 months to reassess recurrence frequency—consider restarting after two or more recurrences

Genital herpes, reduction of transmission (administered on expert advice)
▸ BY MOUTH
  ▹ Adult: 500 mg once daily, to be taken by the infected partner

Prevention of cytomegalovirus disease following solid organ transplantation when valganciclovir or ganciclovir cannot be used
▸ BY MOUTH
  ▹ Adult: 2 g 4 times a day usually for 90 days, preferably starting within 72 hours of transplantation

- **CAUTIONS** Elderly (risk of neurological reactions) · maintain adequate hydration (especially with high doses)
- **INTERACTIONS** → Appendix 1: valaciclovir
- **SIDE-EFFECTS**
▸ **Common or very common** Diarrhoea · dizziness · headache · nausea · photosensitivity reaction · skin reactions · vomiting
▸ **Uncommon** Abdominal discomfort · agitation · confusion · dyspnoea · haematuria · hallucination · leucopenia · level of consciousness decreased · renal pain · thrombocytopenia · tremor
▸ **Rare or very rare** Angioedema · ataxia · coma · delirium · dysarthria · encephalopathy · nephrolithiasis · psychosis · renal impairment · seizure
▸ **Frequency not known** Microangiopathic haemolytic anaemia
  SIDE-EFFECTS, FURTHER INFORMATION Neurological reactions more frequent with higher doses.
- **PREGNANCY** Not known to be harmful—manufacturers advise use only when potential benefit outweighs risk.
- **BREAST FEEDING** Significant amount in milk after systemic administration—not known to be harmful but manufacturer advises caution.
- **HEPATIC IMPAIRMENT** Manufacturer advises caution with doses of 4 g or more per day (no information available).
- **RENAL IMPAIRMENT** Maintain adequate hydration.
  Dose adjustments ▸ In adults For *herpes zoster*, 1 g every 12 hours if eGFR 30–50 mL/minute/1.73 m^2 (1 g every 24 hours if eGFR 10– 30 mL/minute/1.73 m^2; 500 mg every 24 hours if eGFR less than 10 mL/minute/1.73 m^2). For *treatment of herpes simplex*, 500 mg (1 g in immunocompromised or HIV-positive patients) every 24 hours if eGFR less than 30 mL/minute/1.73 m^2. For *treatment of herpes labialis*, if eGFR 30–50 mL/minute/1.73 m^2, initially 1 g, then 1 g 12 hours after initial dose (if eGFR 10–30 mL/minute/1.73 m^2, initially 500 mg, then 500 mg 12 hours after initial dose; if eGFR less than 10 mL/minute/1.73 m^2, 500 mg as a single dose). For *suppression of herpes simplex*, 250 mg (500 mg in immunocompromised or HIV-positive patients) every 24 hours if eGFR less than 30 mL/minute/1.73 m^2. For *reduction of genital herpes transmission*, 250 mg every 24 hours if eGFR less than 15 mL/minute/1.73 m^2. Reduce dose according to eGFR for *cytomegalovirus prophylaxis* following solid organ transplantation (consult product literature).
  ▸ In children For *treatment of herpes labialis*, if estimated glomerular filtration rate 30–50 mL/minute/1.73 m^2, initially 1 g, then 1 g 12 hours after initial dose (if estimated glomerular filtration rate 10–30 mL/minute/1.73 m^2, initially 500 mg, then 500 mg 12 hours after initial dose; if estimated glomerular

5

Infection

filtration rate less than 10 mL/minute/1.73 m^2, 500 mg as a single dose).

- **PRESCRIBING AND DISPENSING INFORMATION** Valaciclovir is a pro-drug of aciclovir.

- **MEDICINAL FORMS** There can be variation in the licensing of different medicines containing the same drug. Forms available from special-order manufacturers include: oral suspension

Tablet

CAUTIONARY AND ADVISORY LABELS 9
  ▸ Valaciclovir (Non-proprietary)
    Valaciclovir (as Valaciclovir hydrochloride) 500 mg Valaciclovir 500mg tablets | 10 tablet [PoM] £24.11 DT = £24.11 | 42 tablet [PoM] £101.26
  ▸ Valtrex (GlaxoSmithKline UK Ltd)
    Valaciclovir (as Valaciclovir hydrochloride) 250 mg Valtrex 250mg tablets | 60 tablet [PoM] £123.28 DT = £123.28
    Valaciclovir (as Valaciclovir hydrochloride) 500 mg Valtrex 500mg tablets | 10 tablet [PoM] £20.59 DT = £24.11 | 42 tablet [PoM] £86.30

6.4a Cytomegalovirus infections

ANTIVIRALS ⟩ NUCLEOSIDE ANALOGUES

Cidofovir

20-Mar-2019

- **DRUG ACTION** Cidofovir is a selective inhibitor of human cytomegalovirus (HCMV) DNA polymerase which inhibits viral DNA synthesis and thereby suppresses HCMV replication.

- **INDICATIONS AND DOSE**

Cytomegalovirus retinitis in patients with AIDS (in combination with probenecid) (specialist use only)
  ▸ **BY INTRAVENOUS INFUSION**
  ▸ **Adult:** Initially 5 mg/kg once weekly for 2 weeks, then maintenance 5 mg/kg every 2 weeks, maintenance treatment to be started 2 weeks after completion of induction treatment

- **CONTRA-INDICATIONS** Concomitant administration with potentially nephrotoxic drugs—discontinue potentially nephrotoxic drugs at least 7 days before starting cidofovir · patients unable to receive probenecid

- **CAUTIONS** Diabetes mellitus (increased risk of ocular hypotony) · ensure concomitant use of probenecid and Sodium Chloride 0.9%

  CAUTIONS, FURTHER INFORMATION
  ▸ Probenecid and Sodium Chloride 0.9% Manufacturer advises oral probenecid and intravenous Sodium Chloride 0.9% must be administered with each cidofovir dose to prevent nephrotoxicity (consult cidofovir product literature for information on probenecid dosing and recommendations on intravenous hydration); see *Prescribing and dispensing information* for details on obtaining probenecid.

- **INTERACTIONS** → Appendix 1: cidofovir

- **SIDE-EFFECTS**
  ▸ **Common or very common** Alopecia · asthenia · chills · diarrhoea · dyspnoea · eye inflammation · fever · headache · nausea · neutropenia · ocular hypotony · proteinuria · rash · renal failure · vomiting
  ▸ **Uncommon** Fanconi syndrome acquired
  ▸ **Frequency not known** Hearing impairment · nephrotoxicity · pancreatitis

  SIDE-EFFECTS, FURTHER INFORMATION Manufacturer advises intravenous sodium chloride 0.9% prehydration and concomitant oral probenecid for prevention of nephrotoxicity; consider treatment interruption, or discontinuation if changes in renal function occur—consult product literature.

- **CONCEPTION AND CONTRACEPTION** Manufacturer advises ensure effective contraception during and after treatment in women; men should be advised to use barrier contraception during and for 3 months after treatment. Cidofovir may cause impaired fertility in males—reduced testes weight and hyposermia observed in *animal* studies.

- **PREGNANCY** Manufacturer advises avoid—toxicity in *animal* studies.

- **BREAST FEEDING** Manufacturer advises avoid (no information available).

- **HEPATIC IMPAIRMENT** Manufacturer advises caution (no information available).

- **RENAL IMPAIRMENT** Manufacturer advises avoid if creatinine clearance is less than or equal to 55 mL/minute or if proteinuria is greater than or equal to 100 mg/dL.

- **MONITORING REQUIREMENTS**
  ▸ Manufacturer advises monitor serum creatinine, urine protein levels, and white blood cell count before each cidofovir dose.
  ▸ Manufacturer advises regular eye examinations (increased risk of iritis, ocular hypotony, and uveitis).

- **DIRECTIONS FOR ADMINISTRATION** Manufacturer advises for *intravenous infusion*, dilute with 100 mL Sodium Chloride 0.9% and mix thoroughly; give at a constant rate over 1 hour via an infusion pump.

- **PRESCRIBING AND DISPENSING INFORMATION** Probenecid is available from 'special-order' manufacturers or specialist importing companies—in case of difficulties, the cidofovir manufacturer (Tillomed) advises contacting their local representative. See probenecid product literature for prescribing information for probenecid, including information on interactions.

- **HANDLING AND STORAGE**
  Caution in handling Manufacturer advises cidofovir should be considered a potential carcinogen and must be handled with caution (consult product literature); if contact with skin or mucous membranes occurs, wash thoroughly with water.

- **MEDICINAL FORMS** There can be variation in the licensing of different medicines containing the same drug.
Solution for infusion
ELECTROLYTES: May contain Sodium
  ▸ Cidofovir (non-proprietary) ▼
    Cidofovir 75 mg per 1 ml Cidofovir 375mg/5ml concentrate for solution for infusion vials | 1 vial [PoM] [⊠]

Ganciclovir

15-Dec-2020

- **INDICATIONS AND DOSE**

Prevention of cytomegalovirus disease [pre-emptive therapy in patients with drug-induced immunosuppression]
  ▸ **BY INTRAVENOUS INFUSION**
  ▸ **Adult:** Initially 5 mg/kg every 12 hours for 7–14 days, then maintenance 6 mg/kg once daily, on 5 days of the week, alternatively maintenance 5 mg/kg once daily

Prevention of cytomegalovirus disease [universal prophylaxis in patients with drug-induced immunosuppression]
  ▸ **BY INTRAVENOUS INFUSION**
  ▸ **Adult:** 6 mg/kg once daily, on 5 days of the week, alternatively 5 mg/kg once daily

Treatment of cytomegalovirus disease [in immunocompromised patients]
  ▸ **BY INTRAVENOUS INFUSION**
  ▸ **Adult:** Initially 5 mg/kg every 12 hours for 14–21 days, then maintenance 6 mg/kg once daily, on 5 days of the week, alternatively maintenance 5 mg/kg once daily, maintenance only for patients at risk of relapse; if

disease progresses initial induction treatment may be repeated

- **CONTRA-INDICATIONS** Abnormally low haemoglobin count (consult product literature) · abnormally low neutrophil count (consult product literature) · abnormally low platelet count (consult product literature)
- **CAUTIONS** History of cytopenia · potential carcinogen (including long-term carcinogenicity) · potential teratogen (including long-term teratogenicity) · radiotherapy
- **INTERACTIONS** → Appendix 1: ganciclovir
- **SIDE-EFFECTS**
▶ **Common or very common** Anaemia · anxiety · appetite decreased · arthralgia · asthenia · bone marrow disorders · chest pain · chills · confusion · constipation · cough · depression · diarrhoea · dizziness · dysphagia · dyspnoea · ear pain · eye disorders · eye inflammation · eye pain · fever · flatulence · gastrointestinal discomfort · headache · hepatic function abnormal · increased risk of infection · insomnia · leucopenia · malaise · muscle complaints · nausea · neutropenia · night sweats · pain · peripheral neuropathy · renal impairment · seizure · sensation abnormal · sepsis · skin reactions · taste altered · thinking abnormal · thrombocytopenia · vomiting · weight decreased
▶ **Uncommon** Alopecia · arrhythmia · deafness · haematuria · hypotension · infertility male · oral ulceration · pancreatitis · psychotic disorder · tremor · visual impairment
▶ **Rare or very rare** Agranulocytosis · hallucination
- **ALLERGY AND CROSS-SENSITIVITY** [EvGr] Contra-indicated in patients hypersensitive to valganciclovir.
  Caution in patients hypersensitive to aciclovir, valaciclovir, or famciclovir. ⊛
- **CONCEPTION AND CONTRACEPTION** Manufacturer advises women of childbearing potential should use effective contraception during and for at least 30 days after treatment; men with partners of childbearing potential should be advised to use barrier contraception during and for at least 90 days after treatment. Ganciclovir may cause temporary or permanent inhibition of spermatogenesis— impaired fertility observed in *animal* studies.
- **PREGNANCY** Manufacturer advises avoid unless potential benefit outweighs risk—teratogenicity in *animal* studies.
- **BREAST FEEDING** Manufacturer advises avoid—present in milk in *animal* studies.
- **RENAL IMPAIRMENT**
  Dose adjustments Manufacturer advises reduce dose for patients receiving mg/kg dosing if creatinine clearance less than 70 mL/minute—consult product literature.
- **MONITORING REQUIREMENTS** Monitor full blood count closely (severe deterioration may require correction and possibly treatment interruption).
- **DIRECTIONS FOR ADMINISTRATION** Manufacturer advises, for *intravenous infusion*, give intermittently in Glucose 5% or Sodium Chloride 0.9%. Reconstitute with Water for Injections (500 mg/10 mL) then dilute requisite dose to a concentration of not more than 10 mg/mL with infusion fluid; give over 1 hour into a vein with adequate flow, preferably using a plastic cannula.
- **HANDLING AND STORAGE**
  Caution in handling Ganciclovir is a potential teratogen and carcinogen. Manufacturer advises avoid inhalation of the powder or direct contact of the powder or reconstituted solution with the skin or mucous membranes; if contact occurs, wash thoroughly with soap and water; rinse eyes thoroughly with plain water.

- **MEDICINAL FORMS** There can be variation in the licensing of different medicines containing the same drug.
  Powder for solution for infusion
  ELECTROLYTES: May contain Sodium
  ▶ Ganciclovir (Non-proprietary)
  Ganciclovir (as Ganciclovir sodium) 500 mg Ganciclovir 500mg powder for concentrate for solution for infusion vials | 5 vial [PoM] £115.00–£125.95 (Hospital only) | 5 vial [PoM] £125.95
  ▶ Cymevene (Cheplapharm Arzneimittel GmbH)
  Ganciclovir (as Ganciclovir sodium) 500 mg Cymevene 500mg powder for concentrate for solution for infusion vials | 5 vial [PoM] £148.83 (Hospital only)

Valganciclovir
15-Dec-2020

- **INDICATIONS AND DOSE**
  Cytomegalovirus retinitis [induction and maintenance treatment in patients with AIDS]
  ▶ BY MOUTH
  ▶ Adult: Initially 900 mg twice daily for 21 days, then maintenance 900 mg daily, induction regimen may be repeated if retinitis progresses

  Prevention of cytomegalovirus disease [following solid organ transplantation from a cytomegalovirus positive donor]
  ▶ BY MOUTH
  ▶ Adult: 900 mg daily for 100 days (for 100–200 days following kidney transplantation), to be started within 10 days of transplantation

  DOSE EQUIVALENCE AND CONVERSION
  ▶ Oral valganciclovir 900 mg twice daily is equivalent to intravenous ganciclovir 5 mg/kg twice daily.

- **CONTRA-INDICATIONS** Abnormally low haemoglobin count (consult product literature) · abnormally low neutrophil count (consult product literature) · abnormally low platelet count (consult product literature)
- **CAUTIONS** History of cytopenia · potential carcinogen (including long-term carcinogenicity) · potential teratogen (including long-term teratogenicity) · radiotherapy
- **INTERACTIONS** → Appendix 1: valganciclovir
- **SIDE-EFFECTS**
▶ **Common or very common** Anaemia · anxiety · appetite decreased · arthralgia · asthenia · bone marrow disorders · chest pain · confusion · constipation · cough · depression · diarrhoea · dizziness · dysphagia · dyspnoea · ear pain · eye disorders · eye inflammation · eye pain · flatulence · gastrointestinal discomfort · headache · hepatic function abnormal · increased risk of infection · insomnia · leucopenia · malaise · muscle complaints · nausea · neutropenia · night sweats · pain · peripheral neuropathy · renal impairment · seizure · sensation abnormal · sepsis · skin reactions · taste altered · thinking abnormal · thrombocytopenia · vomiting · weight decreased
▶ **Uncommon** Alopecia · arrhythmia · deafness · haematuria · hallucination · hypotension · infertility male · oral ulceration · pancreatitis · psychotic disorder · tremor · visual impairment
- **ALLERGY AND CROSS-SENSITIVITY** [EvGr] Contra-indicated in patients hypersensitive to ganciclovir.
  Caution in patients hypersensitive to aciclovir, valaciclovir, or famciclovir. ⊛
- **CONCEPTION AND CONTRACEPTION** Manufacturer advises women of childbearing potential should use effective contraception during and for at least 30 days after treatment; men with partners of childbearing potential should be advised to use barrier contraception during and for at least 90 days after treatment. *Ganciclovir* may cause temporary or permanent inhibition of spermatogenesis— impaired fertility observed in *animal* studies.

- **PREGNANCY** Manufacturer advises avoid unless potential benefit outweighs risk—teratogenicity observed with *ganciclovir* in *animal* studies.
- **BREAST FEEDING** Manufacturer advises avoid— *ganciclovir* present in milk in *animal* studies.
- **RENAL IMPAIRMENT**
  Dose adjustments Manufacturer advises reduce dose if creatinine clearance less than 60 mL/minute—consult product literature.
- **MONITORING REQUIREMENTS** Monitor full blood count closely (severe deterioration may require correction and possibly treatment interruption).
- **PRESCRIBING AND DISPENSING INFORMATION** Valganciclovir is a pro-drug of ganciclovir.
  Flavours of oral liquid formulations may include tutti-frutti.
- **HANDLING AND STORAGE** Manufacturer advises reconstituted powder for oral solution should be stored in a refrigerator (2–8°C) for up to 49 days.
  Caution in handling Valganciclovir is a potential teratogen and carcinogen. Manufacturer advises caution when handling the powder, reconstituted solution, or broken tablets and avoid inhalation of powder; if contact with skin or mucous membranes occurs, wash thoroughly with soap and water; rinse eyes thoroughly with plain water.

- **MEDICINAL FORMS** There can be variation in the licensing of different medicines containing the same drug. Forms available from special-order manufacturers include: oral solution
  Oral solution
  CAUTIONARY AND ADVISORY LABELS 21
  ‣ Valcyte (Roche Products Ltd)
  Valganciclovir (as Valganciclovir hydrochloride) 50 mg per 1 ml Valcyte 50mg/ml oral solution sugar-free | 100 ml PoM £230.32 DT = £230.32
  Tablet
  CAUTIONARY AND ADVISORY LABELS 21
  ‣ Valganciclovir (Non-proprietary)
  Valganciclovir (as Valganciclovir hydrochloride)
  450 mg Valganciclovir 450mg tablets | 60 tablet PoM £865.17–£1,081.46 DT = £1,027.40
  ‣ Valcyte (Roche Products Ltd)
  Valganciclovir (as Valganciclovir hydrochloride) 450 mg Valcyte 450mg tablets | 60 tablet PoM £1,081.46 DT = £1,027.40

ANTIVIRALS > OTHER

Foscarnet sodium

08-Oct-2020

- **INDICATIONS AND DOSE**
Cytomegalovirus disease
  ▸ BY INTRAVENOUS INFUSION
  ‣ Adult: Initially 60 mg/kg every 8 hours for 2–3 weeks, alternatively initially 90 mg/kg every 12 hours for 2–3 weeks, then maintenance 60 mg/kg daily, then increased if tolerated to 90–120 mg/kg daily, if disease progresses on maintenance dose, repeat induction regimen

Mucocutaneous herpes simplex virus infections unresponsive to aciclovir in immunocompromised patients
  ▸ BY INTRAVENOUS INFUSION
  ‣ Adult: 40 mg/kg every 8 hours for 2–3 weeks or until lesions heal

- **UNLICENSED USE** Licensed for CMV retinitis in AIDS patients only. Foscarnet doses in BNF may differ from those in product literature.
- **CAUTIONS** Conditions where excess sodium should be avoided · ensure adequate hydration
- **INTERACTIONS** → Appendix 1: foscarnet

- **SIDE-EFFECTS**
  ▸ **Common or very common** Aggression · anaemia · anxiety · appetite decreased · arrhythmias · asthenia · chest pain · chills · confusion · constipation · coordination abnormal · dehydration · depression · diarrhoea · dizziness · electrolyte imbalance · fever · gastrointestinal discomfort · genital discomfort (due to high concentrations excreted in urine) · genital ulceration (due to high concentrations excreted in urine) · haemorrhage · headache · hepatic function abnormal · hypertension · hypotension · leucopenia · malaise · muscle contractions involuntary · myalgia · nausea (reduce infusion rate) · neutropenia · numbness · oedema · palpitations · pancreatitis · paraesthesia (reduce infusion rate) · peripheral neuropathy · proteinuria · renal impairment · seizure · sepsis · skin reactions · thrombocytopenia · thrombophlebitis · tremor · urinary disorders · vomiting
  ▸ **Uncommon** Acidosis · angioedema · glomerulonephritis · nephropathy · pancytopenia
  ▸ **Frequency not known** Anaphylactoid reaction · diabetes insipidus · muscle weakness · myopathy · oesophageal ulcer · QT interval prolongation · renal pain · renal tubular acidosis · severe cutaneous adverse reactions (SCARs)
- **CONCEPTION AND CONTRACEPTION** Men should avoid fathering a child during and for 6 months after treatment.
- **PREGNANCY** Manufacturer advises avoid.
- **BREAST FEEDING** Avoid—present in milk in *animal* studies.
- **RENAL IMPAIRMENT**
  Dose adjustments Reduce dose; consult product literature.
- **MONITORING REQUIREMENTS**
  ▸ Monitor electrolytes, particularly calcium and magnesium.
  ▸ Monitor serum creatinine every second day during induction and every week during maintenance.
- **DIRECTIONS FOR ADMINISTRATION** For *intravenous infusion* (*Foscavir®*), manufacturer advises give intermittently in Glucose 5% or Sodium Chloride 0.9%; dilute to a concentration of 12 mg/mL for infusion into peripheral vein (undiluted solution *via* central venous line only); infuse over at least 1 hour (infuse doses greater than 60 mg/kg over 2 hours).

- **MEDICINAL FORMS** There can be variation in the licensing of different medicines containing the same drug.
  Solution for infusion
  ELECTROLYTES: May contain Sodium
  ‣ Foscavir (Clinigen Healthcare Ltd)
  Foscarnet sodium 24 mg per 1 ml Foscavir 6g/250ml solution for infusion bottles | 1 bottle PoM £119.85 (Hospital only)

Letermovir

31-Aug-2020

- **DRUG ACTION** Letermovir is a cytomegalovirus DNA terminase complex inhibitor that interferes with cytomegalovirus genome formation and virion maturation.

- **INDICATIONS AND DOSE**
Prevention of cytomegalovirus reactivation and disease [in recipients of an allogeneic haematopoietic stem cell transplant who are seropositive for the human cytomegalovirus] (initiated by a specialist)
  ▸ BY MOUTH
  ‣ Adult: 480 mg once daily for 100 days post-transplant, start within 28 days post-transplant, treatment beyond 100 days may be considered in some patients—consult product literature
  DOSE ADJUSTMENTS DUE TO INTERACTIONS
  ▸ Manufacturer advises reduce dose to 240 mg once daily with concurrent use of ciclosporin.

- **INTERACTIONS** → Appendix 1: letermovir

● SIDE-EFFECTS
► **Common or very common** Diarrhoea · nausea · vomiting
► **Uncommon** Abdominal pain · appetite decreased · fatigue · headache · muscle spasms · peripheral oedema · taste altered · vertigo

● CONCEPTION AND CONTRACEPTION The effect on human fertility is not known—impairment of fertility has been observed in *animal* studies.

● PREGNANCY Manufacturer advises avoid—toxicity in *animal* studies.

● BREAST FEEDING Manufacturer advises avoid—present in milk in *animal* studies.

● HEPATIC IMPAIRMENT Manufacturer advises avoid in moderate impairment in those with co-existing moderate or severe renal impairment, and in severe impairment (risk of increased exposure).

● NATIONAL FUNDING/ACCESS DECISIONS
For full details see funding body website
NICE decisions
► Letermovir for preventing cytomegalovirus disease after a stem cell transplant (July 2019) NICE TA591 Recommended
Scottish Medicines Consortium (SMC) decisions
► Letermovir (*Prevymis*®) for prophylaxis of cytomegalovirus (CMV) reactivation and disease in adult CMV-seropositive recipients [R+] of an allogeneic haematopoietic stem cell transplant (March 2019) SMC No. 1338/18 Recommended

● MEDICINAL FORMS There can be variation in the licensing of different medicines containing the same drug.
Tablet
CAUTIONARY AND ADVISORY LABELS 25
► Prevymis (Merck Sharp & Dohme Ltd) ▼
　Letermovir 240 mg Prevymis 240mg tablets | 28 tablet [PoM] £3,723.16 (Hospital only)

6.5　HIV infection

HIV infection

HIV infection　　　　　　　　　　　　　　　　01-Sep-2020

Overview

The human immunodeficiency virus (HIV) is a retrovirus that causes immunodeficiency by infecting and destroying cells of the immune system, particularly the CD4 cells. Acquired immune deficiency syndrome (AIDS) occurs when the number of CD4 cells fall to below 200 cells/microlitre; opportunistic infections and malignancies (AIDS-defining illnesses) can develop. The prognosis of HIV and AIDS has greatly improved due to more effective and better tolerated antiretroviral therapy (ART). The greatest risk to excess mortality and morbidity is delayed HIV diagnosis and treatment.

Aims of treatment

Treatment aims to achieve an undetectable viral load, to preserve immune function, to reduce the mortality and morbidity associated with chronic HIV infection, and to reduce onward transmission of HIV, whilst minimising drug toxicity. Treatment with a combination of ART aims to improve the physical and psychological well-being of infected people.

Initiation of treatment

[EvGr] All patients with suspected or diagnosed HIV should be reviewed promptly by a HIV specialist.

All patients diagnosed as being HIV positive should be offered immediate treatment, irrespective of CD4 cell counts. ⟨A⟩ Commitment to, and strict adherence to treatment over many years is required. Low adherence can be associated with drug resistance, progression to AIDS, and

death. The treatment regimen should take into account dosing convenience, potential drug interactions, clinical symptoms, and comorbidities.

[EvGr] Treatment of HIV infection in *treatment-naive* patients is initiated with a combination of two nucleoside reverse transcriptase inhibitors (NRTIs) as a backbone regimen plus *one* of the following as a third drug: an integrase inhibitor (INI), a non-nucleoside reverse transcriptase inhibitor (NNRTI), *or* a boosted protease inhibitor (PI).

The regimen of choice contains a backbone of emtricitabine p. 689 and either tenofovir disoproxil p. 692 or tenofovir alafenamide p. 663. An alternative backbone regimen is abacavir p. 685 and lamivudine p. 691. The third drug of choice is either ritonavir p. 698-boosted atazanavir p. 694, or ritonavir-boosted darunavir p. 695, or dolutegravir p. 680, or cobicistat p. 699-boosted elvitegravir p. 682, or raltegravir p. 682, or rilpivirine p. 685. Efavirenz p. 683 may be used as an alternative third drug.

Patients who require treatment for both HIV and chronic hepatitis B should be treated with antivirals active against both diseases as part of fully suppressive combination ART. Regimens of choice are tenofovir disoproxil and emtricitabine, or tenofovir alafenamide p. 663 and emtricitabine. ⟨A⟩ For further information see British HIV Association guidelines for the treatment of HIV-1-positive adults with antiretroviral therapy available at www.bhiva.org/guidelines.

Switching therapy

[EvGr] Deterioration of the condition (including clinical, virological, and CD4 cell count changes) may require a change in therapy. The choice of an alternative regimen should be guided by factors such as the response to previous treatment, tolerability, drug-drug interactions and the possibility of drug resistance. ⟨A⟩ For further information see British HIV Association guidelines for the treatment of HIV-1-positive adults with antiretroviral therapy available at www.bhiva.org/guidelines.

HIV infection in pregnancy

[EvGr] Management of HIV infection in pregnancy should focus on the well-being of the women living with HIV, by ensuring that their ART regimen maximally suppresses viral replication as early as possible (if possible before conception) in order to minimise vertical transmission of HIV. Information on the teratogenic potential of most antiretroviral drugs is limited, however, all pregnant women living with HIV who conceive whilst on effective ART should continue this treatment throughout their pregnancy. All other women should start ART during their pregnancy. The recommended regimen is a NRTI backbone of either tenofovir disoproxil or abacavir with either emtricitabine or lamivudine; the third drug should be efavirenz or ritonavir-boosted atazanavir. All treatment options require careful assessment by a specialist. ⟨A⟩ For further information, including alternative ART options, see British HIV Association guidelines for the management of HIV in pregnancy and postpartum available at www.bhiva.org/guidelines.

[EvGr] Pregnancies in women with HIV and babies born to them should be reported prospectively to the National Study of HIV in Pregnancy and Childhood at www.ucl.ac.uk/nshpc/ **and** to the Antiretroviral Pregnancy Registry at www.apregistry.com. ⟨A⟩

HIV infection and breast-feeding

[EvGr] Breast-feeding by HIV-positive mothers may cause HIV infection in the infant and should be avoided. ⟨A⟩ For further information see British HIV Association guidelines management of HIV in pregnancy and postpartum at www.bhiva.org/guidelines.

5

Infection

5

Infection

HIV infection, pre-exposure prophylaxis

The risk of acquiring HIV is increased in:

- men or transgender individuals who have unprotected anal intercourse with men;
- sexual partners of people who are HIV-positive with a detectable viral load; and
- HIV-negative heterosexual individuals who have unprotected intercourse with a HIV-positive person, and are likely to repeat this with the same person or another person with a similar status.

EvGr Emtricitabine with tenofovir disoproxil p. 690 may be appropriate for pre-exposure prophylaxis to reduce the risk of sexually acquired HIV-1 infection in combination with safer sex practices in adults at high risk. Tenofovir disoproxil alone is an alternative for HIV-negative heterosexual individuals when emtricitabine is contra-indicated. Ⓐ For further information see British HIV Association and British Association for Sexual Health and HIV guidelines on the use of HIV pre-exposure prophylaxis (PrEP) available at: www.bhiva.org/guidelines.

HIV infection, post-exposure prophylaxis

The Department of Health advises prompt prophylaxis with antiretroviral drugs [unlicensed indication] may be appropriate following exposure to HIV-contaminated material. Immediate expert advice should be sought in such cases. National guidelines on post-exposure prophylaxis for healthcare workers have been developed (by the Chief Medical Officer's Expert Advisory Group on AIDS), www.gov.uk/government/publications/eaga-guidance-on-hiv-post-exposure-prophylaxis and local ones may also be available.

EvGr Prompt prophylaxis with antiretroviral drugs [unlicensed indication] may also be appropriate following potential sexual exposure to HIV where there is a significant risk of viral transmission. The recommended treatment for post-exposure prophylaxis is emtricitabine with tenofovir disoproxil plus raltegravir for 28 days. Ⓐ For further information see British Association for Sexual Health and HIV guidelines for the use of HIV post-exposure prophylaxis following sexual exposure available at www.bashh.org.

Drug treatment

Drugs that are licensed for the treatment of HIV/AIDS are listed below according to drug class.

Nucleoside reverse transcriptase inhibitors (NRTI or 'nucleoside analogue'): abacavir (ABC); emtricitabine (FTC); lamivudine (3TC); tenofovir alafenamide fumarate (TAF) p. 663, tenofovir disoproxil fumarate (TDF), and zidovudine (AZT) p. 693.

Non-nucleoside reverse transcriptase inhibitors (NNRTI): doravirine (DOR) p. 683, efavirenz (EFV), etravirine (ETR) p. 684, nevirapine (NVP) p. 684, and rilpivirine (RPV) p. 685.

Protease inhibitors (PI): atazanavir (ATZ), darunavir (DRV), fosamprenavir (FOS-APV) p. 697, lopinavir (LPV), ritonavir (RTV), saquinavir (SQV) p. 698, and tipranavir (TPV) p. 698.

CCR5 antagonists: maraviroc (MVC) p. 699.

Integrase inhibitors (INI): bictegravir (BIC), dolutegravir below (DTG), elvitegravir (EVG) p. 682, and raltegravir (RAL).

Fusion inhibitors: enfuvirtide below (T-20).

Pharmacokinetic enhancers: cobicistat (c) p. 699, and low-dose ritonavir (r). They boost the concentrations of other antiretrovirals metabolised by CYP3A4, but have no antiretroviral activity themselves.

Enfuvirtide

04-Sep-2020

- **DRUG ACTION** Enfuvirtide inhibits the fusion of HIV to the host cell.

- **INDICATIONS AND DOSE**

HIV infection in combination with other antiretroviral drugs for resistant infection or for patients intolerant to other antiretroviral regimens
  ‣ BY SUBCUTANEOUS INJECTION
  ‣ Adult: 90 mg twice daily

- **SIDE-EFFECTS**
  ‣ **Common or very common** Anxiety · appetite decreased · asthenia · concentration impaired · conjunctivitis · diabetes mellitus · gastrooesophageal reflux disease · haematuria · hypertriglyceridaemia · increased risk of infection · influenza like illness · irritability · lymphadenopathy · myalgia · nasal congestion · nephrolithiasis · nightmare · numbness · pancreatitis · peripheral neuropathy · skin papilloma · skin reactions · tremor · vertigo · weight decreased
  ‣ **Frequency not known** Diarrhoea · hypersensitivity · immune reconstitution inflammatory syndrome · nausea · osteonecrosis

  SIDE-EFFECTS, FURTHER INFORMATION **Hypersensitivity** Hypersensitivity reactions including rash, fever, nausea, vomiting, chills, rigors, low blood pressure, respiratory distress, glomerulonephritis, and raised liver enzymes reported; discontinue immediately if any signs or symptoms of systemic hypersensitivity develop and do not rechallenge.

  Osteonecrosis Osteonecrosis has been reported in patients with advanced HIV disease or following long-term exposure to combination antiretroviral therapy.

- **PREGNANCY** Manufacturer advises use only if potential benefit outweighs risk.

- **HEPATIC IMPAIRMENT** Manufacturer advises caution (no information available); increased risk of hepatic side effects in patients with chronic hepatitis B or C.

- **DIRECTIONS FOR ADMINISTRATION** For *subcutaneous injection*, manufacturer advises reconstitute with 1.1 mL Water for Injections and allow to stand (for up to 45 minutes) to dissolve; do **not** shake or invert vial.

- **PATIENT AND CARER ADVICE**
  Hypersensitivity reactions Patients or carers should be told how to recognise signs of hypersensitivity, and advised to discontinue treatment and seek immediate medical attention if symptoms develop.

- **MEDICINAL FORMS** There can be variation in the licensing of different medicines containing the same drug.
  Powder and solvent for solution for injection
  ELECTROLYTES: May contain Sodium
  ‣ Fuzeon (Roche Products Ltd)
    Enfuvirtide 108 mg Fuzeon 108mg powder and solvent for solution for injection vials | 60 vial PoM £1,081.57 (Hospital only)

Dolutegravir

13-Nov-2020

- **DRUG ACTION** Dolutegravir is an inhibitor of HIV integrase.

- **INDICATIONS AND DOSE**

HIV infection without resistance to other inhibitors of HIV integrase, in combination with other antiretroviral drugs
  ‣ BY MOUTH
  ‣ Adult: 50 mg once daily

HIV infection in patients where resistance to other inhibitors of HIV integrase suspected, in combination with other antiretroviral drugs
▶ BY MOUTH
▶ Adult: 50 mg twice daily, dose to be taken with food

HIV infection in combination with other antiretroviral drugs (with concomitant carbamazepine, efavirenz, etravirine (without boosted protease inhibitors, but see also Interactions), fosphenytoin, phenobarbital, phenytoin, primidone, nevirapine, oxcarbazepine, St John's wort, rifampicin, or tipranavir)
▶ BY MOUTH
▶ Adult: 50 mg twice daily, avoid concomitant use with these drugs if resistance to other inhibitors of HIV integrase suspected

---

IMPORTANT SAFETY INFORMATION

MHRA/CHM ADVICE: DOLUTEGRAVIR (*TIVICAY*®, *TRIUMEQ*®, *JULUCA*®): UPDATED ADVICE ON INCREASED RISK OF NEURAL TUBE DEFECTS (OCTOBER 2020)

The MHRA has updated its safety recommendations based on an ongoing European review evaluating cases of neural tube defects in babies born to mothers who became pregnant during dolutegravir treatment that found a smaller increased risk than previously thought, almost comparable to other HIV drugs.

Healthcare professionals are advised to counsel women of childbearing potential on the possible risk of neural tube defects with dolutegravir, including consideration of effective contraceptive measures. The benefits and risks of continuing treatment in women who are trying to become pregnant should be discussed with the patient. If pregnancy is confirmed in the first trimester during treatment, the benefits and risks of continuing dolutegravir versus switching to another antiretroviral regimen should also be discussed, considering the gestational age and the critical time period of neural tube defect development.

● INTERACTIONS → Appendix 1: dolutegravir

● SIDE-EFFECTS
▶ **Common or very common** Anxiety · depression · diarrhoea · dizziness · fatigue · flatulence · gastrointestinal discomfort · headache · nausea · skin reactions · sleep disorders · vomiting
▶ **Uncommon** Arthralgia · hepatic disorders · hypersensitivity · immune reconstitution inflammatory syndrome · myalgia · suicidal behaviours

SIDE-EFFECTS, FURTHER INFORMATION **Hypersensitivity** Hypersensitivity reactions (including severe rash, or rash accompanied by fever, malaise, arthralgia, myalgia, blistering, oral lesions, conjunctivitis, angioedema, eosinophilia, or raised liver enzymes) reported uncommonly. Discontinue immediately if any sign or symptoms of hypersensitivity reactions develop.

Osteonecrosis Osteonecrosis has been reported in patients with advanced HIV disease or following long-term exposure to combination antiretroviral therapy.

● PREGNANCY EvGr May be used during the second and third trimester—expected benefit outweighs potential risk, see also *Important Safety Information*. ⓜ

● HEPATIC IMPAIRMENT Manufacturer advises caution in severe impairment—no information available.

● PATIENT AND CARER ADVICE Patients or carers should be given advice on how to administer dolutegravir tablets.
Missed doses If a dose is more than 20 hours late on the once daily regimen (or more than 8 hours late on the twice daily regimen), the missed dose should not be taken and the next dose should be taken at the normal time.

● NATIONAL FUNDING/ACCESS DECISIONS
For full details see funding body website
Scottish Medicines Consortium (SMC) decisions
▶ Dolutegravir (*Tivicay*®) for use in combination with other antiretroviral medicinal products for the treatment of Human Immunodeficiency Virus (HIV) infected adults (May 2014) SMC No. 961/14 Recommended

All Wales Medicines Strategy Group (AWMSG) decisions
▶ Dolutegravir (*Tivicay*®) for the treatment of Human Immunodeficiency Virus (HIV) infected adults in combination with other anti-retroviral medicinal products (October 2017) AWMSG No. 3373 Recommended

● MEDICINAL FORMS There can be variation in the licensing of different medicines containing the same drug.
Tablet
▶ Tivicay (ViiV Healthcare UK Ltd)
Dolutegravir (as Dolutegravir sodium) 10 mg Tivicay 10mg tablets | 30 tablet [PoM] £99.75 DT = £99.75 (Hospital only)
Dolutegravir (as Dolutegravir sodium) 25 mg Tivicay 25mg tablets | 30 tablet [PoM] £249.38 DT = £249.38 (Hospital only)
Dolutegravir (as Dolutegravir sodium) 50 mg Tivicay 50mg tablets | 30 tablet [PoM] £498.75 DT = £498.75 (Hospital only)

Combinations available: *Abacavir with dolutegravir and lamivudine*, p. 686 · *Lamivudine with dolutegravir*, p. 691

Dolutegravir with rilpivirine   19-Aug-2020

The properties listed below are those particular to the combination only. For the properties of the components please consider, dolutegravir p. 680, rilpivirine p. 685.

● INDICATIONS AND DOSE

HIV-1 infection (initiated by a specialist)
▶ BY MOUTH
▶ Adult: 50/25 mg once daily

DOSE EQUIVALENCE AND CONVERSION
▶ Dose expressed as x/y mg dolutegravir/rilpivirine.

● INTERACTIONS → Appendix 1: dolutegravir · NNRTIs

● PATIENT AND CARER ADVICE
Missed doses If a dose is more than 12 hours late, the missed dose should not be taken and the next dose should be taken at the normal time.
Driving and skilled tasks Manufacturer advises patients and carers should be counselled on the effects on driving and performance of skilled tasks—increased risk of dizziness and drowsiness.

● NATIONAL FUNDING/ACCESS DECISIONS
For full details see funding body website
Scottish Medicines Consortium (SMC) decisions
▶ Dolutegravir / rilpivirine film-coated tablet (*Juluca*®) for the treatment of human immunodeficiency virus type 1 (HIV-1) infection in adults who are virologically suppressed (HIV-1 RNA <50 copies/mL) on a stable antiretroviral regimen for at least six months with no history of virological failure and no known or suspected resistance to any non-nucleoside reverse transcriptase inhibitor (NNRTI) or integrase strand transfer inhibitor (INSTI) (September 2018) SMC No. SMC2091 Recommended

All Wales Medicines Strategy Group (AWMSG) decisions
▶ Dolutegravir / rilpivirine (*Juluca*®) for treatment of human immunodeficiency virus type 1 (HIV-1) infection in adults who are virologically suppressed (HIV-1 RNA <50 copies/mL) on stable antiretroviral regimen for at least six months with no history of virological failure and no known or suspected resistance to any non-nucleoside reverse transcriptase inhibitor or integrase inhibitor (December 2018) AWMSG No 2850 Recommended

- MEDICINAL FORMS There can be variation in the licensing of different medicines containing the same drug.

Tablet
CAUTIONARY AND ADVISORY LABELS 21
▸ Juluca (ViiV Healthcare UK Ltd) ▼
  Rilpivirine (as Rilpivirine hydrochloride) 25 mg, Dolutegravir (as Dolutegravir sodium) 50 mg Juluca 50mg/25mg tablets | 30 tablet [PoM] £699.02 (Hospital only)

Elvitegravir

14-Jul-2018

- DRUG ACTION Elvitegravir is an inhibitor of HIV integrase, which is an enzyme required for viral replication.

- **INDICATIONS AND DOSE**

HIV infection without resistance to other inhibitors of HIV integrase, in combination with low-dose ritonavir and atazanavir or lopinavir
▸ BY MOUTH
  ▸ Adult: 85 mg once daily, take at the same time as a once daily ritonavir-boosted regimen or with the first dose of a twice daily ritonavir-boosted regimen

HIV infection without resistance to other inhibitors of HIV integrase, in combination with low-dose ritonavir and darunavir or fosamprenavir
▸ BY MOUTH
  ▸ Adult: 150 mg once daily, take with the first dose of a twice daily ritonavir-boosted regimen

- CAUTIONS Elderly—limited information available
- INTERACTIONS → Appendix 1: elvitegravir
- SIDE-EFFECTS
▸ **Common or very common** Diarrhoea · fatigue · headache · nausea · rash · vomiting
▸ **Uncommon** Depression · dizziness · drowsiness · flatulence · gastrointestinal discomfort · insomnia · paraesthesia · suicidal ideation (in patients with history of depression or psychiatric illness) · taste altered
▸ **Frequency not known** Hyperglycaemia · osteonecrosis · weight increased

- CONCEPTION AND CONTRACEPTION Manufacturer advises women of child-bearing potential should use effective contraception during treatment (if using a hormonal contraceptive, it must contain norgestimate as the progestogen and at least 30 micrograms ethinylestradiol).
- PREGNANCY Manufacturer advises avoid unless essential—limited data available.
- PATIENT AND CARER ADVICE
Missed doses Manufacturer advises if a dose is more than 18 hours late, the missed dose should not be taken and the next dose should be taken at the normal time. If vomiting occurs within 1 hour of taking a dose, a replacement dose should be taken.

- MEDICINAL FORMS No licensed medicines listed.

  Combinations available: *Elvitegravir with cobicistat, emtricitabine and tenofovir alafenamide*, p. 687 · *Elvitegravir with cobicistat, emtricitabine and tenofovir disoproxil*, p. 688

Raltegravir

10-Nov-2020

- DRUG ACTION Raltegravir is an inhibitor of HIV integrase.

- **INDICATIONS AND DOSE**

HIV-1 infection (initiated by a specialist)
▸ BY MOUTH USING TABLETS
  ▸ Adult: 400 mg twice daily, alternatively 1200 mg once daily, once daily dosing for use in patients who are treatment naive or virologically suppressed on an initial regimen of 400 mg twice daily—use 600 mg tablets only

- CONTRA-INDICATIONS Pre-term neonates—no information available
- CAUTIONS Psychiatric illness (may exacerbate underlying illness including depression) · risk factors for myopathy · risk factors for rhabdomyolysis
- INTERACTIONS → Appendix 1: raltegravir
- SIDE-EFFECTS
▸ **Common or very common** Akathisia · appetite abnormal · asthenia · behaviour abnormal · depression · diarrhoea · dizziness · fever · gastrointestinal discomfort · gastrointestinal disorders · headaches · nausea · skin reactions · sleep disorders · vertigo · vomiting
▸ **Uncommon** Alopecia · anaemia · anxiety · arrhythmias · arthralgia · arthritis · body fat disorder · burping · cachexia · chest discomfort · chills · cognitive disorder · concentration impaired · confusion · constipation · diabetes mellitus · drowsiness · dry mouth · dyslipidaemia · dysphonia · erectile dysfunction · feeling jittery · glossitis · gynaecomastia · haemorrhage · hepatic disorders · hot flush · hyperglycaemia · hypersensitivity · hypertension · immune reconstitution inflammatory syndrome · increased risk of infection · lipodystrophy · lymph node abscess · lymphatic abnormalities · malaise · memory loss · menopausal symptoms · mood altered · myalgia · myopathy · nasal congestion · nephritis · nephrolithiasis · nerve disorders · neutropenia · nocturia · odynophagia · oedema · osteopenia · pain · palpitations · pancreatitis acute · polydipsia · psychiatric disorder · renal cyst · renal impairment · sensation abnormal · severe cutaneous adverse reactions (SCARs) · skin papilloma · submandibular mass · suicidal behaviours · sweat changes · taste altered · tendinitis · thrombocytopenia · tinnitus · tremor · visual impairment · weight increased
▸ **Frequency not known** Osteonecrosis

SIDE-EFFECTS, FURTHER INFORMATION Rash occurs commonly. Discontinue if severe rash or rash accompanied by fever, malaise, arthralgia, myalgia, blistering, mouth ulceration, conjunctivitis, angioedema, hepatitis, or eosinophilia.

- PREGNANCY Manufacturer advises avoid—toxicity in *animal* studies.
- HEPATIC IMPAIRMENT Manufacturer advises caution in severe impairment (no information available), and in patients with chronic hepatitis B or C (consider interrupting or discontinuing treatment if impairment worsens; increased risk of hepatic side-effects).
- PRESCRIBING AND DISPENSING INFORMATION Dispense raltegravir chewable tablets in original container (contains desiccant).
- NATIONAL FUNDING/ACCESS DECISIONS
For full details see funding body website
Scottish Medicines Consortium (SMC) decisions
▸ Raltegravir (*Isentress*®) for the treatment of HIV in adults (May 2010) SMC No. 613/10 Recommended with restrictions
▸ Raltegravir 600 mg film-coated tablets (*Isentress*®) in combination with other anti-retroviral medicinal products for the treatment of human immunodeficiency virus (HIV-1) infection in adults and paediatric patients weighing at least 40 kg (November 2017) SMC No. 1280/17 Recommended with restrictions

- MEDICINAL FORMS There can be variation in the licensing of different medicines containing the same drug.
Tablet
CAUTIONARY AND ADVISORY LABELS 25
▸ Isentress (Merck Sharp & Dohme Ltd)
  Raltegravir 400 mg Isentress 400mg tablets | 60 tablet [PoM] £471.41 DT = £471.41 (Hospital only)
  Raltegravir 600 mg Isentress 600mg tablets | 60 tablet [PoM] £471.41 DT = £471.41 (Hospital only)

5

Infection

ANTIVIRALS > NON-NUCLEOSIDE REVERSE TRANSCRIPTASE INHIBITORS

Doravirine

29-Oct-2020

● **INDICATIONS AND DOSE**

HIV-1 infection in combination with other antiretroviral drugs (initiated by a specialist)
▶ BY MOUTH
▶ Adult: 100 mg once daily
DOSE ADJUSTMENTS DUE TO INTERACTIONS
▶ Manufacturer advises if concurrent use of moderate inducers of CYP3A4, dabrafenib, modafinil, or telotristat ethyl is unavoidable, increase dose to 100 mg twice daily. Manufacturer advises 100 mg twice daily with rifabutin.

● INTERACTIONS → Appendix 1: NNRTIs

● SIDE-EFFECTS
▶ **Common or very common** Asthenia · diarrhoea · dizziness · drowsiness · gastrointestinal discomfort · gastrointestinal disorders · headache · hepatocellular injury · nausea · skin reactions · sleep disorders · vomiting
▶ **Uncommon** Anxiety · arthralgia · concentration impaired · confusion · constipation · depression · electrolyte imbalance · hypertension · malaise · memory loss · mood altered · muscle tone increased · myalgia · paraesthesia · suicidal ideation
▶ **Rare or very rare** Acute kidney injury · adjustment disorder · aggression · chest pain · chills · dyspnoea · hallucination · pain · rash pustular · renal disorder · thirst · tonsillar hypertrophy · urolithiases

● PREGNANCY Manufacturer advises avoid—no information available.

● HEPATIC IMPAIRMENT Manufacturer advises caution in severe impairment (no information available).

● PATIENT AND CARER ADVICE
Missed doses If a dose is more than 12 hours late, the missed dose should not be taken and the next dose should be taken at the normal time.
Driving and skilled tasks Manufacturer advises patients and carers should be counselled on the effects on driving and performance of skilled tasks—increased risk of fatigue, dizziness, and somnolence.

● NATIONAL FUNDING/ACCESS DECISIONS
For full details see funding body website
All Wales Medicines Strategy Group (AWMSG) decisions
▶ Doravirine (*Pifeltro*®) in combination with other antiretroviral medicinal products, for the treatment of adults infected with HIV-1 without past or present evidence of resistance to the NNRTI class (September 2020) AWMSG No. 3109 Recommended

● MEDICINAL FORMS There can be variation in the licensing of different medicines containing the same drug.
Tablet
CAUTIONARY AND ADVISORY LABELS 25, 3
▶ Pifeltro (Merck Sharp & Dohme Ltd) ▼
Doravirine 100 mg Pifeltro 100mg tablets | 30 tablet [PoM] £471.41 (Hospital only)

Combinations available: *Lamivudine with tenofovir disoproxil and doravirine*, p. 692

Efavirenz

02-Sep-2020

● **INDICATIONS AND DOSE**

HIV infection in combination with other antiretroviral drugs
▶ BY MOUTH USING CAPSULES
▶ Adult: 600 mg once daily
▶ BY MOUTH USING TABLETS
▶ Adult: 600 mg once daily

● CAUTIONS Acute porphyrias p. 1107 · elderly · history of psychiatric disorders · history of seizures · risk of QT interval prolongation

● INTERACTIONS → Appendix 1: NNRTIs

● SIDE-EFFECTS
▶ **Common or very common** Abdominal pain · anxiety · concentration impaired · depression · diarrhoea · dizziness · drowsiness · dyslipidaemia · fatigue · headache · movement disorders · nausea · skin reactions · sleep disorders · vomiting
▶ **Uncommon** Behaviour abnormal · confusion · flushing · gynaecomastia · hallucination · hepatic disorders · memory loss · mood altered · pancreatitis · psychosis · seizure · Stevens-Johnson syndrome · suicidal behaviours · thinking abnormal · tinnitus · tremor · vertigo · vision blurred
▶ **Rare or very rare** Delusions · photosensitivity reaction
▶ **Frequency not known** Immune reconstitution inflammatory syndrome · osteonecrosis
SIDE-EFFECTS, FURTHER INFORMATION **Rash** Rash, usually in the first 2 weeks, is the most common side-effect; discontinue if severe rash with blistering, desquamation, mucosal involvement or fever; if rash mild or moderate, may continue without interruption—usually resolves within 1 month.
CNS effects Administration at bedtime especially in first 2–4 weeks reduces CNS effects.
Abnormal hepatic function Manufacturer advises interrupt or discontinue treatment if transaminases more than 5 times the upper limit of normal.

● PREGNANCY Reports of neural tube defects when used in first trimester.

● HEPATIC IMPAIRMENT Greater risk of hepatic side-effects in chronic hepatitis B or C. Manufacturer advises avoid in severe impairment (limited information available).

● RENAL IMPAIRMENT Manufacturer advises caution in severe renal failure—no information available.

● MONITORING REQUIREMENTS Monitor liver function if receiving other hepatotoxic drugs.

● DIRECTIONS FOR ADMINISTRATION Manufacturer advises for patients who cannot swallow capsules, the capsule may be opened and contents added to a small amount of food—consult product literature. No additional food should be consumed for up to 2 hours after administration of efavirenz.

● PATIENT AND CARER ADVICE
Psychiatric disorders Patients or their carers should be advised to seek immediate medical attention if symptoms such as severe depression, psychosis or suicidal ideation occur.

● MEDICINAL FORMS There can be variation in the licensing of different medicines containing the same drug.
Tablet
CAUTIONARY AND ADVISORY LABELS 23
▶ Efavirenz (Non-proprietary)
Efavirenz 600 mg Efavirenz 600mg tablets | 30 tablet [PoM] £31.35-£452.94 (Hospital only)
▶ Sustiva (Bristol-Myers Squibb Pharmaceuticals Ltd)
Efavirenz 600 mg Sustiva 600mg tablets | 30 tablet [PoM] (Hospital only)

Capsule

CAUTIONARY AND ADVISORY LABELS 23

‣ Sustiva (Bristol-Myers Squibb Pharmaceuticals Ltd)
Efavirenz 50 mg Sustiva 50mg capsules | 30 capsule $\boxed{\text{PoM}}$ £16.73 (Hospital only)
Efavirenz 100 mg Sustiva 100mg capsules | 30 capsule $\boxed{\text{PoM}}$ £33.41 (Hospital only)
Efavirenz 200 mg Sustiva 200mg capsules | 90 capsule $\boxed{\text{PoM}}$ £200.27 (Hospital only)

Combinations available: *Efavirenz with emtricitabine and tenofovir disoproxil*, p. 687

Etravirine

04-Sep-2020

● **INDICATIONS AND DOSE**

HIV infection resistant to other non-nucleoside reverse transcriptase inhibitor and protease inhibitors in combination with other antiretroviral drugs (including a boosted protease inhibitor)

‣ BY MOUTH

‣ Adult: 200 mg twice daily, to be taken after food

● CONTRA-INDICATIONS Acute porphyrias p. 1107

● INTERACTIONS → Appendix 1: NNRTIs

● SIDE-EFFECTS

‣ **Common or very common** Diabetes mellitus · diarrhoea · headache · hyperglycaemia · myocardial infarction · nausea · skin reactions · vomiting

‣ **Uncommon** Angioedema · bronchospasm · dry mouth · dyslipidaemia · gynaecomastia · haematemesis · hepatic disorders · hyperhidrosis · hypersomnia · numbness · pancreatitis · sluggishness · vision blurred

‣ **Rare or very rare** Severe cutaneous adverse reactions (SCARs)

‣ **Frequency not known** Haemorrhagic stroke · osteonecrosis · weight increased

SIDE-EFFECTS, FURTHER INFORMATION **Hypersensitivity reactions** Rash, usually in the second week, is the most common side-effect and appears more frequently in females. Life-threatening hypersensitivity reactions reported usually during week 3–6 of treatment and characterised by rash, eosinophilia, and systemic symptoms (including fever, general malaise, myalgia, arthralgia, blistering, oral lesions, conjunctivitis, and hepatitis). Discontinue permanently if hypersensitivity reaction or severe rash develop. If rash mild or moderate (without signs of hypersensitivity reaction), may continue without interruption—usually resolves within 2 weeks.

● HEPATIC IMPAIRMENT Manufacturer advises caution in moderate impairment and in patients with hepatitis B or C (increased risk of hepatic side effects); avoid in severe impairment (no information available).

● DIRECTIONS FOR ADMINISTRATION Manufacturer advises patients with swallowing difficulties may disperse tablets in a glass of water just before administration.

● PRESCRIBING AND DISPENSING INFORMATION Dispense in original container (contains desiccant).

● PATIENT AND CARER ADVICE
Hypersensitivity reactions Patients or carers should be told how to recognise hypersensitivity reactions and advised to seek immediate medical attention if hypersensitivity reaction or severe rash develop.
Missed doses If a dose is more than 6 hours late, the missed dose should not be taken and the next dose should be taken at the normal time.

● MEDICINAL FORMS There can be variation in the licensing of different medicines containing the same drug.

Tablet

CAUTIONARY AND ADVISORY LABELS 21

‣ Intelence (Janssen-Cilag Ltd)
Etravirine 100 mg Intelence 100mg tablets | 120 tablet $\boxed{\text{PoM}}$ £301.27 (Hospital only)
Etravirine 200 mg Intelence 200mg tablets | 60 tablet $\boxed{\text{PoM}}$ £301.27 (Hospital only)

Nevirapine

22-Jun-2020

● **INDICATIONS AND DOSE**

HIV infection in combination with other antiretroviral drugs (initial dose)

‣ BY MOUTH USING IMMEDIATE-RELEASE MEDICINES

‣ Adult: Initially 200 mg once daily for first 14 days, initial dose titration using 'immediate-release' preparation should not exceed 28 days; if rash occurs and is not resolved within 28 days, alternative treatment should be sought. If treatment interrupted for more than 7 days, restart using the lower dose of the 'immediate-release' preparation for the first 14 days as for new treatment

HIV infection in combination with other antiretroviral drugs (maintenance dose following initial dose titration if no rash present)

‣ BY MOUTH USING IMMEDIATE-RELEASE MEDICINES

‣ Adult: 200 mg twice daily

‣ BY MOUTH USING MODIFIED-RELEASE MEDICINES

‣ Adult: 400 mg once daily

● CONTRA-INDICATIONS Acute porphyrias p. 1107 · post-exposure prophylaxis

● CAUTIONS Females (at greater risk of hepatic side effects) · high CD4 cell count (at greater risk of hepatic side effects)

CAUTIONS, FURTHER INFORMATION

‣ Hepatic effects Patients with chronic hepatitis B or C, high CD4 cell count, and women are at increased risk of hepatic side effects—if plasma HIV-1 RNA detectable, manufacturer advises avoid in women with CD4 cell count greater than 250 cells/mm^3 or in men with CD4 cell count greater than 400 cells/mm^3 unless potential benefit outweighs risk.

● INTERACTIONS → Appendix 1: NNRTIs

● SIDE-EFFECTS

‣ **Common or very common** Abdominal pain · angioedema · diarrhoea · fatigue · fever · headache · hepatic disorders · hypersensitivity · hypertransaminasaemia · nausea · skin reactions · vomiting

‣ **Uncommon** Anaemia · arthralgia · myalgia · severe cutaneous adverse reactions (SCARs)

‣ **Frequency not known** Eosinophilia · osteonecrosis · weight increased

SIDE-EFFECTS, FURTHER INFORMATION **Hepatic effects** Potentially life-threatening hepatotoxicity including fatal fulminant hepatitis reported usually in first 6 weeks; discontinue permanently if abnormalities in liver function tests accompanied by hypersensitivity reaction (rash, fever, arthralgia, myalgia, lymphadenopathy, hepatitis, renal impairment, eosinophilia, granulocytopenia); suspend if severe abnormalities in liver function tests but no hypersensitivity reaction—discontinue permanently if significant liver function abnormalities recur; monitor patient closely if mild to moderate abnormalities in liver function tests with no hypersensitivity reaction.

Rash Rash, usually in first 6 weeks, is most common side-effect; incidence reduced if introduced at low dose and dose increased gradually (after 14 days); Discontinue permanently if severe rash or if rash accompanied by blistering, oral lesions, conjunctivitis, facial oedema, general malaise or hypersensitivity reactions; if rash mild or moderate may continue without interruption but dose should not be increased until rash resolves.

Osteonecrosis Osteonecrosis has been reported in patients with advanced HIV disease or following long-term exposure to combination antiretroviral therapy.

● HEPATIC IMPAIRMENT For *modified-release* preparations, manufacturer advises avoid (no information available). For *immediate-release* preparations, manufacturer advises caution in moderate impairment and chronic hepatitis (increased risk of hepatic side-effects); consider interrupting or discontinuing treatment if hepatic function worsens; avoid in severe impairment (no information available).

● RENAL IMPAIRMENT Manufacturer advises avoid modified-release preparation—no information available.

● MONITORING REQUIREMENTS
▸ Hepatic disease Close monitoring of liver function required during first 18 weeks; monitor liver function before treatment then every 2 weeks for 2 months then after 1 month and then regularly.
▸ Rash Monitor closely for skin reactions during first 18 weeks.

● PATIENT AND CARER ADVICE
Hypersensitivity reactions Patients or carers should be told how to recognise hypersensitivity reactions and advised to discontinue treatment and seek immediate medical attention if severe skin reaction, hypersensitivity reactions, or symptoms of hepatitis develop.
Missed doses If a dose is more than 8 hours late with the 'immediate-release' preparation (or more than 12 hours late with the modified-release preparation), the missed dose should not be taken and the next dose should be taken at the usual time.

● MEDICINAL FORMS There can be variation in the licensing of different medicines containing the same drug.
Oral suspension
▸ Viramune (Boehringer Ingelheim Ltd)
  Nevirapine (as Nevirapine hemihydrate) 10 mg per 1 ml Viramune 50mg/5ml oral suspension | 240 ml [PoM] £50.40 (Hospital only)
Modified-release tablet
CAUTIONARY AND ADVISORY LABELS 25
▸ Nevirapine (Non-proprietary)
  Nevirapine 400 mg Nevirapine 400mg modified-release tablets | 30 tablet [PoM] £52.13–£170.00 DT = £81.75 (Hospital only)
▸ Viramune (Boehringer Ingelheim Ltd)
  Nevirapine 100 mg Viramune 100mg modified-release tablets | 90 tablet [PoM] £127.50 (Hospital only)
Tablet
▸ Nevirapine (Non-proprietary)
  Nevirapine 200 mg Nevirapine 200mg tablets | 60 tablet [PoM] £21.45–£170.00 (Hospital only)

Rilpivirine

22-Oct-2020

● **INDICATIONS AND DOSE**
HIV infection in combination with other antiretroviral drugs in patients not previously treated with antiretroviral therapy and if plasma HIV-1 RNA concentration less than or equal to 100 000 copies/mL
▸ BY MOUTH
▸ Adult: 25 mg once daily

● CAUTIONS Acute porphyrias p. 1107
● INTERACTIONS → Appendix 1: NNRTIs
● SIDE-EFFECTS
▸ **Common or very common** Appetite decreased · depression · dizziness · drowsiness · dry mouth · fatigue · gastrointestinal discomfort · headache · nausea · rash · sleep disorders · vomiting

▸ **Uncommon** Immune reconstitution inflammatory syndrome

● PREGNANCY Manufacturer advises avoid unless essential— no information available.

● HEPATIC IMPAIRMENT Manufacturer advises caution in moderate impairment (limited information available); avoid in severe impairment (no information available).

● RENAL IMPAIRMENT Manufacturer advises caution in severe impairment.

● PATIENT AND CARER ADVICE Patients or carers should be given advice on how to administer rilpivirine tablets.
Missed doses If a dose is more than 12 hours late, the missed dose should not be taken and the next dose should be taken at the normal time.

● MEDICINAL FORMS There can be variation in the licensing of different medicines containing the same drug.
Tablet
CAUTIONARY AND ADVISORY LABELS 3, 21, 25
▸ Edurant (Janssen-Cilag Ltd)
  Rilpivirine (as Rilpivirine hydrochloride) 25 mg Edurant 25mg tablets | 30 tablet [PoM] £200.27 (Hospital only)

Combinations available: *Dolutegravir with rilpivirine,* p. 681 · *Emtricitabine with rilpivirine and tenofovir alafenamide,* p. 689 · *Emtricitabine with rilpivirine and tenofovir disoproxil,* p. 690

ANTIVIRALS ❭ NUCLEOSIDE REVERSE TRANSCRIPTASE INHIBITORS

Nucleoside reverse transcriptase inhibitors

● SIDE-EFFECTS
▸ **Common or very common** Abdominal pain · anaemia (may require transfusion) · asthenia · diarrhoea · dizziness · fever · flatulence · headache · insomnia · nausea · neutropenia · skin reactions · vomiting
▸ **Uncommon** Angioedema · pancreatitis
▸ **Rare or very rare** Lactic acidosis
▸ **Frequency not known** Immune reconstitution inflammatory syndrome · osteonecrosis · weight increased
SIDE-EFFECTS, FURTHER INFORMATION Osteonecrosis has been reported in patients with advanced HIV disease or following long-term exposure to combination antiretroviral therapy.

● PREGNANCY
Monitoring Mitochondrial dysfunction has been reported in infants exposed to nucleoside reverse transcriptase inhibitors in utero; the main effects include haematological, metabolic, and neurological disorders; all infants whose mothers received nucleoside reverse transcriptase inhibitors during pregnancy should be monitored for relevant signs or symptoms.

● HEPATIC IMPAIRMENT In general, manufacturers advise caution in patients with chronic hepatitis B or C (increased risk of hepatic side-effects).

◤ above

Abacavir

17-Nov-2020

● **INDICATIONS AND DOSE**
HIV infection in combination with other antiretroviral drugs
▸ BY MOUTH
▸ Adult: 600 mg daily in 1–2 divided doses

● CAUTIONS HIV load greater than 100 000 copies/mᵀ patients at high risk of cardiovascular disease
● INTERACTIONS → Appendix 1: NRTIs

5

Infection

- SIDE-EFFECTS
- ▶ **Common or very common** Appetite decreased · lethargy
- ▶ **Rare or very rare** Severe cutaneous adverse reactions (SCARs)
- ▶ **Frequency not known** Hypersensitivity

  SIDE-EFFECTS, FURTHER INFORMATION Life-threatening hypersensitivity reactions have been reported-characterised by fever or rash and possibly nausea, vomiting, diarrhoea, abdominal pain, dyspnoea, cough, lethargy, malaise, headache, and myalgia; less frequently mouth ulceration, oedema, hypotension, sore throat, acute respiratory distress syndrome, anaphylaxis, paraesthesia, arthralgia, conjunctivitis, lymphadenopathy, lymphocytopenia and renal failure; rarely myolysis. Laboratory abnormalities may include raised liver function tests and creatine kinase; symptoms usually appear in the first 6 weeks, but may occur at any time. Discontinue immediately if any symptom of hypersensitivity develops and do not rechallenge (risk of more severe hypersensitivity reaction).

- ALLERGY AND CROSS-SENSITIVITY EvGr Caution—increased risk of hypersensitivity reaction in presence of HLA-B*5701 allele. ⟨M⟩

- HEPATIC IMPAIRMENT Manufacturer advises caution in mild impairment; consider avoiding in moderate to severe impairment (no information available).

- RENAL IMPAIRMENT Manufacturer advises avoid in end-stage renal disease.

- PRE-TREATMENT SCREENING Test for HLA-B*5701 allele before treatment or if restarting treatment and HLA-B*5701 status not known.

- MONITORING REQUIREMENTS Monitor for symptoms of hypersensitivity reaction every 2 weeks for 2 months.

- PRESCRIBING AND DISPENSING INFORMATION Flavours of oral liquid formulations may include banana, or strawberry.

- PATIENT AND CARER ADVICE Patients and their carers should be told the importance of regular dosing (intermittent therapy may increase the risk of sensitisation), how to recognise signs of hypersensitivity, and advised to seek immediate medical attention if symptoms develop or before re-starting treatment.

  Patients should be provided with an alert card and advised to keep it with them at all times.

- MEDICINAL FORMS There can be variation in the licensing of different medicines containing the same drug.

Oral solution

EXCIPIENTS: May contain Propylene glycol
- ▶ Ziagen (ViiV Healthcare UK Ltd)
  Abacavir (as Abacavir sulfate) 20 mg per 1 ml Ziagen 20mg/ml oral solution sugar-free | 240 ml PoM £55.72 (Hospital only)

Tablet
- ▶ Abacavir (Non-proprietary)
  Abacavir (as Abacavir sulfate) 300 mg Abacavir 300mg tablets | 60 tablet PoM £177.60–£177.61 (Hospital only)
- ▶ Ziagen (ViiV Healthcare UK Ltd)
  Abacavir (as Abacavir sulfate) 300 mg Ziagen 300mg tablets | 60 tablet PoM £208.95 (Hospital only)

Abacavir with dolutegravir and lamivudine

27-Aug-2020

The properties listed below are those particular to the combination only. For the properties of the components please consider, abacavir p. 685, lamivudine p. 691, dolutegravir p. 680.

- INDICATIONS AND DOSE
HIV infection
- ▶ BY MOUTH
- ▶ Adult (body-weight 40 kg and above): 1 tablet once daily

- INTERACTIONS → Appendix 1: dolutegravir · NRTIs

- RENAL IMPAIRMENT Avoid *Triumeq* ® if eGFR less than 50 mL/minute/1.73 m² (consult product literature).

- PATIENT AND CARER ADVICE
Missed doses If a dose is more than 20 hours late, the missed dose should not be taken and the next dose should be taken at the normal time.

- MEDICINAL FORMS There can be variation in the licensing of different medicines containing the same drug.
Tablet
- ▶ Triumeq (ViiV Healthcare UK Ltd)
  Dolutegravir (as Dolutegravir sodium) 50 mg, Lamivudine 300 mg, Abacavir (as Abacavir sulfate) 600 mg Triumeq 50mg/600mg/300mg tablets | 30 tablet PoM £798.16 (Hospital only)

Abacavir with lamivudine

The properties listed below are those particular to the combination only. For the properties of the components please consider, abacavir p. 685, lamivudine p. 691.

- INDICATIONS AND DOSE
HIV infection in combination with other antiretrovirals
- ▶ BY MOUTH
- ▶ Adult (body-weight 40 kg and above): 1 tablet once daily

- INTERACTIONS → Appendix 1: NRTIs

- RENAL IMPAIRMENT Avoid *Kivexa* ® if eGFR less than 50 mL/minute/1.73 m² (consult product literature).

- MEDICINAL FORMS There can be variation in the licensing of different medicines containing the same drug.
Tablet
- ▶ Abacavir with lamivudine (Non-proprietary)
  Lamivudine 300 mg, Abacavir 600 mg Abacavir 600mg / Lamivudine 300mg tablets | 30 tablet PoM £352.25 DT = £190.00 (Hospital only)
- ▶ Kivexa (ViiV Healthcare UK Ltd)
  Lamivudine 300 mg, Abacavir 600 mg Kivexa 600mg/300mg tablets | 30 tablet PoM £352.25 DT = £190.00 (Hospital only)

Abacavir with lamivudine and zidovudine

The properties listed below are those particular to the combination only. For the properties of the components please consider, abacavir p. 685, lamivudine p. 691, zidovudine p. 693.

- INDICATIONS AND DOSE
HIV infection (use only if patient is stabilised for 6–8 weeks on the individual components in the same proportions)
- ▶ BY MOUTH
- ▶ Adult: 1 tablet twice daily

- INTERACTIONS → Appendix 1: NRTIs

- RENAL IMPAIRMENT Avoid *Trizivir*® if eGFR less than 50 mL/minute/1.73 m² (consult product literature).

- MEDICINAL FORMS There can be variation in the licensing of different medicines containing the same drug.
  Tablet
  ▶ Trizivir (ViiV Healthcare UK Ltd)
    Lamivudine 150 mg, Abacavir (as Abacavir sulfate) 300 mg, Zidovudine 300 mg Trizivir tablets | 60 tablet [PoM] £509.06 (Hospital only)

Bictegravir with emtricitabine and tenofovir alafenamide
20-Oct-2020

The properties listed below are those particular to the combination only. For the properties of the components please consider, emtricitabine p. 689, tenofovir alafenamide p. 663.

- INDICATIONS AND DOSE
  HIV-1 infection (initiated by a specialist)
  ▶ BY MOUTH
  ▶ Adult: 1 tablet once daily

- INTERACTIONS → Appendix 1: bictegravir · NRTIs · tenofovir alafenamide

- SIDE-EFFECTS
- **Common or very common** Depression · diarrhoea · dizziness · fatigue · headache · nausea · sleep disorders
- **Uncommon** Anaemia · angioedema · anxiety · arthralgia · flatulence · gastrointestinal discomfort · hyperbilirubinaemia · skin reactions · suicidal behaviour · vomiting

- PREGNANCY Manufacturer advises use only if potential benefit outweighs risk.

- HEPATIC IMPAIRMENT Manufacturer advises avoid in severe impairment—no information available.

- RENAL IMPAIRMENT Manufacturer advises avoid if creatinine clearance is less than 30 mL/minute—limited information available.

- PATIENT AND CARER ADVICE
  Missed doses Manufacturer advises if a dose is more than 18 hours late, the missed dose should not be taken and the next dose should be taken at the normal time.

- NATIONAL FUNDING/ACCESS DECISIONS
  For full details see funding body website
  Scottish Medicines Consortium (SMC) decisions
  ▶ Bictegravir-emtricitabine-tenofovir alafenamide (*Biktarvy*®) for the treatment of adults infected with HIV-1 without any known mutations associated with resistance to the individual components (September 2018) SMC No. SMC2093 Recommended
  All Wales Medicines Strategy Group (AWMSG) decisions
  ▶ Bictegravir/emtricitabine/tenofovir alafenamide (*Biktarvy*®) for the treatment of adults infected with human immunodeficiency virus-1 (HIV-1) without present or past evidence of viral resistance to the integrase inhibitor class, emtricitabine or tenofovir (December 2018) AWMSG No. 3414 Recommended with restrictions

- MEDICINAL FORMS There can be variation in the licensing of different medicines containing the same drug.
  Tablet
  CAUTIONARY AND ADVISORY LABELS 25
  ▶ Biktarvy (Gilead Sciences Ireland UC) ▼
    Tenofovir alafenamide (as Tenofovir alafenamide fumarate) 25 mg, Bictegravir 50 mg, Emtricitabine 200 mg Biktarvy 50mg/200mg/25mg tablets | 30 tablet [PoM] £879.51 (Hospital only)

Efavirenz with emtricitabine and tenofovir disoproxil
02-Sep-2020

The properties listed below are those particular to the combination only. For the properties of the components please consider, tenofovir disoproxil p. 692, efavirenz p. 683, emtricitabine p. 689.

- INDICATIONS AND DOSE
  HIV infection stabilised on antiretroviral therapy for more than 3 months
  ▶ BY MOUTH
  ▶ Adult: 1 tablet once daily

- INTERACTIONS → Appendix 1: NNRTIs · NRTIs · tenofovir disoproxil

- HEPATIC IMPAIRMENT Manufacturer advises caution in mild impairment; avoid in moderate to severe impairment (increased risk of hepatic side-effects).

- RENAL IMPAIRMENT Avoid *Atripla*® if eGFR less than 50 mL/minute/1.73 m².

- PATIENT AND CARER ADVICE
  Missed doses If a dose is more than 12 hours late, the missed dose should not be taken and the next dose should be taken at the normal time.

- MEDICINAL FORMS There can be variation in the licensing of different medicines containing the same drug.
  Tablet
  CAUTIONARY AND ADVISORY LABELS 23, 25
  ▶ Efavirenz with emtricitabine and tenofovir disoproxil (Non-proprietary)
    Emtricitabine 200 mg, Tenofovir disoproxil (as Tenofovir disoproxil fumarate) 245 mg, Efavirenz 600 mg Efavirenz 600mg / Emtricitabine 200mg / Tenofovir disoproxil 245mg tablets | 30 tablet [PoM] £479.58–£532.87 (Hospital only)
  ▶ Atripla (Gilead Sciences Ireland UC)
    Emtricitabine 200 mg, Tenofovir disoproxil (as Tenofovir disoproxil fumarate) 245 mg, Efavirenz 600 mg Atripla 600mg/200mg/245mg tablets | 30 tablet [PoM] £532.87 (Hospital only)

Elvitegravir with cobicistat, emtricitabine and tenofovir alafenamide
22-Oct-2020

The properties listed below are those particular to the combination only. For the properties of the components please consider, emtricitabine p. 689, elvitegravir p. 682, cobicistat p. 699, tenofovir alafenamide p. 663.

- INDICATIONS AND DOSE
  HIV-1 infection (specialist use only)
  ▶ BY MOUTH
  ▶ Adult: 1 tablet once daily

> **IMPORTANT SAFETY INFORMATION**
>
> MHRA/CHM ADVICE: ELVITEGRAVIR BOOSTED WITH COBICISTAT: AVOID USE IN PREGNANCY DUE TO RISK OF TREATMENT FAILURE AND MATERNAL-TO-CHILD TRANSMISSION OF HIV-1 (APRIL 2019)
> Pharmacokinetic data show mean exposure of elvitegravir boosted with cobicistat (available in combination in *Genvoya*® and *Stribild*®) to be lower during the second and third trimesters of pregnancy than postpartum. Low elvitegravir exposure may be associated with an increased risk of treatment failure and an increased risk of HIV-1 transmission to the unborn child. For further information, see *Pregnancy*.

- INTERACTIONS → Appendix 1: cobicistat · elvitegra NRTIs · tenofovir alafenamide

- **SIDE-EFFECTS**
  - ▶ **Common or very common** Abnormal dreams · diarrhoea · dizziness · fatigue · flatulence · gastrointestinal discomfort · headache · nausea · skin reactions · vomiting
  - ▶ **Uncommon** Anaemia · depression · suicidal behaviours
  - ▶ **Frequency not known** Nephrotoxicity · osteonecrosis · weight increased
- **CONCEPTION AND CONTRACEPTION** Manufacturer advises effective contraception in women of childbearing potential; if using a hormonal contraceptive, it must contain drospirenone or norgestimate as the progestogen and at least 30 micrograms ethinylestradiol.
- **PREGNANCY** Manufacturer advises not to be initiated during pregnancy due to low elvitegravir exposure; women who become pregnant during therapy should be switched to an alternative regimen.
- **HEPATIC IMPAIRMENT** Manufacturer advises caution (increased risk of hepatic side-effects); avoid in severe impairment (no information available).
- **RENAL IMPAIRMENT** Manufacturer advises avoid if creatinine clearance less than 30 mL/minute—limited information available.
- **PRESCRIBING AND DISPENSING INFORMATION** Dispense in original container—contains desiccant.
- ▶ **PATIENT AND CARER ADVICE**
  Missed doses Manufacturer advises if a dose is more than 18 hours late, the missed dose should not be taken and the next dose should be taken at the normal time.
  Driving and skilled tasks Manufacturer advises patients and carers should be counselled on the effects on driving and performance of skilled tasks—increased risk of dizziness.
- **NATIONAL FUNDING/ACCESS DECISIONS**
  For full details see funding body website

  Scottish Medicines Consortium (SMC) decisions
  - ▶ Elvitegravir, cobicistat, emtricitabine, tenofovir alafenamide (*Genvoya*®) for the treatment of adults and adolescents (aged 12 years and older with body weight at least 35 kg) infected with human immunodeficiency virus-1 (HIV-1) without any known mutations associated with resistance to the integrase inhibitor class, emtricitabine or tenofovir (May 2016) SMC No. 1142/16 Recommended

  All Wales Medicines Strategy Group (AWMSG) decisions
  - ▶ Elvitegravir / cobicistat / emtricitabine / tenofovir alafenamide (*Genvoya*®) for the treatment of adults and adolescents (aged 12 years and older with body weight at least 35 kg) infected with human immunodeficiency virus-1 (HIV-1) without any known mutations associated with resistance to the integrase inhibitor class, emtricitabine or tenofovir (July 2016) AWMSG No. 2248 Recommended

- **MEDICINAL FORMS** There can be variation in the licensing of different medicines containing the same drug.

  Tablet
  CAUTIONARY AND ADVISORY LABELS 21
  - ▶ Genvoya (Gilead Sciences Ireland UC)
    Tenofovir alafenamide 10 mg, Cobicistat 150 mg, Elvitegravir 150 mg, Emtricitabine 200 mg Genvoya 150mg/150mg/200mg/10mg tablets | 30 tablet [PoM] £879.51 (Hospital only)

Elvitegravir with cobicistat, emtricitabine and tenofovir disoproxil

22-May-2019

The properties listed below are those particular to the combination only. For the properties of the components please consider, tenofovir disoproxil p. 692, emtricitabine p. 689, cobicistat p. 699, elvitegravir p. 682.

- **INDICATIONS AND DOSE**
  HIV infection
  - ▶ BY MOUTH
  - ▶ Adult: 1 tablet once daily

> **IMPORTANT SAFETY INFORMATION**
> MHRA/CHM ADVICE: ELVITEGRAVIR BOOSTED WITH COBICISTAT: AVOID USE IN PREGNANCY DUE TO RISK OF TREATMENT FAILURE AND MATERNAL-TO-CHILD TRANSMISSION OF HIV-1 (APRIL 2019)
> Pharmacokinetic data show mean exposure of elvitegravir boosted with cobicistat (available in combination in *Genvoya*® and *Stribild*®) to be lower during the second and third trimesters of pregnancy than postpartum. Low elvitegravir exposure may be associated with an increased risk of treatment failure and an increased risk of HIV-1 transmission to the unborn child. For further information, see *Pregnancy*.

- **INTERACTIONS** → Appendix 1: cobicistat · elvitegravir · NRTIs · tenofovir disoproxil
- **SIDE-EFFECTS**
  - ▶ **Common or very common** Appetite decreased · asthenia · constipation · diarrhoea · dizziness · electrolyte imbalance · flatulence · gastrointestinal discomfort · headache · hyperbilirubinaemia · hyperglycaemia · hypersensitivity · hypertriglyceridaemia · nausea · neutropenia · pain · rash pustular · skin reactions · sleep disorders · vomiting
  - ▶ **Uncommon** Anaemia · angioedema · depression (in patients with history of depression or psychiatric illness) · muscle weakness · myopathy · pancreatitis · proteinuria · renal failure · renal tubular disorders · suicidal ideation (in patients with history of depression or psychiatric illness)
  - ▶ **Rare or very rare** Acute tubular necrosis · hepatic disorders · lactic acidosis · nephritis · nephrogenic diabetes insipidus · osteomalacia
  - ▶ **Frequency not known** Autoimmune disorder · Grave's disease · inflammation · osteonecrosis · weight increased
- **CONCEPTION AND CONTRACEPTION** Women of child-bearing potential should use effective contraception during treatment (if using a hormonal contraceptive, it must contain norgestimate as the progestogen and at least 30 micrograms ethinylestradiol).
- **PREGNANCY** Manufacturer advises not to be initiated during pregnancy due to low elvitegravir exposure; women who become pregnant during therapy should be switched to an alternative regimen.
- **HEPATIC IMPAIRMENT** Manufacturer advises caution (increased risk of hepatic side-effects); avoid in severe impairment (no information available).
- **RENAL IMPAIRMENT** If eGFR less than 90 mL/minute/1.73 m², only *initiate Stribild*® if other treatments cannot be used (avoid *initiating Stribild*® if eGFR less than 70 mL/minute/1.73 m²); if eGFR less than 70 mL/minute/1.73 m², only *continue Stribild*® if potential benefit outweighs risk (discontinue *Stribild*® if eGFR less than 50 mL/minute/1.73 m²).
- **MONITORING REQUIREMENTS** Test urine glucose before treatment, then every 4 weeks for 1 year and then every 3 months.
- **PRESCRIBING AND DISPENSING INFORMATION** Dispense in original container (contains desiccant).

- **PATIENT AND CARER ADVICE** Patients or carers should be given advice on how to administer *Stribild*®.
  Missed doses If a dose is more than 18 hours late, the missed dose should not be taken and the next dose should be taken at the normal time.

- **MEDICINAL FORMS** There can be variation in the licensing of different medicines containing the same drug.

  Tablet
  CAUTIONARY AND ADVISORY LABELS 21
  ▸ Stribild (Gilead Sciences Ireland UC)
    Cobicistat 150 mg, Elvitegravir 150 mg, Emtricitabine 200 mg, Tenofovir disoproxil (as Tenofovir disoproxil fumarate) 245 mg Stribild 150mg/150mg/200mg/245mg tablets | 30 tablet [PoM] £879.51 (Hospital only)

▶ 685

Emtricitabine

04-Sep-2020

(FTC)

- **INDICATIONS AND DOSE**

  HIV infection in combination with other antiretroviral drugs
  ▸ BY MOUTH USING CAPSULES
  ▸ Adult: 200 mg once daily
  ▸ BY MOUTH USING ORAL SOLUTION
  ▸ Adult: 240 mg once daily

  DOSE EQUIVALENCE AND CONVERSION
  ▸ 240 mg oral solution ≡ 200 mg capsule; where appropriate the capsule may be used instead of the oral solution.

- **SIDE-EFFECTS**
  ▸ **Common or very common** Abnormal dreams · dyspepsia · hyperbilirubinaemia · hyperglycaemia · hypersensitivity · hypertriglyceridaemia · pain · rash pustular

- **HEPATIC IMPAIRMENT**
  Monitoring On discontinuation, monitor patients with hepatitis B (risk of exacerbation of hepatitis).

- **RENAL IMPAIRMENT**
  Dose adjustments Reduce dose if eGFR less than 50 mL/minute/1.73 m²; consult product literature.

- **PRESCRIBING AND DISPENSING INFORMATION** Flavours of oral liquid formulations may include candy.

- **PATIENT AND CARER ADVICE**
  Missed doses If a dose is more than 12 hours late, the missed dose should not be taken and the next dose should be taken at the normal time.

- **MEDICINAL FORMS** There can be variation in the licensing of different medicines containing the same drug.

  Oral solution
  ELECTROLYTES: May contain Sodium
  ▸ Emtriva (Gilead Sciences Ireland UC)
    Emtricitabine 10 mg per 1 ml Emtriva 10mg/ml oral solution sugar-free | 170 ml [PoM] £39.53 (Hospital only)

  Capsule
  ▸ Emtriva (Gilead Sciences Ireland UC)
    Emtricitabine 200 mg Emtriva 200mg capsules | 30 capsule [PoM] £138.98 (Hospital only)

  Combinations available: *Darunavir with cobicistat, emtricitabine and tenofovir alafenamide*, p. 696

Emtricitabine with rilpivirine and tenofovir alafenamide

21-Aug-2020

The properties listed below are those particular to the combination only. For the properties of the components please consider, emtricitabine above, rilpivirine p. 685, tenofovir alafenamide p. 663.

- **INDICATIONS AND DOSE**

  HIV infection in patients with plasma HIV-1 RNA concentration of 100 000 copies/mL or less (specialist use only)
  ▸ BY MOUTH
  ▸ Adult: 1 tablet once daily

- **INTERACTIONS** → Appendix 1: NNRTIs · NRTIs · tenofovir alafenamide

- **SIDE-EFFECTS**
  ▸ **Common or very common** Appetite decreased · depression · diarrhoea · dizziness · drowsiness · dry mouth · fatigue · flatulence · gastrointestinal discomfort · headache · nausea · skin reactions · sleep disorders · vomiting
  ▸ **Uncommon** Anaemia · angioedema · arthralgia · immune reconstitution inflammatory syndrome
  ▸ **Frequency not known** Conjunctivitis · drug reaction with eosinophilia and systemic symptoms (DRESS) · eosinophilia · fever · osteonecrosis · QT interval prolongation · weight increased

  SIDE-EFFECTS, FURTHER INFORMATION Systemic symptoms reported with severe skin reactions include fever, blisters, conjunctivitis, angioedema, elevated liver function tests, and eosinophilia.

- **HEPATIC IMPAIRMENT** Manufacturer advises caution in moderate impairment (increased risk of hepatic side-effects); avoid in severe impairment (no information available).

- **RENAL IMPAIRMENT** Manufacturer advises avoid if creatinine clearance less than 30 mL/minute—no information available.

- **PATIENT AND CARER ADVICE**
  Vomiting Manufacturer advises if vomiting occurs within 4 hours of taking a dose, a replacement dose should be taken.
  Driving and skilled tasks Manufacturer advises patients and carers should be counselled on the effects on driving and performance of skilled tasks—increased risk of dizziness.

- **NATIONAL FUNDING/ACCESS DECISIONS**
  For full details see funding body website

  Scottish Medicines Consortium (SMC) decisions
  ▸ Emtricitabine/rilpivirine/tenofovir alafenamide (*Odesfey*®) for the treatment of HIV-1 without known mutations associated with resistance to the non nucleoside reverse transcriptase inhibitor class, tenofovir or emtricitabine, and with a viral load HIV-1 RNA of 100,000 copies/mL or less (October 2016) SMC No. 1189/16 Recommended

  All Wales Medicines Strategy Group (AWMSG) decisions
  ▸ Emtricitabine/rilpivirine/tenofovir alafenamide (*Odesfey*®) for the treatment of HIV-1 without known mutations associated with resistance to the non-nucleoside reverse transcriptase inhibitor class, tenofovir or emtricitabine, and with a viral load HIV-1 RNA of 100,000 copies/mL or less (November 2016) AWMSG No. 3031 Recommended

- **MEDICINAL FORMS** There can be variation in the licensing of different medicines containing the same drug.

  Tablet
  CAUTIONARY AND ADVISORY LABELS 3, 21
  ▸ Odesfey (Gilead Sciences Ireland UC) ▼
    Rilpivirine (as Rilpivirine hydrochloride) 25 mg, Tenofovir alafenamide (as Tenofovir alafenamide fumarate) 25 mg, Emtricitabine 200 mg Odesfey 200mg/25mg/25mg tablets | 30 tablet [PoM] £525.95 (Hospital only)

5

Infection

Emtricitabine with rilpivirine and tenofovir disoproxil

04-Sep-2020

The properties listed below are those particular to the combination only. For the properties of the components please consider, tenofovir disoproxil p. 692, emtricitabine p. 689, rilpivirine p. 685.

● **INDICATIONS AND DOSE**

HIV infection in patients with plasma HIV-1 RNA concentration less than 100 000 copies/mL
▸ BY MOUTH
▸ Adult: 1 tablet once daily

● **INTERACTIONS** → Appendix 1: NNRTIs · NRTIs · tenofovir disoproxil

● **HEPATIC IMPAIRMENT** Manufacturer advises caution in moderate impairment (increased risk of hepatic side-effects); avoid in severe impairment (no information available).

● **RENAL IMPAIRMENT** Avoid *Eviplera* ® if eGFR less than 50 mL/minute/1.73 m².

● **PATIENT AND CARER ADVICE** Patients or carers should be given advice on how to administer *Eviplera* ®.
Missed doses If a dose is more than 12 hours late, the missed dose should not be taken and the next dose should be taken at the normal time.

● **MEDICINAL FORMS** There can be variation in the licensing of different medicines containing the same drug.
Tablet
CAUTIONARY AND ADVISORY LABELS 21, 25
▸ Eviplera (Gilead Sciences Ireland UC)
Rilpivirine (as Rilpivirine hydrochloride) 25 mg, Emtricitabine 200 mg, Tenofovir disoproxil (as Tenofovir disoproxil fumarate) 245 mg Eviplera 200mg/25mg/245mg tablets | 30 tablet [PoM] £525.95 (Hospital only)

Emtricitabine with tenofovir alafenamide

21-Aug-2020

The properties listed below are those particular to the combination only. For the properties of the components please consider, emtricitabine p. 689, tenofovir alafenamide p. 663.

● **INDICATIONS AND DOSE**

HIV infection in combination with other antiretroviral drugs (specialist use only)
▸ BY MOUTH
▸ Adult: 200/10–200/25 mg once daily, dose is dependent on drug regimen—consult product literature

DOSE EQUIVALENCE AND CONVERSION
▸ Dose expressed as x/y mg emtricitabine/tenofovir alafenamide.

● **INTERACTIONS** → Appendix 1: NRTIs · tenofovir alafenamide

● **SIDE-EFFECTS**
▸ **Common or very common** Abnormal dreams · diarrhoea · dizziness · fatigue · flatulence · gastrointestinal discomfort · headache · nausea · skin reactions · vomiting
▸ **Uncommon** Anaemia · arthralgia
▸ **Frequency not known** Angioedema · osteonecrosis

● **HEPATIC IMPAIRMENT** Manufacturer advises caution (increased risk of hepatic side-effects).

● **RENAL IMPAIRMENT** Manufacturer advises avoid if creatinine clearance less than 30 mL/minute—limited information available.

● **PATIENT AND CARER ADVICE**
Driving and skilled tasks Manufacturer advises patients and carers should be counselled on the effects on driving and performance of skilled tasks—increased risk of dizziness.

● **NATIONAL FUNDING/ACCESS DECISIONS**
For full details see funding body website
Scottish Medicines Consortium (SMC) decisions
▸ Emtricitabine / tenofovir alafenamide (*Descovy* ®) in combination with other antiretroviral agents for the treatment of adults and adolescents (aged 12 years and older with body weight at least 35kg) infected with human immunodeficiency virus type 1 (August 2016) SMC No. 1169/16 Recommended
All Wales Medicines Strategy Group (AWMSG) decisions
▸ Emtricitabine / tenofovir alafenamide (*Descovy* ®) for treatment of adults and adolescents (aged 12 years and older with body weight at least 35 kg) infected with human immunodeficiency virus type 1 (HIV 1) (October 2016) AWMSG No. 2771 Recommended

● **MEDICINAL FORMS** There can be variation in the licensing of different medicines containing the same drug.
Tablet
▸ Descovy (Gilead Sciences Ireland UC) ▼
Tenofovir alafenamide (as Tenofovir alafenamide fumarate) 25 mg, Emtricitabine 200 mg Descovy 200mg/25mg tablets | 30 tablet [PoM] £355.73 DT = £355.73 (Hospital only)
Tenofovir alafenamide (as Tenofovir alafenamide fumarate) 10 mg, Emtricitabine 200 mg Descovy 200mg/10mg tablets | 30 tablet [PoM] £355.73 DT = £355.73 (Hospital only)

Emtricitabine with tenofovir disoproxil

12-Oct-2020

The properties listed below are those particular to the combination only. For the properties of the components please consider, tenofovir disoproxil p. 692, emtricitabine p. 689.

● **INDICATIONS AND DOSE**

HIV-1 infection (initiated by a specialist)
▸ BY MOUTH
▸ Adult: 200/245 mg once daily

Pre-exposure prophylaxis of HIV-1 infection (initiated by a specialist)
▸ BY MOUTH
▸ Adult: 200/245 mg once daily

DOSE EQUIVALENCE AND CONVERSION
▸ Dose expressed as x/y mg emtricitabine/tenofovir disoproxil.

● **INTERACTIONS** → Appendix 1: NRTIs · tenofovir disoproxil

● **HEPATIC IMPAIRMENT** Manufacturer advises caution (increased risk of hepatic side-effects).

● **RENAL IMPAIRMENT**
▸ When used for HIV-1 infection Manufacturer advises avoid in severe impairment.
▸ When used for Pre-exposure prophylaxis of HIV-1 infection Manufacturer advises avoid if creatinine clearance less than 60 mL/minute.
Dose adjustments
▸ When used for HIV-1 infection Manufacturer advises use normal dose every 2 days in moderate impairment.

● **DIRECTIONS FOR ADMINISTRATION** Patients with swallowing difficulties may disperse tablet in half a glass of water, orange juice, or grape juice.

● **PATIENT AND CARER ADVICE** Patients or carers should be given advice on how to administer emtricitabine with tenofovir tablets.

Missed doses If a dose is more than 12 hours late, the missed dose should not be taken and the next dose should be taken at the normal time.

● NATIONAL FUNDING/ACCESS DECISIONS
For full details see funding body website

Scottish Medicines Consortium (SMC) decisions

▸ Emtricitabine/tenofovir disoproxil (*Truvada*®) in combination with safer sex practices for pre-exposure prophylaxis to reduce the risk of sexually acquired HIV-1 infection in adults at high risk (April 2017) SMC No. 1225/17 Recommended

All Wales Medicines Strategy Group (AWMSG) decisions

▸ Emtricitabine/tenofovir disoproxil in combination with safer sex practices for pre-exposure prophylaxis to reduce the risk of sexually acquired HIV-1 infection in adults at high risk (June 2020) AWMSG No. 4623 Recommended

● MEDICINAL FORMS There can be variation in the licensing of different medicines containing the same drug.

Tablet

CAUTIONARY AND ADVISORY LABELS 21

▸ Emtricitabine with tenofovir disoproxil (Non-proprietary)
Emtricitabine 200 mg, Tenofovir disoproxil (as Tenofovir disoproxil fumarate) 245 mg Emtricitabine 200mg / Tenofovir 245mg tablets | 30 tablet [PoM] £78.06–£355.73 DT = £355.73 (Hospital only)

▸ Ictastan (Actavis UK Ltd)
Emtricitabine 200 mg, Tenofovir disoproxil (as Tenofovir disoproxil fumarate) 245 mg Ictastan 200mg/245mg tablets | 30 tablet [PoM] £355.72 DT = £355.73 (Hospital only)

▸ Truvada (Gilead Sciences Ireland UC)
Emtricitabine 200 mg, Tenofovir disoproxil (as Tenofovir disoproxil fumarate) 245 mg Truvada 200mg/245mg tablets | 30 tablet [PoM] £355.73 DT = £355.73 (Hospital only)

⌐ 685

Lamivudine

08-Jun-2020

(3TC)

● **INDICATIONS AND DOSE**

EPIVIR® ORAL SOLUTION

HIV infection in combination with other antiretroviral drugs

▸ BY MOUTH

▸ **Adult:** 150 mg every 12 hours, alternatively 300 mg once daily

EPIVIR® TABLETS

HIV infection in combination with other antiretroviral drugs

▸ BY MOUTH

▸ **Adult:** 150 mg every 12 hours, alternatively 300 mg once daily

ZEFFIX®

Chronic hepatitis B infection either with compensated liver disease (with evidence of viral replication and histology of active liver inflammation or fibrosis) when first-line treatments cannot be used, or (in combination with another antiviral drug without cross-resistance to lamivudine) with decompensated liver disease

▸ BY MOUTH

▸ **Adult:** 100 mg once daily, patients receiving lamivudine for concomitant HIV infection should continue to receive lamivudine in a dose appropriate for HIV infection

● CAUTIONS Recurrent hepatitis in patients with chronic hepatitis B may occur on discontinuation of lamivudine

● INTERACTIONS → Appendix 1: NRTIs

● SIDE-EFFECTS

▸ **Common or very common** Alopecia · arthralgia · cough · gastrointestinal discomfort · hepatic disorders · malaise · muscle complaints · myopathy · nasal disorder

▸ **Uncommon** Thrombocytopenia

▸ **Rare or very rare** Paraesthesia · peripheral neuropathy · pure red cell aplasia

▸ **Frequency not known** Respiratory tract infection · throat complaints

● BREAST FEEDING Can be used with caution in women infected with chronic hepatitis B alone, providing that adequate measures are taken to prevent hepatitis B infection in infants.

● RENAL IMPAIRMENT

Dose adjustments Reduce dose if eGFR less than 50 mL/minute/1.73 m^2; consult product literature.

● MONITORING REQUIREMENTS When treating chronic hepatitis B with lamivudine, monitor liver function tests every 3 months, and viral markers of hepatitis B every 3–6 months, more frequently in patients with advanced liver disease or following transplantation (monitoring to continue for at least 1 year after discontinuation— recurrent hepatitis may occur on discontinuation).

● PRESCRIBING AND DISPENSING INFORMATION Flavours of oral liquid formulations may include banana and strawberry.

● MEDICINAL FORMS There can be variation in the licensing of different medicines containing the same drug.

Oral solution

EXCIPIENTS: May contain Sucrose

▸ Epivir (ViiV Healthcare UK Ltd)
Lamivudine 10 mg per 1 ml Epivir 50mg/5ml oral solution | 240 ml [PoM] £39.01 (Hospital only)

Tablet

▸ Epivir (ViiV Healthcare UK Ltd)
Lamivudine 150 mg Epivir 150mg tablets | 60 tablet [PoM] £143.32 DT = £143.32 (Hospital only)
Lamivudine 300 mg Epivir 300mg tablets | 30 tablet [PoM] £157.51 DT = £157.51 (Hospital only)

▸ Zeffix (GlaxoSmithKline UK Ltd)
Lamivudine 100 mg Zeffix 100mg tablets | 28 tablet [PoM] £78.09 DT = £74.17 (Hospital only)

Lamivudine with dolutegravir

23-Oct-2020

The properties listed below are those particular to the combination only. For the properties of the components please consider, lamivudine above, dolutegravir p. 680.

● **INDICATIONS AND DOSE**

HIV-1 infection

▸ BY MOUTH

▸ **Adult:** 300/50 mg once daily

DOSE EQUIVALENCE AND CONVERSION

▸ Dose expressed as x/y mg lamivudine/dolutegravir.

● INTERACTIONS → Appendix 1: dolutegravir · NRTIs

● RENAL IMPAIRMENT Manufacturer advises avoid if creatinine clearance less than 50 mL/minute.

● PATIENT AND CARER ADVICE

Missed doses Manufacturer advises if a dose is more than 20 hours late, the missed dose should not be taken and the next dose should be taken at the normal time.

● NATIONAL FUNDING/ACCESS DECISIONS
For full details see funding body website

Scottish Medicines Consortium (SMC) decisions

▸ Dolutegravir / lamivudine (*Dovato*®) for treatment of Human Immunodeficiency Virus type 1 (HIV-1) infection in adults and adolescents above 12 years of age weighing at least 40 kg, with no known or suspected resistance to the integrase inhibitor class, or lamivudine (September 2019) SMC No. SMC2205 Recommended

All Wales Medicines Strategy Group (AWMSG) decisions

▸ Dolutegravir / lamivudine (*Dovato*®) for treatment of Human Immunodeficiency Virus type 1 (HIV-1) infection in adults and adolescents above 12 years of age weighing at least 40 kg, with no known or suspected resistance to the integrase inhibitor class, or lamivudine (February 2020) AWMSG No. 3659 Recommended

- MEDICINAL FORMS There can be variation in the licensing of different medicines containing the same drug.
  Tablet
  ‣ Lamivudine with dolutegravir (Non-proprietary)
  Dolutegravir (as Dolutegravir sodium) 50 mg, Lamivudine 300 mg Dovato 50mg/300mg tablets | 30 tablet [PoM] £656.26 (Hospital only)

Lamivudine with tenofovir disoproxil

11-Nov-2019

The properties listed below are those particular to the combination only. For the properties of the components please consider, lamivudine p. 691, tenofovir disoproxil below.

- ● INDICATIONS AND DOSE

HIV-1 infection in combination with other antiretroviral drugs (initiated by a specialist)
‣ BY MOUTH
‣ Adult: 300/245 mg once daily
DOSE EQUIVALENCE AND CONVERSION
‣ Dose expressed as x/y mg lamivudine/tenofovir disoproxil.

- CAUTIONS Elderly (no information available)
- INTERACTIONS → Appendix 1: NRTIs · tenofovir disoproxil
- ALLERGY AND CROSS-SENSITIVITY Manufacturer advises contra-indicated in patients with hypersensitivity to peanut or soya products.
- RENAL IMPAIRMENT Manufacturer advises avoid if creatinine clearance less than 50 mL/minute (consult product literature).
- PATIENT AND CARER ADVICE
  Driving and skilled tasks Manufacturer advises patients should be counselled on the effects on driving and performance of skilled tasks—increased risk of dizziness.
- MEDICINAL FORMS There can be variation in the licensing of different medicines containing the same drug.
  Tablet
  CAUTIONARY AND ADVISORY LABELS 21
  EXCIPIENTS: May contain Lecithin
  ‣ Lamivudine with tenofovir disoproxil (Non-proprietary)
  Tenofovir disoproxil (as Tenofovir disoproxil fumarate) 245 mg, Lamivudine 300 mg Lamivudine 300mg / Tenofovir disoproxil 245mg tablets | 30 tablet [PoM] £9.99 (Hospital only) | 90 tablet [PoM] £29.97 (Hospital only)

Lamivudine with tenofovir disoproxil and doravirine

02-Oct-2020

The properties listed below are those particular to the combination only. For the properties of the components please consider, lamivudine p. 691, tenofovir disoproxil below, doravirine p. 683.

- ● INDICATIONS AND DOSE

HIV-1 infection (initiated by a specialist)
‣ BY MOUTH
‣ Adult: 1 tablet once daily
DOSE ADJUSTMENTS DUE TO INTERACTIONS
‣ Manufacturer advises if concurrent use of moderate inducers of CYP3A4, dabrafenib, modafinil or telotristat ethyl is unavoidable, increase doravirine

dose to 100 mg twice daily. Manufacturer advises increasing doravirine dose to 100 mg twice daily with rifabutin. The extra doravirine 100 mg dose should be taken approximately 12 hours after the dose of *Delstrigo®*.

- INTERACTIONS → Appendix 1: NNRTIs · NRTIs · tenofovir disoproxil
- PREGNANCY Manufacturer advises avoid.
- HEPATIC IMPAIRMENT Manufacturer advises caution in severe impairment—no information available.
- RENAL IMPAIRMENT Manufacturer advises avoid if creatinine clearance less than 50 mL/minute.
- PATIENT AND CARER ADVICE
  Missed doses If a dose is more than 12 hours late, the missed dose should not be taken and the next dose should be taken at the normal time.
  Driving and skilled tasks Manufacturer advises patients and carers should be counselled on the effects on driving and performance of skilled tasks—increased risk of fatigue, dizziness, and somnolence.
- NATIONAL FUNDING/ACCESS DECISIONS
  For full details see funding body website
  All Wales Medicines Strategy Group (AWMSG) decisions
  ‣ Doravirine / lamivudine / tenofovir disoproxil fumarate (*Delstrigo®*) for the treatment of adults infected with HIV-1 without past or present evidence of resistance to the NNRTI class, lamivudine, or tenofovir (September 2020) AWMSG No. 3648 Recommended
- MEDICINAL FORMS There can be variation in the licensing of different medicines containing the same drug.
  Tablet
  CAUTIONARY AND ADVISORY LABELS 25, 3
  ‣ Delstrigo (Merck Sharp & Dohme Ltd) ▼
  Doravirine 100 mg, Tenofovir disoproxil (as Tenofovir disoproxil fumarate) 245 mg, Lamivudine 300 mg Delstrigo 100mg/300mg/245mg tablets | 30 tablet [PoM] £578.55 (Hospital only)

F 685

Tenofovir disoproxil

03-Sep-2020

- ● INDICATIONS AND DOSE

HIV infection in combination with other antiretroviral drugs | Chronic hepatitis B infection with compensated liver disease (with evidence of viral replication, and histologically documented active liver inflammation or fibrosis) | Chronic hepatitis B infection with decompensated liver disease
‣ BY MOUTH
‣ Adult: 245 mg once daily
DOSE EQUIVALENCE AND CONVERSION
‣ 7.5 scoops of granules contains approx. 245 mg tenofovir disoproxil (as fumarate).

- INTERACTIONS → Appendix 1: tenofovir disoproxil
- SIDE-EFFECTS
- **Common or very common** Abdominal distension
- **Uncommon** Proximal renal tubulopathy
- **Rare or very rare** Acute tubular necrosis · hepatic disorders · nephritis · nephrogenic diabetes insipidus · renal impairment
- HEPATIC IMPAIRMENT Manufacturer advises caution in decompensated hepatic disease (limited information available).
- RENAL IMPAIRMENT
  Dose adjustments *Granules*: 132 mg once daily if eGFR 30–50 mL/minute/1.73 m^2; 66 mg once daily if eGFR 20–30 mL/minute/1.73 m^2; 33 mg once daily if eGFR 10–20 mL/minute/1.73 m^2.

Tablets: 245 mg every 2 days if eGFR 30–50 mL/minute/1.73 m^2; 245 mg every 3–4 days if eGFR 10–30 mL/minute/1.73 m^2.

Monitoring Monitor renal function—interrupt treatment if further deterioration.

● MONITORING REQUIREMENTS
▶ Test renal function and serum phosphate before treatment, then every 4 weeks (more frequently if at increased risk of renal impairment) for 1 year and then every 3 months, interrupt treatment if renal function deteriorates or serum phosphate decreases.
▶ When treating chronic hepatitis B with tenofovir, monitor liver function tests every 3 months and viral markers for hepatitis B every 3–6 months during treatment (continue monitoring for at least 1 year after discontinuation—recurrent hepatitis may occur on discontinuation).

● DIRECTIONS FOR ADMINISTRATION *Granules*: Manufacturer advises mix 1 scoop of granules with 1 tablespoon of soft food (e.g. yoghurt, apple sauce) and take immediately without chewing. Do **not** mix granules with liquids.

● PATIENT AND CARER ADVICE Patients or carers should be given advice on how to administer tenofovir granules. **Missed doses** If a dose is more than 12 hours late, the missed dose should not be taken and the next dose should be taken at the normal time.

● NATIONAL FUNDING/ACCESS DECISIONS
For full details see funding body website
NICE decisions
▶ Tenofovir disoproxil for the treatment of chronic hepatitis B (July 2009) NICE TA173 Recommended

● MEDICINAL FORMS There can be variation in the licensing of different medicines containing the same drug.

Granules
CAUTIONARY AND ADVISORY LABELS 21
▶ Viread (Gilead Sciences Ireland UC)
Tenofovir disoproxil (as Tenofovir disoproxil fumarate) 33 mg per 1 gram Viread 33mg/g granules | 60 gram PoM £54.50 (Hospital only)

Tablet
CAUTIONARY AND ADVISORY LABELS 21
▶ Tenofovir disoproxil (Non-proprietary)
Tenofovir disoproxil 245 mg Tenofovir 245mg tablets | 30 tablet PoM £27.49–£204.39 DT = £27.49 (Hospital only)
▶ Viread (Gilead Sciences Ireland UC)
Tenofovir disoproxil (as Tenofovir disoproxil fumarate) 123 mg Viread 123mg tablets | 30 tablet PoM £102.60 DT = £102.60 (Hospital only)
Tenofovir disoproxil (as Tenofovir disoproxil fumarate) 163 mg Viread 163mg tablets | 30 tablet PoM £135.98 DT = £135.98 (Hospital only)
Tenofovir disoproxil (as Tenofovir disoproxil fumarate) 204 mg Viread 204mg tablets | 30 tablet PoM £170.19 DT = £170.19 (Hospital only)
Tenofovir disoproxil 245 mg Viread 245mg tablets | 30 tablet PoM £204.39 DT = £27.49 (Hospital only)

F 685

Zidovudine

17-Jul-2020

(Azidothymidine; AZT)

● INDICATIONS AND DOSE
HIV infection in combination with other antiretroviral drugs
▶ BY MOUTH
▶ Adult: 250–300 mg twice daily
Prevention of maternal-fetal HIV transmission
▶ BY MOUTH, OR BY INTRAVENOUS INFUSION
▶ Adult: Seek specialist advice (combination therapy preferred) (consult local protocol)

HIV infection in combination with other antiretroviral drugs in patients temporarily unable to take zidovudine by mouth
▶ BY INTRAVENOUS INFUSION
▶ Adult: 0.8–1 mg/kg every 4 hours usually for not more than 2 weeks, dose approximating to 1.2–1.5 mg/kg every 4 hours by mouth

● CONTRA-INDICATIONS Abnormally low haemoglobin concentration (consult product literature) · abnormally low neutrophil counts (consult product literature)

● CAUTIONS Elderly · lactic acidosis · risk of haematological toxicity particularly with high dose and advanced disease · vitamin B$_{12}$ deficiency (increased risk of neutropenia)
CAUTIONS, FURTHER INFORMATION
▶ Lactic acidosis Lactic acidosis associated with hepatomegaly and hepatic steatosis has been reported with zidovudine. Use with caution in patients with hepatomegaly, hepatitis, or other risk factors for liver disease and hepatic steatosis (including obesity and alcohol abuse). Manufacturer advises discontinue treatment if symptoms of hyperlactataemia, lactic acidosis, progressive hepatomegaly or rapid deterioration of liver function become apparent.

● INTERACTIONS → Appendix 1: NRTIs

● SIDE-EFFECTS
▶ **Common or very common** Leucopenia · malaise · myalgia
▶ **Uncommon** Bone marrow disorders · dyspnoea · generalised pain · myopathy · thrombocytopenia
▶ **Rare or very rare** Alertness decreased · anxiety · appetite decreased · cardiomyopathy · chest pain · chills · cough · depression · drowsiness · dyspepsia · gynaecomastia · hepatic disorders · hyperhidrosis · influenza like illness · nail discolouration · oral discolouration · paraesthesia · pure red cell aplasia · seizure · taste altered · urinary frequency increased
▶ **Frequency not known** Lipoatrophy
SIDE-EFFECTS, FURTHER INFORMATION **Anaemia and myelosuppression** If anaemia or myelosuppression occur, reduce dose or interrupt treatment according to product literature, or consider other treatment.
Lipodystrophy syndrome Metabolic effects may occur with zidovudine; plasma lipids and blood glucose concentrations should be measured routinely.

● HEPATIC IMPAIRMENT Manufacturer advises caution in moderate to severe impairment (increased risk of accumulation).
Dose adjustments Manufacturer advises consider dose reduction in moderate to severe impairment—consult product literature.

● RENAL IMPAIRMENT
Dose adjustments Reduce oral dose to 300–400 mg daily in divided doses or intravenous dose to 1 mg/kg 3–4 times daily if eGFR is less than 10 mL/minute/1.73 m^2.

● MONITORING REQUIREMENTS Monitor full blood count after 4 weeks of treatment, then every 3 months.

● DIRECTIONS FOR ADMINISTRATION
▶ With intravenous use For *intermittent intravenous infusion*, manufacturer advises dilute to a concentration of 2 mg/mL or 4 mg/mL with Glucose 5% and give over 1 hour.

● PRESCRIBING AND DISPENSING INFORMATION The abbreviation AZT which is sometimes used for zidovudine has also been used for another drug.

● MEDICINAL FORMS There can be variation in the licensing of different medicines containing the same drug.

Solution for infusion
▶ Retrovir (ViiV Healthcare UK Ltd)
Zidovudine 10 mg per 1 ml Retrovir IV 200mg/20ml concentrate for solution for infusion vials | 5 vial PoM £52.48 (Hospital only)

5

Infection

Oral solution

▸ Retrovir (ViiV Healthcare UK Ltd)
Zidovudine 10 mg per 1 ml Retrovir 100mg/10ml oral solution sugar-free | 200 ml [PoM] £20.91 (Hospital only)

Capsule

▸ Zidovudine (Non-proprietary)
Zidovudine 100 mg Zidovudine 100mg capsules | 60 capsule [PoM] £53.31 (Hospital only)
Zidovudine 250 mg Zidovudine 250mg capsules | 60 capsule [PoM] £13.32 (Hospital only)

▸ Retrovir (ViiV Healthcare UK Ltd)
Zidovudine 100 mg Retrovir 100mg capsules | 100 capsule [PoM] £104.54 (Hospital only)
Zidovudine 250 mg Retrovir 250mg capsules | 40 capsule [PoM] £104.54 (Hospital only)

Zidovudine with lamivudine
21-Jul-2020

The properties listed below are those particular to the combination only. For the properties of the components please consider, zidovudine p. 693, lamivudine p. 691.

● **INDICATIONS AND DOSE**

HIV infection in combination with other antiretroviral drugs

▸ BY MOUTH
▸ Adult: 1 tablet twice daily

● INTERACTIONS → Appendix 1: NRTIs

● RENAL IMPAIRMENT Avoid if eGFR less than 50 mL/minute/1.73 m^2 (consult product literature).

● DIRECTIONS FOR ADMINISTRATION

COMBIVIR® TABLETS Manufacturer advises tablets may be crushed and mixed with semi-solid food or liquid just before administration.

● MEDICINAL FORMS There can be variation in the licensing of different medicines containing the same drug.

Tablet

▸ Zidovudine with lamivudine (Non-proprietary)
Lamivudine 150 mg, Zidovudine 300 mg Zidovudine 300mg / Lamivudine 150mg tablets | 60 tablet [PoM] £240.10-£255.10 DT = £300.12 (Hospital only)
▸ Combivir (ViiV Healthcare UK Ltd)
Lamivudine 150 mg, Zidovudine 300 mg Combivir 150mg/300mg tablets | 60 tablet [PoM] £300.12 DT = £300.12 (Hospital only)

ANTIVIRALS ❭ PROTEASE INHIBITORS, HIV

Protease inhibitors

● CONTRA-INDICATIONS Acute porphyrias p. 1107
● CAUTIONS Haemophilia (increased risk of bleeding)
● SIDE-EFFECTS
▸ **Common or very common** Alopecia · anaemia · angioedema · anxiety · appetite abnormal · arthralgia · asthenia · diabetes mellitus · diarrhoea · dizziness · dry mouth · dyslipidaemia · dyspnoea · fever · gastrointestinal discomfort · gastrointestinal disorders · headache · hepatic disorders · hypersensitivity · hypertension · malaise · muscle complaints · nausea · neutropenia · oral ulceration · pancreatitis · peripheral neuropathy · seizure · skin reactions · sleep disorders · taste altered · vomiting
▸ **Uncommon** Drowsiness · immune reconstitution inflammatory syndrome · osteonecrosis · Stevens-Johnson syndrome · weight increased
● HEPATIC IMPAIRMENT In general, manufacturers advise use with caution in patients with chronic hepatitis B or C (increased risk of hepatic side-effects).

Atazanavir
15-Dec-2020

● **INDICATIONS AND DOSE**

HIV infection in combination with other antiretroviral drugs—with low-dose ritonavir

▸ BY MOUTH
▸ Adult: 300 mg once daily

HIV infection in combination with other antiretroviral drugs—with cobicistat

▸ BY MOUTH
▸ Adult: 300 mg once daily

● CAUTIONS Cardiac conduction disorders · electrolyte disturbances · predisposition to QT interval prolongation

● INTERACTIONS → Appendix 1: HIV-protease inhibitors

● SIDE-EFFECTS
▸ **Uncommon** Chest pain · chronic kidney disease · depression · disorientation · drug reaction with eosinophilia and systemic symptoms (DRESS) · gallbladder disorders · gynaecomastia · haematuria · memory loss · myopathy · nephritis tubulointerstitial · nephrolithiasis · proteinuria · syncope · torsade de pointes · urinary frequency increased
▸ **Rare or very rare** Gait abnormal · oedema · palpitations · QT interval prolongation · renal pain · vasodilation
SIDE-EFFECTS, FURTHER INFORMATION Mild to moderate rash occurs commonly, usually within the first 3 weeks of therapy. Severe rash occurs less frequently and may be accompanied by systemic symptoms. Discontinue if severe rash develops.

● PREGNANCY [EvGr] Theoretical risk of hyperbilirubinaemia in neonate if used at term. ⓜ For use with cobicistat, see atazanavir with cobicistat below.
Monitoring In pregnancy, monitor viral load and plasma-atazanavir concentration during third trimester.

● HEPATIC IMPAIRMENT Manufacturer advises caution in mild impairment; avoid in moderate to severe impairment (no information available).

● MEDICINAL FORMS There can be variation in the licensing of different medicines containing the same drug.

Capsule

CAUTIONARY AND ADVISORY LABELS 5, 21

▸ Atazanavir (Non-proprietary)
Atazanavir (as Atazanavir sulfate) 150 mg Atazanavir 150mg capsules | 60 capsule [PoM] £303.38 (Hospital only)
Atazanavir (as Atazanavir sulfate) 200 mg Atazanavir 200mg capsules | 60 capsule [PoM] £303.37-£303.38 (Hospital only)
Atazanavir (as Atazanavir sulfate) 300 mg Atazanavir 300mg capsules | 30 capsule [PoM] £257.87-£303.38 (Hospital only)
▸ Reyataz (Bristol-Myers Squibb Pharmaceuticals Ltd)
Atazanavir (as Atazanavir sulfate) 150 mg Reyataz 150mg capsules | 60 capsule [PoM] £303.38 (Hospital only)
Atazanavir (as Atazanavir sulfate) 200 mg Reyataz 200mg capsules | 60 capsule [PoM] £303.38 (Hospital only)
Atazanavir (as Atazanavir sulfate) 300 mg Reyataz 300mg capsules | 30 capsule [PoM] £303.38 (Hospital only)

Atazanavir with cobicistat
15-Dec-2020

The properties listed below are those particular to the combination only. For the properties of the components please consider, atazanavir above, cobicistat p. 699.

● **INDICATIONS AND DOSE**

HIV infection, in combination with other antiretroviral drugs (initiated by a specialist)

▸ BY MOUTH
▸ Adult: 300/150 mg once daily

DOSE EQUIVALENCE AND CONVERSION

▸ Dose expressed as x/y mg of atazanavir/cobicistat.

- **CONTRA-INDICATIONS** Haemodialysis
- **INTERACTIONS** → Appendix 1: cobicistat · HIV-protease inhibitors
- **PREGNANCY** EvGr Not to be initiated during pregnancy due to low atazanavir exposure; women who become pregnant during therapy should be switched to an alternative regimen. Darunavir with ritonavir may be considered as an alternative. Ⓜ

- **MEDICINAL FORMS** There can be variation in the licensing of different medicines containing the same drug.

Tablet

CAUTIONARY AND ADVISORY LABELS 5, 21
▸ Evotaz (Bristol-Myers Squibb Pharmaceuticals Ltd)
Cobicistat 150 mg, Atazanavir (as Atazanavir sulfate) 300 mg Evotaz 300mg/150mg tablets | 30 tablet PoM £323.38 (Hospital only)

◀ 694

Darunavir

15-Dec-2020

- **INDICATIONS AND DOSE**

HIV infection in combination with other antiretroviral drugs in patients previously treated with antiretroviral therapy—with low-dose ritonavir
▸ BY MOUTH
▸ Adult: 600 mg twice daily, alternatively 800 mg once daily, once daily dose only to be used if no resistance to darunavir, if plasma HIV-RNA concentration less than 100 000 copies/mL, and if CD4 cell count greater than 100 cells × 10^6/litre

HIV infection in combination with other antiretroviral drugs in patients previously treated with antiretroviral therapy—with cobicistat
▸ BY MOUTH
▸ Adult: 800 mg once daily, dose appropriate if no resistance to darunavir, if plasma HIV-RNA concentration less than 100 000 copies/mL, and if CD4 cell count greater than 100 cells × 10^6/litre

HIV infection in combination with other antiretroviral drugs in patients not previously treated with antiretroviral therapy—with low-dose ritonavir
▸ BY MOUTH
▸ Adult: 800 mg once daily

HIV infection in combination with other antiretroviral drugs in patients not previously treated with antiretroviral therapy—with cobicistat
▸ BY MOUTH
▸ Adult: 800 mg once daily

- **INTERACTIONS** → Appendix 1: HIV-protease inhibitors
- **SIDE-EFFECTS**
▸ **Uncommon** Angina pectoris · arrhythmias · burping · chest pain · concentration impaired · confusion · constipation · cough · depression · dry eye · eye erythema · feeling hot · flushing · gout · gynaecomastia · haemorrhage · herpes simplex · hyperglycaemia · hypothyroidism · leucopenia · memory loss · mood altered · muscle weakness · myocardial infarction · nail discolouration · nephrolithiasis · oral disorders · osteoporosis · pain · peripheral oedema · polydipsia · QT interval prolongation · renal impairment · sensation abnormal · sexual dysfunction · sweat changes · throat irritation · thrombocytopenia · urinary disorders · urine abnormalities · vertigo
▸ **Rare or very rare** Arthritis · chills · feeling abnormal · joint stiffness · musculoskeletal stiffness · palpitations · rhinorrhoea · severe cutaneous adverse reactions (SCARs) · syncope · visual impairment
  SIDE-EFFECTS, FURTHER INFORMATION Mild to moderate rash occurs commonly, usually within the first 4 weeks of therapy and resolves without stopping treatment. Severe skin rash (including Stevens-Johnson syndrome and toxic

epidermal necrolysis) occurs less frequently and may be accompanied by fever, malaise, arthralgia, myalgia, oral lesions, conjunctivitis, hepatitis, or eosinophilia; treatment should be stopped if this develops.

- **ALLERGY AND CROSS-SENSITIVITY** EvGr Use with caution in patients with sulfonamide sensitivity. Ⓜ
- **PREGNANCY** Manufacturer advises use only if potential benefit outweighs risk; if required, use the twice daily dose regimen. For use with cobicistat, see darunavir with cobicistat below or darunavir with cobicistat, emtricitabine and tenofovir alafenamide p. 696.
- **HEPATIC IMPAIRMENT** Manufacturer advises caution in mild to moderate impairment; avoid in severe impairment (no information available).
- **MONITORING REQUIREMENTS** Monitor liver function before and during treatment.
- **PRESCRIBING AND DISPENSING INFORMATION** Flavours of oral liquid formulations may include strawberry.
- **PATIENT AND CARER ADVICE**
  Vomiting EvGr If vomiting occurs more than 4 hours after a dose is taken, the missed dose should not be taken and the next dose should be taken at the normal time. Ⓜ
  Missed doses EvGr If a dose is more than 6 hours late on the twice-daily regimen (or more than 12 hours late on the once-daily regimen), the missed dose should not be taken and the next dose should be taken at the normal time. Ⓜ

- **MEDICINAL FORMS** There can be variation in the licensing of different medicines containing the same drug.

Oral suspension

CAUTIONARY AND ADVISORY LABELS 21
▸ Prezista (Janssen-Cilag Ltd)
Darunavir (as Darunavir ethanolate) 100 mg per 1 ml Prezista 100mg/ml oral suspension sugar-free | 200 ml PoM £248.17 (Hospital only)

Tablet

CAUTIONARY AND ADVISORY LABELS 21
▸ Darunavir (Non-proprietary)
Darunavir (as Darunavir ethanolate) 400 mg Darunavir 400mg tablets | 60 tablet PoM £297.80 (Hospital only)
Darunavir (as Darunavir ethanolate) 600 mg Darunavir 600mg tablets | 60 tablet PoM £379.67–£446.70 (Hospital only)
Darunavir (as Darunavir ethanolate) 800 mg Darunavir 800mg tablets | 30 tablet PoM £253.13–£297.80 DT = £268.02 (Hospital only)
▸ Prezista (Janssen-Cilag Ltd)
Darunavir (as Darunavir ethanolate) 75 mg Prezista 75mg tablets | 480 tablet PoM £446.70 (Hospital only)
Darunavir (as Darunavir ethanolate) 150 mg Prezista 150mg tablets | 240 tablet PoM £446.70 (Hospital only)
Darunavir (as Darunavir ethanolate) 400 mg Prezista 400mg tablets | 60 tablet PoM £297.80 (Hospital only)
Darunavir (as Darunavir ethanolate) 600 mg Prezista 600mg tablets | 60 tablet PoM £446.70 (Hospital only)
Darunavir (as Darunavir ethanolate) 800 mg Prezista 800mg tablets | 30 tablet PoM £297.80 DT = £268.02 (Hospital only)

Darunavir with cobicistat

09-Dec-2020

The properties listed below are those particular to the combination only. For the properties of the components please consider, cobicistat p. 699, darunavir above.

- **INDICATIONS AND DOSE**

HIV infection, in combination with other antiretroviral drugs (initiated by a specialist)
▸ BY MOUTH
▸ Adult: 800/150 mg once daily

continued →

5

Infection

5

Infection

IMPORTANT SAFETY INFORMATION

MHRA/CHM ADVICE: DARUNAVIR BOOSTED WITH COBICISTAT: AVOID USE IN PREGNANCY DUE TO RISK OF TREATMENT FAILURE AND MATERNAL-TO-CHILD TRANSMISSION OF HIV-1 (JULY 2018)

Pharmacokinetic data show mean exposure of darunavir boosted with cobicistat (available in combination in *Rezolsta*® and *Symtuza*®) to be lower during the second and third trimesters of pregnancy than during 6–12 weeks postpartum. Low darunavir exposure may be associated with an increased risk of treatment failure and an increased risk of HIV-1 transmission to the unborn child. For further information, see *Pregnancy*.

● CONTRA-INDICATIONS Treatment-experienced patients with 1 or more darunavir resistance-associated mutations, plasma HIV-RNA concentration of 100 000 copies/mL or greater, or CD4 count less than 100 cells × 10⁶/litre

● CAUTIONS Elderly

● INTERACTIONS → Appendix 1: cobicistat · HIV-protease inhibitors

● PREGNANCY Manufacturer advises not to be initiated during pregnancy due to low darunavir exposure; women who become pregnant during therapy should be switched to an alternative regimen. Darunavir with ritonavir may be considered as an alternative.

● NATIONAL FUNDING/ACCESS DECISIONS
For full details see funding body website

Scottish Medicines Consortium (SMC) decisions
▸ Darunavir/cobicistat (*Rezolsta*®) in combination with other antiretroviral medicinal products for the treatment of human immunodeficiency virus-1 (HIV-1) infection in adults aged 18 years or older. Genotypic testing should guide its use (August 2015) SMC No. 1081/15 Recommended

All Wales Medicines Strategy Group (AWMSG) decisions
▸ Darunavir with cobicistat (*Rezolsta*®) in combination with other antiretroviral medicinal products for the treatment of human immunodeficiency virus-1 (HIV-1) infection in adults and adolescents (aged 12 years and older with body weight at least 40 kg) (November 2020) AWMSG No. 3779 Recommended

● MEDICINAL FORMS There can be variation in the licensing of different medicines containing the same drug.
Tablet
CAUTIONARY AND ADVISORY LABELS 21
▸ Rezolsta (Janssen-Cilag Ltd)
Cobicistat 150 mg, Darunavir (as Darunavir ethanolate) 800 mg Rezolsta 800mg/150mg tablets | 30 tablet [PoM] £317.24 (Hospital only)

Darunavir with cobicistat, emtricitabine and tenofovir alafenamide

22-Oct-2020

The properties listed below are those particular to the combination only. For the properties of the components please consider, darunavir p. 695, cobicistat p. 699, emtricitabine p. 689, tenofovir alafenamide p. 663.

● INDICATIONS AND DOSE

HIV infection (initiated by a specialist)
▸ BY MOUTH
 ▸ Adult: 1 tablet once daily

IMPORTANT SAFETY INFORMATION

MHRA/CHM ADVICE: DARUNAVIR BOOSTED WITH COBICISTAT: AVOID USE IN PREGNANCY DUE TO RISK OF TREATMENT FAILURE AND MATERNAL-TO-CHILD TRANSMISSION OF HIV-1 (JULY 2018)

Pharmacokinetic data show mean exposure of darunavir boosted with cobicistat (available in combination in *Rezolsta*® and *Symtuza*®) to be lower during the second and third trimesters of pregnancy than during 6–12 weeks postpartum. Low darunavir exposure may be associated with an increased risk of treatment failure and an increased risk of HIV-1 transmission to the unborn child. For further information, see *Pregnancy*.

● INTERACTIONS → Appendix 1: cobicistat · HIV-protease inhibitors · NRTIs · tenofovir alafenamide

● PREGNANCY Manufacturer advises not to be initiated during pregnancy due to low darunavir exposure; women who become pregnant during therapy should be switched to an alternative regimen.

● RENAL IMPAIRMENT Manufacturer advises avoid if eGFR less than 30 mL/minute/1.73 m²—no information available.

● PATIENT AND CARER ADVICE
Driving and skilled tasks Manufacturer advises patients and carers should be counselled on the effects on driving and performance of skilled tasks—increased risk of dizziness.

● NATIONAL FUNDING/ACCESS DECISIONS
For full details see funding body website

Scottish Medicines Consortium (SMC) decisions
▸ Darunavir, cobicistat, emtricitabine, tenofovir alafenamide (*Symtuza*®) for the treatment of human immunodeficiency virus type 1 (HIV-1) infection in adults and adolescents (aged 12 years and older with body weight at least 40 kg) (January 2018) SMC No. 1290/18 Recommended

All Wales Medicines Strategy Group (AWMSG) decisions
▸ Darunavir / cobicistat / emtricitabine / tenofovir alafenamide (*Symtuza*®) for the treatment of human immunodeficiency virus type 1 (HIV-1) infection in adults and adolescents (aged 12 years and older with body weight at least 40 kg) (March 2018) AWMSG No. 2418 Recommended

● MEDICINAL FORMS There can be variation in the licensing of different medicines containing the same drug.
Tablet
CAUTIONARY AND ADVISORY LABELS 21
▸ Symtuza (Janssen-Cilag Ltd) ▼
Tenofovir alafenamide (as Tenofovir alafenamide fumarate) 10 mg, Cobicistat 150 mg, Emtricitabine 200 mg, Darunavir (as Darunavir ethanolate) 800 mg Symtuza 800mg/150mg/200mg/10mg tablets | 30 tablet [PoM] £672.97 (Hospital only)

Fosamprenavir

03-Aug-2020

⬤ **DRUG ACTION** Fosamprenavir is a pro-drug of amprenavir.

⬤ **INDICATIONS AND DOSE**

HIV infection in combination with other antiretroviral drugs—with low-dose ritonavir

▸ BY MOUTH
▸ Adult: 700 mg twice daily

DOSE EQUIVALENCE AND CONVERSION
▸ 700 mg fosamprenavir is equivalent to approximately 600 mg amprenavir.

⬤ **INTERACTIONS** → Appendix 1: HIV-protease inhibitors

⬤ **SIDE-EFFECTS**
▸ **Common or very common** Oral paraesthesia

SIDE-EFFECTS, FURTHER INFORMATION Rash may occur, usually in the second week of therapy; discontinue permanently if severe rash with systemic or allergic symptoms or, mucosal involvement; if rash mild or moderate, may continue without interruption—usually resolves and may respond to antihistamines.

⬤ **PREGNANCY** Toxicity in *animal* studies; manufacturer advises use only if potential benefit outweighs risk.

⬤ **HEPATIC IMPAIRMENT** Manufacturer advises caution.
Dose adjustments Manufacturer advises dose reduction to 450 mg twice daily in moderate impairment and 300 mg twice daily in severe impairment.

⬤ **DIRECTIONS FOR ADMINISTRATION** Manufacturer advises in adults, oral suspension should be taken on an empty stomach.

⬤ **PRESCRIBING AND DISPENSING INFORMATION** Flavours of oral liquid formulations may include grape, bubblegum, or peppermint.

⬤ **PATIENT AND CARER ADVICE** Patients or carers should be given advice on how to administer fosamprenavir oral suspension.

⬤ **MEDICINAL FORMS** There can be variation in the licensing of different medicines containing the same drug.

Oral suspension
EXCIPIENTS: May contain Propylene glycol
▸ Telzir (ViiV Healthcare UK Ltd)
  Fosamprenavir (as Fosamprenavir calcium) 50 mg per 1 ml Telzir 50mg/ml oral suspension | 225 ml [PoM] £69.06 (Hospital only)

Tablet
▸ Telzir (ViiV Healthcare UK Ltd)
  Fosamprenavir (as Fosamprenavir calcium) 700 mg Telzir 700mg tablets | 60 tablet [PoM] £258.97 (Hospital only)

Lopinavir with ritonavir

22-Oct-2020

⬤ **INDICATIONS AND DOSE**

HIV infection in combination with other antiretroviral drugs

▸ BY MOUTH USING TABLETS
▸ Adult: 400/100 mg twice daily, alternatively 800/200 mg once daily, once daily dose to be used only in adults with a HIV strain that has less than 3 mutations to protease inhibitors
▸ BY MOUTH USING ORAL SOLUTION
▸ Adult: 5 mL twice daily

DOSE EQUIVALENCE AND CONVERSION
▸ Oral solution contains 400 mg lopinavir, 100 mg ritonavir/5 mL (or 80 mg lopinavir, 20 mg ritonavir/mL).

⬤ **CAUTIONS** Cardiac conduction disorders · pancreatitis · patients at high risk of cardiovascular disease · structural heart disease

⬤ **INTERACTIONS** → Appendix 1: HIV-protease inhibitors

⬤ **SIDE-EFFECTS**
▸ **Common or very common** Increased risk of infection · leucopenia · lymphadenopathy · menstrual cycle irregularities · migraine · muscle weakness · myopathy · night sweats · pain · sexual dysfunction
▸ **Uncommon** Atherosclerosis · atrioventricular block · cholangitis · constipation · deep vein thrombosis · haemorrhage · hyperbilirubinaemia · hypogonadism · myocardial infarction · nephritis · stomatitis · stroke · tinnitus · tremor · tricuspid valve incompetence · vasculitis · vertigo · visual impairment

SIDE-EFFECTS, FURTHER INFORMATION Signs and symptoms suggestive of pancreatitis (including raised serum lipase) should be evaluated—discontinue if pancreatitis diagnosed.

⬤ **PREGNANCY** For *tablets*, manufacturer advises only use if potential benefit outweighs risk—toxicity in *animal* studies (recommendation also supported by specialist sources). Avoid *oral solution* due to high alcohol and propylene glycol content.

⬤ **HEPATIC IMPAIRMENT** For *oral solution*, manufacturer advises avoid due to propylene glycol content (risk of toxicity). For *tablets*, manufacturer advises avoid in severe impairment (no information available).

⬤ **RENAL IMPAIRMENT** Avoid *oral solution* due to high propylene glycol content.

⬤ **MONITORING REQUIREMENTS**
▸ Manufacturer advises monitor liver function before and during treatment.
▸ For *oral solution*, manufacturer advises monitor for signs of alcohol and propylene glycol toxicity (particularly in infants).

⬤ **PRESCRIBING AND DISPENSING INFORMATION** For *oral solution*, manufacturer advises high alcohol (42 % v/v) and propylene glycol content—consider total amounts from all medicines that are to be given to infants in order to avoid toxicity; caution in patients for which consumption may be harmful.

⬤ **PATIENT AND CARER ADVICE** Oral solution tastes bitter.

⬤ **NATIONAL FUNDING/ACCESS DECISIONS**
For full details see funding body website

Scottish Medicines Consortium (SMC) decisions
▸ Lopinavir 200 mg, ritonavir 50 mg tablet (*Kaletra*®) for the treatment of HIV-1 infected adults and children above the age of 2 years in combination with other antiretroviral agents (November 2006) SMC No. 326/06 Recommended

⬤ **MEDICINAL FORMS** There can be variation in the licensing of different medicines containing the same drug.

Oral solution
CAUTIONARY AND ADVISORY LABELS 21
EXCIPIENTS: May contain Alcohol, propylene glycol
▸ Kaletra (AbbVie Ltd)
  Ritonavir 20 mg per 1 ml, Lopinavir 80 mg per 1 ml Kaletra 80mg/20mg/1ml oral solution | 120 ml [PoM] £122.96 (Hospital only) | 300 ml [PoM] £307.39 (Hospital only)

Tablet
CAUTIONARY AND ADVISORY LABELS 25
▸ Lopinavir with ritonavir (Non-proprietary)
  Ritonavir 50 mg, Lopinavir 200 mg Lopinavir 200mg / Ritonavir 50mg tablets | 120 tablet [PoM] £242.60-£285.40 (Hospital only)
▸ Kaletra (AbbVie Ltd)
  Ritonavir 25 mg, Lopinavir 100 mg Kaletra 100mg/25mg tablets | 60 tablet [PoM] £76.85 (Hospital only)
  Ritonavir 50 mg, Lopinavir 200 mg Kaletra 200mg/50mg tablets | 120 tablet [PoM] £285.41 (Hospital only)

5

Infection

Ritonavir

F 694

16-Jun-2020

- **INDICATIONS AND DOSE**

HIV infection in combination with other antiretroviral drugs (high-dose ritonavir)
- ▶ BY MOUTH
- ▶ Adult: Initially 300 mg every 12 hours for 3 days, increased in steps of 100 mg every 12 hours over not longer than 14 days; increased to 600 mg every 12 hours

Low-dose booster to increase effect of other protease inhibitors
- ▶ BY MOUTH
- ▶ Adult: 100–200 mg 1–2 times a day

- **CAUTIONS** Cardiac conduction disorders · pancreatitis · structural heart disease
- **INTERACTIONS** → Appendix 1: HIV-protease inhibitors
- **SIDE-EFFECTS**
- ▶ **Common or very common** Back pain · concentration impaired · confusion · cough · dehydration · feeling hot · flushing · gastrointestinal haemorrhage · gout · hypotension · menorrhagia · myopathy · oedema · oral paraesthesia · oropharyngeal pain · paraesthesia · peripheral coldness · pharyngitis · renal impairment · syncope · thrombocytopenia · urinary frequency increased · vision blurred
- ▶ **Uncommon** Myocardial infarction
- ▶ **Rare or very rare** Hyperglycaemia · toxic epidermal necrolysis

 SIDE-EFFECTS, FURTHER INFORMATION Signs and symptoms suggestive of pancreatitis (including raised serum lipase) should be evaluated — discontinue if pancreatitis diagnosed.

- **PREGNANCY**
 Dose adjustments Only use low-dose booster to increase the effect of other protease inhibitors.
- **HEPATIC IMPAIRMENT** When used as a *low-dose booster*, manufacturer advises caution in severe impairment; avoid in decompensated liver disease. When used in *high-doses*, manufacturer advises avoid in severe impairment.
 Dose adjustments Manufacturer advises consult product literature of co-administered protease inhibitor.

- **MEDICINAL FORMS** There can be variation in the licensing of different medicines containing the same drug.
 Tablet
 CAUTIONARY AND ADVISORY LABELS 21, 25
- ▶ Ritonavir (Non-proprietary)
 Ritonavir 100 mg Ritonavir 100mg tablets | 30 tablet [PoM] £16.52–£19.44 (Hospital only)
- ▶ Norvir (AbbVie Ltd)
 Ritonavir 100 mg Norvir 100mg tablets | 30 tablet [PoM] £19.44 (Hospital only)

Saquinavir

F 694

01-Jun-2020

- **INDICATIONS AND DOSE**

HIV infection in combination with other antiretrovirals in patients previously treated with antiretroviral therapy—with low-dose ritonavir
- ▶ BY MOUTH
- ▶ Adult: 1 g every 12 hours

HIV infection in combination with other antiretrovirals in patients not previously treated with antiretroviral therapy—with low-dose ritonavir
- ▶ BY MOUTH
- ▶ Adult: 500 mg every 12 hours for 7 days, then increased to 1 g every 12 hours

- **CONTRA-INDICATIONS** Bradycardia · congenital QT prolongation · electrolyte disturbances · heart failure with reduced ventricular ejection fraction · history of symptomatic arrhythmias
- **INTERACTIONS** → Appendix 1: HIV-protease inhibitors
- **SIDE-EFFECTS**
- ▶ **Common or very common** Burping · constipation · dry lips · libido decreased · lipoatrophy · paraesthesia
- ▶ **Uncommon** Mucosal ulceration · renal impairment · visual impairment
- ▶ **Frequency not known** QT interval prolongation

- **HEPATIC IMPAIRMENT** Manufacturer advises caution in moderate impairment (limited information available); avoid in decompensated liver disease.
- **RENAL IMPAIRMENT** Use with caution if eGFR less than 30 mL/minute/1.73 m^2.
- **MONITORING REQUIREMENTS** Monitor ECG before starting treatment (do not initiate treatment if QT interval over 450 milliseconds); if baseline QT interval less than 450 milliseconds, monitor ECG during treatment (particularly 10 days after starting treatment in patients not previously treated with antiretroviral therapy)— discontinue if QT interval increases over 480 milliseconds, if QT interval more than 20 milliseconds above baseline, if prolongation of PR interval, or if arrhythmias occur.
- **PATIENT AND CARER ADVICE**
 Arrhythmias Patients should be told how to recognise signs of arrhythmia and advised to seek medical attention if symptoms such as palpitation or syncope develop.

- **MEDICINAL FORMS** There can be variation in the licensing of different medicines containing the same drug.
 Tablet
 CAUTIONARY AND ADVISORY LABELS 21
- ▶ Invirase (Roche Products Ltd)
 Saquinavir (as Saquinavir mesilate) 500 mg Invirase 500mg tablets | 120 tablet [PoM] £251.26 (Hospital only)

Tipranavir

F 694

05-Jun-2020

- **INDICATIONS AND DOSE**

HIV infection resistant to other protease inhibitors, in combination with other antiretroviral drugs in patients previously treated with antiretrovirals–with low-dose ritonavir
- ▶ BY MOUTH USING CAPSULES
- ▶ Adult: 500 mg twice daily

- **CAUTIONS** Abnormal liver function tests and/or signs or symptoms of liver injury (consider delaying treatment if serum transaminases are greater than 5 times the upper limit of normal—consult product literature) · patients at risk of increased bleeding from trauma, surgery or other pathological conditions
- **INTERACTIONS** → Appendix 1: HIV-protease inhibitors
- **SIDE-EFFECTS**
- ▶ **Uncommon** Hyperamylasaemia · hyperglycaemia · influenza like illness · renal failure · thrombocytopenia
- ▶ **Rare or very rare** Dehydration · hyperbilirubinaemia · intracranial haemorrhage
- ▶ **Frequency not known** Bleeding tendency
 SIDE-EFFECTS, FURTHER INFORMATION Potentially life-threatening hepatotoxicity reported. Discontinue if signs or symptoms of hepatitis develop or if liver-function abnormality develops (consult product literature).
- **PREGNANCY** Manufacturer advises use only if potential benefit outweighs risk—toxicity in *animal* studies.
- **HEPATIC IMPAIRMENT** Manufacturer advises caution in mild impairment (risk of increased exposure)—monitor liver function before treatment, then every two weeks for

3 months, then monthly until 48 weeks, then every 8 to 12 weeks thereafter, and discontinue if liver function worsens; avoid in moderate to severe impairment.

● MONITORING REQUIREMENTS Monitor liver function before treatment, then every 2 weeks for 1 month, then every 4 weeks until 24 weeks, then every 8 to 12 weeks thereafter.

● MEDICINAL FORMS There can be variation in the licensing of different medicines containing the same drug.

Capsule

CAUTIONARY AND ADVISORY LABELS 5, 21
EXCIPIENTS: May contain Ethanol
▸ Aptivus (Boehringer Ingelheim Ltd)
Tipranavir 250 mg Aptivus 250mg capsules | 120 capsule PoM
£441.00 (Hospital only)

ANTIVIRALS ⟩ OTHER

Maraviroc
31-Aug-2020

● DRUG ACTION Maraviroc is an antagonist of the CCR5 chemokine receptor.

● **INDICATIONS AND DOSE**

CCR5-tropic HIV infection in combination with other antiretroviral drugs in patients previously treated with antiretrovirals
▸ BY MOUTH
▸ Adult: 300 mg twice daily

● CAUTIONS Cardiovascular disease
● INTERACTIONS → Appendix 1: maraviroc
● SIDE-EFFECTS
▸ **Common or very common** Abdominal pain · anaemia · appetite decreased · asthenia · depression · diarrhoea · flatulence · headache · insomnia · nausea · rash
▸ **Uncommon** Hyperbilirubinaemia · increased risk of infection · myopathy · postural hypotension · proteinuria · renal failure · seizure
▸ **Rare or very rare** Angina pectoris · granulocytopenia · hepatic disorders · metastases · neoplasms · pancytopenia · severe cutaneous adverse reactions (SCARs)
▸ **Frequency not known** Fever · hypersensitivity · immune reconstitution inflammatory syndrome · organ dysfunction · osteonecrosis

SIDE-EFFECTS, FURTHER INFORMATION **Osteonecrosis**
Osteonecrosis has been reported in patients with advanced HIV disease or following long-term exposure to combination antiretroviral therapy.
   Hepatotoxicity Manufacturer advises consider discontinuation if signs or symptoms of acute hepatitis, or increased liver transaminases with systemic symptoms of hypersensitivity occur.

● PREGNANCY Manufacturer advises use only if potential benefit outweighs risk—toxicity in *animal* studies.

● HEPATIC IMPAIRMENT Manufacturer advises caution in impairment and in patients with chronic hepatitis (increased risk of hepatic side-effects; limited information available).

● RENAL IMPAIRMENT If eGFR less than 80 mL/minute/1.73 m², consult product literature.

● NATIONAL FUNDING/ACCESS DECISIONS
For full details see funding body website
Scottish Medicines Consortium (SMC) decisions
▸ Maraviroc (*Celsentri*®) for treatment-experienced adult patients infected with only CCR5-tropic HIV-1 detectable (October 2008) SMC No. 458/08 Not recommended

● MEDICINAL FORMS There can be variation in the licensing of different medicines containing the same drug.
Tablet
▸ Celsentri (ViiV Healthcare UK Ltd)
Maraviroc 25 mg Celsentri 25mg tablets | 120 tablet PoM £147.09
DT = £147.09 (Hospital only)
Maraviroc 75 mg Celsentri 75mg tablets | 120 tablet PoM £441.27
DT = £441.27 (Hospital only)
Maraviroc 150 mg Celsentri 150mg tablets | 60 tablet PoM
£519.14 DT = £519.14 (Hospital only)
Maraviroc 300 mg Celsentri 300mg tablets | 60 tablet PoM
£519.14 DT = £519.14 (Hospital only)

PHARMACOKINETIC ENHANCERS

Cobicistat
08-Dec-2020

● **INDICATIONS AND DOSE**

Pharmacokinetic enhancer used to increase the effect of atazanavir or darunavir
▸ BY MOUTH
▸ Adult: 150 mg once daily

● INTERACTIONS → Appendix 1: cobicistat
● PREGNANCY EvGr Not to be initiated during pregnancy.
Ⓜ For use with atazanavir, see atazanavir with cobicistat p. 694. For use with darunavir, see darunavir with cobicistat p. 695 or darunavir with cobicistat, emtricitabine and tenofovir alafenamide p. 696. For use with elvitegravir, see elvitegravir with cobicistat, emtricitabine and tenofovir disoproxil p. 688 or elvitegravir with cobicistat, emtricitabine and tenofovir alafenamide p. 687.

● HEPATIC IMPAIRMENT Manufacturer advises avoid in severe impairment—no information available.

● RENAL IMPAIRMENT No dose adjustment required; inhibits tubular secretion of creatinine; when any co-administered drug requires dose adjustment based on renal function, avoid initiating cobicistat if eGFR less than 70 mL/minute/1.73 m².

● PRESCRIBING AND DISPENSING INFORMATION Dispense in original container (contains desiccant).

● PATIENT AND CARER ADVICE
Missed doses If a dose is more than 12 hours late, the missed dose should not be taken and the next dose should be taken at the normal time.

● MEDICINAL FORMS There can be variation in the licensing of different medicines containing the same drug.
Tablet
CAUTIONARY AND ADVISORY LABELS 21
▸ Tybost (Gilead Sciences Ireland UC)
Cobicistat 150 mg Tybost 150mg tablets | 30 tablet PoM £21.38
(Hospital only)

Combinations available: *Atazanavir with cobicistat*, p. 694 · *Darunavir with cobicistat*, p. 695 · *Darunavir with cobicistat, emtricitabine and tenofovir alafenamide*, p. 696 · *Elvitegravir with cobicistat, emtricitabine and tenofovir alafenamide*, p. 687 · *Elvitegravir with cobicistat, emtricitabine and tenofovir disoproxil*, p. 688

6.6 Influenza

Influenza
07-Apr-2020

Description of condition

Influenza is a highly infectious, acute respiratory infection caused by influenza viruses, of which there are three types (A, B, and C). Influenza A is more virulent and occurs more frequently; influenza B presents a milder course of disease but still has the potential to cause outbreaks; and

5

Infection

influenza C causes mild or asymptomatic disease, similar to the common cold. Types A and B can be further categorised into subtypes depending on their principle H and N antigens. Transmission occurs via droplets, aerosols, or direct contact with respiratory secretions from an infected person, and the usual incubation period is 1–3 days.

Symptoms usually appear suddenly and may include chills, fever, headache, extreme fatigue, and myalgia. Dry cough, sore throat and nasal congestion may also be present. Complications are usually respiratory in nature and may include bronchitis, secondary bacterial pneumonia, or otitis media (in children); non-respiratory complications are rarer, and may be cardiac or neurological in nature.

Although influenza is usually self-limiting with recovery occurring within 2–7 days, it can be severe in some patients. Influenza is classified as uncomplicated or complicated, with the latter described as either requiring hospitalisation, having signs or symptoms of a lower respiratory-tract infection, central nervous system involvement, or exacerbation of an underlying condition. The risk of more serious illness is greater for those in at-risk groups, such as children aged under 6 months; pregnant females (including females up to 2 weeks post-partum); adults aged over 65 years; patients with long-term conditions such as respiratory, renal, hepatic, neurological or cardiac disease, diabetes mellitus, or morbid obesity (BMI $\geq$ 40 kg/m^2); or those with severe immunosuppression.

For further information on at-risk groups, see **Public Health England (PHE) guidance on use of antiviral agents for the treatment and prophylaxis of seasonal influenza** (see *Useful resources*).

Aims of treatment

The management of influenza aims to reduce the duration and severity of illness, reduce the risk of complications, and to prevent infection.

Management

The antivirals oseltamivir p. 701 and zanamivir p. 702 are used for both treatment and post-exposure prophylaxis of influenza, although there is evidence that some strains of influenza are more likely to develop resistance to oseltamivir. In general, the risk of developing oseltamivir resistance is considered to be greater for influenza A(H1N1) pdm09 compared to other strains (such as influenza A(H3N2) and influenza B), with the risk of resistance being higher in patients who are severely immunosuppressed. Specialist advice regarding the management of influenza for individual patients can be obtained from local infection specialists where required. Additional advice can also be obtained from PHE's regional public health virologist and Respiratory Virus Unit. A consultant microbiologist or virologist can be consulted for advice on the resistance risk of individual influenza subtypes, and information on the dominant circulating strain can be found in PHE's weekly influenza reports at: www.gov.uk/government/collections/weekly-national-flu-reports.

Amantadine hydrochloride is not recommended for the treatment or post-exposure prophylaxis of influenza A.

Treatment of suspected or confirmed influenza

Where treatment with oseltamivir is indicated, it should be started as soon as possible, ideally within 48 hours of symptom onset. There is evidence to suggest that the risk of mortality may be reduced even if treatment is started up to 5 days after symptom onset; treatment initiation beyond 48 hours of onset is unlicensed and clinical judgement should be used. Where treatment with inhaled zanamivir is indicated, it should also be started as soon as possible, ideally within 48 hours (36 hours in children) of symptom onset; treatment initiation beyond this time is unlicensed and clinical judgement should be used. Where treatment with intravenous zanamivir is indicated, it should be

commenced as soon as possible and within 6 days of symptom onset.

Uncomplicated influenza

Patients with uncomplicated influenza are usually managed in the community or accident and emergency departments. All patients should be advised about the symptoms of complicated influenza and to seek medical attention if their condition worsens.

For patients who are otherwise healthy (excluding pregnant females), no antiviral treatment is usually needed. For those considered to be at serious risk of developing complications, offer oseltamivir.

For patients in an at-risk group (including pregnant females but excluding those who are severely immunosuppressed), offer oseltamivir—do not wait for laboratory test results to treat. For pregnant females who meet additional criteria for requiring zanamivir first-line, treatment should be discussed with a local infection specialist. For further information, see **PHE guidance on use of antiviral agents for the treatment and prophylaxis of seasonal influenza** (see *Useful resources*).

For severely immunosuppressed patients, consider the subtype of influenza causing the infection, or if not yet known, take into account the current dominant circulating strain. Offer oseltamivir first-line unless the strain has a higher risk for oseltamivir resistance, in which case inhaled zanamivir should be offered. For patients unable to use inhaled zanamivir due to underlying severe respiratory disease or inability to use the device (including children under 5 years), offer oseltamivir and assess response to therapy.

For patients with suspected or confirmed oseltamivir resistant influenza, offer inhaled zanamivir. For patients unable to use inhaled zanamivir, consider intravenous zanamivir [unlicensed indication].

Complicated influenza

All patients should be tested and treated, often in hospital— do not wait for laboratory test results to treat. For patients who are not severely immunosuppressed, oseltamivir should be offered first-line. If there is a risk of reduced gastrointestinal absorption, or if initial oseltamivir treatment is unsuccessful, offer inhaled zanamivir. For pregnant females who meet additional criteria for requiring zanamivir first-line, treatment should be discussed with a local infection specialist. For further information, see **PHE guidance on use of antiviral agents for the treatment and prophylaxis of seasonal influenza** (see *Useful resources*).

For severely immunosuppressed patients, consider the dominant circulating strain of influenza to guide treatment. Offer oseltamivir first-line unless the strain has a higher risk for developing oseltamivir resistance, in which case inhaled zanamivir should be offered.

For patients with suspected or confirmed oseltamivir resistant influenza, offer inhaled zanamivir.

For patients unable to use inhaled zanamivir, or for those with severe complicated illness such as multi-organ failure, consider intravenous zanamivir.

Post-exposure prophylaxis

Contacts in an at-risk group who are not adequately protected through vaccination (either due to infection by a different circulating strain or exposure within 14 days post-vaccination), should be offered prophylaxis following exposure to a person in the same household or residential setting with influenza-like illness (when influenza is circulating). Certain populations that are susceptible to localised outbreaks (such as those in care homes, prisons or detention centres), may be considered for antiviral prophylaxis regardless of vaccination status. For information on prophylaxis in these settings, refer to individual guidelines available at: www.gov.uk/government/collections/seasonal-influenza-guidance-data-and-analysis.

Prophylaxis should be started as soon as possible following exposure—ideally within 48 hours for oseltamivir below and 36 hours for inhaled zanamivir p. 702. Initiation beyond these times is unlicensed and specialist advice should be sought.

For patients in an at-risk group (including pregnant females but excluding severely immunosuppressed patients and children aged under 5 years), offer oseltamivir first-line regardless of the risk for resistance of the circulating or index case strain. For pregnant females who meet additional criteria for requiring zanamivir first-line, treatment should be discussed with a local infection specialist. For patients exposed to a strain with suspected or confirmed oseltamivir resistance, offer inhaled zanamivir.

For severely immunosuppressed patients (excluding children aged under 5 years), offer oseltamivir if the risk for oseltamivir resistance is low. However, if the risk for oseltamivir resistance is high, suspected or confirmed, offer inhaled zanamivir. For patients at higher risk of oseltamivir resistance who are unable to use inhaled zanamivir (due to underlying severe respiratory disease or inability to use the device), offer oseltamivir and advise patients to seek immediate medical attention if symptoms develop subsequently. For patients exposed to suspected or confirmed oseltamivir resistant influenza who are unable to use inhaled zanamivir, specialist advice should be sought and patients monitored closely for influenza-like illness, with arrangements made for prompt treatment if symptoms develop.

For children aged under 5 years in an at-risk group (including severely immunosuppressed children), offer oseltamivir first-line regardless of the risk of resistance for the circulating or index case strain. However, if the child is exposed to suspected or confirmed oseltamivir resistant influenza, monitor closely for influenza-like illness and promptly commence treatment if symptoms develop (see *Treatment of suspected or confirmed influenza*); seek specialist advise if the child is severely immunosuppressed.

Specialist advice is available through local health protection teams and public health virologists.

For further information, see **PHE guidance on use of antiviral agents for the treatment and prophylaxis of seasonal influenza** (see *Useful resources*).

For information on vaccination against influenza, see Influenza vaccine p. 1348.

Useful Resources

Recommendations reflect *PHE guidance on use of antiviral agents for the treatment and prophylaxis of seasonal influenza.* Public Health England. September 2019.
www.gov.uk/government/publications/influenza-treatment-and-prophylaxis-using-anti-viral-agents

> **Other drugs used for Influenza** Amantadine hydrochloride, p. 438

ANTIVIRALS > INFLUENZA > NEURAMINIDASE INHIBITORS

Oseltamivir

23-Sep-2020

- **DRUG ACTION** Reduces replication of influenza A and B viruses by inhibiting viral neuraminidase.

- **INDICATIONS AND DOSE**
Prevention of influenza
▸ BY MOUTH
▸ Child 1–11 months: 3 mg/kg once daily for 10 days for post-exposure prophylaxis
▸ Child 1–12 years (body-weight up to 15 kg): 30 mg once daily for 10 days for post-exposure prophylaxis; for up

to 6 weeks (or up to 12 weeks if immunocompromised) during an epidemic
▸ Child 1–12 years (body-weight 16–23 kg): 45 mg once daily for 10 days for post-exposure prophylaxis; for up to 6 weeks (or up to 12 weeks if immunocompromised) during an epidemic
▸ Child 1–12 years (body-weight 24–40 kg): 60 mg once daily for 10 days for post-exposure prophylaxis; for up to 6 weeks (or up to 12 weeks if immunocompromised) during an epidemic
▸ Child 1–12 years (body-weight 41 kg and above): 75 mg once daily for 10 days for post-exposure prophylaxis; for up to 6 weeks (or up to 12 weeks if immunocompromised) during an epidemic
▸ Child 13–17 years (body-weight 24–40 kg): 60 mg once daily for 10 days for post-exposure prophylaxis; for up to 6 weeks (or up to 12 weeks if immunocompromised) during an epidemic
▸ Child 13–17 years (body-weight 41 kg and above): 75 mg once daily for 10 days for post-exposure prophylaxis; for up to 6 weeks (or up to 12 weeks if immunocompromised) during an epidemic
▸ Adult (body-weight 24–40 kg): 60 mg once daily for 10 days for post-exposure prophylaxis; for up to 6 weeks (or up to 12 weeks if immunocompromised) during an epidemic
▸ Adult (body-weight 41 kg and above): 75 mg once daily for 10 days for post-exposure prophylaxis; for up to 6 weeks (or up to 12 weeks if immunocompromised) during an epidemic

Treatment of influenza
▸ BY MOUTH
▸ Child 1–11 months: 3 mg/kg twice daily for 5 days (10 days if immunocompromised)
▸ Child 1–12 years (body-weight 10–15 kg): 30 mg twice daily for 5 days (10 days if immunocompromised)
▸ Child 1–12 years (body-weight 16–23 kg): 45 mg twice daily for 5 days (10 days if immunocompromised)
▸ Child 1–12 years (body-weight 24–40 kg): 60 mg twice daily for 5 days (10 days if immunocompromised)
▸ Child 1–12 years (body-weight 41 kg and above): 75 mg twice daily for 5 days (10 days if immunocompromised)
▸ Child 13–17 years (body-weight 24–40 kg): 60 mg twice daily for 5 days (10 days if immunocompromised)
▸ Child 13–17 years (body-weight 41 kg and above): 75 mg twice daily for 5 days (10 days if immunocompromised)
▸ Adult (body-weight 24–40 kg): 60 mg twice daily for 5 days (10 days if immunocompromised)
▸ Adult (body-weight 41 kg and above): 75 mg twice daily for 5 days (10 days if immunocompromised)

- **UNLICENSED USE** Public Health England advises oseltamivir is used in the doses provided in *BNF for Children* for the prevention of influenza in children 1–12 years of age weighing less than 10 kg, but these are not licensed.

- **INTERACTIONS** → Appendix 1: oseltamivir

- **SIDE-EFFECTS**
▸ **Common or very common** Dizziness · gastrointestinal discomfort · herpes simplex · nausea · sleep disorders · vertigo · vomiting
▸ **Uncommon** Arrhythmia · consciousness impaired (in adults) · seizure · skin reactions
▸ **Rare or very rare** Angioedema · anxiety · behaviour abnormal · confusion · delirium · delusions · haemorrhage · hallucination · hepatic disorders · self-injurious behaviour · severe cutaneous adverse reactions (SCARs) · thrombocytopenia · visual impairment

- **PREGNANCY** Although safety data are limited, oseltamivir can be used in women who are pregnant when the potential benefit outweighs the risk (e.g. during a pandemic).

5

Infection

- **BREAST FEEDING** Although safety data are limited, oseltamivir can be used in women who are breast-feeding when the potential benefit outweighs the risk (e.g. during a pandemic). Oseltamivir is the preferred drug in women who are breast-feeding.
- **RENAL IMPAIRMENT**
  ‣ In adults Avoid for *treatment* and *prevention* if eGFR less than 10 mL/minute/1.73 m^2.
  ‣ In children Avoid for *treatment* and *prevention* if estimated glomerular filtration rate less than 10 mL/minute/1.73 m^2.
  Dose adjustments ‣ In adults For *treatment*, use 30 mg twice daily if eGFR 30–60 mL/minute/1.73 m^2 (30 mg once daily if eGFR 10–30 mL/minute/1.73 m^2). For *prevention*, use 30 mg once daily if eGFR 30–60 mL/minute/1.73 m^2 (30 mg every 48 hours if eGFR 10–30 mL/minute/1.73 m^2).
  ‣ In children For *treatment*, use 40% of normal dose twice daily if estimated glomerular filtration rate 30–60 mL/minute/1.73 m^2 (40% of normal dose once daily if estimated glomerular filtration rate 10–30 mL/minute/1.73 m^2). For *prevention*, use 40% of normal dose once daily if estimated glomerular filtration rate 30–60 mL/minute/1.73 m^2 (40% of normal dose every 48 hours if estimated glomerular filtration rate 10–30 mL/minute/1.73 m^2).
- **DIRECTIONS FOR ADMINISTRATION** If suspension not available, manufacturer advises capsules can be opened and the contents mixed with a small amount of sweetened food, such as sugar water or chocolate syrup, just before administration.
- **PRESCRIBING AND DISPENSING INFORMATION** Flavours of oral liquid formulations may include tutti-frutti.
  Public Health England advises that oseltamivir oral suspension should be reserved for children under the age of 1 year. Children over 1 year of age, adults with swallowing difficulties, and those receiving nasogastric oseltamivir, should use capsules which can be opened and mixed into an appropriate sugary liquid.
- **PATIENT AND CARER ADVICE**
  Medicines for Children leaflet: Oseltamivir for influenza (flu) www.medicinesforchildren.org.uk/oseltamivir-influenza-flu
- **NATIONAL FUNDING/ACCESS DECISIONS**
  For full details see funding body website
  NICE decisions
  ‣ Oseltamivir, zanamivir, and amantadine for prophylaxis of influenza (September 2008) NICE TA158 Recommended with restrictions
  ‣ Oseltamivir, zanamivir, and amantadine for treatment of influenza (February 2009) NICE TA168 Recommended with restrictions
  NHS restrictions *Tamiflu*® is not prescribable in NHS primary care except for the treatment and prophylaxis of influenza as indicated in the NICE guidance; endorse prescription 'SLS'.

- **MEDICINAL FORMS** There can be variation in the licensing of different medicines containing the same drug. Forms available from special-order manufacturers include: oral suspension, oral solution

Oral suspension
CAUTIONARY AND ADVISORY LABELS 9
EXCIPIENTS: May contain Sorbitol
‣ Tamiflu (Roche Products Ltd)
Oseltamivir (as Oseltamivir phosphate) 6 mg per 1 ml Tamiflu 6mg/ml oral suspension sugar-free | 65 ml [PoM] £10.27 DT = £10.27

Capsule
CAUTIONARY AND ADVISORY LABELS 9
‣ Oseltamivir (Non-proprietary)
Oseltamivir (as Oseltamivir phosphate) 30 mg Oseltamivir 30mg capsules | 10 capsule [PoM] £6.50 DT = £7.71
Oseltamivir (as Oseltamivir phosphate) 75 mg Oseltamivir 75mg capsules | 10 capsule [PoM] £12.33 DT = £15.41

‣ Tamiflu (Roche Products Ltd)
Oseltamivir (as Oseltamivir phosphate) 30 mg Tamiflu 30mg capsules | 10 capsule [PoM] £7.71 DT = £7.71
Oseltamivir (as Oseltamivir phosphate) 45 mg Tamiflu 45mg capsules | 10 capsule [PoM] £15.41 DT = £15.41
Oseltamivir (as Oseltamivir phosphate) 75 mg Tamiflu 75mg capsules | 10 capsule [PoM] £15.41 DT = £15.41

Zanamivir

28-Oct-2020

- **DRUG ACTION** Reduces replication of influenza A and B viruses by inhibiting viral neuraminidase.

- **INDICATIONS AND DOSE**
Post-exposure prophylaxis of influenza
  ‣ BY INHALATION OF POWDER
  ‣ Child 5–17 years: 10 mg once daily for 10 days
  ‣ Adult: 10 mg once daily for 10 days
Prevention of influenza during an epidemic
  ‣ BY INHALATION OF POWDER
  ‣ Child 5–17 years: 10 mg once daily for up to 28 days
  ‣ Adult: 10 mg once daily for up to 28 days
Treatment of influenza
  ‣ BY INHALATION OF POWDER
  ‣ Child 5–17 years: 10 mg twice daily for 5 days
  ‣ Adult: 10 mg twice daily for 5 days
Treatment of influenza [complicated and potentially life-threatening, resistant to other treatments, and/or other treatments are unsuitable] | Treatment of influenza [uncomplicated, resistant to other treatments, and inhaled formulation unsuitable]
  ‣ BY INTRAVENOUS INFUSION
  ‣ Child 6 months–5 years: 14 mg/kg twice daily for 5 to 10 days
  ‣ Child 6–17 years: 12 mg/kg twice daily (max. per dose 600 mg) for 5 to 10 days
  ‣ Adult: 600 mg twice daily for 5 to 10 days

- **UNLICENSED USE** Public Health England advises intravenous zanamivir may be used for the treatment of uncomplicated influenza, but it is not licensed for this indication.
- **CAUTIONS**
  ‣ When used by inhalation Asthma · chronic pulmonary disease · uncontrolled chronic illness
  CAUTIONS, FURTHER INFORMATION
  ‣ Asthma and chronic pulmonary disease
  ‣ When used by inhalation Risk of bronchospasm—short-acting bronchodilator should be available. Avoid in severe asthma unless close monitoring possible and appropriate facilities available to treat bronchospasm.
- **SIDE-EFFECTS**
  GENERAL SIDE-EFFECTS
  ‣ **Common or very common** Skin reactions
  ‣ **Uncommon** Oropharyngeal oedema · severe cutaneous adverse reactions (SCARs)
  ‣ **Rare or very rare** Face oedema
  ‣ **Frequency not known** Behaviour abnormal · delirium · hallucination · level of consciousness decreased · seizure
  SPECIFIC SIDE-EFFECTS
  ‣ **Common or very common**
  ‣ With intravenous use Diarrhoea · hepatocellular injury
  ‣ **Uncommon**
  ‣ When used by inhalation Bronchospasm · dehydration · dyspnoea · presyncope · throat tightness
  ‣ **Frequency not known**
  ‣ When used by inhalation Psychiatric disorder
  SIDE-EFFECTS, FURTHER INFORMATION Neurological and psychiatric disorders occur more commonly in children and adolescents.

● PREGNANCY Manufacturer advises avoid unless potential benefit outweighs risk (e.g. during a pandemic)—limited information available; *animal* studies do not indicate toxicity.

● BREAST FEEDING Manufacturer advises use only if potential benefit outweighs risk (e.g. during a pandemic)—limited information available; present in low levels in milk in *animal* studies.

● RENAL IMPAIRMENT

Dose adjustments ▸ With intravenous use Manufacturer advises reduce dose if creatinine clearance less than 80 mL/minute—consult product literature for details.

● DIRECTIONS FOR ADMINISTRATION
▸ When used by inhalation Manufacturer advises other inhaled drugs should be administered before zanamivir.
▸ With intravenous use Manufacturer advises for *intermittent intravenous infusion*, give undiluted or dilute to a concentration of not less than 200 micrograms/mL with Sodium Chloride 0.9%; give over 30 minutes.

● PRESCRIBING AND DISPENSING INFORMATION
▸ When used by inhalation Except for the treatment and prophylaxis of influenza as indicated in the NICE guidance; endorse prescription 'SLS'.

● NATIONAL FUNDING/ACCESS DECISIONS
For full details see funding body website

NICE decisions
▸ **Oseltamivir, zanamivir, and amantadine for prophylaxis of influenza (September 2008)** NICE TA158 Recommended with restrictions
▸ **Oseltamivir, zanamivir, and amantadine for treatment of influenza (February 2009)** NICE TA168 Recommended with restrictions

Scottish Medicines Consortium (SMC) decisions
▸ Zanamivir (*Dectova* ®) for the treatment of complicated and potentially life-threatening influenza A or B virus infection in patients (aged 6 months and older) when the patient's influenza virus is known or suspected to be resistant to anti-influenza medicinal products other than zanamivir, and/or other anti-viral medicinal products for treatment of influenza, including inhaled zanamivir, are not suitable for the individual patient (December 2019) SMC No. SMC2204 Recommended

All Wales Medicines Strategy Group (AWMSG) decisions
▸ Zanamivir (*Dectova* ®) for the treatment of complicated and potentially life-threatening influenza A or B virus infection in patients (aged 6 months and older) when the patient's influenza virus is known or suspected to be resistant to anti-influenza medicinal products other than zanamivir, and/or other anti-viral medicinal products for treatment of influenza, including inhaled zanamivir, are not suitable for the individual patient (October 2019) AWMSG No. 4130 Recommended

● MEDICINAL FORMS There can be variation in the licensing of different medicines containing the same drug.

Solution for infusion
ELECTROLYTES: May contain Sodium
▸ Dectova (GlaxoSmithKline UK Ltd)' ▼
Zanamivir 10 mg per 1 ml Dectova 200mg/20ml solution for infusion vials | 1 vial PoM £27.83

Inhalation powder
▸ Relenza (GlaxoSmithKline UK Ltd)
Zanamivir 5 mg Relenza 5mg inhalation powder blisters with Diskhaler | 20 blister PoM £16.36 DT = £16.36

6.7 Respiratory syncytial virus

Respiratory syncytial virus

Management in children
Ribavirin p. 666 is licensed for administration by inhalation for the treatment of severe bronchiolitis caused by the respiratory syncytial virus (RSV) in infants, especially when they have other serious diseases. However, there is no evidence that ribavirin produces clinically relevant benefit in RSV bronchiolitis.

Palivizumab below is a monoclonal antibody licensed for preventing serious lower respiratory-tract disease caused by respiratory syncytial virus in children at high risk of the disease; it should be prescribed under specialist supervision and on the basis of the likelihood of hospitalisation. Palivizumab is recommended for:

● children under 9 months of age with chronic lung disease (defined as requiring oxygen for at least 28 days from birth) and who were born preterm; and

● children under 6 months of age with haemodynamically significant, acyanotic congenital heart disease who were born preterm.

Palivizumab should be considered for:

● children under 2 years of age with severe combined immunodeficiency syndrome;

● children under 1 year of age who require long-term ventilation;

● children 1–2 years of age who require long-term ventilation and have an additional co-morbidity (including cardiac disease or pulmonary hypertension).

For details of the preterm age groups included in the recommendations, see *Immunisation against Infectious Disease* (2006), available at www.gov.uk/dh.

DRUGS FOR RESPIRATORY DISEASES ›
MONOCLONAL ANTIBODIES

Palivizumab
14-Dec-2020

● INDICATIONS AND DOSE

Prevention of serious lower respiratory-tract disease caused by respiratory syncytial virus in children at high risk of the disease (under expert supervision)
▸ BY INTRAMUSCULAR INJECTION
▸ Child 1–23 months: 15 mg/kg once a month, preferably injected in the anterolateral thigh, to be administered during season of RSV risk, injection volume over 1 mL should be divided between 2 or more sites

Prevention of serious lower respiratory-tract disease caused by respiratory syncytial virus in children at high risk of the disease and undergoing cardiac bypass surgery (under expert supervision)
▸ BY INTRAMUSCULAR INJECTION
▸ Child 1–23 months: Initially 15 mg/kg, to be administered as soon as stable after surgery, preferably in the anterolateral thigh, then 15 mg/kg once a month, preferably injected in the anterolateral thigh, to be administered during season of RSV risk, injection volume over 1 mL should be divided between 2 or more sites

● UNLICENSED USE Licensed for the prevention of serious lower respiratory-tract disease caused by respiratory syncytial virus (RSV) in children under 6 months of age (at the start of the RSV season) and born at less than 35 weeks corrected gestational age, or in children under 2 years of age who have received treatment for bronchopulmonary

5

Infection

Infection

5

dysplasia in the last 6 months, or in children under 2 years of age with haemodynamically significant congenital heart disease.

- CAUTIONS Moderate to severe acute infection · moderate to severe febrile illness · serum-palivizumab concentration may be reduced after cardiac surgery · thrombocytopenia
- SIDE-EFFECTS
- ▶ **Common or very common** Apnoea
- ▶ **Uncommon** Seizure · thrombocytopenia · urticaria
- ▶ **Frequency not known** Hypersensitivity
- ALLERGY AND CROSS-SENSITIVITY PHE advises avoid if previous anaphylactic reaction to another humanised monoclonal antibody.

- MEDICINAL FORMS There can be variation in the licensing of different medicines containing the same drug.

Solution for injection
- ▶ Synagis (AbbVie Ltd)
  Palivizumab 100 mg per 1 ml Synagis 100mg/1ml solution for injection vials | 1 vial PoM £563.64
  Synagis 50mg/0.5ml solution for injection vials | 1 vial PoM £306.34

Chapter 6
Endocrine system

CONTENTS

Endocrine system

6

1   Antidiuretic hormone disorders

Posterior pituitary hormones and antagonists

14-Sep-2020

Posterior pituitary hormones

Diabetes insipidus
Vasopressin p. 708 (antidiuretic hormone, ADH) is used in the treatment of *pituitary* ('cranial') *diabetes insipidus* as is its analogue desmopressin p. 706. Dosage is tailored to produce a slight diuresis every 24 hours to avoid water intoxication. Treatment may be required for a limited period only in diabetes insipidus following trauma or pituitary surgery.

Desmopressin is more potent and has a longer duration of action than vasopressin; unlike vasopressin it has no vasoconstrictor effect. It is given by mouth or intranasally for maintenance therapy, and by injection in the postoperative period or in unconscious patients. Desmopressin is also used in the differential diagnosis of diabetes insipidus. Following a dose intramuscularly or intranasally, restoration of the ability to concentrate urine after water deprivation confirms a diagnosis of cranial diabetes insipidus. Failure to respond occurs in nephrogenic diabetes insipidus.

In *nephrogenic* and *partial pituitary diabetes insipidus* benefit may be gained from the paradoxical antidiuretic effect of thiazides.

Carbamazepine p. 327 is sometimes useful in partial pituitary diabetes insipidus [unlicensed]; it may act by sensitising the renal tubules to the action of remaining endogenous vasopressin. The MHRA/CHM have released important safety information on the use of antiepileptic drugs and the risk of suicidal thoughts and behaviour. For further information, see Epilepsy p. 321.

Other uses
Desmopressin is also used to boost factor VIII concentration in mild to moderate haemophilia and in von Willebrand's disease; it is also used to test fibrinolytic response. Desmopressin may also have a role in nocturnal enuresis.

Vasopressin infusion is used to control variceal bleeding in portal hypertension, prior to more definitive treatment and with variable results. Terlipressin acetate, a derivative of vasopressin with reportedly less pressor and antidiuretic activity, is used similarly.

Oxytocin p. 868, another posterior pituitary hormone, is indicated in obstetrics.

Antidiuretic hormone antagonists

Demeclocycline hydrochloride p. 600 can be used in the treatment of hyponatraemia resulting from inappropriate secretion of antidiuretic hormone, if fluid restriction alone does not restore sodium concentration or is not tolerable. Demeclocycline hydrochloride is thought to act by directly blocking the renal tubular effect of antidiuretic hormone.

Tolvaptan p. 708 is a vasopressin V_2-receptor antagonist licensed for the treatment of hyponatraemia secondary to syndrome of inappropriate antidiuretic hormone secretion; treatment duration with tolvaptan is determined by the underlying disease and its treatment.

Rapid correction of hyponatraemia during tolvaptan therapy can cause osmotic demyelination, leading to serious neurological events; close monitoring of serum sodium concentration and fluid balance is essential.

1.1   Diabetes insipidus

Other drugs used for Diabetes insipidus Chlortalidone, p. 246

PITUITARY AND HYPOTHALAMIC HORMONES AND ANALOGUES >VASOPRESSIN AND ANALOGUES

Desmopressin
01-Dec-2020

- **DRUG ACTION** Desmopressin is an analogue of vasopressin.

- **INDICATIONS AND DOSE**

Diabetes insipidus, treatment
▸ BY MOUTH
  ▸ Child 1-23 months: Initially 10 micrograms 2–3 times a day, adjusted according to response; usual dose 30–150 micrograms daily
  ▸ Child 2-11 years: Initially 50 micrograms 2–3 times a day, adjusted according to response; usual dose 100–800 micrograms daily
  ▸ Child 12-17 years: Initially 100 micrograms 2–3 times a day, adjusted according to response; usual dose 0.2–1.2 mg daily
  ▸ Adult: Initially 100 micrograms 3 times a day; maintenance 100–200 micrograms 3 times a day; usual dose 0.2–1.2 mg daily
▸ BY SUBLINGUAL ADMINISTRATION
  ▸ Child 2-17 years: Initially 60 micrograms 3 times a day, adjusted according to response; usual dose 40–240 micrograms 3 times a day
  ▸ Adult: Initially 60 micrograms 3 times a day, adjusted according to response; usual dose 40–240 micrograms 3 times a day
▸ BY INTRANASAL ADMINISTRATION
  ▸ Child 1-23 months: Initially 2.5–5 micrograms 1–2 times a day, adjusted according to response
  ▸ Child 2-11 years: Initially 5–20 micrograms 1–2 times a day, adjusted according to response
  ▸ Child 12-17 years: Initially 10–20 micrograms 1–2 times a day, adjusted according to response
  ▸ Adult: 10–40 micrograms daily in 1–2 divided doses
▸ BY SUBCUTANEOUS INJECTION, OR BY INTRAVENOUS INJECTION, OR BY INTRAMUSCULAR INJECTION
  ▸ Adult: 1–4 micrograms daily

Primary nocturnal enuresis
▸ BY MOUTH
  ▸ Child 5-17 years: 200 micrograms once daily, only increased to 400 micrograms if lower dose not effective; withdraw for at least 1 week for reassessment after 3 months, dose to be taken at bedtime, limit fluid intake from 1 hour before to 8 hours after administration
  ▸ Adult 18-65 years: 200 micrograms once daily, only increased to 400 micrograms if lower dose not effective; withdraw for at least 1 week for reassessment after 3 months, dose to be taken at bedtime, limit fluid intake from 1 hour before to 8 hours after administration
▸ BY SUBLINGUAL ADMINISTRATION
  ▸ Child 5-17 years: 120 micrograms once daily, increased if necessary to 240 micrograms once daily, dose to be taken at bedtime, limit fluid intake from 1 hour before to 8 hours after administration, dose to be increased only if lower dose not effective, reassess after 3 months by withdrawing treatment for at least 1 week
  ▸ Adult 18-65 years: 120 micrograms once daily, increased if necessary to 240 micrograms once daily, dose to be taken at bedtime, limit fluid intake from 1 hour before to 8 hours after administration, dose to be increased only if lower dose not effective, reassess after 3 months by withdrawing treatment for at least 1 week

Postoperative polyuria or polydipsia
▸ BY MOUTH
  ▸ Adult: Dose to be adjusted according to urine osmolality

Polyuria or polydipsia after hypophysectomy
▸ BY SUBLINGUAL ADMINISTRATION
  ▸ Adult: Dose to be adjusted according to urine osmolality

Idiopathic nocturnal polyuria in females
▸ BY SUBLINGUAL ADMINISTRATION
  ▸ Adult: 25 micrograms daily, to be taken 1 hour before bedtime

Idiopathic nocturnal polyuria in males
▸ BY SUBLINGUAL ADMINISTRATION
  ▸ Adult: 50 micrograms daily, to be taken 1 hour before bedtime

Diabetes insipidus, diagnosis (water deprivation test)
▸ BY INTRANASAL ADMINISTRATION
  ▸ Adult: 20 micrograms, limit fluid intake to 500 mL from 1 hour before to 8 hours after administration
▸ BY INTRAMUSCULAR INJECTION, OR BY SUBCUTANEOUS INJECTION
  ▸ Adult: 2 micrograms for 1 dose, limit fluid intake to 500 mL from 1 hour before to 8 hours after administration

Nocturia associated with multiple sclerosis (when other treatments have failed)
▸ BY INTRANASAL ADMINISTRATION
  ▸ Adult 18-65 years: 10–20 micrograms once daily, to be taken at bedtime, dose not to be repeated within 24 hours, limit fluid intake from 1 hour before to 8 hours after administration

Renal function testing
▸ BY INTRANASAL ADMINISTRATION
  ▸ Adult: 40 micrograms, empty bladder at time of administration and limit fluid intake to 500 mL from 1 hour before until 8 hours after administration to avoid fluid overload
▸ BY SUBCUTANEOUS INJECTION, OR BY INTRAMUSCULAR INJECTION
  ▸ Adult: 2 micrograms, empty bladder at time of administration and restrict fluid intake to 500 mL from 1 hour before until 8 hours after administration to avoid fluid overload

Mild to moderate haemophilia and von Willebrand's disease
▸ BY INTRANASAL ADMINISTRATION
  ▸ Adult: 300 micrograms every 12 hours if required, one 150 microgram spray into each nostril, 30 minutes before surgery or when bleeding, dose may alternatively be repeated at intervals of at least 3 days, if self-administered
▸ BY INTRAVENOUS INFUSION, OR BY SUBCUTANEOUS INJECTION
  ▸ Adult: 300 nanograms/kg for 1 dose, to be administered immediately before surgery or after trauma; may be repeated at intervals of 12 hours

Fibrinolytic response testing
▸ BY INTRANASAL ADMINISTRATION
  ▸ Adult: 300 micrograms, blood to be sampled after 1 hour for fibrinolytic activity, one 150 microgram spray to be administered into each nostril
▸ BY SUBCUTANEOUS INJECTION, OR BY INTRAVENOUS INJECTION
  ▸ Adult: 300 nanograms/kg for 1 dose, blood to be sampled after 20 minutes for fibrinolytic activity

Lumbar-puncture-associated headache
▸ BY INTRAMUSCULAR INJECTION, OR BY SUBCUTANEOUS INJECTION
  ▸ Adult: (consult product literature)

- UNLICENSED USE
▸ In children Consult product literature for individual preparations. Oral use of *DDAVP* intravenous injection is not licensed.
- CONTRA-INDICATIONS Cardiac insufficiency · conditions treated with diuretics · history of hyponatraemia · polydipsia in alcohol dependence · psychogenic polydipsia · syndrome of inappropriate ADH secretion · von Willebrand's Disease Type IIB (may result in pseudothrombocytopenia)
- CAUTIONS

GENERAL CAUTIONS Asthma · avoid fluid overload · cardiovascular disease (not indicated for nocturnal enuresis or nocturia) · conditions which might be aggravated by water retention · cystic fibrosis · elderly (avoid for primary nocturnal enuresis and nocturia associated with multiple sclerosis in those over 65 years) · epilepsy · heart failure · hypertension (not indicated for nocturnal enuresis or nocturia) · migraine · nocturia—limit fluid intake to minimum from 1 hour before dose until 8 hours afterwards · nocturnal enuresis—limit fluid intake to minimum from 1 hour before dose until 8 hours afterwards

SPECIFIC CAUTIONS
▸ With intranasal use should not be given intranasally for nocturnal enuresis due to an increased incidence of side-effects

CAUTIONS, FURTHER INFORMATION Elderly patients are at increased risk of hyponatraemia and renal impairment—manufacturer advises measure baseline serum sodium concentration, then monitor regularly during treatment; discontinue treatment if levels fall below the normal range. Review treatment if no therapeutic benefit after 3 months.

- INTERACTIONS → Appendix 1: desmopressin
- SIDE-EFFECTS

GENERAL SIDE-EFFECTS
▸ **Common or very common** Hyponatraemia (on administration without restricting fluid intake) · nausea
▸ **Frequency not known** Abdominal pain · aggression (in children) · allergic dermatitis · emotional disorder · fluid retention · headache · hyponatraemic seizure · vomiting · weight increased

SPECIFIC SIDE-EFFECTS
▸ With intranasal use Epistaxis · nasal congestion · rhinitis
▸ With intravenous use Vasodilation

SIDE-EFFECTS, FURTHER INFORMATION Manufacturer advises avoiding concomitant use of drugs which increase secretion of vasopressin (e.g. tricyclic antidepressants)—increases risk of hyponatraemia.

- PREGNANCY Small oxytocic effect in third trimester; increased risk of pre-eclampsia.
- BREAST FEEDING Amount too small to be harmful.
- RENAL IMPAIRMENT Use with caution; antidiuretic effect may be reduced.
- MONITORING REQUIREMENTS In *nocturia*, periodic blood pressure and weight checks are needed to monitor for fluid overload.
- DIRECTIONS FOR ADMINISTRATION Desmopressin oral lyophilisates are for sublingual administration.
  Expert sources advise *DDAVP*® and *Desmotabs*® tablets may be crushed.
  Expert sources advise *DDAVP*® intranasal solution may be diluted with Sodium Chloride 0.9% to a concentration of 10 micrograms/mL.
  Expert sources advise *DDAVP*® injection may be administered orally.

▸ With intravenous use For *intravenous infusion* (*DDAVP*®, *Octim*®), give intermittently in Sodium chloride 0.9%; dilute with 50 mL and give over 20 minutes.

- PRESCRIBING AND DISPENSING INFORMATION Oral, intranasal, intravenous, subcutaneous and intramuscular doses are expressed as desmopressin acetate; sublingual doses are expressed as desmopressin base.
  Children requiring an intranasal dose of less than 10 micrograms should be given *DDAVP*® intranasal solution.
- PATIENT AND CARER ADVICE
Hyponatraemic convulsions Patients being treated for primary nocturnal enuresis should be warned to avoid fluid overload (including during swimming) and to stop taking desmopressin during an episode of vomiting or diarrhoea (until fluid balance normal).
Medicines for Children leaflet: Desmopressin for bedwetting www.medicinesforchildren.org.uk/desmopressin-bedwetting-0
- NATIONAL FUNDING/ACCESS DECISIONS
For full details see funding body website
Scottish Medicines Consortium (SMC) decisions
▸ **Desmopressin oral lyophilisate (*Noqdirna*®) for symptomatic treatment of nocturia due to idiopathic nocturnal polyuria in adults (August 2017)** SMC No. 1218/17 Recommended with restrictions
All Wales Medicines Strategy Group (AWMSG) decisions
▸ **Desmopressin acetate (*Noqdirna*®) for treatment of nocturia due to idiopathic nocturnal polyuria in adults (October 2017)** AWMSG No. 3282 Recommended with restrictions

- MEDICINAL FORMS There can be variation in the licensing of different medicines containing the same drug. Forms available from special-order manufacturers include: capsule, oral suspension, oral solution, spray, nasal drops

Tablet
▸ Desmopressin (Non-proprietary)
  Desmopressin acetate 100 microgram Desmopressin 100microgram tablets | 90 tablet [PoM] £76.62 DT = £63.09
  Desmopressin acetate 200 microgram Desmopressin 200microgram tablets | 30 tablet [PoM] £28.50 DT = £27.62
▸ DDAVP (Ferring Pharmaceuticals Ltd)
  Desmopressin acetate 100 microgram DDAVP 0.1mg tablets | 90 tablet [PoM] £44.12 DT = £63.09
  Desmopressin acetate 200 microgram DDAVP 0.2mg tablets | 90 tablet [PoM] £88.23
▸ Desmotabs (Ferring Pharmaceuticals Ltd)
  Desmopressin acetate 200 microgram Desmotabs 0.2mg tablets | 30 tablet [PoM] £29.43 DT = £27.62

Solution for injection
▸ DDAVP (Ferring Pharmaceuticals Ltd)
  Desmopressin acetate 4 microgram per 1 ml DDAVP 4micrograms/1ml solution for injection ampoules | 10 ampoule [PoM] £13.16 DT = £13.16
▸ Octim (Ferring Pharmaceuticals Ltd)
  Desmopressin acetate 15 microgram per 1 ml Octim 15micrograms/1ml solution for injection ampoules | 10 ampoule [PoM] £192.20

Spray
▸ Desmopressin (Non-proprietary)
  Desmopressin acetate 10 microgram per 1 dose Desmopressin 10micrograms/dose nasal spray | 60 dose [PoM] £27.00 DT = £18.08
▸ Desmospray (Ferring Pharmaceuticals Ltd, Imported (Germany))
  Desmopressin acetate 2.5 microgram per 1 dose Desmospray 2.5micrograms/dose nasal spray | 50 dose 🅂
  Desmopressin acetate 10 microgram per 1 dose Desmospray 10micrograms/dose nasal spray | 60 dose [PoM] £25.02 DT = £18.08
▸ Octim (Ferring Pharmaceuticals Ltd)
  Desmopressin acetate 150 microgram per 1 dose Octim 150micrograms/dose nasal spray | 25 dose [PoM] £576.60 DT = £576.60

6

Endocrine system

Oral lyophilisate
CAUTIONARY AND ADVISORY LABELS 26
▸ DDAVP Melt (Ferring Pharmaceuticals Ltd)
Desmopressin (as Desmopressin acetate) 60 microgram DDAVP
Melt 60microgram oral lyophilisates sugar-free | 100 tablet [PoM]
£50.53 DT = £50.53
Desmopressin (as Desmopressin acetate) 120 microgram DDAVP
Melt 120microgram oral lyophilisates sugar-free | 100 tablet [PoM]
£101.07 DT = £101.07
Desmopressin (as Desmopressin acetate) 240 microgram DDAVP
Melt 240microgram oral lyophilisates sugar-free | 100 tablet [PoM]
£202.14
▸ DesmoMelt (Ferring Pharmaceuticals Ltd)
Desmopressin (as Desmopressin acetate)
120 microgram DesmoMelt 120microgram oral lyophilisates sugar-
free | 30 tablet [PoM] £30.34 DT = £30.34
Desmopressin (as Desmopressin acetate)
240 microgram DesmoMelt 240microgram oral lyophilisates sugar-
free | 30 tablet [PoM] £60.68 DT = £60.68
▸ Noqdirna (Ferring Pharmaceuticals Ltd)
Desmopressin (as Desmopressin acetate) 25 microgram Noqdirna
25microgram oral lyophilisates sugar-free | 30 tablet [PoM] £15.16 DT
= £15.16
Desmopressin (as Desmopressin acetate)
50 microgram Noqdirna 50microgram oral lyophilisates sugar-free
| 30 tablet [PoM] £15.16 DT = £15.16

Nasal drops
▸ DDAVP (Ferring Pharmaceuticals Ltd)
Desmopressin acetate 100 microgram per 1 ml DDAVP
100micrograms/ml intranasal solution | 2.5 ml [PoM] [℥] DT = £9.72

Vasopressin
16-Jul-2020

● **INDICATIONS AND DOSE**
Pituitary diabetes insipidus
▸ BY INTRAMUSCULAR INJECTION, OR BY SUBCUTANEOUS
INJECTION
▸ Adult: 5–20 units every 4 hours
Initial control of oesophageal variceal bleeding
▸ BY INTRAVENOUS INFUSION
▸ Adult: 20 units, dose to be administered over
15 minutes

● CONTRA-INDICATIONS Chronic nephritis (until reasonable
blood nitrogen concentrations attained) · vascular disease
(especially disease of coronary arteries) unless extreme
caution

● CAUTIONS Asthma · avoid fluid overload · conditions which
might be aggravated by water retention · epilepsy · heart
failure · hypertension · migraine

● SIDE-EFFECTS Abdominal pain · angina pectoris ·
bronchospasm · cardiac arrest · chest pain · diarrhoea ·
flatulence · fluid imbalance · gangrene · headache ·
hyperhidrosis · hypertension · musculoskeletal chest pain ·
nausea · pallor · peripheral ischaemia · tremor · urticaria ·
vertigo · vomiting

● PREGNANCY Oxytocic effect in third trimester.

● BREAST FEEDING Not known to be harmful.

● DIRECTIONS FOR ADMINISTRATION
▸ With intravenous use For *intravenous infusion* (argipressin),
manufacturer advises give intermittently in Glucose 5%;
suggested concentration 20 units/100mL given over
15 minutes.

● MEDICINAL FORMS There can be variation in the licensing of
different medicines containing the same drug. Forms available
from special-order manufacturers include: solution for
injection

Solution for injection
▸ Argipressin (Advanz Pharma)
Argipressin 20 unit per 1 ml Argipressin 20units/1ml solution for
injection ampoules | 10 ampoule [PoM] £754.86–£950.00 (Hospital
only)

1.2 Syndrome of inappropriate antidiuretic hormone secretion

> Other drugs used for Syndrome of inappropriate
> antidiuretic hormone secretion Demeclocycline
> hydrochloride, p. 600

DIURETICS 〉 SELECTIVE VASOPRESSIN V$_2$-
RECEPTOR ANTAGONISTS

Tolvaptan
14-May-2020

● **DRUG ACTION** Tolvaptan is a vasopressin V$_2$-receptor
antagonist.

● **INDICATIONS AND DOSE**
JINARC®
**Autosomal dominant polycystic kidney disease in adults
with CKD stage 1 to 4 at initiation of treatment with
evidence of rapidly progressing disease (initiated by a
specialist)**
▸ BY MOUTH
▸ Adult: Initially 60 mg daily in 2 divided doses for at
least a week, 45 mg in the morning before breakfast,
and then 15 mg taken 8 hours later; increased to 90 mg
daily in 2 divided doses for at least a week, 60 mg in the
morning before breakfast, and then 30 mg taken
8 hours later, then increased if tolerated to 120 mg
daily in 2 divided doses, 90 mg in the morning before
breakfast, and then 30 mg taken 8 hours later, dose
titration should be performed cautiously; patients may
down-titrate to lower doses based on tolerability
DOSE ADJUSTMENTS DUE TO INTERACTIONS
▸ For *Jinarc*®, manufacturer advises reduce dose with
concurrent use of potent CYP3A4 inhibitors—if daily
dose 90 mg or 120 mg, reduce to 30 mg once daily (can
be further reduced to 15 mg once daily if not tolerated);
if daily dose 60 mg, reduce to 15 mg once daily.
Manufacturer also advises reduce dose with concurrent
use of moderate CYP3A4 inhibitors or ciprofloxacin—if
daily dose 120 mg, reduce to 60 mg daily (45 mg in
morning and 15 mg taken 8 hours later); if daily dose
90 mg, reduce to 45 mg daily (30 mg in morning and
15 mg taken 8 hours later); if daily dose 60 mg, reduce
to 30 mg daily (15 mg in morning and 15 mg taken
8 hours later).
SAMSCA®
**Hyponatraemia secondary to syndrome of inappropriate
antidiuretic hormone secretion (initiated in hospital or
under specialist supervision)**
▸ BY MOUTH
▸ Adult: Initially 15 mg once daily, increased if necessary
up to 60 mg once daily, a reduced starting dose of
7.5 mg once daily should be considered for patients at
risk of overly rapid correction of serum-sodium
concentration

● CONTRA-INDICATIONS Anuria · hypernatraemia ·
hypovolaemic hyponatraemia · impaired perception of
thirst · volume depletion

● CAUTIONS

GENERAL CAUTIONS Abnormal liver function tests and/or
signs or symptoms of liver injury (do not initiate if the
criteria for permanent discontinuation are met—consult
product literature) · diabetes mellitus · patients at risk of

dehydration (ensure adequate fluid intake) · urinary outflow obstruction (increased risk of acute retention)

SPECIFIC CAUTIONS

▸ When used for autosomal dominant polycystic kidney disease serum-sodium abnormalities (correct before treatment initiation)

▸ When used for hyponatraemia secondary to syndrome of inappropriate antidiuretic hormone secretion patients at risk of demyelination syndromes (e.g hypoxia, alcoholism and malnutrition)

● INTERACTIONS → Appendix 1: tolvaptan

● SIDE-EFFECTS

▸ **Common or very common** Appetite decreased · asthenia · constipation · dehydration · diarrhoea · dizziness · dry mouth · dyspnoea · gastrointestinal discomfort · gastrooesophageal reflux disease · gout · headache · hepatic disorders · hyperglycaemia · hypernatraemia · hyperuricaemia · insomnia · muscle spasms · palpitations · polydipsia · skin reactions · thirst · urinary disorders · weight decreased

▸ **Frequency not known** Acute hepatic failure (cases requiring liver transplantation reported)

SIDE-EFFECTS, FURTHER INFORMATION Interrupt treatment and perform liver-function tests promptly if symptoms of hepatic impairment occur (anorexia, nausea, vomiting, fatigue, abdominal pain, jaundice, dark urine, pruritus)—consult product literature.

● PREGNANCY Avoid—toxicity in *animal* studies.

● BREAST FEEDING Avoid—present in milk in *animal* studies.

● HEPATIC IMPAIRMENT Manufacturer advises caution in severe impairment; avoid if abnormal liver-function tests and/or signs or symptoms of liver injury meet the requirements for permanent discontinuation—consult product literature.

● RENAL IMPAIRMENT No information available in severe impairment.

● MONITORING REQUIREMENTS

▸ Manufacturer advises monitor volume, fluid and electrolyte status (risk of dehydration); monitor electrolytes at least every 3 months during long-term therapy.

▸ When used for Autosomal dominant polycystic kidney disease Manufacturer advises monitor liver function tests and for symptoms of liver injury. Liver enzymes and bilirubin must be measured and reviewed before treatment initiation, monthly for 18 months, and every 3 months thereafter; interrupt treatment if abnormalities occur—consult product literature for further information including the criteria for permanent discontinuation. Manufacturer advises evaluate uric acid concentration before treatment initiation and as clinically indicated during treatment; monitor urine osmolality periodically.

▸ When used for Hyponatraemia secondary to syndrome of inappropriate antidiuretic hormone secretion Manufacturer advises monitor liver function tests and for symptoms of liver injury; interrupt treatment if abnormalities occur. Manufacturer advises monitor serum-sodium concentration no later than 6 hours after treatment initiation, then monitor serum-sodium and volume status at least every 6 hours during the first 1–2 days of treatment and until dose stabilised. If serum-sodium correction exceeds 6 mmol/litre during the first 6 hours or 8 mmol/litre in the first 6–12 hours, frequency of monitoring should be increased; interrupt or discontinue treatment if serum-sodium increases by 12 mmol/litre or greater in 24 hours or 18 mmol/litre or greater in 48 hours.

● PRESCRIBING AND DISPENSING INFORMATION The manufacturer of *Jinarc®* has provided training materials for healthcare professionals to use prior to prescribing tolvaptan in order to minimise the risk of irreversible

hepatotoxicity and to highlight the importance of pregnancy prevention.

● PATIENT AND CARER ADVICE For *Jinarc®*, morning dose to be taken 30 minutes before food, second dose can be taken with or without food.

Risk minimisation materials For *Jinarc®*, a patient brochure and alert card should be provided.

● NATIONAL FUNDING/ACCESS DECISIONS For full details see funding body website

NICE decisions

▸ Tolvaptan for treating autosomal dominant polycystic kidney disease (October 2015) NICE TA358 Recommended with restrictions

● MEDICINAL FORMS There can be variation in the licensing of different medicines containing the same drug.

Tablet

CAUTIONARY AND ADVISORY LABELS 27

▸ Jinarc (Otsuka Pharmaceuticals (U.K.) Ltd) ▼

Tolvaptan 15 mg Jinarc 15mg tablets | 7 tablet [PoM] £302.05 (Hospital only)

Tolvaptan 30 mg Jinarc 30mg tablets | 7 tablet [PoM] £302.05 (Hospital only)

Tolvaptan 45 mg Jinarc 45mg tablets | 7 tablet [PoM] 🚫

Tolvaptan 60 mg Jinarc 60mg tablets | 7 tablet [PoM] 🚫

Tolvaptan 90 mg Jinarc 90mg tablets | 7 tablet [PoM] 🚫

▸ Samsca (Otsuka Pharmaceuticals (U.K.) Ltd)

Tolvaptan 15 mg Samsca 15mg tablets | 10 tablet [PoM] £746.80

Tolvaptan 30 mg Samsca 30mg tablets | 10 tablet [PoM] £746.80

2 Corticosteroid responsive conditions

CORTICOSTEROIDS

Corticosteroids, general use   07-Oct-2020

Overview

Dosages of corticosteroids vary widely in different diseases and in different patients. If the use of a corticosteroid can save or prolong life, as in exfoliative dermatitis, pemphigus, acute leukaemia or acute transplant rejection, high doses may need to be given, because the complications of therapy are likely to be less serious than the effects of the disease itself.

When long-term corticosteroid therapy is used in some chronic diseases, the adverse effects of treatment may become greater than the disabilities caused by the disease. To minimise side-effects the maintenance dose should be kept as low as possible.

When potentially less harmful measures are ineffective, corticosteroids are used topically for the treatment of inflammatory conditions of the skin. Corticosteroids should be avoided or used only under specialist supervision in psoriasis.

Corticosteroids are used both topically (by rectum) and systemically (by mouth or intravenously) in the management of ulcerative colitis and Crohn's disease. They are also included in locally applied creams for haemorrhoids.

Use can be made of the mineralocorticoid activity of fludrocortisone acetate p. 715 to treat postural hypotension in autonomic neuropathy.

High-dose corticosteroids should be avoided for the management of septic shock. However, there is evidence that administration of lower doses of hydrocortisone p. 716 and fludrocortisone acetate is of benefit in adrenal insufficiency resulting from septic shock.

Dexamethasone p. 714 and betamethasone p. 713 have little if any mineralocorticoid action and their long duration of action makes them particularly suitable for suppressing

6

Endocrine system

corticotropin secretion in congenital adrenal hyperplasia where the dose should be tailored to clinical response and by measurement of adrenal androgens and 17-hydroxyprogesterone. In common with all glucocorticoids their suppressive action on the hypothalamic- pituitary-adrenal axis is greatest and most prolonged when they are given at night. In most individuals a single dose of dexamethasone at night, is sufficient to inhibit corticotropin secretion for 24 hours. This is the basis of the 'overnight dexamethasone suppression test' for diagnosing Cushing's syndrome.

Betamethasone and dexamethasone are also appropriate for conditions where water retention would be a disadvantage.

A corticosteroid may be used in the management of raised intracranial pressure or cerebral oedema that occurs as a result of malignancy (see Prescribing in palliative care p. 28). However, a corticosteroid should not be used for the management of head injury or stroke because it is unlikely to be of benefit and may even be harmful.

In acute hypersensitivity reactions, such as angioedema of the upper respiratory tract and anaphylaxis, corticosteroids are indicated as an adjunct to emergency treatment with adrenaline/epinephrine p. 238. In such cases hydrocortisone (as sodium succinate) by intravenous injection may be required.

EvGr Corticosteroids are preferably used by inhalation in the management of asthma and chronic obstructive pulmonary disease (COPD). Systemic therapy along with bronchodilators is required for treatment of acute asthma attacks, in some very severe cases of chronic asthma, and exacerbations of COPD. A

Corticosteroids may also be useful in conditions such as autoimmune hepatitis, rheumatoid arthritis and sarcoidosis; they may also lead to remissions of acquired haemolytic anaemia, and some cases of the nephrotic syndrome (particularly in children) and thrombocytopenic purpura.

Corticosteroids can improve the prognosis of serious conditions such as systemic lupus erythematosus, temporal arteritis, and polyarteritis nodosa; the effects of the disease process may be suppressed and symptoms relieved, but the underlying condition is not cured, although it may ultimately remit. It is usual to begin therapy in these conditions at fairly high dose, and then to reduce the dose to the lowest commensurate with disease control.

For other references to the use of corticosteroids see: Prescribing in Palliative Care, immunosuppression, rheumatic diseases, eye, otitis externa allergic rhinitis, and aphthous ulcers.

Side-effects

MHRA/CHM advice: Corticosteroids: rare risk of central serous chorioretinopathy with local as well as systemic administration (August 2017)
Central serous chorioretinopathy is a retinal disorder that has been linked to the systemic use of corticosteroids. Recently, it has also been reported after local administration of corticosteroids via inhaled and intranasal, epidural, intra-articular, topical dermal, and periocular routes. The MHRA recommends that patients should be advised to report any blurred vision or other visual disturbances with corticosteroid treatment given by any route; consider referral to an ophthalmologist for evaluation of possible causes if a patient presents with vision problems.

Overdosage or prolonged use can exaggerate some of the normal physiological actions of corticosteroids leading to mineralocorticoid and glucocorticoid side-effects.

Mineralocorticoid side effects
- hypertension
- sodium retention
- water retention
- potassium loss
- calcium loss

Mineralocorticoid side effects are most marked with fludrocortisone, but are significant with hydrocortisone, corticotropin, and tetracosactide. Mineralocorticoid actions are negligible with the high potency glucocorticoids, betamethasone and dexamethasone, and occur only slightly with methylprednisolone, prednisolone, and triamcinolone.

Glucocorticoid side effects
- diabetes
- osteoporosis, which is a danger, particularly in the elderly, as it can result in osteoporotic fractures for example of the hip or vertebrae
- in addition high doses are associated with avascular necrosis of the femoral head
- muscle wasting (proximal myopathy) can also occur
- corticosteroid therapy is also weakly linked with peptic ulceration and perforation
- psychiatric reactions may also occur

Managing side-effects
Side-effects can be minimised by using lowest effective dose for minimum period possible. The suppressive action of a corticosteroid on cortisol secretion is least when it is given as a single dose in the morning. In an attempt to reduce pituitary-adrenal suppression further, the total dose for two days can sometimes be taken as a single dose on alternate days; alternate-day administration has not been very successful in the management of asthma. Pituitary-adrenal suppression can also be reduced by means of intermittent therapy with short courses. In some conditions it may be possible to reduce the dose of corticosteroid by adding a small dose of an immunosuppressive drug.

For information on the cessation of oral corticosteroid treatment, see *Treatment cessation*, for systemic corticosteroids (e.g. prednisolone p. 718).

Whenever possible *local treatment* with creams, intra-articular injections, inhalations, eye-drops, or enemas should be used in preference to *systemic treatment*.

Inhaled corticosteroids have considerably fewer systemic effects than oral corticosteroids, but adverse effects including adrenal suppression have been reported. Use of other corticosteroid therapy (including topical) or concurrent use of drugs which inhibit corticosteroid metabolism should be taken into account when assessing systemic risk.

NHS Improvement Patient Safety Alert: Steroid Emergency Card to support early recognition and treatment of adrenal crisis in adults (August 2020)

A patient-held **Steroid Emergency Card** has been developed for patients with adrenal insufficiency and steroid dependence who are at risk of adrenal crisis. It aims to support healthcare staff with the early recognition of patients at risk of adrenal crisis and the emergency treatment of adrenal crisis. All eligible patients should be issued a Steroid Emergency Card. Providers that treat patients with acute physical illness or trauma, or who may require emergency treatment, elective surgery, or other invasive procedures, should establish processes to check for risk of adrenal crisis and confirm if the patient has a Steroid Emergency Card. For further information, see NHS Improvement Patient Safety Alert: **Steroid Emergency Card to support early recognition and treatment of adrenal crisis in adults** (available at: www.england.nhs.uk/publication/national-patient-safety-alert-steroid-emergency-card-to-support-early-recognition-and-treatment-of-adrenal-crisis-in-adults/).

The Royal College of Physicians Patient Safety Committee and Society for Endocrinology Clinical Committee have published national guidance that accompanies the Steroid Emergency Card. For further information, see Royal College of Physicians Patient Safety Committee and Society for Endocrinology Clinical Committee: **Guidance for the prevention and emergency management of adult**

patients with adrenal insufficiency (available at: www.rcpjournals.org/content/clinmedicine/20/4/371).

The Steroid Treatment Card is unaffected by the introduction of the Steroid Emergency Card. For further information on the Steroid Emergency Card and Steroid Treatment Card, see *Patient and Carer advice* in individual drug monographs.

Corticosteroids, replacement therapy

18-Sep-2020

Overview

The adrenal cortex normally secretes hydrocortisone p. 716 (cortisol) which has glucocorticoid activity and weak mineralocorticoid activity. It also secretes the mineralocorticoid aldosterone.

In deficiency states, physiological replacement is best achieved with a combination of hydrocortisone and the mineralocorticoid fludrocortisone acetate p. 715; hydrocortisone alone does not usually provide sufficient mineralocorticoid activity for complete replacement.

In *Addison's disease* or following adrenalectomy, hydrocortisone by mouth is usually required. This is given in 2 doses, the larger in the morning and the smaller in the evening, mimicking the normal diurnal rhythm of cortisol secretion. The optimum daily dose is determined on the basis of clinical response. Glucocorticoid therapy is supplemented by fludrocortisone acetate.

In *adrenal crisis*, parenteral hydrocortisone is given.

In *hypopituitarism*, glucocorticoids should be given as in adrenal insufficiency, but since production of aldosterone is also regulated by the renin-angiotensin system a mineralocorticoid is not usually required. Additional replacement therapy with levothyroxine sodium p. 817 and sex hormones should be given as indicated by the pattern of hormone deficiency.

Glucocorticoid therapy

Glucocorticoid and mineralocorticoid activity

In comparing the relative potencies of corticosteroids in terms of their anti-inflammatory (glucocorticoid) effects it should be borne in mind that high glucocorticoid activity in itself is of no advantage unless it is accompanied by relatively low mineralocorticoid activity (see Disadvantages of Corticosteroids). The mineralocorticoid activity of fludrocortisone acetate p. 715 is so high that its anti-inflammatory activity is of no clinical relevance.

Equivalent anti-inflammatory doses of corticosteroids

This table takes no account of mineralocorticoid effects, nor does it take account of variations in duration of action

Prednisolone 5 mg	
≡	Betamethasone 750 micrograms
≡	Deflazacort 6 mg
≡	Dexamethasone 750 micrograms
≡	Hydrocortisone 20 mg
≡	Methylprednisolone 4 mg
≡	Prednisone 5 mg
≡	Triamcinolone 4 mg

The relatively high mineralocorticoid activity of hydrocortisone p. 716, and the resulting fluid retention, makes it unsuitable for disease suppression on a long-term basis. However, hydrocortisone can be used for adrenal replacement therapy. Hydrocortisone is used on a short-term basis by intravenous injection for the emergency management of some conditions. The relatively moderate anti-inflammatory potency of hydrocortisone also makes it a useful topical corticosteroid for the management of inflammatory skin conditions because side-effects (both topical and systemic) are less marked.

Prednisolone p. 718 and prednisone have predominantly glucocorticoid activity. Prednisolone is the corticosteroid most commonly used by mouth for long-term disease suppression.

Betamethasone p. 713 and dexamethasone p. 714 have very high glucocorticoid activity in conjunction with insignificant mineralocorticoid activity. This makes them particularly suitable for high-dose therapy in conditions where fluid retention would be a disadvantage.

Betamethasone and dexamethasone also have a long duration of action and this, coupled with their lack of mineralocorticoid action, makes them particularly suitable for conditions which require suppression of corticotropin (corticotrophin) secretion (e.g. congenital adrenal hyperplasia).

Some esters of betamethasone and of beclometasone dipropionate p. 48 (beclometasone) exert a considerably more marked topical effect (e.g. on the skin or the lungs) than when given by mouth; use is made of this to obtain topical effects whilst minimising systemic side-effects (e.g. for skin applications and asthma inhalations).

Deflazacort p. 714 has a high glucocorticoid activity; it is derived from prednisolone.

Corticosteroids (systemic)

IMPORTANT SAFETY INFORMATION

MHRA/CHM ADVICE: CORTICOSTEROIDS: RARE RISK OF CENTRAL SEROUS CHORIORETINOPATHY WITH LOCAL AS WELL AS SYSTEMIC ADMINISTRATION (AUGUST 2017)

Central serous chorioretinopathy is a retinal disorder that has been linked to the systemic use of corticosteroids. Recently, it has also been reported after local administration of corticosteroids via inhaled and intranasal, epidural, intra-articular, topical dermal, and periocular routes. The MHRA recommends that patients should be advised to report any blurred vision or other visual disturbances with corticosteroid treatment given by any route; consider referral to an ophthalmologist for evaluation of possible causes if a patient presents with vision problems.

NHS IMPROVEMENT PATIENT SAFETY ALERT: STEROID EMERGENCY CARD TO SUPPORT EARLY RECOGNITION AND TREATMENT OF ADRENAL CRISIS IN ADULTS (AUGUST 2020)

A patient-held **Steroid Emergency Card** has been developed for patients with adrenal insufficiency and steroid dependence who are at risk of adrenal crisis. It aims to support healthcare staff with the early recognition of patients at risk of adrenal crisis and the emergency treatment of adrenal crisis. All eligible patients should be issued a Steroid Emergency Card. Providers that treat patients with acute physical illness or trauma, or who may require emergency treatment, elective surgery, or other invasive procedures, should establish processes to check for risk of adrenal crisis and confirm if the patient has a Steroid Emergency Card.

● CONTRA-INDICATIONS Avoid injections containing benzyl alcohol in neonates · avoid live virus vaccines in those receiving immunosuppressive doses (serum antibody

6

Endocrine system

response diminished) · systemic infection (unless specific therapy given)

CONTRA-INDICATIONS, FURTHER INFORMATION For further information on contra-indications associated with intra-articular, intradermal and intralesional preparations, consult product literature.

- CAUTIONS Congestive heart failure · diabetes mellitus (including a family history of) · diverticulitis · epilepsy · glaucoma (including a family history of or susceptibility to) · history of steroid myopathy · history of tuberculosis or X-ray changes (frequent monitoring required) · hypertension · hypothyroidism · infection (particularly untreated) · long-term use · myasthenia gravis · ocular herpes simplex (risk of corneal perforation) · osteoporosis (in children) · osteoporosis (post-menopausal women and the elderly at risk) · peptic ulcer · psychiatric reactions · recent intestinal anastomoses · recent myocardial infarction (rupture reported) · severe affective disorders (particularly if history of steroid-induced psychosis) · thromboembolic disorders · ulcerative colitis

CAUTIONS, FURTHER INFORMATION For further information on cautions associated with intra-articular, intradermal and intralesional preparations, consult product literature.

▸ Elderly Prescription potentially inappropriate (STOPP criteria):
  - if used instead of inhaled corticosteroids for maintenance therapy in moderate to severe COPD (unnecessary exposure to long-term side-effects)
  - as long-term (longer than 3 months) monotherapy for rheumatoid arthritis (risk of side-effects)
  - for treatment of osteoarthritis other than for periodic intra-articular injections for monoarticular pain (risk of side-effects)
  - with concurrent NSAIDs without proton pump inhibitor prophylaxis (increased risk of peptic ulcer disease)

  See also Prescribing in the elderly p. 33.

- SIDE-EFFECTS
▸ **Common or very common** Anxiety · behaviour abnormal · cataract subcapsular · cognitive impairment · Cushing's syndrome · electrolyte imbalance · fatigue · fluid retention · gastrointestinal discomfort · headache · healing impaired · hirsutism · hypertension · increased risk of infection · menstrual cycle irregularities · mood altered · nausea · osteoporosis · peptic ulcer · psychotic disorder · skin reactions · sleep disorders · weight increased
▸ **Uncommon** Adrenal suppression · alkalosis hypokalaemic · appetite increased · bone fractures · diabetic control impaired · eye disorders · glaucoma · haemorrhage · heart failure · hyperhidrosis · hypotension · leucocytosis · myopathy · osteonecrosis · pancreatitis · papilloedema · seizure · thromboembolism · tuberculosis reactivation · vertigo · vision blurred
▸ **Rare or very rare** Malaise · tendon rupture
▸ **Frequency not known** Chorioretinopathy · growth retardation (very common in children) · intracranial pressure increased with papilloedema (usually after withdrawal) · telangiectasia

SIDE-EFFECTS, FURTHER INFORMATION **Adrenal suppression** During prolonged therapy with corticosteroids, particularly with systemic use, adrenal atrophy develops and can persist for years after stopping. Abrupt withdrawal after a prolonged period can lead to acute adrenal insufficiency, hypotension, or death. To compensate for a diminished adrenocortical response caused by prolonged corticosteroid treatment, any significant intercurrent illness, trauma, or surgical procedure requires a temporary increase in corticosteroid dose, or if already stopped, a temporary reintroduction of corticosteroid treatment.

Infections Prolonged courses of corticosteroids increase susceptibility to infections and severity of infections; clinical presentation of infections may also be atypical. Serious infections e.g. septicaemia and tuberculosis may reach an advanced stage before being recognised, and amoebiasis or strongyloidiasis may be activated or exacerbated (exclude before initiating a corticosteroid in those at risk or with suggestive symptoms). Fungal or viral ocular infections may also be exacerbated.

Chickenpox Unless they have had chickenpox, patients receiving oral or parenteral corticosteroids for purposes other than replacement should be regarded as being at risk of severe chickenpox. Manifestations of fulminant illness include pneumonia, hepatitis and disseminated intravascular coagulation; rash is not necessarily a prominent feature. Passive immunisation with varicella–zoster immunoglobulin is needed for exposed non–immune patients receiving systemic corticosteroids or for those who have used them within the previous 3 months. Confirmed chickenpox warrants specialist care and urgent treatment. Corticosteroids should not be stopped and dosage may need to be increased.

Measles Patients taking corticosteroids should be advised to take particular care to avoid exposure to measles and to seek immediate medical advice if exposure occurs. Prophylaxis with intramuscular normal immunoglobulin may be needed.

Psychiatric reactions Systemic corticosteroids, particularly in high doses, are linked to psychiatric reactions including euphoria, insomnia, irritability, mood lability, suicidal thoughts, psychotic reactions, and behavioural disturbances. These reactions frequently subside on reducing the dose or discontinuing the corticosteroid but they may also require specific management. Patients should be advised to seek medical advice if psychiatric symptoms (especially depression and suicidal thoughts) occur and they should also be alert to the rare possibility of such reactions during withdrawal of corticosteroid treatment. Systemic corticosteroids should be prescribed with care in those predisposed to psychiatric reactions, including those who have previously suffered corticosteroid–induced psychosis, or who have a personal or family history of psychiatric disorders.

- PREGNANCY The benefit of treatment with corticosteroids during pregnancy outweighs the risk. Corticosteroid cover is required during labour. Following a review of the data on the safety of systemic corticosteroids used in pregnancy and breast-feeding the CSM (May 1998) concluded that corticosteroids vary in their ability to cross the placenta but there is no convincing evidence that systemic corticosteroids increase the incidence of congenital abnormalities such as cleft palate or lip. When administration is prolonged or repeated during pregnancy, systemic corticosteroids increase the risk of intra-uterine growth restriction; there is no evidence of intra-uterine growth restriction following short-term treatment (e.g. prophylactic treatment for neonatal respiratory distress syndrome). Any adrenal suppression in the neonate following prenatal exposure usually resolves spontaneously after birth and is rarely clinically important.
  Monitoring Pregnant women with fluid retention should be monitored closely when given systemic corticosteroids.

- BREAST FEEDING The benefit of treatment with corticosteroids during breast-feeding outweighs the risk.

- HEPATIC IMPAIRMENT In general, manufacturers advise caution (risk of increased exposure).

- RENAL IMPAIRMENT Use by oral and injectable routes should be undertaken with caution.

- MONITORING REQUIREMENTS
▸ In children The height and weight of children receiving prolonged treatment with corticosteroids should be

monitored annually; if growth is slowed, referral to a paediatrician should be considered.

● **EFFECT ON LABORATORY TESTS** May suppress skin test reactions.

● **TREATMENT CESSATION**

▸ In adults Abrupt withdrawal after a prolonged period can lead to acute adrenal insufficiency, hypotension or death. Withdrawal can also be associated with fever, myalgia, arthralgia, rhinitis, conjunctivitis, painful itchy skin nodules and weight loss. The magnitude and speed of dose reduction in corticosteroid withdrawal should be determined on a case-by-case basis, taking into consideration the underlying condition that is being treated, and individual patient factors such as the likelihood of relapse and the duration of corticosteroid treatment. *Gradual* withdrawal of systemic corticosteroids should be considered in those whose disease is unlikely to relapse and have:

● received more than 40 mg prednisolone (or equivalent) daily for more than 1 week;
● been given repeat doses in the evening;
● received more than 3 weeks' treatment;
● recently received repeated courses (particularly if taken for longer than 3 weeks);
● taken a short course within 1 year of stopping long-term therapy;
● other possible causes of adrenal suppression.

Systemic corticosteroids may be stopped abruptly in those whose disease is unlikely to relapse *and* who have received treatment for 3 weeks or less *and* who are not included in the patient groups described above.

During corticosteroid withdrawal the dose may be reduced rapidly down to physiological doses (equivalent to prednisolone 7.5 mg daily) and then reduced more slowly. Assessment of the disease may be needed during withdrawal to ensure that relapse does not occur.

▸ In children The magnitude and speed of dose reduction in corticosteroid withdrawal should be determined on a case-by-case basis, taking into consideration the underlying condition that is being treated, and individual patient factors such as the likelihood of relapse and the duration of corticosteroid treatment. *Gradual* withdrawal of systemic corticosteroids should be considered in those whose disease is unlikely to relapse and have:

● received more than 40 mg prednisolone (or equivalent) daily for more than 1 week *or* 2 mg/kg daily for 1 week *or* 1 mg/kg daily for 1 month;
● been given repeat doses in the evening;
● received more than 3 weeks' treatment;
● recently received repeated courses (particularly if taken for longer than 3 weeks);
● taken a short course within 1 year of stopping long-term therapy;
● other possible causes of adrenal suppression.

Systemic corticosteroids may be stopped abruptly in those whose disease is unlikely to relapse *and* who have received treatment for 3 weeks or less *and* who are not included in the patient groups described above.

During corticosteroid withdrawal the dose may be reduced rapidly down to physiological doses (equivalent to prednisolone 2–2.5 mg/m^2 daily) and then reduced more slowly. Assessment of the disease may be needed during withdrawal to ensure that relapse does not occur.

● **PATIENT AND CARER ADVICE**

Advice for patients Patients on long-term corticosteroid treatment should carry a Steroid Treatment Card which gives guidance on minimising risk and provides details of prescriber, drug, dosage and duration of treatment.

A patient information leaflet should be supplied to every patient when a systemic corticosteroid is prescribed. Patients should especially be advised of the following:

● **Immunosuppression** Prolonged courses of corticosteroids can increase susceptibility to infection and serious infections can go unrecognised. Unless already immune, patients are at risk of severe **chickenpox** and should avoid close contact with people who have chickenpox or shingles. Similarly, precautions should also be taken against contracting **measles**;
● **Adrenal suppression** If the corticosteroid is given for longer than 3 weeks, treatment must not be stopped abruptly. Adrenal suppression can last for a year or more after stopping treatment and the patient must mention the course of corticosteroid when receiving treatment for any illness or injury;
● **Mood and behaviour changes** Corticosteroid treatment, especially with high doses, can alter mood and behaviour early in treatment—the patient can become confused, irritable and suffer from delusion and suicidal thoughts. These effects can also occur when corticosteroid treatment is being withdrawn. Medical advice should be sought if worrying psychological changes occur;
● **Other serious effects** Serious gastro-intestinal, musculoskeletal, and ophthalmic effects which require medical help can also occur.

Steroid Treatment Card Steroid Treatment Cards should be issued where appropriate to support communication of the risks associated with treatment. Steroid treatment cards are available for purchase from the NHS Print online ordering portal www.nhsforms.co.uk

GP practices can obtain supplies through Primary Care Support England. NHS Trusts can order supplies via the online ordering portal.

In **Scotland**, steroid treatment cards can be obtained from APS Group Scotland by emailing stockorders.dppas@apsgroup.co.uk or by fax on 0131 629 9967.

Steroid Emergency Card

▸ In adults Steroid Emergency Cards should be issued to patients with adrenal insufficiency and steroid dependence for whom missed doses, illness or surgery puts them at risk of adrenal crisis. The card includes a management summary for the emergency treatment of adrenal crisis and can be issued by any healthcare professional managing patients with adrenal insufficiency or prescribing steroids.

Steroid Emergency Cards are available for purchase from the NHS print online ordering portal www.nhsforms.co.uk or Primary Care Support England (PCSE) online.

◤ 711

Betamethasone   07-Dec-2020

● **DRUG ACTION** Betamethasone has very high glucocorticoid activity and insignificant mineralocorticoid activity.

● **INDICATIONS AND DOSE**

Suppression of inflammatory and allergic disorders | Congenital adrenal hyperplasia

▸ BY MOUTH
▸ Adult: Usual dose 0.5–5 mg daily
▸ BY INTRAMUSCULAR INJECTION, OR BY SLOW INTRAVENOUS INJECTION, OR BY INTRAVENOUS INFUSION
▸ Adult: 4–20 mg, repeated up to 4 times in 24 hours

● **INTERACTIONS** → Appendix 1: corticosteroids

● **SIDE-EFFECTS** Hiccups · myocardial rupture (following recent myocardial infarction) · oedema · Stevens-Johnson syndrome

● **PREGNANCY** Readily crosses the placenta. Transient effect on fetal movements and heart rate.

● DIRECTIONS FOR ADMINISTRATION
▸ With intravenous use For *intravenous infusion* (as sodium phosphate) (*Betnesol*®), give continuously or intermittently *or via* drip tubing *in* Glucose 5% *or* Sodium chloride 0.9%.

● PATIENT AND CARER ADVICE
▸ With oral use Patient counselling is advised for betamethasone soluble tablets (steroid card).

● MEDICINAL FORMS There can be variation in the licensing of different medicines containing the same drug.

Soluble tablet
CAUTIONARY AND ADVISORY LABELS 10, 13, 21 (not for use as mouthwash for oral ulceration)
▸ Betamethasone (Non-proprietary)
Betamethasone (as Betamethasone sodium phosphate) 500 microgram Betamethasone 500microgram soluble tablets sugar free sugar-free | 100 tablet [PoM] £58.15 DT = £58.15

Solution for injection
CAUTIONARY AND ADVISORY LABELS 10
▸ Betamethasone (Non-proprietary)
Betamethasone (as Betamethasone sodium phosphate) 4 mg per 1 ml Betamethasone 4mg/1ml solution for injection ampoules | 5 ampoule [PoM] £38.58 DT = £38.33

▸F 711

▎Deflazacort
25-Sep-2020

● DRUG ACTION Deflazacort is derived from prednisolone; it has predominantly glucocorticoid activity.

● INDICATIONS AND DOSE
Suppression of inflammatory and allergic disorders
▸ BY MOUTH
▸ Adult: Maintenance 3–18 mg daily
Suppression of inflammatory and allergic disorders (acute disorders)
▸ BY MOUTH
▸ Adult: Initially up to 120 mg daily
Inflammatory and allergic disorders
▸ BY MOUTH
▸ Child 1 month–11 years: 0.25–1.5 mg/kg once daily or on alternate days; increased if necessary up to 2.4 mg/kg daily (max. per dose 120 mg), in emergency situations
▸ Child 12-17 years: 3–18 mg once daily or on alternate days; increased if necessary up to 2.4 mg/kg daily (max. per dose 120 mg), in emergency situations

● INTERACTIONS → Appendix 1: corticosteroids

● SIDE-EFFECTS
▸ Uncommon Oedema

● HEPATIC IMPAIRMENT
Dose adjustments Manufacturer advises adjust to the minimum effective dose.

● PATIENT AND CARER ADVICE Patient counselling is advised for deflazacort tablets (steroid card).

● MEDICINAL FORMS There can be variation in the licensing of different medicines containing the same drug. Forms available from special-order manufacturers include: tablet
Tablet
CAUTIONARY AND ADVISORY LABELS 5, 10
▸ Calcort (Sanofi)
Deflazacort 6 mg Calcort 6mg tablets | 60 tablet [PoM] £15.82 DT = £15.82

▸F 711

▎Dexamethasone
18-Nov-2020

● DRUG ACTION Dexamethasone has very high glucocorticoid activity and insignificant mineralocorticoid activity.

● INDICATIONS AND DOSE
Suppression of inflammatory and allergic disorders
▸ BY MOUTH
▸ Adult: 0.5–10 mg daily
Mild croup
▸ BY MOUTH
▸ Child: 150 micrograms/kg for 1 dose
Severe croup (or mild croup that might cause complications)
▸ INITIALLY BY MOUTH
▸ Child: Initially 150 micrograms/kg for 1 dose, to be given before transfer to hospital, then (by mouth or by intravenous injection) 150 micrograms/kg, then (by mouth or by intravenous injection) 150 micrograms/kg after 12 hours if required
Congenital adrenal hyperplasia (under expert supervision)
▸ BY MOUTH
▸ Adult: Consult specialist for advice on dosing
▸ BY INTRAMUSCULAR INJECTION, OR BY SLOW INTRAVENOUS INJECTION, OR BY INTRAVENOUS INFUSION
▸ Adult: Consult specialist for advice on dosing
Overnight dexamethasone suppression test
▸ BY MOUTH
▸ Adult: 1 mg for 1 dose, to be given at night
Adjunctive treatment of bacterial meningitis (starting before or with first dose of antibacterial)
▸ BY INTRAVENOUS INJECTION
▸ Adult: 8.3 mg every 6 hours for 4 days
Symptom control of anorexia in palliative care
▸ Adult: 2–4 mg daily
Dysphagia due to obstruction by tumour in palliative care
▸ Adult: 8 mg daily
Dyspnoea due to bronchospasm or partial obstruction in palliative care
▸ Adult: 4–8 mg daily
Adjunct in the treatment of nausea and vomiting in palliative care
▸ BY MOUTH
▸ Adult: 8–16 mg daily
Headaches due to raised intracranial pressure in palliative care
▸ Adult: 16 mg daily for 4–5 days, then reduced to 4–6 mg daily, reduce dose if possible. To be given before 6pm to reduce the risk of insomnia
Pain due to nerve compression in palliative care
▸ Adult: 8 mg daily
Cerebral oedema associated with malignancy
▸ BY MOUTH
▸ Adult: 0.5–10 mg daily
Cerebral oedema
▸ INITIALLY BY INTRAVENOUS INJECTION
▸ Adult: Initially 8–16 mg for 1 dose, then (by intramuscular injection or by intravenous injection) 5 mg every 6 hours until adequate response achieved then taper-off gradually, use the 3.8 mg/mL injection preparation for this dose
Cerebral oedema associated with malignancy
▸ INITIALLY BY INTRAVENOUS INJECTION
▸ Adult: Initially 8.3 mg for 1 dose, then (by intramuscular injection) 3.3 mg every 6 hours as required for 2–4 days, subsequently, reduce dose gradually and stop over 5–7 days, use the 3.3 mg/mL injection preparation for this dose

Severe or critical COVID-19
- ▶ BY MOUTH, OR BY INTRAVENOUS INJECTION
- ▶ Adult: 6 mg once daily for 7–10 days

- ● UNLICENSED USE
- ▶ With intravenous use Consult product literature; not licensed for use in bacterial meningitis.
- ● INTERACTIONS → Appendix 1: corticosteroids
- ● SIDE-EFFECTS
- ▶ With oral use Hiccups · hyperglycaemia · myocardial rupture (following recent myocardial infarction) · protein catabolism
- ▶ With parenteral use Perineal irritation (may occur following the intravenous injection of large doses of the phosphate ester)
- ● PREGNANCY Dexamethasone readily crosses the placenta.
- ● DIRECTIONS FOR ADMINISTRATION
- ▶ With oral use in children For administration *by mouth* tablets may be dispersed in water or injection solution given by mouth.
- ▶ With intravenous use in children For *intravenous infusion* dilute with Glucose 5% or Sodium Chloride 0.9%; give over 15–20 minutes.
- ▶ With intravenous use in adults For *intravenous infusion* (*Dexamethasone*, Hospira) give continuously *or* intermittently *or via* drip tubing *in* Glucose 5% *or* Sodium Chloride 0.9%.
- ● PRESCRIBING AND DISPENSING INFORMATION
Dexamethasone 3.8 mg/mL Injection has replaced dexamethasone 4 mg/mL Injection. All dosage recommendations for intravenous, intramuscular, intrarticular use or local infiltration; are given in units of dexamethasone base.

  Palliative care For further information on the use of dexamethasone in palliative care, see www.medicinescomplete.com/#/content/palliative/systemic-corticosteroids.
- ● PATIENT AND CARER ADVICE
Medicines for Children leaflet: Dexamethasone for croup www.medicinesforchildren.org.uk/dexamethasone-croup-0

- ● MEDICINAL FORMS There can be variation in the licensing of different medicines containing the same drug. Forms available from special-order manufacturers include: capsule, oral suspension, oral solution

Soluble tablet
- ▶ Dexamethasone (Non-proprietary)
  Dexamethasone (as Dexamethasone sodium phosphate) 2 mg Dexamethasone 2mg soluble tablets sugar free sugar-free | 50 tablet [PoM] £30.01 DT = £30.01
  Dexamethasone (as Dexamethasone sodium phosphate) 4 mg Dexamethasone 4mg soluble tablets sugar free sugar-free | 50 tablet [PoM] £60.01 DT = £60.01
  Dexamethasone (as Dexamethasone sodium phosphate) 8 mg Dexamethasone 8mg soluble tablets sugar free sugar-free | 50 tablet [PoM] £120.01 DT = £120.01
- ▶ Glensoludex (Glenmark Pharmaceuticals Europe Ltd)
  Dexamethasone (as Dexamethasone sodium phosphate) 2 mg Glensoludex 2mg soluble tablets sugar-free | 50 tablet [PoM] £10.00 DT = £30.01
  Dexamethasone (as Dexamethasone sodium phosphate) 4 mg Glensoludex 4mg soluble tablets sugar-free | 50 tablet [PoM] £20.00 DT = £60.01
  Dexamethasone (as Dexamethasone sodium phosphate) 8 mg Glensoludex 8mg soluble tablets sugar-free | 50 tablet [PoM] £40.00 DT = £120.01

Tablet
CAUTIONARY AND ADVISORY LABELS 10, 21
- ▶ Dexamethasone (Non-proprietary)
  Dexamethasone 500 microgram Dexamethasone 500microgram tablets | 28 tablet [PoM] £54.24 DT = £5.91 | 30 tablet [PoM] £6.33–£64.82
  Dexamethasone 2 mg Dexamethasone 2mg tablets | 50 tablet [PoM] £49.00 DT = £4.80 | 100 tablet [PoM] £11.93–£98.00
  Dexamethasone 4 mg Dexamethasone 4mg tablets | 50 tablet [PoM] £85.00 DT = £83.35 | 100 tablet [PoM] £166.70–£169.40
- ▶ Neofordex (Aspire Pharma Ltd)
  Dexamethasone 40 mg Neofordex 40mg tablets | 10 tablet [PoM] £200.00 DT = £200.00

Solution for injection
CAUTIONARY AND ADVISORY LABELS 10
- ▶ Dexamethasone (Non-proprietary)
  Dexamethasone (as Dexamethasone sodium phosphate) 3.3 mg per 1 ml Dexamethasone (base) 6.6mg/2ml solution for injection ampoules | 10 ampoule [PoM] £22.00–£24.04 DT = £24.04 Dexamethasone (base) 6.6mg/2ml solution for injection vials | 5 vial [PoM] £24.00 DT = £24.00 Dexamethasone (base) 3.3mg/1ml solution for injection ampoules | 5 ampoule [PoM] £12.00 | 10 ampoule [PoM] £12.00–£23.85 DT = £23.85
  Dexamethasone (as Dexamethasone sodium phosphate) 3.8 mg per 1 ml Dexamethasone (base) 3.8mg/1ml solution for injection vials | 10 vial [PoM] £19.99–£20.00 DT = £20.00

Oral solution
CAUTIONARY AND ADVISORY LABELS 10, 21
- ▶ Dexamethasone (Non-proprietary)
  Dexamethasone (as Dexamethasone sodium phosphate) 400 microgram per 1 ml Dexamethasone 2mg/5ml oral solution sugar free sugar-free | 150 ml [PoM] £42.30 DT = £42.30
  Dexamethasone (as Dexamethasone sodium phosphate) 2 mg per 1 ml Dexamethasone 10mg/5ml oral solution sugar free sugar-free | 50 ml [PoM] £24.95 sugar-free | 150 ml [PoM] £101.40 DT = £94.44
  Dexamethasone (as Dexamethasone sodium phosphate) 4 mg per 1 ml Dexamethasone 20mg/5ml oral solution sugar-free | 50 ml [PoM] £49.50 DT = £49.50
- ▶ Dexsol (Rosemont Pharmaceuticals Ltd)
  Dexamethasone (as Dexamethasone sodium phosphate) 400 microgram per 1 ml Dexsol 2mg/5ml oral solution sugar-free | 75 ml [PoM] £21.15 sugar-free | 150 ml [PoM] £42.30 DT = £42.30
- ▶ Martapan (Martindale Pharmaceuticals Ltd)
  Dexamethasone (as Dexamethasone sodium phosphate) 400 microgram per 1 ml Martapan 2mg/5ml oral solution sugar-free | 150 ml [PoM] £35.96 DT = £42.30

F 711

Fludrocortisone acetate
25-Sep-2020

- ● DRUG ACTION Fludrocortisone has very high mineralocorticoid activity and insignificant glucocorticoid activity.

- ● INDICATIONS AND DOSE
Neuropathic postural hypotension
- ▶ BY MOUTH
- ▶ Adult: 100–400 micrograms daily
Mineralocorticoid replacement in adrenocortical insufficiency
- ▶ BY MOUTH
- ▶ Adult: 50–300 micrograms once daily
Adrenocortical insufficiency resulting from septic shock (in combination with hydrocortisone)
- ▶ BY MOUTH
- ▶ Adult: 50 micrograms daily

- ● UNLICENSED USE Not licensed for use in neuropathic postural hypotension.
- ● INTERACTIONS → Appendix 1: corticosteroids
- ● SIDE-EFFECTS Conjunctivitis · idiopathic intracranial hypertension · muscle weakness · thrombophlebitis
- ● HEPATIC IMPAIRMENT
Monitoring Monitor patient closely in hepatic impairment.

6

Endocrine system

- MEDICINAL FORMS There can be variation in the licensing of different medicines containing the same drug. Forms available from special-order manufacturers include: tablet, capsule, oral suspension

Tablet

CAUTIONARY AND ADVISORY LABELS 10
- Fludrocortisone acetate (Non-proprietary)
  Fludrocortisone acetate 100 microgram Fludrocortisone 100microgram tablets | 30 tablet [PoM] £13.60 DT = £13.15 | 100 tablet [PoM] £12.00

⌐ 711

Hydrocortisone

23-Nov-2020

- DRUG ACTION Hydrocortisone has equal glucocorticoid and mineralocorticoid activity.

● INDICATIONS AND DOSE

Thyrotoxic crisis (thyroid storm)
- BY INTRAVENOUS INJECTION
- Adult: 100 mg every 6 hours, to be administered as sodium succinate

Adrenocortical insufficiency resulting from septic shock
- BY INTRAVENOUS INJECTION
- Adult: 50 mg every 6 hours, given in combination with fludrocortisone

Acute hypersensitivity reactions such as angioedema of the upper respiratory tract and anaphylaxis (adjunct to adrenaline)
- BY INTRAVENOUS INJECTION
- Adult: 100–300 mg, to be administered as sodium succinate

Corticosteroid replacement, in patients who have taken more than 10 mg prednisolone daily (or equivalent) within 3 months of minor surgery under general anaesthesia
- BY INTRAVENOUS INJECTION, OR BY INTRAVENOUS INFUSION
- Adult: Initially 25–50 mg, to be administered at induction of surgery, the patient's usual oral corticosteroid dose is recommenced after surgery

Corticosteroid replacement, in patients who have taken more than 10 mg prednisolone daily (or equivalent) within 3 months of moderate or major surgery
- INITIALLY BY INTRAVENOUS INJECTION, OR BY INTRAVENOUS INFUSION
- Adult: Initially 25–50 mg, to be administered at induction of surgery (following usual oral corticosteroid dose on the morning of surgery), followed by (by intravenous injection) 25–50 mg 3 times a day for 24 hours after moderate surgery and for 48–72 hours after major surgery

Adrenocortical insufficiency in Addison's disease or following adrenalectomy
- BY MOUTH USING IMMEDIATE-RELEASE MEDICINES
- Adult: 20–30 mg daily in 2 divided doses, the larger dose to be given in the morning and the smaller in the evening, mimicking the normal diurnal rhythm of cortisol secretion, the optimum daily dose is determined on the basis of clinical response

Adrenal crisis
- INITIALLY BY INTRAMUSCULAR INJECTION, OR BY INTRAVENOUS INJECTION
- Adult: Initially 100 mg, then (by continuous intravenous infusion) 200 mg every 24 hours, diluted in Glucose 5%, alternatively (by intramuscular injection or by intravenous injection) 50 mg every 6 hours, dose increased to 100 mg every 6 hours in patients who are severely obese

Severe inflammatory bowel disease
- BY SLOW INTRAVENOUS INJECTION, OR BY INTRAVENOUS INFUSION
- Adult: 100–500 mg 3–4 times a day or when required

Replacement in adrenocortical insufficiency
- BY MOUTH USING MODIFIED-RELEASE MEDICINES
- Adult: 20–30 mg once daily, adjusted according to response, dose to be taken in the morning
- BY MOUTH USING IMMEDIATE-RELEASE MEDICINES
- Adult: 20–30 mg daily in divided doses, adjusted according to response

Acute hypersensitivity reactions | Angioedema
- BY INTRAMUSCULAR INJECTION, OR BY INTRAVENOUS INJECTION
- Child 1-5 months: Initially 25 mg 3 times a day, adjusted according to response
- Child 6 months-5 years: Initially 50 mg 3 times a day, adjusted according to response
- Child 6-11 years: Initially 100 mg 3 times a day, adjusted according to response
- Child 12-17 years: Initially 200 mg 3 times a day, adjusted according to response

Severe acute asthma | Life-threatening acute asthma
- BY INTRAVENOUS INJECTION
- Child 1 month-1 year: 4 mg/kg every 6 hours (max. per dose 100 mg), alternatively 25 mg every 6 hours until conversion to oral prednisolone is possible, dose given, preferably, as sodium succinate
- Child 2-4 years: 4 mg/kg every 6 hours (max. per dose 100 mg), alternatively 50 mg every 6 hours until conversion to oral prednisolone is possible, dose given, preferably, as sodium succinate
- Child 5-11 years: 4 mg/kg every 6 hours (max. per dose 100 mg), alternatively 100 mg every 6 hours until conversion to oral prednisolone is possible, dose given, preferably, as sodium succinate
- Child 12-17 years: 4 mg/kg every 6 hours (max. per dose 100 mg), alternatively 100 mg every 6 hours until conversion to oral prednisolone is possible, dose given, preferably, as sodium succinate
- Adult: 100 mg every 6 hours until conversion to oral prednisolone is possible, dose given, preferably, as sodium succinate

Severe or critical COVID-19
- BY INTRAVENOUS INJECTION, OR BY INTRAVENOUS INFUSION
- Adult: 50 mg every 8 hours for 7–10 days; may be continued for up to 28 days in patients with septic shock

DOSE EQUIVALENCE AND CONVERSION
- With oral use
- When switching from immediate-release hydrocortisone tablets to modified release *Plenadren®* use same total daily dose. Bioavailability of *Plenadren®* lower than immediate release tablets—monitor clinical response.

- INTERACTIONS → Appendix 1: corticosteroids
- SIDE-EFFECTS
- With oral use Dyslipidaemia · myocardial rupture (following recent myocardial infarction) · oedema
- With parenteral use Hiccups · Kaposi's sarcoma · lipomatosis · myocardial rupture (following recent myocardial infarction)
- DIRECTIONS FOR ADMINISTRATION
- With intravenous use in children For *intravenous administration*, dilute with Glucose 5% or Sodium Chloride 0.9%. For *intermittent infusion* give over 20–30 minutes.
- With intravenous use in adults For *intravenous infusion* (*SoluCortef®*), give continuously or intermittently or via drip tubing in Glucose 5% or Sodium chloride 0.9%.

- **PATIENT AND CARER ADVICE** Patient counselling is advised for hydrocortisone tablets and injections (steroid card).
- **NATIONAL FUNDING/ACCESS DECISIONS**
  For full details see funding body website
  Scottish Medicines Consortium (SMC) decisions
- ▶ Hydrocortisone (*Plenadren*®) for the treatment of adrenal insufficiency in adults (December 2016) SMC No. 848/12 Not recommended
- **LESS SUITABLE FOR PRESCRIBING**
- ▶ With intravenous use Hydrocortisone as the sodium phosphate is less suitable for prescribing as paraesthesia and pain (particularly in the perineal region) may follow intravenous injection.
- **EXCEPTIONS TO LEGAL CATEGORY**
- ▶ With intramuscular use or intravenous use Prescription only medicine restriction does not apply where administration is for saving life in emergency.

- **MEDICINAL FORMS** There can be variation in the licensing of different medicines containing the same drug. Forms available from special-order manufacturers include: capsule, oral suspension, oral solution, liquid
  Modified-release tablet
  CAUTIONARY AND ADVISORY LABELS 10, 22, 25
  - ▶ Plenadren (Shire Pharmaceuticals Ltd)
    Hydrocortisone 5 mg Plenadren 5mg modified-release tablets | 50 tablet PoM £242.50 DT = £242.50
    Hydrocortisone 20 mg Plenadren 20mg modified-release tablets | 50 tablet PoM £400.00 DT = £400.00
  Soluble tablet
  - ▶ Hydrocortisone (Non-proprietary)
    Hydrocortisone (as Hydrocortisone sodium phosphate)
    10 mg Hydrocortisone 10mg soluble tablets sugar free sugar-free | 30 tablet PoM £37.50 DT = £37.50
  Tablet
  CAUTIONARY AND ADVISORY LABELS 10, 21
  - ▶ Hydrocortisone (Non-proprietary)
    Hydrocortisone 10 mg Hydrocortisone 10mg tablets | 30 tablet PoM £84.45 DT = £5.26
    Hydrocortisone 20 mg Hydrocortisone 20mg tablets | 30 tablet PoM £147.26 DT = £3.67
  - ▶ Hydventia (OcXia)
    Hydrocortisone 10 mg Hydventia 10mg tablets | 30 tablet PoM £10.47 DT = £5.26
    Hydrocortisone 20 mg Hydventia 20mg tablets | 30 tablet PoM £20.94 DT = £3.67
  Powder for solution for injection
  - ▶ Hydrocortisone (Non-proprietary)
    Hydrocortisone (as Hydrocortisone sodium succinate)
    100 mg Hydrocortisone sodium succinate 100mg powder for solution for injection vials | 10 vial PoM £11.00 DT = £9.17
  - ▶ Solu-Cortef (Pfizer Ltd)
    Hydrocortisone (as Hydrocortisone sodium succinate)
    100 mg Solu-Cortef 100mg powder for solution for injection vials | 10 vial PoM £9.17 DT = £9.17
  Powder and solvent for solution for injection
  CAUTIONARY AND ADVISORY LABELS 10
  - ▶ Solu-Cortef (Pfizer Ltd)
    Hydrocortisone (as Hydrocortisone sodium succinate)
    100 mg Solu-Cortef 100mg powder and solvent for solution for injection vials | 1 vial PoM £1.16 DT = £1.16
  Solution for injection
  CAUTIONARY AND ADVISORY LABELS 10
  - ▶ Hydrocortisone (Non-proprietary)
    Hydrocortisone (as Hydrocortisone sodium phosphate) 100 mg per 1 ml Hydrocortisone sodium phosphate 100mg/1ml solution for injection ampoules | 5 ampoule PoM £10.60 DT = £10.60

F 711

Methylprednisolone
25-Sep-2020

- **DRUG ACTION** Methylprednisolone exerts predominantly glucocorticoid effects with minimal mineralcorticoid effects.

- **INDICATIONS AND DOSE**
  Suppression of inflammatory and allergic disorders | Cerebral oedema associated with malignancy
  - ▶ BY MOUTH
  - ▶ Adult: Initially 2–40 mg daily
  - ▶ BY INTRAMUSCULAR INJECTION, OR BY SLOW INTRAVENOUS INJECTION, OR BY INTRAVENOUS INFUSION
  - ▶ Adult: Initially 10–500 mg
  Treatment of graft rejection reactions
  - ▶ BY INTRAVENOUS INFUSION
  - ▶ Adult: Up to 1 g daily for up to 3 days
  Treatment of relapse in multiple sclerosis
  - ▶ BY MOUTH
  - ▶ Adult: 500 mg once daily for 5 days
  Treatment of relapse in multiple sclerosis (when oral steroids have failed or have not been tolerated, or in those who require hospital admission)
  - ▶ BY INTRAVENOUS INFUSION
  - ▶ Adult: 1 g once daily for 3–5 days
  DEPO-MEDRONE®
  Suppression of inflammatory and allergic disorders
  - ▶ BY DEEP INTRAMUSCULAR INJECTION
  - ▶ Adult: 40–120 mg, then 40–120 mg after 2–3 weeks if required, to be injected into the gluteal muscle

- **UNLICENSED USE**
  - ▶ With intravenous use or oral use EvGr Not licensed for use by mouth for the treatment of multiple sclerosis relapse. Not licensed for use by intravenous infusion for the treatment of multiple sclerosis relapse for durations longer than 3 days. A Methylprednisolone doses in the BNF may differ from those in product literature.

> **IMPORTANT SAFETY INFORMATION**
>
> MHRA/CHM ADVICE: METHYLPREDNISOLONE INJECTABLE MEDICINE CONTAINING LACTOSE (*SOLU-MEDRONE*® 40 MG): DO NOT USE IN PATIENTS WITH COWS' MILK ALLERGY (OCTOBER 2017)
>
> ▶ With intramuscular use or intravenous use
> An EU-wide review has concluded that *Solu-Medrone*® 40 mg may contain trace amounts of milk proteins and should not be used in patients with a known or suspected allergy to cows' milk. Serious allergic reactions, including bronchospasm and anaphylaxis, have been reported in patients allergic to cows' milk proteins. If a patient's symptoms worsen or new allergic symptoms occur, administration should be stopped and the patient treated accordingly.

- **CAUTIONS**
  - ▶ With intravenous use Rapid intravenous administration of large doses associated with cardiovascular collapse
  - ▶ With systemic use Systemic sclerosis (increased incidence of scleroderma renal crisis)
- **INTERACTIONS** → Appendix 1: corticosteroids
- **SIDE-EFFECTS**
  - ▶ **Common or very common**
  - ▶ With oral use Depressed mood
  - ▶ **Frequency not known**
  - ▶ With oral use Confusion · delusions · diarrhoea · dizziness · dyslipidaemia · hallucination · hiccups · Kaposi's sarcoma · lipomatosis · myocardial rupture (following recent myocardial infarction) · oedema · schizophrenia · suicidal ideation · withdrawal syndrome

6

Endocrine system

Endocrine system

6

▸ With parenteral use Confusion · delusions · depressed mood · diarrhoea · dizziness · dyslipidaemia · hallucination · hiccups · Kaposi's sarcoma · lipomatosis · oedema · schizophrenia · suicidal thoughts · vomiting · withdrawal syndrome

● MONITORING REQUIREMENTS Manufacturer advises monitor blood pressure and renal function (s-creatinine) routinely in patients with systemic sclerosis—increased incidence of scleroderma renal crisis.

● DIRECTIONS FOR ADMINISTRATION

▸ With intravenous use For *intravenous infusion* (as sodium succinate) (*Solu-Medrone*®), give continuously *or* intermittently *or via* drip tubing in Glucose 5% *or* Sodium chloride 0.9%. Reconstitute initially with water for injections; doses up to 250 mg should be given over at least 5 minutes, high doses over at least 30 minutes.

● PATIENT AND CARER ADVICE Patient counselling is advised for methylprednisolone tablets and injections (steroid card).

● MEDICINAL FORMS There can be variation in the licensing of different medicines containing the same drug. Forms available from special-order manufacturers include: oral suspension

Powder and solvent for solution for injection
CAUTIONARY AND ADVISORY LABELS 10
▸ Solu-Medrone (Pfizer Ltd)
Methylprednisolone (as Methylprednisolone sodium succinate) 40 mg Solu-Medrone 40mg powder and solvent for solution for injection vials | 1 vial [PoM] £1.58
Methylprednisolone (as Methylprednisolone sodium succinate) 125 mg Solu-Medrone 125mg powder and solvent for solution for injection vials | 1 vial [PoM] £4.75
Methylprednisolone (as Methylprednisolone sodium succinate) 500 mg Solu-Medrone 500mg powder and solvent for solution for injection vials | 1 vial [PoM] £9.60
Methylprednisolone (as Methylprednisolone sodium succinate) 1 gram Solu-Medrone 1g powder and solvent for solution for injection vials | 1 vial [PoM] £17.30

Tablet
CAUTIONARY AND ADVISORY LABELS 10, 21
▸ Medrone (Pfizer Ltd)
Methylprednisolone 2 mg Medrone 2mg tablets | 30 tablet [PoM] £3.88 DT = £3.88
Methylprednisolone 4 mg Medrone 4mg tablets | 30 tablet [PoM] £6.19 DT = £6.19
Methylprednisolone 16 mg Medrone 16mg tablets | 30 tablet [PoM] £17.17 DT = £17.17
Methylprednisolone 100 mg Medrone 100mg tablets | 20 tablet [PoM] £48.32 DT = £48.32

Suspension for injection
CAUTIONARY AND ADVISORY LABELS 10
▸ Depo-Medrone (Pfizer Ltd)
Methylprednisolone acetate 40 mg per 1 ml Depo-Medrone 40mg/1ml suspension for injection vials | 1 vial [PoM] £3.44 DT = £3.44 | 10 vial [PoM] £34.04
Depo-Medrone 80mg/2ml suspension for injection vials | 1 vial £6.18 DT = £6.18 | 10 vial [PoM] £61.39
Depo-Medrone 120mg/3ml suspension for injection vials | 1 vial [PoM] £8.96 DT = £8.96 | 10 vial [PoM] £88.81

◀ 711

Prednisolone

06-Oct-2020

● DRUG ACTION Prednisolone exerts predominantly glucocorticoid effects with minimal mineralocorticoid effects.

● INDICATIONS AND DOSE

Acute exacerbation of chronic obstructive pulmonary disease (if increased breathlessness interferes with daily activities)
▸ BY MOUTH
▸ Adult: 30 mg daily for 7–14 days

Severe croup (before transfer to hospital) | Mild croup that might cause complications (before transfer to hospital)
▸ BY MOUTH
▸ Child: 1–2 mg/kg

Mild to moderate acute asthma (when oral corticosteroid taken for more than a few days) | Severe or life-threatening acute asthma (when oral corticosteroid taken for more than a few days)
▸ BY MOUTH
▸ Child 1 month–11 years: 2 mg/kg once daily (max. per dose 60 mg) for up to 3 days, longer if necessary

Mild to moderate acute asthma | Severe or life-threatening acute asthma
▸ BY MOUTH
▸ Child 1 month–11 years: 1–2 mg/kg once daily (max. per dose 40 mg) for up to 3 days, longer if necessary
▸ Child 12–17 years: 40–50 mg daily for at least 5 days
▸ Adult: 40–50 mg daily for at least 5 days

Suppression of inflammatory and allergic disorders
▸ BY MOUTH
▸ Adult: Initially 10–20 mg daily, dose preferably taken in the morning after breakfast, can often be reduced within a few days but may need to be continued for several weeks or months; maintenance 2.5–15 mg daily, higher doses may be needed; cushingoid side-effects increasingly likely with doses above 7.5 mg daily
▸ BY INTRAMUSCULAR INJECTION
▸ Adult: 25–100 mg 1–2 times a week, as prednisolone acetate

Suppression of inflammatory and allergic disorders (initial dose in severe disease)
▸ BY MOUTH
▸ Adult: Initially up to 60 mg daily, dose preferably taken in the morning after breakfast, can often be reduced within a few days but may need to be continued for several weeks or months

Idiopathic thrombocytopenic purpura
▸ BY MOUTH
▸ Adult: 1 mg/kg daily, gradually reduce dose over several weeks

Ulcerative colitis | Crohn's disease
▸ BY MOUTH
▸ Adult: Initially 20–40 mg daily until remission occurs, followed by reducing doses, up to 60 mg daily, may be used in some cases, doses preferably taken in the morning after breakfast

Neuritic pain or weakness heralding rapid onset of permanent nerve damage (during reversal reactions multibacillary leprosy)
▸ BY MOUTH
▸ Adult: Initially 40–60 mg daily, dose to be instituted at once

Generalised myasthenia gravis (when given on alternate days)
▸ BY MOUTH
▸ Adult: Initially 10 mg once daily on alternate days, then increased in steps of 10 mg once daily on alternate days, increased to 1–1.5 mg/kg once daily on alternate days (max. per dose 100 mg)

Generalised myasthenia gravis in ventilated patients (when given on alternate days)
▸ BY MOUTH
▸ Adult: Initially 1.5 mg/kg once daily on alternate days (max. per dose 100 mg)

Generalised myasthenia gravis (when giving daily)
▸ BY MOUTH
▸ Adult: Initially 5 mg daily, increased in steps of 5 mg daily. maintenance 60–80 mg daily, alternatively maintenance 0.75–1 mg/kg daily, ventilated patients may be started on 1.5 mg/kg (max. 100 mg) on alternate days

Ocular myasthenia
▸ BY MOUTH
▸ Adult: Usual dose 10–40 mg once daily on alternate days, reduce to minimum effective dose

Reduction in rate of joint destruction in moderate to severe rheumatoid arthritis of less than 2 years' duration
▸ BY MOUTH
▸ Adult: 7.5 mg daily

Polymyalgia rheumatica
▸ BY MOUTH
▸ Adult: 10–15 mg daily until remission of disease activity; maintenance 7.5–10 mg daily, reduce gradually until remission of disease. Many patients require treatment for at least 2 years and in some patients it may be necessary to continue long term low-dose corticosteroid treatment

Giant cell (temporal) arteritis
▸ BY MOUTH
▸ Adult: 40–60 mg daily until remission of disease activity, the higher dose being used if visual symptoms occur; maintenance 7.5–10 mg daily, reduce gradually to maintenance dose. Many patients require treatment for at least 2 years and in some patients it may be necessary to continue long term low-dose corticosteroid treatment

Polyarteritis nodosa | Polymyositis | Systemic lupus erythematosus
▸ BY MOUTH
▸ Adult: Initially 60 mg daily, to be reduced gradually; maintenance 10–15 mg daily

Symptom control of anorexia in palliative care
▸ BY MOUTH
▸ Adult: 15–30 mg daily

Pneumocystis pneumonia in moderate to severe infections associated with HIV infection
▸ BY MOUTH
▸ Adult: 50–80 mg daily for 5 days, the dose is then reduced to complete 21 days of treatment, corticosteroid treatment should ideally be started at the same time as the anti-pneumocystis therapy and certainly no later than 24–72 hours afterwards. The corticosteroid should be withdrawn before anti-pneumocystis treatment is complete

Short-term prophylaxis of episodic cluster headache as monotherapy or in combination with verapamil during verapamil titration
▸ BY MOUTH
▸ Adult: 60–100 mg once daily for 2–5 days, then reduced in steps of 10 mg every 2–3 days until prednisolone is discontinued

Proctitis
▸ BY RECTUM USING RECTAL FOAM
▸ Adult: 1 metered application 1–2 times a day for 2 weeks, continued for further 2 weeks if good response, to be inserted into the rectum, 1 metered application contains 20 mg prednisolone
▸ BY RECTUM USING SUPPOSITORIES
▸ Adult: 5 mg twice daily, to be inserted in to the rectum morning and night, after a bowel movement

Distal ulcerative colitis
▸ BY RECTUM USING RECTAL FOAM
▸ Adult: 1 metered application 1–2 times a day for 2 weeks, continued for further 2 weeks if good response, to be inserted into the rectum, 1 metered application contains 20 mg prednisolone

Rectal complications of Crohn's disease
▸ BY RECTUM USING SUPPOSITORIES
▸ Adult: 5 mg twice daily, to be inserted in to the rectum morning and night, after a bowel movement

Rectal and rectosigmoidal ulcerative colitis | Rectal and rectosigmoidal Crohn's disease
▸ BY RECTUM USING ENEMA
▸ Adult: 20 mg daily for 2–4 weeks, continued if response good, to be used at bedtime

---

IMPORTANT SAFETY INFORMATION

SAFE PRACTICE
▸ With systemic use
Prednisolone has been confused with propranolol; care must be taken to ensure the correct drug is prescribed and dispensed.

● CONTRA-INDICATIONS
▸ With rectal use Abdominal or local infection · bowel perforation · extensive fistulas · intestinal obstruction · recent intestinal anastomoses

● CAUTIONS
▸ With rectal use Systemic absorption may occur with rectal preparations
▸ With systemic use Duchenne's muscular dystrophy (possible transient rhabdomyolysis and myoglobinuria following strenuous physical activity) · systemic sclerosis (increased incidence of scleroderma renal crisis with a daily dose of 15 mg or more)

● INTERACTIONS → Appendix 1: corticosteroids

● SIDE-EFFECTS
▸ With intramuscular use Diarrhoea · dizziness · hiccups · Kaposi's sarcoma · myocardial rupture (following recent myocardial infarction) · scleroderma renal crisis · vomiting
▸ With oral use Diarrhoea · dizziness · dyslipidaemia · lipomatosis · protein catabolism · scleroderma renal crisis

● PREGNANCY As it crosses the placenta 88% of prednisolone is inactivated.
Monitoring ▸ With systemic use Pregnant women with fluid retention should be monitored closely.

● BREAST FEEDING Prednisolone appears in small amounts in breast milk but maternal doses of up to 40 mg daily are unlikely to cause systemic effects in the infant.
Monitoring ▸ With systemic use Infant should be monitored for adrenal suppression if mother is taking a dose higher than 40 mg.

● MONITORING REQUIREMENTS
▸ With systemic use Manufacturer advises monitor blood pressure and renal function (s-creatinine) routinely in patients with systemic sclerosis—increased incidence of scleroderma renal crisis.

● PRESCRIBING AND DISPENSING INFORMATION
Palliative care For further information on the use of prednisolone in palliative care, see www.medicinescomplete. com/#/content/palliative/systemic-corticosteroids.

● PATIENT AND CARER ADVICE
Medicines for Children leaflet: Prednisolone for asthma
▸ With oral use www.medicinesforchildren.org.uk/prednisolone-asthma

● MEDICINAL FORMS There can be variation in the licensing of different medicines containing the same drug. Forms available from special-order manufacturers include: oral suspension, oral solution, enema

Foam
▸ Prednisolone (Non-proprietary)
Prednisolone (as Prednisolone sodium metasulfobenzoate) 20 mg per 1 application Prednisolone 20mg/application foam enema | 14 dose [PoM] £187.00 DT = £187.00

Endocrine system

6

Gastro-resistant tablet

CAUTIONARY AND ADVISORY LABELS 5, 10, 25

▸ Prednisolone (Non-proprietary)

Prednisolone 1 mg Prednisolone 1mg gastro-resistant tablets |
30 tablet PoM £6.48 DT = £5.17

Prednisolone 2.5 mg Prednisolone 2.5mg gastro-resistant tablets |
28 tablet PoM £1.35 DT = £1.35 | 30 tablet PoM £1.23–£1.45

Prednisolone 5 mg Prednisolone 5mg gastro-resistant tablets |
28 tablet PoM £3.79 DT = £1.68 | 30 tablet PoM £1.80–£4.06

▸ Dilacort (Teva UK Ltd, Crescent Pharma Ltd)

Prednisolone 2.5 mg Dilacort 2.5mg gastro-resistant tablets |
28 tablet PoM £1.14–£1.85 DT = £1.35

Prednisolone 5 mg Dilacort 5mg gastro-resistant tablets |
28 tablet PoM £1.95 DT = £1.68

Soluble tablet

CAUTIONARY AND ADVISORY LABELS 10, 13, 21

▸ Prednisolone (Non-proprietary)

Prednisolone (as Prednisolone sodium phosphate)
5 mg Prednisolone 5mg soluble tablets | 30 tablet PoM £53.48 DT =
£11.63

Tablet

CAUTIONARY AND ADVISORY LABELS 10, 21

▸ Prednisolone (Non-proprietary)

Prednisolone 1 mg Prednisolone 1mg tablets | 28 tablet PoM
£1.31 DT = £0.89

Prednisolone 2.5 mg Prednisolone 2.5mg tablets | 28 tablet PoM
£3.91 DT = £3.91

Prednisolone 5 mg Prednisolone 5mg tablets | 28 tablet PoM
£9.86 DT = £1.45

Prednisolone 10 mg Prednisolone 10mg tablets | 28 tablet PoM
£9.66 DT = £15.62

Prednisolone 20 mg Prednisolone 20mg tablets | 28 tablet PoM
£19.45 DT = £31.24

Prednisolone 25 mg Prednisolone 25mg tablets | 56 tablet PoM
£78.09 DT = £78.09

Prednisolone 30 mg Prednisolone 30mg tablets | 28 tablet PoM
£29.12 DT = £46.86

▸ Pevanti (Advanz Pharma)

Prednisolone 2.5 mg Pevanti 2.5mg tablets | 30 tablet PoM £1.42

Prednisolone 5 mg Pevanti 5mg tablets | 30 tablet PoM £0.95

Prednisolone 10 mg Pevanti 10mg tablets | 30 tablet PoM £1.90

Prednisolone 20 mg Pevanti 20mg tablets | 30 tablet PoM £3.80

Prednisolone 25 mg Pevanti 25mg tablets | 56 tablet PoM £40.00
DT = £78.09

Suppository

▸ Prednisolone (Non-proprietary)

Prednisolone (as Prednisolone sodium phosphate)
5 mg Prednisolone sodium phosphate 5mg suppositories |
10 suppository PoM £114.05 DT = £111.51

Oral solution

CAUTIONARY AND ADVISORY LABELS 10

▸ Prednisolone (Non-proprietary)

Prednisolone 1 mg per 1 ml Prednisolone 5mg/5ml oral solution unit
dose | 10 unit dose PoM £11.41 DT = £11.41

Prednisolone 10 mg per 1 ml Prednisolone 10mg/ml oral solution
sugar free sugar-free | 30 ml PoM £55.50 DT = £55.50

Enema

▸ Prednisolone (Non-proprietary)

Prednisolone sodium phosphate 200 microgram per
1 ml Prednisolone 20mg/100ml rectal solution | 7 enema PoM
£14.95 DT = £14.95

⌐ 711

⎸ Triamcinolone acetonide

25-Sep-2020

● DRUG ACTION Triamcinolone exerts predominantly
glucocorticoid effects with minimal mineralcorticoid
effect.

● INDICATIONS AND DOSE

Suppression of inflammatory and allergic disorders

▸ BY DEEP INTRAMUSCULAR INJECTION

▸ Adult: 40 mg (max. per dose 100 mg), repeated if
necessary, dose given for depot effect, to be
administered into gluteal muscle; repeated at intervals
according to patient's response

● CAUTIONS High dosage (may cause proximal myopathy),
avoid in chronic therapy

● INTERACTIONS → Appendix 1: corticosteroids

● SIDE-EFFECTS

▸ **Uncommon** Dizziness · flushing · hyperglycaemia

● PATIENT AND CARER ADVICE Patient counselling is advised
for triamcinolone acetonide injection (steroid card).

● MEDICINAL FORMS There can be variation in the licensing of
different medicines containing the same drug.

Suspension for injection

CAUTIONARY AND ADVISORY LABELS 10

EXCIPIENTS: May contain Benzyl alcohol

▸ Adcortyl Intra-articular / Intradermal (Bristol-Myers Squibb
Pharmaceuticals Ltd)

Triamcinolone acetonide 10 mg per 1 ml Adcortyl Intra-articular /
Intradermal 50mg/5ml suspension for injection vials | 1 vial PoM
£3.63 DT = £3.63

▸ Kenalog (Bristol-Myers Squibb Pharmaceuticals Ltd)

Triamcinolone acetonide 40 mg per 1 ml Kenalog Intra-articular /
Intramuscular 40mg/1ml suspension for injection vials | 5 vial PoM
£7.45 DT = £7.45

2.1 Cushing's syndrome and disease

Cushing's Syndrome

Management

Most types of *Cushing's syndrome* are treated surgically, that
which occasionally accompanies carcinoma of the bronchus
is not usually amenable to surgery. Metyrapone p. 721 has
been found helpful in controlling the symptoms of the
disease; it is also used in other forms of Cushing's syndrome
to prepare the patient for surgery.

The dosages of metyrapone used are either low, and
tailored to cortisol production, or high, in which case
corticosteroid replacement therapy is also needed.

Ketoconazole below may have a direct effect on
corticotropic tumour cells in patients with Cushing's disease.
It is used under specialist supervision for treatment of
endogenous Cushing's syndrome.

Other drugs used for Cushing's syndrome and disease
Pasireotide, p. 995

ENZYME INHIBITORS

⎸ Ketoconazole

04-Feb-2020

● DRUG ACTION An imidazole derivative which acts as a
potent inhibitor of cortisol and aldosterone synthesis by
inhibiting the activity of 17α-hydroxylase,
11-hydroxylation steps and at higher doses the cholesterol
side-chain cleavage enzyme. It also inhibits the activity of
adrenal C17-20 lyase enzymes resulting in androgen
synthesis inhibition, and may have a direct effect on
corticotropic tumour cells in patients with Cushing's
disease.

● INDICATIONS AND DOSE

Endogenous Cushing's syndrome (specialist use only)

▸ BY MOUTH

▸ Adult: Initially 400–600 mg daily in 2–3 divided doses,
increased to 800–1200 mg daily; maintenance
400–800 mg daily in 2–3 divided doses, for dose
titrations in patients with established dose,
adjustments in adrenal insufficiency, or concomitant

corticosteroid replacement therapy, consult product literature; maximum 1200 mg per day

DOSE ADJUSTMENTS DUE TO INTERACTIONS
▸ Manufacturer advises max. dose 200 mg daily with concurrent use of cobicistat.

IMPORTANT SAFETY INFORMATION

CHMP ADVICE: KETOCONAZOLE (JULY 2013)

The CHMP has recommended that the marketing authorisation for oral ketoconazole to treat fungal infections should be suspended. The CHMP concluded that the risk of hepatotoxicity associated with oral ketoconazole is greater than the benefit in treating fungal infections. Doctors should review patients who are being treated with oral ketoconazole for fungal infections, with a view to stopping treatment or choosing an alternative treatment. Patients with a prescription of oral ketoconazole for fungal infections should be referred back to their doctors.

Oral ketoconazole for Cushing's syndrome and topical products containing ketoconazole are not affected by this advice.

● CONTRA-INDICATIONS Acquired QTc prolongation · Acute porphyrias p. 1107 · avoid concomitant use of hepatotoxic drugs · congenital QTc prolongation
● CAUTIONS Pre-treatment liver enzymes should not exceed 2 times the normal upper limit · risk of adrenal insufficiency
● INTERACTIONS → Appendix 1: antifungals, azoles
● SIDE-EFFECTS
▸ Common or very common Adrenal insufficiency · diarrhoea · gastrointestinal discomfort · nausea · skin reactions · vomiting
▸ Uncommon Allergic conditions · alopecia · angioedema · asthenia · dizziness · drowsiness · headache · thrombocytopenia
▸ Rare or very rare Fever · hepatic disorders · taste altered
▸ Frequency not known Alcohol intolerance · appetite abnormal · arthralgia · azoospermia · dry mouth · epistaxis · flatulence · fontanelle bulging · gynaecomastia · hot flush · insomnia · intracranial pressure increased · malaise · menstrual disorder · myalgia · nervousness · papilloedema · paraesthesia · peripheral oedema · photophobia · photosensitivity reaction · tongue discolouration

SIDE-EFFECTS, FURTHER INFORMATION Potentially life-threatening hepatotoxicity reported rarely with oral use. Manufacturer advises reduce dose if hepatic enzymes increased to less than 3 times the upper limit of normal—consult product literature; discontinue permanently if hepatic enzymes at least 3 times the upper limit of normal.
● CONCEPTION AND CONTRACEPTION Effective contraception must be used in women of child-bearing potential.
● PREGNANCY Manufacturer advises avoid—teratogenic in *animal* studies.
● BREAST FEEDING Manufacturer advises avoid—present in breast milk.
● HEPATIC IMPAIRMENT Manufacturer advises avoid.
● MONITORING REQUIREMENTS
▸ Monitor ECG before and one week after initiation, and then as clinically indicated thereafter.
▸ Adrenal insufficiency Monitor adrenal function within one week of initiation, then regularly thereafter. When cortisol levels are normalised or close to target and effective dose established, monitor every 3–6 months as there is a risk of autoimmune disease development or exacerbation after normalisation of cortisol levels. If symptoms suggestive of adrenal insufficiency such as fatigue, anorexia, nausea, vomiting, hypotension, hyponatraemia, hyperkalaemia,

and/or hypoglycaemia occur, measure cortisol levels and discontinue treatment temporarily (can be resumed thereafter at lower dose) or reduce dose and if necessary, initiate corticosteroid substitution.
▸ Hepatotoxicity Monitor liver function before initiation of treatment, then weekly for 1 month after initiation, then monthly for 6 months—more frequently if dose adjusted or abnormal liver function detected.
● PATIENT AND CARER ADVICE Patients or their carers should be told how to recognise signs of liver disorder, and advised to discontinue treatment and seek prompt medical attention if symptoms such as anorexia, nausea, vomiting, fatigue, jaundice, abdominal pain, or dark urine develop. Patients or their carers should also be told how to recognise signs of adrenal insufficiency.

Driving and skilled tasks Dizziness and somnolence may affect the performance of skilled tasks (e.g. driving).

● MEDICINAL FORMS There can be variation in the licensing of different medicines containing the same drug. Forms available from special-order manufacturers include: oral suspension

Tablet

CAUTIONARY AND ADVISORY LABELS 2, 5, 21
▸ Ketoconazole (non-proprietary) ▼

Ketoconazole 200 mg Ketoconazole 200mg tablets | 60 tablet (PoM) £480.00 DT = £480.00

Metyrapone

14-Dec-2020

● DRUG ACTION Metyrapone is a competitive inhibitor of 11β-hydroxylation in the adrenal cortex; the resulting inhibition of cortisol (and to a lesser extent aldosterone) production leads to an increase in ACTH production which, in turn, leads to increased synthesis and release of cortisol precursors. Metyrapone may be used as a test of anterior pituitary function.

● INDICATIONS AND DOSE

Differential diagnosis of ACTH-dependent Cushing's syndrome (specialist supervision in hospital)
▸ BY MOUTH
▸ Adult: 750 mg every 4 hours for 6 doses

Management of Cushing's syndrome (specialist supervision in hospital)
▸ BY MOUTH
▸ Adult: Usual dose 0.25–6 g daily, dose to be tailored to cortisol production, dose is either low, and tailored to cortisol production, or high, in which case corticosteroid replacement therapy is also needed

Resistant oedema due to increased aldosterone secretion in cirrhosis, nephrotic syndrome, and congestive heart failure (with glucocorticoid replacement therapy) (specialist supervision in hospital)
▸ BY MOUTH
▸ Adult: 3 g daily in divided doses

● CONTRA-INDICATIONS Adrenocortical insufficiency
● CAUTIONS Avoid in Acute porphyrias p. 1107 · gross hypopituitarism (risk of precipitating acute adrenal failure) · hypertension on long-term administration · hypothyroidism (delayed response)
● INTERACTIONS → Appendix 1: metyrapone
● SIDE-EFFECTS
▸ Common or very common Dizziness · headache · hypotension · nausea · sedation · vomiting
▸ Rare or very rare Abdominal pain · adrenal insufficiency · allergic dermatitis · hirsutism
▸ Frequency not known Alopecia · bone marrow failure · hypertension
● PREGNANCY Avoid (may impair biosynthesis of fetal-placental steroids).

- BREAST FEEDING Avoid—no information available.
- HEPATIC IMPAIRMENT Manufacturer advises caution (risk of delayed response).
- PATIENT AND CARER ADVICE
  Driving and skilled tasks Drowsiness may affect the performance of skilled tasks (e.g. driving).

- MEDICINAL FORMS There can be variation in the licensing of different medicines containing the same drug.
  Capsule
  CAUTIONARY AND ADVISORY LABELS 21
  ► Metopirone (HRA Pharma UK Ltd)
  Metyrapone 250 mg Metopirone 250mg capsules | 100 capsule [PoM] £363.66 DT = £363.66

3 Diabetes mellitus and hypoglycaemia

3.1 Diabetes mellitus

Diabetes

05-Jun-2017

Description of condition

Diabetes mellitus is a group of metabolic disorders in which persistent hyperglycaemia is caused by deficient insulin secretion or by resistance to the action of insulin. This leads to the abnormalities of carbohydrate, fat and protein metabolism that are characteristic of diabetes mellitus.

Type 1 diabetes mellitus p. 723 and Type 2 diabetes mellitus p. 726 are the two most common classifications of diabetes. Other common types of diabetes are gestational diabetes (develops during pregnancy and resolves after delivery) and secondary diabetes (may be caused by pancreatic damage, hepatic cirrhosis, or endocrine disease). Treatment with endocrine, antiviral, or antipsychotic drugs may also cause secondary diabetes.

Driving

Drivers with diabetes may be required to notify the Driver and Vehicle Licensing Agency (DVLA) of their condition depending on their treatment, the type of licence they hold, and whether they have diabetic complications (including episodes of hypoglycaemia). All drivers who are treated with insulin must inform the DVLA, with some exceptions for temporary treatment. Detailed guidance on notification requirements, eligibility to drive, and precautions required, is available from the DVLA at www.gov.uk/guidance/diabetes-mellitus-assessing-fitness-to-drive.

Advice from the DVLA

The DVLA recommends (2018) that drivers with diabetes need to be particularly careful to avoid hypoglycaemia and should be informed of the warning signs and actions to take. Drivers treated with insulin should always carry a glucose meter and blood-glucose strips when driving, and check their blood-glucose concentration no more than 2 hours before driving and every 2 hours while driving. More frequent self-monitoring may be required if, for any reason, there is a greater risk of hypoglycaemia, such as after physical activity or altered meal routine.

Blood-glucose should always be above 5 mmol/litre while driving. If blood-glucose falls to 5 mmol/litre or below, a snack should be taken. Drivers treated with insulin should ensure that a supply of fast-acting carbohydrate is always available in the vehicle. If blood-glucose is less than 4 mmol/litre, or warning signs of hypoglycaemia develop, the driver should not drive. If already driving, the driver should:

- stop the vehicle in a safe place;

- switch off the engine, remove keys from the ignition, and move from the driver's seat;
- eat or drink a suitable source of sugar;
- wait until 45 minutes after blood-glucose has returned to normal, before continuing journey.

Drivers must not drive if hypoglycaemia awareness has been lost and the DVLA must be notified; driving may resume if a medical report confirms that awareness has been regained.

Depending on the type of licence, notification and monitoring may also be necessary for drivers taking oral antidiabetic drugs, particularly those which carry a risk of hypoglycaemia (e.g. sulfonylureas, nateglinide p. 742, repaglinide p. 742).

Note: additional criteria apply for drivers of large goods or passenger carrying vehicles—consult DVLA guidance.

Alcohol

Alcohol can make the signs of hypoglycaemia less clear, and can cause delayed hypoglycaemia; specialist sources recommend that patients with diabetes should drink alcohol only in moderation, and when accompanied by food.

Oral glucose tolerance tests

The oral glucose tolerance test is used mainly for diagnosis of impaired glucose tolerance; it is **not** recommended or necessary for routine diagnostic use when severe symptoms of hyperglycaemia are present. In patients who have less severe symptoms and a blood-glucose concentration that does not establish or exclude diabetes (e.g. impaired fasting glycaemia), an oral glucose tolerance test may be required. It is also used to establish the presence of gestational diabetes.

An oral glucose tolerance test involves measuring the blood-glucose concentration after fasting, and then 2 hours after drinking a standard anhydrous glucose drink. Anhydrous glucose may alternatively be given as the appropriate amount of *Polycal*® or as *Rapilose*® OGTT oral solution.

HbA1c measurement

Glycated haemoglobin (HbA1c) forms when red blood cells are exposed to glucose in the plasma. The HbA1c test reflects average plasma glucose over the previous 2 to 3 months and provides a good indicator of glycaemic control. Unlike the oral glucose tolerance test, an HbA1c test can be performed at any time of the day and does not require any special preparation such as fasting.

HbA1c values are expressed in *mmol of glycated haemoglobin per mol of haemoglobin (mmol/mol)*, a standardised unit specific for HbA1c created by the International Federation of Clinical Chemistry and Laboratory Medicine (IFCC). HbA1c values were previously aligned to the assay used in the Diabetes Control and Complications Trial (DCCT) and expressed as a percentage.

Equivalent values	
IFCC-HbA1c (mmol/mol)	DCCT-HbA1c (%)
42	6.0
48	6.5
53	7.0
59	7.5
64	8.0
69	8.5
75	9.0

Diagnosis

The HbA1c test is used for monitoring glycaemic control in both Type 1 diabetes p. 723 and Type 2 diabetes p. 726 and is now also used for diagnosis of type 2 diabetes. [EvGr] HbA1c should not be used for diagnosis in those with suspected type 1 diabetes, in children, during pregnancy, or in women who are up to two months postpartum. It should also not be used for patients who have:

- had symptoms of diabetes for less than 2 months;
- a high diabetes risk and are acutely ill;
- treatment with medication that may cause hyperglycaemia;
- Acute pancreatic damage;
- end-stage chronic kidney disease;
- HIV infection.

HbA1c used for diagnosis of diabetes should be interpreted with caution in patients with abnormal haemoglobin, anaemia, altered red cell lifespan, or who have had a recent blood transfusion. ⟨A⟩

Monitoring

⟨EvGr⟩ HbA1c is also a reliable predictor of microvascular and macrovascular complications and mortality. Lower HbA1c is associated with a lower risk of long term vascular complications and patients should be supported to aim for an individualised HbA1c target (see Type 1 diabetes below and Type 2 diabetes p. 726).

HbA1c should usually be measured in patients with type 1 diabetes every 3 to 6 months, and more frequently if blood-glucose control is thought to be changing rapidly. Patients with type 2 diabetes should be monitored every 3 to 6 months until HbA1c and medication are stable when monitoring can be reduced to every 6 months. ⟨A⟩

HbA1c monitoring is invalid for patients with disturbed erythrocyte turnover or for patients with a lack of, or abnormal haemoglobin. In these cases, quality-controlled plasma glucose profiles, total glycated haemoglobin estimation (if there is abnormal haemoglobin), or fructosamine estimation can be used.

Laboratory measurement of fructosamine concentration measures the glycated fraction of all plasma proteins over the previous 14 to 21 days but is a less accurate measure of glycaemic control than HbA1c.

Advanced Pharmacy Services

Patients with diabetes may be eligible for the New Medicines Service / Medicines Use Review service provided by a community pharmacist. For further information, see *Advanced Pharmacy Services* in Medicines optimisation p. 18.

Type 1 diabetes
05-Jun-2017

Description of condition

Type 1 diabetes describes an absolute insulin deficiency in which there is little or no endogenous insulin secretory capacity due to destruction of insulin-producing beta-cells in the pancreatic islets of Langerhans. This form of the disease has an auto-immune basis in most cases, and it can occur at any age, but most commonly before adulthood.

Loss of insulin secretion results in hyperglycaemia and other metabolic abnormalities. If poorly managed, the resulting tissue damage has both short-term and long-term adverse effects on health; this can result in retinopathy, nephropathy, neuropathy, premature cardiovascular disease, and peripheral arterial disease.

Typical features in adult patients presenting with type 1 diabetes are hyperglycaemia (random plasma-glucose concentration above 11 mmol/litre), ketosis, rapid weight loss, a body mass index below 25 kg/m^2, age younger than 50 years, and a personal/family history of autoimmune disease (though not all features may be present).

Aims of treatment

Treatment is aimed at using insulin regimens to achieve as optimal a level of blood-glucose control as is feasible, while avoiding or reducing the frequency of hypoglycaemic

episodes, in order to minimise the risk of long-term microvascular and macrovascular complications.

Disability from complications can often be prevented by early detection and active management of the disease (see Diabetic complications p. 728). ⟨EvGr⟩ The target for glycaemic control should be individualised for each patient, considering factors such as daily activities, aspirations, likelihood of complications, adherence to treatment, comorbidities, occupation and history of hypoglycaemia.

A target HbA1c concentration of 48 mmol/mol (6.5%) or lower is recommended in patients with type 1 diabetes. Blood-glucose concentration should be monitored at least four times a day, including before each meal and before bed. ⟨A⟩ Patients should aim for:

- ⟨EvGr⟩ a fasting blood-glucose concentration of 5–7 mmol/litre on waking;
- a blood-glucose concentration of 4–7 mmol/litre before meals at other times of the day;
- a blood-glucose concentration of 5–9 mmol/litre at least 90 minutes after eating;
- a blood-glucose concentration of at least 5 mmol/litre when driving. ⟨A⟩

Overview

⟨EvGr⟩ Type 1 diabetes requires insulin replacement, supported by active management of other cardiovascular risk factors, such as hypertension and high circulating lipids (see Diabetic complications p. 728). ⟨A⟩ Insulin replacement therapy aims to recreate normal fluctuations in circulating insulin concentrations while supporting a flexible lifestyle with minimal restrictions. Flexible insulin therapy usually involves self-injecting multiple daily doses of insulin, with doses adjusted according to planned exercise, intended food intake and other factors, including current blood-glucose, which the patient needs to test on a regular basis.

⟨EvGr⟩ Patients who have a BMI of 25 kg/m^2 or above (23 kg/m^2 or above for patients of South Asian or related ethnicity) who wish to improve their blood-glucose control while minimising their effective insulin dose, may benefit from metformin hydrochloride p. 732 [unlicensed indication] as an addition to insulin therapy.

Dietary control is important in both type 1 and type 2 diabetes and patients should receive advice from a dietitian. Dietary advice should include information on weight control, cardiovascular risk, hyperglycaemic effects of different foods and appropriate changes in insulin doses according to food intake. Healthy eating can reduce cardiovascular risk and dietary modifications may be recommended to account for various associated features of diabetes such as excess weight and obesity, low body-weight, eating disorders, hypertension and renal failure. Patients with type 1 diabetes should be offered carbohydrate-counting training as part of a structured education programme. ⟨A⟩

Insulin therapy in type 1 diabetes

⟨EvGr⟩ All patients with type 1 diabetes require insulin therapy (**see also Insulin p. 725**). Treatment should be initiated and managed by clinicians with relevant expertise; there are several different types of regimens. ⟨A⟩

Multiple daily injection basal-bolus insulin regimens

One or more separate daily injections of intermediate-acting insulin or long-acting insulin analogue as the basal insulin; alongside multiple bolus injections of short-acting insulin before meals. This regimen offers flexibility to tailor insulin therapy with the carbohydrate load of each meal.

Mixed (biphasic) regimen

One, two, or three insulin injections per day of short-acting insulin mixed with intermediate-acting insulin. The insulin preparations may be mixed by the patient at the time of injection, or a premixed product can be used.

Endocrine system

6

Continuous subcutaneous insulin infusion (insulin pump)

A regular or continuous amount of insulin (usually in the form of a rapid-acting insulin analogue or soluble insulin), delivered by a programmable pump and insulin storage reservoir via a subcutaneous needle or cannula.

Recommended insulin regimens

[EvGr] Patients with type 1 diabetes should be offered multiple daily injection basal-bolus insulin regimens as the **first-line choice**. Twice-daily insulin detemir p. 757 should be offered as the long-acting basal insulin therapy. Once-daily insulin glargine p. 758 may be prescribed if insulin detemir is not tolerated, or if a twice-daily regimen is not acceptable to the patient. Insulin detemir may also be offered as an alternative once-daily regimen.

Patients who are using alternative basal regimens may continue if agreed targets are being achieved; other basal insulin regimens should be considered only if the recommended regimens do not deliver agreed targets. Non-basal-bolus insulin regimens (e.g. twice-daily mixed [biphasic], basal-only, or bolus-only regimens) are **not** recommended for adults with *newly diagnosed* type 1 diabetes.

A rapid-acting insulin analogue is recommended as the bolus or mealtime insulin replacement, rather than soluble human insulin or animal insulin (rarely used). The rapid-acting insulin analogue should be injected before meals—routine use after meals should be discouraged. Patients who have a strong preference for an alternative mealtime insulin should be offered their preferred insulin.

Alternatively, if a multiple daily injection basal-bolus regimen is not possible, a twice-daily mixed insulin regimen should be considered if it is preferred.

In patients who are using a twice-daily *human* insulin mixed regimen and have hypoglycaemia that affects their quality of life, a trial of a twice-daily analogue mixed insulin regimen should be considered.

Continuous subcutaneous insulin infusion (insulin pump) therapy, should only be offered to adults who suffer disabling hypoglycaemia, or, who have high HbA1c concentrations (69 mmol/mol [8.5%] or above) with multiple daily injection therapy (including, if appropriate, the use of long-acting insulin analogues) despite a high level of care. Insulin pump therapy should be initiated by a specialist team. [A]

Insulin requirements

[EvGr] The dosage of insulin must be determined individually for each patient and should be adjusted as necessary according to the results of regular monitoring of blood-glucose concentrations. [A]

Persistent poor glucose control, leading to erratic insulin requirements or episodes of hypoglycaemia, may be due to many factors, including adherence, injection technique, injection site problems, blood-glucose monitoring skills, lifestyle issues (including diet, exercise and alcohol intake), psychological issues, and organic causes such as renal disease, thyroid disorders, coeliac disease, Addison's disease or gastroparesis.

Infection, stress, accidental or surgical trauma can all increase the required insulin dose. Insulin requirements may be decreased (and therefore susceptibility to hypoglycaemia increased) by physical activity, intercurrent illness, reduced food intake, impaired renal function, and in certain endocrine disorders.

Risks of hypoglycaemia with insulin

[EvGr] Hypoglycaemia is an inevitable adverse effect of insulin treatment, and patients should be advised of the warning signs and actions to take (for guidance on management, see Hypoglycaemia p. 763).

Impaired awareness of hypoglycaemia can occur when the ability to recognise usual symptoms is lost, or when the symptoms are blunted or no longer present. Patients'

awareness of hypoglycaemia should be assessed annually using the Gold score or the Clarke score. [A]

An increase in the frequency of hypoglycaemic episodes may reduce the warning symptoms experienced by the patient. Impaired awareness of symptoms below 3 mmol/litre is associated with a significantly increased risk of severe hypoglycaemia. Beta-blockers can also blunt hypoglycaemic awareness, by reducing warning signs such as tremor.

Loss of warning of hypoglycaemia among insulin-treated patients can be a serious hazard, especially for drivers and those in dangerous occupations. Advice should be given in line with the Driver and Vehicle Licensing Agency (DVLA) guidance (see *Driving* under Diabetes p. 722).

[EvGr] To restore the warning signs, episodes of hypoglycaemia must be minimised. Insulin regimens, doses and blood-glucose targets should be reviewed and continuous subcutaneous insulin infusion therapy and real-time continuous blood-glucose monitoring should be considered. Patients should receive structured education to ensure they are following the principles of a flexible insulin regimen correctly, with additional education regarding avoiding and treating hypoglycaemia for those who continue to have impaired awareness. Relaxation of individualised blood-glucose targets should be avoided as a strategy to improve impaired awareness of symptoms. If recurrent severe episodes of hypoglycaemia continue despite appropriate interventions, the patient should be referred to a specialist centre. [A]

There is conflicting evidence regarding reports that some patients may experience loss of awareness of hypoglycaemia after transfer from animal to human insulin; clinical studies do not confirm that human insulin decreases hypoglycaemia awareness.

Manufacturers advise any switch between brands or formulation of insulin (including switching from animal to human insulin) should be done under strict supervision; a change in dose may be required.

Hypodermic equipment

[EvGr] Patients should be advised on the safe disposal of lancets, single-use syringes, and needles, and should be provided with suitable disposal containers. Arrangements should be made for the suitable disposal of these containers. [A]

Lancets, needles, syringes, and accessories are listed under Hypodermic Equipment in Part IXA of the Drug Tariff (Part III of the Northern Ireland Drug Tariff, Part 3 of the Scottish Drug Tariff). The Drug Tariffs can be accessed online at:

- National Health Service Drug Tariff for England and Wales:
  www.nhsbsa.nhs.uk/pharmacies-gp-practices-and-appliance-contractors/drug-tariff
- Health and Personal Social Services for Northern Ireland Drug Tariff:
  www.hscbusiness.hscni.net/services/2034.htm
- Scottish Drug Tariff:
  www.isdscotland.org/Health-Topics/Prescribing-and-Medicines/Scottish-Drug-Tariff

Useful Resources

Type 1 diabetes in adults: diagnosis and management. National Institute for Health and Care Excellence. Clinical guideline NG17. August 2015.
www.nice.org.uk/guidance/ng17

Insulin

05-Jun-2017

Overview

For recommended insulin regimens see Type 1 diabetes p. 723 and Type 2 diabetes p. 726.

Insulin is a polypeptide hormone secreted by pancreatic beta-cells. Insulin increases glucose uptake by adipose tissue and muscles, and suppresses hepatic glucose release. The role of insulin is to lower blood-glucose concentrations in order to prevent hyperglycaemia and its associated microvascular, macrovascular and metabolic complications.

The natural profile of insulin secretion in the body consists of basal insulin (a low and steady secretion of background insulin that controls the glucose continuously released from the liver) and meal-time bolus insulin (secreted in response to glucose absorbed from food and drink).

Sources of insulin

Three types of insulin are available in the UK: human insulin, human insulin analogues, and animal insulin. Animal insulins are extracted and purified from animal sources (bovine or porcine insulin). Although widely used in the past, animal insulins are no longer initiated in people with diabetes but may still be used by some adult patients who cannot, or do not wish to, change to human insulins.

Human insulins are produced by recombinant DNA technology and have the same amino acid sequence as endogenous human insulin. Human insulin analogues are produced in the same way as human insulins, but the insulin is modified to produce a desired kinetic characteristic, such as an extended duration of action or faster absorption and onset of action.

Immunological resistance to insulin is uncommon and true insulin allergy is rare. Human insulin and insulin analogues are less immunogenic than animal insulins.

Administration of insulin

Insulin is inactivated by gastro-intestinal enzymes and must therefore be given by injection; the subcutaneous route is ideal in most circumstances. Insulin should be injected into a body area with plenty of subcutaneous fat—usually the abdomen (fastest absorption rate) or outer thighs/buttocks (slower absorption compared with the abdomen or inner thighs).

Absorption from a limb site can vary considerably (by as much as 20–40%) day-to-day, particularly in children. Local tissue reactions, changes in insulin sensitivity, injection site, blood flow, depth of injection, and the amount of insulin injected can all affect the rate of absorption. Increased blood flow around the injection site due to exercise can also increase insulin absorption.

EvGr Lipohypertrophy can occur due to repeatedly injecting into the same small area, and can cause erratic absorption of insulin, and contribute to poor glycaemic control. Patients should be advised not to use affected areas for further injection until the skin has recovered. Lipohypertrophy can be minimised by using different injection sites in rotation. Injection sites should be checked for signs of infection, swelling, bruising, and lipohypertrophy before administration. ◁A▷

Insulin preparations

Insulin preparations can be broadly categorised into three groups based on their time-action profiles: short-acting insulins (including soluble insulin and rapid-acting insulins), intermediate-acting insulins and long-acting insulins. The duration of action of each particular type of insulin varies considerably from one patient to another, and needs to be assessed individually.

Short-acting insulins

Short-acting insulins have a short duration and a relatively rapid onset of action, to replicate the insulin normally produced by the body in response to glucose absorbed from a meal. These are available as soluble Insulin above (human and, bovine or porcine insulin—both rarely used), and the rapid-acting insulin analogues (insulin aspart p. 753, insulin glulisine p. 754 and insulin lispro p. 755).

Soluble insulin

Soluble insulin is usually given subcutaneously but some preparations can be given intravenously and intramuscularly. For maintenance regimens, it is usual to inject the insulin 15 to 30 minutes before meals, depending on the insulin preparation used.

When injected subcutaneously, soluble insulin has a rapid onset of action (30 to 60 minutes), a peak action between 1 and 4 hours, and a duration of action of up to 9 hours.

When injected intravenously, soluble insulin has a short half-life of only a few minutes and its onset of action is instantaneous.

Soluble insulin administered intravenously is the most appropriate form of insulin for use in diabetic emergencies e.g. Diabetic ketoacidosis p. 728 and peri-operatively.

Rapid-acting insulin

Insulin aspart, insulin glulisine, and insulin lispro have a faster onset of action (within 15 minutes) and shorter duration of action (approximately 2–5 hours) than soluble insulin, and are usually given by subcutaneous injection.

EvGr For maintenance regimens, these insulins should ideally be injected immediately before meals. Rapid-acting insulin, administered before meals, has an advantage over short-acting soluble insulin in terms of improved glucose control, reduction of HbA1c, and reduction in the incidence of severe hypoglycaemia, including nocturnal hypoglycaemia.

The routine use of *post-meal* injections of rapid-acting insulin should be avoided—when given during or after meals, they are associated with poorer glucose control, an increased risk of high postprandial-glucose concentration, and subsequent hypoglycaemia. ◁A▷

Intermediate-acting insulin

Intermediate-acting insulins (isophane insulin p. 756) have an intermediate duration of action, designed to mimic the effect of endogenous basal insulin. When given by subcutaneous injection, they have an onset of action of approximately 1–2 hours, a maximal effect at 3–12 hours, and a duration of action of 11–24 hours.

Isophane insulin is a suspension of insulin with protamine; it may be given as one or more daily injections alongside separate meal-time short-acting insulin injections, or mixed with a short-acting (soluble or rapid-acting) insulin in the same syringe—for recommended insulin regimens see Type 1 diabetes p. 723 and Type 2 diabetes p. 726. Isophane insulin may be mixed with a short-acting insulin by the patient, or a pre-mixed biphasic insulin can be supplied (biphasic isophane insulin p. 755, biphasic insulin aspart p. 756 and biphasic insulin lispro p. 756).

Biphasic insulins (biphasic isophane insulin, biphasic insulin aspart, biphasic insulin lispro) are pre-mixed insulin preparations containing various combinations of short-acting insulin (soluble insulin or rapid-acting analogue insulin) and an intermediate-acting insulin.

The percentage of short-acting insulin varies from 15% to 50%. These preparations should be administered by subcutaneous injection immediately before a meal.

Long-acting insulin

Like intermediate-acting insulins, the long-acting insulins (protamine zinc insulin, insulin zinc suspension, insulin detemir p. 757, insulin glargine p. 758 and insulin degludec p. 757) mimic endogenous basal insulin secretion, but their duration of action may last up to 36 hours. They achieve a steady-state level after 2–4 days to produce a constant level of insulin.

Insulin glargine and insulin degludec are given once daily and insulin detemir is given once or twice daily according to individual requirements. The older long-acting insulins, (insulin zinc suspension and protamine zinc insulin) are now rarely prescribed.

Type 2 diabetes

10-May-2018

Description of condition

Type 2 diabetes is a chronic metabolic condition characterised by insulin resistance. Insufficient pancreatic insulin production also occurs progressively over time, resulting in hyperglycaemia.

It is commonly associated with obesity, physical inactivity, raised blood pressure, dyslipidaemia and a tendency to develop thrombosis; therefore it increases cardiovascular risk. It is associated with long-term microvascular and macrovascular complications, together with reduced quality of life and life expectancy.

Type 2 diabetes typically develops later in life but is increasingly diagnosed in children, despite previously being considered a disease of adulthood.

Aims of treatment

Treatment is aimed at minimising the risk of long-term microvascular and macrovascular complications by effective blood-glucose control and maintenance of HbA1c at or below the target value set for each individual patient.

Overview

[EvGr] Weight loss, smoking cessation and regular exercise can help to reduce hyperglycaemia and reduce cardiovascular risk, and should be encouraged (with input from a dietitian where appropriate). For guidance on reducing cardiovascular risk, see Cardiovascular disease risk assessment and prevention p. 203. Antidiabetic drugs should be prescribed to augment lifestyle interventions, when these changes are not adequate to control blood-glucose alone. ⟨A⟩

Antidiabetic drugs

There are several classes of non-insulin antidiabetic drugs available for the treatment of type 2 diabetes. [EvGr] The choice of drug should be based on effectiveness, safety, tolerability and should also take into consideration the patient's comorbidities and concomitant medication. For recommended treatment regimens and the place in therapy of each drug, see Drug treatment, antidiabetic drugs (below). ⟨A⟩

Metformin hydrochloride p. 732 has an anti-hyperglycaemic effect, lowering both basal and postprandial blood-glucose concentrations. It does not stimulate insulin secretion and therefore, when given alone, does not cause hypoglycaemia. [EvGr] The dose of standard-release metformin hydrochloride should be increased gradually to minimise the risk of gastro-intestinal side effects. Modified-release metformin hydrochloride should be offered if standard treatment is not tolerated. ⟨A⟩

The **sulfonylureas** (glibenclamide p. 749, gliclazide p. 749, glimepiride p. 750, glipizide p. 750, tolbutamide p. 750) may cause hypoglycaemia; it is more likely with long-acting sulfonylureas such as glibenclamide, which have been associated with severe, prolonged and sometimes fatal cases of hypoglycaemia. Sulfonylureas are also associated with modest weight gain, probably due to increased plasma-insulin concentrations.

Acarbose p. 731 has a poorer anti-hyperglycaemic effect than many other antidiabetic drugs, including the sulfonylureas, metformin hydrochloride, and pioglitazone p. 751.

The meglitinides, nateglinide p. 742 and repaglinide p. 742, have a rapid onset of action and short duration of activity. These drugs can be used flexibly around mealtimes and adjusted to fit around individual eating habits which may be beneficial for some patients, but generally are a less preferred option than the sulfonylureas.

The thiazolidinedione, pioglitazone, is associated with several long-term risks and its ongoing benefit to the patient should be reviewed regularly and treatment stopped if response is insufficient (see Important safety information under pioglitazone).

The dipeptidylpeptidase-4 inhibitors (gliptins), alogliptin p. 733, linagliptin p. 734, sitagliptin p. 736, saxagliptin p. 734, and vildagliptin p. 736, do not appear to be associated with weight gain and have less incidence of hypoglycaemia than the sulfonylureas.

The sodium glucose co-transporter 2 inhibitors, canagliflozin p. 743, dapagliflozin p. 744, and empagliflozin p. 746, may be suitable for some patients when first-line options are not appropriate. [EvGr] Canagliflozin and empagliflozin can be beneficial in patients with type 2 diabetes and established cardiovascular disease. ⟨A⟩ Sodium glucose co-transporter 2 inhibitors are associated with a risk of diabetic ketoacidosis.

The glucagon-like peptide-1 receptor agonists, dulaglutide p. 737, exenatide p. 738, liraglutide p. 739 and lixisenatide p. 740, should be reserved for combination therapy when other treatment options have failed. [EvGr] Liraglutide has proven cardiovascular benefit and should be considered in patients with type 2 diabetes and established cardiovascular disease. ⟨A⟩

Polycystic ovary syndrome

[EvGr] Metformin hydrochloride (initiated by a specialist) is prescribed as an insulin sensitising drug in women with polycystic ovary syndrome who are not planning pregnancy [unlicensed indication]. ⟨A⟩ Long-term benefit or superiority over other treatment options has not been confirmed by good quality evidence. Metformin hydrochloride may improve short-term insulin sensitivity and reduce androgen concentrations, but there is insufficient supporting evidence that metformin improves weight gain, hirsutism, acne or regulation of the menstrual cycle. Treatment should only be initiated by a specialist. Metformin hydrochloride does not exert a hypoglycaemic action in non-diabetic patients except in overdose.

Drug treatment, antidiabetic drugs

[EvGr] Type 2 diabetes should initially be treated with a single oral antidiabetic drug. A target HbA1c concentration of 48 mmol/mol (6.5%) is generally recommended when type 2 diabetes is managed by diet and lifestyle alone or when combined with a single antidiabetic drug not associated with hypoglycaemia (such as metformin hydrochloride). Adults prescribed a single drug associated with hypoglycaemia (such as a sulphonylurea), or two or more antidiabetic drugs in combination, should usually aim for an HbA1c concentration of 53 mmol/mol (7.0%). Targets may differ and should be individualised and agreed with each patient.

Note: Consider relaxing the target HbA1c level on a case-by-case basis, with particular consideration for people who are older, frail, or where tight blood-glucose control is not appropriate or poses a high risk of the consequences of hypoglycaemia.

If HbA1c concentrations are poorly controlled despite treatment with a single drug (usually considered to be a rise of HbA1c to 58 mmol/mol (7.5%) or higher), the drug treatment should be intensified, alongside reinforcement of advice regarding diet, lifestyle, and adherence to drug treatment.

When two or more antidiabetic drugs are prescribed, an HbA1c concentration target of 53 mmol/mol (7.0%) is recommended for patients in which it is appropriate, but a relaxation of the target may be more appropriate in some individual cases (for example, those at high risk of the consequences of hypoglycaemia, poor life expectancy, or significant comorbidities). Ⓐ

Initial treatment
Ⓔⱽᴳʳ Metformin hydrochloride is recommended as the first choice for initial treatment for all patients, due to its positive effect on weight loss, reduced risk of hypoglycaemic events and the additional long-term cardiovascular benefits associated with its use. Ⓐ

If metformin is contra-indicated or not tolerated, see *Alternative non-metformin regimens* below.

First intensification of treatment
Ⓔⱽᴳʳ If metformin hydrochloride (alongside modification to diet) does not control HbA1c to below the agreed threshold, treatment should be intensified, and metformin hydrochloride combined with one of the following:
- a sulfonylurea (glibenclamide, gliclazide, glimepiride, glipizide, tolbutamide);
- Pioglitazone;
- a dipeptidylpeptidase-4 inhibitor (linagliptin, saxagliptin, sitagliptin, or vildagliptin);
- a sodium glucose co-transporter 2 inhibitor (canagliflozin, dapagliflozin or empagliflozin) only when sulfonylureas are contra-indicated or not tolerated, or if the patient is at significant risk of hypoglycaemia or its consequences. Ⓐ

Ⓔⱽᴳʳ Elderly patients or those with renal impairment are at particular risk of hypoglycaemia; if a sulfonylurea is indicated, a shorter-acting sulfonylurea, such as gliclazide p. 749 or tolbutamide p. 750 should be prescribed. Ⓔ

The place in therapy of alogliptin p. 733 (a dipeptidylpeptidase-4 inhibitor) is not yet known.

Second intensification of treatment
Ⓔⱽᴳʳ If dual therapy is unsuccessful, treatment should be intensified again, and one of the following triple therapy regimens prescribed:
- Metformin hydrochloride p. 732 and a dipeptidylpeptidase-4 inhibitor and a sulfonylurea;
- Metformin hydrochloride and pioglitazone p. 751 and a sulfonylurea;
- Metformin hydrochloride and a sulfonylurea and one of the sodium glucose co-transporter 2 inhibitors;
- Metformin hydrochloride and pioglitazone and a sodium glucose co-transporter 2 inhibitor (canagliflozin p. 743 or empagliflozin p. 746; note that dapagliflozin is not recommended in a triple therapy regimen with pioglitazone).

Alternatively, it may be appropriate to start **insulin**-based treatment at this stage—see *Drug treatment, insulin*. Ⓐ

Glucagon-like peptide-1 receptor agonists
Ⓔⱽᴳʳ If triple therapy with metformin hydrochloride and two other oral drugs is tried and is not effective, not tolerated or contra-indicated, a **glucagon-like peptide-1 receptor agonist** may be prescribed as part of a triple combination regimen with metformin hydrochloride and a sulfonylurea.

These should only be prescribed for patients who have a BMI of 35 kg/m^2 *or above* (adjusted for ethnicity) **and** who also have specific psychological or medical problems associated with obesity; **or** for those who have a BMI *lower* than 35 kg/m^2 but for whom insulin therapy would have significant occupational implications **or** if the weight loss associated with glucagon-like peptide-1 receptor agonists would benefit other significant obesity-related comorbidities.

After 6 months, the drug should be reviewed and only continued if there has been a beneficial metabolic response (a reduction of at least 11 mmol/mol [1.0%] in HbA1c and a weight loss of at least 3% of initial body-weight).

Insulin should only be prescribed in combination with a glucagon-like peptide-1 receptor agonist under specialist care advice and with ongoing support from a consultant-led multidisciplinary team. Ⓐ

Alternative non-metformin regimens
Ⓔⱽᴳʳ If metformin is contra-indicated or not tolerated, initial treatment should be single therapy with:
- a sulfonylurea (glibenclamide p. 749, gliclazide, glimepiride p. 750, glipizide p. 750, or tolbutamide) (first choice), or
- a dipeptidyl peptidase-4 inhibitor (linagliptin p. 734, saxagliptin p. 734, sitagliptin p. 736, or vildagliptin p. 736), or
- Pioglitazone. Ⓐ

The **sodium glucose co-transporter 2 inhibitors** canagliflozin, dapagliflozin p. 744, or empagliflozin are also options for **monotherapy** when metformin is contra-indicated or not tolerated, only if a dipeptidylpeptidase-4 inhibitor would otherwise be prescribed and neither a sulfonylurea nor pioglitazone is appropriate.

Ⓔⱽᴳʳ Repaglinide p. 742 is also an effective alternative option for single therapy, but it has a limited role in treatment because, should an intensification of treatment be required, it is not licensed to be used in any combination other than with metformin hydrochloride; it would therefore require a complete change of treatment in those patients who have started it due to intolerance or contra-indication to metformin. Ⓐ

Intensification
Ⓔⱽᴳʳ If the initial single drug does not control HbA1c to below the agreed threshold, treatment should be intensified and one of the following dual combinations prescribed:
- a dipeptidylpeptidase-4 inhibitor and pioglitazone;
- a dipeptidylpeptidase-4 inhibitor and a sulfonylurea; or
- Pioglitazone and a sulfonylurea.

If dual therapy does not provide adequate glucose control, insulin-based treatment should be considered—see *Drug treatment, insulin*. Ⓐ

Drug treatment, insulin
Ⓔⱽᴳʳ When indicated for intensification, insulin (see also, Insulin p. 725) should be started with a structured support programme covering insulin dose titration, injection technique, self-monitoring, and knowledge of dietary effects and glucose control. Metformin hydrochloride should be continued unless it is contra-indicated or not tolerated. Other antidiabetic drugs should be reviewed and stopped if necessary.

Recommended insulin regimens include:
- human isophane insulin p. 756 injected once or twice daily, according to requirements;
- a human isophane insulin in combination with a short-acting insulin, administered either separately or as a pre-mixed (biphasic) human insulin preparation (this may be particularly appropriate if HbA1c is 75 mmol/mol (9.0%) or higher);
- Insulin detemir p. 757 or insulin glargine p. 758 as an alternative to human isophane insulin. This can be preferable if a *once daily* injection would be beneficial (for example if assistance is required to inject insulin), or if recurrent symptomatic hypoglycaemic episodes are problematic, or if the patient would otherwise need twice-daily human isophane insulin injections in combination with oral glucose-lowering drugs. Also consider switching to insulin detemir or insulin glargine from human isophane insulin if significant hypoglycaemia is problematic, or in patients who cannot use the device needed to inject human isophane insulin;
- biphasic preparations (pre-mixed) that include a short-acting human *analogue* insulin (rather than short-acting human *soluble insulin*) can be preferable for patients who prefer injecting insulin immediately before a meal, or if

6

Endocrine system

Endocrine system

6

hypoglycaemia is a problem, or if blood-glucose concentrations rise markedly after meals.

When starting insulin therapy, bedtime basal insulin should be initiated and the dose titrated against morning (fasting) glucose. Patients who are prescribed a basal insulin regimen (human isophane insulin, insulin detemir or insulin glargine) should be monitored for the need for short-acting insulin before meals (or a biphasic insulin preparation).

Patients who are prescribed a biphasic insulin should be monitored for the need for a further injection of short-acting insulin before meals or for a change to a basal-bolus regimen with human isophane insulin or insulin detemir or insulin glargine if blood-glucose control remains inadequate. ⟨A⟩

Advanced Pharmacy Services

Patients with type 2 diabetes may be eligible for the New Medicines Service / Medicines Use Review service provided by a community pharmacist. For further information, see *Advanced Pharmacy Services* in Medicines optimisation p. 18.

Useful Resources

Type 2 diabetes in adults: management. National Institute for Health and Care Excellence. Clinical guideline NG28. December 2015.
www.nice.org.uk/guidance/ng28

Pharmacological management of glycaemic control in people with type 2 diabetes. Scottish Intercollegiate Guidelines Network. Clinical guideline 154. November 2017.
www.sign.ac.uk/assets/sign154.pdf

Patient decision aid: Type 2 diabetes in adults: controlling your blood glucose by taking a second medicine—what are your options? National Institute for Health and Care Excellence. December 2015.
www.nice.org.uk/about/what-we-do/our-programmes/nice-guidance/nice-guidelines/shared-decision-making

Diabetic complications

06-Oct-2020

See also

Diabetes p. 722
    Type 1 diabetes p. 723
    Type 2 diabetes p. 726
    Diabetic foot infections, antibacterial therapy p. 534. For guidance on other diabetic foot problems, see NICE guideline **Diabetic foot problems** at:
www.nice.org.uk/guidance/ng19

Diabetes and cardiovascular disease

Diabetes is a strong risk factor for cardiovascular disease. EvGr Other risk factors for cardiovascular disease that should also be addressed are: smoking, hypertension, obesity, and dyslipidaemia. ⟨A⟩ Cardiovascular risk in patients with diabetes can be further reduced by the use of an ACE inhibitor (or an angiotensin-II receptor antagonist) and lipid-regulating drugs. For full guidance on the assessment and prevention of cardiovascular disease, see Cardiovascular disease risk assessment and prevention p. 203.

Diabetic nephropathy

EvGr In diabetic patients with nephropathy, blood pressure should be reduced to the lowest achievable level to slow the rate of decline of glomerular filtration rate and reduce proteinuria. Provided there are no contra-indications, all diabetic patients with nephropathy causing proteinuria or with established microalbuminuria should be treated with an ACE inhibitor or an angiotensin-II receptor antagonist, even if the blood pressure is normal. ACE inhibitors or angiotensin-II receptor antagonists should also be given as monotherapy, or combined therapy, in patients with chronic

kidney disease and proteinuria, to reduce the rate of progression of chronic kidney disease. ⟨A⟩

ACE inhibitors can potentiate the hypoglycaemic effect of insulin and oral antidiabetic drugs; this effect is more likely during the first weeks of combined treatment and in patients with renal impairment.

See also treatment of hypertension in diabetes in Hypertension p. 153.

Diabetic neuropathy

EvGr Optimal diabetic control is beneficial for the management of painful neuropathy. Monotherapy with antidepressant drugs, including tricyclics (such as amitriptyline hydrochloride p. 392 and imipramine hydrochloride p. 396 [unlicensed use]), duloxetine p. 387, and venlafaxine p. 388 [unlicensed use] should be considered in patients for the treatment of painful diabetic peripheral neuropathy. Antiepileptic drugs, such as pregabalin p. 342 and gabapentin p. 332, can also be considered. Opioid analgesics in combination with gabapentin can be considered if pain is not controlled with monotherapy. ⟨A⟩ The MHRA/CHM have released important safety information on antiepileptic drugs and the risk of suicidal thoughts and behaviour, see Epilepsy p. 321; and on opioids and the risk of dependence and addiction, see *Important safety information* in individual drug monographs.

In *autonomic neuropathy*, diabetic diarrhoea can often be managed by tetracycline p. 604 [unlicensed use], or codeine phosphate p. 475 as the best alternative; other antidiarrhoeal preparations can also be tried. Erythromycin p. 572 (especially when given intravenously) may be beneficial for gastroparesis [unlicensed use].

In *neuropathic postural hypotension*, increased salt intake and the use of the mineralcorticoid fludrocortisone acetate p. 715 [unlicensed use] may help by increasing plasma volume, but uncomfortable oedema is a common side-effect. Fludrocortisone can also be combined with flurbiprofen p. 1185 and ephedrine hydrochloride p. 287 [both unlicensed]. Midodrine [unlicensed], an alpha agonist, may also be useful in postural hypotension.

Gustatory sweating can be treated with an antimuscarinic such as propantheline bromide p. 94; side-effects are common. See also, the management of hyperhidrosis (Hyperhidrosis p. 1307).

In some patients with *neuropathic oedema*, ephedrine hydrochloride [unlicensed use] offers effective relief.

See also the management of Erectile dysfunction p. 858.

Visual impairment

EvGr Optimal diabetic control (HbA1c ideally around 7% or 53 mmol/mol) and blood pressure control (<130/80 mmHg) should be maintained to prevent onset and progression of diabetic eye disease. ⟨A⟩

Diabetic ketoacidosis

Management

The management of diabetic ketoacidosis involves the replacement of fluid and electrolytes and the administration of insulin. Guidelines for the Management of Diabetic Ketoacidosis in Adults, published by the Joint British Diabetes Societies Inpatient Care Group (available at www.diabetes.org.uk/Professionals/Position-statements-reports/Specialist-care-for-children-and-adults-and-complications/The-Management-of-Diabetic-Ketoacidosis-in-Adults/), should be followed.

- To restore circulating volume if systolic blood pressure is below 90 mmHg (adjusted for age, sex, and medication as appropriate), give 500 mL **sodium chloride 0.9%** by

intravenous infusion over 10–15 minutes; repeat if blood pressure remains below 90 mmHg and seek senior medical advice.
- When blood pressure is over 90 mmHg, **sodium chloride 0.9%** should be given by intravenous infusion at a rate that replaces deficit and provides maintenance; see guideline or suggested regimen.
- Include **potassium chloride** in the fluids unless anuria is suspected; adjust according to plasma-potassium concentration (measure at 60 minutes, 2 hours, and 2 hourly thereafter; measure hourly if outside the normal range).
- Start an intravenous insulin infusion: **soluble insulin** should be diluted (and **mixed thoroughly**) with **sodium chloride 0.9%** intravenous infusion to a concentration of 1 unit/mL; infuse at a fixed rate of 0.1 units/kg/hour.
- Established subcutaneous therapy with long-acting insulin analogues (insulin detemir p. 757 or insulin glargine p. 758) should be continued during treatment of diabetic ketoacidosis.
- Monitor blood-ketone and blood-glucose concentrations hourly and adjust the insulin infusion rate accordingly. Blood-ketone concentration should fall by at least 0.5 mmol/litre/hour and blood-glucose concentration should fall by at least 3 mmol/litre/hour.
- Once blood-glucose concentration falls below 14 mmol/litre, **glucose 10%** should be given by intravenous infusion (into a large vein through a large-gauge needle) at a rate of 125 mL/hour, in addition to the **sodium chloride 0.9% infusion**.
- Continue insulin infusion until blood-ketone concentration is below 0.3 mmol/litre, blood pH is above 7.3 *and* the patient is able to eat and drink; ideally give subcutaneous fast-acting insulin and a meal, and stop the insulin infusion 1 hour later.

The management of hyperosmolar hyperglycaemic state or hyperosmolar hyperglycaemic nonketotic coma is similar to that of diabetic ketoacidosis, although lower rates of insulin infusion are usually necessary and slower rehydration may be required.

Diabetes, surgery and medical illness
05-Jun-2017

Management of diabetes during surgery

Peri-operative management of blood-glucose concentrations depends on factors including the required duration of fasting, timing of surgery (morning or afternoon), usual treatment regimen (insulin, antidiabetic drugs or diet), prior glycaemic control, other co-morbidities, and the likelihood that the patient will be capable of self-managing their diabetes in the immediate post-operative period. EvGr All patients should have emergency treatment for hypoglycaemia written on their drug chart on admission. Ⓔ

Note: The following recommendations provide general guidance for the management of diabetes during surgery. **Local protocols and guidelines should be followed where they exist.**

Use of insulin during surgery
Elective surgery—minor procedures in patients with good glycaemic control

EvGr Patients usually treated with insulin who have good glycaemic control (HbA1c less than 69 mmol/mol or 8.5 %) and are undergoing *minor procedures*, can be managed during the operative period by adjustment of their usual insulin regimen, which should be adjusted depending on the type of insulin usually prescribed, following detailed local protocols (which should also include intravenous fluid management, monitoring and control of electrolytes and avoidance of hyperchloraemic metabolic acidosis). On the day before the

surgery, the patient's usual insulin should be given as normal, other than once daily long-acting insulin analogues, which should be given at a dose reduced by 20 %. Ⓔ

Elective surgery—major procedures or poor glycaemic control
EvGr Patients usually treated with insulin, who are either undergoing *major procedures* (surgery requiring a long fasting period of more than one missed meal) or whose diabetes is poorly controlled, will usually require a variable rate intravenous insulin infusion (continued until the patient is eating/drinking and stabilised on their previous glucose-lowering medication).

The aim is to achieve and maintain glucose concentration within the usual target range (6–10 mmol/litre; but up to 12 mmol/litre is acceptable) by infusing a constant rate of glucose-containing fluid as a substrate, while also infusing insulin at a variable rate. Detailed local protocols should be consulted. In general, the following steps should be followed:

- on the *day before surgery*, once daily long-acting insulin analogues should be given at 80 % of the usual dose; otherwise the patient's usual insulin should be given as normal;
- on the *day of surgery and throughout the intra-operative period,* once daily long-acting insulin analogues should be continued at 80 % of the usual dose; all other insulin should be stopped until the patient is eating and drinking again after surgery;
- on the *day of surgery*, start an intravenous substrate infusion of potassium chloride with glucose and sodium chloride p. 1088 (based on serum electrolytes which must be measured frequently), and infuse at a rate appropriate to the patient's fluid requirements. To prevent hypoglycaemia, this infusion must **not** be stopped while the insulin infusion is running;
- a variable rate intravenous insulin infusion of soluble human insulin p. 753 in sodium chloride 0.9 % p. 1089 (made either according to locally agreed protocols or using prefilled syringes) should be given via a syringe pump at an initial infusion rate determined by bedside capillary blood-glucose measurement. Hourly blood-glucose measurement should be taken to ensure that the intravenous insulin infusion rate is correct for at least the first 12 hours; the insulin infusion rate should be adjusted according to local protocol to maintain blood-glucose concentrations within the usual target range (6–10 mmol/litre; up to 12 mmol/litre is acceptable);
- intravenous glucose 20 % p. 1090 should be given if blood-glucose drops below 6 mmol/litre, and blood-glucose checked every hour, to prevent a drop below 4 mmol/litre. If blood-glucose drops below 4 mmol/litre, intravenous glucose 20 % should be adjusted and blood-glucose checked every 15 minutes, until blood-glucose is above 6 mmol/litre (testing can then revert to hourly). If blood-glucose rises above 12 mmol/litre, check ketones and consider other signs of diabetic ketoacidosis (see Diabetic ketoacidosis p. 728).

Conversion back to a subcutaneous insulin should not begin until the patient can eat and drink without nausea or vomiting. Once the patient's previous insulin regimen is re-started, the usual insulin dose may require adjustment, as insulin requirements can change due to post-operative stress, infection or altered food intake.

Previous subcutaneous basal-bolus regimens, should be restarted when the first postoperative meal-time insulin dose is due (e.g. with breakfast or lunch); doses may need adjustment due to postoperative stress, infection or altered food intake. The variable rate intravenous insulin infusion and intravenous fluids should be continued until 30–60 minutes **after** the first meal-time short-acting insulin dose. If the patient was previously on a **long-acting insulin analogue**, this should have been continued throughout the operative period at 80 % of the normal dose, and should now

6

Endocrine system

just continue at that same dose until the patient leaves hospital; only the short-acting insulin needs to be restarted as above.

Previous subcutaneous twice-daily mixed insulin regimens, should be restarted before breakfast or an evening meal (not at any other time). The variable rate intravenous insulin infusion should be maintained for 30–60 minutes after the first subcutaneous insulin dose has been given.

Patients who were **previously managed with a continuous subcutaneous insulin infusion** should be referred to a specialist team. The subcutaneous infusion should be restarted at the normal basal rate, not at bedtime, and the insulin infusion continued until the next meal bolus has been given.

Patients **not previously prescribed insulin**, who are to start a subcutaneous insulin regimen post-surgery, should have an insulin dose calculated with advice from a specialist diabetes team, considering the patient's sensitivity to insulin, degree of glycaemic control, weight, age, and the average hourly insulin dose used in the peri-operative period. ⓔ

Emergency surgery

EvGr Patients with diabetes (type 1 and 2) requiring emergency surgery, should always have their blood-glucose, blood or urinary ketone concentration, serum electrolytes and serum bicarbonate checked before surgery. If ketones are high or bicarbonate is low, blood gases should also be checked. If ketoacidosis is present, recommendations for Diabetic ketoacidosis p. 728 should be followed immediately, and surgery delayed if possible. If there is no acidosis, intravenous fluids and an insulin infusion should be started and managed as for *major elective surgery* (above). ⓔ

Use of antidiabetic drugs during surgery

EvGr Manipulation of antidiabetic drug may **not** be appropriate for all surgery or for all patients; particularly when fasting time is more than one missed meal, in patients with poor glycaemic control, and when there is risk of renal injury. In these cases, a *variable rate intravenous insulin infusion* p. 753 should be used for *major elective surgery* (above), and usual antidiabetic medication adjusted in the peri-operative period. Insulin is almost always required in medical and surgical emergencies.

When insulin is required and given during surgery, acarbose p. 731, meglitinides, sulfonylureas, pioglitazone p. 751, dipeptidyl peptidase-4 inhibitors (gliptins) and sodium glucose co-transporter 2 inhibitors should be stopped once the insulin infusion is commenced and not restarted until the patient is eating and drinking normally. Glucagon-like peptide-1 receptor agonists can be continued as normal during the insulin infusion.

If elective *minor surgical procedures* only require a short-fasting period (just one missed meal), it may be possible to adjust antidiabetic drugs to avoid a switch to a variable rate intravenous insulin infusion; normal drug treatment can continue.

In suitable cases, acarbose, nateglinide p. 742 and repaglinide p. 742 can be continued with just the dose omitted on the morning of surgery if fasting (the morning dose may be given if the patient is not fasting and surgery is in the afternoon).

Pioglitazone, **dipeptidylpeptidase-4 inhibitors (gliptins)** and **glucagon-like peptide-1 receptor agonists** can be taken as normal during the whole peri-operative period.

Sodium glucose co-transporter 2 inhibitors should be omitted on the day of surgery and not restarted until the patient is stable; their use during periods of dehydration and acute illness is associated with an increased risk of developing diabetic ketoacidosis.

Sulfonylureas are associated with hypoglycaemia in the fasted state and therefore should always be omitted on the

day of surgery until the patient is eating and drinking again. Capillary blood-glucose should be checked hourly. If hyperglycaemia occurs, an appropriate dose of subcutaneous rapid-acting insulin may be given. A second dose may be given 2 hours later, and a variable rate intravenous insulin infusion considered if hyperglycaemia persists.

Metformin hydrochloride p. 732 is renally excreted; renal impairment may lead to accumulation and lactic acidosis during surgery. If only one meal will be missed during surgery, and the patient has an eGFR greater than 60 mL/minute/1.73m^2 and a low risk of acute kidney injury (and the procedure does not involve administration of contrast media), it may be possible to continue metformin hydrochloride throughout the peri-operative period—just the lunchtime dose should be omitted if the usual dose is prescribed three times a day.

If the patient will miss more than one meal or there is significant risk of the patient developing acute kidney injury, metformin hydrochloride should be stopped when the pre-operative fast begins. A variable rate intravenous insulin infusion should be started if the metformin hydrochloride dose is more than once daily. Otherwise insulin should only be started if blood-glucose concentration is greater than 12 mmol/litre on two consecutive occasions. Metformin should not be recommended until the patient is eating and drinking again, and normal renal function has been assured.

There is no need to stop metformin hydrochloride after contrast medium in patients missing only one meal or who have an eGFR greater than 60 mL/minute/1.73m^2. If contrast medium is to be used, and eGFR is less than 60 mL/minute/1.73m^2, metformin should be omitted on the day of the procedure and for the following 48 hours. ⓔ

Use of antidiabetic drugs during medical illness

Manufacturers of some antidiabetic drugs recommend that they may need to be replaced temporarily with insulin during intercurrent illness when the drug is unlikely to control hyperglycaemia (such as myocardial infarction, coma, severe infection, trauma and other medical emergencies). Consult individual product literature.

Sodium glucose co-transporter 2 inhibitors are associated with increased risk of developing diabetic ketoacidosis during periods of dehydration, stress, surgery, trauma, acute medical illness or any other catabolic state, and should be used with caution during these times. The MHRA has advised (2016) that these drugs should be temporarily stopped in patients who are hospitalised for acute serious illness until the patient is medically stable.

Diabetes, pregnancy and breast-feeding

01-Aug-2017

Description of condition

Diabetes in pregnancy is associated with increased risks to the woman (such as pre-eclampsia and rapidly worsening retinopathy), and to the developing fetus, compared with pregnancy in non-diabetic women. Effective blood-glucose control before conception and throughout pregnancy reduces (but does not eliminate) the risk of adverse outcomes such as miscarriage, congenital malformation, stillbirth, and neonatal death.

Management of pre-existing diabetes

EvGr Women with pre-existing diabetes who are planning on becoming pregnant should aim to keep their HbA1c concentration below 48 mmol/mol (6.5%) if possible without causing problematic hypoglycaemia. Any reduction towards this target is likely to reduce the risk of congenital malformations in the newborn.

Women with pre-existing diabetes who are planning to become pregnant should be advised to take folic acid at the dose for women who are at high-risk of conceiving a child with a neural tube defect, see folic acid p. 1071. ⓐ

Overview

Oral antidiabetic drugs

EvGr All oral antidiabetic drugs, except metformin hydrochloride p. 732, should be discontinued before pregnancy (or as soon as an unplanned pregnancy is identified) and substituted with insulin therapy. Women with diabetes may be treated with metformin hydrochloride [unlicensed in type 1 diabetes] as an adjunct or alternative to insulin in the preconception period and during pregnancy, when the likely benefits from improved blood-glucose control outweigh the potential for harm. Metformin hydrochloride can be continued, or glibenclamide p. 749 resumed, immediately after birth and during breast-feeding for those with pre-existing Type 2 diabetes p. 726. All other antidiabetic drugs should be avoided while breast-feeding. ⓐ

Insulin

Limited evidence suggests that the rapid-acting insulin analogues (insulin aspart p. 753 and insulin lispro p. 755) can be associated with fewer episodes of hypoglycaemia, a reduction in postprandial glucose excursions and an improvement in overall glycaemic control compared with regular human insulin.

EvGr Isophane insulin p. 756 is the first-choice for long-acting insulin during pregnancy, however in women who have good blood-glucose control before pregnancy with the long-acting insulin analogues (insulin detemir p. 757 or insulin glargine p. 758), it may be appropriate to continue using them throughout pregnancy.

Continuous subcutaneous insulin infusion p. 753 (insulin pump therapy) may be appropriate for pregnant women who have difficulty achieving glycaemic control with multiple daily injections of insulin p. 753 without significant disabling hypoglycaemia.

All women treated with insulin p. 753 during pregnancy should be aware of the risks of hypoglycaemia, particularly in the first trimester, and should be advised to always carry a fast-acting form of glucose, such as dextrose tablets or a glucose-containing drink. Pregnant women with Type 1 diabetes p. 723 should also be prescribed glucagon p. 764 for use if needed.

Women with pre-existing diabetes treated with insulin p. 753 during pregnancy are at increased risk of hypoglycaemia in the postnatal period and should reduce their insulin immediately after birth. Blood-glucose levels should be monitored carefully to establish the appropriate dose. ⓐ

Medication for diabetic complications

EvGr Angiotensin-converting enzyme inhibitors and angiotensin II receptor antagonists should be discontinued and replaced with an alternative antihypertensive suitable for use in pregnancy before conception or as soon as pregnancy is confirmed (see *Hypertension in pregnancy* under Hypertension p. 153). Statins should not be prescribed during pregnancy and should be discontinued before a planned pregnancy. ⓐ

Gestational diabetes

EvGr Women with gestational diabetes who have a fasting plasma glucose below 7 mmol/litre at diagnosis, should first attempt a change in diet and exercise alone in order to reduce blood-glucose. If blood-glucose targets are not met within 1 to 2 weeks, metformin hydrochloride p. 732 may be prescribed [unlicensed use]. Insulin p. 753 may be prescribed if metformin is contra-indicated or not acceptable, and may also be added to treatment if metformin is not effective alone.

Women who have a fasting plasma glucose above 7 mmol/litre at diagnosis should be treated with insulin immediately, with or without metformin hydrochloride, in addition to a change in diet and exercise.

Women who have a fasting plasma glucose between 6 and 6.9 mmol/litre alongside complications such as macrosomia or hydramnios should be considered for immediate insulin treatment, with or without metformin hydrochloride.

Glibenclamide p. 749 [unlicensed use] may be considered for women from 11 weeks gestation (after organogenesis) who cannot tolerate metformin, or for those in whom metformin is not effective and do not wish to have insulin therapy.

Women with gestational diabetes should discontinue hypoglycaemic treatment immediately after giving birth. ⓐ

Useful Resources

Management of diabetes. Scottish Intercollegiate Guidelines Network. Clinical guideline 116. March 2010 (updated November 2017).
www.sign.ac.uk/assets/sign116.pdf

Diabetes in pregnancy: management from preconception to the postnatal period. National Institute for Health and Care Excellence. Clinical guideline NG3. February 2015.
www.nice.org.uk/guidance/ng3

BLOOD GLUCOSE LOWERING DRUGS > ALPHA GLUCOSIDASE INHIBITORS

Acarbose
27-Aug-2020

- **DRUG ACTION** Acarbose, an inhibitor of intestinal alpha glucosidases, delays the digestion and absorption of starch and sucrose; it has a small but significant effect in lowering blood glucose.

- **INDICATIONS AND DOSE**

Diabetes mellitus inadequately controlled by diet or by diet with oral antidiabetic drugs
  ▶ BY MOUTH
  ▸ Adult: Initially 50 mg daily, then increased to 50 mg 3 times a day for 6–8 weeks, then increased if necessary to 100 mg 3 times a day (max. per dose 200 mg 3 times a day)

- **CONTRA-INDICATIONS** Disorders of digestion or absorption · hernia (condition may deteriorate) · inflammatory bowel disease · predisposition to intestinal obstruction

- **CAUTIONS** May enhance hypoglycaemic effects of insulin and sulfonylureas (hypoglycaemic episodes may be treated with oral glucose but not with sucrose)

- **INTERACTIONS** → Appendix 1: acarbose

- **SIDE-EFFECTS**
  ▶ **Common or very common** Diarrhoea (may need to reduce dose) · gastrointestinal discomfort · gastrointestinal disorders
  ▶ **Uncommon** Nausea · vomiting
  ▶ **Rare or very rare** Hepatic disorders · oedema
  ▶ **Frequency not known** Acute generalised exanthematous pustulosis (AGEP) · thrombocytopenia

  SIDE-EFFECTS, FURTHER INFORMATION Antacids containing magnesium and aluminium salts unlikely to be beneficial for treating side-effects.

- **PREGNANCY** Avoid.

- **BREAST FEEDING** Avoid.

- **HEPATIC IMPAIRMENT** Manufacturer advises avoid in severe impairment.

- **RENAL IMPAIRMENT** Avoid if eGFR less than 25 mL/minute/1.73 m^2.

- **MONITORING REQUIREMENTS** Monitor liver function.

- **DIRECTIONS FOR ADMINISTRATION** Manufacturer advises tablets should be chewed with first mouthful of food or swallowed whole with a little liquid immediately before food.

- PATIENT AND CARER ADVICE Antacids unlikely to be beneficial for treating side-effects. To counteract possible hypoglycaemia, patients receiving insulin or a sulfonylurea as well as acarbose need to carry glucose (not sucrose—acarbose interferes with sucrose absorption). Patients should be given advice on how to administer acarbose tablets.

- MEDICINAL FORMS There can be variation in the licensing of different medicines containing the same drug.

Tablet
  ‣ Acarbose (Non-proprietary)
    Acarbose 50 mg Acarbose 50mg tablets | 90 tablet [PoM] £14.58 DT = £14.58
    Acarbose 100 mg Acarbose 100mg tablets | 90 tablet [PoM] £25.29 DT = £25.29

BLOOD GLUCOSE LOWERING DRUGS ›
BIGUANIDES

Metformin hydrochloride
10-Nov-2020

- DRUG ACTION Metformin exerts its effect mainly by decreasing gluconeogenesis and by increasing peripheral utilisation of glucose; since it acts only in the presence of endogenous insulin it is effective only if there are some residual functioning pancreatic islet cells.

- ● INDICATIONS AND DOSE

Type 2 diabetes mellitus [monotherapy or in combination with other antidiabetic drugs (including insulin)]
  ‣ BY MOUTH USING IMMEDIATE-RELEASE MEDICINES
  ‣ Child 10–17 years (specialist use only): Initially 500 mg once daily, dose to be adjusted according to response at intervals of at least 1 week, maximum daily dose to be given in 2–3 divided doses; maximum 2 g per day
  ‣ Adult: Initially 500 mg once daily for at least 1 week, dose to be taken with breakfast, then 500 mg twice daily for at least 1 week, dose to be taken with breakfast and evening meal, then 500 mg 3 times a day, dose to be taken with breakfast, lunch and evening meal; maximum 2 g per day
  ‣ BY MOUTH USING MODIFIED-RELEASE MEDICINES
  ‣ Adult: Initially 500 mg once daily, then increased if necessary up to 2 g once daily, dose increased gradually, every 10–15 days, dose to be taken with evening meal, alternatively increased to 1 g twice daily, dose to be taken with meals, alternative dose only to be used if control not achieved with once daily dose regimen. If control still not achieved then change to standard release tablets

Type 2 diabetes mellitus [reduction in risk or delay of onset]
  ‣ BY MOUTH USING MODIFIED-RELEASE MEDICINES
  ‣ Adult 18–74 years: Initially 500 mg once daily, then increased if necessary up to 2 g once daily, dose increased gradually, every 10–15 days, dose to be taken with evening meal, for further information on risk factors—consult product literature

Polycystic ovary syndrome
  ‣ BY MOUTH USING IMMEDIATE-RELEASE MEDICINES
  ‣ Adult: Initially 500 mg once daily for 1 week, dose to be taken with breakfast, then 500 mg twice daily for 1 week, dose to be taken with breakfast and evening meal, then 1.5–1.7 g daily in 2–3 divided doses

- ● UNLICENSED USE
  ‣ In adults [EvGr] Based on clinical experience of increased side-effects, maximum dose for metformin immediate-release medicines in BNF Publications differs from product licence. ⓔ Not licensed for polycystic ovary syndrome.

- CONTRA-INDICATIONS Acute metabolic acidosis (including lactic acidosis and diabetic ketoacidosis)

- CAUTIONS Risk factors for lactic acidosis
  CAUTIONS, FURTHER INFORMATION
  ‣ Risk factors for lactic acidosis Manufacturer advises caution in chronic stable heart failure (monitor cardiac function), and concomitant use of drugs that can acutely impair renal function; interrupt treatment if dehydration occurs, and avoid in conditions that can acutely worsen renal function, or cause tissue hypoxia.
  ‣ Elderly Prescription potentially inappropriate (STOPP criteria) if eGFR less than 30 mL/minute/1.73 m² (risk of lactic acidosis). See also Prescribing in the elderly p. 33.

- INTERACTIONS → Appendix 1: metformin

- SIDE-EFFECTS
  ‣ Common or very common Abdominal pain · appetite decreased · diarrhoea (usually transient) · gastrointestinal disorder · nausea · taste altered · vomiting
  ‣ Rare or very rare Hepatitis · lactic acidosis (discontinue) · skin reactions · vitamin B12 absorption decreased
  SIDE-EFFECTS, FURTHER INFORMATION Gastro-intestinal side-effects are initially common with metformin, and may persist in some patients, particularly when very high doses are given. A slow increase in dose may improve tolerability.

- PREGNANCY Can be used in pregnancy for both pre-existing and gestational diabetes. Women with gestational diabetes should discontinue treatment after giving birth.

- BREAST FEEDING May be used during breast-feeding in women with pre-existing diabetes.

- HEPATIC IMPAIRMENT Withdraw if tissue hypoxia likely.

- RENAL IMPAIRMENT
  ‣ In adults Manufacturer advises avoid if eGFR is less than 30 mL/minute/1.73 m².
  ‣ In children Manufacturer advises avoid if estimated glomerular filtration rate is less than 30 mL/minute/1.73 m².
  Dose adjustments ‣ In children Manufacturer advises consider dose reduction in moderate impairment.
  ‣ In adults Manufacturer advises reduce dose in moderate impairment—consult product literature.

- MONITORING REQUIREMENTS Determine renal function before treatment and at least annually (at least twice a year in patients with additional risk factors for renal impairment, or if deterioration suspected).

- PRESCRIBING AND DISPENSING INFORMATION
  ‣ In adults Patients taking up to 2 g daily of the standard-release metformin may start with the same daily dose of metformin modified release; not suitable if dose of standard-release tablets more than 2 g daily.

- PATIENT AND CARER ADVICE Manufacturer advises that patients and their carers should be informed of the risk of lactic acidosis and told to seek immediate medical attention if symptoms such as dyspnoea, muscle cramps, abdominal pain, hypothermia, or asthenia occur.
  Medicines for Children leaflet: Metformin for diabetes www.medicinesforchildren.org.uk/metformin-diabetes

- NATIONAL FUNDING/ACCESS DECISIONS
  GLUCOPHAGE ® SR For full details see funding body website

  Scottish Medicines Consortium (SMC) decisions
  ‣ Metformin hydrochloride (*Glucophage SR* ®) for type 2 diabetes mellitus (October 2009) SMC No. 148/04 Recommended with restrictions

- MEDICINAL FORMS There can be variation in the licensing of different medicines containing the same drug. Forms available from special-order manufacturers include: capsule, oral suspension, oral solution

Modified-release tablet

CAUTIONARY AND ADVISORY LABELS 21, 25
► Metformin hydrochloride (Non-proprietary)
  Metformin hydrochloride 500 mg Metformin 500mg modified-release tablets | 28 tablet [PoM] £2.51 | 56 tablet [PoM] [▲] DT = £4.00
  Metformin hydrochloride 750 mg Metformin 750mg modified-release tablets | 56 tablet [PoM] [▲] DT = £6.40
  Metformin hydrochloride 1 gram Metformin 1g modified-release tablets | 56 tablet [PoM] [▲] DT = £6.40
► Diagemet XL (Genus Pharmaceuticals Ltd)
  Metformin hydrochloride 500 mg Diagemet XL 500mg tablets | 28 tablet [PoM] £1.49
► Glucient SR (Consilient Health Ltd)
  Metformin hydrochloride 500 mg Glucient SR 500mg tablets | 28 tablet [PoM] £2.51 | 56 tablet [PoM] £5.03 DT = £4.00
  Metformin hydrochloride 750 mg Glucient SR 750mg tablets | 28 tablet [PoM] £3.20
  Metformin hydrochloride 1 gram Glucient SR 1000mg tablets | 28 tablet [PoM] £4.26 | 56 tablet [PoM] £8.52 DT = £6.40
► Glucophage SR (Merck Serono Ltd)
  Metformin hydrochloride 500 mg Glucophage SR 500mg tablets | 28 tablet [PoM] £1.99 | 56 tablet [PoM] £4.00 DT = £4.00
  Metformin hydrochloride 750 mg Glucophage SR 750mg tablets | 28 tablet [PoM] £3.20 | 56 tablet [PoM] £6.40 DT = £6.40
  Metformin hydrochloride 1 gram Glucophage SR 1000mg tablets | 28 tablet [PoM] £3.20 | 56 tablet [PoM] £6.40 DT = £6.40
► Meijumet (Medreich Plc)
  Metformin hydrochloride 500 mg Meijumet 500mg modified-release tablets | 28 tablet [PoM] £2.00 | 56 tablet [PoM] £4.00 DT = £4.00
  Metformin hydrochloride 750 mg Meijumet 750mg modified-release tablets | 28 tablet [PoM] £3.20 | 56 tablet [PoM] £6.40 DT = £6.40
  Metformin hydrochloride 1 gram Meijumet 1000mg modified-release tablets | 28 tablet [PoM] £3.20 | 56 tablet [PoM] £6.40 DT = £6.40
► Metabet SR (Morningside Healthcare Ltd)
  Metformin hydrochloride 500 mg Metabet SR 500mg tablets | 28 tablet [PoM] £2.61 | 56 tablet [PoM] £5.22 DT = £4.00
  Metformin hydrochloride 1 gram Metabet SR 1000mg tablets | 28 tablet [PoM] £4.53 | 56 tablet [PoM] £9.06 DT = £6.40
► Metuxtan SR (Accord Healthcare Ltd)
  Metformin hydrochloride 500 mg Metuxtan SR 500mg tablets | 28 tablet [PoM] £1.99 | 56 tablet [PoM] £5.32 DT = £4.00
► Sukkarto SR (Morningside Healthcare Ltd)
  Metformin hydrochloride 500 mg Sukkarto SR 500mg tablets | 56 tablet [PoM] £2.38 DT = £4.00
  Metformin hydrochloride 750 mg Sukkarto SR 750mg tablets | 56 tablet [PoM] £2.87 DT = £6.40
  Metformin hydrochloride 1 gram Sukkarto SR 1000mg tablets | 56 tablet [PoM] £3.82 DT = £6.40
► Yaltormin SR (Wockhardt UK Ltd)
  Metformin hydrochloride 500 mg Yaltormin SR 500mg tablets | 28 tablet [PoM] £1.20 | 56 tablet [PoM] £2.39 DT = £4.00
  Metformin hydrochloride 750 mg Yaltormin SR 750mg tablets | 28 tablet [PoM] £1.44 | 56 tablet [PoM] £2.88 DT = £6.40
  Metformin hydrochloride 1 gram Yaltormin SR 1000mg tablets | 28 tablet [PoM] £1.92 | 56 tablet [PoM] £3.83 DT = £6.40

Tablet

CAUTIONARY AND ADVISORY LABELS 21
► Metformin hydrochloride (Non-proprietary)
  Metformin hydrochloride 500 mg Metformin 500mg tablets | 28 tablet [PoM] £2.88 DT = £1.61 | 84 tablet [PoM] £2.30–£4.83 | 500 tablet [PoM] £28.75
  Metformin hydrochloride 850 mg Metformin 850mg tablets | 56 tablet [PoM] £2.85 DT = £2.07 | 300 tablet [PoM] £11.09
► Glucophage (Merck Serono Ltd)
  Metformin hydrochloride 500 mg Glucophage 500mg tablets | 84 tablet [PoM] £2.88
  Metformin hydrochloride 850 mg Glucophage 850mg tablets | 56 tablet [PoM] £3.20 DT = £2.07

Oral solution

CAUTIONARY AND ADVISORY LABELS 21
► Metformin hydrochloride (Non-proprietary)
  Metformin hydrochloride 100 mg per 1 ml Metformin 500mg/5ml oral solution sugar free sugar-free | 100 ml [PoM] £4.41–£5.97 sugar-free | 150 ml [PoM] £60.00 DT = £6.61
  Metformin hydrochloride 170 mg per 1 ml Metformin 850mg/5ml oral solution sugar free sugar-free | 150 ml [PoM] £19.95 DT = £19.95
  Metformin hydrochloride 200 mg per 1 ml Metformin 1g/5ml oral solution sugar free sugar-free | 150 ml [PoM] £24.00 DT = £24.00

Combinations available: *Alogliptin with metformin*, p. 734 · *Canagliflozin with metformin*, p. 744 · *Dapagliflozin with metformin*, p. 745 · *Empagliflozin with metformin*, p. 747 · *Linagliptin with metformin*, p. 734 · *Pioglitazone with metformin*, p. 752 · *Saxagliptin with metformin*, p. 735 · *Sitagliptin with metformin*, p. 736 · *Vildagliptin with metformin*, p. 737

BLOOD GLUCOSE LOWERING DRUGS ›
DIPEPTIDYLPEPTIDASE-4 INHIBITORS (GLIPTINS)

| Alogliptin
17-Nov-2020

- DRUG ACTION Inhibits dipeptidylpeptidase-4 to increase insulin secretion and lower glucagon secretion.

- ● INDICATIONS AND DOSE

  Type 2 diabetes mellitus in combination with other antidiabetic drugs (including insulin) if existing treatment fails to achieve adequate glycaemic control
  ► BY MOUTH
  ► Adult: 25 mg once daily, for further information on use with other antidiabetic drugs—consult product literature

  DOSE ADJUSTMENTS DUE TO INTERACTIONS
  ► Dose of concomitant sulfonylurea or insulin may need to be reduced.
  ► Caution with use in combination with both metformin and pioglitazone—risk of hypoglycaemia (dose of metformin or pioglitazone may need to be reduced).

- CONTRA-INDICATIONS Ketoacidosis

- CAUTIONS History of pancreatitis · not recommended in moderate to severe heart failure (limited experience)

- INTERACTIONS → Appendix 1: dipeptidylpeptidase-4 inhibitors

- SIDE-EFFECTS
  ► **Common or very common** Abdominal pain · gastrooesophageal reflux disease · headache · increased risk of infection · skin reactions
  ► **Frequency not known** Angioedema · hepatic function abnormal · pancreatitis acute · Stevens-Johnson syndrome
  SIDE-EFFECTS, FURTHER INFORMATION Discontinue if symptoms of acute pancreatitis occur such as persistent, severe abdominal pain.

- ALLERGY AND CROSS-SENSITIVITY [EvGr] Contra-indicated if history of serious hypersensitivity to dipeptidylpeptidase-4 inhibitors. ⟨M⟩

- PREGNANCY Manufacturer advises avoid—no information available.

- BREAST FEEDING Avoid—present in milk in *animal* studies.

- HEPATIC IMPAIRMENT Manufacturer advises avoid in severe impairment—no information available.

- RENAL IMPAIRMENT Use with caution if eGFR less than 30 mL/minute/1.73 m^2.
  Dose adjustments Reduce dose to 12.5 mg once daily if eGFR 30–50 mL/minute/1.73 m^2.
  Reduce dose to 6.25 mg once daily if eGFR less than 30 mL/minute/1.73 m^2.

- MONITORING REQUIREMENTS Determine renal function before treatment and periodically thereafter.

6

Endocrine system

- MEDICINAL FORMS There can be variation in the licensing of different medicines containing the same drug.

Tablet
- Vipidia (Takeda UK Ltd)
  Alogliptin (as Alogliptin benzoate) 6.25 mg Vipidia 6.25mg tablets | 28 tablet [PoM] £26.60 DT = £26.60
  Alogliptin (as Alogliptin benzoate) 12.5 mg Vipidia 12.5mg tablets | 28 tablet [PoM] £26.60 DT = £26.60
  Alogliptin (as Alogliptin benzoate) 25 mg Vipidia 25mg tablets | 28 tablet [PoM] £26.60 DT = £26.60

Alogliptin with metformin
03-Feb-2020

The properties listed below are those particular to the combination only. For the properties of the components please consider, alogliptin p. 733, metformin hydrochloride p. 732.

- INDICATIONS AND DOSE

Type 2 diabetes mellitus not controlled by metformin alone or by metformin in combination with either pioglitazone or insulin
- BY MOUTH
- Adult: 1 tablet twice daily, based on patient's current metformin dose

- INTERACTIONS → Appendix 1: dipeptidylpeptidase-4 inhibitors · metformin

- MEDICINAL FORMS There can be variation in the licensing of different medicines containing the same drug.

Tablet
CAUTIONARY AND ADVISORY LABELS 21
- Vipdomet (Takeda UK Ltd)
  Alogliptin (as Alogliptin benzoate) 12.5 mg, Metformin hydrochloride 1 gram Vipdomet 12.5mg/1000mg tablets | 56 tablet [PoM] £26.60 DT = £26.60

Linagliptin
16-Oct-2020

- DRUG ACTION Inhibits dipeptidylpeptidase-4 to increase insulin secretion and lower glucagon secretion.

- INDICATIONS AND DOSE

Type 2 diabetes mellitus as monotherapy (if metformin inappropriate), or in combination with other antidiabetic drugs (including insulin) if existing treatment fails to achieve adequate glycaemic control
- BY MOUTH
- Adult: 5 mg once daily, for further information on use with other antidiabetic drugs—consult product literature

DOSE ADJUSTMENTS DUE TO INTERACTIONS
- Dose of concomitant sulfonylurea or insulin may need to be reduced.

- INTERACTIONS → Appendix 1: dipeptidylpeptidase-4 inhibitors

- SIDE-EFFECTS
- **Uncommon** Cough · nasopharyngitis
- **Rare or very rare** Angioedema · skin reactions
- **Frequency not known** Pancreatitis

SIDE-EFFECTS, FURTHER INFORMATION Discontinue if symptoms of acute pancreatitis occur such as persistent, severe abdominal pain.

- PREGNANCY Avoid—no information available.
- BREAST FEEDING Avoid—present in milk in *animal* studies.
- NATIONAL FUNDING/ACCESS DECISIONS
  For full details see funding body website

Scottish Medicines Consortium (SMC) decisions
- Linagliptin (*Trajenta*®) for the treatment of type 2 diabetes mellitus to improve glycaemic control in adults (January 2012) SMC No. 746/11 Recommended with restrictions
- Linagliptin (*Trajenta*®) for the treatment of type 2 diabetes mellitus to improve glycaemic control in adults in combination with insulin or without metformin, when this regimen alone, with diet and exercise, does not provide adequate glycaemic control (May 2015) SMC No. 850/13 Recommended

- MEDICINAL FORMS There can be variation in the licensing of different medicines containing the same drug.

Tablet
- Trajenta (Boehringer Ingelheim Ltd)
  Linagliptin 5 mg Trajenta 5mg tablets | 28 tablet [PoM] £33.26 DT = £33.26

Combinations available: *Empagliflozin with linagliptin*, p. 747

Linagliptin with metformin
20-Nov-2020

The properties listed below are those particular to the combination only. For the properties of the components please consider, linagliptin above, metformin hydrochloride p. 732.

- INDICATIONS AND DOSE

Type 2 diabetes mellitus not controlled by metformin alone or by metformin in combination with either a sulfonylurea or insulin
- BY MOUTH
- Adult: 1 tablet twice daily, based on patient's current metformin dose

- INTERACTIONS → Appendix 1: dipeptidylpeptidase-4 inhibitors · metformin

- NATIONAL FUNDING/ACCESS DECISIONS
  For full details see funding body website
Scottish Medicines Consortium (SMC) decisions
- Linagliptin with metformin (*Jentadueto*®) for the treatment of adult patients with type 2 diabetes mellitus in combination with insulin (i.e. triple combination therapy) as an adjunct to diet and exercise to improve glycaemic control when insulin and metformin do not provide adequate glycaemic control (June 2015) SMC No. 1057/15 Recommended with restrictions

- MEDICINAL FORMS There can be variation in the licensing of different medicines containing the same drug.

Tablet
CAUTIONARY AND ADVISORY LABELS 21
- Jentadueto (Boehringer Ingelheim Ltd)
  Linagliptin 2.5 mg, Metformin hydrochloride 850 mg Jentadueto 2.5mg/850mg tablets | 56 tablet [PoM] £33.26 DT = £33.26
  Linagliptin 2.5 mg, Metformin hydrochloride 1000 mg Jentadueto 2.5mg/1000mg tablets | 56 tablet [PoM] £33.26 DT = £33.26

Saxagliptin
02-Dec-2020

- DRUG ACTION Inhibits dipeptidylpeptidase-4 to increase insulin secretion and lower glucagon secretion.

- INDICATIONS AND DOSE

Type 2 diabetes mellitus as monotherapy (if metformin inappropriate), or in combination with other antidiabetic drugs (including insulin) if existing treatment fails to achieve adequate glycaemic control
- BY MOUTH
- Adult: 5 mg once daily, for further information on use with other antidiabetic drugs—consult product literature

DOSE ADJUSTMENTS DUE TO INTERACTIONS
▶ Dose of concomitant sulfonylurea or insulin may need to be reduced.

● CAUTIONS Elderly · history of pancreatitis · moderate to severe heart failure (limited experience)

● INTERACTIONS → Appendix 1: dipeptidylpeptidase-4 inhibitors

● SIDE-EFFECTS
▶ Common or very common Abdominal pain · dizziness · fatigue · headache · increased risk of infection · skin reactions · vomiting
▶ Uncommon Pancreatitis
▶ Rare or very rare Angioedema
▶ Frequency not known Constipation · nausea
SIDE-EFFECTS, FURTHER INFORMATION Discontinue if symptoms of acute pancreatitis occur such as persistent, severe abdominal pain.

● ALLERGY AND CROSS-SENSITIVITY EvGr Contra-indicated if patient has a history of serious hypersensitivity to dipeptidylpeptidase-4 inhibitors. Ⓜ

● PREGNANCY Avoid unless essential—toxicity in *animal* studies.

● BREAST FEEDING Avoid—present in milk in *animal* studies.

● HEPATIC IMPAIRMENT Manufacturer advises caution in moderate impairment; avoid in severe impairment (risk of increased exposure).

● RENAL IMPAIRMENT Use with caution in severe impairment.
Dose adjustments Reduce dose to 2.5 mg once daily in moderate to severe impairment.

● MONITORING REQUIREMENTS Determine renal function before treatment and periodically thereafter.

● NATIONAL FUNDING/ACCESS DECISIONS
For full details see funding body website
Scottish Medicines Consortium (SMC) decisions
▶ Saxagliptin (*Onglyza*®) in adults with type 2 diabetes mellitus to improve glycaemic control as triple oral therapy in combination with metformin plus a sulfonylurea when this regimen alone, with diet and exercise, does not provide adequate glycaemic control (December 2013) SMC No. 918/13 Recommended with restrictions

● MEDICINAL FORMS There can be variation in the licensing of different medicines containing the same drug.
Tablet
▶ Onglyza (AstraZeneca UK Ltd)
Saxagliptin (as Saxagliptin hydrochloride) 2.5 mg Onglyza 2.5mg tablets | 28 tablet PoM £31.60 DT = £31.60
Saxagliptin (as Saxagliptin hydrochloride) 5 mg Onglyza 5mg tablets | 28 tablet PoM £31.60 DT = £31.60

Saxagliptin with dapagliflozin   25-Aug-2020

The properties listed below are those particular to the combination only. For the properties of the components please consider, saxagliptin p. 734, dapagliflozin p. 744.

● INDICATIONS AND DOSE
Type 2 diabetes mellitus not controlled by metformin and/or a sulfonylurea with either saxagliptin or dapagliflozin
▶ BY MOUTH
▶ Adult 18–74 years: 5/10 mg once daily
▶ Adult 75 years and over: Initiation not recommended
DOSE ADJUSTMENTS DUE TO INTERACTIONS
▶ Dose of concomitant sulfonylurea may need to be reduced.
DOSE EQUIVALENCE AND CONVERSION
▶ Dose expressed as *x/y* mg saxagliptin/dapagliflozin.

● INTERACTIONS → Appendix 1: dipeptidylpeptidase-4 inhibitors · sodium glucose co-transporter 2 inhibitors

● HEPATIC IMPAIRMENT Manufacturer advises caution in moderate impairment; avoid in severe impairment.

● RENAL IMPAIRMENT
Dose adjustments Manufacturer advises avoid if eGFR less than 60 mL/minute/1.73 m² (ineffective).

● PATIENT AND CARER ADVICE
Missed doses Manufacturer advises if a dose is more than 12 hours late, the missed dose should not be taken and the next dose should be taken at the normal time.

● NATIONAL FUNDING/ACCESS DECISIONS
For full details see funding body website
Scottish Medicines Consortium (SMC) decisions
▶ Saxagliptin/dapagliflozin (*Qtern*®) in adults with type 2 diabetes mellitus: to improve glycaemic control when metformin and/or sulfonylurea and one of the monocomponents of *Qtern*® do not provide adequate glycaemic control; when already being treated with the free combination of dapagliflozin and saxagliptin (July 2017) SMC No. 1255/17 Recommended with restrictions

● MEDICINAL FORMS There can be variation in the licensing of different medicines containing the same drug.
Tablet
▶ Qtern (AstraZeneca UK Ltd)
Saxagliptin (as Saxagliptin hydrochloride) 5 mg, Dapagliflozin (as Dapagliflozin propanediol monohydrate) 10 mg Qtern 5mg/10mg tablets | 28 tablet PoM £49.56 DT = £49.56

Saxagliptin with metformin   25-Aug-2020

The properties listed below are those particular to the combination only. For the properties of the components please consider, saxagliptin p. 734, metformin hydrochloride p. 732.

● INDICATIONS AND DOSE
Type 2 diabetes mellitus not controlled by metformin alone or by metformin in combination with either a sulfonylurea or insulin
▶ BY MOUTH
▶ Adult: 1 tablet twice daily, based on patient's current metformin dose

● INTERACTIONS → Appendix 1: dipeptidylpeptidase-4 inhibitors · metformin

● NATIONAL FUNDING/ACCESS DECISIONS
For full details see funding body website
Scottish Medicines Consortium (SMC) decisions
▶ Saxagliptin with metformin (*Komboglyze*®) as an adjunct to diet and exercise to improve glycaemic control in adults with type 2 diabetes mellitus inadequately controlled on their maximally tolerated dose of metformin alone or those already being treated with the combination of saxagliptin and metformin as separate tablets (June 2013) SMC No. 870/13 Recommended with restrictions

● MEDICINAL FORMS There can be variation in the licensing of different medicines containing the same drug.
Tablet
CAUTIONARY AND ADVISORY LABELS 21
▶ Komboglyze (AstraZeneca UK Ltd)
Saxagliptin (as Saxagliptin hydrochloride) 2.5 mg, Metformin hydrochloride 850 mg Komboglyze 2.5mg/850mg tablets | 56 tablet PoM £31.60 DT = £31.60
Saxagliptin (as Saxagliptin hydrochloride) 2.5 mg, Metformin hydrochloride 1 gram Komboglyze 2.5mg/1000mg tablets | 56 tablet PoM £31.60 DT = £31.60

Sitagliptin

11-Nov-2020

- DRUG ACTION Inhibits dipeptidylpeptidase-4 to increase insulin secretion and lower glucagon secretion.

- INDICATIONS AND DOSE

Type 2 diabetes mellitus as monotherapy (if metformin inappropriate), or in combination with other antidiabetic drugs (including insulin) if existing treatment fails to achieve adequate glycaemic control
▸ BY MOUTH
▸ Adult: 100 mg once daily, for further information on use with other antidiabetic drugs—consult product literature

DOSE ADJUSTMENTS DUE TO INTERACTIONS
▸ Dose of concomitant sulfonylurea or insulin may need to be reduced.

- CONTRA-INDICATIONS Ketoacidosis
- INTERACTIONS → Appendix 1: dipeptidylpeptidase-4 inhibitors
- SIDE-EFFECTS
▸ Common or very common Headache
▸ Uncommon Constipation · dizziness · skin reactions
▸ Frequency not known Angioedema · back pain · cutaneous vasculitis · interstitial lung disease · joint disorders · myalgia · pancreatitis acute · renal impairment · Stevens-Johnson syndrome · vomiting

SIDE-EFFECTS, FURTHER INFORMATION Discontinue if symptoms of acute pancreatitis occur such as persistent, severe abdominal pain.

- PREGNANCY Avoid—toxicity in *animal* studies.
- BREAST FEEDING Avoid—present in milk in *animal* studies.
- RENAL IMPAIRMENT
Dose adjustments Manufacturer advises reduce dose to 50 mg once daily if eGFR 30–45 mL/minute/1.73 m². Manufacturer advises reduce dose to 25 mg once daily if eGFR less than 30 mL/minute/1.73 m².
- NATIONAL FUNDING/ACCESS DECISIONS
For full details see funding body website
Scottish Medicines Consortium (SMC) decisions
▸ Sitagliptin (*Januvia*®) as monotherapy for type 2 diabetes mellitus (July 2010) SMC No. 607/10 Recommended with restrictions
▸ Sitagliptin (*Januvia*®) for the treatment of type 2 diabetes mellitus to improve glycaemic control in adults as add-on to insulin (with or without metformin) when diet and exercise plus stable dose of insulin do not provide adequate glycaemic control (September 2015) SMC No. 1083/15 Recommended

- MEDICINAL FORMS There can be variation in the licensing of different medicines containing the same drug.
Tablet
▸ Januvia (Merck Sharp & Dohme Ltd)
Sitagliptin (as Sitagliptin phosphate) 25 mg Januvia 25mg tablets | 28 tablet [PoM] £33.26 DT = £33.26
Sitagliptin (as Sitagliptin phosphate) 50 mg Januvia 50mg tablets | 28 tablet [PoM] £33.26 DT = £33.26
Sitagliptin (as Sitagliptin phosphate) 100 mg Januvia 100mg tablets | 28 tablet [PoM] £33.26 DT = £33.26

Sitagliptin with metformin

18-Nov-2020

The properties listed below are those particular to the combination only. For the properties of the components please consider, sitagliptin above, metformin hydrochloride p. 732.

- INDICATIONS AND DOSE

Type 2 diabetes mellitus not controlled by metformin alone or by metformin in combination with either a sulfonylurea or pioglitazone or insulin
▸ BY MOUTH
▸ Adult: 1 tablet twice daily

- INTERACTIONS → Appendix 1: dipeptidylpeptidase-4 inhibitors · metformin
- NATIONAL FUNDING/ACCESS DECISIONS
For full details see funding body website
Scottish Medicines Consortium (SMC) decisions
▸ Sitagliptin/metformin (*Janumet*®) for type 2 diabetes (May 2010) SMC No. 492/08 Recommended with restrictions
▸ Sitagliptin/metformin (*Janumet*®) in combination with a sulfonylurea (i.e. triple combination therapy) as an adjunct to diet and exercise in patients inadequately controlled on their maximal tolerated dose of metformin and a sulfonylurea (August 2010) SMC No. 627/10 Recommended

- MEDICINAL FORMS There can be variation in the licensing of different medicines containing the same drug.
Tablet
CAUTIONARY AND ADVISORY LABELS 21
▸ Janumet (Merck Sharp & Dohme Ltd)
Sitagliptin (as Sitagliptin phosphate) 50 mg, Metformin hydrochloride 1 gram Janumet 50mg/1000mg tablets | 56 tablet [PoM] £33.26 DT = £33.26

Vildagliptin

19-Nov-2020

- DRUG ACTION Inhibits dipeptidylpeptidase-4 to increase insulin secretion and lower glucagon secretion.

- INDICATIONS AND DOSE

Type 2 diabetes mellitus as monotherapy (if metformin inappropriate), or in combination with other antidiabetic drugs (including insulin) if existing treatment fails to achieve adequate glycaemic control
▸ BY MOUTH
▸ Adult: 50 mg twice daily, reduce dose to 50 mg once daily in the morning when used in dual combination with a sulfonylurea. For further information on use with other antidiabetic drugs—consult product literature

DOSE ADJUSTMENTS DUE TO INTERACTIONS
▸ Dose of concomitant sulfonylurea or insulin may need to be reduced.

- CONTRA-INDICATIONS Ketoacidosis
- CAUTIONS History of pancreatitis · manufacturer advises avoid in severe heart failure—no information available
- INTERACTIONS → Appendix 1: dipeptidylpeptidase-4 inhibitors
- SIDE-EFFECTS
▸ Common or very common Dizziness
▸ Uncommon Arthralgia · constipation · headache · hypoglycaemia · peripheral oedema
▸ Rare or very rare Increased risk of infection
▸ Frequency not known Hepatitis · myalgia · pancreatitis · skin reactions

SIDE-EFFECTS, FURTHER INFORMATION **Pancreatitis**
Discontinue if symptoms of acute pancreatitis occur, such as persistent severe abdominal pain.

Liver toxicity Rare reports of liver dysfunction; discontinue if jaundice or other signs of liver dysfunction occur.

- PREGNANCY Avoid—toxicity in *animal* studies.
- BREAST FEEDING Avoid—present in milk in *animal* studies.
- HEPATIC IMPAIRMENT Manufacturer advises avoid.
- RENAL IMPAIRMENT
  Dose adjustments Reduce dose to 50 mg once daily if eGFR less than 50 mL/minute/1.73 m².
- MONITORING REQUIREMENTS Monitor liver function before treatment and every 3 months for first year and periodically thereafter.
- PATIENT AND CARER ADVICE
  Liver toxicity Patients should be advised to seek prompt medical attention if symptoms such as nausea, vomiting, abdominal pain, fatigue, and dark urine develop.
- NATIONAL FUNDING/ACCESS DECISIONS
  For full details see funding body website
  Scottish Medicines Consortium (SMC) decisions
  ‣ Vildagliptin (*Galvus*®) for the treatment of type 2 diabetes mellitus [as dual oral therapy in combination with metformin] (April 2008) SMC No. 435/07 Recommended with restrictions
  ‣ Vildagliptin (*Galvus*®) for the treatment of type 2 diabetes mellitus [as dual oral therapy in combination with a sulphonylurea] (October 2009) SMC No. 571/09 Recommended
  ‣ Vildagliptin (*Galvus*®) as monotherapy for the treatment of type 2 diabetes mellitus, in patients inadequately controlled by diet and exercise alone and for whom metformin is inappropriate due to contra-indications or intolerance (January 2013) SMC No. 826/12 Recommended with restrictions
  ‣ Vildagliptin (*Galvus*®) for the treatment of type 2 diabetes mellitus in adults as triple oral therapy in combination with a sulphonylurea and metformin when diet and exercise plus dual therapy with these medicinal products do not provide adequate glycaemic control (December 2013) SMC No. 875/13 Recommended with restrictions

- MEDICINAL FORMS There can be variation in the licensing of different medicines containing the same drug.
  Tablet
  ‣ Galvus (Novartis Pharmaceuticals UK Ltd)
    Vildagliptin 50 mg Galvus 50mg tablets | 56 tablet [PoM] £33.35 DT = £33.35

Vildagliptin with metformin   16-Nov-2020

The properties listed below are those particular to the combination only. For the properties of the components please consider, vildagliptin p. 736, metformin hydrochloride p. 732.

- INDICATIONS AND DOSE
  Type 2 diabetes mellitus not controlled by metformin alone or by metformin in combination with either a sulfonylurea or insulin
  ‣ BY MOUTH
  ‣ Adult: 1 tablet twice daily, based on patient's current metformin dose

- INTERACTIONS → Appendix 1: dipeptidylpeptidase-4 inhibitors · metformin
- NATIONAL FUNDING/ACCESS DECISIONS
  For full details see funding body website
  Scottish Medicines Consortium (SMC) decisions
  ‣ Vildagliptin with metformin (*Eucreas*®) for the treatment of type 2 diabetes (July 2008) SMC No. 477/08 Recommended with restrictions

- MEDICINAL FORMS There can be variation in the licensing of different medicines containing the same drug.
  Tablet
  CAUTIONARY AND ADVISORY LABELS 21
  ‣ Eucreas (Novartis Pharmaceuticals UK Ltd)
    Vildagliptin 50 mg, Metformin hydrochloride 850 mg Eucreas 50mg/850mg tablets | 60 tablet [PoM] £35.68 DT = £35.68
    Vildagliptin 50 mg, Metformin hydrochloride 1 gram Eucreas 50mg/1000mg tablets | 60 tablet [PoM] £35.68 DT = £35.68

BLOOD GLUCOSE LOWERING DRUGS ›
GLUCAGON-LIKE PEPTIDE-1 RECEPTOR AGONISTS

Dulaglutide   04-Nov-2020

- DRUG ACTION Dulaglutide is a long-acting glucagon-like peptide 1 (GLP-1) receptor agonist that augments glucose-dependent insulin secretion, and slows gastric emptying.

- INDICATIONS AND DOSE
  Type 2 diabetes mellitus as monotherapy if metformin inappropriate
  ‣ BY SUBCUTANEOUS INJECTION
  ‣ Adult: 0.75 mg once weekly
  Type 2 diabetes mellitus in combination with insulin or other antidiabetic drugs (if existing treatment fails to achieve adequate glycaemic control)
  ‣ BY SUBCUTANEOUS INJECTION
  ‣ Adult: 1.5 mg once weekly
  DOSE ADJUSTMENTS DUE TO INTERACTIONS
  ‣ Dose of concomitant insulin or drugs that stimulate insulin secretion may need to be reduced.

IMPORTANT SAFETY INFORMATION
MHRA/CHM ADVICE: GLP-1 RECEPTOR AGONISTS: REPORTS OF DIABETIC KETOACIDOSIS WHEN CONCOMITANT INSULIN WAS RAPIDLY REDUCED OR DISCONTINUED (JUNE 2019)
Serious and life-threatening cases of diabetic ketoacidosis have been reported in patients with type 2 diabetes mellitus on a combination of a glucagon-like peptide-1 (GLP-1) receptor agonist and insulin, particularly after discontinuation or rapid dose reduction of concomitant insulin. Healthcare professionals are advised that any dose reduction of insulin should be done in a stepwise manner with careful blood glucose self-monitoring, particularly when GLP-1 receptor agonist therapy is initiated. Patients should be informed of the risk factors for and signs and symptoms of diabetic ketoacidosis, and advised to seek immediate medical attention if these develop.

- CONTRA-INDICATIONS Severe gastro-intestinal disease—no information available
- INTERACTIONS → Appendix 1: glucagon-like peptide-1 receptor agonists
- SIDE-EFFECTS
  ‣ **Common or very common** Appetite decreased · atrioventricular block · burping · constipation · diarrhoea · fatigue · gastrointestinal discomfort · gastrointestinal disorders · hypoglycaemia · nausea · sinus tachycardia · vomiting
  ‣ **Rare or very rare** Anaphylactic reaction · angioedema · pancreatitis acute (discontinue)
- PREGNANCY Manufacturer advises avoid—toxicity in *animal* studies.
- BREAST FEEDING Manufacturer advises avoid— no information available.
- HANDLING AND STORAGE **Refrigerated storage** is usually necessary (2 °C – 8 °C). Once in use, may be stored unrefrigerated for up to 14 days at a temperature not above 30 °C.

6

Endocrine system

- PATIENT AND CARER ADVICE Patients or carers should be given advice on how to administer dulaglutide injection. Acute pancreatitis Patients should be told how to recognise signs and symptoms of acute pancreatitis and advised to seek medical attention if symptoms such as persistent, severe abdominal pain develop.
  Missed doses If a dose is missed, it should be administered as soon as possible only if there are at least 3 days until the next scheduled dose; if less than 3 days remain before the next scheduled dose, the missed dose should not be taken and the next dose should be taken at the normal time.
- NATIONAL FUNDING/ACCESS DECISIONS
  For full details see funding body website
  Scottish Medicines Consortium (SMC) decisions
  ‣ Dulaglutide (*Trulicity*®) for use in adults with type 2 diabetes mellitus to improve glycaemic control as add-on therapy in combination with other glucose-lowering medicinal products including insulin, when these, together with diet and exercise, do not provide adequate glycaemic control (January 2016) SMC No. 1110/15 Recommended with restrictions

- MEDICINAL FORMS There can be variation in the licensing of different medicines containing the same drug.
  Solution for injection
  ‣ Trulicity (Eli Lilly and Company Ltd)
  Dulaglutide 1.5 mg per 1 ml Trulicity 0.75mg/0.5ml solution for injection pre-filled pens | 4 pre-filled disposable injection [PoM]
  £73.25 DT = £73.25
  Dulaglutide 3 mg per 1 ml Trulicity 1.5mg/0.5ml solution for injection pre-filled pens | 4 pre-filled disposable injection [PoM]
  £73.25 DT = £73.25

Exenatide

09-Nov-2020

- DRUG ACTION Binds to, and activates, the GLP-1 (glucagon-like peptide-1) receptor to increase insulin secretion, suppresses glucagon secretion, and slows gastric emptying.

- INDICATIONS AND DOSE
  Type 2 diabetes mellitus in combination with metformin or a sulfonylurea, or both, or with pioglitazone, or with both metformin and pioglitazone, in patients who have not achieved adequate glycaemic control with these drugs alone or in combination
  ‣ BY SUBCUTANEOUS INJECTION USING IMMEDIATE-RELEASE MEDICINES
  ‣ Adult: Initially 5 micrograms twice daily for at least 1 month, then increased if necessary up to 10 micrograms twice daily, dose to be taken within 1 hour before 2 main meals (at least 6 hours apart)
  ‣ BY SUBCUTANEOUS INJECTION USING MODIFIED-RELEASE MEDICINES
  ‣ Adult: 2 mg once weekly

  Type 2 diabetes mellitus in combination with basal insulin alone or with metformin or pioglitazone (or both)
  ‣ BY SUBCUTANEOUS INJECTION USING IMMEDIATE-RELEASE MEDICINES
  ‣ Adult: Initially 5 micrograms twice daily for at least 1 month, then increased if necessary up to 10 micrograms twice daily, dose to be taken within 1 hour before 2 main meals (at least 6 hours apart)

  DOSE ADJUSTMENTS DUE TO INTERACTIONS
  ‣ Dose of concomitant sulfonylurea may need to be reduced.

PHARMACOKINETICS
‣ Effect of *modified-release* exenatide injection (*Bydureon*®) may persist for 10 weeks after discontinuation.

IMPORTANT SAFETY INFORMATION

MHRA/CHM ADVICE: GLP-1 RECEPTOR AGONISTS: REPORTS OF DIABETIC KETOACIDOSIS WHEN CONCOMITANT INSULIN WAS RAPIDLY REDUCED OR DISCONTINUED (JUNE 2019)
Serious and life-threatening cases of diabetic ketoacidosis have been reported in patients with type 2 diabetes mellitus on a combination of a glucagon-like peptide-1 (GLP-1) receptor agonist and insulin, particularly after discontinuation or rapid dose reduction of concomitant insulin. Healthcare professionals are advised that any dose reduction of insulin should be done in a stepwise manner with careful blood glucose self-monitoring, particularly when GLP-1 receptor agonist therapy is initiated. Patients should be informed of the risk factors for and signs and symptoms of diabetic ketoacidosis, and advised to seek immediate medical attention if these develop.

- CONTRA-INDICATIONS Ketoacidosis · severe gastrointestinal disease
- CAUTIONS Elderly · may cause weight loss greater than 1.5 kg weekly · pancreatitis
- INTERACTIONS → Appendix 1: glucagon-like peptide-1 receptor agonists
- SIDE-EFFECTS
  ‣ **Common or very common** Appetite decreased · asthenia · constipation · diarrhoea · dizziness · gastrointestinal discomfort · gastrointestinal disorders · headache · nausea · skin reactions · vomiting
  ‣ **Uncommon** Alopecia · burping · drowsiness · hyperhidrosis · renal impairment · taste altered
  ‣ **Frequency not known** Angioedema · pancreatitis acute
  SIDE-EFFECTS, FURTHER INFORMATION Severe pancreatitis (sometimes fatal), including haemorrhagic or necrotising pancreatitis, has been reported rarely; discontinue permanently if diagnosed.
- CONCEPTION AND CONTRACEPTION Women of child-bearing age should use effective contraception during treatment with modified-release exenatide and for 12 weeks after discontinuation.
- PREGNANCY Avoid—toxicity in *animal* studies.
- BREAST FEEDING Avoid—no information available.
- RENAL IMPAIRMENT For *standard-release* injection, use with caution if eGFR 30–50 mL/minute/1.73 m². For *standard-release* injection, avoid if eGFR less than 30 mL/minute/1.73 m². For *modified-release* injection, avoid if eGFR less than 50 mL/minute/1.73 m².
- PATIENT AND CARER ADVICE Patients changing from standard-release to modified-release exenatide formulation may experience initial transient increase in blood glucose. Some oral medications should be taken at least 1 hour before or 4 hours after exenatide injection—consult product literature for details. Patients or their carers should be told how to recognise signs and symptoms of pancreatitis and advised to seek prompt medical attention if symptoms such as abdominal pain, nausea, and vomiting develop.
  Missed doses If a dose of the immediate-release medicine is missed, continue with the next scheduled dose—do not administer **after** a meal.
- NATIONAL FUNDING/ACCESS DECISIONS
  For full details see funding body website

Scottish Medicines Consortium (SMC) decisions

▸ Exenatide (*Byetta*®) for the treatment of type 2 diabetes mellitus (July 2007) SMC No. 376/07 Recommended with restrictions

▸ Exenatide (*Byetta*®) for the treatment of type 2 diabetes mellitus in combination with metformin and a thiazolidinedione (March 2011) SMC No. 684/11 Recommended with restrictions

▸ Exenatide (*Bydureon*®) for the treatment of type 2 diabetes mellitus (January 2012) SMC No. 748/11 Recommended with restrictions

▸ Exenatide (*Byetta*®) as adjunctive therapy to basal insulin with or without metformin and/or pioglitazone in adults with type 2 diabetes who have not achieved adequate glycaemic control with these agents (June 2012) SMC No. 785/12 Recommended

● MEDICINAL FORMS There can be variation in the licensing of different medicines containing the same drug.

Solution for injection
CAUTIONARY AND ADVISORY LABELS 10
▸ Byetta (AstraZeneca UK Ltd)
　Exenatide 250 microgram per 1 ml Byetta 5micrograms/0.02ml solution for injection 1.2ml pre-filled pens | 1 pre-filled disposable injection PoM £81.89 DT = £81.89
　Byetta 10micrograms/0.04ml solution for injection 2.4ml pre-filled pens | 1 pre-filled disposable injection PoM £81.89 DT = £81.89

Powder and solvent for prolonged-release suspension for injection
CAUTIONARY AND ADVISORY LABELS 10
▸ Bydureon (AstraZeneca UK Ltd)
　Exenatide 2 mg Bydureon 2mg powder and solvent for prolonged-release suspension for injection pre-filled pens | 4 pre-filled disposable injection PoM £73.36 DT = £73.36

Liraglutide
　　　　　　　　　　　　　　　　　　　　　　06-Nov-2020

● DRUG ACTION Liraglutide binds to, and activates, the GLP-1 (glucagon-like peptide-1) receptor to increase insulin secretion, suppresses glucagon secretion, and slows gastric emptying.

● INDICATIONS AND DOSE

SAXENDA ®

Adjunct in weight management [in conjunction with dietary measures and increased physical activity in individuals with a body mass index (BMI) of 30 kg/m² or more, or in individuals with a BMI of 27 kg/m² or more in the presence of at least one weight-related co-morbidity]
▸ BY SUBCUTANEOUS INJECTION
▸ Adult: Initially 0.6 mg once daily, then increased in steps of 0.6 mg, dose to be increased at intervals of at least 1 week; consider discontinuation if escalation to the next dose is not tolerated for 2 consecutive weeks. Discontinue if at least 5% of initial body-weight has not been lost after 12 weeks at maximum dose; maximum 3 mg per day

VICTOZA ®

Type 2 diabetes mellitus [monotherapy (if metformin inappropriate), or in combination with other antidiabetic drugs]
▸ BY SUBCUTANEOUS INJECTION
▸ Adult: Initially 0.6 mg once daily for at least 1 week, then increased to 1.2 mg once daily for at least 1 week, then increased if necessary to 1.8 mg once daily, for information on use with other antidiabetic drugs—consult product literature

DOSE ADJUSTMENTS DUE TO INTERACTIONS
▸ Dose of concomitant insulin or sulfonylurea may need to be reduced.

IMPORTANT SAFETY INFORMATION
MHRA/CHM ADVICE: GLP-1 RECEPTOR AGONISTS: REPORTS OF DIABETIC KETOACIDOSIS WHEN CONCOMITANT INSULIN WAS RAPIDLY REDUCED OR DISCONTINUED (JUNE 2019)
▸ When used for Type 2 diabetes mellitus
Serious and life-threatening cases of diabetic ketoacidosis have been reported in patients with type 2 diabetes mellitus on a combination of a glucagon-like peptide-1 (GLP-1) receptor agonist and insulin, particularly after discontinuation or rapid dose reduction of concomitant insulin. Healthcare professionals are advised that any dose reduction of insulin should be done in a stepwise manner with careful blood glucose self-monitoring, particularly when GLP-1 receptor agonist therapy is initiated. Patients should be informed of the risk factors for and signs and symptoms of diabetic ketoacidosis, and advised to seek immediate medical attention if these develop.

● CONTRA-INDICATIONS Diabetic gastroparesis · inflammatory bowel disease
SAXENDA ® Concomitant use with other products for weight management · elderly 75 years or over (limited information) · obesity secondary to endocrinological or eating disorders
VICTOZA ® Diabetic ketoacidosis

● CAUTIONS Severe congestive heart failure (no information available) · thyroid disease

● INTERACTIONS → Appendix 1: glucagon-like peptide-1 receptor agonists

● SIDE-EFFECTS
▸ **Common or very common** Appetite decreased · asthenia · burping · constipation · diarrhoea · dizziness · dry mouth · gallbladder disorders · gastrointestinal discomfort · gastrointestinal disorders · headache · increased risk of infection · insomnia · nausea · skin reactions · taste altered · toothache · vomiting
▸ **Uncommon** Dehydration · malaise · pancreatitis · renal impairment · tachycardia
▸ **Frequency not known** Angioedema · dyspnoea · hypotension · oedema · palpitations · pancreatitis acute (discontinue permanently) · thyroid disorder
SIDE-EFFECTS, FURTHER INFORMATION Discontinue if symptoms of acute pancreatitis occur, such as persistent, severe abdominal pain.

● PREGNANCY Manufacturer advises avoid—toxicity in *animal* studies (recommendation also supported by tertiary sources).

● BREAST FEEDING Manufacturer advises avoid—no information available; *animal* studies suggest that transfer into milk is low, but excretion into human milk not known (a tertiary source confirms lack of information in human lactation, but also states that risk to infants appears to be negligible. EvGr Blood glucose monitoring of the infant should be considered). ⓓ

● HEPATIC IMPAIRMENT
SAXENDA ® Manufacturer advises use with caution in mild to moderate impairment; avoid in severe impairment (risk of decreased exposure).
VICTOZA ® Manufacturer advises avoid in severe impairment (risk of decreased exposure).

● RENAL IMPAIRMENT
SAXENDA ® Manufacturer advises avoid if creatinine clearance less than 30 mL/minute.
VICTOZA ® Manufacturer advises avoid in end-stage renal disease.

6

Endocrine system

- HANDLING AND STORAGE Manufacturer advises store in a refrigerator (2–8°C)—after first use can also be stored below 30°C and used within 1 month; keep cap on pen to protect from light.
- PATIENT AND CARER ADVICE Manufacturer advises patients and their carers should be told how to recognise signs and symptoms of acute pancreatitis and advised to seek immediate medical attention if symptoms develop. Manufacturer advises patients and their carers should be informed of the potential risk of dehydration in relation to gastro-intestinal side-effects and advised to take precautions to avoid fluid depletion; they should also be informed of the symptoms of cholelithiasis and cholecystitis, and of increased heart rate.

  SAXENDA® **Missed doses** Manufacturer advises if a dose is more than 12 hours late, the missed dose should not be taken and the next dose should be taken at the normal time.
- MEDICINAL FORMS There can be variation in the licensing of different medicines containing the same drug.

  Solution for injection
  - ▸ Saxenda (Novo Nordisk Ltd)
    Liraglutide 6 mg per 1 ml Saxenda 6mg/ml solution for injection 3ml pre-filled pens | 3 pre-filled disposable injection PoM £117.72 | 5 pre-filled disposable injection PoM £196.20
  - ▸ Victoza (Novo Nordisk Ltd)
    Liraglutide 6 mg per 1 ml Victoza 6mg/ml solution for injection 3ml pre-filled pens | 2 pre-filled disposable injection PoM £78.48 DT = £78.48 | 3 pre-filled disposable injection PoM £117.72

  Combinations available: *Insulin degludec with liraglutide,* p. 757

Lixisenatide

10-Nov-2020

- DRUG ACTION Binds to, and activates, the GLP-1 (glucagon-like peptide-1) receptor to increase insulin secretion, suppresses glucagon secretion, and slows gastric emptying.

- INDICATIONS AND DOSE

  Type 2 diabetes mellitus in combination with oral antidiabetic drugs (e.g. metformin, pioglitazone, or a sulfonylurea) or basal insulin, or both, when adequate glycaemic control has not been achieved with these drugs
  - ▸ BY SUBCUTANEOUS INJECTION
  - ▸ Adult: Initially 10 micrograms once daily for 14 days, then increased to 20 micrograms once daily, dose to be taken within 1 hour before the first meal of the day or the evening meal

  DOSE ADJUSTMENTS DUE TO INTERACTIONS
  - ▸ Dose of concomitant sulfonylurea or insulin may need to be reduced.

IMPORTANT SAFETY INFORMATION

MHRA/CHM ADVICE: GLP-1 RECEPTOR AGONISTS: REPORTS OF DIABETIC KETOACIDOSIS WHEN CONCOMITANT INSULIN WAS RAPIDLY REDUCED OR DISCONTINUED (JUNE 2019)

Serious and life-threatening cases of diabetic ketoacidosis have been reported in patients with type 2 diabetes mellitus on a combination of insulin and the glucagon-like peptide-1 (GLP-1) receptor agonist exenatide, liraglutide, or dulaglutide, particularly after discontinuation or rapid dose reduction of concomitant insulin. The MHRA has not currently received any UK reports of diabetic ketoacidosis with the GLP-1 receptor agonists lixisenatide and semaglutide but this risk cannot be excluded. Healthcare professionals are advised that any dose reduction of insulin should be done in a stepwise manner with careful blood glucose self-monitoring, particularly when GLP-1 receptor agonist

---

therapy is initiated. Patients should be informed of the risk factors for and signs and symptoms of diabetic ketoacidosis, and advised to seek immediate medical attention if these develop.

- CONTRA-INDICATIONS Ketoacidosis · severe gastro-intestinal disease
- CAUTIONS History of pancreatitis
- INTERACTIONS → Appendix 1: glucagon-like peptide-1 receptor agonists
- SIDE-EFFECTS
  - ▸ **Common or very common** Back pain · cystitis · diarrhoea · dizziness · drowsiness · dyspepsia · headache · increased risk of infection · nausea · vomiting
  - ▸ **Uncommon** Urticaria
  - ▸ **Frequency not known** Pancreatitis acute

  SIDE-EFFECTS, FURTHER INFORMATION Manufacturer advises discontinue if symptoms of acute pancreatitis occur, such as persistent, severe abdominal pain.
- CONCEPTION AND CONTRACEPTION Women of child-bearing age should use effective contraception.
- PREGNANCY Avoid—toxicity in *animal* studies.
- BREAST FEEDING Avoid—no information available.
- RENAL IMPAIRMENT Use with caution if eGFR 30–50 mL/minute/1.73 m². Avoid if eGFR less than 30 mL/minute/1.73 m²—no information available.
- PATIENT AND CARER ADVICE Some oral medications should be taken at least 1 hour before or 4 hours after lixisenatide injection—consult product literature for details.
  Missed doses If a dose is missed, inject within 1 hour before the next meal—do not administer **after** a meal.
- NATIONAL FUNDING/ACCESS DECISIONS
  For full details see funding body website

  Scottish Medicines Consortium (SMC) decisions
  - ▸ Lixisenatide (*Lyxumia*®) for the treatment of adults with type 2 diabetes mellitus to achieve glycaemic control in combination with oral glucose-lowering medicinal products and/or basal insulin when these, together with diet and exercise, do not provide adequate glycaemic control (September 2013) SMC No. 903/13 Recommended with restrictions

---

- MEDICINAL FORMS There can be variation in the licensing of different medicines containing the same drug.

  Solution for injection
  CAUTIONARY AND ADVISORY LABELS 10
  - ▸ Lyxumia (Sanofi)
    Lixisenatide 50 microgram per 1 ml Lyxumia 10micrograms/0.2ml solution for injection 3ml pre-filled pens | 1 pre-filled disposable injection PoM £31.67 DT = £31.67
    Lixisenatide 100 microgram per 1 ml Lyxumia 20micrograms/0.2ml solution for injection 3ml pre-filled pens | 2 pre-filled disposable injection PoM £57.93 DT = £57.93

  Combinations available: *Insulin glargine with lixisenatide,* p. 758

Semaglutide

10-Nov-2020

- **DRUG ACTION** Semaglutide binds to, and activates, the GLP-1 (glucagon-like peptide-1) receptor to increase insulin secretion, suppress glucagon secretion, and slow gastric emptying.

- **INDICATIONS AND DOSE**

Type 2 diabetes mellitus [monotherapy (if metformin inappropriate) or in combination with other antidiabetic drugs]
▸ BY SUBCUTANEOUS INJECTION
▸ Adult: Initially 0.25 mg once weekly for 4 weeks, then increased to 0.5 mg once weekly for at least 4 weeks, then increased if necessary to 1 mg once weekly, for information on use with other antidiabetic drugs—consult product literature
▸ BY MOUTH
▸ Adult: Initially 3 mg once daily for 1 month, then increased to 7 mg once daily for at least 1 month, then increased if necessary to 14 mg once daily, dose to be taken on an empty stomach, for information on use with other antidiabetic drugs—consult product literature, one 14 mg tablet should be used to achieve a 14 mg dose; use of two 7 mg tablets to achieve a 14 mg dose has not been studied and is therefore not recommended; maximum 14 mg per day

DOSE ADJUSTMENTS DUE TO INTERACTIONS
▸ Manufacturer advises dose of concomitant insulin or sulfonylurea may need to be reduced.

DOSE EQUIVALENCE AND CONVERSION
▸ Oral semaglutide 14 mg once daily is comparable to subcutaneous semaglutide 0.5 mg once weekly. Due to the high pharmacokinetic variability of oral semaglutide, the effect of switching between oral and subcutaneous semaglutide cannot easily be predicted.

IMPORTANT SAFETY INFORMATION
MHRA/CHM ADVICE: GLP-1 RECEPTOR AGONISTS: REPORTS OF DIABETIC KETOACIDOSIS WHEN CONCOMITANT INSULIN WAS RAPIDLY REDUCED OR DISCONTINUED (JUNE 2019)
Serious and life-threatening cases of diabetic ketoacidosis have been reported in patients with type 2 diabetes mellitus on a combination of insulin and the glucagon-like peptide-1 (GLP-1) receptor agonist exenatide, liraglutide, or dulaglutide, particularly after discontinuation or rapid dose reduction of concomitant insulin. The MHRA has not currently received any UK reports of diabetic ketoacidosis with the GLP-1 receptor agonists lixisenatide and semaglutide but this risk cannot be excluded. Healthcare professionals are advised that any dose reduction of insulin should be done in a stepwise manner with careful blood glucose self-monitoring, particularly when GLP-1 receptor agonist therapy is initiated. Patients should be informed of the risk factors for and signs and symptoms of diabetic ketoacidosis, and advised to seek immediate medical attention if these develop.

- **CONTRA-INDICATIONS** Diabetic ketoacidosis
- **CAUTIONS** Diabetic retinopathy (in patients treated with insulin) · history of pancreatitis · severe congestive heart failure (no information available)
- **INTERACTIONS** → Appendix 1: glucagon-like peptide-1 receptor agonists
- **SIDE-EFFECTS**
▸ **Common or very common** Appetite decreased · burping · cholelithiasis · constipation · diarrhoea · dizziness · fatigue · gastrointestinal discomfort · gastrointestinal disorders · hypoglycaemia (in combination with insulin or sulfonylurea) · nausea · vomiting · weight decreased

▸ **Uncommon** Pancreatitis acute · taste altered
SIDE-EFFECTS, FURTHER INFORMATION Discontinue if symptoms of acute pancreatitis occur, such as persistent, severe abdominal pain.

- **CONCEPTION AND CONTRACEPTION** Manufacturer advises women of childbearing potential should use effective contraception during and for at least two months after stopping treatment.
- **PREGNANCY** Manufacturer advises avoid—toxicity in *animal* studies.
- **BREAST FEEDING** Manufacturer advises avoid—present in milk in *animal* studies.
- **HEPATIC IMPAIRMENT** Manufacturer advises caution (limited information in severe impairment).
- **RENAL IMPAIRMENT** Manufacturer advises avoid in end-stage renal disease.
- **DIRECTIONS FOR ADMINISTRATION**
▸ With oral use Manufacturer advises tablets should be taken whole on an empty stomach, with a sip of water (up to half a glass, equivalent to 120 mL). Patients should wait at least 30 minutes after a dose before eating, drinking, or taking other oral medicines—intake with food or large volumes of water decreases the absorption of semaglutide.
- **PRESCRIBING AND DISPENSING INFORMATION** Semaglutide is a biological medicine. Biological medicines must be prescribed and dispensed by brand name, see *Biological medicines* and *Biosimilar medicines*, under Guidance on prescribing p. 1; manufacturer advises to record the brand name and batch number after each administration.
- **HANDLING AND STORAGE**
▸ With subcutaneous use Manufacturer advises store injection pens in a refrigerator (2–8°C)—after first use can also be stored below 30°C; keep cap on pen to protect from light.
- **PATIENT AND CARER ADVICE**
▸ With oral use Patients or carers should be given advice on how to administer semaglutide tablets.
▸ Acute pancreatitis Manufacturer advises patients and their carers should be told how to recognise signs and symptoms of acute pancreatitis and advised to seek immediate medical attention if symptoms develop.
Missed doses ▸ With subcutaneous use Manufacturer advises if a dose is more than 5 days late, the missed dose should not be taken and the next dose should be administered at the normal time.
▸ With oral use Manufacturer advises if a dose is missed, the missed dose should not be taken and the next dose should be taken at the normal time.
- **NATIONAL FUNDING/ACCESS DECISIONS**
For full details see funding body website
Scottish Medicines Consortium (SMC) decisions
▸ Semaglutide (*Ozempic*®) for the treatment of adults with insufficiently controlled type 2 diabetes mellitus as an adjunct to diet and exercise (January 2019) SMC No. SMC2092 Recommended with restrictions
▸ Semaglutide (*Rybelsus*®) for the treatment of adults with insufficiently controlled type 2 diabetes to improve glycaemic control as an adjunct to diet and exercise: as monotherapy when metformin is considered inappropriate due to intolerance or contra-indications; or in combination with other medicinal products for the treatment of diabetes (September 2020) SMC No. SMC2287 Recommended with restrictions

- **MEDICINAL FORMS** There can be variation in the licensing of different medicines containing the same drug.
Solution for injection
▸ Ozempic (Novo Nordisk Ltd) ▼
  Semaglutide 1.34 mg per 1 ml Ozempic 0.25mg/0.19ml solution for injection 1.5ml pre-filled pens | 1 pre-filled disposable injection PoM
  £73.25 DT = £73.25

6

Endocrine system

Ozempic 0.5mg/0.37ml solution for injection 1.5ml pre-filled pens | 1 pre-filled disposable injection [PoM] £73.25 DT = £73.25
Ozempic 1mg/0.74ml solution for injection 3ml pre-filled pens | 1 pre-filled disposable injection [PoM] £73.25 DT = £73.25

Tablet

CAUTIONARY AND ADVISORY LABELS 25
▸ Rybelsus (Novo Nordisk Ltd) ▼
Semaglutide 3 mg Rybelsus 3mg tablets | 30 tablet [PoM] £78.48
Semaglutide 7 mg Rybelsus 7mg tablets | 30 tablet [PoM] £78.48
Semaglutide 14 mg Rybelsus 14mg tablets | 30 tablet [PoM] £78.48

BLOOD GLUCOSE LOWERING DRUGS ›
MEGLITINIDES

Nateglinide

25-Feb-2020

● DRUG ACTION Nateglinide stimulates insulin secretion.

● **INDICATIONS AND DOSE**

Type 2 diabetes mellitus in combination with metformin when metformin alone inadequate
▸ BY MOUTH
▸ Adult: Initially 60 mg 3 times a day (max. per dose 180 mg), adjusted according to response, to be taken within 30 minutes before main meals

● CONTRA-INDICATIONS Ketoacidosis
● CAUTIONS Debilitated patients · elderly · malnourished patients

CAUTIONS, FURTHER INFORMATION Manufacturer advises patients exposed to stress (including fever, trauma, infection or surgery) may require treatment interruption and temporary replacement with insulin to maintain glycaemic control.

● INTERACTIONS → Appendix 1: meglitinides
● SIDE-EFFECTS
▸ **Common or very common** Diarrhoea · gastrointestinal discomfort · hypoglycaemia · nausea
▸ **Uncommon** Vomiting
▸ **Rare or very rare** Skin reactions
▸ **Frequency not known** Appetite increased · dizziness · fatigue · muscle weakness · palpitations · sweating abnormal · tremor
● PREGNANCY Avoid—toxicity in *animal* studies.
● BREAST FEEDING Avoid—present in milk in *animal* studies.
● HEPATIC IMPAIRMENT Manufacturer advises caution in moderate impairment; avoid in severe impairment (no information available).
● PATIENT AND CARER ADVICE
Driving and skilled tasks Drivers need to be particularly careful to avoid hypoglycaemia and should be warned of the problems.

● MEDICINAL FORMS No licensed medicines listed.

Repaglinide

14-Feb-2020

● DRUG ACTION Repaglinide stimulates insulin secretion.

● **INDICATIONS AND DOSE**

Type 2 diabetes mellitus (as monotherapy or in combination with metformin when metformin alone inadequate)
▸ BY MOUTH
▸ Adult: Initially 500 micrograms (max. per dose 4 mg), adjusted according to response, dose to be taken within 30 minutes before main meals and adjusted at intervals of 1–2 weeks; maximum 16 mg per day

Type 2 diabetes mellitus (as monotherapy or in combination with metformin when metformin alone inadequate), if transferring from another oral antidiabetic drug
▸ BY MOUTH
▸ Adult: Initially 1 mg (max. per dose 4 mg), adjusted according to response, dose to be taken within 30 minutes before main meals and adjusted at intervals of 1–2 weeks; maximum 16 mg per day

● CONTRA-INDICATIONS Ketoacidosis
● CAUTIONS Debilitated patients · elderly (no information available) · malnourished patients

CAUTIONS, FURTHER INFORMATION Manufacturer advises patients exposed to stress (including fever, trauma, infection or surgery) may require treatment interruption and temporary replacement with insulin to maintain glycaemic control.

● INTERACTIONS → Appendix 1: meglitinides
● SIDE-EFFECTS
▸ **Common or very common** Abdominal pain · diarrhoea · hypoglycaemia
▸ **Rare or very rare** Cardiovascular disease · constipation · hepatic function abnormal · vasculitis · vision disorders · vomiting
▸ **Frequency not known** Acute coronary syndrome · hypoglycaemic coma · nausea · skin reactions
● PREGNANCY Avoid.
● BREAST FEEDING Avoid—present in milk in *animal* studies.
● HEPATIC IMPAIRMENT Manufacturer advises avoid in severe impairment (risk of increased exposure).
● RENAL IMPAIRMENT Use with caution.
● PATIENT AND CARER ADVICE
Driving and skilled tasks Drivers need to be particularly careful to avoid hypoglycaemia and should be warned of the problems.

● MEDICINAL FORMS There can be variation in the licensing of different medicines containing the same drug.
Tablet
▸ Repaglinide (Non-proprietary)
Repaglinide 500 microgram Repaglinide 500microgram tablets | 30 tablet [PoM] £0.91–£3.33 | 90 tablet [PoM] £10.00 DT = £4.34
Repaglinide 1 mg Repaglinide 1mg tablets | 30 tablet [PoM] £2.00–£3.53 | 90 tablet [PoM] £10.58 DT = £6.00
Repaglinide 2 mg Repaglinide 2mg tablets | 90 tablet [PoM] £10.50 DT = £3.98
▸ Enyglid (Consilient Health Ltd)
Repaglinide 500 microgram Enyglid 0.5mg tablets | 30 tablet [PoM] £3.33 | 90 tablet [PoM] £9.99 DT = £4.34
Repaglinide 1 mg Enyglid 1mg tablets | 30 tablet [PoM] £3.33 | 90 tablet [PoM] £9.99 DT = £6.00
Repaglinide 2 mg Enyglid 2mg tablets | 90 tablet [PoM] £9.99 DT = £3.98
▸ Prandin (Novo Nordisk Ltd)
Repaglinide 500 microgram Prandin 0.5mg tablets | 30 tablet [PoM] £3.92
Repaglinide 1 mg Prandin 1mg tablets | 30 tablet [PoM] £3.92
Repaglinide 2 mg Prandin 2mg tablets | 90 tablet [PoM] £11.76 DT = £3.98

BLOOD GLUCOSE LOWERING DRUGS ⟩ SODIUM
GLUCOSE CO-TRANSPORTER 2 INHIBITORS

Canagliflozin
15-Sep-2020

- **DRUG ACTION** Reversibly inhibits sodium-glucose co-
transporter 2 (SGLT2) in the renal proximal convoluted
tubule to reduce glucose reabsorption and increase urinary
glucose excretion.

- **INDICATIONS AND DOSE**

**Type 2 diabetes mellitus as monotherapy (if metformin
inappropriate)** | **Type 2 diabetes mellitus in combination
with insulin or other antidiabetic drugs (if existing
treatment fails to achieve adequate glycaemic control)**
▸ BY MOUTH
▸ Adult: 100 mg once daily; increased if tolerated to
300 mg once daily if required, dose to be taken
preferably before breakfast
DOSE ADJUSTMENTS DUE TO INTERACTIONS
▸ Manufacturer advises increase dose if tolerated to
300 mg once daily with concurrent use of rifampicin.
▸ Dose of concomitant insulin or drugs that stimulate
insulin secretion may need to be reduced.

IMPORTANT SAFETY INFORMATION

MHRA/CHM ADVICE (UPDATED APRIL 2016): RISK OF DIABETIC
KETOACIDOSIS WITH SODIUM-GLUCOSE CO-TRANSPORTER 2
(SGLT2) INHIBITORS (CANAGLIFLOZIN, DAPAGLIFLOZIN OR
EMPAGLIFLOZIN)
A review by the European Medicines Agency has
concluded that serious, life-threatening, and fatal cases
of diabetic ketoacidosis (DKA) have been reported rarely
in patients taking an SGLT2 inhibitor. In several cases,
the presentation of DKA was atypical with patients
having only moderately elevated blood glucose levels,
and some of them occurred during off-label use.
  To minimise the risk of such effects when treating
patients with a SGLT2 inhibitor, the European Medicines
Agency has issued the following advice:
- inform patients of the signs and symptoms of DKA,
(including rapid weight loss, nausea or vomiting,
abdominal pain, fast and deep breathing, sleepiness, a
sweet smell to the breath, a sweet or metallic taste in
the mouth, or a different odour to urine or sweat), and
advise them to seek immediate medical advice if they
develop any of these
- test for raised ketones in patients with signs and
symptoms of DKA, even if plasma glucose levels are
near-normal
- use canagliflozin with caution in patients with risk
factors for DKA, (including a low beta cell reserve,
conditions leading to restricted food intake or severe
dehydration, sudden reduction in insulin, increased
insulin requirements due to acute illness, surgery or
alcohol abuse), and discuss these risk factors with
patients
- discontinue treatment if DKA is suspected or
diagnosed
- do not restart treatment with any SGLT2 inhibitor in
patients who experienced DKA during use, unless
another cause for DKA was identified and resolved
- interrupt SGLT2 inhibitor treatment in patients who
are hospitalised for major surgery or acute serious
illnesses; treatment may be restarted once the
patient's condition has stabilised

MHRA/CHM ADVICE: SGLT2 INHIBITORS: MONITOR KETONES IN
BLOOD DURING TREATMENT INTERRUPTION FOR SURGICAL
PROCEDURES OR ACUTE SERIOUS MEDICAL ILLNESS (MARCH
2020)
New recommendations have been issued following a
European review of peri-operative diabetic ketoacidosis

in patients taking SGLT2 inhibitors. Healthcare
professionals are advised to monitor ketone levels
during SGLT2 inhibitor treatment interruption in
patients who have been hospitalised for major surgery or
acute serious illness—measurement of blood ketone
levels is preferred to urine. Treatment may be restarted
once ketone levels are normal and the patient's
condition has stabilised.

MHRA/CHM ADVICE (UPDATED MARCH 2017): INCREASED RISK OF
LOWER-LIMB AMPUTATION (MAINLY TOES)
Canagliflozin may increase the risk of lower-limb
amputation (mainly toes) in patients with type 2
diabetes. Preventive foot care is important for all
patients with diabetes. The MHRA has issued the
following advice while clinical trials are ongoing:
- consider stopping canagliflozin if a patient develops a
significant lower limb complication (e.g. skin ulcer,
osteomyelitis, or gangrene)
- carefully monitor patients who have risk factors for
amputation (e.g. previous amputations, existing
peripheral vascular disease, or neuropathy)
- monitor all patients for signs and symptoms of water
or salt loss; ensure patients stay sufficiently hydrated
to prevent volume depletion in line with the
manufacturer's recommendations
- advise patients to stay well hydrated, carry out routine
preventive foot care, and seek medical advice promptly
if they develop skin ulceration, discolouration, or new
pain or tenderness
- start treatment for foot problems (e.g. ulceration,
infection, or new pain or tenderness) as early as
possible
- continue to follow standard treatment guidelines for
routine preventive foot care for people with diabetes.

MHRA/CHM ADVICE: SGLT2 INHIBITORS: REPORTS OF FOURNIER'S
GANGRENE (NECROTISING FASCIITIS OF THE GENITALIA OR
PERINEUM) (FEBRUARY 2019)
Fournier's gangrene, a rare but serious and potentially
life-threatening infection, has been associated with the
use of sodium-glucose co-transporter 2 (SGLT2)
inhibitors. If Fournier's gangrene is suspected, stop the
SGLT2 inhibitor and urgently start treatment (including
antibiotics and surgical debridement).
  Patients should be advised to seek urgent medical
attention if they experience severe pain, tenderness,
erythema, or swelling in the genital or perineal area,
accompanied by fever or malaise—urogenital infection
or perineal abscess may precede necrotising fasciitis.

- **CONTRA-INDICATIONS** Ketoacidosis
- **CAUTIONS** Elderly (risk of volume depletion) · elevated
haematocrit · hypotension · risk of volume depletion
CAUTIONS, FURTHER INFORMATION
▸ Volume depletion Correct hypovolaemia before starting
treatment.
- **INTERACTIONS** → Appendix 1: sodium glucose co-
transporter 2 inhibitors
- **SIDE-EFFECTS**
▸ **Common or very common** Balanoposthitis · constipation ·
dyslipidaemia · hypoglycaemia (in combination with
insulin or sulfonylurea) · increased risk of infection ·
nausea · thirst · urinary disorders · urosepsis
▸ **Uncommon** Dehydration · dizziness postural · hypotension
· lower limb amputations · renal failure · skin reactions ·
syncope
▸ **Rare or very rare** Anaphylactic reaction · angioedema ·
diabetic ketoacidosis (discontinue immediately)
▸ **Frequency not known** Fournier's gangrene (discontinue
and initiate treatment promptly)
SIDE-EFFECTS, FURTHER INFORMATION Consider
interrupting treatment if volume depletion occurs.

- PREGNANCY Avoid—toxicity in *animal* studies.
- BREAST FEEDING Avoid—present in milk in *animal* studies.
- HEPATIC IMPAIRMENT Manufacturer advises avoid in severe impairment—no information available.
- RENAL IMPAIRMENT Avoid initiation if eGFR less than 60 mL/minute/1.73 m². Avoid if eGFR less than 45 mL/minute/1.73 m².
  Dose adjustments Reduce dose to 100 mg once daily if eGFR falls persistently below 60 mL/minute/1.73 m² and existing canagliflozin treatment tolerated.
  Monitoring Monitor renal function at least twice a year in moderate impairment.
- MONITORING REQUIREMENTS Determine renal function before treatment and at least annually thereafter, and before initiation of concomitant drugs that reduce renal function and periodically thereafter.
- PATIENT AND CARER ADVICE Patients should be advised to report symptoms of volume depletion including postural hypotension and dizziness. Patients should be informed of the signs and symptoms of diabetic ketoacidosis, see MHRA advice.
- NATIONAL FUNDING/ACCESS DECISIONS
  For full details see funding body website
  NICE decisions
  ▸ Canagliflozin, dapagliflozin and empagliflozin as monotherapies for treating type 2 diabetes (May 2016) NICE TA390 Recommended with restrictions
  ▸ Canagliflozin in combination therapy for treating type 2 diabetes (June 2014) NICE TA315 Recommended with restrictions
- MEDICINAL FORMS There can be variation in the licensing of different medicines containing the same drug.
  Tablet
  ▸ Invokana (Napp Pharmaceuticals Ltd)
  Canagliflozin (as Canagliflozin hemihydrate) 100 mg Invokana 100mg tablets | 30 tablet [PoM] £39.20 DT = £39.20
  Canagliflozin (as Canagliflozin hemihydrate) 300 mg Invokana 300mg tablets | 30 tablet [PoM] £39.20 DT = £39.20

Canagliflozin with metformin
21-Aug-2020

The properties listed below are those particular to the combination only. For the properties of the components please consider, canagliflozin p. 743, metformin hydrochloride p. 732.

- ● INDICATIONS AND DOSE
  Type 2 diabetes mellitus not controlled by metformin alone or by metformin in combination with insulin or other antidiabetic drugs
  ▸ BY MOUTH
  ▸ Adult: 1 tablet twice daily, dose based on patient's current metformin dose, daily dose of metformin should not exceed 2 g
  DOSE ADJUSTMENTS DUE TO INTERACTIONS
  ▸ Dose of concomitant insulin or drugs that stimulate insulin secretion may need to be reduced.
- INTERACTIONS → Appendix 1: metformin · sodium glucose co-transporter 2 inhibitors
- RENAL IMPAIRMENT Avoid if eGFR less than 60 mL/minute/1.73 m².
- NATIONAL FUNDING/ACCESS DECISIONS
  For full details see funding body website
  Scottish Medicines Consortium (SMC) decisions
  ▸ Canagliflozin plus metformin (*Vokanamet®*) in adults aged 18 years and older with type 2 diabetes mellitus as an adjunct to diet and exercise to improve glycaemic control (January 2015) SMC No. 1019/14 Recommended with restrictions

- MEDICINAL FORMS There can be variation in the licensing of different medicines containing the same drug.
  Tablet
  CAUTIONARY AND ADVISORY LABELS 21
  ▸ Vokanamet (Napp Pharmaceuticals Ltd)
  Canagliflozin (as Canagliflozin hemihydrate) 50 mg, Metformin hydrochloride 850 mg Vokanamet 50mg/850mg tablets | 60 tablet [PoM] £39.20 DT = £39.20
  Canagliflozin (as Canagliflozin hemihydrate) 50 mg, Metformin hydrochloride 1 gram Vokanamet 50mg/1000mg tablets | 60 tablet [PoM] £39.20 DT = £39.20

Dapagliflozin
04-Nov-2020

- DRUG ACTION Reversibly inhibits sodium-glucose co-transporter 2 (SGLT2) in the renal proximal convoluted tubule to reduce glucose reabsorption and increase urinary glucose excretion.

- ● INDICATIONS AND DOSE
  Type 2 diabetes mellitus [as monotherapy if metformin inappropriate] | Type 2 diabetes mellitus [in combination with insulin or other antidiabetic drugs]
  ▸ BY MOUTH
  ▸ Adult: 10 mg once daily
  Type 1 diabetes mellitus [as an adjunct to insulin in patients with a BMI greater than or equal to 27 kg/m², when insulin alone fails to achieve adequate glycaemic control]
  ▸ BY MOUTH
  ▸ Adult: 5 mg once daily
  DOSE ADJUSTMENTS DUE TO INTERACTIONS
  ▸ Dose of concomitant insulin or drugs that stimulate insulin secretion may need to be reduced (risk of hypoglycaemia)—consult product literature.

IMPORTANT SAFETY INFORMATION

MHRA/CHM ADVICE (UPDATED APRIL 2016): RISK OF DIABETIC KETOACIDOSIS WITH SODIUM-GLUCOSE CO-TRANSPORTER 2 (SGLT2) INHIBITORS (CANAGLIFLOZIN, DAPAGLIFLOZIN OR EMPAGLIFLOZIN)

A review by the European Medicines Agency has concluded that serious, life-threatening, and fatal cases of diabetic ketoacidosis (DKA) have been reported rarely in patients taking an SGLT2 inhibitor. In several cases, the presentation of DKA was atypical with patients having only moderately elevated blood glucose levels, and some of them occurred during off-label use.

To minimise the risk of such effects when treating patients with a SGLT2 inhibitor, the European Medicines Agency has issued the following advice:
- inform patients of the signs and symptoms of DKA, (including rapid weight loss, nausea or vomiting, abdominal pain, fast and deep breathing, sleepiness, a sweet smell to the breath, a sweet or metallic taste in the mouth, or a different odour to urine or sweat), and advise them to seek immediate medical advice if they develop any of these
- test for raised ketones in patients with signs and symptoms of DKA, even if plasma glucose levels are near-normal
- use dapagliflozin with caution in patients with risk factors for DKA, (including a low beta cell reserve, conditions leading to restricted food intake or severe dehydration, sudden reduction in insulin, increased insulin requirements due to acute illness, surgery or alcohol abuse), and discuss these risk factors with patients
- discontinue treatment if DKA is suspected or diagnosed

- do not restart treatment with any SGLT2 inhibitor in patients who experienced DKA during use, unless another cause for DKA was identified and resolved
- interrupt SGLT2 inhibitor treatment in patients who are hospitalised for major surgery or acute serious illnesses; treatment may be restarted once the patient's condition has stabilised

MHRA/CHM ADVICE: SGLT2 INHIBITORS: MONITOR KETONES IN BLOOD DURING TREATMENT INTERRUPTION FOR SURGICAL PROCEDURES OR ACUTE SERIOUS MEDICAL ILLNESS (MARCH 2020)

New recommendations have been issued following a European review of peri-operative diabetic ketoacidosis in patients taking SGLT2 inhibitors. Healthcare professionals are advised to monitor ketone levels during SGLT2 inhibitor treatment interruption in patients who have been hospitalised for major surgery or acute serious illness—measurement of blood ketone levels is preferred to urine. Treatment may be restarted once ketone levels are normal and the patient's condition has stabilised.

MHRA/CHM ADVICE: SGLT2 INHIBITORS: REPORTS OF FOURNIER'S GANGRENE (NECROTISING FASCIITIS OF THE GENITALIA OR PERINEUM) (FEBRUARY 2019)

Fournier's gangrene, a rare but serious and potentially life-threatening infection, has been associated with the use of sodium-glucose co-transporter 2 (SGLT2) inhibitors. If Fournier's gangrene is suspected, stop the SGLT2 inhibitor and urgently start treatment (including antibiotics and surgical debridement).

Patients should be advised to seek urgent medical attention if they experience severe pain, tenderness, erythema, or swelling in the genital or perineal area, accompanied by fever or malaise—urogenital infection or perineal abscess may precede necrotising fasciitis.

- CONTRA-INDICATIONS
▸ When used for type 1 diabetes mellitus High risk of diabetic ketoacidosis (consult product literature)
- CAUTIONS Elderly (risk of volume depletion) · hypotension · raised haematocrit · risk of volume depletion

CAUTIONS, FURTHER INFORMATION
▸ Volume depletion Correct hypovolaemia before starting treatment.
- INTERACTIONS → Appendix 1: sodium glucose co-transporter 2 inhibitors
- SIDE-EFFECTS
▸ **Common or very common** Back pain · balanoposthitis · diabetic ketoacidosis (discontinue immediately) · dizziness · dyslipidaemia · hypoglycaemia (in combination with insulin or sulfonylurea) · increased risk of infection · rash · urinary disorders
▸ **Uncommon** Constipation · dry mouth · genital pruritus · hypovolaemia · thirst · vulvovaginal pruritus · weight decreased
▸ **Rare or very rare** Angioedema · Fournier's gangrene (discontinue and initiate treatment promptly)

SIDE-EFFECTS, FURTHER INFORMATION Interrupt treatment if volume depletion occurs.
- PREGNANCY Avoid—toxicity in *animal* studies.
- BREAST FEEDING Avoid—present in milk in *animal* studies.
- HEPATIC IMPAIRMENT Manufacturer advises caution in severe impairment (risk of increased exposure, limited information available).
Dose adjustments
▸ When used for Type 2 diabetes mellitus Manufacturer advises initially 5 mg daily in severe impairment, increased if tolerated to 10 mg daily.
- RENAL IMPAIRMENT Manufacturer advises avoid initiation if eGFR less than 60 mL/minute/1.73 m^2 (reduced efficacy).

Manufacturer advises avoid if eGFR persistently less than 45 mL/minute/1.73 m^2 (reduced efficacy). If eGFR less than 60 mL/minute/1.73 m^2 manufacturer advises monitor renal function at least 2–4 times per year.
- MONITORING REQUIREMENTS
▸ Manufacturer advises monitor renal function before treatment, and at least annually thereafter.
▸ When used for Type 1 diabetes mellitus Manufacturer advises patients should monitor ketone levels before starting and during treatment (blood ketone levels are preferred to urine)—consult product literature.
- PATIENT AND CARER ADVICE Patients should be informed of the signs and symptoms of diabetic ketoacidosis, see MHRA advice.
- NATIONAL FUNDING/ACCESS DECISIONS
For full details see funding body website
NICE decisions
▸ Dapagliflozin in combination therapy for treating type 2 diabetes (updated November 2016) NICE TA288 Recommended with restrictions
▸ Canagliflozin, dapagliflozin and empagliflozin as monotherapies for treating type 2 diabetes (May 2016) NICE TA390 Recommended with restrictions
▸ Dapagliflozin in triple therapy for treating type 2 diabetes (November 2016) NICE TA418 Recommended with restrictions
▸ Dapagliflozin with insulin for treating type 1 diabetes (updated February 2020) NICE TA597 Recommended with restrictions
Scottish Medicines Consortium (SMC) decisions
▸ Dapagliflozin (*Forxiga*®) in adults for the treatment of insufficiently controlled T1DM as an adjunct to insulin in patients with BMI ≥ 27 kg/m^2, when insulin alone does not provide adequate glycaemic control despite optimal insulin therapy (September 2019) SMC No. SMC2185 Recommended

- MEDICINAL FORMS There can be variation in the licensing of different medicines containing the same drug.
Tablet
▸ Forxiga (AstraZeneca UK Ltd)
   Dapagliflozin (as Dapagliflozin propanediol monohydrate) **5 mg** Forxiga 5mg tablets | 28 tablet [PoM] £36.59 DT = £36.59
   Dapagliflozin (as Dapagliflozin propanediol monohydrate) **10 mg** Forxiga 10mg tablets | 28 tablet [PoM] £36.59 DT = £36.59

Combinations available: *Saxagliptin with dapagliflozin*, p. 735

Dapagliflozin with metformin   04-Nov-2020

The properties listed below are those particular to the combination only. For the properties of the components please consider, dapagliflozin p. 744, metformin hydrochloride p. 732.

- INDICATIONS AND DOSE

Type 2 diabetes mellitus [not controlled by metformin alone, or by metformin in combination with other antidiabetic drugs (including insulin)]
▸ BY MOUTH
▸ Adult: 1 tablet twice daily, based on patient's current metformin dose

- INTERACTIONS → Appendix 1: metformin · sodium glucose co-transporter 2 inhibitors
- HEPATIC IMPAIRMENT Manufacturer advises avoid (increased risk of lactic acidosis).
- NATIONAL FUNDING/ACCESS DECISIONS
For full details see funding body website
Scottish Medicines Consortium (SMC) decisions
▸ Dapagliflozin with metformin (*Xigduo*®) for use in adults with type 2 diabetes mellitus as an adjunct to diet and exercise to improve glycaemic control: in patients inadequately controlled on their maximally tolerated dose of

6

Endocrine system

metformin alone; in combination with other glucose-lowering medicinal products, including insulin, in patients inadequately controlled with metformin and these medicinal products; in patients already being treated with the combination of dapagliflozin and metformin as separate tablets (August 2014) SMC No. 983/14 Recommended with restrictions

- MEDICINAL FORMS There can be variation in the licensing of different medicines containing the same drug.

Tablet
CAUTIONARY AND ADVISORY LABELS 21
- Xigduo (AstraZeneca UK Ltd)
  Dapagliflozin (as Dapagliflozin propanediol monohydrate) 5 mg, Metformin hydrochloride 850 mg Xigduo 5mg/850mg tablets | 56 tablet [PoM] £36.59 DT = £36.59
  Dapagliflozin (as Dapagliflozin propanediol monohydrate) 5 mg, Metformin hydrochloride 1 gram Xigduo 5mg/1000mg tablets | 56 tablet [PoM] £36.59 DT = £36.59

Empagliflozin

15-Sep-2020

- DRUG ACTION Reversibly inhibits sodium-glucose co-transporter 2 (SGLT2) in the renal proximal convoluted tubule to reduce glucose reabsorption and increase urinary glucose excretion.

- INDICATIONS AND DOSE

Type 2 diabetes mellitus as monotherapy (if metformin inappropriate) | Type 2 diabetes mellitus in combination with insulin or other antidiabetic drugs (if existing treatment fails to achieve adequate glycaemic control)
- BY MOUTH
- Adult 18–84 years: 10 mg once daily, increased to 25 mg once daily if necessary and if tolerated
- Adult 85 years and over: Initiation not recommended
DOSE ADJUSTMENTS DUE TO INTERACTIONS
- Dose of concomitant insulin or drugs that stimulate insulin secretion may need to be reduced.

IMPORTANT SAFETY INFORMATION

MHRA/CHM ADVICE (UPDATED APRIL 2016): RISK OF DIABETIC KETOACIDOSIS WITH SODIUM-GLUCOSE CO-TRANSPORTER 2 (SGLT2) INHIBITORS (CANAGLIFLOZIN, DAPAGLIFLOZIN OR EMPAGLIFLOZIN)

A review by the European Medicines Agency has concluded that serious, life-threatening, and fatal cases of diabetic ketoacidosis (DKA) have been reported rarely in patients taking an SGLT2 inhibitor. In several cases, the presentation of DKA was atypical with patients having only moderately elevated blood glucose levels, and some of them occurred during off-label use.

To minimise the risk of such effects when treating patients with a SGLT2 inhibitor, the European Medicines Agency has issued the following advice:
- inform patients of the signs and symptoms of DKA, (including rapid weight loss, nausea or vomiting, abdominal pain, fast and deep breathing, sleepiness, a sweet smell to the breath, a sweet or metallic taste in the mouth, or a different odour to urine or sweat), and advise them to seek immediate medical advice if they develop any of these
- test for raised ketones in patients with signs and symptoms of DKA, even if plasma glucose levels are near-normal
- use empagliflozin with caution in patients with risk factors for DKA, (including a low beta cell reserve, conditions leading to restricted food intake or severe dehydration, sudden reduction in insulin, increased insulin requirements due to acute illness, surgery or alcohol abuse), and discuss these risk factors with patients

- discontinue treatment if DKA is suspected or diagnosed
- do not restart treatment with any SGLT2 inhibitor in patients who experienced DKA during use, unless another cause for DKA was identified and resolved
- interrupt SGLT2 inhibitor treatment in patients who are hospitalised for major surgery or acute serious illnesses; treatment may be restarted once the patient's condition has stabilised

MHRA/CHM ADVICE: SGLT2 INHIBITORS: MONITOR KETONES IN BLOOD DURING TREATMENT INTERRUPTION FOR SURGICAL PROCEDURES OR ACUTE SERIOUS MEDICAL ILLNESS (MARCH 2020)

New recommendations have been issued following a European review of peri-operative diabetic ketoacidosis in patients taking SGLT2 inhibitors. Healthcare professionals are advised to monitor ketone levels during SGLT2 inhibitor treatment interruption in patients who have been hospitalised for major surgery or acute serious illness—measurement of blood ketone levels is preferred to urine. Treatment may be restarted once ketone levels are normal and the patient's condition has stabilised.

MHRA/CHM ADVICE: SGLT2 INHIBITORS: REPORTS OF FOURNIER'S GANGRENE (NECROTISING FASCIITIS OF THE GENITALIA OR PERINEUM) (FEBRUARY 2019)

Fournier's gangrene, a rare but serious and potentially life-threatening infection, has been associated with the use of sodium-glucose co-transporter 2 (SGLT2) inhibitors. If Fournier's gangrene is suspected, stop the SGLT2 inhibitor and urgently start treatment (including antibiotics and surgical debridement).

Patients should be advised to seek urgent medical attention if they experience severe pain, tenderness, erythema, or swelling in the genital or perineal area, accompanied by fever or malaise—urogenital infection or perineal abscess may precede necrotising fasciitis.

- CONTRA-INDICATIONS Diabetic ketoacidosis
- CAUTIONS Complicated urinary tract infections—consider temporarily interrupting treatment · elderly (risk of volume depletion) · hypotension · risk of volume depletion
CAUTIONS, FURTHER INFORMATION
- Volume depletion Manufacturer advises correct hypovolaemia before starting treatment. Consider interrupting treatment if volume depletion occurs.
- INTERACTIONS → Appendix 1: sodium glucose co-transporter 2 inhibitors
- SIDE-EFFECTS
- Common or very common Balanoposthitis · hypoglycaemia (in combination with insulin or sulfonylurea) · increased risk of infection · skin reactions · thirst · urinary disorders · urosepsis
- Uncommon Hypovolaemia
- Rare or very rare Diabetic ketoacidosis (discontinue immediately)
- Frequency not known Angioedema · Fournier's gangrene (discontinue and initiate treatment promptly)
- PREGNANCY Manufacturer advises avoid—toxicity in *animal* studies.
- BREAST FEEDING Manufacturer advises avoid—present in milk in *animal* studies.
- HEPATIC IMPAIRMENT Manufacturer advises avoid in severe impairment—no information available.
- RENAL IMPAIRMENT Avoid initiation if eGFR below 60 mL/minute/1.73 m^2. Avoid if eGFR is persistently below 45 mL/minute/1.73 m^2.
  Dose adjustments Reduce dose to 10 mg once daily if eGFR falls persistently below 60 mL/minute/1.73 m^2.
- MONITORING REQUIREMENTS Determine renal function before treatment and before initiation of concomitant

drugs that may reduce renal function, then at least annually thereafter.

- **PATIENT AND CARER ADVICE** Patients should be informed of the signs and symptoms of diabetic ketoacidosis, see MHRA advice.
- **NATIONAL FUNDING/ACCESS DECISIONS** For full details see funding body website

NICE decisions

▸ Canagliflozin, dapagliflozin and empagliflozin as monotherapies for treating type 2 diabetes (May 2016) NICE TA390 Recommended with restrictions

▸ Empagliflozin in combination therapy for treating type 2 diabetes (March 2015) NICE TA336 Recommended with restrictions

- **MEDICINAL FORMS** There can be variation in the licensing of different medicines containing the same drug.

Tablet
▸ Jardiance (Boehringer Ingelheim Ltd)
  Empagliflozin 10 mg Jardiance 10mg tablets | 28 tablet `PoM`
  £36.59 DT = £36.59
  Empagliflozin 25 mg Jardiance 25mg tablets | 28 tablet `PoM`
  £36.59 DT = £36.59

Empagliflozin with linagliptin   04-Nov-2020

The properties listed below are those particular to the combination only. For the properties of the components please consider, empagliflozin p. 746, linagliptin p. 734.

- **INDICATIONS AND DOSE**

Type 2 diabetes mellitus [not controlled by metformin and/or a sulfonylurea with either empagliflozin or linagliptin]
▸ BY MOUTH
▸ Adult 18–74 years: 10/5 mg once daily, increased to 25/5 mg once daily if necessary and if tolerated
▸ Adult 75 years and over: Initiation not recommended

DOSE ADJUSTMENTS DUE TO INTERACTIONS
▸ Dose of concomitant insulin or drugs that stimulate insulin secretion may need to be reduced.

DOSE EQUIVALENCE AND CONVERSION
▸ Dose expressed as x/y mg of empagliflozin/linagliptin.

- **INTERACTIONS** → Appendix 1: dipeptidylpeptidase-4 inhibitors · sodium glucose co-transporter 2 inhibitors
- **PATIENT AND CARER ADVICE**
Missed doses Manufacturer advises if a dose is more than 12 hours late, the missed dose should not be taken and the next dose should be taken at the normal time.
- **NATIONAL FUNDING/ACCESS DECISIONS** For full details see funding body website

Scottish Medicines Consortium (SMC) decisions
▸ Empagliflozin with linagliptin (*Glyxambi®*) is indicated in adults aged 18 years and older with type 2 diabetes mellitus: to improve glycaemic control when metformin and/or sulphonylurea (SU) and one of the monocomponents of *Glyxambi®* do not provide adequate glycaemic control; or when already being treated with the free combination of empagliflozin and linagliptin (August 2019) SMC No. SMC1236/17 Recommended with restrictions

- **MEDICINAL FORMS** There can be variation in the licensing of different medicines containing the same drug.

Tablet
▸ Glyxambi (Boehringer Ingelheim Ltd) ▼
  Linagliptin 5 mg, Empagliflozin 10 mg Glyxambi 10mg/5mg tablets
  | 28 tablet `PoM` £55.88 DT = £55.88
  Linagliptin 5 mg, Empagliflozin 25 mg Glyxambi 25mg/5mg tablets
  | 28 tablet `PoM` £55.88 DT = £55.88

Empagliflozin with metformin   09-Nov-2020

The properties listed below are those particular to the combination only. For the properties of the components please consider, empagliflozin p. 746, metformin hydrochloride p. 732.

- **INDICATIONS AND DOSE**

Type 2 diabetes mellitus not controlled by metformin alone or by metformin in combination with other antidiabetic drugs or insulin
▸ BY MOUTH
▸ Adult 18–84 years: 5/850–5/1000 mg twice daily, based on patient's current metformin dose, increased if necessary to 12.5/850–12.5/1000 mg twice daily
▸ BY MOUTH
▸ Adult 85 years and over: Initiation not recommended

DOSE ADJUSTMENTS DUE TO INTERACTIONS
▸ Dose of concomitant insulin or drugs that stimulate insulin secretion may need to be reduced.

DOSE EQUIVALENCE AND CONVERSION
▸ The proportions are expressed in the form "x"/"y" where "x" and "y" are the strengths in milligrams of empagliflozin and metformin respectively.

- **INTERACTIONS** → Appendix 1: metformin · sodium glucose co-transporter 2 inhibitors
- **NATIONAL FUNDING/ACCESS DECISIONS** For full details see funding body website

Scottish Medicines Consortium (SMC) decisions
▸ Empagliflozin with metformin (*Synjardy®*) in adults with type 2 diabetes mellitus as an adjunct to diet and exercise to improve glycaemic control: in patients inadequately controlled on their maximally tolerated dose of metformin alone; in patients inadequately controlled with metformin in combination with other glucose-lowering medicinal products, including insulin; in patients already being treated with the combination of empagliflozin and metformin as separate tablets (October 2015) SMC No. 1092/15 Recommended with restrictions

- **MEDICINAL FORMS** There can be variation in the licensing of different medicines containing the same drug.

Tablet
CAUTIONARY AND ADVISORY LABELS 21
▸ Synjardy (Boehringer Ingelheim Ltd)
  Empagliflozin 12.5 mg, Metformin hydrochloride 850 mg Synjardy 12.5mg/850mg tablets | 56 tablet `PoM` £36.59 DT = £36.59
  Empagliflozin 5 mg, Metformin hydrochloride 850 mg Synjardy 5mg/850mg tablets | 56 tablet `PoM` £36.59 DT = £36.59
  Empagliflozin 12.5 mg, Metformin hydrochloride 1 gram Synjardy 12.5mg/1000mg tablets | 56 tablet `PoM` £36.59 DT = £36.59
  Empagliflozin 5 mg, Metformin hydrochloride 1 gram Synjardy 5mg/1000mg tablets | 56 tablet `PoM` £36.59 DT = £36.59

Ertugliflozin   04-Nov-2020

- **DRUG ACTION** Reversibly inhibits sodium-glucose co-transporter 2 (SGLT2) in the renal proximal convoluted tubule to reduce glucose reabsorption and increase urinary glucose excretion.

- **INDICATIONS AND DOSE**

Type 2 diabetes mellitus as monotherapy (if metformin inappropriate) | Type 2 diabetes mellitus in combination with insulin or other antidiabetic drugs (if existing treatment fails to achieve adequate glycaemic control)
▸ BY MOUTH
▸ Adult: 5 mg once daily; increased to 15 mg once daily if necessary and if tolerated, dose to be taken in the morning

continued →

6

Endocrine system

6

Endocrine system

DOSE ADJUSTMENTS DUE TO INTERACTIONS
▶ Manufacturer advises dose of concomitant insulin or drugs that stimulate insulin secretion may need to be reduced.

IMPORTANT SAFETY INFORMATION

MHRA/CHM ADVICE (UPDATED APRIL 2016): RISK OF DIABETIC KETOACIDOSIS WITH SODIUM-GLUCOSE CO-TRANSPORTER 2 (SGLT2) INHIBITORS

A review by the European Medicines Agency has concluded that serious, life-threatening, and fatal cases of diabetic ketoacidosis (DKA) have been reported rarely in patients taking an SGLT2 inhibitor. In several cases, the presentation of DKA was atypical with patients having only moderately elevated blood glucose levels, and some of them occurred during off-label use.

To minimise the risk of such effects when treating patients with a SGLT2 inhibitor, the European Medicines Agency has issued the following advice:
- inform patients of the signs and symptoms of DKA, (including rapid weight loss, nausea or vomiting, abdominal pain, fast and deep breathing, sleepiness, a sweet smell to the breath, a sweet or metallic taste in the mouth, or a different odour to urine or sweat), and advise them to seek immediate medical advice if they develop any of these
- test for raised ketones in patients with signs and symptoms of DKA, even if plasma glucose levels are near-normal
- use ertugliflozin with caution in patients with risk factors for DKA, (including a low beta cell reserve, conditions leading to restricted food intake or severe dehydration, sudden reduction in insulin, increased insulin requirements due to acute illness, surgery or alcohol abuse), and discuss these risk factors with patients
- discontinue treatment if DKA is suspected or diagnosed
- do not restart treatment with any SGLT2 inhibitor in patients who experienced DKA during use, unless another cause for DKA was identified and resolved
- interrupt SGLT2 inhibitor treatment in patients who are hospitalised for major surgery or acute serious illnesses; treatment may be restarted once the patient's condition has stabilised

MHRA/CHM ADVICE: SGLT2 INHIBITORS: MONITOR KETONES IN BLOOD DURING TREATMENT INTERRUPTION FOR SURGICAL PROCEDURES OR ACUTE SERIOUS MEDICAL ILLNESS (MARCH 2020)

New recommendations have been issued following a European review of peri-operative diabetic ketoacidosis in patients taking SGLT2 inhibitors. Healthcare professionals are advised to monitor ketone levels during SGLT2 inhibitor treatment interruption in patients who have been hospitalised for major surgery or acute serious illness—measurement of blood ketone levels is preferred to urine. Treatment may be restarted once ketone levels are normal and the patient's condition has stabilised.

MHRA/CHM ADVICE: SGLT2 INHIBITORS: REPORTS OF FOURNIER'S GANGRENE (NECROTISING FASCIITIS OF THE GENITALIA OR PERINEUM) (FEBRUARY 2019)

Fournier's gangrene, a rare but serious and potentially life-threatening infection, has been associated with the use of sodium-glucose co-transporter 2 (SGLT2) inhibitors. If Fournier's gangrene is suspected, stop the SGLT2 inhibitor and urgently start treatment (including antibiotics and surgical debridement).

Patients should be advised to seek urgent medical attention if they experience severe pain, tenderness, erythema, or swelling in the genital or perineal area,

accompanied by fever or malaise—urogenital infection or perineal abscess may precede necrotising fasciitis.

- **CONTRA-INDICATIONS** Diabetic ketoacidosis
- **CAUTIONS** Dehydration · elderly (risk of volume depletion) · history of hypotension

CAUTIONS, FURTHER INFORMATION
▶ Volume depletion Manufacturer advises correct hypovolaemia before starting treatment—consider interrupting treatment if volume depletion occurs.

- **INTERACTIONS** → Appendix 1: sodium glucose co-transporter 2 inhibitors

- **SIDE-EFFECTS**
  ▶ **Common or very common** Hypoglycaemia (in combination with insulin or sulfonylurea) · hypovolaemia · increased risk of infection · polydipsia · thirst · urinary disorders · vulvovaginal pruritus
  ▶ **Rare or very rare** Diabetic ketoacidosis (discontinue immediately)
  ▶ **Frequency not known** Fournier's gangrene (discontinue and initiate treatment promptly) · lower limb amputations · phimosis

SIDE-EFFECTS, FURTHER INFORMATION Consider interrupting treatment if volume depletion occurs.

- **PREGNANCY** Manufacturer advises avoid—toxicity in *animal* studies.

- **BREAST FEEDING** Manufacturer advises avoid—present in milk in *animal* studies.

- **HEPATIC IMPAIRMENT** Manufacturer advises avoid in severe impairment (no information available).

- **RENAL IMPAIRMENT** Manufacturer advises avoid initiation if eGFR less than 60 mL/minute/1.73 m². Manufacturer advises frequent monitoring of renal function required if eGFR less than 60 mL/minute/1.73 m². Manufacturer advises avoid if eGFR is persistently less than 45 mL/minute/1.73 m².

- **MONITORING REQUIREMENTS**
  ▶ Manufacturer advises to determine renal function before treatment and periodically thereafter.
  ▶ Manufacturer advises monitor volume status and electrolytes during treatment in patients at risk of volume depletion.

- **PATIENT AND CARER ADVICE** Manufacturer advises that patients should be informed of the signs and symptoms of diabetic ketoacidosis, see MHRA advice.

- **NATIONAL FUNDING/ACCESS DECISIONS**
  For full details see funding body website
  NICE decisions
  ▶ Ertugliflozin as monotherapy or with metformin for treating type 2 diabetes (March 2019) NICE TA572 Recommended with restrictions
  ▶ Ertugliflozin with metformin and a dipeptidyl peptidase-4 inhibitor for treating type 2 diabetes (June 2019) NICE TA583 Recommended with restrictions
  Scottish Medicines Consortium (SMC) decisions
  ▶ Ertugliflozin (*Steglatro*®) in adults with type 2 diabetes mellitus as an adjunct to diet and exercise to improve glycaemic control: as monotherapy in patients for whom the use of metformin is considered inappropriate due to intolerance or contra-indications; in addition to other medicinal products for the treatment of diabetes (January 2019) SMC No. SMC2102 Recommended with restrictions

- **MEDICINAL FORMS** There can be variation in the licensing of different medicines containing the same drug.
  Tablet
  ▶ Steglatro (Merck Sharp & Dohme Ltd) ▼
  Ertugliflozin (as Ertugliflozin L-pyroglutamic acid) 5 mg Steglatro 5mg tablets | 28 tablet [PoM] £29.40 DT = £29.40

Ertugliflozin (as Ertugliflozin L-pyroglutamic acid)
15 mg Steglatro 15mg tablets | 28 tablet [PoM] £29.40 DT = £29.40

BLOOD GLUCOSE LOWERING DRUGS >
SULFONYLUREAS

Sulfonylureas

- **DRUG ACTION** The sulfonylureas act mainly by augmenting insulin secretion and consequently are effective only when some residual pancreatic beta-cell activity is present; during long-term administration they also have an extrapancreatic action.
- **CONTRA-INDICATIONS** Presence of ketoacidosis
- **CAUTIONS** Can encourage weight gain · elderly · G6PD deficiency

  CAUTIONS, FURTHER INFORMATION
  ▸ **Elderly** Prescription potentially inappropriate (STOPP criteria) if prescribed a **long-acting** sulfonylurea (e.g. glibenclamide, chlorpropamide, glimepiride) in type 2 diabetes mellitus (risk of prolonged hypoglycaemia). See also Prescribing in the elderly p. 33.
- **SIDE-EFFECTS**
  ▸ **Common or very common** Abdominal pain · diarrhoea · hypoglycaemia · nausea
  ▸ **Uncommon** Hepatic disorders · vomiting
  ▸ **Rare or very rare** Agranulocytosis · erythropenia · granulocytopenia · haemolytic anaemia · leucopenia · pancytopenia · thrombocytopenia
  ▸ **Frequency not known** Allergic dermatitis (usually in the first 6–8 weeks of therapy) · constipation · photosensitivity reaction · skin reactions · visual impairment
- **HEPATIC IMPAIRMENT** In general, manufacturers advise avoid in severe impairment (increased risk of hypoglycaemia).
- **RENAL IMPAIRMENT** Sulfonylureas should be used with care in those with mild to moderate renal impairment, because of the hazard of hypoglycaemia. Care is required to use the lowest dose that adequately controls blood glucose. Avoid where possible in severe renal impairment.
- **PATIENT AND CARER ADVICE** The risk of hypoglycaemia associated with sulfonylureas should be discussed with the patient, especially when concomitant glucose-lowering drugs are prescribed.
  Driving and skilled tasks Drivers need to be particularly careful to avoid hypoglycaemia and should be warned of the problems.

  ⌐ above

Glibenclamide

16-Dec-2019

- **INDICATIONS AND DOSE**
  Type 2 diabetes mellitus
  ▸ BY MOUTH USING TABLETS
  ▸ Adult: Initially 5 mg daily, adjusted according to response, dose to be taken with or immediately after breakfast; maximum 15 mg per day
  ▸ Elderly: 2.5 mg daily, adjusted according to response, dose to be taken with or immediately after breakfast; maximum 15 mg per day
- **UNLICENSED USE** Not licensed for use in breast feeding women with pre-existing diabetes. Not licensed for use in gestational diabetes.
- **CONTRA-INDICATIONS** Avoid where possible in Acute porphyrias p. 1107
- **INTERACTIONS** → Appendix 1: sulfonylureas
- **SIDE-EFFECTS** Appetite abnormal · bone marrow disorders · epigastric discomfort · erythema nodosum · fever · gastrointestinal disorder · hypereosinophilia · SIADH ·

Stevens-Johnson syndrome · taste metallic · vision disorders · weight increased
- **PREGNANCY** The use of sulfonylureas in pregnancy should generally be avoided because of the risk of neonatal hypoglycaemia; however, glibenclamide can be used during the second and third trimesters of pregnancy in women with gestational diabetes.
- **BREAST FEEDING** Glibenclamide can be used during breast-feeding in women with pre-existing diabetes.
- **MEDICINAL FORMS** No licensed medicines listed.

  ⌐ above

Gliclazide

10-Mar-2020

- **INDICATIONS AND DOSE**
  Type 2 diabetes mellitus
  ▸ BY MOUTH USING IMMEDIATE-RELEASE MEDICINES
  ▸ Adult: Initially 40–80 mg daily, adjusted according to response, increased if necessary up to 160 mg once daily, dose to be taken with breakfast, doses higher than 160 mg to be given in divided doses; maximum 320 mg per day
  ▸ BY MOUTH USING MODIFIED-RELEASE MEDICINES
  ▸ Adult: Initially 30 mg daily, dose to be taken with breakfast, adjust dose according to response every 4 weeks (after 2 weeks if no decrease in blood glucose); maximum 120 mg per day

  DOSE EQUIVALENCE AND CONVERSION
  ▸ Gliclazide modified release 30 mg may be considered to be approximately equivalent in therapeutic effect to standard formulation gliclazide 80 mg.

- **CONTRA-INDICATIONS** Avoid where possible in Acute porphyrias p. 1107
- **INTERACTIONS** → Appendix 1: sulfonylureas
- **SIDE-EFFECTS** Anaemia · angioedema · dyspepsia · gastrointestinal disorder · hypersensitivity vasculitis · hyponatraemia · severe cutaneous adverse reactions (SCARs)
- **PREGNANCY** The use of sulfonylureas in pregnancy should generally be avoided because of the risk of neonatal hypoglycaemia.
- **BREAST FEEDING** Avoid—theoretical possibility of hypoglycaemia in the infant.
- **RENAL IMPAIRMENT** If necessary, gliclazide which is principally metabolised in the liver, can be used in renal impairment but careful monitoring of blood-glucose concentration is essential.

- **MEDICINAL FORMS** There can be variation in the licensing of different medicines containing the same drug. Forms available from special-order manufacturers include: oral suspension
  Modified-release tablet
  CAUTIONARY AND ADVISORY LABELS 25
  ▸ Lamzarin (Key Pharmaceuticals Ltd)
    Gliclazide 30 mg Lamzarin 30mg modified-release tablets | 28 tablet [PoM] £2.81 DT = £2.81 | 56 tablet [PoM] £5.62
    Gliclazide 60 mg Lamzarin 60mg modified-release tablets | 28 tablet [PoM] £4.77 DT = £4.77
  ▸ Bilxona (Accord Healthcare Ltd)
    Gliclazide 30 mg Bilxona 30mg modified-release tablets | 28 tablet [PoM] £1.63 DT = £2.81 | 56 tablet [PoM] £3.27
    Gliclazide 60 mg Bilxona 60mg modified-release tablets | 28 tablet [PoM] £3.27 DT = £4.77 | 56 tablet [PoM] £6.55
  ▸ Dacadis MR (Mylan)
    Gliclazide 30 mg Dacadis MR 30mg tablets | 28 tablet [PoM] £2.81 DT = £2.81 | 56 tablet [PoM] £5.62
  ▸ Diamicron MR (Servier Laboratories Ltd)
    Gliclazide 30 mg Diamicron 30mg MR tablets | 28 tablet [PoM] £2.81 DT = £2.81 | 56 tablet [PoM] £5.62

6

Endocrine system

▸ Edicil MR (Teva UK Ltd)
Gliclazide 30 mg Edicil MR 30mg tablets | 28 tablet [PoM] £2.62 DT
= £2.81 | 56 tablet [PoM] £5.24
▸ Laaglyda MR (Consilient Health Ltd)
Gliclazide 60 mg Laaglyda MR 60mg tablets | 28 tablet [PoM] £4.77
DT = £4.77
▸ Nazdol MR (Consilient Health Ltd)
Gliclazide 30 mg Nazdol MR 30mg tablets | 28 tablet [PoM] £2.35 DT
= £2.81 | 56 tablet [PoM] £4.92
▸ Vamju (Advanz Pharma)
Gliclazide 30 mg Vamju 30mg modified-release tablets |
28 tablet [PoM] £1.64 DT = £2.81 | 56 tablet [PoM] £3.28
Gliclazide 60 mg Vamju 60mg modified-release tablets |
28 tablet [PoM] £3.28 DT = £4.77
▸ Ziclaseg (Lupin Healthcare (UK) Ltd)
Gliclazide 30 mg Ziclaseg 30mg modified-release tablets |
28 tablet [PoM] £2.38 DT = £2.81 | 56 tablet [PoM] £4.77
▸ Zicron PR (Bristol Laboratories Ltd)
Gliclazide 30 mg Zicron PR 30mg tablets | 28 tablet [PoM] £1.95 DT
= £2.81 | 56 tablet [PoM] £3.90

Tablet
▸ Gliclazide (Non-proprietary)
Gliclazide 40 mg Gliclazide 40mg tablets | 28 tablet [PoM] £3.19 DT
= £1.56
Gliclazide 80 mg Gliclazide 80mg tablets | 28 tablet [PoM] £1.80 DT
= £1.14 | 60 tablet [PoM] £0.81-£2.44
▸ Diamicron (Servier Laboratories Ltd)
Gliclazide 80 mg Diamicron 80mg tablets | 60 tablet [PoM] £4.38
▸ Glydex (Medreich Plc)
Gliclazide 160 mg Glydex 160mg tablets | 28 tablet [PoM] £3.27
▸ Zicron (Bristol Laboratories Ltd)
Gliclazide 40 mg Zicron 40mg tablets | 28 tablet [PoM] £3.36 DT =
£1.56

Glimepiride

F 749

27-Feb-2020

● **INDICATIONS AND DOSE**
Type 2 diabetes mellitus
▸ BY MOUTH
▸ Adult: Initially 1 mg daily, adjusted according to
response, then increased in steps of 1 mg every
1–2 weeks, increased to 4 mg daily, dose to be taken
shortly before or with first main meal, the daily dose
may be increased further, in exceptional
circumstances; maximum 6 mg per day

● CAUTIONS
▸ Porphyria Sulfonylureas should be avoided where possible
in Acute porphyrias p. 1107 but glimepiride is thought to
be safe.

● INTERACTIONS → Appendix 1: sulfonylureas

● SIDE-EFFECTS
▸ **Rare or very rare** Gastrointestinal discomfort ·
hypersensitivity vasculitis
▸ **Frequency not known** Drug cross-reactivity

● PREGNANCY The use of sulfonylureas in pregnancy should
generally be avoided because of the risk of neonatal
hypoglycaemia.

● BREAST FEEDING Avoid—theoretical possibility of
hypoglycaemia in the infant.

● MONITORING REQUIREMENTS Manufacturer recommends
regular hepatic and haematological monitoring but limited
evidence of clinical value.

● MEDICINAL FORMS There can be variation in the licensing of
different medicines containing the same drug. Forms
available from special-order manufacturers include: oral suspension, oral
solution
Tablet
▸ Glimepiride (Non-proprietary)
Glimepiride 1 mg Glimepiride 1mg tablets | 30 tablet [PoM] £4.33
DT = £1.63
Glimepiride 2 mg Glimepiride 2mg tablets | 30 tablet [PoM] £7.13
DT = £1.87

Glimepiride 3 mg Glimepiride 3mg tablets | 30 tablet [PoM] £10.75
DT = £2.08
Glimepiride 4 mg Glimepiride 4mg tablets | 30 tablet [PoM] £14.24
DT = £2.60

Glipizide

F 749

27-Feb-2020

● **INDICATIONS AND DOSE**
Type 2 diabetes mellitus
▸ BY MOUTH
▸ Adult: Initially 2.5–5 mg daily, adjusted according to
response, dose to be taken shortly before breakfast or
lunch, doses up to 15 mg may be given as a single dose,
higher doses to be given in divided doses; maximum
20 mg per day

● CAUTIONS
▸ Porphyria Sulfonylureas should be avoided where possible
in Acute porphyrias p. 1107 but glipizide is thought to be
safe.

● INTERACTIONS → Appendix 1: sulfonylureas

● SIDE-EFFECTS
▸ **Common or very common** Abdominal pain upper
▸ **Uncommon** Dizziness · drowsiness · tremor · vision
disorders
▸ **Frequency not known** Confusion · headache ·
hyponatraemia · malaise

● PREGNANCY The use of sulfonylureas in pregnancy should
generally be avoided because of the risk of neonatal
hypoglycaemia.

● BREAST FEEDING Avoid—theoretical possibility of
hypoglycaemia in the infant.

● HEPATIC IMPAIRMENT Manufacturer advises caution in
mild to moderate impairment.
Dose adjustments Manufacturer advises consider initial
dose of 2.5 mg daily and conservative maintenance dosing
in mild to moderate impairment.

● MEDICINAL FORMS There can be variation in the licensing of
different medicines containing the same drug.
Tablet
▸ Glipizide (Non-proprietary)
Glipizide 5 mg Glipizide 5mg tablets | 28 tablet [PoM] £3.32 DT =
£2.75 | 56 tablet [PoM] £2.14-£6.53
▸ Minodiab (Pfizer Ltd)
Glipizide 5 mg Minodiab 5mg tablets | 28 tablet [PoM] £1.26 DT =
£2.75

Tolbutamide

F 749

● **INDICATIONS AND DOSE**
Type 2 diabetes mellitus
▸ BY MOUTH
▸ Adult: 0.5–1.5 g daily in divided doses, dose to be taken
with or immediately after meals, alternatively 0.5–1.5 g
once daily, dose to be taken with or immediately after
breakfast; maximum 2 g per day

● CONTRA-INDICATIONS Avoid where possible in Acute
porphyrias p. 1107

● INTERACTIONS → Appendix 1: sulfonylureas

● SIDE-EFFECTS
▸ **Rare or very rare** Aplastic anaemia · blood disorder
▸ **Frequency not known** Alcohol intolerance · appetite
abnormal · erythema multiforme (usually in the first
6–8 weeks of therapy) · exfoliative dermatitis (usually in
the first 6–8 weeks of therapy) · fever (usually in the first
6–8 weeks of therapy) · headache · hypersensitivity
(usually in the first 6–8 weeks of therapy) · paraesthesia ·
tinnitus · weight increased

- **PREGNANCY** The use of sulfonylureas in pregnancy should generally be avoided because of the risk of neonatal hypoglycaemia.
- **BREAST FEEDING** The use of sulfonylureas in breast-feeding should be avoided because there is a theoretical possibility of hypoglycaemia in the infant.
- **RENAL IMPAIRMENT** If necessary, the short-acting drug tolbutamide can be used in renal impairment but careful monitoring of blood-glucose concentration is essential.

- **MEDICINAL FORMS** There can be variation in the licensing of different medicines containing the same drug. Forms available from special-order manufacturers include: oral suspension

Tablet
▸ Tolbutamide (Non-proprietary)
Tolbutamide 500 mg Tolbutamide 500mg tablets | 28 tablet [PoM]
£34.88 DT = £7.38 | 112 tablet [PoM] £35.80

BLOOD GLUCOSE LOWERING DRUGS ⟩
THIAZOLIDINEDIONES

❙ Pioglitazone   31-Mar-2020

- **DRUG ACTION** The thiazolidinedione, pioglitazone, reduces peripheral insulin resistance, leading to a reduction of blood-glucose concentration.

- ● **INDICATIONS AND DOSE**

Type 2 diabetes mellitus (alone or combined with metformin or a sulfonylurea, or with both, or with insulin)
▸ BY MOUTH
▸ Adult: Initially 15–30 mg once daily, adjusted according to response to 45 mg once daily, in elderly patients, initiate with lowest possible dose and increase gradually; review treatment after 3–6 months and regularly thereafter

DOSE ADJUSTMENTS DUE TO INTERACTIONS
▸ Dose of concomitant sulfonylurea or insulin may need to be reduced.

IMPORTANT SAFETY INFORMATION
MHRA/CHM ADVICE: PIOGLITAZONE CARDIOVASCULAR SAFETY (DECEMBER 2007 AND JANUARY 2011)
Incidence of heart failure is increased when pioglitazone is combined with insulin especially in patients with predisposing factors e.g. previous myocardial infarction. Patients who take pioglitazone should be closely monitored for signs of heart failure; treatment should be discontinued if any deterioration in cardiac status occurs.
  Pioglitazone should not be used in patients with heart failure or a history of heart failure.

PIOGLITAZONE: RISK OF BLADDER CANCER (JULY 2011)
The European Medicines Agency has advised that there is a small increased risk of bladder cancer associated with pioglitazone use. However, in patients who respond adequately to treatment, the benefits of pioglitazone continue to outweigh the risks.
  Pioglitazone should not be used in patients with active bladder cancer or a past history of bladder cancer, or in those who have uninvestigated macroscopic haematuria. Pioglitazone should be used with caution in elderly patients as the risk of bladder cancer increases with age.
  Before initiating treatment with pioglitazone, patients should be assessed for risk factors of bladder cancer (including age, smoking status, exposure to certain occupational or chemotherapy agents, or previous radiation therapy to the pelvic region) and any macroscopic haematuria should be investigated. The safety and efficacy of pioglitazone should be reviewed

after 3–6 months and pioglitazone should be stopped in patients who do not respond adequately to treatment.
  Patients already receiving treatment with pioglitazone should be assessed for risk factors of bladder cancer and treatment should be reviewed after 3–6 months, as above.
  Patients should be advised to report promptly any haematuria, dysuria, or urinary urgency during treatment.

- **CONTRA-INDICATIONS** History of heart failure · previous or active bladder cancer · uninvestigated macroscopic haematuria
- **CAUTIONS** Concomitant use with insulin (risk of heart failure) · elderly (increased risk of heart failure, fractures, and bladder cancer) · increased risk of bone fractures, particularly in women · risk factors for bladder cancer · risk factors for heart failure

CAUTIONS, FURTHER INFORMATION
▸ Elderly For thiazolidenediones, prescription potentially inappropriate (STOPP criteria) in patients with heart failure (risk of exacerbation).
    See also Prescribing in the elderly p. 33.
- **INTERACTIONS** → Appendix 1: pioglitazone
- **SIDE-EFFECTS**
▸ **Common or very common** Bone fracture · increased risk of infection · numbness · visual impairment · weight increased
▸ **Uncommon** Bladder cancer · insomnia
▸ **Frequency not known** Macular oedema
    SIDE-EFFECTS, FURTHER INFORMATION Rare reports of liver dysfunction; discontinue if jaundice occurs.
- **PREGNANCY** Avoid—toxicity in *animal* studies.
- **BREAST FEEDING** Avoid—present in milk in *animal* studies.
- **HEPATIC IMPAIRMENT** Manufacturer advises avoid.
- **MONITORING REQUIREMENTS** Monitor liver function before treatment and periodically thereafter.
- **PATIENT AND CARER ADVICE**
    Liver toxicity Patients should be advised to seek immediate medical attention if symptoms such as nausea, vomiting, abdominal pain, fatigue and dark urine develop.
- **NATIONAL FUNDING/ACCESS DECISIONS**
    For full details see funding body website
    Scottish Medicines Consortium (SMC) decisions
▸ Pioglitazone (*Actos®*) in combination with metformin and a sulfonylurea for type 2 diabetes mellitus (March 2007)
    SMC No. 354/07 Recommended with restrictions

- **MEDICINAL FORMS** There can be variation in the licensing of different medicines containing the same drug. Forms available from special-order manufacturers include: oral suspension
Tablet
▸ Pioglitazone (Non-proprietary)
    Pioglitazone (as Pioglitazone hydrochloride) 15 mg Pioglitazone 15mg tablets | 28 tablet [PoM] £25.83 DT = £1.69
    Pioglitazone (as Pioglitazone hydrochloride) 30 mg Pioglitazone 30mg tablets | 28 tablet [PoM] £35.89 DT = £2.08
    Pioglitazone (as Pioglitazone hydrochloride) 45 mg Pioglitazone 45mg tablets | 28 tablet [PoM] £39.55 DT = £2.37
▸ Actos (Takeda UK Ltd)
    Pioglitazone (as Pioglitazone hydrochloride) 15 mg Actos 15mg tablets | 28 tablet [PoM] £25.83 DT = £1.69
    Pioglitazone (as Pioglitazone hydrochloride) 30 mg Actos 30mg tablets | 28 tablet [PoM] £35.89 DT = £2.08
    Pioglitazone (as Pioglitazone hydrochloride) 45 mg Actos 45mg tablets | 28 tablet [PoM] £39.55 DT = £2.37
▸ Glidipion (Actavis UK Ltd)
    Pioglitazone (as Pioglitazone hydrochloride) 45 mg Glidipion 45mg tablets | 28 tablet [PoM] £39.55 DT = £2.37

6

Endocrine system

Endocrine system

6

Pioglitazone with metformin   03-Feb-2020

The properties listed below are those particular to the combination only. For the properties of the components please consider, pioglitazone p. 751, metformin hydrochloride p. 732.

- **INDICATIONS AND DOSE**

Type 2 diabetes not controlled by metformin alone
- ▸ BY MOUTH
- ▸ **Adult:** 1 tablet twice daily, titration with the individual components (pioglitazone and metformin) desirable before initiation

- **INTERACTIONS** → Appendix 1: metformin · pioglitazone

- **MEDICINAL FORMS** There can be variation in the licensing of different medicines containing the same drug.

Tablet
CAUTIONARY AND ADVISORY LABELS 21
- ▸ Pioglitazone with metformin (Non-proprietary)
  Pioglitazone (as Pioglitazone hydrochloride) 15 mg, Metformin hydrochloride 850 mg Pioglitazone 15mg / Metformin 850mg tablets | 56 tablet [PoM] £34.10 DT = £29.31
- ▸ Competact (Takeda UK Ltd)
  Pioglitazone (as Pioglitazone hydrochloride) 15 mg, Metformin hydrochloride 850 mg Competact 15mg/850mg tablets | 56 tablet [PoM] £35.89 DT = £29.31

INSULINS

Insulins

of hypoglycaemia; blood glucose should be closely monitored after changing injection site, and dose adjustment of insulin or other antidiabetic medication may be required.

- **SIDE-EFFECTS**
- ▸ **Common or very common** Oedema
- ▸ **Uncommon** Lipodystrophy
- ▸ **Frequency not known** Cutaneous amyloidosis
  Overdose Overdose causes hypoglycaemia.

- **PREGNANCY**
  Dose adjustments During pregnancy, insulin requirements may alter and doses should be assessed frequently by an experienced diabetes physician.
  The dose of insulin generally needs to be increased in the second and third trimesters of pregnancy.

- **BREAST FEEDING**
  Dose adjustments During breast-feeding, insulin requirements may alter and doses should be assessed frequently by an experienced diabetes physician.

- **HEPATIC IMPAIRMENT** Insulin requirements may be decreased.

- **RENAL IMPAIRMENT** The compensatory response to hypoglycaemia is impaired in renal impairment.
  Dose adjustments Insulin requirements may decrease in patients with renal impairment and therefore dose reduction may be necessary.

- **MONITORING REQUIREMENTS**
- ▸ Many patients now monitor their own blood-glucose concentrations; all carers and children need to be trained to do this.
- ▸ Since blood-glucose concentration varies substantially throughout the day, 'normoglycaemia' cannot always be achieved throughout a 24-hour period without causing damaging hypoglycaemia.
- ▸ In adults It is therefore best to recommend that patients should maintain a blood-glucose concentration of between 4 and 9 mmol/litre for most of the time (4–7 mmol/litre before meals and less than 9 mmol/litre after meals).
- ▸ In children It is therefore best to recommend that children should maintain a blood-glucose concentration of between 4 and 10 mmol/litre for most of the time (4–8 mmol/litre before meals and less than 10 mmol/litre after meals).
  While accepting that on occasions, for brief periods, the blood-glucose concentration will be above these values; strenuous efforts should be made to prevent it from falling below 4 mmol/litre. Patients using multiple injection regimens should understand how to adjust their insulin dose according to their carbohydrate intake. With fixed-dose insulin regimens, the carbohydrate intake needs to be regulated, and should be distributed throughout the day to match the insulin regimen. The intake of energy and of simple and complex carbohydrates should be adequate to allow normal growth and development but obesity must be avoided.

- **DIRECTIONS FOR ADMINISTRATION** Insulin is generally given by *subcutaneous injection*; the injection site should be rotated to prevent lipodystrophy and cutaneous amyloidosis. Injection devices ('pens'), which hold the insulin in a cartridge and meter the required dose, are convenient to use. Insulin syringes (for use with needles) are required for insulins not available in cartridge form, but are less popular with children and carers.

- **PRESCRIBING AND DISPENSING INFORMATION** Show container to patient or carer and confirm the expected version is dispensed.
  Units The word 'unit' should **not** be abbreviated.

- **PATIENT AND CARER ADVICE**
  Hypoglycaemia Hypoglycaemia is a potential problem with insulin therapy. All patients must be carefully instructed

on how to avoid it; this involves appropriate adjustment of insulin type, dose and frequency together with suitable timing and quantity of meals and snacks.

Insulin Passport Insulin Passports and patient information booklets should be offered to patients receiving insulin. The Insulin Passport provides a record of the patient's current insulin preparations and contains a section for emergency information. The patient information booklet provides advice on the safe use of insulin. They are available for purchase from:

3M Security Print and Systems Limited
Gorse Street, Chadderton
Oldham
OL9 9QH
Tel: 0845 610 1112

GP practices can obtain supplies through their Local Area Team stores.

NHS Trusts can order supplies from www.nhsforms.co.uk/ or by emailing nhsforms@mmm.com. Further information is available at www.npsa.nhs.uk.

Driving and skilled tasks Drivers need to be particularly careful to avoid hypoglycaemia and should be warned of the problems.

INSULINS > RAPID-ACTING
▸ F 752

Insulin

(Insulin Injection; Neutral Insulin; Soluble Insulin—short acting)

● **INDICATIONS AND DOSE**

Diabetes mellitus
▸ BY SUBCUTANEOUS INJECTION, OR BY INTRAMUSCULAR INJECTION, OR BY INTRAVENOUS INJECTION, OR BY INTRAVENOUS INFUSION
▸ Adult: According to requirements

Diabetic ketoacidosis | Diabetes during surgery
▸ BY INTRAVENOUS INFUSION
▸ Adult: (consult local protocol)

● INTERACTIONS → Appendix 1: insulin

● SIDE-EFFECTS
▸ **Uncommon** Skin reactions
▸ **Rare or very rare** Refraction disorder

● DIRECTIONS FOR ADMINISTRATION Short-acting injectable insulins can be given by continuous subcutaneous infusion using a portable infusion pump. This device delivers a continuous basal insulin infusion and patient-activated bolus doses at meal times. This technique can be useful for patients who suffer recurrent hypoglycaemia or marked morning rise in blood-glucose concentration despite optimised multiple-injection regimens. Patients on subcutaneous insulin infusion must be highly motivated, able to monitor their blood-glucose concentration, and have expert training, advice and supervision from an experienced healthcare team. Some insulin preparations are not recommended for use in subcutaneous insulin infusion pumps—may precipitate in catheter or needle—consult product literature.
▸ With intravenous use For *intravenous infusion* give continuously in Sodium chloride 0.9%. Adsorbed to some extent by plastic infusion set; ensure insulin is not injected into 'dead space' of injection port of the infusion bag.

● PRESCRIBING AND DISPENSING INFORMATION A sterile solution of insulin (i.e. bovine or porcine) or of human insulin; pH 6.6–8.0.

● NATIONAL FUNDING/ACCESS DECISIONS
For full details see funding body website

NICE decisions
▸ Continuous subcutaneous insulin infusion for the treatment of diabetes mellitus (type 1) (July 2008) NICE TA151 Recommended

● MEDICINAL FORMS There can be variation in the licensing of different medicines containing the same drug. Forms available from special-order manufacturers include: solution for injection, solution for infusion

Solution for injection
▸ Actrapid (Novo Nordisk Ltd)
Insulin human (as Insulin soluble human) 100 unit per 1 ml Actrapid 100units/ml solution for injection 10ml vials | 1 vial PoM £7.48 DT = £15.68
▸ Humulin R (Imported (United States))
Insulin human 500 unit per 1 ml Humulin R 500units/ml solution for injection 20ml vials | 1 vial PoM
Humulin R KwikPen 500units/ml solution for injection 3ml pre-filled pens | 2 pre-filled disposable injection PoM Ⓢ
▸ Humulin S (Eli Lilly and Company Ltd)
Insulin human (as Insulin soluble human) 100 unit per 1 ml Humulin S 100units/ml solution for injection 10ml vials | 1 vial PoM £15.68 DT = £15.68
Humulin S 100units/ml solution for injection 3ml cartridges | 5 cartridge PoM £19.08 DT = £19.08
▸ Hypurin Porcine Neutral (Wockhardt UK Ltd)
Insulin porcine (as Insulin soluble porcine) 100 unit per 1 ml Hypurin Porcine Neutral 100units/ml solution for injection 10ml vials | 1 vial PoM £37.87 DT = £37.87
Hypurin Porcine Neutral 100units/ml solution for injection 3ml cartridges | 5 cartridge PoM £56.81 DT = £56.81
▸ Insuman Infusat (Sanofi)
Insulin human 100 unit per 1 ml Insuman Infusat 100units/ml solution for injection 3.15ml cartridges | 5 cartridge PoM £250.00 DT = £250.00
▸ Insuman Rapid (Sanofi)
Insulin human (as Insulin soluble human) 100 unit per 1 ml Insuman Rapid 100units/ml solution for injection 3ml cartridges | 5 cartridge PoM £17.50 DT = £19.08

Combinations available: *Biphasic insulin aspart*, p. 756 · *Biphasic insulin lispro*, p. 756 · *Biphasic isophane insulin*, p. 755 · *Insulin degludec*, p. 757 · *Insulin degludec with liraglutide*, p. 757 · *Insulin detemir*, p. 757 · *Insulin glargine*, p. 758 · *Insulin glargine with lixisenatide*, p. 758 · *Isophane insulin*, p. 756
▸ F 752

Insulin aspart
28-Jul-2020

(Recombinant human insulin analogue—short acting)

● **INDICATIONS AND DOSE**

FIASP ®

Diabetes mellitus
▸ BY SUBCUTANEOUS INJECTION
▸ Child 1–17 years: Administer immediately before meals or when necessary shortly after meals, according to requirements
▸ Adult: Administer immediately before meals or when necessary shortly after meals, according to requirements
▸ BY SUBCUTANEOUS INFUSION, OR BY INTRAVENOUS INFUSION
▸ Child 1–17 years: According to requirements
▸ Adult: According to requirements

NOVORAPID ®

Diabetes mellitus
▸ BY SUBCUTANEOUS INJECTION
▸ Child: Administer immediately before meals or when necessary shortly after meals, according to requirements
▸ Adult: Administer immediately before meals or when necessary shortly after meals, according to requirements

continued →

6

Endocrine system

▸ BY SUBCUTANEOUS INFUSION, OR BY INTRAVENOUS INFUSION
- ▸ Child: According to requirements
- ▸ Adult: According to requirements

PHARMACOKINETICS
- ▸ *Fiasp*® and *NovoRapid*® are **not** interchangeable due to differences in bioavailability; *Fiasp*® has a quicker onset of action and shorter duration.

● UNLICENSED USE
- ▸ In children Not licensed for use in children under 1 year.

● INTERACTIONS → Appendix 1: insulin

● SIDE-EFFECTS
- ▸ **Common or very common** Skin reactions
- ▸ **Uncommon** Refraction disorder

● PREGNANCY Not known to be harmful—may be used during pregnancy.

● BREAST FEEDING Not known to be harmful—may be used during lactation.

● DIRECTIONS FOR ADMINISTRATION Short-acting injectable insulins can be given by continuous subcutaneous infusion using a portable infusion pump. This device delivers a continuous basal insulin infusion and patient-activated bolus doses at meal times. This technique can be useful for patients who suffer recurrent hypoglycaemia or marked morning rise in blood-glucose concentration despite optimised multiple-injection regimens. Patients on subcutaneous insulin infusion must be highly motivated, able to monitor their blood-glucose concentration, and have expert training, advice and supervision from an experienced healthcare team.

Manufacturer advises for *intravenous infusion* of *Fiasp*®, give continuously in Glucose 5% or Sodium Chloride 0.9%; dilute to 0.5-1 unit/mL with infusion fluid.

Manufacturer advises for *intravenous infusion* of *NovoRapid*®, give continuously in Glucose 5% or Sodium Chloride 0.9%; dilute to 0.05-1 unit/mL with infusion fluid; adsorbed to some extent by plastics of infusion set.

● PRESCRIBING AND DISPENSING INFORMATION Insulin aspart is a biological medicine. Biological medicines must be prescribed and dispensed by brand name, see *Biological medicines* and *Biosimilar medicines*, under Guidance on prescribing p. 1. Dose adjustments and close metabolic monitoring is recommended if switching between insulin aspart preparations.

● NATIONAL FUNDING/ACCESS DECISIONS
For full details see funding body website

NICE decisions
- ▸ Continuous subcutaneous insulin infusion for the treatment of diabetes mellitus (type 1) (July 2008) NICE TA151 Recommended

Scottish Medicines Consortium (SMC) decisions
- ▸ Insulin aspart (*Fiasp*®) for the treatment of diabetes mellitus in adults (April 2017) SMC No. 1227/17 Recommended

● MEDICINAL FORMS There can be variation in the licensing of different medicines containing the same drug.

Solution for injection
- ▸ Fiasp (Novo Nordisk Ltd) ▼
  Insulin aspart 100 unit per 1 ml Fiasp 100units/ml solution for injection 10ml vials | 1 vial [PoM] £14.08 DT = £14.08
- ▸ Fiasp FlexTouch (Novo Nordisk Ltd) ▼
  Insulin aspart 100 unit per 1 ml Fiasp FlexTouch 100units/ml solution for injection 3ml pre-filled pens | 5 pre-filled disposable injection [PoM] £30.60 DT = £30.60
- ▸ Fiasp Penfill (Novo Nordisk Ltd) ▼
  Insulin aspart 100 unit per 1 ml Fiasp Penfill 100units/ml solution for injection 3ml cartridges | 5 cartridge [PoM] £28.31 DT = £28.31
- ▸ NovoRapid (Novo Nordisk Ltd)
  Insulin aspart 100 unit per 1 ml NovoRapid 100units/ml solution for injection 10ml vials | 1 vial [PoM] £14.08 DT = £14.08

- ▸ NovoRapid FlexPen (Novo Nordisk Ltd)
  Insulin aspart 100 unit per 1 ml NovoRapid FlexPen 100units/ml solution for injection 3ml pre-filled pens | 5 pre-filled disposable injection [PoM] £30.60 DT = £30.60
- ▸ NovoRapid FlexTouch (Novo Nordisk Ltd)
  Insulin aspart 100 unit per 1 ml NovoRapid FlexTouch 100units/ml solution for injection 3ml pre-filled pens | 5 pre-filled disposable injection [PoM] £32.13 DT = £30.60
- ▸ NovoRapid Penfill (Novo Nordisk Ltd)
  Insulin aspart 100 unit per 1 ml NovoRapid Penfill 100units/ml solution for injection 3ml cartridges | 5 cartridge [PoM] £28.31 DT = £28.31
- ▸ NovoRapid PumpCart (Novo Nordisk Ltd)
  Insulin aspart 100 unit per 1 ml NovoRapid PumpCart 100units/ml solution for injection 1.6ml cartridges | 5 cartridge [PoM] £15.10 DT = £15.10

F 752

Insulin glulisine

27-Jul-2018

(Recombinant human insulin analogue—short acting)

● INDICATIONS AND DOSE
Diabetes mellitus
- ▸ BY SUBCUTANEOUS INJECTION
- ▸ Child: Administer immediately before meals or when necessary shortly after meals, according to requirements
- ▸ Adult: Administer immediately before meals or when necessary shortly after meals, according to requirements
- ▸ BY SUBCUTANEOUS INFUSION, OR BY INTRAVENOUS INFUSION
- ▸ Child: According to requirements
- ▸ Adult: According to requirements

● UNLICENSED USE
- ▸ In children Not licensed for children under 6 years.

● INTERACTIONS → Appendix 1: insulin

● DIRECTIONS FOR ADMINISTRATION Short-acting injectable insulins can be given by continuous subcutaneous infusion using a portable infusion pump. This device delivers a continuous basal insulin infusion and patient-activated bolus doses at meal times. This technique can be useful for patients who suffer recurrent hypoglycaemia or marked morning rise in blood-glucose concentration despite optimised multiple-injection regimens. Patients on subcutaneous insulin infusion must be highly motivated, able to monitor their blood-glucose concentration, and have expert training, advice and supervision from an experienced healthcare team.

With intravenous use in adults For *intravenous infusion* (*Apidra*®), give continuously in Sodium chloride 0.9%; dilute to 1 unit/mL with infusion fluid; use a co-extruded polyolefin/polyamide plastic infusion bag with a dedicated infusion line.

● NATIONAL FUNDING/ACCESS DECISIONS
For full details see funding body website

NICE decisions
- ▸ Continuous subcutaneous insulin infusion for the treatment of diabetes mellitus (type 1) (July 2008) NICE TA151 Recommended

Scottish Medicines Consortium (SMC) decisions
- ▸ Insulin glulisine (*Apidra*®) for adolescents and children with diabetes mellitus (November 2008) SMC No. 512/08 Recommended with restrictions

● MEDICINAL FORMS There can be variation in the licensing of different medicines containing the same drug.

Solution for injection
- ▸ Apidra (Sanofi)
  Insulin glulisine 100 unit per 1 ml Apidra 100units/ml solution for injection 3ml cartridges | 5 cartridge [PoM] £28.30 DT = £28.30

Apidra 100units/ml solution for injection 10ml vials | 1 vial [PoM]
£16.00 DT = £16.00
▸ **Apidra SoloStar** (Sanofi)
Insulin glulisine 100 unit per 1 ml Apidra 100units/ml solution for
injection 3ml pre-filled SoloStar pens | 5 pre-filled disposable
injection [PoM] £28.30 DT = £28.30

F 752

Insulin lispro   18-Feb-2020

(Recombinant human insulin analogue—short
acting)

● **INDICATIONS AND DOSE**
Diabetes mellitus
▸ BY SUBCUTANEOUS INJECTION
▸ **Child 2–17 years:** Administer shortly before meals or
when necessary shortly after meals, according to
requirements
▸ **Adult:** Administer shortly before meals or when
necessary shortly after meals, according to
requirements
▸ BY SUBCUTANEOUS INFUSION, OR BY INTRAVENOUS INFUSION,
OR BY INTRAVENOUS INJECTION
▸ **Child 2–17 years:** According to requirements
▸ **Adult:** According to requirements

● INTERACTIONS → Appendix 1: insulin
● PREGNANCY Not known to be harmful—may be used
during pregnancy.
● BREAST FEEDING Not known to be harmful—may be used
during lactation.
● DIRECTIONS FOR ADMINISTRATION Short-acting injectable
insulins can be given by continuous subcutaneous infusion
using a portable infusion pump. This device delivers a
continuous basal insulin infusion and patient-activated
bolus doses at meal times. This technique can be useful for
patients who suffer recurrent hypoglycaemia or marked
morning rise in blood-glucose concentration despite
optimised multiple-injection regimens (see also NICE
guidance, below). Patients on subcutaneous insulin
infusion must be highly motivated, able to monitor their
blood-glucose concentration, and have expert training,
advice and supervision from an experienced healthcare
team.
▸ **With intravenous use in adults** For *intravenous infusion* give
continuously in Glucose 5% or Sodium chloride 0.9%.
Adsorbed to some extent by plastics of infusion set.
▸ **With intravenous use in children** For *intravenous infusion*,
dilute to a concentration of 0.1–1 unit/mL with Glucose
5% or Sodium Chloride 0.9% and mix thoroughly; insulin
may be adsorbed by plastics, flush giving set with 5 mL of
infusion fluid containing insulin.
● PRESCRIBING AND DISPENSING INFORMATION Insulin
lispro is a biological medicine. Biological medicines must
be prescribed and dispensed by brand name, see *Biological
medicines* and *Biosimilar medicines*, under Guidance on
prescribing p. 1.
● NATIONAL FUNDING/ACCESS DECISIONS
For full details see funding body website
NICE decisions
▸ **Continuous subcutaneous insulin infusion for the treatment of
diabetes mellitus (type 1) (July 2008)** NICE TA151
Recommended

● MEDICINAL FORMS There can be variation in the licensing of
different medicines containing the same drug.
Solution for injection
▸ Insulin lispro (non-proprietary) ▼
Insulin lispro 100 unit per 1 ml Insulin lispro Sanofi 100units/ml
solution for injection 3ml cartridges | 5 cartridge [PoM] £21.23 DT =
£28.31

Insulin lispro Sanofi 100units/ml solution for injection 10ml vials |
1 vial [PoM] £14.12 DT = £16.61
Insulin lispro Sanofi 100units/ml solution for injection 3ml pre-filled
pens | 5 pre-filled disposable injection [PoM] £22.10 DT = £29.46
Insulin lispro 200 unit per 1 ml Lyumjev KwikPen 200units/ml
solution for injection 3ml pre-filled pens | 5 pre-filled disposable
injection [PoM] £58.92 DT = £58.92
▸ Humalog (Eli Lilly and Company Ltd)
Insulin lispro 100 unit per 1 ml Humalog 100units/ml solution for
injection 10ml vials | 1 vial [PoM] £16.61 DT = £16.61
Humalog 100units/ml solution for injection 3ml cartridges |
5 cartridge [PoM] £28.31 DT = £28.31
▸ Humalog Junior KwikPen (Eli Lilly and Company Ltd)
Insulin lispro 100 unit per 1 ml Humalog Junior KwikPen
100units/ml solution for injection 3ml pre-filled pens | 5 pre-filled
disposable injection [PoM] £29.46 DT = £29.46
▸ Humalog KwikPen (Eli Lilly and Company Ltd)
Insulin lispro 100 unit per 1 ml Humalog KwikPen 100units/ml
solution for injection 3ml pre-filled pens | 5 pre-filled disposable
injection [PoM] £29.46 DT = £29.46
Insulin lispro 200 unit per 1 ml Humalog KwikPen 200units/ml
solution for injection 3ml pre-filled pens | 5 pre-filled disposable
injection [PoM] £58.92 DT = £58.92
▸ Lyumjev (Eli Lilly and Company Ltd)
Insulin lispro 100 unit per 1 ml Lyumjev Junior KwikPen
100units/ml solution for injection 3ml pre-filled pens | 5 pre-filled
disposable injection [PoM] £29.46 DT = £29.46
Lyumjev KwikPen 100units/ml solution for injection 3ml pre-filled pens
| 5 pre-filled disposable injection [PoM] £29.46 DT = £29.46
Lyumjev 100units/ml solution for injection 10ml vials | 1 vial [PoM]
£16.61 DT = £16.61
Lyumjev 100units/ml solution for injection 3ml cartridges |
5 cartridge [PoM] £28.31 DT = £28.31

INSULINS 〉 INTERMEDIATE-ACTING

F 752

Biphasic isophane insulin

(Biphasic Isophane Insulin Injection— intermediate
acting)

● **INDICATIONS AND DOSE**
Diabetes mellitus
▸ BY SUBCUTANEOUS INJECTION
▸ **Child:** According to requirements
▸ **Adult:** According to requirements

● INTERACTIONS → Appendix 1: insulin
● SIDE-EFFECTS
▸ **Rare or very rare** Angioedema
▸ **Frequency not known** Hypokalaemia · weight increased
● PRESCRIBING AND DISPENSING INFORMATION A sterile
buffered suspension of either porcine or human insulin
complexed with protamine sulfate (or another suitable
protamine) in a solution of insulin of the same species.
Check product container—the proportions of the two
components should be checked carefully (the order in
which the proportions are stated may not be the same in
other countries).

● MEDICINAL FORMS There can be variation in the licensing of
different medicines containing the same drug.
Suspension for injection
▸ Humulin M3 (Eli Lilly and Company Ltd)
**Insulin human (as Insulin soluble human) 30 unit per 1 ml,
Insulin human (as Insulin isophane human) 70 unit per
1 ml** Humulin M3 100units/ml suspension for injection 3ml cartridges
| 5 cartridge [PoM] £19.08 DT = £19.08
Humulin M3 100units/ml suspension for injection 10ml vials |
1 vial [PoM] £15.68 DT = £15.68
▸ Humulin M3 KwikPen (Eli Lilly and Company Ltd)
**Insulin human (as Insulin soluble human) 30 unit per 1 ml,
Insulin human (as Insulin isophane human) 70 unit per
1 ml** Humulin M3 KwikPen 100units/ml suspension for injection 3ml
pre-filled pens | 5 pre-filled disposable injection [PoM] £21.70 DT =
£21.70

▸ Hypurin Porcine 30/70 Mix (Wockhardt UK Ltd)
Insulin porcine (as Insulin soluble porcine) 30 unit per 1 ml, Insulin porcine (as Insulin isophane porcine) 70 unit per 1 ml Hypurin Porcine 30/70 Mix 100units/ml suspension for injection 3ml cartridges | 5 cartridge [PoM] £56.81 DT = £56.81
Hypurin Porcine 30/70 Mix 100units/ml suspension for injection 10ml vials | 1 vial [PoM] £37.87 DT = £37.87

▸ Insuman Comb 15 (Sanofi)
Insulin human (as Insulin soluble human) 15 unit per 1 ml, Insulin human (as Insulin isophane human) 85 unit per 1 ml Insuman Comb 15 100units/ml suspension for injection 3ml cartridges | 5 cartridge [PoM] £17.50 DT = £17.50

▸ Insuman Comb 25 (Sanofi)
Insulin human (as Insulin soluble human) 25 unit per 1 ml, Insulin human (as Insulin isophane human) 75 unit per 1 ml Insuman Comb 25 100units/ml suspension for injection 5ml vials | 1 vial [PoM] £5.61
Insuman Comb 25 100units/ml suspension for injection 3ml cartridges | 5 cartridge [PoM] £17.50 DT = £17.50
Insuman Comb 25 100units/ml suspension for injection 3ml pre-filled SoloStar pens | 5 pre-filled disposable injection [PoM] £19.80 DT = £19.80

▸ Insuman Comb 50 (Sanofi)
Insulin human (as Insulin isophane human) 50 unit per 1 ml, Insulin human (as Insulin soluble human) 50 unit per 1 ml Insuman Comb 50 100units/ml suspension for injection 3ml cartridges | 5 cartridge [PoM] £17.50 DT = £17.50

▌**Isophane insulin**   F 752

(Isophane Insulin Injection; Isophane Protamine Insulin Injection; Isophane Insulin (NPH)—intermediate acting)

● **INDICATIONS AND DOSE**
Diabetes mellitus
▸ BY SUBCUTANEOUS INJECTION
▸ Child: According to requirements
▸ Adult: According to requirements

● INTERACTIONS → Appendix 1: insulin
● PREGNANCY Recommended where longer-acting insulins are needed.
● PRESCRIBING AND DISPENSING INFORMATION A sterile suspension of bovine or porcine insulin or of human insulin in the form of a complex obtained by the addition of protamine sulfate or another suitable protamine.

● MEDICINAL FORMS There can be variation in the licensing of different medicines containing the same drug.
Suspension for injection
▸ Humulin I (Eli Lilly and Company Ltd)
Insulin human (as Insulin isophane human) 100 unit per 1 ml Humulin I 100units/ml suspension for injection 10ml vials | 1 vial [PoM] £15.68 DT = £15.68
Humulin I 100units/ml suspension for injection 3ml cartridges | 5 cartridge [PoM] £19.08 DT = £19.08

▸ Humulin I KwikPen (Eli Lilly and Company Ltd)
Insulin human (as Insulin isophane human) 100 unit per 1 ml Humulin I KwikPen 100units/ml suspension for injection 3ml pre-filled pens | 5 pre-filled disposable injection [PoM] £21.70 DT = £21.70

▸ Hypurin Porcine Isophane (Wockhardt UK Ltd)
Insulin porcine (as Insulin isophane porcine) 100 unit per 1 ml Hypurin Porcine Isophane 100units/ml suspension for injection 3ml cartridges | 5 cartridge [PoM] £56.81 DT = £56.81
Hypurin Porcine Isophane 100units/ml suspension for injection 10ml vials | 1 vial [PoM] £37.87 DT = £37.87

▸ Insulatard (Novo Nordisk Ltd)
Insulin human (as Insulin isophane human) 100 unit per 1 ml Insulatard 100units/ml suspension for injection 10ml vials | 1 vial [PoM] £7.48 DT = £15.68

▸ Insulatard InnoLet (Novo Nordisk Ltd)
Insulin human (as Insulin isophane human) 100 unit per 1 ml Insulatard InnoLet 100units/ml suspension for injection 3ml pre-filled pens | 5 pre-filled disposable injection [PoM] £20.40 DT = £21.70

▸ Insulatard Penfill (Novo Nordisk Ltd)
Insulin human (as Insulin isophane human) 100 unit per 1 ml Insulatard Penfill 100units/ml suspension for injection 3ml cartridges | 5 cartridge [PoM] £22.90 DT = £19.08

▸ Insuman Basal (Sanofi)
Insulin human (as Insulin isophane human) 100 unit per 1 ml Insuman Basal 100units/ml suspension for injection 5ml vials | 1 vial [PoM] £5.61
Insuman Basal 100units/ml suspension for injection 3ml cartridges | 5 cartridge [PoM] £17.50 DT = £19.08

▸ Insuman Basal SoloStar (Sanofi)
Insulin human (as Insulin isophane human) 100 unit per 1 ml Insuman Basal 100units/ml suspension for injection 3ml pre-filled SoloStar pens | 5 pre-filled disposable injection [PoM] £19.80 DT = £21.70

INSULINS ⟩ INTERMEDIATE-ACTING COMBINED WITH RAPID-ACTING

▌**Biphasic insulin aspart**   F 752

(Intermediate-acting insulin)

● **INDICATIONS AND DOSE**
Diabetes mellitus
▸ BY SUBCUTANEOUS INJECTION
▸ Child: Administer up to 10 minutes before or soon after a meal, according to requirements
▸ Adult: Administer up to 10 minutes before or soon after a meal, according to requirements

● INTERACTIONS → Appendix 1: insulin
● SIDE-EFFECTS
▸ Uncommon Skin reactions
● PRESCRIBING AND DISPENSING INFORMATION Check product container—the proportions of the two components should be checked carefully (the order in which the proportions are stated may not be the same in other countries).

● MEDICINAL FORMS There can be variation in the licensing of different medicines containing the same drug.
Suspension for injection
▸ NovoMix 30 FlexPen (Novo Nordisk Ltd)
Insulin aspart 30 unit per 1 ml, Insulin aspart (as Insulin aspart protamine) 70 unit per 1 ml NovoMix 30 FlexPen 100units/ml suspension for injection 3ml pre-filled pens | 5 pre-filled disposable injection [PoM] £29.89 DT = £29.89

▸ NovoMix 30 Penfill (Novo Nordisk Ltd)
Insulin aspart 30 unit per 1 ml, Insulin aspart (as Insulin aspart protamine) 70 unit per 1 ml NovoMix 30 Penfill 100units/ml suspension for injection 3ml cartridges | 5 cartridge [PoM] £28.79 DT = £28.79

▌**Biphasic insulin lispro**   F 752
                                                          03-Feb-2020

(Intermediate-acting insulin)

● **INDICATIONS AND DOSE**
Diabetes mellitus
▸ BY SUBCUTANEOUS INJECTION
▸ Child: Administer up to 15 minutes before or soon after a meal, according to requirements
▸ Adult: Administer up to 15 minutes before or soon after a meal, according to requirements

● CAUTIONS Children under 12 years (use only if benefit likely compared to soluble insulin)
● INTERACTIONS → Appendix 1: insulin
● PRESCRIBING AND DISPENSING INFORMATION Check product container—the proportions of the two components should be checked carefully (the order in which the proportions are stated may not be the same in other countries).

● MEDICINAL FORMS There can be variation in the licensing of different medicines containing the same drug.

Suspension for injection

▸ Humalog Mix25 (Eli Lilly and Company Ltd)
Insulin lispro 25 unit per 1 ml, Insulin lispro (as Insulin lispro protamine) 75 unit per 1 ml Humalog Mix25 100units/ml suspension for injection 10ml vials | 1 vial PoM £16.61 DT = £16.61
Humalog Mix25 100units/ml suspension for injection 3ml cartridges | 5 cartridge PoM £29.46 DT = £29.46

▸ Humalog Mix25 KwikPen (Eli Lilly and Company Ltd)
Insulin lispro 25 unit per 1 ml, Insulin lispro (as Insulin lispro protamine) 75 unit per 1 ml Humalog Mix25 KwikPen 100units/ml suspension for injection 3ml pre-filled pens | 5 pre-filled disposable injection PoM £30.98 DT = £30.98

▸ Humalog Mix50 (Eli Lilly and Company Ltd)
Insulin lispro 50 unit per 1 ml, Insulin lispro (as Insulin lispro protamine) 50 unit per 1 ml Humalog Mix50 100units/ml suspension for injection 3ml cartridges | 5 cartridge PoM £29.46 DT = £29.46

▸ Humalog Mix50 KwikPen (Eli Lilly and Company Ltd)
Insulin lispro 50 unit per 1 ml, Insulin lispro (as Insulin lispro protamine) 50 unit per 1 ml Humalog Mix50 KwikPen 100units/ml suspension for injection 3ml pre-filled pens | 5 pre-filled disposable injection PoM £30.98 DT = £30.98

INSULINS ⟩ LONG-ACTING

🏷 752

Insulin degludec
                        22-Oct-2020

(Recombinant human insulin analogue—long acting)

● INDICATIONS AND DOSE

Diabetes mellitus
▸ BY SUBCUTANEOUS INJECTION
▹ **Child 1–17 years:** Dose to be given according to requirements
▹ **Adult:** Dose to be given according to requirements

● INTERACTIONS → Appendix 1: insulin

● SIDE-EFFECTS
▸ Rare or very rare Urticaria

● PREGNANCY Evidence of the safety of long-acting insulin analogues in pregnancy is limited, therefore isophane insulin is recommended where longer-acting insulins are needed; insulin detemir may also be considered.

● PRESCRIBING AND DISPENSING INFORMATION Insulin degludec (*Tresiba*®) is available in strengths of 100 units/mL (allows 1-unit dose adjustment) and 200 units/mL (allows 2-unit dose adjustment)—ensure correct strength prescribed.

● NATIONAL FUNDING/ACCESS DECISIONS
For full details see funding body website
All Wales Medicines Strategy Group (AWMSG) decisions
▸ Insulin degludec (*Tresiba*®) for treatment of diabetes mellitus in adult patients where treatment with a basal insulin analogue is considered appropriate (October 2016) AWMSG No. 3158 Recommended with restrictions
▸ Insulin degludec (*Tresiba*®) for treatment of diabetes mellitus in adolescents and children from the age of 1 year where treatment with a basal insulin analogue is considered appropriate (October 2016) AWMSG No. 3158 Not recommended

● MEDICINAL FORMS There can be variation in the licensing of different medicines containing the same drug.

Solution for injection

▸ Tresiba FlexTouch (Novo Nordisk Ltd)
Insulin degludec 100 unit per 1 ml Tresiba FlexTouch 100units/ml solution for injection 3ml pre-filled pens | 5 pre-filled disposable injection PoM £46.60 DT = £46.60
Insulin degludec 200 unit per 1 ml Tresiba FlexTouch 200units/ml solution for injection 3ml pre-filled pens | 3 pre-filled disposable injection PoM £55.92 DT = £55.92

▸ Tresiba Penfill (Novo Nordisk Ltd)
Insulin degludec 100 unit per 1 ml Tresiba Penfill 100units/ml solution for injection 3ml cartridges | 5 cartridge PoM £46.60 DT = £46.60

Insulin degludec with liraglutide
                22-Oct-2020

The properties listed below are those particular to the combination only. For the properties of the components please consider, insulin degludec above, liraglutide p. 739.

● INDICATIONS AND DOSE

As add-on to oral antidiabetics in type 2 diabetes mellitus not controlled by oral antidiabetics alone
▸ BY SUBCUTANEOUS INJECTION
▹ **Adult:** Initially 10 dose-steps once daily, adjusted according to response; maximum 50 dose-steps per day

When transferring from basal insulin in type 2 diabetes mellitus not controlled by oral antidiabetics in combination with basal insulin
▸ BY SUBCUTANEOUS INJECTION
▹ **Adult:** Initially 16 dose-steps once daily, adjusted according to response; maximum 50 dose-steps per day

● INTERACTIONS → Appendix 1: glucagon-like peptide-1 receptor agonists · insulin

● PATIENT AND CARER ADVICE Counselling advised on administration. Show container to patient and confirm that patient is expecting the version dispensed.

● NATIONAL FUNDING/ACCESS DECISIONS
For full details see funding body website
Scottish Medicines Consortium (SMC) decisions
▸ Insulin degludec/liraglutide (*Xultophy*®) for treatment of adults with type 2 diabetes mellitus to improve glycaemic control in combination with oral glucose-lowering medicinal products when these alone or combined with a GLP-1 receptor agonist or with basal insulin do not provide adequate glycaemic control (October 2015) SMC No. 1088/15 Recommended with restrictions

● MEDICINAL FORMS There can be variation in the licensing of different medicines containing the same drug.

Solution for injection

▸ Xultophy (Novo Nordisk Ltd)
Liraglutide 3.6 mg per 1 ml, Insulin degludec 100 unit per 1 ml Xultophy 100units/ml / 3.6mg/ml solution for injection 3ml pre-filled pens | 3 pre-filled disposable injection PoM £95.53 DT = £95.53

🏷 752

Insulin detemir
                        24-Nov-2020

(Recombinant human insulin analogue—long acting)

● INDICATIONS AND DOSE

Diabetes mellitus
▸ BY SUBCUTANEOUS INJECTION
▹ **Child 1–17 years:** According to requirements
▹ **Adult:** According to requirements

● INTERACTIONS → Appendix 1: insulin

● SIDE-EFFECTS
▸ Uncommon Refraction disorder

● PREGNANCY Evidence of the safety of long-acting insulin analogues in pregnancy is limited, therefore isophane insulin p. 756 is recommended where longer-acting insulins are needed; insulin detemir may also be considered where longer-acting insulins are needed.

● NATIONAL FUNDING/ACCESS DECISIONS
For full details see funding body website

6

Endocrine system

6

Endocrine system

Scottish Medicines Consortium (SMC) decisions
▸ Insulin detemir (*Levemir*®) for the treatment of diabetes mellitus (March 2016) SMC No. 1126/16 Recommended with restrictions

● MEDICINAL FORMS There can be variation in the licensing of different medicines containing the same drug.
Solution for injection
▸ Levemir FlexPen (Novo Nordisk Ltd)
Insulin detemir 100 unit per 1 ml Levemir FlexPen 100units/ml solution for injection 3ml pre-filled pens | 5 pre-filled disposable injection [PoM] £42.00 DT = £42.00
▸ Levemir InnoLet (Novo Nordisk Ltd)
Insulin detemir 100 unit per 1 ml Levemir InnoLet 100units/ml solution for injection 3ml pre-filled pens | 5 pre-filled disposable injection [PoM] £44.85 DT = £42.00
▸ Levemir Penfill (Novo Nordisk Ltd)
Insulin detemir 100 unit per 1 ml Levemir Penfill 100units/ml solution for injection 3ml cartridges | 5 cartridge [PoM] £42.00 DT = £42.00

▸❘ 752

Insulin glargine
18-Nov-2020

(Recombinant human insulin analogue—long acting)

● INDICATIONS AND DOSE
Diabetes mellitus
▸ BY SUBCUTANEOUS INJECTION
▸ Child 2-17 years: According to requirements
▸ Adult: According to requirements

TOUJEO®
Diabetes mellitus
▸ BY SUBCUTANEOUS INJECTION
▸ Adult: According to requirements

● INTERACTIONS → Appendix 1: insulin
● SIDE-EFFECTS
▸ Rare or very rare Myalgia · sodium retention · taste altered
● PREGNANCY Evidence of the safety of long-acting insulin analogues in pregnancy is limited, therefore isophane insulin is recommended where longer-acting insulins are needed; insulin detemir may also be considered.
● PRESCRIBING AND DISPENSING INFORMATION Insulin glargine is a biological medicine. Biological medicines must be prescribed and dispensed by brand name, see *Biological medicines* and *Biosimilar medicines*, under Guidance on prescribing p. 1. Dose adjustments and close metabolic monitoring is recommended if switching between insulin glargine preparations.
● NATIONAL FUNDING/ACCESS DECISIONS
For full details see funding body website
Scottish Medicines Consortium (SMC) decisions
▸ Insulin glargine (*Lantus*®) for the treatment of diabetes mellitus in adults, adolescents and children aged 2 years and above (April 2013) SMC No. 860/13 Recommended with restrictions
▸ Insulin glargine (*Toujeo*®) for the treatment of type 1 or type 2 diabetes mellitus in adults aged 18 years and above (September 2015) SMC No. 1078/15 Recommended with restrictions

● MEDICINAL FORMS There can be variation in the licensing of different medicines containing the same drug.
Solution for injection
▸ Abasaglar (Eli Lilly and Company Ltd)
Insulin glargine 100 unit per 1 ml Abasaglar 100units/ml solution for injection 3ml cartridges | 5 cartridge [PoM] £35.28 DT = £37.77
▸ Abasaglar KwikPen (Eli Lilly and Company Ltd)
Insulin glargine 100 unit per 1 ml Abasaglar KwikPen 100units/ml solution for injection 3ml pre-filled pens | 5 pre-filled disposable injection [PoM] £35.28 DT = £37.77

▸ Lantus (Sanofi)
Insulin glargine 100 unit per 1 ml Lantus 100units/ml solution for injection 3ml cartridges | 5 cartridge [PoM] £37.77 DT = £37.77
Lantus 100units/ml solution for injection 3ml pre-filled SoloStar pens | 5 pre-filled disposable injection [PoM] £37.77 DT = £37.77
Lantus 100units/ml solution for injection 10ml vials | 1 vial [PoM] £27.92 DT = £27.92
▸ Semglee (Mylan) ▼
Insulin glargine 100 unit per 1 ml Semglee 100units/ml solution for injection 3ml pre-filled pens | 5 pre-filled disposable injection [PoM] £29.99 DT = £37.77
▸ Toujeo (Sanofi)
Insulin glargine 300 unit per 1 ml Toujeo 300units/ml solution for injection 1.5ml pre-filled SoloStar pens | 3 pre-filled disposable injection [PoM] £32.14 DT = £32.14
▸ Toujeo DoubleStar (Sanofi)
Insulin glargine 300 unit per 1 ml Toujeo 300units/ml solution for injection 3ml pre-filled DoubleStar pens | 3 pre-filled disposable injection [PoM] £64.27 DT = £64.27

Insulin glargine with lixisenatide
09-Nov-2020

The properties listed below are those particular to the combination only. For the properties of the components please consider, insulin glargine above, lixisenatide p. 740.

● INDICATIONS AND DOSE
Type 2 diabetes mellitus [in combination with metformin]
▸ BY SUBCUTANEOUS INJECTION
▸ Adult: (consult product literature)

● INTERACTIONS → Appendix 1: glucagon-like peptide-1 receptor agonists · insulin
● PRESCRIBING AND DISPENSING INFORMATION *Suliqua*® is available in two pen strengths, providing different dosing options. To avoid medication errors, the prescriber must ensure that the correct strength and number of dose steps is prescribed. The manufacturer of *Suliqua*® has provided a healthcare professional guide and letter which includes important information on dosing.
● PATIENT AND CARER ADVICE Manufacturer advises check pen label before each administration to avoid medication error.
A patient guide should be provided.
● NATIONAL FUNDING/ACCESS DECISIONS
For full details see funding body website
Scottish Medicines Consortium (SMC) decisions
▸ Insulin glargine with lixisenatide (*Suliqua*®) in combination with metformin for the treatment of adults with type II diabetes mellitus (T2DM), to improve glycaemic control when this has not been provided by metformin alone or metformin combined with another oral glucose-lowering medicinal product or with basal insulin (April 2020) SMC No. SMC2235 Recommended with restrictions

● MEDICINAL FORMS There can be variation in the licensing of different medicines containing the same drug.
Solution for injection
CAUTIONARY AND ADVISORY LABELS 10
▸ Suliqua (Sanofi) ▼
Lixisenatide 33 microgram per 1 ml, Insulin glargine 100 unit per 1 ml Suliqua 100units/ml / 33micrograms/ml solution for injection 3ml pre-filled SoloStar pens | 3 pre-filled disposable injection [PoM] £48.60 DT = £48.60
Lixisenatide 50 microgram per 1 ml, Insulin glargine 100 unit per 1 ml Suliqua 100units/ml / 50micrograms/ml solution for injection 3ml pre-filled SoloStar pens | 3 pre-filled disposable injection [PoM] £67.50 DT = £67.50

3.1a Diabetes, diagnosis and monitoring

Diabetes mellitus, diagnostic and monitoring devices

Urinalysis: urinary glucose

Reagent strips are available for measuring for glucose in the urine. Tests for ketones by patients are rarely required unless they become unwell—see Blood Monitoring.

Microalbuminuria can be detected with *Micral-Test II*® but this should be followed by confirmation in the laboratory, since false positive results are common.

Blood glucose monitoring

Blood glucose monitoring using a meter gives a direct measure of the glucose concentration at the time of the test and can detect hypoglycaemia as well as hyperglycaemia. Patients should be properly trained in the use of blood glucose monitoring systems and to take appropriate action on the results obtained. Inadequate understanding of the normal fluctuations in blood glucose can lead to confusion and inappropriate action.

Patients using multiple injection regimens should understand how to adjust their insulin dose according to their carbohydrate intake. With fixed-dose insulin regimens, the carbohydrate intake needs to be regulated, and should be distributed throughout the day to match the insulin regimen.

Self-monitoring of blood-glucose concentration is appropriate for patients with type 2 diabetes:

- who are treated with insulin;
- who are treated with oral hypoglycaemic drugs e.g. sulfonylureas, to provide information on hypoglycaemia;
- to monitor changes in blood-glucose concentration resulting from changes in lifestyle or medication, and during intercurrent illness;
- to ensure safe blood-glucose concentration during activities, including driving.

In the UK blood-glucose concentration is expressed in mmol/litre and Diabetes UK advises that these units should be used for self-monitoring of blood glucose. In other European countries units of mg/100 mL (or mg/dL) are commonly used.

It is advisable to check that the meter is pre-set in the correct units.

If the patient is unwell and diabetic ketoacidosis is suspected, blood **ketones** should be measured according to local guidelines. Patients and their carers should be trained in the use of blood ketone monitoring systems and to take appropriate action on the results obtained, including when to seek medical attention.

> **Other drugs used for Diabetes, diagnosis and monitoring**
> Glucose, p. 1090

❚ Blood glucose testing strips

- ● BLOOD GLUCOSE TESTING STRIPS

4SURE testing strips (Nipro Diagnostics (UK) Ltd)
50 strip · NHS indicative price = £8.99 · Drug Tariff (Part IXr)

Accu-Chek Inform II testing strips (Roche Diagnostics Ltd)
50 strip · No NHS indicative price available · Drug Tariff (Part IXr)

Active testing strips (Roche Diabetes Care Ltd)
50 strip · NHS indicative price = £10.03 · Drug Tariff (Part IXr)

Advocate Redi-Code+ testing strips (Diabetes Care Technology Ltd)
50 strip · NHS indicative price = £9.95 · Drug Tariff (Part IXr)

AutoSense testing strips (Advance Diagnostic Products (NI) Ltd)
25 strip · NHS indicative price = £4.50 · Drug Tariff (Part IXr)

Aviva testing strips (Roche Diabetes Care Ltd)
50 strip · NHS indicative price = £16.21 · Drug Tariff (Part IXr)

BGStar testing strips (Sanofi)
50 strip · NHS indicative price = £14.73 · Drug Tariff (Part IXr)

Betachek C50 cassette (National Diagnostic Products)
100 device · NHS indicative price = £29.98 · Drug Tariff (Part IXr)

Betachek G5 testing strips (National Diagnostic Products)
50 strip · NHS indicative price = £14.19 · Drug Tariff (Part IXr)

Betachek Visual testing strips (National Diagnostic Products)
50 strip · NHS indicative price = £6.80 · Drug Tariff (Part IXr)

Breeze 2 testing discs (Bayer Plc)
50 strip · NHS indicative price = £15.00 · Drug Tariff (Part IXr)

CareSens N testing strips (Spirit Healthcare Ltd)
50 strip · NHS indicative price = £12.75 · Drug Tariff (Part IXr)

CareSens PRO testing strips (Spirit Healthcare Ltd)
50 strip · NHS indicative price = £9.95 · Drug Tariff (Part IXr)

Contour Next testing strips (Ascensia Diabetes Care UK Ltd)
50 strip · NHS indicative price = £15.16 · Drug Tariff (Part IXr)

Contour Plus testing strips (Ascensia Diabetes Care UK Ltd)
50 strip · NHS indicative price = £8.50 · Drug Tariff (Part IXr)

Contour TS testing strips (Ascensia Diabetes Care UK Ltd)
50 strip · NHS indicative price = £9.60 · Drug Tariff (Part IXr)

Contour testing strips (Ascensia Diabetes Care UK Ltd)
50 strip · NHS indicative price = £9.99 · Drug Tariff (Part IXr)

Dario Lite testing strips (LabStyle Innovations Ltd)
50 strip · NHS indicative price = £9.95 · Drug Tariff (Part IXr)

Dario testing strips (LabStyle Innovations Ltd)
50 strip · NHS indicative price = £14.95 · Drug Tariff (Part IXr)

Element testing strips (Neon Diagnostics Ltd)
50 strip · NHS indicative price = £9.89 · Drug Tariff (Part IXr)

Finetest Lite testing strips (Neon Diagnostics Ltd)
50 strip · NHS indicative price = £5.95 · Drug Tariff (Part IXr)

Fora Advanced pro GD40 testing strips (B.Braun Medical Ltd)
50 strip · NHS indicative price = £9.25 · Drug Tariff (Part IXr)

FreeStyle Lite testing strips (Abbott Laboratories Ltd)
50 strip · NHS indicative price = £16.41 · Drug Tariff (Part IXr)

FreeStyle Optium H testing strips (Abbott Laboratories Ltd)
100 strip · No NHS indicative price available · Drug Tariff (Part IXr)

FreeStyle Optium Neo H testing strips (Abbott Laboratories Ltd)
100 strip · No NHS indicative price available · Drug Tariff (Part IXr)

FreeStyle Optium testing strips (Abbott Laboratories Ltd)
50 strip · NHS indicative price = £16.30 · Drug Tariff (Part IXr)

FreeStyle Precision Pro testing strips (Abbott Laboratories Ltd)
100 strip · No NHS indicative price available · Drug Tariff (Part IXr)

FreeStyle testing strips (Abbott Laboratories Ltd)
50 strip · NHS indicative price = £16.40 · Drug Tariff (Part IXr)

GluNEO testing strips (Neon Diagnostics Ltd)
50 strip · NHS indicative price = £9.89 · Drug Tariff (Part IXr)

GlucoDock testing strips (Medisana Healthcare (UK) Ltd)
50 strip · NHS indicative price = £14.90 · Drug Tariff (Part IXr)

GlucoLab testing strips (Neon Diagnostics Ltd)
50 strip · NHS indicative price = £9.89 · Drug Tariff (Part IXr)

GlucoMen LX Sensor testing strips (A. Menarini Diagnostics Ltd)
50 strip · NHS indicative price = £15.76 · Drug Tariff (Part IXr)

GlucoMen areo Sensor testing strips (A. Menarini Diagnostics Ltd)
50 strip · NHS indicative price = £8.25 · Drug Tariff (Part IXr)

GlucoRx GO Professional testing strips (GlucoRx Ltd)
50 strip · NHS indicative price = £9.95 · Drug Tariff (Part IXr)

GlucoRx GO testing strips (GlucoRx Ltd)
50 strip · NHS indicative price = £9.95 · Drug Tariff (Part IXr)

GlucoRx HCT Glucose testing strips (GlucoRx Ltd)
50 strip · NHS indicative price = £8.95 · Drug Tariff (Part IXr)

GlucoRx Nexus testing strips (GlucoRx Ltd)
50 strip · NHS indicative price = £8.95 · Drug Tariff (Part IXr)

GlucoRx Q testing strips (GlucoRx Ltd)
50 strip · NHS indicative price = £5.45 · Drug Tariff (Part IXr)

6

Endocrine system

Meters and test strips

Meter (all NHS)	Type of monitoring	Compatible test strips	Test strip net price	Sensitivity range (mmol/litre)	Manufacturer
Accu-Chek® Active	Blood glucose	Active®	50 strip= £10.03	0.6- 33.3 mmol/litre	Roche Diabetes Care Ltd
Accu-Chek® Advantage Meter no longer available	Blood glucose	Advantage Plus®	50 strip= £0.00	0.6- 33.3 mmol/litre	Roche Diabetes Care Ltd
Accu-Chek® Aviva	Blood glucose	Aviva®	50 strip= £16.21	0.6- 33.3 mmol/litre	Roche Diabetes Care Ltd
Accu-Chek® Aviva Expert	Blood glucose	Aviva®	50 strip= £16.21	0.6- 33.3 mmol/litre	Roche Diabetes Care Ltd
Accu-Chek® Compact Plus Meter no longer available	Blood glucose	Compact®	3 × 17 strips= £0.00	0.6- 33.3 mmol/litre	Roche Diabetes Care Ltd
Accu-Chek® Mobile	Blood glucose	Mobile®	100 device= £0.00	0.3- 33.3 mmol/litre	Roche Diabetes Care Ltd
Accu-Chek® Aviva Nano	Blood glucose	Aviva®	50 strip= £16.21	0.6- 33.3 mmol/litre	Roche Diabetes Care Ltd
BGStar® Free of charge from diabetes healthcare professionals	Blood glucose	BGStar®	50 strip= £14.73	1.1- 33.3 mmol/litre	Sanofi
Breeze 2®	Blood glucose	Breeze 2®	50 strip= £15.00	0.6- 33.3 mmol/litre	Bayer Plc
CareSens N® Free of charge from diabetes healthcare professionals	Blood glucose	CareSens N®	50 strip= £12.75	1.1- 33.3 mmol/litre	Spirit Healthcare Ltd
Contour®	Blood glucose	Contour®	50 strip= £9.99	0.6- 33.3 mmol/litre	Ascensia Diabetes Care UK Ltd
Contour® XT	Blood glucose	Contour® Next	50 strip= £15.16	0.6- 33.3 mmol/litre	Ascensia Diabetes Care UK Ltd
Element®	Blood glucose	Element®	50 strip= £9.89	0.55- 33.3 mmol/litre	Neon Diagnostics Ltd
FreeStyle® Meter no longer available	Blood glucose	FreeStyle®	50 strip= £16.40	1.1- 27.8 mmol/litre	Abbott Laboratories Ltd
FreeStyle Freedom® Meter no longer available	Blood glucose	FreeStyle®	50 strip= £16.40	1.1- 27.8 mmol/litre	Abbott Laboratories Ltd
FreeStyle Freedom Lite®	Blood glucose	FreeStyle Lite®	50 strip= £16.41	1.1- 27.8 mmol/litre	Abbott Laboratories Ltd
FreeStyle InsuLinx®	Blood glucose	FreeStyle Lite®	50 strip= £16.41	1.1- 27.8 mmol/litre	Abbott Laboratories Ltd
FreeStyle Lite®	Blood glucose	FreeStyle Lite®	50 strip= £16.41	1.1- 27.8 mmol/litre	Abbott Laboratories Ltd
FreeStyle Mini® Meter no longer available	Blood glucose	FreeStyle®	50 strip= £16.40	1.1- 27.8 mmol/litre	Abbott Laboratories Ltd
FreeStyle Optium®	Blood glucose	FreeStyle Optium®	50 strip= £16.30	1.1- 27.8 mmol/litre	Abbott Laboratories Ltd
FreeStyle Optium®	Blood ketones	FreeStyle Optium®β-ketone	10 strip= £21.94	0- 8.0 mmol/litre	Abbott Laboratories Ltd
FreeStyle Optium Neo®	Blood glucose	FreeStyle Optium®	50 strip= £16.30	1.1- 27.8 mmol/litre	Abbott Laboratories Ltd
FreeStyle Optium Neo®	Blood ketones	FreeStyle Optium®β-ketone	10 strip= £21.94	0- 8.0 mmol/litre	Abbott Laboratories Ltd
GlucoDock® module	Blood glucose	GlucoDock®	50 strip= £14.90	1.1- 33.3 mmol/litre For use with iPhone®, iPod touch®, and iPad®	Medisana Healthcare (UK) Ltd
GlucoLab®	Blood glucose	GlucoLab®	50 strip= £9.89	0.55- 33.3 mmol/litre	Neon Diagnostics Ltd

Meter (all [NHS])	Type of monitoring	Compatible test strips	Test strip net price	Sensitivity range (mmol/litre)	Manufacturer
GlucoMen® GM	Blood glucose	GlucoMen® GM	50 strip= £0.00	0.6- 33.3 mmol/litre	A. Menarini Diagnostics Ltd
GlucoMen® LX	Blood glucose	GlucoMen® LX Sensor	50 strip= £15.76	1.1- 33.3 mmol/litre	A. Menarini Diagnostics Ltd
GlucoMen® LX Plus	Blood glucose	GlucoMen® LX Sensor	50 strip= £15.76	1.1- 33.3 mmol/litre	A. Menarini Diagnostics Ltd
GlucoMen® LX Plus	Blood ketones	GlucoMen® LX Ketone	10 strip= £21.06	0- 0.8 mmol/litre	A. Menarini Diagnostics Ltd
GlucoMen® Visio	Blood glucose	GlucoMen® Visio Sensor	50 strip= £0.00	1.1- 33.3 mmol/litre	A. Menarini Diagnostics Ltd
GlucoRx® Free of charge from diabetes healthcare professionals	Blood glucose	GlucoRx®	50 strip= £5.45	1.1- 33.3 mmol/litre	GlucoRx Ltd
GlucoRx Nexus® Free of charge from diabetes healthcare professionals	Blood glucose	GlucoRx Nexus®	50 strip= £8.95	1.1- 33.3 mmol/litre	GlucoRx Ltd
Glucotrend® Meter no longer available	Blood glucose	Active®	50 strip= £10.03	0.6- 33.3 mmol/litre	Roche Diabetes Care Ltd
iBGStar®	Blood glucose	BGStar®	50 strip= £14.73	1.1- 33.3 mmol/litre	Sanofi
IME-DC®	Blood glucose	IME-DC®	50 strip= £14.10	1.1- 33.3 mmol/litre	Arctic Medical Ltd
Mendor Discreet®	Blood glucose	Mendor Discreet®	50 strip= £14.75	1.1- 33.3 mmol/litre	SpringMed Solutions Ltd
Microdot®+ Free of charge from diabetes healthcare professionals	Blood glucose	Microdot®+	50 strip= £9.49	1.1- 29.2 mmol/litre	Cambridge Sensors Ltd
MyGlucoHealth®	Blood glucose	MyGlucoHealth®	50 strip= £15.50	0.6- 33.3 mmol/litre	Entra Health Systems Ltd
Omnitest® 3	Blood glucose	Omnitest® 3	50 strip= £9.89	0.6- 33.3 mmol/litre	B.Braun Medical Ltd
One Touch Ultra® Meter no longer available	Blood glucose	One Touch Ultra®	50 strip= £0.00	1.1- 33.3 mmol/litre	LifeScan
One Touch Ultra 2® Free of charge from diabetes healthcare professionals	Blood glucose	One Touch Ultra®	50 strip= £0.00	1.1- 33.3 mmol/litre	LifeScan
One Touch UltraEasy® Free of charge from diabetes healthcare professionals	Blood glucose	One Touch Ultra®	50 strip= £0.00	1.1- 33.3 mmol/litre	LifeScan
One Touch UltraSmart® Free of charge from diabetes healthcare professionals	Blood glucose	One Touch Ultra®	50 strip= £0.00	1.1- 33.3 mmol/litre	LifeScan
One Touch® VerioPro Free of charge from diabetes healthcare professionals	Blood glucose	One Touch Verio	50 strip= £15.12	1.1- 33.3 mmol/litre	LifeScan
One Touch® Vita Free of charge from diabetes healthcare professionals	Blood glucose	One Touch® Vita	50 strip= £0.00	1.1- 33.3 mmol/litre	LifeScan
SD CodeFree®	Blood glucose	SD CodeFree®	50 strip= £6.99	0.6- 33.3 mmol/litre	SD Biosensor Inc
Sensocard Plus® Meter no longer available	Blood glucose	Sensocard®	50 strip= £16.30	1.1- 33.3 mmol/litre	BBI Healthcare Ltd

6

Endocrine system

Meter (all NHS)	Type of monitoring	Compatible test strips	Test strip net price	Sensitivity range (mmol/litre)	Manufacturer
SuperCheck2® Free of charge from diabetes healthcare professionals	Blood glucose	SuperCheck2®	50 strip= £0.00	1.1- 33.3 mmol/litre	Apollo Medical Technologies Ltd
TRUEone® All-in-one test strips and meter	Blood glucose	TRUEone®	50 strip= £0.00	1.1- 33.3 mmol/litre	Nipro Diagnostics (UK) Ltd
TRUEresult® Free of charge from diabetes healthcare professionals	Blood glucose	TRUEresult®	50 strip= £0.00	1.1- 33.3 mmol/litre	Nipro Diagnostics (UK) Ltd
TRUEresult twist® Free of charge from diabetes healthcare professionals	Blood glucose	TRUEresult®	50 strip= £0.00	1.1- 33.3 mmol/litre	Nipro Diagnostics (UK) Ltd
TRUEtrack® Free of charge from diabetes healthcare professionals	Blood glucose	TRUEtrack®	50 strip= £0.00	1.1- 33.3 mmol/litre	Nipro Diagnostics (UK) Ltd
TRUEyou mini®	Blood glucose	TRUEyou®	50 strip= £7.95	1.1- 33.3 mmol/litre	Trividia Health UK Ltd
WaveSense JAZZ® Free of charge from diabetes healthcare professionals	Blood glucose	WaveSense JAZZ®	50 strip= £8.74	1.1- 33.3 mmol/litre	AgaMatrix Europe Ltd

GlucoZen.auto testing strips (GlucoZen Ltd)
50 strip · NHS indicative price = £7.64 · Drug Tariff (Part IXr)100 strip · NHS indicative price = £10.85 · Drug Tariff (Part IXr)

Glucoflex-R testing strips (Bio-Diagnostics Ltd)
50 strip · NHS indicative price = £6.75 · Drug Tariff (Part IXr)

Guide testing strips (Roche Diabetes Care Ltd)
50 strip · NHS indicative price = £16.21 · Drug Tariff (Part IXr)

IME-DC testing strips (Arctic Medical Ltd)
50 strip · NHS indicative price = £14.10 · Drug Tariff (Part IXr)

Kinetik Wellbeing testing strips (Kinetik Medical Devices Ltd)
50 strip · NHS indicative price = £8.49 · Drug Tariff (Part IXr)100 strip · NHS indicative price = £13.98 · Drug Tariff (Part IXr)

MODZ testing strips (Modz Oy)
50 strip · NHS indicative price = £14.00 · Drug Tariff (Part IXr)

MediSense SoftSense testing strips (Abbott Laboratories Ltd)
50 strip · NHS indicative price = £15.05 · Drug Tariff (Part IXr)

MediTouch 2 testing strips (Medisana Healthcare (UK) Ltd)
50 strip · NHS indicative price = £12.49 · Drug Tariff (Part IXr)

MediTouch testing strips (Medisana Healthcare (UK) Ltd)
50 strip · NHS indicative price = £14.90 · Drug Tariff (Part IXr)

Mendor Discreet testing strips (SpringMed Solutions Ltd)
50 strip · NHS indicative price = £14.75 · Drug Tariff (Part IXr)

Microdot Max testing strips (Cambridge Sensors Ltd)
50 strip · NHS indicative price = £7.49 · Drug Tariff (Part IXr)

Microdot+ testing strips (Cambridge Sensors Ltd)
50 strip · NHS indicative price = £9.49 · Drug Tariff (Part IXr)

Mobile cassette (Roche Diabetes Care Ltd)
50 device · NHS indicative price = £9.99 · Drug Tariff (Part IXr)

Myglucohealth testing strips (Entra Health Systems Ltd)
50 strip · NHS indicative price = £15.50 · Drug Tariff (Part IXr)

Mylife Pura testing strips (Ypsomed Ltd)
50 strip · NHS indicative price = £9.50 · Drug Tariff (Part IXr)

Mylife Unio testing strips (Ypsomed Ltd)
50 strip · NHS indicative price = £9.50 · Drug Tariff (Part IXr)

OKmeter Core testing strips (Syringa UK Ltd)
50 strip · NHS indicative price = £9.90 · Drug Tariff (Part IXr)

Oh'Care Lite testing strips (Neon Diagnostics Ltd)
50 strip · NHS indicative price = £8.88 · Drug Tariff (Part IXr)

Omnitest 3 testing strips (B.Braun Medical Ltd)
50 strip · NHS indicative price = £9.89 · Drug Tariff (Part IXr)

Omnitest 5 testing strips (B.Braun Medical Ltd)
50 strip · NHS indicative price = £9.89 · Drug Tariff (Part IXr)

On Call Extra testing strips (Acon Laboratories, Inc)
50 strip · NHS indicative price = £7.50 · Drug Tariff (Part IXr)

On Call Sure testing strips (Acon Laboratories, Inc)
50 strip · NHS indicative price = £9.20 · Drug Tariff (Part IXr)

On-Call Advanced testing strips (Point Of Care Testing Ltd)
50 strip · NHS indicative price = £13.65 · Drug Tariff (Part IXr)

OneTouch Select Plus testing strips (LifeScan)
50 strip · NHS indicative price = £9.99 · Drug Tariff (Part IXr)

OneTouch Verio testing strips (LifeScan)
50 strip · NHS indicative price = £15.12 · Drug Tariff (Part IXr)

Performa testing strips (Roche Diabetes Care Ltd)
50 strip · NHS indicative price = £7.50 · Drug Tariff (Part IXr)

SD CodeFree testing strips (SD Biosensor Inc)
50 strip · NHS indicative price = £6.99 · Drug Tariff (Part IXr)

SURESIGN Resure testing strips (Ciga Healthcare Ltd)
50 strip · NHS indicative price = £8.49 · Drug Tariff (Part IXr)

Sensocard testing strips (BBI Healthcare Ltd)
50 strip · NHS indicative price = £16.30 · Drug Tariff (Part IXr)

StatStrip testing strips (Nova Biomedical)
50 strip · No NHS indicative price available · Drug Tariff (Part IXr)

TEE2 testing strips (Spirit Healthcare Ltd)
50 strip · NHS indicative price = £7.75 · Drug Tariff (Part IXr)

TRUEyou testing strips (Trividia Health UK Ltd)
50 strip · NHS indicative price = £7.95 · Drug Tariff (Part IXr)

True Metrix testing strips (Trividia Health UK Ltd)
50 strip · NHS indicative price = £6.95 · Drug Tariff (Part IXr)100 strip · NHS indicative price = £12.50 · Drug Tariff (Part IXr)

VivaChek Ino testing strips (JR Biomedical Ltd)
50 strip · NHS indicative price = £8.99 · Drug Tariff (Part IXr)

WaveSense JAZZ Duo testing strips (AgaMatrix Europe Ltd)
50 strip · NHS indicative price = £8.74 · Drug Tariff (Part IXr)

WaveSense JAZZ testing strips (AgaMatrix Europe Ltd)
50 strip · NHS indicative price = £8.74 · Drug Tariff (Part IXr)

Xceed Precision Pro testing strips (Abbott Laboratories Ltd)
10 strip · No NHS indicative price available50 strip · No NHS indicative price available · Drug Tariff (Part IXr)100 strip · No NHS indicative price available · Drug Tariff (Part IXr)

palmdoc iCare Advanced Solo testing strips (Palmdoc Ltd)
50 strip · NHS indicative price = £13.50 · Drug Tariff (Part IXr)

palmdoc iCare Advanced testing strips (Palmdoc Ltd)
50 strip · NHS indicative price = £9.70 · Drug Tariff (Part IXr)

palmdoc testing strips (Palmdoc Ltd)
50 strip · NHS indicative price = £5.90 · Drug Tariff (Part IXr)

Blood ketones testing strips

- BLOOD KETONES TESTING STRIPS

4SURE beta-ketone testing strips (Nipro Diagnostics (UK) Ltd)
10 strip · NHS indicative price = £9.92 · Drug Tariff (Part IXr)

Fora Advanced pro GD40 Ketone testing strips (B.Braun Medical Ltd)10 strip · NHS indicative price = £9.25 · Drug Tariff (Part IXr)

FreeStyle Optium H beta-ketone testing strips (Abbott Laboratories Ltd)10 strip · No NHS indicative price available · Drug Tariff (Part IXr)

FreeStyle Optium beta-ketone testing strips (Abbott Laboratories Ltd)10 strip · NHS indicative price = £21.94 · Drug Tariff (Part IXr)

FreeStyle Precision Pro beta-ketone testing strips (Abbott Laboratories Ltd)50 strip · No NHS indicative price available

GlucoMen LX beta-ketone testing strips (A. Menarini Diagnostics Ltd)10 strip · NHS indicative price = £21.06 · Drug Tariff (Part IXr)

GlucoMen areo Ketone Sensor testing strips (A. Menarini Diagnostics Ltd)10 strip · NHS indicative price = £9.95 · Drug Tariff (Part IXr)

GlucoRx HCT Ketone testing strips (GlucoRx Ltd)10 strip · NHS indicative price = £9.95 · Drug Tariff (Part IXr)

KetoSens testing strips (Spirit Healthcare Ltd)10 strip · NHS indicative price = £9.95 · Drug Tariff (Part IXr)

StatStrip beta-ketone testing strips (Nova Biomedical)50 strip · No NHS indicative price available

Xceed Precision Pro beta-ketone testing strips (Abbott Laboratories Ltd)10 strip · No NHS indicative price available · Drug Tariff (Part IXr)50 strip · No NHS indicative price available100 strip · No NHS indicative price available

Glucose interstitial fluid detection sensors

- GLUCOSE INTERSTITIAL FLUID DETECTION SENSORS

FreeStyle Libre 2 Sensor (Abbott Laboratories Ltd)
1 kit · NHS indicative price = £35.00 · Drug Tariff (Part IXa)

FreeStyle Libre Sensor (Abbott Laboratories Ltd)
1 kit · NHS indicative price = £35.00 · Drug Tariff (Part IXa)

Hypodermic insulin injection pens

- HYPODERMIC INSULIN INJECTION PENS

AUTOPEN® 24

Autopen® 24 (for use with Sanofi- Aventis 3-mL insulin cartridges), allowing 1-unit dosage adjustment, max. 21 units (single-unit version) or 2-unit dosage adjustment, max. 42 units (2- unit version).

Autopen 24 hypodermic insulin injection pen reusable for 3ml cartridge 1 unit dial up / range 1-21 units (Owen Mumford Ltd)
1 device · NHS indicative price = £16.89 · Drug Tariff (Part IXa)

Autopen 24 hypodermic insulin injection pen reusable for 3ml cartridge 2 unit dial up / range 2-42 units (Owen Mumford Ltd)
1 device · NHS indicative price = £16.89 · Drug Tariff (Part IXa)

AUTOPEN® CLASSIC

Autopen® *Classic* (for use with Lilly and Wockhardt 3-mL insulin cartridges), allowing 1-unit dosage adjustment, max. 21 units (single-unit version) or 2-unit dosage adjustment, max. 42 units (2-unit version).

Autopen Classic hypodermic insulin injection pen reusable for 3ml cartridge 1 unit dial up / range 1-21 units (Owen Mumford Ltd)
1 device · NHS indicative price = £17.15 · Drug Tariff (Part IXa)

Autopen Classic hypodermic insulin injection pen reusable for 3ml cartridge 2 unit dial up / range 2-42 units (Owen Mumford Ltd)
1 device · NHS indicative price = £17.15 · Drug Tariff (Part IXa)

CLIKSTAR®

For use with *Lantus*®, *Apidra*®, and *Insuman*® 3-mL insulin cartridges; allowing 1-unit dose adjustment, max. 80 units.

HUMAPEN® LUXURA HD

For use with *Humulin*® and *Humalog*® 3-mL cartridges; allowing 0.5-unit dosage adjustment, max. 30 units.

HumaPen Luxura HD hypodermic insulin injection pen reusable for 3ml cartridge 0.5 unit dial up / range 1-30 units (Eli Lilly and Company Ltd)
1 device · NHS indicative price = £27.01 · Drug Tariff (Part IXa)

NOVOPEN® 4

For use with *Penfill*® 3-mL insulin cartridges; allowing 1-unit dosage adjustment, max. 60 units.

Needle free insulin delivery systems

- NEEDLE FREE INSULIN DELIVERY SYSTEMS

INSUJET®

For use with any 10-mL vial or 3-mL cartridge of insulin, allowing 1-unit dosage adjustment, max 40 units. Available as *starter set* (*InsuJet*® device, nozzle cap, nozzle and piston, 1 × 10-mL adaptor, 1 × 3-mL adaptor, 1 cartridge cap removal key), *nozzle pack* (15 nozzles), *cartridge adaptor pack* (15 adaptors), or *vial adaptor pack* (15 adaptors).

InsuJet starter set (Spirit Healthcare Ltd)
1 pack · NHS indicative price = £90.00 · Drug Tariff (Part IXa)

Urine glucose testing strips

- URINE GLUCOSE TESTING STRIPS

Diastix testing strips (Ascensia Diabetes Care UK Ltd)
50 strip · NHS indicative price = £2.89 · Drug Tariff (Part IXr)

Medi-Test Glucose testing strips (BHR Pharmaceuticals Ltd)
50 strip · NHS indicative price = £2.36 · Drug Tariff (Part IXr)

Urine ketone testing strips

- URINE KETONES TESTING STRIPS

GlucoRx KetoRx Sticks 2GK testing strips (GlucoRx Ltd)
50 strip · NHS indicative price = £2.25 · Drug Tariff (Part IXr)

Ketostix testing strips (Ascensia Diabetes Care UK Ltd)
50 strip · NHS indicative price = £3.06 · Drug Tariff (Part IXr)

Urine protein testing strips

- URINE PROTEIN TESTING STRIPS

Albustix testing strips (Siemens Medical Solutions Diagnostics Ltd)
50 strip · NHS indicative price = £4.10 · Drug Tariff (Part IXr)

Medi-Test Protein 2 testing strips (BHR Pharmaceuticals Ltd)
50 strip · NHS indicative price = £3.31 · Drug Tariff (Part IXr)

3.2 Hypoglycaemia

Hypoglycaemia

20-Apr-2020

Description of condition

Hypoglycaemia is a lower than normal blood-glucose concentration. It results from an imbalance between glucose supply, glucose utilisation, and existing insulin concentration. It can be defined as 'mild' if the episode is self-treated and 'severe' if assistance is required. For the purposes of hospital inpatients diagnosed with diabetes, anyone with a blood-glucose concentration less than 4 mmol/litre should be treated.

Hypoglycaemia is the most common side-effect of insulin and sulfonylureas in the treatment of all types of diabetes mellitus and presents a major barrier to satisfactory long-term glycaemic control. Metformin hydrochloride p. 732, pioglitazone p. 751, the dipeptidylpeptidase-4 inhibitors (gliptins), sodium-glucose co-transporter-2 inhibitors, and glucagon-like peptide-1 receptor agonists, prescribed without insulin or sulfonylurea therapy, are unlikely to result in hypoglycaemia. Hypoglycaemia should be excluded in any person with diabetes who is acutely unwell, drowsy, unconscious, unable to co-operate, or presenting with aggressive behaviour or seizures.

Treatment of hypoglycaemia

For a quick reference resource with doses for the treatment of hypoglycaemia, see *Hypoglycaemia* in *Medical emergencies in the community*, inside back pages.

[EvGr] Adults with symptoms of hypoglycaemia who have a blood-glucose concentration greater than 4 mmol/litre, should be treated with a small carbohydrate snack such as a slice of bread or a normal meal, if due.

Any patient with a blood-glucose concentration less than 4 mmol/litre, with or without symptoms, and who is **conscious and able to swallow**, should have 15–20 g of fast-acting carbohydrate. This is available in approximately 3–4 heaped teaspoonfuls of sugar dissolved in water, 4–7 glucose tablets, or 150–200 mL of pure fruit juice. Orange juice should not be given to patients following a low-potassium diet due to chronic kidney disease, and sugar dissolved in water is not effective for patients taking acarbose which prevents the breakdown of sucrose to glucose. ⓔ[EvGr] Chocolates and biscuits should be avoided if possible, because they have a lower sugar content and their high fat content may delay stomach emptying. ⓐ Proprietary products of fast-acting carbohydrate, as glucose 40% gel (e.g. *Glucogel®*, *Dextrogel®*, or *Rapilose gel®*, see glucose p. 1090) are available for patients to keep at hand in case of hypoglycaemia; [EvGr] 2 tubes should be taken.

If necessary, repeat treatment after 10–15 minutes, up to a maximum of 3 treatments in total. Once blood-glucose concentration is above 4 mmol/litre and the patient has recovered, a snack providing a long-acting carbohydrate should be given to prevent blood glucose from falling again (e.g. two biscuits, one slice of bread, 200–300 mL of milk (not soya or other forms of 'alternative' milk, e.g. almond or coconut), or a normal carbohydrate-containing meal if due). Insulin should not be omitted if due, but the dose regimen may need review.

Hypoglycaemia which does not respond (blood-glucose concentration remains below 4 mmol/litre after 30–45 minutes or after 3 treatment cycles), should be treated with intramuscular glucagon below or glucose 10% intravenous infusion. In alcoholic patients, thiamine supplementation should be given with, or following, the administration of intravenous glucose to minimise the risk of Wernicke's encephalopathy. ⓔ

Glucagon is a polypeptide hormone produced by the alpha cells of the islets of Langerhans, which increases blood-glucose concentration by mobilising glycogen stored in the liver. The manufacturer advises that it is ineffective in patients whose liver glycogen is depleted, therefore should not be used in anyone who has fasted for a prolonged period or has adrenal insufficiency, chronic hypoglycaemia, or alcohol-induced hypoglycaemia. [EvGr] Glucagon may also be less effective in patients taking a sulfonylurea; in these cases, intravenous glucose will be required. ⓔ

[EvGr] In an emergency, if the patient has a decreased level of consciousness caused by hypoglycaemia, intramuscular glucagon can be given by a family member or friend who has been shown how to use it. ⓐ[EvGr] If glucagon is not effective after 10 minutes, glucose 10% intravenous infusion should be given. ⓔ

Hypoglycaemia which causes **unconsciousness** is an emergency. [EvGr] Patients who are unconscious, having seizures, or who are very aggressive, should have any intravenous insulin stopped, and be treated initially with glucagon. If glucagon is unsuitable, or there is no response after 10 minutes, glucose 10% intravenous infusion, or alternatively glucose 20% intravenous infusion should be given. ⓔ Glucose 50% intravenous infusion is not recommended as it is hypertonic, thus increases the risk of extravasation injury, and is viscous, making administration difficult.

[EvGr] A long-acting carbohydrate should be given as soon as possible once the patient has recovered and their blood-glucose concentration is above 4 mmol/litre (e.g. two biscuits, one slice of bread, 200–300 mL of milk (not soya or other forms of 'alternative' milk, e.g. almond or coconut), or a normal carbohydrate-containing meal if due). Patients who have received glucagon require a larger portion of long-acting carbohydrate to replenish glycogen stores (e.g. four biscuits, two slices of bread, 400–600 mL of milk (not soya or other forms of 'alternative' milk, e.g. almond or coconut), or a normal carbohydrate containing meal if due). Glucose 10% intravenous infusion should be given to patients who are nil by mouth.

If an insulin injection is due, it should **not** be omitted; however, a review of the usual insulin regimen may be required. Patients who self-manage their insulin pump may need to adjust their pump infusion rate. If the patient was on intravenous insulin, continue to check blood-glucose concentration every 15 minutes until above 3.5 mmol/litre, then re-start intravenous insulin after review of the dose regimen. Concurrent glucose 10% intravenous infusion should be considered. ⓔ

Hypoglycaemia caused by a sulfonylurea or long-acting insulin, may persist for up to 24–36 hours following the last dose, especially if there is concurrent renal impairment.

[EvGr] Blood-glucose monitoring should be continued for at least 24–48 hours. ⓔ

GLYCOGENOLYTIC HORMONES

Glucagon

20-Jul-2020

● **INDICATIONS AND DOSE**

Diabetic hypoglycaemia

▸ BY SUBCUTANEOUS INJECTION, OR BY INTRAMUSCULAR INJECTION

▹ Child 1 month-8 years (body-weight up to 25 kg):
500 micrograms, if no response within 10 minutes intravenous glucose must be given

▹ Child 9-17 years (body-weight 25 kg and above): 1 mg, if no response within 10 minutes intravenous glucose must be given

▹ Adult: 1 mg, if no response within 10 minutes intravenous glucose must be given

Beta-blocker poisoning (cardiogenic shock unresponsive to atropine)

▸ INITIALLY BY INTRAVENOUS INJECTION

▹ Child: 50–150 micrograms/kg (max. per dose 10 mg), to be administered in glucose 5% (with precautions to protect the airway in case of vomiting), followed by (by intravenous infusion) 50 micrograms/kg/hour

▹ Adult: 2–10 mg, to be administered in glucose 5% (with precautions to protect the airway in case of vomiting), followed by (by intravenous infusion) 50 micrograms/kg/hour

Diagnostic aid

▸ BY INTRAVENOUS INJECTION, OR BY INTRAMUSCULAR INJECTION

▹ Adult: (consult product literature)

DOSE EQUIVALENCE AND CONVERSION

▸ 1 unit of glucagon = 1 mg of glucagon.

- **UNLICENSED USE** Dose and indication for cardiogenic shock unresponsive to atropine in beta-blocker overdose not licensed.
- **CONTRA-INDICATIONS** Phaeochromocytoma
- **CAUTIONS** Glucagonoma · ineffective in chronic hypoglycaemia, starvation, and adrenal insufficiency · insulinoma
- **INTERACTIONS** → Appendix 1: glucagon
- **SIDE-EFFECTS**
  - ▶ **Common or very common** Nausea
  - ▶ **Uncommon** Vomiting
  - ▶ **Rare or very rare** Abdominal pain · hypertension · hypotension · tachycardia
- **DIRECTIONS FOR ADMINISTRATION**
  - ▶ With intravenous use in children When administered by *continuous intravenous infusion*, expert sources advise do not add to infusion fluids containing calcium—precipitation may occur.
- **PATIENT AND CARER ADVICE**
  Medicines for Children leaflet: Glucagon for hypoglycaemia
  www.medicinesforchildren.org.uk/glucagon-hypoglycaemia
- **EXCEPTIONS TO LEGAL CATEGORY** Prescription-only medicine restriction does not apply where administration is for saving life in emergency.

- **MEDICINAL FORMS** There can be variation in the licensing of different medicines containing the same drug.
  Powder and solvent for solution for injection
  - ▶ GlucaGen Hypokit (Novo Nordisk Ltd)
    Glucagon hydrochloride 1 mg GlucaGen Hypokit 1mg powder and solvent for solution for injection | 1 vial [PoM] £11.52 DT = £11.52

3.2a Chronic hypoglycaemia

GLYCOGENOLYTIC HORMONES

| Diazoxide

- **INDICATIONS AND DOSE**
  Chronic intractable hypoglycaemia
  ▶ BY MOUTH
  - ▶ Adult: Initially 5 mg/kg daily in 2–3 divided doses, adjusted according to response; maintenance 3–8 mg/kg daily in 2–3 divided doses
- **CAUTIONS** Aortic coarctation · aortic stenosis · arteriovenous shunt · heart failure · hyperuricaemia · impaired cardiac circulation · impaired cerebral circulation
- **INTERACTIONS** → Appendix 1: diazoxide
- **SIDE-EFFECTS** Abdominal pain · albuminuria · appetite decreased (long term use) · arrhythmia · azotaemia · cardiomegaly · cataract · constipation · diabetic hyperosmolar coma · diarrhoea · dizziness · dyspnoea · eosinophilia · extrapyramidal symptoms · fever · fluid retention · galactorrhoea · haemorrhage · headache · heart failure · hirsutism · hyperglycaemia · hyperuricaemia (long term use) · hypogammaglobulinaemia · hypotension · ileus · ketoacidosis · leucopenia · libido decreased · musculoskeletal pain · nausea · nephritic syndrome · oculogyric crisis · pancreatitis · parkinsonism · pulmonary hypertension · skin reactions · sodium retention · taste altered · thrombocytopenia · tinnitus · vision disorders · voice alteration (long term use) · vomiting
- **PREGNANCY** Use only if essential; alopecia and hypertrichosis reported in neonates with prolonged use; may inhibit uterine activity during labour.
- **BREAST FEEDING** Manufacturer advises avoid—no information available.

- **RENAL IMPAIRMENT**
  Dose adjustments Dose reduction may be required.
- **MONITORING REQUIREMENTS**
  - ▶ Monitor blood pressure.
  - ▶ Monitor white cell and platelet count during prolonged use.

- **MEDICINAL FORMS** There can be variation in the licensing of different medicines containing the same drug. Forms available from special-order manufacturers include: capsule, oral suspension, oral solution
  Tablet
  - ▶ Eudemine (RPH Pharmaceuticals AB)
    Diazoxide 50 mg Eudemine 50mg tablets | 100 tablet [PoM] £72.55 DT = £72.55
  Capsule
  - ▶ Proglycem (Imported (Germany))
    Diazoxide 25 mg Proglycem 25 capsules | 100 capsule [PoM] [℞]

6

Endocrine system

4 Disorders of bone metabolism

Osteoporosis
05-Aug-2020

Description of condition
Osteoporosis is a progressive bone disease characterised by low bone mass measured by bone mineral density (BMD), and microarchitectural deterioration of bone tissue. This leads to an increased risk of fragility fractures (fractures resulting from low-level trauma). Osteoporosis is considered severe if there have been one or more fragility fractures.

Osteoporosis occurs most commonly in postmenopausal women, men over 50 years, and in patients taking long-term oral corticosteroids (glucocorticoids). Other risk factors for osteoporosis include increasing age, vitamin D deficiency and low calcium intake, lack of physical activity, low body mass index (BMI), cigarette smoking, excess alcohol intake, parental history of hip fractures, a previous fracture at a site characteristic of osteoporotic fractures, and early menopause. Some diseases are also known to be associated with osteoporosis such as rheumatoid arthritis and diabetes. Certain medications may also increase the risk of fracture in some patients, through mechanisms such as induction of liver enzymes which interfere with vitamin D metabolism.

Aims of treatment
A combination of lifestyle changes and drug treatment aims to prevent fragility fractures in patients with osteoporosis.

Lifestyle changes
[EvGr] Patients should be encouraged to increase their level of physical activity, stop smoking, maintain a normal BMI level (between 20–25 kg/m^2), and reduce their alcohol intake to improve their bone health and reduce the risk of fragility fractures. ⚘ For guidance on stopping smoking, see Smoking cessation p. 519.

[EvGr] Patients at risk of osteoporosis should also ensure an adequate intake of calcium and vitamin D. Calcium should preferably be obtained through increasing dietary intake; supplements may be used if necessary. A daily dietary supplement of vitamin D may be considered for those at increased risk of deficiency.

Elderly patients, especially those who are housebound or live in residential or nursing homes, are at high risk of vitamin D deficiency and may benefit from calcium and vitamin D treatment. ⚘ Elderly patients also have an increased risk of falls (see Prescribing in the elderly p. 33).

Drug treatment

EvGr Choice of treatment is generally determined by the spectrum of anti-fracture effects across skeletal sites, patient preference and suitability. A

Some recommendations on the management of osteoporosis from the National Osteoporosis Guideline Group (NOGG)—Clinical guideline for the prevention and treatment of osteoporosis (July 2019), and Scottish Intercollegiate Guidelines Network (SIGN)—Management of osteoporosis and the prevention of fragility fractures (SIGN 142, June 2020) differ. Recommendations in BNF publications are based on the NOGG guideline, and differences with SIGN (2020) have been highlighted.

Postmenopausal osteoporosis

EvGr The oral bisphosphonates alendronic acid p. 768 and risedronate sodium p. 770, are considered as first-line options for most patients with postmenopausal osteoporosis due to their broad spectrum of anti-fracture efficacy. Alendronic acid and risedronate sodium have been shown to reduce occurrence of vertebral, non-vertebral and hip fractures. SIGN (2020) also recommend that oral ibandronic acid p. 769 may be considered as an alternative. Intravenous bisphosphonates, or denosumab p. 774 are alternative options for women who are intolerant of oral bisphosphonates or in whom they are unsuitable, with raloxifene hydrochloride p. 797 or strontium ranelate p. 773 as additional options.

Hormone replacement therapy (HRT) may also be considered as an additional option, but its use is generally restricted to younger postmenopausal women with menopausal symptoms who are at high risk of fractures. This is due to the risk of adverse effects such as cardiovascular disease and cancer in older postmenopausal women and women on long-term HRT therapy. SIGN (2020) also recommend tibolone p. 802 as an option in younger postmenopausal women, particularly those with menopausal symptoms.

Teriparatide p. 774 is reserved for postmenopausal women with severe osteoporosis at very high risk, particularly for vertebral fractures. Its duration of treatment is limited to 24 months. SIGN (2020) also recommend the use of teriparatide over oral bisphosphonates in postmenopausal women with at least two moderate or one severe low-trauma vertebral fracture. A

Glucocorticoid-induced osteoporosis

Glucocorticoid treatment is strongly associated with bone loss and increased risk of fractures. The greatest rate of bone loss occurs early after initiation of glucocorticoids and increases with dose and duration of therapy. EvGr Bone-protection treatment should be started at the onset of glucocorticoid treatment in patients who are at a high risk of fracture.

Women aged ≥70 years, or with a previous fragility fracture, or taking large doses of glucocorticoids (prednisolone ≥7.5 mg daily or equivalent) should be considered for bone-protection treatment. Men aged ≥70 years with a previous fragility fracture, or taking large doses of glucocorticoids, should also be considered for treatment. For some premenopausal women and younger men (particularly those with a previous history of fracture or receiving high doses of glucocorticoids), bone-protection treatment may be appropriate. SIGN (2020) recommends that bone-protection treatment should be considered in men and women taking large doses of glucocorticoids (prednisolone ≥7.5 mg daily or equivalent) for 3 months or longer.

The oral bisphosphonates alendronic acid or risedronate sodium are first-line treatment options. Zoledronic acid p. 772, denosumab or teriparatide are alternative options in patients intolerant of oral bisphosphonates or in whom they are unsuitable.

If glucocorticoid treatment is stopped, the need to continue bone-protection treatment should be reviewed. However, bone-protection treatment should be continued with long-term glucocorticoid treatment. Complex cases of glucocorticoid-induced osteoporosis should be referred to a specialist. A

Osteoporosis in men

EvGr The oral bisphosphonates alendronic acid or risedronate sodium, are recommended as first-line treatments for osteoporosis in men. Zoledronic acid or denosumab are alternatives in men who are intolerant of oral bisphosphonates or in whom they are unsuitable; teriparatide or strontium ranelate are additional options. A

Men having androgen deprivation therapy for prostate cancer have an increased fracture risk. EvGr Fracture risk assessment should be considered in men when starting this therapy. A bisphosphonate can be offered to men with confirmed osteoporosis; denosumab may be considered as an alternative if bisphosphonates are unsuitable or not tolerated. A

Bisphosphonates: treatment duration

EvGr Some patients may benefit from a bisphosphonate-free period as their therapeutic effects last for some time after cessation of treatment, although there is limited evidence to support this.

Bisphosphonate treatment should be reviewed after 5 years of treatment with alendronic acid, risedronate sodium or ibandronic acid, and after 3 years of treatment with zoledronic acid. Based on fracture-risk assessment, continuation beyond this period can generally be recommended for patients who are over 75 years of age, have a history of previous hip or vertebral fracture, have had one or more fragility fractures during treatment, or who are taking long-term glucocorticoid treatment. Due to limited evidence, recommendations on duration are based on limited extension studies in postmenopausal women. There is no evidence for treatment beyond 10 years; management of these patients should be on a case-by-case basis with specialist input as appropriate. A

Useful Resources

Clinical guideline for the prevention and treatment of osteoporosis. The National Osteoporosis Guideline Group (NOGG). 2017 (updated July 2019).
www.sheffield.ac.uk/NOGG/downloads.html

Management of osteoporosis and the prevention of fragility fractures. Scottish Intercollegiate Guidelines Network. Clinical guideline 142. June 2020.
www.sign.ac.uk/media/1741/sign142.pdf

> **Other drugs used for Disorders of bone metabolism**
> Calcitriol, p. 1133

ANABOLIC STEROIDS

Nandrolone

26-Oct-2020

● **INDICATIONS AND DOSE**

Osteoporosis in postmenopausal women (but not recommended)
▸ BY DEEP INTRAMUSCULAR INJECTION
▸ Adult (female): 50 mg every 3 weeks.

● CONTRA-INDICATIONS Acute porphyrias p. 1107
● CAUTIONS Cardiac impairment · diabetes mellitus · epilepsy · hypertension · migraine · skeletal metastases (risk of hypercalcaemia)
● INTERACTIONS → Appendix 1: nandrolone
● SIDE-EFFECTS Clitoris enlarged · dysphonia · hepatic disorders · hepatic neoplasm · hirsutism · hypertension ·

libido increased · nausea · oedema · skin reactions · sodium retention · urine flow decreased · virilism (with high doses including voice changes - sometimes irreversible)

● HEPATIC IMPAIRMENT Manufacturer advises caution in severe impairment (discontinue treatment if hepatic function worsens or if oedema, with or without congestive heart failure, develops).

● RENAL IMPAIRMENT Use with caution—may cause sodium and water retention.

● LESS SUITABLE FOR PRESCRIBING Nandrolone injection is less suitable for prescribing.

● MEDICINAL FORMS There can be variation in the licensing of different medicines containing the same drug.
Solution for injection
EXCIPIENTS: May contain Arachis (peanut) oil, benzyl alcohol
▸ Deca-Durabolin (Aspen Pharma Trading Ltd)
Nandrolone decanoate 50 mg per 1 ml Deca-Durabolin 50mg/1ml
solution for injection ampoules | 1 ampoule [PoM] £3.17 [CD4-2]

BISPHOSPHONATES

Bisphosphonates 🅖

● DRUG ACTION Bisphosphonates are adsorbed onto hydroxyapatite crystals in bone, slowing both their rate of growth and dissolution, and therefore reducing the rate of bone turnover.

IMPORTANT SAFETY INFORMATION

MHRA/CHM ADVICE: BISPHOSPHONATES: ATYPICAL FEMORAL FRACTURES (JUNE 2011)
Atypical femoral fractures have been reported rarely with bisphosphonate treatment, mainly in patients receiving long-term treatment for osteoporosis.

The need to continue bisphosphonate treatment for osteoporosis should be re-evaluated periodically based on an assessment of the benefits and risks of treatment for individual patients, particularly after 5 or more years of use.

Patients should be advised to report any thigh, hip, or groin pain during treatment with a bisphosphonate.

Discontinuation of bisphosphonate treatment in patients suspected to have an atypical femoral fracture should be considered after an assessment of the benefits and risks of continued treatment.

MHRA/CHM ADVICE: BISPHOSPHONATES: OSTEONECROSIS OF THE JAW (NOVEMBER 2009) AND INTRAVENOUS BISPHOSPHONATES: OSTEONECROSIS OF THE JAW—FURTHER MEASURES TO MINIMISE RISK (JULY 2015)
The risk of osteonecrosis of the jaw is substantially greater for patients receiving intravenous bisphosphonates in the treatment of cancer than for patients receiving oral bisphosphonates for osteoporosis or Paget's disease.

Risk factors for developing osteonecrosis of the jaw that should be considered are: potency of bisphosphonate (highest for zoledronate), route of administration, cumulative dose, duration and type of malignant disease, concomitant treatment, smoking, comorbid conditions, and history of dental disease.

All patients with cancer and patients with poor dental status should have a dental check-up (and any necessary remedial work should be performed) before bisphosphonate treatment, or as soon as possible after starting treatment. Patients should also maintain good oral hygiene, receive routine dental check-ups, and report any oral symptoms such as dental mobility, pain, or swelling, non-healing sores or discharge to a doctor and dentist during treatment.

Before prescribing an intravenous bisphosphonate, patients should be given a patient reminder card and informed of the risk of osteonecrosis of the jaw. Advise patients to tell their doctor if they have any problems with their mouth or teeth before starting treatment, and if the patient wears dentures, they should make sure their dentures fit properly. Patients should tell their doctor and dentist that they are receiving an intravenous bisphosphonate if they need dental treatment or dental surgery.

Guidance for dentists in primary care is included in *Oral Health Management of Patients Prescribed Bisphosphonates: Dental Clinical Guidance*, Scottish Dental Clinical Effectiveness Programme, April 2011 (available at www.sdcep.org.uk).

MHRA/CHM ADVICE: BISPHOSPHONATES: OSTEONECROSIS OF THE EXTERNAL AUDITORY CANAL (DECEMBER 2015)
Benign idiopathic osteonecrosis of the external auditory canal has been reported very rarely with bisphosphonate treatment, mainly in patients receiving long-term therapy (2 years or longer).

The possibility of osteonecrosis of the external auditory canal should be considered in patients receiving bisphosphonates who present with ear symptoms, including chronic ear infections, or suspected cholesteatoma.

Risk factors for developing osteonecrosis of the external auditory canal include: steroid use, chemotherapy, infection, an ear operation, or cotton-bud use.

Patients should be advised to report any ear pain, discharge from the ear, or an ear infection during treatment with a bisphosphonate.

● CAUTIONS
▸ Elderly with oral use Prescription potentially inappropriate (STOPP criteria) in patients with a current or recent history of upper gastrointestinal disease or bleeding (risk of relapse/exacerbation of oesophagitis, oesophageal ulcer or oesophageal stricture). See also Prescribing in the elderly p. 33.

● SIDE-EFFECTS
▸ **Common or very common** Alopecia · anaemia · arthralgia · asthenia · constipation · diarrhoea · dizziness · dysphagia · electrolyte imbalance · eye inflammation · fever · gastritis · gastrointestinal discomfort · headache · influenza like illness · malaise · myalgia · nausea · oesophageal ulcer (discontinue) · oesophagitis (discontinue) · pain · peripheral oedema · renal impairment · skin reactions · taste altered · vomiting
▸ **Uncommon** Anaphylactic reaction · angioedema · bronchospasm · oesophageal stenosis (discontinue) · osteonecrosis
▸ **Rare or very rare** Atypical femur fracture · Stevens-Johnson syndrome

● PATIENT AND CARER ADVICE
Atypical femoral fractures Patients should be advised to report any thigh, hip, or groin pain during treatment with a bisphosphonate.
Osteonecrosis of the jaw During bisphosphonate treatment patients should maintain good oral hygiene, receive routine dental check-ups, and report any oral symptoms.
Osteonecrosis of the external auditory canal Patients should be advised to report any ear pain, discharge from ear or an ear infection during treatment with a bisphosphonate.

Alendronic acid

F 767

02-Nov-2020

(Alendronate)

● INDICATIONS AND DOSE

Treatment of postmenopausal osteoporosis
▸ BY MOUTH
▸ Adult (female): 10 mg daily, alternatively 70 mg once weekly.

Treatment of osteoporosis in men
▸ BY MOUTH
▸ Adult (male): 10 mg daily.

Prevention and treatment of corticosteroid-induced osteoporosis in postmenopausal women not receiving hormone replacement therapy
▸ BY MOUTH
▸ Adult (female): 10 mg daily.

● CONTRA-INDICATIONS Abnormalities of oesophagus · hypocalcaemia · other factors which delay emptying (e.g. stricture or achalasia)

● CAUTIONS Active gastro-intestinal bleeding · atypical femoral fractures · duodenitis · dysphagia · exclude other causes of osteoporosis · gastritis · history (within 1 year) of ulcers · surgery of the upper gastro-intestinal tract · symptomatic oesophageal disease · ulcers · upper gastro-intestinal disorders

● INTERACTIONS → Appendix 1: bisphosphonates

● SIDE-EFFECTS
▸ **Common or very common** Gastrointestinal disorders · joint swelling · vertigo
▸ **Uncommon** Haemorrhage
▸ **Rare or very rare** Femoral stress fracture · oropharyngeal ulceration · photosensitivity reaction · severe cutaneous adverse reactions (SCARs)

SIDE-EFFECTS, FURTHER INFORMATION Severe oesophageal reactions (oesophagitis, oesophageal ulcers, oesophageal stricture and oesophageal erosions) have been reported; patients should be advised to stop taking the tablets and to seek medical attention if they develop symptoms of oesophageal irritation such as dysphagia, new or worsening heartburn, pain on swallowing or retrosternal pain.

● PREGNANCY Avoid.

● BREAST FEEDING Manufacturer advises avoid—no information available.

● RENAL IMPAIRMENT Avoid if eGFR less than 35 mL/minute/1.73 m^2.

● MONITORING REQUIREMENTS Correct disturbances of calcium and mineral metabolism (e.g. vitamin-D deficiency, hypocalcaemia) before starting treatment. Monitor serum-calcium concentration during treatment.

● DIRECTIONS FOR ADMINISTRATION Manufacturer advises tablets should be swallowed whole and oral solution should be swallowed as a single 100 mL dose. Doses should be taken with plenty of water while sitting or standing, on an empty stomach at least 30 minutes before breakfast (or another oral medicine); patient should stand or sit upright for at least 30 minutes after administration.

● PATIENT AND CARER ADVICE Patients or their carers should be given advice on how to administer alendronic acid tablets and oral solution.
Oesophageal reactions Patients (or their carers) should be advised to stop taking alendronic acid and to seek medical attention if they develop symptoms of oesophageal irritation such as dysphagia, new or worsening heartburn, pain on swallowing or retrosternal pain.

● NATIONAL FUNDING/ACCESS DECISIONS
For full details see funding body website

NICE decisions
▸ Bisphosphonates for treating osteoporosis (updated July 2019) NICE TA464 Recommended with restrictions
Scottish Medicines Consortium (SMC) decisions
▸ Alendronic acid (*Binosto*®) for the treatment of postmenopausal osteoporosis (April 2016) SMC No. 1137/16 Recommended with restrictions

● MEDICINAL FORMS There can be variation in the licensing of different medicines containing the same drug. Forms available from special-order manufacturers include: oral solution

Oral solution
▸ Alendronic acid (Non-proprietary)
Alendronic acid 700 microgram per 1 ml Alendronic acid 70mg/100ml oral solution unit dose sugar free sugar-free | 4 unit dose [PoM] £28.58 DT = £28.58

Effervescent tablet
▸ Binosto (Thornton & Ross Ltd)
Alendronic acid (as Alendronate sodium) 70 mg Binosto 70mg effervescent tablets sugar-free | 4 tablet [PoM] £22.80 DT = £22.80

Tablet
▸ Alendronic acid (Non-proprietary)
Alendronic acid (as Alendronate sodium) 10 mg Alendronic acid 10mg tablets | 28 tablet [PoM] £8.93 DT = £4.79
Alendronic acid (as Alendronate sodium) 70 mg Alendronic acid 70mg tablets | 4 tablet [PoM] £22.80 DT = £0.96
▸ Fosamax Once Weekly (Merck Sharp & Dohme Ltd)
Alendronic acid (as Alendronate sodium) 70 mg Fosamax Once Weekly 70mg tablets | 4 tablet [PoM] £22.80 DT = £0.96

Alendronic acid with colecalciferol

12-Nov-2020

The properties listed below are those particular to the combination only. For the properties of the components please consider, alendronic acid above, colecalciferol p. 1133.

● INDICATIONS AND DOSE

Treatment of postmenopausal osteoporosis in women at risk of vitamin D deficiency
▸ BY MOUTH
▸ Adult (female): 1 tablet once weekly.

● INTERACTIONS → Appendix 1: bisphosphonates · vitamin D substances

● DIRECTIONS FOR ADMINISTRATION Manufacturer advises tablets should be swallowed whole with plenty of water while sitting or standing; to be taken on an empty stomach at least 30 minutes before breakfast (or another oral medicine); patient should stand or sit upright for at least 30 minutes after taking tablet.

● PATIENT AND CARER ADVICE Patients or carers should be given advice on how to administer alendronic acid with colecalciferol tablets.

● MEDICINAL FORMS There can be variation in the licensing of different medicines containing the same drug.

Tablet
▸ Alendronic acid with colecalciferol (Non-proprietary)
Colecalciferol 70 microgram, Alendronic acid (as Alendronate sodium) 70 mg Alendronic acid 70mg / Colecalciferol 70microgram tablets | 4 tablet [PoM] £22.80 DT = £22.80
▸ Bentexo (Consilient Health Ltd)
Colecalciferol 140 microgram, Alendronic acid (as Alendronate sodium) 70 mg Bentexo 70mg/5,600unit tablets | 4 tablet [PoM] £4.25 DT = £4.25
▸ Fosavance (Merck Sharp & Dohme Ltd)
Colecalciferol 70 microgram, Alendronic acid (as Alendronate sodium) 70 mg Fosavance tablets | 4 tablet [PoM] £22.80 DT = £22.80

Ibandronic acid

F 767
12-Nov-2020

- **INDICATIONS AND DOSE**

Reduction of bone damage in bone metastases in breast cancer

▸ INITIALLY BY MOUTH
▸ Adult: 50 mg daily, alternatively (by intravenous infusion) 6 mg every 3–4 weeks

Hypercalcaemia of malignancy

▸ BY INTRAVENOUS INFUSION
▸ Adult: 2–4 mg as a single infusion, dose to be adjusted according to serum calcium concentration

Treatment of postmenopausal osteoporosis

▸ INITIALLY BY MOUTH
▸ Adult (female): 150 mg once a month, alternatively (by intravenous injection) 3 mg every 3 months, to be administered over 15–30 seconds.

- **CONTRA-INDICATIONS**

GENERAL CONTRA-INDICATIONS Hypocalcaemia

SPECIFIC CONTRA-INDICATIONS
▸ With oral use Abnormalities of the oesophagus · other factors which delay emptying (e.g. stricture or achalasia)

- **CAUTIONS**

GENERAL CAUTIONS Atypical femoral fractures

SPECIFIC CAUTIONS
▸ With intravenous use Cardiac disease (avoid fluid overload)
▸ With oral use Upper gastro-intestinal disorders

- **INTERACTIONS** → Appendix 1: bisphosphonates

- **SIDE-EFFECTS**

GENERAL SIDE-EFFECTS
▸ **Common or very common** Face oedema
▸ **Uncommon** Asthma exacerbated

SPECIFIC SIDE-EFFECTS
▸ **Common or very common**
▸ With intravenous use Bundle branch block · cataract · increased risk of infection · joint disorder · oral disorders · osteoarthritis · parathyroid disorder · thirst
▸ With oral use Acute phase reaction · gastrointestinal disorders · muscle cramps · musculoskeletal stiffness
▸ **Uncommon**
▸ With intravenous use Acrochordon · affective disorder · altered smell sensation · anxiety · blood disorder · cardiovascular disorder · cerebrovascular disorder · cholelithiasis · cystitis · deafness · hyperaesthesia · hypothermia · injury · memory loss · migraine · muscle tone increased · myocardial ischaemia · palpitations · pelvic pain · pulmonary oedema · radiculopathy · renal cyst · sleep disorder · stridor · urinary retention · weight decreased
▸ **Rare or very rare**
▸ With intravenous use Hypersensitivity
▸ **Frequency not known**
▸ With oral use Oesophagitis erosive (discontinue)

- **PREGNANCY** Avoid.

- **BREAST FEEDING** Avoid—present in milk in *animal* studies.

- **RENAL IMPAIRMENT** When used for postmenopausal osteoporosis, avoid if eGFR less than 30 mL/minute/1.73 m^2.
Dose adjustments ▸ With intravenous use When used for bone metastases, if eGFR 30–50 mL/minute/1.73 m^2 reduce dose to 4 mg and infuse over 1 hour; if eGFR less than 30 mL/minute/1.73 m^2 reduce dose to 2 mg and infuse over 1 hour.
▸ With oral use When used for bone metastases, if eGFR 30–50 mL/minute/1.73 m^2 reduce dose to 50 mg on alternative days; if eGFR less than 30 mL/minute/1.73 m^2 reduce dose to 50 mg once weekly.

- **MONITORING REQUIREMENTS** Monitor renal function and serum calcium, phosphate and magnesium.

- **DIRECTIONS FOR ADMINISTRATION** Tablets should be swallowed whole with plenty of water while sitting or standing; to be taken on an empty stomach at least 30 minutes (for most ibandronic acid tablets, 50 mg) or 1 hour (for *Bonviva*® tablets, 150 mg) before first food or drink (other than water) of the day, or another oral medicine; patient should stand or sit upright for at least 1 hour after taking tablet.
For *intravenous infusion* (*Bondronat*®), give intermittently in Glucose 5% or Sodium chloride 0.9%; dilute requisite dose in 500 mL infusion fluid and give over 1–2 hours.

- **PATIENT AND CARER ADVICE** Patients or carers should be given advice on how to administer ibandronic acid tablets.
Oesophageal reactions Patients and carers should be advised to stop tablets and seek medical attention for symptoms of oesophageal irritation such as dysphagia, pain on swallowing, retrosternal pain, or heartburn.
Patient reminder card A patient reminder card should be provided to patients receiving intravenous ibandronic acid (risk of osteonecrosis of the jaw).

- **NATIONAL FUNDING/ACCESS DECISIONS**
For full details see funding body website

NICE decisions
▸ **Bisphosphonates for treating osteoporosis (updated July 2019)** NICE TA464 Recommended with restrictions

- **MEDICINAL FORMS** There can be variation in the licensing of different medicines containing the same drug.

Solution for injection
▸ Ibandronic acid (Non-proprietary)
  Ibandronic acid (as Ibandronic sodium monohydrate) 1 mg per 1 ml Ibandronic acid 3mg/3ml solution for injection pre-filled syringes | 1 pre-filled disposable injection PoM £37.85–£65.20 DT = £51.58 | 1 pre-filled disposable injection PoM £65.40 DT = £51.58 (Hospital only)
▸ Bonviva (Atnahs Pharma UK Ltd)
  Ibandronic acid (as Ibandronic sodium monohydrate) 1 mg per 1 ml Bonviva 3mg/3ml solution for injection pre-filled syringes | 1 pre-filled disposable injection PoM £68.64 DT = £51.58

Solution for infusion
▸ Ibandronic acid (Non-proprietary)
  Ibandronic acid (as Ibandronic sodium monohydrate) 1 mg per 1 ml Ibandronic acid 6mg/6ml concentrate for solution for infusion vials | 1 vial PoM £130.42 (Hospital only)
  Ibandronic acid 2mg/2ml concentrate for solution for infusion vials | 1 vial PoM £43.60 (Hospital only)
▸ Bondronat (Atnahs Pharma UK Ltd)
  Ibandronic acid (as Ibandronic sodium monohydrate) 1 mg per 1 ml Bondronat 2mg/2ml concentrate for solution for infusion vials | 1 vial PoM £89.36 (Hospital only)
  Bondronat 6mg/6ml concentrate for solution for infusion vials | 1 vial PoM £183.69 (Hospital only)

Tablet
▸ Ibandronic acid (Non-proprietary)
  Ibandronic acid (as Ibandronic sodium monohydrate) 50 mg Ibandronic acid 50mg tablets | 28 tablet PoM £186.69 DT = £47.39
  Ibandronic acid (as Ibandronic sodium monohydrate) 150 mg Ibandronic acid 150mg tablets | 1 tablet PoM £18.40 DT = £4.49 | 3 tablet PoM £3.09–£55.21
▸ Bondronat (Atnahs Pharma UK Ltd)
  Ibandronic acid (as Ibandronic sodium monohydrate) 50 mg Bondronat 50mg tablets | 28 tablet PoM £183.69 DT = £47.39
▸ Bonviva (Atnahs Pharma UK Ltd)
  Ibandronic acid (as Ibandronic sodium monohydrate) 150 mg Bonviva 150mg tablets | 1 tablet PoM £18.40 DT = £4.49
▸ Iasibon (Aspire Pharma Ltd)
  Ibandronic acid (as Ibandronic sodium monohydrate) 50 mg Iasibon 50mg tablets | 28 tablet PoM £174.50 DT = £47.39

Endocrine system

6

▸ Quodixor (Aspire Pharma Ltd)
Ibandronic acid (as Ibandronic sodium monohydrate)
150 mg Quodixor 150mg tablets | 1 tablet PoM £18.40 DT = £4.49

⌐ 767

Pamidronate disodium

28-Jul-2020

(Formerly called aminohydroxypropylidenediphosphonate disodium (APD))

● **INDICATIONS AND DOSE**

Hypercalcaemia of malignancy
▸ BY INTRAVENOUS INFUSION
▸ Adult: 15–60 mg, to be given (via cannula in a relatively large vein) as a single infusion or in divided doses over 2–4 days, dose adjusted according to serum calcium concentration; maximum 90 mg per course

Osteolytic lesions and bone pain in bone metastases associated with breast cancer or multiple myeloma
▸ BY INTRAVENOUS INFUSION
▸ Adult: 90 mg every 4 weeks, to be administered via cannula in a relatively large vein, dose may alternatively be administered every 3 weeks, to coincide with chemotherapy in breast cancer

Paget's disease of bone
▸ BY INTRAVENOUS INFUSION
▸ Adult: 30 mg every week for a 6 week course (total dose 180 mg), alternatively initially 30 mg once weekly for 1 week, then increased to 60 mg every 2 weeks (max. per dose 60 mg) for a 6 week course (total dose 210 mg), to be administered via cannula in a relatively large vein, course may be repeated every 3 months; maximum 360 mg per course

● CAUTIONS Atypical femoral fractures · cardiac disease (especially in elderly) · ensure adequate hydration · previous thyroid surgery (risk of hypocalcaemia)

● INTERACTIONS → Appendix 1: bisphosphonates

● SIDE-EFFECTS
▸ **Common or very common** Appetite decreased · chills · decreased leucocytes · drowsiness · flushing · hypertension · insomnia · paraesthesia · tetany · thrombocytopenia
▸ **Uncommon** Agitation · dyspnoea · hypotension · muscle cramps · seizure
▸ **Rare or very rare** Confusion · glomerulonephritis · haematuria · heart failure · nephritis tubulointerstitial · nephrotic syndrome · oedema · pulmonary oedema · reactivation of infections · renal disorder exacerbated · renal tubular disorder · respiratory disorders · visual hallucinations · xanthopsia
▸ **Frequency not known** Atrial fibrillation

SIDE-EFFECTS, FURTHER INFORMATION Oral supplements are advised to minimise potential risk of hypocalcaemia for those with mainly lytic bone metastases or multiple myeloma at risk of calcium or vitamin D deficiency (e.g. through malabsorption or lack of exposure to sunlight) and in those with Paget's disease.

● PREGNANCY Avoid—toxicity in *animal* studies.

● BREAST FEEDING Avoid.

● HEPATIC IMPAIRMENT Manufacturer advises caution in severe hepatic impairment (no information available).

● RENAL IMPAIRMENT
Dose adjustments Max. infusion rate 20 mg/hour. Avoid if eGFR less than 30 mL/minute/1.73 m^2, except in life-threatening hypercalcaemia if benefit outweighs risk.
   If renal function deteriorates in patients with bone metastases, withhold dose until serum creatinine returns to within 10% of baseline value.

● MONITORING REQUIREMENTS
▸ Monitor serum electrolytes, calcium and phosphate—possibility of convulsions due to electrolyte changes.
▸ Assess renal function before each dose.

● DIRECTIONS FOR ADMINISTRATION For *slow intravenous infusion* (*Pamidronate disodium*, Hospira, Medac, Wockhardt), manufacturer advises give intermittently in Glucose 5% or Sodium chloride 0.9%; give at a rate not exceeding 1 mg/minute; not to be given with infusion fluids containing calcium. For *Pamidronate disodium* (Medac, Hospira, Wockhardt), manufacturer advises dilute with infusion fluid to a concentration of not more than 90 mg in 250 mL.

● PATIENT AND CARER ADVICE A patient reminder card should be provided (risk of osteonecrosis of the jaw).
Driving and skilled tasks Patients should be warned against performing skilled tasks (e.g. cycling, driving or operating machinery) immediately after treatment (somnolence or dizziness can occur).

● MEDICINAL FORMS There can be variation in the licensing of different medicines containing the same drug.
Solution for infusion
▸ Pamidronate disodium (Non-proprietary)
   Pamidronate disodium 3 mg per 1 ml Pamidronate disodium 15mg/5ml solution for infusion vials | 1 vial PoM £27.50 (Hospital only) | 5 vial PoM £149.15 (Hospital only)
   Pamidronate disodium 30mg/10ml solution for infusion vials | 1 vial PoM £55.00–£59.66 (Hospital only)
   Pamidronate disodium 60mg/20ml solution for infusion vials | 1 vial PoM £110.00 (Hospital only)
   Pamidronate disodium 90mg/30ml solution for infusion vials | 1 vial PoM £165.00 (Hospital only)
   Pamidronate disodium 9 mg per 1 ml Pamidronate disodium 90mg/10ml solution for infusion vials | 1 vial PoM £170.45 (Hospital only)
   Pamidronate disodium 15 mg per 1 ml Pamidronate disodium 60mg/4ml solution for infusion ampoules | 1 ampoule PoM £119.32
   Pamidronate disodium 15mg/1ml solution for infusion ampoules | 4 ampoule PoM £119.32
   Pamidronate disodium 90mg/6ml solution for infusion ampoules | 1 ampoule PoM £170.46
   Pamidronate disodium 30mg/2ml solution for infusion ampoules | 2 ampoule PoM £119.32

⌐ 767

Risedronate sodium

17-Aug-2020

● **INDICATIONS AND DOSE**

Paget's disease of bone
▸ BY MOUTH
▸ Adult: 30 mg daily for 2 months, course may be repeated if necessary after at least 2 months

Treatment of postmenopausal osteoporosis to reduce risk of vertebral or hip fractures
▸ BY MOUTH
▸ Adult (female): 5 mg daily, alternatively 35 mg once weekly.

Prevention of osteoporosis (including corticosteroid-induced osteoporosis) in postmenopausal women
▸ BY MOUTH
▸ Adult (female): 5 mg daily.

Treatment of osteoporosis in men at high risk of fractures
▸ BY MOUTH
▸ Adult (male): 35 mg once weekly.

● CONTRA-INDICATIONS Hypocalcaemia

● CAUTIONS Atypical femoral fractures · oesophageal abnormalities · other factors which delay transit or emptying (e.g. stricture or achalasia) · upper gastro-intestinal disorders

● INTERACTIONS → Appendix 1: bisphosphonates

● SIDE-EFFECTS
▸ **Uncommon** Gastrointestinal disorders

▸ **Rare or very rare** Glossitis

▸ **Frequency not known** Amblyopia · apnoea · chest pain · corneal lesion · dry eye · hypersensitivity · hypersensitivity vasculitis · increased risk of infection · leg cramps · liver disorder · muscle weakness · neoplasms · nocturia · tinnitus · toxic epidermal necrolysis · weight decreased

● PREGNANCY Avoid.

● BREAST FEEDING Avoid.

● RENAL IMPAIRMENT Avoid if eGFR less than 30 mL/minute/1.73 m².

● MONITORING REQUIREMENTS

▸ Correct hypocalcaemia before starting.

▸ Correct other disturbances of bone and mineral metabolism (e.g. vitamin-D deficiency) at onset of treatment.

● DIRECTIONS FOR ADMINISTRATION Manufacturer advises swallow tablets whole with full glass of water; on rising, take on an empty stomach at least 30 minutes before first food or drink of the day **or**, if taking at any other time of the day, avoid food and drink for at least 2 hours before or after risedronate (particularly avoid calcium-containing products e.g. milk; also avoid iron and mineral supplements and antacids); stand or sit upright for at least 30 minutes; do not take tablets at bedtime or before rising.

● PATIENT AND CARER ADVICE Patients or carers should be given advice on how to administer risedronate sodium tablets.
Oesophageal reactions Patients should be advised to stop taking the tablets and seek medical attention if they develop symptoms of oesophageal irritation such as dysphagia, pain on swallowing, retrosternal pain, or heartburn.

● NATIONAL FUNDING/ACCESS DECISIONS
For full details see funding body website

NICE decisions

▸ Bisphosphonates for treating osteoporosis (updated July 2019) NICE TA464 Recommended with restrictions

● MEDICINAL FORMS There can be variation in the licensing of different medicines containing the same drug. Forms available from special-order manufacturers include: oral suspension, oral solution

Tablet

▸ Risedronate sodium (Non-proprietary)
Risedronate sodium 5 mg Risedronate sodium 5mg tablets | 28 tablet PoM £24.78 DT = £18.88
Risedronate sodium 30 mg Risedronate sodium 30mg tablets | 28 tablet PoM £155.28 DT = £155.28
Risedronate sodium 35 mg Risedronate sodium 35mg tablets | 4 tablet PoM £19.12 DT = £5.21

▸ Actonel (Warner Chilcott UK Ltd, Teva UK Ltd)
Risedronate sodium 5 mg Actonel 5mg tablets | 28 tablet PoM £17.99 DT = £18.88
Risedronate sodium 35 mg Actonel Once a Week 35mg tablets | 4 tablet PoM £19.12 DT = £5.21
Actonel 35mg tablets | 4 tablet PoM Ⓢ DT = £5.21

Risedronate with calcium carbonate and colecalciferol
09-Nov-2020

The properties listed below are those particular to the combination only. For the properties of the components please consider, risedronate sodium p. 770, calcium carbonate p. 1095, colecalciferol p. 1133.

● INDICATIONS AND DOSE

Treatment of postmenopausal osteoporosis to reduce risk of vertebral or hip fractures

▸ BY MOUTH

▸ Adult: 1 tablet once weekly on day 1 of the weekly cycle, followed by 1 sachet daily on days 2–6 of the weekly cycle

● INTERACTIONS → Appendix 1: bisphosphonates · calcium salts · vitamin D substances

● DIRECTIONS FOR ADMINISTRATION Manufacturer advises tablets should be swallowed whole with plenty of water while sitting or standing; to be taken on an empty stomach at least 30 minutes before breakfast (or another oral medicine); patient should stand or sit upright for at least 30 minutes after taking tablet. Manufacturer advises granules should be stirred into a glass of water and after dissolution complete taken immediately.

● PRESCRIBING AND DISPENSING INFORMATION *Actonel Combi®* effervescent granules contain calcium carbonate 2.5 g (calcium 1 g or Ca²⁺ 25 mmol) and colecalciferol 22 micrograms (880 units)/sachet.

● PATIENT AND CARER ADVICE Patients or carers should be given advice on how to administer risedronate with calcium carbonate and colecalciferol tablets and granules.

● MEDICINAL FORMS There can be variation in the licensing of different medicines containing the same drug.

Tablet/Granules

▸ Actonel Combi (Theramex HQ UK Ltd)
Actonel Combi 35mg tablets and 1000mg/880unit effervescent granules sachets | 4 week supply PoM £19.12

�⧫ 767

Sodium clodronate
20-Jul-2020

● INDICATIONS AND DOSE

Osteolytic lesions, hypercalcaemia and bone pain associated with skeletal metastases in patients with breast cancer or multiple myeloma

▸ BY MOUTH

▸ Adult: 1.6 g daily in 1–2 divided doses, then increased if necessary up to 3.2 g daily in 2 divided doses

LORON 520®

Osteolytic lesions, hypercalcaemia and bone pain associated with skeletal metastases in patients with breast cancer or multiple myeloma

▸ BY MOUTH

▸ Adult: Initially 2 tablets daily in 1–2 divided doses, increased if necessary up to 4 tablets daily

● CONTRA-INDICATIONS Acute severe gastro-intestinal inflammatory conditions

● CAUTIONS Atypical femoral fractures · maintain adequate fluid intake during treatment · upper gastro-intestinal disorders

● INTERACTIONS → Appendix 1: bisphosphonates

● SIDE-EFFECTS Proteinuria · respiratory disorder

● PREGNANCY Avoid.

● BREAST FEEDING Manufacturer advises avoid—no information available.

● RENAL IMPAIRMENT Avoid if eGFR less than 10 mL/minute/1.73 m².
Dose adjustments Max. initial dose 1200 mg daily if eGFR 30-50 mL/minute/1.73m².
Use half normal dose if eGFR 10–30 mL/minute/1.73 m².

● MONITORING REQUIREMENTS Monitor renal function, serum calcium and serum phosphate before and during treatment.

● DIRECTIONS FOR ADMINISTRATION Manufacturer advises avoid food or fluids (other than plain water) for 2 hours before and 1 hour after treatment, particularly calcium-containing products e.g. milk; also avoid iron and mineral supplements and antacids; maintain adequate fluid intake.

● PATIENT AND CARER ADVICE Patients or carers should be given advice on how to administer sodium clodronate capsules and tablets.

6

Endocrine system

- MEDICINAL FORMS There can be variation in the licensing of different medicines containing the same drug.

Tablet

CAUTIONARY AND ADVISORY LABELS 10

▸ Clasteon (Kent Pharmaceuticals Ltd)
Sodium clodronate 800 mg Clasteon 800mg tablets | 60 tablet [PoM] £146.43 DT = £146.43

▸ Loron (Intrapharm Laboratories Ltd)
Sodium clodronate 520 mg Loron 520mg tablets | 60 tablet [PoM] £114.44 DT = £114.44

Capsule

▸ Sodium clodronate (Non-proprietary)
Sodium clodronate 400 mg Sodium clodronate 400mg capsules | 30 capsule [PoM] £34.96 | 120 capsule [PoM] £139.83 DT = £139.83

▸ Clasteon (Kent Pharmaceuticals Ltd)
Sodium clodronate 400 mg Clasteon 400mg capsules | 30 capsule [PoM] £34.96 | 120 capsule [PoM] £139.83 DT = £139.83

F 767

Zoledronic acid

05-Nov-2020

- INDICATIONS AND DOSE

Prevention of skeletal related events in advanced malignancies involving bone (specialist use only)

▸ BY INTRAVENOUS INFUSION

▸ Adult: 4 mg every 3–4 weeks, calcium 500 mg daily and vitamin D 400 units daily should also be taken

Tumour-induced hypercalcaemia (specialist use only)

▸ BY INTRAVENOUS INFUSION

▸ Adult: 4 mg for 1 dose

Paget's disease of bone (specialist use only)

▸ BY INTRAVENOUS INFUSION

▸ Adult: 5 mg for 1 dose, at least 500 mg elemental calcium twice daily (with vitamin D) for at least 10 days is recommended following infusion

Osteoporosis (including corticosteroid-induced osteoporosis) in men and postmenopausal women

▸ BY INTRAVENOUS INFUSION

▸ Adult: 5 mg once yearly as a single dose, in patients with a recent low-trauma hip fracture, the dose should be given at least 2 weeks after hip fracture repair; before first infusion give 50 000–125 000 units of vitamin D

Fracture prevention in osteopenia [hip or femoral neck]

▸ BY INTRAVENOUS INFUSION

▸ Elderly (female): 5 mg once every 18 months as a single dose.

- UNLICENSED USE [EvGr] Zoledronic acid is used for fracture prevention in women with osteopenia, ⟨A⟩ but is not licensed for this indication.
- CAUTIONS Atypical femoral fractures · cardiac disease (avoid fluid overload) · concomitant medicines that affect renal function
- INTERACTIONS → Appendix 1: bisphosphonates
- SIDE-EFFECTS
- ▸ **Common or very common** Appetite decreased · chills · flushing
- ▸ **Uncommon** Anaphylactic shock · anxiety · arrhythmias · chest pain · circulatory collapse · cough · drowsiness · dry mouth · dyspnoea · haematuria · hyperhidrosis · hypertension · hypotension · leucopenia · muscle spasms · proteinuria · respiratory disorders · sensation abnormal · sleep disorder · stomatitis · syncope · thrombocytopenia · tremor · vision blurred · weight increased
- ▸ **Rare or very rare** Confusion · Fanconi syndrome acquired · pancytopenia
- ▸ **Frequency not known** Acute phase reaction

SIDE-EFFECTS, FURTHER INFORMATION Renal impairment and renal failure have been reported; ensure patient is hydrated before each dose and assess renal function.

- CONCEPTION AND CONTRACEPTION Contra-indicated in women of child-bearing potential.
- PREGNANCY Avoid—toxicity in *animal* studies.
- BREAST FEEDING Avoid—no information available.
- HEPATIC IMPAIRMENT Manufacturer advises caution in severe hepatic impairment (limited information available).
- RENAL IMPAIRMENT Avoid in tumour-induced hypercalcaemia if serum creatinine above 400 micromol/litre. Avoid in advanced malignancies involving bone if eGFR less than 30 mL/minute/1.73 m^2 (or if serum creatinine greater than 265 micromol/litre). Avoid in Paget's disease, treatment of postmenopausal osteoporosis and osteoporosis in men if eGFR less than 35 mL/minute/1.73 m^2.

Dose adjustments In advanced malignancies involving bone, if eGFR 50–60 mL/minute/1.73 m^2 reduce dose to 3.5 mg every 3–4 weeks; if eGFR 40–50 mL/minute/1.73 m^2 reduce dose to 3.3 mg every 3–4 weeks; if eGFR 30–40 mL/minute/1.73 m^2 reduce dose to 3 mg every 3–4 weeks; if renal function deteriorates in patients with bone metastases, withhold dose until serum creatinine returns to within 10% of baseline value.

- MONITORING REQUIREMENTS
- ▸ Correct disturbances of calcium metabolism (e.g. vitamin D deficiency, hypocalcaemia) before starting. Monitor serum electrolytes, calcium, phosphate and magnesium.
- ▸ Monitor renal function in patients at risk, such as those with pre-existing renal impairment, those of advanced age, those taking concomitant nephrotoxic drugs or diuretics, or those who are dehydrated.

- DIRECTIONS FOR ADMINISTRATION
- ▸ When used for Prevention of skeletal related events in advanced malignancies involving bone or Tumour-induced hypercalcaemia For *intravenous infusion*, infuse over at least 15 minutes; administer as a single intravenous solution in a separate infusion line. If using 4 *mg/5 mL concentrate for solution for infusion* or preparing a reduced dose of 4 *mg/100 mL solution for infusion* for patients with renal impairment, dilute requisite dose according to product literature.
- ▸ When used for Paget's disease of bone or Osteoporosis (including corticosteroid-induced osteoporosis) in men and postmenopausal women For *intravenous infusion*, give via a vented infusion line over at least 15 minutes.

- PATIENT AND CARER ADVICE A patient reminder card should be provided (risk of osteonecrosis of the jaw).

- NATIONAL FUNDING/ACCESS DECISIONS For full details see funding body website

NICE decisions

▸ Bisphosphonates for treating osteoporosis (updated July 2019) NICE TA464 Recommended with restrictions

Scottish Medicines Consortium (SMC) decisions

▸ Zoledronic acid (*Zometa*®) for patients with breast cancer and multiple myeloma (May 2003) SMC No. 29/02 Recommended with restrictions

▸ Zoledronic acid (*Aclasta*®) for Paget's disease of bone (October 2006) SMC No. 317/06 Recommended

▸ Zoledronic acid (*Aclasta*®) for the treatment of osteoporosis in postmenopausal women at increased risk of fractures (March 2008) SMC No. 447/08 Recommended with restrictions

- MEDICINAL FORMS There can be variation in the licensing of different medicines containing the same drug.

Infusion

▸ Zoledronic acid (Non-proprietary)
Zoledronic acid (as Zoledronic acid monohydrate) 40 microgram per 1 ml Zoledronic acid 4mg/100ml infusion bags | 1 bag [PoM] £174.14 (Hospital only)
Zoledronic acid (as Zoledronic acid monohydrate) 50 microgram per 1 ml Zoledronic acid 5mg/100ml infusion bags | 1 bag [PoM] £217.68 (Hospital only)

▸ Aclasta (Novartis Pharmaceuticals UK Ltd)
Zoledronic acid (as Zoledronic acid monohydrate) 50 microgram per 1 ml Aclasta 5mg/100ml infusion bottles | 1 bottle PoM
£253.38

▸ Zometa (Novartis Pharmaceuticals UK Ltd)
Zoledronic acid (as Zoledronic acid monohydrate) 40 microgram per 1 ml Zometa 4mg/100ml infusion bottles | 1 bottle PoM
£174.14

Solution for infusion

▸ Zoledronic acid (Non-proprietary)
Zoledronic acid (as Zoledronic acid monohydrate) 40 microgram per 1 ml Zoledronic acid 4mg/100ml solution for infusion vials |
1 vial PoM £85.00–£174.14 (Hospital only)
Zoledronic acid (as Zoledronic acid monohydrate) 50 microgram per 1 ml Zoledronic acid 5mg/100ml solution for infusion vials |
1 vial PoM £85.00–£266.72 (Hospital only)
Zoledronic acid (as Zoledronic acid monohydrate)
800 microgram per 1 ml Zoledronic acid 4mg/5ml concentrate for solution for infusion vials | 1 vial PoM £30.00–£233.40 (Hospital only) | 5 vial PoM £25.00 (Hospital only)
Zoledronic acid 4mg/5ml solution for infusion vials | 1 vial PoM
£9.75 (Hospital only)

▸ Zometa (Novartis Pharmaceuticals UK Ltd)
Zoledronic acid (as Zoledronic acid monohydrate)
800 microgram per 1 ml Zometa 4mg/5ml solution for infusion vials
| 1 vial PoM £174.14 (Hospital only)

CALCIUM REGULATING DRUGS > BONE
RESORPTION INHIBITORS

Calcitonin (salmon)   28-Jul-2020

(Salcatonin)

● **INDICATIONS AND DOSE**

Hypercalcaemia of malignancy
▸ BY SUBCUTANEOUS INJECTION, OR BY INTRAMUSCULAR
INJECTION
▸ Adult: 100 units every 6–8 hours (max. per dose
400 units every 6–8 hours), adjusted according to
response
▸ BY INTRAVENOUS INFUSION
▸ Adult: Up to 10 units/kg, in severe or emergency cases,
to be administered by slow intravenous infusion over at
least 6 hours

Paget's disease of bone
▸ BY SUBCUTANEOUS INJECTION, OR BY INTRAMUSCULAR
INJECTION
▸ Adult: 100 units daily, adjusted according to response
for maximum 3 months (6 months in exceptional
circumstances), a minimum dosage regimen of 50 units
three times a week has been shown to achieve clinical
and biochemical improvement

Prevention of acute bone loss due to sudden immobility
▸ BY SUBCUTANEOUS INJECTION, OR BY INTRAMUSCULAR
INJECTION
▸ Adult: Initially 100 units daily in 1–2 divided doses,
then reduced to 50 units daily at the start of
mobilisation, usual duration of treatment is 2 weeks;
maximum 4 weeks

● CONTRA-INDICATIONS Hypocalcaemia
● CAUTIONS History of allergy (skin test advised) · risk of
malignancy—avoid prolonged use (use lowest effective
dose for shortest possible time)
● INTERACTIONS → Appendix 1: calcitonins
● SIDE-EFFECTS
▸ **Common or very common** Abdominal pain · arthralgia ·
diarrhoea · dizziness · fatigue · flushing · headache ·
musculoskeletal pain · nausea · secondary malignancy
(long term use) · taste altered · vomiting
▸ **Uncommon** Hypersensitivity · hypertension · influenza like
illness · oedema · polyuria · skin reactions · visual
impairment

▸ **Rare or very rare** Bronchospasm · throat swelling · tongue
swelling
▸ **Frequency not known** Hypocalcaemia · tremor
● PREGNANCY Avoid unless potential benefit outweighs risk
(toxicity in *animal* studies).
● BREAST FEEDING Avoid; inhibits lactation in *animals*.
● RENAL IMPAIRMENT Use with caution.
● DIRECTIONS FOR ADMINISTRATION
▸ With intravenous use For *intravenous infusion*, manufacturer
advises give intermittently in Sodium Chloride 0.9%.
Diluted solution given without delay. Dilute in 500 mL give
over at least 6 hours; glass or hard plastic containers
should not be used.

● MEDICINAL FORMS There can be variation in the licensing of
different medicines containing the same drug.

Solution for injection

▸ Calcitonin (salmon) (Non-proprietary)
Calcitonin (salmon) 50 unit per 1 ml Calcitonin (salmon)
50units/1ml solution for injection ampoules | 5 ampoule PoM
£167.50 DT = £167.50
Calcitonin (salmon) 100 unit per 1 ml Calcitonin (salmon)
100units/1ml solution for injection ampoules | 5 ampoule PoM
£220.00 DT = £220.00
Calcitonin (salmon) 200 unit per 1 ml Calcitonin (salmon)
400units/2ml solution for injection vials | 1 vial PoM £352.00 DT =
£352.00

Strontium ranelate   09-Oct-2020

● DRUG ACTION Strontium ranelate stimulates bone
formation and reduces bone resorption.

● **INDICATIONS AND DOSE**

**Severe osteoporosis in men and postmenopausal women
at increased risk of fractures [when other treatments
are contra-indicated or not tolerated] (initiated by a
specialist)**
▸ BY MOUTH
▸ Adult: 2 g once daily, dose to be taken in water and at
bedtime

● CONTRA-INDICATIONS Cerebrovascular disease · current or
previous venous thromboembolic event · ischaemic heart
disease · peripheral arterial disease · temporary or
permanent immobilisation · uncontrolled hypertension
● CAUTIONS Risk factors for cardiovascular disease—assess
before and every 6–12 months during treatment · Risk
factors for venous thromboembolism (discontinue in
patients who become immobile)
CAUTIONS, FURTHER INFORMATION
▸ Risk of cardiovascular events Manufacturer advises treatment
should be stopped if ischaemic heart disease, peripheral
arterial disease, or cerebrovascular disease develops, or if
hypertension is uncontrolled.
● INTERACTIONS → Appendix 1: strontium
● SIDE-EFFECTS
▸ **Common or very common** Angioedema · arthralgia ·
bronchial hyperreactivity · consciousness impaired ·
constipation · diarrhoea · dizziness · embolism and
thrombosis · gastrointestinal discomfort · gastrointestinal
disorders · headache · hepatitis · hypercholesterolaemia ·
insomnia · memory loss · muscle complaints · myocardial
infarction · nausea · pain · paraesthesia · peripheral oedema
· skin reactions · vertigo · vomiting
▸ **Uncommon** Alopecia · confusion · dry mouth · fever ·
lymphadenopathy · malaise · oral disorders · seizure
▸ **Rare or very rare** Bone marrow failure · eosinophilia ·
severe cutaneous adverse reactions (SCARs)
● PREGNANCY Manufacturer advises avoid—toxicity in
animal studies.

6

Endocrine system

- **BREAST FEEDING** Manufacturer advises avoid—data suggest present in human milk.
- **RENAL IMPAIRMENT** Manufacturer advises avoid if creatinine clearance less than 30 mL/minute.
- **EFFECT ON LABORATORY TESTS** Manufacturer advises may interfere with colorimetric assay of calcium in blood and urine—consult product literature.
- **DIRECTIONS FOR ADMINISTRATION** Granules should be stirred into at least 30mL of water, and taken immediately at bedtime on an empty stomach; avoid food for at least 2 hours before treatment, particularly calcium-containing products e.g. milk.
- **PATIENT AND CARER ADVICE** Patients or carers should be given advice on how to administer strontium ranelate granules.
  Severe allergic reactions Patients should be advised to stop taking strontium ranelate and consult their doctor immediately if skin rash develops.

- **MEDICINAL FORMS** There can be variation in the licensing of different medicines containing the same drug.
  Granules
  EXCIPIENTS: May contain Aspartame
  ‣ Strontium ranelate (Non-proprietary)
  Strontium ranelate 2 gram Strontium ranelate 2g granules sachets sugar free sugar-free | 28 sachet [PoM] £149.91 DT = £149.91

CALCIUM REGULATING DRUGS > PARATHYROID HORMONES AND ANALOGUES

Teriparatide

10-Jul-2020

- **INDICATIONS AND DOSE**

Treatment of osteoporosis in postmenopausal women and in men at increased risk of fractures | Treatment of corticosteroid-induced osteoporosis
  ‣ BY SUBCUTANEOUS INJECTION
  ‣ **Adult:** 20 micrograms daily for maximum duration of treatment 24 months (course not to be repeated)

- **CONTRA-INDICATIONS** Bone metastases · hyperparathyroidism · metabolic bone diseases · Paget's disease · pre-existing hypercalcaemia · previous radiation therapy to the skeleton · skeletal malignancies · unexplained raised alkaline phosphatase
- **SIDE-EFFECTS**
  ‣ **Common or very common** Anaemia · asthenia · chest pain · gastrointestinal disorders · headache · hypercholesterolaemia · hyperhidrosis · hypotension · muscle complaints · palpitations · sciatica · skin reactions · syncope · vomiting
  ‣ **Uncommon** Arthralgia · back pain · emphysema · hypercalcaemia · hyperuricaemia · nephrolithiasis · tachycardia · urinary disorders · weight increased
  ‣ **Rare or very rare** Oedema · renal impairment
- **PREGNANCY** Avoid.
- **BREAST FEEDING** Avoid.
- **RENAL IMPAIRMENT** Caution in moderate impairment; avoid if severe.
- **PRESCRIBING AND DISPENSING INFORMATION** Teriparatide is a biological medicine. Biological medicines must be prescribed and dispensed by brand name, see *Biological medicines* and *Biosimilar medicines*, under Guidance on prescribing p. 1.
- **NATIONAL FUNDING/ACCESS DECISIONS**
  For full details see funding body website
  NICE decisions
  ‣ Raloxifene and teriparatide for the secondary prevention of osteoporotic fragility fractures in postmenopausal women

(updated February 2018) NICE TA161 Recommended with restrictions

- **MEDICINAL FORMS** There can be variation in the licensing of different medicines containing the same drug.
  Solution for injection
  ‣ Teriparatide (non-proprietary) ▼
  Teriparatide 250 microgram per 1 ml Terrosa 20micrograms/80microlitres solution for injection 2.4ml cartridge with pen | 1 cartridge [PoM] £239.25
  Movymia 20micrograms/80microlitres solution for injection 2.4ml cartridge | 1 cartridge [PoM] £235.00
  Terrosa 20micrograms/80microlitres solution for injection 2.4ml cartridge | 1 cartridge [PoM] £239.25 | 3 cartridge [PoM] £717.75
  Teriparatide 600micrograms/2.4ml solution for injection pre-filled disposable devices | 1 pre-filled disposable injection [PoM] £231.10 DT = £271.88 (Hospital only)
  Movymia 20micrograms/80microlitres solution for injection 2.4ml cartridge with pen | 1 cartridge [PoM] £235.00
  ‣ Forsteo (Eli Lilly and Company Ltd)
  Teriparatide 250 microgram per 1 ml Forsteo 20micrograms/80microlitres solution for injection 2.4ml pre-filled pens | 1 pre-filled disposable injection [PoM] £271.88 DT = £271.88

DRUGS AFFECTING BONE STRUCTURE AND MINERALISATION > MONOCLONAL ANTIBODIES

Denosumab

04-Nov-2020

- **DRUG ACTION** Denosumab is a human monoclonal antibody that inhibits osteoclast formation, function, and survival, thereby decreasing bone resorption.

- **INDICATIONS AND DOSE**
  PROLIA ®

Osteoporosis in postmenopausal women and in men at increased risk of fractures | Bone loss associated with hormone ablation in men with prostate cancer at increased risk of fractures | Bone loss associated with long-term systemic glucocorticoid therapy in patients at increased risk of fracture
  ‣ BY SUBCUTANEOUS INJECTION
  ‣ **Adult:** 60 mg every 6 months, supplement with calcium and Vitamin D, to be administered into the thigh, abdomen or upper arm

  XGEVA ®

Prevention of skeletal related events in patients with bone metastases
  ‣ BY SUBCUTANEOUS INJECTION
  ‣ **Adult:** 120 mg every 4 weeks, supplementation of at least calcium 500 mg and Vitamin D 400 units daily should also be taken unless hypercalcaemia is present, to be administered into the thigh, abdomen or upper arm

Giant cell tumour of bone that is unresectable or where surgical resection is likely to result in severe morbidity
  ‣ BY SUBCUTANEOUS INJECTION
  ‣ **Adult:** 120 mg every 4 weeks, give additional dose on days 8 and 15 of the first month of treatment only, supplementation of at least calcium 500 mg and Vitamin D 400 units daily should also be taken unless hypercalcaemia is present, to be administered into the thigh, abdomen or upper arm

---

IMPORTANT SAFETY INFORMATION
MHRA/CHM ADVICE: DENOSUMAB: ATYPICAL FEMORAL FRACTURES (FEBRUARY 2013)
Atypical femoral fractures have been reported rarely in patients receiving denosumab for the long-term treatment (2.5 or more years) of postmenopausal osteoporosis.

Patients should be advised to report any new or unusual thigh, hip, or groin pain during treatment with denosumab.

Discontinuation of denosumab in patients suspected to have an atypical femoral fracture should be considered after an assessment of the benefits and risks of continued treatment.

MHRA/CHM ADVICE: DENOSUMAB: MINIMISING THE RISK OF OSTEONECROSIS OF THE JAW; MONITORING FOR HYPOCALCAEMIA—UPDATED RECOMMENDATIONS (SEPTEMBER 2014) AND DENOSUMAB: OSTEONECROSIS OF THE JAW—FURTHER MEASURES TO MINIMISE RISK (JULY 2015)

Denosumab is associated with a risk of osteonecrosis of the jaw (ONJ) and with a risk of hypocalcaemia.

Osteonecrosis of the jaw Osteonecrosis of the jaw is a well-known and common side-effect in patients receiving denosumab 120 mg for cancer. Risk factors include smoking, old age, poor oral hygiene, invasive dental procedures (including tooth extractions, dental implants, oral surgery), comorbidity (including dental disease, anaemia, coagulopathy, infection), advanced cancer, previous treatment with bisphosphonates, and concomitant treatments (including chemotherapy, anti-angiogenic biologics, corticosteroids, and radiotherapy to head and neck). The following precautions are now recommended to reduce the risk of ONJ:

Denosumab 120 mg (cancer indication)
- A dental examination and appropriate preventative dentistry before starting treatment are now recommended for all patients
- Do not start denosumab in patients with a dental or jaw condition requiring surgery, or in patients who have unhealed lesions from dental or oral surgery

Denosumab 60 mg (osteoporosis indication)
- Check for ONJ risk factors before starting treatment. A dental examination and appropriate preventative dentistry are now recommended for patients with risk factors

All patients should be given a patient reminder card and informed of the risk of ONJ. Advise patients to tell their doctor if they have any problems with their mouth or teeth before starting treatment, if they wear dentures they should make sure their dentures fit properly before starting treatment, to maintain good oral hygiene, receive routine dental check-ups during treatment, and immediately report any oral symptoms such as dental mobility, pain, swelling, non-healing sores or discharge to a doctor and dentist. Patients should tell their doctor and dentist that they are receiving denosumab if they need dental treatment or dental surgery.

Hypocalcaemia Denosumab is associated with a risk of hypocalcaemia. This risk increases with the degree of renal impairment. Hypocalcaemia usually occurs in the first weeks of denosumab treatment, but it can also occur later in treatment.

Plasma-calcium concentration monitoring is recommended for denosumab 120 mg (cancer indication):
- before the first dose
- within two weeks after the initial dose
- if suspected symptoms of hypocalcaemia occur
- consider monitoring more frequently in patients with risk factors for hypocalcaemia (e.g. severe renal impairment, creatinine clearance less than 30 mL/minute)

Plasma-calcium concentration monitoring is recommended for denosumab 60 mg (osteoporosis indication):
- before each dose
- within two weeks after the initial dose in patients with risk factors for hypocalcaemia (e.g. severe renal impairment, creatinine clearance less than 30 mL/minute)
- if suspected symptoms of hypocalcaemia occur

All patients should be advised to report symptoms of hypocalcaemia to their doctor (e.g. muscle spasms, twitches, cramps, numbness or tingling in the fingers, toes, or around the mouth).

MHRA/CHM ADVICE: DENOSUMAB: REPORTS OF OSTEONECROSIS OF THE EXTERNAL AUDITORY CANAL (JUNE 2017)

Osteonecrosis of the external auditory canal has been reported with denosumab and this should be considered in patients who present with ear symptoms including chronic ear infections or in those with suspected cholesteatoma. Possible risk factors include steroid use and chemotherapy, with or without local risk factors such as infection or trauma. The MHRA recommends advising patients to report any ear pain, discharge from the ear, or an ear infection during denosumab treatment.

MHRA/CHM ADVICE: DENOSUMAB (XGEVA®) FOR GIANT CELL TUMOUR OF BONE: RISK OF CLINICALLY SIGNIFICANT HYPERCALCAEMIA FOLLOWING DISCONTINUATION (JUNE 2018)

Cases of clinically significant hypercalcaemia (rebound hypercalcaemia) have been reported up to 9 months after discontinuation of denosumab treatment for giant cell tumour of bone. The MHRA recommends that prescribers should monitor patients for signs and symptoms of hypercalcaemia after discontinuation, consider periodic assessment of serum calcium, re-evaluate the patient's calcium and vitamin D supplementation requirements, and advise patients to report symptoms of hypercalcaemia.

Denosumab is not recommended in patients with growing skeletons.

MHRA/CHM ADVICE: DENOSUMAB (XGEVA®) FOR ADVANCED MALIGNANCIES INVOLVING BONE: STUDY DATA SHOW NEW PRIMARY MALIGNANCIES REPORTED MORE FREQUENTLY COMPARED TO ZOLEDRONIC ACID (ZOLEDRONATE) (JUNE 2018)

A pooled analysis has shown an increased rate of new primary malignancies in patients given Xgeva® (1-year cumulative incidence 1.1%) compared with those given zoledronic acid (0.6%), when used for the prevention of skeletal-related events with advanced malignancies involving bone. No treatment-related pattern in individual cancers or cancer groupings were apparent.

MHRA/CHM ADVICE: DENOSUMAB 60 MG (PROLIA®): INCREASED RISK OF MULTIPLE VERTEBRAL FRACTURES AFTER STOPPING OR DELAYING ONGOING TREATMENT (AUGUST 2020)

Cases of multiple vertebral fractures have been reported in patients within 18 months of discontinuation or interruption of ongoing denosumab 60 mg treatment for osteoporosis. The MHRA advises healthcare professionals not to discontinue denosumab without a specialist review, and to evaluate patients' individual risk and benefit factors before initiating treatment, particularly in those at increased risk of vertebral fractures (such as patients with previous vertebral fracture). Healthcare professionals should re-evaluate the need for continued treatment periodically based on expected benefits and potential risks of treatment on an individual basis, particularly after 5 or more years of use.

- CONTRA-INDICATIONS Hypocalcaemia
  XGEVA® Unhealed lesions from dental or oral surgery
- CAUTIONS Risk factors for osteonecrosis of the external auditory canal · risk factors for osteonecrosis of the jaw—consider temporary interruption of denosumab if occurs during treatment
  PROLIA®
  ▸ When used for osteoporosis in postmenopausal women Rebound increase in bone turnover on discontinuation (increased risk of fracture)

6

Endocrine system

Endocrine system

6

‣ Rebound increase in bone turnover on discontinuation
‣ When used for osteoporosis in postmenopausal women EvGr
Following discontinuation, transition to an alternative antiresorptive therapy should be considered to prevent rebound increase in bone turnover, bone loss and increased fracture risk. Ⓐ

● SIDE-EFFECTS
‣ **Common or very common** Abdominal discomfort · cataract · constipation · hypocalcaemia (including fatal cases) · increased risk of infection · pain · sciatica · second primary malignancy · skin reactions
‣ **Uncommon** Cellulitis (seek prompt medical attention) · hypercalcaemia (on discontinuation)
‣ **Rare or very rare** Atypical femur fracture · hypersensitivity · osteonecrosis

● CONCEPTION AND CONTRACEPTION Ensure effective contraception in women of child-bearing potential, during treatment and for at least 5 months after stopping treatment.

● PREGNANCY Manufacturer advises avoid—toxicity in *animal* studies; risk of toxicity increases with each trimester.

● BREAST FEEDING Manufacturer advises avoid.

● RENAL IMPAIRMENT Increased risk of hypocalcaemia if creatinine clearance less than 30 mL/minute.

● MONITORING REQUIREMENTS Correct hypocalcaemia and vitamin D deficiency before starting. Monitor plasma-calcium concentration during therapy.

● PATIENT AND CARER ADVICE
Atypical femoral fractures Patients should be advised to report any new or unusual thigh, hip, or groin pain during treatment with denosumab.
Osteonecrosis of the jaw All patients should be informed to maintain good oral hygiene, receive routine dental check-ups, and immediately report any oral symptoms such as dental mobility, pain, or swelling to a doctor and dentist.
Hypocalcaemia All patients should be advised to report symptoms of hypocalcaemia to their doctor (e.g. muscle spasms, twitches, cramps, numbness or tingling in the fingers, toes, or around the mouth).
Patient reminder card A patient reminder card should be provided (risk of osteonecrosis of the jaw).

PROLIA ®
Missed doses
‣ When used for osteoporosis in postmenopausal women EvGr
Treatment should be given within 1 month of scheduled date. Ⓐ

● NATIONAL FUNDING/ACCESS DECISIONS
For full details see funding body website
NICE decisions
‣ **Denosumab for the prevention of osteoporotic fractures in postmenopausal women (October 2010)** NICE TA204 Recommended with restrictions
‣ **Denosumab for the prevention of skeletal-related events in adults with bone metastases from solid tumours (October 2012)** NICE TA265 Recommended with restrictions
Scottish Medicines Consortium (SMC) decisions
‣ **Denosumab (*Prolia*®) for osteoporosis in postmenopausal women at increased risk of fractures (December 2010)** SMC No. 651/10 Recommended with restrictions

● MEDICINAL FORMS There can be variation in the licensing of different medicines containing the same drug.
Solution for injection
CAUTIONARY AND ADVISORY LABELS 10
EXCIPIENTS: May contain Sorbitol
‣ Prolia (Amgen Ltd)
Denosumab 60 mg per 1 ml Prolia 60mg/1ml solution for injection pre-filled syringes | 1 pre-filled disposable injection PoM £183.00 DT = £183.00

‣ Xgeva (Amgen Ltd)
Denosumab 70 mg per 1 ml Xgeva 120mg/1.7ml solution for injection vials | 1 vial PoM £309.86 DT = £309.86

Romosozumab
03-Dec-2020

● DRUG ACTION Romosozumab is a humanised monoclonal antibody that inhibits sclerostin, thereby increasing bone formation and decreasing bone resorption.

● INDICATIONS AND DOSE
Severe osteoporosis in postmenopausal women at increased risk of fractures (specialist use only)
‣ BY SUBCUTANEOUS INJECTION
‣ Adult: 210 mg once a month for 12 months, supplement with calcium and vitamin D, to be administered as two consecutive 105 mg injections at different injection sites into the thigh, abdomen or upper arm

● CONTRA-INDICATIONS History of myocardial infarction or stroke—discontinue if occurs during treatment · hypocalcaemia

● CAUTIONS Risk factors for cardiovascular disease · risk factors for osteonecrosis of the jaw—consider temporary interruption of romosozumab if occurs during treatment

● SIDE-EFFECTS
‣ **Common or very common** Arthralgia · headache · hypersensitivity · increased risk of infection · muscle spasms · neck pain · skin reactions
‣ **Uncommon** Cataract · hypocalcaemia · myocardial infarction · stroke
‣ **Rare or very rare** Angioedema
‣ **Frequency not known** Atypical femur fracture · cardiovascular event · osteonecrosis of jaw

● RENAL IMPAIRMENT Manufacturer advises monitor serum calcium concentration in patients with severe renal impairment, or in those receiving dialysis—increased risk of hypocalcaemia.

● MONITORING REQUIREMENTS Manufacturer advises to correct hypocalcaemia before therapy is initiated. Monitor for signs and symptoms of hypocalcaemia during therapy.

● PRESCRIBING AND DISPENSING INFORMATION
Romosozumab is a biological medicine. Biological medicines must be prescribed and dispensed by brand name, see *Biological medicines* and *Biosimilar medicines*, under Guidance on prescribing p. 1.
The manufacturer of *Evenity*® has provided a *Prescriber Guide*.

● HANDLING AND STORAGE Manufacturer advises store in a refrigerator (2-8°C) and protect from light—consult product literature for further information regarding storage outside the refrigerator.

● PATIENT AND CARER ADVICE
Atypical femoral fractures Manufacturer advises patients should be advised to report any new or unusual thigh, hip, or groin pain during treatment.
Osteonecrosis of the jaw Manufacturer advises patients should be informed to maintain good oral hygiene, receive routine dental check-ups, and immediately report any oral symptoms such as dental mobility, pain, or swelling.
Hypocalcaemia Manufacturer advises patients should be advised to report symptoms of hypocalcaemia.
Patients should receive a package leaflet and patient alert card.

● NATIONAL FUNDING/ACCESS DECISIONS
For full details see funding body website
Scottish Medicines Consortium (SMC) decisions
‣ Romosozumab (*Evenity*®) for the treatment of severe osteoporosis in postmenopausal women at high risk of

fracture (November 2020) SMC No. SMC2280 Recommended
with restrictions

- MEDICINAL FORMS There can be variation in the licensing of
different medicines containing the same drug.

Solution for injection

EXCIPIENTS: May contain Polysorbates

- Evenity (UCB Pharma Ltd) ▼
  Romosozumab 90 mg per 1 ml Evenity 105mg/1.17ml solution for
  injection pre-filled pens | 2 pre-filled disposable injection [PoM]
  £427.75

5 Dopamine responsive conditions

DOPAMINERGIC DRUGS > DOPAMINE RECEPTOR
AGONISTS

Dopamine-receptor agonists

Overview

Bromocriptine p. 440 is used for the treatment of
galactorrhoea, and for the treatment of prolactinomas (when
it reduces both plasma prolactin concentration and tumour
size). Bromocriptine also inhibits the release of growth
hormone and is sometimes used in the treatment of
acromegaly, but somatostatin analogues (such as octreotide
p. 993) are more effective.

Cabergoline p. 441 has similar side-effects to
bromocriptine, however patients intolerant of bromocriptine
may be able to tolerate cabergoline (and *vice versa*).

Quinagolide below has actions and uses similar to those of
ergot-derived dopamine agonists, but its side-effects differ
slightly.

Suppression of lactation

Although bromocriptine and cabergoline are licensed to
suppress lactation, they are **not** recommended for routine
suppression (or for the relief of symptoms of postpartum
pain and engorgement) that can be adequately treated with
simple analgesics and breast support. If a dopamine-receptor
agonist is required, cabergoline is preferred. Quinagolide is
not licensed for the suppression of lactation.

Quinagolide

- DRUG ACTION Quinagolide is a non-ergot dopamine D_2
agonist.

- INDICATIONS AND DOSE

Hyperprolactinaemia

▸ BY MOUTH

▸ Adult: Initially 25 micrograms once daily for 3 days,
dose to be taken at bedtime, increased in steps of
25 micrograms every 3 days; usual dose
75–150 micrograms daily, for doses higher than
300 micrograms daily increase in steps of
75–150 micrograms at intervals of not less than
4 weeks

- UNLICENSED USE Not licensed for the suppression of
lactation.

- CAUTIONS Acute porphyrias p. 1107 · history of psychotic
illness · history of serious mental disorders

CAUTIONS, FURTHER INFORMATION

▸ Hyperprolactinemic patients In hyperprolactinaemic patients,
the source of the hyperprolactinaemia should be
established (i.e. exclude pituitary tumour before
treatment).

- INTERACTIONS → Appendix 1: dopamine receptor agonists
- SIDE-EFFECTS
▸ **Common or very common** Abdominal pain · appetite
decreased · constipation · diarrhoea · dizziness · fatigue ·
flushing · headache · hypotension · insomnia · nasal
congestion · nausea · oedema · syncope · vomiting
▸ **Rare or very rare** Acute psychosis · drowsiness
- ALLERGY AND CROSS-SENSITIVITY Quinagolide should not
be used in patients with hypersensitivity to quinagolide
(does not apply to hypersensitivity to ergot alkaloids).
- CONCEPTION AND CONTRACEPTION Advise non-hormonal
contraception if pregnancy not desired.
- PREGNANCY Discontinue when pregnancy confirmed
unless medical reason for continuing (specialist advice
needed).
- BREAST FEEDING Suppresses lactation.
- HEPATIC IMPAIRMENT Manufacturer advises avoid (no
information available).
- RENAL IMPAIRMENT Avoid—no information available.
- MONITORING REQUIREMENTS Monitor blood pressure for a
few days after starting treatment and following dosage
increase.
- PATIENT AND CARER ADVICE

Driving and skilled tasks

Sudden onset of sleep Excessive daytime sleepiness and
sudden onset of sleep can occur with dopamine-receptor
agonists.

Patients starting treatment with these drugs should be
warned of the risk and of the need to exercise caution
when driving or operating machinery. Those who have
experienced excessive sedation or sudden onset of sleep
should refrain from driving or operating machines until
these effects have stopped occurring.

Management of excessive daytime sleepiness should
focus on the identification of an underlying cause, such as
depression or concomitant medication. Patients should be
counselled on improving sleep behaviour.

Hypotensive reactions Hypotensive reactions can be
disturbing in some patients during the first few days of
treatment with dopamine-receptor agonists, particular
care should be exercised when driving or operating
machinery.

- MEDICINAL FORMS There can be variation in the licensing of
different medicines containing the same drug.

Tablet

CAUTIONARY AND ADVISORY LABELS 10, 21

▸ Quinagolide (Non-proprietary)
  Quinagolide 50microgram tablets and Quinagolide 25microgram
  tablets | 6 tablet [PoM] £30.00–£37.50 DT = £37.50
  Quinagolide (as Quinagolide hydrochloride)
  25 microgram Quinagolide 25microgram tablets | 3 tablet [PoM] 🛇
  Quinagolide (as Quinagolide hydrochloride)
  50 microgram Quinagolide 50microgram tablets | 3 tablet [PoM] 🛇
  Quinagolide (as Quinagolide hydrochloride)
  75 microgram Quinagolide 75microgram tablets | 30 tablet [PoM]
  £82.50 DT = £82.48
▸ Norprolac (Ferring Pharmaceuticals Ltd)
  Quinagolide (as Quinagolide hydrochloride)
  25 microgram Norprolac 25microgram tablets | 3 tablet [PoM] 🛇
  Quinagolide (as Quinagolide hydrochloride)
  50 microgram Norprolac 50microgram tablets | 3 tablet [PoM] 🛇

6

Endocrine system

6 Gonadotrophin responsive conditions

Gonadotrophins

Gonadotrophin-affecting drugs

Danazol p. 783 is licensed for the treatment of *endometriosis* and for the relief of severe pain and tenderness in *benign fibrocystic breast disease* where other measures have proved unsatisfactory. It may also be effective in the long-term management of *hereditary angioedema* [unlicensed indication].

Cetrorelix below and ganirelix below are luteinising hormone releasing hormone antagonists, which inhibit the release of gonadotrophins (luteinising hormone and follicle stimulating hormone). They are used in the treatment of infertility by assisted reproductive techniques.

Gonadorelin analogues

Gonadorelin analogues are used in the treatment of endometriosis, precocious puberty, infertility, male hypersexuality with severe sexual deviation, anaemia due to uterine fibroids (together with iron supplementation), breast cancer, prostate cancer and before intra-uterine surgery. Use of leuprorelin acetate and triptorelin for 3 to 4 months before surgery reduces the uterine volume, fibroid size and associated bleeding.

Breast pain (mastalgia)

Once any serious underlying cause for breast pain has been ruled out, most women will respond to reassurance and reduction in dietary fat; withdrawal of an oral contraceptive or of hormone replacement therapy may help to resolve the pain.

Mild, non-cyclical breast pain is treated with simple analgesics; moderate to severe pain, cyclical pain or symptoms that persist for longer than 6 months may require specific drug treatment.

Danazol is licensed for the relief of severe pain and tenderness in benign fibrocystic breast disease which has not responded to other treatment.

Tamoxifen p. 996 may be a useful adjunct in the treatment of mastalgia [unlicensed indication] especially when symptoms can definitely be related to cyclic oestrogen production; it may be given on the days of the cycle when symptoms are predicted.

Treatment for breast pain should be reviewed after 6 months and continued if necessary. Symptoms recur in about 50% of women within 2 years of withdrawal of therapy but may be less severe.

PITUITARY AND HYPOTHALAMIC HORMONES AND ANALOGUES > ANTI-GONADOTROPHIN-RELEASING HORMONES

▌ Cetrorelix

15-Jun-2018

● **INDICATIONS AND DOSE**

Adjunct in the treatment of female infertility (initiated under specialist supervision)
▸ BY SUBCUTANEOUS INJECTION
▸ Adult (female): 250 micrograms once daily, dose to be administered in the morning, starting on day 5 or 6 of ovarian stimulation with gonadotrophins (or each evening starting on day 5 of ovarian stimulation), continue throughout administration of gonadotrophin including day of ovulation induction (or evening before ovulation induction), dose to be injected into the lower abdominal wall.

● SIDE-EFFECTS
▸ **Common or very common** Ovarian hyperstimulation syndrome
▸ **Uncommon** Headache · hypersensitivity · nausea
● PREGNANCY Avoid in confirmed pregnancy.
● BREAST FEEDING Avoid.
● HEPATIC IMPAIRMENT Manufacturer advises use with caution—no information available.
● RENAL IMPAIRMENT Avoid in moderate or severe renal impairment.
● MEDICINAL FORMS There can be variation in the licensing of different medicines containing the same drug.

Powder and solvent for solution for injection
▸ Cetrotide (Merck Serono Ltd)
Cetrorelix (as Cetrorelix acetate) 250 microgram Cetrotide 250microgram powder and solvent for solution for injection vials | 1 vial [PoM] £27.13 DT = £27.13

▌ Ganirelix

● **INDICATIONS AND DOSE**

Adjunct in the treatment of female infertility (initiated under specialist supervision)
▸ BY SUBCUTANEOUS INJECTION
▸ Adult: 250 micrograms once daily, dose to be administered in the morning (or each afternoon) starting on day 5 or day 6 of ovarian stimulation with gonadotrophins, continue throughout administration of gonadotrophins including day of ovulation induction (if administering in afternoon, give last dose in afternoon before ovulation induction), dose to be injected preferably into the upper leg (rotate injection sites to prevent lipoatrophy)

● SIDE-EFFECTS
▸ **Common or very common** Skin reactions
▸ **Uncommon** Headache · malaise · nausea
▸ **Rare or very rare** Dyspnoea · facial swelling · hypersensitivity
▸ **Frequency not known** Abdominal distension · ovarian hyperstimulation syndrome · pelvic pain
● PREGNANCY Avoid in confirmed pregnancy—toxicity in *animal* studies.
● BREAST FEEDING Avoid—no information available.
● HEPATIC IMPAIRMENT Manufacturer advises avoid in moderate to severe impairment (no information available).
● RENAL IMPAIRMENT Avoid in moderate to severe renal impairment.
● MEDICINAL FORMS There can be variation in the licensing of different medicines containing the same drug.

Solution for injection
▸ Fyremadel (Ferring Pharmaceuticals Ltd)
Ganirelix 500 microgram per 1 ml Fyremadel 250micrograms/0.5ml solution for injection pre-filled syringes | 1 pre-filled disposable injection [PoM] ⊠

PITUITARY AND HYPOTHALAMIC HORMONES AND ANALOGUES > GONADOTROPHIN-RELEASING HORMONES

Buserelin

04-Sep-2020

- **DRUG ACTION** Administration of gonadorelin analogues produces an initial phase of stimulation; continued administration is followed by down-regulation of gonadotrophin-releasing hormone receptors, thereby reducing the release of gonadotrophins (follicle stimulating hormone and luteinising hormone) which in turn leads to inhibition of androgen and oestrogen production.

- **INDICATIONS AND DOSE**

Endometriosis

▶ **BY INTRANASAL ADMINISTRATION**
▶ Adult: 300 micrograms 3 times a day maximum duration of treatment 6 months (do not repeat), to be started on days 1 or 2 of menstruation; administer one 150 microgram spray into each nostril

Pituitary desensitisation before induction of ovulation by gonadotrophins for in vitro fertilisation (under expert supervision)

▶ **BY SUBCUTANEOUS INJECTION**
▶ Adult: 200–500 micrograms once daily, increased if necessary up to 500 micrograms twice daily, starting in early follicular phase (day 1) or, after exclusion of pregnancy, in midluteal phase (day 21) and continued until down-regulation achieved (usually 1–3 weeks) then maintained during gonadotrophin administration (stopping gonadotrophin and buserelin on administration of chorionic gonadotrophin at appropriate stage of follicular development)
▶ **BY INTRANASAL ADMINISTRATION**
▶ Adult: 150–300 micrograms 4 times a day, (150 micrograms equivalent to one spray), to be administered during waking hours. Start in early follicular phase (day 1) or, after exclusion of pregnancy, in the midluteal phase (day 21) and continued until down-regulation achieved (usually about 2–3 weeks) then maintained during gonadotrophin administration (stopping gonadotrophin and buserelin on administration of chorionic gonadotrophin at appropriate stage of follicular development)

Advanced prostate cancer

▶ **INITIALLY BY SUBCUTANEOUS INJECTION**
▶ Adult: 500 micrograms every 8 hours for 7 days, then (by intranasal administration) 200 micrograms 6 times a day, (a single 100 microgram spray to be administered into each nostril)

- **CONTRA-INDICATIONS**
▶ When used for endometriosis Undiagnosed vaginal bleeding · use longer than 6 months (do not repeat)
▶ When used for pituitary desensitisation Undiagnosed vaginal bleeding

- **CAUTIONS** Depression · diabetes · hypertension · patients with metabolic bone disease (decrease in bone mineral density can occur) · polycystic ovarian disease

- **SIDE-EFFECTS**

GENERAL SIDE-EFFECTS

▶ **Common or very common** Depression · mood altered
▶ **Rare or very rare** Auditory disorder · hypotension · leucopenia · pituitary tumour benign · thrombocytopenia · tinnitus
▶ **Frequency not known** Alopecia · anxiety · appetite change · breast abnormalities · broken nails · concentration impaired · constipation · diarrhoea · dizziness · drowsiness ·

dry eye · dysuria · embolism and thrombosis · fatigue · feeling of pressure behind the eyes · follicle recruitment increased · galactorrhoea · gastrointestinal discomfort · gynaecomastia · hair changes · headache · hot flush · hydronephrosis · hyperhidrosis · increased risk of fracture · lymphostasis · memory loss · menopausal symptoms · menstrual cycle irregularities · muscle weakness in legs · musculoskeletal discomfort · nausea · oedema · osteoporosis · ovarian and fallopian tube disorders · pain · painful sexual intercourse · palpitations · paraesthesia · QT interval prolongation · sexual dysfunction · shock · skin reactions · sleep disorder · testicular atrophy · thirst · tumour activation temporary · uterine leiomyoma degeneration · vision disorders · vomiting · vulvovaginal disorders · weight changes

SPECIFIC SIDE-EFFECTS
▶ With intranasal use Altered smell sensation · epistaxis · hoarseness · nasal irritation · taste altered

SIDE-EFFECTS, FURTHER INFORMATION During the initial stage (1–2 weeks) increased production of testosterone may be associated with progression of prostate cancer. In susceptible patients this tumour 'flare' may cause spinal cord compression, ureteric obstruction or increased bone pain.

- **CONCEPTION AND CONTRACEPTION** Non-hormonal, barrier methods of contraception should be used during entire treatment period. Pregnancy should be excluded before treatment, the first injection should be given during menstruation or shortly afterwards or use barrier contraception for 1 month beforehand.

- **PREGNANCY** Avoid.

- **BREAST FEEDING** Avoid.

- **DIRECTIONS FOR ADMINISTRATION**
▶ With intranasal use Manufacturer advises avoid use of nasal decongestants before and for at least 30 minutes after treatment.
▶ With subcutaneous use Rotate injection site to prevent atrophy and nodule formation.

- **PATIENT AND CARER ADVICE** Patients or carers should be given advice on how to administer buserelin nasal spray.

- **MEDICINAL FORMS** There can be variation in the licensing of different medicines containing the same drug.

Solution for injection

▶ Suprecur (Cheplapharm Arzneimittel GmbH)
Buserelin (as Buserelin acetate) 1 mg per 1 ml Suprecur 5.5mg/5.5ml solution for injection vials | 2 vial PoM £33.02
▶ Suprefact (Cheplapharm Arzneimittel GmbH)
Buserelin (as Buserelin acetate) 1 mg per 1 ml Suprefact 5.5mg/5.5ml solution for injection vials | 2 vial PoM £34.37

Spray

▶ Suprecur (Cheplapharm Arzneimittel GmbH)
Buserelin (as Buserelin acetate) 150 microgram per 1 dose Suprecur 150micrograms/dose nasal spray | 168 dose PoM £105.16 DT = £105.16
▶ Suprefact (Cheplapharm Arzneimittel GmbH)
Buserelin (as Buserelin acetate) 100 microgram per 1 dose Suprefact 100micrograms/dose nasal spray | 336 dose PoM £122.24 DT = £122.24

Endocrine system

6

Goserelin

24-Jul-2020

- **DRUG ACTION** Administration of gonadorelin analogues produces an initial phase of stimulation; continued administration is followed by down-regulation of gonadotrophin-releasing hormone receptors, thereby reducing the release of gonadotrophins (follicle stimulating hormone and luteinising hormone) which in turn leads to inhibition of androgen and oestrogen production.

- **INDICATIONS AND DOSE**

ZOLADEX LA ®

Locally advanced prostate cancer as an alternative to surgical castration | Adjuvant treatment to radiotherapy or radical prostatectomy in patients with high-risk localised or locally advanced prostate cancer | Neoadjuvant treatment prior to radiotherapy in patients with high-risk localised or locally advanced prostate cancer | Metastatic prostate cancer
  - ▸ BY SUBCUTANEOUS INJECTION
  - ▸ Adult: 10.8 mg every 12 weeks, to be administered into the anterior abdominal wall

ZOLADEX ®

Locally advanced prostate cancer as an alternative to surgical castration | Adjuvant treatment to radiotherapy or radical prostatectomy in patients with high-risk localised or locally advanced prostate cancer | Neoadjuvant treatment prior to radiotherapy in patients with high-risk localised or locally advanced prostate cancer | Metastatic prostate cancer | Advanced breast cancer | Oestrogen-receptor-positive early breast cancer
  - ▸ BY SUBCUTANEOUS INJECTION
  - ▸ Adult: 3.6 mg every 28 days, to be administered into the anterior abdominal wall

Endometriosis
  - ▸ BY SUBCUTANEOUS INJECTION
  - ▸ Adult: 3.6 mg every 28 days maximum duration of treatment 6 months (do not repeat), to be administered into the anterior abdominal wall

Endometrial thinning before intra-uterine surgery
  - ▸ BY SUBCUTANEOUS INJECTION
  - ▸ Adult: 3.6 mg, dose may be repeated after 28 days if uterus is large or to allow flexible surgical timing, to be administered into the anterior abdominal wall

Before surgery in women who have anaemia due to uterine fibroids
  - ▸ BY SUBCUTANEOUS INJECTION
  - ▸ Adult: 3.6 mg every 28 days maximum duration of treatment 3 months, to be given with supplementary iron, to be administered into the anterior abdominal wall

Pituitary desensitisation before induction of ovulation by gonadotrophins for in vitro fertilisation (after exclusion of pregnancy) (under expert supervision)
  - ▸ BY SUBCUTANEOUS INJECTION
  - ▸ Adult: 3.6 mg, dose given to achieve pituitary down-regulation (usually 1–3 weeks) then gonadotrophin is administered (stopping gonadotrophin on administration of chorionic gonadotrophin at appropriate stage of follicular development), to be administered into the anterior abdominal wall

- **CONTRA-INDICATIONS** Undiagnosed vaginal bleeding · use longer than 6 months in endometriosis (do not repeat)
- **CAUTIONS** Depression · diabetes · hypertension · patients with metabolic bone disease (decrease in bone mineral density can occur) · polycystic ovarian disease · risk of spinal cord compression in men · risk of ureteric obstruction in men

- **SIDE-EFFECTS**
  - ▸ **Common or very common** Alopecia · arthralgia · bone pain · breast abnormalities · depression · glucose tolerance impaired · gynaecomastia · headache · heart failure · hot flush · hyperhidrosis · mood altered · myocardial infarction · neoplasm complications · paraesthesia · sexual dysfunction · skin reactions · spinal cord compression · vulvovaginal disorders · weight increased
  - ▸ **Uncommon** Hypercalcaemia (in women) · ureteral obstruction
  - ▸ **Rare or very rare** Ovarian and fallopian tube disorders · pituitary haemorrhage · pituitary tumour · psychotic disorder
  - ▸ **Frequency not known** Abdominal cramps · body hair change · constipation · diarrhoea · fatigue · hepatic function abnormal · interstitial pneumonia · muscle complaints · nausea · nervousness · peripheral oedema (when used for gynaecological conditions) · premature menopause · pulmonary embolism · QT interval prolongation · sleep disorder · uterine leiomyoma degeneration · voice alteration · vomiting · vulvovaginal infection · withdrawal bleed

  SIDE-EFFECTS, FURTHER INFORMATION Tumour flare can occur when androgen deprivation therapy is initiated.

- **CONCEPTION AND CONTRACEPTION** Non-hormonal, barrier methods of contraception should be used during entire treatment period. Pregnancy should be excluded before treatment, the first injection should be given during menstruation or shortly afterwards or use barrier contraception for 1 month beforehand.

- **PREGNANCY** Avoid.
- **BREAST FEEDING** Avoid.
- **MONITORING REQUIREMENTS** Men at risk of tumour 'flare' should be monitored closely during the first month of therapy for prostate cancer.
- **DIRECTIONS FOR ADMINISTRATION** Rotate injection site to prevent atrophy and nodule formation.

- **MEDICINAL FORMS** There can be variation in the licensing of different medicines containing the same drug.

  Implant
  - ▸ Zoladex (AstraZeneca UK Ltd)
    Goserelin (as Goserelin acetate) 3.6 mg Zoladex 3.6mg implant SafeSystem pre-filled syringes | 1 pre-filled disposable injection [PoM] £70.00 DT = £70.00
  - ▸ Zoladex LA (AstraZeneca UK Ltd)
    Goserelin (as Goserelin acetate) 10.8 mg Zoladex LA 10.8mg implant SafeSystem pre-filled syringes | 1 pre-filled disposable injection [PoM] £235.00 DT = £235.00

Leuprorelin acetate

20-Jul-2020

- **DRUG ACTION** Administration of gonadorelin analogues produces an initial phase of stimulation; continued administration is followed by down-regulation of gonadotrophin-releasing hormone receptors, thereby reducing the release of gonadotrophins (follicle stimulating hormone and luteinising hormone) which in turn leads to inhibition of androgen and oestrogen production.

- **INDICATIONS AND DOSE**

PROSTAP 3 DCS ®

Prostate cancer (specialist use only)
  - ▸ BY SUBCUTANEOUS INJECTION
  - ▸ Adult: 11.25 mg every 3 months

Endometriosis (specialist use only)
  - ▸ BY INTRAMUSCULAR INJECTION
  - ▸ Adult: 11.25 mg every 3 months for maximum duration of 6 months (not to be repeated), to be started during first 5 days of menstrual cycle

Pre- and perimenopausal breast cancer (specialist use only)
▶ BY SUBCUTANEOUS INJECTION
▸ Adult: 11.25 mg every 3 months, for further information on use with adjuvant treatments, consult product literature

PROSTAP SR DCS ®

Prostate cancer (specialist use only)
▶ BY SUBCUTANEOUS INJECTION, OR BY INTRAMUSCULAR INJECTION
▸ Adult: 3.75 mg every month

Endometriosis (specialist use only)
▶ BY SUBCUTANEOUS INJECTION, OR BY INTRAMUSCULAR INJECTION
▸ Adult: 3.75 mg every month for maximum duration of 6 months (not to be repeated), to be started during first 5 days of menstrual cycle

Endometrial thinning before intra-uterine surgery (specialist use only)
▶ BY SUBCUTANEOUS INJECTION, OR BY INTRAMUSCULAR INJECTION
▸ Adult: 3.75 mg for 1 dose, dose to be given as a single dose between day 3 and 5 of menstrual cycle, 5–6 weeks before surgery

Reduction of size of uterine fibroids and of associated bleeding before surgery (specialist use only)
▶ BY SUBCUTANEOUS INJECTION, OR BY INTRAMUSCULAR INJECTION
▸ Adult: 3.75 mg every month usually for 3–4 months (maximum 6 months)

Preservation of ovarian function (specialist use only)
▶ BY SUBCUTANEOUS INJECTION, OR BY INTRAMUSCULAR INJECTION
▸ Adult: Initially 3.75 mg as a single dose 2 weeks before starting chemotherapy, followed by 3.75 mg every month for the duration of chemotherapy treatment

Pre- and perimenopausal breast cancer (specialist use only)
▶ BY SUBCUTANEOUS INJECTION
▸ Adult: 3.75 mg every month, for further information on use with adjuvant treatments, consult product literature

STALADEX ® 10.72MG

Prostate cancer (specialist use only)
▶ BY SUBCUTANEOUS INJECTION
▸ Adult: 10.72 mg every 3 months, to be administered under the skin of the abdomen

● CONTRA-INDICATIONS
GENERAL CONTRA-INDICATIONS Undiagnosed vaginal bleeding
SPECIFIC CONTRA-INDICATIONS
▸ When used for endometriosis Use longer than 6 months (do not repeat)
● CAUTIONS Diabetes · family history of osteoporosis · patients with metabolic bone disease (decrease in bone mineral density can occur) · risk of spinal cord compression in men with prostate cancer · risk of ureteric obstruction in men with prostate cancer
● SIDE-EFFECTS
▸ **Common or very common** Appetite decreased · arthralgia · bone pain · breast abnormalities · depression · dizziness · fatigue · gynaecomastia · headache · hepatic disorders · hot flush · hyperhidrosis · injection site necrosis · insomnia · mood altered · muscle weakness · nausea · paraesthesia · peripheral oedema · sexual dysfunction · testicular atrophy · vulvovaginal dryness · weight change
▸ **Uncommon** Alopecia · diarrhoea · fever · myalgia · palpitations · visual impairment · vomiting

▸ **Rare or very rare** Haemorrhage
▸ **Frequency not known** Anaemia · glucose tolerance impaired · hypertension · hypotension · interstitial lung disease · leucopenia · paralysis · pulmonary embolism · QT interval prolongation · seizure · spinal fracture · thrombocytopenia · urinary tract obstruction

SIDE-EFFECTS, FURTHER INFORMATION In prostate cancer, during the initial stage (1–2 weeks) increased production of testosterone may be associated with progression of prostate cancer. In susceptible patients this tumour 'flare' may cause spinal cord compression, ureteric obstruction or increased bone pain.

● CONCEPTION AND CONTRACEPTION Non-hormonal, barrier methods of contraception should be used during entire treatment period. Pregnancy should be excluded before treatment, the first injection should be given during menstruation or shortly afterwards or use barrier contraception for 1 month beforehand.
● PREGNANCY Avoid—teratogenic in *animal* studies.
● BREAST FEEDING Avoid.
● MONITORING REQUIREMENTS
▸ Monitor liver function.
▸ Monitor prostate-specific antigen serum levels.
● DIRECTIONS FOR ADMINISTRATION Rotate injection site to prevent atrophy and nodule formation.

● MEDICINAL FORMS There can be variation in the licensing of different medicines containing the same drug.
Implant
▸ Staladex (Typharm Ltd)
Leuprorelin (as Leuprorelin acetate) 10.72 mg　Staladex 10.72mg implant pre-filled syringes | 1 pre-filled disposable injection [PoM] £208.79

Powder and solvent for suspension for injection
▸ Prostap 3 DCS (Takeda UK Ltd)
Leuprorelin acetate 11.25 mg　Prostap 3 DCS 11.25mg powder and solvent for suspension for injection pre-filled syringes | 1 pre-filled disposable injection [PoM] £225.72 DT = £225.72
▸ Prostap SR DCS (Takeda UK Ltd)
Leuprorelin acetate 3.75 mg　Prostap SR DCS 3.75mg powder and solvent for suspension for injection pre-filled syringes | 1 pre-filled disposable injection [PoM] £75.24 DT = £75.24

Nafarelin　　　　　　　　　　　　　04-Aug-2020

● DRUG ACTION Administration of gonadorelin analogues produces an initial phase of stimulation; continued administration is followed by down-regulation of gonadotrophin-releasing hormone receptors, thereby reducing the release of gonadotrophins (follicle stimulating hormone and luteinising hormone) which in turn leads to inhibition of androgen and oestrogen production.

● INDICATIONS AND DOSE
Endometriosis
▶ BY INTRANASAL ADMINISTRATION
▸ Adult (female): 200 micrograms twice daily for maximum 6 months (do not repeat), one spray in one nostril in the morning, and one spray in the other nostril in the evening (starting on days 2–4 of menstruation)

Pituitary desensitisation before induction of ovulation by gonadotrophins for in vitro fertilisation (under expert supervision)
▶ BY INTRANASAL ADMINISTRATION
▸ Adult: 400 micrograms twice daily, one spray in each nostril, to be started in early follicular phase (day 2) or, after exclusion of pregnancy, in midluteal phase (day 21) and continued until down regulation achieved (usually within 4 weeks) then maintained　　　continued →

(usually for 8–12 days) during gonadotrophin administration (stopping gonadotrophin and nafarelin on administration of chorionic gonadotrophin at follicular maturity), discontinue if down-regulation not achieved within 12 weeks

- CONTRA-INDICATIONS Undiagnosed vaginal bleeding · use longer than 6 months in the treatment of endometriosis (do not repeat)
- CAUTIONS Patients with metabolic bone disease (decrease in bone mineral density can occur)
- SIDE-EFFECTS
▸ **Common or very common** Artificial menopause · breast abnormalities · chest pain · depression · dyspnoea · emotional lability · headaches · hirsutism · hot flush · hypersensitivity · hypertension · hypotension · insomnia · myalgia · oedema · oestrogen deficiency · paraesthesia · rhinitis · seborrhoea · sexual dysfunction · skin reactions · uterine haemorrhage · vulvovaginal dryness · weight changes
▸ **Uncommon** Alopecia · arthralgia · ovarian cyst (may require discontinuation)
▸ **Frequency not known** Ovarian hyperstimulation syndrome · palpitations · vision blurred
- CONCEPTION AND CONTRACEPTION Non-hormonal, barrier methods of contraception should be used during entire treatment period. Pregnancy should be excluded before treatment, the first dose should be given during menstruation or shortly afterwards or use barrier contraception for 1 month beforehand.
- PREGNANCY Avoid.
- BREAST FEEDING Avoid.
- DIRECTIONS FOR ADMINISTRATION Manufacturer advises avoid use of nasal decongestants before and for at least 30 minutes after treatment; repeat dose if sneezing occurs during or immediately after administration.
- PATIENT AND CARER ADVICE Patients or carers should be given advice on how to administer nafarelin nasal spray.

- MEDICINAL FORMS There can be variation in the licensing of different medicines containing the same drug.
  Spray
  CAUTIONARY AND ADVISORY LABELS 10
  ▸ Synarel (Pfizer Ltd)
  Nafarelin (as Nafarelin acetate) 200 microgram per 1 dose Synarel 200micrograms/dose nasal spray | 60 dose [PoM] £52.43 DT = £52.43

Triptorelin

20-Aug-2020

- DRUG ACTION Administration of gonadorelin analogues produces an initial phase of stimulation; continued administration is followed by down-regulation of gonadotrophin-releasing hormone receptors, thereby reducing the release of gonadotrophins (follicle stimulating hormone and luteinising hormone) which in turn leads to inhibition of androgen and oestrogen production.

- ● INDICATIONS AND DOSE

DECAPEPTYL ® SR 11.25MG

Advanced prostate cancer (specialist use only)
▸ BY INTRAMUSCULAR INJECTION
▸ Adult: 11.25 mg every 3 months

Endometriosis
▸ BY INTRAMUSCULAR INJECTION
▸ Adult: 11.25 mg every 3 months for maximum 6 months (not to be repeated), to be started during first 5 days of menstrual cycle

DECAPEPTYL ® SR 22.5MG

Advanced prostate cancer (specialist use only)
▸ BY INTRAMUSCULAR INJECTION
▸ Adult: 22.5 mg every 6 months

DECAPEPTYL ® SR 3MG

Advanced prostate cancer (specialist use only)
▸ BY INTRAMUSCULAR INJECTION
▸ Adult: 3 mg every 4 weeks

Endometriosis
▸ BY INTRAMUSCULAR INJECTION
▸ Adult: 3 mg every 4 weeks maximum duration of 6 months (not to be repeated), to be started during first 5 days of menstrual cycle

Reduction in size of uterine fibroids
▸ BY INTRAMUSCULAR INJECTION
▸ Adult: 3 mg every 4 weeks for at least 3 months, maximum duration of treatment 6 months (not to be repeated), to be started during first 5 days of menstrual cycle

Premenopausal breast cancer [as combination therapy] (specialist use only)
▸ BY INTRAMUSCULAR INJECTION
▸ Adult: 3 mg every 4 weeks for up to 5 years, initiated 6–8 weeks before starting aromatase inhibitor—for further information, consult product literature

GONAPEPTYL DEPOT ®

Advanced prostate cancer
▸ BY SUBCUTANEOUS INJECTION, OR BY DEEP INTRAMUSCULAR INJECTION
▸ Adult: 3.75 mg every 4 weeks

Endometriosis | Reduction in size of uterine fibroids
▸ BY SUBCUTANEOUS INJECTION, OR BY DEEP INTRAMUSCULAR INJECTION
▸ Adult: 3.75 mg every 4 weeks maximum duration of 6 months (not to be repeated), to be started during first 5 days of menstrual cycle

SALVACYL ®

Male hypersexuality with severe sexual deviation
▸ BY INTRAMUSCULAR INJECTION
▸ Adult: 11.25 mg every 12 weeks

- CONTRA-INDICATIONS In endometriosis do not use for longer than 6 months (do not repeat) · undiagnosed vaginal bleeding
  SALVACYL ® Severe osteoporosis
- CAUTIONS
  GENERAL CAUTIONS History of depression · patients with metabolic bone disease (decrease in bone mineral density can occur)
  SPECIFIC CAUTIONS
  ▸ When used for breast cancer Risk factors for osteoporosis
  ▸ When used for prostate cancer Risk factors for osteoporosis · risk of spinal cord compression in men · risk of ureteric obstruction in men
  SALVACYL ® Increased risk of sensitivity to restored testosterone if treatment interrupted—consider administration of an antiandrogen before stopping treatment · transient increase in serum testosterone occurs on initiation—consider administration of an anti-androgen
- SIDE-EFFECTS
  GENERAL SIDE-EFFECTS
  ▸ **Common or very common** Anxiety · asthenia · depression · diabetes mellitus · dizziness · dry mouth · embolism · gastrointestinal discomfort · gynaecomastia · haemorrhage · headache · hot flush · hyperhidrosis · hypersensitivity · hypertension · joint disorders · menstrual cycle irregularities · mood altered · muscle complaints · nausea ·

oedema · ovarian and fallopian tube disorders · pain · painful sexual intercourse · pelvic pain · sexual dysfunction · skin reactions · sleep disorders · weight changes
▶ **Uncommon** Alopecia · appetite abnormal · asthma exacerbated · chills · confusion · constipation · diarrhoea · drowsiness · dyspnoea · flatulence · gout · muscle weakness · taste altered · testicular disorders · tinnitus · vertigo · vision disorders · vomiting
▶ **Rare or very rare** Abnormal sensation in eye · chest pain · difficulty standing · fever · hypotension · influenza like illness · musculoskeletal stiffness · nasopharyngitis · orthopnoea · osteoarthritis · QT interval prolongation
▶ **Frequency not known** Angioedema · malaise

SPECIFIC SIDE-EFFECTS
▶ **Common or very common**
▶ With intramuscular use Bone disorders · bone fracture · breast abnormalities · glucose tolerance impaired · hyperglycaemia · musculoskeletal disorder · seborrhoea · sensation abnormal · urinary disorders · vulvovaginal disorders
▶ With subcutaneous use Dysuria · vulvovaginal dryness
▶ **Uncommon**
▶ With intramuscular use Broken nails · central nervous system haemorrhage · cerebral ischaemia · concentration impaired · cystocele · dry eye · fluid retention · hirsutism · hyperlipidaemia · memory impairment · myocardial ischaemia · oral ulceration · palpitations · syncope · thrombocytosis · tremor
▶ With subcutaneous use Paraesthesia
▶ **Frequency not known**
▶ With subcutaneous use Bone disorder · breast pain · memory loss

SIDE-EFFECTS, FURTHER INFORMATION During the initial stage increased production of testosterone may be associated with progression of prostate cancer. In susceptible patients this tumour 'flare' may cause spinal cord compression, ureteric obstruction or increased pain.

● CONCEPTION AND CONTRACEPTION Non-hormonal, barrier methods of contraception should be used during entire treatment period. Pregnancy should be excluded before treatment, the first injection should be given during menstruation or shortly afterwards or use barrier contraception for 1 month beforehand.

● PREGNANCY Avoid.

● BREAST FEEDING Avoid.

● MONITORING REQUIREMENTS
▶ When used for Prostate cancer Men at risk of tumour 'flare' should be monitored closely during the first month of therapy.

● DIRECTIONS FOR ADMINISTRATION Rotate injection site to prevent atrophy and nodule formation.

● PRESCRIBING AND DISPENSING INFORMATION
DECAPEPTYL ® SR 22.5MG Each vial includes an overage to allow accurate administration of a 22.5 mg dose.

DECAPEPTYL ® SR 3MG Each vial includes an overage to allow accurate administration of 3 mg dose.

DECAPEPTYL ® SR 11.25MG Each vial includes an overage to allow accurate administration of an 11.25 mg dose.

● NATIONAL FUNDING/ACCESS DECISIONS
For full details see funding body website
Scottish Medicines Consortium (SMC) decisions
▶ Triptorelin (*Decapeptyl® SR* 3 mg) as adjuvant treatment, in combination with tamoxifen or an aromatase inhibitor, of endocrine responsive early stage breast cancer in women at high risk of recurrence who are confirmed as premenopausal after completion of chemotherapy (October 2019) SMC No. SMC2186 Recommended

All Wales Medicines Strategy Group (AWMSG) decisions
▶ Triptorelin (*Decapeptyl® SR*) as adjuvant treatment to radiotherapy in patients with high-risk localised or locally

advanced prostate cancer and as neoadjuvant treatment prior to radiotherapy in patients with high-risk localised or locally advanced prostate cancer (March 2017) AWMSG No. 1658 Recommended

● MEDICINAL FORMS There can be variation in the licensing of different medicines containing the same drug.
Powder and solvent for suspension for injection
▶ Decapeptyl SR (Ipsen Ltd)
Triptorelin (as Triptorelin acetate) 3 mg Decapeptyl SR 3mg powder and solvent for suspension for injection vials | 1 vial PoM £69.00 DT = £69.00
Triptorelin 11.25 mg Decapeptyl SR 11.25mg powder and solvent for suspension for injection vials | 1 vial PoM £207.00 DT = £207.00
Triptorelin (as Triptorelin embonate) 22.5 mg Decapeptyl SR 22.5mg powder and solvent for suspension for injection vials | 1 vial PoM £414.00 DT = £414.00
▶ Gonapeptyl Depot (Ferring Pharmaceuticals Ltd)
Triptorelin (as Triptorelin acetate) 3.75 mg Gonapeptyl Depot 3.75mg powder and solvent for suspension for injection pre-filled syringes | 1 pre-filled disposable injection PoM £81.69 DT = £81.69
▶ Salvacyl (Ipsen Ltd)
Triptorelin 11.25 mg Salvacyl 11.25mg powder and solvent for suspension for injection vials | 1 vial PoM £248.00 DT = £207.00

6.1 Hereditary angioedema

PITUITARY AND HYPOTHALAMIC HORMONES AND ANALOGUES > ANTI-GONADOTROPHIN-RELEASING HORMONES

Danazol
08-Mar-2017

● DRUG ACTION Danazol inhibits pituitary gonadotrophins; it combines androgenic activity with antioestrogenic and antiprogestogenic activity.

● INDICATIONS AND DOSE
Endometriosis
▶ BY MOUTH
▶ Adult: 200–800 mg daily in up to 4 divided doses usually for 3–6 months, dose to be adjusted to achieve amenorrhoea, in women of child-bearing potential, treatment should start during menstruation, preferably on day 1
Severe pain and tenderness in benign fibrocystic breast disease not responding to other treatment
▶ BY MOUTH
▶ Adult: 300 mg daily in divided doses usually for 3–6 months, in women of child-bearing potential, treatment should start during menstruation, preferably on day 1
Hereditary angioedema
▶ BY MOUTH
▶ Adult: Initially 100–200 mg daily, dose to be reduced according to response, in women of child-bearing potential, treatment should start during menstruation, preferably on day 1

● UNLICENSED USE Not licensed for use in hereditary angioedema.

● CONTRA-INDICATIONS Acute porphyrias p. 1107 · androgen-dependent tumours · thromboembolic disease · undiagnosed genital bleeding

● CAUTIONS Cardiac impairment (avoid if severe) · diabetes mellitus · elderly · epilepsy · history of thrombosis or thromboembolic disease · hypertension · lipoprotein disorder · migraine · polycythaemia

● INTERACTIONS → Appendix 1: danazol

● SIDE-EFFECTS Alopecia · aminolevulinic acid synthetase induction · anxiety · appetite increased · breast atrophy · carpal tunnel syndrome · clitoris enlarged · contact lens intolerance · cutaneous lupus erythematosus · depressed mood · dizziness · embolism and thrombosis · emotional lability · eosinophilia · epigastric pain · epilepsy exacerbated · face oedema · fatigue · fever · fluid retention · flushing · glucose tolerance impaired · haematuria · headaches · hepatic disorders · hirsutism · hypertension · idiopathic intracranial hypertension · insulin resistance · joint disorders · leucopenia · libido disorder · menstrual cycle irregularities · muscle contractions involuntary · muscle cramps · myocardial infarction · nausea · neoplasms · pain · palpitations · pancreatitis · photosensitivity reaction · polycythaemia · respiratory disorders · seborrhoea · skin reactions · speech pitch disorder · spermatogenesis reduced · splenic peliosis · tachycardia · throat pain · thrombocytopenia · tremor · vertigo · vision disorders · voice alteration · vulvovaginal disorders · weight increased

SIDE-EFFECTS, FURTHER INFORMATION Withdraw if virilisation effects occur—may be irreversible on continued use.

- CONCEPTION AND CONTRACEPTION Ensure patients with amenorrhoea are not pregnant. Non-hormonal contraceptive methods should be used, if appropriate.
- PREGNANCY Avoid; has weak androgenic effects and virilisation of female fetus reported.
- BREAST FEEDING No data available but avoid because of possible androgenic effects in infant.
- HEPATIC IMPAIRMENT Manufacturer advises caution; avoid in marked impairment.
- RENAL IMPAIRMENT Caution in renal impairment (avoid if severe).
- MONITORING REQUIREMENTS Manufacturer advises periodic monitoring of hepatic function and haematological state (including biannual hepatic ultrasonography for treatment exceeding 6 months or repeated courses of treatment).

- MEDICINAL FORMS Forms available from special-order manufacturers include: capsule

7 Hypothalamic and anterior pituitary hormone related disorders

Hypothalamic and anterior pituitary hormones

Anterior pituitary hormones

Corticotrophins
Tetracosactide below (tetracosactrin), an analogue of corticotropin (ACTH), is used to test adrenocortical function; failure of the plasma cortisol concentration to rise after administration of tetracosactide indicates adrenocortical insufficiency.

Both corticotropin and tetracosactide were formerly used as alternatives to corticosteroids in conditions such as Crohn's disease; their value was limited by the variable and unpredictable therapeutic response and by the waning of their effect with time.

Gonadotrophins
Follicle-stimulating hormone (FSH) and luteinising hormone (LH) together, or follicle-stimulating hormone alone (as in **follitropin**), are used in the treatment of infertility in women with proven hypopituitarism or who have not responded to clomifene citrate p. 808, or in superovulation

treatment for assisted conception (such as *in vitro* fertilisation).

The gonadotrophins are also occasionally used in the treatment of hypogonadotrophic hypogonadism and associated oligospermia. There is no justification for their use in primary gonadal failure.

Growth hormone
Growth hormone is used to treat deficiency of the hormone in children and in adults. In children it is used in Prader-Willi syndrome, Turner syndrome, chronic renal insufficiency, short children considered small for gestational age at birth, and short stature homeobox-containing gene (SHOX) deficiency.

Growth hormone of human origin (HGH; somatotrophin) has been replaced by a growth hormone of human sequence, somatropin p. 789, produced using recombinant DNA technology.

Mecasermin, a human insulin-like growth factor-I (rhIGF-I), is licensed to treat growth failure in children and adolescents with severe primary insulin-like growth factor-I deficiency.

Hypothalamic hormones
Gonadorelin p. 785 when injected intravenously in normal subjects leads to a rapid rise in plasma concentrations of both luteinising hormone (LH) and follicle-stimulating hormone (FSH). It has not proved to be very helpful, however, in distinguishing hypothalamic from pituitary lesions. **Gonadorelin analogues** are indicated in endometriosis and infertility and in breast and prostate cancer.

7.1 Adrenocortical function testing

PITUITARY AND HYPOTHALAMIC HORMONES AND ANALOGUES > CORTICOTROPHINS

Tetracosactide
02-Dec-2020
(Tetracosactrin)

- INDICATIONS AND DOSE

Diagnosis of adrenocortical insufficiency (diagnostic 30-minute test)
▸ BY INTRAVENOUS INJECTION, OR BY INTRAMUSCULAR INJECTION
▹ Adult: 250 micrograms for 1 dose

Diagnosis of adrenocortical insufficiency (diagnostic 5-hour test)
▸ BY INTRAMUSCULAR INJECTION USING DEPOT INJECTION
▹ Adult: 1 mg for 1 dose

Alternative to corticosteroids in conditions such as Crohn's disease or rheumatoid arthritis (formerly used but value was limited by the variable and unpredictable therapeutic response and by the waning of effect with time)
▸ BY INTRAMUSCULAR INJECTION USING DEPOT INJECTION
▹ Adult: Initially 1 mg daily, alternatively initially 1 mg every 12 hours, (in acute cases), then reduced to 1 mg every 2–3 days, followed by 1 mg once weekly, alternatively 500 micrograms every 2–3 days

- CONTRA-INDICATIONS Acute psychosis · adrenogenital syndrome · allergic disorders · asthma · avoid injections containing benzyl alcohol in neonates · Cushing's syndrome · infectious diseases · peptic ulcer · primary adrenocortical insufficiency · refractory heart failure

- CAUTIONS Active infectious diseases (should not be used unless adequate disease-specific therapy is being given) · active systemic diseases (should not be used unless adequate disease-specific therapy is being given) · diabetes mellitus · diverticulitis · history of asthma · history of atopic allergy · history of eczema · history of hayfever · history of hypersensitivity · hypertension · latent amoebiasis (may become activated) · latent tuberculosis (may become activated) · myasthenia gravis · ocular herpes simplex · osteoporosis · predisposition to thromboembolic · pscyhological disturbances may be triggered · recent intestinal anastomosis · reduced immune response (should not be used unless adequate disease-specific therapy is being given) · ulcerative colitis

  CAUTIONS, FURTHER INFORMATION
  - Risk of anaphylaxis Should only be administered under medical supervision. Consult product literature.
  - Hypertension Patients already receiving medication for moderate to severe hypertension must have their dosage adjusted if treatment started.
  - Diabetes mellitus Patients already receiving medication for diabetes mellitus must have their dosage adjusted if treatment started.

- SIDE-EFFECTS Abdominal distension · abscess · adrenocortical unresponsiveness · angioedema · appetite increased · bone fractures · congestive heart failure · Cushing's syndrome · diabetes mellitus exacerbated · dizziness · dyspnoea · electrolyte imbalance · exophthalmos · fluid retention · flushing · gastrointestinal disorders · glaucoma · growth retardation · haemorrhage · headache · healing impaired · hirsutism · hyperglycaemia · hyperhidrosis · hypersensitivity (may be more severe in patients susceptible to allergies, especially asthma) · hypertension · idiopathic intracranial hypertension exacerbated · increased risk of infection · leucocytosis · malaise · menstruation irregular · muscle weakness · myopathy · nausea · osteonecrosis · osteoporosis · pancreatitis · papilloedema · pituitary unresponsiveness · posterior subcapsular cataract · protein catabolism · psychiatric disorder · seizure · skin reactions · tendon rupture · thromboembolism · vasculitis necrotising · vertigo · vomiting · weight increased

- ALLERGY AND CROSS-SENSITIVITY Ⓔⱽᴳʳ Contra-indicated in patients with history of hypersensitivity to tetracosactide/corticotrophins or excipients. Ⓜ

- PREGNANCY Avoid (but may be used diagnostically if essential).

- BREAST FEEDING Avoid (but may be used diagnostically if essential).

- HEPATIC IMPAIRMENT For *depot injection*, manufacturer advises caution in cirrhosis (may enhance effect of tetracosactide therapy).

- RENAL IMPAIRMENT Use with caution in patients with renal impairment.

- EFFECT ON LABORATORY TESTS May suppress skin test reactions.
  Post administration total plasma cortisol levels during 30-minute test for diagnosis of adrenocotical insufficiency might be misleading due to altered cortisol binding globulin levels in some special clinical situations including, patients on oral contraceptives, post-operative patients, critical illness, severe liver disease and nephrotic syndrome.

- MEDICINAL FORMS There can be variation in the licensing of different medicines containing the same drug.
  Solution for injection
  - Synacthen (Atnahs Pharma UK Ltd)
    Tetracosactide acetate 250 microgram per 1 ml Synacthen 250micrograms/1ml solution for injection ampoules | 1 ampoule PoM £38.00 DT = £38.00

Suspension for injection
EXCIPIENTS: May contain Benzyl alcohol
- Synacthen Depot (Atnahs Pharma UK Ltd)
  Tetracosactide acetate 1 mg per 1 ml Synacthen Depot 1mg/1ml suspension for injection ampoules | 1 ampoule PoM £346.28 DT = £346.28

7.2 Assessment of pituitary function

PITUITARY AND HYPOTHALAMIC HORMONES AND ANALOGUES > GONADOTROPHIN-RELEASING HORMONES

▍Gonadorelin

(Gonadotrophin-releasing hormone; GnRH; LH–RH)

- ● INDICATIONS AND DOSE
  Assessment of pituitary function
  - ▸ BY SUBCUTANEOUS INJECTION, OR BY INTRAVENOUS INJECTION
  - ▸ Adult: 100 micrograms for 1 dose

- CAUTIONS Pituitary adenoma

- SIDE-EFFECTS
  - ▸ Uncommon Pain · skin reactions · swelling
  - ▸ Rare or very rare Abdominal discomfort · bronchospasm · dizziness · eye erythema · flushing · headache · nausea · tachycardia
  - ▸ Frequency not known Menorrhagia · sepsis · thrombophlebitis

- PREGNANCY Avoid.

- BREAST FEEDING Avoid.

- MEDICINAL FORMS There can be variation in the licensing of different medicines containing the same drug.
  Powder for solution for injection
  - Gonadorelin (Non-proprietary)
    Gonadorelin (as Gonadorelin hydrochloride)
    100 microgram Gonadorelin 100microgram powder for solution for injection vials | 1 vial PoM £75.00 (Hospital only)

7.3 Gonadotrophin replacement therapy

GONADOTROPHINS

▍Choriogonadotropin alfa

(Human chorionic gonadotropin)　　　　　22-May-2020

- ● INDICATIONS AND DOSE
  Treatment of infertility in women with proven hypopituitarism or who have not responded to clomifene | **Superovulation treatment for assisted conception (such as in vitro fertilisation)**
  - ▸ BY SUBCUTANEOUS INJECTION
  - ▸ Adult (female): Adjusted according to response.

- CONTRA-INDICATIONS Active thromboembolic disorders · ectopic pregnancy in previous 3 months · hypothalamus malignancy · mammary malignancy · ovarian enlargement or cyst (unless caused by polycystic ovarian disease) · ovarian malignancy · pituitary malignancy · undiagnosed vaginal bleeding · uterine malignancy

- CAUTIONS Acute porphyrias p. 1107

- SIDE-EFFECTS
- ▶ **Common or very common** Abdominal pain · fatigue · headache · nausea · ovarian hyperstimulation syndrome · vomiting
- ▶ **Uncommon** Breast pain · depression · diarrhoea · irritability · restlessness
- ▶ **Rare or very rare** Rash · shock · thromboembolism

- MEDICINAL FORMS There can be variation in the licensing of different medicines containing the same drug.
  Solution for injection
  - ▶ Ovitrelle (Merck Serono Ltd)
    Choriogonadotropin alfa 500 microgram per 1 ml Ovitrelle 250micrograms/0.5ml solution for injection pre-filled syringes | 1 pre-filled disposable injection PoM £37.66 DT = £37.66 CD4–2
    Ovitrelle 250micrograms/0.5ml solution for injection pre-filled pens | 1 pre-filled disposable injection PoM £37.66 DT = £37.66 CD4–2

Follitropin alfa

06-Oct-2020

(Recombinant human follicle stimulating hormone)

- INDICATIONS AND DOSE

Infertility in women with proven hypopituitarism or who have not responded to clomifene | Superovulation treatment for assisted conception (such as in vitro fertilisation)
- ▶ BY SUBCUTANEOUS INJECTION
- ▶ Adult (female): Adjusted according to response.

Hypogonadotrophic hypogonadism
- ▶ BY SUBCUTANEOUS INJECTION
- ▶ Adult (male): (consult product literature).

- CONTRA-INDICATIONS Ovarian cysts (not caused by polycystic ovarian syndrome) · ovarian enlargement (not caused by polycystic ovarian syndrome) · tumours of breast · tumours of hypothalamus · tumours of ovaries · tumours of pituitary · tumours of prostate · tumours of testes · tumours of uterus · vaginal bleeding of unknown cause
- CAUTIONS Acute porphyrias p. 1107 · history of tubal disease
- SIDE-EFFECTS
- ▶ **Common or very common** Acne · diarrhoea · gastrointestinal discomfort · gynaecomastia · headache · nausea · ovarian and fallopian tube disorders · varicocele · vomiting · weight increased
- ▶ **Rare or very rare** Asthma exacerbated · thromboembolism
- PREGNANCY Avoid.
- BREAST FEEDING Avoid.
- PRESCRIBING AND DISPENSING INFORMATION Follitropin alfa is a biological medicine. Biological medicines must be prescribed and dispensed by brand name, see *Biological medicines* and *Biosimilar medicines*, under Guidance on prescribing p. 1.
- PATIENT AND CARER ADVICE
  Conception and contraception Patients planning to conceive should be warned that there is a risk of multiple pregnancy.

- MEDICINAL FORMS There can be variation in the licensing of different medicines containing the same drug.
  Solution for injection
  - ▶ Bemfola (Gedeon Richter (UK) Ltd)
    Follitropin alfa 600 unit per 1 ml Bemfola 75units/0.125ml solution for injection pre-filled pens | 1 pre-filled disposable injection PoM £23.50 DT = £23.50
    Bemfola 225units/0.375ml solution for injection pre-filled pens | 1 pre-filled disposable injection PoM £70.50 DT = £70.50
    Bemfola 450units/0.75ml solution for injection pre-filled pens | 1 pre-filled disposable injection PoM £141.00 DT = £169.20
    Bemfola 300units/0.5ml solution for injection pre-filled pens | 1 pre-filled disposable injection PoM £94.00 DT = £112.80

Bemfola 150units/0.25ml solution for injection pre-filled pens | 1 pre-filled disposable injection PoM £47.00 DT = £47.00
- ▶ Gonal-f (Merck Serono Ltd)
  Follitropin alfa 600 unit per 1 ml Gonal-f 900units/1.5ml solution for injection pre-filled pens | 1 pre-filled disposable injection PoM £338.40 DT = £338.40
  Gonal-f 300units/0.5ml solution for injection pre-filled pens | 1 pre-filled disposable injection PoM £112.80 DT = £112.80
  Gonal-f 450units/0.75ml solution for injection pre-filled pens | 1 pre-filled disposable injection PoM £169.20 DT = £169.20
- ▶ Ovaleap (Theramex HQ UK Ltd)
  Follitropin alfa 600 unit per 1 ml Ovaleap 450units/0.75ml solution for injection cartridges | 1 cartridge PoM £141.00
  Ovaleap 900units/1.5ml solution for injection cartridges | 1 cartridge PoM £282.00
  Ovaleap 300units/0.5ml solution for injection cartridges | 1 cartridge PoM £94.00

Powder and solvent for solution for injection
- ▶ Gonal-f (Merck Serono Ltd)
  Follitropin alfa 75 unit Gonal-f 75unit powder and solvent for solution for injection vials | 1 vial PoM £25.22 DT = £25.22
  Follitropin alfa 450 unit Gonal-f 450unit powder and solvent for solution for injection vials | 1 vial PoM £151.32 DT = £151.32
  Follitropin alfa 1050 unit Gonal-f 1,050unit powder and solvent for solution for injection vials | 1 vial PoM £353.06 DT = £353.06

Follitropin alfa with lutropin alfa

22-May-2020

The properties listed below are those particular to the combination only. For the properties of the components please consider, follitropin alfa above, lutropin alfa p. 787.

- INDICATIONS AND DOSE

Infertility in women with proven hypopituitarism or who have not responded to clomifene | Superovulation treatment for assisted conception (such as in vitro fertilisation)
- ▶ BY SUBCUTANEOUS INJECTION
- ▶ Adult (female): Adjusted according to response.

- MEDICINAL FORMS There can be variation in the licensing of different medicines containing the same drug.
  Powder and solvent for solution for injection
  ELECTROLYTES: May contain Sodium
  - ▶ Pergoveris (Merck Serono Ltd)
    Lutropin alfa 75 unit, Follitropin alfa 150 unit Pergoveris 150unit/75unit powder and solvent for solution for injection vials | 1 vial PoM £72.35

Follitropin delta

06-Sep-2017

- DRUG ACTION Follitropin delta is a recombinant human follicle stimulating hormone, which causes development of multiple mature follicles.

- INDICATIONS AND DOSE

Superovulation treatment for assisted conception (such as in vitro fertilisation) (initiated under specialist supervision)
- ▶ BY SUBCUTANEOUS INJECTION
- ▶ Adult (female): Initial dosing based on serum anti-Müllerian hormone concentration and body-weight—consult product literature.

- CONTRA-INDICATIONS Ovarian cysts (not caused by polycystic ovarian syndrome) · ovarian enlargement (not caused by polycystic ovarian syndrome) · tumours of breast · tumours of hypothalamus · tumours of ovaries · tumours of pituitary · tumours of uterus · vaginal bleeding of unknown cause
- CAUTIONS Acute porphyrias p. 1107 · history of tubal disease (increased risk of ectopic pregnancy)

- SIDE-EFFECTS
▸ **Common or very common** Fatigue · headache · nausea · ovarian and fallopian tube disorders · pelvic disorders · uterine pain
▸ **Uncommon** Abdominal discomfort · breast abnormalities · constipation · diarrhoea · dizziness · drowsiness · mood swings · vaginal haemorrhage · vomiting
▸ **Rare or very rare** Thromboembolism
  SIDE-EFFECTS, FURTHER INFORMATION If ovarian hyperstimulation syndrome occurs, the patient should be advised to withhold hCG and avoid intercourse or use barrier contraceptive methods for at least 4 days.
- PREGNANCY Manufacturer advises avoid—not indicated during pregnancy.
- BREAST FEEDING Manufacturer advises avoid—not indicated during breastfeeding.
- MONITORING REQUIREMENTS Manufacturer advises regular monitoring of ovarian response with ultrasound alone, or in combination with serum estradiol levels. Frequent monitoring of follicular development is required to reduce the risk of ovarian hyperstimulation syndrome during treatment, and for at least 2 weeks after triggering of final follicular maturation—consult product literature.
- DIRECTIONS FOR ADMINISTRATION Manufacturer recommends the cartridge should be used with the *Rekovelle*® injection pen. The first injection should be performed under direct medical supervision; self-administration should only be performed by patients who are well motivated, adequately trained and have access to expert advice.
- PRESCRIBING AND DISPENSING INFORMATION Follitropin delta is a biological medicine. Biological medicines must be prescribed and dispensed by brand name, see *Biological medicines* and *Biosimilar medicines*, under Guidance on prescribing p. 1.
- HANDLING AND STORAGE Manufacturer advises store in a refrigerator (2–8 °C)—consult product literature for further information regarding storage conditions outside refrigerator.
- PATIENT AND CARER ADVICE
  Conception and contraception Manufacturer advises that patients planning to conceive should be warned that there is a risk of multiple pregnancy.

- MEDICINAL FORMS There can be variation in the licensing of different medicines containing the same drug.
  Solution for injection
  ▸ Follitropin delta (non-proprietary) ▼
    Follitropin delta 33.33 microgram per 1 ml Rekovelle 36micrograms/1.08ml solution for injection pre-filled pens | 1 pre-filled disposable injection [PoM] £354.94
    Rekovelle 72micrograms/2.16 ml solution for injection pre-filled pens | 1 pre-filled disposable injection [PoM] £709.89
    Rekovelle 12micrograms/0.36ml solution for injection pre-filled pens | 1 pre-filled disposable injection [PoM] £118.31
  ▸ Rekovelle (Ferring Pharmaceuticals Ltd) ▼
    Follitropin delta 33.33 microgram per 1 ml Rekovelle 12micrograms/0.36ml solution for injection cartridges | 1 cartridge [PoM] £118.31
    Rekovelle 36micrograms/1.08ml solution for injection cartridges | 1 cartridge [PoM] £354.94
    Rekovelle 72micrograms/2.16ml solution for injection cartridges | 1 cartridge [PoM] £709.89

Lutropin alfa

22-May-2020

(Recombinant human luteinising hormone)

- INDICATIONS AND DOSE
  Treatment of infertility in women with proven hypopituitarism or who have not responded to clomifene (in conjunction with follicle-stimulating hormone) | Superovulation treatment for assisted conception (such as in vitro fertilisation) (in conjunction with follicle-stimulating hormone)
  ▸ BY SUBCUTANEOUS INJECTION
  ▸ Adult (female): Adjusted according to response.

- CONTRA-INDICATIONS Mammary carcinoma · ovarian carcinoma · ovarian enlargement or cyst (unless caused by polycystic ovarian disease) · tumours of hypothalamus · tumours of pituitary · undiagnosed vaginal bleeding · uterine carcinoma
- CAUTIONS Acute porphyrias p. 1107
- SIDE-EFFECTS
▸ **Common or very common** Breast pain · diarrhoea · gastrointestinal discomfort · headache · nausea · ovarian and fallopian tube disorders · pelvic pain · vomiting
▸ **Rare or very rare** Thromboembolism

- MEDICINAL FORMS There can be variation in the licensing of different medicines containing the same drug.
  Powder and solvent for solution for injection
  ▸ Luveris (Merck Serono Ltd)
    Lutropin alfa 75 unit Luveris 75unit powder and solvent for solution for injection vials | 1 vial [PoM] £31.38

Menotrophin

06-Oct-2020

- INDICATIONS AND DOSE
  Infertility in women with proven hypopituitarism or who have not responded to clomifene | Superovulation treatment for assisted conception (such as in vitro fertilisation)
  ▸ BY SUBCUTANEOUS INJECTION, OR BY DEEP INTRAMUSCULAR INJECTION
  ▸ Adult (female): Adjusted according to response.
  Hypogonadotrophic hypogonadism
  ▸ BY DEEP INTRAMUSCULAR INJECTION, OR BY SUBCUTANEOUS INJECTION
  ▸ Adult (male): (consult product literature).

- CONTRA-INDICATIONS Ovarian cysts (not caused by polycystic ovarian syndrome) · ovarian enlargement (not caused by polycystic ovarian syndrome) · tumours of breast · tumours of hypothalamus · tumours of ovaries · tumours of pituitary · tumours of prostate · tumours of testes · tumours of uterus · vaginal bleeding of unknown cause
- CAUTIONS Acute porphyrias p. 1107 · history of tubal disease
- SIDE-EFFECTS
▸ **Common or very common** Gastrointestinal discomfort · headache · nausea · ovarian and fallopian tube disorders · pelvic pain · uterine pain
▸ **Uncommon** Breast abnormalities · diarrhoea · dizziness · fatigue · hot flush · vomiting
▸ **Rare or very rare** Skin reactions
▸ **Frequency not known** Arthralgia · pain · thromboembolism · vision disorder
- PREGNANCY Avoid.
- BREAST FEEDING Avoid.
- PRESCRIBING AND DISPENSING INFORMATION
  Menotrophin is purified extract of human post-menopausal urine containing follicle-stimulating hormone (FSH) and luteinising hormone (LH) in a ratio of 1:1

- PATIENT AND CARER ADVICE
Conception and contraception Patients planning to conceive should be warned that there is a risk of multiple pregnancy.

- MEDICINAL FORMS There can be variation in the licensing of different medicines containing the same drug.
Powder and solvent for solution for injection
  ‣ Menopur (Ferring Pharmaceuticals Ltd)
  Menotrophin 75 unit Menopur 75unit powder and solvent for solution for injection vials | 10 vial [PoM] £180.18 DT = £180.18
  Menotrophin 150 unit Menopur 150unit powder and solvent for solution for injection vials | 10 vial [PoM] £360.36 DT = £360.36
  Menotrophin 600 unit Menopur 600unit powder and solvent for solution for injection vials | 1 vial [PoM] £144.14 DT = £144.14
  Menotrophin 1200 unit Menopur 1,200unit powder and solvent for solution for injection vials | 1 vial [PoM] £288.29 DT = £288.29
  ‣ Meriofert (Pharmasure Ltd)
  Menotrophin 75 unit Meriofert 75unit powder and solvent for solution for injection vials | 10 vial [PoM] £279.00 DT = £180.18
  Menotrophin 150 unit Meriofert 150unit powder and solvent for solution for injection vials | 10 vial [PoM] £558.00 DT = £360.36

Urofollitropin

02-Sep-2020

- INDICATIONS AND DOSE
Infertility in women with proven hypopituitarism or who have not responded to clomifene | Superovulation treatment for assisted conception (such as in vitro fertilisation)
  ‣ BY SUBCUTANEOUS INJECTION, OR BY DEEP INTRAMUSCULAR INJECTION
  ‣ Adult (female): Adjusted according to response.

- CONTRA-INDICATIONS Ovarian cysts (not caused by polycystic ovarian syndrome) · tumours of breast · tumours of hypothalamus · tumours of ovaries · tumours of pituitary · tumours of uterus · vaginal bleeding of unknown cause

- CAUTIONS Acute porphyrias p. 1107

- SIDE-EFFECTS
▸ Common or very common Breast tenderness · constipation · diarrhoea · gastrointestinal discomfort · headache · hot flush · increased risk of infection · muscle spasms · nausea · ovarian hyperstimulation syndrome · pain · pelvic pain · rash · vaginal discharge · vaginal haemorrhage · vomiting

- PREGNANCY Avoid.

- BREAST FEEDING Avoid.

- PRESCRIBING AND DISPENSING INFORMATION
Urofollitropin is purified extract of human post-menopausal urine containing follicle-stimulating hormone (FSH).

- PATIENT AND CARER ADVICE
Conception and contraception Patients planning to conceive should be warned that there is a risk of multiple pregnancy.

- MEDICINAL FORMS There can be variation in the licensing of different medicines containing the same drug.
Powder and solvent for solution for injection
  ‣ Fostimon (Pharmasure Ltd)
  Follicle stimulating hormone human (as Urofollitropin) 75 unit Fostimon 75unit powder and solvent for solution for injection vials | 10 vial [PoM] £279.00
  Follicle stimulating hormone human (as Urofollitropin) 150 unit Fostimon 150unit powder and solvent for solution for injection vials | 10 vial [PoM] £558.00

7.4 Growth hormone disorders

PITUITARY AND HYPOTHALAMIC HORMONES AND ANALOGUES ⟩ GROWTH HORMONE RECEPTOR ANTAGONISTS

Pegvisomant

20-Aug-2020

- DRUG ACTION Pegvisomant is a genetically modified analogue of human growth hormone and is a highly selective growth hormone receptor antagonist.

- INDICATIONS AND DOSE
Treatment of acromegaly in patients with inadequate response to surgery, radiation, or both, and to treatment with somatostatin analogues (initiated by a specialist)
  ‣ BY SUBCUTANEOUS INJECTION
  ‣ Adult: Initially 80 mg for 1 dose, followed by 10 mg daily, then increased in steps of 5 mg daily, adjusted according to response; maximum 30 mg per day

- CAUTIONS Abnormal liver function tests and/or signs or symptoms of liver injury (further investigations may be required before treatment initiation—consult product literature) · diabetes mellitus (adjustment of antidiabetic therapy may be necessary)

- SIDE-EFFECTS
▸ Common or very common Arthralgia · arthritis · asthenia · constipation · diarrhoea · dizziness · drowsiness · dyslipidaemia · dyspnoea · eye pain · fever · gastrointestinal discomfort · gastrointestinal disorders · haemorrhage · headaches · hyperglycaemia · hypertension · hypoglycaemia · influenza like illness · lipohypertrophy · myalgia · nausea · numbness · oedema · skin reactions · sleep disorders · sweat changes · tremor · vomiting · weight increased
▸ Uncommon Apathy · confusion · dry mouth · eye strain · feeling abnormal · healing impaired · hunger · leucocytosis · leucopenia · libido increased · memory loss · Meniere's disease · oral disorders · panic attack · polyuria · proteinuria · renal impairment · taste altered · thrombocytopenia
▸ Frequency not known Anger · angioedema · hepatic function abnormal · laryngospasm

SIDE-EFFECTS, FURTHER INFORMATION **Injection-site reactions** Rotate injection sites to avoid lipohypertrophy.
Abnormal hepatic function Manufacturer advises interrupt treatment if liver function tests at least 5 times the upper limit of normal *or* transaminase levels at least 3 times the upper limit of normal **and** blood bilirubin increased—consult product literature. Discontinue if liver injury is confirmed.

- CONCEPTION AND CONTRACEPTION Possible increase in female fertility.

- PREGNANCY Avoid.

- BREAST FEEDING Avoid.

- HEPATIC IMPAIRMENT Manufacturer advises caution (no information available); temporary or permanent withdrawal may be needed—consult product literature.

- MONITORING REQUIREMENTS
▸ Manufacturer advises assess liver function tests before treatment initiation and monitor liver function tests during treatment—consult product literature.
▸ Manufacturer advises monitor serum IGF-I concentrations.

- NATIONAL FUNDING/ACCESS DECISIONS
For full details see funding body website

Scottish Medicines Consortium (SMC) decisions
▸ Pegvisomant (*Somavert*®) for the treatment of adult patients with acromegaly who have had an inadequate response to

surgery and/or radiation therapy and in whom an appropriate medical treatment with somatostatin analogues did not normalize insulin-like growth factor type 1 (IGF-1) concentrations or was not tolerated (November 2017) SMC No. 158/05 Recommended

All Wales Medicines Strategy Group (AWMSG) decisions
▶ Pegvisomant (*Somavert*®) for the treatment of adult patients with acromegaly who have had an inadequate response to surgery and/or radiation therapy and in whom an appropriate medical treatment with somatostatin analogues did not normalise insulin-like growth factor-1 (IGF-1) concentrations or was not tolerated (November 2017) AWMSG No. 3545 Recommended

● MEDICINAL FORMS There can be variation in the licensing of different medicines containing the same drug.
Powder and solvent for solution for injection
▶ Somavert (Pfizer Ltd)
Pegvisomant 10 mg Somavert 10mg powder and solvent for solution for injection vials | 30 vial PoM £1,500.00 (Hospital only)
Pegvisomant 15 mg Somavert 15mg powder and solvent for solution for injection vials | 30 vial PoM £2,250.00 (Hospital only)
Pegvisomant 20 mg Somavert 20mg powder and solvent for solution for injection vials | 1 vial PoM £100.00 (Hospital only) | 30 vial PoM £3,000.00 (Hospital only)
Pegvisomant 25 mg Somavert 25mg powder and solvent for solution for injection vials | 30 vial PoM £3,750.00 (Hospital only)
Pegvisomant 30 mg Somavert 30mg powder and solvent for solution for injection vials | 30 vial PoM £4,500.00 (Hospital only)

PITUITARY AND HYPOTHALAMIC HORMONES AND ANALOGUES > HUMAN GROWTH HORMONES

Somatropin
22-Jul-2020
(Recombinant Human Growth Hormone)

● **INDICATIONS AND DOSE**
Gonadal dysgenesis (Turner syndrome)
▶ BY SUBCUTANEOUS INJECTION
▶ Adult: 1.4 mg/m^2 daily, alternatively 45–50 micrograms/kg daily
Deficiency of growth hormone
▶ BY SUBCUTANEOUS INJECTION
▶ Adult: Initially 150–300 micrograms daily, then increased if necessary up to 1 mg daily, dose to be increased gradually, use minimum effective dose (requirements may decrease with age)
DOSE EQUIVALENCE AND CONVERSION
▶ Dose formerly expressed in units; somatropin 1 mg ≡ 3 units.

● CONTRA-INDICATIONS Evidence of tumour activity (complete antitumour therapy and ensure intracranial lesions inactive before starting) · not to be used after renal transplantation · severe obesity in Prader-Willi syndrome · severe respiratory impairment in Prader-Willi syndrome
● CAUTIONS Diabetes mellitus (adjustment of antidiabetic therapy may be necessary) · disorders of the epiphysis of the hip (monitor for limping) · history of malignant disease · hypoadrenalism (initiation or adjustment of glucocorticoid replacement therapy may be necessary) · hypothyroidism—manufacturers recommend periodic thyroid function tests but limited evidence of clinical value · initiation of treatment close to puberty not recommended in child born small for corrected gestational age · papilloedema · relative deficiencies of other pituitary hormones · resolved intracranial hypertension (monitor closely) · Silver-Russell syndrome
● INTERACTIONS → Appendix 1: somatropin

● SIDE-EFFECTS
▶ **Common or very common** Carpal tunnel syndrome · fluid retention · headache · joint disorders · lipoatrophy · myalgia · oedema · paraesthesia
▶ **Uncommon** Gynaecomastia · idiopathic intracranial hypertension
▶ **Rare or very rare** Hyperglycaemia · hyperinsulinism · hypothyroidism · osteonecrosis of femur · pancreatitis · slipped capital femoral epiphysis
▶ **Frequency not known** Leukaemia · musculoskeletal stiffness
SIDE-EFFECTS, FURTHER INFORMATION Funduscopy for papilloedema recommended if severe or recurrent headache, visual problems, nausea and vomiting occur—if papilloedema confirmed consider benign intracranial hypertension (rare cases reported).
● PREGNANCY Discontinue if pregnancy occurs—no information available.
● BREAST FEEDING No information available. Absorption from milk unlikely.
● DIRECTIONS FOR ADMINISTRATION Rotate subcutaneous injection sites to prevent lipoatrophy.
● PRESCRIBING AND DISPENSING INFORMATION Somatropin is a biological medicine. Biological medicines must be prescribed and dispensed by brand name, see *Biological medicines* and *Biosimilar medicines*, under Guidance on prescribing p. 1.
SAIZEN® SOLUTION FOR INJECTION For use with *cool.click*® needle-free autoinjector device or *easypod*® autoinjector device (non-NHS but available free of charge from clinics).
NORDITROPIN® PREPARATIONS Cartridges are for use with appropriate *NordiPen*® device (non-NHS but available free of charge from clinics).
Multidose disposable prefilled pens for use with *NovoFine*® or *NovoTwist*® needles.
OMNITROPE® For use with *Omnitrope Pen 5*® and *Omnitrope Pen 10*® devices (non-NHS but available free of charge from clinics).
NUTROPINAQ® For use with *NutropinAq*® Pen device (non-NHS but available free of charge from clinics).
ZOMACTON® 4 mg vial for use with *ZomaJet 2*® Vision needle-free device (non-NHS but available free of charge from clinics) or with needles and syringes.
10 mg vial for use with *ZomaJet Vision X*® needle-free device (non-NHS but available free of charge from clinics) or with needles and syringes.
SAIZEN® POWDER AND SOLVENT FOR SOLUTION FOR INJECTION For use with *one. click*® autoinjector device or *cool.click*® needle-free autoinjector device or *easypod*® autoinjector device (non-NHS but available free of charge from clinics).
GENOTROPIN® PREPARATIONS Cartridges are for use with *Genotropin*® Pen device (non-NHS but available free of charge from clinics).
● NATIONAL FUNDING/ACCESS DECISIONS
For full details see funding body website
NICE decisions
▶ Somatropin for adults with growth hormone deficiency (August 2003) NICE TA64 Recommended with restrictions
● MEDICINAL FORMS There can be variation in the licensing of different medicines containing the same drug.
Solution for injection
EXCIPIENTS: May contain Benzyl alcohol
▶ Norditropin FlexPro (Novo Nordisk Ltd)
Somatropin (epr) 3.3 mg per 1 ml Norditropin FlexPro 5mg/1.5ml solution for injection pre-filled pens | 1 pre-filled disposable injection PoM £106.35 DT = £115.90 CD4-2

Somatropin (epr) 6.7 mg per 1 ml Norditropin FlexPro 10mg/1.5ml solution for injection pre-filled pens | 1 pre-filled disposable injection [PoM] £212.70 DT = £231.80 [CD4-2]

Somatropin (epr) 10 mg per 1 ml Norditropin FlexPro 15mg/1.5ml solution for injection pre-filled pens | 1 pre-filled disposable injection [PoM] £319.05 DT = £347.70 [CD4-2]

▸ Norditropin NordiFlex (Novo Nordisk Ltd)

Somatropin (epr) 3.3 mg per 1 ml Norditropin NordiFlex 5mg/1.5ml solution for injection pre-filled pens | 1 pre-filled disposable injection [PoM] £115.90 DT = £115.90 [CD4-2]

Somatropin (epr) 6.7 mg per 1 ml Norditropin NordiFlex 10mg/1.5ml solution for injection pre-filled pens | 1 pre-filled disposable injection [PoM] £231.80 DT = £231.80 [CD4-2]

Somatropin (epr) 10 mg per 1 ml Norditropin NordiFlex 15mg/1.5ml solution for injection pre-filled pens | 1 pre-filled disposable injection [PoM] £347.70 DT = £347.70 [CD4-2]

▸ Norditropin SimpleXx (Novo Nordisk Ltd)

Somatropin (epr) 3.3 mg per 1 ml Norditropin SimpleXx 5mg/1.5ml solution for injection cartridges | 1 cartridge [PoM] £106.35 DT = £106.35 [CD4-2]

Somatropin (epr) 6.7 mg per 1 ml Norditropin SimpleXx 10mg/1.5ml solution for injection cartridges | 1 cartridge [PoM] £212.70 DT = £212.70 [CD4-2]

Somatropin (epr) 10 mg per 1 ml Norditropin SimpleXx 15mg/1.5ml solution for injection cartridges | 1 cartridge [PoM] £319.05 DT = £319.05 [CD4-2]

▸ NutropinAq (Ipsen Ltd)

Somatropin (rbe) 5 mg per 1 ml NutropinAq 10mg/2ml solution for injection cartridges | 1 cartridge [PoM] £203.00 DT = £203.00 [CD4-2] | 3 cartridge [PoM] £609.00 DT = £609.00 [CD4-2]

▸ Omnitrope (Sandoz Ltd)

Somatropin (rbe) 3.333 mg per 1 ml Omnitrope Pen 5 5mg/1.5ml solution for injection cartridges | 5 cartridge [PoM] £368.74 DT = £368.74 [CD4-2]

▸ Omnitrope SurePal (Sandoz Ltd)

Somatropin (rbe) 3.333 mg per 1 ml Omnitrope SurePal 5 5mg/1.5ml solution for injection cartridges | 5 cartridge [PoM] £368.74 DT = £368.74 [CD4-2]

Somatropin (rbe) 6.667 mg per 1 ml Omnitrope SurePal 10 10mg/1.5ml solution for injection cartridges | 5 cartridge [PoM] £737.49 DT = £737.49 [CD4-2]

Somatropin (rbe) 10 mg per 1 ml Omnitrope SurePal 15 15mg/1.5ml solution for injection cartridges | 5 cartridge [PoM] £1,106.22 DT = £1,106.22 [CD4-2]

▸ Saizen (Merck Serono Ltd)

Somatropin (rmc) 5.825 mg per 1 ml Saizen 6mg/1.03ml solution for injection cartridges | 1 cartridge [PoM] £139.08 DT = £139.08 [CD4-2]

Somatropin (rmc) 8 mg per 1 ml Saizen 12mg/1.5ml solution for injection cartridges | 1 cartridge [PoM] £278.16 DT = £278.16 [CD4-2] Saizen 20mg/2.5ml solution for injection cartridges | 1 cartridge [PoM] £463.60 DT = £463.60 [CD4-2]

Powder and solvent for solution for injection

EXCIPIENTS: May contain Benzyl alcohol

▸ Genotropin (Pfizer Ltd)

Somatropin (rbe) 5.3 mg Genotropin 5.3mg powder and solvent for solution for injection cartridges | 1 cartridge [PoM] £92.15 DT = £92.15 [CD4-2]

Somatropin (rbe) 12 mg Genotropin 12mg powder and solvent for solution for injection cartridges | 1 cartridge [PoM] £208.65 DT = £208.65 [CD4-2]

▸ Genotropin GoQuick (Pfizer Ltd)

Somatropin (rbe) 5.3 mg Genotropin GoQuick 5.3mg powder and solvent for solution for injection pre-filled pens | 1 pre-filled disposable injection [PoM] £92.15 DT = £92.15 [CD4-2]

Somatropin (rbe) 12 mg Genotropin GoQuick 12mg powder and solvent for solution for injection pre-filled pens | 1 pre-filled disposable injection [PoM] £208.65 DT = £208.65 [CD4-2]

▸ Genotropin MiniQuick (Pfizer Ltd)

Somatropin (rbe) 200 microgram Genotropin MiniQuick 200microgram powder and solvent for solution for injection pre-filled disposable devices | 7 pre-filled disposable injection [PoM] £24.35 DT = £24.35 [CD4-2]

Somatropin (rbe) 400 microgram Genotropin MiniQuick 400microgram powder and solvent for solution for injection pre-filled disposable devices | 7 pre-filled disposable injection [PoM] £48.68 DT = £48.68 [CD4-2]

Somatropin (rbe) 600 microgram Genotropin MiniQuick 600microgram powder and solvent for solution for injection pre-filled disposable devices | 7 pre-filled disposable injection [PoM] £73.03 DT = £73.03 [CD4-2]

Somatropin (rbe) 800 microgram Genotropin MiniQuick 800microgram powder and solvent for solution for injection pre-filled disposable devices | 7 pre-filled disposable injection [PoM] £97.37 DT = £97.37 [CD4-2]

Somatropin (rbe) 1 mg Genotropin MiniQuick 1mg powder and solvent for solution for injection pre-filled disposable devices | 7 pre-filled disposable injection [PoM] £121.71 DT = £121.71 [CD4-2]

Somatropin (rbe) 1.2 mg Genotropin MiniQuick 1.2mg powder and solvent for solution for injection pre-filled disposable devices | 7 pre-filled disposable injection [PoM] £146.06 DT = £146.06 [CD4-2]

Somatropin (rbe) 1.4 mg Genotropin MiniQuick 1.4mg powder and solvent for solution for injection pre-filled disposable devices | 7 pre-filled disposable injection [PoM] £170.39 DT = £170.39 [CD4-2]

Somatropin (rbe) 1.6 mg Genotropin MiniQuick 1.6mg powder and solvent for solution for injection pre-filled disposable devices | 7 pre-filled disposable injection [PoM] £194.74 DT = £194.74 [CD4-2]

Somatropin (rbe) 1.8 mg Genotropin MiniQuick 1.8mg powder and solvent for solution for injection pre-filled disposable devices | 7 pre-filled disposable injection [PoM] £219.08 DT = £219.08 [CD4-2]

Somatropin (rbe) 2 mg Genotropin MiniQuick 2mg powder and solvent for solution for injection pre-filled disposable devices | 7 pre-filled disposable injection [PoM] £243.42 DT = £243.42 [CD4-2]

▸ Humatrope (Eli Lilly and Company Ltd)

Somatropin (rbe) 6 mg Humatrope 6mg powder and solvent for solution for injection cartridges | 1 cartridge [PoM] £108.00 DT = £108.00 [CD4-2]

Somatropin (rbe) 12 mg Humatrope 12mg powder and solvent for solution for injection cartridges | 1 cartridge [PoM] £216.00 DT = £208.65 [CD4-2]

Somatropin (rbe) 24 mg Humatrope 24mg powder and solvent for solution for injection cartridges | 1 cartridge [PoM] £432.00 DT = £432.00 [CD4-2]

▸ Saizen (Merck Serono Ltd)

Somatropin (rmc) 8 mg Saizen 8mg click.easy powder and solvent for solution for injection vials | 1 vial [PoM] £185.44 DT = £185.44 [CD4-2]

▸ Zomacton (Ferring Pharmaceuticals Ltd)

Somatropin (rbe) 4 mg Zomacton 4mg powder and solvent for solution for injection vials | 1 vial [PoM] £68.28 DT = £68.28 [CD4-2]

Somatropin (rbe) 10 mg Zomacton 10mg powder and solvent for solution for injection vials | 1 vial [PoM] £170.70 DT = £170.70 [CD4-2]

8 Sex hormone responsive conditions

Sex hormones

20-Nov-2020

Oestrogens and HRT

Oestrogens are necessary for the development of female secondary sexual characteristics; they also stimulate myometrial hypertrophy with endometrial hyperplasia.

In terms of oestrogenic activity *natural oestrogens* (estradiol p. 798 (oestradiol), estrone (oestrone), and estriol p. 878 (oestriol)) have a more appropriate profile for hormone replacement therapy (HRT) than *synthetic oestrogens* (ethinylestradiol p. 802 (ethinyloestradiol) and mestranol). Tibolone p. 802 has oestrogenic, progestogenic and weak androgenic activity.

Oestrogen therapy is given cyclically or continuously for a number of gynaecological conditions. If long-term therapy is required in women with a uterus, a progestogen should normally be added to reduce the risk of cystic hyperplasia of the endometrium (or of endometriotic foci in women who have had a hysterectomy) and possible transformation to cancer.

Oestrogens are no longer used to suppress lactation because of their association with thromboembolism.

Hormone replacement therapy

Hormone replacement therapy (HRT) with small doses of an oestrogen (together with a progestogen in women with a uterus) is appropriate for alleviating menopausal symptoms such as vaginal atrophy or vasomotor instability. Oestrogen given systemically in the perimenopausal and postmenopausal period or tibolone given in the postmenopausal period also diminish postmenopausal osteoporosis but other drugs are preferred; for further information, see Osteoporosis p. 765. Menopausal atrophic vaginitis may respond to a short course of a topical vaginal oestrogen preparation used for a few weeks and repeated if necessary.

Systemic therapy with an oestrogen or drugs with oestrogenic properties alleviates the symptoms of oestrogen deficiency such as vasomotor symptoms. Tibolone combines oestrogenic and progestogenic activity with weak androgenic activity; it is given continuously, without cyclical progestogen.

HRT may be used in women with early natural or surgical menopause (before age 45 years), since they are at high risk of osteoporosis. For early menopause, HRT can be given until the approximate age of natural menopause (i.e. until age 50 years). Alternatives to HRT should be considered if osteoporosis is the main concern.

Clonidine hydrochloride p. 159 may be used to reduce vasomotor symptoms in women who cannot take an oestrogen, but clonidine hydrochloride may cause unacceptable side-effects.

HRT increases the risk of venous thromboembolism, stroke, endometrial cancer (reduced by a progestogen), breast cancer, and ovarian cancer; there is an increased risk of coronary heart disease in women who start combined HRT more than 10 years after menopause. For details of these risks see HRT Risk table.

The Medicines and Healthcare products Regulatory Agency (MHRA) advises that HRT should only be prescribed to relieve post-menopausal symptoms that are adversely affecting quality of life and treatment should be reviewed regularly to ensure the minimum effective dose is used for the shortest duration. For osteoporosis, consider alternative treatments. HRT does not prevent coronary heart disease or protect against a decline in cognitive function and it should not be prescribed for these purposes. Experience of treating women over 65 years with HRT is limited.

For the treatment of menopausal symptoms the benefits of short-term HRT outweigh the risks in the majority of women, especially in those aged under 60 years.

For the treatment of menopausal symptoms in women with breast cancer see Breast cancer p. 986.

Risk of breast cancer

All types of *systemic* (oral or transdermal) HRT treatment increase the risk of breast cancer after 1 year of use. This risk is higher for combined oestrogen-progestogen HRT (particularly for continuous HRT preparations where both oestrogen and progestogen are taken throughout each month) than for oestrogen-only HRT, but is irrespective of the type of oestrogen or progestogen. Longer duration of HRT use (but not the age at which HRT is started) further increases risk.

Although the risk of breast cancer is lower after stopping HRT than it is during current use, the excess risk persists for more than 10 years after stopping compared with women who have never used HRT. Vaginal preparations containing low doses of oestrogen to treat local symptoms are not thought to be associated with an effect on breast cancer risk.

The MHRA advises discussing the updated information on the risk of breast cancer with women who use or are considering starting HRT, at their next routine appointment. The MHRA advises encouraging current and past HRT users to be vigilant for signs of breast cancer and to attend routine breast screening. If a decision is made to stop treatment, in the absence of contra-indications, the MHRA recommends this should be done gradually to minimise recurrence of menopausal symptoms. For more information, see estradiol p. 798, conjugated oestrogens (equine) p. 797 and the MHRA Drug Safety Update: www.gov.uk/drug-safety-update/hormone-replacement-therapy-hrt-further-information-on-the-known-increased-risk-of-breast-cancer-with-hrt-and-its-persistence-after-stopping.

Radiological detection of breast cancer can be made more difficult as mammographic density can increase with HRT use especially oestrogen-progestogen combined treatment, but this is not thought to be the case with tibolone p. 802.

Tibolone p. 802 has also been associated with an increased risk of breast cancer during treatment, although the extent of risk and its persistence after stopping is currently inconclusive.

Risk of endometrial cancer

The increased risk of endometrial cancer depends on the dose and duration of oestrogen-only HRT. In women with a uterus, the addition of a progestogen cyclically (for at least 10 days per 28-day cycle) reduces the additional risk of endometrial cancer; this additional risk is eliminated if a progestogen is given continuously. However, this should be weighed against the increased risk of breast cancer.

The risk of endometrial cancer in women who have not used HRT increases with body mass index (BMI); the increased risk of endometrial cancer in users of oestrogen-only HRT or tibolone is more apparent in women who are not overweight.

Evidence suggests an increased risk of endometrial cancer with tibolone. After 2.7 years of use (in women of average age 68 years), 1 extra case of endometrial hyperplasia and 4 extra cases of endometrial cancer were diagnosed compared with placebo users.

Risk of ovarian cancer

Long-term use of combined HRT or oestrogen-only HRT is associated with a small increased risk of ovarian cancer; this excess risk disappears within a few years of stopping.

Risk of venous thromboembolism

Women using combined or oestrogen-only HRT are at an increased risk of deep vein thrombosis and of pulmonary embolism especially in the first year of use. In women who have predisposing factors (such as a personal or family history of deep vein thrombosis or pulmonary embolism, severe varicose veins, obesity, trauma, or prolonged bed-rest) it is prudent to review the need for HRT, as in some cases the risks of HRT may exceed the benefits. Travel involving prolonged immobility further increases the risk of deep vein thrombosis.

Although the level of risk of thromboembolism associated with non-oral routes of administration of HRT has not been established, it may be lower for the transdermal route.

Limited data does not suggest an increased risk of thromboembolism with tibolone compared with combined HRT or women not taking HRT.

Risk of stroke

Risk of stroke increases with age, therefore older women have a greater absolute risk of stroke. Combined HRT or oestrogen-only HRT slightly increases the risk of stroke.

Tibolone increases the risk of stroke about 2.2 times from the first year of treatment; risk of stroke is age-dependent and therefore the absolute risk of stroke with tibolone increases with age.

Risk of coronary heart disease

HRT does not prevent coronary heart disease and should not be prescribed for this purpose. There is an increased risk of coronary heart disease in women who start combined HRT more than 10 years after menopause. Although very little information is available on the risk of coronary heart disease in younger women who start HRT close to the menopause, studies suggest a lower relative risk compared with older women.

There is insufficient data to draw a conclusion on the risk of coronary heart disease with tibolone.

6

Endocrine system

6

Endocrine system

Choice

The choice of HRT for an individual depends on an overall balance of indication, risk, and convenience. A woman with a uterus normally requires oestrogen with cyclical progestogen for the last 12 to 14 days of the cycle or a preparation which involves continuous administration of an oestrogen and a progestogen (or one which provides both oestrogenic and progestogenic activity in a single preparation). Continuous combined preparations or tibolone p. 802 are **not suitable** for use in the perimenopause or within 12 months of the last menstrual period; women who use such preparations may bleed irregularly in the early stages of treatment—if bleeding continues endometrial abnormality should be ruled out and consideration given to changing to cyclical HRT.

An oestrogen alone is suitable for continuous use in women without a uterus. However, in endometriosis, endometrial foci may remain despite hysterectomy and the addition of a progestogen should be considered in these circumstances.

An oestrogen may be given by mouth or by transdermal administration, which avoids first-pass metabolism.

Table 1: Summary of HRT risks and benefits* during current use and current use plus post-treatment from age of menopause up to age 69 years, per 1000 women with 5 years or 10 years use of HRT

	Risks over 5 years use (with no use or 5 years current HRT use)		Total risks up to age 69 (after no use or after 5 years HRT use[†])		Risks over 10 years (with no use or 10 years current HRT use)		Total risks up to age 69 (after no use or after 10 years HRT use[†])	
	Cases per 1000 women with no HRT use	Extra cases per 1000 women using HRT	Cases per 1000 women with no HRT use	Extra cases per 1000 women using HRT	Cases per 1000 women with no HRT use	Extra cases per 1000 women using HRT	Cases per 1000 women with no HRT use	Extra cases per 1000 women using HRT
Risks associated with **combined estrogen-progestogen HRT**								
Breast cancer	13	+8	63	+17	27	+20	63	+34
Sequential HRT	13	+7	63	+14	27	+17	63	+29
Continuous combined HRT	13	+10	63	+20	27	+25	63	+40
Endometrial cancer	2	-	10	-	4	-	10	-
Ovarian cancer	2	+ <1	10	+ <1	4	+1	10	+1
Venous thromboembolism (VTE)[§]	5	+7	26	+7	8	+13	26	+13
Stroke	4	+1	26	+1	8	+2	26	+2
Coronary heart disease (CHD)	14	-	88	-	28	-	88	-
Fracture of femur	1.5	-	12	-	1	-	12	-
Risks associated with **estrogen-only HRT**								
Breast cancer	13	+3	63	+5	27	+7	63	+11
Endometrial cancer	2	+4	10	+4	4	+32	10	+32
Ovarian cancer	2	+ <1	10	+ <1	4	+1	10	+1
Venous thromboembolism (VTE)[§]	5	+2	26	+2	10	+3	26	+3
Stroke	4	+1	26	+1	8	+2	26	+2
Coronary heart disease (CHD)	14	-	88	-	28	-	88	-
Fracture of femur	0.5	-	12	-	1	-	12	-

*Menopausal symptom relief is not included in this table, but is a key benefit of HRT and will play a major part in the decision to prescribe HRT.
[†]Best estimates based on relative risks of HRT use from age 50 (see DSU table 2 for relative risks). For breast cancer this includes cases diagnosed during current HRT use and diagnosed after HRT use until age 69 years; for other risks, this assumes no residual effects after stopping HRT use.
[§]Latest evidence suggests that transdermal HRT products have a lower risk of VTE than oral preparations.

Reproduced with permission of the MHRA under the terms of the Open Government Licence (OGL) v3.0

Table 2: Detailed summary of relative and absolute risks and benefits during current use from age of menopause and up to age 69, per 1000 women with 5 years or 10 years use of HRT

	Duration of HRT use (years)	Total cases per 1000 women with no HRT use* (RR= 1)	Total cases (range) per 1000 women using HRT†	Extra cases per 1000 women using HRT	Risk ratio (RR) (95% CI)‡
Risks associated with combined estrogen–progestogen HRT					
Cancer risks					
Breast cancer					
Overall combined HRT					
Current use from age 50	5	13	21	+8	1.62
	10	27	47	+20	1.74
Total risk from age 50 to 69 (HRT use + past use)	5	63	80	+17	1.27
	10	63	97	+34	1.54
Sequential HRT					
Current use from age 50	5	13	20	+7	1.54
	10	27	44	+17	1.63
Total risk from age 50 to 69 (HRT use + past use)	5	63	77	+14	1.22
	10	63	92	+29	1.46
Continuous combined HRT					
Current use from age 50	5	13	23	+10	1.77
	10	27	52	+25	1.93
Total risk to from age 50 to 69 (HRT use + past use)	5	63	83	+20	1.32
	10	63	103	+40	1.63
Endometrial Cancer					
age 50–59	5	2	2 (2–3)	NS	1·0 (0·8–1·2)[4]
	10	4	4 (4–5)	NS	1·1 (0·9–1·2)
age 60–69	5	3	3 (2–4)	NS	1·0 (0·8–1·2)[4]
	10	6	7 (5–7)	NS	1·1 (0·9–1·2)
Ovarian Cancer					
age 50–59	5	2	2 (2–3)	+ <1	1.1 (1.0–1.3)
	10	4	5 (4–6)	+1	1·3 (1·1–1·5)
age 60–69	5	3	3 (3–4)	+ <1	1.1 (1.0–1.3)
	10	6	8 (7–9)	+2	1·3 (1·1–1·5)
Cardiovascular risks					
Venous thromboembolism (VTE)§					
age 50–59	5	5	12 (10–15)	+7	2·3 (1·8–3·0)
age 60–69	5	8	18 (15–24)	+10	
Stroke					
age 50–59	5	4	5 (5–6)	+1	1.3 (1.1–1.4)
age 60–69	5	9	12 (10–13)	+3	
Coronary heart disease (CHD)					
age 50–59	5	9	12 (7–19)	NS	1·3 (0·8–2·1)
age 60–69	5	18	18 (13–25)	NS	1·0 (0·7–1·4)
age 70–79	5	29	44 (29–61)	+15	1·5 (1·0–2·1)
Benefits⏃					
Fracture of femur					
age 50–59	5	1.5	1 (0.8–1.5)	NS	0·7 (0·5–1.0)
age 60-69	5	5.5	4 (3-5.5)	NS	

6

Endocrine system

	Duration of HRT use (years)	Total cases per 1000 women with no HRT use* (RR= 1)	Total cases (range) per 1000 women using HRT†	Extra cases per 1000 women using HRT	Risk ratio (RR) (95% CI)‡
Risks associated with estrogen-only HRT use					
Cancer risks					
Breast cancer					
Current use from age 50	5	13	16	+3	1.2
	10	27	34	+7	1.33
Total risk from age 50 to age 69 (HRT use + past use)	5	63	68	+5	1.08
	10	63	74	+11	1.17
Endometrial cancer					
age 50–59	5	2	6 (5–7)	+4	3.0 (2.5–3.6)
	10	4	36 (25–52)	+32	9.0 (6.3–12.9)
age 60–69	5	3	9 (8–11)	+6	3.0 (2.5–3.6)
	10	6	54 (38–77)	+48	9.0 (6.3–12.9)
Ovarian cancer					
age 50–59	5	2	2	+ <1	1.1 (1.0–1.3)
	10	4	5 (5–6)	+1	1·3 (1·2–1·5)
age 60–69	5	3	3	+ <1	1.1 (1.0–1.3)
	10	6	8 (7–9)	+2	1·3 (1·2–1·5)
Cardiovascular risks					
Venous thromboembolism (VTE)					
age 50–59	5	5	7 (5–9)	+2	1.3 (1.0–1.7)
age 60–69	5	8	10 (8–14)	+2	
Stroke					
age 50–59	5	4	5 (5–6)	+1	1.3 (1.0–1.4)
age 60–69	5	9	12 (10–13)	+3	
Coronary heart disease (CHD)					
age 50–59	5	14	8 (6–15)	NS	0·6 (0·4–1·1)
age 60–69	5	31	28 (22–37)	NS	0·9 (0·7–1·2)
age 70–79	5	44	48 (35–66)	NS	1·1 (0·8–1·5)
Benefits⌠					
Fracture of femur					
age 50–59	5	0.5	0.3 (0.2–0.5)	0	0·6 (0·4–0·9)
age 60-69	5	5.5	3 (2–5)	−2	

* Background incidence from: Hospital Admissions in England (HES) for stroke and VTE; placebo arms of Women's Health Initiative (WHI) trial for coronary heart disease (CHD) and fracture; the International Agency Research on Cancer (IARC) for ovarian cancer and endometrial cancer; and from Office for National Statistics (ONS) for England for 2015, calculated for never-users in the Collaborative Group on Hormonal Factors in Breast Cancer meta-analysis for breast cancer.

† Best estimate and range based on relative risk and 95% confidence intervals (CI).

‡ Risk ratios and 95% CI from: meta-analysis of prospective observational studies for breast cancer (95% CI not available); meta-analyses of RCTs and observational studies for endometrial cancer, ovarian cancer and VTE; meta-analyses of randomised controlled trials (RCTs) for stroke; and from WHI trial for CHD and fracture risk.

§ Latest evidence suggests that transdermal HRT products have a lower risk of VTE than oral preparations.

⌠ Menopausal symptom relief is not included in this table but is a key benefit of HRT and will play a major part in the decision to prescribe HRT.

NS=non-significant difference.

Reproduced with permission of the MHRA under the terms of the Open Government Licence (OGL) v3.0

Considerations in the elderly

The use of oestrogens in elderly patients is potentially inappropriate (STOPP criteria) if prescribed in patients with a history of breast cancer or venous thromboembolism (increased risk of recurrence). Oral oestrogens may be inappropriate if prescribed without concurrent progestogen in those with an intact uterus (risk of endometrial cancer).

For further information, see *STOPP/START criteria* in Prescribing in the elderly p. 33.

Surgery

Major surgery under general anaesthesia, including orthopaedic and vascular leg surgery, is a predisposing factor for venous thromboembolism and it may be prudent to stop HRT 4−6 weeks before surgery; it should be restarted only after full mobilisation. If HRT is continued or if discontinuation is not possible (e.g. in non-elective surgery), prophylaxis with unfractionated or low molecular weight heparin and graduated compression hosiery is advised.

Reasons to stop HRT

Hormone replacement therapy should be stopped (pending investigation and treatment), if any of the following occur:

- sudden severe chest pain (even if not radiating to left arm);
- sudden breathlessness (or cough with blood-stained sputum);
- unexplained swelling or severe pain in calf of one leg;
- severe stomach pain;
- serious neurological effects including unusual severe, prolonged headache especially if first time or getting progressively worse or sudden partial or complete loss of vision or sudden disturbance of hearing or other perceptual disorders or dysphasia or bad fainting attack or collapse or first unexplained epileptic seizure or weakness, motor disturbances, very marked numbness suddenly affecting one side or one part of body;
- hepatitis, jaundice, liver enlargement;
- blood pressure above systolic 160 mmHg or diastolic 95 mmHg;
- prolonged immobility after surgery or leg injury;
- detection of a risk factor which contra-indicates treatment.

Ethinylestradiol

Ethinylestradiol p. 802 (ethinyloestradiol) is licensed for short-term treatment of symptoms of oestrogen deficiency, for osteoporosis prophylaxis if other drugs cannot be used and for the treatment of female hypogonadism and menstrual disorders.

Ethinylestradiol is occasionally used under **specialist supervision** for the management of *hereditary haemorrhagic telangiectasia* (but evidence of benefit is limited). It is also used licensed for the palliative treatment of prostate cancer.

Raloxifene

Raloxifene hydrochloride p. 797 is licensed for the treatment and prevention of *postmenopausal osteoporosis*; unlike hormone replacement therapy, raloxifene hydrochloride does not reduce menopausal vasomotor symptoms.

Progestogens and progesterone receptor modulators

There are two main groups of progestogen, progesterone and its analogues (dydrogesterone and medroxyprogesterone acetate p. 856) and testosterone analogues (norethisterone p. 806 and norgestrel). The newer progestogens (desogestrel p. 851, norgestimate, and gestodene) are all derivatives of norgestrel; levonorgestrel p. 852 is the active isomer of norgestrel and has twice its potency. Progesterone p. 807 and its analogues are less androgenic than the testosterone derivatives and neither progesterone nor dydrogesterone causes virilisation.

Where endometriosis requires drug treatment, it may respond to a progestogen, e.g. norethisterone, administered on a continuous basis. Danazol p. 783 and gonadorelin analogues are also available.

Although oral progestogens have been used widely for menorrhagia (see Heavy menstrual bleeding p. 796) they are relatively ineffective compared with tranexamic acid p. 118 or, particularly where dysmenorrhoea is also a factor, mefenamic acid p. 1191; the levonorgestrel-releasing intra-uterine system may be particularly useful for women also requiring contraception. Oral progestogens have also been used for severe dysmenorrhoea, but where contraception is also required in younger women the best choice is a combined oral contraceptive.

Progestogens have also been advocated for the alleviation of premenstrual symptoms, but no convincing physiological basis for such treatment has been shown.

Progestogens have been used for the prevention of miscarriage in women with a history of recurrent miscarriage but there is no evidence of benefit and they are **not** recommended for this purpose. In pregnant women with antiphospholipid antibody syndrome who have suffered recurrent miscarriage, administration of low-dose aspirin p. 132 and a prophylactic dose of a low molecular weight heparin may decrease the risk of fetal loss (use under specialist supervision only).

Hormone replacement therapy

In women with a uterus a progestogen needs to be added to long-term oestrogen therapy for hormone replacement, to prevent cystic hyperplasia of the endometrium and possible transformation to cancer; it can be added on a cyclical or a continuous basis. Combined packs incorporating suitable progestogen tablets are available.

Oral contraception

Desogestrel p. 851, gestodene, levonorgestrel p. 852, norethisterone p. 806, and norgestimate are used in combined oral contraceptives and in progestogen-only contraceptives.

Cancer

Progestogens also have a role in neoplastic disease.

Progesterone receptor modulators

Ulipristal acetate p. 851 is a progesterone receptor modulator with a partial progesterone antagonist effect. Ulipristal acetate is used as an hormonal emergency contraceptive.

Endometriosis

19-Sep-2017

Description of condition

Endometriosis is the growth of endometrial-like tissue outside the uterus. Endometriosis is a condition affecting women mainly of reproductive age and, although its exact cause is unknown, it is an oestrogen-dependent condition and is associated with menstruation. Endometriosis is typically associated with symptoms such as pelvic pain, painful periods and subfertility. Women with endometriosis report pain, which can be frequent, chronic and severe, as well as tiredness, more sick days, and a significant physical, sexual, psychological and social impact. Endometriosis is an important cause of subfertility and this can also have a significant effect on quality of life.

Women may also have endometriosis without symptoms, so it is difficult to know how common the disease is in the population. It is also unclear whether endometriosis is always progressive or can remain stable or improve with time.

6

Endocrine system

Aims of treatment

The aim of treatment is to reduce the severity of symptoms, improve the quality of life, and to improve fertility if this is affected.

Drug treatment

Management options for endometriosis include drug treatment and surgery. Most drug treatments for endometriosis work by suppressing ovarian function and are contraceptive. Surgical treatment aims to remove or destroy endometriotic lesions. The choice of treatment depends on the woman's preferences and priorities in terms of pain management and fertility.

EvGr A short trial (such as 3 months) of paracetamol or an NSAID alone or in combination should be considered for first-line management of endometriosis-related pain. If pain relief is inadequate, consider other forms of pain management and referral for further assessment.

Hormonal treatment (with a combined oral contraceptive or a progestogen) should be offered to women with suspected, confirmed or recurrent endometriosis. The patient should be informed that hormonal treatment for endometriosis can reduce pain and has no permanent negative effect on subsequent fertility. If initial hormonal treatment for endometriosis is not effective, not tolerated or is contra-indicated, the woman should be referred to a gynaecologist or specialist endometriosis service for possible further treatment, which could include other hormonal treatments or surgery. Ⓐ For use of drugs to treat neuropathic pain, see Neuropathic pain.

Surgery

EvGr Women with suspected or confirmed endometriosis should be asked about their symptoms, preferences and priorities with respect to pain and fertility, to guide surgical decision-making. For deep endometriosis involving the bowel, bladder or ureter, gonadotropin-releasing hormones given for 3 months before surgery should be considered. Excision rather than ablation should be considered to treat endometriomas, taking into account the woman's desire for fertility and her ovarian reserve. After laparoscopic excision or ablation of endometriosis, consider hormonal treatment (with, for example, a combined hormonal contraceptive), to prolong the benefits of surgery and manage symptoms.

A hysterectomy may be indicated if, for example, the woman has adenomyosis or heavy menstrual bleeding that has not responded to other treatments. Ⓐ

Surgical management if fertility is a priority

EvGr If fertility is a priority, the management of endometriosis-related subfertility should have multidisciplinary involvement with input from a fertility specialist. Women with endometriosis who are trying to conceive should not be offered hormonal treatment, because it does not improve spontaneous pregnancy rates. Ⓐ

Useful Resources

Endometriosis: diagnosis and management. National Institute for Health and Care Excellence. NICE guidance 73. February 2017.
www.nice.org.uk/guidance/ng73

Patient decision aid: Hormone treatment for endometriosis symptoms—what are my options? National Institute for Health and Care Excellence. September 2017.
www.nice.org.uk/about/what-we-do/our-programmes/nice-guidance/nice-guidelines/shared-decision-making

Heavy menstrual bleeding

20-Nov-2020

Description of condition

Heavy menstrual bleeding, also known as menorrhagia, is excessive menstrual blood loss of 80 mL or more, and/or for a duration of more than 7 days, which results in the need to change menstrual products every 1–2 hours. Heavy menstrual bleeding occurs regularly, every 24–35 days.

Drug treatment

EvGr The choice of treatment should be guided by the presence or absence of fibroids (including size, number and location), polyps, endometrial pathology or adenomyosis, other symptoms (such as pressure or pain), co-morbidities, and patient preference.

In females with heavy menstrual bleeding and unidentified pathology, fibroids less than 3 cm in diameter causing no distortion of the uterine cavity, or suspected or diagnosed adenomyosis, a levonorgestrel-releasing intra-uterine system p. 852 is the first-line treatment option. Patients should be advised that irregular menstrual bleeding can occur particularly during the first months of use and that the full benefit of treatment may take at least 6 months.

If a levonorgestrel-releasing intra-uterine system p. 852 is unsuitable, either tranexamic acid p. 118, an NSAID, a combined hormonal contraceptive, or a cyclical oral progestogen should be considered. Progestogen-only contraceptives may suppress menstruation and be beneficial to females with heavy menstrual bleeding. A non-hormonal treatment is recommended in patients actively trying to conceive.

If drug treatment is unsuccessful or declined by the patient, or if symptoms are severe, referral to a specialist for alternative drug treatment or surgery should be considered.

In females with fibroids of 3 cm or more in diameter, referral to a specialist should be considered. Treatment options include tranexamic acid, an NSAID, a levonorgestrel-releasing intra-uterine system p. 852, a combined hormonal contraceptive, a cyclical oral progestogen, uterine artery embolisation, or surgery. Treatment choice depends on the size, number and location of the fibroids, and severity of symptoms. If drug treatment is required while investigations and definitive treatment is being organised, either tranexamic acid, or an NSAID, or both, can be given.

The effectiveness of drug treatment for heavy menstrual bleeding may be limited in females with fibroids that are substantially greater than 3 cm in diameter. Treatment with a gonadotrophin-releasing hormone analogue before hysterectomy and myomectomy should be considered if uterine fibroids are causing an enlarged or distorted uterus. Ⓐ

Useful Resources

Heavy menstrual bleeding: assessment and management. National Institute for Health and Care Excellence. NICE guideline 88. March 2018 (updated March 2020).
www.nice.org.uk/guidance/ng88

8.1 Female sex hormone responsive conditions

> **Other drugs used for Female sex hormone responsive conditions** Clonidine hydrochloride, p. 159

CALCIUM REGULATING DRUGS > BONE
RESORPTION INHIBITORS

Raloxifene hydrochloride
20-Jan-2020

● **INDICATIONS AND DOSE**

Treatment and prevention of postmenopausal osteoporosis
▶ BY MOUTH
▸ Adult: 60 mg once daily

Breast cancer [chemoprevention in postmenopausal women at moderate to high risk] (initiated under specialist supervision)
▶ BY MOUTH
▸ Adult: 60 mg once daily for 5 years

● UNLICENSED USE Not licensed for chemoprevention of breast cancer in the UK. Licensed for this indication in USA.

● CONTRA-INDICATIONS Cholestasis · endometrial cancer · history of venous thromboembolism · undiagnosed uterine bleeding

● CAUTIONS Avoid in Acute porphyrias p. 1107 · breast cancer (manufacturer advises avoid during treatment for breast cancer) · history of oestrogen-induced hypertriglyceridaemia (monitor serum triglycerides) · risk factors for stroke · risk factors for venous thromboembolism (discontinue if prolonged immobilisation)

● INTERACTIONS → Appendix 1: raloxifene

● SIDE-EFFECTS
▸ **Common or very common** Influenza · leg cramps · peripheral oedema · vasodilation
▸ **Uncommon** Embolism and thrombosis
▸ **Rare or very rare** Breast abnormalities · gastrointestinal discomfort · gastrointestinal disorder · headaches · nausea · rash · thrombocytopenia · vomiting

● HEPATIC IMPAIRMENT Manufacturer advises avoid (risk of increased exposure).

● RENAL IMPAIRMENT Caution in mild to moderate impairment. Avoid in severe impairment.

● NATIONAL FUNDING/ACCESS DECISIONS
For full details see funding body website

NICE decisions
▸ **Raloxifene for the primary prevention of osteoporotic fragility fractures in postmenopausal women (updated February 2018)** NICE TA160 Not recommended
▸ **Raloxifene and teriparatide for the secondary prevention of osteoporotic fragility fractures in postmenopausal women (updated February 2018)** NICE TA161 Recommended with restrictions

● MEDICINAL FORMS There can be variation in the licensing of different medicines containing the same drug.

Tablet
▸ Raloxifene hydrochloride (Non-proprietary)
Raloxifene hydrochloride 60 mg Raloxifene 60mg tablets |
28 tablet [PoM] £17.06 DT = £3.81 | 84 tablet [PoM] £11.43
▸ Evista (Daiichi Sankyo UK Ltd)
Raloxifene hydrochloride 60 mg Evista 60mg tablets |
28 tablet [PoM] £17.06 DT = £3.81

OESTROGENS

Conjugated oestrogens (equine)
14-Dec-2020

● **INDICATIONS AND DOSE**
PREMARIN® TABLETS

Menopausal symptoms
▶ BY MOUTH
▸ Adult: 0.3–1.25 mg daily continuously; with cyclical progestogen for 12–14 days of each cycle in women with a uterus

Postmenopausal osteoporosis prophylaxis
▶ BY MOUTH
▸ Adult: 0.625–1.25 mg daily continuously; with cyclical progestogen for 12–14 days of each cycle in women with a uterus

---

IMPORTANT SAFETY INFORMATION
MHRA/CHM ADVICE: HORMONE REPLACEMENT THERAPY (HRT): FURTHER INFORMATION ON THE KNOWN INCREASED RISK OF BREAST CANCER WITH HRT AND ITS PERSISTENCE AFTER STOPPING (SEPTEMBER 2019)
Data from a meta-analysis of more than 100 000 women with breast cancer have confirmed that the risk of breast cancer is increased with the use of all forms of systemic HRT, except vaginal oestrogens, for longer than 1 year. Findings have shown that the risk increases further with longer duration of use, is higher for combined oestrogen-progestogen HRT than with oestrogen-only HRT, and persists for more than 10 years after stopping HRT. Healthcare professionals are advised to only prescribe HRT for the relief of postmenopausal symptoms that adversely affect quality of life, and to regularly review patients to ensure that it is used for the shortest time and at the lowest dose. Patients currently and previously on HRT should be informed of the risk and to be vigilant for signs of breast cancer; they should also be encouraged to attend breast screening appointments.

● CONTRA-INDICATIONS Active arterial thromboembolic disease (e.g. angina or myocardial infarction) · history of breast cancer · history of venous thromboembolism · liver disease (where liver function tests have failed to return to normal) · oestrogen-dependent cancer · recent arterial thromboembolic disease (e.g. angina or myocardial infarction) · thrombophilic disorder · undiagnosed vaginal bleeding · untreated endometrial hyperplasia

● CAUTIONS Acute porphyrias p. 1107 · diabetes (increased risk of heart disease) · factors predisposing to thromboembolism · history of breast nodules (closely monitor breast status—risk of breast cancer) · history of endometrial hyperplasia · history of fibrocystic disease (closely monitor breast status—risk of breast cancer) · hypophyseal tumours · increased risk of gall-bladder disease reported · migraine · migraine-like headaches · presence of antiphospholipid antibodies (increased risk of thrombotic events) · risk factors for oestrogen-dependent tumours (e.g. breast cancer in first-degree relative) · risk of breast cancer · symptoms of endometriosis may be exacerbated · uterine fibroids may increase in size

CAUTIONS, FURTHER INFORMATION
▸ Risk of breast cancer HRT use is associated with an increased risk of breast cancer—see *Important safety information.*

Radiological detection of breast cancer can be made more difficult as mammographic density can increase with HRT use.

▸ **Risk of endometrial cancer** The increased risk of endometrial cancer depends on the dose and duration of oestrogen-only HRT.

In women with a uterus, the addition of a progestogen cyclically (for at least 10 days per 28-day cycle) reduces the additional risk of endometrial cancer; this additional risk is eliminated if a progestogen is given continuously. However, this should be weighed against the increased risk of breast cancer.

▸ **Risk of ovarian cancer** Long-term use of combined HRT or oestrogen-only HRT is associated with a small increased risk of ovarian cancer. This excess risk disappears within a few years of stopping.

▸ **Risk of venous thromboembolism** Women using combined or oestrogen-only HRT are at an increased risk of deep vein thrombosis and of pulmonary embolism especially in the first year of use.

In *women who have predisposing factors* (such as a personal or family history of deep vein thrombosis or pulmonary embolism, severe varicose veins, obesity, trauma, or prolonged bed-rest) it is prudent to review the need for HRT, as in some cases the risks of HRT may exceed the benefits.

Travel involving prolonged immobility further increases the risk of deep vein thrombosis.

▸ **Risk of stroke** Risk of stroke increases with age, therefore older women have a greater absolute risk of stroke. Combined HRT or oestrogen-only HRT increases the risk of stroke.

▸ **Risk of coronary heart disease** HRT does not prevent coronary heart disease and should not be prescribed for this purpose. There is an increased risk of coronary heart disease in women who start combined HRT more than 10 years after menopause. Although very little information is available on the risk of coronary heart disease in younger women who start HRT close to the menopause, studies suggest a lower relative risk compared with older women.

● **INTERACTIONS** → Appendix 1: hormone replacement therapy

● **SIDE-EFFECTS**

▸ **Common or very common** Alopecia · arthralgia · breast abnormalities · depression · leg cramps · menstrual cycle irregularities · vaginal discharge · weight changes

▸ **Uncommon** Anxiety · cervical abnormalities · contact lens intolerance · dizziness · embolism and thrombosis · gallbladder disorder · gastrointestinal discomfort · headaches · hirsutism · libido disorder · mood altered · nausea · oedema · skin reactions · vulvovaginal candidiasis

▸ **Rare or very rare** Angioedema · asthma exacerbated · cerebrovascular insufficiency · chorea exacerbated · colitis ischaemic · epilepsy exacerbated · galactorrhoea · glucose tolerance impaired · hypocalcaemia · jaundice cholestatic · myocardial infarction · neoplasms · pancreatitis · pelvic pain · vomiting

▸ **Frequency not known** Endometrial hyperplasia · erythema nodosum

SIDE-EFFECTS, FURTHER INFORMATION Cyclical HRT (where a progestogen is taken for 12–14 days of each 28-day oestrogen treatment cycle) usually results in regular withdrawal bleeding towards the end of the progestogen. Continuous combined HRT commonly produces irregular breakthrough bleeding in the first 4–6 months of treatment. Bleeding beyond 6 months or after a spell of amenorrhoea requires further investigation to exclude serious gynaecological pathology.

● **CONCEPTION AND CONTRACEPTION** HRT does **not** provide contraception and a woman is considered potentially fertile for 2 years after her last menstrual period if she is under 50 years, and for 1 year if she is over 50 years. A woman who is under 50 years and free of all risk factors for venous and arterial disease can use a low-oestrogen combined oral contraceptive pill to provide both relief of menopausal symptoms and contraception; it is recommended that the oral contraceptive be stopped at 50 years of age since there are more suitable alternatives. If any potentially fertile woman needs HRT, non-hormonal contraceptive measures (such as condoms) are necessary. Measurement of follicle-stimulating hormone can help to determine fertility, but high measurements alone (particularly in women aged under 50 years) do not necessarily preclude the possibility of becoming pregnant.

● **PREGNANCY** Manufacturer advises avoid—not indicated during pregnancy.

● **BREAST FEEDING** Avoid until weaning or for 6 months after birth (adverse effects on lactation).

● **HEPATIC IMPAIRMENT** Manufacturer advises caution; avoid in acute or active disease.

● **PATIENT AND CARER ADVICE**
Information sheet The MHRA has provided a patient information sheet to aid healthcare professionals when counselling women on the risk of breast cancer with HRT use.

● **MEDICINAL FORMS** There can be variation in the licensing of different medicines containing the same drug.
Tablet
▸ Premarin (Pfizer Ltd)
Conjugated oestrogens **300 microgram** Premarin 0.3mg tablets | 84 tablet [PoM] £6.07 DT = £6.07
Conjugated oestrogens **625 microgram** Premarin 0.625mg tablets | 84 tablet [PoM] £4.02 DT = £4.02
Conjugated oestrogens **1.25 mg** Premarin 1.25mg tablets | 84 tablet [PoM] £3.58 DT = £3.58

Combinations available: *Conjugated oestrogens with medroxyprogesterone,* p. 803

Estradiol

14-Dec-2020

● **INDICATIONS AND DOSE**

BEDOL ®

Menopausal symptoms | Osteoporosis prophylaxis
▸ BY MOUTH
▸ **Adult:** 2 mg daily, started on day 1–5 of menstruation (or at any time if cycles have ceased or are infrequent), to be taken with cyclical progestogen for 12–14 days of each cycle in women with a uterus

ELLESTE SOLO ® MX

Menopausal symptoms
▸ BY TRANSDERMAL APPLICATION
▸ **Adult:** Apply 1 patch twice weekly continuously, started within 5 days of onset of menstruation (or at any time if cycles have ceased or are infrequent), to be used with cyclical progestogen for 12–14 days of each cycle in women with a uterus, initiate therapy with *MX* 40, subsequently adjust according to response

Osteoporosis prophylaxis
▸ BY TRANSDERMAL APPLICATION
▸ **Adult:** Apply 1 patch twice weekly continuously, started within 5 days of onset of menstruation (or at any time if cycles have ceased or are infrequent), to be used with cyclical progestogen for 12–14 days of each cycle in women with a uterus, initiate therapy with *MX* 80, subsequently adjust according to response

ELLESTE-SOLO ® 1-MG

Menopausal symptoms
▸ BY MOUTH
▸ **Adult:** 1 mg daily, starting on day 1 of menstruation (or at any time if cycles have ceased or are infrequent), to be taken with cyclical progestogen for 12–14 days of each cycle in women with a uterus

ELLESTE-SOLO ® 2-MG

Menopausal symptoms not controlled with lower strength | Osteoporosis prophylaxis

▸ BY MOUTH

▸ **Adult:** 2 mg daily, started on day 1 of menstruation (or at any time if cycles have ceased or are infrequent), to be given with cyclical progestogen for 12–14 days of each cycle in women with a uterus

ESTRADERM MX ®

Menopausal symptoms

▸ BY TRANSDERMAL APPLICATION

▸ **Adult:** Apply 1 patch twice weekly continuously, started within 5 days of onset of menstruation (or at any time if cycles have ceased or are infrequent), to be used with cyclical progestogen for at least 12 days of each cycle in women with a uterus, initiate therapy with *MX25* for first 3 months; subsequently adjust according to response

Osteoporosis prophylaxis

▸ BY TRANSDERMAL APPLICATION

▸ **Adult:** Apply 1 patch twice weekly continuously, started within 5 days of onset of menstruation (or at any time if cycles have ceased or are infrequent), to be used with cyclical progestogen for at least 12 days of each cycle in women with a uterus, initiate therapy with *MX50*; subsequently adjust according to response

ESTRADOT ®

Menopausal symptoms

▸ BY TRANSDERMAL APPLICATION

▸ **Adult:** Apply 1 patch twice weekly continuously, to be used with cyclical progestogen for 12–14 days of each cycle in women with a uterus, initiate therapy with 25 *patch* for 3 months; subsequently adjust according to response

Osteoporosis prophylaxis

▸ BY TRANSDERMAL APPLICATION

▸ **Adult:** Apply 1 patch twice weekly continuously, to be used with cyclical progestogen for 12–14 days of each cycle in women with a uterus, initiate therapy with 50 *patch*; subsequently adjust according to response

EVOREL ®

Menopausal symptoms | Osteoporosis prophylaxis

▸ BY TRANSDERMAL APPLICATION

▸ **Adult:** Apply 1 patch twice weekly continuously, started within 5 days of onset of menstruation (or at any time if cycles have ceased or are infrequent), to be used with cyclical progestogen for 12–14 days of each cycle in women with a uterus, therapy should be initiated with *Evorel* 50 patch; subsequently adjust according to response; dose may be reduced to *Evorel* 25 patch after first month if necessary for menopausal symptoms **only**

FEMSEVEN ®

Menopausal symptoms | Osteoporosis prophylaxis

▸ BY TRANSDERMAL APPLICATION

▸ **Adult:** Apply 1 patch once weekly continuously, to be used with cyclical progestogen for 12–14 days of each cycle in women with a uterus, initiate therapy with *FemSeven* 50 patches for the first few months, subsequently adjust according to response

LENZETTO ®

Menopausal symptoms

▸ BY TRANSDERMAL APPLICATION

▸ **Adult:** Initially 1 spray daily, applied to the dry and healthy skin of the forearm, or alternatively the inner thigh, to be used with cyclical progestogen for 12–14 days of each cycle in women with a uterus, dose increase should be made only after at least 4 weeks of continuous treatmentIncreased if necessary to 2 sprays daily (max. per dose 3 sprays daily)

OESTROGEL ®

Menopausal symptoms

▸ TO THE SKIN

▸ **Adult:** Apply 1.5 mg once daily continuously, increased if necessary up to 3 mg after 1 month continuously, to be applied over a large area, to be used with cyclical progestogen for at least 12 days of each cycle in women with a uterus. If switching from cyclical HRT, start at end of regimen; otherwise start at any time

Osteoporosis prophylaxis

▸ TO THE SKIN

▸ **Adult:** Apply 1.5 mg once daily continuously, to be applied over a large area, to be used with cyclical progestogen for at least 12 days of each cycle in women with a uterus. If switching from cyclical HRT, start at end of regimen; otherwise start at any time

DOSE EQUIVALENCE AND CONVERSION

▸ For *Oestrogel* ®: 2 measures is equivalent to estradiol 1.5 mg.

PROGYNOVA ®

Menopausal symptoms

▸ BY MOUTH

▸ **Adult:** 1–2 mg daily continuously, to be started on day 1 of menstruation (or at any time if cycles have ceased or are infrequent), to be taken with cyclical progestogen for 12–14 days of each cycle in women with a uterus

Osteoporosis prophylaxis

▸ BY MOUTH

▸ **Adult:** 2 mg daily continuously, to be taken with cyclical progestogen for 12–14 days of each cycle in women with a uterus

PROGYNOVA ® TS

Menopausal symptoms | Osteoporosis prophylaxis

▸ BY TRANSDERMAL APPLICATION

▸ **Adult:** Apply 1 patch once weekly continuously, alternatively apply 1 patch once weekly for 3 weeks, followed by a 7-day patch-free interval (cyclical), to be used with cyclical progestogen for 12–14 days of each cycle in women with a uterus, initiate therapy with *Progynova TS* 50, subsequently adjust according to response, women receiving *Progynova TS* 100 patches for menopausal symptoms may continue with this strength for osteoporosis prophylaxis

SANDRENA ®

Menopausal symptoms

▸ TO THE SKIN

▸ **Adult:** Apply 1 mg once daily, to be applied over area 1–2 times size of hand; with cyclical progestogen for 12–14 days of each cycle in women with a uterus, dose may be adjusted after 2–3 cycles to lowest effective dose; usual dose 0.5–1.5 mg daily

ZUMENON ®

Menopausal symptoms

▸ BY MOUTH

▸ **Adult:** Initially 1 mg daily, to be started on day 1 of menstruation (or any time if cycles have ceased or are infrequent), increased if necessary to 2 mg daily, to be taken with a cyclical progestogen for 12–14 days of each cycle in women with a uterus continued →

Osteoporosis prophylaxis

► BY MOUTH

► Adult: 2 mg daily, to be taken with a cyclical progestogen for 12–14 days of each cycle in women with a uterus

---

IMPORTANT SAFETY INFORMATION

MHRA/CHM ADVICE: HORMONE REPLACEMENT THERAPY (HRT): FURTHER INFORMATION ON THE KNOWN INCREASED RISK OF BREAST CANCER WITH HRT AND ITS PERSISTENCE AFTER STOPPING (SEPTEMBER 2019)

► With oral use or topical use or transdermal use

Data from a meta-analysis of more than 100 000 women with breast cancer have confirmed that the risk of breast cancer is increased with the use of all forms of systemic HRT, except vaginal oestrogens, for longer than 1 year. Findings have shown that the risk increases further with longer duration of use, is higher for combined oestrogen-progestogen HRT than with oestrogen-only HRT, and persists for more than 10 years after stopping HRT. Healthcare professionals are advised to only prescribe HRT for the relief of postmenopausal symptoms that adversely affect quality of life, and to regularly review patients to ensure that it is used for the shortest time and at the lowest dose. Patients currently and previously on HRT should be informed of the risk and to be vigilant for signs of breast cancer; they should also be encouraged to attend breast screening appointments.

● CONTRA-INDICATIONS Active arterial thromboembolic disease (e.g. angina or myocardial infarction) · history of breast cancer · history of venous thromboembolism · oestrogen-dependent cancer · recent arterial thromboembolic disease (e.g. angina or myocardial infarction) · thrombophilic disorder · undiagnosed vaginal bleeding · untreated endometrial hyperplasia

● CAUTIONS Acute porphyrias p. 1107 · diabetes (increased risk of heart disease) · factors predisposing to thromboembolism · history of breast nodules—closely monitor breast status (risk of breast cancer) · history of endometrial hyperplasia · history of fibrocystic disease— closely monitor breast status (risk of breast cancer) · hypophyseal tumours · increased risk of gall-bladder disease · migraine (or migraine-like headaches) · presence of antiphospholipid antibodies (increased risk of thrombotic events) · prolonged exposure to unopposed oestrogens may increase risk of developing endometrial cancer · risk factors for oestrogen-dependent tumours (e.g. breast cancer in first-degree relative) · symptoms of endometriosis may be exacerbated · uterine fibroids may increase in size

CAUTIONS, FURTHER INFORMATION

► Risk of endometrial cancer The increased risk of endometrial cancer depends on the dose and duration of oestrogen-only HRT.

In women with a uterus using *systemic* preparations, the addition of a progestogen cyclically (for at least 10 days per 28-day cycle) reduces the additional risk of endometrial cancer; this additional risk is eliminated if a progestogen is given continuously. However, this should be weighed against the increased risk of breast cancer.

► Risk of ovarian cancer Long-term use of combined HRT or oestrogen-only HRT is associated with a small increased risk of ovarian cancer. This excess risk disappears within a few years of stopping.

► Risk of venous thromboembolism Women using combined or oestrogen-only HRT are at an increased risk of deep vein thrombosis and of pulmonary embolism especially in the first year of use.

In *women who have predisposing factors* (such as a personal or family history of deep vein thrombosis or pulmonary embolism, severe varicose veins, obesity, trauma, or prolonged bed-rest) it is prudent to review the need for HRT, as in some cases the risks of HRT may exceed the benefits.

Travel involving prolonged immobility further increases the risk of deep vein thrombosis.

► Risk of stroke Risk of stroke increases with age, therefore older women have a greater absolute risk of stroke. Combined HRT or oestrogen-only HRT increases the risk of stroke.

► Risk of coronary heart disease HRT does not prevent coronary heart disease and should not be prescribed for this purpose. There is an increased risk of coronary heart disease in women who start combined HRT more than 10 years after menopause. Although very little information is available on the risk of coronary heart disease in younger women who start HRT close to the menopause, studies suggest a lower relative risk compared with older women.

► Risk of breast cancer with systemic use HRT use is associated with an increased risk of breast cancer—see *Important safety information*. Radiological detection of breast cancer can be made more difficult as mammographic density can increase with HRT use.

● INTERACTIONS → Appendix 1: hormone replacement therapy

● SIDE-EFFECTS

GENERAL SIDE-EFFECTS

► **Common or very common** Headaches · nausea · skin reactions

► **Uncommon** Hypertension

SPECIFIC SIDE-EFFECTS

► **Common or very common**

► With oral use Asthenia · gastrointestinal discomfort · gastrointestinal disorders · haemorrhage · menstrual cycle irregularities · muscle complaints · pelvic pain · weight changes

► With transdermal use Abdominal pain · breast abnormalities · menstrual cycle irregularities · uterine disorders · vaginal discharge · weight changes

► **Uncommon**

► With oral use Anxiety · back pain · breast abnormalities · cervical abnormalities · cystitis-like symptom · depression · dizziness · embolism and thrombosis · erythema nodosum · gallbladder disorder · oedema · palpitations · peripheral vascular disease · tumour growth · visual impairment · vulvovaginal candidiasis

► With transdermal use Asthenia · breast neoplasm benign · depression · flatulence · increased risk of infection · leiomyoma · mood swings · venous thromboembolism · vertigo · vomiting

► **Rare or very rare**

► With oral use Angioedema · cerebrovascular insufficiency · chorea · contact lens intolerance · haemolytic anaemia · hepatic disorders · hirsutism · malaise · myocardial infarction · sexual dysfunction · steepening of corneal curvature · vaginal discharge · vomiting

► With transdermal use Epilepsy exacerbated · galactorrhoea · glucose tolerance impaired · libido disorder

► **Frequency not known**

► With oral use Carbohydrate metabolism change · epilepsy exacerbated · hypertriglyceridaemia · increased risk of coronary artery disease · neoplasms · pancreatitis · systemic lupus erythematosus (SLE)

SIDE-EFFECTS, FURTHER INFORMATION Cyclical HRT (where a progestogen is taken for 12–14 days of each 28-day oestrogen treatment cycle) usually results in regular withdrawal bleeding towards the end of the progestogen. Continuous combined HRT commonly produces irregular breakthrough bleeding in the first 4–6 months of treatment. Bleeding beyond 6 months or after a spell of amenorrhoea requires further investigation to exclude serious gynaecological pathology.

- CONCEPTION AND CONTRACEPTION HRT does **not** provide contraception and a woman is considered potentially fertile for 2 years after her last menstrual period if she is under 50 years, and for 1 year if she is over 50 years. A woman who is under 50 years and free of all risk factors for venous and arterial disease can use a low-oestrogen combined oral contraceptive pill to provide both relief of menopausal symptoms and contraception; it is recommended that the oral contraceptive be stopped at 50 years of age since there are more suitable alternatives. If any potentially fertile woman needs HRT, non-hormonal contraceptive measures (such as condoms) are necessary. Measurement of follicle-stimulating hormone can help to determine fertility, but high measurements alone (particularly in women aged under 50 years) do not necessarily preclude the possibility of becoming pregnant.
- PREGNANCY Not known to be harmful.
- BREAST FEEDING Avoid; adverse effects on lactation.
- HEPATIC IMPAIRMENT Manufacturer advises caution; avoid in acute or active disease.
- MONITORING REQUIREMENTS
- History of breast nodules or fibrocystic disease—closely monitor breast status (risk of breast cancer).
- The endometrial safety of long-term or repeated use of topical vaginal oestrogens is uncertain; treatment should be reviewed at least annually, with special consideration given to any symptoms of endometrial hyperplasia or carcinoma.
- DIRECTIONS FOR ADMINISTRATION
- With transdermal use Manufacturer advises patch should be removed after 3–4 days (or once a week in case of 7-day patch) and replaced with fresh patch on slightly different site; recommended sites: clean, dry, unbroken areas of skin on trunk below waistline; not to be applied on or near breasts or under waistband. If patch falls off in bath allow skin to cool before applying new patch.
- PATIENT AND CARER ADVICE
- With transdermal use Patient counselling is advised for estradiol patches and spray (administration).
- With topical use Patient counselling is advised for estradiol gels (administration).
Information sheet
- With oral use or topical use or transdermal use The MHRA has provided a patient information sheet to aid healthcare professionals when counselling women on the risk of breast cancer with HRT use.

LENZETTO ® ► With transdermal use Apply to dry, healthy skin of the inner forearm or alternatively the inner thigh and allow to dry for 2 minutes before covering with clothing. Avoid skin contact with another person (particularly children) or pets and avoid washing the area for at least 1 hour after application. If a sunscreen is needed, apply at least 1 hour before Lenzetto ®.

OESTROGEL ® ► With topical use Apply gel to clean, dry, intact skin such as arms, shoulders or inner thighs and allow to dry for 5 minutes before covering with clothing. Not to be applied on or near breasts or on vulval region. Avoid skin contact with another person (particularly male) and avoid other skin products or washing the area for at least 1 hour after application.

SANDRENA ® ► With topical use Apply gel to intact areas of skin such as lower trunk or thighs, using right and left sides on alternate days. Wash hands after application. Not to be applied on the breasts or face and avoid contact with eyes. Allow area of application to dry for 5 minutes and do not wash area for at least 1 hour.

- MEDICINAL FORMS There can be variation in the licensing of different medicines containing the same drug.

Tablet
► Bedol (ReSource Medical UK Ltd)
Estradiol 2 mg Bedol 2mg tablets | 84 tablet [PoM] £5.07 DT = £5.06
► Elleste Solo (Mylan)
Estradiol 1 mg Elleste Solo 1mg tablets | 84 tablet [PoM] £5.06 DT = £5.06
Estradiol 2 mg Elleste Solo 2mg tablets | 84 tablet [PoM] £5.06 DT = £5.06
► Progynova (Bayer Plc)
Estradiol valerate 1 mg Progynova 1mg tablets | 84 tablet [PoM] £7.30 DT = £7.30
Estradiol valerate 2 mg Progynova 2mg tablets | 84 tablet [PoM] £7.30 DT = £7.30
► Zumenon (Mylan)
Estradiol 1 mg Zumenon 1mg tablets | 84 tablet [PoM] £6.89 DT = £5.06
Estradiol 2 mg Zumenon 2mg tablets | 84 tablet [PoM] £6.89 DT = £5.06

Spray
CAUTIONARY AND ADVISORY LABELS 15
EXCIPIENTS: May contain Ethanol
► Lenzetto (Gedeon Richter (UK) Ltd)
Estradiol (as Estradiol hemihydrate) 1.53 mg Lenzetto 1.53mg/dose transdermal spray | 56 dose [PoM] £6.90 | 168 dose [PoM] £20.70

Transdermal patch
► Elleste Solo MX (Mylan)
Estradiol 40 microgram per 24 hour Elleste Solo MX 40 transdermal patches | 8 patch [PoM] £5.19 DT = £5.19
Estradiol 80 microgram per 24 hour Elleste Solo MX 80 transdermal patches | 8 patch [PoM] £5.99 DT = £5.99
► Estraderm MX (Norgine Pharmaceuticals Ltd)
Estradiol 25 microgram per 24 hour Estraderm MX 25 patches | 8 patch [PoM] £5.50 DT = £3.42 | 24 patch [PoM] £16.46 DT = £16.46
Estradiol 50 microgram per 24 hour Estraderm MX 50 patches | 8 patch [PoM] £5.51 DT = £3.88 | 24 patch [PoM] £16.46 DT = £11.66
Estradiol 75 microgram per 24 hour Estraderm MX 75 patches | 8 patch [PoM] £6.42 DT = £4.12 | 24 patch [PoM] £19.27
Estradiol 100 microgram per 24 hour Estraderm MX 100 patches | 8 patch [PoM] £6.66 DT = £4.28 | 24 patch [PoM] £19.99 DT = £19.99
► Estradot (Novartis Pharmaceuticals UK Ltd)
Estradiol 25 microgram per 24 hour Estradot 25micrograms/24hours patches | 8 patch [PoM] £5.99 DT = £3.42
Estradiol 37.5 microgram per 24 hour Estradot 37.5micrograms/24hours patches | 8 patch [PoM] £6.00 DT = £6.00
Estradiol 50 microgram per 24 hour Estradot 50micrograms/24hours patches | 8 patch [PoM] £6.02 DT = £3.88
Estradiol 75 microgram per 24 hour Estradot 75micrograms/24hours patches | 8 patch [PoM] £7.00 DT = £4.12
Estradiol 100 microgram per 24 hour Estradot 100micrograms/24hours patches | 8 patch [PoM] £7.27 DT = £4.28
► Evorel (Theramex HQ UK Ltd)
Estradiol 25 microgram per 24 hour Evorel 25 patches | 8 patch [PoM] £3.42 DT = £3.42
Estradiol 50 microgram per 24 hour Evorel 50 patches | 4 patch [PoM] £3.88 DT = £3.88 | 8 patch [PoM] £3.88 DT = £3.88 | 24 patch [PoM] £11.66 DT = £11.66
Estradiol 75 microgram per 24 hour Evorel 75 patches | 8 patch [PoM] £4.12 DT = £4.12
Estradiol 100 microgram per 24 hour Evorel 100 patches | 8 patch [PoM] £4.28 DT = £4.28
► FemSeven (Theramex HQ UK Ltd)
Estradiol 50 microgram per 24 hour FemSeven 50 patches | 4 patch [PoM] £6.04 DT = £6.04 | 12 patch [PoM] £18.02 DT = £18.02
Estradiol 75 microgram per 24 hour FemSeven 75 patches | 4 patch [PoM] £6.98
Estradiol 100 microgram per 24 hour FemSeven 100 patches | 4 patch [PoM] £7.28 DT = £7.28
► Progynova TS (Bayer Plc)
Estradiol 50 microgram per 24 hour Progynova TS 50micrograms/24hours transdermal patches | 12 patch [PoM] £18.90 DT = £18.02
Estradiol 100 microgram per 24 hour Progynova TS 100micrograms/24hours transdermal patches | 12 patch [PoM] £20.70 DT = £20.70

Endocrine system

6

Gel

EXCIPIENTS: May contain Propylene glycol

▸ Oestrogel (Besins Healthcare (UK) Ltd)

Estradiol 600 microgram per 1 gram Oestrogel Pump-Pack 0.06% gel | 80 gram [PoM] £4.80 DT = £4.80

▸ Sandrena (Orion Pharma (UK) Ltd)

Estradiol (as Estradiol hemihydrate) 500 microgram Sandrena 500microgram gel sachets | 28 sachet [PoM] £5.08 DT = £5.08

Estradiol (as Estradiol hemihydrate) 1 mg Sandrena 1mg gel sachets | 28 sachet [PoM] £5.85 DT = £5.85 | 91 sachet [PoM] £17.57

Combinations available: *Estradiol with dydrogesterone*, p. 803 · *Estradiol with levonorgestrel*, p. 804 · *Estradiol with medroxyprogesterone*, p. 804 · *Estradiol with norethisterone*, p. 804

Ethinylestradiol

22-May-2020

(Ethinyloestradiol)

● **INDICATIONS AND DOSE**

Short-term treatment of symptoms of oestrogen deficiency | Osteoporosis prophylaxis if other drugs cannot be used

▸ BY MOUTH

▸ Adult (female): 10–50 micrograms daily for 21 days, repeated after 7-day tablet-free period, to be given with progestogen for 12–14 days per cycle in women with intact uterus.

Female hypogonadism

▸ BY MOUTH

▸ Adult (female): 10–50 micrograms daily usually on cyclical basis, initial oestrogen therapy should be followed by combined oestrogen and progestogen therapy.

Menstrual disorders

▸ BY MOUTH

▸ Adult (female): 20–50 micrograms daily from day 5 to 25 of each cycle, to be given with progestogen, added either throughout the cycle or from day 15 to 25.

Palliative treatment of prostate cancer

▸ BY MOUTH

▸ Adult (male): 0.15–1.5 mg daily.

● CONTRA-INDICATIONS Active or recent arterial thromboembolic disease (e.g. angina or myocardial infarction) · Acute porphyrias p. 1107 · history of breast cancer · history of venous thromboembolism · liver disease (where liver function tests have failed to return to normal) · oestrogen-dependent cancer · thrombophilic disorder · undiagnosed vaginal bleeding · untreated endometrial hyperplasia

CONTRA-INDICATIONS, FURTHER INFORMATION

▸ Combined hormonal contraception For more information on contra-indications for ethinylestradiol in *contraception* see combined hormonal contraceptive preparations containing ethinylestradiol.

▸ Hormone replacement therapy For more information on contra-indications for hormone replacement therapy see Sex hormones p. 790

● CAUTIONS Cardiovascular disease (risk of fluid retention) · diabetes (increased risk of heart disease) · history of breast nodules or fibrocystic disease—closely monitor breast status (risk of breast cancer) · history of endometrial hyperplasia · history of hypertriglyceridaemia (increased risk of pancreatitis) · hypophyseal tumours · increased risk of gall-bladder disease · migraine (migraine-like headaches) · presence of antiphospholipid antibodies (increased risk of thrombotic events) · prolonged exposure to unopposed oestrogens may increase risk of developing endometrial cancer · risk factors for oestrogen-dependent tumours (e.g. breast cancer in first-degree relative) · risk

factors for venous thromboembolism · symptoms of endometriosis may be exacerbated · uterine fibroids may increase in size

CAUTIONS, FURTHER INFORMATION

▸ Combined hormonal contraception For more information on cautions for ethinylestradiol in *contraception* see combined hormonal contraceptive preparations containing ethinylestradiol.

▸ Hormone replacement therapy For more information on cautions for hormone replacement therapy see Sex hormones p. 790

● INTERACTIONS → Appendix 1: hormone replacement therapy

● SIDE-EFFECTS Breast abnormalities · cervical mucus increased · cholelithiasis · contact lens intolerance · depression · electrolyte imbalance · embolism and thrombosis · erythema nodosum · feminisation · fluid retention · headaches · hypertension · jaundice cholestatic · metrorrhagia · mood altered · myocardial infarction · nausea · neoplasms · skin reactions · stroke · uterine disorders · vomiting · weight change

SIDE-EFFECTS, FURTHER INFORMATION Cyclical HRT (where a progestogen is taken for 12–14 days of each 28-day oestrogen treatment cycle) usually results in regular withdrawal bleeding towards the end of the progestogen. Continuous combined HRT commonly produces irregular breakthrough bleeding in the first 4–6 months of treatment. Bleeding beyond 6 months or after a spell of amenorrhoea requires further investigation to exclude serious gynaecological pathology.

● PREGNANCY Not known to be harmful.

● BREAST FEEDING Avoid until weaning or for 6 months after birth (adverse effects on lactation).

● HEPATIC IMPAIRMENT Manufacturer advises caution; avoid in acute or active disease.

● MEDICINAL FORMS There can be variation in the licensing of different medicines containing the same drug. Forms available from special-order manufacturers include: tablet, capsule, oral suspension

Tablet

▸ Ethinylestradiol (Non-proprietary)

Ethinylestradiol 1 mg Ethinylestradiol 1mg tablets | 28 tablet [PoM] £200.00 DT = £200.00

Tibolone

26-Jun-2020

● **INDICATIONS AND DOSE**

Short-term treatment of symptoms of oestrogen deficiency (including women being treated with gonadotrophin releasing hormone analogues) | Osteoporosis prophylaxis in women at high risk of fractures when other prophylaxis contra-indicated or not tolerated

▸ BY MOUTH

▸ Adult: 2.5 mg daily

● CONTRA-INDICATIONS Acute porphyrias p. 1107 · history of arterial thromboembolic disease (e.g. angina, myocardial infarction, stroke or TIA) · history of breast cancer · history of venous thromboembolism · liver disease (where liver function tests have failed to return to normal) · oestrogen-dependent cancer · thrombophilic disorder · uninvestigated or undiagnosed vaginal bleeding · untreated endometrial hyperplasia

● CAUTIONS Diabetes (increased risk of heart disease) · epilepsy · factors predisposing to thromboembolism · history of breast nodules—closely monitor breast status (risk of breast cancer) · history of endometrial hyperplasia · history of fibrocystic disease—closely monitor breast status (risk of breast cancer) · hypertriglyceridaemia ·

hypophyseal tumours · migraine (or migraine-like headaches) · presence of antiphospholipid antibodies (increased risk of thrombotic events) · prolonged exposure to unopposed oestrogens may increase risk of developing endometrial cancer · risk factors for oestrogen-dependent tumours (e.g. breast cancer in first-degree relative) · risk of stroke

● INTERACTIONS → Appendix 1: tibolone

● SIDE-EFFECTS

▶ **Common or very common** Breast abnormalities · cervical dysplasia · endometrial thickening · gastrointestinal discomfort · genital abnormalities · hair growth abnormal · increased risk of infection · pelvic pain · postmenopausal haemorrhage · vaginal discharge · vaginal haemorrhage · weight increased

▶ **Uncommon** Oedema · skin reactions

▶ **Frequency not known** Arthralgia · dementia · depression · dizziness · erythema nodosum · gallbladder disorder · headaches · increased risk of ischaemic stroke · myalgia · neoplasms · vision disorders

SIDE-EFFECTS, FURTHER INFORMATION **Vaginal bleeding** Investigate for endometrial cancer if bleeding continues beyond 6 months or after stopping treatment.

Reasons to withdraw treatment Withdraw treatment if signs of thromboembolic disease, abnormal liver function tests, or signs of cholestatic jaundice.

● PREGNANCY Avoid; toxicity in *animal* studies.

● BREAST FEEDING Avoid.

● HEPATIC IMPAIRMENT Manufacturer advises caution; avoid in acute disease.

● RENAL IMPAIRMENT

Monitoring Patients with renal impairment should be closely monitored (risk of fluid retention).

● PRESCRIBING AND DISPENSING INFORMATION Unsuitable for use in the premenopause (unless being treated with gonadotrophin-releasing hormone analogue) and as (or with) an oral contraceptive.

Also unsuitable for use within 12 months of last menstrual period (may cause irregular bleeding).

If transferring from cyclical HRT, start at end of regimen; if transferring from continuous-combined HRT, start at any time.

● MEDICINAL FORMS There can be variation in the licensing of different medicines containing the same drug.

Tablet

▶ Tibolone (Non-proprietary)

Tibolone 2.5 mg Tibolone 2.5mg tablets | 28 tablet [PoM] £10.36 DT = £7.28 | 84 tablet [PoM] £21.84-£31.08

▶ Livial (Merck Sharp & Dohme Ltd)

Tibolone 2.5 mg Livial 2.5mg tablets | 28 tablet [PoM] £10.36 DT = £7.28 | 84 tablet [PoM] £31.08

OESTROGENS COMBINED WITH PROGESTOGENS

Conjugated oestrogens with medroxyprogesterone

The properties listed below are those particular to the combination only. For the properties of the components please consider, conjugated oestrogens (equine) p. 797, medroxyprogesterone acetate p. 856.

● INDICATIONS AND DOSE

PREMIQUE ® LOW DOSE TABLETS

Menopausal symptoms in women with a uterus

▶ BY MOUTH

▶ Adult: 1 tablet daily continuously

● INTERACTIONS → Appendix 1: hormone replacement therapy · medroxyprogesterone

● MEDICINAL FORMS There can be variation in the licensing of different medicines containing the same drug.

Modified-release tablet

▶ Premique (Pfizer Ltd)

Conjugated oestrogens 300 microgram, Medroxyprogesterone acetate 1.5 mg Premique Low Dose 0.3mg/1.5mg modified-release tablets | 84 tablet [PoM] £6.52 DT = £6.52

Estradiol with dydrogesterone   21-May-2020

The properties listed below are those particular to the combination only. For the properties of the components please consider, estradiol p. 798.

● INDICATIONS AND DOSE

FEMOSTON ® 1 MG/10 MG

Menopausal symptoms in women with a uterus

▶ BY MOUTH

▶ Adult: 1 tablet daily for 14 days, white tablet to be taken and started within 5 days of onset of menstruation (or any time if cycles have ceased or are infrequent), then 1 tablet daily for 14 days, grey tablet to be taken, subsequent courses repeated without interval, *Femoston* ® 1 *mg*/10 *mg* given initially and *Femoston* ® 2 *mg*/10 *mg* substituted if symptoms not controlled

Osteoporosis prophylaxis in women with a uterus

▶ BY MOUTH

▶ Adult: 1 tablet daily for 14 days, white tablet to be taken and started within 5 days of onset of menstruation (or any time if cycles have ceased or are infrequent), then 1 tablet daily for 14 days, grey tablet to be taken, subsequent courses repeated without interval

FEMOSTON ® 2 MG/10 MG

Menopausal symptoms in women with a uterus

▶ BY MOUTH

▶ Adult: 1 tablet daily for 14 days, red tablet to be taken and started within 5 days of onset of menstruation (or any time if cycles have ceased or are infrequent), then 1 tablet daily for 14 days, yellow tablet to be taken, subsequent courses repeated without interval, *Femoston* ® 1 *mg*/10 *mg* given initially and *Femoston* ® 2 *mg*/10 *mg* substituted if symptoms not controlled

Osteoporosis prophylaxis in women with a uterus

▶ BY MOUTH

▶ Adult: 1 tablet daily for 14 days, red tablet to be taken and started within 5 days of onset of menstruation (or any time if cycles have ceased or are infrequent), then 1 tablet daily for 14 days, yellow tablet to be taken, subsequent courses repeated without interval

FEMOSTON ®-CONTI 0.5 MG/2.5MG

Menopausal symptoms in women with a uterus whose last menstrual period occurred over 12 months previously

▶ BY MOUTH

▶ Adult: 1 tablet daily continuously, if changing from cyclical HRT begin treatment the day after finishing oestrogen plus progestogen phase   continued →

6

Endocrine system

FEMOSTON ®-CONTI 1 MG/5MG

Menopausal symptoms in women with a uterus whose last menstrual period occurred over 12 months previously | Osteoporosis prophylaxis in women with a uterus whose last menstrual period occurred over 12 months previously
‣ BY MOUTH
‣ Adult: 1 tablet daily continuously, if changing from cyclical HRT begin treatment the day after finishing oestrogen plus progestogen phase

● INTERACTIONS → Appendix 1: hormone replacement therapy
● SIDE-EFFECTS
‣ **Common or very common** Asthenia · breast abnormalities · cervical abnormalities · depression · dizziness · flatulence · gastrointestinal discomfort · headaches · malaise · menstrual cycle irregularities · nausea · nervousness · pain · pelvic pain · peripheral oedema · postmenopausal haemorrhage · skin reactions · vomiting · vulvovaginal candidiasis · weight changes
‣ **Uncommon** Cystitis-like symptom · embolism and thrombosis · gallbladder disorder · hepatic function abnormal · hypertension · libido disorder · peripheral vascular disease · tumour growth · varicose veins
‣ **Rare or very rare** Angioedema · myocardial infarction
‣ **Frequency not known** Chorea · contact lens intolerance · dementia · epilepsy exacerbated · erythema nodosum · haemolytic anaemia · hypertriglyceridaemia · leg cramps · neoplasms · pancreatitis · steepening of corneal curvature · systemic lupus erythematosus (SLE) · urinary incontinence
● HEPATIC IMPAIRMENT Manufacturer advises caution; avoid in acute or active disease.
● RENAL IMPAIRMENT Use with caution.

● MEDICINAL FORMS There can be variation in the licensing of different medicines containing the same drug.
Tablet
‣ Femoston 1/10 (Mylan)
Femoston 1/10mg tablets | 84 tablet [PoM] £16.16
‣ Femoston 2/10 (Mylan)
Femoston 2/10mg tablets | 84 tablet [PoM] £16.16
‣ Femoston-conti (Mylan)
Estradiol 500 microgram, Dydrogesterone 2.5 mg Femoston-conti 0.5mg/2.5mg tablets | 84 tablet [PoM] £24.43 DT = £24.43
Estradiol 1 mg, Dydrogesterone 5 mg Femoston-conti 1mg/5mg tablets | 84 tablet [PoM] £24.43 DT = £24.43

Estradiol with levonorgestrel

The properties listed below are those particular to the combination only. For the properties of the components please consider, estradiol p. 798, levonorgestrel p. 852.

● INDICATIONS AND DOSE
FEMSEVEN CONTI ®
Menopausal symptoms in women with a uterus whose last menstrual period occurred over 12 months previously
‣ BY TRANSDERMAL APPLICATION
‣ Adult: Apply 1 patch once weekly continuously
FEMSEVEN SEQUI ®
Menopausal symptoms in women with a uterus
‣ BY TRANSDERMAL APPLICATION
‣ Adult: Apply 1 patch once weekly for 2 weeks, phase 1 patches to be applied, then apply 1 patch once weekly for 2 weeks, phase 2 patches to be applied, subsequent courses are repeated without interval

● INTERACTIONS → Appendix 1: hormone replacement therapy · levonorgestrel
● PATIENT AND CARER ADVICE Patient counselling is advised for estradiol with levonorgestrel patches (application).

● MEDICINAL FORMS There can be variation in the licensing of different medicines containing the same drug.
Transdermal patch
‣ FemSeven Conti (Theramex HQ UK Ltd)
Levonorgestrel 7 microgram per 24 hour, Estradiol 50 microgram per 24 hour FemSeven Conti patches | 4 patch [PoM] £15.48 DT = £15.48 | 12 patch [PoM] £44.12 DT = £44.12
‣ FemSeven Sequi (Theramex HQ UK Ltd)
FemSeven Sequi patches | 4 patch [PoM] £13.18 | 12 patch [PoM] £37.54

Estradiol with medroxyprogesterone

The properties listed below are those particular to the combination only. For the properties of the components please consider, estradiol p. 798, medroxyprogesterone acetate p. 856.

● INDICATIONS AND DOSE
INDIVINA ® TABLETS
Menopausal symptoms in women with a uterus whose last menstrual period occurred over 3 years previously | Osteoporosis prophylaxis in women with a uterus whose last menstrual period occurred over 3 years previously
‣ BY MOUTH
‣ Adult: Initially 1/2.5 mg daily taken continuously, adjust according to response, to be started at end of scheduled bleed if changing from cyclical HRT
TRIDESTRA ®
Menopausal symptoms in women with a uterus | Osteoporosis prophylaxis in women with a uterus
‣ BY MOUTH
‣ Adult: 1 tablet daily for 70 days, white tablet to be taken, then 1 tablet daily for 14 days, blue tablet to be taken, then 1 tablet daily for 7 days, yellow tablet to be taken, subsequent courses are repeated without interval

● INTERACTIONS → Appendix 1: hormone replacement therapy · medroxyprogesterone

● MEDICINAL FORMS There can be variation in the licensing of different medicines containing the same drug.
Tablet
‣ Indivina (Orion Pharma (UK) Ltd)
Estradiol valerate 1 mg, Medroxyprogesterone acetate 2.5 mg Indivina 1mg/2.5mg tablets | 84 tablet [PoM] £20.58 DT = £20.58
Estradiol valerate 2 mg, Medroxyprogesterone acetate 5 mg Indivina 2mg/5mg tablets | 84 tablet [PoM] £20.58 DT = £20.58
Estradiol valerate 1 mg, Medroxyprogesterone acetate 5 mg Indivina 1mg/5mg tablets | 84 tablet [PoM] £20.58 DT = £20.58
‣ Tridestra (Orion Pharma (UK) Ltd)
Tridestra tablets | 91 tablet [PoM] £20.49

Estradiol with norethisterone   11-Dec-2020

The properties listed below are those particular to the combination only. For the properties of the components please consider, estradiol p. 798, norethisterone p. 806.

● INDICATIONS AND DOSE
CLINORETTE ®
Menopausal symptoms in women with a uterus
‣ BY MOUTH
‣ Adult: 1 tablet daily for 16 days, white tablet to be taken, starting on day 5 of menstruation (or at any time if cycles have ceased or are infrequent), then 1 tablet daily for 12 days, pink tablet to be taken, subsequent courses repeated without interval

ELLESTE-DUET ® 1-MG

Menopausal symptoms

▸ BY MOUTH
▸ Adult: 1 tablet daily for 16 days, white tablet to be taken and started on day 1 of menstruation (or at any time if cycles have ceased or are infrequent), then 1 tablet daily for 12 days, green tablet to be taken, subsequent courses are repeated without interval

ELLESTE-DUET ® 2-MG

Menopausal symptoms | Osteoporosis prophylaxis

▸ BY MOUTH
▸ Adult: 1 tablet daily for 16 days, orange tablet to be taken, to be started on day 1 of menstruation (or at any time if cycles have ceased or are infrequent), then 1 tablet daily for 12 days, grey tablet to be taken, subsequent courses are repeated without interval

ELLESTE-DUET ® CONTI

Menopausal symptoms in women whose last menstrual period occurred over 12 months previously | Osteoporosis prophylaxis

▸ BY MOUTH
▸ Adult: 1 tablet daily continuously, to be started at end of scheduled bleed if changing from cyclical HRT

EVOREL ® CONTI

Menopausal symptoms in women whose last menstrual period occurred over 18 months previously | Osteoporosis prophylaxis

▸ BY TRANSDERMAL APPLICATION
▸ Adult: Apply 1 patch twice weekly continuously, to be started at end of scheduled bleed if changing from cyclical HRT

EVOREL ® SEQUI

Menopausal symptoms | Osteoporosis prophylaxis

▸ BY TRANSDERMAL APPLICATION
▸ Adult: Apply 1 patch twice weekly for 2 weeks, *Evorel* ® 50 patch to be applied and started within 5 days of onset of menstruation (or at any time if cycles have ceased or are infrequent), then apply 1 patch twice weekly for the following 2 weeks, *Evorel* ® Conti patch to be applied, subsequent courses are repeated without interval.

KLIOFEM ®

Menopausal symptoms in women with a uterus whose last menstrual period occurred over 12 months previously | Osteoporosis prophylaxis in women with a uterus

▸ BY MOUTH
▸ Adult: 1 tablet daily continuously, to be started at end of scheduled bleed if changing from cyclical HRT

KLIOVANCE ®

Menopausal symptoms in women with a uterus whose last menstrual period occurred over 12 months previously | Osteoporosis prophylaxis in women with a uterus

▸ BY MOUTH
▸ Adult: 1 tablet daily continuously, to be started at end of scheduled bleed if changing from cyclical HRT

NOVOFEM ®

Menopausal symptoms in women whose last menstrual period occurred over 6 months previously | Osteoporosis prophylaxis

▸ BY MOUTH
▸ Adult: 1 tablet daily for 16 days, red tablet to be taken, then 1 tablet daily for 12 days, white tablet to be taken, subsequent courses are repeated without interval; start treatment with red tablet at any time or if changing from cyclical HRT, start treatment the day after finishing previous regimen

TRISEQUENS ®

Menopausal symptoms in women whose last menstrual period occurred over 6 months previously | Osteoporosis prophylaxis

▸ BY MOUTH
▸ Adult: 1 tablet daily for 12 days, blue tablet to be taken, followed by 1 tablet daily for 10 days, white tablet to be taken, then 1 tablet daily for 6 days, red tablet to be taken, subsequent courses are repeated without interval; start treatment with blue tablet at any time or if changing from cyclical HRT, start treatment the day after finishing previous regimen

● INTERACTIONS → Appendix 1: hormone replacement therapy · norethisterone

● PATIENT AND CARER ADVICE

EVOREL ® SEQUI Patients and carers should be advised on the application of *Evorel*® Sequi patches.

● MEDICINAL FORMS There can be variation in the licensing of different medicines containing the same drug.

Tablet

▸ Clinorette (ReSource Medical UK Ltd)
  Clinorette tablets | 84 tablet `PoM` £9.23
▸ Elleste Duet (Mylan)
  Elleste Duet 1mg tablets | 84 tablet `PoM` £9.20
  Elleste Duet 2mg tablets | 84 tablet `PoM` £9.20
  Norethisterone acetate 1 mg, Estradiol 2 mg Elleste Duet Conti tablets | 84 tablet `PoM` £17.02 DT = £17.02
▸ Kliofem (Novo Nordisk Ltd)
  Norethisterone acetate 1 mg, Estradiol 2 mg Kliofem tablets | 84 tablet `PoM` £11.43 DT = £17.02
▸ Kliovance (Novo Nordisk Ltd)
  Norethisterone acetate 500 microgram, Estradiol 1 mg Kliovance tablets | 84 tablet `PoM` £13.20 DT = £13.20
▸ Novofem (Novo Nordisk Ltd)
  Novofem tablets | 84 tablet `PoM` £11.43
▸ Trisequens (Novo Nordisk Ltd)
  Trisequens tablets | 84 tablet `PoM` £11.10

Transdermal patch

▸ Evorel Conti (Theramex HQ UK Ltd)
  Estradiol 50 microgram per 24 hour, Norethisterone acetate 170 microgram per 24 hour Evorel Conti patches | 8 patch `PoM` £13.00 | 24 patch `PoM` £37.22 DT = £37.22
▸ Evorel Sequi (Theramex HQ UK Ltd)
  Evorel Sequi patches | 8 patch `PoM` £11.09

PROGESTOGENS

Dienogest
17-Feb-2020

● DRUG ACTION Dienogest is a nortestosterone derivative that has a progestogenic effect in the uterus, reducing the production of estradiol and thereby suppressing the formation of endometriotic lesions.

● INDICATIONS AND DOSE

Endometriosis

▸ BY MOUTH
▸ Females of childbearing potential: 2 mg once daily, can be started on any day of cycle, dose should be taken continuously at the same time each day

● CONTRA-INDICATIONS Arterial disease (past or present) · cardiovascular disease (past or present) · diabetes with vascular involvement · liver tumours (past or present) · sex hormone-dependent malignancies (confirmed or suspected) · undiagnosed vaginal bleeding · venous thromboembolism (active)

● CAUTIONS Diabetes (progestogens can decrease glucose tolerance—monitor patient closely) · history of depression · history of ectopic pregnancy · history of gestational diabetes · patients at risk of osteoporosis · patients at risk of venous thromboembolism

6

Endocrine system

Endocrine system

6

CAUTIONS, FURTHER INFORMATION
▶ **Immobilisation** Manufacturer advises to discontinue treatment during prolonged immobilisation. For elective surgery, treatment should be discontinued at least 4 weeks before surgery; treatment may be restarted 2 weeks after complete remobilisation.
● INTERACTIONS → Appendix 1: dienogest
● SIDE-EFFECTS
▶ **Common or very common** Alopecia · anxiety · asthenic conditions · breast abnormalities · depression · gastrointestinal discomfort · gastrointestinal disorders · haemorrhage · headaches · hot flush · libido loss · mood altered · nausea · ovarian cyst · pain · skin reactions · sleep disorder · vomiting · vulvovaginal disorders · weight changes
▶ **Uncommon** Anaemia · appetite increased · autonomic dysfunction · broken nails · circulatory system disorder · concentration impaired · constipation · dandruff · diarrhoea · dry eye · dyspnoea · genital discharge · hair changes · hyperhidrosis · hypotension · increased risk of infection · limb discomfort · muscle spasms · oedema · palpitations · pelvic pain · photosensitivity reaction · tinnitus
▶ **Frequency not known** Glucose tolerance impaired · insulin resistance · menstrual cycle irregularities
● CONCEPTION AND CONTRACEPTION Manufacturer advises that, if contraception is required, females of childbearing potential should use non-hormonal contraception during treatment. The menstrual cycle usually returns to normal within 2 months after stopping treatment.
● BREAST FEEDING Manufacturer advises avoid—present in milk in *animal* studies.
● HEPATIC IMPAIRMENT Manufacturer advises avoid in severe impairment (no information available).
● PATIENT AND CARER ADVICE Manufacturer advises patients with a history of chloasma gravidarum to avoid sunlight or UV radiation exposure during treatment.
Missed doses Manufacturer advises if one or more tablets are missed, or if vomiting and/or diarrhoea occurs within 3–4 hours of taking a tablet, another tablet should be taken as soon as possible and the next dose taken at the normal time.

● MEDICINAL FORMS There can be variation in the licensing of different medicines containing the same drug.
Tablet
▶ Zalkya (Stragen UK Ltd)
Dienogest 2 mg Zalkya 2mg tablets | 28 tablet [PoM] £20.68

Norethisterone

24-Apr-2020

● INDICATIONS AND DOSE
Endometriosis
▶ BY MOUTH
▶ Adult: 10–15 mg daily for 4–6 months or longer, to be started on day 5 of cycle; increased to 20–25 mg daily if required, dose only increased if spotting occurs and reduced once bleeding has stopped
Dysfunctional uterine bleeding (to arrest bleeding) | Menorrhagia (to arrest bleeding)
▶ BY MOUTH
▶ Adult: 5 mg 3 times a day for 10 days
Dysfunctional uterine bleeding (to prevent bleeding) | Menorrhagia (to prevent bleeding)
▶ BY MOUTH
▶ Adult: 5 mg twice daily, to be taken from day 19 to day 26 of cycle

Dysmenorrhoea
▶ BY MOUTH
▶ Adult: 5 mg 3 times a day for 3–4 cycles, to be taken from day 5–24 of cycle
Premenstrual syndrome (but not recommended)
▶ BY MOUTH
▶ Adult: 5 mg 2–3 times a day for several cycles, to be taken from day 19–26 of cycle
Postponement of menstruation
▶ BY MOUTH
▶ Females of childbearing potential: 5 mg 3 times a day, to be started 3 days before expected onset (menstruation occurs 2–3 days after stopping)
Breast cancer
▶ BY MOUTH
▶ Adult: 40 mg daily, increased if necessary to 60 mg daily
Short-term contraception
▶ BY DEEP INTRAMUSCULAR INJECTION
▶ Females of childbearing potential: 200 mg, to be administered within first 5 days of cycle or immediately after parturition (duration 8 weeks). To be injected into the gluteal muscle, then 200 mg after 8 weeks if required
Contraception
▶ BY MOUTH
▶ Females of childbearing potential: 350 micrograms daily, dose to be taken at same time each day, starting on day 1 of cycle then continuously, if administration delayed for 3 hours or more it should be regarded as a 'missed pill'

● CONTRA-INDICATIONS
GENERAL CONTRA-INDICATIONS Acute porphyrias p. 1107 · current breast cancer (unless progestogens are being used in the management of this condition) · history during pregnancy of idiopathic jaundice (non-contraceptive indications) · history during pregnancy of pemphigoid gestationis (non-contraceptive indications) · history during pregnancy of severe pruritus (non-contraceptive indications)
SPECIFIC CONTRA-INDICATIONS
▶ With oral use History of thromboembolism (non-contraceptive indications) · undiagnosed vaginal bleeding (non-contraceptive indications)
● CAUTIONS
GENERAL CAUTIONS Cardiac dysfunction · conditions that may worsen with fluid retention · diabetes (progestogens can decrease glucose tolerance—monitor patient closely) · history of breast cancer—seek specialist advice before use · hypertension · liver tumours—seek specialist advice before use · migraine · multiple risk factors for cardiovascular disease—seek specialist advice before intramuscular use · positive antiphospholipid antibodies · rheumatoid arthritis · risk factors for venous thromboembolism · systemic lupus erythematosus
SPECIFIC CAUTIONS
▶ With intramuscular use Cervical cancer
▶ When used for Contraception History of stroke (including transient ischaemic attack)—seek specialist advice before intramuscular use · ischaemic heart disease—seek specialist advice before intramuscular use · undiagnosed vaginal bleeding—seek specialist advice before intramuscular use
▶ With oral use for Contraception Malabsorption syndromes
CAUTIONS, FURTHER INFORMATION
▶ Breast cancer risk with contraceptive use There is a small increase in the risk of having breast cancer diagnosed in women using, or who have recently used, a progestogen-only contraceptive pill; this relative risk may be due to an

earlier diagnosis. The most important risk factor appears to be the age at which the contraceptive is stopped rather than the duration of use; the risk disappears gradually during the 10 years after stopping and there is no excess risk by 10 years. A possible small increase in the risk of breast cancer should be weighed against the benefits.

- INTERACTIONS → Appendix 1: norethisterone

- SIDE-EFFECTS

GENERAL SIDE-EFFECTS
- **Common or very common** Menstrual cycle irregularities
- **Uncommon** Breast tenderness
- **Frequency not known** Hepatic cancer · thromboembolism

SPECIFIC SIDE-EFFECTS
- **Common or very common**
- With intramuscular use Dizziness · haemorrhage · headache · hypersensitivity · nausea · skin reactions · weight increased
- **Uncommon**
- With intramuscular use Abdominal distension · depressed mood
- **Frequency not known**
- With oral use Appetite change · depression · fatigue · gastrointestinal disorder · headaches · hypertension · libido disorder · nervousness · rash · weight change

- PREGNANCY
- With oral use Masculinisation of female fetuses and other defects reported with non-contraceptive use.

- BREAST FEEDING Progestogen-only contraceptives do not affect lactation. Higher doses (used in malignant conditions) may suppress lactation and alter milk composition—use lowest effective dose.
- With intramuscular use Withhold breast-feeding for neonates with severe or persistent jaundice requiring medical treatment.

- HEPATIC IMPAIRMENT Manufacturers advise caution; avoid in severe or active disease.
- When used for breast cancer Manufacturer advises avoid.

- RENAL IMPAIRMENT Use with caution in non-contraceptive indications.

- PATIENT AND CARER ADVICE
- Diarrhoea and vomiting with oral contraceptives Vomiting and persistent, severe diarrhoea can interfere with the absorption of oral progestogen-only contraceptives. If vomiting occurs within 2 hours of taking an oral progestogen-only contraceptive, another pill should be taken as soon as possible. If a replacement pill is not taken within 3 hours of the normal time for taking the progestogen-only pill, or in cases of persistent vomiting or very severe diarrhoea, additional precautions should be used during illness and for 2 days after recovery.
- Starting routine for oral contraceptives One tablet daily, on a continuous basis, starting on day 1 of cycle and taken at the same time each day (if delayed by longer than 3 hours contraceptive protection may be lost). Additional contraceptive precautions are not required if norethisterone is started up to and including day 5 of the menstrual cycle; if started after this time, additional contraceptive precautions are required for 2 days.
- Changing from a combined oral contraceptive Start on the day following completion of the combined oral contraceptive course without a break (or in the case of ED tablets omitting the inactive ones).
- After childbirth Oral progestogen-only contraceptives can be started up to and including day 21 postpartum without the need for additional contraceptive precautions. If started more than 21 days postpartum, additional contraceptive precautions are required for 2 days.
- Contraceptives by injection Full counselling backed by *patient information leaflet* required before administration—likelihood of menstrual disturbance and the potential for a delay in return to full fertility. Delayed return of fertility and irregular cycles may occur after discontinuation of

treatment but there is no evidence of permanent infertility.

Missed doses Missed oral contraceptive pill The following advice is recommended: 'If you forget a pill, take it as soon as you remember and carry on with the next pill at the right time. If the pill was more than 3 hours overdue you are not protected. Continue normal pill-taking but you must also use another method, such as the condom, for the next 2 days.'

The Faculty of Sexual and Reproductive Healthcare recommends emergency contraception if one or more progestogen-only contraceptive tablets are missed or taken more than 3 hours late and unprotected intercourse has occurred before 2 further tablets have been correctly taken.

- MEDICINAL FORMS There can be variation in the licensing of different medicines containing the same drug. Forms available from special-order manufacturers include: oral suspension

Solution for injection
- Noristerat (Bayer Plc)
  Norethisterone enantate 200 mg per 1 ml Noristerat 200mg/1ml solution for injection ampoules | 1 ampoule [PoM] £4.05 DT = £4.05

Tablet
- Norethisterone (Non-proprietary)
  Norethisterone 5 mg Norethisterone 5mg tablets | 30 tablet [PoM] £4.15 DT = £2.74
- Noriday (Pfizer Ltd)
  Norethisterone 350 microgram Noriday 350microgram tablets | 84 tablet [PoM] £2.10 DT = £2.10
- Primolut N (Bayer Plc)
  Norethisterone 5 mg Primolut N 5mg tablets | 30 tablet [PoM] £2.26 DT = £2.74
- Utovlan (Pfizer Ltd)
  Norethisterone 5 mg Utovlan 5mg tablets | 30 tablet [PoM] £1.40 DT = £2.74 | 90 tablet [PoM] £4.21

Combinations available: *Estradiol with norethisterone,* p. 804

Progesterone

02-Dec-2020

- **INDICATIONS AND DOSE**

CRINONE® VAGINAL GEL

Infertility due to inadequate luteal phase
- BY VAGINA
- Adult: 1 applicatorful daily, to be started either after documented ovulation or on day 18–21 of cycle, in vitro fertilisation, daily application continued for 30 days after laboratory evidence of pregnancy

CYCLOGEST® PESSARIES

Premenstrual syndrome | Post-natal depression
- BY VAGINA, OR BY RECTUM
- Adult: 200–800 mg daily, doses above 200 mg to be given in 2 divided doses, for premenstrual syndrome start on day 12–14 and continue until onset of menstruation (but not recommended); rectally if barrier methods of contraception are used, in patients who have recently given birth or in those who suffer from vaginal infection or recurrent cystitis

LUBION®

Supplementation of luteal phase during assisted reproductive technology (ART) treatment in women for whom vaginal preparations are inappropriate
- BY SUBCUTANEOUS INJECTION, OR BY INTRAMUSCULAR INJECTION
- Adult: 25 mg once daily from day of oocyte retrieval up to week 12 of pregnancy

continued →

6

Endocrine system

6

Endocrine system

LUTIGEST ®

Luteal support as part of an Assisted Reproductive Technology (ART) treatment programme
▸ BY VAGINA
▸ Adult: 100 mg 3 times a day, to be started the day after oocyte retrieval, and continued for 30 days once pregnancy is confirmed

UTROGESTAN ® CAPSULES

Progestogenic opposition of oestrogen HRT
▸ BY MOUTH
▸ Adult: 200 mg once daily on days 15–26 of each 28-day oestrogen HRT cycle, alternatively 100 mg once daily on days 1–25 of each 28-day oestrogen HRT cycle

UTROGESTAN ® VAGINAL CAPSULES

Supplementation of luteal phase during assisted reproductive technology (ART) cycles
▸ BY VAGINA
▸ Adult: 1 capsule 3 times a day from day of embryo transfer until at least week 7 of pregnancy up to week 12 of pregnancy

● CONTRA-INDICATIONS Acute porphyrias p. 1107 · breast cancer · genital cancer · history during pregnancy of idiopathic jaundice · history during pregnancy of pemphigoid gestationis · history during pregnancy of severe pruritus · history of thromboembolism · missed miscarriage · thrombophlebitis · undiagnosed vaginal bleeding

● CAUTIONS Conditions that may worsen with fluid retention · diabetes (progestogens can decrease glucose tolerance—monitor patient closely) · history of depression · migraine · risk factors for thromboembolism

● SIDE-EFFECTS
▸ **Common or very common**
▸ With oral use Headache · menstrual cycle irregularities
▸ With vaginal use Breast pain · drowsiness · gastrointestinal discomfort
▸ **Uncommon**
▸ With oral use Breast pain · constipation · diarrhoea · dizziness · drowsiness · jaundice cholestatic · skin reactions · vomiting
▸ **Rare or very rare**
▸ With oral use Depression · nausea
▸ **Frequency not known**
▸ With intramuscular use Alopecia · breast changes · cervical abnormalities · depression · drowsiness · fever · hirsutism · insomnia · jaundice cholestatic · menstrual cycle irregularities · nausea · oedema · protein catabolism · skin reactions · weight increased
▸ With rectal use Diarrhoea · flatulence
▸ With vaginal use Leakage of the pessary base · menstrual cycle irregularities · vulvovaginal pain

● ALLERGY AND CROSS-SENSITIVITY For *Utrogestan*® *oral and vaginal capsules*, manufacturer advises contra-indicated in patients with hypersensitivity to soy or peanut products—contains soya lecithin.

● PREGNANCY Not known to be harmful.

● BREAST FEEDING Avoid—present in milk.

● HEPATIC IMPAIRMENT Manufacturer advises caution; avoid in severe impairment. For *Utrogestan*® *oral capsules*, manufacturer advises avoid in acute or active liver disease. For *Crinone*® *vaginal gel*, manufacturer advises caution in severe impairment.

● RENAL IMPAIRMENT Use with caution.

● DIRECTIONS FOR ADMINISTRATION
▸ With oral use Manufacturer advises capsules should be taken at bedtime on an empty stomach.

● PATIENT AND CARER ADVICE
▸ With oral use Patient counselling is advised for progesterone capsules (administration).

● NATIONAL FUNDING/ACCESS DECISIONS
LUTIGEST ® For full details see funding body website
Scottish Medicines Consortium (SMC) decisions
▸ Progesterone (*Lutigest*®) for luteal support as part of an assisted reproductive technology (ART) treatment program for infertile women (October 2016) SMC No. 1185/16 Recommended

LUBION ® For full details see funding body website
Scottish Medicines Consortium (SMC) decisions
▸ Progesterone (*Lubion*®) is indicated in adults for luteal support as part of an Assisted Reproductive Technology (ART) treatment program in infertile women who are unable to use or tolerate vaginal preparations (July 2018) SMC No. SMC2017 Recommended

UTROGESTAN ® VAGINAL CAPSULES For full details see funding body website
Scottish Medicines Consortium (SMC) decisions
▸ Micronised progesterone (*Utrogestan Vaginal*®) in women for supplementation of the luteal phase during Assisted Reproductive Technology (ART) cycles (May 2017) SMC No. 935/13 Recommended

● LESS SUITABLE FOR PRESCRIBING
▸ With vaginal use Progesterone pessaries are less suitable for prescribing.

● MEDICINAL FORMS There can be variation in the licensing of different medicines containing the same drug.

Pessary
▸ Cyclogest (L.D. Collins & Co. Ltd)
 Progesterone 200 mg Cyclogest 200mg pessaries | 15 pessary [PoM] £8.95 DT = £8.95
 Progesterone 400 mg Cyclogest 400mg pessaries | 15 pessary [PoM] £12.96 DT = £12.96
▸ Lutigest (Ferring Pharmaceuticals Ltd)
 Progesterone 100 mg Lutigest 100mg vaginal tablets | 21 pessary [PoM] £19.50 DT = £19.50

Vaginal gel
▸ Crinone (Merck Serono Ltd)
 Progesterone 80 mg per 1 gram Crinone 8% progesterone vaginal gel | 15 unit dose [PoM] £30.83 DT = £30.83

Capsule
▸ Utrogestan (Besins Healthcare (UK) Ltd)
 Progesterone 100 mg Utrogestan 100mg capsules | 30 capsule [PoM] £5.13 DT = £5.13
 Progesterone 200 mg Utrogestan 200mg vaginal capsules with applicators | 21 capsule [PoM] £21.00 DT = £21.00

8.1a Anti-oestrogens

OVULATION STIMULANTS

Clomifene citrate
23-Nov-2020

(Clomiphene citrate)

● DRUG ACTION Anti-oestrogen which induces gonadotrophin release by occupying oestrogen receptors in the hypothalamus, thereby interfering with feedback mechanisms; chorionic gonadotrophin is sometimes used as an adjunct.

● INDICATIONS AND DOSE
Female infertility due to ovulatory dysfunction
▸ BY MOUTH
▸ Adult (female): 50 mg once daily for 5 days, to be started at any time if no recent uterine bleeding or on or around the fifth day of cycle if progestogen-induced bleeding is planned or if spontaneous uterine bleeding

occurs, then 100 mg once daily if required for 5 days, this second course to be given at least 30 days after the first course, only in the absence of ovulation; most patients who are going to respond will do so to first course, 3 courses should constitute adequate therapeutic trial; long-term cyclical therapy not recommended (beyond a total of 6 cycles).

> **IMPORTANT SAFETY INFORMATION**
> Manufacturer advises clomifene should not normally be used for longer than 6 cycles (possible increased risk of ovarian cancer).

- CONTRA-INDICATIONS Abnormal uterine bleeding of undetermined cause · hormone-dependent tumours · ovarian cysts
- CAUTIONS Ectopic pregnancy · incidence of multiple births increased · ovarian hyperstimulation syndrome · polycystic ovary syndrome (cysts may enlarge during treatment, also risk of exaggerated response to usual doses) · uterine fibroids
- SIDE-EFFECTS Abdominal distension · alopecia · angioedema · anxiety · breast tenderness · cataract · cerebral thrombosis · depression · disorientation · dizziness · fatigue · headache · hot flush · hypertriglyceridaemia · insomnia · jaundice cholestatic · menstrual cycle irregularities · mood altered · nausea · neoplasms · nervous system disorders · optic neuritis · ovarian and fallopian tube disorders · palpitations · pancreatitis · paraesthesia · psychosis · seizure · skin reactions · speech disorder · stroke · syncope · tachycardia · uterine disorders · vertigo · vision disorders · visual impairment (discontinue and initiate ophthalmological examination) · vomiting
- CONCEPTION AND CONTRACEPTION Exclude pregnancy before treatment.
- PREGNANCY Possible effects on fetal development.
- BREAST FEEDING May inhibit lactation.
- HEPATIC IMPAIRMENT Manufacturer advises avoid in liver disease or history of liver dysfunction.
- PATIENT AND CARER ADVICE
  Conception and contraception Patients planning to conceive should be warned that there is a risk of multiple pregnancy (*rarely* more than twins).

- MEDICINAL FORMS There can be variation in the licensing of different medicines containing the same drug.

Tablet
- Clomifene citrate (Non-proprietary)
  Clomifene citrate 50 mg Clomifene 50mg tablets | 30 tablet [PoM] £13.97 DT = £10.15
- Clomid (Sanofi)
  Clomifene citrate 50 mg Clomid 50mg tablets | 30 tablet [PoM] £10.15 DT = £10.15

8.2 Male sex hormone responsive conditions

Androgens, anti-androgens and anabolic steroids

14-Aug-2020

Androgens

Androgens cause masculinisation; they may be used as replacement therapy in castrated adults and in those who are hypogonadal due to either pituitary or testicular disease. In the normal male they inhibit pituitary gonadotrophin secretion and depress spermatogenesis. Androgens also have

an anabolic action which led to the development of anabolic steroids.

Androgens are useless as a treatment of impotence and impaired spermatogenesis unless there is associated hypogonadism; they should not be given until the hypogonadism has been properly investigated. Treatment should be under expert supervision.

When given to patients with hypopituitarism they can lead to normal sexual development and potency but not to fertility. If fertility is desired, the usual treatment is with gonadotrophins or pulsatile gonadotrophin-releasing hormone which will stimulate spermatogenesis as well as androgen production.

Intramuscular depot preparations of **testosterone esters** are preferred for replacement therapy. Testosterone enantate, propionate or undecanoate, or alternatively *Sustanon*®, which consists of a mixture of testosterone esters and has a longer duration of action, may be used.

Anti-androgens

Cyproterone acetate

Cyproterone acetate p. 812 is an anti-androgen used in the treatment of severe hypersexuality and sexual deviation in the male. It inhibits spermatogenesis and produces reversible infertility (but is not a male contraceptive); abnormal sperm forms are produced. Fully informed consent is recommended and an initial spermatogram. As hepatic tumours have been produced in *animal* studies, careful consideration should be given to the risk/benefit ratio before treatment. Cyproterone acetate is also licensed for use alone in patients with metastatic prostate cancer refractory to gonadorelin analogue therapy, and has been used as an adjunct in prostatic cancer and in the treatment of acne and hirsutism in women.

The MHRA/CHM have released important safety information on the use of cyproterone acetate and risk of meningioma. For further information, see *Important safety information* for cyproterone acetate.

Dutasteride and finasteride

Dutasteride p. 831 and finasteride p. 832 are alternatives to alpha-blockers particularly in men with a significantly enlarged prostate. Finasteride is also licensed for use with doxazosin p. 827 in the management of benign prostatic hyperplasia.

A low strength of finasteride is licensed for treating male-pattern baldness in men.

Anabolic steroids

Anabolic steroids have some androgenic activity but they cause less virilisation than androgens in women. They are used in the treatment of some *aplastic anaemias*. Anabolic steroids have been given for osteoporosis in women but they are no longer advocated for this purpose.

The protein-building properties of anabolic steroids have not proved beneficial in the clinical setting. Their use as body builders or tonics is unjustified; some athletes abuse them.

ANDROGENS

Androgens

- CONTRA-INDICATIONS Breast cancer in males · history of liver tumours · hypercalcaemia · prostate cancer
- CAUTIONS Cardiac impairment · diabetes mellitus · elderly · epilepsy · hypertension · ischaemic heart disease · migraine · pre-pubertal boys (fusion of epiphyses is hastened and may result in short stature)—statural growth and sexual development should be monitored · risk factors for venous thromboembolism · skeletal metastases—risk of hypercalcaemia or hypercalciuria (if this occurs, treat appropriately and restart treatment once normal serum

6

Endocrine system

calcium concentration restored) · sleep apnoea · stop treatment or reduce dose if severe polycythaemia occurs · thrombophilia—increased risk of thrombosis · tumours—risk of hypercalcaemia or hypercalciuria (if this occurs, treat appropriately and restart treatment once normal serum calcium concentration restored)

CAUTIONS, FURTHER INFORMATION
▶ **Elderly** Prescription potentially inappropriate (STOPP criteria) in the absence of primary or secondary hypogonadism (risk of androgen toxicity; no proven benefit outside of the hypogonadism indication).
See also Prescribing in the elderly p. 33.

● SIDE-EFFECTS
▶ **Common or very common** Hot flush · hypertension · polycythaemia · prostate abnormalities · skin reactions · weight increased
▶ **Uncommon** Alopecia · asthenia · behaviour abnormal · depression · dizziness · dyspnoea · dysuria · gynaecomastia · headache · hyperhidrosis · insomnia · nausea · sexual dysfunction
▶ **Rare or very rare** Pulmonary oil microembolism
▶ **Frequency not known** Anxiety · epiphyses premature fusion · fluid retention · jaundice · oedema · oligozoospermia · paraesthesia · precocious puberty · prostate cancer · seborrhoea · sleep apnoea · urinary tract obstruction

SIDE-EFFECTS, FURTHER INFORMATION Stop treatment or reduce dose if severe polycythaemia occurs.

● PREGNANCY Avoid—causes masculinisation of female fetus.

● BREAST FEEDING Avoid.

● HEPATIC IMPAIRMENT In general, manufacturers advise caution (increased risk of fluid retention and heart failure).

● RENAL IMPAIRMENT Caution—potential for fluid retention.

● MONITORING REQUIREMENTS
▶ Monitor haematocrit and haemoglobulin before treatment, every three months for the first year, and yearly thereafter.
▶ Monitor prostate and PSA in men over 45 years.

● PATIENT AND CARER ADVICE
Androgenic effects in women Women should be advised to report any signs of virilisation e.g. deepening of the voice or hirsutism.

F 809

Testosterone

12-Nov-2020

● INDICATIONS AND DOSE
Low sexual desire in postmenopausal women (administered on expert advice)
▶ BY TRANSDERMAL APPLICATION
▶ **Adult:** Apply 50 mg every week, the contents of a 5-g sachet or 5-g tube (containing 50 mg/5 g of testosterone) to be divided for daily dosing and applied to non-hair areas, such as the abdomen or upper thighs, over the period of 1 week

TESTAVAN ®
Hypogonadism due to androgen deficiency in men
▶ BY TRANSDERMAL APPLICATION
▶ **Adult:** Apply 23 mg once daily; increased in steps of 23 mg, adjusted according to response; maximum 69 mg per day

DOSE EQUIVALENCE AND CONVERSION
▶ For *Testavan* ® One pump actuation delivers 1.15 g of gel containing 23 mg of testosterone.

TESTIM ®
Hypogonadism due to testosterone deficiency in men
▶ BY TRANSDERMAL APPLICATION
▶ **Adult:** Apply 50 mg once daily, subsequent application adjusted according to response; maximum 100 mg per day

DOSE EQUIVALENCE AND CONVERSION
▶ For *Testim* ® One tube of 5 g contains 50 mg testosterone.

TESTOGEL ® 16.2MG/G
Hypogonadism due to androgen deficiency in men
▶ BY TRANSDERMAL APPLICATION
▶ **Adult:** Apply 40.5 mg once daily; increased in steps of 20.25 mg, adjusted according to response; maximum 81 mg per day

DOSE EQUIVALENCE AND CONVERSION
▶ For *Testogel* ® 16.2mg/g One pump actuation delivers 1.25 g of gel containing 20.25 mg of testosterone.

TESTOGEL ® 50MG/5G
Hypogonadism due to androgen deficiency in men
▶ BY TRANSDERMAL APPLICATION
▶ **Adult:** Apply 50 mg once daily; increased in steps of 25 mg, adjusted according to response; maximum 100 mg per day

DOSE EQUIVALENCE AND CONVERSION
▶ For *Testogel* ® 50mg/5g One sachet of 5 g contains 50 mg of testosterone.

TOSTRAN ®
Hypogonadism due to testosterone deficiency in men
▶ BY TRANSDERMAL APPLICATION
▶ **Adult:** Apply 60 mg once daily, subsequent application adjusted according to response; maximum 80 mg per day

DOSE EQUIVALENCE AND CONVERSION
▶ For *Tostran* ® 1 g of gel contains 20 mg testosterone.

● UNLICENSED USE [EvGr] Testosterone is used for the treatment of low sexual desire in postmenopausal women, Ⓔ but is not licensed for this indication.

● SIDE-EFFECTS
▶ **Common or very common** Hypertriglyceridaemia
▶ **Frequency not known** Anaemia · deep vein thrombosis · electrolyte imbalance · frontal balding (in women) · hair growth unwanted (in women) · hypertrichosis · malaise · muscle cramps · musculoskeletal pain · testicular disorder · vasodilation · voice lowered (in women)

SIDE-EFFECTS, FURTHER INFORMATION **When used for low sexual desire in post-menopausal women** The long-term effects of testosterone in this patient group are largely unknown, but side-effects can include growth of unwanted hair, frontal balding and deepening of the voice.

● DIRECTIONS FOR ADMINISTRATION Manufacturer advises avoid skin contact with gel application sites to prevent testosterone transfer to other people, especially pregnant women and children—consult product literature.

TOSTRAN ® Manufacturer advises apply gel on clean, dry, intact skin of abdomen or both inner thighs, preferably in the morning. Gently rub in with a finger until dry before dressing. Wash hands with soap and water after applying gel; avoid washing application site for at least 2 hours. Not to be applied on genital area.

TESTOGEL ® 50MG/5G Manufacturer advises apply thin layer of gel on clean, dry, healthy skin such as shoulders, arms or abdomen, immediately after sachet is opened. Not to be applied on genital area as high alcohol content may cause local irritation. Allow to dry for 3–5 minutes before dressing. Wash hands with soap and water after applying gel, avoid shower or bath for at least 6 hours.

TESTIM ® Manufacturer advises squeeze entire content of tube on to one palm and apply as a thin layer on clean, dry, healthy skin of shoulder or upper arm, preferably in the morning after washing or bathing (if 2 tubes required use 1 per shoulder or upper arm); rub in and allow to dry before putting on clothing to cover site; wash hands with soap after application; avoid washing application site for at least 6 hours.

TESTOGEL ® 16.2MG/G Apply thin layer of gel on clean, dry, healthy skin over right and left upper arms and shoulders. Not to be applied on genital area as high alcohol content may cause local irritation. Allow to dry for 3–5 minutes before dressing. Wash hands with soap and water after applying gel, and cover the site with clothing once gel dried; avoid shower or bath for at least 2 hours.

TESTAVAN ® Manufacturer advises apply one pump actuation of gel evenly onto clean, dry, intact skin over upper arm and shoulder using the applicator, without getting any gel on the hands—repeat on opposite upper arm and shoulder if two pump actuations are required, and repeat again on initial upper arm and shoulder if three pump actuations are required. Allow to dry completely before dressing and cover application site with clothing. Wash hands with soap and water immediately if gel was touched during application; avoid shower or bath for at least 2 hours.

- PATIENT AND CARER ADVICE Patient or carer should be given advice on how to administer testosterone gel.
- NATIONAL FUNDING/ACCESS DECISIONS
  For full details see funding body website
  Scottish Medicines Consortium (SMC) decisions
- Testosterone (*Testavan*®) as replacement therapy for adult male hypogonadism, when testosterone deficiency has been confirmed by clinical features and biochemical tests (April 2019) SMC No. SMC2152 Recommended with restrictions

- MEDICINAL FORMS There can be variation in the licensing of different medicines containing the same drug.
  Gel
  CAUTIONARY AND ADVISORY LABELS 15
  EXCIPIENTS: May contain Butylated hydroxytoluene, propylene glycol
  ▸ Testavan (Ferring Pharmaceuticals Ltd)
  Testosterone 20 mg per 1 gram Testavan 20mg/g transdermal gel | 85.5 gram [PoM] £25.22 DT = £25.22 [CD4-2]
  ▸ Testim (Endo Ventures Ltd)
  Testosterone 50 mg Testim 50mg/5g gel | 30 tube [PoM] £30.50 DT = £30.50 [CD4-2]
  ▸ Testogel (Besins Healthcare (UK) Ltd)
  Testosterone 50 mg Testogel 50mg/5g gel sachets | 30 sachet [PoM] £31.11 DT = £31.11 [CD4-2]
  Testosterone 16.2 mg per 1 gram Testogel 16.2mg/g gel | 88 gram [PoM] £31.11 DT = £31.11 [CD4-2]
  ▸ Tostran (Kyowa Kirin Ltd)
  Testosterone 20 mg per 1 gram Tostran 2% gel | 60 gram [PoM] £28.63 DT = £28.63 [CD4-2]

Testosterone decanoate, isocaproate, phenylpropionate and propionate

14-Jul-2020

The properties listed below are those particular to the combination only. For the properties of the components please consider, testosterone propionate below.

- INDICATIONS AND DOSE
  Androgen deficiency
  ▸ BY DEEP INTRAMUSCULAR INJECTION
  ▸ Adult: 1 mL every 3 weeks, adjusted according to response

DOSE EQUIVALENCE AND CONVERSION
▸ Each 1 mL dose of *Sustanon*® 250 solution for injection contains 100 mg testosterone decanoate, 60 mg testosterone isocaproate, 60 mg testosterone phenylpropionate and 30 mg testosterone propionate.

- MEDICINAL FORMS There can be variation in the licensing of different medicines containing the same drug.
  Solution for injection
  EXCIPIENTS: May contain Arachis (peanut) oil, benzyl alcohol
  ▸ Sustanon (Aspen Pharma Trading Ltd)
  Testosterone propionate 30 mg per 1 ml, Testosterone isocaproate 60 mg per 1 ml, Testosterone phenylpropionate 60 mg per 1 ml, Testosterone decanoate 100 mg per 1 ml Sustanon 250mg/1ml solution for injection ampoules | 1 ampoule [PoM] £2.45 [CD4-2]

⊩ 809

Testosterone enantate
13-May-2020

- **INDICATIONS AND DOSE**
  Hypogonadism
  ▸ BY SLOW INTRAMUSCULAR INJECTION
  ▸ Adult: Initially 250 mg every 2–3 weeks; maintenance 250 mg every 3–6 weeks
  Breast cancer
  ▸ BY SLOW INTRAMUSCULAR INJECTION
  ▸ Adult: 250 mg every 2–3 weeks

- UNLICENSED USE Not licensed for use in breast cancer.
- SIDE-EFFECTS Bone formation increased · circulatory system disorder · gastrointestinal disorder · gastrointestinal haemorrhage · hepatomegaly · hypercalcaemia · neoplasms · spermatogenesis abnormal

- MEDICINAL FORMS There can be variation in the licensing of different medicines containing the same drug.
  Solution for injection
  ▸ Testosterone enantate (Non-proprietary)
  Testosterone enantate 250 mg per 1 ml Testosterone enantate 250mg/1ml solution for injection ampoules | 3 ampoule [PoM] £83.74–£87.73 DT = £85.74 [CD4-2]

⊩ 809

Testosterone propionate
13-May-2020

- **INDICATIONS AND DOSE**
  Androgen deficiency
  ▸ BY INTRAMUSCULAR INJECTION
  ▸ Adult: 50 mg 2–3 times a week
  Delayed puberty in males
  ▸ BY INTRAMUSCULAR INJECTION
  ▸ Adult: 50 mg once weekly
  Breast cancer in women
  ▸ BY INTRAMUSCULAR INJECTION
  ▸ Adult: 100 mg 2–3 times a week

- MEDICINAL FORMS Forms available from special-order manufacturers include: solution for injection

⊩ 809

Testosterone undecanoate
13-May-2020

- **INDICATIONS AND DOSE**
  Androgen deficiency
  ▸ BY MOUTH
  ▸ Adult: 120–160 mg daily for 2–3 weeks; maintenance 40–120 mg daily continued →

6

Endocrine system

6

Endocrine system

Hypogonadism
▶ BY DEEP INTRAMUSCULAR INJECTION
▶ Adult (male): 1 g every 10–14 weeks, to be given over 2 minutes, if necessary, second dose may be given after 6 weeks to achieve rapid steady state plasma testosterone levels and then every 10–14 weeks.

● SIDE-EFFECTS
GENERAL SIDE-EFFECTS
▶ **Uncommon** Diarrhoea · mood altered
SPECIFIC SIDE-EFFECTS
▶ **Uncommon**
▶ With intramuscular use Appetite increased · arthralgia · breast abnormalities · cardiovascular disorder · cough · dysphonia · hypercholesterolaemia · increased risk of infection · migraine · muscle complaints · musculoskeletal stiffness · night sweats · pain in extremity · snoring · testicular disorders · tremor · urinary disorders · urinary tract disorder
▶ **Frequency not known**
▶ With intramuscular use Hair growth increased · spermatogenesis reduced
▶ With oral use Azoospermia · fluid imbalance · gastrointestinal discomfort · hepatic function abnormal · lipid metabolism change · myalgia

● MEDICINAL FORMS There can be variation in the licensing of different medicines containing the same drug.
Solution for injection
▶ Nebido (Bayer Plc)
Testosterone undecanoate 250 mg per 1 ml Nebido 1000mg/4ml solution for injection vials | 1 vial [PoM] £87.11 DT = £87.11 [CD4-2]

8.2a Male sex hormone antagonism

ANTI-ANDROGENS

Cyproterone acetate

01-Dec-2020

● INDICATIONS AND DOSE
Hyper-sexuality in males | Sexual deviation in males
▶ BY MOUTH
▶ Adult: 50 mg twice daily, to be taken after food
Prevention of tumour flare with initial gonadorelin analogue therapy
▶ BY MOUTH
▶ Adult (male): 200 mg daily in 2–3 divided doses for 5–7 days before initiation of gonadorelin analogue, followed by 200 mg daily in 2–3 divided doses for 3–4 weeks after initiation of gonadorelin analogue; maximum 300 mg per day.
Long-term palliative therapy where gonadorelin analogues or orchidectomy contra-indicated, not tolerated, or where oral therapy preferred
▶ BY MOUTH
▶ Adult (male): 200–300 mg daily in 2–3 divided doses.
Hot flushes with gonadorelin analogue therapy or after orchidectomy
▶ BY MOUTH
▶ Adult (male): Initially 50 mg daily, then adjusted according to response to 50–150 mg daily in 1–3 divided doses.

IMPORTANT SAFETY INFORMATION
MHRA/CHM ADVICE: CYPROTERONE ACETATE: NEW ADVICE TO MINIMISE RISK OF MENINGIOMA (JUNE 2020)
Cyproterone acetate has been associated with an overall rare, but cumulative dose-dependent, increased risk of

meningioma (single and multiple), mainly at doses of 25 mg/day and higher. Healthcare professionals are advised to monitor patients for meningiomas, and to permanently discontinue treatment if diagnosed. Use of cyproterone acetate, including co-cyprindiol, for all indications is contra-indicated in those with meningioma or a history of meningioma. Treatment with high doses of cyproterone acetate for any indication, except prostate cancer, should be restricted to when alternative treatments or interventions are unavailable or considered inappropriate.

● CONTRA-INDICATIONS
GENERAL CONTRA-INDICATIONS Dubin-Johnson syndrome · existing or history of thromboembolic disorders · malignant diseases (except for carcinoma of the prostate) · meningioma or history of meningioma · previous or existing liver tumours (not due to metastases from carcinoma of the prostate) · Rotor syndrome · wasting diseases (except for inoperable carcinoma of the prostate)
SPECIFIC CONTRA-INDICATIONS
▶ When used for hypersexuality Severe depression · severe diabetes (with vascular changes) · sickle-cell anaemia
● CAUTIONS Diabetes mellitus · in prostate cancer, severe depression · in prostate cancer, sickle-cell anaemia · ineffective for male hypersexuality in chronic alcoholism (relevance to prostate cancer not known)
● INTERACTIONS → Appendix 1: anti-androgens
● SIDE-EFFECTS
▶ **Common or very common** Depressed mood · dyspnoea · fatigue · gynaecomastia · hepatic disorders · hot flush · hyperhidrosis · nipple pain · restlessness · weight change
▶ **Uncommon** Skin reactions
▶ **Rare or very rare** Galactorrhoea · meningioma (increased risk with increasing cumulative dose) · neoplasms
▶ **Frequency not known** Adrenocortical suppression · anaemia · azoospermia · hair changes · hypotrichosis · osteoporosis · sebaceous gland underactivity (may clear acne) · thromboembolism

SIDE-EFFECTS, FURTHER INFORMATION Direct hepatic toxicity including jaundice, hepatitis and hepatic failure have been reported (fatalities reported, usually after several months, at dosages of 100 mg and above). If hepatotoxicity is confirmed, cyproterone should normally be withdrawn unless the hepatotoxicity can be explained by another cause such as metastatic disease (in which case cyproterone should be continued only if the perceived benefit exceeds the risk).

● HEPATIC IMPAIRMENT Manufacturer advises avoid (unless used for prostate cancer).
● MONITORING REQUIREMENTS
▶ Monitor blood counts initially and throughout treatment.
▶ Monitor adrenocortical function regularly.
▶ Monitor hepatic function regularly—liver function tests should be performed before and regularly during treatment and whenever symptoms suggestive of hepatotoxicity occur.
● PATIENT AND CARER ADVICE
Driving and skilled tasks Fatigue and lassitude may impair performance of skilled tasks (e.g. driving).

● MEDICINAL FORMS There can be variation in the licensing of different medicines containing the same drug. Forms available from special-order manufacturers include: tablet, capsule, oral suspension, oral solution
Tablet
CAUTIONARY AND ADVISORY LABELS 21
▶ Cyproterone acetate (Non-proprietary)
Cyproterone acetate 50 mg Cyproterone 50mg tablets | 56 tablet [PoM] £48.95 DT = £33.74
Cyproterone acetate 100 mg Cyproterone 100mg tablets | 84 tablet [PoM] £132.57 DT = £64.55

▸ Androcur (Bayer Plc)
Cyproterone acetate 50 mg Androcur 50mg tablets |
60 tablet [PoM] £31.34
▸ Cyprostat (Bayer Plc)
Cyproterone acetate 50 mg Cyprostat 50mg tablets |
160 tablet [PoM] £82.86
Cyproterone acetate 100 mg Cyprostat 100mg tablets |
80 tablet [PoM] £82.86

9   Thyroid disorders

PITUITARY AND HYPOTHALAMIC HORMONES AND ANALOGUES >THYROID STIMULATING HORMONES

| Thyrotropin alfa   02-Dec-2020

(Recombinant human thyroid stimulating hormone; rhTSH)

● DRUG ACTION Thyrotropin alfa is a recombinant form of thyrotrophin (thyroid stimulating hormone).

● INDICATIONS AND DOSE
Detection of thyroid remnants and thyroid cancer in post-thyroidectomy patients, together with serum thyroglobulin testing (with or without radioiodine imaging) | To increase radio-iodine uptake for the ablation of thyroid remnant tissue in suitable post-thyroidectomy patients
▸ BY INTRAMUSCULAR INJECTION
▸ Adult: 900 micrograms every 24 hours for 2 doses, dose to be administered into the gluteal muscle, consult product literature for further information on indications and dose

● CAUTIONS Presence of thyroglobulin autoantibodies may give false negative results

● SIDE-EFFECTS
▸ **Common or very common** Asthenia · dizziness · headache · nausea · vomiting
▸ **Uncommon** Chills · diarrhoea · feeling hot · fever · flushing · hypersensitivity · influenza · influenza like illness · pain · paraesthesia · pulmonary reaction · skin reactions · taste altered
▸ **Rare or very rare** Atrial fibrillation · hyperthyroidism
▸ **Frequency not known** Arthralgia · dyspnoea · goitre · hyperhidrosis · myalgia · neoplasm complications · palpitations · residual metastases enlarged · stroke · tremor

● ALLERGY AND CROSS-SENSITIVITY [EvGr] Contra-indicated if previous hypersensitivity to bovine or human thyrotrophin. ⓐ

● PREGNANCY Avoid.

● BREAST FEEDING Avoid.

● MEDICINAL FORMS There can be variation in the licensing of different medicines containing the same drug.
Powder for solution for injection
▸ Thyrogen (Genzyme Therapeutics Ltd)
Thyrotropin alfa 900 microgram Thyrogen 900microgram powder for solution for injection vials | 2 vial [PoM] £583.04

9.1   Hyperthyroidism

Hyperthyroidism   09-Dec-2019

Description of condition

Hyperthyroidism results from the excessive production and secretion of thyroid hormones leading to thyrotoxicosis (an excess of circulating thyroid hormones). Signs and symptoms of hyperthyroidism include a goitre, hyperactivity, disturbed sleep, fatigue, palpitations, anxiety, heat intolerance, increased appetite with unintentional weight loss, and diarrhoea. Complications include Graves' orbitopathy, thyroid storm (thyrotoxic crisis), pregnancy complications, reduced bone mineral density, heart failure, and atrial fibrillation. Risk factors include smoking, a family history of thyroid disease, co-existent autoimmune conditions, and low iodine intake.

Primary hyperthyroidism refers to when the condition arises from the thyroid gland rather than due to a pituitary or hypothalamic disorder. It is mainly caused by Graves' disease (an autoimmune disorder mediated by antibodies that stimulate the thyroid-stimulating hormone (TSH) receptor). Other causes include toxic nodular goitre (autonomously functioning thyroid nodules that secrete excess thyroid hormone), or drug-induced thyrotoxicosis.

Primary hyperthyroidism is more common in females than males and can be classified as either overt or subclinical; both of which may or may not be symptomatic. Overt hyperthyroidism is characterised by TSH levels below the reference range and free thyroxine (FT4) and/or free tri-iodothyronine (FT3) levels above the reference range. In subclinical hyperthyroidism, TSH is suppressed but FT4 and FT3 are within the reference range.

Thyrotoxicosis can also occur without hyperthyroidism; this is usually transient, and can occur due to excess intake of levothyroxine or over-the-counter supplements containing thyroid hormone, or thyroiditis.

Aims of treatment

Treatment aims to alleviate symptoms, align thyroid function tests within or close to the reference range, and to reduce the risk of long-term complications.

Non-drug treatment

[EvGr] Radioactive iodine or surgery (such as total thyroidectomy or hemithyroidectomy) may be considered by specialists in the management of Graves' disease or toxic nodular goitre. Whilst awaiting these treatments, antithyroid drugs should be offered to control hyperthyroidism, see *Graves' disease* and *Toxic nodular goitre* in *Primary hyperthyroidism*. ⓐ

Primary Hyperthyroidism

[EvGr] Patients with symptoms of thyroid storm should be treated as a medical emergency. Refer patients urgently to an endocrinologist if a pituitary or hypothalamic disorder is suspected, and refer or discuss with an endocrinologist all patients with new-onset hyperthyroidism (base urgency on clinical judgement). If malignancy is suspected, refer patients using a suspected cancer pathway.

Explain to patients, and their family or carers if appropriate, that:
● Some patients may feel well even when their thyroid function tests are outside the reference range;
● Even when they have no symptoms, treatment may be advised to reduce the risk of long-term complications;
● Symptoms may lag behind treatment changes for several weeks to months.

Consider antithyroid drugs alongside supportive treatment (for example, beta-blockers) for patients with hyperthyroidism awaiting specialist assessment and further treatment. Carbimazole p. 814 is the recommended choice of antithyroid drug, with propylthiouracil p. 815 considered for those in whom carbimazole is unsuitable. For further information, see *Graves' disease* and *Toxic nodular goitre*.

Before starting antithyroid drugs, check full blood count and liver function tests. ⓐ

The MHRA/CHM have released important safety information regarding the use of carbimazole p. 814 and the risk of acute pancreatitis. For further information, see *Important safety information* for carbimazole below.

For guidance on follow up and monitoring of hyperthyroidism, see NICE guideline: **Thyroid disease** (see *Useful resources*).

Graves' disease

EvGr Under specialist care, radioactive iodine is recommended as first-line definitive treatment unless it is unsuitable or remission is likely to be achieved with antithyroid drugs. For patients in whom an antithyroid drug is likely to achieve remission (such as in mild and uncomplicated cases), a choice of either carbimazole below or radioactive iodine should be offered. Carbimazole below should be offered as first-line definitive treatment if radioactive iodine and surgery are unsuitable treatment options.

Offer carbimazole below as a 12–18 month course using either a block and replace regimen (combination of fixed high-dose carbimazole with levothyroxine sodium p. 817), or a titration regimen (dose based on thyroid function tests), and review the need for further treatment. If patients have persistent or relapsed hyperthyroidism despite antithyroid drug treatment, consider radioactive iodine or surgery.

Consider propylthiouracil for patients who experience side-effects to carbimazole below, are pregnant or are trying to conceive within the following 6 months, or have a history of pancreatitis.

If agranulocytosis develops during antithyroid treatment, stop and do not restart treatment. Ⓐ

Toxic nodular goitre

EvGr Under specialist care, radioactive iodine is recommended as first-line definitive treatment for patients with hyperthyroidism secondary to multiple nodules; offer total thyroidectomy or life-long antithyroid drugs if radioactive iodine is unsuitable. For patients with hyperthyroidism secondary to a single nodule, offer radioactive iodine or surgery (hemithyroidectomy) as first-line definitive treatment; if these options are unsuitable, offer life-long antithyroid drugs. Consider treatment with a titration regimen of carbimazole below when offering life-long antithyroid drugs.

Consider propylthiouracil for patients who experience side-effects to carbimazole, are pregnant or are trying to conceive within the following 6 months, or have a history of pancreatitis.

If agranulocytosis develops during antithyroid treatment, stop and do not restart treatment. Ⓐ

Subclinical hyperthyroidism

EvGr For patients who have 2 TSH readings lower than 0.1 mIU/litre at least 3 months apart and evidence of thyroid disease or symptoms of thyrotoxicosis, consider seeking specialist advice.

Consider measuring TSH every 6 months for patients with untreated subclinical hyperthyroidism. For further information on monitoring in subclinical hyperthyroidism, see NICE guideline: **Thyroid disease** (see *Useful resources*). Ⓐ

Thyrotoxicosis without hyperthyroidism

EvGr Transient thyrotoxicosis without hyperthyroidism usually only needs supportive treatment (for example, beta-blockers). Ⓐ

Hyperthyroidism in pregnancy

EvGr Females with hyperthyroidism who are planning a pregnancy should be referred to an endocrinologist and advised to use effective contraception until specialist advice has been sought; advise patients to seek immediate medical advice if pregnancy is suspected or confirmed. All pregnant females should be referred urgently to a specialist. If there is uncertainty whether current antithyroid drug treatment should be continued or changed, or if the patient has adrenergic symptoms (such as tremor or tachycardia), seek urgent advice from an endocrinologist whilst awaiting specialist assessment. Pregnant females with severe signs and symptoms of hyperthyroidism (such as thyroid storm) should be admitted to hospital. Females who have recently received radioactive iodine should be advised to avoid becoming pregnant for at least 6 months after treatment. Ⓐ

The MHRA/CHM have released important safety information regarding the use of carbimazole below, with strengthened advice on contraception due to an increased risk of congenital malformations. For further information, see *Conception and contraception, Pregnancy,* and *Important safety information* for carbimazole below.

Useful Resources

Thyroid disease: assessment and management. National Institute for Health and Care Excellence. NICE guideline 145. November 2019, updated February 2020.
www.nice.org.uk/guidance/ng145

> **Other drugs used for Hyperthyroidism** Metoprolol tartrate, p. 169 · Nadolol, p. 164 · Propranolol hydrochloride, p. 164

ANTITHYROID DRUGS › SULFUR-CONTAINING IMIDAZOLES

Carbimazole

02-Sep-2020

● **INDICATIONS AND DOSE**

Hyperthyroidism

▸ BY MOUTH

▸ **Adult:** 15–40 mg daily continue until the patient becomes euthyroid, usually after 4 to 8 weeks, higher doses should be prescribed under specialist supervision only, then reduced to 5–15 mg daily, reduce dose gradually, therapy usually given for 12 to 18 months

Hyperthyroidism (blocking-replacement regimen) in combination with levothyroxine

▸ BY MOUTH

▸ **Adult:** 40–60 mg daily, therapy usually given for 18 months

DOSE EQUIVALENCE AND CONVERSION

▸ When substituting, carbimazole 1 mg is considered equivalent to propylthiouracil 10 mg but the dose may need adjusting according to response.

> **IMPORTANT SAFETY INFORMATION**
>
> NEUTROPENIA AND AGRANULOCYTOSIS
> Manufacturer advises of the importance of recognising bone marrow suppression induced by carbimazole and the need to stop treatment promptly.
> ● Patient should be asked to report symptoms and signs suggestive of infection, especially sore throat.
> ● A white blood cell count should be performed if there is any clinical evidence of infection.
> ● Carbimazole should be stopped promptly if there is clinical or laboratory evidence of neutropenia.
>
> MHRA/CHM ADVICE: CARBIMAZOLE: INCREASED RISK OF CONGENITAL MALFORMATIONS; STRENGTHENED ADVICE ON CONTRACEPTION (FEBRUARY 2019)
> Carbimazole is associated with an increased risk of congenital malformations when used during pregnancy, especially in the first trimester and at high doses (daily dose of 15 mg or more).
> Women of childbearing potential should use effective contraception during treatment with carbimazole. It should only be considered in pregnancy after a thorough benefit-risk assessment, and at the lowest effective dose without additional administration of thyroid

hormones—close maternal, fetal, and neonatal monitoring is recommended.

MHRA/CHM ADVICE: CARBIMAZOLE: RISK OF ACUTE PANCREATITIS (FEBRUARY 2019)
Cases of acute pancreatitis have been reported during treatment with carbimazole. It should be stopped immediately and permanently if acute pancreatitis occurs.

Carbimazole should not be used in patients with a history of acute pancreatitis associated with previous treatment—re-exposure may result in life-threatening acute pancreatitis with a decreased time to onset.

● CONTRA-INDICATIONS Severe blood disorders
● INTERACTIONS → Appendix 1: carbimazole
● SIDE-EFFECTS
▶ Rare or very rare Bone marrow disorders · haemolytic anaemia · severe cutaneous adverse reactions (SCARs) · thrombocytopenia
▶ Frequency not known Agranulocytosis · alopecia · angioedema · dyspepsia · eosinophilia · fever · gastrointestinal disorder · generalised lymphadenopathy · haemorrhage · headache · hepatic disorders · insulin autoimmune syndrome · leucopenia · malaise · myopathy · nausea · nerve disorders · neutropenia · pancreatitis acute (discontinue permanently) · salivary gland enlargement · skin reactions · taste loss
● CONCEPTION AND CONTRACEPTION The MHRA advises that females of childbearing potential should use effective contraception during treatment.
● PREGNANCY The MHRA advises consider use only after a thorough benefit-risk assessment. See *Important Safety Information* for further information.
● BREAST FEEDING Present in breast milk but this does not preclude breast-feeding as long as neonatal development is closely monitored and the lowest effective dose is used. Amount in milk may be sufficient to affect neonatal thyroid function therefore lowest effective dose should be used.
● HEPATIC IMPAIRMENT Manufacturer advises use with caution in mild to moderate insufficiency—half-life may be prolonged; avoid in severe insufficiency.
● PATIENT AND CARER ADVICE Warn patient or carers to tell doctor **immediately** if sore throat, mouth ulcers, bruising, fever, malaise, or non-specific illness develops.

● MEDICINAL FORMS There can be variation in the licensing of different medicines containing the same drug. Forms available from special-order manufacturers include: capsule, oral suspension, oral solution

Tablet
▶ Carbimazole (Non-proprietary)
   Carbimazole 5 mg Carbimazole 5mg tablets | 100 tablet [PoM] £84.80 DT = £3.81
   Carbimazole 10 mg Carbimazole 10mg tablets | 100 tablet [PoM] £104.08 DT = £81.32
   Carbimazole 15 mg Carbimazole 15mg tablets | 100 tablet [PoM] £156.13 DT = £127.03
   Carbimazole 20 mg Carbimazole 20mg tablets | 100 tablet [PoM] £208.17 DT = £15.65

ANTITHYROID DRUGS > THIOURACILS

Propylthiouracil

● **INDICATIONS AND DOSE**
Hyperthyroidism
▶ BY MOUTH
▶ Adult: Initially 200–400 mg daily in divided doses until the patient becomes euthyroid, then reduced to

50–150 mg daily in divided doses, initial dose should be gradually reduced to the maintenance dose

DOSE EQUIVALENCE AND CONVERSION
▶ When substituting, carbimazole 1 mg is considered equivalent to propylthiouracil 10 mg but the dose may need adjusting according to response.

● INTERACTIONS → Appendix 1: propylthiouracil
● SIDE-EFFECTS
▶ Rare or very rare Agranulocytosis · bone marrow disorders · glomerulonephritis acute · hearing impairment · leucopenia · thrombocytopenia · vomiting
▶ Frequency not known Alopecia · arthralgia · arthritis · encephalopathy · fever · gastrointestinal disorder · haemorrhage · headache · hepatic disorders · hypoprothrombinaemia · interstitial pneumonitis · lupus-like syndrome · lymphadenopathy · myopathy · nausea · nephritis · skin reactions · taste altered · vasculitis

SIDE-EFFECTS, FURTHER INFORMATION Severe hepatic reactions have been reported, including fatal cases and cases requiring liver transplant—discontinue if significant liver-enzyme abnormalities develop.

● PREGNANCY Propylthiouracil can be given but the blocking-replacement regimen is **not** suitable. Propylthiouracil crosses the placenta and in high doses may cause fetal goitre and hypothyroidism—the lowest dose that will control the hyperthyroid state should be used (requirements in Graves' disease tend to fall during pregnancy).
● BREAST FEEDING Present in breast milk but this does not preclude breast-feeding as long as neonatal development is closely monitored and the lowest effective dose is used. Amount in milk probably too small to affect infant; high doses may affect neonatal thyroid function.
  Monitoring Monitor infant's thyroid status.
● HEPATIC IMPAIRMENT Manufacturer advises caution (risk of increased half life).
  Dose adjustments Manufacturer advises consider dose reduction.
● RENAL IMPAIRMENT
  Dose adjustments Use three-quarters normal dose if eGFR 10–50 mL/minute/1.73 m^2.
  Use half normal dose if eGFR less than 10 mL/minute/1.73 m^2.
● MONITORING REQUIREMENTS Monitor for hepatotoxicity.
● PATIENT AND CARER ADVICE Patients should be told how to recognise signs of liver disorder and advised to seek prompt medical attention if symptoms such as anorexia, nausea, vomiting, fatigue, abdominal pain, jaundice, dark urine, or pruritus develop.

● MEDICINAL FORMS There can be variation in the licensing of different medicines containing the same drug. Forms available from special-order manufacturers include: oral suspension, oral solution

Tablet
▶ Propylthiouracil (Non-proprietary)
   Propylthiouracil 50 mg Propylthiouracil 50mg tablets | 56 tablet [PoM] £57.58 DT = £8.11 | 100 tablet [PoM] £14.48–£115.98

VITAMINS AND TRACE ELEMENTS

Iodide with iodine

(Lugol's Solution; Aqueous Iodine Oral Solution)

● **INDICATIONS AND DOSE**
Thyrotoxicosis (pre-operative)
▶ BY MOUTH USING ORAL SOLUTION
▶ Adult: 0.1–0.3 mL 3 times a day

continued →

6

Endocrine system

6

Endocrine system

DOSE EQUIVALENCE AND CONVERSION
▸ Doses based on the use of an aqueous oral solution containing iodine 50 mg/mL and potassium iodide 100 mg/mL.

- CAUTIONS Not for long-term treatment
- SIDE-EFFECTS Conjunctivitis · depression (long term use) · erectile dysfunction (long term use) · excessive tearing · headache · hypersensitivity · increased risk of infection · influenza like illness · insomnia (long term use) · rash · salivary gland pain
- PREGNANCY Neonatal goitre and hypothyroidism.
- BREAST FEEDING Stop breast-feeding. Danger of neonatal hypothyroidism or goitre. Appears to be concentrated in milk.
- DIRECTIONS FOR ADMINISTRATION For oral solution, dilute well with milk or water.

- MEDICINAL FORMS Forms available from special-order manufacturers include: oral solution

9.2 Hypothyroidism

Hypothyroidism

09-Dec-2019

Description of condition

Hypothyroidism results from the underproduction and secretion of thyroid hormones. Signs and symptoms of hypothyroidism include fatigue, weight gain, constipation, menstrual irregularities, depression, dry skin, intolerance to the cold, and reduced body and scalp hair. Complications include dyslipidaemia, coronary heart disease, heart failure, impaired fertility, pregnancy complications, impaired concentration and/or memory, and rarely myxoedema coma (which is a life-threatening medical emergency).

Primary hypothyroidism refers to when the condition arises from the thyroid gland and may be caused by iodine deficiency, autoimmune disease (such as Hashimoto's thyroiditis), radiotherapy, surgery or drugs, rather than due to a pituitary or hypothalamic disorder (secondary hypothyroidism).

Primary hypothyroidism is more common in females than males and can be classified as either overt or subclinical; both of which may or may not be symptomatic. Overt hypothyroidism is characterised by thyroid stimulating hormone (TSH) levels above the reference range and free thyroxine (FT4) levels below the reference range. In subclinical hypothyroidism, TSH levels are above the reference range but FT4 and free tri-iodothyronine (FT3) levels are within the reference range. In pregnancy, it is defined as overt based on elevated TSH levels (using trimester-specific reference ranges) regardless of FT4 levels.

Aims of treatment

The aims of treatment are to alleviate symptoms, align thyroid function tests within or close to the reference range, and to reduce the risk of long-term complications.

Management of primary hypothyroidism

EvGr Explain to patients, and their family or carers if appropriate, that:

- Some patients may feel well even when their thyroid function tests are outside the reference range;
- Even when they have no symptoms, treatment may be advised to reduce the risk of long-term complications;
- Symptoms may lag behind treatment changes for several weeks to months. Ⓐ

Overt hypothyroidism

EvGr Offer levothyroxine sodium p. 817 as first-line treatment and aim to maintain thyroid-stimulating hormone (TSH) levels within the reference range. If symptoms persist, even after achieving normal TSH levels, consider adjusting the dose to achieve optimal well-being whilst avoiding doses that cause TSH suppression or thyrotoxicosis.

For patients whose TSH level was very high before starting treatment or who have had a prolonged period of untreated disease, the TSH level can take up to 6 months to return to the reference range.

Consider measuring TSH levels every 3 months until a stable level has been achieved, then yearly thereafter. Monitoring free thyroxine (FT4) should also be considered in those who continue to be symptomatic.

Due to the uncertainty around the long-term adverse effects and the insufficient evidence of benefit over levothyroxine monotherapy, the use of natural thyroid extract is not recommended. Liothyronine (either alone or in combination with levothyroxine) is not routinely recommended for the same reasons. NHS England's specialist pharmacy service have produced guidance on the prescribing of liothyronine, for further information see: www.sps.nhs.uk/articles/updated-rmoc-guidance-prescribing-of-liothyronine/. Ⓐ

Subclinical hypothyroidism

EvGr When considering whether to start treatment for subclinical hypothyroidism, take into account features suggesting underlying thyroid disease.

For patients who have a TSH level of 10 mIU/L or higher on 2 separate occasions 3 months apart, consider levothyroxine sodium p. 817. If symptoms persist, even after achieving normal TSH levels, consider adjusting the dose to achieve optimal well-being whilst avoiding doses that cause TSH suppression or thyrotoxicosis.

For patients whose TSH level was very high before starting treatment or who have had a prolonged period of untreated disease, the TSH level can take up to 6 months to return to the reference range.

For patients in whom treatment is started, consider measuring TSH levels every 3 months until a stable level has been achieved, then yearly thereafter. Monitoring free thyroxine (FT4) should also be considered in those who continue to be symptomatic.

For symptomatic patients aged under 65 years with a TSH level above the reference range, but lower than 10 mIU/L on 2 separate occasions 3 months apart, consider a 6-month trial of levothyroxine sodium p. 817. If symptoms do not improve after starting levothyroxine, re-measure TSH and if the level remains elevated, adjust the dose. If symptoms persist when serum TSH is within the reference range, consider stopping levothyroxine and follow the recommendations on *Monitoring untreated subclinical hypothyroidism and monitoring after stopping treatment* in the NICE guideline: **Thyroid disease** (see *Useful resources*). Ⓐ

Management of secondary hypothyroidism

EvGr If secondary hypothyroidism is suspected, refer the patient urgently to an endocrinologist to assess the underlying cause. Ⓐ

Hypothyroidism in pregnancy

EvGr Refer all females with hypothyroidism who are planning a pregnancy or are pregnant, to an endocrinologist. For those planning a pregnancy and whose thyroid function tests (TFTs) are not within the reference range, advise delaying conception until stabilised on levothyroxine sodium p. 817 treatment. If there is any uncertainty about treatment initiation or dosing, discuss this with an endocrinologist whilst awaiting review.

TFTs may produce misleading results in pregnancy and trimester-related reference ranges should be used. If pregnancy is confirmed, urgently measure TFTs; discuss the initiation, or changes to levothyroxine sodium below treatment and TFT monitoring with an endocrinologist whilst awaiting review, to reduce the risk of obstetric and neonatal complications. Ⓐ

Useful Resources

Thyroid disease: assessment and management. National Institute for Health and Care Excellence. NICE guideline 145. November 2019, updated February 2020 www.nice.org.uk/guidance/ng145

THYROID HORMONES

| Levothyroxine sodium | 12-May-2020 |

(Thyroxine sodium)

● **INDICATIONS AND DOSE**
Primary hypothyroidism
▸ BY MOUTH
▸ **Adult:** Initially 1.6 micrograms/kg once daily, adjusted according to response, round dose to the nearest 25 micrograms, dose to be taken preferably 30–60 minutes before breakfast, caffeine-containing liquids (e.g. coffee, tea), or other medication
▸ **Elderly:** Initially 25–50 micrograms once daily; adjusted in steps of 25 micrograms every 4 weeks, adjusted according to response; maintenance 50–200 micrograms once daily, dose to be taken preferably 30–60 minutes before breakfast, caffeine-containing liquids (e.g. coffee, tea), or other medication

Primary hypothyroidism in patients with cardiac disease
▸ BY MOUTH
▸ **Adult:** Initially 25–50 micrograms once daily; adjusted in steps of 25 micrograms every 4 weeks, adjusted according to response; maintenance 50–200 micrograms once daily, dose to be taken preferably 30–60 minutes before breakfast, caffeine-containing liquids (e.g. coffee, tea), or other medication

Hyperthyroidism (blocking-replacement regimen) in combination with carbimazole
▸ BY MOUTH
▸ **Adult:** 50–150 micrograms daily therapy usually given for 18 months

● **UNLICENSED USE** [EvGr] Levothyroxine is used in the doses provided in the BNF for the treatment of primary hypothyroidism, Ⓐ but these may differ from those licensed.

● **CONTRA-INDICATIONS** Thyrotoxicosis

● **CAUTIONS** Cardiovascular disorders · diabetes insipidus · diabetes mellitus (dose of antidiabetic drugs including insulin may need to be increased) · elderly · hypertension · long-standing hypothyroidism · myocardial infarction · myocardial insufficiency · panhypopituitarism (initiate corticosteroid therapy before starting levothyroxine) · predisposition to adrenal insufficiency (initiate corticosteroid therapy before starting levothyroxine)

CAUTIONS, FURTHER INFORMATION
▸ Cardiovascular disorders Baseline ECG is valuable because changes induced by hypothyroidism can be confused with ischaemia.

● **INTERACTIONS** → Appendix 1: thyroid hormones

● **SIDE-EFFECTS** Angina pectoris · anxiety · arrhythmias · arthralgia · diarrhoea · dyspnoea · fever · flushing · headache · hyperhidrosis · insomnia · malaise · menstruation irregular · muscle spasms · muscle weakness · oedema · palpitations · skin reactions · thyrotoxic crisis · tremor · vomiting · weight decreased

SIDE-EFFECTS, FURTHER INFORMATION **Initial dosage in patients with cardiovascular disorders** If metabolism increases too rapidly (causing diarrhoea, nervousness, rapid pulse, insomnia, tremors and sometimes anginal pain where there is latent myocardial ischaemia), reduce dose or withhold for 1–2 days and start again at a lower dose.

● PREGNANCY Levothyroxine may cross the placenta. Excessive or insufficient maternal thyroid hormones can be detrimental to fetus.
Dose adjustments Levothyroxine requirement may increase during pregnancy.
Monitoring Assess maternal thyroid function before conception (if possible), at diagnosis of pregnancy, at antenatal booking, during both the second and third trimesters, and after delivery (more frequent monitoring required on initiation or adjustment of levothyroxine).

● BREAST FEEDING Amount too small to affect tests for neonatal hypothyroidism.

● **MONITORING REQUIREMENTS**
▸ When used for Primary hypothyroidism [EvGr] Consider measuring thyroid stimulating hormone (TSH) level every three months until stabilised (two similar measurements within the reference range, 3 months apart), then yearly thereafter. Consider measuring free thyroxine (FT4) if symptoms of hypothyroidism persist after starting levothyroxine. Ⓐ

● MEDICINAL FORMS There can be variation in the licensing of different medicines containing the same drug. Forms available from special-order manufacturers include: capsule, oral suspension, oral solution

Tablet
▸ Levothyroxine sodium (Non-proprietary)
Levothyroxine sodium anhydrous 12.5 microgram Levothyroxine sodium 12.5microgram tablets | 28 tablet [PoM] £12.49 DT = £12.48
Levothyroxine sodium anhydrous 25 microgram Levothyroxine sodium 25microgram tablets | 28 tablet [PoM] £3.05 DT = £1.53 | 500 tablet [PoM] £41.61–£54.46
Levothyroxine sodium 25microgram tablets lactose free | 100 tablet [PoM] 🅂
Levothyroxine sodium anhydrous 50 microgram Levothyroxine sodium 50microgram tablets lactose free | 100 tablet [PoM] 🅂
Levothyroxine sodium 50microgram tablets | 28 tablet [PoM] £1.50 DT = £1.21 | 1000 tablet [PoM] £35.36–£48.00
Levothyroxine sodium anhydrous 75 microgram Levothyroxine sodium 75microgram tablets | 28 tablet [PoM] £4.00 DT = £3.07
Levothyroxine sodium anhydrous 100 microgram Levothyroxine sodium 100microgram tablets lactose free | 100 tablet [PoM] 🅂
Levothyroxine sodium 100microgram tablets | 28 tablet [PoM] £1.77 DT = £1.24 | 1000 tablet [PoM] £35.36–£48.00
▸ Eltroxin (Advanz Pharma)
Levothyroxine sodium anhydrous 25 microgram Eltroxin 25microgram tablets | 28 tablet [PoM] £2.54 DT = £1.53
Levothyroxine sodium anhydrous 50 microgram Eltroxin 50microgram tablets | 28 tablet [PoM] £1.77 DT = £1.21
Levothyroxine sodium anhydrous 100 microgram Eltroxin 100microgram tablets | 28 tablet [PoM] £1.78 DT = £1.24

Oral solution
▸ Levothyroxine sodium (Non-proprietary)
Levothyroxine sodium anhydrous 5 microgram per 1 ml Levothyroxine sodium 25micrograms/5ml oral solution sugar free sugar-free | 100 ml [PoM] £118.63 DT = £94.99
Levothyroxine sodium anhydrous 10 microgram per 1 ml Levothyroxine sodium 50micrograms/5ml oral solution sugar free sugar-free | 100 ml [PoM] £96.36 DT = £94.63
Levothyroxine sodium anhydrous 20 microgram per 1 ml Levothyroxine sodium 100micrograms/5ml oral solution sugar free sugar-free | 100 ml [PoM] £165.00 DT = £164.99
Levothyroxine sodium anhydrous 25 microgram per 1 ml Levothyroxine sodium 125micrograms/5ml oral solution sugar free sugar-free | 100 ml [PoM] £185.00 DT = £185.00

Capsule
▸ Tirosint (Imported (United States))
Levothyroxine sodium anhydrous 25 microgram Tirosint 25microgram capsules | 28 capsule [PoM] 🅂

6

Endocrine system

Levothyroxine sodium anhydrous 50 microgram Tirosint
50microgram capsules | 28 capsule [PoM] Ⓢ
Levothyroxine sodium anhydrous 100 microgram Tirosint
100microgram capsules | 28 capsule [PoM] Ⓢ

Liothyronine sodium

08-Jul-2019

(L-Tri-iodothyronine sodium)

● **INDICATIONS AND DOSE**

Hypothyroidism

▶ **BY MOUTH**
▶ Adult: Initially 10–20 micrograms daily; increased to
60 micrograms daily in 2–3 divided doses, dose should
be increased gradually, smaller initial doses given for
the elderly

Hypothyroid coma

▶ **BY SLOW INTRAVENOUS INJECTION**
▶ Adult: 5–20 micrograms every 12 hours, increased to
5–20 micrograms every 4 hours if required,
alternatively initially 50 micrograms for 1 dose, then
25 micrograms every 8 hours, reduced to
25 micrograms twice daily

DOSE EQUIVALENCE AND CONVERSION

▶ 20–25 micrograms of liothyronine sodium is equivalent
to approximately 100 micrograms of levothyroxine
sodium.
▶ Brands without a UK licence may not be bioequivalent
and dose adjustment may be necessary.

● **CONTRA-INDICATIONS** Thyrotoxicosis

● **CAUTIONS** Cardiovascular disorders · diabetes insipidus ·
diabetes mellitus (dose of antidiabetic drugs including
insulin may need to be increased) · elderly · hypertension ·
long-standing hypothyroidism · myocardial infarction ·
myocardial insufficiency · panhypopituitarism (initiate
corticosteroid therapy before starting liothyronine) ·
predisposition to adrenal insufficiency (initiate
corticosteroid therapy before starting liothyronine)

CAUTIONS, FURTHER INFORMATION

▶ Cardiovascular disorders Baseline ECG is valuable because
changes induced by hypothyroidism can be confused with
ischaemia.

● **INTERACTIONS** → Appendix 1: thyroid hormones

● **SIDE-EFFECTS**

GENERAL SIDE-EFFECTS

Angina pectoris · anxiety · arrhythmias · diarrhoea · fever ·
flushing · headache · hyperhidrosis · insomnia · muscle
cramps · muscle weakness · palpitations · tremor · vomiting
· weight decreased

SPECIFIC SIDE-EFFECTS

▶ With intravenous use Menstruation irregular
▶ With oral use Heat intolerance

SIDE-EFFECTS, FURTHER INFORMATION **Initial dosage in
patients with cardiovascular disorders** If metabolism
increases too rapidly (causing diarrhoea, nervousness,
rapid pulse, insomnia, tremors and sometimes anginal
pain where there is latent myocardial ischaemia), reduce
dose or withhold for 1–2 days and start again at a lower
dose.

● **PREGNANCY** Does not cross the placenta in significant
amounts. Excessive or insufficient maternal thyroid
hormones can be detrimental to fetus.
Dose adjustments Liothyronine requirement may increase
during pregnancy.
Monitoring Assess maternal thyroid function before
conception (if possible), at diagnosis of pregnancy, at
antenatal booking, during both the second and third
trimesters, and after delivery (more frequent monitoring
required on initiation or adjustment of liothyronine).

● **BREAST FEEDING** Amount too small to affect tests for
neonatal hypothyroidism.

● **PRESCRIBING AND DISPENSING INFORMATION**
Switching to a different brand Patients switched to a different
brand should be monitored (particularly if pregnant or if
heart disease present) as brands without a UK licence may
not be bioequivalent. Pregnant women or those with heart
disease should undergo an early review of thyroid status,
and other patients should have thyroid function assessed if
experiencing a significant change in symptoms. If
liothyronine is continued long-term, thyroid function tests
should be repeated 1–2 months after any change in brand.

● **MEDICINAL FORMS** There can be variation in the licensing of
different medicines containing the same drug. Forms available
from special-order manufacturers include: tablet, capsule, oral
suspension, oral solution, solution for injection

Tablet

▶ Liothyronine sodium (Non-proprietary)
Liothyronine sodium 5 microgram Liothyronine 5microgram
tablets | 28 tablet [PoM] £98.00 DT = £98.00
Liothyronine sodium 10 microgram Liothyronine 10microgram
tablets | 28 tablet [PoM] £148.00 DT = £148.00
Liothyronine sodium 20 microgram Liothyronine 20microgram
tablets | 28 tablet [PoM] £245.29 DT = £121.19
▶ Cytomel (Imported (United States))
Liothyronine sodium 25 microgram Cytomel 25microgram tablets
| 100 tablet [PoM] Ⓢ

Powder for solution for injection

▶ Liothyronine sodium (Non-proprietary)
Liothyronine sodium 20 microgram Liothyronine 20microgram
powder for solution for injection vials | 5 vial [PoM] £1,567.50 DT =
£1,567.50

Chapter 7
Genito-urinary system

CONTENTS

1 Bladder and urinary disorders

1.1 Urinary frequency, enuresis, and incontinence

Urinary incontinence and pelvic organ prolapse in women
16-Jun-2019

Description of condition

Urinary incontinence is the involuntary leakage of urine and can range in severity and nature. It can impact the person, as well as their families and carers, and can be detrimental to an individual's physical, psychological, and social well-being. Urinary incontinence can be the result of functional abnormalities in the lower urinary tract, or due to other illnesses. It can be sub-classified into four main types: stress, urgency, mixed, and overflow incontinence.

Stress incontinence is the involuntary leakage on effort or exertion, or on sneezing or coughing, and is associated with the loss of pelvic floor support and/or damage to the urethral sphincter.

Urgency incontinence is involuntary leakage which is accompanied, or immediately preceded by a sudden compelling desire to pass urine that is difficult to delay. It is often part of a larger symptom complex known as overactive bladder syndrome. This syndrome is defined as urinary urgency, which may or may not be accompanied by urgency incontinence, but is usually associated with increased frequency and nocturia. The symptoms are thought to be caused by involuntary contractions of the detrusor muscle.

Mixed incontinence is involuntary leakage associated with both urgency and stress, however, one type tends to be predominant.

Overflow incontinence is a complication of chronic urinary retention and occurs when a person cannot empty their bladder completely and it becomes over distended. This may result in continuous, or frequent loss of small quantities of urine. For further information, see Urinary retention p. 826.

Other types include continuous urinary incontinence, where there is constant leakage of urine which may be due to the severity of the persons' condition or may be due to an underlying cause, such as a fistula. Incontinence may also be situational, for example during sexual intercourse or when a person is giggling.

The main risk factor for developing any type of incontinence is older age; this is due to the physiological changes that occur with natural aging. Some other risk factors for *stress* incontinence include pregnancy, vaginal delivery, obesity, constipation, family history, smoking, lack of supporting tissue (such as in prolapse or hysterectomy) and use of some drugs such as ACE inhibitors (can cause cough) and alpha-adrenergic blockers (relax the bladder outlet and urethra).

Some conditions can increase detrusor muscle overactivity and therefore worsen *urgency* incontinence. These include conditions that affect the lower urinary tract such as; Urinary-tract infections p. 626, urinary obstruction, or oestrogen deficiency, those affecting the nervous system such as; stroke, dementia, and Parkinson's disease, and systemic conditions such as; diabetes mellitus or hypercalcaemia. Side-effects of some drugs may also increase detrusor muscle overactivity or indirectly contribute to urgency incontinence; these include cholinesterase inhibitors, drugs that cause constipation, and those with anticholinergic effects. Diuretics, alcohol, and caffeine all increase urine production and can cause polyuria, frequency, urgency, and nocturia.

Aims of treatment

Manage urinary incontinence and the symptoms of overactive bladder syndrome.

Non-drug treatment

EvGr Women with urinary incontinence should modify their fluid intake, and if their BMI is 30 kg/m^2 or greater, be advised to lose weight. For those with an overactive bladder, a reduction in caffeine intake should be trialled.

Absorbent products, hand-held urinals and toileting aids should not be used to treat urinary incontinence, unless the person has severe cognitive or mobility impairment that may prevent further treatment. They may be used in some women as a coping strategy whilst awaiting treatment, as an adjunct to ongoing therapy, or as long-term management after all treatment options have been considered; their use should be reviewed at least annually. Intravaginal and intraurethral devices should only be used when required to prevent leakage at specific times, for example during exercise.

Surgical management may be an option for some women and will depend on a number of factors. Discussion around the details of the procedures and subsequent shared decision making should be carried out. Ⓐ

Urgency incontinence
[EvGr] Women should be offered bladder training for at least 6 weeks as first-line treatment. If frequency is a problem and satisfactory benefit from bladder training is not achieved, drug treatment for an overactive bladder should be added. Ⓐ

Stress incontinence
[EvGr] Women should trial supervised pelvic floor muscle training for at least 3 months, which should include at least 8 contractions performed 3 times per day. Ⓐ

Mixed incontinence
[EvGr] Women should trial both bladder training for at least 6 weeks and supervised pelvic floor muscle training for at least 3 months, which should include at least 8 contractions performed 3 times per day. If frequency is a problem and satisfactory benefit from bladder training is not achieved, drug treatment for an overactive bladder should be added. Ⓐ

Drug treatment

[EvGr] When considering drug treatment in women with incontinence exclude any possible causes, including drugs or conditions that may exacerbate incontinence or overactive bladder.

A urine dipstick test should be performed in all women presenting with incontinence to test for active infection or haematuria, and analysed along with the patients symptoms. For further information, see Urinary-tract infections p. 626. Women should be referred to a specialist if there is:
- persistent bladder or urethral pain;
- pelvic mass that is clinically benign;
- associated faecal incontinence;
- suspected neurological disease, or urogenital fistulae;
- history of previous incontinence surgery, pelvic cancer surgery or pelvic radiation damage;
- recurrent or persistant UTI for those aged over 60; Ⓐ see Urinary-tract infections p. 626
- [EvGr] palpable bladder after voiding, or symptoms of voiding difficulty.

Urgent referral should occur in women aged 45 years or older if there is unexplained visible haematuria without UTI, or visible haematuria persisting or recurring despite successful treatment of UTI. Urgent referral is also required in women aged 60 years or older with unexplained non-visible haematuria and either dysuria or raised white cell count. Ⓐ

Urgency incontinence
[EvGr] An anticholinergic drug should be considered for women who have trialled bladder training, where frequency is a problem and symptoms persist. Consider the total anticholinergic load, coexisting conditions, such as cognitive impairment or poor bladder emptying, and the risk of side-effects when offering anticholinergic medicine. When prescribing an anticholinergic in those with dementia, see Dementia p. 316. Immediate release oxybutynin hydrochloride p. 822, immediate release tolterodine tartrate p. 824, or darifenacin p. 821 can be used first-line. Immediate release oxybutynin should not be used in frail, older women at risk of sudden deterioration in their physical or mental health. The lowest dose should be used and titrated upwards if necessary. *Transdermal* oxybutynin

hydrochloride p. 822 may be used in those unable to tolerate oral treatment. Mirabegron p. 825 may be used if treatment with an anticholinergic is contra-indicated, ineffective, or not tolerated, for further information, see *National funding/access decisions* in mirabegron.

Treatment should be reviewed after 4 weeks, or sooner if required. If treatment is effective review the woman again at 12 weeks, then annually thereafter, or every 6 months if the woman is over 75 years of age. If treatment has not been effective or is not tolerated an alternative anticholinergic drug can be used, the current dose adjusted or, mirabegron trialled; review again after 4 weeks. Alternative anticholinergics include, an untried first-line drug, or one of the following; fesoterodine fumarate p. 822, propiverine hydrochloride p. 823, solifenacin succinate p. 824, trospium chloride p. 825, or an *extended release* formulation of either oxybutynin hydrochloride or tolterodine tartrate. Women who have tried taking medicine for overactive bladder, but treatment has failed, should be referred to secondary care, where treatment with botulinum toxin type A p. 428 or surgical methods may be considered.

Flavoxate hydrochloride p. 822, propantheline bromide p. 94, or imipramine hydrochloride p. 396 should not be used as treatment options.

In women who have troublesome nocturia, desmopressin p. 706 may also be used. *Intravaginal* oestrogen therapy can be used in those women who are post-menopausal and have vaginal atrophy. Treatment with an intravaginal oestrogen should be reviewed at least annually to re-assess the need for continued treatment and monitor for symptoms of endometrial hyperplasia or carcinoma. Ⓐ

Stress incontinence
[EvGr] Duloxetine p. 387 is **not** recommended as first-line treatment for women with stress incontinence. It may be used second-line where conservative treatment including pelvic floor training has failed, and only if surgery is not appropriate or the woman prefers pharmacological treatment, but should not be offered routinely. Ⓐ

Mixed incontinence
Women with mixed urinary incontinence should be treated according to the predominant type, refer to *Urgency incontinence* or *Stress incontinence* for drug treatment options.

Pelvic organ prolapse

Pelvic organ prolapse is the symptomatic descent of part of the wall of the vagina or uterus. Symptoms can include a vaginal bulge or sensation of something coming down, urinary, bowel and sexual symptoms, and pelvic and back pain. These can all affect a woman's quality of life.

[EvGr] Women who present to primary care with symptoms, or an incidental finding of vaginal prolapse should be examined to rule out pelvic mass or other pathology, and a full history taken. Treatment preferences should be discussed and referral made where necessary. Women in secondary care should be considered for referral to a clinician with expertise in prolapse if experiencing incidental symptoms, or on incidental finding of vaginal prolapse. A validated pelvic floor symptom questionnaire may aid assessment and decision making.

Women should be given advice on minimising heavy lifting, preventing or treating constipation, and if their BMI is 30 kg/m² or greater, encouraged to lose weight. A programme of supervised pelvic floor muscle training for at least 16 weeks may also be tried for some women.

A vaginal oestrogen may be used for women with prolapse and signs of vaginal atrophy, an oestrogen-releasing ring may be more appropriate for those women who have cognitive or physical impairments.

A vaginal pessary may be used alone, or in conjunction with pelvic floor muscle training for those with symptomatic pelvic organ prolapse. Surgical management may be required in women whose symptoms have not improved with non-surgical methods, or who have declined non-surgical treatment. Ⓐ

Nocturnal enuresis in children

23-May-2017

Description of condition

Nocturnal enuresis is the involuntary discharge of urine during sleep, which is common in young children. Children are generally expected to be dry by a developmental age of 5 years, and historically it has been common practice to consider children for treatment only when they reach 7 years; however, symptoms may still persist in a small proportion by the age of 10 years.

Treatment

Children under 5 years
EvGr For children under 5 years, treatment is usually unnecessary as the condition is likely to resolve spontaneously. Reassurance and advice can be useful for some families. Ⓐ

Non Drug Treatment
EvGr Initially, advice should be given on fluid intake, diet, toileting behaviour, and use of reward systems. For children who do not respond to this advice (more than 1–2 wet beds per week), an enuresis alarm should be the recommended treatment for motivated, well-supported children. Alarms in children under 7 years should be considered depending on the child's maturity, motivation and understanding of the alarm. Alarms have a lower relapse rate than drug treatment when discontinued.

Treatment using an alarm should be reviewed after 4 weeks and continued until a minimum of 2 weeks' uninterrupted dry nights have been achieved. If complete dryness is not achieved after 3 months but the condition is still improving and the child remains motivated to use the alarm, it is recommended to continue the treatment. Combined treatment with desmopressin p. 706, or the use of desmopressin alone, is recommended if the initial alarm treatment is unsuccessful or it is no longer appropriate or desirable. Ⓐ

Drug Treatment
EvGr Treatment with oral or sublingual desmopressin is recommended for children over 5 years of age when alarm use is inappropriate or undesirable, or when rapid or short-term results are the priority (for example, to cover periods away from home). Desmopressin alone can also be used if there has been a partial response to a combination of desmopressin and an alarm following initial treatment with an alarm alone. Treatment should be assessed after 4 weeks and continued for 3 months if there are signs of response. Repeated courses of desmopressin can be used in responsive children who experience repeated recurrences of bedwetting, but should be withdrawn **gradually** at regular intervals (for 1 week every 3 months) for full reassessment.

Under specialist supervision, nocturnal enuresis associated with daytime symptoms (overactive bladder) can be managed with desmopressin alone or in combination with an antimuscarinic drug (such as oxybutynin hydrochloride p. 822 or tolterodine tartrate p. 824 [unlicensed indication]). Treatment should be continued for 3 months; the course can be repeated if necessary.

The tricyclic antidepressant imipramine hydrochloride p. 396 can be considered for children who have not responded to all other treatments and have undergone specialist assessment, however relapse is common after withdrawal and children and their carers should be aware of the dangers of overdose. Initial treatment should continue for 3 months; further courses can be considered following a medical review every 3 months. Tricyclic antidepressants should be withdrawn gradually. Ⓐ

Useful Resources

Bedwetting in under 19s. National Institute for Health and Care Excellence. Clinical guideline CG111. October 2010. www.nice.org.uk/guidance/cg111

ANTIMUSCARINICS

Antimuscarinics (systemic)

- CONTRA-INDICATIONS Angle-closure glaucoma · gastro-intestinal obstruction · intestinal atony · myasthenia gravis (but some antimuscarinics may be used to decrease muscarinic side-effects of anticholinesterases) · paralytic ileus · pyloric stenosis · severe ulcerative colitis · significant bladder outflow obstruction · toxic megacolon · urinary retention
- CAUTIONS Acute myocardial infarction (in adults) · arrhythmias (may be worsened) · autonomic neuropathy · cardiac insufficiency (due to association with tachycardia) · cardiac surgery (due to association with tachycardia) · children (increased risk of side-effects) · conditions characterised by tachycardia · congestive heart failure (may be worsened) · coronary artery disease (may be worsened) · diarrhoea · elderly (especially if frail) · gastro-oesophageal reflux disease · hiatus hernia with reflux oesophagitis · hypertension · hyperthyroidism (due to association with tachycardia) · individuals susceptible to angle-closure glaucoma · prostatic hyperplasia · pyrexia · ulcerative colitis

CAUTIONS, FURTHER INFORMATION
▸ Elderly Prescription potentially inappropriate (STOPP criteria):
  - to treat extrapyramidal side-effects of antipsychotic medications (risk of antimuscarinic toxicity)
  - with delirium or dementia (risk of exacerbation of cognitive impairment), narrow-angle glaucoma (risk of acute exacerbation of glaucoma), or chronic prostatism (risk of urinary retention)
  - if two or more antimuscarinic drugs prescribed concomitantly (risk of increased antimuscarinic toxicity)
  See also Prescribing in the elderly p. 33.

- SIDE-EFFECTS
▸ Common or very common Constipation · dizziness · drowsiness · dry mouth · dyspepsia · flushing · headache · nausea · palpitations · skin reactions · tachycardia · urinary disorders · vision disorders · vomiting
▸ Rare or very rare Angioedema · confusion (more common in elderly)
- PATIENT AND CARER ADVICE
  Driving and skilled tasks Antimuscarinics can affect the performance of skilled tasks (e.g. driving).

ANTIMUSCARINICS ❯ URINARY

▸ᴳ above

Darifenacin
13-May-2020

- INDICATIONS AND DOSE
  Urinary frequency | Urinary urgency | Incontinence
  ▸ BY MOUTH
  ▸ Adult: Initially 7.5 mg once daily, increased if necessary to 15 mg after 2 weeks

- INTERACTIONS → Appendix 1: darifenacin
- SIDE-EFFECTS
▸ Common or very common Abdominal pain · dry eye · nasal dryness

7

Genito-urinary system

Genito-urinary system

7

▸ **Uncommon** Asthenia · bladder pain · cough · diarrhoea · dyspnoea · erectile dysfunction · flatulence · hyperhidrosis · hypertension · increased risk of infection · injury · insomnia · oedema · oral ulceration · taste altered · thinking abnormal · urinary tract disorder

● PREGNANCY Manufacturer advises avoid—toxicity in *animal* studies.

● BREAST FEEDING Present in milk in *animal* studies—manufacturer advises caution.

● HEPATIC IMPAIRMENT Manufacturer advises caution in moderate impairment; avoid in severe impairment (risk of increased exposure).
Dose adjustments Manufacturer advises maximum 7.5 mg daily in moderate impairment.

● PRESCRIBING AND DISPENSING INFORMATION The need for continuing therapy for urinary incontinence should be reviewed every 4–6 weeks until symptoms stabilise, and then every 6–12 months.

● MEDICINAL FORMS There can be variation in the licensing of different medicines containing the same drug.
Modified-release tablet
CAUTIONARY AND ADVISORY LABELS 3, 25
▸ Emselex (Norgine Pharmaceuticals Ltd)
Darifenacin (as Darifenacin hydrobromide) 7.5 mg Emselex 7.5mg modified-release tablets | 28 tablet [PoM] £25.48 DT = £25.48
Darifenacin (as Darifenacin hydrobromide) 15 mg Emselex 15mg modified-release tablets | 28 tablet [PoM] £25.48 DT = £25.48

F 821

Fesoterodine fumarate

06-Nov-2020

● INDICATIONS AND DOSE

Urinary frequency | Urinary urgency | Urge incontinence
▸ BY MOUTH
▸ Adult: 4 mg once daily, increased if necessary up to 8 mg once daily

DOSE ADJUSTMENTS DUE TO INTERACTIONS
▸ Manufacturer advises max. 4 mg daily with concurrent use of potent inhibitors of CYP3A4; avoid concurrent use in patients who also have hepatic or renal impairment.
▸ For dose adjustments with concurrent use of moderate inhibitors of CYP3A4 in patients with hepatic or renal impairment, consult product literature.

● INTERACTIONS → Appendix 1: fesoterodine

● SIDE-EFFECTS
▸ **Common or very common** Diarrhoea · dry eye · gastrointestinal discomfort · insomnia · throat complaints
▸ **Uncommon** Cough · fatigue · gastrointestinal disorders · nasal dryness · taste altered · urinary tract infection · vertigo

● PREGNANCY Manufacturer advises avoid—toxicity in *animal* studies.

● BREAST FEEDING Manufacturer advises avoid—no information available.

● HEPATIC IMPAIRMENT Manufacturer advises caution in mild to moderate impairment; avoid in severe impairment (no information available).
Dose adjustments Manufacturer advises increase dose cautiously in mild impairment; maximum 4 mg daily in moderate impairment.

● RENAL IMPAIRMENT
Dose adjustments Increase dose cautiously if eGFR 30–80 mL/minute/1.73m^2; max. 4 mg daily if eGFR less than 30 mL/minute/1.73m^2.

● PRESCRIBING AND DISPENSING INFORMATION The need for continuing therapy for urinary incontinence should be reviewed every 4–6 weeks until symptoms stabilise, and then every 6–12 months.

● NATIONAL FUNDING/ACCESS DECISIONS
For full details see funding body website
Scottish Medicines Consortium (SMC) decisions
▸ Fesoterodine fumarate (*Toviaz*®) for treatment of the symptoms of increased urinary frequency (and/or urgency incontinence) that may occur in patients with overactive bladder (OAB) syndrome (July 2008) SMC No. 480/08 Recommended with restrictions

● MEDICINAL FORMS There can be variation in the licensing of different medicines containing the same drug.
Modified-release tablet
CAUTIONARY AND ADVISORY LABELS 3, 25
▸ Toviaz (Pfizer Ltd)
Fesoterodine fumarate 4 mg Toviaz 4mg modified-release tablets | 28 tablet [PoM] £25.78 DT = £25.78
Fesoterodine fumarate 8 mg Toviaz 8mg modified-release tablets | 28 tablet [PoM] £25.78 DT = £25.78

F 821

Flavoxate hydrochloride

13-May-2020

● INDICATIONS AND DOSE

Urinary frequency | Urinary incontinence | Dysuria | Urinary urgency | Bladder spasm due to catheterisation, cytoscopy, or surgery
▸ BY MOUTH
▸ Adult: 200 mg 3 times a day

● CONTRA-INDICATIONS Gastro-intestinal haemorrhage

● INTERACTIONS → Appendix 1: flavoxate

● SIDE-EFFECTS Diarrhoea · dysphagia · eosinophilia · fatigue · hyperpyrexia · hypersensitivity · leucopenia · nervousness · vertigo

● PREGNANCY Manufacturer advises avoid unless no safer alternative.

● BREAST FEEDING Manufacturer advises caution—no information available.

● PRESCRIBING AND DISPENSING INFORMATION The need for continuing therapy for urinary incontinence should be reviewed every 4–6 weeks until symptoms stabilise, and then every 6–12 months.

● MEDICINAL FORMS There can be variation in the licensing of different medicines containing the same drug. Forms available from special-order manufacturers include: oral suspension, oral solution
Tablet
CAUTIONARY AND ADVISORY LABELS 3
▸ Urispas (Recordati Pharmaceuticals Ltd)
Flavoxate hydrochloride 200 mg Urispas 200 tablets | 90 tablet [PoM] £11.67 DT = £11.67

F 821

Oxybutynin hydrochloride

12-Nov-2020

● INDICATIONS AND DOSE

Urinary frequency | Urinary urgency | Urinary incontinence | Neurogenic bladder instability
▸ BY MOUTH USING IMMEDIATE-RELEASE MEDICINES
▸ Child 5-11 years: Initially 2.5–3 mg twice daily, increased to 5 mg 2–3 times a day
▸ Child 12-17 years: Initially 5 mg 2–3 times a day, increased if necessary up to 5 mg 4 times a day
▸ Adult: Initially 5 mg 2–3 times a day, increased if necessary up to 5 mg 4 times a day
▸ Elderly: Initially 2.5–3 mg twice daily, increased if tolerated to 5 mg twice daily, adjusted according to response

▸ BY MOUTH USING MODIFIED-RELEASE TABLETS
▸ Child 5–17 years: Initially 5 mg once daily, adjusted in steps of 5 mg every week, adjusted according to response; maximum 15 mg per day
▸ Adult: Initially 5 mg once daily, increased in steps of 5 mg every week, adjusted according to response; maximum 20 mg per day

Urinary frequency | Urinary urgency | Urinary incontinence
▸ BY TRANSDERMAL APPLICATION USING PATCHES
▸ Adult: Apply 1 patch twice weekly, patch is to be applied to clean, dry unbroken skin on abdomen, hip or buttock. Patch should be removed every 3–4 days and site replacement patch on a different area. The same area should be avoided for 7 days

Nocturnal enuresis associated with overactive bladder
▸ BY MOUTH USING IMMEDIATE-RELEASE MEDICINES
▸ Child 5–17 years: 2.5–3 mg twice daily, increased to 5 mg 2–3 times a day, last dose to be taken before bedtime
▸ BY MOUTH USING MODIFIED-RELEASE TABLETS
▸ Child 5–17 years: Initially 5 mg once daily, adjusted in steps of 5 mg every week, adjusted according to response; maximum 15 mg per day

DOSE EQUIVALENCE AND CONVERSION
▸ Patients taking immediate-release oxybutynin may be transferred to the nearest equivalent daily dose of *Lyrinel* ® XL

● CAUTIONS Acute porphyrias p. 1107
● INTERACTIONS → Appendix 1: oxybutynin
● SIDE-EFFECTS
  GENERAL SIDE-EFFECTS
▸ **Common or very common** Diarrhoea
  SPECIFIC SIDE-EFFECTS
▸ **Common or very common**
▸ With oral use Dry eye
▸ With transdermal use Gastrointestinal discomfort · increased risk of infection
▸ **Uncommon**
▸ With oral use Abdominal discomfort · appetite decreased · dysphagia
▸ With transdermal use Back pain · hot flush · injury
▸ **Frequency not known**
▸ With oral use Anxiety · arrhythmia · cognitive disorder · depressive symptom · drug dependence · gastrointestinal disorders · glaucoma · hallucination · heat stroke · hypohidrosis · mydriasis · nightmare · paranoia · photosensitivity reaction · seizure · urinary tract infection
● PREGNANCY Manufacturers advise avoid unless essential—toxicity in *animal* studies.
● BREAST FEEDING Manufacturers advise avoid—present in milk in *animal* studies.
● HEPATIC IMPAIRMENT Manufacturer advises caution.
● RENAL IMPAIRMENT Manufacturer advises caution.
● DIRECTIONS FOR ADMINISTRATION
▸ With transdermal use Manufacturer advises apply patches to clean, dry, unbroken skin on abdomen, hip or buttock; remove after every 3–4 days and site replacement patch on a different area (avoid using same area for 7 days).
● PRESCRIBING AND DISPENSING INFORMATION
▸ In adults The need for continuing therapy for urinary incontinence should be reviewed every 4–6 weeks until symptoms stabilise, and then every 6–12 months.
▸ In children The need for therapy for urinary indications should be reviewed soon after it has been commenced and then at regular intervals; a response usually occurs within 6 months but may take longer.

● PATIENT AND CARER ADVICE
▸ With transdermal use Patients or carers should be given advice on how to administer oxybutynin transdermal patches.
  Medicines for Children leaflet: Oxybutynin for daytime urinary symptoms www.medicinesforchildren.org.uk/oxybutynin-daytime-urinary-symptoms
● NATIONAL FUNDING/ACCESS DECISIONS
  For full details see funding body website
  Scottish Medicines Consortium (SMC) decisions
▸ Oxybutynin (*Kentera* ®) for treatment of urge incontinence and/or increased urinary frequency and urgency (August 2005) SMC No. 190/05 Recommended with restrictions

● MEDICINAL FORMS There can be variation in the licensing of different medicines containing the same drug. Forms available from special-order manufacturers include: oral suspension, oral solution

Modified-release tablet
CAUTIONARY AND ADVISORY LABELS 3, 25
▸ Lyrinel XL (Janssen-Cilag Ltd)
  Oxybutynin hydrochloride 5 mg Lyrinel XL 5mg tablets | 30 tablet [PoM] £13.77 DT = £13.77
  Oxybutynin hydrochloride 10 mg Lyrinel XL 10mg tablets | 30 tablet [PoM] £27.54 DT = £27.54

Tablet
CAUTIONARY AND ADVISORY LABELS 3
▸ Oxybutynin hydrochloride (Non-proprietary)
  Oxybutynin hydrochloride 2.5 mg Oxybutynin 2.5mg tablets | 56 tablet [PoM] £6.58 DT = £1.86 | 84 tablet [PoM] £2.78–£7.71
  Oxybutynin hydrochloride 3 mg Oxybutynin 3mg tablets | 56 tablet [PoM] £17.91 DT = £17.91
  Oxybutynin hydrochloride 5 mg Oxybutynin 5mg tablets | 56 tablet [PoM] £13.85 DT = £2.00 | 84 tablet [PoM] £2.99–£20.77
▸ Ditropan (Cheplapharm Arzneimittel GmbH)
  Oxybutynin hydrochloride 2.5 mg Ditropan 2.5mg tablets | 84 tablet [PoM] £1.60
  Oxybutynin hydrochloride 5 mg Ditropan 5mg tablets | 84 tablet [PoM] £2.90

Oral solution
CAUTIONARY AND ADVISORY LABELS 3
▸ Oxybutynin hydrochloride (Non-proprietary)
  Oxybutynin hydrochloride 500 microgram per 1 ml Oxybutynin 2.5mg/5ml oral solution sugar free sugar-free | 150 ml [PoM] £214.84 DT = £214.84
  Oxybutynin hydrochloride 1 mg per 1 ml Oxybutynin 5mg/5ml oral solution sugar free sugar-free | 150 ml [PoM] £235.53 DT = £235.53

Transdermal patch
CAUTIONARY AND ADVISORY LABELS 3
▸ Kentera (Orion Pharma (UK) Ltd)
  Oxybutynin 3.9 mg per 24 hour Kentera 3.9mg/24hours patches | 8 patch [PoM] £27.20 DT = £27.20

F 821

Propiverine hydrochloride

● INDICATIONS AND DOSE
Urinary frequency, urgency and incontinence associated with overactive bladder
▸ BY MOUTH USING IMMEDIATE-RELEASE MEDICINES
▸ Adult: 15 mg 1–2 times a day, increased if necessary up to 15 mg 3 times a day
▸ BY MOUTH USING MODIFIED-RELEASE CAPSULES
▸ Adult: 30 mg once daily

Urinary frequency, urgency and incontinence associated with neurogenic bladder instability
▸ BY MOUTH USING IMMEDIATE-RELEASE MEDICINES
▸ Adult: 15 mg 3 times a day

● INTERACTIONS → Appendix 1: propiverine
● SIDE-EFFECTS
▸ **Common or very common** Abdominal pain · fatigue
▸ **Uncommon** Taste altered · tremor
▸ **Rare or very rare** Restlessness
▸ **Frequency not known** Hallucination

- PREGNANCY Manufacturer advises avoid (restriction of skeletal development in *animals*).
- BREAST FEEDING Manufacturer advises avoid—present in milk in *animal* studies.
- HEPATIC IMPAIRMENT Manufacturer advises caution in mild impairment; avoid in moderate to severe impairment (no information available).
- RENAL IMPAIRMENT Manufacturer advises caution in mild or moderate impairment.
  Dose adjustments Max. daily dose 30 mg if eGFR less than 30 mL/minute/1.73m².
- PRESCRIBING AND DISPENSING INFORMATION The need for continuing therapy for urinary incontinence should be reviewed every 4–6 weeks until symptoms stabilise, and then every 6–12 months.

- MEDICINAL FORMS There can be variation in the licensing of different medicines containing the same drug.
  Modified-release capsule
  CAUTIONARY AND ADVISORY LABELS 3, 25
  ‣ Detrunorm XL (Advanz Pharma)
  Propiverine hydrochloride 30 mg Detrunorm XL 30mg capsules | 28 capsule [PoM] £24.45 DT = £24.45
  Propiverine hydrochloride 45 mg Detrunorm XL 45mg capsules | 28 capsule [PoM] £27.90 DT = £27.90
  Tablet
  CAUTIONARY AND ADVISORY LABELS 3
  ‣ Propiverine hydrochloride (Non-proprietary)
  Propiverine hydrochloride 15 mg Propiverine 15mg tablets | 56 tablet [PoM] £39.46 DT = £35.10
  ‣ Detrunorm (Advanz Pharma)
  Propiverine hydrochloride 15 mg Detrunorm 15mg tablets | 56 tablet [PoM] £18.00 DT = £35.10

[F 821]

Solifenacin succinate

23-Jul-2020

- **INDICATIONS AND DOSE**

Urinary frequency | Urinary urgency | Urinary incontinence
‣ BY MOUTH
‣ Adult: 5 mg once daily, increased if necessary to 10 mg once daily

DOSE ADJUSTMENTS DUE TO INTERACTIONS
‣ Manufacturer advises maximum 5 mg once daily with concurrent use of potent inhibitors of CYP3A4; avoid concurrent use in patients who also have moderate hepatic impairment or severe renal impairment.

- CAUTIONS Susceptibility to QT-interval prolongation
- INTERACTIONS → Appendix 1: solifenacin
- SIDE-EFFECTS
‣ **Common or very common** Gastrointestinal discomfort
‣ **Uncommon** Cystitis · dry eye · dry throat · fatigue · gastrointestinal disorders · nasal dryness · peripheral oedema · taste altered · urinary tract infection
‣ **Rare or very rare** Hallucination
‣ **Frequency not known** Anaphylactic reaction · appetite decreased · arrhythmias · delirium · dysphonia · glaucoma · hyperkalaemia · liver disorder · muscle weakness · QT interval prolongation · renal impairment
- PREGNANCY Manufacturer advises caution—no information available.
- BREAST FEEDING Manufacturer advises avoid—present in milk in *animal* studies.
- HEPATIC IMPAIRMENT Manufacturer advises caution in moderate impairment (risk of increased half-life); avoid in severe impairment (no information available).
  Dose adjustments Manufacturer advises maximum 5 mg once daily in moderate impairment.
- RENAL IMPAIRMENT Manufacturer advises caution in severe impairment.

  Dose adjustments Manufacturer advises maximum 5 mg once daily if creatinine clearance 30 mL/minute or less.
- DIRECTIONS FOR ADMINISTRATION Manufacturer advises for *oral suspension*, doses should be followed by a glass of water—ingestion with food or other drinks may lead to the release of solifenacin in the mouth, causing a bitter taste and numbness in the mouth.
- PRESCRIBING AND DISPENSING INFORMATION The need for continuing therapy for urinary incontinence should be reviewed every 4–6 weeks until symptoms stabilise, and then every 6–12 months.

- MEDICINAL FORMS There can be variation in the licensing of different medicines containing the same drug. Forms available from special-order manufacturers include: oral suspension, oral solution
  Oral solution
  ‣ Solifenacin succinate (Non-proprietary)
  Solifenacin succinate 1 mg per 1 ml Solifenacin 5mg/5ml oral solution sugar free sugar-free | 150 ml [PoM] £27.62
  Oral suspension
  CAUTIONARY AND ADVISORY LABELS 3
  EXCIPIENTS: May contain Ethanol, hydroxybenzoates (parabens), propylene glycol
  ‣ Vesicare (Astellas Pharma Ltd)
  Solifenacin succinate 1 mg per 1 ml Vesicare 1mg/ml oral suspension sugar-free | 150 ml [PoM] £27.62 DT = £27.62
  Tablet
  CAUTIONARY AND ADVISORY LABELS 3
  ‣ Solifenacin succinate (Non-proprietary)
  Solifenacin succinate 5 mg Solifenacin 5mg tablets | 30 tablet [PoM] £27.62 DT = £2.64 | 250 tablet [PoM] £29.17-£230.17
  Solifenacin succinate 10 mg Solifenacin 10mg tablets | 30 tablet [PoM] £35.91 DT = £3.13 | 100 tablet [PoM] £119.70 | 250 tablet [PoM] £41.75-£299.25
  ‣ Vesicare (Astellas Pharma Ltd)
  Solifenacin succinate 5 mg Vesicare 5mg tablets | 30 tablet [PoM] £27.62 DT = £2.64
  Solifenacin succinate 10 mg Vesicare 10mg tablets | 30 tablet [PoM] £35.91 DT = £3.13

[F 821]

Tolterodine tartrate

20-Jan-2020

- **INDICATIONS AND DOSE**

Urinary frequency | Urinary urgency | Urinary incontinence
‣ BY MOUTH USING IMMEDIATE-RELEASE MEDICINES
‣ Adult: 2 mg twice daily, reduced if not tolerated to 1 mg twice daily
‣ BY MOUTH USING MODIFIED-RELEASE CAPSULES
‣ Adult: 4 mg once daily

- CAUTIONS History of QT-interval prolongation
- INTERACTIONS → Appendix 1: tolterodine
- SIDE-EFFECTS
‣ **Common or very common** Abdominal pain · bronchitis · chest pain · diarrhoea · dry eye · fatigue · gastrointestinal disorders · paraesthesia · peripheral oedema · vertigo · weight increased
‣ **Uncommon** Arrhythmia · heart failure · memory loss · nervousness
‣ **Frequency not known** Hallucination
- PREGNANCY Manufacturer advises avoid—toxicity in *animal* studies.
- BREAST FEEDING Manufacturer advises avoid—no information available.
- HEPATIC IMPAIRMENT Manufacturer advises caution (risk of increased exposure).
  Dose adjustments For *immediate-release medicines*, manufacturer advises dose reduction to 1 mg twice daily.
  For *modified-release capsules*, manufacturer advises dose reduction to 2 mg once daily.

- RENAL IMPAIRMENT Manufacturer advises caution (risk of increased exposure)
  Dose adjustments For *immediate-release medicines*, manufacturer advises dose reduction to 1 mg twice daily if GFR less than or equal to 30 mL/minute.
  For *modified-release capsules*, manufacturer advises dose reduction to 2 mg once daily if GFR less than or equal to 30 mL/minute.
- PRESCRIBING AND DISPENSING INFORMATION The need for continuing therapy for urinary incontinence should be reviewed every 4–6 weeks until symptoms stabilise, and then every 6–12 months.

- MEDICINAL FORMS There can be variation in the licensing of different medicines containing the same drug. Forms available from special-order manufacturers include: oral suspension, oral solution, powder

Tablet
CAUTIONARY AND ADVISORY LABELS 3
▸ Tolterodine tartrate (Non-proprietary)
  Tolterodine tartrate 1 mg Tolterodine 1mg tablets | 56 tablet [PoM] £29.03 DT = £13.48
  Tolterodine tartrate 2 mg Tolterodine 2mg tablets | 56 tablet [PoM] £30.56 DT = £14.89
▸ Detrusitol (Upjohn UK Ltd)
  Tolterodine tartrate 1 mg Detrusitol 1mg tablets | 56 tablet [PoM] £29.03 DT = £13.48
  Tolterodine tartrate 2 mg Detrusitol 2mg tablets | 56 tablet [PoM] £30.56 DT = £14.89

Modified-release capsule
CAUTIONARY AND ADVISORY LABELS 3, 25
▸ Blerone XL (Zentiva)
  Tolterodine tartrate 4 mg Blerone XL 4mg capsules | 28 capsule [PoM] £9.59 DT = £25.78
▸ Detrusitol XL (Upjohn UK Ltd)
  Tolterodine tartrate 4 mg Detrusitol XL 4mg capsules | 28 capsule [PoM] £25.78 DT = £25.78
▸ Inconex XL (Sandoz Ltd)
  Tolterodine tartrate 4 mg Inconex XL 4mg capsules | 28 capsule [PoM] £21.91 DT = £25.78
▸ Mariosea XL (Teva UK Ltd)
  Tolterodine tartrate 2 mg Mariosea XL 2mg capsules | 28 capsule [PoM] £11.59 DT = £11.60
  Tolterodine tartrate 4 mg Mariosea XL 4mg capsules | 28 capsule [PoM] £12.79 DT = £25.78
▸ Neditol XL (Aspire Pharma Ltd)
  Tolterodine tartrate 2 mg Neditol XL 2mg capsules | 28 capsule [PoM] £11.60 DT = £11.60
  Tolterodine tartrate 4 mg Neditol XL 4mg capsules | 28 capsule [PoM] £12.89 DT = £25.78
▸ Preblacon XL (Accord Healthcare Ltd)
  Tolterodine tartrate 4 mg Preblacon XL 4mg capsules | 28 capsule [PoM] £25.78 DT = £25.78
▸ Santizor XL (Upjohn UK Ltd)
  Tolterodine tartrate 4 mg Santizor XL 4mg capsules | 28 capsule [PoM] £25.78 DT = £25.78
▸ Tolthen XL (Northumbria Pharma Ltd)
  Tolterodine tartrate 2 mg Tolthen XL 2mg capsules | 28 capsule [PoM] £11.60 DT = £11.60
  Tolterma XL 2mg capsules | 28 capsule [PoM] £24.36 DT = £11.60
  Tolterodine tartrate 4 mg Tolthen XL 4mg capsules | 28 capsule [PoM] £12.89 DT = £25.78
  Tolterma XL 4mg capsules | 28 capsule [PoM] £25.78 DT = £25.78

⊩ 821

Trospium chloride
11-May-2018

- **INDICATIONS AND DOSE**
Urinary frequency | Urinary urgency | Urge incontinence
  ▸ BY MOUTH USING IMMEDIATE-RELEASE MEDICINES
  ▸ Adult: 20 mg twice daily, to be taken before food
  ▸ BY MOUTH USING MODIFIED-RELEASE MEDICINES
  ▸ Adult: 60 mg once daily

- INTERACTIONS → Appendix 1: trospium
- SIDE-EFFECTS
- **Common or very common** Abdominal pain

▸ **Uncommon** Chest pain · diarrhoea · flatulence
▸ **Rare or very rare** Arthralgia · asthenia · dyspnoea · myalgia
▸ **Frequency not known** Agitation · anaphylactic reaction · hallucination · severe cutaneous adverse reactions (SCARs)
- PREGNANCY Manufacturer advises caution.
- BREAST FEEDING Manufacturer advises caution.
- HEPATIC IMPAIRMENT Manufacturer advises caution in mild to moderate impairment; avoid in severe impairment (no information available).
- RENAL IMPAIRMENT Use with caution. Avoid *Regurin® XL*.
  Dose adjustments Reduce dose to 20 mg once daily or 20 mg on alternate days if eGFR 10–30 mL/minute/1.73m^2.
- PRESCRIBING AND DISPENSING INFORMATION The need for continuing therapy for urinary incontinence should be reviewed every 4–6 weeks until symptoms stabilise, and then every 6–12 months.

- MEDICINAL FORMS There can be variation in the licensing of different medicines containing the same drug. Forms available from special-order manufacturers include: oral solution

Modified-release capsule
CAUTIONARY AND ADVISORY LABELS 23, 25
▸ Regurin XL (Contura Ltd)
  Trospium chloride 60 mg Regurin XL 60mg capsules | 28 capsule [PoM] £23.05 DT = £23.05

Tablet
CAUTIONARY AND ADVISORY LABELS 23
▸ Trospium chloride (Non-proprietary)
  Trospium chloride 20 mg Trospium chloride 20mg tablets | 60 tablet [PoM] £6.81 DT = £4.56
▸ Flotros (Galen Ltd)
  Trospium chloride 20 mg Flotros 20mg tablets | 60 tablet [PoM] £18.20 DT = £4.56
▸ Regurin (Mylan)
  Trospium chloride 20 mg Regurin 20mg tablets | 60 tablet [PoM] £26.00 DT = £4.56
▸ Uraplex (Contura Ltd)
  Trospium chloride 20 mg Uraplex 20mg tablets | 60 tablet [PoM] £26.00 DT = £4.56

BETA₃-ADRENOCEPTOR AGONISTS

Mirabegron
23-Nov-2020

- **INDICATIONS AND DOSE**
Urinary frequency, urgency, and urge incontinence
  ▸ BY MOUTH
  ▸ Adult: 50 mg once daily

DOSE ADJUSTMENTS DUE TO INTERACTIONS
  ▸ Manufacturer advises reduce dose to 25 mg once daily in patients with mild hepatic impairment with concurrent use of potent inhibitors of CYP3A4; avoid in moderate impairment.
  ▸ Manufacturer advises reduce dose to 25 mg once daily if eGFR 30–89 mL/minute/1.73 m^2 with concurrent use of potent inhibitors of CYP3A4; avoid if eGFR less than 30 mL/minute/1.73 m^2.

- CONTRA-INDICATIONS Severe uncontrolled hypertension (systolic blood pressure ≥180 mmHg or diastolic blood pressure ≥110 mmHg)
- CAUTIONS History of QT-interval prolongation · stage 2 hypertension
- INTERACTIONS → Appendix 1: mirabegron
- SIDE-EFFECTS
▸ **Common or very common** Arrhythmias · constipation · diarrhoea · dizziness · headache · increased risk of infection · nausea
▸ **Uncommon** Cystitis · dyspepsia · gastritis · joint swelling · palpitations · skin reactions · vulvovaginal pruritus

▶ **Rare or very rare** Angioedema · eyelid oedema · hypersensitivity vasculitis · hypertensive crisis · lip swelling · urinary retention
▶ **Frequency not known** Insomnia

● CONCEPTION AND CONTRACEPTION Contraception advised in women of child-bearing potential.

● PREGNANCY Avoid—toxicity in *animal* studies.

● BREAST FEEDING Avoid—present in milk in *animal* studies.

● HEPATIC IMPAIRMENT Manufacturer advises caution in moderate impairment (risk of increased exposure); avoid in severe impairment (no information available).
Dose adjustments Manufacturer advises dose reduction to 25 mg once daily in moderate impairment.

● RENAL IMPAIRMENT Avoid if eGFR less than 15 mL/minute/1.73 m^2—no information available.
Dose adjustments Reduce dose to 25 mg once daily if eGFR 15–29 mL/minute/1.73 m^2.

● MONITORING REQUIREMENTS Blood pressure should be monitored before starting treatment and regularly during treatment, especially in patients with pre-existing hypertension.

● NATIONAL FUNDING/ACCESS DECISIONS
For full details see funding body website
NICE decisions
▶ **Mirabegron for treating symptoms of overactive bladder (June 2013)** NICE TA290 Recommended with restrictions

● MEDICINAL FORMS There can be variation in the licensing of different medicines containing the same drug.
Modified-release tablet
CAUTIONARY AND ADVISORY LABELS 25
▶ Betmiga (Astellas Pharma Ltd)
Mirabegron 25 mg Betmiga 25mg modified-release tablets | 30 tablet [PoM] £29.00 DT = £29.00
Mirabegron 50 mg Betmiga 50mg modified-release tablets | 30 tablet [PoM] £29.00 DT = £29.00

1.2 Urinary retention

Urinary retention

31-May-2017

Description of condition

Urinary retention is the inability to voluntarily urinate. It may be secondary to urethral blockage, drug treatment (such as use of antimuscarinic drugs, sympathomimetics, tricyclic antidepressants), conditions that reduce detrusor contractions or interfere with relaxation of the urethra, neurogenic causes, or it may occur postpartum or postoperatively.

Acute urinary retention is a medical emergency characterised by the abrupt development of the inability to pass urine (over a period of hours).

Chronic urinary retention is the gradual (over months or years) development of the inability to empty the bladder completely, characterised by a residual volume greater than one litre or associated with the presence of a distended or palpable bladder.

Urinary retention due to benign prostatic hyperplasia

The most common cause of urinary retention in men is benign prostatic hyperplasia. Men with an enlarged prostate can have lower urinary tract symptoms associated with obstruction, such as urinary retention (acute or chronic), frequency, urgency or nocturia.

Treatment

Treatment of urinary retention depends on the underlying condition. Catheterisation is used to relieve acute painful urinary retention or when no cause can be found. Surgical procedures or dilatation are often used to correct mechanical outflow obstructions.

Acute urinary retention

[EvGr] Acute retention is painful and requires immediate treatment by catheterisation. Before the catheter is removed an alpha-adrenoceptor blocker (such as alfuzosin hydrochloride p. 827, doxazosin p. 827, tamsulosin hydrochloride p. 829, prazosin p. 829, indoramin p. 828 or terazosin p. 830) should be given for at least two days to manage acute urinary retention Ⓐ.

Chronic urinary retention

[EvGr] In patients with chronic urinary retention, intermittent bladder catheterisation should be offered before an indwelling catheter. Catheters may be used as a long-term solution where persistent urinary retention is causing incontinence, infection, or renal dysfunction and a surgical solution is not feasible. Ⓐ Their use is associated with an increased risk of adverse events including recurrent urinary infections, trauma to the urethra, pain, and stone formation.

[EvGr] In men who have symptoms that are bothersome, drug treatment should only be offered when other conservative management options have failed. Men with moderate-to-severe symptoms should be offered an alpha-adrenoceptor blocker (alfuzosin hydrochloride, doxazosin, tamsulosin hydrochloride or terazosin). Treatment should initially be reviewed after 4–6 weeks and then every 6–12 months. Ⓐ

The parasympathomimetic bethanechol chloride p. 831 increases detrusor muscle contraction. It is licensed for acute postoperative, postpartum and neurogenic urinary retention but its use has largely been superseded by catheterisation.

Urinary retention due to benign prostatic hyperplasia

In patients with benign prostatic hyperplasia, treatment is influenced by the severity of symptoms and their effect on the patient's quality of life. [EvGr] Watchful waiting is suitable for men with symptoms that are not troublesome and in those who have not yet developed complications of benign prostatic hyperplasia such as renal impairment, urinary retention or recurrent infection.

The recommended treatment of benign prostatic hyperplasia is usually an alpha-adrenoceptor blocker. The alpha$_1$-selective adrenoceptor blockers relax smooth muscle in benign prostatic hyperplasia producing an increase in urinary flow-rate and an improvement in obstructive symptoms.

In patients with an enlarged prostate, a raised prostate specific antigen concentration, and who are considered to be at high risk of progression (such as the elderly), a 5α-reductase inhibitor (such as finasteride p. 832 or dutasteride p. 831) should be used. A combination of an alpha-adrenoceptor blocker and a 5α-reductase inhibitor can be offered if symptoms remain a problem.

Surgery is recommended for men with more severe symptoms that do not respond to drug therapy, or who have complications such as acute urinary retention, haematuria, renal failure, bladder calculi or recurrent urinary-tract infection. Ⓐ

Related drugs

Other drugs used for urinary retention: neostigmine p. 1170, pyridostigmine bromide p. 1171.

Useful Resources

Lower urinary tract symptoms in men. National Institute for Health and Care Excellence. Clinical guideline CG97. May 2010 (updated June 2015).
www.nice.org.uk/guidance/cg97

Other drugs used for Urinary retention Tadalafil, p. 861

ALPHA-ADRENOCEPTOR BLOCKERS

Alfuzosin hydrochloride
03-Sep-2020

- **INDICATIONS AND DOSE**

Benign prostatic hyperplasia
▸ BY MOUTH USING IMMEDIATE-RELEASE MEDICINES
▸ Adult: 2.5 mg 3 times a day; maximum 10 mg per day
▸ Elderly: Initially 2.5 mg twice daily, adjusted according to response; maximum 10 mg per day
▸ BY MOUTH USING MODIFIED-RELEASE MEDICINES
▸ Adult: 10 mg once daily

Acute urinary retention associated with benign prostatic hyperplasia
▸ BY MOUTH USING MODIFIED-RELEASE TABLETS
▸ Elderly: 10 mg once daily for 2–3 days during catheterisation and for one day after removal; max. 4 days

- CONTRA-INDICATIONS Avoid if history of micturition syncope · avoid if history of postural hypotension
- CAUTIONS Acute heart failure · cerebrovascular disease · concomitant antihypertensives (reduced dosage and specialist supervision may be required) · discontinue if angina worsens · elderly · history of QT-interval prolongation · patients undergoing cataract surgery (risk of intra-operative floppy iris syndrome)

CAUTIONS, FURTHER INFORMATION
▸ Elderly For alpha$_1$-selective adrenoceptor blockers, prescription potentially inappropriate (STOPP criteria):
  • in those with symptomatic orthostatic hypotension or micturition syncope (risk of precipitating recurrent syncope)
  • in those with persistent postural hypotension i.e. recurrent drop in systolic blood pressure $\geq$ 20 mmHg (risk of syncope and falls).
  See also Prescribing in the elderly p. 33.

- INTERACTIONS → Appendix 1: alpha blockers
- SIDE-EFFECTS
▸ **Common or very common** Asthenia · diarrhoea · dizziness · dry mouth · headache · malaise · nausea · postural hypotension · vertigo · vomiting
▸ **Uncommon** Abdominal pain · arrhythmias · chest pain · drowsiness · flushing · oedema · palpitations · rhinitis · skin reactions · syncope · visual impairment
▸ **Rare or very rare** Angina pectoris · angioedema
▸ **Frequency not known** Cerebral ischaemia · floppy iris syndrome · hepatic disorders · neutropenia · priapism · thrombocytopenia

SIDE-EFFECTS, FURTHER INFORMATION First dose may cause collapse due to hypotensive effect (therefore should be taken on retiring to bed). Patient should be warned to lie down if symptoms such as dizziness, fatigue or sweating develop, and to remain lying down until they abate completely.

- HEPATIC IMPAIRMENT For *immediate-release* preparations manufacturer advises caution in mild to moderate hepatic failure; avoid in severe hepatic failure (risk of increased half-life). For *modified-release* preparations manufacturer advises avoid in hepatic failure.
Dose adjustments For *immediate-release* preparations manufacturer advises initial dose of 2.5 mg once daily, increased to 2.5 mg twice daily according to response in mild to moderate hepatic failure.

- RENAL IMPAIRMENT Manufacturers advise avoid use of modified-release preparations if eGFR less than 30 mL/minute/1.73 m² as limited experience.
Dose adjustments Initial dose 2.5 mg twice daily and adjust according to response.

- PATIENT AND CARER ADVICE Patient should be counselled on the first dose effect.
Driving and skilled tasks May affect performance of skilled tasks e.g. driving.

- MEDICINAL FORMS There can be variation in the licensing of different medicines containing the same drug. Forms available from special-order manufacturers include: oral solution

Modified-release tablet
CAUTIONARY AND ADVISORY LABELS 21, 25
▸ Besavar XL (Zentiva)
  Alfuzosin hydrochloride 10 mg Besavar XL 10mg tablets | 30 tablet [PoM] £4.62 DT = £12.51
▸ Fuzatal XL (Teva UK Ltd)
  Alfuzosin hydrochloride 10 mg Fuzatal XL 10mg tablets | 30 tablet [PoM] £12.76 DT = £12.51
▸ Vasran XL (Ranbaxy (UK) Ltd)
  Alfuzosin hydrochloride 10 mg Vasran XL 10mg tablets | 30 tablet [PoM] £11.48 DT = £12.51
▸ Xatral XL (Sanofi)
  Alfuzosin hydrochloride 10 mg Xatral XL 10mg tablets | 30 tablet [PoM] £12.51 DT = £12.51
▸ Zochek (Milpharm Ltd)
  Alfuzosin hydrochloride 10 mg Zochek 10mg modified-release tablets | 30 tablet [PoM] £12.51 DT = £12.51

Tablet
▸ Alfuzosin hydrochloride (Non-proprietary)
  Alfuzosin hydrochloride 2.5 mg Alfuzosin 2.5mg tablets | 60 tablet [PoM] £21.20 DT = £1.70
▸ Xatral (Sanofi)
  Alfuzosin hydrochloride 2.5 mg Xatral 2.5mg tablets | 60 tablet [PoM] £20.37 DT = £1.70

Doxazosin
02-Sep-2020

- **INDICATIONS AND DOSE**

Hypertension
▸ BY MOUTH USING IMMEDIATE-RELEASE MEDICINES
▸ Adult: Initially 1 mg once daily for 1–2 weeks, then increased to 2 mg once daily, then increased if necessary to 4 mg once daily; maximum 16 mg per day
▸ BY MOUTH USING MODIFIED-RELEASE MEDICINES
▸ Adult: Initially 4 mg once daily, dose can be adjusted after 4 weeks, then increased if necessary to 8 mg once daily

Benign prostatic hyperplasia
▸ BY MOUTH USING IMMEDIATE-RELEASE MEDICINES
▸ Adult: Initially 1 mg daily, dose may be doubled at intervals of 1–2 weeks according to response; usual maintenance 2–4 mg daily; maximum 8 mg per day
▸ BY MOUTH USING MODIFIED-RELEASE MEDICINES
▸ Adult: Initially 4 mg once daily, dose can be adjusted after 4 weeks, then increased if necessary to 8 mg once daily

DOSE EQUIVALENCE AND CONVERSION
▸ Patients stabilised on immediate-release doxazosin can be transferred to the equivalent dose of modified-release doxazosin.

- CONTRA-INDICATIONS History of micturition syncope (in patients with benign prostatic hypertrophy) · history of postural hypotension · monotherapy in patients with overflow bladder or anuria
- CAUTIONS Care with initial dose (postural hypotension) · cataract surgery (risk of intra-operative floppy iris syndrome) · elderly · heart failure · pulmonary oedema due to aortic or mitral stenosis
- INTERACTIONS → Appendix 1: alpha blockers
- SIDE-EFFECTS
▸ **Common or very common** Arrhythmias · asthenia · chest pain · cough · cystitis · dizziness · drowsiness · dry mouth · dyspnoea · gastrointestinal discomfort · headache · hypotension · increased risk of infection · influenza like

7

Genito-urinary system

illness · muscle complaints · nausea · oedema · pain · palpitations · skin reactions · urinary disorders · vertigo
▶ **Uncommon** Angina pectoris · anxiety · appetite abnormal · arthralgia · constipation · depression · diarrhoea · gastrointestinal disorders · gout · haemorrhage · insomnia · myocardial infarction · sensation abnormal · sexual dysfunction · stroke · syncope · tinnitus · tremor · vomiting · weight increased
▶ **Rare or very rare** Alopecia · bronchospasm · flushing · gynaecomastia · hepatic disorders · leucopenia · malaise · muscle weakness · thrombocytopenia · vision blurred
▶ **Frequency not known** Floppy iris syndrome
● PREGNANCY No evidence of teratogenicity; manufacturers advise use only when potential benefit outweighs risk.
● BREAST FEEDING Accumulates in milk in *animal* studies—manufacturer advises avoid.
● HEPATIC IMPAIRMENT Manufacturer advises caution in mild to moderate impairment (limited information available); avoid in severe impairment (no information available).
● PATIENT AND CARER ADVICE Patient counselling is advised for doxazosin tablets (initial dose).
Driving and skilled tasks May affect performance of skilled tasks e.g. driving.

● MEDICINAL FORMS There can be variation in the licensing of different medicines containing the same drug. Forms available from special-order manufacturers include: capsule, oral suspension, oral solution

Modified-release tablet
CAUTIONARY AND ADVISORY LABELS 25
▶ Cardura XL (Upjohn UK Ltd)
  Doxazosin (as Doxazosin mesilate) 4 mg Cardura XL 4mg tablets | 28 tablet [PoM] £5.00 DT = £5.00
  Doxazosin (as Doxazosin mesilate) 8 mg Cardura XL 8mg tablets | 28 tablet [PoM] £9.98 DT = £9.98
▶ Doxadura XL (Dexcel-Pharma Ltd)
  Doxazosin (as Doxazosin mesilate) 4 mg Doxadura XL 4mg tablets | 28 tablet [PoM] £4.75 DT = £5.00
▶ Larbex XL (Teva UK Ltd)
  Doxazosin (as Doxazosin mesilate) 4 mg Larbex XL 4mg tablets | 28 tablet [PoM] £6.08 DT = £5.00
▶ Raporsin XL (Actavis UK Ltd)
  Doxazosin (as Doxazosin mesilate) 4 mg Raporsin XL 4mg tablets | 28 tablet [PoM] £5.70 DT = £5.00
▶ Slocinx XL (Zentiva)
  Doxazosin (as Doxazosin mesilate) 4 mg Slocinx XL 4mg tablets | 28 tablet [PoM] £5.96 DT = £5.00

Tablet
▶ Doxazosin (Non-proprietary)
  Doxazosin (as Doxazosin mesilate) 1 mg Doxazosin 1mg tablets | 28 tablet [PoM] £10.56 DT = £1.00
  Doxazosin (as Doxazosin mesilate) 2 mg Doxazosin 2mg tablets | 28 tablet [PoM] £14.08 DT = £1.04
  Doxazosin (as Doxazosin mesilate) 4 mg Doxazosin 4mg tablets | 28 tablet [PoM] £14.08 DT = £1.20
  Doxazosin (as Doxazosin mesilate) 8 mg Doxazosin 8mg tablets | 28 tablet [PoM] £6.25–£8.25 DT = £6.36
▶ Cardura (Upjohn UK Ltd)
  Doxazosin (as Doxazosin mesilate) 1 mg Cardura 1mg tablets | 28 tablet [PoM] £10.56 DT = £1.00
  Doxazosin (as Doxazosin mesilate) 2 mg Cardura 2mg tablets | 28 tablet [PoM] £14.08 DT = £1.04
▶ Doxadura (Dexcel-Pharma Ltd)
  Doxazosin (as Doxazosin mesilate) 4 mg Doxadura 4mg tablets | 28 tablet [PoM] £1.11 DT = £1.20

Indoramin

15-Oct-2020

● **INDICATIONS AND DOSE**
Hypertension
▶ BY MOUTH
▶ **Adult:** Initially 25 mg twice daily, increased in steps of 25–50 mg every 2 weeks, maximum daily dose should be given in divided doses; maximum 200 mg per day

Benign prostatic hyperplasia
▶ BY MOUTH
▶ **Adult:** 20 mg twice daily, increased in steps of 20 mg every 2 weeks if required, increased if necessary up to 100 mg daily in divided doses
▶ **Elderly:** 20 mg daily may be adequate, dose to be taken at night

DOSE ADJUSTMENTS DUE TO INTERACTIONS
▶ Caution with concomitant antihypertensives in benign prostatic hyperplasia—reduced dosage and specialist supervision may be required.

● CONTRA-INDICATIONS Established heart failure · history micturition syncope (when used for benign prostatic hyperplasia) · history of postural hypotension (when used for benign prostatic hyperplasia)
● CAUTIONS Cataract surgery (risk of intra-operative floppy iris syndrome) · control incipient heart failure before initiating indoramin · elderly · epilepsy (convulsions in *animal* studies) · history of depression · Parkinson's disease (extrapyramidal disorders reported)

CAUTIONS, FURTHER INFORMATION
▶ Elderly For alpha$_1$-selective adrenoceptor blockers, prescription potentially inappropriate (STOPP criteria):
  ● in those with symptomatic orthostatic hypotension or micturition syncope (risk of precipitating recurrent syncope)
  ● in those with persistent postural hypotension i.e. recurrent drop in systolic blood pressure ≥ 20 mmHg (risk of syncope and falls).
See also Prescribing in the elderly p. 33.

● INTERACTIONS → Appendix 1: alpha blockers
● SIDE-EFFECTS
▶ **Rare or very rare** Parkinson's disease exacerbated
▶ **Frequency not known** Depression · dizziness · drowsiness · dry mouth · ejaculation failure · fatigue · headache · nasal congestion · weight increased
● PREGNANCY No evidence of teratogenicity; manufacturers advise use only when potential benefit outweighs risk.
● BREAST FEEDING No information available.
● HEPATIC IMPAIRMENT Manufacturer advises caution.
● RENAL IMPAIRMENT Manufacturer advises caution.
● PATIENT AND CARER ADVICE
Driving and skilled tasks Drowsiness may affect performance of skilled tasks (e.g. driving); effects of alcohol may be enhanced.

● MEDICINAL FORMS There can be variation in the licensing of different medicines containing the same drug.
Tablet
CAUTIONARY AND ADVISORY LABELS 2
▶ Indoramin (Non-proprietary)
  Indoramin (as Indoramin hydrochloride) 20 mg Indoramin 20mg tablets | 60 tablet [PoM] £61.00 DT = £13.47
  Indoramin (as Indoramin hydrochloride) 25 mg Indoramin 25mg tablets | 84 tablet [PoM] £60.26 DT = £60.26
▶ Doralese Tiltab (Chemidex Pharma Ltd)
  Indoramin (as Indoramin hydrochloride) 20 mg Doralese Tiltab 20mg tablets | 60 tablet [PoM] £11.44 DT = £13.47

Prazosin

16-Nov-2020

- ● **INDICATIONS AND DOSE**

Hypertension

▶ BY MOUTH

▶ Adult: Initially 500 micrograms 2–3 times a day for 3–7 days, the initial dose should be taken on retiring to bed at night to avoid collapse, increased to 1 mg 2–3 times a day for a further 3–7 days, then increased if necessary up to 20 mg daily in divided doses

Congestive heart failure (rarely used)

▶ BY MOUTH

▶ Adult: 500 micrograms 2–4 times a day, initial dose to be taken at bedtime, then increased to 4 mg daily in divided doses; maintenance 4–20 mg daily in divided doses

Raynaud's syndrome (but efficacy not established)

▶ BY MOUTH

▶ Adult: Initially 500 micrograms twice daily, initial dose to be taken at bedtime, dose may be increased after 3–7 days, then increased if necessary to 1–2 mg twice daily

Benign prostatic hyperplasia

▶ BY MOUTH

▶ Adult: Initially 500 micrograms twice daily for 3–7 days, subsequent doses should be adjusted according to response, maintenance 2 mg twice daily, initiate with lowest possible dose in elderly patients

DOSE ADJUSTMENTS DUE TO INTERACTIONS

▶ Caution with concomitant antihypertensives in benign prostatic hyperplasia—reduced dosage and specialist supervision may be required.

- ● CONTRA-INDICATIONS History of micturition syncope (in patients with benign prostatic hyperplasia) · history of postural hypotension · not recommended for congestive heart failure due to mechanical obstruction (e.g. aortic stenosis)

- ● CAUTIONS Cataract surgery (risk of intra-operative floppy iris syndrome) · elderly · first dose hypotension

CAUTIONS, FURTHER INFORMATION

▶ Elderly For alpha$_1$-selective adrenoceptor blockers, prescription potentially inappropriate (STOPP criteria):

- ● in those with symptomatic orthostatic hypotension or micturition syncope (risk of precipitating recurrent syncope)

- ● in those with persistent postural hypotension i.e. recurrent drop in systolic blood pressure ≥ 20 mmHg (risk of syncope and falls). See also Prescribing in the elderly p. 33.

- ● INTERACTIONS → Appendix 1: alpha blockers

- ● SIDE-EFFECTS

▶ **Common or very common** Asthenia · constipation · depression · diarrhoea · dizziness · drowsiness · dry mouth · dyspnoea · headache · nasal congestion · nausea · nervousness · oedema · palpitations · postural hypotension · sexual dysfunction · skin reactions · syncope · urinary disorders · vertigo · vision blurred · vomiting

▶ **Uncommon** Angina pectoris · arrhythmias · arthralgia · epistaxis · eye pain · eye redness · gastrointestinal discomfort · hyperhidrosis · paraesthesia · sleep disorders · tinnitus

▶ **Rare or very rare** Alopecia · fever · flushing · gynaecomastia · hallucination · hepatic function abnormal · pain · pancreatitis · vasculitis

- ● PREGNANCY No evidence of teratogenicity; manufacturers advise use only when potential benefit outweighs risk.

- ● BREAST FEEDING Present in milk, amount probably too small to be harmful; manufacturer advises use with caution.

- ● HEPATIC IMPAIRMENT Manufacturer advises caution (no information available).

Dose adjustments Manufacturer advises initial dose reduction to 500 micrograms daily; increased with caution.

- ● RENAL IMPAIRMENT

Dose adjustments Initially 500 micrograms daily in moderate to severe impairment; increased with caution.

- ● PATIENT AND CARER ADVICE

First dose effect First dose may cause collapse due to hypotensive effect (therefore should be taken on retiring to bed). Patients should be warned to lie down if symptoms such as dizziness, fatigue or sweating develop, and to remain lying down until they abate completely.

Driving and skilled tasks May affect performance of skilled tasks e.g. driving.

- ● MEDICINAL FORMS There can be variation in the licensing of different medicines containing the same drug. Forms available from special-order manufacturers include: tablet, oral suspension, oral solution

Tablet

▶ Hypovase (Pfizer Ltd)

Prazosin (as Prazosin hydrochloride) 500 microgram Hypovase 500microgram tablets | 60 tablet [PoM] £2.69 DT = £2.69

Prazosin (as Prazosin hydrochloride) 1 mg Hypovase 1mg tablets | 60 tablet [PoM] £3.46 DT = £3.46

▶ Minipress (Imported (Australia))

Prazosin (as Prazosin hydrochloride) 2 mg Minipress 2mg tablets | 100 tablet [PoM] ⊠

Prazosin (as Prazosin hydrochloride) 5 mg Minipress 5mg tablets | 100 tablet [PoM] ⊠

Tamsulosin hydrochloride

15-Oct-2020

- ● **INDICATIONS AND DOSE**

Benign prostatic hyperplasia

▶ BY MOUTH USING MODIFIED-RELEASE MEDICINES

▶ Adult: 400 micrograms once daily

- ● CONTRA-INDICATIONS History of micturition syncope · history of postural hypotension

- ● CAUTIONS Care with initial dose (postural hypotension) · cataract surgery (risk of intra-operative floppy iris syndrome) · concomitant antihypertensives (reduced dosage and specialist supervision may be required) · elderly

CAUTIONS, FURTHER INFORMATION

▶ Elderly For alpha$_1$-selective adrenoceptor blockers, prescription potentially inappropriate (STOPP criteria):

- ● in those with symptomatic orthostatic hypotension or micturition syncope (risk of precipitating recurrent syncope)

- ● in those with persistent postural hypotension i.e. recurrent drop in systolic blood pressure ≥ 20 mmHg (risk of syncope and falls). See also Prescribing in the elderly p. 33.

- ● INTERACTIONS → Appendix 1: alpha blockers

- ● SIDE-EFFECTS

▶ **Common or very common** Dizziness · sexual dysfunction

▶ **Uncommon** Asthenia · constipation · diarrhoea · headache · nausea · palpitations · postural hypotension · rhinitis · skin reactions · vomiting

▶ **Rare or very rare** Angioedema · Stevens-Johnson syndrome · syncope

▶ **Frequency not known** Dry mouth · epistaxis · vision disorders

- ● HEPATIC IMPAIRMENT Manufacturer advises avoid in severe impairment.

- ● RENAL IMPAIRMENT Use with caution if eGFR less than 10 mL/minute/1.73 m^2.

7

Genito-urinary system

● **PATIENT AND CARER ADVICE**
Driving and skilled tasks May affect performance of skilled tasks e.g. driving.

● **EXCEPTIONS TO LEGAL CATEGORY** Tamsulosin hydrochloride 400 microgram capsules can be sold to the public for the treatment of functional symptoms of benign prostatic hyperplasia in men aged 45–75 years to be taken for up to 6 weeks before clinical assessment by a doctor.

● **MEDICINAL FORMS** There can be variation in the licensing of different medicines containing the same drug.
Modified-release tablet
CAUTIONARY AND ADVISORY LABELS 25
▸ Cositam XL (Consilient Health Ltd)
Tamsulosin hydrochloride 400 microgram Cositam XL 400microgram tablets | 30 tablet [PoM] £8.89 DT = £10.47
▸ Faramsil (Sandoz Ltd)
Tamsulosin hydrochloride 400 microgram Faramsil 400microgram modified-release tablets | 30 tablet [PoM] £8.89 DT = £10.47
▸ Flectone XL (Teva UK Ltd)
Tamsulosin hydrochloride 400 microgram Flectone XL 400microgram tablets | 30 tablet [PoM] £9.95 DT = £10.47
▸ Flomaxtra XL (Astellas Pharma Ltd)
Tamsulosin hydrochloride 400 microgram Flomaxtra XL 400microgram tablets | 30 tablet [PoM] £10.47 DT = £10.47
Modified-release capsule
CAUTIONARY AND ADVISORY LABELS 25
▸ Tamsulosin hydrochloride (Non-proprietary)
Tamsulosin hydrochloride 400 microgram Tamsulosin 400microgram modified-release capsules | 30 capsule [PoM] £2.86–£3.80 DT = £2.90 | 200 capsule [PoM] £67.60
▸ Contiflo XL (Ranbaxy (UK) Ltd)
Tamsulosin hydrochloride 400 microgram Contiflo XL 400microgram capsules | 30 capsule [PoM] £7.44 DT = £2.90
▸ Flomax MR (Sanofi)
Tamsulosin hydrochloride 400 microgram Flomax Relief MR 400microgram capsules | 14 capsule [P] £5.58 | 28 capsule [P] £10.55
▸ Losinate MR (Consilient Health Ltd)
Tamsulosin hydrochloride 400 microgram Losinate MR 400microgram capsules | 30 capsule [PoM] £10.14 DT = £2.90
▸ Pamsvax XL (Accord Healthcare Ltd, Almus Pharmaceuticals Ltd)
Tamsulosin hydrochloride 400 microgram Pamsvax XL 400microgram capsules | 30 capsule [PoM] £1.28 DT = £2.90
▸ Petyme MR (Teva UK Ltd)
Tamsulosin hydrochloride 400 microgram Petyme 400microgram MR capsules | 30 capsule [PoM] £4.06 DT = £2.90
▸ Tabphyn MR (Genus Pharmaceuticals Ltd)
Tamsulosin hydrochloride 400 microgram Tabphyn MR 400microgram capsules | 30 capsule [PoM] £4.45 DT = £2.90
▸ Tamfrex XL (Milpharm Ltd)
Tamsulosin hydrochloride 400 microgram Tamfrex XL 400microgram capsules | 30 capsule [PoM] £28.51 DT = £2.90
▸ Tamsumac (Macleods Pharma UK Ltd)
Tamsulosin hydrochloride 400 microgram Tamsumac 0.4mg modified-release capsules | 30 capsule [PoM] £3.87 DT = £2.90
▸ Tamurex (Somex Pharma)
Tamsulosin hydrochloride 400 microgram Tamurex 400microgram modified-release capsules | 30 capsule [PoM] £3.87 DT = £2.90

Tamsulosin with dutasteride
03-Nov-2020

The properties listed below are those particular to the combination only. For the properties of the components please consider, tamsulosin hydrochloride p. 829, dutasteride p. 831.

● **INDICATIONS AND DOSE**
Benign prostatic hyperplasia
▸ BY MOUTH
▸ Adult (male): 1 capsule daily.

● **INTERACTIONS** → Appendix 1: alpha blockers · dutasteride

● **PATIENT AND CARER ADVICE**
Driving and skilled tasks May affect performance of skilled tasks e.g. driving.

● **MEDICINAL FORMS** There can be variation in the licensing of different medicines containing the same drug.
Capsule
CAUTIONARY AND ADVISORY LABELS 25
▸ Tamsulosin with dutasteride (Non-proprietary)
Tamsulosin hydrochloride 400 microgram, Dutasteride 500 microgram Dutrozen 0.5mg/0.4mg capsules | 30 capsule [PoM] £18.81 DT = £10.06
Tamsulosin 400microgram / Dutasteride 500microgram capsules | 30 capsule [PoM] £10.05–£19.80 DT = £10.06
▸ Combodart (GlaxoSmithKline UK Ltd)
Tamsulosin hydrochloride 400 microgram, Dutasteride 500 microgram Combodart 0.5mg/0.4mg capsules | 30 capsule [PoM] £19.80 DT = £10.06

Tamsulosin with solifenacin
13-May-2020

The properties listed below are those particular to the combination only. For the properties of the components please consider, tamsulosin hydrochloride p. 829, solifenacin succinate p. 824.

● **INDICATIONS AND DOSE**
Moderate to severe urinary frequency, urgency, and obstructive symptoms associated with benign prostatic hyperplasia when monotherapy ineffective
▸ BY MOUTH
▸ Adult (male): 1 tablet daily.

DOSE ADJUSTMENTS DUE TO INTERACTIONS
▸ Manufacturer advises max. 1 *Vesomni*® tablet daily with concurrent use of potent inhibitors of CYP3A4; avoid concurrent use in patients who also have moderate hepatic impairment, severe renal impairment, are poor metabolisers of CYP2D6, or in patients also taking a potent inhibitor of CYP2D6.

● **INTERACTIONS** → Appendix 1: alpha blockers · solifenacin
● **HEPATIC IMPAIRMENT** Manufacturer advises caution in moderate impairment; avoid in severe impairment (no information available).
Dose adjustments Manufacturer advises max. 1 *Vesomni*® tablet daily in moderate impairment.
● **RENAL IMPAIRMENT**
Dose adjustments Max. 1 *Vesomni*® tablet daily if eGFR less than 30 mL/minute/1.73 m².

● **MEDICINAL FORMS** There can be variation in the licensing of different medicines containing the same drug.
Modified-release tablet
CAUTIONARY AND ADVISORY LABELS 3, 25
▸ Vesomni (Astellas Pharma Ltd)
Tamsulosin hydrochloride 400 microgram, Solifenacin succinate 6 mg Vesomni 6mg/0.4mg modified-release tablets | 30 tablet [PoM] £27.62 DT = £27.62

Terazosin
26-Oct-2020

● **INDICATIONS AND DOSE**
Mild to moderate hypertension
▸ BY MOUTH
▸ Adult: 1 mg daily for 7 days, then increased if necessary to 2 mg daily, dose should be taken at bedtime; maintenance 2–10 mg once daily, doses above 20 mg rarely improve efficacy
Benign prostatic hyperplasia
▸ BY MOUTH
▸ Adult: Initially 1 mg daily, dose should be taken at bedtime, if necessary dose may be doubled at intervals of 1–2 weeks according to response; maintenance 5–10 mg daily; maximum 10 mg per day

- CONTRA-INDICATIONS History of micturition syncope (in benign prostatic hyperplasia) · history of postural hypotension (in benign prostatic hyperplasia)
- CAUTIONS Cataract surgery (risk of intra-operative floppy iris syndrome) · elderly · first dose
  CAUTIONS, FURTHER INFORMATION
▶ First dose First dose may cause collapse due to hypotension within 30–90 minutes, therefore should be taken on retiring to bed; may also occur with rapid dose increase.
▶ Elderly For alpha$_1$-selective adrenoceptor blockers, prescription potentially inappropriate (STOPP criteria):
  - in those with symptomatic orthostatic hypotension or micturition syncope (risk of precipitating recurrent syncope)
  - in those with persistent postural hypotension i.e. recurrent drop in systolic blood pressure $\geq$ 20 mmHg (risk of syncope and falls).
  See also Prescribing in the elderly p. 33.
- INTERACTIONS → Appendix 1: alpha blockers
- SIDE-EFFECTS Angioedema · anxiety · arrhythmias · arthritis · asthenia · chest pain · conjunctivitis · constipation · cough · depression · diarrhoea · dizziness · drowsiness · dry mouth · dyspnoea · epistaxis · fever · flatulence · gastrointestinal discomfort · gout · headache · hyperhidrosis · increased risk of infection · insomnia · joint disorders · myalgia · nasal congestion · nausea · oedema · pain · palpitations · paraesthesia · postural hypotension · sexual dysfunction · skin reactions · syncope · thrombocytopenia · tinnitus · urinary disorders · vasodilation · vertigo · vision disorders · vomiting · weight increased
- PREGNANCY No evidence of teratogenicity; manufacturers advise use only when potential benefit outweighs risk.
- BREAST FEEDING No information available.
- PATIENT AND CARER ADVICE Patient counselling is advised for terazosin tablets (initial dose).
  First dose effect First dose may cause collapse due to hypotensive effect (therefore there should be taken on retiring to bed). Patient should be warned to lie down if symptoms such as dizziness, fatigue or sweating develop, and to remain lying down until they abate completely.
  Driving and skilled tasks May affect performance of skilled tasks e.g. driving.

- MEDICINAL FORMS There can be variation in the licensing of different medicines containing the same drug.
  Tablet
  ▶ Terazosin (Non-proprietary)
    Terazosin (as Terazosin hydrochloride) 2 mg Terazosin 2mg tablets | 28 tablet [PoM] £3.10 DT = £2.66
    Terazosin (as Terazosin hydrochloride) 5 mg Terazosin 5mg tablets | 28 tablet [PoM] £5.95 DT = £5.00
    Terazosin (as Terazosin hydrochloride) 10 mg Terazosin 10mg tablets | 28 tablet [PoM] £8.11 DT = £8.09
  ▶ Hytrin (Advanz Pharma)
    Terazosin (as Terazosin hydrochloride) 1 mg Hytrin 1mg tablets | 7 tablet [PoM] 🅰
    Terazosin (as Terazosin hydrochloride) 2 mg Hytrin 2mg tablets | 28 tablet [PoM] £2.20 DT = £2.66
    Terazosin (as Terazosin hydrochloride) 5 mg Hytrin 5mg tablets | 28 tablet [PoM] £4.13 DT = £5.00
    Terazosin (as Terazosin hydrochloride) 10 mg Hytrin 10mg tablets | 28 tablet [PoM] £7.87 DT = £8.09
    Hytrin BPH tablets starter pack | 28 tablet [PoM] £10.97
    Hytrin tablets starter pack | 28 tablet [PoM] £13.00

CHOLINE ESTERS

Bethanechol chloride 09-Dec-2020

- ● **INDICATIONS AND DOSE**
  Urinary retention
  ▶ BY MOUTH
  ▶ Adult: 10–25 mg 3–4 times a day, to be taken 30 minutes before food

- CONTRA-INDICATIONS Bradycardia · conditions where increased motility of the gastro-intestinal tract could be harmful · conditions where increased motility of the urinary tract could be harmful · epilepsy · heart block · hyperthyroidism · hypotension · intestinal obstruction · obstructive airways disease · parkinsonism · peptic ulcer · recent myocardial infarction · urinary obstruction
- CAUTIONS Autonomic neuropathy (use lower initial dose)
- SIDE-EFFECTS Abdominal pain · hyperhidrosis · nausea · vomiting
- PREGNANCY Manufacturer advises avoid—no information available.
- BREAST FEEDING Manufacturer advises avoid; gastrointestinal disturbances in infant reported.
- LESS SUITABLE FOR PRESCRIBING Less suitable for prescribing.

- MEDICINAL FORMS There can be variation in the licensing of different medicines containing the same drug. Forms available from special-order manufacturers include: oral suspension, oral solution
  Tablet
  CAUTIONARY AND ADVISORY LABELS 22
  ▶ Myotonine (Glenwood GmbH)
    Bethanechol chloride 10 mg Myotonine 10mg tablets | 100 tablet [PoM] £18.51 DT = £18.51
    Bethanechol chloride 25 mg Myotonine 25mg tablets | 100 tablet [PoM] £27.26 DT = £27.26

5α-REDUCTASE INHIBITORS

Dutasteride 02-Sep-2020

- DRUG ACTION A specific inhibitor of the enzyme 5α-reductase, which metabolises testosterone into the more potent androgen, dihydrotestosterone.

- ● **INDICATIONS AND DOSE**
  Benign prostatic hyperplasia
  ▶ BY MOUTH
  ▶ Adult: 500 micrograms daily, review treatment at 3–6 months and then every 6–12 months (may require several months treatment before benefit is obtained)

- INTERACTIONS → Appendix 1: dutasteride
- SIDE-EFFECTS
  ▶ **Common or very common** Breast disorder · sexual dysfunction
  ▶ **Uncommon** Alopecia · hypertrichosis
  ▶ **Frequency not known** Angioedema · depressed mood · hypersensitivity · localised oedema · skin reactions · testicular disorders
- CONCEPTION AND CONTRACEPTION Dutasteride is excreted in semen and use of a condom is recommended if sexual partner is pregnant or likely to become pregnant.
- HEPATIC IMPAIRMENT Manufacturer advises caution in mild to moderate impairment; avoid in severe impairment (no information available).
- MONITORING REQUIREMENTS Manufacturer advises that patients should be regularly evaluated for prostate cancer.

7

Genito-urinary system

- **EFFECT ON LABORATORY TESTS** May decrease serum concentration of prostate cancer markers such as prostate-specific antigen; reference values may need adjustment.
- **HANDLING AND STORAGE** Women of childbearing potential should avoid handling leaking capsules of dutasteride.
- **PATIENT AND CARER ADVICE** Cases of male breast cancer have been reported. Patients or their carers should be told to promptly report to their doctor any changes in breast tissue such as lumps, pain, or nipple discharge.

- **MEDICINAL FORMS** There can be variation in the licensing of different medicines containing the same drug. Forms available from special-order manufacturers include: oral solution

Capsule

CAUTIONARY AND ADVISORY LABELS 25
‣ Dutasteride (Non-proprietary)
  Dutasteride 500 microgram Dutasteride 500microgram capsules | 30 capsule [PoM] £19.99 DT = £2.90
‣ Avodart (GlaxoSmithKline UK Ltd)
  Dutasteride 500 microgram Avodart 500microgram capsules | 30 capsule [PoM] £14.60 DT = £2.90
‣ Zepron (Ennogen Healthcare Ltd)
  Zepron 500microgram capsules | 30 capsule [PoM] £3.21 DT = £2.90

Combinations available: *Tamsulosin with dutasteride,* p. 830

Finasteride

04-Sep-2020

- **DRUG ACTION** A specific inhibitor of the enzyme 5α-reductase, which metabolises testosterone into the more potent androgen, dihydrotestosterone.

- **INDICATIONS AND DOSE**

Benign prostatic hyperplasia
‣ BY MOUTH
‣ Adult: 5 mg daily, review treatment at 3–6 months and then every 6–12 months (may require several months treatment before benefit is obtained)

Androgenetic alopecia in men
‣ BY MOUTH
‣ Adult: 1 mg daily, continuous use for 3–6 months is required before benefit is seen, and effects are reversed 6–12 months after treatment is discontinued

---

IMPORTANT SAFETY INFORMATION

MHRA/CHM ADVICE: RARE REPORTS OF DEPRESSION AND SUICIDAL THOUGHTS (MAY 2017)

The MHRA has received reports of depression and, in rare cases, suicidal thoughts in men taking finasteride (*Propecia*®) for male pattern hair loss; depression is also associated with *Proscar*® for benign prostatic hyperplasia. Patients should be advised to stop finasteride immediately and inform a healthcare professional if they develop depression.

- **CAUTIONS** Obstructive uropathy
- **SIDE-EFFECTS**
‣ **Common or very common** Sexual dysfunction
‣ **Uncommon** Breast abnormalities · skin reactions
‣ **Frequency not known** Angioedema · depression · infertility male · palpitations · testicular pain
- **CONCEPTION AND CONTRACEPTION** Finasteride is excreted in semen and use of a condom is recommended if sexual partner is pregnant or likely to become pregnant.
- **EFFECT ON LABORATORY TESTS** Decreases serum concentration of prostate cancer markers such as prostate-specific antigen; reference values may need adjustment.
- **HANDLING AND STORAGE** Women of childbearing potential should avoid handling crushed or broken tablets of finasteride.

- **PATIENT AND CARER ADVICE** Cases of male breast cancer have been reported. Patients or their carers should be told to promptly report to their doctor any changes in breast tissue such as lumps, pain, or nipple discharge.

- **NATIONAL FUNDING/ACCESS DECISIONS**
  NHS restrictions Finasteride is not prescribable in NHS primary care for the treatment of androgenetic alopecia in men.

- **MEDICINAL FORMS** There can be variation in the licensing of different medicines containing the same drug. Forms available from special-order manufacturers include: oral suspension, powder

Tablet

CAUTIONARY AND ADVISORY LABELS 25
‣ Finasteride (Non-proprietary)
  Finasteride 1 mg Finasteride 1mg tablets | 28 tablet [PoM] £6.00–£28.63 | 84 tablet [PoM] £88.40
  Finasteride 5 mg Finasteride 5mg tablets | 28 tablet [PoM] £13.94 DT = £1.49
‣ Propecia (Merck Sharp & Dohme Ltd)
  Finasteride 1 mg Propecia 1mg tablets | 28 tablet [PoM] £33.68 | 84 tablet [PoM] £88.40
‣ Proscar (Merck Sharp & Dohme Ltd)
  Finasteride 5 mg Proscar 5mg tablets | 28 tablet [PoM] £13.94 DT = £1.49 | 30 tablet [PoM] £14.94

1.3 Urolithiasis

Renal and ureteric stones

03-Apr-2019

Description of condition

Renal and ureteric stones are crystalline calculi that may form anywhere in the upper urinary tract. They are often asymptomatic but may cause pain when they move or obstruct the flow of urine. Most stones are composed of calcium salts (calcium oxalate, calcium phosphate or both). The rest are composed of struvite, uric acid, cystine and other substances. Patients are susceptible to stone formation when there is a decrease in urine volume and/or an excess of stone forming substances in the urine.

The following are risk factors that have been associated with stone formation: dehydration, change in urine pH, males aged between 40–60 years, positive family history, obesity, urinary anatomical abnormalities, and excessive dietary intake of oxalate, urate, sodium, and animal protein. Certain diseases which alter urinary volume, pH, and concentrations of certain ions (such as calcium, phosphate, oxalate, sodium, and uric acid) may also increase the risk of stone formation. Certain drugs such as calcium or vitamin D supplements, protease inhibitors, or diuretics may also increase the risk of stone formation.

Symptoms of acute renal or ureteric stones can include an abrupt onset of severe unilateral abdominal pain radiating to the groin (known as renal colic) that may be accompanied with nausea, vomiting, haematuria, increased urinary frequency, dysuria and fever (if concomitant urinary infection is present).

Stones can pass spontaneously and will depend on a number of factors, including the size of the stone (stones greater than 6 mm have a very low chance of spontaneous passage), the location (distal ureteral stones are more likely to pass than proximal ureteral stones), and the degree of obstruction.

Aims of treatment

[EvGr] The aim of treatment is to improve the detection, clearance and prevention of renal and ureteric stones thereby reducing pain and improving quality of life. ◇A

Non-drug treatment

[EvGr] Consider watchful waiting for asymptomatic renal stones if they are less than 5mm in diameter. If they are larger; the risk and benefit of this option should be discussed with the patient.

Options for surgical stone removal should be discussed by the specialist hospital team depending on severity of obstruction, patient factors, size and site of stone. Options include shockwave lithotripsy, percutaneous nephrolithotomy and ureteroscopy.

Consider stone analysis and measure serum calcium in patients with recurring renal or ureteric stones.

Along with maintaining a healthy lifestyle, advise patients to drink 2.5–3 litres of water a day with the addition of fresh lemon juice and to avoid carbonated drinks. Maintain a normal daily calcium intake of 700–1,200mg and salt intake of no more than 6g a day. For patients with recurrent calcium stones avoid excessive intake of oxalate-rich products, such as rhubarb, spinach, cocoa, tea, nuts, soy products, strawberries, and wheat bran. For patients with recurrent uric acid stones, avoid excessive dietary intake of urate rich products, such as liver, kidney, calf thymus, poultry skin, and certain fish (herring with skin, sardines and anchovies). ⒶA

Pain Management

[EvGr] Offer NSAIDs as first line treatment for the management of pain associated with suspected renal colic or renal and ureteric stones. If NSAIDs are contra-indicated or not sufficiently controlling the pain, consider intravenous paracetamol. Subsequently, opioids can be used if both paracetamol and NSAIDs are contra-indicated or not sufficiently controlling the pain. Do not offer antispasmodics to patients with suspected renal colic. ⒶA

Medical Expulsive Therapy

[EvGr] Consider alpha-adrenoceptor blockers for patients with distal ureteric stones less than 10mm in diameter. Alpha-adrenoceptor blockers may also be considered as adjunctive therapy for patients having shockwave lithotripsy for ureteric stones less than 10mm. ⒶA

Prevention of recurrence of stones

[EvGr] Alongside lifestyle advice, consider potassium citrate [unlicensed] in patients with recurrent stones composed of at least 50% calcium oxalate. Thiazides [unlicensed] may be given if patients also have hypercalciuria after restricting their sodium intake to no more than 6g a day. ⒶA

1.4 Urological pain

Urological pain

03-Apr-2019

Treatment

Lidocaine hydrochloride gel is a useful topical application in *urethral pain* or to relieve the discomfort of catheterisation.

For information on the management of pain in renal and ureteric stones, see Renal and ureteric stones p. 832.

Alkalinisation of urine

Alkalinisation of urine can be undertaken with potassium citrate. The alkalinising action may relieve the discomfort of *cystitis* caused by lower urinary tract infections. Sodium bicarbonate p. 1086 is used as a urinary alkalinising agent in some metabolic and renal disorders.

ALKALISING DRUGS › URINARY

Citric acid with potassium citrate

12-May-2020

● **INDICATIONS AND DOSE**

Relief of discomfort in mild urinary-tract infections | Alkalinisation of urine

▶ BY MOUTH USING ORAL SOLUTION
  ▸ Adult: 10 mL 3 times a day, diluted well with water

● CAUTIONS Cardiac disease · elderly
● INTERACTIONS → Appendix 1: potassium citrate
● SIDE-EFFECTS Hyperkalaemia · nausea · vomiting
● RENAL IMPAIRMENT Avoid in severe impairment.
  Monitoring Close monitoring required in renal impairment—high risk of hyperkalaemia.
● PRESCRIBING AND DISPENSING INFORMATION When prepared extemporaneously, the BP states Potassium Citrate Mixture BP consists of potassium citrate 30%, citric acid monohydrate 5% in a suitable vehicle with a lemon flavour. Extemporaneous preparations should be recently prepared according to the following formula: potassium citrate 3 g, citric acid monohydrate 500 mg, syrup 2.5 mL, quillaia tincture 0.1 mL, lemon spirit 0.05 mL, double-strength chloroform water 3 mL, water to 10 mL. Contains about 28 mmol K^+/10 mL.
● EXCEPTIONS TO LEGAL CATEGORY Proprietary brands of potassium citrate are on sale to the public for the relief of discomfort in mild urinary-tract infections.

● MEDICINAL FORMS There can be variation in the licensing of different medicines containing the same drug.
  Oral solution
  CAUTIONARY AND ADVISORY LABELS 27
  ▸ Citric acid with potassium citrate (Non-proprietary)
    Citric acid monohydrate 50 mg per 1 ml, Potassium citrate 300 mg per 1 ml Potassium citrate mixture | 200 ml Ⓟ £1.38 DT = £1.38

Sodium citrate

18-May-2020

● **INDICATIONS AND DOSE**

Bladder washouts

▶ Adult: (consult product literature)

Relief of discomfort in mild urinary-tract infections

▶ BY MOUTH
  ▸ Adult: (consult product literature)

Constipation (dose approved for use by community practitioner nurse prescribers)

▶ BY RECTUM
  ▸ Child 3–17 years: 5 mL for 1 dose
  ▸ Adult: 5 mL for 1 dose

MICOLETTE ®

Constipation

▶ BY RECTUM
  ▸ Child 3–17 years: 5–10 mL for 1 dose
  ▸ Adult: 5–10 mL for 1 dose

MICRALAX ®

Constipation

▶ BY RECTUM
  ▸ Child 3–17 years: 5 mL for 1 dose
  ▸ Adult: 5 mL for 1 dose

RELAXIT ®

Constipation

▶ BY RECTUM
  ▸ Child 1 month–2 years: 5 mL for 1 dose, insert only half the nozzle length   continued →

▸ Child 3-17 years: 5 mL for 1 dose
▸ Adult: 5 mL for 1 dose

● CONTRA-INDICATIONS
▸ With oral use Conditions where excess sodium or glucose should be avoided (e.g. cardiac disease, hypertension, patients on a sodium-restricted diet or diabetes)
▸ With rectal use Acute gastro-intestinal conditions
● CAUTIONS
▸ With oral use Elderly
▸ With rectal use Debilitated patients (in adults) · sodium and water retention in susceptible individuals
● INTERACTIONS → Appendix 1: sodium citrate
● SIDE-EFFECTS Polyuria
● PREGNANCY
▸ With oral use Use with caution.
● RENAL IMPAIRMENT
▸ With oral use In patients with fluid retention, avoid antacids containing large amounts of sodium.
● PRESCRIBING AND DISPENSING INFORMATION Sodium citrate 300 mmol/litre (88.2 mg/mL) oral solution is licensed for use before general anaesthesia for caesarean section (available from Viridian).
● EXCEPTIONS TO LEGAL CATEGORY Proprietary brands of sodium citrate are on sale to the public for the relief of discomfort in mild urinary-tract infections.

● MEDICINAL FORMS There can be variation in the licensing of different medicines containing the same drug. Forms available from special-order manufacturers include: oral solution
Granules
▸ Sodium citrate (Non-proprietary)
    Sodium citrate 4 gram Cystitis Relief 4g oral granules sachets | 6 sachet [GSL] £2.38 DT = £2.38
▸ Brands may include CanesOasis, Cystocalm
Oral solution
▸ Sodium citrate (Non-proprietary)
    Sodium citrate 88.23 mg per 1 ml Sodium citrate 0.3M oral solution | 30 ml [PoM] £4.70 DT = £4.70
Powder
▸ Numark (Numark Ltd)
    Sodium citrate 4 gram Numark cystitis treatment 4g oral powder sachets | 6 sachet [GSL] £1.65 DT = £1.65
▸ Sodium citrate (Non-proprietary)
    Sodium citrate 1 mg per 1 mg Sodium citrate powder | 500 gram [GSL] £7.49 DT = £7.49
Irrigation solution
▸ Sodium citrate (Non-proprietary)
    Sodium citrate 3% irrigation solution 1litre bags | 1 bag [S]
Enema
▸ Micolette Micro-enema (Pinewood Healthcare)
    Sodium citrate 90 mg per 1 ml Micolette Micro-enema 5ml | 12 enema [P] £4.50
▸ Micralax Micro-enema (RPH Pharmaceuticals AB)
    Sodium citrate 90 mg per 1 ml Micralax Micro-enema 5ml | 12 enema [P] £4.87
▸ Relaxit (Supra Enterprises Ltd)
    Sodium citrate 90 mg per 1 ml Relaxit Micro-enema 5ml | 12 enema £5.21

HEPARINOIDS

| **Pentosan polysulfate sodium** 27-Aug-2020

● INDICATIONS AND DOSE
Bladder pain syndrome
▸ BY MOUTH
▸ Adult: 100 mg 3 times a day, review treatment after 6 months and discontinue if no response

---

IMPORTANT SAFETY INFORMATION
MHRA/CHM ADVICE (UPDATED SEPTEMBER 2019): *ELMIRON®* (PENTOSAN POLYSULFATE SODIUM): RARE RISK OF PIGMENTARY MACULOPATHY
Cases of pigmentary maculopathy have been reported rarely with pentosan polysulfate sodium, especially after long-term use at high doses. Healthcare professionals are advised that patients should have regular ophthalmic examinations during treatment, and to consider stopping treatment if pigmentary maculopathy develops. Patients should be advised to seek immediate medical attention if visual changes occur.

● CONTRA-INDICATIONS Active bleeding
● CAUTIONS Patients at increased risk of bleeding
● SIDE-EFFECTS
▸ **Common or very common** Alopecia · asthenia · back pain · diarrhoea · dizziness · gastrointestinal discomfort · haemorrhage · headache · increased risk of infection · nausea · pelvic pain · peripheral oedema
▸ **Uncommon** Amblyopia · anaemia · appetite decreased · arthralgia · constipation · depression · dyspnoea · emotional lability · eye disorders · flatulence · hyperhidrosis · hyperkinesia · insomnia · leucopenia · melanocytic naevus size increased · myalgia · oral ulceration · paraesthesia · photosensitivity reaction · skin reactions · thrombocytopenia · tinnitus · vomiting · weight changes
▸ **Frequency not known** Coagulation disorder · hepatic function abnormal
● PREGNANCY Manufacturer advises avoid—no information available.
● BREAST FEEDING Manufacturer advises avoid—no information available.
● HEPATIC IMPAIRMENT Manufacturer advises caution—evidence of hepatic involvement in elimination.
● RENAL IMPAIRMENT Manufacturer advises caution—evidence of renal involvement in elimination.
● MONITORING REQUIREMENTS Manufacturer advises careful monitoring in patients with history of heparin or pentosan polysulfate sodium induced thrombocytopenia.
● NATIONAL FUNDING/ACCESS DECISIONS
For full details see funding body website
NICE decisions
▸ Pentosan polysulfate sodium for treating bladder pain syndrome (November 2019) NICE TA610 Recommended with restrictions
Scottish Medicines Consortium (SMC) decisions
▸ Pentosan polysulfate sodium (*Elmiron®*) for the treatment of adults with bladder pain syndrome characterised by either glomerulations or Hunner's lesions with moderate to severe pain, urgency and frequency of micturition (November 2019) SMC No. SMC2194 Recommended

- MEDICINAL FORMS There can be variation in the licensing of different medicines containing the same drug.
  Capsule
  CAUTIONARY AND ADVISORY LABELS 23
  ► Fibrase (Imported (Italy))
    Pentosan polysulfate sodium 50 mg Fibrase 50mg capsules | 50 capsule PoM 🔲
  ► Elmiron (Sovereign Medical Ltd, Consilient Health Ltd)
    Pentosan polysulfate sodium 100 mg Elmiron 100mg capsules | 90 capsule PoM £450.00–£699.40 DT = £450.00

TERPENES

Anethol with borneol, camphene, cineole, fenchone and pinene

- **INDICATIONS AND DOSE**
  Urolithiasis for the expulsion of calculi
  ► BY MOUTH
  ► Adult: 1–2 capsules 3–4 times a day, to be taken before food

- LESS SUITABLE FOR PRESCRIBING Preparation is less suitable for prescribing.

- MEDICINAL FORMS There can be variation in the licensing of different medicines containing the same drug.
  Capsule
  CAUTIONARY AND ADVISORY LABELS 25
  ► Rowatinex (Meadow Laboratories Ltd)
    Cineole 3 mg, Anethol 4 mg, Fenchone 4 mg, Borneol 10 mg, Camphene 15 mg, Pinene 31 mg Rowatinex capsules | 50 capsule PoM £7.35

2   Bladder instillations and urological surgery

Bladder instillations and urological surgery

19-Jul-2020

Bladder infection

Chlorhexidine solution p. 1255 given as bladder irrigation is licensed for the management of common infections of the bladder in patients with an indwelling urinary catheter. Chlorhexidine has broad spectrum activity against many Gram-positive and Gram-negative bacteria but it is ineffective against most *Pseudomonas spp.* Solutions containing chlorhexidine 1 in 5000 (0.02%) are used but they may irritate the mucosa and cause burning on micturition (in which case they should be discontinued). Sterile sodium chloride solution 0.9% (physiological saline) p. 1089 is licensed for use as a routine mechanical irrigant to flush out debris, small blood clots, or tissue in catheters.

Continuous bladder irrigation with amphotericin B (*Fungizone*®) 50 micrograms/mL p. 632 is licensed to treat some fungal infections (e.g. candiduria).

Bladder cancer

Bladder instillations of doxorubicin hydrochloride p. 946 and mitomycin p. 963 are licensed for the management of superficial bladder tumours. Such instillations reduce systemic side-effects; adverse effects on the bladder (e.g. micturition disorders and reduction in bladder capacity) may occur. Instillation of epirubicin hydrochloride p. 947 is also licensed for the treatment and prophylaxis of certain forms of superficial bladder cancer.

Instillation of BCG (Bacillus Calmette-Guérin p. 1001), a live attenuated strain derived from *Mycobacterium bovis*, is

licensed for the treatment of primary or recurrent bladder carcinoma *in-situ* and for the prevention of recurrence following transurethral resection.

Urological surgery

Glycine irrigation solution 1.5% below is licensed for use in transurethral surgical procedures such as prostatic resection; EvGr sterile sodium chloride solution 0.9% (physiological saline) is used for irrigation in percutaneous renal surgery (e.g. nephrolithotomy, ureteroscopy). ⟨A⟩

> **Other drugs used for Bladder instillations and urological surgery** Sodium citrate, p. 833

ANTISEPTICS AND DISINFECTANTS

Chlorhexidine with lidocaine

The properties listed below are those particular to the combination only. For the properties of the components please consider, chlorhexidine p. 1255, lidocaine hydrochloride p. 111.

- **INDICATIONS AND DOSE**
  Urethral sounding and catheterisation
  ► BY URETHRAL APPLICATION
  ► Adult: 6–11 mL

  Cystoscopy
  ► BY URETHRAL APPLICATION
  ► Adult: 11 mL, then 6–11 mL if required

  Surface anaesthesia (dose approved for use by community practitioner nurse prescribers) (on doctor's advice only)
  ► BY URETHRAL APPLICATION
  ► Adult: 6–11 mL

- INTERACTIONS → Appendix 1: antiarrhythmics

- MEDICINAL FORMS There can be variation in the licensing of different medicines containing the same drug.
  Gel
  EXCIPIENTS: May contain Hydroxybenzoates (parabens)
  ► Instillagel (CliniMed Ltd)
    Chlorhexidine gluconate 500 microgram per 1 ml, Lidocaine hydrochloride 20 mg per 1 ml Instillagel gel | 60 ml Ⓟ £10.50 DT = £10.50 | 110 ml Ⓟ £11.00 DT = £11.00

IRRIGATING SOLUTIONS

Glycine

23-Nov-2020

- **INDICATIONS AND DOSE**
  Bladder irrigation during urological surgery | Irrigation for transurethral resection of the prostate gland and bladder tumours
  ► Adult: (consult product literature)

- CAUTIONS
  CAUTIONS, FURTHER INFORMATION
  ► Urological surgery There is a high risk of fluid absorption from the irrigant used in endoscopic surgery within the urinary tract.

- SIDE-EFFECTS Cardiovascular disorder · electrolyte depletion · fluid overload · pulmonary disorder · seizure · vision blurred

- MEDICINAL FORMS There can be variation in the licensing of different medicines containing the same drug.
  Irrigation solution
  ► Glycine (Non-proprietary)
    Glycine 1.5% irrigation solution 3litre Easyflow bags | 1 bag 🔲
    Glycine 1.5% irrigation solution 1litre Flowfusor bottles | 1 bottle 🔲
    Glycine 1.5% irrigation solution 1litre Easyflow bags | 1 bag 🔲
    Glycine 1.5% irrigation solution 2litre Flowfusor bottles | 1 bottle 🔲

Catheter maintenance solutions

- CATHETER MAINTENANCE SOLUTIONS

OptiFlo G citric acid 3.23% catheter maintenance solution
(Bard Ltd)
50 ml · NHS indicative price = £3.70 · Drug Tariff (Part IXa)100 ml · NHS indicative price = £3.70 · Drug Tariff (Part IXa)

OptiFlo R citric acid 6% catheter maintenance solution (Bard Ltd)
50 ml · NHS indicative price = £3.70 · Drug Tariff (Part IXa)100 ml · NHS indicative price = £3.70 · Drug Tariff (Part IXa)

Uro-Tainer PHMB polihexanide 0.02% catheter maintenance solution (B.Braun Medical Ltd)
100 ml · NHS indicative price = £3.49 · Drug Tariff (Part IXa)

Uro-Tainer Twin Solutio R citric acid 6% catheter maintenance solution (B.Braun Medical Ltd)
60 ml · NHS indicative price = £4.94 · Drug Tariff (Part IXa)

Uro-Tainer Twin Suby G citric acid 3.23% catheter maintenance solution (B.Braun Medical Ltd)
60 ml · NHS indicative price = £4.94 · Drug Tariff (Part IXa)

UroFlush G citric acid 3.23% catheter maintenance solution
(TriOn Pharma Ltd)
50 ml · NHS indicative price = £3.15 · Drug Tariff (Part IXa)100 ml · NHS indicative price = £3.15 · Drug Tariff (Part IXa)

UroFlush R citric acid 6% catheter maintenance solution (TriOn Pharma Ltd)
50 ml · NHS indicative price = £3.15 · Drug Tariff (Part IXa)100 ml · NHS indicative price = £3.15 · Drug Tariff (Part IXa)

OptiFlo S saline 0.9% catheter maintenance solution (Bard Ltd)
Sodium chloride 9 mg per 1 ml 50 ml · NHS indicative price = £3.49 · Drug Tariff (Part IXa)100 ml · NHS indicative price = £3.49 · Drug Tariff (Part IXa)

Uro-Tainer M sodium chloride 0.9% catheter maintenance solution (B.Braun Medical Ltd) Sodium chloride 9 mg per 1 ml 50 ml · No NHS indicative price available · Drug Tariff (Part IXa)100 ml · No NHS indicative price available · Drug Tariff (Part IXa)

Uro-Tainer sodium chloride 0.9% catheter maintenance solution (B.Braun Medical Ltd) Sodium chloride 9 mg per 1 ml 50 ml · NHS indicative price = £3.61 · Drug Tariff (Part IXa)100 ml · NHS indicative price = £3.61 · Drug Tariff (Part IXa)

UroFlush Saline 0.9% catheter maintenance solution (TriOn Pharma Ltd) Sodium chloride 9 mg per 1 ml 50 ml · NHS indicative price = £3.15 · Drug Tariff (Part IXa)100 ml · NHS indicative price = £3.15 · Drug Tariff (Part IXa)

3   Contraception

Contraceptives, hormonal   16-Apr-2019

Overview

Hormonal contraception includes combined hormonal contraception (containing an oestrogen and a progestogen) and progestogen-only contraception.

[EvGr] When prescribing contraception, information should be given on all available methods taking into consideration medical eligibility. This should include contraceptive effectiveness (including factors that alter efficacy), non-contraceptive benefits, health risks, and side effects to allow an informed decision to be made on the most suitable choice. ⬨

In adolescents, hormonal contraception is used after menarche. When prescribing contraception for females under 16 years of age, it is considered good practice for health professionals to follow the criteria in the Department of Health Guidance (July 2004), commonly known as the Fraser Guidelines available at tinyurl.com/yy3hl2gt.

The UK Medical Eligibility Criteria for Contraceptive Use (available at www.fsrh.org) is published by the Faculty of Sexual and Reproductive Healthcare (FSRH); it categorises the risks of using contraceptive methods with pre-existing medical conditions.

Contraception in patients taking medication with teratogenic potential: FSRH (February 2018) and MHRA (May 2019) guidance

Females of childbearing potential should be advised to use highly effective contraception if they or their male partners are taking known teratogenic drugs or drugs with potential teratogenic effects. Highly effective contraception should be used both during treatment and for the recommended duration after discontinuation to avoid unintended pregnancy. Pregnancy testing should be performed before treatment initiation to exclude pregnancy and repeat testing may be required.

Methods of contraception considered to be 'highly effective' include the long-acting reversible contraceptives (LARC) copper intra-uterine device (Cu-IUD), levonorgestrel intra-uterine system (LNG-IUS) and progestogen-only implant (IMP), and male and female sterilisation. For more information see the FSRH CEU statement (www.fsrh.org/standards-and-guidance/documents/fsrh-ceu-statement-contraception-for-women-using-known/), MHRA drug safety update (www.gov.uk/drug-safety-update/medicines-with-teratogenic-potential-what-is-effective-contraception-and-how-often-is-pregnancy-testing-needed), and the UK teratogenic information service (www.uktis.org).

Combined hormonal contraceptives

Combined hormonal contraceptives (CHC) are available as tablets (COC), transdermal patches (CTP), and vaginal rings (CVR). They are highly user-dependant methods where the failure rate if used perfectly (i.e. correctly and consistently) is less than 1%. Certain factors such as the person's weight, malabsorption (COC only), and drug interactions may contribute to contraceptive failure. Prescriptions of up to 12 months' supply for CHC initiation or continuation may be appropriate to avoid unwanted discontinuation and increased risk of pregnancy.

[EvGr] It is recommended that combined hormonal contraceptives are not continued beyond 50 years of age as safer alternatives exist. ⬨

CHC use may be associated with some health benefits such as:

- Reduced risk of ovarian, endometrial and colorectal cancer;
- Predictable bleeding patterns;
- Reduced dysmenorrhoea and menorrhagia;
- Management of symptoms of polycystic ovary syndrome (PCOS), endometriosis and premenstrual syndrome;
- Improvement of acne;
- Reduced menopausal symptoms;
- Maintaining bone mineral density in peri-menopausal females under the age of 50 years.

The use of CHC is, however also associated with health risks. For information on these risks, and further information on the benefits, see FSRH clinical guideline: **Combined Hormonal Contraception** (see *Useful resources*).

For information on advice to give to patients on switching between CHC and other contraception, and the management of incorrect CHC use, see FSRH clinical guidance: **Combined Hormonal Contraception** and **Incorrect use of Combined Hormonal Contraception** (see *Useful resources*).

Preparation choice

Combined oral contraceptives (COCs) containing a fixed amount of an oestrogen and a progestogen in each active tablet are termed 'monophasic'; those with varying amounts of the two hormones are termed 'multiphasic'.

Combined oral contraceptives usually contain ethinylestradiol as the oestrogen component; mestranol and estradiol are also used. The ethinylestradiol content of COCs range from 20–40 micrograms. [EvGr] A monophasic preparation containing 30 micrograms or less of ethinylestradiol in combination with levonorgestrel or norethisterone (to minimise cardiovascular risk), is generally used as the first line option. However, choice should be made taking into account the patients medical history, personal preference, previous contraceptive experience, and any age related considerations.

Due to potential reduced efficacy, non-oral CHC should be considered if there are concerns over absorption. In females who weigh 90 kg or more, consider non-topical options or use additional precautions with CTP. Ⓐ

Combined Oral Contraceptives Monophasic 21-day preparations

Oestrogen content	Progestogen content	Brand
Ethinylestradiol 20 micrograms	Desogestrel 150 micrograms	Gedarel® 20/150
Ethinylestradiol 20 micrograms	Desogestrel 150 micrograms	Mercilon®
Ethinylestradiol 20 micrograms	Gestodene 75 micrograms	Femodette®
Ethinylestradiol 20 micrograms	Gestodene 75 micrograms	Millinette® 20/75
Ethinylestradiol 20 micrograms	Gestodene 75 micrograms	Sunya® 20/75
Ethinylestradiol 20 micrograms	Norethisterone acetate 1 mg	Loestrin® 20
Ethinylestradiol 30 micrograms	Desogestrel 150 micrograms	Gedarel® 30/150
Ethinylestradiol 30 micrograms	Desogestrel 150 micrograms	Marvelon®
Ethinylestradiol 30 micrograms	Drospirenone 3 mg	Yasmin®
Ethinylestradiol 30 micrograms	Gestodene 75 micrograms	Femodene®
Ethinylestradiol 30 micrograms	Gestodene 75 micrograms	Katya® 30/75
Ethinylestradiol 30 micrograms	Gestodene 75 micrograms	Millinette® 30/75
Ethinylestradiol 30 micrograms	Levonorgestrel 150 micrograms	Levest®
Ethinylestradiol 30 micrograms	Levonorgestrel 150 micrograms	Microgynon® 30
Ethinylestradiol 30 micrograms	Levonorgestrel 150 micrograms	Ovranette®
Ethinylestradiol 30 micrograms	Levonorgestrel 150 micrograms	Rigevidon®
Ethinylestradiol 30 micrograms	Norethisterone acetate 1.5 mg	Loestrin® 30
Ethinylestradiol 35 micrograms	Norgestimate 250 micrograms	Cilest®
Ethinylestradiol 35 micrograms	Norethisterone 500 micrograms	Brevinor®
Ethinylestradiol 35 micrograms	Norethisterone 1 mg	Norimin®
Mestranol 50 micrograms	Norethisterone 1 mg	Norinyl-1®

Combined Oral Contraceptives Monophasic 28-day preparations

Oestrogen content	Progestogen content	Brand
Ethinylestradiol 30 micrograms	Gestodene 75 micrograms	Femodene® ED
Ethinylestradiol 30 micrograms	Levonorgestrel 150 micrograms	Microgynon® 30 ED
Estradiol (as hemihydrate) 1.5 mg	Nomegestrol acetate 2.5 mg	Zoely®

Combined Oral Contraceptives Multiphasic 21-day preparations

Oestrogen content	Progestogen content	Brand
Ethinylestradiol 30 micrograms	Levonorgestrel 50 micrograms	
Ethinylestradiol 40 micrograms	Levonorgestrel 75 micrograms	Logynon®
Ethinylestradiol 30 micrograms	Levonorgestrel 125 micrograms	
Ethinylestradiol 30 micrograms	Levonorgestrel 50 micrograms	
Ethinylestradiol 40 micrograms	Levonorgestrel 75 micrograms	TriRegol®
Ethinylestradiol 30 micrograms	Levonorgestrel 125 micrograms	
Ethinylestradiol 35 micrograms	Norethisterone 500 micrograms	
Ethinylestradiol 35 micrograms	Norethisterone 1 mg	Synphase®
Ethinylestradiol 35 micrograms	Norethisterone 500 micrograms	

Combined Oral Contraceptives Multiphasic 28-day preparations

Oestrogen content	Progestogen content	Brand
Ethinylestradiol 30 micrograms	Levonorgestrel 50 micrograms	
Ethinylestradiol 40 micrograms	Levonorgestrel 75 micrograms	Logynon® ED
Ethinylestradiol 30 micrograms	Levonorgestrel 125 micrograms	
Estradiol valerate 3 mg		
Estradiol valerate 2 mg	Dienogest 2 mg	
Estradiol valerate 2 mg	Dienogest 3 mg	Qlaira®
Estradiol valerate 1 mg		

Regimen choice

ᴇᴠɢʀ Information should be given to females on both the traditional 21 day CHC regimen with a monthly withdrawal bleed during the 7 day hormone free interval (HFI), and 'tailored' CHC regimens [unlicensed use]. Tailored CHC regimens can only be used with monophasic CHC containing ethinylestradiol [unlicensed use]; they offer the choice of either a shortened, or less frequent, or no hormone free interval based on the person's preference.

7

Genito-urinary system

The following tailored regimens may be used [unlicensed use]:

- Shortened HFI: 21 days of continuous use followed by a 4 day HFI;
- Extended use (tricycling): 9 weeks of continuous use followed by a 4 or 7 day HFI;
- Flexible extended use: continuous use for 21 days or more followed by a 4 day HFI when breakthrough bleeding occurs;
- Continuous use: continuous CHC use with no HFI. ⓐ

Withdrawal bleeds do not represent physiological menstruation and there is no difference in efficacy or safety of using the traditional 21 day regimen, which mimics the natural menstrual cycle, over using extended or continuous regimens. Use of the traditional regimen may be associated with disadvantages such as heavy or painful withdrawal bleeds, headaches, mood changes, and increased risk of incorrect use with subsequent unplanned pregnancy. EvGr Withdrawal bleeds during traditional CHC use has been reported in women who are pregnant and should therefore not be relied on as reassurance of a person's pregnancy status. ⓐ

Follow up

EvGr A review of continued medical eligibility, satisfaction and adherence, drug interactions, and consideration of alternative contraception should be undertaken annually. Body mass index and blood pressure should also be checked annually. ⓐ

Surgery

The manufacturers of CHC recommend that CHC use should be discontinued at least 4 weeks prior to major elective surgery, any surgery to the legs or pelvis, or surgery that involves prolonged immobilisation of a lower limb. An alternative method of contraception should be used to prevent unintentional pregnancy, and CHC may be recommenced 2 weeks after full remobilisation. When discontinuation is not possible, e.g. after trauma or if a patient admitted for an elective procedure is still on CHC, thromboprophylaxis should be considered.

When to seek further advice

EvGr All females should be advised to seek advice from a healthcare professional if they experience any troublesome side effects, have a significant health event, start any new medication, would like to discontinue CHC, or to discuss alternative methods at any time. For further information, see FSRH guidance **Combined Hormonal Contraception** (refer to *Useful resources* below). ⓐ

Progestogen-only contraceptives

Oral progestogen-only contraceptives

Oral progestogen-only preparations alter cervical mucus to prevent sperm penetration and may inhibit ovulation in some women; oral desogestrel-only preparations consistently inhibit ovulation and this is their primary mechanism of action. There is insufficient clinical trial evidence to compare the efficacy of oral progestogen-only contraceptives with each other or with combined hormonal contraceptives. Progestogen-only contraceptives offer a suitable alternative to combined hormonal contraceptives when oestrogens are contra-indicated.

Parenteral progestogen-only contraceptives

Medroxyprogesterone acetate (*Depo-Provera®, SAYANA PRESS®*) p. 856 is a long-acting progestogen given by injection; it is at least as effective as the combined oral preparations but because of its prolonged action it should never be given without *full counselling backed by the patient information leaflet.* It may be used as a short-term or long-term contraceptive for women who have been counselled about the likelihood of menstrual disturbance and the potential for a delay in return to full fertility. Delayed return

of fertility and irregular cycles may occur after discontinuation of treatment but there is no evidence of permanent infertility. Troublesome bleeding has been reported in patients given medroxyprogesterone acetate in the immediate puerperium; delaying the first injection until 6 weeks after birth may minimise bleeding problems. If the woman is not breast-feeding, the first injection may be given within 5 days postpartum (she should be warned that the risk of troublesome bleeding may be increased).

- In adolescents, medroxyprogesterone acetate (*Depo-Provera®, SAYANA PRESS®*) should be used only when other methods of contraception are inappropriate;
- in all women, the benefits of using medroxyprogesterone acetate beyond 2 years should be evaluated against the risks;
- in women with risk factors for osteoporosis, a method of contraception other than medroxyprogesterone acetate should be considered.

Norethisterone enantate (*Noristerat®*) is a long-acting progestogen given as an oily injection which provides contraception for 8 weeks; it is used as short-term interim contraception e.g. before vasectomy becomes effective.

An **etonogestrel-releasing implant** (*Nexplanon®*) is also available. It is a highly effective long-acting contraceptive, consisting of a single flexible rod that is inserted subdermally into the lower surface of the upper arm and provides contraception for up to 3 years. The manufacturer advises that in heavier women, blood-etonogestrel concentrations are lower and therefore the implant may not provide effective contraception during the third year; they advise that earlier replacement may be considered in such patients—however, evidence to support this recommendation is lacking. Local reactions such as bruising and itching can occur at the insertion site. The contraceptive effect of etonogestrel is rapidly reversed on removal of the implant.

Intra-uterine progestogen-only device

The progestogen-only intra-uterine systems *Mirena®*, *Jaydess®* and *Levosert®* release levonorgestrel p. 852 directly into the uterine cavity. *Mirena®* is licensed for use as a contraceptive, for the treatment of primary menorrhagia and for the prevention of endometrial hyperplasia during oestrogen replacement therapy. *Jaydess®* and *Levosert®* are licensed for contraception, and *Levosert®* is additionally licensed for the treatment of menorrhagia. These may therefore be a contraceptive method of choice for women who have excessively heavy menses.

The effects of the progestogen-only intra-uterine system are mainly local and hormonal including prevention of endometrial proliferation, thickening of cervical mucus, and suppression of ovulation in some women (in some cycles). In addition to the progestogenic activity, the intra-uterine system itself may contribute slightly to the contraceptive effect. Return of fertility after removal is rapid and appears to be complete.

Advantages of the progestogen-only intra-uterine system over copper intra-uterine devices are that there may be an improvement in any dysmenorrhoea and a reduction in blood loss; there is also evidence that the frequency of pelvic inflammatory disease may be reduced (particularly in the youngest age groups who are most at risk).

In primary menorrhagia, menstrual bleeding is reduced significantly within 3–6 months of inserting the progestogen-only intra-uterine system, probably because it prevents endometrial proliferation. Another treatment should be considered if menorrhagia does not improve within this time.

Surgery

All progestogen-only contraceptives (including those given by injection) are suitable for use as an alternative to combined hormonal contraceptives before major elective surgery, before all surgery to the legs, or before surgery which involves prolonged immobilisation of a lower limb.

Useful resources

FSRH guideline: Combined Hormonal Contraception. The Faculty of Sexual & Reproductive Healthcare. February 2019.

www.fsrh.org/standards-and-guidance/documents/combined-hormonal-contraception/

FSRH CEU guidance: Recommended actions after incorrect use of combined hormonal contraception (e.g. late or missed pills, ring and patch). The Faculty of Sexual & Reproductive Healthcare. March 2020.

www.fsrh.org/documents/fsrh-ceu-guidance-recommended-actions-after-incorrect-use-of/

Contraceptives, non-hormonal

13-Oct-2020

Contraception in patients taking medication with teratogenic potential: FSRH (February 2018) and MHRA (March 2019) guidance

Females of childbearing potential should be advised to use highly effective contraception if they or their male partners are taking known teratogenic drugs or drugs with potential teratogenic effects. Highly effective contraception should be used both during treatment and for the recommended duration after discontinuation to avoid unintended pregnancy. Pregnancy testing should be performed before treatment initiation to exclude pregnancy and repeat testing may be required.

Methods of contraception considered to be 'highly effective' include the long-acting reversible contraceptives (LARC) copper intra-uterine device (Cu-IUD), levonorgestrel intra-uterine system (LNG-IUS) and progestogen-only implant (IMP), and male and female sterilisation. For more information see the FSRH CEU statement (www.fsrh.org/standards-and-guidance/documents/fsrh-ceu-statement-contraception-for-women-using-known/), MHRA drug safety update (www.gov.uk/drug-safety-update/medicines-with-teratogenic-potential-what-is-effective-contraception-and-how-often-is-pregnancy-testing-needed), and the UK teratology information service (www.uktis.org).

Barrier methods

Barrier methods include condoms (male and female), diaphragms and cervical caps. Male condoms are less effective than some other contraception methods but are effective when used consistently and correctly, and provide significant protection against some sexually transmitted infections (STIs). Female condoms are also available; they are pre-lubricated with a non-spermicidal lubricant.

There is no evidence that condoms lubricated with spermicide provide additional protection against pregnancy or STIs. ⟨EvGr⟩ Diaphragms and caps must be used in conjunction with a **spermicide** and should not be removed until at least 6 hours after the last episode of intercourse. ⟨A⟩

Spermicidal contraceptives

Spermicidal contraceptives are useful additional safeguards but do **not** give adequate protection if used alone. They have two components: a spermicide and a vehicle for its delivery (e.g. vaginal gel). ⟨EvGr⟩ They are suitable for use with barrier methods, such as diaphragms or caps; however, spermicidal contraceptives are not recommended for use with condoms, as there is no evidence of any additional protection compared with non-spermicidal lubricants.

Spermicidal contraceptives are not suitable for use in those with or at high risk of sexually transmitted infections (including HIV); ⟨A⟩ high frequency use of the spermicide nonoxinol '9' p. 858 has been associated with genital lesions, which may increase the risk of acquiring these infections.

Contraceptive devices

Intra-uterine devices

⟨EvGr⟩ The intra-uterine device (IUD) is a suitable contraceptive for women of all ages irrespective of parity; ⟨A⟩ however they may be unsuitable in women with certain conditions such as those with pelvic inflammatory disease or unexplained vaginal bleeding. The UK Medical Eligibility Criteria for Contraceptive Use (published by FSRH) provides guidance on safe use of contraceptive methods including restrictions for intra-uterine devices; full guidance is available at www.fsrh.org.

⟨EvGr⟩ Fertility declines with age and therefore a copper intra-uterine device which is fitted in a woman over the age of 40, may remain in the uterus until menopause. ⟨A⟩

The most effective intra-uterine devices have at least 380 mm^2 of copper and have banded copper on the transverse arms. Other smaller devices have been introduced to minimise side-effects.

Caution with oil-based lubricants

Products such as petroleum jelly (*Vaseline*®), baby oil and oil-based vaginal and rectal preparations are likely to damage condoms, contraceptive diaphragms and caps made from latex rubber, and may render them less effective as a barrier method of contraception and as a protection from sexually transmitted infections (including HIV).

Emergency contraception

31-Aug-2017

Overview

⟨EvGr⟩ Emergency contraception is intended for occasional use, to reduce the risk of pregnancy after unprotected sexual intercourse. It does not replace effective regular contraception.

Women who do not wish to conceive should be offered emergency contraception after unprotected sexual intercourse that has taken place on any day of a natural menstrual cycle. Emergency contraception should also be offered after unprotected intercourse from day 21 after childbirth (unless the criteria for lactational amenorrhoea are met), and from day 5 after abortion, miscarriage, ectopic pregnancy or uterine evacuation for gestational trophoblastic disease.

Emergency contraception should also be offered to women if their regular contraception has been compromised or has been used incorrectly. ⟨A⟩

Emergency contraceptive methods

Copper intra-uterine devices

⟨EvGr⟩ Insertion of a copper intra-uterine device (see intra-uterine contraceptive devices (copper) p. 849) is the most effective form of emergency contraception and should be offered (if appropriate) to all women who have had unprotected sexual intercourse and do not want to conceive. A copper intra-uterine contraceptive device can be inserted up to 120 hours (5 days) after unprotected intercourse or up to 5 days after the earliest likely calculated ovulation (i.e. within the minimum period before implantation), regardless of the number of episodes of unprotected intercourse earlier in the cycle. Antibacterial cover should be considered for copper intra-uterine contraceptive device insertion if there is a significant risk of sexually transmitted infection that could be associated with ascending pelvic infection.

A copper intra-uterine device is not known to be affected by body mass index (BMI) or body-weight or by other drugs. ⟨A⟩

Hormonal methods

EvGr Hormonal emergency contraceptives (includes levonorgestrel p. 852 and ulipristal acetate p. 851) should be offered as soon as possible after unprotected intercourse if a copper intra-uterine device is not appropriate or is not acceptable to the patient; either drug should be taken as soon as possible after unprotected intercourse to increase efficacy. Hormonal emergency contraception administered after ovulation is ineffective.

Levonorgestrel is effective if taken within 72 hours (3 days) of unprotected intercourse and may also be used between 72 and 96 hours after unprotected intercourse [unlicensed use], but efficacy decreases with time. Ulipristal acetate is effective if taken within 120 hours (5 days) of unprotected intercourse. Ulipristal acetate has been demonstrated to be more effective than levonorgestrel for emergency contraception.

It is possible that a higher body-weight or BMI could reduce the effectiveness of oral emergency contraception, particularly levonorgestrel; if BMI is greater than 26 kg/m² or body-weight is greater than 70 kg, it is recommended that either ulipristal acetate or a double dose of levonorgestrel [unlicensed indication] (see *Emergency contraception* under levonorgestrel) is given. It is unknown which is more effective.

Ulipristal acetate should be considered as the first-line hormonal emergency contraceptive for a woman who has had unprotected intercourse 96–120 hours ago (even if she has also had unprotected intercourse within the last 96 hours). It should also be considered first line for a woman who has had unprotected sexual intercourse within the last 5 days if it is likely to have taken place during the 5 days before the estimated day of ovulation. ⒶΔ

Hormonal emergency contraception interactions
See Contraceptives, interactions below.

Starting hormonal contraception after emergency hormonal contraception

Emergency hormonal contraception methods do **not** provide ongoing contraception. EvGr After taking levonorgestrel, women should start suitable hormonal contraception immediately. They must use condoms reliably or abstain from intercourse until contraception becomes effective.

Women should wait 5 days after taking ulipristal acetate before starting suitable hormonal contraception. Women must use condoms reliably or abstain from intercourse during the 5 day waiting period and also until their contraceptive method is effective. ⒶΔ

The copper intra-uterine device immediately provides effective ongoing contraception.

Useful Resources

Emergency Contraception. The Faculty of Sexual and Reproductive Healthcare. Clinical guidance. March 2017. www.fsrh.org/standards-and-guidance/documents/ceu-clinical-guidance-emergency-contraception-march-2017

Contraceptives, interactions   06-Jun-2017

Overview

The effectiveness of *combined* oral contraceptives, *progestogen-only* oral contraceptives, contraceptive patches, vaginal rings, and emergency hormonal contraception can be considerably reduced by interaction with drugs that induce hepatic enzyme activity (e.g. carbamazepine p. 327, eslicarbazepine acetate, nevirapine p. 684, oxcarbazepine p. 338, phenytoin p. 340, phenobarbital p. 353, primidone p. 354, ritonavir p. 698, St John's wort, topiramate p. 349 and, above all, rifabutin p. 612 and rifampicin p. 619). and possibly also griseofulvin p. 640. A condom together with a long-acting method (such as an injectable contraceptive)

may be more suitable for patients with HIV infection or at risk of HIV infection; advice on the possibility of interaction with antiretroviral drugs should be sought from HIV specialists.

For further information on other drug interactions with hormonal contraceptives, see the *Interactions* section of the relevant drug monograph.

Combined hormonal contraceptives interactions

Women using combined hormonal contraceptive patches, vaginal rings or oral tablets who require enzyme-inducing drugs or griseofulvin should be advised to change to a reliable contraceptive method that is unaffected by enzyme-inducers, such as some parenteral progestogen-only contraceptives (medroxyprogesterone acetate p. 856 and norethisterone p. 806) or intra-uterine devices (levonorgestrel p. 852; see also Contraceptives, non-hormonal p. 839). This should be continued for the duration of treatment and for four weeks after stopping. If a change in contraceptive method is undesirable or inappropriate the following options should be discussed:

Short course (2 months or less) of an enzyme-inducing drug
Continuing the combined hormonal contraceptive method may be appropriate if used in combination with consistent and careful use of condoms for the duration of treatment and for four weeks after stopping the enzyme-inducing drug.

Long-term course (over 2 months) of an enzyme-inducing drug (except rifampicin or rifabutin) or a course of griseofulvin
Use a monophasic combined oral contraceptive at a dose of ethinylestradiol 50 micrograms or more daily p. 802 [unlicensed use] and use either an extended or a 'tricycling' regimen (i.e. taking three packets of monophasic tablets without a break followed by a shortened tablet-free interval of four days [unlicensed use]); continue for the duration of treatment with the interacting drug and for four weeks after stopping.

If breakthrough bleeding occurs (and all other causes are ruled out) it is recommended that the dose of ethinylestradiol is increased by increments of 10 micrograms up to a maximum of 70 micrograms daily [unlicensed use] on specialist advice, or to use additional precautions, or to change to a method unaffected by the interacting drugs.

Use of contraceptive patches and vaginal rings (including concurrent use of two patches or two vaginal rings) is not recommended for women taking enzyme-inducing drugs over a long period.

Long-term course (over 2 months) of rifampicin or rifabutin
An alternative method of contraception (such as an IUD) is **always** recommended because they are such potent enzyme-inducing drugs; the alternative method of contraception should be continued for four weeks after stopping the enzyme-inducing drug.

Antibacterials that do not induce liver enzymes
It is recommended that no additional contraceptive precautions are required when *combined* oral contraceptives, contraceptive patches or vaginal rings are used with antibacterials that do not induce liver enzymes, unless diarrhoea or vomiting occur. These recommendations should be discussed with the woman.

There had been concerns that some antibacterials that do not induce liver enzymes (e.g. ampicillin p. 584, doxycycline p. 601) reduce the efficacy of *combined* oral contraceptives by impairing the bacterial flora responsible for recycling ethinylestradiol from the large bowel. However, there is a lack of evidence to support this interaction.

Oral progestogen-only contraceptives interactions
Effectiveness of oral progestogen-only preparations is not affected by antibacterials that do not induce liver enzymes. The efficacy of oral progestogen-only preparations is, however, reduced by enzyme-inducing drugs or griseofulvin and an alternative contraceptive method, unaffected by the

interacting drug, is recommended during treatment with an interacting drug and for at least 4 weeks afterwards.

For a short course of an enzyme-inducing drug (less than two months), continuing the progestogen-only oral method may be appropriate if used in combination with consistent and careful use of condoms for the duration of treatment and for four weeks after stopping the enzyme-inducing drug.

Parenteral progestogen-only contraceptives interactions Effectiveness of parenteral progestogen-only contraceptives is not affected by antibacterials that do not induce liver enzymes. The effectiveness of intramuscular norethisterone injection and intramuscular and subcutaneous medroxyprogesterone acetate injections is not affected by enzyme-inducing drugs and they may be continued as normal during courses of these drugs.

Effectiveness of the etonogestrel-releasing implant p. 855 may be reduced by enzyme-inducing drugs or griseofulvin and an alternative contraceptive method, unaffected by the interacting drug, is recommended during treatment with the interacting drug and for at least 4 weeks after stopping.

For a short course of an enzyme-inducing drug, if a change in contraceptive method is undesirable or inappropriate, continued contraception with the implant may be appropriate if used in combination with consistent and careful use of condoms for the duration of treatment and for 4 weeks after stopping the enzyme-inducing drug.

Hormonal emergency contraception interactions
The effectiveness of levonorgestrel and ulipristal acetate p. 851 is reduced in women taking enzyme-inducing drugs or griseofulvin (and for at least 4 weeks after stopping). EvGr A copper intra-uterine device can be offered instead. If the copper intra-uterine device is declined or unsuitable, the dose of levonorgestrel should be increased (See *Dose adjustments due to interactions* under levonorgestrel). There is no need to increase the dose for emergency contraception if the patient is taking antibacterials that are not enzyme inducers. ⓐ

The effectiveness of ulipristal acetate for emergency contraception in women using drugs that increase gastric pH has not been studied. Levonorgestrel or a copper intra-uterine device should be considered as alternatives.

EvGr Hormonal contraception should not be newly initiated in a patient until five days after administration of ulipristal acetate as emergency hormonal contraception—the contraceptive effect of ulipristal acetate will be reduced. Consistent and careful use of condoms is recommended.

Ulipristal acetate can be used as emergency hormonal contraception more than once in the same cycle. ⓐ Conversely, manufacturer advises that use of levonorgestrel as emergency contraception more than once in the same cycle is not advisable due to increased risk of side-effects (such as menstrual irregularities).

EvGr Levonorgestrel should not be used (as emergency hormonal contraception) within 5 days of administration of ulipristal acetate (as emergency hormonal contraception), as the contraceptive effect of ulipristal acetate may be reduced by progestogens.

Ulipristal acetate is not recommend for use in women who have severe asthma treated by oral corticosteroids, due to the antiglucocorticoid effect of ulipristal acetate. ⓐ

Useful Resources

Drug interactions with hormonal contraception. The Faculty of Sexual and Reproductive Healthcare. Clinical guidance. January 2018.
www.fsrh.org/standards-and-guidance/current-clinical-guidance/drug-interactions

Emergency Contraception. The Faculty of Sexual and Reproductive Healthcare. FSRH guideline. December 2017.
www.fsrh.org/documents/ceu-clinical-guidance-emergency-contraception-march-2017/

3.1 Contraception, combined

OESTROGENS COMBINED WITH PROGESTOGENS

Combined hormonal contraceptives

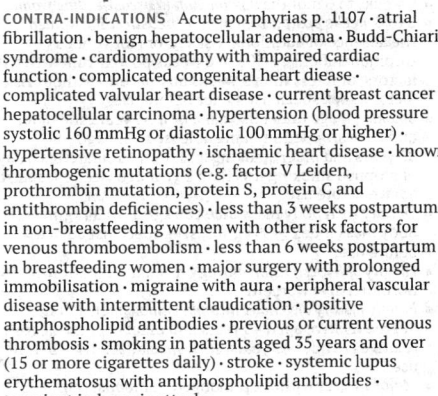

- **CONTRA-INDICATIONS** Acute porphyrias p. 1107 · atrial fibrillation · benign hepatocellular adenoma · Budd-Chiari syndrome · cardiomyopathy with impaired cardiac function · complicated congenital heart disease · complicated valvular heart disease · current breast cancer · hepatocellular carcinoma · hypertension (blood pressure systolic 160 mmHg or diastolic 100 mmHg or higher) · hypertensive retinopathy · ischaemic heart disease · known thrombogenic mutations (e.g. factor V Leiden, prothrombin mutation, protein S, protein C and antithrombin deficiencies) · less than 3 weeks postpartum in non-breastfeeding women with other risk factors for venous thromboembolism · less than 6 weeks postpartum in breastfeeding women · major surgery with prolonged immobilisation · migraine with aura · peripheral vascular disease with intermittent claudication · positive antiphospholipid antibodies · previous or current venous thrombosis · smoking in patients aged 35 years and over (15 or more cigarettes daily) · stroke · systemic lupus erythematosus with antiphospholipid antibodies · transient ischaemic attack

- **CAUTIONS**

  GENERAL CAUTIONS Carrier of breast cancer gene mutations e.g. BRCA1, BRCA2—seek specialist advice before use · cervical intraepithelial neoplasia or cancer · cholestasis during pregnancy · cholestasis with previous use of combined hormonal contraception—seek specialist advice before use · focal nodular hyperplasia · gallbladder disease—if medically treated or current, seek specialist advice before use · history of breast cancer—seek specialist advice before use · history of negative mood changes induced by hormonal contraceptive (a product containing an alternative progestogen may be tried) · inflammatory bowel disease · organ transplantation—when complicated, seek specialist advice before use · personal or family history of hypertriglyceridaemia (increased risk of pancreatitis) · prolactinoma—seek specialist advice before use · risk factors for cardiovascular disease · risk factors for venous thromboembolism · sickle-cell disease · undiagnosed mass or breast symptoms during combined hormonal contraception treatment—if symptoms exist prior to initiation, seek specialist advice before use · undiagnosed vaginal bleeding · viral hepatitis during combined hormonal contraception treatment—if condition exists prior to initiation, seek specialist advice before use

  SPECIFIC CAUTIONS

  ▸ With oral use bariatric surgery with body mass index 30 kg/m² to 34 kg/m² (possible reduction in contraceptive efficacy)—if body mass index $\geq$ 35 kg/m², seek specialist advice before use · severe diarrhoea (possible reduction in contraceptive efficacy) · vomiting (possible reduction in contraceptive efficacy)

  CAUTIONS, FURTHER INFORMATION

  ▸ Risk of venous thromboembolism There is an increased risk of venous thromboembolic disease in users of combined hormonal contraceptives particularly during the first year and possibly after restarting combined hormonal contraceptives following a break of four weeks or more. This risk is smaller than that associated with pregnancy and the postpartum period. In all cases the risk of venous thromboembolism increases with age and in the presence of other risk factors, such as obesity. The risk also varies depending on the type of progestogen and oestrogen dose.

▸ Risk factors for venous thromboembolism Use with **caution** if any of following factors present and **avoid or seek specialist advice** if multiple risk factors present (for risk factors where treatment with combined hormonal contraceptives should be avoided, see *Contra-indications*)

- *Age* 40 years and older—if 50 years and older, seek specialist advice before use;
- 6 weeks to 6 months *postpartum in breastfeeding women*;
- 3 to 6 weeks *postpartum in non-breastfeeding women* in the absence of additional risk factors for venous thromboembolism—if 3 to 6 weeks postpartum with risk factors, or if less than 3 weeks postpartum without risk factors, seek specialist advice before use;
- *Smoking* if age under 35 years, or if 35 years and older and have stopped smoking at least 1 year ago—if 35 years and older smoking less than 15 cigarettes a day or stopped smoking less than 1 year ago, seek specialist advice before use;
- *Obesity* with body mass index 30 kg/m^2 to 34 kg/m^2—if body mass index $\geq$ 35 kg/m^2, seek specialist advice before use;
- *History of hypertension during pregnancy* in currently normotensive women;
- *Family history of venous thromboembolism* in a first-degree relative aged 45 years and older—if first-degree relative is under 45 years, seek specialist advice before use;
- *Major surgery* without prolonged immobilsation;
- *Long-term immobility* (e.g. wheelchair use, debilitating illness)—seek specialist advice before use;
- *Superficial venous thrombosis*;
- *Uncomplicated valvular heart disease*;
- *Uncomplicated congenital heart disease*;
- *Cardiomyopathy* with normal cardiac function;
- *Long QT syndrome*;
- *Systemic lupus erythematosus* with no antiphospholipid antibodies;
- *High altitudes*: women travelling above 4500 m or 14500 feet for more than 1 week should consider alternative contraceptive methods (risk of thrombosis).

Combined Hormonal Contraception and Risk of Venous Thromboembolism

Progestogen in Combined Hormonal Contraceptive	Estimated incidence per 10 000 women per year of use
Non-pregnant, not using combined hormonal contraception	2
Levonorgesterol[1]	5–7
Norgestimate[1]	5–7
Norethisterone[1]	5–7
Etonogestrel[1]	6–12
Norelgestromin[1]	6–12
Gestodene[1]	9–12
Desogestrel[1]	9–12
Drospirenone[1]	9–12
Dienogest[2]	Not known—insufficient data
Nomegestrol[2]	Not known—insufficient data

[1] Combined with ethinylestradiol [2] Combined with estradiol

▸ Risk of cardiovascular disease Combined hormonal contraceptives also slightly increase the risk of *cardiovascular disease* such as myocardial infarction and ischaemic stroke; risk appears to be greater with higher oestrogen doses.

▸ Risk factors for cardiovascular disease Use with **caution** if any one of following factors present but **avoid or seek specialist advice** if multiple risk factors present (for risk factors where treatment with combined hormonal contraceptives should be avoided, see *Contra-indications*)

- *Age* 40 years and older—if 50 years and older, seek specialist advice before use;
- *Smoking* if age under 35 years, or if 35 years and older and have stopped smoking at least 1 year ago—if 35 years and older smoking less than 15 cigarettes a day, or stopped smoking less than 1 year ago, seek specialist advice before use;
- *Hypertension* if adequately controlled or if blood pressure systolic 140–159 *mmHg* or diastolic 90–99 *mmHg*, seek specialist advice before use;
- *History of hypertension during pregnancy* in currently normotensive women;
- *Dyslipidaemias*;
- *Non-migrainous headache (mild or severe)* during combined hormonal contraceptive use;
- *Migraine without aura* prior to initiation of combined hormonal contraceptives—if *migraine without aura* occurs during combined hormonal contraceptive use or when history of *migraine with aura* is 5 or more years ago, seek specialist advice;
- *Idiopathic intracranial hypertension*
- *Uncomplicated valvular heart disease*;
- *Uncomplicated congenital heart disease*;
- *Cardiomyopathy* with normal cardiac function;
- *Long QT syndrome*;
- *Diabetes mellitus*—if vascular disease present, seek specialist advice before use;
- *Rheumatoid arthritis*;
- *Systemic lupus erythematosus* without antiphospholipid antibodies.

● SIDE-EFFECTS

▸ **Common or very common** Acne · fluid retention · headaches · metrorrhagia · nausea · weight increased

▸ **Uncommon** Alopecia · hypertension

▸ **Rare or very rare** Venous thromboembolism

SIDE-EFFECTS, FURTHER INFORMATION

Breast cancer There is a small increase in the risk of having breast cancer diagnosed in women taking the combined oral contraceptive pill; this relative risk may be due to an earlier diagnosis. In users of combined oral contraceptive pills the cancers are more likely to be localised to the breast. The most important factor for diagnosing breast cancer appears to be the age at which the contraceptive is stopped rather than the duration of use; any increase in the rate of diagnosis diminishes gradually during the 10 years after stopping and disappears by 10 years.

Cervical cancer Use of combined oral contraceptives for 5 years or longer is associated with a small increased risk of cervical cancer; the risk diminishes after stopping and disappears by about 10 years. The possible small increase in the risk of breast cancer and cervical cancer should be weighed against the protective effect against cancers of the ovary and endometrium.

● PREGNANCY Not known to be harmful.

● BREAST FEEDING Avoid until weaning or for 6 months after birth (adverse effects on lactation).

● HEPATIC IMPAIRMENT In general, manufacturer advises caution; avoid in acute disease, severe chronic disease, or liver tumour.

● DIRECTIONS FOR ADMINISTRATION

▸ With oral use Each tablet should be taken at approximately same time each day; if delayed, contraceptive protection may be lost. FSRH advises if reasonably certain woman is not pregnant, first course can be started on any day of cycle—if starting on day 6 of cycle or later, additional precautions (barrier methods) necessary during first 7 days; for estradiol-containing preparations, additional precautions (barrier methods) necessary for 7 days (9 days for *Qlaira*®) if started after day 1 of cycle.

Changing to combined preparation containing different progestogen

▸ With oral use FSRH advises if previous contraceptive used correctly, or pregnancy can reasonably be excluded, start the first active tablet of new brand immediately. Consult product literature for requirements of specific preparations.

Changing from progestogen-only tablet

▸ With oral use FSRH advises if previous contraceptive used correctly, or pregnancy can reasonably be excluded, start new brand immediately, additional precautions (barrier methods) necessary for first 7 days (9 days for *Qlaira*®).

Secondary amenorrhoea (exclude pregnancy)

▸ With oral use FSRH advises start any day, additional precautions (barrier methods) necessary during first 7 days (9 days for *Qlaira*®).

After childbirth (not breast-feeding)

▸ With oral use FSRH advises start 3 weeks after childbirth except on specialist advice in the absence of additional risk factors for thromboembolism, or 6 weeks after childbirth in the presence of additional risk factors for thromboembolism (increased risk of thrombosis if started earlier); additional precautions (barrier methods) necessary for first 7 days (9 days for *Qlaira*®).

After abortion, miscarriage, ectopic pregnancy or gestational trophoblastic disease

▸ With oral use FSRH advises additional contraceptive precautions (barrier methods) required for 7 days if started after day 5 following treatment; for estradiol-containing preparations, additional contraceptive precautions (barrier methods) required for 7 days (9 days for *Qlaira*®) if started after day 1 following treatment.

● **PATIENT AND CARER ADVICE**

Travel Women taking oral contraceptives or using the patch or vaginal ring are at an increased risk of deep vein thrombosis during travel involving long periods of immobility (over 3 hours). The risk may be reduced by appropriate exercise during the journey and possibly by wearing graduated compression hosiery.

Diarrhoea and vomiting

▸ With oral use Vomiting and severe diarrhoea can interfere with the absorption of combined oral contraceptives. The FSRH advises following the instructions for missed pills if vomiting occurs within 3 hours of taking a combined oral contraceptive or severe diarrhoea occurs for more than 24 hours. Use of non-oral contraception should be considered if diarrhoea or vomiting persist.

Missed doses

▸ With oral use The critical time for loss of contraceptive protection is when a pill is omitted at the *beginning* or *end* of a cycle (which lengthens the pill-free interval). If a woman forgets to take a pill, it should be taken as soon as she remembers, and the next one taken at the normal time (even if this means taking 2 pills together). A missed pill is one that is 24 or more hours late. If a woman misses only one pill, she should take an active pill as soon as she remembers and then resume normal pill-taking. No additional precautions are necessary. If a woman misses 2 or more pills (especially from the first 7 in a packet), she may not be protected. She should take an active pill as soon as she remembers and then resume normal pill-taking. In addition, she must either abstain from sex or use an additional method of contraception such as a condom for the next 7 days. If these 7 days run beyond the end of the packet, the next packet should be started at once, omitting the pill-free interval (or, in the case of

everyday (ED) pills, omitting the 7 inactive tablets). Emergency contraception is recommended if 2 or more combined oral contraceptive tablets are missed from the first 7 tablets in a packet and unprotected intercourse has occurred since finishing the last packet.

◢ 841

Dienogest with estradiol valerate

13-Sep-2020

● **INDICATIONS AND DOSE**

Contraception with 28-day combined preparations | Menstrual symptoms with 28-day combined preparations

▸ BY MOUTH

▸ Females of childbearing potential: 1 active tablet daily for 26 days, followed by 1 inactive tablet daily for 2 days, to be started on day 1 of cycle with first active tablet (withdrawal bleeding may occur during the 2-day interval of inactive tablets); subsequent courses repeated without interval

● **INTERACTIONS** → Appendix 1: combined hormonal contraceptives

● **SIDE-EFFECTS**

▸ **Common or very common** Breast abnormalities · gastrointestinal discomfort · increased risk of infection · menstrual cycle irregularities

▸ **Uncommon** Appetite increased · cervical abnormalities · crying · depression · diarrhoea · dizziness · fatigue · haemorrhage · hot flush · hyperhidrosis · mood altered · muscle spasms · neoplasms · oedema · ovarian and fallopian tube disorders · painful sexual intercourse · pelvic disorders · sexual dysfunction · skin reactions · sleep disorders · uterine cramps · vomiting · vulvovaginal disorders · weight decreased

▸ **Rare or very rare** Aggression · anxiety · arterial thromboembolism · asthma · chest pain · cholecystitis chronic · concentration impaired · constipation · contact lens intolerance · dry eye · dry mouth · dyspnoea · eye swelling · fever · galactorrhoea · gastrooesophageal reflux disease · genital discharge · hair changes · hypertriglyceridaemia · hypotension · lymphadenopathy · malaise · myocardial infarction · pain · palpitations · paraesthesia · seborrhoea · sensation of pressure · urinary tract pain · vascular disorders · vertigo

● **DIRECTIONS FOR ADMINISTRATION**

Changing to *Qlaira*® Start the first active *Qlaira*® tablet on the day after taking the last active tablet of the previous brand.

● **PATIENT AND CARER ADVICE**

Diarrhoea and vomiting In cases of persistent vomiting or severe diarrhoea lasting more than 12 hours in women taking *Qlaira*®, refer to product literature.

Missed doses A missed pill for a patient taking *Qlaira*® is one that is 12 hours or more late; for information on how to manage missed pills in women taking *Qlaira*®, refer to product literature.

● **MEDICINAL FORMS** There can be variation in the licensing of different medicines containing the same drug.

Tablet

▸ Qlaira (Bayer Plc)
Qlaira tablets | 84 tablet [PoM] £25.18

7

Genito-urinary system

Estradiol with nomegestrol

F 841

13-Sep-2020

- **INDICATIONS AND DOSE**

Contraception

▶ BY MOUTH
  ▶ Females of childbearing potential: 1 active tablet daily for 24 days, followed by 1 inactive tablet daily for 4 days, to be started on day 1 of cycle with first active tablet (withdrawal bleeding occurs when inactive tablets being taken); subsequent courses repeated without interval

- **INTERACTIONS** → Appendix 1: combined hormonal contraceptives

- **SIDE-EFFECTS**
▶ **Common or very common** Breast abnormalities · depression · menstrual cycle irregularities · mood altered · pelvic pain · sexual dysfunction
▶ **Uncommon** Abdominal distension · appetite abnormal · galactorrhoea · hot flush · hyperhidrosis · oedema · painful sexual intercourse · seborrhoea · sensation of pressure · skin reactions · uterine cramps · vulvovaginal disorders
▶ **Rare or very rare** Cerebrovascular insufficiency · concentration impaired · contact lens intolerance · dry eye · dry mouth · gallbladder disorders · hypertrichosis

- **PREGNANCY** Toxicity in *animal* studies.

- **DIRECTIONS FOR ADMINISTRATION** *Zoely®* *(every day (ED) combined (monophasic) preparation)*, 1 *active* tablet daily for 24 days, followed by 1 *inactive* tablet daily for 4 days, starting on day 1 of cycle with first *active* tablet; subsequent courses repeated without interval (withdrawal bleeding occurs when *inactive* tablets being taken). Changing to *Zoely®* Start the first active *Zoely®* tablet on the day after taking the last active tablet of the previous brand or, at the latest, the day after the tablet-free or inactive tablet interval of the previous brand.

- **PATIENT AND CARER ADVICE**
Diarrhoea and vomiting In cases of persistent vomiting or severe diarrhoea lasting more than 12 hours in women taking *Zoely®*, refer to product literature.
Missed doses A missed pill for a patient taking *Zoely®* is one that is 12 hours or more late; for information on how to manage missed pills in women taking *Zoely®*, refer to product literature.

- **MEDICINAL FORMS** There can be variation in the licensing of different medicines containing the same drug.

Tablet
▶ Zoely (Theramex HQ UK Ltd) ▼
  Estradiol (as Estradiol hemihydrate) 1.5 mg, Nomegestrol acetate 2.5 mg Zoely 2.5mg/1.5mg tablets | 84 tablet [PoM] £19.80 DT = £19.80

Ethinylestradiol with desogestrel

F 841

- **INDICATIONS AND DOSE**

Menstrual symptoms with 21-day combined preparations
▶ BY MOUTH
  ▶ Females of childbearing potential: 1 tablet once daily for 21 days; subsequent courses repeated after 7-day interval, withdrawal bleeding occurs during the 7-day interval, if reasonably certain woman is not pregnant, first course can be started on any day of cycle—if starting on day 6 of cycle or later, additional precautions (barrier methods) necessary during first 7 days, tablets should be taken at approximately the same time each day

Contraception with 21-day combined preparations
▶ BY MOUTH
  ▶ Females of childbearing potential: 1 tablet once daily for 21 days; subsequent courses repeated after hormone-free interval, withdrawal bleeding occurs during the hormone-free interval, if reasonably certain woman is not pregnant, first course can be started on any day of cycle—if starting on day 6 of cycle or later, additional precautions (barrier methods) necessary during first 7 days, tablets should be taken at approximately the same time each day, see Contraceptives, hormonal p. 836 for recommendations from the FSRH on 'traditional' and 'tailored' regimens in which there is a shortened, less frequent, or no hormone-free interval.

- **INTERACTIONS** → Appendix 1: combined hormonal contraceptives · desogestrel

- **MEDICINAL FORMS** There can be variation in the licensing of different medicines containing the same drug.

Tablet
▶ Bimizza (Morningside Healthcare Ltd)
  Ethinylestradiol 20 microgram, Desogestrel 150 microgram Bimizza 150microgram/20microgram tablets | 63 tablet [PoM] £5.04 DT = £5.08
▶ Cimizt (Morningside Healthcare Ltd)
  Ethinylestradiol 30 microgram, Desogestrel 150 microgram Cimizt 30microgram/150microgram tablets | 63 tablet [PoM] £3.80 DT = £4.19
▶ Gedarel (Consilient Health Ltd)
  Ethinylestradiol 20 microgram, Desogestrel 150 microgram Gedarel 20microgram/150microgram tablets | 63 tablet [PoM] £5.08 DT = £5.08
  Ethinylestradiol 30 microgram, Desogestrel 150 microgram Gedarel 30microgram/150microgram tablets | 63 tablet [PoM] £4.19 DT = £4.19
▶ Marvelon (Merck Sharp & Dohme Ltd)
  Ethinylestradiol 30 microgram, Desogestrel 150 microgram Marvelon tablets | 63 tablet [PoM] £7.10 DT = £4.19
▶ Mercilon (Merck Sharp & Dohme Ltd)
  Ethinylestradiol 20 microgram, Desogestrel 150 microgram Mercilon 150microgram/20microgram tablets | 63 tablet [PoM] £8.44 DT = £5.08

Ethinylestradiol with drospirenone

F 841

- **INDICATIONS AND DOSE**

Menstrual symptoms with 21-day combined preparations
▶ BY MOUTH
  ▶ Females of childbearing potential: 1 tablet once daily for 21 days; subsequent courses repeated after 7-day interval, withdrawal bleeding occurs during the 7-day interval

Contraception with 21-day combined preparations
▶ BY MOUTH
  ▶ Females of childbearing potential: 1 tablet once daily for 21 days; subsequent courses repeated after hormone-free interval, withdrawal bleeding occurs during the hormone-free interval, see Contraceptives, hormonal p. 836 for recommendations from the FSRH on 'traditional' and 'tailored' regimens in which there is a shortened, less frequent, or no hormone-free interval.

Menstrual symptoms with 28-day combined preparations
▶ BY MOUTH
  ▶ Females of childbearing potential: 1 active tablet once daily for 24 days, followed by 1 inactive tablet once daily for 4 days, to be started on day 1 of cycle with first active tablet (withdrawal bleeding may occur during the 4-day interval of inactive tablets); subsequent courses repeated without interval

Contraception with 28-day combined preparations
▸ BY MOUTH
▸ Females of childbearing potential: 1 active tablet once daily for 24 days, followed by 1 inactive tablet once daily for 4 days, to be started on day 1 of cycle with first active tablet (withdrawal bleeding may occur during the 4-day interval of inactive tablets); subsequent courses repeated without interval, see Contraceptives, hormonal p. 836 for recommendations from the FSRH on 'tailored' regimens in which there is a shortened, less frequent, or no interval where *inactive* tablets are taken.

● INTERACTIONS → Appendix 1: combined hormonal contraceptives · drospirenone
● SIDE-EFFECTS
▸ Common or very common Breast abnormalities · depressed mood · increased risk of infection · menstrual disorder · vaginal discharge
▸ Uncommon Diarrhoea · hypotension · sexual dysfunction · skin reactions · vomiting · weight decreased
▸ Rare or very rare Arterial thromboembolism · asthma · erythema nodosum · hearing impairment
● PATIENT AND CARER ADVICE
Pill-free interval Withdrawal bleeding can occur during the 7-day tablet-free interval.

● MEDICINAL FORMS There can be variation in the licensing of different medicines containing the same drug.
Tablet
▸ Ethinylestradiol with drospirenone (Non-proprietary)
Ethinylestradiol 20 microgram, Drospirenone 3 mg Ethinylestradiol 20microgram / Drospirenone 3mg tablets | 84 tablet [PoM] [S] DT = £14.70
▸ Dretine (Theramex HQ UK Ltd)
Ethinylestradiol 30 microgram, Drospirenone 3 mg Dretine 0.03mg/3mg tablets | 63 tablet [PoM] £8.34 DT = £14.70
▸ ELOINE (Bayer Plc)
Ethinylestradiol 20 microgram, Drospirenone 3 mg Eloine 0.02mg/3mg tablets | 84 tablet [PoM] £14.70 DT = £14.70
▸ Lucette (Consilient Health Ltd)
Ethinylestradiol 30 microgram, Drospirenone 3 mg Lucette 0.03mg/3mg tablets | 63 tablet [PoM] £9.35 DT = £14.70
▸ Yacella (Morningside Healthcare Ltd)
Ethinylestradiol 30 microgram, Drospirenone 3 mg Yacella 0.03mg/3mg tablets | 63 tablet [PoM] £8.30 DT = £14.70
▸ Yasmin (Bayer Plc)
Ethinylestradiol 30 microgram, Drospirenone 3 mg Yasmin tablets | 63 tablet [PoM] £14.70 DT = £14.70
▸ Yiznell (Lupin Healthcare (UK) Ltd)
Ethinylestradiol 30 microgram, Drospirenone 3 mg Yiznell 0.03mg/3mg tablets | 63 tablet [PoM] £8.30 DT = £14.70

F 841

Ethinylestradiol with etonogestrel
13-Sep-2020

● INDICATIONS AND DOSE
Menstrual symptoms
▸ BY VAGINA
▸ Females of childbearing potential: 1 unit, insert the ring into the vagina on day 1 of cycle and leave in for 3 weeks; remove ring on day 22; subsequent courses repeated after 7-day ring free interval (during which withdrawal bleeding occurs)

Contraception
▸ BY VAGINA
▸ Females of childbearing potential: 1 unit, insert the ring into the vagina on day 1 of cycle and leave in for 3 weeks; remove ring on day 22; subsequent courses repeated after 7-day ring free interval (during which withdrawal bleeding occurs), see Contraceptives, hormonal p. 836 for recommendations from the FSRH

on 'tailored' regimens in which there is a shortened, less frequent, or no ring-free interval.

● INTERACTIONS → Appendix 1: combined hormonal contraceptives · etonogestrel
● DIRECTIONS FOR ADMINISTRATION
Changing from combined hormonal contraception to vaginal ring Manufacturer advises insert ring at the latest on the day after the usual tablet-free, patch-free, or inactive-tablet interval. If previous contraceptive used correctly, or pregnancy can reasonably be excluded, can switch to ring on any day of cycle.
Changing from progestogen-only method to vaginal ring From an implant or intra-uterine progestogen-only device, manufacturer advises insert ring on the day implant or intra-uterine progestogen-only device removed; from an injection, insert ring when next injection due; from oral preparation, first ring may be inserted on any day after stopping pill. For all methods additional precautions (barrier methods) should be used concurrently for first 7 days.
● PATIENT AND CARER ADVICE Patients or carers should be given advice on how to administer vaginal ring.
Counselling The presence of the ring should be checked regularly.
Missed doses
Expulsion, delayed insertion or removal, or broken vaginal ring If the vaginal ring is expelled for *less than* 3 *hours*, rinse the ring with cool water and reinsert immediately; no additional contraception is needed.

If the ring remains outside the vagina for *more than* 3 *hours* or if the user does not know when the ring was expelled, contraceptive protection may be reduced:
● If ring expelled during week 1 or 2 of cycle, rinse ring with cool water and reinsert; use additional precautions (barrier methods) for next 7 days;
● If ring expelled during week 3 of cycle, either insert a new ring to start a new cycle *or* allow a withdrawal bleed and insert a new ring no later than 7 days after ring was expelled; latter option only available if ring was used continuously for at least 7 days before expulsion.
If insertion of a new ring at the start of a new cycle is delayed, contraceptive protection is lost. A new ring should be inserted as soon as possible; additional precautions (barrier methods) should be used for the first 7 days of the new cycle. If intercourse occurred during the extended ring-free interval, pregnancy should be considered.

No additional contraception is required if removal of the ring is delayed by up to 1 week (4 weeks of continuous use). The 7-day ring-free interval should be observed and subsequently a new ring should be inserted. Contraceptive protection may be reduced with continuous use of the ring for more than 4 weeks—pregnancy should be ruled out before inserting a new ring.

If the ring breaks during use, remove it and insert a new ring immediately; additional precautions (barrier methods) should be used for the first 7 days of the new cycle.

● MEDICINAL FORMS There can be variation in the licensing of different medicines containing the same drug.
Vaginal delivery system
▸ NuvaRing (Merck Sharp & Dohme Ltd)
Ethinylestradiol 2.7 mg, Etonogestrel 11.7 mg NuvaRing 0.12mg/0.015mg per day vaginal delivery system | 3 system [PoM] £29.70 DT = £29.70
▸ SyreniRing (Crescent Pharma Ltd)
Ethinylestradiol 2.7 mg, Etonogestrel 11.7 mg SyreniRing 0.12mg/0.015mg per day vaginal delivery system | 3 system [PoM] £23.76 DT = £29.70

7

Ethinylestradiol with gestodene

F 841

● **INDICATIONS AND DOSE**

Menstrual symptoms with 21-day combined preparations
▶ BY MOUTH
▶ Females of childbearing potential: 1 tablet once daily for 21 days; subsequent courses repeated after 7-day interval, withdrawal bleeding occurs during the 7-day interval, if reasonably certain woman is not pregnant, first course can be started on any day of cycle—if starting on day 6 of cycle or later, additional precautions (barrier methods) necessary during first 7 days, tablets should be taken at approximately the same time each day

Contraception with 21-day combined preparations
▶ BY MOUTH
▶ Females of childbearing potential: 1 tablet once daily for 21 days; subsequent courses repeated after hormone-free interval, withdrawal bleeding occurs during the hormone-free interval, if reasonably certain woman is not pregnant, first course can be started on any day of cycle—if starting on day 6 of cycle or later, additional precautions (barrier methods) necessary during first 7 days, tablets should be taken at approximately the same time each day, see Contraceptives, hormonal p. 836 for recommendations from the FSRH on 'traditional' and 'tailored' regimens in which there is a shortened, less frequent, or no hormone-free interval.

Menstrual symptoms with 28-day combined preparations
▶ BY MOUTH
▶ Females of childbearing potential: 1 active tablet once daily for 21 days, followed by 1 inactive tablet daily for 7 days; subsequent courses repeated without interval, withdrawal bleeding occurs during the 7-day interval of *inactive* tablets being taken, if reasonably certain woman is not pregnant, first course can be started on any day of cycle—if starting on day 6 of cycle or later, additional precautions (barrier methods) necessary during first 7 days, tablets should be taken at approximately the same time each day

Contraception with 28-day combined preparations
▶ BY MOUTH
▶ Females of childbearing potential: 1 active tablet once daily for 21 days, followed by 1 inactive tablet daily for 7 days; subsequent courses repeated without interval, withdrawal bleeding occurs during the interval of *inactive* tablets being taken, if reasonably certain woman is not pregnant, first course can be started on any day of cycle—if starting on day 6 of cycle or later, additional precautions (barrier methods) necessary during first 7 days, tablets should be taken at approximately the same time each day, see Contraceptives, hormonal p. 836 for recommendations from the FSRH on 'tailored' regimens in which *inactive* tablets are taken for a shortened, less frequent, or absent interval.

● **INTERACTIONS** → Appendix 1: combined hormonal contraceptives

● **SIDE-EFFECTS**
▶ **Common or very common** Abdominal pain · breast abnormalities · depression · dizziness · increased risk of infection · menstrual cycle irregularities · mood swings · nervousness · vaginal discharge
▶ **Uncommon** Appetite abnormal · diarrhoea · hirsutism · hypertriglyceridaemia · sexual dysfunction · skin reactions · vomiting
▶ **Rare or very rare** Angioedema · chorea exacerbated · ear disorders · embolism and thrombosis · erythema nodosum · eye irritation · gallbladder disorders · gastrointestinal disorders · haemolytic uraemic syndrome · hepatic disorders · hypersensitivity · inflammatory bowel disease · neoplasms · optic neuritis · pancreatitis · systemic lupus erythematosus exacerbated · varicose veins exacerbated · weight decreased

● **MEDICINAL FORMS** There can be variation in the licensing of different medicines containing the same drug.

Tablet
▶ Ethinylestradiol with gestodene (Non-proprietary)
Ethinylestradiol 30 microgram, Gestodene 50 microgram Ethinylestradiol 30microgram / Gestodene 50microgram tablets | 18 tablet [PoM] Ⓢ
Ethinylestradiol 40 microgram, Gestodene 70 microgram Ethinylestradiol 40microgram / Gestodene 70microgram tablets | 15 tablet [PoM] Ⓢ
Ethinylestradiol 30 microgram, Gestodene 100 microgram Ethinylestradiol 30microgram / Gestodene 100microgram tablets | 30 tablet [PoM] Ⓢ
▶ Akizza (Morningside Healthcare Ltd)
Ethinylestradiol 20 microgram, Gestodene 75 microgram Akizza 75microgram/20microgram tablets | 63 tablet [PoM] £6.73 DT = £8.85
Ethinylestradiol 30 microgram, Gestodene 75 microgram Akizza 75microgram/30microgram tablets | 63 tablet [PoM] £8.85 DT = £6.73
▶ Femodene (Bayer Plc)
Ethinylestradiol 30 microgram, Gestodene 75 microgram Femodene tablets | 63 tablet [PoM] £6.73 DT = £6.73
▶ Femodette (Bayer Plc)
Ethinylestradiol 20 microgram, Gestodene 75 microgram Femodette tablets | 63 tablet [PoM] £8.85 DT = £8.85
▶ Katya (Stragen UK Ltd)
Ethinylestradiol 30 microgram, Gestodene 75 microgram Katya 30/75 tablets | 63 tablet [PoM] £5.03 DT = £6.73
▶ Millinette (Consilient Health Ltd)
Ethinylestradiol 30 microgram, Gestodene 75 microgram Millinette 30microgram/75microgram tablets | 63 tablet [PoM] £4.12 DT = £6.73
Ethinylestradiol 20 microgram, Gestodene 75 microgram Millinette 20microgram/75microgram tablets | 63 tablet [PoM] £5.41 DT = £8.85
▶ Sunya (Stragen UK Ltd)
Ethinylestradiol 20 microgram, Gestodene 75 microgram Sunya 20/75 tablets | 63 tablet [PoM] £6.62 DT = £8.85

Ethinylestradiol with levonorgestrel

F 841

● **INDICATIONS AND DOSE**

Menstrual symptoms with 21-day combined preparations
▶ BY MOUTH
▶ Females of childbearing potential: 1 tablet once daily for 21 days; subsequent courses repeated after 7-day interval, withdrawal bleeding occurs during the 7-day interval, if reasonably certain woman is not pregnant, first course can be started on any day of cycle—if starting on day 6 of cycle or later, additional precautions (barrier methods) necessary during first 7 days, tablets should be taken at approximately the same time each day

Contraception with 21-day combined preparations
▶ BY MOUTH
▶ Females of childbearing potential: 1 tablet once daily for 21 days; subsequent courses repeated after hormone-free interval, withdrawal bleeding occurs during the hormone-free interval, if reasonably certain woman is not pregnant, first course can be started on any day of cycle—if starting on day 6 of cycle or later, additional precautions (barrier methods) necessary during first 7 days, tablets should be taken at approximately the same time each day, see Contraceptives, hormonal p. 836 for recommendations from the FSRH on 'traditional' and 'tailored' regimens in which there is a shortened, less frequent, or no hormone-free interval.

Menstrual symptoms with 28-day combined preparations

▶ BY MOUTH

▶ Females of childbearing potential: 1 active tablet once daily for 21 days, followed by 1 inactive tablet once daily for 7 days, withdrawal bleeding occurs during the 7-day interval of *inactive* tablets being taken, if reasonably certain woman is not pregnant, first course can be started on any day of cycle—if starting on day 6 of cycle or later, additional precautions (barrier methods) necessary during first 7 days, tablets should be taken at approximately the same time each day. Subsequent courses repeated without interval

Contraception with 28-day combined preparations

▶ BY MOUTH

▶ Females of childbearing potential: 1 active tablet once daily for 21 days, followed by 1 inactive tablet once daily for 7 days, withdrawal bleeding occurs during the interval of *inactive* tablets being taken, if reasonably certain woman is not pregnant, first course can be started on any day of cycle—if starting on day 6 of cycle or later, additional precautions (barrier methods) necessary during first 7 days, tablets should be taken at approximately the same time each day. Subsequent courses repeated without interval, see Contraceptives, hormonal p. 836 for recommendations from the FSRH on 'tailored' regimens in which there is a shortened, less frequent, or no interval where *inactive* tablets are taken.

● INTERACTIONS → Appendix 1: combined hormonal contraceptives · levonorgestrel

● MEDICINAL FORMS There can be variation in the licensing of different medicines containing the same drug.

Tablet

▶ Ethinylestradiol with levonorgestrel (Non-proprietary)
  Ethinylestradiol 30 microgram, Levonorgestrel 50 microgram Ethinylestradiol 30microgram / Levonorgestrel 50microgram tablets | 6 tablet [PoM] ⬛
  Ethinylestradiol 40 microgram, Levonorgestrel 75 microgram Ethinylestradiol 40microgram / Levonorgestrel 75microgram tablets | 5 tablet [PoM] ⬛
  Ethinylestradiol 30 microgram, Levonorgestrel 125 microgram Ethinylestradiol 30microgram / Levonorgestrel 125microgram tablets | 10 tablet [PoM] ⬛

▶ Ambelina (Crescent Pharma Ltd)
  Ethinylestradiol 30 microgram, Levonorgestrel 150 microgram Ambelina 150microgram/30microgram tablets | 63 tablet [PoM] £2.60 DT = £2.82

▶ Elevin (MedRx Licences Ltd)
  Ethinylestradiol 30 microgram, Levonorgestrel 150 microgram Elevin 150microgram/30microgram tablets | 63 tablet [PoM] £29.25 DT = £2.82

▶ Levest (Morningside Healthcare Ltd)
  Ethinylestradiol 30 microgram, Levonorgestrel 150 microgram Levest 150/30 tablets | 21 tablet [PoM] £0.85 (Hospital only) | 63 tablet [PoM] £1.80 DT = £2.82

▶ Maexeni (Lupin Healthcare (UK) Ltd)
  Ethinylestradiol 30 microgram, Levonorgestrel 150 microgram Maexeni 150microgram/30microgram tablets | 63 tablet [PoM] £1.88 DT = £2.82

▶ Microgynon 30 (Bayer Plc)
  Ethinylestradiol 30 microgram, Levonorgestrel 150 microgram Microgynon 30 tablets | 63 tablet [PoM] £2.82 DT = £2.82

▶ Ovranette (Pfizer Ltd)
  Ethinylestradiol 30 microgram, Levonorgestrel 150 microgram Ovranette 150microgram/30microgram tablets | 63 tablet [PoM] £2.20 DT = £2.82

▶ Rigevidon (Consilient Health Ltd)
  Ethinylestradiol 30 microgram, Levonorgestrel 150 microgram Rigevidon tablets | 63 tablet [PoM] £1.89 DT = £2.82

⌐ F 841

Ethinylestradiol with norelgestromin

05-Nov-2020

● INDICATIONS AND DOSE

Menstrual symptoms

▶ BY TRANSDERMAL APPLICATION

▶ Females of childbearing potential: Apply 1 patch once weekly for 3 weeks, apply first patch on day 1 of cycle, change patch on days 8 and 15; remove third patch on day 22 and apply new patch after 7-day patch-free interval to start subsequent contraceptive cycle, subsequent courses repeated after a 7-day patch free interval (during which withdrawal bleeding occurs)

Contraception

▶ BY TRANSDERMAL APPLICATION

▶ Females of childbearing potential: Apply 1 patch once weekly for 3 weeks, apply first patch on day 1 of cycle, change patch on days 8 and 15; remove third patch on day 22 and apply new patch after a patch-free interval to start subsequent contraceptive cycle, subsequent courses repeated after a patch-free interval (during which withdrawal bleeding occurs), see Contraceptives, hormonal p. 836 for recommendations from the FSRH on 'traditional' and 'tailored' regimens in which there is a shortened, less frequent, or no patch-free interval.

● CAUTIONS Body-weight 90 kg and above (possible reduction in contraceptive efficacy)

● INTERACTIONS → Appendix 1: combined hormonal contraceptives

● SIDE-EFFECTS

▶ **Common or very common** Anxiety · breast abnormalities · diarrhoea · dizziness · fatigue · gastrointestinal discomfort · increased risk of infection · malaise · menstrual cycle irregularities · mood altered · muscle spasms · skin reactions · uterine cramps · vaginal haemorrhage · vomiting · vulvovaginal disorders

▶ **Uncommon** Appetite increased · dyslipidaemia · insomnia · lactation disorders · oedema · photosensitivity reaction · sexual dysfunction

▶ **Rare or very rare** Embolism and thrombosis · gallbladder disorders · genital discharge · neoplasms · stroke · swelling

▶ **Frequency not known** Anger · angioedema · cervical dysplasia · colitis · contact lens intolerance · erythema nodosum · hepatic disorders · hyperglycaemia · intracranial haemorrhage · myocardial infarction · pulmonary artery thrombosis · taste altered

● DIRECTIONS FOR ADMINISTRATION Manufacturer advises adhesives or bandages should not be used to hold patch in place. If no longer sticky do not reapply but use a new patch.
  Changing to a transdermal combined hormonal contraceptive
  Changing from combined oral contraception
  Manufacturer advises apply patch on the first day of withdrawal bleeding; if no withdrawal bleeding within 5 days of taking last *active* tablet, rule out pregnancy before applying first patch. Unless patch is applied on first day of withdrawal bleeding, additional precautions (barrier methods) should be used concurrently for first 7 days.
  Changing from progestogen-only method
  Manufacturer advises
  ● from an implant, apply first patch on the day implant removed
  ● from an injection, apply first patch when next injection due
  ● from oral progestogen, first patch may be applied on any day after stopping pill
  For all methods additional precautions (barrier methods) should be used concurrently for first 7 days.

Genito-urinary system

7

After childbirth (not breast-feeding) Manufacturer advises start 4 weeks after birth; if started later than 4 weeks after birth additional precautions (barrier methods) should be used for first 7 days.

After abortion or miscarriage Manufacturer advises before 20 weeks' gestation start immediately; no additional contraception required if started immediately. After 20 weeks' gestation start on day 21 after abortion or on the first day of first spontaneous menstruation; additional precautions (barrier methods) should be used for first 7 days after applying the patch.

- PATIENT AND CARER ADVICE Patients and carers should be given advice on how to administer patches.

Travel Women using patches are at an increased risk of deep vein thrombosis during travel involving long periods of immobility (over 3 hours). The risk may be reduced by appropriate exercise during the journey and possibly by wearing graduated compression hosiery.

Missed doses

Delayed application or detached patch If a patch is partly detached for less than 24 hours, reapply to the same site or replace with a new patch immediately; no additional contraception is needed and the next patch should be applied on the usual 'change day'. If a patch remains detached for more than 24 hours or if the user is not aware when the patch became detached, then stop the current contraceptive cycle and start a new cycle by applying a new patch, giving a new 'Day 1'; an additional non-hormonal contraceptive must be used concurrently for the first 7 days of the new cycle.

If application of a new patch at the start of a new cycle is delayed, contraceptive protection is lost. A new patch should be applied as soon as remembered giving a new 'Day 1'; additional non-hormonal methods of contraception should be used for the first 7 days of the new cycle. If application of a patch in the middle of the cycle is delayed (i.e. the patch is not changed on day 8 or day 15):

- for up to 48 hours, apply a new patch immediately; next patch 'change day' remains the same and no additional contraception is required.
- for more than 48 hours, contraceptive protection may have been lost. Stop the current cycle and start a new 4-week cycle immediately by applying a new patch giving a new 'Day 1'; additional non-hormonal contraception should be used for the first 7 days of the new cycle.

If the patch is not removed at the end of the cycle (day 22), remove it as soon as possible and start the next cycle on the usual 'change day', the day after day 28; no additional contraception is required.

- NATIONAL FUNDING/ACCESS DECISIONS
For full details see funding body website

Scottish Medicines Consortium (SMC) decisions
- Ethinylestradiol with norelgestromin (*Evra*®) for use as female contraception (September 2003) SMC No. 48/03 Recommended with restrictions

- MEDICINAL FORMS There can be variation in the licensing of different medicines containing the same drug.
Transdermal patch
- Evra (Janssen-Cilag Ltd)
Ethinylestradiol 33.9 microgram per 24 hour, Norelgestromin 203 microgram per 24 hour Evra transdermal patches | 9 patch [PoM] £19.51 DT = £19.51

F 841

Ethinylestradiol with norethisterone

- INDICATIONS AND DOSE
Menstrual symptoms with 21-day combined preparations
- BY MOUTH
- Females of childbearing potential: 1 tablet once daily for 21 days; subsequent courses repeated after 7-day interval, withdrawal bleeding occurs during the 7-day interval, if reasonably certain woman is not pregnant, first course can be started on any day of cycle—if starting on day 6 of cycle or later, additional precautions (barrier methods) necessary during first 7 days, tablets should be taken at approximately the same time each day

Contraception with 21-day combined preparations
- BY MOUTH
- Females of childbearing potential: 1 tablet once daily for 21 days; subsequent courses repeated after hormone-free interval, withdrawal bleeding occurs during the hormone-free interval, if reasonably certain woman is not pregnant, first course can be started on any day of cycle—if starting on day 6 of cycle or later, additional precautions (barrier methods) necessary during first 7 days, tablets should be taken at approximately the same time each day, see Contraceptives, hormonal p. 836 for recommendations from the FSRH on 'traditional' and 'tailored' regimens in which there is a shortened, less frequent, or no hormone-free interval.

- INTERACTIONS → Appendix 1: combined hormonal contraceptives · norethisterone

- MEDICINAL FORMS There can be variation in the licensing of different medicines containing the same drug.
Tablet
- Ethinylestradiol with norethisterone (Non-proprietary)
Ethinylestradiol 35 microgram, Norethisterone 500 microgram Ethinylestradiol 35microgram / Norethisterone 500microgram tablets | 5 tablet [PoM] 🛆
Ethinylestradiol 35 microgram, Norethisterone 750 microgram Ethinylestradiol 35microgram / Norethisterone 750microgram tablets | 21 tablet [PoM] 🛆
Ethinylestradiol 35 microgram, Norethisterone 1 mg Ethinylestradiol 35microgram / Norethisterone 1mg tablets | 9 tablet [PoM] 🛆
- Brevinor (Pfizer Ltd)
Ethinylestradiol 35 microgram, Norethisterone 500 microgram Brevinor 500microgram/35microgram tablets | 63 tablet [PoM] £1.99 DT = £1.99
- Norimin (Pfizer Ltd)
Ethinylestradiol 35 microgram, Norethisterone 1 mg Norimin 1mg/35microgram tablets | 63 tablet [PoM] £2.28 DT = £2.28

F 841

Ethinylestradiol with norgestimate

- INDICATIONS AND DOSE
Menstrual symptoms with 21-day combined preparations
- BY MOUTH
- Females of childbearing potential: 1 tablet once daily for 21 days; subsequent courses repeated after 7-day interval, withdrawal bleeding occurs during the 7-day interval, if reasonably certain woman is not pregnant, first course can be started on any day of cycle—if starting on day 6 of cycle or later, additional precautions (barrier methods) necessary during first 7 days, tablets should be taken at approximately the same time each day

Contraception with 21-day combined preparations
- BY MOUTH
- Females of childbearing potential: 1 tablet once daily for 21 days; subsequent courses repeated after hormone-free interval, withdrawal bleeding occurs during the

hormone-free interval, if reasonably certain woman is not pregnant, first course can be started on any day of cycle—if starting on day 6 of cycle or later, additional precautions (barrier methods) necessary during first 7 days, tablets should be taken at approximately the same time each day, see Contraceptives, hormonal p. 836 for recommendations from the FSRH on 'traditional' and 'tailored' regimens in which there is a shortened, less frequent, or no hormone-free interval.

● INTERACTIONS → Appendix 1: combined hormonal contraceptives

● SIDE-EFFECTS

● **Common or very common** Anxiety · asthenic conditions · breast abnormalities · chest pain · constipation · depression · diarrhoea · dizziness · gastrointestinal discomfort · gastrointestinal disorders · genital discharge · hypersensitivity · increased risk of infection · insomnia · menstrual cycle irregularities · mood altered · muscle complaints · oedema · pain · skin reactions · vomiting

● **Uncommon** Appetite abnormal · cervical dysplasia · dry eye · dyspnoea · embolism and thrombosis · hirsutism · hot flush · libido disorder · ovarian cyst · palpitations · paraesthesia · syncope · visual impairment · vulvovaginal disorders · weight changes

● **Rare or very rare** Hepatic disorders · pancreatitis · photosensitivity reaction · sweat changes · tachycardia · vertigo

● **Frequency not known** Angioedema · contact lens intolerance · dyslipidaemia · erythema nodosum · neoplasms · seizure · suppressed lactation

● MEDICINAL FORMS There can be variation in the licensing of different medicines containing the same drug.

Tablet
▸ Cilique (Consilient Health Ltd)
 Ethinylestradiol 35 microgram, Norgestimate
 250 microgram Cilique 250microgram/35microgram tablets |
 63 tablet [PoM] £4.65 DT = £4.65
▸ Lizinna (Morningside Healthcare Ltd)
 Ethinylestradiol 35 microgram, Norgestimate
 250 microgram Lizinna 250microgram/35microgram tablets |
 63 tablet [PoM] £4.64 DT = £4.65

⌐ 841

Norethisterone with mestranol

● INDICATIONS AND DOSE

Contraception | Menstrual symptoms
▸ BY MOUTH
▸ Females of childbearing potential: 1 tablet once daily for 21 days; subsequent courses repeated after 7-day interval, withdrawal bleeding can occur during the 7-day interval, if reasonably certain woman is not pregnant, first course can be started on any day of cycle—if starting on day 6 or later, additional precautions (barrier methods) necessary during first 7 days, tablets should be taken at the same time each day

● INTERACTIONS → Appendix 1: combined hormonal contraceptives · norethisterone

● SIDE-EFFECTS Appetite change · breast tenderness · depression · gastrointestinal disorder · libido disorder · metabolic disorders · uterine leiomyoma exacerbated

● MEDICINAL FORMS There can be variation in the licensing of different medicines containing the same drug.

Tablet
▸ Norinyl-1 (Pfizer Ltd)
 Mestranol 50 microgram, Norethisterone 1 mg Norinyl-1 tablets |
 63 tablet [PoM] £2.19 DT = £2.19

3.2 Contraception, devices

Other drugs used for Contraception, devices
Levonorgestrel, p. 852

CONTRACEPTIVE DEVICES

Intra-uterine contraceptive devices (copper)
24-Nov-2020

● INDICATIONS AND DOSE

Contraception
▸ BY INTRA-UTERINE ADMINISTRATION
▸ Females of childbearing potential: (consult product literature)

IMPORTANT SAFETY INFORMATION
MHRA/CHM ADVICE (JUNE 2015) INTRA-UTERINE CONTRACEPTION: UTERINE PERFORATION—UPDATED INFORMATION ON RISK FACTORS
Uterine perforation most often occurs during insertion, but might not be detected until sometime later. The risk of uterine perforation is increased when the device is inserted up to 36 weeks postpartum or in patients who are breastfeeding. Before inserting an intra-uterine contraceptive device, inform patients that perforation occurs in approximately 1 in every 1000 insertions and signs and symptoms include:
 ● severe pelvic pain after insertion (worse than period cramps);
 ● pain or increased bleeding after insertion which continues for more than a few weeks;
 ● sudden changes in periods;
 ● pain during intercourse;
 ● unable to feel the threads.
Patients should be informed on how to check their threads and to arrange a check-up if threads cannot be felt, especially if they also have significant pain. Partial perforation may occur even if the threads can be seen; consider this if there is severe pain following insertion and perform an ultrasound.

● CONTRA-INDICATIONS Active trophoblastic disease (until return to normal of urine and plasma-gonadotrophin concentration) · genital malignancy · medical diathermy · pelvic inflammatory disease · post-abortion sepsis · postpartum sepsis · recent sexually transmitted infection (if not fully investigated and treated) · severe anaemia · unexplained uterine bleeding · Wilson's disease

● CAUTIONS Anaemia · anatomical abnormalities—seek specialist advice · anticoagulant therapy · cardiac disease—seek specialist advice · endometriosis · epilepsy (risk of seizure at time of insertion) · immunosuppression (risk of infection)—seek specialist advice · menorrhagia (progestogen intra-uterine system might be preferable) · postpartum—seek specialist advice · risk of sexually transmitted infections · severe primary dysmenorrhoea · young age

CAUTIONS, FURTHER INFORMATION The Faculty of Sexual and Reproductive Healthcare advises if removal is after day 3 of the menstrual cycle, intercourse should be avoided or another method of contraception used for at least 7 days before removal of device—emergency contraception may need to be considered if recent intercourse has occurred and the intra-uterine device is removed after day 3 of the menstrual cycle.
▸ Sexually transmitted infections and pelvic inflammatory disease The main excess risk of pelvic infection occurs in

the first 20 days after insertion and is believed to be related to existing carriage of a sexually transmitted infection. Women are considered to be at a higher risk of sexually transmitted infections if:
- they are under 25 years old *or*
- they are over 25 years old *and*
  - have a new partner *or*
  - have had more than one partner in the past year *or*
  - their regular partner has other partners.

The Faculty of Sexual and Reproductive Healthcare advises pre-insertion screening (for chlamydia and, depending on sexual history and local prevalence of disease, *Neisseria gonorrhoeae*) be performed in these women. If results are unavailable at the time of fitting an intra-uterine device for emergency contraception, consider appropriate prophylactic antibacterial cover. The woman should be advised to attend *as an emergency* if she experiences sustained pain during the next 20 days.

- SIDE-EFFECTS Device complications · epilepsy (on insertion) · haemorrhage (on insertion) · hypersensitivity · menstrual cycle irregularities · pain (on insertion— alleviated by NSAID such as ibuprofen 30 minutes before insertion) · pelvic infection exacerbated · presyncope (on insertion) · uterine injuries

  SIDE-EFFECTS, FURTHER INFORMATION Advise the patient to seek medical attention promptly in case of significant symptoms—very small risk of uterine perforation, ectopic pregnancy and pelvic inflammatory disease.

- ALLERGY AND CROSS-SENSITIVITY [EvGr] Contra-indicated if patient has a copper allergy. ⟨M⟩

- PREGNANCY If an intra-uterine device fails and the woman wishes to continue to full-term the device should be removed in the first trimester if possible. Remove device; if pregnancy occurs, increased likelihood that it may be ectopic.

- BREAST FEEDING Not known to be harmful.

- MONITORING REQUIREMENTS Gynaecological examination before insertion, 6–8 weeks after insertion, then annually.

- DIRECTIONS FOR ADMINISTRATION The healthcare professional inserting (or removing) the device should be fully trained in the technique and should provide full counselling backed, where available, by the patient information leaflet.

- PRESCRIBING AND DISPENSING INFORMATION

  TT380 ® SLIMLINE For uterine length 6.5–9 cm; replacement every 10 years.

  LOAD ® 375 For uterine length over 7 cm; replacement every 5 years.

  NOVAPLUS T 380 ® AG '*Mini*' size for minimum uterine length 5 cm; '*Normal*' size for uterine length 6.5–9 cm; replacement every 5 years.

  MULTILOAD ® CU375 For uterine length 6–9 cm; replacement every 5 years.

  GYNEFIX ® Suitable for all uterine sizes; replacement every 5 years.

  IUB BALLERINE MIDI ® For uterine length over 6 cm; replacement every 5 years.

  UT380 STANDARD ® For uterine length 6.5–9 cm; replacement every 5 years.

  UT380 SHORT ® For uterine length 5–7 cm; replacement every 5 years.

  MULTI-SAFE ® 375 For uterine length 6–9 cm; replacement every 5 years.

  ANCORA ® 375 CU For uterine length over 6.5 cm; replacement every 5 years.

  T-SAFE ® 380A QL For uterine length 6.5–9 cm; replacement every 10 years.

NEO-SAFE ® T380 For uterine length 6.5–9 cm; replacement every 5 years.

MINI TT380 ® SLIMLINE For minimum uterine length 5 cm; replacement every 5 years.

COPPER T380 A ® For uterine length 6.5–9 cm; replacement every 10 years.

NOVAPLUS T 380 ® CU '*Mini*' size for minimum uterine length 5 cm; '*Normal*' size for uterine length 6.5–9 cm; replacement every 5 years.

NOVA-T ® 380 For uterine length 6.5–9 cm; replacement every 5 years.

FLEXI-T ®+ 380 For uterine length over 6 cm; replacement every 5 years.

FLEXI-T ® 300 For uterine length over 5 cm; replacement every 5 years.

- MEDICINAL FORMS There can be variation in the licensing of different medicines containing the same drug.

Intra-uterine contraceptive devices

▸ Intra-uterine contraceptive devices (R.F. Medical Supplies Ltd, Farla Medical Ltd, Durbin Plc, Williams Medical Supplies Ltd, Bayer Plc, Organon Laboratories Ltd)
  Copper T380 A intra-uterine contraceptive device | 1 device £8.95
  Steriload intra-uterine contraceptive device | 1 device £9.65
  Load 375 intra-uterine contraceptive device | 1 device £8.52
  Novaplus T 380 Ag intra-uterine contraceptive device mini | 1 device £12.50
  T-Safe 380A QL intra-uterine contraceptive device | 1 device £10.55
  UT380 Standard intra-uterine contraceptive device | 1 device £11.22
  Nova-T 380 intra-uterine contraceptive device | 1 device £15.20
  Flexi-T+ 380 intra-uterine contraceptive device | 1 device £10.06
  Mini TT380 Slimline intra-uterine contraceptive device | 1 device £12.46
  Flexi-T 300 intra-uterine contraceptive device | 1 device £9.47
  Multi-Safe 375 intra-uterine contraceptive device | 1 device £8.96
  Multiload Cu375 intra-uterine contraceptive device | 1 device £9.24
  Optima TCu 380A intra-uterine contraceptive device | 1 device £9.65
  Novaplus T 380 Ag intra-uterine contraceptive device normal | 1 device £12.50
  GyneFix intra-uterine contraceptive device | 1 device £27.11
  Novaplus T 380 Cu intra-uterine contraceptive device mini | 1 device £10.95
  TT380 Slimline intra-uterine contraceptive device | 1 device £12.46
  Ancora 375 Cu intra-uterine contraceptive device | 1 device £7.95
  Novaplus T 380 Cu intra-uterine contraceptive device normal | 1 device £10.95
  Neo-Safe T380 intra-uterine contraceptive device | 1 device £13.40
  UT380 Short intra-uterine contraceptive device | 1 device £11.22

Silicone contraceptive pessaries

- SILICONE CONTRACEPTIVE PESSARIES

  FemCap 22mm (Durbin Plc)
  1 device · NHS indicative price = £15.29 · Drug Tariff (Part IXa)

  FemCap 26mm (Durbin Plc)
  1 device · NHS indicative price = £15.29 · Drug Tariff (Part IXa)

  FemCap 30mm (Durbin Plc)
  1 device · NHS indicative price = £15.29 · Drug Tariff (Part IXa)

3.3 Contraception, emergency

Other drugs used for Contraception, emergency Intra-uterine contraceptive devices (copper), p. 849 · Levonorgestrel, p. 852

PROGESTERONE RECEPTOR MODULATORS

Ulipristal acetate
19-Nov-2020

- **DRUG ACTION** Ulipristal acetate is a synthetic, selective progesterone receptor modulator with a partial progesterone antagonist effect.

- **INDICATIONS AND DOSE**

Emergency contraception
- ▶ BY MOUTH
- ▶ Females of childbearing potential: 30 mg for 1 dose, to be taken as soon as possible after coitus, but no later than after 120 hours

---

IMPORTANT SAFETY INFORMATION

MHRA/CHM ADVICE: *ESMYA*® (ULIPRISTAL ACETATE): SUSPENSION OF THE LICENCE DUE TO RISK OF SERIOUS LIVER INJURY (MARCH 2020)

Rare but serious cases of liver injury, including hepatic failure requiring liver transplantation, have been reported worldwide in women treated with *Esmya*® for symptoms of uterine fibroids. The licence of *Esmya*® has been suspended while a safety review is carried out, following a further case of liver injury requiring transplantation despite liver function monitoring. Healthcare professionals are advised not to start *Esmya*® in new patients and to stop treatment in current patients; alternative treatment options for uterine fibroids should be considered. Liver function tests should be performed 2–4 weeks after stopping treatment, and patients advised to be vigilant for the signs and symptoms of liver injury and to seek immediate medical advice if these occur, even if 1–2 months after stopping treatment. There are currently no concerns with the use of the emergency contraceptive *ellaOne*®—see *Indications and Dose*.

- **CAUTIONS** Uncontrolled severe asthma
- **INTERACTIONS** → Appendix 1: ulipristal
- **SIDE-EFFECTS**
- ▶ **Common or very common** Back pain · breast tenderness · dizziness · fatigue · gastrointestinal discomfort · headaches · menstrual cycle irregularities · mood altered · myalgia · nausea · pelvic pain · vomiting
- ▶ **Uncommon** Anxiety · appetite disorder · chills · concentration impaired · diarrhoea · drowsiness · dry mouth · fever · flatulence · hot flush · increased risk of infection · insomnia · libido disorder · malaise · skin reactions · vision disorders · vulvovaginal disorders
- ▶ **Rare or very rare** Abnormal sensation in eye · disorientation · dry throat · eye erythema · genital pruritus · ovarian cyst ruptured · painful sexual intercourse · syncope · taste altered · thirst · tremor · vertigo
- **PREGNANCY** Limited information available—if pregnancy occurs, manufacturer advises report to the *ellaOne*® pregnancy registry.
- **BREAST FEEDING** Manufacturer advises avoid for 1 week after administration—present in milk.
- **HEPATIC IMPAIRMENT** Manufacturer advises avoid in severe impairment (no information available).
- **PATIENT AND CARER ADVICE** When prescribing or supplying hormonal emergency contraception, manufacturer advises women should be told:
  - if vomiting occurs within 3 hours of taking a dose, a replacement dose should be taken;
  - that their next period may be early or late;
  - to seek medical attention promptly if any lower abdominal pain occurs because this could signify an ectopic pregnancy.

The Faculty of Sexual and Reproductive Healthcare also advises women should be told:
- that a barrier method of contraception needs to be used—see Emergency contraception p. 839 for further information;
- that a pregnancy test should be performed if the next menstrual period is delayed by more than 7 days, is lighter than usual, or is associated with abdominal pain that is not typical of the woman's usual dysmenorrhoea;
- that a pregnancy test should be performed if hormonal contraception is started soon after use of emergency contraception even if they have bleeding; bleeding associated with the contraceptive method may not represent menstruation.

- **MEDICINAL FORMS** There can be variation in the licensing of different medicines containing the same drug.

Tablet
- ▶ Ellaone (HRA Pharma UK Ltd)
  Ulipristal acetate 30 mg   EllaOne 30mg tablets | 1 tablet Ⓟ £14.05
  DT = £14.05

3.4 Contraception, oral progestogen-only

Other drugs used for Contraception, oral progestogen-only Norethisterone, p. 806

PROGESTOGENS

Desogestrel
04-Nov-2020

- **INDICATIONS AND DOSE**

Contraception
- ▶ BY MOUTH
- ▶ Females of childbearing potential: 75 micrograms daily, dose to be taken at same time each day, starting on day 1 of cycle then continuously, if administration delayed for 12 hours or more it should be regarded as a 'missed pill'

- **CONTRA-INDICATIONS** Acute porphyrias p. 1107 · current breast cancer
- **CAUTIONS** Cardiac dysfunction · diabetes (progestogens can decrease glucose tolerance—monitor patient closely) · history of breast cancer—seek specialist advice before use · history of stroke (including transient ischaemic attack) · history of venous thromboembolism · ischaemic heart disease · liver tumours—seek specialist advice before use · malabsorption states · migraine with aura · multiple risk factors for cardiovascular disease · positive antiphospholipid antibodies · rheumatoid arthritis · systemic lupus erythematosus · undiagnosed vaginal bleeding
- **INTERACTIONS** → Appendix 1: desogestrel
- **SIDE-EFFECTS**
- ▶ **Common or very common** Breast abnormalities · depressed mood · headache · libido decreased · menstrual cycle irregularities · mood altered · nausea · skin reactions · weight increased
- ▶ **Uncommon** Alopecia · contact lens intolerance · fatigue · ovarian cyst · vomiting · vulvovaginal infection
- ▶ **Rare or very rare** Erythema nodosum
- ▶ **Frequency not known** Angioedema · embolism and thrombosis · neoplasms

  SIDE-EFFECTS, FURTHER INFORMATION The benefits of using progestogen-only contraceptives (POCs), such as desogestrel, should be weighed against the possible risks for each individual woman.

7

Genito-urinary system

There is a small increase in the risk of having breast cancer diagnosed in women using a combined oral contraceptive pill (COC); this relative risk may be due to an earlier diagnosis, biological effects of the pill or a combination of both. This increased risk is related to the age of the woman using the COC rather than the duration of use and disappears gradually within 10 years after discontinuation.

The risk of breast cancer in users of POCs is possibly of similar magnitude as that associated with COCs, however the evidence is less conclusive.

Available evidence does not support an association between the use of a progestegen-only contraceptive pill and breast cancer. Any increased risk is likely to be small and reduces gradually during the 10 years after stopping; there is no excess risk 10 years after stopping. The older age at which the contraceptive is stopped appears to have a greater influence on increased risk rather than the duration of use.

● PREGNANCY Not known to be harmful.

● BREAST FEEDING Progestogen-only contraceptives do not affect lactation.

● HEPATIC IMPAIRMENT Manufacturer advises caution; avoid in severe or active disease.

● PATIENT AND CARER ADVICE
Surgery All progestogen-only contraceptives are suitable for use as an alternative to combined hormonal contraceptives before major elective surgery, before all surgery to the legs, or before surgery which involves prolonged immobilisation of a lower limb.

Starting routine One tablet daily, on a continuous basis, starting on day 1 of cycle and taken at the same time each day (if delayed by longer than 12 hours contraceptive protection may be lost). Additional contraceptive precautions are not required if desogestrel is started up to and including day 5 of the menstrual cycle; if started after this time, additional contraceptive precautions are required for 2 days.

Changing from a combined oral contraceptive Start on the day following completion of the combined oral contraceptive course without a break (or in the case of ED tablets omitting the inactive ones).

After childbirth Oral progestogen-only contraceptives can be started up to and including day 21 postpartum without the need for additional contraceptive precautions. If started more than 21 days postpartum, additional contraceptive precautions are required for 2 days.

Diarrhoea and vomiting Vomiting and persistent, severe diarrhoea can interfere with the absorption of oral progestogen-only contraceptives. If vomiting occurs within 2 hours of taking desogestrel, another pill should be taken as soon as possible. If a replacement pill is not taken within 12 hours of the normal time for taking desogestrel, or in cases of persistent vomiting or very severe diarrhoea, additional precautions should be used during illness and for 2 days after recovery.

Missed doses The following advice is recommended: 'If you forget a pill, take it as soon as you remember and carry on with the next pill at the right time. If the pill was more than 12 hours overdue you are not protected. Continue normal pill-taking but you must also use another method, such as the condom, for the next 2 days'.

The Faculty of Sexual and Reproductive Healthcare recommends emergency contraception if one or more tablets are missed or taken more than 12 hours late and unprotected intercourse has occurred before 2 further tablets have been correctly taken.

● NATIONAL FUNDING/ACCESS DECISIONS
For full details see funding body website

Scottish Medicines Consortium (SMC) decisions
▸ Desogestrel (*Cerazette®*) for use as contraception (September 2003) SMC No. 36/03 Recommended with restrictions

● MEDICINAL FORMS There can be variation in the licensing of different medicines containing the same drug.

Tablet
▸ Desogestrel (Non-proprietary)
  Desogestrel 75 microgram Desogestrel 75microgram tablets | 84 tablet [PoM] £9.55 DT = £2.86
▸ Cerazette (Merck Sharp & Dohme Ltd)
  Desogestrel 75 microgram Cerazette 75microgram tablets | 84 tablet [PoM] £9.55 DT = £2.86
▸ Cerelle (Consilient Health Ltd)
  Desogestrel 75 microgram Cerelle 75microgram tablets | 84 tablet [PoM] £3.50 DT = £2.86
▸ Desomono (MedRx Licences Ltd)
  Desogestrel 75 microgram Desomono 75microgram tablets | 84 tablet [PoM] £6.50 DT = £2.86
▸ Desorex (Somex Pharma)
  Desogestrel 75 microgram Desorex 75microgram tablets | 84 tablet [PoM] £2.45 DT = £2.86
▸ Feanolla (Lupin Healthcare (UK) Ltd)
  Desogestrel 75 microgram Feanolla 75microgram tablets | 84 tablet [PoM] £3.49 DT = £2.86
▸ Moonia (Stragen UK Ltd)
  Desogestrel 75 microgram Moonia 75microgram tablets | 84 tablet [PoM] [℞] DT = £2.86
▸ Zelleta (Morningside Healthcare Ltd)
  Desogestrel 75 microgram Zelleta 75microgram tablets | 84 tablet [PoM] £2.98 DT = £2.86

Levonorgestrel
09-Nov-2020

● INDICATIONS AND DOSE
Emergency contraception
▸ BY MOUTH
▸ Females of childbearing potential: 1.5 mg for 1 dose, taken as soon as possible after coitus, preferably within 12 hours and no later than after 72 hours (may also be used between 72–96 hours after coitus but efficacy decreases with time), alternatively 3 mg for 1 dose, taken as soon as possible after coitus, preferably within 12 hours and no later than after 72 hours (may also be used between 72–96 hours after coitus but efficacy decreases with time). Higher dose should be considered for patients with body-weight over 70 kg or BMI over 26 kg/m^2

Contraception
▸ BY MOUTH
▸ Females of childbearing potential: 30 micrograms daily starting on day 1 of the cycle then continuously, dose is to be taken at the same time each day, if administration delayed for 3 hours or more it should be regarded as a "missed pill"

JAYDESS® 13.5MG INTRA-UTERINE DEVICE
Contraception
▸ BY INTRA-UTERINE ADMINISTRATION
▸ Females of childbearing potential: Insert into uterine cavity within 7 days of onset of menstruation, or any time if replacement (additional precautions (e.g. barrier methods) advised for at least 7 days before), or any time if reasonably certain woman is not pregnant and there is no risk of conception (additional precautions (e.g. barrier methods) necessary for next 7 days), or immediately following termination of pregnancy below 24 weeks' gestation; postpartum insertions should be delayed until at least 4 weeks after delivery; effective for 3 years

KYLEENA ® 19.5MG INTRA-UTERINE DEVICE

Contraception

▶ BY INTRA-UTERINE ADMINISTRATION

▶ Females of childbearing potential: Insert into uterine cavity within 7 days of onset of menstruation, or any time if replacement (additional precautions (e.g. barrier methods) advised for at least 7 days before), or any time if reasonably certain woman is not pregnant and there is no risk of conception (additional precautions (e.g. barrier methods) necessary for next 7 days), or immediately following termination of pregnancy below 24 weeks' gestation; postpartum insertions should be delayed until at least 4 weeks after delivery; effective for 5 years

LEVOSERT ® 20MICROGRAMS/24HOURS INTRA-UTERINE DEVICE

Contraception | Menorrhagia

▶ BY INTRA-UTERINE ADMINISTRATION

▶ Females of childbearing potential: Insert into uterine cavity within 7 days of onset of menstruation, or any time if replacement (additional precautions (e.g. barrier methods) advised for at least 7 days before), or any time if reasonably certain woman is not pregnant and there is no risk of conception (additional precautions (e.g. barrier methods) necessary for next 7 days), or immediately following termination of pregnancy below 24 weeks' gestation; postpartum insertions should be delayed until at least 4 weeks after delivery; effective for 5 years

MIRENA ® 20MICROGRAMS/24HOURS INTRA-UTERINE DEVICE

Contraception | Menorrhagia

▶ BY INTRA-UTERINE ADMINISTRATION

▶ Females of childbearing potential: Insert into uterine cavity within 7 days of onset of menstruation, or any time if replacement (additional precautions (e.g. barrier methods) advised for at least 7 days before), or any time if reasonably certain woman is not pregnant and there is no risk of conception (additional precautions (e.g. barrier methods) necessary for next 7 days), or immediately following termination of pregnancy below 24 weeks' gestation; postpartum insertions should be delayed until at least 4 weeks after delivery; effective for 5 years

Prevention of endometrial hyperplasia during oestrogen replacement therapy

▶ BY INTRA-UTERINE ADMINISTRATION

▶ Females of childbearing potential: Insert during last days of menstruation or withdrawal bleeding or at any time if amenorrhoeic; effective for 4 years

DOSE ADJUSTMENTS DUE TO INTERACTIONS

▶ When used orally as an emergency contraceptive, the effectiveness of levonorgestrel is reduced in women taking enzyme-inducing drugs (and for up to 4 weeks after stopping); a copper intra-uterine device should preferably be used instead. If the copper intra-uterine device is undesirable or inappropriate, the dose of levonorgestrel should be increased to a total of 3 mg taken as a single dose; pregnancy should be excluded following use, and medical advice sought if pregnancy occurs.

▶ There is no need to increase the dose for emergency contraception if the patient is taking antibacterials that are not enzyme inducers.

▶ With the progestogen-only intra-uterine device, levonorgestrel is released close to the site of the main contraceptive action (on cervical mucus and endometrium) and therefore progestogenic side-effects and interactions are less likely; in particular, enzyme-inducing drugs are unlikely to significantly reduce the contraceptive effect of the progestogen-only intra-uterine system and additional contraceptive precautions are not required.

● UNLICENSED USE

▶ With intra-uterine use The Faculty of Sexual and Reproductive Healthcare (FSRH) advises levonorgestrel is used as detailed below, although these situations are considered unlicensed:
  ● Insertion at any time if reasonably certain the woman is not pregnant or at risk of pregnancy;
  ● Additional precautions (e.g. barrier methods) for at least 7 days before replacement even if immediate replacement is intended;
  ● Insertion immediately following termination of pregnancy below 24 weeks' gestation;
  ● Postpartum insertions 4 weeks after delivery.

▶ With oral use The FSRH advises levonorgestrel is used as detailed below, although these situations are considered unlicensed:
  ● Higher dose option for emergency contraception in patients with body-weight over 70 kg or BMI over 26 kg/m^2;
  ● Use for emergency contraception between 72–96 hours after coitus.

▶ With intra-uterine use or oral use in children Consult product literature for licensing status of individual preparations.

IMPORTANT SAFETY INFORMATION

MHRA/CHM ADVICE (JUNE 2015) INTRA-UTERINE CONTRACEPTION: UTERINE PERFORATION—UPDATED INFORMATION ON RISK FACTORS

Uterine perforation most often occurs during insertion, but might not be detected until sometime later. The risk of uterine perforation is increased when the device is inserted up to 36 weeks postpartum or in patients who are breastfeeding. Before inserting an intra-uterine contraceptive device, inform patients that perforation occurs in approximately 1 in every 1000 insertions and signs and symptoms include:
● severe pelvic pain after insertion (worse than period cramps);
● pain or increased bleeding after insertion which continues for more than a few weeks;
● sudden changes in periods;
● pain during intercourse;
● unable to feel the threads.
Patients should be informed on how to check their threads and to arrange a check-up if threads cannot be felt, especially if they also have significant pain. Partial perforation may occur even if the threads can be seen; consider this if there is severe pain following insertion and perform an ultrasound.

● CONTRA-INDICATIONS

GENERAL CONTRA-INDICATIONS

Current breast cancer (use with caution for emergency contraception)

SPECIFIC CONTRA-INDICATIONS

▶ With intra-uterine use Active trophoblastic disease (until return to normal of urine- and plasma-gonadotrophin concentration) · acute malignancies affecting the blood (use with caution in remission) · not suitable for emergency contraception · pelvic inflammatory disease · post-abortion sepsis · postpartum sepsis · recent sexually transmitted infection (if not fully investigated and treated) · unexplained uterine bleeding · uterine or cervical malignancy

▶ With oral use Acute porphyrias p. 1107

● CAUTIONS

GENERAL CAUTIONS Cardiac disease—seek specialist advice for intra-uterine insertion · diabetes · history of breast cancer—seek specialist advice before use · history of stroke (including transient ischaemic attack) · history of venous thromboembolism · ischaemic heart disease · migraine · multiple risk factors for cardiovascular disease · positive antiphospholipid antibodies · rheumatoid arthritis · systemic lupus erythematosus

SPECIFIC CAUTIONS

‣ With intra-uterine use Anatomical abnormalities—seek specialist advice before use · cervical intraepithelial neoplasia · epilepsy (risk of seizure at time of insertion) · immunosuppression (risk of infection)—seek specialist advice before use · postpartum—seek specialist advice before use · risk of sexually transmitted infections · young age

‣ With oral use Malabsorption states

‣ With oral use for contraception Undiagnosed vaginal bleeding

CAUTIONS, FURTHER INFORMATION

‣ With intra-uterine use The Faculty of Sexual and Reproductive Healthcare advises intercourse should be avoided or another method of contraception used for at least 7 days before removal of intra-uterine device—emergency contraception may need to be considered if recent intercourse has occurred and the intra-uterine device is removed.

‣ Sexually transmitted infections and pelvic inflammatory disease

‣ With intra-uterine use The main excess risk of pelvic infection occurs in the first 20 days after insertion and is believed to be related to existing carriage of a sexually transmitted infection. Women are considered to be at a higher risk of sexually transmitted infections if:

- they are under 25 years old *or*
- they are over 25 years old *and*
- have a new partner *or*
- have had more than one partner in the past year *or*
- their regular partner has other partners.

The Faculty of Sexual and Reproductive Healthcare advises pre-insertion screening (for chlamydia and, depending on sexual history and local prevalence of disease, *Neisseria gonorrhoeae*) be performed in these women. The woman should be advised to attend *as an emergency* if she experiences sustained pain during the next 20 days.

MIRENA ® 20 MICROGRAMS/24 HOURS INTRA-UTERINE DEVICE Advanced uterine atrophy

● INTERACTIONS → Appendix 1: levonorgestrel

● SIDE-EFFECTS

GENERAL SIDE-EFFECTS

▶ **Common or very common** Gastrointestinal discomfort · headaches · menstrual cycle irregularities · nausea · skin reactions

SPECIFIC SIDE-EFFECTS

▶ **Common or very common**

‣ With intra-uterine use Back pain · breast abnormalities · depression · device expulsion · hirsutism · increased risk of infection · libido decreased · nervousness · ovarian cyst · pelvic disorders · uterine haemorrhage (on insertion) · vaginal haemorrhage (on insertion) · vulvovaginal disorders · weight increased

‣ With oral use Breast tenderness · diarrhoea · dizziness · fatigue · haemorrhage · vomiting

▶ **Uncommon**

‣ With intra-uterine use Alopecia · endometritis · oedema · uterine rupture

▶ **Rare or very rare**

‣ With oral use Face oedema · pelvic pain

▶ **Frequency not known**

‣ With oral use Cerebrovascular insufficiency · depressed mood · diabetes mellitus · embolism and thrombosis · neoplasms · sexual dysfunction · weight changes

SIDE-EFFECTS, FURTHER INFORMATION

Breast cancer There is a small increase in the risk of having breast cancer diagnosed in women using, or who have recently used, a progestogen-only contraceptive pill;

this relative risk may be due to an earlier diagnosis. The most important risk factor appears to be the age at which the contraceptive is stopped rather than the duration of use; the risk disappears gradually during the 10 years after stopping and there is no excess risk by 10 years. A possible small increase in the risk of breast cancer should be weighed against the benefits.

With intra-uterine use There is no evidence of an association between the levonorgestrel intra-uterine system and breast cancer. The levonorgestrel intra-uterine system should be avoided in patients with a history of breast cancer; any consideration of it's use should be by a specialist in contraception and in consultation with the patients cancer specialist.

Patients should be informed about the device that has been inserted and when it should be removed or replaced (including refering them to a patient information leaflet and other sources of information).

Patients may experience irregular, prolonged or infrequent menstrual bleeding in the 3–6 months following insertion; bleeding pattern improves with time but persists in some patients.

Progestogenic side-effects resolve with time (after the first few months).

● PREGNANCY

‣ With oral use Not known to be harmful.

‣ With intra-uterine use If an intra-uterine device fails and the woman wishes to continue to full-term the device should be removed in the first trimester if possible. Avoid; if pregnancy occurs remove intra-uterine system.

● BREAST FEEDING Progestogen-only contraceptives do not affect lactation.

● HEPATIC IMPAIRMENT

‣ With intra-uterine use or oral use for Contraception Manufacturer advises avoid in liver tumour.

‣ With oral use for Contraception or Emergency contraception Manufacturer advises avoid in severe impairment.

‣ With intra-uterine use Manufacturer advises avoid in acute hepatic disease or in severe impairment (no information available)—consult product literature.

● MONITORING REQUIREMENTS

‣ With intra-uterine use Gynaecological examination before insertion, 4–6 weeks after insertion, then annually.

● DIRECTIONS FOR ADMINISTRATION

‣ With intra-uterine use The doctor or nurse administering (or removing) the system should be fully trained in the technique and should provide full counselling reinforced by the patient information leaflet.

● PRESCRIBING AND DISPENSING INFORMATION

‣ With intra-uterine use Levonorgestrel-releasing intra-uterine devices vary in licensed indication, duration of use and insertion technique—the MHRA recommends to prescribe and dispense by brand name to avoid inadvertent switching.

● PATIENT AND CARER ADVICE

Diarrhoea and vomiting with use as an oral contraceptive Vomiting and persistent, severe diarrhoea can interfere with the absorption of oral progestogen-only contraceptives. If vomiting occurs within 2 hours of taking an oral progestogen-only contraceptive, another pill should be taken as soon as possible. If a replacement pill is not taken within 3 hours of the normal time for taking the progestogen-only pill, or in cases of persistent vomiting or very severe diarrhoea, additional precautions should be used during illness and for 2 days after recovery.

Starting routine

‣ With oral use for Contraception One tablet daily, on a continuous basis, starting on day 1 of cycle and taken at the same time each day (if delayed by longer than 3 hours contraceptive protection may be lost). Additional contraceptive precautions are not required if levonorgestrel is started up to and including day 5 of the menstrual cycle; if started after this time, additional contraceptive precautions are required for 2 days.

Changing from a combined oral contraceptive Start on the day following completion of the combined oral contraceptive course without a break (or in the case of ED tablets omitting the inactive ones).

After childbirth Oral progestogen-only contraceptives can be started up to and including day 21 postpartum without the need for additional contraceptive precautions. If started more than 21 days postpartum, additional contraceptive precautions are required for 2 days.

▸ **With oral use for Emergency contraception** When prescribing or supplying hormonal emergency contraception, manufacturer advises women should be told:
- if vomiting occurs within 3 hours, a replacement dose should be taken;
- that their next period may be early or late;
- to seek medical attention promptly if any lower abdominal pain occurs because this could signify an ectopic pregnancy.

The Faculty of Sexual and Reproductive Healthcare also advises women should be told:
- that a barrier method of contraception needs to be used—see Emergency contraception p. 839 for further information;
- that a pregnancy test should be performed if the next menstrual period is delayed by more than 7 days, is lighter than usual, or is associated with abdominal pain that is not typical of the woman's usual dysmenorrhoea;
- that a pregnancy test should be performed if hormonal contraception is started soon after use of emergency contraception even if they have bleeding; bleeding associated with the contraceptive method may not represent menstruation.

▸ **With intra-uterine use** Counsel women on the signs, symptoms and risks of perforation and ectopic pregnancy.

Missed doses When used as an oral contraceptive, the following advice is recommended 'If you forget a pill, take it as soon as you remember and carry on with the next pill at the right time. If the pill was more than 3 hours overdue you are not protected. Continue normal pill-taking but you must also use another method, such as the condom, for the next 2 days'.

The Faculty of Sexual and Reproductive Healthcare recommends emergency contraception if one or more progestogen-only contraceptive tablets are missed or taken more than 3 hours late and unprotected intercourse has occurred before 2 further tablets have been correctly taken.

● NATIONAL FUNDING/ACCESS DECISIONS
For full details see funding body website

Scottish Medicines Consortium (SMC) decisions
▸ Levonorgestrel (*Kyleena*®) for contraception for up to 5 years (February 2018) SMC No. 1299/18 Recommended

All Wales Medicines Strategy Group (AWMSG) decisions
▸ Levonorgestrel (*Kyleena*®) for contraception for up to 5 years (September 2018) AWMSG No. 3582 Recommended

● EXCEPTIONS TO LEGAL CATEGORY *Levonelle*® *One Step* can be sold to women over 16 years; when supplying emergency contraception to the public, pharmacists should refer to guidance issued by the Royal Pharmaceutical Society.

● MEDICINAL FORMS There can be variation in the licensing of different medicines containing the same drug.

Intra-uterine device
▸ Jaydess (Bayer Plc) ▼
  Levonorgestrel 13.5 mg Jaydess 13.5mg intra-uterine device | 1 device [PoM] £69.22 DT = £69.22

▸ Kyleena (Bayer Plc)
  Levonorgestrel 19.5 mg Kyleena 19.5mg intra-uterine device | 1 device [PoM] £76.00 DT = £76.00
▸ Levosert (Gedeon Richter (UK) Ltd)
  Levonorgestrel 20 microgram per 24 hour Levosert 20micrograms/24hours intra-uterine device | 1 device [PoM] £66.00 DT = £88.00
▸ Mirena (Bayer Plc)
  Levonorgestrel 20 microgram per 24 hour Mirena 20micrograms/24hours intra-uterine device | 1 device [PoM] £88.00 DT = £88.00

Tablet
▸ Levonorgestrel (Non-proprietary)
  Levonorgestrel 1.5 mg Levonorgestrel 1.5mg tablets | 1 tablet [P] £13.83 DT = £5.20 | 1 tablet [PoM] £3.74–£5.20 DT = £5.20
▸ Emerres (Morningside Healthcare Ltd)
  Levonorgestrel 1.5 mg Emerres Una 1.5mg tablets | 1 tablet [P] £13.83 DT = £5.20
  Emerres 1.5mg tablets | 1 tablet [PoM] £3.65 DT = £5.20
▸ Ezinelle (Mylan)
  Levonorgestrel 1.5 mg Ezinelle 1.5mg tablets | 1 tablet [P] £9.64 DT = £5.20
▸ Levonelle (Bayer Plc)
  Levonorgestrel 1.5 mg Levonelle 1500microgram tablets | 1 tablet [PoM] £5.20 DT = £5.20
▸ Levonelle One Step (Bayer Plc)
  Levonorgestrel 1.5 mg Levonelle One Step 1.5mg tablets | 1 tablet [P] £13.83 DT = £5.20
▸ Melkine (Crescent Pharma Ltd)
  Levonorgestrel 1.5 mg Melkine 1.5mg tablets | 1 tablet [PoM] £4.16 DT = £5.20
▸ Norgeston (Bayer Plc)
  Levonorgestrel 30 microgram Norgeston 30microgram tablets | 35 tablet [PoM] £0.92 DT = £0.92
▸ Upostelle (Gedeon Richter (UK) Ltd)
  Levonorgestrel 1.5 mg Upostelle 1500microgram tablets | 1 tablet [PoM] £3.75 DT = £5.20

3.5   Contraception, parenteral progestogen-only

> Other drugs used for Contraception, parenteral progestogen-only Norethisterone, p. 806

PROGESTOGENS

Etonogestrel
09-Nov-2020

● INDICATIONS AND DOSE

Contraception (no hormonal contraceptive use in previous month)
▸ BY SUBDERMAL IMPLANTATION
▸ Females of childbearing potential: 1 implant inserted during first 5 days of cycle, implant should be removed within 3 years of insertion

Contraception (postpartum)
▸ BY SUBDERMAL IMPLANTATION
▸ Females of childbearing potential: 1 implant to be inserted 21–28 days after delivery (delay until 28 days postpartum if breast-feeding), implant should be removed within 3 years of insertion

Contraception following abortion or miscarriage in the second trimester
▸ BY SUBDERMAL IMPLANTATION
▸ Females of childbearing potential: 1 implant to be inserted 21–28 days after abortion or miscarriage, implant should be removed within 3 years of insertion

continued →

Genito-urinary system

7

Contraception following abortion or miscarriage in the first trimester
▶ BY SUBDERMAL IMPLANTATION
  ▸ Females of childbearing potential: 1 implant to be inserted within 5 days after abortion or miscarriage, implant should be removed within 3 years of insertion

Contraception (changing from other hormonal contraceptive)
▶ BY SUBDERMAL IMPLANTATION
  ▸ Females of childbearing potential: Implant should be removed within 3 years of insertion (consult product literature)

● UNLICENSED USE *Nexplanon®* not licensed for use in females outside of the age range 18–40 years.

┌───┐
IMPORTANT SAFETY INFORMATION

MHRA/CHM ADVICE (UPDATED FEBRUARY 2020): *NEXPLANON®* (ETONOGESTREL) CONTRACEPTIVE IMPLANTS: NEW INSERTION SITE TO REDUCE RARE RISK OF NEUROVASCULAR INJURY AND IMPLANT MIGRATION

There have been reports of neurovascular injury and migration of *Nexplanon®* implants from the insertion site to the vasculature, including the pulmonary artery in rare cases. Correct subdermal insertion by an appropriately trained and accredited healthcare professional is recommended to reduce the risk of these events. Healthcare professionals are advised to review the updated guidance from the manufacturer and the statement from the Faculty of Sexual and Reproductive Healthcare (FSRH) on how to correctly insert the implant. Patients should be advised on how to locate the implant, informed to check this occasionally and report any concerns. An implant that cannot be palpated at its insertion site should be located and removed as soon as possible; if unable to locate implant within the arm, the MHRA recommends using chest imaging. Implants inserted at a previous site that can be palpated should not pose a risk and should only be replaced if there are issues with its location or if a routine replacement is due.
└───┘

● CONTRA-INDICATIONS Acute porphyrias p. 1107 · current breast cancer

● CAUTIONS Cardiac dysfunction · cervical cancer · diabetes (progestogens can decrease glucose tolerance—monitor patient closely) · history of breast cancer—seek specialist advice before use · history of stroke (including transient ischaemic attack) · history of venous thromboembolism · ischaemic heart disease · liver tumours—seek specialist advice before use · migraine · multiple risk factors for cardiovascular disease · positive antiphospholipid antibodies · rheumatoid arthritis · systemic lupus erythematosus · undiagnosed vaginal bleeding—seek specialist advice before use

● INTERACTIONS → Appendix 1: etonogestrel

● SIDE-EFFECTS
▶ **Common or very common** Abdominal pain · alopecia · anxiety · appetite increased · breast abnormalities · depressed mood · dizziness · emotional lability · fatigue · flatulence · headaches · hot flush · increased risk of infection · influenza like illness · libido decreased · menstrual cycle irregularities · nausea · ovarian cyst · pain · skin reactions · weight changes
▶ **Uncommon** Arthralgia · constipation · diarrhoea · drowsiness · dysuria · fever · galactorrhoea · genital abnormalities · hypertrichosis · insomnia · myalgia · oedema · vomiting · vulvovaginal discomfort
▶ **Frequency not known** Abscess · angioedema · embolism and thrombosis · haemorrhage · insulin resistance · neoplasms · paraesthesia · seborrhoea

SIDE-EFFECTS, FURTHER INFORMATION The benefits of using progestogen-only contraceptives (POCs), such as

etonogestrel, should be weighed against the possible risks for each individual woman.

There is a small increase in the risk of having breast cancer diagnosed in women using a combined oral contraceptive pill (COC); this relative risk may be due to an earlier diagnosis, biological effects of the pill or a combination of both. This increased risk is related to the age of the woman using the COC rather than the duration of use and disappears gradually within 10 years after discontinuation.

The risk of breast cancer in users of POCs is possibly of similar magnitude as that associated with COCs, however the evidence is less conclusive.

● PREGNANCY Not known to be harmful, remove implant if pregnancy occurs.

● BREAST FEEDING Progestogen-only contraceptives do not affect lactation.

● DIRECTIONS FOR ADMINISTRATION The doctor or nurse administering (or removing) the system should be fully trained in the technique and should provide full counselling reinforced by the patient information leaflet.

● PATIENT AND CARER ADVICE Full counselling backed by patient information leaflet required before administration.

● MEDICINAL FORMS There can be variation in the licensing of different medicines containing the same drug.
Implant
  ▸ Nexplanon (Merck Sharp & Dohme Ltd)
    Etonogestrel 68 mg Nexplanon 68mg implant | 1 device [PoM]
    £83.43 DT = £83.43

Medroxyprogesterone acetate · 27-Apr-2020

● INDICATIONS AND DOSE
Dysfunctional uterine bleeding
▶ BY MOUTH
  ▸ Adult: 2.5–10 mg daily for 5–10 days, repeated for 2 cycles, begin treatment on day 16–21 of cycle

Secondary amenorrhoea
▶ BY MOUTH
  ▸ Adult: 2.5–10 mg daily for 5–10 days, repeated for 3 cycles, begin treatment on day 16–21 of cycle

Mild to moderate endometriosis
▶ BY MOUTH
  ▸ Adult: 10 mg 3 times a day for 90 consecutive days, begin treatment on day 1 of cycle

Progestogenic opposition of oestrogen HRT
▶ BY MOUTH
  ▸ Adult: 10 mg daily for the last 14 days of each 28-day oestrogen HRT cycle

Endometrial cancer | Renal cell cancer
▶ BY MOUTH
  ▸ Adult: 200–600 mg daily

Breast cancer
▶ BY MOUTH
  ▸ Adult: 0.4–1.5 g daily

Contraception
▶ BY DEEP INTRAMUSCULAR INJECTION
  ▸ Females of childbearing potential: 150 mg, to be administered within the first 5 days of cycle or within first 5 days after parturition (delay until 6 weeks after parturition if breast-feeding)
▶ BY SUBCUTANEOUS INJECTION
  ▸ Females of childbearing potential: 104 mg, to be administered within first 5 days of cycle or within 5 days postpartum (delay until 6 weeks postpartum if breast-feeding), injected into anterior thigh or abdomen, dose only suitable if no hormonal contraceptive use in previous month

Long-term contraception
▶ BY DEEP INTRAMUSCULAR INJECTION
▶ Females of childbearing potential: 150 mg every 12 months, first dose to be administered within the first 5 days of cycle or within first 5 days after parturition (delay until 6 weeks after parturition if breast-feeding)
▶ BY SUBCUTANEOUS INJECTION
▶ Females of childbearing potential: 104 mg every 13 weeks, first dose to be administered within first 5 days of cycle or within 5 days postpartum (delay until 6 weeks postpartum if breast-feeding), injected into anterior thigh or abdomen, dose only suitable if no hormonal contraceptive use in previous month

Contraception (when patient changing from other hormonal contraceptive)
▶ BY SUBCUTANEOUS INJECTION
▶ Females of childbearing potential: (consult product literature)

Hot flushes caused by long-term androgen suppression in men with prostate cancer
▶ BY MOUTH
▶ Adult: 20 mg once daily initially for 10 weeks, evaluate effect at the end of the treatment period

● UNLICENSED USE [EvGr] Medroxyprogesterone acetate is used for the treatment of hot flushes caused by long-term androgen suppression in men, ◁Ⓐ but it is not licensed for this indication.
● CONTRA-INDICATIONS
GENERAL CONTRA-INDICATIONS
Acute porphyrias p. 1107 · current breast cancer (unless progestogens are being used in the management of this condition)
SPECIFIC CONTRA-INDICATIONS
▶ With oral use History of thromboembolism · undiagnosed vaginal bleeding
● CAUTIONS
GENERAL CAUTIONS Cardiac dysfunction · conditions that may worsen with fluid retention · diabetes (progestogens can decrease glucose tolerance—monitor patient closely) · history of breast cancer—seek specialist advice before use · hypertension · liver tumours—seek specialist advice before use · migraine · positive antiphospholipid antibodies · rheumatoid arthritis · risk factors for thromboembolism · systemic lupus erythematosus
SPECIFIC CAUTIONS
▶ With intramuscular use or subcutaneous use Cervical cancer · history of stroke (including transient ischaemic attack)— seek specialist advice before use · history of venous thromboembolism · ischaemic heart disease—seek specialist advice before use · multiple risk factors for cardiovascular disease—seek specialist advice before use · undiagnosed vaginal bleeding—seek specialist advice before use
▶ With oral use History of depression
● INTERACTIONS → Appendix 1: medroxyprogesterone
● SIDE-EFFECTS
GENERAL SIDE-EFFECTS
▶ **Common or very common** Alopecia · breast abnormalities · depression · dizziness · fluid retention · insomnia · menstrual cycle irregularities · nausea · sexual dysfunction · skin reactions · weight changes
▶ **Uncommon** Drowsiness · embolism and thrombosis · fever · galactorrhoea · hirsutism · muscle spasms · tachycardia
SPECIFIC SIDE-EFFECTS
▶ **Common or very common**
▶ With oral use Appetite increased · cervical abnormalities · constipation · fatigue · headache · hyperhidrosis · hypersensitivity · nervousness · oedema · tremor · vomiting

▶ With parenteral use Anxiety · asthenia · gastrointestinal discomfort · headaches · mood altered · pain · vulvovaginal infection
▶ **Uncommon**
▶ With oral use Congestive heart failure · corticoid-like effects · diabetes mellitus exacerbated · diarrhoea · dry mouth · euphoric mood · hypercalcaemia
▶ With parenteral use Appetite abnormal · arthralgia · hot flush · hypertension · ovarian cyst · painful sexual intercourse · uterine haemorrhage · varicose veins · vertigo · vulvovaginal disorders
▶ **Rare or very rare**
▶ With oral use Cerebral infarction · jaundice · malaise · myocardial infarction
▶ With parenteral use Breast cancer · lipodystrophy
▶ **Frequency not known**
▶ With oral use Adrenergic-like effects · cataract diabetic · concentration impaired · confusion · glycosuria · palpitations · visual impairment (discontinue if papilloedema or retinal vascular lesions)
▶ With parenteral use Hepatic disorders · osteoporosis · osteoporotic fractures · seizure
SIDE-EFFECTS, FURTHER INFORMATION
With oral use In general, side effects may be more common with high doses such as those used in malignant disease.
With parenteral use Reduction in bone mineral density is greater with increasing duration of use. The loss is mostly recovered on discontinuation.
● CONCEPTION AND CONTRACEPTION
▶ With intramuscular use If interval between dose is greater than 12 weeks and 5 days (in long-term contraception), rule out pregnancy before next injection and advise patient to use additional contraceptive measures (e.g. barrier) for 14 days after the injection.
▶ With subcutaneous use If interval between dose is greater than 13 weeks and 7 days (in long-term contraception), rule out pregnancy before next injection.
● PREGNANCY
▶ With oral use Avoid—genital malformations and cardiac defects reported.
▶ With intramuscular use or subcutaneous use Not known to be harmful.
● BREAST FEEDING Present in milk—no adverse effects reported. Progestogen-only contraceptives do not affect lactation.
▶ With intramuscular use or subcutaneous use The manufacturers advise that in women who are breast-feeding, the first dose should be delayed until 6 weeks after birth; however, evidence suggests no harmful effect to infant if given earlier. The benefits of using medroxyprogesterone acetate in breast-feeding women outweigh any risks.
● HEPATIC IMPAIRMENT
▶ With oral use Manufacturer advises caution; avoid in acute or active disease.
▶ With intramuscular use or subcutaneous use Manufacturer advises caution; avoid in severe or active disease.
● RENAL IMPAIRMENT
▶ When used for Mild to moderate endometriosis or Progestogenic opposition of oestrogen HRT or Dysfunctional uterine bleeding or Secondary amenorrhoea Use with caution.
● PATIENT AND CARER ADVICE
▶ With intramuscular use or subcutaneous use Full counselling backed by *patient information leaflet* required before administration—likelihood of menstrual disturbance and the potential for a delay in return to full fertility. Delayed return of fertility and irregular cycles may occur after discontinuation of treatment but there is no evidence of permanent infertility.

- MEDICINAL FORMS There can be variation in the licensing of different medicines containing the same drug. Forms available from special-order manufacturers include: oral suspension, oral solution

Tablet

▸ Climanor (ReSource Medical UK Ltd)
Medroxyprogesterone acetate 5 mg Climanor 5mg tablets |
28 tablet [PoM] £3.27
▸ Provera (Pfizer Ltd)
Medroxyprogesterone acetate 2.5 mg Provera 2.5mg tablets |
30 tablet [PoM] £1.84 DT = £1.84
Medroxyprogesterone acetate 5 mg Provera 5mg tablets |
10 tablet [PoM] £1.23 DT = £1.23 | 100 tablet [PoM] £12.32
Medroxyprogesterone acetate 10 mg Provera 10mg tablets |
10 tablet [PoM] £2.47 | 90 tablet [PoM] £22.16 DT = £22.16 |
100 tablet [PoM] £24.73
Medroxyprogesterone acetate 100 mg Provera 100mg tablets |
60 tablet [PoM] £29.98 | 100 tablet [PoM] £49.94 DT = £49.94
Medroxyprogesterone acetate 200 mg Provera 200mg tablets |
30 tablet [PoM] £29.65 DT = £29.65
Medroxyprogesterone acetate 400 mg Provera 400mg tablets |
30 tablet [PoM] £58.67 DT = £58.67

Suspension for injection

▸ Depo-Provera (Pfizer Ltd)
Medroxyprogesterone acetate 150 mg per 1 ml Depo-Provera
150mg/1ml suspension for injection vials | 1 vial [PoM] £6.01
Depo-Provera 150mg/1ml suspension for injection pre-filled syringes
| 1 pre-filled disposable injection [PoM] £6.01 DT = £6.01
▸ Sayana Press (Pfizer Ltd)
Medroxyprogesterone acetate 160 mg per 1 ml Sayana Press
104mg/0.65 ml suspension for injection pre-filled disposable devices
| 1 pre-filled disposable injection [PoM] £6.90 DT = £6.90

3.6 Contraception, spermicidal

SPERMICIDALS

Nonoxinol

- INDICATIONS AND DOSE

Spermicidal contraceptive in conjunction with barrier methods of contraception such as diaphragms or caps

▸ BY VAGINA
▸ Females of childbearing potential: (consult product literature)

- SIDE-EFFECTS Genital erosion · increased risk of HIV infection · pain · paraesthesia · skin reactions · vaginal redness

SIDE-EFFECTS, FURTHER INFORMATION High frequency use of the spermicide nonoxinol-9 has been associated with genital lesions, which may increase the risk of acquiring sexually transmitted infections.

- CONCEPTION AND CONTRACEPTION No evidence of harm to diaphragms.
- PREGNANCY Toxicity in *animal* studies.
- BREAST FEEDING Present in milk in *animal* studies.

- MEDICINAL FORMS There can be variation in the licensing of different medicines containing the same drug.

Gel

EXCIPIENTS: May contain Hydroxybenzoates (parabens), propylene glycol, sorbic acid

▸ Gygel (Marlborough Pharmaceuticals Ltd)
Nonoxinol-9 20 mg per 1 ml Gygel 2% contraceptive jelly |
81 gram [GSL] £11.00 DT = £11.00

---

4 Erectile and ejaculatory conditions

4.1 Erectile dysfunction

Erectile dysfunction

06-Mar-2017

Description of condition

Erectile dysfunction (impotence) is the persistent inability to attain and maintain an erection that is sufficient to permit satisfactory sexual performance. It can have physical or psychological causes. Erectile dysfunction can also be a side-effect of drugs such as antihypertensives, antidepressants, antipsychotics, cytotoxic drugs and recreational drugs (including alcohol).

Risk factors for erectile dysfunction include sedentary lifestyle, obesity, smoking, hypercholesterolaemia and metabolic syndrome. Erectile dysfunction increases the risk of cardiovascular disease. All men with unexplained erectile dysfunction should be evaluated for the presence of cardiovascular risk factors and any identified risk should be addressed.

Drug treatment

[EvGr] The recommended approach for the management of erectile dysfunction is a combination of drug treatment and lifestyle changes (including regular exercise, reduction in body mass index, Smoking cessation p. 519, and reduced alcohol consumption).

An oral phosphodiesterase type-5 inhibitor is the first-line drug treatment for erectile dysfunction, regardless of the cause. Ⓐ These drugs act by increasing the blood flow to the penis. They do not initiate an erection—sexual stimulation is required.

The choice of oral phosphodiesterase type-5 inhibitor depends on the frequency of intercourse and response to treatment. [EvGr] Avanafil p. 859, sildenafil p. 860 and vardenafil p. 862 are short-acting drugs and are suitable for occasional use as required. Tadalafil p. 861 is a longer-acting drug. It can be used as required, but can also be used as a regular lower daily dose to allow for spontaneous (rather than scheduled) sexual activity or in those who have frequent sexual activity. A patient with erectile dysfunction should receive six doses of an individual phosphodiesterase type-5 inhibitor at the maximum dose (with sexual stimulation) before being classified as a non-responder. Patients who fail to respond to the maximum dose of at least two different phosphodiesterase type-5 inhibitors should be referred to a specialist.

Intracavernosal, intraurethral or topical application of alprostadil (prostaglandin E₁) p. 863 is recommended as second-line therapy under careful medical supervision. Intracavernosal or intraurethral preparations can also be used to aid diagnosis. Ⓐ

Priapism associated with alprostadil

Manufacturers advise that patients should seek medical help if a prolonged erection lasting four hours or more occurs; application of an ice pack to the upper-inner thigh (alternating between the left and right thighs every two minutes for up to ten minutes) may result in reflex opening of the venous valves.

If priapism has lasted more than six hours, treatment should not be delayed; manufacturer advises management as follows:

- Initial therapy by penile aspiration: using aseptic technique, 20–50mL of blood should be aspirated using a 19–21 gauge butterfly needle inserted into the *corpus cavernosum*; if necessary the procedure may be repeated on the opposite side;

Lavage: if initial aspiration is unsuccessful, a second 19–21 gauge butterfly needle can be inserted into the opposite *corpus cavernosum*; sterile physiological saline can be injected through the first needle and drained through the second;

If aspiration and lavage of are unsuccessful, intracavernosal injection of a sympathomimetic with action on alpha-adrenergic receptors can be given, with continuous monitoring of blood pressure and pulse— see phenylephrine hydrochloride p. 866 [unlicensed indication], adrenaline/epinephrine p. 865 [unlicensed indication], and metaraminol p. 865 [unlicensed indication]. Extreme **caution** is required in patients with coronary heart disease, hypertension, cerebral ischaemia and in patients taking a monoamine-oxidase inhibitor (facilities for managing hypertensive crisis should be available when administered to patients taking MAOIs);

If necessary the sympathomimetic injections can be followed by further aspiration of blood through the same butterfly needle;

If administration of a sympathomimetic drug is unsuccessful, urgent referral for surgical management is required.

Prescribing on the NHS

Some drug treatments for erectile dysfunction may only be prescribed on the NHS under certain circumstances; for details see the criteria listed in part XVIIIB of the Drug Tariff (Part XIb of the Northern Ireland Drug Tariff, Part 12 of the Scottish Drug Tariff). The Drug Tariffs can be accessed online at: National Health Service Drug Tariff for England and Wales: see www.nhsbsa.nhs.uk/pharmacies-gp-practices-and-appliance-contractors/drug-tariff.

Health and Personal Social Services for Northern Ireland Drug Tariff: www.hscbusiness.hscni.net/services/2034.htm.

Scottish Drug Tariff: www.isdscotland.org/Health-Topics/Prescribing-and-Medicines/Scottish-Drug-Tariff/.

Related drugs

Other drugs used for Erectile dysfunction: aviptadil with phentolamine mesilate p. 866.

PHOSPHODIESTERASE TYPE-5 INHIBITORS

Avanafil　　　　　　　　　　　　　　　　16-Nov-2020

- **INDICATIONS AND DOSE**

Erectile dysfunction
▶ BY MOUTH
- Adult: Initially 100 mg, to be taken approximately 15–30 minutes before sexual activity, then adjusted according to response to 50–200 mg (max. per dose 200 mg), to be taken as a single dose as needed; maximum 1 dose per day

Erectile dysfunction in patients on alpha-blocker therapy
▶ BY MOUTH
- Adult: Initially 50 mg, to be taken approximately 15–30 minutes before sexual activity, then adjusted according to response to 50–200 mg (max. per dose 200 mg), to be taken as a single dose as needed; maximum 1 dose per day

DOSE ADJUSTMENTS DUE TO INTERACTIONS
▶ Manufacturer advises max. 100 mg once every 48 hours with concurrent use of moderate inhibitors of CYP3A4.

- CONTRA-INDICATIONS Avoid if systolic blood pressure below 90 mmHg (no information available) · blood pressure >170/100 mmHg · hereditary degenerative retinal disorders · history of non-arteritic anterior ischaemic optic neuropathy · life-threatening arrhythmia in previous 6 months · mild to severe heart failure · patients in whom vasodilation or sexual activity are inadvisable · recent

history of myocardial infarction · recent history of stroke · recent unstable angina

- CAUTIONS Active peptic ulceration · anatomical deformation of the penis (e.g. angulation, cavernosal fibrosis, Peyronie's disease) · bleeding disorders · cardiovascular disease · left ventricular outflow obstruction · predisposition to priapism (e.g. in sickle-cell disease, multiple myeloma, or leukaemia)

CAUTIONS, FURTHER INFORMATION
▶ Elderly For phosphodiesterase type-5 inhibitors, prescription potentially inappropriate (STOPP criteria) in severe heart failure characterised by hypotension i.e. systolic blood pressure less than 90 mmHg, or concurrent nitrate therapy for angina (risk of cardiovascular collapse). See also Prescribing in the elderly p. 33.

- INTERACTIONS → Appendix 1: phosphodiesterase type-5 inhibitors

- SIDE-EFFECTS
▶ **Common or very common** Headaches · nasal complaints · vasodilation
▶ **Uncommon** Asthenia · dizziness · drowsiness · dyspnoea exertional · gastrointestinal discomfort · muscle complaints · nausea · pain · palpitations · respiratory disorders · vision blurred · vomiting
▶ **Rare or very rare** Akathisia · angina pectoris · chest pain · diarrhoea · dry mouth · emotional disorder · gastritis · genital pruritus · gout · haematuria · hypertension · increased risk of infection · influenza like illness · insomnia · penis disorder · peripheral oedema · rash · seasonal allergy · sexual dysfunction · tachycardia · urinary frequency increased · weight increased

- HEPATIC IMPAIRMENT Manufacturer advises avoid in severe impairment.
  Dose adjustments Manufacturer advises use lowest effective initial dose in mild to moderate impairment and adjust according to tolerance.

- RENAL IMPAIRMENT Avoid if eGFR less than 30 mL/minute/1.73 m^2.

- PATIENT AND CARER ADVICE Onset of effect may be delayed if taken with food.

- NATIONAL FUNDING/ACCESS DECISIONS
  For full details see funding body website
  Scottish Medicines Consortium (SMC) decisions
  ▶ Avanafil (*Spedra®*) for the treatment of erectile dysfunction (ED) in adult men (September 2015) SMC No. 980/14 Not recommended
  All Wales Medicines Strategy Group (AWMSG) decisions
  ▶ Avanafil (*Spedra®*) for the treatment of erectile dysfunction in adult men (July 2015) AWMSG No. 1261 Recommended
  NHS restrictions *Spedra®* is not prescribable in NHS primary care for the treatment of erectile dysfunction except in men who meet the criteria listed in part XVIIIB of the Drug Tariff. The prescription must be endorsed 'SLS'. For more information see *Prices in the BNF*, under How to use the BNF.

- MEDICINAL FORMS There can be variation in the licensing of different medicines containing the same drug.
  Tablet
  ▶ Spedra (A. Menarini Farmaceutica Internazionale SRL)
  Avanafil 50 mg Spedra 50mg tablets | 4 tablet P͟o͟M £10.94 DT = £10.94 | 8 tablet P͟o͟M £19.70 DT = £19.70
  Avanafil 100 mg Spedra 100mg tablets | 4 tablet P͟o͟M £14.08 DT = £14.08 | 8 tablet P͟o͟M £26.26 DT = £26.26
  Avanafil 200 mg Spedra 200mg tablets | 4 tablet P͟o͟M £21.90 DT = £21.90 | 8 tablet P͟o͟M £39.40 DT = £39.40

7

Genito-urinary system

▌Sildenafil

04-Nov-2020

- **INDICATIONS AND DOSE**

Pulmonary arterial hypertension (initiated under specialist supervision)
- ▸ BY MOUTH
- ▸ Adult: 20 mg 3 times a day
- ▸ BY INTRAVENOUS INJECTION
- ▸ Adult: 10 mg 3 times a day, use intravenous route when the oral route is not appropriate

Erectile dysfunction
- ▸ BY MOUTH
- ▸ Adult: Initially 50 mg, to be taken approximately 1 hour before sexual activity, adjusted according to response to 25–100 mg (max. per dose 100 mg) as required, to be taken as a single dose; maximum 1 dose per day

Digital ulcers [associated with systemic sclerosis]
- ▸ BY MOUTH
- ▸ Adult: 25 mg 3 times a day, increased to 50 mg 3 times a day

DOSE ADJUSTMENTS DUE TO INTERACTIONS
▸ When used for Erectile dysfunction Manufacturer advises a starting dose of 25 mg with concurrent use of moderate and potent inhibitors of CYP3A4. Manufacturer advises if concurrent use of ritonavir is unavoidable, the max. dose should not exceed 25 mg within 48 hours.
▸ With oral use for Pulmonary arterial hypertension Manufacturer advises reduce dose to 20 mg twice daily with concurrent use of moderate inhibitors of CYP3A4. Manufacturer advises reduce dose to 20 mg once daily with concurrent use of some potent inhibitors of CYP3A4 (avoid with ketoconazole, itraconazole and ritonavir).
▸ With intravenous use for Pulmonary arterial hypertension Manufacturer advises reduce dose to 10 mg twice daily with concurrent use of moderate inhibitors of CYP3A4. Manufacturer advises reduce dose to 10 mg once daily with concurrent use of some potent inhibitors of CYP3A4 (avoid with ketoconazole, itraconazole and ritonavir).

- **UNLICENSED USE** [EvGr] Sildenafil is used for the treatment of digital ulcer, ◀E▶ but is not licensed for this indication.
- **CONTRA-INDICATIONS**

GENERAL CONTRA-INDICATIONS
Hereditary degenerative retinal disorders · history of non-arteritic anterior ischaemic optic neuropathy · recent history of myocardial infarction · recent history of stroke

SPECIFIC CONTRA-INDICATIONS
▸ When used for erectile dysfunction Avoid if systolic blood pressure below 90 mmHg (no information available) · patients in whom vasodilation or sexual activity are inadvisable · recent unstable angina
▸ When used for pulmonary arterial hypertension Sickle-cell anaemia

- **CAUTIONS**

GENERAL CAUTIONS Active peptic ulceration · anatomical deformation of the penis (e.g. angulation, cavernosal fibrosis, Peyronie's disease) · autonomic dysfunction · bleeding disorders · cardiovascular disease · left ventricular outflow obstruction · predisposition to priapism (e.g. in sickle-cell disease, multiple myeloma, or leukaemia)

SPECIFIC CAUTIONS
▸ When used for pulmonary arterial hypertension Hypotension (avoid if systolic blood pressure below 90 mmHg) · intravascular volume depletion · pulmonary veno-occlusive disease

CAUTIONS, FURTHER INFORMATION
▸ Elderly For phosphodiesterase type-5 inhibitors, prescription potentially inappropriate (STOPP criteria) in severe heart failure characterised by hypotension i.e.

systolic blood pressure less than 90 mmHg, or concurrent nitrate therapy for angina (risk of cardiovascular collapse). See also Prescribing in the elderly p. 33.

- **INTERACTIONS** → Appendix 1: phosphodiesterase type-5 inhibitors
- **SIDE-EFFECTS**
▸ **Common or very common** Alopecia · anaemia · anxiety · cough · diarrhoea · dizziness · fluid retention · gastrointestinal discomfort · gastrointestinal disorders · headaches · increased risk of infection · insomnia · nasal complaints · nausea · night sweats · pain · skin reactions · tremor · vasodilation · vision disorders
▸ **Uncommon** Arrhythmias · chest pain · drowsiness · dry eye · dry mouth · eye discomfort · eye disorders · eye inflammation · fatigue · feeling hot · gynaecomastia · haemorrhage · hypertension · hypotension · myalgia · numbness · palpitations · sinus congestion · tinnitus · vertigo · vomiting
▸ **Rare or very rare** Acute coronary syndrome · arteriosclerotic retinopathy · cerebrovascular insufficiency · glaucoma · haematospermia · hearing impairment · irritability · optic neuropathy (discontinue if sudden visual impairment occurs) · oral hypoaesthesia · priapism · retinal occlusion · scleral discolouration · seizure · severe cutaneous adverse reactions (SCARs) · sudden cardiac death · syncope · throat tightness

- **PREGNANCY** Use only if potential benefit outweighs risk—no evidence of harm in *animal* studies.
- **BREAST FEEDING** Manufacturer advises avoid—no information available.
- **HEPATIC IMPAIRMENT** Manufacturer advises caution in mild to moderate impairment; avoid in severe impairment (no information available).

Dose adjustments
▸ With intravenous use for Pulmonary arterial hypertension Manufacturer advises if usual dose not tolerated, consider dose reduction to 10 mg twice daily in mild to moderate impairment.
▸ With oral use for Pulmonary arterial hypertension Manufacturer advises if usual dose not tolerated, consider dose reduction to 20 mg twice daily in mild to moderate impairment.
▸ When used for Erectile dysfunction Manufacturer advises consider initial dose reduction to 25 mg in mild to moderate impairment; adjust according to response.

- **RENAL IMPAIRMENT**
Dose adjustments Use initial dose of 25 mg in erectile dysfunction if eGFR less than 30 mL/minute/1.73 m².
   In pulmonary hypertension, if usual dose not tolerated, reduce *oral* dose to 20 mg twice daily and *intravenous* dose to 10 mg twice daily.

- **TREATMENT CESSATION**
▸ When used for Pulmonary arterial hypertension Consider gradual withdrawal.

- **PATIENT AND CARER ADVICE**
▸ When used for Erectile dysfunction Onset of effect may be delayed if taken with food.

- **NATIONAL FUNDING/ACCESS DECISIONS**
For full details see funding body website
Scottish Medicines Consortium (SMC) decisions
▸ Sildenafil tablets (*Revatio®*) for the treatment of pulmonary arterial hypertension (February 2010) SMC No. 596/10 Recommended with restrictions
▸ Sildenafil injection (*Revatio®*) for the treatment of pulmonary arterial hypertension (PAH) in patients who are unable to take sildenafil orally (March 2011) SMC No. 688/11 Recommended with restrictions
NHS restrictions *Viagra®* is not prescribable in NHS primary care for treatment of erectile dysfunction except in men who meet the criteria listed in part XVIIIB of the

Drug Tariff (Part XIb of the Northern Ireland Drug Tariff, Part 12 of the Scottish Drug Tariff). The prescription must be endorsed 'SLS'. For more information see *Prices in the BNF*, under How to use the BNF.

● MEDICINAL FORMS There can be variation in the licensing of different medicines containing the same drug. Forms available from special-order manufacturers include: oral suspension, oral solution

Tablet

▸ Sildenafil (Non-proprietary)

Sildenafil (as Sildenafil citrate) 20 mg Sildenafil 20mg tablets | 90 tablet PoM £424.01–£446.33 DT = £446.33

Sildenafil (as Sildenafil citrate) 25 mg Sildenafil 25mg tablets | 4 tablet PoM £16.59 DT = £0.96 | 8 tablet PoM £1.92–£33.19

Sildenafil (as Sildenafil citrate) 50 mg Sildenafil 50mg tablets | 4 tablet PoM £21.27 DT = £1.15 | 8 tablet PoM £1.26–£42.54

Sildenafil (as Sildenafil citrate) 100 mg Sildenafil 100mg tablets | 4 tablet PoM £23.50 DT = £1.25 | 8 tablet PoM £1.44–£46.99

▸ Granpidam (Accord Healthcare Ltd)

Sildenafil (as Sildenafil citrate) 20 mg Granpidam 20mg tablets | 90 tablet PoM £424.01 DT = £446.33

▸ Mysildecard (Mylan)

Sildenafil (as Sildenafil citrate) 20 mg Mysildecard 20mg tablets | 90 tablet PoM £379.38 DT = £446.33

▸ Revatio (Upjohn UK Ltd)

Sildenafil (as Sildenafil citrate) 20 mg Revatio 20mg tablets | 90 tablet PoM £446.33 DT = £446.33

▸ Viagra (Upjohn UK Ltd)

Sildenafil (as Sildenafil citrate) 25 mg Viagra 25mg tablets | 4 tablet PoM £16.59 DT = £0.96 | 8 tablet PoM £33.19

Sildenafil (as Sildenafil citrate) 50 mg Viagra 50mg tablets | 4 tablet PoM £21.27 DT = £1.15 | 8 tablet PoM £42.54

Sildenafil (as Sildenafil citrate) 100 mg Viagra 100mg tablets | 4 tablet PoM £23.50 DT = £1.25 | 8 tablet PoM £46.99

▸ Vizarsin (Consilient Health Ltd)

Sildenafil (as Sildenafil citrate) 25 mg Vizarsin 25mg tablets | 4 tablet PoM £14.10 DT = £0.96

Sildenafil (as Sildenafil citrate) 50 mg Vizarsin 50mg tablets | 4 tablet PoM £18.07 DT = £1.15

Sildenafil (as Sildenafil citrate) 100 mg Vizarsin 100mg tablets | 4 tablet PoM £19.97 DT = £1.25

Solution for injection

▸ Revatio (Upjohn UK Ltd)

Sildenafil (as Sildenafil citrate).8 mg per 1 ml Revatio 10mg/12.5ml solution for injection vials | 1 vial PoM £45.28 (Hospital only)

Oral suspension

▸ Revatio (Upjohn UK Ltd)

Sildenafil (as Sildenafil citrate) 10 mg per 1 ml Revatio 10mg/ml oral suspension sugar-free | 112 ml PoM £186.75 DT = £186.75

Tadalafil

16-Nov-2020

● INDICATIONS AND DOSE

Pulmonary arterial hypertension (initiated under specialist supervision)

▸ BY MOUTH

▸ Adult: 40 mg once daily

Erectile dysfunction

▸ BY MOUTH

▸ Adult: Initially 10 mg (max. per dose 20 mg), to be taken at least 30 minutes before sexual activity, subsequent doses adjusted according to response, the effect of intermittent dosing may persist for longer than 24 hours, continuous daily use not recommended; maximum 1 dose per day

Erectile dysfunction; for patients who anticipate sexual activity at least twice a week

▸ BY MOUTH

▸ Adult: 5 mg once daily, reduced to 2.5 mg once daily, adjusted according to response

Benign prostatic hyperplasia

▸ BY MOUTH

▸ Adult: 5 mg once daily

● CONTRA-INDICATIONS

GENERAL CONTRA-INDICATIONS
Acute myocardial infarction in past 90 days · history of non-arteritic anterior ischaemic optic neuropathy · hypotension (avoid if systolic blood pressure below 90 mmHg)

SPECIFIC CONTRA-INDICATIONS

▸ When used for benign prostatic hyperplasia or erectile dysfunction Mild to severe heart failure · patients in whom vasodilation or sexual activity are inadvisable · recent stroke · uncontrolled arrhythmias · uncontrolled hypertension · unstable angina

● CAUTIONS

▸ When used for benign prostatic hyperplasia or erectile dysfunction Anatomical deformation of the penis (e.g. angulation, cavernosal fibrosis, Peyronie's disease) · cardiovascular disease · left ventricular outflow obstruction · predisposition to priapism (e.g. in sickle-cell disease, multiple myeloma, or leukaemia)

▸ When used for pulmonary arterial hypertension Anatomical deformation of the penis · aortic and mitral valve disease · congestive cardiomyopathy · coronary artery disease · hereditary degenerative retinal disorders · left ventricular dysfunction · life-threatening arrhythmias · pericardial constriction · predisposition to priapism · pulmonary veno-occlusive disease · uncontrolled hypertension

CAUTIONS, FURTHER INFORMATION

▸ Elderly For phosphodiesterase type-5 inhibitors, prescription potentially inappropriate (STOPP criteria) in severe heart failure characterised by hypotension i.e. systolic blood pressure less than 90 mmHg, or concurrent nitrate therapy for angina (risk of cardiovascular collapse).
See also Prescribing in the elderly p. 33.

● INTERACTIONS → Appendix 1: phosphodiesterase type-5 inhibitors

● SIDE-EFFECTS

▸ **Common or very common** Flushing · gastrointestinal discomfort · headaches · myalgia · nasal congestion · pain

▸ **Uncommon** Arrhythmias · chest pain · dizziness · dyspnoea · eye pain · fatigue · gastrooesophageal reflux disease · haemorrhage · hypertension · hypotension · nausea · oedema · palpitations · skin reactions · tinnitus · vision disorders · vomiting

▸ **Rare or very rare** Acute coronary syndrome · angioedema · cerebrovascular insufficiency · eye erythema · eye swelling · haematospermia · hyperhidrosis · memory loss · optic neuropathy (discontinue if sudden visual impairment occurs) · priapism · retinal occlusion · seizure · Stevens-Johnson syndrome · sudden cardiac death · sudden hearing loss (discontinue drug and seek medical advice) · syncope

● PREGNANCY Manufacturer advises avoid.

● BREAST FEEDING Manufacturer advises avoid—present in milk in *animal* studies.

● HEPATIC IMPAIRMENT

▸ When used for Pulmonary arterial hypertension Manufacturer advises caution in mild to moderate impairment (limited information available); avoid in severe impairment (no information available).

▸ When used for Benign prostatic hyperplasia or Erectile dysfunction Manufacturer advises caution for regular once-daily dosing (no information available), and in severe impairment for intermittent use (limited information available).

Dose adjustments

▸ When used for Pulmonary arterial hypertension Manufacturer advises consider initial dose reduction to 20 mg once daily in mild to moderate impairment.

▸ When used for Erectile dysfunction Manufacturer advises dose of 10 mg for intermittent use (no information available for higher doses).

7

Genito-urinary system

- **RENAL IMPAIRMENT**
  - When used for Pulmonary arterial hypertension Manufacturer advises avoid in severe impairment.
  - When used for Erectile dysfunction or Benign prostatic hyperplasia Manufacturer advises avoid regular once-daily dosing in severe impairment.
  - **Dose adjustments**
    - When used for Pulmonary arterial hypertension Manufacturer advises initial dose of 20 mg once daily in mild-to-moderate impairment; dose may be increased to 40 mg once daily if tolerated.
    - When used for Erectile dysfunction Manufacturer advises maximum dose of 10 mg for intermittent use in severe impairment.

- **NATIONAL FUNDING/ACCESS DECISIONS**
  For full details see funding body website
  Scottish Medicines Consortium (SMC) decisions
  - Tadalafil (*Adcirca*®) for the treatment of pulmonary arterial hypertension (PAH) classified as WHO functional class II and III, to improve exercise capacity (July 2012) SMC No. 710/11
    Recommended with restrictions
    NHS restrictions *Cialis*® is not prescribable in NHS primary care for the treatment of erectile dysfunction except in men who meet the criteria listed in part XVIIIB of the Drug Tariff (Part XIb of the Northern Ireland Drug Tariff, Part 12 of the Scottish Drug Tariff). The prescription must be endorsed 'SLS'. For more information see *Prices in the BNF*, under How to use the BNF.

- **MEDICINAL FORMS** There can be variation in the licensing of different medicines containing the same drug.
  Tablet
  - Tadalafil (Non-proprietary)
    Tadalafil 2.5 mg Tadalafil 2.5mg tablets | 28 tablet [PoM] £52.24 DT = £36.81
    Tadalafil 5 mg Tadalafil 5mg tablets | 28 tablet [PoM] £54.99 DT = £6.27
    Tadalafil 10 mg Tadalafil 10mg tablets | 4 tablet [PoM] £28.88 DT = £1.47
    Tadalafil 20 mg Tadalafil 20mg tablets | 4 tablet [PoM] £54.99 DT = £1.89 | 8 tablet [PoM] £3.78–£109.98 | 56 tablet [PoM] £283.99–£390.00
  - Adcirca (Eli Lilly and Company Ltd)
    Tadalafil 20 mg Adcirca 20mg tablets | 56 tablet [PoM] £491.22
  - Cialis (Eli Lilly and Company Ltd)
    Tadalafil 2.5 mg Cialis 2.5mg tablets | 28 tablet [PoM] £54.99 DT = £36.81
    Tadalafil 5 mg Cialis 5mg tablets | 28 tablet [PoM] £54.99 DT = £6.27
    Tadalafil 10 mg Cialis 10mg tablets | 4 tablet [PoM] £28.88 DT = £1.47
    Tadalafil 20 mg Cialis 20mg tablets | 4 tablet [PoM] £28.88 DT = £1.89 | 8 tablet [PoM] £57.76
  - Talmanco (Mylan)
    Tadalafil 20 mg Talmanco 20mg tablets | 56 tablet [PoM] £417.54

| Vardenafil

16-Nov-2020

- **INDICATIONS AND DOSE**
  Erectile dysfunction
  ▶ BY MOUTH USING TABLETS
  - Adult: Initially 10 mg (max. per dose 20 mg), to be taken approximately 25–60 minutes before sexual activity, subsequent doses adjusted according to response, onset of effect may be delayed if taken with high-fat meal; maximum 1 dose per day
  ▶ BY MOUTH USING ORODISPERSIBLE TABLET
  - Adult: 10 mg, to be taken approximately 25–60 minutes before sexual activity; maximum 10 mg per day

Erectile dysfunction (patients on alpha-blocker therapy)
▶ BY MOUTH USING TABLETS
- Adult: Initially 5 mg (max. per dose 20 mg), to be taken approximately 25–60 minutes before sexual activity, subsequent doses adjusted according to response, onset of effect may be delayed if taken with high-fat meal; maximum 1 dose per day
DOSE EQUIVALENCE AND CONVERSION
- *Levitra*® 10 mg orodispersible tablets and *Levitra*® 10 mg film coated tablets are **not** bioequivalent.

- **CONTRA-INDICATIONS** Avoid if systolic blood pressure below 90 mmHg · hereditary degenerative retinal disorders · myocardial infarction · patients in whom vasodilation or sexual activity is inadvisable · previous history of non-arteritic anterior ischaemic optic neuropathy · recent stroke · unstable angina

- **CAUTIONS** Active peptic ulceration · anatomical deformation of the penis (e.g. angulation, cavernosal fibrosis, Peyronie's disease) · bleeding disorders · cardiovascular disease · elderly · left ventricular outflow obstruction · predisposition to priapism (e.g. in sickle-cell disease, multiple myeloma, or leukaemia) · susceptibility to prolongation of QT interval
  CAUTIONS, FURTHER INFORMATION
  - Elderly For phosphodiesterase type-5 inhibitors, prescription potentially inappropriate (STOPP criteria) in severe heart failure characterised by hypotension i.e. systolic blood pressure less than 90 mmHg, or concurrent nitrate therapy for angina (risk of cardiovascular collapse). See also Prescribing in the elderly p. 33.

- **INTERACTIONS** → Appendix 1: phosphodiesterase type-5 inhibitors

- **SIDE-EFFECTS**
  - **Common or very common** Dizziness · flushing · gastrointestinal discomfort · headache · nasal congestion
  - **Uncommon** Allergic oedema · angioedema · arrhythmias · back pain · diarrhoea · drowsiness · dry mouth · dyspnoea · eye discomfort · eye disorders · gastrointestinal disorders · malaise · muscle complaints · muscle tone increased · nausea · palpitations · sensation abnormal · sinus congestion · skin reactions · sleep disorder · tinnitus · vertigo · vision disorders · vomiting
  - **Rare or very rare** Angina pectoris · anxiety · chest pain · conjunctivitis · haemorrhage · hypertension · hypotension · memory loss · myocardial infarction · photosensitivity reaction · priapism · seizure · syncope
  - **Frequency not known** Haematospermia · optic neuropathy (discontinue if sudden visual impairment occurs) · QT interval prolongation · sudden hearing loss

- **HEPATIC IMPAIRMENT** For *film-coated tablets*, manufacturer advises caution in mild to moderate impairment; avoid in severe impairment.
  For *orodispersible tablets*, manufacturer advises caution in mild impairment; avoid in moderate to severe impairment.
  Dose adjustments For *film-coated tablets*, manufacturer advises initial dose reduction to 5 mg in mild to moderate impairment, increase according to response; max. 10 mg in moderate impairment.
  For *orodispersible tablets*, manufacturer advises initial dose reduction to 5 mg using *film-coated tablets* in mild impairment, increase according to response.

- **RENAL IMPAIRMENT** Orodispersible tablets not suitable if eGFR less than 30 mL/minute/1.73 m².
  Dose adjustments Initial dose 5 mg if eGFR less than 30 mL/minute/1.73 m².

- **PRESCRIBING AND DISPENSING INFORMATION**
  Orodispersible tablets not suitable for initiation of therapy in patients taking alpha-blockers.

NATIONAL FUNDING/ACCESS DECISIONS
For full details see funding body website

Scottish Medicines Consortium (SMC) decisions
Vardenafil orodispersible tablet (*Levitra*®) for the treatment of erectile dysfunction (October 2011) SMC No. 727/11
Recommended with restrictions
NHS restrictions *Levitra*® is not prescribable in NHS primary care for the treatment of erectile dysfunction except in men who meet the criteria listed in part XVIIIB of the Drug Tariff (Part XIb of the Northern Ireland Drug Tariff, Part 12 of the Scottish Drug Tariff). The prescription must be endorsed 'SLS'. For more information see *Prices in the BNF*, under How to use the BNF.

▶ MEDICINAL FORMS There can be variation in the licensing of different medicines containing the same drug.

Orodispersible tablet
EXCIPIENTS: May contain Aspartame
▶ Vardenafil (Non-proprietary)
 Vardenafil (as Vardenafil hydrochloride trihydrate)
 10 mg Vardenafil 10mg orodispersible tablets sugar free sugar-free | 4 tablet [PoM] £19.67 DT = £19.67
▶ Levitra (Bayer Plc)
 Vardenafil (as Vardenafil hydrochloride trihydrate) 10 mg Levitra 10mg orodispersible tablets sugar-free | 4 tablet [PoM] £19.67 DT = £19.67

Tablet
▶ Vardenafil (Non-proprietary)
 Vardenafil (as Vardenafil hydrochloride trihydrate)
 5 mg Vardenafil 5mg tablets | 4 tablet [PoM] £11.35 DT = £8.70 | 8 tablet [PoM] £11.36–£16.62
 Vardenafil (as Vardenafil hydrochloride trihydrate)
 10 mg Vardenafil 10mg tablets | 4 tablet [PoM] £20.02 DT = £15.35 | 8 tablet [PoM] £20.02–£29.57
 Vardenafil (as Vardenafil hydrochloride trihydrate)
 20 mg Vardenafil 20mg tablets | 4 tablet [PoM] £24.30 DT = £8.20 | 8 tablet [PoM] £16.40–£48.60
▶ Levitra (Bayer Plc)
 Vardenafil (as Vardenafil hydrochloride trihydrate) 5 mg Levitra 5mg tablets | 4 tablet [PoM] £8.32 DT = £8.70
 Vardenafil (as Vardenafil hydrochloride trihydrate) 10 mg Levitra 10mg tablets | 4 tablet [PoM] £14.78 DT = £15.35 | 8 tablet [PoM] £29.57
 Vardenafil (as Vardenafil hydrochloride trihydrate)
 20 mg Levitra 20mg tablets | 4 tablet [PoM] £24.30 DT = £8.20 | 8 tablet [PoM] £48.60

PROSTAGLANDINS AND ANALOGUES

Alprostadil
20-Jul-2020

● **INDICATIONS AND DOSE**

Erectile dysfunction (initiated under specialist supervision)
▶ BY URETHRAL APPLICATION
▶ Adult: Initially 250 micrograms, adjusted according to response; usual dose 0.125–1 mg; maximum 2 doses per day; maximum 7 doses per week

Aid to diagnosis of erectile dysfunction
▶ BY URETHRAL APPLICATION
▶ Adult: 500 micrograms for 1 dose

Erectile dysfunction
▶ TO THE SKIN
▶ Adult: Apply 300 micrograms, to the tip of the penis, 5–30 minutes before sexual activity; max 1 dose in 24 hours not more than 2–3 times per week

CAVERJECT®

Erectile dysfunction
▶ BY INTRACAVERNOSAL INJECTION
▶ Adult: Initially 2.5 micrograms for 1 dose (first dose), followed by 5 micrograms for 1 dose (second dose), to be given if some response to first dose, alternatively 7.5 micrograms for 1 dose (second dose), to be given if

no response to first dose, then increased in steps of 5–10 micrograms, to obtain a dose suitable for producing erection lasting not more than 1 hour; if no response to dose then next higher dose can be given within 1 hour, if there is a response the next dose should not be given for at least 24 hours; usual dose 5–20 micrograms (max. per dose 60 micrograms), maximum frequency of injection not more than 3 times per week with at least 24 hour interval between injections

Erectile dysfunction associated with neurological dysfunction
▶ BY INTRACAVERNOSAL INJECTION
▶ Adult: Initially 1.25 micrograms for 1 dose (first dose), then 2.5 micrograms for 1 dose (second dose), then 5 micrograms for 1 dose (third dose), increased in steps of 5–10 micrograms, to obtain a dose suitable for producing erection lasting not more than 1 hour; if no response to dose then next higher dose can be given within 1 hour, if there is a response the next dose should not be given for at least 24 hours; usual dose 5–20 micrograms (max. per dose 60 micrograms), maximum frequency of injection not more than 3 times per week with at least 24 hour interval between injections

Aid to diagnosis
▶ BY INTRACAVERNOSAL INJECTION
▶ Adult: 10–20 micrograms for 1 dose (consult product literature)

Aid to diagnosis where evidence of neurological dysfunction
▶ BY INTRACAVERNOSAL INJECTION
▶ Adult: Initially 5 micrograms (max. per dose 10 micrograms) for 1 dose, (consult product literature)

CAVERJECT® DUAL CHAMBER

Erectile dysfunction
▶ BY INTRACAVERNOSAL INJECTION
▶ Adult: Initially 2.5 micrograms for 1 dose (first dose), followed by 5 micrograms for 1 dose (second dose), to be given if some response to first dose, alternatively 7.5 micrograms for 1 dose (second dose), to be given if no response to first dose, then increased in steps of 5–10 micrograms, to obtain a dose suitable for producing erection lasting not more than 1 hour; if no response to dose then next higher dose can be given within 1 hour, if there is a response the next dose should not be given for at least 24 hours; usual dose 5–20 micrograms (max. per dose 60 micrograms), maximum frequency of injection not more than 3 times per week with at least 24 hour interval between injections

Erectile dysfunction associated with neurological dysfunction
▶ BY INTRACAVERNOSAL INJECTION
▶ Adult: Initially 1.25 micrograms for 1 dose (first dose), then 2.5 micrograms for 1 dose (second dose), then 5 micrograms for 1 dose (third dose), increased in steps of 5–10 micrograms, to obtain a dose suitable for producing erection lasting not more than 1 hour; if no response to dose then next higher dose can be given within 1 hour, if there is a response the next dose should not be given for at least 24 hours; usual dose 5–20 micrograms (max. per dose 60 micrograms), maximum frequency of injection not more than 3 times per week with at least 24 hour interval between injections

Aid to diagnosis
▶ BY INTRACAVERNOSAL INJECTION
▶ Adult: 10–20 micrograms for 1 dose (consult product literature)

continued →

Aid to diagnosis where evidence of neurological dysfunction

▸ BY INTRACAVERNOSAL INJECTION
▸ Adult: Initially 5 micrograms (max. per dose 10 micrograms) for 1 dose, (consult product literature)

VIRIDAL ® DUO

Neurogenic erectile dysfunction

▸ BY INTRACAVERNOSAL INJECTION
▸ Adult: Initially 1.25 micrograms, increased in steps of 2.5–5 micrograms, to obtain dose suitable for producing erection not lasting more than 1 hour; usual dose 10–20 micrograms (max. per dose 40 micrograms), maximum frequency of injection not more than 3 times per week with at least 24 hour interval between injections; reduce dose if erection lasts longer than 2 hours

Erectile dysfunction

▸ BY INTRACAVERNOSAL INJECTION
▸ Adult: Initially 2.5 micrograms, increased in steps of 2.5–5 micrograms, to obtain dose suitable for producing erection not lasting more than 1 hour; usual dose 10–20 micrograms (max. per dose 40 micrograms), maximum frequency of injection not more than 3 times per week with at least 24 hour interval between injections; reduce dose if erection lasts longer than 2 hours

● CONTRA-INDICATIONS

GENERAL CONTRA-INDICATIONS
Not for use in patients with penile implants or when sexual activity medically inadvisable (e.g. orthostatic hypotension, myocardial infarction, and syncope) · not for use with other agents for erectile dysfunction · predisposition to prolonged erection (as in thrombocytaemia, polycythaemia, sickle cell anaemia, multiple myeloma or leukaemia) · urethral application contra-indicated in balanitis · urethral application contra-indicated in severe curvature · urethral application contra-indicated in severe hypospadia · urethral application contra-indicated in urethral stricture · urethral application contra-indicated in urethritis

SPECIFIC CONTRA-INDICATIONS
▸ With topical use Balanitis · severe curvature · severe hypospadia · urethral stricture · urethritis

● CAUTIONS Anatomical deformations of penis (painful erection more likely)—follow up regularly to detect signs of penile fibrosis (consider discontinuation if angulation, cavernosal fibrosis or Peyronie's disease develop) · priapism (patients should be instructed to report any erection lasting 4 hours or longer) · risk factors for cardiovascular disorders · risk factors for cerebrovascular disorders

● INTERACTIONS → Appendix 1: alprostadil

● SIDE-EFFECTS

▸ **Common or very common**
▸ With intracavernosal use Haemorrhage · muscle spasms · penile disorders · sexual dysfunction · skin reactions
▸ With topical use Balanoposthitis · genital abnormalities · penile disorders · rash · sexual dysfunction · urinary tract pain
▸ With urethral use Dizziness · haemorrhage · headache · hypotension · muscle spasms · penile disorders · sexual dysfunction · urethral burning
▸ **Uncommon**
▸ With intracavernosal use Asthenia · balanoposthitis · dry mouth · extrasystole · hyperhidrosis · hypotension · increased risk of infection · inflammation · mydriasis · nausea · oedema · pelvic pain · peripheral vascular disease · presyncope · scrotal disorders · sensation abnormal ·

spermatocele · testicular disorders · urinary disorders · vascular disorders · vasodilation
▸ With topical use Dizziness · hyperaesthesia · hypotension · pain in extremity · scrotal pain · syncope · urinary tract disorders
▸ With urethral use Balanoposthitis · hyperhidrosis · increased risk of infection · leg pain · nausea · pelvic pain · perineal pain · peripheral vascular disease · scrotal disorders · sensation abnormal · skin reactions · spermatocele · syncope · testicular disorders · urinary disorders · vascular disorders · vasodilation
▸ **Frequency not known**
▸ With intracavernosal use Myocardial ischaemia · stroke
▸ With intravenous use Peripheral oedema

● CONCEPTION AND CONTRACEPTION
▸ With urethral use If partner is pregnant, barrier contraception should be used. No evidence of harm to latex condoms and diaphragms.
▸ With topical use Condoms should be used to avoid exposure to women of child-bearing age, pregnant or lactating women. No evidence of harm to latex condoms.

● DIRECTIONS FOR ADMINISTRATION
▸ With intracavernosal use Manufacturer advises the first dose of the intracavernosal injection must be given by medically trained personnel; self-administration may only be undertaken after proper training.
▸ With urethral use Manufacturer advises during initiation of treatment the urethral application should be used under medical supervision; self-administration may only be undertaken after proper training.

● PATIENT AND CARER ADVICE Patients should be instructed to report any erection lasting 4 hours or longer.
▸ With topical use Counsel patients that condoms should be used to avoid local reactions and exposure of alprostadil to women of childbearing age, pregnant, or lactating women.

● NATIONAL FUNDING/ACCESS DECISIONS
NHS restrictions *Caverject®*, *Viridal® Duo*, *Vitaros®* and *MUSE®* are not prescribable in NHS primary care for the treatment of erectile dysfunction except in men who meet the criteria listed in part XVIIIB of the Drug Tariff (Part XIb of the Northern Ireland Drug Tariff, Part 12 of the Scottish Drug Tariff). The prescription must be endorsed 'SLS'. For more information see *Prices in the BNF*, under *How to use BNF publications*.

● MEDICINAL FORMS There can be variation in the licensing of different medicines containing the same drug.

Stick
▸ Muse (Mylan)
  Alprostadil 500 microgram Muse 500microgram urethral sticks | 1 applicator [PoM] £11.30 DT = £11.30 | 6 applicator [PoM] £67.79
  Alprostadil 1 mg Muse 1000microgram urethral sticks | 1 applicator [PoM] £11.56 DT = £11.56 | 6 applicator [PoM] £65.67

Cream
▸ Vitaros (Ferring Pharmaceuticals Ltd)
  Alprostadil 3 mg per 1 gram Vitaros 3mg/g cream | 4 applicator [PoM] £40.00 DT = £40.00

Powder and solvent for solution for injection
▸ Caverject (Pfizer Ltd)
  Alprostadil 10 microgram Caverject 10microgram powder and solvent for solution for injection vials | 1 vial [PoM] £9.24 DT = £9.24
  Caverject Dual Chamber 10microgram powder and solvent for solution for injection | 2 pre-filled disposable injection [PoM] £14.70 DT = £14.70
  Alprostadil 20 microgram Caverject Dual Chamber 20microgram powder and solvent for solution for injection | 2 pre-filled disposable injection [PoM] £19.00 DT = £19.00
  Caverject 20microgram powder and solvent for solution for injection vials | 1 vial [PoM] £11.94 DT = £11.94
  Alprostadil 40 microgram Caverject 40microgram powder and solvent for solution for injection vials | 1 vial [PoM] £21.58 DT = £21.58

▶ Viridal (UCB Pharma Ltd)
Alprostadil 10 microgram Viridal Duo Starter Pack 10microgram powder and solvent for solution for injection cartridges with device | 2 cartridge [PoM] £20.13 DT = £20.13
Viridal Duo Continuation Pack 10microgram powder and solvent for solution for injection cartridges | 2 cartridge [PoM] £16.55 DT = £16.55
Alprostadil 20 microgram Viridal Duo Starter Pack 20microgram powder and solvent for solution for injection cartridges with device | 2 cartridge [PoM] £24.54 DT = £24.54
Viridal Duo Continuation Pack 20microgram powder and solvent for solution for injection cartridges | 2 cartridge [PoM] £21.39 DT = £21.39
Alprostadil 40 microgram Viridal Duo Starter Pack 40microgram powder and solvent for solution for injection cartridges with device | 2 cartridge [PoM] £29.83 DT = £29.83
Viridal Duo Continuation Pack 40microgram powder and solvent for solution for injection cartridges | 2 cartridge [PoM] £27.22 DT = £27.22

SYMPATHOMIMETICS > VASOCONSTRICTOR

Adrenaline/epinephrine

21-May-2020

● DRUG ACTION Acts on both alpha and beta receptors and increases both heart rate and contractility (beta$_1$ effects); it can cause peripheral vasodilation (a beta$_2$ effect) or vasoconstriction (an alpha effect).

● **INDICATIONS AND DOSE**

Priapism associated with alprostadil, if aspiration and lavage of corpora are unsuccessful (alternative to phenylephrine or metaraminol)
▶ BY INTRACAVERNOSAL INJECTION
▶ Adult: 10–20 micrograms every 5–10 minutes, using a 20 microgram/mL solution, **Important:** if suitable strength of adrenaline not available may be specially prepared by diluting 0.1 mL of the adrenaline 1 in 1000 (1 mg/mL) injection to 5 mL with sodium chloride 0.9%, continuously monitor blood pressure and pulse; maximum 100 micrograms per course

● UNLICENSED USE The use of adrenaline for the treatment of priapism is an unlicensed indication.

● CAUTIONS Arteriosclerosis · arrhythmias · cerebrovascular disease · cor pulmonale · diabetes mellitus · elderly · hypercalcaemia · hyperreflexia · hypertension · hyperthyroidism · hypokalaemia · ischaemic heart disease · obstructive cardiomyopathy · occlusive vascular disease · organic brain damage · phaeochromocytoma · prostate disorders · psychoneurosis · severe angina · susceptibility to angle-closure glaucoma
CAUTIONS, FURTHER INFORMATION Cautions listed are only for non-life-threatening situations.

● INTERACTIONS → Appendix 1: sympathomimetics, vasoconstrictor

● SIDE-EFFECTS
▶ Rare or very rare Cardiomyopathy
▶ **Frequency not known** Angina pectoris · angle closure glaucoma · anxiety · appetite decreased · arrhythmias · asthenia · CNS haemorrhage · confusion · dizziness · dry mouth · dyspnoea · headache · hepatic necrosis · hyperglycaemia · hyperhidrosis · hypersalivation · hypertension (increased risk of cerebral haemorrhage) · hypokalaemia · injection site necrosis · insomnia · intestinal necrosis · metabolic acidosis · mydriasis · myocardial infarction · nausea · pallor · palpitations · peripheral coldness · psychosis · pulmonary oedema (on excessive dosage or extreme sensitivity) · renal necrosis · soft tissue necrosis · tremor · urinary disorders · vomiting

● RENAL IMPAIRMENT Manufacturers advise use with caution in severe impairment.

● MONITORING REQUIREMENTS Monitor blood pressure and ECG.

● MEDICINAL FORMS There can be variation in the licensing of different medicines containing the same drug. Forms available from special-order manufacturers include: solution for injection

Solution for injection
EXCIPIENTS: May contain Sulfites
▶ Adrenaline/epinephrine (Non-proprietary)
Adrenaline 100 microgram per 1 ml Adrenaline (base) 100micrograms/1ml (1 in 10,000) dilute solution for injection ampoules | 10 ampoule [PoM] £92.59
Adrenaline (base) 1mg/10ml (1 in 10,000) dilute solution for injection pre-filled syringes | 1 pre-filled disposable injection [PoM] £7.21 |
1 pre-filled disposable injection [PoM] £6.87–£18.00 (Hospital only) |
10 pre-filled disposable injection [PoM] £180.00 (Hospital only)
Adrenaline (as Adrenaline acid tartrate) 100 microgram per 1 ml Adrenaline (base) 1mg/10ml (1 in 10,000) dilute solution for injection ampoules | 10 ampoule [PoM] £107.30
Adrenaline (base) 500micrograms/5ml (1 in 10,000) dilute solution for injection ampoules | 10 ampoule [PoM] £98.64
Adrenaline 1 mg per 1 ml Adrenaline (base) 10mg/10ml (1 in 1,000) solution for injection ampoules | 10 ampoule [PoM] £111.32 DT = £111.32
Adrenaline (base) for anaphylaxis 1mg/1ml (1 in 1,000) solution for injection pre-filled syringes | 1 pre-filled disposable injection [PoM] £12.47 DT = £16.68
Adrenaline (base) 1mg/1ml (1 in 1,000) solution for injection pre-filled syringes | 1 pre-filled disposable injection [PoM] £11.88–£14.47 DT = £16.68
Adrenaline (as Adrenaline acid tartrate) 1 mg per 1 ml Adrenaline (base) 5mg/5ml (1 in 1,000) solution for injection ampoules | 10 ampoule [PoM] £113.49 DT = £113.49
Adrenaline (base) 500micrograms/0.5ml (1 in 1,000) solution for injection ampoules | 10 ampoule [PoM] £90.85–£93.06 DT = £90.85
Adrenaline (base) 1mg/1ml (1 in 1,000) solution for injection ampoules | 10 ampoule [PoM] £6.00–£10.50 DT = £10.34

Metaraminol

28-Apr-2020

● **INDICATIONS AND DOSE**

Priapism (alternative to intracavernosal injections of phenylephrine and adrenaline)
▶ BY INTRACAVERNOSAL INJECTION
▶ Adult: 1 mg every 15 minutes

● UNLICENSED USE Use for priapism is an unlicensed indication.

● CAUTIONS Associated with fatal hypertensive crises · cirrhosis · coronary vascular thrombosis · diabetes mellitus · elderly · extravasation at injection site may cause necrosis · following myocardial infarction · hypercapnia · hypertension · hyperthyroidism · hypoxia · mesenteric vascular thrombosis · peripheral vascular thrombosis · Prinzmetal's variant angina · uncorrected hypovolaemia

● INTERACTIONS → Appendix 1: sympathomimetics, vasoconstrictor

● SIDE-EFFECTS
▶ **Common or very common** Headache · hypertension
▶ **Rare or very rare** Skin exfoliation · soft tissue necrosis
▶ **Frequency not known** Abscess · arrhythmias · nausea · palpitations · peripheral ischaemia

● MONITORING REQUIREMENTS Monitor blood pressure and rate of flow frequently.

● DIRECTIONS FOR ADMINISTRATION For *intracavernosal injection*, dilute 1 mg (0.1 mL of 10 mg/mL) metaraminol injection to 50 mL with Sodium chloride injection 0.9% and give carefully by slow injection into the corpora in 5 mL injections.

- MEDICINAL FORMS There can be variation in the licensing of different medicines containing the same drug. Forms available from special-order manufacturers include: solution for injection

Solution for injection
- ▸ Metaraminol (Non-proprietary)
  Metaraminol (as Metaraminol tartrate) 500 microgram per 1 ml Metaraminol 2.5mg/5ml solution for injection ampoules | 10 ampoule [PoM] £37.40
  Metaraminol 5mg/10ml solution for injection ampoules | 10 ampoule [PoM] £76.10
  Metaraminol (as Metaraminol tartrate) 10 mg per 1 ml Metaraminol 10mg/1ml solution for injection ampoules | 10 ampoule [PoM] £21.50

Phenylephrine hydrochloride

- INDICATIONS AND DOSE

Priapism associated with alprostadil, if aspiration and lavage of the corpora are unsuccessful (alternative to adrenaline or metaraminol)
- ▸ BY INTRACAVERNOSAL INJECTION
- ▸ Adult: 100–200 micrograms every 5–10 minutes, dose to be administered using a 200 micrograms/mL solution; maximum 1 mg per course

- UNLICENSED USE Use of phenylephrine hydrochloride injection in priapism is an unlicensed indication.
- CONTRA-INDICATIONS Hypertension
- INTERACTIONS → Appendix 1: sympathomimetics, vasoconstrictor
- SIDE-EFFECTS Angle closure glaucoma · anxiety · appetite decreased · arrhythmias · asthenia · confusion · dyspnoea · headache · hypertension · hypoxia · insomnia · nausea · palpitations · peripheral ischaemia · psychosis · tremor · urinary retention · vomiting
- DIRECTIONS FOR ADMINISTRATION For *intracavernosal injection*, if suitable strength of phenylephrine injection is not available, it may be specially prepared by diluting 0.1 mL of the phenylephrine 1% (10 mg/mL) injection to 5 mL with sodium chloride 0.9%.
- MEDICINAL FORMS There can be variation in the licensing of different medicines containing the same drug. Forms available from special-order manufacturers include: solution for injection

Solution for injection
- ▸ Phenylephrine hydrochloride (Non-proprietary)
  Phenylephrine (as Phenylephrine hydrochloride) 50 microgram per 1 ml Phenylephrine 500micrograms/10ml solution for injection pre-filled syringes | 1 pre-filled disposable injection [PoM] £15.00 | 10 pre-filled disposable injection [PoM] £150.00
  Phenylephrine hydrochloride 100 microgram per 1 ml Phenylephrine 1mg/10ml solution for injection ampoules | 10 ampoule [PoM] £42.00
  Phenylephrine hydrochloride 10 mg per 1 ml Phenylephrine 10mg/1ml solution for injection ampoules | 10 ampoule [PoM] £99.12
  Phenylephrine 10mg/1ml concentrate for solution for injection ampoules | 10 ampoule [PoM] £99.12

VASODILATORS ⟩ PERIPHERAL VASODILATORS

Aviptadil with phentolamine mesilate

16-Oct-2020

- DRUG ACTION Phentolamine is a short-acting alpha-adrenoceptor antagonist that acts directly on vascular smooth muscle, resulting in vasodilatation; aviptadil is a vasoactive intestinal polypeptide that acts as a smooth muscle relaxant.

- INDICATIONS AND DOSE

Erectile dysfunction
- ▸ BY INTRACAVERNOSAL INJECTION
- ▸ Adult: 25/2000 micrograms, frequency of injection should not exceed once daily or three times weekly, duration of erection should not exceed 1 hour

DOSE EQUIVALENCE AND CONVERSION
- ▸ Dose expressed as x/y micrograms of aviptadil/phentolamine.

- CONTRA-INDICATIONS Anatomical deformation of the penis (e.g. angulation, cavernosal fibrosis, Peyronie's disease) · not for use with other agents for erectile dysfunction · patients for whom sexual activity is inadvisable · penile implants · predisposition to priapism (e.g. in sickle cell anaemia or trait, multiple myeloma, or leukaemia)
- CAUTIONS Concomitant treatment with anticoagulants (potential increased risk of bleeding) · history of psychiatric disorder or addiction (potential for abuse) · severe cardiovascular disease · severe cerebrovascular disease
- SIDE-EFFECTS
- ▸ **Common or very common** Bruising · flushing
- ▸ **Uncommon** Dizziness · haematoma · headache · palpitations · tachycardia
- ▸ **Rare or very rare** Angina pectoris · myocardial infarction · penile fibrosis (following multiple injections) · penile nodules · sexual dysfunction
- MONITORING REQUIREMENTS Manufacturer advises monitor regularly (e.g. every 3 months), particularly in the initial stages of self-injection therapy; careful examination of the penis is recommended to detect signs of penile fibrosis or Peyronie's disease—discontinue treatment in patients who develop penile angulation, cavernosal fibrosis, or Peyronie's disease.
- DIRECTIONS FOR ADMINISTRATION Manufacturer advises that the initial injections of *Invicorp*® must be administered by medically trained personnel; self-administration may only be undertaken after proper training.
- HANDLING AND STORAGE Manufacturer advises store in a refrigerator (2–8°C).
- PATIENT AND CARER ADVICE Manufacturer advises that patients should be instructed to report any erection lasting 4 hours or longer.
- NATIONAL FUNDING/ACCESS DECISIONS For full details see funding body website

  Scottish Medicines Consortium (SMC) decisions
- ▸ Aviptadil/phentolamine mesilate (*Invicorp*®) for the symptomatic treatment of erectile dysfunction in adult males due to neurogenic, vasculogenic, psychogenic, or mixed aetiology (December 2017) SMC No. 1284/17 Recommended with restrictions

  All Wales Medicines Strategy Group (AWMSG) decisions
- ▸ Aviptadil/phentolamine mesilate (*Invicorp*®) for the symptomatic treatment of erectile dysfunction in adult males due to neurogenic, vasculogenic, psychogenic, or mixed

aetiology (July 2017) AWMSG No. 3435 Recommended with restrictions

- MEDICINAL FORMS There can be variation in the licensing of different medicines containing the same drug.

  Solution for injection
  ▸ Invicorp (Evolan Pharma AB)
    Aviptadil 71.43 microgram per 1 ml, Phentolamine mesilate 5.71 mg per 1 ml Invicorp 25micrograms/2mg/0.35ml solution for injection ampoules | 5 ampoule [PoM] £47.50 DT = £47.50

4.2 Premature ejaculation

Premature ejaculation

01-Aug-2017

Description of condition

Premature ejaculation is a common male sexual disorder characterised by brief ejaculatory latency, loss of control, and psychological distress.

Treatment

[EvGr] Non-drug treatment (including psychosexual counselling, education, and behavioural treatments) are recommended in patients for whom premature ejaculation causes few (if any) problems or in patients who prefer not to take drug treatment. These techniques can also be used in addition to a drug treatment.

For patients with life-long premature ejaculation, drug treatment is the recommended approach. ⒶDapoxetine below, a short-acting selective serotonin re-uptake inhibitor, is licensed to be used when required for this condition (not continuous daily use).

[EvGr] Other selective serotonin re-uptake inhibitors (citalopram p. 384, fluoxetine p. 385, fluvoxamine maleate p. 386, escitalopram p. 384, paroxetine p. 386, sertraline p. 387 [unlicensed indications]) and the tricyclic antidepressant clomipramine [unlicensed indication] have been widely used as regular, daily treatment. Caution is suggested in prescribing selective serotonin re-uptake inhibitors for young adolescents with premature ejaculation, and to men who also have a depressive disorder, particularly when associated with suicidal ideation. Ejaculation delay may start a few days after the start of treatment, but it is more evident after 1 to 2 weeks, since receptor desensitisation requires time to occur.

If premature ejaculation is secondary to Erectile dysfunction p. 858, the erectile dysfunction should be treated first. Ⓐ

Topical anaesthetic preparations for the management of premature ejaculation are available without prescription.

> **Other drugs used for Premature ejaculation** Lidocaine with prilocaine, p. 1408

SELECTIVE SEROTONIN RE-UPTAKE INHIBITORS

▌**Dapoxetine**   19-Oct-2020

- DRUG ACTION Dapoxetine is a short-acting selective serotonin re-uptake inhibitor.

- INDICATIONS AND DOSE

  Premature ejaculation in men who meet all the following criteria: poor control over ejaculation, a history of premature ejaculation over the past 6 months, marked distress or interpersonal difficulty as a consequence of premature ejaculation, and an intravaginal ejaculatory latency time of less than two minutes
  ▸ BY MOUTH
  ▸ Adult: Initially 30 mg, to be taken approximately 1–3 hours before sexual activity, subsequent doses adjusted according to response; review treatment after 4 weeks (or 6 doses) and at least every 6 months thereafter, not recommended for adults 65 years and over; maximum 1 dose per day; maximum 60 mg per day

  DOSE ADJUSTMENTS DUE TO INTERACTIONS
  ▸ Manufacturer advises max. dose 30 mg with concurrent use of moderate inhibitors of CYP3A4 except in patients verified to be extensive CYP2D6 metabolisers where manufacturer recommends max. dose 60 mg.
  ▸ Manufacturer advises avoid with concurrent use of potent inhibitors of CYP3A4 except in patients verified to be extensive CYP2D6 metabolisers where manufacturer recommends max. dose 30 mg.

- CONTRA-INDICATIONS History of bipolar disorder · history of mania · history of severe depression · history of syncope · postural hypotension · significant cardiac disease · uncontrolled epilepsy

- CAUTIONS Bleeding disorders · epilepsy (discontinue if convulsions develop) · susceptibility to angle-closure glaucoma

- INTERACTIONS → Appendix 1: SSRIs

- SIDE-EFFECTS
  ▸ **Common or very common** Anxiety · asthenia · concentration impaired · constipation · diarrhoea · dizziness · drowsiness · dry mouth · gastrointestinal discomfort · gastrointestinal disorders · headache · hypotension · mood altered · nausea · paraesthesia · sexual dysfunction · sinus congestion · sleep disorders · sweat changes · syncope · tinnitus · tremor · vasodilation · vision blurred · vomiting · yawning
  ▸ **Uncommon** Akathisia · arrhythmias · behaviour abnormal · confusion · depression · eye pain · feeling abnormal · feeling hot · hypertension · level of consciousness decreased · mydriasis · pruritus · taste altered · thinking abnormal · vertigo
  SIDE-EFFECTS, FURTHER INFORMATION Discontinue if psychiatric disorder develops.

- HEPATIC IMPAIRMENT Manufacturer advises avoid in moderate to severe impairment.

- RENAL IMPAIRMENT Use with caution if eGFR 30–80 mL/minute/1.73 m^2; avoid if eGFR less than 30 mL/minute/1.73 m^2.

- PRE-TREATMENT SCREENING Test for postural hypotension before starting treatment.

- TREATMENT CESSATION The dose should preferably be reduced gradually over about 4 weeks, or longer if withdrawal symptoms emerge (6 months in patients who have been on long-term maintenance treatment).

- PATIENT AND CARER ADVICE
  Postural hypotension and syncope Patients should be advised to maintain hydration and to sit or lie down until

prodromal symptoms such as nausea, dizziness, and sweating abate.

- MEDICINAL FORMS There can be variation in the licensing of different medicines containing the same drug.
Tablet
CAUTIONARY AND ADVISORY LABELS 2, 25
▸ Priligy (A. Menarini Farmaceutica Internazionale SRL)
Dapoxetine 30 mg Priligy 30mg tablets | 3 tablet [PoM] £14.71 DT = £14.71 | 6 tablet [PoM] £26.48 DT = £26.48
Dapoxetine 60 mg Priligy 60mg tablets | 3 tablet [PoM] £19.12 DT = £19.12 | 6 tablet [PoM] £34.42 DT = £34.42

5 Obstetrics

Obstetrics

16-Jun-2020

Prostaglandins and oxytocics

Prostaglandins and oxytocics are used to induce abortion, or induce or augment labour, and to minimise blood loss from the placental site. They include oxytocin below, carbetocin p. 871, ergometrine maleate p. 870, and the prostaglandins. All induce uterine contractions with varying degrees of force, frequency, and duration.

Induction of abortion

[EvGr] Pre-treatment with mifepristone p. 872 can facilitate the process of medical abortion. [A] It sensitises the uterus to subsequent administration of a prostaglandin and, therefore, abortion occurs in a shorter time and with a lower dose of prostaglandin.

[EvGr] The prostaglandin misoprostol p. 873 is given by mouth, buccally, sublingually, or vaginally, to induce medical abortion following sequential use with mifepristone; it is also used for cervical priming before surgical abortion. [A]

Gemeprost p. 873, a prostaglandin administered vaginally as pessaries, is licensed for the medical induction of abortion in the second trimester of pregnancy; it is also licensed to soften and dilate the cervix before surgical abortion in early pregnancy.

Induction and augmentation of labour

Dinoprostone p. 869 is available as vaginal tablets and vaginal gels for the induction of labour.

Oxytocin is licensed for induction or augmentation of labour, usually in conjunction with amniotomy; it is administered by slow intravenous infusion, using an infusion pump. Uterine activity must be monitored carefully and hyperstimulation avoided. Large doses of oxytocin may result in excessive fluid retention.

[EvGr] Mifepristone and misoprostol [unlicensed indication] can be given for the induction of labour in women who have intra-uterine fetal death. [A]

Prevention and treatment of haemorrhage

[EvGr] Active management of the third stage of labour reduces the risk of postpartum haemorrhage. Prophylactic oxytocin is given by intramuscular injection [unlicensed] on delivery of the anterior shoulder or, at the latest, immediately after the baby is delivered. Alternatively, ergometrine with oxytocin p. 870 can be given by intramuscular injection in the absence of hypertension; [A] oxytocin alone causes less nausea, vomiting, and hypertension than when given with ergometrine maleate.

[EvGr] Oxytocic drugs are used to treat postpartum haemorrhage caused by uterine atony; treatment options include oxytocin, ergometrine maleate, or a combination of ergometrine with oxytocin p. 870. Carboprost p. 871 and misoprostol [unlicensed] are alternative options. [A]

Ectopic pregnancy

[EvGr] Systemic methotrexate p. 957 [unlicensed indication] is used for the management of ectopic pregnancy. [A]

Myometrial relaxants

Tocolytic drugs postpone premature labour and they are used with the aim of reducing harm to the child. The greatest benefit is gained by using the delay to administer corticosteroid therapy or to implement other measures which improve perinatal health (including transfer to a unit with neonatal intensive care facility).

[EvGr] Women between 24 and 33 weeks of gestation who have intact membranes and are in suspected or diagnosed premature labour can be given nifedipine p. 176 [unlicensed indication] for tocolysis. An oxytocin receptor antagonist (such as atosiban p. 871) is an alternative if nifedipine is contra-indicated or unsuitable.

The beta₂ agonists salbutamol p. 269 and terbutaline sulfate p. 271 are no longer recommended for inhibiting uncomplicated premature labour. [A] Use of high-dose short acting beta₂ agonists in obstetric indications has been associated with serious, sometimes fatal cardiovascular events in the mother and fetus, particularly when used for a prolonged period of time.

Useful resources

Abortion care. National Institute for Health and Care Excellence. NICE guideline 140. September 2019.
www.nice.org.uk/guidance/ng140

Intrapartum care for healthy women and babies. National Institute for Health and Care Excellence. Clinical guideline 190. December 2014 (updated February 2017).
www.nice.org.uk/guidance/cg190

Inducing labour. National Institute for Health and Care Excellence. Clinical guideline 70. July 2008.
www.nice.org.uk/guidance/CG70

Preterm labour and birth. National Institute for Health and Care Excellence. NICE guideline 25. November 2015 (updated August 2019).
www.nice.org.uk/guidance/ng25

5.1 Induction of labour

> **Other drugs used for Induction of labour** Misoprostol, p. 873

OXYTOCIN AND ANALOGUES

Oxytocin

11-Oct-2020

- INDICATIONS AND DOSE

Induction of labour for medical reasons | Stimulation of labour in hypotonic uterine inertia
▸ BY INTRAVENOUS INFUSION
▸ Adult: Initially 0.001–0.004 unit/minute, not to be started for at least 6 hours after administration of vaginal prostaglandin, dose increased at intervals of at least 30 minutes until a maximum of 3–4 contractions occur every 10 minutes (0.01 units/minute is often adequate) up to max. 0.02 units/minute, if regular contractions not established after a total 5 units, stop induction attempt (may be repeated next day starting again at 0.001–0.004 units/minute)

Caesarean section
▸ BY SLOW INTRAVENOUS INJECTION
▸ Adult: 5 units immediately after delivery

Prevention of postpartum haemorrhage after delivery of placenta
▸ BY SLOW INTRAVENOUS INJECTION
▸ Adult: 5 units, if infusion previously used for induction or enhancement of labour, increase rate during third stage and for next few hours
▸ BY INTRAMUSCULAR INJECTION
▸ Adult: 10 units, can be used instead of oxytocin with ergometrine (*Syntometrine ®*).

Treatment of postpartum haemorrhage
▸ BY SLOW INTRAVENOUS INJECTION
▸ Adult: 5 units, repeated if necessary

Treatment of severe cases of postpartum haemorrhage (following intravenous injection)
▸ BY INTRAVENOUS INFUSION
▸ Adult: 40 units, given in 500 mL infusion fluid given at a rate sufficient to control uterine atony

Incomplete, inevitable, or missed miscarriage
▸ INITIALLY BY SLOW INTRAVENOUS INJECTION
▸ Adult: 5 units, followed by (by intravenous infusion) 0.02–0.04 unit/minute if required, the rate of infusion can be faster if necessary

● UNLICENSED USE Oxytocin doses in the BNF may differ from those in the product literature. Administration by intramuscular injection is an unlicensed use.

┌───┐
IMPORTANT SAFETY INFORMATION
Prolonged intravenous administration at high doses with large volume of fluid (which is possible in inevitable or missed miscarriage or postpartum haemorrhage) may cause water intoxication with hyponatraemia. To avoid: manufacturer advises use electrolyte-containing diluent (i.e. not glucose), increase oxytocin concentration to reduce fluid, restrict fluid intake by mouth; monitor fluid and electrolytes.
└───┘

● CONTRA-INDICATIONS Any condition where spontaneous labour inadvisable · any condition where vaginal delivery inadvisable · avoid intravenous injection during labour · avoid prolonged administration in oxytocin-resistant uterine inertia · avoid rapid intravenous injection (may transiently reduce blood pressure) · fetal distress (discontinue immediately if this occurs) · hypertonic uterine contractions (discontinue immediately if this occurs) · severe cardiovascular disease · severe pre-eclamptic toxaemia

● CAUTIONS Avoid large infusion volumes and restrict fluid intake by mouth (risk of hyponatraemia and water-intoxication) · enhancement of labour—presence of borderline cephalopelvic disproportion (avoid if significant) · history of lower-uterine segment caesarean section · induction of labour—presence of borderline cephalopelvic disproportion (avoid if significant) · mild pregnancy-induced cardiac disease · mild pregnancy-induced hypertension · moderate pregnancy-induced cardiac disease · moderate pregnancy-induced hypertension · risk factors for disseminated intravascular coagulation · secondary uterine inertia · women over 35 years

● SIDE-EFFECTS
▸ **Common or very common** Arrhythmias · headache · nausea · vomiting
▸ **Rare or very rare** Dyspnoea · hypotension · rash
▸ **Frequency not known** Angioedema · disseminated intravascular coagulation · electrolyte imbalance · flushing · haemorrhage · myocardial ischaemia · pulmonary oedema · QT interval prolongation · uterine rupture · water intoxication

SIDE-EFFECTS, FURTHER INFORMATION Avoid rapid intravenous injection (may transiently reduce blood pressure).
 Uterine hyperstimulation -usually with excessive doses—may cause fetal distress, asphyxia, and death, or may lead to hypertonicity, tetanic contractions, soft-tissue damage or uterine rupture.
Overdose Placental abruption and amniotic fluid embolism reported on overdose.

● MONITORING REQUIREMENTS
▸ Careful monitoring of fetal heart rate and uterine motility essential for dose titration.
▸ Monitor for disseminated intravascular coagulation after parturition.

● DIRECTIONS FOR ADMINISTRATION For *intravenous infusion* (*Syntocinon ®*), manufacturer advises give continuously in Glucose 5% *or* Sodium chloride 0.9%. Preferably given *via* a variable-speed infusion pump in a concentration appropriate to the pump; if given by drip infusion for *induction* or *enhancement of labour*, dilute 5 units in 500 mL infusion fluid or for higher doses, 10 units in 500 mL. EvGr For *treatment of postpartum uterine haemorrhage* dilute 40 units in 500 mL infusion fluid. ⚠ If high doses given for prolonged period (e.g. for inevitable or missed abortion or for postpartum haemorrhage), manufacturer advises use low volume of an electrolyte-containing infusion fluid (not Glucose 5%) given at higher concentration than for induction or enhancement of labour; close attention to patient's fluid and electrolyte status essential.

● MEDICINAL FORMS There can be variation in the licensing of different medicines containing the same drug. Forms available from special-order manufacturers include: infusion, solution for infusion

Solution for injection
▸ Oxytocin (Non-proprietary)
 Oxytocin 5 unit per 1 ml Oxytocin 5units/1ml solution for injection ampoules | 10 ampoule [PoM] £8.03
 Oxytocin 10 unit per 1 ml Oxytocin 10units/1ml solution for infusion ampoules | 5 ampoule [PoM] £15.00 | 10 ampoule [PoM] £20.00
 Oxytocin 10units/1ml concentrate for solution for infusion ampoules | 5 ampoule [PoM] £4.55 | 10 ampoule [PoM] £9.00
 Oxytocin 10units/1ml solution for injection ampoules | 5 ampoule [PoM] [S] (Hospital only)
▸ Syntocinon (Mylan)
 Oxytocin 5 unit per 1 ml Syntocinon 5units/1ml solution for injection ampoules | 5 ampoule [PoM] £4.01 (Hospital only)
 Oxytocin 10 unit per 1 ml Syntocinon 10units/1ml solution for injection ampoules | 5 ampoule [PoM] £4.53 (Hospital only)

PROSTAGLANDINS AND ANALOGUES

┃ **Dinoprostone**   20-Apr-2020

● INDICATIONS AND DOSE
PROPESS ®
Cervical ripening and induction of labour at term
▸ BY VAGINA
▸ Adult: 1 pessary, insert pessary (in retrieval device) high into posterior fornix and remove when cervical ripening adequate; if oxytocin necessary, remove 30 minutes before oxytocin infusion; remove if cervical ripening inadequate after 24 hours (dose not to be repeated)

PROSTIN E2 ® VAGINAL GEL
Induction of labour
▸ BY VAGINA
▸ Adult: 1 mg, inserted high into the posterior fornix (avoid administration into the cervical canal), followed by 1–2 mg after 6 hours if required; maximum 3 mg per course continued →

7

Genito-urinary system

Induction of labour (unfavourable primigravida)

▸ BY VAGINA

▸ Adult: 2 mg, inserted high into the posterior fornix (avoid administration into the cervical canal), followed by 1–2 mg if required, after 6 hours; maximum 4 mg per course

PROSTIN E2 ® VAGINAL TABLETS

Induction of labour

▸ BY VAGINA

▸ Adult: 3 mg, inserted high into the posterior fornix, followed by 3 mg after 6–8 hours, to be given if labour not established; maximum 6 mg per course

DOSE EQUIVALENCE AND CONVERSION

▸ *Prostin E2 Vaginal tablets* and *Vaginal Gel* are not bioequivalent.

● CONTRA-INDICATIONS Active cardiac disease · active pulmonary disease · avoid extra-amniotic route in cervicitis or vaginitis · fetal distress · fetal malpresentation · grand multiparas · history of caesarean section · history of difficult or traumatic delivery · history of major uterine surgery · major cephalopelvic disproportion · multiple pregnancy · placenta praevia or unexplained vaginal bleeding during pregnancy · ruptured membranes · untreated pelvic infection

● CAUTIONS Effect of oxytocin enhanced · history of asthma · history of epilepsy · history of glaucoma and raised intra-ocular pressure · hypertension · risk factors for disseminated intravascular coagulation · uterine rupture · uterine scarring

● SIDE-EFFECTS

▸ **Uncommon** Amniotic cavity infection · febrile disorders · headache · hyperbilirubinaemia neonatal · hypotension · pruritus · uterine atony · vaginal burning

▸ **Frequency not known** Abdominal pain · diarrhoea · disseminated intravascular coagulation · genital oedema · nausea · uterine rupture · vomiting

● HEPATIC IMPAIRMENT Manufacturer advises avoid.

● RENAL IMPAIRMENT Manufacturers advise avoid.

● MONITORING REQUIREMENTS

▸ Monitor for disseminated intravascular coagulation after parturition.

▸ Monitor uterine activity and fetal status (particular care if history of uterine hypertony).

▸ Care needed in monitoring uterine activity when used in sequence following oxytocin.

● PRESCRIBING AND DISPENSING INFORMATION **Important:** Do not confuse dose of *Prostin E2* ®**vaginal gel** with that of *Prostin E2* ®**vaginal tablets**—not bioequivalent.

● MEDICINAL FORMS There can be variation in the licensing of different medicines containing the same drug.

Pessary

▸ Prostin E2 (Pfizer Ltd)

Dinoprostone 3 mg Prostin E2 3mg vaginal tablets | 8 pessary PoM £106.23 (Hospital only)

Vaginal gel

▸ Prostin E2 (Pfizer Ltd)

Dinoprostone 400 microgram per 1 ml Prostin E2 1mg vaginal gel | 2.5 ml PoM £13.28 (Hospital only)

Dinoprostone 800 microgram per 1 ml Prostin E2 2mg vaginal gel | 2.5 ml PoM £13.28 (Hospital only)

Vaginal device

▸ Propess (Ferring Pharmaceuticals Ltd)

Dinoprostone 10 mg Propess 10mg vaginal delivery system | 5 device PoM £165.00

5.2 Postpartum haemorrhage

Other drugs used for Postpartum haemorrhage Oxytocin, p. 868

ERGOT ALKALOIDS

Ergometrine maleate

20-Apr-2020

● **INDICATIONS AND DOSE**

Postpartum haemorrhage caused by uterine atony

▸ BY INTRAMUSCULAR INJECTION, OR BY SLOW INTRAVENOUS INJECTION

▸ Adult: 250–500 micrograms

● CONTRA-INDICATIONS Eclampsia · first stage of labour · induction of labour · second stage of labour · sepsis · severe cardiac disease · severe hypertension · vascular disease

● CAUTIONS Acute porphyrias p. 1107 · cardiac disease · hypertension · multiple pregnancy · risk of hypertension associated with intravenous administration

● INTERACTIONS → Appendix 1: ergometrine

● SIDE-EFFECTS Abdominal pain · arrhythmias · chest pain · coronary vasospasm · dizziness · dyspnoea · headache · hypertension · myocardial infarction · nausea · palpitations · pulmonary oedema · rash · tinnitus · vasoconstriction · vomiting

● HEPATIC IMPAIRMENT Manufacturer advises caution in mild to moderate impairment; avoid in severe impairment.

● RENAL IMPAIRMENT Manufacturer advises caution in mild or moderate impairment. Manufacturer advises avoid in severe impairment.

● MEDICINAL FORMS There can be variation in the licensing of different medicines containing the same drug.

Solution for injection

▸ Ergometrine maleate (Non-proprietary)

Ergometrine maleate 500 microgram per 1 ml Ergometrine 500micrograms/1ml solution for injection ampoules | 10 ampoule PoM £15.00

Ergometrine with oxytocin

22-Apr-2020

The properties listed below are those particular to the combination only. For the properties of the components please consider, ergometrine maleate above, oxytocin p. 868.

● **INDICATIONS AND DOSE**

Active management of the third stage of labour | Postpartum haemorrhage caused by uterine atony

▸ BY INTRAMUSCULAR INJECTION

▸ Adult: 1 mL for one dose

▸ BY INTRAVENOUS INJECTION

▸ Adult: No longer recommended

Bleeding due to incomplete miscarriage or abortion

▸ BY INTRAMUSCULAR INJECTION

▸ Adult: Adjusted according to response to, the patient's condition and blood loss

● INTERACTIONS → Appendix 1: ergometrine

● MEDICINAL FORMS There can be variation in the licensing of different medicines containing the same drug.

Solution for injection

▸ Syntometrine (Alliance Pharmaceuticals Ltd)

Ergometrine maleate 500 microgram per 1 ml, Oxytocin 5 unit per 1 ml Syntometrine 500micrograms/1ml solution for injection ampoules | 5 ampoule PoM £7.87

OXYTOCIN AND ANALOGUES

Carbetocin

26-Aug-2020

- **INDICATIONS AND DOSE**

Prevention of uterine atony after caesarean section
▶ BY SLOW INTRAVENOUS INJECTION
▶ Adult: 100 micrograms for 1 dose, to be given over
  1 minute, administer as soon as possible after delivery,
  preferably before removal of placenta

- CONTRA-INDICATIONS Eclampsia · epilepsy · pre-eclampsia
- CAUTIONS Asthma · cardiovascular disease (avoid if
  severe) · hyponatraemia · migraine
- SIDE-EFFECTS
▶ **Common or very common** Chest pain · chills · dizziness ·
  dyspnoea · feeling hot · flushing · headache · hypotension ·
  nausea · pain · pruritus · taste metallic · tremor · vomiting
▶ **Frequency not known** Hyperhidrosis · tachycardia
- HEPATIC IMPAIRMENT Manufacturer advises avoid in
  hepatic disease.
- RENAL IMPAIRMENT Manufacturer advises avoid.
- NATIONAL FUNDING/ACCESS DECISIONS
  For full details see funding body website
  Scottish Medicines Consortium (SMC) decisions
▶ Carbetocin (*Pabal*®) for the prevention of uterine atony
  following delivery of the infant by Caesarean section under
  epidural or spinal anaesthesia (January 2018) SMC No. 309/06
  Not recommended
- MEDICINAL FORMS There can be variation in the licensing of
  different medicines containing the same drug.
  Solution for injection
▶ Pabal (Ferring Pharmaceuticals Ltd)
  Carbetocin 100 microgram per 1 ml Pabal 100micrograms/1ml
  solution for injection vials | 5 vial [PoM] £88.20 (Hospital only)

PROSTAGLANDINS AND ANALOGUES

Carboprost

20-Apr-2020

- **INDICATIONS AND DOSE**

**Postpartum haemorrhage due to uterine atony in patients
unresponsive to ergometrine and oxytocin**
▶ BY DEEP INTRAMUSCULAR INJECTION
▶ Adult: 250 micrograms, repeated if necessary, to be
  given at intervals of not less than 15 minutes. Total
  dose should not exceed 2 mg (8 doses)

- CONTRA-INDICATIONS Cardiac disease · pulmonary disease
  · untreated pelvic infection
- CAUTIONS Excessive dosage may cause uterine rupture ·
  history of anaemia · history of asthma · history of diabetes ·
  history of epilepsy · history of glaucoma · history of
  hypertension · history of hypotension · history of jaundice ·
  history of raised intra-ocular pressure · uterine scars
- SIDE-EFFECTS
▶ **Common or very common** Chills · cough · diarrhoea ·
  headache · nausea · uterine disorders · vasodilation ·
  vomiting
▶ **Uncommon** Abdominal pain upper · asthma · back pain ·
  breast tenderness · chest discomfort · dizziness ·
  drowsiness · dry mouth · dyspnoea · eye pain · haemorrhage
  · hiccups · hyperhidrosis · hypertension · increased risk of
  infection · movement disorders · muscle complaints ·
  paraesthesia · pelvic pain · respiratory disorders · septic
  shock · sleep disorder · syncope · tachycardia · taste altered
  · tinnitus · uterine injuries · vertigo · vision blurred
▶ **Frequency not known** Anxiety · asthenia · blepharospasm ·
  choking sensation · palpitations · rash · thirst · throat
  complaints · thyrotoxic crisis

- HEPATIC IMPAIRMENT Manufacturer advises avoid in
  active hepatic disease.
- RENAL IMPAIRMENT Manufacturer advises avoid.
- MEDICINAL FORMS There can be variation in the licensing of
  different medicines containing the same drug.
  Solution for injection
▶ Hemabate (Pfizer Ltd)
  Carboprost (as Carboprost trometamol) 250 microgram per
  1 ml Hemabate 250micrograms/1ml solution for injection ampoules
  | 10 ampoule [PoM] £182.01 (Hospital only)

5.3 Premature labour

Other drugs used for Premature labour Indometacin,
p. 1189 · Nifedipine, p. 176 · Salbutamol, p. 269 · Terbutaline
sulfate, p. 271

OXYTOCIN RECEPTOR ANTAGONISTS

Atosiban

23-Nov-2020

- **INDICATIONS AND DOSE**

**Uncomplicated premature labour between 24 and
33 weeks of gestation**
▶ INITIALLY BY INTRAVENOUS INJECTION
▶ Adult: Initially 6.75 mg over 1 minute, then (by
  intravenous infusion) 18 mg/hour for 3 hours, then (by
  intravenous infusion) reduced to 6 mg/hour for up to
  45 hours. Maximum duration of treatment is 48 hours

- CONTRA-INDICATIONS Abnormal fetal heart rate · abruptio
  placenta · antepartum haemorrhage (requiring immediate
  delivery) · eclampsia · intra-uterine fetal death · intra-
  uterine infection · placenta praevia · premature rupture of
  membranes after 30 weeks' gestation · severe pre-
  eclampsia
- CAUTIONS Intra-uterine growth restriction
- SIDE-EFFECTS
▶ **Common or very common** Dizziness · headache · hot flush ·
  hyperglycaemia · hypotension · nausea · tachycardia ·
  vomiting
▶ **Uncommon** Fever · insomnia · skin reactions
▶ **Rare or very rare** Uterine atony · uterine haemorrhage
▶ **Frequency not known** Dyspnoea · pulmonary oedema
- HEPATIC IMPAIRMENT Manufacturer advises caution—no
  information available.
- RENAL IMPAIRMENT No information available.
- MONITORING REQUIREMENTS Monitor blood loss after
  delivery.
- DIRECTIONS FOR ADMINISTRATION For *intravenous infusion*
  (*Tractocile*® concentrate for intravenous infusion),
  manufacturer advises give continuously *in* Glucose 5% *or*
  Sodium chloride 0.9%. Withdraw 10 mL infusion fluid from
  100-mL bag and replace with 10 mL atosiban concentrate
  (7.5 mg/mL) to produce a final concentration of
  750 micrograms/mL.

- MEDICINAL FORMS There can be variation in the licensing of
  different medicines containing the same drug.
  Solution for injection
▶ Atosiban (Non-proprietary)
  Atosiban (as Atosiban acetate) 7.5 mg per 1 ml Atosiban
  6.75mg/0.9ml solution for injection pre-filled syringes | 1 pre-filled
  disposable injection [PoM] £18.41 (Hospital only)
▶ Tractocile (Ferring Pharmaceuticals Ltd)
  Atosiban (as Atosiban acetate) 7.5 mg per 1 ml Tractocile
  6.75mg/0.9ml solution for injection vials | 1 vial [PoM] £18.41
  (Hospital only)

Solution for infusion

▶ Atosiban (Non-proprietary)

Atosiban (as Atosiban acetate) 7.5 mg per 1 ml Atosiban 37.5mg/5ml concentrate for solution for infusion vials | 1 vial [PoM] £50.18–£52.82 (Hospital only)

Atosiban 6.75mg/0.9ml solution for injection ampoules | 1 ampoule [PoM] £17.99 (Hospital only)

▶ Tractocile (Ferring Pharmaceuticals Ltd)

Atosiban (as Atosiban acetate) 7.5 mg per 1 ml Tractocile 37.5mg/5ml solution for infusion vials | 1 vial [PoM] £52.82 (Hospital only)

5.4 Termination of pregnancy

PROGESTERONE RECEPTOR MODULATORS

Mifepristone

● DRUG ACTION Mifepristone, an antiprogestogenic steroid, sensitises the myometrium to prostaglandin-induced contractions and ripens the cervix.

● INDICATIONS AND DOSE

Cervical ripening before mechanical cervical dilatation for termination of pregnancy of up to 84 days gestation (under close medical supervision)

▶ BY MOUTH

▶ Adult: 200 mg for 1 dose, to be taken 36-48 hours before procedure

Labour induction in fetal death in utero where prostaglandin or oxytocin inappropriate (under close medical supervision)

▶ BY MOUTH

▶ Adult: 600 mg once daily for 2 days, if labour not started within 72 hours of first dose, another method should be used

Medical termination of intra-uterine pregnancy of up to 49 days gestation (under close medical supervision)

▶ BY MOUTH

▶ Adult: 600 mg for 1 dose, dose followed 36–48 hours later (unless abortion already complete) by gemeprost 1 mg by vagina or misoprostol 400 micrograms by mouth, alternatively 200 mg for 1 dose, dose followed 36–48 hours later (unless abortion already complete) by gemeprost 1 mg by vagina; observe for at least 3 hours (or until bleeding or pain at acceptable level); follow-up visit within 2 weeks to verify complete expulsion and to assess vaginal bleeding

Medical termination of intra-uterine pregnancy of 50–63 days gestation (under close medical supervision)

▶ BY MOUTH

▶ Adult: 600 mg for 1 dose, alternatively 200 mg for 1 dose, dose followed 36–48 hours later (unless abortion already complete) by gemeprost 1 mg by vagina; observe for at least 3 hours (or until bleeding or pain at acceptable level); follow-up visit within 2 weeks to verify complete expulsion and to assess vaginal bleeding

Termination of pregnancy of 13–24 weeks gestation (in combination with a prostaglandin) (under close medical supervision)

▶ BY MOUTH

▶ Adult: 600 mg for 1 dose, alternatively 200 mg for 1 dose, dose followed 36–48 hours later by gemeprost 1 mg by vagina every 3 hours up to max. 5 mg or misoprostol; if abortion does not occur, 24 hours after start of treatment repeat course of gemeprost 1 mg by vagina up to max. 5 mg; follow-up visit after appropriate interval to assess vaginal bleeding recommended

● CONTRA-INDICATIONS Acute porphyrias p. 1107 · chronic adrenal failure · suspected ectopic pregnancy (use other specific means of termination) · uncontrolled severe asthma

● CAUTIONS Adrenal suppression (may require corticosteroid) · anticoagulant therapy · asthma (avoid if severe and uncontrolled) · existing cardiovascular disease · haemorrhagic disorders · history of endocarditis · prosthetic heart valve · risk factors for cardiovascular disease

● INTERACTIONS → Appendix 1: mifepristone

● SIDE-EFFECTS

▶ **Common or very common** Abdominal cramps · diarrhoea · infection · nausea · pelvic inflammatory disease · uterine disorders · vaginal haemorrhage (sometimes severe) · vomiting

▶ **Uncommon** Hypotension

▶ **Rare or very rare** Angioedema · chills · dizziness · erythema nodosum · fever · headache · hot flush · malaise · skin reactions · toxic epidermal necrolysis · toxic shock syndrome · uterine rupture

● HEPATIC IMPAIRMENT Manufacturer advises avoid in hepatic failure (no information available).

● RENAL IMPAIRMENT Manufacturer advises avoid.

● MONITORING REQUIREMENTS Careful monitoring of blood pressure and pulse essential for 3 hours after administration of gemeprost pessary (risk of profound hypotension).

● PRESCRIBING AND DISPENSING INFORMATION Supplied to NHS hospitals and premises approved under Abortion Act 1967.

● PATIENT AND CARER ADVICE Patient information leaflet to be provided.

● MEDICINAL FORMS There can be variation in the licensing of different medicines containing the same drug.

Tablet

CAUTIONARY AND ADVISORY LABELS 10

▶ Mifepristone (Non-proprietary)

Mifepristone 200 mg Mifepristone 200mg tablets | 1 tablet [PoM] £10.14

▶ Mifegyne (Nordic Pharma Ltd)

Mifepristone 200 mg Mifegyne 200mg tablets | 3 tablet [PoM] £52.66 (Hospital only)

Mifepristone and misoprostol   02-Jun-2020

The properties listed below are those particular to the combination only. For the properties of the components please consider, misoprostol p. 873, mifepristone above.

● INDICATIONS AND DOSE

Medical termination of intra-uterine pregnancy of up to 63 days gestation (under close medical supervision)

▶ BY MOUTH, OR BY VAGINA

▶ Adult: (consult product literature)

● INTERACTIONS → Appendix 1: mifepristone

● SIDE-EFFECTS

▶ **Common or very common** Diarrhoea · gastrointestinal discomfort · haemorrhage · nausea · uterine disorders · vomiting

▶ **Uncommon** Infection · skin reactions

▶ **Rare or very rare** Chills · dizziness · erythema nodosum · fever · headache · hot flush · hypotension · malaise · toxic epidermal necrolysis · uterine rupture

▶ **Frequency not known** Pelvic inflammatory disease · toxic shock syndrome

● PATIENT AND CARER ADVICE Patient information leaflet to be provided.

● MEDICINAL FORMS There can be variation in the licensing of different medicines containing the same drug.

Tablet
▸ Medabon Combipack (Sun Pharmaceutical Industries Europe B.V.)
Medabon Combipack tablets | 1 pack PoM £17.00 (Hospital only)

PROSTAGLANDINS AND ANALOGUES

Gemeprost

20-Apr-2020

● **INDICATIONS AND DOSE**

Cervical ripening prior to first trimester surgical abortion
▸ BY VAGINA
▸ Adult: 1 mg, dose to be inserted into posterior fornix 3 hours before surgery

Second trimester abortion
▸ BY VAGINA
▸ Adult: 1 mg every 3 hours for maximum 5 administrations, to be inserted into posterior fornix, second course may begin 24 hours after start of treatment (if treatment fails, pregnancy should be terminated by another method)

Second trimester intra-uterine death
▸ BY VAGINA
▸ Adult: 1 mg every 3 hours for maximum 5 administrations only, to be inserted into posterior fornix

Medical termination of intra-uterine pregnancy of up to 49 days gestation following mifepristone | Medical termination of intra-uterine pregnancy of 50–63 days gestation following mifepristone
▸ BY VAGINA
▸ Adult: 1 mg

Termination of pregnancy of 13–24 weeks gestation (in combination with a prostaglandin) following mifepristone
▸ BY VAGINA
▸ Adult: 1 mg every 3 hours, if abortion does not occur, 24 hours after start of treatment repeat course of gemeprost 1 mg by vagina up to max. 5 mg; follow-up visit after appropriate interval to assess vaginal bleeding recommended, careful monitoring of blood pressure and pulse essential for 3 hours after administration of gemeprost pessary (risk of profound hypotension); maximum 5 mg per course

● CONTRA-INDICATIONS Placenta praevia · unexplained vaginal bleeding · uterine scarring

● CAUTIONS Cardiovascular insufficiency · cervicitis · obstructive airways disease · raised intra-ocular pressure · vaginitis

● SIDE-EFFECTS Back pain · chest pain · chills · coronary vasospasm · diarrhoea · dizziness · dyspnoea · fever · flushing · headache · hypotension · muscle weakness · myocardial infarction · nausea · palpitations · uterine pain · uterine rupture · vaginal haemorrhage · vomiting

● RENAL IMPAIRMENT Manufacturer advises avoid.

● MONITORING REQUIREMENTS
▸ If used in combination with mifepristone, carefully monitor blood pressure and pulse for 3 hours.
▸ When used for second trimester intra-uterine death, monitor for coagulopathy during treatment.

● MEDICINAL FORMS There can be variation in the licensing of different medicines containing the same drug.

Pessary
▸ Cervagem (Sanofi)
Gemeprost 1 mg Cervagem 1mg pessaries | 5 pessary PoM ⚠
(Hospital only)

Misoprostol

20-Apr-2020

● DRUG ACTION Misoprostol is a synthetic prostaglandin analogue that acts as a potent uterine stimulant.

● **INDICATIONS AND DOSE**

Termination of pregnancy following mifepristone (gestation up to 49 days)
▸ BY MOUTH
▸ Adult: 400 micrograms for 1 dose, dose to be given 24–48 hours after mifepristone

Termination of pregnancy following mifepristone (gestation 50 to 63 days)
▸ INITIALLY BY VAGINA, OR BY BUCCAL ADMINISTRATION, OR BY SUBLINGUAL ADMINISTRATION
▸ Adult: 800 micrograms for 1 dose, dose to be given 24–48 hours after mifepristone, if abortion has not occurred 4 hours after first misoprostol dose a further dose may be given, (by mouth or by vagina) 400 micrograms for 1 dose

Termination of pregnancy following mifepristone (gestation of 9 to 13 weeks)
▸ INITIALLY BY VAGINA
▸ Adult: 800 micrograms for 1 dose, dose to be given 36–48 hours after mifepristone, followed by (by vagina or by mouth) 400 micrograms every 3 hours if required for a maximum of 4 doses

Termination of pregnancy following mifepristone (gestation of 13 to 24 weeks)
▸ INITIALLY BY VAGINA
▸ Adult: 800 micrograms for 1 dose, dose to be given 36–48 hours after mifepristone, followed by (by vagina or by mouth) 400 micrograms every 3 hours if required for a maximum of 4 doses, if abortion has not occurred 3 hours after the last dose of misoprostol, a further dose of mifepristone may be given, and misoprostol may be recommenced 12 hours later

MYSODELLE ® VAGINAL DELIVERY SYSTEM

Induction of labour (specialist supervision in hospital)
▸ BY VAGINA
▸ Adult: 200 micrograms for 1 dose, to be inserted (in vaginal delivery system) high into posterior fornix; if oxytocin required, remove at least 30 minutes before oxytocin administration, for information on when to remove the delivery system—consult product literature

● UNLICENSED USE Misoprostol doses for termination of pregnancy may differ from those in product literature.

> **IMPORTANT SAFETY INFORMATION**
>
> MHRA/CHM ADVICE: MISOPROSTOL VAGINAL DELIVERY SYSTEM (MYSODELLE ®): REPORTS OF EXCESSIVE UTERINE CONTRACTIONS (TACHYSYSTOLE) UNRESPONSIVE TO TOCOLYTIC TREATMENT (FEBRUARY 2018)
> Mysodelle ® can cause excessive uterine tachysystole that may not respond to tocolytic treatment. Monitor patients closely and remove the vaginal delivery system immediately in cases of excessive or prolonged uterine contractions, at the onset of labour, or if there is clinical concern for mother or baby.
>   Be prepared to administer tocolytic therapy—if needed, it can be administered immediately after removal of Mysodelle ®.

● CONTRA-INDICATIONS
MYSODELLE ® VAGINAL DELIVERY SYSTEM Before 36 weeks' gestation · chorioamnionitis (unless adequate prior treatment initiated) · fetal malpresentation · placenta praevia · suspicion or evidence of fetal compromise · unexplained vaginal bleeding after 24 weeks gestation · uterine abnormality · uterine scar

Genito-urinary system

7

- CAUTIONS
  ▸ When used for termination of pregnancy Cardiovascular disease · risk factors for cardiovascular disease

  MYSODELLE ® VAGINAL DELIVERY SYSTEM Modified Bishop score greater than 4

- SIDE-EFFECTS
  ▸ **Common or very common** Nausea · neonatal respiratory depression · rash · transient tachypnoea of the newborn · vomiting
  ▸ **Uncommon** Genital pruritus · hypoxic-ischaemic encephalopathy · uterine rupture

- BREAST FEEDING Manufacturer advises avoid—present in milk, and may cause diarrhoea in nursing infants. EvGr Tertiary sources state present in milk but amount probably too small to be harmful; to further reduce risk following termination of pregnancy, consider interrupting breastfeeding for 5 hours after a dose. ◑

- HANDLING AND STORAGE
  MYSODELLE ® VAGINAL DELIVERY SYSTEM Manufacturer advises store in a freezer (-10 to -25°C); no thawing required prior to use.

- PATIENT AND CARER ADVICE
  Driving and skilled tasks Manufacturer advises patients should be cautioned on the effects on driving and performance of skilled tasks—increased risk of dizziness.

- MEDICINAL FORMS There can be variation in the licensing of different medicines containing the same drug.
  Vaginal delivery system
  ▸ Mysodelle (Ferring Pharmaceuticals Ltd)
  Misoprostol 7 microgram per 1 hour Mysodelle 200micrograms vaginal delivery system | 5 unit PoM £465.00

  Tablet
  CAUTIONARY AND ADVISORY LABELS 21
  ▸ Misoprostol (Non-proprietary)
  Misoprostol 200 microgram Misoprostol 200microgram vaginal tablets | 4 tablet PoM ⚠ (Hospital only)
  ▸ Topogyne (Nordic Pharma Ltd)
  Misoprostol 400 microgram Topogyne 400microgram tablets | 1 tablet PoM £9.00 (Hospital only) | 16 tablet £128.00 (Hospital only)

  Combinations available: *Mifepristone and misoprostol*, p. 872

6 Vaginal and vulval conditions

Vaginal and vulval conditions

Management

Symptoms are often restricted to the vulva, but infections almost invariably involve the vagina which should also be treated. Applications to the vulva alone are likely to give only symptomatic relief without cure.

Aqueous medicated douches may disturb normal vaginal acidity and bacterial flora.

Topical anaesthetic agents give only symptomatic relief and may cause sensitivity reactions. They are indicated only in cases of pruritus where specific local causes have been excluded.

Systemic drugs are required in the treatment of infections such as gonorrhoea and syphilis.

Vaginal and vulval changes

Topical HRT for vaginal atrophy

A cream containing an oestrogen may be applied on a short-term basis to improve the vaginal epithelium in *menopausal atrophic vaginitis*. It is **important** to bear in mind that topical oestrogens should be used in the **smallest effective** amount

to minimise systemic effects. Modified-release vaginal tablets and an impregnated vaginal ring are now also available.

The risk of endometrial hyperplasia and carcinoma is increased when *systemic* oestrogens are administered alone for prolonged periods. The endometrial safety of long-term or repeated use of *topical* vaginal oestrogens is uncertain; treatment should be reviewed at least annually, with special consideration given to any symptoms of endometrial hyperplasia or carcinoma.

Topical oestrogens are also used in postmenopausal women before vaginal surgery for prolapse when there is epithelial atrophy.

Non-hormonal preparations for vaginal atrophy

Several non-hormonal vaginal moisturisers are available and some are prescribable on the NHS (consult Drug Tariff).

Vaginal and vulval infections

Effective specific treatments are available for the common vaginal infections.

Fungal infections

Candidal vulvitis can be treated locally with cream, but is almost invariably associated with vaginal infection which should also be treated. *Vaginal candidiasis* is treated primarily with antifungal pessaries or cream inserted high into the vagina (including during menstruation). Single-dose preparations offer an advantage when compliance is a problem. Local irritation may occur on application of vaginal antifungal products.

Imidazole drugs (clotrimazole p. 876, econazole nitrate p. 876, fenticonazole, and miconazole p. 877) are effective against candida in short courses of 1 to 14 days according to the preparation used; treatment can be repeated if initial course fails to control symptoms or if symptoms recur. Vaginal applications may be supplemented with antifungal cream for vulvitis and to treat other superficial sites of infection.

Oral treatment of vaginal infection with fluconazole p. 634 or itraconazole p. 636 is also effective.

Vulvovaginal candidiasis in pregnancy

Vulvovaginal candidiasis is common during pregnancy and can be treated with vaginal application of an imidazole (such as clotrimazole), and a topical imidazole cream for vulvitis. Pregnant women need a longer duration of treatment, usually about 7 days, to clear the infection. Oral antifungal treatment should be avoided during pregnancy.

Recurrent vulvovaginal candidiasis

Recurrence of vulvovaginal candidiasis is particularly likely if there are predisposing factors, such as antibacterial therapy, pregnancy, diabetes mellitus, or possibly oral contraceptive use. Reservoirs of infection may also lead to recontamination and should be treated; these include other skin sites such as the digits, nail beds, and umbilicus as well as the gastro-intestinal tract and the bladder. The partner may also be the source of reinfection and, if symptomatic, should be treated with a topical imidazole cream at the same time.

Treatment against candida may need to be extended for 6 months in recurrent vulvovaginal candidiasis.

Other infections

Trichomonal infections commonly involve the lower urinary tract as well as the genital system and need systemic treatment with metronidazole p. 575 or tinidazole p. 577.

Bacterial infections with Gram-negative organisms are particularly common in association with gynaecological operations and trauma. Metronidazole is effective against certain Gram-negative organisms, especially *Bacteroides* spp. and can be used prophylactically in gynaecological surgery.

Clindamycin cream p. 875 and metronidazole gel are indicated for bacterial vaginosis.

Vaginal preparations intended to restore normal acidity may prevent recurrence of vaginal infections and permit the re-establishment of the normal vaginal flora.

The antiviral drugs aciclovir p. 672, famciclovir p. 674, and valaciclovir p. 675 can be used in the treatment of genital infection due to *herpes simplex virus*, the HSV type 2 being a major cause of genital ulceration; they have a beneficial effect on virus shedding and healing, generally giving relief from pain and other symptoms.

6.1   Vaginal and vulval infections

6.1a   Vaginal and vulval bacterial infections

ANTIBACTERIALS › LINCOSAMIDES

Clindamycin

25-Nov-2020

● **INDICATIONS AND DOSE**

DALACIN ® 2% CREAM

Bacterial vaginosis

▸ BY VAGINA
▸ **Adult:** 1 applicatorful daily for 3–7 nights, dose to be administered at night

DOSE EQUIVALENCE AND CONVERSION

▸ 1 applicatorful delivers a 5 g dose of clindamycin 2%.

● INTERACTIONS → Appendix 1: clindamycin

● SIDE-EFFECTS

▸ **Common or very common** Skin reactions
▸ **Frequency not known** Constipation · diarrhoea (discontinue) · dizziness · gastrointestinal discomfort · headache · increased risk of infection · nausea · vertigo · vomiting · vulvovaginal irritation

SIDE-EFFECTS, FURTHER INFORMATION Clindamycin 2% cream is poorly absorbed into the blood—low risk of systemic effects.

● CONCEPTION AND CONTRACEPTION

DALACIN ® 2% CREAM Damages latex condoms and diaphragms.

● PRESCRIBING AND DISPENSING INFORMATION For choice of antibacterial therapy, see Genital system infections, antibacterial therapy p. 536.

● MEDICINAL FORMS There can be variation in the licensing of different medicines containing the same drug.

Cream

EXCIPIENTS: May contain Benzyl alcohol, cetostearyl alcohol (including cetyl and stearyl alcohol), polysorbates, propylene glycol

▸ Dalacin (Pfizer Ltd)
    Clindamycin (as Clindamycin phosphate) 20 mg per 1 gram Dalacin 2% cream | 40 gram [PoM] £10.86 DT = £10.86

ANTISEPTICS AND DISINFECTANTS

Dequalinium chloride

20-Aug-2020

● DRUG ACTION Dequalinium chloride is a bactericidal anti-infective which causes bacterial cell death by increasing cell permeability and reducing enzyme activity.

● **INDICATIONS AND DOSE**

Bacterial vaginosis

▸ BY VAGINA
▸ **Adult 18–55 years:** 10 mg once daily for 6 days, inserted at night

● CONTRA-INDICATIONS Vaginal ulceration

● SIDE-EFFECTS

▸ **Common or very common** Increased risk of infection · vulvovaginal disorders
▸ **Uncommon** Haemorrhage · headache · nausea
▸ **Frequency not known** Cystitis · fever

● CONCEPTION AND CONTRACEPTION Does not affect efficacy of latex condoms; however, manufacturer advises avoid use of non-latex condoms and intravaginal devices—no information available.

● PREGNANCY Manufacturer advises avoid unless essential—limited information available.

● NATIONAL FUNDING/ACCESS DECISIONS
For full details see funding body website
Scottish Medicines Consortium (SMC) decisions
▸ Dequalinium chloride (*Fluomizin*®) for treatment of bacterial vaginosis (November 2016) SMC No. 1194/16 Recommended with restrictions
All Wales Medicines Strategy Group (AWMSG) decisions
▸ Dequalinium chloride (*Fluomizin*®) for treatment of bacterial vaginosis after initial treatment is ineffective or not tolerated as an alternative option to clindamycin vaginal cream (November 2016) AWMSG No. 2775 Recommended with restrictions

● MEDICINAL FORMS There can be variation in the licensing of different medicines containing the same drug.

Tablet

▸ Fluomizin (KoRa Healthcare)
    Dequalinium chloride 10 mg Fluomizin 10mg vaginal tablets | 6 tablet [PoM] £6.95 DT = £6.95

CARBOXYLIC ACIDS

Lactic acid

24-Nov-2020

● **INDICATIONS AND DOSE**

BALANCE ACTIV RX ® GEL

Prevention of bacterial vaginosis

▸ BY VAGINA
▸ **Adult:** 5 mL 1–2 times a week, insert the content of 1 tube (5 mL)

RELACTAGEL ® GEL

Prevention of bacterial vaginosis

▸ BY VAGINA
▸ **Adult:** 5 mL daily for 2–3 nights after menstruation, insert the contents of one tube

Treatment of bacterial vaginosis

▸ BY VAGINA
▸ **Adult:** 5 mL daily for 7 nights, insert the contents of one tube

● ALLERGY AND CROSS-SENSITIVITY [EvGr] Contra-indicated in shellfish allergy. ⟨M⟩

● CONCEPTION AND CONTRACEPTION

RELACTAGEL ® GEL Not recommended if trying to conceive.

● MEDICINAL FORMS There can be variation in the licensing of different medicines containing the same drug.

Gel

EXCIPIENTS: May contain Propylene glycol

▸ Balance Activ (BBI Healthcare Ltd)
    Balance Activ BV vaginal pH correction gel | 7 device £5.25
▸ Relactagel (KoRa Healthcare)
    Relactagel vaginal pH correction gel | 7 device £5.25

7

Genito-urinary system

6.1b Vaginal and vulval fungal infections

Other drugs used for Vaginal and vulval fungal infections
Fluconazole, p. 634 · Itraconazole, p. 636

ANTIFUNGALS > IMIDAZOLE ANTIFUNGALS

Clotrimazole

10-Mar-2020

● **INDICATIONS AND DOSE**

Superficial sites of infection in vaginal and vulval candidiasis (dose for 1% or 2% cream)
▸ BY VAGINA USING CREAM
▸ Adult: Apply 2–3 times a day, to be applied to anogenital area

Vaginal candidiasis (dose for 10% intravaginal cream)
▸ BY VAGINA USING VAGINAL CREAM
▸ Adult: 5 g for 1 dose, one applicatorful to be inserted into the vagina at night, dose can be repeated once if necessary

Vaginal candidiasis
▸ BY VAGINA USING PESSARIES
▸ Adult: 200 mg for 3 nights, course can be repeated once if necessary, alternatively 100 mg for 6 nights, course can be repeated once if necessary, alternatively 500 mg for 1 night, dose can be repeated once if necessary

Recurrent vulvovaginal candidiasis
▸ BY VAGINA USING PESSARIES
▸ Adult: 500 mg every week for 6 months, dose to be administered following topical imidazole for 10–14 days

● INTERACTIONS → Appendix 1: antifungals, azoles

● SIDE-EFFECTS Abdominal pain · discomfort · genital peeling · oedema · paraesthesia · pelvic pain · skin reactions · vaginal haemorrhage

● CONCEPTION AND CONTRACEPTION Cream and pessaries may damage latex condoms and diaphragms.

● PREGNANCY
Dose adjustments Pregnant women need a longer duration of treatment, usually about 7 days, to clear the infection. Oral antifungal treatment should be avoided during pregnancy.

● EXCEPTIONS TO LEGAL CATEGORY Brands for sale to the public include *Canesten*® Internal Cream.

● MEDICINAL FORMS There can be variation in the licensing of different medicines containing the same drug.
Pessary
EXCIPIENTS: May contain Benzyl alcohol, cetostearyl alcohol (including cetyl and stearyl alcohol), polysorbates
▸ Canesten (clotrimazole) (Bayer Plc)
Clotrimazole 100 mg Canesten 100mg pessaries | 6 pessary P £3.85 DT = £3.85
Clotrimazole 200 mg Canesten 200mg pessaries | 3 pessary P £3.41 DT = £3.41
Clotrimazole 500 mg Canesten 500mg Soft Gel pessaries | 1 pessary P £6.99 DT = £5.48
Canesten Vaginal 500mg pessaries | 1 pessary PoM £2.00 DT = £5.48
Cream
EXCIPIENTS: May contain Benzyl alcohol, cetostearyl alcohol (including cetyl and stearyl alcohol), polysorbates
▸ Clotrimazole (Non-proprietary)
Clotrimazole 10 mg per 1 gram Clotrimazole 1% cream | 20 gram P £1.80 DT = £1.38 | 50 gram P £3.67 DT = £3.45
▸ Canesten (clotrimazole) (Bayer Plc)
Clotrimazole 10 mg per 1 gram Canesten 1% cream | 20 gram P £2.20 DT = £1.38 | 50 gram P £3.64 DT = £3.45
Canesten Antifungal 1% cream | 20 gram P £1.85 DT = £1.38

Clotrimazole 20 mg per 1 gram Canesten 2% thrush cream | 20 gram P £4.76 DT = £4.76
Clotrimazole 100 mg per 1 gram Canesten 10% VC cream | 5 gram PoM £4.50 DT = £6.23

Econazole nitrate

08-May-2020

● **INDICATIONS AND DOSE**

GYNO-PEVARYL® ONCE

Vaginal and vulval candidiasis
▸ BY VAGINA
▸ Adult: 1 pessary for 1 dose, pessary to be inserted at night, dose to be repeated once if necessary

GYNO-PEVARYL® CREAM

Vaginal and vulval candidiasis
▸ INITIALLY BY VAGINA USING VAGINAL CREAM
▸ Adult: 1 applicatorful daily for at least 14 days, dose to be inserted vaginally at night and (to the skin) apply daily for at least 14 days, to be applied to vulva at night, course can be repeated once if necessary

GYNO-PEVARYL® PESSARY

Vaginal and vulval candidiasis
▸ BY VAGINA
▸ Adult: 1 pessary daily for 3 days, pessary to be inserted at night, course can be repeated once if necessary

● SIDE-EFFECTS
GENERAL SIDE-EFFECTS
▸ **Common or very common** Skin reactions
▸ **Uncommon** Vaginal burning
▸ **Frequency not known** Angioedema
SIDE-EFFECTS, FURTHER INFORMATION Treatment should be discontinued if side-effects are severe.

● CONCEPTION AND CONTRACEPTION Cream and pessaries damage latex condoms and diaphragms.

● PREGNANCY Pregnant women need a longer duration of treatment, usually about 7 days, to clear the infection.

● MEDICINAL FORMS There can be variation in the licensing of different medicines containing the same drug.
Pessary
▸ Gyno-Pevaryl (Janssen-Cilag Ltd)
Econazole nitrate 150 mg Gyno-Pevaryl 150mg vaginal pessaries | 3 pessary PoM £4.17 DT = £4.17
Cream
EXCIPIENTS: May contain Butylated hydroxyanisole, fragrances
▸ Gyno-Pevaryl (Janssen-Cilag Ltd)
Econazole nitrate 10 mg per 1 gram Gyno-Pevaryl 1% cream | 30 gram PoM £3.78 DT = £3.78

Ketoconazole

04-Feb-2020

● **INDICATIONS AND DOSE**

Vaginal and vulva candidiasis
▸ BY VAGINA USING CREAM
▸ Adult: Apply 1–2 times a day, to be applied to the anogenital area

● CONTRA-INDICATIONS Acute porphyrias p. 1107

● INTERACTIONS → Appendix 1: antifungals, azoles

● SIDE-EFFECTS
▸ **Common or very common** Skin reactions
▸ **Uncommon** Alopecia · angioedema
▸ **Rare or very rare** Taste altered

● CONCEPTION AND CONTRACEPTION Effect on latex condoms and diaphragms not yet known.

- **MEDICINAL FORMS** There can be variation in the licensing of different medicines containing the same drug.

Cream

EXCIPIENTS: May contain Cetostearyl alcohol (including cetyl and stearyl alcohol), polysorbates, propylene glycol

▸ Nizoral (Janssen-Cilag Ltd)
   Ketoconazole 20 mg per 1 gram Nizoral 2% cream | 30 gram [PoM]
   £4.24 DT = £4.24

Miconazole
24-Jul-2020

- **INDICATIONS AND DOSE**

Vaginal and vulval candidiasis
▸ BY VAGINA USING VAGINAL CREAM
▸ Adult: 1 applicatorful once daily for 7 days, to be inserted into the vagina before bedtime, course can be repeated once if necessary

Superficial sites of infection in vaginal and vulval candidiasis | Vulvitis
▸ BY VAGINA USING VAGINAL CREAM
▸ Adult: Apply twice daily, apply to the anogenital area

- **CAUTIONS** Avoid in Acute porphyrias p. 1107
- **INTERACTIONS** → Appendix 1: antifungals, azoles
- **SIDE-EFFECTS**
▸ **Common or very common** Dysmenorrhoea · skin reactions · vulvovaginal disorders
▸ **Frequency not known** Abdominal pain · angioedema · dysuria · headache · nausea · pelvic cramps · urinary tract infection · vaginal haemorrhage
- **CONCEPTION AND CONTRACEPTION** Gyno-Daktarin® damages latex condoms and diaphragms.
- **PREGNANCY** Pregnant women need a longer duration of treatment, usually about 7 days, to clear the infection.
- **BREAST FEEDING** Manufacturer advises caution—no information available.

- **MEDICINAL FORMS** There can be variation in the licensing of different medicines containing the same drug.

Cream

EXCIPIENTS: May contain Butylated hydroxyanisole
▸ Gyno-Daktarin (Janssen-Cilag Ltd)
   Miconazole nitrate 20 mg per 1 gram Gyno-Daktarin 2% vaginal cream | 78 gram [PoM] £4.33 DT = £4.33

6.2 Vaginal atrophy

OESTROGENS

Estradiol
20-Aug-2020

- **INDICATIONS AND DOSE**

ESTRING®

Postmenopausal urogenital conditions (not suitable for vasomotor symptoms or osteoporosis prophylaxis)
▸ BY VAGINA
▸ Adult: To be inserted into upper third of vagina and worn continuously; replace after 3 months; max. duration of continuous treatment 2 years

VAGIFEM®

Improve the vaginal epithelium in menopausal atrophic vaginitis
▸ BY VAGINA
▸ Adult: 1 tablet daily for 2 weeks, then reduced to 1 tablet twice weekly

- **CONTRA-INDICATIONS** Active arterial thromboembolic disease (e.g. angina or myocardial infarction) · history of breast cancer · history of venous thromboembolism ·

oestrogen-dependent cancer · recent arterial thromboembolic disease (e.g. angina or myocardial infarction) · thrombophilic disorder · undiagnosed vaginal bleeding · untreated endometrial hyperplasia

- **CAUTIONS** Acute porphyrias p. 1107 · diabetes (increased risk of heart disease) · factors predisposing to thromboembolism · history of breast nodules—closely monitor breast status (risk of breast cancer) · history of endometrial hyperplasia · history of fibrocystic disease—closely monitor breast status (risk of breast cancer) · hypophyseal tumours · increased risk of gall-bladder disease · migraine (or migraine-like headaches) · presence of antiphospholipid antibodies (increased risk of thrombotic events) · prolonged exposure to unopposed oestrogens may increase risk of developing endometrial cancer · review treatment at least annually to assess need for continued treatment · risk factors for oestrogen-dependent tumours (e.g. breast cancer in first-degree relative) · symptoms of endometriosis may be exacerbated · uterine fibroids may increase in size

CAUTIONS, FURTHER INFORMATION

▸ Risk of endometrial cancer The increased risk of endometrial cancer depends on the dose and duration of oestrogen-only HRT.
▸ Risk of ovarian cancer Long-term use of combined HRT or oestrogen-only HRT is associated with a small increased risk of ovarian cancer. This excess risk disappears within a few years of stopping.
▸ Risk of venous thromboembolism Women using combined or oestrogen-only HRT are at an increased risk of deep vein thrombosis and of pulmonary embolism especially in the first year of use.

   In women who have predisposing factors (such as a personal or family history of deep vein thrombosis or pulmonary embolism, severe varicose veins, obesity, trauma, or prolonged bed-rest) it is prudent to review the need for HRT, as in some cases the risks of HRT may exceed the benefits.

   Travel involving prolonged immobility further increases the risk of deep vein thrombosis.
▸ Risk of stroke Risk of stroke increases with age, therefore older women have a greater absolute risk of stroke. Combined HRT or oestrogen-only HRT increases the risk of stroke.
▸ Risk of coronary heart disease HRT does not prevent coronary heart disease and should not be prescribed for this purpose. There is an increased risk of coronary heart disease in women who start combined HRT more than 10 years after menopause. Although very little information is available on the risk of coronary heart disease in younger women who start HRT close to the menopause, studies suggest a lower relative risk compared with older women.

- **INTERACTIONS** → Appendix 1: hormone replacement therapy
- **SIDE-EFFECTS**
▸ **Common or very common** Abdominal pain · headaches · nausea · skin reactions · vaginal haemorrhage · vulvovaginal disorders
▸ **Uncommon** Hypertension · vulvovaginal fungal infection · weight increased
▸ **Rare or very rare** Diarrhoea · embolism and thrombosis · endometrial hyperplasia · fluid retention · genital pruritus · increased risk of ischaemic stroke · insomnia · neoplasm malignant · neoplasms · vaginismus
- **CONCEPTION AND CONTRACEPTION** HRT does **not** provide contraception and a woman is considered potentially fertile for 2 years after her last menstrual period if she is under 50 years, and for 1 year if she is over 50 years. A woman who is under 50 years and free of all risk factors for venous and arterial disease can use a low-oestrogen

7

Genito-urinary system

combined oral contraceptive pill to provide both relief of menopausal symptoms and contraception; it is recommended that the oral contraceptive be stopped at 50 years of age since there are more suitable alternatives. If any potentially fertile woman needs HRT, non-hormonal contraceptive measures (such as condoms) are necessary. Measurement of follicle-stimulating hormone can help to determine fertility, but high measurements alone (particularly in women aged under 50 years) do not necessarily preclude the possibility of becoming pregnant.

VAGIFEM ® No evidence of damage to latex condoms and diaphragms.

● PREGNANCY Not known to be harmful.

● BREAST FEEDING Avoid; adverse effects on lactation.

● HEPATIC IMPAIRMENT Manufacturer advises caution; avoid in acute or active disease.

● MONITORING REQUIREMENTS
▶ History of breast nodules or fibrocystic disease—closely monitor breast status (risk of breast cancer).
▶ The endometrial safety of long-term or repeated use of topical vaginal oestrogens is uncertain; treatment should be reviewed at least annually, with special consideration given to any symptoms of endometrial hyperplasia or carcinoma.

● MEDICINAL FORMS There can be variation in the licensing of different medicines containing the same drug.

Pessary
▶ Vagifem (Novo Nordisk Ltd)
Estradiol 10 microgram Vagifem 10microgram vaginal tablets | 24 pessary [PoM] £16.72 DT = £16.72

Vaginal delivery system
CAUTIONARY AND ADVISORY LABELS 10
▶ Estring (Pfizer Ltd)
Estradiol (as Estradiol hemihydrate) 7.5 microgram per 24 hour Estring 7.5micrograms/24hours vaginal delivery system | 1 device [PoM] £31.42 DT = £31.42

Estriol
20-May-2020

● INDICATIONS AND DOSE
Vaginal atrophy in postmenopausal women
▶ INITIALLY BY VAGINA USING VAGINAL CREAM, OR BY VAGINA USING VAGINAL GEL
▶ Adult: Apply 1 applicatorful daily for 3–4 weeks, then (by vagina) reduced to 1 applicatorful twice weekly, to be applied at bedtime, treatment should be evaluated after 12 weeks

Vaginal atrophy in postmenopausal women
▶ INITIALLY BY VAGINA USING PESSARIES
▶ Adult: 1 pessary daily for 3 weeks, then (by vagina) 1 pessary twice weekly, to be inserted at bedtime

OVESTIN ®
Vaginal surgery for prolapse when there is epithelial atrophy in postmenopausal women (before surgery)
▶ BY VAGINA
▶ Adult: Apply 1 applicatorful daily for 2 weeks before surgery, resume 2 weeks after surgery

DOSE EQUIVALENCE AND CONVERSION
▶ For *Ovestin* ® cream, 1 applicatorful contains 500 micrograms estriol; for *Blissel* ® gel, 1 applicatorful contains 50 micrograms estriol; for *Imvaggis* ® pessary, 1 pessary contains 30 micrograms estriol.

● CONTRA-INDICATIONS Active arterial thromboembolic disease (e.g. angina or myocardial infarction) · history of breast cancer · history of venous thromboembolism · oestrogen-dependent cancer · recent arterial thromboembolic disease (e.g. angina or myocardial

infarction) · thrombophilic disorder · undiagnosed vaginal bleeding · untreated endometrial hyperplasia

● CAUTIONS Acute porphyrias p. 1107 · diabetes (increased risk of heart disease) · factors predisposing to thromboembolism · history of breast nodules—closely monitor breast status (risk of breast cancer) · history of endometrial hyperplasia · history of fibrocystic disease—closely monitor breast status (risk of breast cancer) · hypophyseal tumours · increased risk of gall-bladder disease · migraine (or migraine-like headaches) · presence of antiphospholipid antibodies (increased risk of thrombotic events) · prolonged exposure to unopposed oestrogens may increase risk of developing endometrial cancer · review treatment at least annually to assess need for continued treatment · risk factors for oestrogen-dependent tumours (e.g. breast cancer in first-degree relative) · symptoms of endometriosis may be exacerbated · uterine fibroids may increase in size

CAUTIONS, FURTHER INFORMATION
▶ Risk of endometrial cancer The increased risk of endometrial cancer depends on the dose and duration of oestrogen-only HRT.
▶ Risk of ovarian cancer Long-term use of combined HRT or oestrogen-only HRT is associated with a small increased risk of ovarian cancer. This excess risk disappears within a few years of stopping.
▶ Risk of venous thromboembolism Women using combined or oestrogen-only HRT are at an increased risk of deep vein thrombosis and of pulmonary embolism especially in the first year of use.
   In *women who have predisposing factors* (such as a personal or family history of deep vein thrombosis or pulmonary embolism, severe varicose veins, obesity, trauma, or prolonged bed-rest) it is prudent to review the need for HRT, as in some cases the risks of HRT may exceed the benefits.
   Travel involving prolonged immobility further increases the risk of deep vein thrombosis.
▶ Risk of stroke Risk of stroke increases with age, therefore older women have a greater absolute risk of stroke. Combined HRT or oestrogen-only HRT increases the risk of stroke.
▶ Risk of coronary heart disease HRT does not prevent coronary heart disease and should not be prescribed for this purpose. There is an increased risk of coronary heart disease in women who start combined HRT more than 10 years after menopause. Although very little information is available on the risk of coronary heart disease in younger women who start HRT close to the menopause, studies suggest a lower relative risk compared with older women.

● INTERACTIONS → Appendix 1: hormone replacement therapy

● SIDE-EFFECTS
▶ Common or very common Dysuria · genital abnormalities · skin reactions · vulvovaginal disorders
▶ Uncommon Anorectal discomfort · candida infection · headache · pelvic pain
▶ Frequency not known Breast abnormalities · cervical mucus increased · dementia · erythema nodosum · gallbladder disorder · increased risk of coronary artery disease · increased risk of ischaemic stroke · increased risk of venous thromboembolism · nausea · neoplasms · vaginal haemorrhage · vomiting

● CONCEPTION AND CONTRACEPTION *Imvaggis* ® pessary may damage latex condoms (decreases tensile strength).
OVESTIN ® Effect on latex condoms and diaphragms not yet known.

● PREGNANCY Not known to be harmful.

● BREAST FEEDING Avoid; adverse effects on lactation.

- HEPATIC IMPAIRMENT Manufacturer advises caution; avoid in acute or active disease.
- RENAL IMPAIRMENT Manufacturer advises caution in renal disease. Evidence for caution is unsatisfactory and many women with these conditions may stand to benefit from HRT.
- MONITORING REQUIREMENTS
- Closely monitor breast status if history of breast nodules or fibrocystic disease (risk of breast cancer).
- The endometrial safety of long-term or repeated use of topical vaginal oestrogens is uncertain; treatment should be reviewed at least annually, with special consideration given to any symptoms of endometrial hyperplasia or carcinoma.

- MEDICINAL FORMS There can be variation in the licensing of different medicines containing the same drug.

Pessary
EXCIPIENTS: May contain Butylated hydroxytoluene
- Imvaggis (Besins Healthcare (UK) Ltd)
 Estriol 30 microgram Imvaggis 0.03mg pessaries |
 24 pessary PoM £13.38 DT = £13.38

Cream
EXCIPIENTS: May contain Arachis (peanut) oil, cetostearyl alcohol (including cetyl and stearyl alcohol), polysorbates
- Estriol (Non-proprietary)
 Estriol 100 microgram per 1 gram Estriol 0.01% cream |
 80 gram PoM Ⓢ
- Ovestin (Aspen Pharma Trading Ltd)
 Estriol 1 mg per 1 gram Ovestin 1mg cream | 15 gram PoM £4.45
 DT = £4.45

Vaginal gel
EXCIPIENTS: May contain Hydroxybenzoates (parabens)
- Estriol (Non-proprietary)
 Estriol 50 microgram per 1 gram Blissel 50micrograms/g vaginal gel with applicator | 30 gram PoM £18.90 DT = £18.90

Prasterone   20-May-2019

- DRUG ACTION Prasterone is biochemically and biologically identical to endogenous dehydroepiandrosterone (DHEA), and is converted to oestrogens and androgens.

- INDICATIONS AND DOSE

Vulvar and vaginal atrophy [in postmenopausal women with moderate to severe symptoms]
- BY VAGINA USING PESSARIES
- Adult: 6.5 mg once daily, at bedtime. Treatment should be reassessed at least every 6 months

- CONTRA-INDICATIONS Active or recent arterial thromboembolic disease (e.g. angina or myocardial infarction) · acute liver disease · acute porphyrias p. 1107 · history of breast cancer · history of liver disease (where liver function tests have failed to return to normal) · oestrogen-dependent cancer · thrombophilic disorder · undiagnosed vaginal bleeding · untreated endometrial hyperplasia · venous thromboembolism

- CAUTIONS Assess need for continued treatment at least every 6 months · cholelithiasis · diabetes mellitus · factors predisposing to thromboembolism · history of endometrial hyperplasia · hypertriglyceridaemia · liver disorders (discontinue if jaundice or deterioration in liver function occurs during treatment) · migraine (or migraine-like headaches) · prolonged exposure to unopposed oestrogens may increase risk of developing endometrial cancer · risk factors for oestrogen-dependent tumours (e.g. breast cancer in first-degree relative) · symptoms of endometriosis may be exacerbated · uterine fibroids may increase in size

CAUTIONS, FURTHER INFORMATION
- Risk of endometrial cancer The increased risk of endometrial cancer depends on the dose and duration of oestrogen-only HRT.
 Bleeding or spotting occurring during treatment should be investigated.
 For oestrogen products for vaginal application, where systemic exposure to oestrogen remains within the normal postmenopausal range, it is not recommended to add a progestogen.
- Risk of ovarian cancer Long-term use of combined HRT or oestrogen-only HRT is associated with a small increased risk of ovarian cancer. This excess risk disappears within a few years of stopping.
- Risk of venous thromboembolism Women using combined or oestrogen-only HRT are at an increased risk of deep vein thrombosis and of pulmonary embolism especially in the first year of use.
 In *women who have predisposing factors* (such as a personal or family history of deep vein thrombosis or pulmonary embolism, severe varicose veins, obesity, trauma, major surgery or prolonged bed-rest) it is prudent to review the need for HRT, as in some cases the risks of HRT may exceed the benefits.
 Travel involving prolonged immobility further increases the risk of deep vein thrombosis.
- Risk of stroke Risk of stroke increases with age, therefore older women have a greater absolute risk of stroke. Combined HRT or oestrogen-only HRT slightly increases the risk of stroke.
- Other conditions The product literature advises caution in other conditions including hypertension, asthma, epilepsy, otosclerosis, and systemic lupus erythematosus. Evidence for caution in these conditions is unsatisfactory and many women with these conditions may stand to benefit from HRT.

- SIDE-EFFECTS
- **Common or very common** Cervical abnormalities · weight change
- **Uncommon** Breast neoplasm benign · uterine polyp

- CONCEPTION AND CONTRACEPTION Manufacturer advises avoid use with condoms, diaphragms or cervical caps made of latex—may damage rubber.

- PREGNANCY Manufacturer advises avoid—no information available.

- BREAST FEEDING Manufacturer advises avoid—no information available.

- PATIENT AND CARER ADVICE
Missed doses Manufacturer advises if a dose is more than 16 hours late, the missed dose should not be taken and the next dose should be taken at the normal time.

- MEDICINAL FORMS There can be variation in the licensing of different medicines containing the same drug.
Pessary
- Intrarosa (Theramex HQ UK Ltd) ▼
 Prasterone 6.5 mg Intrarosa 6.5mg pessaries | 28 pessary PoM £15.94 DT = £15.94 CD4-2

Genito-urinary system

7

SELECTIVE OESTROGEN RECEPTOR MODULATORS

Ospemifene

31-Aug-2020

- DRUG ACTION Ospemifene is a selective oestrogen receptor modulator that has an oestrogen-like effect in the vagina, increasing the cellular maturation and mucification of the vaginal epithelium.

- INDICATIONS AND DOSE

Moderate to severe symptomatic vulvar and vaginal atrophy [in post-menopausal women who are not candidates for local vaginal oestrogen therapy]
  - BY MOUTH
  - Adult: 60 mg once daily

- CONTRA-INDICATIONS Breast cancer (suspected or actively treated) · endometrial hyperplasia · history of venous thromboembolism · sex-hormone dependent malignancy (suspected or active) · unexplained vaginal bleeding

- CAUTIONS Risk factors for stroke · risk factors for venous thromboembolism (discontinue if prolonged immobilisation)

- INTERACTIONS → Appendix 1: ospemifene

- SIDE-EFFECTS
  - **Common or very common** Genital discharge · hot flush · increased risk of infection · muscle spasms · skin reactions · vaginal discharge · vaginal haemorrhage
  - **Uncommon** Endometrial thickening · hypersensitivity · tongue swelling

- PREGNANCY Manufacturer advises avoid—toxicity in *animal* studies.

- HEPATIC IMPAIRMENT Manufacturer advises avoid in severe impairment—no information available.

- PATIENT AND CARER ADVICE Manufacturer advises patients and their carers should be advised to seek immediate medical attention if they experience symptoms of thromboembolism (such as sudden chest pain, dyspnoea or swelling of a leg).

- NATIONAL FUNDING/ACCESS DECISIONS
  For full details see funding body website

  Scottish Medicines Consortium (SMC) decisions
  - Ospemifene (*Senshio*®) for the treatment of moderate to severe symptomatic vulvar and vaginal atrophy in post-menopausal women who are not candidates for local vaginal oestrogen therapy (September 2019) SMC No. SMC2170 Recommended

- MEDICINAL FORMS There can be variation in the licensing of different medicines containing the same drug.

  Tablet
  CAUTIONARY AND ADVISORY LABELS 21
  - Senshio (Shionogi Ltd) ▼
    Ospemifene 60 mg Senshio 60mg tablets | 28 tablet PoM £39.50
    DT = £39.50

Chapter 8
Immune system and malignant disease

CONTENTS

Immune system

1 Immune system disorders and transplantation

Immune response   29-Jun-2020

Inflammatory bowel disease

Azathioprine p. 882, ciclosporin p. 884, mercaptopurine
p. 956, and methotrexate p. 957 have a role in the treatment
of inflammatory bowel disease.

Folic acid p. 1071 should be given to reduce the possibility
of methotrexate toxicity [unlicensed indication]. Folic acid is
usually given weekly on a different day to the methotrexate;
alternative regimens may be used in some settings.

Immunosuppressant therapy

Immunosuppressants are used to suppress rejection in organ
transplant recipients and to treat a variety of chronic
inflammatory and autoimmune diseases. Solid organ
transplant patients are maintained on drug regimens, which
may include antiproliferative drugs (azathioprine or
mycophenolate mofetil p. 891), calcineurin inhibitors
(ciclosporin or tacrolimus p. 887), corticosteroids, or
sirolimus p. 886. Choice is dependent on the type of organ,
time after transplantation, and clinical condition of the
patient. Specialist management is required and other
immunomodulators may be used to initiate treatment or to
treat rejection.

Impaired immune responsiveness

Modification of tissue reactions caused by corticosteroids
and other immunosuppressants may result in the rapid
spread of infection. Corticosteroids may suppress clinical
signs of infection and allow diseases such as septicaemia or
tuberculosis to reach an advanced stage before being
recognised— **important**: normal immunoglobulin
administration should be considered as soon as possible
after measles exposure, and varicella-zoster
immunoglobulin p. 1337 or an antiviral [unlicensed] may be
required for individuals exposed to varicella (chickenpox) or
herpes zoster (shingles); for further information, see
Immunoglobulins p. 1331. Wherever possible, immunisation
or additional booster doses for individuals with
immunosuppression should be carried out either before
immunosuppression occurs or deferred until an

improvement in immunity has been seen. Specialist advice
should be sought on the use of live vaccines for those being
treated with immunosuppressive drugs.

Antiproliferative immunosuppressants

Azathioprine is widely used for transplant recipients and it is
also used to treat a number of auto-immune conditions,
usually when corticosteroid therapy alone provides
inadequate control. It is metabolised to mercaptopurine, and
doses should be reduced when allopurinol p. 1166 is given
concurrently.

Mycophenolate mofetil is metabolised to mycophenolic
acid which has a more selective mode of action than
azathioprine.

There is evidence that compared with similar regimens
incorporating azathioprine, mycophenolate mofetil reduces
the risk of acute rejection episodes; the risk of opportunistic
infections (particularly due to tissue-invasive
cytomegalovirus) and the occurrence of blood disorders such
as leucopenia may be higher.

Cyclophosphamide p. 938 is less commonly prescribed as
an immunosuppressant.

Corticosteroids and other immunosuppressants

Prednisolone p. 718 is widely used in oncology. It has a
marked antitumour effect in acute lymphoblastic leukaemia,
Hodgkin's disease, and the non-Hodgkin lymphomas. It has
a role in the palliation of symptomatic end-stage malignant
disease when it may enhance appetite and produce a sense of
well-being.

The corticosteroids are also powerful
immunosuppressants. They are used to prevent organ
transplant rejection, and in high dose to treat rejection
episodes.

Ciclosporin a calcineurin inhibitor, is a potent
immunosuppressant which is virtually non-myelotoxic but
markedly nephrotoxic. It has an important role in organ and
tissue transplantation, for prevention of graft rejection
following bone marrow, kidney, liver, pancreas, heart, lung,
and heart-lung transplantation, and for prophylaxis and
treatment of graft-versus-host disease.

Tacrolimus is also a calcineurin inhibitor. Although not
chemically related to ciclosporin it has a similar mode of
action and side-effects, but the incidence of neurotoxicity
appears to be greater; cardiomyopathy has also been
reported. Disturbance of glucose metabolism also appears to
be significant.

Sirolimus is a non-calcineurin inhibiting
immunosuppressant licensed for renal transplantation.

Basiliximab p. 890 is used for prophylaxis of acute rejection in allogeneic renal transplantation. It is given with ciclosporin and corticosteroid immunosuppression regimens; its use should be confined to specialist centres.

Belatacept p. 893 is a fusion protein and co-stimulation blocker that prevents T-cell activation; it is licensed for prophylaxis of graft rejection in adults undergoing renal transplantation who are seropositive for the Epstein-Barr virus. It is used with interleukin-2 receptor antagonist induction, in combination with corticosteroids and a mycophenolic acid.

Antithymocyte immunoglobulin (rabbit) below is licensed for the prophylaxis of organ rejection in renal and heart allograft recipients and for the treatment of corticosteroid-resistant allograft rejection in renal transplantation. Tolerability is increased by pretreatment with an intravenous corticosteroid and antihistamine; an antipyretic drug such as paracetamol may also be beneficial.

> **Other drugs used for Immune system disorders and transplantation** Anakinra, p. 1147 · Chloroquine, p. 655 · Everolimus, p. 1025 · Hydroxychloroquine sulfate, p. 1144 · Rituximab, p. 927

IMMUNE SERA AND IMMUNOGLOBULINS >
IMMUNOGLOBULINS

Antithymocyte immunoglobulin (rabbit)

17-Jul-2020

● **INDICATIONS AND DOSE**

Prophylaxis of organ rejection in heart allograft recipients
▸ BY INTRAVENOUS INFUSION
▸ Adult: 1–2.5 mg/kg daily for 3–5 days, to be given over at least 6 hours

Prophylaxis of organ rejection in renal allograft recipients
▸ BY INTRAVENOUS INFUSION
▸ Adult: 1–1.5 mg/kg daily for 3–9 days, to be given over at least 6 hours

Treatment of corticosteroid-resistant allograft rejection in renal transplantation
▸ BY INTRAVENOUS INFUSION
▸ Adult: 1.5 mg/kg daily for 7–14 days, to be given over at least 6 hours

DOSES AT EXTREMES OF BODY-WEIGHT
▸ To avoid excessive dosage in obese patients, calculate dose on the basis of ideal body weight.

● **CONTRA-INDICATIONS** Infection
● **INTERACTIONS** → Appendix 1: immunoglobulins
● **SIDE-EFFECTS**
▸ **Common or very common** Chills · diarrhoea · dysphagia · dyspnoea · fever · hypotension · infection · lymphopenia · myalgia · nausea · neoplasm malignant · neoplasms · neutropenia · reactivation of infection · secondary malignancy · sepsis · skin reactions · thrombocytopenia · vomiting
▸ **Uncommon** Cytokine release syndrome · hepatic disorders · hypersensitivity · infusion related reaction

SIDE-EFFECTS, FURTHER INFORMATION Tolerability is increased by pretreatment with an intravenous corticosteroid and antihistamine; an antipyretic drug such as paracetamol may also be beneficial.

● **PREGNANCY** Manufacturer advises use only if potential benefit outweighs risk—no information available.
● **BREAST FEEDING** Manufacturer advises avoid—no information available.
● **MONITORING REQUIREMENTS** Monitor blood count.

● **DIRECTIONS FOR ADMINISTRATION** For *continuous intravenous infusion* (*Thymoglobuline*®), manufacturer advises give in Glucose 5% or Sodium chloride 0.9%; reconstitute each vial with 5 mL water for injections to produce a solution of 5 mg/mL; gently rotate to dissolve. Dilute requisite dose with infusion fluid to a total volume of 50–500 mL (usually 50 mL/vial); begin infusion immediately after dilution; give through an in-line filter (pore size 0.22 micron); not to be given with unfractionated heparin and hydrocortisone in glucose infusion—precipitation reported.

● **NATIONAL FUNDING/ACCESS DECISIONS** For full details see funding body website

NICE decisions
▸ **Immunosuppressive therapy for kidney transplant in adults (October 2017)** NICE TA481 Not recommended

● **MEDICINAL FORMS** There can be variation in the licensing of different medicines containing the same drug.

Solution for infusion
▸ Grafalon (Imported (Germany))
  Antithymocyte immunoglobulin (rabbit) 20 mg per 1 ml Grafalon 100mg/5ml concentrate for solution for infusion vials | 1 vial PoM $\boxed{\text{S}}$

Powder and solvent for solution for infusion
▸ Thymoglobulin (Sanofi)
  Antithymocyte immunoglobulin (rabbit) 25 mg Thymoglobuline 25mg powder and solvent for solution for infusion vials | 1 vial PoM £158.77 (Hospital only)

IMMUNOSUPPRESSANTS > ANTIMETABOLITES

Azathioprine

16-Dec-2020

● **DRUG ACTION** Azathioprine is metabolised to mercaptopurine.

● **INDICATIONS AND DOSE**

Severe acute Crohn's disease | Maintenance of remission of Crohn's disease | Maintenance of remission of acute ulcerative colitis
▸ BY MOUTH
▸ Adult: 2–2.5 mg/kg daily, some patients may respond to lower doses

Rheumatoid arthritis that has not responded to other disease-modifying drugs | Severe systemic lupus erythematosus and other connective tissue disorders | Polymyositis in cases of corticosteroid resistance
▸ BY MOUTH
▸ Adult: Initially up to 2.5 mg/kg daily in divided doses, adjusted according to response, rarely more than 3 mg/kg daily; maintenance 1–3 mg/kg daily, consider withdrawal if no improvement within 3 months

Autoimmune conditions
▸ BY MOUTH, OR BY INTRAVENOUS INJECTION, OR BY INTRAVENOUS INFUSION
▸ Adult: 1–3 mg/kg daily, adjusted according to response, consider withdrawal if no improvement within 3 months, oral administration preferable, if not possible then can be given by intravenous injection (intravenous solution very irritant) *or* by intravenous infusion

Suppression of transplant rejection
▸ BY MOUTH, OR BY INTRAVENOUS INJECTION, OR BY INTRAVENOUS INFUSION
▸ Adult: 1–2.5 mg/kg daily, adjusted according to response, oral administration preferable, if not possible then can be given by intravenous injection (intravenous solution very irritant) *or* by intravenous infusion

Severe refractory eczema, normal or high TPMT activity
▸ BY MOUTH
▸ Adult: 1–3 mg/kg daily

Severe refractory eczema, intermediate TPMT activity
▶ BY MOUTH
▶ Adult: 0.5–1.5 mg/kg daily
Generalised myasthenia gravis
▶ BY MOUTH, OR BY INTRAVENOUS INJECTION, OR BY
  INTRAVENOUS INFUSION
▶ Adult: Initially 0.5–1 mg/kg daily, then increased to
  2–2.5 mg/kg daily, dose is increased over 3–4 weeks,
  azathioprine is usually started at the same time as the
  corticosteroid and allows a lower maintenance dose of
  the corticosteroid to be used, oral administration
  preferable, if not possible then can be given by
  intravenous injection (intravenous solution very
  irritant) or by intravenous infusion
DOSE ADJUSTMENTS DUE TO INTERACTIONS
▶ Manufacturer advises reduce dose to one-quarter of
  the usual dose with concurrent use of allopurinol.

● UNLICENSED USE Azathioprine doses given in BNF for
  suppression of transplant rejection and autoimmune
  conditions may differ from those in product literature.
  Use for severe refractory eczema is unlicensed.
● CONTRA-INDICATIONS
▶ When used for severe refractory eczema absent thiopurine
  methyltransferase (TPMT) activity · very low thiopurine
  methyltransferase (TPMT) activity
● CAUTIONS Reduce dose in elderly · reduced thiopurine
  methyltransferase activity
● INTERACTIONS → Appendix 1: azathioprine
● SIDE-EFFECTS
GENERAL SIDE-EFFECTS
▶ **Common or very common** Bone marrow depression (dose-
  related) · increased risk of infection · leucopenia ·
  pancreatitis · thrombocytopenia
▶ **Uncommon** Anaemia · hepatic disorders · hypersensitivity
▶ **Rare or very rare** Agranulocytosis · alopecia · bone marrow
  disorders · diarrhoea · gastrointestinal disorders ·
  neoplasms · photosensitivity reaction · pneumonitis ·
  severe cutaneous adverse reactions (SCARs)
▶ **Frequency not known** Nodular regenerative hyperplasia ·
  sinusoidal obstruction syndrome
SPECIFIC SIDE-EFFECTS
▶ With oral use Nausea
SIDE-EFFECTS, FURTHER INFORMATION Side-effects may
require drug withdrawal.
  Hypersensitivity reactions Hypersensitivity reactions
(including malaise, dizziness, vomiting, diarrhoea, fever,
rigors, myalgia, arthralgia, rash, hypotension and renal
dysfunction) call for immediate withdrawal.
  Neutropenia and thrombocytopenia Neutropenia is
dose-dependent. Management of neutropenia and
thrombocytopenia requires careful monitoring and dose
adjustment.
  Nausea Nausea is common early in the course of
treatment and usually resolves after a few weeks without
an alteration in dose. Moderate nausea can be managed by
using divided daily doses, taking doses after food,
prescribing concurrent antiemetics or temporarily
reducing the dose.
● ALLERGY AND CROSS-SENSITIVITY EvGr Contra-indicated
  in hypersensitivity to mercaptopurine. ◈
● PREGNANCY Transplant patients immunosuppressed with
  azathioprine should not discontinue it on becoming
  pregnant. However, there have been reports of premature
  birth and low birth-weight following exposure to
  azathioprine, particularly in combination with
  corticosteroids. Spontaneous abortion has been reported
  following maternal or paternal exposure. Azathioprine is
  teratogenic in animal studies. The use of azathioprine
  during pregnancy needs to be supervised in specialist

units. Treatment should not generally be initiated during
pregnancy.
● BREAST FEEDING Present in milk in low concentration. No
  evidence of harm in small studies—use if potential benefit
  outweighs risk.
● HEPATIC IMPAIRMENT Manufacturer advises caution
  (impaired metabolism)—monitor liver function and
  complete blood count more frequently in those with severe
  impairment.
  Dose adjustments Manufacturer advises use doses at lower
  end of the dose range in hepatic failure; reduce dose if
  hepatic or haematological toxicity occur.
● RENAL IMPAIRMENT
  Dose adjustments Reduce dose.
● PRE-TREATMENT SCREENING
  Thiopurine methyltransferase The enzyme thiopurine
  methyltransferase (TPMT) metabolises thiopurine drugs
  (azathioprine, mercaptopurine, tioguanine); the risk of
  myelosuppression is increased in patients with reduced
  activity of the enzyme, particularly for the few individuals
  in whom TPMT activity is undetectable. Manufacturer
  advises consider measuring TPMT activity before starting
  azathioprine, mercaptopurine, or tioguanine therapy. Seek
  specialist advice for those with reduced or absent TPMT
  activity.
● MONITORING REQUIREMENTS
▶ Monitor for toxicity throughout treatment.
▶ Monitor full blood count weekly (more frequently with
  higher doses or if severe renal impairment) for first
  4 weeks (manufacturer advises weekly monitoring for
  8 weeks but evidence of practical value unsatisfactory),
  thereafter reduce frequency of monitoring to at least every
  3 months.
▶ Blood tests and monitoring for signs of myelosuppression
  are essential in long-term treatment.
● DIRECTIONS FOR ADMINISTRATION
▶ With intravenous use For intravenous injection, manufacturer
  advises give over at least 1 minute (followed by 50 mL
  sodium chloride intravenous infusion). For intravenous
  infusion (Imuran®), manufacturer advises reconstitute
  50 mg with 5–15 mL Water for Injections; dilute requisite
  dose to a volume of 20–200 mL with infusion fluid. Expert
  sources advise give in Glucose 5% or Sodium Chloride
  0.9%. Intravenous injection is alkaline and very irritant.
  Manufacturer advises intravenous route should therefore
  be used **only** if oral route not feasible.
● PATIENT AND CARER ADVICE
  Bone marrow suppression Patients and their carers should be
  warned to report immediately any signs or symptoms of
  bone marrow suppression e.g. inexplicable bruising or
  bleeding, infection.

● MEDICINAL FORMS There can be variation in the licensing of
  different medicines containing the same drug. Forms available
  from special-order manufacturers include: capsule, oral
  suspension, oral solution
Tablet
CAUTIONARY AND ADVISORY LABELS 21
  ▶ Azathioprine (Non-proprietary)
    Azathioprine 25 mg Azathioprine 25mg tablets | 28 tablet PoM
    £5.52 DT = £2.05 | 100 tablet PoM £7.32–£33.26
    Azathioprine 50 mg Azathioprine 50mg tablets | 56 tablet PoM
    £5.50 DT = £2.75 | 100 tablet PoM £4.91–£16.55
  ▶ Azapress (Ennogen Pharma Ltd)
    Azathioprine 50 mg Azapress 50mg tablets | 56 tablet PoM £2.83
    DT = £2.75
  ▶ Imuran (Aspen Pharma Trading Ltd)
    Azathioprine 25 mg Imuran 25mg tablets | 100 tablet PoM £10.99
    Azathioprine 50 mg Imuran 50mg tablets | 100 tablet PoM £7.99
Powder for solution for injection
  ▶ Imuran (Aspen Pharma Trading Ltd)
    Azathioprine 50 mg Imuran 50mg powder for solution for injection
    vials | 1 vial PoM £15.38 DT = £15.38

8

Immune system and malignant disease

Ciclosporin

16-Nov-2020

(Cyclosporin)

- **DRUG ACTION** Ciclosporin inhibits production and release of lymphokines, thereby suppressing cell-mediated immune response.

- **INDICATIONS AND DOSE**

Severe acute ulcerative colitis refractory to corticosteroid treatment
▸ BY CONTINUOUS INTRAVENOUS INFUSION
▸ Adult: 2 mg/kg, to be given over 24 hours, dose adjusted according to blood-ciclosporin concentration and response

Severe active rheumatoid arthritis (administered on expert advice)
▸ BY MOUTH
▸ Adult: Initially 1.5 mg/kg twice daily, increased if necessary up to 2.5 mg/kg twice daily after 6 weeks, dose increases should be made gradually, for maintenance treatment, titrate dose individually to the lowest effective dose according to tolerability, treatment may be required for up to 12 weeks

Severe active rheumatoid arthritis [in combination with low-dose methotrexate, when methotrexate monotherapy has been ineffective] (administered on expert advice)
▸ BY MOUTH
▸ Adult: Initially 1.25 mg/kg twice daily, increased if necessary up to 2.5 mg/kg twice daily after 6 weeks, dose increases should be made gradually, for maintenance treatment, titrate dose individually to the lowest effective dose according to tolerability, treatment may be required for up to 12 weeks

Short-term treatment of severe atopic dermatitis where conventional therapy ineffective or inappropriate (administered on expert advice)
▸ BY MOUTH
▸ Adult: Initially 1.25 mg/kg twice daily (max. per dose 2.5 mg/kg twice daily) usual maximum duration of 8 weeks but may be used for longer under specialist supervision, if good initial response not achieved within 2 weeks, increase dose rapidly up to maximum

Short-term treatment of very severe atopic dermatitis where conventional therapy ineffective or inappropriate (administered on expert advice)
▸ BY MOUTH
▸ Adult: 2.5 mg/kg twice daily usual maximum duration of 8 weeks but may be used for longer under specialist supervision

Severe psoriasis where conventional therapy ineffective or inappropriate (administered on expert advice)
▸ BY MOUTH
▸ Adult: Initially 1.25 mg/kg twice daily (max. per dose 2.5 mg/kg twice daily), increased gradually to maximum if no improvement within 1 month, initial dose of 2.5 mg/kg twice daily justified if condition requires rapid improvement; discontinue if inadequate response after 3 months at the optimum dose; max. duration of treatment usually 1 year unless other treatments cannot be used

Organ transplantation (used alone)
▸ BY MOUTH
▸ Adult: 10–15 mg/kg, to be administered 4–12 hours before transplantation, followed by 10–15 mg/kg daily for 1–2 weeks postoperatively, then maintenance 2–6 mg/kg daily, reduce dose gradually to

maintenance. Dose should be adjusted according to blood-ciclosporin concentration and renal function; dose is lower if given concomitantly with other immunosuppressant therapy (e.g. corticosteroids); if necessary one-third corresponding oral dose can be given by intravenous infusion over 2–6 hours

Bone-marrow transplantation | Prevention and treatment of graft-versus-host disease
▸ INITIALLY BY INTRAVENOUS INFUSION
▸ Adult: 3–5 mg/kg daily, to be administered over 2–6 hours from day before transplantation to 2 weeks postoperatively, alternatively (by mouth) initially 12.5–15 mg/kg daily, then (by mouth) 12.5 mg/kg daily for 3-6 months and then tailed off (may take up to a year after transplantation)

Nephrotic syndrome
▸ BY MOUTH
▸ Adult: 5 mg/kg daily in 2 divided doses, for maintenance reduce to lowest effective dose according to proteinuria and serum creatinine measurements; discontinue after 3 months if no improvement in glomerulonephritis or glomerulosclerosis (after 6 months in membranous glomerulonephritis)

DOSE ADJUSTMENTS DUE TO INTERACTIONS
▸ With oral use Manufacturer advises increase dose by 50% or switch to intravenous administration with concurrent use of octreotide.

- **UNLICENSED USE** Not licensed for use in severe acute ulcerative colitis refractory to corticosteroid treatment.

> IMPORTANT SAFETY INFORMATION
>
> MHRA/CHM ADVICE: CICLOSPORIN MUST BE PRESCRIBED AND DISPENSED BY BRAND NAME (DECEMBER 2009)
>
> Patients should be stabilised on a particular brand of oral ciclosporin because switching between formulations without close monitoring may lead to clinically important changes in blood-ciclosporin concentration.

- **CONTRA-INDICATIONS** Malignancy (in non-transplant indications) · uncontrolled hypertension (in non-transplant indications) · uncontrolled infections (in non-transplant indications)

- **CAUTIONS** Elderly—monitor renal function · hyperuricaemia · in atopic dermatitis, active herpes simplex infections—allow infection to clear before starting (if they occur during treatment withdraw if severe) · in atopic dermatitis, *Staphylococcus aureus* skin infections—not absolute contra-indication providing controlled (but avoid erythromycin unless no other alternative) · in psoriasis treat, patients with malignant or pre-malignant conditions of skin only after appropriate treatment (and if no other option) · in uveitis, Behcet's syndrome (monitor neurological status) · lymphoproliferative disorders (discontinue treatment) · malignancy

CAUTIONS, FURTHER INFORMATION
▸ Malignancy In psoriasis, exclude malignancies (including those of skin and cervix) before starting (biopsy any lesions not typical of psoriasis) and treat patients with malignant or pre-malignant conditions of skin only after appropriate treatment (and if no other option); discontinue if lymphoproliferative disorder develops.

- **INTERACTIONS** → Appendix 1: ciclosporin

- **SIDE-EFFECTS**

GENERAL SIDE-EFFECTS
▸ **Common or very common** Eye inflammation

SPECIFIC SIDE-EFFECTS
▸ **Common or very common** Appetite decreased · diarrhoea · electrolyte imbalance · fatigue · fever · flushing · gastrointestinal discomfort · gingival hyperplasia · hair changes · headaches · hepatic disorders · hyperglycaemia ·

hyperlipidaemia · hypertension · hyperuricaemia · leucopenia · muscle complaints · nausea · paraesthesia · peptic ulcer · renal impairment (renal structural changes on long-term administration) · seizure · skin reactions · tremor · vomiting
▶ **Uncommon** Anaemia · encephalopathy · oedema · thrombocytopenia · weight increased
▶ **Rare or very rare** Gynaecomastia · haemolytic anaemia · idiopathic intracranial hypertension · menstrual disorder · multifocal motor neuropathy · muscle weakness · myopathy · pancreatitis
▶ **Frequency not known** Pain in extremity · thrombotic microangiopathy
● PREGNANCY Crosses placenta; manufacturer advises avoid unless potential benefit outweighs risk—toxicity in *animal* studies.
● BREAST FEEDING Manufacturer advises avoid—present in milk.
● HEPATIC IMPAIRMENT Manufacturer advises caution in severe impairment (risk of increased exposure).
Dose adjustments Manufacturer advises consider dose reduction in severe impairment to maintain blood-ciclosporin concentration in target range—monitor until concentration stable.
● RENAL IMPAIRMENT
Dose adjustments In non-transplant indications, manufacturer advises establishing baseline renal function before initiation of treatment; if baseline function is impaired in non-transplant indications, except nephrotic syndrome—avoid. In nephrotic syndrome, manufacturer advises initial dose should not exceed 2.5 mg/kg daily in patients with baseline renal impairment. *During treatment* for non-transplant indications, manufacturer recommends if eGFR decreases by more than 25% below baseline on more than one measurement, reduce dose by 25–50%. If the eGFR decrease from baseline exceeds 35%, further dose reduction should be considered (even if within normal range); discontinue if reduction not successful within 1 month.
● MONITORING REQUIREMENTS Monitor whole blood ciclosporin concentration (trough level dependent on indication—consult local treatment protocol for details). Dermatological and physical examination, including blood pressure and renal function measurements required at least twice before starting treatment for psoriasis or atopic dermatitis. Monitor liver function. Monitor serum potassium, especially in renal dysfunction (risk of hyperkalaemia). Monitor serum magnesium. Measure blood lipids before treatment and after the first month of treatment. In psoriasis and atopic dermatitis monitor serum creatinine every 2 weeks for first 3 months then every month. Investigate lymphadenopathy that persists despite improvement in atopic dermatitis. Monitor kidney function—dose dependent increase in serum creatinine and urea during first few weeks may necessitate dose reduction in transplant patients (exclude rejection if kidney transplant) or discontinuation in non-transplant patients. Monitor blood pressure—discontinue if hypertension develops that cannot be controlled by antihypertensives. In long-term management of nephrotic syndrome, perform renal biopsies at yearly intervals. In rheumatoid arthritis measure serum creatinine at least twice before treatment. During treatment, monitor serum creatinine every 2 weeks for first 3 months, then every month for a further 3 months, then every 4–8 weeks depending on the stability of the disease, concomitant medication, and concomitant diseases (or more frequently if dose increased or concomitant NSAIDs introduced or increased). Monitor hepatic function if concomitant NSAIDs given.

● DIRECTIONS FOR ADMINISTRATION
▶ With oral use Manufacturer advises mix solution with orange or apple juice, or other soft drink (to improve taste) immediately before taking (and rinse with more to ensure total dose). Do not mix with grapefruit juice. Total daily dose should be taken in 2 divided doses.
▶ With intravenous use For *intravenous infusion (Sandimmun* ®), manufacturer advises give intermittently *or* continuously *in* Glucose 5% *or* Sodium Chloride 0.9%; dilute to a concentration of 50 mg in 20–100 mL; give intermittent infusion over 2–6 hours; not to be used with PVC equipment. Observe patient for signs of anaphylaxis for at least 30 minutes after starting infusion and at frequent intervals thereafter.
● PRESCRIBING AND DISPENSING INFORMATION
Brand name prescribing Prescribing and dispensing of ciclosporin should be by brand name to avoid inadvertent switching. If it is necessary to switch a patient to a different brand of ciclosporin, the patient should be monitored closely for changes in blood-ciclosporin concentration, serum creatinine, blood pressure, and transplant function (for transplant indications). *Sandimmun* ® capsules and oral solution are available direct from Novartis for patients who cannot be transferred to a different oral preparation.
● PATIENT AND CARER ADVICE Patients and carers should be counselled on the administration of different formulations of ciclosporin. Manufacturer advises avoid excessive exposure to UV light, including sunlight. In psoriasis and atopic dermatitis, avoid use of UVB or PUVA.

● MEDICINAL FORMS There can be variation in the licensing of different medicines containing the same drug.
Solution for infusion
CAUTIONARY AND ADVISORY LABELS 11
EXCIPIENTS: May contain Alcohol, polyoxyl castor oils
▶ Sandimmun (Novartis Pharmaceuticals UK Ltd)
Ciclosporin 50 mg per 1 ml Sandimmun 250mg/5ml concentrate for solution for infusion ampoules | 10 ampoule [PoM] £110.05
Sandimmun 50mg/1ml concentrate for solution for infusion ampoules | 10 ampoule [PoM] £23.23
Oral solution
CAUTIONARY AND ADVISORY LABELS 11
EXCIPIENTS: May contain Alcohol, propylene glycol
▶ Capsorin (Morningside Healthcare Ltd)
Ciclosporin 100 mg per 1 ml Capsorin 100mg/ml oral solution sugar-free | 50 ml [PoM] £86.96 DT = £164.72
▶ Neoral (Novartis Pharmaceuticals UK Ltd)
Ciclosporin 100 mg per 1 ml Neoral 100mg/ml oral solution sugar-free | 50 ml [PoM] £102.30 DT = £164.72
▶ Sandimmun (Novartis Pharmaceuticals UK Ltd)
Ciclosporin 100 mg per 1 ml Sandimmun 100mg/ml oral solution sugar-free | 50 ml [PoM] £164.72 DT = £164.72
Capsule
CAUTIONARY AND ADVISORY LABELS 11
EXCIPIENTS: May contain Ethanol, ethyl lactate, propylene glycol
▶ Ciclosporin (Non-proprietary)
Ciclosporin 25 mg Ciclosporin 25mg capsules | 30 capsule [PoM] 🔲 DT = £18.37
Ciclosporin 50 mg Ciclosporin 50mg capsules | 30 capsule [PoM] 🔲 DT = £35.97
Ciclosporin 100 mg Ciclosporin 100mg capsules | 30 capsule [PoM] 🔲 DT = £68.28
▶ Capimune (Mylan)
Ciclosporin 25 mg Capimune 25mg capsules | 30 capsule [PoM] £13.05 DT = £18.37
Ciclosporin 50 mg Capimune 50mg capsules | 30 capsule [PoM] £25.50 DT = £35.97
Ciclosporin 100 mg Capimune 100mg capsules | 30 capsule [PoM] £48.50 DT = £68.28
▶ Capsorin (Morningside Healthcare Ltd)
Ciclosporin 25 mg Capsorin 25mg capsules | 30 capsule [PoM] £11.14 DT = £18.37
Ciclosporin 50 mg Capsorin 50mg capsules | 30 capsule [PoM] £21.80 DT = £35.97

Immune system and malignant disease

Ciclosporin 100 mg Capsorin 100mg capsules | 30 capsule [PoM]
£41.59 DT = £68.28

▸ Deximune (Dexcel-Pharma Ltd)

Ciclosporin 25 mg Deximune 25mg capsules | 30 capsule [PoM]
£13.06 DT = £18.37

Ciclosporin 50 mg Deximune 50mg capsules | 30 capsule [PoM]
£25.60 DT = £35.97

Ciclosporin 100 mg Deximune 100mg capsules | 30 capsule [PoM]
£48.90 DT = £68.28

▸ Neoral (Novartis Pharmaceuticals UK Ltd)

Ciclosporin 10 mg Neoral 10mg capsules | 60 capsule [PoM] £18.25
DT = £18.25

Ciclosporin 25 mg Neoral 25mg capsules | 30 capsule [PoM] £18.37
DT = £18.37

Ciclosporin 50 mg Neoral 50mg capsules | 30 capsule [PoM] £35.97
DT = £35.97

Ciclosporin 100 mg Neoral 100mg capsules | 30 capsule [PoM]
£68.28 DT = £68.28

▸ Sandimmun (Novartis Pharmaceuticals UK Ltd)

Ciclosporin 25 mg Sandimmun 25mg capsules | 30 capsule [PoM]
£29.58 DT = £18.37

Ciclosporin 50 mg Sandimmun 50mg capsules | 30 capsule [PoM]
£57.92 DT = £35.97

Ciclosporin 100 mg Sandimmun 100mg capsules | 30 capsule [PoM]
£109.93 DT = £68.28

▸ Vanquoral (Teva UK Ltd)

Ciclosporin 10 mg Vanquoral 10mg capsules | 60 capsule [PoM]
£12.75 DT = £18.25

Ciclosporin 25 mg Vanquoral 25mg capsules | 30 capsule [PoM]
£13.05 DT = £18.37

Ciclosporin 50 mg Vanquoral 50mg capsules | 30 capsule [PoM]
£25.59 DT = £35.97

Ciclosporin 100 mg Vanquoral 100mg capsules | 30 capsule [PoM]
£48.89 DT = £68.28

| Sirolimus

21-Jul-2020

● DRUG ACTION Sirolimus is a non-calcineurin inhibiting
immunosuppressant.

● **INDICATIONS AND DOSE**

**Prophylaxis of organ rejection in kidney allograft
recipients**

▸ BY MOUTH

▸ **Adult:** Initially 6 mg for 1 dose, to be given after
surgery once wound has healed, then 2 mg once daily;
to be given in combination with ciclosporin and
corticosteroid for 2–3 months (sirolimus doses should
be given 4 hours after ciclosporin), ciclosporin should
then be withdrawn over 4–8 weeks (if not possible,
sirolimus should be discontinued and an alternate
immunosuppressive regimen used), dose to be adjusted
according to whole blood-sirolimus trough
concentration

DOSE EQUIVALENCE AND CONVERSION

▸ The 500 microgram tablet is not bioequivalent to the
1 mg and 2 mg tablets. Multiples of 500 microgram
tablets should **not** be used as a substitute for other
tablet strengths.

● CAUTIONS Hyperlipidaemia · increased susceptibility to
infection (especially urinary-tract infection) · increased
susceptibility to lymphoma and other malignancies,
particularly of the skin (limit exposure to UV light)

● INTERACTIONS → Appendix 1: sirolimus

● SIDE-EFFECTS

▸ **Common or very common** Abdominal pain · anaemia ·
arthralgia · ascites · constipation · diabetes mellitus ·
diarrhoea · dyslipidaemia · electrolyte imbalance ·
embolism and thrombosis · fever · haemolytic uraemic
syndrome · haemorrhage · headache · healing impaired ·
hyperglycaemia · hypertension · increased risk of infection
· leucopenia · lymphatic vessel disorders · menstrual cycle
irregularities · nausea · neoplasms · neutropenia · oedema ·
osteonecrosis · ovarian cyst · pain · pancreatitis ·

pericardial effusion · proteinuria · respiratory disorders ·
sepsis · skin reactions · stomatitis · tachycardia ·
thrombocytopenia

▸ **Uncommon** Antibiotic associated colitis · focal segmental
glomerulosclerosis · hepatic failure · nephrotic syndrome ·
pancytopenia · post transplant lymphoproliferative
disorder

▸ **Frequency not known** Posterior reversible encephalopathy
syndrome (PRES)

● CONCEPTION AND CONTRACEPTION Effective
contraception must be used during treatment and for
12 weeks after stopping.

● PREGNANCY Avoid unless essential—toxicity in *animal*
studies.

● BREAST FEEDING Discontinue breast-feeding.

● HEPATIC IMPAIRMENT Manufacturer advises caution (risk
of increased exposure).

Dose adjustments Manufacturer advises maintenance dose
reduction of approx. 50% in severe impairment—monitor
whole blood-sirolimus trough concentration every
5–7 days until 3 consecutive measurements have shown
stable blood-sirolimus concentration.

● MONITORING REQUIREMENTS

▸ Monitor whole blood-sirolimus trough concentration
(Afro-Caribbean patients may require higher doses).

▸ Manufacturer advises pre-dose ('trough') whole blood-
sirolimus concentration (using **chromatographic** assay)
when used with ciclosporin should be
4–12 micrograms/litre (local treatment protocols may
differ); after withdrawal of ciclosporin pre-dose whole
blood-sirolimus concentration should be
12–20 micrograms/litre (local treatment protocols may
differ).

▸ Close monitoring of whole blood-sirolimus concentration
required if concomitant treatment with potent inducers or
inhibitors of metabolism and after discontinuing them, or
if ciclosporin dose reduced significantly or stopped.

▸ When changing between oral solution and tablets,
measurement of whole blood 'trough' sirolimus
concentration after 1–2 weeks is recommended.

▸ Therapeutic drug monitoring assays Sirolimus whole-blood
concentration is measured using either high performance
liquid chromatography (HPLC) or immunoassay. Switching
between different immunoassays or between an
immunoassay and HPLC can lead to clinically significant
differences in results and therefore incorrect dose
adjustments. Adjustment to the target therapeutic dose
range should be made with knowledge of the assay used
and corresponding reference range.

▸ Monitor kidney function when given with ciclosporin;
monitor lipids; monitor urine proteins.

● DIRECTIONS FOR ADMINISTRATION Manufacturer advises
food may affect absorption (take at the same time with
respect to food). Sirolimus oral solution should be mixed
with at least 60 mL water or orange juice in a glass or
plastic container immediately before taking; refill
container with at least 120 mL of water or orange juice and
drink immediately (to ensure total dose). Do not mix with
any other liquids.

● PATIENT AND CARER ADVICE Patient or carers should be
given advice on how to administer sirolimus.
Patients should be advised to avoid excessive exposure
to UV light.

● NATIONAL FUNDING/ACCESS DECISIONS
For full details see funding body website

NICE decisions

▸ **Immunosuppressive therapy for kidney transplant in adults
(October 2017)** NICE TA481 Not recommended

- MEDICINAL FORMS There can be variation in the licensing of different medicines containing the same drug.

Oral solution
EXCIPIENTS: May contain Ethanol
▸ Rapamune (Pfizer Ltd)
   Sirolimus 1 mg per 1 ml Rapamune 1mg/ml oral solution sugar-free | 60 ml [PoM] £162.41 DT = £162.41

Tablet
▸ Rapamune (Pfizer Ltd)
   Sirolimus 500 microgram Rapamune 0.5mg tablets | 30 tablet [PoM] £69.00 DT = £69.00
   Sirolimus 1 mg Rapamune 1mg tablets | 30 tablet [PoM] £86.49 DT = £86.49
   Sirolimus 2 mg Rapamune 2mg tablets | 30 tablet [PoM] £172.98 DT = £172.98

Tacrolimus

02-Dec-2020

- DRUG ACTION Tacrolimus is a calcineurin inhibitor.

- INDICATIONS AND DOSE

ADOPORT ®

Prophylaxis of graft rejection following liver transplantation, starting 12 hours after transplantation
▸ BY MOUTH
▸ Adult: Initially 100–200 micrograms/kg daily in 2 divided doses

Prophylaxis of graft rejection following kidney transplantation, starting within 24 hours of transplantation
▸ BY MOUTH
▸ Adult: Initially 200–300 micrograms/kg daily in 2 divided doses

Prophylaxis of graft rejection following heart transplantation following antibody induction, starting within 5 days of transplantation
▸ BY MOUTH
▸ Adult: Initially 75 micrograms/kg daily in 2 divided doses

Prophylaxis of graft rejection following heart transplantation without antibody induction, starting within 12 hours of transplantation
▸ BY MOUTH
▸ Adult: Initially 75 micrograms/kg daily in 2 divided doses

Allograft rejection resistant to conventional immunosuppressive therapy
▸ BY MOUTH
▸ Adult: Seek specialist advice

ADVAGRAF ®

Prophylaxis of graft rejection following liver transplantation, starting 12–18 hours after transplantation
▸ BY MOUTH
▸ Adult: Initially 100–200 micrograms/kg once daily, to be taken in the morning

Prophylaxis of graft rejection following kidney transplantation, starting within 24 hours of transplantation
▸ BY MOUTH
▸ Adult: Initially 200–300 micrograms/kg once daily, to be taken in the morning

Allograft rejection resistant to conventional immunosuppressive therapy
▸ BY MOUTH
▸ Adult: Seek specialist advice

ENVARSUS ® MODIFIED-RELEASE TABLETS

Prophylaxis of graft rejection following liver transplantation, starting within 24 hours of transplantation
▸ BY MOUTH
▸ Adult: Initially 110–130 micrograms/kg once daily, to be taken in the morning

Prophylaxis of graft rejection following renal transplantation, starting within 24 hours of transplantation
▸ BY MOUTH
▸ Adult: Initially 170 micrograms/kg once daily, to be taken in the morning

Rejection therapy
▸ BY MOUTH
▸ Adult: Seek specialist advice

MODIGRAF ®

Prophylaxis of graft rejection following liver transplantation, starting 12 hours after transplantation
▸ BY MOUTH
▸ Adult: Initially 100–200 micrograms/kg daily in 2 divided doses

Prophylaxis of graft rejection following kidney transplantation, starting within 24 hours of transplantation
▸ BY MOUTH
▸ Adult: Initially 200–300 micrograms/kg daily in 2 divided doses

Prophylaxis of graft rejection following heart transplantation following antibody induction, starting within 5 days of transplantation
▸ BY MOUTH
▸ Adult: Initially 75 micrograms/kg daily in 2 divided doses

Prophylaxis of graft rejection following heart transplantation without antibody induction, starting within 12 hours of transplantation
▸ BY MOUTH
▸ Adult: Initially 75 micrograms/kg daily in 2 divided doses

Rejection therapy
▸ BY MOUTH
▸ Adult: Seek specialist advice

PROGRAF ® CAPSULES

Prophylaxis of graft rejection following liver transplantation, starting 12 hours after transplantation
▸ BY MOUTH
▸ Adult: Initially 100–200 micrograms/kg daily in 2 divided doses

Prophylaxis of graft rejection following kidney transplantation, starting within 24 hours of transplantation
▸ BY MOUTH
▸ Adult: Initially 200–300 micrograms/kg daily in 2 divided doses

Prophylaxis of graft rejection following heart transplantation following antibody induction, starting within 5 days of transplantation
▸ BY MOUTH
▸ Adult: Initially 75 micrograms/kg daily in 2 divided doses

Prophylaxis of graft rejection following heart transplantation without antibody induction, starting within 12 hours of transplantation
▸ BY MOUTH
▸ Adult: Initially 75 micrograms/kg daily in 2 divided doses

continued →

Allograft rejection resistant to conventional immunosuppressive therapy
▸ BY MOUTH
▸ Adult: Seek specialist advice

PROGRAF ® INFUSION

Prophylaxis of graft rejection following liver transplantation, starting 12 hours after transplantation when oral route not appropriate
▸ BY INTRAVENOUS INFUSION
▸ Adult: Initially 10–50 micrograms/kg daily for up to 7 days (then transfer to oral therapy), dose to be administered over 24 hours

Prophylaxis of graft rejection following kidney transplantation, starting within 24 hours of transplantation when oral route not appropriate
▸ BY INTRAVENOUS INFUSION
▸ Adult: Initially 50–100 micrograms/kg daily for up to 7 days (then transfer to oral therapy), dose to be administered over 24 hours

Prophylaxis of graft rejection following heart transplantation following antibody induction, starting within 5 days of transplantation
▸ BY INTRAVENOUS INFUSION
▸ Adult: Initially 10–20 micrograms/kg daily for up to 7 days (then transfer to oral therapy), dose to be administered over 24 hours

Prophylaxis of graft rejection following heart transplantation without antibody induction, starting within 12 hours of transplantation
▸ BY INTRAVENOUS INFUSION
▸ Adult: Initially 10–20 micrograms/kg daily for up to 7 days (then transfer to oral therapy), dose to be administered over 24 hours

Allograft rejection resistant to conventional immunosuppressive therapy
▸ BY CONTINUOUS INTRAVENOUS INFUSION
▸ Adult: Seek specialist advice (consult local protocol)

DOSE EQUIVALENCE AND CONVERSION
▸ For *Prograf*®: Intravenous and oral doses are **not** interchangeable due to differences in bioavailability. Follow correct dosing recommendations for the dosage form when switching formulations.

TACNI ®

Prophylaxis of graft rejection following liver transplantation, starting 12 hours after transplantation
▸ BY MOUTH
▸ Adult: Initially 100–200 micrograms/kg daily in 2 divided doses

Prophylaxis of graft rejection following kidney transplantation, starting within 24 hours of transplantation
▸ BY MOUTH
▸ Adult: Initially 200–300 micrograms/kg daily in 2 divided doses

Prophylaxis of graft rejection following heart transplantation following antibody induction, starting within 5 days of transplantation
▸ BY MOUTH
▸ Adult: Initially 75 micrograms/kg daily in 2 divided doses

Prophylaxis of graft rejection following heart transplantation without antibody induction, starting within 12 hours of transplantation
▸ BY MOUTH
▸ Adult: Initially 75 micrograms/kg daily in 2 divided doses

Allograft rejection resistant to conventional immunosuppressive therapy
▸ BY MOUTH
▸ Adult: Seek specialist advice

> **IMPORTANT SAFETY INFORMATION**
>
> MHRA/CHM ADVICE: ORAL TACROLIMUS PRODUCTS: PRESCRIBE AND DISPENSE BY BRAND NAME ONLY, TO MINIMISE THE RISK OF INADVERTENT SWITCHING BETWEEN PRODUCTS, WHICH HAS BEEN ASSOCIATED WITH REPORTS OF TOXICITY AND GRAFT REJECTION (JUNE 2012)
>
> Inadvertent switching between oral tacrolimus products has been associated with reports of toxicity and graft rejection. To ensure maintenance of therapeutic response when a patient is stabilised on a particular brand, oral tacrolimus products should be prescribed and dispensed by brand name only.
> - *Adoport*®, *Prograf*®, *Capexion*® and *Tacni*® are immediate-release capsules that are taken twice daily, once in the morning and once in the evening;
> - *Modigraf*® granules are used to prepare an immediate-release oral suspension which is taken twice daily, once in the morning and once in the evening;
> - *Advagraf*® is a prolonged-release capsule that is taken once daily in the morning.
>
> Switching between tacrolimus brands requires careful supervision and therapeutic monitoring by an appropriate specialist.
> Important: *Envarsus*® is not interchangeable with other oral tacrolimus containing products; the MHRA has advised (June 2012) that oral tacrolimus products should be prescribed and dispensed by brand only.

● CAUTIONS Increased risk of infections · lymphoproliferative disorders · malignancies · neurotoxicity · QT-interval prolongation · UV light (avoid excessive exposure to sunlight and sunlamps)

● INTERACTIONS → Appendix 1: tacrolimus

● SIDE-EFFECTS

GENERAL SIDE-EFFECTS
▸ **Common or very common** Alopecia · anaemia · anxiety · appetite decreased · arrhythmias · ascites · asthenic conditions · bile duct disorders · confusion · consciousness impaired · constipation · coronary artery disease · cough · depression · diabetes mellitus · diarrhoea · dizziness · dysgraphia · dyslipidaemia · dyspnoea · electrolyte imbalance · embolism and thrombosis · eye disorder · febrile disorders · fluid imbalance · gastrointestinal discomfort · gastrointestinal disorders · gastrointestinal inflammatory disorders · haemorrhage · hallucination · headache · hepatic disorders · hyperglycaemia · hyperhidrosis · hypertension · hyperuricaemia · hypotension · increased risk of infection · ischaemia · joint disorders · leucocytosis · leucopenia · metabolic acidosis · mood altered · muscle spasms · nasal complaints · nausea · nephropathy · nervous system disorder · oedema · oral disorders · pain · peripheral neuropathy · peripheral vascular disease · primary transplant dysfunction · psychiatric disorder · renal impairment · renal tubular necrosis · respiratory disorders · seizure · sensation abnormal · skin reactions · sleep disorders · temperature sensation altered · thrombocytopenia · tinnitus · tremor · urinary tract disorder · urine abnormal · vision disorders · vomiting · weight changes
▸ **Uncommon** Asthma · cardiac arrest · cardiomyopathy · cataract · central nervous system haemorrhage · chest discomfort · coagulation disorders · coma · dysmenorrhoea · encephalopathy · feeling abnormal · haemolytic anaemia · hearing impairment · heart failure · hypoglycaemia · hypoproteinaemia · influenza like illness · memory loss · multi organ failure · neutropenia · palpitations ·

pancreatitis · pancytopenia · paralysis · paresis · photosensitivity reaction · psychotic disorder · shock · speech disorder · stroke · ventricular hypertrophy

▸ **Rare or very rare** Fall · hirsutism · mobility decreased · muscle tone increased · muscle weakness · pancreatic pseudocyst · pericardial effusion · QT interval prolongation · severe cutaneous adverse reactions (SCARs) · sinusoidal obstruction syndrome · thirst · ulcer

▸ **Frequency not known** Agranulocytosis · neoplasm malignant · neoplasms · polyomavirus-associated nephropathy · progressive multifocal leukoencephalopathy (PML) · pure red cell aplasia

SPECIFIC SIDE-EFFECTS

▸ **With intravenous use** Anaphylactoid reaction (due to excipient)

SIDE-EFFECTS, FURTHER INFORMATION Cardiomyopathy has been reported to occur primarily in children with tacrolimus blood trough concentrations much higher than the recommended maximum levels. Patients should be monitored by echocardiography for hypertrophic changes—consider dose reduction or discontinuation if these occur.

● ALLERGY AND CROSS-SENSITIVITY [EvGr] Contra-indicated if history of hypersensitivity to macrolides. ⓜ

● CONCEPTION AND CONTRACEPTION Exclude pregnancy before treatment.

● PREGNANCY Avoid unless potential benefit outweighs risk—crosses the placenta and risk of premature delivery, intra-uterine growth restriction, and hyperkalaemia.

● BREAST FEEDING Avoid—present in breast milk (following systemic administration).

● HEPATIC IMPAIRMENT Manufacturer advises caution in severe impairment.
Dose adjustments Manufacturer advises consider dose reduction in severe impairment.

● MONITORING REQUIREMENTS

▸ After initial dosing, and for maintenance treatment, tacrolimus doses should be adjusted according to whole-blood concentration. Monitor whole blood-tacrolimus trough concentration (especially during episodes of diarrhoea)—consult local treatment protocol for details.

▸ Monitor blood pressure, ECG (for hypertrophic changes—risk of cardiomyopathy), fasting blood-glucose concentration, haematological and neurological (including visual) and coagulation parameters, electrolytes, hepatic and renal function.

● DIRECTIONS FOR ADMINISTRATION

▸ **With intravenous use** For *intravenous infusion (Prograf®)*; manufacturer advises give continuously in Glucose 5% *or* Sodium Chloride 0.9%. Dilute concentrate in infusion fluid to a final concentration of 4–100 micrograms/mL; give over 24 hours. Tacrolimus is incompatible with PVC.

● PATIENT AND CARER ADVICE Avoid excessive exposure to UV light including sunlight.
Driving and skilled tasks May affect performance of skilled tasks (e.g. driving).

● NATIONAL FUNDING/ACCESS DECISIONS
For full details see funding body website

NICE decisions

▸ **Immunosuppressive therapy for kidney transplant in adults [for immediate-release tacrolimus] (October 2017)** NICE TA481 Recommended with restrictions

▸ **Immunosuppressive therapy for kidney transplant in adults [for prolonged-release tacrolimus] (October 2017)** NICE TA481 Not recommended

Scottish Medicines Consortium (SMC) decisions

▸ Tacrolimus granules for suspension (*Modigraf®*) for prophylaxis of transplant rejection in adult and paediatric, kidney, liver or heart allograft recipients or for treatment of allograft rejection resistant to treatment with other

immunosuppressive medicinal products in adult and paediatric patients (December 2010) SMC No. 657/10 Recommended with restrictions

▸ Tacrolimus (*Envarsus®*) for prophylaxis of transplant rejection in adult kidney or liver allograft recipients and treatment of allograft rejection resistant to treatment with other immunosuppressive medicinal products in adult patients (April 2015) SMC No. 1041/15 Recommended

● MEDICINAL FORMS There can be variation in the licensing of different medicines containing the same drug.

Modified-release tablet

▸ Envarsus (Chiesi Ltd)
Tacrolimus (as Tacrolimus monohydrate)
750 microgram Envarsus 750microgram modified-release tablets | 30 tablet [PoM] £44.33 DT = £44.33
Tacrolimus (as Tacrolimus monohydrate) 1 mg Envarsus 1mg modified-release tablets | 30 tablet [PoM] £59.10 DT = £59.10
Tacrolimus (as Tacrolimus monohydrate) 4 mg Envarsus 4mg modified-release tablets | 30 tablet [PoM] £236.40 DT = £236.40

Granules
CAUTIONARY AND ADVISORY LABELS 13, 23

▸ Modigraf (Astellas Pharma Ltd)
Tacrolimus (as Tacrolimus monohydrate)
200 microgram Modigraf 0.2mg granules sachets sugar-free | 50 sachet [PoM] £71.30 DT = £71.30
Tacrolimus (as Tacrolimus monohydrate) 1 mg Modigraf 1mg granules sachets sugar-free | 50 sachet [PoM] £356.65 DT = £356.65

Modified-release capsule
CAUTIONARY AND ADVISORY LABELS 23, 25

▸ Advagraf (Astellas Pharma Ltd)
Tacrolimus (as Tacrolimus monohydrate)
500 microgram Advagraf 0.5mg modified-release capsules | 50 capsule [PoM] £35.79 DT = £35.79
Tacrolimus (as Tacrolimus monohydrate) 1 mg Advagraf 1mg modified-release capsules | 50 capsule [PoM] £71.59 DT = £71.59 | 100 capsule [PoM] £143.17 DT = £143.17
Tacrolimus (as Tacrolimus monohydrate) 3 mg Advagraf 3mg modified-release capsules | 50 capsule [PoM] £214.76 DT = £214.76
Tacrolimus (as Tacrolimus monohydrate) 5 mg Advagraf 5mg modified-release capsules | 50 capsule [PoM] £266.92 DT = £266.92

Solution for infusion
EXCIPIENTS: May contain Polyoxyl castor oils

▸ Prograf (Astellas Pharma Ltd)
Tacrolimus 5 mg per 1 ml Prograf 5mg/1ml solution for infusion ampoules | 10 ampoule [PoM] £584.51

Capsule
CAUTIONARY AND ADVISORY LABELS 23

▸ Adoport (Sandoz Ltd)
Tacrolimus 500 microgram Adoport 0.5mg capsules | 50 capsule [PoM] £42.92 DT = £61.88
Tacrolimus 1 mg Adoport 1mg capsules | 50 capsule [PoM] £55.69 DT = £80.28 | 100 capsule [PoM] £111.36
Tacrolimus 5 mg Adoport 5mg capsules | 50 capsule [PoM] £205.74 DT = £296.58

▸ Prograf (Astellas Pharma Ltd)
Tacrolimus 500 microgram Prograf 500microgram capsules | 50 capsule [PoM] £61.88 DT = £61.88
Tacrolimus 1 mg Prograf 1mg capsules | 50 capsule [PoM] £80.28 DT = £80.28 | 100 capsule [PoM] £160.54
Tacrolimus 5 mg Prograf 5mg capsules | 50 capsule [PoM] £296.58 DT = £296.58

8

Immune system and malignant disease

IMMUNOSUPPRESSANTS > MONOCLONAL ANTIBODIES

Canakinumab

20-Jun-2019

- **DRUG ACTION** Canakinumab is a recombinant human monoclonal antibody that selectively inhibits interleukin-1 beta receptor binding.

- **INDICATIONS AND DOSE**

Gouty arthritis [in patients whose condition has not responded adequately to treatment with NSAIDs or colchicine, or in those with contra-indications or intolerances to them, and in whom repeated courses of corticosteroids are inappropriate]

▸ BY SUBCUTANEOUS INJECTION

▸ Adult: 150 mg for 1 dose, in patients who respond, dose may be repeated after at least 12 weeks if symptoms recur, to be administered to the upper thigh, abdomen, upper arm or buttocks

Cryopyrin-associated periodic syndromes (specialist use only)

▸ BY SUBCUTANEOUS INJECTION

▸ Adult (body-weight 41 kg and above): 150 mg every 8 weeks, to be administered to the upper thigh, abdomen, upper arm or buttocks, additional doses may be considered if clinical response not achieved within 7 days—consult product literature

Tumour necrosis factor receptor associated periodic syndrome (specialist use only) | Hyperimmunoglobulin D syndrome (specialist use only) | Familial Mediterranean fever (specialist use only)

▸ BY SUBCUTANEOUS INJECTION

▸ Adult (body-weight 41 kg and above): 150 mg every 4 weeks, to be administered to the upper thigh, abdomen, upper arm or buttocks, a second dose may be considered if clinical response not achieved within 7 days—consult product literature

Still's disease (specialist use only)

▸ BY SUBCUTANEOUS INJECTION

▸ Adult: 4 mg/kg every 4 weeks (max. per dose 300 mg), to be administered to the upper thigh, abdomen, upper arm or buttocks

- **CONTRA-INDICATIONS** Active severe infection · leucopenia · neutropenia

- **CAUTIONS** History of recurrent infection · latent and active tuberculosis · predisposition to infection

CAUTIONS, FURTHER INFORMATION

▸ Vaccinations Patients should receive all recommended vaccinations (including pneumococcal and inactivated influenza vaccine) before starting treatment; avoid live vaccines unless potential benefit outweighs risk—consult product literature for further information.

- **INTERACTIONS** → Appendix 1: monoclonal antibodies

- **SIDE-EFFECTS**

▸ **Common or very common** Abdominal pain upper · arthralgia · asthenia · dizziness · increased risk of infection · leucopenia · neutropenia · pain · proteinuria · vertigo

▸ **Uncommon** Gastrooesophageal reflux disease

- **CONCEPTION AND CONTRACEPTION** Effective contraception required during treatment and for up to 3 months after last dose.

- **PREGNANCY** Manufacturer advises avoid unless potential benefit outweighs risk.

- **BREAST FEEDING** Consider if benefit outweighs risk—not known if present in human milk.

- **RENAL IMPAIRMENT** Limited information available but manufacturer advises no dose adjustment required.

- **PRE-TREATMENT SCREENING** Patients should be evaluated for latent and active tuberculosis before starting treatment.

- **MONITORING REQUIREMENTS**

▸ Manufacturer advises monitor full blood count including neutrophil count before starting treatment, 1–2 months after starting treatment, and periodically thereafter.

▸ Manufacturer advises monitor for signs and symptoms of infection (including tuberculosis) during and after treatment.

- **HANDLING AND STORAGE** Manufacturer advises store in a refrigerator (2–8 °C).

- **PATIENT AND CARER ADVICE** Manufacturer advises patients and carers should be instructed to seek medical advice if signs or symptoms suggestive of tuberculosis (including persistent cough, weight loss and subfebrile temperature) occur.

Driving and skilled tasks Manufacturer advises patients and carers should be counselled on the effects on driving and performance of skilled tasks—increased risk of dizziness and drowsiness.

- **MEDICINAL FORMS** There can be variation in the licensing of different medicines containing the same drug.

Solution for injection

▸ Ilaris (Novartis Pharmaceuticals UK Ltd)
Canakinumab 150 mg per 1 ml Ilaris 150mg/1ml solution for injection vials | 1 vial [PoM] £9,927.80

IMMUNOSUPPRESSANTS > MONOCLONAL ANTIBODIES > ANTI-LYMPHOCYTE

Basiliximab

17-Jul-2020

- **DRUG ACTION** Basiliximab is a monoclonal antibody that acts as an interleukin-2 receptor antagonist and prevents T-lymphocyte proliferation.

- **INDICATIONS AND DOSE**

Prophylaxis of acute rejection in allogeneic renal transplantation used in combination with ciclosporin and corticosteroid-containing immunosuppression regimens (specialist use only)

▸ BY INTRAVENOUS INJECTION, OR BY INTRAVENOUS INFUSION

▸ Adult: Initially 20 mg, administered within 2 hours before transplant surgery, followed by 20 mg after 4 days, dose to be administered after surgery, withhold second dose if severe hypersensitivity or graft loss occurs

- **CAUTIONS** Off-label use in cardiac transplantation—increased risk of serious cardiac side-effects

- **INTERACTIONS** → Appendix 1: monoclonal antibodies

- **SIDE-EFFECTS** Anaemia · capillary leak syndrome · constipation · cytokine release syndrome · diarrhoea · dyspnoea · electrolyte imbalance · headache · heart failure · hypercholesterolaemia · hypersensitivity · hypertension · hypotension · increased risk of infection · myocardial infarction · nausea · pain · peripheral oedema · post procedural wound complication · pulmonary oedema · respiratory disorders · skin reactions · sneezing · tachycardia · weight increased

- **CONCEPTION AND CONTRACEPTION** Adequate contraception must be used during treatment and for 16 weeks after last dose.

- **PREGNANCY** Manufacturer advises avoid—no information available.

- **BREAST FEEDING** Manufacturer advises avoid—no information available.

- **DIRECTIONS FOR ADMINISTRATION** For *intravenous infusion* (*Simulect*®), manufacturer advises give intermittently in

Glucose 5% or Sodium chloride 0.9%; reconstitute 10 mg with 2.5 mL water for injections then dilute to at least 25 mL with infusion fluid; reconstitute 20 mg with 5 mL water for injections then dilute to at least 50 mL with infusion fluid; give over 20-30 minutes.

- NATIONAL FUNDING/ACCESS DECISIONS
  For full details see funding body website
  NICE decisions
- ► Immunosuppressive therapy for kidney transplant in adults (October 2017) NICE TA481 Recommended

- MEDICINAL FORMS There can be variation in the licensing of different medicines containing the same drug.
  Powder and solvent for solution for injection
  ▸ Simulect (Novartis Pharmaceuticals UK Ltd)
  Basiliximab 10 mg Simulect 10mg powder and solvent for solution for injection vials | 1 vial [PoM] £758.69 (Hospital only)
  Basiliximab 20 mg Simulect 20mg powder and solvent for solution for injection vials | 1 vial [PoM] £842.38 (Hospital only)

Belimumab
29-Oct-2020

- ● INDICATIONS AND DOSE
  Adjunctive therapy in patients with active, autoantibody-positive systemic lupus erythematosus with a high degree of disease activity despite standard therapy
  ▸ BY INTRAVENOUS INFUSION
  ▸ Adult: 10 mg/kg every 2 weeks for 3 doses, then 10 mg/kg every 4 weeks, review treatment if no response within 6 months

---

IMPORTANT SAFETY INFORMATION

MHRA/CHM ADVICE: BELIMUMAB (*BENLYSTA*®): INCREASED RISK OF SERIOUS PSYCHIATRIC EVENTS SEEN IN CLINICAL TRIALS (APRIL 2019)

Clinical trials show an increased risk of depression, suicidal ideation or behaviour, or self-injury in patients with systemic lupus erythematosus on belimumab. Healthcare professionals should assess patients for these risks before starting treatment, monitor for new or worsening signs of these risks during treatment, and advise patients to seek immediate medical attention if new or worsening symptoms occur.

- CAUTIONS Do not initiate until active infections controlled · history or development of malignancy · predisposition to infection
- INTERACTIONS → Appendix 1: monoclonal antibodies
- SIDE-EFFECTS
  ▸ **Common or very common** Depression · diarrhoea · fever · hypersensitivity · increased risk of infection · infusion related reaction · leucopenia · migraine · nausea · pain in extremity
  ▸ **Uncommon** Angioedema · skin reactions · suicidal behaviours
  ▸ **Frequency not known** Progressive multifocal leukoencephalopathy (PML) · psychiatric disorder · self-injurious behaviour
  SIDE-EFFECTS, FURTHER INFORMATION Infusion-related side-effects are reported commonly, including severe or life-threatening hypersensitivity and infusion reactions. Premedication with an antihistamine, with or without an antipyretic may be considered.
- CONCEPTION AND CONTRACEPTION Manufacturer advises adequate contraception during treatment and for at least 4 months after last dose.
- PREGNANCY Avoid unless essential.
- BREAST FEEDING Avoid—present in milk in *animal* studies.
- RENAL IMPAIRMENT Caution in severe impairment—no information available.

- MONITORING REQUIREMENTS Delay in the onset of acute hypersensitivity reactions has been observed; patients should remain under clinical supervision for several hours following at least the first 2 infusions.
- DIRECTIONS FOR ADMINISTRATION For *intravenous infusion* (*Benlysta*®), manufacturer advises give intermittently in Sodium chloride 0.9%; reconstitute with water for injections (120 mg in 1.5 mL, 400 mg in 4.8 mL) to produce a solution containing 80 mg/mL; gently swirl vial for 60 seconds, then allow to stand; swirl vial (without shaking) for 60 seconds every 5 minutes until dissolved; dilute requisite dose with infusion fluid to a final volume of 250 mL and give over 1 hour.
- PRESCRIBING AND DISPENSING INFORMATION Belimumab is a biological medicine. Biological medicines must be prescribed and dispensed by brand name, see *Biological medicines* and *Biosimilar medicines*, under Guidance on prescribing p. 1; manufacturer advises to record the brand name and batch number after each administration.
- NATIONAL FUNDING/ACCESS DECISIONS
  For full details see funding body website
  NICE decisions
  ▸ Belimumab for treating active autoantibody-positive systemic lupus erythematosus (June 2016) NICE TA397 Recommended with restrictions
  Scottish Medicines Consortium (SMC) decisions
  ▸ Belimumab (*Benlysta*®) as add-on therapy in adult patients with active, autoantibody-positive systemic lupus erythematosus (SLE) with a high degree of disease activity (e.g. positive anti-dsDNA and low complement) despite standard therapy (May 2017) SMC No. 775/12 Recommended with restrictions

- MEDICINAL FORMS There can be variation in the licensing of different medicines containing the same drug.
  Powder for solution for infusion
  ▸ Benlysta (GlaxoSmithKline UK Ltd) ▼
  Belimumab 120 mg Benlysta 120mg powder for concentrate for solution for infusion vials | 1 vial [PoM] £121.50 (Hospital only)
  Belimumab 400 mg Benlysta 400mg powder for concentrate for solution for infusion vials | 1 vial [PoM] £405.00 (Hospital only)

IMMUNOSUPPRESSANTS › PURINE SYNTHESIS INHIBITORS

Mycophenolate mofetil
26-Nov-2020

- ● INDICATIONS AND DOSE
  Prophylaxis of acute rejection in renal transplantation (in combination with a corticosteroid and ciclosporin) (under expert supervision)
  ▸ BY MOUTH
  ▸ Adult: 1 g twice daily, to be started within 72 hours of transplantation
  ▸ BY INTRAVENOUS INFUSION
  ▸ Adult: 1 g twice daily for maximum 14 days, then transfer to oral therapy, to be started within 24 hours of transplantation

  Prophylaxis of acute rejection in cardiac transplantation (in combination with ciclosporin and corticosteroids) (under expert supervision)
  ▸ BY MOUTH
  ▸ Adult: 1.5 g twice daily, to be started within 5 days of transplantation

  Prophylaxis of acute rejection in hepatic transplantation (in combination with ciclosporin and corticosteroids) (under expert supervision)
  ▸ INITIALLY BY INTRAVENOUS INFUSION
  ▸ Adult: 1 g twice daily for 4 days, up to a maximum of 14 days, to be started within 24 hours of continued →

transplantation, then (by mouth) 1.5 g twice daily, the dose route should be changed as soon as is tolerated

CEPTAVA ®

Renal transplantation (specialist use only)
▶ BY MOUTH
▶ Adult: 720 mg twice daily, to be started within 72 hours of transplantation

DOSE EQUIVALENCE AND CONVERSION
▶ For *Ceptava*®: Mycophenolic acid 720 mg is approximately equivalent to mycophenolate mofetil 1 g but avoid unnecessary switching because of pharmacokinetic differences.

MYFORTIC ®

Renal transplantation (specialist use only)
▶ BY MOUTH
▶ Adult: 720 mg twice daily, to be started within 72 hours of transplantation

DOSE EQUIVALENCE AND CONVERSION
▶ For *Myfortic*®: Mycophenolic acid 720 mg is approximately equivalent to mycophenolate mofetil 1 g but avoid unnecessary switching because of pharmacokinetic differences.

IMPORTANT SAFETY INFORMATION
MHRA/CHM ADVICE: MYCOPHENOLATE MOFETIL, MYCOPHENOLIC ACID: UPDATED CONTRACEPTION ADVICE FOR MALE PATIENTS (FEBRUARY 2018)
Available clinical evidence does not indicate an increased risk of malformations or miscarriage in pregnancies where the father was taking mycophenolate medicines, however mycophenolate mofetil and mycophenolic acid are genotoxic and a risk cannot be fully excluded; for further information, see Conception and contraception and Patient and carer advice.

● CAUTIONS Active serious gastro-intestinal disease (risk of haemorrhage, ulceration and perforation) · children (higher incidence of side-effects may call for temporary reduction of dose or interruption) · delayed graft function · elderly (increased risk of infection, gastro-intestinal haemorrhage and pulmonary oedema) · increased susceptibility to skin cancer (avoid exposure to strong sunlight) · risk of hypogammaglobulinaemia or bronchiectasis when used in combination with other immunosuppressants

CAUTIONS, FURTHER INFORMATION
▶ Hypogammaglobulinaemia or bronchiectasis Measure serum immunoglobulin levels if recurrent infections develop, and consider bronchiectasis or pulmonary fibrosis if persistent respiratory symptoms such as cough and dyspnoea develop.

● INTERACTIONS → Appendix 1: mycophenolate

● SIDE-EFFECTS

GENERAL SIDE-EFFECTS
▶ **Common or very common** Acidosis · alopecia · anaemia · appetite decreased · arthralgia · asthenia · bone marrow disorders · chills · constipation · cough · depression · diarrhoea · drowsiness · dyslipidaemia · dyspnoea · electrolyte imbalance · fever · gastrointestinal discomfort · gastrointestinal disorders · gastrointestinal haemorrhage · headache · hyperglycaemia · hypertension · hypotension · increased risk of infection · insomnia · leucocytosis · leucopenia · malaise · nausea · neoplasms · oedema · oral disorders · pain · pancreatitis · paraesthesia · renal impairment · respiratory disorders · seizure · sepsis · skin reactions · tachycardia · thinking abnormal · thrombocytopenia · tremor · vomiting · weight decreased
▶ **Uncommon** Agranulocytosis
▶ **Frequency not known** Endocarditis · hypogammaglobulinaemia · malignancy · meningitis ·

neutropenia · polyomavirus-associated nephropathy · progressive multifocal leukoencephalopathy (PML) · pure red cell aplasia

SPECIFIC SIDE-EFFECTS
▶ **Common or very common**
▶ With intravenous use Hepatitis · muscle tone increased
▶ With oral use Anxiety · burping · confusion · dizziness · gout · hepatic disorders · hyperbilirubinaemia · hyperuricaemia · neuromuscular dysfunction · taste altered · vasodilation

SIDE-EFFECTS, FURTHER INFORMATION Cases of pure red cell aplasia have been reported with mycophenolate mofetil; dose reduction or discontinuation should be considered under specialist supervision.

● CONCEPTION AND CONTRACEPTION
Pregnancy prevention The MHRA advises to exclude pregnancy in females of child-bearing potential before treatment—2 pregnancy tests 8–10 days apart are recommended. Women should use at least 1 method of effective contraception before and during treatment, and for 6 weeks after discontinuation—2 methods of effective contraception are preferred. Male patients or their female partner should use effective contraception during treatment and for 90 days after discontinuation.

● PREGNANCY Avoid unless no suitable alternative—congenital malformations and spontaneous abortions reported.

● BREAST FEEDING Manufacturer advises avoid—present in milk in *animal* studies.

● RENAL IMPAIRMENT No data available in cardiac or hepatic transplant patients with renal impairment.

● MONITORING REQUIREMENTS Monitor full blood count every week for 4 weeks then twice a month for 2 months then every month in the first year (consider interrupting treatment if neutropenia develops).

● DIRECTIONS FOR ADMINISTRATION
▶ With intravenous use For *intravenous infusion* (*CellCept*®), manufacturer advises give intermittently in Glucose 5%; reconstitute each 500–mg vial with 14 mL glucose 5% and dilute the contents of 2 vials in 140 mL infusion fluid; give over 2 hours.

● PATIENT AND CARER ADVICE
Pregnancy prevention advice The MHRA advises that prescribers should ensure that female patients understand the need to comply with the pregnancy prevention advice, and they should be informed to seek immediate medical attention if there is a possibility of pregnancy; male patients planning to conceive children should be informed of the implications of both immunosuppression and the effect of the prescribed medications on the pregnancy. Bone marrow suppression Patients should be warned to report immediately any signs or symptoms of bone marrow suppression e.g. infection or inexplicable bruising or bleeding.

● NATIONAL FUNDING/ACCESS DECISIONS
For full details see funding body website
NICE decisions
▶ Immunosuppressive therapy for kidney transplant in adults [mycophenolate mofetil, when used as part of an immunosuppressive regimen, as an initial option] (October 2017) NICE TA481 Recommended
▶ Immunosuppressive therapy for kidney transplant in adults [mycophenolate sodium (*Ceptava*®, *Myfortic*®) as an initial treatment] (October 2017) NICE TA481 Not recommended

● MEDICINAL FORMS There can be variation in the licensing of different medicines containing the same drug. Forms available from special-order manufacturers include: oral suspension

Gastro-resistant tablet
CAUTIONARY AND ADVISORY LABELS 25
▸ Mycophenolate mofetil (Non-proprietary)
Mycophenolic acid (as Mycophenolate sodium)
180 mg Mycophenolic acid 180mg gastro-resistant tablets | 120 tablet PoM £96.72 DT = £96.72
Mycophenolic acid (as Mycophenolate sodium)
360 mg Mycophenolic acid 360mg gastro-resistant tablets | 120 tablet PoM £193.43 DT = £193.43
▸ Ceptava (Sandoz Ltd)
Mycophenolic acid (as Mycophenolate sodium) 180 mg Ceptava 180mg gastro-resistant tablets | 120 tablet PoM £77.38 DT = £96.72
Mycophenolic acid (as Mycophenolate sodium) 360 mg Ceptava 360mg gastro-resistant tablets | 120 tablet PoM £154.75 DT = £193.43
▸ Myfortic (Novartis Pharmaceuticals UK Ltd)
Mycophenolic acid (as Mycophenolate sodium) 180 mg Myfortic 180mg gastro-resistant tablets | 120 tablet PoM £96.72 DT = £96.72
Mycophenolic acid (as Mycophenolate sodium) 360 mg Myfortic 360mg gastro-resistant tablets | 120 tablet PoM £193.43 DT = £193.43

Tablet
▸ Mycophenolate mofetil (Non-proprietary)
Mycophenolate mofetil 500 mg Mycophenolate mofetil 500mg tablets | 50 tablet PoM £10.44 DT = £6.21
▸ CellCept (Roche Products Ltd)
Mycophenolate mofetil 500 mg CellCept 500mg tablets | 50 tablet PoM £82.26 DT = £6.21
▸ Myfenax (Teva UK Ltd)
Mycophenolate mofetil 500 mg Myfenax 500mg tablets | 50 tablet PoM £78.15 DT = £6.21

Oral suspension
EXCIPIENTS: May contain Aspartame
▸ CellCept (Roche Products Ltd)
Mycophenolate mofetil 200 mg per 1 ml CellCept 1g/5ml oral suspension sugar-free | 175 ml PoM £115.16 DT = £115.16

Powder for solution for infusion
▸ Mycophenolate mofetil (Non-proprietary)
Mycophenolate mofetil (as Mycophenolate mofetil hydrochloride) 500 mg Mycophenolate mofetil 500mg powder for concentrate for solution for infusion vials | 4 vial PoM £34.67 (Hospital only)
▸ CellCept (Roche Products Ltd)
Mycophenolate mofetil (as Mycophenolate mofetil hydrochloride) 500 mg CellCept 500mg powder for solution for infusion vials | 4 vial PoM £36.49 (Hospital only)

Capsule
▸ Mycophenolate mofetil (Non-proprietary)
Mycophenolate mofetil 250 mg Mycophenolate mofetil 250mg capsules | 100 capsule PoM £21.23 DT = £21.64 | 300 capsule PoM £56.25
▸ CellCept (Roche Products Ltd)
Mycophenolate mofetil 250 mg CellCept 250mg capsules | 100 capsule PoM £82.26 DT = £21.64
▸ Myfenax (Teva UK Ltd)
Mycophenolate mofetil 250 mg Myfenax 250mg capsules | 100 capsule PoM £78.15 DT = £21.64

IMMUNOSUPPRESSANTS ›T-CELL ACTIVATION INHIBITORS

| **Belatacept** | 01-Sep-2020 |

● INDICATIONS AND DOSE
Prophylaxis of graft rejection in adults undergoing renal transplantation who are seropositive for the Epstein-Barr virus
▸ BY INTRAVENOUS INFUSION
▸ Adult: (consult product literature)

● CAUTIONS Increased risk of acute graft rejection—with tapering of corticosteroid, particularly in patients with high immunologic risk · increased risk of infection · latent and active tuberculosis · risk factors for post-transplant lymphoproliferative disorder

● INTERACTIONS → Appendix 1: belatacept

● SIDE-EFFECTS
▸ **Common or very common** Acidosis · alopecia · anaemia · angina pectoris · arrhythmias · arterial fibrosis · cataract · chest pain · constipation · cough · Cushing's syndrome · decreased leucocytes · diabetes mellitus · diarrhoea · dizziness · dyslipidaemia · dyspnoea · ear pain · electrolyte imbalance · embolism and thrombosis · eye erythema · fatigue · fever · fluid imbalance · gastrointestinal discomfort · gastrointestinal disorders · haemorrhage · headaches · healing impaired · heart failure · hepatic disorders · hypercapnia · hyperglycaemia · hypertension · hypoproteinaemia · hypotension · increased risk of infection · intervertebral disc disorder · joint disorders · lethargy · leucocytosis · lymphocele · malaise · muscle complaints · muscle weakness · nausea · neoplasms · nerve disorders · neutropenia · oral disorders · oropharyngeal complaints · osteoarthritis · pain · paraesthesia · peripheral oedema · polyomavirus infections · pulmonary oedema · red blood cell abnormalities · renal disorders · renal tubular necrosis · respiratory disorders · scrotal disorders · sepsis · shock · skin reactions · stroke · sweat changes · syncope · thrombocytopenia · tinnitus · transplant rejection · tremor · urinary disorders · urine abnormalities · vascular disorders · ventricular hypertrophy · vertigo · vesicoureteric reflux · vision disorders · vomiting · weight changes
▸ **Uncommon** Acute coronary syndrome · adrenal insufficiency · agranulocytosis · alkalosis · anxiety · aortic valve disease · appetite decreased · arterial stenosis · atrioventricular block · attention deficit/hyperactivity disorder · bone disorders · bone fracture · breast mass · broken nails · cervical dysplasia · cholelithiasis · cognitive disorder · demyelination · depression · diabetic foot · diabetic ketoacidosis · disease recurrence · dysphonia · encephalopathy · endocarditis · eye inflammation · facial paralysis · facial swelling · feeling hot · fibrosis · flushing · haemolysis · hair changes · hearing impairment · hemiparesis · hypercoagulation · hypogammaglobulinaemia · infertility · inflammation · infusion related reaction · intermittent claudication · intracranial pressure increased · lymphangitis · memory loss · mood altered · nephritis · nephrosclerosis · pancreatitis · penile ulceration · post procedural haematoma · procedural complications · progressive multifocal leukoencephalopathy (PML) · pulmonary hypertension · renal tubular atrophy · restless legs · seasonal allergy · seizure · sexual dysfunction · sleep apnoea · sleep disorders · taste altered · tendon rupture · testicular pain · ulcer · vitamin D deficiency · vulvovaginal disorders · wound dehiscence

SIDE-EFFECTS, FURTHER INFORMATION Side effects are reported when used in combination with basiliximab, mycophenolate mofetil and corticosteroids.

● CONCEPTION AND CONTRACEPTION Adequate contraception must be used during treatment and for up to 8 weeks after last dose.

● PREGNANCY Use only if essential.

● BREAST FEEDING Avoid—no information available.

● PRE-TREATMENT SCREENING Patients should be evaluated for latent and active tuberculosis before starting treatment.

● MONITORING REQUIREMENTS Patients should be monitored for signs and symptoms of tuberculosis during and after treatment.

● PATIENT AND CARER ADVICE Patients should be advised to avoid excessive exposure to UV light including sunlight.

● NATIONAL FUNDING/ACCESS DECISIONS
For full details see funding body website

NICE decisions

▶ **Immunosuppressive therapy for kidney transplant in adults (October 2017) NICE TA481** Not recommended

● MEDICINAL FORMS There can be variation in the licensing of different medicines containing the same drug.

Powder for solution for infusion

▶ Nulojix (Bristol-Myers Squibb Pharmaceuticals Ltd)
Belatacept 250 mg Nulojix 250mg powder for concentrate for solution for infusion vials | 1 vial [PoM] £354.52 (Hospital only) | 2 vial [PoM] £709.04 (Hospital only)

1.1 Multiple sclerosis

Multiple sclerosis

14-Sep-2020

Description of condition

Multiple sclerosis is a chronic, immune-mediated, demyelinating inflammatory condition of the central nervous system, which affects the brain, optic nerves and spinal cord, and leads to progressive severe disability.

Relapsing-remitting multiple sclerosis is the most common pattern of the disease. It is characterised by periods of exacerbation of symptoms (relapses) followed by unpredictable periods of stability (remission). The severity and frequency of relapses varies greatly between patients, but on average occur once or twice per year. This clinical pattern often develops into *secondary-progressive* multiple sclerosis, with progressive disability unrelated to relapses. Most patients develop secondary progressive disease 6–10 years after onset.

Primary-progressive multiple sclerosis follows a gradual course, with the development of symptoms that worsen over time, without relapses and remissions.

Progressive-relapsing multiple sclerosis follows a course of steadily worsening neurological function from onset, in addition to acute relapses.

Disease activity in relapsing-remitting multiple sclerosis

Active disease is defined as at least two clinically significant relapses occurring within the last 2 years. *Highly active* disease is characterised by an unchanged/increased relapse rate or by ongoing severe relapses compared with the previous year, despite treatment with interferon beta p. 896. *Rapidly-evolving severe* relapsing-remitting multiple sclerosis is defined by two or more disabling relapses in 1 year, and one or more gadolinium-enhancing lesions on brain magnetic resonance imaging (MRI) or a significant increase in T2 lesion load compared with a previous MRI.

Aims of treatment

There is no cure for multiple sclerosis. The overall aims of treatment are to modify the course of the disease and manage symptoms, in order to improve quality of life. Treatment is aimed at reducing the frequency and duration of relapses and at preventing or slowing disability.

Drug treatment

Shared decision-making between the patient and their clinicians is particularly important in the treatment of multiple sclerosis, due to the unpredictability of the condition and the lack of evidence of long-term benefit of treatments. [EvGr] A discussion about treatment options, disease activity, risk, and benefit should take place to ensure that treatment choices are right for the patient and their circumstances. ⟨A⟩ The choice of drug also depends on the patient's disability status, individual tolerance, disease severity and disease activity (see *Disease activity in relapsing-remitting multiple sclerosis* above). [EvGr] Treatment should be initiated as early as possible, under the supervision of a specialist. ⟨A⟩

Note: NHS England (May 2014) has provided guidance on the use of interferon beta, glatiramer acetate p. 897, fingolimod p. 899 and natalizumab p. 905 for the treatment of multiple sclerosis in England, see *Useful resources* below. This Clinical Commissioning Policy outlines the funding arrangements and the criteria for initiating and discontinuing these treatment options. See also *National funding/access decisions*, under individual monographs for teriflunomide p. 906, dimethyl fumarate p. 898 and alemtuzumab p. 904.

Low levels of vitamin D are believed to be a risk factor for developing multiple sclerosis. Patients with diagnosed multiple sclerosis are usually given regular vitamin D after assessment of their serum levels of vitamin D, but there is insufficient evidence to support its use as a treatment for multiple sclerosis. [EvGr] Patients should not be offered vitamin D solely for the purpose of treating multiple sclerosis. ⟨A⟩

Relapsing-remitting multiple sclerosis

[EvGr] Disease-modifying drugs are the recommended treatment for patients presenting with *active* relapsing-remitting multiple sclerosis. Interferon beta and glatiramer acetate may be the preferred choice for some patients, due to their established safety profile, and the long term clinical experience associated with their use. ⟨A⟩ Peginterferon beta-1a p. 897 requires less frequent administration and is available as an alternative to the non-pegylated interferon beta therapies.

Teriflunomide and dimethyl fumarate are treatment options for patients with *active* disease. [EvGr] They may be preferred due to their oral route of administration. ⟨A⟩ There is insufficient evidence for the use of either drug to treat *highly active* or *rapidly-evolving severe* relapsing-remitting multiple sclerosis.

[EvGr] More active disease may be treated with natalizumab or alemtuzumab. The MHRA has released restrictions on the use of alemtuzumab due to reports of serious cardiovascular and immune-mediated reactions, see *Important safety information* in the alemtuzumab drug monograph. Natalizumab may be preferred due to the complex safety profile associated with alemtuzumab. Natalizumab is only recommended for the treatment of *rapidly-evolving severe* relapsing-remitting multiple sclerosis.

Fingolimod is also taken by the oral route and is the recommended treatment for patients with *highly active* disease. ⟨A⟩ The NHS England Clinical Commissioning Policy (see *Useful resources* below) advises that fingolimod is a suitable alternative for patients receiving natalizumab who are at high risk of developing progressive multifocal leukoencephalopathy (defined as patients previously exposed to the JC virus or who are receiving immunosuppressants or who have been receiving treatment with natalizumab for more than 2 years).

Secondary progressive multiple sclerosis

Currently, only interferon beta 1b is licensed for use in secondary progressive multiple sclerosis. Interferon beta 1b reduces the risk of relapse and of short-term relapse-related disability, but does not prevent the development of permanent physical disability or retard progression once it is established. Therefore its role in secondary progressive disease is limited.

Primary progressive multiple sclerosis

Currently there are no effective disease-modifying treatments licensed for primary progressive multiple sclerosis. Interferon beta [unlicensed indication] has been used, but there is limited evidence to support its use due to the lack of a significant reduction in disability progression.

Progressive-relapsing multiple sclerosis

There are no specific treatment options for this type of multiple sclerosis. None of the currently licensed disease-modifying drugs are recommended in non-relapsing progressive disease.

Management of symptoms

Other than episodes of neurological dysfunction, chronic symptoms (such as fatigue, spasticity, visual problems, and emotional lability) produce much of the disability in multiple sclerosis. EvGr Smoking may increase the progression of disability in multiple sclerosis, and Smoking cessation p. 519 should be encouraged. Ⓐ

Relapses

Suspected relapses should be referred to a specialist for diagnosis and treatment. EvGr Corticosteroids are recommended for reducing inflammation and accelerating recovery in acute relapses of relapsing-remitting multiple sclerosis. Oral methylprednisolone p. 717 is recommended as the first-line option. Intravenous methylprednisolone should be considered as an alternative if oral methylprednisolone has failed or is not tolerated or if hospitalisation is required. Ⓐ

Fatigue and impaired mobility

EvGr Regular exercise may have beneficial effects on mobility and fatigue in patients with multiple sclerosis, and should be encouraged. Cognitive behavioural techniques for fatigue should also be considered in combination with exercise. Amantadine hydrochloride p. 438 [unlicensed indication] may be used to treat fatigue related to multiple sclerosis. Vitamin B_{12} injections are **not** recommended as a treatment for fatigue in patients with multiple sclerosis. Ⓐ Fampridine below is licensed for the improvement of walking in patients with multiple sclerosis who have a walking disability. EvGr NICE do not consider it to be a cost-effective treatment and do not recommend its use. Ⓐ

Spasticity

Many factors may aggravate spasticity in multiple sclerosis, including constipation, infection, poor mobility aids, pressure ulcers, posture and pain. EvGr These causes should be managed appropriately. The first-line drugs for managing spasticity in multiple sclerosis are baclofen p. 1173 or gabapentin p. 332 [unlicensed indication] (for important safety information, released by the MHRA/CHM, on the use of antiepileptic drugs and the risk of suicidal thoughts and behaviour, see Epilepsy p. 321). They may be used cautiously in combination if the individual drugs are ineffective or if side effects prevent an increase in the dose of either drug. Tizanidine p. 1175 or dantrolene sodium p. 1400 are second-line options; benzodiazepines may be used as third-line therapy and may also be effective in treating nocturnal spasms. A 4-week trial of cannabis extract p. 1172 can be offered as adjunctive treatment for moderate to severe spasticity in multiple sclerosis if other pharmacological treatments are not effective. Treatment with cannabis extract should be initiated and supervised by a specialist. For funding/access information, see NICE clinical guideline: **Cannabis-based medicinal products** (see *Useful resources*). Ⓐ

Oscillopsia

EvGr Gabapentin [unlicensed indication] is the first-line treatment for oscillopsia (for important safety information, released by the MHRA/CHM, on the use of antiepileptic drugs and the risk of suicidal thoughts and behaviour, see Epilepsy p. 321.); memantine hydrochloride p. 320 [unlicensed indication] is the second-line option. Ⓐ

Emotional lability

EvGr Amitriptyline hydrochloride p. 392 [unlicensed indication] may be used to treat emotional lability in patients with multiple sclerosis. Ⓐ

Useful Resources

Clinical Commissioning Policy: disease modifying therapies for patients with multiple sclerosis. NHS England. May 2014. www.england.nhs.uk/commissioning/spec-services/npc-crg/group-d/d04/

Multiple sclerosis in adults: management. National Institute for Health and Care Excellence. Clinical guideline 186. October 2014.
www.nice.org.uk/guidance/cg186

Cannabis-based medicinal products. National Institute for Health and Care Excellence. Clinical guideline 144. November 2019.
www.nice.org.uk/guidance/ng144

> **Other drugs used for Multiple sclerosis** Cladribine, p. 951

CHOLINERGIC RECEPTOR STIMULATING DRUGS

▌Fampridine

19-Aug-2020

- **INDICATIONS AND DOSE**

Improvement of walking disability in multiple sclerosis (specialist use only)
▸ BY MOUTH
▸ Adult: 10 mg every 12 hours, discontinue treatment if no improvement within 2 weeks

- CONTRA-INDICATIONS History of seizures (discontinue treatment if seizures occur)
- CAUTIONS Atrioventricular conduction disorders · predisposition to seizures · sinoatrial conduction disorders · symptomatic cardiac rhythm disorders
- INTERACTIONS → Appendix 1: fampridine
- SIDE-EFFECTS
▸ **Common or very common** Anxiety · asthenia · balance impaired · constipation · dizziness · dyspepsia · dyspnoea · headache · insomnia · laryngeal pain · nausea · pain · palpitations · paraesthesia · tremor · urinary tract infection · vomiting
▸ **Uncommon** Seizure · skin reactions · tachycardia
- PREGNANCY Avoid—toxicity in *animal* studies.
- BREAST FEEDING Avoid—no information available.
- RENAL IMPAIRMENT Avoid if eGFR less than 80 mL/minute/1.73 m^2.
- PRESCRIBING AND DISPENSING INFORMATION Dispense in original container (pack contains a desiccant) and discard any tablets remaining 7 days after opening.
- NATIONAL FUNDING/ACCESS DECISIONS
For full details see funding body website
Scottish Medicines Consortium (SMC) decisions
▸ Fampridine (*Fampyra*®) for the improvement of walking in adult patients with multiple sclerosis (MS) with walking disability (EDSS [expanded disability status scale] 4 to 7) (April 2020) SMC No. SMC2253 Recommended
All Wales Medicines Strategy Group (AWMSG) decisions
▸ Fampridine (*Fampyra*®) for improvement of walking in adult patients with multiple sclerosis with walking disability (Expanded Disability Status Scale 4 to 7) (December 2019) AWMSG No. 3942 Recommended

- MEDICINAL FORMS There can be variation in the licensing of different medicines containing the same drug. Forms available from special-order manufacturers include: capsule
Modified-release tablet
CAUTIONARY AND ADVISORY LABELS 23, 25
▸ Fampyra (Biogen Idec Ltd)
Fampridine 10 mg Fampyra 10mg modified-release tablets | 28 tablet PoM £181.00 (Hospital only) | 56 tablet PoM £362.00 (Hospital only)

8

Immune system and malignant disease

IMMUNOSTIMULANTS > INTERFERONS

Interferon beta

26-Nov-2020

● INDICATIONS AND DOSE

AVONEX ® INJECTION

For relapsing, remitting multiple sclerosis | For a single demyelinating event with an active inflammatory process (if severe enough to require intravenous corticosteroid and patient at high risk of developing multiple sclerosis)
▸ BY INTRAMUSCULAR INJECTION
▸ Adult: (consult product literature)

BETAFERON ® INJECTION

For relapsing, remitting multiple sclerosis | For secondary progressive multiple sclerosis with active disease | For a single demyelinating event with an active inflammatory process (if severe enough to require intravenous corticosteroid and patient at high risk of developing multiple sclerosis)
▸ BY SUBCUTANEOUS INJECTION
▸ Adult: (consult product literature)

EXTAVIA ®

For relapsing, remitting multiple sclerosis | For secondary progressive multiple sclerosis with active disease | For a single demyelinating event with an active inflammatory process (if severe enough to require intravenous corticosteroid and patient at high risk of developing multiple sclerosis)
▸ BY SUBCUTANEOUS INJECTION
▸ Adult: (consult product literature)

REBIF ® CARTRIDGE

For relapsing, remitting multiple sclerosis | For a single demyelinating event with an active inflammatory process (if at high risk of developing multiple sclerosis)
▸ BY SUBCUTANEOUS INJECTION
▸ Adult: (consult product literature)

REBIF ® PRE-FILLED PEN AND SYRINGE

For relapsing, remitting multiple sclerosis | For a single demyelinating event with an active inflammatory process (if at high risk of developing multiple sclerosis)
▸ BY SUBCUTANEOUS INJECTION
▸ Adult: (consult product literature)

● CONTRA-INDICATIONS Severe depressive illness
CONTRA-INDICATIONS, FURTHER INFORMATION Consult product literature for further information on contra-indications.

● CAUTIONS History of cardiac disorders · history of depressive disorders (avoid in severe depression or in those with suicidal ideation) · history of seizures · history of severe myelosupression
CAUTIONS, FURTHER INFORMATION Consult product literature for further information on cautions.

● INTERACTIONS → Appendix 1: interferons

● SIDE-EFFECTS
GENERAL SIDE-EFFECTS
▸ **Common or very common** Alopecia · appetite decreased · arthralgia · asthenia · chills · confusion · depression · diarrhoea · fever · headaches · hypothyroidism · influenza like illness (decreasing over time) · insomnia · malaise · menstrual cycle irregularities · nausea · pain · skin reactions · vasodilation · vomiting · weight changes
▸ **Uncommon** Emotional lability · glomerulosclerosis · hepatic disorders · nephrotic syndrome · seizure · thrombocytopenia

▸ **Rare or very rare** Cardiomyopathy · dyspnoea · haemolytic uraemic syndrome · hyperthyroidism · thrombotic microangiopathy
▸ **Frequency not known** Anxiety · chest pain · dizziness · injection site necrosis · muscle weakness · palpitations · pulmonary arterial hypertension
SPECIFIC SIDE-EFFECTS
▸ **Common or very common**
▸ With intramuscular use Muscle complaints · musculoskeletal stiffness · neuromuscular dysfunction · rhinorrhoea · sensation abnormal · sweat changes
▸ With subcutaneous use Anaemia · tachycardia
▸ **Uncommon**
▸ With subcutaneous use Suicide attempt
▸ **Rare or very rare**
▸ With subcutaneous use Bronchospasm · pancreatitis · thyroid disorder
▸ **Frequency not known**
▸ With intramuscular use Angioedema · arrhythmias · arthritis · congestive heart failure · hypersensitivity · neurological effects · pancytopenia · psychosis · suicide · syncope · systemic lupus erythematosus (SLE)
▸ With subcutaneous use Abdominal pain · abscess · capillary leak syndrome · conjunctivitis · constipation · cough aggravated · ear pain · erectile dysfunction · eye disorder · hyperhidrosis · hypertension · increased risk of infection · lupus-like syndrome · lymphadenopathy · muscle tone increased · myalgia · paraesthesia · peripheral oedema · urinary disorders · visual impairment

● PREGNANCY Manufacturer advises use if clinically needed—possible toxicity in *animal* studies, but limited human data do not suggest an increased risk.

● BREAST FEEDING Manufacturer advises suitable for use during breast feeding—amount in milk probably too small to be harmful (recommendation also supported by specialist sources).

● HEPATIC IMPAIRMENT Manufacturer advises caution; avoid in decompensated liver disease.

● RENAL IMPAIRMENT Manufacturer advises caution in severe impairment.

● MONITORING REQUIREMENTS
▸ Liver Function Manufacturer advises monitor liver function at baseline, then 1 month, 3 months and 6 months after initiation of therapy. Consider dose reduction if alanine aminotransferase (ALT) exceeds 5 times the upper limit of normal (consult product literature).
▸ Thrombotic Microangiopathy Manufacturer advises patients should be monitored for clinical features of thrombotic microangiopathy (TMA), including thrombocytopenia, new onset hypertension, fever, central nervous system symptoms (e.g. confusion and paresis), and impaired renal function. Any signs of TMA should be investigated fully and, if diagnosed, interferon beta should be stopped immediately and treatment for TMA promptly initiated (consult product literature for details).
▸ Nephrotic Syndrome Manufacturer advises patients should also be monitored for signs and symptoms of nephrotic syndrome, including oedema, proteinuria, and impaired renal function—monitor renal function periodically. If nephrotic syndrome develops, treat promptly and consider stopping interferon beta treatment.
▸ Thyroid Function Manufacturer advises baseline thyroid function tests and repeat if signs or symptoms of thyroid dysfunction occur.

● PRESCRIBING AND DISPENSING INFORMATION Interferon beta is a biological medicine. Biological medicines must be prescribed and dispensed by brand name, see *Biological medicines* and *Biosimilar medicines*, under Guidance on prescribing p. 1; manufacturer advises to record the brand name and batch number after each administration.

NATIONAL FUNDING/ACCESS DECISIONS
For full details see funding body website

NICE decisions

▸ Beta interferons [*Avonex*®, *Extavia*®, *Rebif*®] and glatiramer acetate for treating multiple sclerosis (June 2018) NICE TA527 Recommended with restrictions

▸ Beta interferons [*Betaferon*®] and glatiramer acetate for treating multiple sclerosis (June 2018) NICE TA527 Not recommended

NHS restrictions

NHS England Clinical Commissioning Policy NHS England (May 2014) has provided guidance on the use of interferon beta p. 896 for the treatment of multiple sclerosis in England. An NHS England Clinical Commissioning Policy outlines the funding arrangements and the criteria for initiating and discontinuing this treatment option, see www.england.nhs.uk/commissioning/spec-services/npc-crg/group-d/d04.

● MEDICINAL FORMS There can be variation in the licensing of different medicines containing the same drug.

Solution for injection

EXCIPIENTS: May contain Benzyl alcohol

▸ Avonex (Biogen Idec Ltd)

Interferon beta-1a 12 mega unit per 1 ml Avonex 30micrograms/0.5ml (6million units) solution for injection pre-filled syringes | 4 pre-filled disposable injection PoM £654.00 | 12 pre-filled disposable injection PoM £1,962.00
Avonex 30micrograms/0.5ml (6million units) solution for injection pre-filled pens | 4 pre-filled disposable injection PoM £654.00 | 12 pre-filled disposable injection PoM £1,962.00

▸ Rebif (Merck Serono Ltd)

Interferon beta-1a 12 mega unit per 1 ml Rebif 22micrograms/0.5ml (6million units) solution for injection pre-filled syringes | 12 pre-filled disposable injection PoM £613.52
Rebif 22micrograms/0.5ml (6million units) solution for injection 1.5ml cartridges | 4 cartridge PoM £613.52
Rebif 8.8micrograms/0.2ml (2.4million units) solution for injection pre-filled syringes | 6 pre-filled disposable injection PoM 🛇
Rebif 22micrograms/0.5ml (6million units) solution for injection pre-filled pens | 12 pre-filled disposable injection PoM £613.52

Interferon beta-1a 24 mega unit per 1 ml Rebif 44micrograms/0.5ml (12million units) solution for injection pre-filled syringes | 12 pre-filled disposable injection PoM £813.21
Rebif 44micrograms/0.5ml (12million units) solution for injection pre-filled pens | 12 pre-filled disposable injection PoM £813.21
Rebif 44micrograms/0.5ml (12million units) solution for injection 1.5ml cartridges | 4 cartridge PoM £813.21

Powder and solvent for solution for injection

▸ Betaferon (Bayer Plc)

Interferon beta-1b 300 microgram Betaferon 300microgram powder and solvent for solution for injection vials | 15 vial PoM £596.63 DT = £596.63 (Hospital only)

▸ Extavia (Novartis Pharmaceuticals UK Ltd)

Interferon beta-1b 300 microgram Extavia 300microgram powder and solvent for solution for injection vials | 15 vial PoM £596.63 DT = £596.63 (Hospital only)

Peginterferon beta-1a   31-Jul-2018

● DRUG ACTION Peginterferon beta-1a is a polyethylene glycol-conjugated ('pegylated') derivative of interferon beta; pegylation increases the persistence of interferon in the blood.

● **INDICATIONS AND DOSE**

Treatment of relapsing, remitting multiple sclerosis
▸ BY SUBCUTANEOUS INJECTION
▸ Adult: (consult product literature)

● CONTRA-INDICATIONS Severe depression · suicidal ideation

● CAUTIONS History of cardiac disorders · history of depressive disorders (avoid in severe depression or in those with suicidal ideation) · history of seizures · history of severe myelosuppression

CAUTIONS, FURTHER INFORMATION Consult product literature for further information about cautions.

● SIDE-EFFECTS

▸ Common or very common Arthralgia · asthenia · chills · depression · fever · headache · hyperthermia · influenza like illness · myalgia · nausea · pain · skin reactions · vomiting

▸ Uncommon Seizure · thrombocytopenia

▸ Rare or very rare Glomerulosclerosis · haemolytic uraemic syndrome · injection site necrosis · nephrotic syndrome · thrombotic microangiopathy

▸ Frequency not known Pulmonary arterial hypertension

● CONCEPTION AND CONTRACEPTION Effective contraception required during treatment—consult product literature.

● PREGNANCY Do not initiate during pregnancy. Avoid unless potential benefit outweighs risk.

● BREAST FEEDING Avoid—no information available.

● HEPATIC IMPAIRMENT Manufacturer advises caution in severe hepatic impairment.

● RENAL IMPAIRMENT Caution in severe renal impairment.

● MONITORING REQUIREMENTS

▸ Monitor for signs of hepatic injury—hepatic failure has been reported rarely.

▸ Thrombotic microangiopathy Patients should be monitored for clinical features of thrombotic microangiopathy (TMA), including thrombocytopenia, new onset hypertension, fever, central nervous system symptoms (e.g. confusion and paresis), and impaired renal function. Any signs of TMA should be investigated fully and, if diagnosed, interferon beta should be stopped immediately and treatment for TMA promptly initiated (consult product literature for details).

▸ Nephrotic syndrome Patients should also be monitored for signs and symptoms of nephrotic syndrome, including oedema, proteinuria, and impaired renal function—monitor renal function periodically. If nephrotic syndrome develops, treat promptly and consider stopping interferon beta treatment.

● NATIONAL FUNDING/ACCESS DECISIONS
For full details see funding body website

NICE decisions

▸ Peginterferon beta-1a for treating relapsing–remitting multiple sclerosis (February 2020) NICE TA624 Recommended

● MEDICINAL FORMS There can be variation in the licensing of different medicines containing the same drug.

Solution for injection

▸ Plegridy (Biogen Idec Ltd)

Interferon beta-1a (as Peginterferon beta-1a) 126 microgram per 1 ml Plegridy 63micrograms/0.5ml solution for injection pre-filled pens | 1 pre-filled disposable injection PoM 🛇

Interferon beta-1a (as Peginterferon beta-1a) 188 microgram per 1 ml Plegridy 94micrograms/0.5ml solution for injection pre-filled pens | 1 pre-filled disposable injection PoM 🛇

Interferon beta-1a (as Peginterferon beta-1a) 250 microgram per 1 ml Plegridy 125micrograms/0.5ml solution for injection pre-filled pens | 2 pre-filled disposable injection PoM £654.00 (Hospital only)

IMMUNOSTIMULANTS ⟩ OTHER

Glatiramer acetate   06-Nov-2020

● DRUG ACTION Glatiramer is an immunomodulating drug comprising synthetic polypeptides.

● **INDICATIONS AND DOSE**

Multiple sclerosis [relapsing-remitting] (initiated under specialist supervision)
▸ BY SUBCUTANEOUS INJECTION
▸ Adult: 20 mg once daily, alternatively 40 mg 3 times a week, doses to be separated by an interval of at least 48 hours

- CAUTIONS Cardiac disorders
- SIDE-EFFECTS
- ▶ **Common or very common** Anxiety · appetite decreased · arrhythmias · asthenia · chest pain · chills · constipation · cough · depression · dyspepsia · dysphagia · dyspnoea (may occur within minutes of injection) · ear disorder · eye disorders · fever · gastrointestinal disorders · headaches · hyperhidrosis · hypersensitivity · increased risk of infection · joint disorders · local reaction · lymphadenopathy · nausea · neoplasms · neuromuscular dysfunction · oedema · oral disorders · pain · palpitations · rhinitis seasonal · skin reactions · speech disorder · syncope · taste altered · tremor · urinary disorders · vasodilation · vision disorders · vomiting · weight increased
- ▶ **Uncommon** Abnormal dreams · abscess · alcohol intolerance · angioedema · apnoea · arthritis · breast engorgement · burping · cataract · choking sensation · cholelithiasis · cognitive disorder · confusion · cyst · dry eye · dysgraphia · dyslexia · erythema nodosum · goitre · gout · haemorrhage · hallucination · hangover · hepatic disorders · hostility · hyperlipidaemia · hyperthyroidism · hypothermia · immediate post-injection reaction · inflammation · injection site necrosis · leucocytosis · leucopenia · mood altered · movement disorders · mucous membrane disorder · muscle atrophy · nephrolithiasis · nerve disorders · paralysis · pelvic prolapse · personality disorder · post vaccination syndrome · prostatic disorder · respiratory disorders · seizure · sexual dysfunction · skin nodule · splenomegaly · stupor · suicide attempt · testicular disorder · thrombocytopenia · urinary tract disorder · urine abnormal · varicose veins · vulvovaginal disorder
- PREGNANCY Manufacturer advises avoid—no information available.
- BREAST FEEDING Manufacturer advises caution—no information available.
- RENAL IMPAIRMENT No information available—manufacturer advises caution.
- NATIONAL FUNDING/ACCESS DECISIONS
  For full details see funding body website
  NICE decisions
- ▶ **Beta interferons and glatiramer acetate for treating multiple sclerosis (June 2018)** NICE TA527 Recommended with restrictions

  Scottish Medicines Consortium (SMC) decisions
- ▶ Glatiramer acetate 40 mg/mL (*Copaxone*®) for the treatment of relapsing forms of multiple sclerosis (MS) (December 2015) SMC No. 1108/15 Recommended
  NHS restrictions
  NHS England Clinical Commissioning Policy NHS England (May 2014) has provided guidance on the use of glatiramer acetate for the treatment of multiple sclerosis in England. An NHS England Clinical Commissioning Policy outlines the funding arrangements and the criteria for initiating and discontinuing this treatment option, see www.england. nhs.uk/commissioning/spec-services/npc-crg/group-d/d04.

- MEDICINAL FORMS There can be variation in the licensing of different medicines containing the same drug.
  Solution for injection
  - ▶ Brabio (Mylan)
    Glatiramer acetate 20 mg per 1 ml Brabio 20mg/1ml solution for injection pre-filled syringes | 28 pre-filled disposable injection PoM £462.56 DT = £513.95
    Glatiramer acetate 40 mg per 1 ml Brabio 40mg/1ml solution for injection pre-filled syringes | 12 pre-filled disposable injection PoM £462.56 DT = £513.95
  - ▶ Copaxone (Teva UK Ltd)
    Glatiramer acetate 20 mg per 1 ml Copaxone 20mg/1ml solution for injection pre-filled syringes | 28 pre-filled disposable injection PoM £513.95 DT = £513.95
    Glatiramer acetate 40 mg per 1 ml Copaxone 40mg/1ml solution for injection pre-filled syringes | 12 pre-filled disposable injection PoM £513.95 DT = £513.95

IMMUNOSUPPRESSANTS ›
IMMUNOMODULATING DRUGS

Dimethyl fumarate
04-Nov-2020

- DRUG ACTION Dimethyl fumarate has immunomodulatory and anti-inflammatory properties.

- **INDICATIONS AND DOSE**
  SKILARENCE ®
  Plaque psoriasis [moderate-to-severe] (under expert supervision)
  - ▶ BY MOUTH
    - ▶ Adult: Initially 30 mg once daily for 1 week, dose to be taken in the evening, then increased in steps of 30 mg every week for 3 weeks, then increased in steps of 120 mg every week for 5 weeks, for further information on the dose titration and administration schedule, advice on establishing a maintenance dose, and for dose adjustments due to side-effects, consult product literature; maximum 720 mg per day

  TECFIDERA ®
  Multiple sclerosis [relapsing-remitting] (initiated by a specialist)
  - ▶ BY MOUTH
    - ▶ Adult: Initially 120 mg twice daily for 7 days, then increased to 240 mg twice daily, for dose adjustments due to side effects—consult product literature

- CONTRA-INDICATIONS
  SKILARENCE ® Do not initiate if leucocyte count below 3×10^9/litre · do not initiate if lymphocyte count below 1×10^9/litre · do not initiate if pathological haematological abnormalities identified · severe gastro-intestinal disorders
- CAUTIONS Reduced lymphocyte count
  TECFIDERA ® Serious infection (do not initiate until infection resolved; consider suspending treatment if infection develops) · severe active gastro-intestinal disease
  SKILARENCE ® Significant infection (consider avoiding initiation until infection resolved and suspending treatment if infection develops)
- INTERACTIONS → Appendix 1: dimethyl fumarate
- SIDE-EFFECTS
- ▶ **Common or very common** Appetite decreased · asthenia · constipation · decreased leucocytes · diarrhoea · eosinophilia · feeling hot · flatulence · gastrointestinal discomfort · headache · leucocytosis · nausea · paraesthesia · skin reactions · vasodilation · vomiting
- ▶ **Uncommon** Dizziness · proteinuria
- ▶ **Rare or very rare** Acute lymphocytic leukaemia · pancytopenia
- ▶ **Frequency not known** Progressive multifocal leukoencephalopathy (PML) · renal failure
  SIDE-EFFECTS, FURTHER INFORMATION Severe prolonged lymphopenia reported, and patients are exposed to a potential risk of PML. Treatment should be stopped immediately if PML is suspected.
- PREGNANCY
  TECFIDERA ® Manufacturer advises avoid unless essential and potential benefit outweighs risk—toxicity in *animal* studies.
  SKILARENCE ® Manufacturer advises avoid—toxicity in *animal* studies.
- BREAST FEEDING Manufacturer advises avoid.
- HEPATIC IMPAIRMENT
  TECFIDERA ® Manufacturer advises caution in severe impairment (no information available).

SKILARENCE ® Manufacturer advises avoid in severe impairment (no information available).

● RENAL IMPAIRMENT

TECFIDERA ® Manufacturer advises caution in severe impairment—no information available.

SKILARENCE ® Manufacturer advises avoid in severe impairment—no information available.

● MONITORING REQUIREMENTS

▶ Manufacturer advises monitor full blood count before treatment initiation then every 3 months thereafter—consult product information for further information.

▶ Manufacturer advises monitor patient closely for features of progressive multifocal leukoencephalopathy (PML) (e.g. signs and symptoms of neurological dysfunction) and other opportunistic infections.

▶ Manufacturer advises monitor renal and hepatic function before treatment initiation and during treatment—consult product literature for further information.

▶ Manufacturer of *Tecfidera* ® advises perform a baseline MRI as a reference and repeat as required during treatment.

● PRESCRIBING AND DISPENSING INFORMATION

SKILARENCE ® The manufacturer of *Skilarence* ® has provided a *Healthcare Professional Guideline*, which includes important safety information on the risk of serious infections.

● PATIENT AND CARER ADVICE Manufacturer advises patients and their carers should be informed of the possibility of experiencing symptoms of flushing; they should also be advised to report symptoms of infection to their doctor. The MHRA recommends that patients and their carers should be counselled on the risk of progressive multifocal leukoencephalopathy and advised to seek immediate medical attention if symptoms develop.

● NATIONAL FUNDING/ACCESS DECISIONS

TECFIDERA ® For full details see funding body website

NICE decisions

▶ Dimethyl fumarate (*Tecfidera* ®) for treating relapsing-remitting multiple sclerosis (August 2014) NICE TA320 Recommended with restrictions

Scottish Medicines Consortium (SMC) decisions

▶ Dimethyl fumarate (*Tecfidera* ®) for the treatment of adult patients with relapsing remitting multiple sclerosis (April 2014) SMC No. 886/13 Recommended

SKILARENCE ® For full details see funding body website

NICE decisions

▶ Dimethyl fumarate for treating moderate-to-severe plaque psoriasis (September 2017) NICE TA475 Recommended with restrictions

Scottish Medicines Consortium (SMC) decisions

▶ Dimethyl fumarate (*Skilarence* ®) for the treatment of moderate to severe plaque psoriasis in adults in need of systemic medicinal therapy (April 2018) SMC No. 1313/18 Recommended with restrictions

● MEDICINAL FORMS There can be variation in the licensing of different medicines containing the same drug.

Gastro-resistant capsule

CAUTIONARY AND ADVISORY LABELS 21, 25

▶ Tecfidera (Biogen Idec Ltd)
Dimethyl fumarate 120mg Tecfidera 120mg gastro-resistant capsules | 14 capsule [PoM] £343.00
Dimethyl fumarate 240mg Tecfidera 240mg gastro-resistant capsules | 56 capsule [PoM] £1,373.00

Gastro-resistant tablet

CAUTIONARY AND ADVISORY LABELS 21, 25

▶ Skilarence (Almirall Ltd)
Dimethyl fumarate 30 mg Skilarence 30mg gastro-resistant tablets | 42 tablet [PoM] £89.04 DT = £89.04 | 210 tablet £445.20
Dimethyl fumarate 120 mg Skilarence 120mg gastro-resistant tablets | 90 tablet [PoM] £190.80 DT = £190.80 | 180 tablet [PoM] £381.60 DT = £381.60

Fingolimod

16-Nov-2020

● DRUG ACTION Fingolimod is a sphingosine-1-phosphate receptor modulator, which prevents movement of lymphocytes out of lymph nodes, thereby limiting inflammation in the central nervous system.

● INDICATIONS AND DOSE

Multiple sclerosis (initiated by a specialist)

▶ BY MOUTH

▶ Adult: 500 micrograms once daily

IMPORTANT SAFETY INFORMATION

MHRA/CHM ADVICE: FINGOLIMOD—NOT RECOMMENDED FOR PATIENTS AT KNOWN RISK OF CARDIOVASCULAR EVENTS. ADVICE FOR EXTENDED MONITORING FOR THOSE WITH SIGNIFICANT BRADYCARDIA OR HEART BLOCK AFTER THE FIRST DOSE AND FOLLOWING TREATMENT INTERRUPTION (JANUARY 2013)

Fingolimod is known to cause transient bradycardias and heart block after the first dose—see *Cautions*, *Contra-indications*, and *Monitoring* for further information.

MHRA/CHM ADVICE: FINGOLIMOD: NEW CONTRA-INDICATIONS IN RELATION TO CARDIAC RISK (DECEMBER 2017)

Fingolimod can cause persistent bradycardia, which can increase the risk of serious cardiac arrhythmias. New contra-indications have been introduced for patients with pre-existing cardiac disorders—see *Contra-indications* for further information.

MHRA/CHM ADVICE: MULTIPLE SCLEROSIS THERAPIES: SIGNAL OF REBOUND EFFECT AFTER STOPPING OR SWITCHING THERAPY (APRIL 2017)

A signal of rebound syndrome in multiple sclerosis patients whose treatment with fingolimod was stopped or switched to other treatments has been reported in two recently published articles. The MHRA advise to be vigilant for such events and report any suspected adverse effects relating to fingolimod, or other treatments for multiple sclerosis, via the Yellow Card Scheme, while this report is under investigation.

MHRA/CHM ADVICE: FINGOLIMOD: UPDATED ADVICE ABOUT RISK OF CANCERS AND SERIOUS INFECTIONS (DECEMBER 2017)

Fingolimod has an immunosuppressive effect and can increase the risk of skin cancers and lymphoma. Following a recent EU review, the MHRA has recommended the following strengthened warnings:

● re-assess the benefit-risk balance of fingolimod therapy in individual patients, particularly those with additional risk factors for malignancy—either closely monitor for skin cancers or consider discontinuation on a case-by-case basis

● examine all patients for skin lesions before they start fingolimod and then re-examine at least every 6 to 12 months

● advise patients to protect themselves against UV radiation exposure and seek urgent medical advice if they notice any skin lesions

● refer patients with suspicious lesions to a dermatologist

Fingolimod has also been associated with risk of fatal fungal infections and reports of progressive multifocal leukoencephalopathy (PML)—see *Monitoring* and *Side effects* for further information.

MHRA/CHM ADVICE: FINGOLIMOD (*GILENYA* ®): INCREASED RISK OF CONGENITAL MALFORMATIONS; NEW CONTRA-INDICATION DURING PREGNANCY AND IN WOMEN OF CHILDBEARING POTENTIAL NOT USING EFFECTIVE CONTRACEPTION (SEPTEMBER 2019)

An increased risk of major congenital malformations, including cardiac, renal, and musculoskeletal defects, has been associated with the use of fingolimod in pregnancy. Females of childbearing potential must use effective contraception during, and for 2 months after stopping, treatment. Healthcare professionals are advised that fingolimod is contra-indicated in pregnancy and that female patients should be informed of the risk of congenital malformations and given a pregnancy-specific patient reminder card. Pregnancy should be excluded before starting treatment, and pregnancy testing repeated at suitable intervals during treatment. Fingolimod should be stopped 2 months before planning a pregnancy. If a female taking fingolimod becomes pregnant, treatment should be stopped immediately, and the patient referred to an obstetrician for close monitoring. Exposed pregnancies should be enrolled on the pregnancy registry.

● CONTRA-INDICATIONS Active malignancies · baseline QTc interval 500 milliseconds or greater · cerebrovascular disease (including transient ischaemic attack) in the previous 6 months · decompensated heart failure (requiring inpatient treatment) in the previous 6 months · heart failure in the previous 6 months (New York Heart Association class III/IV) · increased risk for opportunistic infections (including immunosuppression) · myocardial infarction in the previous 6 months · second-degree Mobitz type II atrioventricular block or third-degree AV block, or sick-sinus syndrome, if the patient does not have a pacemaker · severe active infection · severe cardiac arrhythmias requiring treatment with class Ia or class III anti-arrhythmic drugs · unstable angina in the previous 6 months

● CAUTIONS Check varicella zoster virus status—consult product literature for further information · chronic obstructive pulmonary disease · elderly (limited information available) · history of myocardial infarction · history of symptomatic bradycardia or recurrent syncope · patients receiving anti-arrhythmic or heart-rate lowering drugs, including beta-blockers and heart rate-lowering calcium-channel blockers (seek advice from cardiologist regarding switching to alternative drugs, or appropriate monitoring if unable to switch) · pulmonary fibrosis · severe respiratory disease · severe sleep apnoea · significant QT prolongation (QTc greater than 470 milliseconds in women, or QTc greater than 450 milliseconds in men); if QTc 500 milliseconds or greater—see Contra-indications · susceptibility to QT-interval prolongation (including electrolyte disturbances) · uncontrolled hypertension

CAUTIONS, FURTHER INFORMATION
▸ **Washout period** A washout period is recommended when switching treatment from some disease modifying therapies—consult product literature for further information.
▸ **Bradycardia and cardiac rhythm disturbance** Fingolimod may cause transient bradycardia, atrioventricular conduction delays and heart block after the first dose. Fingolimod is not recommended in patients with the cardiovascular risks listed above unless the anticipated benefits outweigh the potential risks, and advice from a cardiologist (including monitoring advice) is sought before initiation.

● INTERACTIONS → Appendix 1: fingolimod

● SIDE-EFFECTS
▸ **Common or very common** Alopecia · arthralgia · asthenia · atrioventricular block · back pain · bradycardia · cough · decreased leucocytes · depression · diarrhoea · dizziness · dyspnoea · headaches · hypertension · increased risk of infection · myalgia · neoplasms · skin reactions · vision blurred · weight decreased
▸ **Uncommon** Macular oedema · nausea · seizures · thrombocytopenia
▸ **Rare or very rare** Posterior reversible encephalopathy syndrome (PRES)

▸ **Frequency not known** Autoimmune haemolytic anaemia · haemophagocytic lymphohistiocytosis · peripheral oedema · progressive multifocal leukoencephalopathy (PML)

SIDE-EFFECTS, FURTHER INFORMATION **Basal-cell carcinoma** Patients should be advised to seek medical advice if they have any signs of basal-cell carcinoma including skin nodules, patches or open sores that do not heal within weeks.

Progressive multifocal leukoencephalopathy (PML) and other opportunistic infections Patients should be advised to seek medical attention if they have any signs of PML or any other infections. Suspension of treatment should be considered if a patient develops a severe infection, taking into consideration the risk-benefit.

● CONCEPTION AND CONTRACEPTION Manufacturer advises females of childbearing potential should use effective contraception during treatment and for 2 months after last treatment—see *Important safety information* for further information.

● PREGNANCY Manufacturer advises avoid—teratogenic.

● BREAST FEEDING Avoid.

● HEPATIC IMPAIRMENT Manufacturer advises caution when initiating treatment in mild to moderate impairment; avoid in severe impairment.

● MONITORING REQUIREMENTS
▸ **All** patients receiving fingolimod should be monitored at treatment initiation, (first dose monitoring—before, during and after dose), and after treatment interruption (see note below); monitoring should include:
▸ **Pre-treatment**
  ● an ECG and blood pressure measurement before starting
▸ **During the first 6 hours of treatment**
  ● continuous ECG monitoring for 6 hours
  ● blood pressure and heart rate measurement every hour
▸ **After 6 hours of treatment**
  ● a further ECG and blood pressure measurement
▸ If heart rate at the end of the 6 hour period is at its lowest since fingolimod was first administered, monitoring should be extended by at least 2 hours and until heart rate increases.
▸ If post-dose bradyarrhythmia-related symptoms occur, appropriate clinical management should be initiated and monitoring should be continued until the symptoms have resolved. If pharmacological intervention is required during the first-dose monitoring, overnight monitoring should follow, and the first-dose monitoring should then be repeated after the second dose.
▸ If after 6 hours, the heart rate is less than 45 beats per minute, or the ECG shows new onset second degree or higher grade AV block, or a QTc interval of 500 milliseconds or greater, monitoring should be extended (at least overnight, until side-effect resolution).
▸ The occurrence at any time of third degree AV block requires extended monitoring (at least overnight, until side-effect resolution).
▸ In case of T-wave inversion, ensure there are no associated signs or symptoms of myocardial ischaemia—if suspected seek advice from a cardiologist.
▸ **Note**
▸ First dose monitoring as above **should be repeated** in all patients whose treatment is interrupted for:
  ● 1 day or more during the first 2 weeks of treatment
  ● more than 7 days during weeks 3 and 4 of treatment
  ● more than 2 weeks after one month of treatment
▸ If the treatment interruption is of shorter duration than the above, treatment should be continued with the next dose as planned.
▸ Manufacturer advises eye examination recommended 3–4 months after initiation of treatment (and before initiation of treatment in patients with diabetes or history of uveitis).

▸ Manufacturer advises skin examination for skin lesions before starting treatment and then every 6 to 12 months thereafter or as clinically indicated.

▸ Monitor hepatic transaminases before treatment, then every 3 months for 1 year, then periodically thereafter.

▸ Monitor full blood count before treatment, at 3 months, then at least yearly thereafter and if signs of infection (interrupt treatment if lymphocyte count reduced)—consult product literature.

▸ Monitor for signs and symptoms of haemophagocytic syndrome (including pyrexia, asthenia, hepato-splenomegaly and adenopathy—may be associated with hepatic failure and respiratory distress; also progressive cytopenia, elevated serum-ferritin concentrations, hypertriglyceridaemia, hypofibrinogenaemia, coagulopathy, hepatic cytolysis, hyponatraemia)—initiate treatment immediately.

▸ Manufacturer advises to monitor routine MRI for lesions suggestive of progressive multifocal leukoencephalopathy (PML), particularly in patients considered at increased risk; monitor for signs and symptoms of new neurological dysfunction.

● PRESCRIBING AND DISPENSING INFORMATION The manufacturer of *Gilenya®* has provided a *Prescriber's checklist*.

● PATIENT AND CARER ADVICE
Patient reminder card Patients should be given a patient reminder card.
    Female patients of childbearing potential should also be given a pregnancy-specific patient reminder card.

▪ NATIONAL FUNDING/ACCESS DECISIONS
For full details see funding body website

NICE decisions
▸ **Fingolimod for the treatment of highly active relapsing-remitting multiple sclerosis (April 2012)** NICE TA254
Recommended with restrictions

Scottish Medicines Consortium (SMC) decisions
▸ Fingolimod (*Gilenya®*) as a single disease modifying therapy in highly active relapsing remitting multiple sclerosis [in patients with high disease activity despite treatment with a beta-interferon with an unchanged or increased relapse rate or ongoing severe relapses as compared to the previous year] (September 2012) SMC No. 763/12 Recommended with restrictions
▸ Fingolimod (*Gilenya®*) as a single disease modifying therapy in highly active relapsing remitting multiple sclerosis [for patients with rapidly evolving severe relapsing remitting multiple sclerosis] (October 2014) SMC No. 992/14 Recommended with restrictions
▸ Fingolimod (*Gilenya®*) as a single disease modifying therapy in highly active relapsing remitting multiple sclerosis for patients with high disease activity despite treatment with at least one disease modifying therapy (April 2015) SMC No. 1038/15 Recommended

All Wales Medicines Strategy Group (AWMSG) decisions
▸ Fingolimod (*Gilenya®*) as a single disease modifying therapy in highly active relapsing remitting multiple sclerosis in adults with rapidly evolving severe relapsing remitting multiple sclerosis (January 2017) AWMSG No. 3135 Recommended

NHS restrictions
NHS England Clinical Commissioning Policy NHS England (May 2014) has provided guidance on the use of fingolimod for the treatment of multiple sclerosis in England. An NHS England Clinical Commissioning Policy outlines the funding arrangements and the criteria for initiating and discontinuing this treatment option, see www.england.nhs.uk/commissioning/spec-services/npc-crg/group-d/d04/.

● MEDICINAL FORMS There can be variation in the licensing of different medicines containing the same drug.

Capsule
▸ Gilenya (Novartis Pharmaceuticals UK Ltd) ▼
Fingolimod (as Fingolimod hydrochloride)
250 microgram Gilenya 0.25mg capsules | 28 capsule [PoM] £1,470.00
Fingolimod (as Fingolimod hydrochloride)
500 microgram Gilenya 0.5mg capsules | 7 capsule [PoM] £367.50 | 28 capsule [PoM] £1,470.00 DT = £1,470.00

Ozanimod

02-Dec-2020

● DRUG ACTION Ozanimod is a sphingosine-1-phosphate receptor modulator, which prevents movement of lymphocytes out of lymph nodes, thereby limiting inflammation in the central nervous system.

● INDICATIONS AND DOSE
Multiple sclerosis (initiated by a specialist)
▸ BY MOUTH
▸ Adult: Initially 0.23 mg once daily on days 1–4, then increased to 0.46 mg once daily on days 5–7, then increased to 0.92 mg once daily from day 8 onwards, the same dose escalation regimen is recommended when treatment is interrupted for 1 day or more during the first 14 days of treatment, for more than 7 consecutive days between days 15–28, or for more than 14 consecutive days after day 28. For interruptions of shorter duration, treatment may be continued with the next planned dose

● CONTRA-INDICATIONS Active malignancy · decompensated heart failure (requiring inpatient treatment) in the previous 6 months · heart failure (New York Heart Association class III or IV) in the previous 6 months · immunodeficiency · myocardial infarction in the previous 6 months · phototherapy with UV-B radiation or PUVA-photochemotherapy (increased risk of cutaneous neoplasm) · posterior reversible encephalopathy syndrome (suspected or confirmed) · progressive multifocal leukoencephalopathy · second-degree Mobitz type II atrioventricular (AV) block, third-degree AV block, or sick sinus syndrome, if the patient does not have a pacemaker · severe active infection · stroke (including transient ischaemic attack) in the previous 6 months · unstable angina in the previous 6 months

● CAUTIONS Administration of vaccinations · cerebrovascular disease · chronic obstructive pulmonary disease · diabetes mellitus (increased risk of macular oedema) · elderly (limited information available) · heart failure · immunosuppression or other risk factors for infection · myocardial infarction · patients receiving QT-prolonging or heart rate-lowering drugs, including beta-blockers and heart rate-lowering calcium-channel blockers · pulmonary fibrosis · recurrent syncope · retinal disease (increased risk of macular oedema) · risk of discontinuation effects, including disease rebound · second-degree Mobitz type I atrioventricular block · severe respiratory disease · severe untreated sleep apnoea · significant QT prolongation (QTc greater than 500 milliseconds) · sinus bradycardia (heart rate below 55 beats per minute) · uncontrolled hypertension · uveitis (increased risk of macular oedema)

CAUTIONS, FURTHER INFORMATION
▸ Bradycardia and cardiac rhythm disturbance [EvGr] Ozanimod may cause transient bradycardia, atrioventricular conduction delays and heart block after the first dose. It is not recommended in patients with a history of symptomatic bradycardia or recurrent syncope, uncontrolled hypertension, severe untreated sleep apnoea, or significant QT prolongation or other risk factors for QT

prolongation unless the anticipated benefits outweigh the potential risks, and advice from a cardiologist (including monitoring advice) is sought before initiation. ⟨M⟩

▸ Vaccinations [EvGr] Vaccination may be less effective during and for up to 3 months after treatment. Live attenuated vaccines should be avoided during and for 3 months after treatment; if they are required they should be given at least 1 month prior to initiation. Immunisation against varicella zoster is recommended prior to treatment in those without documented immunity. ⟨M⟩

● INTERACTIONS → Appendix 1: ozanimod

● SIDE-EFFECTS

▸ **Common or very common** Bradycardia · hypertension · increased risk of infection · lymphopenia · postural hypotension

● CONCEPTION AND CONTRACEPTION [EvGr] Exclude pregnancy before treatment; females of childbearing potential should use effective contraception during treatment and for 3 months after last dose. ⟨M⟩

● PREGNANCY [EvGr] Avoid—toxicity in *animal* studies. ⟨M⟩

● BREAST FEEDING [EvGr] Avoid—present in milk in *animal* studies. ⟨M⟩

● HEPATIC IMPAIRMENT [EvGr] Avoid in severe impairment (no information available). ⟨M⟩

● MONITORING REQUIREMENTS

▸ [EvGr] Patients with certain pre-existing cardiac conditions should be monitored for bradycardia for 6 hours after the first dose. An ECG should be obtained before dosing and after 6 hours ⟨M⟩—consult product literature for further information.

▸ [EvGr] Monitor blood pressure regularly during treatment.

▸ Monitor hepatic transaminases and bilirubin before initiation of treatment and then at months 1, 3, 6, 9 and 12 and periodically thereafter (interrupt treatment if significant liver injury occurs: liver transaminases above 5 times the upper limit of normal).

▸ Monitor full blood count before initiation and periodically during treatment (interrupt treatment if lymphocyte count reduced) ⟨M⟩—consult product literature.

▸ [EvGr] Eye examination recommended in patients with diabetes or history of uveitis or retinal disease before initiation and periodically during treatment (interrupt treatment if macular oedema occurs). ⟨M⟩

● PRESCRIBING AND DISPENSING INFORMATION The manufacturer of *Zeposia*® has provided a *Prescriber's Checklist*.

● PATIENT AND CARER ADVICE Patients should be advised to avoid exposure to sunlight without protection. Patients should be advised to promptly report symptoms of infection.
Patient reminder card Patients should be given a *Patient/Caregiver Guide*.
Female patients of childbearing potential should be given a *Pregnancy Reminder Card*.

● MEDICINAL FORMS There can be variation in the licensing of different medicines containing the same drug.
Capsule
EXCIPIENTS: May contain Gelatin

▸ Zeposia (Bristol-Myers Squibb Pharmaceuticals Ltd) ▼
Ozanimod (as Ozanimod hydrochloride) 230 microgram Zeposia 0.23mg capsules | 4 capsule [PoM] Ⓢ (Hospital only)
Ozanimod (as Ozanimod hydrochloride) 460 microgram Zeposia 0.46mg capsules | 3 capsule [PoM] Ⓢ (Hospital only)
Ozanimod (as Ozanimod hydrochloride) 920 microgram Zeposia 0.92mg capsules | 28 capsule [PoM] £1,373.00 (Hospital only)

Siponimod

03-Dec-2020

● DRUG ACTION Siponimod is a sphingosine-1-phosphate receptor modulator, which prevents movement of lymphocytes out of lymph nodes, thereby limiting inflammation in the central nervous system.

● INDICATIONS AND DOSE

Multiple sclerosis [secondary progressive, with active disease] (initiated by a specialist)

▸ BY MOUTH

▸ Adult: Initially 0.25 mg once daily on days 1 and 2, followed by 0.5 mg once daily on day 3, followed by 0.75 mg once daily on day 4, followed by 1.25 mg once daily on day 5, dose to be taken in the morning for the first 5 days; maintenance 2 mg once daily from day 6 onwards, in patients with a CYP2C9*1*3 or CYP2C9*2*3 genotype a reduced maintenance dose of 1 mg once daily is used from day 6 onwards. For dose adjustments based on lymphocyte count—consult product literature

● CONTRA-INDICATIONS Active malignancies · cryptococcal meningitis · decompensated heart failure (requiring inpatient treatment) in the previous 6 months · heart failure in the previous 6 months (New York Heart Association class III or IV) · immunodeficiency syndrome · macular oedema · myocardial infarction in the previous 6 months · patients homozygous for CYP2C9*3*3 genotype (poor metabolisers) · phototherapy with UV-B radiation or PUVA-photochemotherapy (increased risk of cutaneous neoplasms) · progressive multifocal leukoencephalopathy · second-degree Mobitz type II atrioventricular block or third-degree AV block, or sick-sinus syndrome, if the patient does not have a pacemaker · severe active infection · stroke (including transient ischaemic attack) in the previous 6 months · unstable angina pectoris in the previous 6 months

● CAUTIONS Administration of vaccinations (may be less effective during siponimod treatment—consult product literature for further information) · diabetes mellitus (increased risk of macular oedema) · elderly (limited information available) · exposure to sunlight (increased risk of cutaneous neoplasms) · first- or second-degree Mobitz type I atrioventricular block · heart failure (New York Heart Association class I and II) · myocardial infarction · patients receiving QT-prolonging or heart rate-lowering drugs, including beta-blockers and heart rate-lowering calcium-channel blockers (seek advice from cardiologist regarding switching to alternative drugs or appropriate monitoring) · recurrent syncope · retinal disease (increased risk of macular oedema) · risk of discontinuation effects, including disease rebound · severe sleep apnoea · significant QT prolongation (QTc greater than 500 milliseconds) · sinus bradycardia (heart rate below 55 beats per minute) · uncontrolled hypertension · uveitis (increased risk of macular oedema)

CAUTIONS, FURTHER INFORMATION

▸ Bradycardia and cardiac rhythm disturbance Siponimod may cause transient bradycardia, atrioventricular conduction delays and heart block after the first dose. Siponimod is not recommended in patients with a history of symptomatic bradycardia or recurrent syncope, uncontrolled hypertension, severe untreated sleep apnoea, or significant QT prolongation unless the anticipated benefits outweigh the potential risks, and advice from a cardiologist (including monitoring advice) is sought before initiation.

● INTERACTIONS → Appendix 1: siponimod

● SIDE-EFFECTS

▸ **Common or very common** Arrhythmias · asthenia · cardiac conduction disorders · diarrhoea · dizziness · headache ·

hypertension · increased risk of infection · lymphopenia · macular oedema · nausea · neoplasms · pain in extremity · peripheral oedema · seizure · tremor
▸ **Frequency not known** Meningitis cryptococcal · vision disorders
● ALLERGY AND CROSS-SENSITIVITY Manufacturer advises contra-indicated in patients with hypersensitivity to peanut or soya products.
● CONCEPTION AND CONTRACEPTION Manufacturer advises exclude pregnancy before treatment; females of childbearing potential should use effective contraception during treatment and for 10 days after last dose.
● PREGNANCY Manufacturer advises avoid—toxicity in *animal* studies.
● BREAST FEEDING Manufacturer advises avoid—present in milk in *animal* studies.
● HEPATIC IMPAIRMENT Manufacturer advises caution when initiating treatment in mild to moderate impairment; avoid in severe impairment.
● PRE-TREATMENT SCREENING Manufacturer advises CYP2C9 genotyping before treatment initiation—consult product literature. Manufacturer advises check varicella zoster virus status in patients with unconfirmed or incomplete vaccination history. A full course of vaccination against varicella zoster is required 1 month before initiating treatment in antibody-negative patients.
● MONITORING REQUIREMENTS
▸ Manufacturer advises regular monitoring of heart rate, particularly during treatment initiation, and of blood pressure.
▸ Manufacturer advises patients with certain pre-existing cardiac conditions should be monitored for bradycardia for 6 hours after the first dose. An ECG should be obtained before dosing and after 6 hours—consult product literature for further information.
▸ Manufacturer advises monitor full blood count before initiation and periodically during treatment (reduce dosage or interrupt treatment if lymphocyte count reduced)—consult product literature.
▸ Manufacturer advises monitor hepatic transaminases and bilirubin before initiation of treatment and then as clinically indicated (interrupt treatment if significant liver injury occurs).
▸ Manufacturer advises eye examination recommended 3–4 months after initiation of treatment (and before initiation of treatment in patients with diabetes or history of uveitis or retinal disease).
● PRESCRIBING AND DISPENSING INFORMATION The manufacturer of *Mayzent*® has provided a *Physician Education Pack*.
● PATIENT AND CARER ADVICE Manufacturer advises patients to avoid exposure to sunlight without protection. Manufacturer advises patients should promptly report symptoms of infection.
Missed doses Manufacturer advises if a dose is missed during treatment initiation (days 1–6), the initial titration regimen should be restarted. If a maintenance dose is missed (after day 6), the missed dose should not be taken, and the next dose should be taken at the normal time. If 4 or more consecutive doses are missed, the initial titration regimen should be used to restart treatment.
Driving and skilled tasks Manufacturer advises patients should be counselled on the effects on driving and performance of skilled tasks—increased risk of dizziness during treatment initiation.
● NATIONAL FUNDING/ACCESS DECISIONS For full details see funding body website
NICE decisions
▸ **Siponimod for treating secondary progressive multiple sclerosis (November 2020)** NICE TA656 Recommended

Scottish Medicines Consortium (SMC) decisions
▸ **Siponimod (***Mayzent***®) for the treatment of adult patients with secondary progressive multiple sclerosis (SPMS) with active disease evidenced by relapses or imaging features of inflammatory activity (October 2020)** SMC No. SMC2265 Recommended

● MEDICINAL FORMS There can be variation in the licensing of different medicines containing the same drug.
Tablet
EXCIPIENTS: May contain Lecithin
▸ Mayzent (Novartis Pharmaceuticals UK Ltd) ▼
Siponimod (as Siponimod fumaric acid) 250 microgram Mayzent 0.25mg tablets | 12 tablet [PoM] £294.32 (Hospital only) | 120 tablet [PoM] £1,765.96 (Hospital only)
Siponimod (as Siponimod fumaric acid) 2 mg Mayzent 2mg tablets | 28 tablet [PoM] £1,648.23 (Hospital only)

IMMUNOSUPPRESSANTS ❭ MONOCLONAL ANTIBODIES ❭ ANTI-LYMPHOCYTE

Anti-lymphocyte monoclonal antibodies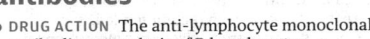

● DRUG ACTION The anti-lymphocyte monoclonal antibodies cause lysis of B lymphocytes.

> **IMPORTANT SAFETY INFORMATION**
> All anti-lymphocyte monoclonal antibodies should be given under the supervision of an experienced specialist, in an environment where full resuscitation facilities are immediately available.

● SIDE-EFFECTS
▸ **Common or very common** Alopecia · anaemia · anaphylactic reaction · arthralgia · asthenia · conjunctivitis · constipation · cough · depression · diarrhoea · fever · headache · hypersensitivity (discontinue permanently) · increased risk of infection · infusion related reaction · leucopenia · myocardial infarction · neutropenia · night sweats · pain · thrombocytopenia · vomiting
▸ **Uncommon** Haemolytic anaemia · progressive multifocal leukoencephalopathy (PML)
▸ **Rare or very rare** Hepatitis B reactivation
SIDE-EFFECTS, FURTHER INFORMATION **Infusion-related side-effects** In rare cases infusion reactions may be fatal. Infusion-related side-effects occur predominantly during the first infusion. Patients should receive premedication before administration of anti-lymphocyte monoclonal antibodies to reduce these effects—consult product literature for details of individual regimens. The infusion may have to be stopped temporarily and the infusion-related effects treated—consult product literature for appropriate management.
Cytokine release syndrome Fatalities following severe cytokine release syndrome (characterised by severe dyspnoea) and associated with features of tumour lysis syndrome have occurred after infusions of anti-lymphocyte monoclonal antibodies. Patients with a high tumour burden as well as those with pulmonary insufficiency or infiltration are at increased risk and should be monitored very closely (and a slower rate of infusion considered).
● PRE-TREATMENT SCREENING All patients should be screened for hepatitis B before treatment.
● MONITORING REQUIREMENTS Patients should also be monitored for cytopenias—consult product literature for specific recommendations.

8 Immune system and malignant disease

Alemtuzumab

06-Oct-2020

F 903

● **INDICATIONS AND DOSE**

Treatment of adults with relapsing-remitting multiple sclerosis with active disease defined by clinical or imaging features

▶ BY INTRAVENOUS INFUSION
▶ Adult: (consult product literature)

● UNLICENSED USE Although no longer licensed for oncological and transplant indications, alemtuzumab is also available through a patient access programme for these indications.

IMPORTANT SAFETY INFORMATION

MHRA/CHM ADVICE (UPDATED FEBRUARY 2020): *LEMTRADA*® (ALEMTUZUMAB): UPDATED RESTRICTIONS AND STRENGTHENED MONITORING REQUIREMENTS FOLLOWING REVIEW OF SERIOUS CARDIOVASCULAR AND IMMUNE-MEDIATED REACTIONS

Following a review of alemtuzumab by the European Medicines Agency, a revised indication, additional contra-indications (see *Contra-indications*), and strengthened monitoring requirements before, during, and after treatment have been recommended. Healthcare professionals are advised that alemtuzumab should only be used for the treatment of patients with relapsing-remitting multiple sclerosis (RRMS) that is highly active despite a full and adequate course of treatment with at least one disease-modifying agent, or in patients with rapidly evolving severe RRMS.

Healthcare professionals should monitor patients before, during, and after treatment for cardiovascular reactions and non-immune thrombocytopenia (see *Monitoring requirements*). Patients should be informed of serious cardiovascular symptoms that can occur within a few days of treatment, signs of autoimmune disorders that can occur 48 months or more after treatment, and symptoms of hepatic injury; immediate medical attention should be sought by patients if they experience any of these symptoms.

● CONTRA-INDICATIONS Angina (past history) · autoimmune diseases (excluding multiple sclerosis) · cervicocephalic arterial dissection (past history) · clotting abnormalities (including patients on anticoagulant therapy) · human immunodeficiency virus · hypertension (uncontrolled) · myocardial infarction (past history) · severe active infection (until complete resolution) · stroke (past history)

● CAUTIONS Hepatitis B carriers · hepatitis C carriers · not recommended for inactive disease · not recommended for stable disease · patients should receive oral prophylaxis for herpes infection starting on the first day of treatment and continuing for at least a month following each treatment course · pretreatment before administration is required (consult product literature)

CAUTIONS, FURTHER INFORMATION For full details of cautions, consult product literature.

▶ Autoimmune mediated conditions The risk of autoimmune mediated conditions may increase during treatment, including immune thrombocytopenic purpura, thyroid disorders, nephropathies, cytopenias, autoimmune hepatitis, and acquired haemophilia A. Manufacturer advises monitoring for autoimmune mediated conditions throughout the course of treatment (consult product literature).

● INTERACTIONS → Appendix 1: monoclonal antibodies

● SIDE-EFFECTS

▶ **Common or very common** Abdominal pain · anxiety · asthma · cytokine release syndrome · endocrine ophthalmopathy · goitre · haemorrhage · hiccups · hyperhidrosis · hyperthyroidism · hypothyroidism ·

influenza like illness · leucocytosis · lymphadenopathy · lymphopenia · malaise · meningitis · menstrual cycle irregularities · multiple sclerosis exacerbated · muscle complaints · muscle weakness · neoplasms · nephropathy · oropharyngeal pain · peripheral oedema · sensation abnormal · skin reactions · stomatitis · thyroiditis · tremor · urine abnormalities · vertigo · vision disorders

▶ **Uncommon** Acquired haemophilia · appetite decreased · cervical dysplasia · dry mouth · dysphagia · ear pain · facial swelling · gallbladder disorders · gastrointestinal disorders · Goodpasture's syndrome · limb discomfort · musculoskeletal stiffness · nephrolithiasis · pancytopenia · pneumonitis · tension headache · throat irritation · weight changes

▶ **Rare or very rare** Haemophagocytic lymphohistiocytosis

▶ **Frequency not known** Artery dissection · cerebrovascular insufficiency · hepatitis autoimmune (including fatal cases) · liver injury · myocardial ischaemia · reactivation of infections · thyroid disorder autoimmune

● CONCEPTION AND CONTRACEPTION Women of childbearing potential should use effective contraception during and for 4 months after treatment.

● PREGNANCY Manufacturer advises avoid unless potential benefit outweighs risk—toxicity in *animal* studies. Autoimmune thyroid disease during treatment may affect fetus (consult product literature).

● BREAST FEEDING Manufacturer advises avoid during and for 4 months after each treatment course unless potential benefit outweighs risk.

● PRE-TREATMENT SCREENING Screening patients at high risk of hepatitis B or C is recommended before treatment. All patients should be evaluated for active or latent tuberculosis before starting treatment.

● MONITORING REQUIREMENTS

▶ The MHRA advises to check liver, thyroid, and kidney function, urinalysis with microscopy, blood counts, and vital signs (including blood pressure, heart rate, and ECG) before infusions.

▶ The MHRA advises monitor blood pressure and heart rate continuously or at least once every hour during infusions—discontinue infusion if severe adverse reactions occur.

▶ The MHRA advises monitor patients for infusion-related reactions for at least 2 hours after infusions; patients should be informed of the risk of delayed infusion-related reactions and to seek immediate medical attention if these occur.

▶ The MHRA advises monitor platelet counts after treatment—consult product literature.

▶ For further information on monitoring, see *Important safety information*.

▶ HPV screening should be carried out annually in female patients.

● PRESCRIBING AND DISPENSING INFORMATION All patients should receive oral prophylaxis for herpes infection starting on the first day of treatment and continuing for at least a month following each treatment course.

● PATIENT AND CARER ADVICE Patients should be provided with a patient alert card and patient guide.

● NATIONAL FUNDING/ACCESS DECISIONS
For full details see funding body website

NICE decisions

▶ Alemtuzumab for treating relapsing-remitting multiple sclerosis (May 2014) NICE TA312 Recommended

● MEDICINAL FORMS There can be variation in the licensing of different medicines containing the same drug.

Solution for infusion

▶ Lemtrada (Genzyme Therapeutics Ltd) ▼
Alemtuzumab 10 mg per 1 ml Lemtrada 12mg/1.2ml concentrate for solution for infusion vials | 1 vial [PoM] £7,045.00 (Hospital only)

Natalizumab

▶ 903

06-Oct-2020

● INDICATIONS AND DOSE

Highly active relapsing-remitting multiple sclerosis despite treatment with at least one disease-modifying drug, or those patients with rapidly-evolving severe relapsing-remitting multiple sclerosis (initiated under specialist supervision)
▶ BY INTRAVENOUS INFUSION
▶ Adult 18-65 years: 300 mg every 4 weeks, consider discontinuing treatment if no response after 6 months

● CONTRA-INDICATIONS Active infection · active malignancies (except cutaneous basal cell carcinoma) · immunosuppression · progressive multifocal leucoencephalopathy

● CAUTIONS
Progressive Multifocal Leucoencephalopathy Natalizumab is associated with an increased risk of opportunistic infection and progressive multifocal leucoencephalopathy (PML) caused by JC virus. The risk of developing PML increases with the presence of anti-JCV antibodies, previous use of immunosuppressant therapy, and treatment duration (especially beyond 2 years of treatment). Patients with all three risk factors should only be treated with natalizumab if the benefits of treatment outweigh the risks. Manufacturer advises treatment should be suspended until PML has been excluded. Manufacturer also advises if a patient develops an opportunistic infection or PML, natalizumab should be permanently discontinued.
For information on cautions consult product literature.

● INTERACTIONS → Appendix 1: monoclonal antibodies

● SIDE-EFFECTS Acute retinal necrosis · basophil count increased · eosinophilia · hyperbilirubinaemia · JC virus granule cell neuronopathy · liver injury · meningitis herpes · nucleated red cells

SIDE-EFFECTS, FURTHER INFORMATION **Progressive Multifocal Leukoencephalopathy (PML)** If suspected, treatment should be suspended until PML has been excluded. If a patient develops an opportunistic infection or PML, natalizumab should be permanently discontinued.
Liver injury Discontinue treatment if significant liver injury occurs.
Infusion-related reactions Infusion-related reactions including dizziness, nausea, urticaria, chills, vomiting and flushing have been reported either during infusion or within 1 hour after completion of infusion.

● PREGNANCY Avoid unless essential—toxicity in *animal* studies.

● BREAST FEEDING Present in milk in *animal* studies—avoid.

● PRE-TREATMENT SCREENING
Progressive Multifocal Leucoencephalopathy A magnetic resonance image (MRI) scan is recommended before starting treatment with natalizumab.
Testing for serum anti-JCV antibodies before starting treatment or in those with unknown antibody status already receiving natalizumab is recommended and should be repeated every 6 months (consult product literature for full details).

● MONITORING REQUIREMENTS
▶ Monitor liver function.
▶ Progressive Multifocal Leucoencephalopathy A magnetic resonance image (MRI) scan is recommended annually. Patients should be monitored for new or worsening neurological symptoms, and for cognitive and psychiatric signs of PML.
All patients should continue to be monitored for signs and symptoms that may be suggestive of PML for approximately 6 months following discontinuation of treatment.

▶ Hypersensitivity reactions Patients should be observed for hypersensitivity reactions, including anaphylaxis, during the infusion and for 1 hour after completion of the infusion.

● DIRECTIONS FOR ADMINISTRATION For *intravenous infusion* (*Tysabri*®), manufacturer advises give intermittently in Sodium chloride 0.9%; dilute 300 mg in 100 ml infusion fluid; gently invert to mix, do not shake. Use within 8 hours of dilution and give over 1 hour.

● PATIENT AND CARER ADVICE
Hypersensitivity reactions Patients should be told the importance of uninterrupted dosing, particularly in the early months of treatment (intermittent therapy may increase risk of sensitisation).
Progressive Multifocal Leucoencephalopathy Patients should be informed about the risks of PML before starting treatment with natalizumab and again after 2 years; they should be given an alert card which includes information about the symptoms of PML.
Liver toxicity Advise patients to seek immediate medical attention if symptoms such as jaundice or dark urine develop.
Alert card A patient alert card should be provided.

● NATIONAL FUNDING/ACCESS DECISIONS
For full details see funding body website
NICE decisions
▶ Natalizumab for the treatment of adults with highly active relapsing-remitting multiple sclerosis (August 2007) NICE TA127 Recommended with restrictions
Scottish Medicines Consortium (SMC) decisions
▶ Natalizumab (*Tysabri*®) for use as single disease modifying therapy in highly active relapsing remitting multiple sclerosis (RRMS) (September 2007) SMC No. 329/06 Recommended with restrictions
NHS restrictions
NHS England Clinical Commissioning Policy NHS England (May 2014) has provided guidance on the use of natalizumab for the treatment of multiple sclerosis in England. An NHS England Clinical Commissioning Policy outlines the funding arrangements and the criteria for initiating and discontinuing this treatment option, see www.england.nhs.uk/commissioning/spec-services/npc-crg/group-d/d04/.

● MEDICINAL FORMS There can be variation in the licensing of different medicines containing the same drug.
Solution for infusion
ELECTROLYTES: May contain Sodium
▶ Tysabri (Biogen Idec Ltd) ▼
    Natalizumab 20 mg per 1 ml Tysabri 300mg/15ml concentrate for solution for infusion vials | 1 vial [PoM] £1,130.00 (Hospital only)

Ocrelizumab

▶ 903

11-Nov-2020

● INDICATIONS AND DOSE

Multiple sclerosis (specialist use only)
▶ BY INTRAVENOUS INFUSION
▶ Adult: Initially 300 mg, then 300 mg after 2 weeks; maintenance 600 mg every 6 months, the first maintenance dose should be given 6 months after the first initial dose; a minimum interval of 5 months should be maintained between each maintenance dose, for dose interruption, adjustment of infusion rate or discontinuation of treatment due to infusion-related reactions or side-effects—consult product literature

● CONTRA-INDICATIONS Active infection · active malignancies · severely immunocompromised patients

● CAUTIONS Complete required vaccinations at least 6 weeks before treatment initiation · hepatitis B reactivation

● INTERACTIONS → Appendix 1: monoclonal antibodies

8

Immune system and malignant disease

- SIDE-EFFECTS
  ‣ **Common or very common** Catarrh
  ‣ **Frequency not known** Malignancy
- CONCEPTION AND CONTRACEPTION Manufacturer advises women of childbearing potential should use contraception during treatment and for 12 months after the last dose.
- PREGNANCY Manufacturer advises avoid unless potential benefit outweighs risk—limited information available; monitor infants for B-cell depletion.
- BREAST FEEDING Manufacturer advises avoid—present in milk in *animal* studies.
- MONITORING REQUIREMENTS
  ‣ Manufacturer advises monitor for signs and symptoms of progressive multifocal leucoencephalopathy (PML) (including any new onset or worsening of neurological symptoms)—if PML is suspected, interrupt treatment; discontinue treatment permanently if PML is confirmed.
  ‣ Manufacturer advises monitor for infusion-related reactions during the infusion and observe patients for 1 hour after completion of the infusion—if severe pulmonary symptoms occur, permanently discontinue treatment.
- PRESCRIBING AND DISPENSING INFORMATION Manufacturer advises to record the batch number after each administration.
- HANDLING AND STORAGE Manufacturer advises store in a refrigerator (2–8°C)—consult product literature for further information regarding storage conditions after preparation of the infusion.
- PATIENT AND CARER ADVICE Manufacturer advises patients and carers should be advised that infusion-related reactions can occur within 24 hours of infusion.
- NATIONAL FUNDING/ACCESS DECISIONS
  For full details see funding body website

  NICE decisions
  ‣ **Ocrelizumab for treating relapsing-remitting multiple sclerosis (July 2018)** NICE TA533 Recommended with restrictions
  ‣ **Ocrelizumab for treating primary progressive multiple sclerosis (June 2019)** NICE TA585 Recommended with restrictions

  Scottish Medicines Consortium (SMC) decisions
  ‣ **Ocrelizumab (*Ocrevus*®) for the treatment of adult patients with relapsing forms of multiple sclerosis (RMS) with active disease defined by clinical or imaging features (December 2018)** SMC No. SMC2121 Recommended with restrictions
  ‣ **Ocrelizumab (*Ocrevus*®) for treatment of adult patients with early primary progressive multiple sclerosis (PPMS) in terms of disease duration and level of disability, and with imaging features characteristic of inflammatory activity (January 2020)** SMC No. SMC2223 Recommended

- MEDICINAL FORMS There can be variation in the licensing of different medicines containing the same drug.

  Solution for infusion
  ‣ Ocrevus (Roche Products Ltd) ▼
    Ocrelizumab 30 mg per 1 ml Ocrevus 300mg/10ml concentrate for solution for infusion vials | 1 vial [PoM] £4,790.00

IMMUNOSUPPRESSANTS 〉 PYRIMIDINE SYNTHESIS INHIBITORS

Teriflunomide

25-Jul-2018

- DRUG ACTION Teriflunomide is a metabolite of leflunomide which has immunomodulating and anti-inflammatory properties.

● INDICATIONS AND DOSE

Treatment of relapsing-remitting multiple sclerosis (initiated under specialist supervision)
‣ BY MOUTH
  ‣ Adult: 14 mg once daily

- CONTRA-INDICATIONS Anaemia · leucopenia · neutropenia · serious infection · severe hypoproteinaemia · severe immunodeficiency · significantly impaired bone-marrow function · thrombocytopenia
- CAUTIONS Adult over 65 years · anaemia · dyspnoea—assess for interstitial lung disease and consider suspending treatment · hypoproteinaemia (avoid if severe) · impaired bone-marrow function (avoid if severe) · latent tuberculosis · leucopenia · persistent cough—assess for interstitial lung disease and consider suspending treatment · severe infection—delay or suspend treatment until resolved · significant alcohol consumption · signs or symptoms of serious skin reactions (including ulcerative stomatitis, Stevens-Johnson syndrome, and toxic epidermal necrolysis)—discontinue treatment · switching between other immunomodulating drugs · thrombocytopenia
- INTERACTIONS → Appendix 1: teriflunomide
- SIDE-EFFECTS
  ‣ **Common or very common** Abdominal pain upper · alopecia · anaemia · anxiety · arthralgia · cystitis · diarrhoea · headache · hypersensitivity · hypertension · increased risk of infection · menorrhagia · myalgia · nausea · nerve disorders · neutropenia · oral disorders · pain · palpitations · sensation abnormal · skin reactions · urinary frequency increased · vomiting · weight decreased
  ‣ **Uncommon** Thrombocytopenia
  ‣ **Frequency not known** Asthenia · hepatitis acute · interstitial lung disease · nail disorder · pancreatitis · sepsis

  SIDE-EFFECTS, FURTHER INFORMATION **Hepatic injury** Discontinue treatment if signs or symptoms of hepatic injury, or if liver enzymes exceed 3 times the upper limit of reference range.

    Important: accelerated elimination procedure recommended following discontinuation due to serious adverse effects (consult product literature).

- CONCEPTION AND CONTRACEPTION Effective contraception essential for women of child-bearing potential during treatment and for up to 2 years after treatment. In patients undergoing treatment with teriflunomide that are planning to conceive, the accelerated elimination procedure should be used prior to conception. Use of non-oral contraception is recommended during the accelerated elimination procedure—consult product literature.
- PREGNANCY Avoid—toxicity in animal studies.
- BREAST FEEDING Present in milk in *animal* studies—manufacturer advises avoid.
- HEPATIC IMPAIRMENT Manufacturer advises avoid in severe impairment.
- MONITORING REQUIREMENTS
  ‣ Monitor full blood count (including differential white cell count and platelet count) before treatment and as clinically indicated during treatment.
  ‣ Monitor blood pressure before treatment and periodically thereafter.

▶ Hepatic monitoring Monitor liver function before treatment and every 2 weeks for first 6 months then every 8 weeks thereafter or as clinically indicated (pre-existing liver disease may increase risk). Increase to weekly monitoring if alanine aminotransferase (ALT) is 2–3 times the upper limit of reference range; discontinue treatment if signs or symptoms of hepatic injury, or if liver enzymes exceed 3 times the upper limit of reference range.

● TREATMENT CESSATION
Accelerated elimination procedures To aid drug elimination in case of serious adverse effect or before conception, stop treatment and give *either* colestyramine p. 212 *or* charcoal, activated p. 1421. After the accelerated elimination procedure a plasma concentration of less than 20 micrograms/litre (measured on 2 occasions at least 14 days apart) and a waiting period of one and a half months are necessary before conception.

● NATIONAL FUNDING/ACCESS DECISIONS
For full details see funding body website
NICE decisions
▶ Teriflunomide for treating relapsing-remitting multiple sclerosis (January 2014) NICE TA303 Recommended with restrictions
Scottish Medicines Consortium (SMC) decisions
▶ Teriflunomide (*Aubagio*®) for adults with relapsing-remitting multiple sclerosis (March 2014) SMC No. 940/14 Recommended with restrictions

● MEDICINAL FORMS There can be variation in the licensing of different medicines containing the same drug.
Tablet
▶ Aubagio (Genzyme Therapeutics Ltd)
Teriflunomide 14 mg Aubagio 14mg tablets | 28 tablet PoM
£1,037.84

Malignant disease

1   Antibody responsive malignancy

ANTINEOPLASTIC DRUGS > MONOCLONAL ANTIBODIES

Atezolizumab   03-Dec-2020

● DRUG ACTION Atezolizumab is a monoclonal antibody, which binds to the programmed death-ligand 1 (PD-L1), thereby reactivating the immune response to tumour cells.

● INDICATIONS AND DOSE
Urothelial carcinoma (specialist use only) | Non-small cell lung cancer (specialist use only) | Small cell lung cancer (specialist use only) | Breast cancer (specialist use only)
▶ BY INTRAVENOUS INFUSION
▶ Adult: (consult product literature)

● CAUTIONS Abnormal thyroid function—manufacturer advises to consider appropriate treatment · patients may need pre-medication to minimise the development of infusion-related reactions—consult product literature

● INTERACTIONS → Appendix 1: monoclonal antibodies

● SIDE-EFFECTS
▶ Common or very common Abdominal pain · appetite decreased · arthralgia · ascites · asthenia · chills · cough · cystitis · cytokine release syndrome · diarrhoea · dysphagia · dyspnoea · electrolyte imbalance · euthyroid sick syndrome · eye disorders · fever · gastrointestinal disorders · goitre · hepatic disorders · hyperglycaemia ·

hypersensitivity · hypotension · hypothyroidism · hypoxia · increased risk of infection · influenza like illness · infusion related reaction · myalgia · myxoedema · nasal congestion · nausea · oesophageal varices · oesophageal varices haemorrhage · oropharyngeal complaints · pain · radiation pneumonitis · respiratory disorders · skin reactions · skin ulcer · throat irritation · thrombocytopenia · thyroid disorder · thyroiditis · toxic epidermal necrolysis · ulcerative colitis · vomiting
▶ Uncommon Adrenal hypofunction · connective tissue disorders · diabetes mellitus · diabetic ketoacidosis · hyperthyroidism · ketoacidosis · meningitis · muscle abscess · myopathy · nerve disorders · pancreatitis · photophobia
▶ Rare or very rare Hypophysitis · myocarditis · nephritis · neuromuscular dysfunction · temperature regulation disorder

SIDE-EFFECTS, FURTHER INFORMATION **Immune-related reactions** Manufacturer advises most immune-related adverse reactions are reversible and managed by temporarily stopping treatment and administration of a corticosteroid—consult product literature.
    Infusion-related reactions Manufacturer advises permanently discontinue treatment in patients with severe infusion reactions.

● CONCEPTION AND CONTRACEPTION Manufacturer advises effective contraception in women of childbearing potential, during treatment and for 5 months after stopping treatment. See also *Pregnancy and reproductive function* in Cytotoxic drugs p. 932.

● PREGNANCY Manufacturer advises avoid unless essential—no information available. See also *Pregnancy and reproductive function* in Cytotoxic drugs p. 932.

● BREAST FEEDING Manufacturer advises avoid—no information available.

● MONITORING REQUIREMENTS Manufacturer advises monitor for signs and symptoms of infusion- and immune-related reactions—consult product literature.

● PRESCRIBING AND DISPENSING INFORMATION
Manufacturer advises to record the brand name and batch number after each administration.
    All prescribers should be familiar with the *Physician Information and Management Guidelines* provided by the manufacturer.

● HANDLING AND STORAGE Manufacturer advises store in a refrigerator (2–8°C); consult product literature for storage conditions after dilution.

● PATIENT AND CARER ADVICE An alert card should be provided.
Driving and skilled tasks Manufacturer advises patients should be counselled on the effects on driving and performance of skilled tasks—increased risk of drowsiness.

● NATIONAL FUNDING/ACCESS DECISIONS
For full details see funding body website
NICE decisions
▶ Atezolizumab for untreated PD-L1-positive locally advanced or metastatic urothelial cancer when cisplatin is unsuitable (updated July 2018) NICE TA492 Recommended with restrictions
▶ Atezolizumab for treating locally advanced or metastatic urothelial carcinoma after platinum-containing chemotherapy (June 2018) NICE TA525 Recommended with restrictions
▶ Atezolizumab for treating locally advanced or metastatic non-small-cell lung cancer after chemotherapy (May 2018) NICE TA520 Recommended with restrictions
▶ Atezolizumab in combination for treating metastatic non-squamous non-small-cell lung cancer (June 2019) NICE TA584 Recommended with restrictions

8

Immune system and malignant disease

▶ Atezolizumab with carboplatin and etoposide for untreated extensive-stage small-cell lung cancer (July 2020) NICE TA638 Recommended with restrictions
▶ Atezolizumab with nab-paclitaxel for untreated PD-L1-positive, locally advanced or metastatic, triple-negative breast cancer (July 2020) NICE TA639 Recommended

Scottish Medicines Consortium (SMC) decisions
▶ Atezolizumab (*Tecentriq*®) for the treatment of adult patients with locally advanced or metastatic non-small cell lung cancer (NSCLC) after prior chemotherapy. Patients with EGFR activating mutations or ALK-positive tumour mutations should also have received targeted therapy before receiving *Tecentriq*® (July 2018) SMC No. 1336/18 Recommended with restrictions
▶ Atezolizumab (*Tecentriq*®), in combination with bevacizumab, paclitaxel and carboplatin, is indicated for the first-line treatment of adult patients with metastatic non-squamous non-small cell lung cancer (NSCLC) (November 2019) SMC No. SMC2208 Not recommended
▶ Atezolizumab (*Tecentriq*®) in combination with carboplatin and etoposide, is indicated for the first-line treatment of adult patients with extensive-stage small cell lung cancer (November 2020) SMC No. SMC2279 Recommended
▶ Atezolizumab (*Tecentriq*®) as monotherapy for the treatment of adult patients with locally advanced or metastatic urothelial carcinoma: after prior platinum-containing chemotherapy, or who are considered cisplatin ineligible (November 2018) SMC No. SMC2103 Not recommended
▶ Atezolizumab (*Tecentriq*®) in combination with nab-paclitaxel for the treatment of adult patients with unresectable locally advanced or metastatic triple-negative breast cancer whose tumours have PD-L1 expression at a level of 1% or more and who have not received prior chemotherapy for metastatic disease (November 2020) SMC No. SMC2267 Recommended

● MEDICINAL FORMS There can be variation in the licensing of different medicines containing the same drug.
Solution for infusion
EXCIPIENTS: May contain Polysorbates, sucrose
▶ Tecentriq (Roche Products Ltd) ▼
Atezolizumab 60 mg per 1 ml Tecentriq 840mg/14ml concentrate for solution for infusion vials | 1 vial PoM £2,665.38
Tecentriq 1200mg/20ml concentrate for solution for infusion vials | 1 vial PoM £3,807.69

▌Avelumab

10-Nov-2020

● DRUG ACTION Avelumab is a monoclonal antibody, which binds to the programmed death-1 (PD-1) receptor, thereby potentiating an immune response to tumour cells.

● **INDICATIONS AND DOSE**

Metastatic Merkel cell carcinoma (specialist use only)
▶ BY INTRAVENOUS INFUSION
▶ Adult: 800 mg every 2 weeks, for information on dose delay or interruption due to side-effects and infusion-related reactions—consult product literature

Advanced renal cell carcinoma (specialist use only)
▶ BY INTRAVENOUS INFUSION
▶ Adult: 800 mg every 2 weeks, for information on dose delay or interruption due to side-effects and infusion-related reactions—consult product literature

● CAUTIONS Patients should receive pre-medication to minimise the development of adverse reactions (consult product literature)

● INTERACTIONS → Appendix 1: monoclonal antibodies

● SIDE-EFFECTS
▶ Common or very common Abdominal pain · anaemia · appetite decreased · arthralgia · asthenia · back pain · chills · constipation · cough · diarrhoea · dizziness · dry mouth · dyspnoea · fever · headache · hypertension · hypotension ·

hypothyroidism · influenza like illness · infusion related reaction · lymphopenia · myalgia · nausea · nerve disorders · peripheral oedema · pneumonitis · skin reactions · vomiting · weight decreased
▶ Uncommon Adrenal insufficiency · diabetes mellitus · eosinophilia · flushing · gastrointestinal disorders · hepatic disorders · hypersensitivity · hyperthyroidism · hypopituitarism · myositis · nephritis · systemic inflammatory response syndrome · thrombocytopenia · thyroiditis · uveitis
▶ Rare or very rare Myocarditis · pancreatitis
▶ Frequency not known Endocrine disorders

SIDE-EFFECTS, FURTHER INFORMATION **Infusion-related reactions** For treatment modifications in patients with grade 1 or 2 infusion-related reactions, consult product literature. Manufacturer advises permanently discontinue treatment in patients with grade 3 or 4 infusion-related reaction.

Immune-related reactions Most immune-related adverse reactions are reversible and managed by temporarily stopping treatment and administration of a corticosteroid—consult product literature for further information.

● CONCEPTION AND CONTRACEPTION Manufacturer advises women of child-bearing potential should use effective contraception during treatment and for at least 1 month after stopping treatment.

● PREGNANCY Manufacturer advises avoid unless essential—no information available. See also *Pregnancy and reproductive function* in Cytotoxic drugs p. 932.

● BREAST FEEDING Manufacturer advises avoid during treatment and for at least 1 month after stopping treatment—no information available.

● MONITORING REQUIREMENTS Manufacturer advises monitor for signs and symptoms of infusion- and immune-related reactions.

● DIRECTIONS FOR ADMINISTRATION Manufacturer advises for *intermittent intravenous infusion* (*Bavencio*®), dilute requisite dose with Sodium Chloride 0.9%; give over 60 minutes via a separate line using a low-protein binding 0.2 micron filter.

● HANDLING AND STORAGE Manufacturer advises store in a refrigerator (2–8 °C)—consult product literature for storage conditions after preparation of the infusion.

● NATIONAL FUNDING/ACCESS DECISIONS
For full details see funding body website

NICE decisions
▶ Avelumab for treating metastatic Merkel cell carcinoma (April 2018) NICE TA517 Recommended with restrictions
▶ Avelumab with axitinib for untreated advanced renal cell carcinoma (September 2020) NICE TA645 Recommended

Scottish Medicines Consortium (SMC) decisions
▶ Avelumab (*Bavencio*®) as monotherapy for the treatment of adult patients with metastatic Merkel cell carcinoma (May 2018) SMC No. 1315/18 Recommended
▶ Avelumab (*Bavencio*®) in combination with axitinib for the first-line treatment of adult patients with advanced renal cell carcinoma (October 2020) SMC No. SMC2248 Recommended

● MEDICINAL FORMS There can be variation in the licensing of different medicines containing the same drug.
Solution for infusion
▶ Bavencio (Merck Serono Ltd) ▼
Avelumab 20 mg per 1 ml Bavencio 200mg/10ml concentrate for solution for infusion vials | 1 vial PoM £768.00

Bevacizumab

28-Sep-2020

- **DRUG ACTION** Bevacizumab is a monoclonal antibody that inhibits vascular endothelial growth factor.

- **INDICATIONS AND DOSE**

  Colorectal cancer (specialist use only) | Breast cancer (specialist use only) | Renal cell carcinoma (specialist use only) | Non-small cell lung cancer (specialist use only) | Epithelial ovarian cancer (specialist use only) | Fallopian tube cancer (specialist use only) | Primary peritoneal cancer (specialist use only) | Carcinoma of the cervix (specialist use only)

  ▸ BY INTRAVENOUS INFUSION
  ▸ Adult: (consult product literature)

IMPORTANT SAFETY INFORMATION

MHRA/CHM ADVICE: BEVACIZUMAB AND SUNITINIB: RISK OF OSTEONECROSIS OF THE JAW (JANUARY 2011)

Treatment with bevacizumab or sunitinib may be a risk factor for the development of osteonecrosis of the jaw.

Patients treated with bevacizumab or sunitinib, who have previously received bisphosphonates, or are treated concurrently with bisphosphonates, may be particularly at risk.

Dental examination and appropriate preventive dentistry should be considered before treatment with bevacizumab or sunitinib.

If possible, invasive dental procedures should be avoided in patients treated with bevacizumab or sunitinib who have previously received, or who are currently receiving, intravenous bisphosphonates.

MHRA/CHM ADVICE: SYSTEMICALLY ADMINISTERED VEGF PATHWAY INHIBITORS: RISK OF ANEURYSM AND ARTERY DISSECTION (JULY 2020)

A European review of worldwide data concluded that systemically administered VEGF pathway inhibitors may lead to aneurysm and artery dissection in patients with or without hypertension. Some fatal cases have been reported, mainly in relation to aortic aneurysm rupture and aortic dissection. The MHRA advises healthcare professionals to carefully consider the risk of aneurysm and artery dissection in patients with risk factors before initiating treatment with bevacizumab; any modifiable risk factors (such as smoking and hypertension) should be reduced as much as possible. Patients should be monitored and treated for hypertension as required.

- CAUTIONS Elective surgery (withhold treatment and avoid for at least 28 days after major surgery or until wound fully healed) · history of cardiovascular disease (increased risk of cardiovascular events, especially in the elderly) · history of hypertension (increased risk of proteinuria—discontinue if nephrotic syndrome) · increased risk of fistulas (discontinue permanently if tracheo-oesophageal or grade 4 fistula develops) · increased risk of haemorrhage · increased risk of tumour-associated haemorrhage · intra-abdominal inflammation (risk of gastro-intestinal perforation and gall bladder perforation) · risk factors for aneurysm or artery dissection · risk factors for arterial thromboembolism · uncontrolled hypertension · untreated CNS metastases

  CAUTIONS, FURTHER INFORMATION
  ▸ Monitoring of blood pressure The MHRA advises to monitor blood pressure regularly—consult product literature if hypertension occurs during treatment.

- INTERACTIONS → Appendix 1: monoclonal antibodies

- SIDE-EFFECTS
  ▸ Common or very common Abscess · anaemia · appetite decreased · arthralgia · asthenia · congestive heart failure · constipation · cough · decreased leucocytes · dehydration ·

diarrhoea · drowsiness · dysarthria · dysphonia · dyspnoea · electrolyte imbalance · embolism and thrombosis · eye disorders · fever · fistula · gastrointestinal discomfort · gastrointestinal disorders · haemorrhage · headache · healing impaired · hypersensitivity · hypertension · hypoxia · increased risk of infection · infusion related reaction · mucositis · muscle weakness · myalgia · nausea · neutropenia · ovarian failure · pain · pelvic pain · peripheral neuropathy · proteinuria · rectovaginal fistula · sepsis · skin reactions · stomatitis · stroke · supraventricular tachycardia · syncope · taste altered · thrombocytopenia · vomiting · weight decreased

  ▸ Rare or very rare Encephalopathy · necrotising fasciitis (discontinue and initiate treatment promptly)
  ▸ Frequency not known Aneurysm · artery dissection · chest pain · chills · flushing · gallbladder perforation · hyperglycaemia · hypotension · nasal septum perforation · osteonecrosis of jaw · pulmonary hypertension · renal thrombotic microangiopathy

- CONCEPTION AND CONTRACEPTION Effective contraception required during and for at least 6 months after treatment in women.

- PREGNANCY Avoid—toxicity in *animal* studies. See also *Pregnancy and reproductive function* in Cytotoxic drugs p. 932.

- BREAST FEEDING Manufacturer advises avoid breast-feeding during and for at least 6 months after treatment.

- MONITORING REQUIREMENTS
  ▸ Monitor for necrotising fasciitis (usually secondary to wound healing complications, gastro-intestinal perforation or fistula formation)—discontinue and initiate treatment promptly.
  ▸ Monitor for congestive heart failure.
  ▸ Monitor for posterior reversible encephalopathy syndrome (presenting as seizures, headache, altered mental status, visual disturbance or cortical blindness, with or without hypertension).
  ▸ Consider dental check-up before initiating treatment (risk of osteonecrosis of the jaw).

- NATIONAL FUNDING/ACCESS DECISIONS
  For full details see funding body website

  NICE decisions
  ▸ **Bevacizumab and cetuximab for the treatment of metastatic colorectal cancer (January 2007)** NICE TA118 Not recommended
  ▸ **Bevacizumab in combination with oxaliplatin and either fluorouracil plus folinic acid or capecitabine for the treatment of metastatic colorectal cancer (December 2010)** NICE TA212 Not recommended
  ▸ **Cetuximab, bevacizumab and panitumumab for the treatment of metastatic colorectal cancer after first-line chemotherapy (January 2012)** NICE TA242 Not recommended
  ▸ **Bevacizumab (first-line), sorafenib (first and second-line), sunitinib (second-line) and temsirolimus (first-line) for the treatment of advanced and/or metastatic renal cell carcinoma (August 2009)** NICE TA178 Not recommended
  ▸ **Bevacizumab in combination with a taxane for the first-line treatment of metastatic breast cancer (February 2011)** NICE TA214 Not recommended
  ▸ **Bevacizumab in combination with capecitabine for the first-line treatment of metastatic breast cancer (August 2012)** NICE TA263 Not recommended
  ▸ **Bevacizumab in combination with paclitaxel and carboplatin for the first-line treatment of advanced ovarian cancer (May 2013)** NICE TA284 Not recommended
  ▸ **Bevacizumab in combination with gemcitabine and carboplatin for the treatment of the first recurrence of platinum-sensitive advanced ovarian cancer (May 2013)** NICE TA285 Not recommended

8

Immune system and malignant disease

Scottish Medicines Consortium (SMC) decisions

▶ Bevacizumab (*Avastin* ®) in combination with capecitabine for first-line treatment of metastatic breast cancer (May 2012) SMC No. 778/12 Not recommended

▶ Bevacizumab (*Avastin* ®) in combination with paclitaxel, topotecan, or pegylated liposomal doxorubicin for the treatment of platinum-resistant recurrent ovarian, fallopian tube, or primary peritoneal cancer (September 2015) SMC No. 1063/15 Recommended with restrictions

▶ Bevacizumab (*Avastin* ®) in combination with carboplatin and paclitaxel, for the front-line treatment of advanced (International Federation of Gynaecology and Obstetrics (FIGO) stages IIIB, IIIC and IV) epithelial ovarian, fallopian tube, or primary peritoneal cancer (November 2015) SMC No. 806/12 Recommended with restrictions

All Wales Medicines Strategy Group (AWMSG) decisions

▶ Bevacizumab (*Avastin* ®) in combination with paclitaxel and cisplatin, or, alternatively, paclitaxel and topotecan in patients who cannot receive platinum therapy, for the treatment of adult patients with persistent, recurrent, or metastatic carcinoma of the cervix (September 2017) AWMSG No. 2166 Not recommended

● MEDICINAL FORMS There can be variation in the licensing of different medicines containing the same drug. Forms available from special-order manufacturers include: solution for injection

Solution for infusion

▶ Avastin (Roche Products Ltd)
Bevacizumab 25 mg per 1 ml Avastin 400mg/16ml solution for infusion vials | 1 vial [PoM] £924.40 (Hospital only)
Avastin 100mg/4ml solution for infusion vials | 1 vial [PoM] £242.66 (Hospital only)

▶ Aybintio (Organon Pharma (UK) Ltd) ▼
Bevacizumab 25 mg per 1 ml Aybintio 100mg/4ml solution for infusion vials | 1 vial [PoM] £218.39 (Hospital only)
Aybintio 400mg/16ml solution for infusion vials | 1 vial [PoM] £831.96 (Hospital only)

▶ Zirabev (Pfizer Ltd) ▼
Bevacizumab 25 mg per 1 ml Zirabev 100mg/4ml solution for infusion vials | 1 vial [PoM] £225.67 (Hospital only)
Zirabev 400mg/16ml solution for infusion vials | 1 vial [PoM] £902.70 (Hospital only)

Blinatumomab

24-Nov-2020

● DRUG ACTION The anti-lymphocyte monoclonal antibodies cause lysis of B lymphocytes.

● **INDICATIONS AND DOSE**

Relapsed or refractory Philadelphia chromosome-negative acute lymphoblastic leukaemia (initiated by a specialist)

▶ BY CONTINUOUS INTRAVENOUS INFUSION
▶ Adult: (consult product literature)

Philadelphia chromosome-negative acute lymphoblastic leukaemia in complete remission with minimal residual disease (initiated by a specialist)

▶ BY CONTINUOUS INTRAVENOUS INFUSION
▶ Adult (body-weight 45 kg and above): (consult product literature)

● CAUTIONS Aphasia · brain injuries (severe) · cerebellar disease · dementia · elderly—limited information available · epilepsy · paresis · Parkinson's disease · patients may need pre-medication to minimise adverse reactions · psychosis · seizure · severe hepatic impairment · severe renal impairment · stroke

CAUTIONS, FURTHER INFORMATION

▶ Pre-medication Manufacturer advises pre-medication with a corticosteroid and an anti-pyretic—consult product literature.

▶ Neurological events There is potentially a higher risk of neurological events in patients with clinically relevant CNS pathology—manufacturer advises caution.

● INTERACTIONS → Appendix 1: monoclonal antibodies

● SIDE-EFFECTS

▶ **Common or very common** Abdominal pain · anaemia · arrhythmias · ataxia · chest discomfort · chills · cognitive disorder · confusion · constipation · cough · cranial nerve disorder · decreased leucocytes · diarrhoea · dizziness · drowsiness · dyspnoea · encephalopathy · facial swelling · fever · flushing · headache · hyperbilirubinaemia · hypersensitivity · hypertension · hypogammaglobulinaemia · hypoglobulinaemia · hypotension · immune disorder · increased risk of infection · infusion related reaction · insomnia · leucocytosis · memory loss · nausea · neutropenia · oedema · pain · respiratory disorders · seizure · sensation abnormal · sepsis · skin reactions · speech impairment · thrombocytopenia · tremor · tumour lysis syndrome · vomiting · weight increased

▶ **Uncommon** Capillary leak syndrome · haemophagocytic lymphohistiocytosis · lymphadenopathy · pancreatitis

▶ **Frequency not known** Consciousness impaired · psychiatric disorder · viral infection reactivation

SIDE-EFFECTS, FURTHER INFORMATION **Pancreatitis** Life-threatening or fatal cases of pancreatitis have been reported; manufacturer advises monitor for signs and symptoms of pancreatitis during treatment—temporary interruption or discontinuation may be required (consult product literature).

Cytokine release syndrome, infusion-reactions and tumour lysis syndrome Life-threatening (including fatal) cases of cytokine release syndrome and tumour lysis syndrome have been reported in patients taking blinatumomab. Manufacturer advises monitor signs and symptoms of cytokine release syndrome and infusion reactions during treatment; temporary interruption or discontinuation may be required—consult product literature.

● CONCEPTION AND CONTRACEPTION Manufacturer advises effective contraception during treatment and for at least 48 hours after treatment in women of child-bearing potential. See also Pregnancy and reproductive function in Cytotoxic drugs p. 932.

● PREGNANCY Manufacturer advises avoid unless potential benefit outweighs risk—no information available; if exposed during pregnancy, monitor infant for B-cell depletion. See also Pregnancy and reproductive function in Cytotoxic drugs p. 932.

● BREAST FEEDING Manufacturer advises avoid during and for at least 48 hours after treatment—no information available.

● HEPATIC IMPAIRMENT Manufacturer advises caution in severe impairment (no information available).

● RENAL IMPAIRMENT Manufacturer advises caution in severe impairment—no information available.

● MONITORING REQUIREMENTS Manufacturer advises neurological examination prior to the initiation of treatment and continued monitoring during treatment—consult product literature.

● HANDLING AND STORAGE Manufacturer advises store in a refrigerator (2–8°C); consult product literature for storage conditions after reconstitution and dilution.

● PATIENT AND CARER ADVICE A patient alert card should be provided. Educational materials should be provided to patients, carers and healthcare professionals to ensure blinatumomab is used in a safe and effective way, and to prevent the risk of medication errors and neurological events—consult product information.

Driving and skilled tasks Manufacturer advises patients and carers should be counselled about the effects on driving and performance of skilled tasks—increased risk of confusion, disorientation, co-ordination and balance disorders, seizures and disturbances in consciousness.

● NATIONAL FUNDING/ACCESS DECISIONS
For full details see funding body website

NICE decisions
▸ Blinatumomab for previously treated Philadelphia-chromosome-negative acute lymphoblastic leukaemia (June 2017) NICE TA450 Recommended
▸ Blinatumomab for treating acute lymphoblastic leukaemia in remission with minimal residual disease activity (July 2019) NICE TA589 Recommended with restrictions

Scottish Medicines Consortium (SMC) decisions
▸ Blinatumomab (*Blincyto*®) as monotherapy for the treatment of adults with Philadelphia chromosome-negative CD19 positive B-precursor acute lymphoblastic leukaemia in first or second complete remission with minimal residual disease greater than or equal to 0.1% (March 2020) SMC No. SMC2234 Recommended with restrictions

● MEDICINAL FORMS There can be variation in the licensing of different medicines containing the same drug.
Powder for solution for infusion
EXCIPIENTS: May contain Polysorbates
▸ Blincyto (Amgen Ltd) ▾
　Blinatumomab 38.5 microgram Blincyto 38.5micrograms powder for concentrate and solution for solution for infusion vials | 1 vial [PoM] £2,017.00

Brentuximab vedotin
03-Nov-2020

● INDICATIONS AND DOSE

CD30 positive Hodgkin lymphoma (specialist use only) | Systemic anaplastic large cell lymphoma (specialist use only) | CD30 positive cutaneous T-cell lymphoma (specialist use only)
▸ BY INTRAVENOUS INFUSION
▸ Adult: (consult product literature)

● CAUTIONS Elevated BMI—risk of hyperglycaemia · high tumour burden—risk of tumour lysis syndrome · rapidly proliferating tumours—risk of tumour lysis syndrome

● INTERACTIONS → Appendix 1: monoclonal antibodies

● SIDE-EFFECTS
▸ Common or very common Abdominal pain · alopecia · anaemia · arthralgia · back pain · chills · constipation · cough · diarrhoea · dizziness · dyspnoea · fatigue · fever · hyperglycaemia · increased risk of infection · infusion related reaction · myalgia · nausea · nerve disorders · neutropenia · skin reactions · thrombocytopenia · vomiting · weight decreased
▸ Uncommon Anaphylactic reaction · cytomegalovirus infection reactivation · pancreatitis acute · sepsis · severe cutaneous adverse reactions (SCARs) · tumour lysis syndrome
▸ Frequency not known Disease recurrence · gastrointestinal disorders · gastrointestinal haemorrhage · progressive multifocal leukoencephalopathy (PML) · respiratory disorders

● CONCEPTION AND CONTRACEPTION Effective contraception required during treatment and for 6 months after treatment in men and women.

● PREGNANCY Avoid unless potential benefit outweighs risk (toxicity in *animal* studies).

● BREAST FEEDING Avoid—no information available.

● MONITORING REQUIREMENTS
▸ Monitor for symptoms of progressive multifocal leucoencephalopathy (presenting as new or worsening neurological, cognitive or behavioural signs or symptoms).
▸ Monitor for new or worsening abdominal pain—investigate and withhold treatment if acute pancreatitis suspected and discontinue if confirmed (fatal cases reported).
▸ Monitor for pulmonary toxicity—treat symptoms promptly.
▸ Routinely monitor hepatic function.
▸ Monitor for infusion-related (including anaphylactic) reactions.
▸ Monitor for signs of peripheral neuropathy—consult product literature for treatment adjustment.

● NATIONAL FUNDING/ACCESS DECISIONS
For full details see funding body website

NICE decisions
▸ Brentuximab vedotin for treating relapsed or refractory systemic anaplastic large cell lymphoma (October 2017) NICE TA478 Recommended with restrictions
▸ Brentuximab vedotin in combination for untreated systemic anaplastic large cell lymphoma (August 2020) NICE TA641 Recommended
▸ Brentuximab vedotin for treating CD30-positive Hodgkin lymphoma (June 2018) NICE TA524 Recommended with restrictions
▸ Brentuximab vedotin for treating CD30-positive cutaneous T-cell lymphoma (April 2019) NICE TA577 Recommended with restrictions

Scottish Medicines Consortium (SMC) decisions
▸ Brentuximab vedotin (*Adcetris*®) for the treatment of adult patients with CD30-positive cutaneous T-cell lymphoma (CTCL) after at least one prior systemic therapy (January 2020) SMC No. SMC2229 Recommended with restrictions

● MEDICINAL FORMS There can be variation in the licensing of different medicines containing the same drug.
Powder for solution for infusion
EXCIPIENTS: May contain Polysorbates
ELECTROLYTES: May contain Sodium
▸ Adcetris (Takeda UK Ltd) ▾
　Brentuximab vedotin 50 mg Adcetris 50mg powder for concentrate for solution for infusion vials | 1 vial [PoM] £2,500.00

Cemiplimab
27-Aug-2020

● DRUG ACTION Cemiplimab is a human immunoglobulin G4 monoclonal antibody, which binds to the programmed death-1 (PD-1) receptor thereby potentiating an immune response to tumour cells.

● INDICATIONS AND DOSE

Cutaneous squamous cell carcinoma (specialist use only)
▸ BY INTRAVENOUS INFUSION
▸ Adult: 350 mg every 3 weeks, for dose interruption or discontinuation of treatment due to side-effects or infusion-related reactions—consult product literature

● CAUTIONS For full details consult product literature.

● INTERACTIONS → Appendix 1: monoclonal antibodies

● SIDE-EFFECTS
▸ Common or very common Arthralgia · arthritis · asthenia · colitis · diarrhoea · hepatic disorders · hyperthyroidism · hypothyroidism · infusion related reaction · myalgia · pain · pneumonitis · skin reactions · stomatitis
▸ Uncommon Adrenal insufficiency · cardiac inflammation · diabetic ketoacidosis · encephalitis · hypophysitis · immune thrombocytopenic purpura · keratitis · meningitis · muscle weakness · myasthenia gravis · nephritis · nerve disorders · nervous system disorders · Sjögren's syndrome · thyroiditis · type 1 diabetes mellitus · vasculitis

8

Immune system and malignant disease

- **Frequency not known** Encephalitis non-infective · severe cutaneous adverse reactions (SCARs)
- CONCEPTION AND CONTRACEPTION Manufacturer advises females of childbearing potential should use effective contraception during treatment and for at least 4 months after the last dose. See also *Pregnancy and reproductive function* in Cytotoxic drugs p. 932.
- PREGNANCY Manufacturer advises avoid unless potential benefit outweighs risk—no information available. See also *Pregnancy and reproductive function* in Cytotoxic drugs p. 932.
- BREAST FEEDING Manufacturer advises discontinue breast-feeding during treatment and for at least 4 months after stopping—no information available.
- MONITORING REQUIREMENTS Manufacturer advises monitor for signs and symptoms of infusion- and immune-related side-effects—consult product literature.
- DIRECTIONS FOR ADMINISTRATION Manufacturer advises for *intermittent intravenous infusion*, dilute to a concentration between 1 mg/mL and 20 mg/mL with Glucose 5% or Sodium Chloride 0.9%; give over 30 minutes through a low-protein binding in-line or add-on filter (pore size 0.2–5 micron).
- PRESCRIBING AND DISPENSING INFORMATION Cemiplimab is a biological medicine. Biological medicines must be prescribed and dispensed by brand name, see *Biological medicines* and *Biosimilar medicines*, under Guidance on prescribing p. 1; manufacturer advises to record the brand name and batch number after each administration.
  The manufacturer of *Libtayo*® has provided a *Risk minimisation materials* document for healthcare professionals.
- HANDLING AND STORAGE Manufacturer advises store in a refrigerator (2–8°C) and protect from light—consult product literature about storage after preparation of the infusion.
- PATIENT AND CARER ADVICE
  Risk of immune-related side-effects A patient alert card and patient guide should be provided.
- NATIONAL FUNDING/ACCESS DECISIONS
  For full details see funding body website
  NICE decisions
- Cemiplimab for treating metastatic or locally advanced cutaneous squamous cell carcinoma (August 2019) NICE TA592 Recommended with restrictions
  Scottish Medicines Consortium (SMC) decisions
- Cemiplimab (*Libtayo*®) as monotherapy for the treatment of adult patients with metastatic or locally advanced cutaneous squamous cell carcinoma (CSCC) who are not candidates for curative surgery or curative radiation (February 2020) SMC No. SMC2216 Recommended

- MEDICINAL FORMS There can be variation in the licensing of different medicines containing the same drug.
  Solution for infusion
  EXCIPIENTS: May contain L-proline, polysorbates, sucrose
  ‣ Libtayo (Sanofi) ▼
  Cemiplimab 50 mg per 1 ml Libtayo 350mg/7ml concentrate for solution for infusion vials | 1 vial [PoM] £4,650.00 (Hospital only)

Cetuximab

28-Jul-2020

- **INDICATIONS AND DOSE**
  Treatment of wild-type RAS metastatic colorectal cancer in patients with tumours expressing epidermal growth factor receptor, as combination therapy, or as monotherapy if oxaliplatin- and irinotecan-based therapy has failed or if irinotecan is not tolerated |
  Treatment of locally advanced squamous cell cancer of the head and neck (in combination with radiotherapy) |
  Treatment of recurrent or metastatic squamous cell cancer of the head and neck (in combination with platinum-based chemotherapy)
  ‣ BY INTRAVENOUS INFUSION
  ‣ Adult (initiated by a specialist): (consult product literature or local protocols)

IMPORTANT SAFETY INFORMATION
Patients must receive an antihistamine and a corticosteroid at least one hour before infusion. Resuscitation facilities should be available and treatment should be initiated by a specialist.

MHRA/CHM ADVICE: EPIDERMAL GROWTH FACTOR RECEPTOR (EGFR) INHIBITORS: SERIOUS CASES OF KERATITIS AND ULCERATIVE KERATITIS (MAY 2012)
Keratitis and ulcerative keratitis have been reported following treatment with epidermal growth factor receptor (EGFR) inhibitors for cancer (cetuximab, erlotinib, gefitinib and panitumumab). In rare cases, this has resulted in corneal perforation and blindness. Patients undergoing treatment with EGFR inhibitors who present with acute or worsening signs and symptoms suggestive of keratitis should be referred promptly to an ophthalmology specialist. Treatment should be interrupted or discontinued if ulcerative keratitis is diagnosed.

- CONTRA-INDICATIONS *RAS* mutated colorectal tumours (or if *RAS* tumour status unknown)
- CAUTIONS Cardiopulmonary disease · cardiovascular disease · history of keratitis · pulmonary disease— discontinue if interstitial lung disease · risk factors for keratitis · risk factors for ulcerative keratitis (including contact lens use) · severe dry eye
- INTERACTIONS → Appendix 1: monoclonal antibodies
- SIDE-EFFECTS
- ‣ **Common or very common** Appetite decreased · cytokine release syndrome · dehydration · diarrhoea · electrolyte imbalance · eye inflammation · fatigue · headache · infusion related reaction · mucositis · nausea · skin eruption · vomiting
- ‣ **Uncommon** Embolism and thrombosis · interstitial lung disease
- ‣ **Rare or very rare** Severe cutaneous adverse reactions (SCARs)
- ‣ **Frequency not known** Meningitis aseptic · superinfection of skin lesions
- CONCEPTION AND CONTRACEPTION Contraceptive advice required, see *Pregnancy and reproductive function* in Cytotoxic drugs p. 932.
- PREGNANCY Use only if potential benefit outweighs risk— no information available. See also *Pregnancy and reproductive function* in Cytotoxic drugs p. 932.
- BREAST FEEDING Avoid breast-feeding during and for 2 months after treatment—no information available.
- PRE-TREATMENT SCREENING Evidence of non-mutated (wild-type) *RAS* status (at exons 2, 3 and 4 of *KRAS* and *NRAS*) is required before cetuximab is initiated for the treatment of metastatic colorectal cancer, and should be

determined by an experienced laboratory using a validated test method.

- DIRECTIONS FOR ADMINISTRATION Manufacturer advises resuscitation facilities should be available.
- NATIONAL FUNDING/ACCESS DECISIONS For full details see funding body website

NICE decisions
▸ Cetuximab for the treatment of locally advanced squamous cell cancer of the head and neck (June 2008) NICE TA145 Recommended
▸ Cetuximab, bevacizumab and panitumumab for the treatment of metastatic colorectal cancer after first-line chemotherapy (January 2012) NICE TA242 Not recommended
▸ Cetuximab and panitumumab for previously untreated metastatic colorectal cancer (updated September 2017) NICE TA439 Recommended with restrictions
▸ Cetuximab for treating recurrent or metastatic squamous cell cancer of the head and neck (August 2017) NICE TA473 Recommended

- MEDICINAL FORMS There can be variation in the licensing of different medicines containing the same drug.

Solution for infusion
▸ Erbitux (Merck Serono Ltd)
Cetuximab 5 mg per 1 ml Erbitux 100mg/20ml solution for infusion vials | 1 vial [PoM] £178.10 (Hospital only)
Erbitux 500mg/100ml solution for infusion vials | 1 vial [PoM] £890.50 (Hospital only)

Daratumumab
16-Nov-2020

- DRUG ACTION Daratumumab is a monoclonal antibody that binds to CD38, a cell-surface protein, resulting in tumour cell death by immune-mediated actions and apoptosis.

INDICATIONS AND DOSE

Multiple myeloma (specialist use only)
▸ BY INTRAVENOUS INFUSION, OR BY SUBCUTANEOUS INJECTION
▸ Adult: (consult product literature or local protocols)

IMPORTANT SAFETY INFORMATION

MHRA/CHM ADVICE: DARATUMUMAB (*DARZALEX*®): RISK OF REACTIVATION OF HEPATITIS B VIRUS (AUGUST 2019)
An EU cumulative review of worldwide data has identified reports of hepatitis B virus (HBV) reactivation in patients treated with daratumumab, including several fatal cases. Healthcare professionals are advised to screen all patients for hepatitis B before starting treatment; patients with unknown serology already being treated with daratumumab should also be screened. Those with positive serology should be monitored for signs of HBV reactivation during, and for at least 6 months after, treatment; immediate medical attention should be sought if signs and symptoms of HBV reactivation develop. Daratumumab should be stopped in patients with HBV reactivation and appropriate treatment initiated, based on expert advice. Experts should be consulted before resuming daratumumab in patients with adequately controlled viral reactivation.

- CAUTIONS History of obstructive pulmonary disorder (consider additional post-medication—consult product literature) · patients may need pre-medication to minimise adverse reactions · risk of herpes zoster reactivation (consider antiviral prophylaxis)

CAUTIONS, FURTHER INFORMATION
▸ Infusion-related reactions Serious infusion-related reactions can occur following either intravenous or subcutaneous injection, and daratumumab should only be administered

by appropriately trained staff where resuscitation facilities are available; manufacturer advises pre-medication with a corticosteroid, an antihistamine and an anti-pyretic and post-medication with oral corticosteroids—consult product literature. Manufacturer advises patients should be closely monitored for signs of infusion-related reactions during and after administration; in the event of a hypersensitivity reaction, treatment should be stopped immediately and appropriate management initiated.

- INTERACTIONS → Appendix 1: monoclonal antibodies
- SIDE-EFFECTS
▸ **Common or very common**
▸ With intravenous use Pruritus
▸ With parenteral use Anaemia · appetite decreased · arthralgia · asthenia · atrial fibrillation · chills · constipation · cough · decreased leucocytes · dehydration · diarrhoea · dizziness · dyspnoea · fever · headache · hyperglycaemia · hypertension · hypocalcaemia · increased risk of infection · infusion related reaction · insomnia · muscle spasms · nausea · neutropenia · pain · pancreatitis · paraesthesia · peripheral neuropathy · peripheral oedema · pulmonary oedema · rash · sepsis · thrombocytopenia · vomiting
▸ **Uncommon**
▸ With parenteral use Hepatitis B reactivation

SIDE-EFFECTS, FURTHER INFORMATION Manufacturer advises treatment should be immediately interrupted if an infusion-related reaction of any grade or severity occurs—consult product literature for specific management recommendations.

- CONCEPTION AND CONTRACEPTION Manufacturer advises effective contraception in women of childbearing potential during treatment and for 3 months after stopping treatment. See also *Pregnancy and reproductive function* in Cytotoxic drugs p. 932.
- PREGNANCY Manufacturer advises avoid unless potential benefit outweighs risk—no information available. See also *Pregnancy and reproductive function* in Cytotoxic drugs p. 932.
- BREAST FEEDING Manufacturer advises avoid—no information available.
- EFFECT ON LABORATORY TESTS Possible positive indirect Coombs test (may affect antibody screening).
- HANDLING AND STORAGE Manufacturer advises store in a refrigerator at 2–8°C; consult product literature for storage advice following dilution.
- NATIONAL FUNDING/ACCESS DECISIONS For full details see funding body website

NICE decisions
▸ Daratumumab monotherapy for treating relapsed and refractory multiple myeloma (March 2018) NICE TA510 Recommended with restrictions
▸ Daratumumab with bortezomib and dexamethasone for previously treated multiple myeloma (April 2019) NICE TA573 Recommended with restrictions

Scottish Medicines Consortium (SMC) decisions
▸ Daratumumab (*Darzalex*®) as monotherapy, for the treatment of adult patients with relapsed and refractory multiple myeloma, whose prior therapy included a proteasome inhibitor and an immunomodulatory agent and have demonstrated disease progression on the last therapy (October 2017) SMC No. 1205/17 Recommended with restrictions
▸ Daratumumab (*Darzalex*®) in combination with lenalidomide and dexamethasone, or bortezomib and dexamethasone, for the treatment of adult patients with multiple myeloma who have received at least one prior therapy (July 2019) SMC No. SMC2180 Recommended with restrictions
▸ Daratumumab subcutaneous injection (*Darzalex*®) in combination with lenalidomide and dexamethasone, or

...ezomib and dexamethasone, for the treatment of adult patients with multiple myeloma who have received at least one prior therapy (October 2020) SMC No. SMC2301 Recommended with restrictions

▶ **Daratumumab subcutaneous injection (*Darzalex*®) as monotherapy, for the treatment of adult patients with relapsed and refractory multiple myeloma, whose prior therapy included a proteasome inhibitor and an immunomodulatory agent and have demonstrated disease progression on the last therapy (October 2020)** SMC No. SMC2304 Recommended with restrictions

● MEDICINAL FORMS There can be variation in the licensing of different medicines containing the same drug.

Solution for injection
EXCIPIENTS: May contain Polysorbates, sorbitol
▶ Darzalex (Janssen-Cilag Ltd) ▼
Daratumumab 120 mg per 1 ml Darzalex 1800mg/15ml solution for injection vials | 1 vial [PoM] £4,320.00 (Hospital only)

Solution for infusion
EXCIPIENTS: May contain Polysorbates
ELECTROLYTES: May contain Sodium
▶ Darzalex (Janssen-Cilag Ltd) ▼
Daratumumab 20 mg per 1 ml Darzalex 100mg/5ml concentrate for solution for infusion vials | 1 vial [PoM] £360.00 (Hospital only)
Darzalex 400mg/20ml concentrate for solution for infusion vials | 1 vial [PoM] £1,440.00 (Hospital only)

Dinituximab beta

04-Nov-2020

● DRUG ACTION Dinutuximab beta is a chimeric monoclonal antibody; it specifically targets the carbohydrate moiety of disialoganglioside 2, which is overexpressed on neuroblastoma cells.

● INDICATIONS AND DOSE
High-risk neuroblastoma (specialist use only)
▶ BY INTRAVENOUS INFUSION
▶ Adult: (consult product literature)

● CONTRA-INDICATIONS Acute grade 3 or 4, or extensive chronic graft-versus-host disease

● CAUTIONS Avoid vaccinations during and for at least 10 weeks after treatment cessation (increased risk of immune stimulation and neurological toxicity) · ensure absence of systemic infection—any other infection should be controlled before treatment initiation · pre-medication must be administered to minimise the risk of infusion-related reactions and neuropathic pain

CAUTIONS, FURTHER INFORMATION
▶ Pre-medication Severe infusion-related reactions can occur and dinutuximab beta should only be administered when appropriately trained staff and resuscitation facilities are immediately available; manufacturer advises pre-medication with an antihistamine, and to monitor closely, particularly during the first and second treatment course; discontinue immediately if reaction occurs and treat as indicated—consult product literature.
Manufacturer advises pre-medication with non-opioid analgesics, gabapentin and opioids—consult product literature.

● INTERACTIONS → Appendix 1: monoclonal antibodies

● SIDE-EFFECTS
▶ **Common or very common** Abdominal distension · anaemia · anxiety · appetite decreased · ascites · capillary leak syndrome · chills · cough · cytokine release syndrome · decreased leucocytes · device related infection · dizziness · dyspnoea · electrolyte imbalance · eye disorders · eye inflammation · fever · fluid imbalance · gastrointestinal disorders · haematuria · headache · heart failure · hyperhidrosis · hypersensitivity · hypertension · hypertriglyceridaemia · hypoalbuminaemia · hypotension · hypoxia · increased risk of infection · left ventricular

dysfunction · muscle spasms · nausea · neutropenia · oedema · oral disorders · pain · paraesthesia · pericardial effusion · peripheral neuropathy · photosensitivity reaction · pulmonary oedema · renal impairment · respiratory disorders · seizure · sepsis · skin reactions · tachycardia · thrombocytopenia · tremor · urinary retention · urine abnormalities · vision disorders · vomiting · weight changes
▶ **Uncommon** Disseminated intravascular coagulation · eosinophilia · hepatocellular injury · hypovolaemic shock · intracranial pressure increased · peripheral vascular disease · posterior reversible encephalopathy syndrome (PRES)

● CONCEPTION AND CONTRACEPTION Manufacturer advises women of childbearing potential should use contraception during and for 6 months after stopping treatment. See also *Pregnancy and reproductive function* in Cytotoxic drugs p. 932.

● PREGNANCY Manufacturer advises avoid—no information available. See also *Pregnancy and reproductive function* in Cytotoxic drugs p. 932.

● BREAST FEEDING Manufacturer advises avoid during treatment and for 6 months after the last dose—no information available.

● MONITORING REQUIREMENTS
▶ Manufacturer advises pre-treatment evaluation of pulse oximetry, bone marrow function, liver function and renal function—consult product literature for values required for treatment initiation.
▶ Manufacturer advises monitor circulatory and respiratory function—risk of capillary leak syndrome.
▶ Manufacturer advises monitor liver function and electrolytes regularly.

● HANDLING AND STORAGE Manufacturer advises store in a refrigerator (2–8°C)—consult product literature for further information regarding storage conditions outside refrigerator and after preparation of the infusion.

● PATIENT AND CARER ADVICE
Driving and skilled tasks Manufacturer advises patients should not use or drive machines during treatment.

● NATIONAL FUNDING/ACCESS DECISIONS
For full details see funding body website

NICE decisions
▶ Dinutuximab beta for treating neuroblastoma (August 2018) NICE TA538 Recommended with restrictions

Scottish Medicines Consortium (SMC) decisions
▶ Dinutuximab beta (*Qarziba*®) for the treatment of high-risk neuroblastoma in patients aged 12 months and above, who have previously received induction chemotherapy and achieved at least a partial response, followed by myeloablative therapy and stem cell transplantation, as well as patients with history of relapsed or refractory neuroblastoma, with or without residual disease (November 2018) SMC No. SMC2105 Recommended

● MEDICINAL FORMS There can be variation in the licensing of different medicines containing the same drug.

Solution for infusion
▶ Qarziba (EUSA Pharma Ltd) ▼
Dinutuximab beta 4.5 mg per 1 ml Qarziba 20mg/4.5ml concentrate for solution for infusion vials | 1 vial [PoM] £7,610.00 (Hospital only)

Durvalumab

31-Aug-2020

- DRUG ACTION Durvalumab is a human monoclonal antibody that selectively binds to programmed cell death ligand-1 (PD-L1), blocking its interaction with the programmed death-1 (PD-1) receptor and with CD80, and thereby potentiating an immune response to tumour cells.

- INDICATIONS AND DOSE

Non-small cell lung cancer (initiated by a specialist)
▸ BY INTRAVENOUS INFUSION
▸ Adult: 10 mg/kg every 2 weeks, consult product literature for information on dose adjustments based on individual patient safety and tolerability

- INTERACTIONS → Appendix 1: monoclonal antibodies
- SIDE-EFFECTS
▸ **Common or very common** Cough · diarrhoea · dysphonia · dysuria · fever · flank pain · gastrointestinal discomfort · gastrointestinal disorders · hyperthyroidism · hypothyroidism · increased risk of infection · infusion related reaction · myalgia · night sweats · peripheral oedema · respiratory disorders · skin reactions · thyroiditis
▸ **Uncommon** Adrenal insufficiency · glomerulonephritis · hepatic disorders · myopathy · nephritis · type 1 diabetes mellitus
▸ **Rare or very rare** Diabetes insipidus · hypophysitis · hypopituitarism · myocarditis
  SIDE-EFFECTS, FURTHER INFORMATION **Immune-related reactions** Manufacturer advises that most immune-related adverse reactions resolved with appropriate management, including initiation of immunosuppressive treatment and treatment modifications—consult product literature.
  Infusion-related reactions Manufacturer advises to permanently discontinue treatment in patients with severe infusion reactions.

- CONCEPTION AND CONTRACEPTION Manufacturer advises effective contraception in women of childbearing potential during treatment and for at least 3 months after stopping treatment. See also *Pregnancy and reproductive function* in Cytotoxic drugs p. 932.

- PREGNANCY Manufacturer advises avoid—no information available. See also *Pregnancy and reproductive function* in Cytotoxic drugs p. 932.

- BREAST FEEDING Manufacturer advises avoid—no information available.

- MONITORING REQUIREMENTS Manufacturer advises monitor for signs and symptoms of infusion- and immune-related reactions—consult product literature.

- DIRECTIONS FOR ADMINISTRATION Manufacturer advises for *intravenous infusion*, dilute to a concentration between 1 mg/mL and 15 mg/mL with Glucose 5% *or* Sodium Chloride 0.9%; give over 60 minutes through a low-protein binding in-line filter (pore size 0.2 or 0.22 micron).

- HANDLING AND STORAGE Manufacturer advises store in a refrigerator (2–8°C) and protect from light—consult product literature for storage conditions after preparation of the infusion.

- NATIONAL FUNDING/ACCESS DECISIONS
For full details see funding body website

NICE decisions
▸ Durvalumab for treating locally advanced unresectable non-small-cell lung cancer after platinum-based chemoradiation (May 2019) NICE TA578 Recommended with restrictions

Scottish Medicines Consortium (SMC) decisions
▸ Durvalumab (*Imfinzi*®) for locally advanced, unresectable non-small cell lung cancer after platinum-based chemoradiation in adults (June 2019) SMC No. SMC2156 Recommended

- MEDICINAL FORMS There can be variation in the licensing of different medicines containing the same drug.
Solution for infusion
EXCIPIENTS: May contain Polysorbates
▸ Imfinzi (AstraZeneca UK Ltd) ▼
  Durvalumab 50 mg per 1 ml Imfinzi 120mg/2.4ml concentrate for solution for infusion vials | 1 vial [PoM] £592.00
  Imfinzi 500mg/10ml concentrate for solution for infusion vials | 1 vial [PoM] £2,466.00

Elotuzumab

12-Apr-2019

- DRUG ACTION Elotuzumab is a monoclonal antibody that targets the signalling lymphocytic activation molecule family member 7 (SLAMF7) protein, thereby activating natural killer cells and mediating myeloma cell death.

- INDICATIONS AND DOSE

Multiple myeloma in patients who have received at least one prior therapy (in combination with lenalidomide and dexamethasone) (specialist use only)
▸ BY INTRAVENOUS INFUSION
▸ Adult: 10 mg/kg every week, on days 1, 8, 15 and 22 of cycles 1 and 2, then 10 mg/kg every 2 weeks, on days 1 and 15 of subsequent cycles

- CAUTIONS Pre-medication must be administered to minimise the development of infusion-related reactions—consult product literature · secondary primary malignancies
  CAUTIONS, FURTHER INFORMATION
▸ Secondary primary malignancies Manufacturer advises to monitor for the development of secondary primary malignancy before and during treatment with elotuzumab.

- INTERACTIONS → Appendix 1: monoclonal antibodies
- SIDE-EFFECTS
▸ **Common or very common** Chest pain · cough · deep vein thrombosis · diarrhoea · fatigue · fever · headache · hypersensitivity · increased risk of infection · infusion related reaction · lymphopenia · mood altered · night sweats · numbness · oropharyngeal pain · weight decreased
  SIDE-EFFECTS, FURTHER INFORMATION Side-effects reported when used in combination with lenalidomide and dexamethasone or bortezomib and dexamethasone.
  Infusion-related reactions Manufacturer advises for mild-to-moderate infusion reactions interrupt treatment or reduce infusion rate, and monitor closely (consult product literature); permanently discontinue therapy in severe infusion reactions.

- CONCEPTION AND CONTRACEPTION Manufacturer advises effective contraception in men and women of childbearing potential; male patients should continue effective contraceptive measures for 180 days after stopping treatment if their partner is pregnant or of childbearing potential. See also *Pregnancy and reproductive function* in Cytotoxic drugs p. 932.

- PREGNANCY Manufacturer advises avoid unless essential—no information available. See also *Pregnancy and reproductive function* in Cytotoxic drugs p. 932.

- HANDLING AND STORAGE Manufacturer advises store in a refrigerator (2–8°C); consult product literature for storage conditions after preparation of the infusion.

- MEDICINAL FORMS There can be variation in the licensing of different medicines containing the same drug.
Powder for solution for infusion
EXCIPIENTS: May contain Polysorbates, sucrose
▸ Empliciti (Bristol-Myers Squibb Pharmaceuticals Ltd) ▼
  Elotuzumab 300 mg Empliciti 300mg powder for concentrate for solution for infusion vials | 1 vial [PoM] £1,085.00
  Elotuzumab 400 mg Empliciti 400mg powder for concentrate for solution for infusion vials | 1 vial [PoM] £1,446.00

8

Immune system and malignant disease

Gemtuzumab ozogamicin

06-Nov-2020

- **DRUG ACTION** Gemtuzumab ozogamicin is a monoclonal antibody that binds to CD33-expressing tumour cells to induce cell cycle arrest and apoptotic cell death.

- **INDICATIONS AND DOSE**

CD33-positive acute myeloid leukaemia (specialist use only)
  - ▸ BY INTRAVENOUS INFUSION
  - ▸ Adult: (consult product literature)

- **CAUTIONS** Adverse-risk cytogenetics (consider benefits and risks of treatment, consult product literature) · haematopoietic stem cell transplantation (increased risk of hepatotoxicity) · pre-medication recommended to minimise adverse reactions
  CAUTIONS, FURTHER INFORMATION
  - ▸ Pre-medication Serious infusion-related reactions can occur and gemtuzumab ozogamicin should only be administered when appropriately trained staff and resuscitation facilities are immediately available; manufacturer advises pre-medication with a corticosteroid, paracetamol and antihistamine 1 hour prior to dosing, and to take appropriate measures to help prevent the development of tumour lysis-related hyperuricaemia—consult product literature.

- **INTERACTIONS** → Appendix 1: gemtuzumab ozogamicin

- **SIDE-EFFECTS**
  - ▸ **Common or very common** Anaemia · appetite decreased · ascites · chills · constipation · decreased leucocytes · diarrhoea · dyspnoea · fatigue · fever · gastrointestinal discomfort · gastrointestinal disorders · haemorrhage · headache · hepatic disorders · hyperbilirubinaemia · hyperglycaemia · hypertension · hypotension · infection · infusion related reaction (including fatal cases) · multi organ failure · nausea · neutropenia · oedema · pancytopenia · sinusoidal obstruction syndrome · skin reactions · stomatitis · tachycardia · thrombocytopenia · tumour lysis syndrome (including fatal cases) · vomiting
  - ▸ **Frequency not known** Interstitial pneumonia
  SIDE-EFFECTS, FURTHER INFORMATION Infusion-related reactions (including fatal cases) can occur during the first 24 hours after administration. Manufacturer advises interrupt treatment immediately and treat as clinically indicated (consult product literature); permanent discontinuation should be strongly considered in patients who develop signs and symptoms of anaphylaxis.

- **CONCEPTION AND CONTRACEPTION** Manufacturer advises women of childbearing potential should use 2 methods of effective contraception during treatment and for at least 7 months after the last dose; male patients should use 2 methods of effective contraception during treatment and for at least 4 months after the last dose if their partner is of childbearing potential. See also Pregnancy and reproductive function in Cytotoxic drugs p. 932.

- **PREGNANCY** Manufacturer advises avoid unless potential benefit outweighs risk—toxicity in *animal* studies. See also Pregnancy and reproductive function in Cytotoxic drugs p. 932.

- **BREAST FEEDING** Manufacturer advises avoid during treatment and for at least one month after the last dose— no information available.

- **HEPATIC IMPAIRMENT** Manufacturer advises caution in moderate-to-severe impairment—increased risk of developing hepatotoxicity; postpone treatment if serum transaminases (ALT or AST) greater than 2.5 times the upper limit of normal or total bilirubin greater than 2 times the upper limit of normal.

- **MONITORING REQUIREMENTS**
  - ▸ Manufacturer advises monitor complete blood counts prior to each dose as well as signs and symptoms of infection, bleeding and other effects of myelosuppression during treatment; dose interruption or discontinuation of treatment may be required—consult product literature.
  - ▸ Manufacturer advises monitor for signs and symptoms of infusion-related reactions—close clinical monitoring, including pulse, blood pressure and temperature, should be performed during infusion; monitor for signs and symptoms of tumour lysis syndrome.
  - ▸ Manufacturer advises monitor for signs and symptoms of hepatotoxicity (including hepatic veno-occlusive disease); liver tests should be monitored prior to each dose—consult product literature.

- **PRESCRIBING AND DISPENSING INFORMATION** Gemtuzumab ozogamicin is a biological medicine. Biological medicines must be prescribed and dispensed by brand name, see *Biological medicines* and *Biosimilar medicines*, under Guidance on prescribing p. 1.

- **HANDLING AND STORAGE** Manufacturer advises store in a refrigerator (2–8°C) and protect from light—consult product literature for storage conditions after reconstitution and dilution.

- **PATIENT AND CARER ADVICE**
  Driving and skilled tasks Manufacturer advises patients and carers should be counselled on the effects on driving and performance of skilled tasks—increased risk of fatigue and headache.

- **NATIONAL FUNDING/ACCESS DECISIONS**
  For full details see funding body website
  NICE decisions
  - ▸ **Gemtuzumab ozogamicin for untreated acute myeloid leukaemia (November 2018)** NICE TA545 Recommended with restrictions
  Scottish Medicines Consortium (SMC) decisions
  - ▸ **Gemtuzumab ozogamicin (*Mylotarg*®) as combination therapy with daunorubicin and cytarabine for the treatment of patients age 15 years and above with previously untreated, *de novo* CD33-positive acute myeloid leukaemia, except acute promyelocytic leukaemia (October 2018)** SMC No. SMC2089 Recommended with restrictions

- **MEDICINAL FORMS** There can be variation in the licensing of different medicines containing the same drug.
  Powder for solution for infusion
  - ▸ Mylotarg (Pfizer Ltd) ▼
    Gemtuzumab ozogamicin 5 mg Mylotarg 5mg powder for concentrate for solution for infusion vials | 1 vial [PoM] £6,300.00 (Hospital only)

Inotuzumab ozogamicin

09-Nov-2020

- **DRUG ACTION** Inotuzumab ozogamicin is a monoclonal antibody that binds to CD22-expressing tumour cells to induce cell cycle arrest and apoptotic cell death.

- **INDICATIONS AND DOSE**

Monotherapy for relapsed or refractory CD22-positive B cell precursor acute lymphoblastic leukaemia (under expert supervision)
  - ▸ BY INTRAVENOUS INFUSION
  - ▸ Adult: (consult product literature)

- **CONTRA-INDICATIONS** Prior confirmed severe or ongoing sinusoidal obstruction syndrome

- **CAUTIONS** History of, or predisposition to QT-interval prolongation (e.g. electrolyte disturbances, concomitant use of drugs that prolong the QT interval) · patients may need pre-medication to minimise adverse reactions ·

patients undergoing haematopoietic stem cell transplantation (increased risk of hepatotoxicity)

CAUTIONS, FURTHER INFORMATION
▸ **Pre-medication** Manufacturer advises pre-medication with a corticosteroid, antipyretic and antihistamine prior to dosing in all patients and pre-medication to reduce uric acid levels and hydration in patients with a high tumour burden (increased risk of tumour lysis syndrome)—consult product literature.

● INTERACTIONS → Appendix 1: monoclonal antibodies

● SIDE-EFFECTS
▸ **Common or very common** Anaemia · appetite decreased · ascites · bone marrow disorders · central nervous system haemorrhage · chills · constipation · decreased leucocytes · diarrhoea · fatigue · fever · gastrointestinal discomfort · haemorrhage · headache · hyperbilirubinaemia · hypersensitivity · hyperuricaemia · increased risk of infection · infusion related reaction · nausea · neutropenia · QT interval prolongation · sepsis · sinusoidal obstruction syndrome · stomatitis · thrombocytopenia · tumour lysis syndrome · vomiting

SIDE-EFFECTS, FURTHER INFORMATION Manufacturer advises interrupt treatment if an infusion related reaction occurs; depending on the severity, discontinuation of the infusion or administration of steroids and antihistamines should be considered (consult product literature); permanently discontinue treatment in severe or life-threatening infusion reactions.

● CONCEPTION AND CONTRACEPTION Manufacturer advises effective contraception in women of childbearing potential during treatment and for at least 8 months after the last dose; male patients should use effective contraception during treatment and for at least 5 months after the last dose if their partner is of childbearing potential. See also Pregnancy and reproductive function in Cytotoxic drugs p. 932.

● PREGNANCY Manufacturer advises avoid unless potential benefit outweighs risk—toxicity in *animal* studies.

● BREAST FEEDING Manufacturer advises avoid during treatment and for at least two months after the last dose—no information available.

● HEPATIC IMPAIRMENT Manufacturer advises caution if bilirubin and transaminase levels are raised (limited information available); avoid in serious ongoing impairment.
Dose adjustments Manufacturer advises dose interruption or discontinuation according to bilirubin and transaminase levels.

● PRE-TREATMENT SCREENING Manufacturer advises baseline CD22 positivity of greater than 0% is required prior to initiating treatment.

● MONITORING REQUIREMENTS
▸ Manufacturer advises monitor complete blood counts prior to each dose as well as signs and symptoms of infection, bleeding and other effects of myelosuppresion during treatment; dose reduction or interruption or discontinuation of treatment may be required—consult product literature.
▸ Manufacturer advises monitor for signs of infusion related-reactions during and for at least 1 hour after infusion; monitor for signs and symptoms of tumour lysis syndrome.
▸ Manufacturer advises ECG and electrolytes should be monitored prior to the start of treatment and periodically during treatment; monitor for increases in serum amylase and lipase.
▸ Manufacturer advises monitor for signs and symptoms of sinusoidal obstruction syndrome; liver tests should be monitored prior to and following each dose—consult product literature.

● DIRECTIONS FOR ADMINISTRATION Manufacturer advises resuscitation facilities should be available during administration.

● PRESCRIBING AND DISPENSING INFORMATION Inotuzumab ozogamicin is a biological medicine. Biological medicines must be prescribed and dispensed by brand name, see *Biological medicines* and *Biosimilar medicines*, under Guidance on prescribing p. 1; manufacturer advises to record the brand name and batch number after each administration.

● HANDLING AND STORAGE Manufacturer advises store in a refrigerator (2–8°C) and protect from light—consult product literature for storage conditions after reconstitution and dilution.

● PATIENT AND CARER ADVICE
Driving and skilled tasks Manufacturer advises patients and carers should be counselled on the effects on driving and performance of skilled tasks—increased risk of fatigue.

● NATIONAL FUNDING/ACCESS DECISIONS
For full details see funding body website
NICE decisions
▸ Inotuzumab ozogamicin for treating relapsed or refractory B-cell acute lymphoblastic leukaemia (September 2018)
NICE TA541 Recommended with restrictions
Scottish Medicines Consortium (SMC) decisions
▸ Inotuzumab ozogamicin (*Besponsa*®) as monotherapy for the treatment of adults with relapsed or refractory CD22-positive B cell precursor acute lymphoblastic leukaemia (ALL). Adult patients with Philadelphia chromosome positive relapsed or refractory B cell precursor ALL should have failed treatment with at least 1 tyrosine kinase inhibitor (June 2018)
SMC No. 1328/18 Recommended with restrictions

● MEDICINAL FORMS There can be variation in the licensing of different medicines containing the same drug.
Powder for solution for infusion
ELECTROLYTES: May contain Sodium
▸ Besponsa (Pfizer Ltd) ▼
  Inotuzumab ozogamicin 1 mg Besponsa 1mg powder for concentrate for solution for infusion vials | 1 vial [PoM] £8,048.00 (Hospital only)

Ipilimumab
22-Oct-2020

● DRUG ACTION Ipilimumab is a monoclonal antibody which causes T-cell activation resulting in tumour cell death.

● **INDICATIONS AND DOSE**

Melanoma (as monotherapy) (specialist use only)
▸ BY INTRAVENOUS INFUSION
▸ Adult: 3 mg/kg every 3 weeks for 4 doses, for dose interruption or discontinuation of treatment due to immune-related side-effects—consult product literature

Melanoma (in combination with nivolumab) (specialist use only) | Advanced renal cell carcinoma (in combination with nivolumab) (specialist use only)
▸ BY INTRAVENOUS INFUSION
▸ Adult: (consult product literature)

IMPORTANT SAFETY INFORMATION

MHRA/CHM ADVICE: IPILIMUMAB (*YERVOY*®): REPORTS OF CYTOMEGALOVIRUS (CMV) GASTROINTESTINAL INFECTION OR REACTIVATION (JANUARY 2019)

There have been post-marketing cases of gastrointestinal CMV infection or reactivation in ipilimumab-treated patients reported to have corticosteroid-refractory immune-related colitis, including fatal cases.

  Patients should be advised to contact their healthcare professional immediately at the onset of symptoms of colitis. Possible causes, including infections, should be investigated; a stool infection work-up should be performed and patients screened for CMV. For patients with corticosteroid-refractory immune-related colitis, use of an additional immunosuppressive agent should only be considered if other causes are excluded using viral PCR on biopsy, and eliminating other viral, bacterial, and parasitic causes.

- CAUTIONS For full details consult product literature.
- INTERACTIONS → Appendix 1: monoclonal antibodies
- SIDE-EFFECTS
  - ▸ **Common or very common** Alopecia · anaemia · appetite decreased · arthralgia · asthenia · cancer pain · chills · confusion · constipation · cough · dehydration · diarrhoea · dizziness · dyspnoea · electrolyte imbalance · eye discomfort · fever · gastrointestinal discomfort · gastrointestinal disorders · haemorrhage · headache · hepatic disorders · hypophysitis · hypopituitarism · hypotension · hypothyroidism · influenza like illness · lethargy · lymphopenia · mucositis · muscle complaints · nausea · nerve disorders · night sweats · oedema · pain · skin reactions · vasodilation · vision disorders · vomiting · weight decreased
  - ▸ **Uncommon** Adrenal hypofunction · alkalosis · allergic rhinitis · amenorrhoea · arrhythmias · arthritis · brain oedema · depression · dysarthria · eosinophilia · eye inflammation · glomerulonephritis · haemolytic anaemia · hair colour changes · hypersensitivity · hyperthyroidism · hypogonadism · increased risk of infection · infusion related reaction · libido decreased · meningitis · movement disorders · multi organ failure · muscle weakness · myopathy · nephritis autoimmune · neutropenia · pancreatitis · paraneoplastic syndrome · peripheral ischaemia · polymyalgia rheumatica · psychiatric disorder · pulmonary oedema · renal failure · renal tubular acidosis · respiratory disorders · sepsis · severe cutaneous adverse reactions (SCARs) · syncope · systemic inflammatory response syndrome · thrombocytopenia · tremor · tumour lysis syndrome · vascular disorders · vasculitis
  - ▸ **Rare or very rare** Myasthenia gravis · proteinuria · thyroiditis
  - ▸ **Frequency not known** Cytomegalovirus infection reactivation

  SIDE-EFFECTS, FURTHER INFORMATION A corticosteroid can be used after starting ipilimumab, to treat immune-related reactions.

- CONCEPTION AND CONTRACEPTION Use effective contraception.
- PREGNANCY Manufacturer advises avoid unless potential benefit outweighs risk—toxicity in *animal* studies.
- BREAST FEEDING Manufacturer advises avoid—present in milk in *animal* studies.
- HEPATIC IMPAIRMENT Manufacturer advises caution if bilirubin greater than 3 times upper limit of normal range or if transaminases equal to or greater than 5 times upper limit of normal range (limited information available).
- MONITORING REQUIREMENTS
  - ▸ Manufacturer advises monitor liver function tests and thyroid function prior to initiation of treatment and before each dose.
  - ▸ Manufacturer advises monitor for signs or symptoms of immune-related side-effects and gastrointestinal perforation—consult product literature.
- DIRECTIONS FOR ADMINISTRATION Manufacturer advises for *intravenous infusion*, give undiluted or dilute to a concentration of 1–4 mg/mL with Glucose 5% *or* Sodium Chloride 0.9%; give over 90 minutes.

- PRESCRIBING AND DISPENSING INFORMATION Infusion-related side-effects have been reported; premedication with paracetamol and an antihistamine is recommended.
- HANDLING AND STORAGE Manufacturer advises store in a refrigerator (2–8 °C) and protect from light—consult product literature for further information regarding storage conditions outside refrigerator and after preparation of the infusion.
- NATIONAL FUNDING/ACCESS DECISIONS For full details see funding body website

  NICE decisions
  - ▸ Ipilimumab for previously treated advanced (unresectable or metastatic) melanoma (December 2012) NICE TA268 Recommended with restrictions
  - ▸ Ipilimumab for previously untreated advanced (unresectable or metastatic) melanoma (July 2014) NICE TA319 Recommended with restrictions
  - ▸ Nivolumab in combination with ipilimumab for treating advanced melanoma (July 2016) NICE TA400 Recommended with restrictions
  - ▸ Nivolumab with ipilimumab for untreated advanced renal cell carcinoma (May 2019) NICE TA581 Recommended with restrictions

  Scottish Medicines Consortium (SMC) decisions
  - ▸ Ipilimumab (*Yervoy*®) for the treatment of advanced (unresectable or metastatic) melanoma in adults who have received prior therapy (April 2013) SMC No. 779/12 Recommended
  - ▸ Ipilimumab (*Yervoy*®) for the treatment of advanced (unresectable or metastatic) melanoma in adults (first-line use) (November 2014) SMC No. 997/14 Recommended

- MEDICINAL FORMS There can be variation in the licensing of different medicines containing the same drug.

  Solution for infusion
  ELECTROLYTES: May contain Sodium
  - ▸ Yervoy (Bristol-Myers Squibb Pharmaceuticals Ltd)
    Ipilimumab 5 mg per 1 ml Yervoy 50mg/10ml concentrate for solution for infusion vials | 1 vial [PoM] £3,750.00 (Hospital only)
    Yervoy 200mg/40ml concentrate for solution for infusion vials | 1 vial [PoM] £15,000.00 (Hospital only)

Isatuximab

03-Dec-2020

- DRUG ACTION Isatuximab is a monoclonal antibody that binds to CD38, a cell-surface protein, resulting in tumour cell death by immune-mediated actions and apoptosis.

- INDICATIONS AND DOSE

  Multiple myeloma in patients who have received at least two prior therapies (in combination with pomalidomide and dexamethasone) (specialist use only)
  - ▸ BY INTRAVENOUS INFUSION
  - ▸ Adult: 10 mg/kg every week on days 1, 8, 15 and 22 of the first 28-day cycle, then 10 mg/kg every 2 weeks on days 1 and 15 of subsequent 28-day cycles until disease progression or unacceptable toxicity, for dose interruption, adjustment of infusion rate or discontinuation of treatment due to infusion-related reactions or side-effects—consult product literature

- CAUTIONS Pre-medication must be administered to minimise the development of infusion-related reactions—consult product literature · secondary primary malignancies

  CAUTIONS, FURTHER INFORMATION
  - ▸ Infusion-related reactions Serious infusion-related reactions can occur and isatuximab should only be administered when appropriately trained staff and resuscitation facilities are immediately available; manufacturer advises pre-medication with dexamethasone, an antihistamine, an anti-pyretic, and a proton pump inhibitor or H_2-receptor

antagonist—consult product literature. Manufacturer advises patients should be closely monitored for signs of infusion-related reactions during and after administration; in the event of a hypersensitivity reaction, treatment should be stopped immediately and appropriate management initiated—consult product literature.

‣ Secondary primary malignancies Manufacturer advises to monitor for the development of secondary primary malignancy before and during treatment with isatuximab and initiate treatment as indicated.

● SIDE-EFFECTS
▶ **Common or very common** Appetite decreased · atrial fibrillation · diarrhoea · dyspnoea · increased risk of infection · infusion related reaction · nausea · neutropenia · squamous cell carcinoma · vomiting · weight decreased

● CONCEPTION AND CONTRACEPTION Manufacturer advises effective contraception in female patients of childbearing potential during treatment and for 5 months after last treatment. See also *Pregnancy and reproductive function* in Cytotoxic drugs p. 932.

● PREGNANCY Manufacturer advises avoid—no information available. See also *Pregnancy and reproductive function* in Cytotoxic drugs p. 932.

● BREAST FEEDING Manufacturer advises avoid during first few days after birth—possible risk from transfer of antibodies to infant. After this time, use during breast-feeding only if clinically needed.

● EFFECT ON LABORATORY TESTS Manufacturer advises may cause false positive indirect Coombs test—consult product literature. Manufacturer advises may affect accuracy of both serum protein electrophoresis (SPE) and immunofixation (IFE) assays—consult product literature.

● PRESCRIBING AND DISPENSING INFORMATION Isatuximab is a biological medicine. Biological medicines must be prescribed and dispensed by brand name, see *Biological medicines* and *Biosimilar medicines*, under Guidance on prescribing p. 1; manufacturer advises to record the brand name and batch number after each administration.

● HANDLING AND STORAGE Store in a refrigerator (2–8°C) and protect from light—consult product literature for storage conditions after preparation of the infusion.

● NATIONAL FUNDING/ACCESS DECISIONS
For full details see funding body website
NICE decisions
▶ Isatuximab with pomalidomide and dexamethasone for treating relapsed and refractory multiple myeloma (November 2020) NICE TA658 Recommended with restrictions

● MEDICINAL FORMS There can be variation in the licensing of different medicines containing the same drug.
Solution for infusion
EXCIPIENTS: May contain Polysorbates, sucrose
▶ Sarclisa (Sanofi) ▼
Isatuximab 20 mg per 1 ml Sarclisa 500mg/25ml concentrate for solution for infusion vials | 1 vial PoM £2,534.69 (Hospital only)
Sarclisa 100mg/5ml concentrate for solution for infusion vials | 1 vial PoM £506.94 (Hospital only)

Mogamulizumab

17-Apr-2020

● DRUG ACTION Mogamulizumab is a monoclonal antibody, which binds to the CCR4 receptor, thereby potentiating an immune response to cancer cells.

● INDICATIONS AND DOSE
Mycosis fungoides (initiated by a specialist) | Sézary syndrome (initiated by a specialist)
▶ BY INTRAVENOUS INFUSION
▶ Adult: 1 mg/kg every week on days 1, 8, 15 and 22 of the first 28-day cycle, followed by 1 mg/kg every

2 weeks on days 1 and 15 of subsequent 28-day cycles, dose to be administered within 2 days of the scheduled day, for treatment interruption or discontinuation due to side-effects and infusion-related reactions—consult product literature

● CAUTIONS Patients may need pre-medication to minimise infusion-related reactions · risk factors for cardiac disorders · risk of serious infection and/or viral reactivation such as hepatitis B · risk of transplant-related complications

CAUTIONS, FURTHER INFORMATION
▶ Pre-medication Manufacturer advises pre-medication with an antihistamine and an anti-pyretic—consult product literature.
▶ Hepatitis B infection Manufacturer advises patients should be tested for hepatitis B infection before treatment initiation; expert advice on measures against hepatitis B reactivation should be sought for patients with positive hepatitis B serology.
▶ Transplant-related complications Manufacturer advises patients who receive an allogeneic haematopoietic stem cell transplant within 50 days of mogamulizumab treatment are at higher risk of complications, such as severe graft-versus-host disease, and should be closely monitored.

● INTERACTIONS → Appendix 1: monoclonal antibodies

● SIDE-EFFECTS
▶ **Common or very common** Anaemia · constipation · diarrhoea · fatigue · fever · headache · hypothyroidism · increased risk of infection · infusion related reaction · leucopenia · nausea · neutropenia · peripheral oedema · sepsis · skin reactions · stomatitis · thrombocytopenia · vomiting
▶ **Uncommon** Hepatic disorders · tumour lysis syndrome
▶ **Frequency not known** Cardiomyopathy · myocardial infarction · polymyositis · severe cutaneous adverse reactions (SCARs) · viral infection reactivation

● CONCEPTION AND CONTRACEPTION Manufacturer advises effective contraception in male and female patients of childbearing potential during treatment and for at least 6 months after last treatment. See also *Pregnancy and reproductive function* in Cytotoxic drugs p. 932.

● PREGNANCY Manufacturer advises avoid—limited information available. See also *Pregnancy and reproductive function* in Cytotoxic drugs p. 932.

● BREAST FEEDING Manufacturer advises avoid during first few days after birth—possible risk from transfer of antibodies to infant. After this time, use during breast-feeding only if clinically needed.

● MONITORING REQUIREMENTS Manufacturer advises monitor electrolytes, hydration status and renal function, particularly in the first month of treatment—risk of tumour lysis syndrome.

● DIRECTIONS FOR ADMINISTRATION Manufacturer advises for *intravenous infusion* (*Poteligeo*®), dilute to a concentration between 0.1 mg/mL to 3 mg/mL with Sodium Chloride 0.9%; give over at least 60 minutes through a low-protein binding 0.22 micron in-line filter. Resuscitation facilities should be available.

● HANDLING AND STORAGE Store in a refrigerator (2–8°C) and protect from light—consult product literature for storage conditions after preparation of the infusion.

● PATIENT AND CARER ADVICE
Driving and skilled tasks Manufacturer advises patients and carers should be counselled on the effects on driving and performance of skilled tasks—increased risk of fatigue.

● MEDICINAL FORMS There can be variation in the licensing of different medicines containing the same drug.

Solution for infusion
EXCIPIENTS: May contain Polysorbates
‣ Poteligeo (Kyowa Kirin Ltd) ▼
  Mogamulizumab 4 mg per 1 ml Poteligeo 20mg/5ml concentrate for solution for infusion vials | 1 vial [PoM] £1,329.00 (Hospital only)

Necitumumab
21-Feb-2017

● DRUG ACTION Necitumumab is a monoclonal antibody that binds to the epidermal growth factor receptor (EGFR).

● INDICATIONS AND DOSE

Locally advanced or metastatic epidermal growth factor receptor expressing squamous non-small-cell lung cancer, in patients who have not received previous chemotherapy (in combination with gemcitabine and cisplatin) (specialist use only)
‣ BY INTRAVENOUS INFUSION
‣ Adult: 800 mg once daily on days 1 and 8 of a 3-week cycle, for up to 6 cycles, patients whose disease has not progressed after combination therapy may continue with necitumumab monotherapy, for dose adjustments due to infusion-related reactions or skin reactions—consult product literature

● CAUTIONS Cardiorespiratory disorders (no information available) · history of thromboembolic events · patients may need pre-medication to minimise the development of infusion-related and skin reactions (consult product literature) · risk factors for thromboembolic events
CAUTIONS, FURTHER INFORMATION
‣ Thromboembolic events Manufacturer advises that necitumumab should not be administered to patients with multiple risk factors for thromboembolic events unless the benefits outweigh the risks. Thromboprophylaxis should be considered after assessment of a patient's risk factors.

● INTERACTIONS → Appendix 1: monoclonal antibodies

● SIDE-EFFECTS
‣ **Common or very common** Conjunctivitis · dysuria · electrolyte imbalance · embolism and thrombosis · fever · haemorrhage · headache · hypersensitivity · hypomagnesaemia (severe) · increased risk of infection · infusion related reaction · muscle spasms · oral disorders · skin reactions · taste altered · vomiting · weight decreased
‣ **Frequency not known** Cardiac arrest · eyelash trichomegaly

● CONCEPTION AND CONTRACEPTION Manufacturer advises women of child-bearing potential should use effective contraception during and for 3 months after treatment.

● PREGNANCY Manufacturer advises avoid unless potential benefit outweighs risk—limited information available. See also *Pregnancy and reproductive function* in Cytotoxic drugs p. 932.

● BREAST FEEDING Manufacturer advises avoid during treatment and for at least 4 months after the last dose—no information available.

● MONITORING REQUIREMENTS Manufacturer advises monitor patients during and following each infusion for signs of hypersensitivity and infusion-related reactions; monitor electrolytes (including magnesium, potassium and calcium) prior to each infusion and after completion of treatment, until within normal limits—correct any electrolyte disturbance promptly.

● DIRECTIONS FOR ADMINISTRATION Manufacturer advises necitumumab should be given under the supervision of an experienced specialist, in an environment where full resuscitation facilities and resources for the treatment of infusion-related reactions are immediately available.

● HANDLING AND STORAGE Manufacturer advises store in a refrigerator (2–8°C); consult product literature for storage conditions after preparation of the infusion.

● PATIENT AND CARER ADVICE Manufacturer advises patients and their carers should be made aware of the symptoms of thromboembolism and advised to seek medical attention if they experience sudden breathlessness, chest pain, or swelling of a limb.

● NATIONAL FUNDING/ACCESS DECISIONS
For full details see funding body website
NICE decisions
‣ Necitumumab for untreated advanced or metastatic squamous non-small-cell lung cancer (September 2016)
NICE TA411 Not recommended

● MEDICINAL FORMS There can be variation in the licensing of different medicines containing the same drug.
Solution for infusion
ELECTROLYTES: May contain Sodium
‣ Portrazza (Eli Lilly and Company Ltd) ▼
  Necitumumab 16 mg per 1 ml Portrazza 800mg/50ml concentrate for solution for infusion vials | 1 vial [PoM] £1,450.00 (Hospital only)

Nivolumab
19-Nov-2020

● DRUG ACTION Nivolumab is a human immunoglobulin G4 monoclonal antibody, which binds to the programmed death-1 (PD-1) receptor thereby potentiating an immune response to tumour cells.

● INDICATIONS AND DOSE

Melanoma (in combination with ipilimumab) (specialist use only) | Advanced renal cell carcinoma (in combination with ipilimumab) (specialist use only)
‣ BY INTRAVENOUS INFUSION
‣ Adult: (consult product literature)

Melanoma (as monotherapy) (specialist use only) | Advanced renal cell carcinoma (as monotherapy) (specialist use only)
‣ BY INTRAVENOUS INFUSION
‣ Adult: 240 mg every 2 weeks, alternatively 480 mg every 4 weeks, consult product literature for information on dose adjustments based on individual patient safety and tolerability

Non-small cell lung cancer (as monotherapy) (specialist use only) | Urothelial carcinoma (as monotherapy) (specialist use only) | Squamous cell cancer of the head and neck (as monotherapy) (specialist use only) | Classical Hodgkin lymphoma (as monotherapy) (specialist use only)
‣ BY INTRAVENOUS INFUSION
‣ Adult: 240 mg every 2 weeks, consult product literature for information on dose adjustments based on individual patient safety and tolerability

Adjuvant treatment of melanoma (as monotherapy) (specialist use only)
‣ BY INTRAVENOUS INFUSION
‣ Adult: 3 mg/kg every 2 weeks, consult product literature for information on dose adjustments based on individual patient safety and tolerability

---

IMPORTANT SAFETY INFORMATION
MHRA/CHM ADVICE: NIVOLUMAB (*OPDIVO*®): REPORTS OF ORGAN TRANSPLANT REJECTION (JULY 2017)
A European review of worldwide data concluded that nivolumab may increase the risk of rejection in organ transplant recipients. The MHRA recommends considering the benefit of treatment with nivolumab versus the risk of possible organ transplant rejection for each patient.

8

MHRA/CHM ADVICE: NIVOLUMAB (*OPDIVO*®): REPORTS OF CYTOMEGALOVIRUS (CMV) GASTROINTESTINAL INFECTION OR REACTIVATION (OCTOBER 2019)

A European review of worldwide data identified cases suggestive of gastrointestinal CMV infection or reactivation in nivolumab-treated patients, including fatal cases.

Patients should be advised to contact their healthcare professional immediately at the onset of symptoms of colitis. Possible causes, including infections, should be investigated; a stool infection work-up should be performed and patients screened for CMV. For patients with corticosteroid-refractory immune-related colitis, use of an additional immunosuppressive agent should only be considered if other causes are excluded using viral PCR on biopsy, and eliminating other viral, bacterial, and parasitic causes.

- CAUTIONS May increase risk of severe graft-versus-host reaction in patients who have had prior haematopoietic stem cell transplant (particularly in those with a prior history) · patients may need pre-medication to minimise the development of infusion-related reactions
- INTERACTIONS → Appendix 1: monoclonal antibodies
- SIDE-EFFECTS
▸ **Common or very common** Abdominal pain · alopecia · anaemia · appetite decreased · arthralgia · constipation · cough · decreased leucocytes · diarrhoea · dizziness · dry mouth · dyspnoea · electrolyte imbalance · fatigue · fever · gastrointestinal disorders · haemolytic anaemia · headache · hyperglycaemia · hypersensitivity · hypertension · hyperthyroidism · hypoglycaemia · hypothyroidism · increased risk of infection · infusion related reaction · musculoskeletal discomfort · myalgia · nausea · nerve disorders · neutropenia · oedema · pain · respiratory disorders · skin reactions · stomatitis · thrombocytopenia · vomiting · weight decreased
▸ **Uncommon** Adrenal insufficiency · arrhythmias · arthritis · cardiac inflammation · chest pain · connective tissue disorders · dehydration · diabetes mellitus · dry eye · eosinophilia · eye inflammation · hepatic disorders · hypophysitis · hypopituitarism · metabolic acidosis · nephritis tubulointerstitial · pancreatitis · paresis · pericardial disorders · renal impairment · thyroiditis · vasculitis · vision blurred
▸ **Rare or very rare** Demyelination · diabetic ketoacidosis · histiocytic necrotising lymphadenitis · myasthenic syndrome · myopathy · severe cutaneous adverse reactions (SCARs)
▸ **Frequency not known** Cytomegalovirus infection reactivation · haemophagocytic lymphohistiocytosis · hypoparathyroidism · meningitis aseptic · sarcoidosis · solid organ transplant rejection · tumour lysis syndrome

SIDE-EFFECTS, FURTHER INFORMATION **Immune-related reactions** Manufacturer advises that most immune-related adverse reactions improved or resolved with appropriate management, including initiation of corticosteroids and treatment modifications—consult product literature for further information.

Infusion-related reactions Manufacturer advises that patients with mild or moderate infusion reactions may continue treatment with close monitoring and use of pre-medication according to local guidelines; discontinue treatment if severe infusion reactions occur.

- CONCEPTION AND CONTRACEPTION Manufacturer advises effective contraception required during treatment and for at least 5 months after treatment in women of childbearing potential.
- PREGNANCY Manufacturer advises avoid unless potential benefit outweighs risk—toxicity in *animal* studies.

- BREAST FEEDING Manufacturer advises avoid—no information available.
- HEPATIC IMPAIRMENT Manufacturer advises caution in moderate to severe impairment (limited information available).
- MONITORING REQUIREMENTS Manufacturer advises monitor for signs and symptoms of infusion- and immune-related reactions, cardiac and pulmonary reactions, and electrolyte disturbances before and periodically during treatment. Patients should be monitored for adverse reactions for at least 5 months after the last dose.
- DIRECTIONS FOR ADMINISTRATION Manufacturer advises for *intermittent intravenous infusion*, give undiluted or dilute to a concentration of not less than 1 mg/mL with Glucose 5% or Sodium Chloride 0.9%; give over 30 or 60 minutes (depending on dose—consult product literature) through an in-line filter (pore size 0.2–1.2 micron).
- HANDLING AND STORAGE Manufacturer advises store in a refrigerator (2–8 °C)—consult product literature for storage conditions after preparation of the infusion.
- PATIENT AND CARER ADVICE Patients should be provided with a patient alert card with each prescription.
- NATIONAL FUNDING/ACCESS DECISIONS For full details see funding body website

NICE decisions
▸ **Nivolumab for treating advanced (unresectable or metastatic) melanoma (February 2016)** NICE TA384 Recommended
▸ **Nivolumab in combination with ipilimumab for treating advanced melanoma (July 2016)** NICE TA400 Recommended with restrictions
▸ **Nivolumab for adjuvant treatment of completely resected melanoma with lymph node involvement or metastatic disease (January 2019)** NICE TA558 Recommended with restrictions
▸ **Nivolumab for previously treated advanced renal cell carcinoma (updated November 2017)** NICE TA417 Recommended with restrictions
▸ **Nivolumab with ipilimumab for untreated advanced renal cell carcinoma (May 2019)** NICE TA581 Recommended with restrictions
▸ **Nivolumab for treating relapsed or refractory classical Hodgkin lymphoma (updated November 2017)** NICE TA462 Recommended with restrictions
▸ **Nivolumab for previously treated non-squamous non-small-cell lung cancer (November 2017)** NICE TA484 Recommended with restrictions
▸ **Nivolumab for advanced squamous non-small-cell lung cancer after chemotherapy (October 2020)** NICE TA655 Recommended with restrictions
▸ **Nivolumab for treating squamous cell carcinoma of the head and neck after platinum-based chemotherapy (November 2017)** NICE TA490 Recommended with restrictions
▸ **Nivolumab for treating locally advanced unresectable or metastatic urothelial cancer after platinum-containing chemotherapy (July 2018)** NICE TA530 Not recommended

Scottish Medicines Consortium (SMC) decisions
▸ **Nivolumab (*Opdivo*®) for the treatment of locally advanced or metastatic squamous non-small cell lung cancer (NSCLC) after prior chemotherapy in adults (July 2016)** SMC No. 1144/16 Recommended
▸ **Nivolumab (*Opdivo*®) for the treatment of locally advanced or metastatic non-squamous non-small cell lung cancer (NSCLC) after prior chemotherapy in adults (October 2016)** SMC No. 1180/16 Recommended with restrictions
▸ **Nivolumab (*Opdivo*®) for use as monotherapy for the treatment of advanced (unresectable or metastatic) melanoma in adults (August 2016)** SMC No. 1120/16 Recommended with restrictions
▸ **Nivolumab (*Opdivo*®) in combination with ipilimumab for the treatment of advanced (unresectable or metastatic)**

melanoma in adults (November 2016) SMC No. 1187/16 Recommended with restrictions
‣ Nivolumab (*Opdivo*®) as monotherapy for the adjuvant treatment of adults with melanoma with involvement of lymph nodes or metastatic disease who have undergone complete resection (December 2018) SMC No. SMC2112 Recommended
‣ Nivolumab (*Opdivo*®) as monotherapy for the treatment of advanced renal cell carcinoma after prior therapy in adults (June 2017) SMC No. 1188/16 Recommended
‣ Nivolumab (*Opdivo*®) in combination with ipilimumab for the first-line treatment of adult patients with intermediate/poor-risk advanced renal cell carcinoma (June 2019) SMC No. SMC2153 Recommended
‣ Nivolumab (*Opdivo*®) for the treatment of adult patients with relapsed or refractory classical Hodgkin lymphoma (cHL) after autologous stem cell transplant (ASCT) and treatment with brentuximab vedotin (July 2017) SMC No. 1240/17 Recommended
‣ Nivolumab (*Opdivo*®) as monotherapy, for the treatment of squamous cell cancer of the head and neck (SCCHN) in adults progressing on or after platinum-based therapy (September 2017) SMC No. 1261/17 Recommended with restrictions
‣ Nivolumab (*Opdivo*®) as monotherapy for the treatment of locally advanced unresectable or metastatic urothelial carcinoma in adults after failure of prior platinum-containing therapy (January 2018) SMC No. 1285/18 Not recommended

● MEDICINAL FORMS There can be variation in the licensing of different medicines containing the same drug.

Solution for infusion
CAUTIONARY AND ADVISORY LABELS 3
ELECTROLYTES: May contain Sodium
‣ Opdivo (Bristol-Myers Squibb Pharmaceuticals Ltd)
Nivolumab 10 mg per 1 ml Opdivo 40mg/4ml concentrate for solution for infusion vials | 1 vial [PoM] £439.00 (Hospital only)
Opdivo 100mg/10ml concentrate for solution for infusion vials | 1 vial [PoM] £1,097.00 (Hospital only)
Opdivo 240mg/24ml concentrate for solution for infusion vials | 1 vial [PoM] £2,633.00 (Hospital only)

⏾ 903

Obinutuzumab

11-Nov-2020

● INDICATIONS AND DOSE

Treatment of previously untreated chronic lymphocytic leukaemia in patients for whom full-dose fludarabine-based therapy is unsuitable due to co-morbidities | Treatment of previously untreated advanced follicular lymphoma | Treatment of follicular lymphoma in patients who did not respond or who progressed during or up to six months after treatment with rituximab or a rituximab-containing regimen

‣ BY INTRAVENOUS INFUSION
‣ Adult: (consult product literature or local protocols)

● CONTRA-INDICATIONS For obinutuzumab contra-indications, consult product literature.
● CAUTIONS For full details on the cautions of obinutuzumab, consult product literature.
Hepatitis B infection and reactivation Hepatitis B infection and reactivation (including fatal cases) have been reported in patients taking **obinutuzumab**. Manufacturer advises patients with positive hepatitis B serology should be referred to a liver specialist for monitoring and initiation of antiviral therapy before treatment initiation; treatment should not be initiated in patients with evidence of current hepatitis B infection until the infection has been adequately treated. Manufacturer also advises patients should be closely monitored for clinical and laboratory signs of active hepatitis B infection (consult product literature).
● INTERACTIONS → Appendix 1: monoclonal antibodies

● SIDE-EFFECTS
‣ **Common or very common** Arrhythmias · chest pain · dyspepsia · eye erythema · gastrointestinal disorders · heart failure · hypertension · hyperuricaemia · lymph node pain · nasal complaints · skin reactions · squamous cell carcinoma · tumour lysis syndrome · urinary disorders · weight increased
‣ **Frequency not known** Acute coronary syndrome · angina pectoris · chills · dizziness · dyspnoea · flushing · hypotension · nausea · viral infection reactivation

● CONCEPTION AND CONTRACEPTION Use effective contraception during and for 18 months after treatment.
● PREGNANCY Avoid unless potential benefit outweighs risk of B-lymphocyte depletion in fetus.
● BREAST FEEDING Avoid breast-feeding during and for 18 months after treatment—present in milk in *animal* studies.
● MONITORING REQUIREMENTS Patients should be closely monitored for clinical and laboratory signs of active hepatitis B infection during treatment and for up to a year following the last infusion (consult product literature).
● PRESCRIBING AND DISPENSING INFORMATION Infusion related side-effects have been reported; Patients should receive premedication with paracetamol, an antihistamine, and a corticosteroid before each dose—consult product literature for details.
● NATIONAL FUNDING/ACCESS DECISIONS For full details see funding body website
NICE decisions
‣ Obinutuzumab in combination with chlorambucil for untreated chronic lymphocytic leukaemia (June 2015) NICE TA343 Recommended with restrictions
‣ Obinutuzumab for untreated advanced follicular lymphoma (March 2018) NICE TA513 Recommended with restrictions
‣ Obinutuzumab with bendamustine for treating follicular lymphoma after rituximab (May 2020) NICE TA629 Recommended
Scottish Medicines Consortium (SMC) decisions
‣ Obinutuzumab (*Gazyvaro*®) in combination with bendamustine followed by obinutuzumab maintenance is indicated for the treatment of patients with follicular lymphoma who did not respond or who progressed during or up to six months after treatment with rituximab or a rituximab-containing regimen (March 2017) SMC No. 1219/17 Recommended
‣ Obinutuzumab (*Gazyvaro*®) in combination with chemotherapy, followed by maintenance therapy in patients achieving a response, for the treatment of patients with previously untreated advanced follicular lymphoma (FL) (September 2018) SMC No. SMC2015 Not recommended

● MEDICINAL FORMS There can be variation in the licensing of different medicines containing the same drug.
Solution for infusion
‣ Gazyvaro (Roche Products Ltd)
Obinutuzumab 25 mg per 1 ml Gazyvaro 1000mg/40ml concentrate for solution for infusion vials | 1 vial [PoM] £3,312.00 (Hospital only)

Panitumumab

21-Jul-2020

● DRUG ACTION Panitumumab is a monoclonal antibody that binds to the epidermal growth factor receptor (EGFR).

● **INDICATIONS AND DOSE**

Treatment of non-mutated RAS metastatic colorectal cancer (combination therapy) | Treatment of non-mutated RAS metastatic colorectal cancer (monotherapy after failure of fluoropyrimidine-, oxaliplatin-, and irinotecan-containing chemotherapy regimens)
▶ BY INTRAVENOUS INFUSION
▶ Adult: (consult product literature)

IMPORTANT SAFETY INFORMATION
MHRA/CHM ADVICE: SEVERE SKIN REACTIONS
Severe skin reactions have been reported very commonly in patients treated with panitumumab. Patients receiving panitumumab who have severe skin reactions or develop worsening skin reactions should be monitored for the development of inflammatory or infectious sequelae (including cellulitis, sepsis, and necrotising fasciitis). Appropriate treatment should be promptly initiated and panitumumab withheld or discontinued.

MHRA/CHM ADVICE: EPIDERMAL GROWTH FACTOR RECEPTOR (EGFR) INHIBITORS: SERIOUS CASES OF KERATITIS AND ULCERATIVE KERATITIS (MAY 2012)
Keratitis and ulcerative keratitis have been reported following treatment with epidermal growth factor receptor (EGFR) inhibitors for cancer (cetuximab, erlotinib, gefitinib and panitumumab). In rare cases, this has resulted in corneal perforation and blindness. Patients undergoing treatment with EGFR inhibitors who present with acute or worsening signs and symptoms suggestive of keratitis should be referred promptly to an ophthalmology specialist. Treatment should be interrupted or discontinued if ulcerative keratitis is diagnosed.

● CONTRA-INDICATIONS Interstitial pulmonary disease · the combination of panitumumab with oxaliplatin-containing chemotherapy is contra-indicated in patients with mutant *RAS* metastatic colorectal cancer or for whom *RAS* status is unknown

● CAUTIONS History of keratitis · history of severe dry eye · history of ulcerative keratitis · pulmonary disease · risk factors for keratitis · risk factors for severe dry eye · risk factors for ulcerative keratitis (including contact lens use)

● INTERACTIONS → Appendix 1: monoclonal antibodies

● SIDE-EFFECTS
▶ **Common or very common** Alopecia · anaemia · anxiety · appetite decreased · asthenia · chest pain · chills · constipation · cough · dehydration · diarrhoea · dizziness · dry eye · dry mouth · dyspnoea · electrolyte imbalance · embolism and thrombosis · eye discomfort · eye disorders · eye inflammation · fever · flushing · gastrointestinal discomfort · gastrooesophageal reflux disease · haemorrhage · hair changes · headache · hyperglycaemia · hyperhidrosis · hypersensitivity (may be delayed) · hypertension · hypotension · increased risk of infection · insomnia · leucopenia · mucositis · nail disorders · nausea · oral disorders · pain · peripheral oedema · skin reactions · skin ulcer · tachycardia · vomiting · weight decreased
▶ **Uncommon** Angioedema · cyanosis · infusion related reaction · nasal dryness · onycholysis · respiratory disorders · severe cutaneous adverse reactions (SCARs)
▶ **Rare or very rare** Anaphylactic reaction

● CONCEPTION AND CONTRACEPTION Manufacturer advises effective contraception during and for 6 months after treatment.

● PREGNANCY Avoid (toxicity in *animal* studies). See also *Pregnancy and reproductive function* in Cytotoxic drugs p. 932.

● BREAST FEEDING Manufacturer advises avoid breastfeeding during and for 2 months after treatment.

● PRE-TREATMENT SCREENING Evidence of non-mutated *RAS* status (at exons 2, 3 and 4 of *KRAS* and *NRAS*) is required before panitumumab treatment is initiated, and should be determined by an experienced laboratory using a validated test method.

● MONITORING REQUIREMENTS
▶ Monitor for hypomagnesaemia.
▶ Monitor for hypocalcaemia.
▶ Monitor for dermatological reactions including Stevens-Johnson syndrome and toxic epidermal necrolysis (consult product literature).

● NATIONAL FUNDING/ACCESS DECISIONS
For full details see funding body website
NICE decisions
▶ **Cetuximab, bevacizumab and panitumumab for the treatment of metastatic colorectal cancer after first-line chemotherapy (January 2012)** NICE TA242 Not recommended
▶ **Cetuximab and panitumumab for previously untreated metastatic colorectal cancer (updated September 2017)** NICE TA439 Recommended with restrictions

● MEDICINAL FORMS There can be variation in the licensing of different medicines containing the same drug.
Solution for infusion
ELECTROLYTES: May contain Sodium
▶ Vectibix (Amgen Ltd)
Panitumumab 20 mg per 1 ml Vectibix 400mg/20ml concentrate for solution for infusion vials | 1 vial [PoM] £1,517.16 (Hospital only)
Vectibix 100mg/5ml concentrate for solution for infusion vials | 1 vial [PoM] £379.29 (Hospital only)

Pembrolizumab

10-Dec-2020

● DRUG ACTION Pembrolizumab is a monoclonal antibody, which binds to the programmed death-1 (PD-1) receptor, thereby potentiating an immune response to tumour cells.

● **INDICATIONS AND DOSE**

Melanoma (specialist use only) | Non-small cell lung cancer (as monotherapy) (specialist use only) | Urothelial carcinoma (specialist use only) | Classical Hodgkin lymphoma (specialist use only) | Head and neck squamous cell carcinoma (as monotherapy) (specialist use only)
▶ BY INTRAVENOUS INFUSION
▶ Adult: 200 mg every 3 weeks, alternatively 400 mg every 6 weeks, for information on dose delay or interruption due to side-effects and infusion-related reactions—consult product literature

Non-small cell lung cancer (as combination therapy) (specialist use only) | Advanced renal cell carcinoma (as combination therapy) (specialist use only) | Head and neck squamous cell carcinoma (as combination therapy) (specialist use only)
▶ BY INTRAVENOUS INFUSION
▶ Adult: 200 mg every 3 weeks, for information on dose delay or interruption due to side-effects and infusion-related reactions—consult product literature

---

IMPORTANT SAFETY INFORMATION
MHRA/CHM ADVICE: PEMBROLIZUMAB (*KEYTRUDA*®): REPORTS OF ORGAN TRANSPLANT REJECTION (JULY 2017)
A European review of worldwide data concluded that pembrolizumab may increase the risk of rejection in organ transplant recipients. The MHRA recommends considering the benefit of treatment with

8

Immune system and malignant disease

pembrolizumab versus the risk of possible organ transplant rejection for each patient.

- **CAUTIONS** May increase risk of severe graft-versus-host reaction in patients who have had prior haematopoietic stem cell transplant (particularly in those with a prior history) · patients may need pretreatment to minimise the development of adverse reactions (consult product literature)

- **INTERACTIONS** → Appendix 1: monoclonal antibodies

- **SIDE-EFFECTS**
  ▸ **Common or very common** Alopecia · anaemia · appetite decreased · arrhythmias · arthritis · asthenia · chills · constipation · cough · cytokine release syndrome · decreased leucocytes · diarrhoea · dizziness · dry eye · dry mouth · dyspnoea · electrolyte imbalance · enterocolitis haemorrhagic · eye inflammation · eyelid hypopigmentation · fever · fluid imbalance · gastrointestinal discomfort · gastrointestinal disorders · genital abnormalities · headache · hepatic disorders · hypersensitivity · hypertension · hyperthyroidism · hypothyroidism · increased risk of infection · influenza like illness · infusion related reaction · insomnia · joint disorders · lethargy · lip swelling · musculoskeletal discomfort · myalgia · myopathy · myxoedema · nausea · nerve disorders · oedema · pain · polymyalgia rheumatica · pressure ulcer · respiratory disorders · severe cutaneous adverse reactions (SCARs) · skin reactions · taste altered · thrombocytopenia · torticollis · vomiting
  ▸ **Uncommon** Adrenal hypofunction · cardiac inflammation · diabetic ketoacidosis · eosinophilia · epilepsy · glomerulonephritis membranous · hair colour changes · hypophysitis · hypopituitarism · nephritis · nephrotic syndrome · neutropenia · pancreatitis · pericardial effusion · renal impairment · sarcoidosis · tendon disorders · thyroid disorder · thyroiditis · type 1 diabetes mellitus
  ▸ **Rare or very rare** Erythema nodosum · haemolytic anaemia · haemophagocytic lymphohistiocytosis · meningitis · meningitis non-infective · neuromuscular dysfunction · pure red cell aplasia · transverse myelitis
  ▸ **Frequency not known** Solid organ transplant rejection
  SIDE-EFFECTS, FURTHER INFORMATION **Immune-related reactions** Most immune-related adverse reactions are reversible and managed by temporarily stopping treatment and administration of a corticosteroid—consult product literature for further information.
  Infusion-related reactions Manufacturer advises to permanently discontinue treatment in patients with severe infusion reactions.

- **CONCEPTION AND CONTRACEPTION** Manufacturer recommends effective contraception during treatment and for at least 4 months after treatment in women of childbearing potential.

- **PREGNANCY** Manufacturer advises avoid unless potential benefit outweighs risk—no information available

- **BREAST FEEDING** Manufacturer advises avoid—no information available.

- **MONITORING REQUIREMENTS** Manufacturer advises monitor for signs and symptoms of infusion- and immune-related reactions.

- **DIRECTIONS FOR ADMINISTRATION** Manufacturer advises for *intermittent intravenous infusion* (Keytruda®), dilute to a concentration of 1 mg/mL to 10 mg/mL with Glucose 5% or Sodium Chloride 0.9%; give over 30 minutes using a low-protein binding 0.2–5 micron filter.

- **HANDLING AND STORAGE** Manufacturer advises store in a refrigerator at 2–8°C.

- **PATIENT AND CARER ADVICE** Patients should be provided with an alert card and advised to keep it with them at all times.

- **NATIONAL FUNDING/ACCESS DECISIONS**
  For full details see funding body website
  NICE decisions
  ▸ Pembrolizumab for treating advanced melanoma after disease progression with ipilimumab (updated September 2017) NICE TA357 Recommended with restrictions
  ▸ Pembrolizumab for advanced melanoma not previously treated with ipilimumab (updated September 2017) NICE TA366 Recommended with restrictions
  ▸ Pembrolizumab for adjuvant treatment of resected melanoma with high risk of recurrence (December 2018) NICE TA553 Recommended with restrictions
  ▸ Pembrolizumab for treating PD-L1-positive non-small-cell lung cancer after chemotherapy (updated September 2017) NICE TA428 Recommended with restrictions
  ▸ Pembrolizumab for untreated PD-L1-positive metastatic non-small-cell lung cancer (July 2018) NICE TA531 Recommended with restrictions
  ▸ Pembrolizumab with pemetrexed and platinum chemotherapy for untreated, metastatic, non-squamous non-small-cell lung cancer (January 2019) NICE TA557 Recommended with restrictions
  ▸ Pembrolizumab with carboplatin and paclitaxel for untreated metastatic squamous non-small-cell lung cancer (September 2019) NICE TA600 Recommended with restrictions
  ▸ Pembrolizumab for treating locally advanced or metastatic urothelial carcinoma after platinum-containing chemotherapy (April 2018) NICE TA519 Recommended with restrictions
  ▸ Pembrolizumab for untreated PD-L1-positive locally advanced or metastatic urothelial cancer when cisplatin is unsuitable (updated July 2018) NICE TA522 Recommended with restrictions
  ▸ Pembrolizumab for treating relapsed or refractory classical Hodgkin lymphoma [in adults who have had autologous stem cell transplant and brentuximab vedotin] (September 2018) NICE TA540 Not recommended
  ▸ Pembrolizumab for treating relapsed or refractory classical Hodgkin lymphoma [in adults who have had brentuximab vedotin and cannot have autologous stem cell transplant] (September 2018) NICE TA540 Recommended with restrictions
  ▸ Pembrolizumab with axitinib for untreated advanced renal cell carcinoma (September 2020) NICE TA650 Not recommended
  ▸ Pembrolizumab for untreated metastatic or unresectable recurrent head and neck squamous cell carcinoma (November 2020) NICE TA661 Recommended with restrictions
  Scottish Medicines Consortium (SMC) decisions
  ▸ Pembrolizumab (Keytruda®) as monotherapy for the treatment of advanced (unresectable or metastatic) melanoma in adults previously untreated with ipilimumab (November 2015) SMC No. 1086/15 Recommended
  ▸ Pembrolizumab (Keytruda®) as monotherapy for the treatment of advanced (unresectable or metastatic) melanoma in adults previously treated with ipilimumab (December 2016) SMC No. 1087/16 Not recommended
  ▸ Pembrolizumab (Keytruda®) as monotherapy for the adjuvant treatment of adults with stage III melanoma and lymph node involvement who have undergone complete resection (May 2019) SMC No. SMC2144 Recommended
  ▸ Pembrolizumab (Keytruda®) for the treatment of locally advanced or metastatic non small cell lung carcinoma (NSCLC) in adults whose tumours express programmed death ligand 1 (PD-L1) and who have received at least one prior chemotherapy regimen (January 2017) SMC No. 1204/17 Recommended with restrictions
  ▸ Pembrolizumab (Keytruda®) as monotherapy for the first-line treatment of metastatic non small cell lung carcinoma in adults whose tumours express programmed death ligand 1 with a 50% or more tumour proportion score with no epidermal growth factor receptor or anaplastic lymphoma

kinase (ALK)-positive tumour mutations (July 2017) SMC No. 1239/17 Recommended with restrictions

▶ Pembrolizumab (*Keytruda*®) in combination with carboplatin and either paclitaxel or nab-paclitaxel, for the first-line treatment of metastatic squamous non-small cell lung cancer in adults (September 2019) SMC No. SMC2187 Recommended with restrictions

▶ Pembrolizumab (*Keytruda*®) in combination with pemetrexed and platinum chemotherapy for the first-line treatment of metastatic non-squamous non-small cell lung carcinoma in adults whose tumours have no epidermal growth factor receptor or anaplastic lymphoma kinase (ALK)-positive mutations (October 2019) SMC No. SMC2207 Recommended with restrictions

▶ Pembrolizumab (*Keytruda*®) as monotherapy for the treatment of locally advanced or metastatic urothelial carcinoma in adults who have received prior platinum-containing chemotherapy (February 2018) SMC No. 1291/18 Recommended with restrictions

▶ Pembrolizumab (*Keytruda*®) as monotherapy for the treatment of locally advanced or metastatic urothelial carcinoma in adults who are not eligible for cisplatin-containing chemotherapy (first line) (September 2018) SMC No. 1339/18 Not recommended

▶ Pembrolizumab (*Keytruda*®) as monotherapy for the treatment of adult patients with relapsed or refractory classical Hodgkin lymphoma who have failed autologous stem cell transplant and brentuximab vedotin, or who are transplant-ineligible and have failed brentuximab vedotin (March 2018) SMC No. 1296/18 Recommended with restrictions

▶ Pembrolizumab (*Keytruda*®) in combination with axitinib for the first-line treatment of advanced renal cell carcinoma (RCC) in adults (September 2020) SMC No. SMC2247 Recommended with restrictions

▶ Pembrolizumab (*Keytruda*®) as monotherapy or in combination with platinum and 5-fluorouracil chemotherapy, for the first-line treatment of metastatic or unresectable recurrent head and neck squamous cell carcinoma in adults whose tumours express programmed death ligand 1 with a combined positive score of 1 or more (September 2020) SMC No. SMC2257 Recommended with restrictions

● MEDICINAL FORMS There can be variation in the licensing of different medicines containing the same drug.

Solution for infusion

CAUTIONARY AND ADVISORY LABELS 3

▶ Keytruda (Merck Sharp & Dohme Ltd)
Pembrolizumab 25 mg per 1 ml Keytruda 100mg/4ml concentrate for solution for infusion vials | 1 vial PoM £2,630.00 (Hospital only)

| Pertuzumab   10-Nov-2020

● DRUG ACTION Pertuzumab is a recombinant humanised monoclonal antibody, and acts by inhibiting human epidermal growth factor receptor 2 protein (HER2) dimerisation.

● INDICATIONS AND DOSE

HER2-positive early stage breast cancer (in combination with trastuzumab and chemotherapy) | HER2-positive metastatic or locally recurrent unresectable breast cancer (in combination with trastuzumab and docetaxel) (specialist use only)

▶ BY INTRAVENOUS INFUSION
▶ Adult: (consult product literature or local protocols)

● CAUTIONS Conditions that could impair left ventricular function · history of congestive heart failure · impaired left ventricular function · prior anthracycline exposure · radiotherapy to the chest area · recent myocardial infarction · serious cardiac arrhythmia · uncontrolled hypertension

● INTERACTIONS → Appendix 1: monoclonal antibodies

● SIDE-EFFECTS

▶ Common or very common Alopecia · anaemia · appetite decreased · arthralgia · asthenia · chills · congestive heart failure · constipation · cough · cytokine release syndrome · diarrhoea · dizziness · dyspepsia · dyspnoea · excessive tearing · fever · headache · hypersensitivity · increased risk of infection · infusion related reaction · insomnia · left ventricular dysfunction · leucopenia · mucositis · myalgia · nail disorder · nausea · neutropenia · oedema · pain · peripheral neuropathy · respiratory disorders · skin reactions · stomatitis · taste altered · vomiting

SIDE-EFFECTS, FURTHER INFORMATION Side effects mostly described for pertuzumab in combination with trastuzumab and docetaxel.

● CONCEPTION AND CONTRACEPTION Ensure effective contraception during and for six months after treatment in women of childbearing potential.

● PREGNANCY Avoid (toxicity in *animal* studies). Most cytotoxic drugs are teratogenic and should not be administered during pregnancy, especially during the first trimester. Considerable caution is necessary if a pregnant woman presents with cancer requiring chemotherapy, and specialist advice should always be sought.

● BREAST FEEDING Avoid—no information available.

● HEPATIC IMPAIRMENT Manufacturer advises caution (no information available).

● RENAL IMPAIRMENT Caution in severe impairment—no information available.

● MONITORING REQUIREMENTS

▶ Assess for signs and symptoms of congestive heart failure (including left ventricular ejection fraction) before and during treatment—consult product literature, and withhold treatment if necessary.

▶ Monitor for febrile neutropenia.

● DIRECTIONS FOR ADMINISTRATION Manufacturer advises resuscitation facilities should be available.

● NATIONAL FUNDING/ACCESS DECISIONS
For full details see funding body website

NICE decisions

▶ Pertuzumab for the neoadjuvant treatment of HER2-positive breast cancer (December 2016) NICE TA424 Recommended with restrictions

▶ Pertuzumab with trastuzumab and docetaxel for treating HER2-positive breast cancer (March 2018) NICE TA509 Recommended with restrictions

▶ Pertuzumab for adjuvant treatment of HER2-positive early stage breast cancer (March 2019) NICE TA569 Recommended with restrictions

Scottish Medicines Consortium (SMC) decisions

▶ Pertuzumab (*Perjeta*®) for use in combination with trastuzumab and chemotherapy for the neoadjuvant treatment of adult patients with human epidermal growth factor receptor 2 (HER2)-positive, locally advanced, inflammatory, or early stage breast cancer at high risk of recurrence (December 2018) SMC No. SMC2119 Recommended

▶ Pertuzumab (*Perjeta*®) for use in combination with trastuzumab and docetaxel in adult patients with HER2-positive metastatic or locally recurrent unresectable breast cancer, who have not received previous anti-HER2 therapy or chemotherapy for their metastatic disease (January 2019) SMC No. SMC2120 Recommended

▶ Pertuzumab (*Perjeta*®) for use in combination with trastuzumab and chemotherapy for the adjuvant treatment of adult patients with human epidermal growth factor receptor 2 (HER2)-positive early breast cancer (eBC) at high risk of recurrence (September 2020) SMC No. SMC2284 Recommended with restrictions

8

Immune system and malignant disease

- **MEDICINAL FORMS** There can be variation in the licensing of different medicines containing the same drug.
  Solution for infusion
  ▸ Perjeta (Roche Products Ltd)
  Pertuzumab 30 mg per 1 ml Perjeta 420mg/14ml concentrate for solution for infusion vials | 1 vial [PoM] £2,395.00 (Hospital only)

Polatuzumab vedotin

12-Nov-2020

- **DRUG ACTION** Polatuzumab vedotin is an antibody-drug conjugate that contains polatuzumab covalently linked to MMAE, a cytotoxic microtubule disrupting agent.

- ● **INDICATIONS AND DOSE**
  Relapsed or refractory diffuse large B-cell lymphoma (in combination with bendamustine and rituximab) (specialist use only)
  ▸ BY INTRAVENOUS INFUSION
  ▸ Adult: (consult product literature)

- **CONTRA-INDICATIONS** Active severe infection

- **CAUTIONS** High tumour burden—risk of tumour lysis syndrome · patients may need pre-medication to mimimise infusion-related reactions · peripheral neuropathy · rapidly proliferating tumours—risk of tumour lysis syndrome
  CAUTIONS, FURTHER INFORMATION
  ▸ Pre-medication Manufacturer advises pre-medication with an antihistamine and antipyretic to minimise the development of infusion-related reactions—consult product literature.

- **INTERACTIONS** → Appendix 1: monoclonal antibodies

- **SIDE-EFFECTS**
  ▸ **Common or very common** Anaemia · appetite decreased · arthralgia · asthenia · bone marrow disorders · chills · constipation · cough · decreased leucocytes · diarrhoea · dizziness · electrolyte imbalance · fever · gait abnormal · gastrointestinal discomfort · hypoalbuminaemia · increased risk of infection · infusion related reaction · nausea · neutropenia · peripheral neuropathy · pneumonitis · pruritus · sensation abnormal · sepsis · thrombocytopenia · vision blurred · vomiting · weight decreased
  ▸ **Frequency not known** Gastrointestinal toxicity · hepatic disorders · progressive multifocal leukoencephalopathy (PML) · reactivation of infection

- **CONCEPTION AND CONTRACEPTION** Manufacturer advises females of childbearing potential should confirm pregnancy status before treatment and use effective contraception during treatment and for 9 months after last treatment; male patients should use effective contraception during treatment and for 6 months after last treatment if their partner is pregnant or of childbearing potential. See also *Pregnancy and reproductive function* in Cytotoxic drugs p. 932

- **PREGNANCY** Manufacturer advises avoid unless potential benefit outweighs risk—toxicity in *animal* studies. See also *Pregnancy and reproductive function* in Cytotoxic drugs p. 932

- **BREAST FEEDING** Manufacturer advises avoid breast feeding during treatment and for at least 2 months after treatment.

- **HEPATIC IMPAIRMENT** Manufacturer advises avoid in moderate to severe hepatic impairment. Manufacturer advises monitor liver enzymes and bilirubin levels (risk of hepatic toxicity)—consult product literature.

- **RENAL IMPAIRMENT**
  Dose adjustments Manufacturer advises no dose adjustment required if creatinine clearance is more than 30 mL/minute; no established dose if creatinine clearance less than 30 mL/minute—no information available.

- **MONITORING REQUIREMENTS** Manufacturer advises monitor complete blood counts prior to each dose; more frequent monitoring may be required—consult product literature for treatment adjustment.

- **PRESCRIBING AND DISPENSING INFORMATION** Polatuzumab vedotin is a biological medicine. Biological medicines must be prescribed and dispensed by brand name, see *Biological medicines* and *Biosimilar medicines*, under Guidance on prescribing p. 1; manufacturer advises to record the brand name and batch number after each administration.

- **HANDLING AND STORAGE** Store in a refrigerator (2-8°C) and protect from light—consult product literature for further information regarding storage conditions after reconstitution and dilution.

- **PATIENT AND CARER ADVICE**
  Driving and skilled tasks Manufacturer advises patients and carers should be counselled on the effects on driving and other skilled tasks—increased risk of infusion-related reactions, peripheral neuropathy, fatigue, and dizziness.

- **NATIONAL FUNDING/ACCESS DECISIONS** For full details see funding body website

  NICE decisions
  ▸ Polatuzumab vedotin with rituximab and bendamustine for treating relapsed or refractory diffuse large B-cell lymphoma (September 2020) NICE TA649 Recommended

  Scottish Medicines Consortium (SMC) decisions
  ▸ Polatuzumab vedotin (*Polivy*®) in combination with bendamustine and rituximab for the treatment of adult patients with relapsed/refractory diffuse large B-cell lymphoma (DLBCL) who are not candidates for haematopoietic stem cell transplant (September 2020) SMC No. SMC2282 Recommended

- **MEDICINAL FORMS** There can be variation in the licensing of different medicines containing the same drug.
  Powder for solution for infusion
  EXCIPIENTS: May contain Polysorbates, sucrose
  ▸ Polivy (Roche Products Ltd) ▼
  Polatuzumab vedotin 140 mg Polivy 140mg powder for concentrate for solution for infusion vials | 1 vial [PoM] £11,060.00 (Hospital only)

Ramucirumab

20-Aug-2020

- **DRUG ACTION** Ramucirumab is a human monoclonal antibody that binds to the vascular endothelial growth factor receptor-2 (VEGFR-2), inhibiting VEGF-induced angiogenesis.

- ● **INDICATIONS AND DOSE**
  Treatment of advanced gastric cancer or gastro-oesophageal junction adenocarcinoma, in combination with paclitaxel, in patients with disease progression after prior platinum and fluoropyrimidine chemotherapy
  ▸ BY INTRAVENOUS INFUSION
  ▸ Adult: 8 mg/kg on days 1 and 15 of a 28 day cycle, dose to be administered prior to paclitaxel infusion, consult product literature for dose adjustments due to side-effects and infusion-related reactions
  Treatment of advanced gastric cancer or gastro-oesophageal junction adenocarcinoma, as monotherapy, in patients with disease progression after prior platinum or fluoropyrimidine chemotherapy, and for whom treatment in combination with paclitaxel is not appropriate
  ▸ BY INTRAVENOUS INFUSION
  ▸ Adult: 8 mg/kg every 2 weeks, consult product literature for dose adjustments due to side-effects and infusion-related reactions

Treatment of metastatic colorectal cancer, in combination with FOLFIRI (irinotecan, fluorouracil and folinic acid), in patients with disease progression on, or after, prior therapy with bevacizumab, oxaliplatin and a fluoropyrimidine
▸ BY INTRAVENOUS INFUSION
▸ Adult: 8 mg/kg every 2 weeks, dose to be administered prior to FOLFIRI administration, consult product literature for dose adjustments due to side-effects and infusion-related reactions

Treatment of locally advanced or metastatic non-small cell lung cancer, in combination with docetaxel, in patients with disease progression after platinum-based chemotherapy
▸ BY INTRAVENOUS INFUSION
▸ Adult: 10 mg/kg on day 1 of a 21 day cycle, dose to be administered prior to docetaxel infusion, consult product literature for dose adjustments due to side-effects and infusion-related reactions

IMPORTANT SAFETY INFORMATION
MHRA/CHM ADVICE: SYSTEMICALLY ADMINISTERED VEGF PATHWAY INHIBITORS: RISK OF ANEURYSM AND ARTERY DISSECTION (JULY 2020)
A European review of worldwide data concluded that systemically administered VEGF pathway inhibitors may lead to aneurysm and artery dissection in patients with or without hypertension. Some fatal cases have been reported, mainly in relation to aortic aneurysm rupture and aortic dissection. The MHRA advises healthcare professionals to carefully consider the risk of aneurysm and artery dissection in patients with risk factors before initiating treatment with ramucirumab; any modifiable risk factors (such as smoking and hypertension) should be reduced as much as possible. Patients should be monitored and treated for hypertension as required.

● CAUTIONS Elective surgery—discontinue treatment for at least 4 weeks prior to surgery · hypertension · impaired wound healing—discontinue treatment until wound fully healed · pretreatment is recommended to minimise the development of adverse reactions (consult product literature) · risk factors for aneurysm or artery dissection · risk of bleeding
CAUTIONS, FURTHER INFORMATION
▸ Monitoring of blood pressure The MHRA advises to monitor blood pressure regularly—consult product literature if hypertension occurs during treatment.

● INTERACTIONS → Appendix 1: monoclonal antibodies

● SIDE-EFFECTS
▸ Common or very common Arterial thromboembolism · diarrhoea · electrolyte imbalance · epistaxis · gastrointestinal discomfort · gastrointestinal disorders · headache · hepatic coma · hepatic encephalopathy · hepatic pain · hypertension · hypoalbuminaemia · infusion related reaction · nephrotic syndrome · neutropenia · peripheral oedema · proteinuria · rash · thrombocytopenia
▸ Frequency not known Aneurysm · artery dissection · cardiac arrest · cerebrovascular insufficiency · haemangioma · myocardial infarction · thrombotic microangiopathy
SIDE-EFFECTS, FURTHER INFORMATION Infusion-related hypersensitivity reactions have been reported with ramucirumab, particularly during or following the first or second infusion; if the patient experiences a grade 1 or 2 infusion-related reaction, the manufacturer advises to reduce rate of infusion by 50% and give premedication for all subsequent infusions—consult product literature. Manufacturer advises to permanently discontinue treatment in the event of a grade 3 or 4 infusion-related reaction.

● CONCEPTION AND CONTRACEPTION Manufacturer advises effective contraception during treatment and for up to 3 months after treatment in women of childbearing potential.
● PREGNANCY Manufacturer advises avoid unless potential benefit outweighs risk—no information available.
● BREAST FEEDING Manufacturer advises discontinue breast-feeding during treatment and for at least 3 months after treatment—no information available.
● HEPATIC IMPAIRMENT Manufacturer advises caution in severe cirrhosis, cirrhosis with hepatic encephalopathy, cirrhosis with clinically significant ascites, or hepatorenal syndrome (risk of progressive hepatic failure, no information available).
● MONITORING REQUIREMENTS Manufacturer advises monitor for signs of infusion-related hypersensitivity reactions; monitor for development or worsening of proteinuria during treatment—consult product literature; monitor blood counts and coagulation parameters in patients at risk of bleeding.
● DIRECTIONS FOR ADMINISTRATION For *intravenous infusion* (*Cyramza®*), manufacturer advises give intermittently in Sodium chloride 0.9%; dilute requisite dose with infusion fluid to final volume of 250 mL and invert gently to mix. Do not exceed a rate of 25 mg/minute, and give over approximately 60 minutes via an infusion pump using a separate infusion line with a protein sparing 0.22 micron filter.
● PRESCRIBING AND DISPENSING INFORMATION For *Cyramza®*, each 10 mL vial contains sodium 17 mg (equivalent to Na⁺ 0.74 mmol).
● NATIONAL FUNDING/ACCESS DECISIONS
For full details see funding body website
NICE decisions
▸ Ramucirumab for treating advanced gastric cancer or gastro-oesophageal junction adenocarcinoma previously treated with chemotherapy (January 2016) NICE TA378 Not recommended
▸ Ramucirumab for previously treated locally advanced or metastatic non-small-cell lung cancer (August 2016) NICE TA403 Not recommended

● MEDICINAL FORMS There can be variation in the licensing of different medicines containing the same drug.
Solution for infusion
ELECTROLYTES: May contain Sodium
▸ Cyramza (Eli Lilly and Company Ltd)
Ramucirumab 10 mg per 1 ml Cyramza 100mg/10ml concentrate for solution for infusion vials | 1 vial [PoM] £500.00 (Hospital only)
Cyramza 500mg/50ml concentrate for solution for infusion vials | 1 vial [PoM] £2,500.00 (Hospital only)

F 903

Rituximab

16-Nov-2020

● INDICATIONS AND DOSE
Rheumatoid arthritis (specialist use only)
▸ BY INTRAVENOUS INFUSION
▸ Adult: 1 g, then 1 g after 2 weeks, consult product literature for information on retreatment
Non-Hodgkin's lymphoma (specialist use only) | Chronic lymphocytic leukaemia (specialist use only) | Granulomatosis with polyangiitis and microscopic polyangiitis (specialist use only)
▸ BY INTRAVENOUS INFUSION
▸ Adult: (consult product literature)
Non-Hodgkin's lymphoma (specialist use only)
▸ BY SUBCUTANEOUS INJECTION
▸ Adult: (consult product literature)

continued →

Pemphigus vulgaris (specialist use only)
▶ BY INTRAVENOUS INFUSION
  ▶ Adult: 1 g, then 1 g after 2 weeks; maintenance 0.5 g, at months 12 and 18, and then every 6 months thereafter if needed, consult product literature for the treatment of relapse

● CONTRA-INDICATIONS
  GENERAL CONTRA-INDICATIONS
  Severe infection
  SPECIFIC CONTRA-INDICATIONS
  ● When used for Granulomatosis with polyangiitis and microscopic polyangiitis, Pemphigus vulgaris, or Rheumatoid arthritis Severe heart failure · severe, uncontrolled heart disease
  CONTRA-INDICATIONS, FURTHER INFORMATION
  For full details on contra-indications, consult product literature.

● CAUTIONS
  GENERAL CAUTIONS History of cardiovascular disease (exacerbation of angina, arrhythmia, and heart failure have been reported) · patients receiving cardiotoxic chemotherapy (exacerbation of angina, arrhythmia, and heart failure have been reported) · pre-medication recommended to minimise adverse reactions (consult product literature) · predisposition to infection · transient hypotension occurs frequently during infusion (anti-hypertensives may need to be withheld for 12 hours before infusion)
  SPECIFIC CAUTIONS
  ▶ When used for Granulomatosis with polyangiitis and microscopic polyangiitis, or Pemphigus vulgaris *Pneumocystis jirovecii* pneumonia—consult product literature for prophylaxis requirements
  CAUTIONS, FURTHER INFORMATION For full details on cautions, consult product literature or local treatment protocol.
  ▶ Hepatitis B infection and reactivation Hepatitis B infection and reactivation (including fatal cases) have been reported in patients taking **rituximab**. Manufacturer advises patients with positive hepatitis B serology should be referred to a liver specialist for monitoring and initiation of antiviral therapy before treatment initiation; treatment should not be initiated in patients with evidence of current hepatitis B infection until the infection has been adequately treated. Manufacturer also advises patients should be closely monitored for clinical and laboratory signs of active hepatitis B infection (consult product literature).

● INTERACTIONS → Appendix 1: monoclonal antibodies

● SIDE-EFFECTS
  ▶ **Common or very common** Angioedema · anxiety · appetite decreased · arrhythmias · bone marrow disorders · bursitis · cancer pain · cardiac disorder · chest pain · chills · dizziness · dysphagia · dyspnoea · ear pain · electrolyte imbalance · gastrointestinal discomfort · gastrointestinal disorders · hepatitis B · hypercholesterolaemia · hyperglycaemia · hyperhidrosis · hypertension · hypotension · insomnia · lacrimation disorder · malaise · migraine · multi organ failure · muscle complaints · muscle tone increased · nausea · nerve disorders · oedema · oral disorders · osteoarthritis · respiratory disorders · sensation abnormal · sepsis · skin reactions · throat irritation · tinnitus · vasodilation · weight decreased
  ▶ **Uncommon** Asthma · coagulation disorder · heart failure · hypoxia · ischaemic heart disease · lymphadenopathy · taste altered
  ▶ **Rare or very rare** Cytokine release syndrome · facial paralysis · renal failure · Stevens-Johnson syndrome (discontinue) · toxic epidermal necrolysis (discontinue) · tumour lysis syndrome · vasculitis · vision disorders

  ▶ **Frequency not known** Epistaxis · hearing loss · hypogammaglobulinaemia · infective thrombosis · influenza like illness · irritability · muscle weakness · nasal congestion · posterior reversible encephalopathy syndrome (PRES) · psychiatric disorder · seizure · skin papilloma · tremor
  SIDE-EFFECTS, FURTHER INFORMATION Associated with infections, sometimes severe, including tuberculosis, septicaemia, and hepatitis B reactivation.
    Progressive multifocal leucoencephalopathy has been reported in association with rituximab; patients should be monitored for cognitive, neurological, or psychiatric signs and symptoms. If progressive multifocal leucoencephalopathy is suspected, suspend treatment until it has been excluded.

● CONCEPTION AND CONTRACEPTION Effective contraception in females of childbearing potential required during and for 12 months after treatment.

● PREGNANCY Avoid unless potential benefit to mother outweighs risk of B-lymphocyte depletion in fetus.

● BREAST FEEDING Avoid breast-feeding during and for 12 months after treatment.

● MONITORING REQUIREMENTS For full details on monitoring requirements consult product literature.

● DIRECTIONS FOR ADMINISTRATION
  ▶ With intravenous use For *intravenous infusion*, give intermittently in Glucose 5% or Sodium chloride 0.9%; dilute to 1–4 mg/mL and gently invert bag to avoid foaming; for further information, consult product literature.

● PRESCRIBING AND DISPENSING INFORMATION Rituximab is a biological medicine. Biological medicines must be prescribed and dispensed by brand name, see *Biological medicines* and *Biosimilar medicines*, under Guidance on prescribing p. 1.

● PATIENT AND CARER ADVICE
  Alert card
  ▶ When used for Granulomatosis with polyangiitis and microscopic polyangiitis or Rheumatoid arthritis or Pemphigus vulgaris Patients should be provided with a patient alert card with each infusion.

● NATIONAL FUNDING/ACCESS DECISIONS
  For full details see funding body website
  NICE decisions
  ▶ **Rituximab in combination with glucocorticoids for treating anti-neutrophil cytoplasmic antibody-associated vasculitis (March 2014)** NICE TA308 Recommended with restrictions
  ▶ **Adalimumab, etanercept, infliximab, rituximab, and abatacept for the treatment of rheumatoid arthritis after the failure of a TNF inhibitor (August 2010)** NICE TA195 Recommended with restrictions
  ▶ **Rituximab for the first-line treatment of stage III-IV follicular lymphoma (January 2012)** NICE TA243 Recommended
  ▶ **Rituximab for the treatment of relapsed or refractory stage III or IV follicular non-Hodgkin's lymphoma (February 2008)** NICE TA137 Recommended with restrictions
  ▶ **Rituximab for the treatment of relapsed or refractory chronic lymphocytic leukaemia (July 2010)** NICE TA193 Recommended with restrictions
  ▶ **Rituximab for the first-line maintenance treatment of follicular non-Hodgkin's lymphoma (June 2011)** NICE TA226 Recommended
  ▶ **Rituximab for the first-line treatment of chronic lymphocytic leukaemia (July 2009)** NICE TA174 Recommended
  ▶ **Idelalisib for treating chronic lymphocytic leukaemia [in combination with rituximab] (October 2015)** NICE TA359 Recommended
  ▶ **Venetoclax with rituximab for previously treated chronic lymphocytic leukaemia (February 2019)** NICE TA561 Recommended with restrictions

Scottish Medicines Consortium (SMC) decisions

▸ Rituximab (*MabThera*®) for use in combination with glucocorticoids for the induction of remission in adult patients with severe, active granulomatosis with polyangiitis (Wegener' s) and microscopic polyangiitis (September 2013) SMC No. 894/13 Recommended with restrictions

▸ Rituximab (*MabThera*®) subcutaneous injection for the treatment of non-Hodgkin' s lymphoma in adults (July 2014) SMC No. 975/14 Recommended with restrictions

● MEDICINAL FORMS There can be variation in the licensing of different medicines containing the same drug.

Solution for injection

▸ MabThera (Roche Products Ltd)

Rituximab 119.66 mg per 1 ml MabThera 1400mg/11.7ml solution for injection vials | 1 vial PoM £1,344.65 (Hospital only)

Solution for infusion

EXCIPIENTS: May contain Polysorbates
ELECTROLYTES: May contain Sodium

▸ MabThera (Roche Products Ltd)

Rituximab 10 mg per 1 ml MabThera 100mg/10ml concentrate for solution for infusion vials | 2 vial PoM £349.25 (Hospital only)
MabThera 500mg/50ml concentrate for solution for infusion vials | 1 vial PoM £873.15 (Hospital only)

▸ Rixathon (Sandoz Ltd) ▼

Rituximab 10 mg per 1 ml Rixathon 100mg/10ml concentrate for solution for infusion vials | 2 vial PoM £314.33 (Hospital only)
Rixathon 500mg/50ml concentrate for solution for infusion vials | 1 vial PoM £785.84 (Hospital only) | 2 vial PoM £1,571.67 (Hospital only)

▸ Ruxience (Pfizer Ltd) ▼

Rituximab 10 mg per 1 ml Ruxience 100mg/10ml concentrate for solution for infusion vials | 1 vial PoM £157.17 (Hospital only)
Ruxience 500mg/50ml concentrate for solution for infusion vials | 1 vial PoM £785.84 (Hospital only)

▸ Truxima (Napp Pharmaceuticals Ltd) ▼

Rituximab 10 mg per 1 ml Truxima 100mg/10ml concentrate for solution for infusion vials | 2 vial PoM £314.33 (Hospital only)
Truxima 500mg/50ml concentrate for solution for infusion vials | 1 vial PoM £785.84 (Hospital only)

Siltuximab

30-Jul-2020

● DRUG ACTION Siltuximab is a monoclonal antibody that inhibits interleukin-6 receptor binding.

● INDICATIONS AND DOSE

Treatment of multicentric Castleman's disease (MCD) in patients who are human immunodeficiency virus (HIV) negative and human herpesvirus-8 (HHV-8) negative

▸ BY INTRAVENOUS INFUSION
▸ Adult: 11 mg/kg every 3 weeks

● CAUTIONS Patients at increased risk of gastrointestinal perforation—promptly investigate those presenting with symptoms suggestive of gastrointestinal perforation · severe infection—withhold treatment until resolved · treat infection prior to treatment

CAUTIONS, FURTHER INFORMATION

▸ Hypersensitivity reactions Infusion-related side-effects are reported commonly with siltuximab; resuscitation facilities should be available during treatment.

Consult product literature for further information about siltuximab cautions.

● INTERACTIONS → Appendix 1: monoclonal antibodies

● SIDE-EFFECTS

▸ **Common or very common** Abdominal pain · arthralgia · constipation · diarrhoea · dizziness · dyslipidaemia · gastrooesophageal reflux disease · headache · hypersensitivity · hypertension · hyperuricaemia · increased risk of infection · infusion related reaction · localised oedema · nausea · neutropenia · oral ulceration · oropharyngeal pain · pain in extremity · renal impairment ·

skin reactions · thrombocytopenia · vomiting · weight increased

SIDE-EFFECTS, FURTHER INFORMATION Siltuximab therapy should be discontinued permanently in the event of a severe infusion-related reaction, anaphylaxis, a severe allergic reaction, or the occurrence of cytokine-release syndrome. Mild to moderate infusion-related reactions may improve by temporarily reducing the rate or stopping the infusion. When restarting treatment, a reduced infusion rate and the administration of antihistamines, paracetamol, and corticosteroids may be considered. Consider discontinuation of siltuximab if more than 2 doses are delayed due to treatment-related toxicities during the first 48 weeks—for full details consult product literature.

● CONCEPTION AND CONTRACEPTION Women of childbearing potential should use effective contraception during and for 3 months after treatment.

● PREGNANCY Manufacturer advises avoid unless potential benefit outweighs risk.

● BREAST FEEDING Manufacturer advises avoid—no information available.

● HEPATIC IMPAIRMENT Manufacturer advises caution (no information).

● MONITORING REQUIREMENTS

▸ Monitor neutrophil and platelet count, and haemoglobin levels prior to each dose of siltuximab treatment for the first 12 months and thereafter prior to every third dosing cycle. Consider delaying treatment if required neutrophil, platelet, and haemoglobin levels not achieved—consult product literature for details.

▸ Monitor for infection during treatment.

● DIRECTIONS FOR ADMINISTRATION For *intravenous infusion* (*Sylvant*®), manufacturer advises give intermittently *in* Glucose 5%. Allow vials to reach room temperature over approximately 30 minutes, then reconstitute each 100 mg vial with 5.2 mL of water for injection, and each 400 mg vial with 20 mL of water for injection, to produce a 20 mg/mL solution. Gently swirl without shaking to dissolve. Further dilute to 250 mL with glucose 5% and gently mix. Use within 6 hours of dilution and give over 60 minutes using an administration set lined with polyvinyl chloride or polyurethane, through a low-protein binding in-line 0.2 micron filter.

● MEDICINAL FORMS There can be variation in the licensing of different medicines containing the same drug.

Powder for solution for infusion

▸ Sylvant (EUSA Pharma Ltd) ▼

Siltuximab 100 mg Sylvant 100mg powder for concentrate for solution for infusion vials | 1 vial PoM £415.00 (Hospital only)
Siltuximab 400 mg Sylvant 400mg powder for concentrate for solution for infusion vials | 1 vial PoM £1,661.00 (Hospital only)

8

Immune system and malignant disease

Trastuzumab

11-Nov-2020

● **INDICATIONS AND DOSE**

Treatment of early breast cancer which overexpresses human epidermal growth factor receptor-2 (HER2) (initiated by a specialist) | Treatment of metastatic breast cancer in patients with HER2-positive tumours who have not received chemotherapy for metastatic breast cancer and in whom anthracycline treatment is inappropriate (in combination with paclitaxel or docetaxel) (initiated by a specialist) | Treatment of metastatic breast cancer in postmenopausal patients with hormone-receptor positive HER2-positive tumours not previously treated with trastuzumab (in combination with an aromatase inhibitor) (initiated by a specialist)

▸ BY INTRAVENOUS INFUSION, OR BY SUBCUTANEOUS INJECTION
▸ Adult: (consult product literature or local protocols)

Monotherapy for metastatic breast cancer in patients with tumours that overexpress HER2 who have received at least 2 chemotherapy regimens including, where appropriate, an anthracycline and a taxane (initiated by a specialist)

▸ BY INTRAVENOUS INFUSION, OR BY SUBCUTANEOUS INJECTION
▸ Adult: Women with oestrogen-receptor-positive breast cancer should also have received hormonal therapy (consult product literature or local protocols)

Treatment of metastatic gastric cancer in patients with HER2-positive tumours who have not received treatment for metastatic gastric cancer (in combination with capecitabine or fluorouracil and cisplatin) (initiated by a specialist)

▸ BY INTRAVENOUS INFUSION
▸ Adult: (consult product literature or local protocols)

● CONTRA-INDICATIONS Severe dyspnoea at rest
● CAUTIONS Coronary artery disease · elderly · history of hypertension · impaired left ventricular function · symptomatic heart failure · uncontrolled arrhythmias
● INTERACTIONS → Appendix 1: monoclonal antibodies
● SIDE-EFFECTS

▸ **Common or very common** Alopecia · anaemia · angioedema · anxiety · appetite decreased · arrhythmias · arthralgia · arthritis · asthenia · asthma · ataxia · breast abnormalities · cardiomyopathy · chest pain · chills · constipation · cough · cystitis · depression · diarrhoea · dizziness · drowsiness · dry eye · dry mouth · dyspnoea · excessive tearing · eye inflammation · fever · gastrointestinal discomfort · haemorrhage · haemorrhoids · headache · heart failure · hepatic disorders · hyperhidrosis · hypersensitivity · hypotension · increased risk of infection · influenza like illness · infusion related reaction (may be delayed) · insomnia · leucopenia · malaise · mucositis · muscle complaints · muscle tone increased · nail disorders · nausea · neutropenia · oedema · oral disorders · pain · palpitations · pancreatitis · paraesthesia · peripheral neuropathy · renal disorder · respiratory disorders · rhinorrhoea · sepsis · skin reactions · taste altered · thinking abnormal · thrombocytopenia · tremor · vasodilation · vomiting · weight decreased
▸ **Uncommon** Deafness · pericardial effusion
▸ **Rare or very rare** Paresis
▸ **Frequency not known** Brain oedema · cancer progression · cardiogenic shock · glomerulonephritis · hyperkalaemia · hypoprothrombinaemia · hypoxia · pericarditis · pulmonary fibrosis (may be delayed) · pulmonary oedema (may be delayed) · renal failure

● CONCEPTION AND CONTRACEPTION Manufacturer advises effective contraception in women of childbearing potential during and for 7 months after treatment. See also

Pregnancy and reproductive function in Cytotoxic drugs p. 932.

● PREGNANCY Manufacturer advises avoid—oligohydramnios reported. See also *Pregnancy and reproductive function* in Cytotoxic drugs p. 932.
● BREAST FEEDING Avoid breast-feeding during treatment and for 7 months afterwards.
● MONITORING REQUIREMENTS
▸ Cardiotoxicity Monitor cardiac function before and during treatment—for details of monitoring and managing cardiotoxicity, consult product literature.
● DIRECTIONS FOR ADMINISTRATION Resuscitation facilities should be available during administration of trastuzumab.
● PRESCRIBING AND DISPENSING INFORMATION When prescribing, dispensing or administering, check that this is the correct preparation—trastuzumab is **not** interchangeable with trastuzumab emtansine.
    Trastuzumab is a biological medicine. Biological medicines must be prescribed and dispensed by brand name, see *Biological medicines* and *Biosimilar medicines*, under Guidance on prescribing p. 1.
● NATIONAL FUNDING/ACCESS DECISIONS For full details see funding body website

NICE decisions

▸ **Guidance on the use of trastuzumab for the treatment of advanced breast cancer (March 2002)** NICE TA34 Recommended with restrictions
▸ **Lapatinib or trastuzumab in combination with an aromatase inhibitor for the first-line treatment of metastatic hormone-receptor-positive breast cancer that overexpresses HER2 (June 2012)** NICE TA257 Not recommended
▸ **Pertuzumab with trastuzumab and docetaxel for treating HER2-positive breast cancer (March 2018)** NICE TA509 Recommended with restrictions
▸ **Trastuzumab for the treatment of HER2-positive metastatic gastric cancer (November 2010)** NICE TA208 Recommended with restrictions

Scottish Medicines Consortium (SMC) decisions

▸ **Trastuzumab (*Herceptin*®) for the treatment of adult patients with HER2 positive metastatic breast cancer and early breast cancer (January 2014)** SMC No. 928/13 Recommended with restrictions
▸ **Trastuzumab (*Herceptin*®) in combination with capecitabine or fluorouracil and cisplatin for the treatment of patients with HER2 positive metastatic adenocarcinoma of the stomach or gastro-oesophageal junction who have not received prior anti-cancer treatment for their metastatic disease (October 2015)** SMC No. 623/10 Recommended with restrictions

● MEDICINAL FORMS There can be variation in the licensing of different medicines containing the same drug.

Solution for injection
▸ Herceptin (Roche Products Ltd)
    Trastuzumab 120 mg per 1 ml Herceptin 600mg/5ml solution for injection vials | 1 vial [PoM] £1,222.20 (Hospital only)

Powder for solution for infusion
▸ Herceptin (Roche Products Ltd)
    Trastuzumab 150 mg Herceptin 150mg powder for concentrate for solution for infusion vials | 1 vial [PoM] £407.40 (Hospital only)
▸ Herzuma (Napp Pharmaceuticals Ltd) ▼
    Trastuzumab 150 mg Herzuma 150mg powder for concentrate for solution for infusion vials | 1 vial [PoM] £366.66 (Hospital only)
    Trastuzumab 420 mg Herzuma 420mg powder for concentrate for solution for infusion vials | 1 vial [PoM] £1,026.65 (Hospital only)
▸ Kanjinti (Amgen Ltd) ▼
    Trastuzumab 150 mg Kanjinti 150mg powder for concentrate for solution for infusion vials | 1 vial [PoM] £366.66 (Hospital only)
    Trastuzumab 420 mg Kanjinti 420mg powder for concentrate for solution for infusion vials | 1 vial [PoM] £1,026.65 (Hospital only)
▸ Ontruzant (Merck Sharp & Dohme Ltd) ▼
    Trastuzumab 150 mg Ontruzant 150mg powder for concentrate for solution for infusion vials | 1 vial [PoM] £366.66 (Hospital only)

8

Immune system and malignant disease

▸ Trazimera (Pfizer Ltd) ▼
Trastuzumab 150 mg Trazimera 150mg powder for concentrate for
solution for infusion vials | 1 vial [PoM] £366.66 (Hospital only)
▸ Zercepac (Accord Healthcare Ltd) ▼
Trastuzumab 150 mg Zercepac 150mg powder for concentrate for
solution for infusion vials | 1 vial [PoM] £366.65 (Hospital only)
Trastuzumab 420 mg Trazimera 420mg powder for concentrate for
solution for infusion vials | 1 vial [PoM] £1,026.65 (Hospital only)

Trastuzumab emtansine   03-Dec-2020

● DRUG ACTION Trastuzumab emtansine is an antibody-
drug conjugate that contains trastuzumab covalently
linked to DM1, a cytotoxic microtubule inhibitor.

● INDICATIONS AND DOSE
**HER2-positive metastatic breast cancer (specialist use
only) | HER2-positive early breast cancer (specialist use
only)**
▸ BY INTRAVENOUS INFUSION
 ▸ Adult: (consult product literature or local protocols)

● CAUTIONS Dyspnoea at rest—increased risk of pulmonary
events · history of congestive heart failure · patients over
75 years · peripheral neuropathy (temporarily discontinue
treatment—consult product literature) · recent history of
myocardial infarction · recent history of unstable angina ·
risk of left ventricular dysfunction—consult product
literature for specific risks with trastuzumab treatment ·
serious arrhythmias

● INTERACTIONS → Appendix 1: monoclonal antibodies

● SIDE-EFFECTS
▸ **Common or very common** Alopecia · anaemia · arthralgia ·
asthenia · chills · conjunctivitis · constipation · cough ·
diarrhoea · dizziness · dry eye · dry mouth · dyspnoea ·
excessive tearing · fever · gastrointestinal discomfort ·
haemorrhage · headache · hypersensitivity · hypertension ·
hypokalaemia · infusion related reaction · insomnia · left
ventricular dysfunction · leucopenia · memory loss ·
musculoskeletal pain · myalgia · nail disorder · nausea ·
neutropenia · peripheral neuropathy · peripheral oedema ·
skin reactions · stomatitis · taste altered ·
thrombocytopenia · urinary tract infection · vision blurred ·
vomiting
▸ **Uncommon** Hepatic disorders · nodular regenerative
hyperplasia · pneumonitis

● CONCEPTION AND CONTRACEPTION Manufacturer advises
effective contraception must be used during and for
7 months after stopping treatment in women and men. See
also *Pregnancy and reproductive function* in Cytotoxic drugs
p. 932.

● PREGNANCY Manufacturer advises avoid—
oligohydramnios reported with trastuzumab. See also
Pregnancy and reproductive function in Cytotoxic drugs
p. 932.

● BREAST FEEDING Manufacturer advises avoid breast-
feeding during and for 7 months after treatment.

● HEPATIC IMPAIRMENT Manufacturer advises caution—
consult product literature.
Dose adjustments Manufacturer advises dose reduction
according to liver function tests—consult product
literature.

● RENAL IMPAIRMENT No information available—
manufacturer advises caution in severe impairment.

● MONITORING REQUIREMENTS
 ▸ Monitor hepatic function before each dose.
 ▸ Monitor for signs and symptoms of neurotoxicity.
 ▸ Monitor closely for infusion-related and hypersensitivity
reactions.

 ▸ Monitor platelet count before each dose and as clinically
indicated (consult product literature for treatment
modification in thrombocytopenia).
 ▸ Test cardiac function before treatment and regularly
during treatment—delay or discontinue treatment in cases
of left ventricular dysfunction.
 ▸ Monitor for dyspnoea, cough, fatigue and pulmonary
infiltrates—discontinue if interstitial lung disease or
pneumonitis confirmed (fatal cases reported).

● DIRECTIONS FOR ADMINISTRATION Resuscitation facilities
should be available during administration of trastuzumab
emtansine.

● PRESCRIBING AND DISPENSING INFORMATION When
prescribing, dispensing or administering, check that this is
the correct preparation— trastuzumab emtansine and
trastuzumab are **not** interchangeable.
    Trastuzumab emtansine is a biological medicine.
Biological medicines must be prescribed and dispensed by
brand name, see *Biological medicines* and *Biosimilar
medicines*, under Guidance on prescribing p. 1;
manufacturer advises to record the brand name and batch
number after each administration.

● NATIONAL FUNDING/ACCESS DECISIONS
For full details see funding body website
NICE decisions
 ▸ Trastuzumab emtansine for treating HER2-positive advanced
breast cancer after trastuzumab and a taxane (updated
November 2017) NICE TA458 Recommended with restrictions
 ▸ Trastuzumab emtansine for adjuvant treatment of
HER2-positive early breast cancer (June 2020) NICE TA632
Recommended
Scottish Medicines Consortium (SMC) decisions
 ▸ Trastuzumab emtansine (*Kadcyla*®) for HER2-positive,
unresectable locally advanced or metastatic breast cancer
after trastuzumab and a taxane (April 2017) SMC No. 990/14
Recommended
 ▸ Trastuzumab emtansine (*Kadcyla*®) as a single agent, for the
adjuvant treatment of adult patients with HER2-positive early
breast cancer who have residual invasive disease, in the
breast and/or lymph nodes, after neoadjuvant taxane-based
and HER2-targeted therapy (November 2020)
SMC No. SMC2298 Recommended

● MEDICINAL FORMS There can be variation in the licensing of
different medicines containing the same drug.
Powder for solution for infusion
 ▸ Kadcyla (Roche Products Ltd)
Trastuzumab emtansine 100 mg Kadcyla 100mg powder for
concentrate for solution for infusion vials | 1 vial [PoM] £1,641.01
Trastuzumab emtansine 160 mg Kadcyla 160mg powder for
concentrate for solution for infusion vials | 1 vial [PoM] £2,625.62

2   Carcinoid syndrome

ENZYME INHIBITORS

Telotristat ethyl   23-Oct-2020

● DRUG ACTION Telotristat ethyl and its active metabolite
inhibit L-tryptophan hydroxylases TPH-1 and TPH-2
which reduces the production of serotonin, thereby
alleviating symptoms associated with carcinoid syndrome.

● INDICATIONS AND DOSE
Carcinoid syndrome diarrhoea (specialist use only)
 ▸ BY MOUTH
 ▸ Adult: 250 mg 3 times a day, review treatment if no
response after 12 weeks

● INTERACTIONS → Appendix 1: telotristat ethyl

8

Immune system and malignant disease

- SIDE-EFFECTS
- ▶ **Common or very common** Appetite decreased · constipation · fatigue · fever · gastrointestinal discomfort · gastrointestinal disorders · headache · peripheral oedema
- PREGNANCY Manufacturer advises avoid—toxicity in *animal* studies.
- BREAST FEEDING Manufacturer advises avoid—no information available.
- HEPATIC IMPAIRMENT Manufacturer advises caution in mild to moderate impairment; avoid in severe impairment (no information available).
  Dose adjustments Manufacturer advises consider dose reduction to 250 mg twice daily in mild impairment and to 250 mg once daily in moderate impairment, according to tolerability.
- RENAL IMPAIRMENT Manufacturer advises caution in mild-to-moderate impairment; avoid in severe impairment—no information available.
- MONITORING REQUIREMENTS Manufacturer advises monitor liver function at initiation and during treatment as clinically indicated—discontinue if liver injury suspected.
- PATIENT AND CARER ADVICE Manufacturer advises inform patients to report any symptoms of depression or decreased interest.
- NATIONAL FUNDING/ACCESS DECISIONS
  For full details see funding body website
  Scottish Medicines Consortium (SMC) decisions
- ▶ Telotristat ethyl (*Xermelo*®) for the treatment of carcinoid syndrome diarrhoea in combination with somatostatin analogue (SSA) therapy in adults inadequately controlled by SSA therapy (June 2018) SMC No. 1327/18 Recommended with restrictions
  All Wales Medicines Strategy Group (AWMSG) decisions
- ▶ Telotristat ethyl (*Xermelo*®) for the treatment of carcinoid syndrome diarrhoea in combination with somatostatin analogue (SSA) therapy in adults inadequately controlled by SSA therapy (July 2018) AWMSG No. 2037 Recommended with restrictions

- MEDICINAL FORMS There can be variation in the licensing of different medicines containing the same drug.
  Tablet
  CAUTIONARY AND ADVISORY LABELS 3, 21
  ▶ Xermelo (Ipsen Ltd) ▼
  Telotristat ethyl 250 mg Xermelo 250mg tablets | 90 tablet [PoM] £1,120.00

3 Cytotoxic responsive malignancy

Cytotoxic drugs

27-Sep-2018

Overview

The chemotherapy of cancer is complex and should be confined to specialists in oncology. Cytotoxic drugs have both anti-cancer activity and the potential to damage normal tissue; most cytotoxic drugs are teratogenic. Chemotherapy may be given with a curative intent or it may aim to prolong life or to palliate symptoms. In an increasing number of cases chemotherapy may be combined with radiotherapy or surgery or both as either neoadjuvant treatment (initial chemotherapy aimed at shrinking the primary tumour, thereby rendering local therapy less destructive or more effective) or as adjuvant treatment (which follows definitive treatment of the primary disease, when the risk of subclinical metastatic disease is known to be high). All cytotoxic drugs cause side-effects and a balance has to be struck between likely benefit and acceptable toxicity.

Combinations of cytotoxic drugs, as continuous or pulsed cycles of treatment, are frequently more toxic than single drugs but have the advantage in certain tumours of enhanced response, reduced development of drug resistance and increased survival. However for some tumours, single-agent chemotherapy remains the treatment of choice.

Cytotoxic drugs fall into a number of classes, each with characteristic antitumour activity, sites of action, and toxicity. A knowledge of sites of metabolism and excretion is important because impaired drug handling as a result of disease is not uncommon and may result in enhanced toxicity.

Cytotoxic drug handling guidelines

- Trained personnel should reconstitute cytotoxics
- Reconstitution should be carried out in designated pharmacy areas
- Protective clothing (including gloves, gowns, and masks) should be worn
- The eyes should be protected and means of first aid should be specified
- Pregnant staff should avoid exposure to cytotoxic drugs (all females of child-bearing age should be informed of the reproductive hazard)
- Use local procedures for dealing with spillages and safe disposal of waste material, including syringes, containers, and absorbent material
- Staff exposure to cytotoxic drugs should be monitored

Intrathecal chemotherapy

A Health Service Circular (HSC 2008/001) provides guidance on the introduction of safe practice in NHS Trusts where intrathecal chemotherapy is administered; written local guidance covering all aspects of national guidance should be available. Support for training programmes is also available.

Copies, and further information may be obtained from the Department of Health and Social Care website (www.gov.uk/government/organisations/department-of-health-and-social-care).

Safe systems for cytotoxic medicines

NHS cancer networks have been established across the UK to bring together all stakeholders in all sectors of care, to work collaboratively to plan and deliver high quality cancer services for a given population. NHS cancer networks have websites containing information on local chemotherapy services and treatment.

Safe system requirements:

- cytotoxic drugs for the treatment of cancer should be given as part of a wider pathway of care coordinated by a multidisciplinary team
- cytotoxic drugs should be prescribed, dispensed, and administered only in the context of a written protocol or treatment plan
- injectable cytotoxic drugs should only be dispensed if they are prepared for administration
- oral cytotoxic medicines should be dispensed with clear directions for use

Cytotoxic drugs: important safety information

Risk of incorrect dosing of oral anti-cancer medicines
The National Patient Safety Agency has advised (January 2008) that the prescribing and use of oral cytotoxic medicines should be carried out to the same standard as parenteral cytotoxic therapy.

- non-specialists who prescribe or administer on-going oral cytotoxic medication should have access to written protocols and treatment plans, including guidance on the monitoring and treatment of toxicity;

- staff dispensing oral cytotoxic medicines should confirm that the prescribed dose is appropriate for the patient. Patients should have written information that includes details of the intended oral anti-cancer regimen, the treatment plan, and arrangements for monitoring, taken from the original protocol from the initiating hospital. Staff dispensing oral cytotoxic medicines should also have access to this information, and to advice from an experienced cancer pharmacist in the initiating hospital.

Cytotoxic drug doses

Doses of cytotoxic drugs are determined using a variety of different methods including body-surface area or body-weight. Alternatively, doses may be fixed. Doses may be further adjusted following consideration of a patient's neutrophil count, renal and hepatic function, and history of previous adverse effects to the cytotoxic drug. Doses may also differ depending on whether a drug is used alone or in combination.

Because of the complexity of dosage regimens in the treatment of malignant disease, dose statements have been omitted from some of the drug entries in this chapter. However, even where dose statements have been provided, detailed specialist literature, individual hospital chemotherapy protocols, or local cancer networks should be consulted before prescribing, dispensing, or administering cytotoxic drugs.

Prescriptions should **not** be repeated except on the instructions of a specialist.

Cytotoxic drug side-effects

Side-effects common to most cytotoxic drugs are discussed below whilst side-effects characteristic of a particular drug or class of drugs (e.g. neurotoxicity with vinca alkaloids) are mentioned in the appropriate sections. Manufacturers' product literature, hospital-trust protocols, and cancer-network protocols should be consulted for full details of side-effects associated with individual drugs and specific chemotherapy regimes.

Many side-effects of cytotoxic drugs often do not occur at the time of administration, but days or weeks later. It is therefore important that patients and healthcare professionals can identify symptoms that cause concern and can contact an expert for advice. Toxicities should be accurately recorded using a recognised scoring system such as the Common Toxicity Criteria for Adverse Events (CTCAE) developed by the National Cancer Institute.

Extravasation of intravenous drugs

A number of cytotoxic drugs will cause severe local tissue necrosis if leakage into the extravascular compartment occurs. To reduce the risk of extravasation injury it is recommended that cytotoxic drugs are administered by appropriately trained staff. See information on the prevention and management of extravasation injury.

Oral mucositis

A sore mouth is a common complication of cancer chemotherapy; it is most often associated with fluorouracil p. 955, methotrexate p. 957, and the anthracyclines. It is best to prevent the complication. Good oral hygiene (rinsing the mouth frequently and effective brushing of the teeth with a soft brush 2–3 times daily) is probably beneficial. For fluorouracil p. 955, sucking ice chips during short infusions of the drug is also helpful.

Once a sore mouth has developed, treatment is much less effective. Saline mouthwashes should be used but there is no good evidence to support the use of antiseptic or anti-inflammatory mouthwashes. In general, mucositis is self-limiting but with poor oral hygiene it can be a focus for blood-borne infection.

Tumour lysis syndrome

Tumour lysis syndrome occurs secondary to spontaneous or treatment-related rapid destruction of malignant cells. Patients at risk of tumour lysis syndrome include those with non-Hodgkin's lymphoma (especially if high grade and bulky disease), Burkitt's lymphoma, acute lymphoblastic leukaemia and acute myeloid leukaemia (particularly if high white blood cell counts or bulky disease), and occasionally those with solid tumours. Pre-existing hyperuricaemia, dehydration, and renal impairment are also predisposing factors. Features include hyperkalaemia, hyperuricaemia (see below), and hyperphosphataemia with hypocalcaemia; renal damage and arrhythmias can follow. Early identification of patients at risk, and initiation of prophylaxis or therapy for tumour lysis syndrome, is essential.

Hyperuricaemia

Hyperuricaemia, which may be present in high-grade lymphoma and leukaemia, can be markedly worsened by chemotherapy and is associated with acute renal failure. Allopurinol p. 1166 should be started 24 hours before treating such tumours and patients should be adequately hydrated. The dose of mercaptopurine p. 956 or azathioprine p. 882 should be reduced if allopurinol needs to be given concomitantly. Febuxostat p. 1167 may also be used and should be started 2 days before cytotoxic therapy is initiated.

Rasburicase p. 985, a recombinant urate oxidase, is licensed for hyperuricaemia in patients with haematological malignancy. It rapidly reduces plasma-uric acid concentration and may be of particular value in preventing complications following treatment of leukaemias or bulky lymphomas.

Bone-marrow suppression

All cytotoxic drugs except vincristine sulfate p. 972 and bleomycin p. 963 cause bone-marrow suppression. This commonly occurs 7 to 10 days after administration, but is delayed for certain drugs, such as carmustine p. 937, lomustine p. 941, and melphalan p. 941. Peripheral blood counts must be checked before each treatment, and doses should be reduced or therapy delayed if bone-marrow has not recovered.

Cytotoxic drugs may be contra-indicated in patients with acute infection; any infection should be treated before, or when starting, cytotoxic drugs.

Fever in a neutropenic patient (neutrophil count less than 1.06×10^9/litre) requires immediate broad-spectrum antibacterial therapy. Appropriate bacteriological investigations should be conducted as soon as possible. Patients taking cytotoxic drugs who have signs or symptoms of infection should be advised to seek prompt medical attention. All patients should initially be investigated and treated under the supervision of the appropriate oncology or haematology specialist.

In selected patients, the duration and the severity of neutropenia can be reduced by the use of recombinant human granulocyte-colony stimulating factors. Symptomatic anaemia is usually treated with red blood cell transfusions. For guidance on the use of erythropoietins in patients with cancer, see MHRA/CHM advice and NICE guidance.

Alopecia

Reversible hair loss is a common complication, although it varies in degree between drugs and individual patients. No pharmacological methods of preventing this are available.

Thromboembolism

Venous thromboembolism can be a complication of cancer itself, but chemotherapy increases the risk.

Cytotoxic drugs: effect on pregnancy and reproductive function

Most cytotoxic drugs are teratogenic and should not be administered during pregnancy, especially during the first trimester. Considerable caution is necessary if a pregnant woman presents with cancer requiring chemotherapy, and specialist advice should always be sought.

Exclude pregnancy before treatment with cytotoxic drugs. Contraceptive advice should be given before cytotoxic therapy begins- women of childbearing age should use effective contraception during and after treatment.

Regimens that do not contain an alkylating drug or procarbazine may have less effect on fertility, but those with an alkylating drug or procarbazine carry the risk of causing permanent male sterility (there is no effect on potency). Pretreatment counselling and consideration of sperm storage may be appropriate. Women are less severely affected, though the span of reproductive life may be shortened by the onset of a premature menopause. No increase in fetal abnormalities or abortion rate has been recorded in patients who remain fertile after cytotoxic chemotherapy.

Cytotoxic drugs: nausea and vomiting

Nausea and vomiting cause considerable distress to many patients who receive chemotherapy and to a lesser extent abdominal radiotherapy, and may lead to refusal of further treatment; prophylaxis of nausea and vomiting is therefore extremely important. Symptoms may be acute (occurring within 24 hours of treatment), delayed (first occurring more than 24 hours after treatment), or anticipatory (occurring prior to subsequent doses). Delayed and anticipatory symptoms are more difficult to control than acute symptoms and require different management.

Patients vary in their susceptibility to drug-induced nausea and vomiting; those affected more often include women, patients under 50 years of age, anxious patients, and those who experience motion sickness. Susceptibility also increases with repeated exposure to the cytotoxic drug.

Drugs may be divided according to their emetogenic potential and some examples are given below, but the symptoms vary according to the dose, to other drugs administered and to the individual's susceptibility to emetogenic stimuli.

Mildly emetogenic treatment—fluorouracil, etoposide p. 967, methotrexate p. 957 (less than 100 mg/m², low dose in children), the vinca alkaloids, and abdominal radiotherapy.

Moderately emetogenic treatment—the taxanes, doxorubicin hydrochloride p. 946, intermediate and low doses of cyclophosphamide p. 938, mitoxantrone p. 948, and high doses of methotrexate (0.1– 1.2 g/m²).

Highly emetogenic treatment— cisplatin p. 966, dacarbazine p. 939, and high doses of cyclophosphamide.

Prevention of acute symptoms

For patients at *low risk of emesis*, pretreatment with dexamethasone p. 714 or lorazepam p. 357 may be used.

For patients at *high risk of emesis*, a 5HT₃-receptor antagonist, usually given by mouth in combination with dexamethasone and the neurokinin receptor antagonist aprepitant p. 452 is effective.

Prevention of delayed symptoms

For delayed symptoms associated with moderately emetogenic chemotherapy, a combination of dexamethasone and 5HT₃-receptor antagonist is effective; for highly emetogenic chemotherapy, a combination of dexamethasone and aprepitant is effective. Rolapitant and metoclopramide hydrochloride p. 451 are also licensed for delayed chemotherapy-induced nausea and vomiting.

Prevention of anticipatory symptoms

Good symptom control is the best way to prevent anticipatory symptoms. Lorazepam can be helpful for its amnesic, sedative, and anxiolytic effects.

For information on the treatment of nausea and vomiting, see Nausea and labyrinth disorders p. 448.

Treatment of cytotoxic-induced side-effects

Anthracycline side-effects

Anthracycline-induced cardiotoxicity

The anthracycline cytotoxic drugs are associated with dose-related, cumulative, and potentially life-threatening cardiotoxic side-effects.

Anthracycline extravasation

Local guidelines for the management of extravasation should be followed or specialist advice sought.

See further information on the prevention and management of extravasation injury.

Chemotherapy-induced mucositis and myelosuppression

Folinic acid p. 984 (given as calcium folinate) is used to counteract the folate-antagonist action of methotrexate p. 957 and thus speed recovery from methotrexate-induced mucositis or myelosuppression ('folinic acid rescue').

Folinic acid is also used in the management of methotrexate overdose, together with other measures to maintain fluid and electrolyte balance, and to manage possible renal failure.

Folinic acid does not counteract the antibacterial activity of folate antagonists such as trimethoprim p. 610.

When folinic acid and fluorouracil p. 955 are used together in metastatic colorectal cancer the response-rate improves compared to that with fluorouracil alone.

The calcium salt of levofolinic acid p. 985, a single isomer of folinic acid, is also used for rescue therapy following methotrexate administration, for cases of methotrexate overdose, and for use with fluorouracil for colorectal cancer. The dose of calcium levofolinate is generally half that of calcium folinate.

The disodium salts of folinic acid and levofolinic acid are also used for rescue therapy following methotrexate therapy, and for use with fluorouracil for colorectal cancer.

Urothelial toxicity

Haemorrhagic cystitis is a common manifestation of urothelial toxicity which occurs with the oxazaphosphorines, cyclophosphamide p. 938 and ifosfamide p. 940; it is caused by the metabolite acrolein. Mesna p. 984 reacts specifically with this metabolite in the urinary tract, preventing toxicity. Mesna is used routinely (preferably by mouth) in patients receiving ifosfamide, and in patients receiving cyclophosphamide by the intravenous route at a high dose (e.g. more than 2 g) or in those who experienced urothelial toxicity when given cyclophosphamide previously.

Anthracyclines and other cytotoxic antibiotics

Drugs in this group are widely used. Many cytotoxic antibiotics act as radiomimetics and simultaneous use of radiotherapy should be **avoided** because it may markedly increased toxicity. Daunorubicin p. 944, doxorubicin hydrochloride p. 946, epirubicin hydrochloride p. 947 and idarubicin hydrochloride p. 947 are anthracycline antibiotics. Mitoxantrone p. 948 is an anthracycline derivative.

Doxorubicin hydrochloride is available as both *conventional* and *liposomal* formulations. The different formulations vary in their licensed indications, pharmacokinetics, dosage and administration, and are not interchangeable. *Conventional* doxorubicin hydrochloride is used to treat the acute leukaemias, Hodgkin's and non-Hodgkin's lymphomas, paediatric malignancies, and some solid tumours including breast cancer.

Epirubicin hydrochloride is structurally related to doxorubicin hydrochloride and can be used to treat breast cancer.

Idarubicin hydrochloride has general properties similar to those of doxorubicin hydrochloride; it is mostly used in the treatment of haematological malignancies.

Daunorubicin also has general properties similar to those of doxorubicin hydrochloride.

Mitoxantrone is structurally related to doxorubicin hydrochloride.

Pixantrone p. 949 is licensed as monotherapy for the treatment of refractory or multiply relapsed aggressive non-Hodgkin B-cell lymphomas, although the benefits of using it as a fifth-line or greater chemotherapy in refractory patients has not been established.

Bleomycin p. 963 is given intravenously or intramuscularly to treat metastatic germ cell cancer and, in some regimens, non-Hodgkin's lymphoma.

Dactinomycin is principally used to treat paediatric cancers. Its side-effects are similar to those of doxorubicin, except that cardiac toxicity is not a problem.

Mitomycin p. 963 can be given intravenously to treat gastro-intestinal, breast, non-small cell lung, and metastatic pancreatic cancers; and by bladder instillation for superficial bladder tumours. It causes delayed bone marrow toxicity.

Vinca alkaloids

The vinca alkaloids, vinblastine sulfate p. 972, vincristine sulfate p. 972, and vindesine sulfate p. 973, are used to treat a variety of cancers including leukaemias, lymphomas, and some solid tumours. Vinorelbine p. 974 is a semi-synthetic vinca alkaloid. See also, role of vinorelbine in the treatment of breast cancer.

Antimetabolites

Antimetabolites are incorporated into new nuclear material or combine irreversibly with cellular enzymes, preventing normal cellular division.

Alkylating drugs

Extensive experience is available with these drugs, which are among the most widely used in cancer chemotherapy. They act by damaging DNA, thus interfering with cell replication.

Cyclophosphamide is used mainly in combination with other agents for treating a wide range of malignancies, including some leukaemias, lymphomas, and solid tumours. It is given by mouth or intravenously; it is inactive until metabolised by the liver.

Ifosfamide is related to cyclophosphamide and is given intravenously.

Melphalan p. 941 is licensed for the treatment of multiple myeloma, polycythaemia vera, childhood neuroblastoma, advanced ovarian adenocarcinoma, and advanced breast cancer. However, in practice, melphalan is rarely used for ovarian adenocarcinoma; it is no longer used for advanced breast cancer. Melphalan is also licensed for regional arterial perfusion in localised malignant melanoma of the extremities and localised soft-tissue sarcoma of the extremities.

Lomustine p. 941 is a lipid-soluble nitrosourea and the drug is given at intervals of 4 to 6 weeks.

Carmustine p. 937 has similar activity to lomustine; it is given to patients with multiple myeloma, non-Hodgkin's lymphomas, Hodgkin's disease, and brain tumours. Carmustine implants are licensed for intralesional use in adults for the treatment of recurrent glioblastoma multiforme as an adjunct to surgery. Carmustine implants are also licensed for high-grade malignant glioma as adjunctive treatment to surgery and radiotherapy.

Estramustine phosphate p. 940 is a combination of an oestrogen and chlormethine used predominantly in prostate cancer. It is given by mouth and has both an antimitotic

effect and (by reducing testosterone concentration) a hormonal effect.

Mitobronitol is occasionally used to treat chronic myeloid leukaemia; it is available on a named-patient basis from specialist importing companies.

ANTINEOPLASTIC DRUGS > ALKYLATING AGENTS

| Bendamustine hydrochloride   07-Jul-2020

● INDICATIONS AND DOSE

Treatment of chronic lymphocytic leukaemia | Treatment of non-Hodgkin's lymphoma | Treatment of multiple myeloma

▸ BY INTRAVENOUS INFUSION
▸ Adult: (consult local protocol)

IMPORTANT SAFETY INFORMATION

MHRA/CHM ADVICE: BENDAMUSTINE (*LEVACT*®): INCREASED MORTALITY OBSERVED IN RECENT CLINICAL STUDIES IN OFF-LABEL USE; MONITOR FOR OPPORTUNISTIC INFECTIONS, HEPATITIS B REACTIVATION (JULY 2017)

Recent clinical trials have shown increased mortality when bendamustine was used in combination treatments outside its approved indications. In addition, a recent European review of post-marketing data has suggested that the risk of opportunistic infections for all patients receiving bendamustine treatment may be greater than previously recognised.

The MHRA recommends monitoring patients for opportunistic infections as well as cardiac, neurological, and respiratory adverse events; known carriers of hepatitis B virus (HBV) should be monitored for signs and symptoms of active HBV infection. Patients should be advised to report promptly new signs of infection; consider discontinuing bendamustine if there are signs of opportunistic infections.

● CONTRA-INDICATIONS Jaundice · low leucocyte count · low platelet count · major surgery less than 30 days before start of treatment · severe bone marrow suppression

● CAUTIONS Cardiac disorders—monitor serum potassium and ECG

● INTERACTIONS → Appendix 1: alkylating agents

● SIDE-EFFECTS

▸ **Common or very common** Alopecia · amenorrhoea · anaemia · angina pectoris · appetite decreased · arrhythmias · cardiac disorder · chills · constipation · decreased leucocytes · dehydration · diarrhoea · dizziness · fatigue · fever · haemorrhage · headache · hepatitis B reactivation · hypersensitivity · hypertension · hypokalaemia · hypotension · increased risk of infection · insomnia · mucositis · nausea · neutropenia · pain · palpitations · respiratory disorders · skin reactions · stomatitis · thrombocytopenia · tumour lysis syndrome · vomiting

▸ **Uncommon** Bone marrow disorders · heart failure · myocardial infarction · neoplasms · pericardial effusion

▸ **Rare or very rare** Anticholinergic syndrome · aphonia · ataxia · circulatory collapse · drowsiness · haemolysis · hyperhidrosis · infertility · multi organ failure · nervous system disorder · paraesthesia · peripheral neuropathy · sepsis · taste altered

▸ **Frequency not known** Extravasation necrosis · hepatic failure · necrosis · renal failure · severe cutaneous adverse reactions (SCARs)

SIDE-EFFECTS, FURTHER INFORMATION **Secondary malignancy** Use of bendamustine is associated with an increased incidence of acute leukaemias.

Infections Serious and fatal infections are reported, including opportunistic infections such as Pneumocystis

8

Immune system and malignant disease

jirovecii pneumonia (PJP), varicella zoster virus (VZV) and cytomegalovirus (CMV)—manufacturer advises monitoring for respiratory signs and symptoms throughout treatment; patients should be advised to report new signs of infection, including fever or respiratory symptoms, promptly. Reactivation of hepatitis B is reported in patients who are chronic carriers of the virus—manufacturer advises monitoring for signs and symptoms of active hepatitis B during treatment and for several months after stopping treatment.

- CONCEPTION AND CONTRACEPTION Effective contraception is required during treatment in men or women, and for 6 months after treatment in men. See also *Pregnancy and reproductive function* in Cytotoxic drugs p. 932.

- PREGNANCY Avoid (teratogenic and mutagenic in *animal* studies). See also *Pregnancy and reproductive function* in Cytotoxic drugs p. 932.

- BREAST FEEDING Discontinue breast-feeding.

- HEPATIC IMPAIRMENT Manufacturer advises avoid in severe impairment—no information available.
  Dose adjustments Manufacturer advises reduce dose by 30% in moderate impairment.

- RENAL IMPAIRMENT No information available on use in patients with creatinine clearance less than 10 mL/minute.

- NATIONAL FUNDING/ACCESS DECISIONS
  For full details see funding body website
  NICE decisions
  ▶ **Bendamustine for the first-line treatment of chronic lymphocytic leukaemia (February 2011)** NICE TA216 Recommended
  ▶ **Obinutuzumab with bendamustine for treating follicular lymphoma refractory to rituximab (August 2017)** NICE TA472 Recommended with restrictions
  Scottish Medicines Consortium (SMC) decisions
  ▶ **Bendamustine hydrochloride (*Levact®*) for chronic lymphocytic leukaemia (CLL) (April 2011)** SMC No. 694/11 Recommended

- MEDICINAL FORMS There can be variation in the licensing of different medicines containing the same drug.
  Powder for solution for infusion
  ▶ Bendamustine hydrochloride (Non-proprietary)
  Bendamustine hydrochloride 25 mg Bendamustine 25mg powder for concentrate for solution for infusion vials | 1 vial [PoM] £65.98 | 5 vial [PoM] £27.75–£347.26 (Hospital only) | 20 vial [PoM] £1,241.14 (Hospital only)
  Bendamustine hydrochloride 100 mg Bendamustine 100mg powder for concentrate for solution for infusion vials | 1 vial [PoM] £23.55 (Hospital only) | 1 vial [PoM] £262.02 | 5 vial [PoM] £1,241.14–£1,379.04 (Hospital only)

Busulfan

08-Jul-2020

(Busulphan)

- INDICATIONS AND DOSE
Chronic myeloid leukaemia, induction of remission
  ▶ BY MOUTH
  ▶ Adult: 60 micrograms/kg daily (max. per dose 4 mg); maintenance 0.5–2 mg daily

Conditioning treatment before haematopoietic progenitor cell transplantation
  ▶ BY MOUTH, OR BY INTRAVENOUS INFUSION
  ▶ Adult: (consult local protocol)

Conditioning treatment before haematopoietic progenitor cell transplantation in patients who are candidates for a reduced-intensity conditioning (RIC) regimen
  ▶ BY INTRAVENOUS INFUSION
  ▶ Adult: (consult local protocol)

DOSES AT EXTREMES OF BODY-WEIGHT
▶ Dose may need to be calculated based on body surface area or adjusted ideal body weight in obese patients— consult product literature.

IMPORTANT SAFETY INFORMATION
RISKS OF INCORRECT DOSING OF ORAL ANTI-CANCER MEDICINES
See Cytotoxic drugs p. 932.

- CAUTIONS Avoid in Acute porphyrias p. 1107 · high dose (antiepileptic prophylaxis required) · history of seizures (antiepileptic prophylaxis required) · ineffective once in blast crisis phase · previous progenitor cell transplant (increased risk of hepatic veno-occlusive disease) · previous radiation therapy (increased risk of hepatic veno-occlusive disease) · risk of second malignancy · three or more cycles of chemotherapy (increased risk of hepatic veno-occlusive disease)

- INTERACTIONS → Appendix 1: alkylating agents

- SIDE-EFFECTS
  GENERAL SIDE-EFFECTS
  ▶ **Common or very common** Alopecia · diarrhoea · hepatic disorders · nausea · respiratory disorders · sinusoidal obstruction syndrome · skin reactions · thrombocytopenia · vomiting
  ▶ **Uncommon** Seizure
  ▶ **Rare or very rare** Cataract · eye disorders
  SPECIFIC SIDE-EFFECTS
  ▶ **Common or very common**
  ▶ With intravenous use Anaemia · anxiety · appetite decreased · arrhythmias · arthralgia · ascites · asthenia · asthma · cardiomegaly · chest pain · chills · confusion · constipation · cough · depression · dizziness · dyspnoea · dysuria · electrolyte imbalance · embolism and thrombosis · fever · gastrointestinal discomfort · gastrointestinal disorders · haemorrhage · headache · hiccups · hyperglycaemia · hypersensitivity · hypertension · hypoalbuminaemia · hypotension · increased risk of infection · insomnia · mucositis · myalgia · nervous system disorder · neutropenia · oedema · pain · pancytopenia · pericardial effusion · pericarditis · reactivation of infections · renal disorder · renal impairment · stomatitis · vasodilation · weight increased
  ▶ With oral use Amenorrhoea (may be reversible) · azoospermia · bone marrow disorders · cardiac tamponade · delayed puberty · hyperbilirubinaemia · infertility male · leucopenia · leukaemia · menopausal symptoms · oral disorders · ovarian and fallopian tube disorders · testicular atrophy
  ▶ **Uncommon**
  ▶ With intravenous use Capillary leak syndrome · delirium · encephalopathy · hallucination · hypoxia · intracranial haemorrhage
  ▶ **Rare or very rare**
  ▶ With oral use Dry mouth · erythema nodosum · gynaecomastia · myasthenia gravis · radiation injury · Sjögren's syndrome
  ▶ **Frequency not known**
  ▶ With intravenous use Hypogonadism · ovarian failure · premature menopause · sepsis
  SIDE-EFFECTS, FURTHER INFORMATION **Lung toxicity** Discontinue if lung toxicity develops.
  Secondary malignancy Use of busulfan is associated with an increased incidence of secondary malignancy.

- CONCEPTION AND CONTRACEPTION Manufacturers advise effective contraception during and for 6 months after treatment in men or women. See also *Pregnancy and reproductive function* in Cytotoxic drugs p. 932.

PREGNANCY Avoid (teratogenic in *animals*). See also *Pregnancy and reproductive function* in Cytotoxic drugs p. 932.

BREAST FEEDING Discontinue breast-feeding.

HEPATIC IMPAIRMENT Manufacturer advises caution (no information available)—monitor hepatic function, especially following transplant (consult product literature).

MONITORING REQUIREMENTS
Monitor cardiac and liver function.
Frequent blood tests are necessary because excessive myelosuppression may result in irreversible bone-marrow aplasia.

MEDICINAL FORMS There can be variation in the licensing of different medicines containing the same drug. Forms available from special-order manufacturers include: capsule, oral suspension, oral solution

Tablet
▶ Busulfan (Non-proprietary)
  Busulfan 2 mg Busulfan 2mg tablets | 25 tablet [PoM] £69.02 DT = £69.02

Solution for infusion
▶ Busulfan (Non-proprietary)
  Busulfan 6 mg per 1 ml Busulfan 60mg/10ml concentrate for solution for infusion vials | 8 vial [PoM] £1,529.50–£2,157.52 (Hospital only)
▶ Busilvex (Pierre Fabre Ltd)
  Busulfan 6 mg per 1 ml Busilvex 60mg/10ml concentrate for solution for infusion ampoules | 8 ampoule [PoM] £1,610.00 (Hospital only)

Carmustine

13-Jul-2020

● INDICATIONS AND DOSE

Brain tumours | Multiple myeloma | Non-Hodgkin's lymphomas | Hodgkin's disease
▶ BY INTRAVENOUS INFUSION
▶ Adult: (consult product literature)

Recurrent glioblastoma multiforme as an adjunct to surgery | High-grade malignant glioma as adjunctive treatment to surgery and radiotherapy
▶ BY INTRALESIONAL IMPLANTATION
▶ Adult: (consult product literature)

● CAUTIONS Avoid in Acute porphyrias p. 1107

● INTERACTIONS → Appendix 1: alkylating agents

● SIDE-EFFECTS

GENERAL SIDE-EFFECTS
▶ **Common or very common** Alopecia · anaemia · ataxia · constipation · diarrhoea · dizziness · headache · nausea · seizures · vomiting

SPECIFIC SIDE-EFFECTS
▶ **Common or very common**
▶ When used by implant Abdominal pain · abscess · anxiety · asthenia · chest pain · coma · confusion · conjunctival oedema · depression · diabetes mellitus · drowsiness · dysphagia · electrolyte imbalance · embolism and thrombosis · eye pain · faecal incontinence · fever · gait abnormal · haemorrhage · hallucination · healing impaired · hydrocephalus · hyperglycaemia · hypersensitivity · hypertension · hypotension · increased risk of infection · injury · insomnia · intracranial pressure increased · leucocytosis · memory loss · meningitis · oedema · pain · paralysis · paranoia · peripheral neuropathy · personality disorder · rash · sensation abnormal · sepsis · speech impairment · stupor · thinking abnormal · thrombocytopenia · tremor · urinary incontinence · vision disorders
▶ With intravenous use Acute leukaemia · appetite decreased · bone marrow depression · encephalopathy (with high

doses) · hepatotoxicity · myelodysplastic syndrome (following long term use) · ocular toxicity · respiratory disorders · retinal haemorrhage · stomatitis
▶ **Uncommon**
▶ When used by implant Cerebral infarction · intracranial haemorrhage
▶ **Rare or very rare**
▶ With intravenous use Gynaecomastia · nephrotoxicity (cumulative) · peripheral vascular disease (with high doses)
▶ **Frequency not known**
▶ With intravenous use Infertility · myalgia

SIDE-EFFECTS, FURTHER INFORMATION **Pulmonary toxicity** Lung infiltration, pulmonary fibrosis, pneumonitis, and interstitial lung disease have been reported with intravenous use, some of which have been fatal. These appear to be dose-related, cumulative, and may be delayed.

Hepatotoxicity Hepatotoxicity has been reported to occur with high intravenous doses, and may be delayed up to 60 days after administration; usually reversible.

● CONCEPTION AND CONTRACEPTION Manufacturer advises effective contraception during treatment in men or women. See also *Pregnancy and reproductive function* in Cytotoxic drugs p. 932.

● PREGNANCY Avoid (teratogenic and embryotoxic in *animals*). See also *Pregnancy and reproductive function* in Cytotoxic drugs p. 932.

● BREAST FEEDING Discontinue breast-feeding.

● HANDLING AND STORAGE For intravenous infusion, manufacturer advises store in a refrigerator (2–8°C) and protect from light. For intralesional implant, manufacturer advises store in a freezer (–20°C)—consult product literature for further information regarding storage outside freezer.

● NATIONAL FUNDING/ACCESS DECISIONS
For full details see funding body website

NICE decisions
▶ **Carmustine implants and temozolomide for the treatment of newly diagnosed high-grade glioma (June 2007)** NICE TA121 Recommended with restrictions

● MEDICINAL FORMS There can be variation in the licensing of different medicines containing the same drug.

Implant
▶ Gliadel (Eisai Ltd)
  Carmustine 7.7 mg Gliadel 7.7mg implant | 8 device [PoM] £5,203.00 (Hospital only)

Chlorambucil

13-Jul-2020

● INDICATIONS AND DOSE

Some lymphomas and chronic leukaemias (used either alone or in combination therapy)
▶ BY MOUTH
▶ Adult: (consult local protocol)

IMPORTANT SAFETY INFORMATION
RISKS OF INCORRECT DOSING OF ORAL ANTI-CANCER MEDICINES
See Cytotoxic drugs p. 932.

● CAUTIONS Children with nephrotic syndrome (increased seizure risk) · history of epilepsy (increased seizure risk)

● INTERACTIONS → Appendix 1: alkylating agents

● SIDE-EFFECTS
▶ **Common or very common** Anaemia · bone marrow disorders · diarrhoea · gastrointestinal disorder · leucopenia · nausea · neoplasms · neutropenia · oral ulceration · seizures · thrombocytopenia · vomiting
▶ **Uncommon** Skin reactions

▸ **Rare or very rare** Cystitis · fever · hepatic disorders · movement disorders · muscle twitching · peripheral neuropathy · respiratory disorders · severe cutaneous adverse reactions (SCARs) · tremor
▸ **Frequency not known** Amenorrhoea · azoospermia

SIDE-EFFECTS, FURTHER INFORMATION **Secondary malignancy** Use of chlorambucil is associated with an increased incidence of acute leukaemia, particularly with prolonged use.

Skin reactions Manufacturer advises assessing continued use if rash occurs—has been reported to progress to Stevens-Johnson syndrome and toxic epidermal necrolysis.

● CONCEPTION AND CONTRACEPTION Contraceptive advice required, see *Pregnancy and reproductive function* in Cytotoxic drugs p. 932.
● PREGNANCY Avoid. See also *Pregnancy and reproductive function* in Cytotoxic drugs p. 932.
● BREAST FEEDING Discontinue breast-feeding.
● HEPATIC IMPAIRMENT Manufacturer advises caution—monitor for signs and symptoms of toxicity.
Dose adjustments Manufacturer advises consider dose reduction in severe impairment—limited information available.
● NATIONAL FUNDING/ACCESS DECISIONS
For full details see funding body website
NICE decisions
▸ Obinutuzumab in combination with chlorambucil for untreated chronic lymphocytic leukaemia (June 2015) NICE TA343 Recommended with restrictions
▸ Ofatumumab in combination with chlorambucil or bendamustine for untreated chronic lymphocytic leukaemia (June 2015) NICE TA344 Recommended with restrictions

● MEDICINAL FORMS There can be variation in the licensing of different medicines containing the same drug.
Tablet
▸ Chlorambucil (Non-proprietary)
Chlorambucil 2 mg Chlorambucil 2mg tablets | 25 tablet [PoM] £42.87 DT = £42.87

Chlormethine

23-Aug-2019

● DRUG ACTION Chlormethine is an alkylating agent which inhibits rapidly proliferating cells.

● INDICATIONS AND DOSE

Mycosis fungoides (initiated by a specialist)
▸ TO THE SKIN
▸ Adult: Apply once daily, apply thinly to the affected areas, for dose adjustments due to side-effects of the skin—consult product literature

● CAUTIONS Avoid contact with mucous membranes
● INTERACTIONS → Appendix 1: chlormethine
● SIDE-EFFECTS
▸ **Common or very common** Hypersensitivity · skin infection · skin reactions · skin ulcer
● CONCEPTION AND CONTRACEPTION Manufacturer advises contraception in women of child-bearing potential during treatment. See also *Pregnancy and reproductive function* in Cytotoxic drugs p. 932.
● PREGNANCY Manufacturer advises avoid—toxicity in *animal* studies following systemic administration. See also *Pregnancy and reproductive function* in Cytotoxic drugs p. 932
● BREAST FEEDING Manufacturer advises avoid—no information available.
● DIRECTIONS FOR ADMINISTRATION Manufacturer advises apply to dry skin at least 4 hours before or 30 minutes after

showering or washing. The treated area should be allowed to dry for 5 to 10 minutes.
● HANDLING AND STORAGE Manufacturer advises store in a refrigerator (2–8 °C)—consult product literature for storage in a freezer.
● PATIENT AND CARER ADVICE Patients and carers should be advised to wash hands after each application and should wear nitrile gloves for each application. If non-affected areas are exposed, these areas should be washed. Occlusive dressings should not be applied over the treated area.

● MEDICINAL FORMS There can be variation in the licensing of different medicines containing the same drug.
Gel
EXCIPIENTS: May contain Butylated hydroxytoluene, propylene glycol
▸ Ledaga (Recordati Rare Diseases UK Ltd)
Chlormethine hydrochloride 160 microgram per 1 gram Ledaga 160micrograms/g gel | 60 gram [PoM] £1,000.00

Cyclophosphamide

11-Aug-2020

● INDICATIONS AND DOSE

Rheumatoid arthritis with severe systemic manifestations
▸ BY MOUTH
▸ Adult: 1–1.5 mg/kg daily

Severe systemic rheumatoid arthritis | Other connective tissue diseases (especially with active vasculitis)
▸ BY INTRAVENOUS INJECTION
▸ Adult: 0.5–1 g every 2 weeks, then reduced to 0.5–1 g every month, frequency adjusted according to clinical response and haematological monitoring. To be given with prophylactic mesna

Used, mainly in combination with other agents for treating a wide range of malignancies, including some leukaemias, lymphomas, and solid tumours
▸ BY MOUTH, OR BY INTRAVENOUS INFUSION
▸ Adult: (consult local protocol)

● UNLICENSED USE Not licensed for rheumatoid arthritis with severe systemic manifestations.

> IMPORTANT SAFETY INFORMATION
> RISKS OF INCORRECT DOSING OF ORAL ANTI-CANCER MEDICINES
> See Cytotoxic drugs p. 932.

● CAUTIONS Avoid in Acute porphyrias p. 1107 · diabetes mellitus · haemorrhagic cystitis · previous or concurrent mediastinal irradiation—risk of cardiotoxicity
● INTERACTIONS → Appendix 1: alkylating agents
● SIDE-EFFECTS
GENERAL SIDE-EFFECTS
▸ **Common or very common** Agranulocytosis · alopecia · anaemia · asthenia · bone marrow disorders · cystitis · decreased leucocytes · fever · haemolytic uraemic syndrome · haemorrhage · hepatic disorders · immunosuppression · increased risk of infection · mucosal abnormalities · neutropenia · progressive multifocal leukoencephalopathy (PML) · reactivation of infections · sperm abnormalities · thrombocytopenia
▸ **Uncommon** Appetite decreased · embolism and thrombosis · flushing · hypersensitivity · ovarian and fallopian tube disorders · sepsis
▸ **Rare or very rare** Bladder disorders · chest pain · confusion · constipation · diarrhoea · disseminated intravascular coagulation · dizziness · eye inflammation · fluid imbalance · headache · hyponatraemia · menstrual cycle irregularities · nail discolouration · nausea · neoplasms · oral disorders · pancreatitis acute · renal failure · secondary neoplasm · seizure · severe cutaneous adverse reactions (SCARs) · SIADH · skin reactions · visual impairment · vomiting

▶ **Frequency not known** Abdominal pain · altered smell sensation · arrhythmias · arthralgia · ascites · cardiac inflammation · cardiogenic shock · cardiomyopathy · cough · deafness · dyspnoea · encephalopathy · excessive tearing · facial swelling · gastrointestinal disorders · heart failure · hyperhidrosis · hypoxia · infertility · influenza like illness · multi organ failure · muscle complaints · myelopathy · myocardial infarction · nasal complaints · nephropathy · nerve disorders · neuralgia · neurotoxicity · oedema · oropharyngeal pain · palpitations · pericardial effusion · peripheral ischaemia · pulmonary hypertension · pulmonary oedema · QT interval prolongation · radiation injuries · renal tubular disorder · renal tubular necrosis · respiratory disorders · rhabdomyolysis · scleroderma · sensation abnormal · sinusoidal obstruction syndrome · taste altered · testicular atrophy · tinnitus · tremor · tumour lysis syndrome · vasculitis

SPECIFIC SIDE-EFFECTS

▶ With intravenous use Infusion site necrosis · injection site necrosis

SIDE-EFFECTS, FURTHER INFORMATION **Haemorrhagic cystitis** A urinary metabolite of cyclophosphamide, acrolein, can cause haemorrhagic cystitis; this is a rare but serious complication that may be prevented by increasing fluid intake for 24–48 hours after intravenous injection. Mesna can also help prevent cystitis when high-dose therapy (e.g. more than 2 g intravenously) is used or when the patient is considered to be at high risk of cystitis (e.g. because of pelvic irradiation).

Secondary malignancy As with all cytotoxic therapy, treatment with cyclophosphamide is associated with an increased incidence of secondary malignancies.

● CONCEPTION AND CONTRACEPTION Manufacturer advises effective contraception during and for at least 3 months after treatment in men or women. See also *Pregnancy and reproductive function* in Cytotoxic drugs p. 932.

● PREGNANCY Avoid. See also *Pregnancy and reproductive function* in Cytotoxic drugs p. 932.

● BREAST FEEDING Discontinue breast-feeding during and for 36 hours after stopping treatment.

● HEPATIC IMPAIRMENT Manufacturer advises caution (risk of decreased cyclophosphamide activation and increased risk of veno-occlusive liver disease).
Dose adjustments Manufacturer advises consider dose adjustment in severe impairment—consult product literature.

● RENAL IMPAIRMENT
Dose adjustments Reduce dose if serum creatinine concentration greater than 120 micromol/litre.

● DIRECTIONS FOR ADMINISTRATION

▶ With intravenous use For *intravenous infusion* (cyclophosphamide injection; *Baxter*), manufacturer advises give via drip tubing in Glucose 5% or Sodium Chloride 0.9%; reconstitute 500 mg with 25 mL Sodium Chloride 0.9%; reconstitute 1 g with 50 mL Sodium Chloride 0.9%.

● MEDICINAL FORMS There can be variation in the licensing of different medicines containing the same drug. Forms available from special-order manufacturers include: tablet, oral suspension, oral solution, solution for injection, solution for infusion

Tablet
CAUTIONARY AND ADVISORY LABELS 25, 27
▶ Cyclophosphamide (Non-proprietary)
Cyclophosphamide (as Cyclophosphamide monohydrate)
50 mg Cyclophosphamide 50mg tablets | 100 tablet [PoM] £139.00
DT = £139.00
▶ Cytoxan (Imported (United States))
Cyclophosphamide 25 mg Cytoxan 25mg tablets |
100 tablet [PoM] [▣]

Powder for solution for injection
▶ Cyclophosphamide (Non-proprietary)
Cyclophosphamide (as Cyclophosphamide monohydrate)
500 mg Cyclophosphamide 500mg powder for solution for injection vials | 1 vial [PoM] £9.20–£9.66 (Hospital only)
Cyclophosphamide (as Cyclophosphamide monohydrate)
1 gram Cyclophosphamide 1g powder for solution for injection vials | 1 vial [PoM] £10.66–£17.91 (Hospital only)
Cyclophosphamide (as Cyclophosphamide monohydrate)
2 gram Cyclophosphamide 2g powder for solution for injection vials | 1 vial [PoM] £31.64 (Hospital only)

Dacarbazine
14-Jul-2020

● **INDICATIONS AND DOSE**
Metastatic melanoma | Soft-tissue sarcomas (combination therapy) | Hodgkin's disease (combination therapy)
▶ BY INTRAVENOUS INFUSION, OR BY INTRAVENOUS INJECTION
▶ Adult: (consult local protocol)

● CAUTIONS Caution in handling—irritant to tissues

● INTERACTIONS → Appendix 1: alkylating agents

● SIDE-EFFECTS
▶ **Common or very common** Anaemia · appetite decreased · leucopenia · nausea · thrombocytopenia · vomiting
▶ **Uncommon** Alopecia · infection · influenza like illness · photosensitivity reaction · skin reactions
▶ **Rare or very rare** Agranulocytosis · confusion · diarrhoea · flushing · headache · hepatic disorders · lethargy · pancytopenia · paraesthesia · renal impairment · seizure · visual impairment

● CONCEPTION AND CONTRACEPTION Ensure effective contraception during and for at least 6 months after treatment in men or women. See also *Pregnancy and reproductive function* in Cytotoxic drugs p. 932.

● PREGNANCY Avoid (carcinogenic and teratogenic in *animal* studies). See also *Pregnancy and reproductive function* in Cytotoxic drugs p. 932.

● BREAST FEEDING Discontinue breast-feeding.

● HEPATIC IMPAIRMENT Avoid in severe impairment.
Dose adjustments Dose reduction may be required in combined renal and hepatic impairment.

● RENAL IMPAIRMENT Avoid in severe impairment.
Dose adjustments Dose reduction may be required in combined renal and hepatic impairment.

● PRESCRIBING AND DISPENSING INFORMATION Dacarbazine is a component of a commonly used combination for Hodgkin's disease (ABVD—doxorubicin [previously *Adriamycin*®], bleomycin, vinblastine, and dacarbazine).

● MEDICINAL FORMS There can be variation in the licensing of different medicines containing the same drug.
Powder for solution for infusion
▶ Dacarbazine (Non-proprietary)
Dacarbazine (as Dacarbazine citrate) 500 mg Dacarbazine 500mg powder for solution for infusion vials | 1 vial [PoM] £37.50
Dacarbazine (as Dacarbazine citrate) 1 gram Dacarbazine 1g powder for solution for infusion vials | 1 vial [PoM] £70.00
Powder for solution for injection
▶ Dacarbazine (Non-proprietary)
Dacarbazine (as Dacarbazine citrate) 100 mg Dacarbazine 100mg powder for solution for injection vials | 10 vial [PoM] £90.00
Dacarbazine (as Dacarbazine citrate) 200 mg Dacarbazine 200mg powder for solution for injection vials | 10 vial [PoM] £160.00

8

Immune system and malignant disease

Estramustine phosphate

04-Sep-2020

- **INDICATIONS AND DOSE**

Prostate cancer
- ▸ BY MOUTH
- ▸ Adult: Initially 560–840 mg daily in divided doses; maintenance 140–1400 mg daily in divided doses

> IMPORTANT SAFETY INFORMATION
> RISKS OF INCORRECT DOSING OF ORAL ANTI-CANCER MEDICINES
> See Cytotoxic drugs p. 932.

- CONTRA-INDICATIONS Peptic ulceration · severe cardiovascular disease · thromboembolic disorders
- CAUTIONS Cardiovascular disease · cerebrovascular disease · conditions which might be aggravated by fluid retention (such as epilepsy or migraine) · congestive heart failure · diabetes · hypercalcaemia · hypertension · metabolic bone disease
- INTERACTIONS → Appendix 1: alkylating agents
- SIDE-EFFECTS
- ▸ **Common or very common** Anaemia · congestive heart failure · diarrhoea · embolism · fluid retention · gynaecomastia · headache · hepatic function abnormal · lethargy · leucopenia · myocardial infarction · nausea · thrombocytopenia · vomiting
- ▸ **Frequency not known** Allergic dermatitis · angioedema · confusion · depression · erectile dysfunction · hypertension · muscle weakness · myocardial ischaemia
- CONCEPTION AND CONTRACEPTION Men should use effective contraceptive methods during treatment. See also *Pregnancy and reproductive function* in Cytotoxic drugs p. 932.
- HEPATIC IMPAIRMENT Manufacturer advises caution— monitor hepatic function; avoid in severe impairment.
- RENAL IMPAIRMENT Manufacturer advises caution.
- DIRECTIONS FOR ADMINISTRATION Manufacturer advises each dose should be taken not less than 1 hour before or 2 hours after meals and should not be taken with products containing calcium, magnesium or aluminium, including dairy products and antacid medication.
- PATIENT AND CARER ADVICE Patients should be given advice on how to administer estramustine capsules.

- MEDICINAL FORMS There can be variation in the licensing of different medicines containing the same drug.

Capsule

CAUTIONARY AND ADVISORY LABELS 5, 23
- ▸ Estracyt (Pfizer Ltd)
  Estramustine phosphate (as Estramustine sodium phosphate) 140 mg Estracyt 140mg capsules | 100 capsule [PoM] £171.28 DT = £171.28

Ifosfamide

15-Jul-2020

- **INDICATIONS AND DOSE**

Malignant disease
- ▸ BY INTRAVENOUS INFUSION
- ▸ Adult: (consult local protocol)

- CONTRA-INDICATIONS Acute infection · cystitis · urinary-tract obstruction · urothelial damage
- CAUTIONS Avoid in Acute porphyrias p. 1107 · cardiac disease
- INTERACTIONS → Appendix 1: alkylating agents
- SIDE-EFFECTS
- ▸ **Common or very common** Alopecia · appetite decreased · bone marrow disorders · haemorrhage · hepatic disorders ·

infection · leucopenia · nausea · reactivation of infection · renal impairment · thrombocytopenia · vomiting
- ▸ **Uncommon** Cardiotoxicity · diarrhoea · hypotension · oral disorders
- ▸ **Rare or very rare** Skin reactions
- ▸ **Frequency not known** Abdominal pain · agranulocytosis · amenorrhoea · anaemia · angina pectoris · angioedema · arrhythmias · arthralgia · asterixis · behaviour abnormal · blood disorders · bone disorders · cancer progression · capillary leak syndrome · cardiac arrest · cardiomyopathy · chills · conjunctivitis · constipation · cough · deafness · delirium · delusions · disseminated intravascular coagulation · dysarthria · dyspnoea · electrolyte imbalance · embolism and thrombosis · encephalopathy · eye irritation · fatigue · fever · flushing · gait abnormal · gastrointestinal disorders · growth retardation · haemolytic anaemia · heart failure · hyperglycaemia · hyperhidrosis · hyperphosphaturia · hypertension · hypoxia · immunosuppression · infertility · malaise · mania · memory loss · metabolic acidosis · movement disorders · mucosal ulceration · multi organ failure · muscle complaints · myocardial infarction · nail disorder · neoplasms · nephritis tubulointerstitial · nephrogenic diabetes insipidus · neurotoxicity · oedema · ovarian and fallopian tube disorders · pain · pancreatitis · panic attack · peripheral neuropathy · polydipsia · premature menopause · psychiatric disorders · pulmonary hypertension · pulmonary oedema · radiation recall reaction · respiratory disorders · rhabdomyolysis · secondary malignancy · sensation abnormal · sepsis · severe cutaneous adverse reactions (SCARs) · SIADH · sinusoidal obstruction syndrome · sperm abnormalities · status epilepticus · tinnitus · tumour lysis syndrome · urinary disorders · vasculitis · vertigo · visual impairment

SIDE-EFFECTS, FURTHER INFORMATION **Urothelial toxicity** Mesna is routinely given with ifosfamide to reduce urothelial toxicity.

Secondary malignancy Use of ifosfamide is associated with an increased incidence of acute leukaemia.

- CONCEPTION AND CONTRACEPTION Manufacturer advises adequate contraception during and for at least 6 months after treatment in men or women. See also *Pregnancy and reproductive function* in Cytotoxic drugs p. 932.
- PREGNANCY Avoid (teratogenic and carcinogenic in *animals*). See also *Pregnancy and reproductive function* in Cytotoxic drugs p. 932.
- BREAST FEEDING Discontinue breast-feeding.
- HEPATIC IMPAIRMENT Manufacturer advises avoid.
- RENAL IMPAIRMENT Avoid if serum creatinine concentration greater than 120 micromol/litre.
- MONITORING REQUIREMENTS Ensure satisfactory electrolyte balance and renal function before each course (risk of tubular dysfunction, Fanconi's syndrome or diabetes insipidus if renal toxicity not treated promptly).

- MEDICINAL FORMS There can be variation in the licensing of different medicines containing the same drug.

Powder for solution for injection
- ▸ Ifosfamide (Non-proprietary)
  Ifosfamide 1 gram Ifosfamide 1g powder for concentrate for solution for injection vials | 1 vial [PoM] £115.79-£119.27
  Ifosfamide 2 gram Ifosfamide 2g powder for concentrate for solution for injection vials | 1 vial [PoM] £228.09-£234.94

Lomustine

08-Jul-2019

- DRUG ACTION Lomustine is a lipid-soluble nitrosourea.

- INDICATIONS AND DOSE

Hodgkin's disease resistant to conventional therapy | Malignant melanoma | Certain solid tumours
- ▸ BY MOUTH
- ▸ Adult: 120–130 mg/m^2 every 6–8 weeks, dose is for when lomustine is used alone

> IMPORTANT SAFETY INFORMATION
> RISKS OF INCORRECT DOSING OF ORAL ANTI-CANCER MEDICINES
> See Cytotoxic drugs p. 932.

- CONTRA-INDICATIONS Coeliac disease
- INTERACTIONS → Appendix 1: alkylating agents
- SIDE-EFFECTS
- ▸ **Common or very common** Leucopenia
- ▸ **Frequency not known** Alopecia · anaemia · apathy · appetite decreased · azotaemia · bone marrow failure (delayed) · confusion · coordination abnormal · diarrhoea · hepatic disorders · lethargy · nausea · neoplasms · neurological effects · renal disorders · renal impairment · respiratory disorders · speech impairment · stomatitis · thrombocytopenia · vision loss (irreversible) · vomiting
  SIDE-EFFECTS, FURTHER INFORMATION Prolonged use of lomustine is associated with an increased incidence of acute leukaemias.
- CONCEPTION AND CONTRACEPTION Manufacturer advises effective contraception during and for at least 6 months after treatment in men *and women. See also Pregnancy and reproductive function* in Cytotoxic drugs p. 932.
- PREGNANCY Avoid. See also *Pregnancy and reproductive function* in Cytotoxic drugs p. 932.
- BREAST FEEDING Discontinue breast-feeding.
- RENAL IMPAIRMENT Avoid in severe impairment.
- PRESCRIBING AND DISPENSING INFORMATION The brand name *CCNU*® has been used for lomustine capsules.

- MEDICINAL FORMS There can be variation in the licensing of different medicines containing the same drug. Forms available from special-order manufacturers include: capsule
Capsule
- ▸ Lomustine (Non-proprietary)
  Lomustine 40 mg Lomustine 40mg capsules | 20 capsule [PoM] £780.82
- ▸ CeeNU (Imported (United States))
  Lomustine 10 mg CeeNU 10mg capsules | 20 capsule [PoM] [℞]
  Lomustine 100 mg CeeNU 100mg capsules | 20 capsule [PoM] [℞]

Melphalan

15-Jul-2020

- INDICATIONS AND DOSE

Multiple myeloma
- ▸ BY MOUTH
- ▸ Adult: 150 micrograms/kg daily for 4 days, dose to be repeated every 6 weeks, dose may vary according to regimen
- ▸ BY INTRAVENOUS INJECTION, OR BY INTRAVENOUS INFUSION
- ▸ Adult: (consult product literature)

Polycythaemia vera
- ▸ BY MOUTH
- ▸ Adult: Initially 6–10 mg daily for 5-7 days, then reduced to 2–4 mg daily until satisfactory response, then reduced to 2–6 mg once weekly

Localised malignant melanoma of the extremities | Localised soft-tissue sarcoma of the extremities
- ▸ BY REGIONAL ARTERIAL PERFUSION
- ▸ Adult: (consult local protocol)

> IMPORTANT SAFETY INFORMATION
> RISKS OF INCORRECT DOSING OF ORAL ANTI-CANCER MEDICINES
> See Cytotoxic drugs p. 932.

- CAUTIONS Consider use of prophylactic anti-infective agents · for high-dose intravenous administration establish adequate hydration · haematopoietic stem cell transplantation essential for high dose treatment (consult local treatment protocol for details)
- INTERACTIONS → Appendix 1: alkylating agents
- SIDE-EFFECTS
  GENERAL SIDE-EFFECTS
- ▸ **Common or very common** Alopecia · anaemia · bone marrow depression (delayed) · diarrhoea · nausea · stomatitis · thrombocytopenia · vomiting
- ▸ **Rare or very rare** Haemolytic anaemia · hepatic disorders · respiratory disorders · skin reactions
  SPECIFIC SIDE-EFFECTS
- ▸ **Common or very common**
- ▸ With oral use Leucopenia
- ▸ With parenteral use Feeling hot · myalgia · myopathy · paraesthesia
- ▸ **Rare or very rare**
- ▸ With parenteral use Peripheral vascular disease
  SIDE-EFFECTS, FURTHER INFORMATION **Secondary malignancy** Use of melphalan is associated with an increased incidence of acute leukaemias.
- CONCEPTION AND CONTRACEPTION Manufacturer advises adequate contraception during treatment in men *or women. See also Pregnancy and reproductive function* in Cytotoxic drugs p. 932.
- PREGNANCY Avoid. See also *Pregnancy and reproductive function* in Cytotoxic drugs p. 932.
- BREAST FEEDING Discontinue breast-feeding.
- RENAL IMPAIRMENT
  Dose adjustments Reduce dose initially (consult product literature).
- MONITORING REQUIREMENTS Monitor full blood count before and throughout treatment.

- MEDICINAL FORMS There can be variation in the licensing of different medicines containing the same drug.
Powder and solvent for solution for injection
- ▸ Melphalan (Non-proprietary)
  Melphalan (as Melphalan hydrochloride) 50 mg Melphalan 50mg powder and solvent for solution for injection vials | 1 vial [PoM] £137.37 (Hospital only)
Tablet
- ▸ Melphalan (Non-proprietary)
  Melphalan 2 mg Melphalan 2mg tablets | 25 tablet [PoM] £45.38 DT = £45.38

Streptozocin

09-Oct-2018

- DRUG ACTION Streptozocin is an antibiotic antineoplastic nitrosourea.

- INDICATIONS AND DOSE

Neuroendocrine tumours of pancreatic origin (specialist use only)
- ▸ BY INTRAVENOUS INFUSION
- ▸ Adult: (consult product literature)

- **CAUTIONS** Antiemetic pre-medication recommended ·
  avoid extravasation (risk of tissue necrosis) · elderly ·
  hyperhydration required (consult product literature)
- **INTERACTIONS** → Appendix 1: streptozocin
- **SIDE-EFFECTS**
  ‣ **Common or very common** Acute kidney injury · diarrhoea ·
    nausea · nephropathy · renal tubular injury · urinary
    disorder · urine abnormalities · vomiting
  ‣ **Frequency not known** Confusion · depression ·
    extravasation necrosis · fever · glucose tolerance impaired ·
    hepatotoxicity · hypoalbuminaemia · lethargy
- **CONCEPTION AND CONTRACEPTION** Manufacturer advises
  women of childbearing potential should use effective
  contraception during treatment and for 30 days after last
  treatment; male patients should use effective
  contraception during treatment and for 90 days after last
  treatment if their partner is of childbearing potential. See
  also *Pregnancy and reproductive function* in Cytotoxic drugs
  p. 932.
- **PREGNANCY** Manufacturer advises avoid unless potential
  benefit outweighs risk—toxicity in *animal* studies. See also
  Pregnancy and reproductive function in Cytotoxic drugs
  p. 932.
- **BREAST FEEDING** Manufacturer advises avoid—no
  information available.
- **HEPATIC IMPAIRMENT** Manufacturer advises caution.
  Dose adjustments Manufacturer advises consider dose
  reduction.
- **RENAL IMPAIRMENT** Manufacturer advises caution—
  evaluate benefit/risk ratio if eGFR
  30–45 mL/minute/1.73 m^2; avoid if eGFR less than
  30 mL/minute/1.73 m^2.
  Dose adjustments Manufacturer advises reduce dose if
  eGFR 46–60 mL/minute/1.73 m^2—consult product
  literature.
- **MONITORING REQUIREMENTS**
  ‣ Manufacturer advises monitor renal function (plasma
    creatinine and eGFR derived from the MDRD formula)
    immediately before treatment initiation and 2 weeks after
    each course of therapy; proteinuria and serum electrolytes
    should also be monitored before treatment initiation and
    2–4 weeks after the last cycle of treatment.
  ‣ Manufacturer advises monitor liver function tests, blood
    glucose levels and complete blood counts regularly.
- **HANDLING AND STORAGE** Manufacturer advises store in a
  refrigerator (2–8°C) and protect from light—consult
  product literature for storage conditions after
  reconstitution and dilution.

- **MEDICINAL FORMS** There can be variation in the licensing of
  different medicines containing the same drug.
  Powder for solution for infusion
  ‣ Zanosar (Intrapharm Laboratories Ltd)
    Streptozocin 1 gram Zanosar 1g powder for concentrate for solution
    for infusion vials | 1 vial [PoM] £570.00

Temozolomide

15-Jul-2020

- **DRUG ACTION** Temozolomide is structurally related to
  dacarbazine.

- **INDICATIONS AND DOSE**
  **Newly diagnosed glioblastoma multiforme in adults (in
  combination with radiotherapy) and subsequently as
  monotherapy | Second-line treatment of malignant
  glioma in adults**
  ‣ BY MOUTH
  ‣ Adult: (consult product literature)

IMPORTANT SAFETY INFORMATION
RISKS OF INCORRECT DOSING OF ORAL ANTI-CANCER MEDICINES
See Cytotoxic drugs p. 932.

- **CAUTIONS** *Pneumocystis jirovecii* pneumonia—consult
  product literature for monitoring and prophylaxis
  requirements
- **INTERACTIONS** → Appendix 1: alkylating agents
- **SIDE-EFFECTS**
  ‣ **Common or very common** Alopecia · anxiety · appetite
    decreased · arthralgia · asthenia · chills · concentration
    impaired · confusion · constipation · cough · decreased
    leucocytes · diarrhoea · dizziness · drowsiness · dysphagia ·
    dyspnoea · emotional lability · fever · gastrointestinal
    discomfort · haemorrhage · headache · hearing impairment
    · hemiparesis · hyperglycaemia · hypersensitivity ·
    increased risk of infection · insomnia · level of
    consciousness decreased · malaise · memory loss ·
    movement disorders · muscle weakness · nausea ·
    neutropenia · oedema · pain · peripheral neuropathy ·
    radiation injury · seizures · sensation abnormal · skin
    reactions · speech impairment · stomatitis · taste altered ·
    thrombocytopenia · tremor · urinary disorders · vision
    disorders · vomiting · weight changes
  ‣ **Uncommon** Altered smell sensation · anaemia · behaviour
    disorder · bone marrow disorders · cognitive impairment ·
    condition aggravated · Cushing's syndrome · depression ·
    diabetes insipidus · ear pain · erectile dysfunction · eye
    pain · gait abnormal · hallucination · hepatic disorders ·
    hyperacusia · hyperbilirubinaemia · hypertension ·
    hypokalaemia · intracranial haemorrhage · myalgia ·
    myopathy · nasal congestion · nervous system disorder ·
    palpitations · photosensitivity reaction · reactivation of
    infections · thirst · tinnitus · tongue discolouration ·
    vasodilation
  ‣ **Rare or very rare** Neoplasms · respiratory disorders ·
    secondary malignancy · severe cutaneous adverse
    reactions (SCARs)
- **CONCEPTION AND CONTRACEPTION** Manufacturer advises
  adequate contraception during treatment. Men should
  avoid fathering a child during and for at least 6 months
  after treatment. See also *Pregnancy and reproductive
  function* in Cytotoxic drugs p. 932.
- **PREGNANCY** Avoid (teratogenic and embryotoxic in *animal*
  studies). See also *Pregnancy and reproductive function* in
  Cytotoxic drugs p. 932.
- **BREAST FEEDING** Discontinue breast-feeding.
- **HEPATIC IMPAIRMENT** Manufacturer advises caution in
  severe impairment (no information available).
- **RENAL IMPAIRMENT** Manufacturer advises caution—no
  information available.
- **MONITORING REQUIREMENTS**
  ‣ Monitor liver function before treatment initiation, after
    each treatment cycle and midway through 42-day
    treatment cycles—consider the balance of benefits and
    risks of treatment if results are abnormal at any point
    (fatal liver injury reported).

► Monitor for myelodysplastic syndrome.
► Monitor for secondary malignancies.

● NATIONAL FUNDING/ACCESS DECISIONS
For full details see funding body website

NICE decisions

► **Temozolomide for the treatment of recurrent malignant glioma (brain cancer) (April 2001)** NICE TA23 Recommended with restrictions

► **Carmustine implants and temozolomide for the treatment of newly diagnosed high-grade glioma (June 2007)** NICE TA121 Recommended with restrictions

● MEDICINAL FORMS There can be variation in the licensing of different medicines containing the same drug. Forms available from special-order manufacturers include: oral suspension

Capsule

CAUTIONARY AND ADVISORY LABELS 23, 25

► Temozolomide (Non-proprietary)
Temozolomide 5 mg Temozolomide 5mg capsules | 5 capsule PoM £10.06–£16.00 (Hospital only)
Temozolomide 20 mg Temozolomide 20mg capsules | 5 capsule PoM £40.23–£65.00 (Hospital only)
Temozolomide 100 mg Temozolomide 100mg capsules | 5 capsule PoM £201.18–£325.00 (Hospital only)
Temozolomide 140 mg Temozolomide 140mg capsules | 5 capsule PoM £296.47–£465.00 (Hospital only)
Temozolomide 180 mg Temozolomide 180mg capsules | 5 capsule PoM £381.18–£586.00 (Hospital only)
Temozolomide 250 mg Temozolomide 250mg capsules | 5 capsule PoM £529.42–£814.00 (Hospital only)

► Temodal (Merck Sharp & Dohme Ltd)
Temozolomide 5 mg Temodal 5mg capsules | 5 capsule PoM £10.59 (Hospital only)
Temozolomide 20 mg Temodal 20mg capsules | 5 capsule PoM £42.35 (Hospital only)
Temozolomide 100 mg Temodal 100mg capsules | 5 capsule PoM £211.77 (Hospital only)
Temozolomide 140 mg Temodal 140mg capsules | 5 capsule PoM £296.48 (Hospital only)
Temozolomide 180 mg Temodal 180mg capsules | 5 capsule PoM £381.19 (Hospital only)
Temozolomide 250 mg Temodal 250mg capsules | 5 capsule PoM £529.43 (Hospital only)

Thiotepa

16-Nov-2020

● **INDICATIONS AND DOSE**

Conditioning treatment before haematopoietic stem cell transplantation in the treatment of haematological disease or solid tumours, in combination with other chemotherapy

► BY INTRAVENOUS INFUSION
► Adult: (consult local protocol)

● CAUTIONS Avoid in Acute porphyrias p. 1107 · cardiac disease

● INTERACTIONS → Appendix 1: alkylating agents

● SIDE-EFFECTS

► **Common or very common** Alopecia · amenorrhoea · anaemia · anxiety · appetite decreased · arrhythmias · arthralgia · asthenia · azoospermia · cataract · chills · cognitive disorder · confusion · conjunctivitis · constipation · cough · cystitis · delirium · diarrhoea · dizziness · dysuria · embolism · encephalopathy · extrapyramidal symptoms · fever · gastrointestinal discomfort · gastrointestinal disorders · generalised oedema · graft versus host disease · haemorrhage · headache · hearing impairment · heart failure · hepatic disorders · hyperglycaemia · hypersensitivity · hypertension · hypopituitarism · increased risk of infection · infertility · intracranial aneurysm · intracranial haemorrhage · leucopenia · lymphoedema · menopausal symptoms · mucositis · multi organ failure · myalgia · nausea · neutropenia · ototoxicity · pain · pancytopenia ·

paraesthesia · psychiatric disorder · pulmonary oedema · renal impairment · respiratory disorders · secondary malignancy · seizure · sepsis · sinusoidal obstruction syndrome · skin reactions · stomatitis · thrombocytopenia · toxic shock syndrome · vision blurred · vomiting · weight increased

► **Uncommon** Cardiomyopathy · hallucination · hypoxia · myocarditis

► **Frequency not known** Severe cutaneous adverse reactions (SCARs)

● CONCEPTION AND CONTRACEPTION Contraceptive advice required, see *Pregnancy and reproductive function* in Cytotoxic drugs p. 932.

● PREGNANCY Avoid (teratogenic and embryotoxic in *animals*). See also *Pregnancy and reproductive function* in Cytotoxic drugs p. 932.

● BREAST FEEDING Discontinue breast-feeding.

● NATIONAL FUNDING/ACCESS DECISIONS
For full details see funding body website

Scottish Medicines Consortium (SMC) decisions

► **Thiotepa** (*Tepadina*®) in combination with other chemotherapy as conditioning treatment in adults or children with haematological diseases, or solid tumours prior to haematopoietic stem cell transplantation (July 2012) SMC No. 790/12 Not recommended

● MEDICINAL FORMS There can be variation in the licensing of different medicines containing the same drug.

Powder for solution for infusion

► Tepadina (Adienne Pharma & Biotech)
Thiotepa 15 mg Tepadina 15mg powder for concentrate for solution for infusion vials | 1 vial PoM £123.00 (Hospital only)
Thiotepa 100 mg Tepadina 100mg powder for concentrate for solution for infusion vials | 1 vial PoM £736.00 (Hospital only)

Treosulfan

24-Sep-2020

● **INDICATIONS AND DOSE**

Ovarian cancer

► BY MOUTH, OR BY INTRAVENOUS INJECTION, OR BY INTRAVENOUS INFUSION, OR BY INTRAPERITONEAL INSTILLATION
► Adult: (consult product literature)

TRECONDI®

Conditioning treatment before allogeneic haematopoietic stem cell transplantation in patients with malignant disease (in combination with other chemotherapy) (specialist use only)

► BY INTRAVENOUS INFUSION
► Adult: (consult product literature)

Conditioning treatment before allogeneic haematopoietic stem cell transplantation in patients with non-malignant disease (in combination with other chemotherapy) (specialist use only)

► BY INTRAVENOUS INFUSION
► Adult: (consult product literature)

IMPORTANT SAFETY INFORMATION
RISKS OF INCORRECT DOSING OF ORAL ANTI-CANCER MEDICINES
See Cytotoxic drugs p. 932.

● CONTRA-INDICATIONS
GENERAL CONTRA-INDICATIONS
Concomitant use of live vaccines
SPECIFIC CONTRA-INDICATIONS

► When used for conditioning treatment before allogeneic haematopoietic stem cell transplantation Active uncontrolled infection · Fanconi anaemia and other DNA repair disorders · severe concomitant cardiac, lung, liver and renal impairment

● CAUTIONS Avoid in Acute porphyrias p. 1107

● INTERACTIONS → Appendix 1: alkylating agents

● SIDE-EFFECTS

GENERAL SIDE-EFFECTS

▶ **Common or very common** Alopecia · anaemia · bone marrow disorders · leucopenia · nausea · sepsis · skin reactions · thrombocytopenia · vomiting

▶ **Uncommon** Neoplasms · respiratory disorders · treatment related secondary malignancy

▶ **Rare or very rare** Addison's disease · cardiomyopathy · hypoglycaemia · influenza like illness · paraesthesia · pneumonia · scleroderma

SPECIFIC SIDE-EFFECTS

▶ **Common or very common**

▶ With intravenous use Appetite decreased · arrhythmia · arthralgia · asthenia · chills · constipation · diarrhoea · dizziness · dysphagia · dyspnoea · febrile neutropenia · fever · flushing · gastrointestinal discomfort · gastrointestinal disorders · haemorrhage · headache · hypersensitivity · hypertension · insomnia · lethargy · myalgia · oedema · oral disorders · pain · renal impairment · weight changes

▶ **Uncommon**

▶ With intravenous use Confusion · cough · dry mouth · hepatic disorders · hiccups · hyperglycaemia · hyperhidrosis · hypotension · laryngeal pain · oesophageal pain · peripheral neuropathy · sinusoidal obstruction syndrome

▶ With oral use Stomatitis

▶ **Rare or very rare**

▶ With intravenous use Inflammation localised

▶ With oral use Cystitis haemorrhagic

▶ **Frequency not known**

▶ With intravenous use Acidosis · agitation · amenorrhoea · cardiac arrest · cystitis · dry eye · dysphonia · dysuria · electrolyte imbalance · embolism · encephalopathy · extrapyramidal symptoms · feeling cold · glucose tolerance impaired · heart failure · hypoxia · intracranial haemorrhage · muscle weakness · myocardial infarction · oropharyngeal pain · ovarian suppression · pericardial effusion · skin ulcer · syncope

SIDE-EFFECTS, FURTHER INFORMATION Prolonged use of treosulfan is associated with an increased incidence of acute non-lymphocytic leukaemia.

● CONCEPTION AND CONTRACEPTION Manufacturer advises females of childbearing potential and male patients with partners of childbearing potential should use effective contraception during and for 6 months after treatment. See also *Pregnancy and reproductive function* in Cytotoxic drugs p. 932.

● PREGNANCY Manufacturer advises avoid—no information available. See also *Pregnancy and reproductive function* in Cytotoxic drugs p. 932.

● BREAST FEEDING Manufacturer advises avoid—no information available.

● HEPATIC IMPAIRMENT

▶ When used for conditioning treatment before allogeneic haematopoietic stem cell transplantation See *contra-indications* for information relating to severe impairment.

● RENAL IMPAIRMENT

▶ When used for conditioning treatment before allogeneic haematopoietic stem cell transplantation Manufacturer advises caution—treosulfan is excreted renally. See also *contra-indications* for further information relating to severe impairment.

● MONITORING REQUIREMENTS Manufacturer advises monitor full blood counts frequently during treatment.

● PATIENT AND CARER ADVICE

Driving and skilled tasks Patients and carers should be counselled on the effects on driving and performance of skilled tasks—increased risk of nausea, vomiting or dizziness.

● NATIONAL FUNDING/ACCESS DECISIONS

For full details see funding body website

NICE decisions

▶ **Treosulfan with fludarabine for malignant disease before allogeneic stem cell transplant (August 2020)** NICE TA640 Recommended

● MEDICINAL FORMS There can be variation in the licensing of different medicines containing the same drug.

Capsule

CAUTIONARY AND ADVISORY LABELS 25

▶ Treosulfan (Non-proprietary)

Treosulfan 250 mg Treosulfan 250mg capsules | 100 capsule PoM £653.20

Powder for solution for injection

▶ Treosulfan (Non-proprietary)

Treosulfan 1 gram Treosulfan 1g powder for solution for injection vials | 5 vial PoM £494.40

Treosulfan 5 gram Treosulfan 5g powder for solution for injection vials | 5 vial PoM £2,434.25

▶ Trecondi (medac UK)

Treosulfan 1 gram Trecondi 1g powder for solution for infusion | 5 vial PoM £494.40

Treosulfan 5 gram Trecondi 5g powder for solution for infusion | 5 vial PoM £2,434.25

ANTINEOPLASTIC DRUGS > ANTHRACYCLINES AND RELATED DRUGS

Daunorubicin

20-Aug-2020

● **INDICATIONS AND DOSE**

Acute myelogenous leukaemia | Acute lymphocytic leukaemia

▶ BY INTRAVENOUS INFUSION

▶ Adult: (consult local protocol)

Advanced AIDS-related Kaposi's sarcoma (liposomal formulation only)

▶ BY INTRAVENOUS INFUSION

▶ Adult: (consult product literature)

IMPORTANT SAFETY INFORMATION

MHRA/CHM ADVICE: LIPOSOMAL AND LIPID-COMPLEX FORMULATIONS: NAME CHANGE TO REDUCE MEDICATION ERRORS (JULY 2020)

Serious harm and fatal overdoses have occurred following confusion between liposomal, pegylated-liposomal, lipid-complex, and conventional formulations of the same drug substance. Medicines with these formulations will explicitly include 'liposomal', 'pegylated-liposomal', or 'lipid-complex' within their name to reduce the risk of potentially fatal medication errors.

The MHRA reminds healthcare professionals that liposomal, pegylated-liposomal, lipid-complex, and conventional formulations containing the same drug substance are **not** interchangeable. Healthcare professionals are advised to make a clear distinction between formulations when prescribing, dispensing, administering, and communicating about daunorubicin. The product name and dose should be verified before administration and the maximum dose should not be exceeded.

● CONTRA-INDICATIONS Myocardial insufficiency · previous treatment with maximum cumulative doses of daunorubicin or other anthracycline · recent myocardial infarction · severe arrhythmia

- CAUTIONS Caution in handling—irritant to tissues · neutrophil count less than 1500/mm^3
- INTERACTIONS → Appendix 1: anthracyclines
- SIDE-EFFECTS Abdominal pain · alopecia · amenorrhoea · anaemia · arrhythmias · ascites · atrioventricular block · azoospermia · bone marrow disorders · cardiac inflammation · cardiomyopathy · chills · congestive heart failure · cyanosis · death · dehydration · diarrhoea · dyspnoea · extravasation necrosis · fever · flushing · gastrointestinal disorders · haemorrhage · hepatomegaly · hyperpyrexia · hyperuricaemia · hypoxia · infection · ischaemic heart disease · leucopenia · mucositis · myocardial infarction · nail discolouration · nausea · nephropathy · neutropenia · oedema · pain · paraesthesia · pleural effusion · radiation injuries · shock · skin reactions · stomatitis · thrombocytopenia · thrombophlebitis · urine red · venous sclerosis · vomiting

  SIDE-EFFECTS, FURTHER INFORMATION Cardiotoxicity is cumulative and may be irreversible, however responds to treatment if detected early.

- CONCEPTION AND CONTRACEPTION Contraceptive advice required, see *Pregnancy and reproductive function* in Cytotoxic drugs p. 932.
- PREGNANCY Avoid (teratogenic and carcinogenic in *animal* studies). See also *Pregnancy and reproductive function* in Cytotoxic drugs p. 932.
- BREAST FEEDING Discontinue breast-feeding.
- HEPATIC IMPAIRMENT For *solution for infusion* manufacturer advises caution. For *powder for solution for infusion* manufacturer advises caution in mild to moderate impairment; avoid in severe impairment.
  Dose adjustments Manufacturer advises dose reduction according to serum bilirubin concentration—consult product literature.
- RENAL IMPAIRMENT Avoid in severe impairment.
  Dose adjustments Reduce dose by 25% if serum creatinine 105–265 micromol/litre.
  Reduce dose by 50% if serum creatinine greater than 265 micromol/litre.
- MONITORING REQUIREMENTS Cardiac monitoring essential.
- PRESCRIBING AND DISPENSING INFORMATION Daunorubicin is available as *conventional* and *liposomal* formulations. These different formulations vary in their licensed indications, pharmacokinetics, dosage and administration, and are **not** interchangeable.

- MEDICINAL FORMS There can be variation in the licensing of different medicines containing the same drug.
  Solution for infusion
  ▸ DaunoXome (Galen Ltd)
  Daunorubicin (as Daunorubicin hydrochloride citrate liposomal pegylated) 2 mg per 1 ml DaunoXome 50mg/25ml concentrate for solution for infusion vials | 1 vial PoM £250.00
  Powder for solution for infusion
  ▸ Daunorubicin (Non-proprietary)
  Daunorubicin (as Daunorubicin hydrochloride)
  20 mg Daunorubicin 20mg powder for solution for infusion vials | 10 vial PoM £715.00 (Hospital only)

Daunorubicin with cytarabine   02-Sep-2020

The properties listed below are those particular to the combination only. For the properties of the components please consider, daunorubicin p. 944, cytarabine p. 953.

- INDICATIONS AND DOSE
  Acute myeloid leukaemia
  ▸ BY INTRAVENOUS INFUSION
  ▸ Adult: (consult product literature)

IMPORTANT SAFETY INFORMATION

MHRA/CHM ADVICE: LIPOSOMAL AND LIPID-COMPLEX FORMULATIONS: NAME CHANGE TO REDUCE MEDICATION ERRORS (JULY 2020)
Serious harm and fatal overdoses have occurred following confusion between liposomal, pegylated-liposomal, lipid-complex, and conventional formulations of the same drug substance. Medicines with these formulations will explicitly include 'liposomal', 'pegylated-liposomal', or 'lipid-complex' within their name to reduce the risk of potentially fatal medication errors.
The MHRA reminds healthcare professionals that liposomal, pegylated-liposomal, lipid-complex, and conventional formulations containing the same drug substance are **not** interchangeable. Healthcare professionals are advised to make a clear distinction between formulations when prescribing, dispensing, administering, and communicating about daunorubicin with cytarabine. The product name and dose should be verified before administration and the maximum dose should not be exceeded.

- CAUTIONS Wilson's disease or other copper-related disorders (each vial contains 100 mg of copper gluconate, equivalent to 14 mg of elemental copper)
- INTERACTIONS → Appendix 1: anthracyclines · cytarabine
- HEPATIC IMPAIRMENT Manufacturer advises caution in severe impairment.
- RENAL IMPAIRMENT Manufacturer advises caution in severe impairment.
- PRESCRIBING AND DISPENSING INFORMATION Daunorubicin with cytarabine is available as a *liposomal* formulation. This is **not** interchangeable with other daunorubicin- or cytarabine-containing preparations; such preparations differ in their licensed indications, pharmacokinetics, dosage and administration.
- NATIONAL FUNDING/ACCESS DECISIONS
  For full details see funding body website
  NICE decisions
  ▸ Liposomal cytarabine–daunorubicin for untreated acute myeloid leukaemia (December 2018) NICE TA552
  Recommended with restrictions
  Scottish Medicines Consortium (SMC) decisions
  ▸ Liposomal daunorubicin and cytarabine (*Vyxeos*®) for the treatment of adults with newly diagnosed, therapy-related acute myeloid leukaemia (t-AML) or AML with myelodysplasia-related changes (March 2019) SMC No. SMC2130
  Recommended

- MEDICINAL FORMS There can be variation in the licensing of different medicines containing the same drug.
  Powder for solution for infusion
  ▸ Vyxeos (Jazz Pharmaceuticals UK)
  Daunorubicin 44 mg, Cytarabine 100 mg Vyxeos liposomal 44mg/100mg powder for concentrate for solution for infusion vials | 1 vial PoM £4,581.00 (Hospital only)

Doxorubicin hydrochloride

20-Aug-2020

● INDICATIONS AND DOSE

Acute leukaemias | Hodgkin's lymphoma | Non-Hodgkin's lymphoma | Some solid tumours including breast cancer | Advanced soft-tissue sarcoma
- ▸ BY INTRAVENOUS INJECTION
- ▸ Adult: (consult product literature)

Some papillary bladder tumours (bladder instillation) | Recurrent superficial bladder tumours (bladder instillation) | Transitional cell carcinoma (bladder instillation) | Carcinoma in situ (bladder instillation)
- ▸ BY INTRAVESICAL INSTILLATION
- ▸ Adult: (consult product literature)

CAELYX ®

For AIDS-related Kaposi's sarcoma in patients with low CD4 count and extensive mucocutaneous or visceral disease | Advanced ovarian cancer when platinum-based chemotherapy has failed | Progressive multiple myeloma (in combination with bortezomib) in patients who have received at least one prior therapy and who have undergone or are unsuitable for bone-marrow transplantation | Monotherapy for metastatic breast cancer in patients with increased cardiac risk
- ▸ BY INTRAVENOUS INFUSION
- ▸ Adult: (consult product literature)

IMPORTANT SAFETY INFORMATION

MHRA/CHM ADVICE: LIPOSOMAL AND LIPID-COMPLEX FORMULATIONS: NAME CHANGE TO REDUCE MEDICATION ERRORS (JULY 2020)

Serious harm and fatal overdoses have occurred following confusion between liposomal, pegylated-liposomal, lipid-complex, and conventional formulations of the same drug substance. Medicines with these formulations will explicitly include 'liposomal', 'pegylated-liposomal', or 'lipid-complex' within their name to reduce the risk of potentially fatal medication errors.

The MHRA reminds healthcare professionals that liposomal, pegylated-liposomal, lipid-complex, and conventional formulations containing the same drug substance are **not** interchangeable. Healthcare professionals are advised to make a clear distinction between formulations when prescribing, dispensing, administering, and communicating about doxorubicin. The product name and dose should be verified before administration and the maximum dose should not be exceeded.

- ● CONTRA-INDICATIONS Consult product literature
- ● CAUTIONS Cardiac disease · caution in handling—irritant to tissues · consult product literature · elderly · hypertension · previous myocardial irradiation
- ● INTERACTIONS → Appendix 1: anthracyclines
- ● SIDE-EFFECTS
- ▸ Common or very common Alopecia · anaemia · anxiety · appetite decreased · arrhythmias · arthralgia · asthenia · bone marrow depression · breast pain · cachexia · cardiovascular disorder · chest discomfort · chills · constipation · cough · decreased leucocytes · dehydration · depression · diarrhoea · dizziness · drowsiness · dry mouth · dysphagia · dyspnoea · dysuria · electrolyte imbalance · epistaxis · eye inflammation · fever · gastrointestinal discomfort · gastrointestinal disorders · headache · hyperhidrosis · hypersensitivity · hypertension · hyperthermia · hypotension · increased risk of infection · influenza like illness · infusion related reaction · insomnia · malaise · mucosal abnormalities · muscle complaints · muscle tone increased · muscle weakness · nail disorder ·

nausea · nerve disorders · neutropenia · oedema · oral disorders · pain · scrotal erythema · sensation abnormal · sepsis · skin reactions · skin ulcer · syncope · taste altered · thrombocytopenia · vasodilation · vision blurred · vomiting · weight decreased
- ▸ Uncommon Confusion · embolism and thrombosis
- ▸ Rare or very rare Secondary oral neoplasms · severe cutaneous adverse reactions (SCARs)
- ▸ Frequency not known Asthma · congestive heart failure · secondary malignancy · throat tightness

SIDE-EFFECTS, FURTHER INFORMATION Extravasation can cause tissue necrosis.

Cardiomyopathy Higher cumulative doses are associated with cardiomyopathy and it is usual to limit total cumulative doses to 450 mg/m^2.

Liposomal formulations Liposomal formulations of doxorubicin may reduce the incidence of cardiotoxicity and lower the potential for local necrosis, but infusion reactions, sometimes severe, may occur. Hand-foot syndrome (painful, macular reddening skin eruptions) occurs commonly with liposomal doxorubicin and may be dose limiting. It can occur after 2–3 treatment cycles and may be prevented by cooling hands and feet and avoiding socks, gloves, or tight-fitting footwear. It may also occur with non-liposomal formulations.

Elevated bilirubin concentrations Doxorubicin is largely excreted in the bile and an elevated bilirubin concentration is an indication for reducing the dose.

- ● CONCEPTION AND CONTRACEPTION Manufacturer advises effective contraception during and for at least 6 months after treatment in men or women.
- ● PREGNANCY Avoid (teratogenic and toxic in *animal* studies). See also *Pregnancy and reproductive function* in Cytotoxic drugs p. 932.
- ● BREAST FEEDING Discontinue breast-feeding.
- ● HEPATIC IMPAIRMENT For *liposomal formulation*, manufacturer advises caution. For *solution for injection or infusion*, manufacturer advises caution in mild to moderate impairment; avoid in severe impairment.
  Dose adjustments Manufacturer advises dose reduction according to bilirubin concentration.
- ● RENAL IMPAIRMENT Consult product literature in severe impairment.
- ● MONITORING REQUIREMENTS Patients should be assessed before treatment, by echocardiography. Cardiac monitoring during treatment may assist in determining safe dosage.
- ● DIRECTIONS FOR ADMINISTRATION Manufacturer advises *conventional* doxorubicin is given by injection into a fast-running infusion, commonly at 21-day intervals.
- ● PRESCRIBING AND DISPENSING INFORMATION Doxorubicin is available as *conventional*, *liposomal* and *pegylated liposomal* formulations. These different formulations vary in their licensed indications, pharmacokinetics, dosage and administration, and are **not** interchangeable.
- ● NATIONAL FUNDING/ACCESS DECISIONS
  For full details see funding body website

  NICE decisions
- ▸ Topotecan, pegylated liposomal doxorubicin hydrochloride, paclitaxel, trabectedin and gemcitabine for treating recurrent ovarian cancer (April 2016) NICE TA389 Recommended
- ▸ Olaratumab in combination with doxorubicin for treating advanced soft tissue sarcoma (August 2017) NICE TA465 Recommended with restrictions

● MEDICINAL FORMS There can be variation in the licensing of different medicines containing the same drug. Forms available from special-order manufacturers include: solution for injection, solution for infusion

Solution for injection

▸ Doxorubicin hydrochloride (Non-proprietary)

Doxorubicin hydrochloride 2 mg per 1 ml Doxorubicin 50mg/25ml solution for injection Cytosafe vials | 1 vial PoM £103.00 (Hospital only)

Doxorubicin 50mg/25ml solution for infusion vials | 1 vial PoM £103.00 (Hospital only)

Doxorubicin 10mg/5ml solution for injection Cytosafe vials | 1 vial PoM £20.60 (Hospital only)

Doxorubicin 10mg/5ml concentrate for solution for infusion vials | 1 vial PoM £11.55–£19.57 (Hospital only)

Doxorubicin 10mg/5ml solution for infusion vials | 1 vial PoM £20.60 (Hospital only)

Doxorubicin 50mg/25ml solution for injection vials | 1 vial PoM £92.70 (Hospital only)

Doxorubicin 50mg/25ml concentrate for solution for infusion vials | 1 vial PoM £54.00–£97.85 (Hospital only)

Solution for infusion

▸ Doxorubicin hydrochloride (Non-proprietary)

Doxorubicin hydrochloride 2 mg per 1 ml Doxorubicin 200mg/100ml solution for infusion vials | 1 vial PoM £412.00 (Hospital only)

Doxorubicin 20mg/10ml concentrate for solution for infusion vials | 1 vial PoM Ⓢ (Hospital only)

Doxorubicin 100mg/50ml concentrate for solution for infusion vials | 1 vial PoM Ⓢ (Hospital only)

Doxorubicin 200mg/100ml solution for injection Cytosafe vials | 1 vial PoM £412.00 (Hospital only)

Doxorubicin 200mg/100ml concentrate for solution for infusion vials | 1 vial PoM £234.66–£391.40 (Hospital only)

▸ Caelyx (Janssen-Cilag Ltd)

Doxorubicin hydrochloride (as Doxorubicin hydrochloride liposomal pegylated) 2 mg per 1 ml Caelyx pegylated liposomal 50mg/25ml concentrate for solution for infusion vials | 1 vial PoM £712.49

Caelyx pegylated liposomal 20mg/10ml concentrate for solution for infusion vials | 1 vial PoM £360.23

Epirubicin hydrochloride   25-Jun-2020

● **INDICATIONS AND DOSE**

Breast cancer (specialist use only) | Gastric cancer (specialist use only) | Small cell lung cancer (specialist use only) | Ovarian cancer (specialist use only) | Colorectal cancer (specialist use only) | Lymphoma (specialist use only) | Leukaemia (specialist use only) | Multiple myeloma (specialist use only)

▸ BY INTRAVENOUS INJECTION, OR BY INTRAVENOUS INFUSION
▸ Adult: (consult product literature or local protocols)

Bladder cancer (specialist use only)

▸ BY INTRAVESICAL INSTILLATION
▸ Adult: (consult product literature or local protocols)

● CONTRA-INDICATIONS Bladder inflammation or contraction (when used as a bladder instillation) · catheterisation difficulties (when used as a bladder instillation) · haematuria (when used as a bladder instillation) · invasive tumours penetrating the bladder (when used as a bladder instillation) · myocardiopathy · previous treatment with maximum cumulative doses of epirubicin or other anthracycline · recent myocardial infarction · severe arrhythmia · severe myocardial insufficiency · unstable angina · urinary tract infections (when used as a bladder instillation)

● CAUTIONS Caution in handling—irritant to tissues

● INTERACTIONS → Appendix 1: anthracyclines

● SIDE-EFFECTS

▸ **Common or very common**
▸ With intravesical use Chemical cystitis
▸ With parenteral use Alopecia · amenorrhoea · anaemia · appetite decreased · arrhythmias · cardiac conduction

disorders · chills · congestive heart failure · dehydration · diarrhoea · eye inflammation · fever · gastrointestinal discomfort · gastrointestinal disorders · haemorrhage · increased risk of infection · leucopenia · malaise · mucositis · nail discolouration · nausea · neutropenia · oral disorders · skin reactions · thrombocytopenia · urine discolouration · vasodilation · vomiting

▸ **Uncommon**
▸ With parenteral use Asthenia · embolism and thrombosis · sepsis
▸ **Rare or very rare**
▸ With parenteral use Hyperuricaemia
▸ **Frequency not known**
▸ With parenteral use Bone marrow depression · cardiomyopathy · cardiotoxicity · photosensitivity reaction · radiation injuries · shock

SIDE-EFFECTS, FURTHER INFORMATION Manufacturer advises extreme caution with cumulative doses exceeding 900 mg/m^2—risk of congestive heart failure increased.

● CONCEPTION AND CONTRACEPTION Contraceptive advice required, see *Pregnancy and reproductive function* in Cytotoxic drugs p. 932.

● PREGNANCY Avoid (carcinogenic in *animal* studies). See also *Pregnancy and reproductive function* in Cytotoxic drugs p. 932.

● BREAST FEEDING Discontinue breast-feeding.

● HEPATIC IMPAIRMENT Manufacturer advises caution in mild to moderate impairment; avoid in severe impairment. **Dose adjustments** Manufacturer advises dose reduction according to bilirubin level.

● RENAL IMPAIRMENT
Dose adjustments Dose reduction may be necessary in severe impairment.

● MEDICINAL FORMS There can be variation in the licensing of different medicines containing the same drug. Forms available from special-order manufacturers include: solution for injection, solution for infusion

Solution for injection

▸ Epirubicin hydrochloride (Non-proprietary)

Epirubicin hydrochloride 2 mg per 1 ml Epirubicin 10mg/5ml solution for injection vials | 1 vial PoM £17.38–£20.18 (Hospital only)

Epirubicin 50mg/25ml solution for injection vials | 1 vial PoM £86.89–£105.00 (Hospital only)

▸ Pharmorubicin (Pfizer Ltd)

Epirubicin hydrochloride 2 mg per 1 ml Pharmorubicin 50mg/25ml solution for injection Cytosafe vials | 1 vial PoM £106.19 (Hospital only)

Pharmorubicin 10mg/5ml solution for injection Cytosafe vials | 1 vial PoM £21.24 (Hospital only)

Solution for infusion

▸ Epirubicin hydrochloride (Non-proprietary)

Epirubicin hydrochloride 2 mg per 1 ml Epirubicin 200mg/100ml solution for infusion vials | 1 vial PoM £306.20–£366.85 (Hospital only)

Epirubicin 100mg/50ml solution for infusion vials | 1 vial PoM £201.76 (Hospital only)

▸ Pharmorubicin (Pfizer Ltd)

Epirubicin hydrochloride 2 mg per 1 ml Pharmorubicin 200mg/100ml solution for infusion Cytosafe vials | 1 vial PoM £386.16 (Hospital only)

Idarubicin hydrochloride   25-Jun-2020

● **INDICATIONS AND DOSE**

Acute non-lymphocytic leukaemias monotherapy

▸ BY MOUTH
▸ Adult: 30 mg/m^2 daily for 3 days; maximum 400 mg/m^2 per course
continued →

8

Immune system and malignant disease

Acute non-lymphocytic leukaemia in combination therapy
▸ BY MOUTH
▸ Adult: 15–30 mg/m^2 daily for 3 days; maximum 400 mg/m^2 per course

Advanced breast cancer after failure of first-line chemotherapy (not including anthracyclines)— monotherapy
▸ BY MOUTH
▸ Adult: 45 mg/m^2 for 1 dose, repeat treatment every 3–4 weeks, alternatively 15 mg/m^2 daily for 3 consecutive days, repeat treatment every 3–4 weeks; maximum 400 mg/m^2 per course

Acute leukaemias | Advanced breast cancer after failure of first-line chemotherapy (not including anthracyclines)
▸ BY INTRAVENOUS INJECTION
▸ Adult: (consult product literature)

IMPORTANT SAFETY INFORMATION
RISKS OF INCORRECT DOSING OF ORAL ANTI-CANCER MEDICINES See Cytotoxic drugs p. 932.

- CONTRA-INDICATIONS Previous treatment with maximum cumulative dose of idarubicin or other anthracycline · recent myocardial infarction · severe arrhythmias · severe myocardial insufficiency
- CAUTIONS Caution in handling—irritant to tissues
- INTERACTIONS → Appendix 1: anthracyclines
- SIDE-EFFECTS

  GENERAL SIDE-EFFECTS
  ▸ **Common or very common** Alopecia · anaemia · appetite decreased · arrhythmias · cardiomyopathy · chills · congestive heart failure · diarrhoea · embolism and thrombosis · fever · haemorrhage · headache · increased risk of infection · leucopenia · nausea · neutropenia · skin reactions · stomatitis · thrombocytopenia · urine red · vomiting
  ▸ **Uncommon** Dehydration · gastrointestinal disorders · hyperuricaemia · leukaemia secondary · myocardial infarction · nail discolouration · sepsis · shock · soft tissue necrosis
  ▸ **Rare or very rare** Cardiac conduction disorders · cardiac inflammation · flushing · intracranial haemorrhage
  ▸ **Frequency not known** Bone marrow disorders · tumour lysis syndrome

  SPECIFIC SIDE-EFFECTS
  ▸ **Common or very common**
  ▸ With intravenous use Abdominal pain · mucosal abnormalities · paraesthesia · radiation injuries
  ▸ With oral use Gastrointestinal discomfort · mucositis · radiation skin sensitivity
- CONCEPTION AND CONTRACEPTION Contraceptive advice required, see *Pregnancy and reproductive function* in Cytotoxic drugs p. 932.
- PREGNANCY Avoid (teratogenic and toxic in *animal* studies). See also *Pregnancy and reproductive function* in Cytotoxic drugs p. 932.
- BREAST FEEDING Discontinue breast-feeding.
- HEPATIC IMPAIRMENT Manufacturer advises caution in mild to moderate impairment; avoid in severe impairment.
  Dose adjustments Manufacturer advises consider dose reduction in mild to moderate impairment—consult product literature.
- RENAL IMPAIRMENT Avoid in severe impairment.
  Dose adjustments Reduce dose.

- MEDICINAL FORMS There can be variation in the licensing of different medicines containing the same drug.
  Capsule
  CAUTIONARY AND ADVISORY LABELS 25
  ▸ Zavedos (Pfizer Ltd)
  Idarubicin hydrochloride 5 mg Zavedos 5mg capsules | 1 capsule [PoM] £41.47
  Idarubicin hydrochloride 10 mg Zavedos 10mg capsules | 1 capsule [PoM] £69.12
  Powder for solution for injection
  ▸ Zavedos (Pfizer Ltd)
  Idarubicin hydrochloride 5 mg Zavedos 5mg powder for solution for injection vials | 1 vial [PoM] £87.36 (Hospital only)
  Idarubicin hydrochloride 10 mg Zavedos 10mg powder for solution for injection vials | 1 vial [PoM] £174.72 (Hospital only)

Mitoxantrone

25-Jun-2020

(Mitozantrone)

- **INDICATIONS AND DOSE**

Metastatic breast cancer | Non-Hodgkin's lymphoma | Adult acute non-lymphocytic leukaemia | Non-resectable primary hepatocellular carcinoma
▸ BY INTRAVENOUS INFUSION
▸ Adult: (consult local protocol)

- CAUTIONS Caution in handling—irritant to tissues · intrathecal administration not recommended
- INTERACTIONS → Appendix 1: anthracyclines
- SIDE-EFFECTS Abdominal pain · acute leukaemia · alopecia · amenorrhoea · anxiety · appetite decreased · arrhythmia · asthenia · bone marrow depression · confusion · constipation · diarrhoea · drowsiness · dyspnoea · fever · gastrointestinal haemorrhage · heart failure · mucositis · nail discolouration · nail dystrophy · nausea · neurological effects · paraesthesia · scleral discolouration · skin discolouration · stomatitis · thrombocytopenia · urine blue · vomiting

  SIDE-EFFECTS, FURTHER INFORMATION Cardiac examinations are recommended after a cumulative dose of 160mg/m^2.
- CONCEPTION AND CONTRACEPTION Manufacturer advises effective contraception during and for at least 6 months after treatment in men or women.
- PREGNANCY Avoid. See also *Pregnancy and reproductive function* in Cytotoxic drugs p. 932.
- BREAST FEEDING Discontinue breast-feeding.
- HEPATIC IMPAIRMENT Manufacturer advises caution (limited information available).
  Dose adjustments Manufacturer advises consider dose reduction.

- MEDICINAL FORMS There can be variation in the licensing of different medicines containing the same drug.
  Solution for infusion
  ▸ Mitoxantrone (Non-proprietary)
  Mitoxantrone (as Mitoxantrone hydrochloride) 2 mg per 1 ml Mitoxantrone 20mg/10ml concentrate for solution for infusion vials | 1 vial [PoM] £51.43–£121.85 (Hospital only) | 1 vial [PoM] £51.43
  ▸ Onkotrone (Baxter Healthcare Ltd)
  Mitoxantrone (as Mitoxantrone hydrochloride) 2 mg per 1 ml Onkotrone 20mg/10ml solution for infusion vials | 1 vial [PoM] £103.57 (Hospital only)
  Onkotrone 25mg/12.5ml solution for infusion vials | 1 vial [PoM] £129.48

Pixantrone

<small>25-Jun-2020</small>

● **INDICATIONS AND DOSE**

Treatment of refractory or multiply relapsed aggressive non-Hodgkin B-cell lymphomas (monotherapy)

▶ BY INTRAVENOUS INFUSION

▶ Adult: (consult product literature)

● CONTRA-INDICATIONS Active severe infection · risk factors for severe infection

● CAUTIONS Active cardiovascular disease · cardiac risk factors · caution in handling—irritant to tissues · concurrent radiotherapy to the mediastinal area · history of cardiovascular disease · previous radiotherapy to the mediastinal area · previous therapy with anthracenediones · previous therapy with anthracyclines

● INTERACTIONS → Appendix 1: anthracyclines

● SIDE-EFFECTS

▶ **Common or very common** Alopecia · anaemia · appetite decreased · arrhythmias · asthenia · blood disorder · bundle branch block · cancer progression · cardiac disorder (during or following treatment) · chest pain · congestive heart failure · constipation · cough · decreased leucocytes · diarrhoea · drowsiness · dry mouth · dyspnoea · electrolyte imbalance · eye inflammation · fever · gastrointestinal discomfort · haemorrhage · headache · hypotension · increased risk of infection · left ventricular dysfunction · mucositis · nail disorder · nausea · neutropenia · oedema · oral disorders · pain · paraesthesia · proteinuria · secondary malignancy · skin reactions · taste altered · thrombocytopenia · urine discolouration · vascular disorders · vomiting

▶ **Uncommon** Anxiety · arthralgia · arthritis · bone marrow failure · chills · dizziness · dry eye · eosinophilia · hyperbilirubinaemia · hyperuricaemia · local reaction · meningitis · muscle weakness · musculoskeletal stiffness · night sweats · oesophagitis · oliguria · respiratory disorders · rhinorrhoea · septic shock · skin ulcer · sleep disorders · spontaneous penile erection · vertigo · weight decreased

● CONCEPTION AND CONTRACEPTION Ensure effective contraception during and for at least 6 months after treatment in men or women.

● PREGNANCY Manufacturer advises avoid—toxicity in *animal* studies. See also *Pregnancy and reproductive function* in Cytotoxic drugs p. 932.

● BREAST FEEDING Manufacturer advises avoid—no information available.

● HEPATIC IMPAIRMENT Manufacturer advises caution in mild to moderate impairment; avoid in severe impairment (no information available).

● RENAL IMPAIRMENT No information available—manufacturer advises caution.

● MONITORING REQUIREMENTS

▶ Baseline investigations should include a full blood count, assessment of cardiac function measured by left ventricular ejection fraction, and measurement of serum concentrations of total bilirubin and total creatinine.

▶ Full blood count and cardiac function should be monitored throughout treatment.

● PATIENT AND CARER ADVICE

Photosensitivity Photosensitivity is a theoretical risk and patients should be advised to follow sun protection strategies.

■ NATIONAL FUNDING/ACCESS DECISIONS

For full details see funding body website

NICE decisions

▶ **Pixantrone monotherapy for treating multiply relapsed or refractory aggressive non-Hodgkin's B-cell lymphoma (February 2014)** NICE TA306 Recommended with restrictions

● MEDICINAL FORMS There can be variation in the licensing of different medicines containing the same drug.

Powder for solution for infusion

ELECTROLYTES: May contain Sodium

▶ Pixuvri (Servier Laboratories Ltd)

Pixantrone (as Pixantrone dimaleate) 29 mg Pixuvri 29mg powder for concentrate for solution for infusion vials | 1 vial PoM £553.50

ANTINEOPLASTIC DRUGS > ANTIMETABOLITES

Azacitidine

<small>17-Jun-2020</small>

● DRUG ACTION Azacitidine is a pyrimidine analogue.

● **INDICATIONS AND DOSE**

Treatment of intermediate-2 and high-risk myelodysplastic syndromes, chronic myelomonocytic leukaemia, and acute myeloid leukaemia, in adults who are not eligible for haemotopoietic stem cell transplantation

▶ BY SUBCUTANEOUS INJECTION

▶ Adult: (consult local protocol)

● CONTRA-INDICATIONS Advanced malignant hepatic tumour

● CAUTIONS History of severe congestive heart failure · unstable cardiac disease (consider cardiopulmonary assessment before and during treatment) · unstable pulmonary disease (consider cardiopulmonary assessment before and during treatment)

● INTERACTIONS → Appendix 1: azacitidine

● SIDE-EFFECTS

▶ **Common or very common** Alopecia · anaemia · anxiety · appetite decreased · arthralgia · asthenia · bone marrow disorders · chest pain · chills · confusion · constipation · dehydration · diarrhoea · dizziness · drowsiness · dyspnoea · fever · gastrointestinal discomfort · haemorrhage · headache · hypertension · hypokalaemia · hypotension · increased risk of infection · induration · inflammation · insomnia · intracranial haemorrhage · laryngeal pain · leucopenia · malaise · muscle complaints · nausea · neutropenia · pain · renal failure · respiratory disorders · sepsis · skin reactions · stomatitis · syncope · thrombocytopenia · vomiting · weight decreased

▶ **Uncommon** Hepatic coma · hepatic failure · pyoderma gangrenosum · renal tubular acidosis

▶ **Rare or very rare** Injection site necrosis · tumour lysis syndrome

● CONCEPTION AND CONTRACEPTION Manufacturer advises effective contraception during and for 3 months after treatment in men or women.

● PREGNANCY Avoid (toxicity in *animal* studies). See also *Pregnancy and reproductive function* in Cytotoxic drugs p. 932.

● BREAST FEEDING Discontinue breast-feeding.

● HEPATIC IMPAIRMENT Manufacturer advises caution in severe impairment (no information available)—monitor for adverse drug reactions.

Dose adjustments Manufacturer advises consider dose reduction—consult local protocol.

● RENAL IMPAIRMENT

Dose adjustments Delay next treatment cycle if serum-creatinine or blood urea nitrogen greater than twice baseline value and above the upper level of normal until values return to normal or baseline, and then reduce dose by 50% on the next treatment cycle.

Reduce dose by 50% on the next treatment cycle if serum-bicarbonate concentration less than 20 mmol/litre.

● MONITORING REQUIREMENTS
▶ Monitor liver function tests, serum creatinine, and serum bicarbonate before initiation of treatment and before each treatment cycle.
▶ Monitor full blood count before initiation of treatment, before each treatment cycle, and as clinically indicated.
▶ Monitor for bleeding.

● NATIONAL FUNDING/ACCESS DECISIONS
For full details see funding body website
NICE decisions
▶ Azacitidine for treating acute myeloid leukaemia with more than 30% bone marrow blasts (July 2016) NICE TA399 Not recommended
▶ Azacitidine for the treatment of myelodysplastic syndromes, chronic myelomonocytic leukaemia and acute myeloid leukaemia (March 2011) NICE TA218 Recommended with restrictions

● MEDICINAL FORMS There can be variation in the licensing of different medicines containing the same drug.
Powder for suspension for injection
▶ Azacitidine (Non-proprietary)
Azacitidine 100 mg Azacitidine 100mg powder for suspension for injection vials | 1 vial [PoM] £220.00–£321.00 (Hospital only)
▶ Vidaza (Celgene Ltd)
Azacitidine 100 mg Vidaza 100mg powder for suspension for injection vials | 1 vial [PoM] £321.00

Capecitabine

16-Nov-2020

● DRUG ACTION Capecitabine is metabolised to fluorouracil.

● INDICATIONS AND DOSE
Stage III colon cancer, adjuvant following surgery (monotherapy)
▶ BY MOUTH
▶ Adult: 1.25 g/m^2 twice daily for 14 days, subsequent courses repeated after a 7-day interval, recommended duration of treatment is 6 months, adjust dose according to tolerability—consult product literature

Stage III colon cancer, adjuvant following surgery (combination therapy)
▶ BY MOUTH
▶ Adult: 0.8–1 g/m^2 twice daily for 14 days, subsequent courses repeated after a 7-day interval, recommended duration of treatment is 6 months, adjust dose according to tolerability—consult product literature

Metastatic colorectal cancer (monotherapy)
▶ BY MOUTH
▶ Adult: 1.25 g/m^2 twice daily for 14 days, subsequent courses repeated after a 7-day interval, adjust dose according to tolerability—consult product literature

Metastatic colorectal cancer (combination therapy)
▶ BY MOUTH
▶ Adult: 0.8–1 g/m^2 twice daily for 14 days, subsequent courses repeated after a 7-day interval, adjust dose according to tolerability—consult product literature

Advanced gastric cancer (first-line treatment in combination with a platinum based regimen)
▶ BY MOUTH
▶ Adult: 0.8–1 g/m^2 twice daily for 14 days, subsequent courses repeated after a 7-day interval, alternatively 625 mg/m^2 twice daily given continuously, adjust dose according to tolerability—consult product literature

Locally advanced or metastatic breast cancer (second-line treatment as monotherapy after failure of a taxane and anthracycline regimen or where further anthracycline treatment is not indicated) | Locally advanced or metastatic breast cancer (second-line treatment, in combination with docetaxel, where previous therapy included an anthracycline)
▶ BY MOUTH
▶ Adult: 1.25 g/m^2 twice daily for 14 days, subsequent courses repeated after a 7-day interval, adjust dose according to tolerability—consult product literature

> **IMPORTANT SAFETY INFORMATION**
> RISKS OF INCORRECT DOSING OF ORAL ANTI-CANCER MEDICINES
> See Cytotoxic drugs p. 932.
>
> MHRA/CHM ADVICE: 5-FLUOROURACIL (INTRAVENOUS), CAPECITABINE, TEGAFUR: DPD TESTING RECOMMENDED BEFORE INITIATION TO IDENTIFY PATIENTS AT INCREASED RISK OF SEVERE AND FATAL TOXICITY (OCTOBER 2020)
> Patients with partial or complete dihydropyrimidine dehydrogenase (DPD) deficiency are at increased risk of severe and fatal toxicity during treatment with fluoropyrimidines. Healthcare professionals are advised to test all patients for DPD deficiency before initiating treatment and confirm their, including family, history of complete or partial DPD deficiency. Capecitabine is contra-indicated in patients with known complete DPD deficiency; in those with partial DPD deficiency, a reduced starting dose is recommended. Patients should be monitored for toxicity, particularly during the first cycle of treatment or after a dose increase; severe toxicity can occur even in those with negative test results for DPD deficiency. Healthcare professionals should also counsel patients on the benefits and risks of their treatment and ensure they are provided with the patient information leaflet.

● CONTRA-INDICATIONS Complete dihydropyrimidine dehydrogenase deficiency (increased risk of severe, life-threatening, or fatal toxicity)—consult product literature

● CAUTIONS Diabetes mellitus · diarrhoea or dehydration—consult product literature for guidance on dose modification and treatment interruption · electrolyte disturbances · history of angina pectoris · history of arrhythmias · history of significant cardiovascular disease · nervous system disease · partial dihydropyrimidine dehydrogenase deficiency—consult product literature

● INTERACTIONS → Appendix 1: capecitabine

● SIDE-EFFECTS
▶ Common or very common Alopecia · anaemia · appetite abnormal · asthenia · chest pain · constipation · cough · dehydration · depression · diarrhoea · dizziness · dry mouth · dyspnoea · embolism and thrombosis · eye disorders · eye inflammation · eye irritation · fever · gastrointestinal discomfort · gastrointestinal disorders · haemorrhage · headache · hyperbilirubinaemia · increased risk of infection · insomnia · joint disorders · lethargy · malaise · nail disorder · nausea · neutropenia · oedema · pain · rhinorrhoea · sensation abnormal · skin reactions · stomatitis · taste altered · vomiting · weight decreased
▶ Uncommon Acute coronary syndrome · aphasia · arrhythmias · ascites · asthma · chills · confusion · diabetes mellitus · dysphagia · ear pain · facial swelling · haemolytic anaemia · hepatic disorders · hot flush · hydronephrosis · hypertension · hypertriglyceridaemia · hypokalaemia · hypotension · influenza like illness · ischaemic heart disease · leucopenia · libido decreased · lipoma · malnutrition · memory loss · movement disorders · muscle weakness · musculoskeletal stiffness · palpitations · pancytopenia · panic attack · peripheral coldness · peripheral neuropathy · photosensitivity reaction ·

pneumothorax · radiation recall reaction · sepsis · skin ulcer · syncope · thrombocytopenia · urinary disorders · vertigo · vision disorders
▸ **Rare or very rare** Cutaneous lupus erythematosus · encephalopathy · QT interval prolongation · severe cutaneous adverse reactions (SCARs) · vasospasm
▸ **Frequency not known** Cardiomyopathy · heart failure · sudden death

● CONCEPTION AND CONTRACEPTION Contraceptive advice required, see *Pregnancy and reproductive function* in Cytotoxic drugs p. 932.

● PREGNANCY Avoid (teratogenic in *animal* studies). See also *Pregnancy and reproductive function* in Cytotoxic drugs p. 932.

● BREAST FEEDING Discontinue breast-feeding.

● HEPATIC IMPAIRMENT Manufacturer advises monitor liver function in mild-to-moderate dysfunction—consult product literature for guidance on treatment interruption; avoid in severe impairment.

● RENAL IMPAIRMENT Avoid if creatinine clearance less than 30 mL/minute.
Dose adjustments Reduce starting dose of $1.25 \, \mathrm{g/m^2}$ to 75% if creatinine clearance 30–50 mL/minute.

● MONITORING REQUIREMENTS
▸ Monitor plasma-calcium concentration.
▸ Monitor for eye disorders (including keratitis and corneal disorders).
▸ Severe skin reactions Monitor for symptoms of severe skin reactions (including Stevens-Johnson syndrome and toxic epidermal necrolysis)—permanently discontinue treatment immediately if symptoms occur.
▸ Hand-foot syndrome Monitor for symptoms of hand-foot syndrome—interrupt treatment if significant syndrome occurs and refer to product literature.

● NATIONAL FUNDING/ACCESS DECISIONS
For full details see funding body website

NICE decisions
▸ **Bevacizumab in combination with capecitabine for the first-line treatment of metastatic breast cancer (August 2012)** NICE TA263 Not recommended
▸ **Bevacizumab in combination with oxaliplatin and either fluorouracil plus folinic acid or capecitabine for the treatment of metastatic colorectal cancer (December 2010)** NICE TA212 Not recommended
▸ **Capecitabine for the treatment of advanced gastric cancer (July 2010)** NICE TA191 Recommended
▸ **Capecitabine and tegafur with uracil for metastatic colorectal cancer (May 2003)** NICE TA61 Recommended
▸ **Capecitabine and oxaliplatin in the adjuvant treatment of stage III (Dukes' C) colon cancer (April 2006)** NICE TA100 Recommended

● MEDICINAL FORMS There can be variation in the licensing of different medicines containing the same drug.

Tablet
CAUTIONARY AND ADVISORY LABELS 21
▸ Capecitabine (Non-proprietary)
Capecitabine 150 mg Capecitabine 150mg tablets | 60 tablet PoM £30.00 DT = £30.00 | 60 tablet PoM £38.02 DT = £30.00 (Hospital only)
Capecitabine 300 mg Capecitabine 300mg tablets | 60 tablet PoM £76.04 DT = £76.04 (Hospital only)
Capecitabine 500 mg Capecitabine 500mg tablets | 120 tablet PoM £225.72 DT = £225.72 | 120 tablet PoM £240.00–£265.55 DT = £225.72 (Hospital only)
▸ Xeloda (Roche Products Ltd)
Capecitabine 150 mg Xeloda 150mg tablets | 60 tablet PoM £40.02 DT = £30.00
Capecitabine 500 mg Xeloda 500mg tablets | 120 tablet PoM £265.55 DT = £225.72

Cladribine

● DRUG ACTION Cladribine is a nucleoside analogue that is cytotoxic particularly to lymphocytes and monocytes, inhibiting both DNA synthesis and repair. Its effect on B- and T-lymphocytes is thought to interrupt the cascade of immune events central to multiple sclerosis.

● INDICATIONS AND DOSE
Hairy cell leukaemia (specialist use only)
▸ BY SUBCUTANEOUS INJECTION, OR BY INTRAVENOUS INFUSION
▸ Adult: (consult product literature or local protocols)
B-cell chronic lymphocytic leukaemia (specialist use only)
▸ BY INTRAVENOUS INFUSION
▸ Adult: (consult product literature or local protocols)
Highly active relapsing-remitting multiple sclerosis (specialist use only)
▸ BY MOUTH
▸ Adult: (consult product literature or local protocols)

> IMPORTANT SAFETY INFORMATION
> MHRA/CHM ADVICE: CLADRIBINE FOR LEUKAEMIA: REPORTS OF PROGRESSIVE MULTIFOCAL ENCEPHALOPATHY (PML); STOP TREATMENT IF PML SUSPECTED (DECEMBER 2017)
> The MHRA is aware of 3 confirmed cases of progressive multifocal encephalopathy (PML) that developed 6 months to several years after cladribine treatment for haematological conditions. An association between cladribine and prolonged lymphopenia has been reported.
> PML should be considered in the differential diagnosis for patients with new or worsening neurological signs or symptoms. Patients should be monitored for signs and symptoms of new neurological dysfunction, and advised to seek urgent medical attention if they experience symptoms—stop treatment immediately if PML is suspected and ensure specialist investigation is received.

● CONTRA-INDICATIONS
▸ With oral use Active chronic hepatitis · active chronic tuberculosis · active malignancy · HIV infection · immunocompromised patients

● CAUTIONS
GENERAL CAUTIONS Acute infection · use irradiated blood only (haematology consultation advised)
SPECIFIC CAUTIONS
▸ With intravenous use or subcutaneous use High tumour burden—consult product literature · symptomatic or severe bone marrow depression
▸ With oral use No prior exposure to varicella zoster virus · prior malignancy (consider if potential benefit outweighs risk)
CAUTIONS, FURTHER INFORMATION
▸ Immunosuppressive effect of cladribine
▸ With intravenous use or subcutaneous use Cladribine has potent and prolonged myelosuppressive and immunosuppressive effects. Patients treated with cladribine are more prone to serious bacterial, opportunistic fungal, and viral infections, and prophylactic therapy should be considered in those at risk. Acute infections should be treated before initiating cladribine. To prevent potentially fatal transfusion-related graft-versus-host reaction, only irradiated blood products should be administered. Prescribers should consult specialist literature when using highly immunosuppressive drugs.
▸ Varicella zoster virus
▸ With oral use Manufacturer advises vaccination prior to initiation of therapy in patients who have no history of exposure to varicella zoster virus; delay treatment for 4–6 weeks after vaccination.

Immune system and malignant disease

8

- INTERACTIONS → Appendix 1: cladribine
- SIDE-EFFECTS
  GENERAL SIDE-EFFECTS
- ▶ **Common or very common** Increased risk of infection
  SPECIFIC SIDE-EFFECTS
- ▶ **Common or very common**
- ▶ With intravenous use Anaemia · anxiety · appetite decreased · arrhythmias · arthritis · asthenia · chest pain · chills · confusion · conjunctivitis · constipation · cough · diarrhoea · dizziness · dyspnoea · febrile neutropenia · fever · flatulence · gastrointestinal discomfort · haemolytic anaemia · headache · hyperhidrosis · hypersensitivity · insomnia · joint disorders · malaise · muscle weakness · myalgia · myocardial ischaemia · nausea · neoplasms · oedema · pain · renal impairment · respiratory disorders · secondary malignancy · septic shock · skin reactions · thrombocytopenia · vomiting
- ▶ With oral use Alopecia · lymphopenia · rash
- ▶ With subcutaneous use Anaemia · anxiety · appetite decreased · arrhythmias · arthralgia · arthritis · asthenia · bone marrow disorders · chills · constipation · cough · diarrhoea · dizziness · dyspnoea · fever · gastrointestinal disorders · gastrointestinal pain · haemorrhage · headache · hyperhidrosis · hypotension · immunosuppression · insomnia · lymphopenia · malaise · mucositis · myalgia · myocardial ischaemia · nausea · neutropenia · oedema · pain · respiratory disorders · secondary malignancy · sepsis · skin reactions · thrombocytopenia · vomiting
- ▶ **Uncommon**
- ▶ With intravenous use Bone marrow disorders · hypereosinophilia · level of consciousness decreased · nerve disorders · neurotoxicity (with high doses) · paralysis · paraparesis · Stevens-Johnson syndrome · tumour lysis syndrome
- ▶ With subcutaneous use Ataxia · cachexia · confusion · drowsiness · eye inflammation · haemolytic anaemia · paraesthesia · polyneuropathy
- ▶ **Rare or very rare**
- ▶ With intravenous use Heart failure
- ▶ With subcutaneous use Amyloidosis · cholecystitis · depression · dysphagia · epilepsy · graft versus host disease · heart failure · hepatic failure · hypereosinophilia · pulmonary embolism · renal failure · severe cutaneous adverse reactions (SCARs) · speech disorder · tumour lysis syndrome
- ▶ **Frequency not known**
- ▶ With oral use Malignancy
- CONCEPTION AND CONTRACEPTION Manufacturer advises effective contraception during treatment and for at least 6 months after the last dose in men and women of childbearing potential.
- ▶ With oral use Manufacturer advises exclude pregnancy before each treatment course; if using a hormonal contraceptive, a barrier method should also be used for at least 4 weeks after the last dose of each course.
- PREGNANCY Manufacturer advises avoid—teratogenic in *animal* studies. See also *Pregnancy and reproductive function* in Cytotoxic drugs p. 932.
- BREAST FEEDING
- ▶ With intravenous use or subcutaneous use Manufacturer advises avoid during treatment and for 6 months after the last dose—no information available.
- ▶ With oral use Manufacturer advises avoid during treatment and for 1 week after the last dose—no information available.
- HEPATIC IMPAIRMENT
- ▶ With intravenous use Manufacturer advises caution (limited information available).
- ▶ With subcutaneous use Manufacturer advises caution in mild impairment; avoid in moderate to severe impairment (no information available).

- ▶ With oral use Manufacturer advises avoid in moderate to severe impairment (no information available).
- RENAL IMPAIRMENT
- ▶ With subcutaneous use Manufacturer advises caution in mild impairment; avoid in moderate-to-severe impairment.
- ▶ With oral use Manufacturer advises avoid in moderate-to-severe impairment—no information available.
- ▶ With intravenous use Manufacturer advises caution—limited information available.
- PRE-TREATMENT SCREENING
- ▶ With oral use Manufacturer advises exclude HIV infection, active or latent tuberculosis and active or latent hepatitis before starting each treatment course—delay treatment until infection adequately treated.
- MONITORING REQUIREMENTS
- ▶ Manufacturer advises monitor for malignancy—follow routine cancer screening guidelines.
- ▶ Manufacturer advises monitor for progressive multifocal leucoencephalopathy—perform a baseline MRI.
- ▶ Manufacturer advises monitor for haemolysis in patients who are or who become Coombs' positive.
- ▶ Manufacturer advises haematological monitoring required—consult product literature.
- ▶ With intravenous use or subcutaneous use Renal and hepatic function should be monitored periodically as clinically indicated.
- DIRECTIONS FOR ADMINISTRATION *Litak®* for subcutaneous use only—no dilution required; manufacturer advises patients may self-administer, after appropriate training.
  Leustat® for infusion use only.
- HANDLING AND STORAGE
  LITAK® Manufacturer advises store in a refrigerator (2–8°C).
  LEUSTAT® Manufacturer advises store in a refrigerator (2–8°C).
- PATIENT AND CARER ADVICE
  Driving and skilled tasks
  - ▶ With intravenous use or subcutaneous use Manufacturer advises patients and carers should be counselled on the effects on driving and performance of skilled tasks—increased risk of dizziness and drowsiness.
- NATIONAL FUNDING/ACCESS DECISIONS
  For full details see funding body website
  NICE decisions
  - ▶ Cladribine for treating relapsing–remitting multiple sclerosis (December 2019) NICE TA616 Recommended with restrictions
  Scottish Medicines Consortium (SMC) decisions
  - ▶ Cladribine (*Mavenclad®*) for the treatment of adult patients with highly active relapsing multiple sclerosis (MS) as defined by clinical or imaging features (February 2018) SMC No. 1300/18 Recommended with restrictions

- MEDICINAL FORMS There can be variation in the licensing of different medicines containing the same drug.
  Solution for injection
  - ▶ Litak (Lipomed GmbH)
    Cladribine 2 mg per 1 ml Litak 10mg/5ml solution for injection vials | 1 vial (PoM) £165.00 (Hospital only)
  Solution for infusion
  ELECTROLYTES: May contain Sodium
  - ▶ Leustat (Janssen-Cilag Ltd)
    Cladribine 1 mg per 1 ml Leustat 10mg/10ml solution for infusion vials | 1 vial (PoM) £159.70
  Tablet
  - ▶ Mavenclad (Merck Serono Ltd)
    Cladribine 10 mg Mavenclad 10mg tablets | 1 tablet (PoM) £2,047.24 | 4 tablet (PoM) £8,188.97 | 6 tablet (PoM) £12,283.46

Clofarabine

17-Jun-2020

- **INDICATIONS AND DOSE**

Relapsed or refractory acute lymphoblastic leukaemia in patients who have received at least two previous regimens
▸ BY INTRAVENOUS INFUSION
▸ Adult 18-20 years: (consult local protocol)

- CAUTIONS Cardiac disease
- INTERACTIONS → Appendix 1: clofarabine
- SIDE-EFFECTS
▸ **Common or very common** Alopecia · anxiety · appetite decreased · arthralgia · capillary leak syndrome · chills · cough · dehydration · diarrhoea · dizziness · drowsiness · dyspnoea · fatigue · feeling abnormal · feeling hot · fever · flushing · gastrointestinal discomfort · haemorrhage · headache · hearing impairment · hepatic disorders · hyperbilirubinaemia · hyperhidrosis · hypersensitivity · hypotension · increased risk of infection · irritability · mucositis · multi organ failure · myalgia · nausea · neutropenia · oedema · oral disorders · pain · paraesthesia · pericardial effusion · peripheral neuropathy · psychiatric disorder · renal impairment · respiratory disorders · sepsis · sinusoidal obstruction syndrome · skin reactions · systemic inflammatory response syndrome · tachycardia · tremor · tumour lysis syndrome · vomiting · weight decreased
▸ **Frequency not known** Antibiotic associated colitis · gastrointestinal disorders · hyponatraemia · pancreatitis · severe cutaneous adverse reactions (SCARs)
- CONCEPTION AND CONTRACEPTION Contraceptive advice required, see *Pregnancy and reproductive function* in Cytotoxic drugs p. 932.
- PREGNANCY Manufacturer advises avoid (teratogenic in *animal* studies). See also *Pregnancy and reproductive function* in Cytotoxic drugs p. 932.
- BREAST FEEDING Discontinue breast-feeding.
- HEPATIC IMPAIRMENT Manufacturer advises use with caution in mild-to-moderate impairment; avoid in severe impairment—no information available.
- RENAL IMPAIRMENT Manufacturer advises caution in mild to moderate impairment. Avoid in severe impairment.

- MEDICINAL FORMS There can be variation in the licensing of different medicines containing the same drug.
Solution for infusion
ELECTROLYTES: May contain Sodium
▸ Clofarabine (Non-proprietary)
  Clofarabine 1 mg per 1 ml Clofarabine 20mg/20ml concentrate for solution for infusion vials | 1 vial PoM £1,326.18 (Hospital only)
▸ Evoltra (Sanofi) ▼
  Clofarabine 1 mg per 1 ml Evoltra 20mg/20ml concentrate for solution for infusion vials | 1 vial PoM £1,326.18 (Hospital only)

❙ Cytarabine

14-Dec-2020

- DRUG ACTION Cytarabine acts by interfering with pyrimidine synthesis.

- **INDICATIONS AND DOSE**

Induction of remission of acute myeloblastic leukaemia
▸ BY INTRAVENOUS INFUSION, OR BY INTRAVENOUS INJECTION, OR BY SUBCUTANEOUS INJECTION
▸ Adult: (consult local protocol)

Lymphomatous meningitis
▸ BY INTRATHECAL INJECTION
▸ Adult: (consult local protocol)

> IMPORTANT SAFETY INFORMATION
> Not all cytarabine preparations can be given by intrathecal injection—consult product literature.

- INTERACTIONS → Appendix 1: cytarabine
- SIDE-EFFECTS
▸ **Common or very common** Alopecia · anaemia · appetite decreased · consciousness impaired · diarrhoea · dysarthria · dysphagia · eye disorders · eye inflammation · eye stinging · fever · gastrointestinal discomfort · gastrointestinal disorders · haemorrhagic conjunctivitis (consider prophylactic corticosteroid eye drops) · hyperuricaemia · leucopenia · nausea · oral disorders · renal impairment · skin reactions · thrombocytopenia · urinary retention · vasculitis · vision disorders · vomiting
▸ **Uncommon** Arthralgia · dyspnoea · headache · increased risk of infection · myalgia · nerve disorders · pain · paralysis · pericarditis · sepsis · skin ulcer · throat pain
▸ **Rare or very rare** Arrhythmias
▸ **Frequency not known** Acute respiratory distress syndrome (ARDS) · amenorrhoea · ataxia · azoospermia · bone marrow disorders · cardiomyopathy · cerebellar dysfunction · chest pain · coma · confusion · cytarabine syndrome · dizziness · drowsiness · haemorrhage · hepatic disorders · hyperbilirubinaemia · neurotoxicity · neurotoxicity rash · neutropenia · pancreatitis · personality change · pulmonary oedema · reticulocytopenia · rhabdomyolysis · seizure · tremor
- CONCEPTION AND CONTRACEPTION Contraceptive advice required, see *Pregnancy and reproductive function* in Cytotoxic drugs p. 932.
- PREGNANCY Avoid (teratogenic in *animal* studies). See also *Pregnancy and reproductive function* in Cytotoxic drugs p. 932.
- BREAST FEEDING Discontinue breast-feeding.
- HEPATIC IMPAIRMENT Manufacturer advises caution (increased risk of CNS toxicity).
Dose adjustments Manufacturer advises dose reduction—consult product literature.
- MONITORING REQUIREMENTS
▸ Haematological monitoring Cytarabine is a potent myelosuppressant and requires careful haematological monitoring.
- MEDICINAL FORMS There can be variation in the licensing of different medicines containing the same drug. Forms available from special-order manufacturers include: solution for injection
Solution for injection
▸ Cytarabine (Non-proprietary)
  Cytarabine 20 mg per 1 ml Cytarabine 500mg/25ml solution for injection vials | 1 vial PoM £19.50 (Hospital only)
  Cytarabine 100mg/5ml solution for injection vials | 5 vial PoM £30.00 (Hospital only)
  Cytarabine 500mg/25ml solution for injection Cytosafe vials | 1 vial PoM £19.50 (Hospital only)
  Cytarabine 100 mg per 1 ml Cytarabine 1g/10ml solution for injection Cytosafe vials | 1 vial PoM £39.00 (Hospital only)
  Cytarabine 1g/10ml solution for injection vials | 1 vial PoM £37.05-£52.27 (Hospital only)
  Cytarabine 500mg/5ml solution for injection vials | 5 vial PoM £89.78-£100.00 (Hospital only)
  Cytarabine 100mg/1ml solution for injection vials | 5 vial PoM £26.93 (Hospital only)
  Cytarabine 2g/20ml solution for injection Cytosafe vials | 1 vial PoM £77.50 (Hospital only)
  Cytarabine 2g/20ml solution for injection vials | 1 vial PoM £73.63-£103.87 (Hospital only)

Combinations available: *Daunorubicin with cytarabine*, p. 945

8

Immune system and malignant disease

Decitabine

17-Jun-2020

- DRUG ACTION Decitabine is a pyrimidine analogue.

- **INDICATIONS AND DOSE**

Treatment of newly diagnosed acute myeloid leukaemia in patients over 65 years of age who are not candidates for standard induction chemotherapy
- ▶ BY INTRAVENOUS INFUSION
- ▶ Elderly: (consult local protocol)

- CAUTIONS History of severe congestive heart failure · history of unstable cardiac disease
- INTERACTIONS → Appendix 1: decitabine
- SIDE-EFFECTS
- ▶ **Common or very common** Anaemia · diarrhoea · epistaxis · fever · headache · hypersensitivity · increased risk of infection · leucopenia · nausea · neutropenia · sepsis · stomatitis · thrombocytopenia · vomiting
- ▶ **Uncommon** Acute febrile neutrophilic dermatosis · pancytopenia
- ▶ **Frequency not known** Gastrointestinal disorders · interstitial lung disease

- CONCEPTION AND CONTRACEPTION Men must avoid fathering a child during and for 3 months after treatment.
- PREGNANCY Avoid (teratogenic in *animal* studies). See also *Pregnancy and reproductive function* in Cytotoxic drugs p. 932.
- BREAST FEEDING Discontinue breast-feeding.
- HEPATIC IMPAIRMENT Manufacturer advises caution—no information available.
- RENAL IMPAIRMENT Manufacturer advises caution if creatinine clearance less than 30 mL/minute—no information available.

- MEDICINAL FORMS There can be variation in the licensing of different medicines containing the same drug.
Powder for solution for infusion
ELECTROLYTES: May contain Potassium, sodium
- ▶ Dacogen (Janssen-Cilag Ltd)
Decitabine 50 mg Dacogen 50mg powder for concentrate for solution for infusion vials | 1 vial [PoM] £970.86

Fludarabine phosphate

05-Nov-2020

- **INDICATIONS AND DOSE**

Initial treatment of advanced B-cell chronic lymphocytic leukaemia (CLL) or after first line treatment in patients with sufficient bone-marrow reserves
- ▶ BY MOUTH
- ▶ Adult: 40 mg/m^2 for 5 days every 28 days, usually given for 6 cycles
- ▶ BY INTRAVENOUS INJECTION, OR BY INTRAVENOUS INFUSION
- ▶ Adult: (consult product literature)

IMPORTANT SAFETY INFORMATION
RISKS OF INCORRECT DOSING OF ORAL ANTI-CANCER MEDICINES
See Cytotoxic drugs p. 932.

- CONTRA-INDICATIONS Haemolytic anaemia
- CAUTIONS Increased susceptibility to skin cancer · worsening of existing skin cancer
CAUTIONS, FURTHER INFORMATION
- ▶ Immunosuppression Fludarabine has a potent immunosuppressive effect. Patients treated with fludarabine are more prone to serious bacterial, opportunistic fungal, and viral infections, and prophylactic therapy can be used in those at risk. Co-trimoxazole is licensed for the prevention of pneumocystis infection.

To prevent potentially fatal transfusion-related graft-versus-host reaction, manufacturer advises only irradiated blood products should be administered.

- INTERACTIONS → Appendix 1: fludarabine
- SIDE-EFFECTS
GENERAL SIDE-EFFECTS
- ▶ **Common or very common** Anaemia · appetite decreased · asthenia · bone marrow depression (may be cumulative) · chills · cough · diarrhoea · fever · increased risk of infection · malaise · mucositis · nausea · neoplasms · nerve disorders · neutropenia · oedema · stomatitis · thrombocytopenia · vision disorders · vomiting
- ▶ **Uncommon** Autoimmune disorder · confusion · dyspnoea · haemorrhage · respiratory disorders · tumour lysis syndrome
- ▶ **Rare or very rare** Agitation · arrhythmia · coma · heart failure · seizure · severe cutaneous adverse reactions (SCARs)
SPECIFIC SIDE-EFFECTS
- ▶ **Common or very common**
- ▶ With oral use Progressive multifocal leukoencephalopathy (PML) · skin reactions · viral infection reactivation
- ▶ With parenteral use Rash
- ▶ **Uncommon**
- ▶ With oral use Acquired haemophilia · crystalluria · electrolyte imbalance · haemolytic anaemia · hyperuricaemia · metabolic acidosis · renal failure
- ▶ **Frequency not known**
- ▶ With parenteral use Encephalopathy · intracranial haemorrhage

- CONCEPTION AND CONTRACEPTION Manufacturer advises effective contraception during and for at least 6 months after treatment in men or women.
- PREGNANCY Avoid (embryotoxic and teratogenic in *animal* studies). See also *Pregnancy and reproductive function* in Cytotoxic drugs p. 932.
- BREAST FEEDING Discontinue breast-feeding.
- RENAL IMPAIRMENT Avoid if creatinine clearance less than 30 mL/minute.
Dose adjustments Reduce dose by up to 50% if creatinine clearance 30–70 mL/minute.
- MONITORING REQUIREMENTS
- ▶ Monitor for signs of haemolysis.
- ▶ Monitor for neurological toxicity.
- ▶ Assess creatinine clearance in patients over 65 years before treatment initiation.
- DIRECTIONS FOR ADMINISTRATION Manufacturer advises concentrate for intravenous injection or infusion must be diluted before administration (consult product literature).
- NATIONAL FUNDING/ACCESS DECISIONS
For full details see funding body website

NICE decisions
- ▶ Fludarabine monotherapy for the first-line treatment of chronic lymphocytic leukaemia (February 2007) NICE TA119 Not recommended
- ▶ Fludarabine for B-cell chronic lymphocytic leukaemia (September 2001) NICE TA29 Recommended
Scottish Medicines Consortium (SMC) decisions
- ▶ Fludarabine phosphate (*Fludara*®) for B-cell chronic lymphocytic leukaemia (November 2006) SMC No. 176/05 Recommended with restrictions

- MEDICINAL FORMS There can be variation in the licensing of different medicines containing the same drug.
Solution for injection
- ▶ Fludarabine phosphate (Non-proprietary)
Fludarabine phosphate 25 mg per 1 ml Fludarabine phosphate 50mg/2ml concentrate for solution for injection vials | 1 vial [PoM] £155.00–£156.00 (Hospital only)

Tablet
▸ Fludara (Sanofi)
Fludarabine phosphate 10 mg Fludara 10mg tablets |
15 tablet PoM £302.48 (Hospital only) | 20 tablet PoM £403.31
(Hospital only)
Powder for solution for injection
▸ Fludarabine phosphate (Non-proprietary)
Fludarabine phosphate 50 mg Fludarabine phosphate 50mg
powder for solution for injection vials | 1 vial PoM £155.00 (Hospital
only)
▸ Fludara (Sanofi)
Fludarabine phosphate 50 mg Fludara 50mg powder for solution
for injection vials | 5 vial PoM £735.34 (Hospital only)

Fluorouracil

11-Aug-2020

● **INDICATIONS AND DOSE**
**Treatment of some solid tumours including gastro-
intestinal tract cancers and breast cancer | In
combination with folinic acid in advanced colorectal
cancer**
▸ BY INTRAVENOUS INJECTION, OR BY INTRAVENOUS INFUSION,
OR BY INTRA-ARTERIAL INFUSION
▸ Adult: (consult product literature)

IMPORTANT SAFETY INFORMATION
MHRA/CHM ADVICE: 5-FLUOROURACIL (INTRAVENOUS),
CAPECITABINE, TEGAFUR: DPD TESTING RECOMMENDED BEFORE
INITIATION TO IDENTIFY PATIENTS AT INCREASED RISK OF SEVERE
AND FATAL TOXICITY (OCTOBER 2020)
▸ With intravenous use
Patients with partial or complete dihydropyrimidine
dehydrogenase (DPD) deficiency are at increased risk of
severe and fatal toxicity during treatment with
fluoropyrimidines. Healthcare professionals are advised
to test all patients for DPD deficiency before initiating
treatment and confirm their, including family, history of
complete or partial DPD deficiency. Fluorouracil is
contra-indicated in patients with known complete DPD
deficiency; in those with partial DPD deficiency, a
reduced starting dose is recommended. Patients should
be monitored for toxicity, particularly during the first
cycle of treatment or after a dose increase; severe
toxicity can occur even in those with negative test
results for DPD deficiency. Therapeutic drug monitoring
may improve clinical outcomes in patients receiving
continuous fluorouracil infusions. Healthcare
professionals should also counsel patients on the
benefits and risks of their treatment and ensure they are
provided with the patient information leaflet.

● CONTRA-INDICATIONS Bone marrow depression (after
treatment with radiotherapy or other antineoplastic
agents) · complete or near complete absence of
dihydropyrimidine dehydrogenase activity (increased risk
of severe, life-threatening, or fatal toxicity)—consult
product literature · serious infections
● CAUTIONS History of heart disease · partial
dihydropyrimidine dehydrogenase deficiency—consult
product literature
● INTERACTIONS → Appendix 1: fluorouracil
● SIDE-EFFECTS
▸ **Common or very common** Agranulocytosis · alopecia ·
anaemia · anal inflammation · appetite decreased ·
asthenia · bone marrow disorders · bronchospasm ·
diarrhoea · gastrointestinal disorders · haemorrhage · hand
and foot syndrome (long term use) · healing impaired ·
immunosuppression · increased risk of infection ·
ischaemic heart disease · leucopenia · malaise · mucositis ·
nausea · neutropenia · skin reactions · stomatitis ·
thrombocytopenia · vomiting

▸ **Uncommon** Arrhythmias · cardiac inflammation ·
cardiogenic shock · cardiomyopathy congestive ·
dehydration · dizziness · drowsiness · euphoric mood · eye
disorders · eye inflammation · headache · heart failure ·
hepatic disorders · hypotension · movement disorders ·
myocardial infarction · nail discolouration · nail disorders ·
nerve disorders · ovulation disorder · parkinsonism ·
photosensitivity reaction · sepsis · spermatogenesis
disorder · vision disorders
▸ **Rare or very rare** Biliary sclerosis · cardiac arrest · cerebral
ischaemia · cholecystitis · coma · confusion · embolism and
thrombosis · encephalopathy · fever · muscle weakness ·
peripheral vascular disease · renal failure · seizure · speech
impairment · sudden cardiac death
▸ **Frequency not known** Vein discolouration
● CONCEPTION AND CONTRACEPTION Contraceptive advice
required, see *Pregnancy and reproductive function* in
Cytotoxic drugs p. 932.
● PREGNANCY Avoid (teratogenic). See also *Pregnancy and
reproductive function* in Cytotoxic drugs p. 932.
● BREAST FEEDING Discontinue breast-feeding.
● HEPATIC IMPAIRMENT Manufacturer advises caution
(increased risk of hyperammonaemia and
hyperammonaemic encephalopathy).
Dose adjustments Manufacturer advises consider dose
reduction.
● RENAL IMPAIRMENT Manufacturer advises caution
(increased risk of hyperammonaemia and
hyperammonaemic encephalopathy).
Dose adjustments Manufacturer advises consider dose
reduction.
● PRE-TREATMENT SCREENING Manufacturer advises
genotyping of the DPYD gene to identify patients at
increased risk for severe toxicity—consult product
literature.
● MONITORING REQUIREMENTS Manufacturer advises
monitor cardiac function regularly
● HANDLING AND STORAGE Caution in handling—irritant to
tissues.

● MEDICINAL FORMS There can be variation in the licensing of
different medicines containing the same drug. Forms available
from special-order manufacturers include: solution for
injection
Solution for injection
▸ Fluorouracil (Non-proprietary)
Fluorouracil (as Fluorouracil sodium) 25 mg per 1 ml Fluorouracil
500mg/20ml solution for injection vials | 10 vial PoM £64.00
(Hospital only)
Fluorouracil (as Fluorouracil sodium) 50 mg per 1 ml Fluorouracil
1g/20ml solution for injection vials | 1 vial PoM £12.16 (Hospital
only) | 1 vial PoM £12.80
Fluorouracil 500mg/10ml solution for injection vials | 1 vial PoM
£6.08-£6.40 (Hospital only) | 5 vial PoM £32.00 (Hospital only)
Solution for infusion
▸ Fluorouracil (Non-proprietary)
Fluorouracil (as Fluorouracil sodium) 25 mg per 1 ml Fluorouracil
2.5g/100ml solution for infusion vials | 1 vial PoM £32.00 (Hospital
only)
Fluorouracil (as Fluorouracil sodium) 50 mg per 1 ml Fluorouracil
5g/100ml solution for infusion vials | 1 vial PoM £60.80-£64.00
(Hospital only)
Fluorouracil 2.5g/50ml solution for infusion vials | 1 vial PoM
£30.40-£32.00 (Hospital only)

8

Immune system and malignant disease

Gemcitabine

06-Nov-2020

- **INDICATIONS AND DOSE**

First-line treatment for locally advanced or metastatic non-small cell lung cancer (as monotherapy in elderly patients and in palliative treatment; otherwise in combination with cisplatin) | Treatment of locally advanced or metastatic pancreatic cancer | Treatment of advanced or metastatic bladder cancer (in combination with cisplatin) | Treatment of locally advanced or metastatic epithelial ovarian cancer which has relapsed after a recurrence-free interval of at least 6 months following previous platinum-based therapy (in combination with carboplatin) | Treatment of metastatic breast cancer which has relapsed after previous chemotherapy including an anthracycline (in combination with paclitaxel)
  - ▸ BY INTRAVENOUS INFUSION
  - ▸ Adult: (consult local protocol)

- INTERACTIONS → Appendix 1: gemcitabine
- SIDE-EFFECTS
  - ▸ **Common or very common** Alopecia · anaemia · appetite decreased · asthenia · back pain · bone marrow depression · chills · constipation · cough · diarrhoea · drowsiness · dyspnoea · fever · haematuria · headache · hyperhidrosis · influenza like illness · insomnia · leucopenia · myalgia · nausea · neutropenia · oedema · oral disorders · proteinuria · rhinitis · skin reactions · thrombocytopenia · vomiting
  - ▸ **Uncommon** Respiratory disorders
  - ▸ **Rare or very rare** Capillary leak syndrome · hypotension · myocardial infarction · posterior reversible encephalopathy syndrome (PRES) · severe cutaneous adverse reactions (SCARs) · skin ulcer · thrombocytosis
  - ▸ **Frequency not known** Arrhythmias · colitis ischaemic · gangrene · haemolytic uraemic syndrome · heart failure · hepatic disorders · pulmonary oedema · radiation injuries · renal failure · stroke · vasculitis

    SIDE-EFFECTS, FURTHER INFORMATION Gemcitabine should be discontinued if signs of microangiopathic haemolytic anaemia occur.
- CONCEPTION AND CONTRACEPTION Manufacturer advises effective contraception during treatment. Men must avoid fathering a child during and for 6 months after treatment.
- PREGNANCY Avoid (teratogenic in *animal* studies). See *Pregnancy and reproductive function* in Cytotoxic drugs p. 932.
- BREAST FEEDING Discontinue breast-feeding.
- HEPATIC IMPAIRMENT Manufacturer advises caution (limited information available).
- RENAL IMPAIRMENT Manufacturer advises caution.
- NATIONAL FUNDING/ACCESS DECISIONS
  For full details see funding body website

  NICE decisions
  - ▸ **Gemcitabine for the treatment of pancreatic cancer (May 2001)** NICE TA25 Recommended
  - ▸ **Gemcitabine for the treatment of metastatic breast cancer (January 2007)** NICE TA116 Recommended with restrictions
  - ▸ **Bevacizumab in combination with gemcitabine and carboplatin for treating the first recurrence of platinum-sensitive advanced ovarian cancer (May 2013)** NICE TA285 Not recommended
  - ▸ **Topotecan, pegylated liposomal doxorubicin hydrochloride, paclitaxel, trabectedin and gemcitabine for treating recurrent ovarian cancer (April 2016)** NICE TA389 Not recommended
  - ▸ **Paclitaxel as albumin-bound nanoparticles with gemcitabine for untreated metastatic pancreatic cancer (September 2017)** NICE TA476 Recommended with restrictions

- MEDICINAL FORMS There can be variation in the licensing of different medicines containing the same drug.

  Solution for infusion
  - ▸ Gemcitabine (Non-proprietary)

    Gemcitabine (as Gemcitabine hydrochloride) 10 mg per 1 ml Gemcitabine 1.6g/160ml infusion bags | 1 bag [PoM] £140.00
    Gemcitabine 2.2g/220ml infusion bags | 1 bag [PoM] £200.00
    Gemcitabine 2g/200ml infusion bags | 1 bag [PoM] £180.00
    Gemcitabine 1.2g/120ml infusion bags | 1 bag [PoM] £120.00
    Gemcitabine 1.8g/180ml infusion bags | 1 bag [PoM] £160.00
    Gemcitabine 1.4g/140ml infusion bags | 1 bag [PoM] [⊠]

    Gemcitabine (as Gemcitabine hydrochloride) 38 mg per 1 ml Gemcitabine 1g/26.3ml concentrate for solution for infusion vials | 1 vial [PoM] £160.30 (Hospital only)
    Gemcitabine 2g/52.6ml concentrate for solution for infusion vials | 1 vial [PoM] £320.63 (Hospital only)
    Gemcitabine 200mg/5.26ml concentrate for solution for infusion vials | 1 vial [PoM] £32.09 (Hospital only)

    Gemcitabine (as Gemcitabine hydrochloride) 100 mg per 1 ml Gemcitabine 2g/20ml concentrate for solution for infusion vials | 1 vial [PoM] £26.86 (Hospital only)
    Gemcitabine 1g/10ml concentrate for solution for infusion vials | 1 vial [PoM] £13.09 (Hospital only)
    Gemcitabine 200mg/2ml concentrate for solution for infusion vials | 1 vial [PoM] £6.40 (Hospital only)

  Powder for solution for infusion
  - ▸ Gemcitabine (Non-proprietary)

    Gemcitabine (as Gemcitabine hydrochloride) 200 mg Gemcitabine 200mg powder for solution for infusion vials | 1 vial [PoM] £32.00-£32.55 (Hospital only)

    Gemcitabine (as Gemcitabine hydrochloride) 1 gram Gemcitabine 1g powder for solution for infusion vials | 1 vial [PoM] £155.67-£162.76 (Hospital only)

    Gemcitabine (as Gemcitabine hydrochloride) 2 gram Gemcitabine 2g powder for solution for infusion vials | 1 vial [PoM] £324.00-£413.51 (Hospital only)

Mercaptopurine

23-Jun-2020

(6-Mercaptopurine)

- **INDICATIONS AND DOSE**

Severe acute Crohn's disease | Maintenance of remission of Crohn's disease | Ulcerative colitis
  - ▸ BY MOUTH
  - ▸ Adult: 1–1.5 mg/kg daily, some patients may respond to lower doses

Acute leukaemias | Chronic myeloid leukaemia
  - ▸ BY MOUTH USING TABLETS
  - ▸ Adult: Initially 2.5 mg/kg daily, adjusted according to response, alternatively initially 50–75 mg/m² daily, adjusted according to response
  - ▸ BY MOUTH USING ORAL SUSPENSION
  - ▸ Adult: Initially 25–75 mg/m² daily, adjusted according to response

  DOSE ADJUSTMENTS DUE TO INTERACTIONS
  - ▸ Manufacturer advises reduce dose to one-quarter of the usual dose with concurrent use of allopurinol.

  DOSE EQUIVALENCE AND CONVERSION
  - ▸ Mercaptopurine tablets and *Xaluprine*® oral suspension are **not** bioequivalent, haematological monitoring is advised when switching formulations.

- UNLICENSED USE Not licensed for use in severe ulcerative colitis and Crohn's disease.

  ┌───┐
  IMPORTANT SAFETY INFORMATION
  SAFE PRACTICE
  Mercaptopurine has been confused with mercaptamine; care must be taken to ensure the correct drug is prescribed and dispensed.

  RISKS OF INCORRECT DOSING OF ORAL ANTI-CANCER MEDICINES
  See Cytotoxic drugs p. 932.
  └───┘

- **CONTRA-INDICATIONS**
‣ When used for non-cancer indications Absent thiopurine methyltransferase activity
- **CAUTIONS** Reduced thiopurine methyltransferase activity
CAUTIONS, FURTHER INFORMATION
‣ Thiopurine methyltransferase The enzyme thiopurine methyltransferase (TPMT) metabolises thiopurine drugs (azathioprine, mercaptopurine, tioguanine); the risk of myelosuppression is increased in patients with reduced activity of the enzyme, particularly for the few individuals in whom TPMT activity is undetectable. Those with reduced TPMT activity may be treated under specialist supervision.
- **INTERACTIONS** → Appendix 1: mercaptopurine
- **SIDE-EFFECTS**
‣ **Common or very common** Anaemia · appetite decreased · bone marrow depression · diarrhoea · hepatic disorders · hepatotoxicity (more common at high doses) · leucopenia · nausea · oral disorders · pancreatitis · thrombocytopenia · vomiting
‣ **Uncommon** Arthralgia · fever · increased risk of infection · neutropenia · rash
‣ **Rare or very rare** Alopecia · face oedema · intestinal ulcer · neoplasms · oligozoospermia
‣ **Frequency not known** Photosensitivity reaction
- **CONCEPTION AND CONTRACEPTION** Contraceptive advice required, see *Pregnancy and reproductive function* in Cytotoxic drugs p. 932.
- **PREGNANCY** Avoid (teratogenic). See also *Pregnancy and reproductive function* in Cytotoxic drugs p. 932.
- **BREAST FEEDING** Discontinue breast-feeding.
- **HEPATIC IMPAIRMENT** Manufacturer advises caution (risk of increased exposure).
Dose adjustments Manufacturer advises consider dose reduction.
- **RENAL IMPAIRMENT**
Dose adjustments Reduce dose.
- **PRE-TREATMENT SCREENING** Manufacturer advises consider measuring thiopurine methyltransferase (TPMT) activity before starting mercaptopurine therapy.
- **MONITORING REQUIREMENTS** Monitor liver function.
- **PRESCRIBING AND DISPENSING INFORMATION** Flavours of oral liquid formulations may include raspberry.

- **MEDICINAL FORMS** There can be variation in the licensing of different medicines containing the same drug. Forms available from special-order manufacturers include: tablet, capsule, oral suspension

Oral suspension
EXCIPIENTS: May contain Aspartame
‣ Xaluprine (Nova Laboratories Ltd)
Mercaptopurine 20 mg per 1 ml Xaluprine 20mg/ml oral suspension | 100 ml [PoM] £170.00 DT = £170.00

Tablet
‣ Mercaptopurine (Non-proprietary)
Mercaptopurine 50 mg Mercaptopurine 50mg tablets | 25 tablet [PoM] £49.15 DT = £49.15
‣ Mercaptopurine (Imported (Germany))
Mercaptopurine 10 mg Mercaptopurine 10mg tablets | 100 tablet [PoM] [⤫]

Methotrexate

02-Oct-2020

- **DRUG ACTION** Methotrexate inhibits the enzyme dihydrofolate reductase, essential for the synthesis of purines and pyrimidines.

- **INDICATIONS AND DOSE**
Severe Crohn's disease
‣ BY INTRAMUSCULAR INJECTION
‣ Adult: Initially 25 mg once weekly until remission induced; maintenance 15 mg once weekly
Maintenance of remission of severe Crohn's disease
‣ BY MOUTH
‣ Adult: 10–25 mg once weekly
Moderate to severe active rheumatoid arthritis
‣ BY MOUTH
‣ Adult: 7.5 mg once weekly, adjusted according to response; maximum 20 mg per week
Severe active rheumatoid arthritis
‣ BY INTRAMUSCULAR INJECTION, OR BY SUBCUTANEOUS INJECTION
‣ Adult: Initially 7.5 mg once weekly, then increased in steps of 2.5 mg once weekly, adjusted according to response; maximum 25 mg per week
Neoplastic diseases
‣ BY MOUTH, OR BY INTRAVENOUS INJECTION, OR BY INTRAVENOUS INFUSION, OR BY INTRA-ARTERIAL INFUSION, OR BY INTRAMUSCULAR INJECTION, OR BY INTRATHECAL INJECTION
‣ Adult: (consult product literature)
Severe psoriasis unresponsive to conventional therapy (specialist use only)
‣ BY MOUTH, OR BY INTRAMUSCULAR INJECTION, OR BY INTRAVENOUS INJECTION, OR BY SUBCUTANEOUS INJECTION
‣ Adult: Initially 2.5–10 mg once weekly, then increased in steps of 2.5–5 mg, adjusted according to response, dose to be adjusted at intervals of at least 1 week; usual dose 7.5–15 mg once weekly, stop treatment if inadequate response after 3 months at the optimum dose; maximum 30 mg per week

- **UNLICENSED USE** Not licensed for use in severe Crohn's disease.

IMPORTANT SAFETY INFORMATION
MHRA/CHM ADVICE: METHOTREXATE ONCE-WEEKLY FOR AUTOIMMUNE DISEASES: NEW MEASURES TO REDUCE RISK OF FATAL OVERDOSE DUE TO INADVERTENT DAILY INSTEAD OF WEEKLY DOSING (SEPTEMBER 2020)
‣ With oral use
Methotrexate should be taken **once a week** in autoimmune conditions and, less commonly, in some cancer therapy regimens. A European review highlighted continued reports of inadvertent overdose due to more frequent dosing (including daily administration), which has resulted in some fatalities. Subsequently, new measures have been implemented by the MHRA. Prescribers are advised to:
- ensure patients can understand and comply with once-weekly dosing before prescribing methotrexate, decide with the patient which day of the week they will take their dose, and note this down in full on the prescription;
- consider the patient's overall polypharmacy burden when deciding which formulation to prescribe, especially in those with a high pill burden;
- inform patients and carers of the potentially fatal risk of accidental overdose if methotrexate is taken more frequently than once a week, and reaffirm that it should not be taken daily;
- advise patients and carers to seek immediate medical attention if overdose is suspected.

The MHRA further advises dispensers to remind patients of the once-weekly dosing and the risks of potentially fatal overdose if they take more than directed. Where possible, the day of the week for dosing should be written in full in the space provided on the outer packaging. Patients should be encouraged to write the day of the week for dosing in their patient alert card and carry it with them.

- CONTRA-INDICATIONS Active infection · ascites · immunodeficiency syndromes · significant pleural effusion
- CAUTIONS Photosensitivity—psoriasis lesions aggravated by UV radiation (skin ulceration reported) · dehydration (increased risk of toxicity) · diarrhoea · extreme caution in blood disorders (avoid if severe) · peptic ulceration (avoid in active disease) · risk of accumulation in pleural effusion or ascites—drain before treatment · ulcerative colitis · ulcerative stomatitis

CAUTIONS, FURTHER INFORMATION
- Blood count Bone marrow suppression can occur abruptly; factors likely to increase toxicity include advanced age, renal impairment, and concomitant use with another anti-folate drug (e.g. trimethoprim). Manufacturer advises a clinically significant drop in white cell count or platelet count calls for immediate withdrawal of methotrexate and introduction of supportive therapy.
- Gastro-intestinal toxicity Manufacturer advises withdraw treatment if stomatitis or diarrhoea develops—may be first sign of gastro-intestinal toxicity.
- Liver toxicity Liver cirrhosis reported. Manufacturer advises treatment should not be started or should be discontinued if any abnormality of liver function or liver biopsy is present or develops during therapy. Abnormalities can return to normal within 2 weeks after which treatment may be recommenced if judged appropriate. Persistent increases in liver transaminases may necessitate dose reduction or discontinuation.
- Pulmonary toxicity Pulmonary toxicity may be a special problem in rheumatoid arthritis. Manufacturer advises patients to seek medical attention if dyspnoea, cough or fever develops; monitor for symptoms at each visit—discontinue if pneumonitis suspected.
- INTERACTIONS → Appendix 1: methotrexate
- SIDE-EFFECTS
- Common or very common
- With intrathecal use Necrotising demyelinating leukoencephalopathy · neurotoxicity
- With oral use Anaemia · appetite decreased · diarrhoea · drowsiness · fatigue · gastrointestinal discomfort · headache · increased risk of infection · leucopenia · nausea · oral disorders · respiratory disorders · skin reactions · throat ulcer · thrombocytopenia · vomiting
- With parenteral use Anaemia · appetite decreased · chest pain · cough · diarrhoea · drowsiness · dyspnoea · fatigue · fever · gastrointestinal discomfort · headache · leucopenia · malaise · nausea · oral disorders · respiratory disorders · skin reactions · throat complaints · thrombocytopenia · vomiting
- Uncommon
- With oral use Agranulocytosis · alopecia · arthralgia · bone marrow disorders · chills · confusion · cystitis · depression · diabetes mellitus · dysuria · fever · gastrointestinal disorders · haemorrhage · healing impaired · hepatic disorders · myalgia · neoplasms · nephropathy · osteoporosis · photosensitivity reaction · rheumatoid arthritis aggravated · seizure · severe cutaneous adverse reactions (SCARs) · vasculitis · vertigo · vulvovaginal disorders
- With parenteral use Agranulocytosis · alopecia · arthralgia · bone marrow disorders · confusion · cystitis · depression · diabetes mellitus · drug toxicity · dysuria · gastrointestinal

disorders · haemorrhage · healing impaired · hepatic disorders · increased risk of infection · lipoatrophy · local reaction · myalgia · neoplasms · osteoporosis · pain · paraesthesia · photosensitivity reaction · rheumatoid arthritis aggravated · seizure · severe cutaneous adverse reactions (SCARs) · sterile abscess · vasculitis · vertigo · vulvovaginal disorders
- Rare or very rare
- With oral use Azotaemia · brain oedema · cognitive impairment · conjunctivitis · cough · dyspnoea · eosinophilia · gynaecomastia · hypotension · immune deficiency · infertility · insomnia · lymphadenopathy · meningitis aseptic · menstrual disorder · mood altered · muscle weakness · nail discolouration · neutropenia · oligozoospermia · pain · pancreatitis · paresis · pericardial disorders · pericarditis · proteinuria · psychosis · radiation injuries · renal impairment · retinopathy · sensation abnormal · sepsis · sexual dysfunction · speech impairment · stress fracture · taste metallic · telangiectasia · tinnitus · visual impairment
- With parenteral use Apnoea · asthma-like conditions · azotaemia · conjunctivitis · embolism and thrombosis · eosinophilia · gynaecomastia · hypotension · immune deficiency · infertility · influenza like illness · insomnia · lymphadenopathy · meningism · meningitis aseptic · menstrual disorder · mood altered · muscle weakness · nail discolouration · necrosis · neutropenia · paralysis · pericardial disorders · pericarditis · proteinuria · reactivation of infection · renal impairment · retinopathy · sepsis · sexual dysfunction · sperm abnormalities · stress fracture · taste altered · telangiectasia · vision disorders
- Frequency not known
- With oral use Encephalopathy
- With parenteral use Aphasia · chills · cognitive disorder · defective oogenesis · dizziness · hemiparesis · leukoencephalopathy · metabolic change · mucositis · nephropathy · pancreatitis · pulmonary oedema · skin ulcer · sudden death · tinnitus

SIDE-EFFECTS, FURTHER INFORMATION Give folic acid to reduce side-effects. Folic acid decreases mucosal and gastrointestinal side-effects of methotrexate and may prevent hepatotoxicity; there is no evidence of a reduction in haematological side-effects.

Withdraw treatment if ulcerative stomatitis develops—may be first sign of gastro-intestinal toxicity.

Treatment with folinic acid (as calcium folinate) may be required in acute toxicity.

- CONCEPTION AND CONTRACEPTION Manufacturer advises effective contraception during and for at least 6 months after treatment in men and women.
- PREGNANCY Avoid (teratogenic; fertility may be reduced during therapy but this may be reversible).
- BREAST FEEDING Discontinue breast-feeding—present in milk.
- HEPATIC IMPAIRMENT When used for malignancy, avoid in severe hepatic impairment—consult local treatment protocol for details. Avoid with hepatic impairment in non-malignant conditions—dose-related toxicity.
- RENAL IMPAIRMENT Risk of nephrotoxicity at high doses. Avoid in severe impairment.
  Dose adjustments Reduce dose.
- PRE-TREATMENT SCREENING Exclude pregnancy before treatment.
  Patients should have full blood count and renal and liver function tests before starting treatment.
- MONITORING REQUIREMENTS
- In view of reports of blood dyscrasias (including fatalities) and liver cirrhosis with low-dose methotrexate patients should:
  - have full blood count and renal and liver function tests repeated every 1–2 weeks until therapy stabilised,

thereafter patients should be monitored every 2–3 months.
● be advised to report all symptoms and signs suggestive of infection, especially sore throat

► Local protocols for frequency of monitoring may vary.

► Treatment with folinic acid (as calcium folinate) may be required in acute toxicity.

● PRESCRIBING AND DISPENSING INFORMATION Folinic acid following methotrexate administration helps to prevent methotrexate-induced mucositis and myelosuppression.

The licensed routes of administration for parenteral preparations vary—further information can be found in the product literature for the individual preparations.

● PATIENT AND CARER ADVICE Patients and their carers should be warned to report immediately the onset of any feature of blood disorders (e.g. sore throat, bruising, and mouth ulcers), liver toxicity (e.g. nausea, vomiting, abdominal discomfort and dark urine), and respiratory effects (e.g. shortness of breath).

Patients should be advised to avoid self-medication with over-the-counter aspirin or ibuprofen.

Patients should be counselled on the dose, treatment booklet, and the use of NSAIDs.

► With oral use A patient alert card should be provided to patients on once-weekly dosing—see also *Important safety information*.

Methotrexate treatment booklets Methotrexate treatment booklets should be issued where appropriate.

In **England**, **Wales**, and **Northern Ireland**, they are available for purchase from:

3M Security Print and Systems Limited
Gorse Street, Chadderton
Oldham
OL9 9QH
Tel: 0845 610 1112

GP practices can obtain supplies through their Local Area Team stores.

NHS Hospitals can order supplies from www.nhsforms.co. uk or by emailing nhsforms@mmm.com.

In **Scotland**, treatment booklets can be obtained by emailing stockorders.dppas@theapsgroup.com or by fax on 0131 629 9967.

These booklets include advice for adults taking oral methotrexate for inflammatory conditions, and a section for recording results of blood tests and dosage information.

● MEDICINAL FORMS There can be variation in the licensing of different medicines containing the same drug. Forms available from special-order manufacturers include: oral suspension, oral solution, solution for injection

Tablet
► Methotrexate (Non-proprietary)
Methotrexate 2.5 mg Methotrexate 2.5mg tablets | 24 tablet PoM £1.29–£3.55 | 28 tablet PoM £3.82 DT = £2.56 | 100 tablet PoM £5.39–£14.10
Methotrexate 10 mg Methotrexate 10mg tablets | 100 tablet PoM £55.74 DT = £54.32
► Maxtrex (Pfizer Ltd)
Methotrexate 2.5 mg Maxtrex 2.5mg tablets | 24 tablet PoM £2.39 | 100 tablet PoM £9.96
Methotrexate 10 mg Maxtrex 10mg tablets | 100 tablet PoM £45.16 DT = £54.32

Solution for injection
► Methotrexate (Non-proprietary)
Methotrexate (as Methotrexate sodium) 2.5 mg per 1 ml Methotrexate 5mg/2ml solution for injection vials | 5 vial PoM £36.00 (Hospital only)
Methotrexate (as Methotrexate sodium) 25 mg per 1 ml Methotrexate 1g/40ml solution for injection vials | 1 vial PoM £1,452.55 (Hospital only)
Methotrexate 500mg/20ml solution for injection vials | 1 vial PoM £48.00–£726.28 (Hospital only)

Methotrexate 50mg/2ml solution for injection vials | 1 vial PoM £72.63 (Hospital only) | 5 vial PoM £35.00 (Hospital only)
Methotrexate 50 mg per 1 ml Methofill 30mg/0.6ml solution for injection pre-filled syringes | 1 pre-filled disposable injection PoM £14.55
Methotrexate (as Methotrexate sodium) 50 mg per 1 ml Methofill 15mg/0.3ml solution for injection pre-filled syringes | 1 pre-filled disposable injection PoM £12.40 DT = £12.40
Methofill 25mg/0.5ml solution for injection pre-filled syringes | 1 pre-filled disposable injection PoM £14.24 DT = £14.24
Methofill 10mg/0.2ml solution for injection pre-filled syringes | 1 pre-filled disposable injection PoM £11.25 DT = £11.25
Methofill 7.5mg/0.15ml solution for injection pre-filled syringes | 1 pre-filled disposable injection PoM £10.86 DT = £10.86
Methofill 17.5mg/0.35ml solution for injection pre-filled syringes | 1 pre-filled disposable injection PoM £13.24 DT = £13.24
Methofill 27.5mg/0.55ml solution for injection pre-filled syringes | 1 pre-filled disposable injection PoM £14.49
Methofill 22.5mg/0.45ml solution for injection pre-filled syringes | 1 pre-filled disposable injection PoM £14.10 DT = £14.10
Methofill 12.5mg/0.25ml solution for injection pre-filled syringes | 1 pre-filled disposable injection PoM £12.34 DT = £12.34
Methofill 20mg/0.4ml solution for injection pre-filled syringes | 1 pre-filled disposable injection PoM £13.55 DT = £13.55
Methotrexate (as Methotrexate sodium) 100 mg per 1 ml Methotrexate 1g/10ml solution for injection vials | 1 vial PoM £80.75–£85.00 (Hospital only)
► Methofill (Accord Healthcare Ltd)
Methotrexate 50 mg per 1 ml Methofill 12.5mg/0.25ml solution for injection pre-filled injector | 1 pre-filled disposable injection PoM £14.34 DT = £14.35
Methofill 22.5mg/0.45ml solution for injection pre-filled injector | 1 pre-filled disposable injection PoM £16.10 DT = £16.11
Methofill 30mg/0.6ml solution for injection pre-filled injector | 1 pre-filled disposable injection PoM £16.55 DT = £16.56
Methofill 27.5mg/0.55ml solution for injection pre-filled injector | 1 pre-filled disposable injection PoM £16.49 DT = £16.50
Methofill 7.5mg/0.15ml solution for injection pre-filled injector | 1 pre-filled disposable injection PoM £12.86 DT = £12.87
Methofill 20mg/0.4ml solution for injection pre-filled injector | 1 pre-filled disposable injection PoM £15.55 DT = £15.56
Methofill 10mg/0.2ml solution for injection pre-filled injector | 1 pre-filled disposable injection PoM £13.25 DT = £13.26
Methofill 15mg/0.3ml solution for injection pre-filled injector | 1 pre-filled disposable injection PoM £14.40 DT = £14.41
Methofill 17.5mg/0.35ml solution for injection pre-filled injector | 1 pre-filled disposable injection PoM £15.24 DT = £15.25
Methofill 25mg/0.5ml solution for injection pre-filled injector | 1 pre-filled disposable injection PoM £16.12 DT = £16.13
► Metoject PEN (medac UK)
Methotrexate 50 mg per 1 ml Metoject PEN 27.5mg/0.55ml solution for injection pre-filled pens | 1 pre-filled disposable injection PoM £16.50 DT = £16.50
Metoject PEN 17.5mg/0.35ml solution for injection pre-filled pens | 1 pre-filled disposable injection PoM £15.25 DT = £15.25
Metoject PEN 30mg/0.6ml solution for injection pre-filled pens | 1 pre-filled disposable injection PoM £16.56 DT = £16.56
Metoject PEN 12.5mg/0.25ml solution for injection pre-filled pens | 1 pre-filled disposable injection PoM £14.35 DT = £14.35
Metoject PEN 10mg/0.2ml solution for injection pre-filled pens | 1 pre-filled disposable injection PoM £13.26 DT = £13.26
Metoject PEN 15mg/0.3ml solution for injection pre-filled pens | 1 pre-filled disposable injection PoM £14.41 DT = £14.41
Metoject PEN 22.5mg/0.45ml solution for injection pre-filled pens | 1 pre-filled disposable injection PoM £16.11 DT = £16.11
Metoject PEN 7.5mg/0.15ml solution for injection pre-filled pens | 1 pre-filled disposable injection PoM £12.87 DT = £12.87
Metoject PEN 25mg/0.5ml solution for injection pre-filled pens | 1 pre-filled disposable injection PoM £16.13 DT = £16.13
Metoject PEN 20mg/0.4ml solution for injection pre-filled pens | 1 pre-filled disposable injection PoM £15.56 DT = £15.56
► Nordimet (Nordic Pharma Ltd)
Methotrexate 25 mg per 1 ml Nordimet 15mg/0.6ml solution for injection pre-filled pens | 1 pre-filled disposable injection PoM £14.92 DT = £14.92
Nordimet 20mg/0.8ml solution for injection pre-filled pens | 1 pre-filled disposable injection PoM £16.06 DT = £16.06
Nordimet 22.5mg/0.9ml solution for injection pre-filled pens | 1 pre-filled disposable injection PoM £16.61 DT = £16.61
Nordimet 12.5mg/0.5ml solution for injection pre-filled pens | 1 pre-filled disposable injection PoM £14.85 DT = £14.85
Nordimet 10mg/0.4ml solution for injection pre-filled pens | 1 pre-filled disposable injection PoM £13.77 DT = £13.77

8

Immune system and malignant disease

Nordimet 17.5mg/0.7ml solution for injection pre-filled pens | 1 pre-filled disposable injection [PoM] £15.75 DT = £15.75
Nordimet 25mg/1ml solution for injection pre-filled pens | 1 pre-filled disposable injection [PoM] £16.64 DT = £16.64
Nordimet 7.5mg/0.3ml solution for injection pre-filled pens | 1 pre-filled disposable injection [PoM] £13.37 DT = £13.37

▸ Zlatal (Nordic Pharma Ltd)
Methotrexate (as Methotrexate sodium) 25 mg per 1 ml Zlatal 17.5mg/0.7ml solution for injection pre-filled syringes | 1 pre-filled disposable injection [PoM] £15.75 DT = £15.75
Zlatal 10mg/0.4ml solution for injection pre-filled syringes | 1 pre-filled disposable injection [PoM] £13.77 DT = £13.77
Zlatal 25mg/1ml solution for injection pre-filled syringes | 1 pre-filled disposable injection [PoM] £16.64 DT = £16.64
Zlatal 20mg/0.8ml solution for injection pre-filled syringes | 1 pre-filled disposable injection [PoM] £16.06 DT = £16.06
Zlatal 12.5mg/0.5ml solution for injection pre-filled syringes | 1 pre-filled disposable injection [PoM] £14.85 DT = £14.85
Zlatal 7.5mg/0.3ml solution for injection pre-filled syringes | 1 pre-filled disposable injection [PoM] £13.37 DT = £13.37
Zlatal 22.5mg/0.9ml solution for injection pre-filled syringes | 1 pre-filled disposable injection [PoM] £16.61 DT = £16.61
Zlatal 15mg/0.6ml solution for injection pre-filled syringes | 1 pre-filled disposable injection [PoM] £14.92 DT = £14.92

Solution for infusion
▸ Methotrexate (Non-proprietary)
Methotrexate (as Methotrexate sodium) 100 mg per 1 ml Methotrexate 5g/50ml solution for infusion vials | 1 vial [PoM] £380.00–£400.00 (Hospital only)

Oral solution
▸ Methotrexate (Non-proprietary)
Methotrexate (as Methotrexate sodium) 2 mg per 1 ml Methotrexate 2mg/ml oral solution sugar free sugar-free | 35 ml [PoM] £114.00 DT = £95.00 sugar-free | 65 ml [PoM] £125.00 DT = £125.00

▸ Jylamvo (Intrapharm Laboratories Ltd)
Methotrexate (as Methotrexate sodium) 2 mg per 1 ml Jylamvo 2mg/ml oral solution sugar-free | 60 ml [PoM] £112.50

Nelarabine

10-Nov-2020

● **INDICATIONS AND DOSE**

T-cell acute lymphoblastic leukaemia and T-cell lymphoblastic lymphoma in patients who have relapsed or who are refractory after receiving at least two previous regimens
▸ BY INTRAVENOUS INFUSION
▸ Adult: (consult local protocol)

● CAUTIONS Previous or concurrent craniospinal irradiation (increased risk of neurotoxicity) · previous or concurrent intrathecal chemotherapy (increased risk of neurotoxicity)

● INTERACTIONS → Appendix 1: nelarabine

● SIDE-EFFECTS
▸ **Common or very common** Abdominal pain · anaemia · appetite decreased · arthralgia · asthenia · confusion · constipation · cough · diarrhoea · dizziness · drowsiness · dyspnoea · electrolyte imbalance · fever · gait abnormal · headache · hyperbilirubinaemia · hypotension · increased risk of infection · leucopenia · memory loss · movement disorders · muscle weakness · myalgia · nausea · neutropenia · oedema · pain · peripheral neuropathy · respiratory disorders · seizures · sensation abnormal · sepsis · stomatitis · taste altered · thrombocytopenia · tremor · tumour lysis syndrome · vision blurred · vomiting
▸ **Rare or very rare** Rhabdomyolysis
▸ **Frequency not known** Progressive multifocal leukoencephalopathy (PML)

SIDE-EFFECTS, FURTHER INFORMATION If neurotoxicity occurs, treatment should be discontinued.

● CONCEPTION AND CONTRACEPTION Manufacturer advises effective contraception during and for at least 3 months after treatment in men and women.

● PREGNANCY Avoid (toxicity in *animal* studies). See also *Pregnancy and reproductive function* in Cytotoxic drugs p. 932.

● BREAST FEEDING Discontinue breast-feeding.

● MONITORING REQUIREMENTS
▸ Neurotoxicity Close monitoring for neurological events is strongly recommended—discontinue if neurotoxicty occurs.

● PATIENT AND CARER ADVICE
Driving and skilled tasks Drowsiness may affect performance of skilled tasks (e.g. cycling or driving).

● NATIONAL FUNDING/ACCESS DECISIONS
For full details see funding body website
Scottish Medicines Consortium (SMC) decisions
▸ Nelarabine (*Atriance*®) for the treatment of patients with T-cell acute lymphoblastic leukaemia (T-ALL) and T-cell lymphoblastic lymphoma (T-LBL) (April 2008) SMC No. 454/08 Recommended with restrictions

● MEDICINAL FORMS There can be variation in the licensing of different medicines containing the same drug.
Solution for infusion
ELECTROLYTES: May contain Sodium
▸ Atriance (Novartis Pharmaceuticals UK Ltd) ▼
Nelarabine 5 mg per 1 ml Atriance 250mg/50ml solution for infusion vials | 6 vial [PoM] £1,332.00 (Hospital only)

Pemetrexed

10-Nov-2020

● **DRUG ACTION** Pemetrexed inhibits thymidylate transferase and other folate-dependent enzymes.

● **INDICATIONS AND DOSE**

Treatment of unresectable malignant pleural mesothelioma which has not previously been treated with chemotherapy (in combination with cisplatin) | **First-line treatment of locally advanced or metastatic non-small cell lung cancer other than predominantly squamous cell histology (in combination with cisplatin)** | **Second-line treatment of locally advanced or metastatic non-small cell lung cancer other than predominantly squamous cell histology (monotherapy)** | **Maintenance treatment in locally advanced or metastatic non-small cell lung cancer other than predominantly squamous cell histology that has not progressed immediately following platinum-based chemotherapy (monotherapy)**
▸ BY INTRAVENOUS INFUSION
▸ Adult: (consult local protocol)

● CAUTIONS Diabetes · history of cardiovascular disease · prophylactic folic acid supplementation required (consult product literature) · prophylactic vitamin B_{12} supplementation required (consult product literature)

● INTERACTIONS → Appendix 1: pemetrexed

● SIDE-EFFECTS
▸ **Common or very common** Appetite decreased · fatigue · mucositis · nausea · neuropathy sensory · oedema · pain · renal disorder · skin reactions · stomatitis · vomiting

● CONCEPTION AND CONTRACEPTION Manufacturer advises effective contraception during treatment. Men must avoid fathering a child during and for 6 months after treatment.

● PREGNANCY Avoid (toxicity in *animal* studies). See also *Pregnancy and reproductive function* in Cytotoxic drugs p. 932.

● BREAST FEEDING Discontinue breast-feeding.

● RENAL IMPAIRMENT Manufacturer advises avoid if creatinine clearance less than 45 mL/minute—no information available.

● NATIONAL FUNDING/ACCESS DECISIONS
For full details see funding body website

NICE decisions
▶ Pemetrexed for the treatment of non-small cell lung cancer (August 2007) NICE TA124 Not recommended
▶ Pemetrexed for the first-line treatment of non-small cell lung cancer (September 2009) NICE TA181 Recommended with restrictions
▶ Pemetrexed maintenance treatment for non-squamous non-small cell lung cancer after pemetrexed and cisplatin (August 2016) NICE TA402 Recommended with restrictions
▶ Pemetrexed for the maintenance treatment of non-small-cell lung cancer (updated August 2017) NICE TA190 Recommended
▶ Pemetrexed for the treatment of malignant pleural mesothelioma (January 2008) NICE TA135 Recommended with restrictions

Scottish Medicines Consortium (SMC) decisions
▶ Pemetrexed (*Alimta*®) as monotherapy for the second line treatment of patients with locally advanced or metastatic non-small cell lung cancer other than predominantly squamous cell histology (September 2008) SMC No. 342/07 Recommended with restrictions
▶ Pemetrexed (*Alimta*®) for the first line treatment of patients with locally advanced or metastatic non-small cell lung cancer (February 2010) SMC No. 531/09 Recommended with restrictions
▶ Pemetrexed (*Alimta*®) as monotherapy for the maintenance treatment of locally advanced or metastatic non-small cell lung cancer other than predominantly squamous cell histology in patients whose disease has not progressed immediately following platinum-based chemotherapy (December 2014) SMC No. 770/12 Recommended

● MEDICINAL FORMS There can be variation in the licensing of different medicines containing the same drug.

Powder for solution for infusion
ELECTROLYTES: May contain Sodium
▶ Pemetrexed (Non-proprietary)
  Pemetrexed (as Pemetrexed disodium) 100 mg Pemetrexed 100mg powder for concentrate for solution for infusion vials | 1 vial PoM £125.00–£185.22 (Hospital only)
  Pemetrexed (as Pemetrexed disodium) 500 mg Pemetrexed 500mg powder for concentrate for solution for infusion vials | 1 vial PoM £450.00–£926.10 (Hospital only)
▶ Alimta (Eli Lilly and Company Ltd)
  Pemetrexed (as Pemetrexed disodium) 100 mg Alimta 100mg powder for concentrate for solution for infusion vials | 1 vial PoM £160.00 (Hospital only)
  Pemetrexed (as Pemetrexed disodium) 500 mg Alimta 500mg powder for concentrate for solution for infusion vials | 1 vial PoM £800.00 (Hospital only)

Tegafur with gimeracil and oteracil

17-Nov-2020

● DRUG ACTION Tegafur is a prodrug of fluorouracil. Gimeracil inhibits the degradation of fluorouracil and oteracil decreases the activity of fluorouracil in normal gastrointestinal mucosa.

● INDICATIONS AND DOSE
Treatment of advanced gastric cancer when used in combination with cisplatin
▶ BY MOUTH
▶ Adult: (consult local protocol)

IMPORTANT SAFETY INFORMATION
RISKS OF INCORRECT DOSING OF ORAL ANTI-CANCER MEDICINES
See Cytotoxic drugs p. 932.

MHRA/CHM ADVICE: 5-FLUOROURACIL (INTRAVENOUS), CAPECITABINE, TEGAFUR: DPD TESTING RECOMMENDED BEFORE INITIATION TO IDENTIFY PATIENTS AT INCREASED RISK OF SEVERE AND FATAL TOXICITY (OCTOBER 2020)
Patients with partial or complete dihydropyrimidine dehydrogenase (DPD) deficiency are at increased risk of

severe and fatal toxicity during treatment with fluoropyrimidines. Healthcare professionals are advised to test all patients for DPD deficiency before initiating treatment and confirm their, including family, history of complete or partial DPD deficiency. Tegafur with gimeracil and oteracil is contra-indicated in patients with known complete DPD deficiency; in those with partial DPD deficiency, a reduced starting dose is recommended. Patients should be monitored for toxicity, particularly during the first cycle of treatment or after a dose increase; severe toxicity can occur even in those with negative test results for DPD deficiency. Healthcare professionals should also counsel patients on the benefits and risks of their treatment and ensure they are provided with the patient information leaflet.

● CONTRA-INDICATIONS Complete dihydropyrimidine dehydrogenase deficiency (increased risk of severe, life-threatening, or fatal toxicity)—consult product literature

● CAUTIONS Partial dihydropyrimidine dehydrogenase deficiency

● INTERACTIONS → Appendix 1: tegafur

● SIDE-EFFECTS
▶ **Common or very common** Anaemia · appetite abnormal · asthenia · constipation · cough · decreased leucocytes · dehydration · diarrhoea · dizziness · dry mouth · dysphagia · dyspnoea · electrolyte imbalance · embolism and thrombosis · eye disorders · eye inflammation · gastrointestinal discomfort · gastrointestinal disorders · haemorrhage · headache · hearing impairment · hiccups · hyperbilirubinaemia · hypertension · hypoproteinaemia · hypotension · insomnia · nausea · nerve disorders · neutropenia · oral disorders · taste altered · thrombocytopenia · vision disorders · vomiting
▶ **Uncommon** Aerophagia · allergic rhinitis · alopecia · angina pectoris · anxiety · aphasia · arrhythmias · ascites · breast abnormalities · burping · cerebrovascular insufficiency · chills · coagulation disorders · confusion · depression · drowsiness · dysphonia · ear discomfort · encephalopathy · eosinophilia · fever · gout · hallucination · heart failure · hemiparesis · hyperaemia · hyperglobulinaemia · hyperglycaemia · hyperlipidaemia · hypertrichosis · hypovolaemic shock · increased leucocytes · increased risk of infection · joint disorders · limb discomfort · loss of consciousness · memory loss · movement disorders · mucositis · muscle complaints · muscle weakness · myocardial infarction · nail disorders · nasal complaints · neoplasm complications · nephrotoxicity · oedema · oesophageal spasm · pain · palpitations · pancytopenia · pericardial effusion · personality disorder · renal impairment · seizure · sensation abnormal · sepsis · sexual dysfunction · skin reactions · smell altered · sweat changes · syncope · throat complaints · thrombocytosis · tremor · urinary frequency increased · vasodilation · vertigo · weight changes
▶ **Rare or very rare** Acute hepatic failure · chest discomfort · feeling cold · interstitial lung disease · local swelling · malaise · multi organ failure · pancreatitis acute · photosensitivity reaction · rhabdomyolysis · severe cutaneous adverse reactions (SCARs)

● CONCEPTION AND CONTRACEPTION Manufacturer advises effective contraception during and for up to 6 months after treatment.

● PREGNANCY Avoid. See also *Pregnancy and reproductive function* in Cytotoxic drugs p. 932.

● BREAST FEEDING Discontinue breast-feeding.

● RENAL IMPAIRMENT Manufacturer advises avoid if creatinine clearance less than 30 mL/minute.
  Dose adjustments Reduce dose if creatinine clearance 30–50 mL/minute—consult product literature.

8

Immune system and malignant disease

● NATIONAL FUNDING/ACCESS DECISIONS
For full details see funding body website
Scottish Medicines Consortium (SMC) decisions
▸ Tegafur with gimeracil and oteracil (*Teysuno*®) for the
treatment of advanced gastric cancer when given in
combination with cisplatin (September 2012) SMC No. 802/12
Recommended with restrictions

● MEDICINAL FORMS There can be variation in the licensing of
different medicines containing the same drug.
Capsule
CAUTIONARY AND ADVISORY LABELS 23
▸ Teysuno (Nordic Pharma Ltd)
**Gimeracil 4.35 mg, Oteracil (as Oteracil potassium) 11.8 mg,
Tegafur 15 mg** Teysuno 15mg/4.35mg/11.8mg capsules |
126 capsule PoM £279.72
**Gimeracil 5.8 mg, Oteracil (as Oteracil potassium) 15.8 mg,
Tegafur 20 mg** Teysuno 20mg/5.8mg/15.8mg capsules |
84 capsule PoM £248.40

Tioguanine

(Thioguanine)

27-Jul-2020

● INDICATIONS AND DOSE

Acute leukaemia | Chronic myeloid leukaemia
▸ BY MOUTH
▸ Adult: 100–200 mg/m^2 daily, can be given at various
stages of treatment in short-term cycles

IMPORTANT SAFETY INFORMATION
RISKS OF INCORRECT DOSING OF ORAL ANTI-CANCER MEDICINES
See Cytotoxic drugs p. 932.

● CAUTIONS Thiopurine methyltransferase status
CAUTIONS, FURTHER INFORMATION
▸ Thiopurine methyltransferase The enzyme thiopurine
methyltransferase (TPMT) metabolises thiopurine drugs
(azathioprine, mercaptopurine, tioguanine); the risk of
myelosuppression is increased in patients with reduced
activity of the enzyme, particularly for the few individuals
in whom TPMT activity is undetectable. Those with
reduced TPMT activity may be treated under specialist
supervision.
▸ Long-term therapy Manufacturer advises long-term therapy
is no longer recommended because of the high risk of liver
toxicity.
● INTERACTIONS → Appendix 1: tioguanine
● SIDE-EFFECTS
▸ Common or very common Bone marrow failure ·
gastrointestinal disorders · hepatic disorders ·
hyperbilirubinaemia · hyperuricaemia · hyperuricosuria ·
nodular regenerative hyperplasia · oesophageal varices ·
sinusoidal obstruction syndrome · splenomegaly ·
stomatitis · thrombocytopenia · uric acid nephropathy ·
weight increased
▸ Frequency not known Photosensitivity reaction
● CONCEPTION AND CONTRACEPTION Ensure effective
contraception during treatment in men or women.
● PREGNANCY Avoid (teratogenicity reported when men
receiving tioguanine have fathered children). See also
Pregnancy and reproductive function in Cytotoxic drugs
p. 932.
● BREAST FEEDING Discontinue breast-feeding.
● HEPATIC IMPAIRMENT Manufacturer advises caution.
Dose adjustments Manufacturer advises consider dose
reduction.

● RENAL IMPAIRMENT
Dose adjustments Reduce dose.
● PRE-TREATMENT SCREENING Manufacturer advises
consider measuring thiopurine methyltransferase (TPMT)
activity before starting tioguanine therapy.
● MONITORING REQUIREMENTS Monitor liver function
weekly—discontinue if liver toxicity develops.

● MEDICINAL FORMS There can be variation in the licensing of
different medicines containing the same drug. Forms available
from special-order manufacturers include: capsule
Tablet
▸ Tioguanine (Non-proprietary)
Tioguanine 40 mg Tioguanine 40mg tablets | 25 tablet PoM
£109.57 DT = £109.57

Trifluridine with tipiracil

02-Sep-2020

● DRUG ACTION Trifluridine is an antimetabolite that
interferes with cancer cell DNA synthesis and inhibits cell
proliferation; tipiracil is a TPase inhibitor that boosts
trifluridine concentrations.

● INDICATIONS AND DOSE

**Metastatic colorectal cancer, in patients previously
treated with (or unsuitable for treatment with) available
therapies including fluoropyrimidine-, oxaliplatin-, and
irinotecan-based chemotherapies, or anti-vascular
endothelial growth factor (VEGF) agents, or anti-
epidermal growth factor receptor (EGFR) agents
(specialist use only)**
▸ BY MOUTH
▸ Adult: Initially 35 mg/m^2 twice daily (max. per dose
80 mg), given on days 1 to 5 and days 8 to 12 of each
28-day cycle, consult product literature for further
information on dose adjustment

IMPORTANT SAFETY INFORMATION
RISKS OF INCORRECT DOSING OF ORAL ANTI-CANCER MEDICINES
See Cytotoxic drugs p. 932.

● SIDE-EFFECTS
▸ Common or very common Alopecia · anaemia · appetite
decreased · asthenia · constipation · cough · decreased
leucocytes · diarrhoea · dizziness · dyspnoea · fever ·
flushing · gastrointestinal discomfort · headache ·
hyperbilirubinaemia · hypoalbuminaemia · increased
leucocytes · increased risk of infection · insomnia · malaise
· mucositis · nausea · neutropenia · oedema · oral disorders
· peripheral neuropathy · skin reactions · taste altered ·
thrombocytopenia · urine abnormalities · vomiting · weight
decreased
▸ Uncommon Angina pectoris · anxiety · arrhythmia · ascites ·
bile duct disorders · cancer pain · cataract · conjunctivitis ·
cystitis · dehydration · dry eye · dysphonia · ear discomfort ·
electrolyte imbalance · embolism and thrombosis ·
erythropenia · feeling of body temperature change ·
gastrointestinal disorders · gout · haemorrhage ·
hepatotoxicity · hyperglycaemia · hyperhidrosis ·
hypertension · hypotension · joint disorders · lethargy ·
menstrual disorder · muscle complaints · muscle weakness
· nail disorder · neurotoxicity · oropharyngeal pain · pain ·
palpitations · pancreatitis acute · pancytopenia ·
photosensitivity reaction · pleural effusion · QT interval
prolongation · renal failure · rhinorrhoea · sensation
abnormal · sensation of pressure · septic shock (including
fatal cases) · syncope · urinary disorder · vertigo · vision
disorders
● CONCEPTION AND CONTRACEPTION Manufacturer advises
effective contraception in women of child-bearing
potential and in men with a partner of child-bearing

potential, during treatment and for 6 months after stopping treatment. Manufacturer also advises use of an additional barrier method in women using hormonal contraceptives—effect of trifluridine with tipiracil on hormonal contraception unknown.

- PREGNANCY Manufacturer advises avoid unless essential—reproductive toxicity in *animal* studies.
- BREAST FEEDING Manufacturer advises avoid—present in milk in *animal* studies.
- HEPATIC IMPAIRMENT Manufacturer advises avoid in moderate to severe impairment (limited information available).
- RENAL IMPAIRMENT Manufacturer advises caution if eGFR 30–59 mL/minute/1.73 m² —monitor for haematological toxicities; manufacturer advises avoid if eGFR less than 30 mL/minute/ 1.73m² —no information available.
- MONITORING REQUIREMENTS Manufacturer advises obtain baseline blood cell counts before and during treatment; monitor closely for myelosuppression. Manufacturer also advises monitoring for proteinuria before and during treatment.
- NATIONAL FUNDING/ACCESS DECISIONS For full details see funding body website

NICE decisions
▸ Trifluridine with tipiracil for previously treated metastatic colorectal cancer (August 2016) NICE TA405 Recommended with restrictions

Scottish Medicines Consortium (SMC) decisions
▸ Trifluridine / tipiracil (*Lonsurf*®) for the treatment of adult patients with metastatic colorectal cancer who have been previously treated with, or are not considered candidates for, available therapies including fluoropyrimidine-, oxaliplatin- and irinotecan-based chemotherapies, anti vascular endothelial growth factor agents, and anti-epidermal growth factor receptor agents (February 2017) SMC No. 1221/17 Recommended

- MEDICINAL FORMS There can be variation in the licensing of different medicines containing the same drug.

Tablet
CAUTIONARY AND ADVISORY LABELS 21
▸ Lonsurf (Servier Laboratories Ltd) ▼
Tipiracil (as Tipiracil hydrochloride) 6.14 mg, Trifluridine 15 mg Lonsurf 15mg/6.14mg tablets | 20 tablet PoM £500.00 | 60 tablet PoM £1,500.00
Tipiracil (as Tipiracil hydrochloride) 8.19 mg, Trifluridine 20 mg Lonsurf 20mg/8.19mg tablets | 20 tablet PoM £666.67 | 60 tablet PoM £2,000.00

ANTINEOPLASTIC DRUGS > CYTOTOXIC ANTIBIOTICS AND RELATED SUBSTANCES

Bleomycin
28-Jul-2020

- INDICATIONS AND DOSE

Squamous cell carcinoma | Metastatic germ cell cancer | Non-Hodgkin's lymphoma
▸ BY INTRAMUSCULAR INJECTION, OR BY INTRAVENOUS INJECTION, OR BY INTRAVENOUS INFUSION, OR BY INTRA-ARTERIAL INFUSION, OR BY LOCAL INFILTRATION
▸ Adult: (consult product literature or local protocols)

- CONTRA-INDICATIONS Acute pulmonary infection · significantly reduced lung function
- CAUTIONS Caution in handling—irritant to tissues · risk factors for pulmonary toxicity
- INTERACTIONS → Appendix 1: bleomycin
- SIDE-EFFECTS
▸ **Common or very common** Alopecia · angular stomatitis · appetite decreased · chills · fever (after administration) · haemorrhage · headache · interstitial pneumonia ·

leucopenia · malaise · nail discolouration · nail disorder · nausea · pain · pulmonary fibrosis (dose-related) · scleroderma · skin reactions · stomatitis · vomiting · weight decreased
▸ **Uncommon** Diarrhoea · dizziness · hepatocellular injury · oliguria · shock · urinary disorders · vein wall hypertrophy · venous stenosis

SIDE-EFFECTS, FURTHER INFORMATION **Progressive pulmonary fibrosis** Progressive pulmonary fibrosis is dose-related, and may occur at lower doses in the elderly. Suspicious chest X-ray changes are an indication to stop therapy with this drug.
Pulmonary toxicity Patients who have received bleomycin may be at risk of developing pulmonary toxicity if exposed to high inspired oxygen concentrations, for example peri-operatively, or during lung function testing.

- CONCEPTION AND CONTRACEPTION Contraceptive advice required, see *Pregnancy and reproductive function* in Cytotoxic drugs p. 932.
- PREGNANCY Avoid (teratogenic and carcinogenic in *animal* studies). See also *Pregnancy and reproductive function* in Cytotoxic drugs p. 932
- BREAST FEEDING Discontinue breast feeding.
- RENAL IMPAIRMENT
Dose adjustments Reduce dose by half if serum creatinine 177–354 micromol/litre; reduce dose further if serum-creatinine greater than 354 micromol/litre.
- PRESCRIBING AND DISPENSING INFORMATION To conform to the European Pharmacopoeia vials previously labelled as containing '15 units' of bleomycin are now labelled as containing 15 000 units. The amount of bleomycin in the vial has not changed.
- MEDICINAL FORMS There can be variation in the licensing of different medicines containing the same drug.

Powder for solution for injection
▸ Bleo-Kyowa (Kyowa Kirin Ltd)
Bleomycin (as Bleomycin sulfate) 15000 unit Bleo-Kyowa 15,000unit powder for solution for injection vials | 10 vial PoM £190.60

Mitomycin
28-Jul-2020

- INDICATIONS AND DOSE

Recurrent superficial bladder tumours (bladder instillation)
▸ BY INTRAVESICAL INSTILLATION
▸ Adult: (consult product literature or local protocols)

Upper gastro-intestinal cancer (specialist use only) | Breast cancer (specialist use only) | Non-small cell lung cancer (specialist use only) | Pancreatic cancer (specialist use only)
▸ BY INTRAVENOUS INJECTION
▸ Adult: (consult product literature or local protocols)

> **IMPORTANT SAFETY INFORMATION**
> MHRA/CHM ADVICE: *MITOMYCIN-C KYOWA* ® 40 MG RESTRICTED TO INTRAVESICAL ADMINISTRATION ONLY FOR TREATMENT OF SUPERFICIAL BLADDER CANCER (SEPTEMBER 2019)
> Sub-visible particles, at levels above specification limits, have been observed after reconstitution of *Mitomycin-C Kyowa*® 40 mg; healthcare professionals are advised that its use has been restricted to the treatment of superficial bladder cancer via the intravesical route only.

- CAUTIONS Caution in handling—irritant to tissues
- INTERACTIONS → Appendix 1: mitomycin

Immune system and malignant disease

8

- SIDE-EFFECTS
  GENERAL SIDE-EFFECTS
  ▶ **Common or very common** Bone marrow disorders · cough · cystitis · haemorrhage · leucopenia · malaise · nausea · respiratory disorders · skin reactions · thrombocytopenia · vomiting
  ▶ **Uncommon** Alopecia · appetite decreased · diarrhoea · fever
  ▶ **Rare or very rare** Hepatic disorders · increased risk of infection · renal disorder · sepsis
  ▶ **Frequency not known** Anaemia · asthenia · chills · constipation · eosinophilia · erythropenia · flushing · hypertension · lethargy · neutropenia · oedema · weight decreased

  SPECIFIC SIDE-EFFECTS
  ▶ **Common or very common**
  ▶ With intravenous use Dyspnoea · extravasation necrosis · glomerulonephropathy · nephropathy · renal impairment
  ▶ With intravesical use Hypersensitivity · urinary disorders · urinary tract discomfort
  ▶ **Uncommon**
  ▶ With intravenous use Mucositis · oral disorders
  ▶ **Rare or very rare**
  ▶ With intravenous use Haemolytic anaemia · heart failure · pulmonary hypertension · sinusoidal obstruction syndrome
  ▶ With intravesical use Acute kidney injury · bladder disorders · urinary tract stenosis
  ▶ **Frequency not known**
  ▶ With intravenous use Abdominal discomfort · cholecystitis · injection site necrosis · neoplasms · shock · urine abnormalities · vascular pain
  ▶ With intravesical use Pain · penile necrosis · proteinuria · pulmonary oedema · ulcer
  SIDE-EFFECTS, FURTHER INFORMATION Mitomycin is usually administered at 6-weekly intervals because it causes delayed bone-marrow toxicity. Prolonged use may result in a cumulative effect.

- CONCEPTION AND CONTRACEPTION Contraceptive advice required, see *Pregnancy and reproductive function* in Cytotoxic drugs p. 932.

- PREGNANCY Avoid (teratogenic in *animal* studies). See also *Pregnancy and reproductive function* in Cytotoxic drugs p. 932.

- BREAST FEEDING Discontinue breast-feeding.

- MEDICINAL FORMS There can be variation in the licensing of different medicines containing the same drug.
  Powder for solution for injection
  ▶ Mitomycin (Non-proprietary)
    Mitomycin 40 mg Mitomycin 40mg powder for solution for injection vials | 1 vial PoM £75.89 (Hospital only)
  ▶ Mitomycin (Imported (United States))
    Mitomycin 5 mg Mitomycin 5mg powder for solution for injection vials | 1 vial PoM Ⓢ (Hospital only)
  ▶ Mitocin (Vygoris Ltd)
    Mitomycin 20 mg Mitocin 20mg powder for solution for injection vials | 1 vial PoM £39.00 (Hospital only)
  Powder and solvent for intravesical solution
  ELECTROLYTES: May contain Sodium
  ▶ Mitomycin (Non-proprietary)
    Mitomycin 40 mg Mitomycin 40mg powder and solvent for intravesical solution vials | 1 vial PoM £135.00

Pentostatin

28-Jul-2020

- **INDICATIONS AND DOSE**
  Hairy cell leukaemia (initiated in specialist centres)
  ▶ BY INTRAVENOUS INJECTION, OR BY INTRAVENOUS INFUSION
  ▶ Adult: To be given on alternate weeks (consult product literature)

- INTERACTIONS → Appendix 1: pentostatin

- SIDE-EFFECTS
  ▶ **Common or very common** Agranulocytosis · alopecia · amenorrhoea · anaemia · angina pectoris · anxiety · appetite decreased · arrhythmias · arthritis · asthenia · asthma · atrioventricular block · blood disorder · bone disorder · bone marrow disorders · breast mass · cardiac arrest · chest pain · chills · confusion · constipation · cough · deafness · death · depersonalisation · depression · diarrhoea · dizziness · drowsiness · dry eye · dry mouth · dysarthria · dysphagia · dyspnoea · ear pain · electrolyte imbalance · embolism and thrombosis · emotional lability · eosinophilia · eye disorders · eye inflammation · eye pain · febrile neutropenia · fever · fluid imbalance · flushing · gastrointestinal discomfort · gastrointestinal disorders · gout · graft versus host disease · haemorrhage · hallucination · hangover · headaches · heart failure · hostility · hyperbilirubinaemia · hyperglycaemia · hyperhidrosis · hypersensitivity · hypertension · hypotension · increased risk of infection · influenza like illness · jaundice · joint disorders · leucopenia · lymphadenopathy · malaise · memory loss · meningism · movement disorders · muscle complaints · nausea · neoplasms · nephrolithiasis · nephropathy · nerve disorders · neurotoxicity (withhold or discontinue) · oedema · oral disorders · pain · paralysis · pericardial effusion · photosensitivity reaction · pulmonary oedema · rash (withhold if severe) · renal impairment · respiratory disorders · retinopathy · seborrhoea · seizures · sensation abnormal · sepsis · sexual dysfunction · skin reactions · sleep disorders · splenomegaly · syncope · taste altered · thinking abnormal · thrombocytopenia · tinnitus · tremor · urinary disorders · urogenital disorder · vasculitis · vertigo · vision disorders · vomiting · weight changes
  ▶ **Uncommon** Angioedema · antibiotic associated colitis · capillary leak syndrome · cardiomyopathy · cystitis · haemolytic anaemia · mucositis · multi organ failure · myocardial infarction · pure red cell aplasia · transplant failure · tumour lysis syndrome
  ▶ **Rare or very rare** Dementia · pericarditis · shock · Stevens-Johnson syndrome · systemic inflammatory response syndrome
  SIDE-EFFECTS, FURTHER INFORMATION Pentostatin can cause myelosuppression, immunosuppression, and a number of other side-effects that may be severe. Treatment should be withheld in patients who develop a severe rash, and withheld or discontinued in patients showing signs of neurotoxicity.

- CONCEPTION AND CONTRACEPTION Manufacturer advises that men should not father children during and for 6 months after treatment.

- PREGNANCY Avoid (teratogenic in *animal* studies). See also *Pregnancy and reproductive function* in Cytotoxic drugs p. 932.

- BREAST FEEDING Discontinue breast-feeding.

- HEPATIC IMPAIRMENT Manufacturer advises caution (limited information available).

- RENAL IMPAIRMENT Avoid if creatinine clearance less than 60 mL/minute.

- MEDICINAL FORMS There can be variation in the licensing of different medicines containing the same drug.
  Powder for solution for injection
  ▶ Nipent (Pfizer Ltd)
    Pentostatin 10 mg Nipent 10mg powder for solution for injection vials | 1 vial PoM £734.21 (Hospital only)

ANTINEOPLASTIC DRUGS > PLANT ALKALOIDS

Trabectedin

07-Dec-2020

● **INDICATIONS AND DOSE**

Treatment of advanced soft-tissue sarcoma when treatment with anthracyclines and ifosfamide has failed or is contra-indicated | Treatment of relapsed platinum-sensitive ovarian cancer (in combination with pegylated liposomal doxorubicin)
▶ BY INTRAVENOUS INFUSION
▶ Adult: (consult product literature or local protocols)

● CONTRA-INDICATIONS Elevated creatine phosphokinase (consult product literature)

● INTERACTIONS → Appendix 1: trabectedin

● SIDE-EFFECTS
▶ **Common or very common** Alopecia · anaemia · appetite decreased · arthralgia · asthenia · back pain · constipation · cough · dehydration · diarrhoea · dizziness · dyspnoea · fever · flushing · gastrointestinal discomfort · headache · hyperbilirubinaemia · hypersensitivity · hypokalaemia · hypotension · infection · insomnia · leucopenia · mucositis · myalgia · nausea · neutropenia · oedema · paraesthesia · peripheral neuropathy · skin reactions · stomatitis · taste altered · thrombocytopenia · vomiting · weight decreased
▶ **Uncommon** Capillary leak syndrome · septic shock
▶ **Rare or very rare** Hepatic failure
▶ **Frequency not known** Extravasation necrosis · rhabdomyolysis

SIDE-EFFECTS, FURTHER INFORMATION A corticosteroid, such as dexamethasone by intravenous infusion, must be given 30 minutes before therapy for its antiemetic and hepatoprotective effects (consult product literature).

● CONCEPTION AND CONTRACEPTION Effective contraception recommended during and for at least 3 months after treatment in women and during and for at least 5 months after treatment in men.

● PREGNANCY See *Pregnancy and reproductive function* in Cytotoxic drugs p. 932.

● BREAST FEEDING Manufacturer advises avoid breast-feeding during and for 3 months after treatment.

● HEPATIC IMPAIRMENT Manufacturer advises caution (risk of increased exposure).
Dose adjustments Manufacturer advises consider dose reduction.

● RENAL IMPAIRMENT Avoid monotherapy if creatinine clearance less than 30 mL/minute. Avoid combination regimens if creatinine clearance less than 60 mL/minute.

● MONITORING REQUIREMENTS
▶ Specific haematological, renal and hepatic parameters must be monitored and within certain ranges prior to starting treatment and repeated weekly during the first 2 cycles and at least once between treatments in subsequent cycles—consult product literature for full details.
▶ Monitor for signs and symptoms of rhabdomyolysis (including myelotoxicity, severe liver function disorder, renal failure, muscle weakness or pain)—monitor creatine phosphokinase closely and discontinue treatment (consult product literature).

● NATIONAL FUNDING/ACCESS DECISIONS
For full details see funding body website
NICE decisions
▶ Trabectedin for the treatment of advanced soft tissue sarcoma (February 2010) NICE TA185 Recommended with restrictions
▶ Topotecan, pegylated liposomal doxorubicin hydrochloride, paclitaxel, trabectedin and gemcitabine for treating recurrent ovarian cancer (April 2016) NICE TA389 Not recommended

Scottish Medicines Consortium (SMC) decisions
▶ Trabectedin (*Yondelis*®) for the treatment of adult patients with advanced soft tissue sarcoma, after failure of anthracyclines and ifosfamide, or who are unsuited to receive these agents (November 2020) SMC No. SMC2283 Recommended

● MEDICINAL FORMS There can be variation in the licensing of different medicines containing the same drug.
Powder for solution for infusion
▶ Yondelis (Immedica Pharma AB)
Trabectedin 250 microgram Yondelis 0.25mg powder for concentrate for solution for infusion vials | 1 vial [PoM] £363.00 (Hospital only)
Trabectedin 1 mg Yondelis 1mg powder for concentrate for solution for infusion vials | 1 vial [PoM] £1,366.00 (Hospital only)

ANTINEOPLASTIC DRUGS > PLATINUM COMPOUNDS

Carboplatin

08-Mar-2019

● **INDICATIONS AND DOSE**

Advanced ovarian cancer [epithelial origin] | Small cell lung cancer | High risk seminoma (stage I) testicular germ cell tumours [adjuvant treatment]
▶ BY INTRAVENOUS INFUSION
▶ Adult: (consult product literature)

● INTERACTIONS → Appendix 1: platinum compounds

● SIDE-EFFECTS
▶ **Common or very common** Alopecia · anaemia · asthenia · cardiovascular disorder · constipation · diarrhoea · gastrointestinal discomfort · haemorrhage · hypersensitivity · increased risk of infection · leucopenia · mucosal abnormalities · musculoskeletal disorder · nausea · neutropenia · ototoxicity · peripheral neuropathy · reflexes decreased · respiratory disorders · sensation abnormal · skin reactions · taste altered · thrombocytopenia · urogenital disorder · vision disorders · vomiting
▶ **Rare or very rare** Angioedema
▶ **Frequency not known** Appetite decreased · bone marrow failure · chills · dehydration · embolism · encephalopathy · extravasation necrosis · fever · haemolytic uraemic syndrome · heart failure · hypertension · hyponatraemia · hypotension · injection site necrosis · malaise · pancreatitis · stomatitis · stroke · treatment related secondary malignancy · tumour lysis syndrome

● CONCEPTION AND CONTRACEPTION Contraceptive advice required, see *Pregnancy and reproductive function* in Cytotoxic drugs p. 932.

● PREGNANCY Avoid (teratogenic and embryotoxic in *animal* studies). See also *Pregnancy and reproductive function* in Cytotoxic drugs p. 932.

● BREAST FEEDING Discontinue breast-feeding.

● RENAL IMPAIRMENT Avoid if creatinine clearance less than 20 mL/minute.
Dose adjustments Reduce dose.
Monitoring Monitor haematological parameters in renal impairment.
Monitor renal function in renal impairment.

● PRESCRIBING AND DISPENSING INFORMATION Carboplatin can be given in an outpatient setting.

● NATIONAL FUNDING/ACCESS DECISIONS
For full details see funding body website
NICE decisions
▶ Bevacizumab in combination with paclitaxel and carboplatin for the first-line treatment of advanced ovarian cancer (May 2013) NICE TA284 Not recommended

▸ Bevacizumab in combination with gemcitabine and carboplatin for treating the first recurrence of platinum-sensitive advanced ovarian cancer (May 2013) NICE TA285 Not recommended

● MEDICINAL FORMS There can be variation in the licensing of different medicines containing the same drug.
Solution for infusion
▸ Carboplatin (Non-proprietary)
Carboplatin 10 mg per 1 ml Carboplatin 50mg/5ml concentrate for solution for infusion vials | 1 vial [PoM] £20.20–£21.70 (Hospital only)
Carboplatin 150mg/15ml concentrate for solution for infusion | 1 vial [PoM] £56.06–£60.59 (Hospital only)
Carboplatin 600mg/60ml concentrate for solution for infusion | 1 vial [PoM] £232.64–£256.08 (Hospital only)
Carboplatin 600mg/60ml solution for infusion vials | 1 vial [PoM] £260.00 (Hospital only)
Carboplatin 450mg/45ml concentrate for solution for infusion | 1 vial [PoM] £166.32–£181.77 (Hospital only)
Carboplatin 450mg/45ml solution for infusion vials | 1 vial [PoM] £197.48 (Hospital only)
Carboplatin 150mg/15ml solution for infusion vials | 1 vial [PoM] £65.83 (Hospital only)
Carboplatin 50mg/5ml solution for infusion vials | 1 vial [PoM] £22.86 (Hospital only)

Cisplatin

13-Aug-2020

● INDICATIONS AND DOSE
Treatment of testicular, lung, cervical, bladder, head and neck, and ovarian cancer (alone or in combination)
▸ BY INTRAVENOUS INFUSION
▸ Adult: (consult product literature)

● CAUTIONS Manufacturer advises cisplatin requires intensive intravenous hydration and treatment may be complicated by severe nausea and vomiting.
● INTERACTIONS → Appendix 1: platinum compounds
● SIDE-EFFECTS
▸ **Common or very common** Anaemia · arrhythmias · bone marrow failure · electrolyte imbalance · extravasation necrosis · fever · leucopenia · nephrotoxicity (dose-related and potentially cumulative) · sepsis · thrombocytopenia
▸ **Uncommon** Anaphylactoid reaction · ototoxicity (dose-related and potentially cumulative) · spermatogenesis abnormal
▸ **Rare or very rare** Acute leukaemia · cardiac arrest · encephalopathy · myocardial infarction · nerve disorders · seizure · stomatitis
▸ **Frequency not known** Alopecia · appetite decreased · asthenia · autonomic dysfunction · cardiac disorder · cerebrovascular insufficiency · deafness · dehydration · diarrhoea · haemolytic anaemia · hiccups · hyperuricaemia · infection · Lhermitte's sign · malaise · muscle spasms · myelopathy · nausea · papilloedema · pulmonary embolism · rash · Raynaud's phenomenon · renal impairment · renal tubular disorder · retinal discolouration · SIADH · taste loss · tetany · thrombotic microangiopathy · tinnitus · vision disorders · vomiting
● CONCEPTION AND CONTRACEPTION Manufacturer advises effective contraception during and for at least 6 months after treatment in men or women.
● PREGNANCY Avoid (teratogenic and toxic in *animal* studies. See also *Pregnancy and reproductive function* in Cytotoxic drugs p. 932.
● BREAST FEEDING Discontinue breast-feeding.
● RENAL IMPAIRMENT Avoid if possible—nephrotoxic.
● MONITORING REQUIREMENTS
▸ Monitor full blood count.
▸ Monitor audiology.
▸ Monitor plasma electrolytes.
▸ Nephrotoxicity Monitoring of renal function is essential.

● MEDICINAL FORMS There can be variation in the licensing of different medicines containing the same drug.
Solution for infusion
▸ Cisplatin (Non-proprietary)
Cisplatin 1 mg per 1 ml Cisplatin 50mg/50ml concentrate for solution for infusion vials | 1 vial [PoM] £24.50–£28.11 DT = £19.50 (Hospital only)
Cisplatin 100mg/100ml solution for infusion vials | 1 vial [PoM] £50.22 DT = £51.54 (Hospital only)
Cisplatin 50mg/50ml solution for infusion vials | 1 vial [PoM] £25.37–£28.11 DT = £19.50 (Hospital only)
Cisplatin 10mg/10ml concentrate for solution for infusion vials | 1 vial [PoM] £5.36–£5.90 (Hospital only)
Cisplatin 100mg/100ml concentrate for solution for infusion vials | 1 vial [PoM] £50.22–£55.64 DT = £51.54 (Hospital only)

Oxaliplatin

● INDICATIONS AND DOSE
Treatment of metastatic colorectal cancer (in combination with fluorouracil and folinic acid) | Treatment of colon cancer after resection of the primary tumour (adjuvant treatment)
▸ BY INTRAVENOUS INFUSION
▸ Adult: (consult product literature)

● CONTRA-INDICATIONS Peripheral neuropathy with functional impairment
● INTERACTIONS → Appendix 1: platinum compounds
● SIDE-EFFECTS
▸ **Common or very common** Alopecia · anaemia · appetite decreased · arthralgia · asthenia · chills · conjunctivitis · constipation · cough · decreased leucocytes · dehydration · depression · diarrhoea · dizziness · dyspnoea · electrolyte imbalance · embolism and thrombosis · fever · flushing · gastrointestinal discomfort · gastrointestinal disorders · haemorrhage · headache · hiccups · hyperglycaemia · hyperhidrosis · hypersensitivity · hypertension · increased risk of infection · insomnia · meningism · mucositis · nail disorder · nausea · necrosis · nerve disorders · neutropenia · neutropenic sepsis · pain · peripheral neuropathy (dose-limiting) · sensation abnormal · skin reactions · stomatitis · taste altered · thrombocytopenia · urinary disorders · vision disorders · vomiting · weight changes
▸ **Uncommon** Metabolic acidosis · nervousness · ototoxicity
▸ **Rare or very rare** Acute kidney injury · acute tubular necrosis · antibiotic associated colitis · deafness · disseminated intravascular coagulation · dysarthria · haemolytic anaemia · hepatic disorders · immuno-allergic thrombocytopenia · nephritis acute interstitial · nodular regenerative hyperplasia · pancreatitis · posterior reversible encephalopathy syndrome (PRES) (with oxaliplatin combination chemotherapy) · respiratory disorders · sinusoidal obstruction syndrome · vision loss (reversible on discontinuation)
▸ **Frequency not known** Autoimmune pancytopenia · chest discomfort · dysphagia · extravasation necrosis · gait abnormal · hypersensitivity vasculitis · movement disorders · muscle complaints · muscle contractions involuntary · QT interval prolongation · rhabdomyolysis · throat complaints

SIDE-EFFECTS, FURTHER INFORMATION Neurotoxicity is dose limiting.
Respiratory symptoms If unexplained respiratory symptoms occur, oxaliplatin should be discontinued until investigations exclude interstitial lung disease and pulmonary fibrosis.

● CONCEPTION AND CONTRACEPTION Effective contraception required during and for 4 months after treatment in women and 6 months after treatment in men.

● PREGNANCY Manufacturer advises avoid—toxicity in *animal* studies. See also *Pregnancy and reproductive function* in Cytotoxic drugs p. 932.

● BREAST FEEDING Discontinue breast-feeding.

● RENAL IMPAIRMENT Avoid if creatinine clearance less than 30 mL/minute.

Dose adjustments Reduce dose in mild to moderate impairment (consult product literature).

● NATIONAL FUNDING/ACCESS DECISIONS
For full details see funding body website

NICE decisions

▶ **Capecitabine and oxaliplatin in the adjuvant treatment of stage III (Dukes' C) colon cancer (April 2006)** NICE TA100 Recommended

▶ **Irinotecan, oxaliplatin, and raltitrexed for advanced colorectal cancer (August 2005)** NICE TA93 Recommended with restrictions

● MEDICINAL FORMS There can be variation in the licensing of different medicines containing the same drug.

Solution for infusion
▶ Oxaliplatin (Non-proprietary)
Oxaliplatin 5 mg per 1 ml Oxaliplatin 50mg/10ml concentrate for solution for infusion vials | 1 vial [PoM] £146.80-£163.78 (Hospital only)
Oxaliplatin 100mg/20ml concentrate for solution for infusion vials | 1 vial [PoM] £289.50-£327.98 (Hospital only)
Oxaliplatin 200mg/40ml concentrate for solution for infusion vials | 1 vial [PoM] £591.26-£655.96 (Hospital only)

ANTINEOPLASTIC DRUGS 〉 PODOPHYLLOTOXIN DERIVATIVES

Etoposide

03-Aug-2020

● **INDICATIONS AND DOSE**

Small cell carcinoma of the bronchus, the lymphomas and testicular cancer
▶ BY MOUTH
▶ Adult: 120–240 mg/m^2 daily for 5 days
▶ BY INTRAVENOUS INFUSION
▶ Adult: (consult product literature)

IMPORTANT SAFETY INFORMATION
RISKS OF INCORRECT DOSING OF ORAL ANTI-CANCER MEDICINES
See Cytotoxic drugs p. 932.

● INTERACTIONS → Appendix 1: etoposide

● SIDE-EFFECTS

GENERAL SIDE-EFFECTS
▶ **Common or very common** Abdominal pain · acute leukaemia · alopecia · anaemia · appetite decreased · arrhythmia · asthenia · bone marrow depression · constipation · diarrhoea · dizziness · hepatotoxicity · hypertension · leucopenia · malaise · mucositis · myocardial infarction · nausea · neutropenia · skin reactions · thrombocytopenia · vomiting
▶ **Uncommon** Nerve disorders
▶ **Rare or very rare** Dysphagia · neurotoxicity · radiation recall reaction · respiratory disorders · seizure · severe cutaneous adverse reactions (SCARs) · taste altered · vision loss

SPECIFIC SIDE-EFFECTS
● **Common or very common**
▶ With intravenous use Anaphylactic reaction · hypotension · infection
▶ With oral use Oesophagitis · stomatitis · transient systolic hypotension
● **Uncommon**
▶ With intravenous use Haemorrhage

▶ **Rare or very rare**
▶ With intravenous use Fever
▶ With oral use Drowsiness
▶ **Frequency not known**
▶ With intravenous use Angioedema · extravasation necrosis · infertility · tumour lysis syndrome

● CONCEPTION AND CONTRACEPTION Contraceptive advice required, see *Pregnancy and reproductive function* in Cytotoxic drugs p. 932.

● PREGNANCY Avoid (teratogenic in *animal* studies). See also *Pregnancy and reproductive function* in Cytotoxic drugs p. 932.

● BREAST FEEDING Discontinue breast-feeding.

● HEPATIC IMPAIRMENT Manufacturer advises caution (increased risk of accumulation).

● RENAL IMPAIRMENT
Dose adjustments Consider dose reduction—consult local treatment protocol for details.

● DIRECTIONS FOR ADMINISTRATION Manufacturer advises etoposide is given by slow intravenous infusion. It may also be given by mouth, but it is unpredictably absorbed.

● MEDICINAL FORMS There can be variation in the licensing of different medicines containing the same drug.

Solution for infusion
▶ Etoposide (Non-proprietary)
Etoposide 20 mg per 1 ml Etoposide 100mg/5ml concentrate for solution for infusion vials | 1 vial [PoM] £11.50-£16.29 (Hospital only)
Etoposide 200mg/10ml concentrate for solution for infusion vials | 1 vial [PoM] [▨] (Hospital only)
Etoposide 500mg/25ml concentrate for solution for infusion vials | 1 vial [PoM] £60.70-£81.42 (Hospital only)

Capsule
CAUTIONARY AND ADVISORY LABELS 23
▶ Vepesid (Cheplapharm Arzneimittel GmbH)
Etoposide 50 mg Vepesid 50mg capsules | 20 capsule [PoM] £99.82
Etoposide 100 mg Vepesid 100mg capsules | 10 capsule [PoM] £87.23

Powder for solution for injection
▶ Etopophos (Cheplapharm Arzneimittel GmbH)
Etoposide (as Etoposide phosphate) 100 mg Etopophos 100mg powder for solution for injection vials | 10 vial [PoM] £261.68

ANTINEOPLASTIC DRUGS 〉TAXANES

Cabazitaxel

04-Nov-2020

● **INDICATIONS AND DOSE**

Treatment of hormone refractory metastatic prostate cancer in patients who have previously been treated with a docetaxel-containing regimen (in combination with prednisone or prednisolone)
▶ BY INTRAVENOUS INFUSION
▶ Adult: (consult product literature or local protocols)

● CAUTIONS Avoid in Acute porphyrias p. 1107 · consult product literature

● INTERACTIONS → Appendix 1: taxanes

● SIDE-EFFECTS
▶ **Common or very common** Acute kidney injury · alopecia · anaemia · anxiety · appetite decreased · arrhythmias · arthralgia · asthenia · chest pain · chills · confusion · conjunctivitis · constipation · cough · cystitis · deep vein thrombosis · dehydration · diarrhoea · dizziness · dry mouth · dyspnoea · excessive tearing · fever · gastrointestinal discomfort · gastrointestinal disorders · haemorrhage · headache · hydronephrosis · hyperglycaemia · hypersensitivity · hypertension · hypokalaemia · hypotension · increased risk of infection · lethargy · leucopenia · malaise · mucositis · muscle complaints · nausea · nerve disorders · neutropenia · oedema · oropharyngeal pain · pain · pelvic pain · renal colic · renal

failure (fatal cases of renal failure reported) · sensation abnormal · sepsis · skin reactions · taste altered · thrombocytopenia · tinnitus · ureteral obstruction · urinary disorders · vasodilation · vertigo · vomiting · weight decreased

▶ **Frequency not known** Respiratory disorders

SIDE-EFFECTS, FURTHER INFORMATION Manufacturer advises pretreatment with a corticosteroid, antihistamine and histamine H2-receptor antagonist to reduce the risk and severity of hypersensitivity reactions.

● CONCEPTION AND CONTRACEPTION Ensure effective contraception during treatment (women) and for up to 6 months after treatment (men).

● PREGNANCY See also *Pregnancy and reproductive function* in Cytotoxic drugs p. 932.

● BREAST FEEDING Discontinue breast-feeding.

● HEPATIC IMPAIRMENT Manufacturer advises caution in mild to moderate impairment; avoid in severe impairment.
Dose adjustments Manufacturer advises dose reduction in mild to moderate impairment—consult product literature.

● RENAL IMPAIRMENT Use with caution if creatinine clearance less than 50 mL/minute.

● MONITORING REQUIREMENTS Monitor electrolytes—correct dehydration.

● DIRECTIONS FOR ADMINISTRATION Intravenous infusion incompatible with PVC.

● NATIONAL FUNDING/ACCESS DECISIONS
For full details see funding body website
NICE decisions
▶ Cabazitaxel for hormone-relapsed metastatic prostate cancer treated with docetaxel (updated August 2016) NICE TA391 Recommended with restrictions
Scottish Medicines Consortium (SMC) decisions
▶ Cabazitaxel (*Jevtana®*) in combination with prednisone or prednisolone is indicated for the treatment of adult patients with hormone refractory metastatic prostate cancer previously treated with a docetaxel-containing regimen (December 2016) SMC No. 735/11 Recommended with restrictions

● MEDICINAL FORMS There can be variation in the licensing of different medicines containing the same drug.
Solution for infusion
EXCIPIENTS: May contain Ethanol
▶ Jevtana (Sanofi)
Cabazitaxel 40 mg per 1 ml JEVTANA 60mg/1.5ml concentrate and solvent for solution for infusion vials | 1 vial PoM £3,696.00 (Hospital only)

Docetaxel

06-Jul-2020

● INDICATIONS AND DOSE

Adjuvant treatment of operable node-positive and operable node-negative breast cancer (in combination with doxorubicin and cyclophosphamide) | Initial chemotherapy of locally advanced or metastatic breast cancer (with doxorubicin) | Locally advanced or metastatic breast cancer where cytotoxic chemotherapy with an anthracycline or an alkylating drug has failed (monotherapy) | Locally advanced or metastatic breast cancer where cytotoxic chemotherapy with an anthracycline has failed (with capecitabine) | Initial chemotherapy of metastatic breast cancer which overexpresses human epidermal growth factor-2 (with trastuzumab) | Locally advanced or metastatic non-small cell lung cancer where previous chemotherapy has failed | Initial chemotherapy of unresectable, locally advanced or metastatic non-small cell lung cancer (with cisplatin) | Hormone-resistant metastatic prostate cancer (in combination with prednisone or prednisolone) | Initial treatment of metastatic gastric adenocarcinoma, including adenocarcinoma of the gastro-oesophageal junction (with cisplatin and fluorouracil) | Induction treatment of locally advanced squamous cell carcinoma of the head and neck (with cisplatin and fluorouracil)
▶ BY INTRAVENOUS INFUSION
▶ Adult: (consult product literature or local protocols)

● CAUTIONS Avoid in Acute porphyrias p. 1107 · consult product literature
● INTERACTIONS → Appendix 1: taxanes
● SIDE-EFFECTS
▶ **Common or very common** Abdominal pain · alopecia · anaemia · appetite decreased · arrhythmia · arthralgia · asthenia · constipation · diarrhoea · dyspnoea · fluid imbalance · haemorrhage · hypersensitivity · hypertension · hypotension · increased risk of infection · myalgia · nail disorders · nausea · neutropenia · pain · peripheral neuropathy · sepsis · skin reactions · stomatitis · taste altered · thrombocytopenia · vomiting
▶ **Uncommon** Gastrointestinal disorders · heart failure
▶ **Frequency not known** Ascites · bone marrow depression · chest tightness · chills · cutaneous lupus erythematosus · disseminated intravascular coagulation · eye disorders · eye inflammation · fever · hearing impairment · hepatitis · hyponatraemia · loss of consciousness · multi organ failure · myocardial infarction · nail discolouration · neurotoxicity · ototoxicity · pericardial effusion · peripheral lymphoedema · peripheral oedema · pulmonary oedema · radiation injuries · renal impairment · respiratory disorders · sclerodermal-like changes · seizure · sensation abnormal · severe cutaneous adverse reactions (SCARs) · vasodilation · venous thromboembolism · vision disorders · weight increased

SIDE-EFFECTS, FURTHER INFORMATION Pretreatment with dexamethasone by mouth is recommended for reducing fluid retention and hypersensitivity reactions.

● CONCEPTION AND CONTRACEPTION Manufacturer advises effective contraception for men and women during treatment, and for at least 6 months after stopping treatment in men.

● PREGNANCY Avoid (toxicity in *animal* studies). See also *Pregnancy and reproductive function* in Cytotoxic drugs p. 932.

● BREAST FEEDING Discontinue breast-feeding.

● HEPATIC IMPAIRMENT Manufacturer advises caution in mild to moderate and to avoid in severe impairment.
Dose adjustments Manufacturer advises dose reduction according to liver function tests in mild to moderate impairment —consult product literature.
Monitoring Monitor liver function in hepatic impairment.

● NATIONAL FUNDING/ACCESS DECISIONS
For full details see funding body website

NICE decisions

▶ Docetaxel for the treatment of hormone-refractory metastatic prostate cancer (June 2006) NICE TA101 Recommended
▶ Pertuzumab with trastuzumab and docetaxel for treating HER2-positive breast cancer (March 2018) NICE TA509 Recommended with restrictions

● MEDICINAL FORMS There can be variation in the licensing of different medicines containing the same drug.

Solution for infusion
EXCIPIENTS: May contain Ethanol
▶ Docetaxel (Non-proprietary)
Docetaxel 10 mg per 1 ml Docetaxel 80mg/8ml concentrate for solution for infusion vials | 1 vial [PoM] £534.75 (Hospital only)
Docetaxel 160mg/16ml concentrate for solution for infusion vials | 1 vial [PoM] £1,069.50 (Hospital only)
Docetaxel 20mg/2ml concentrate for solution for infusion vials | 1 vial [PoM] £162.75 (Hospital only)
Docetaxel 20 mg per 1 ml Docetaxel 80mg/4ml concentrate for solution for infusion vials | 1 vial [PoM] £51.00–£710.26 (Hospital only)
Docetaxel 160mg/8ml concentrate for solution for infusion vials | 1 vial [PoM] £101.25–£1,206.08 (Hospital only)
Docetaxel 20mg/1ml concentrate for solution for infusion vials | 1 vial [PoM] £15.00–£204.20 (Hospital only)

Paclitaxel
11-Nov-2020

● DRUG ACTION Paclitaxel is a member of the taxane group of drugs.

● **INDICATIONS AND DOSE**

Treatment of ovarian cancer (advanced or residual disease following laparotomy) in combination with cisplatin (conventional paclitaxel only) | Treatment of metastatic ovarian cancer where platinum-containing therapy has failed (conventional paclitaxel only) | Treatment of locally advanced breast cancer (in combination with other cytotoxics) or metastatic breast cancer (in combination with other cytotoxics or alone if other cytotoxics have failed or are inappropriate) (conventional paclitaxel only) | Adjuvant treatment of node-positive breast cancer following treatment with anthracycline and cyclophosphamide (conventional paclitaxel only) | Treatment of non-small cell lung cancer (in combination with cisplatin) when surgery or radiotherapy not appropriate (conventional paclitaxel only) | Treatment of advanced AIDS-related Kaposi's sarcoma where liposomal anthracycline therapy has failed (conventional paclitaxel only) | Monotherapy of metastatic breast cancer when first-line treatment has failed and standard, anthracycline-containing therapy is not indicated (albumin-bound paclitaxel only) | In combination with gemcitabine for the first-line treatment of metastatic adenocarcinoma of the pancreas (albumin-bound paclitaxel only)
▶ BY INTRAVENOUS INFUSION
▶ Adult: (consult product literature or local protocols)

● CAUTIONS Avoid in Acute porphyrias p. 1107 · consult product literature · patients aged over 75 years with metastatic adenocarcinoma of the pancreas

● INTERACTIONS → Appendix 1: taxanes

● SIDE-EFFECTS

▶ **Common or very common** Alopecia · anaemia · anxiety · appetite decreased · arrhythmias · arthralgia · asthenia · bone marrow disorders · chest discomfort · chills · constipation · cough · decreased leucocytes · depression · diarrhoea · dizziness · drowsiness · dry eye · dyspnoea · electrolyte imbalance · excessive tearing · extravasation necrosis · eye inflammation · fever · fluid imbalance ·

gastrointestinal discomfort · gastrointestinal disorders · haemorrhage · headache · hyperpyrexia · hypertension · increased risk of infection · influenza like illness · insomnia · laryngeal pain · lymphoedema · malaise · movement disorders · mucositis · muscle complaints · nail discolouration · nail disorders · nasal complaints · nausea · nerve disorders · neutropenia · oedema · oral disorders · pain · respiratory disorders · sensation abnormal · skin reactions · taste altered · thrombocytopenia · vasodilation · vertigo · vision disorders · vomiting · weight changes

▶ **Uncommon** Allergic rhinitis · breast pain · catheter related infection · dry mouth · dysphagia · ear pain · embolism and thrombosis · eye discomfort · facial swelling · gait abnormal · hepatomegaly · hoarseness · hyperglycaemia · hypoalbuminaemia · hypoglycaemia · hypotension · limb discomfort · muscle weakness · neoplasm complications · peripheral coldness · photosensitivity reaction · polydipsia · reflexes abnormal · sepsis · sweat changes · swelling · syncope · tinnitus · tremor · urinary disorders

▶ **Rare or very rare** Atrioventricular block · cardiac arrest · congestive heart failure · left ventricular dysfunction · radiation injuries · severe cutaneous adverse reactions (SCARs)

SIDE-EFFECTS, FURTHER INFORMATION Manufacturer advises routine premedication with a corticosteroid, an antihistamine and a histamine H2-receptor antagonist is recommended to prevent severe hypersensitivity reactions; hypersensitivity reactions may occur rarely despite premedication.

● CONCEPTION AND CONTRACEPTION Ensure effective contraception during and for at least 6 months after treatment in men or women.

● PREGNANCY Avoid (toxicity in *animal* studies). See also *Pregnancy and reproductive function* in Cytotoxic drugs p. 932.

● BREAST FEEDING Discontinue breast-feeding.

● HEPATIC IMPAIRMENT (Consult product literature)

● MONITORING REQUIREMENTS
▶ Cardiac monitoring should be undertaken, particularly if patients have underlying cardiac disease or previous exposure to anthracyclines.
▶ Patients should be monitored for signs and symptoms of pneumonitis and sepsis.

● PRESCRIBING AND DISPENSING INFORMATION Paclitaxel is available as both conventional and albumin-bound formulations. The different formulations vary in their licensed indications, pharmacokinetics, dosage and administration, and are not interchangeable.
Prescribers should specify the brand to be dispensed.

● NATIONAL FUNDING/ACCESS DECISIONS
For full details see funding body website

NICE decisions
▶ Guidance on the use of paclitaxel in the treatment of ovarian cancer (updated May 2005) NICE TA55 Recommended
▶ Bevacizumab in combination with paclitaxel and carboplatin for the first-line treatment of advanced ovarian cancer (May 2013) NICE TA284 Not recommended
▶ Topotecan, pegylated liposomal doxorubicin hydrochloride, paclitaxel, trabectedin and gemcitabine for treating recurrent ovarian cancer (April 2016) NICE TA389 Recommended
▶ Paclitaxel as albumin-bound nanoparticles with gemcitabine for untreated metastatic pancreatic cancer (September 2017) NICE TA476 Recommended with restrictions

Scottish Medicines Consortium (SMC) decisions
▶ Paclitaxel albumin (*Abraxane®*) for the treatment of metastatic breast cancer (April 2010) SMC No. 556/09 Recommended with restrictions
▶ Paclitaxel albumin (*Abraxane®*) in combination with gemcitabine for the first-line treatment of adult patients with

8

Immune system and malignant disease

metastatic adenocarcinoma of the pancreas (February 2015) SMC No. 968/14 Recommended

- MEDICINAL FORMS There can be variation in the licensing of different medicines containing the same drug.

Solution for infusion
EXCIPIENTS: May contain Polyoxyl castor oils
▸ Paclitaxel (Non-proprietary)
Paclitaxel 6 mg per 1 ml Paclitaxel 150mg/25ml concentrate for solution for infusion vials | 1 vial [PoM] £300.52-£561.00 (Hospital only)
Paclitaxel 30mg/5ml concentrate for solution for infusion vials | 1 vial [PoM] £35.00-£120.03 (Hospital only)
Paclitaxel 300mg/50ml concentrate for solution for infusion vials | 1 vial [PoM] £192.50-£1,122.00 (Hospital only)
Paclitaxel 100mg/16.7ml concentrate for solution for infusion vials | 1 vial [PoM] £87.50-£374.00 (Hospital only)

Powder for suspension for infusion
ELECTROLYTES: May contain Sodium
▸ Abraxane (Celgene Ltd)
Paclitaxel albumin 100 mg Abraxane 100mg powder for suspension for infusion vials | 1 vial [PoM] £246.00 (Hospital only)

ANTINEOPLASTIC DRUGS ＞ TOPOISOMERASE I INHIBITORS

Irinotecan hydrochloride
26-Aug-2020

- DRUG ACTION Irinotecan inhibits topoisomerase I, an enzyme involved in DNA replication.

- ● INDICATIONS AND DOSE

Metastatic colorectal cancer in combination with fluorouracil and folinic acid or as monotherapy when treatment containing fluorouracil has failed | Treatment of epidermal growth factor receptor-expressing metastatic colorectal cancer after failure of chemotherapy that has included irinotecan (in combination with cetuximab) | First-line treatment of metastatic carcinoma of the colon or rectum (in combination with fluorouracil, folinic acid and bevacizumab) | First-line treatment of metastatic colorectal carcinoma (in combination with capecitabine with or without bevacizumab)
▸ BY INTRAVENOUS INFUSION
▸ Adult: (consult product literature or local protocols)

Metastatic adenocarcinoma of the pancreas in patients who have progressed following gemcitabine based therapy (in combination with fluorouracil and leucovorin) (specialist use only)
▸ BY INTRAVENOUS INFUSION USING LIPID FORMULATION
▸ Adult: (consult product literature or local protocols)

IMPORTANT SAFETY INFORMATION

MHRA/CHM ADVICE: *ONIVYDE*® (IRINOTECAN, LIPOSOMAL FORMULATIONS): REPORTS OF SERIOUS AND FATAL THROMBOEMBOLIC EVENTS (MARCH 2019)
Onivyde® has been associated with reports of serious thromboembolic events, such as pulmonary embolism, venous thrombosis, and arterial thromboembolism. Healthcare professionals are advised to obtain a thorough medical history to identify patients with multiple risk factors. Patients should be advised to seek medical advice immediately if signs or symptoms of thromboembolism occur, such as sudden pain and swelling in a leg or an arm, sudden onset of coughing, chest pain or difficulty breathing.

MHRA/CHM ADVICE: LIPOSOMAL AND LIPID-COMPLEX FORMULATIONS: NAME CHANGE TO REDUCE MEDICATION ERRORS (JULY 2020)
Serious harm and fatal overdoses have occurred following confusion between liposomal, pegylated-liposomal, lipid-complex, and conventional formulations of the same drug substance. Medicines with

---

these formulations will explicitly include 'liposomal', 'pegylated-liposomal', or 'lipid-complex' within their name to reduce the risk of potentially fatal medication errors.

The MHRA reminds healthcare professionals that liposomal, pegylated-liposomal, lipid-complex, and conventional formulations containing the same drug substance are **not** interchangeable. Healthcare professionals are advised to make a clear distinction between formulations when prescribing, dispensing, administering, and communicating about irinotecan. The product name and dose should be verified before administration and the maximum dose should not be exceeded.

- CONTRA-INDICATIONS Bowel obstruction · chronic inflammatory bowel disease
- CAUTIONS Raised plasma-bilirubin concentration · risk factors for cardiac disease · risk factors for pulmonary toxicity · underweight patients (increased risk of adverse events)
- INTERACTIONS → Appendix 1: irinotecan
- SIDE-EFFECTS
▸ **Common or very common** Alopecia · anaemia (dose-limiting) · appetite decreased · asthenia · cholinergic syndrome · constipation · decreased leucocytes · diarrhoea (delayed diarrhoea requires prompt treatment) · dizziness · dysphonia · dyspnoea · electrolyte imbalance · embolism and thrombosis · febrile neutropenia (dose-limiting) · fever · fluid imbalance · gastrointestinal discomfort · gastrointestinal disorders · hypoalbuminaemia · hypoglycaemia · hypotension · increased risk of infection · infusion related reaction · insomnia · mucositis · nausea · neutropenia (dose-limiting) · oedema · renal impairment · sepsis · stomatitis · taste altered · thrombocytopenia (dose-limiting) · vomiting · weight decreased
▸ **Uncommon** Hypersensitivity · hypoxia · nail discolouration · skin reactions
▸ **Frequency not known** Antibiotic associated colitis · circulatory collapse · gastrointestinal haemorrhage · hiccups · hypertension · interstitial lung disease · muscle cramps · paraesthesia · speech disorder · ulcerative colitis
- CONCEPTION AND CONTRACEPTION For *conventional* formulations, manufacturer advises effective contraception during treatment and for up to 1 month after treatment in women of child-bearing potential, and up to 3 months after treatment in men. For *liposomal* formulations, manufacturer advises effective contraception during treatment and for up to 1 month after treatment in women of child-bearing potential, and up to 4 months after treatment in men.
- PREGNANCY Manufacturer advises avoid unless essential—toxicity in *animal* studies. See also Pregnancy and reproductive function in Cytotoxic drugs p. 932.
- BREAST FEEDING For *conventional* formulations, manufacturer advises avoid. For *liposomal* formulations, manufacturer advises avoid until one month after the last dose—no information available.
- HEPATIC IMPAIRMENT For *conventional* formulations, manufacturer advises caution if bilirubin concentration 1.5–3 times the upper limit of normal (risk of decreased clearance)—monitor liver function at baseline and before each cycle; avoid if bilirubin concentration greater than 3 times the upper limit of normal (no information available for combination therapy). For *liposomal* formulations, manufacturer advises caution; avoid if bilirubin greater than 2 mg/dL, or if transaminases are greater than 2.5 times the upper limit of normal, or greater than 5 times the upper limit of normal if liver metastasis present (limited information available).

Dose adjustments For *conventional* formulations, manufacturer advises dose reduction—consult product literature.

- **RENAL IMPAIRMENT** For *conventional* formulations, manufacturer advises avoid—no information available. For *liposomal* formulations, manufacturer advises avoid in severe impairment—no information available.

- **MONITORING REQUIREMENTS** Manufacturer advises monitor for respiratory symptoms in patients with risk factors for interstitial lung disease before and during treatment; monitor complete blood count weekly during treatment.

- **PRESCRIBING AND DISPENSING INFORMATION** Irinotecan is available as both *conventional* and *liposomal* formulations. These different formulations vary in their licensed indications, pharmacokinetics, dosage and administration, and are **not** interchangeable.

- **PATIENT AND CARER ADVICE**
Driving and skilled tasks Manufacturer advises patients and carers should be counselled on the effects on driving and performance of skilled tasks—increased risk of dizziness and visual disturbances within 24 hours of administration.

- **NATIONAL FUNDING/ACCESS DECISIONS**
For full details see funding body website
NICE decisions
- **Pegylated liposomal irinotecan for treating pancreatic cancer after gemcitabine (April 2017)** NICE TA440 Not recommended
Scottish Medicines Consortium (SMC) decisions
- Liposomal irinotecan (*Onivyde*®) for treatment of metastatic adenocarcinoma of the pancreas, in combination with fluorouracil (5-FU) and leucovorin (folinic acid), in adult patients who have progressed following gemcitabine based therapy (March 2017) SMC No. 1217/17 Not recommended

- **MEDICINAL FORMS** There can be variation in the licensing of different medicines containing the same drug.
Solution for infusion
ELECTROLYTES: May contain Sodium
- Irinotecan hydrochloride (Non-proprietary)
Irinotecan hydrochloride trihydrate 20 mg per 1 ml Irinotecan 500mg/25ml concentrate for solution for infusion vials | 1 vial [PoM] £172.50–£767.36 (Hospital only)
Irinotecan 40mg/2ml concentrate for solution for infusion vials | 1 vial [PoM] £15.00–£54.84 (Hospital only)
Irinotecan 300mg/15ml concentrate for solution for infusion vials | 1 vial [PoM] £110.00–£403.34 (Hospital only)
Irinotecan 100mg/5ml concentrate for solution for infusion vials | 1 vial [PoM] £48.00–£134.46 (Hospital only)
- Campto (Pfizer Ltd)
Irinotecan hydrochloride trihydrate 20 mg per 1 ml Campto 100mg/5ml concentrate for solution for infusion vials | 1 vial [PoM] £130.00 (Hospital only)
Campto 40mg/2ml concentrate for solution for infusion vials | 1 vial [PoM] £53.00 (Hospital only)
Campto 300mg/15ml concentrate for solution for infusion vials | 1 vial [PoM] £390.00 (Hospital only)
- Onivyde (Servier Laboratories Ltd)
Irinotecan (as Irinotecan sucrosofate salt pegylated liposomal) 4.3 mg per 1 ml Onivyde pegylated liposomal 43mg/10ml concentrate for solution for infusion vials | 1 vial [PoM] £615.35 (Hospital only)

Topotecan

24-Aug-2020

- **DRUG ACTION** Topotecan inhibits topoisomerase I, an enzyme involved in DNA replication.

- **INDICATIONS AND DOSE**

Metastatic ovarian cancer when first-line or subsequent treatment has failed | Treatment of recurrent carcinoma of the cervix, after radiotherapy, and for patients with stage IVB disease (in combination with cisplatin)
▸ BY INTRAVENOUS INFUSION
▸ Adult: (consult product literature or local protocols)

Relapsed small-cell lung cancer when retreatment with the first-line regimen is considered inappropriate
▸ BY INTRAVENOUS INFUSION, OR BY MOUTH
▸ Adult: (consult product literature or local protocols)

> **IMPORTANT SAFETY INFORMATION**
> RISKS OF INCORRECT DOSING OF ORAL ANTI-CANCER MEDICINES
> See Cytotoxic drugs p. 932.

- **INTERACTIONS** → Appendix 1: topotecan
- **SIDE-EFFECTS**
▸ **Common or very common** Alopecia · anaemia · appetite decreased · asthenia · colitis neutropenic · constipation · diarrhoea · fever · gastrointestinal discomfort · hyperbilirubinaemia · hypersensitivity · infection · leucopenia · malaise · mucositis · nausea · neutropenia · pancytopenia · sepsis · skin reactions · thrombocytopenia · vomiting
▸ **Rare or very rare** Angioedema · interstitial lung disease
▸ **Frequency not known** Bone marrow depression (dose-limiting) · haemorrhage

- **CONCEPTION AND CONTRACEPTION** Contraceptive advice required, see *Pregnancy and reproductive function* in Cytotoxic drugs p. 932.

- **PREGNANCY** Avoid (teratogenicity and fetal loss in *animal* studies). See also *Pregnancy and reproductive function* in Cytotoxic drugs p. 932.

- **BREAST FEEDING** Discontinue breast-feeding.

- **HEPATIC IMPAIRMENT** Manufacturer advises avoid in severe impairment (limited information available).

- **RENAL IMPAIRMENT** Avoid infusion if creatinine clearance less than 20 mL/minute. Avoid oral route if creatinine clearance less than 60 mL/minute.
Dose adjustments Reduce dose.

- **NATIONAL FUNDING/ACCESS DECISIONS**
For full details see funding body website
NICE decisions
- **Topotecan for the treatment of recurrent and stage IVB cervical cancer (October 2009)** NICE TA183 Recommended
- **Topotecan for the treatment of relapsed small-cell lung cancer (November 2009)** NICE TA184 Recommended
- **Topotecan, pegylated liposomal doxorubicin hydrochloride, paclitaxel, trabectedin and gemcitabine for treating recurrent ovarian cancer (April 2016)** NICE TA389 Not recommended
Scottish Medicines Consortium (SMC) decisions
- **Topotecan (*Hycamtin*®) in combination with cisplatin for patients with carcinoma of the cervix recurrent after radiotherapy and for patients with stage IVB disease (December 2007)** SMC No. 421/07 Recommended with restrictions

- **MEDICINAL FORMS** There can be variation in the licensing of different medicines containing the same drug.
Solution for infusion
- Topotecan (Non-proprietary)
Topotecan (as Topotecan hydrochloride) 1 mg per 1 ml Topotecan 4mg/4ml concentrate for solution for infusion vials | 1 vial [PoM] £290.00 | 5 vial [PoM] £1,453.10 (Hospital only)

Topotecan 1mg/1ml concentrate for solution for infusion vials |
1 vial [PoM] £97.00

Powder for solution for infusion
▸ Hycamtin (Novartis Pharmaceuticals UK Ltd)
Topotecan (as Topotecan hydrochloride) 1 mg Hycamtin 1mg
powder for concentrate for solution for infusion vials | 1 vial [PoM]
£97.65
Topotecan (as Topotecan hydrochloride) 4 mg Hycamtin 4mg
powder for concentrate for solution for infusion vials | 1 vial
£348.76 (Hospital only)

Capsule
CAUTIONARY AND ADVISORY LABELS 25
▸ Hycamtin (Novartis Pharmaceuticals UK Ltd)
Topotecan (as Topotecan hydrochloride)
250 microgram Hycamtin 0.25mg capsules | 10 capsule [PoM]
£75.00
Topotecan (as Topotecan hydrochloride) 1 mg Hycamtin 1mg
capsules | 10 capsule [PoM] £360.00

ANTINEOPLASTIC DRUGS > VINCA ALKALOIDS

Vinblastine sulfate
02-Jul-2020

● **INDICATIONS AND DOSE**
Variety of cancers including leukaemias, lymphomas, and
some solid tumours (e.g. breast and lung cancer)
▸ Adult: (consult product literature)

IMPORTANT SAFETY INFORMATION
Vinblastine is for **intravenous administration only**.
Inadvertent intrathecal administration can cause severe
neurotoxicity, which is usually fatal.
  The National Patient Safety Agency has advised
(August 2008) that adult and teenage patients treated in
an adult or adolescent unit should receive their vinca
alkaloid dose in a 50 mL minibag. Teenagers and children
treated in a child unit may receive their vinca alkaloid
dose in a syringe.

● CONTRA-INDICATIONS Intrathecal injection **contra-**
indicated.
● CAUTIONS Caution in handling—irritant to tissues
● INTERACTIONS → Appendix 1: vinca alkaloids
● SIDE-EFFECTS
▸ **Rare or very rare** Hearing impairment · nerve disorders ·
vestibular damage
▸ **Frequency not known** Abdominal pain · alopecia
(reversible) · anaemia · appetite decreased · asthenia ·
balance impaired · cancer pain · constipation · depression ·
diarrhoea · dizziness · dyspnoea · haemorrhage · headache ·
hypertension · ileus · increased risk of infection ·
leucopenia (dose-limiting) · malaise · myalgia · myocardial
infarction · nausea · nystagmus · oral blistering · pain ·
Raynaud's phenomenon · reflexes absent · respiratory
disorders · seizure · sensation abnormal · SIADH · skin
reactions · stroke · thrombocytopenia · vertigo · vomiting
● CONCEPTION AND CONTRACEPTION Contraceptive advice
required, see *Pregnancy and reproductive function* in
Cytotoxic drugs p. 932.
● PREGNANCY Avoid (limited experience suggests fetal
harm; teratogenic in *animal* studies). See also *Pregnancy*
and reproductive function in Cytotoxic drugs p. 932.
● BREAST FEEDING Discontinue breast-feeding.
● HEPATIC IMPAIRMENT Manufacturer advises caution in
significantly impaired hepatic or biliary function.
Dose adjustments Manufacturer advises consider initial
dose reduction in significantly impaired hepatic or biliary
function.

● MEDICINAL FORMS There can be variation in the licensing of
different medicines containing the same drug.
Solution for injection
▸ Vinblastine sulfate (Non-proprietary)
Vinblastine sulfate 1 mg per 1 ml Vinblastine 10mg/10ml solution
for injection vials | 5 vial [PoM] £85.00 (Hospital only)

Vincristine sulfate
03-Jul-2020

● **INDICATIONS AND DOSE**
Variety of cancers including leukaemias, lymphomas, and
some solid tumours (e.g. breast and lung cancer)
▸ Adult: (consult local protocol)

IMPORTANT SAFETY INFORMATION
Vincristine injections are for **intravenous**
administration only. Inadvertent intrathecal
administration can cause severe neurotoxicity, which is
usually fatal.
  The National Patient Safety Agency has advised
(August 2008) that adult and teenage patients treated in
an adult or adolescent unit should receive their vinca
alkaloid dose in a 50 mL minibag. Teenagers and children
treated in a child unit may receive their vinca alkaloid
dose in a syringe.

● CONTRA-INDICATIONS Intrathecal injection **contra-**
indicated.
● CAUTIONS Caution in handling—irritant to tissues · ileus ·
neuromuscular disease
● INTERACTIONS → Appendix 1: vinca alkaloids
● SIDE-EFFECTS
▸ **Rare or very rare** Hypersensitivity · rash · SIADH
▸ **Frequency not known** Abdominal cramps · adrenal disorder
· alopecia · anaemia · appetite decreased · azotaemia ·
bladder atony · bronchospasm · connective tissue disorders
· constipation · coronary artery disease · dehydration ·
diarrhoea · dizziness · dyspnoea · eighth cranial nerve
damage · eye disorders · fever · gait abnormalities ·
gastrointestinal disorders · haemolytic anaemia · headache
· hearing impairment · hypertension · hyponatraemia ·
hypotension · infection · leucopenia · movement disorders ·
muscle atrophy · myalgia · myocardial infarction · nausea ·
neuromuscular effects (dose-limiting) · neutropenia ·
oedema · oral ulceration · pain · paralysis · paresis · reflexes
absent · renal disorder · secondary malignancy · sensation
abnormal · sepsis · throat pain · thrombocytopenia · urinary
disorders · vertigo · vestibular damage · vision loss ·
vomiting · weight decreased

SIDE-EFFECTS, FURTHER INFORMATION **Bronchospasm**
Severe bronchospasm following administration is more
common when used in combination with mitomycin-C.
  Neurotoxicity Sensory and motor neuropathies are
common and are cumulative. Manufacturer advises
monitoring patients for symptoms of neuropathy, such as
hypoesthesia, hyperesthesia, paresthesia, hyporeflexia,
areflexia, neuralgia, jaw pain, decreased vibratory sense,
cranial neuropathy, ileus, burning sensation, arthralgia,
myalgia, muscle spasm, or weakness, both before and
during treatment—requires dose reduction, treatment
interruption or treatment discontinuation, depending on
severity.
  Motor weakness can also occur and dose reduction or
discontinuation of therapy may be appropriate if motor
weakness increases. Recovery from neurotoxic effects is
usually slow but complete.

● CONCEPTION AND CONTRACEPTION Contraceptive advice
required, see *Pregnancy and reproductive function* in
Cytotoxic drugs p. 932.

Immune system and malignant disease

- **PREGNANCY** Avoid (teratogenicity and fetal loss in *animal* studies). See also *Pregnancy and reproductive function* in Cytotoxic drugs p. 932.
- **BREAST FEEDING** Discontinue breast-feeding.
- **HEPATIC IMPAIRMENT** Manufacturer advises caution. **Dose adjustments** Manufacturer advises dose reduction.
- **MEDICINAL FORMS** There can be variation in the licensing of different medicines containing the same drug.
  Solution for injection
  ‣ Vincristine sulfate (Non-proprietary)
    Vincristine sulfate 1 mg per 1 ml Vincristine 1mg/1ml solution for injection vials | 1 vial PoM £13.47 (Hospital only) | 5 vial PoM £67.35 (Hospital only)
    Vincristine 2mg/2ml solution for injection vials | 1 vial PoM £26.66 (Hospital only) | 5 vial PoM £133.30 (Hospital only)
    Vincristine 5mg/5ml solution for injection vials | 5 vial PoM £329.50 (Hospital only)

Vindesine sulfate
03-Jul-2020

- **INDICATIONS AND DOSE**

Variety of cancers including leukaemias, lymphomas, and some solid tumours (e.g. breast and lung cancer)
‣ Adult: (consult product literature)

> **IMPORTANT SAFETY INFORMATION**
> Vindesine injections are for **intravenous administration only**. Inadvertent intrathecal administration can cause severe neurotoxicity, which is usually fatal.
> The National Patient Safety Agency has advised (August 2008) that adult and teenage patients treated in an adult or adolescent unit should receive their vinca alkaloid dose in a 50 mL minibag. Teenagers and children treated in a child unit may receive their vinca alkaloid dose in a syringe.

- **CONTRA-INDICATIONS** Intrathecal injection **contra-indicated**.
- **CAUTIONS** Caution in handling—irritant to tissues · neuromuscular disease
- **INTERACTIONS** → Appendix 1: vinca alkaloids
- **SIDE-EFFECTS**
‣ **Common or very common** Alopecia
‣ **Frequency not known** Anaemia · appetite decreased · asthenia · balance impaired · cellulitis · chills · constipation · depression · diarrhoea · dizziness · dysphagia · fever · gastrointestinal discomfort · gastrointestinal disorders · granulocytopenia (dose-limiting) · headache · hearing impairment · malaise · nausea · nerve disorders · nystagmus · oral disorders · pain · peroneal nerve palsy · rash maculopapular · reflexes absent · seizure · sensation abnormal · thrombocytopenia · thrombocytosis · vertigo · vestibular damage · vision loss · vomiting
SIDE-EFFECTS, FURTHER INFORMATION Neurotoxicity, usually as peripheral or autonomic neuropathy; it occurs less often with vindesine than with vincristine. Patients with neurotoxicity commonly have peripheral paraesthesia, loss of deep tendon reflexes; and ototoxicity has been reported. There have been instances in which neurotoxicity has made it necessary to reduce the dosage or temporarily discontinue use of vindesine.

- **CONCEPTION AND CONTRACEPTION** Contraceptive advice required, see *Pregnancy and reproductive function* in Cytotoxic drugs p. 932.
- **PREGNANCY** Avoid (teratogenic in *animal* studies). See also *Pregnancy and reproductive function* in Cytotoxic drugs p. 932.
- **BREAST FEEDING** Discontinue breast-feeding.

- **HEPATIC IMPAIRMENT** Manufacturer advises caution. **Dose adjustments** Manufacturer advises consider initial dose reduction in significant impairment.

- **MEDICINAL FORMS** There can be variation in the licensing of different medicines containing the same drug.
  Powder for solution for injection
  ‣ Eldisine (Genus Pharmaceuticals Ltd)
    Vindesine sulfate 5 mg Eldisine 5mg powder for solution for injection vials | 1 vial PoM £78.30 (Hospital only)

Vinflunine
03-Jul-2020

- **INDICATIONS AND DOSE**

Treatment of advanced or metastatic transitional cell carcinoma of the urothelial tract after failure of a platinum-containing regimen (monotherapy)
‣ Adult: (consult local protocol)

> **IMPORTANT SAFETY INFORMATION**
> Vinflunine injections are for **intravenous administration only**. Inadvertent intrathecal administration can cause severe neurotoxicity, which is usually fatal.
> The National Patient Safety Agency has advised (August 2008) that adult and teenage patients treated in an adult or adolescent unit should receive their vinca alkaloid dose in a 50 mL minibag. Teenagers and children treated in a child unit may receive their vinca alkaloid dose in a syringe.

- **CONTRA-INDICATIONS** Intrathecal injection **contra-indicated**.
- **CAUTIONS** Cardiovascular disease · QT-interval prolongation (avoid hypokalaemia)
- **INTERACTIONS** → Appendix 1: vinca alkaloids
- **SIDE-EFFECTS**
‣ **Common or very common** Alopecia · anaemia · appetite decreased · arthralgia · asthenia · chest pain · chills · constipation · cough · dehydration · diarrhoea · dizziness · dyspnoea · ear pain · fever · gastrointestinal discomfort · gastrointestinal disorders · headache · hyperhidrosis · hypersensitivity · hypertension · hyponatraemia · hypotension · increased risk of infection · insomnia · leucopenia · muscle weakness · myalgia · nausea · neutropenia · oedema · oral disorders · pain · peripheral neuropathy · skin reactions · swallowing difficulty · syncope · tachycardia · taste altered · thrombocytopenia · venous thrombosis · vomiting · weight changes
‣ **Uncommon** Acute respiratory distress syndrome (ARDS) · cancer pain · laryngeal pain · myocardial infarction · myocardial ischaemia · neutropenic sepsis · renal failure · SIADH · tinnitus · vertigo · visual impairment
‣ **Rare or very rare** Posterior reversible encephalopathy syndrome (PRES)

- **CONCEPTION AND CONTRACEPTION** Manufacturer advises effective contraception during and for up to 3 months after treatment.
- **PREGNANCY** Avoid unless essential—teratogenicity and embryotoxicity in *animal* studies. See also *Pregnancy and reproductive function* in Cytotoxic drugs p. 932.
- **BREAST FEEDING** Discontinue breast-feeding.
- **HEPATIC IMPAIRMENT** Manufacturer advises caution (no information available in severe impairment). **Dose adjustments** Manufacturer advises dose reduction.
- **RENAL IMPAIRMENT** **Dose adjustments** Reduce dose if creatinine clearance less than 60 mL/minute—consult product literature.
- **NATIONAL FUNDING/ACCESS DECISIONS** For full details see funding body website

8

Immune system and malignant disease

NICE decisions

▶ Vinflunine for the treatment of advanced or metastatic transitional cell carcinoma of the urothelial tract (January 2013) NICE TA272 Not recommended

● MEDICINAL FORMS There can be variation in the licensing of different medicines containing the same drug.

Solution for infusion

▶ Javlor (Pierre Fabre Ltd)
Vinflunine (as Vinflunine ditartrate) 25 mg per 1 ml Javlor 250mg/10ml concentrate for solution for infusion vials | 1 vial [PoM] £1,062.50
Javlor 50mg/2ml concentrate for solution for infusion vials | 1 vial [PoM] £212.50

Vinorelbine

04-Jul-2020

● DRUG ACTION Vinorelbine is a semi-synthetic vinca alkaloid.

● **INDICATIONS AND DOSE**

Advanced breast cancer | Advanced non-small cell lung cancer

▶ BY MOUTH
▶ Adult: 60 mg/m^2 once weekly for 3 weeks, then increased if tolerated to 80 mg/m^2 once weekly (max. per dose 160 mg once weekly)
▶ BY INTRAVENOUS INJECTION, OR BY INTRAVENOUS INFUSION
▶ Adult: (consult product literature)

IMPORTANT SAFETY INFORMATION

Vinorelbine injections are for **intravenous administration only**. Inadvertent intrathecal administration can cause severe neurotoxicity, which is usually fatal.

The National Patient Safety Agency has advised (August 2008) that adult and teenage patients treated in an adult or adolescent unit should receive their vinca alkaloid dose in a 50 mL minibag. Teenagers and children treated in a child unit may receive their vinca alkaloid dose in a syringe.

RISKS OF INCORRECT DOSING OF ORAL ANTI-CANCER MEDICINES See Cytotoxic drugs p. 932.

● CONTRA-INDICATIONS
GENERAL CONTRA-INDICATIONS
Concurrent radiotherapy if treating the liver
SPECIFIC CONTRA-INDICATIONS
▶ With oral use Long-term oxygen therapy · previous significant surgical resection of small bowel · previous significant surgical resection of stomach
CONTRA-INDICATIONS, FURTHER INFORMATION
Intrathecal injection **contra-indicated**.

● CAUTIONS Caution in handling—irritant to tissues · ischaemic heart disease

● INTERACTIONS → Appendix 1: vinca alkaloids

● SIDE-EFFECTS
GENERAL SIDE-EFFECTS
▶ **Common or very common** Alopecia · anaemia · appetite decreased · arthralgia · bone marrow depression (dose-limiting) · constipation · diarrhoea · dyspnoea · fever · hypertension · hypotension · increased risk of infection · leucopenia · myalgia · nausea · neutropenia (dose-limiting) · pain · reflexes absent · stomatitis · thrombocytopenia · vomiting
▶ **Uncommon** Flushing · peripheral coldness · respiratory disorders · sepsis
▶ **Rare or very rare** Circulatory collapse · hyponatraemia · myocardial infarction · pancreatitis
▶ **Frequency not known** SIADH

SPECIFIC SIDE-EFFECTS
▶ **Common or very common**
▶ With intravenous use Asthenia · cancer pain · chest pain · muscle weakness in legs · nervous system disorder · vein discolouration
▶ With oral use Abdominal pain · chills · cough · dizziness · dysphagia · dysuria · fatigue · gastrointestinal disorders · headache · insomnia · liver disorder · neuromuscular disorders · sensory disorder · skin eruption · taste altered · urogenital disorder · vision disorder · weight changes
▶ **Uncommon**
▶ With intravenous use Paraesthesia
▶ With oral use Ataxia
▶ **Rare or very rare**
▶ With intravenous use Arrhythmias · ischaemic heart disease · necrosis · palpitations · paralytic ileus · skin reactions
▶ **Frequency not known**
▶ With intravenous use Febrile neutropenia
▶ With oral use Gastrointestinal haemorrhage · hypersensitivity

SIDE-EFFECTS, FURTHER INFORMATION **Bronchospasm** Severe bronchospasm following administration of the vinca alkaloids is more common when used in combination with mitomycin-C.

Neurotoxicity Neurotoxicity reported in clinical trials, most commonly as constipation, paresthesia, hypersthesia, and hyporeflexia.

● CONCEPTION AND CONTRACEPTION Manufacturer advises effective contraception during and for 3 months after treatment; men must avoid fathering a child during and for at least 3 months after treatment.

● PREGNANCY Avoid unless essential (teratogenicity, and fetal loss in *animal* studies). See also *Pregnancy and reproductive function* in Cytotoxic drugs p. 932.

● BREAST FEEDING Discontinue breast-feeding.

● HEPATIC IMPAIRMENT
▶ With oral use Manufacturer advises caution in moderate impairment; avoid in severe impairment (no information available).
▶ With intravenous use Manufacturer advises caution in severe impairment.
Dose adjustments
▶ With oral use Manufacturer advises dose reduction in moderate impairment—consult product literature.
▶ With intravenous use Manufacturer advises dose reduction in severe impairment.

● MEDICINAL FORMS There can be variation in the licensing of different medicines containing the same drug.

Solution for infusion

▶ Vinorelbine (Non-proprietary)
Vinorelbine (as Vinorelbine tartrate) 10 mg per 1 ml Vinorelbine 50mg/5ml concentrate for solution for infusion vials | 1 vial [PoM] £139.00 (Hospital only) | 1 vial [PoM] £139.00 | 10 vial [PoM] £1,539.80 (Hospital only)
Vinorelbine 10mg/1ml concentrate for solution for infusion vials | 1 vial [PoM] £29.00 (Hospital only) | 1 vial [PoM] £29.00 | 10 vial [PoM] £329.50 (Hospital only)
▶ Navelbine (Pierre Fabre Ltd)
Vinorelbine (as Vinorelbine tartrate) 10 mg per 1 ml Navelbine 10mg/1ml concentrate for solution for infusion vials | 10 vial [PoM] £297.45 (Hospital only)
Navelbine 50mg/5ml concentrate for solution for infusion vials | 10 vial [PoM] £1,399.79 (Hospital only)

Capsule
CAUTIONARY AND ADVISORY LABELS 21, 25
▶ Vinorelbine (Non-proprietary)
Vinorelbine (as Vinorelbine tartrate) 20 mg Vinorelbine 20mg capsules | 1 capsule [PoM] £43.98 (Hospital only)
Vinorelbine (as Vinorelbine tartrate) 30 mg Vinorelbine 30mg capsules | 1 capsule [PoM] £65.98 (Hospital only)
Vinorelbine (as Vinorelbine tartrate) 80 mg Vinorelbine 80mg capsules | 1 capsule [PoM] £175.92 (Hospital only)

▶ Navelbine (Pierre Fabre Ltd)
Vinorelbine (as Vinorelbine tartrate) 20 mg Navelbine 20mg
capsules | 1 capsule [PoM] £43.98 (Hospital only)
Vinorelbine (as Vinorelbine tartrate) 30 mg Navelbine 30mg
capsules | 1 capsule [PoM] £65.98 (Hospital only)
Vinorelbine (as Vinorelbine tartrate) 80 mg Navelbine 80mg
capsules | 1 capsule [PoM] £175.92 (Hospital only)

ANTINEOPLASTIC DRUGS > OTHER

Amsacrine
11-Sep-2018

● **INDICATIONS AND DOSE**

Acute leukaemia (refractory to anthracycline chemotherapy used alone or in combination with other chemotherapy agents) (specialist use only)
▶ BY INTRAVENOUS INFUSION
▶ Adult: (consult product literature)

● CAUTIONS Hypokalaemia—increased risk of ventricular fibrillation (correct hypokalaemia before initiating treatment)

● INTERACTIONS → Appendix 1: amsacrine

● SIDE-EFFECTS
▶ **Common or very common** Abdominal pain · alopecia · arrhythmias · bone marrow disorders · cardiotoxicity · congestive heart failure · diarrhoea · dyspnoea · emotional lability · fever · generalised tonic-clonic seizure · haemorrhage · hepatic disorders · hypokalaemia · hypotension · infection · nausea · necrosis · skin reactions · stomatitis · thrombocytopenia · vomiting
▶ **Rare or very rare** Anaemia · cardiomyopathy · confusion · dizziness · granulocytopenia · headache · lethargy · leucopenia · numbness · peripheral neuropathy · proteinuria · renal impairment · visual impairment · weight changes
▶ **Frequency not known** Cardiac arrest · hyperuricaemia

● CONCEPTION AND CONTRACEPTION Manufacturer advises effective contraception during and for 3 months after treatment in women of child-bearing potential, and during and for 6 months after treatment in men.

● PREGNANCY Manufacturer advises avoid—toxicity in *animal* studies. See also *Pregnancy and reproductive function* in Cytotoxic drugs p. 932.

● BREAST FEEDING Manufacturer advises avoid—no information available.

● HEPATIC IMPAIRMENT Manufacturer advises caution (increased risk of toxicity).
Dose adjustments Manufacturer advises consider dose reduction (consult product literature).

● RENAL IMPAIRMENT Manufacturer advises monitor renal function at baseline and during treatment—increased risk of toxicity.
Dose adjustments Manufacturer advises consider dose reduction in renal impairment.

● MONITORING REQUIREMENTS
▶ Manufacturer advises monitor full blood count, liver function and renal function regularly; electrolytes should be re-evaluated prior to each treatment.
▶ Manufacturer advises monitor for cardiotoxicity during treatment.

● MEDICINAL FORMS There can be variation in the licensing of different medicines containing the same drug.
Solution for infusion
▶ Amsidine (Eurocept International bv)
Amsacrine 50 mg per 1 ml Amsidine 75mg/1.5ml solution for infusion ampoules and diluent | 6 ampoule [PoM] £1,200.00 (Hospital only)

Arsenic trioxide
15-Oct-2020

● **INDICATIONS AND DOSE**

Acute promyelocytic leukaemia (specialist use only)
▶ BY INTRAVENOUS INFUSION
▶ Adult: (consult product literature or local protocols)

● CAUTIONS Hypokalaemia (correct before treatment) · hypomagnesaemia (correct before treatment) · previous treatment with anthracyclines (increased risk of QT interval prolongation) · vitamin B_1 deficiency (risk of encephalopathy)

● INTERACTIONS → Appendix 1: arsenic trioxide

● SIDE-EFFECTS
▶ **Common or very common** Abdominal pain · alveolar haemorrhage · anaemia · arrhythmias · arthralgia · chest pain · chills · diarrhoea · differentiation syndrome · dizziness · dyspnoea · electrolyte imbalance · fatigue · fever · headache · hyperbilirubinaemia · hyperglycaemia · hypotension · hypoxia · increased risk of infection · ketoacidosis · leucocytosis · myalgia · nausea · neutropenia · oedema · pain · pancytopenia · paraesthesia · pericardial effusion · QT interval prolongation · renal failure · respiratory disorders · seizure · skin reactions · thrombocytopenia · vasculitis · vision blurred · vomiting · weight increased
▶ **Frequency not known** Confusion · decreased leucocytes · encephalopathy · fluid imbalance · heart failure · hepatotoxicity · peripheral neuropathy · sepsis

SIDE-EFFECTS, FURTHER INFORMATION Signs and symptoms of differentiation syndrome (leucocyte activation syndrome) include unexplained fever, dyspnoea, weight gain, pulmonary infiltrates, pleural or pericardial effusions, with or without leucocytosis—treat with high dose corticosteroids, consult product literature.

● CONCEPTION AND CONTRACEPTION Manufacturer advises effective contraception during treatment in men and women.

● PREGNANCY Avoid (teratogenic and embryotoxic in *animal* studies). See also *Pregnancy and reproductive function* in Cytotoxic drugs p. 932.

● BREAST FEEDING Discontinue breast-feeding.

● HEPATIC IMPAIRMENT Manufacturer advises use with caution—no information available.

● RENAL IMPAIRMENT Manufacturer advises caution— limited information available.

● MONITORING REQUIREMENTS ECG required before and during treatment—consult product literature.

● NATIONAL FUNDING/ACCESS DECISIONS
For full details see funding body website
NICE decisions
▶ Arsenic trioxide for treating acute promyelocytic leukaemia (June 2018) NICE TA526 Recommended
Scottish Medicines Consortium (SMC) decisions
▶ Arsenic trioxide (*Trisenox*®) for newly diagnosed, low-to-intermediate risk acute promyelocytic leukaemia (July 2019) SMC No. SMC2181 Recommended

● MEDICINAL FORMS There can be variation in the licensing of different medicines containing the same drug.
Solution for infusion
▶ Arsenic trioxide (Non-proprietary)
Arsenic trioxide 1 mg per 1 ml Arsenic 10mg/10ml concentrate for solution for infusion vials | 10 vial [PoM] £2,295.00–£2,700.00 (Hospital only)
Arsenic 10mg/10ml solution for infusion ampoules | 10 ampoule [PoM] £2,920.00 (Hospital only)
Arsenic 10mg/10ml concentrate for solution for infusion ampoules | 10 ampoule [PoM] £2,920.00 (Hospital only)

8

Immune system and malignant disease

▶ Trisenox (Teva UK Ltd)
Arsenic trioxide 2 mg per 1 ml Trisenox 12mg/6ml concentrate for
solution for infusion vials | 10 vial [PoM] £2,480.00 (Hospital only)

Asparaginase
03-Nov-2020

- **DRUG ACTION** Asparaginase is an enzyme which acts by
breaking down L-asparagine to aspartic acid and ammonia,
this disrupts protein synthesis of tumour cells.

- ● **INDICATIONS AND DOSE**

**Acute lymphoblastic leukaemia (in combination with
other antineoplastic drugs) (specialist use only)**
  - ▶ BY INTRAVENOUS INFUSION
  - ▶ Adult: 5000 units/m^2 every 3 days

- **CONTRA-INDICATIONS** History of pancreatitis related to
asparaginase therapy · history of serious haemorrhage
related to asparaginase therapy · history of serious
thrombosis related to asparaginase therapy · pancreatitis ·
pre-existing known coagulopathy

- **CAUTIONS** Diabetes (may raise blood glucose) ·
hypersensitivity reactions · hypertriglyceridaemia
(severe)—increased risk of acute pancreatitis
  CAUTIONS, FURTHER INFORMATION
  ▶ Hypersensitivity reactions Serious hypersensitivity reactions,
  including life-threatening anaphylaxis, can occur—
  asparaginase should only be administered when
  appropriately trained staff and resuscitation facilities are
  immediately available; in the event of a hypersensitivity
  reaction, treatment should be stopped immediately and
  appropriate management initiated. Manufacturer advises
  an intracutaneous or small intravenous test dose can be
  used but is of limited value for predicting which patients
  will experience an allergic reaction.

- **INTERACTIONS** → Appendix 1: asparaginase

- **SIDE-EFFECTS**
  ▶ **Common or very common** Abdominal pain · agitation ·
  anaemia · angioedema · appetite decreased · arthralgia ·
  back pain · bronchospasm · confusion · depression ·
  diarrhoea · disseminated intravascular coagulation ·
  dizziness · drowsiness · dyspnoea · embolism and
  thrombosis · fatigue · flushing · haemorrhage ·
  hallucination · hyperglycaemia · hypersensitivity ·
  hypoalbuminaemia · hypoglycaemia · hypotension ·
  increased risk of infection · leucopenia · nausea ·
  neurological effects · oedema · pancreatitis · skin reactions
  · thrombocytopenia · vomiting · weight decreased
  ▶ **Uncommon** Headache · hyperammonaemia ·
  hyperuricaemia
  ▶ **Rare or very rare** Coma · consciousness impaired · diabetic
  ketoacidosis · hepatic disorders · hyperparathyroidism ·
  hypoparathyroidism · ischaemic stroke · necrotising
  pancreatitis · pancreatic pseudocyst · posterior reversible
  encephalopathy syndrome (PRES) · seizure · tremor
  SIDE-EFFECTS, FURTHER INFORMATION There have been
  rare reports of cholestasis, icterus, hepatic cell necrosis
  and hepatic failure with fatal outcome; manufacturer
  advises interrupt treatment if these symptoms develop.

- **CONCEPTION AND CONTRACEPTION** Manufacturer advises
effective contraception in men and women of childbearing potential during treatment and for at least
3 months after last dose; asparaginase may reduce
effectiveness of oral contraceptives—additional
precautions (e.g. barrier method) are required, see also
Pregnancy and reproductive function in Cytotoxic drugs
p. 932.

- **PREGNANCY** Manufacturer advises avoid unless
essential—toxicity in *animal* studies. See also *Pregnancy
and reproductive function* in Cytotoxic drugs p. 932.

- **BREAST FEEDING** Manufacturer advises avoid—no
information available.

- **HEPATIC IMPAIRMENT** Manufacturer advises avoid in
severe impairment—no information available.

- **MONITORING REQUIREMENTS**
  ▶ Manufacturer advises monitor trough serum asparaginase
  levels 3 days after administration; consider switching to a
  different asparaginase preparation if target levels not
  reached—seek expert advice.
  ▶ Manufacturer advises monitor bilirubin, hepatic
  transaminases, and coagulation parameters before and
  during treatment; in addition, monitor plasma and urinary
  glucose, amylase, lipase, triglycerides, cholesterol and
  serum protein levels during treatment.

- **HANDLING AND STORAGE** Manufacturer advises store in a
refrigerator (2–8°C)—consult product literature for storage
conditions after reconstitution and dilution.

- **PATIENT AND CARER ADVICE**
  Driving and skilled tasks Manufacturer advises
  asparaginase has moderate influence on driving and
  performance of skilled tasks—increased risk of dizziness
  and somnolence.

- **NATIONAL FUNDING/ACCESS DECISIONS**
  For full details see funding body website
  Scottish Medicines Consortium (SMC) decisions
  ▶ Asparaginase (*Spectrila*®) as a component of antineoplastic
  combination therapy for the treatment of acute lymphoblastic
  leukaemia in paediatric patients from birth to 18 years and
  adult patients (April 2018) SMC No. 1319/18 Recommended

- **MEDICINAL FORMS** No licensed medicines listed.

Crisantaspase
07-Aug-2020

- **DRUG ACTION** Crisantaspase is the enzyme asparaginase
produced by *Erwinia chrysanthemi.*

- ● **INDICATIONS AND DOSE**

Acute lymphoblastic leukaemia
  - ▶ BY INTRAMUSCULAR INJECTION, OR BY SUBCUTANEOUS
    INJECTION, OR BY INTRAVENOUS INJECTION
  - ▶ Adult: (consult product literature)

- **CONTRA-INDICATIONS** History of pancreatitis related to
asparaginase therapy

- **CAUTIONS** Diabetes (may raise blood glucose)

- **INTERACTIONS** → Appendix 1: crisantaspase

- **SIDE-EFFECTS**
  ▶ **Common or very common** Chills · coagulation disorders ·
  confusion · diarrhoea · dizziness · drowsiness · dyspnoea ·
  face oedema · fever · headache · hepatic disorders ·
  hypersensitivity · limb swelling · lip swelling ·
  neurotoxicity · pain · pallor · pancreatitis · seizures · skin
  reactions · thrombosis
  ▶ **Uncommon** Hyperglycaemia · hyperlipidaemia · hypoxia ·
  increased risk of infection · respiratory disorders
  ▶ **Rare or very rare** Arthritis reactive · coma · diabetic
  ketoacidosis · dysphagia · dysphasia · encephalopathy ·
  haemorrhage · level of consciousness decreased · myalgia ·
  myocardial infarction · necrotising pancreatitis ·
  neutropenia · paresis · sepsis · thrombocytopenia
  ▶ **Frequency not known** Abdominal pain · flushing ·
  hyperammonaemia · hypertension · hypotension · nausea ·
  pseudocyst · vomiting

- **CONCEPTION AND CONTRACEPTION** Contraceptive advice
required, see *Pregnancy and reproductive function* in
Cytotoxic drugs p. 932.

- **PREGNANCY** Avoid. See also, *Pregnancy and reproductive
function* in Cytotoxic drugs p. 932.

- **BREAST FEEDING** Discontinue breast-feeding.

● DIRECTIONS FOR ADMINISTRATION Manufacturer advises facilities for the management of anaphylaxis should be available.

● MEDICINAL FORMS There can be variation in the licensing of different medicines containing the same drug.
Powder for solution for injection
▶ Erwinase (Jazz Pharmaceuticals UK)
 Crisantaspase 10000 unit Erwinase 10,000unit powder for solution for injection vials | 5 vial [PoM] £3,065.00

Eribulin   04-Nov-2020

● INDICATIONS AND DOSE
Treatment of locally advanced or metastatic breast cancer when the disease has progressed after treatment with at least 1 chemotherapy regimen for advanced disease
▶ BY INTRAVENOUS INJECTION
▶ Adult: Give on day 1 and day 8 of a 21-day cycle, previous therapy should have included an anthracycline and a taxane in either the adjuvant or metastatic setting unless the patient is unsuitable for these treatments (consult local protocol)

● CONTRA-INDICATIONS Congenital long QT syndrome
● CAUTIONS Bradyarrhythmias (increased susceptibility to QT-interval prolongation) · congestive heart failure (increased susceptibility to QT-interval prolongation) · electrolyte disturbances (increased susceptibility to QT-interval prolongation) · susceptibility to QT-interval prolongation

● INTERACTIONS → Appendix 1: eribulin

● SIDE-EFFECTS
▶ **Common or very common** Alopecia · anaemia · appetite decreased · arthralgia · asthenia · chest pain · chills · conjunctivitis · constipation · cough · decreased leucocytes · dehydration · depression · diarrhoea · dizziness · dry mouth · dyspnoea · dysuria · electrolyte imbalance · embolism and thrombosis · excessive tearing · fever · gastrointestinal discomfort · gastrooesophageal reflux disease · haemorrhage · headache · hot flush · hyperbilirubinaemia · hyperglycaemia · increased risk of infection · influenza like illness · insomnia · lethargy · mucositis · muscle complaints · muscle weakness · nail disorder · nausea · nerve disorders · neurotoxicity · neutropenia · oral disorders · oropharyngeal pain · pain · peripheral oedema · rhinorrhoea · sensation abnormal · skin reactions · sweat changes · tachycardia · taste altered · thrombocytopenia · tinnitus · vertigo · vomiting · weight decreased
▶ **Uncommon** Angioedema · hepatotoxicity · interstitial lung disease · pancreatitis · proteinuria · renal failure · sepsis
▶ **Rare or very rare** Disseminated intravascular coagulation
▶ **Frequency not known** QT interval prolongation · severe cutaneous adverse reactions (SCARs)

● CONCEPTION AND CONTRACEPTION Ensure effective contraception during and for up to 3 months after treatment in men or women.
● PREGNANCY Avoid unless essential (teratogenic in *animal* studies). See also *Pregnancy and reproductive function* in Cytotoxic drugs p. 932.
● BREAST FEEDING Discontinue breast-feeding.
● HEPATIC IMPAIRMENT Manufacturer advises caution (increased risk of neutropenia).
Dose adjustments Manufacturer advises dose reduction—consult product literature.
● RENAL IMPAIRMENT
Dose adjustments Consider dose reduction if creatinine clearance less than 40 mL/minute.

● MONITORING REQUIREMENTS
▶ Monitor for signs of peripheral neuropathy—severe peripheral neurotoxicity requires treatment delay or dose reduction (consult product literature).
▶ ECG monitoring recommended in patients prescribed concomitant use of drugs that prolong the QT-interval or who are susceptible to QT-interval prolongation.
▶ Monitor electrolytes periodically.
● NATIONAL FUNDING/ACCESS DECISIONS
For full details see funding body website
NICE decisions
▶ Eribulin for treating locally advanced or metastatic breast cancer after 2 or more chemotherapy regimens (December 2016) NICE TA423 Recommended with restrictions
▶ Eribulin for treating locally advanced or metastatic breast cancer after 1 chemotherapy regimen (March 2018) NICE TA515 Not recommended
Scottish Medicines Consortium (SMC) decisions
▶ Eribulin (*Halaven*®) for the treatment of adult patients with locally advanced or metastatic breast cancer who have progressed after at least one chemotherapeutic regimen for advanced disease (March 2016) SMC No. 1065/15 Recommended with restrictions

● MEDICINAL FORMS There can be variation in the licensing of different medicines containing the same drug.
Solution for injection
EXCIPIENTS: May contain Ethanol
▶ Halaven (Eisai Ltd)
 Eribulin.44 mg per 1 ml Halaven 0.88mg/2ml solution for injection vials | 1 vial [PoM] £361.00 (Hospital only)

Hydroxycarbamide   04-Sep-2020
(Hydroxyurea)

● INDICATIONS AND DOSE
Polycythaemia vera (specialist use only)
▶ BY MOUTH
▶ Adult: Initially 15–20 mg/kg daily, adjusted according to response, for information on dose adjustment based on haematocrit and platelet count—consult product literature; usual dose 500–1000 mg daily, dosage should be based on actual or ideal body weight, whichever is less
Essential thrombocythaemia (specialist use only)
▶ BY MOUTH
▶ Adult: Initially 15 mg/kg daily, adjusted according to response, for information on dose adjustment based on platelet count and white cell count—consult product literature, dosage should be based on actual or ideal body weight, whichever is less
Chronic myeloid leukaemia (specialist use only)
▶ BY MOUTH
▶ Adult: Initially 40 mg/kg daily, then reduced to 20 mg/kg daily, adjusted according to response, for information on dose adjustment based on white cell count—consult product literature, dosage should be based on actual or ideal body weight, whichever is less
HYDREA®
Chronic myeloid leukaemia (specialist use only) | Cancer of the cervix (specialist use only)
▶ BY MOUTH
▶ Adult: 20–30 mg/kg daily, alternatively 80 mg/kg every 3 days, for information on dose adjustment based on platelet count, white cell count and actual or ideal body weight—consult product literature   continued →

8

Immune system and malignant disease

SIKLOS®

Sickle-cell disease [prevention of recurrent vaso-occlusive crises] (initiated by a specialist)
▸ BY MOUTH
▸ Adult: Initially 15 mg/kg daily, increased in steps of 2.5–5 mg/kg daily, dose to be increased every 12 weeks according to response; usual dose 15–30 mg/kg daily; maximum 35 mg/kg per day

XROMI®

Sickle-cell disease [prevention of vaso-occlusive complications] (specialist use only)
▸ BY MOUTH
▸ Adult: Initially 15 mg/kg daily, increased in steps of 5 mg/kg daily, dose to be increased every 8 weeks according to response; usual maintenance 20–25 mg/kg daily; maximum 35 mg/kg per day

> IMPORTANT SAFETY INFORMATION
> RISKS OF INCORRECT DOSING OF ORAL ANTI-CANCER MEDICINES
> See Cytotoxic drugs p. 932.

- CAUTIONS Leg ulcers (review treatment if cutaneous vasculitic ulcerations develop)
- INTERACTIONS → Appendix 1: hydroxycarbamide
- SIDE-EFFECTS
▸ **Common or very common** Alopecia · anaemia · appetite decreased · asthenia · bone marrow disorders · chills · constipation · cutaneous vasculitis · dermatomyositis · diarrhoea · disorientation · dizziness · drowsiness · dyspnoea · dysuria · fever · gastrointestinal discomfort · haemorrhage · hallucination · headache · hepatic disorders · leucopenia · malaise · mucositis · nail discolouration · nail disorder · nausea · neoplasms · neutropenia · oral disorders · pancreatitis · peripheral neuropathy · pulmonary oedema · red blood cell abnormalities · respiratory disorders · seizure · skin reactions · skin ulcers · sperm abnormalities · thrombocytopenia · vomiting
▸ **Rare or very rare** Cutaneous lupus erythematosus · gangrene · systemic lupus erythematosus (SLE)
▸ **Frequency not known** Amenorrhoea · gastrointestinal disorders · hypomagnesaemia · Parvovirus B19 infection · vitamin D deficiency · weight increased
- CONCEPTION AND CONTRACEPTION Manufacturer advises effective contraception before and during treatment.
- PREGNANCY Avoid (teratogenic in *animal* studies). See also *Pregnancy and reproductive function* in Cytotoxic drugs p. 932.
- BREAST FEEDING Discontinue breast-feeding.
- HEPATIC IMPAIRMENT Manufacturer advises caution in mild to moderate impairment; avoid in severe impairment (unless used for malignant conditions).
- RENAL IMPAIRMENT In sickle-cell disease, avoid if eGFR less than 30 mL/minute/1.73 m². Use with caution in malignant disease.
  Dose adjustments In sickle-cell disease, reduce initial dose by 50% if eGFR less than 60 mL/minute/1.73 m².
- MONITORING REQUIREMENTS
▸ Monitor renal and hepatic function before and during treatment.
▸ Monitor full blood count before treatment, and repeatedly throughout use; in sickle-cell disease monitor every 2 weeks for the first 2 months and then every 2 to 3 months thereafter (or every 2 weeks if on maximum dose).
▸ Patients receiving long-term therapy for malignant disease should be monitored for secondary malignancies.
- PATIENT AND CARER ADVICE Patients receiving long-term therapy with hydroxycarbamide should be advised to protect skin from sun exposure.

- NATIONAL FUNDING/ACCESS DECISIONS
  For full details see funding body website
  Scottish Medicines Consortium (SMC) decisions
▸ Hydroxycarbamide oral solution (*Xromi*®) for the prevention of vaso-occlusive complications of sickle-cell disease in patients over 2 years of age (August 2020) SMC No. SMC2271 Recommended with restrictions

  All Wales Medicines Strategy Group (AWMSG) decisions
▸ Hydroxycarbamide oral solution (*Xromi*®) for the prevention of vaso-occlusive complications of sickle-cell disease in patients over 2 years of age (August 2020) AWMSG No. 4264 Recommended with restrictions

- MEDICINAL FORMS There can be variation in the licensing of different medicines containing the same drug. Forms available from special-order manufacturers include: capsule, oral suspension, oral solution
  Oral solution
  CAUTIONARY AND ADVISORY LABELS 27
  EXCIPIENTS: May contain Hydroxybenzoates (parabens)
▸ Xromi (Nova Laboratories Ltd)
  Hydroxycarbamide 100 mg per 1 ml Xromi 100mg/ml oral solution sugar-free | 150 ml [PoM] £250.00 DT = £250.00
  Tablet
▸ Siklos (Masters Pharmaceuticals Ltd)
  Hydroxycarbamide 100 mg Siklos 100mg tablets | 60 tablet [PoM] £100.00 DT = £100.00
  Hydroxycarbamide 1 gram Siklos 1000mg tablets | 30 tablet [PoM] £500.00 DT = £500.00
  Capsule
▸ Hydroxycarbamide (Non-proprietary)
  Hydroxycarbamide 500 mg Hydroxycarbamide 500mg capsules | 100 capsule [PoM] £86.00 DT = £12.14
▸ Droxia (Imported (United States))
  Hydroxycarbamide 300 mg Droxia 300mg capsules | 60 capsule [PoM] [℞]
▸ Hydrea (Bristol-Myers Squibb Pharmaceuticals Ltd)
  Hydroxycarbamide 500 mg Hydrea 500mg capsules | 100 capsule [PoM] £10.47 DT = £12.14

| Mitotane

20-Jul-2020

- DRUG ACTION Mitotane selectively inhibits the activity of the adrenal cortex, necessitating corticosteroid replacement therapy.

- INDICATIONS AND DOSE
  Symptomatic treatment of advanced or inoperable adrenocortical carcinoma
▸ BY MOUTH
▸ Adult: Initially 2–3 g daily in 2–3 divided doses adjusted according to plasma-concentration monitoring, in severe illness initial dose can be increased up to 6 g daily, reduce dose or interrupt treatment if signs of toxicity, discontinue if inadequate response after 3 months

> IMPORTANT SAFETY INFORMATION
> RISKS OF INCORRECT DOSING OF ORAL ANTI-CANCER MEDICINES
> See Cytotoxic drugs p. 932.

- CAUTIONS Avoid in Acute porphyrias p. 1107 · risk of accumulation in overweight patients
- INTERACTIONS → Appendix 1: mitotane
- SIDE-EFFECTS
▸ **Common or very common** Adrenal insufficiency · anaemia · appetite decreased · asthenia · cognitive impairment · confusion · diarrhoea · dizziness · drowsiness · dyslipidaemia · gastrointestinal discomfort · gynaecomastia · headache · hepatic disorders · leucopenia · movement disorders · mucositis · muscle weakness · nausea · paraesthesia · polyneuropathy · rash · thrombocytopenia · vertigo · vomiting

- **Frequency not known** Encephalopathy · eye disorders · flushing · fungal infection · generalised pain · growth retardation · haemorrhage · hyperpyrexia · hypersalivation · hypertension · hypothyroidism · hypouricaemia · lens opacity · neuro-psychological retardation · ovarian cyst · postural hypotension · proteinuria · taste altered · thyroid disorder · vision disorders
- CONCEPTION AND CONTRACEPTION Contraceptive advice required, see *Pregnancy and reproductive* function in Cytotoxic drugs p. 932.
- PREGNANCY Manufacturer advises avoid. See also *Pregnancy and reproductive function* in Cytotoxic drugs p. 932.
- BREAST FEEDING Discontinue breast-feeding.
- HEPATIC IMPAIRMENT Manufacturer advises caution in mild to moderate impairment; avoid in severe impairment (limited information available).
  Monitoring In mild to moderate hepatic impairment, monitoring of plasma-mitotane concentration is recommended.
- RENAL IMPAIRMENT Manufacturer advises caution in mild to moderate impairment. Avoid in severe impairment.
  Monitoring In mild to moderate renal impairment, monitoring of plasma-mitotane concentration is recommended.
- MONITORING REQUIREMENTS
  ▸ Plasma-mitotane concentration for optimum response 14–20 mg/litre.
  ▸ Monitor plasma-mitotane concentration—consult product literature.
- PRESCRIBING AND DISPENSING INFORMATION Corticosteroid replacement therapy Corticosteroid replacement therapy is necessary with treatment with mitotane. The dose of glucocorticoid should be increased in case of shock, trauma, or infection.
- PATIENT AND CARER ADVICE Patients should be warned to contact doctor immediately if injury, infection, or illness occurs (because of risk of acute adrenal insufficiency).
  Driving and skilled tasks Central nervous system toxicity may affect performance of skilled tasks (e.g. driving).

- MEDICINAL FORMS There can be variation in the licensing of different medicines containing the same drug.
  Tablet
  CAUTIONARY AND ADVISORY LABELS 2, 10, 21
  ▸ Lysodren (HRA Pharma UK Ltd)
  Mitotane 500 mg Lysodren 500mg tablets | 100 tablet PoM
  £590.97 DT = £590.97

Panobinostat   28-Jul-2020

- DRUG ACTION Panobinostat is a histone deacetylase inhibitor, which promotes cell-cycle arrest and apoptosis of tumour cells via multiple pathways.

- INDICATIONS AND DOSE
  Treatment of relapsed or refractory multiple myeloma (in combination with bortezomib and dexamethasone), in patients who have received at least two prior regimens, including bortezomib and an immunomodulatory agent
  ▸ BY MOUTH
  ▸ Adult 18–74 years: 20 mg once daily, on days 1, 3, 5, 8, 10 and 12 of a 21-day cycle for 8 cycles. Patients with clinical benefit should continue treatment for 8 additional cycles; total duration 16 cycles (48 weeks), for doses of dexamethasone and bortezomib, or dose adjustment due to side-effects—consult product literature
  ▸ Adult 75 years and over: 20 mg once daily, on days 1, 3, 5, 8, 10 and 12 of a 21-day cycle for 8 cycles. Patients

with clinical benefit should continue treatment for 8 additional cycles; total duration 16 cycles (48 weeks), alternatively initially 15 mg once daily, on days 1, 3, 5, 8, 10 and 12 of a 21-day cycle for 1 cycle, increased if tolerated to 20 mg once daily, on days 1, 3, 5, 8, 10 and 12 of a 21-day cycle for 7 subsequent cycles, patients with clinical benefit should continue treatment for 8 additional cycles; total duration 16 cycles (48 weeks), lower dose may be used for the first cycle depending on patient's condition and co-morbidities, for doses of dexamethasone and bortezomib, or dose adjustment due to side-effects—consult product literature
DOSE ADJUSTMENTS DUE TO INTERACTIONS
  ▸ Manufacturer advises reduce dose to 10 mg with concurrent use of potent inhibitors of CYP3A4; if the potent inhibitor of CYP3A4 is to be continued, consider increasing the dose to 15 mg if tolerated.
  ▸ Manufacturer advises avoid potent inhibitors of CYP3A4 if possible in patients taking a reduced panobinostat dose due to side-effects, or in those with hepatic impairment.

  > **IMPORTANT SAFETY INFORMATION**
  > RISKS OF INCORRECT DOSING OF ORAL ANTI-CANCER MEDICINES
  > See Cytotoxic drugs p. 932.

- CAUTIONS Coagulation disorders · elderly · QT-interval prolongation · risk factors for QT-interval prolongation
  CAUTIONS, FURTHER INFORMATION
  ▸ Risk factors for QT-interval prolongation Patients at risk of developing QT-interval prolongation include those with long QT syndrome, or uncontrolled or significant cardiac disease.
- INTERACTIONS → Appendix 1: panobinostat
- SIDE-EFFECTS
  ▸ **Common or very common** Anaemia · antibiotic associated colitis · appetite decreased · arrhythmias · asthenia · cheilitis · chills · cough · decreased leucocytes · diarrhoea · dizziness · dry mouth · dyspnoea · electrolyte imbalance · fever · fluid imbalance · gastrointestinal discomfort · gastrointestinal disorders · haemorrhage · headache · hepatic disorders · hyperbilirubinaemia · hyperglycaemia · hypertension · hyperuricaemia · hypoalbuminaemia · hypotension · hypothyroidism · increased risk of infection · insomnia · intracranial haemorrhage · joint swelling · malaise · nausea · neutropenia · palpitations · pancytopenia · peripheral oedema · QT interval prolongation · renal failure · respiratory disorders · sepsis · skin reactions · syncope · taste altered · thrombocytopenia · tremor · urinary incontinence · vomiting · weight decreased
  ▸ **Uncommon** Haemorrhagic shock · myocardial infarction
  SIDE-EFFECTS, FURTHER INFORMATION Side-effects are reported when used in combination with bortezomib and dexamethasone.
  Gastro-intestinal disorders Manufacturer advises that patients are treated with anti-diarrhoeals, or any additional treatment, in accordance with local treatment guidelines at the first sign of abdominal cramping or onset of diarrhoea.
- CONCEPTION AND CONTRACEPTION Manufacturer advises exclude pregnancy before starting treatment in women of child-bearing potential, and ensure highly effective contraception used during treatment and for 3 months after last dose. Women using hormonal contraceptives should also use a barrier method of contraception. Highly effective contraception also required for men and their female partners during treatment and for 6 months after last dose.
- PREGNANCY Manufacturer advises avoid unless potential benefit outweighs risk—toxicity in *animal* studies. See also

Pregnancy and reproductive function in Cytotoxic drugs p. 932.

- BREAST FEEDING Manufacturer advises avoid—no information available.
- HEPATIC IMPAIRMENT Manufacturer advises caution in mild and moderate impairment (risk of increased exposure); avoid in severe impairment (no information available).

  Dose adjustments In mild impairment, manufacturer advises dose reduction to 15 mg for the first treatment cycle, dose may be increased to 20 mg based on patient tolerability; in moderate impairment, manufacturer advises dose reduction to 10 mg for the first treatment cycle, dose may be increased to 15 mg based on patient tolerability.
- MONITORING REQUIREMENTS
  ‣ Manufacturer advises monitor full blood count before treatment, then frequently during treatment; reduce dose or interrupt treatment if thrombocytopenia or neutropenia occur—consult product literature.
  ‣ Manufacturer advises monitor ECG before treatment and repeat periodically before each treatment cycle; QTcF should be <480 milliseconds before treatment initiation—consult product literature.
  ‣ Manufacturer advises monitor electrolytes before treatment and periodically as clinically indicated, especially in patients with diarrhoea; monitor thyroid and pituitary function (free T4 and TSH) as clinically indicated; monitor hepatic function before treatment and regularly during treatment as clinically indicated.
  ‣ Manufacturer advises monitor patients over 65 years more frequently, especially for thrombocytopenia and gastro-intestinal toxicity.
- PATIENT AND CARER ADVICE Manufacturer advises that patients and their carers should be told to seek medical advice if severe gastro-intestinal toxicity occurs.
  Missed doses Manufacturer advises if a dose is missed, it can be taken up to 12 hours after the specified dose time.
  Driving and skilled tasks Dizziness may affect performance of skilled tasks (e.g. driving).
- NATIONAL FUNDING/ACCESS DECISIONS
  For full details see funding body website
  NICE decisions
  ‣ **Panobinostat for treating multiple myeloma after at least 2 previous treatments (January 2016)** NICE TA380
  Recommended with restrictions

- MEDICINAL FORMS There can be variation in the licensing of different medicines containing the same drug.
  Capsule
  CAUTIONARY AND ADVISORY LABELS 25
  ‣ Farydak (Durbin Plc)
  Panobinostat (as Panobinostat lactate anhydrous) 10 mg Farydak 10mg capsules | 6 capsule [PoM] £3,492.00
  Panobinostat (as Panobinostat lactate anhydrous) 15 mg Farydak 15mg capsules | 6 capsule [PoM] £3,492.00
  Panobinostat (as Panobinostat lactate anhydrous) 20 mg Farydak 20mg capsules | 6 capsule [PoM] £4,656.00

Pegaspargase
25-Aug-2020

- DRUG ACTION Pegaspargase breaks down the amino acid L-asparagine, thereby interfering with the growth of malignant cells, which are unable to synthesise L-asparagine.

- INDICATIONS AND DOSE
  Acute lymphoblastic leukaemia (in combination with other antineoplastic drugs) (specialist use only)
  ‣ BY INTRAMUSCULAR INJECTION, OR BY INTRAVENOUS INFUSION
  ‣ Adult 18–21 years: 2500 units/m^2 every 14 days
  ‣ Adult 22 years and over: 2000 units/m^2 every 14 days

- CONTRA-INDICATIONS History of pancreatitis · history of serious haemorrhagic event with previous L-asparaginase therapy · history of serious thrombosis with previous L-asparaginase therapy
- CAUTIONS Concomitant use of other hepatotoxic drugs (particularly in pre-existing hepatic impairment)—monitor hepatic function · diabetes (may raise blood glucose) · hypersensitivity reactions · marked decrease of leukocyte count at start of treatment is possible—may be associated with significant rise in serum uric acid and development of uric acid nephropathy
  CAUTIONS, FURTHER INFORMATION
  ‣ Hypersensitivity reactions Serious hypersensitivity reactions, including life-threatening anaphylaxis, can occur—pegaspargase should only be administered when appropriately trained staff and resuscitation facilities are immediately available; manufacturer advises patients should be closely monitored for signs of hypersensitivity during treatment and for an hour after administration. In the event of a hypersensitivity reaction, treatment should be stopped immediately and appropriate management initiated.
- INTERACTIONS → Appendix 1: pegaspargase
- SIDE-EFFECTS
  ‣ **Common or very common** Abdominal pain · anaemia · appetite decreased · ascites · bone marrow disorders · coagulation disorders · diarrhoea · dyslipidaemia · embolism and thrombosis · febrile neutropenia · hepatic disorders · hyperglycaemia · hypersensitivity · hypoalbuminaemia · hypokalaemia · hypoxia · increased risk of infection · nausea · pain in extremity · pancreatitis (discontinue if suspected and do not restart if confirmed) · peripheral neuropathy · seizure · sepsis · skin reactions · stomatitis · syncope · vomiting · weight decreased
  ‣ **Rare or very rare** Haemorrhage · necrotising pancreatitis · posterior reversible encephalopathy syndrome (PRES)
  ‣ **Frequency not known** Acute kidney injury · confusion · diabetic ketoacidosis · drowsiness · fever · hyperammonaemia (monitor if symptoms present) · hypoglycaemia · pancreatic pseudocyst · stroke · toxic epidermal necrolysis · tremor
  SIDE-EFFECTS, FURTHER INFORMATION There have been rare reports of cholestasis, icterus, hepatic cell necrosis and hepatic failure with fatal outcome in patients receiving pegaspargase.
- CONCEPTION AND CONTRACEPTION Manufacturer advises effective contraception in men and women of child-bearing potential during treatment and for at least 6 months after discontinuing treatment; pegaspargase may reduce effectiveness of oral contraceptives—additional precautions (e.g. barrier method) are required, see also *Pregnancy and reproductive function* in Cytotoxic drugs p. 932.
- PREGNANCY Manufacturer advises avoid unless essential. See also *Pregnancy and reproductive function* in Cytotoxic drugs p. 932.
- BREAST FEEDING Manufacturer advises avoid—no information available.
- HEPATIC IMPAIRMENT Manufacturer advises avoid in severe impairment.
- MONITORING REQUIREMENTS
  ‣ Manufacturer advises trough serum asparaginase activity levels may be measured before the next administration of pegaspargase; consider switching to a different asparaginase preparation if target levels not reached—seek expert advice.
  ‣ Manufacturer advises monitor plasma and urine glucose levels during treatment; monitor coagulation profile at baseline and periodically during and after treatment (particularly with concomitant use of other drugs that inhibit coagulation); monitor serum amylase.

- **DIRECTIONS FOR ADMINISTRATION** Manufacturer advises *for intramuscular injection*, volumes over 3 mL must be divided between more than one site.
- **HANDLING AND STORAGE** Manufacturer advises store in a refrigerator between 2–8°C.
- **PATIENT AND CARER ADVICE**
Pancreatitis Manufacturer advises patients and carers should be told how to recognise signs and symptoms of pancreatitis and advised to seek medical attention if symptoms such as persistent, severe abdominal pain develop.
Driving and skilled tasks Manufacturer advises patients and carers should be counselled on the effects on driving and performance of skilled tasks—increased risk of confusion and somnolence.
- **NATIONAL FUNDING/ACCESS DECISIONS**
For full details see funding body website
NICE decisions
▶ Pegaspargase for treating acute lymphoblastic leukaemia (September 2016) NICE TA408 Recommended
Scottish Medicines Consortium (SMC) decisions
▶ Pegaspargase (*Oncaspar*®) as a component of antineoplastic combination therapy in acute lymphoblastic leukaemia (ALL) in paediatric patients from birth to 18 years, and adult patients (November 2016) SMC No. 1197/16 Recommended
- **MEDICINAL FORMS** There can be variation in the licensing of different medicines containing the same drug.
Solution for injection
▶ Oncaspar (Servier Laboratories Ltd) ▼
Pegaspargase 750 unit per 1 ml Oncaspar 3,750units/5ml solution for injection vials | 1 vial [PoM] £1,296.19
Powder for solution for injection
▶ Oncaspar (Servier Laboratories Ltd) ▼
Pegaspargase 3750 unit Oncaspar 3,750unit powder for solution for injection vials | 1 vial [PoM] £1,296.19 (Hospital only)

Procarbazine

21-Jul-2020

- **DRUG ACTION** Procarbazine is a mild monoamine-oxidase inhibitor.

- **INDICATIONS AND DOSE**
Hodgkin's lymphoma
▶ BY MOUTH
▶ Adult: (consult local protocol)

IMPORTANT SAFETY INFORMATION
RISKS OF INCORRECT DOSING OF ORAL ANTI-CANCER MEDICINES
See Cytotoxic drugs p. 932.

- **CONTRA-INDICATIONS** Pre-existing severe leucopenia · pre-existing severe thrombocytopenia
- **CAUTIONS** Cardiovascular disease · cerebrovascular disease · epilepsy · phaeochromocytoma · procarbazine is a mild monoamineoxidase inhibitor (dietary restriction is rarely considered necessary)
- **INTERACTIONS** → Appendix 1: procarbazine
- **SIDE-EFFECTS**
▶ **Common or very common** Appetite decreased
▶ **Frequency not known** Azoospermia · hepatic disorders · infection · lethargy · leucopenia · nausea · neutropenia · ovarian failure · pneumonitis · skin reactions · thrombocytopenia · vomiting
- **CONCEPTION AND CONTRACEPTION** Contraceptive advice required, see *Pregnancy and reproductive function* in Cytotoxic drugs p. 932.
- **PREGNANCY** Avoid (teratogenic in *animal* studies and isolated reports in humans). See also *Pregnancy and reproductive function* in Cytotoxic drugs p. 932.

- **BREAST FEEDING** Discontinue breast-feeding.
- **HEPATIC IMPAIRMENT** Manufacturer advises caution in mild to moderate impairment; avoid in severe impairment.
- **RENAL IMPAIRMENT** Caution in mild to moderate impairment. Avoid in severe impairment.

- **MEDICINAL FORMS** There can be variation in the licensing of different medicines containing the same drug.
Capsule
CAUTIONARY AND ADVISORY LABELS 4
▶ Procarbazine (Non-proprietary)
Procarbazine (as Procarbazine hydrochloride)
50 mg Procarbazine 50mg capsules | 50 capsule [PoM] £411.35–£479.63 DT = £445.49

Raltitrexed

28-Jul-2020

- **DRUG ACTION** Raltitrexed is a thymidylate synthase inhibitor.

- **INDICATIONS AND DOSE**
Palliation of advanced colorectal cancer when fluorouracil and folinic acid cannot be used
▶ BY INTRAVENOUS INFUSION
▶ Adult: (consult local protocol)
- **INTERACTIONS** → Appendix 1: raltitrexed
- **SIDE-EFFECTS**
▶ **Common or very common** Alopecia · anaemia · appetite decreased · arthralgia · asthenia · cellulitis · conjunctivitis · constipation · dehydration · diarrhoea · fever · gastrointestinal discomfort · headache · hyperbilirubinaemia · hyperhidrosis · influenza like illness · leucopenia · malaise · mucositis · muscle cramps · muscle tone increased · nausea · neutropenia · oral disorders · pain · peripheral oedema · sepsis · skin reactions · taste altered · thrombocytopenia · vomiting · weight decreased
▶ **Frequency not known** Gastrointestinal haemorrhage
- **CONCEPTION AND CONTRACEPTION** Ensure effective contraception during and for at least 6 months after treatment in men or women.
- **PREGNANCY** See *Pregnancy and reproductive function* in Cytotoxic drugs p. 932.
- **BREAST FEEDING** Discontinue breast-feeding.
- **HEPATIC IMPAIRMENT** Manufacturer advises caution in mild to moderate impairment; avoid in severe impairment, jaundice or decompensated disease (no information available).
- **RENAL IMPAIRMENT** Avoid if creatinine clearance less than 25 mL/minute.
Dose adjustments Reduce dose and increase dosing interval if creatinine clearance less than 65 mL/minute (consult product literature).

- **MEDICINAL FORMS** There can be variation in the licensing of different medicines containing the same drug.
Powder for solution for infusion
▶ Tomudex (Pfizer Ltd)
Raltitrexed 2 mg Tomudex 2mg powder for solution for infusion vials | 1 vial [PoM] £148.75 (Hospital only)

8

Immune system and malignant disease

RETINOID AND RELATED DRUGS

Bexarotene

20-Nov-2020

- **DRUG ACTION** Bexarotene is an agonist at the retinoid X receptor, which is involved in the regulation of cell differentiation and proliferation. Bexarotene can cause regression of cutaneous T-cell lymphoma.

● INDICATIONS AND DOSE

Skin manifestations of cutaneous T-cell lymphoma refractory to previous systemic treatment

▸ BY MOUTH
▸ Adult: Initially 300 mg/m² once daily, adjusted according to response, to be taken with a meal

---

IMPORTANT SAFETY INFORMATION

RISKS OF INCORRECT DOSING OF ORAL ANTI-CANCER MEDICINES
See Cytotoxic drugs p. 932.

MHRA/CHM ADVICE: ORAL RETINOID MEDICINES: REVISED AND SIMPLIFIED PREGNANCY PREVENTION EDUCATIONAL MATERIALS FOR HEALTHCARE PROFESSIONALS AND WOMEN (JUNE 2019)
Materials to support the Pregnancy Prevention Programme in women and girls of childbearing potential taking oral acitretin, alitretinoin, or isotretinoin have been updated. Oral tretinoin and bexarotene do not have a Pregnancy Prevention Programme in light of their oncology indication and specialist care setting. However, healthcare professionals are advised that these medicines are extremely teratogenic and product information should be consulted for contraceptive and pregnancy testing requirements when used in females of childbearing potential.

Neuropsychiatric reactions have been reported in patients taking oral retinoids. Healthcare professionals are advised to monitor patients for signs of depression or suicidal ideation and refer for appropriate treatment, if necessary; particular care is needed in those with a history of depression. Patients should be advised to speak to their doctor if they experience any changes in mood or behaviour, and encouraged to ask family and friends to look out for any change in mood.

- **CONTRA-INDICATIONS** History of pancreatitis · hypervitaminosis A · uncontrolled hyperlipidaemia · uncontrolled hypothyroidism
- **CAUTIONS** Avoid in Acute porphyrias p. 1107 · history of depression (risk of neuropsychiatric reactions) · hyperlipidaemia · hypothyroidism
- **INTERACTIONS** → Appendix 1: retinoids
- **SIDE-EFFECTS**
▸ **Common or very common** Alopecia · anaemia · appetite decreased · arthralgia · asthenia · chills · constipation · deafness · diarrhoea · dizziness · dry eye · dry mouth · dyslipidaemia · eye disorders · gastrointestinal discomfort · gastrointestinal disorders · headaches · hyperhidrosis · hypersensitivity · hypoproteinaemia · hypothyroidism · increased risk of infection · insomnia · leucopenia · lymphadenopathy · muscle complaints · nausea · oedema · oral disorders · pain · pseudolymphoma · sensation abnormal · skin nodule · skin reactions · skin ulcer · thyroid disorder · vomiting · weight changes
▸ **Uncommon** Albuminuria · anxiety · arrhythmias · ataxia · blood disorder · cataract · coagulation disorder · depression · ear disorder · eosinophilia · eye inflammation · fever · gout · haemorrhage · hair disorder · hepatic failure · hyperbilirubinaemia · hypertension · hyperthyroidism · increased leucocytes · mucous membrane disorder · muscle weakness · nail disorder · neoplasms · nerve disorders · pancreatitis · renal impairment · serous drainage ·

thrombocytopenia · thrombocytosis · varicose veins · vasodilation · vertigo · vision disorders
▸ **Frequency not known** Burping · chest pain · confusion · cough aggravated · dehydration · drowsiness · dysphagia · dyspnoea · emotional lability · hypercalcaemia · hyperuricaemia · libido decreased · muscle tone increased · pelvic pain · peripheral vascular disease · red blood cell abnormality · taste altered · thirst · tinnitus · white blood cell abnormalities

- **ALLERGY AND CROSS-SENSITIVITY** EvGr Caution—hypersensitivity to retinoids. ⓜ
- **CONCEPTION AND CONTRACEPTION** Manufacturer advises effective contraception during and for at least 1 month after treatment in men and women.
- **PREGNANCY** Avoid. See also *Pregnancy and reproductive function* in Cytotoxic drugs p. 932.
- **BREAST FEEDING** Discontinue breast-feeding.
- **HEPATIC IMPAIRMENT** Manufacturer advises avoid in hepatic insufficiency.
- **PATIENT AND CARER ADVICE**
Risk of neuropsychiatric reactions The MHRA advises patients and carers to seek medical attention if changes in mood or behaviour occur.
- **NATIONAL FUNDING/ACCESS DECISIONS**
For full details see funding body website
Scottish Medicines Consortium (SMC) decisions
▸ Bexarotene (*Targretin*®) for skin manifestations of advanced stage cutaneous T-cell lymphoma (November 2002)
SMC No. 14/02 Recommended with restrictions
- **MEDICINAL FORMS** There can be variation in the licensing of different medicines containing the same drug.
Capsule
▸ Targretin (Eisai Ltd)
Bexarotene 75 mg Targretin 75mg capsules | 100 capsule PoM
£937.50

Tretinoin

15-Jan-2020

● INDICATIONS AND DOSE

Induction of remission in acute promyelocytic leukaemia (used in previously untreated patients as well as in those who have relapsed after standard chemotherapy or who are refractory to it)

▸ BY MOUTH
▸ Adult: 45 mg/m² daily in 2 divided doses maximum duration of treatment is 90 days, consult product literature for details of concomitant chemotherapy

---

IMPORTANT SAFETY INFORMATION

MHRA/CHM ADVICE: ORAL RETINOID MEDICINES: REVISED AND SIMPLIFIED PREGNANCY PREVENTION EDUCATIONAL MATERIALS FOR HEALTHCARE PROFESSIONALS AND WOMEN (JUNE 2019)
Materials to support the Pregnancy Prevention Programme in women and girls of childbearing potential taking oral acitretin, alitretinoin, or isotretinoin have been updated. Oral tretinoin and bexarotene do not have a Pregnancy Prevention Programme in light of their oncology indication and specialist care setting. However, healthcare professionals are advised that these medicines are extremely teratogenic and product information should be consulted for contraceptive and pregnancy testing requirements when used in females of childbearing potential.

Neuropsychiatric reactions have been reported in patients taking oral retinoids. Healthcare professionals are advised to monitor patients for signs of depression or suicidal ideation and refer for appropriate treatment, if necessary; particular care is needed in those with a history of depression. Patients should be advised to speak to their doctor if they experience any changes in mood or behaviour, and encouraged to ask family and friends to look out for any change in mood.

- CAUTIONS History of depression (risk of neuropsychiatric reactions) · increased risk of thromboembolism during first month of treatment
- INTERACTIONS → Appendix 1: retinoids
- SIDE-EFFECTS
- ▶ **Common or very common** Abdominal pain · alopecia · anxiety · appetite decreased · arrhythmia · asthma · bone pain · cheilitis · chest pain · chills · confusion · constipation · depression · diarrhoea · dizziness · dry mouth · flushing · headache · hearing impairment · hyperhidrosis · insomnia · intracranial pressure increased · malaise · nasal dryness · nausea · pancreatitis · paraesthesia · respiratory disorders · skin reactions · visual impairment · vomiting
- ▶ **Frequency not known** Embolism and thrombosis · erythema nodosum · genital ulceration · hepatotoxicity · hypercalcaemia · increased leucocytes · myocardial infarction · myositis · necrotising fasciitis · QT interval prolongation · stroke · thrombocytosis · vasculitis
  SIDE-EFFECTS, FURTHER INFORMATION **Retinoic acid syndrome** Fever, dyspnoea, acute respiratory distress, pulmonary infiltrates, pleural effusion, hyperleucocytosis, hypotension, oedema, weight gain, hepatic, renal and multi-organ failure requires immediate treatment— consult product literature.
- CONCEPTION AND CONTRACEPTION Effective contraception must be used for at least 1 month before oral treatment, during treatment and for at least 1 month after stopping (oral progestogen-only contraceptives not considered effective).
- PREGNANCY Teratogenic. See *Pregnancy and reproductive function* in Cytotoxic drugs p. 932.
- BREAST FEEDING Avoid (discontinue breast-feeding).
- HEPATIC IMPAIRMENT Manufacturer advises caution. **Dose adjustments** Manufacturer advises dose reduction to 25 mg/m².
- RENAL IMPAIRMENT **Dose adjustments** Reduce dose to 25 mg/m².
- MONITORING REQUIREMENTS Monitor haematological and coagulation profile, liver function, serum calcium and plasma lipids before and during treatment.
- PRESCRIBING AND DISPENSING INFORMATION Tretinoin is the acid form of vitamin A.
- PATIENT AND CARER ADVICE **Risk of neuropsychiatric reactions** The MHRA advises patients and carers to seek medical attention if changes in mood or behaviour occur.

- MEDICINAL FORMS There can be variation in the licensing of different medicines containing the same drug.
  Capsule
  CAUTIONARY AND ADVISORY LABELS 21, 25
  ▶ Tretinoin (Non-proprietary)
  Tretinoin 10 mg Tretinoin 10mg capsules | 100 capsule [PoM] £325.00 DT = £300.00

3.1 Cytotoxic drug-induced side effects

ANTIDOTES AND CHELATORS > IRON CHELATORS

Dexrazoxane

23-Nov-2020

- DRUG ACTION Dexrazoxane is an iron chelator.

- INDICATIONS AND DOSE
  CARDIOXANE ®
  Prevention of chronic cumulative cardiotoxicity caused by doxorubicin or epirubicin treatment in advanced or metastatic breast cancer patients who have received a prior cumulative dose of 300 mg/m² of doxorubicin or a prior cumulative dose of 540 mg/m² of epirubicin when further anthracycline treatment is required
  ▶ BY INTRAVENOUS INFUSION
  ▶ Adult: Administer 10 times the doxorubicin-equivalent dose or 10 times the epirubicin-equivalent dose, dose to be given 30 minutes before anthracycline administration

  SAVENE ®
  Anthracycline extravasation
  ▶ BY INTRAVENOUS INFUSION
  ▶ Adult: Initially 1 g/m² daily (max. per dose 2 g) for 2 days, then 500 mg/m² for 1 day, first dose to be given as soon as possible and within 6 hours after injury

- CONTRA-INDICATIONS Children
- CAUTIONS Myelosuppression (effects may be additive to those of chemotherapy)
  CARDIOXANE ® Heart failure—no information available · myocardial infarction in previous 12 months—no information available · symptomatic valvular heart disease—no information available · uncontrolled angina— no information available
- INTERACTIONS → Appendix 1: iron chelators
- SIDE-EFFECTS
- ▶ **Common or very common** Alopecia · anaemia · appetite decreased · asthenia · constipation · cough · diarrhoea · dizziness · drowsiness · dry mouth · dyspnoea · embolism and thrombosis · fever · gastrointestinal discomfort · headache · increased risk of infection · leucopenia · myalgia · nail disorder · nausea · neutropenia · peripheral neuropathy · peripheral oedema · post procedural infection · sensation abnormal · skin reactions · stomatitis · syncope · tachycardia · thrombocytopenia · tremor · vaginal haemorrhage · vomiting · weight decreased · wound complications
- ▶ **Uncommon** Acute myeloid leukaemia · lymphoedema · sepsis · thirst · vertigo
- ▶ **Frequency not known** Anaphylactic reaction
- CONCEPTION AND CONTRACEPTION Ensure effective contraception during and for at least 3 months after treatment in men and women.
- PREGNANCY Avoid unless essential (toxicity in *animal* studies).
- BREAST FEEDING Discontinue breast-feeding.
- HEPATIC IMPAIRMENT
  CARDIOXANE ® Manufacturer advises caution (no information available).
  Dose adjustments Manufacturer advises if anthracycline dose is reduced, reduce the *Cardioxane* ® dose by a similar ratio.
  SAVENE ® Manufacturer advises avoid (no information available).

8

Immune system and malignant disease

Immune system and malignant disease

8

- **RENAL IMPAIRMENT**
CARDIOXANE ® **Dose adjustments** Manufacturer advises reduce dose by 50% if creatinine clearance less than 40 mL/minute.
SAVENE ® Manufacturer advises avoid—risk of accumulation.

- **MONITORING REQUIREMENTS**
  ▸ Monitor full blood count.
  ▸ Monitor for cardiac toxicity.
  ▸ Monitor liver function.

- **DIRECTIONS FOR ADMINISTRATION**
CARDIOXANE ® For *intravenous infusion*, give intermittently *in* Compound sodium lactate; reconstitute each vial with 25 mL water for injections and dilute each vial with 25–100 mL infusion fluid; give requisite dose over 15 minutes.
SAVENE ® For *intravenous infusion*, give intermittently *in* diluent; reconstitute each 500-mg vial with 25 mL of diluent; dilute requisite dose further in remaining diluent and give over 1–2 hours into a large vein in an area other than the one affected. Local coolants such as ice packs should be removed at least 15 minutes before administration.

- **MEDICINAL FORMS** There can be variation in the licensing of different medicines containing the same drug.
Powder for solution for infusion
  ▸ Cardioxane (Clinigen Healthcare Ltd)
  Dexrazoxane 500 mg Cardioxane 500mg powder for solution for infusion vials | 1 vial PoM £156.57
Powder and solvent for solution for infusion
ELECTROLYTES: May contain Potassium, sodium
  ▸ Savene (Clinigen Healthcare Ltd)
  Dexrazoxane 500 mg Savene 500mg powder for concentrate and solvent for solution for infusion vials | 10 vial PoM 🔲

DETOXIFYING DRUGS > UROPROTECTIVE DRUGS

Mesna

16-Dec-2020

- **INDICATIONS AND DOSE**
Cytotoxic induced urothelial toxicity
  ▸ BY MOUTH, OR BY INTRAVENOUS INJECTION
  ▸ Adult: Dose to be calculated according to oxazaphosphorine (cyclophosphamide or ifosfamide) treatment (consult product literature)

- **SIDE-EFFECTS**
  ▸ **Common or very common** Appetite decreased · arthralgia · asthenia · chest pain · chills · concentration impaired · conjunctivitis · constipation · cough · dehydration · diarrhoea · dizziness · drowsiness · dry mouth · dyspnoea · dysuria · fever · flatulence · flushing · gastrointestinal discomfort · haemorrhage · headache · hyperhidrosis · influenza like illness · laryngeal discomfort · lymphadenopathy · malaise · mucosal irritation · myalgia · nasal congestion · nausea · oral irritation · pain · palpitations · respiratory disorders · sensation abnormal · skin reactions · sleep disorders · syncope · vision disorders · vomiting
  ▸ **Frequency not known** Acute kidney injury · angioedema · drug reaction with eosinophilia and systemic symptoms (DRESS) · hypotension · hypoxia · oedema · tachycardia · ulcer

- **ALLERGY AND CROSS-SENSITIVITY** EvGr Caution if history of hypersensitivity to thiol-containing compounds. ⓜ

- **PREGNANCY** Not known to be harmful. See also *Pregnancy and reproductive function* in Cytotoxic drugs p. 932.

- **EFFECT ON LABORATORY TESTS** False positive urinary ketones. False positive or false negative urinary erythrocytes.

- **DIRECTIONS FOR ADMINISTRATION** Manufacturer advises for administration *by mouth*, injection solution may be given in a flavoured drink such as orange juice or cola which may be stored in a refrigerator for up to 24 hours in a sealed container.

- **MEDICINAL FORMS** There can be variation in the licensing of different medicines containing the same drug. Forms available from special-order manufacturers include: oral solution
Solution for injection
  ▸ Mesna (Non-proprietary)
  Mesna 100 mg per 1 ml Mesna 1g/10ml solution for injection ampoules | 15 ampoule PoM £441.15-£447.15
  Mesna 400mg/4ml solution for injection ampoules | 5 ampoule PoM £17.00 | 15 ampoule PoM £201.15
Tablet
  ▸ Mesna (Non-proprietary)
  Mesna 400 mg Mesna 400mg tablets | 10 tablet PoM £134.30
  Mesna 600 mg Mesna 600mg tablets | 10 tablet PoM £190.60

VITAMINS AND TRACE ELEMENTS > FOLATES

Folinic acid

12-Apr-2019

- **INDICATIONS AND DOSE**
Prevention of methotrexate-induced adverse effects
  ▸ BY INTRAMUSCULAR INJECTION, OR BY INTRAVENOUS INJECTION, OR BY INTRAVENOUS INFUSION
  ▸ Adult: 15 mg every 6 hours for 24 hours, to be started usually 12–24 hours after start of methotrexate infusion, dose may be continued by mouth, consult local treatment protocol for further information
Suspected methotrexate overdosage
  ▸ BY INTRAVENOUS INJECTION, OR BY INTRAVENOUS INFUSION
  ▸ Adult: Initial dose equal to or exceeding dose of methotrexate, to be given at a maximum rate of 160 mg/minute, consult poisons information centres for advice on continuing management
Adjunct to fluorouracil in colorectal cancer
  ▸ BY SLOW INTRAVENOUS INJECTION
  ▸ Adult: (consult product literature)
SODIOFOLIN ®
As an antidote to methotrexate
  ▸ BY INTRAVENOUS INFUSION, OR BY INTRAVENOUS INJECTION
  ▸ Adult: (consult product literature)
Adjunct to fluorouracil in colorectal cancer
  ▸ BY INTRAVENOUS INJECTION, OR BY INTRAVENOUS INFUSION
  ▸ Adult: (consult product literature)

- **CONTRA-INDICATIONS** Intrathecal injection

- **CAUTIONS** Avoid simultaneous administration of methotrexate · **not** indicated for pernicious anaemia or other megaloblastic anaemias caused by vitamin B_{12} deficiency

- **INTERACTIONS** → Appendix 1: folates

- **SIDE-EFFECTS**
  ▸ **Common or very common**
  ▸ With intravenous use Bone marrow failure · dehydration · diarrhoea · mucositis · nausea · oral disorders · skin reactions · vomiting
  ▸ **Uncommon** Fever
  ▸ **Rare or very rare**
  ▸ With intramuscular use Agitation (with high doses) · depression (with high doses) · epilepsy exacerbated · gastrointestinal disorder · insomnia (with high doses) · urticaria
  ▸ With intravenous use Agitation (with high doses) · depression (with high doses) · epilepsy exacerbated · gastrointestinal disorder · insomnia (with high doses) · sensitisation
  ▸ **Frequency not known**
  ▸ With intravenous use Hyperammonaemia

- PREGNANCY Not known to be harmful; benefit outweighs risk.
- BREAST FEEDING Presence in milk unknown but benefit outweighs risk.
- NATIONAL FUNDING/ACCESS DECISIONS For full details see funding body website

NICE decisions

▶ Bevacizumab in combination with oxaliplatin and either fluorouracil plus folinic acid or capecitabine for the treatment of metastatic colorectal cancer (December 2010) NICE TA212 Not recommended

- MEDICINAL FORMS There can be variation in the licensing of different medicines containing the same drug.

Solution for injection

▶ Folinic acid (Non-proprietary)

  Folinic acid (as Calcium folinate) 7.5 mg per 1 ml Calcium folinate 15mg/2ml solution for injection ampoules | 5 ampoule PoM £39.00 DT = £39.00 (Hospital only)

  Folinic acid (as Calcium folinate) 10 mg per 1 ml Calcium folinate 350mg/35ml solution for injection vials | 10 vial PoM £1,277.60 (Hospital only)

  Calcium folinate 50mg/5ml solution for injection vials | 1 vial PoM £20.00 (Hospital only)

  Calcium folinate 300mg/30ml solution for injection vials | 1 vial PoM £100.00 (Hospital only)

  Calcium folinate 100mg/10ml solution for injection vials | 1 vial PoM £37.50 (Hospital only) | 10 vial PoM £404.50 (Hospital only)

▶ Sodiofolin (medac UK)

  Folinic acid (as Disodium folinate) 50 mg per 1 ml Sodiofolin 400mg/8ml solution for injection vials | 1 vial PoM £126.25 (Hospital only)

  Sodiofolin 100mg/2ml solution for injection vials | 1 vial PoM £35.09 (Hospital only)

Levofolinic acid

18-May-2020

- DRUG ACTION Levofolinic acid is an isomer of folinic acid.

● INDICATIONS AND DOSE

Prevention of methotrexate-induced adverse effects

▶ BY INTRAMUSCULAR INJECTION, OR BY INTRAVENOUS INJECTION, OR BY INTRAVENOUS INFUSION

▶ Adult: Usual dose 7.5 mg every 6 hours for 10 doses, usually started 12–24 hours after beginning of methotrexate infusion

Suspected methotrexate overdosage

▶ BY INTRAVENOUS INFUSION, OR BY INTRAVENOUS INJECTION

▶ Adult: Initial dose at least 50% of the dose of methotrexate, intravenous infusion to be administered at a maximum rate of 160 mg/minute, consult poisons information centres for advice on continuing management

Adjunct to fluorouracil in colorectal cancer

▶ BY SLOW INTRAVENOUS INJECTION

▶ Adult: (consult product literature)

- CONTRA-INDICATIONS Intrathecal injection
- CAUTIONS Avoid simultaneous administration of methotrexate · **not** indicated for pernicious anaemia or other megaloblastic anaemias caused by vitamin B₁₂ deficiency
- INTERACTIONS → Appendix 1: folates
- SIDE-EFFECTS
▶ Common or very common Dehydration · diarrhoea · mucosal toxicity · nausea · vomiting
▶ Uncommon Fever
▶ Rare or very rare Agitation (with high doses) · depression (with high doses) · epilepsy exacerbated · gastrointestinal disorder · insomnia (with high doses) · urticaria
- PREGNANCY Not known to be harmful; benefit outweighs risk.

- BREAST FEEDING Presence in milk unknown but benefit outweighs risk.
- MEDICINAL FORMS There can be variation in the licensing of different medicines containing the same drug.

Solution for injection

▶ Levofolinic acid (Non-proprietary)

  Levofolinic acid (as Disodium levofolinate) 50 mg per 1 ml Levofolinic acid 50mg/1ml solution for injection vials | 1 vial PoM £24.70 (Hospital only)

  Levofolinic acid 200mg/4ml solution for injection vials | 1 vial PoM £80.40 (Hospital only)

▶ Isovorin (Pfizer Ltd)

  Levofolinic acid (as Calcium levofolinate) 10 mg per 1 ml Isovorin 175mg/17.5ml solution for injection vials | 1 vial PoM £81.33 (Hospital only)

  Isovorin 25mg/2.5ml solution for injection vials | 1 vial PoM £11.62 (Hospital only)

3.1a Hyperuricaemia associated with cytotoxic drugs

Other drugs used for Hyperuricaemia associated with cytotoxic drugs Allopurinol, p. 1166 · Febuxostat, p. 1167

DETOXIFYING DRUGS ⟩ URATE OXIDASES

Rasburicase

21-Nov-2020

● INDICATIONS AND DOSE

Prophylaxis and treatment of acute hyperuricaemia, before and during initiation of chemotherapy, in patients with haematological malignancy and high tumour burden at risk of rapid lysis

▶ BY INTRAVENOUS INFUSION

▶ Adult: 200 micrograms/kg once daily for up to 7 days according to plasma-uric acid concentration

- CONTRA-INDICATIONS G6PD deficiency
- CAUTIONS Atopic allergies
- SIDE-EFFECTS
▶ Common or very common Diarrhoea · fever · headache · nausea · skin reactions · vomiting
▶ Uncommon Bronchospasm · haemolysis · haemolytic anaemia · hypersensitivity · hypotension · methaemoglobinaemia · seizure
▶ Rare or very rare Rhinitis
▶ Frequency not known Muscle contractions involuntary
- PREGNANCY Manufacturer advises avoid—no information available.
- BREAST FEEDING Manufacturer advises avoid—no information available.
- MONITORING REQUIREMENTS Monitor closely for hypersensitivity.
- EFFECT ON LABORATORY TESTS May interfere with test for uric acid—consult product literature.
- DIRECTIONS FOR ADMINISTRATION For *intravenous infusion* (*Fasturtec®*), manufacturer advises give intermittently in Sodium chloride 0.9%; reconstitute with solvent provided; gently swirl vial without shaking to dissolve; dilute requisite dose to 50 mL with infusion fluid and give over 30 minutes.
- MEDICINAL FORMS There can be variation in the licensing of different medicines containing the same drug.

Powder and solvent for solution for infusion

▶ Fasturtec (Sanofi)

  Rasburicase 1.5 mg Fasturtec 1.5mg powder and solvent for solution for infusion vials | 3 vial PoM £208.39 (Hospital only)

Rasburicase 7.5 mg Fasturtec 7.5mg powder and solvent for solution for infusion vials | 1 vial [PoM] £347.32 (Hospital only)

4 Hormone responsive malignancy

Breast cancer

14-Sep-2020

Description of condition

Breast cancer is the most common form of malignancy in women, especially in those aged over 50 years. Established risk factors include age, early onset of menstruation, late menopause, older age at first completed pregnancy, and a family history of breast cancer. The use of oral contraceptives or hormone replacement therapy (HRT) is also associated with an increased risk of breast cancer.

Breast cancer in men is rare. Although risk factors are not fully understood, it may be associated with abnormalities of sex hormone metabolism, including those caused by liver disease or testicular trauma, genetic predisposition, and environmental risk factors such as industrial exposure to chronic heat.

Additional risk factors include obesity and alcohol consumption.

Physical activity and breast-feeding protect against breast cancer.

Non-invasive breast cancer, also known as ductal carcinoma *in situ*, is when the cancer remains localised in the ducts. However, in most cases, the cancer is invasive at the time of diagnosis, which means that malignant cells are liable to spread beyond the immediate area of the tumour. Invasive breast cancer, where malignant cells spread beyond the ducts, can be defined as early breast cancer (stage I/II), locally advanced disease (stage III) and advanced disease (stage IV).

Aims of treatment

Reducing mortality, increasing progression-free and disease-free survival and improving quality of life are the main aims of treatment, and are dependent on the stage of the disease.

Surgery and radiotherapy aim to remove the tumour mass, whilst adjuvant drug therapy (drug treatment following surgery) aims to reduce the risk of disease recurrence and the risk of developing invasive disease. Neoadjuvant drug therapy (drug treatment before surgery) aims to reduce the size of the tumour to allow breast-conserving surgery to be possible and to reduce axillary lymph node involvement. Advanced breast cancer is not curable, and treatment aims to prolong survival, relieve symptoms and improve quality of life.

Overview

The management of patients with breast cancer involves surgery, radiotherapy, drug therapy, or a combination of these. The course of the disease and the therapeutic approach vary depending on the characteristics of the cancer. Factors such as patient age, menopausal status, tumour size and grade, involvement of axillary lymph nodes or skin, and the presence of hormone receptors within the tumour, may inform the extent and aggressiveness of the disease. [EvGr] The risks and benefits of each therapy should be discussed with the patient before being started. Ⓐ

Early and locally advanced breast cancer

For operable breast cancer, treatment involves surgery to the breast (breast-conserving surgery or mastectomy) and to the axillary lymph nodes, with or without radiotherapy to reduce local recurrence rates. This is often followed by adjuvant drug therapy to eradicate the micro-metastases that cause relapses. [EvGr] In women with invasive breast cancer, radiotherapy is recommended after breast-conserving surgery with clear margins (no cancer cells are found at the edges of the removed tissue), as it reduces local recurrence rates. However, the use of radiotherapy may be omitted if risk of local recurrence is very low and the woman is willing to take adjuvant endocrine therapy for a minimum of 5 years. Radiotherapy is also recommended after mastectomy in patients with node-positive invasive breast cancer or involved resection margins (cancer cells are found at the edges of the removed tissue). It should also be considered in patients with node-negative T3 or T4 invasive breast cancer. Ⓐ

Adjuvant drug therapy

Adjuvant drug therapy may include the use of chemotherapy, endocrine therapy, biological therapy, or bisphosphonate therapy. [EvGr] The decision to use adjuvant drug therapy should be based on the risks and benefits of treatment, disease prognosis and predictive factors such as oestrogen receptor (ER), progesterone receptor (PR), and human epidermal growth factor receptor 2 (HER2) status of the primary tumour.

In women with invasive breast cancer in only one breast who have not received treatment, including the use of neoadjuvant chemotherapy, NICE clinical guideline 101 recommends the use of the PREDICT tool to estimate prognosis and the absolute benefits of adjuvant therapy (www.predict.nhs.uk). Ⓐ

Chemotherapy

[EvGr] Adjuvant anthracycline–taxane combination chemotherapy is recommended in patients with invasive breast cancer who are at sufficient risk of disease recurrence to require chemotherapy. Ⓐ The choice of chemotherapy regimen is usually guided by local policy, Cancer Alliances, and the National Cancer Drugs Fund list.

Biological therapy

[EvGr] Trastuzumab p. 930 should be offered to patients with tumour size T1c and above HER2-positive invasive breast cancer, in combination with surgery, chemotherapy, or radiotherapy. It should also be considered in patients with a smaller tumour size (T1a or T1b) depending on their co-morbidities, prognosis, and possible toxicity with concomitant chemotherapy. Cardiac function should be regularly assessed in patients receiving trastuzumab p. 930, and particular caution should be taken in patients with underlying cardiac disease (consult product literature for further details). Ⓐ

Endocrine therapy

[EvGr] Tamoxifen p. 996 should be used as initial adjuvant endocrine therapy in men and premenopausal women with oestrogen-receptor-positive breast cancer. In addition, ovarian function suppression with a gonadotropin-releasing hormone (GnRH) should be considered in premenopausal women, taking into account the risk of temporary menopause. Ⓐ Ovarian function suppression aims to stop the production of circulating oestrogen, which can stimulate breast cancer progression. It may be most beneficial in women who are at sufficient risk of disease recurrence to have been offered chemotherapy.

[EvGr] In postmenopausal women with oestrogen-receptor positive invasive breast cancer who are at medium or high-risk of disease recurrence, an aromatase inhibitor should be given as first-line therapy. Alternatively, tamoxifen should be given if an aromatase inhibitor is not tolerated or is contra-indicated, or if the risk of disease recurrence is low. Ⓐ

Extended endocrine therapy

[EvGr] Extended endocrine therapy (total duration longer than 5 years) with an aromatase inhibitor [unlicensed indication] should be offered to postmenopausal women with oestrogen-receptor-positive invasive breast cancer at medium or high-risk of disease recurrence who have been taking tamoxifen for 2 to 5 years. Extended therapy should also be considered in postmenopausal women at low risk of disease recurrence.

Extended tamoxifen therapy for longer than 5 years can also be considered in both premenopausal and postmenopausal women with oestrogen-receptor-positive invasive breast cancer. ⒶA

Endocrine therapy for ductal carcinoma in situ

EvGr Following breast-conserving surgery, endocrine therapy should be offered to women with oestrogen-positive ductal carcinoma *in situ*, if radiotherapy is recommended but not given. If radiotherapy is **not** recommended, the use of endocrine therapy should also be considered. ⒶA

Bisphosphonate therapy

Zoledronic acid p. 772 and sodium clodronate p. 771 have been shown to improve disease-free survival and overall survival in postmenopausal women with node-positive invasive breast cancer. However, there is insufficient evidence to recommend their use in premenopausal women.

EvGr Intravenous zoledronic acid [unlicensed indication] or oral sodium clodronate [unlicensed indication] should be offered to postmenopausal women with lymph-node-positive invasive breast cancer. Treatment should be considered in those with lymph-node-negative invasive breast cancer who are at high-risk of recurrence.

Bisphosphonate therapy is also recommended in women at high-risk of osteoporosis due to the use of aromatase inhibitors in postmenopausal women, or in women with treatment-induced premature menopause. For further information, see Guidance for the management of breast cancer treatment-induced bone loss: a consensus position statement from a UK expert group, 2008. ⒶA

Neoadjuvant drug therapy

Neoadjuvant drug therapy may involve the use of chemotherapy or endocrine therapy.

Chemotherapy

EvGr Neoadjuvant chemotherapy should be offered to reduce tumour size in patients with oestrogen-receptor-negative invasive breast cancer. In patients with oestrogen-receptor-positive invasive breast cancer, chemotherapy should be considered. In patients with HER2-positive invasive breast cancer, neoadjuvant chemotherapy should be offered in combination with trastuzumab p. 930 and pertuzumab p. 925.

A chemotherapy regimen containing both a platinum [unlicensed indication] and an anthracycline should be considered in patients with triple-negative invasive breast cancer (oestrogen-receptor-negative, progesterone-receptor negative and HER2-negative). ⒶA

Endocrine therapy

EvGr If chemotherapy is not indicated, neoadjuvant endocrine therapy should be considered as an alternative in postmenopausal women with oestrogen-receptor-positive invasive breast cancer. ⒶA Chemotherapy and endocrine therapy are equally effective in postmenopausal women in terms of breast-conservation and shrinking of the tumour. Although chemotherapy is more effective than endocrine therapy at shrinking the tumour in premenopausal women, some tumours may respond to endocrine treatment.

Advanced breast cancer

Treatment of advanced breast cancer depends on the patient's treatment history, disease severity, and oestrogen receptor and HER2 status.

Endocrine therapy

EvGr For the majority of patients with oestrogen-receptor-positive advanced breast cancer, endocrine therapy is recommended as first-line treatment. Aromatase inhibitors should be offered to postmenopausal women with no

previous history of endocrine treatment, or to those previously treated with tamoxifen p. 996.

Tamoxifen in combination with ovarian function suppression should be offered as first-line treatment to pre- and perimenopausal women with oestrogen-receptor-positive advanced breast cancer not previously treated with tamoxifen.

Ovarian function suppression should be offered to pre- and perimenopausal women who have had disease progression despite treatment with tamoxifen.

Tamoxifen should be offered as first-line treatment to men with oestrogen-receptor-positive advanced breast cancer. ⒶA

Chemotherapy

EvGr Chemotherapy should be offered as first-line treatment in patients with oestrogen-receptor-positive advanced breast cancer that is imminently life-threatening or requires early relief of symptoms because of significant visceral organ involvement. Once chemotherapy treatment is completed, endocrine therapy should be offered. ⒶA The choice of chemotherapy regimen is usually guided by local policy, Cancer Alliances, and the National Cancer Drugs Fund list.

Biological therapy

EvGr Trastuzumab is recommended for the treatment of HER2-positive advanced breast cancer. It is used in combination with paclitaxel p. 969 in those who have not received chemotherapy for metastatic breast cancer, and as monotherapy for patients who have received at least two chemotherapy regimens for metastatic breast cancer (see trastuzumab *National funding/access decisions*). ⒶA

Bisphosphonate therapy

EvGr The use of bisphosphonates should be considered in patients with metastatic breast cancer to reduce pain and prevent skeletal complications of bone metastases. ⒶA

Familial breast cancer

EvGr Chemoprevention should be offered to all women who have been identified as being at high-risk of developing breast cancer. Chemoprevention should also be considered in women at moderate-risk. Other strategies to reduce breast cancer risk should also be considered, for example bilateral mastectomy or bilateral oophorectomy. Women who were at high-risk of breast cancer and have undergone a bilateral mastectomy should not receive chemoprevention. ⒶA

Treatment options for chemoprevention

EvGr Chemoprevention should only be continued for 5 years.

Tamoxifen is recommended for premenopausal women who do not have a history of, or increased risk of thromboembolic disease or endometrial cancer.

Anastrozole p. 997 [unlicensed indication] is recommended in postmenopausal women who do not have severe osteoporosis, see Osteoporosis p. 765. In women who have severe osteoporosis, or who do not wish to take anastrozole, treatment with tamoxifen can be given, provided there is no history, or increased risk of thromboembolic disease or endometrial cancer. Alternatively, raloxifene hydrochloride p. 797 is an option [unlicensed indication] in postmenopausal women with a uterus who do not wish to take tamoxifen, unless there is a history or increased risk of thromboembolic disease. ⒶA

Treatment of menopausal symptoms

EvGr Some treatments used in the management of breast cancer, such as tamoxifen or ovarian function suppression may lead to menopausal symptoms or early menopause, and women should be counselled about these side-effects prior to starting any of these treatments.

Women diagnosed with breast cancer should discontinue their hormone replacement therapy (HRT) because of possible tumour stimulation and interference with adjuvant endocrine therapy. HRT should not be offered routinely to

8

Immune system and malignant disease

women with menopausal symptoms if they have a history of breast cancer; however, in exceptional circumstances, HRT can be offered to women with severe menopausal symptoms once the associated risks have been discussed.

Selective serotonin re-uptake inhibitor (SSRIs) antidepressants may be offered to relieve menopausal symptoms such as hot flushes in women with breast cancer who are not taking tamoxifen. Ⓐ Clonidine hydrochloride p. 159, venlafaxine p. 388 [unlicensed indication] and gabapentin p. 332 [unlicensed indication] are sometimes used for the treatment of hot flushes in women with breast cancer after discussion with the patient and information given about side effects. The MHRA/CHM have released important safety information on the use of antiepileptic drugs and the risk of suicidal thoughts and behaviour. For further information, see Epilepsy p. 321.

Useful Resources

Early and locally advanced breast cancer: diagnosis and management. National Institute for Health and Care Excellence. Clinical guideline 101. July 2018.
www.nice.org.uk/guidance/ng101

Advanced breast cancer: diagnosis and treatment. National Institute for Health and Care Excellence. Clinical guideline 81. August 2017.
www.nice.org.uk/guidance/cg81

Familial breast cancer: classification, care and managing breast cancer and related risks in people with a family history of breast cancer. National Institute for Health and Care Excellence. Clinical guideline 164. June 2013 (updated March 2017).
www.nice.org.uk/guidance/cg164

Guidance for the management of breast cancer treatment-induced bone loss: a consensus position statement from a UK expert group, 2008.
nos.org.uk/media/98027/bone-health-guidelines-breast-cancer-treatments.pdf

Patient decision aids: Taking a medicine to reduce the chance of developing breast cancer: postmenopausal women at moderately increased risk; Taking a medicine to reduce the chance of developing breast cancer: postmenopausal women at high risk. National Institute for Health and Care Excellence. March 2017.
www.nice.org.uk/about/what-we-do/our-programmes/nice-guidance/nice-guidelines/shared-decision-making

Prostate cancer

14-Aug-2020

Description of condition

Prostate cancer is the most common form of cancer affecting men. It can also affect transgender women, as the prostate is usually conserved after gender-confirming surgery. The main risk factors are age (most cases being diagnosed in men over 70 years of age), ethnicity (more common in black African-Caribbean men), obesity, and a familial component. Prostate cancer is usually slow-growing and asymptomatic at diagnosis, however, the presenting symptoms of advanced disease are usually urinary outflow obstruction, or, pelvic or back pain due to bone metastases. Treatment decisions are guided by baseline prostate specific antigen (PSA) levels, tumour grade (Gleason score), the stage of the tumour, the patient's life expectancy (based on age and comorbid conditions), treatment morbidity, and patient preference.

Aims of treatment

Reducing mortality, increasing progression-free and disease-free survival and improving quality of life are the main aims of treatment, and are dependent on the stage of disease.

Watchful waiting or active surveillance aim to monitor for disease progression, while radical treatments such as prostatectomy and radiotherapy aim to eliminate the

malignancy. Hormone therapy and chemotherapy aim to slow the progression of prostate cancer and to control symptoms. In metastatic disease, treatment is aimed at prolonging survival and relieving symptoms.

Overview

[EvGr] Treatment options for patients with prostate cancer include watchful waiting, active surveillance, prostatectomy, radiotherapy (such as external beam), brachytherapy, hormone therapy, and chemotherapy. The benefits and risks of each option should be discussed with patients. Ⓐ

Watchful waiting is a strategy for 'controlling' rather than 'curing' prostate cancer and is aimed at patients in whom curative treatment is unsuitable or declined. It involves monitoring for disease progression and is often suitable in patients not likely to suffer significant morbidity from their prostate cancer. Active surveillance, a 'curative' strategy, is aimed at patients who do not wish to have immediate treatment. It involves the deferred use of radical treatment until disease progression occurs or until the patient requests treatment. For information on monitoring in watchful waiting or the protocol for active surveillance, see NICE clinical guideline **Prostate cancer** (see *Useful resources*).

[EvGr] At any stage of care, when moving from active surveillance to radical treatment, patient preferences, comorbidities and life expectancy should be taken into account. Ⓐ

Hormone therapy includes anti-androgen therapy—to block the effects of androgens, androgen deprivation therapy such as a luteinising hormone-releasing hormone (LHRH) agonist, or a gonadorelin antagonist—to reduce androgen levels, and bilateral orchidectomy—to remove the endogenous supply of androgens.

In patients with localised prostate cancer, the choice of treatment is guided by whether the disease is considered low, intermediate, or high risk according to the Gleason score, the serum PSA level, and the tumour clinical stage. High risk localised prostate cancer is also included in the definition of locally advanced prostate cancer. For further information on risk stratification, see NICE clinical guideline **Prostate cancer** (see *Useful resources*).

Localised or locally advanced prostate cancer

[EvGr] In patients with **low-risk localised prostate cancer**, offer a choice between active surveillance, radical prostatectomy or radiotherapy.

Radical treatment should be offered to patients with localised prostate cancer undergoing active surveillance who show evidence of disease progression.

In patients with **intermediate-risk localised prostate cancer**, radical treatments (prostatectomy or radiotherapy) should be offered, and for those who decline them, active surveillance can be considered.

In patients with **high-risk localised prostate cancer** (when there is a realistic prospect of long-term disease control), and in those with **locally advanced disease**, radical prostatectomy or radiotherapy should be offered.

In patients with **intermediate-risk** and **high-risk localised prostate cancer** who have chosen radical radiotherapy, this should be offered in combination with androgen deprivation therapy. Androgen deprivation therapy should be given for 6 months before, during or after radiotherapy; in patients with **high-risk localised prostate cancer**, consider continuing therapy for up to 3 years. Brachytherapy in combination with radiotherapy can also be considered in these patients.

In patients with newly diagnosed **non-metastatic prostate cancer** discuss the option of chemotherapy with docetaxel p. 968 [unlicensed indication] if they are starting long term androgen deprivation therapy, have no significant co-morbidities and have high-risk disease.

Pelvic radiotherapy should be considered in those with **locally advanced prostate cancer** who have a higher than

15% risk of pelvic lymph node involvement and are to receive neoadjuvant hormonal therapy and radical radiotherapy. Ⓐ

Metastatic prostate cancer

EvGr Patients with newly diagnosed **metastatic prostate cancer** who do not have significant comorbidities, should be offered chemotherapy with docetaxel.

Bilateral orchidectomy should be offered to all patients with **metastatic prostate cancer** as an alternative to continuous LHRH agonist treatment. Anti-androgen monotherapy with bicalutamide p. 990 [unlicensed indication] can be offered to those who are willing to accept the adverse impact on overall survival and gynaecomastia, in the hope of retaining sexual function. However, if satisfactory sexual function is not maintained, stop bicalutamide and start androgen deprivation therapy.

Abiraterone acetate below (in combination with prednisone or prednisolone p. 718) and enzalutamide p. 991 are both recommended as options for the treatment of **hormone-relapsed metastatic prostate cancer** in patients who have no or mild symptoms after androgen deprivation therapy has failed, and before chemotherapy is indicated.

In patients with **hormone-relapsed metastatic prostate cancer**, chemotherapy with docetaxel can be used. It is recommended that treatment with docetaxel is stopped after 10 cycles, or if severe adverse events occur, or if there is evidence of disease progression.

Abiraterone acetate (in combination with prednisone or prednisolone) and enzalutamide are also recommended in **hormone-relapsed metastatic prostate cancer** if disease has progressed during or after treatment with a docetaxel-containing chemotherapy regimen.

In patients with **hormone-relapsed metastatic prostate cancer**, a corticosteroid such as dexamethasone p. 714 can be offered as third line therapy after androgen deprivation therapy and anti-androgen therapy.

In patients with **hormone-relapsed metastatic prostate cancer**, zoledronic acid p. 772 can be considered to prevent or reduce skeletal-related events.

Bisphosphonates can be considered for pain relief in **hormone-relapsed metastatic prostate cancer** when other treatments have failed to give satisfactory pain relief. Ⓐ

Management of side-effects of treatment

EvGr Patients should be informed about the side-effects of treatment; particularly urinary and sexual dysfunction, loss of fertility, radiation-induced enteropathy, osteoporosis, gynaecomastia, fatigue, and hot flushes. Ⓐ

Tumour flare due to an initial surge in testosterone concentrations has been reported in the initial stages of treatment with LHRH agonists; the manufacturers advise that the use of prophylactic anti-androgen therapy (such as cyproterone acetate p. 812) should be considered.

EvGr Medroxyprogesterone acetate p. 856 [unlicensed indication] can be used, initially for up to 10 weeks, to manage troublesome hot flushes caused by long-term androgen suppression; cyproterone acetate can be considered as an alternative if medroxyprogesterone acetate is not effective or not tolerated. Ⓐ

The MHRA/CHM have issued important safety information on the use of cyproterone acetate and risk of meningioma. For further information, see *Important safety information* for cyproterone acetate.

EvGr Patients who experience loss of sexual function should have access to specialist erectile dysfunction services and be considered for treatment with a phosphodiesterase type-5 inhibitor.

Patients who are on androgen deprivation therapy should be offered a supervised exercise program (at least twice a week for 12 weeks) to reduce fatigue and improve quality of life.

A bisphosphonate should be offered to patients who have osteoporosis and who are having androgen deprivation

therapy; denosumab p. 774 is an alternative if bisphosphonates are not appropriate.

Although there is limited evidence, intermittent therapy may be considered for patients who are having long-term androgen deprivation therapy to reduce side-effects.

Gynaecomastia can occur with long-term (longer than 6 months) bicalutamide p. 990 treatment. Prophylactic radiotherapy (within the first month of treatment) should be offered; or if radiotherapy is unsuccessful, weekly tamoxifen p. 996 [unlicensed indication] can be considered. Ⓐ

Useful Resources

Prostate cancer: diagnosis and management. National Institute for Health and Care Excellence. NICE guideline 131. May 2019.
www.nice.org.uk/guidance/ng131

Other drugs used for Hormone responsive malignancy
Buserelin, p. 779 · Ethinylestradiol, p. 802 · Goserelin, p. 780 · Leuprorelin acetate, p. 780 · Norethisterone, p. 806 · Triptorelin, p. 782

ANTINEOPLASTIC DRUGS > ANTI-ANDROGENS

Abiraterone acetate

02-Nov-2020

● **INDICATIONS AND DOSE**

Metastatic castration-resistant prostate cancer in patients whose disease has progressed during or after treatment with a docetaxel-containing chemotherapy regimen (in combination with prednisone or prednisolone) | Metastatic castration-resistant prostate cancer in patients who are asymptomatic or mildly symptomatic after failure of androgen deprivation therapy in whom chemotherapy is not yet clinically indicated (in combination with prednisone or prednisolone) | High risk metastatic hormone-sensitive prostate cancer in newly diagnosed patients (in combination with androgen deprivation therapy, and prednisone or prednisolone)

▶ BY MOUTH
▶ Adult: 1 g once daily, for dose of concurrent prednisone or prednisolone—consult product literature

● CAUTIONS Diabetes (increased risk of hyperglycaemia—monitor blood sugar frequently) · history of cardiovascular disease

CAUTIONS, FURTHER INFORMATION
▶ Cardiovascular disease Manufacturer advises correct hypertension and hypokalaemia before treatment (if significant risk of congestive heart failure, such as history of cardiac failure, uncontrolled hypertension or cardiac events, consult product literature for management and increased monitoring).

● INTERACTIONS → Appendix 1: anti-androgens

● SIDE-EFFECTS
▶ **Common or very common** Angina pectoris · arrhythmias · bone fracture · diarrhoea · dyspepsia · haematuria · heart failure · hepatic disorders · hypertension · hypertriglyceridaemia · hypokalaemia · left ventricular dysfunction · osteoporosis · peripheral oedema · rash · sepsis · urinary tract infection
▶ **Uncommon** Adrenal insufficiency · myopathy
▶ **Rare or very rare** Alveolitis allergic
▶ **Frequency not known** Myocardial infarction · QT interval prolongation

● CONCEPTION AND CONTRACEPTION Men should use condoms if their partner is pregnant, and use condoms in combination with another effective contraceptive method if their partner is of child-bearing potential—toxicity in *animal* studies.

- HEPATIC IMPAIRMENT Manufacturer advises use with caution in moderate impairment and only if benefit clearly outweighs risk; avoid in severe impairment.
- RENAL IMPAIRMENT Use with caution in severe impairment—no information available.
- MONITORING REQUIREMENTS
  - ▶ Monitor blood pressure, serum potassium concentration, and fluid balance before treatment, and at least monthly during treatment—consult product literature for management of hypertension, hypokalaemia and oedema.
  - ▶ Monitor liver function before treatment, then every 2 weeks for the first 3 months of treatment, then monthly thereafter—interrupt treatment if serum alanine aminotransferase or aspartate aminotransferase greater than 5 times the upper limit (consult product literature for details of restarting treatment at a lower dose) and discontinue permanently if 20 times the upper limit.
- NATIONAL FUNDING/ACCESS DECISIONS
  For full details see funding body website
  NICE decisions
  - ▶ Abiraterone for castration-resistant metastatic prostate cancer previously treated with a docetaxel-containing regimen (updated July 2016) NICE TA259 Recommended with restrictions
  - ▶ Abiraterone for treating metastatic hormone-relapsed prostate cancer before chemotherapy is indicated (updated July 2016) NICE TA387 Recommended with restrictions
  Scottish Medicines Consortium (SMC) decisions
  - ▶ Abiraterone acetate (*Zytiga*®) with prednisone or prednisolone for the treatment of metastatic castration-resistant prostate cancer (mCRPC) in adult men whose disease has progressed on or after a docetaxel-based chemotherapy regimen (August 2012) SMC No. 764/12 Recommended with restrictions
  - ▶ Abiraterone acetate (*Zytiga*®) is indicated with prednisone or prednisolone for the treatment of metastatic castration-resistant prostate cancer (mCRPC) in adult men who are asymptomatic or mildly symptomatic after failure of androgen deprivation therapy in whom chemotherapy is not yet clinically indicated (October 2015) SMC No. 873/13 Recommended
  - ▶ Abiraterone acetate (*Zytiga*®) with prednisone or prednisolone for the treatment of adult men with newly diagnosed high-risk metastatic hormone-sensitive prostate cancer (mHSPC) in combination with androgen deprivation therapy (ADT) (January 2020) SMC No. SMC2215 Recommended
- MEDICINAL FORMS There can be variation in the licensing of different medicines containing the same drug.
  Tablet
  CAUTIONARY AND ADVISORY LABELS 23
  - ▶ Zytiga (Janssen-Cilag Ltd)
    Abiraterone acetate 500 mg Zytiga 500mg tablets | 56 tablet [PoM] £2,735.00

Apalutamide
23-Apr-2019

- DRUG ACTION Apalutamide is an androgen receptor inhibitor that decreases tumour cell proliferation and increases apoptosis.

- INDICATIONS AND DOSE
  Prostate cancer (specialist use only)
  - ▶ BY MOUTH
  - ▶ Adult: 240 mg once daily, for dose adjustments due to side-effects—consult product literature
- CONTRA-INDICATIONS History or risk of seizures
- CAUTIONS History or risk of QT-interval prolongation · recent cardiovascular disease

- INTERACTIONS → Appendix 1: anti-androgens
- SIDE-EFFECTS
  - ▶ **Common or very common** Arthralgia · autoimmune thyroiditis · bone fractures · conjunctivitis · costal cartilage fracture · dyslipidaemia · fall · fatigue · genital rash · hypothyroidism · oral disorders · rash pustular · sacrum fracture · skin reactions · weight decreased
  - ▶ **Uncommon** Seizure (discontinue permanently)
  - ▶ **Frequency not known** QT interval prolongation
- CONCEPTION AND CONTRACEPTION Manufacturer advises men should use condoms in combination with another highly effective contraceptive method during treatment and for 3 months after stopping treatment if their partner is of childbearing potential.
- HEPATIC IMPAIRMENT Manufacturer advises avoid in severe impairment (no information available).
- RENAL IMPAIRMENT Manufacturer advises caution in severe impairment (no information available).

- MEDICINAL FORMS There can be variation in the licensing of different medicines containing the same drug.
  Tablet
  - ▶ Erleada (Janssen-Cilag Ltd) ▼
    Apalutamide 60 mg Erleada 60mg tablets | 112 tablet [PoM] £2,735.00

Bicalutamide
01-Sep-2020

- INDICATIONS AND DOSE
  Locally advanced prostate cancer at high risk of disease progression either alone or as adjuvant treatment to prostatectomy or radiotherapy | Locally advanced, non-metastatic prostate cancer when surgical castration or other medical intervention inappropriate
  - ▶ BY MOUTH
  - ▶ Adult: 150 mg once daily
  Advanced prostate cancer, in combination with gonadorelin analogue or surgical castration
  - ▶ BY MOUTH
  - ▶ Adult: 50 mg once daily, to be started at the same time as surgical castration or at least 3 days before gonadorelin therapy
  Prostate cancer (metastatic) with the aim of retaining sexual function.
  - ▶ BY MOUTH
  - ▶ Adult: 150 mg once daily
- UNLICENSED USE [EvGr] Bicalutamide is used in prostate cancer (metastatic) with the aim of retaining sexual function, ⚠ but it is not licensed for this indication.
- CAUTIONS Risk of photosensitivity—avoid excessive exposure to UV light and sunlight
- INTERACTIONS → Appendix 1: anti-androgens
- SIDE-EFFECTS
  - ▶ **Common or very common** Alopecia · anaemia · appetite decreased · asthenia · breast tenderness · chest pain · constipation · depression · dizziness · drowsiness · flatulence · gastrointestinal discomfort · gynaecomastia · haematuria · hair changes · hepatic disorders · hot flush · hypertransaminasaemia · nausea · oedema · sexual dysfunction · skin reactions · weight increased
  - ▶ **Uncommon** Angioedema · interstitial lung disease
  - ▶ **Rare or very rare** Photosensitivity reaction
  - ▶ **Frequency not known** QT interval prolongation
- HEPATIC IMPAIRMENT Manufacturer advises caution in moderate to severe impairment (increased risk of accumulation).
- MONITORING REQUIREMENTS Consider periodic liver function tests.

- PATIENT AND CARER ADVICE
Risk of photosensitivity Patients should be advised to consider the use of sunscreen.

- MEDICINAL FORMS There can be variation in the licensing of different medicines containing the same drug. Forms available from special-order manufacturers include: oral suspension

Tablet
‣ Bicalutamide (Non-proprietary)
Bicalutamide 50 mg Bicalutamide 50mg tablets | 28 tablet `PoM`
£95.83 DT = £4.09
Bicalutamide 150 mg Bicalutamide 150mg tablets | 28 tablet `PoM`
£192.00 DT = £6.23
‣ Casodex (AstraZeneca UK Ltd)
Bicalutamide 50 mg Casodex 50mg tablets | 28 tablet `PoM`
£119.79 DT = £4.09
Bicalutamide 150 mg Casodex 150mg tablets | 28 tablet `PoM`
£240.00 DT = £6.23

Darolutamide
03-Dec-2020

- DRUG ACTION Darolutamide is an androgen receptor inhibitor that decreases tumour cell proliferation.

- INDICATIONS AND DOSE
Prostate cancer (specialist use only)
▸ BY MOUTH
‣ Adult: 600 mg twice daily, for dose adjustments or interruption due to side-effects—consult product literature

- CAUTIONS History or risk of QT-interval prolongation · recent cardiovascular disease

- INTERACTIONS → Appendix 1: anti-androgens

- SIDE-EFFECTS
▸ **Common or very common** Acute coronary syndrome · asthenia · atherosclerosis coronary artery · bone fracture · cardiogenic shock · heart failure · ischaemic heart disease · lethargy · malaise · pain · rash
▸ **Frequency not known** Neutropenia

- CONCEPTION AND CONTRACEPTION Manufacturer advises men use condoms during and for 1 week after stopping treatment if their partner is pregnant, and highly effective contraception if their partner is of childbearing potential.

- HEPATIC IMPAIRMENT Manufacturer advises caution in moderate and severe impairment.
Dose adjustments Manufacturer advises reduce initial dose in moderate or severe impairment to 300 mg twice daily.

- RENAL IMPAIRMENT Manufacturer advises caution in severe impairment.
Dose adjustments Manufacturer advises reduce initial dose in severe impairment to 300 mg twice daily.

- NATIONAL FUNDING/ACCESS DECISIONS
For full details see funding body website
NICE decisions
▸ **Darolutamide with androgen deprivation therapy for treating hormone-relapsed non-metastatic prostate cancer (November 2020)** NICE TA660 Recommended
Scottish Medicines Consortium (SMC) decisions
▸ Darolutamide (*Nubeqa*®) for the treatment of adult men with non-metastatic castration-resistant prostate cancer who are at high risk of developing metastatic disease (November 2020) SMC No. SMC2297 Recommended

- MEDICINAL FORMS There can be variation in the licensing of different medicines containing the same drug.
Tablet
CAUTIONARY AND ADVISORY LABELS 21
▸ Nubeqa (Bayer Plc) ▼
Darolutamide 300 mg Nubeqa 300mg tablets | 112 tablet `PoM`
£4,040.00 (Hospital only)

Enzalutamide
27-Aug-2020

- INDICATIONS AND DOSE
Castration-resistant prostate cancer (specialist use only)
▸ BY MOUTH
‣ Adult: 160 mg once daily, for dose adjustments due to side-effects—consult product literature
DOSE ADJUSTMENTS DUE TO INTERACTIONS
▸ Manufacturer advises if concurrent use of potent inhibitors of CYP2C8 is unavoidable, reduce dose to 80 mg daily.

- CAUTIONS History or risk of QT-interval prolongation · history or risk of seizure · recent cardiovascular disease

- INTERACTIONS → Appendix 1: anti-androgens

- SIDE-EFFECTS
▸ **Common or very common** Acute coronary syndrome · anxiety · asthenia · atherosclerosis coronary artery · bone fracture · concentration impaired · fall · gynaecomastia · headache · hot flush · hypertension · ischaemic heart disease · memory loss · restless legs · skin reactions
▸ **Uncommon** Cognitive disorder · leucopenia · neutropenia · seizures · visual hallucinations
▸ **Frequency not known** Back pain · diarrhoea · face oedema · muscle complaints · muscle weakness · nausea · oral disorders · posterior reversible encephalopathy syndrome (PRES) · QT interval prolongation · throat oedema · thrombocytopenia · vomiting

- CONCEPTION AND CONTRACEPTION Men should use condoms during treatment and for 3 months after stopping treatment if their partner is pregnant, and use condoms in combination with another effective contraceptive method if their partner is of child-bearing potential—toxicity in *animal* studies.

- RENAL IMPAIRMENT Caution in severe impairment—no information available.

- PATIENT AND CARER ADVICE
Missed doses Manufacturer advises if a dose is not taken at the usual time, the missed dose should be taken as close as possible to the usual time; if a dose is missed entirely for the day, the missed dose should be taken the following day at the usual dose.
Driving and skilled tasks Manufacturer advises patients and carers should be counselled on the effects on driving and performance of skilled tasks—risk of psychiatric or neurological events, including seizures.

- NATIONAL FUNDING/ACCESS DECISIONS
For full details see funding body website
NICE decisions
▸ **Enzalutamide for metastatic hormone-relapsed prostate cancer previously treated with a docetaxel-containing regimen (July 2014)** NICE TA316 Recommended with restrictions
▸ **Enzalutamide for treating metastatic hormone-relapsed prostate cancer before chemotherapy is indicated (January 2016)** NICE TA377 Recommended with restrictions
▸ **Enzalutamide for hormone-relapsed non-metastatic prostate cancer (May 2019)** NICE TA580 Not recommended
Scottish Medicines Consortium (SMC) decisions
▸ Enzalutamide (*Xtandi*®) for the treatment of adult men with high-risk non-metastatic castration-resistant prostate cancer (October 2019) SMC No. SMC2195 Not recommended

- MEDICINAL FORMS There can be variation in the licensing of different medicines containing the same drug.
Tablet
CAUTIONARY AND ADVISORY LABELS 25
▸ Xtandi (Astellas Pharma Ltd)
Enzalutamide 40 mg Xtandi 40mg tablets | 112 tablet `PoM`
£2,734.67

8

Immune system and malignant disease

Flutamide

04-Jun-2020

● **INDICATIONS AND DOSE**

Advanced prostate cancer | Metastatic prostate cancer refractory to gonadorelin analogue therapy (monotherapy)
▶ BY MOUTH
▶ Adult: 250 mg 3 times a day

● CONTRA-INDICATIONS Do not initiate if serum transaminases greater than 2–3 times the upper limit of normal

● CAUTIONS Avoid excessive alcohol consumption · avoid in Acute porphyrias p. 1107 · cardiac disease (oedema reported) · diabetes (decreased tolerance to glucose)

● INTERACTIONS → Appendix 1: anti-androgens

● SIDE-EFFECTS
▶ **Common or very common** Appetite abnormal · asthenia · breast abnormalities · diarrhoea · drowsiness · galactorrhoea · gynaecomastia · hepatic function abnormal (sometimes fatal) · hepatitis (sometimes fatal) · insomnia · nausea · vomiting
▶ **Rare or very rare** Alopecia · anxiety · breast neoplasm · cardiovascular disorder · chest pain · constipation · cough · depression · dizziness · dyspnoea · gastrointestinal discomfort · gastrointestinal disorders · hair growth abnormal · headache · herpes zoster · hot flush · hypertension · interstitial pneumonitis · libido decreased · lupus-like syndrome · lymphoedema · malaise · muscle cramps · oedema · photosensitivity reaction · skin reactions · thirst · vision blurred
▶ **Frequency not known** QT interval prolongation

● HEPATIC IMPAIRMENT Manufacturer advises caution.

● RENAL IMPAIRMENT Manufacturer advises caution.

● MONITORING REQUIREMENTS
▶ Manufacturer advises monitor liver function before starting treatment, monthly for the first 4 months, and thereafter as clinically indicated.
▶ Manufacturer advises monitor bone mineral density before starting treatment, after 1 year of treatment, and thereafter as clinically indicated.
▶ Manufacturer advises monitor for respiratory symptoms during the first few weeks of treatment (interstitial pneumonitis reported).

● PATIENT AND CARER ADVICE Manufacturer advises patients and their carers should be told to discontinue treatment and seek immediate medical attention if signs or symptoms of hepatic toxicity occur.

● MEDICINAL FORMS There can be variation in the licensing of different medicines containing the same drug.
Tablet
▶ Flutamide (Non-proprietary)
Flutamide 250 mg Flutamide 250mg tablets | 84 tablet [PoM] £106.23 DT = £106.23

OESTROGENS

Diethylstilbestrol

21-May-2020

(Stilboestrol)

● **INDICATIONS AND DOSE**

Breast cancer in postmenopausal women
▶ BY MOUTH
▶ Adult: 10–20 mg daily
Prostate cancer
▶ BY MOUTH
▶ Adult: 1–3 mg daily

● CAUTIONS Cardiovascular disease

● SIDE-EFFECTS Bone pain (in breast cancer) · breast abnormalities · cervical mucus increased · cholelithiasis · contact lens intolerance · depression · erectile dysfunction · erythema nodosum · feminisation · fluid retention · gynaecomastia · headaches · hypercalcaemia (in breast cancer) · hypertension · increased risk of thrombosis · jaundice cholestatic · mood altered · nausea · neoplasms · skin reactions · sodium retention · testicular atrophy · uterine disorders · vomiting · weight changes · withdrawal bleed

● PREGNANCY In first trimester, high doses associated with vaginal carcinoma, urogenital abnormalities, and reduced fertility in female offspring. Increased risk of hypospadias in male offspring.

● HEPATIC IMPAIRMENT Manufacturer advises caution in mild to moderate impairment; avoid in severe or active impairment.

● MEDICINAL FORMS There can be variation in the licensing of different medicines containing the same drug.
Tablet
▶ Diethylstilbestrol (Non-proprietary)
Diethylstilbestrol 1 mg Diethylstilbestrol 1mg tablets | 28 tablet [PoM] £115.26 DT = £115.23

PITUITARY AND HYPOTHALAMIC HORMONES AND ANALOGUES > ANTI-GONADOTROPHIN-RELEASING HORMONES

Degarelix

08-Feb-2019

● **INDICATIONS AND DOSE**

Advanced hormone-dependent prostate cancer
▶ BY SUBCUTANEOUS INJECTION
▶ Adult: Initially 240 mg, to be administered as 2 injections of 120 mg, then 80 mg every 28 days, dose to be administered into the abdominal region

● CAUTIONS Diabetes · susceptibility to QT-interval prolongation

● SIDE-EFFECTS
▶ **Common or very common** Anaemia · chills · diarrhoea · dizziness · fatigue · fever · gynaecomastia · headache · hot flush · influenza like illness · insomnia · musculoskeletal discomfort · musculoskeletal pain · nausea · sexual dysfunction · skin reactions · sweat changes · testicular disorders · weight changes
▶ **Uncommon** Alopecia · appetite decreased · arrhythmias · bone disorders · breast pain · cognitive impairment · constipation · depression · diabetes mellitus · dry mouth · dyspnoea · gastrointestinal discomfort · genital discomfort · hyperglycaemia · hypertension · hypotension · joint disorders · malaise · muscle spasms · muscle weakness · numbness · palpitations · pelvic pain · peripheral oedema · QT interval prolongation · renal impairment · urinary disorders · vision blurred · vomiting
▶ **Rare or very rare** Febrile neutropenia · heart failure · injection site necrosis · myocardial infarction

● HEPATIC IMPAIRMENT Manufacturer advises caution (limited information available)—monitor liver function.

● RENAL IMPAIRMENT Manufacturer advises caution in severe impairment—no information available.

● MONITORING REQUIREMENTS Monitor bone density.

● NATIONAL FUNDING/ACCESS DECISIONS
For full details see funding body website
NICE decisions
▶ Degarelix for treating advanced hormone-dependent prostate cancer (August 2016) NICE TA404 Recommended with restrictions

● MEDICINAL FORMS There can be variation in the licensing of different medicines containing the same drug.

Powder and solvent for solution for injection
▸ Firmagon (Ferring Pharmaceuticals Ltd)
Degarelix (as Degarelix acetate) 80 mg Firmagon 80mg powder and solvent for solution for injection vials | 1 vial [PoM] £129.37 DT = £129.37
Degarelix (as Degarelix acetate) 120 mg Firmagon 120mg powder and solvent for solution for injection vials | 2 vial [PoM] £260.00 DT = £260.00

PITUITARY AND HYPOTHALAMIC HORMONES AND ANALOGUES ⟩ SOMATOSTATIN ANALOGUES

Somatostatin analogues   🔵

● CAUTIONS Diabetes mellitus (antidiabetic requirements may be reduced) · insulinoma (increased depth and duration of hypoglycaemia may occur—observe patients and monitor blood glucose levels when initiating treatment and changing doses) · may cause growth hormone-secreting pituitary tumour expansion during treatment (causing serious complications)

● SIDE-EFFECTS
▸ **Common or very common** Alopecia · appetite decreased · asthenia · cholecystitis · cholelithiasis (following long term use) · cholestasis · constipation · diabetes mellitus · diarrhoea · dizziness · gastrointestinal discomfort · gastrointestinal disorders · glucose tolerance impaired (following long term use) · headache · hyperglycaemia (long term use) · hypoglycaemia · myalgia · nausea · pruritus · sinus bradycardia · vomiting

● MONITORING REQUIREMENTS
▸ Monitor for signs of tumour expansion (e.g. visual field defects).
▸ Ultrasound examination of the gallbladder is recommended before treatment and at intervals of 6–12 months during treatment.

● DIRECTIONS FOR ADMINISTRATION Injection sites should be rotated.

🏳 above

┃ Lanreotide
13-Aug-2020

● **INDICATIONS AND DOSE**
SOMATULINE AUTOGEL ®

Acromegaly (if somatostatin analogue not given previously)
▸ BY DEEP SUBCUTANEOUS INJECTION
▸ Adult: Initially 60 mg every 28 days, adjusted according to response, (consult product literature), for patients treated previously with somatostatin analogue, consult product literature for initial dose, dose to be given in the gluteal region

Neuroendocrine (particularly carcinoid) tumours
▸ BY DEEP SUBCUTANEOUS INJECTION
▸ Adult: Initially 60–120 mg every 28 days, adjusted according to response, dose to be given in the gluteal region

Unresectable locally advanced or metastatic gastroenteropancreatic neuroendocrine tumours of midgut, pancreatic or unknown origin where hindgut sites of origin have been excluded
▸ BY DEEP SUBCUTANEOUS INJECTION
▸ Adult: 120 mg every 28 days

SOMATULINE LA ®

Acromegaly and neuroendocrine (particularly carcinoid) tumours
▸ BY INTRAMUSCULAR INJECTION
▸ Adult: Initially 30 mg every 14 days, increased to 30 mg every 7–10 days, adjusted according to response

Thyroid tumours
▸ BY INTRAMUSCULAR INJECTION
▸ Adult: Initially 30 mg every 14 days, increased to 30 mg every 10 days, adjusted according to response

● CAUTIONS Cardiac disorders (including bradycardia) · patients with carcinoid tumours—exclude the presence of an obstructive intestinal tumour before treatment

● INTERACTIONS → Appendix 1: lanreotide

● SIDE-EFFECTS
▸ **Common or very common** Biliary dilatation · lethargy · musculoskeletal pain · weight decreased
▸ **Uncommon** Hot flush · insomnia
▸ **Frequency not known** Pancreatitis

● PREGNANCY Manufacturer advises use only if potential benefit outweighs risk.

● BREAST FEEDING Manufacturer advises caution—no information available.

● MONITORING REQUIREMENTS Monitor for hypothyroidism when clinically indicated.

● NATIONAL FUNDING/ACCESS DECISIONS
For full details see funding body website
All Wales Medicines Strategy Group (AWMSG) decisions
▸ Lanreotide (*Somatuline Autogel*) for treatment of grade 1 and a subset of grade 2 (Ki67 index up to 10 %) gastroenteropancreatic neuroendocrine tumours (GEP-NETs) of midgut, pancreatic or unknown origin where hindgut sites of origin have been excluded, in adult patients with unresectable locally advanced or metastatic disease (September 2018) AWMSG No. 1988 Recommended

● MEDICINAL FORMS There can be variation in the licensing of different medicines containing the same drug.

Solution for injection
▸ Somatuline Autogel (Ipsen Ltd)
Lanreotide (as Lanreotide acetate) 120 mg per 1 ml Somatuline Autogel 60mg/0.5ml solution for injection pre-filled syringes with safety system | 1 pre-filled disposable injection [PoM] £551.00 DT = £551.00
Lanreotide (as Lanreotide acetate) 180 mg per 1 ml Somatuline Autogel 90mg/0.5ml solution for injection pre-filled syringes with safety system | 1 pre-filled disposable injection [PoM] £736.00 DT = £736.00
Lanreotide (as Lanreotide acetate) 240 mg per 1 ml Somatuline Autogel 120mg/0.5ml solution for injection pre-filled syringes with safety system | 1 pre-filled disposable injection [PoM] £937.00 DT = £937.00

Powder and solvent for suspension for injection
▸ Somatuline LA (Ipsen Ltd)
Lanreotide (as Lanreotide acetate) 30 mg Somatuline LA 30mg powder and solvent for suspension for injection vials | 1 vial [PoM] £323.00 DT = £323.00

🏳 above

┃ Octreotide
14-Sep-2020

● **INDICATIONS AND DOSE**

Symptoms associated with carcinoid tumours with features of carcinoid syndrome, VIPomas, glucagonomas
▸ BY SUBCUTANEOUS INJECTION
▸ Adult: Initially 50 micrograms 1–2 times a day, adjusted according to response; increased to 200 micrograms 3 times a day, higher doses may be required exceptionally; maintenance doses are variable; in carcinoid tumours, discontinue after 1 week if no effect, if rapid response continued →

required, initial dose may be given by intravenous injection (with ECG monitoring and after dilution)

Acromegaly, short-term treatment before pituitary surgery or long-term treatment in those inadequately controlled by other treatment or until radiotherapy becomes fully effective
‣ BY SUBCUTANEOUS INJECTION
‣ Adult: 100–200 micrograms 3 times a day, discontinue if no improvement within 3 months

Prevention of complications following pancreatic surgery
‣ BY SUBCUTANEOUS INJECTION
‣ Adult: (consult product literature)

Test dose before use of depot preparation
‣ BY SUBCUTANEOUS INJECTION
‣ Adult: Test dose 50–100 micrograms for 1 dose, test dose should be given if subcutanous octreotide not previously given

Acromegaly | Neuroendocrine (particularly carcinoid) tumour adequately controlled by subcutaneous octreotide
‣ BY DEEP INTRAMUSCULAR INJECTION USING DEPOT INJECTION
‣ Adult: Initially 20 mg every 4 weeks for 3 months then adjusted according to response, increased if necessary up to 30 mg every 4 weeks, to be administered into the gluteal muscle, for *acromegaly*, start depot 1 day after the last dose of subcutaneous octreotide, for *neuroendocrine tumours*, continue subcutaneous octreotide for 2 weeks after first dose of depot octreotide

Advanced neuroendocrine tumours of the midgut, or tumours of unknown primary origin where non-midgut sites of origin have been excluded
‣ BY DEEP INTRAMUSCULAR INJECTION USING DEPOT INJECTION
‣ Adult: 30 mg every 4 weeks

Reduce intestinal secretions in palliative care | Reduce vomiting due to bowel obstruction in palliative care
‣ BY CONTINUOUS SUBCUTANEOUS INFUSION
‣ Adult: 0.25–0.5 mg/24 hours (max. per dose 0.75 mg/24 hours), occasionally doses higher than the maximum are sometimes required

● INTERACTIONS → Appendix 1: octreotide

● SIDE-EFFECTS
‣ **Common or very common** Arrhythmias · biliary sludge · dyspnoea · hyperbilirubinaemia · hypothyroidism · skin reactions · thyroid disorder
‣ **Uncommon** Dehydration
‣ **Frequency not known** Hepatic disorders · pancreatitis acute (after administration) · thrombocytopenia

SIDE-EFFECTS, FURTHER INFORMATION Administering non-depot injections of octreotide between meals and at bedtime may reduce gastrointestinal side-effects.

● CONCEPTION AND CONTRACEPTION Effective contraception required during treatment.

● PREGNANCY Possible effect on fetal growth; manufacturer advises use only if potential benefit outweighs risk.

● BREAST FEEDING Manufacturer advises avoid—present in milk in *animal* studies.

● HEPATIC IMPAIRMENT Manufacturer advises caution (risk of increased half-life in cirrhosis).
Dose adjustments Manufacturer advises consider dose reduction—consult product literature.

● MONITORING REQUIREMENTS
‣ Monitor thyroid function on long-term therapy.
‣ Monitor liver function.
‣ With intravenous use ECG monitoring required with intravenous administration.

● TREATMENT CESSATION Avoid abrupt withdrawal of short-acting subcutaneous octreotide (associated with biliary colic and pancreatitis).

● DIRECTIONS FOR ADMINISTRATION For *intravenous injection or intravenous infusion*, manufacturer advises dilute requisite dose to a ratio of at least 1:1 and up to a maximum of 1:9 by volume with Sodium Chloride 0.9%.

● PRESCRIBING AND DISPENSING INFORMATION
Palliative care For further information on the use of octreotide in palliative care, see www.medicinescomplete.com/#/content/palliative/octreotide.

● NATIONAL FUNDING/ACCESS DECISIONS
For full details see funding body website
All Wales Medicines Strategy Group (AWMSG) decisions
‣ Octreotide (*Sandostatin® LAR®*) for the treatment of patients with advanced neuroendocrine tumours of the midgut or of unknown primary origin where non-midgut sites of origin have been excluded (September 2018) AWMSG No. 3732 Recommended

● MEDICINAL FORMS There can be variation in the licensing of different medicines containing the same drug.
Solution for injection
‣ Octreotide (Non-proprietary)
Octreotide (as Octreotide acetate) 50 microgram per 1 ml Octreotide 50micrograms/1ml solution for injection pre-filled syringes | 5 pre-filled disposable injection (PoM) £18.85–£18.88 DT = £18.88
Octreotide 50micrograms/1ml solution for injection ampoules | 5 ampoule (PoM) £2.97–£18.60 DT = £14.87
Octreotide 50micrograms/1ml solution for injection vials | 5 vial (PoM) £22.00
Octreotide (as Octreotide acetate) 100 microgram per 1 ml Octreotide 100micrograms/1ml solution for injection ampoules | 5 ampoule (PoM) £32.65 DT = £27.97
Octreotide 100micrograms/1ml solution for injection pre-filled syringes | 5 pre-filled disposable injection (PoM) £30.33–£32.90 DT = £30.33
Octreotide 100micrograms/1ml solution for injection vials | 5 vial (PoM) £32.65 DT = £32.65
Octreotide (as Octreotide acetate) 200 microgram per 1 ml Octreotide 1mg/5ml solution for injection vials | 1 vial (PoM) £65.00 DT = £65.00
Octreotide (as Octreotide acetate) 500 microgram per 1 ml Octreotide 500micrograms/1ml solution for injection vials | 5 vial (PoM) £158.25 DT = £158.25
Octreotide 500micrograms/1ml solution for injection ampoules | 5 ampoule (PoM) £27.09–£169.35 DT = £135.47
Octreotide 500micrograms/1ml solution for injection pre-filled syringes | 5 pre-filled disposable injection (PoM) £154.22–£169.00 DT = £154.22
‣ Sandostatin (Novartis Pharmaceuticals UK Ltd)
Octreotide (as Octreotide acetate) 50 microgram per 1 ml Sandostatin 50micrograms/1ml solution for injection ampoules | 5 ampoule (PoM) £14.87 DT = £14.87
Octreotide (as Octreotide acetate) 100 microgram per 1 ml Sandostatin 100micrograms/1ml solution for injection ampoules | 5 ampoule (PoM) £27.97 DT = £27.97
Octreotide (as Octreotide acetate) 500 microgram per 1 ml Sandostatin 500micrograms/1ml solution for injection ampoules | 5 ampoule (PoM) £135.47 DT = £135.47

Powder and solvent for suspension for injection
‣ Olatuton (Teva UK Ltd)
Octreotide (as Octreotide acetate) 10 mg Olatuton 10mg powder and solvent for prolonged-release suspension for injection vials | 1 vial (PoM) £494.74 DT = £549.71
Octreotide (as Octreotide acetate) 20 mg Olatuton 20mg powder and solvent for prolonged-release suspension for injection vials | 1 vial (PoM) £719.40 DT = £799.33
Octreotide (as Octreotide acetate) 30 mg Olatuton 30mg powder and solvent for prolonged-release suspension for injection vials | 1 vial (PoM) £898.57 DT = £998.41
‣ Sandostatin LAR (Novartis Pharmaceuticals UK Ltd)
Octreotide (as Octreotide acetate) 10 mg Sandostatin LAR 10mg powder and solvent for suspension for injection vials | 1 vial (PoM) £549.71 DT = £549.71
Octreotide (as Octreotide acetate) 20 mg Sandostatin LAR 20mg powder and solvent for suspension for injection vials | 1 vial (PoM) £799.33 DT = £799.33

Octreotide (as Octreotide acetate) 30 mg Sandostatin LAR 30mg
powder and solvent for suspension for injection vials | 1 vial PoM
£998.41 DT = £998.41

⚑ 993

Pasireotide

02-Mar-2018

● **INDICATIONS AND DOSE**

Cushing's disease [when surgery has failed or is inappropriate]

▶ BY SUBCUTANEOUS INJECTION

▶ **Adult:** Initially 600 micrograms twice daily for 2 months, then increased if necessary to 900 micrograms twice daily, consider discontinuation if no response after 2 months of treatment, for dose adjustment due to side-effects—consult product literature

▶ BY DEEP INTRAMUSCULAR INJECTION

▶ **Adult:** Initially 10 mg every 4 weeks, increased if necessary up to 40 mg every 4 weeks, dose may be titrated every 2–4 months based on response and tolerability, consider discontinuation if no clinical benefit observed, for dose adjustment due to side-effects—consult product literature

Acromegaly [when surgery has failed or is inappropriate, and control with another somatostatin analogue is inadequate]

▶ BY DEEP INTRAMUSCULAR INJECTION

▶ **Adult:** Initially 40 mg every 4 weeks, increased if necessary up to 60 mg every 4 weeks, dose may be increased if levels of growth hormone and/or insulin-like growth factor-1 are not fully controlled after 3 months of initial dosing, for dose adjustment due to side-effects—consult product literature

● CAUTIONS Cardiac disorders (including bradycardia) · susceptibility to QT-interval prolongation (including electrolyte disturbances)

● INTERACTIONS → Appendix 1: pasireotide

● SIDE-EFFECTS

▶ **Common or very common** Adrenal insufficiency · arthralgia · hypotension · QT interval prolongation

▶ **Uncommon** Anaemia

● PREGNANCY Manufacturer advises avoid—toxicity in *animal* studies.

● BREAST FEEDING Manufacturer advises avoid—present in milk in *animal* studies.

● HEPATIC IMPAIRMENT Manufacturer advises caution in moderate impairment (risk of increased exposure); avoid in severe impairment.

Dose adjustments

▶ With subcutaneous use for Cushing's disease Manufacturer advises reduce initial dose to 300 micrograms twice daily (max. dose 600 micrograms twice daily) in moderate impairment.

▶ With intramuscular use for Cushing's disease Manufacturer advises max. dose 20 mg every four weeks in moderate impairment.

▶ When used for Acromegaly Manufacturer advises reduce initial dose to 20 mg every four weeks (max. dose 40 mg every four weeks) in moderate impairment.

● RENAL IMPAIRMENT Manufacturer advises caution in severe impairment—increased plasma-pasireotide exposure.

● MONITORING REQUIREMENTS

▶ Manufacturer advises consider monitoring pituitary function before treatment initiation and periodically thereafter.

▶ With subcutaneous use Manufacturer advises monitor liver function before treatment initiation, after 1, 2, 4, 8, and 12 weeks of treatment, and thereafter as clinically

indicated. Manufacturer advises assess glycaemic status before treatment initiation, weekly for the first 2–3 months of treatment, over the first 2–4 weeks after any dose increase, periodically thereafter, and 3 months after treatment is complete—if glycaemic control is poor, diabetes management and monitoring should be intensified before and during treatment. Manufacturer advises monitor ECG and electrolytes before treatment initiation, after one week of treatment, and periodically thereafter.

▶ With intramuscular use Manufacturer advises monitor liver function before treatment initiation, after the first 2–3 weeks of treatment, then monthly for 3 months, and thereafter as clinically indicated. Manufacturer advises assess glycaemic status before treatment initiation, weekly for the first 3 months of treatment, over the first 4–6 weeks after any dose increase, periodically thereafter, and 3 months after treatment is complete—if glycaemic control is poor, diabetes management and monitoring should be intensified before and during treatment. Manufacturer advises monitor ECG and electrolytes before treatment initiation, after 3 weeks of treatment, and periodically thereafter.

● PRESCRIBING AND DISPENSING INFORMATION
Switching between formulations

▶ When used for Cushing's disease There are no clinical data available on switching between formulations; if a switch is required, manufacturer advises to maintain an interval of at least 28 days between the last intramuscular injection and the first subcutaneous injection—for further information, consult product literature.

● PATIENT AND CARER ADVICE Manufacturer advises patients and their carers should be informed of the signs and symptoms of hypocortisolism (including weakness, fatigue, anorexia, nausea, vomiting, hypotension, hyperkalaemia, hyponatraemia, hypoglycaemia).

Driving and skilled tasks Manufacturer advises patients and carers should be counselled on the effects on driving and performance of skilled tasks—increased risk of fatigue and dizziness.

● MEDICINAL FORMS There can be variation in the licensing of different medicines containing the same drug.

Solution for injection

▶ Signifor (Recordati Rare Diseases UK Ltd)
Pasireotide (as Pasireotide diaspartate) 300 microgram per 1 ml Signifor 0.3mg/1ml solution for injection ampoules | 60 ampoule PoM £2,800.00
Pasireotide (as Pasireotide diaspartate) 600 microgram per 1 ml Signifor 0.6mg/1ml solution for injection ampoules | 60 ampoule PoM £3,240.00
Pasireotide (as Pasireotide diaspartate) 900 microgram per 1 ml Signifor 0.9mg/1ml solution for injection ampoules | 60 ampoule PoM £3,240.00

Powder and solvent for suspension for injection

▶ Signifor (Recordati Rare Diseases UK Ltd)
Pasireotide (as Pasireotide pamoate) 10 mg Signifor 10mg powder and solvent for suspension for injection vials | 1 vial PoM £2,300.00
Pasireotide (as Pasireotide pamoate) 20 mg Signifor 20mg powder and solvent for suspension for injection vials | 1 vial PoM £2,300.00
Pasireotide (as Pasireotide pamoate) 30 mg Signifor 30mg powder and solvent for suspension for injection vials | 1 vial PoM £2,300.00
Pasireotide (as Pasireotide pamoate) 40 mg Signifor 40mg powder and solvent for suspension for injection vials | 1 vial PoM £2,300.00
Pasireotide (as Pasireotide pamoate) 60 mg Signifor 60mg powder and solvent for suspension for injection vials | 1 vial PoM £2,300.00

8

Immune system and malignant disease

PROGESTOGENS

Megestrol acetate

31-Jan-2020

● **INDICATIONS AND DOSE**

Treatment of breast cancer
▸ BY MOUTH
▸ Adult: 160 mg once daily

● CONTRA-INDICATIONS Acute porphyrias p. 1107
● CAUTIONS Elderly · history of thrombophlebitis
● SIDE-EFFECTS
▸ **Common or very common** Adrenal insufficiency · alopecia · appetite increased · asthenia · carpal tunnel syndrome · constipation · Cushing's syndrome · diabetes mellitus · diarrhoea · dyspnoea · embolism and thrombosis · erectile dysfunction · flatulence · glucose tolerance impaired · heart failure · hot flush · hypercalcaemia · hyperglycaemia · hypertension · lethargy · menorrhagia · mood altered · nausea · oedema · pain · skin reactions · tumour flare · urinary frequency increased · vomiting · weight increased
● PREGNANCY Avoid. Reversible feminisation of male fetuses reported in *animal* studies. Risk of hypospadias in male fetuses and masculinisation of female fetuses.
● BREAST FEEDING Discontinue breast-feeding.
● HEPATIC IMPAIRMENT Manufacturer advises caution in severe impairment.

● MEDICINAL FORMS There can be variation in the licensing of different medicines containing the same drug. Forms available from special-order manufacturers include: tablet, capsule, oral suspension

Oral suspension
▸ Megestrol (Imported (United States))
  Megestrol acetate 40 mg per 1 ml Megestrol 200mg/5ml oral suspension | 240 ml [PoM] [⊠]
Tablet
▸ Megestrol (Imported (United States))
  Megestrol acetate 40 mg Megestrol 40mg tablets | 100 tablet [⊠]
▸ Megace (Bausch & Lomb UK Ltd)
  Megestrol acetate 160 mg Megace 160mg tablets | 30 tablet [PoM]
  £19.52 DT = £19.52

4.1 Hormone responsive breast cancer

ANTINEOPLASTIC DRUGS ⟩ ANTI-OESTROGENS

Fulvestrant

16-Jul-2020

● **INDICATIONS AND DOSE**

Oestrogen-receptor-positive breast cancer
▸ BY DEEP INTRAMUSCULAR INJECTION
▸ Adult: 500 mg every 2 weeks for the first 3 doses, then 500 mg every month, to be administered into the buttock

● INTERACTIONS → Appendix 1: fulvestrant
● SIDE-EFFECTS
▸ **Common or very common** Appetite decreased · arthralgia · asthenia · diarrhoea · headache · hot flush · hypersensitivity · increased risk of infection · nausea · pain · rash · vaginal haemorrhage · venous thromboembolism · vomiting
▸ **Uncommon** Hepatic disorders · vaginal discharge
▸ **Frequency not known** Myalgia
● PREGNANCY Manufacturer advises avoid—increased incidence of fetal abnormalities and death in *animal* studies.

● BREAST FEEDING Manufacturer advises avoid—present in milk in *animal* studies.
● HEPATIC IMPAIRMENT Manufacturer advises caution in mild to moderate impairment—risk of increased exposure; avoid in severe impairment—no information available.
● RENAL IMPAIRMENT Manufacturer advises caution if creatinine clearance less than 30 mL/minute—no information available.
● DIRECTIONS FOR ADMINISTRATION Manufacturer advises 500 mg dose should be administered as one 250-mg injection (slowly over 1–2 minutes) into each buttock.
● NATIONAL FUNDING/ACCESS DECISIONS
For full details see funding body website

NICE decisions
▸ Fulvestrant for untreated locally advanced or metastatic oestrogen-receptor positive breast cancer (January 2018) NICE TA503 Not recommended

● MEDICINAL FORMS There can be variation in the licensing of different medicines containing the same drug.
Solution for injection
▸ Fulvestrant (Non-proprietary)
  Fulvestrant 50 mg per 1 ml Fulvestrant 250mg/5ml solution for injection pre-filled syringes | 2 pre-filled disposable injection [PoM] £444.05 DT = £522.41 (Hospital only)
▸ Faslodex (AstraZeneca UK Ltd)
  Fulvestrant 50 mg per 1 ml Faslodex 250mg/5ml solution for injection pre-filled syringes | 2 pre-filled disposable injection [PoM] £522.41 DT = £522.41

Tamoxifen

28-Jul-2020

● DRUG ACTION An anti-oestrogen which induces gonadotrophin release by occupying oestrogen receptors in the hypothalamus, thereby interfering with feedback mechanisms; chorionic gonadotrophin is sometimes used as an adjunct in the treatment of female infertility.

● **INDICATIONS AND DOSE**

Pre- and perimenopausal women with oestrogen-receptor-positive breast cancer not previously treated with tamoxifen
▸ BY MOUTH
▸ Adult: 20 mg daily
Anovulatory infertility
▸ BY MOUTH
▸ Adult: Initially 20 mg daily on days 2, 3, 4 and 5 of cycle, if necessary the daily dose may be increased to 40 mg then 80 mg for subsequent courses; if cycles irregular, start initial course on any day, with subsequent course starting 45 days later or on day 2 of cycle if menstruation occurs
Gynaecomastia [prevention in men undergoing long-term bicalutamide treatment, if radiotherapy unsuccessful]
▸ BY MOUTH
▸ Adult: 20 mg once weekly
Breast cancer [chemoprevention in women at moderate-to-high risk]
▸ BY MOUTH
▸ Adult: 20 mg daily for 5 years

● UNLICENSED USE Tamoxifen may be used as detailed below, although these situations are considered outside the scope of its licence:
  ● [EvGr] the prevention of gynaecomastia in men ⟨Ⓐ⟩.
● CONTRA-INDICATIONS Treatment of infertility contra-indicated if personal or family history of idiopathic venous thromboembolism or genetic predisposition to thromboembolism
● CAUTIONS Acute porphyrias p. 1107
● INTERACTIONS → Appendix 1: tamoxifen

- SIDE-EFFECTS
▶ **Common or very common** Alopecia · anaemia · cataract · cerebral ischaemia · constipation · diarrhoea · dizziness · embolism and thrombosis · fatigue · fluid retention · headache · hepatic disorders · hot flush · hypersensitivity · hypertriglyceridaemia · muscle complaints · nausea · neoplasms · retinopathy · sensation abnormal · skin reactions · taste altered · uterine disorders · vaginal haemorrhage · vomiting · vulvovaginal disorders
▶ **Uncommon** Hypercalcaemia · interstitial pneumonitis · leucopenia · pancreatitis · thrombocytopenia · vision disorders
▶ **Rare or very rare** Agranulocytosis · angioedema · corneal changes · cutaneous lupus erythematosus · cutaneous vasculitis · cystic ovarian swelling · nerve disorders · neutropenia · radiation recall reaction · Stevens-Johnson syndrome · tumour flare
▶ **Frequency not known** Amenorrhoea
SIDE-EFFECTS, FURTHER INFORMATION **Endometrial changes** Increased endometrial changes, including hyperplasia, polyps, cancer, and uterine sarcoma reported; prompt investigation required if abnormal vaginal bleeding including menstrual irregularities, vaginal discharge, and pelvic pain or pressure in those receiving (or who have received) tamoxifen.

Risk of thromboembolism Tamoxifen can increase the risk of thromboembolism particularly during and immediately after major surgery or periods of immobility (consider interrupting treatment and initiating anticoagulant measures).

- CONCEPTION AND CONTRACEPTION Unless being used in the treatment of female infertility, effective contraception must be used during treatment and for 2 months after stopping. Patients being treated for infertility should be warned that there is a risk of multiple pregnancy (*rarely* more than twins).
- PREGNANCY Avoid—possible effects on fetal development.
- BREAST FEEDING Suppresses lactation. Avoid unless potential benefit outweighs risk.
- PRESCRIBING AND DISPENSING INFORMATION
Patient decision aids Taking tamoxifen to reduce the chance of developing breast cancer: premenopausal women at moderately increased risk; Taking tamoxifen to reduce the chance of developing breast cancer: premenopausal women at high risk. National Institute for Health and Care Excellence. March 2017.
www.nice.org.uk/about/what-we-do/our-programmes/nice-guidance/nice-guidelines/shared-decision-making
- PATIENT AND CARER ADVICE
Endometrial changes Patients should be informed of the risk of endometrial cancer and told to report relevant symptoms promptly.
Thromboembolism Patients should be made aware of the symptoms of thromboembolism and advised to report sudden breathlessness and any pain in the calf of one leg.

- MEDICINAL FORMS There can be variation in the licensing of different medicines containing the same drug. Forms available from special-order manufacturers include: oral suspension, oral solution

Oral solution
▶ Tamoxifen (Non-proprietary)
Tamoxifen (as Tamoxifen citrate) 2 mg per 1 ml Tamoxifen 10mg/5ml oral solution sugar free sugar-free | 150 ml PoM £39.14 DT = £39.02

Tablet
▶ Tamoxifen (Non-proprietary)
Tamoxifen (as Tamoxifen citrate) 10 mg Tamoxifen 10mg tablets | 30 tablet PoM £47.21 DT = £38.03
Tamoxifen (as Tamoxifen citrate) 20 mg Tamoxifen 20mg tablets | 30 tablet PoM £15.37 DT = £7.25
Tamoxifen (as Tamoxifen citrate) 40 mg Tamoxifen 40mg tablets | 30 tablet PoM £76.74 DT = £75.15

Toremifene   25-Aug-2020

- INDICATIONS AND DOSE
Hormone-dependent metastatic breast cancer in postmenopausal women
▶ BY MOUTH
▶ Adult: 60 mg daily

- CONTRA-INDICATIONS Bradycardia · electrolyte disturbances (particularly uncorrected hypokalaemia) · endometrial hyperplasia · heart failure with reduced left-ventricular ejection fraction · history of arrhythmias · QT prolongation
- CAUTIONS Avoid in Acute porphyrias p. 1107 · history of severe thromboembolic disease
- INTERACTIONS → Appendix 1: toremifene
- SIDE-EFFECTS
▶ **Common or very common** Dizziness · fatigue · hot flush · hyperhidrosis · nausea · oedema · skin reactions · vaginal discharge · vomiting
▶ **Uncommon** Appetite decreased · constipation · depression · dyspnoea · headache · insomnia · thromboembolism · uterine disorders · weight increased
▶ **Rare or very rare** Alopecia · corneal opacity · endometrial cancer · hepatic disorders · uterine haemorrhage · vertigo
▶ **Frequency not known** Anaemia · leucopenia · thrombocytopenia
SIDE-EFFECTS, FURTHER INFORMATION Increased endometrial changes, including hyperplasia, polyps and cancer reported.
- PREGNANCY Avoid.
- BREAST FEEDING Avoid.
- HEPATIC IMPAIRMENT Manufacturer advises caution; avoid in severe hepatic failure (risk of decreased elimination).

- MEDICINAL FORMS There can be variation in the licensing of different medicines containing the same drug.
Tablet
▶ Fareston (Orion Pharma (UK) Ltd)
Toremifene (as Toremifene citrate) 60 mg Fareston 60mg tablets | 30 tablet PoM £29.08 DT = £29.08

HORMONE ANTAGONISTS AND RELATED AGENTS > AROMATASE INHIBITORS

Anastrozole   16-Oct-2020

- INDICATIONS AND DOSE
Adjuvant treatment of oestrogen-receptor-positive early invasive breast cancer in postmenopausal women | Adjuvant treatment of oestrogen-receptor-positive early breast cancer in postmenopausal women following 2–3 years of tamoxifen therapy | Advanced breast cancer in postmenopausal women which is oestrogen-receptor-positive or responsive to tamoxifen
▶ BY MOUTH
▶ Adult: 1 mg daily

Breast cancer [chemoprevention in postmenopausal women at moderate to high risk] (initiated under specialist supervision)
▶ BY MOUTH
▶ Adult: 1 mg daily for 5 years

- UNLICENSED USE EvGr Anastrozole is used for chemoprevention of breast cancer, ⓔ but it is not licensed for this indication.
- CONTRA-INDICATIONS Not for premenopausal women
- CAUTIONS Susceptibility to osteoporosis

8

Immune system and malignant disease

● SIDE-EFFECTS
▸ **Common or very common** Alopecia · appetite decreased · arthritis · asthenia · bone pain · carpal tunnel syndrome · diarrhoea · drowsiness · headache · hot flush · hypercholesterolaemia · hypersensitivity · joint disorders · myalgia · nausea · osteoporosis · sensation abnormal · skin reactions · taste altered · vaginal haemorrhage · vomiting · vulvovaginal dryness
▸ **Uncommon** Hepatitis · hypercalcaemia · trigger finger
▸ **Rare or very rare** Angioedema · Stevens-Johnson syndrome · vasculitis
▸ **Frequency not known** Mood altered
● PREGNANCY Avoid.
● BREAST FEEDING Avoid.
● HEPATIC IMPAIRMENT Manufacturer advises use with caution in moderate-to-severe impairment.
● RENAL IMPAIRMENT Avoid if creatinine clearance less than 20 mL/minute.
● PRE-TREATMENT SCREENING Laboratory test for menopause if doubt.
● MONITORING REQUIREMENTS
▸ Osteoporosis Assess bone mineral density before treatment and at regular intervals.
● PATIENT AND CARER ADVICE
Driving and skilled tasks Asthenia and drowsiness may affect ability to drive or operate machinery.
● NATIONAL FUNDING/ACCESS DECISIONS
For full details see funding body website
Scottish Medicines Consortium (SMC) decisions
▸ Anastrozole (*Arimidex*®) for the adjuvant treatment of postmenopausal women with oestrogen receptor-positive early invasive breast cancer (September 2005) SMC No. 198/05 Recommended with restrictions
▸ Anastrozole (*Arimidex*®) for early breast cancer in hormone receptor-positive postmenopausal women who have received 2 to 3 years of adjuvant tamoxifen (November 2006) SMC No. 322/06 Recommended with restrictions
● MEDICINAL FORMS There can be variation in the licensing of different medicines containing the same drug.
Tablet
▸ Anastrozole (Non-proprietary)
Anastrozole 1 mg Anastrozole 1mg tablets | 28 tablet [PoM] £68.56 DT = £1.80
▸ Arimidex (AstraZeneca UK Ltd)
Anastrozole 1 mg Arimidex 1mg tablets | 28 tablet [PoM] £68.56 DT = £1.80

Exemestane

08-Feb-2019

● INDICATIONS AND DOSE
Adjuvant treatment of oestrogen-receptor-positive early breast cancer in postmenopausal women following 2–3 years of tamoxifen therapy | Advanced breast cancer in postmenopausal women in whom anti-oestrogen therapy has failed
▸ BY MOUTH
▸ Adult: 25 mg daily

● CONTRA-INDICATIONS Not indicated for premenopausal women
● INTERACTIONS → Appendix 1: exemestane
● SIDE-EFFECTS
▸ **Common or very common** Alopecia · appetite decreased · arthralgia · asthenia · bone fracture · carpal tunnel syndrome · constipation · depression · diarrhoea · dizziness · gastrointestinal discomfort · headache · hot flush · hyperhidrosis · insomnia · leucopenia · nausea · osteoporosis · pain · paraesthesia · peripheral oedema · skin reactions · thrombocytopenia · vomiting

▸ **Rare or very rare** Acute generalised exanthematous pustulosis (AGEP) · drowsiness · hepatic disorders
● PREGNANCY Avoid.
● BREAST FEEDING Avoid.
● HEPATIC IMPAIRMENT Manufacturer advises caution.
● RENAL IMPAIRMENT Manufacturer advises caution.

● MEDICINAL FORMS There can be variation in the licensing of different medicines containing the same drug.
Tablet
CAUTIONARY AND ADVISORY LABELS 21
▸ Exemestane (Non-proprietary)
Exemestane 25 mg Exemestane 25mg tablets | 30 tablet [PoM] £88.80 DT = £20.98
▸ Aromasin (Pfizer Ltd)
Exemestane 25 mg Aromasin 25mg tablets | 30 tablet [PoM] £88.80 DT = £20.98

Letrozole

01-Aug-2018

● INDICATIONS AND DOSE
First-line treatment in postmenopausal women with hormone-dependent advanced breast cancer | Adjuvant treatment of oestrogen-receptor-positive invasive early breast cancer in postmenopausal women | Advanced breast cancer in postmenopausal women (naturally or artificially induced menopause) in whom other anti-oestrogen therapy has failed | Extended adjuvant treatment of hormone-dependent invasive breast cancer in postmenopausal women who have received standard adjuvant tamoxifen therapy for 5 years | Neo-adjuvant treatment in postmenopausal women with localised hormone-receptor-positive, human epidermal growth factor-2 negative breast cancer where chemotherapy is not suitable and surgery not yet indicated
▸ BY MOUTH
▸ Adult: 2.5 mg daily

● CONTRA-INDICATIONS Not indicated for premenopausal women
● CAUTIONS Susceptibility to osteoporosis
● SIDE-EFFECTS
▸ **Common or very common** Alopecia · appetite abnormal · arthralgia · asthenia · bone fracture · bone pain · constipation · depression · diarrhoea · dizziness · gastrointestinal discomfort · headache · hot flush · hypercholesterolaemia · hyperhidrosis · hypertension · malaise · myalgia · nausea · oedema · osteoporosis · skin reactions · vaginal haemorrhage · vomiting · weight changes
▸ **Uncommon** Anxiety · arthritis · breast pain · cancer pain · carpal tunnel syndrome · cataract · cerebrovascular insufficiency · cough · drowsiness · dry mouth · dysaesthesia · dyspnoea · embolism and thrombosis · eye irritation · fever · insomnia · irritability · ischaemic heart disease · leucopenia · memory loss · mucosal dryness · myocardial infarction · palpitations · stomatitis · tachycardia · taste altered · thirst · urinary frequency increased · urinary tract infection · vision blurred · vulvovaginal disorders
▸ **Frequency not known** Angioedema · hepatitis · toxic epidermal necrolysis · trigger finger
● CONCEPTION AND CONTRACEPTION Manufacturer advises effective contraception required until postmenopausal status fully established (return of ovarian function reported in postmenopausal women).
● PREGNANCY Avoid (isolated cases of birth defects reported).
● BREAST FEEDING Manufacturer advises avoid.

8

Immune system and malignant disease

HEPATIC IMPAIRMENT Manufacturer advises caution in severe impairment (increased exposure and half-life).

RENAL IMPAIRMENT Manufacturer advises caution if creatinine clearance less than 10 mL/minute.

MONITORING REQUIREMENTS
Osteoporosis Assess bone mineral density before treatment and at regular intervals.

MEDICINAL FORMS There can be variation in the licensing of different medicines containing the same drug.

Tablet

▸ Letrozole (Non-proprietary)
Letrozole 2.5 mg Letrozole 2.5mg tablets | 14 tablet [PoM] £49.90
DT = £1.38 | 28 tablet [PoM] £2.04–£84.86

▸ Femara (Novartis Pharmaceuticals UK Ltd)
Letrozole 2.5 mg Femara 2.5mg tablets | 30 tablet [PoM] £90.92

5   Immunotherapy responsive malignancy

ANTINEOPLASTIC DRUGS ⟩ ANTINEOPLASTICS, OTHER

▎Talimogene laherparepvec   25-Jul-2018

● DRUG ACTION Talimogene laherparepvec is an oncolytic immunotherapy derived from herpes simplex virus type-1 which causes tumour lysis and the release of tumour-derived antigens.

● **INDICATIONS AND DOSE**

Unresectable metastatic melanoma with no bone, brain, or visceral disease

▸ BY INTRALESIONAL INJECTION
▸ Adult: (consult product literature)

● CONTRA-INDICATIONS Severely immunocompromised patients

CONTRA-INDICATIONS, FURTHER INFORMATION
Manufacturer advises avoid in patients who are severely immunocompromised, for example, those with severe congenital or acquired cellular and/or humoral immune deficiency—may be at increased risk of disseminated herpetic infection.

● CAUTIONS Administration of antivirals (may interfere with effectiveness of *Imlygic*®) · autoimmune disease · immunocompromised patients · multiple myeloma (risk of plasmacytoma at injection site)

CAUTIONS, FURTHER INFORMATION
▸ Immunocompromised patients Manufacturer advises caution in patients who are immunocompromised, for example, those with HIV/AIDS, leukaemia, lymphoma, common variable immunodeficiency, or in those who require chronic high-dose steroids or other immunosuppressive agents—risk of disseminated herpetic infection.

● SIDE-EFFECTS
▸ **Common or very common** Anaemia · anxiety · arthralgia · chills · confusion · constipation · cough · deep vein thrombosis · dehydration · depression · diarrhoea · dizziness · dyspnoea exertional · ear pain · fatigue · fever · flushing · gastrointestinal discomfort · headache · hypertension · immune-mediated events · increased risk of infection · influenza like illness · insomnia · malaise · myalgia · nausea · neoplasm complications · oropharyngeal pain · pain · peripheral oedema · procedural pain · secretion discharge · skin reactions · tachycardia · vomiting · weight decreased · wound complications

▸ **Uncommon** Glomerulonephritis · injection site plasmacytoma · post procedural infection · respiratory disorders · vasculitis

SIDE-EFFECTS, FURTHER INFORMATION Necrosis or ulceration of tumour tissue may occur, and impaired healing at the injection site has been reported. Manufacturer advises careful wound care and infection precautions; if persistent infection or delayed healing develops, the risks and benefits of continuing treatment should be considered.

● CONCEPTION AND CONTRACEPTION Manufacturer advises use of latex condoms.

● PREGNANCY Manufacturer advises avoid—no information available.

● BREAST FEEDING Manufacturer advises avoid—no information available.

● DIRECTIONS FOR ADMINISTRATION Consult product literature for information on injection technique.

● HANDLING AND STORAGE Manufacturer advises caution in handling—risk of accidental exposure; avoid preparation or administration if immunocompromised or pregnant. For further information, see the *Physician's Brochure* provided by the manufacturer. Store and transport frozen at -90°C to -70°C—consult product literature for further information on thawing and storage after thawing.

● PATIENT AND CARER ADVICE Manufacturer advises that patients and carers should be informed about the risks of treatment, advised to avoid touching or scratching injection sites, and to keep these sites covered with occlusive dressings. Close contacts should avoid direct contact with injected lesions or body fluids of treated patients during treatment and for up to 30 days after last treatment—if exposed, clean the affected area and seek medical attention if symptoms of herpetic infection develop; close contacts who are immunocompromised or pregnant should not be exposed to potentially contaminated materials. For further information, see the *Information for Patients and Close Contacts* provided by the manufacturer.

Provide patient alert card—record batch number for each administration of *Imlygic*®.

Driving and skilled tasks Manufacturer advises that patients and their carers should be counselled on the effects on driving and performance of skilled tasks—risk of dizziness and confusion.

● NATIONAL FUNDING/ACCESS DECISIONS
For full details see funding body website

NICE decisions

▸ **Talimogene laherparepvec for treating unresectable metastatic melanoma (September 2016) NICE TA410** Recommended

● MEDICINAL FORMS There can be variation in the licensing of different medicines containing the same drug.

Solution for injection
EXCIPIENTS: May contain Sorbitol
ELECTROLYTES: May contain Sodium

▸ Imlygic (Amgen Ltd) ▼
Talimogene laherparepvec 1 million plaque forming units per 1 ml Imlygic 1million plaque forming units/1ml solution for injection vials | 1 vial [PoM] £1,670.00
Talimogene laherparepvec 100 million plaque forming units per 1 ml Imlygic 100million plaque forming units/1ml solution for injection vials | 1 vial [PoM] £1,670.00

Immune system and malignant disease

Interferon gamma-1b

(Immune interferon)

- **INDICATIONS AND DOSE**

To reduce the frequency of serious infection in chronic granulomatous disease
- ▶ BY SUBCUTANEOUS INJECTION
  - ▸ Adult: 50 micrograms/m^2 3 times a week

To reduce the frequency of serious infection in severe malignant osteopetrosis
- ▶ BY SUBCUTANEOUS INJECTION
  - ▸ Adult: 50 micrograms/m^2 3 times a week

- **CONTRA-INDICATIONS** Simultaneous administration of foreign proteins including immunological products (such as vaccines)—risk of exaggerated immune response
- **CAUTIONS** Arrhythmias · cardiac disease · congestive heart failure · ischaemia · seizure disorders (including seizures associated with fever)
- **SIDE-EFFECTS**
  - ▶ **Common or very common** Abdominal pain · arthralgia · back pain · chills · depression · diarrhoea · fatigue · fever · headache · nausea · rash · vomiting
  - ▶ **Frequency not known** Atrioventricular block · chest discomfort · confusion · connective tissue disorders · embolism and thrombosis · gait abnormal · gastrointestinal haemorrhage · hallucination · heart failure · hepatic failure · hypertriglyceridaemia · hypoglycaemia · hyponatraemia · hypotension · influenza like illness · myocardial infarction · neutropenia · pancreatitis · parkinsonism · proteinuria · renal failure · respiratory disorders · seizure · syncope · systemic lupus erythematosus (SLE) · tachycardia · thrombocytopenia · transient ischaemic attack
- **CONCEPTION AND CONTRACEPTION** Effective contraception required during treatment—consult product literature.
- **PREGNANCY** Manufacturers recommend avoid unless potential benefit outweighs risk (toxicity in *animal* studies).
- **BREAST FEEDING** Manufacturers advise avoid—no information available.
- **HEPATIC IMPAIRMENT** Manufacturer advises caution in severe impairment (increased risk of accumulation).
- **RENAL IMPAIRMENT** Manufacturer advises caution in severe impairment—risk of accumulation.
- **MONITORING REQUIREMENTS** Monitor before and during treatment: haematological tests (including full blood count, differential white cell count, and platelet count), blood chemistry tests (including renal and liver function tests) and urinalysis.

- **MEDICINAL FORMS** There can be variation in the licensing of different medicines containing the same drug.
  Solution for injection
  - ▸ Immukin (Clinigen Healthcare Ltd)
    Interferon gamma-1b (recombinant human) 200 microgram per 1 ml Immukin 100micrograms/0.5ml solution for injection vials | 6 vial [PoM] £450.00

Aldesleukin

24-Jul-2020

- **DRUG ACTION** Aldesleukin produces tumour shrinkage in a small proportion of patients, but it has not been shown to increase survival.

- **INDICATIONS AND DOSE**

Metastatic renal cell carcinoma (specialist use only)
- ▶ BY SUBCUTANEOUS INJECTION, OR BY INTRAVENOUS INFUSION
  - ▸ Adult: (consult product literature)

- **UNLICENSED USE** Aldesleukin is not licensed for use in patients in whom all three of the following prognostic factors are present: performance status of Eastern Co-operative Oncology Group of 1 or greater, more than one organ with metastatic disease sites, and a period of less than 24 months between initial diagnosis of primary tumour and date of evaluation of treatment.
- **CONTRA-INDICATIONS** Consult product literature
- **CAUTIONS** Consult product literature
- **INTERACTIONS** → Appendix 1: aldesleukin
- **SIDE-EFFECTS**
  - ▶ **Common or very common** Acidosis · alopecia · anaemia · anxiety · appetite decreased · arrhythmias · arthralgia · ascites · asthenia · cardiovascular disorders · chest pain · chills · coagulation disorders · confusion · conjunctivitis · constipation · cough · cyanosis · dehydration · depression · diarrhoea · dizziness · drowsiness · dyspepsia · dysphagia · dyspnoea · electrolyte imbalance · eosinophilia · fever · gastrointestinal disorders · haemorrhage · hallucination · headache · heart failure · hepatic disorders · hyperbilirubinaemia · hyperglycaemia · hyperhidrosis · hypertension · hyperthyroidism · hypotension · hypothermia · hypothyroidism · hypoxia · increased risk of infection · insomnia · irritability · ischaemic heart disease · leucopenia · malaise · mucositis · myalgia · nasal congestion · nausea · nerve disorders · oedema · oral disorders · pain · palpitations · paraesthesia · pulmonary oedema · renal impairment · respiratory disorders · sepsis · skin reactions · speech disorder · syncope · taste loss · thrombocytopenia · vomiting · weight changes
  - ▶ **Uncommon** Angioedema · cardiac arrest · cardiac inflammation · cardiomyopathy · coma · embolism and thrombosis · hypoglycaemia · muscle weakness · myopathy · neutropenia · pancreatitis · paralysis · pericardial disorders · seizure
  - ▶ **Rare or very rare** Agranulocytosis · aplastic anaemia · cholecystitis · Crohn's disease aggravated · diabetes mellitus · haemolytic anaemia · injection site necrosis · Stevens-Johnson syndrome · ventricular dysfunction
  - ▶ **Frequency not known** Capillary leak syndrome · immune complex RPGN · inflammatory arthritis · intracranial haemorrhage · leukoencephalopathy · myocardial infarction · oculo-bulbar myasthenia gravis · psychiatric disorder · stroke · thyroiditis · vasculitis cerebral
- **CONCEPTION AND CONTRACEPTION** Ensure effective contraception during treatment in men and women.
- **PREGNANCY** Use only if potential benefit outweighs risk (toxicity in *animal* studies). See also *Pregnancy and reproductive function* in Cytotoxic drugs p. 932.
- **BREAST FEEDING** Discontinue breast-feeding.
- **DIRECTIONS FOR ADMINISTRATION** Intravenous infusion is associated with increased risk of capillary leak syndrome (which can cause pulmonary oedema and hypotension), compared to subcutaneous injection.

● MEDICINAL FORMS There can be variation in the licensing of different medicines containing the same drug.

Powder for solution for injection

▸ Proleukin (Clinigen Healthcare Ltd)
Aldesleukin 18 mega unit Proleukin 18million unit powder for solution for injection vials | 1 vial [PoM] £112.00 | 10 vial [PoM] £1,036.00

IMMUNOSTIMULANTS ⟩ OTHER

Bacillus Calmette-Guérin

● DRUG ACTION Bacillus Calmette-Guérin is a live attenuated strain derived from *Mycobacterium bovis*.

● INDICATIONS AND DOSE

Bladder instillation for the treatment of primary or recurrent bladder carcinoma and for the prevention of recurrence following transurethral resection

▸ BY INTRAVESICAL INSTILLATION
▸ Adult: (consult product literature)

● CONTRA-INDICATIONS Fever of unknown origin · HIV infection · impaired immune response · severe haematuria · tuberculosis · urinary-tract infection

● CAUTIONS Bladder injury (delay administration until mucosal damage healed) · traumatic catheterisation (delay administration until mucosal damage healed) · urethral injury (delay administration until mucosal damage healed)

● SIDE-EFFECTS

▸ **Common or very common** Appetite decreased · arthritis · bladder cramps · bladder disorders · cardiovascular event · chills · cystitis · diarrhoea · fatigue · fever · haematuria · hepatic disorders · increased risk of infection · joint disorders · malaise · myalgia · nausea · pain · skin reactions · urinary disorders · vomiting

▸ **Uncommon** Abdominal pain · anaemia · coagulation disorder · constipation · dizziness · genital pain · headache · leucopenia · mucositis · nephrotoxicity · stomatitis · thrombocytopenia · tissue in urine · ulcer · ureteral obstruction

▸ **Frequency not known** Erythema nodosum · eye disorders · eye inflammation · glomerulonephritis · influenza like illness · interstitial lung disease · nephritis · renal abscess · renal failure

● PREGNANCY Avoid.

● BREAST FEEDING Avoid.

● PRE-TREATMENT SCREENING Screen for active tuberculosis (contra-indicated if tuberculosis confirmed).

● MEDICINAL FORMS There can be variation in the licensing of different medicines containing the same drug.

Powder for reconstitution for instillation

▸ OncoTICE (Merck Sharp & Dohme Ltd)
TICE strain Bacillus of Calmette-Guerin 12.5 mg OncoTICE 12.5mg powder for reconstitution for instillation vials | 1 vial [PoM] £71.61 (Hospital only)

Mifamurtide   02-Sep-2020

● INDICATIONS AND DOSE

Treatment of high-grade, resectable, non-metastatic osteosarcoma after complete surgical resection (in combination with chemotherapy)

▸ BY INTRAVENOUS INFUSION
▸ Adult: Infusion to be given over 1 hour (consult product literature or local protocols)

● UNLICENSED USE Not licensed for use in patients over 30 years of age at initial diagnosis.

● CAUTIONS Asthma—consider prophylactic bronchodilator therapy · chronic obstructive pulmonary disease—consider prophylactic bronchodilator therapy · history of autoimmune disease · history of collagen disease · history of inflammatory disease

● INTERACTIONS → Appendix 1: mifamurtide

● SIDE-EFFECTS

▸ **Common or very common** Alopecia · anaemia · anxiety · appetite decreased · arthralgia · asthenia · cancer pain · chest discomfort · chills · confusion · constipation · cough · cyanosis · dehydration · depression · diarrhoea · dizziness · drowsiness · dysmenorrhoea · dyspnoea · feeling cold · fever · flushing · gastrointestinal discomfort · haemorrhage · headache · hearing loss · hepatic pain · hyperhidrosis · hypertension · hypokalaemia · hypotension · hypothermia · increased risk of infection · insomnia · laryngeal pain · leucopenia · malaise · mucositis · muscle complaints · musculoskeletal stiffness · nasal congestion · nausea · neutropenia · oedema · pain · pallor · palpitations · respiratory disorders · sensation abnormal · sepsis · skin reactions · tachycardia · thrombocytopenia · tinnitus · tremor · urinary disorders · vertigo · vision blurred · vomiting · weight decreased

● CONCEPTION AND CONTRACEPTION Effective contraception required.

● PREGNANCY Avoid.

● BREAST FEEDING Avoid—no information available.

● HEPATIC IMPAIRMENT Manufacturer advises caution in moderate impairment (risk of increased half-life and exposure); avoid in severe impairment (no information available).

● RENAL IMPAIRMENT Use with caution—no information available.

● MONITORING REQUIREMENTS

▸ Monitor renal function, hepatic function and clotting parameters.

▸ Monitor patients with history of venous thrombosis, vasculitis, or unstable cardiovascular disorders for persistent or worsening symptoms during administration—consult product literature.

● NATIONAL FUNDING/ACCESS DECISIONS
For full details see funding body website

NICE decisions

▸ **Mifamurtide for the treatment of osteosarcoma (October 2011) NICE TA235 Recommended**

● MEDICINAL FORMS There can be variation in the licensing of different medicines containing the same drug.

Powder for suspension for infusion

▸ Mepact (Takeda UK Ltd)
Mifamurtide 4 mg Mepact 4mg powder for suspension for infusion vials | 1 vial [PoM] £2,375.00

IMMUNOSUPPRESSANTS ⟩ THALIDOMIDE AND RELATED ANALOGUES

Lenalidomide   19-Nov-2020

● DRUG ACTION Lenalidomide is an immunomodulating drug with anti-neoplastic, anti-angiogenic, and pro-erythropoietic properties.

● INDICATIONS AND DOSE

Newly diagnosed multiple myeloma in patients who have undergone autologous stem cell transplantation (specialist use only)

▸ BY MOUTH
▸ Adult: 10 mg once daily for 28 consecutive days of repeated 28-day cycles; increased if tolerated to 15 mg once daily, after 3 cycles, for dose adjustments due to side-effects—consult product literature   continued →

8

Immune system and malignant disease

Newly diagnosed multiple myeloma in patients not eligible for transplant (in combination with dexamethasone) (specialist use only) | Multiple myeloma in patients who have received at least one prior therapy (in combination with dexamethasone) (specialist use only)
▸ BY MOUTH
▸ Adult: 25 mg once daily for 21 consecutive days of repeated 28-day cycles, for doses of dexamethasone, and dose adjustments due to side-effects—consult product literature

Newly diagnosed multiple myeloma in patients not eligible for transplant (in combination with melphalan and prednisone) (specialist use only)
▸ BY MOUTH
▸ Adult: 10 mg once daily for 21 consecutive days of repeated 28-day cycles for up to 9 cycles, patients who complete 9 cycles or are intolerant to combination therapy should continue treatment with lenalidomide as monotherapy, for doses of melphalan and prednisone, and dose adjustments due to side-effects—consult product literature

Newly diagnosed multiple myeloma in patients not eligible for transplant (in combination with bortezomib and dexamethasone) (specialist use only)
▸ BY MOUTH
▸ Adult: 25 mg once daily for 14 consecutive days of repeated 21-day cycles for up to 8 cycles, followed by 25 mg once daily for 21 consecutive days of repeated 28-day cycles (in combination with dexamethasone alone), for doses of bortezomib and dexamethasone, and dose adjustments due to side-effects—consult product literature

Myelodysplastic syndromes (specialist use only)
▸ BY MOUTH
▸ Adult: 10 mg once daily for 21 consecutive days of repeated 28-day cycles, for dose adjustments due to side-effects—consult product literature

Mantle cell lymphoma (specialist use only)
▸ BY MOUTH
▸ Adult: 25 mg once daily for 21 consecutive days of repeated 28-day cycles, for dose adjustments due to side-effects—consult product literature

Follicular lymphoma (in combination with rituximab) (specialist use only)
▸ BY MOUTH
▸ Adult: 20 mg once daily for 21 consecutive days of repeated 28-day cycles for up to 12 cycles, for doses of rituximab, and dose adjustments due to side-effects—consult product literature

---

IMPORTANT SAFETY INFORMATION

MHRA/CHM ADVICE: IMMUNOMODULATORY DRUGS AND PREGNANCY PREVENTION: TEMPORARY ADVICE FOR MANAGEMENT DURING CORONAVIRUS (COVID-19) (MAY 2020)
The MHRA has issued temporary guidance for female patients on lenalidomide during the coronavirus (COVID-19) pandemic to support adherence to the Pregnancy Prevention Programme (see *Conception and contraception*), particularly for those who are shielding due to other health conditions, and should be followed until further notice.

● CAUTIONS High tumour burden—risk of tumour lysis syndrome · patients with risk factors for myocardial infarction

CAUTIONS, FURTHER INFORMATION
▸ Thromboembolism Risk factors for thromboembolism (such as smoking, hypertension, hyperlipidaemia) should be minimised and thromboprophylaxis should be considered in patients with multiple risk factors.

▸ Second primary malignancy Patients should be carefully evaluated before and during treatment with lenalidomide using routine cancer screening for occurrence of second primary malignancy and treatment should be instituted as indicated.

● INTERACTIONS → Appendix 1: lenalidomide

● SIDE-EFFECTS
▸ **Common or very common** Anaemia · appetite decreased · arthralgia · asthenia · atrial fibrillation · chills · constipation · cough · decreased leucocytes · dehydration · diarrhoea · dizziness · dry mouth · dyspnoea · electrolyte imbalance · embolism and thrombosis · fall · fever · gastrointestinal discomfort · haemorrhage · headache · heart failure · hyperglycaemia · hypertension · hyperthyroidism · hypotension · hypothyroidism · increased risk of infection · influenza like illness · insomnia · iron overload · lethargy · mood altered · muscle complaints · muscle weakness · myocardial infarction · nausea · neoplasms · nerve disorders · neutropenia · night sweats · pain · pancytopenia · paraesthesia · peripheral oedema · renal failure · respiratory disorders · rhinorrhoea · sepsis · skin reactions · taste altered · thrombocytopenia · toothache · tumour flare · vertigo · vomiting · weight decreased
▸ **Uncommon** Angioedema
▸ **Rare or very rare** Hypersensitivity · severe cutaneous adverse reactions (SCARs) · tumour lysis syndrome
▸ **Frequency not known** Acquired haemophilia · gastrointestinal disorders · hepatic disorders · hypersensitivity vasculitis · pancreatitis · progressive multifocal leukoencephalopathy (PML) · reactivation of infections · solid organ transplant rejection

SIDE-EFFECTS, FURTHER INFORMATION If rash occurs, treatment should be discontinued and only restarted following appropriate clinical evaluation.
  Discontinue permanently if angioedema, exfoliative or bullous rash, or if Stevens-Johnson syndrome or toxic epidermal necrolysis is suspected.

● CONCEPTION AND CONTRACEPTION For women of child-bearing potential, pregnancy must be excluded before starting treatment with lenalidomide (perform pregnancy test on initiation or within 3 days prior to initiation). Women must practise effective contraception at least 1 month before, during, and for at least 1 month after treatment, including during dose interruptions (oral combined hormonal contraceptives and copper-releasing intra-uterine devices not recommended) and men should use condoms during treatment, during dose interruption, and for at least 1 week after stopping if their partner is pregnant or is of childbearing potential and not using effective contraception. Patients, prescribers and pharmacists must comply with pregnancy prevention measures as specified in the manufacturer's Pregnancy Prevention Programme.

● PREGNANCY **Important: teratogenic risk.** Lenalidomide is structurally related to thalidomide and there is a risk of teratogenesis.

● BREAST FEEDING Discontinue breast-feeding—no information available.

● RENAL IMPAIRMENT
Dose adjustments Reduce dose in moderate to severe impairment—consult product literature.

● MONITORING REQUIREMENTS
▸ Monitor full blood count (including differential white cell count, platelet count, haemoglobin, and haematocrit) and liver function before treatment, then every week for the first 8 weeks, then monthly thereafter (reduce dose or interrupt treatment if neutropenia, thrombocytopenia or impaired liver function develop—consult product literature).

- Monitor for arterial or venous thromboembolism (if thromboembolic event occurs, discontinue lenalidomide and treat with standard anticoagulation therapy; lenalidomide may be restarted with continued anticoagulation therapy once thromboembolic event resolved—consult product literature).
- Monitor thyroid function.
- Monitor for signs and symptoms of peripheral neuropathy.
- Monitor visual ability regularly (risk of cataract).
- Hepatic disorders Liver function should be monitored particularly when there is history of, or concurrent viral liver infection, or when lenalidomide is combined with drugs known to be associated with liver dysfunction (e.g. paracetamol).

- ● PRESCRIBING AND DISPENSING INFORMATION Patient, prescriber, and supplying pharmacy must comply with a pregnancy prevention programme. Every prescription must be accompanied by a completed Prescription Authorisation Form.

- ● PATIENT AND CARER ADVICE
  Thromboembolism Patients and their carers should be made aware of the symptoms of thromboembolism and advised to report sudden breathlessness, chest pain, or swelling of a limb.
  Neutropenia and thrombocytopenia Patients and their carers should be made aware of the symptoms of neutropenia and advised to seek medical advice if symptoms suggestive of neutropenia (such as fever, sore throat) or of thrombocytopenia (such as bleeding) develop.
  Conception and contraception Patient counselling is advised for lenalidomide capsules (pregnancy and contraception).

- ● NATIONAL FUNDING/ACCESS DECISIONS
  For full details see funding body website
  NICE decisions
- ▶ Lenalidomide for treating myelodysplastic syndromes associated with an isolated deletion 5q cytogenetic abnormality (updated June 2019) NICE TA322 Recommended with restrictions
- ▶ Lenalidomide for the treatment of multiple myeloma in people who have received at least 2 prior therapies (updated June 2019) NICE TA171 Recommended with restrictions
- ▶ Ixazomib with lenalidomide and dexamethasone for treating relapsed or refractory multiple myeloma (February 2018) NICE TA505 Recommended with restrictions
- ▶ Lenalidomide plus dexamethasone for multiple myeloma after 1 treatment with bortezomib (June 2019) NICE TA586 Recommended with restrictions
- ▶ Lenalidomide plus dexamethasone for previously untreated multiple myeloma (June 2019) NICE TA587 Recommended with restrictions
- ▶ Lenalidomide with rituximab for previously treated follicular lymphoma (April 2020) NICE TA627 Recommended
  Scottish Medicines Consortium (SMC) decisions
- ▶ Lenalidomide (*Revlimid*®) for third line treatment of multiple myeloma (May 2010) SMC No. 441/08 Recommended with restrictions
- ▶ Lenalidomide (*Revlimid*®) in combination with dexamethasone, for the treatment of multiple myeloma in adult patients who have received at least one prior therapy (April 2014) SMC No. 441/08 Recommended with restrictions
- ▶ Lenalidomide (*Revlimid*®) for the treatment of adult patients with previously untreated multiple myeloma who are not eligible for transplant (December 2015) SMC No. 1096/15 Recommended with restrictions
- ▶ Lenalidomide (*Revlimid*®) as monotherapy for the maintenance treatment of adult patients with newly diagnosed multiple myeloma who have undergone autologous stem cell transplantation (October 2020) SMC No. SMC2289 Recommended

- ▶ Lenalidomide (*Revlimid*®) in combination with rituximab (anti-CD20 antibody) for the treatment of adult patients with previously treated follicular lymphoma (Grade 1 to 3a) (October 2020) SMC No. SMC2281 Recommended

- ● MEDICINAL FORMS There can be variation in the licensing of different medicines containing the same drug.
  Capsule
  CAUTIONARY AND ADVISORY LABELS 25
  ▶ Revlimid (Celgene Ltd) ▼
  Lenalidomide 2.5 mg Revlimid 2.5mg capsules | 21 capsule [PoM]
  £3,426.00 DT = £3,426.00
  Lenalidomide 5 mg Revlimid 5mg capsules | 21 capsule [PoM]
  £3,570.00 DT = £3,570.00
  Lenalidomide 7.5 mg Revlimid 7.5mg capsules | 21 capsule [PoM]
  £3,675.00 DT = £3,675.00
  Lenalidomide 10 mg Revlimid 10mg capsules | 21 capsule [PoM]
  £3,780.00 DT = £3,780.00
  Lenalidomide 15 mg Revlimid 15mg capsules | 21 capsule [PoM]
  £3,969.00 DT = £3,969.00
  Lenalidomide 20 mg Revlimid 20mg capsules | 21 capsule [PoM]
  £4,168.50 DT = £4,168.50
  Lenalidomide 25 mg Revlimid 25mg capsules | 21 capsule [PoM]
  £4,368.00 DT = £4,368.00

Pomalidomide   05-Nov-2020

- ● DRUG ACTION Pomalidomide is structurally related to thalidomide and has immunomodulatory properties and direct anti-myeloma tumoricidal activity.

- ● INDICATIONS AND DOSE
  Treatment of relapsed and refractory multiple myeloma in patients who have received at least two prior treatment regimens, including both lenalidomide and bortezomib, and who have had disease progression during the last treatment (in combination with dexamethasone)
  ▶ BY MOUTH
  ▶ Adult: 4 mg once daily for 21 consecutive days of repeated 28–day cycles, for doses of dexamethasone and dose adjustment due to side effects—consult product literature

  DOSE ADJUSTMENTS DUE TO INTERACTIONS
  ▶ Manufacturer advises halve dose with concurrent use of potent inhibitors of CYP1A2 and ciprofloxacin.

  > IMPORTANT SAFETY INFORMATION
  > MHRA/CHM ADVICE: RISK OF HEPATITIS B REACTIVATION (MAY 2016)
  > An EU wide review has concluded that pomalidomide can cause hepatitis B reactivation; the MHRA recommends to establish hepatitis B virus status in all patients before initiation of treatment.
  >
  > MHRA/CHM ADVICE: IMMUNOMODULATORY DRUGS AND PREGNANCY PREVENTION: TEMPORARY ADVICE FOR MANAGEMENT DURING CORONAVIRUS (COVID-19) (MAY 2020)
  > The MHRA has issued temporary guidance for female patients on pomalidomide during the coronavirus (COVID-19) pandemic to support adherence to the Pregnancy Prevention Programme (see *Conception and contraception*), particularly for those who are shielding due to other health conditions, and should be followed until further notice.

- ● CAUTIONS Cardiac disease · cardiac risk factors · hepatitis B infection · high tumour burden—risk of tumour lysis syndrome · interstitial lung disease—discontinue if suspected · peripheral neuropathy
  CAUTIONS, FURTHER INFORMATION
  ▶ **Thromboembolism** Risk factors for thromboembolism (such as smoking, hypertension, hyperlipidaemia) should be

8

Immune system and malignant disease

minimised. Thromboprophylaxis should be considered, particularly in patients with additional risk factors.
▸ Second primary malignancy Patients should be carefully evaluated before and during treatment with pomalidomide using routine cancer screening for occurrence of second primary malignancy and treatment should be instituted as indicated.
▸ Hepatitis B infection The MHRA advises that those with a history of hepatitis B infection should be closely monitored for signs and symptoms of active infection throughout treatment; expert advice should be sought for patients who test positive for active infection.
● INTERACTIONS → Appendix 1: pomalidomide
● SIDE-EFFECTS
▸ **Common or very common** Anaemia · angioedema · appetite decreased · atrial fibrillation · cataract · Clostridioides difficile colitis · confusion · constipation · cough · decreased leucocytes · depression · diarrhoea · dizziness · dry mouth · dyspnoea · electrolyte imbalance · embolism and thrombosis · fall · fatigue · fever · gastrointestinal discomfort · haemorrhage · heart failure · hyperglycaemia · hypertension · hyperuricaemia · hypotension · increased risk of infection · insomnia · intracranial haemorrhage · level of consciousness decreased · muscle spasms · muscle weakness · myocardial infarction · nausea · neoplasms · neutropenia · oedema · pain · pancytopenia · paraesthesia · pelvic pain · peripheral neuropathy · renal impairment · respiratory disorders · sepsis · skin reactions · stomatitis · syncope · taste altered · thrombocytopenia · tremor · urinary retention · vertigo · vomiting · weight decreased
▸ **Uncommon** Hepatitis · hyperbilirubinaemia · stroke · tumour lysis syndrome
▸ **Frequency not known** Hepatitis B reactivation · severe cutaneous adverse reactions (SCARs)
● CONCEPTION AND CONTRACEPTION For women of child-bearing potential, pregnancy must be excluded before starting treatment with pomalidomide (perform pregnancy test on initiation or within 3 days prior to initiation). Women must practise effective contraception at least 1 month before, during, and for at least 1 month after treatment, including during dose interruptions (oral combined hormonal contraceptives and copper-releasing intra-uterine devices not recommended) and men should use condoms during treatment, during dose interruption, and for at least 1 week after stopping if their partner is pregnant or is of childbearing potential and not using effective contraception. Patients, prescribers and pharmacists must comply with pregnancy prevention measures as specified in the manufacturer's Pregnancy Prevention Programme.
● PREGNANCY **Important: teratogenic risk.**
● BREAST FEEDING Avoid—present in milk in *animal* studies.
● HEPATIC IMPAIRMENT Manufacturer advises caution (risk of increased exposure).
● RENAL IMPAIRMENT Manufacturer advises caution—no information available.
● MONITORING REQUIREMENTS
▸ Maufacturer advises monitor full blood count before treatment, then every week for the first 8 weeks, then monthly thereafter (reduce dose or interrupt treatment if neutropenia or thrombocytopenia develop—consult product literature).
▸ Manufacturer advises monitor for arterial or venous thromboembolism.
▸ Manufacturer advises monitor for signs and symptoms of cardiac failure.
▸ Manufacturer advises monitor for acute onset or unexplained worsening of respiratory symptoms.
▸ Manufacturer advises monitor liver function for 6 months after initiation, then as clinically indicated.

● PRESCRIBING AND DISPENSING INFORMATION Patient, prescriber, and supplying pharmacy must comply with a pregnancy prevention programme. Every prescription must be accompanied by a completed Prescription Authorisation Form.
● PATIENT AND CARER ADVICE Patients and their carers should be made aware of the symptoms of thromboembolism and advised to report sudden breathlessness, chest pain, or swelling of a limb.
   Patients and their carers should be made aware of the symptoms of neutropenia and advised to seek medical advice if symptoms suggestive of neutropenia (such as fever, sore throat) or of thrombocytopenia (such as bleeding) develop.
Conception and contraception Patient counselling is advised for pomalidomide capsules (pregnancy and contraception).
● NATIONAL FUNDING/ACCESS DECISIONS For full details see funding body website
NICE decisions
▸ Pomalidomide for multiple myeloma previously treated with lenalidomide and bortezomib (January 2017) NICE TA427 Recommended with restrictions

● MEDICINAL FORMS There can be variation in the licensing of different medicines containing the same drug.
Capsule
CAUTIONARY AND ADVISORY LABELS 3, 25
EXCIPIENTS: May contain Propylene glycol
▸ Imnovid (Celgene Ltd) ▼
  Pomalidomide 1 mg Imnovid 1mg capsules | 21 capsule [PoM] £8,884.00
  Pomalidomide 2 mg Imnovid 2mg capsules | 21 capsule [PoM] £8,884.00
  Pomalidomide 3 mg Imnovid 3mg capsules | 21 capsule [PoM] £8,884.00
  Pomalidomide 4 mg Imnovid 4mg capsules | 21 capsule [PoM] £8,884.00

Thalidomide

03-Sep-2020

● DRUG ACTION Thalidomide has immunomodulatory and anti-inflammatory activity.

● INDICATIONS AND DOSE
First-line treatment for untreated multiple myeloma, in patients aged 65 years and over, or for those not eligible for high-dose chemotherapy (for example, patients with significant co-morbidity such as cardiac risk factors) in combination with melphalan and prednisolone
▸ BY MOUTH
▸ Adult 18–75 years: 200 mg once daily for 6–week cycle for a maximum of 12 cycles, dose to be taken at bedtime
▸ Adult 76 years and over: 100 mg once daily for 6–week cycle for a maximum of 12 cycles, dose to be taken at bedtime

IMPORTANT SAFETY INFORMATION
MHRA/CHM ADVICE: IMMUNOMODULATORY DRUGS AND PREGNANCY PREVENTION: TEMPORARY ADVICE FOR MANAGEMENT DURING CORONAVIRUS (COVID-19) (MAY 2020)
The MHRA has issued temporary guidance for female patients on thalidomide during the coronavirus (COVID-19) pandemic to support adherence to the Pregnancy Prevention Programme (see *Conception and contraception*), particularly for those who are shielding due to other health conditions, and should be followed until further notice.

● CAUTIONS High tumour burden—risk of tumour lysis syndrome · patients aged 76 years and over—increased risk of serious side-effects

CAUTIONS, FURTHER INFORMATION

▸ Thromboembolism Risk factors for thromboembolism (such as smoking, hypertension, hyperlipidaemia) should be minimised. Thromboprophylaxis is recommended for at least the first 5 months of treatment, especially in patients with additional thrombotic risk factors.

▸ Second primary malignancy Patients should be carefully evaluated before and during treatment with thalidomide using routine cancer screening for occurrence of second primary malignancy and treatment should be instituted as indicated.

▸ Peripheral neuropathy Patients with pre-existing peripheral neuropathy should not be treated with thalidomide unless the potential clinical benefits outweigh the risk.

● INTERACTIONS → Appendix 1: thalidomide

● SIDE-EFFECTS

▸ **Common or very common** Anaemia · arrhythmias · asthenia · confusion · constipation · decreased leucocytes · depression · dizziness · drowsiness · dry mouth · dyspnoea · embolism and thrombosis · fever · heart failure · increased risk of infection · malaise · movement disorders · neutropenia · peripheral neuropathy · peripheral oedema · respiratory disorders · sensation abnormal · skin reactions · thrombocytopenia · tremor · vomiting

▸ **Frequency not known** Atrioventricular block · gastrointestinal disorders · gastrointestinal haemorrhage · hearing impairment · hypothyroidism · liver disorder · menstrual cycle irregularities · myocardial infarction · neoplasms · pancreatitis · pancytopenia · posterior reversible encephalopathy syndrome (PRES) · pulmonary hypertension · reactivation of infections · renal failure · seizure · sexual dysfunction · toxic epidermal necrolysis · tumour lysis syndrome

SIDE-EFFECTS, FURTHER INFORMATION **Rash** If rash occurs, treatment should be discontinued and only restarted following appropriate clinical evaluation.

　Peripheral neuropathy If symptoms suggestive of peripheral neuropathy develop (such as paraesthesia, abnormal coordination, or weakness) dose reduction, dose interruption, or treatment discontinuation may be necessary—consult product literature.

● CONCEPTION AND CONTRACEPTION For women of child-bearing potential, pregnancy must be excluded before starting treatment with thalidomide (perform pregnancy test on initiation or within 3 days prior to initiation). Women must practise effective contraception at least 1 month before, during, and for at least 1 month after treatment, including during dose interruptions (oral combined hormonal contraceptives and copper-releasing intra-uterine devices not recommended) and men should use condoms during treatment, during dose interruption, and for at least 1 week after stopping if their partner is pregnant or is of childbearing potential and not using effective contraception. Patients, prescribers and pharmacists must comply with pregnancy prevention measures as specified in the manufacturer's Pregnancy Prevention Programme.

● PREGNANCY **Important: teratogenic risk.**

● BREAST FEEDING Avoid—present in milk in *animal* studies.

● HEPATIC IMPAIRMENT Manufacturer advises caution in severe impairment (no information available).

● RENAL IMPAIRMENT Caution in severe impairment—no information available.

● MONITORING REQUIREMENTS

▸ Monitor white blood cell count (including differential count) and platelet count (reduce dose or interrupt

treatment if neutropenia or thrombocytopenia develop—consult product literature).

▸ Monitor for arterial or venous thromboembolism.

▸ Monitor patients for signs and symptoms of peripheral neuropathy.

▸ Hepatic disorder Liver function should be monitored, particularly when there is history of, or concurrent viral liver infection, or when thalidomide is combined with drugs known to be associated with liver dysfunction (e.g. paracetamol).

● PRESCRIBING AND DISPENSING INFORMATION Patient, prescriber, and supplying pharmacy must comply with a pregnancy prevention programme. Every prescription must be accompanied by a complete Prescription Authorisation Form.

● PATIENT AND CARER ADVICE Patients and their carers should be made aware of the symptoms of thromboembolism and advised to report sudden breathlessness, chest pain, or swelling of a limb.

　Patients and their carers should be made aware of the symptoms of neutropenia and advised to seek medical advice if symptoms suggestive of neutropenia (such as fever, sore throat) or of thrombocytopenia (such as bleeding) develop.

　Patients and their carers should be advised to seek medical advice if symptoms of peripheral neuropathy such as paraesthesia, abnormal coordination, or weakness develop.

Conception and contraception Patient counselling advised for thalidomide capsules (pregnancy and contraception).

● NATIONAL FUNDING/ACCESS DECISIONS
For full details see funding body website

NICE decisions

▸ **Bortezomib and thalidomide for the first-line treatment of multiple myeloma (July 2011)** NICE TA228 Recommended

● MEDICINAL FORMS There can be variation in the licensing of different medicines containing the same drug. Forms available from special-order manufacturers include: tablet, oral suspension, oral solution

Tablet
▸ Talidex (Special Order)
　Thalidomide 25 mg Talidex 25mg tablets | 30 tablet 🔒

Capsule
CAUTIONARY AND ADVISORY LABELS 2
▸ Thalidomide (Non-proprietary)
　Thalidomide 50 mg Thalidomide Celgene 50mg capsules | 28 capsule [PoM] £298.48

6　Photodynamic therapy responsive malignancy

PHOTOSENSITISERS

Porfimer sodium　　　　　27-May-2020

● DRUG ACTION Porfimer sodium accumulates in malignant tissue and is activated by laser light to produce a cytotoxic effect.

● INDICATIONS AND DOSE

Photodynamic therapy of non-small cell lung cancer and obstructing oesophageal cancer
▸ BY SLOW INTRAVENOUS INJECTION
▸ Adult: (consult product literature)

● CONTRA-INDICATIONS Acute porphyrias p. 1107 · broncho-oesophageal fistula · tracheo-oesophageal fistula

- SIDE-EFFECTS
▸ **Common or very common** Anaemia · anxiety · appetite decreased · arrhythmias · asthenia · chest discomfort · confusion · constipation · cough · diarrhoea · dyspnoea · fever · fluid imbalance · gastrointestinal discomfort · gastrointestinal disorders · haemorrhage · heart failure · hypertension · hypotension · increased risk of infection · insomnia · nausea · oedema · oesophageal disorder · pain · photosensitivity reaction (sunscreens ineffective) · respiratory disorders · sepsis · swallowing difficulty · tracheo-oesophageal fistula · vomiting · weight decreased
▸ **Frequency not known** Angina pectoris · angioedema · atrioventricular block · bladder spasm · cataract · chills · dizziness · embolism and thrombosis · erythropenia · eye discomfort · eye disorders · hepatic disorders · hiccups · hydronephrosis · hypocalcaemia · laryngotracheal oedema · leucocytosis · malaise · myocardial infarction · numbness · oral disorders · pancreatitis · pulmonary oedema · skin reactions · swelling · syncope · urinary disorders · vision disorders
- PREGNANCY Manufacturer advises avoid unless essential.
- BREAST FEEDING No information available—manufacturer advises avoid.
- HEPATIC IMPAIRMENT Manufacturer advises caution in mild to moderate impairment (may increase duration of photosensitivity); avoid in severe impairment (no information available).
- PATIENT AND CARER ADVICE
Photosensitivity Avoid exposure of skin and eyes to direct sunlight or bright indoor light for at least 30 days.
- MEDICINAL FORMS There can be variation in the licensing of different medicines containing the same drug.
Powder for solution for injection
▸ Photofrin (Axcan Pharma Inc, Pinnacle Biologics BV)
Porfimer sodium 15 mg Photofrin 15mg powder for solution for injection vials | 1 vial PoM ⓢ (Hospital only)
Porfimer sodium 75 mg Photofrin 75mg powder for solution for injection vials | 1 vial PoM £1,011.00 (Hospital only)

Temoporfin
03-Sep-2020

- DRUG ACTION Temoporfin accumulates in malignant tissue and is activated by laser light to produce a cytotoxic effect.

● INDICATIONS AND DOSE

Photodynamic therapy of advanced head and neck squamous cell carcinoma refractory to, or unsuitable for, other treatments
▸ BY SLOW INTRAVENOUS INJECTION
▸ Adult: (consult product literature)

- CONTRA-INDICATIONS Acute porphyrias p. 1107 · concomitant photosensitising treatment · diseases exacerbated by light · elective surgery · ophthalmic slit-lamp examination for 30 days after administration
- SIDE-EFFECTS
▸ **Common or very common** Anaemia · constipation · dizziness · dysphagia · fever · haemorrhage · headache · local infection · nausea · oedema · oral disorders · pain · paraesthesia · photosensitivity reaction (sunscreens ineffective) · skin reactions · stomatitis necrotising · sunburn · vomiting
▸ **Frequency not known** Fistula · obstructive airway disorder · sepsis · vascular rupture
- CONCEPTION AND CONTRACEPTION Manufacturer advises avoid pregnancy for at least 3 months after treatment.
- PREGNANCY Toxicity in *animal* studies. See also Pregnancy and reproductive function in Cytotoxic drugs p. 932.

- BREAST FEEDING Manufacturer advises avoid breastfeeding for at least 1 month after treatment—no information available.
- PATIENT AND CARER ADVICE
Photosensitivity Avoid exposure of skin and eyes to direct sunlight or bright indoor light for at least 15 days after administration.
Avoid prolonged exposure of injection site arm to direct sunlight for 6 months after administration.
If extravasation occurs protect area from light for at least 3 months.
- MEDICINAL FORMS There can be variation in the licensing of different medicines containing the same drug.
Solution for injection
▸ Foscan (Biolitec Pharma Ltd)
Temoporfin 1 mg per 1 ml Foscan 3mg/3ml solution for injection vials | 1 vial PoM £1,800.00 (Hospital only)
Foscan 6mg/6ml solution for injection vials | 1 vial PoM £3,400.00 (Hospital only)

7 Targeted therapy responsive malignancy

ANTINEOPLASTIC DRUGS > PROTEASOME INHIBITORS

Bortezomib
03-Nov-2020

- DRUG ACTION Bortezomib is a proteasome inhibitor.

● INDICATIONS AND DOSE

Multiple myeloma (specialist use only) | Mantle cell lymphoma (specialist use only)
▸ BY INTRAVENOUS INJECTION, OR BY SUBCUTANEOUS INJECTION
▸ Adult: (consult product literature or local protocols)

IMPORTANT SAFETY INFORMATION
Bortezomib injection is for **intravenous or subcutaneous administration** only. Inadvertent intrathecal administration with fatal outcome has been reported.

- CONTRA-INDICATIONS Acute diffuse infiltrative pulmonary disease · pericardial disease
- CAUTIONS Amyloidosis · cardiovascular disease · consider antiviral prophylaxis for herpes zoster infection · dehydration · diabetes (may affect blood glucose) · history of syncope · pulmonary disease · risk factors for seizures · risk of neuropathy—consult product literature
- INTERACTIONS → Appendix 1: bortezomib
- SIDE-EFFECTS
▸ **Common or very common** Anaemia · anxiety · appetite abnormal · arrhythmias · asthenia · chills · constipation · cough · decreased leucocytes · diabetes mellitus · diarrhoea · dizziness · dysphagia · dyspnoea · electrolyte imbalance · encephalopathy · enzyme abnormality · eye inflammation · fever · fluid imbalance · gastrointestinal discomfort · gastrointestinal disorders · haemorrhage · hair disorder · headaches · hearing impairment · heart failure · hepatic disorders · hiccups · hyperbilirubinaemia · hypersensitivity · hypertension · hypotension · increased risk of infection · ischaemic heart disease · lethargy · loss of consciousness · malaise · mood altered · muscle complaints · muscle weakness · nausea · nerve disorders · neuromuscular dysfunction · neutropenia · oedema · oral disorders · oropharyngeal complaints · pain · renal impairment · sensation abnormal · sepsis · skin reactions · sleep disorder · syncope · taste altered · thrombocytopenia · tinnitus ·

ventricular dysfunction · vertigo · vision disorders · vomiting · weight changes
Uncommon Altered smell sensation · angioedema · antibiotic associated colitis · arthritis · azotaemia · cardiac arrest · cardiomyopathy · cardiovascular disorder · cerebrovascular insufficiency · chest discomfort · circulation impaired · circulatory collapse · coagulation disorders · concentration impaired · confusion · Cushing's syndrome · dry eye · dysphonia · ear discomfort · embolism and thrombosis · eye discomfort · eye disorders · failure to thrive · gait abnormal · gas exchange abnormal · genital pain · haemolytic anaemia · hallucination · hyperthyroidism · increased leucocytes · injury · irritable bowel syndrome · joint disorders · lymphadenopathy · memory loss · movement disorders · mucous membrane disorder · myopathy · neurotoxicity · palpitations · pancreatitis · pancytopenia · pericardial disorders · pericarditis · posterior reversible encephalopathy syndrome (PRES) (discontinue) · proteinuria · psychiatric disorders · psychotic disorder · pulmonary hypertension · pulmonary oedema · reflexes abnormal · respiratory disorders · rhinorrhoea · seizure · sensation of pressure · severe cutaneous adverse reactions (SCARs) · sexual dysfunction · shock · SIADH · skin mass · skin ulcers · speech disorder · sweat changes · temperature sensation altered · thirst change · tremor · tumour lysis syndrome · urinary disorders · urinary tract disorder · vascular disorders · vasculitis · vasodilation
▸ **Rare or very rare** Acidosis · acute coronary syndrome · alcohol intolerance · amyloidosis · apnoea · ascites · atrioventricular block · bladder irritation · blood disorders · bone disorder · bone fracture · brain oedema · breast disorder · cardiac valve disorder · cholelithiasis · CNS haemorrhage · cognitive disorder · coma · coronary artery insufficiency · delirium · drooling · ear disorder · erythromelalgia · fistula · gout · healing impaired · hypothyroidism · inflammation · lymphoedema · macrophage activation · mass · meningitis · metabolic disorder · multi organ failure · nail disorder · neoplasm malignant · neoplasms · nervous system disorder · paralysis · paresis · pelvic pain · perforation · photosensitivity reaction · platelet abnormalities · procedural complications · prostatitis · radiation injury · seborrhoea · sudden death · suicidal ideation · testicular disorders · throat complaints · ulcer · vaginal ulceration · venous insufficiency · vitamin deficiencies
▸ **Frequency not known** Herpes zoster reactivation · JC virus infection · progressive multifocal leukoencephalopathy (PML)
● CONCEPTION AND CONTRACEPTION Manufacturer advises effective contraception during and for 3 months after treatment in men or women.
● PREGNANCY Toxicity in *animal* studies. See also *Pregnancy and reproductive function* in Cytotoxic drugs p. 932.
● BREAST FEEDING Discontinue breast-feeding.
● HEPATIC IMPAIRMENT Manufacturer advises caution in moderate to severe impairment—monitor for toxicity.
Dose adjustments Manufacturer advises reduce dose in moderate to severe impairment—consult product literature.
● RENAL IMPAIRMENT No information available for creatinine clearance less than 20 mL/minute/1.73 m^2.
● MONITORING REQUIREMENTS
▸ Monitor blood-glucose concentration in patients on oral antidiabetics.
▸ Monitor for symptoms of progressive multifocal leucoencephalopathy (presenting as new or worsening neurological signs or symptoms)—discontinue treatment if diagnosed.

▸ Chest x-ray recommended before treatment to monitor for pulmonary disease—discontinue if interstitial lung disease develops.
● NATIONAL FUNDING/ACCESS DECISIONS
For full details see funding body website
NICE decisions
▸ **Bortezomib for previously untreated mantle cell lymphoma (December 2015)** NICE TA370 Recommended
▸ **Bortezomib for induction therapy in multiple myeloma before high-dose chemotherapy and autologous stem cell transplantation (April 2014)** NICE TA311 Recommended
▸ **Bortezomib and thalidomide for the first-line treatment of multiple myeloma (July 2011)** NICE TA228 Recommended with restrictions
▸ **Bortezomib monotherapy for relapsed multiple myeloma (October 2007)** NICE TA129 Recommended with restrictions
Scottish Medicines Consortium (SMC) decisions
▸ Bortezomib (*Velcade*®) in combination with dexamethasone, or with dexamethasone and thalidomide, for the induction treatment of adult patients with previously untreated multiple myeloma who are eligible for high-dose chemotherapy with haematopoietic stem cell transplantation (January 2014) SMC No. 927/13 Recommended with restrictions

● MEDICINAL FORMS There can be variation in the licensing of different medicines containing the same drug. Forms available from special-order manufacturers include: solution for injection

Solution for injection
▸ Bortezomib (Non-proprietary)
  Bortezomib 2.5 mg per 1 ml Bortezomib 3.5mg/1.4ml solution for injection vials | 1 vial PoM £495.55 (Hospital only)
Powder for solution for injection
▸ Bortezomib (Non-proprietary)
  Bortezomib 1 mg Bortezomib 1mg powder for solution for injection vials | 1 vial PoM £217.82 (Hospital only)
  Bortezomib 2.5 mg Bortezomib 2.5mg powder for solution for injection vials | 1 vial PoM £544.56 (Hospital only)
  Bortezomib 3.5 mg Bortezomib 3.5mg powder for solution for injection vials | 1 vial PoM £533.67-£762.38 (Hospital only)
▸ Velcade (Janssen-Cilag Ltd)
  Bortezomib 3.5 mg Velcade 3.5mg powder for solution for injection vials | 1 vial PoM £762.38 (Hospital only)

Carfilzomib
03-Dec-2020

● DRUG ACTION Carfilzomib is an irreversible selective proteasome inhibitor that disrupts tumour cell turnover and induces apoptosis.

● INDICATIONS AND DOSE
Treatment of multiple myeloma in patients who have received at least one prior therapy (in combination with dexamethasone, or with dexamethasone and lenalidomide) (specialist use only)
▸ BY INTRAVENOUS INFUSION
▸ Adult: (consult product literature or local protocols)

IMPORTANT SAFETY INFORMATION
MHRA/CHM ADVICE: CARFILZOMIB (*KYPROLIS*®): REMINDER OF RISK OF POTENTIALLY FATAL CARDIAC EVENTS (AUGUST 2019)
Cases of cardiac arrest, cardiac failure, and myocardial infarction, including fatalities, have been reported in patients with or without pre-existing cardiac disorders receiving carfilzomib. Healthcare professionals are advised to monitor patients for signs and symptoms of cardiac disorders before and during carfilzomib treatment. Carfilzomib should be discontinued if severe or life-threatening cardiac events occur; restarting treatment may be considered at a lower dose once the condition is controlled and the patient is stable.

MHRA/CHM ADVICE: CARFILZOMIB (*KYPROLIS*®): RISK OF REACTIVATION OF HEPATITIS B VIRUS (NOVEMBER 2019)

An EU review of worldwide data has identified reports of hepatitis B virus (HBV) reactivation in patients treated with carfilzomib. Healthcare professionals are advised to screen all patients for HBV before initiating treatment; those with unknown serology already being treated with carfilzomib should also be screened. Patients with positive serology should be considered for antiviral prophylaxis, and be monitored for signs of HBV reactivation during and after treatment; immediate medical attention should be sought if signs and symptoms of HBV reactivation develop. Experts should be consulted for advice about HBV treatment and the continuation, interruption, or resumption of carfilzomib in patients with HBV reactivation.

- CAUTIONS Elderly (over 75 years)—higher incidence of adverse effects · ensure adequate hydration · infusion-related reactions · recent history of myocardial infarction · risk of cardiac failure · risk of herpes zoster reactivation · uncontrolled angina · uncontrolled arrhythmias

  CAUTIONS, FURTHER INFORMATION
  ▸ Infusion-related reactions Manufacturer advises premedication with dexamethasone to reduce incidence and severity of infusion-related reactions.
  ▸ Risk of herpes zoster reactivation Manufacturer advises consider antiviral prophylaxis for herpes zoster infection.

- INTERACTIONS → Appendix 1: carfilzomib

- SIDE-EFFECTS
  ▸ Common or very common Anaemia · anxiety · appetite decreased · arrhythmias · arthralgia · asthenia · cataract · chest pain · chills · confusion · constipation · cough · decreased leucocytes · dehydration · diarrhoea · dizziness · dysphonia · dyspnoea · electrolyte imbalance · embolism and thrombosis · fever · flushing · gastrointestinal discomfort · haemorrhage · headache · heart failure · hyperbilirubinaemia · hyperglycaemia · hyperhidrosis · hypertension · hyperuricaemia · hypoalbuminaemia · hypotension · increased risk of infection · influenza like illness · infusion related reaction · insomnia · malaise · muscle complaints · muscle weakness · myocardial infarction · nausea · neutropenia · oropharyngeal pain · pain · palpitations · peripheral neuropathy · peripheral oedema · pulmonary hypertension · pulmonary oedema · renal impairment · respiratory disorders · sensation abnormal · sepsis · skin reactions · thrombocytopenia · tinnitus · toothache · vision blurred · vomiting
  ▸ Uncommon Cardiac arrest · cardiomyopathy · Clostridioides difficile colitis · gastrointestinal perforation · haemolytic uraemic syndrome · hepatic disorders · hepatitis B reactivation · intracranial haemorrhage · multiple organ dysfunction syndrome · myocardial ischaemia · pericardial effusion · pericarditis · stroke · tumour lysis syndrome
  ▸ Rare or very rare Angioedema · posterior reversible encephalopathy syndrome (PRES) · thrombotic microangiopathy
  ▸ Frequency not known Progressive multifocal leukoencephalopathy (PML) · QT interval prolongation

- CONCEPTION AND CONTRACEPTION Manufacturer recommends effective contraception during and for 1 month after treatment in women of childbearing potential; hormonal contraceptives associated with a risk of thrombosis should be avoided. Male patients should use effective contraception during and for 3 months after treatment if their partner is pregnant or of childbearing potential. See also *Pregnancy and reproductive function* in Cytotoxic drugs p. 932.

- PREGNANCY Manufacturer advises avoid unless potential benefit outweighs risk—toxicity in *animal* studies. See also

Pregnancy and reproductive function in Cytotoxic drugs p. 932.

- BREAST FEEDING Manufacturer advises avoid during and for at least 2 days after treatment—no information available.

- HEPATIC IMPAIRMENT Manufacturer advises caution (increased risk of side-effects), particularly in moderate to severe impairment (limited information available).

- RENAL IMPAIRMENT Manufacturer advises caution—increased incidence of adverse effects.

- MONITORING REQUIREMENTS Manufacturer advises monitoring of the following patient parameters: serum potassium concentration at least monthly; signs and symptoms of fluid overload, especially in those at risk of cardiac failure; renal function at treatment initiation and at least monthly during treatment—consider dose modification; hepatic function at treatment initiation and monthly during treatment—consider dose modification; platelet count and blood pressure. Also monitor for signs and symptoms of thrombotic microangiopathy.

- HANDLING AND STORAGE Manufacturer advises store in a refrigerator at 2–8°C.

- PATIENT AND CARER ADVICE Manufacturer advises that patients and carers are warned to report signs and symptoms of thromboembolism (such as dyspnoea, chest pain, arm or leg swelling or pain).
  Driving and skilled tasks Patients and their carers should be counselled on the effects on driving and skilled tasks—increased risk of dizziness, hypotension and blurred vision.

- NATIONAL FUNDING/ACCESS DECISIONS
  For full details see funding body website
  NICE decisions
  ▸ Carfilzomib for previously treated multiple myeloma (November 2020) NICE TA657 Recommended with restrictions

  Scottish Medicines Consortium (SMC) decisions
  ▸ Carfilzomib (*Kyprolis*®) in combination with lenalidomide and dexamethasone for the treatment of adult patients with multiple myeloma who have received at least one prior therapy [see also SMC2290] (January 2017) SMC No. 1171/16 Not recommended
  ▸ Carfilzomib (*Kyprolis*®) in combination with dexamethasone alone for the treatment of adult patients with multiple myeloma who have received at least one prior therapy (August 2017) SMC No. 1242/17 Recommended
  ▸ Carfilzomib (*Kyprolis*®) in combination with lenalidomide and dexamethasone for the treatment of adult patients with multiple myeloma who have received at least one prior therapy [for patients who have received only one prior therapy] (October 2020) SMC No. SMC2290 Recommended

- MEDICINAL FORMS There can be variation in the licensing of different medicines containing the same drug.
  Powder for solution for infusion
  ELECTROLYTES: May contain Sodium
  ▸ Kyprolis (Amgen Ltd) ▼
  Carfilzomib 10 mg Kyprolis 10mg powder for solution for infusion vials | 1 vial [PoM] £176.00
  Carfilzomib 30 mg Kyprolis 30mg powder for solution for infusion vials | 1 vial [PoM] £528.00
  Carfilzomib 60 mg Kyprolis 60mg powder for solution for infusion vials | 1 vial [PoM] £1,056.00

Ixazomib

21-Mar-2018

● DRUG ACTION Ixazomib is a proteasome inhibitor.

● **INDICATIONS AND DOSE**

Multiple myeloma in patients who have received at least one prior therapy, in combination with lenalidomide and dexamethasone (specialist use only)

▸ BY MOUTH
▸ Adult: 4 mg once weekly on days 1, 8, and 15 of a 28-day treatment cycle, for dose adjustments due to side-effects, consult product literature

---

IMPORTANT SAFETY INFORMATION

RISKS OF INCORRECT DOSING OF ORAL ANTI-CANCER MEDICINES
See Cytotoxic drugs p. 932.

● CAUTIONS Risk of herpes zoster reactivation
CAUTIONS, FURTHER INFORMATION
▸ Herpes zoster reactivation Manufacturer advises consider concomitant antiviral prophylaxis to decrease the risk of herpes zoster reactivation.

● INTERACTIONS → Appendix 1: ixazomib

● SIDE-EFFECTS
▸ **Common or very common** Back pain · constipation · diarrhoea · increased risk of infection · nausea · neutropenia · peripheral neuropathy (monitor for symptoms) · peripheral oedema · rash · thrombocytopenia · vomiting
▸ **Frequency not known** Posterior reversible encephalopathy syndrome (PRES) (discontinue)

● CONCEPTION AND CONTRACEPTION Manufacturer advises effective contraception in women of child-bearing potential and in men with a partner of child-bearing potential, during treatment and for at least 90 days after stopping treatment; additional barrier method recommended in women using hormonal contraceptives.

● PREGNANCY Manufacturer advises avoid—toxicity in *animal* studies. See also *Pregnancy and reproductive function* in Cytotoxic drugs p. 932.

● BREAST FEEDING Manufacturer advises avoid—no information available.

● HEPATIC IMPAIRMENT Manufacturer advises caution in moderate to severe impairment (risk of increased exposure).
Dose adjustments Manufacturer advises dose reduction to 3 mg in moderate to severe impairment.

● RENAL IMPAIRMENT
Dose adjustments Manufacturer advises reduce dose to 3 mg in severe impairment (creatinine clearance less than 30 mL/min).

● MONITORING REQUIREMENTS Manufacturer advises to monitor hepatic function regularly and adjust dose accordingly—consult product literature.

● PATIENT AND CARER ADVICE
Missed doses Manufacturer advises if less than 72 hours remain before the next scheduled dose, the missed dose should not be taken and the next dose should be taken at the normal time.

● NATIONAL FUNDING/ACCESS DECISIONS
For full details see funding body website

NICE decisions
▸ **Ixazomib with lenalidomide and dexamethasone for treating relapsed or refractory multiple myeloma (February 2018)**
NICE TA505 Recommended with restrictions

● MEDICINAL FORMS There can be variation in the licensing of different medicines containing the same drug.
Capsule
CAUTIONARY AND ADVISORY LABELS 23, 25
▸ Ninlaro (Takeda UK Ltd) ▼
Ixazomib (as Ixazomib citrate) 2.3 mg Ninlaro 2.3mg capsules |
3 capsule PoM £6,336.00
Ixazomib (as Ixazomib citrate) 3 mg Ninlaro 3mg capsules |
3 capsule PoM £6,336.00
Ixazomib (as Ixazomib citrate) 4 mg Ninlaro 4mg capsules |
3 capsule PoM £6,336.00

ANTINEOPLASTIC DRUGS 〉 PROTEIN KINASE INHIBITORS

Abemaciclib

02-Nov-2020

● DRUG ACTION Abemaciclib is a selective inhibitor of cyclin-dependent kinases 4 and 6, which leads to disruption of cancer cell proliferation.

● **INDICATIONS AND DOSE**

Locally advanced or metastatic breast cancer (initiated by a specialist)

▸ BY MOUTH
▸ Adult: 150 mg twice daily, for dose adjustments due to side-effects—consult product literature
DOSE ADJUSTMENTS DUE TO INTERACTIONS
▸ Manufacturer advises if concomitant use with potent CYP3A4 inhibitors is unavoidable, reduce abemaciclib dose to 100 mg twice daily; in those already taking a reduced dose, consult product literature. If the CYP3A4 inhibitor is stopped, increase the abemaciclib dose (after 3–5 half lives of the inhibitor) to the dose used before starting the CYP3A4 inhibitor.

IMPORTANT SAFETY INFORMATION

RISKS OF INCORRECT DOSING OF ORAL ANTI-CANCER MEDICINES
See Cytotoxic drugs p. 932.

● INTERACTIONS → Appendix 1: abemaciclib

● SIDE-EFFECTS
▸ **Common or very common** Alopecia · anaemia · appetite decreased · decreased leucocytes · diarrhoea · dizziness · embolism and thrombosis · excessive tearing · fatigue · fever · infection · muscle weakness · nausea · neutropenia · skin reactions · taste altered · thrombocytopenia · vomiting

● CONCEPTION AND CONTRACEPTION Manufacturer advises highly effective contraception in women of childbearing potential during treatment and for at least 3 weeks after completing treatment. See also *Pregnancy and reproductive function* in Cytotoxic drugs p. 932.

● PREGNANCY Manufacturer advises avoid—toxicity in *animal* studies. See also *Pregnancy and reproductive function* in Cytotoxic drugs p. 932.

● BREAST FEEDING Manufacturer advises avoid—no information available.

● HEPATIC IMPAIRMENT Manufacturer advises caution in severe impairment. Temporary or permanent withdrawal may be needed following increases in aminotransferases—consult product literature.
Dose adjustments Manufacturer advises dose reduction to 150 mg once daily in severe impairment.

● RENAL IMPAIRMENT Manufacturer advises caution in severe impairment—monitor for signs of toxicity.

● MONITORING REQUIREMENTS Manufacturer advises monitor full blood count, and alanine and aspartate aminotransferases before starting treatment, every 2 weeks for the first 2 months, monthly for the following 2 months, and as clinically indicated thereafter.

8

Immune system and malignant disease

- NATIONAL FUNDING/ACCESS DECISIONS
For full details see funding body website
NICE decisions
▸ Abemaciclib with an aromatase inhibitor for previously untreated, hormone receptor-positive, HER2-negative, locally advanced or metastatic breast cancer (February 2019) NICE TA563 Recommended with restrictions
▸ Abemaciclib with fulvestrant for treating hormone receptor-positive, HER2-negative advanced breast cancer after endocrine therapy (May 2019) NICE TA579 Recommended with restrictions

Scottish Medicines Consortium (SMC) decisions
▸ Abemaciclib (*Verzenios*®) for the treatment of women with hormone receptor (HR) positive, human epidermal growth factor receptor 2 (HER2) negative locally advanced or metastatic breast cancer in combination with an aromatase inhibitor as initial endocrine-based therapy, or in women who have received prior endocrine therapy (May 2019) SMC No. SMC2135 Recommended
▸ Abemaciclib (*Verzenios*®) for the treatment of women with hormone receptor (HR) positive, human epidermal growth factor receptor 2 (HER2) negative locally advanced or metastatic breast cancer in combination with fulvestrant as initial endocrine-based therapy or in women who have received prior endocrine therapy (May 2019) SMC No. SMC2179 Recommended with restrictions

- MEDICINAL FORMS There can be variation in the licensing of different medicines containing the same drug.
Tablet
CAUTIONARY AND ADVISORY LABELS 3, 25
▸ Verzenios (Eli Lilly and Company Ltd) ▼
Abemaciclib 50 mg Verzenios 50mg tablets | 28 tablet [PoM]
£1,475.00 (Hospital only) | 56 tablet [PoM] £2,950.00 (Hospital only)
Abemaciclib 100 mg Verzenios 100mg tablets | 28 tablet [PoM]
£1,475.00 (Hospital only) | 56 tablet [PoM] £2,950.00 (Hospital only)
Abemaciclib 150 mg Verzenios 150mg tablets | 28 tablet [PoM]
£1,475.00 (Hospital only) | 56 tablet [PoM] £2,950.00 (Hospital only)

Acalabrutinib

04-Dec-2020

- DRUG ACTION Acalabrutinib is a tyrosine kinase inihibitor.

- INDICATIONS AND DOSE
Chronic lymphocytic leukaemia (specialist use only)
▸ BY MOUTH
▸ Adult: 100 mg twice daily, doses should be taken approximately 12 hours apart, for dose adjustment, interruption, or treatment discontinuation due to side-effects—consult product literature

---
IMPORTANT SAFETY INFORMATION
RISKS OF INCORRECT DOSING OF ORAL ANTI-CANCER MEDICINES
See Cytotoxic drugs p. 932.

- CAUTIONS Exposure to sun (risk of skin cancer)—protect skin from exposure to sun · patients at high risk for thromboembolic disease—consider alternative treatment options to acalabrutinib · patients at increased risk for opportunistic infections—consider prophylaxis and monitor for signs and symptoms of infection · risk of haemorrhage—consider withholding acalabrutinib treatment for at least 3 days before and after surgery
- INTERACTIONS → Appendix 1: acalabrutinib
- SIDE-EFFECTS
▸ **Common or very common** Abdominal pain · anaemia · arrhythmias · arthralgia · asthenia · constipation · diarrhoea · dizziness · haemorrhage · headache · increased risk of infection · intracranial haemorrhage · musculoskeletal pain · nausea · neutropenia · second primary malignancy · skin reactions · thrombocytopenia · vomiting

▸ **Uncommon** Hepatitis B reactivation · lymphocytosis · tumour lysis syndrome
▸ **Frequency not known** Cough · leucopenia · progressive multifocal leukoencephalopathy (PML) · sepsis
- PREGNANCY [EvGr] Avoid unless potential benefit outweighs risk—toxicity in *animal* studies. ⓂSee also *Pregnancy and reproductive function* in Cytotoxic drugs p. 932.
- BREAST FEEDING [EvGr] Avoid breast feeding during treatment and for 2 days after the last dose—present in milk in *animal* studies. Ⓜ
- HEPATIC IMPAIRMENT [EvGr] Caution in moderate impairment; avoid in severe impairment (risk of increased exposure). Ⓜ
- RENAL IMPAIRMENT [EvGr] Caution in severe impairment (no information available). Ⓜ
- PRE-TREATMENT SCREENING Patients should be evaluated for hepatitis B virus status before starting treatment—consult product literature.
- PATIENT AND CARER ADVICE
Missed doses [EvGr] If a dose is more than 3 hours late, the missed dose should not be taken and the next dose should be taken at the normal time. Ⓜ
Driving and skilled tasks [EvGr] Patients and carers should be counselled on the effects on driving and performance of skilled tasks—increased risk of dizziness and fatigue. Ⓜ

- MEDICINAL FORMS There can be variation in the licensing of different medicines containing the same drug.
Capsule
CAUTIONARY AND ADVISORY LABELS 25
▸ Calquence (AstraZeneca UK Ltd) ▼
Acalabrutinib 100 mg Calquence 100mg capsules |
60 capsule [PoM] £5,059.00 (Hospital only)

Afatinib

03-Sep-2020

- DRUG ACTION Afatinib is a protein kinase inhibitor.

- INDICATIONS AND DOSE
Treatment of locally advanced or metastatic non-small cell lung cancer with activating epidermal growth factor receptor (EGFR) mutations, in patients who have not previously been treated with EGFR tyrosine kinase inhibitor
▸ BY MOUTH
▸ Adult: 40 mg once daily; increased if tolerated to up to 50 mg once daily, dose increase may be considered after 3 weeks at initial dose; consult product literature for details on dosing and dose adjustment due to side effects

---
IMPORTANT SAFETY INFORMATION
RISKS OF INCORRECT DOSING OF ORAL ANTI-CANCER MEDICINES
See Cytotoxic drugs p. 932.

- CAUTIONS Cardiac risk factors · conditions which may affect left ventricular ejection fraction—consider cardiac monitoring, including assessment of left ventricular ejection fraction, at baseline and during treatment · diarrhoea—proactive management recommended (consult product literature) · exposure to sun (protect skin from exposure to sun) · history of keratitis · new pulmonary symptoms (including dyspnoea, cough, fever)—interrupt treatment until interstitial lung disease is excluded · severe dry eyes · signs and symptoms of keratitis—promptly refer to ophthalmologist for assessment · signs and symptoms of skin reaction—treat promptly and interrupt afatinib treatment if severe or if Stevens-Johnson syndrome suspected (consult product literature) · ulcerative keratitis · use of contact lenses · worsening pulmonary symptoms (including dyspnoea, cough, fever)—interrupt treatment until interstitial lung disease is excluded

● INTERACTIONS → Appendix 1: afatinib

● SIDE-EFFECTS

► **Common or very common** Appetite decreased · cystitis · dehydration · diarrhoea · dry eye · dyspepsia · epistaxis · eye inflammation · fever · hypokalaemia · muscle spasms · nausea · oral disorders · paronychia · renal impairment · rhinorrhoea · skin reactions · taste altered · vomiting · weight decreased

► **Uncommon** Interstitial lung disease · pancreatitis

► **Rare or very rare** Severe cutaneous adverse reactions (SCARs)

● CONCEPTION AND CONTRACEPTION Ensure effective contraception during and for at least one month after treatment in women of childbearing potential.

● PREGNANCY Manufacturer advises avoid. See also *Pregnancy and reproductive function* in Cytotoxic drugs p. 932.

● BREAST FEEDING Manufacturer advises avoid—present in milk in *animal* studies.

● HEPATIC IMPAIRMENT Manufacturer advises caution in mild to moderate impairment; avoid in severe impairment (no information available).

Dose adjustments Manufacturer advises consider dose interruption if hepatic function worsens in mild to moderate impairment—consult product literature.

● RENAL IMPAIRMENT Manufacturer advises avoid in severe renal impairment.

● DIRECTIONS FOR ADMINISTRATION Manufacturer advises tablets should be taken whole on an empty stomach. Food should not be consumed for at least 3 hours before and at least 1 hour after each dose.

Giotrif® tablets may be dispersed in approximately 100 mL of noncarbonated water by stirring occasionally for up to 15 minutes (must not be crushed). The dispersion should be swallowed immediately, and the glass rinsed with the same volume of water which should also be swallowed. The dispersion can also be administered via a gastric tube.

● PATIENT AND CARER ADVICE Patient counselling advised (administration).

Driving and skilled tasks Ocular adverse reactions may affect performance of skilled tasks e.g. driving.

● NATIONAL FUNDING/ACCESS DECISIONS For full details see funding body website

NICE decisions

► Afatinib for treating epidermal growth factor receptor mutation-positive locally advanced or metastatic non-small-cell lung cancer (April 2014) NICE TA310 Recommended with restrictions

● MEDICINAL FORMS There can be variation in the licensing of different medicines containing the same drug.

Tablet

CAUTIONARY AND ADVISORY LABELS 25

► Giotrif (Boehringer Ingelheim Ltd)
Afatinib (as Afatinib dimaleate) 20 mg Giotrif 20mg tablets |
28 tablet PoM £2,023.28
Afatinib (as Afatinib dimaleate) 30 mg Giotrif 30mg tablets |
28 tablet PoM £2,023.28
Afatinib (as Afatinib dimaleate) 40 mg Giotrif 40mg tablets |
28 tablet PoM £2,023.28
Afatinib (as Afatinib dimaleate) 50 mg Giotrif 50mg tablets |
28 tablet PoM £2,023.28

Alectinib
31-Aug-2020

● DRUG ACTION Alectinib is a tyrosine kinase inhibitor.

● INDICATIONS AND DOSE

Anaplastic lymphoma kinase (ALK)-positive advanced non-small cell lung cancer (specialist use only)

► BY MOUTH

► Adult: 600 mg twice daily, for dose adjustments due to side-effects—consult product literature

IMPORTANT SAFETY INFORMATION
RISKS OF INCORRECT DOSING OF ORAL ANTI-CANCER MEDICINES
See Cytotoxic drugs p. 932.

● INTERACTIONS → Appendix 1: alectinib

● SIDE-EFFECTS

► **Common or very common** Anaemia · arrhythmias · constipation · diarrhoea · eye disorders · eye inflammation · hyperbilirubinaemia · musculoskeletal pain · myalgia · nausea · oedema · photosensitivity reaction · skin reactions · vision disorders · vomiting

► **Uncommon** Drug-induced liver injury · respiratory disorders

● CONCEPTION AND CONTRACEPTION Manufacturer advises women of child-bearing potential should use effective contraception during and for at least 3 months after stopping treatment.

● PREGNANCY Manufacturer advises avoid—toxicity in *animal* studies. See also *Pregnancy and reproductive function* in Cytotoxic drugs p. 932.

● BREAST FEEDING Manufacturer advises avoid—no information available.

● HEPATIC IMPAIRMENT

Dose adjustments Manufacturer advises reduce dose to 450 mg twice daily in severe impairment.

● MONITORING REQUIREMENTS

► Manufacturer advises monitor creatine phosphokinase every 2 weeks for the first month and as clinically indicated thereafter in patients reporting symptoms of myalgia.

► Manufacturer advises monitor heart rate and blood pressure as clinically indicated.

► Manufacturer advises monitor liver function at baseline then every 2 weeks during the first 3 months of treatment and periodically thereafter as clinically indicated; more frequent monitoring should be performed in patients who develop aminotransferase and bilirubin elevations.

► Manufacturer advises monitor for symptoms of interstitial lung disease and pneumonitis.

● PATIENT AND CARER ADVICE

Photosensitivity Manufacturer advises patients should use a broad spectrum sunscreen and lip balm and be advised to avoid prolonged sun exposure during treatment, and for 7 days after discontinuation.

Myalgia Manufacturer advises patients should advised to report any unexplained muscle pain, tenderness or weakness.

Vomiting Manufacturer advises if vomiting occurs after taking tablets, no additional dose should be taken on that day and the next dose should be taken at the usual time.

Missed doses Manufacturer advises if a dose is more than 6 hours late, the missed dose should not be taken and the next dose should be taken at the normal time.

Driving and skilled tasks Manufacturer advises patients and carers should be counselled on the effects on driving and performance of skilled tasks—increased risk of symptomatic bradycardia and vision disorders.

● NATIONAL FUNDING/ACCESS DECISIONS For full details see funding body website

8

Immune system and malignant disease

NICE decisions
▶ Alectinib (*Alecensa*®) for untreated ALK-positive advanced non-small cell lung cancer (August 2018) NICE TA536
Recommended
Scottish Medicines Consortium (SMC) decisions
▶ Alectinib hydrochloride (*Alecensa*®) as monotherapy for the first-line treatment of adult patients with anaplastic lymphoma kinase (ALK)-positive advanced non-small cell lung cancer (NSCLC) (August 2018) SMC No. SMC2012
Recommended

● MEDICINAL FORMS There can be variation in the licensing of different medicines containing the same drug.
Capsule
CAUTIONARY AND ADVISORY LABELS 11, 21
ELECTROLYTES: May contain Sodium
▶ Alecensa (Roche Products Ltd) ▼
  Alectinib (as Alectinib hydrochloride) 150 mg Alecensa 150mg capsules | 224 capsule [PoM] £5,032.00

Alpelisib

20-Oct-2020

● DRUG ACTION Alpelisib is an alpha-specific class 1 protein kinase inhibitor.

● INDICATIONS AND DOSE
Locally advanced or metastatic breast cancer (in combination with fulvestrant) [in postmenopausal women and men] (initiated by a specialist)
▶ BY MOUTH
▶ Adult: 300 mg once daily, for dose adjustments, treatment interruption, or discontinuation due to side-effects—consult product literature

> IMPORTANT SAFETY INFORMATION
> RISKS OF INCORRECT DOSING OF ORAL ANTI-CANCER MEDICINES
> See Cytotoxic drugs p. 932.

● CONTRA-INDICATIONS History of severe cutaneous reactions · osteonecrosis of the jaw
● CAUTIONS History of diabetes mellitus (risk of hyperglycaemia)
● INTERACTIONS → Appendix 1: alpelisib
● SIDE-EFFECTS
▶ Common or very common Acute kidney injury · alopecia · anaemia · appetite decreased · asthenia · dehydration · diarrhoea · dry eye · dry mouth · electrolyte imbalance · eyelid oedema · facial swelling · fever · gastrointestinal discomfort · headache · hypersensitivity · hypertension · increased risk of infection · insomnia · lymphoedema · mucosal abnormalities · muscle complaints · nausea · oedema · oral disorders · osteonecrosis of jaw · respiratory disorders · skin reactions · taste altered · urosepsis · vision blurred · vomiting · vulvovaginal dryness · weight decreased
▶ Uncommon Diabetic ketoacidosis · ketoacidosis · pancreatitis · severe cutaneous adverse reactions (SCARs)
▶ Frequency not known Hyperglycaemia
● CONCEPTION AND CONTRACEPTION Manufacturer advises male patients should use effective contraception during treatment and for one week after last dose if their partner is pregnant or of childbearing potential. See also *Pregnancy and reproductive function* in Cytotoxic drugs p. 932. The effect on human fertility is not known—impairment of fertility has been observed in *animal* studies.
● RENAL IMPAIRMENT Manufacturer advises use with caution in severe renal impairment—no information available.
● MONITORING REQUIREMENTS Manufacturer advises assess fasting plasma glucose and HbA1c levels before

initiation and monitor frequently in the first 4 weeks of treatment—consult product literature.
● PATIENT AND CARER ADVICE
Vomiting Manufacturer advises if vomiting occurs after taking tablets, no additional dose should be taken on that day and the next dose should be taken at the usual time.
Missed doses Manufacturer advises if dose is more than 9 hours late, the missed dose should not be taken and the next dose should be taken at the usual time.
Driving and skilled tasks Manufacturer advises patients and carers should be cautioned on the effects on driving and performance of skilled tasks—increased risk of fatigue or blurred vision.

● MEDICINAL FORMS There can be variation in the licensing of different medicines containing the same drug.
Tablet
CAUTIONARY AND ADVISORY LABELS 25, 21
▶ Piqray (Novartis Pharmaceuticals UK Ltd) ▼
  Alpelisib 50 mg Piqray 50mg tablets | 28 tablet [PoM] 🅧 (Hospital only)
  Alpelisib 150 mg Piqray 150mg tablets | 56 tablet [PoM] £4,082.14 (Hospital only)
  Alpelisib 200 mg Piqray 200mg tablets | 28 tablet [PoM] £4,082.14 (Hospital only)

Avapritinib

17-Nov-2020

● DRUG ACTION Avapritinib is a tyrosine kinase inhibitor.

● INDICATIONS AND DOSE
Gastro-intestinal stromal tumours (initiated by a specialist)
▶ BY MOUTH
▶ Adult: 300 mg once daily, for dose adjustments, treatment interruption, or discontinuation due to side-effects—consult product literature
DOSE ADJUSTMENTS DUE TO INTERACTIONS
▶ [EvGr] If concurrent use of moderate CYP3A4 inhibitors is unavoidable, decrease the initial avapritinib dose to 100 mg once daily. ◁ⓜ

> IMPORTANT SAFETY INFORMATION
> RISKS OF INCORRECT DOSING OF ORAL ANTI-CANCER MEDICINES
> See Cytotoxic drugs p. 932.

● CAUTIONS Risk factors for haemorrhage · susceptibility to QT-interval prolongation
● INTERACTIONS → Appendix 1: avapritinib
● SIDE-EFFECTS
▶ Common or very common Abdominal pain · acute kidney injury · alopecia · anaemia · anxiety · appetite decreased · arthralgia · ascites · asthenia · back pain · CNS haemorrhage · cognitive impairment · concentration impaired · confusion · constipation · cough · dementia · depression · diarrhoea · dizziness · drowsiness · dry mouth · dysphagia · dyspnoea · electrolyte imbalance · excessive tearing · eye inflammation · facial swelling · feeling cold · fever · fluid imbalance · gastrointestinal disorders · haemorrhage · hair colour changes · headache · hyperbilirubinaemia · hypertension · hypoalbuminaemia · insomnia · malaise · memory impairment · movement disorders · muscle complaints · nasal congestion · nausea · oedema · oral disorders · peripheral neuropathy · peripheral swelling · photosensitivity reaction · psychiatric disorder · QT interval prolongation · respiratory disorders · skin reactions · speech impairment · taste altered · thrombocytopenia · tremor · vertigo · vision disorders · vomiting · weight changes
▶ Uncommon Encephalopathy · pericardial effusion · tumour haemorrhage

▸ CONCEPTION AND CONTRACEPTION [EvGr] Females of childbearing potential should use effective contraception during treatment and for one month after last treatment. See also *Pregnancy and reproductive function* in Cytotoxic drugs p. 932. ⟨M⟩

▸ PREGNANCY [EvGr] Avoid—toxicity in *animal* studies. See also *Pregnancy and reproductive function* in Cytotoxic drugs p. 932. ⟨M⟩

▸ BREAST FEEDING [EvGr] Avoid during treatment and for at least 2 weeks after the last dose—no information available. ⟨M⟩

▸ HEPATIC IMPAIRMENT [EvGr] Avoid in severe impairment (no information available). ⟨M⟩

▸ RENAL IMPAIRMENT [EvGr] Avoid in severe impairment or end-stage renal disease (no information available). ⟨M⟩

▸ PATIENT AND CARER ADVICE
Vomiting [EvGr] If vomiting occurs after taking tablets, no additional dose should be taken on that day and the next dose should be taken at the usual time. ⟨M⟩
Photosensitivity [EvGr] Avoid or minimise exposure to direct sunlight; patients should be advised to use a high protection sunscreen and wear protective clothing. ⟨M⟩
Missed doses [EvGr] If a dose is more than 16 hours late, the missed dose should not be taken and the next dose should be taken at the usual time. ⟨M⟩
Driving and skilled tasks [EvGr] Patients and carers should be cautioned on the effects on driving and performance of skilled tasks—increased risk of cognitive effects. ⟨M⟩

● MEDICINAL FORMS There can be variation in the licensing of different medicines containing the same drug.
Tablet
CAUTIONARY AND ADVISORY LABELS 23, 25
▸ Ayvakyt (Blueprint Medicines (UK) Ltd) ▼
Avapritinib 100 mg Ayvakyt 100mg tablets | 30 tablet [PoM] £26,667.00 (Hospital only)
Avapritinib 200 mg Ayvakyt 200mg tablets | 30 tablet [PoM] £26,667.00 (Hospital only)
Avapritinib 300 mg Ayvakyt 300mg tablets | 30 tablet [PoM] £26,667.00 (Hospital only)

Axitinib
15-Oct-2020

● DRUG ACTION Axitinib is a tyrosine kinase inhibitor.

● INDICATIONS AND DOSE
Advanced renal cell carcinoma (specialist use only)
▸ BY MOUTH
▸ Adult: (consult product literature)

IMPORTANT SAFETY INFORMATION
MHRA/CHM ADVICE: SYSTEMICALLY ADMINISTERED VEGF PATHWAY INHIBITORS: RISK OF ANEURYSM AND ARTERY DISSECTION (JULY 2020)
A European review of worldwide data concluded that systemically administered VEGF pathway inhibitors may lead to aneurysm and artery dissection in patients with or without hypertension. Some fatal cases have been reported, mainly in relation to aortic aneurysm rupture and aortic dissection. The MHRA advises healthcare professionals to carefully consider the risk of aneurysm and artery dissection in patients with risk factors before initiating treatment with axitinib; any modifiable risk factors (such as smoking and hypertension) should be reduced as much as possible. Patients should be monitored and treated for hypertension as required.

RISKS OF INCORRECT DOSING OF ORAL ANTI-CANCER MEDICINES
See Cytotoxic drugs p. 932.

● CONTRA-INDICATIONS Recent active gastro-intestinal bleeding · untreated brain metastases

● CAUTIONS Hypertension · risk factors for aneurysm or artery dissection
CAUTIONS, FURTHER INFORMATION
▸ Monitoring of blood pressure The MHRA advises to monitor blood pressure regularly—consult product literature if hypertension occurs during treatment.

● INTERACTIONS → Appendix 1: axitinib

● SIDE-EFFECTS
▸ **Common or very common** Alopecia · anaemia · appetite decreased · arthralgia · asthenia · constipation · cough · dehydration · diarrhoea · dizziness · dysphonia · dyspnoea · electrolyte imbalance · embolism and thrombosis · gastrointestinal discomfort · gastrointestinal disorders · haemorrhage · headache · heart failure · hyperbilirubinaemia · hypertension · hyperthyroidism · hypothyroidism · mucositis · myalgia · nausea · oral disorders · oropharyngeal pain · pain in extremity · polycythaemia · proteinuria · renal failure · skin reactions · taste altered · thrombocytopenia · tinnitus · vomiting · weight decreased
▸ **Uncommon** Leucopenia · neutropenia · posterior reversible encephalopathy syndrome (PRES)
▸ **Frequency not known** Aneurysm · artery dissection

● CONCEPTION AND CONTRACEPTION Effective contraception required during and for up to 1 week after treatment.

● PREGNANCY Manufacturer advises avoid unless potential benefit outweighs risk (toxicity in *animal* studies). See also *Pregnancy and reproductive function* in Cytotoxic drugs p. 932.

● HEPATIC IMPAIRMENT Manufacturer advises avoid in severe impairment—no information available.
Dose adjustments Manufacturer advises reduce dose in moderate impairment.

● MONITORING REQUIREMENTS
▸ Monitor for thyroid dysfunction.
▸ Monitor haemoglobin or haematocrit before and during treatment.
▸ Monitor for symptoms of gastro-intestinal perforation.
▸ Monitor for symptoms of fistula.
▸ Monitor for proteinuria before and during treatment.
▸ Monitor liver function before and during treatment.

● NATIONAL FUNDING/ACCESS DECISIONS
For full details see funding body website
NICE decisions
▸ Axitinib for treating advanced renal cell carcinoma after failure of prior systemic treatment (February 2015) NICE TA333 Recommended with restrictions
▸ Avelumab with axitinib for untreated advanced renal cell carcinoma (September 2020) NICE TA645 Recommended
▸ Pembrolizumab with axitinib for untreated advanced renal cell carcinoma (September 2020) NICE TA650 Not recommended

● MEDICINAL FORMS There can be variation in the licensing of different medicines containing the same drug.
Tablet
CAUTIONARY AND ADVISORY LABELS 25
▸ Inlyta (Pfizer Ltd)
Axitinib 1 mg Inlyta 1mg tablets | 56 tablet [PoM] £703.40 (Hospital only)
Axitinib 3 mg Inlyta 3mg tablets | 56 tablet [PoM] £2,110.20 (Hospital only)
Axitinib 5 mg Inlyta 5mg tablets | 56 tablet [PoM] £3,517.00 (Hospital only)
Axitinib 7 mg Inlyta 7mg tablets | 56 tablet [PoM] £4,923.80 (Hospital only)

8

Immune system and malignant disease

Binimetinib

05-Mar-2019

- **DRUG ACTION** Binimetinib inhibits the mitogen-activated protein kinase (MAPK) pathway, specifically mitogen-activated extracellular kinases MEK 1 and 2, thereby inhibiting BRAF V600 mutation-positive cell growth.

  - **INDICATIONS AND DOSE**

  Unresectable or metastatic melanoma with a BRAF V600 mutation (in combination with encorafenib) (specialist use only)
  ▶ BY MOUTH
  ▸ Adult: 45 mg twice daily, for dose adjustments due to side-effects, consult product literature

---

IMPORTANT SAFETY INFORMATION

RISKS OF INCORRECT DOSING OF ORAL ANTI-CANCER MEDICINES
See Cytotoxic drugs p. 932.

- **CONTRA-INDICATIONS** History of retinal vein occlusion
- **CAUTIONS** Left ventricular dysfunction (ejection fraction below 50%, or below the institutional lower limits of normal) · neuromuscular conditions associated with elevated creatine kinase and rhabdomyolysis · risk factors for retinal vein occlusion · risk factors for venous thromboembolism
- **SIDE-EFFECTS**
- ▶ **Common or very common** Alopecia · anaemia · angioedema · arthralgia · constipation · detachment of retinal pigment epithelium · diarrhoea · dizziness · embolism and thrombosis · eye inflammation · fatigue · fever · fluid retention · gastrointestinal discomfort · gastrointestinal disorders · haemorrhage · headache · heart failure · hypersensitivity · hypersensitivity vasculitis · hypertension · intracranial haemorrhage · left ventricular dysfunction · lip squamous cell carcinoma · muscle complaints · muscle weakness · myopathy · nausea · neoplasms · nerve disorders · oedema · pain · panniculitis · photosensitivity reaction · renal failure · skin reactions · taste altered · ulcerative colitis · vision disorders · vomiting
- ▶ **Uncommon** Facial paralysis · pancreatitis · paresis
- ▶ **Frequency not known** Respiratory disorders · retinal occlusion (discontinue permanently)
- **CONCEPTION AND CONTRACEPTION** Manufacturer advises women of child-bearing potential should use effective contraception during and for at least one month after stopping treatment.
- **PREGNANCY** Manufacturer advises avoid—toxicity in *animal* studies. See also *Pregnancy and reproductive function* in Cytotoxic drugs p. 932.
- **BREAST FEEDING** Manufacturer advises avoid—no information available.
- **HEPATIC IMPAIRMENT** Manufacturer advises avoid in moderate or severe impairment (increased exposure).
- **MONITORING REQUIREMENTS**
- ▶ Manufacturer advises monitor liver function before treatment, at least monthly during the first 6 months, and thereafter as clinically indicated.
- ▶ Manufacturer advises assess left ventricular ejection fraction before treatment, one month after starting treatment, then every 3 months or more frequently as clinically indicated.
- ▶ Manufacturer advises monitor for visual disturbances.
- ▶ Manufacturer advises monitor blood pressure before and during treatment.
- ▶ Manufacturer advises monitor creatine kinase and creatinine levels monthly during the first 6 months of treatment, and as clinically indicated.

- **PATIENT AND CARER ADVICE**
  Missed doses Manufacturer advises if a dose is more than 6 hours late, the missed dose should not be taken and the next dose should be taken at the normal time.
  Driving and skilled tasks Manufacturer advises patients and carers should be counselled on the effects on driving and performance of skilled tasks—increased risk of visual disturbances.
- **NATIONAL FUNDING/ACCESS DECISIONS**
  For full details see funding body website
  NICE decisions
- ▶ Encorafenib with binimetinib for unresectable or metastatic BRAF V600 mutation-positive melanoma (February 2019) NICE TA562 Recommended with restrictions
- **MEDICINAL FORMS** There can be variation in the licensing of different medicines containing the same drug.
  Tablet
  CAUTIONARY AND ADVISORY LABELS 3, 25
- ▸ Mektovi (Pierre Fabre Ltd) ▼
  Binimetinib 15 mg Mektovi 15mg tablets | 84 tablet [PoM]
  £2,240.00 (Hospital only)

Bosutinib

05-Dec-2019

- **INDICATIONS AND DOSE**

  Previously treated chronic, accelerated and blast phase Philadelphia chromosome-positive chronic myeloid leukaemia (specialist use only)
  ▶ BY MOUTH
  ▸ Adult: 500 mg once daily, consult product literature for dose adjustment due to side-effects, or incomplete haematologic response by week 8, or incomplete cytogenetic response by week 12

  Newly-diagnosed chronic phase Philadelphia chromosome-positive chronic myeloid leukaemia (specialist use only)
  ▶ BY MOUTH
  ▸ Adult: 400 mg once daily, consult product literature for dose adjustment due to side-effects, or failure to demonstrate breakpoint cluster region-Abelson (BCR-ABL) transcripts ≤10% by month 3

IMPORTANT SAFETY INFORMATION

RISKS OF INCORRECT DOSING OF ORAL ANTI-CANCER MEDICINES
See Cytotoxic drugs p. 932.

MHRA/CHM ADVICE (MAY 2016): RISK OF HEPATITIS B VIRUS REACTIVATION WITH BCR-ABL TYROSINE KINASE INHIBITORS
An EU wide review has concluded that bosutinib can cause hepatitis B reactivation; the MHRA recommends establishing hepatitis B virus status in all patients before initiation of treatment.

- **CAUTIONS** Cardiac disease · hepatitis B infection · history of pancreatitis—withhold treatment if lipase elevated and abdominal symptoms occur · history of QT prolongation—monitor ECG and correct hypokalaemia and hypomagnesaemia before and during treatment · recent cardiac event—monitor ECG and correct hypokalaemia and hypomagnesaemia before and during treatment · risk factors for QT prolongation—monitor ECG and correct hypokalaemia and hypomagnesaemia before and during treatment · significant gastrointestinal disorder
  CAUTIONS, FURTHER INFORMATION
- ▶ Hepatitis B infection The MHRA advises that patients who are carriers of hepatitis B virus should be closely monitored for signs and symptoms of active infection throughout treatment and for several months after stopping treatment; expert advice should be sought for

patients who test positive for hepatitis B virus and in those with active infection.

- **INTERACTIONS** → Appendix 1: bosutinib
- **SIDE-EFFECTS**
- ▶ **Common or very common** Anaemia · appetite decreased · arthralgia · asthenia · chest discomfort · cough · dehydration · diarrhoea · dizziness · dyspnoea · electrolyte imbalance · fever · gastritis · gastrointestinal discomfort · haemorrhage · headache · hepatic disorders · hyperbilirubinaemia · hyperlipasaemia · hypertension · increased risk of infection · leucopenia · long QT syndrome · malaise · myalgia · nausea · neutropenia · oedema · pain · pericardial effusion · QT interval prolongation · renal impairment · respiratory disorders · skin reactions · taste altered · thrombocytopenia · tinnitus · vomiting
- ▶ **Uncommon** Pancreatitis · pericarditis · pulmonary hypertension · pulmonary oedema · tumour lysis syndrome
- ▶ **Frequency not known** Hepatitis B reactivation · severe cutaneous adverse reactions (SCARs)
- **CONCEPTION AND CONTRACEPTION** Effective contraception required during treatment in women.
- **PREGNANCY** Avoid—toxicity in *animal* studies. See also *Pregnancy and reproductive function* in Cytotoxic drugs p. 932.
- **BREAST FEEDING** Manufacturer advises avoid—no information available.
- **HEPATIC IMPAIRMENT** Manufacturer advises avoid.
- **RENAL IMPAIRMENT**
  Dose adjustments For *chronic, accelerated and blast phase Philadelphia chromosome-positive chronic myeloid leukaemia,* manufacturer advises reduce dose to 400 mg in moderate impairment; reduce dose to 300 mg in severe impairment; consult product literature for dose adjustment due to side-effects, or incomplete haematological, cytogenetic, or molecular response.
  For *newly-diagnosed chronic phase Philadelphia chromosome-positive chronic myeloid leukaemia,* manufacturer advises reduce dose to 300 mg in moderate impairment; reduce dose to 200 mg in severe impairment; consult product literature for dose adjustment due to side-effects, or incomplete haematological, cytogenetic, or molecular response.
- **MONITORING REQUIREMENTS**
- ▶ Manufacturer advises monitor liver function before treatment initiation, then monthly for the first 3 months and thereafter as clinically indicated—consult product literature for management of raised transaminases.
- ▶ Manufacturer advises monitor full blood count weekly for the first month and then monthly thereafter or as clinically indicated.
- ▶ Manufacturer advises monitor for signs and symptoms of fluid retention (including pericardial effusion, pleural effusion and pulmonary oedema).
- **NATIONAL FUNDING/ACCESS DECISIONS**
  For full details see funding body website
  NICE decisions
- ▶ Bosutinib for previously treated chronic myeloid leukaemia (August 2016) NICE TA401 Recommended with restrictions

- **MEDICINAL FORMS** There can be variation in the licensing of different medicines containing the same drug.

Tablet
CAUTIONARY AND ADVISORY LABELS 21
- ▶ Bosulif (Pfizer Ltd) ▼
  Bosutinib 100 mg Bosulif 100mg tablets | 28 tablet [PoM] £859.17 (Hospital only)
  Bosutinib 400 mg Bosulif 400mg tablets | 28 tablet [PoM] £3,436.67 (Hospital only)
  Bosutinib 500 mg Bosulif 500mg tablets | 28 tablet [PoM] £3,436.67 (Hospital only)

Brigatinib   20-Oct-2020

- **DRUG ACTION** Brigatinib is a tyrosine kinase inhibitor.

- **INDICATIONS AND DOSE**
  Anaplastic lymphoma kinase (ALK)-positive advanced non-small cell lung cancer previously treated with crizotinib (specialist use only)
  ▶ BY MOUTH
  ▶ Adult: Initially 90 mg once daily for 7 days, then increased to 180 mg once daily, for dose adjustments due to dose interruption or side-effects—consult product literature
  DOSE ADJUSTMENTS DUE TO INTERACTIONS
  ▶ Manufacturer advises if concomitant use with potent CYP3A4 inhibitors is unavoidable, reduce brigatinib dose to 90 mg once daily; in those starting treatment or already taking a reduced dose, consult product literature.

> **IMPORTANT SAFETY INFORMATION**
> RISKS OF INCORRECT DOSING OF ORAL ANTI-CANCER MEDICINES
> See Cytotoxic drugs p. 932.

- **INTERACTIONS** → Appendix 1: brigatinib
- **SIDE-EFFECTS**
- ▶ **Common or very common** Anaemia · appetite decreased · arrhythmias · arthralgia · asthenia · cataract · chest discomfort · constipation · cough · diarrhoea · dizziness · dry mouth · dyspnoea · electrolyte imbalance · eye disorders · eye inflammation · facial swelling · fever · flatulence · gastrointestinal discomfort · glaucoma · headaches · hyperbilirubinaemia · hyperglycaemia · hyperinsulinaemia · hypertension · increased risk of infection · insomnia · memory loss · muscle complaints · musculoskeletal discomfort · nausea · nerve disorders · neurotoxicity · oedema · oral disorders · pain · palpitations · peripheral swelling · photosensitivity reaction · QT interval prolongation · respiratory disorders · sensation abnormal · skin reactions · taste altered · vision disorders · vomiting · weight decreased
- ▶ **Uncommon** Pancreatitis
- **CONCEPTION AND CONTRACEPTION** Manufacturer advises effective non-hormonal contraception in females of childbearing potential during and for at least 4 months after treatment. Male patients with partners of childbearing potential should use effective contraception during and for at least 3 months after treatment.
- **PREGNANCY** Manufacturer advises avoid unless potential benefit outweighs risk—toxicity in *animal* studies. See also *Pregnancy and reproductive function* in Cytotoxic drugs p. 932.
- **BREAST FEEDING** Manufacturer advises avoid—no information available.
- **HEPATIC IMPAIRMENT** Manufacturer advises caution in severe impairment.
  Dose adjustments Manufacturer advises dose reduction to 60 mg once daily for 7 days, then increase to 120 mg once daily in severe impairment.
- **RENAL IMPAIRMENT** Manufacturer advises caution in severe impairment.
  Dose adjustments Manufacturer advises dose reduction to 60 mg once daily for 7 days, then increase to 90 mg once daily in severe impairment.
- **MONITORING REQUIREMENTS**
- ▶ Manufacturer advises monitor for new or worsening respiratory symptoms, particularly in the first week of treatment—promptly investigate if pneumonitis suspected (consult product literature).

8

Immune system and malignant disease

▸ Manufacturer advises monitor blood pressure, heart rate, creatine phosphokinase, amylase, and lipase regularly.
▸ Manufacturer advises monitor liver function at baseline, then every 2 weeks during the first 3 months of treatment, and periodically thereafter.
▸ Manufacturer advises monitor fasting serum glucose at baseline and periodically thereafter.

● PATIENT AND CARER ADVICE Manufacturer advises patients and carers should be told to report symptoms of visual disturbance, or unexplained muscle pain, tenderness, or weakness.
Driving and skilled tasks Manufacturer advises patients and carers should be counselled on the effects on driving and performance of skilled tasks—increased risk of visual disturbance, dizziness, or fatigue.

● NATIONAL FUNDING/ACCESS DECISIONS
For full details see funding body website
NICE decisions
▸ Brigatinib for treating ALK-positive advanced non-small-cell lung cancer after crizotinib (March 2019) NICE TA571
Recommended with restrictions
Scottish Medicines Consortium (SMC) decisions
▸ Brigatinib (*Alunbrig*®) as monotherapy for the treatment of adult patients with anaplastic lymphoma kinase positive (ALK+) advanced non-small cell lung cancer (NSCLC) previously treated with crizotinib (June 2019) SMC No. SMC2147
Recommended

● MEDICINAL FORMS There can be variation in the licensing of different medicines containing the same drug.
Tablet
CAUTIONARY AND ADVISORY LABELS 25
▸ Alunbrig (Takeda UK Ltd) ▼
Brigatinib 30 mg Alunbrig 30mg tablets | 28 tablet PoM £1,225.00
Brigatinib 90 mg Alunbrig 90mg tablets | 28 tablet PoM £3,675.00
Brigatinib 180 mg Alunbrig 180mg tablets | 28 tablet PoM £4,900.00

Cabozantinib

04-Sep-2020

● DRUG ACTION Cabozantinib is an inhibitor of several protein kinases.

INDICATIONS AND DOSE

Treatment of progressive, unresectable locally advanced or metastatic medullary thyroid carcinoma (initiated by a specialist)
▸ BY MOUTH USING CAPSULES
▸ Adult: 140 mg once daily, for dose adjustment or treatment interruption due to side-effects, consult product literature (closely monitor for first 8 weeks of therapy)

Advanced renal cell carcinoma (initiated by a specialist)
▸ BY MOUTH USING TABLETS
▸ Adult: 60 mg once daily, for dose adjustment or treatment interruption due to side-effects, consult product literature (closely monitor for first 8 weeks of therapy)

DOSE EQUIVALENCE AND CONVERSION
▸ Cabozantinib tablets and capsules are not bioequivalent—consult product literature when switching formulations.

IMPORTANT SAFETY INFORMATION

MHRA/CHM ADVICE: SYSTEMICALLY ADMINISTERED VEGF PATHWAY INHIBITORS: RISK OF ANEURYSM AND ARTERY DISSECTION (JULY 2020)
A European review of worldwide data concluded that systemically administered VEGF pathway inhibitors may lead to aneurysm and artery dissection in patients with or without hypertension. Some fatal cases have been reported, mainly in relation to aortic aneurysm rupture and aortic dissection. The MHRA advises healthcare professionals to carefully consider the risk of aneurysm and artery dissection in patients with risk factors before initiating treatment with cabozantinib; any modifiable risk factors (such as smoking and hypertension) should be reduced as much as possible. Patients should be monitored and treated for hypertension as required.

RISKS OF INCORRECT DOSING OF ORAL ANTI-CANCER MEDICINES
See Cytotoxic drugs p. 932.

● CONTRA-INDICATIONS Reversible posterior leucoencephalopathy syndrome

● CAUTIONS Hypertension · palmar-plantar erythrodysaesthesia syndrome—consider treatment interruption if severe and restart at a lower dose when resolved to grade 1 · patients at increased risk of fistulas—consult product literature · patients at increased risk of gastro-intestinal perforation—consult product literature · patients at increased risk of intra-abdominal abscess—consult product literature · patients at risk of haemorrhage (including tumour involvement of the trachea or bronchi)—discontinue if symptoms develop · patients at risk of thromboembolic events including myocardial infarction—discontinue if symptoms develop · risk factors for aneurysm or artery dissection · risk of osteonecrosis of the jaw · susceptibility to QT-interval prolongation (e.g. cardiac disease, electrolyte disturbances, bradycardia, concomitant use of drugs that prolong the QT interval)—monitor ECG and electrolytes periodically

CAUTIONS, FURTHER INFORMATION
▸ Elective surgery Withhold treatment for at least 28 days before elective surgery and restart only if adequate wound healing—discontinue in patients with wound healing complications requiring medical intervention.
▸ Risk of osteonecrosis of the jaw Discontinue treatment at least 28 days before elective invasive dental procedures—monitor for symptoms before and during treatment and discontinue if osteonecrosis develops.
▸ Monitoring of blood pressure The MHRA advises to monitor blood pressure regularly—consult product literature if hypertension occurs during treatment.

● INTERACTIONS → Appendix 1: cabozantinib

● SIDE-EFFECTS
▸ **Common or very common** Abscess · alopecia · anxiety · appetite decreased · arrhythmias · arthralgia · asthenia · chills · cholelithiasis · confusion · constipation · dehydration · depression · diarrhoea · dizziness · dysphagia · dysphonia · dysuria · ear pain · electrolyte imbalance · embolism and thrombosis · fistula · gastrointestinal discomfort · gastrointestinal disorders · haemorrhage · hair changes · headache · healing impaired · hyperbilirubinaemia · hypertension · hypoalbuminaemia · hypotension · hypothyroidism · increased risk of infection · lymphopenia · mucositis · muscle spasms · nausea · neutropenia · oedema · oral disorders · oropharyngeal pain · osteonecrosis of jaw · pain · pallor · pancreatitis · paraesthesia · peripheral coldness · peripheral neuropathy · proteinuria · respiratory disorders · skin reactions · stroke · taste altered · thrombocytopenia · tinnitus · tracheo-oesophageal fistula · tremor · vision blurred · vomiting · weight decreased
▸ **Uncommon** Abnormal dreams · acute kidney injury · amenorrhoea · angina pectoris · ataxia · cataract · concentration impaired · conjunctivitis · cyst · delirium · encephalopathy · hearing impairment · loss of consciousness · rhabdomyolysis · skin ulcer · speech disorder · telangiectasia · throat oedema
▸ **Frequency not known** Aneurysm · artery dissection · myocardial infarction

- CONCEPTION AND CONTRACEPTION Patients and their sexual partners must use effective contraception (in addition to barrier method) during treatment and for at least 4 months after the last dose.
- PREGNANCY Manufacturer advises avoid unless potential benefit outweighs risk—toxicity in *animal* studies. See also *Pregnancy and reproductive function* in Cytotoxic drugs p. 932.
- BREAST FEEDING Manufacturer advises discontinue breast-feeding during treatment and for at least 4 months after the last dose.
- HEPATIC IMPAIRMENT For *capsules* manufacturer advises caution in mild to moderate impairment (risk of increased exposure); avoid in severe impairment (no information available). For *tablets* manufacturer advises caution in moderate impairment (limited information available); avoid in severe impairment (no information available). **Dose adjustments** For *capsules* manufacturer advises dose reduction to 60 mg once daily in mild to moderate impairment.
- RENAL IMPAIRMENT Manufacturer advises caution in renal impairment. Avoid in severe impairment.
- MONITORING REQUIREMENTS Monitor urine protein regularly and discontinue if nephrotic syndrome develops.
- PATIENT AND CARER ADVICE Food should not be consumed for at least 2 hours before and at least 1 hour after each dose.
  Driving and skilled tasks Fatigue and weakness may affect performance of skilled tasks e.g. driving.
- NATIONAL FUNDING/ACCESS DECISIONS
  For full details see funding body website
  NICE decisions
  ‣ Cabozantinib for previously treated advanced renal cell carcinoma (August 2017) NICE TA463 Recommended
  ‣ Cabozantinib for untreated advanced renal cell carcinoma (October 2018) NICE TA542 Recommended with restrictions
  ‣ Cabozantinib for treating medullary thyroid cancer (March 2018) NICE TA516 Recommended with restrictions
  Scottish Medicines Consortium (SMC) decisions
  ‣ Cabozantinib (*Cabometyx*®) for the treatment of advanced renal cell carcinoma (RCC) in adults following prior vascular endothelial growth factor (VEGF)-targeted therapy (June 2017) SMC No. 1234/17 Recommended
  ‣ Cabozantinib (*Cabometyx*®) for treatment of advanced renal cell carcinoma (RCC) in treatment-naïve adults with intermediate or poor risk per IMDC criteria (February 2019) SMC No. SMC2136 Not recommended

- MEDICINAL FORMS There can be variation in the licensing of different medicines containing the same drug.

  Tablet
  CAUTIONARY AND ADVISORY LABELS 23, 25
  ‣ Cabometyx (Ipsen Ltd) ▼
  Cabozantinib (as Cabozantinib s-malate) 20 mg Cabometyx 20mg tablets | 30 tablet [PoM] £5,143.00
  Cabozantinib (as Cabozantinib s-malate) 40 mg Cabometyx 40mg tablets | 30 tablet [PoM] £5,143.00
  Cabozantinib (as Cabozantinib s-malate) 60 mg Cabometyx 60mg tablets | 30 tablet [PoM] £5,143.00

  Capsule
  CAUTIONARY AND ADVISORY LABELS 23, 25
  ‣ Cometriq (Ipsen Ltd) ▼
  Cabozantinib (as Cabozantinib s-malate) 20 mg Cometriq 20mg capsules | 84 capsule [PoM] £4,800.00
  Cabozantinib (as Cabozantinib s-malate) 80 mg Cometriq 80mg capsules | 7 capsule [PoM] ⓧ
  Cometriq 20mg capsules and Cometriq 80mg capsules | 56 capsule [PoM] £4,800.00 | 112 capsule [PoM] £4,800.00

Ceritinib
16-Nov-2020

- DRUG ACTION Ceritinib is a tyrosine kinase inhibitor, with particular activity against anaplastic lymphoma kinase (ALK).

- INDICATIONS AND DOSE
  First-line treatment of anaplastic lymphoma kinase (ALK)-positive advanced non-small cell lung cancer (specialist use only) | Anaplastic lymphoma kinase (ALK)-positive advanced non-small cell lung cancer previously treated with crizotinib (specialist use only)
  ▸ BY MOUTH
  ▸ Adult: 450 mg once daily, dose interruption, dose reduction or discontinuation may be required based on individual safety and tolerability—consult product literature; discontinue treatment if patient unable to tolerate at least 150 mg daily
  DOSE ADJUSTMENTS DUE TO INTERACTIONS
  ▸ Manufacturer advises if concurrent use of potent inhibitors of CYP3A4 is unavoidable, reduce the dose by one-third (rounded to the nearest multiple of the 150 mg dosage form).

  IMPORTANT SAFETY INFORMATION
  RISKS OF INCORRECT DOSING OF ORAL ANTI-CANCER MEDICINES
  See Cytotoxic drugs p. 932.

- CONTRA-INDICATIONS Congenital long QT syndrome
- CAUTIONS Diabetes mellitus · history of or susceptibility to QT-interval prolongation
  CAUTIONS, FURTHER INFORMATION
  ▸ QT-interval prolongation QT-interval prolongation has been observed in clinical studies, which may lead to an increased risk for ventricular tachyarrhythmias (e.g. torsade de pointes) or sudden death. Risk factors include pre-existing bradycardia, other relevant pre-existing cardiac disease or electrolyte disturbances; manufacturer advises to monitor ECG and electrolytes periodically.
- INTERACTIONS → Appendix 1: ceritinib
- SIDE-EFFECTS
  ▸ Common or very common Anaemia · appetite decreased · arrhythmias · asthenia · azotaemia · constipation · diarrhoea · dysphagia · gastrointestinal discomfort · gastrooesophageal reflux disease · hepatic disorders · hyperbilirubinaemia · hyperglycaemia · hypophosphataemia · nausea · oesophageal disorder · pericardial effusion · pericarditis · QT interval prolongation · renal impairment · respiratory disorders · skin reactions · vision disorders · vitreous floater · vomiting · weight decreased
  ▸ Uncommon Pancreatitis
  SIDE-EFFECTS, FURTHER INFORMATION **Gastro-intestinal effects** Manufacturer advises monitor for signs of gastro-intestinal toxicity and consider dose reduction or discontinuation of treatment.
  Interstitial lung disease Manufacturer advises monitor patients who exhibit pulmonary symptoms and consider dose reduction or discontinuation of treatment.
- CONCEPTION AND CONTRACEPTION Manufacturer recommends effective contraception in women of childbearing potential during treatment and for up to 3 months after discontinuation of treatment.
- PREGNANCY Manufacturer advises avoid unless essential—no information available. See also *Pregnancy and reproductive function* in Cytotoxic drugs p. 932.
- BREAST FEEDING Manufacturer advises avoid—no information available.

8   Immune system and malignant disease

- HEPATIC IMPAIRMENT Manufacturer advises caution in severe impairment (limited information available).
  Dose adjustments Manufacturer advises reduce dose by approx. 33% in severe impairment (round to the nearest multiple of the 150 mg dosage strength).
- RENAL IMPAIRMENT Manufacturer advises caution in severe impairment—no information available.
- MONITORING REQUIREMENTS
  ‣ Manufacturer advises monitor fasting plasma-glucose concentration, amylase and lipase levels before treatment initiation and periodically thereafter as clinically indicated.
  ‣ Manufacturer advises measure baseline liver function, then monitor every 2 weeks for the first three months of treatment and monthly thereafter; if transaminases are elevated, more frequent monitoring should be performed as clinically indicated.
  ‣ Manufacturer advises monitor for pulmonary symptoms indicative of interstitial lung disease and pneumonitis—discontinue treatment if diagnosis confirmed; also monitor heart rate and blood pressure regularly.
- DIRECTIONS FOR ADMINISTRATION Manufacturer advises *Zykadia*® tablets should be taken with food at the same time each day—consult product literature for dosing information if patients are unable to take tablets with food.
- PATIENT AND CARER ADVICE Patients and carers should be counselled on the administration of tablets.
  Missed doses Manufacturer advises if a patient vomits during a course of treatment or if a dose is more than 12 hours late, the replacement or missed dose should not be taken and the next dose should be taken at the normal time.
  Driving and skilled tasks Manufacturer advises patients and their carers should be counselled on the effects on driving and skilled tasks—increased risk of fatigue and vision disorders.
- NATIONAL FUNDING/ACCESS DECISIONS
  For full details see funding body website
  NICE decisions
  ‣ Ceritinib for previously treated anaplastic lymphoma kinase-positive non-small cell lung cancer (June 2016) NICE TA395 Recommended with restrictions
  ‣ Ceritinib for untreated ALK-positive non-small cell lung cancer (January 2018) NICE TA500 Recommended with restrictions
  Scottish Medicines Consortium (SMC) decisions
  ‣ Ceritinib (*Zykadia*®) for treatment of adult patients with anaplastic lymphoma kinase (ALK)-positive advanced non-small cell lung cancer (NSCLC) previously treated with crizotinib (December 2015) SMC No. 1097/15 Recommended

- MEDICINAL FORMS There can be variation in the licensing of different medicines containing the same drug.
  Tablet
  CAUTIONARY AND ADVISORY LABELS 21, 25
  ‣ Zykadia (Novartis Pharmaceuticals UK Ltd) ▼
  Ceritinib 150 mg Zykadia 150mg tablets | 84 tablet [PoM] £2,757.13

Cobimetinib

11-Feb-2019

- DRUG ACTION Cobimetinib is a mitogen-activated protein kinase (MAPK) inhibitor.
- INDICATIONS AND DOSE
  Treatment of BRAF V600 mutation-positive unresectable or metastatic melanoma (in combination with vemurafenib) (specialist use only)
  ‣ BY MOUTH
  ‣ Adult: 60 mg once daily for 21 days; subsequent cycles repeated after a 7-day interval, for dose adjustment due to side-effects—consult product literature

---

IMPORTANT SAFETY INFORMATION
RISKS OF INCORRECT DOSING OF ORAL ANTI-CANCER MEDICINES
See Cytotoxic drugs p. 932.

- CAUTIONS Left ventricular dysfunction · risk factors for bleeding
- INTERACTIONS → Appendix 1: cobimetinib
- SIDE-EFFECTS
  ‣ **Common or very common** Anaemia · basal cell carcinoma · chills · dehydration · diarrhoea · electrolyte imbalance · fever · haemorrhage · hyperglycaemia · hypertension · nausea · photosensitivity · pneumonitis · retinal detachment · retinopathy · skin reactions · sunburn · vision disorders · vomiting
  ‣ **Uncommon** Rhabdomyolysis
  ‣ **Frequency not known** Intracranial haemorrhage
- CONCEPTION AND CONTRACEPTION Manufacturer advises use of two effective contraceptive methods during treatment and for at least 3 months after stopping treatment.
- PREGNANCY Manufacturer advises avoid unless essential—toxicity in *animal* studies. See also *Pregnancy and reproductive function* in Cytotoxic drugs p. 932.
- BREAST FEEDING Manufacturer advises avoid—no information available.
- HEPATIC IMPAIRMENT Manufacturer advises caution.
- RENAL IMPAIRMENT Manufacturer advises caution in severe impairment—limited information available.
- MONITORING REQUIREMENTS
  ‣ Creatine kinase elevation Manufacturer advises baseline creatine kinase and creatinine levels should be measured before starting treatment, and then at monthly intervals during treatment or as clinically indicated—consult product literature if elevated.
  ‣ Left ventricular function Manufacturer advises ejection fraction should be evaluated before initiation of treatment, then after the first month of treatment and at least every 3 months thereafter (or as clinically indicated) until treatment discontinuation.
  ‣ Liver function Manufacturer advises liver function should be evaluated before initiation of treatment and monthly thereafter (or more frequently as clinically indicated).
  ‣ Visual disturbances Manufacturer advises assess for new or worsening visual disturbances at each visit; if symptoms of new or worsening visual disturbances are identified, an ophthalmologic examination is recommended.
- PATIENT AND CARER ADVICE
  Vomiting Manufacturer advises if vomiting occurs after taking tablets, no additional dose should be taken on that day and the next dose should be taken at the usual time.
  Missed doses Manufacturer advises if a dose is more than 12 hours late, the missed dose should not be taken and the next dose should be taken at the normal time.
  Driving and skilled tasks Manufacturer advises patients should be counselled on the effects on driving and

performance of skilled tasks—increased risk of visual disturbances.

- NATIONAL FUNDING/ACCESS DECISIONS
For full details see funding body website
  NICE decisions
  ▸ **Cobimetinib in combination with vemurafenib for treating unresectable or metastatic BRAF V600 mutation-positive melanoma (October 2016)** NICE TA414 Not recommended

- MEDICINAL FORMS There can be variation in the licensing of different medicines containing the same drug.
  Tablet
  ▸ Cotellic (Roche Products Ltd)
    Cobimetinib (as Cobimetinib hemifumarate) 20 mg Cotellic 20mg tablets | 63 tablet [PoM] £4,275.67

Crizotinib

31-Aug-2020

- DRUG ACTION Crizotinib is a tyrosine kinase inhibitor.

- INDICATIONS AND DOSE
Anaplastic lymphoma kinase (ALK)-positive advanced non-small cell lung cancer (specialist use only) | ROS1-positive advanced non-small cell lung cancer (specialist use only)
  ▸ BY MOUTH
  ▸ Adult: 250 mg twice daily, consult product literature for information on dose adjustments based on individual patient safety and tolerability

---

IMPORTANT SAFETY INFORMATION
RISKS OF INCORRECT DOSING OF ORAL ANTI-CANCER MEDICINES
See Cytotoxic drugs p. 932.

MHRA/CHM ADVICE (NOVEMBER 2015): RISK OF CARDIAC FAILURE
Severe, sometimes fatal cases of cardiac failure have been reported in patients treated with crizotinib. The MHRA has issued the following advice:
- monitor all patients for signs and symptoms of heart failure (including dyspnoea, oedema, or rapid weight gain from fluid retention)
- consider reducing the dose, or interrupting or stopping treatment if symptoms of heart failure occur

---

- CAUTIONS History of diverticulitis (risk of gastro-intestinal perforation—discontinue treatment if gastrointestinal perforation occurs) · metastases of gastrointestinal tract (risk of gastro-intestinal perforation—discontinue treatment if gastrointestinal perforation occurs) · patients with susceptibility to QT-prolongation (including bradycardia, history of cardiac disease, concomitant use of drugs that prolong QT interval, and electrolyte disturbances)—periodic renal monitoring required · risk of gastro-intestinal perforation—discontinue treatment if gastrointestinal perforation occurs · vision disorders reported—consider full ophthalmological evaluation if vision disorder worsens or persists

CAUTIONS, FURTHER INFORMATION
▸ Fatal interstitial lung disease and pneumonitis Fatal interstitial lung disease and pneumonitis reported (monitor patients with pulmonary symptoms, withdraw treatment if suspected, and permanently discontinue treatment if diagnosed).

- INTERACTIONS → Appendix 1: crizotinib

- SIDE-EFFECTS
▸ **Common or very common** Anaemia · appetite decreased · arrhythmias · constipation · diarrhoea · dizziness · fatigue · gait abnormal · gastrointestinal discomfort · gastrointestinal disorders · heart failure · hepatic function abnormal · hypogonadism · hypophosphataemia · leucopenia · local swelling · movement disorders · muscle

atrophy · muscle tone decreased · muscle weakness · nausea · nerve disorders · neuralgia · neurotoxicity · neutropenia · oedema · periorbital oedema · peroneal nerve palsy · pulmonary oedema · QT interval prolongation · renal abscess · renal cyst · respiratory disorders · sensation abnormal · skin reactions · syncope · taste altered · vision disorders · vitreous floater · vomiting
▸ **Uncommon** Gastrointestinal perforation (including fatal cases) · hepatic failure (including fatal cases) · renal impairment

SIDE-EFFECTS, FURTHER INFORMATION Consider reducing the dose, or interrupting or stopping treatment if symptoms of cardiac failure occur.

- CONCEPTION AND CONTRACEPTION Ensure effective contraception during and for at least 90 days after treatment.

- PREGNANCY Avoid (toxicity in *animal* studies). See also *Pregnancy and reproductive function* in Cytotoxic drugs p. 932.

- BREAST FEEDING Avoid—no information available.

- HEPATIC IMPAIRMENT Manufacturer advises use with caution.
  Dose adjustments Manufacturer advises reduce dose in moderate to severe impairment—consult product literature.

- RENAL IMPAIRMENT
  Dose adjustments Reduce dose to 250 mg once daily in severe impairment not requiring peritoneal dialysis or hemodialysis, may be increased to 200 mg twice daily after at least 4 weeks, based on individual assessment of safety and tolerability.

- MONITORING REQUIREMENTS Monitor liver function once a week during the first 2 months of treatment, then at least monthly thereafter and as clinically indicated. Monitor ECG and electrolytes (correct if abnormal) in all patients before starting treatment, then periodically and as clinically indicated thereafter. Monitor for signs and symptoms of treatment emergent bradycardia (including syncope, dizziness and hypotension)—monitor blood pressure and heart rate regularly.

- PATIENT AND CARER ADVICE Counsel all patients on the early signs and symptoms of gastrointestinal perforation—advice to seek immediate medical attention.
  Driving and skilled tasks Symptomatic bradycardia (including syncope, dizziness and hypotension), vision disorder and fatigue may affect performance of skilled tasks (e.g. driving or operating machinery).

- NATIONAL FUNDING/ACCESS DECISIONS
For full details see funding body website
  NICE decisions
  ▸ **Crizotinib for untreated anaplastic lymphoma kinase-positive advanced non-small-cell lung cancer (September 2016)** NICE TA406 Recommended with restrictions
  ▸ **Crizotinib for previously treated anaplastic lymphoma kinase-positive advanced non-small-cell lung cancer (December 2016)** NICE TA422 Recommended with restrictions
  ▸ **Crizotinib for treating ROS1-positive advanced non-small-cell lung cancer (July 2018)** NICE TA529 Recommended with restrictions
  Scottish Medicines Consortium (SMC) decisions
  ▸ **Crizotinib (*Xalkori*®) for treatment of adults with ROS1-positive advanced non-small cell lung cancer (June 2018)** SMC No. 1329/18 Recommended

- MEDICINAL FORMS There can be variation in the licensing of different medicines containing the same drug.
  Capsule
  CAUTIONARY AND ADVISORY LABELS 25
  ▸ Xalkori (Pfizer Ltd)
    Crizotinib 200 mg Xalkori 200mg capsules | 60 capsule [PoM] £4,689.00 (Hospital only)

Crizotinib 250 mg Xalkori 250mg capsules | 60 capsule PoM
£4,689.00 (Hospital only)

Dabrafenib

21-Aug-2020

- DRUG ACTION Dabrafenib is a BRAF kinase inhibitor, which inhibits BRAF V600 mutation-positive melanoma cell growth.

- INDICATIONS AND DOSE

Unresectable or metastatic melanoma with a BRAF V600 mutation (as monotherapy or in combination with trametinib) (specialist use only) | Advanced non-small cell lung cancer with a BRAF V600 mutation (in combination with trametinib) (specialist use only)
  ▶ BY MOUTH
    ▸ Adult: 150 mg every 12 hours, for dose adjustments due to side-effects, consult product literature

Adjuvant treatment of stage III melanoma with a BRAF V600 mutation following complete resection (in combination with trametinib) (specialist use only)
  ▶ BY MOUTH
    ▸ Adult: 150 mg every 12 hours for 12 months, for dose adjustments due to side-effects, consult product literature

> IMPORTANT SAFETY INFORMATION
> RISKS OF INCORRECT DOSING OF ORAL ANTI-CANCER MEDICINES
> See Cytotoxic drugs p. 932.

- CONTRA-INDICATIONS BRAF wild-type melanoma · BRAF wild-type non-small cell lung cancer
- CAUTIONS Elderly (more frequent dose adjustments may be required) · prior or concurrent cancer associated with RAS mutations—risk of secondary or recurrent malignancy
- INTERACTIONS → Appendix 1: dabrafenib
- SIDE-EFFECTS
  ▶ **Common or very common** Alopecia · appetite decreased · arthralgia · asthenia · chills · constipation · cough · diarrhoea · fever · headache · hyperglycaemia · hypophosphataemia · influenza like illness · myalgia · nausea · neoplasms · pain in extremity · photosensitivity reaction · skin reactions · vomiting
  ▶ **Uncommon** Nephritis · pancreatitis · panniculitis · renal impairment · uveitis
  SIDE-EFFECTS, FURTHER INFORMATION Additional side-effects reported when used in combination with trametinib include dizziness, hyperhidrosis, hyponatraemia, hypotension, leucopenia, muscle spasms, myocarditis, neutropenia, night sweats, and thrombocytopenia.
- CONCEPTION AND CONTRACEPTION Manufacturer advises women of child-bearing potential should use effective non-hormonal contraception during and for 4 weeks after stopping treatment.
- PREGNANCY Manufacturer advises avoid unless potential benefit outweighs risk—toxicity in *animal* studies. See also *Pregnancy and reproductive function* in Cytotoxic drugs p. 932.
- BREAST FEEDING Manufacturer advises avoid—no information available.
- HEPATIC IMPAIRMENT Manufacturer advises caution in moderate to severe impairment—no information available.
- RENAL IMPAIRMENT Manufacturer advises caution in severe impairment—no information available.
- MONITORING REQUIREMENTS Manufacturer advises assess for cutaneous squamous cell carcinoma and new primary melanoma before treatment, monthly during treatment, and for 6 months after discontinuation or until initiation of alternative treatment; assess and monitor for non-

cutaneous secondary or recurrent malignancy before, during, and for 6 months after discontinuation or until initiation of alternative treatment—consult product literature; monitor full blood count as clinically indicated; monitor for ophthalmologic reactions including uveitis, iridocyclitis and iritis; monitor serum creatinine.
- PATIENT AND CARER ADVICE Manufacturer advises patients should be informed to immediately report new skin lesions—risk of cutaneous squamous cell carcinoma and new primary melanoma.
  Missed doses Manufacturer advises if a dose is more than 6 hours late, the missed dose should not be taken and the next dose should be taken at the normal time.
  Driving and skilled tasks Manufacturer advises patients and carers should be counselled on the effects on driving and performance of skilled tasks—increased risk of ocular adverse reactions.
- NATIONAL FUNDING/ACCESS DECISIONS
  For full details see funding body website
  NICE decisions
  ▶ Dabrafenib for treating unresectable or metastatic BRAF V600 mutation-positive melanoma (October 2014) NICE TA321 Recommended with restrictions
  ▶ Trametinib in combination with dabrafenib for treating unresectable or metastatic melanoma (June 2016) NICE TA396 Recommended with restrictions
  ▶ Dabrafenib with trametinib for adjuvant treatment of resected BRAF V600 mutation-positive melanoma (October 2018) NICE TA544 Recommended with restrictions
  Scottish Medicines Consortium (SMC) decisions
  ▶ Dabrafenib (*Tafinlar*®) for the monotherapy of adult patients with unresectable or metastatic melanoma with a BRAF V600 mutation (March 2015) SMC No. 1023/15 Recommended with restrictions
  ▶ Dabrafenib (*Tafinlar*®) in combination with trametinib for the adjuvant treatment of adult patients with Stage III melanoma with a BRAF V600 mutation, following complete resection (February 2019) SMC No. SMC2131 Recommended

- MEDICINAL FORMS There can be variation in the licensing of different medicines containing the same drug.
  Capsule
  CAUTIONARY AND ADVISORY LABELS 3, 23, 25
  ▸ Tafinlar (Novartis Pharmaceuticals UK Ltd)
    Dabrafenib (as Dabrafenib mesilate) 50 mg Tafinlar 50mg capsules | 28 capsule PoM £933.33 (Hospital only)
    Dabrafenib (as Dabrafenib mesilate) 75 mg Tafinlar 75mg capsules | 28 capsule PoM £1,400.00 (Hospital only)

Dacomitinib

31-Aug-2020

- DRUG ACTION Dacomitinib is a tyrosine kinase inhibitor that inhibits epidermal growth factor receptor (EGFR).

- INDICATIONS AND DOSE

Non-small cell lung cancer with activating epidermal growth factor receptor (EGFR) mutations (specialist use only)
  ▶ BY MOUTH
    ▸ Adult: 45 mg once daily, for dose adjustments, treatment interruption or discontinuation due to side-effects—consult product literature

- INTERACTIONS → Appendix 1: dacomitinib
- SIDE-EFFECTS
  ▶ **Common or very common** Alopecia · appetite decreased · asthenia · dehydration · diarrhoea · dry eye · dry mouth · eye inflammation · hypertrichosis · hypokalaemia · increased risk of infection · interstitial lung disease (discontinue permanently) · mucositis · nail discolouration · nail disorders · nausea · oral disorders · oropharyngeal

pain · pneumonitis (discontinue permanently) · skin reactions · taste altered · vomiting · weight decreased

- CONCEPTION AND CONTRACEPTION Manufacturer advises females of childbearing potential should use effective contraception during treatment and for at least 17 days after stopping treatment.
- PREGNANCY Manufacturer advises avoid. See also *Pregnancy and reproductive function* in Cytotoxic drugs p. 932.
- BREAST FEEDING Manufacturer advises avoid—no information available.
- HEPATIC IMPAIRMENT Manufacturer advises avoid in severe impairment (no information available).
- RENAL IMPAIRMENT Manufacturer advises caution in severe impairment (no information available).
- MONITORING REQUIREMENTS Manufacturer advises monitor liver function periodically—interrupt treatment if severe changes in liver function occur.
- PATIENT AND CARER ADVICE
  Photosensitivity Manufacturer advises patients should wear protective clothing and apply sunscreen before sun exposure.
  Driving and skilled tasks Manufacturer advises patients and carers should be cautioned on the effects on driving and performance of skilled tasks—increased risk of fatigue and ocular side-effects.
- NATIONAL FUNDING/ACCESS DECISIONS
  For full details see funding body website
  NICE decisions
  ▸ Dacomitinib for untreated EGFR mutation-positive non-small cell lung cancer (August 2019) NICE TA595 Recommended
  Scottish Medicines Consortium (SMC) decisions
  ▸ Dacomitinib (*Vizimpro*®) as monotherapy for the first-line treatment of adult patients with locally advanced or metastatic non-small cell lung cancer (NSCLC) with epidermal growth factor receptor (EGFR)-activating mutations (September 2019) SMC No. SMC2184 Recommended
- MEDICINAL FORMS There can be variation in the licensing of different medicines containing the same drug.
  Tablet
  ▸ Vizimpro (Pfizer Ltd) ▼
    Dacomitinib (as Dacomitinib monohydrate) 15 mg Vizimpro 15mg tablets | 30 tablet [PoM] £2,703.00 (Hospital only)
    Dacomitinib (as Dacomitinib monohydrate) 30 mg Vizimpro 30mg tablets | 30 tablet [PoM] £2,703.00 (Hospital only)
    Dacomitinib (as Dacomitinib monohydrate) 45 mg Vizimpro 45mg tablets | 30 tablet [PoM] £2,703.00 (Hospital only)

Dasatinib
24-Nov-2020

- DRUG ACTION Dasatinib is a tyrosine kinase inhibitor.

- INDICATIONS AND DOSE

Chronic phase chronic myeloid leukaemia (initiated by a specialist)
▸ BY MOUTH USING TABLETS
▸ Adult: 100 mg once daily, then increased if necessary up to 140 mg once daily, for dose adjustment due to side-effects—consult product literature
▸ BY MOUTH USING ORAL SUSPENSION
▸ Adult (body-weight 30-44 kg): 105 mg once daily, adjust dose based on changes in body-weight every 3 months or more often if necessary; for dose escalation, or dose adjustment due to side-effects—consult product literature
▸ Adult (body-weight 45 kg and above): 120 mg once daily, adjust dose based on changes in body-weight every 3 months or more often if necessary; for dose

escalation, or dose adjustment due to side-effects—consult product literature

Accelerated and blast phase chronic myeloid leukaemia [resistant or intolerant to prior therapy] (initiated by a specialist) | Acute lymphoblastic leukaemia [resistant or intolerant to prior therapy] (initiated by a specialist)
▸ BY MOUTH USING TABLETS
▸ Adult: 140 mg once daily, then increased if necessary up to 180 mg once daily, for dose adjustment due to side-effects—consult product literature

DOSE EQUIVALENCE AND CONVERSION
▸ *Sprycel*® film-coated tablets and *Sprycel*® powder for oral suspension are **not** bioequivalent. Follow correct dosing recommendations for the dosage form when switching formulations.

> IMPORTANT SAFETY INFORMATION
> RISKS OF INCORRECT DOSING OF ORAL ANTI-CANCER MEDICINES See Cytotoxic drugs p. 932.
> MHRA/CHM ADVICE (MAY 2016): RISK OF HEPATITIS B VIRUS REACTIVATION WITH BCR-ABL TYROSINE KINASE INHIBITORS
> An EU wide review has concluded that dasatinib can cause hepatitis B reactivation; the MHRA recommends establishing hepatitis B virus status in all patients before initiation of treatment.

- CAUTIONS Hepatitis B infection · risk of cardiac dysfunction (monitor closely) · susceptibility to QT-interval prolongation (correct hypokalaemia or hypomagnesaemia before starting treatment)
  CAUTIONS, FURTHER INFORMATION
  ▸ Hepatitis B infection The MHRA advises that patients who are carriers of hepatitis B virus should be closely monitored for signs and symptoms of active infection throughout treatment and for several months after stopping treatment; expert advice should be sought for patients who test positive for hepatitis B virus and in those with active infection.
- INTERACTIONS → Appendix 1: dasatinib
- SIDE-EFFECTS
  ▸ **Common or very common** Alopecia · anaemia · appetite abnormal · arrhythmias · arthralgia · asthenia · bone marrow depression · cardiac disorder · cardiomyopathy · chest pain · chills · constipation · cough · depression · diarrhoea · dizziness · drowsiness · dry eye · dyspnoea · eye inflammation · facial swelling · fever · fluid imbalance · flushing · gastrointestinal discomfort · gastrointestinal disorders · genital abnormalities · haemorrhage · headache · heart failure · hypertension · hyperuricaemia · increased risk of infection · insomnia · milia · mucositis · muscle complaints · muscle weakness · musculoskeletal stiffness · myocardial dysfunction · nausea · nerve disorders · neutropenia · oedema · oral disorders · pain · palpitations · pericardial effusion · perinephric effusion · peripheral swelling · pulmonary hypertension · pulmonary oedema · respiratory disorders · sepsis · skin reactions · sweat changes · taste altered · thrombocytopenia · tinnitus · vision disorders · vomiting · weight changes
  ▸ **Uncommon** Acute coronary syndrome · anxiety · arthritis · ascites · asthma · cardiac inflammation · cardiomegaly · cerebrovascular insufficiency · cholecystitis · CNS haemorrhage · confusion · dysphagia · embolism and thrombosis · emotional lability · excessive tearing · gynaecomastia · hair disorder · hearing loss · hepatic disorders · hypercholesterolaemia · hypoalbuminaemia · hypotension · hypothyroidism · ischaemic heart disease · libido decreased · lymphadenopathy · lymphopenia · malaise · memory loss · menstrual disorder · movement disorders · myopathy · nail disorder · osteonecrosis · pancreatitis · panniculitis · penile disorders · photosensitivity reaction · proteinuria · QT interval

prolongation · renal impairment · scrotal oedema · skin ulcer · syncope · tendinitis · testicular swelling · tremor · tumour lysis syndrome · urinary frequency increased · vertigo · vulvovaginal swelling
▶ **Rare or very rare** Cardiac arrest · dementia · diabetes mellitus · epiphyses delayed fusion · facial paralysis · gait abnormal · growth retardation · hypersensitivity vasculitis · hyperthyroidism · pure red cell aplasia · seizure · thyroiditis
▶ **Frequency not known** Hepatitis B reactivation · nephrotic syndrome · Stevens-Johnson syndrome · thrombotic microangiopathy

● CONCEPTION AND CONTRACEPTION Effective contraception required during treatment.
● PREGNANCY Manufacturer advises avoid unless potential benefit outweighs risk—toxicity in *animal* studies. See also *Pregnancy and reproductive function* in Cytotoxic drugs p. 932.
● BREAST FEEDING Discontinue breast-feeding.
● HEPATIC IMPAIRMENT Manufacturer advises caution.
● MONITORING REQUIREMENTS
▶ Manufacturer advises evaluate for signs and symptoms of underlying cardiopulmonary disease before initiation of therapy—echocardiography should be performed at treatment initiation in patients with symptoms of cardiac disease and considered for patients with risk factors for cardiac or pulmonary disease.
▶ Manufacturer advises monitor patients with risk factors or a history of cardiac disease for signs or symptoms of cardiac dysfunction during treatment.
▶ When used for Accelerated or blast phase chronic myeloid leukaemia or Acute lymphoblastic leukaemia Manufacturer advises monitor full blood count weekly for the first 2 months, then monthly or as clinically indicated thereafter.
▶ When used for Chronic phase chronic myeloid leukaemia Manufacturer advises monitor full blood count every 2 weeks for 3 months, then every 3 months or as clinically indicated thereafter.
● NATIONAL FUNDING/ACCESS DECISIONS
For full details see funding body website
NICE decisions
▶ **Dasatinib, nilotinib and imatinib for untreated chronic myeloid leukaemia (CML) (December 2016)** NICE TA426 Recommended with restrictions
▶ **Dasatinib, nilotinib and high-dose imatinib for treating imatinib-resistant or intolerant chronic myeloid leukaemia (CML) (December 2016)** NICE TA425 Recommended with restrictions
Scottish Medicines Consortium (SMC) decisions
▶ Dasatinib (*Sprycel*®) tablets for the treatment of adult patients with chronic, accelerated or blast phase chronic myelogenous leukaemia (CML) with resistance or intolerance to prior therapy including imatinib mesilate (September 2016) SMC No. 370/07 Recommended
▶ Dasatinib (*Sprycel*®) tablets for the treatment of adult patients with newly diagnosed Philadelphia chromosome positive (Ph+) chronic myelogenous leukaemia (CML) in the chronic phase (September 2016) SMC No. 1170/16 Recommended

● MEDICINAL FORMS There can be variation in the licensing of different medicines containing the same drug.
Oral suspension
EXCIPIENTS: May contain Benzyl alcohol, sucrose
▶ Sprycel (Bristol-Myers Squibb Pharmaceuticals Ltd)
Dasatinib (as Dasatinib monohydrate) 10 mg per 1 ml Sprycel 10mg/ml oral suspension | 99 ml [PoM] £626.74
Tablet
CAUTIONARY AND ADVISORY LABELS 25
▶ Dasatinib (Non-proprietary)
Dasatinib (as Dasatinib monohydrate) 20 mg Dasatinib 20mg tablets | 60 tablet [PoM] £650.00 DT = £1,252.48

Dasatinib (as Dasatinib monohydrate) 50 mg Dasatinib 50mg tablets | 60 tablet [PoM] £1,200.00 DT = £2,504.96
Dasatinib (as Dasatinib monohydrate) 80 mg Dasatinib 80mg tablets | 30 tablet [PoM] £1,200.00 DT = £2,504.96
Dasatinib (as Dasatinib monohydrate) 100 mg Dasatinib 100mg tablets | 30 tablet [PoM] £1,200.00 DT = £2,504.96
Dasatinib (as Dasatinib monohydrate) 140 mg Dasatinib 140mg tablets | 30 tablet [PoM] £1,200.00 DT = £2,504.96
▶ Sprycel (Bristol-Myers Squibb Pharmaceuticals Ltd)
Dasatinib (as Dasatinib monohydrate) 20 mg Sprycel 20mg tablets | 60 tablet [PoM] £1,252.48 DT = £1,252.48
Dasatinib (as Dasatinib monohydrate) 50 mg Sprycel 50mg tablets | 60 tablet [PoM] £2,504.96 DT = £2,504.96
Dasatinib (as Dasatinib monohydrate) 80 mg Sprycel 80mg tablets | 30 tablet [PoM] £2,504.96 DT = £2,504.96
Dasatinib (as Dasatinib monohydrate) 100 mg Sprycel 100mg tablets | 30 tablet [PoM] £2,504.96 DT = £2,504.96
Dasatinib (as Dasatinib monohydrate) 140 mg Sprycel 140mg tablets | 30 tablet [PoM] £2,504.96 DT = £2,504.96

Encorafenib

05-Nov-2020

● DRUG ACTION Encorafenib inhibits the mitogen-activated protein kinase (MAPK) pathway, specifically BRAF kinase, thereby inhibiting BRAF V600 mutation-positive cell growth.

● INDICATIONS AND DOSE
Unresectable or metastatic melanoma with a BRAF V600 mutation (in combination with binimetinib) (specialist use only)
▶ BY MOUTH
▶ Adult: 450 mg once daily, for dose adjustments due to side-effects, consult product literature

---
IMPORTANT SAFETY INFORMATION
RISKS OF INCORRECT DOSING OF ORAL ANTI-CANCER MEDICINES
See Cytotoxic drugs p. 932.

● CONTRA-INDICATIONS BRAF wild-type malignant melanoma
● CAUTIONS Prior or concurrent cancer associated with RAS mutation · risk factors for QT-interval prolongation
● INTERACTIONS → Appendix 1: encorafenib
● SIDE-EFFECTS
▶ **Common or very common** Alopecia · anaemia · angioedema · appetite decreased · arrhythmias · arthralgia · arthritis · constipation · detachment of retinal pigment epithelium · diarrhoea · dizziness · embolism and thrombosis · eye inflammation · facial paralysis · fatigue · fever · fluid retention · gastrointestinal discomfort · gastrointestinal disorders · haemorrhage · headache · heart failure · hypersensitivity · hypersensitivity vasculitis · hypertension · insomnia · intracranial haemorrhage · left ventricular dysfunction · lip squamous cell carcinoma · muscle complaints · muscle weakness · myopathy · nausea · neoplasms · nerve disorders · oedema · pain · panniculitis · paresis · photosensitivity reaction · renal impairment · skin reactions · taste altered · ulcerative colitis · vision disorders · vomiting
▶ **Uncommon** Pancreatitis
▶ **Frequency not known** QT interval prolongation
● CONCEPTION AND CONTRACEPTION Manufacturer advises women of child-bearing potential should use effective contraception during and for at least one month after stopping treatment; additional barrier method recommended in women using hormonal contraceptives.
● PREGNANCY Manufacturer advises avoid—toxicity in *animal* studies. See also *Pregnancy and reproductive function* in Cytotoxic drugs p. 932.
● BREAST FEEDING Manufacturer advises avoid—no information available.

HEPATIC IMPAIRMENT Manufacturer advises caution in mild impairment (increased exposure); avoid in moderate or severe impairment (no information available).
Dose adjustments Manufacturer advises dose reduction to 300 mg once daily in mild impairment.

RENAL IMPAIRMENT Manufacturer advises caution in severe impairment (no information available).

● MONITORING REQUIREMENTS
▶ Manufacturer advises assess for cutaneous squamous cell carcinoma and new primary melanoma before treatment, every 2 months during treatment, and for up to 6 months after discontinuation; assess for non-cutaneous malignancy and monitor full blood count before, during, and after treatment discontinuation as clinically indicated—consult product literature.
▶ Manufacturer advises monitor liver function before treatment, at least monthly during the first 6 months, and thereafter as clinically indicated.
▶ Manufacturer advises assess ECG before treatment, one month after starting treatment, then every 3 months or more frequently as clinically indicated.
▶ Manufacturer advises monitor blood creatinine levels as clinically indicated.
▶ Manufacturer advises monitor for ophthalmologic reactions including uveitis, iridocyclitis, and iritis.

● PATIENT AND CARER ADVICE Manufacturer advises patients should be informed to immediately report new skin lesions—risk of cutaneous squamous cell carcinoma and new primary melanoma.
Missed doses Manufacturer advises if a dose is more than 12 hours late, the missed dose should not be taken and the next dose should be taken at the normal time.
Driving and skilled tasks Manufacturer advises patients and carers should be counselled on the effects on driving and performance of skilled tasks—increased risk of visual disturbances.

● NATIONAL FUNDING/ACCESS DECISIONS
For full details see funding body website

NICE decisions
▶ **Encorafenib with binimetinib for unresectable or metastatic BRAF V600 mutation-positive melanoma (February 2019)** NICE TA562 Recommended with restrictions

Scottish Medicines Consortium (SMC) decisions
▶ **Encorafenib (Braftovi®) in combination with binimetinib for the treatment of adult patients with unresectable or metastatic melanoma with a BRAF V600 mutation (February 2020)** SMC No. SMC2238 Recommended

● MEDICINAL FORMS There can be variation in the licensing of different medicines containing the same drug.

Capsule
CAUTIONARY AND ADVISORY LABELS 3, 25
▶ Braftovi (Pierre Fabre Ltd) ▼
Encorafenib 50 mg Braftovi 50mg capsules | 28 capsule [PoM] £622.22 (Hospital only)
Encorafenib 75 mg Braftovi 75mg capsules | 42 capsule [PoM] £1,400.00 (Hospital only)

Entrectinib
25-Sep-2020

● DRUG ACTION Entrectinib is a tropomyosin receptor kinase inhibitor.

● INDICATIONS AND DOSE
Solid tumours with neurotrophic tyrosine receptor kinase gene fusion (initiated by a specialist)
▶ BY MOUTH
▶ Adult: 600 mg once daily, for dose adjustments, treatment interruption, or discontinuation due to side-effects—consult product literature

ROS1-positive advanced non-small cell lung cancer (initiated by a specialist)
▶ BY MOUTH
▶ Adult: 600 mg once daily, for dose adjustments, treatment interruption, or discontinuation due to side-effects—consult product literature

DOSE ADJUSTMENTS DUE TO INTERACTIONS
▶ Manufacturer advises if concomitant use with potent CYP3A4 inhibitors is unavoidable, reduce entrectinib dose to 100 mg once daily; if concomitant use with moderate CYP3A4 inhibitors is unavoidable, reduce entrectinib dose to 200 mg once daily.

● CONTRA-INDICATIONS Congenital long QT syndrome

● CAUTIONS Susceptibility to QT-interval prolongation · symptoms or risk factors for congestive heart failure (assess left ventricular ejection fraction before initiation)

CAUTIONS, FURTHER INFORMATION
▶ QT-interval prolongation QT-interval prolongation has been observed in clinical studies. Manufacturer advises avoid in patients with pre-existing risk factors; if potential benefit outweighs risk in this patient group, additional monitoring should be considered. Monitor ECG and electrolytes in **all** patients before treatment, after 1 month, and periodically as clinically indicated (treatment not recommended if QT interval greater than 450 milliseconds at baseline)—consult product literature if QT-interval prolongation occurs during treatment.

● INTERACTIONS → Appendix 1: entrectinib

● SIDE-EFFECTS
▶ **Common or very common** Abdominal pain · anaemia · anxiety · appetite decreased · arthralgia · asthenia · bone fractures · cognitive disorder · concentration impaired · confusion · constipation · cough · delirium · depression · diarrhoea · dizziness · drowsiness · dysphagia · dyspnoea · fever · fluid imbalance · gait abnormal · hallucinations · headache · heart failure · hyperuricaemia · hypotension · increased risk of infection · memory impairment · mood altered · movement disorders · muscle weakness · myalgia · nausea · neutropenia · oedema · pain · peripheral neuropathy · peripheral swelling · photosensitivity reaction · pleural effusion · psychiatric disorders · pulmonary oedema · QT interval prolongation · sensation abnormal · skin reactions · sleep disorders · syncope · taste altered · urinary disorders · vertigo · vision disorders · vomiting · weight increased
▶ **Uncommon** Tumour lysis syndrome

● CONCEPTION AND CONTRACEPTION Manufacturer advises females of childbearing potential should use effective contraception during treatment and for 5 weeks after last treatment; male patients should use effective contraception during treatment and for 3 months after last treatment if their partner is of childbearing potential. Additional barrier method recommended in females using hormonal contraceptives. See also *Pregnancy and reproductive function* in Cytotoxic drugs p. 932.

● PREGNANCY Manufacturer advises avoid—limited information available. See also *Pregnancy and reproductive function* in Cytotoxic drugs p. 932.

● BREAST FEEDING Manufacturer advises avoid—no information available.

● PATIENT AND CARER ADVICE
Missed doses Manufacturer advises if a dose is more than 12 hours late, the missed dose should not be taken and the next dose should be taken at the normal time. If vomiting occurs immediately after a dose is taken, patients may repeat the dose.
Driving and skilled tasks Manufacturer advises patients and carers should be counselled on the effects on driving and

8

Immune system and malignant disease

performance of skilled tasks—increased risk of cognitive disorders, syncope, blurred vision, or dizziness.

● NATIONAL FUNDING/ACCESS DECISIONS
For full details see funding body website

NICE decisions
▶ **Entrectinib for treating ROS1-positive advanced non-small-cell lung cancer (August 2020)** NICE TA643 Recommended
▶ **Entrectinib for treating NTRK fusion-positive solid tumours (August 2020)** NICE TA644 Recommended

● MEDICINAL FORMS There can be variation in the licensing of different medicines containing the same drug.

Capsule
CAUTIONARY AND ADVISORY LABELS 25
▶ Rozlytrek (Roche Products Ltd) ▼
    Entrectinib 100 mg Rozlytrek 100mg capsules | 30 capsule [PoM] £860.00 (Hospital only)
    Entrectinib 200 mg Rozlytrek 200mg capsules | 90 capsule [PoM] £5,160.00 (Hospital only)

Erlotinib

26-Nov-2020

● DRUG ACTION Erlotinib is a tyrosine kinase inhibitor.

● **INDICATIONS AND DOSE**

Treatment of locally advanced or metastatic non-small cell lung cancer after failure of previous chemotherapy | Monotherapy for maintenance treatment of locally advanced or metastatic non-small cell lung cancer with stable disease after four cycles of platinum-based chemotherapy
▶ BY MOUTH
▶ Adult: 150 mg once daily

Treatment of metastatic pancreatic cancer (in combination with gemcitabine)
▶ BY MOUTH
▶ Adult: 100 mg once daily

DOSE ADJUSTMENTS DUE TO INTERACTIONS
▶ Manufacturer advises if concurrent use of potent inducers of CYP3A4 is unavoidable, increase dose to 300 mg daily, if well tolerated for more than 2 weeks, further increase to 450 mg daily could be considered with close monitoring.

IMPORTANT SAFETY INFORMATION

MHRA/CHM ADVICE: EPIDERMAL GROWTH FACTOR RECEPTOR (EGFR) INHIBITORS: SERIOUS CASES OF KERATITIS AND ULCERATIVE KERATITIS (MAY 2012)

Keratitis and ulcerative keratitis have been reported following treatment with epidermal growth factor receptor (EGFR) inhibitors for cancer (cetuximab, erlotinib, gefitinib and panitumumab). In rare cases, this has resulted in corneal perforation and blindness. Patients undergoing treatment with EGFR inhibitors who present with acute or worsening signs and symptoms suggestive of keratitis should be referred promptly to an ophthalmology specialist. Treatment should be interrupted or discontinued if ulcerative keratitis is diagnosed.

RISKS OF INCORRECT DOSING OF ORAL ANTI-CANCER MEDICINES
See Cytotoxic drugs p. 932.

● CAUTIONS
▶ Smoking Dose adjustment may be necessary if smoking started or stopped during treatment.

● INTERACTIONS → Appendix 1: erlotinib

● SIDE-EFFECTS
▶ **Common or very common** Alopecia · diarrhoea · eye inflammation · haemorrhage · increased risk of infection · renal failure · skin reactions

▶ **Uncommon** Brittle nails · eye disorders · gastrointestinal disorders · hair changes · interstitial lung disease · nephritis · proteinuria
▶ **Rare or very rare** Hepatic failure · severe cutaneous adverse reactions (SCARs)
▶ **Frequency not known** Appetite decreased · chills · cough · depression · dyspnoea · fatigue · fever · gastrointestinal discomfort · headache · nausea · neuropathy sensory · stomatitis · vomiting · weight decreased

● CONCEPTION AND CONTRACEPTION Effective contraception required during and for at least 2 weeks after treatment.

● PREGNANCY Manufacturer advises avoid—toxicity in *animal* studies. See also *Pregnancy and reproductive function* in Cytotoxic drugs p. 932.

● BREAST FEEDING Manufacturer advises avoid breast-feeding during treatment and for at least 2 weeks after the last dose.

● HEPATIC IMPAIRMENT Manufacturer advises caution in mild to moderate impairment—monitor liver function and interrupt treatment if changes in liver function are severe (increased risk of hepatic failure); avoid in severe impairment—no information available.
Dose adjustments Manufacturer advises consider dose reduction or interruption if serious adverse effects occur.

● RENAL IMPAIRMENT Manufacturer advises avoid in severe impairment.

● NATIONAL FUNDING/ACCESS DECISIONS
For full details see funding body website

NICE decisions
▶ **Erlotinib monotherapy for maintenance treatment of non-small-cell lung cancer (June 2011)** NICE TA227 Not recommended
▶ **Erlotinib for the first-line treatment of locally advanced or metastatic EGFR mutation-positive non-small-cell lung cancer (June 2012)** NICE TA258 Recommended with restrictions
▶ **Erlotinib and gefitinib for treating non-small-cell lung cancer that has progressed after prior chemotherapy [in patients with tumours that are EGFR-TK mutation-negative] (December 2015)** NICE TA374 Not recommended
▶ **Erlotinib and gefitinib for treating non-small-cell lung cancer that has progressed after prior chemotherapy [in patients with tumours of unknown EGFR-TK mutation status] (December 2015)** NICE TA374 Recommended with restrictions

● MEDICINAL FORMS There can be variation in the licensing of different medicines containing the same drug.

Tablet
CAUTIONARY AND ADVISORY LABELS 23
▶ Erlotinib (Non-proprietary)
    Erlotinib (as Erlotinib hydrochloride) 25 mg Erlotinib 25mg tablets | 30 tablet [PoM] £169.50–£378.33 | 30 tablet [PoM] £139.00–£378.33 (Hospital only)
    Erlotinib (as Erlotinib hydrochloride) 100 mg Erlotinib 100mg tablets | 30 tablet [PoM] £704.00–£1,324.24 | 30 tablet [PoM] £378.33–£704.00 (Hospital only)
    Erlotinib (as Erlotinib hydrochloride) 150 mg Erlotinib 150mg tablets | 30 tablet [PoM] £815.00–£1,631.59 | 30 tablet [PoM] £378.33–£815.00 (Hospital only)
▶ Tarceva (Roche Products Ltd)
    Erlotinib (as Erlotinib hydrochloride) 25 mg Tarceva 25mg tablets | 30 tablet [PoM] £378.33
    Erlotinib (as Erlotinib hydrochloride) 100 mg Tarceva 100mg tablets | 30 tablet [PoM] £1,324.14
    Erlotinib (as Erlotinib hydrochloride) 150 mg Tarceva 150mg tablets | 30 tablet [PoM] £1,631.53

Everolimus

20-Nov-2020

● DRUG ACTION Everolimus is a protein kinase inhibitor.

● INDICATIONS AND DOSE

**Neuroendocrine tumours of pancreatic origin |
Neuroendocrine tumours of gastro-intestinal origin**
▸ BY MOUTH
▸ Adult: 10 mg once daily, for dose interruption or
adjustments due to side effects—consult product
literature

AFINITOR ®

**Neuroendocrine tumours of pancreatic origin |
Neuroendocrine tumours of lung origin | Neuroendocrine
tumours of gastro-intestinal origin | Renal cell carcinoma
| Hormone-receptor positive HER2-negative breast
cancer [in combination with exemestane]**
▸ BY MOUTH
▸ Adult: 10 mg once daily, for dose interruption or
adjustments due to side-effects—consult product
literature

CERTICAN ®

Liver transplantation
▸ BY MOUTH
▸ Adult: Initially 1 mg twice daily, to be started
approximately 4 weeks after transplantation;
maintenance, dose adjusted according to response and
whole blood everolimus concentration; dose
adjustments can be made every 4–5 days

Renal transplantation | Heart transplantation
▸ BY MOUTH
▸ Adult: Initially 750 micrograms twice daily, to be
started as soon as possible after transplantation;
maintenance, dose adjusted according to response and
whole blood everolimus concentration; dose
adjustments can be made every 4–5 days

VOTUBIA ® DISPERSIBLE TABLETS

**Subependymal giant cell astrocytoma associated with
tuberous sclerosis complex**
▸ BY MOUTH USING DISPERSIBLE TABLETS
▸ Adult: (consult product literature)

**Adjunctive treatment of refractory partial-onset seizures,
with or without secondary generalisation, associated
with tuberous sclerosis complex**
▸ BY MOUTH USING DISPERSIBLE TABLETS
▸ Adult: (consult product literature)

VOTUBIA ® TABLETS

**Subependymal giant cell astrocytoma associated with
tuberous sclerosis complex**
▸ BY MOUTH USING TABLETS
▸ Adult: (consult product literature)

**Renal angiomyolipoma associated with tuberous sclerosis
complex**
▸ BY MOUTH USING TABLETS
▸ Adult: (consult product literature)

IMPORTANT SAFETY INFORMATION

RISKS OF INCORRECT DOSING OF ORAL ANTI-CANCER MEDICINES
See Cytotoxic drugs p. 932.

MHRA/CHM ADVICE: ANTIEPILEPTICS: RISK OF SUICIDAL
THOUGHTS AND BEHAVIOUR (AUGUST 2008)
See Epilepsy p. 321.

MHRA/CHM ADVICE: ANTIEPILEPTIC DRUGS: UPDATED ADVICE ON
SWITCHING BETWEEN DIFFERENT MANUFACTURERS' PRODUCTS
(NOVEMBER 2017)
See Epilepsy p. 321 and see also *Prescribing and
dispensing information.*

● CAUTIONS History of bleeding disorders · peri-surgical
period (impaired wound healing)
● INTERACTIONS → Appendix 1: everolimus
● SIDE-EFFECTS
▸ **Common or very common** Alopecia · anaemia · appetite
decreased · arthralgia · asthenia · cough · decreased
leucocytes · dehydration · diabetes mellitus · diarrhoea · dry
mouth · dyslipidaemia · dysphagia · dyspnoea · electrolyte
imbalance · eye inflammation · fever · gastrointestinal
discomfort · haemorrhage · headache · hyperglycaemia ·
hypertension · increased risk of infection · insomnia ·
menstrual cycle irregularities · mucositis · nail disorders ·
nausea · neutropenia · oral disorders · peripheral oedema ·
proteinuria · renal impairment · respiratory disorders · skin
reactions · taste altered · thrombocytopenia · vomiting ·
weight decreased
▸ **Uncommon** Congestive heart failure · embolism and
thrombosis · flushing · healing impaired · hepatitis B ·
musculoskeletal chest pain · pancytopenia · sepsis · urinary
frequency increased
▸ **Rare or very rare** Pure red cell aplasia
▸ **Frequency not known** Hepatitis B reactivation · suicidal
behaviours
SIDE-EFFECTS, FURTHER INFORMATION Reduce dose or
discontinue if severe side-effects occur—consult product
literature.
● CONCEPTION AND CONTRACEPTION Effective
contraception must be used during and for up to 8 weeks
after treatment.
● PREGNANCY Manufacturer advises avoid (toxicity in
animal studies). See also *Pregnancy and reproductive
function* in Cytotoxic drugs p. 932.
● BREAST FEEDING Manufacturer advises avoid.
● HEPATIC IMPAIRMENT Consult product literature.
● MONITORING REQUIREMENTS
▸ For *Votubia*® preparations: manufacturer advises
everolimus blood concentration monitoring is required—
consult product literature.
▸ For *Certican*®: manufacturer advises pre-dose ('trough')
whole blood everolimus concentration should be
3–8 nanograms/mL; monitoring should be performed
every 4–5 days (using **chromatographic** assay) after
initiation or dose adjustment until 2 consecutive stable
concentrations; monitor patients with hepatic impairment
taking concomitant strong CYP3A4 inducers and
inhibitors when switching formulation, and/or if
concomitant ciclosporin dose is reduced.
▸ Manufacturer advises monitor blood-glucose
concentration, complete blood count, serum-triglycerides
and serum-cholesterol before treatment and periodically
thereafter.
▸ Manufacturer advises monitor renal function before
treatment and periodically thereafter.
▸ Manufacturer advises monitor for signs and symptoms of
infection before and during treatment.
● DIRECTIONS FOR ADMINISTRATION
VOTUBIA ® DISPERSIBLE TABLETS Manufacturer advises
tablets must be dispersed in water before administration—
consult product literature for details.
VOTUBIA ® TABLETS Manufacturer advises tablets may be
dispersed in approximately 30 mL of water by gently
stirring, immediately before drinking. After solution has
been swallowed, any residue must be re-dispersed in the
same volume of water and swallowed.
● PRESCRIBING AND DISPENSING INFORMATION *Votubia*® is
available as both *tablets* and *dispersible tablets*. These
formulations vary in their licensed indications and are not
interchangeable—consult product literature for
information on switching between formulations.

- **PATIENT AND CARER ADVICE**
  Pneumonitis Non-infectious pneumonitis reported. Manufacturer advises patients and their carers should be informed to seek urgent medical advice if new or worsening respiratory symptoms occur.
  Infections Manufacturer advises patients and their carers should be informed of the risk of infection.
- **NATIONAL FUNDING/ACCESS DECISIONS**
  For full details see funding body website
  NICE decisions
  ▸ Everolimus with exemestane for treating advanced breast cancer after endocrine therapy (December 2016) NICE TA421 Recommended with restrictions
  ▸ Everolimus for advanced renal cell carcinoma after previous treatment (February 2017) NICE TA432 Recommended with restrictions
  ▸ Everolimus and sunitinib for treating unresectable or metastatic neuroendocrine tumours in people with progressive disease (June 2017) NICE TA449 Recommended with restrictions
  VOTUBIA ® DISPERSIBLE TABLETS For full details see funding body website
  Scottish Medicines Consortium (SMC) decisions
  ▸ Everolimus dispersible tablets (*Votubia* ®) for the adjunctive treatment of patients aged 2 years and older whose refractory partial-onset seizures, with or without secondary generalisation, are associated with tuberous sclerosis complex (June 2018) SMC No. 1331/18 Recommended
  AFINITOR ® For full details see funding body website
  NICE decisions
  ▸ Lenvatinib with everolimus for previously treated advanced renal cell carcinoma (January 2018) NICE TA498 Recommended with restrictions
  CERTICAN ® For full details see funding body website
  NICE decisions
  ▸ Everolimus for preventing organ rejection in liver transplantation (July 2015) NICE TA348 Not recommended
  ▸ Immunosuppressive therapy for kidney transplant in adults (October 2017) NICE TA481 Not recommended

- **MEDICINAL FORMS** There can be variation in the licensing of different medicines containing the same drug.
  Dispersible tablet
  CAUTIONARY AND ADVISORY LABELS 13
  ▸ Votubia (Novartis Pharmaceuticals UK Ltd)
  Everolimus 2 mg Votubia 2mg dispersible tablets sugar-free | 30 tablet [PoM] £960.00
  Everolimus 3 mg Votubia 3mg dispersible tablets sugar-free | 30 tablet [PoM] £1,440.00
  Everolimus 5 mg Votubia 5mg dispersible tablets sugar-free | 30 tablet [PoM] £2,250.00
  Tablet
  CAUTIONARY AND ADVISORY LABELS 25
  ▸ Everolimus (Non-proprietary)
  Everolimus 2.5 mg Everolimus 2.5mg tablets | 30 tablet [PoM] £1,150.00
  Everolimus 5 mg Everolimus 5mg tablets | 30 tablet [PoM] £2,200.00
  Everolimus 10 mg Everolimus 10mg tablets | 30 tablet [PoM] £2,920.00
  ▸ Afinitor (Novartis Pharmaceuticals UK Ltd)
  Everolimus 2.5 mg Afinitor 2.5mg tablets | 30 tablet [PoM] £1,200.00
  Everolimus 5 mg Afinitor 5mg tablets | 30 tablet [PoM] £2,250.00
  Everolimus 10 mg Afinitor 10mg tablets | 30 tablet [PoM] £2,673.00
  ▸ Certican (Novartis Pharmaceuticals UK Ltd)
  Everolimus 250 microgram Certican 0.25mg tablets | 60 tablet [PoM] £148.50
  Everolimus 750 microgram Certican 0.75mg tablets | 60 tablet [PoM] £445.20
  ▸ Votubia (Novartis Pharmaceuticals UK Ltd)
  Everolimus 2.5 mg Votubia 2.5mg tablets | 30 tablet [PoM] £1,200.00
  Everolimus 5 mg Votubia 5mg tablets | 30 tablet [PoM] £2,250.00

Everolimus 10 mg Votubia 10mg tablets | 30 tablet [PoM] £2,970.00

Gefitinib

06-Nov-2020

- **DRUG ACTION** Gefitinib is a tyrosine kinase inhibitor.

- **INDICATIONS AND DOSE**
  Treatment of locally advanced or metastatic non-small cell lung cancer with activating mutations of epidermal growth factor receptor
  ▸ BY MOUTH
  ▸ Adult: 250 mg once daily

IMPORTANT SAFETY INFORMATION

MHRA/CHM ADVICE: EPIDERMAL GROWTH FACTOR RECEPTOR (EGFR) INHIBITORS: SERIOUS CASES OF KERATITIS AND ULCERATIVE KERATITIS (MAY 2012)

Keratitis and ulcerative keratitis have been reported following treatment with epidermal growth factor receptor (EGFR) inhibitors for cancer (cetuximab, erlotinib, gefitinib and panitumumab). In rare cases, this has resulted in corneal perforation and blindness. Patients undergoing treatment with EGFR inhibitors who present with acute or worsening signs and symptoms suggestive of keratitis should be referred promptly to an ophthalmology specialist. Treatment should be interrupted or discontinued if ulcerative keratitis is diagnosed.

RISKS OF INCORRECT DOSING OF ORAL ANTI-CANCER MEDICINES
See Cytotoxic drugs p. 932.

- **INTERACTIONS** → Appendix 1: gefitinib
- **SIDE-EFFECTS**
  ▸ **Common or very common** Alopecia · angioedema · appetite decreased · asthenia · cystitis · dehydration · diarrhoea · dry eye · dry mouth · eye inflammation · fever · haemorrhage · hypersensitivity · interstitial lung disease (discontinue) · nail disorder · nausea · proteinuria · rash pustular · skin reactions · stomatitis · vomiting
  ▸ **Uncommon** Corneal erosion · gastrointestinal perforation · hepatic disorders · pancreatitis
  ▸ **Rare or very rare** Cutaneous vasculitis · severe cutaneous adverse reactions (SCARs)
- **CONCEPTION AND CONTRACEPTION** Contraceptive advice required, see *Pregnancy and reproductive function* in Cytotoxic drugs p. 932.
- **PREGNANCY** Manufacturer advises avoid unless essential—toxicity in *animal* studies. See also *Pregnancy and reproductive function* in Cytotoxic drugs p. 932.
- **BREAST FEEDING** Discontinue breast-feeding.
- **HEPATIC IMPAIRMENT** Manufacturer advises caution in moderate to severe impairment due to cirrhosis—monitor for adverse events (risk of increased drug plasma concentrations).
- **RENAL IMPAIRMENT** Manufacturer advises caution if creatinine clearance less than 20 mL/minute.
- **MONITORING REQUIREMENTS**
  ▸ Monitor for worsening of dyspnoea, cough and fever—discontinue if interstitial lung disease confirmed.
  ▸ Monitor liver function—consider discontinuing if severe changes in liver function occur.
- **NATIONAL FUNDING/ACCESS DECISIONS**
  For full details see funding body website
  NICE decisions
  ▸ Gefitinib for the first-line treatment of locally advanced or metastatic non-small-cell lung cancer (July 2010) NICE TA192 Recommended with restrictions
  ▸ Erlotinib and gefitinib for treating non-small-cell lung cancer that has progressed after prior chemotherapy (December 2015) NICE TA374 Not recommended

Scottish Medicines Consortium (SMC) decisions
▸ Gefitinib (*Iressa*®) for the treatment of adult patients with locally advanced or metastatic non-small cell lung cancer with activating mutations of epidermal growth factor receptor tyrosine kinase (December 2015) SMC No. 615/10
Recommended with restrictions

● MEDICINAL FORMS There can be variation in the licensing of different medicines containing the same drug.

Tablet
▸ Gefitinib (Non-proprietary)
Gefitinib 250 mg Gefitinib 250mg tablets | 30 tablet [PoM]
£1,500.00-£2,167.71 | 30 tablet [PoM] £2,166.10 (Hospital only)
▸ Iressa (AstraZeneca UK Ltd)
Gefitinib 250 mg Iressa 250mg tablets | 30 tablet [PoM] £2,167.71

Gilteritinib   06-Nov-2020

● DRUG ACTION Gilteritinib is a FMS-like tyrosine kinase-3 (FLT3) inhibitor.

● **INDICATIONS AND DOSE**
FLT3 mutation-positive acute myeloid leukaemia (specialist use only)
▸ BY MOUTH
▸ Adult: 120 mg once daily, for dose adjustments, treatment interruption, or discontinuation due to side-effects—consult product literature, if no response is observed after 4 weeks, dose may be increased to 200 mg once daily. Up to 6 months treatment may be required before a clinical response is seen

● CAUTIONS Risk factors for QT-interval prolongation (including hypokalaemia or hypomagnesaemia)

● INTERACTIONS → Appendix 1: gilteritinib

● SIDE-EFFECTS
▸ **Common or very common** Acute kidney injury · anaphylactic reaction · arthralgia · asthenia · constipation · cough · diarrhoea · differentiation syndrome · dizziness · dyspnoea · heart failure · hypotension · malaise · myalgia · nausea · pain · pericardial effusion · pericarditis · peripheral oedema · QT interval prolongation
▸ **Uncommon** Posterior reversible encephalopathy syndrome (PRES)
▸ **Frequency not known** Pancreatitis

● CONCEPTION AND CONTRACEPTION Manufacturer advises perform pregnancy test in females of childbearing potential within 7 days prior to treatment initiation; effective contraception should be used during treatment and for at least 6 months after last treatment— additional barrier method recommended in those using hormonal contraceptives. Male patients should use effective contraception during treatment and for at least 4 months after last treatment if their partner is of childbearing potential. See also *Pregnancy and reproductive function* in Cytotoxic drugs p. 932.

● PREGNANCY Manufacturer advises avoid—toxicity in *animal* studies. See also *Pregnancy and reproductive function* in Cytotoxic drugs p. 932.

● BREAST FEEDING Manufacturer advises discontinue breast-feeding during treatment and for at least 2 months after stopping—present in milk in *animal* studies.

● HEPATIC IMPAIRMENT Manufacturer advises avoid in severe impairment (no information available).

● MONITORING REQUIREMENTS
▸ Manufacturer advises monitor blood chemistry, including creatine phosphokinase, before treatment, on day 15 of treatment, and then monthly during treatment.
▸ Manufacturer advises monitor ECG before treatment, on days 8 and 15 of treatment, and then prior to the start of the next three subsequent months of treatment—consult

product literature for dose modifications if QT-interval prolonged.

● PRESCRIBING AND DISPENSING INFORMATION The manufacturer of *Xospata*® has provided a *Risk minimisation materials* document for healthcare professionals.

● PATIENT AND CARER ADVICE
Vomiting Manufacturer advises if vomiting occurs after taking tablets, no additional dose should be taken on that day and the next dose should be taken at the usual time.
A patient alert card should be provided.
Missed doses Manufacturer advises if a dose is missed or not taken at the usual time, the missed dose should be taken as soon as possible on the same day. The next dose should be taken at the usual time.
Driving and skilled tasks Manufacturer advises patients and their carers should be counselled on the effects on driving and performance of skilled tasks—increased risk of dizziness.

● NATIONAL FUNDING/ACCESS DECISIONS
For full details see funding body website
NICE decisions
▸ Gilteritinib for treating relapsed or refractory acute myeloid leukaemia (August 2020) NICE TA642 Recommended
Scottish Medicines Consortium (SMC) decisions
▸ Gilteritinib (*Xospata*®) as monotherapy for the treatment of adult patients who have relapsed or refractory acute myeloid leukaemia with a FLT3 mutation (September 2020) SMC No. SMC2252 Recommended

● MEDICINAL FORMS There can be variation in the licensing of different medicines containing the same drug.

Tablet
CAUTIONARY AND ADVISORY LABELS 25
▸ Xospata (Astellas Pharma Ltd) ▼
Gilteritinib (as Gilteritinib fumarate) 40 mg Xospata 40mg tablets | 84 tablet [PoM] £14,188.00 (Hospital only)

Ibrutinib   06-Nov-2020

● DRUG ACTION Ibrutinib is a tyrosine kinase inhibitor.

● **INDICATIONS AND DOSE**
Mantle cell lymphoma (specialist use only)
▸ BY MOUTH
▸ Adult: 560 mg once daily, for dose adjustments due to side-effects—consult product literature
Chronic lymphocytic leukaemia (specialist use only) | Waldenström's macroglobulinaemia (specialist use only)
▸ BY MOUTH
▸ Adult: 420 mg once daily, for dose adjustments due to side-effects—consult product literature
DOSE ADJUSTMENTS DUE TO INTERACTIONS
▸ Manufacturer advises if concurrent use of moderate inhibitors of CYP3A4, amiodarone or ciprofloxacin is unavoidable, reduce dose to 280 mg once daily.
▸ Manufacturer advises if concurrent use of potent inhibitors of CYP3A4 is unavoidable, reduce dose to 140 mg once daily, or withhold ibrutinib for up to 7 days.

IMPORTANT SAFETY INFORMATION
RISKS OF INCORRECT DOSING OF ORAL ANTI-CANCER MEDICINES
See Cytotoxic drugs p. 932.

MHRA/CHM ADVICE: IBRUTINIB (*IMBRUVICA*®): REPORTS OF VENTRICULAR TACHYARRHYTHMIA; RISK OF HEPATITIS B REACTIVATION AND OF OPPORTUNISTIC INFECTIONS (AUGUST 2017)
Cases of ventricular tachyarrhythmia have been reported with the use of ibrutinib. The MHRA advises that ibrutinib should be temporarily discontinued in patients

who develop symptoms suggestive of ventricular arrhythmia and to assess benefit-risk before restarting therapy.

Hepatitis B virus status should be established before initiating therapy—for patients with positive hepatitis B serology, consultation with a liver disease expert is recommended before the start of treatment; monitor and manage patients according to local protocols to minimise the risk of hepatitis B virus reactivation. Prophylaxis should be considered for those at an increased risk of opportunistic infections.

- CAUTIONS Family history of congenital short QT syndrome · increased lymphocytes—increased risk of leukostasis, consider withholding treatment temporarily and monitor closely · patients at risk from further shortening of QTc interval · personal history of congenital short QT syndrome · risk of haemorrhagic events—withhold ibrutinib treatment for at least 3 to 7 days before and after surgery depending on risk of bleeding
- INTERACTIONS → Appendix 1: ibrutinib
- SIDE-EFFECTS
  ‣ **Common or very common** Arrhythmias · arthralgia · broken nails · CNS haemorrhage · constipation · diarrhoea · dizziness · fever · haemorrhage · headache · hypertension · hyperuricaemia · increased leucocytes · increased risk of infection · interstitial lung disease · muscle spasms · musculoskeletal pain · nausea · neoplasms · neutropenia · peripheral neuropathy · peripheral oedema · sepsis · skin reactions · stomatitis · thrombocytopenia · tumour lysis syndrome · vision blurred · vomiting
  ‣ **Uncommon** Angioedema · hepatitis B reactivation · leukostasis syndrome · panniculitis
  ‣ **Frequency not known** Anaemia · hepatic failure · progressive multifocal leukoencephalopathy (PML) · Stevens-Johnson syndrome
- CONCEPTION AND CONTRACEPTION Highly effective contraception (must include a non-hormonal method) required during and for 3 months after stopping treatment.
- PREGNANCY Manufacturer advises avoid—toxicity in *animal* studies. See also *Pregnancy and reproductive function* in Cytotoxic drugs p. 932.
- BREAST FEEDING Manufacturer advises discontinue breastfeeding—no information available.
- HEPATIC IMPAIRMENT Manufacturer advises avoid in severe impairment (risk of increased exposure)—monitor for toxicity.
  Dose adjustments Manufacturer advises dose reduction to 280 mg daily in mild impairment and to 140 mg daily in moderate impairment with further adjustments if necessary—consult product literature.
- RENAL IMPAIRMENT Use in severe impairment only if benefit outweighs risk and with close monitoring for toxicity.
  Monitoring Maintain hydration and monitor serum creatinine periodically in mild to moderate renal impairment.
- MONITORING REQUIREMENTS
  ‣ Monitor full blood count once a month.
  ‣ Monitor for atrial fibrillation (increased risk in cardiac risk factors, acute infections and history of atrial fibrillation), monitor all patients periodically and complete ECG if arrhythmic symptoms or dyspnoea develop—consult product literature for treatment options.
- NATIONAL FUNDING/ACCESS DECISIONS
  For full details see funding body website
  NICE decisions
  ‣ Ibrutinib for previously treated chronic lymphocytic leukaemia and untreated chronic lymphocytic leukaemia with

17p deletion or TP53 mutation (January 2017) NICE TA429 Recommended with restrictions
‣ Ibrutinib for treating Waldenstrom's macroglobulinaemia (November 2017) NICE TA491 Recommended with restrictions
‣ Ibrutinib for treating relapsed or refractory mantle cell lymphoma (January 2018) NICE TA502 Recommended with restrictions
Scottish Medicines Consortium (SMC) decisions
‣ Ibrutinib (*Imbruvica*®) for the treatment of adult patients with chronic lymphocytic leukaemia who have received at least one prior therapy (April 2017) SMC No. 1151/16 Recommended with restrictions
‣ Ibrutinib (*Imbruvica*®) in combination with rituximab for the treatment of adult patients with Waldenström's macroglobulinaemia (October 2020) SMC No. SMC2259 Recommended with restrictions

- MEDICINAL FORMS There can be variation in the licensing of different medicines containing the same drug.
  Tablet
  CAUTIONARY AND ADVISORY LABELS 25
  ‣ Imbruvica (Janssen-Cilag Ltd)
     Ibrutinib 140 mg Imbruvica 140mg tablets | 28 tablet [PoM] £1,430.80
     Ibrutinib 280 mg Imbruvica 280mg tablets | 28 tablet [PoM] £2,861.60
     Ibrutinib 420 mg Imbruvica 420mg tablets | 28 tablet [PoM] £4,292.40
     Ibrutinib 560 mg Imbruvica 560mg tablets | 28 tablet [PoM] £5,723.20

Idelalisib

16-Oct-2020

- DRUG ACTION Idelalisib is a protein kinase inhibitor.

- INDICATIONS AND DOSE
  Treatment of chronic lymphocytic leukaemia in patients who have received at least one previous therapy, or as first-line treatment in the presence of 17p deletion or TP53 mutation in patients who are not eligible for any other therapies (in combination with rituximab) | Treatment of follicular lymphoma refractory to two lines of treatment (monotherapy)
  ‣ BY MOUTH
  ‣ Adult: 150 mg twice daily, for dose adjustment due to side effects, consult product literature

---

IMPORTANT SAFETY INFORMATION
RISKS OF INCORRECT DOSING OF ORAL ANTI-CANCER MEDICINES
See Cytotoxic drugs p. 932.

MHRA/CHM ADVICE: IDELALISIB (ZYDELIG®): UPDATED INDICATIONS AND ADVICE ON MINIMISING THE RISK OF INFECTION (SEPTEMBER 2016)
In light of a recent safety review the indications for idelalisib have been updated. Manufacturer recommendations regarding monitoring for infection and prophylaxis of *Pneumocystis jirovecii* pneumonia have also been updated. Patients should be advised on the risk of serious or fatal infections during treatment, and idelalisib should not be initiated in patients with any evidence of infection.

- CAUTIONS Active hepatitis · diarrhoea—symptomatic management recommended (consult product literature) · pneumonitis—withhold treatment (consult product literature)
- INTERACTIONS → Appendix 1: idelalisib
- SIDE-EFFECTS
  ‣ **Common or very common** Colitis · diarrhoea · fever · infection · neutropenia · pneumonitis · rash
  ‣ **Rare or very rare** Severe cutaneous adverse reactions (SCARs)

CONCEPTION AND CONTRACEPTION Highly effective contraception (in addition to barrier method) required during and for one month after treatment.

PREGNANCY Manufacturer advises avoid (toxicity in *animal* studies). See also *Pregnancy and reproductive function* in Cytotoxic drugs p. 932.

BREAST FEEDING Manufacturer advises avoid—no information available.

HEPATIC IMPAIRMENT Manufacturer advises caution (risk of increased exposure-limited information available in severe impairment)—monitor for adverse reactions.

MONITORING REQUIREMENTS
Manufacturer advises monitor liver function—consult product literature.
Manufacturer advises monitor for signs and symptoms of infection, including *cytomegalovirus* infection and respiratory infections; new symptoms should be reported promptly. Neutrophil count should be monitored in all patients every 2 weeks for the first 6 months of treatment; patients with neutrophil count <1000 per mm^3 should be monitored weekly.

NATIONAL FUNDING/ACCESS DECISIONS
For full details see funding body website

NICE decisions
Idelalisib for treating chronic lymphocytic leukaemia (October 2015) NICE TA359 Recommended
Idelalisib for treating refractory follicular lymphoma (October 2019) NICE TA604 Not recommended

Scottish Medicines Consortium (SMC) decisions
Idelalisib (*Zydelig*®) in combination with rituximab for the treatment of adult patients with chronic lymphocytic leukaemia (CLL): who have received at least one prior therapy, or as first line treatment in the presence of 17p deletion or TP53 mutation in patients unsuitable for chemo-immunotherapy (March 2015) SMC No. 1026/15 Recommended with restrictions
Idelalisib (*Zydelig*®) as monotherapy for the treatment of adult patients with follicular lymphoma (FL) that is refractory to two prior lines of treatment (May 2015) SMC No. 1039/15 Recommended with restrictions

MEDICINAL FORMS There can be variation in the licensing of different medicines containing the same drug.

Tablet
CAUTIONARY AND ADVISORY LABELS 25
Zydelig (Gilead Sciences Ireland UC)
Idelalisib 100 mg Zydelig 100mg tablets | 60 tablet $\boxed{\text{PoM}}$ £3,114.75 (Hospital only)
Idelalisib 150 mg Zydelig 150mg tablets | 60 tablet $\boxed{\text{PoM}}$ £3,114.75 (Hospital only)

Imatinib
27-Jul-2020

DRUG ACTION Imatinib is a tyrosine kinase inhibitor.

INDICATIONS AND DOSE
Treatment of chronic myeloid leukaemia in chronic phase after failure with interferon alfa
▶ BY MOUTH
▶ Adult: 400 mg once daily, increased if necessary up to 800 mg daily in 2 divided doses

Treatment of chronic myeloid leukaemia in accelerated phase, or in blast crisis
▶ BY MOUTH
▶ Adult: 600 mg once daily, then increased if necessary up to 800 mg daily in 2 divided doses

Treatment of newly diagnosed acute lymphoblastic leukaemia (in combination with other chemotherapy) | Monotherapy for relapsed or refractory acute lymphoblastic leukaemia
▶ BY MOUTH
▶ Adult: 600 mg once daily

Treatment of c-kit (CD117)-positive unresectable or metastatic malignant gastro-intestinal stromal tumours (GIST) | Adjuvant treatment following resection of c-kit (CD117)-positive GIST, in patients at significant risk of relapse | Treatment of myelodysplastic/myeloproliferative diseases associated with platelet-derived growth factor receptor gene rearrangement
▶ BY MOUTH
▶ Adult: 400 mg once daily

Treatment of unresectable dermatofibrosarcoma protuberans | Recurrent or metastatic dermatofibrosarcoma protuberans, in patients who cannot have surgery
▶ BY MOUTH
▶ Adult: 800 mg daily in 2 divided doses

Treatment of advanced hypereosinophilic syndrome and chronic eosinophilic leukaemia
▶ BY MOUTH
▶ Adult: 100–400 mg once daily

IMPORTANT SAFETY INFORMATION
RISKS OF INCORRECT DOSING OF ORAL ANTI-CANCER MEDICINES
See Cytotoxic drugs p. 932.
MHRA/CHM ADVICE (MAY 2016): RISK OF HEPATITIS B VIRUS REACTIVATION WITH BCR-ABL TYROSINE KINASE INHIBITORS
An EU wide review has concluded that imatinib can cause hepatitis B reactivation; the MHRA recommends establishing hepatitis B virus status in all patients before initiation of treatment.

CAUTIONS Cardiac disease · hepatitis B infection · history of renal failure · risk factors for heart failure
CAUTIONS, FURTHER INFORMATION
▶ Hepatitis B infection The MHRA advises that patients who are carriers of hepatitis B virus should be closely monitored for signs and symptoms of active infection throughout treatment and for several months after stopping treatment; expert advice should be sought for patients who test positive for hepatitis B virus and in those with active infection.

INTERACTIONS → Appendix 1: imatinib

SIDE-EFFECTS
▶ Common or very common Alopecia · anaemia · appetite abnormal · asthenia · bone marrow disorders · chills · constipation · cough · diarrhoea · dizziness · dry eye · dry mouth · dyspnoea · excessive tearing · eye inflammation · fever · fluid imbalance · flushing · gastrointestinal discomfort · gastrointestinal disorders · haemorrhage · headaches · insomnia · joint disorders · muscle complaints · nausea · neutropenia · oedema · pain · photosensitivity reaction · sensation abnormal · skin reactions · sweat changes · taste altered · thrombocytopenia · vision blurred · vomiting · weight changes
▶ Uncommon Anxiety · arrhythmias · ascites · breast abnormalities · broken nails · burping · chest pain · CNS haemorrhage · congestive heart failure · depression · drowsiness · dysphagia · electrolyte imbalance · eosinophilia · eye discomfort · gout · gynaecomastia · hearing loss · hepatic disorders · hyperbilirubinaemia · hyperglycaemia · hypertension · hyperuricaemia · hypotension · increased risk of infection · laryngeal pain · lymphadenopathy · lymphopenia · malaise · memory loss · menstrual cycle irregularities · nerve disorders · oral

8

Immune system and malignant disease

disorders · palpitations · pancreatitis · peripheral coldness · pulmonary oedema · Raynaud's phenomenon · renal impairment · renal pain · respiratory disorders · restless legs · scrotal oedema · sepsis · sexual dysfunction · syncope · thrombocytosis · tinnitus · tremor · urinary frequency increased · vertigo

▸ **Rare or very rare** Angina pectoris · angioedema · arthritis · cardiac arrest · cataract · confusion · glaucoma · haemolytic anaemia · haemorrhagic ovarian cyst · hepatic failure (including fatal cases) · hypersensitivity vasculitis · inflammatory bowel disease · intracranial pressure increased · muscle weakness · myocardial infarction · myopathy · nail discolouration · pericardial disorders · pulmonary hypertension · seizure · severe cutaneous adverse reactions (SCARs) · thrombotic microangiopathy · tumour lysis syndrome

▸ **Frequency not known** Embolism and thrombosis · hepatitis B reactivation · neoplasm complications · osteonecrosis · pericarditis

● CONCEPTION AND CONTRACEPTION Effective contraception required during treatment.

● PREGNANCY Manufacturer advises avoid unless potential benefit outweighs risk. See also *Pregnancy and reproductive function* in Cytotoxic drugs p. 932.

● BREAST FEEDING Discontinue breast-feeding.

● HEPATIC IMPAIRMENT Manufacturer advises caution.
Dose adjustments Manufacturer advises max. 400 mg once daily; consider further dose reduction if not tolerated—consult product literature.

● RENAL IMPAIRMENT
Dose adjustments Maximum starting dose 400 mg daily if creatinine clearance less than 60 mL/minute; reduce dose further if not tolerated.

● MONITORING REQUIREMENTS
▸ Monitor for gastrointestinal haemorrhage.
▸ Monitor complete blood counts regularly.
▸ Monitor for fluid retention.
▸ Monitor liver function.
▸ Monitor growth in children (may cause growth retardation).

● DIRECTIONS FOR ADMINISTRATION Manufacturer advises tablets may be dispersed in water or apple juice.

● PATIENT AND CARER ADVICE Patients or carers should be given advice on how to administer imatinib tablets.

● NATIONAL FUNDING/ACCESS DECISIONS
For full details see funding body website
NICE decisions
▸ **Imatinib for the adjuvant treatment of gastro-intestinal stromal tumours (November 2014)** NICE TA326 Recommended
▸ **Imatinib for chronic myeloid leukaemia (updated January 2016)** NICE TA70 Recommended
▸ **Imatinib for the treatment of unresectable and/or metastatic gastro-intestinal stromal tumours (updated November 2010)** NICE TA86 Recommended with restrictions
▸ **Imatinib for the treatment of unresectable and/or metastatic gastro-intestinal stromal tumours (November 2010)** NICE TA209 Not recommended
▸ **Dasatinib, nilotinib and imatinib for untreated chronic myeloid leukaemia (CML) (December 2016)** NICE TA426 Recommended
▸ **Dasatinib, nilotinib and high-dose imatinib for treating imatinib-resistant or intolerant chronic myeloid leukaemia (CML) (December 2016)** NICE TA425 Not recommended
Scottish Medicines Consortium (SMC) decisions
▸ Imatinib (*Glivec*®) for chronic myeloid leukaemia (January 2003) SMC No. 26/02 Recommended with restrictions
▸ Imatinib (*Glivec*®) for the adjuvant treatment of gastrointestinal stromal tumours (September 2010) SMC No. 584/09 Recommended with restrictions

● MEDICINAL FORMS There can be variation in the licensing of different medicines containing the same drug.
Tablet
CAUTIONARY AND ADVISORY LABELS 21, 27
▸ Imatinib (Non-proprietary)
Imatinib (as Imatinib mesilate) 100 mg Imatinib 100mg tablets | 60 tablet PoM £104.49 DT = £478.08 (Hospital only) | 60 tablet PoM £973.32 DT = £478.08
Imatinib (as Imatinib mesilate) 400 mg Imatinib 400mg tablets | 30 tablet PoM £208.98 DT = £787.42 (Hospital only) | 30 tablet PoM £1,946.67 DT = £787.42
▸ Glivec (Novartis Pharmaceuticals UK Ltd) ▼
Imatinib (as Imatinib mesilate) 100 mg Glivec 100mg tablets | 60 tablet PoM £973.32 DT = £478.08
Imatinib (as Imatinib mesilate) 400 mg Glivec 400mg tablets | 30 tablet PoM £1,946.67 DT = £787.42

Lapatinib

23-Jul-2020

● DRUG ACTION Lapatinib is a tyrosine kinase inhibitor.

● INDICATIONS AND DOSE

Treatment of metastatic breast cancer in patients with tumours that overexpress human epidermal growth factor receptor-2 (HER2) with hormone-receptor-negative disease who have had previous treatment with trastuzumab in combination with chemotherapy (in combination with trastuzumab)
▸ BY MOUTH
▸ Adult: 1 g once daily

Treatment of advanced or metastatic breast cancer in patients with tumours that overexpress human epidermal growth factor receptor-2 (HER2), for patients who have had previous treatment with an anthracycline, a taxane, and trastuzumab (in combination with capecitabine)
▸ BY MOUTH
▸ Adult: 1.25 g once daily

Treatment of metastatic breast cancer with tumours that overexpress human epidermal growth factor receptor-2 (HER2), for postmenopausal women with hormone-receptor-positive disease (in combination with an aromatase inhibitor)
▸ BY MOUTH
▸ Adult: 1.5 g once daily

IMPORTANT SAFETY INFORMATION
RISKS OF INCORRECT DOSING OF ORAL ANTI-CANCER MEDICINES
See Cytotoxic drugs p. 932.

● CAUTIONS Diarrhoea—withhold treatment if severe (consult product literature) · low gastric pH (reduced absorption) · susceptibility to QT-interval prolongation (including electrolyte disturbances)

● INTERACTIONS → Appendix 1: lapatinib

● SIDE-EFFECTS
▸ **Common or very common** Alopecia · appetite decreased · arthralgia · asthenia · constipation · cough · dehydration · diarrhoea (treat promptly) · dyspnoea · epistaxis · gastrointestinal discomfort · headache · hepatotoxicity (discontinue permanently if severe) · hot flush · hyperbilirubinaemia · insomnia · mucositis · nail disorder · nausea · pain · paronychia · skin reactions · stomatitis · vomiting
▸ **Uncommon** Respiratory disorders
▸ **Frequency not known** Severe cutaneous adverse reactions (SCARs)

● CONCEPTION AND CONTRACEPTION Contraceptive advice required, see *Pregnancy and reproductive function* in Cytotoxic drugs p. 932.

- **PREGNANCY** Avoid unless potential benefit outweighs risk—toxicity in *animal* studies. See also Pregnancy and reproductive function in Cytotoxic drugs p. 932.
- **BREAST FEEDING** Discontinue breast-feeding.
- **HEPATIC IMPAIRMENT** Manufacturer advises caution in moderate to severe impairment—increased exposure (limited information available).
- **RENAL IMPAIRMENT** Caution in severe impairment—no information available.
- **MONITORING REQUIREMENTS**
  ▸ Monitor left ventricular function.
  ▸ Monitor for pulmonary toxicity.
  ▸ Monitor liver function before treatment and at monthly intervals.
- **DIRECTIONS FOR ADMINISTRATION** Manufacturer advises always take at the same time in relation to food: either one hour before or one hour after food.
- **PATIENT AND CARER ADVICE** Counselling advised (administration). Patients should be advised to report any unexpected changes in bowel habit.
- **NATIONAL FUNDING/ACCESS DECISIONS**
  For full details see funding body website
  NICE decisions
  ▸ **Lapatinib or trastuzumab in combination with an aromatase inhibitor for the first-line treatment of metastatic hormone-receptor-positive breast cancer that overexpresses HER2 (June 2012)** NICE TA257 Not recommended
- **MEDICINAL FORMS** There can be variation in the licensing of different medicines containing the same drug.
  Tablet
  ▸ Tyverb (Novartis Pharmaceuticals UK Ltd)
  Lapatinib (as Lapatinib ditosylate monohydrate) 250 mg Tyverb 250mg tablets | 84 tablet [PoM] £965.16 | 105 tablet [PoM] £1,206.45

Larotrectinib
03-Jun-2020

- **DRUG ACTION** Larotrectinib is a tropomyosin receptor kinase inhibitor.

- **INDICATIONS AND DOSE**
  Solid tumours with neurotrophic tyrosine receptor kinase gene fusion (initiated by a specialist)
  ▸ BY MOUTH
  ▸ **Adult:** 100 mg twice daily, for dose adjustments, treatment interruption, or discontinuation due to side-effects—consult product literature
  DOSE ADJUSTMENTS DUE TO INTERACTIONS
  ▸ Manufacturer advises if concomitant use with potent CYP3A4 inhibitors is unavoidable, reduce dose by 50%.

  > **IMPORTANT SAFETY INFORMATION**
  > RISKS OF INCORRECT DOSING OF ORAL ANTI-CANCER MEDICINES
  > See Cytotoxic drugs p. 932.

- **INTERACTIONS** → Appendix 1: larotrectinib
- **SIDE-EFFECTS**
  ▸ **Common or very common** Anaemia · constipation · dizziness · fatigue · gait abnormal · leucopenia · muscle weakness · myalgia · nausea · neutropenia · paraesthesia · taste altered · vomiting · weight increased
- **CONCEPTION AND CONTRACEPTION** Manufacturer advises effective contraception in females of childbearing potential and in men with a partner of childbearing potential, during treatment and for 1 month after last treatment; additional barrier method recommended in women using hormonal contraceptives. See also *Pregnancy and reproductive function* in Cytotoxic drugs p. 932.

- **PREGNANCY** Manufacturer advises avoid—limited information available. See also *Pregnancy and reproductive function* in Cytotoxic drugs p. 932.
- **BREAST FEEDING** Manufacturer advises avoid during treatment and for 3 days after last treatment—no information available.
- **HEPATIC IMPAIRMENT** Manufacturer advises caution in moderate to severe impairment (increased risk of exposure).
  Dose adjustments Manufacturer advises dose reduction by 50% in moderate to severe impairment.
- **MONITORING REQUIREMENTS** Manufacturer advises monitor liver function (including ALT and AST) at baseline, then monthly during the first 3 months of treatment, and periodically thereafter; more frequent monitoring should be performed in patients who develop transaminase elevations. Treatment should be withheld or permanently discontinued based on severity—consult product literature.
- **HANDLING AND STORAGE** For *oral solution*, manufacturer advises store in a refrigerator (2–8°C).
- **PATIENT AND CARER ADVICE**
  Driving and skilled tasks Manufacturer advises patients and carers should be counselled on the effects on driving and performance of skilled tasks—increased risk of dizziness and fatigue.
- **NATIONAL FUNDING/ACCESS DECISIONS**
  For full details see funding body website
  NICE decisions
  ▸ **Larotrectinib for treating NTRK fusion-positive solid tumours (May 2020)** NICE TA630 Recommended with restrictions

- **MEDICINAL FORMS** There can be variation in the licensing of different medicines containing the same drug.
  Oral solution
  EXCIPIENTS: May contain Hydroxybenzoates (parabens), potassium sorbate, propylene glycol, sorbitol, sucrose
  ▸ Vitrakvi (Bayer Plc) ▼
  Larotrectinib (as Larotrectinib sulfate) 20 mg per 1 ml Vitrakvi 20mg/ml oral solution | 100 ml [PoM] £5,000.00 (Hospital only)

Lenvatinib
10-Nov-2020

- **DRUG ACTION** Lenvatinib is a multireceptor tyrosine kinase inhibitor.

- **INDICATIONS AND DOSE**
  KISPLYX ®
  Advanced renal cell carcinoma following one prior vascular endothelial growth factor-targeted therapy (in combination with everolimus) (specialist use only)
  ▸ BY MOUTH
  ▸ **Adult:** 18 mg once daily, dose should be taken at the same time every day, for dose adjustment due to side-effects—consult product literature
  LENVIMA ®
  Differentiated thyroid carcinoma (specialist use only)
  ▸ BY MOUTH
  ▸ **Adult:** 24 mg once daily, dose should be taken at the same time every day, for dose adjustments due to side-effects—consult product literature
  Hepatocellular carcinoma (specialist use only)
  ▸ BY MOUTH
  ▸ **Adult (body-weight up to 60 kg):** 8 mg once daily, dose should be taken at the same time every day, for dose adjustments due to side-effects—consult product literature
  ▸ **Adult (body-weight 60 kg and above):** 12 mg once daily, dose should be taken at the same time continued →

every day, for dose adjustments due to side-effects—consult product literature

---

IMPORTANT SAFETY INFORMATION

MHRA/CHM ADVICE: SYSTEMICALLY ADMINISTERED VEGF PATHWAY INHIBITORS: RISK OF ANEURYSM AND ARTERY DISSECTION (JULY 2020)

A European review of worldwide data concluded that systemically administered VEGF pathway inhibitors may lead to aneurysm and artery dissection in patients with or without hypertension. Some fatal cases have been reported, mainly in relation to aortic aneurysm rupture and aortic dissection. The MHRA advises healthcare professionals to carefully consider the risk of aneurysm and artery dissection in patients with risk factors before initiating treatment with lenvatinib; any modifiable risk factors (such as smoking and hypertension) should be reduced as much as possible. Patients should be monitored and treated for hypertension as required.

RISKS OF INCORRECT DOSING OF ORAL ANTI-CANCER MEDICINES
See Cytotoxic drugs p. 932.

- CONTRA-INDICATIONS Fistulae
- CAUTIONS Arterial thromboembolism within the previous 6 months · elderly (75 years and over)—reduced tolerability · hypertension · impaired wound healing—consider temporary interruption of treatment for major surgical procedures · risk factors for aneurysm or artery dissection
  CAUTIONS, FURTHER INFORMATION
  ▸ Monitoring of blood pressure The MHRA advises to monitor blood pressure regularly—consult product literature if hypertension occurs during treatment.
- INTERACTIONS → Appendix 1: lenvatinib
- SIDE-EFFECTS
  ▸ **Common or very common** Alopecia · appetite decreased · arthralgia · asthenia · cerebrovascular insufficiency · cholecystitis · constipation · decreased leucocytes · dehydration · diarrhoea · dizziness · dry mouth · dysphonia · electrolyte imbalance · embolism and thrombosis · encephalopathy · gastrointestinal discomfort · gastrointestinal disorders · headache · heart failure · hepatic coma · hepatic disorders · hyperbilirubinaemia · hypercholesterolaemia · hypertension · hypoalbuminaemia · hypotension · hypothyroidism · increased risk of infection · insomnia · malaise · mucositis · myalgia · myocardial infarction · nausea · neutropenia · oral disorders · oropharyngeal complaints · pain · peripheral oedema · proteinuria · QT interval prolongation · renal impairment · renal tubular necrosis · skin reactions · taste altered · thrombocytopenia · vomiting · weight decreased
  ▸ **Uncommon** Healing impaired · nephrotic syndrome · pancreatitis · paresis · pneumothorax · splenic infarction
  ▸ **Frequency not known** Aneurysm · artery dissection · cardiac disorder · cardiogenic shock · fistula
  SIDE-EFFECTS, FURTHER INFORMATION Manufacturer advises gastrointestinal toxicity should be actively managed — dehydration and/or hypovolaemia caused by gastrointestinal toxicity are identified as primary risk factors for renal impairment or failure.
- CONCEPTION AND CONTRACEPTION Manufacturer advises women of child-bearing potential should use highly effective contraception during treatment and for 1 month after the last dose, an additional barrier method of contraception should be used in women using oral hormonal contraceptives. See also *Pregnancy and reproductive function* in Cytotoxic drugs p. 932.
- PREGNANCY Manufacturer advises avoid unless potential benefit outweighs risk—teratogenic in *animal* studies. See also *Pregnancy and reproductive function* in Cytotoxic drugs p. 932.

- BREAST FEEDING Manufacturer advises avoid—present in milk in *animal* studies.
- HEPATIC IMPAIRMENT
  KISPLYX ® Manufacturer advises caution in severe impairment (risk of increased exposure).
  Dose adjustments Manufacturer advises dose reduction to 10 mg once daily in severe impairment.
  LENVIMA ® Manufacturer advises caution.
  ▸ When used for Hepatocellular carcinoma Manufacturer advises avoid in severe impairment (no information available).
  Dose adjustments
  ▸ When used for Differentiated thyroid carcinoma Manufacturer advises dose reduction to 14 mg once daily in severe impairment; further dose adjustments may be necessary based on tolerability—consult product literature.
- RENAL IMPAIRMENT
  KISPLYX ® Manufacturer advises avoid in end-stage renal disease.
  Dose adjustments Manufacturer advises reduce dose to 10 mg once daily in severe impairment; further dose adjustments may be necessary based on individual tolerability—consult product literature.
  LENVIMA ®
  ▸ When used for Differentiated thyroid carcinoma Manufacturer advises caution in severe impairment; avoid in end-stage renal disease.
  ▸ When used for Hepatocellular carcinoma The available data do not allow for a dosing recommendation in severe impairment—consult product literature.
  Dose adjustments
  ▸ When used for Differentiated thyroid carcinoma Manufacturer advises dose reduction to 14 mg once daily in severe impairment; further dose adjustments may be necessary based on tolerability—consult product literature.
- MONITORING REQUIREMENTS
  ▸ Manufacturer advises monitor for signs and symptoms of cardiac decompensation (adjust dose as necessary—consult product literature).
  ▸ Manufacturer advises monitor liver function before treatment, then every 2 weeks for the first 2 months, and then monthly thereafter; monitor urine protein regularly.
  ▸ Manufacturer advises monitor ECG and electrolytes before and periodically during treatment (calcium levels should be monitored at least monthly), correct electrolyte abnormalities prior to treatment; monitor thyroid function before and regularly during treatment.
- DIRECTIONS FOR ADMINISTRATION Manufacturer advises capsules should be swallowed whole. Alternatively, capsules may be added to a tablespoon of water or apple juice in a small glass (without breaking or crushing), allowed to sit for at least 10 minutes, then stirred for at least 3 minutes to dissolve the capsule shells before swallowing; the same amount of liquid should then be added to the glass, swirled a few times, then swallowed.
- PATIENT AND CARER ADVICE
  Missed doses Manufacturer advises if a dose is more than 12 hours late, the missed dose should not be taken and the next dose should be taken at the normal time.
  Driving and skilled tasks Manufacturer advises patients and carers should be counselled on the effects on driving and performance of skilled tasks—increased risk of fatigue and dizziness.
- NATIONAL FUNDING/ACCESS DECISIONS
  For full details see funding body website
  NICE decisions
  ▸ Lenvatinib and sorafenib for treating differentiated thyroid cancer after radioactive iodine (August 2018) NICE TA535 Recommended with restrictions
  ▸ Lenvatinib for untreated advanced hepatocellular carcinoma (December 2018) NICE TA551 Recommended with restrictions

Scottish Medicines Consortium (SMC) decisions

▶ Lenvatinib (*Lenvima*®) as monotherapy for the treatment of adult patients with advanced or unresectable hepatocellular carcinoma (HCC) who have received no prior systemic therapy (April 2019) SMC No. SMC2138 Recommended

▶ Lenvatinib (*Kisplyx*®) in combination with everolimus for the treatment of adult patients with advanced renal cell carcinoma (RCC) following one prior vascular endothelial growth factor (VEGF)-targeted therapy (November 2019) SMC No. SMC2199 Recommended

KISPLYX ® For full details see funding body website

NICE decisions

▶ Lenvatinib with everolimus for previously treated advanced renal cell carcinoma (January 2018) NICE TA498 Recommended with restrictions

LENVIMA ® For full details see funding body website

Scottish Medicines Consortium (SMC) decisions

▶ Lenvatinib (*Lenvima*®) for the treatment of adult patients with progressive, locally advanced or metastatic, differentiated (papillary/follicular/Hürthle cell) thyroid carcinoma (DTC), refractory to radioactive iodine (RAI) (October 2016) SMC No. 1179/16 Recommended

● **MEDICINAL FORMS** There can be variation in the licensing of different medicines containing the same drug.

Capsule

CAUTIONARY AND ADVISORY LABELS 25

▶ Kisplyx (Eisai Ltd) ▼

Lenvatinib (as Lenvatinib mesilate) 4 mg Kisplyx 4mg capsules | 30 capsule PoM £1,437.00 (Hospital only)

Lenvatinib (as Lenvatinib mesilate) 10 mg Kisplyx 10mg capsules | 30 capsule PoM £1,437.00 (Hospital only)

▶ Lenvima (Eisai Ltd) ▼

Lenvatinib (as Lenvatinib mesilate) 4 mg Lenvima 4mg capsules | 30 capsule PoM £1,437.00

Lenvatinib (as Lenvatinib mesilate) 10 mg Lenvima 10mg capsules | 30 capsule PoM £1,437.00

Lorlatinib   27-Aug-2020

● DRUG ACTION Lorlatinib is a tyrosine kinase inhibitor.

● **INDICATIONS AND DOSE**

Anaplastic lymphoma kinase (ALK)-positive advanced non-small cell lung cancer (specialist use only)

▶ BY MOUTH

▶ Adult: 100 mg daily, for dose adjustments due to side-effects—consult product literature

DOSE ADJUSTMENTS DUE TO INTERACTIONS

▶ Manufacturer advises if concomitant use with potent CYP3A4 inhibitors is unavoidable, reduce starting dose to 75 mg once daily.

IMPORTANT SAFETY INFORMATION
RISKS OF INCORRECT DOSING OF ORAL ANTI-CANCER MEDICINES
See Cytotoxic drugs p. 932.

● CAUTIONS Cardiac risk factors or conditions which may affect left ventricular ejection fraction—consider cardiac monitoring, including assessment of left ventricular ejection fraction, at baseline and during treatment · lactose intolerance · worsening respiratory symptoms indicative of interstitial lung disease or pneumonitis (including dyspnoea, cough, and fever)—withhold or permanently discontinue treatment based on severity

● INTERACTIONS → Appendix 1: lorlatinib

● SIDE-EFFECTS

▶ **Common or very common** Anaemia · anxiety · arthralgia · asthenia · behaviour abnormal · cognitive disorder · concentration impaired · confusion · constipation · delirium · dementia · depression · diarrhoea · dyslipidaemia

· gait abnormal · hallucinations · headache · inflammation · learning disability · memory loss · mental impairment (thought disturbance) · mood altered · muscle weakness · myalgia · nausea · nerve disorders · neurotoxicity · oedema · pain · peroneal nerve palsy · respiratory disorders · sensation abnormal · skin reactions · speech impairment · vision disorders · vitreous floater · weight increased

▶ **Frequency not known** Atrioventricular block

● CONCEPTION AND CONTRACEPTION Manufacturer advises females of childbearing potential should use effective non-hormonal contraception during treatment and for 35 days after last treatment; male patients should use effective contraception during treatment and for 14 weeks after last treatment if their partner is pregnant or of childbearing potential. See also *Pregnancy and reproductive function* in Cytotoxic drugs p. 932.

● PREGNANCY Manufacturer advises avoid—toxicity in *animal* studies. See also *Pregnancy and reproductive function* in Cytotoxic drugs p. 932.

● BREAST FEEDING Manufacturer advises avoid during treatment and for 7 days after last treatment—no information available.

● HEPATIC IMPAIRMENT Manufacturer advises avoid in moderate to severe impairment (no information available).

● RENAL IMPAIRMENT Manufacturer advises avoid in severe impairment (limited information available).

● MONITORING REQUIREMENTS

▶ Manufacturer advises monitor serum cholesterol and triglycerides before starting treatment, then at weeks 2, 4, and 8, and regularly thereafter.

▶ Manufacturer advises monitor ECG before starting treatment and monthly thereafter, particularly in patients with predisposing conditions.

▶ Manufacturer advises monitor for lipase and amylase elevations before starting treatment, and regularly thereafter as clinically indicated.

● PATIENT AND CARER ADVICE

Missed doses Manufacturer advises if a dose is more than 20 hours late, the missed dose should not be taken and the next dose should be taken at the normal time.

Driving and skilled tasks Manufacturer advises patients and carers should be counselled on the effects on driving and performance of skilled tasks—increased risk of CNS effects.

● NATIONAL FUNDING/ACCESS DECISIONS
For full details see funding body website

NICE decisions

▶ Lorlatinib for previously treated ALK-positive advanced non-small-cell lung cancer (May 2020) NICE TA628 Recommended

Scottish Medicines Consortium (SMC) decisions

▶ Lorlatinib (*Lorviqua*®) as monotherapy for the treatment of adult patients with anaplastic lymphoma kinase (ALK) positive advanced non-small cell lung cancer whose disease has progressed after alectinib or ceritinib as the first ALK tyrosine kinase inhibitor (TKI) therapy or crizotinib and at least one other ALK TKI (March 2020) SMC No. SMC2239 Recommended

● MEDICINAL FORMS There can be variation in the licensing of different medicines containing the same drug.

Tablet

CAUTIONARY AND ADVISORY LABELS 25

▶ Lorviqua (Pfizer Ltd) ▼

Lorlatinib 25 mg Lorviqua 25mg tablets | 90 tablet PoM £5,283.00 (Hospital only) | 120 tablet PoM £7,044.00 (Hospital only)

Lorlatinib 100 mg Lorviqua 100mg tablets | 30 tablet PoM £5,283.00

Midostaurin

02-Sep-2020

- DRUG ACTION Midostaurin is an inhibitor of multiple tyrosine kinases.

- ● INDICATIONS AND DOSE

Acute myeloid leukaemia (specialist use only)
- ▸ BY MOUTH
- ▸ Adult: 50 mg twice daily, on days 8–21 of induction and consolidation chemotherapy cycles; for administration following consolidation chemotherapy, and dose adjustment or treatment interruption due to side-effects—consult product literature

Aggressive systemic mastocytosis (specialist use only) | Systemic mastocytosis with associated haematological neoplasm (specialist use only) | Mast cell leukaemia (specialist use only)
- ▸ BY MOUTH
- ▸ Adult: 100 mg twice daily, for dose adjustment or treatment interruption due to side-effects—consult product literature

> IMPORTANT SAFETY INFORMATION
> RISKS OF INCORRECT DOSING OF ORAL ANTI-CANCER MEDICINES
> See Cytotoxic drugs p. 932.

- CAUTIONS Active severe infection (control before initiation of monotherapy) · elderly (limited experience) · patients at risk of congestive heart failure · risk factors for QT-interval prolongation
- INTERACTIONS → Appendix 1: midostaurin
- SIDE-EFFECTS
- ▸ **Common or very common** Asthenia · bruising · chills · concentration impaired · constipation · cough · cystitis · diarrhoea · dizziness · dyspepsia · dyspnoea · fall · febrile neutropenia · fever · haemorrhage · headache · hyperglycaemia · hypersensitivity · hypotension · increased risk of infection · nausea · oedema · oropharyngeal pain · respiratory disorders · sepsis · tremor · vertigo · vomiting · weight increased
- ▸ **Frequency not known** Cardiac disorder · congestive heart failure · QT interval prolongation
- CONCEPTION AND CONTRACEPTION Manufacturer advises perform pregnancy test in women of childbearing potential within 7 days prior to treatment initiation; effective contraception must be used during treatment and for at least 4 months after stopping treatment—additional barrier method recommended in women using hormonal contraceptives. See also *Pregnancy and reproductive function* in Cytotoxic drugs p. 932.
- PREGNANCY Manufacturer advises avoid—toxicity in *animal* studies. See also *Pregnancy and reproductive function* in Cytotoxic drugs p. 932.
- BREAST FEEDING Manufacturer advises avoid during treatment and for 4 months after stopping treatment—present in milk in *animal* studies.
- HEPATIC IMPAIRMENT Manufacturer advises caution in severe impairment and monitor for toxicity—no information available.
- RENAL IMPAIRMENT Manufacturer advises caution in severe impairment and monitor for toxicity—limited information available.
- MONITORING REQUIREMENTS
- ▸ Manufacturer advises monitor white blood cell count regularly, especially at treatment initiation; also monitor for signs and symptoms of infection.
- ▸ Manufacturer advises assess left ventricular ejection fraction in patients at risk of congestive heart failure at baseline and during treatment as clinically indicated;

consider performing ECGs if concomitant use with drugs that can prolong QT-interval.
- ▸ Manufacturer advises monitor for pulmonary symptoms indicative of interstitial lung disease or pneumonitis.
- ● NATIONAL FUNDING/ACCESS DECISIONS
For full details see funding body website
NICE decisions
- ▸ Midostaurin for untreated acute myeloid leukaemia (June 2018) NICE TA523 Recommended with restrictions
Scottish Medicines Consortium (SMC) decisions
- ▸ Midostaurin (*Rydapt®*) for treatment of adult patients with newly diagnosed acute myeloid leukaemia who are FLT3 mutation positive in combination with standard daunorubicin and cytarabine induction and high dose cytarabine consolidation chemotherapy, and for patients in complete response followed by midostaurin single agent maintenance therapy (June 2018) SMC No. 1330/18 Recommended

- ● MEDICINAL FORMS There can be variation in the licensing of different medicines containing the same drug.
Capsule
CAUTIONARY AND ADVISORY LABELS 21, 25
EXCIPIENTS: May contain Alcohol
- ▸ Rydapt (Novartis Pharmaceuticals UK Ltd) ▼
Midostaurin 25 mg Rydapt 25mg capsules | 56 capsule PoM £5,609.94

Neratinib

11-Nov-2020

- DRUG ACTION Neratinib is a tyrosine kinase inhibitor.

- ● INDICATIONS AND DOSE

HER2-overexpressed/amplified breast cancer (specialist use only)
- ▸ BY MOUTH
- ▸ Adult: 240 mg once daily for 1 year, dose to be taken with food, preferably in the morning, for dose adjustments due to side-effects—consult product literature

DOSE ADJUSTMENTS DUE TO INTERACTIONS
- ▸ Manufacturer advises if concurrent use of potent CYP3A4 inhibitors is unavoidable, reduce neratinib dose to 40 mg once daily.

- CAUTIONS Cardiac risk factors or conditions which may affect left ventricular ejection fraction—consider cardiac monitoring, including assessment of left ventricular ejection fraction, as clinically indicated · elderly (increased risk of complications of diarrhoea) · gastro-intestinal disorder (significant, chronic) with diarrhoea as a major symptom—no clinical experience
- INTERACTIONS → Appendix 1: neratinib
- SIDE-EFFECTS
- ▸ **Common or very common** Appetite decreased · dehydration · diarrhoea · dry mouth · epistaxis · fatigue · gastrointestinal discomfort · increased risk of infection · mucositis · muscle spasms · nail discolouration · nail disorders · nausea · oral disorders · skin reactions · vomiting · weight decreased
- ▸ **Uncommon** Renal failure

SIDE-EFFECTS, FURTHER INFORMATION Diarrhoea may be severe and associated with dehydration. Diarrhoea is more likely to occur during initiation and may be recurrent. Manufacturer advises prophylactic treatment, with anti-diarrhoeal agent.
- CONCEPTION AND CONTRACEPTION Manufacturer advises females of childbearing potential should use highly effective contraception during treatment and for 1 month after last treatment; an additional barrier method of contraception should be used in females using hormonal contraceptives. Male patients should use effective

contraception during treatment and for 3 months after last treatment if their partner is of childbearing potential. See also *Pregnancy and reproductive function* in Cytotoxic drugs p. 932.

- PREGNANCY Manufacturer advises avoid unless potential benefit outweighs risk—toxicity in *animal* studies. See also *Pregnancy and reproductive function* in Cytotoxic drugs p. 932.
- BREAST FEEDING Manufacturer advises avoid—no information available.
- HEPATIC IMPAIRMENT Manufacturer advises avoid in severe impairment (risk of increased exposure).
- RENAL IMPAIRMENT Manufacturer advises caution in mild to moderate impairment (increased risk of complications of dehydration from diarrhoea); avoid in severe impairment (no information available).
- MONITORING REQUIREMENTS Manufacturer advises monitor liver function (including ALT, AST, and total bilirubin) at 1 week, then monthly for the first 3 months, and every 6 weeks thereafter, during treatment or as clinically indicated. Treatment should be withheld or permanently discontinued, based on severity, in those who develop hepatotoxicity—consult product literature.
- PRESCRIBING AND DISPENSING INFORMATION Prophylactic treatment with an anti-diarrhoeal should be initiated with the first dose, and maintained during the first 1–2 months of treatment—consult product literature.
  The manufacturer of *Nerlynx*® has provided a *Risk minimisation materials* document for healthcare professionals.
- PATIENT AND CARER ADVICE A patient alert card, patient treatment journal, and patient guide should be provided.
  Missed doses Manufacturer advises if a dose is missed, the missed dose should not be taken and the next dose should be taken at the normal time.
  Driving and skilled tasks Manufacturer advises patients and carers should be counselled on the effects on driving and performance of skilled tasks—increased risk of fatigue, dizziness, dehydration, and syncope.
- NATIONAL FUNDING/ACCESS DECISIONS
  For full details see funding body website
  NICE decisions
  ▸ Neratinib for extended adjuvant treatment of hormone receptor-positive, HER2-positive early stage breast cancer after adjuvant trastuzumab (November 2019) NICE TA612 Recommended with restrictions
  Scottish Medicines Consortium (SMC) decisions
  ▸ Neratinib (*Nerlynx*®) for extended adjuvant treatment of adult patients with early-stage hormone receptor positive HER2-overexpressed/amplified breast cancer and who completed adjuvant trastuzumab-based therapy less than one year ago (August 2020) SMC No. SMC2251 Recommended
- MEDICINAL FORMS There can be variation in the licensing of different medicines containing the same drug.

Tablet
CAUTIONARY AND ADVISORY LABELS 21, 25
▸ Nerlynx (Pierre Fabre Ltd) ▼
  Neratinib (as Neratinib maleate) 40 mg Nerlynx 40mg tablets | 180 tablet [PoM] £4,500.00

Nilotinib

- DRUG ACTION Nilotinib is a tyrosine kinase inhibitor.

- INDICATIONS AND DOSE
Newly diagnosed chronic phase Philadelphia chromosome-positive chronic myeloid leukaemia (initiated by a specialist)
▸ BY MOUTH
  ▸ Adult: 300 mg twice daily, for dose adjustments due to side-effects—consult product literature

Chronic and accelerated phase Philadelphia chromosome-positive chronic myeloid leukaemia resistant or intolerant to previous therapy, including imatinib (initiated by a specialist)
▸ BY MOUTH
  ▸ Adult: 400 mg twice daily, for dose adjustments due to side-effects—consult product literature

> **IMPORTANT SAFETY INFORMATION**
> RISKS OF INCORRECT DOSING OF ORAL ANTI-CANCER MEDICINES
> See Cytotoxic drugs p. 932.
>
> MHRA/CHM ADVICE (MAY 2016): RISK OF HEPATITIS B VIRUS REACTIVATION WITH TYROSINE KINASE INHIBITORS
> An EU wide review has concluded that nilotinib can cause hepatitis B virus reactivation; the MHRA recommends establishing hepatitis B virus status in all patients before initiation of treatment.

- CAUTIONS Clinically significant bradycardia · congestive heart failure · hepatitis B infection · history of pancreatitis · recent myocardial infarction · susceptibility to QT-interval prolongation (including electrolyte disturbances) · unstable angina
  CAUTIONS, FURTHER INFORMATION
  ▸ Hepatitis B infection The MHRA advises that patients who are carriers of hepatitis B virus should be closely monitored for signs and symptoms of active infection throughout treatment and for several months after stopping treatment; expert advice should be sought for patients who test positive for hepatitis B virus and in those with active infection.
- INTERACTIONS → Appendix 1: nilotinib
- SIDE-EFFECTS
  ▸ **Common or very common** Alopecia · anaemia · angina pectoris · anxiety · appetite abnormal · arrhythmias · arthralgia · asthenia · bone marrow disorders · cardiac conduction disorders · chest discomfort · constipation · cough · decreased leucocytes · depression · diabetes mellitus · diarrhoea · dizziness · dry eye · dyslipidaemia · dyspnoea · electrolyte imbalance · eosinophilia · eye discomfort · eye disorders · eye inflammation · fever · flushing · gastrointestinal discomfort · gastrointestinal disorders · headaches · hepatic disorders · hyperbilirubinaemia · hyperglycaemia · hypertension · increased risk of infection · insomnia · muscle complaints · muscle weakness · myocardial infarction · nausea · neoplasms · neutropenia · oedema · pain · palpitations · peripheral neuropathy · QT interval prolongation · respiratory disorders · sensation abnormal · skin reactions · sweat changes · taste altered · thrombocytopenia · vertigo · vomiting · weight changes
  ▸ **Uncommon** Atherosclerosis · cerebrovascular insufficiency · chills · cyanosis · erectile dysfunction · gout · haemorrhage · heart failure · hyperaemia · malaise · oral disorders · pancreatitis · peripheral vascular disease · temperature sensation altered · vision disorders
  ▸ **Frequency not known** Breast abnormalities · chorioretinopathy · diastolic dysfunction · dry mouth · facial swelling · gynaecomastia · hepatitis B reactivation · hyperparathyroidism · hyperuricaemia · hypoglycaemia ·

Immune system and malignant disease

lethargy · memory loss · menorrhagia · oesophageal pain · oropharyngeal pain · pericardial effusion · pericarditis · restless legs · sebaceous hyperplasia · syncope · tremor · urinary disorders · urine discolouration

- **CONCEPTION AND CONTRACEPTION** Manufacturer advises highly effective contraception in women of childbearing potential during treatment and for up to two weeks after stopping treatment.
- **PREGNANCY** Manufacturer advises avoid unless potential benefit outweighs risk—toxicity in *animal* studies; see also *Pregnancy and reproductive function* in Cytotoxic drugs p. 932.
- **BREAST FEEDING** Manufacturer advises avoid—present in milk in *animal* studies.
- **HEPATIC IMPAIRMENT** Manufacturer advises caution (risk of increased exposure).
- **MONITORING REQUIREMENTS**
  ‣ Manufacturer advises monitor lipid profiles before initiating treatment, at 3 and 6 months, and then yearly thereafter; monitor blood glucose before initiating treatment and then periodically during treatment, as clinically indicated.
  ‣ Manufacturer advises monitor full blood count every 2 weeks for the first 2 months of treatment, then monthly thereafter, or as clinically indicated.
  ‣ Manufacturer advises perform baseline ECG before treatment and as clinically indicated thereafter; correct any electrolyte disturbances before treatment and monitor periodically during treatment.
  ‣ Manufacturer advises monitor and actively manage cardiovascular risk factors during treatment.
- **DIRECTIONS FOR ADMINISTRATION** Manufacturer advises capsules should either be swallowed whole or the contents of each capsule may be dispersed in one teaspoon of apple sauce and taken immediately.
- **PRESCRIBING AND DISPENSING INFORMATION** All prescribers should be familiar with the *Summary of Key Safety Recommendations for Tasigna* ® *(nilotinib)* provided by the manufacturer.
- **PATIENT AND CARER ADVICE** Manufacturer advises patients and carers should seek immediate medical attention if signs or symptoms of cardiovascular events occur.

  All patients should be provided with the *Important Information About How to Take Your Medication* leaflet provided by the manufacturer.
- **NATIONAL FUNDING/ACCESS DECISIONS**
  For full details see funding body website
  NICE decisions
  ‣ **Dasatinib, nilotinib and imatinib for untreated chronic myeloid leukaemia (CML) (December 2016)** NICE TA426 Recommended with restrictions
  ‣ **Dasatinib, nilotinib and high-dose imatinib for treating imatinib-resistant or intolerant chronic myeloid leukaemia (CML) (December 2016)** NICE TA425 Recommended with restrictions

- **MEDICINAL FORMS** There can be variation in the licensing of different medicines containing the same drug.

  Capsule
  CAUTIONARY AND ADVISORY LABELS 23, 25, 27
  ‣ Tasigna (Novartis Pharmaceuticals UK Ltd)
  Nilotinib (as Nilotinib hydrochloride monohydrate)
  50 mg Tasigna 50mg capsules | 120 capsule PoM £2,432.85 DT = £2,432.85
  Nilotinib (as Nilotinib hydrochloride monohydrate)
  150 mg Tasigna 150mg capsules | 112 capsule PoM £2,432.85 DT = £2,432.85
  Nilotinib (as Nilotinib hydrochloride monohydrate)
  200 mg Tasigna 200mg capsules | 112 capsule PoM £2,432.85 DT = £2,432.85

Nintedanib

02-Dec-2020

- **DRUG ACTION** Nintedanib is a tyrosine protein kinase inhibitor.

● **INDICATIONS AND DOSE**

OFEV ®

Treatment of idiopathic pulmonary fibrosis
‣ BY MOUTH
  ‣ Adult: 150 mg twice daily, reduced if not tolerated to 100 mg twice daily, for dose adjustments due to side-effects, consult product literature

VARGATEF ®

Treatment of locally advanced, metastatic or locally recurrent non-small cell lung cancer of adenocarcinoma histology after first-line chemotherapy (in combination with docetaxel) (initiated under specialist supervision)
‣ BY MOUTH
  ‣ Adult: 200 mg twice daily on days 2–21 of a standard 21 day docetaxel cycle, for treatment following discontinuation of docetaxel and for dose adjustments due to side-effects, consult product literature

---

IMPORTANT SAFETY INFORMATION

MHRA/CHM ADVICE: SYSTEMICALLY ADMINISTERED VEGF PATHWAY INHIBITORS: RISK OF ANEURYSM AND ARTERY DISSECTION (JULY 2020)

A European review of worldwide data concluded that systemically administered VEGF pathway inhibitors may lead to aneurysm and artery dissection in patients with or without hypertension. Some fatal cases have been reported, mainly in relation to aortic aneurysm rupture and aortic dissection. The MHRA advises healthcare professionals to carefully consider the risk of aneurysm and artery dissection in patients with risk factors before initiating treatment with nintedanib; any modifiable risk factors (such as smoking and hypertension) should be reduced as much as possible. Patients should be monitored and treated for hypertension as required.

RISKS OF INCORRECT DOSING OF ORAL ANTI-CANCER MEDICINES
See Cytotoxic drugs p. 932.

- **CAUTIONS** History or risk factors for QT prolongation · hypertension · impaired wound healing · increased risk of bleeding · patients at high risk of cardiovascular disease · previous abdominal surgery · recent history of hollow organ perforation · risk factors for aneurysm or artery dissection · theoretical increased risk of gastrointestinal perforation · theoretical increased risk of venous thromboembolism
  CAUTIONS, FURTHER INFORMATION
  ‣ Monitoring of blood pressure The MHRA advises to monitor blood pressure regularly.
- **INTERACTIONS** → Appendix 1: nintedanib
- **SIDE-EFFECTS**
- **Common or very common** Abdominal pain · abscess · appetite decreased · dehydration · diarrhoea · electrolyte imbalance · haemorrhage · hyperbilirubinaemia · hypertension · mucositis · nausea · neutropenia · peripheral neuropathy · sepsis · skin reactions · stomatitis · thrombocytopenia · venous thromboembolism · vomiting · weight decreased
- **Uncommon** Drug-induced liver injury · gastrointestinal perforation · myocardial infarction · pancreatitis · renal impairment
- **Frequency not known** Aneurysm · artery dissection
- **ALLERGY AND CROSS-SENSITIVITY** EvGr Contra-indicated in patients with peanut or soya hypersensitivity. ⓜ
- **CONCEPTION AND CONTRACEPTION** Manufacturer advises exclude pregnancy before treatment and ensure effective

contraception (in addition to barrier method) during treatment and for at least 3 months after last dose.

- PREGNANCY Manufacturer advises avoid—toxicity in *animal* studies. See also *Pregnancy and reproductive function* in Cytotoxic drugs p. 932.

- BREAST FEEDING Manufacturer advises avoid—present in milk in *animal* studies.

- HEPATIC IMPAIRMENT Manufacturer advises caution in mild impairment (risk of increased exposure); avoid in moderate to severe impairment (limited information available).

OFEV ® **Dose adjustments** Manufacturer advises dose reduction to 100 mg twice daily in mild impairment.

- RENAL IMPAIRMENT Manufacturer advises caution in severe impairment—no information available.

- MONITORING REQUIREMENTS
  - For *Vargatef®*, manufacturer advises monitor full blood count before each treatment cycle and regularly thereafter; monitor hepatic function before each treatment cycle during combination therapy and monthly during monotherapy; monitor renal function during treatment; monitor for thromboembolic events; monitor prothrombin time, INR and for bleeding if used concomitantly with anticoagulants; monitor for cerebral bleeding in patients with stable brain metastases.
  - For *Ofev®* manufacturer advises monitor hepatic function before treatment initiation and during the first month of treatment, then at regular intervals during the subsequent 2 months and as clinically indicated thereafter; monitor renal function during treatment.

- PRESCRIBING AND DISPENSING INFORMATION
VARGATEF ® Not to be taken on the same day as docetaxel therapy.

- NATIONAL FUNDING/ACCESS DECISIONS
For full details see funding body website
NICE decisions
  - Nintedanib for previously treated locally advanced, metastatic, or locally recurrent non-small-cell lung cancer (July 2015) NICE TA347 Recommended with restrictions
  - Nintedanib for treating idiopathic pulmonary fibrosis (January 2016) NICE TA379 Recommended with restrictions

Scottish Medicines Consortium (SMC) decisions
  - Nintedanib (*Ofev®*) in adults for the treatment of idiopathic pulmonary fibrosis (IPF) (October 2015) SMC No. 1076/15 Recommended with restrictions

- MEDICINAL FORMS There can be variation in the licensing of different medicines containing the same drug.

Capsule
CAUTIONARY AND ADVISORY LABELS 25
EXCIPIENTS: May contain Lecithin
  - Ofev (Boehringer Ingelheim Ltd)
    Nintedanib (as Nintedanib esilate) 100 mg Ofev 100mg capsules | 60 capsule PoM £2,151.10 (Hospital only)
    Nintedanib (as Nintedanib esilate) 150 mg Ofev 150mg capsules | 60 capsule PoM £2,151.10 (Hospital only)
  - Vargatef (Boehringer Ingelheim Ltd)
    Nintedanib (as Nintedanib esilate) 100 mg Vargatef 100mg capsules | 120 capsule PoM £2,151.10 (Hospital only)
    Nintedanib (as Nintedanib esilate) 150 mg Vargatef 150mg capsules | 60 capsule PoM £2,151.10 (Hospital only)

Osimertinib

19-Nov-2020

- DRUG ACTION Osimertinib is a tyrosine kinase inhibitor.

- INDICATIONS AND DOSE
Non-small cell lung cancer (initiated by a specialist)
  - BY MOUTH
    - Adult: 80 mg once daily, for dose adjustment, interruption, or treatment discontinuation due to side-effects—consult product literature

IMPORTANT SAFETY INFORMATION
RISKS OF INCORRECT DOSING OF ORAL ANTI-CANCER MEDICINES
See Cytotoxic drugs p. 932.

- CONTRA-INDICATIONS Congenital long QT syndrome

- CAUTIONS Elderly (more frequent dose adjustments may be required) · history of interstitial lung disease · radiation pneumonitis requiring steroid treatment · risk factors for QTc interval prolongation

- INTERACTIONS → Appendix 1: osimertinib

- SIDE-EFFECTS
  - **Common or very common** Diarrhoea · eyelid pruritus · increased risk of infection · nail discolouration · nail disorders · respiratory disorders · skin reactions · stomatitis
  - **Uncommon** Eye disorders · eye inflammation · QT interval prolongation

- CONCEPTION AND CONTRACEPTION Manufacturer advises use of effective, non-hormonal, contraception during and for 2 months after treatment in women, and 4 months after treatment in men.

- PREGNANCY Manufacturer advises avoid unless essential—toxicity in *animal* studies. See also *Pregnancy and reproductive function* in Cytotoxic drugs p. 932.

- BREAST FEEDING Manufacturer advises avoid—may be present in milk based on *animal* studies.

- HEPATIC IMPAIRMENT Manufacturer advises avoid in severe impairment (no information available).

- RENAL IMPAIRMENT Manufacturer advises caution in severe and end-stage impairment—limited information available.

- PRE-TREATMENT SCREENING [EvGr] Evidence of epidermal growth factor receptor (EGFR) mutation positive status is required before osimertinib treatment is initiated, and should be determined by an experienced laboratory using a validated test method. ⟨M⟩

- MONITORING REQUIREMENTS Manufacturer advises monitor ECG and electrolytes periodically in patients with risk factors for QTc interval prolongation; dose adjustment is advised if QTc interval is more than 500 milliseconds on at least 2 separate ECGs—consult product literature.

- DIRECTIONS FOR ADMINISTRATION Manufacturer advises tablet may be dispersed in 50 mL of non-carbonated water, by stirring until dispersed and swallowed immediately (do not crush). The residue must then be re-dispersed in an additional half a glass of water and immediately swallowed. Manufacturer advises if administration via a nasogastric tube is required, the tablet may be dispersed in 15 mL of non-carbonated water, by stirring until dispersed and the residue re-dispersed in an additional 15 mL of water (do not crush). The total 30 mL of liquid should then be administered as per the nasogastric tube manufacturer's instructions with appropriate water flushes; the solution should be administered within 30 minutes of adding the tablets to water.

- PATIENT AND CARER ADVICE
Missed doses Manufacturer advises if a dose is more than 12 hours late, the missed dose should not be taken and the next dose should be taken at the normal time.

- NATIONAL FUNDING/ACCESS DECISIONS
For full details see funding body website
NICE decisions
▶ **Osimertinib for treating EGFR T790M mutation-positive advanced non-small-cell lung cancer (October 2020)** NICE TA653 Recommended with restrictions
▶ **Osimertinib for untreated EGFR mutation-positive non-small-cell lung cancer (October 2020)** NICE TA654 Recommended
Scottish Medicines Consortium (SMC) decisions
▶ Osimertinib (*Tagrisso*®) for the treatment of adult patients with locally advanced or metastatic epidermal growth factor receptor (EGFR) T790M mutation-positive non-small-cell lung cancer (NSCLC) (February 2017) SMC No. 1214/17 Recommended with restrictions
▶ Osimertinib (*Tagrisso*®) as monotherapy for the first-line treatment of adult patients with locally advanced or metastatic non-small cell lung cancer (NSCLC) with activating epidermal growth factor receptor (EGFR) mutations (September 2019) SMC No. SMC2171 Not recommended

- MEDICINAL FORMS There can be variation in the licensing of different medicines containing the same drug.
Tablet
▶ Tagrisso (AstraZeneca UK Ltd) ▼
Osimertinib (as Osimertinib mesylate) 40 mg Tagrisso 40mg tablets | 30 tablet [PoM] £5,770.00
Osimertinib (as Osimertinib mesylate) 80 mg Tagrisso 80mg tablets | 30 tablet [PoM] £5,770.00

Palbociclib

10-Nov-2020

- DRUG ACTION Palbociclib is a highly selective inhibitor of cyclin-dependent kinases 4 and 6, which leads to disruption of cancer cell proliferation.

- **INDICATIONS AND DOSE**

Locally advanced or metastatic breast cancer (initiated by a specialist)
▶ BY MOUTH
▶ Adult: 125 mg once daily for 21 consecutive days of repeated 28 day cycles, for dose adjustments due to side-effects—consult product literature
DOSE ADJUSTMENTS DUE TO INTERACTIONS
▶ Manufacturer advises if concomitant use with potent CYP3A4 inhibitors is unavoidable, reduce palbociclib dose to 75 mg once daily. If the CYP3A4 inhibitor is stopped, increase the palbociclib dose (after 3–5 half lives of the inhibitor) to the dose used before starting the CYP3A4 inhibitor.

> IMPORTANT SAFETY INFORMATION
> RISKS OF INCORRECT DOSING OF ORAL ANTI-CANCER MEDICINES
> See Cytotoxic drugs p. 932.

- INTERACTIONS → Appendix 1: palbociclib
- SIDE-EFFECTS
▶ **Common or very common** Alopecia · anaemia · appetite decreased · asthenia · diarrhoea · dry eye · epistaxis · excessive tearing · fever · infection · leucopenia · mucositis · nausea · neutropenia · oral disorders · oropharyngeal complaints · skin reactions · taste altered · thrombocytopenia · vision blurred · vomiting
SIDE-EFFECTS, FURTHER INFORMATION Side-effects are reported when used in combination with letrozole or fulvestrant.

- CONCEPTION AND CONTRACEPTION Manufacturer advises effective contraception in women of childbearing potential during treatment and for at least 3 weeks after completing treatment. Male patients should use effective contraception during treatment and for at least 14 weeks after completing treatment if their partner is of

childbearing potential. See also Pregnancy and reproductive function in Cytotoxic drugs p. 932.

- PREGNANCY Manufacturer advises avoid—toxicity in *animal* studies. See also Pregnancy and reproductive function in Cytotoxic drugs p. 932.
- BREAST FEEDING Manufacturer advises avoid—no information available.
- HEPATIC IMPAIRMENT Manufacturer advises caution in moderate to severe impairment (risk of increased exposure).
Dose adjustments Manufacturer advises dose reduction to 75 mg once daily in severe impairment.
- RENAL IMPAIRMENT Manufacturer advises caution and monitor closely for signs of toxicity in moderate-to-severe impairment.
- MONITORING REQUIREMENTS Manufacturer advises monitor full blood count prior to starting therapy, at the start of each cycle, on day 14 of the first 2 cycles and as clinically indicated.
- PATIENT AND CARER ADVICE
Missed doses Manufacturer advises to take palbociclib at the same time each day; if a dose is missed, the missed dose should not be taken and the next dose should be taken at the usual time.
- NATIONAL FUNDING/ACCESS DECISIONS
For full details see funding body website
NICE decisions
▶ **Palbociclib with an aromatase inhibitor for previously untreated, hormone receptor-positive, HER2-negative, locally advanced or metastatic breast cancer (December 2017)** NICE TA495 Recommended with restrictions
▶ **Palbociclib with fulvestrant for treating hormone receptor-positive, HER2-negative, advanced breast cancer (January 2020)** NICE TA619 Recommended with restrictions
Scottish Medicines Consortium (SMC) decisions
▶ Palbociclib (*Ibrance*®) for the treatment of hormone receptor (HR)-positive, human epidermal growth factor receptor 2 (HER2)-negative locally advanced or metastatic breast cancer: in combination with an aromatase inhibitor; or in combination with fulvestrant in women who have received prior endocrine therapy (December 2017) SMC No. 1276/17 Recommended with restrictions
▶ Palbociclib (*Ibrance*®) for the treatment of hormone receptor (HR)-positive, human epidermal growth factor receptor 2 (HER2)-negative locally advanced or metastatic breast cancer -in combination with fulvestrant in women who have received prior endocrine therapy (July 2019) SMC No. SMC2149 Recommended

- MEDICINAL FORMS There can be variation in the licensing of different medicines containing the same drug.
Capsule
CAUTIONARY AND ADVISORY LABELS 1, 21, 25
▶ Ibrance (Pfizer Ltd) ▼
Palbociclib 75 mg Ibrance 75mg capsules | 21 capsule [PoM] £2,950.00 (Hospital only) | 63 capsule [PoM] £8,850.00 (Hospital only)
Palbociclib 100 mg Ibrance 100mg capsules | 21 capsule [PoM] £2,950.00 (Hospital only) | 63 capsule [PoM] £8,850.00 (Hospital only)
Palbociclib 125 mg Ibrance 125mg capsules | 21 capsule [PoM] £2,950.00 (Hospital only) | 63 capsule [PoM] £8,850.00 (Hospital only)

Pazopanib
11-Nov-2020

- **DRUG ACTION** Pazopanib is a tyrosine kinase inhibitor.

- **INDICATIONS AND DOSE**

**First-line treatment of advanced renal cell carcinoma |
Treatment of advanced renal cell carcinoma in patients
who have had previous treatment with cytokine therapy**
- ▸ BY MOUTH
- ▸ Adult: 800 mg daily, adjust dose in steps of 200 mg
  according to tolerability; maximum 800 mg per day

**Treatment of selective subtypes of advanced soft-tissue
sarcoma**
- ▸ BY MOUTH
- ▸ Adult: (consult product literature)

DOSE ADJUSTMENTS DUE TO INTERACTIONS
- ▸ Manufacturer advises if concurrent use of potent
  inhibitors of CYP3A4 is unavoidable, reduce dose to
  400 mg daily.

IMPORTANT SAFETY INFORMATION
MHRA/CHM ADVICE: SYSTEMICALLY ADMINISTERED VEGF
PATHWAY INHIBITORS: RISK OF ANEURYSM AND ARTERY
DISSECTION (JULY 2020)
A European review of worldwide data concluded that
systemically administered VEGF pathway inhibitors may
lead to aneurysm and artery dissection in patients with
or without hypertension. Some fatal cases have been
reported, mainly in relation to aortic aneurysm rupture
and aortic dissection. The MHRA advises healthcare
professionals to carefully consider the risk of aneurysm
and artery dissection in patients with risk factors before
initiating treatment with pazopanib; any modifiable risk
factors (such as smoking and hypertension) should be
reduced as much as possible. Patients should be
monitored and treated for hypertension as required.

RISKS OF INCORRECT DOSING OF ORAL ANTI-CANCER MEDICINES
See Cytotoxic drugs p. 932.

- **CAUTIONS** Cardiac disease · hypertension · increased risk
  of gastro-intestinal fistulas · increased risk of gastrointestinal perforation · increased risk of haemorrhage ·
  increased risk of thrombotic microangiopathy—
  permanently discontinue if symptoms develop · ischaemic
  stroke · myocardial infarction · risk factors for aneurysm or
  artery dissection · risk of thrombotic events · susceptibility
  to QT-interval prolongation (including electrolyte
  disturbances) · transient ischaemic attack

CAUTIONS, FURTHER INFORMATION
- ▸ Elective surgery Discontinue treatment 7 days before
  elective surgery and restart only if adequate wound
  healing.
- ▸ Monitoring of blood pressure The MHRA advises to monitor
  blood pressure regularly—consult product literature if
  hypertension occurs during treatment.

- **INTERACTIONS** → Appendix 1: pazopanib

- **SIDE-EFFECTS**
- ▸ **Common or very common** Alopecia · appetite decreased ·
  arthralgia · asthenia · bradycardia · cancer pain · cardiac
  disorder · chest pain · chills · cough · dehydration ·
  diarrhoea · dizziness · drowsiness · dry mouth · dysphonia ·
  dyspnoea · electrolyte imbalance · gastrointestinal
  discomfort · gastrointestinal disorders · haemorrhage · hair
  colour changes · headache · hepatic disorders · hiccups ·
  hyperbilirubinaemia · hyperhidrosis · hypertension ·
  hypoalbuminaemia · hypothyroidism · increased risk of
  infection · insomnia · left ventricular dysfunction ·
  leucopenia · mucosal abnormalities · muscle complaints ·
  musculoskeletal pain · nail disorder · nausea · neutropenia ·
  oedema · oral disorders · peripheral neuropathy ·
  proteinuria · respiratory disorders · sensation abnormal ·

skin reactions · taste altered · thrombocytopenia ·
vasodilation · venous thromboembolism · vision blurred ·
vomiting · weight decreased
- ▸ **Uncommon** Cerebrovascular insufficiency · eye disorders ·
  haemolytic uraemic syndrome · menstrual cycle
  irregularities · myocardial infarction · myocardial
  ischaemia · oropharyngeal pain · pancreatitis ·
  photosensitivity reaction · polycythaemia · QT interval
  prolongation · rhinorrhoea · skin ulcer · thrombotic
  microangiopathy
- ▸ **Rare or very rare** Posterior reversible encephalopathy
  syndrome (PRES)
- ▸ **Frequency not known** Aneurysm · artery dissection

- **CONCEPTION AND CONTRACEPTION** Effective
  contraception advised during treatment.

- **PREGNANCY** Avoid unless potential benefit outweighs
  risk—toxicity in *animal* studies. See also *Pregnancy and
  reproductive function* in Cytotoxic drugs p. 932.

- **BREAST FEEDING** Discontinue breast-feeding.

- **HEPATIC IMPAIRMENT** Manufacturer advises caution in
  mild to moderate impairment; avoid in severe impairment.
  Dose adjustments Manufacturer advises dose reduction to
  200 mg daily in moderate impairment.

- **RENAL IMPAIRMENT** Use with caution if creatinine
  clearance less than 30 mL/minute—no information
  available.

- **MONITORING REQUIREMENTS**
- ▸ Monitor liver function before treatment and at weeks 3, 5,
  7, and 9, then at months 3 and 4, and periodically
  thereafter as clinically indicated—consult product
  literature if elevated liver enzymes observed.
- ▸ Monitor for signs or symptoms of congestive heart
  failure—monitor left ventricular ejection fraction in
  patients at risk of heart failure before and during
  treatment.
- ▸ Monitor for proteinuria.
- ▸ Monitor thyroid function.
- ▸ Monitor for signs and symptoms of posterior reversible
  encephalopathy syndrome (including headache,
  hypertension, seizure, lethargy, confusion, visual and
  neurological disturbances)—permanently discontinue
  treatment if symptoms occur.

- **NATIONAL FUNDING/ACCESS DECISIONS**
  For full details see funding body website

NICE decisions
- ▸ Pazopanib for the first-line treatment of advanced renal cell
  carcinoma (updated August 2013) NICE TA215 Recommended
  with restrictions

Scottish Medicines Consortium (SMC) decisions
- ▸ Pazopanib (*Votrient®*) for the first-line treatment of advanced
  renal cell carcinoma (RCC) and for patients who have received
  prior cytokine therapy for advanced disease (March 2011)
  SMC No. 676/11 Recommended with restrictions
- ▸ Pazopanib (*Votrient®*) for the treatment of adult patients
  with selective subtypes of advanced soft tissue sarcoma (STS)
  who have received prior chemotherapy for metastatic disease
  or who have progressed within 12 months after (neo)adjuvant
  therapy (December 2012) SMC No. 820/12 Not recommended

- **MEDICINAL FORMS** There can be variation in the licensing of
  different medicines containing the same drug.

Tablet
CAUTIONARY AND ADVISORY LABELS 23, 25
- ▸ Votrient (Novartis Pharmaceuticals UK Ltd)
  Pazopanib (as Pazopanib hydrochloride) 200 mg Votrient 200mg
  tablets | 30 tablet PoM £560.50
  Pazopanib (as Pazopanib hydrochloride) 400 mg Votrient 400mg
  tablets | 30 tablet PoM £1,121.00

Ponatinib

21-Aug-2020

● INDICATIONS AND DOSE

Treatment of chronic, accelerated, or blast phase chronic myeloid leukaemia in patients who have the T315I mutation or who have resistance to or intolerance of dasatinib or nilotinib, and for whom subsequent treatment with imatinib is not clinically appropriate | **Treatment of Philadelphia chromosome-positive acute lymphoblastic leukaemia in patients who have the T315I mutation or who have resistance to or intolerance of dasatinib, and for whom subsequent treatment with imatinib is not clinically appropriate**

▶ BY MOUTH

▸ Adult: 45 mg once daily, for dose adjustments due to side-effects or dose reduction due to risk of vascular occlusive events, consult product literature

DOSE ADJUSTMENTS DUE TO INTERACTIONS

▸ Manufacturer advises consider a reduced initial dose of 30 mg daily with concurrent use of potent inhibitors of CYP3A4.

IMPORTANT SAFETY INFORMATION

MHRA/CHM ADVICE: RISK OF HEPATITIS B VIRUS REACTIVATION WITH BCR-ABL TYROSINE KINASE INHIBITORS (MAY 2016)

An EU wide review has concluded that ponatinib can cause hepatitis B reactivation; the MHRA recommends establishing hepatitis B virus status in all patients before initiation of treatment.

MHRA/CHM ADVICE (UPDATED APRIL 2017): PONATINIB: RISK OF VASCULAR OCCLUSIVE EVENTS—UPDATED ADVICE ON POSSIBLE DOSE REDUCTION

The benefits and risks of ponatinib were reviewed by the European Medicines Agency's Committee on Medicinal Products for Human Use in 2014, which recommended that strengthened warnings should be added to the product information aimed at minimising the risk of blood clots and blockages in the arteries. Additional long-term follow-up data are now available that support new advice on dose modification to reduce this risk. The MHRA advises that although the recommended starting dose of ponatinib remains unchanged, prescribers should consider reducing the dose for patients with chronic phase chronic myeloid leukaemia (CP-CML) who have achieved a major cytogenetic response while on treatment. The following factors should be taken into account in the individual patient assessment:

● cardiovascular risk;
● side-effects of ponatinib therapy (including cardiovascular and other dose-related toxicity);
● time to cytogenetic response;
● BCR-ABL transcript levels.

The MHRA recommends close monitoring of response, if dose reduction is undertaken.

MHRA/CHM ADVICE: PONATINIB (*ICLUSIG*®): REPORTS OF POSTERIOR REVERSIBLE ENCEPHALOPATHY SYNDROME (OCTOBER 2018)

Post-marketing cases of posterior reversible encephalopathy syndrome (PRES) have been reported in patients receiving ponatinib.

Treatment should be interrupted if PRES is confirmed and resumed only once the event is resolved and if the benefit of continued treatment outweighs the risk.

Patients should be advised to contact their healthcare professional immediately if they develop sudden-onset severe headache, confusion, seizures, or vision changes.

MHRA/CHM ADVICE: SYSTEMICALLY ADMINISTERED VEGF PATHWAY INHIBITORS: RISK OF ANEURYSM AND ARTERY DISSECTION (JULY 2020)

A European review of worldwide data concluded that systemically administered VEGF pathway inhibitors may lead to aneurysm and artery dissection in patients with or without hypertension. Some fatal cases have been reported, mainly in relation to aortic aneurysm rupture and aortic dissection. The MHRA advises healthcare professionals to carefully consider the risk of aneurysm and artery dissection in patients with risk factors before initiating treatment with ponatinib; any modifiable risk factors (such as smoking and hypertension) should be reduced as much as possible. Patients should be monitored and treated for hypertension as required.

RISKS OF INCORRECT DOSING OF ORAL ANTI-CANCER MEDICINES

See Cytotoxic drugs p. 932.

● CAUTIONS Alcohol abuse—increased risk of pancreatitis · current severe hypertriglyceridaemia—increased risk of pancreatitis · discontinue treatment if a complete haematologic response has not occurred within 3 months · hepatitis B infection · history of myocardial infarction—do not use unless potential benefit outweighs potential risk · history of pancreatitis · history of stroke—do not use unless potential benefit outweighs potential risk · hypertension · risk factors for aneurysm or artery dissection

CAUTIONS, FURTHER INFORMATION

▸ **Cardiovascular status** Assess cardiovascular status before treatment—manage cardiovascular risk factors before and during treatment.

▸ **Hepatitis B infection** The MHRA advises that patients who are carriers of hepatitis B virus should be closely monitored for signs and symptoms of active infection throughout treatment and for several months after stopping treatment; expert advice should be sought for patients who test positive for hepatitis B virus and in those with active infection.

▸ **Monitoring of blood pressure** The MHRA advises to monitor blood pressure regularly—consult product literature if hypertension occurs during treatment.

● INTERACTIONS → Appendix 1: ponatinib

● SIDE-EFFECTS

▸ **Common or very common** Acute coronary syndrome · alopecia · anaemia · appetite decreased · arrhythmias · arthralgia · asthenia · cerebrovascular insufficiency · chills · constipation · cough · diarrhoea · dizziness · dry eye · dry mouth · dysphonia · dyspnoea · electrolyte imbalance · embolism and thrombosis · erectile dysfunction · eye inflammation · febrile neutropenia · fever · fluid imbalance · gastrointestinal discomfort · gastrooesophageal reflux disease · haemorrhage · headaches · heart failure · hyperglycaemia · hypertension · hypertriglyceridaemia · hyperuricaemia · hypothyroidism · increased risk of infection · influenza like illness · insomnia · ischaemic heart disease · lethargy · mass · muscle complaints · nausea · oedema · pain · pancreatitis · pancytopenia · pericardial effusion · peripheral neuropathy · peripheral vascular disease · pleural effusion · pulmonary hypertension · sensation abnormal · sepsis · skin reactions · stomatitis · sweat changes · vasodilation · vision disorders · vomiting · weight decreased

▸ **Uncommon** Cardiac discomfort · cardiomyopathy ischaemic · coronary vasospasm · hepatic disorders · hepatic failure (including fatal cases) · intracranial haemorrhage · left ventricular dysfunction · posterior reversible encephalopathy syndrome (PRES) · renal artery stenosis · splenic infarction · tumour lysis syndrome

▸ **Frequency not known** Aneurysm · artery dissection

● CONCEPTION AND CONTRACEPTION Ensure effective contraception during treatment in men and women; effectiveness of hormonal contraception unknown—alternative or additional methods of contraception should be used.

- PREGNANCY Avoid—toxicity in *animal* studies. See also *Pregnancy and reproductive function* in Cytotoxic drugs p. 932.
- BREAST FEEDING Manufacturer advises discontinue breastfeeding—no information available.
- HEPATIC IMPAIRMENT Manufacturer advises caution.
- RENAL IMPAIRMENT No information available— manufacturer advises caution if creatinine clearance less than 50 mL/minute.
- MONITORING REQUIREMENTS
▸ Manufacturer advises monitor serum lipase every 2 weeks for the first 2 months and periodically thereafter— withhold treatment if lipase elevated and abdominal symptoms occur.
▸ Manufacturer advises a full blood count every 2 weeks for the first 3 months and then monthly thereafter or as clinically indicated.
▸ Manufacturer advises monitor liver function periodically.
▸ Manufacturer advises monitor for vascular occlusion or thromboembolism—interrupt treatment immediately if this occurs.
- NATIONAL FUNDING/ACCESS DECISIONS
For full details see funding body website
NICE decisions
▸ Ponatinib for treating chronic myeloid leukaemia and acute lymphoblastic leukaemia (June 2017) NICE TA451 Recommended

- MEDICINAL FORMS There can be variation in the licensing of different medicines containing the same drug.
Tablet
CAUTIONARY AND ADVISORY LABELS 3, 25
▸ Iclusig (Incyte Biosciences UK Ltd) ▼
Ponatinib (as Ponatinib hydrochloride) 15 mg Iclusig 15mg tablets | 30 tablet PoM £2,525.00
Ponatinib (as Ponatinib hydrochloride) 30 mg Iclusig 30mg tablets | 30 tablet PoM £5,050.00
Ponatinib (as Ponatinib hydrochloride) 45 mg Iclusig 45mg tablets | 30 tablet PoM £5,050.00

Regorafenib

31-Aug-2020

- DRUG ACTION Regorafenib is an inhibitor of several protein kinases.

● **INDICATIONS AND DOSE**

Metastatic colorectal cancer (specialist use only) | Unresectable or metastatic gastrointestinal stromal tumours (specialist use only) | Hepatocellular carcinoma (specialist use only)
▸ BY MOUTH
▸ Adult: 160 mg once daily for 21 consecutive days of repeated 28-day cycles, for dose adjustment due to side effects—consult product literature

IMPORTANT SAFETY INFORMATION
MHRA/CHM ADVICE: SYSTEMICALLY ADMINISTERED VEGF PATHWAY INHIBITORS: RISK OF ANEURYSM AND ARTERY DISSECTION (JULY 2020)
A European review of worldwide data concluded that systemically administered VEGF pathway inhibitors may lead to aneurysm and artery dissection in patients with or without hypertension. Some fatal cases have been reported, mainly in relation to aortic aneurysm rupture and aortic dissection. The MHRA advises healthcare professionals to carefully consider the risk of aneurysm and artery dissection in patients with risk factors before initiating treatment with regorafenib; any modifiable risk factors (such as smoking and hypertension) should be reduced as much as possible. Patients should be monitored and treated for hypertension as required.

RISKS OF INCORRECT DOSING OF ORAL ANTI-CANCER MEDICINES
See Cytotoxic drugs p. 932.

- CAUTIONS Ensure measures to prevent hand-foot skin reaction · Gilbert's syndrome—risk of hyperbilirubinaemia · history of ischaemic heart disease—monitor for signs and symptoms of myocardial ischaemia and interrupt treatment if signs of ischaemia or infarction develop · hypertension · may impair wound healing— withhold treatment for major surgical procedures · predisposition to bleeding · risk factors for aneurysm or artery dissection
CAUTIONS, FURTHER INFORMATION
▸ Monitoring of blood pressure The MHRA advises to monitor blood pressure regularly—consult product literature if hypertension occurs during treatment.
- INTERACTIONS → Appendix 1: regorafenib
- SIDE-EFFECTS
▸ Common or very common Alopecia · anaemia · appetite decreased · asthenia · diarrhoea · dry mouth · dysphonia · electrolyte imbalance · fever · gastrooesophageal reflux disease · headache · hyperbilirubinaemia · hypertension · hyperuricaemia · hypothyroidism · increased risk of infection · leucopenia · mucositis · musculoskeletal stiffness · nausea · pain · proteinuria · skin reactions · stomatitis · taste altered · thrombocytopenia · tremor · vomiting · weight decreased
▸ Uncommon Gastrointestinal fistula (discontinue) · gastrointestinal perforation (including fatal cases, discontinue) · hepatic disorders · myocardial infarction · myocardial ischaemia · nail disorder
▸ Rare or very rare Neoplasms · posterior reversible encephalopathy syndrome (PRES) · severe cutaneous adverse reactions (SCARs)
▸ Frequency not known Aneurysm · artery dissection
- CONCEPTION AND CONTRACEPTION Women of childbearing potential and men must use effective contraception during treatment and up to 8 weeks after last dose.
- PREGNANCY Manufacturer advises avoid unless potential benefit outweighs risk—toxicity in *animal* studies. See also *Pregnancy and reproductive function* in Cytotoxic drugs p. 932.
- BREAST FEEDING Avoid—present in milk in *animal* studies.
- HEPATIC IMPAIRMENT Manufacturer advises caution in moderate impairment (limited information available); avoid in severe impairment (no information available).
- RENAL IMPAIRMENT Caution in severe impairment—no information available.
- MONITORING REQUIREMENTS
▸ Monitor blood count and coagulation parameters and consider permanent discontinuation in event of severe bleeding.
▸ Monitor hepatic function before treatment, then at least every two weeks for the first 2 months, then at least monthly thereafter and as clinically indicated—consult product literature if changes in liver function observed.
▸ Monitor for signs and symptoms of posterior reversible encephalopathy syndrome (including seizure, headache, altered mental status, visual disturbances or cortical blindness, with or without hypertension)—discontinue treatment if symptoms occur.
▸ Monitor biochemical, electrolyte and metabolic parameters during treatment; ensure measures to prevent hand-foot skin reaction—consult product literature if signs or symptoms develop.
- DIRECTIONS FOR ADMINISTRATION Manufacturer advises tablets should be taken at the same time each day, swallowed whole with water after a light meal that contains less than 30% fat.

- PATIENT AND CARER ADVICE Counselling advised (administration).
- NATIONAL FUNDING/ACCESS DECISIONS
  For full details see funding body website

  NICE decisions

  ▸ Regorafenib for previously treated unresectable or metastatic gastrointestinal stromal tumours (November 2017) NICE TA488 Recommended with restrictions
  ▸ Regorafenib for previously treated advanced hepatocellular carcinoma (January 2019) NICE TA555 Recommended with restrictions

  Scottish Medicines Consortium (SMC) decisions

  ▸ Regorafenib (*Stivarga*®) as a monotherapy for the treatment of adult patients with hepatocellular carcinoma (HCC) who have been previously treated with sorafenib (May 2018) SMC No. 1316/18 Recommended

- MEDICINAL FORMS There can be variation in the licensing of different medicines containing the same drug.

  Tablet
  CAUTIONARY AND ADVISORY LABELS 21
  ELECTROLYTES: May contain Sodium
  ▸ Stivarga (Bayer Plc)
  Regorafenib 40 mg Stivarga 40mg tablets | 84 tablet PoM £3,744.00 (Hospital only)

▌Ribociclib

12-Nov-2020

- DRUG ACTION Ribociclib is an inhibitor of cyclin-dependent kinases 4 and 6, which are involved in cancer cell proliferation; their inhibition results in prevention of cancer cell growth.

- **INDICATIONS AND DOSE**

  Locally advanced or metastatic breast cancer (specialist use only)
  ▸ BY MOUTH
  ▸ Adult: 600 mg once daily for 21 consecutive days of repeated 28 day cycles, to be taken at approximately the same time each day, preferably in the morning, for dose adjustments due to side-effects—consult product literature

  DOSE ADJUSTMENTS DUE TO INTERACTIONS
  ▸ Manufacturer advises if concurrent use of potent inhibitors of CYP3A4 is unavoidable, reduce dose to 400 mg once daily; in those already taking 400 mg once daily, reduce dose to 200 mg once daily.

  > IMPORTANT SAFETY INFORMATION
  > RISKS OF INCORRECT DOSING OF ORAL ANTI-CANCER MEDICINES
  > See Cytotoxic drugs p. 932.

- CONTRA-INDICATIONS Pre-existing QTc prolongation · risk factors for QTc prolongation (including concomitant use of drugs known to prolong QTc interval)
- INTERACTIONS → Appendix 1: ribociclib
- SIDE-EFFECTS
  ▸ **Common or very common** Alopecia · anaemia · appetite decreased · asthenia · back pain · constipation · cough · decreased leucocytes · diarrhoea · dizziness · dry eye · dry mouth · dyspnoea · electrolyte imbalance · excessive tearing · fever · gastrointestinal discomfort · headache · hepatic disorders · increased risk of infection · nausea · neutropenia · oropharyngeal pain · peripheral oedema · QT interval prolongation · sepsis · skin reactions · stomatitis · syncope · taste altered · thrombocytopenia · vertigo · vomiting
- ALLERGY AND CROSS-SENSITIVITY Contra-indicated in patients with hypersensitivity to peanut or soya products.

- HEPATIC IMPAIRMENT Manufacturer advises caution in moderate to severe impairment (risk of increased exposure).
  Dose adjustments Manufacturer advises initial dose reduction to 400 mg once daily in moderate to severe impairment.
- RENAL IMPAIRMENT Manufacturer advises use with caution in severe renal impairment—limited information available.
- MONITORING REQUIREMENTS
  ▸ Manufacturer advises to perform full blood counts and liver function tests before initiating treatment, every 2 weeks for the first 2 cycles, at the beginning of the subsequent 4 cycles, and then as clinically indicated thereafter.
  ▸ Manufacturer advises to assess ECG before initiating treatment (only initiate treatment in patients with QTcF values <450 milliseconds); ECG should be repeated at approx. day 14 of the first cycle and at the beginning of the second cycle, then as clinically indicated.
  ▸ Manufacturer advises to monitor serum electrolytes (including potassium, calcium, phosphorus and magnesium) before initiating treatment, at the beginning of the first 6 cycles and then as clinically indicated; any abnormality should be corrected before initiating treatment.
- NATIONAL FUNDING/ACCESS DECISIONS
  For full details see funding body website

  NICE decisions

  ▸ Ribociclib with an aromatase inhibitor for previously untreated, hormone receptor-positive, HER2-negative, locally advanced or metastatic breast cancer (December 2017) NICE TA496 Recommended
  ▸ Ribociclib with fulvestrant for treating hormone receptor-positive, HER2-negative, advanced breast cancer (August 2019) NICE TA593 Recommended with restrictions

  Scottish Medicines Consortium (SMC) decisions

  ▸ Ribociclib (*Kisqali*®) for use in combination with an aromatase inhibitor, for the treatment of postmenopausal women with hormone receptor (HR)-positive, human epidermal growth factor receptor 2 (HER2)-negative locally advanced or metastatic breast cancer as initial endocrine-based therapy (March 2018) SMC No. 1295/18 Recommended
  ▸ Ribociclib (*Kisqali*®) for the treatment of women with hormone receptor (HR)-positive, human epidermal growth factor receptor 2 (HER2)-negative locally advanced or metastatic breast cancer in combination with fulvestrant as initial endocrine-based therapy, or in women who have received prior endocrine therapy (November 2019) SMC No. SMC2198 Recommended with restrictions

- MEDICINAL FORMS There can be variation in the licensing of different medicines containing the same drug.

  Tablet
  CAUTIONARY AND ADVISORY LABELS 3, 25
  ▸ Kisqali (Novartis Pharmaceuticals UK Ltd) ▼
  Ribociclib (as Ribociclib succinate) 200 mg Kisqali 200mg tablets | 21 tablet PoM £983.33 | 42 tablet PoM £1,966.67 | 63 tablet PoM £2,950.00

Ruxolitinib

27-Aug-2020

- **DRUG ACTION** Ruxolitinib is a selective inhibitor of the Janus-associated tyrosine kinases JAK1 and JAK2.

- **INDICATIONS AND DOSE**

Disease-related splenomegaly or symptoms [in patients with primary myelofibrosis, post-polycythaemia vera myelofibrosis, or post-essential thrombocythaemia myelofibrosis] (specialist use only) | Polycythaemia vera [in patients resistant to, or intolerant of, hydroxyurea] (specialist use only)
  - ▸ BY MOUTH
  - ▸ Adult: (consult product literature or local protocols)

IMPORTANT SAFETY INFORMATION

RISKS OF INCORRECT DOSING OF ORAL ANTI-CANCER MEDICINES
See Cytotoxic drugs p. 932.

- **CAUTIONS** Assess risk of developing infection before treatment—do not initiate until active serious infections are resolved

  CAUTIONS, FURTHER INFORMATION
  - ▸ Tuberculosis Patients should be evaluated for latent and active tuberculosis before starting treatment and monitored for signs and symptoms of tuberculosis during treatment.

- **INTERACTIONS** → Appendix 1: ruxolitinib

- **SIDE-EFFECTS**
  - ▸ **Common or very common** Anaemia · bruising · constipation · dizziness · dyslipidaemia · flatulence · haemorrhage · headache · hypertension · increased risk of infection · intracranial haemorrhage · neutropenia · sepsis · thrombocytopenia · weight increased

- **CONCEPTION AND CONTRACEPTION** Contraceptive advice required, see *Pregnancy and reproductive function* in Cytotoxic drugs p. 932.

- **PREGNANCY** Avoid—toxicity in *animal* studies.

- **BREAST FEEDING** Avoid—present in milk in *animal* studies.

- **HEPATIC IMPAIRMENT** Manufacturer advises caution.
  Dose adjustments Manufacturer advises initial dose reduction—consult product literature.

- **RENAL IMPAIRMENT**
  Dose adjustments Reduce dose in severe impairment (consult product literature).

- **MONITORING REQUIREMENTS**
  - ▸ Monitor full blood count (including differential white cell count) before treatment, then every 2–4 weeks until dose stabilised, then as clinically indicated.
  - ▸ Monitor for infection during treatment.
  - ▸ Monitor for symptoms of progressive multifocal leucoencephalopathy (presenting as new or worsening neurological, cognitive or psychiatric signs or symptoms)—withhold treatment if suspected.

- **NATIONAL FUNDING/ACCESS DECISIONS**
  For full details see funding body website

  NICE decisions
  - ▸ Ruxolitinib for treating disease-related splenomegaly or symptoms in adults with myelofibrosis (March 2016) NICE TA386 Recommended with restrictions

  Scottish Medicines Consortium (SMC) decisions
  - ▸ Ruxolitinib (*Jakavi*®) for the treatment of adult patients with polycythaemia vera (PV) who are resistant to or intolerant of hydroxyurea (HU) (December 2019) SMC No. SMC2213 Recommended

- **MEDICINAL FORMS** There can be variation in the licensing of different medicines containing the same drug.
  Tablet
  - ▸ Jakavi (Novartis Pharmaceuticals UK Ltd)
    Ruxolitinib (as Ruxolitinib phosphate) 5 mg Jakavi 5mg tablets | 56 tablet [PoM] £1,428.00 DT = £1,428.00
    Ruxolitinib (as Ruxolitinib phosphate) 10 mg Jakavi 10mg tablets | 56 tablet [PoM] £2,856.00 DT = £2,856.00
    Ruxolitinib (as Ruxolitinib phosphate) 15 mg Jakavi 15mg tablets | 56 tablet [PoM] £2,856.00 DT = £2,856.00
    Ruxolitinib (as Ruxolitinib phosphate) 20 mg Jakavi 20mg tablets | 56 tablet [PoM] £2,856.00 DT = £2,856.00

Sorafenib

13-Nov-2020

- **DRUG ACTION** Sorafenib is an inhibitor of multiple kinases.

- **INDICATIONS AND DOSE**

Treatment of advanced renal cell carcinoma when treatment with interferon alfa or interleukin-2 has failed or is unsuitable | Treatment of progressive, locally advanced, or metastatic, differentiated thyroid carcinoma that is refractory to radioactive iodine | Treatment of hepatocellular carcinoma
  - ▸ BY MOUTH
  - ▸ Adult: 400 mg twice daily, for dose adjustments due to side effects, consult product literature

---

IMPORTANT SAFETY INFORMATION

MHRA/CHM ADVICE: SYSTEMICALLY ADMINISTERED VEGF PATHWAY INHIBITORS: RISK OF ANEURYSM AND ARTERY DISSECTION (JULY 2020)

A European review of worldwide data concluded that systemically administered VEGF pathway inhibitors may lead to aneurysm and artery dissection in patients with or without hypertension. Some fatal cases have been reported, mainly in relation to aortic aneurysm rupture and aortic dissection. The MHRA advises healthcare professionals to carefully consider the risk of aneurysm and artery dissection in patients with risk factors before initiating treatment with sorafenib; any modifiable risk factors (such as smoking and hypertension) should be reduced as much as possible. Patients should be monitored and treated for hypertension as required.

RISKS OF INCORRECT DOSING OF ORAL ANTI-CANCER MEDICINES
See Cytotoxic drugs p. 932.

- **CAUTIONS** Cardiac ischaemia · hypertension · major surgical procedures · potential risk of bleeding—treat tracheal, bronchial, or oesophageal infiltration with localised therapy before initiating sorafenib in patients with differentiated thyroid carcinoma (DTC) and consider permanent withdrawal of sorafenib in any patient that requires medical intervention for bleeding · risk factors for aneurysm or artery dissection · susceptibility to QT-interval prolongation

  CAUTIONS, FURTHER INFORMATION
  - ▸ Monitoring of blood pressure The MHRA advises to monitor blood pressure regularly—consult product literature if hypertension occurs during treatment.

- **INTERACTIONS** → Appendix 1: sorafenib

- **SIDE-EFFECTS**
  - ▸ **Common or very common** Alopecia · anaemia · appetite decreased · arthralgia · asthenia · congestive heart failure · constipation · decreased leucocytes · depression · diarrhoea · dry mouth · dysphagia · dysphonia · electrolyte imbalance · erectile dysfunction · fever · flushing · gastrointestinal discomfort · gastrointestinal disorders · haemorrhage · headache · hypertension · hypothyroidism · increased risk of infection · influenza like illness · intracranial haemorrhage · mucositis · muscle complaints · myocardial

infarction · myocardial ischaemia · nausea · neoplasms · neutropenia · oral disorders · pain · peripheral neuropathy · proteinuria · renal failure · rhinorrhoea · skin reactions · taste altered · thrombocytopenia · tinnitus · vomiting · weight decreased

▶ **Uncommon** Cholangitis · cholecystitis · dehydration · encephalopathy · gynaecomastia · hepatic disorders · hyperthyroidism · pancreatitis · radiation injuries · respiratory disorders

▶ **Rare or very rare** Angioedema · hypersensitivity vasculitis · nephrotic syndrome · QT interval prolongation · rhabdomyolysis · severe cutaneous adverse reactions (SCARs)

▶ **Frequency not known** Aneurysm · artery dissection

● CONCEPTION AND CONTRACEPTION Contraceptive advice required, see *Pregnancy and reproductive function* in Cytotoxic drugs p. 932.

● PREGNANCY Manufacturer advises avoid unless essential—toxicity in *animal* studies. See also *Pregnancy and reproductive function* in Cytotoxic drugs p. 932.

● BREAST FEEDING Discontinue breast-feeding.

● HEPATIC IMPAIRMENT Manufacturer advises caution in severe impairment (no information available).

● MONITORING REQUIREMENTS
▶ Consider periodic monitoring of ECG and electrolytes in patients susceptible to QT-interval prolongation.
▶ Monitor plasma-calcium concentration (increased risk of hypocalcaemia if history of hypoparathyroidism).
▶ Monitor thyroid stimulating hormone in patients with differentiated thyroid carcinoma.

● NATIONAL FUNDING/ACCESS DECISIONS
For full details see funding body website

NICE decisions
▶ Bevacizumab (first-line), sorafenib (first- and second-line), sunitinib (second-line) and temsirolimus (first-line) for the treatment of advanced and/or metastatic renal cell carcinoma (August 2009) NICE TA178 Not recommended
▶ Sorafenib for treating advanced hepatocellular carcinoma (September 2017) NICE TA474 Recommended with restrictions
▶ Lenvatinib and sorafenib for treating differentiated thyroid cancer after radioactive iodine (August 2018) NICE TA535 Recommended with restrictions

Scottish Medicines Consortium (SMC) decisions
▶ Sorafenib (*Nexavar*®) for the treatment of hepatocellular carcinoma (January 2016) SMC No. 482/08 Recommended with restrictions

● MEDICINAL FORMS There can be variation in the licensing of different medicines containing the same drug.
Tablet
CAUTIONARY AND ADVISORY LABELS 23
▶ Nexavar (Bayer Plc)
Sorafenib (as Sorafenib tosylate) 200 mg Nexavar 200mg tablets | 112 tablet [PoM] £3,576.56

Sunitinib

26-Nov-2020

● DRUG ACTION Sunitinib is a tyrosine kinase inhibitor.

● INDICATIONS AND DOSE

Treatment of unresectable or metastatic malignant gastro-intestinal stromal tumours, after failure of imatinib | Treatment of advanced or metastatic renal cell carcinoma
▶ BY MOUTH
▶ Adult: 50 mg once daily for 4 weeks, followed by a 2-week treatment-free period to complete 6-week cycle, adjusted in steps of 12.5 mg, doses adjusted according to tolerability; usual dose 25–75 mg daily

Treatment of unresectable or metastatic pancreatic neuroendocrine tumours
▶ BY MOUTH
▶ Adult: 37.5 mg once daily without treatment-free period; adjusted in steps of 12.5 mg, doses adjusted according to tolerability; maximum 50 mg per day

DOSE ADJUSTMENTS DUE TO INTERACTIONS
▶ Manufacturer advises if concurrent use of potent inducers of CYP3A4 is unavoidable, dose may need to be increased in steps of 12.5 mg to a max. dose of 87.5 mg per day for gastro-intestinal stromal tumours or renal cell carcinoma, or to a max. dose of 62.5 mg per day for pancreatic neuroendocrine tumours.
▶ Manufacturer advises if concurrent use of potent inhibitors of CYP3A4 is unavoidable, dose may need to be decreased to a minimum of 37.5 mg per day for gastrointestinal stromal tumours or renal cell carcinoma, or to a minimum of 25 mg per day for pancreatic neuroendocrine tumours.

IMPORTANT SAFETY INFORMATION
MHRA/CHM ADVICE: BEVACIZUMAB AND SUNITINIB: RISK OF OSTEONECROSIS OF THE JAW (JANUARY 2011)
Treatment with bevacizumab or sunitinib may be a risk factor for the development of osteonecrosis of the jaw.
Patients treated with bevacizumab or sunitinib, who have previously received bisphosphonates, or are treated concurrently with bisphosphonates, may be particularly at risk.
Dental examination and appropriate preventive dentistry should be considered before treatment with bevacizumab or sunitinib.
If possible, invasive dental procedures should be avoided in patients treated with bevacizumab or sunitinib who have previously received, or who are currently receiving, intravenous bisphosphonates.

MHRA/CHM ADVICE: SYSTEMICALLY ADMINISTERED VEGF PATHWAY INHIBITORS: RISK OF ANEURYSM AND ARTERY DISSECTION (JULY 2020)
A European review of worldwide data concluded that systemically administered VEGF pathway inhibitors may lead to aneurysm and artery dissection in patients with or without hypertension. Some fatal cases have been reported, mainly in relation to aortic aneurysm rupture and aortic dissection. The MHRA advises healthcare professionals to carefully consider the risk of aneurysm and artery dissection in patients with risk factors before initiating treatment with sunitinib; any modifiable risk factors (such as smoking and hypertension) should be reduced as much as possible. Patients should be monitored and treated for hypertension as required.

RISKS OF INCORRECT DOSING OF ORAL ANTI-CANCER MEDICINES
See Cytotoxic drugs p. 932.

● CAUTIONS Cardiovascular disease—discontinue if congestive heart failure develops · hypertension · increased risk of bleeding · risk factors for aneurysm or artery dissection · susceptibility to QT-interval prolongation

CAUTIONS, FURTHER INFORMATION
▶ Monitoring of blood pressure The MHRA advises to monitor blood pressure regularly—consult product literature if hypertension occurs during treatment.

● INTERACTIONS → Appendix 1: sunitinib

● SIDE-EFFECTS
▶ **Common or very common** Abscess · alopecia · anaemia · appetite decreased · arthralgia · burping · chest pain · chills · constipation · cough · dehydration · depression · diarrhoea · dizziness · dry mouth · dysphagia · dyspnoea · embolism and thrombosis · excessive tearing · eye inflammation · fatigue · fever · gastrointestinal discomfort · gastrointestinal disorders · haemorrhage · hair colour

changes · headache · hypertension · hypoglycaemia · hypothyroidism · increased risk of infection · influenza like illness · insomnia · leucopenia · mucositis · muscle complaints · muscle weakness · myocardial ischaemia · nail disorder · nasal complaints · nausea · neutropenia · oedema · oral disorders · oropharyngeal pain · pain · peripheral neuropathy · proteinuria · renal impairment · respiratory disorders · sensation abnormal · sepsis · skin reactions · taste altered · thrombocytopenia · urine discolouration · vasodilation · vomiting · weight decreased

▸ **Uncommon** Anal fistula (interrupt treatment) · cardiomyopathy · cerebrovascular insufficiency · cholecystitis · fistula (interrupt treatment) · healing impaired · heart failure · hepatic disorders · hypersensitivity · hyperthyroidism · intracranial haemorrhage · myocardial infarction · osteonecrosis of jaw · pancreatitis · pancytopenia · pericardial effusion · QT interval prolongation · tumour haemorrhage

▸ **Rare or very rare** Angioedema · myopathy · nephrotic syndrome · posterior reversible encephalopathy syndrome (PRES) · pyoderma gangrenosum · severe cutaneous adverse reactions (SCARs) · thrombotic microangiopathy · thyroiditis · torsade de pointes · tumour lysis syndrome

▸ **Frequency not known** Aneurysm · aortic dissection · artery dissection

● CONCEPTION AND CONTRACEPTION Effective contraception required during treatment.

● PREGNANCY Manufacturer advises avoid unless potential benefit outweighs risk—toxicity in *animal* studies. See also *Pregnancy and reproductive function* in Cytotoxic drugs p. 932.

● BREAST FEEDING Discontinue breast-feeding.

● MONITORING REQUIREMENTS Monitor for thyroid dysfunction.

● NATIONAL FUNDING/ACCESS DECISIONS
For full details see funding body website

NICE decisions

▸ Sunitinib for the first-line treatment of advanced and/or metastatic renal cell carcinoma (March 2009) NICE TA169 Recommended

▸ Sunitinib for the treatment of gastrointestinal stromal tumours (September 2009) NICE TA179 Recommended with restrictions

▸ Bevacizumab (first-line), sorafenib (first- and second-line), sunitinib (second-line) and temsirolimus (first-line) for the treatment of advanced and/or metastatic renal cell carcinoma (August 2009) NICE TA178 Not recommended

▸ Everolimus and sunitinib for treating unresectable or metastatic neuroendocrine tumours in people with progressive disease (June 2017) NICE TA449 Recommended

Scottish Medicines Consortium (SMC) decisions

▸ Sunitinib (*Sutent*®) for unresectable and/or metastatic malignant gastrointestinal stromal tumour (GIST) after failure of imatinib mesylate treatment due to resistance or intolerance (November 2009) SMC No. 275/06 Recommended

● MEDICINAL FORMS There can be variation in the licensing of different medicines containing the same drug.

Capsule
CAUTIONARY AND ADVISORY LABELS 14
▸ Sutent (Pfizer Ltd)
     Sunitinib (as Sunitinib malate) 12.5 mg   Sutent 12.5mg capsules | 28 capsule PoM £784.70 (Hospital only)
     Sunitinib (as Sunitinib malate) 25 mg   Sutent 25mg capsules | 28 capsule PoM £1,569.40 (Hospital only)
     Sunitinib (as Sunitinib malate) 50 mg   Sutent 50mg capsules | 28 capsule PoM £3,138.80 (Hospital only)

| Temsirolimus

22-Jun-2020

● DRUG ACTION Temsirolimus is a protein kinase inhibitor.

● **INDICATIONS AND DOSE**

First-line treatment of advanced renal cell carcinoma | Treatment of relapsed or refractory mantle cell lymphoma

▸ BY INTRAVENOUS INFUSION
   ▸ Adult: (consult product literature or local protocols)

● INTERACTIONS → Appendix 1: temsirolimus

● SIDE-EFFECTS

▸ **Common or very common** Abscess · anaemia · anxiety · appetite decreased · arthralgia · asthenia · chest pain · chills · conjunctivitis · constipation · cough · cystitis · decreased leucocytes · dehydration · depression · diabetes mellitus · diarrhoea · dizziness · drowsiness · dyslipidaemia · dysphagia · dyspnoea · electrolyte imbalance · embolism and thrombosis · fever · gastrointestinal discomfort · gastrointestinal disorders · genital oedema · haemorrhage · headache · hypersensitivity · hypertension · increased risk of infection · insomnia · lacrimation disorder · mucositis · myalgia · nail disorder · nausea · neutropenia · oedema · oral disorders · pain · paraesthesia · post procedural infection · renal failure · respiratory disorders · scrotal oedema · sepsis · skin reactions · taste altered · thrombocytopenia · vomiting

▸ **Uncommon** Healing impaired · intracranial haemorrhage · pericardial effusion

SIDE-EFFECTS, FURTHER INFORMATION Hypersensitivity reactions, including some life-threatening and rare fatal reactions, are associated with temsirolimus therapy. Symptoms include flushing, chest pain, dyspnoea, apnoea, hypotension, loss of consciousness, and anaphylaxis. Patients should receive an intravenous dose of antihistamine 30 minutes before starting the temsirolimus infusion. The infusion may have to be stopped temporarily for the treatment of infusion-related effects—consult product literature for appropriate management. If adverse reactions are not managed with dose delays, a dose reduction should be considered—consult product literature.

● CONCEPTION AND CONTRACEPTION Ensure effective contraception during treatment in men and women.

● PREGNANCY Manufacturer advises avoid (toxicity in *animal* studies). See also *Pregnancy and reproductive function* in Cytotoxic drugs p. 932.

● BREAST FEEDING Manufacturer advises discontinue breast-feeding.

● HEPATIC IMPAIRMENT
▸ When used for Renal cell carcinoma Manufacturer advises caution.
▸ When used for Mantle cell lymphoma Manufacturer advises caution in mild impairment; avoid in moderate to severe impairment.

Dose adjustments
   ▸ When used for Renal cell carcinoma Manufacturer advises dose reduction in severe impairment—consult product literature.

● RENAL IMPAIRMENT Manufacturer advises caution in severe impairment—no information available.

● MONITORING REQUIREMENTS
▸ Monitor respiratory function.
▸ Monitor blood lipids.

● NATIONAL FUNDING/ACCESS DECISIONS
For full details see funding body website

NICE decisions

▸ Bevacizumab (first-line), sorafenib (first- and second-line), sunitinib (second-line) and temsirolimus (first-line) for the treatment of advanced and/or metastatic renal cell carcinoma (August 2009) NICE TA178 Not recommended

● MEDICINAL FORMS There can be variation in the licensing of different medicines containing the same drug.

Solution for infusion

EXCIPIENTS: May contain Ethanol, propylene glycol
▸ Torisel (Pfizer Ltd)
Temsirolimus 25 mg per 1 ml Torisel 30mg/1.2ml concentrate for solution for infusion vials and diluent | 1 vial PoM £620.00 (Hospital only)

Tivozanib

11-Nov-2020

● DRUG ACTION Tivozanib is a tyrosine kinase inhibitor.

● **INDICATIONS AND DOSE**

Advanced renal cell carcinoma (specialist use only)
▸ BY MOUTH
▸ Adult: 1340 micrograms once daily for 21 consecutive days of repeated 28 day cycles, for dose adjustments due to side effects—consult product literature

---

IMPORTANT SAFETY INFORMATION

MHRA/CHM ADVICE: SYSTEMICALLY ADMINISTERED VEGF PATHWAY INHIBITORS: RISK OF ANEURYSM AND ARTERY DISSECTION (JULY 2020)

A European review of worldwide data concluded that systemically administered VEGF pathway inhibitors may lead to aneurysm and artery dissection in patients with or without hypertension. Some fatal cases have been reported, mainly in relation to aortic aneurysm rupture and aortic dissection. The MHRA advises healthcare professionals to carefully consider the risk of aneurysm and artery dissection in patients with risk factors before initiating treatment with tivozanib; any modifiable risk factors (such as smoking and hypertension) should be reduced as much as possible. Patients should be monitored and treated for hypertension as required.

RISKS OF INCORRECT DOSING OF ORAL ANTI-CANCER MEDICINES
See Cytotoxic drugs p. 932.

● CAUTIONS History of arterial thromboembolic events · history of bleeding disorders · history of posterior reversible encephalopathy syndrome following tivozanib treatment · history of QT-interval prolongation · history of venous thromboembolic events · hypertension · major surgical procedures—interrupt treatment · patients aged over 65 years—increased risk of adverse effects · pre-existing cardiac disease · risk factors for aneurysm or artery dissection · risk factors for arterial thromboembolic events · risk factors for gastro-intestinal perforation · risk factors for venous thromboembolic events · risk of bleeding

CAUTIONS, FURTHER INFORMATION
▸ Monitoring of blood pressure The MHRA advises to monitor blood pressure regularly—consult product literature if hypertension occurs during treatment.

● INTERACTIONS → Appendix 1: tivozanib

● SIDE-EFFECTS
▸ **Common or very common** Alopecia · anaemia · angina pectoris · appetite decreased · arrhythmias · arthralgia · asthenia · cancer pain · cerebrovascular insufficiency · chest pain · chills · constipation · cough · diarrhoea · dizziness · dry mouth · dysphonia · dyspnoea · embolism and thrombosis · fever · gastrointestinal discomfort · gastrointestinal disorders · haemorrhage · headache · hypertension · hypothermia · hypothyroidism · increased risk of infection · insomnia · ischaemia · myalgia · myocardial infarction · nasal complaints · nausea · nerve disorders · oral disorders · oropharyngeal pain · pain · pancreatitis · peripheral oedema · proteinuria · sensation

abnormal · skin reactions · swallowing difficulty · taste altered · tinnitus · vasodilation · vertigo · vision disorders · vomiting · weight decreased
▸ **Uncommon** Coronary artery insufficiency · ear congestion · excessive tearing · goitre · hyperhidrosis · hyperthyroidism · memory loss · mucositis · muscle weakness · pulmonary oedema · QT interval prolongation · thrombocytopenia · toxic nodular goitre
▸ **Rare or very rare** Posterior reversible encephalopathy syndrome (PRES)
▸ **Frequency not known** Aneurysm · artery dissection · heart failure

● CONCEPTION AND CONTRACEPTION Manufacturer advises effective contraception in men, women of childbearing potential, and their partners during treatment and for at least one month after the last dose; an additional barrier method of contraception should be used in women using hormonal contraceptives. See also *Pregnancy and reproductive function* in Cytotoxic drugs p. 932.

● PREGNANCY Manufacturer advises avoid—toxicity in *animal* studies. See also *Pregnancy and reproductive function* in Cytotoxic drugs p. 932.

● BREAST FEEDING Manufacturer advises avoid—no information available.

● HEPATIC IMPAIRMENT Manufacturer advises caution in mild-to-moderate impairment—monitor patients for tolerability; avoid in severe impairment.
Dose adjustments Manufacturer advises reduce dose to 1340 micrograms on alternate days in moderate impairment—increased risk of adverse effects due to increased exposure.

● RENAL IMPAIRMENT Manufacturer advises caution in severe impairment—limited information available.

● MONITORING REQUIREMENTS
▸ Manufacturer advises perform liver function tests (including ALT, AST and AP) before and during treatment; monitor for proteinuria before treatment and periodically thereafter.
▸ Manufacturer advises monitor for signs or symptoms of cardiac failure during treatment.
▸ Manufacturer advises perform baseline ECG and monitor electrolytes before treatment and as clinically indicated thereafter.
▸ Manufacturer advises monitor thyroid function before treatment and periodically thereafter.
▸ Manufacturer advises monitor for symptoms of gastro-intestinal perforation or fistula.

● NATIONAL FUNDING/ACCESS DECISIONS
For full details see funding body website
NICE decisions
▸ Tivozanib for treating advanced renal cell carcinoma (March 2018) NICE TA512 Recommended with restrictions
Scottish Medicines Consortium (SMC) decisions
▸ Tivozanib (*Fotivda®*) for the first-line treatment of adult patients with advanced renal cell carcinoma (RCC) and for adult patients who are vascular endothelial growth factor receptor and mammalian target of rapamycin pathway inhibitor-naive following disease progression after one prior treatment with cytokine therapy for advanced RCC (July 2018) SMC No. 1335/18 Recommended with restrictions

● MEDICINAL FORMS There can be variation in the licensing of different medicines containing the same drug.

Capsule
CAUTIONARY AND ADVISORY LABELS 25
▸ Fotivda (EUSA Pharma Ltd) ▼
Tivozanib (as Tivozanib hydrochloride monohydrate).89 mg Fotivda 890microgram capsules | 21 capsule PoM £2,052.00 (Hospital only)

Tivozanib (as Tivozanib hydrochloride monohydrate)
1.34 mg Fotivda 1340microgram capsules | 21 capsule [PoM]
£2,052.00 (Hospital only)

Trametinib
16-Nov-2020

● DRUG ACTION Trametinib is a protein kinase inhibitor.

● INDICATIONS AND DOSE
Unresectable or metastatic melanoma with a BRAF V600 mutation (as monotherapy or in combination with dabrafenib) (specialist use only) | Advanced non-small cell lung cancer with a BRAF V600 mutation (in combination with dabrafenib) (specialist use only)
▶ BY MOUTH
▶ Adult: 2 mg once daily, when used in combination with dabrafenib, the dose should be taken at the same time each day with *either* the morning or evening dose of dabrafenib, for dose adjustments due to side-effects, consult product literature

Adjuvant treatment of stage III melanoma with a BRAF V600 mutation following complete resection (in combination with dabrafenib) (specialist use only)
▶ BY MOUTH
▶ Adult: 2 mg once daily for 12 months, the dose should be taken at the same time each day with *either* the morning or evening dose of dabrafenib, for dose adjustments due to side-effects, consult product literature

---

IMPORTANT SAFETY INFORMATION
MHRA/CHM ADVICE (MARCH 2016): TRAMETINIB: RISK OF GASTROINTESTINAL PERFORATION AND COLITIS
A review by EU medicines regulators has concluded that trametinib can cause gastrointestinal perforation or colitis.
Trametinib should be used with caution in patients with risk factors for gastrointestinal perforation, such as gastrointestinal metastases, diverticulitis, or use of concomitant medicines that can cause gastrointestinal perforation. Prescribers should be vigilant for signs and symptoms of gastrointestinal perforation and should advise patients to seek urgent medical attention if they develop severe abdominal pain.

RISKS OF INCORRECT DOSING OF ORAL ANTI-CANCER MEDICINES
See Cytotoxic drugs p. 932.

● CONTRA-INDICATIONS History of retinal vein occlusion
● CAUTIONS Concomitant antiplatelet or anticoagulant therapy—increased risk of haemorrhage · conditions that could impair left ventricular function · elderly (more frequent dose adjustments may be required) · impaired left ventricular function · predisposing factors for retinal vein occlusion · risk factors for gastrointestinal perforation
● INTERACTIONS → Appendix 1: trametinib
● SIDE-EFFECTS
▶ **Common or very common** Abdominal pain · alopecia · anaemia · asthenia · bradycardia · constipation · cough · dehydration · diarrhoea · dry mouth · dyspnoea · eye inflammation · fever · haemorrhage · hypersensitivity · hypertension · increased risk of infection · intracranial haemorrhage · left ventricular dysfunction · lymphoedema · mucositis · nausea · oedema · respiratory disorders · skin reactions · stomatitis · vision disorders · vomiting
▶ **Uncommon** Chorioretinopathy · gastrointestinal disorders · heart failure · retinal detachment · retinal occlusion · rhabdomyolysis
SIDE-EFFECTS, FURTHER INFORMATION Additional side-effects reported when used in combination with dabrafenib include dizziness, hyperhidrosis,

hyponatraemia, hypotension, leucopenia, muscle spasms, myocarditis, neutropenia, night sweats, and thrombocytopenia.

● CONCEPTION AND CONTRACEPTION Manufacturer advises women of child-bearing potential should use highly effective non-hormonal contraception during, and for 4 months after stopping treatment.
● PREGNANCY Manufacturer advises avoid—toxicity in *animal* studies. See also *Pregnancy and reproductive function* in Cytotoxic drugs p. 932.
● BREAST FEEDING Manufacturer advises avoid—no information available.
● HEPATIC IMPAIRMENT Manufacturer advises caution in moderate to severe impairment (no information available).
● RENAL IMPAIRMENT Manufacturer advises caution in severe impairment—no information available.
● MONITORING REQUIREMENTS Manufacturer advises measure blood pressure at baseline and monitor during treatment; evaluate left ventricular ejection fraction before treatment, after one month of treatment, and then approximately every 3 months thereafter; monitor liver function every 4 weeks for 6 months after treatment initiation, and thereafter as clinically indicated.
● HANDLING AND STORAGE Manufacturer advises store in refrigerator (2–8 °C); once opened, bottle may be stored for 30 days at not more than 30 °C.
● PATIENT AND CARER ADVICE Manufacturer advises patients and their carers should be told to seek immediate medical attention if symptoms of pulmonary embolism or deep vein thrombosis occur; patients and their carers should also be reported to report new visual disturbances.
Missed doses Manufacturer advises if a dose is more than 12 hours late, the missed dose should not be taken and the next dose should be taken at the normal time.
Driving and skilled tasks Manufacturer advises patients and carers should be counselled on the effects on driving and performance of skilled tasks—risk of dizziness and visual disturbances.
● NATIONAL FUNDING/ACCESS DECISIONS
For full details see funding body website
NICE decisions
▶ Trametinib in combination with dabrafenib for treating unresectable or metastatic melanoma (June 2016) NICE TA396 Recommended with restrictions
▶ Dabrafenib with trametinib for adjuvant treatment of resected BRAF V600 mutation-positive melanoma (October 2018) NICE TA544 Recommended with restrictions
Scottish Medicines Consortium (SMC) decisions
▶ Trametinib (*Mekinist®*) in combination with dabrafenib for the treatment of adult patients with unresectable or metastatic melanoma with a BRAF V600 mutation (September 2016) SMC No. 1161/16 Recommended with restrictions

● MEDICINAL FORMS There can be variation in the licensing of different medicines containing the same drug.
Tablet
CAUTIONARY AND ADVISORY LABELS 3, 23, 25
▶ Mekinist (Novartis Pharmaceuticals UK Ltd)
Trametinib 500 microgram Mekinist 0.5mg tablets | 7 tablet [PoM]
£280.00 | 30 tablet [PoM] £1,200.00
Trametinib 2 mg Mekinist 2mg tablets | 7 tablet [PoM] £1,120.00 |
30 tablet [PoM] £4,800.00

Vandetanib

02-Sep-2020

- **DRUG ACTION** Vandetanib is a tyrosine kinase inhibitor.

- **INDICATIONS AND DOSE**

Treatment of aggressive and symptomatic medullary thyroid cancer in patients with unresectable locally advanced or metastatic disease
  - ▸ BY MOUTH
  - ▸ Adult: 300 mg once daily, for dose adjustment due to side effects—consult product literature

IMPORTANT SAFETY INFORMATION

MHRA/CHM ADVICE: SYSTEMICALLY ADMINISTERED VEGF PATHWAY INHIBITORS: RISK OF ANEURYSM AND ARTERY DISSECTION (JULY 2020)

A European review of worldwide data concluded that systemically administered VEGF pathway inhibitors may lead to aneurysm and artery dissection in patients with or without hypertension. Some fatal cases have been reported, mainly in relation to aortic aneurysm rupture and aortic dissection. The MHRA advises healthcare professionals to carefully consider the risk of aneurysm and artery dissection in patients with risk factors before initiating treatment with vandetanib; any modifiable risk factors (such as smoking and hypertension) should be reduced as much as possible. Patients should be monitored and treated for hypertension as required.

RISKS OF INCORRECT DOSING OF ORAL ANTI-CANCER MEDICINES
See Cytotoxic drugs p. 932.

- **CONTRA-INDICATIONS** Congenital long QT syndrome · QT interval greater than 480 milliseconds
- **CAUTIONS** Brain metastases (intracranial haemorrhage reported) · electrolyte disturbances · history of torsades de pointes · hypertension · phototoxicity reactions reported (wear protective clothing and/or sunscreen) · risk factors for aneurysm or artery dissection · susceptibility to QT-prolongation

CAUTIONS, FURTHER INFORMATION
- ▸ Monitoring of blood pressure The MHRA advises to monitor blood pressure regularly—consult product literature if hypertension occurs during treatment.
- **INTERACTIONS** → Appendix 1: vandetanib
- **SIDE-EFFECTS**
- ▸ **Common or very common** Alopecia · anxiety · appetite decreased · asthenia · cerebral ischaemia · cholelithiasis · constipation · corneal deposits · cystitis · dehydration · depression · diarrhoea · dizziness · dry eye · dry mouth · dysphagia · electrolyte imbalance · eye disorders · eye inflammation · fever · gastrointestinal discomfort · gastrointestinal disorders · glaucoma · haemorrhage · headache · hyperglycaemia · hypertension · hypothyroidism · increased risk of infection · insomnia · lethargy · loss of consciousness · movement disorders · nail disorder · nausea · nephrolithiasis · oedema · pain · photosensitivity reaction · proteinuria · QT interval prolongation · renal impairment · respiratory disorders · sensation abnormal · sepsis · skin reactions · stomatitis · taste altered · tremor · urinary disorders · vision disorders · vomiting · weight decreased
- ▸ **Uncommon** Arrhythmias · brain oedema · cardiac arrest · cardiac conduction disorder · cataract · healing impaired · heart failure · malnutrition · pancreatitis · posterior reversible encephalopathy syndrome (PRES) · seizure · urine discolouration
- ▸ **Frequency not known** Aneurysm · artery dissection · Stevens-Johnson syndrome
- **CONCEPTION AND CONTRACEPTION** Effective contraception required during and for at least 4 months after treatment.

- **PREGNANCY** Manufacturer advises avoid unless potential benefit outweighs risk. Most cytotoxic drugs are teratogenic and should not be administered during pregnancy, especially during the first trimester. Considerable caution is necessary if a pregnant woman presents with cancer requiring chemotherapy, and specialist advice should always be sought.
- **BREAST FEEDING** Avoid—no information available.
- **HEPATIC IMPAIRMENT** Manufacturer advises avoid if liver function tests exceed specific limits—consult product literature.
- **RENAL IMPAIRMENT** Avoid if creatinine clearance less than 30 mL/minute.
  Dose adjustments Reduce dose to 200 mg if creatinine clearance 30–49 mL/minute.
- **MONITORING REQUIREMENTS** Monitor ECG, serum potassium, calcium, magnesium and thyroid stimulating hormone before treatment, then 1, 3, 6 and 12 weeks after starting treatment and following dose adjustment or interruption, then every 3 months for at least 1 year.
- **DIRECTIONS FOR ADMINISTRATION** Manufacturer advises tablets may be dispersed in half a glass of water by stirring until dispersed (approximately 10 minutes), immediately before drinking (do not crush). After solution has been swallowed, any residue must be re-dispersed in the same volume of water and swallowed. The solution can also be administered via nasogastric or gastrostomy tubes.
- **PATIENT AND CARER ADVICE** Patients or carers should be given advice on how to administer vandetanib tablets. Phototoxicity reactions Patients should be advised to wear protective clothing and/or sunscreen.
  Alert card An alert card should be provided.
- **NATIONAL FUNDING/ACCESS DECISIONS**
  For full details see funding body website
  NICE decisions
  - ▸ Vandetanib for treating medullary thyroid cancer (December 2018) NICE TA550 Not recommended

- **MEDICINAL FORMS** There can be variation in the licensing of different medicines containing the same drug.
  Tablet
  - ▸ Caprelsa (Genzyme Therapeutics Ltd) ▼
    Vandetanib 100 mg Caprelsa 100mg tablets | 30 tablet [PoM]
    £2,500.00
    Vandetanib 300 mg Caprelsa 300mg tablets | 30 tablet [PoM]
    £5,000.00

Vemurafenib

02-Sep-2020

- **DRUG ACTION** Vemurafenib is a BRAF kinase inhibitor.

- **INDICATIONS AND DOSE**

Monotherapy for the treatment of BRAF V600 mutation-positive unresectable or metastatic melanoma
  - ▸ BY MOUTH
  - ▸ Adult: 960 mg twice daily, for dose adjustment due to side effects—consult product literature

IMPORTANT SAFETY INFORMATION

DRUG RASH WITH EOSINOPHILIA AND SYSTEMIC SYMPTOMS (DRESS SYNDROME)

DRESS syndrome has been reported in patients taking vemurafenib. DRESS syndrome starts with rash, fever, swollen glands, and increased white cell count, and it can affect the liver, kidneys and lungs; DRESS can also be fatal.

Patients should be advised to stop taking vemurafenib and consult their doctor immediately if skin rash develops. Treatment with vemurafenib should not be restarted.

MHRA/CHM ADVICE (NOVEMBER 2015): RISK OF POTENTIATION OF RADIATION TOXICITY

Potentiation of radiation toxicity has been reported in patients treated with vemurafenib before, during, or after radiotherapy— use with caution.

RISKS OF INCORRECT DOSING OF ORAL ANTI-CANCER MEDICINES

See Cytotoxic drugs p. 932.

- CONTRA-INDICATIONS Wild-type BRAF malignant melanoma
- CAUTIONS Electrolyte disturbances · prior or concurrent cancer associated with RAS mutation—increased risk of tumour progression · susceptibility to QT-prolongation
- INTERACTIONS → Appendix 1: vemurafenib
- SIDE-EFFECTS
  - ▸ **Common or very common** 7th nerve paralysis · alopecia · appetite decreased · arthralgia · arthritis · asthenia · connective tissue disorders · constipation · cough · diarrhoea · dizziness · eye inflammation · fever · folliculitis · headache · myalgia · nausea · neoplasms · pain · panniculitis · peripheral oedema · photosensitivity reaction · QT interval prolongation · radiation injuries · skin reactions · taste altered · vomiting · weight decreased
  - ▸ **Uncommon** Liver injury · neutropenia · pancreatitis · peripheral neuropathy · retinal occlusion · severe cutaneous adverse reactions (SCARs) · vasculitis
  - ▸ **Rare or very rare** Acute tubular necrosis · nephritis acute interstitial
  - ▸ **Frequency not known** Acute kidney injury
- CONCEPTION AND CONTRACEPTION Effective contraception required during for at least 6 months after treatment.
- PREGNANCY Manufacturer advises avoid unless potential benefit outweighs risk. See also *Pregnancy and reproductive function* in Cytotoxic drugs p. 932.
- BREAST FEEDING Avoid—no information available.
- HEPATIC IMPAIRMENT Manufacturer advises caution in moderate to severe impairment (risk of increased exposure)—monitor ECG monthly during the first 3 months of treatment, followed by at least every 3 months thereafter (if QTc interval is prolonged, consult product literature).
- RENAL IMPAIRMENT Manufacturer advises caution in severe impairment.
- MONITORING REQUIREMENTS
  - ▸ Monitor ECG and electrolytes before treatment, after one month and following dose adjustment (treatment not recommended if QT interval greater than 500 milliseconds at baseline).
  - ▸ Monitor liver function before treatment and periodically thereafter.
  - ▸ Monitor for uveitis, iritis and retinal vein occlusion.
  - ▸ Monitor for cutaneous and non-cutaneous squamous cell carcinoma and new primary melanoma before, during and for up to 6 months after treatment—consult product literature.
- DIRECTIONS FOR ADMINISTRATION Manufacturer advises may be taken with or without food; avoid consistent intake of both daily doses on an empty stomach (may affect absorption).
- PATIENT AND CARER ADVICE Counselling advised (administration).

  Drug rash with eosinophilia and systemic symptoms (DRESS syndrome) Patients should be advised to stop taking vemurafenib and consult their doctor immediately if skin rash develops.
- NATIONAL FUNDING/ACCESS DECISIONS
  For full details see funding body website

NICE decisions
- ▸ Vemurafenib for treating locally advanced or metastatic BRAF V600 mutation-positive malignant melanoma (updated January 2015) NICE TA269 Recommended with restrictions

Scottish Medicines Consortium (SMC) decisions
- ▸ Vemurafenib (*Zelboraf*®) as monotherapy for the treatment of adult patients with BRAF V600 mutation-positive unresectable or metastatic melanoma (December 2013) SMC No. 792/12 Recommended with restrictions

- MEDICINAL FORMS There can be variation in the licensing of different medicines containing the same drug.

Tablet

CAUTIONARY AND ADVISORY LABELS 25
- ▸ Zelboraf (Roche Products Ltd)
  Vemurafenib 240 mg Zelboraf 240mg tablets | 56 tablet PoM £1,750.00 (Hospital only)

ANTINEOPLASTIC DRUGS › OTHER

Glasdegib
22-Oct-2020

- DRUG ACTION Glasdegib is a hedgehog pathway inhibitor.

- INDICATIONS AND DOSE

  Acute myeloid leukaemia [in combination with low-dose cytarabine] (specialist use only)
  - ▸ BY MOUTH
  - ▸ Adult: 100 mg once daily, for dose adjustments, treatment interruption, or discontinuation due to side-effects—consult product literature

  DOSE ADJUSTMENTS DUE TO INTERACTIONS
  - ▸ Manufacturer advises if concurrent use of moderate CYP3A4 inducers, etravirine, or modafinil is unavoidable, double the once-daily dose.

  IMPORTANT SAFETY INFORMATION
  RISKS OF INCORRECT DOSING OF ORAL ANTI-CANCER MEDICINES
  See Cytotoxic drugs p. 932.

- INTERACTIONS → Appendix 1: glasdegib
- SIDE-EFFECTS
  - ▸ **Common or very common** Alopecia · anaemia · appetite decreased · arrhythmias · arthralgia · CNS haemorrhage · constipation · diarrhoea · dyspnoea · eye contusion · fatigue · fever · gastrointestinal discomfort · haemorrhage · increased risk of infection · muscle complaints · muscle contractions involuntary · musculoskeletal pain · nausea · neutropenia · peripheral oedema · QT interval prolongation · sepsis · skin reactions · stomatitis · taste altered · thrombocytopenia · vomiting · weight decreased
- CONCEPTION AND CONTRACEPTION Manufacturer advises females of childbearing potential and male patients with a partner who is pregnant or of childbearing potential should use effective contraception (including condoms in males) during treatment and for at least 30 days after last dose. See also *Pregnancy and reproductive function* in Cytotoxic drugs p. 932. Fertility may be impaired in males and females—consult product literature.
- PREGNANCY Manufacturer advises avoid—embryotoxicity in *animal* studies. See also *Pregnancy and reproductive function* in Cytotoxic drugs p. 932.
- BREAST FEEDING Manufacturer advises avoid during treatment and for at least one week after last dose—no information available.
- RENAL IMPAIRMENT Manufacturer advises use with caution.

  Monitoring Manufacturer advises monitor renal function in patients with pre-existing renal impairment or risk factors for renal dysfunction; assess before initiation and at least once weekly for the first month of treatment.

Monitor electrolytes and renal function once monthly thereafter during treatment.

● **PATIENT AND CARER ADVICE**
Vomiting Manufacturer advises if vomiting occurs after taking tablets, no additional dose should be taken on that day and the next dose should be taken at the usual time.
Missed doses Manufacturer advises if a dose is more than 10 hours late, the missed dose should not be taken and the next dose should be taken at the usual time.
Driving and skilled tasks Manufacturer advises patients and carers should be cautioned on the effects on driving and performance of skilled tasks—increased risk of fatigue, muscle cramps, pain, or nausea.

● **MEDICINAL FORMS** There can be variation in the licensing of different medicines containing the same drug.
Tablet
▸ Daurismo (Pfizer Ltd) ▼
Glasdegib (as Glasdegib maleate) 25 mg Daurismo 25mg tablets | 60 tablet [PoM] £10,517.00 (Hospital only)
Glasdegib (as Glasdegib maleate) 100 mg Daurismo 100mg tablets | 30 tablet [PoM] £10,517.00 (Hospital only)

Niraparib

12-Nov-2020

● **DRUG ACTION** Niraparib is an inhibitor of PARP enzymes which are involved in DNA repair. PARP inhibition results in disruption of cellular homoeostasis and cell death.

● **INDICATIONS AND DOSE**
Ovarian cancer (initiated by a specialist) | Fallopian tube cancer (initiated by a specialist) | Peritoneal cancer (initiated by a specialist)
▸ BY MOUTH
▸ **Adult:** 300 mg once daily, consider initial dose of 200 mg in patients with body-weight less than 58 kg, for dose adjustments due to side-effects—consult product literature

---

IMPORTANT SAFETY INFORMATION

RISKS OF INCORRECT DOSING OF ORAL ANTI-CANCER MEDICINES
See Cytotoxic drugs p. 932.

MHRA/CHM ADVICE: NIRAPARIB (ZEJULA®): REPORTS OF SEVERE HYPERTENSION AND POSTERIOR REVERSIBLE ENCEPHALOPATHY SYNDROME (PRES), PARTICULARLY IN EARLY TREATMENT (OCTOBER 2020)
A European review of niraparib safety data identified worldwide reports of severe hypertension, including rare cases of hypertensive crisis, some with onset in the first month of treatment. Rare cases of PRES have also been reported, mostly associated with hypertension and within the first month of treatment.

Healthcare professionals are advised to control pre-existing hypertension before starting niraparib. Blood pressure should be monitored at least weekly for the first 2 months of treatment, then monthly for the first year, and periodically thereafter. Home blood pressure monitoring may be considered if appropriate; patients should be trained and advised to contact their doctor in case of an increase in blood pressure.

Hypertension during treatment should be managed with antihypertensives; treatment interruption or dose adjustment of niraparib may be required—consult product literature. Niraparib should be discontinued in case of hypertensive crisis or medically significant hypertension that cannot be adequately controlled with antihypertensive therapy. In cases of PRES, niraparib should also be discontinued and patients treated for specific symptoms (including hypertension).

● **CAUTIONS** Pre-existing hypertension (control before treatment initiation)

● **INTERACTIONS** → Appendix 1: niraparib
● **SIDE-EFFECTS**
▸ **Common or very common** Anaemia · anxiety · appetite decreased · arthralgia · asthenia · back pain · conjunctivitis · constipation · cough · depression · diarrhoea · dizziness · dry mouth · dyspnoea · epistaxis · gastrointestinal discomfort · headache · hypertension · hypokalaemia · increased risk of infection · insomnia · leucopenia · mucositis · myalgia · nausea · neutropenia · palpitations · peripheral oedema · photosensitivity reaction · rash · stomatitis · tachycardia · taste altered · thrombocytopenia · vomiting · weight decreased
▸ **Uncommon** Pancytopenia
▸ **Frequency not known** Acute myeloid leukaemia (discontinue permanently) · myelodysplastic syndrome (discontinue permanently) · posterior reversible encephalopathy syndrome (PRES)

● **CONCEPTION AND CONTRACEPTION** Manufacturer advises effective contraception in women of childbearing potential during treatment and for 1 month after receiving the last dose.

● **PREGNANCY** Manufacturer advises avoid—limited information available.

● **BREAST FEEDING** Manufacturer advises avoid during treatment and for 1 month after last dose—no information available.

● **HEPATIC IMPAIRMENT** Manufacturer advises caution in severe impairment (no information available).

● **RENAL IMPAIRMENT** Manufacturer advises caution in severe impairment—no information available.

● **MONITORING REQUIREMENTS**
▸ Manufacturer advises monitor full blood count weekly for the first month of treatment, then monthly for the next 10 months and periodically thereafter.
▸ Manufacturer advises monitor blood pressure weekly for the first 2 months of treatment, then monthly for the first year, and periodically thereafter.

● **PATIENT AND CARER ADVICE**
Driving and skilled tasks Manufacturer advises patients and their carers should be counselled on the effects on driving and skilled tasks—increased risk of dizziness and fatigue.

● **NATIONAL FUNDING/ACCESS DECISIONS**
For full details see funding body website
NICE decisions
▸ Niraparib for maintenance treatment of relapsed, platinum-sensitive ovarian, fallopian tube and peritoneal cancer (July 2018) NICE TA528 Recommended with restrictions
Scottish Medicines Consortium (SMC) decisions
▸ Niraparib tosylate monohydrate (Zejula®) as monotherapy for the maintenance treatment of adult patients with platinum-sensitive relapsed high grade serous epithelial ovarian, fallopian tube, or primary peritoneal cancer who are in response (complete or partial) to platinum-based chemotherapy (August 2018) SMC No. 1341/18 Recommended with restrictions

● **MEDICINAL FORMS** There can be variation in the licensing of different medicines containing the same drug.
Capsule
CAUTIONARY AND ADVISORY LABELS 25
▸ Zejula (GlaxoSmithKline UK Ltd) ▼
Niraparib (as Niraparib tosylate monohydrate) 100 mg Zejula 100mg capsules | 56 capsule [PoM] £4,500.00 (Hospital only) | 84 capsule [PoM] £6,750.00 (Hospital only)

Olaparib

27-Aug-2020

- **DRUG ACTION** Olaparib is a PARP inhibitor. PARP are enzymes that repair damaged DNA in cancer cells and, in the absence of functional BRCA, inhibition of PARP results in an inability of cancer cells to repair. Therefore inhibition of PARP results in an antineoplastic effect.

- **INDICATIONS AND DOSE**

Ovarian cancer (initiated by a specialist) | Fallopian tube cancer (initiated by a specialist) | Peritoneal cancer (initiated by a specialist)

▸ BY MOUTH USING CAPSULES
▸ Adult: 400 mg twice daily, patients should start treatment no later than 8 weeks after completion of their final dose of the platinum-containing regimen, for dose adjustments due to side-effects—consult product literature

▸ BY MOUTH USING TABLETS
▸ Adult: 300 mg twice daily, patients should start treatment no later than 8 weeks after completion of their final dose of the platinum-containing regimen, for dose adjustments due to side-effects—consult product literature

DOSE ADJUSTMENTS DUE TO INTERACTIONS
▸ Manufacturer advises if concurrent use of moderate inhibitors of CYP3A4 is unavoidable, reduce dose of *capsules* to 200 mg twice daily and *tablets* to 150 mg twice daily.
▸ Manufacturer advises if concurrent use of potent inhibitors of CYP3A4 is unavoidable, reduce dose of *capsules* to 150 mg twice daily and *tablets* to 100 mg twice daily.

DOSE EQUIVALENCE AND CONVERSION
▸ Manufacturer advises capsules and tablets are not interchangeable on a milligram-for-milligram basis due to differences in dosing and bioavailability.

IMPORTANT SAFETY INFORMATION

RISKS OF INCORRECT DOSING OF ORAL ANTI-CANCER MEDICINES
See Cytotoxic drugs p. 932.

MHRA/CHM ADVICE: *LYNPARZA*® (OLAPARIB): RISK OF MEDICATION ERRORS WITH NEW PHARMACEUTICAL FORM (MAY 2018)
A tablet formulation of olaparib was approved by the European Commission in May 2018. Capsules and tablets are not to be substituted on a milligram-to-milligram basis due to differences in dosing and bioavailability of each formulation. Prescribers should specify the formulation and dosage of olaparib on each prescription and pharmacists should ensure that the correct formulation and dose is dispensed. Patients should be instructed on the correct dose they should take for their capsules or tablets and if switched, informed of the difference in dosing.

- **INTERACTIONS** → Appendix 1: olaparib

- **SIDE-EFFECTS**
▸ **Common or very common** Agranulocytosis · anaemia · appetite decreased · asthenia · cough · decreased leucocytes · diarrhoea · dizziness · dyspnoea · erythropenia · gastrointestinal discomfort · headache · nausea · neutropenia · neutropenic infection · neutropenic sepsis · oral disorders · skin reactions · taste altered · thrombocytopenia · vomiting
▸ **Frequency not known** Haematotoxicity · neoplasms · pneumonitis

SIDE-EFFECTS, FURTHER INFORMATION **Haematological toxicity** Withhold treatment if severe haematological toxicity develops; further analysis recommended if toxicity still present 4 weeks after treatment withdrawal.

- **Pneumonitis** If dyspnoea, cough and fever, or radiological abnormalities develop, withhold treatment and investigate; if pneumonitis confirmed, discontinue.

- **CONCEPTION AND CONTRACEPTION** Manufacturer advises effective contraception during treatment and for 1 month after receiving the last dose. Consider an additional non-hormonal method of contraception.

- **PREGNANCY** Manufacturer advises avoid—toxicity in *animal* studies.

- **BREAST FEEDING** Manufacturer advises avoid during treatment and for 1 month after last dose—no information available.

- **HEPATIC IMPAIRMENT** Manufacturer advises avoid in severe impairment (no information available).

- **RENAL IMPAIRMENT** Manufacturer advises avoid in severe impairment unless benefit outweighs potential risk—no information available.
Dose adjustments For *capsules*, manufacturer advises reduce dose to 300 mg twice daily in moderate impairment. For *tablets*, manufacturer advises reduce dose to 200 mg twice daily in moderate impairment.

- **MONITORING REQUIREMENTS** Manufacturer advises monitor full blood count before treatment initiation, then every month for the first 12 months of treatment and periodically thereafter.

- **DIRECTIONS FOR ADMINISTRATION** Manufacturer advises *capsules* should be taken at least 1 hour after food, and food should preferably be avoided for up to 2 hours after administration.

- **PATIENT AND CARER ADVICE**
Driving and skilled tasks Manufacturer advises patients should be counselled on the effects on driving and performance of skilled tasks—increased risk of malaise and dizziness.

- **NATIONAL FUNDING/ACCESS DECISIONS**
For full details see funding body website
NICE decisions
▸ Olaparib for maintenance treatment of BRCA mutation-positive advanced ovarian, fallopian tube or peritoneal cancer after response to first-line platinum-based chemotherapy (August 2019) NICE TA598 Recommended with restrictions
▸ Olaparib for maintenance treatment of relapsed platinum-sensitive ovarian, fallopian tube or peritoneal cancer (January 2020) NICE TA620 Recommended with restrictions
Scottish Medicines Consortium (SMC) decisions
▸ Olaparib (*Lynparza*®) as monotherapy for the maintenance treatment of adult patients with platinum-sensitive relapsed BRCA-mutated (germline and/or somatic) high grade serous epithelial ovarian, fallopian tube, or primary peritoneal cancer who are in response (complete response or partial response) to platinum-based chemotherapy (November 2016) SMC No. 1047/15 Recommended
▸ Olaparib (*Lynparza*®) as monotherapy for the maintenance treatment of adult patients with newly diagnosed advanced (FIGO stages III and IV) BRCA1/2-mutated (germline and/or somatic) high-grade epithelial ovarian, fallopian tube or primary peritoneal cancer who are in response (complete or partial) following completion of first line platinum-based chemotherapy (December 2019) SMC No. SMC2209 Recommended

---

- **MEDICINAL FORMS** There can be variation in the licensing of different medicines containing the same drug.

Tablet
CAUTIONARY AND ADVISORY LABELS 25
▸ Lynparza (AstraZeneca UK Ltd)
Olaparib 100 mg Lynparza 100mg tablets | 56 tablet [PoM]
£2,317.50 DT = £2,317.50
Olaparib 150 mg Lynparza 150mg tablets | 56 tablet [PoM]
£2,317.50 DT = £2,317.50

Capsule

▸ Lynparza (AstraZeneca UK Ltd)
Olaparib 50 mg Lynparza 50mg capsules | 448 capsule [PoM]
£3,550.00 DT = £3,550.00

Rucaparib

11-Nov-2020

● **DRUG ACTION** Rucaparib is a PARP inhibitor. PARP are enzymes that repair damaged DNA in cancer cells and, in the absence of functional BRCA, inhibition of PARP results in an inability of cancer cells to repair. Therefore inhibition of PARP results in an antineoplastic effect.

● **INDICATIONS AND DOSE**

Ovarian cancer (initiated by a specialist) | Fallopian tube cancer (initiated by a specialist) | Peritoneal cancer (initiated by a specialist)

▸ BY MOUTH
▸ Adult: 600 mg twice daily, for dose adjustments due to side-effects—consult product literature

---

IMPORTANT SAFETY INFORMATION
RISKS OF INCORRECT DOSING OF ORAL ANTI-CANCER MEDICINES
See Cytotoxic drugs p. 932.

● **INTERACTIONS** → Appendix 1: rucaparib
● **SIDE-EFFECTS**
▸ **Common or very common** Anaemia · appetite decreased · asthenia · decreased leucocytes · diarrhoea · dizziness · dyspepsia · dyspnoea · fever · hypercholesterolaemia · nausea · neutropenia · photosensitivity reaction · skin reactions · taste altered · thrombocytopenia · vomiting
▸ **Uncommon** Acute myeloid leukaemia (discontinue) · myelodysplastic syndrome (discontinue)
▸ **Frequency not known** Memory loss
● **CONCEPTION AND CONTRACEPTION** Manufacturer advises effective contraception in women of childbearing potential during treatment and for 6 months after receiving the last dose.
● **PREGNANCY** Manufacturer advises avoid—toxicity in *animal* studies.
● **BREAST FEEDING** Manufacturer advises avoid during treatment and for 2 weeks after last dose—no information available.
● **HEPATIC IMPAIRMENT** Manufacturer advises avoid in moderate to severe impairment (limited information available).
● **RENAL IMPAIRMENT** Manufacturer advises avoid in severe impairment unless benefit outweighs potential risk—no information available.
● **MONITORING REQUIREMENTS** Manufacturer advises monitor full blood count before treatment initiation, then monthly thereafter.
● **PATIENT AND CARER ADVICE**
Driving and skilled tasks Manufacturer advises patients and their carers should be counselled on the effects on driving and performance of skilled tasks—increased risk of dizziness and fatigue.
● **NATIONAL FUNDING/ACCESS DECISIONS**
For full details see funding body website

NICE decisions
▸ Rucaparib for maintenance treatment of relapsed platinum-sensitive ovarian, fallopian tube or peritoneal cancer (November 2019) NICE TA611 Recommended

Scottish Medicines Consortium (SMC) decisions
▸ Rucaparib (*Rubraca*® as monotherapy for the maintenance treatment of adult patients with platinum-sensitive relapsed high-grade epithelial ovarian, fallopian tube, or primary

peritoneal cancer who are in response (complete or partial) to platinum-based chemotherapy (March 2020) SMC No. SMC2224 Recommended with restrictions

● **MEDICINAL FORMS** There can be variation in the licensing of different medicines containing the same drug.

Tablet
▸ Rubraca (Clovis Oncology UK Ltd) ▼
Rucaparib (as Rucaparib camsilate) 200 mg Rubraca 200mg tablets | 60 tablet [PoM] [℞]
Rucaparib (as Rucaparib camsilate) 250 mg Rubraca 250mg tablets | 60 tablet [PoM] [℞]
Rucaparib (as Rucaparib camsilate) 300 mg Rubraca 300mg tablets | 60 tablet [PoM] [℞]

Talazoparib

23-Oct-2019

● **DRUG ACTION** Talazoparib is a PARP inhibitor. PARP are enzymes that repair damaged DNA in cancer cells and, in the absence of functional BRCA, inhibition of PARP results in an inability of cancer cells to repair. Therefore inhibition of PARP results in an antineoplastic effect.

● **INDICATIONS AND DOSE**

Breast cancer (initiated by a specialist)

▸ BY MOUTH
▸ Adult: 1 mg once daily, for dose adjustments due to side-effects—consult product literature

DOSE ADJUSTMENTS DUE TO INTERACTIONS
▸ Manufacturer advises if concomitant use with P-glycoprotein inhibitors is unavoidable, reduce dose to 750 micrograms once daily.

IMPORTANT SAFETY INFORMATION
RISKS OF INCORRECT DOSING OF ORAL ANTI-CANCER MEDICINES
See Cytotoxic drugs p. 932.

● **INTERACTIONS** → Appendix 1: talazoparib
● **SIDE-EFFECTS**
▸ **Common or very common** Alopecia · anaemia · appetite decreased · asthenia · decreased leucocytes · diarrhoea · dizziness · gastrointestinal discomfort · headache · nausea · neutropenia · stomatitis · taste altered · thrombocytopenia · vomiting
▸ **Frequency not known** Bone marrow depression · neoplasms
● **CONCEPTION AND CONTRACEPTION** Manufacturer advises effective contraception in women of childbearing potential during treatment and for 7 months after receiving the last dose. Male patients should use effective contraception during and for at least 4 months after treatment if their partner is pregnant or of childbearing potential. See also *Pregnancy and reproductive function* in Cytotoxic drugs p. 932.
● **PREGNANCY** Manufacturer advises avoid—toxicity in *animal* studies. See also *Pregnancy and reproductive function* in Cytotoxic drugs p. 932.
● **BREAST FEEDING** Manufacturer advises avoid during treatment and for 1 month after last dose—no information available.
● **HEPATIC IMPAIRMENT** Manufacturer advises avoid in moderate or severe impairment unless benefit outweighs risk (no information available).
● **RENAL IMPAIRMENT** Manufacturer advises avoid if creatinine clearance less than 30 mL/minute unless benefit outweighs risk (no information available).
Dose adjustments Manufacturer advises reduce starting dose to 750 micrograms once daily if creatinine clearance 30–60 mL/minute.
● **MONITORING REQUIREMENTS** Manufacturer advises monitor full blood count before treatment initiation, then monthly thereafter and as clinically indicated.

- PATIENT AND CARER ADVICE
Driving and skilled tasks Manufacturer advises patients and their carers should be counselled on the effects on driving and skilled tasks—increased risk of fatigue and dizziness.

- MEDICINAL FORMS There can be variation in the licensing of different medicines containing the same drug.
Capsule
CAUTIONARY AND ADVISORY LABELS 25
  ▸ Talzenna (Pfizer Ltd) ▼
    Talazoparib (as Talazoparib tosylate) 250 microgram Talzenna 0.25mg capsules | 30 capsule PoM £1,655.00 (Hospital only)
    Talazoparib (as Talazoparib tosylate) 1 mg Talzenna 1mg capsules | 30 capsule PoM £4,965.00 (Hospital only)

Venetoclax   11-Nov-2020

- DRUG ACTION Venetoclax is a potent, selective inhibitor of B-cell lymphoma-2 (BCL-2).

  - INDICATIONS AND DOSE

  Chronic lymphocytic leukaemia in the presence of 17p deletion or TP53 mutation when a B-cell receptor pathway inhibitor is unsuitable or ineffective (specialist use only) | Chronic lymphocytic leukaemia in the absence of 17p deletion or TP53 mutation when both chemo-immunotherapy and a B-cell receptor pathway inhibitor has been ineffective (specialist use only)
  ▸ BY MOUTH
  ▸ Adult: (consult product literature)

  Chronic lymphocytic leukaemia in patients who have received at least one prior therapy [in combination with rituximab] (specialist use only)
  ▸ BY MOUTH
  ▸ Adult: (consult product literature)

  IMPORTANT SAFETY INFORMATION
  RISKS OF INCORRECT DOSING OF ORAL ANTI-CANCER MEDICINES
  See Cytotoxic drugs p. 932.

- CAUTIONS Ensure adequate hydration
- INTERACTIONS → Appendix 1: venetoclax
- SIDE-EFFECTS
  ▸ **Common or very common** Anaemia · constipation · diarrhoea · electrolyte imbalance · fatigue · hyperuricaemia · increased risk of infection · lymphopenia · nausea · neutropenia · tumour lysis syndrome · vomiting
- CONCEPTION AND CONTRACEPTION Manufacturer advises ensure effective, non-hormonal contraception during and for 30 days after treatment in women of child-bearing potential. See also *Pregnancy and reproductive function* in Cytotoxic drugs p. 932.
- PREGNANCY Manufacturer advises avoid—toxicity in *animal* studies. See also *Pregnancy and reproductive function* in Cytotoxic drugs p. 932.
- BREAST FEEDING Manufacturer advises avoid—no information available.
- HEPATIC IMPAIRMENT Manufacturer advises caution in moderate impairment (increased risk of toxicity); avoid in severe impairment (no information available).
- RENAL IMPAIRMENT Manufacturer advises close monitoring (increased risk of tumour lysis syndrome); use only if potential benefit outweighs risk in severe impairment—no information available.
- MONITORING REQUIREMENTS Manufacturer advises monitor renal function before starting treatment.
- PATIENT AND CARER ADVICE
Hydration Manufacturer advises patients should drink 1.5–2 L of water daily, starting 2 days before and throughout the dose-titration phase; intravenous fluids

should be administered for those who cannot maintain an adequate level of oral hydration with consideration of overall risk of tumour lysis syndrome.
Vomiting Manufacturer advises that if vomiting occurs following dose administration, no additional doses should be taken on that day and the next dose should be taken at the normal time.
Missed doses Manufacturer advises that if a dose is more than 8 hours late, the missed dose should not be taken and the next dose should be taken at the normal time.

- NATIONAL FUNDING/ACCESS DECISIONS
For full details see funding body website
NICE decisions
  ▸ Venetoclax for treating chronic lymphocytic leukaemia (November 2017) NICE TA487 Recommended with restrictions
  ▸ Venetoclax with rituximab for previously treated chronic lymphocytic leukaemia (February 2019) NICE TA561 Recommended with restrictions
Scottish Medicines Consortium (SMC) decisions
  ▸ Venetoclax (*Venclyxto*®) as monotherapy for the treatment of chronic lymphocytic leukaemia in the presence of 17p deletion or TP53 mutation in adult patients who are unsuitable for or have failed a B-cell receptor pathway inhibitor, or in the absence of 17p deletion or TP53 mutation in adult patients who have failed both chemoimmunotherapy and a B-cell receptor pathway inhibitor (August 2017) SMC No. 1249/17 Recommended
  ▸ Venetoclax (*Venclyxto*®) in combination with rituximab for the treatment of adult patients with chronic lymphocytic leukaemia (CLL) who have received at least one prior therapy (August 2019) SMC No. SMC2166 Recommended

- MEDICINAL FORMS There can be variation in the licensing of different medicines containing the same drug.
Tablet
CAUTIONARY AND ADVISORY LABELS 21, 25
  ▸ Venclyxto (AbbVie Ltd) ▼
    Venetoclax 10 mg Venclyxto 10mg tablets | 14 tablet PoM £59.87
    Venetoclax 50 mg Venclyxto 50mg tablets | 7 tablet PoM £149.67
    Venetoclax 100 mg Venclyxto 100mg tablets | 7 tablet PoM £299.34 | 14 tablet PoM £598.68 | 112 tablet PoM £4,789.47

Vismodegib   24-Nov-2020

- DRUG ACTION Vismodegib is a hedgehog pathway inhibitor.

  - INDICATIONS AND DOSE

  Symptomatic metastatic basal cell carcinoma | Locally advanced basal cell carcinoma not appropriate for surgery or radiotherapy
  ▸ BY MOUTH
  ▸ Adult: 150 mg once daily

  IMPORTANT SAFETY INFORMATION
  RISKS OF INCORRECT DOSING OF ORAL ANTI-CANCER MEDICINES
  See Cytotoxic drugs p. 932.

- INTERACTIONS → Appendix 1: vismodegib
- SIDE-EFFECTS
  ▸ **Common or very common** Alopecia · amenorrhoea · appetite decreased · arthralgia · asthenia · constipation · dehydration · diarrhoea · gastrointestinal discomfort · hair growth abnormal · muscle complaints · nausea · pain · skin reactions · taste altered · vomiting · weight decreased
  ▸ **Frequency not known** Epiphyses premature fusion
- CONCEPTION AND CONTRACEPTION For women of child-bearing potential, pregnancy must be excluded before initiation of treatment, and monthly during treatment. Women must use two contraceptive methods (including

one highly effective method and one barrier method) during treatment and for 24 months after the final dose of vismodegib. Men must use a condom during treatment and for 2 months after the final dose.

● PREGNANCY **Important: teratogenic risk**—may cause severe birth defects and embryo-fetal death.

● BREAST FEEDING Avoid during treatment and for 24 months after final dose.

● RENAL IMPAIRMENT No information available— manufacturer advises caution in severe impairment.

● PRESCRIBING AND DISPENSING INFORMATION Prescribers and pharmacists must comply with prescribing and dispensing restrictions as specified in the manufacturer's Pregnancy Prevention Programme, and ensure that the patient fully acknowledges the programme's pregnancy prevention measures—consult product literature for further information.

● PATIENT AND CARER ADVICE
Conception and contraception Counselling on pregnancy and contraception advised. Patients must comply with the manufacturer's pregnancy prevention programme.

● NATIONAL FUNDING/ACCESS DECISIONS
For full details see funding body website
NICE decisions
▸ Vismodegib for treating basal cell carcinoma (November 2017) NICE TA489 Not recommended

● MEDICINAL FORMS There can be variation in the licensing of different medicines containing the same drug.
Capsule
CAUTIONARY AND ADVISORY LABELS 25
   ▸ Erivedge (Roche Products Ltd)
   Vismodegib 150 mg Erivedge 150mg capsules | 28 capsule [PoM]
   £6,285.00 (Hospital only)

ANTINEOVASCULARISATION DRUGS ›
VASCULAR ENDOTHELIAL GROWTH FACTOR INHIBITORS

| Aflibercept
15-Oct-2020

● DRUG ACTION Aflibercept is a recombinant fusion protein that acts as a soluble decoy receptor and binds to vascular endothelial growth factors A and B (VEGF-A, VEGF-B) and placental growth factor (PlGF). Aflibercept inhibits the activation of VEGF receptors and the proliferation of endothelial cells, thereby inhibiting the growth of new vessels that supply tumours with oxygen and nutrients.

● INDICATIONS AND DOSE
In combination with irinotecan, fluorouracil and folinic acid (FOLFIRI) chemotherapy, in metastatic colorectal cancer that is resistant to, or has progressed after, an oxaliplatin-containing regimen
   ▸ BY INTRAVENOUS INFUSION
   ▸ Adult: (consult local protocol)

IMPORTANT SAFETY INFORMATION
MHRA/CHM ADVICE: SYSTEMICALLY ADMINISTERED VEGF PATHWAY INHIBITORS: RISK OF ANEURYSM AND ARTERY DISSECTION (JULY 2020)
A European review of worldwide data concluded that systemically administered VEGF pathway inhibitors may lead to aneurysm and artery dissection in patients with or without hypertension. Some fatal cases have been reported, mainly in relation to aortic aneurysm rupture and aortic dissection. The MHRA advises healthcare professionals to carefully consider the risk of aneurysm and artery dissection in patients with risk factors before initiating treatment with aflibercept; any modifiable risk factors (such as smoking and hypertension) should be

reduced as much as possible. Patients should be monitored and treated for hypertension as required.

● CONTRA-INDICATIONS Moderate or severe congestive heart failure · uncontrolled hypertension

● CAUTIONS Febrile neutropenia · history of cardiovascular disease (may be exacerbated by hypertension) · increased risk of haemorrhage (including fatal events) · increased risk of hypertension · increased risk of thromboembolic events (consult product literature if event occurs) · may impair wound healing—withhold treatment for at least 4 weeks before elective surgery and for at least 4 weeks after major surgery, or until wound fully healed · neutropenic infection · risk factors for aneurysm or artery dissection · risk of fistula formation (discontinue if fistula develops) · risk of neutropenia · risk of thrombocytopenia
CAUTIONS, FURTHER INFORMATION
▸ Monitoring of blood pressure The MHRA advises to monitor blood pressure regularly—consult product literature if hypertension occurs during treatment.

● INTERACTIONS → Appendix 1: aflibercept

● SIDE-EFFECTS
▸ **Common or very common** Appetite decreased · asthenic conditions · dehydration · diarrhoea · dysphonia · dyspnoea · embolism and thrombosis · fistula · gastrointestinal discomfort · gastrointestinal disorders · haemorrhage · headache · hypersensitivity · hypertension · increased risk of infection · leucopenia · neutropenia · neutropenic sepsis · oral disorders · oropharyngeal pain · proteinuria · rhinorrhoea · skin reactions · thrombocytopenia · weight decreased
▸ **Uncommon** Healing impaired · heart failure · nephrotic syndrome · osteonecrosis of jaw · posterior reversible encephalopathy syndrome (PRES) · thrombotic microangiopathy
▸ **Frequency not known** Alopecia · anaemia · aneurysm · angina pectoris · artery dissection · cerebrovascular insufficiency · constipation · hyperbilirubinaemia · myocardial infarction · nausea · vomiting · wound complications

● CONCEPTION AND CONTRACEPTION Exclude pregnancy before treatment. Effective contraception required during and for at least 6 months after treatment in men and women. Contraceptive advice should be given to men and women before therapy begins (and should cover the duration of contraception required after therapy has ended).

● PREGNANCY Manufacturer advises avoid—toxicity in *animal* studies. Considerable caution is necessary if a pregnant woman presents with cancer requiring chemotherapy, and specialist advice should always be sought.

● BREAST FEEDING Manufacturer advises avoid—no information available.

● HEPATIC IMPAIRMENT Manufacturer advises caution in severe impairment (no information available).

● RENAL IMPAIRMENT Caution in severe impairment— no information available.

● MONITORING REQUIREMENTS
▸ Monitor for signs and symptoms of gastro-intestinal perforation—discontinue if perforation develops.
▸ Monitor full blood count, including differential count and platelets at baseline and before each treatment cycle.
▸ Monitor for proteinuria before each treatment administration—consult product literature if symptoms develop.
▸ Monitor for signs and symptoms of diarrhoea and dehydration, particularly in elderly—consult product literature if severe diarrhoea occurs.

▶ Monitor for posterior reversible encephalopathy syndrome (presenting as seizures, altered mental status, nausea, vomiting, headache, or visual disturbance).
▶ Monitor for signs and symptoms of cardiac failure and decreased ejection fraction—consider baseline and periodic evaluations of left ventricular function during treatment; discontinue if cardiac failure or decreased ejection fraction develops.

● NATIONAL FUNDING/ACCESS DECISIONS
For full details see funding body website

NICE decisions
▶ **Aflibercept in combination with irinotecan and fluorouracil-based therapy for treating metastatic colorectal cancer that has progressed following prior oxaliplatin-based chemotherapy (March 2014)** NICE TA307 Not recommended

● MEDICINAL FORMS There can be variation in the licensing of different medicines containing the same drug.

Solution for infusion
▶ Zaltrap (Sanofi)
  Aflibercept 25 mg per 1 ml Zaltrap 200mg/8ml concentrate for solution for infusion vials | 1 vial [PoM] £591.30 (Hospital only)
  Zaltrap 100mg/4ml concentrate for solution for infusion vials | 1 vial [PoM] £295.65 (Hospital only)

Chapter 9
Blood and nutrition

CONTENTS

Blood and blood-forming organs

1   Anaemias

Anaemias

Anaemia treatment considerations

Before initiating treatment for anaemia it is essential to determine which type is present. Iron salts may be harmful and result in iron overload if given alone to patients with anaemias other than those due to iron deficiency.

Sickle-cell anaemia

Sickle-cell disease is caused by a structural abnormality of haemoglobin resulting in deformed, less flexible red blood cells. Acute complications in the more severe forms include sickle-cell crisis, where infarction of the microvasculature and blood supply to organs results in severe pain. Sickle-cell crisis requires hospitalisation, intravenous fluids, analgesia and treatment of any concurrent infection. Chronic complications include skin ulceration, renal failure, and increased susceptibility to infection. Pneumococcal vaccine, haemophilus influenzae type b vaccine, an annual influenza vaccine and prophylactic penicillin reduce the risk of infection. Hepatitis B vaccine should be considered if the patient is not immune.

In most forms of sickle-cell disease, varying degrees of haemolytic anaemia are present accompanied by increased erythropoiesis; this may increase folate requirements and folate supplementation may be necessary.

Hydroxycarbamide p. 977 can reduce the frequency of crises and the need for blood transfusions in sickle-cell disease. The beneficial effects of hydroxycarbamide may not become evident for several months.

G6PD deficiency

Glucose 6-phosphate dehydrogenase (G6PD) deficiency is highly prevalent in individuals originating from most parts of Africa, from most parts of Asia, from Oceania, and from Southern Europe; it can also occur, rarely, in any other individuals. G6PD deficiency is more common in males than it is in females.

Individuals with G6PD deficiency are susceptible to developing acute haemolytic anaemia when they take a number of common drugs. They are also susceptible to developing acute haemolytic anaemia when they eat fava beans (broad beans, *Vicia faba*); this is termed *favism* and can be more severe in children or when the fresh fava beans are eaten raw.

When prescribing drugs for patients with G6PD deficiency, the following three points should be kept in mind:

- G6PD deficiency is genetically heterogeneous; susceptibility to the haemolytic risk from drugs varies; thus, a drug found to be safe in some G6PD-deficient individuals may not be equally safe in others;
- manufacturers do not routinely test drugs for their effects in G6PD-deficient individuals;
- the risk and severity of haemolysis is almost always dose-related.

The lists below should be read with these points in mind. Ideally, information about G6PD deficiency should be available before prescribing a drug listed below. However, in the absence of this information, the possibility of haemolysis should be considered, especially if the patient belongs to a group in which G6PD deficiency is common.

A very few G6PD-deficient individuals with chronic non-spherocytic haemolytic anaemia have haemolysis even in the absence of an exogenous trigger. These patients must be regarded as being at high risk of severe exacerbation of haemolysis following administration of any of the drugs listed below.

Drugs with definite risk of haemolysis in most G6PD-deficient individuals

- Dapsone and other sulfones (higher doses for dermatitis herpetiformis more likely to cause problems)
- Fluoroquinolones (including ciprofloxacin, moxifloxacin, norfloxacin, and ofloxacin)
- Methylthioninium chloride
- Niridazole [not on UK market]
- Nitrofurantoin
- Pamaquin [not on UK market]
- Primaquine (30 mg weekly for 8 weeks has been found to be without undue harmful effects in African and Asian people)
- Quinolones (such as nalidixic acid [not on UK market])
- Rasburicase
- Sulfonamides (including co-trimoxazole; some sulfonamides, e.g. sulfadiazine, have been tested and found not to be haemolytic in many G6PD-deficient individuals)

Drugs with possible risk of haemolysis in some G6PD-deficient individuals

- Aspirin (acceptable up to a dose of at least 1 g daily in most G6PD-deficient individuals)
- Chloroquine (acceptable in acute malaria and malaria chemoprophylaxis)
- Menadione, water-soluble derivatives (e.g. menadiol sodium phosphate)
- Quinidine (acceptable in acute malaria) [not on UK market]
- Quinine (acceptable in acute malaria)
- Sulfonylureas

Naphthalene in mothballs also causes haemolysis in individuals with G6PD deficiency.

Hypoplastic, haemolytic, and renal anaemias

Anabolic steroids, pyridoxine hydrochloride p. 1130, antilymphocyte immunoglobulin, rituximab p. 927 [unlicensed indication], and various corticosteroids are used in hypoplastic and haemolytic anaemias.

Antilymphocyte immunoglobulin given intravenously through a central line over 12–18 hours each day for 5 days produces a response in about 50% of cases of acquired *aplastic anaemia*; the response rate may be increased when ciclosporin p. 884 is given as well. Severe reactions are common in the first 2 days and profound immunosuppression can occur; antilymphocyte immunoglobulin should be given under specialist supervision with appropriate resuscitation facilities.

Alternatively, oxymetholone tablets (available from 'special order' manufacturers or specialist importing companies) can be used in aplastic anaemia for 3 to 6 months.

It is unlikely that dietary deprivation of pyridoxine hydrochloride produces clinically relevant haematological effects. However, certain forms of *sideroblastic anaemia* respond to pharmacological doses, possibly reflecting its role as a co-enzyme during haemoglobin synthesis. Pyridoxine hydrochloride is indicated in both *idiopathic acquired* and *hereditary sideroblastic anaemias*. Although complete cures have not been reported, some increase in haemoglobin can occur; the dose required is usually high. *Reversible sideroblastic anaemias* respond to treatment of the underlying cause but in pregnancy, haemolytic anaemias, and alcohol dependence, or during isoniazid p. 624 treatment, pyridoxine hydrochloride is also indicated.

Corticosteroids have an important place in the management of haematological disorders. They include conditions with an *autoimmune haemolytic anaemia*, *immune thrombocytopenias* and *neutropenias*, and *major transfusion reactions*. They are also used in chemotherapy schedules for many types of *lymphoma*, *lymphoid leukaemias*, and *paraproteinaemias*, including *multiple myeloma*.

Erythropoietins

Epoetins (recombinant human erythropoietins) are used to treat the anaemia associated with erythropoietin deficiency in chronic renal failure, to increase the yield of autologous blood in normal individuals and to shorten the period of symptomatic anaemia in patients receiving cytotoxic chemotherapy.

Epoetin beta p. 1061 is also used for the prevention of anaemia in preterm neonates of low birth-weight; only unpreserved formulations should be used in neonates because other preparations may contain benzyl alcohol.

Darbepoetin alfa p. 1058 is a hyperglycosylated derivative of epoetin; it has a longer half life and can be administered less frequently than epoetin.

Methoxy polyethylene glycol-epoetin beta p. 1062 is a continuous erythropoietin receptor activator that is licensed for the treatment of symptomatic anaemia associated with chronic kidney disease. It has a longer duration of action than epoetin.

1.1   Hypoplastic, haemolytic, and renal anaemias

> **Other drugs used for Hypoplastic, haemolytic, and renal anaemias** Eltrombopag, p. 1082

ANABOLIC STEROIDS › ANDROSTAN DERIVATIVES

| Oxymetholone

- ● **INDICATIONS AND DOSE**
  Aplastic anaemia
  ▸ BY MOUTH
  ▸ Adult: 1–5 mg/kg daily for 3 to 6 months

- ● **INTERACTIONS** → Appendix 1: oxymetholone

- ● **MEDICINAL FORMS** There can be variation in the licensing of different medicines containing the same drug. Forms available from special-order manufacturers include: oral suspension
  Capsule
  ▸ Oxymetholone (Non-proprietary)
    Oxymetholone 50 mg Oxymetholone 50mg capsules |
    50 capsule [PoM] £475.00 [CD4-2]

Blood and nutrition   **9**

EPOETINS

Epoetins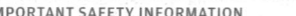

> **IMPORTANT SAFETY INFORMATION**
>
> MHRA/CHM ADVICE: RECOMBINANT HUMAN ERYTHROPOIETINS: VERY RARE RISK OF SEVERE CUTANEOUS ADVERSE REACTIONS (UPDATED JANUARY 2018)
>
> The MHRA is aware of very rare cases of severe cutaneous adverse reactions, including Stevens-Johnson syndrome and toxic epidermal necrolysis, in patients treated with erythropoietins; some cases were fatal. More severe cases were recorded with long-acting agents (darbepoetin alfa and methoxy polyethylene glycol-epoetin beta).
>
> Patients and their carers should be advised of the signs and symptoms of severe skin reactions when starting treatment and instructed to stop treatment and seek immediate medical attention if they develop widespread rash and blistering; these rashes often follow fever or flu-like symptoms—discontinue treatment permanently if such reactions occur.
>
> MHRA/CHM ADVICE (DECEMBER 2007) ERYTHROPOIETINS—HAEMOGLOBIN CONCENTRATION
>
> Overcorrection of haemoglobin concentration in patients with chronic kidney disease may increase the risk of death and serious cardiovascular events, and in patients with cancer may increase the risk of thrombosis and related complications:
>
> - patients should not be treated with erythropoietins for the licensed indications in chronic kidney disease or cancer in patients receiving chemotherapy *unless* symptoms of anaemia are present
> - the haemoglobin concentration should be maintained within the range 10–12 g/100 mL
> - haemoglobin concentrations higher than 12 g/100 mL should be avoided
> - the aim of treatment is to relieve symptoms of anaemia, and in patients with chronic kidney disease to avoid the need for blood transfusion; the haemoglobin concentration should not be increased beyond that which provides adequate control of symptoms of anaemia (in some patients, this may be achieved at concentrations lower than the recommended range)
>
> MHRA/CHM ADVICE (DECEMBER 2007 AND AUGUST 2008) ERYTHROPOIETINS—TUMOUR PROGRESSION AND SURVIVAL IN PATIENTS WITH CANCER
>
> Clinical trial data show an unexplained excess mortality and increased risk of tumour progression in patients with anaemia associated with cancer who have been treated with erythropoietins. Many of these trials used erythropoietins outside of the licensed indications (i.e. overcorrected haemoglobin concentration or given to patients who have not received chemotherapy):
>
> - erythropoietins licensed for the treatment of *symptomatic* anaemia associated with cancer, are licensed only for patients who are receiving chemotherapy
> - the decision to use erythropoietins should be based on an assessment of the benefits and risks for individual patients; blood transfusion may be the preferred treatment for anaemia associated with cancer chemotherapy, particularly in those with a good cancer prognosis

- CONTRA-INDICATIONS Patients unable to receive thromboprophylaxis · pure red cell aplasia following erythropoietin therapy · uncontrolled hypertension
- CAUTIONS Aluminium toxicity (can impair the response to erythropoietin) · concurrent infection (can impair the

response to erythropoietin) · correct factors that contribute to the anaemia of chronic renal failure, such as iron or folate deficiency, before treatment. · during dialysis (increase in unfractionated or low molecular weight heparin dose may be needed) · epilepsy · inadequately treated or poorly controlled blood pressure—interrupt treatment if blood pressure uncontrolled · ischaemic vascular disease · malignant disease · other inflammatory disease (can impair the response to erythropoietin) · risk of thrombosis may be increased when used for anaemia before orthopaedic surgery—avoid in cardiovascular disease including recent myocardial infarction or cerebrovascular accident · risk of thrombosis may be increased when used for anaemia in adults receiving cancer chemotherapy · sickle-cell disease (lower target haemoglobin concentration may be appropriate) · sudden stabbing migraine-like pain (warning of a hypertensive crisis) · thrombocytosis (monitor platelet count for first 8 weeks)

- SIDE-EFFECTS
  - **Common or very common** Arthralgia · embolism and thrombosis · headache · hypertension (dose-dependent) · influenza like illness · skin reactions · stroke
  - **Uncommon** Hypertensive crisis (in isolated patients with normal or low blood pressure) · respiratory tract congestion · seizure
  - **Rare or very rare** Thrombocytosis
  - **Frequency not known** Pure red cell aplasia (more common following subcutaneous administration in patients with chronic renal failure) · severe cutaneous adverse reactions (SCARs)

  SIDE-EFFECTS, FURTHER INFORMATION **Hypertensive crisis** In isolated patients with normal or low blood pressure, hypertensive crisis with encephalopathy-like symptoms and generalised tonic-clonic seizures requiring immediate medical attention has occurred with epoetin.

  Pure red cell aplasia There have been very rare reports of pure red cell aplasia in patients treated with erythropoietins. In patients who develop a lack of efficacy with erythropoietin therapy and with a diagnosis of pure red cell aplasia, treatment with erythropoietins must be discontinued and testing for erythropoietin antibodies considered. Patients who develop pure red cell aplasia should not be switched to another form of erythropoietin.

- MONITORING REQUIREMENTS
  - Monitor closely blood pressure, reticulocyte counts, haemoglobin, and electrolytes—interrupt treatment if blood pressure uncontrolled.
  - Other factors, such as iron or folate deficiency, that contribute to the anaemia of chronic renal failure should be corrected before treatment and monitored during therapy. Supplemental iron may improve the response in resistant patients.

▶ above

Darbepoetin alfa

30-Apr-2019

- INDICATIONS AND DOSE

Symptomatic anaemia associated with chronic renal failure in patients on dialysis

▶ BY SUBCUTANEOUS INJECTION, OR BY INTRAVENOUS INJECTION
▶ Adult: Initially 450 nanograms/kg once weekly, dose to be adjusted according to response by approximately 25% at intervals of at least 4 weeks, maintenance dose to be given once weekly or once every 2 weeks, reduce dose by approximately 25% if rise in haemoglobin concentration exceeds 2 g/100 mL over 4 weeks or if haemoglobin concentration exceeds 12 g/100 mL; if haemoglobin concentration continues to rise, despite dose reduction, suspend treatment until haemoglobin concentration decreases and then restart at a dose

approximately 25% lower than the previous dose, when changing route give same dose then adjust according to weekly or fortnightly haemoglobin measurements, adjust doses not more frequently than every 2 weeks during maintenance treatment

Symptomatic anaemia associated with chronic renal failure in patients not on dialysis
▸ BY SUBCUTANEOUS INJECTION
▸ Adult: Initially 450 nanograms/kg once weekly, alternatively initially 750 nanograms/kg every 2 weeks, dose to be adjusted according to response by approximately 25% at intervals of at least 4 weeks, maintenance dose can be given once weekly, every 2 weeks, or once a month, subcutaneous route preferred in patients not on haemodialysis, reduce dose by approximately 25% if rise in haemoglobin concentration exceeds 2 g/100 mL over 4 weeks or if haemoglobin concentration exceeds 12 g/100 mL; if haemoglobin concentration continues to rise, despite dose reduction, suspend treatment until haemoglobin concentration decreases and then restart at a dose approximately 25% lower than the previous dose, when changing route give same dose then adjust according to weekly or fortnightly haemoglobin measurements, adjust doses not more frequently than every 2 weeks during maintenance treatment

Symptomatic anaemia associated with chronic renal failure in patients not on dialysis
▸ BY INTRAVENOUS INJECTION
▸ Adult: Initially 450 nanograms/kg once weekly, dose to be adjusted according to response by approximately 25% at intervals of at least 4 weeks, maintenance dose given once weekly, subcutaneous route preferred in patients not on haemodialysis, reduce dose by approximately 25% if rise in haemoglobin concentration exceeds 2 g/100 mL over 4 weeks or if haemoglobin concentration exceeds 12 g/100 mL; if haemoglobin concentration continues to rise, despite dose reduction, suspend treatment until haemoglobin concentration decreases and then restart at a dose approximately 25% lower than the previous dose, when changing route give same dose then adjust according to weekly or fortnightly haemoglobin measurements, adjust doses not more frequently than every 2 weeks during maintenance treatment

Symptomatic anaemia in adults with non-myeloid malignancies receiving chemotherapy
▸ BY SUBCUTANEOUS INJECTION
▸ Adult: Initially 6.75 micrograms/kg every 3 weeks, alternatively initially 2.25 micrograms/kg once weekly, if response inadequate after 9 weeks further treatment may not be effective; if adequate response obtained then reduce dose by 25–50%, reduce dose by approximately 25–50% if rise in haemoglobin concentration exceeds 2 g/100 mL over 4 weeks or if haemoglobin concentration exceeds 12 g/100 mL; if haemoglobin concentration continues to rise, despite dose reduction, suspend treatment until haemoglobin concentration decreases and restart at a dose approximately 25% lower than the previous dose. Discontinue approximately 4 weeks after ending chemotherapy

● INTERACTIONS → Appendix 1: darbepoetin alfa
● SIDE-EFFECTS
▸ **Common or very common** Hypersensitivity · oedema
● PREGNANCY No evidence of harm in *animal* studies—manufacturer advises caution.
● BREAST FEEDING Manufacturer advises avoid—no information available.

● HEPATIC IMPAIRMENT Manufacturer advises caution (no information available).
● NATIONAL FUNDING/ACCESS DECISIONS
For full details see funding body website
NICE decisions
▸ Erythropoiesis-stimulating agents (epoetin and darbepoetin) for treating anaemia in people with cancer having chemotherapy (November 2014) NICE TA323 Recommended with restrictions

● MEDICINAL FORMS There can be variation in the licensing of different medicines containing the same drug.
Solution for injection
▸ Aranesp (Amgen Ltd)
Darbepoetin alfa 25 microgram per 1 ml Aranesp 10micrograms/0.4ml solution for injection pre-filled syringes | 4 pre-filled disposable injection [PoM] £58.72 DT = £58.72
Darbepoetin alfa 40 microgram per 1 ml Aranesp 20micrograms/0.5ml solution for injection pre-filled syringes | 4 pre-filled disposable injection [PoM] £117.45 DT = £117.45
Darbepoetin alfa 100 microgram per 1 ml Aranesp 50micrograms/0.5ml solution for injection pre-filled syringes | 4 pre-filled disposable injection [PoM] £293.62 DT = £293.62
Aranesp 40micrograms/0.4ml solution for injection pre-filled syringes | 4 pre-filled disposable injection [PoM] £234.90 DT = £234.90
Aranesp 30micrograms/0.3ml solution for injection pre-filled syringes | 4 pre-filled disposable injection [PoM] £176.17 DT = £176.17
Darbepoetin alfa 200 microgram per 1 ml Aranesp 130micrograms/0.65ml solution for injection pre-filled syringes | 4 pre-filled disposable injection [PoM] £763.42 DT = £763.42
Aranesp 100micrograms/0.5ml solution for injection pre-filled syringes | 4 pre-filled disposable injection [PoM] £587.24 DT = £587.24
Aranesp 60micrograms/0.3ml solution for injection pre-filled syringes | 4 pre-filled disposable injection [PoM] £352.35 DT = £352.35
Aranesp 80micrograms/0.4ml solution for injection pre-filled syringes | 4 pre-filled disposable injection [PoM] £469.79 DT = £469.79
Darbepoetin alfa 500 microgram per 1 ml Aranesp 300micrograms/0.6ml solution for injection pre-filled syringes | 1 pre-filled disposable injection [PoM] £440.43 DT = £440.43
Aranesp 500micrograms/1ml solution for injection pre-filled syringes | 1 pre-filled disposable injection [PoM] £734.05 DT = £734.05
Aranesp 150micrograms/0.3ml solution for injection pre-filled syringes | 4 pre-filled disposable injection [PoM] £880.86 DT = £880.86
▸ Aranesp SureClick (Amgen Ltd)
Darbepoetin alfa 40 microgram per 1 ml Aranesp SureClick 20micrograms/0.5ml solution for injection pre-filled pens | 1 pre-filled disposable injection [PoM] £29.36 DT = £29.36
Darbepoetin alfa 100 microgram per 1 ml Aranesp SureClick 40micrograms/0.4ml solution for injection pre-filled pens | 1 pre-filled disposable injection [PoM] £58.72 DT = £58.72
Aranesp SureClick 80micrograms/0.4ml solution for injection pre-filled pens | 1 pre-filled disposable injection [PoM] £117.45 DT = £117.45
Darbepoetin alfa 200 microgram per 1 ml Aranesp SureClick 100micrograms/0.5ml solution for injection pre-filled pens | 1 pre-filled disposable injection [PoM] £146.81 DT = £146.81
Aranesp SureClick 60micrograms/0.3ml solution for injection pre-filled pens | 1 pre-filled disposable injection [PoM] £88.09 DT = £88.09
Darbepoetin alfa 500 microgram per 1 ml Aranesp SureClick 300micrograms/0.6ml solution for injection pre-filled pens | 1 pre-filled disposable injection [PoM] £440.43 DT = £440.43
Aranesp SureClick 150micrograms/0.3ml solution for injection pre-filled pens | 1 pre-filled disposable injection [PoM] £220.22 DT = £220.22
Aranesp SureClick 500micrograms/1ml solution for injection pre-filled pens | 1 pre-filled disposable injection [PoM] £734.05 DT = £734.05

F 1058

Epoetin alfa
30-Apr-2019

● INDICATIONS AND DOSE
EPREX ® PRE-FILLED SYRINGES
Symptomatic anaemia associated with chronic renal failure in patients on haemodialysis
▸ BY INTRAVENOUS INJECTION, OR BY SUBCUTANEOUS INJECTION
▸ Adult: Initially 50 units/kg 3 times a week, adjusted in steps of 25 units/kg 3 times a week, dose adjusted according to response at intervals of at least continued →

4 weeks; maintenance 75–300 units/kg once weekly, intravenous route preferred, intravenous injection to be given over 1–5 minutes, subcutaneous injection, maximum 1 mL per injection site, maintenance dose can be given as a single dose or in divided doses, reduce dose by approximately 25% if rise in haemoglobin concentration exceeds 2 g/100 mL over 4 weeks or if haemoglobin concentration exceeds 12 g/100 mL; if haemoglobin concentration continues to rise, despite dose reduction, suspend treatment until haemoglobin concentration decreases and then restart at a dose approximately 25% lower than the previous dose

Symptomatic anaemia associated with chronic renal failure in adults on peritoneal dialysis
▸ BY INTRAVENOUS INJECTION, OR BY SUBCUTANEOUS INJECTION
▸ Adult: Initially 50 units/kg twice weekly; maintenance 25–50 units/kg twice weekly, intravenous route preferred, intravenous injection to be given over 1–5 minutes, subcutaneous injection, maximum 1 mL per injection site, reduce dose by approximately 25% if rise in haemoglobin concentration exceeds 2 g/100 mL over 4 weeks or if haemoglobin concentration exceeds 12 g/100 mL; if haemoglobin concentration continues to rise, despite dose reduction, suspend treatment until haemoglobin concentration decreases and then restart at a dose approximately 25% lower than the previous dose

Severe symptomatic anaemia of renal origin in adults with renal insufficiency not yet on dialysis
▸ BY INTRAVENOUS INJECTION, OR BY SUBCUTANEOUS INJECTION
▸ Adult: Initially 50 units/kg 3 times a week, increased in steps of 25 units/kg 3 times a week, adjusted according to response, dose to be increased at intervals of at least 4 weeks; maintenance 17–33 units/kg 3 times a week (max. per dose 200 units/kg 3 times a week), intravenous route preferred, intravenous injection to be given over 1–5 minutes, subcutaneous injection, maximum 1 mL per injection site, reduce dose by approximately 25% if rise in haemoglobin concentration exceeds 2 g/100 mL over 4 weeks or if haemoglobin concentration exceeds 12 g/100 mL; if haemoglobin concentration continues to rise, despite dose reduction, suspend treatment until haemoglobin concentration decreases and then restart at a dose approximately 25% lower than the previous dose

Symptomatic anaemia in adults receiving cancer chemotherapy
▸ BY SUBCUTANEOUS INJECTION
▸ Adult: Initially 150 units/kg 3 times a week, alternatively initially 450 units/kg once weekly, increased to 300 units/kg 3 times a week, increased if appropriate rise in haemoglobin (or reticulocyte count) not achieved after 4 weeks; discontinue if inadequate response after 4 weeks at higher dose, subcutaneous injection maximum 1 mL per injection site, reduce dose by approximately 25–50% if rise in haemoglobin concentration exceeds 2 g/100 mL over 4 weeks or if haemoglobin concentration exceeds 12 g/100 mL; if haemoglobin concentration continues to rise, despite dose reduction, suspend treatment until haemoglobin concentration decreases and then restart at a dose approximately 25% lower than the previous dose. Discontinue approximately 4 weeks after ending chemotherapy

To increase yield of autologous blood (to avoid homologous blood) in predonation programme in moderate anaemia either when large volume of blood required or when sufficient blood cannot be saved for elective major surgery
▸ BY INTRAVENOUS INJECTION
▸ Adult: 600 units/kg twice weekly for 3 weeks before surgery, consult product literature for details and advice on ensuring high iron stores, intravenous injection to be given over 1–5 minutes

Moderate anaemia (haemoglobin concentration 10-13 g/100 mL) before elective orthopaedic surgery in adults with expected moderate blood loss to reduce exposure to allogeneic blood transfusion or if autologous transfusion unavailable
▸ BY SUBCUTANEOUS INJECTION
▸ Adult: 600 units/kg once weekly for 3 weeks before surgery and on day of surgery, alternatively 300 units/kg daily for 15 days starting 10 days before surgery, consult product literature for details, subcutaneous injection maximum 1 mL per injection site

● INTERACTIONS → Appendix 1: epoetin alfa
● SIDE-EFFECTS
▸ **Common or very common** Chills · cough · diarrhoea · fever · myalgia · nausea · pain · peripheral oedema · vomiting
▸ **Uncommon** Hyperkalaemia

● PREGNANCY No evidence of harm. Benefits probably outweigh risk of anaemia and of blood transfusion in pregnancy.

● BREAST FEEDING Unlikely to be present in milk. Minimal effect on infant.

● HEPATIC IMPAIRMENT Manufacturer advises caution in chronic hepatic failure.

● PRESCRIBING AND DISPENSING INFORMATION Epoetin alfa is a biological medicine. Biological medicines must be prescribed and dispensed by brand name, see *Biological medicines* and *Biosimilar medicines*, under Guidance on prescribing p. 1.

● NATIONAL FUNDING/ACCESS DECISIONS
For full details see funding body website

NICE decisions
▸ Erythropoiesis-stimulating agents (epoetin and darbepoetin) for treating anaemia in people with cancer having chemotherapy (November 2014) NICE TA323 Recommended with restrictions

● MEDICINAL FORMS There can be variation in the licensing of different medicines containing the same drug.
Solution for injection
▸ Eprex (Janssen-Cilag Ltd)
   Epoetin alfa 2000 unit per 1 ml Eprex 1,000units/0.5ml solution for injection pre-filled syringes | 6 pre-filled disposable injection [PoM] £33.18 DT = £33.18
   Epoetin alfa 4000 unit per 1 ml Eprex 2,000units/0.5ml solution for injection pre-filled syringes | 6 pre-filled disposable injection [PoM] £66.37 DT = £66.37
   Epoetin alfa 10000 unit per 1 ml Eprex 6,000units/0.6ml solution for injection pre-filled syringes | 6 pre-filled disposable injection [PoM] £199.11 DT = £199.11
   Eprex 4,000units/0.4ml solution for injection pre-filled syringes | 6 pre-filled disposable injection [PoM] £132.74 DT = £132.74
   Eprex 5,000units/0.5ml solution for injection pre-filled syringes | 6 pre-filled disposable injection [PoM] £165.92 DT = £165.92
   Eprex 3,000units/0.3ml solution for injection pre-filled syringes | 6 pre-filled disposable injection [PoM] £99.55 DT = £99.55
   Eprex 10,000units/1ml solution for injection pre-filled syringes | 6 pre-filled disposable injection [PoM] £331.85 DT = £331.85
   Eprex 8,000units/0.8ml solution for injection pre-filled syringes | 6 pre-filled disposable injection [PoM] £265.48 DT = £265.48
   Epoetin alfa 40000 unit per 1 ml Eprex 20,000units/0.5ml solution for injection pre-filled syringes | 1 pre-filled disposable injection [PoM] £110.62 DT = £110.62

Eprex 30,000units/0.75ml solution for injection pre-filled syringes |
1 pre-filled disposable injection [PoM] £199.11 DT = £199.11
Eprex 40,000units/1ml solution for injection pre-filled syringes |
1 pre-filled disposable injection [PoM] £265.48 DT = £265.48

▶ 1058

Epoetin beta

06-Dec-2019

● **INDICATIONS AND DOSE**

Symptomatic anaemia associated with chronic renal failure

▶ BY SUBCUTANEOUS INJECTION

▶ Adult: Initially 20 units/kg 3 times a week for 4 weeks, increased in steps of 20 units/kg 3 times a week, according to response at intervals of 4 weeks, total weekly dose may be divided into daily doses; maintenance dose, initially reduce dose by half then adjust according to response at intervals of 1–2 weeks, total weekly maintenance dose may be given as a single dose or in 3 or 7 divided doses. Subcutaneous route preferred in patients not on haemodialysis. Reduce dose by approximately 25% if rise in haemoglobin concentration exceeds 2 g/100 mL over 4 weeks or if haemoglobin concentration approaches or exceeds 12 g/100 mL; if haemoglobin concentration continues to rise, despite dose reduction, suspend treatment until haemoglobin concentration decreases and then restart at a dose approximately 25% lower than the previous dose; maximum 720 units/kg per week

▶ BY INTRAVENOUS INJECTION

▶ Adult: Initially 40 units/kg 3 times a week for 4 weeks, then increased to 80 units/kg 3 times a week, then increased in steps of 20 units/kg 3 times a week if required, at intervals of 4 weeks; maintenance dose, initially reduce dose by half then adjust according to response at intervals of 1–2 weeks. Intravenous injection to be administered over 2 minutes. Subcutaneous route preferred in patients not on haemodialysis. Reduce dose by approximately 25% if rise in haemoglobin concentration exceeds 2 g/100 mL over 4 weeks or if haemoglobin concentration approaches or exceeds 12 g/100 mL; if haemoglobin concentration continues to rise, despite dose reduction, suspend treatment until haemoglobin concentration decreases and then restart at a dose approximately 25% lower than the previous dose; maximum 720 units/kg per week

Symptomatic anaemia in adults with non-myeloid malignancies receiving chemotherapy

▶ BY SUBCUTANEOUS INJECTION

▶ Adult: Initially 450 units/kg once weekly for 4 weeks, dose to be given weekly as a single dose or in 3–7 divided doses, increase dose after 4 weeks (if a rise in haemoglobin of at least 1 g/100 mL not achieved), increased to 900 units/kg once weekly, dose to be given weekly as a single dose or in 3–7 divided doses, if adequate response obtained reduce dose by 25–50%, discontinue treatment if haemoglobin concentration does not increase by at least 1 g/100 mL after 8 weeks of therapy (response unlikely). Reduce dose by approximately 25–50% if rise in haemoglobin concentration exceeds 2 g/100 mL over 4 weeks or if haemoglobin concentration exceeds 12 g/100 mL; if haemoglobin concentration continues to rise, despite dose reduction, suspend treatment until haemoglobin concentration decreases and then restart at a dose approximately 25% lower than the previous dose. Discontinue approximately 4 weeks after ending chemotherapy; maximum 60 000 units per week

To increase yield of autologous blood (to avoid homologous blood) in predonation programme in moderate anaemia when blood-conserving procedures are insufficient or unavailable

▶ BY INTRAVENOUS INJECTION, OR BY SUBCUTANEOUS INJECTION

▶ Adult: (consult product literature)

● INTERACTIONS → Appendix 1: epoetin beta

● PREGNANCY No evidence of harm. Benefits probably outweigh risk of anaemia and of blood transfusion in pregnancy.

● BREAST FEEDING Unlikely to be present in milk. Minimal effect on infant.

● HEPATIC IMPAIRMENT Manufacturer advises caution in chronic hepatic failure.

● NATIONAL FUNDING/ACCESS DECISIONS
For full details see funding body website

NICE decisions

▶ Erythropoiesis-stimulating agents (epoetin and darbepoetin) for treating anaemia in people with cancer having chemotherapy (November 2014) NICE TA323 Recommended with restrictions

● MEDICINAL FORMS There can be variation in the licensing of different medicines containing the same drug.

Solution for injection
EXCIPIENTS: May contain Phenylalanine

▶ NeoRecormon (Roche Products Ltd)
Epoetin beta 1667 unit per 1 ml NeoRecormon 500units/0.3ml solution for injection pre-filled syringes | 6 pre-filled disposable injection [PoM] £21.05 DT = £21.05
Epoetin beta 6667 unit per 1 ml NeoRecormon 2,000units/0.3ml solution for injection pre-filled syringes | 6 pre-filled disposable injection [PoM] £84.17 DT = £84.17
Epoetin beta 10000 unit per 1 ml NeoRecormon 3,000units/0.3ml solution for injection pre-filled syringes | 6 pre-filled disposable injection [PoM] £126.25 DT = £126.25
Epoetin beta 13333 unit per 1 ml NeoRecormon 4,000units/0.3ml solution for injection pre-filled syringes | 6 pre-filled disposable injection [PoM] £168.34 DT = £168.34
Epoetin beta 16667 unit per 1 ml NeoRecormon 10,000units/0.6ml solution for injection pre-filled syringes | 6 pre-filled disposable injection [PoM] £420.85 DT = £420.85
NeoRecormon 5,000units/0.3ml solution for injection pre-filled syringes | 6 pre-filled disposable injection [PoM] £210.42 DT = £210.42
Epoetin beta 20000 unit per 1 ml NeoRecormon 6,000units/0.3ml solution for injection pre-filled syringes | 6 pre-filled disposable injection [PoM] £252.50 DT = £252.50
Epoetin beta 33333 unit per 1 ml NeoRecormon 20,000units/0.6ml solution for injection pre-filled syringes | 6 pre-filled disposable injection [PoM] £841.71 DT = £841.71
Epoetin beta 50000 unit per 1 ml NeoRecormon 30,000units/0.6ml solution for injection pre-filled syringes | 4 pre-filled disposable injection [PoM] £841.71 DT = £841.71

▶ 1058

Epoetin zeta

30-Apr-2019

● **INDICATIONS AND DOSE**

Symptomatic anaemia associated with chronic renal failure in patients on haemodialysis

▶ BY INTRAVENOUS INJECTION, OR BY SUBCUTANEOUS INJECTION

▶ Adult: Initially 50 units/kg 3 times a week, adjusted according to response, adjusted in steps of 25 units/kg 3 times a week, dose to be adjusted at intervals of at least 4 weeks; maintenance 25–100 units/kg 3 times a week, intravenous injection to be given over 1–5 minutes, if given by subcutaneous injection, a maximum of 1 mL can be given per injection site, avoid increasing haemoglobin concentration at a rate exceeding 2 g/100 mL over 4 weeks

continued →

9

Blood and nutrition

Symptomatic anaemia associated with chronic renal failure in adults on peritoneal dialysis

▸ BY INTRAVENOUS INJECTION, OR BY SUBCUTANEOUS INJECTION
▸ Adult: Initially 50 units/kg twice weekly; maintenance 25–50 units/kg twice weekly, intravenous injection to be given over 1–5 minutes, if given by subcutaneous injection, a maximum of 1 mL can be given per injection site, avoid increasing haemoglobin concentration at a rate exceeding 2 g/100 mL over 4 weeks

Severe symptomatic anaemia of renal origin in adults with renal insufficiency not yet on dialysis

▸ BY INTRAVENOUS INJECTION, OR BY SUBCUTANEOUS INJECTION
▸ Adult: Initially 50 units/kg 3 times a week, adjusted according to response, adjusted in steps of 25 units/kg 3 times a week, dose to be increased at intervals of at least 4 weeks; maintenance 17–33 units/kg 3 times a week (max. per dose 200 units/kg 3 times a week), intravenous injection to be given over 1–5 minutes, if given by subcutaneous injection, a maximum of 1 mL can be given per injection site, avoid increasing haemoglobin concentration at a rate exceeding 2 g/100 mL over 4 weeks

Symptomatic anaemia in adults receiving cancer chemotherapy

▸ BY SUBCUTANEOUS INJECTION
▸ Adult: Initially 150 units/kg 3 times a week, alternatively initially 450 units/kg once weekly, increased to 300 units/kg 3 times a week, only increase dose if appropriate rise in haemoglobin (or reticulocyte count) not achieved after 4 weeks; discontinue if inadequate response after 4 weeks at higher dose, maximum 1 mL per injection site, reduce dose by approximately 25–50% if rise in haemoglobin concentration exceeds 2 g/100 mL over 4 weeks or if haemoglobin concentration exceeds 12 g/100 mL; if haemoglobin concentration continues to rise, suspend treatment until haemoglobin concentration decreases and then restart at a dose approximately 25% lower than the previous dose. Discontinue approximately 4 weeks after ending chemotherapy

To increase yield of autologous blood (to avoid homologous blood) in predonation programme in moderate anaemia either when large volume of blood required or when sufficient blood cannot be saved for elective major surgery

▸ BY INTRAVENOUS INJECTION
▸ Adult: 600 units/kg twice weekly for 3 weeks before surgery, intravenous injection to be given over 1–5 minutes, consult product literature for details and advice on ensuring high iron stores

Moderate anaemia (haemoglobin concentration 10–13 g/100 mL) before elective orthopaedic surgery in adults with expected moderate blood loss to reduce exposure to allogeneic blood transfusion or if autologous transfusion unavailable

▸ BY SUBCUTANEOUS INJECTION
▸ Adult: 600 units/kg every week for 3 weeks before surgery and on day of surgery, alternatively 300 units/kg daily for 15 days starting 10 days before surgery, maximum 1 mL per injection site, consult product literature for details

● INTERACTIONS → Appendix 1: epoetin zeta
● SIDE-EFFECTS
▸ **Common or very common** Asthenia · dizziness
▸ **Uncommon** Intracranial haemorrhage
▸ **Rare or very rare** Angioedema

▸ **Frequency not known** Aneurysm · cerebrovascular insufficiency · hypertensive encephalopathy · myocardial infarction · myocardial ischaemia
● PREGNANCY No evidence of harm. Benefits probably outweigh risk of anaemia and of blood transfusion in pregnancy.
● BREAST FEEDING Unlikely to be present in milk. Minimal effect on infant.
● HEPATIC IMPAIRMENT Manufacturer advises caution in chronic hepatic failure.
● PRESCRIBING AND DISPENSING INFORMATION Epoetin zeta is a biological medicine. Biological medicines must be prescribed and dispensed by brand name, see *Biological medicines* and *Biosimilar medicines*, under Guidance on prescribing p. 1.
● NATIONAL FUNDING/ACCESS DECISIONS For full details see funding body website
NICE decisions
▸ Erythropoiesis-stimulating agents (epoetin and darbepoetin) for treating anaemia in people with cancer having chemotherapy (November 2014) NICE TA323 Recommended with restrictions

● MEDICINAL FORMS There can be variation in the licensing of different medicines containing the same drug.
Solution for injection
EXCIPIENTS: May contain Phenylalanine
▸ Retacrit (Pfizer Ltd)
Epoetin zeta 3333 unit per 1 ml Retacrit 2,000units/0.6ml solution for injection pre-filled syringes | 6 pre-filled disposable injection PoM £57.70 DT = £57.70
Retacrit 3,000units/0.9ml solution for injection pre-filled syringes | 6 pre-filled disposable injection PoM £86.55 DT = £86.55
Retacrit 1,000units/0.3ml solution for injection pre-filled syringes | 6 pre-filled disposable injection PoM £28.85 DT = £28.85
Epoetin zeta 10000 unit per 1 ml Retacrit 6,000units/0.6ml solution for injection pre-filled syringes | 6 pre-filled disposable injection PoM £173.09 DT = £173.09
Retacrit 10,000units/1ml solution for injection pre-filled syringes | 6 pre-filled disposable injection PoM £288.48 DT = £288.48
Retacrit 8,000units/0.8ml solution for injection pre-filled syringes | 6 pre-filled disposable injection PoM £230.79 DT = £230.79
Retacrit 4,000units/0.4ml solution for injection pre-filled syringes | 6 pre-filled disposable injection PoM £115.40 DT = £115.40
Retacrit 5,000units/0.5ml solution for injection pre-filled syringes | 6 pre-filled disposable injection PoM £144.25 DT = £144.25
Epoetin zeta 40000 unit per 1 ml Retacrit 20,000units/0.5ml solution for injection pre-filled syringes | 1 pre-filled disposable injection PoM £96.16 DT = £96.16
Retacrit 40,000units/1ml solution for injection pre-filled syringes | 1 pre-filled disposable injection PoM £193.32 DT = £193.32
Retacrit 30,000units/0.75ml solution for injection pre-filled syringes | 1 pre-filled disposable injection PoM £144.25 DT = £144.25

Methoxy polyethylene glycol-epoetin beta

29-Nov-2017

● INDICATIONS AND DOSE

Symptomatic anaemia associated with chronic kidney disease in patients on dialysis and not currently treated with erythropoietins

▸ BY SUBCUTANEOUS INJECTION, OR BY INTRAVENOUS INJECTION
▸ Adult: Initially 600 nanograms/kg every 2 weeks, subcutaneous route preferred in patients not on haemodialysis, dose to be adjusted according to response at intervals of at least 1 month, maintenance dose of double the previous fortnightly dose may be given once a month if haemoglobin concentration is above 10 g/100 mL, reduce dose by approximately 25% if rate of rise in haemoglobin concentration exceeds 2 g/100 mL in 1 month or if haemoglobin concentration is increasing or approaching 12 g/100 mL; if haemoglobin concentration continues to rise, despite

dose reduction, suspend treatment until haemoglobin concentration decreases and then restart at a dose approximately 25% lower than the previous dose, dose may be increased by approximately 25% if the rate of rise in haemoglobin concentration is less than 1 g/100 mL over 1 month; further increases of approximately 25% may be made at monthly intervals until the individual target haemoglobin concentration is obtained

Symptomatic anaemia associated with chronic kidney disease in patients not on dialysis and not currently treated with erythropoietins

▸ INITIALLY BY SUBCUTANEOUS INJECTION
▸ Adult: Initially 1.2 micrograms/kg every month, alternatively (by subcutaneous injection or by intravenous injection) initially 600 nanograms/kg every 2 weeks, subcutaneous route preferred in patients not on haemodialysis, dose to be adjusted according to response at intervals of at least 1 month, patients treated once every 2 weeks may be given a maintenance dose of double the previous fortnightly dose once a month if haemoglobin concentration is above 10 g/100 mL, reduce dose by approximately 25% if rate of rise in haemoglobin concentration exceeds 2 g/100 mL in 1 month or if haemoglobin concentration is increasing or approaching 12 g/100 mL; if haemoglobin concentration continues to rise, despite dose reduction, suspend treatment until haemoglobin concentration decreases and then restart at a dose approximately 25% lower than the previous dose, dose may be increased by approximately 25% if the rate of rise in haemoglobin concentration is less than 1 g/100 mL over 1 month; further increases of approximately 25% may be made at monthly intervals until the individual target haemoglobin concentration is obtained

Symptomatic anaemia associated with chronic kidney disease in patients currently treated with erythropoietins

▸ BY SUBCUTANEOUS INJECTION, OR BY INTRAVENOUS INJECTION
▸ Adult: (consult product literature)

IMPORTANT SAFETY INFORMATION

MHRA/CHM ADVICE: RECOMBINANT HUMAN ERYTHROPOIETINS: VERY RARE RISK OF SEVERE CUTANEOUS ADVERSE REACTIONS (UPDATED JANUARY 2018)

The MHRA is aware of very rare cases of severe cutaneous adverse reactions, including Stevens-Johnson syndrome and toxic epidermal necrolysis, in patients treated with erythropoietins; some cases were fatal. More severe cases were recorded with long-acting agents (darbepoetin alfa and methoxy polyethylene glycol-epoetin beta).

Patients and their carers should be advised of the signs and symptoms of severe skin reactions when starting treatment and instructed to stop treatment and seek immediate medical attention if they develop widespread rash and blistering; these rashes often follow fever or flu-like symptoms—discontinue treatment permanently if such reactions occur.

MHRA/CHM ADVICE (DECEMBER 2007) ERYTHROPOIETINS—HAEMOGLOBIN CONCENTRATION

Overcorrection of haemoglobin concentration in patients with chronic kidney disease may increase the risk of death and serious cardiovascular events, and in patients with cancer may increase the risk of thrombosis and related complications.

● patients should not be treated with erythropoietins for the licensed indications in chronic kidney disease or cancer in patients receiving chemotherapy *unless* symptoms of anaemia are present

● the haemoglobin concentration should be maintained within the range 10–12 g/100 mL
● haemoglobin concentrations higher than 12 g/100 mL should be avoided
● the aim of treatment is to relieve symptoms of anaemia, and in patients with chronic kidney disease to avoid the need for blood transfusion; the haemoglobin concentration should not be increased beyond that which provides adequate control of symptoms of anaemia (in some patients, this may be achieved at concentrations lower than the recommended range)

● CONTRA-INDICATIONS Pure red cell aplasia following erythropoietin therapy · uncontrolled hypertension

● CAUTIONS Bone marrow fibrosis (can impair the response to erythropoietin) · concurrent infection (can impair the response to erythropoietin) · haematological disease (can impair the response to erythropoietin) · haemolysis (can impair the response to erythropoietin) · inflammatory or traumatic episodes (can impair the response to erythropoietin) · malignant disease · occult blood loss (can impair the response to erythropoietin) · severe aluminium toxicity (can impair the response to erythropoietin)

● INTERACTIONS → Appendix 1: methoxy polyethylene glycol-epoetin beta

● SIDE-EFFECTS
▸ **Common or very common** Hypertension (dose-dependent)
▸ **Uncommon** Embolism and thrombosis · headache
▸ **Rare or very rare** Hot flush · hypertensive encephalopathy · rash maculopapular
▸ **Frequency not known** Pure red cell aplasia (discontinue) · severe cutaneous adverse reactions (SCARs) · thrombocytopenia

● PREGNANCY No evidence of harm in *animal* studies—manufacturer advises caution.

● BREAST FEEDING Manufacturer advises use only if potential benefit outweighs risk—present in milk in *animal* studies.

● RENAL IMPAIRMENT Manufacturer advises caution with escalation of doses in chronic renal failure.

● MONITORING REQUIREMENTS
▸ Manufacturer advises monitor haemoglobin concentration every 2 weeks until stabilised and periodically thereafter—if patient fails to respond, check reticulocyte count, and search for causative factors such as deficiencies of iron, folic acid or vitamin B12, and correct if necessary. Monitor iron status before and during treatment.
▸ Manufacturer advises monitor blood pressure before and during treatment—if inadequately controlled, reduce dose or discontinue treatment.

● PRESCRIBING AND DISPENSING INFORMATION Methoxy polyethylene glycol-epoetin beta is a biological medicine. Biological medicines must be prescribed and dispensed by brand name, see *Biological medicines* and *Biosimilar medicines*, under Guidance on prescribing p. 1.
   The manufacturer of *Mircera*® has provided a *Physician's Guide* which includes important safety information to minimise the risk of pure red cell aplasia.

● MEDICINAL FORMS There can be variation in the licensing of different medicines containing the same drug.

Solution for injection
▸ Mircera (Roche Products Ltd)
   Methoxy polyethylene glycol-epoetin beta 100 microgram per 1 ml Mircera 30micrograms/0.3ml solution for injection pre-filled syringes | 1 pre-filled disposable injection PoM £44.05 DT = £44.05
   Methoxy polyethylene glycol-epoetin beta 166.667 microgram per 1 ml Mircera 50micrograms/0.3ml solution for injection pre-filled syringes | 1 pre-filled disposable injection PoM £73.41 DT = £73.41
   Methoxy polyethylene glycol-epoetin beta 250 microgram per 1 ml Mircera 75micrograms/0.3ml solution for injection pre-filled

9

Blood and nutrition

syringes | 1 pre-filled disposable injection PoM £110.11 DT = £110.11
Methoxy polyethylene glycol-epoetin beta 333.333 microgram per 1 ml Mircera 100micrograms/0.3ml solution for injection pre-filled syringes | 1 pre-filled disposable injection PoM £146.81 DT = £146.81
Methoxy polyethylene glycol-epoetin beta 400 microgram per 1 ml Mircera 120micrograms/0.3ml solution for injection pre-filled syringes | 1 pre-filled disposable injection PoM £176.18 DT = £176.18
Methoxy polyethylene glycol-epoetin beta 500 microgram per 1 ml Mircera 150micrograms/0.3ml solution for injection pre-filled syringes | 1 pre-filled disposable injection PoM £220.22 DT = £220.22
Methoxy polyethylene glycol-epoetin beta 600 microgram per 1 ml Mircera 360micrograms/0.6ml solution for injection pre-filled syringes | 1 pre-filled disposable injection PoM £528.56 DT = £528.56
Methoxy polyethylene glycol-epoetin beta 666.667 microgram per 1 ml Mircera 200micrograms/0.3ml solution for injection pre-filled syringes | 1 pre-filled disposable injection PoM £293.62 DT = £293.62
Methoxy polyethylene glycol-epoetin beta 833.333 microgram per 1 ml Mircera 250micrograms/0.3ml solution for injection pre-filled syringes | 1 pre-filled disposable injection PoM £367.03 DT = £367.03

1.1a Atypical haemolytic uraemic syndrome and paroxysmal nocturnal haemoglobinuria

IMMUNOSUPPRESSANTS › MONOCLONAL ANTIBODIES

Eculizumab
13-Aug-2020

● **DRUG ACTION** Eculizumab, a recombinant monoclonal antibody, inhibits terminal complement activation at the C5 protein and thereby reduces haemolysis and thrombotic microangiopathy.

● **INDICATIONS AND DOSE**

Reduce haemolysis in paroxysmal nocturnal haemoglobinuria (PNH), in those with a history of blood transfusions (under expert supervision)
▶ BY INTRAVENOUS INFUSION
▶ Adult: Initially 600 mg once weekly for 4 weeks, then increased to 900 mg once weekly for 1 week; maintenance 900 mg every 12–16 days

Reduce thrombotic microangiopathy in atypical haemolytic uraemic syndrome (aHUS) (specialist use only)
▶ BY INTRAVENOUS INFUSION
▶ Adult: Initially 900 mg once weekly for 4 weeks, then increased to 1.2 g once weekly for 1 week; maintenance 1.2 g every 12–16 days

● **CONTRA-INDICATIONS** Patients unvaccinated against *Neisseria meningitidis* · unresolved *Neisseria meningitidis* infection

● **CAUTIONS** Active systemic infection
CAUTIONS, FURTHER INFORMATION
▶ **Meningococcal infection** Manufacturer advises vaccinate against *Neisseria meningitidis* at least 2 weeks before treatment (vaccines against serotypes A, C, Y, W135 and B where available, are recommended). Patients receiving eculizumab less than 2 weeks after receiving meningococcal vaccine must be given prophylactic antibiotics until 2 weeks after vaccination. Advise patient to report promptly any signs of meningococcal infection. Other immunisations should also be up to date.

● **INTERACTIONS** → Appendix 1: monoclonal antibodies
● **SIDE-EFFECTS**
▶ **Common or very common** Alopecia · asthenia · chills · cough · decreased leucocytes · diarrhoea · dizziness · fever · gastrointestinal discomfort · headache · hypertension · increased risk of infection · influenza like illness · joint disorders · muscle complaints · nausea · oropharyngeal pain · pain · skin reactions · sleep disorders · taste altered · tremor · vomiting
▶ **Uncommon** Abscess · anxiety · appetite decreased · chest discomfort · constipation · cystitis · depression · dysuria · haemorrhage · hot flush · hyperhidrosis · hypersensitivity · hypotension · meningitis meningococcal · mood swings · nasal complaints · oedema · palpitations · paraesthesia · sepsis · spontaneous penile erection · throat irritation · tinnitus · vascular disorders · vertigo · vision blurred
▶ **Rare or very rare** Abnormal clotting factor · conjunctival irritation · feeling hot · gastrooesophageal reflux disease · gingival discomfort · Grave's disease · infusion related reaction · jaundice · malignant melanoma · menstrual disorder · syncope · urogenital tract gonococcal infection

● CONCEPTION AND CONTRACEPTION Manufacturer advises effective contraception during and for 5 months after treatment.

● PREGNANCY Manufacturer advises use only if potential benefit outweighs risk—limited information available. Eculizumab is an immunoglobulin G (IgG) monoclonal antibody; human IgG antibodies are known to cross the placenta.

● BREAST FEEDING Manufacturer advises use with caution—limited information available; unlikely to be present in milk.

● **MONITORING REQUIREMENTS**
▶ Monitor for 1 hour after infusion.
▶ For *paroxysmal nocturnal haemoglobinuria*, monitor for intravascular haemolysis (including serum-lactate dehydrogenase concentration) during treatment and for at least 8 weeks after discontinuation.
▶ For *atypical haemolytic uraemic syndrome*, monitor for thrombotic microangiopathy (measure platelet count, serum-lactate dehydrogenase concentration, and serum creatinine) during treatment and for at least 12 weeks after discontinuation.

● DIRECTIONS FOR ADMINISTRATION For *intravenous infusion* (*Soliris ®*), manufacturer advises give intermittently in Glucose 5% *or* Sodium chloride 0.9%. Dilute requisite dose to a concentration of 5 mg/mL and mix gently; give over 25–45 minutes (infusion time may be increased to 2 hours if infusion-related reactions occur).

● PRESCRIBING AND DISPENSING INFORMATION Consult product literature for details of supplemental doses with concomitant plasmapheresis, plasma exchange, or plasma infusion.

● PATIENT AND CARER ADVICE Patients or carers should be advised to report promptly any signs of meningococcal infection. Advice about prevention of gonorrhoea should also be given.
A patient information card and a patient safety card should be provided.

● NATIONAL FUNDING/ACCESS DECISIONS
For full details see funding body website
NICE decisions
▶ Eculizumab for treating atypical haemolytic uraemic syndrome (January 2015) NICE HST1 Recommended

● MEDICINAL FORMS There can be variation in the licensing of different medicines containing the same drug.

Solution for infusion
ELECTROLYTES: May contain Sodium
▸ Soliris (Alexion Pharma UK Ltd)
    Eculizumab 10 mg per 1 ml Soliris 300mg/30ml concentrate for solution for infusion vials | 1 vial PoM £3,150.00 (Hospital only)

Ravulizumab

16-Apr-2020

● DRUG ACTION Ravulizumab is a recombinant monoclonal antibody that inhibits terminal complement activation at the C5 protein and thereby reduces haemolysis in paroxysmal nocturnal haemoglobinuria.

● INDICATIONS AND DOSE

Paroxysmal nocturnal haemoglobinuria (under expert supervision)
▸ BY INTRAVENOUS INFUSION
▸ Adult (body-weight 40–59 kg): Loading dose 2.4 g for 1 dose, infused over at least 114 minutes, then maintenance 3 g every 8 weeks, infused over at least 140 minutes. Start maintenance dosing 2 weeks after the loading dose, a maintenance dose (except for the first maintenance dose) may be given up to 7 days before or after the scheduled date; the subsequent dose should be given according to the original schedule
▸ Adult (body-weight 60–99 kg): Loading dose 2.7 g for 1 dose, infused over at least 102 minutes, then maintenance 3.3 g every 8 weeks, infused over at least 120 minutes. Start maintenance dosing 2 weeks after the loading dose, a maintenance dose (except for the first maintenance dose) may be given up to 7 days before or after the scheduled date; the subsequent dose should be given according to the original schedule
▸ Adult (body-weight 100 kg and above): Loading dose 3 g for 1 dose, infused over at least 108 minutes, then maintenance 3.6 g every 8 weeks, infused over at least 132 minutes. Start maintenance dosing 2 weeks after the loading dose, a maintenance dose (except for the first maintenance dose) may be given up to 7 days before or after the scheduled date; the subsequent dose should be given according to the original schedule

DOSE EQUIVALENCE AND CONVERSION
▸ For patients switching from eculizumab to ravulizumab, the initial loading dose of ravulizumab should be administered 2 weeks after the last eculizumab infusion.

● CONTRA-INDICATIONS Patients unvaccinated against *Neisseria meningitidis* · unresolved *Neisseria meningitidis* infection

● CAUTIONS Active systemic infection
CAUTIONS, FURTHER INFORMATION
▸ Meningococcal infection Manufacturer advises vaccinate against *Neisseria meningitidis* at least 2 weeks before treatment (vaccines against serotypes A, C, Y, W135 and B where available, are recommended); revaccinate according to current medical guidelines. Patients receiving ravulizumab less than 2 weeks after receiving meningococcal vaccine must be given prophylactic antibiotics until 2 weeks after vaccination. Advise patient to report promptly any signs of meningococcal infection. Other immunisations should also be up to date.

● SIDE-EFFECTS
▸ Common or very common Arthralgia · asthenia · back pain · chills · diarrhoea · dizziness · fever · gastrointestinal discomfort · headache · increased risk of infection · influenza like illness · meningococcal sepsis · muscle complaints · nausea · skin reactions · vomiting
▸ Frequency not known Infusion related reaction

● CONCEPTION AND CONTRACEPTION Manufacturer advises effective contraception during and for up to 8 months after treatment.

● PREGNANCY Manufacturer advises use only if potential benefit outweighs risk—no information available. Ravulizumab is an immunoglobulin G (IgG) monoclonal antibody; human IgG antibodies are known to cross the placenta.

● BREAST FEEDING Manufacturer advises avoid breast-feeding during and for up to 8 months after treatment—no information available.

● MONITORING REQUIREMENTS Manufacturer advises monitor for intravascular haemolysis (including serum-lactate dehydrogenase concentration) for at least 16 weeks after stopping treatment; consider restarting ravulizumab if haemolysis occurs.

● DIRECTIONS FOR ADMINISTRATION Manufacturer advises for *intravenous infusion* (*Ultomiris* ®), give intermittently in Sodium Chloride 0.9%. Dilute requisite dose with infusion fluid to a final concentration of 5 mg/mL and administer through an in-line filter (0.2 micron).

● PRESCRIBING AND DISPENSING INFORMATION
Ravulizumab is a biological medicine. Biological medicines must be prescribed and dispensed by brand name, see *Biological medicines* and *Biosimilar medicines*, under Guidance on prescribing p. 1.
    The manufacturer of *Ultomiris* ® has provided a *Physician's guide* for healthcare professionals.

● HANDLING AND STORAGE Store in a refrigerator (2-8°C) and protect from light—consult product literature for further information regarding storage outside refrigerator.

● PATIENT AND CARER ADVICE Patients or carers should be advised to report promptly any signs of meningococcal infection. Advice about prevention of gonorrhoea should also be given.
    A patient information card and a patient safety card should be provided.

● MEDICINAL FORMS There can be variation in the licensing of different medicines containing the same drug.

Solution for infusion
EXCIPIENTS: May contain Polysorbates
ELECTROLYTES: May contain Sodium
▸ Ultomiris (Alexion Pharma UK Ltd) ▼
    Ravulizumab 10 mg per 1 ml Ultomiris 300mg/30ml concentrate for solution for infusion vials | 1 vial PoM ⟨S⟩ (Hospital only)

1.2   Iron deficiency anaemia

Anaemia, iron deficiency

01-Sep-2020

Iron deficiency, treatment and prophylaxis

Treatment with an iron preparation is justified only in the presence of a demonstrable iron-deficiency state. Before starting treatment, it is important to exclude any serious underlying cause of the anaemia (e.g. gastric erosion, gastrointestinal cancer).

    Prophylaxis with an iron preparation may be appropriate in malabsorption, menorrhagia, pregnancy, after subtotal or total gastrectomy, in haemodialysis patients, and in the management of low birth-weight infants such as preterm neonates.

    For information on oral and intravenous iron use before and after surgery in patients with iron-deficiency anaemia, see NICE guideline: **Blood transfusion** (available from: www.nice.org.uk/guidance/ng24).

Oral iron
Iron salts should be given by mouth unless there are good reasons for using another route.

9

Blood and nutrition

Ferrous salts show only marginal differences between one another in efficiency of absorption of iron. Haemoglobin regeneration rate is little affected by the type of salt used provided sufficient iron is given, and in most patients the speed of response is not critical. Choice of preparation is thus usually decided by the incidence of side-effects and cost.

The oral dose of elemental iron for iron-deficiency anaemia should be 100 to 200 mg daily. It is customary to give this as dried ferrous sulfate; for prophylaxis of iron-deficiency anaemia, ferrous sulfate may be effective.

Iron content of different iron salts

Iron salt/amount	Content of ferrous iron
ferrous fumarate 200 mg	65 mg
ferrous gluconate 300 mg	35 mg
ferrous sulfate 300 mg	60 mg
ferrous sulfate, dried 200 mg	65 mg

Compound preparations
Preparations containing iron and folic acid p. 1071 are used during pregnancy in women who are at high risk of developing iron and folic acid deficiency; they should be distinguished from those used for the prevention of neural tube defects in women planning a pregnancy.

It is important to note that the small doses of folic acid contained in these preparations are inadequate for the treatment of megaloblastic anaemias.

Some oral preparations contain ascorbic acid p. 1132 to aid absorption of the iron but the therapeutic advantage of such preparations is minimal and cost may be increased.

There is no justification for the inclusion of other ingredients, such as the **B group of vitamins** (except folic acid for pregnant women).

Modified-release preparations
Modified-release preparations of iron are licensed for once-daily dosage, but have no therapeutic advantage and should not be used. These preparations are formulated to release iron gradually; the low incidence of side-effects may reflect the small amounts of iron available for absorption as the iron is carried past the first part of the duodenum into an area of the gut where absorption may be poor.

Parenteral iron
Iron can be administered parenterally as iron dextran p. 1067, iron sucrose p. 1068, ferric carboxymaltose p. 1067, or iron isomaltoside 1000 p. 1067. Parenteral iron is generally reserved for use when oral therapy is unsuccessful because the patient cannot tolerate oral iron, or does not take it reliably, or if there is continuing blood loss, or in malabsorption. Parenteral iron may also have a role in the management of chemotherapy-induced anaemia, when given with erythropoietins, in specific patient groups (see NICE guidance).

Many patients with chronic renal failure who are receiving haemodialysis (and some who are receiving peritoneal dialysis) also require iron by the intravenous route on a regular basis.

With the exception of patients with severe renal failure receiving haemodialysis, parenteral iron does not produce a faster haemoglobin response than oral iron provided that the oral iron preparation is taken reliably and is absorbed adequately. Depending on the preparation used, parenteral iron is given as a total dose or in divided doses. Further treatment should be guided by monitoring haemoglobin and serum iron concentrations.

MINERALS AND TRACE ELEMENTS › IRON, INJECTABLE

Iron (injectable)

> **IMPORTANT SAFETY INFORMATION**
>
> MHRA/CHM ADVICE: SERIOUS HYPERSENSITIVITY REACTIONS WITH INTRAVENOUS IRON (AUGUST 2013)
>
> Serious hypersensitivity reactions, including life-threatening and fatal anaphylactic reactions, have been reported in patients receiving intravenous iron. These reactions can occur even when a previous administration has been tolerated (including a negative test dose). Test doses are no longer recommended and caution is needed with every dose of intravenous iron.
>
> Intravenous iron products should only be administered when appropriately trained staff and resuscitation facilities are immediately available; patients should be closely monitored for signs of hypersensitivity during and for at least 30 minutes after every administration. In the event of a hypersensitivity reaction, treatment should be stopped immediately and appropriate management initiated.
>
> The risk of hypersensitivity is increased in patients with known allergies, immune or inflammatory conditions, or those with a history of severe asthma, eczema, or other atopic allergy; in these patients, intravenous iron should only be used if the benefits outweigh the risks.
>
> Intravenous iron should be avoided in the first trimester of pregnancy and used in the second or third trimesters only if the benefit outweighs the potential risks for both mother and fetus.

- **CONTRA-INDICATIONS** Disturbances in utilisation of iron · iron overload
- **CAUTIONS** Allergic disorders · eczema · hepatic dysfunction · immune conditions · infection (discontinue if ongoing bacteraemia) · inflammatory conditions · oral iron should not be given until 5 days after the last injection · severe asthma
- **SIDE-EFFECTS**
  - ▶ **Common or very common** Dizziness · flushing · headache · hypertension · hypophosphataemia · hypotension · nausea · skin reactions · taste altered
  - ▶ **Uncommon** Arrhythmias · arthralgia · bronchospasm · chest pain · chills · constipation · diarrhoea · dyspnoea · fatigue · fever · gastrointestinal discomfort · hyperhidrosis · hypersensitivity · loss of consciousness · muscle complaints · pain · peripheral oedema · sensation abnormal · vision blurred · vomiting
  - ▶ **Rare or very rare** Angioedema · anxiety · circulatory collapse · influenza like illness · malaise · pallor · palpitations · psychiatric disorder · seizure · syncope · tremor
  - ▶ **Frequency not known** Kounis syndrome

  SIDE-EFFECTS, FURTHER INFORMATION Anaphylactic reactions can occur with parenteral administration of iron complexes and facilities for cardiopulmonary resuscitation must be available.

  Overdose For details on the management of poisoning, see Iron salts, under Emergency treatment of poisoning p. 1413.

Ferric carboxymaltose

☞ 1066

27-Nov-2020

● **INDICATIONS AND DOSE**

Iron-deficiency anaemia

▸ BY SLOW INTRAVENOUS INJECTION, OR BY INTRAVENOUS INFUSION

▸ Adult: Dose calculated according to body-weight and iron deficit (consult product literature)

IMPORTANT SAFETY INFORMATION

MHRA/CHM ADVICE: FERRIC CARBOXYMALTOSE (*FERINJECT* ®): RISK OF SYMPTOMATIC HYPOPHOSPHATAEMIA LEADING TO OSTEOMALACIA AND FRACTURES (NOVEMBER 2020)

A European review of worldwide data concluded that ferric carboxymaltose is associated with hypophosphataemia, resulting in hypophosphataemic osteomalacia and fractures, particularly in patients with existing risk factors and following prolonged exposure to high doses—some cases required clinical intervention, including surgery. The risk of persistent hypophosphatemia and osteomalacia may be higher with ferric carboxymaltose than with other intravenous iron formulations.

 Healthcare professionals are advised to monitor serum phosphate levels in patients requiring multiple high-dose administrations, on long-term treatment, or with pre-existing risk factors for hypophosphataemia. Patients experiencing symptoms of hypophosphataemia (including new musculoskeletal symptoms or worsening tiredness) should seek medical advice—be aware that these symptoms may be confused with those of iron deficiency anaemia. If hypophosphataemia persists, ferric carboxymaltose treatment should be re-evaluated.

● INTERACTIONS → Appendix 1: iron

● SIDE-EFFECTS

▸ **Rare or very rare** Face oedema · flatulence

● PREGNANCY Avoid in first trimester; crosses the placenta in *animal* studies. May influence skeletal development.

● HEPATIC IMPAIRMENT Manufacturer advises caution—monitor iron status to avoid iron overload; avoid where iron overload increases risk of impairment (particularly porphyria cutanea tarda).

● DIRECTIONS FOR ADMINISTRATION For *intravenous infusion* (*Ferinject* ®), manufacturer advises give intermittently in Sodium chloride 0.9%, dilute 200–500 mg in up to 100 mL infusion fluid and give over at least 6 minutes; dilute 0.5–1 g in up to 250 mL infusion fluid and give over at least 15 minutes.

● PRESCRIBING AND DISPENSING INFORMATION A ferric carboxymaltose complex containing 5% (50 mg/mL) of iron.

● MEDICINAL FORMS There can be variation in the licensing of different medicines containing the same drug.

Solution for injection

ELECTROLYTES: May contain Sodium

▸ Ferinject (Vifor Pharma UK Ltd) ▼

Iron (as Ferric carboxymaltose) 50 mg per 1 mL Ferinject 1000mg/20ml solution for injection vials | 1 vial [PoM] £154.23 Ferinject 100mg/2ml solution for injection vials | 5 vial [PoM] £95.50 Ferinject 500mg/10ml solution for injection vials | 5 vial [PoM] £477.50

Iron dextran

☞ 1066

17-Jul-2020

● **INDICATIONS AND DOSE**

Iron-deficiency anaemia

▸ BY DEEP INTRAMUSCULAR INJECTION

▸ Adult: Intramuscular injection to be administered into the gluteal muscle, doses calculated according to body-weight and iron deficit (consult product literature)

▸ BY SLOW INTRAVENOUS INJECTION, OR BY INTRAVENOUS INFUSION

▸ Adult: Doses calculated according to body-weight and iron deficit (consult product literature)

● INTERACTIONS → Appendix 1: iron

● SIDE-EFFECTS

▸ **Uncommon** Feeling hot

▸ **Rare or very rare** Deafness (transient) · haemolysis

▸ **Frequency not known** Injection site necrosis · rheumatoid arthritis aggravated

● PREGNANCY Avoid in first trimester.

● HEPATIC IMPAIRMENT Manufacturer advises avoid in decompensated cirrhosis and hepatitis.

● RENAL IMPAIRMENT Avoid in acute renal failure.

● DIRECTIONS FOR ADMINISTRATION

▸ With intravenous use For *intravenous infusion* (*Cosmofer* ®), manufacturer advises give intermittently in Glucose 5% *or* Sodium chloride 0.9%, dilute 100–200 mg in 100 mL infusion fluid; give 25mg over 15 minutes initially, then give at a rate not exceeding 6.67 mg/minute; *total dose infusion* diluted in 500 mL infusion fluid and given over 4–6 hours (initial dose 25 mg over 15 minutes).

● PRESCRIBING AND DISPENSING INFORMATION A complex of ferric hydroxide with dextran containing 5% (50 mg/mL) of iron.

● MEDICINAL FORMS There can be variation in the licensing of different medicines containing the same drug.

Solution for injection

▸ CosmoFer (Pharmacosmos UK Ltd) ▼

Iron (as Iron dextran) 50 mg per 1 mL CosmoFer 500mg/10ml solution for injection ampoules | 2 ampoule [PoM] £79.70 DT = £79.70 CosmoFer 100mg/2ml solution for injection ampoules | 5 ampoule [PoM] £39.85 DT = £39.85

Iron isomaltoside 1000

☞ 1066

09-Dec-2020

(Ferric derisomaltose)

● **INDICATIONS AND DOSE**

Iron-deficiency anaemia

▸ BY INTRAVENOUS INJECTION

▸ Adult: (consult product literature)

● INTERACTIONS → Appendix 1: iron

● SIDE-EFFECTS

▸ **Uncommon** Fishbane reaction · infection

▸ **Rare or very rare** Dysphonia

● PREGNANCY Avoid in first trimester.

● HEPATIC IMPAIRMENT Manufacturer advises caution in compensated hepatic disease—monitor iron status to avoid iron overload; avoid in decompensated hepatic disease, in hepatitis and where iron overload is a precipitating factor (particularly porphyria cutanea tarda).

● NATIONAL FUNDING/ACCESS DECISIONS

For full details see funding body website

Scottish Medicines Consortium (SMC) decisions

▸ Iron (III) isomaltoside 1000 5% (*Diafer* ®) for iron deficiency in adults with chronic kidney disease (CKD) on dialysis, when oral iron preparations are ineffective or cannot be used (February 2017) SMC No. 1177/16 Recommended

9

Blood and nutrition

- MEDICINAL FORMS There can be variation in the licensing of different medicines containing the same drug.

Solution for injection
- Diafer (Pharmacosmos UK Ltd) ▼
  Iron (as Iron isomaltoside 1000) 50 mg per 1 ml Diafer 100mg/2ml solution for injection ampoules | 25 ampoule PoM £423.75
- Monofer (Pharmacosmos UK Ltd) ▼
  Iron (as Iron isomaltoside 1000) 100 mg per 1 ml Monofer 500mg/5ml solution for injection vials | 5 vial PoM £423.75
  Monofer 100mg/1ml solution for injection vials | 5 vial PoM £84.75
  Monofer 1g/10ml solution for injection vials | 2 vial PoM £339.00

F 1066

Iron sucrose

29-Nov-2019

- **INDICATIONS AND DOSE**
  Iron-deficiency anaemia
  ▸ BY SLOW INTRAVENOUS INJECTION, OR BY INTRAVENOUS INFUSION
  ▸ Adult: Doses calculated according to body-weight and iron deficit (consult product literature)

- INTERACTIONS → Appendix 1: iron

- SIDE-EFFECTS
- ▸ **Uncommon** Asthenia
- ▸ **Rare or very rare** Drowsiness · urine discolouration
- ▸ **Frequency not known** Cold sweat · confusion · level of consciousness decreased · thrombophlebitis

- PREGNANCY Avoid in first trimester.

- HEPATIC IMPAIRMENT Manufacturer advises caution— monitor iron status to avoid iron overload; avoid where iron overload is a precipitating factor (particularly porphyria cutanea tarda).

- DIRECTIONS FOR ADMINISTRATION Manufacturer advises for *intermittent intravenous infusion* (*Venofer®*), dilute to a concentration of 1 mg/mL with Sodium Chloride 0.9%; give at a rate not exceeding 6.67 mg/minute (consult product literature). Manufacturer advises for *slow intravenous injection* (*Venofer®*), give undiluted at a rate of 1 mL/minute; do not exceed 10 mL (200 mg iron) per injection.

- PRESCRIBING AND DISPENSING INFORMATION A complex of ferric hydroxide with sucrose containing 2% (20 mg/mL) of iron.

- MEDICINAL FORMS There can be variation in the licensing of different medicines containing the same drug.
  Solution for injection
  ▸ Venofer (Vifor Pharma UK Ltd) ▼
    Iron (as Iron sucrose) 20 mg per 1 ml Venofer 100mg/5ml solution for injection vials | 5 vial PoM £51.20 DT = £51.20

MINERALS AND TRACE ELEMENTS > IRON, ORAL

Iron (oral)

- CAUTIONS High doses in elderly
  CAUTIONS, FURTHER INFORMATION
  ▸ Elderly Prescription potentially inappropriate (STOPP criteria) at oral doses greater than 200 mg elemental iron daily (no evidence of enhanced iron absorption above these doses). See also Prescribing in the elderly p. 33.

- SIDE-EFFECTS
- ▸ **Common or very common** Constipation · diarrhoea · gastrointestinal discomfort · nausea
- ▸ **Uncommon** Vomiting
- ▸ **Frequency not known** Appetite decreased · faeces discoloured
  SIDE-EFFECTS, FURTHER INFORMATION Iron can be constipating and occasionally lead to faecal impaction. Oral iron, particularly modified-release preparations, can

exacerbate diarrhoea in patients with inflammatory bowel disease; care is also needed in patients with intestinal strictures and diverticular disease.

Overdose For details on the management of poisoning, see Iron salts, under Emergency treatment of poisoning p. 1413.

- MONITORING REQUIREMENTS
- ▸ Therapeutic response The haemoglobin concentration should rise by about 100–200 mg/100 mL (1–2 g/litre) per day *or* 2 g/100 mL (20 g/litre) over 3–4 weeks. When the haemoglobin is in the normal range, treatment should be continued for a further 3 months to replenish the iron stores. Epithelial tissue changes such as atrophic glossitis and koilonychia are usually improved, but the response is often slow.

- PRESCRIBING AND DISPENSING INFORMATION
- ▸ In children Express the dose in terms of elemental iron and iron salt and select the most appropriate preparation; specify both the iron salt and formulation on the prescription. The iron content of artificial formula feeds should also be considered. The most common reason for lack of response in children is poor compliance; poor absorption is rare in children.

- PATIENT AND CARER ADVICE Although iron preparations are best absorbed on an empty stomach they can be taken after food to reduce gastro-intestinal side-effects. May discolour stools.

F above

Ferric maltol

20-Nov-2020

- **INDICATIONS AND DOSE**
  Iron-deficiency anaemia
  ▸ BY MOUTH
  ▸ Adult: 30 mg twice daily continued until iron stores are replenished; usual duration at least 12 weeks

- CONTRA-INDICATIONS Exacerbation of inflammatory bowel disease · haemochromatosis · inflammatory bowel disease with haemoglobin less than 9.5 g/dL · iron overload syndromes · repeated blood transfusions

- INTERACTIONS → Appendix 1: iron

- SIDE-EFFECTS
- ▸ **Common or very common** Flatulence
- ▸ **Uncommon** Headache · joint stiffness · pain in extremity · skin reactions · small intestinal bacterial overgrowth · thirst

- NATIONAL FUNDING/ACCESS DECISIONS
  For full details see funding body website

  Scottish Medicines Consortium (SMC) decisions
  ▸ Ferric maltol (*Feraccru®*) for the treatment of iron deficiency anaemia in adults with inflammatory bowel disease (December 2016) SMC No. 1202/16 Not recommended

  All Wales Medicines Strategy Group (AWMSG) decisions
  ▸ Ferric maltol (*Feraccru®*) for the treatment of iron deficiency anaemia in adults with inflammatory bowel disease (January 2017) AWMSG No. 2631 Not recommended

- MEDICINAL FORMS There can be variation in the licensing of different medicines containing the same drug.
  Capsule
  CAUTIONARY AND ADVISORY LABELS 23
  ▸ Feraccru (Norgine Pharmaceuticals Ltd)
    Iron (as Ferric maltol) 30 mg Feraccru 30mg capsules | 56 capsule PoM £47.60 DT = £47.60

Ferrous fumarate

F 1068

12-Aug-2020

- **INDICATIONS AND DOSE**

Iron-deficiency anaemia (prophylactic)
▶ BY MOUTH USING TABLETS
▸ Child 12–17 years: 210 mg 1–2 times a day
▸ Adult: 210 mg 1–2 times a day
▶ BY MOUTH USING SYRUP
▸ Child 12–17 years: 140 mg twice daily
▸ Adult: 140 mg twice daily

Iron-deficiency anaemia (therapeutic)
▶ BY MOUTH USING TABLETS
▸ Child 12–17 years: 210 mg 2–3 times a day
▸ Adult: 210 mg 2–3 times a day
▶ BY MOUTH USING SYRUP
▸ Child 12–17 years: 280 mg twice daily
▸ Adult: 280 mg twice daily

GALFER® CAPSULES
Iron-deficiency anaemia (prophylactic)
▶ BY MOUTH
▸ Child 12–17 years: 305 mg daily
▸ Adult: 305 mg daily
Iron-deficiency anaemia (therapeutic)
▶ BY MOUTH
▸ Child 12–17 years: 305 mg twice daily
▸ Adult: 305 mg twice daily

GALFER® SYRUP
Iron-deficiency anaemia (prophylaxis)
▶ BY MOUTH
▸ Child 1 month–11 years: 0.25 mL/kilogram twice daily, the total daily dose may alternatively be given in 3 divided doses, prophylactic iron supplementation may be required in babies of low birth-weight who are solely breast-fed; supplementation is started 4–6 weeks after birth and continued until mixed feeding is established; maximum 20 mL per day
▸ Child 12–17 years: 10 mL once daily
▸ Adult: 10 mL once daily
Iron-deficiency anaemia (therapeutic)
▶ BY MOUTH
▸ Child 1 month–11 years: 0.25 mL/kilogram twice daily, the total daily dose may alternatively be given in 3 divided doses; maximum 20 mL per day
▸ Child 12–17 years: 10 mL 1–2 times a day
▸ Adult: 10 mL 1–2 times a day

- **INTERACTIONS** → Appendix 1: iron
- **SIDE-EFFECTS** Faecal impaction · haemosiderosis
- **PRESCRIBING AND DISPENSING INFORMATION** Non-proprietary ferrous fumarate tablets may contain 210 mg (68 mg iron), syrup may contain approx. 140 mg (45 mg iron)/5 mL; *Galfer*® capsules contain ferrous fumarate 305 mg (100 mg iron).
- **PATIENT AND CARER ADVICE**
  Medicines for Children leaflet: Ferrous fumarate for iron-deficiency anaemia www.medicinesforchildren.org.uk/ferrous-fumarate-iron-deficiency-anaemia
- **MEDICINAL FORMS** There can be variation in the licensing of different medicines containing the same drug.
  Oral solution
  ▸ Ferrous fumarate (Non-proprietary)
    Ferrous fumarate 28 mg per 1 ml Ferrous fumarate 140mg/5ml oral solution | 200 ml [P] £3.92 DT = £3.92
  ▸ Galfer (Thornton & Ross Ltd)
    Ferrous fumarate 28 mg per 1 ml Galfer 140mg/5ml syrup sugar-free | 300 ml [P] £5.33 DT = £5.33

Tablet
▸ Ferrous fumarate (Non-proprietary)
  Ferrous fumarate 210 mg Ferrous fumarate 210mg tablets | 84 tablet [P] £3.99 DT = £3.99
  Ferrous fumarate 322 mg Ferrous fumarate 322mg tablets | 28 tablet [PoM] [℞] DT = £1.00
Capsule
▸ Galfer (Thornton & Ross Ltd)
  Ferrous fumarate 305 mg Galfer 305mg capsules | 100 capsule [P] £5.00 DT = £5.00 | 250 capsule [P] £12.50

Ferrous fumarate with folic acid

04-May-2020

The properties listed below are those particular to the combination only. For the properties of the components please consider, ferrous fumarate above, folic acid p. 1071.

- **INDICATIONS AND DOSE**

Iron-deficiency anaemia
▶ BY MOUTH USING CAPSULES
▸ Adult: 1 capsule daily, to be taken before food
▶ BY MOUTH USING TABLETS
▸ Adult: 1 tablet daily

- **INTERACTIONS** → Appendix 1: folates · iron
- **PRESCRIBING AND DISPENSING INFORMATION** *Pregaday*® contains ferrous fumarate 322 mg (100 mg iron), folic acid 350 micrograms; *Galfer FA*® contains ferrous fumarate 305 mg (100 mg iron), folic acid 350 micrograms.
- **MEDICINAL FORMS** There can be variation in the licensing of different medicines containing the same drug.
  Tablet
  ▸ Pregaday (RPH Pharmaceuticals AB)
    Folic acid 350 microgram, Ferrous fumarate 322 mg Pregaday 322mg/350microgram tablets | 28 tablet [P] £1.25 DT = £1.25

F 1068

Ferrous gluconate

10-Mar-2020

- **INDICATIONS AND DOSE**

Prophylaxis of iron-deficiency anaemia
▶ BY MOUTH USING TABLETS
▸ Child 6–11 years: 300–900 mg daily
▸ Child 12–17 years: 600 mg daily
▸ Adult: 600 mg daily

Treatment of iron-deficiency anaemia
▶ BY MOUTH USING TABLETS
▸ Child 6–11 years: 300–900 mg daily
▸ Child 12–17 years: 1.2–1.8 g daily in divided doses
▸ Adult: 1.2–1.8 g daily in divided doses

- **INTERACTIONS** → Appendix 1: iron
- **SIDE-EFFECTS** Gastrointestinal disorders
- **PRESCRIBING AND DISPENSING INFORMATION** Ferrous gluconate 300 mg contains 35 mg iron.
- **PATIENT AND CARER ADVICE**
  Medicines for Children leaflet: Ferrous gluconate for iron-deficiency anaemia www.medicinesforchildren.org.uk/ferrous-gluconate-iron-deficiency-anaemia
- **MEDICINAL FORMS** There can be variation in the licensing of different medicines containing the same drug.
  Tablet
  ▸ Ferrous gluconate (Non-proprietary)
    Ferrous gluconate 300 mg Ferrous gluconate 300mg tablets | 28 tablet [P] £3.35 DT = £1.07 | 1000 tablet [P] £38.21–£119.64

9

Blood and nutrition

Ferrous sulfate

F 1068

30-Sep-2020

- **INDICATIONS AND DOSE**

Iron-deficiency anaemia (prophylactic)
▸ BY MOUTH USING TABLETS
- Child 6-17 years: 200 mg daily
- Adult: 200 mg daily

Iron-deficiency anaemia (therapeutic)
▸ BY MOUTH USING TABLETS
- Child 6-17 years: 200 mg 2–3 times a day
- Adult: 200 mg 2–3 times a day

FEOSPAN ®

Iron-deficiency anaemia
▸ BY MOUTH
- Child 1-17 years: 1 capsule daily, capsule can be opened and sprinkled on food
- Adult: 1–2 capsules daily, capsule can be opened and sprinkled on food

FERROGRAD ®

Iron-deficiency anaemia (prophylactic and therapeutic)
▸ BY MOUTH
- Child 12-17 years: 1 tablet daily
- Adult: 1 tablet daily

IRONORM ® DROPS

Iron-deficiency anaemia (prophylactic)
▸ BY MOUTH
- Adult: 2.4–4.8 mL daily

Iron-deficiency anaemia (therapeutic)
▸ BY MOUTH
- Adult: 4 mL 1–2 times a day

- INTERACTIONS → Appendix 1: iron
- SIDE-EFFECTS Tooth discolouration
- PRESCRIBING AND DISPENSING INFORMATION
Iron content Ferrous sulfate 200 mg is equivalent to 65 mg iron; *Ironorm* ® drops contain ferrous sulfate 125 mg (equivalent to 25 mg iron)/mL; *Feospan* ® spansules contains ferrous sulfate 150 mg (47 mg iron) (spansule (= capsules m/r)); *Ferrograd* ® tablets contain ferrous sulfate 325 mg (105 mg iron).
▸ In adults Modified-release preparations of iron are licensed for once-daily dosage, but have no therapeutic advantage and should not be used. These preparations are formulated to release iron gradually; the low incidence of side-effects may reflect the small amounts of iron available for absorption as the iron is carried past the first part of the duodenum into an area of the gut where absorption may be poor.

- PATIENT AND CARER ADVICE
Medicines for Children leaflet: Ferrous sulfate for iron-deficiency anaemia www.medicinesforchildren.org.uk/ferrous-sulfate-iron-deficiency-anaemia

- NATIONAL FUNDING/ACCESS DECISIONS
NHS restrictions *Feospan* ® is not prescribable in NHS primary care.

- LESS SUITABLE FOR PRESCRIBING *Feospan* ® is less suitable for prescribing. *Ferrograd* ® is less suitable for prescribing.

- MEDICINAL FORMS There can be variation in the licensing of different medicines containing the same drug.
Modified-release tablet
CAUTIONARY AND ADVISORY LABELS 25
▸ Ferrograd (Teofarma)
Ferrous sulfate dried 325 mg Ferrograd 325mg modified-release tablets | 30 tablet DT = £2.58

Tablet
▸ Ferrous sulfate (Non-proprietary)
Ferrous sulfate dried 200 mg Ferrous sulfate 200mg tablets | 28 tablet [P] £8.15 DT = £1.30 | 60 tablet [P] £1.80–£3.05 | 100 tablet [P] £4.32–£5.04 | 1000 tablet [P] £43.21–£46.43
Modified-release capsule
CAUTIONARY AND ADVISORY LABELS 25
▸ Feospan (Intrapharm Laboratories Ltd)
Ferrous sulfate dried 150 mg Feospan 150mg Spansules | 30 capsule [P] £3.95
Oral drops
▸ Ironorm (Wallace Manufacturing Chemists Ltd)
Ferrous sulfate 125 mg per 1 ml Ironorm 125mg/ml oral drops sugar-free | 15 ml [P] £30.00 DT = £30.00

Ferrous sulfate with ascorbic acid

07-May-2020

The properties listed below are those particular to the combination only. For the properties of the components please consider, ferrous sulfate above, ascorbic acid p. 1132.

- **INDICATIONS AND DOSE**

Iron-deficiency anaemia
▸ BY MOUTH USING MODIFIED-RELEASE TABLETS
- Adult: 1 tablet daily, dose to be taken before food

- INTERACTIONS → Appendix 1: ascorbic acid · iron
- NATIONAL FUNDING/ACCESS DECISIONS
NHS restrictions *Ferrograd C* ® is not prescribable in NHS primary care.
- LESS SUITABLE FOR PRESCRIBING *Ferrograd C* ® is less suitable for prescribing.

- MEDICINAL FORMS There can be variation in the licensing of different medicines containing the same drug.
Modified-release tablet
CAUTIONARY AND ADVISORY LABELS 25
▸ Ferrograd C (Teofarma)
Ferrous sulfate dried 325 mg, Ascorbic acid (as Sodium ascorbate) 500 mg Ferrograd C modified-release tablets | 30 tablet [P] £3.20

Ferrous sulfate with folic acid

07-May-2020

The properties listed below are those particular to the combination only. For the properties of the components please consider, ferrous sulfate above, folic acid p. 1071.

- **INDICATIONS AND DOSE**

Iron-deficiency anaemia
▸ BY MOUTH USING MODIFIED-RELEASE TABLETS
- Child 12-17 years: 1 tablet daily, to be taken before food
- Adult: 1 tablet daily, to be taken before food

- INTERACTIONS → Appendix 1: folates · iron
- LESS SUITABLE FOR PRESCRIBING *Ferrograd Folic* ® is less suitable for prescribing.

- MEDICINAL FORMS There can be variation in the licensing of different medicines containing the same drug.
Modified-release tablet
CAUTIONARY AND ADVISORY LABELS 25
▸ Ferrograd Folic (Teofarma)
Folic acid 350 microgram, Ferrous sulfate dried 325 mg Ferrograd Folic 325mg/350microgram modified-release tablets | 30 tablet [P] £2.64 DT = £2.64

Sodium feredetate

F 1068
09-Dec-2020

(Sodium ironedetate)

● INDICATIONS AND DOSE

Iron-deficiency anaemia (therapeutic)
▶ BY MOUTH USING ORAL SOLUTION
▸ Child 1–11 months: Up to 2.5 mL twice daily, smaller doses to be used initially
▸ Child 1–4 years: 2.5 mL 3 times a day
▸ Child 5–11 years: 5 mL 3 times a day
▸ Child 12–17 years: 5 mL 3 times a day, increased to 10 mL 3 times a day, dose to be increased gradually
▸ Adult: 5 mL 3 times a day, increased to 10 mL 3 times a day, dose to be increased gradually

● INTERACTIONS → Appendix 1: iron

● PRESCRIBING AND DISPENSING INFORMATION *Sytron*® contains 207.5 mg sodium feredetate trihydrate, which is equivalent to 27.5 mg of iron/5 mL.

● PATIENT AND CARER ADVICE
Medicines for Children leaflet: Sytron (sodium feredetate) for the treatment of anaemia www.medicinesforchildren.org.uk/sytron-treatment-anaemia

● MEDICINAL FORMS There can be variation in the licensing of different medicines containing the same drug.
Oral solution
EXCIPIENTS: May contain Ethanol, hydroxybenzoates (parabens), sorbitol
▸ SodiFer (Essential-Healthcare Ltd)
Iron (as Sodium feredetate) 5.5 mg per 1 ml SodiFer 190mg/5ml oral solution sugar-free | 500 ml £12.07 DT = £14.95
▸ Sytron (Forum Health Products Ltd)
Iron (as Sodium feredetate) 5.5 mg per 1 ml Sytron oral solution sugar-free | 500 ml P £14.95 DT = £14.95

1.3 Megaloblastic anaemia

Anaemia, megaloblastic

Overview

Most megaloblastic anaemias result from a lack of either vitamin B$_{12}$ or folate, and it is essential to establish in every case which deficiency is present and the underlying cause. In emergencies, when delay might be dangerous, it is sometimes necessary to administer both substances after the bone marrow test while plasma assay results are awaited. Normally, however, appropriate treatment should not be instituted until the results of tests are available.

One cause of megaloblastic anaemia in the UK is *pernicious anaemia* in which lack of gastric intrinsic factor resulting from an autoimmune gastritis causes malabsorption of vitamin B$_{12}$.

Vitamin B$_{12}$ is also needed in the treatment of megaloblastosis caused by *prolonged nitrous oxide anaesthesia*, which inactivates the vitamin, and in the rare syndrome of *congenital transcobalamin II deficiency*.

Vitamin B$_{12}$ should be given prophylactically after *total gastrectomy* or *total ileal resection* (or after *partial gastrectomy* if a vitamin B$_{12}$ absorption test shows vitamin B$_{12}$ malabsorption).

Apart from dietary deficiency, all other causes of vitamin B$_{12}$ deficiency are attributable to malabsorption. There is little place for the use of low-dose vitamin B$_{12}$ orally and none for vitamin B$_{12}$ intrinsic factor complexes given by mouth. Vitamin B$_{12}$ in larger oral doses [unlicensed] may be effective.

Hydroxocobalamin p. 1072 has completely replaced cyanocobalamin p. 1072 as the form of vitamin B$_{12}$ of choice

for therapy; it is retained in the body longer than cyanocobalamin and thus for maintenance therapy can be given at intervals of up to 3 months. Treatment is generally initiated with frequent administration of intramuscular injections to replenish the depleted body stores. Thereafter, maintenance treatment, which is usually for life, can be instituted. There is no evidence that doses larger than those recommended provide any additional benefit in vitamin B$_{12}$ neuropathy.

Folic acid below has few indications for long-term therapy since most causes of folate deficiency are self-limiting or will yield to a short course of treatment. It should not be used in undiagnosed megaloblastic anaemia unless vitamin B$_{12}$ is administered concurrently otherwise neuropathy may be precipitated.

In *folate-deficient megaloblastic anaemia* (e.g. because of poor nutrition, pregnancy, or antiepileptic drugs), daily folic acid supplementation for 4 months brings about haematological remission and replenishes body stores.

For prophylaxis in *chronic haemolytic states*, *malabsorption*, or *in renal dialysis*, folic acid is given daily or sometimes weekly, depending on the diet and the rate of haemolysis.

Folic acid is also used for the prevention of methotrexate-induced side-effects in severe Crohn's disease, rheumatic disease, and severe psoriasis.

Folinic acid p. 984 is also effective in the treatment of folate deficient megaloblastic anaemia but it is generally used in association with cytotoxic drugs; it is given as calcium folinate.

There is **no** justification for prescribing multiple ingredient vitamin preparations containing vitamin B$_{12}$ or folic acid.

For the use of folic acid before and during pregnancy, see Neural tube defects (prevention in pregnancy) p. 1139.

VITAMINS AND TRACE ELEMENTS ⟩ FOLATES

Folic acid

10-Mar-2020

● INDICATIONS AND DOSE

Folate-deficient megaloblastic anaemia
▶ BY MOUTH
▸ Child 1–11 months: Initially 500 micrograms/kg once daily (max. per dose 5 mg) for up to 4 months, doses up to 10 mg daily may be required in malabsorption states
▸ Child 1–17 years: 5 mg daily for 4 months (until term in pregnant women), doses up to 15 mg daily may be required in malabsorption states
▸ Adult: 5 mg daily for 4 months (until term in pregnant women), doses up to 15 mg daily may be required in malabsorption states

Prevention of neural tube defects (in those at a low risk of conceiving a child with a neural tube defect see Neural tube defects (prevention in pregnancy) p. 1139)
▶ BY MOUTH
▸ Females of childbearing potential: 400 micrograms daily, to be taken before conception and until week 12 of pregnancy

Prevention of neural tube defects (in those in the high-risk group who wish to become pregnant or who are at risk of becoming pregnant see Neural tube defects (prevention in pregnancy) p. 1139)
▶ BY MOUTH
▸ Females of childbearing potential: 5 mg daily, to be taken before conception and until week 12 of pregnancy

Prevention of neural tube defects (in those with sickle-cell disease)
▶ BY MOUTH
▸ Females of childbearing potential: 5 mg daily, patient should continue taking their normal dose of

continued →

9

Blood and nutrition

folic acid 5 mg daily (or increase the dose to 5 mg daily) before conception and continue this throughout pregnancy

Prevention of methotrexate-induced side-effects in rheumatic disease
▸ BY MOUTH
▸ Adult: 5 mg once weekly, dose to be taken on a different day to methotrexate dose

Prevention of methotrexate side-effects in severe Crohn's disease | Prevention of methotrexate side-effects in severe psoriasis
▸ BY MOUTH
▸ Adult: 5 mg once weekly, dose to be taken on a different day to methotrexate dose

Prophylaxis in chronic haemolytic states
▸ BY MOUTH
▸ Adult: 5 mg every 1–7 days, frequency dependent on underlying disease

Prophylaxis of folate deficiency in dialysis
▸ BY MOUTH
▸ Child 1 month–11 years: 250 micrograms/kg once daily (max. per dose 10 mg)
▸ Child 12–17 years: 5–10 mg once daily
▸ Adult: 5 mg every 1–7 days

Prophylaxis of folate deficiency in patients receiving parenteral nutrition
▸ BY INTRAVENOUS INFUSION
▸ Adult: 15 mg 1–2 times a week, usually given by *intravenous infusion* in the parenteral nutrition solution

● UNLICENSED USE
▸ In adults Not licensed for prevention of methotrexate-induced side-effects in severe Crohn's disease. Not licensed for prevention of methotrexate-induced side-effects in rheumatic disease. Not licensed for prevention of methotrexate-induced side-effects in severe psoriasis.

● CAUTIONS Should never be given alone for pernicious anaemia (may precipitate subacute combined degeneration of the spinal cord)

● INTERACTIONS → Appendix 1: folates

● SIDE-EFFECTS Abdominal distension · appetite decreased · flatulence · nausea · vitamin B12 deficiency exacerbated

● PATIENT AND CARER ADVICE
Medicines for Children leaflet: Folic acid for megaloblastic anaemia caused by folate deficiency and haemolytic anaemia www.medicinesforchildren.org.uk/folic-acid-megaloblastic-anaemia-caused-folate-deficiency-and-haemolytic-anaemia

● EXCEPTIONS TO LEGAL CATEGORY
▸ With oral use Can be sold to the public provided daily doses do not exceed 500 micrograms.

● MEDICINAL FORMS There can be variation in the licensing of different medicines containing the same drug. Forms available from special-order manufacturers include: capsule, oral suspension, oral solution, solution for injection

Tablet
▸ Folic acid (Non-proprietary)
Folic acid 400 microgram Folic acid 400microgram tablets | 90 tablet PoM Ⓧ DT = £3.52
Folic acid 5 mg Folic acid 5mg tablets | 28 tablet PoM £2.00 DT = £1.12 | 1000 tablet PoM £40.00

Oral solution
▸ Folic acid (Non-proprietary)
Folic acid 500 microgram per 1 ml Folic acid 2.5mg/5ml oral solution sugar free sugar-free | 150 ml PoM £9.16 DT = £9.16 sugar-free | 150 ml £9.16 DT = £9.16
Folic acid 1 mg per 1 ml Folic acid 5mg/5ml oral solution sugar free sugar-free | 150 ml PoM £43.91-£54.72 DT = £54.72
▸ Lexpec (Rosemont Pharmaceuticals Ltd)
Folic acid 500 microgram per 1 ml Lexpec Folic Acid 2.5mg/5ml oral solution sugar-free | 150 ml PoM £9.16 DT = £9.16

VITAMINS AND TRACE ELEMENTS ❭ VITAMIN B GROUP

Cyanocobalamin

29-Mar-2019

● INDICATIONS AND DOSE
Vitamin B₁₂ deficiency of dietary origin
▸ BY MOUTH
▸ Adult: 50–150 micrograms daily, dose to be taken between meals
▸ BY INTRAMUSCULAR INJECTION
▸ Adult: Initially 1 mg every 2–3 days for 11 doses; maintenance 1 mg every month

● PRESCRIBING AND DISPENSING INFORMATION Currently available brands of the tablet may not be suitable for vegans.
The BP directs that when vitamin B₁₂ injection is prescribed or demanded hydroxocobalamin injection shall be dispensed or supplied.

● NATIONAL FUNDING/ACCESS DECISIONS
NHS restrictions *Cyanocobalamin* solution and *Cytamen*® injection are not prescribable in NHS primary care.

● LESS SUITABLE FOR PRESCRIBING Cyanocobalamin is less suitable for prescribing.

● MEDICINAL FORMS There can be variation in the licensing of different medicines containing the same drug.
Solution for injection
▸ Cytamen (RPH Pharmaceuticals AB)
Cyanocobalamin 1 mg per 1 ml Cytamen 1000micrograms/1ml solution for injection ampoules | 5 ampoule PoM £14.50 DT = £14.50
Tablet
▸ Cyanocobalamin (Non-proprietary)
Cyanocobalamin 50 microgram Cyanocobalamin 50microgram tablets | 50 tablet Ⓟ £14.32 DT = £14.32
▸ CyanocoMinn (Essential-Healthcare Ltd)
Cyanocobalamin 100 microgram CyanocoMinn 100microgram tablets | 50 tablet £3.21
▸ Behepan (Imported (Sweden))
Cyanocobalamin 1 mg Behepan 1mg tablets | 100 tablet PoM Ⓧ

Hydroxocobalamin

20-Jul-2017

● INDICATIONS AND DOSE
Prophylaxis of macrocytic anaemias associated with vitamin B₁₂ deficiency
▸ BY INTRAMUSCULAR INJECTION
▸ Adult: 1 mg every 2–3 months

Pernicious anaemia and other macrocytic anaemias without neurological involvement
▸ BY INTRAMUSCULAR INJECTION
▸ Adult: Initially 1 mg 3 times a week for 2 weeks, then 1 mg every 2–3 months

Pernicious anaemia and other macrocytic anaemias with neurological involvement
▸ BY INTRAMUSCULAR INJECTION
▸ Adult: Initially 1 mg once daily on alternate days until no further improvement, then 1 mg every 2 months

Tobacco amblyopia
▸ BY INTRAMUSCULAR INJECTION
▸ Adult: Initially 1 mg daily for 2 weeks, then 1 mg twice weekly until no further improvement, then 1 mg every 1–3 months

Leber's optic atrophy
▸ BY INTRAMUSCULAR INJECTION
▸ Adult: Initially 1 mg daily for 2 weeks, then 1 mg twice weekly until no further improvement, then 1 mg every 1–3 months

CYANOKIT ®

Poisoning with cyanides

▸ **BY INTRAVENOUS INFUSION**

▸ Child (body-weight 5 kg and above): Initially 70 mg/kg (max. per dose 5 g), to be given over 15 minutes, then 70 mg/kg (max. per dose 5 g) if required, this second dose can be given over 15 minutes–2 hours depending on severity of poisoning and patient stability

▸ Adult: Initially 5 g, to be given over 15 minutes, then 5 g if required, this second dose can be given over 15 minutes–2 hours depending on severity of poisoning and patient stability

● **CAUTIONS**

▸ With intramuscular use Should not be given before diagnosis fully established

● **SIDE-EFFECTS**

GENERAL SIDE-EFFECTS

Diarrhoea · dizziness · headache · hot flush · nausea · skin reactions · urine discolouration

SPECIFIC SIDE-EFFECTS

▸ With intramuscular use Arrhythmia · chills · drug fever · hypokalaemia · malaise · pain · thrombocytosis · tremor · vomiting

▸ With intravenous use Angioedema · dysphagia · extrasystole · gastrointestinal discomfort · memory loss · mucosal discolouration red · peripheral oedema · pleural effusion · rash pustular · red discolouration of plasma · restlessness · swelling · throat complaints

● **BREAST FEEDING** Present in milk but not known to be harmful.

● **EFFECT ON LABORATORY TESTS**

▸ With intravenous use Deep red colour of hydroxocobalamin may interfere with laboratory tests.

● **DIRECTIONS FOR ADMINISTRATION**

▸ With intravenous use For *intravenous infusion (Cyanokit)* ®, given intermittently *in* Sodium chloride 0.9%, reconstitute 5 g vial with 200 mL Sodium Chloride 0.9%; gently invert vial for at least 1 minute to mix (do not shake).

● **PRESCRIBING AND DISPENSING INFORMATION**

▸ With intramuscular use The BP directs that when vitamin B_{12} injection is prescribed or demanded, hydroxocobalamin injection shall be dispensed or supplied.

Poisoning by cyanides

▸ With intravenous use *Cyanokit* ® is the only preparation of hydroxocobalamin that is suitable for use in victims of smoke inhalation who show signs of significant cyanide poisoning.

● **NATIONAL FUNDING/ACCESS DECISIONS**

NHS restrictions *Cobalin-H* ® is not prescribable in NHS primary care.

Neo-Cytamen ® is not prescribable in NHS primary care.

● **MEDICINAL FORMS** There can be variation in the licensing of different medicines containing the same drug.

Solution for injection

▸ Hydroxocobalamin (Non-proprietary)
Hydroxocobalamin 1 mg per 1 ml Hydroxocobalamin 1mg/1ml solution for injection ampoules | 5 ampoule [PoM] £12.49 DT = £7.28

▸ Hepavit (Imported (Austria))
Hydroxocobalamin 2.5 mg per 1 ml Hepavit 5mg/2ml solution for injection ampoules | 2 ampoule [PoM] 🚫

▸ Megamilbedoce (Imported (Spain))
Hydroxocobalamin 5 mg per 1 ml Megamilbedoce 10mg/2ml solution for injection ampoules | 10 ampoule [PoM] 🚫

▸ Cobalin (Advanz Pharma)
Hydroxocobalamin 1 mg per 1 ml Cobalin-H 1mg/1ml solution for injection ampoules | 5 ampoule [PoM] £9.50 DT = £7.28

▸ Neo-Cytamen (RPH Pharmaceuticals AB)
Hydroxocobalamin 1 mg per 1 ml Neo-Cytamen 1000micrograms/1ml solution for injection ampoules | 5 ampoule [PoM] £12.49 DT = £7.28

Powder for solution for infusion

▸ Cyanokit (SERB)
Hydroxocobalamin 5 gram Cyanokit 5g powder for solution for infusion vials | 1 vial [PoM] £772.00

2 Iron overload

Iron overload

Overview

Severe tissue iron overload can occur in aplastic and other refractory anaemias, mainly as the result of repeated blood transfusions. It is a particular problem in refractory anaemias with hyperplastic bone marrow, especially *thalassaemia major*, where excessive iron absorption from the gut and inappropriate iron therapy can add to the tissue siderosis.

Iron overload associated with haemochromatosis can be treated with repeated venesection. Venesection may also be used for patients who have received multiple transfusions and whose bone marrow has recovered. Where venesection is contra-indicated, the long-term administration of the iron chelating compound desferrioxamine mesilate p. 1075 is useful. Desferrioxamine mesilate (up to 2 g per unit of blood) may also be given at the time of blood transfusion, provided that the desferrioxamine mesilate is **not** added to the blood and is **not** given through the same line as the blood (but the two may be given through the same cannula).

Iron excretion induced by desferrioxamine mesilate is enhanced by administration of ascorbic acid (vitamin C) p. 1132 daily by mouth; it should be given separately from food since it also enhances iron absorption. Ascorbic acid should not be given to patients with cardiac dysfunction; in patients with normal cardiac function ascorbic acid should be introduced 1 month after starting desferrioxamine mesilate.

Desferrioxamine mesilate infusion can be used to treat *aluminium overload* in dialysis patients; theoretically 100 mg of desferrioxamine binds with 4.1 mg of aluminium.

ANTIDOTES AND CHELATORS ⟩ IRON CHELATORS

▌Deferasirox

23-Nov-2020

● **DRUG ACTION** Deferasirox is an oral iron chelator.

● **INDICATIONS AND DOSE**

Transfusion-related chronic iron overload in patients with beta thalassaemia major who receive frequent blood transfusions (7 mL/kg/month or more of packed red blood cells) (specialist use only)

▸ **BY MOUTH**

▸ Adult: Initially 7–21 mg/kg once daily, dose adjusted according to serum-ferritin concentration and amount of transfused blood—consult product literature, then adjusted in steps of 3.5–7 mg/kg every 3–6 months, maintenance dose adjusted according to serum-ferritin concentration; maximum 28 mg/kg per day; Usual maximum 21 mg/kg   continued →

Transfusion-related chronic iron overload when desferrioxamine is contra-indicated or inadequate in patients with beta thalassaemia major who receive infrequent blood transfusions (less than 7 mL/kg/month of packed red blood cells) (specialist use only) | **Transfusion-related chronic iron overload when desferrioxamine is contra-indicated or inadequate in patients with other anaemias (specialist use only)**

▸ BY MOUTH
▸ Adult: Initially 7–21 mg/kg once daily, dose adjusted according to serum-ferritin concentration and amount of transfused blood—consult product literature, then adjusted in steps of 3.5–7 mg/kg every 3–6 months, maintenance dose adjusted according to serum-ferritin concentration; maximum 28 mg/kg per day; Usual maximum 21 mg/kg

Chronic iron overload when desferrioxamine is contra-indicated or inadequate in non-transfusion-dependent thalassaemia syndromes (specialist use only)

▸ BY MOUTH
▸ Adult: Initially 7 mg/kg once daily, then adjusted in steps of 3.5–7 mg/kg every 3–6 months, maintenance dose adjusted according to serum-ferritin concentration and liver-iron concentration (consult product literature); maximum 14 mg/kg per day

● CAUTIONS Elderly (increased risk of side-effects) · history of liver cirrhosis · not recommended in conditions which may reduce life expectancy (e.g. high-risk myelodysplastic syndromes) · platelet count less than 50x10^9/litre · risk of gastro-intestinal ulceration and haemorrhage · unexplained cytopenia—consider treatment interruption

● INTERACTIONS → Appendix 1: iron chelators

● SIDE-EFFECTS
▸ **Common or very common** Constipation · diarrhoea · gastrointestinal discomfort · headache · nausea · skin reactions · urine abnormalities · vomiting
▸ **Uncommon** Anxiety · cataract · cholelithiasis · dizziness · fatigue · fever · gastrointestinal disorders · gastrointestinal haemorrhage (including fatal cases) · hearing impairment · hepatic disorders · laryngeal pain · maculopathy · oedema · renal tubular disorders · sleep disorder
▸ **Rare or very rare** Optic neuritis · severe cutaneous adverse reactions (SCARs)
▸ **Frequency not known** Acute kidney injury · alopecia · anaemia aggravated · hyperammonaemic encephalopathy · hypersensitivity vasculitis · lens opacity · leucopenia · metabolic acidosis · nephritis tubulointerstitial · nephrolithiasis · neutropenia · pancreatitis acute · pancytopenia · renal tubular necrosis · thrombocytopenia

● PREGNANCY Manufacturer advises avoid unless essential— toxicity in *animal* studies.

● BREAST FEEDING Manufacturer advises avoid—present in milk in *animal* studies.

● HEPATIC IMPAIRMENT Manufacturer advises caution in moderate impairment; avoid in severe impairment.
Dose adjustments Manufacturer advises reduce initial dose considerably then gradually increase to max. 50% of normal dose in moderate impairment.

● RENAL IMPAIRMENT Manufacturer advises avoid if estimated creatinine clearance less than 60 mL/minute.
Dose adjustments Manufacturer advises reduce dose if creatinine clearance less than 90 mL/minute and serum creatinine increased by more than 33% of baseline measurement on 2 consecutive occasions—consult product literature.

● MONITORING REQUIREMENTS Manufacturer advises monitoring of the following patient parameters: baseline serum creatinine twice and creatinine clearance once before initiation of treatment, weekly in the first month after treatment initiation or modification, then monthly

thereafter; proteinuria before treatment initiation then monthly thereafter, and other markers of renal tubular function as needed; liver function before treatment initiation, every 2 weeks during the first month of treatment, then monthly thereafter; eye and ear examinations before treatment and annually during treatment; serum-ferritin concentration monthly.

● DIRECTIONS FOR ADMINISTRATION For *film-coated tablets*, manufacturer advises tablets may be crushed and sprinkled on to soft food (yoghurt or apple sauce), then administered immediately.

● PATIENT AND CARER ADVICE Patient or carers should be given advice on how to administer deferasirox tablets.

● NATIONAL FUNDING/ACCESS DECISIONS
For full details see funding body website
Scottish Medicines Consortium (SMC) decisions
▸ Deferasirox (*Exjade*®) for the treatment of chronic iron overload due to blood transfusions when deferoxamine therapy is contra-indicated or inadequate, in adult and paediatric patients aged 2 years and older with rare acquired or inherited anaemias (January 2017) SMC No. 347/07 Recommended with restrictions
▸ Deferasirox (*Exjade*®) for the treatment of chronic iron overload: due to frequent blood transfusions in patients with beta thalassaemia major aged 6 years and over; due to blood transfusions when deferoxamine therapy is contra-indicated or inadequate in other patient groups (June 2017) SMC No. 1246/17 Recommended with restrictions

● MEDICINAL FORMS There can be variation in the licensing of different medicines containing the same drug.
Tablet
CAUTIONARY AND ADVISORY LABELS 25
▸ Exjade (Novartis Pharmaceuticals UK Ltd) ▼
Deferasirox 90 mg Exjade 90mg tablets | 30 tablet [PoM] £126.00 DT = £126.00
Deferasirox 180 mg Exjade 180mg tablets | 30 tablet [PoM] £252.00 DT = £252.00
Deferasirox 360 mg Exjade 360mg tablets | 30 tablet [PoM] £504.00 DT = £504.00

Deferiprone

01-Sep-2020

● DRUG ACTION Deferiprone is an oral iron chelator.

● INDICATIONS AND DOSE
Treatment of iron overload in patients with thalassaemia major in whom desferrioxamine is contra-indicated or is inadequate
▸ BY MOUTH
▸ Adult: 25 mg/kg 3 times a day; maximum 100 mg/kg per day

● CONTRA-INDICATIONS History of agranulocytosis or recurrent neutropenia

● INTERACTIONS → Appendix 1: iron chelators

● SIDE-EFFECTS
▸ **Common or very common** Abdominal pain (reducing dose and increasing gradually may improve tolerance) · agranulocytosis · appetite increased · arthralgia · diarrhoea (reducing dose and increasing gradually may improve tolerance) · fatigue · headache · nausea (reducing dose and increasing gradually may improve tolerance) · neutropenia · urine discolouration · vomiting (reducing dose and increasing gradually may improve tolerance)
▸ **Frequency not known** Skin reactions · zinc deficiency

● CONCEPTION AND CONTRACEPTION Manufacturer advises avoid before intended conception—teratogenic and embryotoxic in *animal* studies. Contraception advised in females of child-bearing potential.

- **PREGNANCY** Manufacturer advises avoid during pregnancy—teratogenic and embryotoxic in *animal* studies.
- **BREAST FEEDING** Manufacturer advises avoid—no information available.
- **HEPATIC IMPAIRMENT** Manufacturer advises caution (no information available)—monitor hepatic function and consider interrupting treatment if persistent elevation in serum alanine aminotransferase. Manufacturer advises caution in patients with hepatitis C (ensure iron chelation is optimal)—monitor liver histology.
- **RENAL IMPAIRMENT** Manufacturer advises caution—no information available.
- **MONITORING REQUIREMENTS**
- ▶ Monitor neutrophil count weekly and discontinue treatment if neutropenia develops.
- ▶ Monitor plasma-zinc concentration.
- **PATIENT AND CARER ADVICE**
  Blood disorders Patients or their carers should be told how to recognise signs of neutropenia and advised to seek immediate medical attention if symptoms such as fever or sore throat develop.

- **MEDICINAL FORMS** There can be variation in the licensing of different medicines containing the same drug. Forms available from special-order manufacturers include: capsule, oral suspension, oral solution

Oral solution
CAUTIONARY AND ADVISORY LABELS 14
- ▶ Ferriprox (Chiesi Ltd)
  Deferiprone 100 mg per 1 ml Ferriprox 100mg/ml oral solution sugar-free | 500 ml [PoM] £152.39 DT = £152.39

Tablet
CAUTIONARY AND ADVISORY LABELS 14
- ▶ Deferiprone (Non-proprietary)
  Deferiprone 500 mg Deferiprone 500mg tablets | 100 tablet [PoM] £130.00 DT = £130.00
- ▶ Ferriprox (Chiesi Ltd)
  Deferiprone 500 mg Ferriprox 500mg tablets | 100 tablet [PoM] £130.00 DT = £130.00
  Deferiprone 1 gram Ferriprox 1000mg tablets | 50 tablet [PoM] £130.00 DT = £130.00

Desferrioxamine mesilate

23-Nov-2020

(Deferoxamine Mesilate)

- **INDICATIONS AND DOSE**

Iron poisoning
- ▶ BY CONTINUOUS INTRAVENOUS INFUSION
- ▶ Adult: Initially up to 15 mg/kg/hour, max. 80 mg/kg in 24 hours, dose to be reduced after 4–6 hours, in severe cases, higher doses may be given on advice from the National Poisons Information Service

Aluminium overload in dialysis patients
- ▶ BY INTRAVENOUS INFUSION
- ▶ Adult: (consult product literature or local protocols)

Chronic iron overload (low iron overload)
- ▶ BY SUBCUTANEOUS INFUSION
- ▶ Adult: The dose should reflect the degree of iron overload

Chronic iron overload (established overload)
- ▶ BY SUBCUTANEOUS INFUSION
- ▶ Adult: 20–50 mg/kg daily

- **CAUTIONS** Aluminium-related encephalopathy (may exacerbate neurological dysfunction)
- **INTERACTIONS** → Appendix 1: iron chelators

- **SIDE-EFFECTS**
- ▶ **Common or very common** Arthralgia · bone disorder · fever · growth retardation · headache · muscle complaints · nausea · skin reactions
- ▶ **Uncommon** Abdominal pain · asthma · deafness neurosensory · tinnitus · vomiting
- ▶ **Rare or very rare** Angioedema · blood disorder · cataract · diarrhoea · dizziness · encephalopathy · eye disorders · hypersensitivity · hypotension (more common when given too rapidly by intravenous injection) · increased risk of infection · nerve disorders · nervous system disorder · paraesthesia · respiratory disorders · shock · tachycardia · thrombocytopenia · vision disorders
- ▶ **Frequency not known** Acute kidney injury · hypocalcaemia · leucopenia · renal tubular disorder · seizure · urine red

- **PREGNANCY** Teratogenic in *animal* studies. Manufacturer advises use only if potential benefit outweighs risk.
- **BREAST FEEDING** Manufacturer advises use only if potential benefit outweighs risk—no information available.
- **RENAL IMPAIRMENT** Use with caution.
- **MONITORING REQUIREMENTS**
- ▶ Eye and ear examinations before treatment and at 3-month intervals during treatment.
- **DIRECTIONS FOR ADMINISTRATION** For full details and warnings relating to administration, consult product literature.
  For *intravenous infusion (Desferal®)*, give continuously *or* intermittently in Glucose 5% or Sodium chloride 0.9%. Reconstitute with water for injections to a concentration of 100 mg/mL; dilute with infusion fluid.

- **MEDICINAL FORMS** There can be variation in the licensing of different medicines containing the same drug.
  Powder for solution for injection
- ▶ Desferrioxamine mesilate (Non-proprietary)
  Desferrioxamine mesilate 500 mg Desferrioxamine 500mg powder for solution for injection vials | 10 vial [PoM] £46.63 DT = £46.63
  Desferrioxamine mesilate 2 gram Desferrioxamine 2g powder for solution for injection vials | 10 vial [PoM] £186.60
- ▶ Desferal (Novartis Pharmaceuticals UK Ltd)
  Desferrioxamine mesilate 500 mg Desferal 500mg powder for solution for injection vials | 10 vial [PoM] £46.63 DT = £46.63

3 Neutropenia and stem cell mobilisation

3.1 Neutropenia

Neutropenia

Management

Recombinant human granulocyte-colony stimulating factor (rhG-CSF) stimulates the production of neutrophils and may reduce the duration of chemotherapy-induced neutropenia and thereby reduce the incidence of associated sepsis; there is as yet no evidence that it improves overall survival. Filgrastim p. 1076 (unglycosylated rhG-CSF) and lenograstim p. 1077 (glycosylated rhG-CSF) have similar effects; both have been used in a variety of clinical settings, but they do not have any clear-cut routine indications. In congenital neutropenia filgrastim usually increases the neutrophil count with an appropriate clinical response. Pegfilgrastim p. 1078 is a polyethylene glycol-conjugated ('pegylated') derivative of filgrastim; pegylation increases the duration of filgrastim activity. Lipegfilgrastim p. 1077 is a polyethylene glycol-conjugated via a glycine linker derivative of filgrastim.

Granulocyte-colony stimulating factors should only be prescribed by those experienced in their use.

IMMUNOSTIMULANTS > GRANULOCYTE-COLONY STIMULATING FACTORS

Granulocyte-colony stimulating factors

- **DRUG ACTION** Recombinant human granulocyte-colony stimulating factor (rhG-CSF) stimulates the production of neutrophils.
- **CAUTIONS** Malignant myeloid conditions · pre-malignant myeloid conditions · risk of splenomegaly and rupture— spleen size should be monitored · sickle-cell disease

  CAUTIONS, FURTHER INFORMATION
- Acute respiratory distress syndrome There have been reports of pulmonary infiltrates leading to acute respiratory distress syndrome—patients with a recent history of pulmonary infiltrates or pneumonia may be at higher risk.
- **SIDE-EFFECTS**
- **Common or very common** Arthralgia · cutaneous vasculitis · dyspnoea · haemoptysis · headache · hypersensitivity · leucocytosis · pain · spleen abnormalities · thrombocytopenia
- **Uncommon** Acute febrile neutrophilic dermatosis · capillary leak syndrome · hypoxia · pulmonary oedema · respiratory disorders · sickle cell anaemia with crisis

  SIDE-EFFECTS, FURTHER INFORMATION Treatment should be withdrawn in patients who develop signs of pulmonary infiltration.
- **PREGNANCY** Manufacturers advise avoid—toxicity in *animal* studies.
- **BREAST FEEDING** There is no evidence for the use of granulocyte-colony stimulating factors during breast-feeding and manufacturers advise avoiding their use.
- **MONITORING REQUIREMENTS**
- Full blood counts including differential white cell and platelet counts should be monitored.
- Spleen size should be monitored during treatment—risk of splenomegaly and rupture.

▶ above

Filgrastim

24-Jul-2020

(Recombinant human granulocyte-colony stimulating factor; G-CSF)

- **INDICATIONS AND DOSE**

Reduction in duration of neutropenia and incidence of febrile neutropenia in cytotoxic chemotherapy for malignancy (except chronic myeloid leukaemia and myelodysplastic syndromes) (specialist use only)
- BY SUBCUTANEOUS INJECTION, OR BY INTRAVENOUS INFUSION
- Adult: 5 micrograms/kg daily until neutrophil count in normal range, usually for up to 14 days (up to 38 days in acute myeloid leukaemia), to be started at least 24 hours after cytotoxic chemotherapy. Preferably given by subcutaneous injection; if given by intravenous infusion, administer over 30 minutes

Reduction in duration of neutropenia (and associated sequelae) in myeloablative therapy followed by bone-marrow transplantation (specialist use only)
- BY SUBCUTANEOUS INFUSION, OR BY INTRAVENOUS INFUSION
- Adult: 10 micrograms/kg daily, to be started at least 24 hours following cytotoxic chemotherapy and within 24 hours of bone-marrow transplant, then adjusted according to neutrophil count— consult product literature, doses administered over 30 minutes or 24 hours via intravenous route and over 24 hours via subcutaneous route

Mobilisation of peripheral blood progenitor cells for autologous infusion, used alone (specialist use only)
- BY SUBCUTANEOUS INFUSION, OR BY SUBCUTANEOUS INJECTION
- Adult: 10 micrograms/kg daily for 5–7 days, to be administered over 24 hours if given by subcutaneous infusion

Mobilisation of peripheral blood progenitor cells for autologous infusion, used following adjunctive myelosuppressive chemotherapy—to improve yield (specialist use only)
- BY SUBCUTANEOUS INJECTION
- Adult: 5 micrograms/kg daily until neutrophil count in normal range, to be started the day after completing chemotherapy, for timing of leucopheresis, consult product literature

Mobilisation of peripheral blood progenitor cells in normal donors for allogeneic infusion (specialist use only)
- BY SUBCUTANEOUS INJECTION
- Adult 18–59 years: 10 micrograms/kg daily for 4–5 days, for timing of leucopheresis, consult product literature

Severe congenital neutropenia and history of severe or recurrent infections (distinguish carefully from other haematological disorders) (specialist use only)
- BY SUBCUTANEOUS INJECTION
- Adult: Initially 12 micrograms/kg daily, adjusted according to response, can be given in single or divided doses, consult product literature and local protocol

Severe cyclic neutropenia, or idiopathic neutropenia and history of severe or recurrent infections (distinguish carefully from other haematological disorders) (specialist use only)
- BY SUBCUTANEOUS INJECTION
- Adult: Initially 5 micrograms/kg daily, adjusted according to response, can be given in single or divided doses, consult product literature and local protocol

Persistent neutropenia in HIV infection (specialist use only)
- BY SUBCUTANEOUS INJECTION
- Adult: Initially 1 microgram/kg daily, subsequent doses increased as necessary until neutrophil count in normal range, then adjusted to maintain neutrophil count in normal range—consult product literature; maximum 4 micrograms/kg per day

- **CONTRA-INDICATIONS** Severe congenital neutropenia who develop leukaemia or have evidence of leukaemic evolution
- **CAUTIONS** Osteoporotic bone disease (monitor bone density if given for more than 6 months) · secondary acute myeloid leukaemia
- **SIDE-EFFECTS**
- **Common or very common** Anaemia · diarrhoea · dysuria · haemorrhage · hepatomegaly · hyperuricaemia · hypotension · osteoporosis · rash
- **Uncommon** Fluid imbalance · graft versus host disease · peripheral vascular disease · pseudogout · rheumatoid arthritis aggravated · urine abnormalities
- **MONITORING REQUIREMENTS** Regular morphological and cytogenetic bone-marrow examinations recommended in severe congenital neutropenia (possible risk of myelodysplastic syndromes or leukaemia).
- **DIRECTIONS FOR ADMINISTRATION**
- With intravenous use or subcutaneous use For *subcutaneous* or *intravenous infusion*, manufacturer advises give continuously *or* intermittently *in* Glucose 5%; for a filgrastim concentration of less than 1 500 000 units/mL (15 micrograms/mL) albumin solution (human albumin solution) is added to produce a final albumin

concentration of 2 mg/mL; should not be diluted to a filgrastim concentration of less than 200 000 units/mL (2 micrograms/mL) and should not be diluted with sodium chloride solution.

- PRESCRIBING AND DISPENSING INFORMATION Filgrastim is a biological medicine. Biological medicines must be prescribed and dispensed by brand name, see *Biological medicines* and *Biosimilar medicines*, under Guidance on prescribing p. 1.

  1 million units of filgrastim solution for injection contains 10 micrograms filgrastim.

- MEDICINAL FORMS There can be variation in the licensing of different medicines containing the same drug.

  Solution for injection
  - Accofil (Accord Healthcare Ltd)
    Filgrastim 60 mega unit per 1 ml Accofil 30million units/0.5ml solution for injection pre-filled syringes | 5 pre-filled disposable injection [PoM] £284.20 DT = £250.75 (Hospital only)
    Filgrastim 96 mega unit per 1 ml Accofil 48million units/0.5ml solution for injection pre-filled syringes | 5 pre-filled disposable injection [PoM] £455.70 DT = £399.50 (Hospital only)
  - Neupogen (Amgen Ltd)
    Filgrastim 30 mega unit per 1 ml Neupogen 30million units/1ml solution for injection vials | 5 vial [PoM] £263.52 DT = £263.52
  - Neupogen Singleject (Amgen Ltd)
    Filgrastim 60 mega unit per 1 ml Neupogen Singleject 30million units/0.5ml solution for injection pre-filled syringes | 1 pre-filled disposable injection [PoM] £52.70
    Filgrastim 96 mega unit per 1 ml Neupogen Singleject 48million units/0.5ml solution for injection pre-filled syringes | 1 pre-filled disposable injection [PoM] £84.06
  - Nivestim (Pfizer Ltd)
    Filgrastim 60 mega unit per 1 ml Nivestim 30million units/0.5ml solution for injection pre-filled syringes | 5 pre-filled disposable injection [PoM] £246.50 DT = £250.75
    Nivestim 12million units/0.2ml solution for injection pre-filled syringes | 5 pre-filled disposable injection [PoM] £153.00
    Filgrastim 96 mega unit per 1 ml Nivestim 48million units/0.5ml solution for injection pre-filled syringes | 5 pre-filled disposable injection [PoM] £395.25 DT = £399.50
  - Zarzio (Sandoz Ltd)
    Filgrastim 60 mega unit per 1 ml Zarzio 30million units/0.5ml solution for injection pre-filled syringes | 5 pre-filled disposable injection [PoM] £250.75 DT = £250.75
    Filgrastim 96 mega unit per 1 ml Zarzio 48million units/0.5ml solution for injection pre-filled syringes | 5 pre-filled disposable injection [PoM] £399.50 DT = £399.50

⇟ 1076

Lenograstim

20-Jul-2020

(Recombinant human granulocyte-colony stimulating factor; rHuG-CSF)

- INDICATIONS AND DOSE

  Reduction in the duration of neutropenia and associated complications following bone-marrow transplantation for non-myeloid malignancy (specialist use only) | Reduction in the duration of neutropenia and associated complications following peripheral stem cells transplantation for non-myeloid malignancy (specialist use only)
  - BY INTRAVENOUS INFUSION, OR BY SUBCUTANEOUS INJECTION
  - Adult: 150 micrograms/m^2 daily until neutrophil count stable in acceptable range (max. 28 days), to be started the day after transplantation. Intravenous infusion to be given over 30 minutes

Reduction in the duration of neutropenia and associated complications following treatment with cytotoxic chemotherapy associated with a significant incidence of febrile neutropenia (specialist use only)
- BY SUBCUTANEOUS INJECTION
- Adult: 150 micrograms/m^2 daily until neutrophil count stable in acceptable range (max. 28 days), to be started on the day after completion of chemotherapy

Mobilisation of peripheral blood progenitor cells for harvesting and subsequent infusion, used alone (specialist use only)
- BY SUBCUTANEOUS INJECTION
- Adult: 10 micrograms/kg daily for 4–6 days (5–6 days in healthy donors)

Mobilisation of peripheral blood progenitor cells, used following adjunctive myelosuppressive chemotherapy (to improve yield) (specialist use only)
- BY SUBCUTANEOUS INJECTION
- Adult: 150 micrograms/m^2 daily until neutrophil count stable in acceptable range, to be started 1–5 days after completion of chemotherapy, for timing of leucopheresis, consult product literature

- SIDE-EFFECTS
- **Common or very common** Abdominal pain · asthenia
- **Rare or very rare** Erythema nodosum · pyoderma gangrenosum · toxic epidermal necrolysis

- DIRECTIONS FOR ADMINISTRATION
- With intravenous use For *intravenous infusion* (Granocyte$^®$), manufacturer advises give intermittently *in* Glucose 5% *or* Sodium chloride 0.9%; initially reconstitute with 1 mL water for injection provided (do not shake vigorously) then dilute with up to 50 mL infusion fluid for each vial of *Granocyte*-13 or up to 100 mL infusion fluid for *Granocyte*-34; give over 30 minutes.

- PRESCRIBING AND DISPENSING INFORMATION *Granocyte$^®$* solution for injection contains 105 micrograms of lenograstim per 13.4 mega unit vial and 263 micrograms lenograstim per 33.6 mega unit vial.

- MEDICINAL FORMS There can be variation in the licensing of different medicines containing the same drug.

  Powder and solvent for solution for injection
  EXCIPIENTS: May contain Phenylalanine
  - Granocyte (Chugai Pharma UK Ltd)
    Lenograstim 13.4 mega unit Granocyte 13million unit powder and solvent for solution for injection pre-filled syringes | 1 pre-filled disposable injection [PoM] £40.11 DT = £40.11 | 5 pre-filled disposable injection [PoM] £200.55
    Lenograstim 33.6 mega unit Granocyte 34million unit powder and solvent for solution for injection pre-filled syringes | 1 pre-filled disposable injection [PoM] £62.54 DT = £62.54 | 5 pre-filled disposable injection [PoM] £312.69

⇟ 1076

Lipegfilgrastim

10-Jun-2020

(Glycopegylated recombinant methionyl human granulocyte-colony stimulating factor)

- INDICATIONS AND DOSE

  Reduction in duration of neutropenia and incidence of febrile neutropenia in cytotoxic chemotherapy for malignancy (except chronic myeloid leukaemia and myelodysplastic syndromes)
  - BY SUBCUTANEOUS INJECTION
  - Adult (specialist use only): 6 mg, for each chemotherapy cycle, given approximately 24 hours after chemotherapy, dose expressed as filgrastim

- CAUTIONS Myelosuppressive chemotherapy

Blood and nutrition

9

- SIDE-EFFECTS
  ▸ **Common or very common** Chest pain · hypokalaemia · skin eruption

- MEDICINAL FORMS There can be variation in the licensing of different medicines containing the same drug.
  Solution for injection
  ▸ Lonquex (Teva UK Ltd)
    Filgrastim (as Lipegfilgrastim) 10 mg per 1 ml Lonquex 6mg/0.6ml solution for injection pre-filled syringes | 1 pre-filled disposable injection [PoM] £652.06

⚑ 1076

Pegfilgrastim

10-Jun-2020

(Pegylated recombinant methionyl human granulocyte-colony stimulating factor)

- INDICATIONS AND DOSE
Reduction in duration of neutropenia and incidence of febrile neutropenia in cytotoxic chemotherapy for malignancy (except chronic myeloid leukaemia and myelodysplastic syndromes) (specialist use only)
  ▸ BY SUBCUTANEOUS INJECTION
  ▸ Adult: 6 mg for each chemotherapy cycle, to be given at least 24 hours after chemotherapy, dose is expressed as filgrastim

- CAUTIONS Acute leukaemia · myelosuppressive chemotherapy
- SIDE-EFFECTS
  ▸ **Common or very common** Myalgia · nausea
  ▸ **Uncommon** Glomerulonephritis

- MEDICINAL FORMS There can be variation in the licensing of different medicines containing the same drug.
  Solution for injection
  ▸ Neulasta (Amgen Ltd)
    Filgrastim (as Pegfilgrastim) 10 mg per 1 ml Neulasta 6mg/0.6ml solution for injection pre-filled syringes | 1 pre-filled disposable injection [PoM] £686.38
    Neulasta 6mg/0.6ml solution for injection pre-filled syringes with Onpro kit | 1 pre-filled disposable injection [PoM] £686.38 (Hospital only)
  ▸ Pelgraz (Accord Healthcare Ltd) ▼
    Filgrastim (as Pegfilgrastim) 10 mg per 1 ml Pelgraz 6mg/0.6ml solution for injection pre-filled syringes | 1 pre-filled disposable injection [PoM] £686.37 (Hospital only)
  ▸ Pelmeg (Napp Pharmaceuticals Ltd) ▼
    Filgrastim (as Pegfilgrastim) 10 mg per 1 ml Pelmeg 6mg/0.6ml solution for injection pre-filled syringes | 1 pre-filled disposable injection [PoM] £411.83 (Hospital only)
  ▸ Ziextenzo (Sandoz Ltd) ▼
    Filgrastim (as Pegfilgrastim) 10 mg per 1 ml Ziextenzo 6mg/0.6ml solution for injection pre-filled syringes | 1 pre-filled disposable injection [PoM] £617.74

3.2 Stem cell mobilisation

IMMUNOSTIMULANTS ⟩ CHEMOKINE RECEPTOR ANTAGONISTS

Plerixafor

22-Oct-2020

- DRUG ACTION Plerixafor is a chemokine receptor antagonist.

- INDICATIONS AND DOSE
Mobilise haematopoietic stem cells to peripheral blood for collection and subsequent autologous transplantation in patients with lymphoma or multiple myeloma (specialist use only)
  ▸ BY SUBCUTANEOUS INJECTION
  ▸ Adult (body-weight up to 84 kg): 240 micrograms/kg daily, alternatively 20 mg daily usually for 2–4 days (and up to 7 days), to be administered 6–11 hours before initiation of apheresis, dose to be given following 4 days treatment with a granulocyte-colony stimulating factor; maximum 40 mg per day
  ▸ Adult (body-weight 84 kg and above): 240 micrograms/kg daily usually for 2–4 days (and up to 7 days), to be administered 6–11 hours before initiation of apheresis, dose to be given following 4 days treatment with a granulocyte-colony stimulating factor; maximum 40 mg per day

- SIDE-EFFECTS
  ▸ **Common or very common** Arthralgia · constipation · diarrhoea · dizziness · dry mouth · erythema · fatigue · flatulence · gastrointestinal discomfort · headache · hyperhidrosis · malaise · musculoskeletal pain · nausea · oral hypoaesthesia · sleep disorders · vomiting
  ▸ **Frequency not known** Postural hypotension · splenomegaly · syncope

- CONCEPTION AND CONTRACEPTION Use effective contraception during treatment— teratogenic in *animal* studies.

- PREGNANCY Manufacturer advises avoid unless essential— teratogenic in *animal* studies.

- BREAST FEEDING Manufacturer advises avoid—no information available.

- RENAL IMPAIRMENT No information available if creatinine clearance less than 20 mL/minute.
  Dose adjustments Manufacturer advises reduce dose to 160 micrograms/kg (maximum 27 mg) daily if creatinine clearance 20–50 mL/minute.

- MONITORING REQUIREMENTS Monitor platelets and white blood cell count.

- PATIENT AND CARER ADVICE
  Driving and skilled tasks Manufacturer advises patients and carers should be cautioned on the effects on driving and performance of skilled tasks—increased risk of dizziness, fatigue, or vasovagal reactions.

- NATIONAL FUNDING/ACCESS DECISIONS
  For full details see funding body website
  Scottish Medicines Consortium (SMC) decisions
  ▸ Plerixafor (*Mozobil®*) combined with G-CSF to enhance mobilisation of haematopoietic stem cells to the peripheral blood for collection & subsequent autologous transplantation in patients with lymphoma and multiple myeloma (January 2010) SMC No. 594/09 Recommended
  All Wales Medicines Strategy Group (AWMSG) decisions
  ▸ Plerixafor (*Mozobil®*) in combination with G-CSF to enhance mobilisation of haematopoietic stem cells to the peripheral blood for collection and subsequent autologous transplantation in patients with lymphoma and multiple myeloma whose cells mobilise poorly (April 2010) AWMSG No. 249 Recommended with restrictions

- MEDICINAL FORMS There can be variation in the licensing of different medicines containing the same drug.

Solution for injection
- Mozobil (Sanofi)
Plerixafor 20 mg per 1 ml Mozobil 24mg/1.2ml solution for injection vials | 1 vial [PoM] £4,882.77

4 Platelet disorders

4.1 Essential thrombocythaemia

Other drugs used for Essential thrombocythaemia
Hydroxycarbamide, p. 977

ANTITHROMBOTIC DRUGS > CYCLIC AMP PHOSPHODIESTERASE III INHIBITORS

Anagrelide
03-Sep-2020

- **INDICATIONS AND DOSE**

Essential thrombocythaemia in patients at risk of thrombo-haemorrhagic events who have not responded adequately to other drugs or who cannot tolerate other drugs (initiated under specialist supervision)
- BY MOUTH
- Adult: Initially 500 micrograms twice daily, dose to be adjusted at weekly intervals according to response, increased in steps of 500 micrograms daily; usual dose 1–3 mg daily in divided doses (max. per dose 2.5 mg); maximum 10 mg per day

- CAUTIONS Cardiovascular disease—assess cardiac function before and regularly during treatment · concomitant use of drugs that prolong QT-interval—assess cardiac function before and regularly during treatment · risk factors for QT-interval prolongation—assess cardiac function before and regularly during treatment

- INTERACTIONS → Appendix 1: anagrelide

- SIDE-EFFECTS
- **Common or very common** Anaemia · arrhythmias · asthenia · diarrhoea · dizziness · fluid retention · gastrointestinal discomfort · gastrointestinal disorders · headaches · nausea · palpitations · skin reactions · vomiting
- **Uncommon** Alopecia · appetite decreased · arthralgia · chest pain · chills · confusion · congestive heart failure · constipation · depression · dry mouth · dyspnoea · erectile dysfunction · fever · haemorrhage · hypertension · insomnia · malaise · memory loss · myalgia · nervousness · oedema · pain · pancreatitis · pancytopenia · pneumonia · pulmonary hypertension · respiratory disorders · sensation abnormal · syncope · thrombocytopenia · weight changes
- **Rare or very rare** Angina pectoris · cardiomegaly · cardiomyopathy · coordination abnormal · drowsiness · dysarthria · influenza like illness · myocardial infarction · nocturia · pericardial effusion · postural hypotension · renal failure · tinnitus · vasodilation · vision disorders
- **Frequency not known** Hepatitis · nephritis tubulointerstitial

- CONCEPTION AND CONTRACEPTION Effective contraception required during treatment.

- PREGNANCY Manufacturer advises avoid (toxicity in *animal* studies).

- BREAST FEEDING Manufacturer advises avoid—present in milk in *animal* studies.

- HEPATIC IMPAIRMENT Manufacturer advises use with caution in mild impairment; avoid in moderate-to-severe impairment or if serum transaminases exceed 5 times the upper limit of normal.

- RENAL IMPAIRMENT Manufacturer advises avoid if eGFR less than 50 mL/minute/1.73 m^2.

- MONITORING REQUIREMENTS
- Monitor full blood count (monitor platelet count every 2 days for 1 week, then weekly until maintenance dose established).
- Monitor liver function.
- Monitor serum creatinine.
- Monitor urea.
- Monitor electrolytes (including potassium, magnesium and calcium) before and during treatment.

- PATIENT AND CARER ADVICE
Driving and skilled tasks Dizziness may affect performance of skilled tasks (e.g. cycling, driving).

- MEDICINAL FORMS There can be variation in the licensing of different medicines containing the same drug.

Capsule
- Anagrelide (Non-proprietary)
Anagrelide (as Anagrelide hydrochloride)
500 microgram Anagrelide 500microgram capsules | 100 capsule [PoM] £404.57 DT = £404.47
- Xagrid (Shire Pharmaceuticals Ltd)
Anagrelide (as Anagrelide hydrochloride) 500 microgram Xagrid 500microgram capsules | 100 capsule [PoM] £404.57 DT = £404.47

4.2 Thrombocytopenias

ANTIHAEMORRHAGICS > THROMBOPOIETIN RECEPTOR AGONISTS

Avatrombopag
03-Dec-2020

- DRUG ACTION Avatrombopag is a thrombopoietin receptor agonist that binds to and activates the thrombopoietin (TPO) receptor, thereby increasing platelet production.

- **INDICATIONS AND DOSE**

Thrombocytopenia [in patients with chronic liver disease undergoing invasive procedures and platelet count less than 40x10^9/litre] (under expert supervision)
- BY MOUTH
- Adult: 60 mg once daily for 5 days, treatment to be started 10 to 13 days before procedure; procedures to be carried out 5 to 8 days after the last dose of avatrombopag

Thrombocytopenia [in patients with chronic liver disease undergoing invasive procedures and platelet count between 40 to 50x10^9/litre] (under expert supervision)
- BY MOUTH
- Adult: 40 mg once daily for 5 days, treatment to be started 10 to 13 days before procedure; procedures to be carried out 5 to 8 days after the last dose of avatrombopag

- CAUTIONS Administration before laparotomy, thoracotomy, open-heart surgery, craniotomy, or excision of organs (no clinical experience) · risk factors for thromboembolism

- SIDE-EFFECTS
- **Common or very common** Fatigue
- **Uncommon** Anaemia · bone pain · fever · myalgia · portal vein thrombosis

- PREGNANCY [EvGr] Avoid—limited information available. ⟨M⟩

- BREAST FEEDING [EvGr] Avoid—present in milk in *animal* studies. ⟨M⟩

Blood and nutrition

9

- HEPATIC IMPAIRMENT [EvGr] Caution in severe impairment (limited information available). ⓜ
- MONITORING REQUIREMENTS [EvGr] Monitor platelet count before starting treatment and on the day of procedure. ⓜ
- NATIONAL FUNDING/ACCESS DECISIONS
  For full details see funding body website

  NICE decisions
  ▸ Avatrombopag for treating thrombocytopenia in people with chronic liver disease needing a planned invasive procedure (June 2020) NICE TA626 Recommended

- MEDICINAL FORMS There can be variation in the licensing of different medicines containing the same drug.

  Tablet
  CAUTIONARY AND ADVISORY LABELS 21
  ▸ Doptelet (Swedish Orphan Biovitrum Ltd) ▼
  Avatrombopag (as Avatrombopag maleate) 20 mg Doptelet 20mg tablets | 10 tablet [PoM] 💊 (Hospital only)

Lusutrombopag

27-Aug-2020

- DRUG ACTION Lusutrombopag is a thrombopoietin receptor agonist that binds to and activates the thrombopoietin (TPO) receptor, thereby increasing platelet production.

- **INDICATIONS AND DOSE**

  Thrombocytopenia [in patients with chronic liver disease undergoing invasive procedures] (under expert supervision)
  ▸ BY MOUTH
  ▸ **Adult:** 3 mg once daily for 7 days, treatment to be started at least 8 days before procedure; in clinical trials procedures were carried out between 9 to 14 days after starting lusutrombopag

- CAUTIONS Administration before laparotomy, thoracotomy, open-heart surgery, craniotomy, or excision of organs (no clinical experience) · body-weight less than 45kg (limited information available) · history of splenectomy (no clinical experience) · risk factors for thromboembolism
  CAUTIONS, FURTHER INFORMATION
  ▸ Body-weight less than 45kg Monitor platelet count approximately 5 days after the first dose and as necessary thereafter; stop treatment if the platelet count reaches 50×10^9/litre or more and has increased 20×10^9/litre from baseline.

- SIDE-EFFECTS
  ▸ **Common or very common** Headache · nausea · rash
  ▸ **Frequency not known** Embolism and thrombosis

- PREGNANCY Manufacturer advises avoid—no information available.

- BREAST FEEDING Manufacturer advises avoid—present in milk in *animal* studies.

- HEPATIC IMPAIRMENT Manufacturer advises caution in severe impairment (limited information available)— monitor platelet count approximately 5 days after the first dose and as necessary thereafter. Stop treatment if the platelet count reaches 50×10^9/litre or more and has increased 20×10^9/litre from baseline.

- MONITORING REQUIREMENTS Manufacturer advises monitor platelet count prior to procedure; more frequent monitoring may be required in some patients—see *Cautions* and *Hepatic Impairment* for further information.

- NATIONAL FUNDING/ACCESS DECISIONS
  For full details see funding body website

- **NICE decisions**
  ▸ Lusutrombopag for treating thrombocytopenia in people with chronic liver disease needing a planned invasive procedure (January 2020) NICE TA617 Recommended
  Scottish Medicines Consortium (SMC) decisions
  ▸ Lusutrombopag (*Mulpleo*®) for the treatment of severe thrombocytopenia in adult patients with chronic liver disease undergoing invasive procedures (December 2019) SMC No. SMC2227 Recommended

- MEDICINAL FORMS There can be variation in the licensing of different medicines containing the same drug.

  Tablet
  ▸ Mulpleo (Shionogi Ltd) ▼
  Lusutrombopag 3 mg Mulpleo 3mg tablets | 7 tablet [PoM] £800.00

4.2a Acquired thrombotic thrombocytopenic purpura

ANTITHROMBOTIC DRUGS

Caplacizumab

04-Nov-2020

- DRUG ACTION Caplacizumab is a monoclonal antibody fragment (nanobody) that binds to von Willebrand factor, thereby inhibiting platelet adhesion.

- **INDICATIONS AND DOSE**

  Acquired thrombotic thrombocytopenic purpura (specialist use only)
  ▸ INITIALLY BY INTRAVENOUS INJECTION
  ▸ **Adult:** Initially 10 mg for 1 dose, given before plasma exchange, followed by (by subcutaneous injection) 10 mg once daily given after each plasma exchange during, and for 30 days after finishing, daily plasma exchange therapy, treatment may be continued after this if there is evidence of unresolved immunological disease

- CONTRA-INDICATIONS Active bleeding (interrupt treatment)

- CAUTIONS Increased risk of bleeding

- INTERACTIONS → Appendix 1: caplacizumab

- SIDE-EFFECTS
  ▸ **Common or very common** Cerebral infarction · dyspnoea · fatigue · fever · haemorrhage · headache · menorrhagia · myalgia · subarachnoid haemorrhage · urticaria

- PREGNANCY Manufacturer advises avoid—no information available.

- BREAST FEEDING Manufacturer advises avoid—no information available.

- HEPATIC IMPAIRMENT Manufacturer advises caution in severe impairment (no information available).

- DIRECTIONS FOR ADMINISTRATION Manufacturer advises injection into the abdomen. Patients may self-administer *Cablivi*® after appropriate training in subcutaneous injection technique.

- PRESCRIBING AND DISPENSING INFORMATION
  Caplacizumab is a biological medicine. Biological medicines must be prescribed and dispensed by brand name, see *Biological medicines* and *Biosimilar medicines*, under Guidance on prescribing p. 1.

- HANDLING AND STORAGE Manufacturer advises store in a refrigerator (2-8°C) and protect from light—consult product literature for further information regarding storage outside refrigerator.

● PATIENT AND CARER ADVICE
Missed doses Manufacturer advises if a dose is more than
12 hours late, the missed dose should not be given and the
next dose should be given at the normal time.

● NATIONAL FUNDING/ACCESS DECISIONS
For full details see funding body website
Scottish Medicines Consortium (SMC) decisions
▶ Caplacizumab (*Cablivi*®) for the treatment of adults
experiencing an episode of acquired thrombotic
thrombocytopenic purpura (aTTP), in conjunction with plasma
exchange and immunosuppression (September 2020)
SMC No. SMC2266 Recommended

● MEDICINAL FORMS There can be variation in the licensing of
different medicines containing the same drug.
Powder and solvent for solution for injection
EXCIPIENTS: May contain Polysorbates
▶ Cablivi (Sanofi) ▼
   Caplacizumab 10 mg Cablivi 10mg powder and solvent for solution
   for injection vials | 1 vial [PoM] £4,143.00 (Hospital only)

4.2b Immune thrombocytopenia

Immune thrombocytopenic purpura

Overview

Acute immune (idiopathic) thrombocytopenic purpura is
usually self-limiting in children. In adults, immune
thrombocytopenic purpura can be treated with a
corticosteroid, e.g. prednisolone p. 718, gradually reducing
the dose over several weeks. Splenectomy is considered if a
satisfactory platelet count is not achieved or if there is a
relapse on reducing the dose of corticosteroid or
withdrawing it.

Immunoglobulin preparations, are also used in immune
thrombocytopenic purpura or where a temporary rapid rise
in platelets is needed, as in pregnancy or pre-operatively;
they are also used for children often in preference to a
corticosteroid. Anti-D (Rh$_0$) immunoglobulin p. 1333 is
effective in raising the platelet count in about 80% of
unsplenectomised rhesus-positive individuals; its effects
may last longer than normal immunoglobulin p. 1335 for
intravenous use, but further doses are usually required.

Other therapies that have been tried in refractory immune
thrombocytopenic purpura include: azathioprine p. 882,
cyclophosphamide p. 938, vincristine sulfate p. 972,
ciclosporin p. 884, and danazol p. 783. Rituximab p. 927
[unlicensed indication] may also be effective and in some
cases induces prolonged remission. For patients with chronic
severe thrombocytopenia refractory to other therapy,
tranexamic acid p. 118 may be given to reduce the severity of
haemorrhage.

Eltrombopag p. 1082 and romiplostim p. 1083 are
thrombopoietin receptor agonists. They are licensed for the
treatment of chronic immune thrombocytopenic purpura in
patients refractory to other treatments, such as
corticosteroids or immunoglobulins. They should both be
used under the supervision of a specialist.

Fostamatinib
03-Jul-2020

● DRUG ACTION Fostamatinib, through its metabolite R406,
blocks the activity of the spleen tyrosine kinase (SYK)
enzyme, thereby reducing immune-mediated destruction
of platelets.

● INDICATIONS AND DOSE
**Chronic immune thrombocytopenia in patients refractory
to other treatments (under expert supervision)**
▶ BY MOUTH
▶ Adult: Initially 100 mg twice daily; increased if
   tolerated to 150 mg twice daily after 4 weeks, dose to be
   adjusted to achieve a platelet count of 50x10^9/litre or
   more, discontinue if inadequate response after
   12 weeks of treatment, for dose reduction, interruption
   or treatment discontinuation due to side-effects—
   consult product literature

● INTERACTIONS → Appendix 1: fostamatinib

● SIDE-EFFECTS
▶ **Common or very common** Chest pain · diarrhoea · dizziness
   · fatigue · frequent bowel movements · gastrointestinal
   discomfort · hypertension · increased risk of infection ·
   influenza like illness · nausea · neutropenia · skin reactions
   · taste altered
▶ **Frequency not known** Hyperbilirubinaemia · hypoxia ·
   nephrolithiasis · pain in extremity · syncope · toothache

● CONCEPTION AND CONTRACEPTION Manufacturer advises
effective contraception during and for at least 1 month
after stopping treatment in females of childbearing
potential.

● PREGNANCY Manufacturer advises avoid—toxicity in
animal studies.

● BREAST FEEDING Manufacturer advises avoid during and
for at least 1 month after stopping treatment—metabolites
present in milk in *animal* studies.

● HEPATIC IMPAIRMENT Manufacturer advises avoid in
severe impairment; caution in mild to moderate
impairment—monitor liver function monthly during
treatment.
Dose adjustments Manufacturer advises consider dose
reduction, interruption or treatment discontinuation in
mild to moderate impairment—consult product literature.

● MONITORING REQUIREMENTS
▶ Manufacturer advises monitor blood pressure every
   2 weeks until stable, then monthly thereafter;
   antihypertensive therapy can be initiated or adjusted
   during treatment. If increased blood pressure persists,
   consider fostamatinib dose reduction, interruption or
   discontinuation—consult product literature.
▶ Manufacturer advises monitor full blood count, including
   neutrophils and platelet counts, monthly until a stable
   platelet count of at least 50x10^9/litre is reached; monitor
   full blood counts regularly thereafter.
▶ Manufacturer advises monitor for any effects on bone
   remodelling or formation, especially in patients with
   osteoporosis, fractures or young adults where epiphyseal
   fusion has not yet occurred—limited information
   available.

● MEDICINAL FORMS There can be variation in the licensing of
different medicines containing the same drug.
Tablet
▶ Tavlesse (Grifols UK Ltd) ▼
   Fostamatinib (as Fostamatinib disodium hexahydrate)
   100 mg Tavlesse 100mg tablets | 60 tablet [PoM] £3,090.00
   Fostamatinib (as Fostamatinib disodium hexahydrate)
   150 mg Tavlesse 150mg tablets | 60 tablet [PoM] £4,635.00

9

Blood and nutrition

ANTIHAEMORRHAGICS > THROMBOPOIETIN RECEPTOR AGONISTS

Eltrombopag

22-Oct-2020

- **DRUG ACTION** Eltrombopag is a thrombopoietin receptor agonist that binds to and activates the thrombopoietin (TPO) receptor, thereby increasing platelet production.

- **INDICATIONS AND DOSE**

Chronic immune (idiopathic) thrombocytopenic purpura in patients refractory to other treatments (such as corticosteroids or immunoglobulins) (under expert supervision)

▶ BY MOUTH

▶ Adult: Initially 50 mg once daily, dose to be adjusted to achieve a platelet count of 50×10^9/litre or more—consult product literature for dose adjustments, discontinue if inadequate response after 4 weeks treatment at maximum dose; maximum 75 mg per day

▶ Adult (patients of East Asian origin): Initially 25 mg once daily, dose to be adjusted to achieve a platelet count of 50×10^9/litre or more—consult product literature for dose adjustments, discontinue if inadequate response after 4 weeks treatment at maximum dose; maximum 75 mg per day.

Treatment of thrombocytopenia associated with chronic hepatitis C infection, where the degree of thrombocytopenia is the main factor preventing the initiation or limiting the ability to maintain optimal interferon-based therapy (under expert supervision)

▶ BY MOUTH

▶ Adult: Initially 25 mg once daily, dose to be adjusted to achieve a platelet count sufficient to initiate antiviral therapy then a platelet count of $50–75 \times 10^9$/litre during antiviral therapy—consult product literature for dose adjustments, discontinue if inadequate response after 2 weeks treatment at maximum dose; maximum 100 mg per day

Acquired severe aplastic anaemia in patients either refractory to or heavily pretreated with prior immunosuppressive therapy and are unsuitable for haematopoietic stem cell transplantation (under expert supervision)

▶ BY MOUTH

▶ Adult: Initially 50 mg once daily, dose to be adjusted to achieve a platelet count of 50×10^9/litre or more—consult product literature for dose adjustments, discontinue if no haematological response after 16 weeks treatment; maximum 150 mg per day

▶ Adult (patients of East Asian origin): Initially 25 mg once daily, dose to be adjusted to achieve a platelet count of 50×10^9/litre or more—consult product literature for dose adjustments, discontinue if no haematological response after 16 weeks treatment; maximum 150 mg per day.

IMPORTANT SAFETY INFORMATION

MHRA/CHM ADVICE: ELTROMBOPAG (*REVOLADE*®): REPORTS OF INTERFERENCE WITH BILIRUBIN AND CREATININE TEST RESULTS (JULY 2018)

See *Effect on laboratory tests*.

- **CAUTIONS** Patients of East Asian origin · risk factors for thromboembolism

- **INTERACTIONS** → Appendix 1: eltrombopag

- **SIDE-EFFECTS**
▶ **Common or very common** Abnormal loss of weight · alopecia · anaemia · anxiety · appetite abnormal · arthralgia · asthenia · cataract · chest discomfort · chills · concentration impaired · confusion · constipation · cough ·

depression · diarrhoea · dizziness · drowsiness · dry eye · dry mouth · dysphagia · dyspnoea · eye discomfort · eye disorders · fever · gastrointestinal discomfort · gastrointestinal disorders · haemolytic anaemia · haemorrhage · headaches · hepatic disorders · hyperbilirubinaemia · hyperglycaemia · hypoglycaemia · increased risk of infection · influenza like illness · iron overload · lymphopenia · malaise · memory loss · menorrhagia · mood altered · muscle complaints · nasal complaints · nausea · neutropenia · oedema · oral disorders · oropharyngeal complaints · pain · palpitations · QT interval prolongation · sensation abnormal · skin reactions · sleep disorders · splenic infarction · sweat changes · syncope · taste altered · urine discolouration · vertigo · vision disorders · vomiting · weight decreased

▶ **Uncommon** Anisocytosis · arrhythmias · balance impaired · cardiovascular disorder · cyanosis · ear pain · electrolyte imbalance · embolism and thrombosis · eosinophilia · eye inflammation · feeling hot · feeling jittery · food poisoning · gout · hemiparesis · increased leucocytes · lens opacity · muscle weakness · myocardial infarction · nephritis lupus · nerve disorders · rectosigmoid cancer · renal failure · retinal pigment epitheliopathy · sinus disorder · sleep apnoea · speech disorder · sunburn · thrombocytopenia · tremor · urinary disorders · urine abnormalities · vasodilation · wound inflammation

- **CONCEPTION AND CONTRACEPTION** Ensure effective contraception during treatment.

- **PREGNANCY** Avoid—toxicity in *animal* studies.

- **BREAST FEEDING** Manufacturer advises avoid.

- **HEPATIC IMPAIRMENT**
▶ When used for Idiopathic thrombocytopenic purpura Manufacturer advises consider avoiding.
▶ When used for Severe aplastic anaemia Manufacturer advises caution.
▶ When used for Thrombocytopenia associated with chronic hepatitis C infection Manufacturer advises caution (increased risk of hepatic decompensation and thromboembolic events).

Dose adjustments
▶ When used for Idiopathic thrombocytopenic purpura Manufacturer advises initial dose reduction to 25 mg once daily and wait at least 3 weeks before upwards titration of dose.
▶ When used for Severe aplastic anaemia Manufacturer advises initial dose reduction to 25 mg once daily and wait at least 2 weeks before upwards titration of dose.
▶ When used for Thrombocytopenia associated with chronic hepatitis C infection Manufacturer advises initial dose reduction to 25 mg once daily in moderate to severe impairment and wait at least 2 weeks before upwards titration of dose.

- **RENAL IMPAIRMENT** Use with caution.

- **PRE-TREATMENT SCREENING** For *severe aplastic anaemia*, manufacturer advises do not initiate if patients have existing cytogenetic abnormalities of chromosome 7.

- **MONITORING REQUIREMENTS**
▶ Manufacturer advises monitor liver function before treatment, every two weeks when adjusting the dose, and monthly thereafter.
▶ Manufacturer advises regular ophthalmological examinations for cataract formation.
▶ Manufacturer advises peripheral blood smear prior to initiation to establish baseline level of cellular morphologic abnormalities; once stabilised, full blood count with white blood cell count differential should be performed monthly.
▶ For *idiopathic thrombocytopenic purpura*, manufacturer advises monitor full blood count including platelet count and peripheral blood smears every week during treatment until a stable platelet count is reached (50×10^9/litre or more for at least 4 weeks), then monthly thereafter;

monitor platelet count weekly for 4 weeks following treatment discontinuation.

▸ For *severe aplastic anaemia*, manufacturer advises bone marrow examination with aspirations for cytogenetics prior to initiation, at 3 months of treatment and 6 months thereafter.

▸ For *thrombocytopenia associated with chronic hepatitis C infection*, manufacturer advises monitor platelet count every week before and during antiviral treatment until a stable platelet count is reached (50–75x10^9/litre), then monitor full blood count including platelet count and peripheral blood smears monthly thereafter.

● EFFECT ON LABORATORY TESTS Eltrombopag is highly coloured and can cause serum discolouration and interference with total bilirubin and creatinine testing. If laboratory results are inconsistent with clinical observations, manufacturer advises re-testing using another method to help determine the validity of the result.

● DIRECTIONS FOR ADMINISTRATION Manufacturer advises each dose should be taken at least 2 hours before or 4 hours after any dairy products (or foods containing calcium), indigestion remedies, or medicines containing aluminium, calcium, iron, magnesium, zinc, or selenium to reduce possible interference with absorption.

● PATIENT AND CARER ADVICE Patient counselling is advised on how to administer eltrombopag tablets.

● NATIONAL FUNDING/ACCESS DECISIONS
For full details see funding body website

NICE decisions
▸ Eltrombopag for treating chronic immune (idiopathic) thrombocytopenic purpura (updated October 2018) NICE TA293 Recommended with restrictions

Scottish Medicines Consortium (SMC) decisions
▸ Eltrombopag (*Revolade*®) for adult chronic immune (idiopathic) thrombocytopenic purpura (August 2010) SMC No. 625/10 Recommended with restrictions

● MEDICINAL FORMS There can be variation in the licensing of different medicines containing the same drug.

Tablet
▸ Promacta (Imported (United States))
    Eltrombopag (as Eltrombopag olamine) 12.5 mg Promacta 12.5mg tablets | 30 tablet [PoM] [⚠]
▸ Revolade (Novartis Pharmaceuticals UK Ltd)
    Eltrombopag (as Eltrombopag olamine) 25 mg Revolade 25mg tablets | 28 tablet [PoM] £770.00 DT = £770.00
    Eltrombopag (as Eltrombopag olamine) 50 mg Revolade 50mg tablets | 28 tablet [PoM] £1,540.00 DT = £1,540.00
    Eltrombopag (as Eltrombopag olamine) 75 mg Revolade 75mg tablets | 28 tablet [PoM] £2,310.00 DT = £2,310.00

Romiplostim

22-Oct-2020

● DRUG ACTION Romiplostim is an Fc–peptide fusion protein that binds to and activates the thrombopoietin (TPO) receptor, thereby increasing platelet production.

● INDICATIONS AND DOSE

Chronic immune (idiopathic) thrombocytopenic purpura in patients refractory to other treatments (such as corticosteroids or immunoglobulins) (under expert supervision)
▸ BY SUBCUTANEOUS INJECTION
▸ Adult: Initially 1 microgram/kg once weekly, adjusted in steps of 1 microgram/kg once weekly (max. per dose 10 micrograms/kg once weekly) until a stable platelet count of 50x10^9/litre or more is reached, consult product literature for further details of dose adjustments, discontinue treatment if inadequate response after 4 weeks at maximum dose

● CAUTIONS Risk factors for thromboembolism

● SIDE-EFFECTS
▸ **Common or very common** Anaemia · angioedema · arthralgia · asthenia · bone marrow disorders · chills · constipation · diarrhoea · dizziness · embolism and thrombosis · fever · flushing · gastrointestinal discomfort · headaches · hypersensitivity · increased risk of infection · influenza like illness · muscle complaints · nausea · pain · palpitations · peripheral oedema · sensation abnormal · skin reactions · sleep disorders
▸ **Uncommon** Alopecia · appetite decreased · chest pain · clonus · cough · dehydration · depression · dry throat · dysphagia · dyspnoea · erythromelalgia · eye disorders · eye pruritus · feeling hot · feeling jittery · gastrooesophageal reflux disease · gout · haemorrhage · hair growth abnormal · hypotension · irritability · leucocytosis · malaise · muscle weakness · myocardial infarction · nasal complaints · neoplasms · oral disorders · papilloedema · peripheral ischaemia · peripheral neuropathy · photosensitivity reaction · pleuritic pain · portal vein thrombosis · skin nodule · splenomegaly · taste altered · thrombocytosis · tooth discolouration · vertigo · vision disorders · vomiting · weight changes

● PREGNANCY Manufacturer advises avoid—toxicity in *animal* studies.

● BREAST FEEDING Manufacturer advises avoid—no information available.

● HEPATIC IMPAIRMENT Manufacturer advises caution; consider avoiding in moderate to severe impairment (risk of thromboembolic complications).

● RENAL IMPAIRMENT Manufacturer advises caution—no information available.

● MONITORING REQUIREMENTS
▸ Manufacturer advises monitor full blood count and peripheral blood smears for morphological abnormalities before and during treatment.
▸ Manufacturer advises monitor platelet count weekly until platelet count reaches 50x10^9/litre or more for at least 4 weeks without dose adjustment, then monthly thereafter.
▸ Manufacturer advises monitor platelet count following treatment discontinuation—risk of bleeding.

● PATIENT AND CARER ADVICE
Driving and skilled tasks Manufacturer advises that patients and their carers should be counselled on the effects on driving and the performance of skilled tasks—increased risk of dizziness.

● NATIONAL FUNDING/ACCESS DECISIONS
For full details see funding body website

NICE decisions
▸ Romiplostim for the treatment of chronic immune (idiopathic) thrombocytopenic purpura (updated October 2018) NICE TA221 Recommended with restrictions

Scottish Medicines Consortium (SMC) decisions
▸ Romiplostim (*Nplate*®) for adult chronic immune (idiopathic) thrombocytopenic purpura (October 2009) SMC No. 553/09 Recommended with restrictions

● MEDICINAL FORMS There can be variation in the licensing of different medicines containing the same drug.

Powder and solvent for solution for injection
▸ Nplate (Amgen Ltd)
    Romiplostim 250 microgram Nplate 250microgram powder and solvent for solution for injection pre-filled disposable devices | 1 pre-filled disposable injection [PoM] £482.00

Powder for solution for injection
▸ Nplate (Amgen Ltd)
    Romiplostim 125 microgram Nplate 125microgram powder for solution for injection vials | 1 vial [PoM] £241.00

9

Blood and nutrition

Nutrition and metabolic disorders

1 Fluid and electrolyte imbalances

Fluids and electrolytes

Electrolyte replacement therapy

The electrolyte concentrations (intravenous fluid) table and the electrolyte content (gastro-intestinal secretions) table may be helpful in planning replacement electrolyte therapy; faeces, vomit, or aspiration should be saved and analysed where possible if abnormal losses are suspected.

Oral preparations for fluid and electrolyte imbalance

Sodium and potassium salts, may be given by mouth to prevent deficiencies or to treat established deficiencies of mild or moderate degree.

Oral potassium

Compensation for potassium loss is especially necessary:

- in those taking digoxin or anti-arrhythmic drugs, where potassium depletion may induce arrhythmias;
- in patients in whom secondary hyperaldosteronism occurs, e.g. renal artery stenosis, cirrhosis of the liver, the nephrotic syndrome, and severe heart failure;
- in patients with excessive losses of potassium in the faeces, e.g. chronic diarrhoea associated with intestinal malabsorption or laxative abuse.

Measures to compensate for potassium loss may also be required in the elderly since they frequently take inadequate amounts of potassium in the diet (but see **warning** on **renal insufficiency**). Measures may also be required during long-term administration of drugs known to induce potassium loss (e.g. corticosteroids). Potassium supplements are **seldom required** with the small doses of diuretics given to treat hypertension; **potassium-sparing diuretics** (rather than potassium supplements) are recommended for prevention of hypokalaemia due to diuretics such as furosemide p. 243 or the thiazides when these are given to eliminate oedema.

If potassium salts are used for the prevention of hypokalaemia, then doses of potassium chloride daily (in divided doses) by mouth are suitable in patients taking a normal diet. *Smaller doses* must be used if there is *renal insufficiency (common in the elderly)* to reduce the **risk** of **hyperkalaemia**.

Potassium salts cause nausea and vomiting and poor compliance is a major limitation to their effectiveness; when appropriate, potassium-sparing diuretics are preferable.

When there is *established potassium depletion* larger doses may be necessary, the quantity depending on the severity of any continuing potassium loss (monitoring of plasma-potassium concentration and specialist advice would be required). Potassium depletion is frequently associated with chloride depletion and with metabolic alkalosis, and these disorders require correction.

Management of hyperkalaemia

Acute severe hyperkalaemia (plasma-potassium concentration above 6.5 mmol/litre or in the presence of ECG changes) calls for urgent treatment with calcium gluconate 10% p. 1096 by slow intravenous injection, titrated and adjusted to ECG improvement, to temporarily protect against myocardial excitability. An intravenous injection of soluble insulin (5–10 units) with 50 mL glucose 50% p. 1090 given over 5-15 minutes, reduces serum-potassium concentration; this is repeated if necessary or a continuous infusion instituted. Salbutamol p. 269 [unlicensed indication], by nebulisation or slow intravenous injection may also reduce plasma-potassium concentration; it should be used with caution in patients with cardiovascular disease. The correction of causal or compounding acidosis with sodium bicarbonate infusion p. 1086 should be considered (**important**: preparations of sodium bicarbonate and calcium salts should not be administered in the same line—risk of precipitation). Drugs exacerbating hyperkalaemia should be reviewed and stopped as appropriate; occasionally haemodialysis is needed.

Ion-exchange resins may be used to remove excess potassium in *mild hyperkalaemia* or in *moderate hyperkalaemia* when there are no ECG changes.

Oral sodium and water

Sodium chloride p. 1089 is indicated in states of sodium depletion and usually needs to be given intravenously. In chronic conditions associated with mild or moderate degrees of sodium depletion, e.g. in salt-losing bowel or renal disease, oral supplements of sodium chloride or sodium bicarbonate, according to the acid-base status of the patient, may be sufficient.

Oral rehydration therapy (ORT)

As a worldwide problem *diarrhoea* is by far the most important indication for fluid and electrolyte replacement. Intestinal absorption of sodium and water is enhanced by glucose (and other carbohydrates). Replacement of fluid and electrolytes lost through diarrhoea can therefore be achieved by giving solutions containing sodium, potassium, and glucose or another carbohydrate such as rice starch.

Oral rehydration solutions should:

- enhance the absorption of water and electrolytes;
- replace the electrolyte deficit adequately and safely;
- contain an alkalinising agent to counter acidosis;
- be slightly hypo-osmolar (about 250 mmol/litre) to prevent the possible induction of osmotic diarrhoea;
- be simple to use in hospital and at home;
- be palatable and acceptable, especially to children;
- be readily available.

It is the policy of the World Health Organization (WHO) to promote a single oral rehydration solution but to use it flexibly (e.g. by giving extra water between drinks of oral rehydration solution to moderately dehydrated infants).

The WHO oral rehydration salts formulation contains sodium chloride 2.6 g, potassium chloride 1.5 g, sodium citrate 2.9 g, anhydrous glucose 13.5 g. It is dissolved in sufficient water to produce 1 litre (providing Na^+ 75 mmol, K^+ 20 mmol, Cl^- 65 mmol, citrate 10 mmol, glucose 75 mmol/litre). This formulation is recommended by the WHO and the United Nations Children's fund, but it is not commonly used in the UK.

Oral rehydration solutions used in the UK are lower in sodium (50–60 mmol/litre) than the WHO formulation since, in general, patients suffer less severe sodium loss.

Rehydration should be rapid over 3 to 4 hours (except in hypernatraemic dehydration in which case rehydration should occur more slowly over 12 hours). The patient should be reassessed after initial rehydration and if still dehydrated rapid fluid replacement should continue.

Once rehydration is complete further dehydration is prevented by encouraging the patient to drink normal volumes of an appropriate fluid and by replacing continuing losses with an oral rehydration solution; in infants, breast-feeding or formula feeds should be offered between oral rehydration drinks.

Fluids and electrolytes

Electrolyte concentrations—intravenous fluids

Intravenous infusion	Millimoles per litre				
	Na$^+$	K$^+$	HCO$_3^-$	Cl$^-$	Ca^{2+}
Normal plasma values	142	4.5	26	103	2.5
Sodium Chloride 0.9%	150	-	-	150	-
Compound Sodium Lactate (Hartmann's)	131	5	29	111	2
Sodium Chloride 0.18% and Glucose 4% (Adults only)	30	-	-	30	-
Sodium Chloride 0.45% and Glucose 5% (Children only)	75	-	-	75	-
Potassium Chloride 0.15% and Glucose 5% (Children only)	-	20	-	20	-
Potassium Chloride 0.15% and Sodium Chloride 0.9% (Children only)	150	20	-	170	-
Potassium Chloride 0.3% and Glucose 5%	-	40	-	40	-
Potassium Chloride 0.3% and Sodium Chloride 0.9%	150	40	-	190	-
To correct metabolic acidosis					
Sodium Bicarbonate 1.26%	150	-	150	-	-
Sodium Bicarbonate 8.4% for cardiac arrest	1000	-	1000	-	-
Sodium Lactate (m/6)	167	-	167	-	-

Electrolyte content—gastro-intestinal secretions

Type of fluid	Millimoles per litre				
	H$^+$	Na$^+$	K$^+$	HCO$_3^-$	Cl$^-$
Gastric	40–60	20–80	5–20	-	100–150
Biliary	-	120–140	5–15	30–50	80–120
Pancreatic	-	120–140	5–15	70–110	40–80
Small bowel	-	120–140	5–15	20–40	90–130

Oral bicarbonate

Sodium bicarbonate is given by mouth for *chronic acidotic states* such as uraemic acidosis or renal tubular acidosis. The dose for correction of metabolic acidosis is not predictable and the response must be assessed. For severe *metabolic acidosis*, sodium bicarbonate can be given intravenously.

Sodium bicarbonate may also be used to increase the pH of the urine; it is also used in dyspepsia.

Sodium supplements may increase blood pressure or cause fluid retention and pulmonary oedema in those at risk; hypokalaemia may be exacerbated.

Where *hyperchloraemic acidosis* is associated with potassium deficiency, as in some renal tubular and gastrointestinal disorders it may be appropriate to give oral **potassium bicarbonate**, although acute or severe deficiency should be managed by intravenous therapy.

Parenteral preparations for fluid and electrolyte imbalance

Electrolytes and water

Solutions of electrolytes are given intravenously, to meet normal fluid and electrolyte requirements or to replenish substantial deficits or continuing losses, when the patient is nauseated or vomiting and is unable to take adequate amounts by mouth. When intravenous administration is not possible, fluid (as sodium chloride 0.9% p. 1089 or glucose 5% p. 1090) can also be given by subcutaneous infusion (hypodermoclysis).

The nature and severity of the electrolyte imbalance must be assessed from the history and clinical and biochemical investigations. Sodium, potassium, chloride, magnesium, phosphate, and water depletion can occur singly and in combination with or without disturbances of acid-base balance.

Isotonic solutions may be infused safely into a peripheral vein. Solutions more concentrated than plasma, e.g. 20% glucose, are best given through an indwelling catheter positioned in a large vein.

Intravenous sodium

Sodium chloride in isotonic solution provides the most important extracellular ions in near physiological concentrations and is indicated in *sodium depletion*, which can arise from such conditions as gastro-enteritis, diabetic ketoacidosis, ileus, and ascites. In a severe deficit of 4 to 8 litres, 2 to 3 litres of isotonic sodium chloride may be given over 2 to 3 hours; thereafter the infusion can usually be at a slower rate.

Chronic hyponatraemia arising from inappropriate secretion of antidiuretic hormone should ideally be corrected by fluid restriction. However, if sodium chloride is required for acute or chronic hyponatraemia, regardless of the cause, the deficit should be corrected slowly to avoid the risk of osmotic demyelination syndrome and the rise in plasma-sodium concentration should not exceed 10 mmol/litre in 24 hours. In severe hyponatraemia, sodium chloride 1.8% may be used cautiously.

Compound sodium lactate (Hartmann's solution) can be used instead of isotonic sodium chloride solution during or after surgery, or in the initial management of the injured or wounded; it may reduce the risk of hyperchloraemic acidosis.

Sodium chloride with glucose solutions p. 1090 are indicated when there is combined *water and sodium depletion*. A 1:1 mixture of isotonic sodium chloride and 5% glucose allows some of the water (free of sodium) to enter

9

Blood and nutrition

body cells which suffer most from dehydration while the sodium salt with a volume of water determined by the normal plasma Na$^+$ remains extracellular.

Combined sodium, potassium, chloride, and water depletion may occur, for example, with severe diarrhoea or persistent vomiting; replacement is carried out with sodium chloride intravenous infusion 0.9% and glucose intravenous infusion 5% with potassium as appropriate.

Intravenous glucose

Glucose solutions (5%) are used mainly to replace water deficit. Average water requirements in a healthy adult are 1.5 to 2.5 litres daily and this is needed to balance unavoidable losses of water through the skin and lungs and to provide sufficient for urinary excretion. Water depletion (dehydration) tends to occur when these losses are not matched by a comparable intake, as may occur in coma or dysphagia or in the elderly or apathetic who may not drink enough water on their own initiative.

Excessive loss of water without loss of electrolytes is uncommon, occurring in fevers, hyperthyroidism, and in uncommon water-losing renal states such as diabetes insipidus or hypercalcaemia. The volume of glucose solution needed to replace deficits varies with the severity of the disorder, but usually lies within the range of 2 to 6 litres.

Glucose solutions are also used to correct and prevent hypoglycaemia and to provide a source of energy in those too ill to be fed adequately by mouth; glucose solutions are a key component of parenteral nutrition.

Glucose solutions are given in regimens with calcium and insulin for the emergency management of *hyperkalaemia*. They are also given, after correction of hyperglycaemia, during treatment of diabetic ketoacidosis, when they must be accompanied by continuing insulin infusion.

Intravenous potassium

Potassium chloride with sodium chloride intravenous infusion p. 1089 is the initial treatment for the correction of *severe hypokalaemia* and when sufficient potassium cannot be taken by mouth.

Repeated measurement of plasma-potassium concentration is necessary to determine whether further infusions are required and to avoid the development of hyperkalaemia, which is especially likely in renal impairment.

Initial potassium replacement therapy should **not** involve glucose infusions, because glucose may cause a further decrease in the plasma-potassium concentration.

Bicarbonate and lactate

Sodium bicarbonate below is used to control severe *metabolic acidosis* (pH<7.1) particularly that caused by loss of bicarbonate (as in renal tubular acidosis or from excessive gastro-intestinal losses). Mild metabolic acidosis associated with volume depletion should first be managed by appropriate fluid replacement because acidosis usually resolves as tissue and renal perfusion are restored. In more severe metabolic acidosis or when the acidosis remains unresponsive to correction of anoxia or hypovolaemia, sodium bicarbonate (1.26%) can be infused over 3–4 hours with plasma-pH and electrolyte monitoring. In severe shock, for example in cardiac arrest, metabolic acidosis can develop without sodium or volume depletion; in these circumstances sodium bicarbonate is best given as a small volume of hypertonic solution, such as 50 mL of 8.4% solution intravenously.

Sodium lactate intravenous infusion is no longer used in metabolic acidosis because of the risk of producing lactic acidosis, particularly in seriously ill patients with poor tissue perfusion or impaired hepatic function.

For *chronic acidotic states*, sodium bicarbonate can be given by mouth.

Plasma and plasma substitutes

Plasma and plasma substitutes ('colloids') contain large molecules that do not readily leave the intravascular space where they exert osmotic pressure to maintain circulatory volume. Compared to fluids containing electrolytes such as sodium chloride and glucose ('crystalloids'), a smaller volume of colloid is required to produce the same expansion of blood volume, thereby shifting salt and water from the extravascular space. If resuscitation requires a volume of fluid that exceeds the maximum dose of the colloid then crystalloids can be given; packed red cells may also be required.

Albumin solution p. 1097, prepared from whole blood, contain soluble proteins and electrolytes but no clotting factors, blood group antibodies, or plasma cholinesterases; they may be given without regard to the recipient's blood group.

Albumin is usually used after the acute phase of illness, to correct a plasma-volume deficit; hypoalbuminaemia itself is not an appropriate indication. The use of albumin solution in acute plasma or blood loss may be wasteful; plasma substitutes are more appropriate. Concentrated albumin solution (20%) can be used under specialist supervision in patients with an intravascular fluid deficit and oedema because of interstitial fluid overload, to restore intravascular plasma volume with less exacerbation of the salt and water overload than isotonic solutions. Concentrated albumin solution p. 1097 may also be used to obtain a diuresis in hypoalbuminaemic patients (e.g. in hepatic cirrhosis).

Recent evidence does not support the previous view that the use of albumin increases mortality.

Plasma substitutes

Dextran, gelatin p. 1097, and the hydroxyethyl starch, tetrastarch, are macromolecular substances which are metabolised slowly. Dextran and gelatin may be used at the outset to expand and maintain blood volume in shock arising from conditions such as burns or septicaemia; they may also be used as an immediate short-term measure to treat haemorrhage until blood is available. Dextran and gelatin are rarely needed when shock is due to sodium and water depletion because, in these circumstances, the shock responds to water and electrolyte repletion.

Hydroxyethyl starches should only be used for the treatment of hypovolaemia due to acute blood loss when crystalloids alone are not sufficient; they should be used at the lowest effective dose for the first 24 hours of fluid resuscitation.

Plasma substitutes should **not** be used to maintain plasma volume in conditions such as burns or peritonitis where there is loss of plasma protein, water, and electrolytes over periods of several days or weeks. In these situations, plasma or plasma protein fractions containing large amounts of albumin should be given.

Large volumes of *some* plasma substitutes can increase the risk of bleeding through depletion of coagulation factors.

BICARBONATE

I **Sodium bicarbonate**   14-Dec-2020

● **INDICATIONS AND DOSE**

Alkalinisation of urine | Relief of discomfort in mild urinary-tract infections
▸ BY MOUTH
▸ Adult: 3 g every 2 hours until urinary pH exceeds 7, to be dissolved in water

Maintenance of alkaline urine
▸ BY MOUTH
▸ Adult: 5–10 g daily, to be dissolved in water

Chronic acidotic states such as uraemic acidosis or renal tubular acidosis

▸ BY MOUTH

▸ Adult: 4.8 g daily, (57 mmol each of Na^+ and HCO_3^-), higher doses may be required and should be adjusted according to response

Severe metabolic acidosis

▸ BY SLOW INTRAVENOUS INJECTION, OR BY INTRAVENOUS INFUSION

▸ Adult: Administer an amount appropriate to the body base deficit, to be given by slow intravenous injection of a strong solution (up to 8.4%), or by continuous intravenous infusion of a weaker solution (usually 1.26%)

● CONTRA-INDICATIONS
▸ With intravenous use Salt restricted diet

● CAUTIONS Avoid prolonged use in urinary conditions · cardiac disease · elderly · patients on sodium-restricted diet · respiratory acidosis

● INTERACTIONS → Appendix 1: sodium bicarbonate

● SIDE-EFFECTS
▸ With intravenous use Skin exfoliation · soft tissue necrosis · ulcer
▸ With oral use Abdominal cramps · burping · flatulence · hypokalaemia · metabolic alkalosis

● PREGNANCY
▸ With oral use Use with caution in urinary conditions.

● HEPATIC IMPAIRMENT
▸ With oral use Manufacturer advises caution in cirrhosis.

● RENAL IMPAIRMENT
▸ With oral use Avoid (except for specialised role in some forms of renal disease).

● MONITORING REQUIREMENTS
▸ With intravenous use Plasma-pH and electrolytes should be monitored.

● DIRECTIONS FOR ADMINISTRATION
▸ With intravenous use For *slow intravenous injection* use a small volume of hypertonic solution (such as 50 mL of 8.4%). For *continuous intravenous infusion* a weaker solution of 1.26% solution can be infused over 3–4 hours.
▸ With oral use Sodium bicarbonate may affect the stability or absorption of other drugs if administered at the same time. If possible, allow 1–2 hours before administering other drugs orally.

● PRESCRIBING AND DISPENSING INFORMATION
▸ With oral use *Sodium bicarbonate* 500*mg* capsules contain approximately 6 mmol each of Na^+ and HCO_3^-; *Sodium bicarbonate* 600*mg* capsules contain approximately 7 mmol each of Na^+ and HCO_3^-. Oral solutions of sodium bicarbonate are required occasionally; these are available from 'special-order' manufacturers or specialist importing companies; the strength of sodium bicarbonate should be stated on the prescription.
▸ With intravenous use Usual strength Sodium bicarbonate 1.26% (12.6 g, 150 mmol each of Na^+ and HCO_3^-/litre), various other strengths available.

● PATIENT AND CARER ADVICE
▸ With oral use Patients or carers should be given advice on the administration of sodium bicarbonate oral medicines.

● MEDICINAL FORMS There can be variation in the licensing of different medicines containing the same drug. Forms available from special-order manufacturers include: capsule, oral suspension, oral solution, solution for injection, liquid

Tablet
▸ Sodium bicarbonate (Non-proprietary)
Sodium bicarbonate 600 mg Sodium bicarbonate 600mg tablets | 100 tablet GSL £29.75 DT = £26.79

Solution for injection
▸ Sodium bicarbonate (Non-proprietary)
Sodium bicarbonate 84 mg per 1 ml Sodium bicarbonate 8.4% (1mmol/ml) solution for injection 10ml ampoules | 10 ampoule PoM £119.27 DT = £119.27
Sodium bicarbonate 8.4% (1mmol/ml) solution for injection 250ml bottles | 10 bottle PoM £100.00 DT = £100.00
Sodium bicarbonate 8.4% (1mmol/ml) solution for injection 100ml bottles | 10 bottle PoM £100.00 DT = £119.27

Oral solution
▸ Thamicarb (Thame Laboratories Ltd)
Sodium bicarbonate 84 mg per 1 ml Thamicarb 84mg/1ml oral solution sugar-free | 100 ml PoM £39.80 DT = £39.80 sugar-free | 500 ml PoM £199.20 DT = £199.20

Capsule
▸ Sodium bicarbonate (Non-proprietary)
Sodium bicarbonate 500 mg Sodium bicarbonate 500mg capsules | 56 capsule PoM 🄴 DT = £1.71

Infusion
▸ Sodium bicarbonate (Non-proprietary)
Sodium bicarbonate 12.6 mg per 1 ml Polyfusor sodium bicarbonate 1.26% solution for infusion 500ml bottles | 1 bottle PoM £11.98
Sodium bicarbonate 14 mg per 1 ml Polyfusor sodium bicarbonate 1.4% solution for infusion 500ml bottles | 1 bottle PoM £11.98
Sodium bicarbonate 27.4 mg per 1 ml Polyfusor sodium bicarbonate 2.74% solution for infusion 500ml bottles | 1 bottle PoM £11.98
Sodium bicarbonate 42 mg per 1 ml Polyfusor sodium bicarbonate 4.2% solution for infusion 500ml bottles | 1 bottle PoM £11.98
Sodium bicarbonate 84 mg per 1 ml Polyfusor sodium bicarbonate 8.4% solution for infusion 200ml bottles | 1 bottle PoM £11.98

ELECTROLYTES AND MINERALS ⟩ POTASSIUM

Potassium chloride with calcium chloride dihydrate and sodium chloride

(Ringer's solution)

The properties listed below are those particular to the combination only. For the properties of the components please consider, potassium chloride p. 1106, sodium chloride p. 1089.

● INDICATIONS AND DOSE

Electrolyte imbalance

▸ BY INTRAVENOUS INFUSION

▸ Adult: Dosed according to the deficit or daily maintenance requirements (consult product literature)

● INTERACTIONS → Appendix 1: potassium chloride

● PRESCRIBING AND DISPENSING INFORMATION Ringer's solution for injection provides the following ions (in mmol/litre), Ca^{2+} 2.2, K^+ 4, Na^+ 147, Cl^- 156.

● MEDICINAL FORMS There can be variation in the licensing of different medicines containing the same drug.

Infusion
▸ Potassium chloride with calcium chloride dihydrate and sodium chloride (Non-proprietary)
Potassium chloride 300 microgram per 1 ml, Calcium chloride 320 microgram per 1 ml, Sodium chloride 8.6 mg per 1 ml Steriflex No.9 ringers infusion 500ml bags | 1 bag PoM £1.96
Steriflex No.9 ringers infusion 1litre bags | 1 bag PoM £2.22
Polyfusor Ringers solution for infusion 500ml bottles | 1 bottle PoM £3.58

9

Blood and nutrition

Potassium chloride with calcium chloride, sodium chloride and sodium lactate

(Sodium Lactate Intravenous Infusion, Compound; Compound, Hartmann's Solution for Injection; Ringer-Lactate Solution for Injection)

The properties listed below are those particular to the combination only. For the properties of the components please consider, potassium chloride p. 1106, sodium chloride p. 1089, calcium chloride p. 1096.

● **INDICATIONS AND DOSE**

For prophylaxis, and replacement therapy, requiring the use of sodium chloride and lactate, with minimal amounts of calcium and potassium
‣ BY INTRAVENOUS INFUSION
‣ Adult: (consult product literature)

● INTERACTIONS → Appendix 1: calcium salts · potassium chloride

● PRESCRIBING AND DISPENSING INFORMATION Compound sodium lactate intravenous infusion contains Na$^+$ 131 mmol, K$^+$ 5 mmol, Ca^{2+} 2 mmol, HCO$_3^-$ (as lactate) 29 mmol, Cl$^-$ 111 mmol/litre.

● MEDICINAL FORMS There can be variation in the licensing of different medicines containing the same drug.
Infusion
‣ Potassium chloride with calcium chloride, sodium chloride and sodium lactate (Non-proprietary)
Calcium chloride 270 microgram per 1 ml, Potassium chloride 400 microgram per 1 ml, Sodium lactate 3.17 mg per 1 ml, Sodium chloride 6 mg per 1 ml Sodium lactate compound (Hartmann's Solution) infusion 1litre bags | 1 bag [PoM] 🅢

Potassium chloride with glucose

The properties listed below are those particular to the combination only. For the properties of the components please consider, potassium chloride p. 1106, glucose p. 1090.

● **INDICATIONS AND DOSE**

Electrolyte imbalance
‣ BY INTRAVENOUS INFUSION
‣ Adult: Dosed according to the deficit or daily maintenance requirements

● INTERACTIONS → Appendix 1: potassium chloride

● PRESCRIBING AND DISPENSING INFORMATION Potassium chloride 0.3% contains 40 mmol each of K$^+$ and Cl$^-$/litre or 0.15% contains 20 mmol each of K$^+$ and Cl$^-$/litre with 5% of anhydrous glucose.

● MEDICINAL FORMS There can be variation in the licensing of different medicines containing the same drug. Forms available from special-order manufacturers include: infusion, solution for infusion
Infusion
‣ Potassium chloride with glucose (Non-proprietary)
Potassium chloride 3 mg per 1 ml, Glucose anhydrous 50 mg per 1 ml Potassium chloride 0.3% (potassium 40mmol/1litre) / Glucose 5% infusion 1litre bags | 1 bag [PoM] 🅢
Potassium chloride 0.3% (potassium 20mmol/500ml) / Glucose 5% infusion 500ml bags | 1 bag [PoM] 🅢
Potassium chloride 2 mg per 1 ml, Glucose anhydrous 50 mg per 1 ml Steriflex No.29 potassium chloride 0.2% (potassium 27mmol/1litre) / glucose 5% infusion 1litre bags | 1 bag [PoM] £2.20
Steriflex No.29 potassium chloride 0.2% (potassium 13.3mmol/500ml) / glucose 5% infusion 500ml bags | 1 bag [PoM] £1.67
Potassium chloride 1.5 mg per 1 ml, Glucose anhydrous 50 mg per 1 ml Potassium chloride 0.15% (potassium 20mmol/1litre) / Glucose 5% infusion 1litre bags | 1 bag [PoM] 🅢
Potassium chloride 0.15% (potassium 10mmol/500ml) / Glucose 5% infusion 500ml bags | 1 bag [PoM] £1.30

Potassium chloride with glucose and sodium chloride

The properties listed below are those particular to the combination only. For the properties of the components please consider, potassium chloride p. 1106, glucose p. 1090, sodium chloride p. 1089.

● **INDICATIONS AND DOSE**

Electrolyte imbalance
‣ BY INTRAVENOUS INFUSION
‣ Adult: Dosed according to the deficit or daily maintenance requirements

● INTERACTIONS → Appendix 1: potassium chloride

● PRESCRIBING AND DISPENSING INFORMATION Concentration of potassium chloride to be specified by the prescriber (usually K$^+$ 10–40 mmol/litre).

● MEDICINAL FORMS There can be variation in the licensing of different medicines containing the same drug. Forms available from special-order manufacturers include: infusion, solution for infusion
Infusion
‣ Potassium chloride with glucose and sodium chloride (Non-proprietary)
Sodium chloride 1.8 mg per 1 ml, Potassium chloride 3 mg per 1 ml, Glucose anhydrous 40 mg per 1 ml Potassium chloride 0.3% (potassium 20mmol/500ml) / Glucose 4% / Sodium chloride 0.18% infusion 500ml bags | 1 bag [PoM] 🅢
Potassium chloride 0.3% (potassium 40mmol/1litre) / Glucose 4% / Sodium chloride 0.18% infusion 1litre bags | 1 bag [PoM] 🅢
Potassium chloride 1.5 mg per 1 ml, Sodium chloride 1.8 mg per 1 ml, Glucose anhydrous 40 mg per 1 ml Potassium chloride 0.15% (potassium 20mmol/1litre) / Glucose 4% / Sodium chloride 0.18% infusion 1litre bags | 1 bag [PoM] 🅢
Potassium chloride 0.15% (potassium 10mmol/500ml) / Glucose 4% / Sodium chloride 0.18% infusion 500ml bags | 1 bag [PoM] 🅢
Sodium chloride 1.8 mg per 1 ml, Potassium chloride 2 mg per 1 ml, Glucose anhydrous 40 mg per 1 ml Steriflex No.30 potassium chloride 0.2% (potassium 13.3mmol/500ml) / glucose 4% / sodium chloride 0.18% infusion 500ml bags | 1 bag [PoM] £1.67
Steriflex No.30 potassium chloride 0.2% (potassium 27mmol/1litre) / glucose 4% / sodium chloride 0.18% infusion 1litre bags | 1 bag [PoM] £2.20
Potassium chloride 1.5 mg per 1 ml, Sodium chloride 4.5 mg per 1 ml, Glucose anhydrous 50 mg per 1 ml Intraven potassium chloride 0.15% (potassium 10mmol/500ml) / glucose 5% / sodium chloride 0.45% infusion 500ml bags | 1 bag [PoM] £3.76

Potassium chloride with potassium bicarbonate

10-Mar-2020

The properties listed below are those particular to the combination only. For the properties of the components please consider, potassium chloride p. 1106.

● **INDICATIONS AND DOSE**

Potassium depletion
‣ BY MOUTH
‣ Adult: Dosed according to the deficit or daily maintenance requirements (consult product literature)

● INTERACTIONS → Appendix 1: potassium chloride

● PRESCRIBING AND DISPENSING INFORMATION Each *Sando-K*® tablet contains potassium 470 mg (12 mmol of K$^+$) and chloride 285mg (8 mmol of Cl$^-$).

● MEDICINAL FORMS There can be variation in the licensing of different medicines containing the same drug.

Effervescent tablet

CAUTIONARY AND ADVISORY LABELS 13, 21
▸ Sando-K (Alturix Ltd)
    Potassium bicarbonate 400 mg, Potassium chloride 600 mg Sando-K effervescent tablets | 100 tablet P £9.95 DT = £9.95

Potassium chloride with sodium chloride

The properties listed below are those particular to the combination only. For the properties of the components please consider, potassium chloride p. 1106, sodium chloride below.

● **INDICATIONS AND DOSE**

Electrolyte imbalance

▸ BY INTRAVENOUS INFUSION
▸ Adult: Depending on the deficit or the daily maintenance requirements (consult product literature)

● INTERACTIONS → Appendix 1: potassium chloride

● PRESCRIBING AND DISPENSING INFORMATION Potassium chloride 0.15% with sodium chloride 0.9% contains K⁺ 20 mmol, Na⁺ 150 mmol, and Cl⁻ 170 mmol/litre or potassium chloride 0.3% with sodium chloride 0.9% contains K⁺ 40 mmol, Na⁺ 150 mmol, and Cl⁻ 190 mmol/litre.

● MEDICINAL FORMS There can be variation in the licensing of different medicines containing the same drug. Forms available from special-order manufacturers include: infusion, solution for infusion

Infusion

▸ Potassium chloride with sodium chloride (Non-proprietary)
    Potassium chloride 3 mg per 1 ml, Sodium chloride 9 mg per 1 ml Potassium chloride 0.3% (potassium 20mmol/500ml) / Sodium chloride 0.9% infusion 500ml bags | 1 bag PoM 🔲
    Potassium chloride 0.3% (potassium 40mmol/1litre) / Sodium chloride 0.9% infusion 1litre bags | 1 bag PoM 🔲
    Potassium chloride 1.5 mg per 1 ml, Sodium chloride 9 mg per 1 ml Potassium chloride 0.15% (potassium 10mmol/500ml) / Sodium chloride 0.9% infusion 500ml bags | 1 bag PoM 🔲
    Potassium chloride 0.15% (potassium 20mmol/1litre) / Sodium chloride 0.9% infusion 1litre bags | 1 bag PoM 🔲
    Potassium chloride 2 mg per 1 ml, Sodium chloride 9 mg per 1 ml Steriflex No.28 potassium chloride 0.2% (potassium 13.3mmol/500ml) / sodium chloride 0.9% infusion 500ml bags | 1 bag PoM £1.67
    Steriflex No.28 potassium chloride 0.2% (potassium 27mmol/1litre) / sodium chloride 0.9% infusion 1litre bags | 1 bag PoM £2.20

ELECTROLYTES AND MINERALS ⟩ SODIUM CHLORIDE

Sodium chloride   07-Oct-2020

● **INDICATIONS AND DOSE**

Prophylaxis of sodium chloride deficiency

▸ BY MOUTH
▸ Adult: 4–8 tablets daily, to be taken with water, up to maximum 20 tablets daily in severe depletion

Chronic renal salt wasting

▸ BY MOUTH
▸ Adult: Up to 20 tablets daily, to be taken with appropriate fluid intake

Management of diabetic ketoacidosis (to restore circulating volume if systolic blood pressure is below 90 mmHg and adjusted for age, sex, and medication as appropriate)

▸ BY INTRAVENOUS INFUSION
▸ Adult: 500 mL, sodium chloride 0.9% to be given over 10–15 minutes, repeat if blood pressure remains below 90 mmHg and seek senior medical advice, when blood pressure is over 90 mmHg, sodium chloride 0.9% should be given by intravenous infusion at a rate that replaces deficit and provides maintenance, management regimen also includes administration of potassium chloride, soluble insulin, long acting insulin analogues and glucose 10% solution

Diluent for instillation of drugs to the bladder

▸ BY INTRAVESICAL INSTILLATION
▸ Adult: (consult product literature)

● CAUTIONS
▸ With intravenous use Avoid excessive administration · cardiac failure · dilutional hyponatraemia especially in the elderly · hypertension · peripheral oedema · pulmonary oedema · restrict intake in impaired renal function · toxaemia of pregnancy

● SIDE-EFFECTS
▸ With intravenous use Chills · fever · hypervolaemia · hypotension · local reaction · localised pain · paraesthesia · skin reactions · tremor · vascular irritation · venous thrombosis
▸ With oral use Abdominal cramps · acidosis hyperchloraemic · diarrhoea · generalised oedema · hypertension · hypotension · irritability · muscle complaints · nausea · vomiting

● MONITORING REQUIREMENTS
▸ With intravenous use The jugular venous pressure should be assessed, the bases of the lungs should be examined for crepitations, and in elderly or seriously ill patients it is often helpful to monitor the right atrial (central) venous pressure.

● PRESCRIBING AND DISPENSING INFORMATION
▸ With intravenous use Sodium chloride 0.9% intravenous infusion contains Na⁺ and Cl⁻ each 150 mmol/litre. The term 'normal saline' should not be used to describe sodium chloride intravenous infusion 0.9%; the term 'physiological saline' is acceptable but it is preferable to give the composition (i.e. sodium chloride intravenous infusion 0.9%).
▸ With oral use Each Slow Sodium® tablet contains approximately 10 mmol each of Na⁺ and Cl⁻.

● MEDICINAL FORMS There can be variation in the licensing of different medicines containing the same drug. Forms available from special-order manufacturers include: capsule, solution for injection, infusion, solution for infusion

Modified-release tablet

CAUTIONARY AND ADVISORY LABELS 25
▸ Slow Sodium (Alturix Ltd)
    Sodium chloride 600 mg Slow Sodium 600mg tablets | 100 tablet GSL £9.20 DT = £9.20

Solution for injection

▸ Sodium chloride (Non-proprietary)
    Sodium chloride 9 mg per 1 ml Sodium chloride 0.9% solution for injection 50ml vials | 25 vial PoM £85.00–£85.01 DT = £85.01
    Sodium chloride 0.9% solution for injection 10ml ampoules | 10 ampoule PoM £3.24–£3.70 DT = £3.24 | 20 ampoule PoM £10.21 | 50 ampoule PoM £25.50 | 100 ampoule PoM £51.00
    Sodium chloride 0.9% solution for injection 20ml ampoules | 20 ampoule PoM £18.93 DT = £19.87
    Sodium chloride 0.9% solution for injection 2ml ampoules | 10 ampoule PoM £2.33–£2.60 DT = £2.33
    Sodium chloride 0.9% solution for injection 5ml ampoules | 10 ampoule PoM £2.64–£2.80 DT = £2.64 | 50 ampoule PoM £22.00
    Sodium chloride 300 mg per 1 ml Sodium chloride 30% solution for injection 10ml ampoules | 10 ampoule PoM £82.94 DT = £82.76

9

Blood and nutrition

Solution for infusion

► Sodium chloride (Non-proprietary)

Sodium chloride 300 mg per 1 ml Sodium chloride 30% concentrate for solution for infusion 100ml vials | 10 vial [PoM] £61.70 DT = £61.70

Sodium chloride 30% concentrate for solution for infusion 50ml vials | 1 vial [PoM] £15.36 DT = £15.36 | 10 vial [PoM] £85.10 DT = £85.10

Sodium chloride 30% concentrate for solution for infusion 10ml ampoules | 10 ampoule [PoM] £86.80

Infusion

► Sodium chloride (Non-proprietary)

Sodium chloride 1.8 mg per 1 ml Polyfusor O sodium chloride 0.18% infusion 500ml bottles | 1 bottle [PoM] £4.18

Sodium chloride 4.5 mg per 1 ml Sodium chloride 0.45% infusion 500ml bags | 1 bag [PoM] [℞]

Polyfusor SB sodium chloride 0.45% infusion 500ml bottles | 1 bottle [PoM] £3.98

Steriflex No.2 sodium chloride 0.45% infusion 500ml bags | 1 bag [PoM] [℞]

Sodium chloride 9 mg per 1 ml Sodium chloride 0.9% infusion 250ml bags | 1 bag [PoM] [℞]

Sodium chloride 0.9% infusion 1litre bags | 1 bag [PoM] [℞]

Sodium chloride 0.9% infusion 100ml bags | 1 bag [PoM] [℞]

Sodium chloride 0.9% infusion 500ml bags | 1 bag [PoM] [℞]

Sodium chloride 0.9% infusion 50ml bags | 1 bag [PoM] [℞]

Sodium chloride 0.9% infusion 100ml polyethylene bottles | 1 bottle [PoM] £0.55 | 20 bottle [PoM] £11.00

Polyfusor S sodium chloride 0.9% infusion 500ml bottles | 1 bottle [PoM] £2.84 DT = £2.84

Polyfusor S sodium chloride 0.9% infusion 1litre bottles | 1 bottle [PoM] £3.77 DT = £3.77

Sodium chloride 18 mg per 1 ml Polyfusor SC sodium chloride 1.8% infusion 500ml bottles | 1 bottle [PoM] £4.18

Sodium chloride 27 mg per 1 ml Polyfusor SD sodium chloride 2.7% infusion 500ml bottles | 1 bottle [PoM] £4.18

Sodium chloride 50 mg per 1 ml Polyfusor SE sodium chloride 5% infusion 500ml bottles | 1 bottle [PoM] £4.18

Combinations available: *Potassium chloride with calcium chloride dihydrate and sodium chloride,* p. 1087 · *Potassium chloride with calcium chloride, sodium chloride and sodium lactate,* p. 1088 · *Potassium chloride with glucose and sodium chloride,* p. 1088 · *Potassium chloride with sodium chloride,* p. 1089

Sodium chloride with glucose

The properties listed below are those particular to the combination only. For the properties of the components please consider, sodium chloride p. 1089, glucose below.

● **INDICATIONS AND DOSE**

Combined water and sodium depletion

► BY INTRAVENOUS INFUSION

► Adult: (consult product literature)

● MONITORING REQUIREMENTS Maintenance fluid should accurately reflect daily requirements and close monitoring is required to avoid fluid and electrolyte imbalance.

● MEDICINAL FORMS There can be variation in the licensing of different medicines containing the same drug. Forms available from special-order manufacturers include: infusion, solution for infusion

Infusion

► Sodium chloride with glucose (Non-proprietary)

Sodium chloride 4.5 mg per 1 ml, Glucose anhydrous 25 mg per 1 ml Sodium chloride 0.45% / Glucose 2.5% infusion 500ml Viaflo bags | 1 bag [PoM] [℞]

Sodium chloride 1.8 mg per 1 ml, Glucose anhydrous 40 mg per 1 ml Polyfusor T glucose 4% / sodium chloride 0.18% infusion 500ml bottles | 1 bottle [PoM] £2.40 DT = £2.40

Sodium chloride 0.18% / Glucose 4% infusion 500ml bags | 1 bag [PoM] [℞]

Sodium chloride 0.18% / Glucose 4% infusion 1litre bags | 1 bag [PoM] [℞]

Sodium chloride 9 mg per 1 ml, Glucose 50 mg per 1 ml Steriflex No.3 glucose 5% / sodium chloride 0.9% infusion 500ml bags | 1 bag [PoM] £1.47

Steriflex No.3 glucose 5% / sodium chloride 0.9% infusion 1litre bags | 1 bag [PoM] £2.10

Sodium chloride 4.5 mg per 1 ml, Glucose anhydrous 50 mg per 1 ml Steriflex No.45 glucose 5% / sodium chloride 0.45% infusion 500ml bags | 1 bag [PoM] £2.46

Sodium chloride 1.8 mg per 1 ml, Glucose anhydrous 100 mg per 1 ml Steriflex No.19 glucose 10% / sodium chloride 0.18% infusion 500ml bags | 1 bag [PoM] £2.46

NUTRIENTS ❭ SUGARS

Glucose

06-Feb-2020

(Dextrose Monohydrate)

● **INDICATIONS AND DOSE**

Establish presence of gestational diabetes

► BY MOUTH

► Adult: Test dose 75 g, anhydrous glucose to be given to the fasting patient and blood-glucose concentrations measured at intervals, to be given with 200–300 mL fluid

Oral glucose tolerance test

► BY MOUTH

► Adult: Test dose 75 g, anhydrous glucose to be given to the fasting patient and blood-glucose concentrations measured at intervals, to be given with 200–300 mL fluid

Hypoglycaemia

► BY INTRAVENOUS INFUSION

► Child: 500 mg/kg, to be administered as Glucose 10% intravenous infusion into a large vein through a large-gauge needle; care is required since this concentration is irritant

► Adult: 15–20 g, to be administered over 15 minutes as Glucose 10% or 20% intravenous infusion into a large vein through a large-gauge needle; care is required since these concentrations are irritant

Energy source

► BY INTRAVENOUS INFUSION

► Adult: 1–3 litres daily, solution concentration of 20–50% to be administered

Water replacement

► BY INTRAVENOUS INFUSION

► Adult: The volume of glucose solution needed to replace deficits may vary (consult product literature)

Persistent cyanosis (in combination with propranolol) when blood glucose less than 3 mmol/litre (followed by morphine)

► BY INTRAVENOUS INFUSION

► Child: 200 mg/kg, to be administered as Glucose 10% intravenous infusion over 10 minutes

Management of diabetic ketoacidosis

► BY INTRAVENOUS INFUSION

► Child: Glucose 5% or 10% should be added to replacement fluid once blood-glucose concentration falls below 14 mmol/litre

► Adult: Glucose 10% should be given once blood-glucose concentration falls below 14 mmol/litre, to be administered into a large vein through a large-gauge needle at a rate of 125 mL/hour, in addition to the sodium chloride 0.9% infusion

DOSE EQUIVALENCE AND CONVERSION

► 75 g anhydrous glucose is equivalent to Glucose BP 82.5 g.

● CAUTIONS Do not give alone except when there is no significant loss of electrolytes · prolonged administration of glucose solutions without electrolytes can lead to hyponatraemia and other electrolyte disturbances

- SIDE-EFFECTS Chills · electrolyte imbalance · fever · fluid imbalance · hypersensitivity · local reaction · localised pain · polyuria · rash · venous thrombosis

- DIRECTIONS FOR ADMINISTRATION
With intravenous use in children Injections containing more than 10% glucose can be irritant and should be given into a central venous line; however, solutions containing up to 12.5% can be administered for a short period into a peripheral line.

- PRESCRIBING AND DISPENSING INFORMATION Glucose BP is the monohydrate but Glucose Intravenous Infusion BP is a sterile solution of anhydrous glucose or glucose monohydrate, potency being expressed in terms of anhydrous glucose.

- EXCEPTIONS TO LEGAL CATEGORY
With intravenous use Prescription only medicine restriction does not apply to 50% solution where administration is for saving life in emergency.

- MEDICINAL FORMS There can be variation in the licensing of different medicines containing the same drug. Forms available from special-order manufacturers include: oral solution, solution for injection, solution for infusion

Solution for infusion
- Glucose (Non-proprietary)
   Glucose anhydrous 200 mg per 1 ml Glucose 20% solution for infusion 100ml vials | 1 vial [PoM] £6.00
   Glucose anhydrous 500 mg per 1 ml Glucose 50% solution for infusion 20ml ampoules | 10 ampoule [PoM] £14.00 DT = £14.00
   Glucose 50% solution for infusion 50ml vials | 25 vial [PoM] £60.00 DT = £60.00

Oral solution
- Rapilose OGTT (Galen Ltd)
   Glucose 250 mg per 1 ml Rapilose OGTT solution | 300 ml £3.48

Oral gel
- Dextrogel (Neoceuticals Ltd)
   Glucose 400 mg per 1 gram Dextrogel 40% gel | 75 gram £4.30 DT = £7.16 | 80 gram £4.30
- GlucoBoost (Ennogen Healthcare Ltd)
   Glucose 400 mg per 1 gram GlucoBoost 40% gel | 75 gram £5.72 DT = £7.16 | 80 gram £6.11
- GlucoGel (BBI Healthcare Ltd)
   Glucose 400 mg per 1 gram GlucoGel 40% gel berry | 75 gram £7.16 DT = £7.16
   GlucoGel 40% gel original | 75 gram £7.16 DT = £7.16 | 80 gram £6.84
- Rapilose (Galen Ltd)
   Glucose 400 mg per 1 gram Rapilose 40% gel | 75 gram £5.49 DT = £7.16

Infusion
- Glucose (Non-proprietary)
   Glucose anhydrous 50 mg per 1 ml Glucose 5% infusion 500ml bags | 1 bag [PoM] [⚠]
   Glucose 5% infusion 1litre bags | 1 bag [PoM] [⚠]
   Glucose 5% infusion 100ml bags | 1 bag [PoM] [⚠]
   Glucose 5% infusion 250ml bags | 1 bag [PoM] [⚠]
   Polyfusor D glucose 5% infusion 1litre bottles | 1 bottle [PoM] £3.68
   Glucose 5% infusion 50ml bags | 1 bag [PoM] [⚠]
   Polyfusor D glucose 5% infusion 500ml bottles | 1 bottle [PoM] £2.73
   Glucose anhydrous 100 mg per 1 ml Glucose 10% infusion 500ml bags | 1 bag [PoM] [⚠]
   Glucose 10% infusion 1litre bags | 1 bag [PoM] [⚠]
   Glucose anhydrous 200 mg per 1 ml Steriflex No.31 glucose 20% infusion 500ml bags | 1 bag [PoM] £2.64
   Glucose (as Glucose monohydrate) 300 mg per 1 ml Glucose 30% infusion 500ml polyethylene bottles | 10 bottle [PoM] £40.21
   Glucose anhydrous 400 mg per 1 ml Steriflex No.33 glucose 40% infusion 500ml bags | 1 bag [PoM] £2.81
   Glucose anhydrous 500 mg per 1 ml Steriflex No.34 glucose 50% infusion 500ml bags | 1 bag [PoM] £3.11
   Glucose anhydrous 700 mg per 1 ml Glucose 70% concentrate for solution for infusion 500ml Viaflex bags | 1 bag [PoM] [⚠]

Combinations available: *Potassium chloride with glucose,* p. 1088 · *Potassium chloride with glucose and sodium chloride,* p. 1088 · *Sodium chloride with glucose,* p. 1090

ORAL REHYDRATION SALTS

Disodium hydrogen citrate with glucose, potassium chloride and sodium chloride

19-Oct-2020

(Formulated as oral rehydration salts)

- INDICATIONS AND DOSE
Fluid and electrolyte loss in diarrhoea
- BY MOUTH
  - Child 1–11 months: 1–1½ times usual feed volume to be given
  - Child 1–11 years: 200 mL, to be given after every loose motion
  - Child 12–17 years: 200–400 mL, to be given after every loose motion, dose according to fluid loss
  - Adult: 200–400 mL, to be given after every loose motion, dose according to fluid loss

- DIRECTIONS FOR ADMINISTRATION Manufacturer advises reconstitute 1 sachet with 200mL of water (freshly boiled and cooled for infants); 5 sachets reconstituted with 1 litre of water provide Na$^+$ 60 mmol, K$^+$ 20 mmol, Cl$^-$ 60 mmol, citrate 10 mmol, and glucose 90 mmol.

- PRESCRIBING AND DISPENSING INFORMATION Flavours of oral powder formulations may include black currant, citrus, or natural.

- PATIENT AND CARER ADVICE After reconstitution any unused solution should be discarded no later than 1 hour after preparation unless stored in a refrigerator when it may be kept for up to 24 hours.
Medicines for Children leaflet: Oral rehydration salts
www.medicinesforchildren.org.uk/oral-rehydration-salts

- MEDICINAL FORMS There can be variation in the licensing of different medicines containing the same drug.
Powder
- Dioralyte (Sanofi)
   Potassium chloride 300 mg, Sodium chloride 470 mg, Disodium hydrogen citrate 530 mg, Glucose 3.56 gram Dioralyte oral powder sachets citrus | 20 sachet [P] £6.72
   Dioralyte oral powder sachets plain | 20 sachet [P] £6.72
   Dioralyte oral powder sachets blackcurrant | 20 sachet [P] £6.72

Potassium chloride with rice powder, sodium chloride and sodium citrate

19-Oct-2020

(Formulated as oral rehydation salts)

- INDICATIONS AND DOSE
Fluid and electrolyte loss in diarrhoea
- BY MOUTH
  - Adult: 200–400 mL, to be given after every loose motion, dose according to fluid loss

- DIRECTIONS FOR ADMINISTRATION Manufacturer advises reconstitute 1 sachet with 200 mL of water (freshly boiled and cooled for infants); 5 sachets when reconstituted with 1 litre of water provide Na$^+$ 60 mmol, K$^+$ 20 mmol, Cl$^-$ 50 mmol and citrate 10 mmol.

- PRESCRIBING AND DISPENSING INFORMATION Flavours of oral powder formulations may include apricot, black currant, or raspberry.

- PATIENT AND CARER ADVICE Patients and carers should be advised how to reconstitute *Dioralyte*® Relief oral powder. After reconstitution any unused solution should be discarded no later than 1 hour after preparation unless stored in a refrigerator when it may be kept for up to 24 hours.

● MEDICINAL FORMS There can be variation in the licensing of different medicines containing the same drug.

Powder

EXCIPIENTS: May contain Aspartame

▸ Dioralyte Relief (Sanofi)

Potassium chloride 300 mg, Sodium chloride 350 mg, Sodium citrate 580 mg, Rice powder pre-cooked 6 gram Dioralyte Relief oral powder sachets blackcurrant sugar-free | 20 sachet P £7.13

1.1 Calcium imbalance

Calcium imbalance

Calcium supplements

Calcium supplements are usually only required where dietary calcium intake is deficient. This dietary requirement varies with age and is relatively greater in childhood, pregnancy, and lactation, due to an increased demand, and in old age, due to impaired absorption. In osteoporosis, a calcium intake which is double the recommended amount reduces the rate of bone loss. If the actual dietary intake is less than the recommended amount, a supplement of as much as 40 mmol is appropriate.

In severe acute hypocalcaemia or hypocalcaemic tetany, an initial slow intravenous injection of calcium gluconate injection 10% p. 1096 should be given, with plasma-calcium and ECG monitoring (risk of arrhythmias if given too rapidly), and either repeated as required or, if only temporary improvement, followed by a continuous intravenous infusion to prevent recurrence. Calcium chloride injection p. 1096 is also available, but is more irritant; care should be taken to prevent extravasation. Oral supplements of calcium and vitamin D may also be required in persistent hypocalcaemia. Concurrent hypomagnesaemia should be corrected with magnesium sulfate p. 1099.

See the role of calcium gluconate in temporarily reducing the toxic effects of hyperkalaemia.

Severe hypercalcaemia

Severe hypercalcaemia calls for urgent treatment before detailed investigation of the cause. Dehydration should be corrected first with intravenous infusion of sodium chloride **0.9%** p. 1089. Drugs (such as thiazides and vitamin D compounds) which promote hypercalcaemia, should be discontinued and dietary calcium should be restricted.

If *severe hypercalcaemia persists* drugs which inhibit mobilisation of calcium from the skeleton may be required. The **bisphosphonates** are useful and pamidronate disodium p. 770 is probably the most effective.

Corticosteroids are widely given, but may only be useful where hypercalcaemia is due to sarcoidosis or vitamin D intoxication; they often take several days to achieve the desired effect.

Calcitonin (salmon) p. 773 can be used for the treatment of hypercalcaemia associated with malignancy; it is rarely effective where bisphosphonates have failed to reduce serum calcium adequately.

After treatment of severe hypercalcaemia the underlying cause must be established. *Further treatment* is governed by the same principles as for initial therapy. Salt and water depletion and drugs promoting hypercalcaemia should be avoided; oral administration of a bisphosphonate may be useful.

Hypercalciuria

Hypercalciuria should be investigated for an underlying cause, which should be treated. Where a cause is not identified (idiopathic hypercalciuria), the condition is managed by increasing fluid intake and giving bendroflumethiazide p. 180. Reducing dietary calcium intake may be beneficial but severe restriction of calcium intake has not proved beneficial and may even be harmful.

Hyperparathyroidism

07-Jul-2020

Hyperparathyroidism, primary

Primary hyperparathyroidism is a disorder of the parathyroid glands—most commonly caused by a non-cancerous tumour (adenoma) in one of the glands. The resulting excess secretion of parathyroid hormone leads to hypercalcaemia, hypophosphataemia and hypercalciuria. The main symptoms are a result of hypercalcaemia and include thirst, increased urine output, constipation, fatigue and memory impairment. Long term effects include cardiovascular disease, kidney stones, osteoporosis, and fractures.

Primary hyperparathyroidism is one of the leading causes of hypercalcaemia, and one of the most common endocrine disorders. It affects twice as many women than men and can develop at any age—with diagnosis most common in women aged 50 to 60 years.

Aims of treatment

Treatment is focused on cure through surgery; other treatment options aim to reduce long-term complications and improve quality of life.

Non-drug treatment

EvGr Information regarding the advantages and disadvantages of available treatments, ongoing monitoring, and advice on how to reduce the symptoms of primary hyperparathyroidism, should be given to all patients.

Parathyroidectomy surgery is the recommended first-line treatment of primary hyperparathyroidism, with unsuccessful surgery requiring multidisciplinary team review at a specialist centre.

For all patients with primary hyperparathyroidism, Cardiovascular disease risk assessment and prevention p. 203, and assessment of Osteoporosis p. 765 and fracture risk should be carried out. ⒶFor further information on fracture risk assessment, see NICE clinical guideline: **Osteoporosis** (see *Useful resources*).

Women of childbearing age

EvGr For women with primary hyperparathyroidism who are considering pregnancy, parathyroid surgery should be offered; and for pregnant women the management and monitoring of primary hyperparathyroidism should be discussed with a multidisciplinary team at a specialist centre.

Women with primary hyperparathyroidism are at increased risk of hypertensive disease in pregnancy. ⒶFor information on diagnosis and management, see *Hypertension in pregnancy* in Hypertension p. 153.

Drug treatment

EvGr Treatment with cinacalcet p. 1093 may be considered for patients with primary hyperparathyroidism if surgery has been unsuccessful [unlicensed indication], is unsuitable, or has been declined; and they have an elevated albumin-adjusted serum calcium level with or without symptoms of hypercalcaemia.

In secondary care, vitamin D levels should be measured and supplementation with vitamin D (see Vitamins p. 1127) offered for people with a probable diagnosis of primary hyperparathyroidism if needed.

To reduce fracture risk for people with primary hyperparathyroidism who have an increased fracture risk, a bisphosphonate can be considered. Do not offer

1.1a Hypercalcaemia and hypercalciuria

bisphosphonates for chronic hypercalcaemia of primary hyperparathyroidism. Ⓐ

Useful Resources

Hyperparathyroidism (primary): diagnosis, assessment and initial management. National Institute of Health and Care Excellence. NICE guideline 132. May 2019.
www.nice.org.uk/guidance/ng132
   Osteoporosis: assessing the risk of fragility fracture. National Institute for Health and Care Excellence. Clinical guideline 146. February 2017.
www.nice.org.uk/guidance/cg146

CALCIUM REGULATING DRUGS > BONE RESORPTION INHIBITORS

Cinacalcet   22-Jan-2020

- **DRUG ACTION** Cinacalcet reduces parathyroid hormone which leads to a decrease in serum calcium concentrations.

- **INDICATIONS AND DOSE**

   Secondary hyperparathyroidism [in patients with end-stage renal disease on dialysis] (under expert supervision)
   ▸ BY MOUTH
   ▸ Adult: Initially 30 mg once daily, dose to be adjusted every 2–4 weeks according to response; maximum 180 mg per day

   Hypercalcaemia in parathyroid carcinoma | Primary hyperparathyroidism [in patients where parathyroidectomy is inappropriate]
   ▸ BY MOUTH
   ▸ Adult: Initially 30 mg twice daily (max. per dose 90 mg 4 times a day), dose to be adjusted every 2–4 weeks according to response

- **CONTRA-INDICATIONS** Hypocalcaemia
- **CAUTIONS** Conditions that may worsen with a decrease in serum-calcium concentrations · switching from etelcalcetide

   CAUTIONS, FURTHER INFORMATION
   ▸ Conditions that may worsen with a decrease in serum-calcium concentrations Manufacturer advises caution with use in patients with conditions that may worsen with a decrease in serum-calcium concentrations, including predisposition to QT-interval prolongation, history of seizures, and history of impaired cardiac function—serum-calcium concentration should be closely monitored.
   ▸ Switching from etelcalcetide Manufacturer advises that in patients who have discontinued etelcalcetide, do not initiate cinacalcet until at least three subsequent haemodialysis sessions are completed, and serum-calcium concentration is confirmed within normal range.

- **INTERACTIONS** → Appendix 1: cinacalcet
- **SIDE-EFFECTS**
   ▸ **Common or very common** Appetite decreased · asthenia · back pain · constipation · cough · diarrhoea · dizziness · dyspnoea · electrolyte imbalance · gastrointestinal discomfort · headache · hypersensitivity · hypotension · muscle complaints · nausea · paraesthesia · rash · seizure · upper respiratory tract infection · vomiting
   ▸ **Frequency not known** Heart failure aggravated · QT interval prolongation · ventricular arrhythmia

- **PREGNANCY** Manufacturer advises use only if potential benefit outweighs risk—no information available.
- **BREAST FEEDING** Manufacturer advises avoid—present in milk in *animal* studies.
- **HEPATIC IMPAIRMENT** Manufacturer advises caution in moderate to severe impairment.
- **MONITORING REQUIREMENTS**
   ▸ When used for Secondary hyperparathyroidism Manufacturer advises measure serum-calcium concentration before initiation of treatment and within 1 week after starting treatment or adjusting dose, then monthly thereafter. Measure parathyroid hormone concentration 1–4 weeks after starting treatment or adjusting dose, then every 1–3 months.
   ▸ When used for Primary hyperparathyroidism and parathyroid carcinoma Manufacturer advises measure serum-calcium concentration before initiation of treatment and within 1 week after starting treatment or adjusting dose, then every 2–3 months.
- **DIRECTIONS FOR ADMINISTRATION** Manufacturer advises capsules containing granules should be opened and the granules sprinkled on to a small amount of soft food (apple sauce or yogurt) or liquid, then administered immediately. Capsules should not be swallowed whole. For administration advice via nasogastric or gastrostomy tube—consult product literature.
- **PATIENT AND CARER ADVICE** Manufacturer advises patients and their carers should be counselled on the symptoms of hypocalcaemia and importance of serum-calcium monitoring.
   Driving and skilled tasks Manufacturer advises patients and carers should be counselled on the effects on driving and performance of skilled tasks—increased risk of dizziness and seizures.
- **NATIONAL FUNDING/ACCESS DECISIONS** For full details see funding body website

   NICE decisions
   ▸ Cinacalcet for the treatment of secondary hyperparathyroidism in patients with end-stage renal disease on maintenance dialysis therapy (January 2007) NICE TA117 Not recommended
   ▸ Cinacalcet for the treatment of secondary hyperparathyroidism in patients with end-stage renal disease on maintenance dialysis therapy (January 2007) NICE TA117 Recommended with restrictions

- **MEDICINAL FORMS** There can be variation in the licensing of different medicines containing the same drug.
   Granules
   CAUTIONARY AND ADVISORY LABELS 21
   ▸ Mimpara (Amgen Ltd)
   Cinacalcet (as Cinacalcet hydrochloride) 1 mg Mimpara 1mg granules in capsules for opening | 30 capsule PoM £161.16 (Hospital only)
   Cinacalcet (as Cinacalcet hydrochloride) 2.5 mg Mimpara 2.5mg granules in capsules for opening | 30 capsule PoM £161.16 (Hospital only)
   Cinacalcet (as Cinacalcet hydrochloride) 5 mg Mimpara 5mg granules in capsules for opening | 30 capsule PoM £161.16 (Hospital only)
   Tablet
   CAUTIONARY AND ADVISORY LABELS 21
   ▸ Cinacalcet (Non-proprietary)
   Cinacalcet (as Cinacalcet hydrochloride) 30 mg Cinacalcet 30mg tablets | 28 tablet PoM £125.75 DT = £106.89
   Cinacalcet (as Cinacalcet hydrochloride) 60 mg Cinacalcet 60mg tablets | 28 tablet PoM £231.97 DT = £197.17
   Cinacalcet (as Cinacalcet hydrochloride) 90 mg Cinacalcet 90mg tablets | 28 tablet PoM £347.96 DT = £295.77
   ▸ Mimpara (Amgen Ltd)
   Cinacalcet (as Cinacalcet hydrochloride) 30 mg Mimpara 30mg tablets | 28 tablet PoM £125.75 DT = £106.89

Cinacalcet (as Cinacalcet hydrochloride) 60 mg Mimpara 60mg tablets | 28 tablet [PoM] £231.97 DT = £197.17

Cinacalcet (as Cinacalcet hydrochloride) 90 mg Mimpara 90mg tablets | 28 tablet [PoM] £347.96 DT = £295.77

Etelcalcetide

26-Aug-2020

- **DRUG ACTION** Etelcalcetide reduces parathyroid hormone secretion, which leads to a decrease in serum calcium concentrations.

INDICATIONS AND DOSE

Secondary hyperparathyroidism in patients with chronic kidney disease on haemodialysis
- ▸ BY INTRAVENOUS INJECTION
- ▸ Adult: Initially 5 mg 3 times a week, then increased in steps of 2.5–5 mg if required, dose to be increased at intervals of at least 4 weeks; usual maintenance 2.5–15 mg 3 times a week, max. dose 15 mg 3 times a week; consult product literature for information on missed doses, and for dose adjustment due to parathyroid hormone levels or serum-calcium concentrations

- **CAUTIONS** Conditions that may worsen with hypocalcaemia · hypocalcaemia (do not initiate if serum-calcium concentration is less than the lower limit of normal range) · switching from cinacalcet (do not initiate until 7 days after the last dose of cinacalcet)

  CAUTIONS, FURTHER INFORMATION
- ▸ Conditions that may worsen with hypocalcaemia Manufacturer advises caution with use in patients with conditions that may worsen with hypocalcaemia, including predisposition to QT-interval prolongation, history of seizures, and history of congestive heart failure—serum-calcium concentration should be closely monitored.
- **INTERACTIONS** → Appendix 1: etelcalcetide
- **SIDE-EFFECTS**
- ▸ **Common or very common** Diarrhoea · electrolyte imbalance · headache · heart failure aggravated · hypotension · muscle complaints · nausea · paraesthesia · QT interval prolongation · vomiting

  SIDE-EFFECTS, FURTHER INFORMATION Manufacturer advises if formation of anti-etelcalcetide antibodies with a clinically significant effect is suspected, contact manufacturer to discuss antibody testing.
- **PREGNANCY** Manufacturer advises avoid—limited information available.
- **BREAST FEEDING** Manufacturer advises avoid—present in milk in *animal* studies.
- **MONITORING REQUIREMENTS** Manufacturer advises monitor parathyroid hormone level 4 weeks after treatment initiation or dose adjustment and approximately every 1–3 months during maintenance treatment; monitor serum-calcium concentration before treatment initiation, within 1 week of initiation or dose adjustment, and then approximately every 4 weeks during maintenance treatment.
- **HANDLING AND STORAGE** Manufacturer advises store in a refrigerator (2–8°C)—consult product literature for further information regarding storage outside refrigerator.
- **PATIENT AND CARER ADVICE** Manufacturer advises patients and their carers should be told to seek medical advice if symptoms of hypocalcaemia occur.
- **NATIONAL FUNDING/ACCESS DECISIONS** For full details see funding body website

  NICE decisions
- ▸ Etelcalcetide for treating secondary hyperparathyroidism (June 2017) NICE TA448 Recommended with restrictions

  Scottish Medicines Consortium (SMC) decisions
- ▸ Etelcalcetide (*Parsabiv*®) for the treatment of secondary hyperparathyroidism (HPT) in adult patients with chronic kidney disease (CKD) on haemodialysis therapy (September 2017) SMC No. 1262/17 Not recommended

- **MEDICINAL FORMS** There can be variation in the licensing of different medicines containing the same drug.

  Solution for injection
- ▸ Parsabiv (Amgen Ltd) ▼
  Etelcalcetide (as Etelcalcetide hydrochloride) 5 mg per 1 ml Parsabiv 2.5mg/0.5ml solution for injection vials | 6 vial [PoM] £136.87
  Parsabiv 10mg/2ml solution for injection vials | 6 vial [PoM] £327.84
  Parsabiv 5mg/1ml solution for injection vials | 6 vial [PoM] £163.92

1.1b Hypocalcaemia

CALCIUM REGULATING DRUGS > PARATHYROID HORMONES AND ANALOGUES

Parathyroid hormone

21-Nov-2017

(Human recombinant parathyroid hormone)

- **DRUG ACTION** Parathyroid hormone is produced by recombinant DNA technology; endogenous parathyroid hormone is involved in modulating serum calcium and phosphate levels, regulating renal calcium and phosphate excretion, activating vitamin D, and maintaining normal bone turnover.

INDICATIONS AND DOSE

Chronic hypoparathyroidism (specialist use only)
- ▸ BY SUBCUTANEOUS INJECTION
- ▸ Adult: (consult product literature)

- **CONTRA-INDICATIONS** Bone metastases · current or previous radiation therapy to skeleton · increased risk factors for osteosarcoma (including Paget's disease or hereditary disorders) · pseudohypoparathyroidism · skeletal malignancy · unexplained raised levels of bone-specific alkaline phosphatase
- **CAUTIONS** Concomitant use of cardiac glycosides (hypercalcaemia may predispose to digitalis toxicity)—monitor cardiac glycoside levels and check for signs and symptoms of digitalis toxicity · concomitant use of drugs that affect calcium levels · young adults with open epiphyses—increased risk of osteosarcoma
- **INTERACTIONS** → Appendix 1: parathyroid hormone
- **SIDE-EFFECTS**
- ▸ **Common or very common** Abdominal pain upper · anxiety · arthralgia · asthenia · chest pain · cough · diarrhoea · drowsiness · electrolyte imbalance · headache · hypercalciuria · hypertension · insomnia · muscle complaints · nausea · pain · palpitations · sensation abnormal · tetany · thirst · urinary frequency increased · vomiting

  SIDE-EFFECTS, FURTHER INFORMATION Hypercalcaemia is more likely during initial dose titration; if severe hypercalcaemia develops, hydrate and consider suspending treatment (including calcium supplement and active vitamin D).
- **PREGNANCY** Manufacturer advises use only if potential benefit outweighs risk—no information available.
- **BREAST FEEDING** Manufacturer advises avoid—present in milk in *animal* studies.
- **HEPATIC IMPAIRMENT** Manufacturer advises caution in severe impairment (no information available).
- **RENAL IMPAIRMENT** Manufacturer advises caution in severe impairment—no information available.

- **PRE-TREATMENT SCREENING** Manufacturer advises confirm sufficient 25-hydroxyvitamin D stores and normal serum magnesium before treatment.
- **MONITORING REQUIREMENTS**
- Manufacturer advises monitor serum calcium and assess for signs and symptoms of hypocalcaemia and hypercalcaemia—adjust active vitamin D and calcium supplement as necessary; consult product literature.
- Manufacturer advises periodic monitoring of the response of serum calcium to treatment (response may decrease over time—if 25-hydroxyvitamin D is low, supplementation may restore serum calcium response).
- **TREATMENT CESSATION** Abrupt interruption or discontinuation can result in severe hypocalcaemia—manufacturer advises to monitor serum calcium and adjust calcium supplement and active vitamin D treatment.
- **PRESCRIBING AND DISPENSING INFORMATION** Manufacturer advises record the brand name and batch number after each administration.
- **HANDLING AND STORAGE** Manufacturer advises store in a refrigerator (2–8 °C); reconstituted solution may be stored for up to 14 days in a refrigerator, and up to 3 days outside of a refrigerator (below 25 °C), during the 14-day use period.
- **PATIENT AND CARER ADVICE** Patients may self-administer *Natpar*®, after appropriate training in subcutaneous injection technique.
  Missed doses Manufacturer advises missed doses should be administered as soon as possible, and additional treatment with calcium and/or active vitamin D must be taken, based on symptoms of hypocalcaemia.

- **MEDICINAL FORMS** There can be variation in the licensing of different medicines containing the same drug.
  Powder and solvent for solution for injection
  ELECTROLYTES: May contain Sodium
  - Natpar (Shire Pharmaceuticals Ltd) ▼
    Parathyroid hormone 25 microgram Natpar 25micrograms/dose powder and solvent for solution for injection cartridges | 2 cartridge [PoM] £4,880.00
    Parathyroid hormone 50 microgram Natpar 50micrograms/dose powder and solvent for solution for injection cartridges | 2 cartridge [PoM] £4,880.00
    Parathyroid hormone 75 microgram Natpar 75micrograms/dose powder and solvent for solution for injection cartridges | 2 cartridge [PoM] £4,880.00
    Parathyroid hormone 100 microgram Natpar 100micrograms/dose powder and solvent for solution for injection cartridges | 2 cartridge [PoM] £4,880.00

ELECTROLYTES AND MINERALS > CALCIUM

Calcium salts

- **CONTRA-INDICATIONS** Conditions associated with hypercalcaemia (e.g. some forms of malignant disease) · conditions associated with hypercalciuria (e.g. some forms of malignant disease)
- **CAUTIONS** History of nephrolithiasis · sarcoidosis
- **SIDE-EFFECTS**
- **Uncommon** Constipation · diarrhoea · hypercalcaemia · nausea
- **RENAL IMPAIRMENT** Use with caution.

⌐ above

Calcium carbonate

10-Mar-2020

- **INDICATIONS AND DOSE**
  Phosphate binding in renal failure and hyper-phosphataemia
  - BY MOUTH
  - Adult: (consult product literature)

Calcium deficiency
- BY MOUTH
- Adult: (consult product literature)

- **INTERACTIONS** → Appendix 1: calcium salts
- **SIDE-EFFECTS**
- **Uncommon** Hypercalciuria
- **Rare or very rare** Flatulence · gastrointestinal discomfort · milk-alkali syndrome · skin reactions
- **PRESCRIBING AND DISPENSING INFORMATION** *Adcal*® contains calcium carbonate 1.5 g (calcium 600 mg or Ca^{2+} 15 mmol); *Calcichew*® contains calcium carbonate 1.25 g (calcium 500 mg or Ca^{2+} 12.5 mmol); *Calcichew Forte*® contains calcium carbonate 2.5 g (calcium 1 g or Ca^{2+} 25 mmol); *Cacit*® contains calcium carbonate 1.25 g, providing calcium citrate when dispersed in water (calcium 500 mg or Ca^{2+} 12.5 mmol); consult product literature for details of other available products.
  Flavours of chewable tablet formulations may include orange or fruit flavour.

- **MEDICINAL FORMS** There can be variation in the licensing of different medicines containing the same drug. Forms available from special-order manufacturers include: tablet, capsule, oral suspension
  Effervescent tablet
  CAUTIONARY AND ADVISORY LABELS 13
  - Cacit (Accord Healthcare Ltd)
    Calcium carbonate 1.25 gram Cacit 500mg effervescent tablets sugar-free | 76 tablet [P] £11.81 DT = £11.81
  Chewable tablet
  CAUTIONARY AND ADVISORY LABELS 24
  EXCIPIENTS: May contain Aspartame
  - Adcal (Kyowa Kirin Ltd)
    Calcium carbonate 1.5 gram Adcal 1500mg chewable tablets sugar-free | 100 tablet [P] £8.70 DT = £8.70
  - Calcichew (Takeda UK Ltd)
    Calcium carbonate 1.25 gram Calcichew 500mg chewable tablets sugar-free | 100 tablet [P] £9.33 DT = £9.33
    Calcium carbonate 2.5 gram Calcichew Forte chewable tablets sugar-free | 60 tablet [P] £13.16 DT = £13.16
  - Remegel (SSL International Plc)
    Calcium carbonate 800 mg Remegel 800mg chewable tablets mint | 24 tablet [GSL] £2.58
  - Rennie (Bayer Plc)
    Calcium carbonate 500 mg Rennie Orange 500mg chewable tablets | 24 tablet [GSL] £1.59 | 48 tablet [GSL] £2.72 DT = £2.72
  - Setlers Antacid (Thornton & Ross Ltd)
    Calcium carbonate 500 mg Setlers Antacid spearmint chewable tablets | 36 tablet [GSL] £1.40
    Setlers Antacid peppermint chewable tablets | 36 tablet [GSL] £1.40

Calcium carbonate with calcium lactate gluconate

The properties listed below are those particular to the combination only. For the properties of the components please consider, calcium carbonate above.

- **INDICATIONS AND DOSE**
  Calcium deficiency
  - BY MOUTH
  - Adult: Dose according to requirements

- **INTERACTIONS** → Appendix 1: calcium salts
- **PRESCRIBING AND DISPENSING INFORMATION** Each *Sandocal*® tablet contains 1 g calcium (Ca^{2+} 25 mmol); flavours of soluble tablet formulations may include orange.

9

Blood and nutrition

- MEDICINAL FORMS There can be variation in the licensing of different medicines containing the same drug.

Effervescent tablet
CAUTIONARY AND ADVISORY LABELS 13
EXCIPIENTS: May contain Aspartame
- Sandocal (GlaxoSmithKline Consumer Healthcare)
  Calcium carbonate 1.75 gram, Calcium lactate gluconate 2.263 gram Calvive 1000 effervescent tablets sugar-free | 30 tablet P £12.82 DT = £12.82

⚑ 1095

Calcium chloride

28-Jul-2020

- **INDICATIONS AND DOSE**

Severe acute hypocalcaemia or hypocalcaemic tetany
- BY INTRAVENOUS INJECTION
- Adult: Dose according to requirements

- CAUTIONS Avoid in respiratory acidosis · avoid in respiratory failure
- INTERACTIONS → Appendix 1: calcium salts
- SIDE-EFFECTS Soft tissue calcification · taste unpleasant · vasodilation
- DIRECTIONS FOR ADMINISTRATION Care should be taken to avoid extravasation.
- PRESCRIBING AND DISPENSING INFORMATION Non-proprietary *Calcium chloride dihydrate* 7.35%(calcium 20 mg or Ca^{2+} 500 micromol/mL); *Calcium chloride dihydrate* 10%(calcium 27.3 mg or Ca^{2+} 680 micromol/mL); *Calcium chloride dihydrate* 14.7%(calcium 40.1 mg or Ca^{2+} 1000 micromol/mL).
- MEDICINAL FORMS There can be variation in the licensing of different medicines containing the same drug. Forms available from special-order manufacturers include: solution for infusion

Solution for injection
- Calcium chloride (Non-proprietary)
  Calcium chloride dihydrate 100 mg per 1 ml Calcium chloride 10% solution for injection 10ml pre-filled syringes | 1 pre-filled disposable injection PoM £9.89 DT = £9.42
  Calcium chloride dihydrate 147 mg per 1 ml Calcium chloride 14.7% solution for injection 5ml ampoules | 10 ampoule PoM £146.72
  Calcium chloride 14.7% solution for injection 10ml ampoules | 10 ampoule PoM £101.96-£107.06 DT = £101.96

⚑ 1095

Calcium gluconate

20-Nov-2019

- **INDICATIONS AND DOSE**

Severe acute hypocalcaemia or hypocalcaemic tetany
- INITIALLY BY SLOW INTRAVENOUS INJECTION
- Adult: Initially 10−20 mL, calcium gluconate injection 10% (providing approximately 2.25–4.5 mmol of calcium) should be administered with plasma-calcium and ECG monitoring, and either repeated as required or, if only temporary improvement, followed by a continuous intravenous infusion to prevent recurrence, alternatively (by continuous intravenous infusion), initially 50 mL/hour, adjusted according to response, infusion to be administered using 100 mL of calcium gluconate 10% diluted in 1 litre of glucose 5% or sodium chloride 0.9%

Acute severe hyperkalaemia (plasma-potassium concentration above 6.5 mmol/litre or in the presence of ECG changes)
- BY SLOW INTRAVENOUS INJECTION
- Adult: 10−20 mL, calcium gluconate 10% should be administered, dose titrated and adjusted to ECG improvement

Calcium deficiency | Mild asymptomatic hypocalcaemia
- BY MOUTH
- Adult: Dose according to requirements

DOSE EQUIVALENCE AND CONVERSION
- 0.11 mmol/kg is equivalent to 0.5 mL/kg of calcium gluconate 10%.

> IMPORTANT SAFETY INFORMATION
> The MHRA has advised that repeated or prolonged administration of calcium gluconate injection packaged in 10 mL glass containers is contra-indicated in children under 18 years and in patients with renal impairment owing to the risk of aluminium accumulation; in these patients the use of calcium gluconate injection packaged in plastic containers is recommended.

- INTERACTIONS → Appendix 1: calcium salts
- SIDE-EFFECTS

GENERAL SIDE-EFFECTS
Arrhythmias

SPECIFIC SIDE-EFFECTS
- With intravenous use Circulatory collapse · feeling hot · hyperhidrosis · hypotension · vasodilation · vomiting
- With oral use Gastrointestinal disorder

- MONITORING REQUIREMENTS
- With intravenous use Plasma-calcium and ECG monitoring required for administration by slow intravenous injection (risk of arrhythmias if given too rapidly)

- DIRECTIONS FOR ADMINISTRATION
- With intravenous use For continuous intravenous infusion, dilute 100 mL of calcium gluconate 10% in 1 litre of glucose 5% or sodium chloride 0.9% and give at an initial rate of 50 mL/hour adjusted according to response. Avoid bicarbonates, phosphates, or sulfates.

- PRESCRIBING AND DISPENSING INFORMATION Calcium gluconate 1 g contains calcium 89 mg or Ca^{2+} 2.23 mmol.

- MEDICINAL FORMS There can be variation in the licensing of different medicines containing the same drug. Forms available from special-order manufacturers include: tablet, capsule, oral suspension, oral solution, solution for injection, solution for infusion

Solution for injection
- Calcium gluconate (Non-proprietary)
  Calcium gluconate 100 mg per 1 ml Calcium gluconate 10% solution for injection 10ml ampoules | 10 ampoule PoM £12.00-£19.18 DT = £19.18 | 20 ampoule PoM £30.00-£46.00

Effervescent tablet
CAUTIONARY AND ADVISORY LABELS 13
ELECTROLYTES: May contain Sodium
- Calcium gluconate (Non-proprietary)
  Calcium gluconate 1 gram Calcium gluconate 1g effervescent tablets | 28 tablet GSL £16.08 DT = £16.08

⚑ 1095

Calcium lactate

- **INDICATIONS AND DOSE**

Calcium deficiency
- BY MOUTH
- Adult: Dose according to requirements

- INTERACTIONS → Appendix 1: calcium salts

- MEDICINAL FORMS There can be variation in the licensing of different medicines containing the same drug.

Tablet
- Calcium lactate (Non-proprietary)
  Calcium lactate 300 mg Calcium lactate 300mg tablets | 84 tablet ℞ DT = £4.57 | 84 tablet GSL ℞ DT = £4.57

Calcium phosphate

🏳 1095

- **INDICATIONS AND DOSE**

Indications listed in combination monographs (available in the UK only in combination with other drugs)
▸ BY MOUTH
▸ Adult: Doses listed in combination monographs

- **INTERACTIONS** → Appendix 1: calcium salts
- **SIDE-EFFECTS** Epigastric pain · gastrointestinal disorder · hypercalciuria

- **MEDICINAL FORMS** No licensed medicines listed.

1.2 Low blood volume

BLOOD AND RELATED PRODUCTS ⟩ PLASMA PRODUCTS

▌ Albumin solution

30-Jan-2020

(Human Albumin Solution)

- **INDICATIONS AND DOSE**

Acute or sub-acute loss of plasma volume e.g. in burns, pancreatitis, trauma, and complications of surgery (with isotonic solutions) | Plasma exchange (with isotonic solutions) | Severe hypoalbuminaemia associated with low plasma volume and generalised oedema where salt and water restriction with plasma volume expansion are required (with concentrated solutions 20%) | Paracentesis of large volume ascites associated with portal hypertension (with concentrated solutions 20%)
▸ BY INTRAVENOUS INFUSION
▸ Adult: (consult product literature)

- **CAUTIONS** Correct dehydration when administering concentrated solution · history of cardiovascular disease · increased capillary permeability · risk of haemodilution (e.g. severe anaemia or haemorrhagic disorders) · risk of hypervolaemia (e.g. oesophageal varices or pulmonary oedema) · vaccination against hepatitis A and hepatitis B may be required

CAUTIONS, FURTHER INFORMATION
▸ Volume status Manufacturer advises adjust dose and rate of infusion to avoid fluid overload.

- **SIDE-EFFECTS**
▸ **Rare or very rare** Fever · flushing · nausea · shock · urticaria
- **MONITORING REQUIREMENTS** Plasma and plasma substitutes are often used in very ill patients whose condition is unstable. Therefore, close monitoring is required and fluid and electrolyte therapy should be adjusted according to the patient's condition at all times.
- **PRESCRIBING AND DISPENSING INFORMATION** A solution containing protein derived from plasma, serum, or normal placentas; at least 95% of the protein is albumin. The solution may be isotonic (containing 3.5–5% protein) or concentrated (containing 15–25% protein).

- **MEDICINAL FORMS** There can be variation in the licensing of different medicines containing the same drug.

Infusion
▸ Flexbumin (Shire Pharmaceuticals Ltd)
Albumin solution human 200 gram per 1 litre Flexbumin 20% infusion 100ml bags | 1 bag PoM 🔲
Flexbumin 20% infusion 50ml bags | 1 bag PoM 🔲

Solution for infusion
▸ Albunorm (Octapharma Ltd)
Albumin solution human 50 mg per 1 ml Albunorm 5% solution for infusion 250ml bottles | 1 bottle PoM £33.75

Albunorm 5% solution for infusion 100ml bottles | 1 bottle PoM £13.50
Albunorm 5% solution for infusion 500ml bottles | 1 bottle PoM £67.50
Albumin solution human 200 mg per 1 ml Albunorm 20% solution for infusion 100ml bottles | 1 bottle PoM £54.00
Albunorm 20% solution for infusion 50ml bottles | 1 bottle PoM £27.00
▸ Alburex (CSL Behring UK Ltd)
Albumin solution human 50 mg per 1 ml Alburex 5% solution for infusion 500ml vials | 1 vial PoM £67.50
Albumin solution human 200 mg per 1 ml Alburex 20% solution for infusion 100ml vials | 1 vial PoM £54.00
▸ Albutein (Grifols UK Ltd)
Albumin solution human 50 mg per 1 ml Albutein 5% solution for infusion 500ml vials | 1 vial PoM 🔲
Albutein 5% solution for infusion 250ml vials | 1 vial PoM 🔲
Albumin solution human 200 mg per 1 ml Albutein 20% solution for infusion 100ml vials | 1 vial PoM 🔲
Albutein 20% solution for infusion 50ml vials | 1 vial PoM 🔲
▸ Biotest (Biotest (UK) Ltd)
Albumin solution human 50 mg per 1 ml Human Albumin Biotest 5% solution for infusion 250ml vials | 1 vial PoM 🔲
Albumin solution human 200 mg per 1 ml Human Albumin Biotest 20% solution for infusion 50ml vials | 1 vial PoM 🔲
Human Albumin Biotest 20% solution for infusion 100ml vials | 1 vial PoM 🔲
▸ Zenalb (Bio Products Laboratory Ltd)
Albumin solution human 45 mg per 1 ml Zenalb 4.5% solution for infusion 250ml bottles | 1 bottle PoM £27.51
Zenalb 4.5% solution for infusion 500ml bottles | 1 bottle PoM £55.02
Albumin solution human 200 mg per 1 ml Zenalb 20% solution for infusion 100ml bottles | 1 bottle PoM £54.00
Zenalb 20% solution for infusion 50ml bottles | 1 bottle PoM £27.00

PLASMA SUBSTITUTES

▌ Gelatin

- **INDICATIONS AND DOSE**

Low blood volume in hypovolaemic shock, burns and cardiopulmonary bypass
▸ BY INTRAVENOUS INFUSION
▸ Adult: Initially 500–1000 mL, use 3.5–4% solution

- **CAUTIONS** Cardiac disease · severe liver disease
- **SIDE-EFFECTS**
▸ **Rare or very rare** Chills · dyspnoea · fever · hyperhidrosis · hypersensitivity · hypertension · hypotension · hypoxia · tachycardia · tremor · urticaria · wheezing
- **PREGNANCY** Manufacturer of *Geloplasma*® advises avoid at the end of pregnancy.
- **HEPATIC IMPAIRMENT** Manufacturers advise avoid preparations that contain lactate (risk of impaired lactate metabolism).
- **RENAL IMPAIRMENT** Use with caution in renal impairment.
- **MONITORING REQUIREMENTS**
▸ Urine output should be monitored. Care should be taken to avoid haematocrit concentration from falling below 25–30% and the patient should be monitored for hypersensitivity reactions.
▸ Plasma and plasma substitutes are often used in very ill patients whose condition is unstable. Therefore, close monitoring is required and fluid and electrolyte therapy should be adjusted according to the patient's condition at all times.
- **PRESCRIBING AND DISPENSING INFORMATION** The gelatin is partially degraded.
Gelaspan® contains succinylated gelatin (modified fluid gelatin, average molecular weight 26 500) 40 g, Na$^+$ 151 mmol, K$^+$ 4 mmol, Mg^{2+} 1 mmol, Cl$^-$ 103 mmol, Ca^{2+} 1 mmol, acetate 24 mmol/litre; *Gelofusine*® contains succinylated gelatin (modified fluid gelatin, average molecular weight 30 000) 40 g (4%), Na$^+$ 154 mmol,

Cl⁻ 124 mmol/litre; *Geloplasma*® contains partially hydrolysed and succinylated gelatin (modified liquid gelatin) (as anhydrous gelatin) 30 g (3%), Na⁺ 150 mmol, K⁺ 5 mmol, Mg²⁺ 1.5mmol, Cl⁻ 100 mmol, lactate 30 mmol/litre; *Isoplex*® contains succinylated gelatin (modified fluid gelatin, average molecular weight 30 000) 40g (4%), Na⁺ 145 mmol, K⁺ 4 mmol, Mg²⁺ 0.9 mmol, Cl⁻ 105 mmol, lactate 25mmol/litre; *Volplex*® contains succinylated gelatin (modified fluid gelatin, average molecular weight 30 000) 40 g (4%), Na⁺ 154 mmol, Cl⁻ 125 mmol/litre.

- MEDICINAL FORMS There can be variation in the licensing of different medicines containing the same drug.
  Infusion
  ▸ Gelaspan (B.Braun Medical Ltd)
    Gelatin 40 mg per 1 ml Gelaspan 4% infusion 500ml Ecobags | 1 bag PoM £5.95 (Hospital only)
  ▸ Gelofusine (B.Braun Medical Ltd)
    Gelatin 40 mg per 1 ml Gelofusine 4% infusion 1litre Ecobags | 1 bag PoM £9.31
    Gelofusine 4% infusion 500ml Ecobags | 1 bag PoM £4.97 (Hospital only)
  ▸ Geloplasma (Fresenius Kabi Ltd)
    Gelatin 30 mg per 1 ml Geloplasma 3% infusion 500ml Freeflex bags | 20 bag PoM £85.50 (Hospital only)
  ▸ Isoplex (Kent Pharmaceuticals Ltd)
    Gelatin 40 mg per 1 ml Isoplex 4% infusion 500ml bags | 10 bag PoM £75.00 (Hospital only)
  ▸ Volplex (Kent Pharmaceuticals Ltd)
    Gelatin 40 mg per 1 ml Volplex 4% infusion 500ml bags | 10 bag PoM £47.00 (Hospital only)

1.3 Magnesium imbalance

Magnesium imbalance

Overview

Magnesium is an essential constituent of many enzyme systems, particularly those involved in energy generation; the largest stores are in the skeleton.

Magnesium salts are not well absorbed from the gastrointestinal tract, which explains the use of magnesium sulfate p. 1099 as an osmotic laxative.

Magnesium is excreted mainly by the kidneys and is therefore retained in renal failure, but significant *hypermagnesaemia* (causing muscle weakness and arrhythmias) is rare.

Hypomagnesaemia

Since magnesium is secreted in large amounts in the gastro-intestinal fluid, excessive losses in diarrhoea, stoma or fistula are the most common causes of *hypomagnesaemia*; deficiency may also occur in alcoholism or as a result of treatment with certain drugs. Hypomagnesaemia often causes secondary hypocalcaemia, and also hypokalaemia and hyponatraemia.

Symptomatic *hypomagnesaemia* is associated with a deficit of 0.5–1 mmol/kg; up to 160 mmol Mg²⁺ over up to 5 days may be required to replace the deficit (allowing for urinary losses). Magnesium is given initially by intravenous infusion or by intramuscular injection of magnesium sulfate; the intramuscular injection is painful. Plasma magnesium concentration should be measured to determine the rate and duration of infusion and the dose should be reduced in renal impairment. To prevent *recurrence of the deficit*, magnesium may be given by mouth, but there is limited evidence of benefit. Magnesium aspartate powder for oral solution below is available as a licensed preparation and, magnesium glycerophosphate tablets and liquid p. 1099 [unlicensed] are available from 'special-order' manufacturers or specialist importing companies.

Arrhythmias

Magnesium sulfate injection has also been recommended for the emergency treatment of *serious arrhythmias*, especially in the presence of hypokalaemia (when hypomagnesaemia may also be present) and when salvos of rapid ventricular tachycardia show the characteristic twisting wave front known as *torsade de pointes*.

Myocardial infarction

Limited evidence that magnesium sulfate prevents arrhythmias and reperfusion injury in patients with suspected myocardial infarction has not been confirmed by large studies. Routine use of magnesium sulfate for this purpose is not recommended.

Eclampsia and pre-eclampsia

Magnesium sulfate injection is the drug of choice for the treatment of seizures and the prevention of recurrent seizures in women with *eclampsia*. Regimens may vary between hospitals. Calcium gluconate injection p. 1096 is used for the management of magnesium toxicity.

Magnesium sulfate injection is also of benefit in women with *pre-eclampsia* in whom there is concern about developing eclampsia. The patient should be monitored carefully.

1.3a Hypomagnesaemia

ELECTROLYTES AND MINERALS ⟩ MAGNESIUM

❚ Magnesium aspartate   23-Jul-2020

- INDICATIONS AND DOSE
  Treatment and prevention of magnesium deficiency
  ▸ BY MOUTH
  ▸ Adult: 10–20 mmol daily, taken as 1–2 sachets of *Magnaspartate*® powder.

- CONTRA-INDICATIONS Disorders of cardiac conduction
- INTERACTIONS → Appendix 1: magnesium
- SIDE-EFFECTS
  ▸ **Uncommon** Diarrhoea · faeces soft
  ▸ **Rare or very rare** Fatigue · hypermagnesaemia
  ▸ **Frequency not known** Gastrointestinal irritation

  SIDE-EFFECTS, FURTHER INFORMATION Side-effects generally occur at higher doses; if side-effects (such as diarrhoea) occur, consider interrupting treatment and restarting at a reduced dose.

  Overdose Symptoms of hypermagnesaemia may include nausea, vomiting, flushing, thirst, hypotension, drowsiness, confusion, reflexes absent (due to neuromuscular blockade), respiratory depression, speech slurred, diplopia, muscle weakness, arrhythmias, coma, and cardiac arrest.

- RENAL IMPAIRMENT Avoid in severe impairment (eGFR less than 30 mL/minute/1.73m²).
- DIRECTIONS FOR ADMINISTRATION Manufacturer advises dissolve sachet contents in 50–200 mL water, tea or orange juice and take immediately.
- PRESCRIBING AND DISPENSING INFORMATION *Magnaspartate*® contains magnesium aspartate 6.5 g (10 mmol Mg²⁺)/sachet.
- PATIENT AND CARER ADVICE Patients and carers should be given advice on how to administer magnesium aspartate powder.

● MEDICINAL FORMS There can be variation in the licensing of different medicines containing the same drug. Forms available from special-order manufacturers include: powder

Powder

EXCIPIENTS: May contain Sucrose

▸ Magnesiocard (Imported (Germany))

Magnesium (as Magnesium aspartate hydrochloride) 121.5 mg Magnesiocard (magnesium 5mmol) oral powder 5g sachets | 50 sachet🄴

▸ Magnaspartate (KoRa Healthcare)

Magnesium (as Magnesium aspartate) 243 mg Magnaspartate 243mg (magnesium 10mmol) oral powder sachets | 10 sachet PoM £9.45 DT = £9.45

Magnesium glycerophosphate　　05-Nov-2020

● INDICATIONS AND DOSE

Prevent recurrence of magnesium deficit

▸ BY MOUTH

▸ Adult: 24 mmol daily in divided doses, dose expressed as Mg^{2+}

DOSE EQUIVALENCE AND CONVERSION

▸ Magnesium glycerophosphate 1 g is approximately equivalent to Mg^{2+} 4 mmol *or* magnesium 97 mg.

NEOMAG® CHEWABLE TABLETS

Hypomagnesaemia

▸ BY MOUTH

▸ Adult: Initially 1–2 tablets 3 times a day, dose to be adjusted according to the serum total magnesium level

DOSE EQUIVALENCE AND CONVERSION

▸ Each *Neomag*® chewable tablet contains Mg^{2+} 4 mmol *or* magnesium 97 mg.

● UNLICENSED USE Preparations other than *Neomag*® are not licensed for use.

● INTERACTIONS → Appendix 1: magnesium

● SIDE-EFFECTS Diarrhoea · hypermagnesaemia

Overdose Symptoms of hypermagnesaemia may include nausea, vomiting, flushing, thirst, hypotension, drowsiness, confusion, reflexes absent (due to neuromuscular blockade), respiratory depression, speech slurred, diplopia, muscle weakness, arrhythmias, coma, and cardiac arrest.

● RENAL IMPAIRMENT Increased risk of toxicity.
Dose adjustments Avoid or reduce dose.
NEOMAG® CHEWABLE TABLETS Manufacturer advises avoid in severe impairment.

● MONITORING REQUIREMENTS Manufacturer advises to monitor serum magnesium levels every 3–6 months.

● DIRECTIONS FOR ADMINISTRATION
NEOMAG® CHEWABLE TABLETS Manufacturer advises that tablets may be broken into quarters and chewed or swallowed with water.

● NATIONAL FUNDING/ACCESS DECISIONS
NEOMAG® CHEWABLE TABLETS For full details see funding body website

Scottish Medicines Consortium (SMC) decisions

▸ **Magnesium glycerophosphate (*Neomag*®) for use as an oral magnesium supplement for the treatment of patients with chronic magnesium loss, hypomagnesaemia, or drug-induced hypomagnesaemia (September 2017) SMC No. 1267/17 Recommended**

● MEDICINAL FORMS There can be variation in the licensing of different medicines containing the same drug. Forms available from special-order manufacturers include: tablet, capsule, oral suspension, oral solution, powder

Tablet

▸ Mag-4 (Ennogen Healthcare Ltd)

Magnesium (as Magnesium glycerophosphate) 97.2 mg Mag-4 (magnesium 97.2mg (4mmol)) tablets | 30 tablet £84.50

Oral solution

▸ LiquaMag GP (Fontus Health Ltd)

Magnesium (as Magnesium glycerophosphate) 24.25 mg per 1 ml LiquaMag GP (magnesium 121.25mg/5ml (5mmol/5ml)) oral solution sugar-free | 200 ml £49.99

▸ MagnaPhos (TriOn Pharma Ltd)

Magnesium (as Magnesium glycerophosphate) 19.44 mg per 1 ml MagnaPhos 97.2mg/5ml (4mmol/5ml) oral solution | 200 ml £25.64 DT = £25.64

Magnesium (as Magnesium glycerophosphate) 24.25 mg per 1 ml MagnaPhos 121.25mg/5ml (5mmol/5ml) oral solution | 200 ml £37.87 DT = £37.87

Chewable tablet

EXCIPIENTS: May contain Aspartame

▸ Magnesium glycerophosphate (Non-proprietary)

Magnesium (as Magnesium glycerophosphate) 97.2 mg Magnesium glycerophosphate (magnesium 97.2mg (4mmol)) chewable tablets | 50 tablet PoM £22.77

▸ Neomag (Neoceuticals Ltd)

Magnesium (as Magnesium glycerophosphate) 97.2 mg Neomag (magnesium 97mg (4mmol)) chewable tablets | 50 tablet PoM £22.77 DT = £22.75

Capsule

▸ MagnEss Gly (Essential-Healthcare Ltd)

Magnesium (as Magnesium glycerophosphate) 39.5 mg MagnEss Gly 39.5mg (1.6mmol) capsules | 50 capsule £28.17

Magnesium (as Magnesium glycerophosphate) 48.6 mg MagnEss Gly 48.6mg (2mmol) capsules | 50 capsule £35.87

Magnesium (as Magnesium glycerophosphate) 97.2 mg MagnEss Gly 97.2mg (4mmol) capsules | 50 capsule £37.87

▸ MagnaPhos (TriOn Pharma Ltd)

Magnesium (as Magnesium glycerophosphate) 48.6 mg MagnaPhos 48.6mg (2mmol) capsules | 50 capsule £35.87

Magnesium (as Magnesium glycerophosphate) 97.2 mg MagnaPhos 97.2mg (4mmol) capsules | 50 capsule £37.87

Magnesium sulfate　　13-Mar-2020

● INDICATIONS AND DOSE

Severe acute asthma | Continuing respiratory deterioration in anaphylaxis

▸ BY INTRAVENOUS INFUSION

▸ Child 2-17 years: 40 mg/kg (max. per dose 2 g), to be given over 20 minutes

▸ Adult: 1.2–2 g, to be given over 20 minutes

Prevention of seizures in pre-eclampsia

▸ INITIALLY BY INTRAVENOUS INJECTION

▸ Adult: Initially 4 g, to be given over 5–15 minutes, followed by (by intravenous infusion) 1 gram/hour for 24 hours, if seizure occurs, give an additional dose of 2–4 g by intravenous injection over 5–15 minutes

Treatment of seizures and prevention of seizure recurrence in eclampsia

▸ INITIALLY BY INTRAVENOUS INJECTION

▸ Adult: Initially 4 g, to be given over 5–15 minutes, followed by (by intravenous infusion) 1 gram/hour for 24 hours after seizure or delivery (whichever is later), if seizure recurs, give an additional dose of 2–4 g by intravenous injection over 5–15 minutes

Hypomagnesaemia

▸ BY INTRAVENOUS INFUSION, OR BY INTRAMUSCULAR INJECTION

▸ Adult: Up to 40 g, given over a period of up to 5 days, dose given depends on the amount required to replace the deficit (allowing for urinary losses) continued →

Hypomagnesaemia maintenance (e.g. in intravenous nutrition)
▶ BY INTRAVENOUS INFUSION, OR BY INTRAMUSCULAR INJECTION
▸ Adult: 2.5–5 g daily, usual dose 3 g daily

Emergency treatment of serious arrhythmias
▶ BY INTRAVENOUS INJECTION
▸ Adult: 2 g, to be given over 10-15 minutes, dose may be repeated once if necessary

Rapid bowel evacuation (acts in 2–4 hours)
▶ BY MOUTH
▸ Adult: 5–10 g, dose to be mixed in a glass of water, taken preferably before breakfast

DOSE EQUIVALENCE AND CONVERSION
▸ Magnesium sulfate heptahydrate 1 g equivalent to Mg^{2+} approx. 4 mmol.

● UNLICENSED USE Unlicensed indication in severe acute asthma and continuing respiratory deterioration in anaphylaxis.

> IMPORTANT SAFETY INFORMATION
> MHRA/CHM ADVICE: MAGNESIUM SULFATE: RISK OF SKELETAL ADVERSE EFFECTS IN THE NEONATE FOLLOWING PROLONGED OR REPEATED USE IN PREGNANCY (MAY 2019)
> Maternal administration of magnesium sulfate for longer than 5–7 days in pregnancy has been associated with hypocalcaemia, hypermagnesaemia, and skeletal side-effects in neonates. Healthcare professionals are advised to consider monitoring neonates for abnormal calcium and magnesium levels, and skeletal side-effects if maternal treatment with magnesium sulfate during pregnancy is prolonged or repeated beyond current recommendations.

● CONTRA-INDICATIONS
▸ With oral use In rapid bowel evacuation—acute gastro-intestinal conditions
● CAUTIONS
▸ With oral use In rapid bowel evacuation—elderly and debilitated patients
● INTERACTIONS → Appendix 1: magnesium
● SIDE-EFFECTS
▸ **Rare or very rare**
▸ With oral use Paralytic ileus
▸ **Frequency not known**
▸ With intravenous use Bone demineralisation (reported in neonates following prolonged or repeated use in pregnancy) · electrolyte imbalance · osteopenia (reported in neonates following prolonged or repeated use in pregnancy)
▸ With oral use Diarrhoea · gastrointestinal discomfort · hypermagnesaemia

Overdose Symptoms of hypermagnesaemia may include nausea, vomiting, flushing, thirst, hypotension, drowsiness, confusion, reflexes absent (due to neuromuscular blockade), respiratory depression, speech slurred, diplopia, muscle weakness, arrhythmias, coma, and cardiac arrest.

● PREGNANCY For information on the risk of side-effects in neonates following prolonged or repeated maternal use of magnesium sulfate during pregnancy, see *Important Safety Information*.
▸ When used for Hypomagnesaemia or Arrhythmias or Prevention of seizures in pre-eclampsia or Treatment of seizures and prevention of seizure recurrence in eclampsia or Severe acute asthma or Continuing respiratory deterioration in anaphylaxis in adults Not known to be harmful for short-term intravenous administration in eclampsia, but excessive doses in third trimester cause neonatal respiratory depression. Sufficient amount may cross the placenta in mothers treated with

high doses e.g. in pre-eclampsia, causing hypotonia and respiratory depression in newborns.

● HEPATIC IMPAIRMENT Avoid in hepatic coma if risk of renal failure.

● RENAL IMPAIRMENT Increased risk of toxicity.
Dose adjustments Avoid or reduce dose.

● MONITORING REQUIREMENTS Monitor blood pressure, respiratory rate, urinary output and for signs of overdosage (loss of patellar reflexes, weakness, nausea, sensation of warmth, flushing, drowsiness, double vision, and slurred speech).

● DIRECTIONS FOR ADMINISTRATION
▸ With intravenous use In severe hypomagnesaemia administer initially via controlled infusion device (preferably syringe pump). For *intravenous injection*, in arrhythmias, hypomagnesaemia, eclampsia, and pre-eclampsia, give continuously in Glucose 5% or Sodium chloride 0.9%. Concentration of magnesium sulfate heptahydrate should not exceed 20% (200 mg/mL or 0.8 mmol/mL Mg^{2+}); dilute 1 part of magnesium sulfate injection 50% with at least 1.5 parts of water for injections. Max. rate 150 mg/minute (0.6 mmol/minute Mg^{2+}).

● PRESCRIBING AND DISPENSING INFORMATION
▸ With intramuscular use or intravenous use The BP directs that the label states the strength as the % w/v of magnesium sulfate heptahydrate and as the approximate concentration of magnesium ions (Mg^{2+}) in mmol/mL. Magnesium Sulfate Injection BP is a sterile solution of Magnesium Sulfate Heptahydrate.

● EXCEPTIONS TO LEGAL CATEGORY
▸ With oral use Magnesium sulfate is on sale to the public as Epsom Salts.

● MEDICINAL FORMS There can be variation in the licensing of different medicines containing the same drug. Forms available from special-order manufacturers include: capsule, solution for injection, infusion, solution for infusion

Solution for injection
▸ Magnesium sulfate (Non-proprietary)
Magnesium sulfate heptahydrate 500 mg per 1 ml Magnesium sulfate 50% (magnesium 2mmol/ml) solution for injection 10ml ampoules | 10 ampoule [PoM] £21.71–£56.70 DT = £21.71 | 50 ampoule [PoM] £21.71
Magnesium sulfate 50% (magnesium 2mmol/ml) solution for injection 20ml vials | 10 vial [PoM] £63.00
Magnesium sulfate 50% (magnesium 2mmol/ml) solution for injection 5ml ampoules | 10 ampoule [PoM] £46.00–£67.39
Magnesium sulfate 50% (magnesium 2mmol/ml) solution for injection 2ml ampoules | 10 ampoule [PoM] £17.35–£22.70 DT = £17.35

Solution for infusion
▸ Magnesium sulfate (Non-proprietary)
Magnesium sulfate heptahydrate 100 mg per 1 ml Magnesium sulfate 10% (magnesium 0.4mmol/ml) solution for injection 10ml ampoules | 10 ampoule [PoM] £66.26–£88.39 DT = £84.18
Magnesium sulfate 10% (magnesium 0.4mmol/ml) solution for infusion 10ml ampoules | 10 ampoule [PoM] [℞] DT = £84.18 (Hospital only)
Magnesium sulfate heptahydrate 200 mg per 1 ml Magnesium sulfate 20% (magnesium 0.8mmol/ml) solution for infusion 10ml ampoules | 10 ampoule [PoM] [℞] (Hospital only)
Magnesium sulfate heptahydrate 500 mg per 1 ml Magnesium sulfate 50% (magnesium 2mmol/ml) solution for infusion 100ml vials | 10 vial [PoM] £83.10
Magnesium sulfate 50% (magnesium 2mmol/ml) solution for infusion 50ml vials | 10 vial [PoM] £89.00

Powder
▸ Magnesium sulfate (Non-proprietary)
Magnesium sulfate dried 1 mg per 1 mg Magnesium sulfate powder | 300 gram [GSL] £2.09 | 500 gram [GSL] £3.32 DT = £3.32 | 2000 gram [GSL] £5.82 | 5000 gram [GSL] £11.95

1.4 Phosphate imbalance

Phosphate imbalance

Phosphate supplements

Oral phosphate supplements p. 1103 may be required in
addition to vitamin D in a small minority of patients with
hypophosphataemic vitamin D-resistant rickets.

Phosphate infusion is occasionally needed in alcohol
dependence or in phosphate deficiency arising from use of
parenteral nutrition deficient in phosphate supplements;
phosphate depletion also occurs in severe diabetic
ketoacidosis.

For phosphate requirements in total parenteral nutrition
regimens, see Intravenous nutrition p. 1122.

Phosphate-binding agents

Calcium-containing preparations are used as phosphate-
binding agents in the management of hyperphosphataemia
complicating renal failure. Aluminium-containing
preparations are rarely used as phosphate binding agents
and can cause aluminium accumulation.

Sevelamer p. 1102 is licensed for the treatment of
hyperphosphataemia in patients on haemodialysis or
peritoneal dialysis. Sevelamer carbonate is also licensed for
the treatment of patients with chronic kidney disease not on
dialysis who have a serum-phosphate concentration of
1.78 mmol/litre or more.

Lanthanum p. 1102 is licensed for the control of
hyperphosphataemia in patients with chronic renal failure
on haemodialysis or continuous ambulatory peritoneal
dialysis (CAPD), and in patients with chronic kidney disease
not on dialysis who have a serum-phosphate concentration
of 1.78 mmol/litre or more that cannot be controlled by a
low-phosphate diet.

Sucroferric oxyhydroxide p. 1103 is licensed for the control
of hyperphosphataemia in patients with chronic kidney
disease on haemodialysis or peritoneal dialysis. It is used as
part of a multiple therapeutic approach to control the
development of renal bone disease; this could include the
concomitant use of a calcium supplement, a vitamin D
analogue or calcimimetics.

1.4a Hyperphosphataemia

ELECTROLYTES AND MINERALS >
CALCIUM

> ⬛ 1095

Calcium acetate

03-Aug-2020

● **INDICATIONS AND DOSE**

PHOSEX ® TABLETS

Hyperphosphataemia

▶ BY MOUTH

▶ Adult: Initially 1 tablet 3 times a day, to be taken with
meals, dose to be adjusted according to serum-
phosphate concentration, usual dose 4–6 tablets daily
in divided doses, (1 or 2 tablets with each meal);
maximum 12 tablets per day

RENACET ® TABLETS

Hyperphosphataemia

▶ BY MOUTH

▶ Adult: 475–950 mg, to be taken with breakfast and with
snacks, 0.95–2.85 g, to be taken with main meals and
0.95–1.9 g, to be taken with supper, dose to be adjusted
according to serum-phosphate concentration;
maximum 6.65 g per day

● **INTERACTIONS** → Appendix 1: calcium salts

● **SIDE-EFFECTS**

▶ **Uncommon** Vomiting

● **DIRECTIONS FOR ADMINISTRATION**

PHOSEX ® TABLETS Manufacturer advises *Phosex* ® tablets
are taken with meals.

Tablets can be broken to aid swallowing, but not chewed
(bitter taste).

RENACET ® TABLETS Manufacturer advises that other
drugs should be taken 1 to 2 hours before or after *Renacet* ®
to reduce the possible interference with absorption of
other drugs.

Renacet ® tablets are taken with meals.

● **PRESCRIBING AND DISPENSING INFORMATION**

PHOSEX ® TABLETS *Phosex* ® tablets contain calcium
acetate 1 g (equivalent to calcium 250 mg or Ca^{2+}
6.2 mmol).

RENACET ® TABLETS *Renacet* ® tablets contain calcium
acetate 475 mg (equivalent to calcium 120.25 mg or Ca^{2+}
3 mmol).

● **PATIENT AND CARER ADVICE**

PHOSEX ® TABLETS Patients or carers should be given
advice on how to administer *Phosex* ® tablets.

RENACET ® TABLETS Patients or carers should be given
advice on how to administer *Renacet* ® tablets.

● **MEDICINAL FORMS** There can be variation in the licensing of
different medicines containing the same drug.

Tablet

CAUTIONARY AND ADVISORY LABELS 25

▶ Phosex (Pharmacosmos UK Ltd)

Calcium acetate 1 gram Phosex 1g tablets | 180 tablet PoM £19.79
DT = £19.79

▶ Renacet (Stanningley Pharma Ltd)

Calcium acetate 475 mg Renacet 475mg tablets | 200 tablet P
£9.71 DT = £9.71

Calcium acetate 950 mg Renacet 950mg tablets | 200 tablet P
£18.45 DT = £18.45

Combinations available: *Calcium acetate with magnesium
carbonate,* below

PHOSPHATE BINDERS

Calcium acetate with magnesium carbonate

04-Sep-2020

The properties listed below are those particular to the
combination only. For the properties of the components
please consider, calcium acetate above, magnesium
carbonate p. 76.

● **INDICATIONS AND DOSE**

Hyperphosphataemia

▶ BY MOUTH

▶ Adult: Initially 1 tablet 3 times a day, adjusted
according to serum-phosphate concentration, to be
taken with food; usual dose 3–10 tablets daily;
maximum 12 tablets per day

● **CONTRA-INDICATIONS** Hypercalcaemia ·
hypermagnesaemia · myasthenia gravis · third-degree AV
block

● **INTERACTIONS** → Appendix 1: calcium salts · magnesium

● **DIRECTIONS FOR ADMINISTRATION** Manufacturer advises
that other drugs should be taken at least 2 hours before or
3 hours after calcium acetate with magnesium carbonate
to reduce possible interference with absorption of other
drugs.

- PATIENT AND CARER ADVICE Patients or carers should be given advice on how to administer calcium acetate with magnesium carbonate tablets.

- MEDICINAL FORMS There can be variation in the licensing of different medicines containing the same drug.
  Tablet
  CAUTIONARY AND ADVISORY LABELS 25
  ▸ Osvaren (Vifor Fresenius Medical Care Renal Pharma UK Ltd)
  Magnesium carbonate heavy 235 mg, Calcium acetate 435 mg Osvaren 435mg/235mg tablets | 180 tablet [PoM] £24.00 DT = £24.00

Lanthanum

09-Nov-2020

- INDICATIONS AND DOSE

Hyperphosphataemia in patients with chronic renal failure on haemodialysis or continuous ambulatory peritoneal dialysis (CAPD) | Hyperphosphataemia in patients with chronic kidney disease not on dialysis who have a serum-phosphate concentration of 1.78 mmol/litre or more that cannot be controlled by a low-phosphate diet
  ▸ BY MOUTH
  ▸ Adult: 1.5–3 g daily in divided doses, dose to be adjusted according to serum-phosphate concentration every 2–3 weeks, to be taken with or immediately after meals

- CAUTIONS Gastro-intestinal disorders
- INTERACTIONS → Appendix 1: lanthanum
- SIDE-EFFECTS
  ▸ Common or very common Constipation · diarrhoea · electrolyte imbalance · gastrointestinal discomfort · gastrointestinal disorders · headache · nausea · vomiting
  ▸ Uncommon Alopecia · appetite abnormal · arthralgia · asthenia · burping · chest pain · dizziness · dry mouth · eosinophilia · hyperglycaemia · hyperhidrosis · hyperparathyroidism · increased risk of infection · irritable bowel syndrome · malaise · myalgia · oral disorders · osteoporosis · pain · peripheral oedema · taste altered · thirst · vertigo · weight decreased
- PREGNANCY Manufacturer advises avoid—toxicity in *animal* studies.
- BREAST FEEDING Manufacturer advises caution—no information available.
- HEPATIC IMPAIRMENT Manufacturer advises caution (may be excreted in bile—possible risk of slower elimination and increased plasma concentrations in patients with reduced bile flow)—monitor liver function tests.
- DIRECTIONS FOR ADMINISTRATION Manufacturer advises tablets are to be chewed. Manufacturer advises each sachet of powder to be mixed with soft food and consumed within 15 minutes.
- PATIENT AND CARER ADVICE Patient and carers should be given advice on how to administer lanthanum tablets and powder.
- NATIONAL FUNDING/ACCESS DECISIONS
  For full details see funding body website
  Scottish Medicines Consortium (SMC) decisions
  ▸ Lanthanum carbonate chewable tablets (*Fosrenol*®) for the control of hyperphosphataemia in chronic renal failure patients (May 2007) SMC No. 286/06 Recommended with restrictions
  ▸ Lanthanum carbonate chewable tablets (*Fosrenol*®) for the control of hyperphosphataemia in adult patients with chronic renal failure not on dialysis with serum phosphate levels ≥1.78 mmol/L (October 2010) SMC No. 640/10 Not recommended

▸ Lanthanum carbonate oral powder (*Fosrenol*®) for the treatment of hyperphosphataemia in chronic renal failure patients (December 2012) SMC No. 821/12 Recommended with restrictions

- MEDICINAL FORMS There can be variation in the licensing of different medicines containing the same drug.
  Powder
  CAUTIONARY AND ADVISORY LABELS 21
  ▸ Fosrenol (Shire Pharmaceuticals Ltd)
  Lanthanum (as Lanthanum carbonate) 750 mg Fosrenol 750mg oral powder sachets | 90 sachet [PoM] £182.60 DT = £182.60
  Lanthanum (as Lanthanum carbonate) 1 gram Fosrenol 1000mg oral powder sachets | 90 sachet [PoM] £193.59 DT = £193.59
  Chewable tablet
  CAUTIONARY AND ADVISORY LABELS 21
  ▸ Fosrenol (Shire Pharmaceuticals Ltd)
  Lanthanum (as Lanthanum carbonate) 500 mg Fosrenol 500mg chewable tablets | 90 tablet [PoM] £124.06 DT = £124.06
  Lanthanum (as Lanthanum carbonate) 750 mg Fosrenol 750mg chewable tablets | 90 tablet [PoM] £182.60 DT = £182.60
  Lanthanum (as Lanthanum carbonate) 1 gram Fosrenol 1000mg chewable tablets | 90 tablet [PoM] £193.59 DT = £193.59

Sevelamer

12-Nov-2020

- INDICATIONS AND DOSE

RENAGEL ®

Hyperphosphataemia in patients on haemodialysis or peritoneal dialysis
  ▸ BY MOUTH
  ▸ Adult: Initially 2.4–4.8 g daily in 3 divided doses, dose to be given with meals and adjusted according to serum-phosphate concentration; usual dose 2.4–12 g daily in 3 divided doses

RENVELA ® 2.4G ORAL POWDER SACHETS

Hyperphosphataemia in patients on haemodialysis or peritoneal dialysis | Hyperphosphataemia in patients with chronic kidney disease not on dialysis who have a serum-phosphate concentration of 1.78 mmol/litre or more
  ▸ BY MOUTH
  ▸ Adult: Initially 2.4–4.8 g daily in 3 divided doses, dose to be taken with meals and adjusted according to serum-phosphate concentration every 2–4 weeks— consult product literature; usual dose 6 g daily in 3 divided doses

RENVELA ® 800MG TABLETS

Hyperphosphataemia in patients on haemodialysis or peritoneal dialysis | Hyperphosphataemia in patients with chronic kidney disease not on dialysis who have a serum-phosphate concentration of 1.78 mmol/litre or more
  ▸ BY MOUTH
  ▸ Adult: Initially 2.4–4.8 g daily in 3 divided doses, dose to be taken with meals and adjusted according to serum-phosphate concentration every 2–4 weeks; usual dose 6 g daily in 3 divided doses

- CONTRA-INDICATIONS Bowel obstruction
- CAUTIONS Gastro-intestinal disorders
- INTERACTIONS → Appendix 1: sevelamer
- SIDE-EFFECTS
  ▸ Common or very common Constipation · diarrhoea · gastrointestinal discomfort · gastrointestinal disorders · nausea · vomiting
  ▸ Frequency not known Skin reactions
- PREGNANCY Manufacturer advises use only if potential benefit outweighs risk.

9

Blood and nutrition

- BREAST FEEDING
RENAGEL ® Manufacturer advises use only if potential benefit outweighs risk.
RENVELA ® 2.4G ORAL POWDER SACHETS, 800MG TABLETS Unlikely to be present in milk (however, manufacturer advises avoid).

- DIRECTIONS FOR ADMINISTRATION
RENVELA ® 2.4G ORAL POWDER SACHETS Manufacturer advises each sachet should be dispersed in 60 mL water, or mixed with a small amount of cool food (100 g), prior to administration and discarded if unused after 30 minutes.

- PATIENT AND CARER ADVICE
RENVELA ® 2.4G ORAL POWDER SACHETS Patients and carers should be advised on how to administer powder for oral suspension.

- NATIONAL FUNDING/ACCESS DECISIONS
For full details see funding body website
Scottish Medicines Consortium (SMC) decisions
▸ Sevelamer carbonate (*Renvela* ®) for hyperphosphataemia in adult patients receiving haemodialysis (April 2011) SMC No. 641/10 Recommended with restrictions

- MEDICINAL FORMS There can be variation in the licensing of different medicines containing the same drug.
Powder
CAUTIONARY AND ADVISORY LABELS 13
▸ Renvela (Sanofi)
Sevelamer carbonate 2.4 gram Renvela 2.4g oral powder sachets sugar-free | 60 sachet PoM £167.04 DT = £167.04
Tablet
CAUTIONARY AND ADVISORY LABELS 25
EXCIPIENTS: May contain Propylene glycol
▸ Renagel (Sanofi)
Sevelamer 800 mg Renagel 800mg tablets | 180 tablet PoM £167.04 DT = £40.68
▸ Renvela (Sanofi)
Sevelamer 800 mg Renvela 800mg tablets | 180 tablet PoM £167.04 DT = £40.68

Sucroferric oxyhydroxide   24-Jul-2020

- INDICATIONS AND DOSE
Hyperphosphataemia in patients with chronic kidney disease on haemodialysis or peritoneal dialysis
▸ BY MOUTH
▸ Adult: Initially 1.5 g daily in 3 divided doses, dose to be taken with meals, then adjusted in steps of 500 mg every 2–4 weeks, dose adjusted according to serum-phosphate concentration; maintenance 1.5–2 g daily in divided doses; maximum 3 g per day

- CONTRA-INDICATIONS Haemochromatosis · iron accumulation disorders
- CAUTIONS Gastric disorders · hepatic disorders · major gastrointestinal surgery · peritonitis in the last 3 months
- SIDE-EFFECTS
▸ **Common or very common** Constipation · diarrhoea · gastrointestinal discomfort · gastrointestinal disorders · nausea · product taste abnormal · tooth discolouration · vomiting
▸ **Uncommon** Dysphagia · dyspnoea · electrolyte imbalance · fatigue · headache · skin reactions · tongue discolouration
SIDE-EFFECTS, FURTHER INFORMATION Discoloured faeces may mask the visual signs of gastrointestinal bleeding.
- PREGNANCY Manufacturer advises use only if potential benefit outweighs risk—no information available.
- BREAST FEEDING Manufacturer advises avoid—no information available.
- DIRECTIONS FOR ADMINISTRATION Manufacturer advises *Velphoro* ® tablets must be chewed or crushed, not swallowed whole.

- PATIENT AND CARER ADVICE Patients or carers should be counselled on administration of sucroferric oxyhydroxide tablets and advised that this medication can cause discoloured black stools.

- MEDICINAL FORMS There can be variation in the licensing of different medicines containing the same drug.
Chewable tablet
▸ Velphoro (Vifor Fresenius Medical Care Renal Pharma UK Ltd)
Iron (as Sucroferric oxyhydroxide) 500 mg Velphoro 500mg chewable tablets | 90 tablet PoM £179.00 DT = £179.00

1.4b Hypophosphataemia

ELECTROLYTES AND MINERALS ❭ PHOSPHATES

Phosphate   08-Apr-2020

- INDICATIONS AND DOSE
Treatment of moderate to severe hypophosphatemia
▸ BY INTRAVENOUS INFUSION
▸ Adult: (consult product literature)
Established hypophosphataemia (with monobasic potassium phosphate)
▸ BY INTRAVENOUS INFUSION
▸ Adult: 9 mmol every 12 hours, increased if necessary up to 0.5 mmol/kg (max. per dose 50 mmol), increased dose to be used in critically ill patients; dose to be infused over 6–12 hours, according to severity
Vitamin D-resistant hypophosphataemic osteomalacia
▸ BY MOUTH USING EFFERVESCENT TABLETS
▸ Adult: 4–6 tablets daily, using *Phosphate Sandoz* ®.

IMPORTANT SAFETY INFORMATION
▸ With intravenous use
Some phosphate injection preparations also contain potassium. Expert sources advise for peripheral intravenous administration the *concentration* of potassium should not usually exceed 40 mmol/litre; the infusion solution should be **thoroughly mixed**. Local policies on avoiding inadvertent use of potassium concentrate should be followed. The potassium content of some phosphate preparations may also limit the *rate* at which they may be administered.

- CAUTIONS
GENERAL CAUTIONS Cardiac disease · dehydration · diabetes mellitus · sodium and potassium concentrations of preparations
SPECIFIC CAUTIONS
▸ With intravenous use Avoid extravasation · severe tissue necrosis
- SIDE-EFFECTS
▸ With intravenous use Electrolyte imbalance
▸ With oral use Abdominal distress · diarrhoea · nausea
SIDE-EFFECTS, FURTHER INFORMATION Diarrhoea is a common side-effect and should prompt a reduction in dosage.
- RENAL IMPAIRMENT
Dose adjustments Reduce dose.
Monitoring Monitor closely in renal impairment.
- MONITORING REQUIREMENTS It is essential to monitor closely plasma concentrations of calcium, phosphate, potassium, and other electrolytes—excessive doses of phosphates may cause hypocalcaemia and metastatic calcification.
- PRESCRIBING AND DISPENSING INFORMATION *Phosphate Sandoz* ® contains sodium dihydrogen phosphate anhydrous (anhydrous sodium acid phosphate) 1.936 g,

9

Blood and nutrition

sodium bicarbonate 350 mg, potassium bicarbonate 315 mg, equivalent to phosphorus 500 mg (phosphate 16.1 mmol), sodium 468.8 mg (Na^+ 20.4 mmol), potassium 123 mg (K^+ 3.1 mmol); *Polyfusor NA* ® contains Na^+ 162 mmol/litre, K^+ 19 mmol/litre, PO_4^{3-} 100 mmol/litre; non-proprietary *potassium dihydrogen phosphate injection* (potassium acid phosphate) 13.6% may contain 1 mmol/mL phosphate, 1 mmol/mL potassium.

- MEDICINAL FORMS There can be variation in the licensing of different medicines containing the same drug. Forms available from special-order manufacturers include: infusion, solution for infusion

Effervescent tablet
CAUTIONARY AND ADVISORY LABELS 13
‣ Phosphate Sandoz (Alturix Ltd)
Sodium dihydrogen phosphate anhydrous 1.936 gram Phosphate Sandoz effervescent tablets | 100 tablet [PoM] £19.39 DT = £19.39

Solution for infusion
‣ Phosphate (Non-proprietary)
Potassium dihydrogen phosphate 136 mg per 1 ml Potassium dihydrogen phosphate 13.6% (potassium 10mmol/10ml) solution for infusion 10ml ampoules | 10 ampoule [PoM] £117.77–£123.66 DT = £117.77

Infusion
‣ Phosphate (Non-proprietary)
Potassium dihydrogen phosphate 1.295 gram per 1 litre, Disodium hydrogen phosphate anhydrous 5.75 gram per 1 litre Polyfusor NA phosphates infusion 500ml bottles | 1 bottle [PoM] £5.15

1.5 Potassium imbalance

1.5a Hyperkalaemia

Other drugs used for Hyperkalaemia Calcium gluconate, p. 1096

ANTIDOTES AND CHELATORS > CATION EXCHANGE COMPOUNDS

Calcium polystyrene sulfonate   05-Aug-2020

- INDICATIONS AND DOSE
Hyperkalaemia associated with anuria or severe oliguria, and in dialysis patients
‣ BY MOUTH
‣ Adult: 15 g 3–4 times a day
‣ BY RECTUM
‣ Adult: 30 g, retained for 9 hours followed by irrigation to remove resin from colon

- CONTRA-INDICATIONS Hyperparathyroidism · metastatic carcinoma · multiple myeloma · obstructive bowel disease · sarcoidosis
- INTERACTIONS → Appendix 1: polystyrene sulfonate
- SIDE-EFFECTS Appetite decreased · constipation (discontinue—avoid magnesium-containing laxatives) · diarrhoea · electrolyte imbalance · epigastric discomfort · gastrointestinal disorders · gastrointestinal necrosis (in combination with sorbitol) · hypercalcaemia (in dialysed patients and occasionally in those with renal impairment) · increased risk of infection · nausea · vomiting
- PREGNANCY Manufacturers advise use only if potential benefit outweighs risk—no information available.
- BREAST FEEDING Manufacturers advise use only if potential benefit outweighs risk—no information available.

- MONITORING REQUIREMENTS Monitor for electrolyte disturbances (stop if plasma-potassium concentration below 5 mmol/litre).
- DIRECTIONS FOR ADMINISTRATION
‣ With rectal use Manufacturer advises mix each 30 g of resin with 150 mL of water or 10% glucose.

- MEDICINAL FORMS There can be variation in the licensing of different medicines containing the same drug. Forms available from special-order manufacturers include: enema
Powder
CAUTIONARY AND ADVISORY LABELS 13, 21 (Sorbisterit ® powder only)
EXCIPIENTS: May contain Sucrose
‣ Calcium Resonium (Sanofi)
Calcium polystyrene sulfonate 999.34 mg per 1 gram Calcium Resonium powder sugar-free | 300 gram [P] £82.16 DT = £82.16

Patiromer calcium   03-Dec-2020

- DRUG ACTION Patiromer is a non-absorbed cation-exchange polymer that acts as a potassium binder in the gastro-intestinal tract.

- INDICATIONS AND DOSE
Hyperkalaemia
‣ BY MOUTH
‣ Adult: Initially 8.4 g once daily; adjusted in steps of 8.4 g as required, dose adjustments should be made at intervals of at least one week; maximum 25.2 g per day
PHARMACOKINETICS
‣ Onset of action 4–7 hours.

- CAUTIONS Risk factors for hypercalcaemia (calcium partially released from counterion complex) · severe gastro-intestinal disorders (ischaemia, necrosis, and intestinal perforation reported with other potassium binders)
- INTERACTIONS → Appendix 1: patiromer
- SIDE-EFFECTS
‣ Common or very common Abdominal pain · constipation · diarrhoea · flatulence · hypomagnesaemia
‣ Uncommon Nausea · vomiting
- PREGNANCY Manufacturer advises avoid—no information available.
- BREAST FEEDING Manufacturer advises avoid—no information available (although no effects on the infant are anticipated).
- MONITORING REQUIREMENTS Manufacturer advises monitor for electrolyte disturbances, particularly plasma-potassium (as clinically indicated) and plasma-magnesium (continue to monitor for at least 1 month after initiation of treatment).
- DIRECTIONS FOR ADMINISTRATION Manufacturer advises *Veltassa* ® should be mixed with approx. 40 mL of water, then stirred and mixed with a further approx. 40 mL of water; the powder will not dissolve. More water may be added as needed. The mixture should be taken within 1 hour of preparation. Apple juice or cranberry juice may be used instead of water, other liquids should be avoided as they may contain high amounts of potassium.
- HANDLING AND STORAGE Store in a refrigerator (2–8°C) prior to dispensing; once dispensed, patient may store below 25°C for up to 6 months.
- NATIONAL FUNDING/ACCESS DECISIONS
For full details see funding body website
NICE decisions
‣ Patiromer for treating hyperkalaemia (February 2020) NICE TA623 Recommended with restrictions

▶ Patiromer (*Veltassa*®) for the treatment of hyperkalaemia in adults (November 2020) SMC No. SMC2264 Not recommended

● MEDICINAL FORMS There can be variation in the licensing of different medicines containing the same drug.
Powder
CAUTIONARY AND ADVISORY LABELS 13, 21
▶ Veltassa (Vifor Fresenius Medical Care Renal Pharma UK Ltd) ▼
Patiromer calcium (as Patiromer sorbitex calcium)
8.4 gram Veltassa 8.4g oral powder sachets | 30 sachet [PoM]
£172.50 DT = £172.50
Patiromer calcium (as Patiromer sorbitex calcium)
16.8 gram Veltassa 16.8g oral powder sachets | 30 sachet [PoM]
£172.50 DT = £172.50

Sodium polystyrene sulfonate 06-Aug-2020

● INDICATIONS AND DOSE
Hyperkalaemia associated with anuria or severe oliguria, and in dialysis patients
▶ BY MOUTH
▶ Adult: 15 g 3–4 times a day
▶ BY RECTUM
▶ Adult: 30 g, retain for 9 hours followed by irrigation to remove resin from colon

● CONTRA-INDICATIONS Obstructive bowel disease
● CAUTIONS Congestive heart failure · hypertension · oedema
● INTERACTIONS → Appendix 1: polystyrene sulfonate
● SIDE-EFFECTS Appetite decreased · bezoar · constipation (discontinue—avoid magnesium-containing laxatives) · diarrhoea · electrolyte imbalance · epigastric discomfort · gastrointestinal disorders · increased risk of infection · nausea · necrosis (in combination with sorbitol) · vomiting
● PREGNANCY Manufacturers advise use only if potential benefit outweighs risk—no information available.
● BREAST FEEDING Manufacturers advise use only if potential benefit outweighs risk—no information available.
● RENAL IMPAIRMENT Use with caution.
● MONITORING REQUIREMENTS Monitor for electrolyte disturbances (stop if plasma-potassium concentration below 5 mmol/litre).
● DIRECTIONS FOR ADMINISTRATION
▶ With rectal use Manufacturer advises mix each 30 g of resin with 150 mL of water or 10% glucose.
▶ With oral use Manufacturer advises administer dose (powder) in a small amount of water or honey—do not give with fruit juice or squash, which have a high potassium content.

● MEDICINAL FORMS There can be variation in the licensing of different medicines containing the same drug. Forms available from special-order manufacturers include: oral suspension
Powder
CAUTIONARY AND ADVISORY LABELS 13
▶ Resonium A (Sanofi)
Sodium polystyrene sulfonate 999.34 mg per 1 gram Resonium A powder sugar-free | 454 gram [P] £81.11 DT = £81.11

Sodium zirconium cyclosilicate 16-Nov-2020

● DRUG ACTION Sodium zirconium cyclosilicate is a non-absorbed cation-exchange compound that acts as a selective potassium binder in the gastro-intestinal tract.

● INDICATIONS AND DOSE
Hyperkalaemia
▶ BY MOUTH
▶ Adult: Initially 10 g 3 times a day, for up to 72 hours, followed by maintenance 5 g once daily, adjusted according to serum-potassium concentrations. The usual maintenance dose range is 5 g once every other day to 10 g once daily
PHARMACOKINETICS
▶ Onset of action about 1 hour.

● CAUTIONS Abdominal X-ray (sodium zirconium cyclosilicate may be opaque to X-rays)
● INTERACTIONS → Appendix 1: sodium zirconium cyclosilicate
● SIDE-EFFECTS
▶ **Common or very common** Fluid imbalance · oedema · peripheral swelling
▶ **Frequency not known** Constipation · nausea
● PREGNANCY Manufacturer advises avoid—limited information; *animal* studies do not indicate toxicity.
● MONITORING REQUIREMENTS Manufacturer advises monitor serum potassium as clinically indicated.
● DIRECTIONS FOR ADMINISTRATION Manufacturer advises mix the contents of each 5- or 10-g sachet of powder with approx. 45 mL of water and stir well. The powder will not dissolve and the suspension should be taken while it is cloudy; if the powder settles it should be stirred again.
● NATIONAL FUNDING/ACCESS DECISIONS
For full details see funding body website
NICE decisions
▶ Sodium zirconium cyclosilicate for treating hyperkalaemia (September 2019) NICE TA599 Recommended with restrictions
Scottish Medicines Consortium (SMC) decisions
▶ Sodium zirconium cyclosilicate (*Lokelma*®) for the treatment of hyperkalaemia (HK) in adult patients (September 2020) SMC No. SMC2288 Recommended with restrictions

● MEDICINAL FORMS There can be variation in the licensing of different medicines containing the same drug.
Powder
CAUTIONARY AND ADVISORY LABELS 13
▶ Lokelma (AstraZeneca UK Ltd) ▼
Sodium zirconium cyclosilicate 5 gram Lokelma 5g oral powder sachets | 30 sachet [PoM] £213.60
Sodium zirconium cyclosilicate 10 gram Lokelma 10g oral powder sachets | 3 sachet [PoM] £42.72 | 30 sachet [PoM] £427.20

1.5b Hypokalaemia

ELECTROLYTES AND MINERALS ❭ POTASSIUM

Potassium bicarbonate with potassium acid tartrate 03-Aug-2020

● INDICATIONS AND DOSE
Hyperchloraemic acidosis associated with potassium deficiency (as in some renal tubular and gastro-intestinal disorders)
▶ BY MOUTH
▶ Adult: (consult product literature)

9

Blood and nutrition

- CONTRA-INDICATIONS Hypochloraemia · plasma-potassium concentration above 5 mmol/litre
- CAUTIONS Cardiac disease · elderly
- SIDE-EFFECTS Diarrhoea · flatulence · gastrointestinal discomfort · nausea · vomiting
- RENAL IMPAIRMENT Avoid in severe impairment. **Monitoring** Close monitoring required in renal impairment—high risk of hyperkalaemia.
- DIRECTIONS FOR ADMINISTRATION Manufacturer advises tablets to be dissolved in water before administration.
- PRESCRIBING AND DISPENSING INFORMATION These tablets do not contain chloride.

- MEDICINAL FORMS There can be variation in the licensing of different medicines containing the same drug.
  Effervescent tablet
  CAUTIONARY AND ADVISORY LABELS 13, 21
  ▸ Potassium bicarbonate with potassium acid tartrate (Non-proprietary)
  Potassium acid tartrate 300 mg, Potassium bicarbonate 500 mg Potassium (potassium 6.5mmol) effervescent tablets BPC 1968 | 56 tablet [GSL] £91.91

Potassium chloride

20-Nov-2019

- **INDICATIONS AND DOSE**

  Prevention of hypokalaemia (patients with normal diet)
  ▸ BY MOUTH
  ▸ Adult: 2–4 g daily in divided doses

  Electrolyte imbalance
  ▸ BY INTRAVENOUS INFUSION
  ▸ Adult: Dose dependent on deficit or the daily maintenance requirements

> **IMPORTANT SAFETY INFORMATION**
>
> SAFE PRACTICE
> Potassium overdose can be fatal. Ready-mixed infusion solutions containing potassium should be used. Exceptionally, if potassium chloride concentrate is used for preparing an infusion, the infusion solution should be **thoroughly mixed**. Local policies on avoiding inadvertent use of potassium chloride concentrate should be followed.
>
> NHS NEVER EVENT: MIS-SELECTION OF A STRONG POTASSIUM SOLUTION (JANUARY 2018)
> Patients should not be inadvertently given a strong potassium solution ($\geq$10% potassium w/v) intravenously, rather than the intended medication.

- CONTRA-INDICATIONS Plasma-potassium concentration above 5 mmol/litre
- CAUTIONS
  ▸ With intravenous use seek specialist advice in very severe potassium depletion or difficult cases
  ▸ With oral use Cardiac disease · elderly · hiatus hernia (with modified-release preparations) · history of peptic ulcer (with modified-release preparations) · intestinal stricture (with modified-release preparations)
- INTERACTIONS → Appendix 1: potassium chloride
- SIDE-EFFECTS
  GENERAL SIDE-EFFECTS
  Hyperkalaemia
  SPECIFIC SIDE-EFFECTS
  ▸ With oral use Abdominal cramps · diarrhoea · gastrointestinal disorders · nausea · vomiting
- RENAL IMPAIRMENT Avoid in severe impairment.
  Dose adjustments Smaller doses must be used in the prevention of hypokalaemia, to reduce the risk of hyperkalaemia.

Monitoring Close monitoring required in renal impairment—high risk of hyperkalaemia.

- MONITORING REQUIREMENTS
  ▸ Regular monitoring of plasma-potassium concentration is essential in those taking potassium supplements.
  ▸ With intravenous use ECG monitoring should be performed in difficult cases.
- DIRECTIONS FOR ADMINISTRATION
  ▸ With oral use Potassium salts are preferably given as a liquid (or effervescent) preparation, rather than modified-release tablets; they should be given as the chloride (the use of effervescent potassium tablets BPC 1968 should be restricted to *hyperchloraemic* states).
  ▸ With intravenous use Potassium chloride concentrate must be diluted with **not less** than 50 times its volume of sodium chloride intravenous infusion 0.9% or other suitable diluent and **mixed well**. Ready-mixed infusion solutions should be used where possible; alternatively, potassium chloride concentrate as ampoules containing 1.5 g (K^+ 20 mmol) in 10 mL, is **thoroughly mixed** with 500 mL of sodium chloride 0.9% intravenous infusion and given slowly over 2 to 3 hours with specialist advice and ECG monitoring in difficult cases. For *peripheral intravenous infusion*, the concentration of potassium should not usually exceed 40 mmol/L. Higher concentrations of potassium chloride may be given in very severe depletion, but require specialist advice.
- PRESCRIBING AND DISPENSING INFORMATION Kay-Cee-L ® contains 1 mmol/mL each of K^+ and Cl^-.
  Potassium Tablets
  ▸ With oral use Do not confuse Effervescent Potassium Tablets BPC 1968 with effervescent potassium chloride tablets. Effervescent Potassium Tablets BPC 1968 do not contain chloride ions and their use should be restricted to hyperchloraemic states.
- PATIENT AND CARER ADVICE Patient or carers should be given advice on how to administer potassium chloride modified-release tablets.
  Salt substitutes A number of salt substitutes which contain significant amounts of potassium chloride are readily available as health food products (e.g. *LoSalt* ® and *Ruthmol* ®). These should not be used by patients with renal failure as potassium intoxication may result.
- LESS SUITABLE FOR PRESCRIBING Modified-release tablets are less suitable for prescribing. Modified-release preparations should be avoided unless effervescent tablets or liquid preparations inappropriate.

- MEDICINAL FORMS There can be variation in the licensing of different medicines containing the same drug. Forms available from special-order manufacturers include: modified-release tablet, oral solution, solution for injection, infusion, solution for infusion
  Modified-release tablet
  CAUTIONARY AND ADVISORY LABELS 25, 27
  ▸ Potassium chloride (Imported)
  Potassium chloride 600 mg Kaleorid LP 600mg tablets | 30 tablet [PoM] Ⓢ
  Duro-K 600mg tablets | 100 tablet [PoM] Ⓢ
  Solution for infusion
  ▸ Potassium chloride (Non-proprietary)
  Potassium chloride 150 mg per 1 ml Potassium chloride 15% (potassium 20mmol/10ml) solution for infusion 10ml ampoules | 10 ampoule [PoM] £7.00–£10.00 | 20 ampoule [PoM] £6.50–£11.24
  Potassium chloride 200 mg per 1 ml Potassium chloride 20% (potassium 13.3mmol/5ml) solution for infusion 5ml ampoules | 10 ampoule [PoM] £8.00
  Oral solution
  CAUTIONARY AND ADVISORY LABELS 21
  ▸ Kay-Cee-L (Geistlich Sons Ltd)
  Potassium chloride 75 mg per 1 ml Kay-Cee-L syrup sugar-free | 500 ml [P] £8.77 DT = £8.77

Infusion

▸ Potassium chloride (Non-proprietary)

Potassium chloride 30 mg per 1 ml Potassium chloride 3% (potassium 40mmol/100ml) infusion 100ml bags | 1 bag [PoM] [Ⓢ]
Potassium chloride 3% (potassium 20mmol/50ml) infusion 50ml bags | 1 bag [PoM] [Ⓢ]

2 Metabolic disorders
2.1 Acute porphyrias

Acute porphyrias
11-Sep-2020

Overview

The acute porphyrias (acute intermittent porphyria, variegate porphyria, hereditary coproporphyria, and 5-aminolaevulinic acid dehydratase deficiency porphyria) are hereditary disorders of haem biosynthesis; they have a prevalence of about 1 in 75 000 of the population.

Great care must be taken when prescribing for patients with acute porphyria, since certain drugs can induce acute porphyric crises. Since acute porphyrias are hereditary, relatives of affected individuals should be screened and advised about the potential danger of certain drugs.

EvGr Where there is no safe alternative, drug treatment for serious or life-threatening conditions should not be withheld from patients with acute porphyria. Where possible, the clinical situation should be discussed with a porphyria specialist for advice on how to proceed and monitor the patient. In the UK clinical advice can be obtained from the National Acute Porphyria Service or from the UK Porphyria Medicines Information Service (UKPMIS) (see *Useful resources*). Ⓔ

Haem arginate p. 1108 is administered by short intravenous infusion as haem replacement in moderate, severe, or unremitting acute porphyria crises.

In the United Kingdom the National Acute Porphyria Service (NAPS) provides clinical support and treatment with haem arginate from two centres (Cardiff and Vale University Health Board and King's College Hospital) (see *Useful resources*).

Drugs unsafe for use in acute porphyrias

EvGr The following list contains drugs that have been classified as 'unsafe' in porphyria because they have been shown to be porphyrinogenic in animals or in vitro, or have been associated with acute attacks in patients. Absence of a drug from the following lists does not necessarily imply that the drug is safe. For many drugs no information about porphyria is available. Ⓔ

An up-to-date list of drugs considered safe in acute porphyrias is available from the UKPMIS (see *Useful resources*).

Further information may be obtained from the European Porphyria Network (available at: porphyria.eu/) and UKPMIS (see *Useful resources*).

Quite modest changes in chemical structure can lead to changes in porphyrinogenicity but where possible general statements have been made about groups of drugs; these should be checked first.

Unsafe Drug Groups (check first)

- Anabolic steroids
- Antidepressants, MAOIs (contact UKPMIS for advice)
- Antidepressants, Tricyclic and related (contact UKPMIS for advice)
- Barbiturates (includes primidone and thiopental)
- Contraceptives, hormonal (for detailed advice contact UKPMIS or a porphyria specialist)

- Hormone replacement therapy (for detailed advice contact UKPMIS or a porphyria specialist)
- Imidazole antifungals (applies to oral and intravenous use; topical antifungals are thought to be safe due to low systemic exposure)
- Non-nucleoside reverse transcriptase inhibitors (contact UKPMIS for advice)
- Progestogens (for detailed advice contact UKPMIS or a porphyria specialist)
- Protease inhibitors (contact UKPMIS for advice)
- Sulfonamides (includes co-trimoxazole and sulfasalazine)
- Sulfonylureas (glipizide and glimepiride are thought to be safe)
- Taxanes (contact UKPMIS for advice)
- Triazole antifungals (applies to oral and intravenous use; topical antifungals are thought to be safe due to low systemic exposure)

Unsafe Drugs (check groups above first)

- Aceclofenac
- Alcohol
- Amiodarone
- Aprepitant
- Artemether with lumefantrine
- Bexarotene
- Bosentan
- Busulfan
- Carbamazepine
- Chloral hydrate (although evidence of hazard is uncertain, manufacturer advises avoid)
- Chloramphenicol
- Chloroform (small amounts in medicines probably safe)
- Clemastine
- Clindamycin
- Cocaine
- Danazol
- Dapsone
- Diltiazem
- Disopyramide
- Disulfiram
- Ergometrine
- Ergotamine
- Erythromycin
- Etamsylate
- Ethosuximide
- Etomidate
- Flutamide
- Fosaprepitant
- Fosphenytoin
- Griseofulvin
- Hydralazine
- Ifosfamide
- Indapamide
- Isometheptene mucate
- Isoniazid (safety uncertain, contact UKPMIS for advice)
- Ketamine
- Mefenamic acid (safety uncertain, contact UKPMIS for advice)
- Meprobamate
- Methyldopa
- Metolazone
- Metyrapone
- Mifepristone
- Minoxidil (safety uncertain, contact UKPMIS for advice)
- Mitotane
- Nalidixic acid
- Nitrazepam
- Nitrofurantoin
- Orphenadrine
- Oxcarbazepine
- Oxybutynin
- Pentazocine

- Pentoxifylline
- Pergolide
- Phenoxybenzamine
- Phenytoin
- Pivmecillinam
- Pizotifen
- Porfimer
- Raloxifene
- Rifabutin (safety uncertain, contact UKPMIS for advice)
- Rifampicin
- Riluzole
- Risperidone
- Spironolactone
- Sulfinpyrazone
- Tamoxifen
- Temoporfin
- Thiotepa
- Tiagabine
- Tibolone
- Topiramate
- Toremifene
- Trimethoprim
- Valproate
- Verapamil
- Xipamide

Useful Resources

Cardiff and Vale University Health Board National Acute Porphyria Service.
tinyurl.com/y559nmeq
   King's College Hospital National Acute Porphyria Service.
www.kch.nhs.uk/service/a-z/porphyria
   UK Porphyria Medicines Information Service. Drugs in porphyrias.
www.wmic.wales.nhs.uk/specialist-services/drugs-in-porphyria

BLOOD AND RELATED PRODUCTS › HAEM DERIVATIVES

❙ Haem arginate

17-Jul-2020

(Human hemin)

- **INDICATIONS AND DOSE**

Acute porphyrias | Acute intermittent porphyria | Porphyria variegata | Hereditary coproporphyria
▸ BY INTRAVENOUS INFUSION
▸ Adult: Initially 3 mg/kg once daily for 4 days, if response inadequate, repeat 4-day course with close biochemical monitoring; maximum 250 mg per day

- SIDE-EFFECTS
▸ **Common or very common** Poor venous access
▸ **Rare or very rare** Fever
▸ **Frequency not known** Headache · injection site necrosis · skin discolouration · venous thrombosis
- PREGNANCY Manufacturer advises avoid unless essential.
- BREAST FEEDING Manufacturer advises avoid unless essential—no information available.
- DIRECTIONS FOR ADMINISTRATION For *intravenous infusion* (*Normosang®*), manufacturer advises give intermittently in Sodium chloride 0.9%; dilute requisite dose in 100 mL infusion fluid in glass bottle and give over at least 30 minutes through a filter *via* large antebrachial or central vein; administer within 1 hour after dilution.

- MEDICINAL FORMS There can be variation in the licensing of different medicines containing the same drug.
  Solution for infusion
▸ Normosang (Recordati Rare Diseases UK Ltd)
   Haem arginate 25 mg per 1 ml Normosang 250mg/10ml solution for infusion ampoules | 4 ampoule [PoM] £1,737.00

2.2 Amyloidosis

NEUROPROTECTIVE DRUGS

❙ Inotersen

27-Aug-2020

- DRUG ACTION Inotersen is an antisense oligonucleotide inhibitor which inhibits transthyretin production.

- **INDICATIONS AND DOSE**

Stage 1 or stage 2 polyneuropathy in patients with hereditary transthyretin amyloidosis (hATTR) (initiated by a specialist)
▸ BY SUBCUTANEOUS INJECTION
▸ Adult: 284 mg once weekly, for dose adjustments due to side-effects and information on Vitamin A supplementation—consult product literature

- CONTRA-INDICATIONS Patients undergoing liver transplantation (no information available) · platelet count less than 100×10^9/litre before starting treatment · urine protein to creatinine ratio (UPCR) greater than or equal to 113 mg/mmol before starting treatment
- CAUTIONS Concomitant administration with nephrotoxic drugs · elderly · history of major bleeding
- INTERACTIONS → Appendix 1: inotersen
- SIDE-EFFECTS
▸ **Common or very common** Anaemia · appetite decreased · chills · eosinophilia · fever · glomerulonephritis · haematoma · headache · hypotension · influenza like illness · nausea · peripheral oedema · peripheral swelling · proteinuria · renal impairment · skin reactions · thrombocytopenia · vomiting
▸ **Frequency not known** Intracranial haemorrhage · vitamin A deficiency
- CONCEPTION AND CONTRACEPTION Manufacturer advises women of childbearing potential should use effective contraception during treatment; if conception is planned, inotersen and vitamin A supplementation should be stopped and vitamin A levels monitored—consult product literature.
- PREGNANCY Manufacturer advises avoid unless essential (limited information available)—potential teratogenic risk due to unbalanced vitamin A levels, consult product literature.
- BREAST FEEDING Manufacturer advises avoid—present in milk in *animal* studies.
- HEPATIC IMPAIRMENT Manufacturer advises avoid in severe impairment (no information available).
- RENAL IMPAIRMENT Manufacturer advises avoid if eGFR less than 45 mL/minute/1.73 m^2.
- PRE-TREATMENT SCREENING Manufacturer advises plasma vitamin A levels below the lower limit of normal should be corrected and any ocular symptoms or signs of vitamin A deficiency should have resolved before starting treatment.
- MONITORING REQUIREMENTS
▸ Manufacturer advises monitor platelet count before starting treatment, every 2 weeks during treatment, and for 8 weeks after stopping treatment—consult product literature.
▸ Manufacturer advises monitor UPCR and eGFR before starting treatment, every 3 months or more frequently as clinically indicated during treatment, and for 8 weeks after stopping treatment—consult product literature.
▸ Manufacturer advises monitor hepatic enzymes before starting treatment, then 4 months after starting treatment, and annually thereafter or more frequently as clinically indicated.

- **DIRECTIONS FOR ADMINISTRATION** Manufacturer advises to take the syringe out of the refrigerator at least 30 minutes before administration. Patients may self-administer *Tegsedi*® after appropriate training in subcutaneous injection technique.
- **HANDLING AND STORAGE** Manufacturer advises store in a refrigerator (2–8°C) and protect from light—consult product literature for further information regarding storage outside refrigerator.
- **PATIENT AND CARER ADVICE** Manufacturer advises patients should immediately report any signs of unusual or prolonged bleeding, neck stiffness, or atypical severe headache.
  Self-administration Manufacturer advises patients and carers should be given training in subcutaneous injection technique.
  Missed doses If a dose is missed, the next dose should be administered as soon as possible, unless the next scheduled dose is within 2 days, in which case the missed dose should not be taken and the next dose should be taken at the normal time.
- **NATIONAL FUNDING/ACCESS DECISIONS**
  For full details see funding body website
  NICE decisions
  ▸ Inotersen for treating hereditary transthyretin amyloidosis (May 2019) NICE HST9 Recommended
  Scottish Medicines Consortium (SMC) decisions
  ▸ Inotersen (*Tegsedi*®) for the treatment of stage 1 or stage 2 polyneuropathy in adult patients with hereditary transthyretin amyloidosis (hATTR) (August 2019) SMC No. SMC2188 Recommended

- **MEDICINAL FORMS** There can be variation in the licensing of different medicines containing the same drug.
  Solution for injection
  ▸ Tegsedi (Akcea Therapeutics UK Ltd) ▼
  Inotersen (as Inotersen sodium) 189.33 mg per 1 ml Tegsedi 284mg/1.5ml solution for injection pre-filled syringes | 4 pre-filled disposable injection [PoM] £23,700.00

Patisiran   31-Aug-2020

- **DRUG ACTION** Patisiran is a double-stranded small interfering RNA which reduces transthyretin production.

- **INDICATIONS AND DOSE**
  Stage 1 or stage 2 polyneuropathy in patients with hereditary transthyretin amyloidosis (hATTR) (initiated under specialist supervision)
  ▸ **BY INTRAVENOUS INFUSION**
  ▸ **Adult:** 300 micrograms/kg every 3 weeks (max. per dose 30 mg), dosage is based on actual body weight, for information on premedication, vitamin A supplementation, and missed doses—consult product literature

- **SIDE-EFFECTS**
  ▸ **Common or very common** Arthralgia · dyspepsia · dyspnoea · erythema · increased risk of infection · infusion related reaction · muscle spasms · peripheral oedema · vertigo
  ▸ **Frequency not known** Vitamin A deficiency
- **CONCEPTION AND CONTRACEPTION** Manufacturer advises women of childbearing potential should use effective contraception during treatment; if conception is planned, patisiran and vitamin A supplementation should be stopped and vitamin A levels monitored—consult product literature.
- **PREGNANCY** Manufacturer advises avoid unless essential (limited information available)—potential teratogenic risk due to unbalanced vitamin A levels, consult product literature.

- **BREAST FEEDING** Manufacturer advises avoid—present in milk in *animal* studies.
- **HEPATIC IMPAIRMENT** Manufacturer advises caution in moderate or severe impairment (no information available).
- **RENAL IMPAIRMENT** Manufacturer advises caution in severe impairment (no information available).
- **PRE-TREATMENT SCREENING** Manufacturer advises plasma vitamin A levels below the lower limit of normal should be corrected and any ocular symptoms or signs of vitamin A deficiency should be evaluated before starting treatment.
- **DIRECTIONS FOR ADMINISTRATION** Manufacturer advises for *intravenous infusion* (*Onpattro*®), filter through 0.45-micron syringe filter and dilute requisite dose with Sodium Chloride 0.9% to final volume of 200 mL; use a DEHP-free infusion set and give over about 80 minutes through an in-line filter (1.2 micron) at a rate of about 1 mL/minute for the first 15 minutes, then increase to about 3 mL/minute for the remainder of the infusion.
- **PRESCRIBING AND DISPENSING INFORMATION** Manufacturer advises patients should receive pre-medication (to reduce the risk of infusion-related reactions)—consult product literature.
- **HANDLING AND STORAGE** Manufacturer advises store in a refrigerator (2–8°C)—consult product literature for further information regarding storage outside refrigerator.
- **NATIONAL FUNDING/ACCESS DECISIONS**
  For full details see funding body website
  NICE decisions
  ▸ Patisiran for treating hereditary transthyretin amyloidosis (August 2019) NICE HST10 Recommended
  Scottish Medicines Consortium (SMC) decisions
  ▸ Patisiran (*Onpattro*®) for the treatment of hereditary transthyretin-mediated amyloidosis (hATTR amyloidosis) in adult patients with stage 1 or stage 2 polyneuropathy (June 2019) SMC No. SMC2157 Recommended

- **MEDICINAL FORMS** There can be variation in the licensing of different medicines containing the same drug.
  Solution for infusion
  ELECTROLYTES: May contain Sodium
  ▸ Onpattro (Alnylam UK Ltd) ▼
  Patisiran (as Patisiran sodium) 2 mg per 1 ml Onpattro 10mg/5ml concentrate for solution for infusion vials | 1 vial [PoM] £7,676.47

Tafamidis   25-Aug-2020

- **DRUG ACTION** Tafamidis is a transthyretin stabiliser which inhibits amyloid formation, thereby delaying the development of nerve and cardiac muscle damage caused by transthyretin amyloidosis.

- **INDICATIONS AND DOSE**
  Treatment of transthyretin amyloidosis in patients with stage 1 symptomatic polyneuropathy (ATTR-PN) [using 20 mg capsules] (initiated under specialist supervision)
  ▸ **BY MOUTH**
  ▸ **Adult:** 20 mg once daily
  Treatment of wild-type transthyretin amyloidosis in patients with cardiomyopathy (ATTR-CM) [using 61 mg capsules] (initiated under specialist supervision) | Treatment of hereditary transthyretin amyloidosis in patients with cardiomyopathy (ATTR-CM) [using 61 mg capsules] (initiated under specialist supervision)
  ▸ **BY MOUTH**
  ▸ **Adult:** 61 mg once daily
  DOSE EQUIVALENCE AND CONVERSION
  ▸ Each 20 mg capsule contains tafamidis meglumine equivalent to 12.2 mg tafamidis.
  ▸ Each 61 mg capsule contains tafamidis equivalent to 80 mg tafamidis meglumine. continued →

▸ Tafamidis and tafamidis meglumine are not interchangeable on a milligram-for-milligram basis.

● SIDE-EFFECTS
▸ **Common or very common** Abdominal pain upper · diarrhoea · increased risk of infection
▸ **Frequency not known** Flatulence
● CONCEPTION AND CONTRACEPTION Exclude pregnancy before treatment and ensure effective contraception during and for one month after stopping treatment.
● PREGNANCY Avoid (toxicity in *animal* studies).
● BREAST FEEDING Avoid—present in milk in *animal* studies.
● HEPATIC IMPAIRMENT Manufacturer advises caution in severe impairment (no information available).
● PRESCRIBING AND DISPENSING INFORMATION Manufacturer advises tafamidis should be prescribed in addition to standard treatment, but before organ transplantation; it should be discontinued in patients who undergo organ transplantation.
  The manufacturer of *Vyndaqel*® has provided a *Guide for Healthcare Professionals*.
● PATIENT AND CARER ADVICE
Missed doses Manufacturer advises if vomiting occurs after a dose is taken and the intact capsule is identified, another dose can be taken if possible; otherwise the next dose should be taken at the normal time.

● MEDICINAL FORMS There can be variation in the licensing of different medicines containing the same drug.
Capsule
CAUTIONARY AND ADVISORY LABELS 25
EXCIPIENTS: May contain Sorbitol
▸ Vyndaqel (Pfizer Ltd) ▼
Tafamidis meglumine 20 mg Vyndaqel 20mg capsules | 30 capsule [PoM] £10,685.00 (Hospital only)
Tafamidis 61 mg Vyndaqel 61mg capsules | 30 capsule [PoM] £10,685.00 (Hospital only)

2.3 Carnitine deficiency

AMINO ACIDS AND DERIVATIVES

Levocarnitine
(Carnitine)

16-Jul-2020

● INDICATIONS AND DOSE
Primary carnitine deficiency due to inborn errors of metabolism
▸ BY MOUTH
▸ **Adult:** Up to 200 mg/kg daily in 2–4 divided doses; maximum 3 g per day
▸ BY SLOW INTRAVENOUS INJECTION
▸ **Adult:** Up to 100 mg/kg daily in 2–4 divided doses, to be administered over 2–3 minutes
Secondary carnitine deficiency in haemodialysis patients
▸ INITIALLY BY SLOW INTRAVENOUS INJECTION
▸ **Adult:** 20 mg/kg, to be administered over 2–3 minutes, after each dialysis session, dosage adjusted according to plasma-carnitine concentration, then (by mouth) maintenance 1 g daily, administered if benefit is gained from first intravenous course

● CAUTIONS Diabetes mellitus
● SIDE-EFFECTS
▸ **Rare or very rare** Abdominal cramps · diarrhoea · nausea · skin odour abnormal · vomiting
SIDE-EFFECTS, FURTHER INFORMATION Side-effects may be dose-related—monitor tolerance during first week and after any dose increase.

● PREGNANCY Appropriate to use; no evidence of teratogenicity in *animal* studies.
● RENAL IMPAIRMENT Accumulation of metabolites may occur with chronic oral administration in severe impairment.
● MONITORING REQUIREMENTS
▸ Monitoring of free and acyl carnitine in blood and urine recommended.

● MEDICINAL FORMS There can be variation in the licensing of different medicines containing the same drug. Forms available from special-order manufacturers include: capsule
Solution for injection
▸ Carnitor (Logixx Pharma Solutions Ltd)
L-Carnitine 200 mg per 1 ml Carnitor 1g/5ml solution for injection ampoules | 5 ampoule [PoM] £59.50 DT = £59.50
Oral solution
▸ Levocarnitine (Non-proprietary)
L-Carnitine 300 mg per 1 ml Levocarnitine 1.5g/5ml (30%) oral solution paediatric | 20 ml [PoM] £71.40 DT = £71.40 | 40 ml [PoM] £118.00
▸ Carnitor (Logixx Pharma Solutions Ltd)
L-Carnitine 100 mg per 1 ml Carnitor oral single dose 1g solution sugar-free | 10 unit dose [PoM] £35.00 DT = £35.00
Chewable tablet
▸ Carnitor (Logixx Pharma Solutions Ltd)
L-Carnitine 1 gram Carnitor 1g chewable tablets | 10 tablet [PoM] £35.00 DT = £35.00
Capsule
▸ Bio-Carnitine (Pharma Nord (UK) Ltd)
L-Carnitine 250 mg Bio-Carnitine 250mg capsules | 125 capsule £11.06

2.4 Cystinosis

2.4a Nephropathic cystinosis

AMINO ACIDS AND DERIVATIVES

Mercaptamine
(Cysteamine)

17-Nov-2020

● INDICATIONS AND DOSE
Corneal cystine crystal deposits in patients with cystinosis (specialist use only)
▸ TO THE EYE
▸ **Adult:** Apply 1 drop 4 times a day, to be applied to both eyes (minimum 4 hours between doses); dose may be reduced according to response (minimum daily dose 1 drop in each eye)
CYSTAGON ®
Nephropathic cystinosis (specialist use only)
▸ BY MOUTH
▸ **Adult (body-weight 50 kg and above):** Initially one-sixth to one-quarter of the expected maintenance dose, increased gradually over 4–6 weeks to avoid intolerance, dose increased if there is adequate tolerance and the leucocyte-cystine concentration remains above 1 nanomol hemicystine/mg protein, maintenance 500 mg 4 times a day; maximum 1.95 g/m^2 per day
PROCYSBI ®
Nephropathic cystinosis (specialist use only)
▸ BY MOUTH
▸ **Adult:** Initially one-sixth to one-quarter of the expected maintenance dose, increased if there is adequate tolerance and the leucocyte-cystine concentration remains above 1 nanomol hemicystine/mg protein (measured using the mixed leucocyte assay), maintenance 650 mg/m^2 twice daily,

administered every 12 hours; maximum 1.95 g/m^2 per day

> **IMPORTANT SAFETY INFORMATION**
>
> SAFE PRACTICE
>
> Mercaptamine has been confused with mercaptopurine; care must be taken to ensure the correct drug is prescribed and dispensed.

- CAUTIONS
- ▸ When used by eye Contact lens wearers
- ▸ With oral use Dose of phosphate supplement may need to be adjusted if transferring from phosphocysteamine to mercaptamine
- SIDE-EFFECTS
- ▸ **Common or very common**
- ▸ When used by eye Dry eye · eye discomfort · eye disorders · vision blurred
- ▸ With oral use Appetite decreased · asthenia · breath odour · diarrhoea · drowsiness · encephalopathy · fever · gastroenteritis · gastrointestinal discomfort · headache · nausea · skin reactions · vomiting
- ▸ **Uncommon**
- ▸ With oral use Compression fracture · gastrointestinal ulcer · hair colour changes · hallucination · joint hyperextension · leg pain · leucopenia · musculoskeletal disorders · nephrotic syndrome · nervousness · osteopenia · seizure
- ▸ **Frequency not known**
- ▸ With oral use Depression · intracranial pressure increased · papilloedema
- ALLERGY AND CROSS-SENSITIVITY EvGr Contra-indicated if history of hypersensitivity to penicillamine. ⓜ
- PREGNANCY
- ▸ With oral use Manufacturer advises avoid—teratogenic and toxic in *animal* studies.
- BREAST FEEDING
- ▸ With oral use Manufacturer advises avoid—no information available.
- MONITORING REQUIREMENTS
- ▸ With oral use Manufacturer advises leucocyte-cystine concentration, liver function, and haematological monitoring required—consult product literature. Manufacturer advises monitor for skin and bone abnormalities; dose reduction or treatment discontinuation may be required—consult product literature.
- DIRECTIONS FOR ADMINISTRATION

  PROCYSBI ® Manufacturer advises capsules can be opened and contents sprinkled on food, water, acidic fruit juice or administered via an enteral feeding tube—consult product literature. Avoid dairy products and meals (rich in fats and protein) at least 1 hour before and after taking a dose.
- PRESCRIBING AND DISPENSING INFORMATION

  Mercaptamine has a very unpleasant taste and smell, which can affect compliance.
- HANDLING AND STORAGE
- ▸ When used by eye Manufacturer advises store in a refrigerator (2–8°C)—after opening store at room temperature up to 25°C for up to 7 days; protect from light.

  PROCYSBI ® Manufacturer advises store in a refrigerator (2–8°C).
- PATIENT AND CARER ADVICE

  Driving and skilled tasks ▸ With oral use Manufacturer advises patients and carers should be counselled on the effects on driving and performance of skilled tasks—increased risk of drowsiness.

  ▸ When used by eye Manufacturer advises patients and carers should be counselled on the effects on driving and

performance of skilled tasks—increased risk of blurred vision and visual disturbances.

PROCYSBI ® **Missed doses** Manufacturer advises if a dose is within 4 hours of the next dose, the missed dose should not be taken and the next dose should be taken at the normal time.

- NATIONAL FUNDING/ACCESS DECISIONS

  For full details see funding body website

  Scottish Medicines Consortium (SMC) decisions
- ▸ Mercaptamine (*Procysbi* ®) for the treatment of proven nephropathic cystinosis (November 2017) SMC No. 1272/17 Not recommended

- MEDICINAL FORMS There can be variation in the licensing of different medicines containing the same drug. Forms available from special-order manufacturers include: eye drops

Gastro-resistant capsule

CAUTIONARY AND ADVISORY LABELS 25

- ▸ Procysbi (Chiesi Ltd)

  Mercaptamine (as Mercaptamine bitartrate) 25 mg Procysbi 25mg gastro-resistant capsules | 60 capsule PoM £335.97 DT = £335.97

  Mercaptamine (as Mercaptamine bitartrate) 75 mg Procysbi 75mg gastro-resistant capsules | 250 capsule PoM £4,199.65

Eye drops

EXCIPIENTS: May contain Benzalkonium chloride, disodium edetate

- ▸ Cystaran (Imported (United States))

  Mercaptamine (as Mercaptamine hydrochloride) 4.4 mg per 1 ml Cystaran 0.44% eye drops | 15 ml PoM ⚠

- ▸ Cystadrops (Recordati Rare Diseases UK Ltd)

  Mercaptamine (as Mercaptamine hydrochloride) 3.8 mg per 1 ml Cystadrops 3.8mg/ml eye drops | 5 ml PoM £865.00 DT = £865.00

Capsule

CAUTIONARY AND ADVISORY LABELS 21

- ▸ Cystagon (Recordati Rare Diseases UK Ltd)

  Mercaptamine (as Mercaptamine bitartrate) 50 mg Cystagon 50mg capsules | 100 capsule PoM £70.00 DT = £70.00

  Mercaptamine (as Mercaptamine bitartrate) 150 mg Cystagon 150mg capsules | 100 capsule PoM £190.00 DT = £190.00

2.5 Fabry's disease

ENZYMES

Agalsidase alfa

27-Jul-2020

- DRUG ACTION Agalsidase alfa, an enzyme produced by recombinant DNA technology are licensed for long-term enzyme replacement therapy in Fabry's disease (a lysosomal storage disorder caused by deficiency of alpha-galactosidase A).

- **INDICATIONS AND DOSE**

  Fabry's disease (specialist use only)
  - ▸ BY INTRAVENOUS INFUSION
  - ▸ Adult: 200 micrograms/kg every 2 weeks

- INTERACTIONS → Appendix 1: agalsidase alfa
- SIDE-EFFECTS
- ▸ **Common or very common** Arrhythmias · asthenia · chest discomfort · chills · cough · diarrhoea · dizziness · dyspnoea · excessive tearing · fever · flushing · gastrointestinal discomfort · headache · hoarseness · hypersomnia · hypertension · increased risk of infection · influenza like illness · joint disorders · malaise · musculoskeletal discomfort · myalgia · nausea · ototoxicity · pain · palpitations · peripheral oedema · peripheral swelling · rhinorrhoea · sensation abnormal · skin reactions · taste altered · temperature sensation altered · throat complaints · tremor · vomiting
- ▸ **Uncommon** Altered smell sensation · angioedema · hypersensitivity · sensation of pressure

▶ **Frequency not known** Heart failure · hyperhidrosis · hypotension · myocardial ischaemia

SIDE-EFFECTS, FURTHER INFORMATION Infusion-related reactions; manage by interrupting the infusion, or minimise by pre-treatment with an antihistamine or corticosteroid — consult product literature.

● PREGNANCY Use with caution.

● BREAST FEEDING Use with caution—no information available.

● DIRECTIONS FOR ADMINISTRATION Administration for *intravenous infusion*, manufacturer advises give intermittently *in* sodium chloride 0.9%; dilute requisite dose with 100 mL infusion fluid and give over 40 minutes using an in-line filter.

● MEDICINAL FORMS There can be variation in the licensing of different medicines containing the same drug.
Solution for infusion
▶ Replagal (Shire Pharmaceuticals Ltd)
Agalsidase alfa 1 mg per 1 ml Replagal 3.5mg/3.5ml solution for infusion vials | 1 vial PoM £1,049.94

Agalsidase beta

27-Jul-2020

● DRUG ACTION Agalsidase beta, an enzyme produced by recombinant DNA technology are licensed for long-term enzyme replacement therapy in Fabry's disease (a lysosomal storage disorder caused by deficiency of alpha-galactosidase A).

● **INDICATIONS AND DOSE**
Fabry's disease (specialist use only)
▶ BY INTRAVENOUS INFUSION
▶ Adult: 1 mg/kg every 2 weeks

● INTERACTIONS → Appendix 1: agalsidase beta

● SIDE-EFFECTS
▶ **Common or very common** Angioedema · arrhythmias · arthralgia · asthenia · chest discomfort · chills · cough · diarrhoea · dizziness · drowsiness · dyspnoea · eye disorders · fever · gastrointestinal discomfort · headache · hypertension · hyperthermia · hypotension · increased risk of infection · muscle complaints · musculoskeletal stiffness · nasal complaints · nausea · oedema · oral hypoaesthesia · pain · pallor · palpitations · respiratory disorders · sensation abnormal · skin reactions · syncope · temperature sensation altered · throat complaints · tinnitus · vasodilation · vertigo · vomiting
▶ **Uncommon** Dysphagia · ear discomfort · eye pruritus · influenza like illness · malaise · peripheral coldness · tremor
▶ **Frequency not known** Anaphylactoid reaction · hypersensitivity vasculitis · hypoxia

SIDE-EFFECTS, FURTHER INFORMATION Infusion-related reactions; manage by slowing the infusion rate, or minimise by pre-treatment with an antihistamine, antipyretic, or corticosteroid — consult product literature.

● PREGNANCY Use with caution.

● BREAST FEEDING Use with caution—no information available.

● DIRECTIONS FOR ADMINISTRATION For *intravenous infusion*, manufacturer advises give intermittently *in* Sodium chloride 0.9%, reconstitute initially with Water for Injections (5 mg in 1.1 mL, 35 mg in 7.2 mL) to produce a solution containing 5 mg/mL. Dilute with Sodium Chloride 0.9% (for doses less than 35 mg dilute with at least 50 mL; doses 35–70 mg dilute with at least 100 mL; doses 70–100 mg dilute with at least 250 mL; doses greater than 100 mg dilute with 500 mL) and give through an in-line low protein-binding 0.2 micron filter at an initial rate of no more than 15 mg/hour; for subsequent infusions, infusion

rate may be increased gradually once tolerance has been established.

● MEDICINAL FORMS There can be variation in the licensing of different medicines containing the same drug.
Powder for solution for infusion
▶ Fabrazyme (Genzyme Therapeutics Ltd)
Agalsidase beta 5 mg Fabrazyme 5mg powder for solution for infusion vials | 1 vial PoM £315.08
Agalsidase beta 35 mg Fabrazyme 35mg powder for solution for infusion vials | 1 vial PoM £2,196.59

ENZYME STABILISER

Migalastat

09-Sep-2020

● DRUG ACTION Migalastat is a pharmacological chaperone that binds to the active sites of certain mutant forms of alpha-galactosidase A, thereby stabilising these mutant forms in the endoplasmic reticulum, and facilitating normal trafficking to lysosomes.

● **INDICATIONS AND DOSE**
Fabry's disease (specialist use only)
▶ BY MOUTH
▶ Adult: 123 mg once daily on alternate days, take at the same time of day, food should not be consumed at least 2 hours before and after taking migalastat to give a minimum 4 hours fast

● SIDE-EFFECTS
▶ **Common or very common** Constipation · defaecation urgency · depression · diarrhoea · dizziness · dry mouth · dyspnoea · epistaxis · fatigue · gastrointestinal discomfort · headache · muscle complaints · nausea · pain · palpitations · proteinuria · sensation abnormal · skin reactions · torticollis · vertigo · weight increased

● PREGNANCY Manufacturer advises avoid—toxicity in *animal* studies.

● BREAST FEEDING Manufacturer advises avoid—present in milk in *animal* studies.

● RENAL IMPAIRMENT Manufacturer advises avoid if eGFR less than 30 mL/minute/1.73 m^2.

● MONITORING REQUIREMENTS Manufacturer advises monitor renal function, echocardiographic parameters and biochemical markers every 6 months.

● PATIENT AND CARER ADVICE
Missed doses Manufacturer advises if a dose is more than 12 hours late or missed entirely for the day, the missed dose should not be taken and the next dose should be taken on the normal day and at the normal time (not to be taken on 2 consecutive days).

● NATIONAL FUNDING/ACCESS DECISIONS
For full details see funding body website
NICE decisions
▶ Migalastat for treating Fabry disease (February 2017)
NICE HST4 Recommended with restrictions
Scottish Medicines Consortium (SMC) decisions
▶ Migalastat (*Galafold*®) for long-term treatment of adults and adolescents aged 16 years and older with a confirmed diagnosis of Fabry disease (α-galactosidase A deficiency) and who have an amenable mutation (November 2016)
SMC No. 1196/16 Recommended with restrictions

● MEDICINAL FORMS There can be variation in the licensing of different medicines containing the same drug.
Capsule
CAUTIONARY AND ADVISORY LABELS 25
▶ Galafold (Amicus Therapeutics UK Ltd) ▼
Migalastat (as Migalastat hydrochloride) 123 mg Galafold 123mg capsules | 14 capsule PoM £16,153.85

2.6 Gaucher's disease

Other drugs used for Gaucher's disease Miglustat, p. 1117

ENZYME INHIBITORS > GLUCOSYLCERAMIDE
SYNTHASE INHIBITORS

Eliglustat
26-Aug-2020

- **DRUG ACTION** Eliglustat is an inhibitor of
  glucosylceramide synthase.

  - **INDICATIONS AND DOSE**

    **Type 1 Gaucher disease (CYP2D6 poor metabolisers)
    (under expert supervision)**
    - BY MOUTH
    - Adult: 84 mg once daily
    **Type 1 Gaucher disease (CYP2D6 intermediate or
    extensive metabolisers) (under expert supervision)**
    - BY MOUTH
    - Adult: 84 mg twice daily

- **CONTRA-INDICATIONS** Cardiac disease (no information
  available) · concurrent use of Class IA and Class III
  antiarrhythmics · long QT syndrome (no information
  available)
- **INTERACTIONS** → Appendix 1: eliglustat
- **SIDE-EFFECTS**
  - **Common or very common** Arthralgia · constipation · dry
    mouth · dry skin · dyspepsia · dysphagia · fatigue ·
    gastrointestinal disorders · nausea · palpitations · taste
    altered · throat irritation
- **PREGNANCY** Manufacturer advises avoid—limited
  information available.
- **BREAST FEEDING** Manufacturer advises avoid—present in
  milk in *animal* studies.
- **PRE-TREATMENT SCREENING** Manufacturer advises
  CYP2D6 metaboliser status should be determined before
  initiation of treatment.
- **MONITORING REQUIREMENTS**
  - For treatment-naive patients showing less than 20%
    spleen volume reduction after 9 months of treatment,
    manufacturer advises monitor for further improvement or
    consider an alternative treatment.
  - For patients with stable disease who have switched from
    enzyme replacement therapy, manufacturer advises
    monitor for disease progression—consider reinstitution of
    enzyme replacement therapy or an alternative treatment if
    response sub-optimal.
- **PRESCRIBING AND DISPENSING INFORMATION** The
  manufacturer of *Cerdelga*® has provided a *Prescriber Guide*,
  which includes a prescriber checklist.
- **PATIENT AND CARER ADVICE** A patient alert card should be
  provided.
- **NATIONAL FUNDING/ACCESS DECISIONS**
  For full details see funding body website
  NICE decisions
  - Eliglustat for treating type 1 Gaucher disease (June 2017)
    NICE HST5 Recommended
  Scottish Medicines Consortium (SMC) decisions
  - Eliglustat (*Cerdelga*®) for the long-term treatment of adult
    patients with Gaucher disease type 1 (GD1) who are CYP2D6
    poor metabolisers, intermediate metabolisers or extensive
    metabolisers (December 2017) SMC No. 1277/17 Recommended

- **MEDICINAL FORMS** There can be variation in the licensing of
  different medicines containing the same drug.
  Capsule
  CAUTIONARY AND ADVISORY LABELS 10
  - Cerdelga (Sanofi) ▼
    Eliglustat (as Eliglustat tartrate) 84.4 mg Cerdelga 84mg capsules
    | 56 capsule [PoM] £19,164.96

ENZYMES

Imiglucerase
21-Jul-2020

- **DRUG ACTION** Imiglucerase is an enzyme produced by
  recombinant DNA technology that is administered as
  enzyme replacement therapy for non-neurological
  manifestations of type I or type III Gaucher's disease, a
  familial disorder affecting principally the liver, spleen,
  bone marrow, and lymph nodes.

  - **INDICATIONS AND DOSE**

    **Non-neurological manifestations of type I Gaucher's
    disease (specialist use only) | Non-neurological
    manifestations of type III Gaucher's disease (specialist
    use only)**
    - BY INTRAVENOUS INFUSION
    - Adult: Initially 60 units/kg every 2 weeks;
      maintenance, adjusted according to response, doses as
      low as 15 units/kg once every 2 weeks may improve
      haematological parameters and organomegaly

- **SIDE-EFFECTS**
  - **Common or very common** Angioedema · cough · dyspnoea ·
    hypersensitivity · skin reactions
  - **Uncommon** Abdominal cramps · arthralgia · back pain ·
    chest discomfort · chills · cyanosis · diarrhoea · dizziness ·
    fatigue · fever · flushing · headache · hypotension · nausea ·
    paraesthesia · tachycardia · vomiting
- **PREGNANCY** Manufacturer advises use with caution—
  limited information available.
- **BREAST FEEDING** No information available.
- **MONITORING REQUIREMENTS**
  - Monitor for immunoglobulin G (IgG) antibodies to
    imiglucerase.
  - When stabilised, monitor all parameters and response to
    treatment at intervals of 6–12 months.
- **DIRECTIONS FOR ADMINISTRATION** For *intravenous infusion*
  (*Cerezyme*®), manufacturer advises give intermittently in
  Sodium chloride 0.9%; initially reconstitute with water for
  injections (400 units in 10.2 mL) to give 40 units/mL
  solution; dilute requisite dose with infusion fluid to a final
  volume of 100–200 mL and give initial dose at a rate not
  exceeding 0.5 units/kg/minute, subsequent doses to be
  given at a rate not exceeding 1 unit/kg/minute; administer
  within 3 hours after reconstitution.

- **MEDICINAL FORMS** There can be variation in the licensing of
  different medicines containing the same drug.
  Powder for solution for infusion
  ELECTROLYTES: May contain Sodium
  - Cerezyme (Genzyme Therapeutics Ltd)
    Imiglucerase 400 unit Cerezyme 400unit powder for solution for
    infusion vials | 1 vial [PoM] £1,071.29 (Hospital only)

9

Blood and nutrition

Velaglucerase alfa

29-Jul-2020

- **DRUG ACTION** Velaglucerase alfa is an enzyme produced by recombinant DNA technology that is administered as enzyme replacement therapy for the treatment of type I Gaucher's disease.

- ● **INDICATIONS AND DOSE**

Type I Gaucher's disease (specialist use only)
▶ BY INTRAVENOUS INFUSION
▶ Adult: Initially 60 units/kg every 2 weeks; adjusted according to response to 15–60 units/kg every 2 weeks

- ● **SIDE-EFFECTS**
▶ **Common or very common** Arthralgia · asthenia · chest discomfort · dizziness · dyspnoea · fever · flushing · gastrointestinal discomfort · headache · hypersensitivity · hypertension · hypotension · infusion related reaction · nausea · pain · skin reactions · tachycardia
  SIDE-EFFECTS, FURTHER INFORMATION Infusion-related reactions are very common; manage by slowing the infusion rate, or interrupting the infusion, or minimise by pre-treatment with an antihistamine, antipyretic, or corticosteroid—consult product literature.

- **PREGNANCY** Manufacturer advises use with caution—limited information available.

- **BREAST FEEDING** Manufacturer advises use with caution—no information available.

- **MONITORING REQUIREMENTS** Monitor immunoglobulin G (IgG) antibody concentration in severe infusion-related reactions or if there is a lack or loss of effect with velaglucerase alfa.

- **DIRECTIONS FOR ADMINISTRATION** For *intravenous infusion* (*VPRIV®*), manufacturer advises give intermittently *in* Sodium chloride 0.9%; reconstitute each 400-unit vial with 4.3 mL water for injections to produce a 100 units/mL solution; dilute requisite dose in 100 mL infusion fluid; give over 60 minutes through a 0.22 micron filter; start infusion within 24 hours of reconstitution.

- **MEDICINAL FORMS** There can be variation in the licensing of different medicines containing the same drug.
  Powder for solution for infusion
  ELECTROLYTES: May contain Sodium
  ▶ VPRIV (Shire Pharmaceuticals Ltd)
    Velaglucerase alfa 400 unit VPRIV 400units powder for solution for infusion vials | 1 vial [PoM] £1,410.20

2.7 Homocystinuria

METHYL DONORS

Betaine

03-Nov-2020

- ● **INDICATIONS AND DOSE**

Adjunctive treatment of homocystinuria involving deficiencies or defects in cystathionine beta-synthase, 5,10-methylene-tetrahydrofolate reductase, or cobalamin cofactor metabolism (specialist use only)
▶ BY MOUTH
▶ Adult: 3 g twice daily (max. per dose 10 g), adjusted according to response; maximum 20 g per day

- ● **SIDE-EFFECTS**
▶ **Uncommon** Abdominal discomfort · agitation · alopecia · appetite decreased · brain oedema · diarrhoea · glossitis · irritability · nausea · skin reactions · urinary incontinence · vomiting

- **PREGNANCY** Manufacturer advises avoid unless essential—limited information available.

- **BREAST FEEDING** Manufacturer advises caution—no information available.

- **MONITORING REQUIREMENTS** Monitor plasma-methionine concentration before and during treatment—interrupt treatment if symptoms of cerebral oedema occur.

- **DIRECTIONS FOR ADMINISTRATION** Manufacturer advises powder should be mixed with water, juice, milk, formula, or food until completely dissolved and taken immediately; measuring spoons are provided to measure 1 g, 150 mg, and 100 mg of *Cystadane®* powder.

- **PRESCRIBING AND DISPENSING INFORMATION** Betaine should be used in conjunction with dietary restrictions and may be given with supplements of Vitamin B$_{12}$, pyridoxine, and folate under specialist advice.

- **NATIONAL FUNDING/ACCESS DECISIONS** For full details see funding body website
  Scottish Medicines Consortium (SMC) decisions
  ▶ Betaine anhydrous (*Cystadane®*) for the adjunctive treatment of homocystinuria involving deficiencies or defects in cystathionine beta-synthase (CBS), 5,10-methylene-tetrahydrofolate reductase (MTHFR) or cobalamin cofactor metabolism (cbl) (August 2010) SMC No. 407/07
    Recommended with restrictions

- **MEDICINAL FORMS** There can be variation in the licensing of different medicines containing the same drug. Forms available from special-order manufacturers include: tablet, oral solution
  Powder
  ▶ Cystadane (Recordati Rare Diseases UK Ltd)
    Betaine 1 gram per 1 gram Cystadane oral powder | 180 gram [PoM] £347.00 DT = £347.00

2.8 Hypophosphatasia

ENZYMES

Asfotase alfa

04-Dec-2017

- **DRUG ACTION** Asfotase alfa is a human recombinant tissue-nonspecific alkaline phosphatase that promotes mineralisation of the skeleton.

- ● **INDICATIONS AND DOSE**

Paediatric-onset hypophosphatasia (initiated by a specialist)
▶ BY SUBCUTANEOUS INJECTION
▶ Adult: 2 mg/kg 3 times a week, alternatively 1 mg/kg 6 times a week, dosing frequency depends on body-weight—consult product literature for further information

- **CAUTIONS** Hypersensitivity reactions
  CAUTIONS, FURTHER INFORMATION
  ▶ Hypersensitivity reactions Reactions, including signs and symptoms consistent with anaphylaxis, have occurred within minutes of administration and can occur in patients on treatment for more than one year; if these reactions occur, manufacturer advises immediate discontinuation of treatment and initiation of appropriate medical treatment. For information on re-administration, consult product literature.

- ● **SIDE-EFFECTS**
▶ **Common or very common** Bruising tendency · chills · cough · cutis laxa · fever · headache · hypersensitivity · hypocalcaemia · irritability · myalgia · nausea · nephrolithiasis · oral hypoaesthesia · pain · skin reactions · tachycardia · vasodilation · vomiting
  SIDE-EFFECTS, FURTHER INFORMATION Injection-site reactions including hypertrophy, induration, skin discolouration, and cellulitis may occur, particularly in

patients receiving treatment 6 times a week. Manufacturer advises rotation of injection sites to manage these reactions; interrupt treatment if severe reactions occur and administer appropriate medical therapy.

● PREGNANCY Manufacturer advises avoid—no information available.

● BREAST FEEDING Manufacturer advises avoid—no information available.

● MONITORING REQUIREMENTS
▶ Manufacturer advises monitor serum parathyroid hormone and calcium concentrations—supplements of calcium and oral vitamin D may be required.
▶ Manufacturer advises periodic ophthalmological examination and renal ultrasounds.

● DIRECTIONS FOR ADMINISTRATION Manufacturer advises max. 1 mL per injection site; administer multiple injections if more than 1 mL is required—consult product literature.

● HANDLING AND STORAGE Manufacturer advises store in a refrigerator (2–8 °C).

● PATIENT AND CARER ADVICE
Injection guides The manufacturer has produced injection guides for patients and carers to support training given by health care professionals.

● NATIONAL FUNDING/ACCESS DECISIONS
For full details see funding body website
NICE decisions
▶ **Asfotase alfa for treating paediatric-onset hypophosphatasia (August 2017)** NICE HST6 Recommended

● MEDICINAL FORMS There can be variation in the licensing of different medicines containing the same drug.

Solution for injection
▶ Strensiq (Alexion Pharma UK Ltd) ▼
    Asfotase alfa 40 mg per 1 ml Strensiq 18mg/0.45ml solution for injection vials | 12 vial [PoM] £12,700.80 (Hospital only)
    Strensiq 28mg/0.7ml solution for injection vials | 12 vial [PoM] £19,756.80 (Hospital only)
    Strensiq 40mg/1ml solution for injection vials | 12 vial [PoM] £28,224.00 (Hospital only)
    Asfotase alfa 100 mg per 1 ml Strensiq 80mg/0.8ml solution for injection vials | 12 vial [PoM] £56,448.00 (Hospital only)

2.9 Mucopolysaccharidosis

ENZYMES

Elosulfase alfa
24-Jul-2020

● DRUG ACTION Elosulfase alfa is an enzyme produced by recombinant DNA technology that provides replacement therapy in conditions caused by N-acetylgalactosamine-6-sulfatase (GALNS) deficiency.

● INDICATIONS AND DOSE
Mucopolysaccharidosis IVA (specialist use only)
▶ BY INTRAVENOUS INFUSION
▶ Adult: 2 mg/kg once weekly

● CAUTIONS Elderly—no information available · infusion-related reactions

CAUTIONS, FURTHER INFORMATION
▶ Infusion-related reactions Infusion-related reactions can occur; manufacturer advises these may be minimised by pre-treatment with an antihistamine and antipyretic, given 30-60 minutes before treatment. If reaction is severe, stop infusion and start appropriate treatment. Caution and close monitoring is advised during re-administration following a severe reaction.

● SIDE-EFFECTS
▶ **Common or very common** Chills · diarrhoea · dizziness · dyspnoea · fever · gastrointestinal discomfort · headache · hypersensitivity · myalgia · nausea · oropharyngeal pain · vomiting
▶ **Frequency not known** Infusion related reaction

● PREGNANCY Manufacturer advises avoid unless essential—limited information available.

● BREAST FEEDING Manufacturer advises use only if potential benefit outweighs risk—present in milk in *animal* studies.

● DIRECTIONS FOR ADMINISTRATION For *intravenous infusion* (*Vimizim®*), manufacturer advises give intermittently *in* Sodium chloride 0.9%; body-weight under 25 kg, dilute requisite dose to final volume of 100 mL infusion fluid and mix gently, give over 4 hours through in-line filter (0.2 micron) initially at a rate of 3 mL/hour, then increase to a rate of 6 mL/hour after 15 minutes, then increase gradually if tolerated every 15 minutes by 6 mL/hour to max. 36 mL/hour; body-weight 25 kg or over, dilute requisite dose to final volume of 250 mL and mix gently, give over 4 hours through in-line filter (0.2 micron) initially at a rate of 6 mL/hour, then increase to a rate of 12 mL/hour after 15 minutes, then increase gradually if tolerated every 15 minutes by 12 mL/hour to max. 72 mL/hour.

● HANDLING AND STORAGE Manufacturer advises store in a refrigerator at 2–8°C. After dilution use immediately or, if necessary, store at 2-8°C for max. 24 hours, followed by up to 24 hours at 23–27°C.

● PATIENT AND CARER ADVICE
Driving and skilled tasks Manufacturer advises patients and carers should be counselled about the effects on driving and performance of skilled tasks—increased risk of dizziness.

● NATIONAL FUNDING/ACCESS DECISIONS
For full details see funding body website
NICE decisions
▶ **Elosulfase alfa for treating mucopolysaccharidosis type IVa (December 2015)** NICE HST2 Recommended

● MEDICINAL FORMS There can be variation in the licensing of different medicines containing the same drug.

Solution for infusion
EXCIPIENTS: May contain Polysorbates, sorbitol
ELECTROLYTES: May contain Sodium
▶ Vimizim (BioMarin Europe Ltd) ▼
    Elosulfase alfa 1 mg per 1 ml Vimizim 5mg/5ml concentrate for solution for infusion vials | 1 vial [PoM] £750.00

Galsulfase
16-Jul-2020

● DRUG ACTION Galsulfase is a recombinant form of human N-acetylgalactosamine-4-sulfatase.

● INDICATIONS AND DOSE
Mucopolysaccharidosis VI (specialist use only)
▶ BY INTRAVENOUS INFUSION
▶ Adult: 1 mg/kg once weekly

● CAUTIONS Acute febrile illness (consider delaying treatment) · acute respiratory illness (consider delaying treatment) · infusion-related reactions can occur · respiratory disease

● SIDE-EFFECTS
▶ **Common or very common** Abdominal pain · angioedema · apnoea · arthralgia · asthma · chest pain · chills · conjunctivitis · corneal opacity · cough · dyspnoea · ear pain · fever · headache · hearing impairment · hypertension · hypotension · increased risk of infection · malaise · nasal congestion · nausea · pain · reflexes absent · respiratory

disorders · skin reactions · tremor · umbilical hernia · vomiting
▸ **Frequency not known** Arrhythmias · cyanosis · hypoxia · infusion related reaction · nerve disorders · pallor · paraesthesia · shock

SIDE-EFFECTS, FURTHER INFORMATION Infusion-related reactions often occur, they can be managed by slowing the infusion rate or interrupting the infusion, and can be minimised by pre-treatment with an antihistamine and an antipyretic. Recurrent infusion-related reactions may require pre-treatment with a corticosteroid — consult product literature for details.

● **PREGNANCY** Manufacturer advises avoid unless essential.

● **BREAST FEEDING** Manufacturer advises avoid—no information available.

● **DIRECTIONS FOR ADMINISTRATION** For *intravenous infusion* (*Naglazyme*®), manufacturer advises give intermittently *in* Sodium chloride 0.9%; dilute requisite dose with infusion fluid to final volume of 250 mL and mix gently; infuse through a 0.2 micron in-line filter; give approx. 2.5% of the total volume over 1 hour, then infuse remaining volume over next 3 hours; if body-weight under 20 kg at risk of fluid overload, dilute requisite dose in 100 mL infusion fluid and give over at least 4 hours.

● **MEDICINAL FORMS** There can be variation in the licensing of different medicines containing the same drug.
Solution for infusion
▸ Naglazyme (BioMarin Europe Ltd) ▼
Galsulfase 1 mg per 1 ml Naglazyme 5mg/5ml solution for infusion vials | 1 vial (PoM) £982.00

Idursulfase

16-Jul-2020

● **DRUG ACTION** Idursulfase is an enzyme produced by recombinant DNA technology licensed for long-term replacement therapy in mucopolysaccharidosis II (Hunter syndrome), a lysosomal storage disorder caused by deficiency of iduronate-2-sulfatase.

● **INDICATIONS AND DOSE**

Mucopolysaccharidosis II (specialist use only)
▸ BY INTRAVENOUS INFUSION
▸ Adult: 500 micrograms/kg once weekly

● **CAUTIONS** Acute febrile respiratory illness (consider delaying treatment) · infusion-related reactions can occur · severe respiratory disease

● **SIDE-EFFECTS**
▸ **Common or very common** Arrhythmias · arthralgia · chest pain · cough · cyanosis · diarrhoea · dizziness · dyspnoea · fever · flushing · gastrointestinal discomfort · headache · hypertension · hypotension · hypoxia · infusion related reaction · nausea · oedema · respiratory disorders · skin reactions · tongue swelling · tremor · vomiting
▸ **Frequency not known** Hypersensitivity

SIDE-EFFECTS, FURTHER INFORMATION Infusion-related reactions often occur, they can be managed by slowing the infusion rate or interrupting the infusion, and can be minimised by pre-treatment with an antihistamine and an antipyretic. Recurrent infusion-related reactions may require pre-treatment with a corticosteroid—consult product literature for details.

● **CONCEPTION AND CONTRACEPTION** Contra-indicated in women of child-bearing potential.

● **PREGNANCY** Manufacturer advises avoid.

● **BREAST FEEDING** Manufacturer advises avoid—present in milk in *animal* studies.

● **DIRECTIONS FOR ADMINISTRATION** For *intravenous infusion* (*Elaprase*®), manufacturer advises give intermittently *in* Sodium chloride 0.9%; dilute requisite dose in

100 mL infusion fluid and mix gently (do not shake); give over 3 hours (gradually reduced to 1 hour if no infusion-related reactions).

● **MEDICINAL FORMS** There can be variation in the licensing of different medicines containing the same drug.
Solution for infusion
▸ Elaprase (Shire Pharmaceuticals Ltd) ▼
Idursulfase 2 mg per 1 ml Elaprase 6mg/3ml concentrate for solution for infusion vials | 1 vial (PoM) £1,985.00

Laronidase

27-Jul-2020

● **DRUG ACTION** Laronidase is an enzyme produced by recombinant DNA technology licensed for long-term replacement therapy in the treatment of non-neurological manifestations of mucopolysaccharidosis I, a lysosomal storage disorder caused by deficiency of alpha-L-iduronidase.

● **INDICATIONS AND DOSE**

Non-neurological manifestations of mucopolysaccharidosis I (specialist use only)
▸ BY INTRAVENOUS INFUSION
▸ Adult: 100 units/kg once weekly

● **CAUTIONS** Infusion-related reactions can occur

● **INTERACTIONS** → Appendix 1: laronidase

● **SIDE-EFFECTS**
▸ **Common or very common** Abdominal pain · alopecia · anaphylactic reaction · angioedema · chills · cough · diarrhoea · dizziness · dyspnoea · fatigue · fever · flushing · headache · hypotension · influenza like illness · joint disorders · nausea · pain · pallor · paraesthesia · peripheral coldness · respiratory disorders · restlessness · skin reactions · sweat changes · tachycardia · temperature sensation altered · vomiting
▸ **Frequency not known** Cyanosis · hypoxia · oedema

SIDE-EFFECTS, FURTHER INFORMATION Infusion-related reactions often occur, they can be managed by slowing the infusion rate or interrupting the infusion, and can be minimised by pre-treatment with an antihistamine and an antipyretic. Recurrent infusion-related reactions may require pre-treatment with a corticosteroid—consult product literature for details.

● **PREGNANCY** Manufacturer advises avoid unless essential—no information available.

● **BREAST FEEDING** Manufacturer advises avoid—no information available.

● **MONITORING REQUIREMENTS** Monitor immunoglobulin G (IgG) antibody concentration.

● **DIRECTIONS FOR ADMINISTRATION** For *intravenous infusion* (*Aldurazyme*®), manufacturer advises give intermittently in Sodium chloride 0.9%; body-weight under 20 kg, use 100 mL infusion fluid; body-weight over 20 kg use 250 mL infusion fluid; withdraw volume of infusion fluid equivalent to volume of laronidase concentrate being added; give through in-line filter (0.2 micron) initially at a rate of 2 units/kg/hour then increase gradually every 15 minutes to max. 43 units/kg/hour.

● **MEDICINAL FORMS** There can be variation in the licensing of different medicines containing the same drug.
Solution for infusion
ELECTROLYTES: May contain Sodium
▸ Aldurazyme (Genzyme Therapeutics Ltd)
Laronidase 100 unit per 1 ml Aldurazyme 500units/5ml solution for infusion vials | 1 vial (PoM) £444.70

2.10 Niemann-Pick type C disease

ENZYME INHIBITORS > GLUCOSYLCERAMIDE SYNTHASE INHIBITORS

Miglustat

- DRUG ACTION Miglustat is an inhibitor of glucosylceramide synthase.

  - INDICATIONS AND DOSE

  Mild to moderate type I Gaucher's disease for whom enzyme replacement therapy is unsuitable (under expert supervision)
  ▶ BY MOUTH
  ▶ Adult: 100 mg 3 times a day, reduced if not tolerated to 100 mg 1–2 times a day

  Treatment of progressive neurological manifestations of Niemann-Pick type C disease (under expert supervision)
  ▶ BY MOUTH
  ▶ Adult: 200 mg 3 times a day

- SIDE-EFFECTS
  ▶ Common or very common Appetite decreased · asthenia · chills · constipation · depression · diarrhoea · dizziness · flatulence · gastrointestinal discomfort · headache · insomnia · libido decreased · malaise · muscle spasms · muscle weakness · nausea · peripheral neuropathy · sensation abnormal · thrombocytopenia · tremor · vomiting · weight decreased

- CONCEPTION AND CONTRACEPTION Effective contraception must be used during treatment. Men should avoid fathering a child during and for 3 months after treatment.

- PREGNANCY Manufacturer advises avoid—toxicity in *animal* studies.

- BREAST FEEDING Manufacturer advises avoid—no information available.

- HEPATIC IMPAIRMENT Manufacturer advises caution (no information available).

- RENAL IMPAIRMENT Avoid if eGFR less than 30 mL/minute/1.73 m².
  Dose adjustments For Gaucher's disease initially 100 mg twice daily if eGFR 50–70 mL/minute/1.73 m². Initially 100 mg once daily if eGFR 30–50 mL/minute/1.73 m².
  For Niemann-Pick type C disease, initially 200 mg twice daily if eGFR 50–70 mL/minute/1.73 m². Initially 100 mg twice daily if eGFR 30–50 mL/minute/1.73 m²

- MONITORING REQUIREMENTS
  ▶ Monitor cognitive and neurological function.
  ▶ Monitor growth and platelet count in Niemann-Pick type C disease.

- MEDICINAL FORMS There can be variation in the licensing of different medicines containing the same drug.
  Capsule
  ▶ Miglustat (Non-proprietary)
    Miglustat 100 mg Miglustat 100mg capsules | 84 capsule PoM £3,934.00 (Hospital only) | 84 capsule PoM £3,442.00
  ▶ Zavesca (Janssen-Cilag Ltd)
    Miglustat 100 mg Zavesca 100mg capsules | 84 capsule PoM £3,934.17 (Hospital only)

2.11 Pompe disease

ENZYMES

Alglucosidase alfa

17-Jul-2020

- DRUG ACTION Alglucosidase alfa is an enzyme produced by recombinant DNA technology licensed for long-term replacement therapy in Pompe disease, a lysosomal storage disorder caused by deficiency of acid alpha-glucosidase.

  - INDICATIONS AND DOSE

  Pompe disease (specialist use only)
  ▶ BY INTRAVENOUS INFUSION
  ▶ Adult: 20 mg/kg every 2 weeks

- CAUTIONS Cardiac dysfunction · infusion-related reactions—consult product literature · respiratory dysfunction

- SIDE-EFFECTS
  ▶ Common or very common Anxiety · arrhythmias · chest discomfort · chills · cough · cyanosis · diarrhoea · dizziness · fatigue · feeling hot · fever · flushing · hyperhidrosis · hypersensitivity · hypertension · irritability · local swelling · muscle complaints · nausea · oedema · pallor · paraesthesia · respiratory disorders · skin reactions · throat complaints · tremor · vomiting
  ▶ Frequency not known Abdominal pain · angioedema · apnoea · arthralgia · cardiac arrest · dyspnoea · excessive tearing · eye inflammation · headache · hypotension · nephrotic syndrome · peripheral coldness · proteinuria · vasoconstriction

  SIDE-EFFECTS, FURTHER INFORMATION Infusion-related reactions are very common, calling for use of antihistamine, antipyretic, or corticosteroid; consult product literature for details.

- PREGNANCY Toxicity in *animal* studies, but treatment should not be withheld.

- BREAST FEEDING Manufacturer advises avoid—no information available.

- MONITORING REQUIREMENTS
  ▶ Monitor closely if cardiac dysfunction.
  ▶ Monitor closely if respiratory dysfunction.
  ▶ Monitor immunoglobulin G (IgG) antibody concentration.

- DIRECTIONS FOR ADMINISTRATION For *intravenous infusion* (*Myozyme ®*), manufacturer advises give intermittently *in* Sodium chloride 0.9%; reconstitute 50 mg with 10.3 mL water for injections to produce 5 mg/mL solution; gently rotate vial without shaking; dilute requisite dose with infusion fluid to give a final concentration of 0.5–4 mg/mL; give through a low protein-binding in-line filter (0.2 micron) at an initial rate of 1 mg/kg/hour increased by 2 mg/kg/hour every 30 minutes to max. 7 mg/kg/hour.

- MEDICINAL FORMS There can be variation in the licensing of different medicines containing the same drug.
  Powder for solution for infusion
  ▶ Myozyme (Genzyme Therapeutics Ltd)
    Alglucosidase alfa 50 mg Myozyme 50mg powder for concentrate for solution for infusion vials | 1 vial PoM £356.06 (Hospital only)

9

Blood and nutrition

2.12 Tyrosinaemia type I

ENZYME INHIBITORS › 4-HYDROXYPHENYLPYRUVATE DIOXYGENASE INHIBITORS

▌ Nitisinone

(NTBC)

04-Aug-2020

● **INDICATIONS AND DOSE**

Hereditary tyrosinaemia type I (in combination with dietary restriction of tyrosine and phenylalanine) (specialist use only)

▸ BY MOUTH

▸ Adult: Initially 500 micrograms/kg twice daily, adjusted according to response; maximum 2 mg/kg per day

● INTERACTIONS → Appendix 1: nitisinone

● SIDE-EFFECTS

▸ **Common or very common** Corneal opacity · eye inflammation · eye pain · granulocytopenia · leucopenia · photophobia · thrombocytopenia

▸ **Uncommon** Leucocytosis · skin reactions

● PREGNANCY Manufacturer advises avoid unless potential benefit outweighs risk—toxicity in *animal* studies.

● BREAST FEEDING Manufacturer advises avoid—adverse effects in *animal* studies.

● PRE-TREATMENT SCREENING Slit-lamp examination of eyes recommended before treatment.

● MONITORING REQUIREMENTS

▸ Monitor liver function regularly.

▸ Monitor platelet and white blood cell count every 6 months.

● DIRECTIONS FOR ADMINISTRATION Manufacturer advises capsules can be opened and the contents suspended in a small amount of water or formula diet and taken immediately.

● MEDICINAL FORMS There can be variation in the licensing of different medicines containing the same drug.

Oral suspension

▸ Orfadin (Swedish Orphan Biovitrum Ltd)
Nitisinone 4 mg per 1 ml Orfadin 4mg/1ml oral suspension sugar-free | 90 ml P̲o̲M̲ £1,692.00 DT = £1,692.00

Capsule

▸ Nitisinone (Non-proprietary)
Nitisinone 2 mg Nitisinone 2mg capsules | 60 capsule P̲o̲M̲ £423.00
Nitisinone 5 mg Nitisinone 5mg capsules | 60 capsule P̲o̲M̲ £845.25
Nitisinone 10 mg Nitisinone 10mg capsules | 60 capsule P̲o̲M̲ £1,546.50
Nitisinone 20 mg Nitisinone 20mg capsules | 60 capsule P̲o̲M̲ £3,384.00 DT = £3,384.00

▸ Orfadin (Swedish Orphan Biovitrum Ltd)
Nitisinone 2 mg Orfadin 2mg capsules | 60 capsule P̲o̲M̲ £423.00
Nitisinone 5 mg Orfadin 5mg capsules | 60 capsule P̲o̲M̲ £845.25
Nitisinone 10 mg Orfadin 10mg capsules | 60 capsule P̲o̲M̲ £1,546.50
Nitisinone 20 mg Orfadin 20mg capsules | 60 capsule P̲o̲M̲ £3,384.00 DT = £3,384.00

2.13 Urea cycle disorders

AMINO ACIDS AND DERIVATIVES

▌ Carglumic acid

24-Jul-2020

● **INDICATIONS AND DOSE**

Hyperammonaemia due to N-acetylglutamate synthase deficiency (under expert supervision)

▸ BY MOUTH

▸ Adult: Initially 50–125 mg/kg twice daily, to be taken immediately before food, dose adjusted according to plasma–ammonia concentration; maintenance 5–50 mg/kg twice daily, the total daily dose may alternatively be given in 3–4 divided doses

Hyperammonaemia due to organic acidaemia (under expert supervision)

▸ BY MOUTH

▸ Adult: Initially 50–125 mg/kg twice daily, to be taken immediately before food, dose adjusted according to plasma-ammonia concentration, the total daily dose may alternatively be given in 3–4 divided doses

> **IMPORTANT SAFETY INFORMATION**
> EMERGENCY MANAGEMENT OF UREA CYCLE DISORDERS
> For further information on the emergency management of urea cycle disorders consult the British Inherited Metabolic Disease Group (BIMDG) website at www.bimdg.org.uk.

● SIDE-EFFECTS

▸ **Common or very common** Hyperhidrosis

▸ **Uncommon** Bradycardia · diarrhoea · fever · vomiting

▸ **Frequency not known** Rash

● PREGNANCY Manufacturer advises avoid unless essential—no information available.

● BREAST FEEDING Manufacturer advises avoid—present in milk in *animal* studies.

● DIRECTIONS FOR ADMINISTRATION Manufacturer advises dispersible tablets must be dispersed in at least 5–10 mL of water and taken orally immediately, or administered via a nasogastric tube.

● MEDICINAL FORMS There can be variation in the licensing of different medicines containing the same drug.

Dispersible tablet

CAUTIONARY AND ADVISORY LABELS 13

▸ Carglumic acid (Non-proprietary)
Carglumic acid 200 mg Carglumic acid 200mg dispersible tablets sugar free sugar-free | 5 tablet P̲o̲M̲ £218.69 sugar-free | 15 tablet P̲o̲M̲ £625.37 sugar-free | 60 tablet P̲o̲M̲ £2,624.30

▸ Carbaglu (Recordati Rare Diseases UK Ltd)
Carglumic acid 200 mg Carbaglu 200mg dispersible tablets sugar-free | 5 tablet P̲o̲M̲ £299.00 sugar-free | 15 tablet P̲o̲M̲ £897.00 sugar-free | 60 tablet P̲o̲M̲ £3,499.00

▸ Ucedane (Eurocept International bv)
Carglumic acid 200 mg Ucedane 200mg dispersible tablets sugar-free | 12 tablet P̲o̲M̲ £660.00 sugar-free | 60 tablet P̲o̲M̲ £3,300.00

DRUGS FOR METABOLIC DISORDERS >
AMMONIA LOWERING DRUGS

Glycerol phenylbutyrate
18-Nov-2020

- DRUG ACTION Glycerol phenylbutyrate is a nitrogen-binding agent that provides an alternative vehicle for waste nitrogen excretion.

- INDICATIONS AND DOSE

Urea cycle disorders (specialist use only)
▶ BY MOUTH, OR BY GASTROSTOMY TUBE, OR BY NASOGASTRIC TUBE
▸ Adult (body surface area up to 1.3 m²): Initially 9.4 g/m² daily in divided doses, usual maintenance 5.3–12.4 g/m² daily in divided doses, each dose should be rounded up to the nearest 0.5 mL and given with each meal. For dose adjustments based on individual requirements—consult product literature
▸ Adult (body surface area 1.3 m² and above): Initially 8 g/m² daily in divided doses, usual maintenance 5.3–12.4 g/m² daily in divided doses, each dose should be rounded up to the nearest 0.5 mL and given with each meal. For dose adjustments based on individual requirements—consult product literature

DOSE EQUIVALENCE AND CONVERSION
▸ 1 mL of liquid contains 1.1 g of glycerol phenylbutyrate.
▸ For patients switching from sodium phenylbutyrate or sodium benzoate—consult product literature.

IMPORTANT SAFETY INFORMATION
EMERGENCY MANAGEMENT OF UREA CYCLE DISORDERS
For further information on the emergency management of urea cycle disorders consult the British Inherited Metabolic Disease Group (BIMDG) website at www.bimdg.org.uk.

- CONTRA-INDICATIONS Treatment of acute hyperammonaemia
- CAUTIONS Elderly—limited information available · intestinal malabsorption · pancreatic insufficiency
- INTERACTIONS → Appendix 1: glycerol phenylbutyrate
- SIDE-EFFECTS
▶ **Common or very common** Appetite abnormal · constipation · diarrhoea · dizziness · fatigue · food aversion · gastrointestinal discomfort · gastrointestinal disorders · headache · menstrual cycle irregularities · nausea · oral disorders · peripheral oedema · skin reactions · tremor · vomiting
▶ **Uncommon** Akathisia · alopecia · biliary colic · bladder pain · burping · confusion · depressed mood · drowsiness · dry mouth · dysphonia · epistaxis · fever · gastrointestinal infection viral · hot flush · hyperhidrosis · hypoalbuminaemia · hypokalaemia · hypothyroidism · joint swelling · muscle spasms · nasal congestion · oropharyngeal pain · pain · paraesthesia · plantar fasciitis · speech disorder · taste altered · throat irritation · ventricular arrhythmia · weight changes
- PREGNANCY Manufacturer advises avoid unless essential—toxicity in *animal* studies.
- BREAST FEEDING Manufacturer advises avoid—no information available.
- HEPATIC IMPAIRMENT Manufacturer advises caution (risk of increased exposure).
Dose adjustments Manufacturer advises use lowest possible dose—consult product literature.
- RENAL IMPAIRMENT Manufacturer advises use with caution in severe impairment—no information available.
- DIRECTIONS FOR ADMINISTRATION Manufacturer advises may be added to a small amount of apple sauce, ketchup,

or squash puree and used within 2 hours. For administration advice via nasogastric or gastrostomy tube—consult product literature.
- HANDLING AND STORAGE Manufacturer advises discard contents of bottle 14 days after opening.
- PATIENT AND CARER ADVICE
Driving and skilled tasks Manufacturer advises patients and carers should be counselled on the effects on driving and performance of skilled tasks—increased risk of dizziness.
- NATIONAL FUNDING/ACCESS DECISIONS
For full details see funding body website
Scottish Medicines Consortium (SMC) decisions
▸ Glycerol phenylbutyrate (*Ravicti*®) as adjunctive therapy for chronic management of adult and paediatric patients aged 2 months and older with urea cycle disorders who cannot be managed by dietary protein restriction and/or amino acid supplementation alone (August 2018) SMC No. 1342/18 Recommended
All Wales Medicines Strategy Group (AWMSG) decisions
▸ Glycerol phenylbutyrate (*Ravicti*®) as adjunctive therapy for chronic management of patients with urea cycle disorders who cannot be managed by dietary protein restriction and/or amino acid supplementation alone (December 2019) AWMSG No. 2127 Recommended

- MEDICINAL FORMS There can be variation in the licensing of different medicines containing the same drug.
Liquid
▸ Ravicti (Immedica Pharma AB) ▼
   Glycerol phenylbutyrate 1.1 gram per 1 ml Ravicti 1.1g/ml oral liquid | 25 ml [PoM] £161.00

Sodium phenylbutyrate
29-Apr-2020

- INDICATIONS AND DOSE

Long-term treatment of urea cycle disorders (as adjunctive therapy in all patients with neonatal-onset disease and in those with late-onset disease who have a history of hyperammonaemic encephalopathy) (under expert supervision)
▶ BY MOUTH
▸ Adult: 9.9–13 g/m² daily in divided doses, with meals; maximum 20 g per day

IMPORTANT SAFETY INFORMATION
EMERGENCY MANAGEMENT OF UREA CYCLE DISORDERS
For further information on the emergency management of urea cycle disorders consult the British Inherited Metabolic Disease Group (BIMDG) website at www.bimdg.org.uk.

- CAUTIONS Conditions involving sodium retention with oedema (preparations contain significant amounts of sodium) · congestive heart failure (preparations contain significant amounts of sodium)
- INTERACTIONS → Appendix 1: sodium phenylbutyrate
- SIDE-EFFECTS
▶ **Common or very common** Abdominal pain · anaemia · appetite decreased · constipation · depression · headache · irritability · leucocytosis · leucopenia · menstrual cycle irregularities · metabolic acidosis · metabolic alkalosis · nausea · oedema · renal tubular acidosis · skin reactions · syncope · taste altered · thrombocytopenia · thrombocytosis · vomiting · weight increased
▶ **Uncommon** Anorectal haemorrhage · aplastic anaemia · arrhythmia · gastrointestinal disorders · pancreatitis
- CONCEPTION AND CONTRACEPTION Manufacturer advises adequate contraception during administration in women of child-bearing potential.

- PREGNANCY Avoid—toxicity in *animal* studies.
- BREAST FEEDING Manufacturer advises avoid—no information available.
- HEPATIC IMPAIRMENT Manufacturer advises caution.
- RENAL IMPAIRMENT Manufacturer advises use with caution (preparations contain significant amounts of sodium).
- DIRECTIONS FOR ADMINISTRATION Granules should be mixed with food before taking. *Pheburane®* granules must not be administered by nasogastric or gastrostromy tubes.
- MEDICINAL FORMS There can be variation in the licensing of different medicines containing the same drug. Forms available from special-order manufacturers include: capsule, oral suspension, oral solution

Granules
- Pheburane (Eurocept International bv)
Sodium phenylbutyrate 483 mg per 1 gram Pheburane 483mg/g granules | 174 gram [PoM] £331.00

Tablet
- Ammonaps (Immedica Pharma AB)
Sodium phenylbutyrate 500 mg Ammonaps 500mg tablets | 250 tablet [PoM] £493.00 DT = £493.00

2.14 Wilson's disease

Other drugs used for Wilson's disease Penicillamine, p. 1146

ANTIDOTES AND CHELATORS > COPPER ABSORPTION INHIBITORS

Zinc acetate
23-Jul-2020

- DRUG ACTION Zinc prevents the absorption of copper in Wilson's disease.

- INDICATIONS AND DOSE

Wilson's disease (initiated under specialist supervision)
- BY MOUTH
- Adult: 50 mg 3 times a day (max. per dose 50 mg 5 times a day), adjusted according to response

DOSE EQUIVALENCE AND CONVERSION
- Doses expressed as elemental zinc.

PHARMACOKINETICS
- Symptomatic Wilson's disease patients should be treated initially with a chelating agent because zinc has a slow onset of action. When transferring from chelating treatment to zinc maintenance therapy, chelating treatment should be co-administered for 2–3 weeks until zinc produces its maximal effect.

- CAUTIONS Portal hypertension (risk of hepatic decompensation when switching from chelating agent)
- INTERACTIONS → Appendix 1: zinc
- SIDE-EFFECTS
- **Common or very common** Epigastric discomfort (usually transient)
- **Uncommon** Leucopenia · sideroblastic anaemia
- **Frequency not known** Condition aggravated
SIDE-EFFECTS, FURTHER INFORMATION Transient gastric irritation may be reduced if first dose is taken mid-morning or with a little protein.
- PREGNANCY
Dose adjustments Reduce dose to 25 mg 3 times daily adjusted according to plasma-copper concentration and urinary copper excretion.
- BREAST FEEDING Manufacturer advises avoid; present in milk—may cause zinc-induced copper deficiency in infant.

- MONITORING REQUIREMENTS Monitor full blood count and serum cholesterol.

- MEDICINAL FORMS There can be variation in the licensing of different medicines containing the same drug.
Capsule
CAUTIONARY AND ADVISORY LABELS 23
- Wilzin (Recordati Rare Diseases UK Ltd)
Zinc (as Zinc acetate) 25 mg Wilzin 25mg capsules | 250 capsule [PoM] £132.00 DT = £132.00
Zinc (as Zinc acetate) 50 mg Wilzin 50mg capsules | 250 capsule [PoM] £242.00 DT = £242.00

ANTIDOTES AND CHELATORS > COPPER CHELATORS

Trientine dihydrochloride
16-Nov-2020

- INDICATIONS AND DOSE

Wilson's disease in patients intolerant of penicillamine
- BY MOUTH USING CAPSULES
- Adult: 1.2–2.4 g daily in 2–4 divided doses, adjusted according to response, to be taken before food

DOSE EQUIVALENCE AND CONVERSION
- Doses expressed as trientine dihydrochloride.
- Capsules and tablets are not interchangeable on a milligram-for-milligram basis due to differences in bioavailability.

CUPRIOR®

Wilson's disease in patients intolerant of penicillamine
- BY MOUTH USING FILM-COATED TABLETS
- Adult: 450–975 mg daily in 2–4 divided doses, adjusted according to response

DOSE EQUIVALENCE AND CONVERSION
- Each *Cuprior®* tablet contains trientine tetrahydrochloride equivalent to 150 mg of trientine base; doses expressed as trientine base.
- Tablets and capsules are not interchangeable on a milligram-for-milligram basis due to differences in bioavailability.

- INTERACTIONS → Appendix 1: trientine
- SIDE-EFFECTS
- **Common or very common** Nausea
- **Uncommon** Skin reactions
- **Frequency not known** Anaemia · gastrointestinal disorders · neurological deterioration in Wilson's Disease
- PREGNANCY Teratogenic in *animal* studies—use only if benefit outweighs risk.
Monitoring Monitor maternal and neonatal serum-copper concentrations.
- BREAST FEEDING [EvGr] Specialist sources indicate caution—limited information available; effect on copper levels in milk conflicting and impact on infant unknown.

- DIRECTIONS FOR ADMINISTRATION
CUPRIOR® Tablets can be divided into 2 equal halves.
- PRESCRIBING AND DISPENSING INFORMATION Trientine is **not** an alternative to penicillamine for rheumatoid arthritis or cystinuria. Penicillamine-induced systemic lupus erythematosus may not resolve on transfer to trientine.
- HANDLING AND STORAGE Manufacturer advises store *capsules* in a refrigerator (2–8°C)—keep in the original container with the silica gel sachet to protect from moisture.
- NATIONAL FUNDING/ACCESS DECISIONS For full details see funding body website

▸ Trientine tetrahydrochloride (*Cuprior®*) for the treatment of Wilson's disease in adults, adolescents and children aged 5 years and older, intolerant to D-penicillamine therapy (November 2019) SMC No. SMC2222 Recommended

● MEDICINAL FORMS There can be variation in the licensing of different medicines containing the same drug.
Tablet
CAUTIONARY AND ADVISORY LABELS 7, 23
▸ Cuprior (GMP-Orphan UK Ltd)
Trientine tetrahydrochloride 150 mg Cuprior 150mg tablets | 72 tablet [PoM] £2,725.00
Capsule
CAUTIONARY AND ADVISORY LABELS 6, 22
▸ Cufence (Univar Solutions B.V.)
Trientine dihydrochloride 250 mg | 100 capsule [PoM] £3,090.00 DT = £3,090.00
▸ Trientine dihydrochloride (Non-proprietary)
Trientine dihydrochloride 300 mg Trientine dihydrochloride 300mg capsules | 100 capsule [PoM] £3,090.00 DT = £3,090.00

3 Mineral and trace elements deficiencies

3.1 Selenium deficiency

Selenium deficiency

Overview

Selenium deficiency can occur as a result of inadequate diet or prolonged parenteral nutrition. A selenium supplement should not be given unless there is good evidence of deficiency.

VITAMINS AND TRACE ELEMENTS

Selenium

● INDICATIONS AND DOSE
Selenium deficiency
▸ BY MOUTH, OR BY INTRAMUSCULAR INJECTION, OR BY INTRAVENOUS INJECTION
▸ **Adult:** 100–500 micrograms daily

● INTERACTIONS → Appendix 1: selenium

● MEDICINAL FORMS There can be variation in the licensing of different medicines containing the same drug. Forms available from special-order manufacturers include: solution for infusion
Tablet
▸ SelenoPrecise (Pharma Nord (UK) Ltd)
Selenium (as L-Selenomethionine) 100 microgram SelenoPrecise 100microgram tablets | 60 tablet £4.02
L-Selenomethionine 200 microgram SelenoPrecise 200microgram tablets | 60 tablet £4.41 | 150 tablet £8.01
Solution for injection
▸ Selenase (Baxter Healthcare Ltd)
Selenium (as Sodium selenite) 50 microgram per 1 ml Selenase 100micrograms/2ml solution for injection ampoules | 1 ampoule [PoM] ⟨⟩
Selenase 500micrograms/10ml solution for injection vials | 1 vial [PoM] ⟨⟩
Solution for infusion
▸ Selenium (Non-proprietary)
Selenium (as Sodium selenite) 10 microgram per 1 ml Selenium 100micrograms/10ml solution for infusion vials | 10 vial [PoM] ⟨⟩
Oral solution
▸ Selenase (Baxter Healthcare Ltd)
Selenium (as Sodium selenite) 50 microgram per 1 ml Selenase 100micrograms/2ml oral solution 2ml unit dose ampoules | 20 unit dose [P] £20.60 DT = £20.60

Selenase 500micrograms/10ml oral solution unit dose vials | 1 unit dose [P] ⟨⟩
Capsule
▸ Selenium (Non-proprietary)
L-Selenomethionine 200 microgram Selenium 200microgram capsules | 30 capsule £3.20 | 60 capsule £5.79

3.2 Zinc deficiency

Zinc deficiency

Overview

Zinc supplements should not be given unless there is good evidence of deficiency (hypoproteinaemia spuriously lowers plasma-zinc concentration) or in zinc-losing conditions. Zinc deficiency can occur as a result of inadequate diet or malabsorption; excessive loss of zinc can occur in trauma, burns, and protein-losing conditions. A zinc supplement is given until clinical improvement occurs, but it may need to be continued in severe malabsorption, metabolic disorders, or in zinc-losing states.

Zinc is used in the treatment of Wilson's disease and acrodermatitis enteropathica, a rare inherited abnormality of zinc absorption.

Parenteral nutrition regimens usually include trace amounts of zinc. If necessary, further zinc can be added to intravenous feeding regimens.

ELECTROLYTES AND MINERALS ⟩ ZINC

Zinc sulfate

● INDICATIONS AND DOSE
Zinc deficiency or supplementation in zinc-losing conditions
▸ BY MOUTH USING EFFERVESCENT TABLETS
▸ **Child (body-weight up to 10 kg):** 22.5 mg daily, dose to be adjusted as necessary, to be dissolved in water and taken after food, dose expressed as elemental zinc
▸ **Child (body-weight 10–30 kg):** 22.5 mg 1–3 times a day, dose to be adjusted as necessary, to be dissolved in water and taken after food, dose expressed as elemental zinc
▸ **Child (body-weight 31 kg and above):** 45 mg 1–3 times a day, dose to be adjusted as necessary, to be dissolved in water and taken after food, dose expressed as elemental zinc
▸ **Adult (body-weight 31 kg and above):** 45 mg 1–3 times a day, dose to be adjusted as necessary, to be dissolved in water and taken after food, dose expressed as elemental zinc

Additional elemental zinc for intravenous nutrition
▸ BY INTRAVENOUS INJECTION
▸ **Adult:** 6.5 mg daily (Zn^{2+} 100 micromol)

● UNLICENSED USE *Solvazinc®* is not licensed for use in acrodermatitis enteropathica.

● INTERACTIONS → Appendix 1: zinc

● SIDE-EFFECTS Diarrhoea · gastritis · gastrointestinal discomfort · nausea · vomiting

● PREGNANCY Crosses placenta; risk theoretically minimal, but no information available.

● BREAST FEEDING Present in milk; risk theoretically minimal, but no information available.

● RENAL IMPAIRMENT Accumulation may occur in acute renal failure.

● PRESCRIBING AND DISPENSING INFORMATION Each *Solvazinc®* tablet contains zinc sulfate monohydrate 125 mg (45 mg zinc).

9

Blood and nutrition

- MEDICINAL FORMS There can be variation in the licensing of different medicines containing the same drug. Forms available from special-order manufacturers include: oral solution, solution for injection, liquid

Effervescent tablet

CAUTIONARY AND ADVISORY LABELS 13, 21

▸ Solvazinc (Galen Ltd)

Zinc sulfate monohydrate 125 mg Solvazinc 125mg effervescent tablets sugar-free | 90 tablet Ⓟ £17.20 DT = £17.20

4 Nutrition (intravenous)

Intravenous nutrition

Overview

When adequate feeding through the alimentary tract is not possible, nutrients may be given by intravenous infusion. This may be in addition to ordinary oral or tube feeding—**supplemental parenteral nutrition**, or may be the sole source of nutrition— **total parenteral nutrition** (TPN). Indications for this method include preparation of undernourished patients for surgery, chemotherapy, or radiation therapy; severe or prolonged disorders of the gastro-intestinal tract; major surgery, trauma, or burns; prolonged coma or refusal to eat; and some patients with renal or hepatic failure. The composition of proprietary preparations available is given under Proprietary Infusion Fluids for Parenteral Feeding below.

Parenteral nutrition requires the use of a solution containing amino acids, glucose, fat, electrolytes, trace elements, and vitamins. This is now commonly provided by the pharmacy in the form of a 3-litre bag. A single dose of vitamin B_{12}, as hydroxocobalamin p. 1072, is given by intramuscular injection; regular vitamin B_{12} injections are not usually required unless total parenteral nutrition continues for many months. Folic acid p. 1071 is given in a dose of 15 mg once or twice each week, usually in the nutrition solution. Other vitamins are usually given daily; they are generally introduced in the parenteral nutrition solution. Alternatively, if the patient is able to take small amounts by mouth, vitamins may be given orally.

The nutrition solution is infused through a central venous catheter inserted under full surgical precautions. Alternatively, infusion through a peripheral vein may be used for supplementary as well as total parenteral nutrition for periods of up to a month, depending on the availability of peripheral veins; factors prolonging cannula life and preventing thrombophlebitis include the use of soft polyurethane paediatric cannulas and use of feeds of low osmolality and neutral pH. Only nutritional fluids should be given by the dedicated intravenous line.

Proprietary Infusion Fluids for Parenteral Feeding

Preparation	Nitrogen g/litre	[1,2]Energy kJ/litre	K^+	Mg^{2+}	Na^+	Acet⁻	Cl⁻	Other components/litre
			Electrolytes mmol/litre					
Aminoven 25 (Fresenius Kabi Ltd) Net price 500 ml: no price available	25.7	–	–	–	–	–	–	
Clinimix N9G20E (Baxter Healthcare Ltd) Net price (dual compartment bag of amino acids with electrolytes 1000 mL and glucose 20% with calcium 1000 mL) 2 litre: no price available	4.6	1680	30.0	2.5	35.0	50.0	40.0	Ca^{2+} 2.3 mmol, phosphate 15 mmol, anhydrous glucose 100 g
ClinOleic 20% (Baxter Healthcare Ltd) Net price 100 ml: no price available; Net price 500 ml: no price available	–	8360	–	–	–	–	–	purified olive and soya oil 200 g, glycerol 22.5 g, egg phosphatides 12 g
Intralipid 10% (Fresenius Kabi Ltd) Net price 100 ml = £4.12; Net price 500 ml = £9.01	–	4600	–	–	–	–	–	soya oil 100 g, glycerol 22 g, purified egg phospholipids 12 g, phosphate 15 mmol
Intralipid 20% (Fresenius Kabi Ltd) Net price 100 ml = £6.21; Net price 250 ml = £10.16; Net price 500 ml = £13.52	–	8400	–	–	–	–	–	soya oil 200 g, glycerol 22 g, purified egg phospholipids 12 g, phosphate 15 mmol
Kabiven (Fresenius Kabi Ltd) Net price 1.54 litre = £44.09; Net price 2.053 litre = £57.42; Net price 2.566 litre = £59.92	5.3	3275	23.0	4.0	31.0	38.0	45.0	Ca^{2+} 2 mmol, phosphate 9.7 mmol, anhydrous glucose 97 g, soya oil 39 g
Kabiven peripheral (Fresenius Kabi Ltd) Net price (triple compartment bag of amino acids and electrolytes 300 mL, 400 mL, or 500 mL; glucose 885 mL, 1180 mL, or 1475 mL; lipid emulsion 255 mL, 340 mL, or 425 mL) 1.44 litre = £30.77; Net price 1.92 litre = £44.09; Net price 2.4 litre = £55.72	3.75	2625	17.0	2.8	22.0	27.0	33.0	Ca^{2+} 1.4 mmol, phosphate 7.5 mmol, anhydrous glucose 67.5 g, soya oil 35.4 g
Lipidem (B.Braun Medical Ltd) Net price 100 ml = £19.11; Net price 250 ml = £31.85; Net price 500 ml = £40.34	–	7900	–	–	–	–	–	omega-3-acid triglycerides 20 g, soya oil 80 g, medium chain triglycerides 100 g
Lipofundin MCT/LCT 10% (B.Braun Medical Ltd) Net price 500 ml = £13.69	–	4430	–	–	–	–	–	soya oil 50 g, medium-chain triglycerides 50 g

1 1000 kcal = 4200kJ; 1000 kJ = 238.8 kcal. All entries are Prescription-only medicines.
2 Excludes protein- or amino acid-derived energy

Preparation	Nitrogen g/litre	[1,2]Energy kJ/litre	Electrolytes mmol/litre					Other components/litre
			K⁺	Mg²⁺	Na⁺	Acet⁻	Cl⁻	

Preparation	Nitrogen g/litre	Energy kJ/litre	K⁺	Mg²⁺	Na⁺	Acet⁻	Cl⁻	Other components/litre
Lipofundin MCT/LCT 20% (B.Braun Medical Ltd) Net price 100 ml = £13.28; Net price 500 ml = £20.36	–	8000	–	–	–	–	–	soya oil 100 g, medium-chain triglycerides 100 g
Nutriflex basal (B.Braun Medical Ltd) Net price 2 litre = £29.20	4.6	2095	30.0	5.7	49.9	35.0	50.0	Ca²⁺ 3.6 mmol, acid phosphate 12.8 mmol, anhydrous glucose 125 g
Nutriflex peri (B.Braun Medical Ltd) Net price 2 litre = £30.47	5.7	1340	15.0	4.0	27.0	19.5	31.6	Ca²⁺ 2.5 mmol, acid phosphate 5.7 mmol, anhydrous glucose 80 g
Nutriflex plus (B.Braun Medical Ltd) Net price (dual compartment bag of amino acids 400 mL or 800 mL; glucose 600 mL or 1200 mL) 1 litre: no price available; Net price 2 litre = £33.02	6.8	2510	25.0	5.7	37.2	22.9	35.5	Ca²⁺ 3.6 mmol, acid phosphate 20 mmol, anhydrous glucose 150 g
Nutriflex special (B.Braun Medical Ltd) Net price (dual compartment bag of amino acids 500 mL or 750 mL; glucose 500 mL or 750 mL) 1 litre: no price available; Net price 1.5 litre = £27.60	10.0	4020	25.7	5.0	40.5	22.0	49.5	Ca²⁺ 4.1 mmol, acid phosphate 14.7 mmol, anhydrous glucose 240 g
NuTRIflex Lipid peri (B.Braun Medical Ltd) Net price (triple compartment bag of amino acids 500 mL, 750 mL or 1000 mL; glucose 500 mL, 750 mL or 1000 mL; lipid emulsion 20% 250 mL, 375 mL or 500 mL) 1.25 litre = £42.83; Net price 1.875 litre = £54.37; Net price 2.5 litre = £64.22	4.56	2664	24.0	2.4	40.0	32.0	38.4	Ca²⁺ 2.4 mmol, Zn²⁺ 24 micromol, phosphate 6 mmol, anhydrous glucose 64 g, soya oil 20 g, medium-chain triglycerides 20 g
NuTRIflex Lipid plus (B.Braun Medical Ltd) Net price (triple compartment bag of amino acids 500 mL, 750 mL or 1000 mL; glucose 500 mL, 750 mL or 1000 mL; lipid emulsion 20% 250 mL, 375 mL or 500 mL) 1.25 litre = £46.56; Net price 1.875 litre = £59.46; Net price 2.5 litre = £68.39	5.44	3600	28.0	3.2	40.0	36.0	36.0	Ca²⁺ 3.2 mmol, Zn²⁺ 24 micromol, phosphate 12 mmol, anhydrous glucose 120 g, soya oil 20 g, medium-chain triglycerides 20 g
NuTRIflex Lipid plus without Electrolytes (B.Braun Medical Ltd) Net price (triple compartment bag of amino acids 500 mL, 750 mL or 1000 mL; glucose 500 mL, 750 mL or 1000 mL; lipid emulsion 20% 250 mL, 375 mL or 500 mL) 1.25 litre = £46.56; Net price 1.875 litre = £59.45; Net price 2.5 litre = £84.64	5.44	3600	–	–	–	–	–	anhydrous glucose 120 g, soya oil 20 g, medium-chain triglycerides 20 g
NuTRIflex Lipid special (B.Braun Medical Ltd) Net price (triple compartment bag of amino acids 500 mL, 750 mL or 1000 mL; glucose 500 mL, 750 mL or 1000 mL; lipid emulsion 20% 250 mL, 375 mL or 500 mL) 1.25 litre = £56.96; Net price 1.875 litre = £74.62	8.0	4004	37.6	4.24	53.6	48.0	48.0	Ca²⁺ 4.24 mmol, Zn²⁺ 32 micromol, phosphate 16 mmol, anhydrous glucose 144 g, soya oil 20 g, medium-chain triglycerides 20 g
NuTRIflex Lipid special without Electrolytes (B.Braun Medical Ltd) Net price (triple compartment bag of amino acids 500 mL, 750 mL or 1000 mL; glucose 500 mL, 750 mL or 1000 mL; lipid emulsion 20% 250 mL, 375 mL or 500 mL) 1.25 litre = £56.96; Net price 1.875 litre = £74.62	8.0	4004	–	–	–	–	–	anhydrous glucose 144 g, soya oil 20 g, medium-chain triglycerides 20 g

1 1000 kcal = 4200kJ; 1000 kJ = 238.8 kcal. All entries are Prescription-only medicines.
2 Excludes protein- or amino acid-derived energy

9

Blood and nutrition

Preparation	Nitrogen g/litre	[1,2]Energy kJ/litre	Electrolytes mmol/litre					Other components/litre
			K+	Mg2+	Na+	Acet−	Cl−	
NuTRIflex Omega plus (B.Braun Medical Ltd) Net price (triple compartment bag of amino acids 500 mL, 750 mL or 1000 mL; glucose 500 mL, 750 mL or 1000 mL; lipid emulsion 250 mL, 375 mL or 500 mL) 1.25 litre = £47.42; Net price 1.875 litre = £60.57; Net price 2.5 litre = £69.66	5.4	3600	28.0	3.2	40.0	36.0	36.0	Ca^{2+} 3.2 mmol, Zn^{2+} 24 micromol, phosphate 12 mmol, anhydrous glucose 120 g, refined soya oil 16 g, medium-chain triglycerides 20 g, omega-3-acid triglycerides 4 g
NuTRIflex Omega special (B.Braun Medical Ltd) Net price (triple compartment bag of amino acids 250 mL, 500 mL, 750 mL or 1000 mL; glucose 250 mL, 500 mL, 750 mL or 1000 mL; lipid emulsion 125 mL, 250 mL, 375 mL or 500 mL) 625 ml = £43.62; Net price 1.25 litre = £58.01; Net price 1.875 litre = £76.01; Net price 2.5 litre = £89.71	8.0	4004	37.6	4.24	53.6	48.0	48.0	Ca^{2+} 4.24 mmol, Zn^{2+} 30 micromol, phosphate 16 mmol, anhydrous glucose 144 g, refined soya oil 16 g, medium-chain triglycerides 20 g, omega-3-acid triglycerides 4 g
Plasma-Lyte 148 (water) (Baxter Healthcare Ltd) Net price 1 litre: no price available	–	–	5.0	1.5	140.0	27.0	98.0	gluconate 23 mmol
Plasma-Lyte 148 (dextrose 5%) (Baxter Healthcare Ltd) Net price 1 litre: no price available	–	840	5.0	1.5	140.0	27.0	98.0	gluconate 23 mmol, anhydrous glucose 50 g
SMOFlipid (Fresenius Kabi Ltd) Net price 500 ml = £174.30	–	8400	–	–	–	–	–	fish oil 30 g, olive oil 50 g, soya oil 60 g, medium-chain triglycerides 60 g
Synthamin 9 (Baxter Healthcare Ltd) Net price 500 ml: no price available	9.1	–	60.0	5.0	70.0	100.0	70.0	acid phosphate 30 mmol
Synthamin 9 EF (electrolyte-free) (Baxter Healthcare Ltd) Net price 500 ml: no price available; Net price 1 litre: no price available	9.1	–	–	–	–	44.0	22.0	
Synthamin 14 (Baxter Healthcare Ltd) Net price 500 ml: no price available; Net price 1 litre: no price available	14.0	–	60.0	5.0	70.0	140.0	70.0	acid phosphate 30 mmol
Synthamin 14 EF (electrolyte-free) (Baxter Healthcare Ltd) Net price 500 ml: no price available; Net price 1 litre: no price available	14.0	–	–	–	–	68.0	34.0	
Synthamin 17 (Baxter Healthcare Ltd) Net price 500 ml: no price available	16.5	–	60.0	5.0	70.0	150.0	70.0	acid phosphate 30 mmol
Synthamin 17 EF (electrolyte-free) (Baxter Healthcare Ltd) Net price 500 ml: no price available; Net price 3 litre: no price available	16.5	–	–	–	–	82.0	40.0	
Vamin 14 (Fresenius Kabi Ltd) Net price 1 litre = £16.02	13.5	–	50.0	8.0	100.0	135.0	100.0	Ca^{2+} 5 mmol, SO_4^{2-} 8 mmol
Vamin 14 (electrolyte-free) (Fresenius Kabi Ltd) Net price 500 ml = £9.48; Net price 1 litre = £16.02	13.5	–	–	–	–	90.0	–	
Vamin 18 (electrolyte-free) (Fresenius Kabi Ltd) Net price 500 ml = £11.99; Net price 1 litre = £23.38	18.0	–	–	–	–	110.0	–	

1 1000 kcal = 4200kJ; 1000 kJ = 238.8 kcal. All entries are Prescription-only medicines.
2 Excludes protein- or amino acid-derived energy

Before starting, the patient should be well oxygenated with a near normal circulating blood volume and attention should be given to renal function and acid-base status. Appropriate biochemical tests should have been carried out beforehand and serious deficits corrected. Nutritional and electrolyte status must be monitored throughout treatment.

Complications of long-term parenteral nutrition include gall bladder sludging, gall stones, cholestasis and abnormal liver function tests. For details of the prevention and management of parenteral nutrition complications, specialist literature should be consulted.

Protein is given as mixtures of essential and non-essential synthetic L-amino acids. Ideally, all essential amino acids should be included with a wide variety of nonessential ones to provide sufficient nitrogen together with electrolytes. Solutions vary in their composition of amino acids; they often contain an energy source (usually glucose p. 1090) and electrolytes.

Energy is provided in a ratio of 0.6 to 1.1 megajoules (150–250 kcals) per gram of protein nitrogen. Energy requirements must be met if amino acids are to be utilised for tissue maintenance. A mixture of carbohydrate and fat energy sources (usually 30–50% as fat) gives better utilisation of amino acids than glucose alone.

Glucose is the preferred source of carbohydrate, but if more than 180 g is given per day frequent monitoring of blood glucose is required, and insulin may be necessary. Glucose in various strengths from 10 to 50% must be infused through a central venous catheter to avoid thrombosis.

In parenteral nutrition regimens, it is necessary to provide adequate **phosphate** in order to allow phosphorylation of glucose and to prevent hypophosphataemia; between 20 and 30 mmol of phosphate is required daily.

Fructose and sorbitol have been used in an attempt to avoid the problem of hyperosmolar hyperglycaemic non-ketotic acidosis but other metabolic problems may occur, as with xylitol and ethanol which are now rarely used.

Fat emulsions have the advantages of a high energy to fluid volume ratio, neutral pH, and iso-osmolarity with plasma, and provide essential fatty acids. Several days of adaptation may be required to attain maximal utilisation. Reactions include occasional febrile episodes (usually only with 20% emulsions) and rare anaphylactic responses. Interference with biochemical measurements such as those for blood gases and calcium may occur if samples are taken before fat has been cleared. Daily checks are necessary to ensure complete clearance from the plasma in conditions where fat metabolism may be disturbed. **Additives should not be mixed with fat emulsions unless compatibility is known.**

Administration
Because of the complex requirements relating to parenteral nutrition full details relating to administration have been omitted. In all cases *product literature and other specialist literature should be consulted.*

NUTRIENTS ⟩ PARENTERAL NUTRITION

Parenteral nutrition supplements

05-Aug-2020

- ● INDICATIONS AND DOSE
Supplement in intravenous nutrition
  - ▶ BY INTRAVENOUS INFUSION, OR BY SLOW INTRAVENOUS INJECTION
  - ▶ Adult: (consult product literature)

DIPEPTIVEN 20G/100ML CONCENTRATE FOR SOLUTION FOR INFUSION BOTTLES
Amino acid supplement for hypercatabolic or hypermetabolic states
- ▶ BY INTRAVENOUS INFUSION
- ▶ Adult: 300–400 mg/kg daily, dose not to exceed 20% of total amino acid intake

- ● CAUTIONS
Total parenteral nutrition exceeding one month Measure serum manganese concentration and check liver function before commencing treatment and regularly during treatment—discontinue if manganese concentration raised or if cholestasis develops.

- ● DIRECTIONS FOR ADMINISTRATION Because of the complex requirements relating to parenteral nutrition, full details relating to administration have been omitted. In all cases *specialist pharmacy advice, product literature, and other specialist literature should be consulted.* Compatibility with the infusion solution must be ascertained before adding supplementary preparations. **Additives should not be mixed with fat emulsions unless compatibility is known.**

ADDITRACE SOLUTION FOR INFUSION 10ML AMPOULES For addition to *Vamin*® solutions and glucose intravenous infusions.

DIPEPTIVEN 20G/100ML CONCENTRATE FOR SOLUTION FOR INFUSION BOTTLES For addition to infusion solutions containing amino acids.

ADDIPHOS® VIALS For addition to *Vamin*® solutions and glucose intravenous infusions.

DECAN CONCENTRATE FOR SOLUTION FOR INFUSION 40ML BOTTLES For addition to infusion solutions.

TRACUTIL® AMPOULES For addition to infusion solutions.

SOLIVITO N POWDER FOR SOLUTION FOR INFUSION VIALS Dissolve in water for injections or glucose intravenous infusion for adding to glucose intravenous infusion or *Intralipid*®; dissolve in *Vitlipid N*® or *Intralipid*® for adding to *Intralipid*® only.

VITLIPID N ADULT EMULSION FOR INJECTION 10ML AMPOULES For addition to *Intralipid*®.

CERNEVIT® POWDER FOR SOLUTION FOR INJECTION VIALS Dissolve in 5 mL water for injections or Glucose 5% or Sodium Chloride 0.9% for adding to infusion solutions.

- ● PRESCRIBING AND DISPENSING INFORMATION
ADDITRACE SOLUTION FOR INFUSION 10ML AMPOULES For patients over 40 kg.
  Additrace® solution contains traces of Fe^{3+}, Zn^{2+}, Mn^{2+}, Cu^{2+}, Cr^{3+}, Se^{4+}, Mo^{6+}, F^-, I^-.

DIPEPTIVEN 20G/100ML CONCENTRATE FOR SOLUTION FOR INFUSION BOTTLES *Dipeptiven*® solution contains N(2)-L-alanyl-L-glutamine 200 mg/mL (providing L-alanine 82 mg, L-glutamine 134.6 mg).

ADDIPHOS® VIALS *Addiphos*® sterile solution contains phosphate 40 mmol, K^+ 30 mmol, Na^+ 30 mmol/20 mL.

DECAN CONCENTRATE FOR SOLUTION FOR INFUSION 40ML BOTTLES For patients over 40 kg.
  Decan® solution contains trace elements Fe^{2+}, Zn^{2+}, Cu^{2+}, Mn^{2+}, F^-, Co^{2+}, I^-, Se^{4+}, Mo^{6+}, Cr^{3+}.

TRACUTIL® AMPOULES *Tracutil*® solution contains trace elements Fe^{2+}, Zn^{2+}, Mn^{2+}, Cu^{2+}, Cr^{3+}, Se^{4+}, Mo^{6+}, I^-, F^-.

SOLIVITO N POWDER FOR SOLUTION FOR INFUSION VIALS *Solivito N*® powder for reconstitution contains biotin 60 micrograms, cyanocobalamin 5 micrograms, folic acid 400 micrograms, glycine 300 mg, nicotinamide 40 mg, pyridoxine hydrochloride 4.9 mg, riboflavin sodium phosphate 4.9 mg, sodium ascorbate 113 mg, sodium pantothenate 16.5 mg, thiamine mononitrate 3.1 mg.

VITLIPID N ADULT EMULSION FOR INJECTION 10ML
AMPOULES *Vitlipid N*® adult emulsion contains vitamin A
330 units, ergocalciferol 20 units, *dl*-alpha tocopherol
1 unit, phytomenadione 15 micrograms/mL.
  For adults and children over 11 years.

CERNEVIT® POWDER FOR SOLUTION FOR INJECTION
VIALS *Cernevit*® powder for reconstitution contains *dl*-
alpha tocopherol 10.2 mg, ascorbic acid 125 mg, biotin
69 micrograms, colecalciferol 220 units, cyanocobalamin
6 micrograms, folic acid 414 micrograms, nicotinamide
46 mg, pantothenic acid (as dexpanthenol) 17.25 mg,
pyridoxine hydrochloride 5.5 mg, retinol (as palmitate)
3500 units, riboflavin (as dihydrated sodium phosphate)
4.14 mg, thiamine (as cocarboxylase tetrahydrate) 3.51 mg.
  For adults and children over 11 years.

- MEDICINAL FORMS There can be variation in the licensing of
different medicines containing the same drug. Forms available
from special-order manufacturers include: solution for infusion
  Solution for infusion
  ▸ Parenteral nutrition supplements (Non-proprietary)
    Sodium glycerophosphate 216 mg per 1 ml Sodium
    glycerophosphate 4.32g/20ml concentrate for solution for infusion
    vials | 1 vial [PoM] £5.60
  ▸ Additrace (Fresenius Kabi Ltd)
    **Sodium molybdate 4.85 microgram per 1 ml, Chromic chloride
    5.33 microgram per 1 ml, Sodium selenite anhydrous
    6.9 microgram per 1 ml, Potassium iodide 16.6 microgram per
    1 ml, Manganese chloride 99 microgram per 1 ml, Sodium
    fluoride 210 microgram per 1 ml, Copper chloride 340 microgram
    per 1 ml, Ferric chloride hexahydrate 540 microgram per 1 ml,
    Zinc chloride 1.36 mg per 1 ml** Additrace concentrate for solution
    for infusion 10ml ampoules | 1 ampoule [PoM] £1.96
  ▸ Dipeptiven (Fresenius Kabi Ltd)
    N(2)-L-alanyl-L-glutamine 200 mg per 1 ml Dipeptiven 20g/100ml
    concentrate for solution for infusion bottles | 1 bottle [PoM] £25.93
    Dipeptiven 10g/50ml concentrate for solution for infusion bottles |
    1 bottle [PoM] £13.94
  ▸ Tracutil (B.Braun Melsungen AG)
    **Sodium molybdate dihydrate 2.42 microgram per 1 ml, Chromic
    chloride 5.3 microgram per 1 ml, Sodium selenite pentahydrate
    7.89 microgram per 1 ml, Potassium iodide 16.6 microgram per
    1 ml, Sodium fluoride 126 microgram per 1 ml, Manganese
    chloride 197.9 microgram per 1 ml, Copper chloride
    204.6 microgram per 1 ml, Zinc chloride 681.5 microgram per
    1 ml, Ferrous chloride 695.8 microgram per 1 ml** Tracutil
    concentrate for solution for infusion 10ml ampoules |
    5 ampoule [PoM] £7.96
  Powder for solution for infusion
  ▸ Solivito N (Fresenius Kabi Ltd)
    **Cyanocobalamin 5 microgram, Biotin 60 microgram, Folic acid
    400 microgram, Thiamine nitrate 3.1 mg, Pyridoxine
    hydrochloride 4.9 mg, Riboflavin sodium phosphate 4.9 mg,
    Sodium pantothenate 16.5 mg, Nicotinamide 40 mg, Sodium
    ascorbate 113 mg** Solivito N powder for solution for infusion vials |
    1 vial [PoM] £1.97
  Emulsion for injection
  ▸ Vitlipid N Adult (Fresenius Kabi Ltd)
    **Ergocalciferol 500 nanogram per 1 ml, Phytomenadione
    15 microgram per 1 ml, Retinol palmitate 99 microgram per 1 ml,
    Alpha tocopherol 910 microgram per 1 ml** Vitlipid N Adult
    emulsion for infusion 10ml ampoules | 1 ampoule [PoM] £1.97
  Powder for solution for injection
  EXCIPIENTS: May contain Glycocholic acid
  ▸ Cernevit (Baxter Healthcare Ltd)
    **Cyanocobalamin 6 microgram, Biotin 69 microgram, Folic acid
    414 microgram, Thiamine 3.51 mg, Riboflavin (as Riboflavin
    sodium phosphate) 4.14 mg, Pyridoxine (as Pyridoxine
    hydrochloride) 4.53 mg, Pantothenic acid (as Dexpanthenol)
    17.25 mg, Nicotinamide 46 mg, Ascorbic acid 125 mg, Alpha
    tocopherol 11.2 unit, Colecalciferol 220 unit, Retinol
    3500 unit** Cernevit powder for solution for injection vials |
    10 vial [PoM] [Ⓢ]

5   Nutrition (oral)

Enteral nutrition

Overview

The body's reserves of protein rapidly become exhausted in
severely ill patients, especially during chronic illness or in
those with severe burns, extensive trauma, pancreatitis, or
intestinal fistula. Much can be achieved by frequent meals
and by persuading the patient to take supplementary snacks
of ordinary food between the meals.

However, extra calories, protein, other nutrients, and
vitamins are often best given by supplementing ordinary
meals with enteral sip or tube feeds.

When patients cannot feed normally, for example, patients
with severe facial injury, oesophageal obstruction, or coma, a
nutritionally complete diet of enteral feeds must be given.
The advice of a dietitian should be sought to determine the
protein and total energy requirement of the patient and the
form and relative contribution of carbohydrate and fat to the
energy requirements.

Most enteral feeds contain protein derived from cows' milk
or soya. Elemental feeds containing protein hydrolysates or
free amino acids can be used for patients who have
diminished ability to break down protein, for example in
inflammatory bowel disease or pancreatic insufficiency.

Even when nutritionally complete feeds are given, water
and electrolyte balance should be monitored.
Haematological and biochemical parameters should also be
monitored, particularly in clinically unstable patients. Extra
minerals (e.g. magnesium and zinc) may be needed in
patients where gastro-intestinal secretions are being lost.
Additional vitamins may also be needed.

Enteral nutrition in children

Children have special requirements and in most situations
liquid feeds prepared for adults are totally unsuitable—the
advice of a paediatric dietitian should be sought.

5.1   Special diets

Nutrition in special diets

Overview

These are preparations that have been modified to eliminate
a particular constituent from a food or that are nutrient
mixtures formulated as food substitutes for patients who
either cannot tolerate or cannot metabolise certain common
constituents of food. In certain clinical conditions, some
food preparations are regarded as drugs and can be
prescribed within the NHS if they have been approved by the
Advisory Committee on Borderline Substances (ACBS).

Coeliac disease

Coeliac disease is caused by an abnormal immune response
to gluten. For management and further information, see
Coeliac disease p. 40.

Phenylketonuria

Phenylketonuria (hyperphenylalaninaemia, PKU), which
results from the inability to metabolise **phenylalanine**, is
managed by restricting dietary intake of **phenylalanine** to a
small amount sufficient for tissue building and repair.

Sapropterin dihydrochloride p. 1127, a synthetic form of
tetrahydrobiopterin, is licensed as an adjunct to dietary
restriction of **phenylalanine** in the management of patients
with *phenylketonuria* and *tetrahydrobiopterin deficiency*.

Aspartame (used as a sweetener in some foods and medicines) contributes to the **phenylalanine** intake and may affect control of *phenylketonuria*. Where the presence of **aspartame** is specified in the product literature this is indicated in the BNF against the preparation; the patient should be informed of this.

5.1a Phenylketonuria

DRUGS FOR METABOLIC DISORDERS >
TETRAHYDROBIOPTERIN AND DERIVATIVES

Sapropterin dihydrochloride   11-Nov-2020

- **INDICATIONS AND DOSE**

Phenylketonuria (adjunct to dietary restriction of phenylalanine) (specialist use only)
▸ BY MOUTH
  ▸ Adult: Initially 10 mg/kg once daily, adjusted according to response; usual dose 5–20 mg/kg once daily, dose to be taken preferably in the morning

Tetrahydrobiopterin deficiency (adjunct to dietary restriction of phenylalanine) (specialist use only)
▸ BY MOUTH
  ▸ Adult: Initially 2–5 mg/kg once daily, adjusted according to response, dose to be taken preferably in the morning, the total daily dose may alternatively be given in 2–3 divided doses; maximum 20 mg/kg per day

- **CAUTIONS** History of convulsions
- **INTERACTIONS** → Appendix 1: sapropterin
- **SIDE-EFFECTS**
▸ **Common or very common** Cough · diarrhoea · gastrointestinal discomfort · headache · laryngeal pain · nasal complaints · nausea · vomiting
▸ **Frequency not known** Gastrointestinal disorders · rash
- **PREGNANCY** Manufacturer advises caution—consider only if strict dietary management inadequate.
- **BREAST FEEDING** Manufacturer advises avoid—no information available.
- **HEPATIC IMPAIRMENT** Manufacturer advises caution (no information available).
- **RENAL IMPAIRMENT** Manufacturer advises caution—no information available.
- **MONITORING REQUIREMENTS**
▸ Monitor blood-phenylalanine concentration before and after first week of treatment—if unsatisfactory response increase dose at weekly intervals to max. dose and monitor blood-phenylalanine concentration weekly; discontinue treatment if unsatisfactory response after 1 month.
▸ Monitor blood-phenylalanine and tyrosine concentrations 1–2 weeks after dose adjustment and during treatment.
- **DIRECTIONS FOR ADMINISTRATION** Manufacturer advises tablets should be dissolved in water and taken within 20 minutes.
- **PRESCRIBING AND DISPENSING INFORMATION** Sapropterin is a synthetic form of tetrahydrobiopterin.
- **PATIENT AND CARER ADVICE** Patient or carers should be given advice on how to administer sapropterin dihydrochloride dispersible tablets.
- **NATIONAL FUNDING/ACCESS DECISIONS**
For full details see funding body website

Scottish Medicines Consortium (SMC) decisions
▸ Sapropterin (*Kuvan*®) for the treatment of hyperphenylalaninaemia (HPA) in adults and paediatric patients of all ages with phenylketonuria (PKU) who have been shown to be responsive to such treatment (August 2018) SMC No. 558/09 Not recommended

- **MEDICINAL FORMS** There can be variation in the licensing of different medicines containing the same drug.
Soluble tablet
CAUTIONARY AND ADVISORY LABELS 13, 21
▸ Kuvan (BioMarin Europe Ltd)
  Sapropterin dihydrochloride 100 mg Kuvan 100mg soluble tablets sugar-free | 30 tablet PoM £597.22

6   Vitamin deficiency

Vitamins

Overview

Vitamins are used for the prevention and treatment of specific deficiency states or where the diet is known to be inadequate; they may be prescribed in the NHS to prevent or treat deficiency but not as dietary supplements.

Their use as general 'pick-me-ups' is of unproven value and, in the case of preparations containing vitamin A or D, may actually be harmful if patients take more than the prescribed dose. The 'fad' for mega-vitamin therapy with water-soluble vitamins, such as ascorbic acid p. 1132 and pyridoxine hydrochloride p. 1130, is unscientific and can be harmful.

Dietary reference values for vitamins are available in the Department of Health publication:

Dietary Reference Values for Food Energy and Nutrients for the United Kingdom: Report of the Panel on Dietary Reference Values of the Committee on Medical Aspects of Food Policy. *Report on Health and Social Subjects* 41. London: HMSO, 1991.

Dental patients

It is unjustifiable to treat stomatitis or glossitis with mixtures of vitamin preparations; this delays diagnosis and correct treatment.

Most patients who develop a nutritional deficiency despite an adequate intake of vitamins have malabsorption and if this is suspected the patient should be referred to a medical practitioner.

Vitamin A

Deficiency of vitamin A (retinol) p. 1129 is associated with ocular defects (particularly xerophthalmia) and an increased susceptibility to infections, but deficiency is rare in the UK (even in disorders of fat absorption).

Vitamin B group

Deficiency of the B vitamins, other than vitamin B_{12}, is rare in the UK and is usually treated by preparations containing thiamine (B_1) p. 1130, riboflavin (B_2), and nicotinamide p. 1316, which is used in preference to nicotinic acid p. 215, as it does not cause vasodilatation. Other members (or substances traditionally classified as members) of the vitamin B complex such as aminobenzoic acid, biotin, choline, inositol nicotinate p. 248, and pantothenic acid or panthenol may be included in vitamin B preparations but there is no evidence of their value.

The severe deficiency states Wernicke's encephalopathy and Korsakoff's psychosis, especially as seen in chronic alcoholism, are best treated initially by the parenteral administration of B vitamins (*Pabrinex*®), followed by oral administration of thiamine in the longer term. Anaphylaxis has been reported with parenteral B vitamins.

As with other vitamins of the B group, pyridoxine hydrochloride (B_6) deficiency is rare, but it may occur during isoniazid therapy p. 624 or penicillamine treatment p. 1146 in Wilson's disease and is characterised by peripheral neuritis. High doses of pyridoxine hydrochloride are given in some metabolic disorders, such as hyperoxaluria, and it is

9

Blood and nutrition

also used in sideroblastic anaemia. There is evidence to suggest that pyridoxine hydrochloride may provide some benefit in premenstrual syndrome. It has been tried for a wide variety of other disorders, but there is little sound evidence to support the claims of efficacy.

Nicotinic acid inhibits the synthesis of cholesterol and triglyceride. Folic acid p. 1071 and vitamin B_{12} are used in the treatment of megaloblastic anaemia. Folinic acid p. 984 (available as calcium folinate) is used in association with cytotoxic therapy.

Vitamin C

Vitamin C (ascorbic acid) therapy is essential in scurvy, but less florid manifestations of vitamin C deficiency are commonly found, especially in the elderly.

Severe scurvy causes gingival swelling and bleeding margins as well as petechiae on the skin. This is, however, exceedingly rare and a patient with these signs is more likely to have leukaemia. Investigation should not be delayed by a trial period of vitamin treatment.

Claims that vitamin C ameliorates colds or promotes wound healing have not been proven.

Vitamin D

The term Vitamin D is used for a range of compounds which possess the property of preventing or curing rickets. They include ergocalciferol (calciferol, vitamin D_2) p. 1136, colecalciferol (vitamin D_3) p. 1133, dihydrotachysterol p. 1136, alfacalcidol (1α-hydroxycholecalciferol) p. 1132, and calcitriol (1,25-dihydroxycholecalciferol) p. 1133.

Simple vitamin D deficiency can be prevented by taking an oral supplement of ergocalciferol (calciferol, vitamin D_2) or colecalciferol (vitamin D_3) daily. Vitamin D deficiency can occur in people whose exposure to sunlight is limited and in those whose diet is deficient in vitamin D. In these individuals, ergocalciferol or colecalciferol daily by mouth may be given to treat vitamin D deficiency; higher doses may be necessary for *severe* deficiency. Patients who do not respond should be referred to a specialist.

Preparations containing colecalciferol with calcium carbonate p. 1135 are available for the management of combined calcium and vitamin D deficiency, or for those at high risk of deficiency.

Vitamin D deficiency caused by *intestinal malabsorption* or *chronic liver disease* usually requires vitamin D in pharmacological doses.

Vitamin D requires hydroxylation by the kidney to its active form, therefore the hydroxylated derivatives alfacalcidol or calcitriol should be prescribed if patients with *severe renal impairment* require vitamin D therapy. Calcitriol is also licensed for the management of postmenopausal osteoporosis.

Paricalcitol p. 1137, a synthetic vitamin D analogue, is licensed for the prevention and treatment of secondary hyperparathyroidism associated with chronic kidney disease.

Vitamin E

The daily requirement of vitamin E (tocopherol) has not been well defined but is probably 3 to 15 mg daily. There is little evidence that oral supplements of vitamin E are essential in adults, even where there is fat malabsorption secondary to cholestasis. In young children with congenital cholestasis, abnormally low vitamin E concentrations may be found in association with neuromuscular abnormalities, which usually respond only to the parenteral administration of vitamin E.

Vitamin E has been tried for various other conditions but there is little scientific evidence of its value.

Vitamin K

Vitamin K is necessary for the production of blood clotting factors and proteins necessary for the normal calcification of bone.

Because vitamin K is fat soluble, patients with fat malabsorption, especially in biliary obstruction or hepatic disease, may become deficient. Menadiol sodium phosphate p. 1138 is a water-soluble synthetic vitamin K derivative that can be given orally to prevent vitamin K deficiency in malabsorption syndromes.

Oral coumarin anticoagulants act by interfering with vitamin K metabolism in the hepatic cells and their effects can be antagonised by giving vitamin K.

Other compounds

Potassium aminobenzoate p. 1129 has been used in the treatment of various disorders associated with excessive fibrosis such as scleroderma and Peyronie's disease. In Peyronie's disease there is some evidence to support efficacy in reducing progression when given early in the disease; however, there is no evidence for reversal of the condition. The therapeutic value of potassium aminobenzoate p. 1129 in scleroderma is doubtful.

VITAMINS AND TRACE ELEMENTS >
MULTIVITAMINS

| Vitamins A and D
01-Dec-2020

The properties listed below are those particular to the combination only. For the properties of the components please consider, vitamin A p. 1129, colecalciferol p. 1133.

● **INDICATIONS AND DOSE**

Prevention of vitamin A and D deficiency (using 4000 units vitamin A/400 units vitamin D capsules)
▸ BY MOUTH
▹ Child: 1 capsule daily
▹ Adult: (consult product literature)

Prevention of vitamin A and D deficiency (using 4500 units vitamin A/450 units vitamin D_3 capsules)
▸ BY MOUTH
▹ Child 7–17 years: 1 capsule daily, increased if necessary to 2 capsules daily, dose increase to be guided by serum values
▹ Adult: 1 capsule daily, increased if necessary to 2 capsules daily, dose increase to be guided by serum values

DOSE EQUIVALENCE AND CONVERSION
▸ Each 4000 units vitamin A/400 units vitamin D capsule (vitamins A and D capsules BPC 1973) contains the equivalent of 10 micrograms vitamin D.
▸ Each 4500 units vitamin A/450 units vitamin D_3 capsule contains the equivalent of 11 micrograms vitamin D_3.

● **UNLICENSED USE**
▸ In children Vitamins A and D capsules BPC 1973 may be used in children under the age of 6 months for the prevention of vitamin A and D deficiency, but it is not licensed for this age group.

● INTERACTIONS → Appendix 1: vitamin A · vitamin D substances

● SIDE-EFFECTS

Overdose Prolonged excessive ingestion of vitamins A and D can lead to hypervitaminosis.

● BREAST FEEDING Manufacturer advises avoid—present in milk.

● PRESCRIBING AND DISPENSING INFORMATION This drug contains vitamin D; consult individual vitamin D monographs.

- MEDICINAL FORMS There can be variation in the licensing of different medicines containing the same drug.

Capsule

EXCIPIENTS: May contain Gelatin

▸ Vitamins a and d (Non-proprietary)

Vitamin D 400 unit, Vitamin A 4000 unit Vitamins A and D capsules BPC 1973 | 28 capsule £2.81 | 84 capsule £8.42 DT = £8.42

Colecalciferol 450 unit, Retinol palmitate 4500 unit Retinol 4,500unit / Colecalciferol 450unit capsules | 84 capsule Ⓟ £25.95

Vitamins A, C and D

05-May-2020

The properties listed below are those particular to the combination only. For the properties of the components please consider, vitamin A below, ascorbic acid p. 1132.

- **INDICATIONS AND DOSE**

Prevention of vitamin deficiency

▸ BY MOUTH

▸ Child 1 month-4 years: 5 drops daily, 5 drops contain vitamin A approx. 700 units, vitamin D approx. 300 units (7.5 micrograms), ascorbic acid approx. 20 mg

- INTERACTIONS → Appendix 1: ascorbic acid · vitamin A
- PRESCRIBING AND DISPENSING INFORMATION This drug contains vitamin D; consult individual vitamin D monographs.

Available free of charge to children under 4 years in families on the Healthy Start Scheme, or alternatively may be available direct to the public—further information for healthcare professionals can be accessed at www.healthystart.nhs.uk. Beneficiaries can contact their midwife or health visitor for further information on where to obtain supplies.

Healthy Start Vitamins for women (containing ascorbic acid, vitamin D, and folic acid) are also available free of charge to women on the Healthy Start Scheme during pregnancy and until their baby is one year old, or alternatively may be available direct to the public—further information for healthcare professionals can be accessed at www.healthystart.nhs.uk. Beneficiaries can contact their midwife or health visitor for further information on where to obtain supplies.

- MEDICINAL FORMS There can be variation in the licensing of different medicines containing the same drug.

Oral drops

▸ Healthy Start Children's Vitamin (Secretary of State for Health)
Vitamin A and D3 concentrate.55 mg per 1 ml, Sodium ascorbate 18.58 mg per 1 ml, Ascorbic acid 150 mg per 1 ml, Vitamin D 2000 iu per 1 ml, Vitamin A 5000 iu per 1 ml Healthy Start Children's Vitamin drops | 10 ml 🅢

VITAMINS AND TRACE ELEMENTS ❭ VITAMIN A

Vitamin A

(Retinol)

- **INDICATIONS AND DOSE**

Vitamin A deficiency

▸ BY MOUTH

▸ Child 1-11 months: 5000 units daily, to be taken with or after food, higher doses may be used initially for treatment of severe deficiency

▸ Child 1-17 years: 10 000 units daily, to be taken with or after food, higher doses may be used initially for treatment of severe deficiency

- UNLICENSED USE Preparations containing only vitamin A are not licensed.
- INTERACTIONS → Appendix 1: vitamin A

- SIDE-EFFECTS

Overdose Massive overdose can cause rough skin, dry hair, an enlarged liver, and increases in erythrocyte sedimentation rate, serum calcium and serum alkaline phosphatase concentration.

- PREGNANCY Excessive doses may be teratogenic. In view of evidence suggesting that high levels of vitamin A may cause birth defects, women who are (or may become) pregnant are advised not to take vitamin A supplements (including tablets and fish liver oil drops), except on the advice of a doctor or an antenatal clinic; nor should they eat liver or products such as liver paté or liver sausage.
- BREAST FEEDING Theoretical risk of toxicity in infants of mothers taking large doses.
- MONITORING REQUIREMENTS Treatment is sometimes initiated with very high doses of vitamin A and the child should be monitored closely; very high doses are associated with acute toxicity.

- MEDICINAL FORMS There can be variation in the licensing of different medicines containing the same drug. Forms available from special-order manufacturers include: oral drops

Oral drops

▸ Arovit (Imported (Italy))
Vitamin A 150000 unit per 1 ml Arovit 150,000units/ml drops | 7.5 ml PoM 🅢

Combinations available: *Vitamins A and D*, p. 1128 · *Vitamins A, C and D*, above

VITAMINS AND TRACE ELEMENTS ❭ VITAMIN B GROUP

Potassium aminobenzoate

30-Apr-2020

- **INDICATIONS AND DOSE**

Peyronie's disease | Scleroderma

▸ BY MOUTH

▸ Adult: 12 g daily in divided doses, to be taken after food

- CONTRA-INDICATIONS Hyperkalaemia · severe liver damage
- CAUTIONS Interrupt treatment during periods of low food intake (such as fasting, anorexia and nausea)—increased risk of hypoglycaemia
- INTERACTIONS → Appendix 1: potassium aminobenzoate
- SIDE-EFFECTS Hepatitis · hypoglycaemia
- PREGNANCY Manufacturer advises avoid—limited information available.
- BREAST FEEDING Manufacturer advises unknown if excreted in milk—risk to infant cannot be excluded.
- RENAL IMPAIRMENT Manufacturer advises use with caution—increased risk of hyperkalaemia; avoid if GFR less than 45 mL/minute.
- MONITORING REQUIREMENTS Manufacturer advises liver function tests should be performed monthly—discontinue immediately if elevated.

- MEDICINAL FORMS There can be variation in the licensing of different medicines containing the same drug.

Powder

CAUTIONARY AND ADVISORY LABELS 13, 21

▸ Potaba (Neon Healthcare Ltd)
Potassium aminobenzoate 3 gram Potaba 3g sachets | 40 sachet PoM £34.31 DT = £34.31

9

Blood and nutrition

Pyridoxine hydrochloride

(Vitamin B$_6$)

● **INDICATIONS AND DOSE**

Deficiency states
▶ BY MOUTH
▸ Adult: 20–50 mg 1–3 times a day

Isoniazid-induced neuropathy (prophylaxis)
▶ BY MOUTH
▸ Adult: 10–20 mg daily

Isoniazid-induced neuropathy (treatment)
▶ BY MOUTH
▸ Adult: 50 mg 3 times a day

Idiopathic sideroblastic anaemia
▶ BY MOUTH
▸ Adult: 100–400 mg daily in divided doses

Prevention of penicillamine-induced neuropathy in Wilson's disease
▶ BY MOUTH
▸ Adult: 20 mg daily

Premenstrual syndrome
▶ BY MOUTH
▸ Adult: 50–100 mg daily

● UNLICENSED USE Not licensed for prophylaxis of penicillamine-induced neuropathy in Wilson's disease. Not licensed for treatment of premenstrual syndrome.

┌──┐
IMPORTANT SAFETY INFORMATION
Prolonged use of pyridoxine in a dose of 10 mg daily is considered safe but the long-term use of pyridoxine in a dose of 200 mg or more daily has been associated with neuropathy. The safety of long-term pyridoxine supplementation with doses above 10 mg daily has not been established.
└──┘

● SIDE-EFFECTS Peripheral neuritis
Overdose Overdosage induces toxic effects.

● MEDICINAL FORMS There can be variation in the licensing of different medicines containing the same drug. Forms available from special-order manufacturers include: capsule, oral suspension, oral solution

Tablet
▶ Pyridoxine hydrochloride (Non-proprietary)
  Pyridoxine hydrochloride 10 mg Pyridoxine 10mg tablets | 28 tablet [PoM] £16.98–£18.25 DT = £16.98 | 500 tablet £15.99
  Pyridoxine hydrochloride 20 mg Pyridoxine 20mg tablets | 500 tablet [GSL] 🔲
  Pyridoxine hydrochloride 50 mg Pyridoxine 50mg tablets | 28 tablet [PoM] £31.02 DT = £18.90

Oral solution
▶ Pyridoxine hydrochloride (Non-proprietary)
  Pyridoxine hydrochloride 20 mg per 1 ml Apyrid 100mg/5ml oral solution | 100 ml £23.97 DT = £23.88
▶ PyriDose (TriOn Pharma Ltd)
  Pyridoxine hydrochloride 20 mg per 1 ml PyriDose 100mg/5ml oral solution | 100 ml £23.88 DT = £23.88

Capsule
▶ Pyridoxine hydrochloride (Non-proprietary)
  Pyridoxine hydrochloride 100 mg Vitamin B6 100mg capsules | 100 capsule 🔲 | 120 capsule £5.50

Thiamine

(Vitamin B$_1$)

28-Nov-2019

● **INDICATIONS AND DOSE**

Mild deficiency
▶ BY MOUTH
▸ Adult: 25–100 mg daily

Severe deficiency
▶ BY MOUTH
▸ Adult: 200–300 mg daily in divided doses

┌──┐
IMPORTANT SAFETY INFORMATION
MHRA/CHM ADVICE (SEPTEMBER 2007)
Although potentially serious allergic adverse reactions may rarely occur during, or shortly after, parenteral administration, the CHM has recommended that:
● This should not preclude the use of parenteral thiamine in patients where this route of administration is required, particularly in patients at risk of Wernicke-Korsakoff syndrome where treatment with thiamine is essential;
● Intravenous administration should be by infusion over 30 minutes;
● Facilities for treating anaphylaxis (including resuscitation facilities) should be available when parenteral thiamine is administered.
└──┘

● BREAST FEEDING Severely thiamine-deficient mothers should avoid breast-feeding as toxic methyl-glyoxal present in milk.

● MEDICINAL FORMS There can be variation in the licensing of different medicines containing the same drug. Forms available from special-order manufacturers include: oral suspension, oral solution

Modified-release tablet
▶ Athiam (Essential-Healthcare Ltd)
  Thiamine hydrochloride 100 mg Athiam 100mg sustained release tablets | 30 tablet £37.89

Tablet
▶ Thiamine (Non-proprietary)
  Thiamine hydrochloride 25 mg Vitamin B1 25mg tablets | 100 tablet [P] 🔲
  Thiamine hydrochloride 50 mg Thiamine 50mg tablets | 28 tablet [P] £1.34–£1.85 | 100 tablet [P] £6.72 DT = £4.80
  Thiamine hydrochloride 100 mg Thiamine 100mg tablets | 28 tablet [P] £1.89–£6.72 | 100 tablet [P] £11.55 DT = £6.76
▶ Benerva (Teofarma)
  Thiamine hydrochloride 50 mg Benerva 50mg tablets | 100 tablet [P] £4.00 DT = £4.80
  Thiamine hydrochloride 100 mg Benerva 100mg tablets | 100 tablet [P] £6.29 DT = £6.76

Oral solution
▶ Athiam (Essential-Healthcare Ltd)
  Thiamine hydrochloride 20 mg per 1 ml Athiam 100mg/5ml oral solution | 100 ml £23.97 DT = £58.41

Vitamin B complex

01-May-2020

● **INDICATIONS AND DOSE**

Treatment of deficiency
▶ BY MOUTH USING TABLETS
▸ Adult: 1–2 tablets 3 times a day, this dose is for vitamin B compound **strong** tablets

Prophylaxis of deficiency
▶ BY MOUTH USING TABLETS
▸ Adult: 1–3 tablets daily, this dose is for vitamin B compound tablets

● LESS SUITABLE FOR PRESCRIBING Vitamin B compound tablets and vitamin B compound strong tablets are less suitable for prescribing.

● MEDICINAL FORMS There can be variation in the licensing of different medicines containing the same drug.

Tablet
▶ Vitamin b complex (Non-proprietary)
  Riboflavin 1 mg, Thiamine hydrochloride 1 mg, Nicotinamide 15 mg Vitamin B compound tablets | 28 tablet [P] £21.30 DT = £26.63

Pyridoxine hydrochloride 2 mg, Riboflavin 2 mg, Thiamine hydrochloride 5 mg, Nicotinamide 20 mg Vitamin B compound strong tablets | 28 tablet P 🔄 DT = £1.84

Vitamin B substances with ascorbic acid

29-Jul-2020

The properties listed below are those particular to the combination only. For the properties of the components please consider, thiamine p. 1130, ascorbic acid p. 1132.

● **INDICATIONS AND DOSE**

Severe depletion or malabsorption of vitamins B and C postoperatively

▸ BY INTRAVENOUS INFUSION, OR BY DEEP INTRAMUSCULAR INJECTION

▸ Adult: (consult product literature)

Treatment of suspected or established Wernicke's encephalopathy

▸ BY INTRAVENOUS INFUSION

▸ Adult: 2–3 pairs 3 times a day for 3–5 days, followed by 1 pair once daily for a further 3–5 days or for as long as improvement continues

Prophylaxis of Wernicke's encephalopathy [assisted alcohol withdrawal in an inpatient setting]

▸ BY DEEP INTRAMUSCULAR INJECTION

▸ Adult: 1 pair once daily for at least 5 days and up to 7 days if required, give into the gluteal muscle

Severe depletion or malabsorption of vitamins B and C in psychosis following narcosis or electroconvulsive therapy | Severe depletion or malabsorption of vitamins B and C following toxicity from acute infections

▸ BY INTRAVENOUS INFUSION, OR BY DEEP INTRAMUSCULAR INJECTION

▸ Adult: 1 pair twice daily for up to 7 days, give deep intramuscular injection into the gluteal muscle

Severe depletion or malabsorption of vitamins B and C in haemodialysis

▸ BY INTRAVENOUS INFUSION

▸ Adult: 1 pair every 2 weeks

DOSE EQUIVALENCE AND CONVERSION

▸ Dose is expressed in pairs of ampoules.

▸ For *intravenous* administration, 1 pair is one 5 mL ampoule containing thiamine 250 mg, riboflavin 4 mg and pyridoxine 50 mg, and one 5 mL ampoule containing ascorbic acid 500 mg, nicotinamide 160 mg and glucose 1000 mg.

▸ For *intramuscular* administration, 1 pair is one 5 mL ampoule containing thiamine 250 mg, riboflavin 4 mg and pyridoxine 50 mg, and one 2 mL ampoule containing ascorbic acid 500 mg and nicotinamide 160 mg.

● UNLICENSED USE Vitamin B substances with ascorbic acid may be used as detailed below, although these situations are considered outside the scope of its licence:

● EvGr durations and further dosing for treatment of suspected or established Wernicke's encephalopathy

● prophylaxis of Wernicke's encephalopathy ◈

● INTERACTIONS → Appendix 1: ascorbic acid

● DIRECTIONS FOR ADMINISTRATION Manufacturer advises give (*Pabrinex*® I/V High Potency) intermittently *or via* drip tubing in Glucose 5% *or* Sodium chloride 0.9%. Manufacturer advises ampoules contents should be mixed, diluted, and administered without delay; give over 30 minutes. See MHRA/CHM advice in thiamine p. 1130.

● PRESCRIBING AND DISPENSING INFORMATION Some formulations of *Pabrinex*® may contain benzyl alcohol (avoid in neonates). *Pabrinex*® I/M High Potency injection

is for intramuscular use only. *Pabrinex*® I/V High Potency injection is for intravenous use only.

● MEDICINAL FORMS There can be variation in the licensing of different medicines containing the same drug.

Solution for Injection

EXCIPIENTS: May contain Benzyl alcohol

▸ Pabrinex Intramuscular High Potency (Kyowa Kirin Ltd) Pabrinex Intramuscular High Potency solution for injection 5ml and 2ml ampoules | 20 ampoule PoM £22.53 DT = £22.53

▸ Pabrinex Intravenous High Potency (Kyowa Kirin Ltd) Pabrinex Intravenous High Potency solution for injection 5ml and 5ml ampoules | 12 ampoule PoM £16.23

Vitamins with minerals and trace elements

13-May-2020

● **INDICATIONS AND DOSE**

FORCEVAL® CAPSULES

Vitamin and mineral deficiency and as adjunct in synthetic diets

▸ BY MOUTH

▸ Adult: 1 capsule daily, one hour after a meal

KETOVITE® LIQUID

Prevention of vitamin deficiency in disorders of carbohydrate or amino-acid metabolism | Adjunct in restricted, specialised, or synthetic diets

▸ BY MOUTH

▸ Adult: 5 mL daily, use with *Ketovite*® *Tablets* for complete vitamin supplementation.

KETOVITE® TABLETS

Prevention of vitamin deficiency in disorders of carbohydrate or amino-acid metabolism | Adjunct in restricted, specialised, or synthetic diets

▸ BY MOUTH

▸ Adult: 1 tablet 3 times a day, use with *Ketovite*® *Liquid* for complete vitamin supplementation.

● PRESCRIBING AND DISPENSING INFORMATION To avoid potential toxicity, the content of all vitamin preparations, particularly vitamin A, should be considered when used together with other supplements.

● PATIENT AND CARER ADVICE

KETOVITE® LIQUID *Ketovite*® liquid may be mixed with milk, cereal, or fruit juice.

KETOVITE® TABLETS Tablets may be crushed immediately before use.

● MEDICINAL FORMS There can be variation in the licensing of different medicines containing the same drug.

Oral emulsion

▸ Ketovite (Essential Pharmaceuticals Ltd) Cyanocobalamin 2.5 microgram per 1 ml, Choline chloride 30 mg per 1 ml, Ergocalciferol 80 unit per 1 ml, Vitamin A 500 unit per 1 ml Ketovite liquid sugar-free | 150 ml P £119.10

Tablet

▸ Ketovite (Essential Pharmaceuticals Ltd) Biotin 170 microgram, Folic acid 250 microgram, Pyridoxine hydrochloride 330 microgram, Acetomenaphthone 500 microgram, Riboflavin 1 mg, Thiamine hydrochloride 1 mg, Calcium pantothenate 1.16 mg, Nicotinamide 3.3 mg, Alpha tocopheryl acetate 5 mg, Ascorbic acid 16.6 mg, Inositol 50 mg Ketovite tablets | 100 tablet £28.77

Capsule

▸ Forceval (Forum Health Products Ltd) Cyanocobalamin 3 microgram, Selenium 50 microgram, Biotin 100 microgram, Iodine 140 microgram, Chromium 200 microgram, Molybdenum 250 microgram, Folic acid 400 microgram, Thiamine 1.2 mg, Riboflavin 1.6 mg, Copper 2 mg, Pyridoxine 2 mg, Manganese 3 mg, Pantothenic acid 4 mg, Potassium 4 mg, Tocopheryl acetate 10 mg, Iron 12 mg, Zinc

9

Blood and nutrition

15 mg, Nicotinamide 18 mg, Magnesium 30 mg, Ascorbic acid
60 mg, Phosphorus 77 mg, Calcium 100 mg, Ergocalciferol
400 unit, Vitamin A 2500 unit Forceval capsules | 15 capsule [P]
£5.46 | 30 capsule [P] £9.92 | 90 capsule [P] £28.77

VITAMINS AND TRACE ELEMENTS > VITAMIN C

Ascorbic acid

08-Jul-2019

(Vitamin C)

● **INDICATIONS AND DOSE**

Prevention of scurvy
▸ BY MOUTH
  ▸ Adult: 25–75 mg daily

Treatment of scurvy
▸ BY MOUTH
  ▸ Adult: Not less than 250 mg daily in divided doses

● CONTRA-INDICATIONS Hyperoxaluria

● CAUTIONS
▸ Iron overload Ascorbic acid should not be given to patients
  with cardiac dysfunction.
    In patients with normal cardiac function ascorbic acid
  should be introduced 1 month after starting
  desferrioxamine.

● INTERACTIONS → Appendix 1: ascorbic acid

● SIDE-EFFECTS Diarrhoea · gastrointestinal disorder ·
  hyperoxaluria · oxalate nephrolithiasis · polyuria

● PRESCRIBING AND DISPENSING INFORMATION It is rarely
  necessary to prescribe more than 100 mg daily except early
  in the treatment of scurvy.

● MEDICINAL FORMS There can be variation in the licensing of
  different medicines containing the same drug. Forms available
  from special-order manufacturers include: tablet, oral
  suspension, oral solution

Tablet
EXCIPIENTS: May contain Aspartame
▸ Ascorbic acid (Non-proprietary)
  Ascorbic acid 50 mg Ascorbic acid 50mg tablets | 28 tablet [GSL]
  £15.08 DT = £15.08
  Ascorbic acid 100 mg Ascorbic acid 100mg tablets | 28 tablet [GSL]
  £14.30 DT = £14.30
  Ascorbic acid 200 mg Ascorbic acid 200mg tablets | 28 tablet [GSL]
  £19.88 DT = £19.88
  Ascorbic acid 250 mg Ascorbic acid 250mg tablets |
  1000 tablet [PoM] [↯]
  Ascorbic acid 500 mg Ascorbic acid 500mg tablets | 28 tablet [GSL]
  £26.89 DT = £26.89

Chewable tablet
CAUTIONARY AND ADVISORY LABELS 24
EXCIPIENTS: May contain Aspartame
▸ Ascur (Ennogen Healthcare Ltd)
  Ascorbic acid 100 mg Ascur 100mg chewable tablets | 30 tablet
  £3.95
  Ascorbic acid (as Sodium ascorbate) 500 mg Ascur 500mg
  chewable tablets sugar-free | 30 tablet £2.99

Capsule
▸ BioCare (BioCare Ltd)
  Ascorbic acid 500 mg BioCare Vitamin C 500mg capsules |
  60 capsule £7.73 | 180 capsule £19.82

Combinations available: *Vitamin B substances with ascorbic
acid,* p. 1131 · *Vitamins A, C and D,* p. 1129

VITAMINS AND TRACE ELEMENTS > VITAMIN D AND ANALOGUES

Vitamin D and analogues (systemic)

● CONTRA-INDICATIONS Hypercalcaemia · metastatic
  calcification

● SIDE-EFFECTS
▸ **Common or very common** Abdominal pain · headache ·
  hypercalcaemia · hypercalciuria · nausea · skin reactions
▸ **Uncommon** Appetite decreased · arrhythmia · asthenia ·
  constipation · diarrhoea · hypertension · myalgia · thirst ·
  vomiting · weight decreased
▸ **Frequency not known** Polyuria

Overdose Symptoms of overdosage include anorexia,
lassitude, nausea and vomiting, diarrhoea, constipation,
weight loss, polyuria, sweating, headache, thirst, vertigo,
and raised concentrations of calcium and phosphate in
plasma and urine.

● PREGNANCY High doses teratogenic in *animals* but
  therapeutic doses unlikely to be harmful.

● BREAST FEEDING Caution with high doses; may cause
  hypercalcaemia in infant—monitor serum-calcium
  concentration.

● MONITORING REQUIREMENTS **Important**: all patients
  receiving pharmacological doses of vitamin D should have
  their plasma-calcium concentration checked at intervals
  (initially once or twice weekly) and whenever nausea or
  vomiting occur.

⚑ above

Alfacalcidol

22-Jul-2020

(1α-Hydroxycholecalciferol)

● **INDICATIONS AND DOSE**

**Patients with severe renal impairment requiring vitamin
D therapy**
▸ BY MOUTH, OR BY INTRAVENOUS INJECTION
  ▸ Adult: Initially 1 microgram daily, dose to be adjusted
    to avoid hypercalcaemia; maintenance
    0.25–1 microgram daily
  ▸ Elderly: Initially 500 nanograms daily, dose adjusted to
    avoid hypercalcaemia; maintenance 0.25–1 microgram
    daily

**Hypophosphataemic rickets | Persistent hypocalcaemia
due to hypoparathyroidism or
pseudohypoparathyroidism**
▸ BY MOUTH, OR BY INTRAVENOUS INJECTION
  ▸ Child 1 month-11 years: 25–50 nanograms/kg once daily,
    dose to be adjusted as necessary; maximum
    1 microgram per day
  ▸ Child 12-17 years: 1 microgram once daily, dose to be
    adjusted as necessary

**Prevention of vitamin D deficiency in renal or cholestatic
liver disease**
▸ BY MOUTH, OR BY INTRAVENOUS INJECTION
  ▸ Child 1 month-11 years (body-weight up to 20 kg):
    15–30 nanograms/kg once daily (max. per dose
    500 nanograms)
  ▸ Child 1 month-11 years (body-weight 20 kg and above):
    250–500 nanograms once daily, dose to be adjusted as
    necessary
  ▸ Child 12-17 years: 250–500 nanograms once daily, dose
    to be adjusted as necessary

DOSE EQUIVALENCE AND CONVERSION
▸ One drop of alfacalcidol 2 microgram/mL oral drops
  contains approximately 100 nanograms alfacalcidol.

● CAUTIONS Nephrolithiasis · take care to ensure correct
  dose in infants

● INTERACTIONS → Appendix 1: vitamin D substances

● SIDE-EFFECTS
▸ **Common or very common** Abdominal discomfort ·
  hyperphosphataemia · rash pustular
▸ **Uncommon** Malaise · urolithiases
▸ **Rare or very rare** Dizziness
▸ **Frequency not known** Confusion · renal impairment

- RENAL IMPAIRMENT
Monitoring Monitor plasma-calcium concentration in renal impairment.
- MONITORING REQUIREMENTS Monitor plasma-calcium concentration in patients receiving high doses.
- DIRECTIONS FOR ADMINISTRATION
▶ With intravenous use For *injection*, manufacturer advises shake ampoule for at least 5 seconds before use, and give over 30 seconds.

- MEDICINAL FORMS There can be variation in the licensing of different medicines containing the same drug. Forms available from special-order manufacturers include: oral suspension, oral solution

Solution for injection
EXCIPIENTS: May contain Alcohol, propylene glycol
▶ One-Alpha (LEO Pharma)
Alfacalcidol 2 microgram per 1 ml One-Alpha 2micrograms/1ml solution for injection ampoules | 10 ampoule PoM £41.13
One-Alpha 1micrograms/0.5ml solution for injection ampoules | 10 ampoule PoM £21.57
Oral drops
EXCIPIENTS: May contain Alcohol
▶ One-Alpha (LEO Pharma)
Alfacalcidol 2 microgram per 1 ml One-Alpha 2micrograms/ml oral drops sugar-free | 10 ml PoM £21.30 DT = £21.30
Capsule
EXCIPIENTS: May contain Sesame oil
▶ Alfacalcidol (Non-proprietary)
Alfacalcidol 250 nanogram Alfacalcidol 250nanogram capsules | 30 capsule PoM £5.00 DT = £4.93
AlfacalEss 0.25microgram capsules | 30 capsule £1.29 DT = £4.93
Alfacalcidol 500 nanogram Alfacalcidol 500nanogram capsules | 30 capsule PoM £10.00 DT = £9.90
Alfacalcidol 1 microgram Alfacalcidol 1microgram capsules | 30 capsule ⟨S⟩ DT = £4.10 | 30 capsule PoM £14.00 DT = £4.10
▶ One-Alpha (LEO Pharma)
Alfacalcidol 250 nanogram One-Alpha 250nanogram capsules | 30 capsule PoM £3.37 DT = £4.93
Alfacalcidol 500 nanogram One-Alpha 0.5microgram capsules | 30 capsule PoM £6.27 DT = £9.90
Alfacalcidol 1 microgram One-Alpha 1microgram capsules | 30 capsule PoM £8.75 DT = £4.10

F 1132

Calcitriol
12-Oct-2020

(1,25-Dihydroxycholecalciferol)

- INDICATIONS AND DOSE
Renal osteodystrophy
▶ BY MOUTH
▶ Adult: Initially 250 nanograms daily, adjusted in steps of 250 nanograms every 2–4 weeks if required; usual dose 0.5–1 microgram daily
Renal osteodystrophy (in patients with normal or only slightly reduced plasma-calcium concentration)
▶ BY MOUTH
▶ Adult: Initially 250 nanograms once daily on alternate days, adjusted in steps of 250 nanograms every 2–4 weeks if required; usual dose 0.5–1 microgram daily
Established postmenopausal osteoporosis
▶ BY MOUTH
▶ Adult: 250 nanograms twice daily, plasma-calcium concentration and creatinine to be monitored (consult product literature)

- INTERACTIONS → Appendix 1: vitamin D substances
- SIDE-EFFECTS
▶ **Common or very common** Urinary tract infection
▶ **Frequency not known** Abdominal pain upper · apathy · dehydration · drowsiness · fever · growth retardation · muscle weakness · nocturia · paralytic ileus · polydipsia · psychiatric disorder · sensory disorder

- RENAL IMPAIRMENT Manufacturer advises avoid—no information available.
Monitoring Monitor plasma-calcium concentration in renal impairment.
- MONITORING REQUIREMENTS
▶ Monitor plasma calcium, phosphate, and creatinine during dosage titration.
▶ Monitor plasma-calcium concentration in patients receiving high doses.

- MEDICINAL FORMS There can be variation in the licensing of different medicines containing the same drug. Forms available from special-order manufacturers include: oral suspension, oral solution

Oral solution
▶ Rocaltrol (Imported (Switzerland))
Calcitriol 1 microgram per 1 ml Rocaltrol 1micrograms/ml oral solution sugar-free | 10 ml PoM ⟨S⟩
Capsule
▶ Calcitriol (Non-proprietary)
Calcitriol 250 nanogram Calcitriol 250nanogram capsules | 30 capsule PoM £5.41-£18.04
Calcitriol 500 nanogram Calcitriol 500nanogram capsules | 30 capsule PoM £11.93-£32.25
▶ Rocaltrol (Atnahs Pharma UK Ltd)
Calcitriol 250 nanogram Rocaltrol 250nanogram capsules | 100 capsule PoM £18.04 DT = £18.04
Calcitriol 500 nanogram Rocaltrol 500nanogram capsules | 100 capsule PoM £32.25 DT = £32.25

F 1132

Colecalciferol
13-Aug-2020

(Cholecalciferol; Vitamin D_3)

- INDICATIONS AND DOSE
Prevention of vitamin D deficiency
▶ BY MOUTH
▶ Adult: 400 units daily
Treatment of vitamin D deficiency
▶ BY MOUTH
▶ Adult: 800 units daily, higher doses may be necessary for severe deficiency

- INTERACTIONS → Appendix 1: vitamin D substances
- SIDE-EFFECTS Laryngeal oedema
- RENAL IMPAIRMENT
Monitoring Monitor plasma-calcium concentration in renal impairment.
- MONITORING REQUIREMENTS Monitor plasma-calcium concentration in patients receiving high doses.
- DIRECTIONS FOR ADMINISTRATION
INVITA D3 ® ORAL SOLUTION Manufacturer advises may be mixed with a small amount of cold or lukewarm food immediately before administration.

- MEDICINAL FORMS There can be variation in the licensing of different medicines containing the same drug. Forms available from special-order manufacturers include: tablet, capsule, oral suspension, oral solution, oral drops

Tablet
▶ Colecalciferol (Non-proprietary)
Colecalciferol 400 unit Colecalciferol 400unit tablets | 60 tablet £15.50
Colecalciferol 800 unit Colecalciferol 800unit tablets | 30 tablet PoM £4.59 DT = £4.59
Colecalciferol 5000 unit Vitamin D3 High Strength 5,000unit tablets | 60 tablet £5.50
▶ Aciferol D3 (Rhodes Pharma Ltd)
Colecalciferol 2200 unit Aciferol D3 2,200unit tablets | 90 tablet £25.99
Colecalciferol 3000 unit Aciferol D3 3,000unit tablets | 60 tablet £14.99
Colecalciferol 5000 unit Aciferol D3 5,000unit tablets | 60 tablet £19.99

9

Blood and nutrition

Colecalciferol 10000 unit Aciferol D3 10,000unit tablets | 30 tablet £13.99
Colecalciferol 20000 unit Aciferol D3 20,000unit tablets | 30 tablet £18.99

▸ Desunin (Mylan)
Colecalciferol 800 unit Desunin 800unit tablets | 30 tablet [PoM] £3.60 DT = £4.59 | 90 tablet [PoM] £10.17
Colecalciferol 4000 unit Desunin 4,000unit tablets | 70 tablet [PoM] £15.90 DT = £15.90

▸ E-D3 (Ennogen Healthcare Ltd)
Colecalciferol 400 unit E-D3 400unit tablets | 30 tablet £78.50
Colecalciferol 10000 unit E-D3 10,000unit tablets | 30 tablet £95.00
Colecalciferol 20000 unit E-D3 20,000unit tablets | 30 tablet £95.90

▸ Iso D3 (Nutri Advanced Ltd)
Colecalciferol 2000 unit Vitamin D3 + Isoflavones 2,000unit tablets | 90 tablet £18.43

▸ Stexerol-D3 (Kyowa Kirin Ltd)
Colecalciferol 1000 unit Stexerol-D3 1,000unit tablets | 28 tablet [PoM] £2.95 DT = £2.95
Colecalciferol 25000 unit Stexerol-D3 25,000unit tablets | 12 tablet [PoM] £17.00 DT = £17.00

▸ SunVit D3 (SunVit-D3 Ltd)
Colecalciferol 2000 unit SunVit-D3 2,000unit tablets | 28 tablet £3.99
Colecalciferol 3000 unit SunVit-D3 3,000unit tablets | 28 tablet £5.49
Colecalciferol 5000 unit SunVit-D3 5,000unit tablets | 28 tablet £4.99
Colecalciferol 10000 unit SunVit-D3 10,000unit tablets | 28 tablet £6.99
Colecalciferol 20000 unit SunVit-D3 20,000unit tablets | 28 tablet £4.40
Colecalciferol 50000 unit SunVit-D3 50,000unit tablets | 15 tablet £19.99

Oral drops

▸ Colecalciferol (Non-proprietary)
Colecalciferol 1000 unit per 1 ml Vitamin D3 1,000unit oral drops sugar-free | 30 ml £6.76

▸ Colecalciferol (Imported (Germany))
Colecalciferol 20000 unit per 1 ml Vigantol 20,000units/ml oral drops | 10 ml [⊠]

▸ E-D3 (Ennogen Healthcare Ltd)
Colecalciferol 2000 unit per 1 ml E-D3 2,000units/ml oral drops sugar-free | 20 ml [⊠]

▸ Fultium-D3 (Thornton & Ross Ltd)
Colecalciferol 2740 unit per 1 ml Fultium-D3 2,740units/ml oral drops sugar-free | 25 ml [PoM] £10.70 DT = £10.70

▸ InVita D3 (Consilient Health Ltd)
Colecalciferol 2400 unit per 1 ml InVita D3 2,400units/ml oral drops sugar-free | 10 ml [PoM] £3.60 DT = £3.60

▸ Pro D3 (Synergy Biologics Ltd)
Colecalciferol 2000 unit per 1 ml Pro D3 2,000units/ml liquid drops sugar-free | 20 ml £9.80

▸ SunVit D3 (SunVit-D3 Ltd)
Colecalciferol 2000 unit per 1 ml SunVit-D3 2,000units/ml oral drops sugar-free | 20 ml £6.20

▸ Thorens (Galen Ltd)
Colecalciferol 10000 unit per 1 ml Thorens 10,000units/ml oral drops sugar-free | 10 ml [PoM] £5.85 DT = £5.85

Oral solution

CAUTIONARY AND ADVISORY LABELS 21

▸ Colecalciferol (Non-proprietary)
Colecalciferol 3000 unit per 1 ml Colecalciferol 3,000units/ml oral solution | 100 ml [PoM] £144.00 DT = £144.00

▸ Aciferol D3 (Rhodes Pharma Ltd)
Colecalciferol 2000 unit per 1 ml Aciferol D3 2,000units/ml liquid | 100 ml £18.00

▸ Baby D (KoRa Healthcare)
Colecalciferol 1000 unit per 1 ml BabyD 1,000units/ml oral solution | 30 ml £4.50

▸ E-D3 (Ennogen Healthcare Ltd)
Colecalciferol 1000 unit per 1 ml E-D3 1,000units/ml oral solution | 15 ml [⊠]
Colecalciferol 10000 unit per 1 ml E-D3 10,000units/ml oral solution | 10 ml [⊠]

▸ InVita D3 (Consilient Health Ltd)
Colecalciferol 25000 unit per 1 ml InVita D3 25,000units/1ml oral solution sugar-free | 3 ampoule [PoM] £4.45 DT = £4.45
Colecalciferol 50000 unit per 1 ml InVita D3 50,000units/1ml oral solution sugar-free | 3 ampoule [PoM] £6.25 DT = £6.25

▸ Pro D3 (Synergy Biologics Ltd)
Colecalciferol 2000 unit per 1 ml Pro D3 2,000units/ml liquid | 50 ml £16.80 | 100 ml £22.50

▸ SunVit D3 (SunVit-D3 Ltd)
Colecalciferol 2000 unit per 1 ml SunVit-D3 10,000units/5ml oral solution sugar-free | 50 ml £8.90
SunVit-D3 2,000units/ml oral solution sugar-free | 50 ml £8.90

▸ Thorens (Galen Ltd)
Colecalciferol 10000 unit per 1 ml Thorens 25,000units/2.5ml oral solution sugar-free | 2.5 ml [PoM] £1.55 DT = £1.55 sugar-free | 10 ml [PoM] £5.85 DT = £5.85

Chewable tablet

▸ EveryDay-D (Vega Nutritionals Ltd)
Colecalciferol 400 unit EveryDay-D 400unit chewable tablets | 100 tablet £3.22

▸ Urgent-D (Vega Nutritionals Ltd)
Colecalciferol 2000 unit Urgent-D 2,000unit chewable tablets | 60 tablet £4.31

Capsule

CAUTIONARY AND ADVISORY LABELS 25

▸ Colecalciferol (Non-proprietary)
Colecalciferol 800 unit Colecalciferol 800unit capsules | 30 capsule £2.43 DT = £3.60 | 30 capsule [PoM] £3.60 DT = £3.60
Colecalciferol 1000 unit Colecalciferol 1,000unit capsules | 30 capsule [PoM] £10.00 DT = £10.00
Colecalciferol 2500 unit FSC High Strength Vitamin D3 2,500unit capsules | 60 capsule £1.95
Colecalciferol 3200 unit Strivit-D3 3,200unit capsules | 30 capsule [PoM] £9.32 DT = £13.32
Colecalciferol 5000 unit Colecalciferol 5,000unit capsules | 40 capsule [⊠]
Colecalciferol 10000 unit Colecalciferol 10,000unit capsules | 20 capsule [PoM] £9.99
Colecalciferol 20000 unit Colecalciferol 20,000unit capsules | 10 capsule [PoM] £9.67 | 20 capsule [PoM] £20.50–£27.49 | 30 capsule [PoM] £29.00 DT = £29.00
Colecalciferol 25000 unit Thorens 25,000unit capsules | 3 capsule [PoM] £3.16 DT = £3.95 | 12 capsule [PoM] £13.60

▸ Aciferol D3 (Rhodes Pharma Ltd)
Colecalciferol 30000 unit Aciferol D3 30,000unit capsules | 10 capsule £19.99

▸ Bio-Vitamin D3 (Pharma Nord (UK) Ltd)
Colecalciferol 5000 unit Bio-Vitamin D3 5,000unit capsules | 40 capsule £5.51

▸ Cubicole D3 (Cubic Pharmaceuticals Ltd)
Colecalciferol 600 unit Cubicole D3 600unit capsules | 30 capsule £6.95
Colecalciferol 2200 unit Cubicole D3 2,200unit capsules | 30 capsule £8.95
Colecalciferol 3000 unit Cubicole D3 3,000unit capsules | 30 capsule £9.95
Colecalciferol 50000 unit Cubicole D3 50,000unit capsules | 10 capsule £12.95

▸ D-Max (Nutraconcepts Ltd)
Colecalciferol 5000 unit D-Max 5,000unit capsules | 30 capsule £4.85

▸ E-D3 (Ennogen Healthcare Ltd)
Colecalciferol 600 unit E-D3 600unit capsules | 30 capsule £82.10
Colecalciferol 2200 unit E-D3 2,200unit capsules | 30 capsule £86.20
Colecalciferol 2500 unit E-D3 2,500unit capsules | 30 capsule £86.20
Colecalciferol 3000 unit E-D3 3,000unit capsules | 30 capsule £88.60
Colecalciferol 5000 unit E-D3 5,000unit capsules | 30 capsule £94.00
Colecalciferol 30000 unit E-D3 30,000unit capsules | 10 capsule £94.40

▸ Fultium-D3 (Thornton & Ross Ltd)
Colecalciferol 800 unit Fultium-D3 800unit capsules | 30 capsule [PoM] £3.60 DT = £3.60 | 90 capsule [PoM] £8.85
Colecalciferol 3200 unit Fultium-D3 3,200unit capsules | 30 capsule [PoM] £13.32 DT = £13.32 | 90 capsule [PoM] £39.96

Colecalciferol 20000 unit Fultium-D3 20,000unit capsules |
15 capsule [PoM] £17.04 DT = £17.04 | 30 capsule [PoM] £29.00 DT =
£29.00

▸ InVita D3 (Consilient Health Ltd)
Colecalciferol 400 unit InVita D3 400unit capsules |
28 capsule [PoM] £1.85 DT = £1.85
Colecalciferol 800 unit InVita D3 800unit capsules |
28 capsule [PoM] £2.50
Colecalciferol 5600 unit InVita D3 5,600unit capsules |
4 capsule [PoM] £2.50 DT = £2.50
Colecalciferol 25000 unit InVita D3 25,000unit capsules |
3 capsule [PoM] £3.95 DT = £3.95
Colecalciferol 50000 unit InVita D3 50,000unit capsules |
3 capsule [PoM] £4.95 DT = £4.95

▸ Plenachol (Accord Healthcare Ltd)
Colecalciferol 20000 unit Plenachol D3 20,000unit capsules |
10 capsule [PoM] £9.00
Colecalciferol 40000 unit Plenachol D3 40,000unit capsules |
10 capsule [PoM] £15.00 DT = £15.00

▸ Pro D3 (Synergy Biologics Ltd)
Colecalciferol 2500 unit Pro D3 2,500unit capsules | 30 capsule
£9.99
Colecalciferol 30000 unit Pro D3 30,000unit capsules | 10 capsule
£24.99

▸ Strivit-D3 (Strides Pharma UK Ltd)
Colecalciferol 800 unit Strivit-D3 800unit capsules |
30 capsule [PoM] £2.50 DT = £3.60

▸ SunVit D3 (SunVit-D3 Ltd)
Colecalciferol 2200 unit SunVit-D3 2,200unit capsules | 28 capsule
£4.99
Colecalciferol 2500 unit SunVit-D3 2,500unit capsules | 28 capsule
£5.49

Orodispersible tablet
▸ Colecalciferol (Non-proprietary)
Colecalciferol 2000 unit Vitamin D3 Lemon Melts 2,000unit tablets
sugar-free | 120 tablet £5.39

Combinations available: *Vitamins A and D*, p. 1128

Colecalciferol with calcium carbonate

The properties listed below are those particular to the
combination only. For the properties of the components
please consider, colecalciferol p. 1133, calcium carbonate
p. 1095.

● **INDICATIONS AND DOSE**

**Prevention and treatment of vitamin D and calcium
deficiency**
▸ BY MOUTH
▸ **Adult:** Dosed according to the deficit or daily
maintenance requirements (consult product literature)

● INTERACTIONS → Appendix 1: calcium salts · vitamin D
substances

● PRESCRIBING AND DISPENSING INFORMATION *Accrete D3*®
contains calcium carbonate 1.5 g (calcium 600 mg or Ca^{2+}
15 mmol), colecalciferol 10 micrograms (400 units); *Adcal-
D3*® tablets contain calcium carbonate 1.5 g (calcium
600 mg or Ca^{2+} 15 mmol), colecalciferol 10 micrograms
(400 units); *Cacit*® *D3* contains calcium carbonate 1.25 g
(calcium 500 mg or Ca^{2+} 12.5 mmol), colecalciferol
11 micrograms (440 units)/sachet; *Calceos*® contains
calcium carbonate 1.25 g (calcium 500 mg or Ca^{2+}
12.5 mmol), colecalciferol 10 micrograms (400 units);
Calcichew-D3® tablets contain calcium carbonate 1.25 g
(calcium 500 mg or Ca^{2+} 12.5 mmol), colecalciferol
5 micrograms (200 units); *Calcichew-D3*® *Forte* tablets
contain calcium carbonate 1.25 g (calcium 500 mg or Ca^{2+}
12.5 mmol), colecalciferol 10 micrograms (400 units);
Calcichew-D3® 500 mg/400 unit caplets contain calcium
carbonate (calcium 500 mg or Ca^{2+} 12.5 mmol),
colecalciferol 10 micrograms (400 units); *Kalcipos-D*®
contains calcium carbonate (calcium 500 mg or Ca^{2+}
12.5 mmol), colecalciferol 20 micrograms (800 units);
Natecal D3® contains calcium carbonate 1.5 g (calcium

600 mg or Ca^{2+} 15 mmol), colecalciferol 10 micrograms
(400 units); consult product literature for details of other
available products.
Flavours of chewable and soluble forms may include
orange, lemon, aniseed, peppermint, molasses, or tutti-
frutti.

● MEDICINAL FORMS There can be variation in the licensing of
different medicines containing the same drug.

Effervescent granules
CAUTIONARY AND ADVISORY LABELS 13
▸ Colecalciferol with calcium carbonate (Non-proprietary)
**Calcium carbonate 2.5 gram, Colecalciferol
880 unit** Colecalciferol 880unit / Calcium carbonate 2.5g
effervescent granules sachets | 24 sachet [PoM] 🚫
▸ Cacit D3 (Theramex HQ UK Ltd)
Calcium carbonate 1.25 gram, Colecalciferol 440 unit Cacit D3
effervescent granules sachets | 30 sachet [P] £4.06 DT = £4.06

Tablet
EXCIPIENTS: May contain Propylene glycol
▸ Accrete D3 (Thornton & Ross Ltd)
Calcium carbonate 1.5 gram, Colecalciferol 400 unit Accrete
D3 tablets | 60 tablet [P] £2.95 DT = £2.95
▸ Adcal-D3 (Kyowa Kirin Ltd)
Calcium carbonate 750 mg, Colecalciferol 200 unit Adcal-D3
750mg/200unit caplets | 112 tablet [P] £2.95 DT = £2.95

Effervescent tablet
CAUTIONARY AND ADVISORY LABELS 13
▸ ColeKal-D3 (Essential-Healthcare Ltd)
Calcium carbonate 1.5 gram, Colecalciferol 400 unit ColeKal-D3
Dissolve 400unit/1500mg effervescent tablets | 56 tablet £4.97 DT =
£5.99
▸ Adcal-D3 (Kyowa Kirin Ltd)
Calcium carbonate 1.5 gram, Colecalciferol 400 unit Adcal-D3
Dissolve 1500mg/400unit effervescent tablets | 56 tablet [P] £5.99
DT = £5.99

Chewable tablet
CAUTIONARY AND ADVISORY LABELS 24
EXCIPIENTS: May contain Aspartame
▸ Colecalciferol with calcium carbonate (Non-proprietary)
**Calcium carbonate 1.25 gram, Colecalciferol
400 unit** Colecalciferol 400unit / Calcium carbonate 1.25g chewable
tablets | 60 tablet 🚫 DT = £4.24 | 100 tablet £14.75
Calcium carbonate 1.5 gram, Colecalciferol 400 unit
Colecalciferol 400unit / Calcium carbonate 1.5g chewable tablets |
56 tablet [P] £3.65 DT = £3.65 | 60 tablet [P] £4.93
▸ Accrete D3 One a Day (Thornton & Ross Ltd)
Calcium carbonate 2.5 gram, Colecalciferol 880 unit Accrete D3
One a Day 1000mg/880unit chewable tablets | 30 tablet [P] £2.95 DT
= £2.95
▸ Adcal-D3 (Kyowa Kirin Ltd)
Calcium carbonate 1.5 gram, Colecalciferol 400 unit Adcal-D3
Lemon chewable tablets | 56 tablet [P] £3.65 DT = £3.65 |
112 tablet [P] £7.49
Adcal-D3 chewable tablets tutti frutti | 56 tablet [P] £3.65 DT = £3.65
| 112 tablet [P] £7.49
▸ Calceos (Galen Ltd)
Calcium carbonate 1.25 gram, Colecalciferol 400 unit Calceos
500mg/400unit chewable tablets | 60 tablet [P] £3.94 DT = £4.24
▸ Calci-D (Consilient Health Ltd)
Calcium carbonate 2.5 gram, Colecalciferol 1000 iu Calci-D
1000mg/1,000unit chewable tablets | 28 tablet [PoM] £2.25 DT =
£2.25
▸ Calcichew D3 (Takeda UK Ltd)
Calcium carbonate 2.5 gram, Colecalciferol 800 iu Calcichew D3
1000mg/800unit Once Daily chewable tablets | 30 tablet [P] £6.75 DT
= £6.75
Calcium carbonate 1.25 gram, Colecalciferol 200 unit Calcichew
D3 chewable tablets | 100 tablet [P] £7.68 DT = £7.68
▸ Calcichew D3 Forte (Takeda UK Ltd)
Calcium carbonate 1.25 gram, Colecalciferol 400 unit Calcichew
D3 Forte tablets | 60 tablet [P] £4.24 DT = £4.24 |
100 tablet [P] £7.08
▸ Evacal D3 (Teva UK Ltd)
Calcium carbonate 1.5 gram, Colecalciferol 400 unit Evacal D3
1500mg/400unit chewable tablets | 56 tablet [P] £2.75 DT = £3.65 |
112 tablet [P] £5.50

9

Blood and nutrition

▸ Kalcipos-D (Mylan)
  Calcium carbonate 1.25 gram, Colecalciferol 800 unit Kalcipos-D 500mg/800unit chewable tablets | 30 tablet [PoM] £4.21 DT = £4.21
▸ Natecal (Chiesi Ltd)
  Calcium carbonate 1.5 gram, Colecalciferol 400 unit Natecal D3 600mg/400unit chewable tablets | 60 tablet [P] £3.63
▸ TheiCal-D3 (Stirling Anglian Pharmaceuticals Ltd)
  Calcium carbonate 2.5 gram, Colecalciferol 880 unit TheiCal-D3 1000mg/880unit chewable tablets | 30 tablet [P] £2.95 DT = £2.95

Colecalciferol with calcium phosphate

The properties listed below are those particular to the combination only. For the properties of the components please consider, colecalciferol p. 1133, calcium phosphate p. 1097.

● **INDICATIONS AND DOSE**

Calcium and vitamin D deficiency
▸ BY MOUTH
▸ Adult: (consult product literature)

● INTERACTIONS → Appendix 1: calcium salts · vitamin D substances

● MEDICINAL FORMS There can be variation in the licensing of different medicines containing the same drug.
Powder
CAUTIONARY AND ADVISORY LABELS 13, 21
▸ Calfovit D3 (A. Menarini Farmaceutica Internazionale SRL)
  Calcium phosphate 3.1 gram, Colecalciferol 800 unit Calfovit D3 oral powder sachets | 30 sachet [P] £4.32 DT = £4.32

F 1132

Dihydrotachysterol

11-May-2020

● **INDICATIONS AND DOSE**

Acute, chronic, and latent forms of hypocalcaemic tetany due to hypoparathyroidism
▸ BY MOUTH
▸ Adult: (consult product literature)

● INTERACTIONS → Appendix 1: vitamin D substances
● SIDE-EFFECTS Abdominal cramps · apathy · dehydration · paralysis · renal failure · stupor · urinary urgency · vertigo
● RENAL IMPAIRMENT
Monitoring Monitor plasma-calcium concentration in renal impairment.
● MONITORING REQUIREMENTS Monitor plasma-calcium concentration in patients receiving high doses.

● MEDICINAL FORMS There can be variation in the licensing of different medicines containing the same drug.
Oral solution
EXCIPIENTS: May contain Arachis (peanut) oil
▸ AT10 (Intrapharm Laboratories Ltd)
  Dihydrotachysterol 250 microgram per 1 ml AT10 250micrograms/ml oral solution sugar-free | 15 ml [P] £22.87

F 1132

Ergocalciferol

(Calciferol; Vitamin D$_2$)

● **INDICATIONS AND DOSE**

Vitamin D deficiency caused by intestinal malabsorption or chronic liver disease
▸ BY MOUTH
▸ Adult: Up to 40 000 units daily
Hypocalcaemia of hypoparathyroidism to achieve normocalcaemia
▸ BY MOUTH
▸ Adult: Up to 100 000 units daily

Prevention of vitamin D deficiency
▸ BY MOUTH
▸ Adult: 400 units daily
Treatment of vitamin D deficiency
▸ BY MOUTH
▸ Adult: 800 units daily, higher doses may be necessary for severe deficiency

● INTERACTIONS → Appendix 1: vitamin D substances
● RENAL IMPAIRMENT
Monitoring Monitor plasma-calcium concentration in renal impairment.
● MONITORING REQUIREMENTS Monitor plasma-calcium concentration in patients receiving high doses.
● PRESCRIBING AND DISPENSING INFORMATION The BP directs that when calciferol is prescribed or demanded, colecalciferol or ergocalciferol should be dispensed or supplied.
  When the strength of the tablets ordered or prescribed is not clear, the intention of the prescriber with respect to the strength (expressed in micrograms or milligrams per tablet) should be ascertained.

● MEDICINAL FORMS There can be variation in the licensing of different medicines containing the same drug. Forms available from special-order manufacturers include: tablet, capsule, oral suspension, oral solution
Tablet
▸ Ergo-D2 (Ennogen Healthcare Ltd)
  Ergocalciferol 12.5 microgram Ergo-D2 12.5microgram tablets | 30 tablet [S]
▸ Ergoral (Cubic Pharmaceuticals Ltd)
  Ergocalciferol 250 microgram Ergoral D2 10,000unit tablets | 30 tablet £12.95
Oral solution
▸ Ergocalciferol (Non-proprietary)
  Ergocalciferol 1500 unit per 1 ml Uvesterol D 1,500units/ml oral solution sugar-free | 20 ml [PoM] [S]
▸ Eciferol (Rhodes Pharma Ltd)
  Ergocalciferol 3000 unit per 1 ml Eciferol D2 3,000units/ml liquid | 60 ml £55.00 DT = £42.88
Capsule
▸ Eciferol (Rhodes Pharma Ltd)
  Ergocalciferol 1.25 mg Eciferol D2 50,000unit capsules | 10 capsule £29.99
▸ Ergoral (Cubic Pharmaceuticals Ltd)
  Ergocalciferol 1.25 mg Ergoral D2 50,000unit capsules | 10 capsule £19.95

Ergocalciferol with calcium lactate and calcium phosphate

06-Aug-2020

(Calcium and vitamin D)

The properties listed below are those particular to the combination only. For the properties of the components please consider, ergocalciferol above, calcium lactate p. 1096.

● **INDICATIONS AND DOSE**

Prevention of calcium and vitamin D deficiency | Treatment of calcium and vitamin D deficiency
▸ BY MOUTH
▸ Adult: (consult product literature)

● INTERACTIONS → Appendix 1: calcium salts · vitamin D substances
● DIRECTIONS FOR ADMINISTRATION Manufacturer advises tablets may be crushed before administration, or may be chewed.
● PRESCRIBING AND DISPENSING INFORMATION Each tablet contains calcium lactate 300 mg, calcium phosphate 150 mg (calcium 97 mg or Ca^{2+} 2.4 mmol), ergocalciferol 10 micrograms (400 units).

● PATIENT AND CARER ADVICE Patient or carers should be given advice on how to administer calcium and ergocalciferol tablets.

● MEDICINAL FORMS There can be variation in the licensing of different medicines containing the same drug.

Tablet
▸ Ergocalciferol with calcium lactate and calcium phosphate (Non-proprietary)
   Ergocalciferol 10 microgram, Calcium phosphate 150 mg, Calcium lactate 300 mg Calcium and Ergocalciferol tablets | 28 tablet P £40.53 DT = £25.98

> ⚑ 1132

Paricalcitol

24-Jul-2018

● INDICATIONS AND DOSE

Prevention and treatment of secondary hyperparathyroidism associated with chronic kidney disease
▸ BY MOUTH
▸ Adult: (consult product literature)

Prevention and treatment of secondary hyperparathyroidism associated with chronic renal failure in patients on haemodialysis
▸ Adult: To be administered via haemodialysis access (consult product literature)

● INTERACTIONS → Appendix 1: vitamin D substances

● SIDE-EFFECTS

GENERAL SIDE-EFFECTS
▸ **Common or very common** Electrolyte imbalance · hypoparathyroidism · taste altered
▸ **Uncommon** Dizziness · dry mouth · malaise · pain
▸ **Frequency not known** Angioedema · laryngeal oedema

SPECIFIC SIDE-EFFECTS
▸ **Uncommon**
▸ With oral use Breast tenderness · gastrointestinal discomfort · gastrooesophageal reflux disease · muscle spasms · palpitations · peripheral oedema · pneumonia
▸ With parenteral use Alopecia · anaemia · anxiety · asthma · atrial flutter · breast cancer · breast pain · cardiac arrest · cerebrovascular insufficiency · chest pain · coma · condition aggravated · confusion · conjunctivitis · cough · delirium · depersonalisation · dyspepsia · dysphagia · dyspnoea · ear disorder · erectile dysfunction · fever · gait abnormal · gastrointestinal disorders · glaucoma · haemorrhage · hirsutism · hyperhidrosis · hyperparathyroidism · hypertension · increased risk of infection · insomnia · joint disorders · leucopenia · lymphadenopathy · muscle twitching · myoclonus · oedema · pulmonary oedema · sensation abnormal · sepsis · syncope

● PREGNANCY Manufacturer advises avoid—toxicity in *animal* studies.

● BREAST FEEDING Manufacturer advises avoid—no information available.

● MONITORING REQUIREMENTS
▸ Monitor plasma calcium and phosphate during dose titration and at least monthly when stabilised.
▸ Monitor parathyroid hormone concentration.

● MEDICINAL FORMS There can be variation in the licensing of different medicines containing the same drug.

Solution for injection
EXCIPIENTS: May contain Ethanol, propylene glycol
▸ Zemplar (AbbVie Ltd)
   Paricalcitol 5 microgram per 1 ml Zemplar 5micrograms/1ml solution for injection vials | 5 vial PoM £62.00 (Hospital only)

Capsule
EXCIPIENTS: May contain Ethanol
▸ Zemplar (AbbVie Ltd)
   Paricalcitol 1 microgram Zemplar 1microgram capsules | 28 capsule PoM £69.44 DT = £69.44
   Paricalcitol 2 microgram Zemplar 2microgram capsules | 28 capsule PoM £138.88 DT = £138.88

VITAMINS AND TRACE ELEMENTS > VITAMIN E

Alpha tocopherol

06-May-2020

(Tocopherol)

● INDICATIONS AND DOSE

Vitamin E deficiency because of malabsorption in congenital or hereditary chronic cholestasis
▸ BY MOUTH USING ORAL SOLUTION
▸ Child: 17 mg/kg daily, dose to be adjusted as necessary

● CAUTIONS Predisposition to thrombosis

● INTERACTIONS → Appendix 1: vitamin E substances

● SIDE-EFFECTS
▸ **Common or very common** Diarrhoea
▸ **Uncommon** Alopecia · asthenia · headache · skin reactions
▸ **Frequency not known** Abdominal pain

● PREGNANCY Manufacturer advises caution, no evidence of harm in *animal* studies.

● BREAST FEEDING Manufacturer advises use only if potential benefit outweighs risk—no information available.

● HEPATIC IMPAIRMENT Manufacturer advises caution.

● RENAL IMPAIRMENT Manufacturer advises caution. Risk of renal toxicity due to polyethylene glycol content.
   Monitoring Manufacturer advises monitor closely in renal impairment.

● PRESCRIBING AND DISPENSING INFORMATION Tocofersolan is a water-soluble form of D-alpha tocopherol.

● MEDICINAL FORMS There can be variation in the licensing of different medicines containing the same drug.

Oral solution
▸ Vedrop (Recordati Rare Diseases UK Ltd) ▼
   D-alpha tocopherol (as Tocofersolan) 50 mg per 1 ml Vedrop 50mg/ml oral solution sugar-free | 20 ml PoM £54.55 DT = £54.55
   sugar-free | 60 ml PoM £163.65

Alpha tocopheryl acetate

(Tocopherol)

● INDICATIONS AND DOSE

Vitamin E deficiency
▸ BY MOUTH
▸ Child: 2–10 mg/kg daily, increased if necessary up to 20 mg/kg daily

Malabsorption in cystic fibrosis
▸ BY MOUTH
▸ Child 1-11 months: 50 mg once daily, dose to be adjusted as necessary, to be taken with food and pancreatic enzymes
▸ Child 1-11 years: 100 mg once daily, dose to be adjusted as necessary, to be taken with food and pancreatic enzymes
▸ Child 12-17 years: 100–200 mg once daily, dose to be adjusted as necessary, to be taken with food and pancreatic enzymes
▸ Adult: 100–200 mg once daily, dose to be adjusted as necessary, to be taken with food and pancreatic enzymes
continued →

9

Blood and nutrition

Vitamin E deficiency in cholestasis and severe liver disease

▶ BY MOUTH
▶ Child 1 month–11 years: Initially 100 mg daily, adjusted according to response, increased if necessary up to 200 mg/kg daily
▶ Child 12–17 years: Initially 200 mg daily, adjusted according to response, increased if necessary up to 200 mg/kg daily

Malabsorption in abetalipoproteinaemia

▶ BY MOUTH
▶ Adult: 50–100 mg/kg once daily

● CAUTIONS Predisposition to thrombosis
● INTERACTIONS → Appendix 1: vitamin E substances
● SIDE-EFFECTS Abdominal pain (more common at high doses) · bleeding tendency · diarrhoea (more common at high doses) · increased risk of thrombosis
● PREGNANCY No evidence of safety of high doses.
● BREAST FEEDING Excreted in milk; minimal risk, although caution with large doses.
● MONITORING REQUIREMENTS Increased bleeding tendency in vitamin-K deficient patients or those taking anticoagulants (prothrombin time and INR should be monitored).

● MEDICINAL FORMS There can be variation in the licensing of different medicines containing the same drug. Forms available from special-order manufacturers include: chewable tablet

Oral suspension
EXCIPIENTS: May contain Sucrose
▶ Alpha tocopheryl acetate (Non-proprietary)
   Alpha tocopheryl acetate 100 mg per 1 ml Alpha tocopheryl acetate 500mg/5ml oral suspension | 100 ml [GSL] £69.67 DT = £67.21
▶ Liqua-E (TriOn Pharma Ltd)
   Alpha tocopheryl acetate 100 mg per 1 ml Liqua-E 500mg/5ml oral suspension | 100 ml £47.69 DT = £67.21

Chewable tablet
▶ AlphaToc-E (Essential-Healthcare Ltd)
   Alpha tocopheryl acetate 100 mg AlphaToc-E 100mg chewable tablets | 30 tablet £29.67
▶ E-Tabs (Ennogen Healthcare Ltd)
   Alpha tocopheryl acetate 100 mg E-Tabs 100mg chewable tablets | 30 tablet £87.30
▶ Ephynal (Imported (Italy))
   Alpha tocopheryl acetate 100 mg Ephynal 100mg chewable tablets | 30 tablet [℞]

Capsule
▶ Alpha tocopheryl acetate (Non-proprietary)
   Alpha tocopherol 75 unit AlphaToc-E 75unit capsules | 100 capsule £5.83
   Vitamin E 75unit capsules | 100 capsule £13.05
   Alpha tocopherol 200 unit Vitamin E 200unit capsules | 30 capsule £10.05
   Alpha tocopherol 400 unit Vitamin E 400unit capsules | 30 capsule £15.12
▶ E-Caps (Ennogen Healthcare Ltd)
   Alpha tocopherol 75 unit E-Caps 75unit capsules | 100 capsule £109.50
   Alpha tocopherol 100 unit E-Caps 100unit capsules | 30 capsule £84.40
   Alpha tocopherol 200 unit E-Caps 200unit capsules | 30 capsule £89.50
   Alpha tocopherol 400 unit E-Caps 400unit capsules | 30 capsule £128.50
   Alpha tocopherol 1000 unit E-Caps 1,000unit capsules | 30 capsule £130.20
▶ Nutra-E (TriOn Pharma Ltd)
   Alpha tocopherol 75 unit Nutra-E 75unit capsules | 100 capsule £5.86
   Alpha tocopherol 200 unit Nutra-E 200unit capsules | 100 capsule £12.88
   Alpha tocopherol 400 unit Nutra-E 400unit capsules | 100 capsule £19.82

▶ Vita-E (Typharm Ltd)
   Alpha tocopherol 75 unit Vita-E 75unit capsules | 100 capsule £6.99
   Alpha tocopherol 200 unit Vita-E 200unit capsules | 30 capsule £5.35 | 100 capsule £14.99
   Alpha tocopherol 400 unit Vita-E 400unit capsules | 30 capsule £7.99 | 100 capsule £21.85

VITAMINS AND TRACE ELEMENTS ❭ VITAMIN K

Menadiol sodium phosphate

● INDICATIONS AND DOSE

Prevention of Vitamin K deficiency in malabsorption syndromes

▶ BY MOUTH
▶ Adult: 10–40 mg daily, dose to be adjusted as necessary

● CAUTIONS G6PD deficiency (risk of haemolysis) · vitamin E deficiency (risk of haemolysis)
● PREGNANCY Avoid in late pregnancy and labour unless benefit outweighs risk of neonatal haemolytic anaemia, hyperbilirubinaemia, and kernicterus in neonate.

● MEDICINAL FORMS There can be variation in the licensing of different medicines containing the same drug.
Tablet
▶ Menadiol sodium phosphate (Non-proprietary)
   Menadiol phosphate (as Menadiol sodium phosphate)
   10 mg Menadiol 10mg tablets | 100 tablet [℞] £214.71 DT = £214.71

Phytomenadione

15-Sep-2020

(Vitamin K₁)

● INDICATIONS AND DOSE

Major bleeding in patients on warfarin (in combination with dried prothrombin complex or fresh frozen plasma)

▶ BY SLOW INTRAVENOUS INJECTION
▶ Adult: 5 mg for 1 dose, stop warfarin treatment

INR > 8.0 with minor bleeding in patients on warfarin

▶ BY SLOW INTRAVENOUS INJECTION
▶ Adult: 1–3 mg, stop warfarin treatment, dose may be repeated if INR still too high after 24 hours, restart warfarin treatment when INR <5

INR > 8.0 with no bleeding in patients on warfarin

▶ BY MOUTH
▶ Adult: 1–5 mg, intravenous preparation to be used orally, stop warfarin treatment, repeat dose if INR still too high after 24 hours, restart warfarin treatment when INR <5

INR 5.0–8.0 with minor bleeding in patients on warfarin

▶ BY SLOW INTRAVENOUS INJECTION
▶ Adult: 1–3 mg, stop warfarin treatment, restart warfarin treatment when INR <5

Reversal of anticoagulation prior to elective surgery (after warfarin stopped)

▶ BY MOUTH
▶ Adult: 1–5 mg, intravenous preparation to be used orally, dose to be given the day before surgery if INR ≥1.5

Reversal of anticoagulation prior to emergency surgery (when surgery can be delayed 6–12 hours)

▶ BY INTRAVENOUS INJECTION
▶ Adult: 5 mg as a single dose, if surgery cannot be delayed, dried prothrombin complex can be given in addition to phytomenadione and the INR checked before surgery

● UNLICENSED USE Oral use of intravenous preparations is unlicensed.

CAUTIONS Intravenous injections should be given very slowly—risk of vascular collapse

KONAKION ® MM Reduce dose in elderly

PREGNANCY Use if potential benefit outweighs risk.

BREAST FEEDING Present in milk.

HEPATIC IMPAIRMENT

KONAKION ® MM Manufacturer advises caution—monitor INR in patients with severe impairment (contains glycocholic acid which may displace bilirubin).

DIRECTIONS FOR ADMINISTRATION

KONAKION ® MM PAEDIATRIC *Konakion ® MM Paediatric* may be administered *by mouth* or *by intramuscular injection* or *by intravenous injection*. For *intravenous injection*, expert sources advise may be diluted with Glucose 5% if necessary.

KONAKION ® MM *Konakion ® MM* may be administered by slow intravenous injection or by intravenous infusion in glucose 5%; **not** for intramuscular injection. For *intravenous infusion (Konakion ® MM)*, give intermittently in Glucose 5%; dilute with 55 mL; may be injected into lower part of infusion apparatus.

MEDICINAL FORMS There can be variation in the licensing of different medicines containing the same drug. Forms available from special-order manufacturers include: capsule, oral suspension, oral solution

Solution for injection

EXCIPIENTS: May contain Glycocholic acid, lecithin

▸ Konakion MM (Cheplapharm Arzneimittel GmbH)
 Phytomenadione 10 mg per 1 ml Konakion MM Paediatric 2mg/0.2ml solution for injection ampoules | 5 ampoule [PoM] £4.71 DT = £4.71
 Konakion MM 10mg/1ml solution for injection ampoules | 10 ampoule [PoM] £3.78 DT = £3.78

Fertility problems: assessment and treatment. National Institute for Health and Care Excellence. Clinical guideline 156. June 2015.
www.nice.org.uk/guidance/cg156

6.1 Neural tube defects (prevention in pregnancy)

Neural tube defects (prevention in pregnancy)

01-Aug-2017

Description of condition

Neural tube defects represent a group of congenital defects, caused by incomplete closure of the neural tube within 28 days of conception. The most common forms are anencephaly, spina bifida and encephalocele.

The main risk factors are maternal folate deficiency, maternal vitamin B_{12} deficiency, previous history of having an infant with a neural tube defect, smoking, diabetes, obesity, and use of antiepileptic drugs. For information on smoking cessation see Smoking cessation p. 519.

Prevention in pregnancy

[EvGr] Pregnant women or women who wish to become pregnant should be advised to take supplementation with folic acid p. 1071 before conception and until week 12 of pregnancy.

A higher daily dose (see folic acid) is recommended for women at a high risk of conceiving a child with a neural tube defect, including women who have previously had an infant with a neural tube defect, who are receiving antiepileptic medication (see Epilepsy p. 321), or who have diabetes or sickle-cell disease. ⟨A⟩

Useful Resources

Antenatal care for uncomplicated pregnancies. National Institute for Health and Care Excellence. Clinical guideline 62. March 2008 (Updated March 2016).
www.nice.org.uk/guidance/cg62

9

Blood and nutrition

Chapter 10
Musculoskeletal system

1 Arthritis

Osteoarthritis and soft-tissue disorders

Overview

For pain relief in osteoarthritis and soft-tissue disorders, paracetamol p. 464 should be used first and may need to be taken regularly. A topical NSAID or topical capsaicin 0.025% p. 505 should also be considered, particularly in knee or hand osteoarthritis. An oral NSAID can be substituted for, or used in addition to, paracetamol. If further pain relief is required in osteoarthritis, then the addition of an opioid analgesic may be considered, but with a substantial risk of adverse effects; however, an opioid analgesic should be considered before a NSAID in patients taking low-dose aspirin.

Intra-articular corticosteroid injections may produce temporary benefit in osteoarthritis, especially if associated with soft-tissue inflammation.

Non-drug measures, such as weight reduction and exercise, should also be encouraged.

Glucosamine p. 1144 and rubefacients are not recommended for the treatment of osteoarthritis.

Hyaluronic acid and its derivatives are available for osteoarthritis of the knee, but are not recommended. Sodium hyaluronate p. 1214 (*Durolane*®, *Euflexxa*®, *Fermathron*®, *Orthovisc*®, *Ostenil*®, *Ostenil Plus*®, *RenehaVis*®, *Suplasyn*®, *Synocrom*®, *Synopsis*®) or hylan G-F 20 (*Synvisc*®) is injected intra-articularly to supplement natural hyaluronic acid in the synovial fluid. These injections may reduce pain over 1–6 months, but are associated with a short-term increase in knee inflammation. Sodium hyaluronate (*SportVis*®) is also licensed for the relief of pain and optimisation of recovery following ankle sprain, and for the relief of chronic pain and disability associated with tennis elbow.

Rheumatoid arthritis

10-Sep-2018

Description of condition

Rheumatoid arthritis is a chronic systemic inflammatory disease that causes persistent symmetrical joint synovitis (inflammation of the synovial membrane) typically of the small joints of the hands and feet, although any synovial joint can be affected. Synovitis presents as pain and prolonged stiffness that tends to be worse at rest or following periods of inactivity, swelling, tenderness, and heat in the affected joints. Other symptoms of rheumatoid arthritis include rheumatoid nodules and non-specific symptoms such as malaise, fatigue, fever, and weight loss.

As the disease progresses, it can cause joint deformity and affect different organs of the body, such as the heart, lungs, and eyes; therefore early diagnosis and treatment of rheumatoid arthritis is essential to reduce the impact of the disease.

Palindromic rheumatism is a rare form of inflammatory arthritis which causes attacks of joint pain and swelling similar to rheumatoid arthritis, but the joints return to normal in between attacks. Patients with palindromic rheumatism may later develop rheumatoid arthritis.

Aims of treatment

The aims of treatment are to relieve the symptoms of rheumatoid arthritis, achieve disease remission or low disease activity if remission cannot be achieved, and to improve the patient's ability to perform daily activities.

Non-drug treatment

EvGr Patients with rheumatoid arthritis should have access to a multidisciplinary team, and may benefit from physiotherapy to encourage exercise, enhance flexibility of joints and strengthen muscles. Psychological interventions such as relaxation, stress management, and cognitive coping skills to support patients with their perception and management of their disease can also be offered. ◁A▷

Drug treatment

EvGr All patients with suspected persistent synovitis of unknown cause should be referred to a specialist for advice as soon as possible to confirm diagnosis and evaluate disease activity.

In patients with newly diagnosed active rheumatoid arthritis, monotherapy with a conventional disease-modifying antirheumatic drug (DMARD), either oral methotrexate p. 957, leflunomide p. 1145, or sulfasalazine p. 47, should be given as first-line treatment; hydroxychloroquine sulfate p. 1144, a weak DMARD, is an alternative in patients with mild rheumatoid arthritis or those with palindromic rheumatism. Treatment should be started as soon as possible, ideally within 3 months of onset of persistent symptoms, and the dose should be titrated to the maximum tolerated effective dose. ◁A▷

Conventional DMARDs have a slow onset of action and can take 2–3 months to take effect. EvGr Consider short-term bridging treatment with a corticosteroid (by oral, intramuscular, or intra-articular administration) when starting treatment with a new DMARD to provide rapid symptomatic control, while waiting for the DMARD to take effect. Short-term corticosteroids should also be given to rapidly decrease inflammation during flare-ups.

If symptoms of rheumatoid arthritis are inadequately controlled despite dose escalation on DMARD monotherapy, combination therapy with another conventional DMARD (either oral methotrexate p. 957, leflunomide p. 1145, sulfasalazine p. 47, or hydroxychloroquine sulfate p. 1144) should be given.

Treatment with a tumour necrosis factor (TNF) alpha inhibitor (either adalimumab p. 1157, certolizumab pegol p. 1158, etanercept p. 1159, golimumab p. 1161, or infliximab p. 1162), other biological DMARD (either abatacept p. 1156, sarilumab p. 1148, or tocilizumab p. 1150), or targeted synthetic DMARD (either baricitinib p. 1152 or tofacitinib p. 1154) is recommended if there has been an inadequate response to combination therapy with conventional DMARDS. ⟨A⟩ See *National funding/access decisions* for individual drugs for full prescribing information.

EvGr Rituximab p. 927 in combination with methotrexate p. 957 is an alternative option for patients with severe active rheumatoid arthritis who have had an inadequate response to, or are intolerant of other DMARDs, including at least one TNF alpha inhibitor. ⟨A⟩ See *National funding/access decisions* for rituximab p. 927.

EvGr In patients with established rheumatoid arthritis, the long-term use of corticosteroids should only be continued if all other treatments options (including biological and targeted synthetic DMARDs) have been offered.

Patients with active rheumatoid arthritis should be monitored monthly until the treatment target (either remission or low disease activity) has been achieved, and all patients with rheumatoid arthritis should be reviewed annually. In patients who have maintained the treatment target for at least 1 year without corticosteroids, cautiously reducing drug doses to the lowest that are clinically effective, or tapering and stopping at least one drug if the patient is being treated with two or more DMARDs should be considered. ⟨A⟩

Older conventional DMARDs such as sodium aurothiomalate (gold) p. 1147, azathioprine p. 882, ciclosporin p. 884 and penicillamine p. 1146 are no longer commonly used in practice due to the availability of newer, more effective drugs.

Pain relief

EvGr Short-term use of an oral non-steroidal anti-inflammatory drug (NSAID) or a selective cyclo-oxygenase-2 inhibitor should be considered for additional control of pain and stiffness associated with rheumatoid arthritis. Patients should be offered a proton pump inhibitor to minimise associated gastrointestinal adverse effects. In patients already taking low-dose aspirin p. 132, paracetamol p. 464 or a compound analgesic should be considered before giving a NSAID. NSAIDs should be used at the lowest effective dose, and if possible, withdrawn when a good response to DMARDs is achieved. ⟨A⟩

Surgery

EvGr Surgery may be an option for some patients if drug treatment has failed to adequately manage persistent pain due to joint damage or other identifiable soft tissue causes, if there is worsening of joint function, progressive deformity, or persistent localised synovitis. ⟨A⟩

Useful Resources

Rheumatoid arthritis in adults: management. National Institute for Health and Care Excellence. NICE guideline 100. July 2018.
www.nice.org.uk/guidance/ng100

Spondyloarthritis

01-Sep-2017

Description of condition

Spondyloarthritis refers to a group of inflammatory musculoskeletal conditions with shared features which affect both axial and peripheral joints. Most people with these conditions have either axial spondyloarthritis (which includes ankylosing spondylitis and non-radiographic axial spondyloarthritis) or psoriatic arthritis. Axial spondyloarthritis primarily affects the spine, in particular the sacroiliac joint.

Psoriatic arthritis may present in several forms, including involvement of small joints (in the hands and feet), large joints (particularly in the knees), or combinations of both. Psoriatic arthritis may also involve the axial joints, finger and toe joints, and inflammation of the connective tissue between tendon/ligament and bone.

Less common subgroups are enteropathic spondyloarthritis, which is associated with inflammatory bowel disease (Crohn's disease p. 41 and Ulcerative colitis p. 43), and reactive arthritis (a form of peripheral arthritis), which can occur following gastro-intestinal or genito-urinary infections.

Aims of treatment

The aims of treatment are to relieve symptoms, slow the progression of the condition, and improve quality of life.

Non-drug treatment

EvGr Patients who have difficulties with everyday activities should be referred to a specialist therapist (such as a physiotherapist, occupational therapist, hand therapist, orthotist or podiatrist). Hydrotherapy can be considered as an adjunctive therapy to manage pain and maintain or improve function for people with axial spondyloarthritis. ⟨A⟩

Drug treatment

Axial spondyloarthritis

EvGr For pain associated with axial spondyloarthritis, start one of the Non-steroidal anti-inflammatory drugs p. 1176 (NSAIDs) at the lowest effective dose. Clinical assessment, monitoring of risk factors, and the use of gastroprotective treatment should be considered. If an NSAID taken at the maximum tolerated dose for 2–4 weeks does not provide adequate pain relief, consider switching to a different NSAID.

A tumour necrosis factor (TNF) alpha inhibitor (or biological DMARD) such as adalimumab p. 1157, certolizumab pegol p. 1158, etanercept p. 1159, golimumab p. 1161, or infliximab p. 1162 is recommended as an option for treating severe active **ankylosing spondylitis** in patients whose disease has responded inadequately to, or who are intolerant of, NSAIDs.

Secukinumab p. 1149 is recommended as an option for treating active ankylosing spondylitis in patients who have responded inadequately to NSAIDs or TNF-alpha inhibitors (see *National funding/access decisions* under secukinumab p. 1149).

Adalimumab p. 1157, certolizumab pegol p. 1158 and etanercept p. 1159 are also recommended as options for treating severe **non-radiographic axial spondyloarthritis** in patients whose disease has responded inadequately to, or who are intolerant of, NSAIDs.

The choice of treatment should depend on patient preference and extra-articular involvement. The response to treatment should be assessed after 12 weeks and should only be continued if there is clear evidence of response.

Treatment with another TNF-alpha inhibitor is recommended in those who cannot tolerate, or whose disease has not responded to, treatment with the first TNF-alpha inhibitor, or in those whose disease has stopped responding after an initial response. ⟨A⟩

Psoriatic arthritis and other peripheral spondyloarthritides

EvGr Monotherapy with local corticosteroid injections should be considered for non-progressive **monoarthritis** (see Corticosteroids, inflammatory disorders p. 1199).

Standard DMARDs, such as methotrexate p. 957, leflunomide p. 1145 or sulfasalazine p. 47, can be used for patients with peripheral **polyarthritis**, **oligoarthritis**, or persistent or progressive **monoarthritis** associated with peripheral spondyloarthritis.

Standard DMARDs, such as methotrexate p. 957 or leflunomide p. 1145 can also be used for patients with **psoriatic arthritis**.

The choice of DMARD will depend on numerous factors such as the patient's circumstances (such as pregnancy planning and alcohol consumption), comorbidities (such as uveitis, psoriasis and inflammatory bowel disease), and potential side-effects.

If a standard DMARD taken at the maximum tolerated dose for at least 3 months does not provide adequate relief from symptoms, a switch to, or the addition of, another standard DMARD can be considered.

An NSAID can be used as an adjunct to standard DMARDs or biological DMARDs to manage symptoms. If NSAIDs do not provide adequate relief from symptoms, consider corticosteroid injections or short-term oral corticosteroid therapy as an adjunct to standard DMARDs or biological DMARDs to manage symptoms.

If extra-articular disease is adequately controlled by an existing standard DMARD but peripheral spondyloarthritis is not, consider adding another standard DMARD. Ⓐ

Further options for psoriatic arthritis

EvGr The targeted DMARD apremilast p. 1164, used alone or in combination with standard DMARDs, is recommended for the treatment of active and progressive psoriatic arthritis if the patient has peripheral arthritis with 3 or more tender joints and 3 or more swollen joints, and the psoriatic arthritis has not responded to at least 2 standard DMARDs given alone or in combination.

The biological DMARDs etanercept p. 1159, infliximab p. 1162, golimumab p. 1161 and adalimumab p. 1157 (TNF-alpha inhibitors) are recommended for the treatment of active and progressive psoriatic arthritis if the patients has peripheral arthritis with 3 or more tender joints and 3 or more swollen joints, and the psoriatic arthritis has not responded to at least 2 standard DMARDs given alone or in combination.

Ustekinumab p. 1151, alone or in combination with methotrexate, is recommended for treating active psoriatic arthritis when treatment with TNF-alpha inhibitors is contra-indicated but would otherwise be considered or the patient has had treatment with one or more TNF-alpha inhibitors. The response to treatment should be assessed at 24 weeks and should only be continued if there is clear evidence of response. Ⓐ

Reactive arthritis

EvGr After treating the initial infection, do not offer long-term (4 weeks or longer) treatment with an antibacterial solely to manage reactive arthritis caused by a gastro-intestinal or genito-urinary infection. Ⓐ

Useful Resources

Spondyloarthritis in over 16s: diagnosis and management. National Institute for Health and Care Excellence. Clinical Guideline NG65. February 2017.
www.nice.org.uk/guidance/ng65

Rheumatic disease, suppressing drugs

Overview

Certain drugs such as those affecting the immune response can suppress the disease process in *rheumatoid arthritis* and *psoriatic arthritis*, see Rheumatoid arthritis p. 1140 or Spondyloarthritis p. 1141. *Systemic* and *discoid lupus erythematosus* are sometimes treated with chloroquine p. 655 or hydroxychloroquine sulfate p. 1144.

The choice of a disease-modifying antirheumatic drug (DMARD) should take into account co-morbidity and patient preference. Methotrexate p. 957, sulfasalazine p. 47, intramuscular gold, and penicillamine p. 1146 are similar in efficacy. However, methotrexate or sulfasalazine may be better tolerated.

Gold

Gold, given as sodium aurothiomalate p. 1147, is licensed for active progressive rheumatoid arthritis; it must be given by deep intramuscular injection and the area gently massaged. A test dose must be given followed by doses at weekly intervals until there is definite evidence of remission. In patients who do respond, the interval between injections is then gradually increased to 4 weeks and treatment is continued for up to 5 years after complete remission. If relapse occurs the dosage frequency may be immediately increased and only once control has been obtained again should the dosage frequency be decreased; if no response is seen within 2 months, alternative treatment should be sought. It is important to avoid complete relapse since second courses of gold are not usually effective.

Penicillamine

Penicillamine has a similar action to gold. More patients are able to continue treatment than with gold but side-effects are common.

Patients should be warned not to expect improvement for at least 6 to 12 weeks after treatment is initiated. Penicillamine should be discontinued if there is no improvement within 1 year.

Sulfasalazine

Sulfasalazine has a beneficial effect in suppressing the inflammatory activity of rheumatoid arthritis. Sulfasalazine may also be used by specialists, in the management of psoriatic arthritis affecting peripheral joints [unlicensed indication]. Haematological abnormalities occur usually in the first 3 to 6 months of treatment and are reversible on cessation of treatment.

Antimalarials

The antimalarial hydroxychloroquine sulfate is used to treat rheumatoid arthritis of mild inflammatory activity; chloroquine is also licensed for treating inflammatory disorders but is used much less frequently and is generally reserved for use if other drugs have failed.

Chloroquine and hydroxychloroquine sulfate are effective for mild systemic lupus erythematosus, particularly involving the skin and joints. These drugs should not be used for psoriatic arthritis. Chloroquine and hydroxychloroquine sulfate are better tolerated than gold or penicillamine. Retinopathy rarely occurs provided that the recommended doses are not exceeded; in the elderly it is difficult to distinguish drug-induced retinopathy from changes of ageing.

Mepacrine hydrochloride p. 527 is sometimes used in discoid lupus erythematosus [unlicensed].

Drugs affecting the immune response

Methotrexate is a DMARD used in active rheumatoid arthritis. Methotrexate is usually given by mouth once a week, adjusted according to response. In patients who experience mucosal or gastro-intestinal side-effects with methotrexate, folic acid p. 1071 given every week [unlicensed indication], on a different day from the methotrexate, may help to reduce the frequency of such side-effects.

Leflunomide p. 1145 acts on the immune system as a DMARD. Its therapeutic effect starts after 4–6 weeks and improvement may continue for a further 4–6 months.

Drugs that affect the immune response are also used in the management of severe cases of *systemic lupus erythematosus* and other connective tissue disorders. They are often given in conjunction with corticosteroids for patients with severe or progressive renal disease. They may be used in cases of *polymyositis* that are resistant to corticosteroids. They are used for their corticosteroid-sparing effect in patients whose corticosteroid requirements are excessive. Azathioprine p. 882 is usually used.

In the specialist management of psoriatic arthritis affecting peripheral joints, leflunomide, methotrexate, or azathioprine [unlicensed indication] may be used.

Juvenile idiopathic arthritis

Many children with *juvenile idiopathic arthritis* (juvenile chronic arthritis) do not require DMARDs. Methotrexate is effective; sulfasalazine is an alternative [unlicensed indication] but it should be avoided in *systemic-onset juvenile idiopathic arthritis*. Gold and penicillamine are no longer used. Cytokine modulators have a role in *juvenile idiopathic arthritis*.

Cytokine modulators

Cytokine modulators should be used under specialist supervision.

Adalimumab p. 1157, certolizumab pegol p. 1158, etanercept p. 1159, golimumab p. 1161, and infliximab p. 1162 inhibit the activity of tumour necrosis factor alpha (TNF-α).

Adalimumab is licensed for moderate to severe active *rheumatoid arthritis* when response to other DMARDs (including methotrexate) has been inadequate; it is also licensed for severe, active, and progressive disease in adults not previously treated with methotrexate. In the treatment of rheumatoid arthritis, adalimumab should be used in combination with methotrexate, but it can be given alone if methotrexate is inappropriate. Adalimumab is also licensed for the treatment of active and progressive *psoriatic arthritis* and severe active *ankylosing spondylitis* that have not responded adequately to other DMARDs. It is also licensed for the treatment of severe axial spondyloarthritis without radiographic evidence of ankylosing spondylitis but with objective signs of inflammation, in patients who have had an inadequate response to, or are intolerant of NSAIDs. Adalimumab also has a role in inflammatory bowel disease and plaque psoriasis.

Certolizumab pegol is licensed for use in patients with moderate to severe active *rheumatoid arthritis* when response to DMARDs (including methotrexate) has been inadequate. Certolizumab pegol can be used in combination with methotrexate, or as a monotherapy if methotrexate is not tolerated or is contra-indicated. Certolizumab pegol is also licensed for the treatment of severe active *ankylosing spondylitis* in patients who have had an inadequate response to, or are intolerant of NSAIDs. It is also licensed for the treatment of severe active *axial spondyloarthritis*, without radiographic evidence of ankylosing spondylitis but with objective signs of inflammation, in patients who have had an inadequate response to, or are intolerant of NSAIDs.

Etanercept is licensed for the treatment of moderate to severe active *rheumatoid arthritis* either alone or in combination with methotrexate when the response to other DMARDs is inadequate and in severe, active and progressive *rheumatoid arthritis* in patients not previously treated with methotrexate. It is also licensed for the treatment of active and progressive *psoriatic arthritis* inadequately responsive to other DMARDs, and for severe *ankylosing spondylitis* inadequately responsive to conventional therapy. Etanercept also has a role in plaque psoriasis.

Golimumab is licensed in combination with methotrexate for the treatment of moderate to severe active *rheumatoid arthritis* when response to DMARD therapy (including methotrexate) has been inadequate; it is also licensed in combination with methotrexate for patients with severe, active, and progressive rheumatoid arthritis not previously treated with methotrexate p. 957. Golimumab p. 1161 is also licensed for the treatment of active and progressive *psoriatic arthritis*, as monotherapy or in combination with methotrexate, when response to DMARD therapy has been inadequate; it is also licensed for the treatment of severe active *ankylosing spondylitis* when there is an inadequate response to conventional treatment.

Infliximab p. 1162 is licensed for the treatment of active *rheumatoid arthritis* in combination with methotrexate when the response to other DMARDs, including methotrexate, is inadequate; it is also licensed in combination with methotrexate for patients not previously treated with methotrexate or other DMARDs who have severe, active, and progressive rheumatoid arthritis. Infliximab is also licensed for the treatment of *ankylosing spondylitis*, in patients with severe axial symptoms who have not responded adequately to conventional therapy, and in combination with methotrexate (or alone if methotrexate is not tolerated or is contra-indicated) for the treatment of active and progressive *psoriatic arthritis* which has not responded adequately to DMARDs.

Rituximab p. 927 is licensed in combination with methotrexate for the treatment of severe active *rheumatoid arthritis* in patients whose condition has not responded adequately to other DMARDs (including one or more tumour necrosis factor inhibitors) or who are intolerant of them. Rituximab has a role in malignant disease.

Abatacept p. 1156 prevents the full activation of T-lymphocytes. It is licensed for moderate to severe active *rheumatoid arthritis* in combination with methotrexate, in patients unresponsive to other DMARDs (including methotrexate or a tumour necrosis factor (TNF) inhibitor). Abatacept is not recommended for use in combination with TNF inhibitors.

Anakinra p. 1147 inhibits the activity of interleukin-1. Anakinra (in combination with methotrexate) is licensed for the treatment of *rheumatoid arthritis* which has not responded to methotrexate alone. Anakinra is not recommended for the treatment of rheumatoid arthritis except when used in a controlled long-term clinical study. Patients who are already receiving anakinra for rheumatoid arthritis should continue treatment until they and their specialist consider it appropriate to stop.

Baricitinib p. 1152 and tofacitinib p. 1154 are licensed alone or in combination with methotrexate for the treatment of moderate to severe active *rheumatoid arthritis* in patients who have had an inadequate response to, or who are intolerant to, one or more DMARDs.

Belimumab p. 891 inhibits the activity of B-lymphocyte stimulator. Belimumab is licensed as adjunctive therapy in patients with active, autoantibody-positive systemic lupus erythematosus with a high degree of disease activity despite standard therapy.

Sarilumab p. 1148 is a recombinant human monoclonal antibody that specifically binds to interleukin-6 receptors and blocks the activity of pro-inflammatory cytokines; it is licensed alone or in combination with methotrexate for the treatment of moderate to severe active rheumatoid arthritis in patients who have had an inadequate response to, or are intolerant to one or more DMARDs.

Secukinumab p. 1149 inhibits the activity of interleukin-17A. Secukinumab is licensed for the treatment of active *psoriatic arthritis*, in combination with methotrexate or alone, which has not responded adequately to DMARDs; it is also licensed for the treatment of *ankylosing spondylitis*, in patients who have not responded adequately to conventional therapy. Secukinumab also has a role in plaque psoriasis.

Tocilizumab p. 1150 antagonises the actions of interleukin-6. Tocilizumab is licensed for use in patients with moderate to severe active *rheumatoid arthritis* when response to at least one DMARD or tumour necrosis factor inhibitor has been inadequate, or in those who are intolerant of these drugs. Tocilizumab can be used in combination with methotrexate, or as monotherapy if methotrexate is not tolerated or is contra-indicated.

Ustekinumab p. 1151 inhibits the activity of interleukins 12 and 23. It is licensed for the treatment of active *psoriatic arthritis* (in combination with methotrexate or alone) in patients who have had an inadequate response to one or more DMARDs.

> **Other drugs used for Arthritis** Aceclofenac, p. 1177 · Celecoxib, p. 1178 · Cyclophosphamide, p. 938 · Dexibuprofen, p. 1179 · Diclofenac potassium, p. 1180 · Diclofenac sodium, p. 1181 · Etodolac, p. 1183 · Etoricoxib, p. 1184 · Flurbiprofen, p. 1185 · Ibuprofen, p. 1186 · Indometacin, p. 1189 · Ixekizumab, p. 1302 · Ketoprofen, p. 1190 · Mefenamic acid, p. 1191 · Meloxicam, p. 1192 · Nabumetone, p. 1193 · Naproxen, p. 1194 · Piroxicam, p. 1195 · Sulindac, p. 1196 · Tenoxicam, p. 1197 · Tiaprofenic acid, p. 1198

CHONDROPROTECTIVE DRUGS

Glucosamine

24-Nov-2020

● **DRUG ACTION** Glucosamine is a natural substance found in mucopolysaccharides, mucoproteins, and chitin.

● **INDICATIONS AND DOSE**

ALATERIS ®

Symptomatic relief of mild to moderate osteoarthritis of the knee
▸ BY MOUTH
▸ Adult: 1250 mg once daily, review treatment if no benefit after 2–3 months

DOLENIO ®

Symptomatic relief of mild to moderate osteoarthritis of the knee
▸ BY MOUTH
▸ Adult: 1500 mg once daily, review treatment if no benefit after 2–3 months

GLUSARTEL ®

Symptomatic relief of mild to moderate osteoarthritis of the knee
▸ BY MOUTH
▸ Adult: 1500 mg once daily, dose to be dissolved in at least 250 mL of water, review treatment if no benefit after 2–3 months

● **CAUTIONS** Asthma · impaired glucose tolerance · predisposition to cardiovascular disease

● **INTERACTIONS** → Appendix 1: glucosamine

● **SIDE-EFFECTS**
▸ **Common or very common** Constipation · diarrhoea · fatigue · gastrointestinal discomfort · headache · nausea

▸ **Uncommon** Flushing · skin reactions
▸ **Rare or very rare** Jaundice
▸ **Frequency not known** Angioedema · asthma · diabetes mellitus · dizziness · hypercholesterolaemia · oedema · vomiting

● **ALLERGY AND CROSS-SENSITIVITY** [EvGr] Contra-indicated if patient has a shellfish allergy. ⓜ

● **PREGNANCY** Manufacturers advise avoid—no information available.

● **BREAST FEEDING** Manufacturers advise avoid—no information available.

● **MONITORING REQUIREMENTS**
▸ Monitor blood-glucose concentration before treatment and periodically thereafter in patients with impaired glucose tolerance.
▸ Monitor cholesterol in patients with predisposition to cardiovascular disease.

● **NATIONAL FUNDING/ACCESS DECISIONS**
For full details see funding body website

Scottish Medicines Consortium (SMC) decisions
▸ Glucosamine (*Alateris*®) for relief of symptoms in mild to moderate osteoarthritis of the knee (June 2008)
SMC No. 471/08 Not recommended
▸ Glucosamine (*Glusartel*®) for the relief of symptoms in mild to moderate osteoarthritis of the knee (August 2011)
SMC No. 647/10 Not recommended

● **LESS SUITABLE FOR PRESCRIBING** Less suitable for prescribing—the mechanism of action is not understood and there is limited evidence to show it is effective.

● **MEDICINAL FORMS** There can be variation in the licensing of different medicines containing the same drug.

Tablet
ELECTROLYTES: May contain Sodium
▸ Dolenio (Alissa Healthcare Research Ltd)
Dolenio 1500mg tablets | 30 tablet [PoM] £18.20 DT = £18.20

DISEASE-MODIFYING ANTI-RHEUMATIC DRUGS

Hydroxychloroquine sulfate

11-May-2020

● **INDICATIONS AND DOSE**

Active rheumatoid arthritis (administered on expert advice) | Systemic and discoid lupus erythematosus (administered on expert advice) | Dermatological conditions caused or aggravated by sunlight (administered on expert advice)
▸ BY MOUTH
▸ Adult: 200–400 mg daily, daily maximum dose to be based on ideal body-weight; maximum 6.5 mg/kg per day

● **CAUTIONS** Acute porphyrias p. 1107 · diabetes (may lower blood glucose) · G6PD deficiency · maculopathy · may aggravate myasthenia gravis · may exacerbate psoriasis · neurological disorders (especially in those with a history of epilepsy—may lower seizure threshold) · severe gastro-intestinal disorders

CAUTIONS, FURTHER INFORMATION
▸ Monitoring for retinopathy A review group convened by the Royal College of Ophthalmologists has updated guidelines on monitoring for chloroquine and hydroxychloroquine retinopathy (*Hydroxychloroquine and Chloroquine Retinopathy: Recommendations on Monitoring* 2020). Recent data have highlighted that hydroxychloroquine retinopathy is more common than previously reported.
Monitoring recommendations for hydroxychloroquine:
● All patients planning to be on long-term treatment should receive a baseline examination (including fundus photography and spectral domain optical coherence

tomography) within 6–12 months of treatment initiation;

- Annual monitoring is recommended in all patients who have taken hydroxychloroquine for greater than 5 years;
- Annual monitoring may be commenced before 5 years of treatment if additional risk factors for retinal toxicity exist, such as concomitant tamoxifen therapy, impaired renal function (eGFR less than 60 mL/minute/1.73 m^2) or high-dose therapy (greater than 5 mg/kg/day of hydroxychloroquine sulfate).

- **INTERACTIONS** → Appendix 1: hydroxychloroquine
- **SIDE-EFFECTS**
- ► **Common or very common** Abdominal pain · appetite decreased · diarrhoea · emotional lability · headache · nausea · skin reactions · vision disorders · vomiting
- ► **Uncommon** Alopecia · corneal oedema · dizziness · eye disorders · hair colour changes · nervousness · neuromuscular dysfunction · retinopathy · seizure · tinnitus · vertigo
- ► **Frequency not known** Acute hepatic failure · agranulocytosis · anaemia · angioedema · bone marrow disorders · bronchospasm · cardiac conduction disorders · cardiomyopathy · hearing loss · hypoglycaemia · leucopenia · movement disorders · muscle weakness · myopathy · photosensitivity reaction · psychosis · reflexes absent · severe cutaneous adverse reactions (SCARs) · thrombocytopenia · tremor · ventricular hypertrophy

Overdose Hydroxychloroquine is very toxic in overdosage; overdosage is extremely hazardous and difficult to treat. Urgent advice from the National Poisons Information Service is essential. Life-threatening features include arrhythmias (which can have a very rapid onset) and convulsions (which can be intractable).

- **PREGNANCY** It is not necessary to withdraw an antimalarial drug during pregnancy if the rheumatic disease is well controlled; however, the manufacturer of hydroxychloroquine advises avoiding use.
- **BREAST FEEDING** Manufacturer advises use with caution—present in milk in small amounts. Specialist sources indicate risk of accumulation in infant due to long half-life; monitor infant for symptoms of uveitis e.g. eye redness or sensitivity to light.
- **HEPATIC IMPAIRMENT** Manufacturer advises caution. **Dose adjustments** Manufacturer advises consider dose adjustment in severe impairment.
- **RENAL IMPAIRMENT** Manufacturer advises caution. **Monitoring** Monitor plasma-hydroxychloroquine concentration in severe renal impairment.
- **MONITORING REQUIREMENTS** Manufacturer advises regular ophthalmological examination but the evidence of practical value is unsatisfactory (see *Cautions, further information* for advice of the Royal College of Ophthalmologists).
- **PRESCRIBING AND DISPENSING INFORMATION** To avoid excessive dosage in obese patients, the dose of hydroxychloroquine should be calculated on the basis of ideal body-weight.

- **MEDICINAL FORMS** There can be variation in the licensing of different medicines containing the same drug. Forms available from special-order manufacturers include: oral suspension, oral solution

Tablet
CAUTIONARY AND ADVISORY LABELS 21
- ► Hydroxychloroquine sulfate (Non-proprietary)
  Hydroxychloroquine sulfate 200 mg Hydroxychloroquine 200mg tablets | 60 tablet [PoM] £32.49 DT = £7.11
  Hydroxychloroquine sulfate 300 mg Hydroxychloroquine 300mg tablets | 30 tablet [PoM] £17.00
- ► Quinoric (Bristol Laboratories Ltd)
  Hydroxychloroquine sulfate 200 mg Quinoric 200mg tablets | 60 tablet [PoM] £5.10 DT = £7.11

Leflunomide

16-Nov-2020

- **INDICATIONS AND DOSE**
Moderate to severe active rheumatoid arthritis (specialist use only)
  - ► BY MOUTH
    - ► Adult: Initially 100 mg once daily for 3 days, then reduced to 10–20 mg once daily
Active psoriatic arthritis (specialist use only)
  - ► BY MOUTH
    - ► Adult: Initially 100 mg once daily for 3 days, then reduced to 20 mg once daily

- **CONTRA-INDICATIONS** Serious infection · severe hypoproteinaemia · severe immunodeficiency
- **CAUTIONS** Anaemia (avoid if significant and due to causes other than rheumatoid or psoriatic arthritis) · history of tuberculosis · impaired bone-marrow function (avoid if significant and due to causes other than rheumatoid or psoriatic arthritis) · leucopenia (avoid if significant and due to causes other than rheumatoid or psoriatic arthritis) · thrombocytopenia (avoid if significant and due to causes other than rheumatoid or psoriatic arthritis)
- **INTERACTIONS** → Appendix 1: leflunomide
- **SIDE-EFFECTS**
- ► **Common or very common** Abdominal pain · accelerated hair loss · appetite decreased · asthenia · diarrhoea · dizziness · gastrointestinal disorders · headache · leucopenia · nausea · oral disorders · paraesthesia · peripheral neuropathy · skin reactions · tendon disorders · vomiting · weight decreased
- ► **Uncommon** Anaemia · anxiety · electrolyte imbalance · hyperlipidaemia · taste altered · thrombocytopenia
- ► **Rare or very rare** Agranulocytosis · eosinophilia · hepatic disorders · infection · pancreatitis · pancytopenia · respiratory disorders · sepsis · severe cutaneous adverse reactions (SCARs) · vasculitis
- ► **Frequency not known** Cutaneous lupus erythematosus · hypouricaemia · pulmonary hypertension · renal failure
  SIDE-EFFECTS, FURTHER INFORMATION Discontinue treatment and institute washout procedure in case of serious side-effect (consult product literature).
  Hepatotoxicity Potentially life-threatening hepatotoxicity reported usually in the first 6 months. Discontinue treatment (and institute washout procedure—consult product literature) or reduce dose according to liver-function abnormality; if liver-function abnormality persists after dose reduction, discontinue treatment and institute washout procedure.
- **CONCEPTION AND CONTRACEPTION** Effective contraception **essential** during treatment and for at least 2 years after treatment in women and at least 3 months after treatment in men (plasma concentration monitoring required; waiting time before conception may be reduced with washout procedure—consult product literature). The concentration of the active metabolite after washout should be less than 20 micrograms/litre (measured on 2 occasions 14 days apart) in men or women before conception—consult product literature.
- **PREGNANCY** Avoid—active metabolite teratogenic in *animal* studies.
- **BREAST FEEDING** Present in milk in *animal* studies—manufacturer advises avoid.
- **HEPATIC IMPAIRMENT** Manufacturer advises avoid—active metabolite may accumulate.
- **RENAL IMPAIRMENT** Manufacturer advises avoid in moderate or severe impairment—no information available.
- **PRE-TREATMENT SCREENING** Exclude pregnancy before treatment.

10

Musculoskeletal system

● MONITORING REQUIREMENTS
▶ Monitor full blood count (including differential white cell count and platelet count) before treatment and every 2 weeks for 6 months then every 8 weeks.
▶ Monitor liver function before treatment and every 2 weeks for first 6 months then every 8 weeks.
▶ Monitor blood pressure.

● TREATMENT CESSATION
Washout Procedure The active metabolite persists for a long period; to aid drug elimination in case of serious adverse effect, or before starting another disease-modifying antirheumatic drug, or before conception, stop treatment and give *either* colestyramine p. 212 *or* charcoal, activated p. 1421. Procedure may be repeated as necessary.

● MEDICINAL FORMS There can be variation in the licensing of different medicines containing the same drug.

Tablet
CAUTIONARY AND ADVISORY LABELS 4
▶ Leflunomide (Non-proprietary)
Leflunomide 10 mg Leflunomide 10mg tablets | 30 tablet PoM
£46.00 DT = £4.63
Leflunomide 15 mg Leflunomide 15mg tablets | 30 tablet PoM
£46.00 DT = £46.00
Leflunomide 20 mg Leflunomide 20mg tablets | 30 tablet PoM
£61.36 DT = £4.83
▶ Arava (Sanofi)
Leflunomide 10 mg Arava 10mg tablets | 30 tablet PoM £51.13 DT
= £4.63
Leflunomide 20 mg Arava 20mg tablets | 30 tablet PoM £61.36 DT
= £4.83

Penicillamine

08-Dec-2020

● DRUG ACTION Penicillamine aids the elimination of copper ions in Wilson's disease (hepatolenticular degeneration).

● INDICATIONS AND DOSE
Severe active rheumatoid arthritis (administered on expert advice)
▶ BY MOUTH
▶ Adult: Initially 125–250 mg daily for 1 month, then increased in steps of 125–250 mg, at intervals of not less than 4 weeks; maintenance 500–750 mg daily in divided doses, then reduced in steps of 125–250 mg every 12 weeks, dose reduction attempted only if remission sustained for 6 months; maximum 1.5 g per day
▶ Elderly: Initially up to 125 mg daily for 1 month, then increased in steps of up to 125 mg, at intervals of at least 4 weeks; maximum 1 g per day

Wilson's disease
▶ BY MOUTH
▶ Adult: 1.5–2 g daily in divided doses, adjusted according to response, to be taken before food; maintenance 0.75–1 g daily, a dose of 2 g daily should not be continued for more than one year; maximum 2 g per day
▶ Elderly: 20 mg/kg daily in divided doses, adjusted according to response

Autoimmune hepatitis (used rarely; after disease controlled with corticosteroids)
▶ BY MOUTH
▶ Adult: Initially 500 mg daily in divided doses, to be increased slowly over 3 months; maintenance 1.25 g daily

Cystinuria, therapeutic
▶ BY MOUTH
▶ Adult: 1–3 g daily in divided doses, to be adjusted to maintain urinary cystine below 200 mg/litre, to be taken before food

Cystinuria, prophylactic
▶ BY MOUTH
▶ Adult: 0.5–1 g daily, maintain urinary cystine below 300 mg/litre and adequate fluid intake (at least 3 litres daily), to be taken at bedtime
▶ Elderly: Minimum dose to maintain urinary cystine below 200 mg/litre is recommended

● CONTRA-INDICATIONS Lupus erythematosus
● CAUTIONS Neurological involvement in Wilson's disease
● INTERACTIONS → Appendix 1: penicillamine
● SIDE-EFFECTS
▶ **Common or very common** Proteinuria · thrombocytopenia
▶ **Rare or very rare** Alopecia · breast enlargement (males and females) · connective tissue disorders · haematuria (discontinue immediately if cause unknown) · hypersensitivity · oral disorders · skin reactions
▶ **Frequency not known** Agranulocytosis · aplastic anaemia · appetite decreased · fever · glomerulonephritis · Goodpasture's syndrome · haemolytic anaemia · increased risk of infection · jaundice cholestatic · leucopenia · lupus-like syndrome · myasthenia gravis · nausea · nephrotic syndrome · neurological deterioration in Wilson's Disease · neutropenia · pancreatitis · polymyositis · pulmonary haemorrhage · rash (consider dose reduction) · respiratory disorders · Stevens-Johnson syndrome · taste loss (mineral supplements not recommended) · vomiting · yellow nail syndrome

SIDE-EFFECTS, FURTHER INFORMATION Proteinuria occurs in up to 30% of patients—can be a sign of immune-mediated nephropathy. Discontinue immediately if nephrotoxicity occurs.
  Nausea and rash more common early in treatment if full dose used from initiation. Delayed rash can occur after months or years of treatment—manufacturer advises reduce dose.

● ALLERGY AND CROSS-SENSITIVITY Patients who are hypersensitive to penicillin may react rarely to penicillamine.
● PREGNANCY Fetal abnormalities reported rarely; avoid if possible.
● BREAST FEEDING Manufacturer advises avoid unless potential benefit outweighs risk—no information available.
● RENAL IMPAIRMENT
Dose adjustments Reduce dose and monitor renal function or avoid (consult product literature).
● MONITORING REQUIREMENTS
▶ Consider withdrawal if platelet count falls below 120 000/mm^3 or white blood cells below 2500/mm^3 or if 3 successive falls within reference range (can restart at reduced dose when counts return to within reference range but permanent withdrawal necessary if recurrence of leucopenia or thrombocytopenia).
▶ Blood counts, including platelets, and urine examinations should be carried out before starting treatment and then every 1 or 2 weeks for the first 2 months then every 4 weeks to detect blood disorders and proteinuria (they should also be carried out in the week after any dose increase).
▶ A reduction in platelet count calls for discontinuation with subsequent re-introduction at a lower dosage and then, if possible, gradual increase.
▶ Longer intervals may be adequate in cystinuria and Wilson's disease.
● PATIENT AND CARER ADVICE Counselling on the symptoms of blood disorders is advised. Warn patient and carers to tell doctor immediately if sore throat, fever, infection, non-specific illness, unexplained bleeding and bruising, purpura, mouth ulcers, or rashes develop.

- MEDICINAL FORMS There can be variation in the licensing of different medicines containing the same drug. Forms available from special-order manufacturers include: oral solution

Tablet

CAUTIONARY AND ADVISORY LABELS 6, 22
▸ Penicillamine (Non-proprietary)
Penicillamine 125 mg Penicillamine 125mg tablets | 56 tablet [PoM] £62.52 DT = £62.37
Penicillamine 250 mg Penicillamine 250mg tablets | 56 tablet [PoM] £113.70 DT = £113.63

Sodium aurothiomalate
13-Aug-2019

- INDICATIONS AND DOSE

Active progressive rheumatoid arthritis (administered on expert advice)
▸ BY DEEP INTRAMUSCULAR INJECTION
▸ Adult: Test dose 10 mg, followed by 50 mg once weekly until there is definite evidence of remission, then reduced to 50 mg every 4 weeks continued for up to 5 years after complete remission, dose to be reduced gradually. Benefit is not expected until 300–500 mg has been given; it should be discontinued if there is no remission after 1 g has been given

Relapse in patients who have previously received sodium aurothiomalate therapy for active progressive rheumatoid arthritis (administered on expert advice)
▸ BY DEEP INTRAMUSCULAR INJECTION
▸ Adult: 50 mg once weekly until control has been obtained again, then reduced to 50 mg every 4 weeks continued for up to 5 years after complete remission, if no response is seen within 2 months, alternative treatment should be sought

- CONTRA-INDICATIONS Exfoliative dermatitis · history of blood disorders · history of bone marrow aplasia · systemic lupus erythematosus
- CAUTIONS Eczema · elderly · history of enterocolitis · history of urticaria · pulmonary fibrosis
  CAUTIONS, FURTHER INFORMATION Sodium aurothiomalate should be discontinued in the presence of blood disorders, gastro-intestinal bleeding (associated with ulcerative enterocolitis), or unexplained proteinuria (associated with immune complex nephritis) which is repeatedly above 300 mg/litre.
- INTERACTIONS → Appendix 1: gold
- SIDE-EFFECTS Abdominal pain · agranulocytosis · albuminuria · alopecia · asthenia · blood disorder · bone marrow disorders · circulatory collapse · dry cough · dyspnoea · encephalopathy · enterocolitis · eosinophilia · flushing · hepatic disorders · hypersensitivity · hypotension · leucopenia · nephrotic syndrome · nerve disorders · neutropenia · palpitations · respiratory disorders · shock · skin reactions · tachycardia · thrombocytopenia
  SIDE-EFFECTS, FURTHER INFORMATION Rashes with pruritus often occur after 2 to 6 months of treatment and may necessitate discontinuation.
- PREGNANCY Manufacturer advises avoid but limited data suggests usually not necessary to withdraw if condition well controlled.
  Dose adjustments Consider reducing dose and frequency.
- BREAST FEEDING Manufacturer advises avoid—present in milk; theoretical possibility of rashes and idiosyncratic reactions.
- HEPATIC IMPAIRMENT Manufacturer advises avoid in severe impairment.
- RENAL IMPAIRMENT Caution in mild to moderate impairment. Avoid in severe impairment.

- MONITORING REQUIREMENTS
▸ Urine tests and full blood counts (including total and differential white cell and platelet counts) must be performed before starting treatment and before each intramuscular injection.
▸ Monitor for pulmonary fibrosis with annual chest X-ray.
- PATIENT AND CARER ADVICE Patients should be advised to seek prompt medical attention if diarrhoea, sore throat, fever, infection, non-specific illness, unexplained bleeding and bruising, purpura, mouth ulcers, metallic taste, rash, breathlessness, or cough develop.

- MEDICINAL FORMS There can be variation in the licensing of different medicines containing the same drug.

Solution for injection

CAUTIONARY AND ADVISORY LABELS 11
▸ Myocrisin (Sanofi)
Sodium aurothiomalate 20 mg per 1 ml Myocrisin 10mg/0.5ml solution for injection ampoules | 10 ampoule [PoM] £45.55 DT = £45.55
Sodium aurothiomalate 100 mg per 1 ml Myocrisin 50mg/0.5ml solution for injection ampoules | 10 ampoule [PoM] £134.80 DT = £134.80

IMMUNOSUPPRESSANTS 〉 INTERLEUKIN INHIBITORS

Anakinra
21-Aug-2020

- INDICATIONS AND DOSE

Rheumatoid arthritis (in combination with methotrexate) which has not responded to methotrexate alone (specialist use only)
▸ BY SUBCUTANEOUS INJECTION
▸ Adult: 100 mg once daily

Cryopyrin-associated periodic syndromes (specialist use only)
▸ BY SUBCUTANEOUS INJECTION
▸ Adult: 1–2 mg/kg daily, for severe cryopyrin-associated periodic syndromes, usual maintenance is 3–4 mg/kg daily, up to a maximum of 8 mg/kg daily

Still's disease (specialist use only)
▸ BY SUBCUTANEOUS INJECTION
▸ Adult (body-weight up to 49 kg): 1–2 mg/kg daily
▸ Adult (body-weight 50 kg and above): 100 mg daily

- CONTRA-INDICATIONS Active infection · neutropenia (absolute neutrophil count less than 1.5×10^9/litre)—do not initiate · pre-existing malignancy
- CAUTIONS Elderly · history of asthma (increased risk of serious infection) · history of recurrent infection · predisposition to infection
- INTERACTIONS → Appendix 1: anakinra
- SIDE-EFFECTS
▸ **Common or very common** Headache · infection · neutropenia · thrombocytopenia
▸ **Uncommon** Skin reactions
▸ **Frequency not known** Hepatitis
  SIDE-EFFECTS, FURTHER INFORMATION Neutropenia reported commonly—discontinue if neutropenia develops.
- PREGNANCY Manufacturer advises avoid.
- BREAST FEEDING Manufacturer advises avoid—no information available.
- HEPATIC IMPAIRMENT Manufacturer advises caution in severe impairment.
- RENAL IMPAIRMENT Manufacturer advises caution in moderate impairment.
  Dose adjustments Manufacturer advises consider alternate day dosing in severe impairment.

10

Musculoskeletal system

Musculoskeletal system

10

- PRE-TREATMENT SCREENING Manufacturer advises patients should be screened for latent tuberculosis and viral hepatitis prior to initiation of treatment.
- MONITORING REQUIREMENTS
  ‣ Manufacturer advises monitor neutrophil count before treatment, then every month for 6 months, then every 3 months thereafter.
  ‣ When used for Cryopyrin-associated periodic syndromes Manufacturer advises monitor for CNS inflammation (including ear and eye tests) 3 months after starting treatment, then every 6 months until effective treatment doses have been identified, then yearly thereafter.
  ‣ When used for Still's disease Manufacturer advises consider routine monitoring of hepatic enzymes during the first month of treatment.
- PRESCRIBING AND DISPENSING INFORMATION
  ‣ When used for Cryopyrin-associated periodic syndromes or Still's disease The manufacturer of *Kineret*® has provided a *Guide for Healthcare Professionals*.
- PATIENT AND CARER ADVICE
  Blood disorders Patients should be instructed to seek medical advice if symptoms suggestive of neutropenia (such as fever, sore throat, bruising or, bleeding) develop.
  ‣ When used for Still's disease A patient card and patient booklet should be provided.
  ‣ When used for Cryopyrin-associated periodic syndromes A patient booklet should be provided.
- NATIONAL FUNDING/ACCESS DECISIONS
  For full details see funding body website
  Scottish Medicines Consortium (SMC) decisions
  ‣ Anakinra (*Kineret*®) for rheumatoid arthritis (November 2002) SMC No. 05/02 Not recommended
  ‣ Anakinra (*Kineret*®) for the treatment of Still's disease, as monotherapy or in combination with other anti-inflammatory drugs and disease-modifying antirheumatic drugs (October 2018) SMC No. SMC2104 Recommended

- MEDICINAL FORMS There can be variation in the licensing of different medicines containing the same drug.
  Solution for injection
  ‣ Kineret (Swedish Orphan Biovitrum Ltd)
  Anakinra 150 mg per 1 ml Kineret 100mg/0.67ml solution for injection pre-filled syringes | 7 pre-filled disposable injection PoM
  £183.61 DT = £183.61

Sarilumab

11-Nov-2020

- DRUG ACTION Sarilumab is a recombinant human monoclonal antibody that specifically binds to interleukin-6 receptors and blocks the activity of pro-inflammatory cytokines.

- **INDICATIONS AND DOSE**

  Moderate-to-severe active rheumatoid arthritis in patients who have had an inadequate response to, or are intolerant to one or more disease-modifying anti-rheumatic drugs (as monotherapy or in combination with methotrexate) (specialist use only)
  ‣ BY SUBCUTANEOUS INJECTION
  ‣ Adult: 200 mg every 2 weeks, for dose adjustments due to neutropenia, thrombocytopenia, or liver enzyme elevations—consult product literature

- CONTRA-INDICATIONS Do not initiate if absolute neutrophil count less than 2 × 10⁹/litre · do not initiate if platelet count less than 150 × 10³/microlitre · do not initiate if serum transaminases (ALT or AST) greater than 1.5 times the upper limit of normal · severe active infection
- CAUTIONS Chronic or recurrent infection · elderly (increased risk of infection) · history of diverticulitis ·

history of intestinal ulceration · history of serious or opportunistic infection · predisposition to infection
CAUTIONS, FURTHER INFORMATION
  ‣ Infection Manufacturer advises caution in patients who have been exposed to tuberculosis, or who have lived in or travelled to areas of endemic tuberculosis or mycoses. Patients with latent tuberculosis should complete anti-tuberculosis therapy before initiation of sarilumab; consider anti-tuberculosis therapy before initiation of sarilumab in patients with a past history of latent or active tuberculosis in whom an adequate course of treatment cannot be confirmed, and for those with a negative test for latent tuberculosis but have risk factors for tuberculosis—consultation with a tuberculosis specialist may be appropriate.
    Manufacturer advises patients should be brought up-to-date with current immunisation schedule before initiating treatment.
- INTERACTIONS → Appendix 1: monoclonal antibodies
- SIDE-EFFECTS
  ‣ **Common or very common** Dyslipidaemia · increased risk of infection · neutropenia · thrombocytopenia
  ‣ **Frequency not known** Hypersensitivity · skin reactions
- CONCEPTION AND CONTRACEPTION Manufacturer advises effective contraception in women of childbearing potential during treatment and for up to 3 months after treatment.
- PREGNANCY Manufacturer advises avoid unless essential—limited information available.
- BREAST FEEDING Manufacturer advises avoid—no information available.
- HEPATIC IMPAIRMENT Manufacturer advises avoid (no information available).
- PRE-TREATMENT SCREENING Manufacturer advises that patients should be evaluated for tuberculosis before treatment.
- MONITORING REQUIREMENTS
  ‣ Manufacturer advises monitor for signs and symptoms of infection; monitor neutrophil count 4 to 8 weeks after treatment initiation and according to clinical judgement thereafter—discontinue if absolute neutrophil count less than 0.5 × 10⁹/litre.
  ‣ Manufacturer advises monitor platelet count 4 to 8 weeks after treatment initiation and according to clinical judgement thereafter—discontinue if platelet count less than 50 × 10³/microlitre.
  ‣ Manufacturer advises monitor hepatic transaminases (ALT and AST) 4 to 8 weeks after treatment initiation and every 3 months thereafter, and consider other liver function tests if clinically indicated—discontinue if ALT is greater than 5 times the upper limit of normal.
  ‣ Manufacturer advises monitor lipid profile approximately 4 to 8 weeks after treatment initiation and approximately every 6 months thereafter—hyperlipidaemia should be managed according to clinical guidelines.
- DIRECTIONS FOR ADMINISTRATION Manufacturer advises to avoid injecting into areas of the skin that are tender, damaged, or have bruises or scars; patients may self-administer *Kevzara*®, after appropriate training in subcutaneous injection technique.
- PRESCRIBING AND DISPENSING INFORMATION Sarilumab is a biological medicine. Biological medicines must be prescribed and dispensed by brand name, see *Biological medicines* and *Biosimilar medicines*, under Guidance on prescribing p. 1; manufacturer advises to record the brand name and batch number after each administration.
- HANDLING AND STORAGE Manufacturer advises store in a refrigerator (2–8°C) and protect from light—consult product literature for further information regarding storage outside refrigerator.

● PATIENT AND CARER ADVICE Manufacturer advises patients should be advised to seek immediate medical attention if symptoms of a hypersensitivity reaction occur. Self-administration Manufacturer advises patients and their carers should be given training in subcutaneous injection technique if appropriate.
Alert card An alert card should be provided.
Missed doses Manufacturer advises if a dose is more than 3 days late, the missed dose should not be taken and the next dose should be taken at the normal time.

● NATIONAL FUNDING/ACCESS DECISIONS
For full details see funding body website
NICE decisions
▶ Sarilumab for moderate-to-severe rheumatoid arthritis (November 2017) NICE TA485 Recommended with restrictions
Scottish Medicines Consortium (SMC) decisions
▶ Sarilumab (*Kevzara*®) in combination with methotrexate, or as monotherapy for the treatment of moderately to severely active rheumatoid arthritis in adult patients who have responded inadequately to, or who are intolerant to one or more disease modifying anti rheumatic drugs (April 2018) SMC No. 1314/18 Recommended with restrictions

● MEDICINAL FORMS There can be variation in the licensing of different medicines containing the same drug.
Solution for injection
CAUTIONARY AND ADVISORY LABELS 10
▶ Kevzara (Sanofi) ▼
Sarilumab 131.6 mg per 1 ml Kevzara 150mg/1.14ml solution for injection pre-filled syringes | 2 pre-filled disposable injection PoM £912.25
Kevzara 150mg/1.14ml solution for injection pre-filled pens | 2 pre-filled disposable injection PoM £912.25
Sarilumab 175 mg per 1 ml Kevzara 200mg/1.14ml solution for injection pre-filled syringes | 2 pre-filled disposable injection PoM £912.25
Kevzara 200mg/1.14ml solution for injection pre-filled pens | 2 pre-filled disposable injection PoM £912.25

Secukinumab

06-Oct-2020

● DRUG ACTION Secukinumab is a recombinant human monoclonal antibody that selectively binds to cytokine interleukin-17A (IL-17A) and inhibits the release of proinflammatory cytokines and chemokines.

● INDICATIONS AND DOSE
Ankylosing spondylitis (initiated by a specialist)
▶ BY SUBCUTANEOUS INJECTION
▶ Adult: 150 mg every week for 5 doses, then maintenance 150 mg every month, review treatment if no response within 16 weeks of initial dose
Psoriatic arthritis (initiated by a specialist)
▶ BY SUBCUTANEOUS INJECTION
▶ Adult: 150 mg every week for 5 doses, then maintenance 150 mg every month, dose may be increased to 300 mg according to clinical response. Review treatment if no response within 16 weeks of initial dose
Psoriatic arthritis with concomitant moderate to severe plaque psoriasis or if inadequate response to anti-TNFα treatment (initiated by a specialist) | Plaque psoriasis (initiated by a specialist)
▶ BY SUBCUTANEOUS INJECTION
▶ Adult: 300 mg every week for 5 doses, then maintenance 300 mg every month, review treatment if no response within 16 weeks of initial dose

● CONTRA-INDICATIONS Severe active infection

● CAUTIONS Chronic infection · Crohn's disease (monitor for exacerbations) · history of recurrent infection ·

predisposition to infection (discontinue if new serious infection develops)
CAUTIONS, FURTHER INFORMATION
▶ Tuberculosis Manufacturer advises that patients with latent tuberculosis should complete anti-tuberculosis therapy before starting secukinumab.

● INTERACTIONS → Appendix 1: monoclonal antibodies

● SIDE-EFFECTS
▶ **Common or very common** Diarrhoea · increased risk of infection · rhinorrhoea
▶ **Uncommon** Conjunctivitis · neutropenia (usually mild and reversible) · urticaria
▶ **Rare or very rare** Anaphylactic reaction

● CONCEPTION AND CONTRACEPTION Manufacturer advises that women of childbearing potential should use effective contraception during treatment and for at least 20 weeks after stopping treatment.

● PREGNANCY Manufacturer advises avoid—no information available.

● BREAST FEEDING Manufacturer advises avoid during treatment and for up to 20 weeks after discontinuing treatment—no information available.

● DIRECTIONS FOR ADMINISTRATION Manufacturer advises to take the syringe or pen out of the refrigerator 20 minutes before administration and to avoid injecting into areas of the skin that show psoriasis. Patients may self-administer *Cosentyx*® pre-filled pen.

● PATIENT AND CARER ADVICE
Self-administration Patients and their carers should be given training in subcutaneous injection technique.
Infection Patients and their carers should be advised to seek immediate medical attention if symptoms of infection develop during treatment with secukinumab.

● NATIONAL FUNDING/ACCESS DECISIONS
For full details see funding body website
NICE decisions
▶ Secukinumab for treating moderate to severe plaque psoriasis (July 2015) NICE TA350 Recommended with restrictions
▶ Secukinumab for active ankylosing spondylitis after treatment with non-steroidal anti-inflammatory drugs or TNF-alpha inhibitors (September 2016) NICE TA407 Recommended with restrictions
▶ Certolizumab pegol and secukinumab for treating active psoriatic arthritis after inadequate response to DMARDs (May 2017) NICE TA445 Recommended with restrictions
Scottish Medicines Consortium (SMC) decisions
▶ Secukinumab (*Cosentyx*®) for treatment of moderate to severe plaque psoriasis in adults who are candidates for systemic therapy (June 2015) SMC No. 1054/15 Recommended with restrictions

● MEDICINAL FORMS There can be variation in the licensing of different medicines containing the same drug.
Solution for injection
▶ Cosentyx (Novartis Pharmaceuticals UK Ltd)
Secukinumab 150 mg per 1 ml Cosentyx 150mg/1ml solution for injection pre-filled pens | 2 pre-filled disposable injection PoM £1,218.78
Cosentyx 150mg/1ml solution for injection pre-filled syringes | 2 pre-filled disposable injection PoM £1,218.78

10

Musculoskeletal system

Tocilizumab

16-Nov-2020

● INDICATIONS AND DOSE

Rheumatoid arthritis [severe, active and progressive, not previously treated with methotrexate] | Rheumatoid arthritis [moderate-to-severe, in combination with methotrexate or alone if methotrexate inappropriate, when response to at least one disease-modifying antirheumatic drug or tumour necrosis factor inhibitor has been inadequate, or in those who are intolerant of these drugs]

▸ BY INTRAVENOUS INFUSION
▸ Adult: 8 mg/kg every 4 weeks (max. per dose 800 mg), for dose adjustments in patients with liver enzyme abnormalities, or low absolute neutrophil or platelet count—consult product literature
▸ BY SUBCUTANEOUS INJECTION
▸ Adult: 162 mg once weekly, administer to abdomen, thigh or upper arm, for dose adjustments in patients with liver enzyme abnormalities, or low absolute neutrophil or platelet count—consult product literature

Giant cell arteritis [in combination with a tapering course of glucocorticoid or alone following discontinuation of glucocorticoid]

▸ BY SUBCUTANEOUS INJECTION
▸ Adult: 162 mg once weekly, administer to abdomen, thigh or upper arm, for dose adjustments in patients with liver enzyme abnormalities, or low absolute neutrophil or platelet count—consult product literature, not to be used alone for acute relapses; review need for treatment beyond 52 weeks

---

IMPORTANT SAFETY INFORMATION

MHRA/CHM ADVICE: TOCILIZUMAB (*ROACTEMRA*®): RARE RISK OF SERIOUS LIVER INJURY INCLUDING CASES REQUIRING TRANSPLANTATION (JULY 2019)

There have been reports of rare but serious cases of drug-induced liver injury, including acute liver failure and hepatitis, in patients treated with tocilizumab; some cases required liver transplantation. Serious liver injury was reported from 2 weeks to more than 5 years after initiation of tocilizumab.

Healthcare professionals are advised to initiate tocilizumab treatment with caution in patients with hepatic transaminases (ALT or AST) more than 1.5 times the upper limit of normal (ULN); initiation is not recommended in those with ALT or AST more than 5 times the ULN (see *Monitoring requirements*). Patients and their carers should be advised to seek immediate medical attention if signs and symptoms of liver injury, such as tiredness, abdominal pain, and jaundice, occur.

● CONTRA-INDICATIONS Do not initiate if absolute neutrophil count less than 2×10^9/litre · severe active infection
● CAUTIONS History of diverticulitis · history of intestinal ulceration · history of recurrent or chronic infection (interrupt treatment if serious infection occurs) · low absolute neutrophil count · low platelet count · predisposition to infection (interrupt treatment if serious infection occurs)

CAUTIONS, FURTHER INFORMATION
▸ Tuberculosis Patients with latent tuberculosis should be treated with standard therapy before starting tocilizumab.
● INTERACTIONS → Appendix 1: monoclonal antibodies
● SIDE-EFFECTS
▸ **Common or very common** Abdominal pain · conjunctivitis · cough · dizziness · dyslipidaemia · dyspnoea · gastrointestinal disorders · headache · hypersensitivity · hypertension · increased risk of infection · leucopenia ·

neutropenia · oral disorders · peripheral oedema · skin reactions · weight increased
▸ **Uncommon** Hypothyroidism · nephrolithiasis
▸ **Frequency not known** Hepatic disorders · infusion related reaction · interstitial lung disease · pancytopenia · Stevens-Johnson syndrome

SIDE-EFFECTS, FURTHER INFORMATION **Neutrophil and platelet counts** Manufacturer advises discontinue if absolute neutrophil count less than 0.5×10^9/litre or platelet count less than 50×10^3/microlitre.

Abnormal hepatic function Manufacturer advises caution if hepatic enzymes more than 1.5 times the upper limit of normal. Manufacturer advises discontinue if hepatic enzymes more than 5 times the upper limit of normal.

● CONCEPTION AND CONTRACEPTION Effective contraception required during and for 3 months after treatment.
● PREGNANCY Manufacturer advises avoid unless essential—toxicity in *animal* studies.
● BREAST FEEDING Manufacturer advises avoid—no information available.
● HEPATIC IMPAIRMENT Manufacturer advises caution—consult product literature.
● RENAL IMPAIRMENT
▸ With intravenous use Manufacturer advises monitor renal function closely in moderate-to-severe impairment—no information available.
▸ With subcutaneous use Manufacturer advises monitor renal function closely in severe impairment—no information available.
● PRE-TREATMENT SCREENING
Tuberculosis Patients should be evaluated for tuberculosis before treatment.
● MONITORING REQUIREMENTS
▸ Manufacturer advises monitor lipid profile 4–8 weeks after starting treatment and then as indicated.
▸ Manufacturer advises monitor for demyelinating disorders.
▸ Manufacturer advises monitor hepatic transaminases before starting treatment, every 4–8 weeks for first 6 months of treatment, then every 12 weeks thereafter.
▸ Manufacturer advises monitor neutrophil and platelet count before starting treatment, 4–8 weeks after starting treatment and then as indicated.
● DIRECTIONS FOR ADMINISTRATION
▸ With intravenous use For *intravenous infusion*, manufacturer advises give intermittently in Sodium chloride 0.9%; dilute requisite dose to a volume of 100 mL with infusion fluid and give over 1 hour.
▸ With subcutaneous use For *subcutaneous injection*, manufacturer advises rotate injection site and avoid skin that is tender, damaged or scarred. Patients may self-administer RoActemra®, after appropriate training in subcutaneous injection technique.
● PRESCRIBING AND DISPENSING INFORMATION Manufacturer advises to record the brand name and batch number after each administration.
● HANDLING AND STORAGE Manufacturer advises protect from light and store in a refrigerator (2–8 °C)—consult product literature for further information regarding storage conditions outside refrigerator and after preparation of the infusion.
● PATIENT AND CARER ADVICE Manufacturer advises patients and their carers should be advised to seek immediate medical attention if symptoms of infection occur, or if symptoms of diverticular perforation such as abdominal pain, haemorrhage, or fever accompanying change in bowel habits occur.

An alert card should be provided.

Driving and skilled tasks Manufacturer advises patients should be counselled on the effects on driving and performance of skilled tasks—increased risk of dizziness.

● NATIONAL FUNDING/ACCESS DECISIONS
For full details see funding body website

NICE decisions

▸ Adalimumab, etanercept, infliximab, certolizumab pegol, golimumab, tocilizumab and abatacept for rheumatoid arthritis not previously treated with DMARDs or after conventional DMARDs only have failed (January 2016) NICE TA375 Recommended with restrictions

▸ Tocilizumab for the treatment of rheumatoid arthritis (February 2012) NICE TA247 Recommended with restrictions

▸ Tocilizumab for treating giant cell arteritis (April 2018) NICE TA518 Recommended with restrictions

Scottish Medicines Consortium (SMC) decisions

▸ Tocilizumab (*RoActemra*®) for the treatment of Giant Cell Arteritis (GCA) in adult patients (September 2018) SMC No. SMC2014 Recommended with restrictions

● MEDICINAL FORMS There can be variation in the licensing of different medicines containing the same drug.

Solution for injection

▸ RoActemra (Roche Products Ltd)
Tocilizumab 180 mg per 1 ml RoActemra 162mg/0.9ml solution for injection pre-filled syringes | 4 pre-filled disposable injection `PoM` £913.12 DT = £913.12 (Hospital only)
RoActemra 162mg/0.9ml solution for injection pre-filled pens | 4 pre-filled disposable injection `PoM` £913.12 DT = £913.12

Solution for infusion

ELECTROLYTES: May contain Sodium

▸ RoActemra (Roche Products Ltd)
Tocilizumab 20 mg per 1 ml RoActemra 400mg/20ml concentrate for solution for infusion vials | 1 vial `PoM` £512.00 (Hospital only)
RoActemra 200mg/10ml concentrate for solution for infusion vials | 1 vial `PoM` £256.00 (Hospital only)
RoActemra 80mg/4ml concentrate for solution for infusion vials | 1 vial `PoM` £102.40 (Hospital only)

Ustekinumab

25-Nov-2020

● INDICATIONS AND DOSE

Plaque psoriasis (specialist use only)

▸ BY SUBCUTANEOUS INJECTION

▸ Adult (body-weight up to 100 kg): Initially 45 mg, then 45 mg after 4 weeks, then 45 mg every 12 weeks, consider discontinuation if no response within 28 weeks

▸ Adult (body-weight 100 kg and above): Initially 90 mg, then 90 mg after 4 weeks, then 90 mg every 12 weeks, consider discontinuation if no response within 28 weeks

Psoriatic arthritis (specialist use only)

▸ BY SUBCUTANEOUS INJECTION

▸ Adult: Initially 45 mg, then 45 mg after 4 weeks, then 45 mg every 12 weeks, consider discontinuation if no response within 28 weeks, higher doses of 90 mg may be used in patients with body-weight over 100 kg

Crohn's disease (specialist use only) | Ulcerative colitis (specialist use only)

▸ INITIALLY BY INTRAVENOUS INFUSION

▸ Adult (body-weight up to 56 kg): 260 mg, then (by subcutaneous injection) 90 mg after 8 weeks, then (by subcutaneous injection) 90 mg every 12 weeks, if response is inadequate 8 weeks after first subcutaneous dose, or response is lost, dosing frequency may be increased—consult product literature; consider discontinuation if no response within 16 weeks of initial dose or increase in dosing frequency

▸ Adult (body-weight 56-85 kg): 390 mg, then (by subcutaneous injection) 90 mg after 8 weeks, then (by subcutaneous injection) 90 mg every 12 weeks, if response is inadequate 8 weeks after first subcutaneous dose, or response is lost, dosing frequency may be increased—consult product literature; consider discontinuation if no response within 16 weeks of initial dose or increase in dosing frequency

▸ Adult (body-weight 86 kg and above): 520 mg, then (by subcutaneous injection) 90 mg after 8 weeks, then (by subcutaneous injection) 90 mg every 12 weeks, if response is inadequate 8 weeks after first subcutaneous dose, or response is lost, dosing frequency may be increased—consult product literature; consider discontinuation if no response within 16 weeks of initial dose or increase in dosing frequency

● CONTRA-INDICATIONS Active infection

● CAUTIONS Development of malignancy · elderly · history of malignancy · predisposition to infection · start appropriate treatment if widespread erythema and skin exfoliation develop, and stop ustekinumab treatment if exfoliative dermatitis suspected

CAUTIONS, FURTHER INFORMATION

▸ Tuberculosis Active tuberculosis should be treated with standard treatment for at least 2 months before starting ustekinumab. Patients who have previously received adequate treatment for tuberculosis can start ustekinumab but should be monitored every 3 months for possible recurrence. In patients without active tuberculosis but who were previously not treated adequately, chemoprophylaxis should ideally be completed before starting ustekinumab. In patients at high risk of tuberculosis who cannot be assessed by tuberculin skin test, chemoprophylaxis can be given concurrently with ustekinumab.

● INTERACTIONS → Appendix 1: monoclonal antibodies

● SIDE-EFFECTS

▸ **Common or very common** Arthralgia · asthenia · back pain · diarrhoea · dizziness · headache · increased risk of infection · myalgia · nausea · oropharyngeal pain · skin reactions · vomiting

▸ **Uncommon** Depression · facial paralysis · hypersensitivity (may be delayed) · nasal congestion

▸ **Rare or very rare** Respiratory disorders

▸ **Frequency not known** Increased risk of cancer

● CONCEPTION AND CONTRACEPTION Manufacturer advises effective contraception during treatment and for 15 weeks after stopping treatment.

● PREGNANCY Avoid.

● BREAST FEEDING Manufacturer advises avoid—present in milk in *animal* studies.

● PRE-TREATMENT SCREENING
Tuberculosis Patients should be evaluated for tuberculosis before treatment.

● MONITORING REQUIREMENTS

▸ Monitor for non-melanoma skin cancer, especially in patients with a history of PUVA treatment or prolonged immunosuppressant therapy, or those over 60 years of age.

▸ Monitor for signs and symptoms of exfoliative dermatitis or erythrodermic psoriasis.

● DIRECTIONS FOR ADMINISTRATION Manufacturer advises for *intravenous infusion (Stelara*®), give intermittently in Sodium Chloride 0.9%; dilute requisite dose with infusion fluid to final volume of 250 mL and give over at least 1 hour through an in-line low-protein binding filter (pore size 0.2 micron); use within 4 hours of dilution.

● PATIENT AND CARER ADVICE
Exfoliative dermatitis Patients should be advised to seek prompt medical attention if symptoms suggestive of exfoliative dermatitis or erythrodermic psoriasis (such as

10

Musculoskeletal system

increased redness and shedding of skin over a larger area of the body) develop.

Tuberculosis Patients should be advised to seek medical attention if symptoms suggestive of tuberculosis (e.g. persistent cough, weight loss, and fever) develop.

- **NATIONAL FUNDING/ACCESS DECISIONS**
For full details see funding body website

NICE decisions

▶ Ustekinumab for the treatment of adults with moderate to severe psoriasis (updated March 2017) NICE TA180 Recommended with restrictions

▶ Ustekinumab for treating active psoriatic arthritis (updated March 2017) NICE TA340 Recommended with restrictions

▶ Ustekinumab for moderately to severely active Crohn's disease after previous treatment (July 2017) NICE TA456 Recommended

▶ Ustekinumab for treating moderately to severely active ulcerative colitis (June 2020) NICE TA633 Recommended with restrictions

Scottish Medicines Consortium (SMC) decisions

▶ Ustekinumab (*Stelara*®) alone or in combination with methotrexate, for the treatment of active psoriatic arthritis in adult patients when the response to previous non-biological disease-modifying anti-rheumatic drug therapy has been inadequate (March 2014) SMC No. 944/14 Recommended with restrictions

▶ Ustekinumab (*Stelara*®) for the treatment of adult patients with moderately to severely active Crohn's disease who have had an inadequate response with, lost response to, or were intolerant to either conventional therapy or a tumour necrosis factor-alpha antagonist or have medical contra-indications to such therapies (July 2017) SMC No. 1250/17 Recommended

▶ Ustekinumab (*Stelara*®) for the treatment of adult patients with moderately to severely active ulcerative colitis who have had an inadequate response with, lost response to, or were intolerant to either conventional therapy or a biologic or have medical contra-indications to such therapies (April 2020) SMC No. SMC2250 Recommended

- **MEDICINAL FORMS** There can be variation in the licensing of different medicines containing the same drug.

Solution for injection
CAUTIONARY AND ADVISORY LABELS 10

▶ Stelara (Janssen-Cilag Ltd)
Ustekinumab 90 mg per 1 ml Stelara 90mg/1ml solution for injection pre-filled syringes | 1 pre-filled disposable injection PoM £2,147.00 (Hospital only)
Stelara 45mg/0.5ml solution for injection vials | 1 vial PoM £2,147.00 (Hospital only)
Stelara 45mg/0.5ml solution for injection pre-filled syringes | 1 pre-filled disposable injection PoM £2,147.00 (Hospital only)

Solution for infusion
CAUTIONARY AND ADVISORY LABELS 10

▶ Stelara (Janssen-Cilag Ltd)
Ustekinumab 5 mg per 1 ml Stelara 130mg/26ml concentrate for solution for infusion vials | 1 vial PoM £2,147.00 (Hospital only)

IMMUNOSUPPRESSANTS ⟩ JAK INHIBITORS

Baricitinib

03-Nov-2020

- **DRUG ACTION** Baricitinib selectively and reversibly inhibits the Janus-associated tyrosine kinases JAK1 and JAK2.

- **INDICATIONS AND DOSE**

Moderate-to-severe active rheumatoid arthritis in patients who have had an inadequate response to, or are intolerant to, one or more disease-modifying anti-rheumatic drugs (as monotherapy or in combination with methotrexate) (initiated by a specialist)

▶ BY MOUTH

▶ Adult 18–74 years: 4 mg once daily, for dose adjustments due to side-effects or dose reduction due to history of infection or sustained control of disease activity, consult product literature

▶ Adult 75 years and over: 2 mg once daily, for dose adjustments due to side-effects, consult product literature

---

IMPORTANT SAFETY INFORMATION

MHRA/CHM ADVICE: BARICITINIB (*OLUMIANT*®): RISK OF VENOUS THROMBOEMBOLISM (MARCH 2020)

Clinical trial data have shown that baricitinib is associated with an increased frequency of venous thromboembolism (VTE) compared with placebo. Healthcare professionals are advised to use baricitinib with caution in patients with additional risk factors for VTE. Patients should be informed of the signs and symptoms of VTE before starting treatment and advised to seek urgent medical attention if these develop. Baricitinib should be permanently discontinued if clinical features of VTE occur.

MHRA/CHM ADVICE: BARICITINIB (*OLUMIANT*®): INCREASED RISK OF DIVERTICULITIS, PARTICULARLY IN PATIENTS WITH RISK FACTORS (AUGUST 2020)

A European review of worldwide data concluded that baricitinib is associated with an increased risk of diverticulitis. The MHRA recommends healthcare professionals use baricitinib with caution in patients with pre-exisiting diverticular disease, and in patients on long-term concomitant medicines associated with an increased risk of diverticulitis (including non-steroidal anti-inflammatory drugs, corticosteroids, and opioids). Patients should be advised to seek immediate medical attention if they experience severe abdominal pain especially accompanied with fever, nausea and vomiting, or other symptoms of diverticulitis. Prompt evaluation is needed of any patients treated with baricitnib who present with new-onset abdominal signs and symptoms to identify early diverticulitis or gastrointestinal perforation.

- **CONTRA-INDICATIONS** Absolute lymphocyte count less than 0.5×10^9 cells/litre (do not initiate) · absolute neutrophil count less than 1×10^9 cells/litre (do not initiate) · haemoglobin less than 8 g/dL (do not initiate) · tuberculosis (active)

- **CAUTIONS** Active, chronic or recurrent infection (interrupt treatment if no response to standard therapy) · risk of diverticulitis · risk of viral reactivation (consult product literature)

CAUTIONS, FURTHER INFORMATION

▶ Tuberculosis Manufacturer advises consider anti-tuberculosis therapy prior to initiation of baricitinib in patients with previously untreated latent tuberculosis.

- **INTERACTIONS** → Appendix 1: baricitinib

SIDE-EFFECTS

Common or very common Dyslipidaemia · herpes zoster (interrupt treatment) · increased risk of infection · nausea · oropharyngeal pain · thrombocytosis
Uncommon Acne · deep vein thrombosis (discontinue permanently) · neutropenia · pulmonary embolism (discontinue permanently) · weight increased
Frequency not known Venous thromboembolism (discontinue permanently)

CONCEPTION AND CONTRACEPTION Manufacturer advises effective contraception during and for at least 1 week after treatment in women of child-bearing potential.

PREGNANCY Manufacturer advises avoid—toxicity in *animal* studies.

BREAST FEEDING Manufacturer advises avoid—present in milk in *animal* studies.

HEPATIC IMPAIRMENT Manufacturer advises avoid in severe impairment (no information available).

RENAL IMPAIRMENT Manufacturer advises avoid if creatinine clearance less than 30 mL/minute.
Dose adjustments Manufacturer advises reduce dose to 2 mg once daily if creatinine clearance 30–60 mL/minute.

PRE-TREATMENT SCREENING Manufacturer advises patients should be evaluated for tuberculosis and viral hepatitis before treatment.

MONITORING REQUIREMENTS
▸ Manufacturer advises monitor patients with hepatitis B surface antibody and hepatitis B core antibody, without hepatitis B surface antigen, for expression of hepatitis B virus (HBV) DNA—if HBV DNA detected, consult liver specialist for advice.
▸ Manufacturer advises monitor lipid profile 12 weeks after treatment initiation—hyperlipidaemia should be managed according to international clinical guidelines; monitor hepatic transaminases routinely—interrupt treatment if drug-induced liver injury suspected.
▸ Manufacturer advises monitor for haematological abnormalities; interrupt treatment if absolute neutrophil count less than 1×10^9 cells/litre, absolute lymphocyte count less than 0.5×10^9 cells/litre, or haemoglobin less than 8 g/dL—treatment may be restarted when levels return above these values.

NATIONAL FUNDING/ACCESS DECISIONS
For full details see funding body website
NICE decisions
▸ Baricitinib for moderate to severe rheumatoid arthritis (August 2017) NICE TA466 Recommended with restrictions
Scottish Medicines Consortium (SMC) decisions
▸ Baricitinib (*Olumiant®*) for treatment of moderate to severe active rheumatoid arthritis (RA) in adult patients who have responded inadequately to, or who are intolerant to one or more disease-modifying anti-rheumatic drugs (DMARDs). Baricitinib may be used as monotherapy or in combination with methotrexate (September 2017) SMC No. 1265/17 Recommended with restrictions

MEDICINAL FORMS There can be variation in the licensing of different medicines containing the same drug.
Tablet
▸ Olumiant (Eli Lilly and Company Ltd) ▼
  Baricitinib 2 mg Olumiant 2mg tablets | 28 tablet [PoM] £805.56 DT = £805.56
  Baricitinib 4 mg Olumiant 4mg tablets | 28 tablet [PoM] £805.56 DT = £805.56

Filgotinib

19-Nov-2020

DRUG ACTION Filgotinib is a selective inhibitor of the Janus-associated tyrosine kinase JAK1.

INDICATIONS AND DOSE

Rheumatoid arthritis (initiated by a specialist)
▸ BY MOUTH
▸ Adult 18-74 years: 200 mg once daily
▸ Adult 75 years and over: Initially 100 mg once daily, any further dose increase to 200 mg once daily should be based on the particular clinical circumstances of the patient

CONTRA-INDICATIONS Absolute lymphocyte count less than 0.5×10^9 cells/litre · absolute neutrophil count less than 1×10^9 cells/litre · haemoglobin less than 8 g/dL · serious infection (active) · tuberculosis (active)

CAUTIONS 75 years and older · history of serious or opportunistic infection · infection (chronic or recurrent) · malignancy · predisposition to infection · risk factors for venous thromboembolism · risk of viral reactivation · tuberculosis exposure

CAUTIONS, FURTHER INFORMATION
▸ Tuberculosis [EvGr] Anti-tuberculosis therapy should be initiated in patients with latent tuberculosis before starting filgotinib. Use filgotinib with caution in patients who have travelled or resided in areas of endemic tuberculosis or endemic mycoses, or who have had previous exposure to tuberculosis. ◈
▸ Immunisation [EvGr] Patients should receive all recommended vaccinations before starting treatment; live vaccines are not recommended immediately before, or during, treatment. ◈
▸ Venous thromboembolism [EvGr] Use with caution in patients with risk factors for deep-vein thrombosis or pulmonary embolism—discontinue and initiate appropriate treatment promptly. ◈

INTERACTIONS → Appendix 1: filgotinib

SIDE-EFFECTS
▸ **Common or very common** Dizziness · increased risk of infection · nausea
▸ **Uncommon** Hypercholesterolaemia · neutropenia
▸ **Frequency not known** Embolism and thrombosis · malignancy · non-melanoma skin cancer · reactivation of infections

CONCEPTION AND CONTRACEPTION [EvGr] Females of childbearing potential should use effective contraception during and for at least 1 week after stopping treatment. Impaired sperm production, decreased fertility and effects on male reproductive organs were observed in *animal* studies; the effect on humans is unknown (including if reversible)—male patients should be informed of the potential risk of reduced fertility or infertility before initiating treatment. No effects on female fertility were observed in *animal* studies. ◈

PREGNANCY [EvGr] Avoid—toxicity in *animal* studies. ◈

BREAST FEEDING [EvGr] Avoid—no information available. ◈

HEPATIC IMPAIRMENT [EvGr] Avoid in severe impairment (no information available). ◈

RENAL IMPAIRMENT [EvGr] Caution in moderate or severe impairment; avoid in end-stage renal disease (no information available). ◈
Dose adjustments [EvGr] A dose of 100 mg once daily is recommended in moderate or severe impairment. ◈

PRE-TREATMENT SCREENING [EvGr] Patients should be evaluated for tuberculosis and viral hepatitis before treatment. ◈

10

Musculoskeletal system

- MONITORING REQUIREMENTS
- ▶ EvGr Monitor for signs and symptoms of infections (including tuberculosis) during and after treatment—consider treatment interruption until the infection is controlled.
- ▶ Monitor for haematological abnormalities before and during treatment; interrupt treatment if absolute neutrophil count less than 1×10^9 cells/litre, absolute lymphocyte count less than 0.5×10^9 cells/litre, or haemoglobin less than 8 g/dL—treatment may be restarted when levels return above these values.
- ▶ Monitor lipid profile 12 weeks after treatment initiation and as needed thereafter—hyperlipidaemia should be managed according to international clinical guidelines.
- ▶ Monitor for viral reactivation (including viral hepatitis and herpes zoster) during treatment; interrupt treatment if herpes zoster infection develops and resume once resolved.
- ▶ Periodic skin examination is recommended in patients at increased risk for skin cancer. ⓜ

- PRESCRIBING AND DISPENSING INFORMATION The manufacturer of *Jyseleca*® has provided a guide for healthcare professionals.

- PATIENT AND CARER ADVICE For *Jyseleca*®, a patient alert card should be provided.

- MEDICINAL FORMS There can be variation in the licensing of different medicines containing the same drug.

Tablet

CAUTIONARY AND ADVISORY LABELS 25
- ▶ Jyseleca (Gilead Sciences Ireland UC) ▼
  Filgotinib (as Filgotinib maleate) 100 mg Jyseleca 100mg tablets | 30 tablet [PoM] £863.10 (Hospital only)
  Filgotinib (as Filgotinib maleate) 200 mg Jyseleca 200mg tablets | 30 tablet [PoM] £863.10 (Hospital only)

Tofacitinib

10-Nov-2020

- DRUG ACTION Tofacitinib selectively inhibits the Janus-associated tyrosine kinases JAK1 and JAK3.

- INDICATIONS AND DOSE

Moderate to severe active rheumatoid arthritis in patients who have had an inadequate response to, or are intolerant to one or more disease-modifying anti-rheumatic drugs (as monotherapy or in combination with methotrexate) (specialist use only) | Active psoriatic arthritis in patients who have had an inadequate response to, or are intolerant to one or more disease-modifying anti-rheumatic drugs (in combination with methotrexate) (specialist use only)
- ▶ BY MOUTH
- ▶ Adult: 5 mg twice daily, for dose adjustments due to side-effects—consult product literature

Moderate to severe active ulcerative colitis in patients who have had an inadequate or lost response to, or are intolerant to either conventional therapy or a biologic agent (specialist use only)
- ▶ BY MOUTH
- ▶ Adult: Initially 10 mg twice daily for 8 weeks, then maintenance 5 mg twice daily, if an adequate therapeutic response is not achieved after 8 weeks, the initial dose can be extended for an additional 8 weeks, discontinue treatment if no response 16 weeks after initial dose, for dose adjustments due to side-effects, decreased response during maintenance treatment or following treatment interruption—consult product literature

DOSE ADJUSTMENTS DUE TO INTERACTIONS
- ▶ Manufacturer advises reduce dose with concurrent use of potent CYP3A4 inhibitors, or concurrent use of a

moderate CYP3A4 inhibitor and a potent CYP2C19 inhibitor, or concurrent use of drugs which are both moderate CYP3A4 and potent CYP2C19 inhibitors. Dose should be reduced to 5 mg once daily in patients receiving 5 mg twice daily. Dose should be reduced to 5 mg twice daily in patients receiving 10 mg twice daily.

> IMPORTANT SAFETY INFORMATION
>
> MHRA/CHM ADVICE: TOFACITINIB (*XELJANZ*®): NEW MEASURES TO MINIMISE RISK OF VENOUS THROMBOEMBOLISM AND OF SERIOUS AND FATAL INFECTIONS (MARCH 2020)
> New recommendations have been issued following a European safety review that found a dose-dependent increased risk of serious venous thromboembolism (VTE) associated with tofacitinib. Healthcare professionals are advised to use tofacitinib with caution in any patients with known risk factors for VTE, in addition to the underlying disease. In patients with high risk factors being treated for ulcerative colitis, the use of tofacitinib 10 mg twice daily as maintenance treatment is **not** recommended, unless no suitable alternative is available. In **all** patients being treated for rheumatoid or psoriatic arthritis, the recommended daily dose of tofacitinib should not be exceeded— *see Indications and Dose.* Patients should be informed of the signs and symptoms of VTE before starting treatment and advised to seek urgent medical attention if these develop. Tofacitinib should be permanently discontinued if signs of VTE occur.
> Tofacitinib was also found to increase the risk of serious and fatal infections, with higher rates of infections in the elderly. Use of tofacitinib in patients older than 65 years is **not** recommended, unless no suitable alternative is available.

- CONTRA-INDICATIONS Absolute lymphocyte count less than 750 cells/mm³ (do not initiate) · absolute neutrophil count less than 1000 cells/mm³ (do not initiate) · active infection including localised infection · active tuberculosis · haemoglobin less than 9 g/dL (do not initiate) · risk factors for pulmonary embolism (high doses)

- CAUTIONS Active, chronic or recurrent infection · elderly · predisposition to infection · previous or current malignancy · raised serum transaminases (particularly in combination with potentially hepatotoxic drugs) · risk of diverticulitis · risk of gastrointestinal perforation (new onset abdominal signs and symptoms should be evaluated promptly) · risk of viral reactivation (consult product literature)

CAUTIONS, FURTHER INFORMATION Manufacturer advises patients should receive all recommended vaccinations before starting treatment (consider prophylactic varicella zoster vaccination); live vaccines should be given at least 2 weeks, but preferably 4 weeks before treatment initiation—consult product literature.
- ▶ Tuberculosis Manufacturer advises consider anti-tuberculosis therapy prior to initiation of tofacitinib in patients with previously untreated latent tuberculosis.

- INTERACTIONS → Appendix 1: tofacitinib

- SIDE-EFFECTS
- ▶ **Common or very common** Anaemia · cough · diarrhoea · fatigue · fever · gastrointestinal discomfort · gastrointestinal disorders · headache · hypertension · increased risk of infection · joint disorders · nausea · peripheral oedema · skin reactions · vomiting
- ▶ **Uncommon** Decreased leucocytes · dehydration · dyslipidaemia · dyspnoea · hepatic steatosis · insomnia · ligament sprain · muscle strain · musculoskeletal pain · neoplasms · neutropenia · paraesthesia · sinus congestion · tendinitis · venous thromboembolism (discontinue permanently) · weight increased

Rare or very rare Meningitis cryptococcal · sepsis
Frequency not known Angioedema · BK virus infection ·
deep vein thrombosis (discontinue permanently) ·
interstitial lung disease (including fatal cases) ·
malignancy · pulmonary embolism (discontinue
permanently) · reactivation of infections

● CONCEPTION AND CONTRACEPTION Manufacturer advises
effective contraception during and for at least 4 weeks
after treatment in women of child-bearing potential.

● PREGNANCY Manufacturer advises avoid—toxicity in
animal studies.

● BREAST FEEDING Manufacturer advises avoid—present in
milk in *animal* studies.

● HEPATIC IMPAIRMENT Manufacturer advises caution in
moderate impairment; avoid in severe impairment.
Dose adjustments Manufacturer advises dose reduction in
moderate impairment—consult product literature.

● RENAL IMPAIRMENT
Dose adjustments Manufacturer advises reduce dose in
severe impairment —consult product literature.

● PRE-TREATMENT SCREENING Manufacturer advises
patients should be evaluated for tuberculosis and viral
hepatitis before treatment.

● MONITORING REQUIREMENTS
► Manufacturer advises monitor for signs and symptoms of
infection during and after treatment.
► Manufacturer advises periodic skin examination in
patients at increased risk for skin cancer.
► Manufacturer advises monitor liver function routinely;
monitor lipid profile 8 weeks after treatment initiation.
► Manufacturer advises monitor lymphocytes at baseline
and every 3 months thereafter; neutrophils and
haemoglobin should be monitored at baseline, after 4 to
8 weeks of treatment and every 3 months thereafter.

● DIRECTIONS FOR ADMINISTRATION Manufacturer advises
tablets may be crushed and taken with water.

● NATIONAL FUNDING/ACCESS DECISIONS
For full details see funding body website
NICE decisions
► **Tofacitinib for moderate-to-severe rheumatoid arthritis
(October 2017)** NICE TA480 Recommended with restrictions
► **Tofacitinib for treating active psoriatic arthritis after
inadequate response to DMARDs (October 2018)** NICE TA543
Recommended with restrictions
► **Tofacitinib for moderately to severely active ulcerative colitis
(November 2018)** NICE TA547 Recommended with
restrictions
Scottish Medicines Consortium (SMC) decisions
► **Tofacitinib citrate (*Xeljanz*®) in combination with
methotrexate for the treatment of moderate to severe active
rheumatoid arthritis in adult patients who have responded
inadequately to, or who are intolerant to one or more disease-
modifying anti-rheumatic drugs (DMARDs). Tofacitinib can be
given as monotherapy in case of intolerance to methotrexate
or when treatment with methotrexate is inappropriate
(February 2018)** SMC No. 1298/18 Recommended with
restrictions
► **Tofacitinib (*Xeljanz*®) in combination with methotrexate for
the treatment of active psoriatic arthritis in adult patients
who have had an inadequate response or who have been
intolerant to a prior disease-modifying antirheumatic drug
(DMARD) therapy (January 2019)** SMC No. SMC2116
Recommended with restrictions
► **Tofacitinib (*Xeljanz*®) for the treatment of adult patients with
moderately to severely active ulcerative colitis who have had
an inadequate response, lost response, or were intolerant to
either conventional therapy or a biologic agent (February
2019)** SMC No. SMC2122 Recommended

● MEDICINAL FORMS There can be variation in the licensing of
different medicines containing the same drug.
Tablet
► Xeljanz (Pfizer Ltd) ▼
Tofacitinib (as Tofacitinib citrate) 5 mg Xeljanz 5mg tablets |
56 tablet [PoM] £690.03 (Hospital only)
Tofacitinib (as Tofacitinib citrate) 10 mg Xeljanz 10mg tablets |
56 tablet [PoM] £1,380.06 (Hospital only)

Upadacitinib   20-Apr-2020

● DRUG ACTION Upadacitinib is a selective and reversible
inhibitor of the Janus-associated tyrosine kinase JAK1.

● INDICATIONS AND DOSE
Rheumatoid arthritis (specialist use only)
► BY MOUTH
► Adult: 15 mg once daily

> **IMPORTANT SAFETY INFORMATION**
> **MHRA/CHM ADVICE: UPADACITINIB (*RINVOQ*®): ADVICE FOR
> VENOUS THROMBOEMBOLISM (MARCH 2020)**
> Cases of deep vein thrombosis and pulmonary embolism
> have been reported in patients taking upadacitinib.
> Healthcare professionals are advised to use upadacitinib
> with caution in patients with risk factors for VTE.
> Patients should be informed of the signs and symptoms
> of VTE before starting treatment and advised to seek
> urgent medical attention if these develop. Upadacitinib
> should be discontinued if clinical features of VTE occur.

● CONTRA-INDICATIONS Absolute lymphocyte count less
than 500 cells/mm^3 · absolute neutrophil count less than
1000 cells/mm^3 · active serious infection including
localised infection · active tuberculosis · haemoglobin less
than 8 g/dL

● CAUTIONS 75 years and over · chronic or recurrent
infection · history of serious or opportunistic infection ·
known malignancy · patients at high risk for deep-vein
thrombosis or pulmonary embolism · patients who have
travelled or resided in areas of endemic tuberculosis or
endemic mycoses · predisposition to infection · risk of viral
reactivation (consult product literature) · tuberculosis
exposure
CAUTIONS, FURTHER INFORMATION
► Immunisation Manufacturer advises patients should receive
all recommended vaccinations, including prophylactic
varicella zoster vaccination, before starting treatment; live
vaccines are not recommended.
► Tuberculosis Manufacturer advises consider anti-
tuberculosis therapy prior to initiation of upadacitinib in
patients with previously untreated latent tuberculosis or in
patients at risk of tuberculosis infection.

● INTERACTIONS → Appendix 1: upadacitinib

● SIDE-EFFECTS
► **Common or very common** Cough · dyslipidaemia · fever ·
increased risk of infection · nausea · neutropenia ·
oropharyngeal pain · weight increased
► **Frequency not known** Deep vein thrombosis (discontinue
and initiate treatment promptly) · malignancy · meningitis
bacterial · non-melanoma skin cancer · pulmonary
embolism (discontinue and initiate treatment promptly) ·
reactivation of infections · venous thromboembolism
(discontinue and initiate treatment promptly)

● CONCEPTION AND CONTRACEPTION Manufacturer advises
females of childbearing potential should use effective
contraception during and for 4 weeks after treatment.

● PREGNANCY Manufacturer advises avoid—toxicity in
animal studies.

10

Musculoskeletal system

- ● BREAST FEEDING Manufacturer advises avoid—present in milk in *animal* studies.
- ● HEPATIC IMPAIRMENT Manufacturer advises avoid in severe impairment (no information available).
- ● RENAL IMPAIRMENT Manufacturer advises caution in severe impairment (limited information available).
- ● PRE-TREATMENT SCREENING Manufacturer advises patients should be evaluated for tuberculosis and viral hepatitis before treatment.
- ● MONITORING REQUIREMENTS
- ▶ Manufacturer advises monitor for signs and symptoms of infection during and after treatment.
- ▶ Manufacturer advises periodic skin examination in patients at increased risk for skin cancer.
- ▶ Manufacturer advises monitor neutrophils, lymphocytes and haemoglobin before starting treatment, and as clinically indicated thereafter; interrupt treatment if absolute neutrophil count less than 1000 cells/mm^3, absolute lymphocyte count less than 500 cells/mm^3, or haemoglobin less than 8 g/dL—treatment may be restarted when levels return above these values.
- ▶ Manufacturer advises monitor hepatic transaminases before starting treatment, and as clinically indicated thereafter—interrupt treatment if drug-induced liver injury suspected; monitor lipids 12 weeks after starting treatment, and then as clinically indicated.

- ● MEDICINAL FORMS There can be variation in the licensing of different medicines containing the same drug.
  Modified-release tablet
  CAUTIONARY AND ADVISORY LABELS 25
  ▶ Rinvoq (AbbVie Ltd) ▼
  Upadacitinib (as Upadacitinib hemihydrate) 15 mg Rinvoq 15mg modified-release tablets | 28 tablet [PoM] £805.56

IMMUNOSUPPRESSANTS ＞ T-CELL ACTIVATION INHIBITORS

Abatacept

17-Jul-2020

- ● INDICATIONS AND DOSE
  Moderate-to-severe active rheumatoid arthritis (specialist use only) | Active psoriatic arthritis (specialist use only)
  ▶ BY INTRAVENOUS INFUSION
  ▶ Adult (body-weight up to 60 kg): 500 mg every 2 weeks for 3 doses, then 500 mg every 4 weeks, review treatment if no response within 6 months
  ▶ Adult (body-weight 60–100 kg): 750 mg every 2 weeks for 3 doses, then 750 mg every 4 weeks, review treatment if no response within 6 months
  ▶ Adult (body-weight 101 kg and above): 1 g every 2 weeks for 3 doses, then 1 g every 4 weeks, review treatment if no response within 6 months
  Moderate-to-severe active rheumatoid arthritis (specialist use only) | Active psoriatic arthritis (specialist use only)
  ▶ BY SUBCUTANEOUS INJECTION
  ▶ Adult: 125 mg once weekly, review treatment if no response within 6 months, subcutaneous dosing may be initiated with or without an intravenous loading dose—consult product literature

- ● CONTRA-INDICATIONS Severe infection
- ● CAUTIONS Do not initiate until active infections are controlled · elderly (increased risk of side-effects) · predisposition to infection (screen for latent tuberculosis and viral hepatitis) · progressive multifocal leucoencephalopathy (discontinue treatment if neurological symptoms present)
- ● INTERACTIONS → Appendix 1: abatacept

- ● SIDE-EFFECTS
- ▶ **Common or very common** Asthenia · cough · diarrhoea · dizziness · gastrointestinal discomfort · headaches · hypertension · increased risk of infection · nausea · oral ulceration · skin reactions · vomiting
- ▶ **Uncommon** Alopecia · anxiety · arrhythmias · arthralgia · bruising tendency · conjunctivitis · depression · dry eye · dyspnoea · gastritis · hyperhidrosis · hypotension · influenza like illness · leucopenia · menstrual cycle irregularities · neoplasms · pain in extremity · palpitations · paraesthesia · respiratory disorders · sepsis · sleep disorders · throat tightness · thrombocytopenia · vasculitis · vasodilation · vertigo · visual acuity decreased · weight increased
- ▶ **Rare or very rare** Pelvic inflammatory disease
- ● CONCEPTION AND CONTRACEPTION Effective contraception required during treatment and for 14 weeks after last dose.
- ● PREGNANCY Manufacturer advises avoid unless essential.
- ● BREAST FEEDING Present in milk in *animal* studies—manufacturer advises avoid breast-feeding during treatment and for 14 weeks after last dose.
- ● DIRECTIONS FOR ADMINISTRATION For *intravenous infusion*, manufacturer advises give intermittently *in* Sodium chloride 0.9%; reconstitute each vial with 10 mL water for injections using the silicone-free syringe provided; dilute requisite dose in Sodium Chloride 0.9% to 100 mL (using the same silicone-free syringe); give over 30 minutes through a low protein-binding filter (pore size 0.2–1.2 micron).
- ● NATIONAL FUNDING/ACCESS DECISIONS For full details see funding body website
  NICE decisions
- ▶ **Adalimumab, etanercept, infliximab, rituximab, and abatacept for the treatment of rheumatoid arthritis after the failure of a TNF inhibitor (August 2010)** NICE TA195 Recommended
- ▶ **Adalimumab, etanercept, infliximab, certolizumab pegol, golimumab, tocilizumab and abatacept for rheumatoid arthritis not previously treated with DMARDs or after conventional DMARDs only have failed (January 2016)** NICE TA375 Recommended with restrictions

- ● MEDICINAL FORMS There can be variation in the licensing of different medicines containing the same drug.
  Solution for injection
  ▶ Orencia (Bristol-Myers Squibb Pharmaceuticals Ltd)
  Abatacept 125 mg per 1 ml Orencia 50mg/0.4ml solution for injection pre-filled syringes | 4 pre-filled disposable injection [PoM] [⊠] (Hospital only)
  Orencia 87.5mg/0.7ml solution for injection pre-filled syringes | 4 pre-filled disposable injection [PoM] [⊠] (Hospital only)
  Orencia 125mg/1ml solution for injection pre-filled syringes | 4 pre-filled disposable injection [PoM] £1,209.60 DT = £1,209.60 (Hospital only)
  ▶ Orencia ClickJect (Bristol-Myers Squibb Pharmaceuticals Ltd)
  Abatacept 125 mg per 1 ml Orencia ClickJect 125mg/1ml solution for injection pre-filled pens | 4 pre-filled disposable injection [PoM] £1,209.60 DT = £1,209.60
  Powder for solution for infusion
  ELECTROLYTES: May contain Sodium
  ▶ Orencia (Bristol-Myers Squibb Pharmaceuticals Ltd)
  Abatacept 250 mg Orencia 250mg powder for concentrate for solution for infusion vials | 1 vial [PoM] £302.40 (Hospital only)

IMMUNOSUPPRESSANTS 〉 TUMOR NECROSIS FACTOR ALPHA (TNF-α) INHIBITORS

Adalimumab

24-Nov-2020

● INDICATIONS AND DOSE

Plaque psoriasis (initiated by a specialist)

▸ BY SUBCUTANEOUS INJECTION

▸ Adult: Initially 80 mg, then 40 mg every 2 weeks, to be started 1 week after initial dose, review treatment if no response within 16 weeks—consult product literature

Rheumatoid arthritis (initiated by a specialist)

▸ BY SUBCUTANEOUS INJECTION

▸ Adult: 40 mg every 2 weeks, then increased if necessary to 40 mg once weekly, alternatively 80 mg every 2 weeks, dose to be increased only in patients receiving adalimumab alone, review treatment if no response within 12 weeks

Psoriatic arthritis (initiated by a specialist) | Ankylosing spondylitis (initiated by a specialist) | Axial spondyloarthritis (initiated by a specialist)

▸ BY SUBCUTANEOUS INJECTION

▸ Adult: 40 mg every 2 weeks, review treatment if no response within 12 weeks

Crohn's disease (initiated by a specialist)

▸ BY SUBCUTANEOUS INJECTION

▸ Adult: Initially 80 mg, then 40 mg after 2 weeks; maintenance 40 mg every 2 weeks, increased if necessary to 40 mg once weekly, alternatively 80 mg every 2 weeks, review treatment if no response within 12 weeks

Crohn's disease (accelerated regimen) (initiated by a specialist)

▸ BY SUBCUTANEOUS INJECTION

▸ Adult: Initially 160 mg, dose can alternatively be given as divided injections over 2 days, then 80 mg after 2 weeks; maintenance 40 mg every 2 weeks, increased if necessary to 40 mg once weekly, alternatively 80 mg every 2 weeks, review treatment if no response within 12 weeks

Ulcerative colitis (initiated by a specialist)

▸ BY SUBCUTANEOUS INJECTION

▸ Adult: Initially 160 mg, dose can alternatively be given as divided injections over 2 days, then 80 mg after 2 weeks; maintenance 40 mg every 2 weeks, increased if necessary to 40 mg once weekly, alternatively 80 mg every 2 weeks, review treatment if no response within 8 weeks

Hidradenitis suppurativa (initiated by a specialist)

▸ BY SUBCUTANEOUS INJECTION

▸ Adult: Initially 160 mg, dose can alternatively be given as divided injections over 2 days, followed by 80 mg after 2 weeks, then maintenance 40 mg once weekly, after 2 weeks, alternatively 80 mg every 2 weeks, after 2 weeks, review treatment if no response within 12 weeks; if treatment interrupted—consult product literature

Uveitis (initiated by a specialist)

▸ BY SUBCUTANEOUS INJECTION

▸ Adult: Initially 80 mg, then 40 mg after 1 week; maintenance 40 mg every 2 weeks

● CONTRA-INDICATIONS Moderate or severe heart failure · severe infections

● CAUTIONS Demyelinating disorders (risk of exacerbation) · development of malignancy · do not initiate until active infections are controlled (discontinue if new serious infection develops) · hepatitis B virus—monitor for active infection · history of malignancy · mild heart failure (discontinue if symptoms develop or worsen) · predisposition to infection

CAUTIONS, FURTHER INFORMATION

▸ Tuberculosis Active tuberculosis should be treated with standard treatment for at least 2 months before starting adalimumab. Patients who have previously received adequate treatment for tuberculosis can start adalimumab but should be monitored every 3 months for possible recurrence. In patients without active tuberculosis but who were previously not treated adequately, chemoprophylaxis should ideally be completed before starting adalimumab. In patients at high risk of tuberculosis who cannot be assessed by tuberculin skin test, chemoprophylaxis can be given concurrently with adalimumab.

● INTERACTIONS → Appendix 1: monoclonal antibodies

● SIDE-EFFECTS

▸ **Common or very common** Agranulocytosis · alopecia · anaemia · anxiety · arrhythmias · arterial occlusion · asthma · broken nails · chest pain · coagulation disorder · connective tissue disorders · cough · dehydration · depression · dyspnoea · electrolyte imbalance · embolism and thrombosis · eye inflammation · fever · flushing · gastrointestinal discomfort · gastrointestinal disorders · haemorrhage · headaches · healing impaired · hyperglycaemia · hypersensitivity · hypertension · increased risk of infection · insomnia · leucocytosis · leucopenia · mood altered · muscle spasms · musculoskeletal pain · nausea · neoplasms · nerve disorders · neutropenia · oedema · renal impairment · seasonal allergy · sensation abnormal · sepsis · skin reactions · sweat changes · thrombocytopenia · vasculitis · vertigo · vision disorders · vomiting

▸ **Uncommon** Aortic aneurysm · congestive heart failure · deafness · demyelinating disorders · dysphagia · erectile dysfunction · gallbladder disorders · hepatic disorders · inflammation · lupus erythematosus · meningitis viral · myocardial infarction · nocturia · pancreatitis · respiratory disorders · rhabdomyolysis · sarcoidosis · solid organ neoplasm · stroke · tinnitus · tremor

▸ **Rare or very rare** Cardiac arrest · pancytopenia · Stevens-Johnson syndrome

SIDE-EFFECTS, FURTHER INFORMATION Associated with infections, sometimes severe, including tuberculosis, septicaemia, and hepatitis B reactivation.

● CONCEPTION AND CONTRACEPTION Manufacturer advises effective contraception required during treatment and for at least 5 months after last dose.

● PREGNANCY Manufacturer advises use only if potential benefit outweighs risk.

● BREAST FEEDING Manufacturer advises can be used—excreted in breast milk at very low concentrations (limited information available).

● PRE-TREATMENT SCREENING
Tuberculosis Manufacturer advises patients should be evaluated for active and latent tuberculosis before treatment.

● MONITORING REQUIREMENTS

▸ Manufacturer advises monitor for infection before, during, and for 4 months after treatment.

▸ Manufacturer advises monitor for non-melanoma skin cancer before and during treatment, especially in patients with a history of PUVA treatment for psoriasis or extensive immunosuppressant therapy.

▸ *For uveitis*, manufacturer advises patients should be assessed for pre-existing or developing central demyelinating disorders before and at regular intervals during treatment.

● PRESCRIBING AND DISPENSING INFORMATION
Adalimumab is a biological medicine. Biological medicines

10

Musculoskeletal system

must be prescribed and dispensed by brand name, see *Biological medicines* and *Biosimilar medicines*, under Guidance on prescribing p. 1.

- **PATIENT AND CARER ADVICE** When used to treat *hidradenitis suppurativa*, patients and their carers should be advised to use a daily topical antiseptic wash on lesions during treatment with adalimumab.
  Tuberculosis Patients and their carers should be advised to seek medical attention if symptoms suggestive of tuberculosis (e.g. persistent cough, weight loss, and fever) develop.
  Blood disorders Patients and their carers should be advised to seek medical attention if symptoms suggestive of blood disorders (such as fever, sore throat, bruising, or bleeding) develop.
  Alert card An alert card should be provided.
- **NATIONAL FUNDING/ACCESS DECISIONS**
  For full details see funding body website

  NICE decisions
  ▸ **Adalimumab for plaque psoriasis in adults (June 2008)** NICE TA146 Recommended with restrictions
  ▸ **Infliximab and adalimumab for Crohn's disease (May 2010)** NICE TA187 Recommended
  ▸ **Infliximab, adalimumab and golimumab for treating moderately to severely active ulcerative colitis after the failure of conventional therapy (February 2015)** NICE TA329 Recommended with restrictions
  ▸ **Etanercept, infliximab, and adalimumab for the treatment of psoriatic arthritis (August 2010)** NICE TA199 Recommended with restrictions
  ▸ **Adalimumab, etanercept, infliximab, rituximab, and abatacept for the treatment of rheumatoid arthritis after the failure of a TNF inhibitor (August 2010)** NICE TA195 Recommended with restrictions
  ▸ **Adalimumab, etanercept, infliximab, certolizumab pegol, golimumab, tocilizumab and abatacept for rheumatoid arthritis not previously treated with DMARDs or after conventional DMARDs only have failed (January 2016)** NICE TA375 Recommended with restrictions
  ▸ **TNF-alpha inhibitors for ankylosing spondylitis and non-radiographic axial spondyloarthritis (February 2016)** NICE TA383 Recommended
  ▸ **Adalimumab for treating moderate-to-severe hidradenitis suppurativa (June 2016)** NICE TA392 Recommended with restrictions
  ▸ **Adalimumab and dexamethasone for treating non-infectious uveitis (July 2017)** NICE TA460 Recommended

  Scottish Medicines Consortium (SMC) decisions
  ▸ **Adalimumab (*Humira*®) for moderate to severe chronic plaque psoriasis in adult patients (June 2008)** SMC No. 468/08 Recommended with restrictions

- **MEDICINAL FORMS** There can be variation in the licensing of different medicines containing the same drug.

  Solution for injection
  CAUTIONARY AND ADVISORY LABELS 10
  ▸ Amgevita (Amgen Ltd) ▼
  Adalimumab 50 mg per 1 ml Amgevita 20mg/0.4ml solution for injection pre-filled syringes | 1 pre-filled disposable injection [PoM] £158.40
  Amgevita 40mg/0.8ml solution for injection pre-filled syringes | 2 pre-filled disposable injection [PoM] £633.60
  Amgevita 40mg/0.8ml solution for injection pre-filled pens | 2 pre-filled disposable injection [PoM] £633.60
  ▸ Humira (AbbVie Ltd)
  Adalimumab 100 mg per 1 ml Humira 40mg/0.4ml solution for injection pre-filled pens | 2 pre-filled disposable injection [PoM] £704.28 DT = £704.28
  Humira 40mg/0.4ml solution for injection pre-filled syringes | 2 pre-filled disposable injection [PoM] £704.28 DT = £704.28
  Humira 20mg/0.2ml solution for injection pre-filled syringes | 2 pre-filled disposable injection [PoM] £352.14 DT = £352.14
  Humira 80mg/0.8ml solution for injection pre-filled syringes | 1 pre-filled disposable injection [PoM] £704.28

Humira 80mg/0.8ml solution for injection pre-filled pens | 1 pre-filled disposable injection [PoM] £704.28
- ▸ Hyrimoz (Sandoz Ltd) ▼
  Adalimumab 50 mg per 1 ml Hyrimoz 40mg/0.8ml solution for injection pre-filled pens | 2 pre-filled disposable injection [PoM] £646.18
  Hyrimoz 40mg/0.8ml solution for injection pre-filled syringes | 2 pre-filled disposable injection [PoM] £646.18
- ▸ Idacio (Fresenius Kabi Ltd) ▼
  Adalimumab 50 mg per 1 ml Idacio 40mg/0.8ml solution for injection vials | 1 vial [PoM] £316.93
  Idacio 40mg/0.8ml solution for injection pre-filled syringes | 2 pre-filled disposable injection [PoM] £633.86
  Idacio 40mg/0.8ml solution for injection pre-filled pens | 2 pre-filled disposable injection [PoM] £633.86
- ▸ Imraldi (Biogen Idec Ltd) ▼
  Adalimumab 50 mg per 1 ml Imraldi 40mg/0.8ml solution for injection pre-filled pens | 2 pre-filled disposable injection [PoM] £633.85
  Imraldi 40mg/0.8ml solution for injection pre-filled syringes | 2 pre-filled disposable injection [PoM] £633.85

Certolizumab pegol

11-Nov-2020

- **INDICATIONS AND DOSE**

  Moderate to severe active rheumatoid arthritis when response to disease-modifying antirheumatic drugs (including methotrexate) has been inadequate (as monotherapy or in combination with methotrexate) | Severe, active and progressive rheumatoid arthritis in patients not previously treated with methotrexate or other disease-modifying antirheumatic drugs (in combination with methotrexate) | Active psoriatic arthritis when response to disease-modifying antirheumatic drugs has been inadequate (as monotherapy or in combination with methotrexate)
  ▸ BY SUBCUTANEOUS INJECTION
  ▸ Adult: Loading dose 400 mg every 2 weeks for 3 doses, then maintenance 200 mg every 2 weeks, once clinical response is confirmed, an alternative maintenance dosing of 400 mg every 4 weeks can be considered, review treatment if no response within 12 weeks

  Treatment of severe active ankylosing spondylitis in patients who have had an inadequate response to, or are intolerant of NSAIDs | Treatment of severe active axial spondyloarthritis, without radiographic evidence of ankylosing spondylitis but with objective signs of inflammation, in patients who have had an inadequate response to, or are intolerant of NSAIDs
  ▸ BY SUBCUTANEOUS INJECTION
  ▸ Adult: Loading dose 400 mg every 2 weeks for 3 doses, then maintenance 200 mg every 2 weeks, alternatively maintenance 400 mg every 4 weeks, review treatment if no response within 12 weeks

  Moderate to severe plaque psoriasis
  ▸ BY SUBCUTANEOUS INJECTION
  ▸ Adult: Loading dose 400 mg every 2 weeks for 3 doses, then maintenance 200 mg every 2 weeks, an alternative maintenance dosing of 400 mg every 2 weeks can be considered in patients with insufficient response, review treatment if no response within 16 weeks

- **CONTRA-INDICATIONS** Moderate to severe heart failure · severe active infection
- **CAUTIONS** Demyelinating CNS disorders (risk of exacerbation) · do not initiate until active infections are controlled (discontinue if new serious infection develops and until infection controlled) · hepatitis B virus (monitor for active infection) · history or development of malignancy · mild heart failure (discontinue if symptoms develop or worsen) · predisposition to infection

CAUTIONS, FURTHER INFORMATION

Tuberculosis Active tuberculosis should be treated with standard treatment for at least 2 months before starting certolizumab pegol. Patients who have previously received adequate treatment for tuberculosis can start certolizumab pegol but should be monitored every 3 months for possible recurrence. In patients without active tuberculosis but who were previously not treated adequately, chemoprophylaxis should ideally be completed before starting certolizumab pegol. In patients at high risk of tuberculosis who cannot be assessed by tuberculin skin test, chemoprophylaxis can be given concurrently with certolizumab pegol.

● **INTERACTIONS** → Appendix 1: monoclonal antibodies

● SIDE-EFFECTS

● **Common or very common** Abscess · asthenia · decreased leucocytes · eosinophilic disorders · fever · headaches · hepatic disorders · hypertension · increased risk of infection · nausea · neoplasms · neutropenia · pain · sensory disorder · skin reactions

● **Uncommon** Alopecia · anaemia · anxiety · appetite disorder · arrhythmias · ascites · asthma · breast disorder · cardiomyopathy · chills · coronary artery disease · cough · cyst · dizziness · dyslipidaemia · electrolyte imbalance · embolism and thrombosis · eye inflammation · flushing · gastrointestinal discomfort · gastrointestinal disorders · haemorrhage · healing impaired · heart failure · hypercoagulation · hypersensitivity · influenza like illness · lacrimation disorder · lymphadenopathy · menstrual cycle irregularities · mood disorder · muscle disorder · nail disorder · nerve disorders · oedema · oral disorders · oropharyngeal dryness · palpitations · photosensitivity reaction · renal impairment · respiratory disorders · sepsis · skin ulcer · solid organ neoplasm · sweat changes · syncope · systemic lupus erythematosus (SLE) · temperature perception abnormal · thrombocytopenia · thrombocytosis · tinnitus · tremor · urinary tract disorder · vasculitides · vertigo · vision disorders · weight change

▶ **Rare or very rare** Angioedema · atherosclerosis · atrioventricular block · cholelithiasis · cognitive impairment · delirium · fistula · haemosiderosis · hair texture abnormal · movement disorders · nephritis · nephropathy · odynophagia · pancytopenia · panniculitis · pericarditis · polycythaemia · Raynaud's phenomenon · sarcoidosis · seizure · sexual dysfunction · splenomegaly · stroke · suicide attempt · telangiectasia · thyroid disorder

▶ **Frequency not known** Multiple sclerosis

SIDE-EFFECTS, FURTHER INFORMATION Associated with infections, sometimes severe, including tuberculosis, septicaemia, and hepatitis B reactivation.

● CONCEPTION AND CONTRACEPTION Manufacturer advises adequate contraception in women of childbearing potential during treatment and for 5 months after last dose.

● PREGNANCY Manufacturer advises use only if potential benefit outweighs risk—limited information available.

● PRE-TREATMENT SCREENING

Tuberculosis Patients should be evaluated for tuberculosis before treatment.

● MONITORING REQUIREMENTS Monitor for infection before, during, and for 5 months after treatment.

● PATIENT AND CARER ADVICE

Blood disorders Patients should be advised to seek medical attention if symptoms suggestive of blood disorders (such as fever, sore throat, bruising, or bleeding) develop.

Tuberculosis Patients should be advised to seek medical attention if symptoms suggestive of tuberculosis (e.g. persistent cough, weight loss and fever) develop.

Alert card An alert card should be provided.

● NATIONAL FUNDING/ACCESS DECISIONS

For full details see funding body website

NICE decisions

▶ Adalimumab, etanercept, infliximab, certolizumab pegol, golimumab, tocilizumab and abatacept for rheumatoid arthritis not previously treated with DMARDs or after conventional DMARDs only have failed (January 2016) NICE TA375 Recommended with restrictions

▶ TNF-alpha inhibitors for ankylosing spondylitis and non-radiographic axial spondyloarthritis (February 2016) NICE TA383 Recommended

▶ Certolizumab pegol for treating rheumatoid arthritis after inadequate response to a TNF-alpha inhibitor (October 2016) NICE TA415 Recommended with restrictions

▶ Certolizumab pegol and secukinumab for treating active psoriatic arthritis after inadequate response to DMARDs (May 2017) NICE TA445 Recommended with restrictions

▶ Certolizumab pegol for treating moderate to severe plaque psoriasis (April 2019) NICE TA574 Recommended with restrictions

Scottish Medicines Consortium (SMC) decisions

▶ Certolizumab pegol (*Cimzia*®) for the treatment of moderate to severe plaque psoriasis in adults who are candidates for systemic therapy (April 2019) SMC No. SMC2132 Recommended with restrictions

● MEDICINAL FORMS There can be variation in the licensing of different medicines containing the same drug.

Solution for injection

CAUTIONARY AND ADVISORY LABELS 10

▶ Cimzia (UCB Pharma Ltd)

Certolizumab pegol 200 mg per 1 ml Cimzia 200mg/1ml solution for injection in a dose-dispenser cartridge | 2 cartridge [PoM] £715.00 (Hospital only)

Cimzia 200mg/1ml solution for injection pre-filled pens | 2 pre-filled disposable injection [PoM] £715.00

Cimzia 200mg/1ml solution for injection pre-filled syringes | 2 syringe [PoM] £715.00

Etanercept

05-Nov-2020

● INDICATIONS AND DOSE

BENEPALI ® SOLUTION FOR INJECTION

Moderate-to-severe active rheumatoid arthritis (alone or in combination with methotrexate) when the response to other disease-modifying antirheumatic drugs is inadequate | Severe, active and progressive rheumatoid arthritis not previously treated with methotrexate | Active and progressive psoriatic arthritis when the response to other disease-modifying antirheumatic drugs is inadequate | Severe active ankylosing spondylitis when the response to conventional therapy is inadequate | Severe, non-radiographic axial spondyloarthritis when the response to non-steroidal anti-inflammatory drugs is inadequate

▶ BY SUBCUTANEOUS INJECTION

▶ Adult: 50 mg once weekly, review treatment if no response within 12 weeks of initial dose

Moderate-to-severe plaque psoriasis when the response to other systemic therapies or psoralen and ultraviolet-A light (PUVA) is inadequate, or when these therapies cannot be used because of intolerance or contra-indications

▶ BY SUBCUTANEOUS INJECTION

▶ Adult: 50 mg once weekly, alternatively 50 mg twice weekly for up to 12 weeks, followed by 50 mg once weekly if required continue treatment for up to 24 weeks—continuous therapy beyond 24 weeks may be appropriate in some patients (consult product literature), discontinue if no response after 12 weeks

continued →

ENBREL ® POWDER AND SOLVENT FOR SOLUTION FOR INJECTION

Moderate-to-severe active rheumatoid arthritis (alone or in combination with methotrexate) when the response to other disease-modifying antirheumatic drugs is inadequate | Severe, active and progressive rheumatoid arthritis not previously treated with methotrexate | Active and progressive psoriatic arthritis when the response to other disease-modifying antirheumatic drugs is inadequate | Severe active ankylosing spondylitis when the response to conventional therapy is inadequate | Severe, non-radiographic axial spondyloarthritis when the response to non-steroidal anti-inflammatory drugs is inadequate

▸ BY SUBCUTANEOUS INJECTION

▸ Adult: 25 mg twice weekly, alternatively 50 mg once weekly, review treatment if no response within 12 weeks of initial dose

Moderate-to-severe plaque psoriasis when the response to other systemic therapies or psoralen and ultraviolet-A light (PUVA) is inadequate, or when these therapies cannot be used because of intolerance or contra-indications

▸ BY SUBCUTANEOUS INJECTION

▸ Adult: 25 mg twice weekly, alternatively 50 mg once weekly, alternatively 50 mg twice weekly for up to 12 weeks, followed by 25 mg twice weekly, alternatively 50 mg once weekly if required continue treatment for up to 24 weeks—continuous therapy beyond 24 weeks may be appropriate in some patients (consult product literature), discontinue if no response after 12 weeks

ENBREL ® SOLUTION FOR INJECTION

Moderate-to-severe active rheumatoid arthritis (alone or in combination with methotrexate) when the response to other disease-modifying antirheumatic drugs is inadequate | Severe, active and progressive rheumatoid arthritis not previously treated with methotrexate | Active and progressive psoriatic arthritis when the response to other disease-modifying antirheumatic drugs is inadequate | Severe active ankylosing spondylitis when the response to conventional therapy is inadequate | Severe, non-radiographic axial spondyloarthritis when the response to non-steroidal anti-inflammatory drugs is inadequate

▸ BY SUBCUTANEOUS INJECTION

▸ Adult: 25 mg twice weekly, alternatively 50 mg once weekly, review treatment if no response within 12 weeks of initial dose

Moderate-to-severe plaque psoriasis when the response to other systemic therapies or psoralen and ultraviolet-A light (PUVA) is inadequate, or when these therapies cannot be used because of intolerance or contra-indications

▸ BY SUBCUTANEOUS INJECTION

▸ Adult: 25 mg twice weekly, alternatively 50 mg once weekly, alternatively 50 mg twice weekly for up to 12 weeks, followed by 25 mg twice weekly, alternatively 50 mg once weekly if required continue treatment for up to 24 weeks—continuous therapy beyond 24 weeks may be appropriate in some patients (consult product literature), discontinue if no response after 12 weeks

● CONTRA-INDICATIONS Active infection

● CAUTIONS Development of malignancy · diabetes mellitus · heart failure (risk of exacerbation) · hepatitis B virus—monitor for active infection · hepatitis C infection (monitor for worsening infection) · history of blood disorders · history of malignancy · history or increased risk of demyelinating disorders · predisposition to infection (avoid if predisposition to septicaemia) · significant

exposure to herpes zoster virus—interrupt treatment and consider varicella–zoster immunoglobulin

CAUTIONS, FURTHER INFORMATION

▸ Tuberculosis Active tuberculosis should be treated with standard treatment for at least 2 months before starting etanercept. Patients who have previously received adequate treatment for tuberculosis can start etanercept but should be monitored every 3 months for possible recurrence. In patients without active tuberculosis but who were previously not treated adequately, chemoprophylaxis should ideally be completed before starting etanercept. In patients at high risk of tuberculosis who cannot be assessed by tuberculin skin test, chemoprophylaxis can be given concurrently with etanercept.

● INTERACTIONS → Appendix 1: etanercept

● SIDE-EFFECTS

▸ Common or very common Cystitis · fever · hypersensitivity · increased risk of infection · pain · skin reactions · swelling

▸ Uncommon Abscess · bursitis · cholecystitis · diarrhoea · endocarditis · eye inflammation · gastritis · hepatic disorders · myositis · neoplasms · respiratory disorders · sepsis · skin ulcers · thrombocytopenia · vasculitis

▸ Rare or very rare Anaemia · bone marrow disorders · congestive heart failure · cutaneous lupus erythematosus · demyelination · leucopenia · lupus-like syndrome · nerve disorders · neutropenia · sarcoidosis · seizure · severe cutaneous adverse reactions (SCARs) · transverse myelitis

▸ Frequency not known Dermatomyositis exacerbated · hepatitis B reactivation

SIDE-EFFECTS, FURTHER INFORMATION Associated with infections, sometimes severe, including tuberculosis, septicaemia, and hepatitis B reactivation.

● CONCEPTION AND CONTRACEPTION Manufacturer advises effective contraception required during treatment and for 3 weeks after last dose.

● PREGNANCY Avoid—limited information available.

● BREAST FEEDING Manufacturer advises avoid—present in milk in *animal* studies.

● HEPATIC IMPAIRMENT Manufacturer advises caution in moderate to severe alcoholic hepatitis.

● PRE-TREATMENT SCREENING
Tuberculosis Patients should be evaluated for tuberculosis before treatment.

● MONITORING REQUIREMENTS Monitor for skin cancer before and during treatment, particularly in those at risk (including patients with psoriasis or a history of PUVA treatment).

● PRESCRIBING AND DISPENSING INFORMATION Etanercept is a biological medicine. Biological medicines must be prescribed and dispensed by brand name, see *Biological medicines* and *Biosimilar medicines*, under Guidance on prescribing p. 1.

● PATIENT AND CARER ADVICE
Blood disorders Patients and their carers should be advised to seek medical attention if symptoms suggestive of blood disorders (such as fever, sore throat, bruising, or bleeding) develop.
Tuberculosis Patients and their carers should be advised to seek medical attention if symptoms suggestive of tuberculosis (e.g. persistent cough, weight loss, and fever) develop.
Alert card An alert card should be provided.

● NATIONAL FUNDING/ACCESS DECISIONS
For full details see funding body website

NICE decisions

▸ **Etanercept and efalizumab for plaque psoriasis (July 2006)**
NICE TA103 Recommended with restrictions

▸ **Adalimumab, etanercept, infliximab, rituximab, and abatacept for the treatment of rheumatoid arthritis after the** failure of a **TNF inhibitor** (August 2010) NICE TA195 Recommended with restrictions

▸ **Etanercept, infliximab, and adalimumab for the treatment of psoriatic arthritis** (August 2010) NICE TA199 Recommended with restrictions

▸ **Adalimumab, etanercept, infliximab, certolizumab pegol, golimumab, tocilizumab and abatacept for rheumatoid arthritis not previously treated with DMARDs or after conventional DMARDs only have failed** (January 2016) NICE TA375 Recommended with restrictions

▸ **TNF-alpha inhibitors for ankylosing spondylitis and non-radiographic axial spondyloarthritis** (February 2016) NICE TA383 Recommended

● MEDICINAL FORMS There can be variation in the licensing of different medicines containing the same drug.

Solution for injection
CAUTIONARY AND ADVISORY LABELS 10
▸ Benepali (Biogen Idec Ltd) ▼
Etanercept 50 mg per 1 ml Benepali 50mg/1ml solution for injection pre-filled pens | 4 pre-filled disposable injection PoM £656.00 DT = £715.00 (Hospital only)
Benepali 50mg/1ml solution for injection pre-filled syringes | 4 pre-filled disposable injection PoM £656.00 DT = £715.00 (Hospital only)
▸ Enbrel (Pfizer Ltd)
Etanercept 50 mg per 1 ml Enbrel 50mg/1ml solution for injection pre-filled syringes | 4 pre-filled disposable injection PoM £715.00 DT = £715.00 (Hospital only)
Enbrel 25mg/0.5ml solution for injection pre-filled syringes | 4 pre-filled disposable injection PoM £357.50 DT = £357.50 (Hospital only)
▸ Enbrel MyClic (Pfizer Ltd)
Etanercept 50 mg per 1 ml Enbrel 25mg/0.5ml solution for injection pre-filled MyClic pens | 4 pre-filled disposable injection PoM £357.50 (Hospital only)
Enbrel 50mg/1ml solution for injection pre-filled MyClic pens | 4 pre-filled disposable injection PoM £715.00 DT = £715.00 (Hospital only)

Powder and solvent for solution for injection
CAUTIONARY AND ADVISORY LABELS 10
EXCIPIENTS: May contain Benzyl alcohol
▸ Enbrel (Pfizer Ltd)
Etanercept 10 mg Enbrel Paediatric 10mg powder and solvent for solution for injection vials | 4 vial PoM £143.00 (Hospital only)
Etanercept 25 mg Enbrel 25mg powder and solvent for solution for injection vials | 4 vial PoM £357.50 (Hospital only)

Golimumab

06-Nov-2020

● INDICATIONS AND DOSE
Ulcerative colitis (initiated by a specialist)
▸ BY SUBCUTANEOUS INJECTION
▸ **Adult (body-weight up to 80 kg):** Initially 200 mg, then 100 mg after 2 weeks; maintenance 50 mg every 4 weeks, alternatively maintenance 100 mg every 4 weeks, if inadequate response, review treatment if no response after 4 doses
▸ **Adult (body-weight 80 kg and above):** Initially 200 mg, then 100 mg after 2 weeks; maintenance 100 mg every 4 weeks, review treatment if no response after 4 doses

Rheumatoid arthritis (initiated by a specialist) | Psoriatic arthritis (initiated by a specialist) | Ankylosing spondylitis (initiated by a specialist) | Non-radiographic axial spondyloarthritis (initiated by a specialist)
▸ BY SUBCUTANEOUS INJECTION
▸ **Adult (body-weight up to 100 kg):** 50 mg once a month, on the same date each month, review treatment if no response after 3–4 doses
▸ **Adult (body-weight 100 kg and above):** Initially 50 mg once a month for 3–4 doses, on the same date each month, dose may be increased if inadequate response, increased to 100 mg once a month, review treatment if inadequate response to this higher dose after 3–4 doses

● CONTRA-INDICATIONS Moderate or severe heart failure · severe active infection

● CAUTIONS Active infection (do not initiate until active infections are controlled; discontinue if new serious infection develops until infection controlled) · demyelinating disorders (risk of exacerbation) · hepatitis B virus—monitor for active infection · history or development of malignancy · mild heart failure (discontinue if symptoms develop or worsen) · predisposition to infection · risk factors for dysplasia or carcinoma of the colon—screen for dysplasia regularly

CAUTIONS, FURTHER INFORMATION
▸ Tuberculosis Active tuberculosis should be treated with standard treatment for at least 2 months before starting golimumab. Patients who have previously received adequate treatment for tuberculosis can start golimumab but should be monitored every 3 months for possible recurrence. In patients without active tuberculosis but who were previously not treated adequately, chemoprophylaxis should ideally be completed before starting golimumab. In patients at high risk of tuberculosis who cannot be assessed by tuberculin skin test, chemoprophylaxis can be given concurrently with golimumab. Patients who have tested negative for latent tuberculosis, and those who are receiving or who have completed treatment for latent tuberculosis, should be monitored closely for symptoms of active infection.

● INTERACTIONS → Appendix 1: monoclonal antibodies

● SIDE-EFFECTS
▸ **Common or very common** Abscess · alopecia · anaemia · asthenia · asthma · bone fracture · chest discomfort · depression · dizziness · fever · gastrointestinal discomfort · gastrointestinal disorders · gastrointestinal inflammatory disorders · headache · hypersensitivity · hypertension · increased risk of infection · insomnia · nausea · paraesthesia · respiratory disorders · skin reactions · stomatitis
▸ **Uncommon** Arrhythmia · balance impaired · bone marrow disorders · breast disorder · cholelithiasis · constipation · eye inflammation · eye irritation · flushing · goitre · hyperthyroidism · hypothyroidism · leucopenia · liver disorder · menstrual disorder · myocardial ischaemia · neoplasms · sepsis · thrombocytopenia · thrombosis · thyroid disorder · vision disorders
▸ **Rare or very rare** Bladder disorder · congestive heart failure · demyelination · healing impaired · hepatitis B reactivation · lupus-like syndrome · Raynaud's phenomenon · renal disorder · sarcoidosis · taste altered · vasculitis

SIDE-EFFECTS, FURTHER INFORMATION Associated with infections, sometimes severe, including tuberculosis, septicaemia, and hepatitis B reactivation.

● CONCEPTION AND CONTRACEPTION Manufacturer advises adequate contraception during treatment and for at least 6 months after last dose.

● PREGNANCY Use only if essential.

● BREAST FEEDING Manufacturer advises avoid during and for at least 6 months after treatment—present in milk in *animal* studies.

● HEPATIC IMPAIRMENT Manufacturer advises caution (no information available).

● PRE-TREATMENT SCREENING
Tuberculosis Patients should be evaluated for tuberculosis before treatment.

● MONITORING REQUIREMENTS Monitor for infection before, during, and for 5 months after treatment.

● DIRECTIONS FOR ADMINISTRATION For doses requiring multiple injections, each injection should be administered at a different site.

10

Musculoskeletal system

Missed dose If dose administered more than 2 weeks late, manufacturer advises subsequent doses should be administered on the new monthly due date.

● PATIENT AND CARER ADVICE

Tuberculosis All patients and their carers should be advised to seek medical attention if symptoms suggestive of tuberculosis (e.g. persistent cough, weight loss, and fever) develop.

Blood disorders Patients and their carers should be advised to seek medical attention if symptoms suggestive of blood disorders (such as fever, sore throat, bruising, or bleeding) develop.

Alert card An alert card should be provided.

● NATIONAL FUNDING/ACCESS DECISIONS

For full details see funding body website

NICE decisions

▸ Golimumab for the treatment of psoriatic arthritis (April 2011) NICE TA220 Recommended with restrictions

▸ Adalimumab, etanercept, infliximab, certolizumab pegol, golimumab, tocilizumab and abatacept for rheumatoid arthritis not previously treated with DMARDs or after conventional DMARDs only have failed (January 2016) NICE TA375 Recommended with restrictions

▸ Golimumab for the treatment of rheumatoid arthritis after the failure of previous disease-modifying anti-rheumatic drugs (June 2011) NICE TA225 Recommended with restrictions

▸ TNF-alpha inhibitors for ankylosing spondylitis and non-radiographic axial spondyloarthritis (February 2016) NICE TA383 Recommended

▸ Golimumab for treating non-radiographic axial spondyloarthritis (January 2018) NICE TA497 Recommended with restrictions

▸ Infliximab, adalimumab and golimumab for treating moderately to severely active ulcerative colitis after the failure of conventional therapy (February 2015) NICE TA329 Recommended with restrictions

Scottish Medicines Consortium (SMC) decisions

▸ Golimumab 50 mg (*Simponi*®) for the treatment of active and progressive psoriatic arthritis in adult patients (July 2012) SMC No. 674/11 Recommended with restrictions

▸ Golimumab (*Simponi*®) for the treatment of adults with severe non-radiographic axial spondyloarthritis with objective signs of inflammation as indicated by elevated C-reactive protein and/or magnetic resonance imaging (MRI) evidence, who have had an inadequate response to, or are intolerant to non-steroidal anti-inflammatory drugs (February 2016) SMC No. 1124/16 Recommended

● MEDICINAL FORMS There can be variation in the licensing of different medicines containing the same drug.

Solution for injection

CAUTIONARY AND ADVISORY LABELS 10

▸ Simponi (Merck Sharp & Dohme Ltd)

Golimumab 100 mg per 1 ml Simponi 100mg/1ml solution for injection pre-filled pens | 1 pre-filled disposable injection PoM £1,525.94 DT = £1,525.94

Simponi 50mg/0.5ml solution for injection pre-filled syringes | 1 pre-filled disposable injection PoM £762.97 DT = £762.97

Simponi 50mg/0.5ml solution for injection pre-filled pens | 1 pre-filled disposable injection PoM £762.97 DT = £762.97

Infliximab

06-Nov-2020

● INDICATIONS AND DOSE

Active Crohn's disease (under expert supervision)

▸ BY INTRAVENOUS INFUSION

▸ Adult: Initially 5 mg/kg, then 5 mg/kg after 2 weeks, then 5 mg/kg, to be taken at 6 weeks after initial dose if condition has responded; discontinue if no response within 6 weeks of initial infusion (after 2 doses), then

maintenance 5 mg/kg every 8 weeks, maintenance treatment can be restarted after a drug-free interval if symptoms recur within 16 weeks of the last infusion. Consult product literature for dose escalation in selected patients

▸ INITIALLY BY INTRAVENOUS INFUSION

▸ Adult: Initially 5 mg/kg, then (by intravenous infusion) 5 mg/kg after 2 weeks; (by subcutaneous injection) maintenance 120 mg every 2 weeks, subcutaneous maintenance dosing to be started 4 weeks after the second of the initial intravenous infusions if a response has been seen. Discontinue if no response within 6 weeks of the initial infusion (after 2 doses). Treatment can be restarted after a drug-free interval if symptoms recur within 16 weeks of the last dose— consult product literature

Fistulating Crohn's disease (under expert supervision)

▸ BY INTRAVENOUS INFUSION

▸ Adult: Initially 5 mg/kg, then 5 mg/kg, to be taken at week 2 and 6 after initial dose, discontinue if no response after initial 3 doses, then maintenance 5 mg/kg every 8 weeks, maintenance treatment can be restarted after a drug-free interval if symptoms recur within 16 weeks of the last dose

▸ INITIALLY BY INTRAVENOUS INFUSION

▸ Adult: Initially 5 mg/kg, followed by (by intravenous infusion) 5 mg/kg after 2 weeks; (by subcutaneous injection) maintenance 120 mg every 2 weeks, subcutaneous maintenance dosing to be started 4 weeks after the second of the initial intravenous infusions. Discontinue if no response after 6 doses in total. Treatment can be restarted after a drug-free interval if symptoms recur within 16 weeks of the last dose—consult product literature

Active ulcerative colitis (under expert supervision)

▸ BY INTRAVENOUS INFUSION

▸ Adult: Initially 5 mg/kg, then 5 mg/kg, to be taken at week 2 and 6 after initial dose, then 5 mg/kg every 8 weeks, consider discontinuation if no response within 14 weeks after initial infusion (3 doses)

▸ INITIALLY BY INTRAVENOUS INFUSION

▸ Adult: Initially 5 mg/kg, then (by intravenous infusion) 5 mg/kg after 2 weeks; (by subcutaneous injection) maintenance 120 mg every 2 weeks, subcutaneous maintenance dosing to be started 4 weeks after the second of the initial intravenous infusions. Consider discontinuation if no response within 14 weeks (after 6 doses in total)

Rheumatoid arthritis (in combination with methotrexate) (under expert supervision)

▸ BY INTRAVENOUS INFUSION

▸ Adult: Initially 3 mg/kg, then 3 mg/kg, to be taken at week 2 and 6 after initial dose, then 3 mg/kg every 8 weeks, dose to be increased only if response is inadequate after 12 weeks of initial treatment; increased if necessary to 3 mg/kg every 4 weeks, alternatively increased in steps of 1.5 mg/kg every 8 weeks (max. per dose 7.5 mg/kg every 8 weeks), consider discontinuation if no response within 12 weeks of initial infusion (after 3 doses) or after dose adjustment. Maintenance treatment can be restarted after a drug-free interval if symptoms recur within 16 weeks of the last infusion

▸ INITIALLY BY INTRAVENOUS INFUSION

▸ Adult: Initially 3 mg/kg, then (by intravenous infusion) 3 mg/kg after 2 weeks; (by subcutaneous injection) maintenance 120 mg every 2 weeks, subcutaneous maintenance dosing to be started 4 weeks after the second of the initial intravenous infusions. Consider discontinuation if no response within 12 weeks of the initial infusion. Treatment can be restarted after a drug-free interval if symptoms recur within 16 weeks of the last dose—consult product literature

Ankylosing spondylitis (under expert supervision)

▶ BY INTRAVENOUS INFUSION
▸ **Adult:** Initially 5 mg/kg, then 5 mg/kg, to be taken at week 2 and 6 after initial dose, then 5 mg/kg every 6–8 weeks, discontinue if no response by 6 weeks of initial infusion (after 2 doses)
▶ INITIALLY BY INTRAVENOUS INFUSION
▸ **Adult:** Initially 5 mg/kg, followed by (by intravenous infusion) 5 mg/kg after 2 weeks; (by subcutaneous injection) maintenance 120 mg every 2 weeks, subcutaneous maintenance dosing to be started 4 weeks after the second of the initial intravenous infusions. Discontinue if no response within 6 weeks of the initial infusion (after 2 doses)

Psoriatic arthritis (under expert supervision)

▶ BY INTRAVENOUS INFUSION
▸ **Adult:** Initially 5 mg/kg, then 5 mg/kg, to be taken at week 2 and 6 after initial dose, followed by 5 mg/kg every 8 weeks
▶ INITIALLY BY INTRAVENOUS INFUSION
▸ **Adult:** Initially 5 mg/kg, followed by (by intravenous infusion) 5 mg/kg after 2 weeks; (by subcutaneous injection) maintenance 120 mg every 2 weeks, subcutaneous maintenance dosing to be started 4 weeks after the second of the initial intravenous infusions

Plaque psoriasis (under expert supervision)

▶ BY INTRAVENOUS INFUSION
▸ **Adult:** Initially 5 mg/kg, then 5 mg/kg, to be taken at week 2 and 6 after initial dose, then 5 mg/kg every 8 weeks, discontinue if no response after 14 weeks of initial infusion (after 4 doses)
▶ INITIALLY BY INTRAVENOUS INFUSION
▸ **Adult:** Initially 5 mg/kg, followed by (by intravenous infusion) 5 mg/kg after 2 weeks; (by subcutaneous injection) maintenance 120 mg every 2 weeks, subcutaneous maintenance dosing to be started 4 weeks after the second of the initial intravenous infusions. Discontinue if no response after 14 weeks of the initial infusion (after 7 doses in total)

IMPORTANT SAFETY INFORMATION
Adequate resuscitation facilities must be available when infliximab is used.

● CONTRA-INDICATIONS Moderate or severe heart failure · severe infections
● CAUTIONS Demyelinating disorders (risk of exacerbation) · dermatomyositis · development of malignancy · hepatitis B virus—monitor for active infection · history of colon carcinoma (in inflammatory bowel disease) · history of dysplasia (in inflammatory bowel disease) · history of malignancy · history of prolonged immunosuppressant or PUVA treatment in patients with psoriasis · mild heart failure (discontinue if symptoms develop or worsen) · predisposition to infection (discontinue if new serious infection develops) · risk of delayed hypersensitivity reactions if drug-free interval exceeds 16 weeks (re-administration after interval exceeding 16 weeks not recommended)

CAUTIONS, FURTHER INFORMATION
▸ **Infection** Manufacturer advises patients should be up-to-date with current immunisation schedule before initiating treatment.
▸ **Tuberculosis** Manufacturer advises to evaluate patients for active and latent tuberculosis before treatment. Active tuberculosis should be treated with standard treatment for at least 2 months before starting infliximab. If latent tuberculosis is diagnosed, treatment should be started

before commencing treatment with infliximab. Patients who have previously received adequate treatment for tuberculosis can start infliximab but should be monitored every 3 months for possible recurrence. In patients without active tuberculosis but who were previously not treated adequately, chemoprophylaxis should ideally be completed before starting infliximab. In patients at high risk of tuberculosis who cannot be assessed by tuberculin skin test, chemoprophylaxis can be given concurrently with infliximab. Patients should be advised to seek medical attention if symptoms suggestive of tuberculosis develop (e.g. persistent cough, weight loss and fever).
▸ **Hypersensitivity reactions** Hypersensitivity reactions (including fever, chest pain, hypotension, hypertension, dyspnoea, transient visual loss, pruritus, urticaria, serum sickness-like reactions, angioedema, anaphylaxis) reported during or within 1–2 hours after infusion (risk greatest during first or second infusion or in patients who discontinue other immunosuppressants). Manufacturer advises prophylactic antipyretics, antihistamines, or hydrocortisone may be administered.

● INTERACTIONS → Appendix 1: monoclonal antibodies

● SIDE-EFFECTS
▶ **Common or very common** Abscess · alopecia · anaemia · arrhythmias · arthralgia · chest pain · chills · constipation · decreased leucocytes · depression · diarrhoea · dizziness · dyspnoea · eye inflammation · fatigue · fever · gastrointestinal discomfort · gastrointestinal disorders · haemorrhage · headache · hepatic disorders · hyperhidrosis · hypertension · hypotension · increased risk of infection · infusion related reaction · insomnia · lymphadenopathy · myalgia · nausea · neutropenia · oedema · pain · palpitations · respiratory disorders · sensation abnormal · sepsis · skin reactions · vasodilation · vertigo
▶ **Uncommon** Anxiety · cheilitis · cholecystitis · confusion · drowsiness · healing impaired · heart failure · hypersensitivity · lupus erythematosus · lymphocytosis · memory loss · neoplasms · nerve disorders · pancreatitis · peripheral ischaemia · pulmonary oedema · seborrhoea · seizure · syncope · thrombocytopenia · thrombophlebitis
▶ **Rare or very rare** Agranulocytosis · circulatory collapse · cyanosis · demyelinating disorders · granuloma · haemolytic anaemia · hepatitis B reactivation · meningitis · pancytopenia · pericardial effusion · sarcoid-like reaction · severe cutaneous adverse reactions (SCARs) · transverse myelitis · vasculitis · vasospasm
▶ **Frequency not known** Dermatomyositis exacerbated · hepatosplenic T-cell lymphoma (increased risk in inflammatory bowel disease) · myocardial infarction · myocardial ischaemia · sarcoidosis · stroke · vision loss

● CONCEPTION AND CONTRACEPTION Manufacturer advises adequate contraception during and for at least 6 months after last dose.
● PREGNANCY Use only if essential.
● BREAST FEEDING Specialist sources indicate amount present in milk probably too small to be harmful.
● PRE-TREATMENT SCREENING
Tuberculosis Manufacturer advises patients should be evaluated for tuberculosis before treatment.
● MONITORING REQUIREMENTS
▶ Monitor for infection before, during, and for 6 months after treatment.
▶ All patients should be observed carefully for 1–2 hours after infusion and resuscitation equipment should be available for immediate use (risk of hypersensitivity reactions).
▶ Monitor for symptoms of delayed hypersensitivity if re-administered after a prolonged period.
▶ Manufacturer advises periodic skin examination for non-melanoma skin cancer, particularly in patients with risk factors.

10

Musculoskeletal system

- DIRECTIONS FOR ADMINISTRATION For *intravenous infusion* (*Remicade®*), manufacturer advises give intermittently *in* Sodium chloride 0.9%; reconstitute each 100-mg vial with 10 mL water for injections using a 21-gauge or smaller needle; gently swirl vial without shaking to dissolve; allow to stand for 5 minutes; dilute requisite dose with infusion fluid to a final volume of 250 mL and give through a low protein-binding filter (1.2 micron or less) over at least 2 hours (adults over 18 years who have tolerated 3 initial 2-hour infusions may be given subsequent infusions of up to 6 mg/kg over at least 1 hour); start infusion within 3 hours of reconstitution.

- PRESCRIBING AND DISPENSING INFORMATION Infliximab is a biological medicine. Biological medicines must be prescribed and dispensed by brand name, see *Biological medicines* and *Biosimilar medicines*, under Guidance on prescribing p. 1.

- HANDLING AND STORAGE Store in a refrigerator (2–8°C)—consult product literature for further information regarding storage outside refrigerator.

- PATIENT AND CARER ADVICE
  Tuberculosis Patients and carers should be advised to seek medical attention if symptoms suggestive of tuberculosis (e.g. persistent cough, weight loss, and fever) develop.
  Blood disorders Patients and carers should be advised to seek medical attention if symptoms suggestive of blood disorders (such as fever, sore throat, bruising, or bleeding) develop.
  Hypersensitivity reactions Patients and carers should be advised to keep Alert card with them at all times and seek medical advice if symptoms of delayed hypersensitivity develop.
  Self-administration Manufacturer advises patients may self-administer *Remsima®* pre-filled syringes or pens following training in subcutaneous injection technique.
  Alert card An alert card should be provided.
  Driving and skilled tasks Manufacturer advises patients and carers should be counselled on the effects on driving and performance of skilled tasks—increased risk of dizziness.

- NATIONAL FUNDING/ACCESS DECISIONS
  For full details see funding body website
  NICE decisions
  ▸ Infliximab for plaque psoriasis in adults (January 2008) NICE TA134 Recommended with restrictions
  ▸ Infliximab for acute exacerbations of ulcerative colitis (December 2008) NICE TA163 Recommended with restrictions
  ▸ Infliximab and adalimumab for Crohn's disease (May 2010) NICE TA187 Recommended with restrictions
  ▸ Adalimumab, etanercept, infliximab, rituximab, and abatacept for the treatment of rheumatoid arthritis after the failure of a TNF inhibitor (August 2010) NICE TA195 Recommended with restrictions
  ▸ Etanercept, infliximab, and adalimumab for the treatment of psoriatic arthritis (August 2010) NICE TA199 Recommended with restrictions
  ▸ Infliximab, adalimumab and golimumab for treating moderately to severely active ulcerative colitis after the failure of conventional therapy (February 2015) NICE TA329 Recommended with restrictions
  ▸ Adalimumab, etanercept, infliximab, certolizumab pegol, golimumab, tocilizumab and abatacept for rheumatoid arthritis not previously treated with DMARDs or after conventional DMARDs only have failed (January 2016) NICE TA375 Recommended with restrictions
  ▸ TNF-alpha inhibitors for ankylosing spondylitis and non-radiographic axial spondyloarthritis (February 2016) NICE TA383 Recommended

- MEDICINAL FORMS There can be variation in the licensing of different medicines containing the same drug.
  Solution for injection
  CAUTIONARY AND ADVISORY LABELS 10
  EXCIPIENTS: May contain Polysorbates
  ▸ Remsima (Celltrion Healthcare UK Ltd)
  Infliximab 120 mg per 1 ml Remsima 120mg/1ml solution for injection pre-filled syringes | 2 pre-filled disposable injection [PoM] £755.32
  Remsima 120mg/1ml solution for injection pre-filled pens | 2 pre-filled disposable injection [PoM] £755.32
  Powder for solution for infusion
  CAUTIONARY AND ADVISORY LABELS 10
  EXCIPIENTS: May contain Polysorbates
  ▸ Flixabi (Biogen Idec Ltd) ▼
  Infliximab 100 mg Flixabi 100mg powder for concentrate for solution for infusion vials | 1 vial [PoM] £377.00 (Hospital only)
  ▸ Inflectra (Pfizer Ltd)
  Infliximab 100 mg Inflectra 100mg powder for concentrate for solution for infusion vials | 1 vial [PoM] £377.66 (Hospital only)
  ▸ Remicade (Merck Sharp & Dohme Ltd)
  Infliximab 100 mg Remicade 100mg powder for concentrate for solution for infusion vials | 1 vial [PoM] £419.62 (Hospital only)
  ▸ Remsima (Celltrion Healthcare UK Ltd)
  Infliximab 100 mg Remsima 100mg powder for concentrate for solution for infusion vials | 1 vial [PoM] £377.66 (Hospital only)
  ▸ Zessly (Sandoz Ltd) ▼
  Infliximab 100 mg Zessly 100mg powder for concentrate for solution for infusion vials | 1 vial [PoM] £377.66 (Hospital only)

PHOSPHODIESTERASE TYPE-4 INHIBITORS

Apremilast

02-Nov-2020

- DRUG ACTION Apremilast inhibits the activity of phosphodiesterase type-4 (PDE4) which results in suppression of pro-inflammatory mediator synthesis and promotes anti-inflammatory mediators.

- INDICATIONS AND DOSE
  Active psoriatic arthritis (in combination with disease-modifying antirheumatic drugs or alone) in patients who have had an inadequate response or who have been intolerant to a prior disease-modifying antirheumatic drug therapy | Moderate to severe chronic plaque psoriasis that has not responded to standard systemic treatments or photochemotherapy, or when these treatments cannot be used because of intolerance or contra-indications
  ▸ BY MOUTH
  ▸ Adult: Initially 10 mg daily on day 1, then 10 mg twice daily on day 2, then 10 mg in the morning and 20 mg in the evening on day 3, then 20 mg twice daily on day 4, then 20 mg in the morning and 30 mg in the evening on day 5, then maintenance 30 mg twice daily, doses should be taken approximately 12 hours apart; review treatment if no response within 24 weeks of initiation

  IMPORTANT SAFETY INFORMATION
  MHRA/CHM ADVICE (JANUARY 2017): APREMILAST (*OTEZLA®*): RISK OF SUICIDAL THOUGHTS AND BEHAVIOUR
  A review of evidence from clinical trials and postmarketing cases has suggested a causal association between apremilast and suicidal thoughts and behaviour.

- CAUTIONS Concomitant use of drugs likely to cause psychiatric symptoms · history of psychiatric illness · low body-weight—consider discontinuation if weight loss is unexplained or clinically significant

- INTERACTIONS → Appendix 1: phosphodiesterase type-4 inhibitors

- SIDE-EFFECTS
▸ **Common or very common** Appetite decreased · back pain · cough · depression · diarrhoea · fatigue · gastrointestinal discomfort · gastrointestinal disorders · headaches · increased risk of infection · insomnia · nausea · vomiting
▸ **Uncommon** Gastrointestinal haemorrhage · rash · suicidal behaviours · weight decreased

- CONCEPTION AND CONTRACEPTION Exclude pregnancy before treatment and ensure effective contraception during treatment.

- PREGNANCY Avoid—teratogenic in *animal* studies.

- BREAST FEEDING Manufacturer advises avoid—present in milk in *animal* studies.

- RENAL IMPAIRMENT
 Dose adjustments Reduce dose if eGFR less than 30 mL/minute/1.73 m^2; consult product literature for initial dose titration.

- MONITORING REQUIREMENTS
▸ Manufacturer advises monitor body-weight regularly in patients underweight at the start of treatment.
▸ Manufacturer advises monitor for psychiatric symptoms (including depression, suicidal ideation and behaviour)—discontinue treatment if new or worsening psychiatric symptoms are identified.

- PATIENT AND CARER ADVICE Manufacturer advises patients and carers should be instructed to notify the prescriber of any changes in behaviour or mood, and of any suicidal ideation.

- NATIONAL FUNDING/ACCESS DECISIONS
 For full details see funding body website
 NICE decisions
▸ **Apremilast for treating active psoriatic arthritis (February 2017)** NICE TA433 Recommended with restrictions
▸ **Apremilast for treating moderate to severe plaque psoriasis (November 2016)** NICE TA419 Recommended with restrictions
 Scottish Medicines Consortium (SMC) decisions
▸ **Apremilast (*Otezla*®) alone or in combination with disease modifying anti-rheumatic drugs (DMARDs), for the treatment of active psoriatic arthritis (PsA) in adult patients who have had an inadequate response or who have been intolerant to a prior DMARD therapy (June 2015)** SMC No. 1053/15 Recommended with restrictions
▸ **Apremilast (*Otezla*®) for the treatment of moderate to severe chronic plaque psoriasis in adult patients who have failed to respond to or who have a contra-indication to, or are intolerant to other systemic therapy including ciclosporin, methotrexate or psoralen and ultraviolet A light (PUVA) (June 2015)** SMC No. 1052/15 Recommended

- MEDICINAL FORMS There can be variation in the licensing of different medicines containing the same drug.
 Tablet
 CAUTIONARY AND ADVISORY LABELS 25
▸ Otezla (Amgen Ltd)
 Apremilast 10 mg Otezla 10mg tablets | 4 tablet PoM ⊠
 Apremilast 20 mg Otezla 20mg tablets | 4 tablet PoM ⊠
 Apremilast 30 mg Otezla 30mg tablets | 56 tablet PoM £550.00 DT = £550.00

2   Hyperuricaemia and gout

Gout   08-Aug-2020

Overview
Gout is a common form of inflammatory arthritis characterised by raised uric acid concentration in the blood (hyperuricaemia) and the deposition of urate crystals in joints and other tissues. It occurs in three distinct phases—asymptomatic hyperuricaemia, a period of acute attacks followed by variable intervals (months to years) with no symptoms, and a final period of chronic tophaceous gout, where people have nodules affecting joints. EvGr The management of gout in those under 30 years of age requires specialist supervision. Ⓐ

Acute attacks of gout
EvGr Treatment for an acute attack of gout should be started as soon as possible. Acute attacks of gout are usually treated with either colchicine p. 1166 or high doses of an NSAID (excluding aspirin). The choice of drug depends on factors such as patient preference, renal function, and co-morbidities. A gastro-protective drug (such as a proton pump inhibitor) should be co-prescribed in patients using NSAIDs. Ⓐ

The use of colchicine is limited by the development of toxicity at higher doses. However unlike NSAIDs, it does not induce fluid retention; moreover, it can be co-administered with anticoagulants.

EvGr Combination treatment can be considered for acute attacks of gout in patients with inadequate response to monotherapy.

Joint aspiration and intra-articular injection of a corticosteroid can be used in acute monoarticular gout [unlicensed indication]. A short course of oral corticosteroid or a single injection of intramuscular corticosteroid are effective alternatives in those who cannot tolerate NSAIDs or colchicine, and when intra-articular injection is unsuitable.

An interleukin-1 inhibitor, such as canakinumab p. 890, can be considered for treatment of frequent gouty arthritis attacks (at least 3 in the previous 12 months) in patients who have an inadequate response to standard treatment. Ⓐ

Long-term control of gout
EvGr All patients with gout should be offered urate-lowering therapy, particularly in those with frequent recurrence of acute attacks of gout (2 or more in a year), the presence of tophi, or signs of chronic gouty arthritis.

For long-term control of gout, the formation of uric acid from purines may be reduced with xanthine-oxidase inhibitors, allopurinol p. 1166 or febuxostat p. 1167. Allopurinol is recommended as first-line urate-lowering therapy where renal function allows. Febuxostat can be used as an alternative when allopurinol is contra-indicated or not tolerated. Uricosuric drugs, such as sulfinpyrazone or benzbromarone (specialist use–available from 'special-order' manufacturers or specialist importing companies), may be used as urate-lowering therapy in patients who are resistant to or are intolerant of xanthine-oxidase inhibitors; they increase the excretion of uric acid in the urine. Uricosuric drugs may also be used in combination with xanthine-oxidase inhibitors in patients who have an inadequate response to monotherapy.

Urate-lowering therapy is ideally started after the inflammation in an acute attack has settled. The initiation or up-titration of urate-lowering therapy may precipitate an acute attack, and therefore colchicine should be considered as prophylaxis and continued for up to 6 months. A low-dose NSAID with gastro-protection is an alternative in patients who have contra-indications to colchicine. If an acute attack develops during treatment, the urate-lowering therapy should continue at the same dosage and the acute attack treated separately.

Patients with gout and a history of urolithiasis should be advised to ensure adequate daily fluid intake and avoid dehydration. Alkalinisation of the urine with potassium citrate can be considered in recurrent stone formers. Ⓐ

10

Musculoskeletal system

Other drugs used for Hyperuricaemia and gout Diclofenac potassium, p. 1180 · Diclofenac sodium, p. 1181 · Etoricoxib, p. 1184 · Indometacin, p. 1189 · Ketoprofen, p. 1190 · Naproxen, p. 1194 · Naproxen with esomeprazole, p. 1195 · Sulindac, p. 1196

ALKALOIDS > PLANT ALKALOIDS

Colchicine
29-Apr-2020

● **INDICATIONS AND DOSE**

Acute gout
▸ BY MOUTH
▸ Adult: 500 micrograms 2–4 times a day until symptoms relieved, maximum 6 mg per course, do not repeat course within 3 days

Short-term prophylaxis during initial therapy with allopurinol and uricosuric drugs
▸ BY MOUTH
▸ Adult: 500 micrograms twice daily

Prophylaxis of familial Mediterranean fever (recurrent polyserositis)
▸ BY MOUTH
▸ Adult: 0.5–2 mg once daily

DOSE ADJUSTMENTS DUE TO INTERACTIONS
▸ Manufacturer advises reduce dose by half with concurrent use of moderate inhibitors of CYP3A4.
▸ Manufacturer advises reduce dose by 75% (to one quarter of usual dose) with concurrent use of potent inhibitors of CYP3A4 or P-glycoprotein inhibitors; avoid concurrent use in patients with hepatic or renal impairment.

● UNLICENSED USE BNF doses may differ from those in the product literature. Use of colchicine for prophylaxis of familial Mediterranean fever (recurrent polyserositis) is an unlicensed indication.
● CONTRA-INDICATIONS Blood disorders
● CAUTIONS Cardiac disease · elderly · gastro-intestinal disease
CAUTIONS, FURTHER INFORMATION
▸ Elderly Prescription potentially inappropriate (STOPP criteria):
  ● if eGFR less than 10 mL/minute/1.73 m^2 (risk of toxicity)
  ● for chronic treatment of gout where there is no contra-indication to a xanthine-oxidase inhibitor (xanthine-oxidase inhibitors are first choice prophylactic drugs in gout)
See also Prescribing in the elderly p. 33.
● INTERACTIONS → Appendix 1: colchicine
● SIDE-EFFECTS
▸ **Common or very common** Abdominal pain · diarrhoea · nausea · vomiting
▸ **Frequency not known** Agranulocytosis · alopecia · bone marrow disorders · gastrointestinal haemorrhage · kidney injury · liver injury · menstrual cycle irregularities · myopathy · nerve disorders · rash · sperm abnormalities · thrombocytopenia
● PREGNANCY Avoid—teratogenicity in *animal* studies.
● BREAST FEEDING Present in milk but no adverse effects reported. Manufacturers advise caution.
● HEPATIC IMPAIRMENT Manufacturer advises caution in mild to moderate impairment; avoid in severe impairment.
● RENAL IMPAIRMENT Avoid if eGFR less than 10 mL/minute/1.73 m^2.
Dose adjustments Reduce dose or increase dosage interval if eGFR 10–50 mL/minute/1.73 m^2.

● MEDICINAL FORMS There can be variation in the licensing of different medicines containing the same drug.
Tablet
▸ Colchicine (Non-proprietary)
  Colchicine 500 microgram Colchicine 500microgram tablets | 28 tablet [PoM] £1.78–£2.54 | 100 tablet [PoM] £21.95 DT = £6.34

XANTHINE OXIDASE INHIBITORS

Allopurinol
22-May-2020

● **INDICATIONS AND DOSE**

Prophylaxis of gout and of uric acid and calcium oxalate renal stones | Prophylaxis of hyperuricaemia associated with cancer chemotherapy
▸ BY MOUTH
▸ Adult: Initially 100 mg daily, for maintenance adjust dose according to plasma or urinary uric acid concentration, dose to be taken preferably after food

Prophylaxis of gout and of uric acid and calcium oxalate renal stones (usual maintenance in mild conditions) | Prophylaxis of hyperuricaemia associated with cancer chemotherapy (usual maintenance in mild conditions)
▸ BY MOUTH
▸ Adult: 100–200 mg daily, dose to be taken preferably after food

Prophylaxis of gout and of uric acid and calcium oxalate renal stones (usual maintenance in moderately severe conditions) | Prophylaxis of hyperuricaemia associated with cancer chemotherapy (usual maintenance in moderately severe conditions)
▸ BY MOUTH
▸ Adult: 300–600 mg daily in divided doses (max. per dose 300 mg), dose to be taken preferably after food

Prophylaxis of gout and of uric acid and calcium oxalate renal stones (usual maintenance in severe conditions) | Prophylaxis of hyperuricaemia associated with cancer chemotherapy (usual maintenance in severe conditions)
▸ BY MOUTH
▸ Adult: 700–900 mg daily in divided doses (max. per dose 300 mg), dose to be taken preferably after food

● CONTRA-INDICATIONS Not a treatment for acute gout but continue if attack develops when already receiving allopurinol, and treat attack separately
● CAUTIONS Ensure adequate fluid intake (2–3 litres/day) · for hyperuricaemia associated with cancer therapy, allopurinol treatment should be started before cancer therapy
CAUTIONS, FURTHER INFORMATION Administer prophylactic NSAID (*not* aspirin or salicylates) or colchicine until at least 1 month after hyperuricaemia corrected (usually for first 3 months) to avoid precipitating an acute attack.
● INTERACTIONS → Appendix 1: allopurinol
● SIDE-EFFECTS
▸ **Common or very common** Rash (discontinue therapy; if rash mild re-introduce cautiously but discontinue immediately if recurrence)
▸ **Uncommon** Hypersensitivity · nausea · vomiting
▸ **Rare or very rare** Agranulocytosis · alopecia · angina pectoris · angioedema · angioimmunoblastic T-cell lymphoma · aplastic anaemia · asthenia · ataxia · boil · bradycardia · cataract · coma · depression · diabetes mellitus · drowsiness · erectile dysfunction · fever · gastrointestinal disorders · gynaecomastia · haemorrhage · hair colour changes · headache · hepatic disorders · hyperlipidaemia · hypertension · infertility male · maculopathy · malaise · oedema · paraesthesia · paralysis · peripheral neuropathy · severe cutaneous adverse

reactions (SCARs) · skin reactions · stomatitis · taste altered · thrombocytopenia · vertigo · visual impairment

- PREGNANCY Toxicity not reported. Manufacturer advises use only if no safer alternative and disease carries risk for mother or child.
- BREAST FEEDING Present in milk—not known to be harmful.
- HEPATIC IMPAIRMENT Manufacturer advises monitor liver function periodically during early stages of therapy.
  Dose adjustments Manufacturer advises reduce dose.
- RENAL IMPAIRMENT
  Dose adjustments Max. 100 mg daily, increased only if response inadequate; in severe impairment, reduce daily dose below 100 mg, or increase dose interval; if facilities available, adjust dose to maintain plasma-oxipurinol concentration below 100 micromol/litre.

- MEDICINAL FORMS There can be variation in the licensing of different medicines containing the same drug. Forms available from special-order manufacturers include: oral suspension, oral solution, mouthwash
  Tablet
  CAUTIONARY AND ADVISORY LABELS 8, 21, 27
  ▸ Allopurinol (Non-proprietary)
  Allopurinol 100 mg Allopurinol 100mg tablets | 28 tablet [PoM] £2.28 DT = £1.18
  Allopurinol 300 mg Allopurinol 300mg tablets | 28 tablet [PoM] £5.85 DT = £1.79
  ▸ Uricto (Ennogen Pharma Ltd)
  Allopurinol 100 mg Uricto 100mg tablets | 28 tablet [PoM] £0.78 DT = £1.18
  Allopurinol 300 mg Uricto 300mg tablets | 28 tablet [PoM] £1.85 DT = £1.79
  ▸ Zyloric (Aspen Pharma Trading Ltd)
  Allopurinol 100 mg Zyloric 100mg tablets | 100 tablet [PoM] £10.19
  Allopurinol 300 mg Zyloric 300mg tablets | 28 tablet [PoM] £7.31 DT = £1.79

Febuxostat

23-Nov-2020

- **INDICATIONS AND DOSE**
  Treatment of chronic hyperuricaemia in gout
  ▸ BY MOUTH
  ▸ **Adult:** Initially 80 mg once daily, if after 2–4 weeks of initial dose, serum uric acid greater than 6 mg/100 mL then increase dose; increased if necessary to 120 mg once daily

  Prophylaxis and treatment of acute hyperuricaemia with initial chemotherapy for haematologic malignancies
  ▸ BY MOUTH
  ▸ **Adult:** 120 mg once daily, to be started 2 days before start of cytotoxic therapy and continued for 7–9 days, according to chemotherapy duration

IMPORTANT SAFETY INFORMATION
MHRA/CHM ADVICE: SERIOUS HYPERSENSITIVITY REACTIONS (JUNE 2012)
There have been rare but serious reports of hypersensitivity reactions, including Stevens-Johnson syndrome and acute anaphylactic shock with febuxostat. Patients should be advised of the signs and symptoms of severe hypersensitivity; febuxostat must be stopped immediately if these occur (early withdrawal is associated with a better prognosis), and must not be restarted in patients who have ever developed a hypersensitivity reaction to febuxostat. Most cases occur during the first month of treatment; a prior history of hypersensitivity to allopurinol and/or renal disease may indicate potential hypersensitivity to febuxostat.

MHRA/CHM ADVICE: FEBUXOSTAT (ADENURIC®): INCREASED RISK OF CARDIOVASCULAR DEATH AND ALL-CAUSE MORTALITY IN CLINICAL TRIAL IN PATIENTS WITH A HISTORY OF MAJOR CARDIOVASCULAR DISEASE (JULY 2019)
Results from the clinical study (CARES) in patients with gout and a history of major cardiovascular disease showed an increased risk of cardiovascular-related death and all-cause mortality associated with febuxostat compared with allopurinol. Healthcare professionals are advised to avoid treatment with febuxostat in patients with pre-existing major cardiovascular disease (e.g. myocardial infarction, stroke, or unstable angina), unless no other therapy options are appropriate; clinical guidelines for gout recommend treatment with febuxostat only when allopurinol is not tolerated or is contra-indicated.

- CONTRA-INDICATIONS Not a treatment for acute gout but continue if attack develops when already receiving febuxostat, and treat attack separately
- CAUTIONS Major cardiovascular disease, see *Important safety information* · thyroid disorders · transplant recipients
  CAUTIONS, FURTHER INFORMATION [EvGr] Administer prophylactic NSAID (*not* aspirin or salicylates) or colchicine for at least 6 months after starting febuxostat to avoid precipitating an acute attack. ◈
- INTERACTIONS → Appendix 1: febuxostat
- SIDE-EFFECTS
  ▸ **Common or very common** Diarrhoea · gout aggravated · headache · hepatic disorders · nausea · oedema · skin reactions
  ▸ **Uncommon** Altered smell sensation · appetite abnormal · arrhythmias · arthritis · bundle branch block · chest discomfort · cholelithiasis · constipation · cough · diabetes mellitus · dizziness · drowsiness · dry mouth · dyspnoea · fatigue · gastrointestinal discomfort · gastrointestinal disorders · haemorrhage · hemiparesis · hyperlipidaemia · hypertension · increased risk of infection · insomnia · joint disorders · muscle complaints · muscle weakness · musculoskeletal pain · nephrolithiasis · palpitations · proteinuria · renal failure · sensation abnormal · sexual dysfunction · taste altered · urinary disorders · vasodilation · vomiting · weight changes
  ▸ **Rare or very rare** Agranulocytosis · alopecia · angioedema · hyperhidrosis · hypersensitivity · musculoskeletal stiffness · nephritis tubulointerstitial · nervousness · oral ulceration · pancreatitis · pancytopenia · rhabdomyolysis · severe cutaneous adverse reactions (SCARs) · sudden cardiac death · thirst · thrombocytopenia · tinnitus · vision blurred
- PREGNANCY Manufacturer advises avoid—limited information available.
- BREAST FEEDING Manufacturer advises avoid—present in milk in *animal* studies.
- HEPATIC IMPAIRMENT Manufacturer advises caution.
  Dose adjustments Manufacturer advises max. 80 mg daily in mild impairment; no dose information available in moderate to severe impairment.
- RENAL IMPAIRMENT Use with caution if eGFR less than 30 mL/minute/1.73 m^2—no information available.
- PRE-TREATMENT SCREENING Monitor liver function tests before treatment as indicated.
- MONITORING REQUIREMENTS Monitor liver function tests periodically during treatment as indicated.
- NATIONAL FUNDING/ACCESS DECISIONS
  For full details see funding body website
  NICE decisions
  ▸ Febuxostat for the management of hyperuricaemia in patients with gout (December 2008) NICE TA164 Recommended with restrictions

10

Musculoskeletal system

▸ Febuxostat (*Adenuric*®) for the treatment of chronic hyperuricaemia (September 2010) SMC No. 637/10
Recommended with restrictions
▸ Febuxostat (*Adenuric*®) for the prevention and treatment of hyperuricaemia in adult patients undergoing chemotherapy for haematologic malignancies at intermediate to high risk of tumour lysis syndrome (TLS) (June 2016) SMC No. 1153/16
Recommended with restrictions

● MEDICINAL FORMS There can be variation in the licensing of different medicines containing the same drug.

Tablet
▸ Febuxostat (Non-proprietary)
Febuxostat 80 mg Febuxostat 80mg tablets | 28 tablet PoM
£24.36 DT = £4.44
Febuxostat 120 mg Febuxostat 120mg tablets | 28 tablet PoM
£24.36 DT = £24.36
▸ Adenuric (A. Menarini Farmaceutica Internazionale SRL)
Febuxostat 80 mg Adenuric 80mg tablets | 28 tablet PoM | £24.36
DT = £4.44
Febuxostat 120 mg Adenuric 120mg tablets | 28 tablet PoM
£24.36 DT = £24.36

3 Neuromuscular disorders

Neuromuscular disorders

17-Dec-2019

Drugs that enhance neuromuscular transmission

Anticholinesterases are used as first-line treatment in *ocular myasthenia gravis* and as an adjunct to immunosuppressant therapy for *generalised myasthenia gravis*.

Corticosteroids are used when anticholinesterases do not control symptoms completely. A second-line immunosuppressant such as azathioprine p. 882 is frequently used to reduce the dose of corticosteroid.

Plasmapheresis or infusion of intravenous immunoglobulin [unlicensed indication] may induce temporary remission in severe relapses, particularly where bulbar or respiratory function is compromised or before thymectomy.

Anticholinesterases

Anticholinesterase drugs enhance neuromuscular transmission in voluntary and involuntary muscle in myasthenia gravis. Excessive dosage of these drugs can impair neuromuscular transmission and precipitate cholinergic crises by causing a depolarising block. This may be difficult to distinguish from a worsening myasthenic state.

Muscarinic side-effects of anticholinesterases include increased sweating, increased salivary and gastric secretions, increased gastro-intestinal and uterine motility, and bradycardia. These parasympathomimetic effects are antagonised by atropine sulfate p. 1386.

Neostigmine p. 1170 produces a therapeutic effect for up to 4 hours. Its pronounced muscarinic action is a disadvantage, and simultaneous administration of an antimuscarinic drug such as atropine sulfate or propantheline bromide p. 94 may be required to prevent colic, excessive salivation, or diarrhoea. In severe disease neostigmine can be given every 2 hours. The maximum that most patients can tolerate is 180 mg daily.

Pyridostigmine bromide p. 1171 is less powerful and slower in action than neostigmine but it has a longer duration of action. It is preferable to neostigmine because of its smoother action and the need for less frequent dosage. It is particularly preferred in patients whose muscles are weak on waking. It has a comparatively mild gastrointestinal effect but an antimuscarinic drug may still be required.

Neostigmine is also used to reverse the actions of the non-depolarising neuromuscular blocking drugs.

Immunosuppressant therapy

Corticosteroids are established as treatment for myasthenia gravis; although they are commonly given on alternate days there is little evidence of benefit over daily administration. Corticosteroid treatment is usually initiated under in-patient supervision and all patients should receive osteoporosis prophylaxis.

In *generalised myasthenia gravis* prednisolone p. 718 is given. About 10% of patients experience a transient but very serious worsening of symptoms in the first 2–3 weeks, especially if the corticosteroid is started at a high dose. Smaller doses of corticosteroid are usually required in *ocular myasthenia*. Once clinical remission has occurred (usually after 2–6 months), the dose of prednisolone should be reduced slowly to the minimum effective dose.

In generalised myasthenia gravis azathioprine is usually started at the same time as the corticosteroid and it allows a lower maintenance dose of the corticosteroid to be used. Ciclosporin p. 884, methotrexate p. 957, or mycophenolate mofetil p. 891 can be used in patients unresponsive or intolerant to other treatments [unlicensed indications].

Acetylcholine-release enhancers

Amifampridine p. 1171 is licensed for the symptomatic treatment of Lambert-Eaton myasthenic syndrome (LEMS), a rare disorder of neuromuscular transmission.

Fampridine p. 895 is licensed for the improvement of walking in patients with Multiple sclerosis p. 894 who have a walking disability.

Skeletal muscle relaxants

The drugs described are used for the relief of chronic muscle spasm or spasticity associated with Multiple sclerosis p. 894 or other neurological damage; they are not indicated for spasm associated with minor injuries. Baclofen, diazepam, and tizanidine act principally on the central nervous system. Dantrolene has a peripheral site of action; cannabis extract has both a central and a peripheral action. Skeletal muscle relaxants differ in action from the muscle relaxants used in anaesthesia, which block transmission at the neuromuscular junction.

The underlying cause of spasticity should be treated and any aggravating factors (e.g. pressure sores, infection) remedied. Skeletal muscle relaxants are effective in most forms of spasticity except the rare alpha variety. The major disadvantage of treatment with these drugs is that reduction in muscle tone can cause a loss of splinting action of the spastic leg and trunk muscles and sometimes lead to an increase in disability.

Baclofen p. 1173 inhibits transmission at spinal level and also depresses the central nervous system. The dose should be increased slowly to avoid the major side-effects of sedation and muscular hypotonia (other adverse events are uncommon).

Dantrolene sodium p. 1400 acts directly on skeletal muscle and produces fewer central adverse effects making it a drug of choice. The dose should be increased slowly.

Diazepam p. 362 can also be used. Sedation and occasionally extensor hypotonus are disadvantages. Other benzodiazepines also have muscle-relaxant properties. Muscle-relaxant doses of benzodiazepines are similar to anxiolytic doses.

Tizanidine p. 1175 is an alpha$_2$-adrenoceptor agonist indicated for spasticity associated with Multiple sclerosis p. 894 or spinal cord injury.

EvGr Cannabis extract p. 1172 can be trialled as an adjunct treatment for moderate to severe spasticity in multiple sclerosis if other pharmacological treatments are not effective. Treatment must be initiated and supervised by a specialist. For further information see Multiple sclerosis p. 894. ◬

Other muscle relaxants
The clinical efficacy of methocarbamol p. 1174 and
meprobamate p. 365 as muscle relaxants is **not** well
established, although they have been included in compound
analgesic preparations.

NEUROPROTECTIVE DRUGS

▌ Riluzole
21-May-2020

- **INDICATIONS AND DOSE**

**To extend life in patients with amyotrophic lateral
sclerosis, initiated by specialist experienced in the
management of motor neurone disease**
‣ BY MOUTH
‣ Adult: 50 mg twice daily

- **CONTRA-INDICATIONS** Acute porphyrias p. 1107
- **CAUTIONS** History of abnormal hepatic function (consult
product literature for details) · interstitial lung disease
CAUTIONS, FURTHER INFORMATION
‣ Interstitial lung disease Perform chest radiography if
symptoms such as dry cough or dyspnoea develop;
discontinue if interstitial lung disease is diagnosed.
- **INTERACTIONS** → Appendix 1: riluzole
- **SIDE-EFFECTS**
‣ **Common or very common** Abdominal pain · asthenia ·
diarrhoea · dizziness · drowsiness · headache · nausea · oral
paraesthesia · pain · tachycardia · vomiting
‣ **Uncommon** Anaemia · angioedema · interstitial lung
disease · pancreatitis
‣ **Frequency not known** Hepatitis · neutropenia
SIDE-EFFECTS, FURTHER INFORMATION White blood cell
counts should be determined in febrile illness;
neutropenia requires discontinuation of riluzole.
- **PREGNANCY** Avoid—no information available.
- **BREAST FEEDING** Avoid—no information available.
- **HEPATIC IMPAIRMENT** Manufacturer advises avoid (risk of
increased exposure).
- **RENAL IMPAIRMENT** Avoid—no information available.
- **PATIENT AND CARER ADVICE**
Blood disorders Patients or their carers should be told how
to recognise signs of neutropenia and advised to seek
immediate medical attention if symptoms such as fever
occur.
Driving and skilled tasks Dizziness or vertigo may affect
performance of skilled tasks (e.g. driving).
- **NATIONAL FUNDING/ACCESS DECISIONS**
For full details see funding body website
NICE decisions
‣ Guidance on the use of Riluzole (*Rilutek*®) for the treatment
of Motor Neurone Disease (January 2001) NICE TA20
Recommended

- **MEDICINAL FORMS** There can be variation in the licensing of
different medicines containing the same drug. Forms available
from special-order manufacturers include: oral suspension, oral
solution, powder
Oral suspension
‣ Teglutik (Martindale Pharmaceuticals Ltd)
Riluzole 5 mg per 1 ml Teglutik 5mg/1ml oral suspension sugar-free
| 300 ml [PoM] £100.00 DT = £100.00
Tablet
‣ Riluzole (Non-proprietary)
Riluzole 50 mg Riluzole 50mg tablets | 56 tablet [PoM] £320.33 DT =
£16.50
‣ Rilutek (Sanofi)
Riluzole 50 mg Rilutek 50mg tablets | 56 tablet [PoM] £320.33 DT =
£16.50

3.1 Muscular dystrophy

DRUGS FOR NEUROMUSCULAR DISORDERS

▌ Ataluren
02-Nov-2020

- **DRUG ACTION** Ataluren restores the synthesis of
dystrophin by allowing ribosomes to read through
premature stop codons that cause incomplete dystrophin
synthesis in nonsense mutation Duchenne muscular
dystrophy.

- **INDICATIONS AND DOSE**

**Duchenne muscular dystrophy resulting from a nonsense
mutation in the dystrophin gene, in ambulatory patients
(initiated by a specialist)**
‣ BY MOUTH
‣ Adult: (consult product literature)

- **INTERACTIONS** → Appendix 1: ataluren
- **SIDE-EFFECTS**
‣ **Common or very common** Appetite decreased · constipation
· cough · enuresis · fever · flatulence · gastrointestinal
discomfort · haemorrhage · headache · hypertension ·
hypertriglyceridaemia · nausea · pain · skin reactions ·
vomiting · weight decreased
‣ **Frequency not known** Ear infection · malaise
- **PREGNANCY** Manufacturer advises avoid—toxicity in
animal studies.
- **BREAST FEEDING** Manufacturer advises discontinue
breastfeeding—present in milk in *animal* studies.
- **RENAL IMPAIRMENT** Manufacturer advises close
monitoring—safety and efficacy not established.
- **MONITORING REQUIREMENTS** Manufacturer advises
monitor renal function at least every 6–12 months, and
cholesterol and triglyceride concentrations at least
annually.
- **DIRECTIONS FOR ADMINISTRATION** Manufacturer advises
the contents of each sachet should be mixed with at least
30 mL of liquid (water, milk, fruit juice), or 3 tablespoons
of semi-solid food (yoghurt or apple sauce).
- **PATIENT AND CARER ADVICE** Manufacturer advises
patients should maintain adequate hydration during
treatment.
Missed doses Manufacturer advises if a morning or midday
dose is more than 3 hours late, or an evening dose is more
than 6 hours late, the missed dose should not be taken and
the next dose should be taken at the normal time.
- **NATIONAL FUNDING/ACCESS DECISIONS**
For full details see funding body website
NICE decisions
‣ Ataluren for treating Duchenne muscular dystrophy with a
nonsense mutation in the dystrophin gene (July 2016)
NICE HST3 Recommended
Scottish Medicines Consortium (SMC) decisions
‣ Ataluren (*Translarna*®) for the treatment of Duchenne
muscular dystrophy resulting from a nonsense mutation in
the dystrophin gene, in ambulatory patients aged 5 years and
older (April 2016) SMC No. 1131/16 Not recommended

- **MEDICINAL FORMS** There can be variation in the licensing of
different medicines containing the same drug.
Granules
‣ Translarna (PTC Therapeutics Ltd) ▼
Ataluren 125 mg Translarna 125mg granules for oral suspension
sachets | 30 sachet [PoM] £2,532.00
Ataluren 250 mg Translarna 250mg granules for oral suspension
sachets | 30 sachet [PoM] £5,064.00
Ataluren 1 gram Translarna 1,000mg granules for oral suspension
sachets | 30 sachet [PoM] £20,256.00

10

Musculoskeletal system

Musculoskeletal system

10

Nusinersen

11-Nov-2020

- DRUG ACTION Nusinersen is an antisense oligonucleotide that increases the production of survival motor neurone (SMN) protein, thereby helping to compensate for the defect in the SMN1 gene found in 5q spinal muscular atrophy.

● INDICATIONS AND DOSE

5q spinal muscular atrophy (initiated by a specialist)
- ▶ BY INTRATHECAL INJECTION
- ▶ Adult: Initially 12 mg for 4 doses, on days 0, 14, 28 and 63, then 12 mg every 4 months, for advice on missed doses—consult product literature

IMPORTANT SAFETY INFORMATION

MHRA/CHM ADVICE: NUSINERSEN (*SPINRAZA* ®): REPORTS OF COMMUNICATING HYDROCEPHALUS NOT RELATED TO MENINGITIS OR BLEEDING (JULY 2018)
Communicating hydrocephalus not related to meningitis or bleeding has been reported in patients treated with *Spinraza* ®. Patients and caregivers should be informed about the signs and symptoms of hydrocephalus before *Spinraza* ® is started and should be instructed to seek medical attention in case of: persistent vomiting or headache, unexplained decrease in consciousness, and in children increase in head circumference. Patients with signs and symptoms suggestive of hydrocephalus should be further investigated by a physician with expertise in its management.

- CAUTIONS Risk factors for renal toxicity—monitor urine protein (preferably using a first morning urine specimen) · risk factors for thrombocytopenia and coagulation disorders—monitor platelet and coagulation profile before treatment
- PREGNANCY Manufacturer advises avoid—no information available.
- BREAST FEEDING Manufacturer advises avoid—no information available.
- RENAL IMPAIRMENT Manufacturer advises close monitoring—safety and efficacy not established.
- HANDLING AND STORAGE Manufacturer advises store in a refrigerator (2–8 °C); may be stored (in the original carton, protected from light) at or below 30 °C, for up to 14 days.
- NATIONAL FUNDING/ACCESS DECISIONS
  For full details see funding body website
  NICE decisions
- ▶ **Nusinersen for treating spinal muscular atrophy (July 2019)** NICE TA588 Recommended with restrictions

- MEDICINAL FORMS There can be variation in the licensing of different medicines containing the same drug.
  Solution for injection
  - ▶ Spinraza (Biogen Idec Ltd) ▼
    Nusinersen (as Nusinersen sodium) 2.4 mg per 1 ml Spinraza 12mg/5ml solution for injection vials | 1 vial PoM £75,000.00

3.2 Myasthenia gravis and Lambert-Eaton myasthenic syndrome

ANTICHOLINESTERASES

Anticholinesterases

- DRUG ACTION They prolong the action of acetylcholine by inhibiting the action of the enzyme acetylcholinesterase.

- CONTRA-INDICATIONS Intestinal obstruction · urinary obstruction
- CAUTIONS Arrhythmias · asthma (extreme caution) · atropine or other antidote to muscarinic effects may be necessary (particularly when neostigmine is given by injection) but not given routinely because it may mask signs of overdosage · bradycardia · epilepsy · hyperthyroidism · hypotension · parkinsonism · peptic ulceration · recent myocardial infarction · vagotonia

CAUTIONS, FURTHER INFORMATION
- ▶ Elderly Prescription potentially inappropriate (STOPP criteria) in patients with a known history of persistent bradycardia (heart rate less than 60 beats per minute), heart block, or recurrent unexplained syncope, or concurrent treatment with drugs that reduce heart rate (risk of cardiac conduction failure, syncope and injury).
  See also Prescribing in the elderly p. 33.

- SIDE-EFFECTS Abdominal cramps · diarrhoea · excessive tearing · hypersalivation · nausea · vomiting
  Overdose Signs of overdosage include bronchoconstriction, increased bronchial secretions, lacrimation, excessive sweating, involuntary defaecation, involuntary micturition, miosis, nystagmus, bradycardia, heart block, arrhythmias, hypotension, agitation, excessive dreaming, and weakness eventually leading to fasciculation and paralysis.
- PREGNANCY Manufacturer advises use only if potential benefit outweighs risk.
- BREAST FEEDING Amount probably too small to be harmful.

◗ above

Neostigmine

(Neostigmine methylsulfate)

● INDICATIONS AND DOSE

Treatment of myasthenia gravis
- ▶ BY MOUTH
- ▶ Adult: Initially 15–30 mg, dose repeated at suitable intervals throughout the day, total daily dose 75–300 mg, the maximum that most patients can tolerate is 180 mg daily
- ▶ BY SUBCUTANEOUS INJECTION, OR BY INTRAMUSCULAR INJECTION
- ▶ Adult: 1–2.5 mg, dose repeated at suitable intervals throughout the day (usual total daily dose 5–20 mg)

Reversal of non-depolarising (competitive) neuromuscular blockade
- ▶ BY INTRAVENOUS INJECTION
- ▶ Adult: 2.5 mg (max. per dose 5 mg), repeated if necessary after or with glycopyrronium or atropine, to be given over 1 minute

- CAUTIONS
- ▶ With intravenous use Glycopyrronium or atropine should also be given when reversing neuromuscular blockade
- INTERACTIONS → Appendix 1: neostigmine
- SIDE-EFFECTS
- ▶ With parenteral use Intestinal hypermotility · muscle spasms
- RENAL IMPAIRMENT
  Dose adjustments May need dose reduction.

- MEDICINAL FORMS There can be variation in the licensing of different medicines containing the same drug. Forms available from special-order manufacturers include: oral solution
  Solution for injection
  - ▶ Neostigmine (Non-proprietary)
    Neostigmine metilsulfate 2.5 mg per 1 ml Neostigmine 2.5mg/1ml solution for injection ampoules | 10 ampoule PoM £7.50-£7.51 DT = £7.51

Tablet
▸ Neostigmine (Non-proprietary)
Neostigmine bromide 15 mg Neostigmine 15mg tablets |
140 tablet PoM £120.52 DT = £120.52

⚑ 1170

Pyridostigmine bromide

- DRUG ACTION Pyridostigmine bromide has weaker muscarinic action than neostigmine.

- **INDICATIONS AND DOSE**

Myasthenia gravis
▸ INITIALLY BY MOUTH
▸ Adult: 30–120 mg, doses to be given at suitable intervals throughout day; (by mouth) usual dose 0.3–1.2 g daily in divided doses, it is inadvisable to exceed a total daily dose of 450 mg in order to avoid acetylcholine receptor down-regulation; patients requiring doses exceeding 450 mg daily will usually require input from a specialised neuromuscular service. Immunosuppressant therapy is usually considered if the dose of pyridostigmine exceeds 360 mg daily

- INTERACTIONS → Appendix 1: pyridostigmine

- SIDE-EFFECTS Gastrointestinal hypermotility · muscle cramps · rash

- RENAL IMPAIRMENT
Dose adjustments Reduce dose; excreted by kidney.

- MEDICINAL FORMS There can be variation in the licensing of different medicines containing the same drug. Forms available from special-order manufacturers include: tablet, oral suspension, oral solution
Tablet
▸ Pyridostigmine bromide (Non-proprietary)
Pyridostigmine bromide 60 mg Pyridostigmine bromide 60mg tablets | 200 tablet PoM £45.48 DT = £45.00
▸ Mestinon (Mylan)
Pyridostigmine bromide 60 mg Mestinon 60mg tablets | 200 tablet PoM £45.57 DT = £45.00

CHOLINERGIC RECEPTOR STIMULATING DRUGS

▍Amifampridine

31-Aug-2020

- **INDICATIONS AND DOSE**

Symptomatic treatment of Lambert-Eaton myasthenic syndrome (specialist use only)
▸ BY MOUTH
▸ Adult: Initially 15 mg daily in 3 divided doses, then increased in steps of 5 mg every 4–5 days, increased to up to 60 mg daily in 3–4 divided doses (max. per dose 20 mg); maximum 60 mg per day

- CONTRA-INDICATIONS Congenital QT syndromes · epilepsy · uncontrolled asthma

- CAUTIONS Non-paraneoplastic form of Lambert- Eaton myasthenic syndrome

- INTERACTIONS → Appendix 1: amifampridine

- SIDE-EFFECTS
▸ **Common or very common** Dizziness · gastrointestinal discomfort · nausea · oral disorders · peripheral coldness · sensation abnormal · sweat changes
▸ **Frequency not known** Anxiety · arrhythmia · asthenia · asthmatic attack · bronchial secretion increased · cough · diarrhoea · drowsiness · gastrointestinal disorder · headache · movement disorders · palpitations · Raynaud's phenomenon · seizures · sleep disorder · vision blurred

- CONCEPTION AND CONTRACEPTION Ensure effective contraception during treatment in men and women.

- PREGNANCY Manufacturer advises avoid.

- BREAST FEEDING Manufacturer advises avoid—no information available.

- HEPATIC IMPAIRMENT Manufacturer advises caution (risk of increased exposure).
Dose adjustments Manufacturer advises initial dose reduction to 5 mg twice daily in mild impairment, titrate in steps of 5 mg every 7 days.
   Manufacturer advises initial dose reduction to 5 mg once daily in moderate to severe impairment, titrate in steps of 5 mg every 7 days.

- RENAL IMPAIRMENT Use with caution.
Dose adjustments In mild impairment reduce initial dose to 10 mg daily in divided doses, increased in steps of 5 mg every 7 days.
   In moderate or severe impairment reduce initial dose to 5 mg daily in divided doses, increased in steps of 5 mg every 7 days.

- MONITORING REQUIREMENTS Clinical and ECG monitoring required at treatment initiation and yearly thereafter.

- NATIONAL FUNDING/ACCESS DECISIONS
For full details see funding body website
Scottish Medicines Consortium (SMC) decisions
▸ Amifampridine (*Firdapse*®) for the symptomatic treatment of Lambert-Eaton myasthenic syndrome (LEMS) in adults (August 2012) SMC No. 660/10 Not recommended

- MEDICINAL FORMS There can be variation in the licensing of different medicines containing the same drug. Forms available from special-order manufacturers include: tablet
Tablet
CAUTIONARY AND ADVISORY LABELS 3, 21
▸ Firdapse (SERB) ▼
Amifampridine (as Amifampridine phosphate) 10 mg Firdapse 10mg tablets | 100 tablet PoM £1,815.00

3.3 Myotonic disorders

DRUGS FOR NEUROMUSCULAR DISORDERS

▍Mexiletine

27-Aug-2020

- DRUG ACTION Mexiletine is a sodium channel blocker which reduces the delay of muscle relaxation thereby decreasing muscle stiffness.

- **INDICATIONS AND DOSE**

Myotonia in non-dystrophic myotonic disorders
▸ BY MOUTH
▸ Adult: 167 mg once daily for at least 1 week, then increased if necessary to 333 mg daily in divided doses for at least 1 week, then increased if necessary to 500 mg daily in divided doses; maintenance 167–500 mg daily; maximum 500 mg daily

- CONTRA-INDICATIONS Abnormal Q-waves · atrial tachyarrhythmia, fibrillation or flutter · complete heart block or any heart block susceptible to evolve to complete heart block · heart failure (with ejection fraction less than 50%) · history of myocardial infarction · sinus node dysfunction · symptomatic coronary artery disease · ventricular tachyarrhythmia

- CAUTIONS Cardiac disorders other than those contra-indicated · epilepsy (increased risk of seizures)

- INTERACTIONS → Appendix 1: mexiletine

- SIDE-EFFECTS
▸ **Common or very common** Abdominal pain · arrhythmias · asthenia · chest discomfort · drowsiness · headache · hypotension · insomnia · malaise · nausea · pain in extremity · paraesthesia · skin reactions · vasodilation · vertigo · vision disorders
▸ **Uncommon** Seizure · speech disorder

▶ **Rare or very rare** Hepatic disorders · severe cutaneous adverse reactions (SCARs)
▶ **Frequency not known** Atrioventricular block · circulatory collapse · confusion · diarrhoea · gastrointestinal disorders · hallucination · leucopenia · lupus-like syndrome · pulmonary fibrosis · taste altered · thrombocytopenia · vomiting

SIDE-EFFECTS, FURTHER INFORMATION Manufacturer advises evaluation and correction of electrolytes prior to therapy initiation, with monitoring continued throughout treatment with mexiletine, due to possible proarrhythmic effects.

● ALLERGY AND CROSS-SENSITIVITY Manufacturer advises avoid if hypersensitivity to any local anaesthetic.
● PREGNANCY Manufacturer advises avoid—limited information available.
● BREAST FEEDING Manufacturer advises avoid—present in human milk and insufficient information on the effects in infants.
● HEPATIC IMPAIRMENT Manufacturer advises caution in mild or moderate impairment; avoid in severe impairment (limited information available).
Dose adjustments Manufacturer advises any dose increase should only be made after at least 2 weeks of treatment in mild or moderate impairment.
● RENAL IMPAIRMENT Manufacturer advises avoid in severe impairment (limited information available).
● MONITORING REQUIREMENTS
▶ Manufacturer advises cardiac evaluation before starting treatment, within 48 hours of starting treatment, and during treatment (consult product literature).
▶ Manufacturer advises monitor electrolytes before starting treatment and during treatment—imbalances should be corrected.
● DIRECTIONS FOR ADMINISTRATION Manufacturer advises capsules should be swallowed whole with water, while in an upright position. If digestive intolerance occurs, capsules should be taken during a meal.
● PRESCRIBING AND DISPENSING INFORMATION The manufacturer of *Namuscla*® has provided a *Guide for Healthcare Professionals*.
● PATIENT AND CARER ADVICE Manufacturer advises patients and carers should be informed about the presenting symptoms of arrhythmias (e.g. fainting, palpitation, chest pain, shortness of breath, light-headedness, lipothymia, and syncope) and advised to seek immediate medical attention if symptoms develop.
Alert card An alert card should be provided.
Driving and skilled tasks Manufacturer advises patients and carers should be counselled on the effects on driving and performance of skilled tasks—increased risk of fatigue, confusion, and blurred vision.
● NATIONAL FUNDING/ACCESS DECISIONS
For full details see funding body website
Scottish Medicines Consortium (SMC) decisions
▶ Mexiletine (*Namuscla*®) for the symptomatic treatment of myotonia in adult patients with non-dystrophic myotonic disorders (NDM) (March 2020) SMC No. SMC2241 Not recommended

● MEDICINAL FORMS There can be variation in the licensing of different medicines containing the same drug.
Capsule
▶ Namuscla (Lupin Healthcare (UK) Ltd)
Mexiletine (as Mexiletine hydrochloride) 167 mg Namuscla 167mg capsules | 100 capsule [PoM] £5,000.00 DT = £5,000.00

3.4 Nocturnal leg cramps

Nocturnal leg cramps

Quinine salts

Quinine salts p. 658, such as quinine sulfate are effective in reducing the frequency of nocturnal leg cramps by about 25% in ambulatory patients; however, because of potential toxicity, quinine is not recommended for routine treatment and should not be used unless cramps cause regular disruption to sleep. Quinine should only be considered when cramps are very painful or frequent; when other treatable causes of cramp have been excluded; and when non-pharmacological treatments have not worked (e.g. passive stretching exercises). It may take up to 4 weeks for improvement to become apparent; if there is benefit, quinine treatment can be continued. Treatment should be interrupted at intervals of approximately 3 months to assess the need for further quinine treatment. In patients taking quinine long term, a trial discontinuation may be considered. Quinine is toxic in overdosage and accidental fatalities have occurred.

3.5 Spasticity

Other drugs used for Spasticity Dantrolene sodium, p. 1400 · Diazepam, p. 362

CANNABINOIDS

Cannabis extract

20-Nov-2020

The properties listed below are those particular to the combination only. For the properties of the components please consider, cannabidiol p. 326.

● INDICATIONS AND DOSE
Adjunct in moderate to severe spasticity in multiple sclerosis (specialist use only)
▶ BY BUCCAL ADMINISTRATION
▸ Adult: (consult product literature)

● CONTRA-INDICATIONS Family history of psychosis · history of other severe psychiatric disorder · personal history of psychosis
● CAUTIONS History of epilepsy · significant cardiovascular disease
● INTERACTIONS → Appendix 1: cannabidiol · dronabinol
● SIDE-EFFECTS
▶ **Common or very common** Appetite abnormal · balance impaired · concentration impaired · constipation · depression · diarrhoea · disorientation · dizziness · drowsiness · dry mouth · dysarthria · euphoric mood · feeling drunk · malaise · memory loss · nausea · oral disorders · perception altered · taste altered · vertigo · vision blurred · vomiting
▶ **Uncommon** Abdominal pain upper · delusions · hallucinations · hypertension · palpitations · paranoia · pharyngitis · suicidal ideation · syncope · tachycardia · throat irritation · tooth discolouration
● CONCEPTION AND CONTRACEPTION Manufacturer recommends effective contraception during and for 3 months after treatment in men and women.
● PREGNANCY Manufacturer advises use only if potential benefit outweighs risks.
● BREAST FEEDING Avoid—present in milk.

● HEPATIC IMPAIRMENT Manufacturer advises avoid in moderate to severe impairment (risk of accumulation with chronic dosing)—no information available.

● RENAL IMPAIRMENT
Monitoring Manufacturer advises more frequent monitoring in significant renal impairment—possible risk of prolonged or enhanced effect.

● MONITORING REQUIREMENTS Monitor oral mucosa—interrupt treatment if lesions or persistent soreness.

● PATIENT AND CARER ADVICE
Driving and skilled tasks For information on 2015 legislation regarding driving whilst taking certain controlled drugs, including cannabis, see Drugs and driving under Guidance on prescribing p. 1.

● MEDICINAL FORMS There can be variation in the licensing of different medicines containing the same drug.
Spray
EXCIPIENTS: May contain Propylene glycol
▸ Sativex (GW Pharma Ltd)
Cannabidiol 2.5 mg per 1 dose, Dronabinol 2.7 mg per 1 dose Sativex oromucosal spray | 270 dose PoM £300.00 DT = £300.00 CD4–1

MUSCLE RELAXANTS ❯ CENTRALLY ACTING

❚ **Baclofen**   03-Sep-2020

● **INDICATIONS AND DOSE**
Pain of muscle spasm in palliative care
▸ BY MOUTH
▸ Adult: 5–10 mg 3 times a day
Hiccup due to gastric distension in palliative care
▸ BY MOUTH
▸ Adult: 5 mg twice daily
Chronic severe spasticity resulting from disorders such as multiple sclerosis or traumatic partial section of spinal cord
▸ BY MOUTH
▸ Adult: Initially 5 mg 3 times a day, gradually increased; maintenance up to 60 mg daily in divided doses, review treatment if no benefit within 6 weeks of achieving maximum dose; maximum 100 mg per day
Severe chronic spasticity unresponsive to oral antispastic drugs (or where side-effects of oral therapy unacceptable) or as alternative to ablative neurosurgical procedures (specialist use only)
▸ BY INTRATHECAL INJECTION
▸ Adult: Test dose 25–50 micrograms, to be given over at least 1 minute via catheter or lumbar puncture, then increased in steps of 25 micrograms (max. per dose 100 micrograms), not given more often than every 24 hours to determine appropriate dose, then *dose-titration phase*, most often using infusion pump (implanted into chest wall or abdominal wall tissues) to establish maintenance dose (ranging from 12 micrograms to 2 mg daily for spasticity of spinal origin or 22 micrograms to 1.4 mg daily for spasticity of cerebral origin) retaining some spasticity to avoid sensation of paralysis

IMPORTANT SAFETY INFORMATION
Consult product literature for details on test dose and titration—important to monitor patients closely in appropriately equipped and staffed environment during screening and immediately after pump implantation. Resuscitation equipment must be available for immediate use. Treatment with continuous pump-administered intrathecal baclofen should be initiated

within 3 months of a satisfactory response to intrathecal baclofen testing.

● CONTRA-INDICATIONS
▸ With intrathecal use Local infection · systemic infection
▸ With oral use Active peptic ulceration

● CAUTIONS
GENERAL CAUTIONS Cerebrovascular disease · diabetes · elderly · epilepsy · history of peptic ulcer · hypertonic bladder sphincter · Parkinson's disease · psychiatric illness · respiratory impairment
SPECIFIC CAUTIONS
▸ With intrathecal use Coagulation disorders · malnutrition (increased risk of post-surgical complications) · previous spinal fusion procedure

● INTERACTIONS → Appendix 1: baclofen

● SIDE-EFFECTS
GENERAL SIDE-EFFECTS
▸ **Common or very common** Confusion · constipation · depression · diarrhoea · dizziness · drowsiness · dry mouth · euphoric mood · hallucination · headache · hyperhidrosis · hypotension · nausea · paraesthesia · skin reactions · urinary disorders · vision disorders · vomiting
▸ **Uncommon** Bradycardia · hypothermia
▸ **Rare or very rare** Withdrawal syndrome
SPECIFIC SIDE-EFFECTS
▸ **Common or very common**
▸ With intrathecal use Anxiety · appetite decreased · asthenia · chills · dyspnoea · fever · hypersalivation · insomnia · neuromuscular dysfunction · oedema · pain · pneumonia · respiratory disorders · seizure · sexual dysfunction
▸ With oral use Fatigue · gastrointestinal disorder · muscle weakness · myalgia · respiratory depression · sleep disorders
▸ **Uncommon**
▸ With intrathecal use Alopecia · deep vein thrombosis · dehydration · flushing · hypertension · hypogeusia · ileus · memory loss · pallor · paranoia · suicidal behaviours
▸ **Rare or very rare**
▸ With oral use Abdominal pain · erectile dysfunction · hepatic function abnormal · taste altered
▸ **Frequency not known**
▸ With intrathecal use Scoliosis

● PREGNANCY Manufacturer advises use only if potential benefit outweighs risk (toxicity in *animal* studies).

● BREAST FEEDING Present in milk—amount probably too small to be harmful.

● HEPATIC IMPAIRMENT
▸ With oral use Manufacturer advises use with caution—no information available.

● RENAL IMPAIRMENT Excreted by the kidney.
Dose adjustments ▸ With oral use Risk of toxicity—use smaller doses (e.g. 5 mg daily by mouth) and if necessary increase dosage interval; if eGFR less than 15 mL/minute/1.73 m^2 manufacturer advises use by mouth only if potential benefit outweighs risk.

● TREATMENT CESSATION Avoid abrupt withdrawal (risk of hyperactive state, may exacerbate spasticity, and precipitate autonomic dysfunction including hyperthermia, psychiatric reactions and convulsions; to minimise risk, discontinue by gradual dose reduction over at least 1–2 weeks (longer if symptoms occur)).

● PRESCRIBING AND DISPENSING INFORMATION Flavours of oral liquid formulations may include raspberry.
Palliative care For further information on the use of baclofen in palliative care, see www.medicinescomplete.com/#/content/palliative/baclofen.

10

Musculoskeletal system

● PATIENT AND CARER ADVICE
Driving and skilled tasks Drowsiness may affect performance of skilled tasks (e.g. driving); effects of alcohol enhanced.

● MEDICINAL FORMS There can be variation in the licensing of different medicines containing the same drug. Forms available from special-order manufacturers include: oral suspension, oral solution, solution for injection

Tablet
CAUTIONARY AND ADVISORY LABELS 2, 8, 21
EXCIPIENTS: May contain Gluten
▸ Baclofen (Non-proprietary)
  Baclofen 10 mg Baclofen 10mg tablets | 84 tablet [PoM] £9.99 DT = £1.58 | 250 tablet [PoM] £9.75
▸ Lioresal (Novartis Pharmaceuticals UK Ltd)
  Baclofen 10 mg Lioresal 10mg tablets | 100 tablet [PoM] £14.86

Solution for injection
▸ Baclofen (Non-proprietary)
  Baclofen 50 microgram per 1 ml Baclofen 50micrograms/1ml solution for injection ampoules | 10 ampoule [PoM] £25.00
▸ Gablofen (Imported (United States))
  Baclofen 1 mg per 1 ml Gablofen 20mg/20ml solution for injection pre-filled syringes | 1 pre-filled disposable injection [PoM] [⬚]
  Gablofen 20mg/20ml solution for injection vials | 1 vial [PoM] [⬚]
▸ Lioresal (Novartis Pharmaceuticals UK Ltd)
  Baclofen 50 microgram per 1 ml Lioresal Intrathecal 50micrograms/1ml solution for injection ampoules | 1 ampoule [PoM] £3.16 DT = £3.16

Solution for infusion
▸ Baclofen (Non-proprietary)
  Baclofen 500 microgram per 1 ml Baclofen 10mg/20ml solution for infusion ampoules | 1 ampoule [PoM] £50.00 DT = £70.01
  Baclofen 2 mg per 1 ml Baclofen 40mg/20ml solution for infusion ampoules | 1 ampoule [PoM] £250.00
  Baclofen 10mg/5ml solution for infusion ampoules | 10 ampoule [PoM] £500.00
▸ Lioresal (Novartis Pharmaceuticals UK Ltd)
  Baclofen 500 microgram per 1 ml Lioresal Intrathecal 10mg/20ml solution for infusion ampoules | 1 ampoule [PoM] £70.01 DT = £70.01
  Baclofen 2 mg per 1 ml Lioresal Intrathecal 10mg/5ml solution for infusion ampoules | 1 ampoule [PoM] £70.01 DT = £70.01

Oral solution
CAUTIONARY AND ADVISORY LABELS 2, 8, 21
▸ Baclofen (Non-proprietary)
  Baclofen 1 mg per 1 ml Baclofen 5mg/5ml oral solution sugar free sugar-free | 300 ml [PoM] £24.78 DT = £4.64
  Baclofen 2 mg per 1 ml Baclofen 10mg/5ml oral solution sugar free sugar-free | 150 ml [PoM] £10.72
▸ Lioresal (Novartis Pharmaceuticals UK Ltd)
  Baclofen 1 mg per 1 ml Lioresal 5mg/5ml liquid sugar-free | 300 ml [PoM] £10.31 DT = £4.64
▸ Lyflex (Chemidex Pharma Ltd)
  Baclofen 1 mg per 1 ml Lyflex 5mg/5ml oral solution sugar-free | 300 ml [PoM] £7.95 DT = £4.64

Methocarbamol

17-Nov-2020

● INDICATIONS AND DOSE
Short-term symptomatic relief of muscle spasm
▸ BY MOUTH
▸ Adult: 1.5 g 4 times a day; reduced to 750 mg 3 times a day if required
▸ Elderly: Up to 750 mg 4 times a day, dose may be sufficient

● CONTRA-INDICATIONS Brain damage · coma · epilepsy · myasthenia gravis · pre-coma

● INTERACTIONS → Appendix 1: methocarbamol

● SIDE-EFFECTS Angioedema · anxiety · bradycardia · confusion · conjunctivitis · dizziness · drowsiness · dyspepsia · fever · flushing · headache · hepatic disorders · hypotension · insomnia · leucopenia · memory loss · nasal congestion · nausea · seizures · skin reactions · syncope · taste metallic · vertigo · vision disorders · vomiting

● PREGNANCY Manufacturer advises avoid unless potential benefit outweighs risk.

● BREAST FEEDING Present in milk in *animal studies*— manufacturer advises caution.

● HEPATIC IMPAIRMENT Manufacturer advises caution (risk of increased half-life).
Dose adjustments Manufacturer advises consider increasing dose interval in chronic impairment.

● RENAL IMPAIRMENT Manufacturer advises caution.

● PATIENT AND CARER ADVICE
Driving and skilled tasks Drowsiness may affect performance of skilled tasks (e.g. driving); effects of alcohol enhanced.

● LESS SUITABLE FOR PRESCRIBING Less suitable for prescribing.

● MEDICINAL FORMS There can be variation in the licensing of different medicines containing the same drug. Forms available from special-order manufacturers include: oral suspension

Tablet
CAUTIONARY AND ADVISORY LABELS 2
▸ Methocarbamol (Non-proprietary)
  Methocarbamol 750 mg Methocarbamol 750mg tablets | 100 tablet [PoM] £12.71 DT = £10.82
▸ Robaxin (Almirall Ltd)
  Methocarbamol 750 mg Robaxin 750 tablets | 100 tablet [PoM] £12.65 DT = £10.82

Pridinol

17-Nov-2020

● DRUG ACTION Pridinol is a centrally acting muscle relaxant.

● INDICATIONS AND DOSE
Central and peripheral muscle spasms
▸ BY MOUTH
▸ Adult: 1.5–3 mg 3 times a day

● CONTRA-INDICATIONS Arrhythmia · gastrointestinal obstruction · glaucoma · prostatic hypertrophy · urinary retention

● CAUTIONS Elderly (higher or longer-lasting blood levels expected) · hypotension (increased risk of circulatory problems)—take dose after meals

● INTERACTIONS → Appendix 1: pridinol

● SIDE-EFFECTS
▸ **Uncommon** Abdominal pain · anxiety · arrhythmias · asthenia · circulatory collapse · dizziness · dry mouth · headache · hypotension · nausea · speech disorder
▸ **Rare or very rare** Concentration impaired · coordination abnormal · depression · diarrhoea · taste altered · vision disorders · vomiting
▸ **Frequency not known** Constipation · feeling hot · hallucination · muscle weakness · mydriasis · paraesthesia · skin reactions · thirst · tremor · urinary disorder

● PREGNANCY [EvGr] Avoid in the first trimester; thereafter, use only if potential benefit outweighs risk (no information available). ◈

● BREAST FEEDING [EvGr] Avoid—no information available. ◈

● HEPATIC IMPAIRMENT [EvGr] Caution in severe impairment (no information available)—higher or longer-lasting blood levels expected. ◈

● RENAL IMPAIRMENT [EvGr] Caution in severe impairment (no information available)—higher or longer-lasting blood levels expected. ◈

● MEDICINAL FORMS There can be variation in the licensing of different medicines containing the same drug.

Tablet

▸ Myopridin (Mibe Pharma UK Ltd)
  Pridinol (as Pridinol mesilate) 3 mg Myopridin 3mg tablets | 20 tablet PoM £5.36 | 100 tablet PoM £26.16

Tizanidine

24-Nov-2020

● **INDICATIONS AND DOSE**

Spasticity associated with multiple sclerosis or spinal cord injury or disease

▸ BY MOUTH

▸ **Adult:** Initially 2 mg daily, then increased in steps of 2 mg daily in divided doses, increased at intervals of at least 3–4 days and adjust according to response; usual dose up to 24 mg daily in 3–4 divided doses; maximum 36 mg per day

● CAUTIONS Elderly

● INTERACTIONS → Appendix 1: tizanidine

● SIDE-EFFECTS

▸ **Common or very common** Arrhythmias · dizziness · drowsiness · dry mouth · fatigue · hypotension · rebound hypertension

▸ **Rare or very rare** Gastrointestinal disorder · hallucination · hepatic disorders · muscle weakness · nausea · sleep disorders

▸ **Frequency not known** Abdominal pain · accommodation disorder · anxiety · appetite decreased · confusion · headache · QT interval prolongation · skin reactions · vomiting · withdrawal syndrome

SIDE-EFFECTS, FURTHER INFORMATION Treatment should be discontinued if liver enzymes are persistently raised—consult product literature.

● PREGNANCY Avoid (toxicity in *animal* studies).

● BREAST FEEDING Avoid (present in milk in *animal* studies).

● HEPATIC IMPAIRMENT Manufacturer advises avoid in significant impairment.

● RENAL IMPAIRMENT Manufacturer advises caution.

● MONITORING REQUIREMENTS Monitor liver function monthly for first 4 months for doses of 12 mg or higher, and in those who develop unexplained nausea, anorexia or fatigue.

● TREATMENT CESSATION Avoid abrupt withdrawal (risk of rebound hypertension and tachycardia); to minimise risk, discontinue gradually and monitor blood pressure.

● PATIENT AND CARER ADVICE
  Driving and skilled tasks Drowsiness may affect performance of skilled tasks (e.g. driving); effects of alcohol enhanced.

● MEDICINAL FORMS There can be variation in the licensing of different medicines containing the same drug. Forms available from special-order manufacturers include: oral suspension, oral solution

Tablet

CAUTIONARY AND ADVISORY LABELS 2, 8
▸ Tizanidine (Non-proprietary)
  Tizanidine (as Tizanidine hydrochloride) 2 mg Tizanidine 2mg tablets | 120 tablet PoM £28.89 DT = £14.03
  Tizanidine (as Tizanidine hydrochloride) 4 mg Tizanidine 4mg tablets | 120 tablet PoM £40.07 DT = £40.05

---

4 Pain and inflammation in musculoskeletal disorders

Low back pain and sciatica

08-Mar-2017

Description of condition

Low back pain is pain in the lumbosacral area of the back. It can be described as *non-specific*, *mechanical*, *musculoskeletal* or *simple* (if it is not associated with serious or potentially serious causes). Episodes of back pain do not usually last long, with rapid improvements in pain and disability seen within a few weeks to months.

Sciatica (*radicular pain* or *radiculopathy*) is neuropathic leg pain secondary to compressive lumbosacral nerve root pathology.

Non-drug treatment

EvGr Exercise programmes, manual therapy, and psychological therapies should be considered for managing low back pain with or without sciatica.

Spinal decompression may be considered in patients with sciatica when pain and function has not improved with non-surgical treatment (including drug treatment). Ⓐ

Drug treatment

EvGr An oral NSAID (see Non-steroidal anti-inflammatory drugs p. 1176) should be considered for managing acute low back pain, taking into consideration the gastro-intestinal, cardio-renal and hepatic risks associated with NSAIDs; as well as the need for continued monitoring, and the possible need for gastroprotective treatment (for further information, see Peptic ulcer disease p. 77).

A weak opioid, either alone or with paracetamol p. 464, can be used to manage acute low back pain only if an NSAID is contra-indicated, not tolerated or ineffective (see *Opioid analgesics* under Analgesics p. 462). Paracetamol alone is ineffective for managing low back pain. Ⓐ

EvGr Benzodiazepines are sometimes used to manage acute low back pain (particularly in loss of lordosis); however evidence to support their use is very weak. Ⓔ

EvGr In patients with chronic low back pain who have had an inadequate response to non-drug treatment, NSAIDs should be considered as first-line therapy. Opioids should be the last treatment option considered and should be considered only in patients for whom other therapies have failed and only if the potential benefits outweigh the risks for individual patients. If indicated, opioids should only be prescribed for a limited period of time. Long term opioid therapy should be avoided.

Selective serotonin re-uptake inhibitors (SSRIs), serotonin and noradrenaline re-uptake inhibitors (SNRIs), tricyclic antidepressants, and antiepileptic drugs should **not** be offered for managing low back pain.

When non-surgical treatment is ineffective in patients with moderate and severe localised back pain arising from structures supplied by the medial branch nerve, radiofrequency denervation can be considered. Ⓐ

Sciatica

Patients with sciatica may require specific treatment for Neuropathic pain p. 504.

EvGr Patients with acute and severe sciatica may benefit from treatment with epidural injections of local anaesthetic and/or corticosteroid. Ⓐ

Useful Resources

Low back pain and sciatica. National Institute for Health and Care Excellence. Clinical guideline NG59. November 2016. www.nice.org.uk/guidance/ng59

10

Musculoskeletal system

Non-steroidal anti-inflammatory drugs

18-Mar-2020

Therapeutic effects

In *single doses* non-steroidal anti-inflammatory drugs (NSAIDs) have analgesic activity comparable to that of paracetamol p. 464, but paracetamol is preferred, particularly in the elderly.

In regular *full dosage* NSAIDs have both a lasting analgesic and an anti-inflammatory effect which makes them particularly useful for the treatment of continuous or regular pain associated with inflammation. Therefore, although paracetamol often gives adequate pain control in osteoarthritis, NSAIDs are more appropriate than paracetamol or the opioid analgesics in the *inflammatory arthritides* (e.g. rheumatoid arthritis) and in some cases of *advanced osteoarthritis*. NSAIDs can also be of benefit in the less well defined conditions of *back pain* and *soft-tissue disorders*.

Choice

Differences in anti-inflammatory activity between NSAIDs are small, but there is considerable variation in individual response and tolerance to these drugs. About 60% of patients will respond to any NSAID; of the others, those who do not respond to one may well respond to another. Pain relief starts soon after taking the first dose and a full analgesic effect should normally be obtained within a week, whereas an anti-inflammatory effect may not be achieved (or may not be clinically assessable) for up to 3 weeks. If appropriate responses are not obtained within these times, another NSAID should be tried.

NSAIDs reduce the production of prostaglandins by inhibiting the enzyme cyclo-oxygenase. They vary in their selectivity for inhibiting different types of cyclo-oxygenase; selective inhibition of cyclo-oxygenase-2 (COX-2) is associated with less gastro-intestinal intolerance. Several other factors also influence susceptibility to gastrointestinal effects, and a NSAID should be chosen on the basis of the incidence of gastro-intestinal and other side-effects.

Ibuprofen p. 1186 is a propionic acid derivative with anti-inflammatory, analgesic, and antipyretic properties. It has fewer side-effects than other non-selective NSAIDs but its anti-inflammatory properties are weaker. It is unsuitable for conditions where inflammation is prominent. Dexibuprofen p. 1179 is the active enantiomer of ibuprofen. It has similar properties to ibuprofen and is licensed for the relief of mild to moderate pain and inflammation.

Other propionic acid derivatives:

Naproxen p. 1194 is one of the first choices because it combines good efficacy with a low incidence of side-effects (but more than ibuprofen).

Flurbiprofen p. 1185 may be slightly more effective than naproxen, and is associated with slightly more gastro-intestinal side-effects than ibuprofen.

Ketoprofen p. 1190 has anti-inflammatory properties similar to ibuprofen and has more side-effects. Dexketoprofen p. 1180, an isomer of ketoprofen, has been introduced for the short-term relief of mild to moderate pain.

Tiaprofenic acid p. 1198 is as effective as naproxen; it has more side-effects than ibuprofen.

Drugs with properties similar to those of propionic acid derivatives:

Diclofenac sodium p. 1181 and aceclofenac p. 1177 are similar in efficacy to naproxen.

Etodolac p. 1183 is comparable in efficacy to naproxen; it is licensed for symptomatic relief of osteoarthritis and rheumatoid arthritis.

Indometacin p. 1189 has an action equal to or superior to that of naproxen, but with a high incidence of side-effects

including headache, dizziness, and gastro-intestinal disturbances.

Mefenamic acid p. 1191 has minor anti-inflammatory properties. It has occasionally been associated with diarrhoea and haemolytic anaemia which require discontinuation of treatment.

Meloxicam p. 1192 is licensed for the short-term relief of pain in osteoarthritis and for long-term treatment of rheumatoid arthritis and ankylosing spondylitis.

Nabumetone p. 1193 is comparable in effect to naproxen.

Phenylbutazone is licensed for ankylosing spondylitis, but is not recommended because it is associated with serious side-effects, in particular haematological reactions; it should be used only by a specialist in severe cases where other treatments have been found unsuitable.

Piroxicam p. 1195 is as effective as naproxen and has a long duration of action which permits once-daily administration. However, it has more gastro-intestinal side-effects than most other NSAIDs, and is associated with more frequent serious skin reactions.

Sulindac p. 1196 is similar in tolerance to naproxen.

Tenoxicam p. 1197 is similar in activity and tolerance to naproxen. Its long duration of action allows once-daily administration.

Tolfenamic acid p. 496 is licensed for the treatment of migraine.

Ketorolac trometamol p. 1395 and the selective inhibitor of cyclo-oxygenase-2, parecoxib p. 1396, are licensed for the short-term management of postoperative pain.

The selective inhibitors of COX-2, etoricoxib p. 1184 and celecoxib p. 1178, are as effective as non-selective NSAIDs such as diclofenac sodium and naproxen. Although selective inhibitors can cause serious gastro-intestinal events, available evidence appears to indicate that the risk of serious upper gastro-intestinal events is lower with selective inhibitors compared to non-selective NSAIDs; this advantage may be lost in patients who require concomitant low-dose aspirin.

Celecoxib and etoricoxib are licensed for the relief of pain in osteoarthritis, rheumatoid arthritis, and ankylosing spondylitis; etoricoxib is also licensed for the relief of pain from acute gout.

Aspirin p. 132 has been used in high doses to treat rheumatoid arthritis, but other NSAIDs are now preferred.

Dental and orofacial pain

Most mild to moderate dental pain and inflammation is effectively relieved by NSAIDs. Those used for dental pain include ibuprofen, diclofenac sodium, and diclofenac potassium p. 1180.

Considerations in the elderly

The use of NSAIDs in elderly patients is potentially inappropriate (STOPP criteria) if prescribed:

- with a vitamin K antagonist, direct thrombin inhibitor or factor Xa inhibitor in combination (risk of major gastrointestinal bleeding);
- with concurrent antiplatelet agent(s) without proton pump inhibitor (PPI) prophylaxis (increased risk of peptic ulcer disease);
- in a history of peptic ulcer disease or gastrointestinal bleeding, unless with concurrent PPI or H_2-receptor antagonist (risk of peptic ulcer relapse)—not including COX-2 selective NSAIDs;
- with concurrent corticosteroids without PPI prophylaxis (increased risk of peptic ulcer disease);
- in patients with an eGFR less than 50 mL/minute/1.73 m^2 (risk of deterioration in renal function);
- in severe hypertension or severe heart failure (risk of exacerbation);
- for long-term (longer than 3 months) symptom relief of osteoarthritis pain where paracetamol has not been tried

(simple analgesics are preferable and usually as effective for pain relief);

- for chronic treatment of gout where there is no contra-indication to a xanthine-oxidase inhibitor (xanthine-oxidase inhibitors are first choice prophylactic drugs in gout);

- a **COX-2 selective** NSAID in concurrent cardiovascular disease (increased risk of myocardial infarction and stroke).

For further information, see *STOPP/START criteria* in *Prescribing in the elderly* p. 33.

Asthma

Any degree of worsening of asthma may be related to the ingestion of NSAIDs, either prescribed or (in the case of ibuprofen **and** others) purchased over the counter.

NSAIDs and cardiovascular events

All NSAID use (including COX-2 selective inhibitors) can, to varying degrees, be associated with a small increased risk of thrombotic events (e.g. myocardial infarction and stroke) independent of baseline cardiovascular risk factors or duration of NSAID use; however, the greatest risk may be in those receiving high doses long term.

COX-2 selective inhibitors, diclofenac (150 mg daily) and ibuprofen p. 1186 (2.4 g daily) are associated with an increased risk of thrombotic events. Although there are limited data regarding the thrombotic effects of aceclofenac below, treatment advice has been updated in line with diclofenac, based on aceclofenac's structural similarity to diclofenac and its metabolism to diclofenac. The increased risk for diclofenac is similar to that of licensed doses of etoricoxib p. 1184. Naproxen p. 1194 (1 g daily) is associated with a lower thrombotic risk, and low doses of ibuprofen (1.2 g daily or less) have not been associated with an increased risk of myocardial infarction.

The lowest effective dose of NSAID should be prescribed for the shortest period of time to control symptoms and the need for long-term treatment should be reviewed periodically.

NSAIDs and gastro-intestinal events

All NSAIDs are associated with serious gastro-intestinal toxicity; the risk is higher in the elderly. Evidence on the relative safety of non-selective NSAIDs indicates differences in the risks of serious upper gastro-intestinal side-effects—piroxicam p. 1195, ketoprofen p. 1190, and ketorolac trometamol p. 1395 are associated with the highest risk; indometacin p. 1184, diclofenac, and naproxen are associated with intermediate risk, and ibuprofen with the lowest risk (although high doses of ibuprofen have been associated with intermediate risk). Selective inhibitors of COX-2 are associated with a *lower risk* of serious upper gastro-intestinal side-effects than non-selective NSAIDs.

Recommendations are that NSAIDs associated with a low risk e.g. ibuprofen are *generally preferred*, to start at the *lowest recommended dose* **and** not to use more than one oral NSAID at a time.

The combination of a NSAID **and** low-dose aspirin can increase the risk of gastro-intestinal side-effects; this combination should be used only if absolutely necessary **and** the patient should be monitored closely.

While it is preferable to avoid NSAIDs in patients with active or previous gastro-intestinal ulceration or bleeding, and to withdraw them if gastro-intestinal lesions develop, nevertheless patients with serious rheumatic diseases (e.g. rheumatoid arthritis) are usually dependent on NSAIDs for effective relief of pain and stiffness.

Patients at risk of gastro-intestinal ulceration (including the elderly), who need NSAID treatment should receive gastroprotective treatment.

Systemic as well as local effects of NSAIDs contribute to gastro-intestinal damage; taking oral formulations with milk or food, or using enteric-coated formulations, or changing the route of administration may only partially reduce symptoms such as dyspepsia.

NSAIDs and alcohol

Alcohol increases the risk of gastro-intestinal haemorrhage associated with NSAIDs. Specialist sources recommend that concurrent use need not be avoided with moderate alcohol intake, but greater caution is warranted in those who drink more than the recommended daily limits.

Some cases of acute kidney injury have been attributed to use of NSAIDs and acute excessive alcohol consumption.

Advanced Pharmacy Services

Patients taking NSAIDs may be eligible for the Medicines Use Review service provided by a community pharmacist. For further information, see *Advanced Pharmacy Services* in *Medicines optimisation* p. 18.

> **Other drugs used for Pain and inflammation in musculoskeletal disorders** Tramadol with dexketoprofen, p. 493

ANALGESICS ⟩ NON-STEROIDAL ANTI-INFLAMMATORY DRUGS

Aceclofenac
18-Nov-2020

- **INDICATIONS AND DOSE**

Pain and inflammation in rheumatoid arthritis, osteoarthritis and ankylosing spondylitis
▸ BY MOUTH
  ▸ Adult: 100 mg twice daily

- **CONTRA-INDICATIONS** Active bleeding · active gastro-intestinal bleeding · active gastro-intestinal ulceration · bleeding disorders · cerebrovascular disease · history of gastro-intestinal bleeding related to previous NSAID therapy · history of gastro-intestinal perforation related to previous NSAID therapy · history of recurrent gastro-intestinal haemorrhage (two or more distinct episodes) · history of recurrent gastro-intestinal ulceration (two or more distinct episodes) · ischaemic heart disease · mild to severe heart failure · peripheral arterial disease · varicella infection

- **CAUTIONS** Allergic disorders · avoid in Acute porphyrias p. 1107 · cardiac impairment (NSAIDs may impair renal function) · connective-tissue disorders · dehydration (risk of renal impairment) · elderly (risk of serious side-effects and fatalities) · history of cardiac failure · history of cerebrovascular bleeding · history of gastro-intestinal disorders (e.g. ulcerative colitis, Crohn's disease) · hypertension · may mask symptoms of infection · oedema · risk factors for cardiovascular events

- **INTERACTIONS** → Appendix 1: NSAIDs

- **SIDE-EFFECTS**
▸ **Common or very common** Diarrhoea · dizziness · gastrointestinal discomfort · nausea
▸ **Uncommon** Constipation · gastrointestinal disorders · oral disorders · skin reactions · vomiting
▸ **Rare or very rare** Anaemia · angioedema · bone marrow disorders · depression · drowsiness · dyspnoea · fatigue · haemolytic anaemia · haemorrhage · headache · heart failure · hepatic disorders · hyperkalaemia · hypersensitivity · hypertension · inflammatory bowel disease · leg cramps · nephrotic syndrome · neutropenia · oedema · palpitations · pancreatitis · paraesthesia · renal failure (more common in patients with pre-existing renal impairment) · respiratory disorders · severe cutaneous

adverse reactions (SCARs) · sleep disorders · taste altered · thrombocytopenia · tinnitus · tremor · vasculitis · vasodilation · vertigo · visual impairment · weight increased
▶ **Frequency not known** Acute coronary syndrome · agranulocytosis · asthma · confusion · hallucination · increased risk of arterial thromboembolism · increased risk of ischaemic stroke · malaise · meningitis aseptic (patients with connective-tissue disorders such as systemic lupus erythematosus may be especially susceptible) · nephritis tubulointerstitial · optic neuritis · photosensitivity reaction · platelet aggregation inhibition · respiratory tract reaction

SIDE-EFFECTS, FURTHER INFORMATION For information about cardiovascular and gastrointestinal side-effects, and a possible exacerbation of symptoms in asthma, see Non-steroidal anti-inflammatory drugs. p. 1176

● ALLERGY AND CROSS-SENSITIVITY EvGr Contra-indicated in patients with a history of hypersensitivity to aspirin or any other NSAID—which includes those in whom attacks of asthma, angioedema, urticaria or rhinitis have been precipitated by aspirin or any other NSAID. ⓜ

● CONCEPTION AND CONTRACEPTION Caution—long-term use of some NSAIDs is associated with reduced female fertility, which is reversible on stopping treatment.

● PREGNANCY Most manufacturers advise avoiding the use of NSAIDs during pregnancy or avoiding them unless the potential benefit outweighs the risk. NSAIDs should be avoided during the third trimester because use is associated with a risk of closure of fetal ductus arteriosus *in utero* and possibly persistent pulmonary hypertension of the newborn. In addition, the onset of labour may be delayed and its duration may be increased.

● BREAST FEEDING Use with caution during breast-feeding. Manufacturer advises avoid.

● HEPATIC IMPAIRMENT Manufacturer advises caution in mild to moderate impairment; avoid in hepatic failure.
Dose adjustments Manufacturer advises consider initial dose reduction to 100 mg daily in mild to moderate impairment.

● RENAL IMPAIRMENT Avoid if possible or use with caution; avoid in moderate to severe impairment.
Dose adjustments The lowest effective dose should be used for the shortest possible duration.
Monitoring In renal impairment monitor renal function; sodium and water retention may occur and renal function may deteriorate, possibly leading to renal failure.

● MEDICINAL FORMS There can be variation in the licensing of different medicines containing the same drug.

Tablet
CAUTIONARY AND ADVISORY LABELS 21
▶ Aceclofenac (Non-proprietary)
Aceclofenac 100 mg Aceclofenac 100mg tablets | 60 tablet PoM
£8.00 DT = £7.18
▶ Preservex (Almirall Ltd)
Aceclofenac 100 mg Preservex 100mg tablets | 60 tablet PoM
£9.63 DT = £7.18

Celecoxib

18-Nov-2020

● INDICATIONS AND DOSE

Pain and inflammation in osteoarthritis
▶ BY MOUTH
▶ Adult: 200 mg daily in 1–2 divided doses, then increased if necessary to 200 mg twice daily, discontinue if no improvement after 2 weeks on maximum dose

Pain and inflammation in rheumatoid arthritis
▶ BY MOUTH
▶ Adult: 100 mg twice daily, then increased if necessary to 200 mg twice daily, discontinue if no improvement after 2 weeks on maximum dose

Ankylosing spondylitis
▶ BY MOUTH
▶ Adult: 200 mg daily in 1–2 divided doses, then increased if necessary to 400 mg daily in 1–2 divided doses, discontinue if no improvement after 2 weeks on maximum dose

DOSE ADJUSTMENTS DUE TO INTERACTIONS
▶ Manufacturer advises reduce dose by half with concurrent use of fluconazole.

● CONTRA-INDICATIONS Active gastro-intestinal bleeding · active gastro-intestinal ulceration · cerebrovascular disease · inflammatory bowel disease · ischaemic heart disease · mild to severe heart failure · peripheral arterial disease

● CAUTIONS Allergic disorders · cardiac impairment (NSAIDs may impair renal function) · coagulation defects · connective-tissue disorders · dehydration (risk of renal impairment) · elderly (risk of serious side-effects and fatalities) · history of cardiac failure · history of gastro-intestinal disorders · hypertension · left ventricular dysfunction · may mask symptoms of infection · oedema · risk factors for cardiovascular events

● INTERACTIONS → Appendix 1: NSAIDs

● SIDE-EFFECTS
▶ **Common or very common** Angina pectoris · benign prostatic hyperplasia · cough · diarrhoea · dizziness · dysphagia · dyspnoea · fluid retention · gastrointestinal discomfort · gastrointestinal disorders · headache · hypersensitivity · hypertension · increased risk of infection · influenza like illness · injury · insomnia · irritable bowel syndrome · joint disorders · muscle tone increased · myocardial infarction · nausea · nephrolithiasis · oedema · skin reactions · vomiting · weight increased
▶ **Uncommon** Anaemia · anxiety · arrhythmias · breast tenderness · burping · cerebral infarction · chest pain · conjunctivitis · constipation · depression · drowsiness · dysphonia · electrolyte imbalance · embolism and thrombosis · fatigue · haemorrhage · hearing impairment · heart failure · hepatic disorders · lipoma · lower limb fracture · muscle complaints · nocturia · oral disorders · palpitations · paraesthesia · respiratory disorders · tinnitus · vision blurred · vitreous floater
▶ **Rare or very rare** Acute kidney injury (more common in patients with pre-existing renal impairment) · alopecia · angioedema · anosmia · ataxia · confusion · flushing · hallucination · intracranial haemorrhage · leucopenia · meningitis aseptic · menstrual disorder · myositis · nephritis tubulointerstitial · nephropathy · pancreatitis · pancytopenia · photosensitivity reaction · seizures · severe cutaneous adverse events (SCARs) · taste altered · thrombocytopenia · vasculitis
▶ **Frequency not known** Infertility

SIDE-EFFECTS, FURTHER INFORMATION For information about cardiovascular and gastrointestinal side-effects, and a possible exacerbation of symptoms in asthma, see Non-steroidal anti-inflammatory drugs. p. 1176

● ALLERGY AND CROSS-SENSITIVITY EvGr Contra-indicated in patients with a history of hypersensitivity to aspirin or any other NSAID—which includes those in whom attacks of asthma, angioedema, urticaria or rhinitis have been precipitated by aspirin or any other NSAID.
Contra-indicated in patients with sulfonamide sensitivity. ⓜ

● CONCEPTION AND CONTRACEPTION Caution—long-term use of some NSAIDs is associated with reduced female fertility, which is reversible on stopping treatment.

● PREGNANCY Avoid (teratogenic in *animal* studies).

● BREAST FEEDING Avoid—present in milk in *animal* studies.

● HEPATIC IMPAIRMENT Manufacturer advises caution in mild to moderate impairment; avoid in severe impairment (no information available).
Dose adjustments Manufacturer advises initial dose reduction of 50% in moderate impairment.

● RENAL IMPAIRMENT Avoid if possible or use with caution. Avoid if eGFR less than 30 mL/minute/1.73 m^2.
Dose adjustments The lowest effective dose should be used for the shortest possible duration.
Monitoring In renal impairment monitor renal function; sodium and water retention may occur and renal function may deteriorate, possibly leading to renal failure.

● MONITORING REQUIREMENTS Monitor blood pressure before and during treatment.

● MEDICINAL FORMS There can be variation in the licensing of different medicines containing the same drug.

Capsule
▸ Celecoxib (Non-proprietary)
  Celecoxib 100 mg Celecoxib 100mg capsules | 60 capsule PoM
  £21.55 DT = £1.99
  Celecoxib 200 mg Celecoxib 200mg capsules | 30 capsule PoM
  £21.55 DT = £2.30
▸ Celebrex (Upjohn UK Ltd)
  Celecoxib 100 mg Celebrex 100mg capsules | 60 capsule PoM
  £21.55 DT = £1.99
  Celecoxib 200 mg Celebrex 200mg capsules | 30 capsule PoM
  £21.55 DT = £2.30

Dexibuprofen

18-Nov-2020

● **INDICATIONS AND DOSE**

Osteoarthritis
▸ BY MOUTH
▸ Adult: 600–900 mg daily in up to 3 divided doses; increased if necessary up to 1200 mg daily (max. per dose 400 mg)

Dysmenorrhoea
▸ BY MOUTH
▸ Adult: 600–900 mg daily in up to 3 divided doses (max. per dose 400 mg)

Mild-to-moderate pain
▸ BY MOUTH
▸ Adult: 600 mg daily in up to 3 divided doses; increased if necessary up to 1200 mg daily (max. per dose 400 mg), higher dose for short-term use for acute pain

● CONTRA-INDICATIONS Active gastro-intestinal bleeding · active gastro-intestinal ulceration · cerebrovascular bleeding · history of gastro-intestinal bleeding related to previous NSAID therapy · history of gastro-intestinal perforation related to previous NSAID therapy · history of recurrent gastro-intestinal haemorrhage (two or more distinct episodes) · history of recurrent gastro-intestinal ulceration (two or more distinct episodes) · severe heart failure

● CAUTIONS Allergic disorders · cardiac impairment (NSAIDs may impair renal function) · cerebrovascular disease · coagulation defects · congestive heart failure · connective-tissue disorders · Crohn's disease (may be exacerbated) · elderly (risk of serious side-effects and fatalities) · ischaemic heart disease · peripheral arterial disease · risk factors for cardiovascular events · ulcerative colitis (may be exacerbated) · uncontrolled hypertension

CAUTIONS, FURTHER INFORMATION
▸ High-dose dexibuprofen A small increase in cardiovascular risk, similar to the risk associated with cyclo-oxygenase-2 inhibitors and diclofenac, has been reported with high-dose dexibuprofen ($\geq$ 1.2 g daily); use should be avoided in patients with established ischaemic heart disease, peripheral arterial disease, cerebrovascular disease, congestive heart failure (New York Heart Association classification II-III), and uncontrolled hypertension.

● INTERACTIONS → Appendix 1: NSAIDs

● SIDE-EFFECTS
▸ **Common or very common** Diarrhoea · dizziness · drowsiness · fatigue · gastrointestinal discomfort · headache · nausea · skin reactions · vertigo · vomiting
▸ **Uncommon** Angioedema · anxiety · gastrointestinal disorders · haemorrhage · increased risk of infection · insomnia · oral disorders · respiratory disorders · tinnitus · vasculitis · vision disorders
▸ **Rare or very rare** Agranulocytosis · alopecia · asthma · blood disorder · bone marrow disorders · confusion · constipation · depression · fever · granulocytopenia · haemolytic anaemia · hearing impairment · hepatic disorders · hypersensitivity · hypotension · inflammatory bowel disease · irritability · leucopenia · meningitis aseptic (patients with connective-tissue disorders such as systemic lupus erythematosus may be especially susceptible) · nephritis tubulointerstitial · nephrotic syndrome · photosensitivity reaction · psychotic disorder · renal failure (more common in patients with pre-existing renal impairment) · severe cutaneous adverse reactions (SCARs) · shock · tachycardia · thrombocytopenia
▸ **Frequency not known** Fluid retention · generalised oedema · glomerulonephritis · increased risk of arterial thromboembolism · renal impairment · renal papillary necrosis

SIDE-EFFECTS, FURTHER INFORMATION For information about cardiovascular and gastrointestinal side-effects, and a possible exacerbation of symptoms in asthma, see Non-steroidal anti-inflammatory drugs. p. 1176

● ALLERGY AND CROSS-SENSITIVITY EvGr Contra-indicated in patients with a history of hypersensitivity to aspirin or any other NSAID—which includes those in whom attacks of asthma, angioedema, urticaria or rhinitis have been precipitated by aspirin or any other NSAID. ◈

● CONCEPTION AND CONTRACEPTION Caution—long-term use of some NSAIDs is associated with reduced female fertility, which is reversible on stopping treatment.

● PREGNANCY Avoid unless the potential benefit outweighs the risk. Avoid during the third trimester (risk of closure of fetal ductus arteriosus *in utero* and possibly persistent pulmonary hypertension of the newborn); onset of labour may be delayed and duration may be increased.

● BREAST FEEDING Use with caution during breast-feeding. Present in milk—but risk to infant minimal.

● HEPATIC IMPAIRMENT Manufacturer advises caution in mild to moderate impairment; avoid in severe impairment.
Dose adjustments Manufacturer advises initial dose reduction in mild to moderate impairment.

● RENAL IMPAIRMENT Avoid if possible or use with caution. Avoid if eGFR less than 30 mL/minute/1.73 m^2.
Dose adjustments Reduce initial dose.
  The lowest effective dose should be used for the shortest possible duration.
Monitoring Monitor renal function; sodium and water retention may occur and renal function may deteriorate, possibly leading to renal failure.

● MEDICINAL FORMS No licensed medicines listed.

Dexketoprofen

18-Nov-2020

● **INDICATIONS AND DOSE**

Short-term treatment of mild to moderate pain including dysmenorrhoea

▶ BY MOUTH
▶ Adult: 12.5 mg every 4–6 hours, alternatively 25 mg every 8 hours; maximum 75 mg per day
▶ Elderly: 12.5 mg every 4–6 hours, alternatively 25 mg every 8 hours, initial max. 50 mg; maximum 75 mg daily

● **CONTRA-INDICATIONS** Active bleeding or bleeding disorders · active or recurrent gastro-intestinal haemorrhage · active or recurrent gastro-intestinal ulcer · chronic dyspepsia · Crohn's disease · history of NSAID-associated gastro-intestinal bleeding or perforation · known photoallergic or phototoxic reactions during treatment with ketoprofen or fibrates · severe dehydration · severe heart failure · ulcerative colitis · varicella infection

● **CAUTIONS** Allergic disorders · asthma · cerebrovascular disease · coagulation defects · congenital disorder of porphyrin metabolism · congestive heart failure · dehydration · elderly (risk of serious side-effects and fatalities) · following major surgery · haematopoietic disorders · history of cardiac disease (NSAIDs may cause fluid retention and oedema) · history of gastro-intestinal disease · history of gastro-intestinal toxicity · ischaemic heart disease · may mask symptoms of infection · mixed connective-tissue disorders · peripheral arterial disease · risk factors for cardiovascular events · systemic lupus erythematosus · uncontrolled hypertension

● **INTERACTIONS** → Appendix 1: NSAIDs

● **SIDE-EFFECTS**

▶ **Common or very common** Diarrhoea · gastrointestinal discomfort · nausea · vomiting
▶ **Uncommon** Anxiety · asthenia · chills · constipation · dizziness · drowsiness · dry mouth · flushing · gastrointestinal disorders · headache · insomnia · malaise · pain · palpitations · skin reactions · vertigo
▶ **Rare or very rare** Angioedema · appetite decreased · dyspnoea · haemorrhage · hepatic disorders · hyperhidrosis · hypersensitivity · hypertension · hypotension · menstrual disorder · nephritis · nephrotic syndrome · neutropenia · oedema · pancreatitis · paraesthesia · photosensitivity reaction · polyuria · prostatic disorder · respiratory disorders · severe cutaneous adverse reactions (SCARs) · syncope · tachycardia · thrombocytopenia · tinnitus · vision blurred
▶ **Frequency not known** Acute kidney injury (more common in patients with pre-existing renal impairment) · agranulocytosis · anaemia · aplastic anaemia · haemolytic anaemia · inflammatory bowel disease · meningitis aseptic · oral ulceration · platelet aggregation inhibition · renal papillary necrosis

SIDE-EFFECTS, FURTHER INFORMATION For information about cardiovascular and gastrointestinal side-effects, and a possible exacerbation of symptoms in asthma, see Non-steroidal anti-inflammatory drugs. p. 1176

● **ALLERGY AND CROSS-SENSITIVITY** EvGr Contra-indicated in patients with a history of hypersensitivity to aspirin or any other NSAID—which includes those in whom attacks of asthma, angioedema, urticaria or rhinitis have been precipitated by aspirin or any other NSAID. ⓜ

● **CONCEPTION AND CONTRACEPTION** Caution—long-term use of some NSAIDs is associated with reduced female fertility, which is reversible on stopping treatment.

● **PREGNANCY** Avoid unless the potential benefit outweighs the risk. Avoid during the third trimester (risk of closure of fetal ductus arteriosus *in utero* and possibly persistent pulmonary hypertension of the newborn); onset of labour may be delayed and duration may be increased.

● **BREAST FEEDING** Use with caution during breast-feeding. Manufacturer advises avoid—no information available.

● **HEPATIC IMPAIRMENT** Manufacturer advises caution in mild to moderate impairment; avoid in severe impairment. **Dose adjustments** Manufacturer advises initial dose reduction to max. 50 mg daily in mild to moderate impairment.

● **RENAL IMPAIRMENT** Avoid if possible or use with caution. Avoid in moderate to severe impairment. **Dose adjustments** Reduce initial dose to 50 mg daily. The lowest effective dose should be used for the shortest possible duration. **Monitoring** In renal impairment monitor renal function; sodium and water retention may occur and renal function may deteriorate, possibly leading to renal failure.

● **MEDICINAL FORMS** There can be variation in the licensing of different medicines containing the same drug.

Tablet
CAUTIONARY AND ADVISORY LABELS 22
▶ Keral (A. Menarini Farmaceutica Internazionale SRL)
Dexketoprofen (as Dexketoprofen trometamol) 25 mg Keral 25mg tablets | 20 tablet [PoM] £3.67 | 50 tablet [PoM] £9.18 DT = £9.18

Combinations available: *Tramadol with dexketoprofen*, p. 493

Diclofenac potassium

18-Nov-2020

● **INDICATIONS AND DOSE**

Pain and inflammation in rheumatic disease and other musculoskeletal disorders

▶ BY MOUTH
▶ Child 14–17 years: 75–100 mg daily in 2–3 divided doses
▶ Adult: 75–150 mg daily in 2–3 divided doses

Acute gout

▶ BY MOUTH
▶ Adult: 75–150 mg daily in 2–3 divided doses

Postoperative pain

▶ BY MOUTH
▶ Child 9–13 years (body-weight 35 kg and above): Up to 2 mg/kg daily in 3 divided doses; maximum 100 mg per day
▶ Child 14–17 years: 75–100 mg daily in 2–3 divided doses
▶ Adult: 75–150 mg daily in 2–3 divided doses

Migraine

▶ BY MOUTH
▶ Adult: 50 mg, to be given at onset of migraine, then 50 mg after 2 hours if required, then 50 mg after 4–6 hours; maximum 200 mg per day

Fever in ear, nose, or throat infection

▶ BY MOUTH
▶ Child 9–17 years (body-weight 35 kg and above): Up to 2 mg/kg daily in 3 divided doses; maximum 100 mg per day

● **UNLICENSED USE** *Voltarol® Rapid* not licensed for use in children under 14 years or in fever.

● **CONTRA-INDICATIONS** Active gastro-intestinal bleeding · active gastro-intestinal ulceration · cerebrovascular disease · history of gastro-intestinal bleeding related to previous NSAID therapy · history of gastro-intestinal perforation related to previous NSAID therapy · history of recurrent gastro-intestinal haemorrhage (two or more distinct episodes) · history of recurrent gastro-intestinal ulceration (two or more distinct episodes) · ischaemic heart disease · mild to severe heart failure · peripheral arterial disease

● **CAUTIONS** Allergic disorders · cardiac impairment (NSAIDs may impair renal function) · coagulation defects ·

connective-tissue disorders · dehydration (risk of renal impairment) · elderly (risk of serious side-effects and fatalities) · history of cardiac failure · history of gastro-intestinal disorders (e.g. ulcerative colitis, Crohn's disease) · hypertension · may mask symptoms of infection · oedema · risk factors for cardiovascular events

● INTERACTIONS → Appendix 1: NSAIDs

● SIDE-EFFECTS
▸ **Common or very common** Appetite decreased · diarrhoea · dizziness · gastrointestinal discomfort · gastrointestinal disorders · headache · nausea · skin reactions · vertigo · vomiting
▸ **Uncommon** Chest pain · heart failure · myocardial infarction · palpitations
▸ **Rare or very rare** Acute kidney injury · agranulocytosis · alopecia · anaemia · angioedema · anxiety · aplastic anaemia · asthma · confusion · constipation · depression · drowsiness · dyspnoea · erectile dysfunction · fatigue · haemolytic anaemia · haemorrhage · hearing impairment · hepatic disorders · hypersensitivity · hypertension · hypotension · inflammatory bowel disease · irritability · leucopenia · memory loss · meningitis aseptic (patients with connective-tissue disorders such as systemic lupus erythematosus may be especially susceptible) · nephritis tubulointerstitial · nephrotic syndrome · oedema · oesophageal disorder · oral disorders · pancreatitis · photosensitivity reaction · pneumonitis · proteinuria · psychotic disorder · renal papillary necrosis · seizure · sensation abnormal · severe cutaneous adverse reactions (SCARs) · shock · sleep disorders · stroke · taste altered · thrombocytopenia · tinnitus · tremor · vasculitis · vision disorders
▸ **Frequency not known** Hallucination · malaise · optic neuritis

SIDE-EFFECTS, FURTHER INFORMATION For information about cardiovascular and gastrointestinal side-effects, and a possible exacerbation of symptoms in asthma, see Non-steroidal anti-inflammatory drugs.

● ALLERGY AND CROSS-SENSITIVITY EvGr Contra-indicated in patients with a history of hypersensitivity to aspirin or any other NSAID—which includes those in whom attacks of asthma, angioedema, urticaria or rhinitis have been precipitated by aspirin or any other NSAID.

● CONCEPTION AND CONTRACEPTION Caution—long-term use of some NSAIDs is associated with reduced female fertility, which is reversible on stopping treatment.

● PREGNANCY Avoid unless the potential benefit outweighs the risk. Avoid during the third trimester (risk of closure of fetal ductus arteriosus *in utero* and possibly persistent pulmonary hypertension of the newborn); onset of labour may be delayed and duration may be increased.

● BREAST FEEDING Use with caution during breast-feeding. Amount in milk too small to be harmful.

● HEPATIC IMPAIRMENT Manufacturer advises caution in mild to moderate impairment; avoid in severe impairment.

● RENAL IMPAIRMENT Avoid if possible or use with caution. Avoid in severe impairment.
Dose adjustments The lowest effective dose should be used for the shortest possible duration.
Monitoring In renal impairment monitor renal function; sodium and water retention may occur and renal function may deteriorate, possibly leading to renal failure.

● PATIENT AND CARER ADVICE
Medicines for Children leaflet: Diclofenac for pain and inflammation www.medicinesforchildren.org.uk/diclofenac-pain-and-inflammation

● MEDICINAL FORMS There can be variation in the licensing of different medicines containing the same drug.
Tablet
CAUTIONARY AND ADVISORY LABELS 21
▸ Diclofenac potassium (Non-proprietary)
Diclofenac potassium 25 mg Diclofenac potassium 25mg tablets | 28 tablet PoM £3.86 DT = £3.86
Diclofenac potassium 50 mg Diclofenac potassium 50mg tablets | 28 tablet PoM £7.41 DT = £7.41
▸ Voltarol Rapid (Novartis Pharmaceuticals UK Ltd)
Diclofenac potassium 50 mg Voltarol Rapid 50mg tablets | 30 tablet PoM £7.94

Diclofenac sodium
18-Nov-2020

● INDICATIONS AND DOSE

Pain and inflammation in musculoskeletal disorders | Acute gout
▸ BY MOUTH USING IMMEDIATE-RELEASE MEDICINES
▸ Adult: 75–150 mg daily in 2–3 divided doses
▸ BY RECTUM
▸ Adult: 75–150 mg daily in divided doses

Pain and inflammation in rheumatic disease including juvenile idiopathic arthritis
▸ BY MOUTH USING IMMEDIATE-RELEASE MEDICINES
▸ Adult: 75–150 mg daily in 2–3 divided doses
▸ BY RECTUM
▸ Adult: 75–150 mg daily in divided doses

Postoperative pain
▸ BY MOUTH USING IMMEDIATE-RELEASE MEDICINES
▸ Adult: 75–150 mg daily in 2–3 divided doses
▸ BY RECTUM
▸ Adult: 75–150 mg daily in divided doses

DICLOMAX RETARD ®
Pain and inflammation in rheumatic disease (including juvenile idiopathic arthritis) and other musculoskeletal disorders | Acute gout | Postoperative pain
▸ BY MOUTH
▸ Adult: 1 capsule once daily

DICLOMAX SR ®
Pain and inflammation in rheumatic disease (including juvenile idiopathic arthritis) and other musculoskeletal disorders | Acute gout | Postoperative pain
▸ BY MOUTH
▸ Adult: 1 capsule 1–2 times a day, alternatively 2 capsules once daily

MOTIFENE ®
Pain and inflammation in rheumatic disease (including juvenile idiopathic arthritis) and other musculoskeletal disorders | Acute gout | Postoperative pain
▸ BY MOUTH
▸ Adult: 1 capsule 1–2 times a day

VOLTAROL ® 75MG SR TABLETS
Pain and inflammation in rheumatic disease (including juvenile idiopathic arthritis) and other musculoskeletal disorders | Acute gout | Postoperative pain
▸ BY MOUTH
▸ Adult: 1 tablet 1–2 times a day

VOLTAROL ® EMULGEL
Relief of pain in musculoskeletal conditions | Adjunctive treatment in knee or hand osteoarthritis
▸ TO THE SKIN
▸ Adult: Apply 3–4 times a day, therapy should be reviewed after 14 days (or after 28 days for osteoarthritis)

continued →

10

Musculoskeletal system

VOLTAROL® RETARD

Pain and inflammation in rheumatic disease (including juvenile idiopathic arthritis) and other musculoskeletal disorders | Acute gout | Postoperative pain
▸ BY MOUTH
▸ Adult: 1 tablet once daily

VOLTAROL® SOLUTION FOR INJECTION

Postoperative pain
▸ BY DEEP INTRAMUSCULAR INJECTION
▸ Adult: 75 mg 1–2 times a day for maximum 2 days, twice daily administration in severe cases, to be injected into the gluteal muscle

Acute exacerbations of pain
▸ BY DEEP INTRAMUSCULAR INJECTION
▸ Adult: 75 mg 1–2 times a day for maximum 2 days, twice daily administration in severe cases, to be injected into the gluteal muscle

Ureteric colic
▸ BY DEEP INTRAMUSCULAR INJECTION
▸ Adult: 75 mg, then 75 mg after 30 minutes if required

Acute postoperative pain (in hospital setting)
▸ BY INTRAVENOUS INFUSION
▸ Adult: 75 mg, then 75 mg after 4–6 hours if required for maximum 2 days; maximum 150 mg per day

Prevention of postoperative pain (in hospital setting)
▸ BY INTRAVENOUS INFUSION
▸ Adult: Initially 25–50 mg, to be given after surgery over 15–60 minutes, then 5 mg/hour for maximum 2 days; maximum 150 mg per day

● CONTRA-INDICATIONS
▸ With intravenous use Dehydration · history of asthma · history of confirmed or suspected cerebrovascular bleeding · history of haemorrhagic diathesis · hypovolaemia · operations with high risk of haemorrhage
▸ With systemic use Active gastro-intestinal bleeding · active gastro-intestinal ulceration · avoid suppositories in proctitis · cerebrovascular disease · history of gastro-intestinal bleeding related to previous NSAID therapy · history of gastro-intestinal perforation related to previous NSAID therapy · history of recurrent gastro-intestinal haemorrhage (two or more distinct episodes) · history of recurrent gastro-intestinal ulceration (two or more distinct episodes) · ischaemic heart disease · mild to severe heart failure · peripheral arterial disease

● CAUTIONS
▸ With systemic use Allergic disorders · cardiac impairment (NSAIDs may impair renal function) · coagulation defects · connective-tissue disorders · dehydration (risk of renal impairment) · elderly (risk of serious side-effects and fatalities) · history of cardiac failure · history of gastro-intestinal disorders (e.g. ulcerative colitis, Crohn's disease) · hypertension · may mask symptoms of infection · oedema · risk factors for cardiovascular events

● INTERACTIONS → Appendix 1: NSAIDs

● SIDE-EFFECTS
▸ **Common or very common**
▸ With systemic use Appetite decreased · diarrhoea · dizziness · gastrointestinal discomfort · gastrointestinal disorders · headache · nausea · rash (discontinue) · vertigo · vomiting
▸ With topical use Conjunctivitis · muscle tone increased · rash (discontinue) · sensation abnormal · skin ulcer
▸ **Uncommon**
▸ With systemic use Chest pain · heart failure · myocardial infarction · palpitations
▸ With topical use Abdominal pain · alopecia · diarrhoea · eye pain · haemorrhage · lacrimation disorder · nausea · seborrhoea
▸ **Rare or very rare**
▸ With rectal use Ulcerative colitis aggravated

▸ With systemic use Acute kidney injury · agranulocytosis · alopecia · anaemia · angioedema · anxiety · aplastic anaemia · asthma · confusion · constipation · depression · drowsiness · dyspnoea · erectile dysfunction · fatigue · haemolytic anaemia · haemorrhage · hearing impairment · hepatic disorders · hypersensitivity · hypertension · hypotension · irritability · leucopenia · memory loss · meningitis aseptic (patients with connective-tissue disorders such as systemic lupus erythematosus may be especially susceptible) · nephritis tubulointerstitial · nephrotic syndrome · oesophageal disorder · oral disorders · pancreatitis · photosensitivity reaction · pneumonitis · proteinuria · psychotic disorder · renal papillary necrosis · seizure · sensation abnormal · severe cutaneous adverse reactions (SCARs) · shock · sleep disorders · stroke · taste altered · thrombocytopenia · tinnitus · tremor · vasculitis · vision disorders
▸ With topical use Acute kidney injury · angioedema · asthma · photosensitivity reaction · rash pustular
▸ **Frequency not known**
▸ With parenteral use Injection site necrosis
▸ With systemic use Fertility decreased female · fluid retention · hallucination · malaise · optic neuritis · platelet aggregation inhibition
▸ With topical use Hair colour changes
SIDE-EFFECTS, FURTHER INFORMATION Topical application of large amounts of diclofenac can result in systemic effects.
   For information about cardiovascular and gastrointestinal side-effects, and a possible exacerbation of symptoms in asthma, see Non-steroidal anti-inflammatory drugs p. 1176

● ALLERGY AND CROSS-SENSITIVITY EvGr Contra-indicated in patients with a history of hypersensitivity to aspirin or any other NSAID—which includes those in whom attacks of asthma, angioedema, urticaria or rhinitis have been precipitated by aspirin or any other NSAID. Ⓜ

● CONCEPTION AND CONTRACEPTION
▸ With systemic use Caution—long-term use of some NSAIDs is associated with reduced female fertility, which is reversible on stopping treatment.

● PREGNANCY
▸ With systemic use Avoid unless the potential benefit outweighs the risk. Avoid during the third trimester (risk of closure of fetal ductus arteriosus *in utero* and possibly persistent pulmonary hypertension of the newborn); onset of labour may be delayed and duration may be increased.

● BREAST FEEDING
▸ With systemic use Use with caution during breast-feeding. Amount in milk too small to be harmful.

● HEPATIC IMPAIRMENT
▸ With systemic use Manufacturer advises caution in mild to moderate impairment; avoid in severe impairment.

● RENAL IMPAIRMENT
▸ With systemic use Avoid if possible or use with caution. Avoid in severe impairment.
▸ With intravenous use Avoid intravenous use if serum creatinine greater than 160 micromol/litre. Contra-indicated in moderate or severe renal impairment.
Dose adjustments ▸ With systemic use The lowest effective dose should be used for the shortest possible duration.
Monitoring ▸ With systemic use In renal impairment monitor renal function; sodium and water retention may occur and renal function may deteriorate, possibly leading to renal failure.

● DIRECTIONS FOR ADMINISTRATION
▸ With intravenous use For *intravenous infusion* (*Voltarol*®), give continuously or intermittently in Glucose 5% or Sodium chloride 0.9%. Dilute 75 mg with 100–500 mL infusion fluid (previously buffered with 0.5 mL sodium bicarbonate 8.4% solution *or* with

1 mL sodium bicarbonate 4.2% solution). For intermittent infusion give 25–50 mg over 15–60 minutes or 75 mg over 30–120 minutes. For continuous infusion give at a rate of 5 mg/hour.

- PRESCRIBING AND DISPENSING INFORMATION *Voltarol*® dispersible tablets are more suitable for **short-term** use in acute conditions for which treatment required for no more than 3 months (no information on use beyond 3 months).
- PROFESSION SPECIFIC INFORMATION

Dental practitioners' formulary Diclofenac Sodium Tablets may be prescribed.

- MEDICINAL FORMS There can be variation in the licensing of different medicines containing the same drug. Forms available from special-order manufacturers include: dispersible tablet, oral suspension, oral solution

Modified-release tablet
CAUTIONARY AND ADVISORY LABELS 21, 25
- ▸ Dicloflex 75mg SR (Dexcel-Pharma Ltd)
  Diclofenac sodium 75 mg Dicloflex 75mg SR tablets |
  28 tablet [PoM] £9.00 | 56 tablet [PoM] £17.56 DT = £17.56
- ▸ Dicloflex Retard (Dexcel-Pharma Ltd)
  Diclofenac sodium 100 mg Dicloflex Retard 100mg tablets |
  28 tablet [PoM] £11.33 DT = £11.33
- ▸ Diclo-SR (Strides Pharma UK Ltd)
  Diclofenac sodium 75 mg Diclo-SR 75mg tablets | 28 tablet [PoM]
  £6.50 | 56 tablet [PoM] £14.50 DT = £17.56
- ▸ Enstar XL (Ennogen Pharma Ltd)
  Diclofenac sodium 100 mg Enstar XL 100 tablets | 28 tablet [PoM]
  £7.58 DT = £11.33

Gastro-resistant tablet
CAUTIONARY AND ADVISORY LABELS 5, 25
- ▸ Diclofenac sodium (Non-proprietary)
  Diclofenac sodium 25 mg Diclofenac sodium 25mg gastro-resistant
  tablets | 28 tablet [PoM] £8.99 DT = £1.69 | 84 tablet [PoM] £1.50–
  £26.97
  Diclofenac sodium 50 mg Diclofenac sodium 50mg gastro-resistant
  tablets | 28 tablet [PoM] £4.97 DT = £1.37 | 84 tablet [PoM] £4.11–
  £15.00

Suppository
- ▸ Econac (Advanz Pharma)
  Diclofenac sodium 100 mg Econac 100mg suppositories |
  10 suppository [PoM] £3.04 DT = £3.64
- ▸ Voltarol (Novartis Pharmaceuticals UK Ltd)
  Diclofenac sodium 12.5 mg Voltarol 12.5mg suppositories |
  10 suppository [PoM] £0.70 DT = £0.70
  Diclofenac sodium 25 mg Voltarol 25mg suppositories |
  10 suppository [PoM] £1.24 DT = £1.24
  Diclofenac sodium 50 mg Voltarol 50mg suppositories |
  10 suppository [PoM] £2.04 DT = £2.04
  Diclofenac sodium 100 mg Voltarol 100mg suppositories |
  10 suppository [PoM] £3.64 DT = £3.64

Solution for injection
EXCIPIENTS: May contain Benzyl alcohol, propylene glycol
- ▸ Akis (Flynn Pharma Ltd)
  Diclofenac sodium 75 mg per 1 ml Akis 75mg/1ml solution for
  injection ampoules | 5 ampoule [PoM] £24.00 DT = £24.00
- ▸ Voltarol (Novartis Pharmaceuticals UK Ltd)
  Diclofenac sodium 25 mg per 1 ml Voltarol 75mg/3ml solution for
  injection ampoules | 10 ampoule [PoM] £9.91 DT = £9.91

Modified-release capsule
CAUTIONARY AND ADVISORY LABELS 21 (does not apply to Motifene
® 75 mg), 25
EXCIPIENTS: May contain Propylene glycol
- ▸ Diclomax Retard (Galen Ltd)
  Diclofenac sodium 100 mg Diclomax Retard 100mg capsules |
  28 capsule [PoM] £8.20 DT = £8.20
- ▸ Diclomax SR (Galen Ltd)
  Diclofenac sodium 75 mg Diclomax SR 75mg capsules |
  56 capsule [PoM] £11.40 DT = £11.40
- ▸ Motifene (Daiichi Sankyo UK Ltd)
  Diclofenac sodium 75 mg Motifene 75mg modified-release capsules
  | 56 capsule [PoM] £8.00 DT = £8.00

Diclofenac sodium with misoprostol
05-Aug-2020

The properties listed below are those particular to the combination only. For the properties of the components please consider, diclofenac sodium p. 1181, misoprostol p. 82.

- INDICATIONS AND DOSE

ARTHROTEC ® 50/200

Prophylaxis against NSAID-induced gastroduodenal ulceration in patients requiring diclofenac for rheumatoid arthritis or osteoarthritis
- ▸ BY MOUTH
- ▸ **Adult:** 1 tablet 2–3 times a day, take with food

ARTHROTEC ® 75/200

Prophylaxis against NSAID-induced gastroduodenal ulceration in patients requiring diclofenac for rheumatoid arthritis or osteoarthritis
- ▸ BY MOUTH
- ▸ **Adult:** 1 tablet twice daily, take with food

MISOFEN ® 50/200

Prophylaxis against NSAID-induced gastroduodenal ulceration in patients requiring diclofenac for rheumatoid arthritis or osteoarthritis
- ▸ BY MOUTH
- ▸ **Adult:** 1 tablet 2–3 times a day, take with food

MISOFEN ® 75/200

Prophylaxis against NSAID-induced gastroduodenal ulceration in patients requiring diclofenac for rheumatoid arthritis or osteoarthritis
- ▸ BY MOUTH
- ▸ **Adult:** 1 tablet twice daily, take with food

- INTERACTIONS → Appendix 1: NSAIDs

- MEDICINAL FORMS There can be variation in the licensing of different medicines containing the same drug.

Gastro-resistant tablet
CAUTIONARY AND ADVISORY LABELS 21, 25
- ▸ Arthrotec (Pfizer Ltd)
  Misoprostol 200 microgram, Diclofenac sodium 50 mg Arthrotec
  50 gastro-resistant tablets | 60 tablet [PoM] £11.98 DT = £11.98
  Misoprostol 200 microgram, Diclofenac sodium 75 mg Arthrotec
  75 gastro-resistant tablets | 60 tablet [PoM] £15.83 DT = £15.83
- ▸ Misofen (Morningside Healthcare Ltd)
  Misoprostol 200 microgram, Diclofenac sodium 50 mg Misofen
  50mg/200microgram gastro-resistant tablets | 60 tablet [PoM] £11.98
  DT = £11.98
  Misoprostol 200 microgram, Diclofenac sodium 75 mg Misofen
  75mg/200microgram gastro-resistant tablets | 60 tablet [PoM] £15.83
  DT = £15.83

Etodolac
18-Nov-2020

- INDICATIONS AND DOSE

Pain and inflammation in rheumatoid arthritis and osteoarthritis
- ▸ BY MOUTH USING MODIFIED-RELEASE MEDICINES
- ▸ **Adult:** 600 mg once daily

- CONTRA-INDICATIONS Active gastro-intestinal bleeding · active gastro-intestinal ulceration · history of gastro-intestinal bleeding related to previous NSAID therapy · history of gastro-intestinal perforation related to previous NSAID therapy · history of recurrent gastro-intestinal haemorrhage (two or more distinct episodes) · history of recurrent gastro-intestinal ulceration (two or more distinct episodes) · severe heart failure
- CAUTIONS Allergic disorders · cardiac impairment (NSAIDs may impair renal function) · cerebrovascular disease ·

10

Musculoskeletal system

coagulation defects · connective-tissue disorders · dehydration (risk of renal impairment) · elderly (risk of serious side-effects and fatalities) · heart failure · history of gastro-intestinal disorders (e.g. ulcerative colitis, Crohn's disease) · ischaemic heart disease · may mask symptoms of infection · peripheral arterial disease · risk factors for cardiovascular events · uncontrolled hypertension

● INTERACTIONS → Appendix 1: NSAIDs

● SIDE-EFFECTS Agranulocytosis · angioedema · aplastic anaemia · asthenia · asthma · bilirubinuria · bronchospasm · chills · confusion · constipation · Crohn's disease aggravated · depression · diarrhoea · dizziness · drowsiness · dyspnoea · fever · gastrointestinal discomfort · gastrointestinal disorders · haemolytic anaemia · haemorrhage · hallucination · headache · heart failure · hepatic disorders · hypersensitivity · hypertension · insomnia · malaise · meningitis aseptic (patients with connective-tissue disorders such as systemic lupus erythematosus may be especially susceptible) · nausea · nephritic syndrome · nephritis tubulointerstitial · nephrotoxicity · nervousness · neutropenia · oedema · optic neuritis · oral ulceration · palpitations · pancreatitis · paraesthesia · photosensitivity reaction · renal failure (more common in patients with pre-existing renal impairment) · severe cutaneous adverse reactions (SCARs) · skin reactions · thrombocytopenia · tinnitus · tremor · urinary disorders · vasculitis · vertigo · visual impairment · vomiting

SIDE-EFFECTS, FURTHER INFORMATION For information about cardiovascular and gastrointestinal side-effects, and a possible exacerbation of symptoms in asthma, see Non-steroidal anti-inflammatory drugs. p. 1176

● ALLERGY AND CROSS-SENSITIVITY [EvGr] Contra-indicated in patients with a history of hypersensitivity to aspirin or any other NSAID—which includes those in whom attacks of asthma, angioedema, urticaria or rhinitis have been precipitated by aspirin or any other NSAID. ◈

● CONCEPTION AND CONTRACEPTION Caution—long-term use of some NSAIDs is associated with reduced female fertility, which is reversible on stopping treatment.

● PREGNANCY Avoid unless the potential benefit outweighs the risk. Avoid during the third trimester (risk of closure of fetal ductus arteriosus *in utero* and possibly persistent pulmonary hypertension of the newborn); onset of labour may be delayed and duration may be increased.

● BREAST FEEDING Use with caution during breast-feeding. Manufacturer advises avoid.

● HEPATIC IMPAIRMENT Manufacturer advises caution in mild to moderate impairment; avoid in severe impairment.

● RENAL IMPAIRMENT Avoid if possible or use with caution. Avoid in severe impairment.
Dose adjustments The lowest effective dose should be used for the shortest possible duration.
Monitoring In renal impairment monitor renal function; sodium and water retention may occur and renal function may deteriorate, possibly leading to renal failure.

● MEDICINAL FORMS There can be variation in the licensing of different medicines containing the same drug.
Modified-release tablet
CAUTIONARY AND ADVISORY LABELS 25, 21
▸ Etolyn (Mylan)
  Etodolac 600 mg Etolyn 600mg modified-release tablets | 30 tablet [PoM] £12.40 DT = £15.50
▸ Etopan XL (Sun Pharmaceutical Industries Europe B.V.)
  Etodolac 600 mg Etopan XL 600mg tablets | 30 tablet [PoM] £14.60 DT = £15.50
▸ Lodine SR (Almirall Ltd)
  Etodolac 600 mg Lodine SR 600mg tablets | 30 tablet [PoM] £15.50 DT = £15.50

Etoricoxib

18-Nov-2020

● INDICATIONS AND DOSE
Pain and inflammation in osteoarthritis
▸ BY MOUTH
▸ Child 16-17 years: 30 mg once daily, increased if necessary to 60 mg once daily
▸ Adult: 30 mg once daily, increased if necessary to 60 mg once daily

Pain and inflammation in rheumatoid arthritis | Ankylosing spondylitis
▸ BY MOUTH
▸ Child 16-17 years: 60 mg once daily, increased if necessary to 90 mg once daily
▸ Adult: 60 mg once daily, increased if necessary to 90 mg once daily

Acute gout
▸ BY MOUTH
▸ Child 16-17 years: 120 mg once daily for maximum 8 days
▸ Adult: 120 mg once daily for maximum 8 days

● CONTRA-INDICATIONS Active gastro-intestinal bleeding · active gastro-intestinal ulceration · cerebrovascular disease · inflammatory bowel disease · ischaemic heart disease · mild to severe heart failure · peripheral arterial disease · uncontrolled hypertension (persistently above 140/90 mmHg)

● CAUTIONS Allergic disorders · cardiac impairment (NSAIDs may impair renal function) · coagulation defects · connective-tissue disorders · dehydration (risk of renal impairment) · elderly (risk of serious side-effects and fatalities) · history of cardiac failure · history of gastro-intestinal disorders · hypertension · left ventricular dysfunction · may mask symptoms of infection · oedema · risk factors for cardiovascular events

● INTERACTIONS → Appendix 1: NSAIDs

● SIDE-EFFECTS
▸ **Common or very common** Arrhythmias · asthenia · bronchospasm · constipation · diarrhoea · dizziness · fluid retention · gastrointestinal discomfort · gastrointestinal disorders · headache · hypertension · increased risk of infection · influenza like illness · nausea · oedema · oral ulceration · palpitations · skin reactions · vomiting
▸ **Uncommon** Alertness decreased · anaemia · angina pectoris · anxiety · appetite abnormal · cerebrovascular insufficiency · chest pain · congestive heart failure · conjunctivitis · cough · depression · drowsiness · dry mouth · dyspnoea · flushing · haemorrhage · hallucination · hyperkalaemia · hypersensitivity · insomnia · irritable bowel syndrome · leucopenia · myocardial infarction · pancreatitis · proteinuria · renal failure (more common in patients with pre-existing renal impairment) · sensation abnormal · taste altered · thrombocytopenia · tinnitus · vasculitis · vertigo · vision blurred · weight increased
▸ **Rare or very rare** Angioedema · confusion · hepatic disorders · muscle complaints · severe cutaneous adverse reactions (SCARs) · shock
▸ **Frequency not known** Nephritis tubulointerstitial · nephropathy

SIDE-EFFECTS, FURTHER INFORMATION For information about cardiovascular and gastrointestinal side-effects, and a possible exacerbation of symptoms in asthma, see Non-steroidal anti-inflammatory drugs p. 1176

● ALLERGY AND CROSS-SENSITIVITY [EvGr] Contra-indicated in patients with a history of hypersensitivity to aspirin or any other NSAID—which includes those in whom attacks of asthma, angioedema, urticaria or rhinitis have been precipitated by aspirin or any other NSAID. ◈

- CONCEPTION AND CONTRACEPTION Caution—long-term use of some NSAIDs is associated with reduced female fertility, which is reversible on stopping treatment.
- PREGNANCY Manufacturer advises avoid (teratogenic in *animal* studies). Avoid during the third trimester (risk of closure of fetal ductus arteriosus *in utero* and possibly persistent pulmonary hypertension of the newborn); onset of labour may be delayed and duration may be increased.
- BREAST FEEDING Use with caution during breast-feeding. Manufacturer advises avoid—present in milk in *animal* studies.
- HEPATIC IMPAIRMENT Manufacturer advises caution in mild to moderate impairment; avoid in severe impairment (no information available).
  Dose adjustments Manufacturer advises max. 60 mg once daily in mild impairment; max. 30 mg once daily in moderate impairment.
- RENAL IMPAIRMENT Avoid if possible or use with caution.
  ▸ In adults Avoid if eGFR less than 30 mL/minute/1.73 m².
  ▸ In children Avoid if estimated glomerular filtration rate less than 30 mL/minute/1.73 m².
  Dose adjustments The lowest effective dose should be used for the shortest possible duration.
  Monitoring In renal impairment monitor renal function; sodium and water retention may occur and renal function may deteriorate, possibly leading to renal failure.
- MONITORING REQUIREMENTS Monitor blood pressure before treatment, 2 weeks after initiation and periodically during treatment.

- MEDICINAL FORMS There can be variation in the licensing of different medicines containing the same drug.

  Tablet
  ▸ Etoricoxib (Non-proprietary)
  Etoricoxib 30 mg Etoricoxib 30mg tablets | 28 tablet [PoM] £13.99 DT = £5.63
  Etoricoxib 60 mg Etoricoxib 60mg tablets | 28 tablet [PoM] £20.11 DT = £2.77
  Etoricoxib 90 mg Etoricoxib 90mg tablets | 28 tablet [PoM] £22.96 DT = £2.48
  Etoricoxib 120 mg Etoricoxib 120mg tablets | 7 tablet [PoM] £4.82 | 28 tablet [PoM] £24.11 DT = £14.23
  ▸ Arcoxia (Merck Sharp & Dohme Ltd)
  Etoricoxib 30 mg Arcoxia 30mg tablets | 28 tablet [PoM] £13.99 DT = £5.63
  Etoricoxib 60 mg Arcoxia 60mg tablets | 28 tablet [PoM] £20.11 DT = £2.77
  Etoricoxib 90 mg Arcoxia 90mg tablets | 28 tablet [PoM] £22.96 DT = £2.48
  Etoricoxib 120 mg Arcoxia 120mg tablets | 7 tablet [PoM] £6.03 | 28 tablet [PoM] £24.11 DT = £14.23

Felbinac

07-Dec-2020

- DRUG ACTION Felbinac is an active metabolite of the NSAID fenbufen.

- INDICATIONS AND DOSE

  Relief of pain in musculoskeletal conditions | Treatment in knee or hand osteoarthritis (adjunct)
  ▸ TO THE SKIN
  ▸ Adult: Apply 2–4 times a day, therapy should be reviewed after 14 days; maximum 25 g per day

- CAUTIONS Avoid contact with eyes · avoid contact with inflamed or broken skin · avoid contact with mucous membranes · not for use with occlusive dressings · topical application of large amounts can result in systemic effects, including hypersensitivity and asthma (renal disease has also been reported)
- INTERACTIONS → Appendix 1: NSAIDs

- SIDE-EFFECTS Bronchospasm · gastrointestinal disorder · hypersensitivity · paraesthesia · photosensitivity reaction · skin reactions
  SIDE-EFFECTS, FURTHER INFORMATION For information about cardiovascular and gastrointestinal side-effects, and a possible exacerbation of symptoms in asthma, see Non-steroidal anti-inflammatory drugs p. 1176
- ALLERGY AND CROSS-SENSITIVITY [EvGr] Contra-indicated in patients with a history of hypersensitivity to aspirin or any other NSAID—which includes those in whom attacks of asthma, angioedema, urticaria or rhinitis have been precipitated by aspirin or any other NSAID. ⟨⟩
- PREGNANCY Patient packs for topical preparations carry a warning to avoid during pregnancy.
- BREAST FEEDING Patient packs for topical preparations carry a warning to avoid during breast-feeding.
- RENAL IMPAIRMENT Deterioration in renal function has also been reported after topical use.
- DIRECTIONS FOR ADMINISTRATION Manufacturer advises for topical preparations, apply with gentle massage only.
- PATIENT AND CARER ADVICE For topical preparations patients and carers should be advised to wash hands immediately after use.
  Photosensitivity Patients should be advised against excessive exposure to sunlight of area treated in order to avoid possibility of photosensitivity.

- MEDICINAL FORMS There can be variation in the licensing of different medicines containing the same drug.

  Gel
  ▸ Traxam (Advanz Pharma)
  Felbinac 30 mg per 1 gram Traxam 3% gel | 100 gram [PoM] £8.03 DT = £8.03
  Foam
  CAUTIONARY AND ADVISORY LABELS 15
  EXCIPIENTS: May contain Cetostearyl alcohol (including cetyl and stearyl alcohol)
  ▸ Traxam (Advanz Pharma)
  Felbinac 31.7 mg per 1 gram Traxam 3.17% foam | 100 gram [PoM] £8.41 DT = £8.41

Flurbiprofen

18-Nov-2020

- INDICATIONS AND DOSE

  Pain and inflammation in rheumatic disease and other musculoskeletal disorders | Migraine | Postoperative analgesia | Mild to moderate pain
  ▸ BY MOUTH
  ▸ Child 12–17 years: 150–200 mg daily in 2–4 divided doses, then increased to 300 mg daily, dose to be increased only in acute conditions
  ▸ Adult: 150–200 mg daily in 2–4 divided doses, then increased to 300 mg daily, dose to be increased only in acute conditions

  Dysmenorrhoea
  ▸ BY MOUTH
  ▸ Child 12–17 years: Initially 100 mg, then 50–100 mg every 4–6 hours; maximum 300 mg per day
  ▸ Adult: Initially 100 mg, then 50–100 mg every 4–6 hours; maximum 300 mg per day

- CONTRA-INDICATIONS Active gastro-intestinal bleeding · active gastro-intestinal ulceration · Crohn's disease (may be exacerbated) · history of gastro-intestinal bleeding related to previous NSAID therapy · history of gastro-intestinal perforation related to previous NSAID therapy · history of recurrent gastro-intestinal haemorrhage (two or more distinct episodes) · history of recurrent gastro-intestinal ulceration (two or more distinct episodes) · severe heart failure · ulcerative colitis (may be exacerbated)

- CAUTIONS Allergic disorders · cardiac impairment (NSAIDs may impair renal function) · cerebrovascular disease · coagulation defects · connective-tissue disorders · dehydration (risk of renal impairment) · elderly (risk of serious side-effects and fatalities) · heart failure · history of gastro-intestinal disorders · ischaemic heart disease · may mask symptoms of infection · peripheral arterial disease · risk factors for cardiovascular events · uncontrolled hypertension

- INTERACTIONS → Appendix 1: NSAIDs

- SIDE-EFFECTS Agranulocytosis · angioedema · aplastic anaemia · asthma · bronchospasm · confusion · constipation · Crohn's disease · depression · diarrhoea · dizziness · drowsiness · dyspnoea · fatigue · fertility decreased female · gastrointestinal discomfort · gastrointestinal disorders · haemolytic anaemia · haemorrhage · hallucination · headache · heart failure · hepatic disorders · hypersensitivity · hypertension · malaise · meningitis aseptic (patients with connective-tissue disorders such as systemic lupus erythematosus may be especially susceptible) · nausea · nephritis tubulointerstitial · nephropathy · neutropenia · oedema · optic neuritis · oral ulceration · pancreatitis · paraesthesia · photosensitivity reaction · platelet aggregation inhibition · renal failure (more common in patients with pre-existing renal impairment) · respiratory tract reaction · severe cutaneous adverse reactions (SCARs) · skin reactions · stroke · thrombocytopenia · tinnitus · vertigo · visual impairment · vomiting

  SIDE-EFFECTS, FURTHER INFORMATION For information about cardiovascular and gastrointestinal side-effects, and a possible exacerbation of symptoms in asthma, see Non-steroidal anti-inflammatory drugs. p. 1176

- ALLERGY AND CROSS-SENSITIVITY [EvGr] Contra-indicated in patients with a history of hypersensitivity to aspirin or any other NSAID—which includes those in whom attacks of asthma, angioedema, urticaria or rhinitis have been precipitated by aspirin or any other NSAID. Ⓜ

- CONCEPTION AND CONTRACEPTION
- In adults Caution—long-term use of some NSAIDs is associated with reduced female fertility, which is reversible on stopping treatment.

- PREGNANCY Avoid unless the potential benefit outweighs the risk. Avoid during the third trimester (risk of closure of fetal ductus arteriosus *in utero* and possibly persistent pulmonary hypertension of the newborn); onset of labour may be delayed and duration may be increased.

- BREAST FEEDING Use with caution during breast-feeding. Small amount present in milk—manufacturer advises avoid.

- HEPATIC IMPAIRMENT Manufacturer advises caution in mild to moderate impairment; avoid in severe impairment.

- RENAL IMPAIRMENT Avoid if possible or use with caution. Avoid in severe impairment.
  Dose adjustments The lowest effective dose should be used for the shortest possible duration.
  Monitoring In renal impairment monitor renal function; sodium and water retention may occur and renal function may deteriorate, possibly leading to renal failure.

- MEDICINAL FORMS There can be variation in the licensing of different medicines containing the same drug.
  Tablet
  CAUTIONARY AND ADVISORY LABELS 21
  - Flurbiprofen (Non-proprietary)
    Flurbiprofen 50 mg Flurbiprofen 50mg tablets | 100 tablet [PoM]
    £21.30–£51.81 DT = £51.78
    Flurbiprofen 100 mg Flurbiprofen 100mg tablets | 100 tablet [PoM]
    £92.64 DT = £92.58

Ibuprofen

18-Nov-2020

- INDICATIONS AND DOSE

Pain and inflammation in rheumatic disease and other musculoskeletal disorders | Mild to moderate pain including dysmenorrhoea | Postoperative analgesia | Dental pain

- BY MOUTH USING IMMEDIATE-RELEASE MEDICINES
- Adult: Initially 300–400 mg 3–4 times a day; increased if necessary up to 600 mg 4 times a day; maintenance 200–400 mg 3 times a day, may be adequate
- BY MOUTH USING MODIFIED-RELEASE MEDICINES
- Adult: 1.6 g once daily, dose to be taken in the early evening, increased if necessary to 2.4 g daily in 2 divided doses, dose to be increased only in severe cases

Acute migraine

- BY MOUTH USING IMMEDIATE-RELEASE MEDICINES
- Adult: 400–600 mg for 1 dose, to be taken as soon as migraine symptoms develop

Mild to moderate pain | Pain and inflammation of soft-tissue injuries | Pyrexia with discomfort

- BY MOUTH USING IMMEDIATE-RELEASE MEDICINES
- Child 3–5 months: 50 mg 3 times a day, maximum daily dose to be given in 3–4 divided doses; maximum 30 mg/kg per day
- Child 6–11 months: 50 mg 3–4 times a day, maximum daily dose to be given in 3–4 divided doses; maximum 30 mg/kg per day
- Child 1–3 years: 100 mg 3 times a day, maximum daily dose to be given in 3–4 divided doses; maximum 30 mg/kg per day
- Child 4–6 years: 150 mg 3 times a day, maximum daily dose to be given in 3–4 divided doses; maximum 30 mg/kg per day
- Child 7–9 years: 200 mg 3 times a day, maximum daily dose to be given in 3–4 divided doses; maximum 30 mg/kg per day; maximum 2.4 g per day
- Child 10–11 years: 300 mg 3 times a day, maximum daily dose to be given in 3–4 divided doses; maximum 30 mg/kg per day; maximum 2.4 g per day
- Child 12–17 years: Initially 300–400 mg 3–4 times a day; increased if necessary up to 600 mg 4 times a day; maintenance 200–400 mg 3 times a day, may be adequate

Pain and inflammation

- BY MOUTH USING MODIFIED-RELEASE MEDICINES
- Child 12–17 years: 1.6 g once daily, dose preferably taken in the early evening, increased to 2.4 g daily in 2 divided doses, dose to be increased only in severe cases

Pain and inflammation in rheumatic disease including juvenile idiopathic arthritis

- BY MOUTH USING IMMEDIATE-RELEASE MEDICINES
- Child 3 months–17 years: 30–40 mg/kg daily in 3–4 divided doses; maximum 2.4 g per day

Pain and inflammation in systemic juvenile idiopathic arthritis

- BY MOUTH USING IMMEDIATE-RELEASE MEDICINES
- Child 3 months–17 years: Up to 60 mg/kg daily in 4–6 divided doses; maximum 2.4 g per day

Post-immunisation pyrexia in infants (on doctor's advice only)

- BY MOUTH USING IMMEDIATE-RELEASE MEDICINES
- Child 2–3 months: 50 mg for 1 dose, followed by 50 mg after 6 hours if required

Pain relief in musculoskeletal conditions | Treatment in knee or hand osteoarthritis (adjunct)

▸ TO THE SKIN
▸ Adult: Apply up to 3 times a day, ibuprofen gel 5% gel to be administered

Pain and inflammation in rheumatic disease and other musculoskeletal disorders (dose approved for use by community practitioner nurse prescribers) | Mild to moderate pain including dysmenorrhoea (dose approved for use by community practitioner nurse prescribers) | Migraine (dose approved for use by community practitioner nurse prescribers) | Dental pain (dose approved for use by community practitioner nurse prescribers) | Headache (dose approved for use by community practitioner nurse prescribers) | Fever (dose approved for use by community practitioner nurse prescribers) | Symptoms of colds and influenza (dose approved for use by community practitioner nurse prescribers) | Neuralgia (dose approved for use by community practitioner nurse prescribers)

▸ BY MOUTH USING IMMEDIATE-RELEASE MEDICINES
▹ Child 12–17 years: 200–400 mg 3 times a day, if symptoms worsen or persist for more than 3 days refer to doctor
▹ Adult: 200–400 mg 3 times a day, if symptoms worsen or persist for more than 10 days refer to doctor

Mild to moderate pain (dose approved for use by community practitioner nurse prescribers) | Pain and inflammation of soft-tissue injuries (dose approved for use by community practitioner nurse prescribers) | Pyrexia with discomfort (dose approved for use by community practitioner nurse prescribers)

▸ BY MOUTH USING IMMEDIATE-RELEASE MEDICINES
▹ Child 3-5 months (body-weight 5 kg and above): 20–30 mg/kg daily in divided doses, alternatively 50 mg 3 times a day for maximum of 24 hours, refer to doctor if symptoms persist for more than 24 hours
▹ Child 6-11 months: 50 mg 3–4 times a day, refer to doctor if symptoms persist for more than 3 days
▹ Child 1-3 years: 100 mg 3 times a day, refer to doctor if symptoms persist for more than 3 days
▹ Child 4-6 years: 150 mg 3 times a day, refer to doctor if symptoms persist for more than 3 days
▹ Child 7-9 years: 200 mg 3 times a day, refer to doctor if symptoms persist for more than 3 days
▹ Child 10-11 years: 300 mg 3 times a day, refer to doctor if symptoms persist for more than 3 days

Post-immunisation pyrexia in infants (dose approved for use by community practitioner nurse prescribers) (on doctor's advice only)

▸ BY MOUTH USING IMMEDIATE-RELEASE MEDICINES
▹ Child 3 months: 50 mg for 1 dose, followed by 50 mg after 6 hours if required, if pyrexia persists refer to doctor

FENBID ® FORTE

Pain relief in musculoskeletal conditions | Treatment in knee or hand osteoarthritis (adjunct)

▸ TO THE SKIN
▹ Adult: Apply up to 4 times a day, therapy should be reviewed after 14 days

IBUGEL ® FORTE

Pain relief in musculoskeletal conditions | Treatment in knee or hand osteoarthritis (adjunct)

▸ TO THE SKIN
▹ Adult: Apply up to 3 times a day

● UNLICENSED USE
▸ With oral use in children Not licensed for use in children under 3 months or body-weight under 5 kg. Maximum dose for systemic juvenile idiopathic arthritis is unlicensed.

● CONTRA-INDICATIONS
▸ With systemic use Active gastro-intestinal bleeding · active gastro-intestinal ulceration · history of gastro-intestinal bleeding related to previous NSAID therapy · history of gastro-intestinal perforation related to previous NSAID therapy · history of recurrent gastro-intestinal haemorrhage (two or more distinct episodes) · history of recurrent gastro-intestinal ulceration (two or more distinct episodes) · severe heart failure · varicella infection

● CAUTIONS
▸ With systemic use Allergic disorders · cardiac impairment (NSAIDs may impair renal function) · cerebrovascular disease · coagulation defects · connective-tissue disorders · dehydration (risk of renal impairment) · elderly (risk of serious side-effects and fatalities) · heart failure · history of gastro-intestinal disorders (e.g. ulcerative colitis, Crohn's disease) · ischaemic heart disease · may mask symptoms of infection · peripheral arterial disease · risk factors for cardiovascular events · uncontrolled hypertension
▸ With topical use Avoid contact with eyes · avoid contact with inflamed or broken skin · avoid contact with mucous membranes · not for use with occlusive dressings · topical application of large amounts can result in systemic effects, including hypersensitivity and asthma (renal disease has also been reported)

CAUTIONS, FURTHER INFORMATION
▸ High-dose ibuprofen
▸ With oral use A small increase in cardiovascular risk, similar to the risk associated with cyclo-oxygenase-2 inhibitors and diclofenac, has been reported with high-dose ibuprofen (≥ 2.4 g daily); use should be avoided in patients with established ischaemic heart disease, peripheral arterial disease, cerebrovascular disease, congestive heart failure (New York Heart Association classification II-III), and uncontrolled hypertension.
▸ Masking of symptoms of underlying infections
▸ With systemic use Ibuprofen can mask symptoms of infection, which may lead to delayed initiation of appropriate treatment and thereby worsen infection outcome. This has been observed in bacterial community-acquired pneumonia and bacterial complications to varicella. When administered for fever or pain relief in relation to infection, monitoring of infection is advised.

● INTERACTIONS → Appendix 1: NSAIDs
● SIDE-EFFECTS
GENERAL SIDE-EFFECTS
▸ **Uncommon** Gastrointestinal discomfort · hypersensitivity · rash (discontinue) · skin reactions
▸ **Rare or very rare** Angioedema · dyspnoea
▸ **Frequency not known** Asthma
SPECIFIC SIDE-EFFECTS
▸ **Uncommon**
▸ With oral use Headache · nausea
▸ **Rare or very rare**
▸ With oral use Acute kidney injury · agranulocytosis · anaemia · constipation · diarrhoea · gastrointestinal disorders · haemorrhage · leucopenia · liver disorder · meningitis aseptic (patients with connective-tissue disorders such as systemic lupus erythematosus may be especially susceptible) · oedema · oral ulceration · pancytopenia · renal papillary necrosis · severe cutaneous adverse reactions (SCARs) · shock · thrombocytopenia · vomiting
▸ **Frequency not known**
▸ With oral use Crohn's disease · fertility decreased female · fluid retention · heart failure · hypertension · increased risk of arterial thromboembolism · renal failure (more common in patients with pre-existing renal impairment) · respiratory disorders · respiratory tract reaction
▸ With topical use Bronchospasm · renal impairment · toxic epidermal necrolysis

10

Musculoskeletal system

SIDE-EFFECTS, FURTHER INFORMATION For information about cardiovascular and gastrointestinal side-effects, and a possible exacerbation of symptoms in asthma, see Non-steroidal anti-inflammatory drugs. p. 1176

With topical use Topical application of large amounts can result in systemic effects, including hypersensitivity and asthma (renal disease has also been reported).

Overdose Overdosage with ibuprofen may cause nausea, vomiting, epigastric pain, and tinnitus, but more serious toxicity is very uncommon. Charcoal, activated followed by symptomatic measures are indicated if more than 100 mg/kg has been ingested within the preceding hour.

For details on the management of poisoning, see Emergency treatment of poisoning p. 1413.

● ALLERGY AND CROSS-SENSITIVITY [EvGr] Contra-indicated in patients with a history of hypersensitivity to aspirin or any other NSAID—which includes those in whom attacks of asthma, angioedema, urticaria or rhinitis have been precipitated by aspirin or any other NSAID. ⟨M⟩

● CONCEPTION AND CONTRACEPTION
▸ With systemic use in adults Caution—long-term use of some NSAIDs is associated with reduced female fertility, which is reversible on stopping treatment.

● PREGNANCY
▸ With systemic use Avoid unless the potential benefit outweighs the risk. Avoid during the third trimester (risk of closure of fetal ductus arteriosus *in utero* and possibly persistent pulmonary hypertension of the newborn); onset of labour may be delayed and duration may be increased.
▸ With topical use Patient packs for topical preparations carry a warning to avoid during pregnancy.

● BREAST FEEDING
▸ With oral use Use with caution during breast-feeding. Amount too small to be harmful but some manufacturers advise avoid.
▸ With topical use Patient packs for topical preparations carry a warning to avoid during breast-feeding.

● HEPATIC IMPAIRMENT
▸ With oral use Manufacturer advises caution in mild to moderate impairment; avoid in severe impairment.

● RENAL IMPAIRMENT
▸ With oral use Avoid if possible or use with caution. Avoid in severe impairment.
▸ With topical use Deterioration in renal function has also been reported after topical use.
Dose adjustments ▸ With oral use The lowest effective dose should be used for the shortest possible duration.
Monitoring ▸ With systemic use In renal impairment monitor renal function; sodium and water retention may occur and renal function may deteriorate, possibly leading to renal failure.

● DIRECTIONS FOR ADMINISTRATION
▸ With topical use For topical preparations, manufacturer advises apply with gentle massage only.

● PRESCRIBING AND DISPENSING INFORMATION
▸ With oral use Flavours of syrup may include orange.

● PATIENT AND CARER ADVICE
▸ With topical use For topical preparations, patients and their carers should be advised to wash hands immediately after use.
Photosensitivity For topical preparations, patients or their carers should be advised against excessive exposure to sunlight of area treated in order to avoid possibility of photosensitivity.
Medicines for Children leaflet: Ibuprofen for pain and inflammation www.medicinesforchildren.org.uk/ibuprofen-pain-and-inflammation

● PROFESSION SPECIFIC INFORMATION
Dental practitioners' formulary
▸ With oral use Ibuprofen Oral Suspension Sugar-free may be prescribed. Ibuprofen Tablets may be prescribed.

● EXCEPTIONS TO LEGAL CATEGORY
▸ With topical use Smaller pack sizes of gel preparations may be available on sale to the public.
▸ With oral use Oral preparations can be sold to the public in certain circumstances.

● MEDICINAL FORMS There can be variation in the licensing of different medicines containing the same drug. Forms available from special-order manufacturers include: oral suspension

Effervescent granules
CAUTIONARY AND ADVISORY LABELS 13, 21
ELECTROLYTES: May contain Sodium
▸ Brufen (Mylan)
   Ibuprofen 600 mg Brufen 600mg effervescent granules sachets | 20 sachet [PoM] £6.80 DT = £6.80

Modified-release tablet
CAUTIONARY AND ADVISORY LABELS 25, 27
▸ Brufen Retard (Mylan)
   Ibuprofen 800 mg Brufen Retard 800mg tablets | 56 tablet [PoM] £7.74 DT = £7.74

Tablet
CAUTIONARY AND ADVISORY LABELS 21
▸ Ibuprofen (Non-proprietary)
   Ibuprofen 200 mg Ibuprofen 200mg tablets | 16 tablet [P] £0.25 | 24 tablet [P] £1.41 DT = £1.41 | 48 tablet [P] £2.82 | 84 tablet [P] £4.94 DT = £4.94
   Ibuprofen 200mg caplets | 16 tablet [P] £0.25 | 24 tablet [P] [⅀] DT = £1.41
   Ibuprofen 400 mg Ibuprofen 400mg caplets | 24 tablet [P] [⅀] DT = £2.26
   Ibuprofen 400mg tablets | 24 tablet [P] £2.26 DT = £2.26 | 48 tablet [P] £4.52 | 84 tablet [P] £7.91 DT = £7.91
   Ibuprofen 600 mg Ibuprofen 600mg tablets | 84 tablet [PoM] £4.96 DT = £4.96
   Ibuprofen 600mg tablets film coated | 84 tablet [PoM] £4.96 DT = £4.96
▸ Brufen (Mylan)
   Ibuprofen 400 mg Brufen 400mg tablets | 60 tablet [PoM] £4.90
▸ Cuprofen (Reckitt Benckiser Healthcare (UK) Ltd)
   Ibuprofen 400 mg Cuprofen Maximum Strength 400mg tablets | 24 tablet [P] £2.06 DT = £2.26 | 48 tablet [P] £3.49 | 96 tablet [P] £5.49
▸ Feminax Express (Bayer Plc)
   Ibuprofen (as Ibuprofen lysine) 200 mg Feminax Express 342mg tablets | 8 tablet [GSL] £1.76 DT = £1.76 | 16 tablet [GSL] £2.67 DT = £2.67
▸ Ibucalm (Aspar Pharmaceuticals Ltd)
   Ibuprofen 200 mg Ibucalm 200mg tablets | 24 tablet [P] £0.33 DT = £1.41 | 48 tablet [P] £0.62 | 96 tablet [P] £1.15
   Ibuprofen 400 mg Ibucalm 400mg tablets | 24 tablet [P] £0.56 DT = £2.26 | 48 tablet [P] £1.15 | 96 tablet [P] £2.05
▸ Ibular (Ennogen Pharma Ltd)
   Ibuprofen 200 mg Ibular 200mg tablets | 84 tablet [P] £3.26 DT = £4.94
   Ibuprofen 400 mg Ibular 400mg tablets | 84 tablet [P] £2.80 DT = £7.91
▸ Nurofen (Reckitt Benckiser Healthcare (UK) Ltd)
   Ibuprofen 200 mg Nurofen 200mg caplets | 24 tablet [P] £2.71 DT = £1.41
   Nurofen 200mg tablets | 24 tablet [P] £2.58 DT = £1.41 | 48 tablet [P] £4.85 | 96 tablet [P] £7.76
   Ibuprofen (as Ibuprofen lysine) 400 mg Nurofen Maximum Strength Migraine Pain 684mg caplets | 12 tablet [P] £3.68 DT = £3.68
▸ Nurofen Express (Reckitt Benckiser Healthcare (UK) Ltd)
   Ibuprofen (as Ibuprofen sodium dihydrate) 200 mg Nurofen Express 256mg tablets | 16 tablet [GSL] £2.30
   Nurofen Express 256mg caplets | 12 tablet [GSL] £2.11 | 16 tablet [GSL] £2.44
   Ibuprofen (as Ibuprofen lysine) 400 mg Nurofen Express 684mg caplets | 24 tablet [P] £6.40 DT = £6.40
▸ Nurofen Joint & Back Pain Relief (Reckitt Benckiser Healthcare (UK) Ltd)
   Ibuprofen (as Ibuprofen sodium dihydrate) 200 mg Nurofen Joint & Back Pain Relief 256mg caplets | 16 tablet [GSL] £2.44

Nurofen Joint & Back Pain Relief 256mg tablets | 16 tablet GSL £2.30

Ibuprofen (as Ibuprofen sodium dihydrate) 400 mg Nurofen Max Strength Joint & Back Pain Relief 512mg tablets | 24 tablet P £6.46

‣ Nurofen Migraine Pain (Reckitt Benckiser Healthcare (UK) Ltd)
Ibuprofen (as Ibuprofen lysine) 200 mg Nurofen Migraine Pain 342mg tablets | 12 tablet GSL £2.09

Oral suspension

CAUTIONARY AND ADVISORY LABELS 21

‣ Brufen (Mylan)
Ibuprofen 20 mg per 1 ml Brufen 100mg/5ml syrup | 500 ml PoM £8.88 DT = £8.88

‣ Care Ibuprofen for Children (Thornton & Ross Ltd)
Ibuprofen 20 mg per 1 ml Care Ibuprofen for Children 100mg/5ml oral suspension sugar-free | 500 ml PoM £9.00

‣ Nurofen (Reckitt Benckiser Healthcare (UK) Ltd)
Ibuprofen 40 mg per 1 ml Nurofen for Children 200mg/5ml oral suspension orange sugar-free | 100 ml P £4.20 DT = £3.49
Nurofen for Children 200mg/5ml oral suspension strawberry sugar-free | 100 ml P £4.20 DT = £3.49

Modified-release capsule

‣ Nurofen Back Pain SR (Reckitt Benckiser Healthcare (UK) Ltd)
Ibuprofen 300 mg Nurofen Back Pain SR 300mg capsules | 24 capsule P £4.85 DT = £4.85

Chewable capsule

‣ Nurofen (Reckitt Benckiser Healthcare (UK) Ltd)
Ibuprofen 100 mg Nurofen for Children 100mg chewable capsules | 12 capsule P £3.23

Gel

EXCIPIENTS: May contain Benzyl alcohol

‣ Ibuprofen (Non-proprietary)
Ibuprofen 50 mg per 1 gram Mentholatum Ibuprofen 5% gel | 100 gram P £5.01 DT = £2.80
Ibuprofen 5% gel | 30 gram P £1.71 | 50 gram P £1.75 DT = £1.40 | 100 gram P £2.80 DT = £2.80
Ibuprofen 100 mg per 1 gram Ibuprofen 10% gel | 30 gram P £1.74 | 50 gram P £3.32-£3.45 | 100 gram P £5.79 DT = £5.79

‣ Fenbid (Advanz Pharma)
Ibuprofen 100 mg per 1 gram Fenbid Forte 10% gel | 100 gram PoM £3.80 DT = £5.79

‣ Ibugel (Dermal Laboratories Ltd)
Ibuprofen 50 mg per 1 gram Ibugel 5% gel | 100 gram P £4.87 DT = £2.80
Ibuprofen 100 mg per 1 gram Ibugel Forte 10% gel | 100 gram PoM £5.79 DT = £5.79

‣ Ibuleve (Dendron Ltd)
Ibuprofen 50 mg per 1 gram Ibuleve 5% gel | 30 gram P £2.64 | 50 gram P £3.70 DT = £1.40 | 100 gram P £6.80 DT = £2.80

‣ Phorpain (Advanz Pharma)
Ibuprofen 50 mg per 1 gram Phorpain 5% gel | 100 gram P £1.50 DT = £2.80

Capsule

‣ Ibuprofen (Non-proprietary)
Ibuprofen 200 mg Ibuprofen 200mg capsules | 30 capsule P ⚠ DT = £4.85

‣ Flarin (infirst Ltd)
Ibuprofen 200 mg Flarin 200mg capsules | 12 capsule P £3.31 | 30 capsule P £6.22 DT = £4.85

‣ Nurofen Express (Reckitt Benckiser Healthcare (UK) Ltd)
Ibuprofen 200 mg Nurofen Express 200mg liquid capsules | 30 capsule P £4.85 DT = £4.85
Ibuprofen 400 mg Nurofen Express 400mg liquid capsules | 10 capsule P £3.88 | 20 capsule P £6.47 DT = £6.47

Orodispersible tablet

‣ Nurofen Meltlets (Reckitt Benckiser Healthcare (UK) Ltd)
Ibuprofen 200 mg Nurofen Meltlets 200mg tablets sugar-free | 12 tablet GSL £2.58 DT = £2.58

Indometacin

18-Nov-2020

(Indomethacin)

● **INDICATIONS AND DOSE**

Pain and moderate to severe inflammation in rheumatic disease and other musculoskeletal disorders

‣ BY MOUTH USING IMMEDIATE-RELEASE MEDICINES
  ‣ Adult: 50–200 mg daily in divided doses
‣ BY RECTUM
  ‣ Adult: 100 mg 1–2 times a day, dose to be administered at night and in the morning if required, combined oral and rectal treatment maximum total daily dose 150–200 mg
‣ BY MOUTH USING MODIFIED-RELEASE MEDICINES
  ‣ Adult: 75 mg 1–2 times a day

Acute gout

‣ BY MOUTH USING IMMEDIATE-RELEASE MEDICINES
  ‣ Adult: 150–200 mg daily in divided doses
‣ BY RECTUM
  ‣ Adult: 100 mg 1–2 times a day, dose to be administered at night and in the morning if required, combined oral and rectal treatment maximum total daily dose 150–200 mg
‣ BY MOUTH USING MODIFIED-RELEASE MEDICINES
  ‣ Adult: 75 mg 1–2 times a day

Dysmenorrhoea

‣ BY MOUTH USING IMMEDIATE-RELEASE MEDICINES
  ‣ Adult: Up to 75 mg daily
‣ BY RECTUM
  ‣ Adult: 100 mg 1–2 times a day, dose to be administered at night and in the morning if required, combined oral and rectal treatment maximum total daily dose 150–200 mg
‣ BY MOUTH USING MODIFIED-RELEASE MEDICINES
  ‣ Adult: 75 mg daily

● CONTRA-INDICATIONS Active gastro-intestinal bleeding · active gastro-intestinal ulceration · history of gastro-intestinal bleeding related to previous NSAID therapy · history of gastro-intestinal perforation related to previous NSAID therapy · history of recurrent gastro-intestinal haemorrhage (two or more distinct episodes) · history of recurrent gastro-intestinal ulceration (two or more distinct episodes) · severe heart failure

● CAUTIONS

GENERAL CAUTIONS Allergic disorders · cardiac impairment (NSAIDs may impair renal function) · cerebrovascular disease · coagulation defects · connective-tissue disorders · dehydration (risk of renal impairment) · elderly (risk of serious side-effects and fatalities) · epilepsy · heart failure · history of gastro-intestinal disorders (e.g. ulcerative colitis, Crohn's disease) · ischaemic heart disease · may mask symptoms of infection · parkinsonism · peripheral arterial disease · psychiatric disturbances · risk factors for cardiovascular events · uncontrolled hypertension

SPECIFIC CAUTIONS

‣ With rectal use Avoid rectal administration in proctitis · avoid rectal administration in recent rectal bleeding

● INTERACTIONS → Appendix 1: NSAIDs

● SIDE-EFFECTS

GENERAL SIDE-EFFECTS Agranulocytosis · alopecia · anaphylactic reaction · angioedema · anxiety · appetite decreased · arrhythmias · asthma · blood disorder · bone marrow disorders · breast abnormalities · chest pain · coma · confusion · congestive heart failure · constipation · corneal deposits · depression · diarrhoea · disseminated intravascular coagulation · dizziness · drowsiness · dysarthria · erythema nodosum · eye disorder · eye pain · fatigue · fluid retention · flushing · gastrointestinal discomfort · gastrointestinal disorders · gynaecomastia ·

10

Musculoskeletal system

haemolytic anaemia · haemorrhage · hallucination · headache · hearing impairment · hepatic disorders · hyperglycaemia · hyperhidrosis · hyperkalaemia · hypotension · inflammatory bowel disease · insomnia · leucopenia · movement disorders · muscle weakness · nausea · nephritis tubulointerstitial · nephrotic syndrome · oedema · oral disorders · palpitations · pancreatitis · paraesthesia · peripheral neuropathy · photosensitivity reaction · platelet aggregation inhibition · psychiatric disorders · renal failure (more common in patients with pre-existing renal impairment) · respiratory disorders · seizures · severe cutaneous adverse reactions (SCARs) · skin reactions · syncope · thrombocytopenia · tinnitus · urine abnormalities · vasculitis · vertigo · vision disorders · vomiting

SPECIFIC SIDE-EFFECTS

● With oral use Dyspnoea · malaise · pulmonary oedema · sigmoid lesion perforation

SIDE-EFFECTS, FURTHER INFORMATION For information about cardiovascular and gastrointestinal side-effects, and a possible exacerbation of symptoms in asthma, see Non-steroidal anti-inflammatory drugs. p. 1176

● ALLERGY AND CROSS-SENSITIVITY [EvGr] Contra-indicated in patients with a history of hypersensitivity to aspirin or any other NSAID—which includes those in whom attacks of asthma, angioedema, urticaria or rhinitis have been precipitated by aspirin or any other NSAID. Ⓜ

● CONCEPTION AND CONTRACEPTION Caution—long-term use of some NSAIDs is associated with reduced female fertility, which is reversible on stopping treatment.

● PREGNANCY Avoid unless the potential benefit outweighs the risk. Avoid during the third trimester (risk of closure of fetal ductus arteriosus *in utero* and possibly persistent pulmonary hypertension of the newborn); onset of labour may be delayed and duration may be increased.

● BREAST FEEDING Amount probably too small to be harmful—manufacturers advise avoid. Use with caution during breast-feeding.

● HEPATIC IMPAIRMENT Manufacturer advises caution in mild to moderate impairment; avoid in severe impairment (increased risk of gastro-intestinal bleeding and fluid retention).

● RENAL IMPAIRMENT Avoid if possible or use with caution. Avoid in severe impairment.
Dose adjustments The lowest effective dose should be used for the shortest possible duration.
Monitoring In renal impairment monitor renal function; sodium and water retention may occur and renal function may deteriorate, possibly leading to renal failure.

● MONITORING REQUIREMENTS During prolonged therapy ophthalmic and blood examinations particularly advisable.

● PATIENT AND CARER ADVICE
Driving and skilled tasks Dizziness may affect performance of skilled tasks (e.g. driving).

● MEDICINAL FORMS There can be variation in the licensing of different medicines containing the same drug. Forms available from special-order manufacturers include: oral suspension, oral solution

Suppository
▸ Indocid (Aspen Pharma Trading Ltd)
  Indometacin 100 mg Indocid 100mg suppositories | 10 suppository [PoM] £17.61 DT = £17.61

Modified-release capsule
CAUTIONARY AND ADVISORY LABELS 21, 25
▸ Berlind Retard (Tillomed Laboratories Ltd)
  Indometacin 75 mg Berlind 75 Retard capsules | 100 capsule [PoM]
  £8.65 DT = £8.65

Capsule
CAUTIONARY AND ADVISORY LABELS 21
▸ Indometacin (Non-proprietary)
  Indometacin 25 mg Indometacin 25mg capsules | 28 capsule [PoM]
  £1.40 DT = £1.40
  Indometacin 50 mg Indometacin 50mg capsules | 28 capsule [PoM]
  £1.69 DT = £1.69

Ketoprofen

18-Nov-2020

● INDICATIONS AND DOSE

Pain and mild inflammation in rheumatic disease and musculoskeletal conditions | Dysmenorrhoea | Acute gout
▸ BY MOUTH
▸ Adult: 100–200 mg once daily

Relief of pain in rheumatic disease and musculoskeletal conditions
▸ TO THE SKIN
▸ Adult: Apply 2–4 times a day for up to 7 days, ketoprofen 2.5% gel to be administered; maximum 15 g per day

POWERGEL ®

Relief of pain in musculoskeletal conditions | Adjunctive treatment in knee or hand osteoarthritis
▸ TO THE SKIN
▸ Adult: Apply 2–3 times a day for up to max. 10 days

● CONTRA-INDICATIONS
▸ With systemic use Active gastro-intestinal bleeding · active gastro-intestinal ulceration · coagulation disorders · history of gastro-intestinal bleeding · history of gastro-intestinal perforation · history of gastro-intestinal ulceration · severe heart failure

● CAUTIONS
▸ With systemic use Allergic disorders · cardiac impairment (NSAIDs may impair renal function) · cerebrovascular disease · connective-tissue disorders · dehydration (risk of renal impairment) · elderly (risk of serious side-effects and fatalities) · heart failure · history of gastro-intestinal disorders (e.g. ulcerative colitis, Crohn's disease) · ischaemic heart disease · may mask symptoms of infection · peripheral arterial disease · risk factors for cardiovascular events · uncontrolled hypertension
▸ With topical use Avoid contact with eyes · avoid contact with inflamed or broken skin · avoid contact with mucous membranes · not for use with occlusive dressings · topical application of large amounts can result in systemic effects, including hypersensitivity and asthma (renal disease has also been reported)

CAUTIONS, FURTHER INFORMATION
▸ Masking of symptoms of underlying infections
▸ With systemic use Ketoprofen can mask symptoms of infection, which may lead to delayed initiation of appropriate treatment and thereby worsen infection outcome. This has been observed in bacterial community-acquired pneumonia and bacterial complications to varicella. When administered for fever or pain relief in relation to infection, monitoring of infection is advised.

● INTERACTIONS → Appendix 1: NSAIDs

● SIDE-EFFECTS

GENERAL SIDE-EFFECTS
▸ **Uncommon** Diarrhoea · paraesthesia · skin reactions
▸ **Rare or very rare** Hypersensitivity · photosensitivity reaction · renal impairment
▸ **Frequency not known** Angioedema

SPECIFIC SIDE-EFFECTS
▸ **Common or very common**
▸ With oral use Gastrointestinal discomfort · nausea · vomiting

Uncommon

With oral use Constipation · dizziness · drowsiness · fatigue · gastrointestinal disorders · headache · oedema · rash (discontinue)

With topical use Increased risk of infection

Rare or very rare

With oral use Asthma · haemorrhagic anaemia · hepatic disorders · pancreatitis · shock · stomatitis · tinnitus · vision disorders · weight increased

Frequency not known

With oral use Acute kidney injury (more common in patients with pre-existing renal impairment) · agranulocytosis · alopecia · appetite decreased · bone marrow failure · bronchospasm · confusion · Crohn's disease aggravated · depression · dyspnoea · fertility decreased female · haemorrhage · hallucination · hearing impairment · heart failure · hypertension · increased risk of arterial thromboembolism · increased risk of ischaemic stroke · increased risk of myocardial infarction · malaise · meningitis aseptic (patients with connective-tissue disorders such as systemic lupus erythematosus may be especially susceptible) · menometrorrhagia · mood altered · nephritic syndrome · nephritis tubulointerstitial · nephrotic syndrome · neutropenia · optic neuritis · rhinitis · seizure · severe cutaneous adverse reactions (SCARs) · taste altered · thrombocytopenia · vasodilation · vertigo

With topical use Eosinophilia · eyelid oedema · fever · gastrointestinal haemorrhage · lip swelling · peptic ulcer · vasculitis · wound complications

SIDE-EFFECTS, FURTHER INFORMATION Topical application of large amounts can result in systemic effects, including hypersensitivity and asthma (renal disease has also been reported).

For information about cardiovascular and gastrointestinal side-effects, and a possible exacerbation of symptoms in asthma, see Non-steroidal anti-inflammatory drugs p. 1176

● ALLERGY AND CROSS-SENSITIVITY ⟨EvGr⟩ Contra-indicated in patients with a history of hypersensitivity to aspirin or any other NSAID—which includes those in whom attacks of asthma, angioedema, urticaria or rhinitis have been precipitated by aspirin or any other NSAID. ⟨M⟩

● CONCEPTION AND CONTRACEPTION

▸ With systemic use Caution—long-term use of some NSAIDs is associated with reduced female fertility, which is reversible on stopping treatment.

● PREGNANCY

▸ With systemic use Avoid unless the potential benefit outweighs the risk. Avoid during the third trimester (risk of closure of fetal ductus arteriosus *in utero* and possibly persistent pulmonary hypertension of the newborn); onset of labour may be delayed and duration may be increased.

▸ With topical use Patient packs for topical preparations carry a warning to avoid during pregnancy.

● BREAST FEEDING

▸ With systemic use Use with caution during breast-feeding. Amount probably too small to be harmful but manufacturers advise avoid.

▸ With topical use Patient packs for topical preparations carry a warning to avoid during breast-feeding.

● HEPATIC IMPAIRMENT

▸ With systemic use Manufacturer advises caution in mild to moderate impairment; avoid in severe impairment.

▸ With topical use Manufacturer advises caution.

● RENAL IMPAIRMENT

▸ With systemic use Avoid if possible or use with caution. Avoid in severe impairment.

▸ With topical use Deterioration in renal function has also been reported after topical use.

Dose adjustments ▸ With systemic use The lowest effective dose should be used for the shortest possible duration.

Monitoring ▸ With systemic use In renal impairment monitor renal function; sodium and water retention may occur and renal function may deteriorate, possibly leading to renal failure.

● DIRECTIONS FOR ADMINISTRATION

▸ With topical use For topical preparations, manufacturer advises apply with gentle massage only.

● PATIENT AND CARER ADVICE

▸ With topical use For topical preparations, patients and their carers should be advised to wash hands immediately after use.

Photosensitivity

▸ With topical use Patients should be advised against excessive exposure to sunlight of area treated in order to avoid possibility of photosensitivity. Patients should be advised not to expose area treated to sunbeds or sunlight (even on a bright but cloudy day) during, and for two weeks after stopping treatment; treated areas should be protected with clothing.

● EXCEPTIONS TO LEGAL CATEGORY Smaller pack sizes of gel preparations may be available on sale to the public.

● MEDICINAL FORMS There can be variation in the licensing of different medicines containing the same drug. Forms available from special-order manufacturers include: gel

Modified-release capsule

CAUTIONARY AND ADVISORY LABELS 21, 25

▸ Larafen CR (Ennogen Pharma Ltd)

Ketoprofen 200 mg Larafen CR 200mg capsules | 28 capsule PoM £19.08 DT = £23.85

▸ Oruvail (Sanofi)

Ketoprofen 100 mg Oruvail 100 modified-release capsules | 56 capsule PoM £23.93 DT = £23.93

Ketoprofen 200 mg Oruvail 200 modified-release capsules | 28 capsule PoM £23.85 DT = £23.85

▸ Valket Retard (Tillomed Laboratories Ltd)

Ketoprofen 200 mg Valket 200 Retard capsules | 28 capsule PoM £10.70 DT = £23.85

Gel

CAUTIONARY AND ADVISORY LABELS 11

EXCIPIENTS: May contain Ethanol, fragrances

▸ Ketoprofen (Non-proprietary)

Ketoprofen 25 mg per 1 gram Ketoprofen 2.5% gel | 50 gram PoM £1.83 DT = £1.83 | 100 gram PoM £3.66

▸ Oruvail (Sanofi)

Ketoprofen 25 mg per 1 gram Oruvail 2.5% gel | 100 gram PoM £6.84

▸ Powergel (A. Menarini Farmaceutica Internazionale SRL)

Ketoprofen 25 mg per 1 gram Powergel 2.5% gel | 50 gram PoM £3.06 DT = £1.83 | 100 gram PoM £5.89

▸ Tiloket (Tillomed Laboratories Ltd)

Ketoprofen 25 mg per 1 gram Tiloket 2.5% gel | 50 gram PoM £3.00 DT = £1.83 | 100 gram PoM £6.00

Mefenamic acid   18-Nov-2020

● INDICATIONS AND DOSE

Pain and inflammation in rheumatoid arthritis and osteoarthritis | Postoperative pain | Mild to moderate pain

▸ BY MOUTH

▸ Adult: 500 mg 3 times a day

Acute pain including dysmenorrhoea | Menorrhagia

▸ BY MOUTH

▸ Child 12–17 years: 500 mg 3 times a day

▸ Adult: 500 mg 3 times a day

● CONTRA-INDICATIONS Active gastro-intestinal bleeding · active gastro-intestinal ulceration · following coronary artery bypass graft (CABG) surgery · history of gastro-intestinal bleeding related to previous NSAID therapy · history of gastro-intestinal perforation related to previous NSAID therapy · history of recurrent gastro-intestinal haemorrhage (two or more distinct episodes) · history of recurrent gastro-intestinal ulceration (two or more distinct episodes) · inflammatory bowel disease · severe heart failure

- CAUTIONS Acute porphyrias p. 1107 · allergic disorders · cardiac impairment (NSAIDs may impair renal function) · cerebrovascular disease · coagulation defects · connective-tissue disorders · dehydration (risk of renal impairment) · elderly (risk of serious side-effects and fatalities) · epilepsy · heart failure · history of gastro-intestinal disorders (e.g. ulcerative colitis, Crohn's disease) · ischaemic heart disease · may mask symptoms of infection · peripheral arterial disease · risk factors for cardiovascular events · uncontrolled hypertension

- INTERACTIONS → Appendix 1: NSAIDs

- SIDE-EFFECTS Agranulocytosis · anaemia · angioedema · appetite decreased · asthma · bone marrow disorders · confusion · constipation · Crohn's disease · depression · diarrhoea (discontinue) · disseminated intravascular coagulation · dizziness · drowsiness · dyspnoea · dysuria · ear pain · eosinophilia · eye irritation · fatigue · fertility decreased female · gastrointestinal discomfort · gastrointestinal disorders · glomerulonephritis · glucose tolerance impaired · haemolytic anaemia · haemorrhage · hallucination · headache · heart failure · hepatic disorders · hyperhidrosis · hypersensitivity · hypertension · hyponatraemia · hypotension · insomnia · leucopenia · malaise · meningitis aseptic (patients with connective-tissue disorders such as systemic lupus erythematosus may be especially susceptible) · multi organ failure · nausea · nephritis acute interstitial · nephrotic syndrome · nervousness · neutropenia · oedema · optic neuritis · oral ulceration · palpitations · pancreatitis · paraesthesia · photosensitivity reaction · proteinuria · rash (discontinue) · renal failure (more common in patients with pre-existing renal impairment) · renal failure non-oliguric · renal papillary necrosis · respiratory disorders · seizure · sepsis · severe cutaneous adverse reactions (SCARs) · skin reactions · thrombocytopenia · tinnitus · vertigo · vision disorders · vomiting

SIDE-EFFECTS, FURTHER INFORMATION For information about cardiovascular and gastrointestinal side-effects, and a possible exacerbation of symptoms in asthma, see Non-steroidal anti-inflammatory drugs. p. 1176

Overdose Mefenamic acid has important consequences in overdosage because it can cause convulsions, which if prolonged or recurrent, require treatment.

For details on the management of poisoning, see Emergency treatment of poisoning p. 1413, in particular, Convulsions.

- ALLERGY AND CROSS-SENSITIVITY EvGr Contra-indicated in patients with a history of hypersensitivity to aspirin or any other NSAID—which includes those in whom attacks of asthma, angioedema, urticaria or rhinitis have been precipitated by aspirin or any other NSAID. ⓜ

- CONCEPTION AND CONTRACEPTION Caution—long-term use of some NSAIDs is associated with reduced female fertility, which is reversible on stopping treatment.

- PREGNANCY Avoid unless the potential benefit outweighs the risk. Avoid during the third trimester (risk of closure of fetal ductus arteriosus *in utero* and possibly persistent pulmonary hypertension of the newborn); onset of labour may be delayed and duration may be increased.

- BREAST FEEDING Use with caution during breast-feeding. Amount too small to be harmful but manufacturer advises avoid.

- HEPATIC IMPAIRMENT Manufacturer advises caution in mild to moderate impairment; avoid in severe impairment.

- RENAL IMPAIRMENT Avoid if possible or use with caution. Avoid in severe impairment.

Dose adjustments The lowest effective dose should be used for the shortest possible duration.

Monitoring In renal impairment monitor renal function; sodium and water retention may occur and renal function may deteriorate, possibly leading to renal failure.

- MEDICINAL FORMS There can be variation in the licensing of different medicines containing the same drug. Forms available from special-order manufacturers include: oral suspension

Oral suspension

CAUTIONARY AND ADVISORY LABELS 21

EXCIPIENTS: May contain Ethanol

▸ Mefenamic acid (Non-proprietary)
  Mefenamic acid 10 mg per 1 ml Mefenamic acid 50mg/5ml oral suspension | 125 ml PoM £179.00 DT = £179.00

Tablet

CAUTIONARY AND ADVISORY LABELS 21

▸ Mefenamic acid (Non-proprietary)
  Mefenamic acid 500 mg Mefenamic acid 500mg tablets | 28 tablet PoM £60.00 DT = £23.57 | 84 tablet PoM £77.00-£170.00
▸ Ponstan (Chemidex Pharma Ltd)
  Mefenamic acid 500 mg Ponstan Forte 500mg tablets | 100 tablet PoM £15.72

Capsule

CAUTIONARY AND ADVISORY LABELS 21

▸ Mefenamic acid (Non-proprietary)
  Mefenamic acid 250 mg Mefenamic acid 250mg capsules | 100 capsule PoM £60.10 DT = £23.89
▸ Ponstan (Chemidex Pharma Ltd)
  Mefenamic acid 250 mg Ponstan 250mg capsules | 100 capsule PoM £8.17 DT = £23.89

Meloxicam

18-Nov-2020

- **INDICATIONS AND DOSE**

Exacerbation of osteoarthritis (short-term)

▸ BY MOUTH
▸ Child 16–17 years: 7.5 mg once daily, then increased if necessary up to 15 mg once daily
▸ Adult: 7.5 mg once daily, then increased if necessary up to 15 mg once daily

Pain and inflammation in rheumatic disease | Ankylosing spondylitis

▸ BY MOUTH
▸ Child 16–17 years: 15 mg once daily, then reduced to 7.5 mg once daily if required
▸ Adult: 15 mg once daily, then reduced to 7.5 mg once daily if required
▸ Elderly: 7.5 mg once daily

Relief of pain and inflammation in juvenile idiopathic arthritis and other musculoskeletal disorders in children intolerant to other NSAIDs

▸ BY MOUTH
▸ Child 12–17 years (body-weight up to 50 kg): 7.5 mg once daily
▸ Child 12–17 years (body-weight 50 kg and above): 15 mg once daily

- UNLICENSED USE Expert sources advise that meloxicam may be used from the age of 12 years for the treatment of pain and inflammation in juvenile idiopathic arthritis and other musculoskeletal disorders in children intolerant to other NSAIDS, but it is not licensed for this age group.

- CONTRA-INDICATIONS Active gastro-intestinal bleeding · active gastro-intestinal ulceration · following coronary artery bypass graft surgery · history of gastro-intestinal bleeding related to previous NSAID therapy · history of gastro-intestinal perforation related to previous NSAID therapy · history of recurrent gastro-intestinal haemorrhage (two or more distinct episodes) · history of recurrent gastro-intestinal ulceration (two or more distinct episodes) · severe heart failure

CAUTIONS Allergic disorders · cardiac impairment (NSAIDs may impair renal function) · cerebrovascular disease · coagulation defects · connective-tissue disorders · dehydration (risk of renal impairment) · elderly (risk of serious side-effects and fatalities) · heart failure · history of gastro-intestinal disorders (e.g. ulcerative colitis, Crohn's disease) · ischaemic heart disease · may mask symptoms of infection · peripheral arterial disease · risk factors for cardiovascular events · uncontrolled hypertension

INTERACTIONS → Appendix 1: NSAIDs

SIDE-EFFECTS

Common or very common Constipation · diarrhoea · gastrointestinal discomfort · gastrointestinal disorders · headache · nausea · vomiting

Uncommon Anaemia · angioedema · burping · dizziness · drowsiness · electrolyte imbalance · fluid retention · flushing · haemorrhage · hepatic disorders · hypersensitivity · oedema · skin reactions · stomatitis · vertigo

Rare or very rare Acute kidney injury · asthma · conjunctivitis · leucopenia · mood altered · nightmare · palpitations · severe cutaneous adverse reactions (SCARs) · thrombocytopenia · tinnitus · vision disorders

Frequency not known Agranulocytosis · confusion · fertility decreased female · heart failure · increased risk of arterial thromboembolism · nephritis tubulointerstitial · nephrotic syndrome · photosensitivity reaction · renal necrosis

SIDE-EFFECTS, FURTHER INFORMATION For information about cardiovascular and gastrointestinal side-effects, and a possible exacerbation of symptoms in asthma, see Non-steroidal anti-inflammatory drugs. p. 1176

ALLERGY AND CROSS-SENSITIVITY EvGr Contra-indicated in patients with a history of hypersensitivity to aspirin or any other NSAID—which includes those in whom attacks of asthma, angioedema, urticaria or rhinitis have been precipitated by aspirin or any other NSAID. ⓜ

CONCEPTION AND CONTRACEPTION Caution—long-term use of some NSAIDs is associated with reduced female fertility, which is reversible on stopping treatment.

PREGNANCY Avoid unless the potential benefit outweighs the risk. Avoid during the third trimester (risk of closure of fetal ductus arteriosus *in utero* and possibly persistent pulmonary hypertension of the newborn); onset of labour may be delayed and duration may be increased.

BREAST FEEDING Use with caution during breast-feeding. Present in milk in *animal* studies—manufacturer advises avoid.

HEPATIC IMPAIRMENT Manufacturer advises caution in mild to moderate impairment; avoid in severe impairment.

RENAL IMPAIRMENT Avoid if possible or use with caution.
▸ In adults Avoid if eGFR less than 25 mL/minute/1.73 m^2.
▸ In children Avoid if estimated glomerular filtration rate less than 25 mL/minute/1.73 m^2.

Dose adjustments The lowest effective dose should be used for the shortest possible duration.

Monitoring In renal impairment monitor renal function; sodium and water retention may occur and renal function may deteriorate, possibly leading to renal failure.

MEDICINAL FORMS There can be variation in the licensing of different medicines containing the same drug. Forms available from special-order manufacturers include: oral suspension

Orodispersible tablet
▸ Meloxicam (Non-proprietary)
Meloxicam 7.5 mg Meloxicam 7.5mg orodispersible tablets sugar free sugar-free | 30 tablet PoM £25.50 DT = £25.50
Meloxicam 15 mg Meloxicam 15mg orodispersible tablets sugar free sugar-free | 30 tablet PoM £25.50 DT = £25.50

Tablet
CAUTIONARY AND ADVISORY LABELS 21
▸ Meloxicam (Non-proprietary)
Meloxicam 7.5 mg Meloxicam 7.5mg tablets | 30 tablet PoM £3.84 DT = £3.42
Meloxicam 15 mg Meloxicam 15mg tablets | 30 tablet PoM £7.29 DT = £6.11

Nabumetone

18-Nov-2020

● INDICATIONS AND DOSE

Pain and inflammation in osteoarthritis and rheumatoid arthritis
▸ BY MOUTH
▸ Adult: 1 g once daily, dose to be taken at night
▸ Elderly: 0.5–1 g daily

Pain and inflammation in osteoarthritis and rheumatoid arthritis (severe and persistent symptoms)
▸ BY MOUTH
▸ Adult: 0.5–1 g, dose to be taken in the morning and 1 g, dose to be taken at night
▸ Elderly: 0.5–1 g daily

● CONTRA-INDICATIONS Active gastro-intestinal bleeding · active gastro-intestinal ulceration · history of gastro-intestinal bleeding related to previous NSAID therapy · history of gastro-intestinal perforation related to previous NSAID therapy · history of recurrent gastro-intestinal haemorrhage (two or more distinct episodes) · history of recurrent gastro-intestinal ulceration (two or more distinct episodes) · severe heart failure

● CAUTIONS Allergic disorders · cardiac impairment (NSAIDs may impair renal function) · cerebrovascular disease · coagulation defects · connective-tissue disorders · dehydration (risk of renal impairment) · elderly (risk of serious side-effects and fatalities) · heart failure · history of gastro-intestinal disorders (e.g. ulcerative colitis, Crohn's disease) · ischaemic heart disease · may mask symptoms of infection · peripheral arterial disease · risk factors for cardiovascular events · uncontrolled hypertension

● INTERACTIONS → Appendix 1: NSAIDs

● SIDE-EFFECTS
▸ **Common or very common** Constipation · diarrhoea · ear disorder · gastrointestinal discomfort · gastrointestinal disorders · nausea · oedema · skin reactions · tinnitus
▸ **Uncommon** Anxiety · asthenia · confusion · dizziness · drowsiness · dry mouth · dyspnoea · eye disorder · haemorrhage · headache · hyperhidrosis · insomnia · myopathy · oral disorders · paraesthesia · photosensitivity reaction · respiratory disorders · urinary tract disorder · visual impairment · vomiting
▸ **Rare or very rare** Alopecia · angioedema · hepatic disorders · hypersensitivity · menorrhagia · nephrotic syndrome · pancreatitis · renal failure (more common in patients with pre-existing renal impairment) · severe cutaneous adverse reactions (SCARs) · thrombocytopenia
▸ **Frequency not known** Agranulocytosis · aplastic anaemia · asthma · Crohn's disease aggravated · depression · fertility decreased female · haemolytic anaemia · hallucination · heart failure · hypertension · increased risk of arterial thromboembolism · leucopenia · malaise · meningitis aseptic (patients with connective-tissue disorders such as systemic lupus erythematosus may be especially susceptible) · nephritis tubulointerstitial · neutropenia · optic neuritis · vertigo

SIDE-EFFECTS, FURTHER INFORMATION For information about cardiovascular and gastrointestinal side-effects, and a possible exacerbation of symptoms in asthma, see Non-steroidal anti-inflammatory drugs p. 1176

● ALLERGY AND CROSS-SENSITIVITY EvGr Contra-indicated in patients with a history of hypersensitivity to aspirin or

10

Musculoskeletal system

any other NSAID—which includes those in whom attacks of asthma, angioedema, urticaria or rhinitis have been precipitated by aspirin or any other NSAID. (M)

● CONCEPTION AND CONTRACEPTION Caution—long-term use of some NSAIDs is associated with reduced female fertility, which is reversible on stopping treatment.

● PREGNANCY Avoid unless the potential benefit outweighs the risk. Avoid during the third trimester (risk of closure of fetal ductus arteriosus *in utero* and possibly persistent pulmonary hypertension of the newborn); onset of labour may be delayed and duration may be increased.

● BREAST FEEDING Use with caution during breast-feeding. Manufacturer advises avoid.

● HEPATIC IMPAIRMENT Manufacturer advises caution in mild to moderate impairment; avoid in severe impairment.

● RENAL IMPAIRMENT Avoided if possible or use with caution. Avoid in severe impairment.
Dose adjustments The lowest effective dose should be used for the shortest possible duration.
Monitoring In renal impairment monitor renal function; sodium and water retention may occur and renal function may deteriorate, possibly leading to renal failure.

● MEDICINAL FORMS There can be variation in the licensing of different medicines containing the same drug.
Tablet
CAUTIONARY AND ADVISORY LABELS 21
▸ Nabumetone (Non-proprietary)
Nabumetone 500 mg Nabumetone 500mg tablets | 56 tablet [PoM]
£6.90 DT = £6.90

Naproxen

18-Nov-2020

● INDICATIONS AND DOSE

Pain and inflammation in rheumatic disease
▸ BY MOUTH
▸ Adult: 0.5–1 g daily in 1–2 divided doses

Pain and inflammation in musculoskeletal disorders | Dysmenorrhoea
▸ BY MOUTH
▸ Adult: Initially 500 mg, then 250 mg every 6–8 hours as required, maximum dose after the first day 1.25 g daily

Acute gout
▸ BY MOUTH
▸ Adult: Initially 750 mg, then 250 mg every 8 hours until attack has passed

Acute migraine
▸ BY MOUTH
▸ Adult: 500 mg for 1 dose, to be taken in combination with sumatriptan as soon as migraine symptoms develop

● UNLICENSED USE [EvGr] Naproxen is used for the treatment of acute migraine in combination with sumatriptan, (A) but is not licensed for this indication.

● CONTRA-INDICATIONS Active gastro-intestinal bleeding · active gastro-intestinal ulceration · history of gastro-intestinal bleeding related to previous NSAID therapy · history of gastro-intestinal perforation related to previous NSAID therapy · history of recurrent gastro-intestinal haemorrhage (two or more distinct episodes) · history of recurrent gastro-intestinal ulceration (two or more distinct episodes) · severe heart failure

● CAUTIONS Allergic disorders · cardiac impairment (NSAIDs may impair renal function) · cerebrovascular disease · coagulation defects · connective-tissue disorders · dehydration (risk of renal impairment) · elderly (risk of serious side-effects and fatalities) · heart failure · history of gastro-intestinal disorders (e.g. ulcerative colitis, Crohn's disease) · ischaemic heart disease · may mask symptoms of

infection · peripheral arterial disease · risk factors for cardiovascular events · uncontrolled hypertension

● INTERACTIONS → Appendix 1: NSAIDs

● SIDE-EFFECTS Agranulocytosis · alopecia · angioedema · aplastic anaemia · asthma · cognitive impairment · concentration impaired · confusion · constipation · cornea opacity · depression · diarrhoea · dizziness · drowsiness · dyspnoea · erythema nodosum · fatigue · gastrointestinal discomfort · gastrointestinal disorders · glomerulonephriti · haemolytic anaemia · haemorrhage · hallucination · headache · hearing impairment · heart failure · hepatic disorders · hyperhidrosis · hyperkalaemia · hypersensitivity · hypertension · increased risk of arterial thromboembolism · infertility female · inflammatory bowe disease · malaise · meningitis aseptic (patients with connective-tissue disorders such as systemic lupus erythematosus may be especially susceptible) · muscle weakness · myalgia · nausea · nephritis tubulointerstitial · nephropathy · neutropenia · oedema · optic neuritis · oral disorders · palpitations · pancreatitis · papillitis · papilloedema · paraesthesia · photosensitivity reaction · platelet aggregation inhibition · pulmonary oedema · rash pustular · renal failure (more common in patients with pre-existing renal impairment) · renal papillary necrosis · respiratory disorders · seizure · severe cutaneous adverse reactions (SCARs) · skin reactions · sleep disorders · thirst · thrombocytopenia · tinnitus · vasculitis · vertigo · visual impairment · vomiting

SIDE-EFFECTS, FURTHER INFORMATION For information about cardiovascular and gastrointestinal side-effects, and a possible exacerbation of symptoms in asthma, see Non-steroidal anti-inflammatory drugs. p. 1176

● ALLERGY AND CROSS-SENSITIVITY [EvGr] Contra-indicated in patients with a history of hypersensitivity to aspirin or any other NSAID—which includes those in whom attacks of asthma, angioedema, urticaria or rhinitis have been precipitated by aspirin or any other NSAID. (M)

● CONCEPTION AND CONTRACEPTION Caution—long-term use of some NSAIDs is associated with reduced female fertility, which is reversible on stopping treatment.

● PREGNANCY Avoid unless the potential benefit outweighs the risk. Avoid during the third trimester (risk of closure of fetal ductus arteriosus *in utero* and possibly persistent pulmonary hypertension of the newborn); onset of labour may be delayed and duration may be increased.

● BREAST FEEDING Use with caution during breast-feeding. Amount too small to be harmful but manufacturer advises avoid.

● HEPATIC IMPAIRMENT Manufacturer advises caution in mild to moderate impairment; avoid in severe impairment.
Dose adjustments Manufacturer advises consider dose reduction in mild to moderate impairment.

● RENAL IMPAIRMENT Avoid if possible or use with caution. Avoid if eGFR less than 30 mL/minute/1.73 m².
Dose adjustments The lowest effective dose should be used for the shortest possible duration.
Monitoring In renal impairment monitor renal function; sodium and water retention may occur and renal function may deteriorate, possibly leading to renal failure.

● NATIONAL FUNDING/ACCESS DECISIONS
For full details see funding body website
Scottish Medicines Consortium (SMC) decisions
▸ Naproxen (*Stirlescent*®) for the treatment of rheumatoid arthritis, osteoarthritis, ankylosing spondylitis, acute musculoskeletal disorders, dysmenorrhoea and acute gout in adults (June 2016) SMC No. 1154/16 Recommended with restrictions

● EXCEPTIONS TO LEGAL CATEGORY Can be sold to the public for the treatment of primary dysmenorrhoea in women aged 15–50 years subject to max. single dose of 500 mg, max. daily dose of 750 mg for max. 3 days, and a max. pack size of 9 × 250 mg tablets.

● MEDICINAL FORMS There can be variation in the licensing of different medicines containing the same drug. Forms available from special-order manufacturers include: oral suspension

Gastro-resistant tablet

CAUTIONARY AND ADVISORY LABELS 5, 25

▸ Naproxen (Non-proprietary)
Naproxen 250 mg Naproxen 250mg gastro-resistant tablets | 56 tablet [PoM] £10.97 DT = £7.64
Naproxen 375 mg Naproxen 375mg gastro-resistant tablets | 56 tablet [PoM] £27.78 DT = £27.77
Naproxen 500 mg Naproxen 500mg gastro-resistant tablets | 56 tablet [PoM] £23.79 DT = £15.08

▸ Naprosyn EC (Atnahs Pharma UK Ltd)
Naproxen 250 mg Naprosyn EC 250mg tablets | 56 tablet [PoM] £4.29 DT = £7.64
Naproxen 375 mg Naprosyn EC 375mg tablets | 56 tablet [PoM] £6.42 DT = £27.77
Naproxen 500 mg Naprosyn EC 500mg tablets | 56 tablet [PoM] £8.56 DT = £15.08

Tablet

CAUTIONARY AND ADVISORY LABELS 21

▸ Naproxen (Non-proprietary)
Naproxen 250 mg Naproxen 250mg tablets | 28 tablet [PoM] £5.26 DT = £2.49 | 56 tablet [PoM] £4.70
Naproxen 500 mg Naproxen 500mg tablets | 28 tablet [PoM] £8.14 DT = £2.86 | 56 tablet [PoM] £5.71

▸ Naprosyn (Atnahs Pharma UK Ltd)
Naproxen 250 mg Naprosyn 250mg tablets | 56 tablet [PoM] £4.29
Naproxen 500 mg Naprosyn 500mg tablets | 56 tablet [PoM] £8.56

Oral suspension

▸ Naproxen (Non-proprietary)
Naproxen 25 mg per 1 ml Naproxen 25mg/ml oral suspension sugar free sugar-free | 100 ml [PoM] £110.00 DT = £112.25
Naproxen 125mg/5ml oral suspension sugar free sugar-free | 100 ml [PoM] £110.00-£114.50 DT = £112.25
Naproxen 50 mg per 1 ml Naproxen 50mg/ml oral suspension | 100 ml [PoM] £45.01 DT = £45.01

Effervescent tablet

▸ Stirlescent (Stirling Anglian Pharmaceuticals Ltd)
Naproxen 250 mg Stirlescent 250mg effervescent tablets sugar-free | 20 tablet [PoM] £52.72 DT = £52.72

Naproxen with esomeprazole   17-Jul-2020

The properties listed below are those particular to the combination only. For the properties of the components please consider, naproxen p. 1194, esomeprazole p. 83.

● INDICATIONS AND DOSE

Patients requiring naproxen for osteoarthritis, rheumatoid arthritis, or ankylosing spondylitis, who are at risk of NSAID-associated duodenal or gastric ulcer and when treatment with lower doses of naproxen or other NSAIDs ineffective

▸ BY MOUTH
▸ Adult: 500/20 mg twice daily, dose expressed as x/y mg naproxen/esomeprazole

● INTERACTIONS → Appendix 1: NSAIDs · proton pump inhibitors

● PRESCRIBING AND DISPENSING INFORMATION Naproxen component is gastro-resistant.

● MEDICINAL FORMS There can be variation in the licensing of different medicines containing the same drug.

Modified-release tablet

CAUTIONARY AND ADVISORY LABELS 22, 25

▸ Vimovo (AstraZeneca UK Ltd)
Esomeprazole (as Esomeprazole magnesium trihydrate) 20 mg, Naproxen 500 mg Vimovo 500mg/20mg modified-release tablets | 60 tablet [PoM] £14.95 DT = £14.95

Piroxicam   18-Nov-2020

● INDICATIONS AND DOSE

Rheumatoid arthritis (initiated by a specialist) | Osteoarthritis (initiated by a specialist) | Ankylosing spondylitis (initiated by a specialist)

▸ BY MOUTH
▸ Adult: Up to 20 mg once daily

Pain relief in musculoskeletal conditions | Treatment in knee or hand osteoarthritis (adjunct)

▸ TO THE SKIN
▸ Adult: Apply 3–4 times a day, 0.5% gel to be applied; review treatment after 4 weeks

IMPORTANT SAFETY INFORMATION
CHMP ADVICE—PIROXICAM (JUNE 2007)

▸ With systemic use
The CHMP has recommended restrictions on the use of piroxicam because of the increased risk of gastro-intestinal side effects and serious skin reactions. The CHMP has advised that:

● piroxicam should be initiated only by physicians experienced in treating inflammatory or degenerative rheumatic diseases
● piroxicam should not be used as first-line treatment
● in adults, use of piroxicam should be limited to the symptomatic relief of osteoarthritis, rheumatoid arthritis, and ankylosing spondylitis
● piroxicam dose should not exceed 20 mg daily
● piroxicam should no longer be used for the treatment of acute painful and inflammatory conditions
● treatment should be reviewed 2 weeks after initiating piroxicam, and periodically thereafter
● concomitant administration of a gastro-protective agent should be considered.

Topical preparations containing piroxicam are not affected by these restrictions.

● CONTRA-INDICATIONS

▸ With systemic use Active gastro-intestinal bleeding · active gastro-intestinal ulceration · history of gastro-intestinal bleeding · history of gastro-intestinal perforation · history of gastro-intestinal ulceration · inflammatory bowel disease · severe heart failure

● CAUTIONS

▸ With systemic use Allergic disorders · cardiac impairment (NSAIDs may impair renal function) · cerebrovascular disease · coagulation defects · connective-tissue disorders · dehydration (risk of renal impairment) · elderly (risk of serious side-effects and fatalities) · heart failure · history of gastro-intestinal disorders · ischaemic heart disease · may mask symptoms of infection · peripheral arterial disease · risk factors for cardiovascular events · uncontrolled hypertension

▸ With topical use Avoid contact with eyes · avoid contact with inflamed or broken skin · avoid contact with mucous membranes · not for use with occlusive dressings · topical application of large amounts can result in systemic effects, including hypersensitivity and asthma (renal disease has also been reported)

● INTERACTIONS → Appendix 1: NSAIDs

● SIDE-EFFECTS

GENERAL SIDE-EFFECTS

▸ **Common or very common** Gastrointestinal discomfort · gastrointestinal disorders · nausea · skin reactions
▸ **Rare or very rare** Severe cutaneous adverse reactions (SCARs)
▸ **Frequency not known** Bronchospasm · dyspnoea · photosensitivity reaction

10

Musculoskeletal system

SPECIFIC SIDE-EFFECTS
► **Common or very common**
► With oral use Anaemia · appetite decreased · constipation · diarrhoea · dizziness · drowsiness · eosinophilia · headache · hyperglycaemia · leucopenia · oedema · rash (discontinue) · thrombocytopenia · tinnitus · vertigo · vomiting · weight changes
► **Uncommon**
► With oral use Hypoglycaemia · palpitations · stomatitis · vision blurred
► **Rare or very rare**
► With oral use Nephritis tubulointerstitial · nephrotic syndrome · renal failure · renal papillary necrosis
► **Frequency not known**
► With oral use Alopecia · angioedema · aplastic anaemia · confusion · depression · embolism and thrombosis · eye irritation · eye swelling · fertility decreased female · fluid retention · haemolytic anaemia · haemorrhage · hallucination · hearing impairment · heart failure · hepatic disorders · hypersensitivity · hypertension · malaise · mood altered · nervousness · onycholysis · pancreatitis · paraesthesia · sleep disorders · vasculitis

SIDE-EFFECTS, FURTHER INFORMATION For information about cardiovascular and gastrointestinal side-effects, and a possible exacerbation of symptoms in asthma, see Non-steroidal anti-inflammatory drugs. p. 1176
  Topical application of large amounts can result in systemic effects.

● ALLERGY AND CROSS-SENSITIVITY EvGr Contra-indicated in patients with a history of hypersensitivity to aspirin or any other NSAID—which includes those in whom attacks of asthma, angioedema, urticaria or rhinitis have been precipitated by aspirin or any other NSAID. ⓜ

● CONCEPTION AND CONTRACEPTION
► With systemic use Caution—long-term use of some NSAIDs is associated with reduced female fertility, which is reversible on stopping treatment.

● PREGNANCY
► With systemic use Avoid unless the potential benefit outweighs the risk. Avoid during the third trimester (risk of closure of fetal ductus arteriosus *in utero* and possibly persistent pulmonary hypertension of the newborn); onset of labour may be delayed and duration may be increased.
► With topical use Patient packs for topical preparations carry a warning to avoid during pregnancy.

● BREAST FEEDING
► With systemic use Use with caution during breast-feeding. Amount too small to be harmful.
► With topical use Patient packs for topical preparations carry a warning to avoid during breast-feeding.

● HEPATIC IMPAIRMENT
► With oral use Manufacturer advises caution.

● RENAL IMPAIRMENT
► With systemic use Avoid if possible or use with caution.
► With topical use Deterioration in renal function has also been reported after topical use.
  Dose adjustments ► With systemic use The lowest effective dose should be used for the shortest possible duration.
  Monitoring ► With systemic use In renal impairment monitor renal function; sodium and water retention may occur and renal function may deteriorate, possibly leading to renal failure.

● DIRECTIONS FOR ADMINISTRATION Piroxicam orodispersible tablets can be taken by placing on the tongue and allowing to dissolve or by swallowing.
► With topical use For topical preparations, manufacturer advises apply with gentle massage only.

● PRESCRIBING AND DISPENSING INFORMATION
► With topical use Caution—topical preparations not generally suitable for children.

● PATIENT AND CARER ADVICE
► With topical use For topical preparations, patients and their carers should be advised to wash hands immediately after use.
  Photosensitivity
► With topical use Patients should be advised against excessive exposure to sunlight of area treated in order to avoid possibility of photosensitivity.

● LESS SUITABLE FOR PRESCRIBING
► With oral use Piroxicam is less suitable for prescribing.

● MEDICINAL FORMS There can be variation in the licensing of different medicines containing the same drug.
Orodispersible tablet
CAUTIONARY AND ADVISORY LABELS 10, 21
EXCIPIENTS: May contain Aspartame
► Feldene Melt (Pfizer Ltd)
  Piroxicam 20 mg Feldene Melt 20mg tablets sugar-free | 30 tablet PoM £10.53 DT = £10.53
Gel
EXCIPIENTS: May contain Benzyl alcohol, propylene glycol
► Piroxicam (Non-proprietary)
  Piroxicam 5 mg per 1 gram Piroxicam 0.5% gel | 60 gram PoM £3.50 DT = £2.86 | 100 gram PoM £4.80 | 112 gram PoM £5.88 DT = £5.34
► Feldene (Pfizer Ltd)
  Piroxicam 5 mg per 1 gram Feldene 0.5% gel | 60 gram PoM £6.00 DT = £2.86 | 112 gram PoM £9.41 DT = £5.34
Capsule
CAUTIONARY AND ADVISORY LABELS 21
► Piroxicam (Non-proprietary)
  Piroxicam 10 mg Piroxicam 10mg capsules | 56 capsule PoM £5.77 DT = £4.90
  Piroxicam 20 mg Piroxicam 20mg capsules | 28 capsule PoM £5.76 DT = £5.14
► Feldene (Pfizer Ltd)
  Piroxicam 10 mg Feldene 10mg capsules | 30 capsule PoM £3.86
  Piroxicam 20 mg Feldene 20 capsules | 30 capsule PoM £7.71

Sulindac

18-Nov-2020

● INDICATIONS AND DOSE
Pain and inflammation in rheumatic disease and other musculoskeletal disorders | Acute gout
► BY MOUTH
► Adult: 200 mg twice daily for maximum duration 7–10 days in peri-articular disorders, dose may be reduced according to response; acute gout should respond within 7 days; maximum 400 mg per day

● CONTRA-INDICATIONS Active gastro-intestinal bleeding · active gastro-intestinal ulceration · history of gastro-intestinal bleeding related to previous NSAID therapy · history of gastro-intestinal perforation related to previous NSAID therapy · history of recurrent gastro-intestinal haemorrhage (two or more distinct episodes) · history of recurrent gastro-intestinal ulceration (two or more distinct episodes) · severe heart failure

● CAUTIONS Allergic disorders · cardiac impairment (NSAIDs may impair renal function) · cerebrovascular disease · coagulation defects · connective-tissue disorders · dehydration (risk of renal impairment) · elderly (risk of serious side-effects and fatalities) · heart failure · history of gastro-intestinal disorders (e.g. ulcerative colitis, Crohn's disease) · history of renal stones (ensure adequate hydration) · ischaemic heart disease · may mask symptoms of infection · peripheral arterial disease · risk factors for cardiovascular events · uncontrolled hypertension

● INTERACTIONS → Appendix 1: NSAIDs

● SIDE-EFFECTS Acute psychosis · agranulocytosis · alopecia · angioedema · appetite decreased · arrhythmia · asthenia · asthma · bone marrow disorders · cholecystitis · confusion · constipation · Crohn's disease aggravated · depression ·

diarrhoea · dizziness · drowsiness · dyspnoea · dysuria · eye disorder · fever · gastrointestinal discomfort · gastrointestinal disorders · gynaecomastia · haemolytic anaemia · haemorrhage · hallucination · headache · hearing loss · heart failure · hepatic disorders · hyperglycaemia · hyperhidrosis · hyperkalaemia · hypersensitivity · hypersensitivity vasculitis · hypertension · increased risk of arterial thromboembolism · increased risk of infection · insomnia · leucopenia · malaise · meningitis aseptic (patients with connective-tissue disorders such as systemic lupus erythematosus may be especially susceptible) · mucosal abnormalities · muscle weakness · nausea · nephritis tubulointerstitial · nephrotic syndrome · nerve disorders · nervousness · neutropenia · oedema · oral disorders · palpitations · pancreatitis · paraesthesia · photosensitivity reaction · psychiatric disorder · renal impairment · respiratory disorders · seizure · severe cutaneous adverse reactions (SCARs) · skin reactions · syncope · taste altered · thrombocytopenia · tinnitus · urine abnormalities · urine discolouration · vertigo · vision disorders · vomiting

SIDE-EFFECTS, FURTHER INFORMATION   For information about cardiovascular and gastrointestinal side-effects, and a possible exacerbation of symptoms in asthma, see Non-steroidal anti-inflammatory drugs. p. 1176

● ALLERGY AND CROSS-SENSITIVITY   EvGr   Contra-indicated in patients with a history of hypersensitivity to aspirin or any other NSAID—which includes those in whom attacks of asthma, angioedema, urticaria or rhinitis have been precipitated by aspirin or any other NSAID. ◈

● CONCEPTION AND CONTRACEPTION   Caution—long-term use of some NSAIDs is associated with reduced female fertility, which is reversible on stopping treatment.

● PREGNANCY   Avoid unless the potential benefit outweighs the risk. Avoid during the third trimester (risk of closure of fetal ductus arteriosus *in utero* and possibly persistent pulmonary hypertension of the newborn); onset of labour may be delayed and duration may be increased.

● BREAST FEEDING   Use with caution during breast-feeding.

● HEPATIC IMPAIRMENT   Manufacturer advises caution in mild to moderate impairment; avoid in severe impairment.

● RENAL IMPAIRMENT   Avoid if possible or use with caution. Avoid in severe impairment.

Dose adjustments   The lowest effective dose should be used for the shortest possible duration.

Monitoring   In renal impairment monitor renal function; sodium and water retention may occur and renal function may deteriorate, possibly leading to renal failure.

● MEDICINAL FORMS   There can be variation in the licensing of different medicines containing the same drug.

Tablet
CAUTIONARY AND ADVISORY LABELS   21
▸ Sulindac (Non-proprietary)
    Sulindac 100 mg   Sulindac 100mg tablets | 56 tablet PoM   £48.00
    DT = £29.79
    Sulindac 200 mg   Sulindac 200mg tablets | 56 tablet PoM   £96.00
    DT = £38.30

Tenoxicam
                             18-Nov-2020

● INDICATIONS AND DOSE

Pain and inflammation in rheumatic disease
▸ BY MOUTH
▸ Adult: 20 mg once daily
▸ BY INTRAVENOUS INJECTION, OR BY INTRAMUSCULAR INJECTION
▸ Adult: 20 mg once daily as initial treatment for 1–2 days if oral administration not possible

Pain and inflammation in acute musculoskeletal disorders
▸ BY MOUTH
▸ Adult: 20 mg once daily for 7 days; maximum duration of treatment 14 days (including treatment by intravenous or intramuscular injection)
▸ BY INTRAVENOUS INJECTION, OR BY INTRAMUSCULAR INJECTION
▸ Adult: 20 mg once daily as initial treatment for 1–2 days if oral administration not possible

● CONTRA-INDICATIONS   Active gastro-intestinal bleeding · active gastro-intestinal ulceration · history of gastro-intestinal bleeding related to previous NSAID therapy · history of gastro-intestinal perforation related to previous NSAID therapy · history of recurrent gastro-intestinal haemorrhage (two or more distinct episodes) · history of recurrent gastro-intestinal ulceration (two or more distinct episodes) · severe heart failure

● CAUTIONS   Allergic disorders · cardiac impairment (NSAIDs may impair renal function) · cerebrovascular disease · coagulation defects · connective-tissue disorders · dehydration (risk of renal impairment) · elderly (risk of serious side-effects and fatalities) · heart failure · history of gastro-intestinal disorders (e.g. ulcerative colitis, Crohn's disease) · ischaemic heart disease · may mask symptoms of infection · peripheral arterial disease · risk factors for cardiovascular events · uncontrolled hypertension

● INTERACTIONS   → Appendix 1: NSAIDs

● SIDE-EFFECTS
GENERAL SIDE-EFFECTS
▸ **Common or very common**   Constipation · Crohn's disease aggravated · diarrhoea · gastrointestinal discomfort · gastrointestinal disorders · haemorrhage · headache · nausea · vomiting
▸ **Uncommon**   Fatigue · oedema · skin reactions
▸ **Rare or very rare**   Asthma · bronchospasm · depression · dyspnoea · hyperglycaemia · nervousness · palpitations · pancreatitis · severe cutaneous adverse reactions (SCARs) · sleep disorders · vertigo · weight changes
▸ **Frequency not known**   Agranulocytosis · alopecia · anaemia · angioedema · aplastic anaemia · confusion · eosinophilia · fertility decreased female · haemolytic anaemia · nail disorder · nephritis tubulointerstitial · nephropathy · paraesthesia · photosensitivity reaction · platelet aggregation inhibition · purpura non-thrombocytopenic · renal failure (more common in patients with pre-existing renal impairment) · thrombocytopenia · tinnitus · vasculitis · vision disorders

SPECIFIC SIDE-EFFECTS
▸ **Common or very common**
▸ With oral use   Dizziness · dry mouth · oral disorders
▸ **Rare or very rare**
▸ With oral use   Embolism and thrombosis · metabolic disorder
▸ **Frequency not known**
▸ With oral use   Drowsiness · eye irritation · eye swelling
▸ With parenteral use   Appetite decreased · increased risk of arterial thromboembolism · increased risk of ischaemic stroke · increased risk of myocardial infarction · meningitis aseptic (patients with connective-tissue disorders such as systemic lupus erythematosus may be especially susceptible) · neutropenia · oral ulceration

SIDE-EFFECTS, FURTHER INFORMATION   For information about cardiovascular and gastrointestinal side-effects, and a possible exacerbation of symptoms in asthma, see Non-steroidal anti-inflammatory drugs. p. 1176

● ALLERGY AND CROSS-SENSITIVITY   EvGr   Contra-indicated in patients with a history of hypersensitivity to aspirin or any other NSAID—which includes those in whom attacks of asthma, angioedema, urticaria or rhinitis have been precipitated by aspirin or any other NSAID. ⓜ

- CONCEPTION AND CONTRACEPTION Caution—long-term use of some NSAIDs is associated with reduced female fertility, which is reversible on stopping treatment.
- PREGNANCY Avoid unless the potential benefit outweighs the risk. Avoid during the third trimester (risk of closure of fetal ductus arteriosus *in utero* and possibly persistent pulmonary hypertension of the newborn); onset of labour may be delayed and duration may be increased.
- BREAST FEEDING Use with caution during breast-feeding. Present in milk in *animal* studies.
- HEPATIC IMPAIRMENT Manufacturer advises caution in mild to moderate impairment; avoid in severe impairment.
- RENAL IMPAIRMENT Avoid if possible or use with caution. Avoid in severe impairment.
  Dose adjustments The lowest effective dose should be used for the shortest possible duration.
  Monitoring In renal impairment monitor renal function; sodium and water retention may occur and renal function may deteriorate, possibly leading to renal failure.

- MEDICINAL FORMS There can be variation in the licensing of different medicines containing the same drug.
  Powder and solvent for solution for injection
  ‣ Tenoxicam (Non-proprietary)
    Tenoxicam 20 mg Tenoxicam 20mg powder and solvent for solution for injection vials | 1 vial PoM £3.98
  Tablet
  CAUTIONARY AND ADVISORY LABELS 21
  ‣ Mobiflex (Mylan)
    Tenoxicam 20 mg Mobiflex 20mg tablets | 30 tablet PoM £13.42
    DT = £13.42

Tiaprofenic acid

18-Nov-2020

● **INDICATIONS AND DOSE**

Pain and inflammation in rheumatic disease and other musculoskeletal disorders
‣ BY MOUTH
‣ Adult: 300 mg twice daily

IMPORTANT SAFETY INFORMATION

CSM ADVICE

Following reports of **severe cystitis** the CSM has recommended that tiaprofenic acid should not be given to patients with urinary-tract disorders and should be stopped if urinary symptoms develop.

Patients should be advised to stop taking tiaprofenic acid and to report to their doctor promptly if they develop urinary-tract symptoms (such as increased frequency, nocturia, urgency, pain on urinating, or blood in urine).

- CONTRA-INDICATIONS Active bladder disease (or symptoms) · active gastro-intestinal bleeding · active gastro-intestinal ulceration · active prostate disease (or symptoms) · history of gastro-intestinal bleeding related to previous NSAID therapy · history of gastro-intestinal perforation related to previous NSAID therapy · history of recurrent gastro-intestinal haemorrhage (two or more distinct episodes) · history of recurrent gastro-intestinal ulceration (two or more distinct episodes) · history of recurrent urinary-tract disorders (if urinary symptoms develop discontinue immediately and perform urine tests and culture) · severe heart failure
- CAUTIONS Allergic disorders · cardiac impairment (NSAIDs may impair renal function) · cerebrovascular disease · coagulation defects · connective-tissue disorders · dehydration (risk of renal impairment) · elderly (risk of

serious side-effects and fatalities) · heart failure · history of gastro-intestinal disorders (e.g. ulcerative colitis, Crohn's disease) · ischaemic heart disease · may mask symptoms of infection · peripheral arterial disease · risk factors for cardiovascular events · uncontrolled hypertension

- INTERACTIONS → Appendix 1: NSAIDs
- SIDE-EFFECTS Agranulocytosis · alopecia · anaemia · angioedema · aplastic anaemia · appetite decreased · asthma · bladder pain · bronchospasm · confusion · constipation · Crohn's disease aggravated · cystitis · depression · diarrhoea · dizziness · drowsiness · dyspnoea · fatigue · fertility decreased female · fluid retention · gastrointestinal discomfort · gastrointestinal disorders · haemolytic anaemia · haemorrhage · hallucination · headache · heart failure · hepatic disorders · hypersensitivity · hypertension · increased risk of arterial thromboembolism · malaise · meningitis aseptic (patients with connective-tissue disorders such as systemic lupus erythematosus may be especially susceptible) · nausea · nephritis tubulointerstitial · nephropathy · neutropenia · oedema · optic neuritis · oral ulceration · pancreatitis · paraesthesia · photosensitivity reaction · renal failure (more common in patients with pre-existing renal impairment) · severe cutaneous adverse reactions (SCARs) · skin reactions · sodium retention · thrombocytopenia · tinnitus · urinary disorders · urinary tract inflammation · vertigo · visual impairment · vomiting

  SIDE-EFFECTS, FURTHER INFORMATION For information about cardiovascular and gastrointestinal side-effects, and a possible exacerbation of symptoms in asthma, see Non-steroidal anti-inflammatory drugs. p. 1176

- ALLERGY AND CROSS-SENSITIVITY EvGr Contra-indicated in patients with a history of hypersensitivity to aspirin or any other NSAID—which includes those in whom attacks of asthma, angioedema, urticaria or rhinitis have been precipitated by aspirin or any other NSAID. ⓜ
- CONCEPTION AND CONTRACEPTION Caution—long-term use of some NSAIDs is associated with reduced female fertility, which is reversible on stopping treatment.
- PREGNANCY Avoid unless the potential benefit outweighs the risk. Avoid during the third trimester (risk of closure of fetal ductus arteriosus *in utero* and possibly persistent pulmonary hypertension of the newborn); onset of labour may be delayed and duration may be increased.
- BREAST FEEDING Use with caution during breast-feeding. Amount too small to be harmful.
- HEPATIC IMPAIRMENT Manufacturer advises caution in mild to moderate impairment; avoid in severe impairment.
  Dose adjustments In elderly patients, manufacturer advises dose reduction to 200 mg twice daily in mild to moderate impairment.
- RENAL IMPAIRMENT Avoid if possible or use with caution. Avoid in severe impairment.
  Dose adjustments Reduce dose in mild or moderate impairment. The lowest effective dose should be used for the shortest possible duration.
  Monitoring In renal impairment monitor renal function; sodium and water retention may occur and renal function may deteriorate, possibly leading to renal failure.

- MEDICINAL FORMS There can be variation in the licensing of different medicines containing the same drug.
  Tablet
  CAUTIONARY AND ADVISORY LABELS 21
  ‣ Surgam (Sanofi)
    Tiaprofenic acid 300 mg Surgam 300mg tablets | 56 tablet PoM £14.95 DT = £14.95

tendon sheath and not directly into the tendon (due to the absence of a true tendon sheath and a high risk of rupture, the Achilles tendon should not be injected).

Hydrocortisone acetate p. 1200 or one of the synthetic analogues is generally used for local injection. Intra-articular corticosteroid injections can cause flushing and may affect the hyaline cartilage. Each joint should not usually be treated more than 4 times in one year.

Corticosteroid injections are also injected into soft tissues for the treatment of skin lesions.

For further information on corticosteroid use, see Corticosteroids, general use p. 709.

5   Soft tissue and joint disorders

5.1   Local inflammation of joints and soft tissue

> Other drugs used for Local inflammation of joints and soft tissue Prednisolone, p. 718

CORTICOSTEROIDS

Corticosteroids, inflammatory disorders

18-Sep-2020

Systemic corticosteroids

Short-term treatment with corticosteroids can help to rapidly decrease inflammatory symptoms of rheumatoid arthritis. [EvGr] Long-term treatment in patients with established rheumatoid arthritis should only be continued after evaluating the risks and all other treatments have been considered, see Rheumatoid arthritis p. 1140. Ⓐ

Polymyalgia rheumatica and *giant cell (temporal) arteritis* are always treated with corticosteroids. Relapse is common if therapy is stopped prematurely. Many patients require treatment for at least 2 years and in some patients it may be necessary to continue long-term low-dose corticosteroid treatment.

Polyarteritis nodosa and *polymyositis* are usually treated with corticosteroids.

Systemic lupus erythematosus is treated with corticosteroids when necessary using a similar dosage regimen to that for polyarteritis nodosa and polymyositis. Patients with pleurisy, pericarditis, or other systemic manifestations will respond to corticosteroids. It may then be possible to reduce the dosage; alternate-day treatment is sometimes adequate, and the drug may be gradually withdrawn. In some mild cases corticosteroid treatment may be stopped after a few months. Many mild cases of systemic lupus erythematosus do not require corticosteroid treatment. Alternative treatment with anti-inflammatory analgesics, and possibly chloroquine p. 655 or hydroxychloroquine sulfate p. 1144, should be considered.

Ankylosing spondylitis should not be treated with long-term corticosteroids; rarely, pulse doses may be needed and may be useful in extremely active disease that does not respond to conventional treatment.

For further information on corticosteroid use, see Corticosteroids, general use p. 709.

Local corticosteroid injections

Corticosteroids are injected locally for an anti-inflammatory effect. In inflammatory conditions of the joints, particularly in rheumatoid arthritis, they are given by intra-articular injection to relieve pain, increase mobility, and reduce deformity in one or a few joints; they can also provide symptomatic relief while waiting for disease-modifying antirheumatic drugs (DMARDs) to take effect. Full aseptic precautions are essential; infected areas should be avoided. Occasionally an acute inflammatory reaction develops after an intra-articular or soft-tissue injection of a corticosteroid. This may be a reaction to the microcrystalline suspension of the corticosteroid used, but must be distinguished from sepsis introduced into the injection site.

Smaller amounts of corticosteroids may also be injected directly into soft tissues for the relief of inflammation in conditions such as *tennis* or *golfer's elbow* or *compression neuropathies*. In *tendinitis*, injections should be made into the

Dexamethasone

18-Nov-2020

- **DRUG ACTION** Dexamethasone has very high glucocorticoid activity and insignificant mineralocorticoid activity.

- **INDICATIONS AND DOSE**

  Local inflammation of joints
  ▸ BY INTRA-ARTICULAR INJECTION
  ▸ **Adult:** 0.3–3.3 mg, where appropriate, dose may be repeated at intervals of 3–21 days according to response, dose given according to size—consult product literature

  Local inflammation of soft tissues
  ▸ BY LOCAL INFILTRATION
  ▸ **Adult:** 1.7–5 mg, dose given according to size—consult product literature, where appropriate may be repeated at intervals of 3–21 days, use the 3.3 mg/mL injection preparation for this dose

- **INTERACTIONS** → Appendix 1: corticosteroids

- **PREGNANCY** Dexamethasone readily crosses the placenta.

- **PRESCRIBING AND DISPENSING INFORMATION**
  Dexamethasone 3.8 mg/mL Injection has replaced dexamethasone 4 mg/mL Injection. All dosage recommendations for intravenous, intramuscular, intrarticular use or local infiltration; are given in units of dexamethasone base.

- **MEDICINAL FORMS** There can be variation in the licensing of different medicines containing the same drug. Forms available from special-order manufacturers include: capsule, oral suspension, oral solution, eye drops

  Solution for injection
  CAUTIONARY AND ADVISORY LABELS 10
  ▸ Dexamethasone (Non-proprietary)
    Dexamethasone (as Dexamethasone sodium phosphate) 3.3 mg per 1 ml Dexamethasone (base) 6.6mg/2ml solution for injection ampoules | 10 ampoule [PoM] £22.00–£24.04 DT = £24.04
    Dexamethasone (base) 6.6mg/2ml solution for injection vials | 5 vial [PoM] £24.00 DT = £24.00
    Dexamethasone (base) 3.3mg/1ml solution for injection ampoules | 5 ampoule [PoM] £12.00 | 10 ampoule [PoM] £12.00–£23.85 DT = £23.85
    Dexamethasone (as Dexamethasone sodium phosphate) 3.8 mg per 1 ml Dexamethasone (base) 3.8mg/1ml solution for injection vials | 10 vial [PoM] £19.99–£20.00 DT = £20.00

Hydrocortisone

F 711

23-Nov-2020

- DRUG ACTION Hydrocortisone has equal glucocorticoid and mineralocorticoid activity.

- **INDICATIONS AND DOSE**

HYDROCORTISTAB ®

Local inflammation of joints and soft-tissues
- ▸ BY INTRA-ARTICULAR INJECTION
- ▸ Adult: 5–50 mg, select dose according to size of patient and joint; where appropriate dose may be repeated at intervals of 21 days. Not more than 3 joints should be treated on any one day, for details consult product literature

- INTERACTIONS → Appendix 1: corticosteroids
- SIDE-EFFECTS Myocardial rupture (following recent myocardial infarction)

- MEDICINAL FORMS There can be variation in the licensing of different medicines containing the same drug.
Suspension for injection
- ▸ Hydrocortistab (Advanz Pharma)
Hydrocortisone acetate 25 mg per 1 ml Hydrocortistab 25mg/1ml suspension for injection ampoules | 10 ampoule [PoM] £68.72 DT = £68.72

Methylprednisolone

F 711

25-Sep-2020

- DRUG ACTION Methylprednisolone exerts predominantly glucocorticoid effects with minimal mineralcorticoid effects.

- **INDICATIONS AND DOSE**

DEPO-MEDRONE ®

Local inflammation of joints and soft tissues
- ▸ BY INTRA-ARTICULAR INJECTION
- ▸ Adult: 4–80 mg, select dose according to size; where appropriate dose may be repeated at intervals of 7–35 days, for details consult product literature

- INTERACTIONS → Appendix 1: corticosteroids
- SIDE-EFFECTS Angioedema · cataract · confusion · delusions · depressed mood · diarrhoea · dizziness · drug dependence · dyslipidaemia · embolism and thrombosis · epidural lipomatosis · gastrointestinal disorders · glucose tolerance impaired · hallucination · hepatitis · hiccups · hypopituitarism · increased insulin requirement · intracranial pressure increased · memory loss · metabolic acidosis · muscle weakness · myalgia · neuropathic arthropathy · peripheral oedema · psychiatric disorder · schizophrenia exacerbated · sterile abscess · suicidal ideation · vision loss · withdrawal syndrome

- PATIENT AND CARER ADVICE Patient counselling is advised for methylprednisolone tablets and injections (steroid card).

- MEDICINAL FORMS There can be variation in the licensing of different medicines containing the same drug.
Suspension for injection
CAUTIONARY AND ADVISORY LABELS 10
- ▸ Depo-Medrone (Pfizer Ltd)
Methylprednisolone acetate 40 mg per 1 ml Depo-Medrone 40mg/1ml suspension for injection vials | 1 vial [PoM] £3.44 DT = £3.44 | 10 vial [PoM] £34.04
Depo-Medrone 80mg/2ml suspension for injection vials | 1 vial [PoM] £6.18 DT = £6.18 | 10 vial [PoM] £61.39
Depo-Medrone 120mg/3ml suspension for injection vials | 1 vial [PoM] £8.96 DT = £8.96 | 10 vial [PoM] £88.81

Methylprednisolone with lidocaine

The properties listed below are those particular to the combination only. For the properties of the components please consider, methylprednisolone above, lidocaine hydrochloride p. 1406.

- **INDICATIONS AND DOSE**

Local inflammation of joints
- ▸ BY INTRA-ARTICULAR INJECTION
- ▸ Adult: 4–80 mg, dose adjusted according to size; where appropriate may be repeated at intervals of 7–35 days, for details consult product literature

- INTERACTIONS → Appendix 1: antiarrhythmics · corticosteroids

- MEDICINAL FORMS There can be variation in the licensing of different medicines containing the same drug.
Suspension for injection
- ▸ Depo-Medrone with Lidocaine (Pfizer Ltd)
Lidocaine hydrochloride 10 mg per 1 ml, Methylprednisolone acetate 40 mg per 1 ml Depo-Medrone with Lidocaine suspension for injection 2ml vials | 1 vial [PoM] £7.06 DT = £7.06 | 10 vial [PoM] £70.13
Depo-Medrone with Lidocaine suspension for injection 1ml vials | 1 vial [PoM] £3.94 DT = £3.94 | 10 vial [PoM] £38.88

Triamcinolone acetonide

F 711

25-Sep-2020

- DRUG ACTION Triamcinolone exerts predominantly glucocorticoid effects with minimal mineralcorticoid effect.

- **INDICATIONS AND DOSE**

ADCORTYL ® INTRA-ARTICULAR/INTRADERMAL

Local inflammation of joints and soft tissues
- ▸ BY INTRA-ARTICULAR INJECTION
- ▸ Adult: 2.5–15 mg, adjusted according to size (for larger doses use Kenalog ®). Where appropriate dose may be repeated when relapse occurs, for details consult product literature.
- ▸ BY INTRADERMAL INJECTION
- ▸ Adult: 2–3 mg, max. 5 mg at any one site (total max. 30 mg). Where appropriate may be repeated at intervals of 1–2 weeks, for details consult product literature

KENALOG ® VIALS

Local inflammation of joints and soft tissues
- ▸ BY INTRA-ARTICULAR INJECTION
- ▸ Adult: 5–40 mg (max. per dose 80 mg), for further details consult product literature, select dose according to size. For doses below 5 mg use Adcortyl ® Intra-articular/Intradermal injection, where appropriate dose may be repeated when relapse occurs.

- INTERACTIONS → Appendix 1: corticosteroids
- PATIENT AND CARER ADVICE Patient counselling is advised for triamcinolone acetonide injection (steroid card).

- MEDICINAL FORMS There can be variation in the licensing of different medicines containing the same drug.
Suspension for injection
CAUTIONARY AND ADVISORY LABELS 10
EXCIPIENTS: May contain Benzyl alcohol
- ▸ Adcortyl Intra-articular / Intradermal (Bristol-Myers Squibb Pharmaceuticals Ltd)
Triamcinolone acetonide 10 mg per 1 ml Adcortyl Intra-articular / Intradermal 50mg/5ml suspension for injection vials | 1 vial [PoM] £3.63 DT = £3.63
- ▸ Kenalog (Bristol-Myers Squibb Pharmaceuticals Ltd)
Triamcinolone acetonide 40 mg per 1 ml Kenalog Intra-articular / Intramuscular 40mg/1ml suspension for injection vials | 5 vial [PoM] £7.45 DT = £7.45

Triamcinolone hexacetonide

F 711 02-Nov-2020

DRUG ACTION Triamcinolone exerts predominantly glucocorticoid effects with minimal mineralcorticoid effects.

● INDICATIONS AND DOSE

Local inflammation of joints and soft-tissues (for details, consult product literature)

▸ BY INTRA-ARTICULAR INJECTION

▸ Adult: 2–20 mg, adjusted according to size of joint, no more than 2 joints should be treated on any one day, where appropriate, may be repeated at intervals of 3–4 weeks

▸ BY PERI-ARTICULAR INJECTION

▸ Adult: 10–20 mg, adjusted according to size of joint, no more than 2 joints should be treated on any one day

● CONTRA-INDICATIONS Consult product literature

● CAUTIONS Consult product literature

● INTERACTIONS → Appendix 1: corticosteroids

● SIDE-EFFECTS Protein catabolism

● PRESCRIBING AND DISPENSING INFORMATION Various strengths available from 'special order' manufacturers or specialist importing companies.

● MEDICINAL FORMS There can be variation in the licensing of different medicines containing the same drug.

Suspension for injection

EXCIPIENTS: May contain Benzyl alcohol

▸ Triamcinolone hexacetonide (Non-proprietary)

Triamcinolone hexacetonide 20 mg per 1 ml Triamcinolone hexacetonide 20mg/1ml suspension for injection ampoules | 10 ampoule [PoM] £120.00 DT = £120.00

5.2 Soft tissue disorders

Soft-tissue disorders

07-Jul-2020

Extravasation

Local guidelines for the management of extravasation should be followed where they exist or specialist advice sought.

Extravasation injury follows leakage of drugs or intravenous fluids from the veins or inadvertent administration into the subcutaneous or subdermal tissue. It must be dealt with **promptly** to prevent tissue necrosis.

Acidic or alkaline preparations and those with an osmolarity greater than that of plasma can cause extravasation injury; excipients including alcohol and polyethylene glycol have also been implicated. Cytotoxic drugs commonly cause extravasation injury. In addition, certain patients such as the very young and the elderly are at increased risk. Those receiving anticoagulants are more likely to lose blood into surrounding tissues if extravasation occurs, while those receiving sedatives or analgesics may not notice the early signs or symptoms of extravasation.

Extravasation prevention

Precautions should be taken to avoid extravasation; ideally, drugs likely to cause extravasation injury should be given through a central line and patients receiving repeated doses of hazardous drugs peripherally should have the cannula resited at regular intervals. Attention should be paid to the manufacturers' recommendations for administration. Placing a glyceryl trinitrate patch p. 233 distal to the cannula may improve the patency of the vessel in patients with small veins or in those whose veins are prone to collapse.

Patients should be asked to report any pain or burning at the site of injection immediately.

Extravasation management

If extravasation is suspected the infusion should be stopped immediately but the cannula should not be removed until after an attempt has been made to aspirate the area (through the cannula) in order to remove as much of the drug as possible. Aspiration is sometimes possible if the extravasation presents with a raised bleb or blister at the injection site and is surrounded by hardened tissue, but it is often unsuccessful if the tissue is soft or soggy.

Corticosteroids are usually given to treat inflammation, although there is little evidence to support their use in extravasation. Hydrocortisone p. 716 or dexamethasone p. 714 can be given either locally by subcutaneous injection or intravenously at a site distant from the injury.

Antihistamines and **analgesics** may be required for symptom relief.

The management of extravasation beyond these measures is not well standardised and calls for specialist advice. Treatment depends on the nature of the offending substance; one approach is to localise and neutralise the substance whereas another is to spread and dilute it.

The first method may be appropriate following extravasation of vesicant drugs and involves administration of an antidote (if available) and the application of cold compresses 3–4 times a day (consult specialist literature for details of specific antidotes). Spreading and diluting the offending substance involves infiltrating the area with physiological saline, applying warm compresses, elevating the affected limb, and administering hyaluronidase p. 1202. A saline flush-out technique (involving flushing the subcutaneous tissue with physiological saline) may be effective but requires specialist advice. Hyaluronidase should not be administered following extravasation of vesicant drugs (unless it is either specifically indicated or used in the saline flush-out technique). Dexrazoxane p. 983 is licensed for the treatment of anthracycline-induced extravasation.

Enzymes used in soft-tissue disorders

Collagenase

Collagenases are proteolytic enzymes that are derived from the fermentation of *Clostridium histolyticum* and have the ability to break down collagen.

Hyaluronidase

Hyaluronidase is used to render the tissues more readily permeable to injected fluids, e.g. for introduction of fluids by subcutaneous infusion (termed hypodermoclysis).

Rubefacients

Rubefacients act by counter-irritation. Pain, whether superficial or deep-seated, is relieved by any method that itself produces irritation of the skin. Topical rubefacient preparations may contain nicotinate and salicylate compounds, essential oils, capsicum, and camphor.

Topical NSAIDs

The use of a NSAID by mouth is effective for relieving musculoskeletal pain. Topical NSAIDs (e.g. felbinac p. 1185, ibuprofen p. 1186, ketoprofen p. 1190, and piroxicam p. 1195) may provide some relief of pain in musculoskeletal conditions; they can be considered as an adjunctive treatment in knee or hand osteoarthritis.

ENZYMES

| Hyaluronidase

24-Feb-2020

● INDICATIONS AND DOSE

Enhance permeation of subcutaneous or intramuscular injections

▸ BY SUBCUTANEOUS INJECTION, OR BY INTRAMUSCULAR INJECTION
▸ Adult: 1500 units, to be dissolved directly into the solution to be injected (ensure compatibility)

Enhance permeation of local anaesthetics

▸ BY LOCAL INFILTRATION
▸ Adult: 1500 units, to be mixed with the local anaesthetic solution

Enhance permeation of ophthalmic local anaesthetic

▸ TO THE EYE
▸ Adult: 15 units/mL, to be mixed with the local anaesthetic solution

Hypodermoclysis

▸ BY SUBCUTANEOUS INJECTION
▸ Adult: 1500 units, to be dissolved in 1 mL water for injections or 0.9% sodium chloride injection, administered before start of 500–1000 mL infusion fluid

Extravasation

▸ BY LOCAL INFILTRATION
▸ Adult: 1500 units, to be dissolved in 1 mL water for injections or 0.9% sodium chloride and infiltrated into affected area as soon as possible after extravasation

Haematoma

▸ BY LOCAL INFILTRATION
▸ Adult: 1500 units, to be dissolved in 1 mL water for injections or 0.9% sodium chloride and infiltrated into affected area

● CONTRA-INDICATIONS Avoid sites where infection is present · avoid sites where malignancy is present · do not apply direct to cornea · not for anaesthesia in unexplained premature labour · not for intravenous administration · not to be used to enhance the absorption and dispersion of dopamine and/or alpha-adrenoceptor agonists · not to be used to reduce swelling of bites · not to be used to reduce swelling of stings

● CAUTIONS
▸ When used for hypodermoclysis Elderly (control speed and total volume and avoid overhydration especially in renal impairment)

● SIDE-EFFECTS Oedema · periorbital oedema

● MEDICINAL FORMS There can be variation in the licensing of different medicines containing the same drug.

Powder for solution for injection

▸ Hyaluronidase (Non-proprietary)
Hyaluronidase 1500 unit Hyaluronidase 1,500unit powder for solution for injection ampoules | 10 ampoule [PoM] £136.55

Chapter 11
Eye

CONTENTS

11
Eye

Eye

30-Nov-2020

Eye treatment: drug administration

The structure of the eye is divided into two main parts: the anterior segment and the posterior segment. Drugs are most commonly administered to the anterior segment of the eye by topical application in the form of eye drops or ointments. When a higher drug concentration is required, and when wanting to achieve therapeutic drug concentrations to the posterior segment of the eye, administration by intravitreal injection, periocular injection, or by the systemic route may be necessary.

Eye drops and eye ointments

Eye drops are generally instilled into the pocket formed by gently pulling down the lower eyelid, blinking a few times to ensure even spread, and then closing the eye; in neonates and infants it may be more appropriate to administer the drop in the inner angle of the open eye. A small amount of eye ointment is applied similarly; blinking helps to spread it. EvGr Eye drops and ointments may cause temporary blurring of vision. If affected, patients should be warned not to drive or perform other skilled tasks until vision is clear.

When two different eye preparations are used at the same time of day, the patient should leave an interval of at least 5 minutes between the two, to allow the first to be fully absorbed; eye ointment should be applied after drops. Ⓜ

Systemic effects may arise from absorption of drugs into the general circulation either directly from the conjunctival sac or after the excess preparation has drained down through the tear ducts into the nasal cavity. The extent of systemic absorption following ocular administration is highly variable due to a number of factors (e.g. drainage, blink rate, tear turnover). Nasal drainage of drugs is associated with eye drops much more often than with eye ointments. Applying pressure on the lacrimal punctum for at least a minute after administering eye drops reduces nasolacrimal drainage and therefore decreases systemic absorption from the nasal mucosa.

Eye-drop dispenser devices are available to aid the instillation of eye drops from plastic bottles and some are prescribable on the NHS (consult Drug Tariff—see Part IXA - Appliances). Product-specific devices may be supplied by manufacturers—consult individual manufacturers for information. They are particularly useful in patients with poor manual dexterity (e.g. due to arthritis) or reduced vision.

Eye irrigation solutions

These are solutions for the irrigation of the conjunctival sac. They act mechanically to flush out irritants or foreign bodies as a first-aid treatment. Sterile sodium chloride 0.9% solution p. 1214 is usually used. Clean water will suffice in an emergency.

Other preparations administered to the eye

The intravitreal route is used to administer drug into the posterior segment of the eye for conditions such as macular oedema and age-related macular degeneration. The intracameral route can be used to deliver certain drugs to the anterior chamber, for example antibacterials after cataract surgery. These injections should only be used under specialist supervision.

Ophthalmic Specials

The Royal College of Ophthalmologists and the UK Ophthalmic Pharmacy Group have produced the Ophthalmic Special Order Products guidance to help prescribers and pharmacists manage and restrict the use of unlicensed eye preparations. 'Specials' should only be prescribed in situations where a licensed product is not suitable for a patient's needs. The Ophthalmic Special Order Products guidance can be accessed on the Royal College of Ophthalmologists website (www.rcophth.ac.uk).

Preservatives and sensitisers

Information on preservatives and substances identified as skin sensitisers is provided under Excipients statements in Medicinal form entries—see individual drug monographs. Very rarely, cases of corneal calcification have been reported with the use of phosphate-containing eye drops in patients with significantly damaged corneas—consult product literature for further information.

Eye preparations: control of microbial contamination

Preparations for the eye should be sterile when issued. Care should be taken to avoid contamination of the contents during use.

Eye preparations in multiple-application containers for use by the patient *at home* are normally discarded 4 weeks after first opening (unless otherwise stated by the manufacturer).

Multiple application eye preparations for use in *hospital general wards* are also normally discarded 4 weeks after first opening (unless otherwise stated by the manufacturer)— local practice may vary. Individual containers should be provided for each patient. A separate container should be supplied for each eye only if there are special concerns about contamination. Patients admitted with an eye infection should be supplied with a fresh container on admission. On discharge from hospital, eye preparations used during the hospital stay should be assessed for suitability (e.g. period of use, risk of contamination); if unsuitable, a fresh supply should be provided.

During formal *eye examinations* and in *eye surgery*, single-application containers should be used if possible to reduce the risk of contamination. There is a high-risk of cross-contamination in areas such as operating theatres, eye disease clinics, and ophthalmic accident and emergency departments, therefore all containers should be discarded after single patient use whether they are single- or multiple-application containers.

Compared to eye preparations containing a preservative, unpreserved eye preparations may have a shorter period of safe use; consult packaging and see Guidance on the in-use shelf life for eye drops and ointments for more information (www.sps.nhs.uk/articles/guidance-on-in-use-shelf-life-for-eye-drops-and-ointments/).

Contact lenses

Contact lenses are usually worn for their visual corrective function (e.g. myopia, astigmatism). There are two main types of lenses; hard (rigid or gas-permeable rigid) lenses or soft (hydrogel or hydrophilic) lenses. Soft lenses are the most popular type because they tend to be more comfortable, but they may not give the best vision.

Lenses are usually worn for a specified number of hours each day and removed for sleeping unless specifically designed for overnight wear. The risk of infectious and non-infectious keratitis is increased by extended continuous contact lens wear, and poor compliance with directions for use, daily cleaning, and disinfection.

Acanthamoeba keratitis, a painful and severe sight-threatening infection of the cornea, can be associated with ineffective lens cleaning and disinfection, the use of contaminated lens cases, or tap water coming into contact with the lenses. The condition, which is treated promptly by specialists, is especially associated with the use of soft lenses (particularly reusable or extended wear lenses).

Contact lenses and drug treatment

Unless medically indicated, soft lenses should be removed before instillation of the eye preparation. Alternatively, unpreserved drops can be used, as preservatives accumulate in soft lenses and can cause irritation. Eye drops, however, may be instilled while patients are wearing hard contact lenses but removal prior to instillation is still generally advised. Ointment preparations should never be used in conjunction with contact lens wear; oily eye drops can cause lens deposits and should also be avoided.

Many drugs given systemically can also have adverse effects on contact lens wear. These include drugs which can cause corneal oedema (e.g. oral contraceptives–particularly those with a higher oestrogen content), drugs which reduce eye movement and blink reflex (e.g. anxiolytics, sedative hypnotics, antihistamines, and muscle relaxants), drugs which reduce lacrimation (e.g. older generation antihistamines, phenothiazines and related drugs, some beta-blockers, diuretics, and tricyclic antidepressants), and drugs which increase lacrimation (including ephedrine hydrochloride p. 287 and hydralazine hydrochloride p. 194). Other drugs that may affect contact lens wear include isotretinoin p. 1314 (can decrease tolerance to contact lens), aspirin p. 132 (can cause irritation), and rifampicin p. 619 and sulfasalazine p. 47 (can discolour lenses).

1 Allergic and inflammatory eye conditions

Eye, allergy and inflammation

05-Jun-2020

Corticosteroids

Corticosteroids administered locally to the eye or given by mouth are effective for treating anterior segment inflammation, including that which results from surgery.

Topical corticosteroids are applied frequently for the first 24–48 hours; once inflammation is controlled, the frequency of application is reduced. They should normally only be used under expert supervision; three main dangers are associated with their use:

- a 'red eye', when the diagnosis is unconfirmed, may be due to herpes simplex virus, and a corticosteroid may aggravate the condition, leading to corneal ulceration, with possible damage to vision and even loss of the eye. Bacterial, fungal, and amoebic infections pose a similar hazard;
- 'steroid glaucoma' can follow the use of corticosteroid eye preparations in susceptible individuals;
- a 'steroid cataract' can follow prolonged use.

Combination products containing a corticosteroid with an anti-infective drug are sometimes used after ocular surgery to reduce inflammation and prevent infection; use of combination products is otherwise rarely justified.

Systemic corticosteroids may be useful for ocular conditions. The risk of producing a 'steroid cataract' increases with the dose and duration of corticosteroid use.

Intravitreal corticosteroids

An intravitreal implant containing dexamethasone p. 1207 (*Ozurdex*®) is licensed for the treatment of adults with macular oedema following either branch retinal vein occlusion or central retinal vein occlusion; it is also licensed for the treatment of adult patients with inflammation of the posterior segment of the eye presenting as non-infectious uveitis.

An intravitreal implant containing fluocinolone acetonide (*Iluvien*®) p. 1236 is licensed for the treatment of visual impairment associated with chronic diabetic macular oedema which is insufficiently responsive to available therapies; it is also licensed for the prevention of relapse in recurrent non-infectious uveitis affecting the posterior segment of the eye. It should be administered by specialists experienced in the use of intravitreal injections.

Eye care, other anti-inflammatory preparations

Other preparations used for the topical treatment of inflammation and allergic conjunctivitis include antihistamines, lodoxamide p. 1206, and sodium cromoglicate p. 1206.

Eye drops containing antihistamines, such as **antazoline** (with xylometazoline hydrochloride p. 1247 as *Otrivine-Antistin*®), azelastine hydrochloride p. 1205, epinastine hydrochloride p. 1205, ketotifen p. 1205, and olopatadine p. 1206, can be used for allergic conjunctivitis.

Sodium cromoglicate (sodium cromoglycate) and nedocromil sodium eye drops can be useful for vernal keratoconjunctivitis and other allergic forms of conjunctivitis.

Lodoxamide eye drops are used for allergic conjunctival conditions including seasonal allergic conjunctivitis.

Diclofenac sodium eye drops p. 1222 are also licensed for seasonal allergic conjunctivitis.

Non-steroidal anti-inflammatory eye drops are used for the prophylaxis and treatment of inflammation of the eye following surgery or laser treatment.

ciclosporin p. 1209 is licensed for severe keratitis in patients with dry eye disease, which has not improved despite treatment with tear substitutes.

Cenegermin p. 1210 is licensed for moderate to severe neurotrophic keratitis.

4.1   Allergic conjunctivitis

> **Other drugs used for Allergic conjunctivitis** Diclofenac sodium, p. 1222

ANTIHISTAMINES

Antazoline with xylometazoline

06-Apr-2020

● **INDICATIONS AND DOSE**

Allergic conjunctivitis
▸ TO THE EYE
▸ **Child 12-17 years:** Apply 2–3 times a day for maximum 7 days
▸ **Adult:** Apply 2–3 times a day for maximum 7 days

● CAUTIONS Angle-closure glaucoma · cardiovascular disease · diabetes mellitus · hypertension · hyperthyroidism · phaeochromocytoma · urinary retention

● INTERACTIONS → Appendix 1: antihistamines, sedating · sympathomimetics, vasoconstrictor

● SIDE-EFFECTS Drowsiness · eye irritation · headache · hyperhidrosis · hypertension · mydriasis · nausea · palpitations · vascular disorders · vision blurred

SIDE-EFFECTS, FURTHER INFORMATION Absorption of antazoline and xylometazoline may result in systemic side-effects.

● MEDICINAL FORMS There can be variation in the licensing of different medicines containing the same drug.
Eye drops
EXCIPIENTS: May contain Benzalkonium chloride, disodium edetate
▸ Otrivine Antistin (Thea Pharmaceuticals Ltd)
   Xylometazoline hydrochloride 500 microgram per 1 ml, Antazoline sulfate 5 mg per 1 ml Otrivine Antistin 0.5%/0.05% eye drops | 10 ml [P] £3.35 DT = £3.35

Azelastine hydrochloride

11-May-2020

● **INDICATIONS AND DOSE**

Seasonal allergic conjunctivitis
▸ TO THE EYE
▸ **Child 4-17 years:** Apply twice daily, increased if necessary to 4 times a day
▸ **Adult:** Apply twice daily, increased if necessary to 4 times a day

Perennial conjunctivitis
▸ TO THE EYE
▸ **Child 12-17 years:** Apply twice daily; increased if necessary to 4 times a day, maximum duration of treatment 6 weeks
▸ **Adult:** Apply twice daily; increased if necessary to 4 times a day, maximum duration of treatment 6 weeks

● INTERACTIONS → Appendix 1: antihistamines, non-sedating

● SIDE-EFFECTS
▸ **Common or very common** Eye irritation · taste bitter (if applied incorrectly)

● MEDICINAL FORMS There can be variation in the licensing of different medicines containing the same drug.
Eye drops
EXCIPIENTS: May contain Benzalkonium chloride, disodium edetate
▸ Optilast (Mylan)
   Azelastine hydrochloride 500 microgram per 1 ml Optilast 0.05% eye drops | 8 ml [PoM] £6.40 DT = £6.40

Epinastine hydrochloride

26-Mar-2020

● **INDICATIONS AND DOSE**

Seasonal allergic conjunctivitis
▸ TO THE EYE
▸ **Child 12-17 years:** Apply twice daily for maximum 8 weeks
▸ **Adult:** Apply twice daily for maximum 8 weeks

● SIDE-EFFECTS
▸ **Common or very common** Eye discomfort
▸ **Uncommon** Dry eye · eye disorders · headache · nasal irritation · rhinitis · taste altered · visual impairment

● MEDICINAL FORMS There can be variation in the licensing of different medicines containing the same drug.
Eye drops
EXCIPIENTS: May contain Benzalkonium chloride, disodium edetate
▸ Relestat (Allergan Ltd)
   Epinastine hydrochloride 500 microgram per 1 ml Relestat 500micrograms/ml eye drops | 5 ml [PoM] £9.90 DT = £9.90

Ketotifen

14-Dec-2020

● **INDICATIONS AND DOSE**

Seasonal allergic conjunctivitis
▸ TO THE EYE
▸ **Child 3-17 years:** Apply twice daily
▸ **Adult:** Apply twice daily

● INTERACTIONS → Appendix 1: antihistamines, sedating

● SIDE-EFFECTS
▸ **Common or very common** Eye discomfort · eye disorders · eye inflammation
▸ **Uncommon** Conjunctival haemorrhage · drowsiness · dry eye · dry mouth · headache · skin reactions · vision disorders
▸ **Frequency not known** Asthma exacerbated · facial swelling · oedema

● NATIONAL FUNDING/ACCESS DECISIONS
   For full details see funding body website
   All Wales Medicines Strategy Group (AWMSG) decisions
▸ Ketotifen (*Ketofall*®) for symptomatic treatment of seasonal allergic conjunctivitis (June 2020) AWMSG No. 3930 Recommended with restrictions

● MEDICINAL FORMS There can be variation in the licensing of different medicines containing the same drug.
Eye drops
EXCIPIENTS: May contain Benzalkonium chloride
▸ Ketofall (Scope Ophthalmics Ltd)
   Ketotifen (as Ketotifen hydrogen fumarate) 250 microgram per 1 ml Ketofall 0.25mg/ml eye drops 0.4ml unit dose | 30 unit dose [PoM] £6.95 DT = £6.95
▸ Zaditen (Thea Pharmaceuticals Ltd)
   Ketotifen (as Ketotifen fumarate) 250 microgram per 1 ml Zaditen 250micrograms/ml eye drops | 5 ml [PoM] £7.80 DT = £7.80

11

Eye

Olopatadine

25-Mar-2020

● INDICATIONS AND DOSE

Seasonal allergic conjunctivitis
▸ TO THE EYE
▹ Child 3-17 years: Apply twice daily for maximum 4 months
▹ Adult: Apply twice daily for maximum 4 months

● SIDE-EFFECTS
▸ **Common or very common** Asthenia · dry eye · eye discomfort · headache · nasal dryness · taste altered
▸ **Uncommon** Dizziness · eye disorders · eye inflammation · increased risk of infection · numbness · skin reactions · vision disorders
▸ **Frequency not known** Drowsiness · dyspnoea · malaise · nausea · vomiting

● MEDICINAL FORMS There can be variation in the licensing of different medicines containing the same drug.

Eye drops
EXCIPIENTS: May contain Benzalkonium chloride
▹ Olopatadine (Non-proprietary)
Olopatadine (as Olopatadine hydrochloride) 1 mg per 1 ml Olopatadine 1mg/ml eye drops | 5 ml [PoM] £6.09 DT = £4.68
▹ Opatanol (Novartis Pharmaceuticals UK Ltd)
Olopatadine (as Olopatadine hydrochloride) 1 mg per 1 ml Opatanol 1mg/ml eye drops | 5 ml [PoM] £4.68 DT = £4.68

MAST-CELL STABILISERS

Lodoxamide

06-Apr-2020

● INDICATIONS AND DOSE

Allergic conjunctivitis
▸ TO THE EYE
▹ Child 4-17 years: Apply 4 times a day, improvement of symptoms may sometimes require treatment for up to 4 weeks
▹ Adult: Apply 4 times a day, improvement of symptoms may sometimes require treatment for up to 4 weeks

● SIDE-EFFECTS
▸ **Common or very common** Dry eye · eye discomfort · eye disorders · vision disorders
▸ **Uncommon** Corneal deposits · dizziness · eye inflammation · headache · nausea
▸ **Rare or very rare** Nasal complaints · rash · taste altered
● EXCEPTIONS TO LEGAL CATEGORY Lodoxamide 0.1% eye drops can be sold to the public for treatment of allergic conjunctivitis in adults and children over 4 years.

● MEDICINAL FORMS There can be variation in the licensing of different medicines containing the same drug.

Eye drops
EXCIPIENTS: May contain Benzalkonium chloride, disodium edetate
▹ Alomide (Novartis Pharmaceuticals UK Ltd)
Lodoxamide (as Lodoxamide trometamol) 1 mg per 1 ml Alomide 0.1% eye drops | 10 ml [PoM] £5.21 DT = £5.21

Sodium cromoglicate

23-Nov-2020

● INDICATIONS AND DOSE

Allergic conjunctivitis | Seasonal keratoconjunctivitis
▸ TO THE EYE
▹ Child: Apply 4 times a day
▹ Adult: Apply 4 times a day

● SIDE-EFFECTS Eye stinging
● EXCEPTIONS TO LEGAL CATEGORY Sodium cromoglicate 2% eye drops can be sold to the public (in max. pack size of

10 mL) for treatment of acute seasonal and perennial allergic conjunctivitis.

● MEDICINAL FORMS There can be variation in the licensing of different medicines containing the same drug.

Eye drops
▹ Sodium cromoglicate (Non-proprietary)
Sodium cromoglicate 20 mg per 1 ml Sodium cromoglicate 2% eye drops | 13.5 ml [PoM] £13.83 DT = £11.57
Vividrin 2% eye drops 0.5ml unit dose preservative free | 20 unit dose [PoM] ⬛
▹ Opticrom (Sanofi)
Sodium cromoglicate 20 mg per 1 ml Opticrom Aqueous 2% eye drops | 13.5 ml [PoM] £8.03 DT = £11.57

1.2 Inflammatory eye conditions

Other drugs used for Inflammatory eye conditions
Adalimumab, p. 1157 · Fluocinolone acetonide, p. 1236

ANALGESICS ❭ NON-STEROIDAL ANTI-INFLAMMATORY DRUGS

Nepafenac

26-Aug-2020

● INDICATIONS AND DOSE

Prophylaxis and treatment of postoperative pain and inflammation associated with cataract surgery | Reduction in the risk of postoperative macular oedema associated with cataract surgery in diabetic patients
▸ TO THE EYE
▹ Adult: (consult product literature)

● CAUTIONS Avoid sunlight · corneal epithelial breakdown (if evidence of, then discontinue immediately) · may mask symptoms of infection
● INTERACTIONS → Appendix 1: NSAIDs
● SIDE-EFFECTS
▸ **Uncommon** Eye discomfort · eye disorders · eye inflammation
▸ **Rare or very rare** Allergic dermatitis · corneal deposits · dizziness · dry eye · headache · nausea
▸ **Frequency not known** Cutis laxa · vision disorders · vomiting
● NATIONAL FUNDING/ACCESS DECISIONS
For full details see funding body website

Scottish Medicines Consortium (SMC) decisions
▸ Nepafenac (*Nevanac*®) 3 mg/mL eye drops for the reduction in risk of postoperative macular oedema associated with cataract surgery in diabetic patients (May 2017)
SMC No. 1228/17 Recommended

● MEDICINAL FORMS There can be variation in the licensing of different medicines containing the same drug.

Eye drops
EXCIPIENTS: May contain Benzalkonium chloride, disodium edetate
▹ Nevanac (Novartis Pharmaceuticals UK Ltd)
Nepafenac 1 mg per 1 ml Nevanac 1mg/ml eye drops | 5 ml [PoM] £14.92 DT = £14.92
Nepafenac 3 mg per 1 ml Nevanac 3mg/ml eye drops | 3 ml [PoM] £14.92 DT = £14.92

CORTICOSTEROIDS

F 711

Betamethasone

07-Dec-2020

> DRUG ACTION Betamethasone has very high glucocorticoid activity and insignificant mineralocorticoid activity.

● INDICATIONS AND DOSE

Local treatment of inflammation (short-term)

▶ TO THE EYE USING EYE DROP

▶ Child: Apply every 1–2 hours until controlled then reduce frequency

▶ Adult: Apply every 1–2 hours until controlled then reduce frequency

● INTERACTIONS → Appendix 1: corticosteroids

● SIDE-EFFECTS Vision disorders

● MEDICINAL FORMS There can be variation in the licensing of different medicines containing the same drug.

Ear/eye/nose drops solution

EXCIPIENTS: May contain Benzalkonium chloride, disodium edetate

▶ Betnesol (RPH Pharmaceuticals AB)
Betamethasone sodium phosphate 1 mg per 1 ml Betnesol 0.1% eye/ear/nose drops | 10 ml [PoM] £2.32 DT = £2.32

▶ Vistamethasone (Martindale Pharmaceuticals Ltd)
Betamethasone sodium phosphate 1 mg per 1 ml Vistamethasone 0.1% ear/eye/nose drops | 5 ml [PoM] £1.02 | 10 ml [PoM] £1.16 DT = £2.32

Combinations available: *Betamethasone with neomycin,* p. 1208

F 711

Dexamethasone

18-Nov-2020

> DRUG ACTION Dexamethasone has very high glucocorticoid activity and insignificant mineralocorticoid activity.

● INDICATIONS AND DOSE

Local treatment of inflammation (short-term)

▶ TO THE EYE USING EYE DROP

▶ Child: Apply 4–6 times a day

▶ Adult: Apply every 30–60 minutes until controlled, then reduced to 4–6 times a day

Short term local treatment of inflammation (severe conditions)

▶ TO THE EYE USING EYE DROP

▶ Child: Apply every 30–60 minutes until controlled, reduce frequency when control achieved

Macular oedema following either branch retinal vein occlusion or central retinal vein occlusion (specialist use only) | Visual impairment due to diabetic macular oedema in adults who are pseudophakic, or who are insufficiently responsive to, or unsuitable for non-corticosteroid therapy (specialist use only) | For the treatment of inflammation of the posterior segment of the eye presenting as non-infectious uveitis (specialist use only)

▶ BY INTRAVITREAL INJECTION

▶ Adult: 700 micrograms, to be administered into the affected eye, concurrent administration to both eyes not recommended. For further information on pre-treatment, administration and repeat dosing, consult product literature

● UNLICENSED USE *Maxidex*® not licensed for use in children under 2 years. *Dropodex*® not licensed for use in children.

● CONTRA-INDICATIONS

▶ With intravitreal use Active ocular herpes simplex · active or suspected ocular infection · active or suspected periocular infection · rupture of the posterior lens capsule in patients with aphakia, iris or transscleral fixated intra-ocular lens or anterior chamber intra-ocular lens · uncontrolled advanced glaucoma

● CAUTIONS

▶ With intravitreal use history of ocular viral infection (including herpes simplex) · posterior capsule tear or iris defect (risk of implant migration into the anterior chamber which may cause corneal oedema and, in persistent severe cases, the need for corneal transplantation) · retinal vein occlusion with significant retinal ischaemia

● INTERACTIONS → Appendix 1: corticosteroids

● SIDE-EFFECTS

▶ **Common or very common**

▶ When used by eye (topical) Eye discomfort

▶ With intravitreal use Eye discomfort

▶ **Uncommon**

▶ When used by eye (topical) Photophobia · taste altered

▶ With intravitreal use Retinitis necrotising

● PREGNANCY Dexamethasone readily crosses the placenta.

▶ With intravitreal use Manufacturer advises avoid unless potential benefit outweighs risk—no information available.

● BREAST FEEDING

▶ With intravitreal use Manufacturer advises avoid unless potential benefit outweighs risk—no information available.

● MONITORING REQUIREMENTS

▶ With intravitreal use Monitor intra-ocular pressure and for signs of ocular infection. In patients with posterior capsule tear or iris defect monitor for implant migration to allow for; early diagnosis and management.

● PRESCRIBING AND DISPENSING INFORMATION

▶ When used by eye Although multi-dose dexamethasone eye drops commonly contain preservatives, preservative-free unit dose vials may be available.

● NATIONAL FUNDING/ACCESS DECISIONS

For full details see funding body website

NICE decisions

▶ **Dexamethasone intravitreal implant for the treatment of macular oedema secondary to retinal vein occlusion (July 2011)** NICE TA229 Recommended

▶ **Dexamethasone intravitreal implant for treating diabetic macular oedema (July 2015)** NICE TA349 Recommended with restrictions

▶ **Adalimumab and dexamethasone for treating non-infectious uveitis (July 2017)** NICE TA460 Recommended

Scottish Medicines Consortium (SMC) decisions

▶ **Dexamethasone intravitreal implant (*Ozurdex*®) for the treatment of adult patients with macular oedema following either branch retinal vein occlusion (BRVO) or central retinal vein occlusion (CRVO) (June 2012)** SMC No. 652/10 Recommended with restrictions

● MEDICINAL FORMS There can be variation in the licensing of different medicines containing the same drug. Forms available from special-order manufacturers include: eye drops

Eye drops

EXCIPIENTS: May contain Benzalkonium chloride, disodium edetate, polysorbates

▶ Dexamethasone (Non-proprietary)
Dexamethasone sodium phosphate 1 mg per 1 ml Minims dexamethasone 0.1% eye drops 0.5ml unit dose | 20 unit dose [PoM] £11.46 DT = £11.46

▶ Dexafree (Thea Pharmaceuticals Ltd)
Dexamethasone sodium phosphate 1 mg per 1 ml Dexafree 1mg/1ml eye drops 0.4ml unit dose | 30 unit dose [PoM] £9.70

▶ Dropodex (Rayner Pharmaceuticals Ltd)
Dexamethasone sodium phosphate 1 mg per 1 ml Dropodex 0.1% eye drops 0.4ml unit dose | 20 unit dose [PoM] £10.48 DT = £10.48

11

Eye

- Eythalm (Aspire Pharma Ltd)
  Dexamethasone 1 mg per 1 ml Eythalm 1mg/ml eye drops | 6 ml [PoM] £9.75 DT = £9.75
- Maxidex (Novartis Pharmaceuticals UK Ltd)
  Dexamethasone 1 mg per 1 ml Maxidex 0.1% eye drops | 5 ml [PoM] £1.42 DT = £1.42 | 10 ml [PoM] £2.80 DT = £2.80

Implant
- Ozurdex (Allergan Ltd)
  Dexamethasone 700 microgram Ozurdex 700microgram intravitreal implant in applicator | 1 device [PoM] £870.00 (Hospital only)

Combinations available: *Dexamethasone with framycetin sulfate and gramicidin,* p. 1209 · *Dexamethasone with hypromellose, neomycin and polymyxin B sulfate,* p. 1209 · *Dexamethasone with tobramycin,* p. 1209

Eye

Fluorometholone

25-Sep-2020

- **INDICATIONS AND DOSE**

Local treatment of inflammation (short term)
- ▶ TO THE EYE
- ▸ Child 2-17 years: Apply every 1 hour for 24–48 hours, then reduced to 2–4 times a day
- ▸ Adult: Apply every 1 hour for 24–48 hours, then reduced to 2–4 times a day

---

IMPORTANT SAFETY INFORMATION

MHRA/CHM ADVICE: CORTICOSTEROIDS: RARE RISK OF CENTRAL SEROUS CHORIORETINOPATHY WITH LOCAL AS WELL AS SYSTEMIC ADMINISTRATION (AUGUST 2017)

NHS IMPROVEMENT PATIENT SAFETY ALERT: STEROID EMERGENCY CARD TO SUPPORT EARLY RECOGNITION AND TREATMENT OF ADRENAL CRISIS IN ADULTS (AUGUST 2020)
See Corticosteroids, general use p. 709.

- **SIDE-EFFECTS** Cataract · eye discomfort · eye disorders · eye infection · eye inflammation · rash · taste altered · vision disorders

- **MEDICINAL FORMS** There can be variation in the licensing of different medicines containing the same drug.
  Eye drops
  EXCIPIENTS: May contain Benzalkonium chloride, disodium edetate, polysorbates
  - FML Liquifilm (Allergan Ltd)
    Fluorometholone 1 mg per 1 ml FML Liquifilm 0.1% ophthalmic suspension | 5 ml [PoM] £1.71 DT = £1.71 | 10 ml [PoM] £2.95 DT = £2.95

F 711

Hydrocortisone

23-Nov-2020

- **DRUG ACTION** Hydrocortisone has equal glucocorticoid and mineralocorticoid activity.

- **INDICATIONS AND DOSE**

Local treatment of conjunctival inflammation (short-term)
- ▶ TO THE EYE
- ▸ Adult: Apply 2 drops 2–4 times a day for up to 14 days, to avoid relapse, frequency may be gradually reduced to once every other day

- **INTERACTIONS** → Appendix 1: corticosteroids
- **SIDE-EFFECTS** Eye stinging

- **MEDICINAL FORMS** There can be variation in the licensing of different medicines containing the same drug.
  Eye drops
  EXCIPIENTS: May contain Disodium edetate
  - Softacort (Thea Pharmaceuticals Ltd)
    Hydrocortisone sodium phosphate 3.35 mg per 1 ml Softacort 3.35mg/ml eye drops 0.4ml unit dose | 30 unit dose [PoM] £10.99 DT = £10.99

F 711

Prednisolone

06-Oct-2020

- **DRUG ACTION** Prednisolone exerts predominantly glucocorticoid effects with minimal mineralocorticoid effects.

- **INDICATIONS AND DOSE**

Local treatment of inflammation (short-term)
- ▶ TO THE EYE
- ▸ Child: Apply every 1–2 hours until controlled then reduce frequency
- ▸ Adult: Apply every 1–2 hours until controlled then reduce frequency

- **UNLICENSED USE** *Pred Forte®* not licensed for use in children (age range not specified by manufacturer).
- **INTERACTIONS** → Appendix 1: corticosteroids
- **SIDE-EFFECTS** Eye discomfort · taste altered · visual impairment
- **PREGNANCY** As it crosses the placenta 88% of prednisolone is inactivated.
- **PRESCRIBING AND DISPENSING INFORMATION** Although multi-dose prednisolone eye drops commonly contain preservatives, preservative-free unit dose vials may be available.

- **MEDICINAL FORMS** There can be variation in the licensing of different medicines containing the same drug. Forms available from special-order manufacturers include: eye drops
  Eye drops
  EXCIPIENTS: May contain Benzalkonium chloride, disodium edetate, polysorbates
  - Prednisolone (Non-proprietary)
    Prednisolone sodium phosphate 5 mg per 1 ml Minims prednisolone sodium phosphate 0.5% eye drops 0.5ml unit dose | 20 unit dose [PoM] £12.25 DT = £12.25
  - Pred Forte (Allergan Ltd)
    Prednisolone acetate 10 mg per 1 ml Pred Forte 1% eye drops | 5 ml [PoM] £1.82 DT = £1.82 | 10 ml [PoM] £3.66 DT = £3.66
  Ear/eye drops solution
  EXCIPIENTS: May contain Benzalkonium chloride, disodium edetate
  - Prednisolone (Non-proprietary)
    Prednisolone sodium phosphate 5 mg per 1 ml Prednisolone sodium phosphate 0.5% ear/eye drops | 10 ml [PoM] £2.57 DT = £2.57

CORTICOSTEROIDS > COMBINATIONS WITH ANTI-INFECTIVES

Betamethasone with neomycin

18-Nov-2020

The properties listed below are those particular to the combination only. For the properties of the components please consider, betamethasone p. 1207, neomycin sulfate p. 546.

- **INDICATIONS AND DOSE**

Local treatment of eye inflammation and bacterial infection (short-term)
- ▶ TO THE EYE USING EYE DROP
- ▸ Adult: Apply up to 6 times a day

- **INTERACTIONS** → Appendix 1: corticosteroids · neomycin
- **LESS SUITABLE FOR PRESCRIBING** Betamethasone with neomycin eye-drops are less suitable for prescribing.

MEDICINAL FORMS There can be variation in the licensing of different medicines containing the same drug.

Ear/eye/nose drops solution
EXCIPIENTS: May contain Benzalkonium chloride, disodium edetate
▸ Betnesol-N (RPH Pharmaceuticals AB)
   Betamethasone (as Betamethasone sodium phosphate) 1 mg per 1 ml, Neomycin sulfate 5 mg per 1 ml Betnesol-N ear/eye/nose drops | 10 ml PoM £2.39 DT = £2.39

Dexamethasone with framycetin sulfate and gramicidin
25-Sep-2020

The properties listed below are those particular to the combination only. For the properties of the components please consider, dexamethasone p. 1207, framycetin sulfate p. 1239.

● INDICATIONS AND DOSE

Local treatment of inflammation (short-term)
▸ TO THE EYE
▸ Child: Apply 4–6 times a day, may be administered every 30–60 minutes in severe conditions until controlled, then reduce frequency
▸ Adult: Apply 4–6 times a day, may be administered every 30–60 minutes in severe conditions until controlled, then reduce frequency

● CAUTIONS Avoid prolonged use
● INTERACTIONS → Appendix 1: corticosteroids
● LESS SUITABLE FOR PRESCRIBING *Sofradex®* is less suitable for prescribing.

● MEDICINAL FORMS There can be variation in the licensing of different medicines containing the same drug.

Ear/eye drops solution
EXCIPIENTS: May contain Polysorbates
▸ Sofradex (Sanofi)
   Gramicidin 50 microgram per 1 ml, Dexamethasone (as Dexamethasone sodium metasulfobenzoate) 500 microgram per 1 ml, Framycetin sulfate 5 mg per 1 ml Sofradex ear/eye drops | 8 ml PoM £7.50

Dexamethasone with hypromellose, neomycin and polymyxin B sulfate
14-Dec-2020

The properties listed below are those particular to the combination only. For the properties of the components please consider, dexamethasone p. 1207, neomycin sulfate p. 546.

● INDICATIONS AND DOSE

Local treatment of inflammation (short-term)
▸ TO THE EYE USING EYE DROP
▸ Adult: Apply every 30–60 minutes until controlled, then reduced to 4–6 times a day

Local treatment of inflammation (short-term)
▸ TO THE EYE USING EYE OINTMENT
▸ Adult: Apply 3–4 times a day, alternatively, apply at night when used with eye drops

● INTERACTIONS → Appendix 1: corticosteroids · neomycin · polymyxin b
● LESS SUITABLE FOR PRESCRIBING Dexamethasone with neomycin and polymixin B sulfate is less suitable for prescribing.

● MEDICINAL FORMS There can be variation in the licensing of different medicines containing the same drug.

Eye ointment
EXCIPIENTS: May contain Hydroxybenzoates (parabens), woolfat and related substances (including lanolin)
▸ Maxitrol (Novartis Pharmaceuticals UK Ltd)
   Dexamethasone 1 mg per 1 gram, Neomycin (as Neomycin sulfate) 3500 unit per 1 gram, Polymyxin B sulfate 6000 unit per 1 gram Maxitrol eye ointment | 3.5 gram PoM £1.44

Eye drops
EXCIPIENTS: May contain Benzalkonium chloride, polysorbates
▸ Maxitrol (Novartis Pharmaceuticals UK Ltd)
   Dexamethasone 1 mg per 1 ml, Hypromellose 5 mg per 1 ml, Neomycin (as Neomycin sulfate) 3500 unit per 1 ml, Polymyxin B sulfate 6000 unit per 1 ml Maxitrol eye drops | 5 ml PoM £1.68

Dexamethasone with tobramycin

The properties listed below are those particular to the combination only. For the properties of the components please consider, dexamethasone p. 1207, tobramycin p. 1215.

● INDICATIONS AND DOSE

Local treatment of inflammation (short-term)
▸ TO THE EYE
▸ Adult: (consult product literature)

● INTERACTIONS → Appendix 1: aminoglycosides · corticosteroids
● LESS SUITABLE FOR PRESCRIBING Dexamethasone with tobramycin eye-drops are less suitable for prescribing.

● MEDICINAL FORMS There can be variation in the licensing of different medicines containing the same drug.

Eye drops
EXCIPIENTS: May contain Benzalkonium chloride, disodium edetate
▸ Tobradex (Novartis Pharmaceuticals UK Ltd)
   Dexamethasone 1 mg per 1 ml, Tobramycin 3 mg per 1 ml Tobradex 3mg/ml / 1mg/ml eye drops | 5 ml PoM £5.37 DT = £5.37

IMMUNOSUPPRESSANTS ⟩ CALCINEURIN INHIBITORS AND RELATED DRUGS

Ciclosporin
16-Nov-2020

(Cyclosporin)

● DRUG ACTION Ciclosporin inhibits production and release of lymphokines, thereby suppressing cell-mediated immune response.

● INDICATIONS AND DOSE

IKERVIS®

Severe keratitis in dry eye disease that has not responded to treatment with tear substitutes (initiated by a specialist)
▸ TO THE EYE
▸ Adult: Apply 1 drop once daily, to be applied to the affected eye(s) at bedtime, review treatment at least every 6 months

● CONTRA-INDICATIONS Active or suspected ocular or peri-ocular infection · Ocular or peri-ocular malignancies or premalignant conditions
● CAUTIONS Glaucoma—limited information available · history of ocular herpes—no information available
● INTERACTIONS → Appendix 1: ciclosporin
● SIDE-EFFECTS
▸ **Common or very common** Eye discomfort · eye disorders · eye inflammation · vision blurred
▸ **Uncommon** Eye deposit · increased risk of infection

11

Eye

- PREGNANCY Manufacturer advises avoid unless potential benefit outweighs risk—no information available.
- BREAST FEEDING Manufacturer advises avoid—limited information.
- DIRECTIONS FOR ADMINISTRATION Manufacturer advises keep eyes closed for 2 minutes after using eye drops to increase local drug action and reduce systemic absorption.
- PATIENT AND CARER ADVICE
  Driving and skilled tasks Manufacturer advises patients and carers should be counselled on the effects on driving and performance of skilled tasks—increased risk of blurred vision.
- NATIONAL FUNDING/ACCESS DECISIONS
  For full details see funding body website
  NICE decisions
  ▸ Ciclosporin for treating dry eye disease that has not improved despite treatment with artificial tears (December 2015)
  NICE TA369 Recommended
- MEDICINAL FORMS There can be variation in the licensing of different medicines containing the same drug.
  Eye drops
  ▸ Ikervis (Santen UK Ltd)
    Ciclosporin 1 mg per 1 ml Ikervis 0.1% eye drops 0.3ml unit dose | 30 unit dose [PoM] £72.00 DT = £72.00

NERVE GROWTH FACTORS

| Cenegermin

10-Aug-2018

- DRUG ACTION Cenegermin is a recombinant form of human nerve growth factor which allows restoration of corneal integrity; endogenous human nerve growth factor is involved in the differentiation and maintenance of neurons.

- INDICATIONS AND DOSE
  Moderate or severe neurotrophic keratitis (specialist use only)
  ▸ TO THE EYE
  ▸ Adult: Apply 1 drop 6 times a day, to be applied every 2 hours, starting in the morning and completing within 12 hours; treatment should be continued for 8 weeks

- CONTRA-INDICATIONS Eye infection—resolve before initiating treatment (if an infection occurs during treatment, cenegermin should be suspended until infection resolution) · patients requiring immediate corneal surgery (assess for risk of corneal melting or impending perforation before initiating treatment)
- CAUTIONS Ocular cancer—manufacturer recommends monitor for cancer progression before and after treatment
- SIDE-EFFECTS
  ▸ **Common or very common** Eye discomfort · eye disorders · eye inflammation · headache · photophobia
  ▸ **Uncommon** Corneal abscess
  ▸ **Frequency not known** Eye haemorrhage
- PREGNANCY Manufacturer advises avoid—no information available.
- BREAST FEEDING Manufacturer advises avoid—no information available.
- DIRECTIONS FOR ADMINISTRATION Manufacturer advises that other topical ophthalmic preparations should be administered at least 15 minutes before or after use.
- HANDLING AND STORAGE For information on storage of cenegermin, consult product literature.
- PATIENT AND CARER ADVICE Manufacturer advises patients and carers should be counselled on how to administer cenegermin eye drops.
- NATIONAL FUNDING/ACCESS DECISIONS
  For full details see funding body website

NICE decisions
▸ Cenegermin for treating neurotrophic keratitis (July 2018)
NICE TA532 Not recommended

- MEDICINAL FORMS No licensed medicines listed.

1.2a Anterior uveitis

ANTIMUSCARINICS

Antimuscarinics (eye)

- CAUTIONS Children under 3 months owing to the possible association between cycloplegia and the development of amblyopia · darkly pigmented iris is more resistant to pupillary dilatation and caution should be exercised to avoid overdosage · mydriasis can precipitate acute angle-closure glaucoma (usually in those aged over 60 years and hypermetropic (long-sighted), who are predisposed to the condition because of a shallow anterior chamber) · mydriasis can precipitate acute angle-closure glaucoma (usually in those who are predisposed to the condition because of a shallow anterior chamber) (in children) · neonates at increased risk of systemic toxicity (in neonates)
- SIDE-EFFECTS Dizziness · photophobia · skin reactions · tachycardia
- PATIENT AND CARER ADVICE Patients may not be able to undertake skilled tasks until vision clears after mydriasis.

⌐ above

| Atropine sulfate

24-Jul-2020

- INDICATIONS AND DOSE
  Cycloplegia
  ▸ TO THE EYE USING EYE DROP
  ▸ Adult: (consult product literature)
  Anterior uveitis
  ▸ TO THE EYE USING EYE DROP
  ▸ Adult: (consult product literature)

- INTERACTIONS → Appendix 1: atropine
- SIDE-EFFECTS Systemic side-effects can occur.
- PRESCRIBING AND DISPENSING INFORMATION Although multi-dose atropine sulphate eye drops commonly contain preservatives, preservative-free unit dose vials may be available.

- MEDICINAL FORMS There can be variation in the licensing of different medicines containing the same drug. Forms available from special-order manufacturers include: oral suspension, oral solution, solution for injection, solution for infusion, eye drops, eye ointment
  Eye drops
  ▸ Atropine sulfate (Non-proprietary)
    Atropine sulfate 10 mg per 1 ml Atropine 1% eye drops | 10 ml [PoM] £131.89 DT = £131.89
  ▸ Atropine sulfate (Bausch & Lomb UK Ltd)
    Atropine sulfate 10 mg per 1 ml Minims atropine sulfate 1% eye drops 0.5ml unit dose | 20 unit dose [PoM] £15.10 DT = £15.10

⌐ above

| Cyclopentolate hydrochloride

- INDICATIONS AND DOSE
  Cycloplegia
  ▸ TO THE EYE
  ▸ Child 3 months-11 years: Apply 1 drop, 30–60 minutes before examination, using 1% eye drops
  ▸ Child 12-17 years: Apply 1 drop, 30–60 minutes before examination, using 0.5% eye drops

Uveitis

▶ TO THE EYE
▶ Child 3 months-17 years: Apply 1 drop 2–4 times a day, using 0.5% eye drops (1% for deeply pigmented eyes)

Anterior uveitis | Cyclopegia

▶ TO THE EYE
▶ Adult: (consult product literature)

● INTERACTIONS → Appendix 1: cyclopentolate

● SIDE-EFFECTS Abdominal distension (in children) · arrhythmias · behaviour abnormal (in children) · cardio-respiratory distress (in children) · conjunctivitis (on prolonged administration) · constipation · dry mouth · eye oedema (on prolonged administration) · flushing · gastrointestinal disorders · hyperaemia (on prolonged administration) · mydriasis · palpitations · psychotic disorder (in children) · staggering · urinary disorders · vomiting

SIDE-EFFECTS, FURTHER INFORMATION Systemic side-effects can occur, particularly in children and the elderly.

● PRESCRIBING AND DISPENSING INFORMATION Although multi-dose cyclopentolate eye drops commonly contain preservatives, preservative-free unit dose vials may be available.

● MEDICINAL FORMS There can be variation in the licensing of different medicines containing the same drug.

Eye drops
EXCIPIENTS: May contain Benzalkonium chloride
▶ Cyclopentolate hydrochloride (Bausch & Lomb UK Ltd)
Cyclopentolate hydrochloride 5 mg per 1 ml Minims cyclopentolate hydrochloride 0.5% eye drops 0.5ml unit dose | 20 unit dose [PoM] £11.41 DT = £11.41
Cyclopentolate hydrochloride 10 mg per 1 ml Minims cyclopentolate hydrochloride 1% eye drops 0.5ml unit dose | 20 unit dose [PoM] £11.68 DT = £11.68
▶ Mydrilate (Intrapharm Laboratories Ltd)
Cyclopentolate hydrochloride 5 mg per 1 ml Mydrilate 0.5% solution | 5 ml [PoM] £8.08 DT = £8.08
Cyclopentolate hydrochloride 10 mg per 1 ml Mydrilate 1% solution | 5 ml [PoM] £8.08 DT = £8.08

⚑ 1210

Homatropine hydrobromide

● INDICATIONS AND DOSE

Anterior uveitis
▶ TO THE EYE
▶ Adult: (consult product literature)

● INTERACTIONS → Appendix 1: homatropine

● MEDICINAL FORMS Forms available from special-order manufacturers include: eye drops

2   Dry eye conditions

Dry eye

08-Feb-2020

Description of condition

Dry eye presents as chronic soreness and inflammation of ocular surface associated with reduced or abnormal tear secretion (e.g. in Sjögren's syndrome). It often responds to tear replacement therapy in the form of eye drops (preferably preservative-free), eye ointment (used at night), or gels. Choice of preparation is based on the type of dry eye (e.g. aqueous-deficient or evaporative), symptoms, and patient preference.

Drug treatment

[EvGr] Hypromellose p. 1212 is the most frequently used treatment for tear deficiency in patients with mild dry eye. ⓐ Initially, it may need to be instilled frequently (e.g. hourly) for adequate symptom relief, then at a reduced frequency. [EvGr] Carbomers below and polyvinyl alcohol p. 1213 are suitable alternatives. ⓐ The ability of carbomers below and polyvinyl alcohol to cling to the eye surface and their higher viscosity may help reduce frequency of application to 4 times daily. Carbomers below can be less tolerated than hypromellose due to their impact on vision. [EvGr] Preservative-free tear replacement is preferred in cases of frequent and chronic application.

Ocular lubricants containing sodium hyaluronate p. 1214, hydroxypropyl guar, or carmellose sodium p. 1212 can be used for moderate to severe dry eye following a suitable trial (6–8 weeks) of treatment options for mild dry eye.

Eye ointments containing a paraffin (e.g. liquid paraffin with white soft paraffin and wool alcohols p. 1213) can be used in addition to other options to lubricate the eye surface, especially in cases of recurrent corneal epithelial erosion. ⓐ They may cause temporary visual disturbance and are best suited for application before sleep. Ointments should not be used during contact lens wear.

OCULAR LUBRICANTS

Acetylcysteine

05-Oct-2020

● INDICATIONS AND DOSE

Tear deficiency | Impaired or abnormal mucus production
▶ TO THE EYE
▶ Adult: Apply 3–4 times a day

● SIDE-EFFECTS Eye discomfort · eye redness

● MEDICINAL FORMS There can be variation in the licensing of different medicines containing the same drug. Forms available from special-order manufacturers include: eye drops

Eye drops
EXCIPIENTS: May contain Benzalkonium chloride, disodium edetate
▶ Ilube (Rayner Pharmaceuticals Ltd)
Acetylcysteine 50 mg per 1 ml Ilube 5% eye drops | 10 ml [PoM] £33.46 DT = £33.46

Carbomers

27-Mar-2020

(Polyacrylic acid)

● INDICATIONS AND DOSE

Dry eyes including keratoconjunctivitis sicca, unstable tear film
▶ TO THE EYE
▶ Child: Apply 3–4 times a day or when required
▶ Adult: Apply 3–4 times a day or when required

● PRESCRIBING AND DISPENSING INFORMATION Synthetic high molecular weight polymers of acrylic acid cross-linked with either allyl ethers of sucrose or allyl ethers of pentaerithrityl.

● MEDICINAL FORMS There can be variation in the licensing of different medicines containing the same drug.

Eye gel
EXCIPIENTS: May contain Benzalkonium chloride, cetrimide, disodium edetate
▶ Blephagel (Thea Pharmaceuticals Ltd)
Carbomer 3.6 mg per 1 gram Blephagel 0.36% eye gel preservative free | 30 gram £7.53
▶ Liquivisc (Thea Pharmaceuticals Ltd)
Carbomer 974P 2.5 mg per 1 gram Liquivisc 0.25% eye gel | 10 gram [P] £4.50 DT = £4.50

11

Eye

Eye drops

▸ Carbomers (Non-proprietary)
Carbomer 980 2 mg per 1 gram Carbomer 0.2% eye gel | 10 gram £2.80 DT = £2.80
▸ Artelac Nighttime (Bausch & Lomb UK Ltd)
Carbomer 980 2 mg per 1 gram Artelac Nighttime 0.2% eye gel | 10 gram £2.96 DT = £2.80
▸ Clinitas Carbomer (Altacor Ltd)
Carbomer 980 2 mg per 1 gram Clinitas Carbomer 0.2% eye gel | 10 gram £1.49 DT = £2.80
▸ GelTears (Bausch & Lomb UK Ltd)
Carbomer 980 2 mg per 1 gram GelTears 0.2% gel | 10 gram Ⓟ £2.80 DT = £2.80
▸ Lumecare Long Lasting (Medicom Healthcare Ltd)
Carbomer 980 2 mg per 1 gram Lumecare Carbomer 0.2% eye gel | 10 gram £1.53 DT = £2.80
▸ Ocu-Lube Carbomer (Sai-Meds Ltd)
Carbomer 980 2 mg per 1 gram Ocu-Lube Carbomer 0.2% eye gel 0.6ml unit dose preservative free | 30 unit dose £5.25 DT = £5.42
▸ Viscotears (Bausch & Lomb UK Ltd)
Carbomer 980 2 mg per 1 gram Viscotears 2mg/g liquid gel | 10 gram Ⓟ £1.59 DT = £2.80
Viscotears 2mg/g eye gel 0.6ml unit dose | 30 unit dose Ⓟ £5.42 DT = £5.42
▸ Xailin (Visufarma UK Ltd)
Carbomer 980 2 mg per 1 gram Xailin 0.2% eye gel | 10 gram £3.35 DT = £2.80

Carmellose sodium

04-Dec-2020

● **INDICATIONS AND DOSE**

Dry eye conditions
▸ TO THE EYE
▸ Child: Apply as required
▸ Adult: Apply as required

● PRESCRIBING AND DISPENSING INFORMATION Some preparations are contained units which are resealable and may be used for up to 12 hours.

● MEDICINAL FORMS There can be variation in the licensing of different medicines containing the same drug.

Eye drops
▸ Carmellose sodium (Non-proprietary)
Carmellose 0.5% eye drops | 10 ml £7.49
Carmellose 1% eye drops 0.4ml unit dose preservative free | 30 unit dose £3.00 DT = £3.00
Carmellose sodium 5 mg per 1 ml Carmellose 0.5% eye drops 0.4ml unit dose preservative free | 30 unit dose £5.75 DT = £4.80
▸ Carmellose (Aspire Pharma Ltd, Medicom Healthcare Ltd)
PF Drops Carmellose 0.5% eye drops preservative free | 10 ml £7.49
PF Drops Carmellose 1% eye drops preservative free | 10 ml £7.49
Lumecare Advance Carmellose 0.5% eye drops | 10 ml £6.05
▸ Carmize (Aspire Pharma Ltd)
Carmize 1% eye drops | 10 ml £8.49
Carmize 1% eye drops 0.4ml unit dose preservative free | 30 unit dose £3.00 DT = £3.00 | 60 unit dose £6.00
Carmize 0.5% eye drops | 10 ml £7.49
Carmellose sodium 5 mg per 1 ml Carmize 0.5% eye drops 0.4ml unit dose preservative free | 30 unit dose £5.75 DT = £4.80 | 90 unit dose £15.53
▸ Cellusan (Farmigea S.p.A.)
Cellusan 1% eye drops preservative free | 10 ml £4.80
Cellusan Light 0.5% eye drops preservative free | 10 ml £4.80
Cellusan 1% eye drops 0.4ml unit dose preservative free | 30 unit dose £3.00 DT = £3.00
Carmellose sodium 5 mg per 1 ml Cellusan Light 0.5% eye drops 0.4ml unit dose preservative free | 30 unit dose £4.80 DT = £4.80
▸ Celluvisc (Allergan Ltd)
Celluvisc 1% eye drops 0.4ml unit dose | 30 unit dose Ⓟ £3.00 = £3.00 | 60 unit dose Ⓟ £10.99
Carmellose sodium 5 mg per 1 ml Celluvisc 0.5% eye drops 0.4ml unit dose | 30 unit dose Ⓟ £4.80 DT = £4.80 | 90 unit dose Ⓟ £15.53
▸ Lumecare (Carmellose) (Medicom Healthcare Ltd)
Carmellose sodium 5 mg per 1 ml Lumecare Singles Carmellose 0.5% eye drops 0.4ml unit dose | 30 unit dose £3.36 DT = £4.80

▸ Ocu-Lube Carmellose (Sai-Meds Ltd)
Ocu-Lube Carmellose 0.5% eye drops preservative free | 10 ml £7.49
Ocu-Lube Carmellose 1% eye drops preservative free | 10 ml £7.49
▸ Optho-Lique (Essential-Healthcare Ltd)
Optho-Lique 0.5% eye drops | 10 ml £3.73
Optho-Lique Forte 1% eye drops | 10 ml £3.97
▸ Optive (Allergan Ltd)
Optive 0.5% eye drops | 10 ml £7.49
▸ Optive Plus (Allergan Ltd)
Optive Plus 0.5% eye drops | 10 ml £7.49
▸ Tearvis (Sai-Meds Ltd)
Tearvis 1% eye drops | 10 ml £8.49
Tearvis 0.5% eye drops | 10 ml £7.49
▸ Xailin Fresh (Visufarma UK Ltd)
Carmellose sodium 5 mg per 1 ml Xailin Fresh 0.5% eye drops 0.4ml unit dose | 30 unit dose £3.95 DT = £4.80

Hydroxyethylcellulose

23-Mar-2020

● **INDICATIONS AND DOSE**

Tear deficiency
▸ TO THE EYE
▸ Child: Apply as required
▸ Adult: Apply as required

● PRESCRIBING AND DISPENSING INFORMATION Although multi-dose hydroxyethylcellulose eye drops commonly contain preservatives, preservative-free unit dose vials may be available.

● MEDICINAL FORMS There can be variation in the licensing of different medicines containing the same drug.

Eye drops
▸ Artificial tears (Bausch & Lomb UK Ltd)
Hydroxyethylcellulose 4.4 mg per 1 ml Minims artificial tears 0.44% eye drops 0.5ml unit dose | 20 unit dose Ⓟ £9.33 DT = £9.33

Hydroxypropyl guar with polyethylene glycol and propylene glycol

(Formulated as an ocular lubricant)

● **INDICATIONS AND DOSE**

Dry eye conditions
▸ TO THE EYE
▸ Child: Apply as required
▸ Adult: Apply as required

● MEDICINAL FORMS No licensed medicines listed.

Hypromellose

23-Mar-2020

● **INDICATIONS AND DOSE**

Tear deficiency
▸ TO THE EYE
▸ Child: Apply as required
▸ Adult: Apply as required

● PRESCRIBING AND DISPENSING INFORMATION Although multi-dose hypromellose eye drops commonly contain preservatives, preservative-free unit dose vials may be available.

● MEDICINAL FORMS There can be variation in the licensing of different medicines containing the same drug. Forms available from special-order manufacturers include: eye drops

Eye drops
EXCIPIENTS: May contain Benzalkonium chloride, cetrimide, disodium edetate
▸ Hypromellose (Non-proprietary)
Hypromellose 3 mg per 1 ml Hypromellose 0.3% eye drops preservative free | 10 ml £5.75

Hypromellose 0.3% eye drops | 10 ml Ⓟ £1.05 DT = £1.05 | 10 ml £0.99 DT = £1.05
▸ Artelac (Bausch & Lomb UK Ltd)
Hypromellose 3.2 mg per 1 ml Artelac Single Dose Unit 0.32% eye drops 0.5ml unit dose | 30 unit dose Ⓟ £16.95 DT = £16.95
Artelac 0.32% eye drops | 10 ml Ⓟ £4.99 DT = £4.99
▸ Hydromoor (Rayner Pharmaceuticals Ltd)
Hydromoor 0.3% eye drops 0.4ml unit dose preservative free | 30 unit dose £5.75
▸ Hypromellose (Aspire Pharma Ltd)
Hypromellose 3 mg per 1 ml PF Drops Hypromellose 0.3% eye drops preservative free | 10 ml £5.75
▸ Hypromol (Ennogen Healthcare Ltd)
Hypromellose 3 mg per 1 ml Hypromol 0.3% eye drops preservative free | 10 ml £4.55
▸ Isopto Plain (Alcon Eye Care Ltd)
Hypromellose 5 mg per 1 ml Isopto Plain 0.5% eye drops | 10 ml Ⓟ £0.81 DT = £0.81
▸ Lumecare (Hypromellose) (Medicom Healthcare Ltd)
Hypromellose 3 mg per 1 ml Lumecare Hypromellose 0.3% eye drops | 10 ml £1.69 DT = £1.05
▸ Lumecare Tear Drops (Medicom Healthcare Ltd)
Hypromellose 3 mg per 1 ml Lumecare Tear Drops 0.3% eye drops | 10 ml £0.79 DT = £1.05
▸ Mandanol (Hydroxypropyl methylcellulose) (M & A Pharmachem Ltd)
Hypromellose 3 mg per 1 ml Mandanol eye drops | 10 ml £1.33 DT = £1.05
▸ Ocu-Lube (Sai-Meds Ltd)
Hypromellose 3 mg per 1 ml Ocu-Lube 0.3% eye drops preservative free | 10 ml £5.75
▸ Ocufresh (Blumont Healthcare Ltd)
Hypromellose 3 mg per 1 ml Ocufresh 0.3% eye drops | 10 ml £1.50 DT = £1.05
▸ Tear-Lac (Scope Ophthalmics Ltd)
Hypromellose 3 mg per 1 ml Tear-Lac Hypromellose 0.3% eye drops preservative free | 10 ml £5.80
▸ Teardew (Sai-Meds Ltd)
Hypromellose 3 mg per 1 ml Teardew 0.3% eye drops | 10 ml £0.99 DT = £1.05
▸ Xailin Hydrate (Visufarma UK Ltd)
Hypromellose 3 mg per 1 ml Xailin Hydrate 0.3% eye drops preservative free | 10 ml £4.74

Hypromellose with dextran 70   07-Apr-2020

The properties listed below are those particular to the combination only. For the properties of the components please consider, hypromellose p. 1212.

● **INDICATIONS AND DOSE**
Tear deficiency
▸ TO THE EYE
▸ Adult: Apply as required

● MEDICINAL FORMS There can be variation in the licensing of different medicines containing the same drug.
Eye drops
EXCIPIENTS: May contain Benzalkonium chloride, disodium edetate
▸ Tears Naturale (Alcon Eye Care Ltd)
Dextran 70 1 mg per 1 ml, Hypromellose 3 mg per 1 ml Tears Naturale eye drops | 15 ml Ⓟ £1.89 DT = £1.89
Tears Naturale eye drops 0.4ml unit dose | 28 unit dose Ⓟ £13.26 DT = £13.26

Liquid paraffin with white soft paraffin and wool alcohols   26-Nov-2020

● **INDICATIONS AND DOSE**
Dry eye conditions
▸ TO THE EYE
▸ Child: Apply as required, best suited for application before sleep
▸ Adult: Apply as required, best suited for application before sleep

● PATIENT AND CARER ADVICE May cause temporary visual disturbance. Should not be used during contact lens wear.

● MEDICINAL FORMS There can be variation in the licensing of different medicines containing the same drug.
Eye ointment
▸ Liquid paraffin with white soft paraffin and wool alcohols (Non-proprietary)
Xailin Night eye ointment preservative free | 5 gram £2.56
▸ Lacri-Lube (Allergan Ltd)
Wool alcohols 2 mg per 1 gram, Liquid paraffin 425 mg per 1 gram, White soft paraffin 573 mg per 1 gram Lacri-lube eye ointment | 3.5 gram Ⓟ £3.01 | 5 gram Ⓟ £3.98

Paraffin, yellow, soft   23-Nov-2020

● **INDICATIONS AND DOSE**
Eye surface lubrication
▸ TO THE EYE
▸ Child: Apply as required
▸ Adult: Apply as required

● PATIENT AND CARER ADVICE Ophthalmic preparations may cause temporary visual disturbance. Should not be used during contact lens wear.

● MEDICINAL FORMS There can be variation in the licensing of different medicines containing the same drug.
Eye ointment
▸ Paraffin, yellow, soft (Non-proprietary)
Liquid paraffin 100 mg per 1 gram, Wool fat 100 mg per 1 gram, Yellow soft paraffin 800 mg per 1 gram Simple eye ointment | 4 gram Ⓟ £53.73 DT = £53.03

Polyvinyl alcohol   17-Apr-2020

● **INDICATIONS AND DOSE**
Tear deficiency
▸ TO THE EYE
▸ Child: Apply as required
▸ Adult: Apply as required

● PRESCRIBING AND DISPENSING INFORMATION Although multi-dose polyvinyl alcohol eye drops commonly contain preservatives, preservative-free unit dose vials may be available.

● MEDICINAL FORMS There can be variation in the licensing of different medicines containing the same drug. Forms available from special-order manufacturers include: eye drops
Eye drops
EXCIPIENTS: May contain Benzalkonium chloride, disodium edetate
▸ Liquifilm Tears (Allergan Ltd)
Polyvinyl alcohol 14 mg per 1 ml Liquifilm Tears 1.4% eye drops | 15 ml £1.93
Liquifilm Tears 1.4% eye drops 0.4ml unit dose preservative free | 30 unit dose £5.35
▸ Refresh Ophthalmic (Allergan Ltd)
Polyvinyl alcohol 14 mg per 1 ml Refresh Ophthalmic 1.4% eye drops 0.4ml unit dose | 30 unit dose £2.25
▸ Sno Tears (Bausch & Lomb UK Ltd)
Polyvinyl alcohol 14 mg per 1 ml Sno Tears 1.4% eye drops | 10 ml £1.06

11

Eye

Retinol palmitate with white soft paraffin, light liquid paraffin, liquid paraffin and wool fat

(Formulated as an ocular lubricant)

● **INDICATIONS AND DOSE**

Dry eye conditions
▶ TO THE EYE
▶ Adult: (consult product literature)

● MEDICINAL FORMS There can be variation in the licensing of different medicines containing the same drug.
Eye ointment
▶ Retinol palmitate with white soft paraffin, light liquid paraffin, liquid paraffin and wool fat (Non-proprietary)
Hylo Night eye ointment preservative free | 5 gram £2.75
▶ VitA-POS (Scope Ophthalmics Ltd)
VitA-POS eye ointment preservative free | 5 gram £2.75

Sodium chloride

07-Oct-2020

● **INDICATIONS AND DOSE**

Tear deficiency | Ocular lubricants and astringents | Irrigation, including first-aid removal of harmful substances | Intra-ocular or topical irrigation during surgical procedures
▶ TO THE EYE
▶ Child: Apply as required, use 0.9% eye preparations
▶ Adult: Apply as required, use 0.9% eye preparations

Corneal oedema
▶ TO THE EYE
▶ Adult: Use 5% eye preparations (consult product literature)

● PRESCRIBING AND DISPENSING INFORMATION Although multi-dose sodium chloride eye drops commonly contain preservatives, preservative-free unit dose vials may be available.

● MEDICINAL FORMS There can be variation in the licensing of different medicines containing the same drug. Forms available from special-order manufacturers include: eye drops, eye ointment
Eye drops
▶ Sodium chloride (Non-proprietary)
Sodium chloride 50 mg per 1 ml Sodium chloride 5% eye drops | 10 ml £25.25
▶ Hypersal (Ennogen Healthcare Ltd)
Sodium chloride 50 mg per 1 ml Hypersal 5% eye drops | 10 ml £25.25
▶ ODM5 (Kestrel Ophthalmics Ltd)
Sodium chloride 50 mg per 1 ml ODM5 5% eye drops preservative free | 10 ml £24.00 DT = £0.00
▶ Saline (Bausch & Lomb UK Ltd)
Sodium chloride 9 mg per 1 ml Minims saline 0.9% eye drops 0.5ml unit dose | 20 unit dose P £7.43 DT = £7.43
▶ SodiEye (TriOn Pharma Ltd)
SodiEye 5% eye drops 0.5ml unit dose preservative free | 20 unit dose £17.70
Sodium chloride 50 mg per 1 ml SodiEye 5% eye drops preservative free | 10 ml £15.98 DT = £0.00
▶ Sodium chloride (Essential Pharmaceuticals Ltd, Aspire Pharma Ltd)
Sodium chloride 50 mg per 1 ml NaCl 5% eye drops 0.45ml unit dose preservative free | 20 unit dose £14.95
PF Drops Sodium Chloride 5% eye drops preservative free | 10 ml £25.20 DT = £0.00
Eye ointment
▶ Sodium chloride (Non-proprietary)
Sodium chloride 50 mg per 1 ml Sodium chloride 5% eye ointment preservative free | 5 gram £22.50

Sodium hyaluronate

04-Dec-202●

● **INDICATIONS AND DOSE**

Dry eye conditions
▶ TO THE EYE
▶ Adult: Apply as required

● PRESCRIBING AND DISPENSING INFORMATION Some preparations are contained in units which are resealable and may be used for up to 12 hours.
Although multi-dose sodium hyaluronate eye drops commonly contain preservatives, preservative-free unit dose vials may be available.

● MEDICINAL FORMS There can be variation in the licensing of different medicines containing the same drug.
Eye drops
▶ Artelac Rebalance (Bausch & Lomb UK Ltd)
Artelac Rebalance 0.15% eye drops | 10 ml £4.00
▶ Artelac Splash (Bausch & Lomb UK Ltd)
Artelac Splash 0.2% eye drops 0.5ml unit dose | 30 unit dose £7.00 | 60 unit dose £11.20
▶ Blink Intensive (AMO UK Ltd)
Blink Intensive Tears 0.2% eye drops 0.4ml unit dose | 20 unit dose £2.97
Blink Intensive Tears 0.2% eye drops | 10 ml £2.97
▶ Clinitas (Altacor Ltd)
Clinitas Multi 0.4% eye drops preservative free | 10 ml £6.99
Clinitas 0.4% eye drops 0.5ml unit dose | 30 unit dose £5.70
▶ Evolve HA (Medicom Healthcare Ltd)
Evolve HA 0.2% eye drops preservative free | 10 ml £5.99
▶ Hy-Opti (Alissa Healthcare Research Ltd)
Hy-Opti 0.1% eye drops preservative free | 10 ml £8.50
Hy-Opti 0.2% eye drops preservative free | 10 ml £9.50
▶ Hyabak (Thea Pharmaceuticals Ltd)
Hyabak 0.15% eye drops preservative free | 10 ml £7.99
▶ Hycosan (Scope Ophthalmics Ltd)
Hycosan Extra 0.2% eye drops | 7.5 ml 🅢
Hycosan 0.1% eye drops | 7.5 ml 🅢
▶ HydraMed (Farmigea S.p.A.)
HydraMed 0.2% eye drops preservative free | 10 ml £5.60
HydraMed 0.2% eye drops 0.5ml unit dose preservative free | 30 unit dose £5.60
▶ Hylo-Comod (Scope Ophthalmics Ltd)
Hylo-Tear 0.1% eye drops preservative free | 10 ml £8.50
Hylo-Forte 0.2% eye drops preservative free | 10 ml £9.50
▶ Hylo-fresh (Scope Ophthalmics Ltd)
Hylo-Fresh 0.03% eye drops preservative free | 10 ml £4.95
▶ Lubristil (Rayner Pharmaceuticals Ltd)
Lubristil 0.15% eye drops 0.3ml unit dose preservative free | 20 unit dose £4.99
▶ Ocu-Lube HA (Sai-Meds Ltd)
Ocu-Lube HA 0.1% eye drops preservative free | 10 ml £8.00
▶ Ocusan (Agepha Pharma s.r.o.)
Ocusan 0.2% eye drops 0.5ml unit dose | 20 unit dose £5.47
▶ Optive Fusion (Allergan Ltd)
Optive Fusion 0.1% eye drops | 10 ml £7.49
▶ Oxyal (Bausch & Lomb UK Ltd)
Oxyal 0.15% eye drops | 10 ml £4.15
▶ Vismed (TRB Chemidica (UK) Ltd)
Vismed Multi 0.3% eye drops preservative free | 10 ml £8.01
Vismed Multi 0.18% eye drops preservative free | 10 ml £6.87
Vismed 0.18% eye drops 0.3ml unit dose preservative free | 20 ml unit dose £5.14
▶ VisuXL (Visufarma UK Ltd)
VisuXL eye drops preservative free | 10 ml £10.30
▶ Xailin HA (Visufarma UK Ltd)
Xailin HA 0.2% eye drops | 10 ml £7.34
Eye gel
▶ Lubristil (Rayner Pharmaceuticals Ltd)
Lubristil 0.15% eye gel 0.4ml unit dose preservative free | 20 unit dose £6.49
▶ Vismed (TRB Chemidica (UK) Ltd)
Vismed Gel 0.3% eye gel 0.45ml unit dose preservative free | 20 unit dose £6.03

Sodium hyaluronate with trehalose

21-Nov-2017

● **INDICATIONS AND DOSE**

Dry eye conditions

▸ TO THE EYE
▸ Adult: Apply 1 drop 4–6 times a day

● PRESCRIBING AND DISPENSING INFORMATION Sodium hyaluronate and trehalose preparations do not contain preservatives; multi-dose preparation can be used for up to 3 months.

● MEDICINAL FORMS There can be variation in the licensing of different medicines containing the same drug.

Eye drops

▸ Thealoz Duo (Thea Pharmaceuticals Ltd)
Thealoz Duo eye drops preservative free | 10 ml £8.99
Thealoz Duo UD eye drops 0.4ml unit dose preservative free | 30 unit dose £7.07

Soybean oil

● **INDICATIONS AND DOSE**

Dry eye conditions

▸ TO THE EYE
▸ Child: Apply up to 4 times a day
▸ Adult: Apply up to 4 times a day

● MEDICINAL FORMS There can be variation in the licensing of different medicines containing the same drug.

Eye drops

▸ Emustil (Rayner Pharmaceuticals Ltd)
Emustil eye drops 0.3ml unit dose preservative free | 20 unit dose £6.22

3   Eye infections

Eye, infections

07-Jun-2020

Overview

Most acute superficial eye infections can be treated topically with eye drops or ointment. Blepharitis is often caused by staphylococci. Bacterial conjunctivitis is commonly caused by *Streptococcus pneumoniae*, *Staphylococcus aureus*, or *Haemophilus influenzae*. Keratitis may be bacterial, viral, or fungal; it can also be caused by Acanthamoeba (parasite). Endophthalmitis is usually either bacterial or fungal; it can also be non-infective (retention of foreign material).

EvGr Anterior bacterial blepharitis is treated by application of an antibacterial eye ointment (such as chloramphenicol p. 1217) to the conjunctival sac or rubbed into the lid margins, if blepharitis is not controlled by eyelid hygiene alone. Systemic treatment (e.g. tetracyclines in patients over 12 years of age) may be required in patients with posterior blepharitis. Treatments can be intermittently stopped and restarted, based on the severity of the blepharitis and drug tolerance. Ⓐ

Most cases of acute bacterial conjunctivitis are self-limiting and resolve within 5–7 days without treatment. EvGr In severe infection or where rapid resolution is required, treatment with antibacterial eye drops or ointments are used. Ongoing symptoms despite treatment may indicate viral conjunctivitis or the need for a different antibacterial; cultures or referral to a specialist may be required.

Corneal ulcer and keratitis require specialist treatment and may call for hospital admission for intensive therapy.

Endophthalmitis is a medical emergency which also calls for specialist management and may require treatment with antibacterial drugs and steroids. Surgical intervention, such as vitrectomy, is sometimes indicated. Ⓐ

Trachoma which results from chronic infection with *Chlamydia trachomatis* can be treated with azithromycin p. 1216 by mouth [unlicensed indication] as recommended by the World Health Organisation.

For information on the management of ocular herpes, see Herpesvirus infections p. 671.

Fungal infections of the cornea (e.g. fungal keratitis) are rare but can occur particularly in agricultural areas and tropical climates. Antifungal preparations for the eye are not generally available. For information about supply of preparations not commercially available, contact the local Clinical Commissioning Group (CCG), or equivalent in Scotland, Wales, or Northern Ireland, or the nearest hospital ophthalmology unit, or Moorfields Eye Hospital, 162 City Road, London EC1V 2PD (tel. (020) 7253 3411) or www.moorfields.nhs.uk.

3.1   Bacterial eye infection

ANTIBACTERIALS > AMINOGLYCOSIDES

⏻ 544

Gentamicin

04-Dec-2020

● **INDICATIONS AND DOSE**

Bacterial eye infections

▸ TO THE EYE
▸ Child: Apply 1 drop at least every 2 hours in severe infection, reduce frequency as infection is controlled and continue for 48 hours after healing, frequency of eye drops depends on the severity of the infection and the potential for irreversible ocular damage; for less severe infection 3–4 times daily is generally sufficient
▸ Adult: Apply 1 drop at least every 2 hours, reduce frequency as infection is controlled and continue for 48 hours after healing, frequency of eye drops depends on the severity of the infection and the potential for irreversible ocular damage; for less severe infection 3–4 times daily is generally sufficient

● UNLICENSED USE Gentamicin doses in BNF publications may differ from those in product literature.

● INTERACTIONS → Appendix 1: aminoglycosides

● PRESCRIBING AND DISPENSING INFORMATION For choice of antibacterial therapy, see Eye infections, antibacterial therapy p. 535.

Eye drops may be sourced as a manufactured special or from specialist importing companies.

● MEDICINAL FORMS There can be variation in the licensing of different medicines containing the same drug. Forms available from special-order manufacturers include: eye drops

Ear/eye drops solution

EXCIPIENTS: May contain Benzalkonium chloride

▸ Gentamicin (Non-proprietary)
Gentamicin (as Gentamicin sulfate) 3 mg per 1 ml Gentamicin 0.3% ear/eye drops | 10 ml PoM £3.06 DT = £2.78

⏻ 544

Tobramycin

03-Sep-2020

● **INDICATIONS AND DOSE**

Local treatment of infections

▸ TO THE EYE
▸ Child 1-17 years: Apply twice daily for 6–8 days
▸ Adult: Apply twice daily for 6–8 days

continued →

11

Eye

Local treatment of infections (severe infection)
▸ TO THE EYE
▸ Child 1-17 years: Apply 4 times a day for first day, then apply twice daily for 5–7 days
▸ Adult: Apply 4 times a day for first day, then apply twice daily for 5–7 days

● INTERACTIONS → Appendix 1: aminoglycosides

● MEDICINAL FORMS No licensed medicines listed.

ANTIBACTERIALS > CEPHALOSPORINS, SECOND-GENERATION

⟋ 551

Cefuroxime

10-Nov-2020

● INDICATIONS AND DOSE
APROKAM ® INTRACAMERAL INJECTION
Prophylaxis of endophthalmitis after cataract surgery
▸ BY INTRACAMERAL INJECTION
▸ Adult: 1 mg, dose to be injected into the anterior chamber of the eye at the end of cataract surgery

● CAUTIONS
APROKAM ® INTRACAMERAL INJECTION
▸ With intracameral use Combined operations with cataract surgery · complicated cataracts · reduced corneal endothelial cells (less than 2000) · severe risk of infection · severe thyroid disease

● INTERACTIONS → Appendix 1: cephalosporins

● PREGNANCY Not known to be harmful.

● BREAST FEEDING Present in milk in low concentration, but appropriate to use.

● NATIONAL FUNDING/ACCESS DECISIONS
APROKAM ® INTRACAMERAL INJECTION For full details see funding body website
Scottish Medicines Consortium (SMC) decisions
▸ Cefuroxime (*Aprokam*®) for antibiotic prophylaxis of postoperative endophthalmitis after cataract surgery (December 2016) SMC No. 932/13 Recommended
All Wales Medicines Strategy Group (AWMSG) decisions
▸ Cefuroxime (*Aprokam*®) for postoperative endophthalmitis after cataract surgery (August 2017) AWMSG No. 2224 Recommended

● MEDICINAL FORMS
Powder for solution for injection
▸ Aprokam (Thea Pharmaceuticals Ltd)
Cefuroxime (as Cefuroxime sodium) 50 mg Aprokam 50mg powder for solution for injection vials | 10 vial PoM £49.95

ANTIBACTERIALS > MACROLIDES

⟋ 568

Azithromycin

29-Jul-2020

● INDICATIONS AND DOSE
Trachomatous conjunctivitis caused by *Chlamydia trachomatis* | Purulent bacterial conjunctivitis
▸ TO THE EYE
▸ Child: Apply twice daily for 3 days, review if no improvement after 3 days of treatment
▸ Adult: Apply twice daily for 3 days, review if no improvement after 3 days of treatment

● INTERACTIONS → Appendix 1: macrolides

● SIDE-EFFECTS
▸ Common or very common Eye discomfort
▸ Uncommon Eye allergy

● MEDICINAL FORMS There can be variation in the licensing of different medicines containing the same drug.
Eye drops
▸ Azyter (Thea Pharmaceuticals Ltd)
Azithromycin dihydrate 15 mg per 1 gram Azyter 15mg/g eye drops 0.25g unit dose | 6 unit dose PoM £6.99 DT = £6.99

ANTIBACTERIALS > QUINOLONES

⟋ 592

Ciprofloxacin

18-Nov-202●

● INDICATIONS AND DOSE
Superficial bacterial eye infection
▸ TO THE EYE USING EYE DROP
▸ Child: Apply 4 times a day for maximum duration of treatment 21 days
▸ Adult: Apply 4 times a day for maximum duration of treatment 21 days
▸ TO THE EYE USING EYE OINTMENT
▸ Child 1-17 years: Apply 1.25 centimetres 3 times a day for 2 days, then apply 1.25 centimetres twice daily for 5 days
▸ Adult: Apply 1.25 centimetres 3 times a day for 2 days, then apply 1.25 centimetres twice daily for 5 days

Superficial bacterial eye infection (severe infection)
▸ TO THE EYE USING EYE DROP
▸ Child: Apply every 2 hours during waking hours for 2 days, then apply 4 times a day for maximum duration of treatment 21 days
▸ Adult: Apply every 2 hours during waking hours for 2 days, then apply 4 times a day for maximum duration of treatment 21 days

Corneal ulcer
▸ TO THE EYE USING EYE DROP
▸ Child: Apply every 15 minutes for 6 hours, then apply every 30 minutes for the remainder of day 1, then apply every 1 hour on day 2, then apply every 4 hours on days 3–14, maximum duration of treatment 21 days, to be administered throughout the day and night
▸ Adult: Apply every 15 minutes for 6 hours, then apply every 30 minutes for the remainder of day 1, then apply every 1 hour on day 2, then apply every 4 hours on days 3–14, maximum duration of treatment 21 days, to be administered throughout the day and night
▸ TO THE EYE USING EYE OINTMENT
▸ Child 1-17 years: Apply 1.25 centimetres every 1–2 hours for 2 days, then apply 1.25 centimetres every 4 hours for the next 12 days, to be administered throughout the day and night
▸ Adult: Apply 1.25 centimetres every 1–2 hours for 2 days, then apply 1.25 centimetres every 4 hours for the next 12 days, to be administered throughout the day and night

● UNLICENSED USE Eye ointment not licensed for use in children under 1 year.

● INTERACTIONS → Appendix 1: quinolones

● SIDE-EFFECTS
▸ Common or very common Corneal deposits (reversible after completion of treatment)
▸ Rare or very rare Ear pain · increased risk of infection · paranasal sinus hypersecretion

● PREGNANCY Manufacturer advises use only if potential benefit outweighs risk.

● BREAST FEEDING Manufacturer advises caution.

▸ MEDICINAL FORMS There can be variation in the licensing of different medicines containing the same drug. Forms available from special-order manufacturers include: eye drops, eye ointment

Eye drops
EXCIPIENTS: May contain Benzalkonium chloride
▸ Ciloxan (Novartis Pharmaceuticals UK Ltd)
  Ciprofloxacin (as Ciprofloxacin hydrochloride) 3 mg per 1 ml Ciloxan 0.3% eye drops | 5 ml [PoM] £4.70 DT = £4.70

⟶ 592

Levofloxacin
26-Nov-2020

● **INDICATIONS AND DOSE**
Local treatment of eye infections
▸ TO THE EYE
▸ Child 1-17 years: Apply every 2 hours for first 2 days, to be applied maximum 8 times a day, then apply 4 times a day for 3 days
▸ Adult: Apply every 2 hours for first 2 days, to be applied maximum 8 times a day, then apply 4 times a day for 3 days

● INTERACTIONS → Appendix 1: quinolones

● SIDE-EFFECTS
▸ **Uncommon** Rhinitis
▸ **Rare or very rare** Laryngeal oedema

● PREGNANCY Manufacturer advises use only if potential benefit outweighs risk.

● BREAST FEEDING Manufacturer advises use only if potential benefit outweighs risk.

● PRESCRIBING AND DISPENSING INFORMATION Although multi-dose levofloxacin eye drops commonly contain preservatives, preservative-free unit dose vials may be available.

● MEDICINAL FORMS There can be variation in the licensing of different medicines containing the same drug.

Eye drops
EXCIPIENTS: May contain Benzalkonium chloride
▸ Levofloxacin (Non-proprietary)
  Levofloxacin (as Levofloxacin hemihydrate) 5 mg per 1 ml Eyflox 5mg/ml eye drops | 5 ml [PoM] £13.46
  Levofloxacin 5mg/ml eye drops | 5 ml [PoM] £6.95 DT = £8.10 (Hospital only) | 5 ml [PoM] £8.10 DT = £8.10
▸ Oftaquix (Santen UK Ltd)
  Levofloxacin (as Levofloxacin hemihydrate) 5 mg per 1 ml Oftaquix 5mg/ml eye drops 0.3ml unit dose | 30 unit dose [PoM] £17.95 DT = £17.95
  Oftaquix 5mg/ml eye drops | 5 ml [PoM] £6.95 DT = £8.10

⟶ 592

Moxifloxacin
17-Apr-2020

● **INDICATIONS AND DOSE**
Local treatment of infections
▸ TO THE EYE
▸ Child: Apply 3 times a day continue treatment for 2-3 days after infection improves; review if no improvement within 5 days
▸ Adult: Apply 3 times a day continue treatment for 2-3 days after infection improves; review if no improvement within 5 days

● INTERACTIONS → Appendix 1: quinolones

● SIDE-EFFECTS
▸ **Uncommon** Conjunctival haemorrhage
▸ **Rare or very rare** Laryngeal pain · nasal discomfort
▸ **Frequency not known** Corneal deposits

● MEDICINAL FORMS There can be variation in the licensing of different medicines containing the same drug.
Eye drops
▸ Moxivig (Novartis Pharmaceuticals UK Ltd)
  Moxifloxacin (as Moxifloxacin hydrochloride) 5 mg per 1 ml Moxivig 0.5% eye drops | 5 ml [PoM] £9.80 DT = £9.80

⟶ 592

Ofloxacin
26-Aug-2020

● **INDICATIONS AND DOSE**
Local treatment of infections
▸ TO THE EYE
▸ Child 1-17 years: Apply every 2-4 hours for the first 2 days, then reduced to 4 times a day for maximum 10 days treatment
▸ Adult: Apply every 2-4 hours for the first 2 days, then reduced to 4 times a day for maximum 10 days treatment

● CAUTIONS Corneal ulcer (risk of corneal perforation) · epithelial defect (risk of corneal perforation)

● INTERACTIONS → Appendix 1: quinolones

● SIDE-EFFECTS Face oedema · oropharyngeal swelling · tongue swelling

● PREGNANCY Manufacturer advises use only if benefit outweighs risk (systemic quinolones have caused arthropathy in *animal* studies).

● BREAST FEEDING Manufacturer advises avoid.

● PRESCRIBING AND DISPENSING INFORMATION For choice of antibacterial therapy, see Eye, infections p. 1215.

● MEDICINAL FORMS There can be variation in the licensing of different medicines containing the same drug.
Eye drops
EXCIPIENTS: May contain Benzalkonium chloride
▸ Exocin (Allergan Ltd)
  Ofloxacin 3 mg per 1 ml Exocin 0.3% eye drops | 5 ml [PoM] £2.17 DT = £2.17

ANTIBACTERIALS ⟩ OTHER

Chloramphenicol
09-Nov-2020

● DRUG ACTION Chloramphenicol is a potent broad-spectrum antibiotic.

● **INDICATIONS AND DOSE**
Superficial eye infections
▸ TO THE EYE USING EYE DROP
▸ Child: Apply 1 drop every 2 hours then reduce frequency as infection is controlled and continue for 48 hours after healing, frequency dependent on the severity of the infection. For less severe infection 3-4 times daily is generally sufficient
▸ Adult: Apply 1 drop every 2 hours then reduce frequency as infection is controlled and continue for 48 hours after healing, frequency dependent on the severity of the infection. For less severe infection 3-4 times daily is generally sufficient
▸ TO THE EYE USING EYE OINTMENT
▸ Child: Apply daily, to be applied at night (if eye drops used during the day), alternatively apply 3-4 times a day, if ointment used alone
▸ Adult: Apply daily, to be applied at night (if eye drops used during the day), alternatively apply 3-4 times a day, if ointment used alone

● INTERACTIONS → Appendix 1: chloramphenicol

● SIDE-EFFECTS Angioedema · bone marrow disorders · eye stinging · fever · paraesthesia · skin reactions

11

Eye

- PREGNANCY Avoid unless essential—no information on *topical* use but risk of 'neonatal grey-baby syndrome' with *oral* use in third trimester.
- BREAST FEEDING Avoid unless essential— *theoretical* risk of bone-marrow toxicity.
- PRESCRIBING AND DISPENSING INFORMATION Although multi-dose chloramphenicol eye drops commonly contain preservatives, preservative-free unit dose vials may be available.
- PATIENT AND CARER ADVICE
  Medicines for Children leaflet: Chloramphenicol for eye infections www.medicinesforchildren.org.uk/chloramphenicol-eye-infections-0
- EXCEPTIONS TO LEGAL CATEGORY Chloramphenicol 0.5% eye drops (in max. pack size 10 mL) and 1% eye ointment (in max. pack size 4 g) can be sold to the public for treatment of acute bacterial conjunctivitis in adults and children over 2 years; max. duration of treatment 5 days.
- MEDICINAL FORMS There can be variation in the licensing of different medicines containing the same drug.
  Eye drops
  EXCIPIENTS: May contain Phenylmercuric acetate
  ‣ Chloramphenicol (Non-proprietary)
    Chloramphenicol 5 mg per 1 ml Minims chloramphenicol 0.5% eye drops 0.5ml unit dose | 20 unit dose [PoM] £11.43 DT = £11.43
    Chloramphenicol 0.5% eye drops | 10 ml [PoM] £5.45 DT = £5.45
  ‣ Eykappo (Aspire Pharma Ltd)
    Chloramphenicol 5 mg per 1 ml Eykappo 5mg/ml eye drops | 10 ml [PoM] £10.12 DT = £10.12
  Eye ointment
  ‣ Chloramphenicol (Non-proprietary)
    Chloramphenicol 10 mg per 1 gram Chloramphenicol 1% eye ointment | 4 gram [PoM] £2.49 DT = £2.02

Fusidic acid

30-Apr-2020

- DRUG ACTION Fusidic acid and its salts are narrow-spectrum antibiotics used for staphylococcal infections.

- INDICATIONS AND DOSE
  Staphylococcal eye infections
  ‣ TO THE EYE
  ‣ Child: Apply twice daily
  ‣ Adult: Apply twice daily

- INTERACTIONS → Appendix 1: fusidate
- SIDE-EFFECTS
  ‣ **Common or very common** Dry eye · eye discomfort · vision blurred
  ‣ **Uncommon** Crying on application · skin reactions · watering eye
  ‣ **Frequency not known** Angioedema · eye inflammation
- MEDICINAL FORMS There can be variation in the licensing of different medicines containing the same drug.
  Modified-release drops
  EXCIPIENTS: May contain Benzalkonium chloride, disodium edetate
  ‣ Fusidic acid (Non-proprietary)
    Fusidic acid 10 mg per 1 gram Fusidic acid 1% modified-release eye drops | 5 gram [PoM] £35.00 DT = £35.00

ANTIPROTOZOALS > OTHER

Propamidine isetionate

- INDICATIONS AND DOSE
  ***Acanthamoeba keratitis* infections (specialist use only) | Local treatment of eye infections**
  ‣ TO THE EYE USING EYE OINTMENT
  ‣ Adult: Apply 1–2 times a day
  ‣ TO THE EYE USING EYE DROP
  ‣ Adult: Apply up to 4 times a day

- UNLICENSED USE Not licensed for *acanthamoeba keratitis* infections.
- SIDE-EFFECTS Eye discomfort · vision blurred
- PREGNANCY Manufacturer advises avoid unless essential—no information available.
- BREAST FEEDING Manufacturer advises avoid unless essential—no information available.

- MEDICINAL FORMS There can be variation in the licensing of different medicines containing the same drug.
  Eye ointment
  ‣ Golden Eye (dibrompropamidine) (Cambridge Healthcare Supplies Ltd)
    Dibrompropamidine isetionate 1.5 mg per 1 gram Golden Eye 0.15% ointment | 5 gram [P] £4.15 DT = £4.15
  Eye drops
  EXCIPIENTS: May contain Benzalkonium chloride
  ‣ Brolene (Propamidine) (Sanofi)
    Propamidine isetionate 1 mg per 1 ml Brolene 0.1% eye drops | 10 ml [P] £2.80 DT = £2.80
  ‣ Golden Eye (propamidine) (Cambridge Healthcare Supplies Ltd)
    Propamidine isetionate 1 mg per 1 ml Golden Eye 0.1% drops | 10 ml [P] £3.95 DT = £2.80

3.2 Viral eye infection

3.2a Ophthalmic herpes simplex

ANTIVIRALS > NUCLEOSIDE ANALOGUES

Aciclovir

09-Jun-2020

(Acyclovir)

- INDICATIONS AND DOSE
  Herpes simplex infection (local treatment)
  ‣ TO THE EYE USING EYE OINTMENT
  ‣ Child: Apply 1 centimetre 5 times a day continue for at least 3 days after complete healing
  ‣ Adult: Apply 1 centimetre 5 times a day continue for at least 3 days after complete healing

- INTERACTIONS → Appendix 1: aciclovir
- SIDE-EFFECTS
  ‣ **Common or very common** Eye inflammation · eye pain
- PATIENT AND CARER ADVICE
  Medicines for Children leaflet: Aciclovir eye ointment for herpes simplex infections www.medicinesforchildren.org.uk/aciclovir-eye-ointment-herpes-simplex-infection-0

- MEDICINAL FORMS There can be variation in the licensing of different medicines containing the same drug.
  Eye ointment
  ‣ Aciclovir (Non-proprietary)
    Aciclovir 30 mg per 1 gram Aciclovir 3% eye ointment | 4.5 gram [PoM] £45.00 DT = £45.00

Ganciclovir

15-Dec-2020

- INDICATIONS AND DOSE
  Acute herpetic keratitis
  ‣ TO THE EYE
  ‣ Adult: Apply 5 times a day until healing complete, then apply 3 times a day for a further 7 days, treatment does not usually exceed 21 days

- INTERACTIONS → Appendix 1: ganciclovir
- SIDE-EFFECTS
  ‣ **Common or very common** Eye stinging · punctate keratitis
- ALLERGY AND CROSS-SENSITIVITY [EvGr] Contra-indicated in patients hypersensitive to valganciclovir.

Caution in patients hypersensitive to aciclovir, valaciclovir, or famciclovir. ⓜ

● CONCEPTION AND CONTRACEPTION As teratogenicity and impaired fertility observed in animal studies with *oral* and *intravenous* ganciclovir, manufacturer advises women of childbearing potential should use effective contraception during treatment; men with partners of childbearing potential should be advised to use barrier contraception during and for at least 90 days after treatment.

● PREGNANCY Manufacturer advises avoid unless no suitable alternative—limited information available.

● BREAST FEEDING Manufacturer advises avoid unless no suitable alternative—limited information available.

● MEDICINAL FORMS There can be variation in the licensing of different medicines containing the same drug.

Eye gel
EXCIPIENTS: May contain Benzalkonium chloride
▸ Virgan (Thea Pharmaceuticals Ltd)
  Ganciclovir 1.5 mg per 1 gram Virgan 0.15% eye gel | 5 gram PoM
  £19.99 DT = £19.99

4 Eye procedures

Mydriatics and cycloplegics   25-Apr-2020

Overview
Antimuscarinics dilate the pupil and paralyse the ciliary muscle; they vary in potency and duration of action.

Short-acting, relatively weak mydriatics, such as tropicamide below (action lasts for up to 6 hours), facilitate the examination of the fundus of the eye. Longer-acting options include cyclopentolate hydrochloride p. 1210 (complete recovery can take up to 24 hours) or atropine sulfate p. 1210 (action up to 7 days).

Phenylephrine hydrochloride p. 1220 is a sympathomimetic licensed for mydriasis in diagnostic or therapeutic procedures. Mydriasis occurs within 60–90 minutes and lasts up to 5–7 hours.

EvGr Mydriatics and cycloplegics are used in the treatment of anterior uveitis, usually as an adjunct to corticosteroids. Atropine sulfate or cyclopentolate hydrochloride can prevent posterior synechiae and relieve ciliary spasm when used for anterior uveitis. Ⓐ

Other drugs used for Eye procedures Apraclonidine, p. 1232

ANTIMUSCARINICS

▰ 1210

Tropicamide

● INDICATIONS AND DOSE
Funduscopy
▸ TO THE EYE
▸ Child: 0.5% eye drops to be applied 20 minutes before examination
▸ Adult: (consult product literature)

● INTERACTIONS → Appendix 1: tropicamide
● SIDE-EFFECTS Eye erythema · eye irritation (on prolonged administration) · eye pain · headache · hypotension · nausea · syncope · vision blurred
● PRESCRIBING AND DISPENSING INFORMATION Although multi-dose tropicamide eye drops commonly contain preservatives, preservative-free unit dose vials may be available.

● MEDICINAL FORMS There can be variation in the licensing of different medicines containing the same drug.

Eye drops
EXCIPIENTS: May contain Benzalkonium chloride, edetic acid (edta)
▸ Mydriacyl (Alcon Eye Care Ltd)
  Tropicamide 10 mg per 1 ml Mydriacyl 1% eye drops | 5 ml PoM
  £1.60 DT = £1.60
▸ Tropicamide (Bausch & Lomb UK Ltd)
  Tropicamide 5 mg per 1 ml Minims tropicamide 0.5% eye drops
  0.5ml unit dose | 20 unit dose PoM £11.18 DT = £11.18
  Tropicamide 10 mg per 1 ml Minims tropicamide 1% eye drops
  0.5ml unit dose | 20 unit dose PoM £11.31 DT = £11.31

Combinations available: *Phenylephrine with tropicamide,* p. 1220 · *Tropicamide with phenylephrine and lidocaine,* p. 1220

ANTISEPTICS AND DISINFECTANTS ⟩ IODINE PRODUCTS

Povidone-iodine

● INDICATIONS AND DOSE
Cutaneous peri-ocular and conjunctival antisepsis before ocular surgery
▸ TO THE EYE
▸ Adult: Apply, leave for 2 minutes, then irrigate thoroughly with sodium chloride 0.9%

● CONTRA-INDICATIONS Concomitant use of ocular antimicrobial drugs · concomitant use of ocular formulations containing mercury-based preservatives · preterm neonates
● SIDE-EFFECTS
▸ **Rare or very rare** Eye erythema · punctate keratitis
▸ **Frequency not known** Cytotoxicity · eye discolouration
● BREAST FEEDING Avoid regular or excessive use.
● PRESCRIBING AND DISPENSING INFORMATION Although multi-dose povidone iodine eye drops commonly contain preservatives, preservative-free unit dose vials may be available.

● MEDICINAL FORMS There can be variation in the licensing of different medicines containing the same drug. Forms available from special-order manufacturers include: eye drops, eye lotion

Eye drops
▸ Povidone iodine (Bausch & Lomb UK Ltd)
  Povidone-Iodine 50 mg per 1 ml Minims povidone iodine 5% eye drops 0.4ml unit dose | 20 unit dose PoM £16.00 DT = £16.00

DIAGNOSTIC AGENTS ⟩ DYES

Fluorescein sodium

● INDICATIONS AND DOSE
Detection of lesions and foreign bodies
▸ TO THE EYE
▸ Adult: Use sufficient amount to stain damaged areas

● PRESCRIBING AND DISPENSING INFORMATION Although multi-dose fluorescein eye drops commonly contain preservatives, preservative-free unit dose vials may be available.

● MEDICINAL FORMS There can be variation in the licensing of different medicines containing the same drug.

Eye drops
▸ Fluorescein sodium (Bausch & Lomb UK Ltd)
  Fluorescein sodium 10 mg per 1 ml Minims fluorescein sodium 1% eye drops 0.5ml unit dose | 20 unit dose Ⓟ £9.25
  Fluorescein sodium 20 mg per 1 ml Minims fluorescein sodium 2% eye drops 0.5ml unit dose | 20 unit dose Ⓟ £9.25

11
Eye

MIOTICS > PARASYMPATHOMIMETICS

Acetylcholine chloride

- **INDICATIONS AND DOSE**

Cataract surgery | Penetrating keratoplasty | Iridectomy | Anterior segment surgery requiring rapid complete miosis
  ▸ TO THE EYE
  ▸ Adult: (consult product literature)

- **CAUTIONS** Asthma · gastro-intestinal spasm · heart failure · hyperthyroidism · parkinsonism · peptic ulcer · urinary-tract obstruction
- **SIDE-EFFECTS** Bradycardia · corneal decompensation · corneal oedema · dyspnoea · flushing · hyperhidrosis · hypotension
- **PREGNANCY** Avoid unless potential benefit outweighs risk—no information available.
- **BREAST FEEDING** Avoid unless potential benefit outweighs risk—no information available.

- **MEDICINAL FORMS** There can be variation in the licensing of different medicines containing the same drug.
  Irrigation
  ▸ Miochol-E (Bausch & Lomb UK Ltd)
    Acetylcholine chloride 20 mg Miochol-E 20mg powder and solvent for solution for intraocular irrigation vials | 1 vial PoM £7.28
  ▸ Miphtel (Farmigea S.p.A.)
    Acetylcholine chloride 20 mg Miphtel 20mg powder and solvent for solution for intraocular irrigation ampoules | 6 ampoule PoM £43.68 (Hospital only)

SYMPATHOMIMETICS > VASOCONSTRICTOR

Phenylephrine hydrochloride

- **INDICATIONS AND DOSE**

Mydriasis
  ▸ TO THE EYE
  ▸ Child: Apply 1 drop, to be administered before procedure, a drop of proxymetacaine topical anaesthetic may be applied to the eye a few minutes before using phenylephrine to prevent stinging
  ▸ Adult: Apply 1 drop, to be administered before procedure, then apply 1 drop after 60 minutes if required, a drop of topical anaesthetic may be applied to the eye a few minutes before using phenylephrine to prevent stinging

- **CONTRA-INDICATIONS** 10% strength eye drops in children · 10% strength eye drops in elderly · aneurysms · cardiovascular disease · hypertension · thyrotoxicosis
- **CAUTIONS** Asthma · cerebral arteriosclerosis (in adults) · corneal epithelial damage · darkly pigmented iris is more resistant to pupillary dilatation and caution should be exercised to avoid overdosage · diabetes (avoid eye drops in long standing diabetes) · mydriasis can precipitate acute angle-closure glaucoma in a few patients, usually over 60 years and hypermetropic (long-sighted), who are pre-disposed to the condition because of a shallow anterior chamber (in adults) · mydriasis can precipitate acute angle-closure glaucoma in the very few children who are predisposed to the condition because of a shallow anterior chamber · ocular hyperaemia · susceptibility to angle-closure glaucoma
- **INTERACTIONS** → Appendix 1: sympathomimetics, vasoconstrictor
- **SIDE-EFFECTS** Arrhythmias · conjunctivitis allergic · eye discomfort · hypertension · myocardial infarction (usually after use of 10% strength in patients with pre-existing cardiovascular disease) · palpitations · periorbital pallor (in children) · vision disorders

- **PREGNANCY** Use only if potential benefit outweighs risk.
- **BREAST FEEDING** Use only if potential benefit outweighs risk—no information available.
- **PRESCRIBING AND DISPENSING INFORMATION** Although multi-dose phenylephrine eye drops commonly contain preservatives, preservative-free unit dose vials may be available.
- **PATIENT AND CARER ADVICE**
  Driving and skilled tasks Patients should be warned not to undertake skilled tasks (e.g. driving) until vision clears after mydriasis.

- **MEDICINAL FORMS** There can be variation in the licensing of different medicines containing the same drug. Forms available from special-order manufacturers include: eye drops
  Eye drops
  EXCIPIENTS: May contain Disodium edetate, sodium metabisulfite
  ▸ Phenylephrine hydrochloride (Bausch & Lomb UK Ltd)
    Phenylephrine hydrochloride 25 mg per 1 ml Minims phenylephrine hydrochloride 2.5% eye drops 0.5ml unit dose | 20 unit dose P £11.87 DT = £11.87
    Phenylephrine hydrochloride 100 mg per 1 ml Minims phenylephrine hydrochloride 10% eye drops 0.5ml unit dose | 20 unit dose P £11.87 DT = £11.87

Phenylephrine with tropicamide

12-Aug-2020

The properties listed below are those particular to the combination only. For the properties of the components please consider, phenylephrine hydrochloride above, tropicamide p. 1219.

- **INDICATIONS AND DOSE**

Pre-operative mydriasis | Diagnostic procedures when monotherapy insufficient
  ▸ TO THE EYE
  ▸ Adult: One insert to be applied into the lower conjunctival sac up to max. 2 hours before procedure; remove insert within 30 minutes of satisfactory mydriasis, and within 2 hours of application

- **INTERACTIONS** → Appendix 1: sympathomimetics, vasoconstrictor · tropicamide
- **DIRECTIONS FOR ADMINISTRATION** Manufacturer advises patients with severe dry eyes may require a drop of saline to improve insert tolerance.

- **MEDICINAL FORMS** There can be variation in the licensing of different medicines containing the same drug.
  Ophthalmic insert
  ▸ Mydriasert (Thea Pharmaceuticals Ltd)
    Tropicamide.28 mg, Phenylephrine hydrochloride 5.4 mg Mydriasert 5.4mg/0.28mg ophthalmic inserts | 20 insert PoM £84.00

Tropicamide with phenylephrine and lidocaine

17-Aug-2017

- **INDICATIONS AND DOSE**

Mydriasis and intraocular anaesthesia during cataract surgery
  ▸ BY INTRACAMERAL INJECTION
  ▸ Adult: 0.2 mL for 1 dose, to be injected slowly at the start of the surgical procedure

DOSE EQUIVALENCE AND CONVERSION
  ▸ Each 0.2 mL dose of *Mydrane*® solution for injection contains 0.04 mg of tropicamide, 0.62 mg of phenylephrine hydrochloride and 2 mg of lidocaine hydrochloride.

11

Eye

CONTRA-INDICATIONS Cataract surgery combined with vitrectomy · history of acute, narrow-angle glaucoma · shallow anterior chamber

CAUTIONS Conditions where systemic exposure to phenylephrine or lidocaine could be harmful (consult product literature) · risk of floppy iris syndrome (consult product literature)

INTERACTIONS → Appendix 1: antiarrhythmics · sympathomimetics, vasoconstrictor · tropicamide

SIDE-EFFECTS
Uncommon Headache · hyperaemia · hypertension · keratitis

ALLERGY AND CROSS-SENSITIVITY Contra-indicated in patients with known hypersensitivity to amide-type anaesthetics or atropine derivatives.

PREGNANCY Manufacturer advises avoid (systemic uptake after administration cannot be excluded)—insufficient data available for phenylephrine and tropicamide in pregnancy; lidocaine crosses the placenta but is not known to be harmful in *animal* studies.

BREAST FEEDING Manufacturer advises avoid—no data available for phenylephrine or tropicamide; lidocaine present in milk in small amount.

PRE-TREATMENT SCREENING Manufacturer advises patients must have demonstrated, at a previous visit, a satisfactory pupil dilation with topical mydriatic treatment.

PATIENT AND CARER ADVICE
Driving and skilled tasks Manufacturer advises patients should be counselled about the effects on driving and skilled tasks.

MEDICINAL FORMS There can be variation in the licensing of different medicines containing the same drug.
Solution for injection
EXCIPIENTS: May contain Disodium edetate
▸ Mydrane (Thea Pharmaceuticals Ltd)
 Tropicamide 200 microgram per 1 ml, Phenylephrine hydrochloride 3.1 mg per 1 ml, Lidocaine hydrochloride 10 mg per 1 ml Mydrane 0.2mg/ml / 3.1mg/ml / 10mg/ml solution for injection 0.6ml ampoules | 20 ampoule [PoM] £119.95

4.1 Post-operative pain and inflammation

Eye, surgical and peri-operative drug use

Ocular peri-operative drugs

Drugs used to prepare the eye for surgery, drugs that are injected into the anterior chamber at the time of surgery, and those used after eye surgery, are included here.

Cefuroxime p. 1216, administered by intra-ocular injection into the anterior chamber of the eye (intracameral use), is used for the prophylaxis of endophthalmitis after cataract surgery.

Non-steroidal anti-inflammatory eye drops such as diclofenac sodium p. 1222, flurbiprofen p. 1222, ketorolac trometamol p. 1223, and nepafenac p. 1206, are used for the prophylaxis and treatment of inflammation, pain, and other symptoms associated with ocular surgery or laser treatment of the eye. Bromfenac p. 1222 is used for the treatment of postoperative inflammation following cataract surgery. Diclofenac sodium and flurbiprofen are also used to prevent miosis during ocular surgery.

Apraclonidine p. 1232, an alpha$_2$-adrenoreceptor agonist, reduces intra-ocular pressure possibly by reducing the production of aqueous humour. It is used to control increases in intra-ocular pressure associated with ocular surgery and as short-term treatment to reduce intraocular pressure prior to surgery.

Acetylcholine chloride p. 1220, administered into the anterior chamber of the eye during surgery, rapidly produces miosis which lasts approximately 20 minutes. If prolonged miosis is required, it can be applied again.

Intra-ocular sodium hyaluronate p. 1214 and balanced salt solution are used during surgical procedures on the eye.

Povidone-iodine p. 1219 is used for peri-ocular and conjunctival antisepsis before ocular surgery to support postoperative infection control.

Ocular local anaesthetics

Oxybuprocaine hydrochloride below and tetracaine p. 1222 are widely used topical local anaesthetics. Proxymetacaine hydrochloride p. 1222 causes less initial stinging and is useful for children. Oxybuprocaine hydrochloride or a combined preparation of lidocaine hydrochloride p. 1406 and fluorescein sodium p. 1219 is used for tonometry. Tetracaine produces a more profound anaesthesia and is suitable for use before minor surgical procedures, such as the removal of corneal sutures. It has a temporary disruptive effect on the corneal epithelium. Lidocaine hydrochloride, with or without adrenaline/epinephrine p. 238, is injected into the eyelids for minor surgery. Local anaesthetics should never be used for the management of ocular symptoms.

ANAESTHETICS, LOCAL

Fluorescein with lidocaine

● INDICATIONS AND DOSE
Local anaesthesia
▸ TO THE EYE
▸ Adult: Apply as required

● PRESCRIBING AND DISPENSING INFORMATION Although multi-dose lidocaine and fluorescein eye drops commonly contain preservatives, preservative-free unit dose vials may be available.

● MEDICINAL FORMS There can be variation in the licensing of different medicines containing the same drug.
Eye drops
▸ Lidocaine and Fluorescein (Bausch & Lomb UK Ltd)
 Fluorescein sodium 2.5 mg per 1 ml, Lidocaine hydrochloride 40 mg per 1 ml Minims lidocaine and fluorescein eye drops 0.5ml unit dose | 20 unit dose [PoM] £11.69

Oxybuprocaine hydrochloride

(Benoxinate hydrochloride)

● INDICATIONS AND DOSE
Local anaesthetic
▸ TO THE EYE
▸ Adult: Apply as required

● CONTRA-INDICATIONS Avoid in preterm neonates

● INTERACTIONS → Appendix 1: anaesthetics, local

● PRESCRIBING AND DISPENSING INFORMATION Although multi-dose oxybuprocaine eye drops commonly contain preservatives, preservative-free unit dose vials may be available.

11

Eye

● MEDICINAL FORMS There can be variation in the licensing of different medicines containing the same drug.
Eye drops
 ‣ Oxybuprocaine hydrochloride (Bausch & Lomb UK Ltd)
 Oxybuprocaine hydrochloride 4 mg per 1 ml Minims oxybuprocaine hydrochloride 0.4% eye drops 0.5ml unit dose | 20 unit dose [PoM] £10.56

Proxymetacaine hydrochloride

● INDICATIONS AND DOSE

Local anaesthetic
 ▸ TO THE EYE
 ‣ Adult: Apply as required

● INTERACTIONS → Appendix 1: anaesthetics, local
● PRESCRIBING AND DISPENSING INFORMATION Although multi-dose proxymetacaine eye drops commonly contain preservatives, preservative-free unit dose vials may be available.

● MEDICINAL FORMS There can be variation in the licensing of different medicines containing the same drug.
Eye drops
 ‣ Proxymetacaine (Bausch & Lomb UK Ltd)
 Proxymetacaine hydrochloride 5 mg per 1 ml Minims proxymetacaine 0.5% eye drops 0.5ml unit dose | 20 unit dose [PoM] £12.12

Tetracaine

10-Mar-2020

(Amethocaine)

● INDICATIONS AND DOSE

Local anaesthetic
 ▸ TO THE EYE
 ‣ Adult: Apply as required

● INTERACTIONS → Appendix 1: anaesthetics, local
● SIDE-EFFECTS Dermatitis · eye disorders · eye inflammation · paraesthesia
● PRESCRIBING AND DISPENSING INFORMATION Although multi-dose tetracaine eye drops commonly contain preservatives, preservative-free unit dose vials may be available.

● MEDICINAL FORMS There can be variation in the licensing of different medicines containing the same drug.
Eye drops
 ‣ Tetracaine (Non-proprietary)
 Tetracaine hydrochloride 5 mg per 1 ml Minims tetracaine hydrochloride 0.5% eye drops 0.5ml unit dose | 20 unit dose [PoM] £10.57 DT = £10.57
 Tetracaine hydrochloride 10 mg per 1 ml Minims tetracaine hydrochloride 1% eye drops 0.5ml unit dose | 20 unit dose [PoM] £10.57 DT = £10.57

ANALGESICS 〉 NON-STEROIDAL ANTI-INFLAMMATORY DRUGS

Bromfenac

14-Jul-2020

● INDICATIONS AND DOSE

Postoperative inflammation following cataract surgery
 ▸ TO THE EYE
 ‣ Adult: (consult product literature)

● INTERACTIONS → Appendix 1: NSAIDs

● MEDICINAL FORMS There can be variation in the licensing of different medicines containing the same drug.
Eye drops
 EXCIPIENTS: May contain Benzalkonium chloride, disodium edetate, sulfites
 ‣ Yellox (Bausch & Lomb UK Ltd)
 Bromfenac (as Bromfenac sodium sesquihydrate) 900 microgram per 1 ml Yellox 900micrograms/ml eye drops | 5 ml [PoM] £8.50 DT = £8.50

Diclofenac sodium

18-Nov-202●

● INDICATIONS AND DOSE

Inhibition of intra-operative miosis during cataract surgery (but does not possess intrinsic mydriatic properties) | Postoperative inflammation in cataract surgery, strabismus surgery or argon laser trabeculoplasty | Pain in corneal epithelial defects after photorefractive keratectomy, radial keratotomy or accidental trauma | Seasonal allergic conjunctivitis
 ▸ TO THE EYE
 ‣ Adult: (consult product literature)

● INTERACTIONS → Appendix 1: NSAIDs
● SIDE-EFFECTS
 ▸ **Common or very common** Oedema · skin reactions
 ▸ **Rare or very rare** Asthma exacerbated · eye disorders · eye inflammation · hypersensitivity
 ▸ **Frequency not known** Dyspnoea · eye discomfort · rhinitis · vision blurred
● ALLERGY AND CROSS-SENSITIVITY [EvGr] Contra-indicated in patients with a history of hypersensitivity to aspirin or any other NSAID—which includes those in whom attacks of asthma, angioedema, urticaria or rhinitis have been precipitated by aspirin or any other NSAID. ⟨M⟩
● PRESCRIBING AND DISPENSING INFORMATION Although multi-dose diclofenac sodium eye drops commonly contain preservatives, preservative-free unit dose vials may be available.

● MEDICINAL FORMS There can be variation in the licensing of different medicines containing the same drug.
Eye drops
 EXCIPIENTS: May contain Benzalkonium chloride, disodium edetate, propylene glycol
 ‣ Voltarol Ophtha (Thea Pharmaceuticals Ltd)
 Diclofenac sodium 1 mg per 1 ml Voltarol Ophtha 0.1% eye drops 0.3ml unit dose | 5 unit dose [PoM] £4.00 DT = £4.00 | 40 unit dose [PoM] £32.00 DT = £32.00
 ‣ Voltarol Ophtha Multidose (Thea Pharmaceuticals Ltd)
 Diclofenac sodium 1 mg per 1 ml Voltarol Ophtha Multidose 0.1% eye drops | 5 ml [PoM] £6.68 DT = £6.68

Flurbiprofen

18-Nov-2020

● INDICATIONS AND DOSE

Inhibition of intra-operative miosis (but does not possess intrinsic mydriatic properties) | Control of anterior segment inflammation following postoperative and post-laser trabeculoplasty when corticosteroids contra-indicated
 ▸ TO THE EYE
 ‣ Adult: (consult product literature)

● INTERACTIONS → Appendix 1: NSAIDs
● SIDE-EFFECTS
 ▸ **Common or very common** Eye discomfort · haemorrhage
 ▸ **Frequency not known** Eye disorders
● ALLERGY AND CROSS-SENSITIVITY [EvGr] Contra-indicated in patients with a history of hypersensitivity to aspirin or any other NSAID—which includes those in whom attacks

of asthma, angioedema, urticaria or rhinitis have been precipitated by aspirin or any other NSAID. Ⓜ

● MEDICINAL FORMS There can be variation in the licensing of different medicines containing the same drug.

Eye drops
▸ Ocufen (Allergan Ltd)
Flurbiprofen sodium 300 microgram per 1 ml Ocufen 0.03% eye drops 0.4ml unit dose | 40 unit dose [PoM] £37.15 DT = £37.15

Ketorolac trometamol
07-Dec-2020

● INDICATIONS AND DOSE

Prophylaxis and reduction of inflammation and associated symptoms following ocular surgery
▸ TO THE EYE
▸ Adult: (consult product literature)

● CAUTIONS May mask symptoms of infection

● INTERACTIONS → Appendix 1: NSAIDs

● SIDE-EFFECTS
● **Common or very common** Eye discomfort · eye disorders · eye infection · eye inflammation · headache · hypersensitivity · keratic deposits · paraesthesia · retinal haemorrhage · vision disorders
● **Uncommon** Dry eye
● **Frequency not known** Asthma exacerbated · bronchospasm

● ALLERGY AND CROSS-SENSITIVITY [EvGr] Contra-indicated in patients with a history of hypersensitivity to aspirin or any other NSAID—which includes those in whom attacks of asthma, angioedema, urticaria or rhinitis have been precipitated by aspirin or any other NSAID. Ⓜ

● MEDICINAL FORMS There can be variation in the licensing of different medicines containing the same drug.

Eye drops
EXCIPIENTS: May contain Benzalkonium chloride, disodium edetate
▸ Ketorolac trometamol (Non-proprietary)
Ketorolac trometamol 5 mg per 1 ml Ketorolac 0.5% eye drops | 5 ml [PoM] £3.99 DT = £3.99
▸ Acular (Allergan Ltd)
Ketorolac trometamol 5 mg per 1 ml Acular 0.5% eye drops | 5 ml [PoM] £3.00 DT = £3.99

CORTICOSTEROIDS

Loteprednol etabonate
25-Sep-2020

● INDICATIONS AND DOSE

Treatment of post-operative inflammation following ocular surgery
▸ TO THE EYE
▸ Adult: Apply 4 times a day for maximum duration of treatment of 14 days, to be started 24 hours after surgery

IMPORTANT SAFETY INFORMATION
MHRA/CHM ADVICE: CORTICOSTEROIDS: RARE RISK OF CENTRAL SEROUS CHORIORETINOPATHY WITH LOCAL AS WELL AS SYSTEMIC ADMINISTRATION (AUGUST 2017) See Corticosteroids, general use p. 709.
NHS IMPROVEMENT PATIENT SAFETY ALERT: STEROID EMERGENCY CARD TO SUPPORT EARLY RECOGNITION AND TREATMENT OF ADRENAL CRISIS IN ADULTS (AUGUST 2020) See Corticosteroids, general use p. 709.

● SIDE-EFFECTS
● **Common or very common** Dry eye · eye discomfort · eye disorders · headaches
● **Uncommon** Conjunctival oedema · vision disorders
● **Rare or very rare** Breast neoplasm · face oedema · muscle twitching · taste altered

● MEDICINAL FORMS There can be variation in the licensing of different medicines containing the same drug.

Eye drops
EXCIPIENTS: May contain Benzalkonium chloride, disodium edetate
▸ Lotemax (Bausch & Lomb UK Ltd)
Loteprednol etabonate 5 mg per 1 ml Lotemax 0.5% eye drops | 5 ml [PoM] £5.50 DT = £5.50

5   Glaucoma and ocular hypertension

Glaucoma and ocular hypertension
11-Apr-2018

Description of condition
Glaucoma is a group of eye disorders characterised by a loss of visual field associated with pathological cupping of the optic disc and optic nerve damage. While glaucoma is generally linked to raised intra-ocular pressure, which is the main treatable risk factor, it can also occur when the intra-ocular pressure is within the normal range. Other risk factors include age, family history, ethnicity, corticosteroid use, myopia, type 2 diabetes mellitus, cardiovascular disease, and hypertension.

The most common form of glaucoma is chronic open-angle glaucoma (also known as primary open-angle glaucoma) where drainage of the aqueous humour through the trabecular meshwork is restricted, and the angle between the iris and the cornea is normal. Initially, this condition tends to be asymptomatic, however, as glaucoma progresses, patients may present with irreversible sight loss or visual field defects. Patients with ocular hypertension (an intra-ocular pressure greater than 21 mmHg) are at high risk of developing chronic open-angle glaucoma. The diagnosis, monitoring, and management of patients with ocular hypertension, suspected chronic open-angle glaucoma, or chronic open-angle glaucoma should be carried out by a specialist.

Acute angle-closure glaucoma is less common and occurs when the outflow of aqueous humour from the eye is totally obstructed by bowing of the iris against the trabecular meshwork. It is characterised by its abrupt onset of symptoms, and it is a sight-threatening medical emergency that requires urgent reduction of intra-ocular pressure to prevent loss of vision.

Aims of treatment
The aim of treatment is to control intra-ocular pressure to prevent the development or progression of glaucoma and subsequent visual field damage, or sight loss.

Ocular hypertension
[EvGr] A topical prostaglandin analogue, such as latanoprost p. 1228, tafluprost p. 1229, travoprost p. 1230, or bimatoprost p. 1231 (a synthetic prostamide), is recommended as first-line treatment in patients with an intra-ocular pressure of 24 mmHg or greater and who are at risk of visual impairment within their lifetime. When assessing patient's risk of future visual impairment, the level of intra-ocular pressure, central corneal thickness measurement, family history, and life expectancy should be taken into consideration. Patients who are not at risk of visual impairment in their lifetime do not require treatment but should be monitored regularly.

If initial treatment with a topical prostaglandin analogue is not tolerated, an alternative prostaglandin analogue should be tried before switching to a topical beta-blocker such as betaxolol p. 1224, levobunolol hydrochloride p. 1224, or timolol maleate p. 1225). If treatment is still not tolerated, alternative options include carbonic anhydrase inhibitors such as brinzolamide p. 1226 or dorzolamide p. 1227, a topical sympathomimetic such as apraclonidine p. 1232 [unlicensed use] or brimonidine tartrate p. 1232, or a topical miotic such as pilocarpine p. 1228 [unlicensed use], given either as monotherapy or as combination therapy.

Alternatives as either monotherapy or combination therapy with drugs from different therapeutic classes (topical beta-blockers, carbonic anhydrase inhibitors, or topical sympathomimetics), should also be offered to patients with an intra-ocular pressure of 24 mmHg or more whose current treatment is not reducing intra-ocular pressure sufficiently to prevent the risk of progression to sight loss. The patient's adherence and drop instillation technique should also be checked. If drug treatment still does not sufficiently reduce intra-ocular pressure to a satisfactory level, patients should be referred to a consultant ophthalmologist to discuss other options.

Preservative free eye drops should be used in patients who are allergic to preservatives, or those who have clinically significant ocular surface disease and are at high risk of conversion to chronic open-angle glaucoma. ⟨A⟩

Note: based on cost-effective analysis, NICE guidelines 81 recommend treatment with generic prostaglandin analogues as first-line, and non-generic prostaglandin analogues as third - line if topical beta-blocker treatment is ineffective.

Suspected chronic open-angle glaucoma

⟨EvGr⟩ In patients with suspected chronic open-angle glaucoma and an intra-ocular pressure of 24 mmHg or greater, the same treatment recommendations as for the management of ocular hypertension should be followed. Patients with an intra-ocular pressure below 24 mmHg do not require drug treatment, but should be regularly monitored for changes in intra-ocular pressure and visual impairment. ⟨A⟩

Chronic open-angle glaucoma

⟨EvGr⟩ Topical prostaglandin analogues such as latanoprost p. 1228, tafluprost p. 1229, travoprost p. 1230, or bimatoprost p. 1231 (a synthetic prostamide), are used first-line in patients with confirmed chronic open-angle glaucoma. If first-line treatment does not sufficiently reduce intra-ocular pressure and the patient's adherence to treatment and eye drop instillation technique are both satisfactory, treatment with either a topical beta-blocker such as betaxolol below, levobunolol hydrochloride below, and timolol maleate p. 1225, a carbonic anhydrase inhibitor such as brinzolamide p. 1226 or dorzolamide p. 1227, a topical sympathomimetic such as apraclonidine p. 1232 or brimonidine tartrate p. 1232, or a combination of these, should be offered. When a particular drug is not tolerated, another drug from a different therapeutic class can be tried. Preservative free eye drops should be used in patients who are allergic to preservatives, or those who have clinically significant ocular surface disease. Alternative treatment options are laser trabeculoplasty or surgery with pharmacological augmentation (with mitomycin p. 963 [unlicensed indication]).

Patients with *advanced chronic open-angle glaucoma* should be offered surgery with pharmacological augmentation (with mitomycin p. 963 [unlicensed indication]). Treatment with a topical prostaglandin analogue should be initiated and continued until surgery takes place.

If surgery fails to adequately reduce the intra-ocular pressure, alternative options include drug treatment (a combination of topical drugs from different therapeutic classes may be needed), further surgery, laser trabeculoplasty, or cyclodiode laser treatment. ⟨A⟩

Useful Resources

Glaucoma: diagnosis and management. National Institute for Health and Care Excellence. NICE guideline 81. November 2017.
www.nice.org.uk/guidance/ng81

BETA-ADRENOCEPTOR BLOCKERS

Betaxolol

03-Apr-202●

● **INDICATIONS AND DOSE**

Chronic open-angle glaucoma | Ocular hypertension
▸ TO THE EYE
▸ Adult: Apply twice daily

● CONTRA-INDICATIONS Also consider contra-indications listed for systemically administered beta blockers · bradycardia · heart block
● CAUTIONS Patients with corneal disease
CAUTIONS, FURTHER INFORMATION Systemic absorption can follow topical application to the eyes; consider cautions listed for systemically administered beta blockers.
● INTERACTIONS → Appendix 1: beta blockers, selective
● SIDE-EFFECTS
▸ **Common or very common** Eye discomfort · eye disorders · vision disorders
▸ **Uncommon** Dry eye · eye inflammation · rhinitis
▸ **Rare or very rare** Cataract · rhinorrhoea · skin reactions
▸ **Frequency not known** Angioedema · hypersensitivity
SIDE-EFFECTS, FURTHER INFORMATION Systemic absorption can follow topical application to the eyes; consider side effects listed for systemically administered beta blockers.
● PRESCRIBING AND DISPENSING INFORMATION Although multi-dose bextaxolol eye drops commonly contain preservatives, preservative-free unit dose vials may be available.

● MEDICINAL FORMS There can be variation in the licensing of different medicines containing the same drug.
Eye drops
EXCIPIENTS: May contain Benzalkonium chloride, disodium edetate
▸ Betaxolol (Non-proprietary)
  Betaxolol (as Betaxolol hydrochloride) 5 mg per 1 ml Betaxolol 0.5% eye drops | 5 ml [PoM] [N] DT = £1.90
▸ Betoptic (Novartis Pharmaceuticals UK Ltd)
  Betaxolol (as Betaxolol hydrochloride) 2.5 mg per 1 ml Betoptic 0.25% suspension eye drops | 5 ml [PoM] £2.66 DT = £2.66
  Betoptic 0.25% eye drops suspension 0.25ml unit dose | 50 unit dose [PoM] £13.77 DT = £13.77
  Betaxolol (as Betaxolol hydrochloride) 5 mg per 1 ml Betoptic 0.5% eye drops | 5 ml [PoM] £1.90 DT = £1.90

Levobunolol hydrochloride

03-Apr-2020

● **INDICATIONS AND DOSE**

Chronic open-angle glaucoma | Ocular hypertension
▸ TO THE EYE
▸ Adult: Apply 1–2 times a day

● CONTRA-INDICATIONS Also consider contra-indications listed for systemically administered beta blockers · bradycardia · heart block
● CAUTIONS Patients with corneal disease
CAUTIONS, FURTHER INFORMATION Systemic absorption can follow topical application to the eyes; consider cautions listed for systemically administered beta blockers.
● INTERACTIONS → Appendix 1: beta blockers, non-selective

SIDE-EFFECTS

Common or very common Eye discomfort · eye inflammation
Frequency not known Dry eye · eye disorders · eyelid eczema · vision blurred

SIDE-EFFECTS, FURTHER INFORMATION Systemic absorption can follow topical application to the eyes; consider side effects listed for systemically administered beta blockers.

▶ PRESCRIBING AND DISPENSING INFORMATION Although multi-dose (Levobunolol) eye drops commonly contain preservatives, preservative-free unit dose vials may be available.

▶ MEDICINAL FORMS There can be variation in the licensing of different medicines containing the same drug.

Eye drops

EXCIPIENTS: May contain Disodium edetate
▶ Betagan (Allergan Ltd)
    Levobunolol hydrochloride 5 mg per 1 ml Betagan Unit Dose 0.5% eye drops 0.4ml unit dose | 30 dose | PoM | £9.98 DT = £9.98

⬛ 161

Timolol maleate

31-Jul-2019

● INDICATIONS AND DOSE

Chronic open-angle glaucoma | Ocular hypertension
▶ TO THE EYE
▶ Adult: Apply twice daily

TIMOPTOL-LA ®

Reduction of intra-ocular pressure in primary open-angle glaucoma
▶ TO THE EYE
▶ Adult: Apply once daily

TIOPEX ®

Reduction of intra-ocular pressure in primary open-angle glaucoma
▶ TO THE EYE
▶ Adult: Apply once daily, to be applied in the morning

● CONTRA-INDICATIONS Also consider contra-indications listed for systemically administered beta blockers · bradycardia · heart block
● CAUTIONS Consider also cautions listed for systemically administered beta blockers · patients with corneal disease
● INTERACTIONS → Appendix 1: beta blockers, non-selective
● SIDE-EFFECTS
▶ **Common or very common** Eye discomfort · eye disorders · eye inflammation · vision disorders

SIDE-EFFECTS, FURTHER INFORMATION Systemic absorption can follow topical application to the eyes; consider side effects listed for systemically administered beta blockers.

● BREAST FEEDING Manufacturer advises avoidance.
● PRESCRIBING AND DISPENSING INFORMATION Although multi-dose timolol eye drops commonly contain preservatives, preservative-free unit dose vials may be available.
● NATIONAL FUNDING/ACCESS DECISIONS

TIOPEX ® For full details see funding body website
Scottish Medicines Consortium (SMC) decisions
▶ timolol eye gel (*Tiopex*®) for the reduction of the elevated intra-ocular pressure in patients with ocular hypertension or chronic open angle glaucoma.(February 2014) SMC No. 941/14 Recommended with restrictions

● MEDICINAL FORMS There can be variation in the licensing of different medicines containing the same drug.

Eye gel

EXCIPIENTS: May contain Benzododecinium bromide
▶ Timoptol-LA (Santen UK Ltd)
    Timolol (as Timolol maleate) 2.5 mg per 1 ml Timoptol-LA 0.25% ophthalmic gel-forming solution | 2.5 ml | PoM | £3.12 DT = £3.12
    Timolol (as Timolol maleate) 5 mg per 1 ml Timoptol-LA 0.5% ophthalmic gel-forming solution | 2.5 ml | PoM | £3.12 DT = £3.12

Eye drops

EXCIPIENTS: May contain Benzalkonium chloride
▶ Timolol maleate (Non-proprietary)
    Timolol (as Timolol maleate) 2.5 mg per 1 ml Timolol 0.25% eye drops | 5 ml | PoM | £1.58 DT = £1.33
    Timolol (as Timolol maleate) 5 mg per 1 ml Timolol 0.5% eye drops | 5 ml | PoM | £1.34 DT = £1.34
▶ Eysano (Aspire Pharma Ltd)
    Timolol (as Timolol maleate) 2.5 mg per 1 ml Eysano 2.5mg/ml eye drops | 5 ml | PoM | £8.45 DT = £8.45
    Timolol (as Timolol maleate) 5 mg per 1 ml Eysano 5mg/ml eye drops | 5 ml | PoM | £9.65 DT = £9.65
▶ Timoptol (Santen UK Ltd)
    Timolol (as Timolol maleate) 2.5 mg per 1 ml Timoptol 0.25% eye drops | 5 ml | PoM | £3.12 DT = £1.33
    Timolol (as Timolol maleate) 5 mg per 1 ml Timoptol 0.5% eye drops | 5 ml | PoM | £3.12 DT = £1.34
▶ Tiopex (Thea Pharmaceuticals Ltd)
    Timolol (as Timolol maleate) 1 mg per 1 gram Tiopex 1mg/g eye gel 0.4g unit dose | 30 unit dose | PoM | £7.49 DT = £7.49

Combinations available: *Bimatoprost with timolol*, p. 1231 · *Brimonidine with timolol*, p. 1233 · *Brinzolamide with timolol*, p. 1227 · *Dorzolamide with timolol*, p. 1227 · *Latanoprost with timolol*, p. 1229 · *Tafluprost with timolol*, p. 1230 · *Travoprost with timolol*, p. 1230

CARBONIC ANHYDRASE INHIBITORS

Acetazolamide

17-Nov-2020

● INDICATIONS AND DOSE

Reduction of intra-ocular pressure in open-angle glaucoma | Reduction of intra-ocular pressure in secondary glaucoma | Reduction of intra-ocular pressure perioperatively in angle-closure glaucoma
▶ BY MOUTH USING IMMEDIATE-RELEASE MEDICINES, OR BY INTRAVENOUS INJECTION, OR BY INTRAMUSCULAR INJECTION
▶ Adult: 0.25–1 g daily in divided doses, intramuscular injection preferably avoided because of alkalinity

Glaucoma
▶ BY MOUTH USING MODIFIED-RELEASE MEDICINES
▶ Adult: 250–500 mg daily

Epilepsy
▶ BY MOUTH USING IMMEDIATE-RELEASE MEDICINES, OR BY INTRAVENOUS INJECTION, OR BY INTRAMUSCULAR INJECTION
▶ Adult: 0.25–1 g daily in divided doses, intramuscular injection preferably avoided because of alkalinity

---

IMPORTANT SAFETY INFORMATION

MHRA/CHM ADVICE: ANTIEPILEPTICS: RISK OF SUICIDAL THOUGHTS AND BEHAVIOUR (AUGUST 2008)
See Epilepsy p. 321.

MHRA/CHM ADVICE: ANTIEPILEPTIC DRUGS: UPDATED ADVICE ON SWITCHING BETWEEN DIFFERENT MANUFACTURERS' PRODUCTS (NOVEMBER 2017)
See Epilepsy p. 321.

● CONTRA-INDICATIONS Adrenocortical insufficiency · hyperchloraemic acidosis · hypokalaemia · hyponatraemia · long-term administration in chronic angle-closure glaucoma
● CAUTIONS Avoid extravasation at injection site (risk of necrosis) · diabetes mellitus · elderly · impaired alveolar

11

Eye

ventilation (risk of acidosis) · long-term use · pulmonary obstruction (risk of acidosis) · renal calculi

● INTERACTIONS → Appendix 1: acetazolamide

● SIDE-EFFECTS

GENERAL SIDE-EFFECTS

▶ **Common or very common** Haemorrhage · metabolic acidosis · nephrolithiasis · sensation abnormal

▶ **Uncommon** Bone marrow disorders · depression · dizziness · electrolyte imbalance · hearing impairment · hepatic disorders · leucopenia · nausea · renal colic · renal impairment · renal lesions · severe cutaneous adverse reactions (SCARs) · skin reactions · thrombocytopenia · tinnitus · urinary tract discomfort · urine abnormalities · vomiting

▶ **Rare or very rare** Anaphylactic reaction · appetite disorder · confusion · diarrhoea · fatigue · fever · flushing · headache · irritability · libido decreased · paralysis · photosensitivity reaction · seizure

▶ **Frequency not known** Agranulocytosis · drowsiness · myopia · polyuria · suicidal behaviours · taste altered · thirst

SPECIFIC SIDE-EFFECTS

▶ **Uncommon**

▶ With oral use Osteomalacia

▶ **Rare or very rare**

▶ With oral use Ataxia · hyperglycaemia · hypoglycaemia · renal tubular necrosis

▶ **Frequency not known**

▶ With oral use Agitation

SIDE-EFFECTS, FURTHER INFORMATION Acetazolamide is a sulfonamide derivative; blood disorders, rashes, and other sulfonamide-related side-effects occur occasionally — patients should be told to report any unusual skin rash.

If electrolyte disturbances and metabolic acidosis occur, these can be corrected by administering bicarbonate.

● ALLERGY AND CROSS-SENSITIVITY [EvGr] Contra-indicated if history of sulfonamide hypersensitivity. ⟨M⟩

● PREGNANCY Manufacturer advises avoid, especially in first trimester (toxicity in *animal* studies).

● BREAST FEEDING Amount too small to be harmful.

● HEPATIC IMPAIRMENT Manufacturer advises avoid.

● RENAL IMPAIRMENT Avoid — risk of metabolic acidosis.

● MONITORING REQUIREMENTS Monitor blood count and plasma electrolyte concentrations with prolonged use.

● MEDICINAL FORMS There can be variation in the licensing of different medicines containing the same drug. Forms available from special-order manufacturers include: oral suspension, oral solution

Tablet

CAUTIONARY AND ADVISORY LABELS 3

▶ Acetazolamide (Non-proprietary)
  Acetazolamide 250 mg Acetazolamide 250mg tablets | 112 tablet [PoM] £75.36 DT = £8.53

Powder for solution for injection

▶ Diamox (Advanz Pharma)
  Acetazolamide 500 mg Diamox Sodium Parenteral 500mg powder for solution for injection vials | 1 vial [PoM] £14.76

Modified-release capsule

CAUTIONARY AND ADVISORY LABELS 3, 25

▶ Diamox SR (Advanz Pharma)
  Acetazolamide 250 mg Diamox SR 250mg capsules | 30 capsule [PoM] £16.66 DT = £16.66

▶ Eytazox (Teva UK Ltd)
  Acetazolamide 250 mg Eytazox 250mg modified-release capsules | 30 capsule [PoM] £16.60 DT = £16.66

Brinzolamide

20-Nov-202

● INDICATIONS AND DOSE

Reduction of intra-ocular pressure in ocular hypertension and open-angle glaucoma either as adjunct to beta-blockers or prostaglandin analogues or used alone in patients unresponsive to beta-blockers or if beta-blockers contra-indicated

▶ TO THE EYE

▶ Adult: Apply twice daily, then increased if necessary up to 3 times a day

● CONTRA-INDICATIONS Hyperchloraemic acidosis

● CAUTIONS Renal tubular immaturity or abnormality — risk of metabolic acidosis · systemic absorption follows topical application

● INTERACTIONS → Appendix 1: brinzolamide

● SIDE-EFFECTS

▶ **Common or very common** Eye discomfort · eye disorders · taste altered · vision disorders

▶ **Uncommon** Arrhythmias · asthenia · cardio-respiratory distress · chest discomfort · cough · depression · diarrhoea · dizziness · dry eye · dry mouth · dyspnoea · epistaxis · eye deposit · eye inflammation · feeling abnormal · foreign body in eye · gastrointestinal discomfort · gastrointestinal disorders · headache · increased risk of infection · memory loss · motor dysfunction · muscle complaints · nasal complaints · nausea · nervousness · oral disorders · oropharyngeal pain · pain · palpitations · renal pain · scleral discolouration · sensation abnormal · sexual dysfunction · skin reactions · sleep disorders · throat complaints · vomiting

▶ **Rare or very rare** Alopecia · angina pectoris · drowsiness · irritability · optic nerve disorder · respiratory disorders · tinnitus

▶ **Frequency not known** Appetite decreased · arthralgia · asthma · hypertension · malaise · peripheral oedema · tremor · urinary frequency increased · vertigo

SIDE-EFFECTS, FURTHER INFORMATION Systemic absorption can rarely cause sulfonamide-like side-effects and may require discontinuation if severe.

● ALLERGY AND CROSS-SENSITIVITY [EvGr] Contra-indicated if history of sulfonamide hypersensitivity. ⟨M⟩

● PREGNANCY Avoid — toxicity in *animal* studies.

● BREAST FEEDING Use only if benefit outweighs risk.

● HEPATIC IMPAIRMENT Manufacturer advises avoid — no information available.

● RENAL IMPAIRMENT Avoid if eGFR less than 30 mL/minute/1.73 m^2.

● MEDICINAL FORMS There can be variation in the licensing of different medicines containing the same drug.

Eye drops

EXCIPIENTS: May contain Benzalkonium chloride, disodium edetate

▶ Brinzolamide (Non-proprietary)
  Brinzolamide 10 mg per 1 ml Brinzolamide 10mg/ml eye drops | 5 ml [PoM] £7.45 DT = £3.13

▶ Azopt (Novartis Pharmaceuticals UK Ltd)
  Brinzolamide 10 mg per 1 ml Azopt 10mg/ml eye drops | 5 ml [PoM] £6.92 DT = £3.13

Brinzolamide with brimonidine   11-May-2020

The properties listed below are those particular to the combination only. For the properties of the components please consider, brinzolamide p. 1226, brimonidine tartrate p. 1232.

● **INDICATIONS AND DOSE**

Raised intra-ocular pressure in open-angle glaucoma and in ocular hypertension when monotherapy is inadequate
▶ TO THE EYE
▸ Adult: Apply 1 drop twice daily

● INTERACTIONS → Appendix 1: brimonidine · brinzolamide

● MEDICINAL FORMS There can be variation in the licensing of different medicines containing the same drug.
Eye drops
CAUTIONARY AND ADVISORY LABELS 3
EXCIPIENTS: May contain Benzalkonium chloride, propylene glycol
▸ Simbrinza (Novartis Pharmaceuticals UK Ltd)
Brimonidine tartrate 2 mg per 1 ml, Brinzolamide 10 mg per 1 ml Simbrinza 10mg/ml / 2mg/ml eye drops | 5 ml [PoM] £9.23 DT = £9.23

Brinzolamide with timolol   11-May-2020

The properties listed below are those particular to the combination only. For the properties of the components please consider, brinzolamide p. 1226, timolol maleate p. 1225.

● **INDICATIONS AND DOSE**

Raised intra-ocular pressure in open-angle glaucoma or ocular hypertension when beta-blocker alone not adequate
▶ TO THE EYE
▸ Adult: Apply twice daily

● INTERACTIONS → Appendix 1: beta blockers, non-selective · brinzolamide

● MEDICINAL FORMS There can be variation in the licensing of different medicines containing the same drug.
Eye drops
EXCIPIENTS: May contain Benzalkonium chloride, disodium edetate
▸ Brinzolamide with timolol (Non-proprietary)
Timolol (as Timolol maleate) 5 mg per 1 ml, Brinzolamide 10 mg per 1 ml Brinzolamide 10mg/ml / Timolol 5mg/ml eye drops | 5 ml [PoM] £9.39–£13.03 DT = £11.05
▸ Azarga (Novartis Pharmaceuticals UK Ltd)
Timolol (as Timolol maleate) 5 mg per 1 ml, Brinzolamide 10 mg per 1 ml Azarga 10mg/ml / 5mg/ml eye drops | 5 ml [PoM] £11.05 DT = £11.05

Dorzolamide   20-Jan-2020

● **INDICATIONS AND DOSE**

Raised intra-ocular pressure in ocular hypertension used alone in patients unresponsive to beta-blockers or if beta-blockers contra-indicated | Open-angle glaucoma used alone in patients unresponsive to beta-blockers or if beta-blockers contra-indicated | Pseudo-exfoliative glaucoma used alone in patients unresponsive to beta-blockers or if beta-blockers contra-indicated
▶ TO THE EYE
▸ Adult: Apply 3 times a day

Raised intra-ocular pressure in ocular hypertension as adjunct to beta-blocker | Open-angle glaucoma as adjunct to beta-blocker | Pseudo-exfoliative glaucoma as adjunct to beta-blocker
▶ TO THE EYE
▸ Adult: Apply twice daily

● CONTRA-INDICATIONS Hyperchloraemic acidosis

● CAUTIONS Chronic corneal defects · history of intra-ocular surgery · history of renal calculi · low endothelial cell count · systemic absorption follows topical application

● INTERACTIONS → Appendix 1: dorzolamide

● SIDE-EFFECTS
▸ **Common or very common** Asthenia · eye discomfort · eye disorders · eye inflammation · headache · nausea · taste bitter · vision disorders
▸ **Rare or very rare** Angioedema · bronchospasm · dizziness · dry mouth · epistaxis · local reaction · paraesthesia · severe cutaneous adverse reactions (SCARs) · skin reactions · throat irritation · urolithiasis
▸ **Frequency not known** Dyspnoea · palpitations
SIDE-EFFECTS, FURTHER INFORMATION Systemic absorption can cause sulfonamide-like side-effects and may require discontinuation if severe.

● ALLERGY AND CROSS-SENSITIVITY Contra-indicated if history of sulfonamide hypersensitivity.

● PREGNANCY Manufacturer advises avoid—toxicity in *animal* studies.

● BREAST FEEDING Manufacturer advises avoid—no information available.

● HEPATIC IMPAIRMENT Manufacturer advises caution—no information available.

● RENAL IMPAIRMENT Avoid if eGFR less than 30 mL/minute/1.73 m^2.

● PRESCRIBING AND DISPENSING INFORMATION Although multi-dose dorzolamide eye drops commonly contain preservatives, preservative-free unit dose vials may be available.

● MEDICINAL FORMS There can be variation in the licensing of different medicines containing the same drug.
Eye drops
EXCIPIENTS: May contain Benzalkonium chloride
▸ Dorzolamide (Non-proprietary)
Dorzolamide (as Dorzolamide hydrochloride) 20 mg per 1 ml Dorzolamide 20mg/ml eye drops | 5 ml [PoM] £5.69 DT = £2.36
▸ Eydelto (Aspire Pharma Ltd)
Dorzolamide (as Dorzolamide hydrochloride) 20 mg per 1 ml Eydelto 20mg/ml eye drops | 5 ml [PoM] £12.09 DT = £12.09
▸ Trusopt (Santen UK Ltd)
Dorzolamide (as Dorzolamide hydrochloride) 20 mg per 1 ml Trusopt 20mg/ml eye drops 0.2ml unit dose preservative free | 60 unit dose [PoM] £24.18 DT = £24.18
Trusopt 20mg/ml eye drops | 5 ml [PoM] £6.33 DT = £2.36

Dorzolamide with timolol

The properties listed below are those particular to the combination only. For the properties of the components please consider, dorzolamide above, timolol maleate p. 1225.

● **INDICATIONS AND DOSE**

Raised intra-ocular pressure in ocular hypertension when beta-blockers alone not adequate | Raised intra-ocular pressure in open-angle glaucoma when beta-blockers alone not adequate | Raised intra-ocular pressure in pseudo-exfoliative glaucoma when beta-blockers alone not adequate
▶ TO THE EYE
▸ Adult: Apply twice daily

● INTERACTIONS → Appendix 1: beta blockers, non-selective · dorzolamide

● PRESCRIBING AND DISPENSING INFORMATION Although multi-dose dorzolamide with timolol eye drops commonly contain preservatives, preservative-free unit dose vials may be available.

11

Eye

11

Eye

- **MEDICINAL FORMS** There can be variation in the licensing of different medicines containing the same drug.

Eye drops

EXCIPIENTS: May contain Benzalkonium chloride

▸ Dorzolamide with timolol (Non-proprietary)

Timolol (as Timolol maleate) 5 mg per 1 ml, Dorzolamide (as Dorzolamide hydrochloride) 20 mg per 1 ml Dorzolamide 20mg/ml / Timolol 5mg/ml eye drops 0.2ml unit dose preservative free | 60 unit dose [PoM] £34.30 DT = £28.59
Dorzolamide 20mg/ml / Timolol 5mg/ml eye drops | 5 ml [PoM] £27.16 DT = £2.32

▸ Cosopt (Santen UK Ltd)

Timolol (as Timolol maleate) 5 mg per 1 ml, Dorzolamide (as Dorzolamide hydrochloride) 20 mg per 1 ml Cosopt 20mg/ml / 5mg/ml eye drops 0.2ml unit dose preservative free | 60 unit dose [PoM] £28.59 DT = £28.59
Cosopt 20mg/ml / 5mg/ml eye drops | 5 ml [PoM] £10.05 DT = £2.32

▸ Cosopt iMulti (Santen UK Ltd)

Timolol (as Timolol maleate) 5 mg per 1 ml, Dorzolamide (as Dorzolamide hydrochloride) 20 mg per 1 ml Cosopt iMulti 20mg/ml / 5mg/ml eye drops preservative free | 10 ml [PoM] £28.00

▸ Eylamdo (Aspire Pharma Ltd)

Timolol (as Timolol maleate) 5 mg per 1 ml, Dorzolamide (as Dorzolamide hydrochloride) 20 mg per 1 ml Eylamdo 20mg/ml / 5mg/ml eye drops | 5 ml [PoM] £13.99 DT = £13.99

MIOTICS ⟩ PARASYMPATHOMIMETICS

Pilocarpine

31-Oct-2019

- **DRUG ACTION** Pilocarpine acts by opening the inefficient drainage channels in the trabecular meshwork.

- **INDICATIONS AND DOSE**

Primary angle-closure glaucoma | Some secondary glaucomas

▸ TO THE EYE

▸ Adult: Apply up to 4 times a day

- **CONTRA-INDICATIONS** Acute iritis · anterior uveitis · conditions where pupillary constriction is undesirable · some forms of secondary glaucoma (where pupillary constriction is undesirable)

- **CAUTIONS** A darkly pigmented iris may require a higher concentration of the miotic or more frequent administration and care should be taken to avoid overdosage · asthma · cardiac disease · care in conjunctival damage · care in corneal damage · epilepsy · gastro-intestinal spasm · hypertension · hyperthyroidism · hypotension · marked vasomotor instability · Parkinson's disease · peptic ulceration · retinal detachment has occurred in susceptible individuals and those with retinal disease · urinary-tract obstruction

- **INTERACTIONS** → Appendix 1: pilocarpine

- **SIDE-EFFECTS**

▸ **Common or very common** Diarrhoea · headache · hyperhidrosis · hypersalivation · nausea · skin reactions · vision disorders · vomiting

▸ **Frequency not known** Bradycardia · bronchospasm · conjunctival vascular congestion · eye disorder (long term use) · eye disorders · hypotension · lens changes (long term use) · pain · paraesthesia · pulmonary oedema · sensitisation · vitreous haemorrhage

- **PREGNANCY** Avoid unless the potential benefit outweighs risk—limited information available.

- **BREAST FEEDING** Avoid unless the potential benefit outweighs risk—no information available.

- **PRE-TREATMENT SCREENING** Fundus examination is advised before starting treatment with a miotic (retinal detachment has occurred).

- **MONITORING REQUIREMENTS** Intra-ocular pressure and visual fields should be monitored in those with chronic

simple glaucoma and those receiving long-term treatment with a miotic.

- **PRESCRIBING AND DISPENSING INFORMATION** Although multi-dose pilocarpine eye drops commonly contain preservatives, preservative-free unit dose vials may be available.

- **PATIENT AND CARER ADVICE**

Driving and skilled tasks Blurred vision may affect performance of skilled tasks (e.g. driving) particularly at night or in reduced lighting.

- **MEDICINAL FORMS** There can be variation in the licensing of different medicines containing the same drug. Forms available from special-order manufacturers include: eye drops

Eye drops

EXCIPIENTS: May contain Benzalkonium chloride

▸ Pilocarpine (Non-proprietary)

Pilocarpine hydrochloride 10 mg per 1 ml Pilocarpine hydrochloride 1% eye drops | 10 ml [PoM] £23.31 DT = £22.20
Pilocarpine hydrochloride 20 mg per 1 ml Pilocarpine hydrochloride 2% eye drops | 10 ml [PoM] £23.93 DT = £22.79
Pilocarpine hydrochloride 40 mg per 1 ml Pilocarpine hydrochloride 4% eye drops | 10 ml [PoM] £29.82 DT = £28.40

▸ Pilocarpine nitrate (Bausch & Lomb UK Ltd)

Pilocarpine nitrate 20 mg per 1 ml Minims pilocarpine nitrate 2% eye drops 0.5ml unit dose | 20 unit dose [PoM] £12.47 DT = £12.47

PROSTAGLANDINS AND ANALOGUES

Latanoprost

16-Nov-2020

- **INDICATIONS AND DOSE**

Raised intra-ocular pressure in open-angle glaucoma | Ocular hypertension

▸ TO THE EYE

▸ Adult: Apply once daily, to be administered preferably in the evening

> **IMPORTANT SAFETY INFORMATION**
>
> MHRA/CHM ADVICE: LATANOPROST (*XALATAN*®): INCREASED REPORTING OF EYE IRRITATION SINCE REFORMULATION (JULY 2015)
>
> Following reformulation of *Xalatan*®, to allow for long-term storage at room temperature, there has been an increase in the number of reports of eye irritation from across the EU. Patients should be advised to tell their health professional promptly (within a week) if they experience eye irritation (e.g. excessive watering) severe enough to make them consider stopping treatment. Review treatment and prescribe a different formulation if necessary.

- **CONTRA-INDICATIONS** Active herpes simplex keratitis · history of recurrent herpetic keratitis associated with prostaglandin analogues

- **CAUTIONS** Angle-closure glaucoma · aphakia · asthma · contact lens wearers · do not use within 5 minutes of thiomersal-containing preparations · history of significant ocular viral infections · inflammatory ocular conditions (no experience of use) · narrow-angle glaucoma (no experience of use) · neovascular glaucoma (no experience of use) · peri-operative period of cataract surgery · pseudophakia with torn posterior lens capsule or anterior chamber lenses · risk factors for cystoid macular oedema · risk factors for iritis · risk factors for uveitis

- **SIDE-EFFECTS**

▸ **Common or very common** Eye discolouration · eye discomfort · eye disorders · eye inflammation · vision disorders

▸ **Uncommon** Dry eye · rash

▸ **Rare or very rare** Asthma · chest pain · dyspnoea · unstable angina

▶ **Frequency not known** Arthralgia · dizziness · headache · myalgia · ophthalmic herpes simplex · palpitations

● PREGNANCY Manufacturer advises avoid.

● BREAST FEEDING May be present in milk—manufacturer advises avoid.

● PRESCRIBING AND DISPENSING INFORMATION Although multi-dose latanoprost eye drops commonly contain preservatives, preservative-free unit dose vials may be available.

● PATIENT AND CARER ADVICE
Changes in eye colour Before initiating treatment, patients should be warned of a possible change in eye colour as an increase in the brown pigment in the iris can occur, which may be permanent; particular care is required in those with mixed coloured irides and those receiving treatment to one eye only. Changes in eyelashes and vellus hair can also occur, and patients should also be advised to avoid repeated contact of the eye drop solution with skin as this can lead to hair growth or skin pigmentation.

● NATIONAL FUNDING/ACCESS DECISIONS
MONOPOST ® For full details see funding body website
Scottish Medicines Consortium (SMC) decisions
▶ Latanoprost *Monopost*® for the reduction of elevated intraocular pressure in patients with open-angle glaucoma and ocular hypertension (July 2013) SMC No. 879/13 Recommended with restrictions

● MEDICINAL FORMS There can be variation in the licensing of different medicines containing the same drug.
Eye drops
EXCIPIENTS: May contain Benzalkonium chloride
▶ Latanoprost (Non-proprietary)
Latanoprost 50 microgram per 1 ml Latanoprost 50micrograms/ml eye drops | 2.5 ml [PoM] £12.48 DT = £3.12
▶ Medizol (Medicom Healthcare Ltd)
Latanoprost 50 microgram per 1 ml Medizol 0.005% eye drops | 2.5 ml [PoM] Ⓢ DT = £3.12
▶ Monopost (Thea Pharmaceuticals Ltd)
Latanoprost 50 microgram per 1 ml Monopost 50micrograms/ml eye drops 0.2ml unit dose | 30 unit dose [PoM] £8.49 DT = £8.49 | 90 unit dose [PoM] £25.47 DT = £25.47
▶ Xalatan (Upjohn UK Ltd)
Latanoprost 50 microgram per 1 ml Xalatan 50micrograms/ml eye drops | 2.5 ml [PoM] £12.48 DT = £3.12

Latanoprost with timolol
10-Nov-2020

The properties listed below are those particular to the combination only. For the properties of the components please consider, latanoprost p. 1228, timolol maleate p. 1225.

● INDICATIONS AND DOSE
Raised intra-ocular pressure in patients with open-angle glaucoma and ocular hypertension when beta-blocker or prostaglandin analogue alone not adequate
▶ TO THE EYE
▶ Adult: Apply once daily

● INTERACTIONS → Appendix 1: beta blockers, non-selective

● NATIONAL FUNDING/ACCESS DECISIONS
For full details see funding body website
Scottish Medicines Consortium (SMC) decisions
▶ Latanoprost with timolol (*Fixapost*®) for the reduction of intraocular pressure (IOP) in patients with open-angle glaucoma and ocular hypertension who are insufficiently responsive to topical beta-blockers or prostaglandin analogues (May 2019) SMC No. SMC2159 Recommended with restrictions

● MEDICINAL FORMS There can be variation in the licensing of different medicines containing the same drug.
Eye drops
EXCIPIENTS: May contain Benzalkonium chloride
▶ Latanoprost with timolol (Non-proprietary)
Latanoprost 50 microgram per 1 ml, Timolol (as Timolol maleate) 5 mg per 1 ml Latanoprost 50micrograms/ml / Timolol 5mg/ml eye drops | 2.5 ml [PoM] £14.32 DT = £5.84
▶ Fixapost (Thea Pharmaceuticals Ltd)
Latanoprost 50 microgram per 1 ml, Timolol (as Timolol maleate) 5 mg per 1 ml Fixapost 50micrograms/ml / 5mg/ml eye drops 0.2ml unit dose | 30 unit dose [PoM] £13.49 DT = £13.49
▶ Medox (Medicom Healthcare Ltd)
Latanoprost 50 microgram per 1 ml, Timolol (as Timolol maleate) 5 mg per 1 ml Medox 50micrograms/ml / 5mg/ml eye drops | 2.5 ml [PoM] Ⓢ DT = £5.84
▶ Xalacom (Upjohn UK Ltd)
Latanoprost 50 microgram per 1 ml, Timolol (as Timolol maleate) 5 mg per 1 ml Xalacom eye drops | 2.5 ml [PoM] £14.32 DT = £5.84

Tafluprost
16-Nov-2020

● INDICATIONS AND DOSE
Raised intra-ocular pressure in open-angle glaucoma | Ocular hypertension
▶ TO THE EYE
▶ Adult: Apply once daily, to be administered preferably in the evening

● CAUTIONS Angle-closure glaucoma (no experience of use) · aphakia · asthma · congenital glaucoma (no experience of use) · contact lens wearers · inflammatory ocular conditions (no experience of use) · narrow-angle glaucoma (no experience of use) · neovascular glaucoma (no experience of use) · pseudophakia with torn posterior lens capsule or anterior chamber lenses · risk factors for cystoid macular oedema · risk factors for iritis · risk factors for uveitis

● SIDE-EFFECTS
▶ **Common or very common** Dry eye · eye discolouration · eye discomfort · eye disorders · eye inflammation · headache · vision disorders
▶ **Uncommon** Hypertrichosis
▶ **Frequency not known** Asthma exacerbated · dyspnoea

● PREGNANCY Manufacturer advises avoid unless potential benefit outweighs risk—toxicity in *animal* studies.

● BREAST FEEDING Manufacturer advises avoid—present in milk in *animal* studies.

● HEPATIC IMPAIRMENT Manufacturer advises caution (no information available).

● RENAL IMPAIRMENT Use with caution—no information available.

● PRESCRIBING AND DISPENSING INFORMATION Although multi-dose tafluprost eye drops commonly contain preservatives, preservative-free unit dose vials may be available.

● PATIENT AND CARER ADVICE
Changes to eye colour Before initiating treatment, patients should be warned of a possible change in eye colour as an increase in the brown pigment in the iris can occur, which may be permanent; particular care is required in those with mixed coloured irides and those receiving treatment to one eye only. Changes in eyelashes and vellus hair can also occur, and patients should also be advised to avoid repeated contact of the eye drop solution with skin as this can lead to hair growth or skin pigmentation.

11

Eye

● MEDICINAL FORMS There can be variation in the licensing of different medicines containing the same drug.

Eye drops

EXCIPIENTS: May contain Disodium edetate

▸ Saflutan (Santen UK Ltd)

Tafluprost 15 microgram per 1 ml Saflutan 15micrograms/ml eye drops 0.3ml unit dose | 30 unit dose [PoM] £12.20 DT = £12.20
Saflutan 15micrograms/ml eye drops | 3 ml [PoM] £11.39 DT = £11.39

Tafluprost with timolol

16-Nov-2020

The properties listed below are those particular to the combination only. For the properties of the components please consider, tafluprost p. 1229, timolol maleate p. 1225.

● INDICATIONS AND DOSE

Raised intra-ocular pressure in open-angle glaucoma and ocular hypertension when beta-blocker or prostaglandin analogue alone not adequate

▸ TO THE EYE

▸ Adult: Apply 1 drop once daily

● INTERACTIONS → Appendix 1: beta blockers, non-selective

● PATIENT AND CARER ADVICE

Driving and skilled tasks Blurred vision may affect performance of skilled tasks (e.g. driving or operating machinery).

● NATIONAL FUNDING/ACCESS DECISIONS

For full details see funding body website

Scottish Medicines Consortium (SMC) decisions

▸ Tafluprost with timolol (*Taptiqom*®) for reduction of intra-ocular pressure in adult patients with open angle glaucoma or ocular hypertension who are insufficiently responsive to topical monotherapy with beta-blockers or prostaglandin analogues and require a combination therapy, and who would benefit from preservative-free eye drops (September 2015) SMC No. 1085/15 Recommended with restrictions

● MEDICINAL FORMS There can be variation in the licensing of different medicines containing the same drug.

Eye drops

EXCIPIENTS: May contain Disodium edetate

▸ Taptiqom (Santen UK Ltd)

Tafluprost 15 microgram per 1 ml, Timolol (as Timolol maleate) 5 mg per 1 ml Taptiqom 15micrograms/ml / 5mg/ml eye drops 0.3ml unit dose | 30 unit dose [PoM] £14.50 DT = £14.50

Travoprost

03-Sep-2020

● INDICATIONS AND DOSE

Raised intra-ocular pressure in open-angle glaucoma | Ocular hypertension

▸ TO THE EYE

▸ Adult: Apply once daily, to be administered preferably in the evening

● CAUTIONS Angle-closure glaucoma (no experience of use) · aphakia · asthma · congenital glaucoma (no experience of use) · contact lens wearers · inflammatory ocular conditions (no experience of use) · narrow-angle glaucoma (no experience of use) · neovascular glaucoma (no experience of use) · pseudophakia with torn posterior lens capsule or anterior chamber lenses · risk factors for cystoid macular oedema · risk factors for iritis · risk factors for uveitis

● SIDE-EFFECTS

▸ **Common or very common** Dry eye · eye discolouration · eye discomfort · eye disorders

▸ **Uncommon** Cataract · cough · eye inflammation · hair changes · headache · nasal complaints · palpitations · seasonal allergy · skin reactions · throat irritation · vision disorders

▸ **Rare or very rare** Allergic rhinitis · arthralgia · asthenia · asthma · constipation · dizziness · dry mouth · dysphonia · dyspnoea · gastrointestinal disorders · hypertension · hypotension · madarosis · musculoskeletal pain · ophthalmic herpes simplex · oropharyngeal pain · respiratory disorder · taste altered

▸ **Frequency not known** Abdominal pain · anxiety · arrhythmias · chest pain · depression · diarrhoea · epistaxis · insomnia · nausea · tinnitus · urinary disorders · vertigo · vomiting

● PREGNANCY Manufacturer advises avoid unless potential benefit outweighs risk—toxicity in *animal* studies.

● BREAST FEEDING Present in milk in *animal* studies; manufacturer advises avoid.

● PATIENT AND CARER ADVICE

Changes to eye colour Before initiating treatment, patients should be warned of a possible change in eye colour as an increase in the brown pigment in the iris can occur, which may be permanent; particular care is required in those with mixed coloured irides and those receiving treatment to one eye only. Changes in eyelashes and vellus hair can also occur, and patients should also be advised to avoid repeated contact of the eye drop solution with skin as this can lead to hair growth or skin pigmentation.

● MEDICINAL FORMS There can be variation in the licensing of different medicines containing the same drug.

Eye drops

EXCIPIENTS: May contain Propylene glycol

▸ Travoprost (Non-proprietary)

Travoprost 40 microgram per 1 ml Travoprost 40micrograms/ml eye drops | 2.5 ml [PoM] £10.95 DT = £2.43

▸ Bondulc (Accord Healthcare Ltd)

Travoprost 40 microgram per 1 ml Bondulc 40micrograms/ml eye drops | 2.5 ml [PoM] £10.94 DT = £2.43

▸ Travatan (Novartis Pharmaceuticals UK Ltd)

Travoprost 40 microgram per 1 ml Travatan 40micrograms/ml eye drops | 2.5 ml [PoM] £10.95 DT = £2.43

Travoprost with timolol

02-Jun-2020

The properties listed below are those particular to the combination only. For the properties of the components please consider, travoprost above, timolol maleate p. 1225.

● INDICATIONS AND DOSE

Raised intra-ocular pressure in patients with open-angle glaucoma or ocular hypertension when beta-blocker or prostaglandin analogue alone not adequate

▸ TO THE EYE

▸ Adult: Apply once daily

● INTERACTIONS → Appendix 1: beta blockers, non-selective

● MEDICINAL FORMS There can be variation in the licensing of different medicines containing the same drug.

Eye drops

EXCIPIENTS: May contain Propylene glycol

▸ Travoprost with timolol (Non-proprietary)

Travoprost 40 microgram per 1 ml, Timolol (as Timolol maleate) 5 mg per 1 ml Travoprost 40micrograms/ml / Timolol 5mg/ml eye drops | 2.5 ml [PoM] £16.18 DT = £16.17

▸ DuoTrav (Novartis Pharmaceuticals UK Ltd)

Travoprost 40 microgram per 1 ml, Timolol (as Timolol maleate) 5 mg per 1 ml DuoTrav 40micrograms/ml / 5mg/ml eye drops | 2.5 ml [PoM] £13.95 DT = £16.17 | 7.5 ml [PoM] £39.68

PROSTAMIDES

▌Bimatoprost

16-Nov-2020

- ● **INDICATIONS AND DOSE**

Raised intra-ocular pressure in open-angle glaucoma | Ocular hypertension
- ▸ TO THE EYE
- ▸ **Adult:** Apply once daily, to be administered preferably in the evening

- ● CAUTIONS Angle-closure glaucoma (no experience of use) · aphakia · asthma · chronic obstructive pulmonary disease · compromised respiratory function · congenital glaucoma (no experience of use) · contact lens wearers · history of significant ocular viral infections · inflammatory ocular conditions (no experience of use) · narrow-angle glaucoma (no experience of use) · neovascular glaucoma (no experience of use) · predisposition to bradycardia · predisposition to hypotension · pseudophakia with torn posterior lens capsule or anterior chamber lenses · risk factors for cystoid macular oedema · risk factors for iritis · risk factors for uveitis

- ● SIDE-EFFECTS
- ▸ **Common or very common** Dry eye · eye discolouration · eye discomfort · eye disorders · eye inflammation · headache · hypertension · hypertrichosis · skin reactions · vision disorders
- ▸ **Uncommon** Asthenia · dizziness · madarosis · nausea · retinal haemorrhage
- ▸ **Frequency not known** Asthma · bradycardia · dyspnoea · hypotension · reactivation of infection

- ● PREGNANCY Manufacturer advises use only if potential benefit outweighs risk.

- ● BREAST FEEDING Manufacturer advises avoid—present in milk in *animal* studies.

- ● HEPATIC IMPAIRMENT Manufacturer advises use with caution in moderate-to-severe impairment—no information available.

- ● RENAL IMPAIRMENT Use with caution—no information available.

- ● PRESCRIBING AND DISPENSING INFORMATION Although multi-dose bimatoprost eye drops commonly contain preservatives, preservative-free unit dose vials may be available.

- ● PATIENT AND CARER ADVICE
Changes to eye colour Before initiating treatment, patients should be warned of a possible change in eye colour as an increase in the brown pigment in the iris can occur, which may be permanent; particular care is required in those with mixed coloured irides and those receiving treatment to one eye only. Changes in eyelashes and vellus hair can also occur, and patients should also be advised to avoid repeated contact of the eye drop solution with skin as this can lead to hair growth or skin pigmentation.

- ● NATIONAL FUNDING/ACCESS DECISIONS
LUMIGAN ® For full details see funding body website
Scottish Medicines Consortium (SMC) decisions
- ▸ **Bimatoprost 300 micrograms/mL preservative-free eye drops (*Lumigan* ® single-dose eye drops) for reduction of elevated intraocular pressure in chronic open-angle glaucoma and ocular hypertension in adults (as monotherapy or as adjunctive therapy to beta-blockers) (March 2013) SMC No. 839/13 Recommended with restrictions**

- ● MEDICINAL FORMS There can be variation in the licensing of different medicines containing the same drug.
Eye drops
EXCIPIENTS: May contain Benzalkonium chloride
- ▸ Bimatoprost (Non-proprietary)
Bimatoprost 100 microgram per 1 ml Bimatoprost 100micrograms/ml eye drops | 3 ml PoM £14.23 DT = £10.10 | 9 ml PoM £29.86–£30.30
Bimatoprost 300 microgram per 1 ml Bimatoprost 300micrograms/ml eye drops | 3 ml PoM £13.76 DT = £12.36
- ▸ Eyreida (Aspire Pharma Ltd)
Bimatoprost 300 microgram per 1 ml Eyreida 0.3mg/ml eye drops | 3 ml PoM £11.71 DT = £11.71
- ▸ Lumigan (Allergan Ltd)
Bimatoprost 100 microgram per 1 ml Lumigan 100micrograms/ml eye drops | 3 ml PoM £11.71 DT = £10.10 | 9 ml PoM £35.13
Bimatoprost 300 microgram per 1 ml Lumigan 300micrograms/ml eye drops 0.4ml unit dose | 30 unit dose PoM £13.75 DT = £13.75

▌Bimatoprost with timolol

02-Jun-2020

The properties listed below are those particular to the combination only. For the properties of the components please consider, bimatoprost above, timolol maleate p. 1225.

- ● **INDICATIONS AND DOSE**

Raised intra-ocular pressure in patients with open-angle glaucoma or ocular hypertension when beta-blocker or prostaglandin analogue alone not adequate
- ▸ TO THE EYE
- ▸ **Adult:** Apply once daily

- ● INTERACTIONS → Appendix 1: beta blockers, non-selective

- ● NATIONAL FUNDING/ACCESS DECISIONS
GANFORT ® SINGLE USE For full details see funding body website
Scottish Medicines Consortium (SMC) decisions
- ▸ Bimatoprost with timolol (*Ganfort* ®) unit dose eye drops for reduction of intraocular pressure (IOP) in adult patients with open-angle glaucoma or ocular hypertension who are insufficiently responsive to topical beta-blockers or prostaglandin analogues (October 2013) SMC No. 906/13 Recommended with restrictions

- ● MEDICINAL FORMS There can be variation in the licensing of different medicines containing the same drug.
Eye drops
EXCIPIENTS: May contain Benzalkonium chloride
- ▸ Bimatoprost with timolol (Non-proprietary)
Bimatoprost 300 microgram per 1 ml, Timolol (as Timolol maleate) 5 mg per 1 ml Bimatoprost 300micrograms/ml / Timolol 5mg/ml eye drops | 3 ml PoM £14.16–£16.98 DT = £14.16
- ▸ Eyzeetan (Aspire Pharma Ltd)
Eyzeetan 0.3mg/ml / 5mg/ml eye drops preservative free | 3 ml PoM £14.16
- ▸ Ganfort (Allergan Ltd)
Bimatoprost 300 microgram per 1 ml, Timolol (as Timolol maleate) 5 mg per 1 ml Ganfort 0.3mg/ml / 5mg/ml eye drops | 3 ml PoM £14.16 DT = £14.16 | 9 ml PoM £38.15
Ganfort 0.3mg/ml / 5mg/ml eye drops 0.4ml unit dose | 30 unit dose PoM £17.94 DT = £17.94

11

Eye

SYMPATHOMIMETICS ⟩ ALPHA₂-ADRENOCEPTOR AGONISTS

Apraclonidine

03-Sep-2020

- **DRUG ACTION** Apraclonidine is an alpha₂-adrenoceptor agonist that lowers intra-ocular pressure by reducing aqueous humour formation. It is a derivative of clonidine.

- **INDICATIONS AND DOSE**

Control or prevention of postoperative elevation of intra-ocular pressure after anterior segment laser surgery
  - ▸ TO THE EYE
  - ▸ Adult: Apply 1 drop, 1 hour before laser procedure, then 1 drop, immediately after completion of procedure, 1% eye drops to be administered

Short-term adjunctive treatment of chronic glaucoma in patients not adequately controlled by another drug
  - ▸ TO THE EYE
  - ▸ Adult: Apply 1 drop 3 times a day usually for maximum 1 month, 0.5% eye drops to be administered, may not provide additional benefit if patient already using two drugs that suppress the production of aqueous humour

- **CONTRA-INDICATIONS** History of severe or unstable and uncontrolled cardiovascular disease
- **CAUTIONS** Cerebrovascular disease · depression · heart failure · history of angina · hypertension · loss of effect may occur over time · Parkinson's syndrome · Raynaud's syndrome · recent myocardial infarction · reduction in vision in end-stage glaucoma (suspend treatment) · severe coronary insufficiency · thromboangiitis obliterans · vasovagal attack
- **INTERACTIONS** → Appendix 1: apraclonidine
- **SIDE-EFFECTS**
  - ▸ **Common or very common** Eye disorders
  - ▸ **Uncommon** Bradycardia · conjunctival haemorrhage · diarrhoea · dry eye · eye discomfort · eye inflammation · gastrointestinal discomfort · irritability · libido decreased · nasal dryness · palpitations · postural hypotension · sensation abnormal · sleep disorders · syncope · vision disorders · vomiting
  - ▸ **Rare or very rare** Chest pain · dry mouth · fatigue · headache · hyperhidrosis · pain in extremity · pruritus · taste altered · temperature sensation altered

  SIDE-EFFECTS, FURTHER INFORMATION Since absorption may follow topical application, systemic effects may occur– see clonidine hydrochloride p. 159.

  Ocular intolerance Manufacturer advises withdrawal if eye pruritus, ocular hyperaemia, increased lacrimation, or oedema of the eyelids and conjunctiva occur.
- **PREGNANCY** Manufacturer advises avoid—no information available.
- **BREAST FEEDING** Manufacturer advises avoid—no information available.
- **HEPATIC IMPAIRMENT** Manufacturer advises use with caution and monitor, including close monitoring of cardiovascular parameters—no information available.
- **RENAL IMPAIRMENT** Use with caution in chronic renal failure.
- **MONITORING REQUIREMENTS**
  - ▸ Monitor intra-ocular pressure and visual fields.
  - ▸ Monitor for excessive reduction in intra-ocular pressure following peri-operative use.
- **PATIENT AND CARER ADVICE**
  Driving and skilled tasks Drowsiness may affect performance of skilled tasks (e.g. driving).

- **MEDICINAL FORMS** There can be variation in the licensing of different medicines containing the same drug.
  Eye drops
  EXCIPIENTS: May contain Benzalkonium chloride
  - ▸ Iopidine (Novartis Pharmaceuticals UK Ltd)
  Apraclonidine (as Apraclonidine hydrochloride) 5 mg per 1 ml Iopidine 5mg/ml eye drops | 5 ml [PoM] £10.88 DT = £10.88
  Apraclonidine (as Apraclonidine hydrochloride) 10 mg per 1 ml Iopidine 1% eye drops 0.25ml unit dose | 24 unit dose [PoM] £77.85 DT = £77.85

Brimonidine tartrate

19-Nov-2020

- **DRUG ACTION** Brimonidine, an alpha₂-adrenoceptor agonist, is thought to lower intra-ocular pressure by reducing aqueous humour formation and increasing uveoscleral outflow.

- **INDICATIONS AND DOSE**

Raised intra-ocular pressure in open-angle glaucoma in patients for whom beta-blockers are inappropriate | Ocular hypertension in patients for whom beta-blockers are inappropriate | Adjunctive therapy when intra-ocular pressure is inadequately controlled by other antiglaucoma therapy
  - ▸ TO THE EYE
  - ▸ Adult: Apply twice daily

- **CAUTIONS** Cerebral insufficiency · coronary insufficiency · depression · postural hypotension · Raynaud's syndrome · severe cardiovascular disease · thromboangiitis obliterans
- **INTERACTIONS** → Appendix 1: brimonidine
- **SIDE-EFFECTS**
  - ▸ **Common or very common** Asthenia · dizziness · drowsiness · dry eye · dry mouth · eye discomfort · eye disorders · eye inflammation · gastrointestinal disorder · headache · hyperaemia · hypersensitivity · pulmonary reaction · sensation of foreign body · skin reactions · taste altered · vision disorders
  - ▸ **Uncommon** Arrhythmias · nasal dryness · palpitations
  - ▸ **Rare or very rare** Dyspnoea · hypertension · hypotension · insomnia · syncope
  - ▸ **Frequency not known** Face oedema · vasodilation
- **PREGNANCY** Manufacturer advises use only if benefit outweighs risk—limited information available.
- **BREAST FEEDING** Manufacturer advises avoid—no information available.
- **HEPATIC IMPAIRMENT** Manufacturer advises caution (no information available).
- **RENAL IMPAIRMENT** Manufacturer advises use with caution.
- **PATIENT AND CARER ADVICE**
  Driving and skilled tasks Drowsiness or blurred vision may affect performance of skilled tasks (e.g. driving).

- **MEDICINAL FORMS** There can be variation in the licensing of different medicines containing the same drug.
  Eye drops
  EXCIPIENTS: May contain Benzalkonium chloride
  - ▸ Brimonidine tartrate (Non-proprietary)
  Brimonidine tartrate 2 mg per 1 ml Brimonidine 2mg/ml eye drops | 5 ml [PoM] Ⓢ DT = £1.99
  Brimonidine 0.2% eye drops | 5 ml [PoM] £1.99 DT = £1.99
  - ▸ Alphagan (Allergan Ltd)
  Brimonidine tartrate 2 mg per 1 ml Alphagan 0.2% eye drops | 5 ml [PoM] £6.85 DT = £1.99
  - ▸ Brymont (Blumont Pharma Ltd)
  Brimonidine tartrate 2 mg per 1 ml Brymont 2mg/ml eye drops | 5 ml [PoM] £1.50 DT = £1.99

Combinations available: *Brinzolamide with brimonidine,* p. 1227

Brimonidine with timolol
02-Jun-2020

The properties listed below are those particular to the combination only. For the properties of the components please consider, brimonidine tartrate p. 1232, timolol maleate p. 1225.

● **INDICATIONS AND DOSE**

Raised intra-ocular pressure in open-angle glaucoma and for ocular hypertension when beta-blocker alone not adequate
▸ TO THE EYE
▸ Adult: Apply twice daily

● **INTERACTIONS** → Appendix 1: beta blockers, non-selective
· brimonidine

● **MEDICINAL FORMS** There can be variation in the licensing of different medicines containing the same drug.

Eye drops
EXCIPIENTS: May contain Benzalkonium chloride
▸ Brimonidine with timolol (Non-proprietary)
 Brimonidine tartrate 2 mg per 1 ml, Timolol (as Timolol maleate) **5 mg per 1 ml** Brimonidine 2mg/ml / Timolol 5mg/ml eye drops |
 5 ml PoM £8.50 DT = £10.00
▸ Combigan (Allergan Ltd)
 Brimonidine tartrate 2 mg per 1 ml, Timolol (as Timolol maleate) **5 mg per 1 ml** Combigan eye drops | 5 ml PoM £10.00 DT = £10.00
 | 15 ml PoM £27.00

6   Retinal disorders
6.1 Macular degeneration

Age-related macular degeneration
25-Apr-2018

Description of condition

Age-related macular degeneration is a progressive eye condition that affects the central area of the retina (macula). It occurs mainly in people aged 55 years and over and is a common cause of vision loss. The progressive loss of central vision affects the patient's ability to see well enough to recognise faces, drive, and to read and write. Although the exact cause is unknown, known risk factors in addition to increasing age include smoking and a family history of age-related macular degeneration.

There are two types of age-related macular degeneration—dry and wet. Dry (non-neovascular) age-related macular degeneration progresses slowly as extensive wasting of macula cells occurs. Whereas, with wet (neovascular) age-related macular degeneration, new blood vessels develop beneath and within the retina, and can lead to a rapid deterioration of vision. Wet age-related macular degeneration is further classified as *wet-active* (neovascular lesions that may benefit from treatment) and *wet-inactive* (neovascular disease with irreversible structural change).

Aims of treatment

The aim of treatment is to slow down the progression of age-related macular degeneration and central vision loss; treatment is initiated under specialist care.

Treatment

Treatment is dependent on the stage and type of age-related macular degeneration, with drug treatment only recommended in patients with *wet-active* age-related macular degeneration. Counselling and support, advice on Smoking cessation p. 519, and use of visual aids is recommended in all patients with age related macular degeneration as appropriate.

EvGr An intravitreal anti-vascular endothelial growth factor (anti-VEGF), such as aflibercept below, ranibizumab p. 1235, or bevacizumab p. 909 [unlicensed use], is first-line treatment for patients with *wet-active* age-related macular degeneration who have a visual acuity between 6/12 and 6/96. If visual acuity is less than 6/96, anti-VEGF treatment should only be given if the patient's overall visual function is likely to improve (e.g. if the affected eye is the patient's better-seeing eye). Anti-VEGF treatment should only be administered by healthcare professionals experienced in the use of intravitreal injections. See also National funding/access decisions for aflibercept below and ranibizumab p. 1235.

Treatment should be stopped if the patient develops severe, progressive loss of visual acuity despite treatment, or if the patient's age-related macular degeneration develops into *wet-inactive* with no prospect of visual function improvement. A treatment-free period can be considered in patients whose age-related macular degeneration appears to be stable.

Photodynamic therapy alone should not be given to patients with *wet-active* age-related macular degeneration. It can be given as an adjunct to anti-VEGF treatment as a second-line option in the context of a randomised controlled trial. Intravitreal corticosteroids are not recommended in combination with anti-VEGF treatment as there is limited evidence of benefit to a patient's visual acuity.

Patients should be advised to attend routine sight tests, self-monitor, and to report any changes in vision such as appearance of grey patches or blurred vision, straight lines appearing distorted, and objects appearing smaller than normal. ⟨A⟩

Useful Resources

Age-related macular degeneration. National Institute for Health and Care Excellence. NICE guideline 82. January 2018.
www.nice.org.uk/guidance/ng82

ANTINEOVASCULARISATION DRUGS ⟩
VASCULAR ENDOTHELIAL GROWTH FACTOR INHIBITORS

❙ Aflibercept
15-Oct-2020

● **DRUG ACTION** Aflibercept is a recombinant fusion protein that acts as a soluble decoy receptor and binds to vascular endothelial growth factors A and B (VEGF-A, VEGF-B) and placental growth factor (PlGF). Aflibercept inhibits the activation of VEGF receptors and the proliferation of endothelial cells, thereby inhibiting the growth of new vessels.

● **INDICATIONS AND DOSE**

Neovascular (wet) age-related macular degeneration (specialist use only)
▸ BY INTRAVITREAL INJECTION
▸ Adult: Initially 2 mg once a month for 3 months, then 2 mg every 2 months, review treatment frequency after 12 months

Macular oedema secondary to retinal vein occlusion (specialist use only)
▸ BY INTRAVITREAL INJECTION
▸ Adult: Initially 2 mg once a month until maximum visual acuity is achieved or there are no signs of disease activity (discontinue treatment if no improvement in visual and anatomic outcomes)

Diabetic macular oedema (specialist use only)
▸ BY INTRAVITREAL INJECTION
▸ Adult: Initially 2 mg once a month for 5 months, then maintenance 2 mg every 2 months, review   continued →

treatment frequency after 12 months (discontinue treatment if no improvement in visual and anatomic outcomes)

Myopic choroidal neovascularisation (specialist use only)
‣ BY INTRAVITREAL INJECTION
‣ Adult: 2 mg for 1 dose, if visual or anatomic outcomes indicate that disease persists, additional doses may be administered; the interval between 2 doses should be greater than 1 month

● CONTRA-INDICATIONS Clinical signs of irreversible ischaemic visual function loss · ocular or periocular infection · severe intra-ocular inflammation

● CAUTIONS Active systemic infection · diabetic patients with uncontrolled hypertension · discontinue treatment if stage 3 or 4 macular holes develop—consult product literature for full details · discontinue treatment in the event of a retinal break—consult product literature for full details · discontinue treatment in the event of rhegmatogenous retinal detachment—consult product literature for full details · patients at risk of retinal pigment epithelial tear · poorly controlled glaucoma · recent history of myocardial infarction · recent history of stroke · recent history of transient ischaemic attack

CAUTIONS, FURTHER INFORMATION Aflibercept is given by intravitreal injection by specialists experienced in the management of this condition. There is a potential risk of arterial thromboembolic events and non-ocular haemorrhage following the intravitreal injection of vascular endothelial growth factor inhibitors. Endophthalmitis can occur after intravitreal injections—patients should be advised to report any signs of infection immediately.

● INTERACTIONS → Appendix 1: aflibercept

● SIDE-EFFECTS
‣ **Common or very common** Cataract · eye discomfort · eye disorders · eye inflammation · haemorrhage · retinal pigment epithelial tear · vision disorders
‣ **Uncommon** Lens opacity

● CONCEPTION AND CONTRACEPTION Manufacturer recommends women use effective contraception during and for at least 3 months after treatment.

● PREGNANCY Manufacturer advises avoid unless potential benefit outweighs risk.

● BREAST FEEDING Manufacturer advises avoid—no information available.

● HEPATIC IMPAIRMENT Manufacturer advises caution in severe impairment (no information available).

● MONITORING REQUIREMENTS Monitor intra-ocular pressure following injection.

● DIRECTIONS FOR ADMINISTRATION For further information on administration, consult product literature.

● NATIONAL FUNDING/ACCESS DECISIONS
For full details see funding body website

NICE decisions
‣ **Aflibercept solution for injection for treating wet age-related macular degeneration (July 2013)** NICE TA294 Recommended with restrictions
‣ **Aflibercept for treating visual impairment caused by macular oedema secondary to central retinal vein occlusion (February 2014)** NICE TA305 Recommended
‣ **Aflibercept for treating diabetic macular oedema (July 2015)** NICE TA346 Recommended with restrictions
‣ **Aflibercept for treating visual impairment caused by macular oedema after branch retinal vein occlusion (September 2016)** NICE TA409 Recommended with restrictions
‣ **Aflibercept for treating choroidal neovascularisation (November 2017)** NICE TA486 Recommended with restrictions

Scottish Medicines Consortium (SMC) decisions
‣ Aflibercept (*Eylea*®) for adults for the treatment of visual impairment due to myopic choroidal neovascularisation (myopic CNV) (October 2016) SMC No. 1186/16 Recommended

● MEDICINAL FORMS There can be variation in the licensing of different medicines containing the same drug.

Solution for Injection
‣ Eylea (Bayer Plc)
Aflibercept 40 mg per 1 ml Eylea 4mg/100microlitres solution for injection vials | 1 vial (PoM) £816.00
Eylea 3.6mg/90microlitres solution for injection pre-filled syringes | 1 pre-filled disposable injection (PoM) £816.00

Brolucizumab

03-Nov-2020

● DRUG ACTION Brolucizumab is a monoclonal antibody that inhibits vascular endothelial growth factor A (VEGF-A), thereby suppressing endothelial cell proliferation and inhibiting the growth of new vessels and decreasing vascular permeability.

● INDICATIONS AND DOSE

Neovascular (wet) age-related macular degeneration (specialist use only)
‣ BY INTRAVITREAL INJECTION
‣ Adult: Initially 6 mg once a month for the first three doses, to be administered into the affected eye, for continued treatment and subsequent dose intervals—consult product literature, discontinue treatment if no improvement in visual and anatomic outcomes

● CONTRA-INDICATIONS Active intra-ocular inflammation · active or suspected ocular or periocular infection

● CAUTIONS History of myocardial infarction within the past 3 months · history of stroke within the past 3 months · history of transient ischaemic attack within the past 3 months · patients at risk of retinal pigment epithelial tear · poorly controlled glaucoma (do not use while intra-ocular pressure is 30 mmHg or higher) · retinal detachment or macular hole (discontinue treatment if rhegmatogenous retinal detachment or stage 3 or 4 macular holes develop)

CAUTIONS, FURTHER INFORMATION Brolucizumab is given by intravitreal injection by specialists experienced in the management of this condition. There is a potential risk of arterial thromboembolic events and non-ocular haemorrhage following the intravitreal injection of vascular endothelial growth factor inhibitors. Endophthalmitis can occur after intravitreal injections—patients should be advised to report any signs of infection immediately.

● SIDE-EFFECTS
‣ **Common or very common** Cataract · eye discomfort · eye disorders · eye inflammation · haemorrhage · hypersensitivity · retinal pigment epithelial tear · skin reactions · vision disorders
‣ **Uncommon** Embolism and thrombosis
‣ **Frequency not known** Myocardial infarction · stroke

● CONCEPTION AND CONTRACEPTION Manufacturer advises females of childbearing potential to use effective contraception during treatment and for 1 month after treatment.

● PREGNANCY Manufacturer advises avoid unless potential benefit outweighs risk—limited information available.

● BREAST FEEDING Manufacturer advises avoid during and for 1 month after treatment—no information available.

● MONITORING REQUIREMENTS
‣ Manufacturer advises monitor intra-ocular pressure, perfusion of the optic nerve head, and for signs of ocular infection following injection.
‣ Manufacturer advises monitor visual acuity.

- DIRECTIONS FOR ADMINISTRATION For further information on administration, consult product literature.
- PRESCRIBING AND DISPENSING INFORMATION
Brolucizumab is a biological medicine. Biological medicines must be prescribed and dispensed by brand name, see *Biological medicines* and *Biosimilar medicines*, under Guidance on prescribing p. 1; manufacturer advises to record the brand name and batch number after each administration.
- HANDLING AND STORAGE Manufacturer advises store in a refrigerator (2-8°C)—may be stored unopened at room temperature (below 25°C) for up to 24 hours before use; protect from light.
- NATIONAL FUNDING/ACCESS DECISIONS
For full details see funding body website

Scottish Medicines Consortium (SMC) decisions
▶ Brolucizumab (*Beovu*®) for the treatment of neovascular (wet) age-related macular degeneration (wAMD) (September 2020) SMC No. SMC2272 Recommended

- MEDICINAL FORMS There can be variation in the licensing of different medicines containing the same drug.
Solution for injection
EXCIPIENTS: May contain Polysorbates, sucrose
▶ Beovu (Novartis Pharmaceuticals UK Ltd) ▼
Brolucizumab 120 mg per 1 ml Beovu 19.8mg/0.165ml solution for injection pre-filled syringes | 1 pre-filled disposable injection PoM £816.00 (Hospital only)

Ranibizumab
20-Oct-2020

- INDICATIONS AND DOSE
Neovascular (wet) age-related macular degeneration (specialist use only) | Diabetic macular oedema (specialist use only) | Macular oedema secondary to retinal vein occlusion (specialist use only) | Choroidal neovascularisation (specialist use only)
▶ BY INTRAVITREAL INJECTION
▶ Adult: Initially 500 micrograms once a month, to be administered into the affected eye, until maximum visual acuity is achieved or there are no signs of disease activity, for continued treatment and subsequent dose intervals—consult product literature, discontinue treatment if no improvement in visual and anatomic outcomes

Concomitant treatment of diabetic macular oedema, or macular oedema secondary to branch retinal vein occlusion, with laser photocoagulation (specialist use only)
▶ BY INTRAVITREAL INJECTION
▶ Adult: 500 micrograms, to be administered at least 30 minutes after laser photocoagulation

- CONTRA-INDICATIONS Ocular or periocular infection · severe intra-ocular inflammation · signs of irreversible ischaemic visual function loss in patients with retinal vein occlusion (no information available)
- CAUTIONS Active systemic infection · diabetic macular oedema due to type 1 diabetes (limited information available) · diabetic patients with HbA$_{1c}$ over 12% · history of stroke · history of transient ischaemic attack · patients at risk of retinal pigment epithelial tear · previous intravitreal injections · retinal detachment or macular hole (discontinue treatment if rhegmatogenous retinal detachment or stage 3 or 4 macular holes develop) · uncontrolled hypertension

CAUTIONS, FURTHER INFORMATION Ranibizumab is given by intravitreal injection by specialists. There is a potential risk of arterial thromboembolic events and non-ocular haemorrhage following the intravitreal injection of vascular endothelial growth factor inhibitors.

Endophthalmitis can occur after intravitreal injections—patients should be advised to report any signs of infection immediately.

- INTERACTIONS → Appendix 1: ranibizumab
- SIDE-EFFECTS
▶ **Common or very common** Anaemia · anxiety · arthralgia · cataract · cough · dry eye · eye discomfort · eye disorders · eye inflammation · haemorrhage · headache · hypersensitivity · increased risk of infection · lens opacity · nausea · retinal pigment epithelial tear · vision disorders
▶ **Uncommon** Corneal deposits
▶ **Frequency not known** Arterial thromboembolism
- CONCEPTION AND CONTRACEPTION Manufacturer recommends women use effective contraception during and for at least 3 months after treatment.
- PREGNANCY Manufacturer advises avoid unless potential benefit outweighs risk.
- BREAST FEEDING Manufacturer advises avoid—no information available.
- MONITORING REQUIREMENTS
▶ Manufacturer advises monitor intra-ocular pressure, perfusion of the optic nerve head, and for signs of ocular infection following injection.
▶ Manufacturer advises monitor visual acuity.
- DIRECTIONS FOR ADMINISTRATION For further information on administration, consult product literature.
- NATIONAL FUNDING/ACCESS DECISIONS
For full details see funding body website

NICE decisions
▶ Ranibizumab for treating choroidal neovascularisation associated with pathological myopia (November 2013) NICE TA298 Recommended
▶ Ranibizumab for the treating visual impairment caused by macular oedema secondary to retinal vein occlusion (May 2013) NICE TA283 Recommended with restrictions
▶ Ranibizumab for treating diabetic macular oedema (February 2013) NICE TA274 Recommended with restrictions
▶ Ranibizumab and pegaptanib for the treatment of age-related macular degeneration (updated May 2012) NICE TA155 Recommended with restrictions

Scottish Medicines Consortium (SMC) decisions
▶ Ranibizumab (*Lucentis*®) for the treatment of visual impairment due to Diabetic Macular Oedema (December 2012) SMC No. 711/11 Recommended with restrictions
▶ Ranibizumab (*Lucentis*®) for the treatment of visual impairment due to macular oedema secondary to branch retinal vein occlusion (BRVO) in adults (May 2013) SMC No. 732/11 Recommended
▶ Ranibizumab (*Lucentis*®) for treatment of visual impairment due to choroidal neovascularisation secondary to pathologic myopia in adults (November 2013) SMC No. 907/13 Recommended

All Wales Medicines Strategy Group (AWMSG) decisions
▶ Ranibizumab (*Lucentis*®) for treatment of visual impairment in adults due to choroidal neovascularisation and not due to pathological myopia or wet age-related macular degeneration (June 2018) AWMSG No. 3233 Recommended

---

- MEDICINAL FORMS There can be variation in the licensing of different medicines containing the same drug.
Solution for injection
▶ Lucentis (Novartis Pharmaceuticals UK Ltd)
Ranibizumab 10 mg per 1 ml Lucentis 2.3mg/0.23ml solution for injection vials | 1 vial PoM £551.00 (Hospital only)
Lucentis 1.65mg/0.165ml solution for injection pre-filled syringes | 1 pre-filled disposable injection PoM £551.00

11

Eye

PHOTOSENSITISERS

Verteporfin
02-Sep-2020

- DRUG ACTION Following intravenous infusion, verteporfin is activated by local irradiation using non-thermal red light to produce cytotoxic derivatives.

- INDICATIONS AND DOSE

Photodynamic treatment of age-related macular degeneration associated with predominantly classic subfoveal choroidal neovascularisation or with pathological myopia (specialist use only)
  ▸ BY INTRAVENOUS INFUSION
  ▸ Adult: 6 mg/m², dose to be given over 10 minutes

- CONTRA-INDICATIONS Acute porphyrias p. 1107
- CAUTIONS Avoid extravasation · biliary obstruction · photosensitivity
- INTERACTIONS → Appendix 1: verteporfin
- SIDE-EFFECTS
  ▸ **Common or very common** Asthenia · dizziness · dyspnoea · headache · hypercholesterolaemia · hypersensitivity · infusion related chest pain · infusion related reaction · nausea · photosensitivity reaction · syncope · vision disorders
  ▸ **Uncommon** Eye inflammation · fever · haemorrhage · hyperaesthesia · hypertension · pain · retinal detachment · skin reactions
  ▸ **Rare or very rare** Malaise · retinal ischaemia
  ▸ **Frequency not known** Myocardial infarction · retinal pigment epithelial tear
- PREGNANCY Manufacturer advises use only if potential benefit outweighs risk (teratogenic in *animal* studies).
- BREAST FEEDING No information available—manufacturer advises avoid breast-feeding for 48 hours after administration.
- HEPATIC IMPAIRMENT Manufacturer advises caution in moderate impairment and avoid in severe impairment (no information available).
- DIRECTIONS FOR ADMINISTRATION For information on administration and light activation, consult product literature.
    For *intravenous infusion* (*Visudyne®*), manufacturer advises give intermittently in Glucose 5%; reconstitute each 15 mg with 7 ml water for injections to produce a 2 mg/ml solution then dilute requisite dose with infusion fluid to a final volume of 30 mL and give over 10 minutes; protect infusion from light and administer within 4 hours of reconstitution. Incompatible with sodium chloride infusion.
- PATIENT AND CARER ADVICE Photosensitivity—avoid exposure of unprotected skin and eyes to bright light during infusion and for 48 hours afterwards.

- MEDICINAL FORMS There can be variation in the licensing of different medicines containing the same drug.
Powder for solution for infusion
EXCIPIENTS: May contain Butylated hydroxytoluene
  ▸ Visudyne (Cheplapharm Arzneimittel GmbH)
    Verteporfin 15 mg Visudyne 15mg powder for solution for infusion vials | 1 vial PoM £850.00 (Hospital only)

6.2 Macular oedema

Other drugs used for Macular oedema Aflibercept, p. 1233 · Dexamethasone, p. 1207 · Ranibizumab, p. 1235

CORTICOSTEROIDS

Fluocinolone acetonide
05-Nov-2020

- INDICATIONS AND DOSE

Treatment of visual impairment associated with chronic diabetic macular oedema which is insufficiently responsive to available therapies (specialist use only) | Prevention of relapse in recurrent non-infectious uveitis affecting the posterior segment of the eye (specialist use only)
  ▸ BY INTRAVITREAL INJECTION
  ▸ Adult: 190 micrograms, to be administered into the affected eye, concurrent administration to both eyes not recommended. For further information on pre-treatment, administration and repeat dosing, consult product literature

> **IMPORTANT SAFETY INFORMATION**
>
> MHRA/CHM ADVICE: CORTICOSTEROIDS: RARE RISK OF CENTRAL SEROUS CHORIORETINOPATHY WITH LOCAL AS WELL AS SYSTEMIC ADMINISTRATION (AUGUST 2017)
> See Corticosteroids, general use p. 709.
>
> NHS IMPROVEMENT PATIENT SAFETY ALERT: STEROID EMERGENCY CARD TO SUPPORT EARLY RECOGNITION AND TREATMENT OF ADRENAL CRISIS IN ADULTS (AUGUST 2020)
> See Corticosteroids, general use p. 709.

- CONTRA-INDICATIONS Active or suspected ocular infection · active or suspected peri-ocular infection · pre-existing glaucoma
- CAUTIONS Raised baseline intra-ocular pressure
- INTERACTIONS → Appendix 1: fluocinolone
- SIDE-EFFECTS
  ▸ **Common or very common** Cataract · dry eye · eye discomfort · eye disorders · glaucoma · haemorrhage · vision disorders
  ▸ **Uncommon** Corneal deposits · eye inflammation · headache · optic nerve disorder
  ▸ **Frequency not known** Thromboembolism
- PREGNANCY Manufacturer advises avoid unless potential benefit outweighs risk—no information available.
- BREAST FEEDING Manufacturer advises avoid unless essential.
- MONITORING REQUIREMENTS
  ▸ Monitor for raised intra-ocular pressure (particularly if raised at baseline), retinal detachment, endophthalmitis, vitreous haemorrhage or detachment within 2–7 days following the procedure.
  ▸ Monitor intra-ocular pressure at least every 3 months thereafter (for approximately 36 months).
- DIRECTIONS FOR ADMINISTRATION EvGr Concurrent administration to both eyes not recommended. Ⓜ For further information on administration and repeat dosing, consult product literature.
- NATIONAL FUNDING/ACCESS DECISIONS
  For full details see funding body website
  NICE decisions
  ▸ Fluocinolone acetonide intravitreal implant for treating chronic diabetic macular oedema after an inadequate response to prior therapy (November 2013) NICE TA301 Recommended with restrictions
  ▸ Fluocinolone acetonide intravitreal implant for treating chronic diabetic macular oedema in phakic eyes after an inadequate response to previous therapy (November 2019) NICE TA613 Not recommended
  ▸ Fluocinolone acetonide intravitreal implant for treating recurrent non-infectious uveitis (July 2019) NICE TA590 Recommended with restrictions

11

Eye

Scottish Medicines Consortium (SMC) decisions
▸ Fluocinolone acetonide (*Iluvien* ®) for the treatment of vision impairment associated with chronic diabetic macular oedema, considered insufficiently responsive to available therapies (February 2014) SMC No. 864/13 Recommended with restrictions
▸ Fluocinolone acetonide (*Iluvien* ®) for prevention of relapse in recurrent non-infectious uveitis affecting the posterior segment of the eye (September 2020) SMC No. SMC2260 Recommended

● MEDICINAL FORMS There can be variation in the licensing of different medicines containing the same drug.
Implant
▸ Iluvien (Alimera Sciences Ltd)
　Fluocinolone acetonide 190 microgram ILUVIEN 190microgram intravitreal implant in applicator | 1 device [PoM] £5,500.00

6.3 Optic neuropathy

DRUGS FOR METABOLIC DISORDERS ＞
ANTIOXIDANTS

Idebenone

09-Nov-2020

● DRUG ACTION Idebenone is a nootropic and antioxidant that is thought to act by restoring cellular ATP generation, thereby reactivating retinal ganglion cells.

● INDICATIONS AND DOSE
Leber's Hereditary Optic Neuropathy (initiated by a specialist)
▸ BY MOUTH
▸ Adult: 300 mg 3 times a day

● SIDE-EFFECTS
▸ **Common or very common** Cough · diarrhoea · increased risk of infection · pain
▸ **Frequency not known** Agranulocytosis · anaemia · anxiety · appetite decreased · azotaemia · delirium · dizziness · dyspepsia · hallucination · headache · hepatitis · leucopenia · malaise · movement disorders · nausea · neutropenia · poriomania · seizure · skin reactions · stupor · thrombocytopenia · urine discolouration · vomiting
SIDE-EFFECTS, FURTHER INFORMATION The metabolites of idebenone may cause red-brown discolouration of the urine. This effect is harmless, but the manufacturer advises caution as this may mask colour changes due to other causes (e.g. renal or blood disorders).

● PREGNANCY Manufacturer advises avoid unless potential benefit outweighs risk—no information available.
● BREAST FEEDING Manufacturer advises avoid—present in milk in *animal* studies.
● HEPATIC IMPAIRMENT Manufacturer advises caution (no information available).
● RENAL IMPAIRMENT Manufacturer advises use with caution—no information available.
● NATIONAL FUNDING/ACCESS DECISIONS
For full details see funding body website
Scottish Medicines Consortium (SMC) decisions
▸ Idebenone (*Raxone* ®) for the treatment of visual impairment in adolescent and adult patients with Leber's Hereditary Optic Neuropathy (LHON) (May 2017) SMC No. 1226/17 Recommended with restrictions

● MEDICINAL FORMS There can be variation in the licensing of different medicines containing the same drug. Forms available from special-order manufacturers include: tablet
Tablet
CAUTIONARY AND ADVISORY LABELS 14, 21
▸ Raxone (Chiesi Ltd) ▼
　Idebenone 150 mg Raxone 150mg tablets | 180 tablet [PoM] £6,364.00 DT = £6,364.00

6.4 Vitreomacular traction

RECOMBINANT PROTEOLYTIC ENZYMES

Ocriplasmin

03-Aug-2020

● INDICATIONS AND DOSE
Treatment of vitreomacular traction, including when associated with a macular hole of diameter less than or equal to 400 microns (specialist use only)
▸ BY INTRAVITREAL INJECTION
▸ Adult: 125 micrograms for 1 dose, to be administered into the affected eye, concurrent administration to both eyes is not recommended

● CONTRA-INDICATIONS Active or suspected ocular or periocular infection · aphakia · exudative age-related macular degeneration · high myopia · history of rhegmatogenous retinal detachment · ischaemic retinopathies · large diameter macular hole (> 400 microns) · lens zonule instability · proliferative diabetic retinopathy · recent intra-ocular injection (including laser therapy) · recent ocular surgery · retinal vein occlusions · vitreous haemorrhage
● CAUTIONS History of uveitis (including severe active inflammation) · non-proliferative diabetic retinopathy · significant eye trauma
● SIDE-EFFECTS
▸ **Common or very common** Dry eye · eye discomfort · eye disorders · eye inflammation · haemorrhage · retinal pigment epitheliopathy · vision disorders
● PREGNANCY Manufacturer advises use only if potential benefit outweighs risk—no information available.
● BREAST FEEDING Manufacturer advises use only if potential benefit outweighs risk—no information available.
● MONITORING REQUIREMENTS Monitor intra-ocular pressure, visual acuity, and for signs of intra-ocular inflammation or infection following injection.
● DIRECTIONS FOR ADMINISTRATION For further information on administration, consult product literature.
● NATIONAL FUNDING/ACCESS DECISIONS
For full details see funding body website
NICE decisions
▸ Ocriplasmin for treating vitreomacular traction (October 2013) NICE TA297 Recommended with restrictions
Scottish Medicines Consortium (SMC) decisions
▸ Ocriplasmin (*Jetrea* ®) in adults for the treatment of vitreomacular traction, including when associated with macular hole of diameter less than or equal to 400 microns (August 2014) SMC No. 892/13 Recommended with restrictions

● MEDICINAL FORMS There can be variation in the licensing of different medicines containing the same drug.
Solution for injection
▸ Jetrea (Inceptua AB)
　Ocriplasmin 1.25 mg per 1 ml Jetrea 0.375mg/0.3ml solution for injection vials | 1 vial [PoM] £2,500.00 (Hospital only)

11

Eye

Chapter 12
Ear, nose and oropharynx

CONTENTS

Ear

Ear

13-Apr-2020

Otitis externa

Otitis externa refers to inflammation of the external ear canal which in some cases may involve oedema. It is primarily caused by bacterial infection. EvGr It is important to consider underlying otitis media as otitis externa may be secondary to otorrhoea from otitis media.

Any precipitating factors should be managed and cleaning the external ear canal should be considered (using dry swabbing, microsuction, or irrigation techniques) if ear wax or debris are blocking passage of topical medicine (may require specialist referral).

A solution of **acetic acid** 2% acts as an astringent in the external ear canal by reducing the pH and reducing bacterial and fungal cell growth. It may be used to treat mild otitis externa and is comparable to an anti-infective combined with a corticosteroid; efficacy is reduced if treatment extends beyond 1 week.

If infection is present, a topical anti-infective with or without a corticosteroid may be considered. These are used for a minimum of one week but if symptoms persist they can be used until they resolve, up to a maximum of 2 weeks. Prolonged and extensive use of topical anti-infective or corticosteroid treatment may affect the flora in the ear canal, increasing the risk of fungal infections. If a mild to moderate, uncomplicated fungal infection is suspected in the context of chronic otitis externa, a topical antifungal such as clotrimazole 1% solution p. 1241, acetic acid 2% spray [unlicensed indication], or clioquinol and a corticosteroid such as flumetasone pivalate with clioquinol p. 1241 can be offered. Sensitivity to topical ear preparations may also occur, especially with prolonged or recurrent use. Astringent agents such as aluminium acetate ear drops p. 1243 are also available. Ⓐ

In view of reports of ototoxicity, treatment with topical **aminoglycosides** is contra-indicated in patients with a perforated tympanic membrane (eardrum). EvGr However, some specialists do use these drops cautiously in the presence of a perforation or patent grommet in patients with chronic suppurative otitis media and when other measures have failed for otitis externa; treatment should be considered only **by specialists** in the following circumstances:

- drops should only be used in the presence of obvious infection;
- treatment should be for no longer than 2 weeks;
- patients should be counselled on the risk of ototoxicity and given justification for the use of these topical antibiotics;
- baseline audiometry should be performed, if possible, before treatment is commenced.

Clinical expertise and judgement should be used to assess the risk of treatment versus the benefit to the patient in such circumstances. Ⓔ

EvGr For severe pain associated with otitis externa, a simple analgesic, such as paracetamol p. 464 or ibuprofen p. 1186, is usually sufficient; codeine phosphate p. 475 may be used for severe pain. Oral antibacterials are rarely indicated but if they are required, consider seeking specialist advice. A systemic antibacterial may be considered if the infection is spreading outside the ear canal, the patient is systemically unwell, or in a high risk group (e.g. diabetics, immunocompromised patients, patients with severe infection or at high risk of severe infection such as pseudomonal infections). Referral should be considered if there is extensive swelling of the auditory canal. If a systemic antibacterial is required, consider a course of flucloxacillin p. 589, or clarithromycin p. 569 if the patient is penicillin allergic. Ⓐ

Otitis media

Acute otitis media

Acute otitis media is a self-limiting condition that mainly affects children. It is characterised by inflammation in the middle ear associated with effusion and accompanied by the rapid onset of signs and symptoms of an ear infection. The infection can be caused by viruses or bacteria; often both are present simultaneously.

Children with acute otitis media usually present with symptoms such as ear pain, rubbing of the ear, fever, irritability, crying, poor feeding, restlessness at night, cough, or rhinorrhoea. Symptoms usually resolve within 3 to 7 days without antibacterial drugs and they make little difference to the development of complications such as short-term hearing loss, perforated eardrum or recurrent infection. Acute complications such as mastoiditis, meningitis, intracranial abscess, sinus thrombosis, and facial nerve paralysis, are rare.

EvGr Children and their carers should be given advice about the usual duration of acute otitis media, self-care of symptoms such as pain and fever with paracetamol or ibuprofen p. 1186, and when to seek medical help. In children aged 3 years and over who do not have a perforated eardrum, pain can be relieved with anaesthetic ear drops in addition to oral analgesics [unlicensed use]. Children and their carers should be reassured that antibacterial drugs are usually not required.

An immediate antibacterial drug should be given if the child is systemically very unwell, has signs or symptoms of a more serious illness, or is at high risk of complications such as significant heart, lung, renal, liver or neuromuscular disease, immunosuppression, cystic fibrosis, or young children who were born prematurely. An immediate antibacterial drug can also be considered if otorrhoea is present, or in children under 2 years of age with bilateral otitis media. See *Antibacterial therapy for otitis media* in Ear infections, antibacterial therapy p. 534.

Children with acute otitis media associated with a severe systemic infection or acute complications should be referred to hospital. Ⓐ

Otitis media with effusion

Otitis media with effusion (glue ear) is characterised by the collection of fluid within the middle ear without any signs of inflammation. It occurs most frequently in children, often in those aged 2 to 5 years; it is the most common cause of hearing impairment in children. It is more common in children with cleft palate, Down's syndrome, primary ciliary dyskinesia, and allergic rhinitis. EvGr Children with otitis media with effusion should be observed (for 6–12 weeks) as it commonly resolves spontaneously. Systemic antibacterials, antihistamines, mucolytics, decongestants, and corticosteroids are not recommended due to lack of evidence supporting their use. Referral to a specialist in certain circumstances (including in children with Down's syndrome and cleft palate) are warranted to avoid complications such as severe hearing impairment, and communication and developmental difficulties. Ⓐ

Chronic suppurative otitis media

Chronic suppurative otitis media is a chronic inflammation of the middle ear and mastoid cavity, and is thought to be a complication of acute otitis media. The usual presentation is otorrhoea through a tympanic perforation and can involve infection due to a number of different bacteria or fungi. EvGr Referral to an ear, nose and throat specialist is required and treatment is likely to involve antibacterials, corticosteroids (usually topical), and intensive aural cleaning. Ⓐ

Removal of ear wax

Ear wax (cerumen) is a normal bodily secretion which provides a protective film on the lining of the ear canal and need only be removed if it causes hearing loss or interferes with a proper view of the ear drum.

Ear wax can be softened using simple remedies such as **olive oil** ear drops or **almond oil** ear drops; sodium bicarbonate ear drops p. 1244 are also effective, but may cause dryness of the ear canal. The drops can be used three to four times daily for several days. Lying down with the affected ear uppermost, ear drops are instilled before waiting for 5 minutes.

If necessary, wax may be removed by irrigation with water (warmed to body temperature). Ear irrigation is generally best avoided in some cases including in young children (under 12 years of age), in patients unable to co-operate with the procedure, in those with otitis media in the last six weeks, in otitis externa, in patients with cleft palate, a history of ear drum perforation, or previous ear surgery. A person who has hearing in one ear only should not have that ear irrigated because even a very slight risk of damage may lead to permanent deafness.

1   Otitis externa

> **Other drugs used for Otitis externa** Hydrocortisone with miconazole, p. 1296

ANTIBACTERIALS > AMINOGLYCOSIDES

Framycetin sulfate

- **INDICATIONS AND DOSE**

Bacterial infection in otitis externa
▶ TO THE EAR
  ▹ Adult: (consult product literature)

- CONTRA-INDICATIONS   Perforated tympanic membrane
- CAUTIONS   Avoid prolonged use
- MEDICINAL FORMS   No licensed medicines listed.

  Combinations available: *Dexamethasone with framycetin sulfate and gramicidin,* p. 1243

▰ F 544

Gentamicin

04-Dec-2020

- **INDICATIONS AND DOSE**

Bacterial infection in otitis externa
▶ TO THE EAR
  ▹ Child: Apply 2–3 drops 4–5 times a day, (including a dose at bedtime)
  ▹ Adult: Apply 2–3 drops 4–5 times a day, (including a dose at bedtime)

- UNLICENSED USE   Gentamicin doses in BNF publications may differ from those in product literature.
- CONTRA-INDICATIONS   Patent grommet (although may be used by specialists, see Ear p. 1238) · perforated tympanic membrane (although may be used by specialists, see Ear p. 1238)
- CAUTIONS   Avoid prolonged use
- INTERACTIONS   → Appendix 1: aminoglycosides
- PRESCRIBING AND DISPENSING INFORMATION   For choice of antibacterial therapy, see Ear infections, antibacterial therapy p. 534.
- MEDICINAL FORMS   There can be variation in the licensing of different medicines containing the same drug. Forms available from special-order manufacturers include: eye drops

  Ear/eye drops solution
  EXCIPIENTS: May contain Benzalkonium chloride
  ▹ Gentamicin (Non-proprietary)
    Gentamicin (as Gentamicin sulfate) 3 mg per 1 ml   Gentamicin 0.3% ear/eye drops | 10 ml PoM £3.06 DT = £2.78

Gentamicin with hydrocortisone

18-Nov-2020

- **INDICATIONS AND DOSE**

Eczematous inflammation in otitis externa
▶ TO THE EAR
  ▹ Child: Apply 2–4 drops 4–5 times a day, (including a dose at bedtime)
  ▹ Adult: Apply 2–4 drops 4–5 times a day, (including a dose at bedtime)

> **IMPORTANT SAFETY INFORMATION**
>
> MHRA/CHM ADVICE: CORTICOSTEROIDS: RARE RISK OF CENTRAL SEROUS CHORIORETINOPATHY WITH LOCAL AS WELL AS SYSTEMIC ADMINISTRATION (AUGUST 2017)
> See Corticosteroids, general use p. 709.

NHS IMPROVEMENT PATIENT SAFETY ALERT: STEROID EMERGENCY CARD TO SUPPORT EARLY RECOGNITION AND TREATMENT OF ADRENAL CRISIS IN ADULTS (AUGUST 2020) See Corticosteroids, general use p. 709.

- CONTRA-INDICATIONS Patent grommet (although may be used by specialists, see Ear p. 1238) · perforated tympanic membrane (although may be used by specialists, see Ear p. 1238)
- CAUTIONS Avoid prolonged use
- SIDE-EFFECTS Local reaction
- PATIENT AND CARER ADVICE
  Medicines for Children leaflet: Gentamicin and hydrocortisone ear drops for inflammatory ear infections
  www.medicinesforchildren.org.uk/gentamicin-and-hydrocortisone-ear-drops-inflammatory-ear-infections
- MEDICINAL FORMS There can be variation in the licensing of different medicines containing the same drug.
  Ear drops
  EXCIPIENTS: May contain Benzalkonium chloride, disodium edetate
  ▸ Gentamicin with hydrocortisone (Non-proprietary)
  Gentamicin (as Gentamicin sulfate) 3 mg per 1 ml, Hydrocortisone acetate 10 mg per 1 ml Gentamicin 0.3% / Hydrocortisone acetate 1% ear drops | 10 ml [PoM] £33.26 DT = £33.26

Neomycin sulfate

- INDICATIONS AND DOSE

Bacterial infection in otitis externa
▸ TO THE EAR
  ▸ Child: (consult product literature)
  ▸ Adult: (consult product literature)

- CONTRA-INDICATIONS Patent grommet (although may be used by specialists, see Ear p. 1238) · perforated tympanic membrane (although may be used by specialists, see Ear p. 1238)
- CAUTIONS Avoid prolonged use
- INTERACTIONS → Appendix 1: neomycin
- SIDE-EFFECTS Local reaction

- MEDICINAL FORMS No licensed medicines listed.

  Combinations available: _Betamethasone with neomycin_, p. 1242 · _Dexamethasone with glacial acetic acid and neomycin sulfate_, p. 1243 · _Hydrocortisone with neomycin and polymyxin B sulfate_, p. 1243

ANTIBACTERIALS > QUINOLONES

📭 592

Ciprofloxacin

18-Nov-2020

- INDICATIONS AND DOSE

Acute otitis externa
▸ TO THE EAR
  ▸ Child 1-17 years: Apply 0.25 mL twice daily for 7 days, each 0.25 mL dose contains 0.5 mg ciprofloxacin
  ▸ Adult: Apply 0.25 mL twice daily for 7 days, each 0.25 mL dose contains 0.5 mg ciprofloxacin

- CAUTIONS Known (or at risk of) perforated tympanic membrane
- INTERACTIONS → Appendix 1: quinolones

- SIDE-EFFECTS
▸ **Uncommon** Ear pruritus
- PRESCRIBING AND DISPENSING INFORMATION For choice of antibacterial therapy, see Ear infections, antibacterial therapy p. 534.
- HANDLING AND STORAGE Manufacturer advises discard any ampoules remaining 8 days after opening the pouch.
- PATIENT AND CARER ADVICE
  Medicines for Children leaflet: Ciprofloxacin drops for infection www.medicinesforchildren.org.uk/ciprofloxacin-drops-infection
- NATIONAL FUNDING/ACCESS DECISIONS
  For full details see funding body website
  Scottish Medicines Consortium (SMC) decisions
  ▸ Ciprofloxacin (_Cetraxal_®) for the treatment of acute otitis externa in adults and children older than 1 year with an intact tympanic membrane, caused by ciprofloxacin susceptible microorganisms (April 2018) SMC No. 1320/18 Recommended with restrictions
  All Wales Medicines Strategy Group (AWMSG) decisions
  ▸ Ciprofloxacin (_Cetraxal_®) for the treatment of acute otitis externa in adults and children older than 1 year with an intact tympanic membrane, caused by ciprofloxacin susceptible microorganisms (July 2018) AWMSG No. 1343 Recommended

- MEDICINAL FORMS There can be variation in the licensing of different medicines containing the same drug. Forms available from special-order manufacturers include: ear drops
  Ear drops
  ▸ Cetraxal (Aspire Pharma Ltd)
  Ciprofloxacin (as Ciprofloxacin hydrochloride) 2 mg per 1 ml Cetraxal 2mg/ml ear drops 0.25ml unit dose | 15 unit dose [PoM] £6.01 DT = £6.01

  Combinations available: _Ciprofloxacin with dexamethasone_, p. 1242 · _Ciprofloxacin with fluocinolone acetonide_, p. 1242

ANTIBACTERIALS > OTHER

Chloramphenicol

09-Nov-2020

- DRUG ACTION Chloramphenicol is a potent broad-spectrum antibiotic.

- INDICATIONS AND DOSE

Bacterial infection in otitis externa
▸ TO THE EAR
  ▸ Child: Apply 2–3 drops 2–3 times a day
  ▸ Adult: Apply 2–3 drops 2–3 times a day

- CAUTIONS Avoid prolonged use
- INTERACTIONS → Appendix 1: chloramphenicol
- SIDE-EFFECTS Blood disorder · bone marrow depression
- PATIENT AND CARER ADVICE
  Medicines for Children leaflet: Chloramphenicol ear drops for infections (otitis externa) www.medicinesforchildren.org.uk/chloramphenicol-ear-drops-ear-infections-otitis-externa-0
- LESS SUITABLE FOR PRESCRIBING Chloramphenicol ear drops are less suitable for prescribing.

- MEDICINAL FORMS There can be variation in the licensing of different medicines containing the same drug.
  Ear drops
  EXCIPIENTS: May contain Propylene glycol
  ▸ Chloramphenicol (Non-proprietary)
  Chloramphenicol 50 mg per 1 ml Chloramphenicol 5% ear drops | 10 ml [PoM] £102.57 DT = £97.69
  Chloramphenicol 100 mg per 1 ml Chloramphenicol 10% ear drops | 10 ml [PoM] £98.97 DT = £90.03

Clotrimazole

10-Mar-2020

● **INDICATIONS AND DOSE**

Fungal infection in otitis externa
▶ TO THE EAR
▸ Child: Apply 2–3 times a day continue for at least
  14 days after disappearance of infection
▸ Adult: Apply 2–3 times a day continue for at least
  14 days after disappearance of infection

● INTERACTIONS → Appendix 1: antifungals, azoles
● SIDE-EFFECTS Hypersensitivity · oedema · pain ·
  paraesthesia · skin reactions
● PATIENT AND CARER ADVICE
  Medicines for Children leaflet: Clotrimazole for fungal infections
  www.medicinesforchildren.org.uk/clotrimazole-fungal-
  infections

● MEDICINAL FORMS There can be variation in the licensing of
  different medicines containing the same drug. Forms available
  from special-order manufacturers include: powder
  Spray
  CAUTIONARY AND ADVISORY LABELS 15
  EXCIPIENTS: May contain Propylene glycol
  ▸ Canesten (clotrimazole) (Bayer Plc)
    Clotrimazole 10 mg per 1 ml Canesten Dermatological 1% spray |
    40 ml P £4.72 DT = £4.72
  Liquid
  ▸ Canesten (clotrimazole) (Bayer Plc)
    Clotrimazole 10 mg per 1 ml Canesten 1% solution | 20 ml P
    £2.53 DT = £2.53

CORTICOSTEROIDS

▰ 711

Betamethasone

07-Dec-2020

● DRUG ACTION Betamethasone has very high glucocorticoid
  activity and insignificant mineralocorticoid activity.

● **INDICATIONS AND DOSE**

BETNESOL ®

Eczematous inflammation in otitis externa
▶ TO THE EAR
▸ Adult: Apply 2–3 drops every 2–3 hours, reduce
  frequency when relief obtained

VISTAMETHASONE ®

Eczematous inflammation in otitis externa
▶ TO THE EAR
▸ Adult: Apply 2–3 drops every 3–4 hours, reduce
  frequency when relief obtained

● CONTRA-INDICATIONS Avoid alone in the presence of
  untreated infection (combine with suitable anti-infective)
● CAUTIONS Avoid prolonged use
● INTERACTIONS → Appendix 1: corticosteroids

● MEDICINAL FORMS There can be variation in the licensing of
  different medicines containing the same drug.
  Ear/eye/nose drops solution
  EXCIPIENTS: May contain Benzalkonium chloride, disodium edetate
  ▸ Betnesol (RPH Pharmaceuticals AB)
    Betamethasone sodium phosphate 1 mg per 1 ml Betnesol 0.1%
    eye/ear/nose drops | 10 ml PoM £2.32 DT = £2.32
  ▸ Vistamethasone (Martindale Pharmaceuticals Ltd)
    Betamethasone sodium phosphate 1 mg per 1 ml Vistamethasone
    0.1% ear/eye/nose drops | 5 ml PoM £1.02 | 10 ml PoM £1.16 DT =
    £2.32

  Combinations available: *Betamethasone with neomycin*,
  p. 1242

Flumetasone pivalate with clioquinol

25-Sep-2020

● **INDICATIONS AND DOSE**

**Eczematous inflammation in otitis externa | Mild bacterial
or fungal infections in otitis externa**
▶ TO THE EAR
▸ Child 2-17 years: 2–3 drops twice daily for 7–10 days, to
  be instilled into the ear
▸ Adult: 2–3 drops twice daily for 7 days, to be
  instilled into the ear

● **IMPORTANT SAFETY INFORMATION**

  MHRA/CHM ADVICE: CORTICOSTEROIDS: RARE RISK OF CENTRAL
  SEROUS CHORIORETINOPATHY WITH LOCAL AS WELL AS SYSTEMIC
  ADMINISTRATION (AUGUST 2017)
  See Corticosteroids, general use p. 709.

  NHS IMPROVEMENT PATIENT SAFETY ALERT: STEROID
  EMERGENCY CARD TO SUPPORT EARLY RECOGNITION AND
  TREATMENT OF ADRENAL CRISIS IN ADULTS (AUGUST 2020)
  See Corticosteroids, general use p. 709.

● CONTRA-INDICATIONS Iodine sensitivity
● CAUTIONS Avoid prolonged use · manufacturer advises
  avoid in perforated tympanic membrane (but used by
  specialists for short periods)
● SIDE-EFFECTS Paraesthesia · skin reactions
● PATIENT AND CARER ADVICE Clioquinol stains skin and
  clothing

● MEDICINAL FORMS There can be variation in the licensing of
  different medicines containing the same drug.
  Ear drops
  ▸ Flumetasone pivalate with clioquinol (Non-proprietary)
    **Flumetasone pivalate 200 microgram per 1 ml, Clioquinol 10 mg
    per 1 ml** Flumetasone 0.02% / Clioquinol 1% ear drops |
    7.5 ml PoM £11.34 DT = £11.34 | 10 ml PoM £15.13 DT = £15.13

▰ 711

Prednisolone

06-Oct-2020

● DRUG ACTION Prednisolone exerts predominantly
  glucocorticoid effects with minimal mineralocorticoid
  effects.

● **INDICATIONS AND DOSE**

Eczematous inflammation in otitis externa
▶ TO THE EAR
▸ Child: Apply 2–3 drops every 2–3 hours, frequency to
  be reduced when relief obtained
▸ Adult: Apply 2–3 drops every 2–3 hours, frequency to
  be reduced when relief obtained

● CONTRA-INDICATIONS Avoid alone in the presence of
  untreated infection (combine with suitable anti-infective)
● CAUTIONS Avoid prolonged use
● INTERACTIONS → Appendix 1: corticosteroids
● SIDE-EFFECTS Local reaction

● MEDICINAL FORMS There can be variation in the licensing of
  different medicines containing the same drug. Forms available
  from special-order manufacturers include: ear drops
  Ear/eye drops solution
  EXCIPIENTS: May contain Benzalkonium chloride, disodium edetate
  ▸ Prednisolone (Non-proprietary)
    Prednisolone sodium phosphate 5 mg per 1 ml Prednisolone
    sodium phosphate 0.5% ear/eye drops | 10 ml PoM £2.57 DT = £2.57

12

Ear, nose and oropharynx

CORTICOSTEROIDS > CORTICOSTEROID COMBINATIONS WITH ANTI-INFECTIVES

Betamethasone with neomycin
18-Nov-2020

The properties listed below are those particular to the combination only. For the properties of the components please consider, betamethasone p. 1241, neomycin sulfate p. 1240.

- **INDICATIONS AND DOSE**

Eczematous inflammation in otitis externa
▸ TO THE EAR USING EAR DROPS
▸ Child: Apply 2–3 drops 3–4 times a day
▸ Adult: Apply 2–3 drops 3–4 times a day

- **CONTRA-INDICATIONS** Patent grommet (although may be used by specialists, see Ear p. 1238) · perforated tympanic membrane (although may be used by specialists, see Ear p. 1238)
- **CAUTIONS** Avoid prolonged use
- **INTERACTIONS** → Appendix 1: corticosteroids · neomycin

- **MEDICINAL FORMS** There can be variation in the licensing of different medicines containing the same drug.
Ear/eye/nose drops solution
EXCIPIENTS: May contain Benzalkonium chloride, disodium edetate
▸ Betnesol-N (RPH Pharmaceuticals AB)
Betamethasone (as Betamethasone sodium phosphate) 1 mg per 1 ml, Neomycin sulfate 5 mg per 1 ml Betnesol-N ear/eye/nose drops | 10 ml [PoM] £2.39 DT = £2.39

Ciprofloxacin with dexamethasone
04-Nov-2020

The properties listed below are those particular to the combination only. For the properties of the components please consider, dexamethasone p. 714, ciprofloxacin p. 1240.

- **INDICATIONS AND DOSE**

Acute otitis media in patients with tympanostomy tubes
▸ TO THE EAR
▸ Adult: Apply 4 drops twice daily for 7 days
Acute otitis externa
▸ TO THE EAR
▸ Adult: Apply 4 drops twice daily for 7 days

- **CONTRA-INDICATIONS** Fungal ear infections · viral ear infections
- **CAUTIONS** Avoid prolonged use
- **INTERACTIONS** → Appendix 1: corticosteroids · quinolones
- **SIDE-EFFECTS**
▸ **Common or very common** Ear discomfort
▸ **Uncommon** Ear infection fungal · flushing · irritability · malaise · otorrhoea · paraesthesia · skin reactions · taste altered · vomiting
▸ **Rare or very rare** Dizziness · headache · hearing loss · tinnitus
SIDE-EFFECTS, FURTHER INFORMATION Manufacturer advises further evaluation of underlying conditions if otorrhoea persists after a full course, or if at least two episodes of otorrhoea occur within 6 months.
- **PREGNANCY** Manufacturer advises use only if potential benefit outweighs risk—no information available.
- **BREAST FEEDING** Manufacturer advises caution—no information available.
- **PATIENT AND CARER ADVICE** Manufacturer advises counselling on administration.

- **NATIONAL FUNDING/ACCESS DECISIONS**
For full details see funding body website
Scottish Medicines Consortium (SMC) decisions
▸ Ciprofloxacin with dexamethasone (*Cilodex*®) for treatment o the following infections in adults and children: Acute otitis media in patients with tympanostomy tubes (AOMT) (July 2017) SMC No. 1256/17 Recommended with restrictions

- **MEDICINAL FORMS** There can be variation in the licensing of different medicines containing the same drug.
Ear drops
EXCIPIENTS: May contain Benzalkonium chloride, disodium edetate
▸ Ciprofloxacin with dexamethasone (Non-proprietary)
Dexamethasone 1 mg per 1 ml, Ciprofloxacin (as Ciprofloxacin hydrochloride) 3 mg per 1 ml Ciprofloxacin 0.3% / Dexamethasone 0.1% ear drops | 5 ml [PoM] £6.12 DT = £6.12

Ciprofloxacin with fluocinolone acetonide
25-Sep-2020

The properties listed below are those particular to the combination only. For the properties of the components please consider, ciprofloxacin p. 1240.

- **INDICATIONS AND DOSE**

Acute otitis externa | Acute otitis media in patients with tympanostomy tubes
▸ TO THE EAR
▸ Adult: Apply 0.25 mL twice daily for 7 days
DOSE EQUIVALENCE AND CONVERSION
▸ Each 0.25 mL dose contains 0.75 mg ciprofloxacin and 0.0625 mg of fluocinolone acetonide.

> **IMPORTANT SAFETY INFORMATION**
>
> MHRA/CHM ADVICE: CORTICOSTEROIDS: RARE RISK OF CENTRAL SEROUS CHORIORETINOPATHY WITH LOCAL AS WELL AS SYSTEMIC ADMINISTRATION (AUGUST 2017)
> See Corticosteroids, general use p. 709.
>
> NHS IMPROVEMENT PATIENT SAFETY ALERT: STEROID EMERGENCY CARD TO SUPPORT EARLY RECOGNITION AND TREATMENT OF ADRENAL CRISIS IN ADULTS (AUGUST 2020)
> See Corticosteroids, general use p. 709.

- **CONTRA-INDICATIONS** Fungal ear infections · viral ear infections
- **INTERACTIONS** → Appendix 1: fluocinolone · quinolones
- **SIDE-EFFECTS**
▸ **Common or very common** Ear discomfort · taste altered
▸ **Uncommon** Crying · dizziness · fatigue · flushing · headache · hearing impairment · increased risk of infection · irritability · otorrhoea · paraesthesia · skin reactions · tinnitus · tympanic membrane disorder · vomiting
SIDE-EFFECTS, FURTHER INFORMATION Manufacturer advises further evaluation of underlying conditions if otorrhoea persists after a full course, or if at least two episodes of otorrhoea occur within 6 months.
- **PREGNANCY** Manufacturer advises use only if potential benefit outweighs risk—limited information available.
- **BREAST FEEDING** Manufacturer advises caution.
- **PATIENT AND CARER ADVICE** Manufacturer advises counselling on administration.

- **MEDICINAL FORMS** There can be variation in the licensing of different medicines containing the same drug.
Ear drops
EXCIPIENTS: May contain Polysorbates
▸ Cetraxal Plus (Aspire Pharma Ltd)
Fluocinolone acetonide.25 mg per 1 ml, Ciprofloxacin (as Ciprofloxacin hydrochloride) 3 mg per 1 ml Cetraxal Plus 3mg/ml + 0.25mg/ml ear drops 0.25ml unit dose | 15 unit dose [PoM] £6.01 DT = £6.01

Dexamethasone with framycetin sulfate and gramicidin
25-Sep-2020

The properties listed below are those particular to the combination only. For the properties of the components please consider, dexamethasone p. 714, framycetin sulfate p. 1239.

● INDICATIONS AND DOSE

Eczematous inflammation in otitis externa
▸ TO THE EAR
▸ Child: 2–3 drops 3–4 times a day
▸ Adult: 2–3 drops 3–4 times a day

● CAUTIONS Avoid prolonged use

● INTERACTIONS → Appendix 1: corticosteroids

● LESS SUITABLE FOR PRESCRIBING *Sofradex*® is less suitable for prescribing.

● MEDICINAL FORMS There can be variation in the licensing of different medicines containing the same drug.
Ear/Eye drops
EXCIPIENTS: May contain Polysorbates
▸ Sofradex (Sanofi)
Gramicidin 50 microgram per 1 ml, Dexamethasone (as Dexamethasone sodium metasulfobenzoate) 500 microgram per 1 ml, Framycetin sulfate 5 mg per 1 ml Sofradex ear/eye drops | 8 ml PoM £7.50

Dexamethasone with glacial acetic acid and neomycin sulfate
18-Nov-2020

The properties listed below are those particular to the combination only. For the properties of the components please consider, dexamethasone p. 714, neomycin sulfate p. 1240.

● INDICATIONS AND DOSE

Eczematous inflammation in otitis externa
▸ TO THE EAR
▸ Child 2-17 years: Apply 1 spray 3 times a day
▸ Adult: Apply 1 spray 3 times a day

● CONTRA-INDICATIONS Patent grommet (although may be used by specialists, see Ear p. 1238) · perforated tympanic membrane (although may be used by specialists, see Ear p. 1238)

● CAUTIONS Avoid prolonged use

● INTERACTIONS → Appendix 1: corticosteroids · neomycin

● SIDE-EFFECTS Paraesthesia · skin reactions · vision blurred

● MEDICINAL FORMS There can be variation in the licensing of different medicines containing the same drug.
Spray
EXCIPIENTS: May contain Hydroxybenzoates (parabens)
▸ Otomize (Teva UK Ltd)
Dexamethasone 1 mg per 1 gram, Neomycin sulfate 5 mg per 1 gram, Acetic acid glacial 20 mg per 1 gram Otomize ear spray | 5 ml PoM £3.27

Hydrocortisone with neomycin and polymyxin B sulfate
25-Sep-2020

The properties listed below are those particular to the combination only. For the properties of the components please consider, hydrocortisone p. 716, neomycin sulfate p. 1240.

● INDICATIONS AND DOSE

Bacterial infection in otitis externa
▸ TO THE EAR
▸ Child 3-17 years: Apply 3 drops 3–4 times a day for 7 days (review treatment if there is no clinical improvement)
▸ Adult: Apply 3 drops 3–4 times a day for 7 days (review treatment if there is no clinical improvement)

● INTERACTIONS → Appendix 1: corticosteroids · neomycin · polymyxin b

● RENAL IMPAIRMENT Manufacturer advises avoid prolonged, unsupervised use.
Dose adjustments Manufacturer advises reduce dose.

● MEDICINAL FORMS There can be variation in the licensing of different medicines containing the same drug.
Ear drops
EXCIPIENTS: May contain Cetostearyl alcohol (including cetyl and stearyl alcohol), hydroxybenzoates (parabens), polysorbates
▸ Otosporin (Phoenix Labs Ltd)
Hydrocortisone 10 mg per 1 ml, Neomycin sulfate 3400 unit per 1 ml, Polymyxin B sulfate 10000 unit per 1 ml Otosporin ear drops | 10 ml PoM £7.45

DERMATOLOGICAL DRUGS ⟩ ASTRINGENTS

Aluminium acetate

● INDICATIONS AND DOSE

Inflammation in otitis externa
▸ TO THE EAR
▸ Adult: To be inserted into meatus or apply on a ribbon gauze dressing or sponge wick which should be kept saturated with the ear drops

● DIRECTIONS FOR ADMINISTRATION For ear drops 8%— dilute 8 parts aluminium acetate ear drops (13%) with 5 parts purified water. Must be freshly prepared.

● MEDICINAL FORMS Forms available from special-order manufacturers include: ear drops

2 Otitis media

ANALGESICS ⟩ NON-STEROIDAL ANTI-INFLAMMATORY DRUGS

Phenazone with lidocaine
26-Nov-2020

The properties listed below are those particular to the combination only. For the properties of the components please consider, lidocaine hydrochloride p. 111.

● INDICATIONS AND DOSE

Acute otitis media | Barotraumatic otitis
▸ TO THE EAR
▸ Child: Apply 4 drops 2–3 times a day, re-evaluate therapy if symptoms do not improve within 7 days or worsen at any time
▸ Adult: Apply 4 drops 2–3 times a day, re-evaluate therapy if symptoms do not improve within 7 days or worsen at any time

12

Ear, nose and oropharynx

- CONTRA-INDICATIONS Perforated tympanic membrane (risk of ototoxicity)
- INTERACTIONS → Appendix 1: antiarrhythmics · NSAIDs
- SIDE-EFFECTS
► **Rare or very rare** Skin reactions · tympanic membrane hyperaemia
- PREGNANCY [EvGr] Use with caution—no information available but systemic absorption unlikely with intact tympanic membrane. ⟨M⟩
- BREAST FEEDING [EvGr] Use with caution—no information available but systemic absorption unlikely with intact tympanic membrane. ⟨M⟩

- MEDICINAL FORMS There can be variation in the licensing of different medicines containing the same drug.
Ear drops
EXCIPIENTS: May contain Ethanol
► Otigo (Renascience Pharma Ltd)
Lidocaine hydrochloride 10 mg per 1 gram, Phenazone 40 mg per 1 gram Otigo 40mg/g / 10mg/g ear drops | 15 ml [PoM] £8.92

3 Removal of earwax

BICARBONATE

Sodium bicarbonate

14-Dec-2020

- INDICATIONS AND DOSE
Removal of earwax (with 5% ear drop solution)
► TO THE EAR
► Child: (consult product literature)
► Adult: (consult product literature)

- INTERACTIONS → Appendix 1: sodium bicarbonate
- SIDE-EFFECTS Dry ear

- MEDICINAL FORMS There can be variation in the licensing of different medicines containing the same drug.
Ear drops
► Sodium bicarbonate (Non-proprietary)
Sodium bicarbonate 50 mg per 1 ml Sodium bicarbonate 5% ear drops | 10 ml £1.23–£1.25
► KliarVax Sodium Bicarbonate (Essential-Healthcare Ltd)
Sodium bicarbonate 50 mg per 1 ml KliarVax Sodium Bicarbonate ear drops | 10 ml £0.97

SOFTENING DRUGS

Almond oil

04-Aug-2020

- INDICATIONS AND DOSE
Removal of earwax
► TO THE EAR
► Child: Allow drops to warm to room temperature before use (consult product literature)
► Adult: Allow drops to warm to room temperature before use (consult product literature)

- DIRECTIONS FOR ADMINISTRATION Expert sources advise the patient should lie with the affected ear uppermost for 5 to 10 minutes after a generous amount of the softening remedy has been introduced into the ear.

- MEDICINAL FORMS There can be variation in the licensing of different medicines containing the same drug.
Form unstated
► Almond oil (Non-proprietary)
Almond oil 1 ml per 1 ml Almond oil liquid | 50 ml £0.95 DT = £0.95 | 70 ml £0.73–£0.94

Docusate sodium

30-Jul-2020

(Dioctyl sodium sulphosuccinate)

- INDICATIONS AND DOSE
Removal of ear wax
► TO THE EAR
► Adult: (consult product literature)

- INTERACTIONS → Appendix 1: docusate sodium
- SIDE-EFFECTS Skin reactions
- LESS SUITABLE FOR PRESCRIBING Ear drops less suitable for prescribing.

- MEDICINAL FORMS There can be variation in the licensing of different medicines containing the same drug.
Ear drops
EXCIPIENTS: May contain Propylene glycol
► Molcer (Wallace Manufacturing Chemists Ltd)
Docusate sodium 50 mg per 1 ml Molcer ear drops | 15 ml [P] £5.60
► Waxsol (Mylan)
Docusate sodium 5 mg per 1 ml Waxsol ear drops | 10 ml [P] £1.95 DT = £1.95

Olive oil

04-Aug-2020

- INDICATIONS AND DOSE
Removal of earwax
► TO THE EAR
► Child: Apply twice daily for several days (if wax is hard and impacted)
► Adult: Apply twice daily for several days (if wax is hard and impacted)

Removal of earwax (dose approved for use by community practitioner nurse prescribers)
► TO THE EAR
► Child: (consult product literature)
► Adult: (consult product literature)

- DIRECTIONS FOR ADMINISTRATION Expert sources advise the patient should lie with the affected ear uppermost for 5 to 10 minutes after a generous amount of the softening remedy has been introduced into the ear. Allow ear drops to warm to room temperature before use.

- MEDICINAL FORMS There can be variation in the licensing of different medicines containing the same drug.
Spray
► Earol (HL Healthcare Ltd)
Earol olive oil ear spray | 10 ml [⊠]
Ear drops
► Olive oil (Non-proprietary)
Olive oil ear drops | 10 ml £1.35–£1.42
► Arjun (Arjun Products Ltd)
Arjun ear drops | 10 ml £1.26
► Cerumol (olive oil) (Thornton & Ross Ltd)
Cerumol olive oil ear drops | 10 ml [⊠]
► KliarVax (Essential-Healthcare Ltd)
KliarVax Olive Oil ear drops | 10 ml £0.97
► Olive oil (Thornton & Ross Ltd)
Care olive oil ear drops | 10 ml £1.42
► St George's (St Georges Medical Ltd)
Olive oil ear drops | 10 ml £1.40 | 20 ml £2.70

Urea hydrogen peroxide

02-Sep-2020

- INDICATIONS AND DOSE
Softening and removal of earwax
► TO THE EAR
► Adult: (consult product literature)

- PATIENT AND CARER ADVICE The patient should lie with the affected ear uppermost for 5 to 10 minutes after a generous amount of the softening remedy has been introduced into the ear.
- LESS SUITABLE FOR PRESCRIBING Urea-hydrogen peroxide ear drops are less suitable for prescribing.

- MEDICINAL FORMS There can be variation in the licensing of different medicines containing the same drug.

Ear drops
▸ Exterol (Dermal Laboratories Ltd)
   Urea hydrogen peroxide 50 mg per 1 gram Exterol 5% ear drops | 8 ml P £1.75 DT = £2.89
▸ Otex (Dendron Ltd)
   Urea hydrogen peroxide 50 mg per 1 gram Otex 5% ear drops | 8 ml P £2.89 DT = £2.89

Nose

Nose
30-Mar-2020

Rhinitis

Rhinitis may be acute or chronic, allergic or non-allergic. Nasal spray and drop preparations often carry indications for the management of allergic rhinitis and perennial rhinitis. Many nasal preparations contain sympathomimetic drugs which may irritate the nasal mucosa.

Drugs used in nasal allergy

EvGr Sodium chloride 0.9% solution p. 1089 may be used as nasal irrigation in allergic rhinitis for modest symptom reduction, and to reduce the need for other drug treatment.

Mild allergic rhinitis is controlled by **antihistamines** (see under Antihistamines, allergen immunotherapy and allergic emergencies p. 292) or topical **nasal corticosteroids**. Topical antihistamines (e.g. azelastine hydrochloride p. 1248) are faster acting than oral antihistamines and therefore useful for controlling breakthrough symptoms in allergic rhinitis; they are less effective than topical nasal corticosteroids. Topical nasal decongestants can be used for a short period to provide quick relief from congestion and allow penetration of a topical nasal corticosteroid. Systemic nasal decongestants are weakly effective in reducing nasal obstruction but have considerable potential for side-effects, and therefore are not recommended. Sodium cromoglicate is a weakly effective alternative in patients with mild symptoms, sporadic seasonal problems, or limited allergen exposure.

Moderate to severe allergic rhinitis can be relieved by topical **nasal corticosteroids** during periods of allergen exposure. Severe allergic rhinitis causing very disabling symptoms despite conventional treatment may justify the use of **oral corticosteroids** for short periods. In severe cases, oral corticosteroids may also be used in combination with nasal corticosteroids during treatment initiation to relieve severe mucosal oedema and allow the spray to penetrate the nasal cavity.

Nasal ipratropium bromide p. 1249 may be added to allergic rhinitis treatment when watery rhinorrhoea persists despite treatment with topical nasal corticosteroids and antihistamines; it has no effect on other nasal symptoms.

In seasonal allergic rhinitis (e.g. hay fever), treatment should begin 2 to 3 weeks before the season commences and/or exposure to the allergen.

Montelukast p. 285 is less effective than topical nasal corticosteroids but can be used in patients with seasonal allergic rhinitis and concomitant asthma. A

Corticosteroids

EvGr Topical nasal corticosteroid preparations should be avoided in the presence of untreated nasal infections, after

nasal surgery (until healing has occurred), and in pulmonary tuberculosis. Systemic absorption may follow nasal administration particularly if high doses are used or if treatment is prolonged. The extent of absorption varies between steroids; mometasone furoate p. 1251 and fluticasone p. 1251 have negligible systemic absorption, others have modest absorption, whilst betamethasone p. 1250 has high systemic absorption and should only be used short-term. The growth of children receiving treatment with corticosteroids should be monitored; especially in those receiving corticosteroids via multiple routes. A

Nasal polyps

EvGr Patients presenting with nasal polyps should initially be reviewed by an ear, nose and throat specialist. Nasal polyps may be treated with topical nasal corticosteroids (drops or spray). There may be a higher risk of side-effects with use of nasal drops compared to nasal spray due to greater systemic absorption and incorrect administration of drops. To reduce the risk, the drops must be administered with the patient in the 'head down' position. A short course of a systemic corticosteroid can provide symptomatic relief but effects may be temporary and its use is rare due to concerns of systemic side-effects. If systemic corticosteroids are given, they should be used in combination with topical nasal corticosteroids. A

Pregnancy

EvGr If a pregnant woman cannot tolerate the symptoms of allergic rhinitis, treatment may be given. A Although the safety of nasal corticosteroids in pregnancy has not been established through clinical trials, only minimal amounts of nasal corticosteroids are systemically absorbed. Beclometasone dipropionate p. 1249, budesonide p. 1250, and fluticasone are widely used in asthmatic pregnant women; fluticasone has the lowest systemic absorption when used intra-nasally. EvGr Decongestants are not recommended however, some antihistamines and sodium cromoglicate may be used. A

Topical nasal decongestants

The nasal mucosa is sensitive to changes in atmospheric temperature and humidity and these alone may cause slight nasal congestion. EvGr Sodium chloride 0.9% given as nasal drops, spray, or irrigation may relieve nasal congestion.

Steam inhalation may help to relieve congestion but care should be taken to avoid scalding (see under Aromatic inhalations, cough preparations and systemic nasal decongestants p. 312).

Symptoms of nasal congestion associated with allergic rhinitis, the common cold, and sinusitis may be relieved by the short-term use (usually not longer than 7 days) of decongestant nasal drops and sprays. A These all contain sympathomimetic drugs which exert their effect by vasoconstriction of the mucosal blood vessels which in turn reduces oedema of the nasal mucosa. Their use, especially with longer durations, can give rise to rebound congestion (rhinitis medicamentosa) on withdrawal, due to a secondary vasodilatation with a subsequent temporary increase in nasal congestion. This in turn tempts the further use of the decongestant, leading to a vicious cycle of events; tolerance with reduced effect may also be seen with excessive use.

EvGr Non-allergic watery rhinorrhoea often responds to treatment with nasal antimuscarinic ipratropium bromide. A

Nasal preparations for infection

Nasal staphylococci

EvGr Elimination of organisms such as staphylococci from the nasal vestibule can be achieved by the use of antimicrobial preparations such as chlorhexidine with neomycin cream (*Naseptin*®) p. 1248. A nasal ointment containing mupirocin p. 1248 is available if *Naseptin*® is unsuitable or ineffective.

In hospitals or in care establishments, mupirocin nasal ointment can be used for the eradication of nasal carriage of meticillin-resistant *Staphylococcus aureus* (MRSA). ⚠

For information on eradication of MRSA, consult local infection control policy. See also management of MRSA p. 615.

1 Nasal congestion

SYMPATHOMIMETICS ⟩ VASOCONSTRICTOR

Ephedrine hydrochloride

04-Dec-2019

● **INDICATIONS AND DOSE**

Nasal congestion | Sinusitis affecting the maxillary antrum
▸ BY INTRANASAL ADMINISTRATION
▸ **Child 12-17 years:** Apply 1–2 drops up to 4 times a day as required for a maximum of 7 days, to be instilled into each nostril, administer ephedrine 0.5% nasal drops
▸ **Adult:** Apply 1–2 drops up to 4 times a day as required for a maximum of 7 days, to be instilled into each nostril

IMPORTANT SAFETY INFORMATION

CHM/MHRA ADVICE

The CHM/MHRA has stated that non-prescription cough and cold medicines containing ephedrine can be considered for up to 5 days' treatment in children aged 6–12 years after basic principles of best care have been tried; these medicines should not be used in children under 6 years of age.

● **CAUTIONS** Avoid excessive or prolonged use · cardiovascular disease (in children) · diabetes mellitus · elderly · hypertension · hyperthyroidism · ischaemic heart disease (in adults) · prostatic hypertrophy (risk of acute urinary retention) (in adults)
● **INTERACTIONS** → Appendix 1: sympathomimetics, vasoconstrictor
● **SIDE-EFFECTS**
▸ **Common or very common** Anxiety · headache · insomnia · nausea
▸ **Frequency not known** Appetite decreased · arrhythmia · circulation impaired · dermatitis · dizziness · drug dependence · dry mouth · dyspnoea · hallucination · hyperglycaemia · hyperhidrosis · hypersalivation · hypertension · hypokalaemia · hypotension · irritability · muscle weakness · mydriasis · pain · palpitations · paranoia · piloerection · rebound congestion · syncope · thirst · tremor · urinary disorders · vasoconstriction · vasodilation · vomiting
● **PREGNANCY** Manufacturer advises avoid.
● **BREAST FEEDING** Present in milk; manufacturer advises avoid—irritability and disturbed sleep reported.
● **PRESCRIBING AND DISPENSING INFORMATION** For nasal drops, the BP directs that if no strength is specified 0.5% drops should be supplied.
● **PROFESSION SPECIFIC INFORMATION**

Dental practitioners' formulary
Ephedrine nasal drops may be prescribed.
● **EXCEPTIONS TO LEGAL CATEGORY** Ephedrine nasal drops can be sold to the public provided no more than 180 mg of ephedrine base (or salts) are supplied at one time, and pseudoephedrine salts are not supplied at the same time; for conditions that apply to supplies made at the request of a patient, see *Medicines, Ethics and Practice*, London, Pharmaceutical Press (always consult latest edition).

● **MEDICINAL FORMS** There can be variation in the licensing of different medicines containing the same drug. Forms available from special-order manufacturers include: nasal drops
Nasal drops
▸ Ephedrine hydrochloride (Non-proprietary)
  Ephedrine hydrochloride 5 mg per 1 ml Ephedrine 0.5% nasal drops | 10 ml Ⓟ £1.90 DT = £1.90
  Ephedrine hydrochloride 10 mg per 1 ml Ephedrine 1% nasal drops | 10 ml Ⓟ £1.94 DT = £1.94

Pseudoephedrine hydrochloride

06-Apr-2020

● **INDICATIONS AND DOSE**

Congestion of mucous membranes of upper respiratory tract
▸ BY MOUTH
▸ **Child 6-11 years:** 30 mg 3–4 times a day
▸ **Child 12-17 years:** 60 mg 3–4 times a day
▸ **Adult:** 60 mg 3–4 times a day

IMPORTANT SAFETY INFORMATION

MHRA/CHM ADVICE: OVER-THE-COUNTER COUGH AND COLD MEDICINES FOR CHILDREN (APRIL 2009)

Children under 6 years should not be given over-the-counter cough and cold medicines containing pseudoephedrine.

● **CAUTIONS** Diabetes · heart disease · hypertension · hyperthyroidism · ischaemic heart disease (in adults) · prostatic hypertrophy (in adults) · raised intra-ocular pressure (in children) · susceptibility to angle-closure glaucoma (in adults)
● **INTERACTIONS** → Appendix 1: sympathomimetics, vasoconstrictor
● **SIDE-EFFECTS** Angle closure glaucoma · anxiety · arrhythmias · circulation impaired · dry mouth · hallucination · headache · hypertension · irritability · nausea · palpitations · psychotic disorder · skin reactions · sleep disorders · tremor · urinary retention · vomiting
● **PREGNANCY** Defective closure of the abdominal wall (gastroschisis) reported very rarely in newborns after first trimester exposure.
● **BREAST FEEDING** May suppress lactation; avoid if lactation not well established or if milk production insufficient.
● **HEPATIC IMPAIRMENT** Manufacturer advises caution in severe impairment.
● **RENAL IMPAIRMENT** Use with caution in mild to moderate renal impairment. Manufacturer advises avoid in severe renal impairment.
● **LESS SUITABLE FOR PRESCRIBING** Pseudoephedrine hydrochloride is less suitable for prescribing.
● **EXCEPTIONS TO LEGAL CATEGORY** *Galpseud®* and *Sudafed®* can be sold to the public provided no more than 720 mg of pseudoephedrine salts are supplied, and ephedrine base (or salts) are not supplied at the same time; for details see *Medicines, Ethics and Practice*, London, Pharmaceutical Press (always consult latest edition).
● **MEDICINAL FORMS** There can be variation in the licensing of different medicines containing the same drug.
Oral solution
EXCIPIENTS: May contain Alcohol
▸ Galpseud (Thornton & Ross Ltd)
  Pseudoephedrine hydrochloride 6 mg per 1 ml Galpseud 30mg/5ml linctus sugar-free | 2000 ml PoM £14.00
Tablet
▸ Galpseud (Thornton & Ross Ltd)
  Pseudoephedrine hydrochloride 60 mg Galpseud 60mg tablets | 24 tablet PoM £2.25 DT = £2.25

Xylometazoline hydrochloride   13-Feb-2020

● **DRUG ACTION**   Xylometazoline is a sympathomimetic.

● **INDICATIONS AND DOSE**

Nasal congestion

▸ **BY INTRANASAL ADMINISTRATION USING NASAL DROPS**

▸ Child 6–11 years: 1–2 drops 1–2 times a day as required for maximum duration of 5 days, 0.05% solution to be administered into each nostril

▸ Child 12–17 years: 2–3 drops 2–3 times a day as required for maximum duration of 7 days, 0.1% solution to be administered into each nostril

▸ Adult: 2–3 drops 2–3 times a day as required for maximum duration of 7 days, 0.1% solution to be administered into each nostril

▸ **BY INTRANASAL ADMINISTRATION USING NASAL SPRAY**

▸ Child 12–17 years: 1 spray 1–3 times a day as required for maximum duration of 7 days, to be administered into each nostril

▸ Adult: 1 spray 1–3 times a day as required for maximum duration of 7 days, to be administered into each nostril

---

IMPORTANT SAFETY INFORMATION

The CHM/MHRA has stated that non-prescription cough and cold medicines containing oxymetazoline or xylometazoline can be considered for up to 5 days' treatment in children aged 6–12 years after basic principles of best care have been tried; these medicines should not be used in children under 6 years of age.

● **CAUTIONS**   Angle-closure glaucoma · avoid excessive or prolonged use · cardiovascular disease (in children) · diabetes mellitus · elderly · hypertension · hyperthyroidism · ischaemic heart disease (in adults) · prostatic hypertrophy (risk of acute retention) (in adults) · rebound congestion

CAUTIONS, FURTHER INFORMATION

▸ Rebound congestion   Sympathomimetic drugs are of limited value in the treatment of nasal congestion because they can, following prolonged use (more than 7 days), give rise to a rebound congestion (rhinitis medicamentosa) on withdrawal, due to a secondary vasodilatation with a subsequent temporary increase in nasal congestion. This in turn tempts the further use of the decongestant, leading to a vicious cycle of events.

● **INTERACTIONS**   → Appendix 1: sympathomimetics, vasoconstrictor

● **SIDE-EFFECTS**   Cardiovascular effects · headache · hypersensitivity · nasal dryness · nausea · paraesthesia · visual impairment

SIDE-EFFECTS, FURTHER INFORMATION   Use of decongestants in infants and children under 6 years has been associated with agitated psychosis, ataxia, hallucinations, and even death—avoid.

● **PREGNANCY**   Manufacturer advises avoid.

● **BREAST FEEDING**   Manufacturer advises caution—no information available.

● **MEDICINAL FORMS**   There can be variation in the licensing of different medicines containing the same drug.

Spray

▸ Otrivine (GlaxoSmithKline Consumer Healthcare)
Xylometazoline hydrochloride 1 mg per 1 ml   Otrivine Congestion Relief 0.1% nasal spray | 10 ml [GSL] £3.05 DT = £2.18
Otrivine Adult Measured Dose Sinusitis spray | 10 ml [GSL] £2.62 DT = £2.18
Otrivine Allergy Relief 0.1% nasal spray | 10 ml [GSL] £2.62 DT = £2.18
Otrivine Adult nasal spray | 10 ml [GSL] £2.18 DT = £2.18
Otrivine Adult Metered Dose 0.1% nasal spray | 10 ml [GSL] £2.62 DT = £2.18

▸ Sudafed Congestion Relief (McNeil Products Ltd)
Xylometazoline hydrochloride 1 mg per 1 ml   Sudafed Congestion Relief 0.1% nasal spray | 10 ml [GSL] £3.65 DT = £2.18

▸ Sudafed Non-Drowsy Decongestant (xylometazoline) (McNeil Products Ltd)
Xylometazoline hydrochloride 1 mg per 1 ml   Sudafed Blocked Nose 0.1% spray | 15 ml [GSL] £2.91

▸ Sudafed Sinus-Ease (McNeil Products Ltd)
Xylometazoline hydrochloride 1 mg per 1 ml   Sudafed Sinus-Ease 0.1% nasal spray | 15 ml [GSL] £2.96

Nasal drops

▸ Otrivine (GlaxoSmithKline Consumer Healthcare)
Xylometazoline hydrochloride 500 microgram per 1 ml   Otrivine Child nasal drops | 10 ml [P] £1.91 DT = £1.91
Xylometazoline hydrochloride 1 mg per 1 ml   Otrivine Adult 0.1% nasal drops | 10 ml [GSL] £2.18 DT = £2.18

---

2   Nasal infection

Sinusitis (acute)   31-Oct-2017

Description of condition

Sinusitis is an inflammation of the mucosal lining of the paranasal sinuses. Acute sinusitis (rhinosinusitis) is a self-limiting condition usually triggered by a viral upper-respiratory tract infection such as the 'common cold'. Occasionally, acute sinusitis may become complicated by a bacterial infection (see *Antibacterial therapy for acute sinusitis* in Nose infections, antibacterial therapy p. 537).

Patients with acute sinusitis usually present with symptoms of nasal blockage or congestion, nasal discharge, dental or facial pain or pressure, and reduction or loss of the sense of smell.

Symptoms usually improve within 2 to 3 weeks without requiring treatment.

Rarely, acute sinusitis may lead to orbital, intracranial or skeletal complications (e.g. periorbital cellulitis, symptoms or signs of meningitis).

Aims of treatment

Treatment is aimed at managing symptoms including pain, fever, and nasal congestion as well as treatment of bacterial infection if present.

Treatment

[EvGr] Patients presenting with symptoms for around 10 *days or less*, should be given advice about the usual duration of acute sinusitis, self-care of pain or fever with paracetamol p. 464 or ibuprofen p. 1186, and when to seek medical help. Patients should be reassured that antibiotics are usually not required. Some patients may try nasal saline or nasal decongestants, however there is limited evidence to show they help to relieve nasal congestion.

Patients presenting with symptoms for around 10 *days or more* with no improvement could be considered for treatment with a high-dose nasal corticosteroid, such as mometasone furoate p. 1251 [unlicensed use] or fluticasone p. 1251 [unlicensed use] for 14 days. Supply of a back-up antibiotic prescription could be considered and used if symptoms do not improve within 7 days, or if they worsen rapidly or significantly.

If the patient is systemically very unwell, has signs and symptoms of a more serious illness or condition, or is at high-risk of complications, an immediate antibiotic should be given. ⟨A⟩(see *Antibacterial therapy for acute sinusitis* in Nose infections, antibacterial therapy p. 537).

[EvGr] Patients presenting with symptoms of acute sinusitis associated with a severe systemic infection or with orbital or intracranial complications should be referred to hospital. ⟨A⟩

Useful Resources

Sinusitis (acute): antimicrobial prescribing. National Institute for Health and Care Excellence. NICE guideline 79. October 2017.
www.nice.org.uk/guidance/ng79

ANTIBACTERIALS ⟩ AMINOGLYCOSIDES

Chlorhexidine with neomycin

- **INDICATIONS AND DOSE**
Eradication of nasal carriage of staphylococci
  ‣ BY INTRANASAL ADMINISTRATION
  ‣ Child: Apply 4 times a day for 10 days
  ‣ Adult: Apply 4 times a day for 10 days
Preventing nasal carriage of staphylococci
  ‣ BY INTRANASAL ADMINISTRATION
  ‣ Child: Apply twice daily
  ‣ Adult: Apply twice daily

- MEDICINAL FORMS There can be variation in the licensing of different medicines containing the same drug.
Cream
  EXCIPIENTS: May contain Arachis (peanut) oil, cetostearyl alcohol (including cetyl and stearyl alcohol)
  ‣ Naseptin (Alliance Pharmaceuticals Ltd)
    Chlorhexidine hydrochloride 1 mg per 1 gram, Neomycin sulfate 5 mg per 1 gram Naseptin nasal cream | 15 gram [PoM] £1.99 DT = £1.99

ANTIBACTERIALS ⟩ OTHER

Mupirocin

18-May-2020

- **INDICATIONS AND DOSE**
BACTROBAN NASAL ®
For eradication of nasal carriage of staphylococci, including meticillin-resistant *Staphylococcus aureus* (MRSA)
  ‣ BY INTRANASAL ADMINISTRATION
  ‣ Child: Apply 2–3 times a day for 5 days; a sample should be taken 2 days after treatment to confirm eradication. Course may be repeated once if sample positive (and throat not colonised), dose to be applied to the inner surface of each nostril
  ‣ Adult: Apply 2–3 times a day for 5 days; a sample should be taken 2 days after treatment to confirm eradication. Course may be repeated once if sample positive (and throat not colonised), dose to be applied to the inner surface of each nostril

- SIDE-EFFECTS
  ‣ **Common or very common** Skin reactions
  ‣ **Uncommon** Nasal mucosal disorder

- PREGNANCY Manufacturer advises avoid unless potential benefit outweighs risk—no information available.
- BREAST FEEDING No information available.
- RENAL IMPAIRMENT Manufacturer advises caution when mupirocin ointment used in moderate or severe impairment because it contains macrogols (polyethylene glycol).

- MEDICINAL FORMS There can be variation in the licensing of different medicines containing the same drug.
Nasal ointment
  ‣ Bactroban (GlaxoSmithKline UK Ltd)
    Mupirocin (as Mupirocin calcium) 20 mg per 1 gram Bactroban 2% nasal ointment | 3 gram [PoM] £4.24 DT = £4.24

CORTICOSTEROIDS ⟩ CORTICOSTEROID COMBINATIONS WITH ANTI-INFECTIVES

Betamethasone with neomycin

18-Nov-2020

The properties listed below are those particular to the combination only. For the properties of the components please consider, betamethasone p. 1250, neomycin sulfate p. 546.

- **INDICATIONS AND DOSE**
Nasal infection
  ‣ BY INTRANASAL ADMINISTRATION USING NASAL DROPS
  ‣ Child: Apply 2–3 drops 2–3 times a day, to be applied into each nostril
  ‣ Adult: Apply 2–3 drops 2–3 times a day, to be applied into each nostril

- INTERACTIONS → Appendix 1: corticosteroids · neomycin
- LESS SUITABLE FOR PRESCRIBING Betamethasone with neomycin nasal-drops are less suitable for prescribing; there is no evidence that topical anti-infective nasal preparations have any therapeutic value in rhinitis or sinusitis.

- MEDICINAL FORMS There can be variation in the licensing of different medicines containing the same drug.
Ear/eye/nose drops solution
  EXCIPIENTS: May contain Benzalkonium chloride, disodium edetate
  ‣ Betnesol-N (RPH Pharmaceuticals AB)
    Betamethasone (as Betamethasone sodium phosphate) 1 mg per 1 ml, Neomycin sulfate 5 mg per 1 ml Betnesol-N ear/eye/nose drops | 10 ml [PoM] £2.39 DT = £2.39

3 Nasal inflammation, nasal polyps and rhinitis

Other drugs used for Nasal inflammation, nasal polyps and rhinitis Desloratadine, p. 295 · Fexofenadine hydrochloride, p. 296 · Ketotifen, p. 301 · Rupatadine, p. 298 · Sodium cromoglicate, p. 286

ANTIHISTAMINES

Azelastine hydrochloride

11-May-2020

- **INDICATIONS AND DOSE**
Allergic rhinitis
  ‣ BY INTRANASAL ADMINISTRATION
  ‣ Child 6–17 years: 1 spray twice daily, to be administered into each nostril
  ‣ Adult: 1 spray twice daily, to be administered into each nostril

DOSE EQUIVALENCE AND CONVERSION
  ‣ 1 spray equivalent to 140 micrograms.

- INTERACTIONS → Appendix 1: antihistamines, non-sedating
- SIDE-EFFECTS
  ‣ **Common or very common** Taste bitter (if applied incorrectly)
  ‣ **Uncommon** Epistaxis · nasal complaints

- MEDICINAL FORMS There can be variation in the licensing of different medicines containing the same drug.

Spray
▸ Rhinolast (Mylan)
  Azelastine hydrochloride 140 microgram per 1 actuation Rhinolast 140micrograms/dose nasal spray | 22 ml [PoM] £10.50 DT = £10.50

Combinations available: *Fluticasone with azelastine,* p. 1251

ANTIMUSCARINICS

⟋ 261

Ipratropium bromide
20-Jul-2020

- INDICATIONS AND DOSE

Rhinorrhoea associated with allergic and non-allergic rhinitis
▸ BY INTRANASAL ADMINISTRATION
▸ Child 12-17 years: 2 sprays 2–3 times a day, dose to be sprayed into each nostril
▸ Adult: 2 sprays 2–3 times a day, dose to be sprayed into each nostril

DOSE EQUIVALENCE AND CONVERSION
▸ 1 metered spray of nasal spray = 21 micrograms.

- CAUTIONS Avoid spraying near eyes · bladder outflow obstruction · cystic fibrosis · prostatic hyperplasia (in adults) · susceptibility to angle-closure glaucoma
- INTERACTIONS → Appendix 1: ipratropium
- SIDE-EFFECTS
▸ **Common or very common** Epistaxis · gastrointestinal motility disorder · headache · nasal complaints · throat complaints
▸ **Uncommon** Corneal oedema · eye disorders · eye pain · nausea · respiratory disorders · stomatitis · vision disorders
▸ **Rare or very rare** Palpitations
- ALLERGY AND CROSS-SENSITIVITY Contra-indicated in patients with hypersensitivity to atropine or its derivatives.
- PREGNANCY Manufacturer advises only use if potential benefit outweighs the risk.
- BREAST FEEDING No information available—manufacturer advises only use if potential benefit outweighs risk.
- PATIENT AND CARER ADVICE Patients or carers should be counselled on appropriate administration technique and warned against accidental contact with the eye (due to risk of ocular complications).
  Driving and skilled tasks Manufacturer advises patients and carers should be counselled on the effects on driving and performance of skilled tasks—increased risk of dizziness and vision disorders.

- MEDICINAL FORMS There can be variation in the licensing of different medicines containing the same drug.

Spray
EXCIPIENTS: May contain Benzalkonium chloride, disodium edetate
▸ Rinatec (Sanofi)
  Ipratropium bromide 21 microgram per 1 dose Rinatec 21micrograms/dose nasal spray | 180 dose [PoM] £6.54 DT = £6.54

CORTICOSTEROIDS

Corticosteroids (intranasal)

> IMPORTANT SAFETY INFORMATION
> MHRA/CHM ADVICE: CORTICOSTEROIDS: RARE RISK OF CENTRAL SEROUS CHORIORETINOPATHY WITH LOCAL AS WELL AS SYSTEMIC ADMINISTRATION (AUGUST 2017)
> Central serous chorioretinopathy is a retinal disorder that has been linked to the systemic use of corticosteroids. Recently, it has also been reported after local administration of corticosteroids via inhaled and

intranasal, epidural, intra-articular, topical dermal, and periocular routes. The MHRA recommends that patients should be advised to report any blurred vision or other visual disturbances with corticosteroid treatment given by any route; consider referral to an ophthalmologist for evaluation of possible causes if a patient presents with vision problems.

NHS IMPROVEMENT PATIENT SAFETY ALERT: STEROID EMERGENCY CARD TO SUPPORT EARLY RECOGNITION AND TREATMENT OF ADRENAL CRISIS IN ADULTS (AUGUST 2020)
A patient-held **Steroid Emergency Card** has been developed for patients with adrenal insufficiency and steroid dependence who are at risk of adrenal crisis. It aims to support healthcare staff with the early recognition of patients at risk of adrenal crisis and the emergency treatment of adrenal crisis. All eligible patients should be issued a Steroid Emergency Card. Providers that treat patients with acute physical illness or trauma, or who may require emergency treatment, elective surgery, or other invasive procedures, should establish processes to check for risk of adrenal crisis and confirm if the patient has a Steroid Emergency Card.

- CAUTIONS Avoid after nasal surgery (until healing has occurred) · avoid in pulmonary tuberculosis · avoid in the presence of untreated nasal infections · patients transferred from systemic corticosteroids may experience exacerbation of some symptoms
  CAUTIONS, FURTHER INFORMATION
▸ Systemic absorption Systemic absorption may follow nasal administration particularly if high doses are used or if treatment is prolonged; therefore also consider the cautions and side-effects of systemic corticosteroids. The risk of systemic effects may be greater with nasal drops than with nasal sprays; drops are administered incorrectly more often than sprays.
- SIDE-EFFECTS
▸ **Common or very common** Altered smell sensation · epistaxis · headache · nasal complaints · taste altered · throat irritation
▸ **Rare or very rare** Glaucoma · nasal septum perforation (more common following nasal surgery) · vision blurred
  SIDE-EFFECTS, FURTHER INFORMATION Systemic absorption may follow nasal administration particularly if high doses are used or if treatment is prolonged. Therefore also consider the side-effects of systemic corticosteroids.
- MONITORING REQUIREMENTS
▸ In children The height of children receiving prolonged treatment with nasal corticosteroids should be monitored; if growth is slowed, referral to a paediatrician should be considered.

⟋ above

Beclometasone dipropionate
25-Sep-2020

(Beclomethasone dipropionate)

- INDICATIONS AND DOSE

Prophylaxis and treatment of allergic and vasomotor rhinitis
▸ BY INTRANASAL ADMINISTRATION
▸ Child 6-17 years: 100 micrograms twice daily, dose to be administered into each nostril, reduced to 50 micrograms twice daily, dose to be administered into each nostril, dose to be reduced when symptoms controlled; maximum 400 micrograms per day
▸ Adult: 100 micrograms twice daily, dose to be administered into each nostril, reduced to 50 micrograms twice daily, dose to be administered into each nostril, dose to be reduced when symptoms controlled; maximum 400 micrograms per day

12

Ear, nose and oropharynx

- INTERACTIONS → Appendix 1: corticosteroids
- EXCEPTIONS TO LEGAL CATEGORY
▸ In adults Preparations of beclometasone dipropionate can be sold to the public for nasal administration as a nasal spray if supplied for the prevention and treatment of allergic rhinitis in adults over 18 years subject to max. single dose of 100 micrograms per nostril, max. daily dose of 200 micrograms per nostril for max. 3 months, and a pack size of 20 mg.

- MEDICINAL FORMS There can be variation in the licensing of different medicines containing the same drug.
Spray
EXCIPIENTS: May contain Benzalkonium chloride, polysorbates
▸ Beclometasone dipropionate (Non-proprietary)
Beclometasone dipropionate 50 microgram per 1 dose Beclometasone 50micrograms/dose nasal spray | 200 dose [PoM] 🅂 DT = £3.04
▸ Beconase (GlaxoSmithKline UK Ltd, Omega Pharma Ltd)
Beclometasone dipropionate 50 microgram per 1 dose Beconase Aqueous 50micrograms/dose nasal spray | 200 dose [PoM] £2.63 DT = £3.04
▸ Nasobec (Teva UK Ltd)
Beclometasone dipropionate 50 microgram per 1 dose Nasobec Aqueous 50micrograms/dose nasal spray | 200 dose [PoM] £3.06 DT = £3.04

Betamethasone

07-Dec-2020 ℉ 1249

- DRUG ACTION Betamethasone has very high glucocorticoid activity and insignificant mineralocorticoid activity.

- INDICATIONS AND DOSE
BETNESOL ®

Non-infected inflammatory conditions of nose
▸ BY INTRANASAL ADMINISTRATION
▸ Adult: Apply 2–3 drops 2–3 times a day, dose to be applied into each nostril

VISTAMETHASONE ®

Non-infected inflammatory conditions of nose
▸ BY INTRANASAL ADMINISTRATION
▸ Adult: Apply 2–3 drops twice daily, dose to be applied into each nostril

- INTERACTIONS → Appendix 1: corticosteroids

- MEDICINAL FORMS There can be variation in the licensing of different medicines containing the same drug.
Ear/eye/nose drops solution
EXCIPIENTS: May contain Benzalkonium chloride, disodium edetate
▸ Betnesol (RPH Pharmaceuticals AB)
Betamethasone sodium phosphate 1 mg per 1 ml Betnesol 0.1% eye/ear/nose drops | 10 ml [PoM] £2.32 DT = £2.32
▸ Vistamethasone (Martindale Pharmaceuticals Ltd)
Betamethasone sodium phosphate 1 mg per 1 ml Vistamethasone 0.1% ear/eye/nose drops | 5 ml [PoM] £1.02 | 10 ml [PoM] £1.16 DT = £2.32

Budesonide

12-Nov-2020 ℉ 1249

- DRUG ACTION Budesonide is a glucocorticoid, which exerts significant local anti-inflammatory effects.

- INDICATIONS AND DOSE
Allergic rhinitis | Nasal polyps
▸ BY INTRANASAL ADMINISTRATION
▸ Child 6–17 years: 128 micrograms once daily, dose to be administered into each nostril in the morning, alternatively 64 micrograms twice daily, dose to be administered to each nostril, reduce dose when control achieved
▸ Adult: 128 micrograms once daily, dose to be administered into each nostril in the morning,

alternatively 64 micrograms twice daily, dose to be administered to each nostril, reduce dose when control achieved

Prophylaxis and treatment of allergic and vasomotor rhinitis
▸ BY INTRANASAL ADMINISTRATION
▸ Child 12–17 years: Initially 200 micrograms once daily, dose to be administered into each nostril in the morning, alternatively initially 100 micrograms twice daily, dose to be administered to each nostril; reduced to 100 micrograms once daily, dose to be administered into each nostril, dose can be reduced when control achieved
▸ Adult: Initially 200 micrograms once daily, dose to be administered into each nostril in the morning, alternatively initially 100 micrograms twice daily, dose to be administered to each nostril; reduced to 100 micrograms once daily, dose to be administered into each nostril, dose can be reduced when control achieved

Nasal polyps
▸ BY INTRANASAL ADMINISTRATION
▸ Child 12–17 years: 100 micrograms twice daily for up to 3 months, dose to be administered into each nostril
▸ Adult: 100 micrograms twice daily for up to 3 months, dose to be administered into each nostril

RHINOCORT AQUA ®

Rhinitis
▸ BY INTRANASAL ADMINISTRATION
▸ Adult: 128 micrograms once daily, dose to be administered into each nostril in the morning, alternatively 64 micrograms twice daily, dose to be administered into each nostril; reduced to 64 micrograms once daily when control achieved. Use for maximum 3 months, doses to be administered into each nostril

Nasal polyps
▸ BY INTRANASAL ADMINISTRATION
▸ Adult: 64 micrograms twice daily for up to 3 months, dose to be administered into each nostril

- INTERACTIONS → Appendix 1: corticosteroids
- SIDE-EFFECTS
▸ Rare or very rare Adrenal suppression
- EXCEPTIONS TO LEGAL CATEGORY
▸ In adults Preparations of budesonide can be sold to the public for nasal administration as a nasal spray if supplied for the prevention and treatment of seasonal allergic rhinitis in adults over 18 years subject to max. single dose of 200 micrograms per nostril, max. daily dose of 200 micrograms per nostril for max. period of 3 months, and a pack size of 10 mg.

- MEDICINAL FORMS There can be variation in the licensing of different medicines containing the same drug.
Spray
EXCIPIENTS: May contain Disodium edetate, polysorbates, potassium sorbate
▸ Budesonide (Non-proprietary)
Budesonide 64 microgram per 1 dose Budesonide 64micrograms/dose nasal spray | 120 dose [PoM] £5.79 DT = £5.25
Budesonide 100 microgram per 1 dose Budeflam Aquanase 100micrograms/dose nasal spray | 150 dose [PoM] 🅂
▸ Rhinocort (McNeil Products Ltd)
Budesonide 64 microgram per 1 dose Rhinocort Aqua 64 nasal spray | 120 dose [PoM] £3.77 DT = £5.25

Fluticasone

F 1249

25-Sep-2020

● **INDICATIONS AND DOSE**

Prophylaxis and treatment of allergic rhinitis and perennial rhinitis

▸ BY INTRANASAL ADMINISTRATION USING NASAL SPRAY

▸ Child 4–11 years: 50 micrograms once daily, to be administered into each nostril preferably in the morning, increased if necessary to 50 micrograms twice daily

▸ Child 12–17 years: 100 micrograms once daily, to be administered into each nostril preferably in the morning, increased if necessary to 100 micrograms twice daily; reduced to 50 micrograms once daily, dose to be administered into each nostril, dose to be reduced when control achieved

▸ Adult: 100 micrograms once daily, to be administered into each nostril preferably in the morning, increased if necessary to 100 micrograms twice daily; reduced to 50 micrograms once daily, dose to be administered into each nostril, dose to be reduced when control achieved

Nasal polyps

▸ BY INTRANASAL ADMINISTRATION USING NASAL DROPS

▸ Child 16–17 years: 200 micrograms 1–2 times a day, to be administered into each nostril, alternative treatment should be considered if no improvement after 4–6 weeks, (200 micrograms is equivalent to approximately 6 drops)

▸ Adult: 200 micrograms 1–2 times a day, to be administered into each nostril, alternative treatment should be considered if no improvement after 4–6 weeks, (200 micrograms is equivalent to approximately 6 drops)

AVAMYS ® SPRAY

Prophylaxis and treatment of allergic rhinitis

▸ BY INTRANASAL ADMINISTRATION

▸ Child 6–11 years: 27.5 micrograms once daily, dose to be sprayed into each nostril, then increased if necessary to 55 micrograms once daily, dose to be sprayed into each nostril, reduced to 27.5 micrograms once daily, to be sprayed into each nostril, dose to be reduced once control achieved; use minimum effective dose

▸ Child 12–17 years: 55 micrograms once daily, dose to be sprayed into each nostril, reduced to 27.5 micrograms once daily, to be sprayed into each nostril, dose to be reduced once control achieved; use minimum effective dose

▸ Adult: 55 micrograms once daily, dose to be sprayed into each nostril, reduced to 27.5 micrograms once daily, to be sprayed into each nostril, dose to be reduced once control achieved; use minimum effective dose

DOSE EQUIVALENCE AND CONVERSION

▸ For *Avamys* ® *spray*: 1 spray equivalent to 27.5 micrograms.

● INTERACTIONS → Appendix 1: corticosteroids

● SIDE-EFFECTS Adrenal suppression

SIDE-EFFECTS, FURTHER INFORMATION Nasal ulceration occurs commonly with nasal preparations containing fluticasone furoate.

● EXCEPTIONS TO LEGAL CATEGORY

▸ With intranasal use in adults Preparations of fluticasone propionate can be sold to the public for nasal administration (other than by pressurised nasal spray) if supplied for the prevention and treatment of allergic rhinitis in adults over 18 years, subject to max. single dose of 100 micrograms per nostril, max. daily dose of 200 micrograms per nostril for max. 3 months, and a pack size of 3 mg.

● MEDICINAL FORMS There can be variation in the licensing of different medicines containing the same drug.

Spray

EXCIPIENTS: May contain Benzalkonium chloride, disodium edetate, polysorbates

▸ Avamys (GlaxoSmithKline UK Ltd)
  Fluticasone furoate 27.5 microgram per 1 dose Avamys 27.5micrograms/dose nasal spray | 120 dose [PoM] £6.44 DT = £6.44

▸ Flixonase (GlaxoSmithKline Consumer Healthcare, GlaxoSmithKline UK Ltd)
  Fluticasone propionate 50 microgram per 1 dose Flixonase 50micrograms/dose aqueous nasal spray | 150 dose [PoM] £11.01 DT = £7.97

▸ Nasofan (Teva UK Ltd)
  Fluticasone propionate 50 microgram per 1 dose Nasofan 50micrograms/dose aqueous nasal spray | 150 dose [PoM] £8.04 DT = £7.97

Nasal drops

EXCIPIENTS: May contain Polysorbates

▸ Flixonase (GlaxoSmithKline UK Ltd)
  Fluticasone propionate 400 microgram Flixonase Nasule 400microgram/unit dose nasal drops | 28 unit dose [PoM] £12.99 DT = £12.99

Fluticasone with azelastine

The properties listed below are those particular to the combination only. For the properties of the components please consider, fluticasone above, azelastine hydrochloride p. 1248.

● **INDICATIONS AND DOSE**

Moderate to severe seasonal and perennial allergic rhinitis, if monotherapy with antihistamine or corticosteroid is inadequate

▸ BY INTRANASAL ADMINISTRATION

▸ Child 12–17 years: 1 spray twice daily, dose to be administered into each nostril

▸ Adult: 1 spray twice daily, dose to be administered into each nostril

● INTERACTIONS → Appendix 1: antihistamines, non-sedating · corticosteroids

● MEDICINAL FORMS There can be variation in the licensing of different medicines containing the same drug.

Spray

EXCIPIENTS: May contain Benzalkonium chloride, polysorbates

▸ Dymista (Mylan)
  Fluticasone propionate 50 microgram per 1 actuation, Azelastine hydrochloride 137 microgram per 1 actuation Dymista 137micrograms/dose / 50micrograms/dose nasal spray | 120 dose [PoM] £14.80 DT = £14.80

Mometasone furoate

F 1249

10-Nov-2020

● **INDICATIONS AND DOSE**

Prophylaxis and treatment of seasonal allergic or perennial rhinitis

▸ BY INTRANASAL ADMINISTRATION

▸ Child 3–11 years: 50 micrograms daily, dose to be sprayed into each nostril

▸ Child 12–17 years: 100 micrograms daily, increased if necessary up to 200 micrograms daily, dose to be sprayed into each nostril; reduced to 50 micrograms daily, dose to be reduced when control achieved, dose to be sprayed into each nostril

▸ Adult: 100 micrograms daily, increased if necessary up to 200 micrograms daily, dose to be sprayed into each nostril; reduced to 50 micrograms daily, dose to be reduced when control achieved, dose to be sprayed into each nostril

continued →

Ear, nose and oropharynx

Nasal polyps

▶ BY INTRANASAL ADMINISTRATION

▶ **Adult:** Initially 100 micrograms daily for 5–6 weeks, dose to be sprayed into each nostril, then increased if necessary to 100 micrograms twice daily, dose to be sprayed into each nostril, consider alternative treatment if no improvement after further 5–6 weeks, reduce to the lowest effective dose when control achieved

● INTERACTIONS → Appendix 1: corticosteroids

● SIDE-EFFECTS

SIDE-EFFECTS, FURTHER INFORMATION Nasal ulceration occurs commonly with preparations containing mometasone furoate.

● MEDICINAL FORMS There can be variation in the licensing of different medicines containing the same drug.

Spray
EXCIPIENTS: May contain Benzalkonium chloride, polysorbates
▶ Mometasone furoate (Non-proprietary)
Mometasone furoate 50 microgram per 1 dose Mometasone 50micrograms/dose nasal spray | 140 dose [PoM] £6.23 DT = £5.02
▶ Nasonex (Merck Sharp & Dohme Ltd)
Mometasone furoate 50 microgram per 1 dose Nasonex 50micrograms/dose nasal spray | 140 dose [PoM] £7.68 DT = £5.02

⌐ 1249

Triamcinolone acetonide

25-Sep-2020

● DRUG ACTION Triamcinolone exerts predominantly glucocorticoid effects with minimal mineralcorticoid effect.

● **INDICATIONS AND DOSE**

Prophylaxis and treatment of allergic rhinitis
▶ BY INTRANASAL ADMINISTRATION

▶ **Child 6–11 years:** 55 micrograms once daily, dose to be sprayed into each nostril, increased if necessary to 110 micrograms once daily, dose to be sprayed into each nostril; reduced to 55 micrograms once daily, dose to be sprayed into each nostril, reduce dose when control achieved; maximum duration of treatment 3 months

▶ **Child 12–17 years:** 110 micrograms once daily, dose to be sprayed into each nostril, reduced to 55 micrograms once daily, dose to be sprayed into each nostril, reduce dose when control achieved

▶ **Adult:** 110 micrograms once daily, dose to be sprayed into each nostril, reduced to 55 micrograms once daily, dose to be sprayed into each nostril, reduce dose when control achieved

● INTERACTIONS → Appendix 1: corticosteroids

● EXCEPTIONS TO LEGAL CATEGORY

▶ In adults Preparations of triamcinolone acetonide can be sold to the public for nasal administration as a non-pressurised nasal spray if supplied for the symptomatic treatment of seasonal allergic rhinitis in adults over 18 years, subject to maximum daily dose of 110 micrograms per nostril for maximum 3 months, and a pack size of 3.575 mg.

● MEDICINAL FORMS There can be variation in the licensing of different medicines containing the same drug.

Spray
EXCIPIENTS: May contain Benzalkonium chloride, disodium edetate, polysorbates
▶ Nasacort (Sanofi)
Triamcinolone acetonide 55 microgram per 1 dose Nasacort 55micrograms/dose nasal spray | 120 dose [PoM] £7.39 DT = £7.39

Oropharynx

1 Dry mouth

Dry mouth

14-Dec-2020

Overview

Dry mouth (xerostomia) resulting from reduced saliva secretion may be caused by drugs such as antimuscarinics, antihistamines, tricyclic antidepressants, and some diuretics. It can also be caused by irradiation of the head and neck region, dehydration, anxiety, or Sjögren's syndrome. Patients with dry mouth may be at greater risk of developing dental caries, periodontal disease, and oral infections (particularly candidiasis).

[EvGr] Underlying causes of dry mouth such as dehydration, anxiety, infection, or drugs causing dry mouth should be managed if appropriate. Dry mouth may be relieved in many patients by simple measures that stimulate salivation such as frequent sips of cold unsweetened drinks, or sucking pieces of ice or sugar-free fruit pastilles, or chewing sugar-free gum.

An artificial saliva substitute can be considered if simple stimulatory measures are inadequate. ⟨A⟩ The acidic pH of some artificial saliva products may be inappropriate for some patients as it may damage the enamel of natural teeth. Artificial saliva products below are available in oral lozenges, oral gel, oral spray, and pastille forms.

Pilocarpine tablets p. 1254 are licensed for the treatment of xerostomia following irradiation for head and neck cancer, and dry mouth and dry eyes (xerophthalmia) in Sjögren's syndrome. [EvGr] They may take up to 3 months to be effective; treatment should be withdrawn if there is no response within this time. ⟨A⟩

LUBRICANTS

Artificial saliva products

● ARTIFICIAL SALIVA PRODUCTS
AS SALIVA ORTHANA® LOZENGES
Mucin 65 mg, xylitol 59 mg, in a sorbitol basis, pH neutral

● **INDICATIONS AND DOSE**

Dry mouth as a result of having (or having undergone) radiotherapy (ACBS) | Dry mouth as a result of sicca syndrome (ACBS)
▶ BY MOUTH
▶ **Adult:** 1 lozenge as required, allow to dissolve slowly in the mouth

● PRESCRIBING AND DISPENSING INFORMATION *AS Saliva Orthana*® lozenges do not contain fluoride.

AS Saliva Orthana lozenges (CCMed Ltd)
30 lozenge(ACBS) · NHS indicative price = £3.04 · Drug Tariff (Part VIIIA Category C) price = £3.04

AS SALIVA ORTHANA® SPRAY
Gastric mucin (porcine) 3.5%, xylitol 2%, sodium fluoride 4.2 mg/litre, with preservatives and flavouring agents, pH neutral.

● **INDICATIONS AND DOSE**

Symptomatic treatment of dry mouth
▶ BY MOUTH
▶ **Adult:** Apply 2–3 sprays as required, spray onto oral and pharyngeal mucosa

● PROFESSION SPECIFIC INFORMATION

Dental practitioners' formulary
AS Saliva Orthana ® Oral Spray may be prescribed.

AS Saliva Orthana spray (CCMed Ltd)
50 ml · NHS indicative price = £4.92 · Drug Tariff (Part IXa)

BIOXTRA ® GEL
Lactoperoxidase, lactoferrin, lysozyme, whey colostrum, xylitol and other ingredients.

● INDICATIONS AND DOSE

Dry mouth as a result of having (or having undergone) radiotherapy | Dry mouth as a result of sicca syndrome
▶ BY MOUTH
▹ Adult: Apply as required, apply to oral mucosa

● PROFESSION SPECIFIC INFORMATION

Dental practitioners' formulary
BioXtra ® Gel may be prescribed.

BioXtra Dry Mouth oral gel (R.I.S. Products Ltd)
40 ml · NHS indicative price = £3.98 · Drug Tariff (Part IXa)

BIOTENE ORALBALANCE ®
Lactoperoxidase, lactoferrin, lysozyme, glucose oxidase, xylitol in a gel basis

● INDICATIONS AND DOSE

Symptomatic treatment of dry mouth
▶ BY MOUTH
▹ Adult: Apply as required, apply to gums and tongue

● PATIENT AND CARER ADVICE Avoid use with toothpastes containing detergents (including foaming agents).

● PROFESSION SPECIFIC INFORMATION

Dental practitioners' formulary
Biotene Oralbalance ® Saliva Replacement Gel may be prescribed as Artificial Saliva Gel.

Biotene Oralbalance dry mouth saliva replacement gel
(GlaxoSmithKline Consumer Healthcare) Glucose oxidase 12000 unit, Lactoferrin 12 mg, Lactoperoxidase 12000 unit, Muramidase 12 mg 50 gram · NHS indicative price = £4.46 · Drug Tariff (Part IXa)

GLANDOSANE ®
Carmellose sodium 500 mg, sorbitol 1.5 g, potassium chloride 60 mg, sodium chloride 42.2 mg, magnesium chloride 2.6 mg, calcium chloride 7.3 mg, and dipotassium hydrogen phosphate 17.1 mg/50 g, pH 5.75.

● INDICATIONS AND DOSE

Dry mouth as a result of having (or having undergone) radiotherapy (ACBS) | Dry mouth as a result of sicca syndrome (ACBS)
▶ BY MOUTH
▹ Adult: Apply as required, spray onto oral and pharyngeal mucosa

● PROFESSION SPECIFIC INFORMATION

Dental practitioners' formulary
Glandosane ® Aerosol Spray may be prescribed.

Glandosane synthetic saliva spray lemon (Fresenius Kabi Ltd)
50 ml · NHS indicative price = £5.68 · Drug Tariff (Part IXa)

Glandosane synthetic saliva spray natural (Fresenius Kabi Ltd)
50 ml · NHS indicative price = £5.68 · Drug Tariff (Part IXa)

Glandosane synthetic saliva spray peppermint (Fresenius Kabi Ltd) 50 ml · NHS indicative price = £5.68 · Drug Tariff (Part IXa)

ORALIEVE MOISTURISING MOUTH SPRAY
Aqua, glycerin, xylitol, poloxamer 407, sodium benzoate, monosodium phosphate, xanthan gum, aroma, disodium phosphate, benzoic acid, whey protein, lactoferrin, lactoperoxidase, potassium thiocyanate, glucose oxidase, SLS free, alcohol free, pH 5.8

● INDICATIONS AND DOSE

Dry mouth
▶ BY MOUTH
▹ Adult: 1 spray as required, on the inside of each cheek, gums and tongue

Oralieve moisturising mouth spray (Oralieve UK)
50 ml · NHS indicative price = £4.95 · Drug Tariff (Part IXa)

ORALIEVE GEL

● INDICATIONS AND DOSE

Symptomatic treatment of dry mouth
▶ BY MOUTH
▹ Adult: Apply as required, particularly at night, to oral mucosa

● PRESCRIBING AND DISPENSING INFORMATION Contains traces of milk protein and egg white protein.

Oralieve moisturising mouth gel (Oralieve UK)
50 ml · NHS indicative price = £2.96 · Drug Tariff (Part IXa)

SST ®
Sugar-free, citric acid, malic acid and other ingredients in a sorbitol base.

● INDICATIONS AND DOSE

Symptomatic treatment of dry mouth in patients with impaired salivary gland function and patent salivary ducts
▶ BY MOUTH
▹ Adult: 1 tablet as required, allow tablet to dissolve slowly in the mouth

● PROFESSION SPECIFIC INFORMATION

Dental practitioners' formulary
May be prescribed as Saliva Stimulating Tablets.

SST saliva stimulating tablets (Sinclair IS Pharma Plc)
100 tablet · NHS indicative price = £4.86 · Drug Tariff (Part IXa)

SALIVEZE ®
Carmellose sodium (sodium carboxymethylcellulose), calcium chloride, magnesium chloride, potassium chloride, sodium chloride, and dibasic sodium phosphate, pH neutral

● INDICATIONS AND DOSE

Dry mouth as a result of having (or having undergone) radiotherapy (ACBS) | Dry mouth as a result of sicca syndrome (ACBS)
▶ BY MOUTH
▹ Adult: Apply 1 spray as required, spray onto oral mucosa

● PROFESSION SPECIFIC INFORMATION

Dental practitioners' formulary
Saliveze ® Oral Spray may be prescribed.

Saliveze mouth spray (Wyvern Medical Ltd)
50 ml · NHS indicative price = £3.50 · Drug Tariff (Part IXa)

SALIVIX ®
Sugar-free, reddish-amber, acacia, malic acid and other ingredients.

● INDICATIONS AND DOSE

Symptomatic treatment of dry mouth
▶ BY MOUTH USING PASTILLES
▹ Adult: 1 unit as required, suck pastille

● PROFESSION SPECIFIC INFORMATION

Dental practitioners' formulary
Salivix ® Pastilles may be prescribed as Artificial Saliva Pastilles.

12

Ear, nose and oropharynx

Salivix pastilles (Galen Ltd)
50 pastille · NHS indicative price = £3.59 · Drug Tariff (Part IXa)

XEROTIN ®
Sugar-free, water, sorbitol, carmellose
(carboxymethylcellulose), potassium chloride, sodium
chloride, potassium phosphate, magnesium chloride,
calcium chloride and other ingredients, pH neutral.

● INDICATIONS AND DOSE
Symptomatic treatment of dry mouth
▸ BY MOUTH
▸ Adult: 1 spray as required

● PROFESSION SPECIFIC INFORMATION
Dental practitioners' formulary
Xerotin ® Oral Spray may be prescribed as Artificial Saliva
Oral Spray.

Xerotin spray (SePharm UK Ltd)
100 ml · NHS indicative price = £6.86 · Drug Tariff (Part IXa)

PARASYMPATHOMIMETICS

| Pilocarpine   31-Oct-2019

● INDICATIONS AND DOSE
Xerostomia following irradiation for head and neck cancer
▸ BY MOUTH
▸ Adult: 5 mg 3 times a day for 4 weeks, then increased if
tolerated to up to 30 mg daily in divided doses if
required, dose to be taken with or immediately after
meals (last dose always with evening meal), maximum
therapeutic effect normally within 4–8 weeks;
discontinue if no improvement after 2–3 months

Dry mouth and dry eyes in Sjögren's syndrome
▸ BY MOUTH
▸ Adult: 5 mg 4 times a day; increased if tolerated to up
to 30 mg daily in divided doses if required, dose to be
taken with meals and at bedtime, discontinue if no
improvement after 2–3 months

● CONTRA-INDICATIONS Acute iritis · uncontrolled asthma
(increased bronchial secretions and increased airways
resistance) · uncontrolled cardiorenal disease ·
uncontrolled chronic obstructive pulmonary disease
(increased bronchial secretions and increased airways
resistance)

● CAUTIONS Asthma (avoid if uncontrolled) · biliary-tract
disease · cardiovascular disease (avoid if uncontrolled) ·
cholelithiasis · chronic obstructive pulmonary disease
(avoid if uncontrolled) · cognitive disturbances · maintain
adequate fluid intake to avoid dehydration associated with
excessive sweating · peptic ulceration · psychiatric
disturbances · risk of increased renal colic · risk of
increased urethral smooth muscle tone · susceptibility to
angle-closure glaucoma

● INTERACTIONS → Appendix 1: pilocarpine

● SIDE-EFFECTS
▸ **Common or very common** Asthenia · conjunctivitis ·
constipation · diarrhoea · dizziness · excessive tearing · eye
pain · flushing · gastrointestinal discomfort · headache ·
hyperhidrosis · hypersalivation · hypersensitivity ·
hypertension · increased risk of infection · nausea ·
palpitations · skin reactions · urinary disorders · vision
disorders · vomiting
▸ **Uncommon** Gastrointestinal disorders
▸ **Frequency not known** Affective disorder · agitation ·
arrhythmias · atrioventricular block · chills · confusion ·
hallucination · hypotension · memory loss · psychiatric
disorder · respiratory distress · shock · tremor

● PREGNANCY Avoid—smooth muscle stimulant; toxicity in
animal studies.

● BREAST FEEDING Manufacturer advises avoid—present in
milk in *animal* studies.

● HEPATIC IMPAIRMENT Manufacturer advises caution in
moderate to severe cirrhosis.
Dose adjustments Manufacturer advises initial dose
reduction in moderate to severe cirrhosis.

● RENAL IMPAIRMENT Manufacturer advises caution with
tablets.

● PATIENT AND CARER ADVICE
Driving and skilled tasks Blurred vision may affect
performance of skilled tasks (e.g. driving) particularly at
night or in reduced lighting.

● MEDICINAL FORMS There can be variation in the licensing of
different medicines containing the same drug. Forms available
from special-order manufacturers include: oral solution
Tablet
CAUTIONARY AND ADVISORY LABELS 21, 27
▸ Salagen (Norgine Pharmaceuticals Ltd)
Pilocarpine hydrochloride 5 mg Salagen 5mg tablets |
84 tablet [PoM] £41.14 DT = £41.14

2   Oral hygiene

Mouthwashes and other preparations for oropharyngeal use
01-Sep-2020

Lozenges and sprays

[EvGr] Lozenges containing either a local anaesthetic, an
antiseptic, or a non-steroidal anti-inflammatory drug may be
trialled but may only lead to a small reduction in pain.
However, there is no evidence that non-medicated lozenges
and local anaesthetic sprays have a beneficial action on their
own in treating sore throat. [A]

Mouthwashes, gargles, and dentifrices

Expert sources advise that a saline mouthwash may be used
for cleaning or freshening the mouth and can be prepared by
dissolving half a teaspoonful of salt in a glassful of warm
water.
[EvGr] Mouthwashes containing an oxidising agent, such as
hydrogen peroxide p. 1255, may be useful in the treatment of
acute ulcerative gingivitis whilst awaiting to be seen by a
dentist. [A]
Chlorhexidine p. 1255 can be used as a mouthwash, spray,
or gel and is licensed for the management of gingivitis and
maintenance of oral hygiene, particularly where there is a
painful periodontal condition or if the patient is unable to
adequately brush their teeth (e.g. following dental
procedures or due to disability). It is also licensed for the
management of denture stomatitis, aphthous ulcers, oral
candidiasis, and following post-periodontal treatment to
promote healing. Chlorhexidine mouthwash should not be
used for the prevention of endocarditis in patients
undergoing dental procedures.
Chlorhexidine is an effective antiseptic which has the
advantage of inhibiting plaque formation on the teeth but
there is limited evidence to demonstrate efficacy in
preventing dental caries. Public Health England advise to use
other treatments for preventing dental caries, such as
fluoride-based products.
Chlorhexidine is incompatible with anionic agents present
in some toothpastes; it has therefore been suggested to wait
30 minutes between using these two preparations.

ANTISEPTICS AND DISINFECTANTS

Chlorhexidine

01-Sep-2020

● **INDICATIONS AND DOSE**

Oral hygiene and plaque inhibition | Oral candidiasis | Gingivitis | Management of aphthous ulcers

▸ BY MOUTH USING MOUTHWASH

▸ Child: Rinse or gargle 10 mL twice daily (rinse or gargle for about 1 minute)

▸ Adult: Rinse or gargle 10 mL twice daily (rinse or gargle for about 1 minute)

Denture stomatitis

▸ MOUTHWASH

▸ Adult: Cleanse and soak dentures in mouthwash solution for 15 minutes twice daily

Oral hygiene and plaque inhibition and gingivitis

▸ BY MOUTH USING DENTAL GEL

▸ Child: Apply 1–2 times a day, to be brushed on the teeth

▸ Adult: Apply 1–2 times a day, to be brushed on the teeth

Oral candidiasis | Management of aphthous ulcers

▸ BY MOUTH USING DENTAL GEL

▸ Child: Apply 1–2 times a day, to affected areas

▸ Adult: Apply 1–2 times a day, to affected areas

Oral hygiene and plaque inhibition | Oral candidiasis | Gingivitis | Management of aphthous ulcers

▸ BY MOUTH USING OROMUCOSAL SPRAY

▸ Child: Apply up to 12 sprays twice daily as required, to be applied tooth, gingival, or ulcer surfaces

▸ Adult: Apply up to 12 sprays twice daily as required, to be applied tooth, gingival, or ulcer surfaces

Bladder irrigation and catheter patency solutions

▸ BY INTRAVESICAL INSTILLATION

▸ Adult: (consult product literature)

● UNLICENSED USE *Corsodyl* ® not licensed for use in children under 12 years (unless on the advice of a healthcare professional).

● SIDE-EFFECTS

▸ **Common or very common**

▸ With oromucosal use Dry mouth · hypersensitivity · oral disorders · taste altered · tongue discolouration · tooth discolouration

SIDE-EFFECTS, FURTHER INFORMATION If desquamation occurs with mucosal irritation, discontinue treatment.

● PATIENT AND CARER ADVICE

▸ With oral (topical) use Chlorhexidine gluconate may be incompatible with some ingredients in toothpaste; rinse the mouth thoroughly with water between using toothpaste and chlorhexidine-containing product.

● PROFESSION SPECIFIC INFORMATION

Dental practitioners' formulary

Corsodyl ® dental gel may be prescribed as Chlorhexidine Gluconate Gel; *Corsodyl* ® mouthwash may be prescribed as Chlorhexidine Mouthwash; *Corsodyl* ® oral spray may be prescribed as Chlorhexidine Oral Spray.

● MEDICINAL FORMS There can be variation in the licensing of different medicines containing the same drug.

Dental gel

▸ Corsodyl (GlaxoSmithKline Consumer Healthcare)
Chlorhexidine gluconate 10 mg per 1 gram Corsodyl 1% dental gel sugar-free | 50 gram P £2.23 DT = £2.23

Irrigation

▸ Chlorhexidine (Non-proprietary)
Chlorhexidine acetate 200 microgram per 1 ml Chlorhexidine acetate 0.02% catheter maintenance solution | 100 ml P ⊠ DT = £2.70

▸ Uro-Tainer (chlorhexidine) (B.Braun Medical Ltd)
Chlorhexidine acetate 200 microgram per 1 ml Uro-Tainer chlorhexidine 1:5000 catheter maintenance solution | 100 ml P £2.70 DT = £2.70

Mouthwash

▸ Chlorhexidine (Non-proprietary)
Chlorhexidine gluconate 2 mg per 1 ml Chlorhexidine gluconate 0.2% mouthwash aniseed | 300 ml GSL £2.09 DT = £3.10
Chlorhexidine gluconate 0.2% mouthwash natural | 300 ml GSL £4.18 DT = £3.10
Chlorhexidine gluconate 0.2% mouthwash plain | 300 ml GSL £3.10 DT = £3.10
Chlorhexidine gluconate 0.2% mouthwash peppermint | 300 ml GSL £4.18 DT = £3.10
Chlorhexidine gluconate 0.2% mouthwash original | 300 ml GSL £4.18 DT = £3.10

▸ Corsodyl (GlaxoSmithKline Consumer Healthcare)
Chlorhexidine gluconate 2 mg per 1 ml Corsodyl Mint 0.2% mouthwash | 300 ml GSL £2.99 DT = £3.10 | 600 ml GSL £4.50
Corsodyl 0.2% mouthwash aniseed | 300 ml GSL £2.99 DT = £3.10
Corsodyl 0.2% mouthwash alcohol free | 300 ml GSL £3.57 DT = £3.10

▸ Curasept (Curaprox (UK) Ltd)
Chlorhexidine gluconate 2 mg per 1 ml Curasept 0.2% oral rinse | 200 ml ⊠

Irrigation solution

▸ Chlorhexidine (Non-proprietary)
Chlorhexidine acetate 200 microgram per 1 ml Chlorhexidine acetate 0.02% irrigation solution 1litre bottles | 1 bottle P ⊠
Chlorhexidine acetate 500 microgram per 1 ml Chlorhexidine acetate 0.05% irrigation solution 1litre bottles | 1 bottle P ⊠

Hexetidine

06-Aug-2018

● **INDICATIONS AND DOSE**

Oral hygiene

▸ BY MOUTH USING MOUTHWASH

▸ Child 12-17 years: Rinse or gargle 15 mL 2–3 times a day, to be used undiluted

▸ Adult: Rinse or gargle 15 mL 2–3 times a day, to be used undiluted

● SIDE-EFFECTS

▸ **Rare or very rare** Anaesthesia · taste altered

▸ **Frequency not known** Cough · dry mouth · dysphagia · dyspnoea · nausea · salivary gland enlargement · vomiting

● MEDICINAL FORMS There can be variation in the licensing of different medicines containing the same drug.

Mouthwash

▸ Oraldene (McNeil Products Ltd)
Hexetidine 1 mg per 1 ml Oraldene 0.1% mouthwash peppermint sugar-free | 200 ml GSL £2.92 DT = £2.92

Hydrogen peroxide

03-Mar-2020

● DRUG ACTION Hydrogen peroxide is an oxidising agent.

● **INDICATIONS AND DOSE**

Oral hygiene (with hydrogen peroxide 6%)

▸ BY MOUTH USING MOUTHWASH

▸ Child: Rinse or gargle 15 mL 2–3 times a day for 2–3 minutes, to be diluted in half a tumblerful of warm water

▸ Adult: Rinse or gargle 15 mL 2–3 times a day for 2–3 minutes, to be diluted in half a tumblerful of warm water

PEROXYL ®

Oral hygiene

▸ BY MOUTH USING MOUTHWASH

▸ Child 6-17 years: Rinse or gargle 10 mL 3 times a day for about 1 minute, for maximum 7 days, to be used after meals and at bedtime continued →

12

Ear, nose and oropharynx

> Adult: Rinse or gargle 10 mL up to 4 times a day for about 1 minute, to be used after meals and at bedtime

● PRESCRIBING AND DISPENSING INFORMATION When prepared extemporaneously, the BP states Hydrogen Peroxide Mouthwash, BP consists of hydrogen peroxide 6% solution (= approx. 20 volume) BP.

● HANDLING AND STORAGE Hydrogen peroxide bleaches fabric.

● PROFESSION SPECIFIC INFORMATION
Dental practitioners' formulary
Hydrogen Peroxide Mouthwash may be prescribed.

● MEDICINAL FORMS There can be variation in the licensing of different medicines containing the same drug.
Mouthwash
> Peroxyl (Colgate-Palmolive (UK) Ltd)
Hydrogen peroxide 15 mg per 1 ml Peroxyl 1.5% mouthwash sugar-free | 300 ml [GSL] £2.94 DT = £2.94

Sodium bicarbonate with sodium chloride

● INDICATIONS AND DOSE
Oral hygiene
▸ BY MOUTH USING MOUTHWASH
> Adult: (consult product literature)

● DIRECTIONS FOR ADMINISTRATION For mouthwash, extemporaneous preparations should be prepared according to the following formula: sodium chloride 1.5 g, sodium bicarbonate 1 g, concentrated peppermint emulsion 2.5 mL, double-strength chloroform water 50 mL, water to 100 mL. To be diluted with an equal volume of warm water prior to administration.

● PRESCRIBING AND DISPENSING INFORMATION Flavours of mouthwash may include peppermint.

● PROFESSION SPECIFIC INFORMATION
Dental practitioners' formulary
Compound sodium chloride mouthwash may be prescribed.

● MEDICINAL FORMS Forms available from special-order manufacturers include: mouthwash

---

Sodium chloride

07-Oct-2020

● INDICATIONS AND DOSE
Oral hygiene
▸ BY MOUTH USING MOUTHWASH
> Child: Rinse or gargle as required
> Adult: Rinse or gargle as required

● DIRECTIONS FOR ADMINISTRATION Extemporaneous mouthwash preparations should be prepared according to the following formula: sodium chloride 1.5 g, sodium bicarbonate 1 g, concentrated peppermint emulsion 2.5 mL, double-strength chloroform water 50 mL, water to 100 mL. To be diluted with an equal volume of warm water.

● PRESCRIBING AND DISPENSING INFORMATION No mouthwash preparations available—when prepared extemporaneously, the BP states Sodium Chloride Mouthwash, Compound, BP consists of sodium bicarbonate 1%, sodium chloride 1.5% in a suitable vehicle with peppermint flavour.
▸ In children The RCPCH and NPPG recommend that, when a liquid special of sodium chloride is required, the following strength is used: 5 mmol/mL.

● PROFESSION SPECIFIC INFORMATION
Dental practitioners' formulary
Compound Sodium Chloride Mouthwash may be prescribed.

● MEDICINAL FORMS No licensed medicines listed.

2.1 Dental caries

Fluoride

24-Apr-2020

Overview

Fluoride is a naturally occurring mineral found in water supplies in varying amounts and in some foods; it has beneficial topical effects on teeth. Public Health England advise that all adults and children brush their teeth with fluoridated toothpaste at least twice daily to help prevent tooth decay.

Individuals who are either particularly caries prone or medically compromised may be given additional protection. Public Health England recommends the daily use of a fluoride mouthwash in adults and children aged 7 years and over who are causing concern to their dentist (e.g. those with active caries, dry mouth, or special needs). They should be used at a different time to brushing to avoid removal of the beneficial effects of fluoride in toothpaste.

Fluoride varnish is also available and can be applied topically to both primary or permanent teeth. Public Health England recommends that all children aged 3 years and over have fluoride varnish applied (usually twice a year) regardless of their risk of caries. Application of fluoride varnish at least twice a year may also be considered in adults and children aged under 3 years who are causing concern to their dentist.

Useful resources

Delivering better oral health: an evidence-based toolkit for prevention. Public Health England. March 2017.
   www.gov.uk/government/publications/delivering-better-oral-health-an-evidence-based-toolkit-for-prevention

VITAMINS AND TRACE ELEMENTS

Sodium fluoride

25-Nov-2020

● INDICATIONS AND DOSE
Prophylaxis of dental caries for water content less than 300micrograms/litre (0.3 parts per million) of fluoride ion
▸ BY MOUTH USING TABLETS
> Child 6 months–2 years: 250 micrograms daily, doses expressed as fluoride ion (F⁻)
> Child 3–5 years: 500 micrograms daily, doses expressed as fluoride ion (F⁻)
> Child 6–17 years: 1 mg daily, doses expressed as fluoride ion (F⁻)
> Adult: 1 mg daily, doses expressed as fluoride ion (F⁻)

Prophylaxis of dental caries for water content between 300 and 700micrograms/litre (0.3–0.7 parts per million) of fluoride ion
▸ BY MOUTH USING TABLETS
> Child 3–5 years: 250 micrograms daily, doses expressed as fluoride ion (F⁻)
> Child 6–17 years: 500 micrograms daily, doses expressed as fluoride ion (F⁻)
> Adult: 500 micrograms daily, doses expressed as fluoride ion (F⁻)

Prophylaxis of dental caries
▸ BY MOUTH USING MOUTHWASH
▸ Adult: Rinse or gargle 5–10 mL daily
DOSE EQUIVALENCE AND CONVERSION
▸ Sodium fluoride 2.2 mg provides approx. 1 mg fluoride ion.

COLGATE DURAPHAT ® 2800PPM FLUORIDE TOOTHPASTE

Prophylaxis of dental caries
▸ BY MOUTH USING PASTE
▸ Child 10-17 years: Apply 1 centimetre twice daily, to be applied using a toothbrush
▸ Adult: Apply 1 centimetre twice daily, to be applied using a toothbrush

COLGATE DURAPHAT ® 5000PPM FLUORIDE TOOTHPASTE

Prophylaxis of dental caries
▸ BY MOUTH USING PASTE
▸ Child 16-17 years: Apply 2 centimetres 3 times a day, to be applied after meals using a toothbrush
▸ Adult: Apply 2 centimetres 3 times a day, to be applied after meals using a toothbrush

EN-DE-KAY ® FLUORINSE

Prophylaxis of dental caries
▸ BY MOUTH USING MOUTHWASH
▸ Adult: 5 drops daily, dilute 5 drops to 10 mL of water, alternatively 20 drops once weekly, dilute 20 drops to 10 mL

● SIDE-EFFECTS Dental fluorosis
● DIRECTIONS FOR ADMINISTRATION
▸ With oral use Manufacturer advises tablets should be sucked or dissolved in the mouth at a different time of day to tooth brushing.
▸ With oral (topical) use Manufacturer advises for mouthwash, rinse mouth for 1 minute and then spit out.
COLGATE DURAPHAT ® 5000PPM FLUORIDE TOOTHPASTE Manufacturer advises brush teeth for 3 minutes before spitting out.
COLGATE DURAPHAT ® 2800PPM FLUORIDE TOOTHPASTE Manufacturer advises brush teeth for 1 minute before spitting out.

● PRESCRIBING AND DISPENSING INFORMATION Flavours of oral tablet formulations may include orange.

● PATIENT AND CARER ADVICE
Mouthwash Avoid eating, drinking, or rinsing mouth for 15 minutes after use.
COLGATE DURAPHAT ® 5000PPM FLUORIDE TOOTHPASTE Patients or carers should be given advice on how to administer Sodium fluoride toothpaste.
COLGATE DURAPHAT ® 2800PPM FLUORIDE TOOTHPASTE Patients or carers should be given advice on how to administer sodium fluoride toothpaste.
Avoid drinking or rinsing mouth for 30 minutes after use.

● PROFESSION SPECIFIC INFORMATION

Dental practitioners' formulary
Tablets may be prescribed as Sodium Fluoride Tablets.
Oral drops may be prescribed as Sodium Fluoride Oral Drops.
Mouthwashes may be prescribed as Sodium Fluoride Mouthwash 0.05% or Sodium Fluoride Mouthwash 2%.

Dental information
Fluoride mouthwash, oral drops, tablets and toothpaste are prescribable on form FP10D (GP14 in Scotland, WP10D in Wales).
There are also arrangements for health authorities to supply fluoride tablets in the course of pre-school dental schemes, and they may also be supplied in school dental schemes.

Fluoride gels are not prescribable on form FP10D (GP14 in Scotland, WP10D in Wales).
COLGATE DURAPHAT ® 5000PPM FLUORIDE TOOTHPASTE **Dental practitioners' formulary**
May be prescribed as Sodium Fluoride Toothpaste 1.1%.
COLGATE DURAPHAT ® 2800PPM FLUORIDE TOOTHPASTE **Dental practitioners' formulary**
May be prescribed as Sodium Fluoride Toothpaste 0.619%.

● MEDICINAL FORMS There can be variation in the licensing of different medicines containing the same drug.

Tablet
▸ Endekay (Manx Healthcare Ltd)
Sodium fluoride 1.1 mg Endekay Fluotabs 3-6 Years 1.1mg tablets | 200 tablet [P] £2.38 DT = £2.38
Sodium fluoride 2.2 mg Endekay Fluotabs 6+ Years 2.2mg tablets | 200 tablet [P] £2.38 DT = £2.38

Paste
▸ Sodium fluoride (Non-proprietary)
Fluoride (as Sodium fluoride) 2.8 mg per 1 gram Sodium fluoride 0.619% dental paste sugar free sugar-free | 75 ml [PoM] £4.14 DT = £3.52
Fluoride (as Sodium fluoride) 5 mg per 1 gram Sodium fluoride 1.1% dental paste sugar free sugar-free | 51 gram [PoM] £8.28 DT = £6.91
▸ Colgate Duraphat (Colgate-Palmolive (UK) Ltd)
Fluoride (as Sodium fluoride) 2.8 mg per 1 gram Colgate Duraphat 2800ppm fluoride toothpaste sugar-free | 75 ml [PoM] £3.26 DT = £3.52
Fluoride (as Sodium fluoride) 5 mg per 1 gram Colgate Duraphat 5000ppm fluoride toothpaste sugar-free | 51 gram [PoM] £6.50 DT = £6.91

Chewable tablet
▸ Fluor-a-day (DHP Healthcare Ltd)
Sodium fluoride 1.1 mg Fluor-a-day 1.1mg chewable tablets sugar-free | 200 tablet [P] £3.38 DT = £3.38
Sodium fluoride 2.2 mg Fluor-a-day 2.2mg chewable tablets sugar-free | 200 tablet [P] £3.38 DT = £3.38

Mouthwash
▸ Sodium fluoride (Non-proprietary)
Sodium fluoride 500 microgram per 1 ml Sodium fluoride 0.05% mouthwash sugar free sugar-free | 250 ml [GSL] [N] DT = £1.51
▸ Colgate FluoriGard (Colgate-Palmolive (UK) Ltd)
Sodium fluoride 500 microgram per 1 ml Colgate FluoriGard 0.05% daily dental rinse alcohol free sugar-free | 400 ml £2.99
Colgate FluoriGard 0.05% daily dental rinse sugar-free | 400 ml [GSL] £2.99
▸ Endekay (Manx Healthcare Ltd)
Sodium fluoride 500 microgram per 1 ml Endekay 0.05% daily fluoride mouthrinse sugar-free | 250 ml [GSL] £1.51 DT = £1.51 sugar-free | 500 ml [GSL] £2.45

---

3   Oral ulceration and inflammation

Oral ulceration and inflammation
09-Dec-2020

Ulceration and inflammation
Ulceration of the oral mucosa is common and usually transient but may require treatment in some cases. Causes include mechanical trauma, infections, malignant lesions, inflammatory conditions, nutritional deficiencies (e.g. iron, folic acid, vitamin B12), immunodeficiency states, gastro-intestinal disease, and drug therapy (see also *Chemotherapy induced mucositis and myelosuppression* under Cytotoxic drugs p. 932).

Aphthous ulcers are often recurrent and are not associated with an underlying systemic disease; they are small, round or ovoid mouth ulcers with defined margins. Aphthous ulcers may be precipitated by triggers such as certain food and drinks, allergies, anxiety, or hormonal changes. It is important to consider and exclude any possible systemic disease; treatment may include correcting the underlying cause. Treatment aims to relieve pain, reduce ulcer duration, and reduce the frequency of recurrent episodes. Secondary bacterial infections may occur with mucosal ulceration; it can increase discomfort and delay healing.

EvGr Patients with an unexplained mouth ulcer of more than 3 weeks' duration should be referred urgently to a specialist to exclude oral cancer. Ⓐ

Treatment of aphthous ulcers

EvGr Advise patients to avoid known triggers for ulceration, such as oral trauma (e.g. biting during chewing, ill-fitting dentures) or certain food and drinks (e.g. coffee, gluten-containing products). If the ulcers are mild, infrequent, and do not interfere with daily activities (such as eating), treatment may not be required. Ⓐ

Corticosteroids

EvGr Topical corticosteroids are usually considered to be first-line treatment. Ⓐ Expert sources advise that hydrocortisone oromucosal tablets p. 1260, beclometasone dipropionate inhaler p. 1259 [unlicensed indication] sprayed onto the oral mucosa, and betamethasone soluble tablets p. 1260 [unlicensed indication] used as a mouthwash are suitable options.

EvGr A short course of systemic corticosteroids may be prescribed for patients with severe recurrent aphthous ulcers. Ⓐ

Other therapies

EvGr Other therapies that may be used alone or in combination with topical corticosteroids include topical anaesthetics (e.g. lidocaine hydrochloride below), topical analgesics/anti-inflammatory agents (e.g. benzydamine hydrochloride p. 1259), and topical antimicrobial agents (e.g. chlorhexidine mouthwash p. 1255). Ⓐ EvGr Doxycycline p. 1261 [unlicensed indication], rinsed in the mouth and expelled, may be considered for recurrent aphthous ulceration when other treatments are unsuccessful or unsuitable. Ⓔ

Expert sources advise that a saline (with or without sodium bicarbonate) mouthwash may soothe ulcers, help to maintain oral hygiene, and prevent secondary infection. Tepid water appears to be more soothing than cold or warm water.

Expert sources advise that local anaesthetics have a short duration of action; there is limited evidence for their use in the management of oral ulceration. Lidocaine hydrochloride 5% ointment or lozenges containing the local anaesthetic may be applied to the ulcer. Lidocaine hydrochloride 10% solution [unlicensed indication] as spray can be applied thinly to the ulcer using a cotton bud. When local anaesthetics are used in the mouth, care must be taken to avoid causing anaesthesia of the pharynx before meals, as this might lead to choking.

Benzydamine hydrochloride and flurbiprofen p. 1259 are non-steroidal anti-inflammatory drugs (NSAIDs). Benzydamine hydrochloride mouthwash and spray are licensed for the relief of painful inflammatory conditions associated with a variety of ulcerative conditions, as well as for discomfort of tonsillectomy and post-irradiation mucositis. Benzydamine hydrochloride mouthwash should generally be used undiluted; it can be diluted with an equal volume of water if a stinging sensation occurs. Flurbiprofen lozenges are licensed for the relief of sore throat.

Choline salicylate p. 1260 is a derivative of salicylic acid and has some analgesic properties. The dental gel is licensed for pain relief in mouth ulcers including ulcers due to dentures and orthodontic devices.

EvGr Consider offering or advising the use of a vitamin B12 supplement regardless of serum vitamin B12 levels. Ⓐ

ANAESTHETICS, LOCAL

Lidocaine hydrochloride

17-Aug-202

(Lignocaine hydrochloride)

● **INDICATIONS AND DOSE**

Dental practice
▶ BY BUCCAL ADMINISTRATION USING OINTMENT
▸ Adult: Rub gently into dry gum

Relief of pain in oral lesions
▶ TO THE LESION USING OINTMENT
▸ Adult: Apply as required, rub sparingly and gently on affected areas

XYLOCAINE ®

Bronchoscopy | Laryngoscopy | Oesophagoscopy | Endotracheal intubation
▶ TO MUCOUS MEMBRANES
▸ Adult: Up to 20 doses

Dental practice
▶ TO MUCOUS MEMBRANES
▸ Adult: 1–5 doses

Maxillary sinus puncture
▶ TO MUCOUS MEMBRANES
▸ Adult: 3 doses

Relief of pain in oral lesions
▶ TO THE LESION
▸ Adult: Apply thinly to the ulcer using a cotton bud

● UNLICENSED USE Spray not licensed for the relief of pain in oral lesions.

● CAUTIONS Avoid anaesthesia of the pharynx before meals—risk of choking · can damage plastic cuffs of endotracheal tubes

● INTERACTIONS → Appendix 1: antiarrhythmics

● ALLERGY AND CROSS-SENSITIVITY
▸ Hypersensitivity and cross-sensitivity Hypersensitivity reactions occur mainly with the ester-type local anaesthetics, such as tetracaine; reactions are less frequent with the amide types, such as articaine, bupivacaine, levobupivacaine, lidocaine, mepivacaine, prilocaine, and ropivacaine. Cross-sensitivity reactions may be avoided by using the alternative chemical type.

● PREGNANCY Crosses the placenta but not known to be harmful in *animal* studies—use if benefit outweighs risk. When used as a local anaesthetic, large doses can cause fetal bradycardia; if given during delivery can also cause neonatal respiratory depression, hypotonia, or bradycardia after paracervical or epidural block.

● BREAST FEEDING Present in milk but amount too small to be harmful.

● HEPATIC IMPAIRMENT Manufacturer advises caution (risk of increased exposure).

● RENAL IMPAIRMENT Possible accumulation of lidocaine and active metabolite; caution in severe impairment.

● PROFESSION SPECIFIC INFORMATION

Dental practitioners' formulary
Lidocaine ointment 5% may be prescribed. Spray may be prescribed as Lidocaine Spray 10%

XYLOCAINE ® **Dental practitioners' formulary**
May be prescribed as lidocaine spray 10%.

● MEDICINAL FORMS There can be variation in the licensing of different medicines containing the same drug. Forms available from special-order manufacturers include: ointment
Spray
▸ Xylocaine (Aspen Pharma Trading Ltd)
Lidocaine 10 mg per 1 actuation Xylocaine 10mg/dose spray sugar-free | 50 ml P £6.29 DT = £6.29

Ointment

▸ Lidocaine hydrochloride (Non-proprietary)
  Lidocaine hydrochloride 50 mg per 1 gram Lidocaine 5% ointment
  | 15 gram P £9.00 DT = £8.28

ANALGESICS ❭ NON-STEROIDAL ANTI-INFLAMMATORY DRUGS

Benzydamine hydrochloride
21-Aug-2020

● INDICATIONS AND DOSE

Painful inflammatory conditions of oropharynx

▸ TO THE LESION USING MOUTHWASH

▸ Child 13-17 years: Rinse or gargle 15 mL every
  1.5–3 hours as required usually for not more than
  7 days, dilute with an equal volume of water if stinging
  occurs

▸ Adult: Rinse or gargle 15 mL every 1.5–3 hours as
  required usually for not more than 7 days, dilute with
  an equal volume of water if stinging occurs

▸ TO THE LESION USING OROMUCOSAL SPRAY

▸ Child 1 month-5 years (body-weight 4-7 kg): 1 spray every
  1.5–3 hours, to be administered onto the affected area

▸ Child 1 month-5 years (body-weight 8-11 kg): 2 sprays
  every 1.5–3 hours, to be administered onto the affected
  area

▸ Child 1 month-5 years (body-weight 12-15 kg): 3 sprays
  every 1.5–3 hours, to be administered onto the affected
  area

▸ Child 1 month-5 years (body-weight 16 kg and above):
  4 sprays every 1.5–3 hours, to be administered onto the
  affected area

▸ Child 6-11 years: 4 sprays every 1.5–3 hours, to be
  administered onto affected area

▸ Child 12-17 years: 4–8 sprays every 1.5–3 hours, to be
  administered onto affected area

▸ Adult: 4–8 sprays every 1.5–3 hours, to be
  administered onto affected area

● INTERACTIONS → Appendix 1: NSAIDs

● SIDE-EFFECTS

▸ **Uncommon** Oral disorders

▸ **Rare or very rare** Photosensitivity reaction · respiratory
  disorders · skin reactions

▸ **Frequency not known** Angioedema

● PROFESSION SPECIFIC INFORMATION

Dental practitioners' formulary
Benzydamine Oromucosal Spray 0.15% may be prescribed.
Benzydamine mouthwash may be prescribed as
Benzydamine Mouthwash 0.15%.

● MEDICINAL FORMS There can be variation in the licensing of
different medicines containing the same drug.

Spray

▸ Benzydamine hydrochloride (Non-proprietary)
  Benzydamine hydrochloride 1.5 mg per 1 ml Benzydamine 0.15%
  oromucosal spray sugar free sugar-free | 30 ml P £4.24 DT = £2.70

▸ Difflam (Mylan)
  Benzydamine hydrochloride 1.5 mg per 1 ml Difflam 0.15% spray
  sugar-free | 30 ml P £4.24 DT = £2.70

Mouthwash

▸ Benzydamine hydrochloride (Non-proprietary)
  Benzydamine hydrochloride 1.5 mg per 1 ml Benzydamine 0.15%
  mouthwash sugar free sugar-free | 300 ml P £9.75 DT = £9.56

▸ Difflam (Mylan)
  Benzydamine hydrochloride 1.5 mg per 1 ml Difflam Oral Rinse
  0.15% solution sugar-free | 300 ml P £6.50 DT = £9.56
  Difflam 0.15% Sore Throat Rinse sugar-free | 200 ml P £4.64

Diclofenac
28-Aug-2018

● INDICATIONS AND DOSE

**Painful inflammatory conditions of the oral cavity and
throat and/or following dental treatment or dental
extraction**

▸ BY MOUTH USING MOUTHWASH

▸ Adult: Rinse or gargle 15 mL 2–3 times a day for 7 days,
  treatment may be extended to 6 weeks in mucositis
  caused by radiotherapy

● INTERACTIONS → Appendix 1: NSAIDs

● PREGNANCY Manufacturer advises avoid unless essential.

● BREAST FEEDING Manufacturer advises avoid unless
essential.

● DIRECTIONS FOR ADMINISTRATION Manufacturer advises
mouthwash may be diluted with a little water.

● MEDICINAL FORMS There can be variation in the licensing of
different medicines containing the same drug.

Mouthwash
EXCIPIENTS: May contain Sorbitol

▸ Diclofenac (Non-proprietary)
  Diclofenac.74 mg per 1 ml Diclofenac 0.74mg/ml mouthwash sugar
  free sugar-free | 200 ml PoM £12.95 DT = £12.95
  Diclofenac 0.074% mouthwash sugar free sugar-free | 200 ml PoM
  £12.95 DT = £12.95

Flurbiprofen
18-Nov-2020

● INDICATIONS AND DOSE

Relief of sore throat

▸ BY MOUTH USING LOZENGES

▸ Child 12-17 years: 1 lozenge every 3–6 hours for
  maximum 3 days, allow lozenge to dissolve slowly in
  the mouth; maximum 5 lozenges per day

▸ Adult: 1 lozenge every 3–6 hours for maximum 3 days,
  allow lozenge to dissolve slowly in the mouth;
  maximum 5 lozenges per day

● INTERACTIONS → Appendix 1: NSAIDs

● SIDE-EFFECTS Oral ulceration (move lozenge around
mouth) · taste altered

● ALLERGY AND CROSS-SENSITIVITY EvGr Contra-indicated
in patients with a history of hypersensitivity to aspirin or
any other NSAID—which includes those in whom attacks
of asthma, angioedema, urticaria or rhinitis have been
precipitated by aspirin or any other NSAID. ◈

● MEDICINAL FORMS There can be variation in the licensing of
different medicines containing the same drug.

Lozenge

▸ Strefen (Reckitt Benckiser Healthcare (UK) Ltd)
  Flurbiprofen 8.75 mg Strefen Honey and Lemon 8.75mg lozenges |
  16 lozenge P £3.42 DT = £3.42

CORTICOSTEROIDS

⯈ 711

Beclometasone dipropionate
25-Sep-2020

(Beclomethasone dipropionate)

● INDICATIONS AND DOSE

Management of oral ulceration

▸ TO THE LESION

▸ Adult: 50–100 micrograms twice daily, administered
  using an inhaler device

● UNLICENSED USE Use of inhaler is unlicensed for oral
ulceration.

● INTERACTIONS → Appendix 1: corticosteroids

12

Ear, nose and oropharynx

● MEDICINAL FORMS There can be variation in the licensing of different medicines containing the same drug. For preparations, see inhaled beclometasone, p. 273.

F 711

Betamethasone
07-Dec-2020

● DRUG ACTION Betamethasone has very high glucocorticoid activity and insignificant mineralocorticoid activity.

● **INDICATIONS AND DOSE**

Oral ulceration
▸ TO THE LESION USING SOLUBLE TABLETS
▸ Child 12-17 years: 500 micrograms 4 times a day, to be dissolved in 20 mL water and rinsed around the mouth; not to be swallowed
▸ Adult: 500 micrograms 4 times a day, to be dissolved in 20 mL water and rinsed around the mouth; not to be swallowed

● UNLICENSED USE
▸ In children Betamethasone soluble tablets not licensed for use as mouthwash or in oral ulceration.

● CONTRA-INDICATIONS Untreated local infection
● INTERACTIONS → Appendix 1: corticosteroids
● PATIENT AND CARER ADVICE Patient counselling is advised for betamethasone soluble tablets (administration).
● PROFESSION SPECIFIC INFORMATION
Dental practitioners' formulary
Betamethasone Soluble Tablets 500 micrograms may be prescribed.

● MEDICINAL FORMS There can be variation in the licensing of different medicines containing the same drug.
Soluble tablet
CAUTIONARY AND ADVISORY LABELS 10, 13, 21 (not for use as mouthwash for oral ulceration)
▸ Betamethasone (Non-proprietary)
Betamethasone (as Betamethasone sodium phosphate)
500 microgram Betamethasone 500microgram soluble tablets sugar free sugar-free | 100 tablet [PoM] £58.15 DT = £58.15

F 711

Hydrocortisone
23-Nov-2020

● DRUG ACTION Hydrocortisone has equal glucocorticoid and mineralocorticoid activity.

● **INDICATIONS AND DOSE**

Oral and perioral lesions
▸ TO THE LESION USING BUCCAL TABLET
▸ Child 1 month-11 years: Only on medical advice
▸ Child 12-17 years: 1 lozenge 4 times a day, allowed to dissolve slowly in the mouth in contact with the ulcer
▸ Adult: 1 lozenge 4 times a day, allowed to dissolve slowly in the mouth in contact with the ulcer

● UNLICENSED USE *Hydrocortisone mucoadhesive buccal tablets* licensed for use in children (under 12 years—on medical advice only).

> **IMPORTANT SAFETY INFORMATION**
>
> MHRA/CHM ADVICE: HYDROCORTISONE MUCO-ADHESIVE BUCCAL TABLETS: SHOULD NOT BE USED OFF-LABEL FOR ADRENAL INSUFFICIENCY IN CHILDREN DUE TO SERIOUS RISKS (DECEMBER 2018)
> The MHRA has received reports of off-label use of hydrocortisone muco-adhesive buccal tablets for adrenal insufficiency in children. Healthcare professionals are advised that:
> ● hydrocortisone muco-adhesive buccal tablets are indicated only for local use in the mouth for aphthous ulceration and should not be used to treat adrenal insufficiency;

● substitution of licensed oral hydrocortisone formulations with muco-adhesive buccal tablets can result in insufficient cortisol absorption and, in stress situations, life-threatening adrenal crisis;
● only hydrocortisone products licensed for adrenal replacement therapy should be used.

● CONTRA-INDICATIONS Untreated local infection
● INTERACTIONS → Appendix 1: corticosteroids
● PROFESSION SPECIFIC INFORMATION
Dental practitioners' formulary
Mucoadhesive buccal tablets may be prescribed as Hydrocortisone Oromucosal Tablets.

● MEDICINAL FORMS There can be variation in the licensing of different medicines containing the same drug.
Muco-adhesive buccal tablet
▸ Hydrocortisone (Non-proprietary)
Hydrocortisone (as Hydrocortisone sodium succinate)
2.5 mg Hydrocortisone 2.5mg muco-adhesive buccal tablets sugar free sugar-free | 20 tablet [P] £9.87 DT = £9.32

SALICYLIC ACID AND DERIVATIVES

Choline salicylate
23-Nov-2020

● **INDICATIONS AND DOSE**

Mild oral and perioral lesions
▸ TO THE LESION
▸ Child 16-17 years: Apply 0.5 inch, apply with gentle massage, not more often than every 3 hours
▸ Adult: Apply 0.5 inch, apply with gentle massage, not more often than every 3 hours

● CONTRA-INDICATIONS Children under 16 years
CONTRA-INDICATIONS, FURTHER INFORMATION
▸ Reye's syndrome The CHM has advised that topical oral pain relief products containing salicylate salts should not be used in children under 16 years, as a cautionary measure due to the theoretical risk of Reye's syndrome.

● CAUTIONS Frequent application, especially in children, may give rise to salicylate poisoning · not to be applied to dentures—leave at least 30 minutes before re-insertion of dentures (in adults)
● INTERACTIONS → Appendix 1: choline salicylate
● SIDE-EFFECTS Bronchospasm
● PRESCRIBING AND DISPENSING INFORMATION When prepared extemporaneously, the BP states Choline Salicylate Dental Gel, BP consists of choline salicylate 8.7% in a flavoured gel basis.
● PROFESSION SPECIFIC INFORMATION
Dental practitioners' formulary
Choline Salicylate Dental Gel may be prescribed.

● MEDICINAL FORMS There can be variation in the licensing of different medicines containing the same drug.
Oromucosal gel
▸ Bonjela (Reckitt Benckiser Healthcare (UK) Ltd)
Choline salicylate 87 mg per 1 gram Bonjela Cool Mint gel sugar-free | 15 gram [GSL] £3.55 DT = £2.91
Bonjela Original gel sugar-free | 15 gram [GSL] £2.91 DT = £2.91

Salicylic acid with rhubarb extract

23-Nov-2020

- **INDICATIONS AND DOSE**

Mild oral and perioral lesions

▸ TO THE LESION
  - ▸ Child 16–17 years: Apply 3–4 times a day maximum duration 7 days
  - ▸ Adult: Apply 3–4 times a day maximum duration 7 days

- CONTRA-INDICATIONS Children under 16 years

  CONTRA-INDICATIONS, FURTHER INFORMATION
  Reye's syndrome The CHM has advised that topical oral pain relief products containing salicylate salts should not be used in children under 16 years, as a cautionary measure due to the theoretical risk of Reye's syndrome.

- CAUTIONS Frequent application, especially in children, may give rise to salicylate poisoning · not to be applied to dentures—leave at least 30 minutes before re-insertion of dentures (in adults)

- SIDE-EFFECTS
- ▸ **Common or very common** Oral discolouration · tooth discolouration

- PATIENT AND CARER ADVICE May cause temporary discolouration of teeth and oral mucosa.

- MEDICINAL FORMS There can be variation in the licensing of different medicines containing the same drug.

  Paint
  EXCIPIENTS: May contain Ethanol
  - ▸ Pyralvex (Mylan)
    Salicylic acid 10 mg per 1 ml, Rhubarb extract 50 mg per 1 ml Pyralvex solution | 10 ml P £3.25

4   Oropharyngeal bacterial infections

Oropharyngeal infections, antibacterial therapy

Pericoronitis

Antibacterial required only in presence of systemic features of infection, or of trismus, or persistent swelling despite local treatment.

- Metronidazole p. 575, or *alternatively*, amoxicillin p. 582
- ▸ *Suggested duration of treatment* 3 days or until symptoms resolve.

Gingivitis (acute necrotising ulcerative)

Antibacterial required only if systemic features of infection.

- Metronidazole, or *alternatively*, amoxicillin
- ▸ *Suggested duration of treatment* 3 days or until symptoms resolve.

Abscess (periapical or periodontal)

Antibacterial required only in severe disease with cellulitis or if systemic features of infection.

- Amoxicillin, or *alternatively*, metronidazole
- ▸ *Suggested duration of treatment* 5 days.

Periodontitis

Antibacterial used as an adjunct to debridement in severe disease or disease unresponsive to local treatment alone.

- Metronidazole, or *alternatively in adults and children over 12 years*, doxycycline p. 601

Sore throat (acute)

Acute sore throat is usually triggered by a viral infection and is self-limiting. Symptoms can last for around 1 week, and most people will improve within this time without treatment with antibiotics, regardless of the cause.

EvGr Antibacterial therapy is required only in patients with severe systemic symptoms, signs and symptoms of a more serious illness or condition, or those at high risk of complications. Patients with severe systemic infection or severe suppurative complications such as peri-tonsillar abscess (quinsy), acute otitis media, acute sinusitis or cellulitis should be referred to hospital. Ⓐ

- Phenoxymethylpenicillin p. 581
- ▸ *Suggested duration of treatment* 5 to 10 days.
- If *penicillin-allergic*, clarithromycin p. 569 (*or* erythromycin p. 572)
- ▸ *Suggested duration of treatment* 5 days.

ANTIBACTERIALS ⟩ TETRACYCLINES AND RELATED DRUGS

F 600

Doxycycline

02-Sep-2020

- **INDICATIONS AND DOSE**

Treatment of recurrent aphthous ulceration

- ▸ BY MOUTH USING SOLUBLE TABLETS
  - ▸ Child 12–17 years: 100 mg 4 times a day usually for 3 days, dispersible tablet can be stirred into a small amount of water then rinsed around the mouth for 2–3 minutes, it should preferably not be swallowed
  - ▸ Adult: 100 mg 4 times a day usually for 3 days, dispersible tablet can be stirred into a small amount of water then rinsed around the mouth for 2–3 minutes, it should preferably not be swallowed

- UNLICENSED USE Doxycycline may be used as detailed below, although these situations are considered outside the scope of its licence:
  - recurrent aphthous ulceration.

- CAUTIONS Alcohol dependence

- INTERACTIONS → Appendix 1: tetracyclines

- SIDE-EFFECTS
- ▸ **Common or very common** Dyspnoea · hypotension · peripheral oedema · tachycardia
- ▸ **Uncommon** Gastrointestinal discomfort
- ▸ **Rare or very rare** Antibiotic associated colitis · anxiety · arthralgia · flushing · intracranial pressure increased with papilloedema · Jarisch-Herxheimer reaction · myalgia · photoonycholysis · severe cutaneous adverse reactions (SCARs) · skin hyperpigmentation (long term use) · tinnitus · vision disorders

- RENAL IMPAIRMENT Use with caution (avoid excessive doses).

- PATIENT AND CARER ADVICE Counselling on administration advised.
  Photosensitivity Patients should be advised to avoid exposure to sunlight or sun lamps.

- PROFESSION SPECIFIC INFORMATION
  Dental practitioners' formulary
  Dispersible tablets may be prescribed as Dispersible Doxycycline Tablets.

- MEDICINAL FORMS There can be variation in the licensing of different medicines containing the same drug.
  Dispersible tablet
  CAUTIONARY AND ADVISORY LABELS 6, 9, 11, 13
  - ▸ Vibramycin-D (Pfizer Ltd)
    Doxycycline (as Doxycycline monohydrate) 100 mg Vibramycin-D 100mg dispersible tablets sugar-free | 8 tablet PoM £4.91 DT = £4.91

5 Oropharyngeal fungal infections

Oropharyngeal fungal infections

Overview

Fungal infections of the mouth are usually caused by *Candida* spp. (candidiasis or candidosis). Different types of oropharyngeal candidiasis are managed as follows:

Thrush

Acute pseudomembranous candidiasis (thrush), is usually an acute infection but it may persist for months in patients receiving inhaled corticosteroids, cytotoxics or broad-spectrum antibacterials. Thrush also occurs in patients with serious systemic disease associated with reduced immunity such as leukaemia, other malignancies, and HIV infection. Any predisposing condition should be managed appropriately. When thrush is associated with corticosteroid inhalers, rinsing the mouth with water (or cleaning a child's teeth) immediately after using the inhaler may avoid the problem. Treatment with nystatin p. 1263 or miconazole below may be needed. Fluconazole p. 634 is effective for unresponsive infections or if a topical antifungal drug cannot be used or if the patient has dry mouth. Topical therapy may not be adequate in immunocompromised patients and an oral triazole antifungal is preferred.

Acute erythematous candidiasis

Acute erythematous (atrophic) candidiasis is a relatively uncommon condition associated with corticosteroid and broad-spectrum antibacterial use and with HIV disease. It is usually treated with fluconazole.

Denture stomatitis

Patients with denture stomatitis (chronic atrophic candidiasis), should cleanse their dentures thoroughly and leave them out as often as possible during the treatment period. To prevent recurrence of the problem, dentures should not normally be worn at night. New dentures may be required if these measures fail despite good compliance.

Miconazole oral gel can be applied to the fitting surface of the denture before insertion (for short periods only). Denture stomatitis is not always associated with candidiasis and other factors such as mechanical or chemical irritation, bacterial infection, or rarely allergy to the dental base material, may be the cause.

Chronic hyperplastic candidiasis

Chronic hyperplastic candidiasis (candidal leucoplakia) carries an increased risk of malignancy; biopsy is essential—this type of candidiasis may be associated with varying degrees of dysplasia, with oral cancer present in a high proportion of cases. Chronic hyperplastic candidiasis is treated with a systemic antifungal such as fluconazole to eliminate candidal overlay. Patients should avoid the use of tobacco.

Angular cheilitis

Angular cheilitis (angular stomatitis) is characterised by soreness, erythema and fissuring at the angles of the mouth. It is commonly associated with denture stomatitis but may represent a nutritional deficiency or it may be related to orofacial granulomatosis or HIV infection. Both yeasts (*Candida* spp.) and bacteria (*Staphylococcus aureus* and beta-haemolytic streptococci) are commonly involved as interacting, infective factors. A reduction in facial height related to ageing and tooth loss with maceration in the deep occlusive folds that may subsequently arise, predisposes to such infection. While the underlying cause is being identified and treated, it is often helpful to apply miconazole cream or fusidic acid ointment p. 608; if the angular cheilitis

is unresponsive to treatment, hydrocortisone with miconazole cream or ointment p. 1296 can be used.

Immunocompromised patients

See advice on prevention of fungal infections in *Immunocompromised patients* under Antifungals, systemic use p. 629.

Drugs used in oropharyngeal candidiasis

Nystatin is not absorbed from the gastro-intestinal tract and is applied locally (as a suspension) to the mouth for treating local fungal infections. Miconazole is applied locally (as an oral gel) in the mouth but it is absorbed to the extent that potential interactions need to be considered. Miconazole also has some activity against Gram-positive bacteria including streptococci and staphylococci. Fluconazole is given by mouth for infections that do not respond to topical therapy or when topical therapy cannot be used. It is reliably absorbed and effective. Itraconazole p. 636 can be used for fluconazole-resistant infections.

If candidal infection fails to respond to 1 to 2 weeks of treatment with antifungal drugs the patient should be sent for investigation to eliminate the possibility of underlying disease. Persistent infection may also be caused by reinfection from the genito-urinary or gastro-intestinal tract. Infection can be eliminated from these sources by appropriate anticandidal therapy; the patient's partner may also require treatment to prevent reinfection.

Antiseptic mouthwashes are used in the prevention of oral candidiasis in immunocompromised patients and in the treatment of denture stomatitis.

ANTIFUNGALS > IMIDAZOLE ANTIFUNGALS

Miconazole

24-Jul-2020

● **INDICATIONS AND DOSE**

Oral candidiasis

▸ BY MOUTH USING ORAL GEL

▸ Child 2–17 years: 2.5 mL 4 times a day treatment should be continued for at least 7 days after lesions have healed or symptoms have cleared, to be administered after meals, retain near oral lesions before swallowing (dental prostheses and orthodontic appliances should be removed at night and brushed with gel)

▸ Adult: 2.5 mL 4 times a day treatment should be continued for at least 7 days after lesions have healed or symptoms have cleared, to be administered after meals, retain near oral lesions before swallowing (dental prostheses and orthodontic appliances should be removed at night and brushed with gel)

Intestinal candidiasis

▸ BY MOUTH USING ORAL GEL

▸ Child 4 months–17 years: 5 mg/kg 4 times a day (max. per dose 250 mg) treatment should be continued for at least 7 days after lesions have healed or symptoms have cleared

▸ Adult: 5 mg/kg 4 times a day (max. per dose 250 mg) treatment should be continued for at least 7 days after lesions have healed or symptoms have cleared

Prevention and treatment of oral candidiasis (dose approved for use by community practitioner nurse prescribers)

▸ BY MOUTH USING ORAL GEL

▸ Child 4–23 months: 1.25 mL 4 times a day treatment should be continued for at least 7 days after lesions have healed or symptoms have cleared, to be smeared around the inside of the mouth after feeds

▸ Child 2–17 years: 2.5 mL 4 times a day treatment should be continued for at least 7 days after lesions have healed or symptoms have cleared, to be administered after meals, retain near oral lesions before swallowing (dental prostheses and orthodontic appliances should be removed at night and brushed with gel)

▸ Adult: 2.5 mL 4 times a day treatment should be continued for at least 7 days after lesions have healed or symptoms have cleared, to be administered after meals, retain near oral lesions before swallowing (dental prostheses and orthodontic appliances should be removed at night and brushed with gel)

UNLICENSED USE Not licensed for use in children under 4 months of age or during first 5–6 months of life of an infant born pre-term.

CONTRA-INDICATIONS Infants with impaired swallowing reflex

CAUTIONS Avoid in Acute porphyrias p. 1107

INTERACTIONS → Appendix 1: antifungals, azoles

SIDE-EFFECTS
Common or very common Skin reactions
Frequency not known Angioedema

PREGNANCY Manufacturer advises avoid if possible—toxicity at high doses in *animal* studies.

BREAST FEEDING Manufacturer advises caution—no information available.

HEPATIC IMPAIRMENT Manufacturer advises avoid.

DIRECTIONS FOR ADMINISTRATION Manufacturer advises oral gel should be held in mouth, after food.

PRESCRIBING AND DISPENSING INFORMATION Flavours of oral gel may include orange.

PATIENT AND CARER ADVICE Patients or carers should be given advice on how to administer miconazole oromucosal gel.

PROFESSION SPECIFIC INFORMATION
Dental practitioners' formulary
Miconazole Oromucosal Gel may be prescribed.

EXCEPTIONS TO LEGAL CATEGORY
15-g tube of oral gel can be sold to the public.

MEDICINAL FORMS There can be variation in the licensing of different medicines containing the same drug.

Oromucosal gel
CAUTIONARY AND ADVISORY LABELS 9
▸ Daktarin (Johnson & Johnson Ltd, Janssen-Cilag Ltd)
  Miconazole 20 mg per 1 gram Daktarin 20mg/g oromucosal gel sugar-free | 80 gram [PoM] £4.38 DT = £4.38

ANTIFUNGALS > POLYENE ANTIFUNGALS

Nystatin   05-May-2020

● INDICATIONS AND DOSE
Oral candidiasis
▸ BY MOUTH
▸ Child: 100 000 units 4 times a day usually for 7 days, and continued for 48 hours after lesions have resolved
▸ Adult: 100 000 units 4 times a day usually for 7 days, and continued for 48 hours after lesions have resolved

Oral and perioral fungal infections (dose approved for use by community practitioner nurse prescribers)
▸ BY MOUTH
▸ Neonate: 100 000 units 4 times a day usually for 7 days, and continued for 48 hours after lesions have resolved, to be given after feeds.

▸ Child: 100 000 units 4 times a day usually for 7 days, and continued for 48 hours after lesions have resolved
▸ Adult: 100 000 units 4 times a day usually for 7 days, and continued for 48 hours after lesions have resolved

● UNLICENSED USE Suspension not licensed for use in neonates for the treatment of candidiasis but the Department of Health has advised that a Community Practitioner Nurse Prescriber may prescribe nystatin oral

suspension for a neonate, in the doses provided in the BNF, provided that there is a clear diagnosis of oral thrush. The nurse prescriber must only prescribe within their own competence and must accept clinical and medicolegal responsibility for prescribing.

● SIDE-EFFECTS Abdominal distress · angioedema · diarrhoea · face oedema · nausea · sensitisation · skin reactions · Stevens-Johnson syndrome · vomiting

● PATIENT AND CARER ADVICE Counselling advised with oral suspension (use of pipette, hold in mouth, after food). Medicines for Children leaflet: Nystatin for Candida infection www.medicinesforchildren.org.uk/nystatin-candida-infection

● PROFESSION SPECIFIC INFORMATION
Dental practitioners' formulary
Nystatin Oral Suspension may be prescribed.

● MEDICINAL FORMS There can be variation in the licensing of different medicines containing the same drug. Forms available from special-order manufacturers include: tablet, capsule, oral suspension

Oral suspension
CAUTIONARY AND ADVISORY LABELS 9
EXCIPIENTS: May contain Ethanol
▸ Nystatin (Non-proprietary)
  Nystatin 100000 unit per 1 ml Nystatin 100,000units/ml oral suspension | 30 ml [PoM] £3.05 DT = £3.05

6 Oropharyngeal viral infections

Oropharyngeal viral infections

Management
Viral infections are the most common cause of a sore throat. They do not benefit from anti-infective treatment.

The management of primary herpetic gingivostomatitis is a soft diet, adequate fluid intake, and analgesics as required, including local use of benzydamine hydrochloride p. 1259. The use of chlorhexidine mouthwash p. 1255 will control plaque accumulation if toothbrushing is painful and will also help to control secondary infection in general.

In the case of severe herpetic stomatitis, a systemic antiviral such as aciclovir p. 672 is required. Valaciclovir p. 675 and famciclovir p. 674 are suitable alternatives for oral lesions associated with herpes zoster. Aciclovir and valaciclovir are also used for the prevention of frequently recurring herpes simplex lesions of the mouth, particularly when implicated in the initiation of erythema multiforme.

12

Ear, nose and oropharynx

Chapter 13
Skin

CONTENTS

Skin conditions, management

Vehicles

The British Association of Dermatologists list of preferred unlicensed dermatological preparations (specials) is available at www.bad.org.uk/specials.

Both vehicle and active ingredients are important in the treatment of skin conditions; the vehicle alone may have more than a mere placebo effect. The vehicle affects the degree of hydration of the skin, has a mild anti-inflammatory effect, and aids the penetration of active drug.

Applications are usually viscous solutions, emulsions, or suspensions for application to the skin (including the scalp) or nails.

Collodions are painted on the skin and allowed to dry to leave a flexible film over the site of application.

Creams are emulsions of oil and water and are generally well absorbed into the skin. They may contain an antimicrobial preservative unless the active ingredient or basis is intrinsically bactericidal and fungicidal. Generally, creams are cosmetically more acceptable than ointments because they are less greasy and easier to apply.

Gels consist of active ingredients in suitable hydrophilic or hydrophobic bases; they generally have a high water content. Gels are particularly suitable for application to the face and scalp.

Lotions have a cooling effect and may be preferred to ointments or creams for application over a hairy area. Lotions in alcoholic basis can sting if used on broken skin. *Shake lotions* (such as calamine lotion) contain insoluble powders which leave a deposit on the skin surface.

Ointments are greasy preparations which are normally anhydrous and insoluble in water, and are more occlusive than creams. They are particularly suitable for chronic, dry lesions. The most commonly used ointment bases consist of soft paraffin or a combination of soft, liquid, and hard paraffin. Some ointment bases have both *hydrophilic and lipophilic* properties; they may have occlusive properties on the skin surface, encourage hydration, and also be miscible with water; they often have a mild anti-inflammatory effect. *Water-soluble ointments* contain macrogols which are freely soluble in water and are therefore readily washed off; they

have a limited but useful role where ready removal is desirable.

Pastes are stiff preparations containing a high proportion of finely powdered solids such as zinc oxide and starch suspended in an ointment. They are used for circumscribed lesions such as those which occur in lichen simplex, chronic eczema, or psoriasis. They are less occlusive than ointments and can be used to protect inflamed, lichenified, or excoriated skin.

Dusting powders are used only rarely. They reduce friction between opposing skin surfaces. Dusting powders should not be applied to moist areas because they can cake and abrade the skin. Talc is a lubricant but it does not absorb moisture; it can cause respiratory irritation. Starch is less lubricant but absorbs water.

Dilution

The BP directs that creams and ointments should **not** normally be diluted but that should dilution be necessary care should be taken, in particular, to prevent microbial contamination. The appropriate diluent should be used and heating should be avoided during mixing; excessive dilution may affect the stability of some creams. Diluted creams should normally be used within 2 weeks of preparation.

Suitable quantities for prescribing

Suitable quantities of dermatological preparations to be prescribed for specific areas of the body		
Area of body	Creams and Ointments	Lotions
Face	15–30 g	100 ml
Both hands	25–50 g	200 ml
Scalp	50–100 g	200 ml
Both arms or both legs	100–200 g	200 ml
Trunk	400 g	500 ml
Groins and genitalia	15–25 g	100 ml

These amounts are usually suitable for an adult for twice daily application for 1 week. The recommendations do not apply to corticosteroid preparations. For suitable quantities of corticosteroid preparations, see relevant table.

Excipients and sensitisation

Excipients in topical products rarely cause problems. If a patch test indicates allergy to an excipient, products containing the substance should be avoided. The following excipients in topical preparations are associated, rarely, with sensitisation; the presence of these excipients is indicated in the entries for topical products.

- Beeswax
- Benzyl alcohol
- Butylated hydroxyanisole
  Butylated hydroxytoluene
- Cetostearyl alcohol (including cetyl and stearyl alcohol)
- Chlorocresol
- Edetic acid (EDTA)
- Ethylenediamine
- Fragrances
- Hydroxybenzoates (parabens)
  Imidurea
- Isopropyl palmitate
- N-(3-Chloroallyl)hexaminium chloride (quaternium 15)
- Polysorbates
- Propylene glycol
- Sodium metabisulfite
- Sorbic acid
- Wool fat and related substances including lanolin (purified versions of wool fat have reduced the problem)

1   Dry and scaling skin disorders

Emollient and barrier preparations

04-Sep-2020

Borderline substances

The preparations marked 'ACBS' are regarded as drugs when prescribed in accordance with the advice of the Advisory Committee on Borderline Substances for the clinical conditions listed. Prescriptions issued in accordance with this advice and endorsed 'ACBS' will normally not be investigated.

Emollients

Emollients soothe, smooth and hydrate the skin and are indicated for all dry or scaling disorders. Their effects are short lived and they should be applied frequently even after improvement occurs. They are useful in dry and eczematous disorders, and to a lesser extent in psoriasis. The choice of an appropriate emollient will depend on the severity of the condition, patient preference, and the site of application. Some ingredients rarely cause sensitisation and this should be suspected if an eczematous reaction occurs. The use of aqueous cream as a leave-on emollient may increase the risk of skin reactions, particularly in eczema.

Preparations such as **aqueous cream** and **emulsifying ointment** can be used as soap substitutes for hand washing and in the bath; the preparation is rubbed on the skin before rinsing off completely. The addition of a bath oil may also be helpful.

Urea is occasionally used with other topical agents such as corticosteroids to enhance penetration of the skin.

Emollient bath and shower preparations

Emollient bath additives should be added to bath water; hydration can be improved by soaking in the bath for 10–20 minutes. Some bath emollients can be applied to wet skin undiluted and rinsed off. In dry skin conditions soap should be avoided.

The quantities of bath additives recommended for adults are suitable for an adult-size bath. Proportionately less should be used for a child-size bath or a washbasin; recommended bath additive quantities for children reflect this.

MHRA/CHM advice (updated December 2018): Emollients: new information about risk of severe and fatal burns with paraffin-containing and paraffin-free emollients
Emollients are an important and effective treatment for chronic dry skin disorders and people should continue to use these products. However, healthcare professionals must ensure that patients and their carers understand the fire risk associated with the build-up of residue on clothing and bedding and can take action to minimise the risk. There is a fire risk with all paraffin-containing emollients, regardless of paraffin concentration, and it cannot be excluded with paraffin-free emollients. A similar risk may apply to products that are applied to the skin over large body areas, or in large volumes for repeated use for more than a few days.

Healthcare professionals should advise patients not to smoke or go near naked flames because clothing, bedding, dressings, and other fabrics that have been in contact with an emollient or emollient-treated skin can rapidly ignite. Washing these materials at high temperature may reduce emollient build-up but not totally remove it.

The MHRA/CHM (August 2020) have released a toolkit of resources for health and social care professionals to support the safe use of emollients, available at: www.gov.uk/safety-update/emollients-and-risk-of-severe-and-fatal-burns-new-resources-available.

Barrier preparations

Barrier preparations often contain water-repellent substances such as dimeticone (see barrier creams and ointments p. 1266) or other silicones. They are used on the skin around stomas, bedsores, and pressure areas in the elderly where the skin is intact. Where the skin has broken down, barrier preparations have a limited role in protecting adjacent skin. Barrier preparations are not a substitute for adequate nursing care.

Nappy rash

The first line of treatment is to ensure that nappies are changed frequently and that tightly fitting water-proof pants are avoided. The rash may clear when left exposed to the air and a barrier preparation, applied with each nappy change, can be helpful. A mild corticosteroid such as hydrocortisone 0.5% or 1% p. 1291 can be used if inflammation is causing discomfort, but it should be avoided in neonates. The barrier preparation should be applied after the corticosteroid preparation to prevent further damage. Preparations containing hydrocortisone should be applied for no more than a week; the hydrocortisone should be discontinued as soon as the inflammation subsides. The occlusive effect of nappies and waterproof pants may increase absorption of corticosteroids. If the rash is associated with candidal infection, a topical antifungal such as clotrimazole cream p. 1276 can be used. Topical antibacterial preparations can be used if bacterial infection is present; treatment with an oral antibacterial may occasionally be required in severe or recurrent infection. Hydrocortisone may be used in combination with antimicrobial preparations if there is considerable inflammation, erosion, and infection.

13

Skin

DERMATOLOGICAL DRUGS > BARRIER PREPARATIONS

Barrier creams and ointments

13-Feb-2020

● **INDICATIONS AND DOSE**

For use as a barrier preparation
▶ TO THE SKIN
▶ Child: (consult product literature)
▶ Adult: (consult product literature)

● MEDICINAL FORMS There can be variation in the licensing of different medicines containing the same drug.
Ointment
EXCIPIENTS: May contain Woolfat and related substances (including lanolin)
▶ Barrier creams and ointments (Non-proprietary)
Cetostearyl alcohol 20 mg per 1 gram, Zinc oxide 75 mg per 1 gram, Beeswax white 100 mg per 1 gram, Arachis oil 305 mg per 1 gram, Castor oil 500 mg per 1 gram Zinc and Castor oil ointment | 500 gram [GSL] £5.14–£5.15 DT = £5.15
Zinc and Castor oil cream | 100 gram [GSL] £1.46
▶ Metanium (Thornton & Ross Ltd)
Titanium salicylate 30 mg per 1 gram, Titanium peroxide 50 mg per 1 gram, Titanium dioxide 200 mg per 1 gram Metanium Nappy Rash ointment | 30 gram [GSL] £2.24 DT = £2.24
Spray
CAUTIONARY AND ADVISORY LABELS 15
EXCIPIENTS: May contain Cetostearyl alcohol (including cetyl and stearyl alcohol), hydroxybenzoates (parabens), woolfat and related substances (including lanolin)
▶ Sprilon (J M Loveridge Ltd)
Dimeticone 10.4 mg per 1 gram, Zinc oxide 125 mg per 1 gram Sprilon aerosol spray | 115 gram [GSL] £8.90 DT = £8.90
Cream
EXCIPIENTS: May contain Beeswax, butylated hydroxyanisole, butylated hydroxytoluene, cetostearyl alcohol (including cetyl and stearyl alcohol), chlorocresol, fragrances, hydroxybenzoates (parabens), propylene glycol, woolfat and related substances (including lanolin)
▶ Conotrane (Karo Pharma)
Benzalkonium chloride 1 mg per 1 gram, Dimeticone 220 mg per 1 gram Conotrane cream | 100 gram [GSL] £0.88 DT = £0.88 | 500 gram [GSL] £3.51
▶ Drapolene (Supra Enterprises Ltd)
Benzalkonium chloride 100 microgram per 1 gram, Cetrimide 2 mg per 1 gram Drapolene cream | 100 gram [GSL] £2.81 DT = £2.81 | 200 gram [GSL] £3.74 DT = £3.74 | 350 gram [GSL] £4.99 DT = £4.99
▶ Siopel (Derma UK Ltd)
Cetrimide 3 mg per 1 gram, Dimeticone 1000 100 mg per 1 gram Siopel cream | 50 gram [GSL] £4.65 DT = £4.65
▶ Sudocrem (Teva UK Ltd)
Benzyl cinnamate 1.5 mg per 1 gram, Benzyl alcohol 3.9 mg per 1 gram, Benzyl benzoate 10.1 mg per 1 gram, Wool fat hydrous 40 mg per 1 gram, Zinc oxide 152.5 mg per 1 gram Sudocrem antiseptic healing cream | 60 gram [GSL] £1.45 | 125 gram [GSL] £2.15 | 250 gram [GSL] £3.67 | 400 gram [GSL] £5.25

DERMATOLOGICAL DRUGS > EMOLLIENTS

Emollient bath and shower products, antimicrobial-containing

19-Nov-2020

● **INDICATIONS AND DOSE**

DERMOL® 200 SHOWER EMOLLIENT

Dry and pruritic skin conditions including eczema and dermatitis
▶ TO THE SKIN
▶ Child: To be applied to the skin or used as a soap substitute
▶ Adult: To be applied to the skin or used as a soap substitute

DERMOL® 600 BATH EMOLLIENT

Dry and pruritic skin conditions including eczema and dermatitis
▶ TO THE SKIN
▶ Child 1–23 months: 5–15 mL/bath, not to be used undiluted
▶ Child 2–17 years: 15–30 mL/bath, not to be used undiluted
▶ Adult: Up to 30 mL/bath, not to be used undiluted

DERMOL® WASH EMULSION

Dry and pruritic skin conditions including eczema and dermatitis
▶ TO THE SKIN
▶ Child: To be applied to the skin or used as a soap substitute
▶ Adult: To be applied to the skin or used as a soap substitute

EMULSIDERM®

Dry skin conditions including eczema and ichthyosis
▶ TO THE SKIN
▶ Child 1–23 months: 5–10 mL/bath, alternatively, to be rubbed into dry skin until absorbed
▶ Child 2–17 years: 7–30 mL/bath, alternatively, to be rubbed into dry skin until absorbed
▶ Adult: 7–30 mL/bath, alternatively, to be rubbed into dry skin until absorbed

OILATUM® PLUS

Topical treatment of eczema, including eczema at risk from infection
▶ TO THE SKIN
▶ Child 6–11 months: 1 mL/bath, not to be used undiluted
▶ Child 1–17 years: 1–2 capfuls/bath, not to be used undiluted
▶ Adult: 1–2 capfuls/bath, not to be used undiluted

> **IMPORTANT SAFETY INFORMATION**
> These preparations make skin and surfaces slippery—particular care is needed when bathing.
> MHRA/CHM ADVICE (UPDATED DECEMBER 2018): EMOLLIENTS: NEW INFORMATION ABOUT RISK OF SEVERE AND FATAL BURNS WITH PARAFFIN-CONTAINING AND PARAFFIN-FREE EMOLLIENTS See Emollient and barrier preparations p. 1265.

● DIRECTIONS FOR ADMINISTRATION Emollient bath additives should be added to bath water; [EvGr] hydration can be improved by soaking in the bath for 5–20 minutes (consult product literature). Some bath emollients can be applied to wet skin undiluted and rinsed off. ⓜ Emollient preparations contained in tubs should be removed with a clean spoon or spatula to reduce bacterial contamination of the emollient. Emollients should be applied in the direction of hair growth to reduce the risk of folliculitis.
● PRESCRIBING AND DISPENSING INFORMATION Preparations containing an antibacterial should be avoided unless infection is present or is a frequent complication.

● MEDICINAL FORMS There can be variation in the licensing of different medicines containing the same drug.
Bath additive
CAUTIONARY AND ADVISORY LABELS 15
EXCIPIENTS: May contain Acetylated lanolin alcohols, isopropyl palmitate, polysorbates
▶ Dermol 600 (Dermal Laboratories Ltd)
Benzalkonium chloride 5 mg per 1 gram, Isopropyl myristate 250 mg per 1 gram, Liquid paraffin 250 mg per 1 gram Dermol 600 bath emollient | 600 ml [P] £7.55
▶ Emulsiderm (Dermal Laboratories Ltd)
Benzalkonium chloride 5 mg per 1 gram, Isopropyl myristate 250 mg per 1 gram, Liquid paraffin 250 mg per

1 gram Emulsiderm emollient | 300 ml P £3.85 | 1000 ml P £12.00

▸ Oilatum Plus (Thornton & Ross Ltd)
Triclosan 20 mg per 1 gram, Benzalkonium chloride 60 mg per 1 gram, Liquid paraffin light 525 mg per 1 gram Oilatum Plus bath additive | 500 ml GSL £7.94

Liquid
CAUTIONARY AND ADVISORY LABELS 15
EXCIPIENTS: May contain Cetostearyl alcohol (including cetyl and stearyl alcohol)

▸ Dermol 200 (Dermal Laboratories Ltd)
Benzalkonium chloride 1 mg per 1 gram, Chlorhexidine hydrochloride 1 mg per 1 gram, Isopropyl myristate 25 mg per 1 gram, Liquid paraffin 25 mg per 1 gram Dermol 200 shower emollient | 200 ml P £3.55

▸ Dermol Wash (Dermal Laboratories Ltd)
Benzalkonium chloride 1 mg per 1 gram, Chlorhexidine hydrochloride 1 mg per 1 gram, Isopropyl myristate 25 mg per 1 gram, Liquid paraffin 25 mg per 1 gram Dermol Wash cutaneous emulsion | 200 ml P £3.55

Emollient bath and shower products, paraffin-containing

19-Nov-2020

● **INDICATIONS AND DOSE**

Dry skin conditions (using Aqueous Cream BP)
▸ TO THE SKIN
▸ Child: To be used as a soap substitute
▸ Adult: To be used as a soap substitute

AQUAMAX ® WASH

Dry skin conditions
▸ TO THE SKIN
▸ Child: To be applied to wet or dry skin and rinse
▸ Adult: To be applied to wet or dry skin and rinse

CETRABEN ® BATH

Dry skin conditions, including eczema
▸ TO THE SKIN
▸ Child 1 month–11 years: 0.5–1 capful/bath, alternatively, to be applied to wet skin and rinse
▸ Child 12–17 years: 1–2 capfuls/bath, alternatively, to be applied to wet skin and rinse
▸ Adult: 1–2 capfuls/bath, alternatively, to be applied to wet skin and rinse

DERMALO ®

Dermatitis | Dry skin conditions, including ichthyosis
▸ TO THE SKIN
▸ Child 1 month–11 years: 5–10 mL/bath, alternatively, to be applied to wet skin and rinse
▸ Child 12–17 years: 15–20 mL/bath, alternatively, to be applied to wet skin and rinse
▸ Adult: 15–20 mL/bath, alternatively, to be applied to wet skin and rinse

Pruritus of the elderly
▸ TO THE SKIN
▸ Elderly: 15–20 mL/bath, alternatively, to be applied to wet skin and rinse

DOUBLEBASE ® EMOLLIENT BATH ADDITIVE

Dry skin conditions including dermatitis and ichthyosis
▸ TO THE SKIN
▸ Child 1 month–11 years: 5–10 mL/bath
▸ Child 12–17 years: 15–20 mL/bath
▸ Adult: 15–20 mL/bath

Pruritus of the elderly
▸ TO THE SKIN
▸ Elderly: 15–20 mL/bath

DOUBLEBASE ® EMOLLIENT SHOWER GEL

Dry, chapped, or itchy skin conditions
▸ TO THE SKIN
▸ Child: To be applied to wet or dry skin and rinse, or apply to dry skin after showering
▸ Adult: To be applied to wet or dry skin and rinse, or apply to dry skin after showering

DOUBLEBASE ® EMOLLIENT WASH GEL

Dry, chapped, or itchy skin conditions
▸ TO THE SKIN
▸ Child: To be used as a soap substitute
▸ Adult: To be used as a soap substitute

E45 ® BATH OIL

Endogenous and exogenous eczema, xeroderma, and ichthyosis
▸ TO THE SKIN
▸ Child 1 month–11 years: 5–10 mL/bath, alternatively, to be applied to wet skin and rinse
▸ Child 12–17 years: 15 mL/bath, alternatively, to be applied to wet skin and rinse
▸ Adult: 15 mL/bath, alternatively, to be applied to wet skin and rinse

Pruritus of the elderly associated with dry skin
▸ TO THE SKIN
▸ Elderly: 15 mL/bath, alternatively, to be applied to wet skin and rinse

E45 ® WASH CREAM

Endogenous and exogenous eczema, xeroderma, and ichthyosis
▸ TO THE SKIN
▸ Child: To be used as a soap substitute
▸ Adult: To be used as a soap substitute

Pruritus of the elderly associated with dry skin
▸ TO THE SKIN
▸ Elderly: To be used as a soap substitute

HYDROMOL ® BATH AND SHOWER EMOLLIENT

Dry skin conditions | Eczema | Ichthyosis
▸ TO THE SKIN
▸ Child 1 month–11 years: 0.5–2 capfuls/bath, alternatively apply to wet skin and rinse
▸ Child 12–17 years: 1–3 capfuls/bath, alternatively apply to wet skin and rinse
▸ Adult: 1–3 capfuls/bath, alternatively apply to wet skin and rinse

Pruritus of the elderly
▸ TO THE SKIN
▸ Elderly: 1–3 capfuls/bath, alternatively apply to wet skin and rinse

LPL 63.4 ®

Dry skin conditions
▸ TO THE SKIN
▸ Child 1 month–11 years: 0.5–2 capfuls/bath, alternatively, to be applied to wet skin and rinse
▸ Child 12–17 years: 1–3 capfuls/bath, alternatively, to be applied to wet skin and rinse
▸ Adult: 1–3 capfuls/bath, alternatively, to be applied to wet skin and rinse

OILATUM ® EMOLLIENT BATH ADDITIVE

Dry skin conditions including dermatitis and ichthyosis
▸ TO THE SKIN
▸ Child 1 month–11 years: 0.5–2 capfuls/bath, alternatively, to be applied to wet skin and rinse
▸ Child 12–17 years: 1–3 capfuls/bath, alternatively, to be applied to wet skin and rinse
▸ Adult: 1–3 capfuls/bath, alternatively, to be applied to wet skin and rinse

continued →

Pruritus of the elderly

▸ TO THE SKIN

▸ Elderly: 1–3 capfuls/bath, alternatively, to be applied to wet skin and rinse

OILATUM ® JUNIOR BATH ADDITIVE

Dry skin conditions including dermatitis and ichthyosis

▸ TO THE SKIN

▸ Child 1 month-11 years: 0.5–2 capfuls/bath, alternatively, apply to wet skin and rinse

▸ Child 12-17 years: 1–3 capfuls/bath, alternatively, apply to wet skin and rinse

▸ Adult: 1–3 capfuls/bath, alternatively, apply to wet skin and rinse

Pruritus of the elderly

▸ TO THE SKIN

▸ Elderly: 1–3 capfuls/bath, alternatively, apply to wet skin and rinse

QV ® BATH OIL

Dry skin conditions including eczema, psoriasis, ichthyosis, and pruritus

▸ TO THE SKIN

▸ Child 1-11 months: 5 mL/bath, alternatively, to be applied to wet skin and rinse

▸ Child 1-17 years: 10 mL/bath, alternatively, to be applied to wet skin and rinse

▸ Adult: 10 mL/bath, alternatively, to be applied to wet skin and rinse

QV ® GENTLE WASH

Dry skin conditions including eczema, psoriasis, ichthyosis, and pruritus

▸ TO THE SKIN

▸ Child: To be used as a soap substitute

▸ Adult: To be used as a soap substitute

ZEROLATUM ®

Dry skin conditions | Dermatitis | Ichthyosis

▸ TO THE SKIN

▸ Child 1 month-11 years: 5–10 mL/bath

▸ Child 12-17 years: 15–20 mL/bath

▸ Adult: 15–20 mL/bath

Pruritus of the elderly

▸ TO THE SKIN

▸ Elderly: 15–20 mL/bath

IMPORTANT SAFETY INFORMATION

These preparations make the skin and surfaces slippery—particular care is needed when bathing.

MHRA/CHM ADVICE (UPDATED DECEMBER 2018): EMOLLIENTS: NEW INFORMATION ABOUT RISK OF SEVERE AND FATAL BURNS WITH PARAFFIN-CONTAINING AND PARAFFIN-FREE EMOLLIENTS See Emollient and barrier preparations p. 1265.

● DIRECTIONS FOR ADMINISTRATION Emollient bath additives should be added to bath water; EvGr hydration can be improved by soaking in the bath for 5–20 minutes (consult product literature). Some bath emollients can be applied to wet skin undiluted and rinsed off. Emollient preparations contained in tubs should be removed with a clean spoon or spatula to reduce bacterial contamination of the emollient. Emollients should be applied in the direction of hair growth to reduce the risk of folliculitis.

● MEDICINAL FORMS There can be variation in the licensing of different medicines containing the same drug.

Bath additive

CAUTIONARY AND ADVISORY LABELS 15

EXCIPIENTS: May contain Acetylated lanolin alcohols, cetostearyl alcohol (including cetyl and stearyl alcohol), fragrances, isopropyl palmitate

▸ Cetraben (Genus Pharmaceuticals Ltd)

Liquid paraffin light 828 mg per 1 gram Cetraben emollient 82.8% bath additive | 500 ml GSL £5.75 DT = £5.75

▸ Dermalo (Dermal Laboratories Ltd)

Acetylated wool alcohols 50 mg per 1 gram, Liquid paraffin 650 mg per 1 gram Dermalo bath emollient | 500 ml GSL £3.44

▸ Doublebase (Dermal Laboratories Ltd)

Liquid paraffin 650 mg per 1 gram Doublebase emollient bath additive | 500 ml GSL £5.45 DT = £5.45

▸ E45 emollient bath (Forum Health Products Ltd)

E45 emollient bath oil | 500 ml £5.29

▸ Hydromol (Alliance Pharmaceuticals Ltd)

Isopropyl myristate 130 mg per 1 ml, Liquid paraffin light 378 mg per 1 ml Hydromol Bath & Shower emollient | 350 ml £3.91 | 500 ml £4.46 | 1000 ml £8.87

▸ LPL (Huxley Europe Ltd)

Liquid paraffin light 634 mg per 1 ml LPL 63.4 bath additive and emollient | 500 ml £3.13 DT = £5.80

▸ Oilatum (Thornton & Ross Ltd)

Liquid paraffin light 634 mg per 1 ml Oilatum Bath Formula | 150 ml GSL £2.95 DT = £2.95 | 300 ml GSL £5.02 DT = £5.02 Oilatum Emollient | 500 ml GSL £5.80 DT = £5.80

▸ Oilatum junior (Thornton & Ross Ltd)

Liquid paraffin light 634 mg per 1 ml Oilatum Junior bath additive | 150 ml GSL £2.95 DT = £2.95 | 300 ml GSL £5.02 DT = £5.02 | 600 ml GSL £7.34 DT = £7.34

▸ QV (Crawford Healthcare Ltd)

Liquid paraffin light 850.9 mg per 1 gram QV 85.09% bath oil | 250 ml £2.93 | 500 ml £4.79

▸ Zerolatum (Thornton & Ross Ltd)

Acetylated wool alcohols 50 mg per 1 gram, Liquid paraffin 650 mg per 1 gram Zerolatum Emollient bath additive | 500 ml £4.79

Gel

CAUTIONARY AND ADVISORY LABELS 15

EXCIPIENTS: May contain Cetostearyl alcohol (including cetyl and stearyl alcohol)

▸ AproDerm (isopropyl myristate / liquid paraffin) (Fontus Health Ltd)

Isopropyl myristate 150 mg per 1 gram, Liquid paraffin 150 mg per 1 gram AproDerm gel | 100 gram £1.99 DT = £2.65 | 500 gram £3.99 DT = £5.83

▸ Doublebase (Dermal Laboratories Ltd)

Isopropyl myristate 150 mg per 1 gram, Liquid paraffin 150 mg per 1 gram Doublebase Dayleve gel | 100 gram P £2.65 DT = £2.65 | 500 gram P £6.29 DT = £5.83

Doublebase gel | 100 gram P £2.65 DT = £2.65 | 500 gram P £5.83 DT = £5.83 | 1000 gram P £10.98

Doublebase emollient wash gel | 200 gram P £5.21

Doublebase emollient shower gel | 200 gram P £5.21

▸ Exmabase (Ascot Laboratories Ltd)

Isopropyl myristate 150 mg per 1 gram, Liquid paraffin 150 mg per 1 gram Exmabase gel | 500 gram £2.85 DT = £5.83

▸ HypoBase (Galen Ltd)

Isopropyl myristate 150 mg per 1 gram, Liquid paraffin 150 mg per 1 gram HypoBase gel | 500 gram £5.83 DT = £5.83

▸ Isomol (Aspire Pharma Ltd)

Isopropyl myristate 150 mg per 1 gram, Liquid paraffin 150 mg per 1 gram Epimax isomol gel | 100 gram £1.99 = £2.65 | 500 gram £2.92 DT = £5.83

▸ MyriBase (Galen Ltd)

Isopropyl myristate 150 mg per 1 gram, Liquid paraffin 150 mg per 1 gram MyriBase gel | 100 gram £2.12 DT = £2.65 | 500 ml £4.66 MyriBase emollient shower gel | 200 ml £4.17

▸ Oilatum (Thornton & Ross Ltd)

Liquid paraffin light 700 mg per 1 gram Oilatum shower gel fragrance free | 150 gram GSL £5.27 DT = £5.27

▸ Zerodouble (Thornton & Ross Ltd)

Isopropyl myristate 150 mg per 1 gram, Liquid paraffin 150 mg per 1 gram Zerodouble gel | 100 gram £2.25 DT = £2.65 | 500 gram £4.90 DT = £5.83

Cream

CAUTIONARY AND ADVISORY LABELS 15

EXCIPIENTS: May contain Cetostearyl alcohol (including cetyl and stearyl alcohol)

▸ Emollient bath and shower products, paraffin-containing (Non-proprietary)

Phenoxyethanol 10 mg per 1 gram, Liquid paraffin 60 mg per 1 gram, Emulsifying wax 90 mg per 1 gram, White soft paraffin

150 mg per 1 gram, Purified water 690 mg per 1 gram Aqueous cream | 100 gram GSL £1.19 DT = £0.97 | 500 gram GSL £4.85 DT = £4.85

Wash

CAUTIONARY AND ADVISORY LABELS 15

EXCIPIENTS: May contain Cetostearyl alcohol (including cetyl and stearyl alcohol), polysorbates

▸ Aquamax (Intrapharm Laboratories Ltd)
Aquamax wash | 250 gram £2.99

▸ E45 emollient wash (Forum Health Products Ltd)
E45 emollient wash cream | 250 ml £3.30

▸ QV Gentle (Crawford Healthcare Ltd)
QV Gentle wash | 250 ml £3.19 | 500 ml £5.32

Emollient bath and shower products, soya-bean oil-containing

19-Nov-2020

● **INDICATIONS AND DOSE**

BALNEUM ® BATH OIL

Dry skin conditions including those associated with dermatitis and eczema

▸ TO THE SKIN

▸ Child 1-23 months: 5–15 mL/bath, not to be used undiluted

▸ Child 2-17 years: 20–60 mL/bath, not to be used undiluted

▸ Adult: 20–60 mL/bath, not to be used undiluted

BALNEUM ® PLUS BATH OIL

Dry skin conditions including those associated with dermatitis and eczema where pruritus also experienced

▸ TO THE SKIN

▸ Child 1-23 months: 5 mL/bath, alternatively, to be applied to wet skin and rinse

▸ Child 2-17 years: 10–20 mL/bath, alternatively, to be applied to wet skin and rinse

▸ Adult: 20 mL/bath, alternatively, to be applied to wet skin and rinse

ZERONEUM ®

Dry skin conditions, including eczema

▸ TO THE SKIN

▸ Child 1 month-11 years: 5 mL/bath

▸ Child 12-17 years: 20 mL/bath

▸ Adult: 20 mL/bath

IMPORTANT SAFETY INFORMATION

These preparations make skin and surfaces slippery—particular care is needed when bathing.

MHRA/CHM ADVICE (UPDATED DECEMBER 2018): EMOLLIENTS: NEW INFORMATION ABOUT RISK OF SEVERE AND FATAL BURNS WITH PARAFFIN-CONTAINING AND PARAFFIN-FREE EMOLLIENTS
See Emollient and barrier preparations p. 1265.

● DIRECTIONS FOR ADMINISTRATION Emollient bath additives should be added to bath water; EvGr hydration can be improved by soaking in the bath for 5–20 minutes (consult product literature). Some bath emollients can be applied to wet skin undiluted and rinsed off. ◈ Emollient preparations contained in tubs should be removed with a clean spoon or spatula to reduce bacterial contamination of the emollient. Emollients should be applied in the direction of hair growth to reduce the risk of folliculitis.

● MEDICINAL FORMS There can be variation in the licensing of different medicines containing the same drug.

Bath additive

CAUTIONARY AND ADVISORY LABELS 15

EXCIPIENTS: May contain Butylated hydroxytoluene, fragrances, propylene glycol

▸ Balneum (Almirall Ltd)
Lauromacrogols 150 mg per 1 gram, Soya oil 829.5 mg per 1 gram Balneum Plus bath oil | 500 ml GSL £6.66 DT = £6.66

Soya oil 847.5 mg per 1 gram Balneum 84.75% bath oil | 500 ml GSL £5.38 DT = £5.38 | 1000 ml GSL £10.39 DT = £10.39

▸ Zeroneum (Thornton & Ross Ltd)
Soya oil 833.5 mg per 1 gram Zeroneum 83.35% bath additive | 500 ml £4.48

Emollient bath and shower products, tar-containing

19-Nov-2020

● **INDICATIONS AND DOSE**

POLYTAR EMOLLIENT ®

Psoriasis, eczema, atopic and pruritic dermatoses

▸ TO THE SKIN

▸ Adult: 2–4 capfuls/bath, add 15–30 mL to an adult-size bath; soak for 20 minutes

PSORIDERM ® EMULSION

Psoriasis

▸ TO THE SKIN

▸ Adult: Up to 30 mL/bath, use 30mL in adult-size bath, soak for 5 minutes

---

IMPORTANT SAFETY INFORMATION

These preparations make skin and surfaces slippery—particular care is needed when bathing.

MHRA/CHM ADVICE (UPDATED DECEMBER 2018): EMOLLIENTS: NEW INFORMATION ABOUT RISK OF SEVERE AND FATAL BURNS WITH PARAFFIN-CONTAINING AND PARAFFIN-FREE EMOLLIENTS
See Emollient and barrier preparations p. 1265.

● DIRECTIONS FOR ADMINISTRATION Emollient bath additives should be added to bath water; hydration can be improved by soaking in the bath for 5–20 minutes (consult product literature). Some bath emollients can be applied to wet skin undiluted and rinsed off. Emollient preparations contained in tubs should be removed with a clean spoon or spatula to reduce bacterial contamination of the emollient. Emollients should be applied in the direction of hair growth to reduce the risk of folliculitis.

● MEDICINAL FORMS There can be variation in the licensing of different medicines containing the same drug.

Bath additive

CAUTIONARY AND ADVISORY LABELS 15

EXCIPIENTS: May contain Isopropyl palmitate, polysorbates

▸ Psoriderm (Dermal Laboratories Ltd)
Coal tar distilled 400 mg per 1 ml Psoriderm Emulsion 40% bath additive | 200 ml P £2.74 DT = £2.74

Emollient creams and ointments, antimicrobial-containing

19-Nov-2020

● **INDICATIONS AND DOSE**

Dry and pruritic skin conditions including eczema and dermatitis

▸ TO THE SKIN

▸ Child: To be applied to the skin or used as a soap substitute

▸ Adult: To be applied to the skin or used as a soap substitute

---

IMPORTANT SAFETY INFORMATION

These preparations make skin and surfaces slippery—particular care is needed when bathing.

MHRA/CHM ADVICE (UPDATED DECEMBER 2018): EMOLLIENTS: NEW INFORMATION ABOUT RISK OF SEVERE AND FATAL BURNS WITH PARAFFIN-CONTAINING AND PARAFFIN-FREE EMOLLIENTS
See Emollient and barrier preparations p. 1265.

13

Skin

- **DIRECTIONS FOR ADMINISTRATION** Emollients should be applied immediately after washing or bathing to maximise the effect of skin hydration. Emollient preparations contained in tubs should be removed with a clean spoon or spatula to reduce bacterial contamination of the emollient. Emollients should be applied in the direction of hair growth to reduce the risk of folliculitis.
- **PRESCRIBING AND DISPENSING INFORMATION** Preparations containing an antibacterial should be avoided unless infection is present or is a frequent complication.

- **MEDICINAL FORMS** There can be variation in the licensing of different medicines containing the same drug.

Cream

CAUTIONARY AND ADVISORY LABELS 15

EXCIPIENTS: May contain Cetostearyl alcohol (including cetyl and stearyl alcohol)

- Dermol (Dermal Laboratories Ltd)
  Benzalkonium chloride 1 mg per 1 gram, Chlorhexidine hydrochloride 1 mg per 1 gram, Isopropyl myristate 100 mg per 1 gram, Liquid paraffin 100 mg per 1 gram Dermol cream | 100 gram Ⓟ £2.86 | 500 gram Ⓟ £6.63

Liquid

CAUTIONARY AND ADVISORY LABELS 15

EXCIPIENTS: May contain Cetostearyl alcohol (including cetyl and stearyl alcohol)

- Dermol 500 (Dermal Laboratories Ltd)
  Benzalkonium chloride 1 mg per 1 gram, Chlorhexidine hydrochloride 1 mg per 1 gram, Isopropyl myristate 25 mg per 1 gram, Liquid paraffin 25 mg per 1 gram Dermol 500 lotion | 500 ml Ⓟ £6.04

Emollient creams and ointments, colloidal oatmeal-containing
19-Nov-2020

- **INDICATIONS AND DOSE**

Endogenous and exogenous eczema | Xeroderma | Ichthyosis

▸ TO THE SKIN

- Child: (consult product literature)
- Adult: (consult product literature)

Senile pruritus (pruritus of the elderly) associated with dry skin

▸ TO THE SKIN

- Elderly: (consult product literature)

IMPORTANT SAFETY INFORMATION

MHRA/CHM ADVICE (UPDATED DECEMBER 2018): EMOLLIENTS: NEW INFORMATION ABOUT RISK OF SEVERE AND FATAL BURNS WITH PARAFFIN-CONTAINING AND PARAFFIN-FREE EMOLLIENTS See Emollient and barrier preparations p. 1265.

- **DIRECTIONS FOR ADMINISTRATION** Emollients should be applied immediately after washing or bathing to maximise the effect of skin hydration. Emollient preparations contained in tubs should be removed with a clean spoon or spatula to reduce bacterial contamination of the emollient. Emollients should be applied in the direction of hair growth to reduce the risk of folliculitis.

- **MEDICINAL FORMS** There can be variation in the licensing of different medicines containing the same drug.

Lotion/cream

CAUTIONARY AND ADVISORY LABELS 15

EXCIPIENTS: May contain Benzyl alcohol, cetostearyl alcohol (including cetyl and stearyl alcohol), isopropyl palmitate

- Aveeno (Johnson & Johnson Ltd)
  Aveeno lotion | 500 ml(ACBS) £6.66
  Aveeno cream | 100 ml(ACBS) £3.97 | 300 ml(ACBS) £6.80 | 500 ml (ACBS) £6.47

Emollient creams and ointments, paraffin-containing
19-Nov-202

- **INDICATIONS AND DOSE**

Dry skin conditions | Eczema | Psoriasis | Ichthyosis | Pruritus

▸ TO THE SKIN

- Child: (consult product literature)
- Adult: (consult product literature)

IMPORTANT SAFETY INFORMATION

MHRA/CHM ADVICE (UPDATED DECEMBER 2018): EMOLLIENTS: NEW INFORMATION ABOUT RISK OF SEVERE AND FATAL BURNS WITH PARAFFIN-CONTAINING AND PARAFFIN-FREE EMOLLIENTS See Emollient and barrier preparations p. 1265.

- **DIRECTIONS FOR ADMINISTRATION** Emollients should be applied immediately after washing or bathing to maximise the effect of skin hydration. Emollient preparations contained in tubs should be removed with a clean spoon or spatula to reduce bacterial contamination of the emollient. Emollients should be applied in the direction of hair growth to reduce the risk of folliculitis.

- **MEDICINAL FORMS** There can be variation in the licensing of different medicines containing the same drug.

Spray

CAUTIONARY AND ADVISORY LABELS 15

- Dermamist (Alliance Pharmaceuticals Ltd)
  White soft paraffin 100 mg per 1 gram Dermamist 10% spray | 250 ml Ⓟ £5.97 DT = £5.97
- Emollin (C D Medical Ltd)
  Emollin aerosol spray | 150 ml £4.05 | 240 ml £6.48

Gel

CAUTIONARY AND ADVISORY LABELS 15

- AproDerm (isopropyl myristate / liquid paraffin) (Fontus Health Ltd)
  Isopropyl myristate 150 mg per 1 gram, Liquid paraffin 150 mg per 1 gram AproDerm gel | 100 gram £1.99 DT = £2.65 | 500 gram £3.99 DT = £5.83
- Doublebase (Dermal Laboratories Ltd)
  Isopropyl myristate 150 mg per 1 gram, Liquid paraffin 150 mg per 1 gram Doublebase Dayleve gel | 100 gram Ⓟ £2.65 DT = £2.65 | 500 gram Ⓟ £6.29 DT = £5.83
  Doublebase gel | 100 gram Ⓟ £2.65 DT = £2.65 | 500 gram Ⓟ £5.83 DT = £5.83 | 1000 gram Ⓟ £10.98
  Doublebase emollient wash gel | 200 gram Ⓟ £5.21
  Doublebase emollient shower gel | 200 gram Ⓟ £5.21
- Exmabase (Ascot Laboratories Ltd)
  Isopropyl myristate 150 mg per 1 gram, Liquid paraffin 150 mg per 1 gram Exmabase gel | 500 gram £2.85 DT = £5.83
- HypoBase (Galen Ltd)
  Isopropyl myristate 150 mg per 1 gram, Liquid paraffin 150 mg per 1 gram HypoBase gel | 500 gram £5.83 DT = £5.83
- Isomol (Aspire Pharma Ltd)
  Isopropyl myristate 150 mg per 1 gram, Liquid paraffin 150 mg per 1 gram Epimax isomol gel | 100 gram £1.99 DT = £2.65 | 500 gram £2.92 DT = £5.83
- MyriBase (Galen Ltd)
  Isopropyl myristate 150 mg per 1 gram, Liquid paraffin 150 mg per 1 gram MyriBase gel | 100 gram £2.12 DT = £2.65 | 500 ml £4.66
  MyriBase emollient shower gel | 200 ml £4.17
- Zerodouble (Thornton & Ross Ltd)
  Isopropyl myristate 150 mg per 1 gram, Liquid paraffin 150 mg per 1 gram Zerodouble gel | 100 gram £2.25 DT = £2.65 | 500 gram £4.90 DT = £5.83

Cream

CAUTIONARY AND ADVISORY LABELS 15

EXCIPIENTS: May contain Benzyl alcohol, cetostearyl alcohol (including cetyl and stearyl alcohol), chlorocresol, disodium edetate, fragrances, hydroxybenzoates (parabens), polysorbates, propylene glycol, sorbic acid, lanolin

- Cetraben (Thornton & Ross Ltd)
  Liquid paraffin light 105 mg per 1 gram, White soft paraffin 132 mg per 1 gram Cetraben cream | 50 gram £1.40 | 150 gram £3.98 | 500 gram £5.99 | 1050 gram £11.62

▸ Diprobase (Bayer Plc)
Diprobase cream | 50 gram £1.28 | 500 gram £6.32

▸ E45 (Forum Health Products Ltd)
Wool fat 10 mg per 1 gram, Liquid paraffin light 126 mg per 1 gram, White soft paraffin 145 mg per 1 gram E45 cream | 50 gram GSL £1.93 | 125 gram GSL £3.22 | 350 gram GSL £5.81 | 500 gram GSL £5.99

▸ Enopen (Ennogen Healthcare Ltd)
Liquid paraffin light 105 mg per 1 gram, White soft paraffin 132 mg per 1 gram Enopen cream | 50 gram £1.40 | 150 gram £3.98 | 500 gram £5.99 | 1050 gram £11.62

▸ Epaderm (Molnlycke Health Care Ltd)
Epaderm cream | 50 gram £1.71 | 150 gram £3.58 | 500 gram £7.01

▸ Epimax (Aspire Pharma Ltd)
Epimax original cream | 100 gram £0.75 | 500 gram £2.49

▸ ExCetra (Aspire Pharma Ltd)
Liquid paraffin light 105 mg per 1 gram, White soft paraffin 132 mg per 1 gram Epimax excetra cream | 100 gram £1.75 | 500 gram £2.95

▸ ExmaQS (Ascot Laboratories Ltd)
Liquid paraffin light 60 mg per 1 gram, White soft paraffin 150 mg per 1 gram ExmaQS cream | 500 gram £2.95

▸ Exmaben (Ascot Laboratories Ltd)
Liquid paraffin light 105 mg per 1 gram, White soft paraffin 132 mg per 1 gram Exmaben cream | 500 gram £4.25

▸ Exmalatum (Ascot Laboratories Ltd)
Liquid paraffin light 60 mg per 1 gram, White soft paraffin 150 mg per 1 gram Exmalatum cream | 500 gram £4.45

▸ Hydromol (Alliance Pharmaceuticals Ltd)
Sodium lactate 10 mg per 1 gram, Sodium pidolate 25 mg per 1 gram, Isopropyl myristate 50 mg per 1 gram, Liquid paraffin 100 mg per 1 gram Hydromol 2.5% cream | 50 gram £2.25 | 100 gram £4.20 | 500 gram £12.25

▸ Lipobase (Karo Pharma)
Lipobase cream | 50 gram P £1.46

▸ Oilatum (Thornton & Ross Ltd)
Liquid paraffin light 60 mg per 1 gram, White soft paraffin 150 mg per 1 gram Oilatum cream | 150 gram GSL £3.06 DT = £3.06 | 500 ml GSL £5.28 DT = £5.28

▸ Oilatum junior (Thornton & Ross Ltd)
Liquid paraffin light 60 mg per 1 gram, White soft paraffin 150 mg per 1 gram Oilatum Junior cream | 150 gram GSL £3.06 DT = £3.06 | 350 ml GSL £4.65 DT = £4.65 | 500 ml GSL £5.28 DT = £5.28

▸ Soffen (Vitame Ltd)
Liquid paraffin light 105 mg per 1 gram, White soft paraffin 132 mg per 1 gram Soffen cream | 500 gram £4.79

▸ Ultrabase (Derma UK Ltd)
Ultrabase cream | 500 gram GSL £8.67

▸ Unguentum M (Almirall Ltd)
Unguentum M cream | 500 gram GSL £8.48

▸ ZeroAQS (Thornton & Ross Ltd)
ZeroAQS emollient cream | 500 gram £3.29

▸ Zerobase (Thornton & Ross Ltd)
Liquid paraffin 110 mg per 1 gram Zerobase 11% cream | 50 gram £1.04 | 500 gram £5.26

▸ Zerocream (Thornton & Ross Ltd)
Liquid paraffin 126 mg per 1 gram, White soft paraffin 145 mg per 1 gram Zerocream | 50 gram £1.17 | 500 gram £4.08

▸ Zeroguent (Thornton & Ross Ltd)
White soft paraffin 40 mg per 1 gram, Soya oil 50 mg per 1 gram, Liquid paraffin light 80 mg per 1 gram Zeroguent cream | 100 gram £2.33 | 500 gram £6.99

Ointment

CAUTIONARY AND ADVISORY LABELS 15
EXCIPIENTS: May contain Cetostearyl alcohol (including cetyl and stearyl alcohol), polysorbates

▸ Emollient creams and ointments, paraffin-containing (Non-proprietary)
Liquid paraffin 200 mg per 1 gram, Emulsifying wax 300 mg per 1 gram, White soft paraffin 500 mg per 1 gram Emulsifying ointment | 500 gram GSL £4.82
Liquid paraffin 500 mg per 1 gram, White soft paraffin 500 mg per 1 gram White soft paraffin 50% / Liquid paraffin 50% ointment | 250 gram £2.03 | 500 gram £4.32 DT = £4.57 | 500 gram P £4.57 DT = £4.57
Magnesium sulfate dried 5 mg per 1 gram, Phenoxyethanol 10 mg per 1 gram, Wool alcohols ointment 500 mg per 1 gram Hydrous ointment | 500 gram GSL ⬛

White soft paraffin 1 mg per 1 mg White soft paraffin solid | 500 gram GSL £5.18 DT = £4.03 | 4500 gram GSL £22.72
Yellow soft paraffin 1 mg per 1 mg Yellow soft paraffin solid | 15 gram GSL £1.21 | 500 gram GSL £4.26 DT = £4.26 | 4500 gram GSL £21.99

▸ Diprobase (Bayer Plc)
Liquid paraffin 50 mg per 1 gram, White soft paraffin 950 mg per 1 gram Diprobase ointment | 50 gram GSL £1.28 DT = £1.28 | 500 gram GSL £5.99 DT = £5.99

▸ Emelpin (Vitame Ltd)
Emulsifying wax 300 mg per 1 gram, Yellow soft paraffin 300 mg per 1 gram Emelpin ointment | 125 gram £3.08 | 500 gram £3.97

▸ Epaderm (Molnlycke Health Care Ltd)
Emulsifying wax 300 mg per 1 gram, Yellow soft paraffin 300 mg per 1 gram Epaderm ointment | 125 gram £3.88 | 500 gram £6.58 | 1000 gram £12.42

▸ Epaderm Junior (Molnlycke Health Care Ltd)
Emulsifying wax 300 mg per 1 gram, Yellow soft paraffin 300 mg per 1 gram Epaderm Junior ointment | 125 gram £3.85

▸ Fifty:50 (Ennogen Healthcare Ltd)
Liquid paraffin 500 mg per 1 gram, White soft paraffin 500 mg per 1 gram Fifty:50 ointment | 250 gram £1.83 | 500 gram £3.66 DT = £4.57

▸ Hydromol (Alliance Pharmaceuticals Ltd)
Emulsifying wax 300 mg per 1 gram, Yellow soft paraffin 300 mg per 1 gram Hydromol ointment | 100 gram £3.20 | 125 gram £2.92 | 500 gram £4.96 | 1000 gram £8.20

▸ KreaMoint (Essential-Healthcare Ltd)
Liquid paraffin 500 mg per 1 gram, White soft paraffin 500 mg per 1 gram KreaMoint 50:50 ointment | 500 gram £3.17 DT = £4.57

▸ Thirty:30 (Ennogen Healthcare Ltd)
Emulsifying wax 300 mg per 1 gram, Yellow soft paraffin 300 mg per 1 gram Thirty:30 ointment | 125 gram £3.81 | 250 gram £4.29 | 500 gram £6.47

▸ Vaseline (Unilever UK Home & Personal Care)
White soft paraffin 1 mg per 1 mg Vaseline Pure Petroleum jelly | 50 ml GSL ⬛

Liquid

CAUTIONARY AND ADVISORY LABELS 15
EXCIPIENTS: May contain Benzyl alcohol, cetostearyl alcohol (including cetyl and stearyl alcohol), hydroxybenzoates (parabens), isopropyl palmitate

▸ E45 (Forum Health Products Ltd)
E45 lotion | 200 ml £2.45 | 500 ml £4.59

▸ QV (Crawford Healthcare Ltd)
White soft paraffin 50 mg per 1 gram QV 5% skin lotion | 250 ml £3.19 | 500 ml £5.32

Emollients, urea-containing   19-Nov-2020

● DRUG ACTION Urea is a keratin softener and hydrating agent used in the treatment of dry, scaling conditions (including ichthyosis) and may be useful in elderly patients.

● INDICATIONS AND DOSE

AQUADRATE ®

Dry, scaling, and itching skin
▸ TO THE SKIN
▸ Child: Apply twice daily, to be applied thinly
▸ Adult: Apply twice daily, to be applied thinly

BALNEUM ® CREAM

Dry skin conditions
▸ TO THE SKIN
▸ Child: Apply twice daily
▸ Adult: Apply twice daily

BALNEUM ® PLUS CREAM

Dry, scaling, and itching skin
▸ TO THE SKIN
▸ Child: Apply twice daily
▸ Adult: Apply twice daily continued →

13

Skin

CALMURID ®

Dry, scaling, and itching skin

▶ TO THE SKIN

▶ Child: Apply twice daily, apply a thick layer for 3–5 minutes, massage into area, and remove excess. Can be diluted with aqueous cream (life of diluted cream is 14 days). Half-strength cream can be used for 1 week if stinging occurs

▶ Adult: Apply twice daily, apply a thick layer for 3–5 minutes, massage into area, and remove excess. Can be diluted with aqueous cream (life of diluted cream is 14 days). Half-strength cream can be used for 1 week if stinging occurs

DERMATONICS ONCE HEEL BALM ®

Dry skin on soles of feet

▶ TO THE SKIN

▶ Child 12–17 years: Apply once daily

▶ Adult: Apply once daily

E45 ® ITCH RELIEF CREAM

Dry, scaling, and itching skin

▶ TO THE SKIN

▶ Child: Apply twice daily

▶ Adult: Apply twice daily

EUCERIN ® INTENSIVE CREAM

Dry skin conditions including eczema, ichthyosis, xeroderma, and hyperkeratosis

▶ TO THE SKIN

▶ Child: Apply twice daily, to be applied thinly and rubbed into area

▶ Adult: Apply twice daily, to be applied thinly and rubbed into area

EUCERIN ® INTENSIVE LOTION

Dry skin conditions including eczema, ichthyosis, xeroderma, and hyperkeratosis

▶ TO THE SKIN

▶ Child: Apply twice daily, to be applied sparingly and rubbed into area

▶ Adult: Apply twice daily, to be applied sparingly and rubbed into area

FLEXITOL ®

Dry skin on soles of feet and heels

▶ TO THE SKIN

▶ Child 12–17 years: Apply 1–2 times a day

▶ Adult: Apply 1–2 times a day

HYDROMOL ® INTENSIVE

Dry, scaling, and itching skin

▶ TO THE SKIN

▶ Child: Apply twice daily, to be applied thinly

▶ Adult: Apply twice daily, to be applied thinly

IMUDERM ® EMOLLIENT

Dry skin conditions including eczema, psoriasis or dermatitis

▶ TO THE SKIN

▶ Adult: Apply to skin or use as a soap substitute

NUTRAPLUS ®

Dry, scaling, and itching skin

▶ TO THE SKIN

▶ Child: Apply 2–3 times a day

▶ Adult: Apply 2–3 times a day

IMPORTANT SAFETY INFORMATION

MHRA/CHM ADVICE (UPDATED DECEMBER 2018): EMOLLIENTS: NEW INFORMATION ABOUT RISK OF SEVERE AND FATAL BURNS WITH PARAFFIN-CONTAINING AND PARAFFIN-FREE EMOLLIENTS

See Emollient and barrier preparations p. 1265.

● DIRECTIONS FOR ADMINISTRATION Emollients should be applied immediately after washing or bathing to maximise the effect of skin hydration. Emollient preparations contained in tubs should be removed with a clean spoon or spatula to reduce bacterial contamination of the emollient. Emollients should be applied in the direction of hair growth to reduce the risk of folliculitis.

● MEDICINAL FORMS There can be variation in the licensing of different medicines containing the same drug.

Cream

CAUTIONARY AND ADVISORY LABELS 15

EXCIPIENTS: May contain Benzyl alcohol, cetostearyl alcohol (including cetyl and stearyl alcohol), hydroxybenzoates (parabens), isopropyl palmitate, polysorbates, propylene glycol, woolfat and related substance (including lanolin)

▶ Aquadrate (Alliance Pharmaceuticals Ltd)
Urea 100 mg per 1 gram Aquadrate 10% cream | 30 gram £1.64 | 100 gram £4.45

▶ Balneum (Almirall Ltd)
Balneum cream | 50 gram £2.85 | 500 gram £9.97

▶ Balneum Plus (Almirall Ltd)
Lauromacrogols 30 mg per 1 gram, Urea 50 mg per 1 gram Balneum Plus cream | 100 gram GSL £3.29 DT = £4.28 | 500 gram GSL £14.99 DT = £14.99

▶ E45 Itch Relief (Forum Health Products Ltd)
Lauromacrogols 30 mg per 1 gram, Urea 50 mg per 1 gram E45 Itch Relief cream | 50 gram GSL £2.81 DT = £2.81 | 100 gram GSL £4.28 DT = £4.28 | 500 gram GSL £14.99 DT = £14.99

▶ Eucerin Intensive (Beiersdorf UK Ltd)
Urea 100 mg per 1 gram Eucerin Intensive 10% cream | 100 ml GSL £7.59

▶ Hydromol Intensive (Alliance Pharmaceuticals Ltd)
Urea 100 mg per 1 gram Hydromol Intensive 10% cream | 30 gram £1.67 | 100 gram £4.45

▶ imuDERM (CliniSupplies Ltd)
imuDERM emollient | 500 gram £6.62

▶ Nutraplus (Galderma (UK) Ltd)
Urea 100 mg per 1 gram Nutraplus 10% cream | 100 gram P £4.37

Liquid

CAUTIONARY AND ADVISORY LABELS 15

EXCIPIENTS: May contain Benzyl alcohol, isopropyl palmitate

▶ Eucerin Intensive (Beiersdorf UK Ltd)
Urea 100 mg per 1 gram Eucerin Intensive 10% lotion | 250 ml GSL £7.93 DT = £7.93

Balm

CAUTIONARY AND ADVISORY LABELS 15

EXCIPIENTS: May contain Beeswax, benzyl alcohol, cetostearyl alcohol (including cetyl and stearyl alcohol), fragrances, lanolin

▶ Dermatonics Once (Dermatonics Ltd)
Dermatonics Once Heel Balm | 75 ml £3.60 | 200 ml £8.50

▶ Flexitol (Thornton & Ross Ltd)
Flexitol 25% Urea Heel Balm | 40 gram £2.75 | 75 gram £3.80 | 200 gram £9.40 | 500 gram £14.75

---

2   Infections of the skin

Skin infections

22-Mar-2020

Antibacterial preparations for the skin

Cellulitis, *erysipelas*, and *leg ulcer* infections require systemic antibacterial treatment, see Skin infections, antibacterial therapy p. 541.

Impetigo requires topical antiseptic/antibacterial or systemic antibacterial treatment, see Skin infections, antibacterial therapy p. 541.

Although many antibacterial drugs are available in topical preparations, some are potentially hazardous and frequently their use is not necessary if adequate hygienic measures can be taken. Moreover, not all skin conditions that are oozing, crusted, or characterised by pustules are actually infected.

To minimise the development of resistant organisms it is advisable to limit the choice of antibacterials applied

pically to those not used systemically. Unfortunately some
f these, for example neomycin sulfate p. 1274, may cause
ensitisation, and there is cross-sensitivity with other
minoglycoside antibiotics, such as gentamicin p. 545. If
arge areas of skin are being treated, ototoxicity may also be a
azard with aminoglycoside antibiotics, particularly in
hildren, in the elderly, and in those with renal impairment.
esistant organisms are more common in hospitals, and
vhenever possible swabs should be taken for bacteriological
xamination before beginning treatment.

Mupirocin p. 1276 is not related to any other antibacterial
n use; it is effective for skin infections, particularly those
lue to Gram-positive organisms but it is not indicated for
seudomonal infection. Although *Staphylococcus aureus*
trains with low-level resistance to mupirocin are emerging,
t is generally useful in infections resistant to other
ntibacterials. To avoid the development of resistance,
nupirocin or fusidic acid p. 608 should not be used for longer
han 10 days and local microbiology advice should be sought
before using it in hospital. In the presence of mupirocin-
esistant MRSA infection, a topical antiseptic such as
ovidone-iodine p. 1320, chlorhexidine p. 1321, or alcohol
an be used; their use should be discussed with the local
nicrobiologist.

Tedizolid p. 610 is licensed for the treatment of acute
acterial skin and skin structure infections.

Silver sulfadiazine p. 1275 is used in the treatment of
nfected burns.

Antibacterial preparations also used systemically

Fusidic acid is a narrow-spectrum antibacterial used for
staphylococcal infections.

An ointment containing fusidic acid is used in the fissures
of angular cheilitis when associated with staphylococcal
nfection. See Oropharyngeal fungal infections p. 1262 for
further information on angular cheilitis.

Metronidazole p. 1275 is used topically for rosacea and to
reduce the odour associated with anaerobic infections; oral
metronidazole is used to treat wounds infected with
anaerobic bacteria.

Antifungal preparations for the skin

Most localised fungal infections are treated with topical
preparations. To prevent relapse, local antifungal treatment
should be continued for 1–2 weeks after the disappearance
of all signs of infection. Systemic therapy is necessary for
scalp infection or if the skin infection is widespread,
disseminated, or intractable; although topical therapy may
be used to treat some nail infections, systemic therapy is
more effective. Skin scrapings should be examined if
systemic therapy is being considered or where there is doubt
about the diagnosis.

Dermatophytoses

Ringworm infection can affect the scalp (tinea capitis), body
(tinea corporis), groin (tinea cruris), hand (tinea manuum),
foot (tinea pedis, athlete's foot), or nail (tinea unguium).
Scalp infection requires systemic treatment; additional
application of a topical antifungal, during the early stages of
treatment, may reduce the risk of transmission. A topical
antifungal can also be used to treat asymptomatic carriers of
scalp ringworm. Most other local ringworm infections can be
treated adequately with topical antifungal preparations
(including shampoos). The imidazole antifungals
clotrimazole p. 1276, econazole nitrate p. 1277,
ketoconazole p. 1277, and miconazole p. 1277 are all
effective. Terbinafine cream p. 1279 is also effective but it is
more expensive. Other topical antifungals include
griseofulvin p. 1278 and the undecenoates. **Compound
benzoic acid ointment** (Whitfield's ointment) has been
used for ringworm infections but it is cosmetically less
acceptable than proprietary preparations. Topical
preparations for athlete's foot containing **tolnaftate** are on
sale to the public.

Antifungal dusting powders are of little therapeutic value in
the treatment of fungal skin infections and may cause skin
irritation; they may have some role in preventing reinfection.

Antifungal treatment may not be necessary in
asymptomatic patients with tinea infection of the nails. If
treatment is necessary, a systemic antifungal is more
effective than topical therapy. However, topical application
of amorolfine p. 1278 or tioconazole p. 1278 may be useful
for treating early onychomycosis when involvement is
limited to mild distal disease, or for superficial white
onychomycosis, or where there are contra-indications to
systemic therapy.

Pityriasis versicolor

Pityriasis (tinea) versicolor can be treated with ketoconazole
shampoo. Alternatively, **selenium sulfide** shampoo
[unlicensed indication] can be used as a lotion (diluting with
a small amount of water can reduce irritation) and left on the
affected area for 10 minutes before rinsing off; it should be
applied once daily for 7 days, and the course repeated if
necessary.

Topical imidazole antifungals such as clotrimazole,
econazole nitrate, ketoconazole, and miconazole, or topical
terbinafine are alternatives, but large quantities may be
required.

If topical therapy fails, or if the infection is widespread,
pityriasis versicolor is treated systemically with a triazole
antifungal. Relapse is common, especially in the
immunocompromised.

Candidiasis

Candidal skin infections can be treated with a topical
imidazole antifungal, such as clotrimazole, econazole
nitrate, ketoconazole, or miconazole; topical terbinafine is
an alternative. Topical application of nystatin p. 1263 is also
effective for candidiasis but it is ineffective against
dermatophytosis. Refractory candidiasis requires systemic
treatment generally with a triazole such as fluconazole
p. 634; systemic treatment with terbinafine is **not
appropriate** for refractory candidiasis.

Angular cheilitis

Miconazole cream is used in the fissures of angular cheilitis
when associated with *Candida*.

Compound topical preparations

Combination of an imidazole and a mild corticosteroid (such
as hydrocortisone 1% p. 1291) may be of value in the
treatment of eczematous intertrigo and, in the first few days
only, of a severely inflamed patch of ringworm.

Combination of a mild corticosteroid with either an
imidazole or nystatin may be of use in the treatment of
intertrigo associated with candida.

Antiviral preparations for the skin

Aciclovir cream p. 1282 is licensed for the treatment of initial
and recurrent labial and genital *herpes simplex infections*;
treatment should begin as early as possible. Systemic
treatment is necessary for buccal or vaginal infections and
for *herpes zoster* (*shingles*).

Herpes labialis

Aciclovir cream can be used for the treatment of initial and
recurrent labial herpes simplex infections (cold sores). It is
best applied at the earliest possible stage, usually when
prodromal changes of sensation are felt in the lip and before
vesicles appear.

Penciclovir cream is also licensed for the treatment of
herpes labialis; it needs to be applied more frequently than
aciclovir cream p. 1282.

Systemic treatment is necessary if cold sores recur
frequently or for infections in the mouth.

13

Skin

Parasiticidal preparations for the skin

Suitable quantities of parasiticidal preparations

Area of body	Skin creams	Lotions	Cream rinses
Scalp (head lice)		50–100 mL	50–100 mL
Body (scabies)	30–60 g	100 mL	
Body (crab lice)	30–60 g	100 mL	

These amounts are usually suitable for an adult for single application.

Scabies

Permethrin p. 1281 is used for the treatment of *scabies* (*Sarcoptes scabiei*); malathion p. 1281 can be used if permethrin is inappropriate.

Benzyl benzoate p. 1280 is an irritant and should be avoided in children; it is less effective than malathion and permethrin.

Ivermectin p. 643 (available on a named patient basis from 'special-order' manufacturers or specialist importing companies) by mouth has been used, in combination with topical drugs, for the treatment of hyperkeratotic (crusted or 'Norwegian') scabies that does not respond to topical treatment alone; further doses may be required.

Application

Although acaricides have traditionally been applied after a hot bath, this is **not** necessary and there is even evidence that a hot bath may increase absorption into the blood, removing them from their site of action on the skin.

All members of the affected household should be treated simultaneously. Treatment should be applied to the whole body including the scalp, neck, face, and ears. Particular attention should be paid to the webs of the fingers and toes and lotion brushed under the ends of nails. It is now recommended that malathion and permethrin should be applied twice, one week apart; in the case of benzyl benzoate in adults, up to 3 applications on consecutive days may be needed. It is important to warn users to reapply treatment to the hands if they are washed. Patients with hyperkeratotic scabies may require 2 or 3 applications of acaricide on consecutive days to ensure that enough penetrates the skin crusts to kill all the mites.

Itching

The *itch* and *eczema* of scabies persists for some weeks after the infestation has been eliminated and treatment for pruritus and eczema may be required. Application of crotamiton p. 1309 can be used to control itching after treatment with more effective acaricides. A topical corticosteroid may help to reduce itch and inflammation after scabies has been treated successfully; however, persistent symptoms suggest that scabies eradication was not successful. Oral administration of a **sedating antihistamine** at night may also be useful.

Head lice

Dimeticone p. 1281 is effective against head lice (*Pediculus humanus capitis*). It coats head lice and interferes with water balance in lice by preventing the excretion of water; it is less active against eggs and treatment should be repeated after 7 days. Malathion, an organophosphorus insecticide, is an alternative, but resistance has been reported. Benzyl benzoate is licensed for the treatment of head lice but it is less effective than other drugs and not recommended for use in children. Permethrin is active against head lice but the formulation and licensed methods of application of the current products make them unsuitable for the treatment of head lice.

Head lice infestation (pediculosis) should be treated using lotion or liquid formulations only if live lice are present. Shampoos are diluted too much in use to be effective. A contact time of 8–12 hours or overnight treatment is recommended for lotions and liquids; a 2-hour treatment is not sufficient to kill eggs.

In general, a course of treatment for head lice should be 2 applications of product 7 days apart to kill lice emerging from any eggs that survive the first application. All affected household members should be treated simultaneously.

MHRA/CHM advice: Head lice eradication products: risk of serious burns if treated hair is exposed to open flames or other sources of ignition (March 2018)

Some products for the eradication of head lice infestations are combustible/flammable when on the hair and can ignite and cause serious harm in the presence of an open flame or other source of ignition such as when lighting cigarettes.

Patients and carers should be advised on the safe and correct use of head lice eradication treatments and if appropriate, should be advised that they should not smoke around treated hair and that it should be kept away from open flames or other sources of ignition, including in the morning after overnight application until hair is washed.

Wet combing

Head lice can be mechanically removed by combing wet hair meticulously with a plastic detection comb (probably for at least 30 minutes each time) over the whole scalp at 4-day intervals for a minimum of 2 weeks, and continued until no lice are found on 3 consecutive sessions; hair conditioner or vegetable oil can be used to facilitate the process.

Several devices for the removal of head lice such as combs and topical solutions, are available and some are prescribable on the NHS.

The Drug Tariffs can be accessed online at:

- National Health Service Drug Tariff for England and Wales: www.ppa.org.uk/ppa/edt_intro.htm
- Health and Personal Social Services for Northern Ireland Drug Tariff: www.hscbusiness.hscni.net/services/2034.htm
- Scottish Drug Tariff: www.isdscotland.org/Health-topics/Prescribing-and-Medicines/Scottish-Drug-Tariff/

Crab lice

Permethrin and malathion are used to eliminate *crab lice* (*Pthirus pubis*). An aqueous preparation should be applied, allowed to dry naturally and washed off after 12 hours; a second treatment is needed after 7 days to kill lice emerging from surviving eggs. All surfaces of the body should be treated, including the scalp, neck, and face (paying particular attention to the eyebrows and other facial hair). A different insecticide should be used if a course of treatment fails.

2.1 Bacterial skin infections

ANTIBACTERIALS › AMINOGLYCOSIDES

Neomycin sulfate

- **INDICATIONS AND DOSE**

Bacterial skin infections

▸ TO THE SKIN
  ▸ Child: Apply up to 3 times a day, for short-term use only
  ▸ Adult: Apply up to 3 times a day, for short-term use only

- UNLICENSED USE
▸ In children *Neomycin Cream BPC*—no information available.

- CONTRA-INDICATIONS Neonates

- CAUTIONS
  Large areas
▸ In adults If large areas of skin are being treated ototoxicity may be a hazard, particularly in the elderly, and in those with renal impairment.

In children If large areas of skin are being treated ototoxicity may be a hazard in children, particularly in those with renal impairment.

- INTERACTIONS → Appendix 1: neomycin
- SIDE-EFFECTS Sensitisation (cross sensitivity with other aminoglycosides may occur)
- RENAL IMPAIRMENT Ototoxicity may be a hazard if large areas of skin are treated.
- LESS SUITABLE FOR PRESCRIBING Neomycin sulfate cream is less suitable for prescribing.

- MEDICINAL FORMS Forms available from special-order manufacturers include: cream

ANTIBACTERIALS > NITROIMIDAZOLE DERIVATIVES

▌Metronidazole
24-Nov-2020

- DRUG ACTION Metronidazole is an antimicrobial drug with high activity against anaerobic bacteria and protozoa.

- INDICATIONS AND DOSE

ACEA ®
Acute inflammatory exacerbation of rosacea
▸ TO THE SKIN
▸ Adult: Apply twice daily for 8 weeks, to be applied thinly

ANABACT ®
Malodorous fungating tumours and malodorous gravitational and decubitus ulcers
▸ TO THE SKIN
▸ Adult: Apply 1–2 times a day, to be applied to clean wound and covered with non-adherent dressing

METROGEL ®
Acute inflammatory exacerbation of rosacea
▸ TO THE SKIN
▸ Adult: Apply twice daily for 8–9 weeks, to be applied thinly

Malodorous fungating tumours
▸ TO THE SKIN
▸ Adult: Apply 1–2 times a day, to be applied to clean wound and covered with non-adherent dressing

METROSA ®
Acute exacerbation of rosacea
▸ TO THE SKIN
▸ Adult: Apply twice daily for up to 8 weeks, to be applied thinly

ROSICED ®
Inflammatory papules and pustules of rosacea
▸ TO THE SKIN
▸ Adult: Apply twice daily for 6 weeks (longer if necessary)

ROZEX ® CREAM
Inflammatory papules, pustules and erythema of rosacea
▸ TO THE SKIN
▸ Adult: Apply twice daily for 3–4 months

ROZEX ® GEL
Inflammatory papules, pustules and erythema of rosacea
▸ TO THE SKIN
▸ Adult: Apply twice daily for 3–4 months

ZYOMET ®
Acute inflammatory exacerbation of rosacea
▸ TO THE SKIN
▸ Adult: Apply twice daily for 8–9 weeks, to be applied thinly

- CAUTIONS Avoid exposure to strong sunlight or UV light

- INTERACTIONS → Appendix 1: metronidazole
- SIDE-EFFECTS
▸ Common or very common Skin reactions

- MEDICINAL FORMS There can be variation in the licensing of different medicines containing the same drug.

Gel
EXCIPIENTS: May contain Benzyl alcohol, disodium edetate, hydroxybenzoates (parabens), propylene glycol
▸ Acea (Ferndale Pharmaceuticals Ltd)
  Metronidazole 7.5 mg per 1 gram Acea 0.75% gel | 40 gram PoM £9.95 DT = £22.63
▸ Anabact (Cambridge Healthcare Supplies Ltd)
  Metronidazole 7.5 mg per 1 gram Anabact 0.75% gel | 15 gram PoM £5.64 DT = £5.64 | 30 gram PoM £7.89 | 40 gram PoM £15.89 DT = £22.63
▸ Metrogel (Galderma (UK) Ltd)
  Metronidazole 7.5 mg per 1 gram Metrogel 0.75% gel | 40 gram PoM £22.63 DT = £22.63
▸ Metrosa (M & A Pharmachem Ltd)
  Metronidazole 7.5 mg per 1 gram Metrosa 0.75% gel | 30 gram PoM £12.00 | 40 gram PoM £19.90 DT = £22.63
▸ Rozex (Galderma (UK) Ltd)
  Metronidazole 7.5 mg per 1 gram Rozex 0.75% gel | 30 gram PoM £6.60 | 40 gram PoM £9.88 DT = £22.63
▸ Zyomet (Advanz Pharma)
  Metronidazole 7.5 mg per 1 gram Zyomet 0.75% gel | 30 gram PoM £12.00

Cream
EXCIPIENTS: May contain Benzyl alcohol, isopropyl palmitate, propylene glycol
▸ Rosiced (Pierre Fabre Dermo-Cosmetique)
  Metronidazole 7.5 mg per 1 gram Rosiced 0.75% cream | 30 gram PoM £6.60 DT = £6.60
▸ Rozex (Galderma (UK) Ltd)
  Metronidazole 7.5 mg per 1 gram Rozex 0.75% cream | 30 gram PoM £6.60 DT = £6.60 | 40 gram PoM £9.88 DT = £9.88

ANTIBACTERIALS > SULFONAMIDES

▌Silver sulfadiazine
14-Dec-2020

- INDICATIONS AND DOSE
Prophylaxis and treatment of infection in burn wounds
▸ TO THE SKIN
▸ Child: Apply daily, may be applied more frequently if very exudative
▸ Adult: Apply daily, may be applied more frequently if very exudative

For conservative management of finger-tip injuries
▸ TO THE SKIN
▸ Child: Apply every 2–3 days, consult product literature for details
▸ Adult: Apply every 2–3 days, consult product literature for details

Adjunct to prophylaxis of infection in skin graft donor sites and extensive abrasions
▸ TO THE SKIN
▸ Adult: (consult product literature)

Adjunct to short-term treatment of infection in pressure sores
▸ TO THE SKIN
▸ Adult: Apply once daily or on alternate days

As an adjunct to short-term treatment of infection in leg ulcers
▸ TO THE SKIN
▸ Adult: Apply once daily or on alternate days, not recommended if ulcer is very exudative

- UNLICENSED USE
▸ In children No age range specified by manufacturer.
- CONTRA-INDICATIONS Not recommended for neonates
- CAUTIONS G6PD deficiency

13

Skin

CAUTIONS, FURTHER INFORMATION
▶ **Large areas** Plasma-sulfadiazine concentrations may approach therapeutic levels with *side-effects* and *interactions* as for sulfonamides if large areas of skin are treated.

● INTERACTIONS → Appendix 1: silver sulfadiazine

● SIDE-EFFECTS
▶ **Common or very common** Leucopenia · skin reactions
▶ **Rare or very rare** Argyria (following treatment of large areas of skin or long term use) · renal failure

SIDE-EFFECTS, FURTHER INFORMATION Leucopenia developing 2–3 days after starting treatment of burns patients is reported usually to be self-limiting and silver sulfadiazine need not usually be discontinued provided blood counts are monitored carefully to ensure return to normality within a few days.

● ALLERGY AND CROSS-SENSITIVITY EvGr Caution in patients with sensitivity to sulfonamides. ⓜ See, *Cautions, further information.*

● PREGNANCY Risk of neonatal haemolysis and methaemoglobinaemia in third trimester.

● BREAST FEEDING Small risk of kernicterus in jaundiced infants and of haemolysis in G6PD-deficient infants.

● HEPATIC IMPAIRMENT Manufacturer advises caution in significant hepatic impairment.

● RENAL IMPAIRMENT Manufacturer advises caution if significant impairment.

● MONITORING REQUIREMENTS Monitor for leucopenia.

● DIRECTIONS FOR ADMINISTRATION Manufacturer advises apply with sterile applicator.

● MEDICINAL FORMS There can be variation in the licensing of different medicines containing the same drug.
Cream
EXCIPIENTS: May contain Cetostearyl alcohol (including cetyl and stearyl alcohol), polysorbates, propylene glycol
▶ Flamazine (Smith & Nephew Healthcare Ltd)
Sulfadiazine silver 10 mg per 1 gram Flamazine 1% cream | 50 gram PoM £3.85 DT = £3.85 | 250 gram PoM £10.32 DT = £10.32 | 500 gram PoM £18.27 DT = £18.27

ANTIBACTERIALS > OTHER

Mupirocin

18-May-2020

● INDICATIONS AND DOSE

Bacterial skin infections, particularly those caused by Gram-positive organisms (except pseudomonal infection)
▶ TO THE SKIN
▶ **Child:** Apply up to 3 times a day for up to 10 days
▶ **Adult:** Apply up to 3 times a day for up to 10 days

Non-bullous impetigo [in patients who are not systemically unwell or at high risk of complications]
▶ TO THE SKIN
▶ **Child:** Apply 3 times a day for 5–7 days
▶ **Adult:** Apply 3 times a day for 5–7 days

● UNLICENSED USE
▶ In children Mupirocin ointment licensed for use in children (age range not specified by manufacturer). *Bactroban*® cream not recommended for use in children under 1 year.

● SIDE-EFFECTS
▶ **Common or very common** Skin reactions

● PREGNANCY Manufacturer advises avoid unless potential benefit outweighs risk—no information available.

● BREAST FEEDING No information available.

● RENAL IMPAIRMENT Manufacturer advises caution when mupirocin ointment used in moderate or severe

impairment because it contains macrogols (polyethylene glycol).

● PRESCRIBING AND DISPENSING INFORMATION For choice of antibacterial therapy, see Skin infections, antibacterial therapy p. 541.

● MEDICINAL FORMS There can be variation in the licensing of different medicines containing the same drug.
Ointment
▶ Mupirocin (Non-proprietary)
Mupirocin 20 mg per 1 gram Mupirocin 2% ointment | 15 gram PoM £12.50 DT = £5.26
▶ Bactroban (GlaxoSmithKline UK Ltd)
Mupirocin 20 mg per 1 gram Bactroban 2% ointment | 15 gram PoM £5.26 DT = £5.26
Cream
EXCIPIENTS: May contain Benzyl alcohol, cetostearyl alcohol (including cetyl and stearyl alcohol)
▶ Bactroban (GlaxoSmithKline UK Ltd)
Mupirocin (as Mupirocin calcium) 20 mg per 1 gram Bactroban 2% cream | 15 gram PoM £5.26 DT = £5.26

2.2 Fungal skin infections

Other drugs used for Fungal skin infections
Hydrocortisone with clotrimazole, p. 1295

ANTIFUNGALS > IMIDAZOLE ANTIFUNGALS

Clotrimazole

10-Mar-2020

● INDICATIONS AND DOSE

Fungal skin infections
▶ TO THE SKIN
▶ **Child:** Apply 2–3 times a day
▶ **Adult:** Apply 2–3 times a day

● CAUTIONS Contact with eyes and mucous membranes should be avoided

● INTERACTIONS → Appendix 1: antifungals, azoles

● SIDE-EFFECTS Oedema · pain · paraesthesia · skin reactions

● PREGNANCY Minimal absorption from skin; not known to be harmful.

● PRESCRIBING AND DISPENSING INFORMATION Spray may be useful for application of clotrimazole to large or hairy areas of the skin.

● PATIENT AND CARER ADVICE
Medicines for Children leaflet: Clotrimazole for fungal infections www.medicinesforchildren.org.uk/clotrimazole-fungal-infections

● MEDICINAL FORMS There can be variation in the licensing of different medicines containing the same drug.
Cream
EXCIPIENTS: May contain Benzyl alcohol, cetostearyl alcohol (including cetyl and stearyl alcohol), polysorbates
▶ Clotrimazole (Non-proprietary)
Clotrimazole 10 mg per 1 gram Clotrimazole 1% cream | 20 gram P £1.80 DT = £1.38 | 50 gram P £3.67 DT = £3.45
▶ Canesten (clotrimazole) (Bayer Plc)
Clotrimazole 10 mg per 1 gram Canesten 1% cream | 20 gram P £2.20 DT = £1.38 | 50 gram P £3.64 DT = £3.45
Canesten Antifungal 1% cream | 20 gram P £1.85 DT = £1.38
Clotrimazole 20 mg per 1 gram Canesten 2% thrush cream | 20 gram P £4.76 DT = £4.76
Clotrimazole 100 mg per 1 gram Canesten 10% VC cream | 5 gram PoM £4.50 DT = £6.23

Liquid
▶ Canesten (clotrimazole) (Bayer Plc)
  Clotrimazole 10 mg per 1 ml Canesten 1% solution | 20 ml Ⓟ
  £2.53 DT = £2.53

Combinations available: *Hydrocortisone with clotrimazole,*
p. 1295

Econazole nitrate
08-May-2020

● **INDICATIONS AND DOSE**

Fungal skin infections
▶ TO THE SKIN
▶ Child: Apply twice daily
▶ Adult: Apply twice daily

Fungal nail infections
▶ BY TRANSUNGUAL APPLICATION
▶ Child: Apply once daily, applied under occlusive
  dressing
▶ Adult: Apply once daily, applied under occlusive
  dressing

● CAUTIONS Avoid contact with eyes and mucous
  membranes

● SIDE-EFFECTS
▶ **Common or very common** Pain · skin reactions
▶ **Uncommon** Swelling
▶ **Frequency not known** Angioedema

  SIDE-EFFECTS, FURTHER INFORMATION Treatment should
  be discontinued if side-effects are severe.

● PREGNANCY Minimal absorption from skin; not known to
  be harmful.

● PRESCRIBING AND DISPENSING INFORMATION *Pevaryl*® 1%
  cream should be used.

● MEDICINAL FORMS There can be variation in the licensing of
  different medicines containing the same drug.

Cream
EXCIPIENTS: May contain Butylated hydroxyanisole, fragrances
▶ Gyno-Pevaryl (Janssen-Cilag Ltd)
  Econazole nitrate 10 mg per 1 gram Gyno-Pevaryl 1% cream |
  30 gram PoM £3.78 DT = £3.78

Ketoconazole
04-Feb-2020

● **INDICATIONS AND DOSE**

Tinea pedis
▶ TO THE SKIN USING CREAM
▶ Adult: Apply twice daily

Fungal skin infection (not Tinea pedis)
▶ TO THE SKIN USING CREAM
▶ Adult: Apply 1–2 times a day

Treatment of seborrhoeic dermatitis and dandruff
▶ TO THE SKIN USING SHAMPOO
▶ Child 12–17 years: Apply twice weekly for 2–4 weeks,
  leave preparation on for 3–5 minutes before rinsing
▶ Adult: Apply twice weekly for 2–4 weeks, leave
  preparation on for 3–5 minutes before rinsing

Prophylaxis of seborrhoeic dermatitis and dandruff
▶ TO THE SKIN USING SHAMPOO
▶ Child 12–17 years: Apply every 1–2 weeks, leave
  preparation on for 3–5 minutes before rinsing
▶ Adult: Apply every 1–2 weeks, leave preparation on for
  3–5 minutes before rinsing

Treatment of pityriasis versicolor
▶ TO THE SKIN USING SHAMPOO
▶ Child 12–17 years: Apply once daily for maximum 5 days,
  leave preparation on for 3–5 minutes before rinsing
▶ Adult: Apply once daily for maximum 5 days, leave
  preparation on for 3–5 minutes before rinsing

Prophylaxis of pityriasis versicolor
▶ TO THE SKIN USING SHAMPOO
▶ Child 12–17 years: Apply once daily for up to 3 days
  before sun exposure, leave preparation on for
  3–5 minutes before rinsing
▶ Adult: Apply once daily for up to 3 days before sun
  exposure, leave preparation on for 3–5 minutes before
  rinsing

● CONTRA-INDICATIONS Acute porphyrias p. 1107

● CAUTIONS Avoid contact with eyes · avoid contact with
  mucous membranes

● INTERACTIONS → Appendix 1: antifungals, azoles

● SIDE-EFFECTS
▶ **Common or very common** Skin reactions
▶ **Uncommon** Alopecia · angioedema · excessive tearing ·
  folliculitis · hair changes
▶ **Rare or very rare** Eye irritation · taste altered

● NATIONAL FUNDING/ACCESS DECISIONS
  NHS restrictions *Nizoral*® cream is not prescribable in NHS
  primary care except for the treatment of seborrhoeic
  dermatitis and pityriasis versicolor; endorse prescription
  'SLS'.

● EXCEPTIONS TO LEGAL CATEGORY
  A 15-g tube is available for sale to the public for the
  treatment of tinea pedis, tinea cruris, and candidal
  intertrigo.
    Can be sold to the public for the prevention and
  treatment of dandruff and seborrhoeic dermatitis of the
  scalp as a shampoo formulation containing ketoconazole
  maximum 2%, in a pack containing maximum 120 mL and
  labelled to show a maximum frequency of application of
  once every 3 days.

● MEDICINAL FORMS There can be variation in the licensing of
  different medicines containing the same drug.

Cream
EXCIPIENTS: May contain Cetostearyl alcohol (including cetyl and
stearyl alcohol), polysorbates, propylene glycol
▶ Nizoral (Janssen-Cilag Ltd)
  Ketoconazole 20 mg per 1 gram Nizoral 2% cream | 30 gram PoM
  £4.24 DT = £4.24

Shampoo
EXCIPIENTS: May contain Imidurea
▶ Ketoconazole (Non-proprietary)
  Ketoconazole 20 mg per 1 gram Ketoconazole 2% shampoo |
  120 ml PoM £5.62 DT = £5.62
▶ Dandrazol (Transdermal Ltd)
  Ketoconazole 20 mg per 1 gram Dandrazol 2% shampoo |
  120 ml PoM £3.39 DT = £5.62
▶ Nizoral (Thornton & Ross Ltd)
  Ketoconazole 20 mg per 1 gram Nizoral 2% shampoo |
  120 ml PoM £3.59 DT = £5.62

Miconazole
24-Jul-2020

● **INDICATIONS AND DOSE**

Fungal skin infections
▶ TO THE SKIN
▶ Child: Apply twice daily continuing for 10 days after
  lesions have healed
▶ Adult: Apply twice daily continuing for 10 days after
  lesions have healed

Fungal nail infections
▶ TO THE SKIN
▶ Child: Apply 1–2 times a day
▶ Adult: Apply 1–2 times a day

● UNLICENSED USE
▶ In children Licensed for use in children (age range not
  specified by manufacturer).

- **CAUTIONS** Avoid in Acute porphyrias p. 1107 · contact with eyes and mucous membranes should be avoided
- **INTERACTIONS** → Appendix 1: antifungals, azoles
- **SIDE-EFFECTS**
- **Common or very common** Skin reactions
- **Frequency not known** Angioedema
- **PREGNANCY** Absorbed from the skin in small amounts; manufacturer advises caution.
- **BREAST FEEDING** Manufacturer advises caution—no information available.
- **PROFESSION SPECIFIC INFORMATION**
  Dental practitioners' formulary
  Miconazole cream may be prescribed.
- **NATIONAL FUNDING/ACCESS DECISIONS**
  NHS restrictions *Daktarin*® powder and *Daktarin*® cream 15 g is not prescribable in NHS primary care.

- **MEDICINAL FORMS** There can be variation in the licensing of different medicines containing the same drug.
  Cream
  EXCIPIENTS: May contain Butylated hydroxyanisole
  - Daktarin (McNeil Products Ltd, Janssen-Cilag Ltd, Johnson & Johnson Ltd)
    Miconazole nitrate 20 mg per 1 gram Daktarin 2% cream | 15 gram P £2.66 | 30 gram P £1.82 DT = £1.82
  - Gyno-Daktarin (Janssen-Cilag Ltd)
    Miconazole nitrate 20 mg per 1 gram Gyno-Daktarin 2% vaginal cream | 78 gram PoM £4.33 DT = £4.33
  Powder
  - Daktarin (McNeil Products Ltd)
    Miconazole nitrate 20 mg per 1 gram Daktarin 2% powder | 20 gram P £3.13 DT = £3.13

Tioconazole

03-Feb-2020

- **INDICATIONS AND DOSE**
  Fungal nail infection
  - BY TRANSUNGUAL APPLICATION
  - Child: Apply twice daily usually for up to 6 months (may be extended to 12 months), apply to nails and surrounding skin
  - Adult: Apply twice daily usually for up to 6 months (may be extended to 12 months), apply to nails and surrounding skin

- **UNLICENSED USE**
  - In children Licensed for use in children (age range not specified by manufacturer).
- **CAUTIONS** Contact with eyes and mucous membranes should be avoided · use with caution if child likely to suck affected digits (in children)
- **SIDE-EFFECTS**
- **Common or very common** Peripheral oedema
- **Uncommon** Skin reactions
- **Frequency not known** Nail disorder · pain · paraesthesia · periorbital oedema
- **PREGNANCY** Manufacturer advises avoid.

- **MEDICINAL FORMS** There can be variation in the licensing of different medicines containing the same drug.
  Paint
  - Tioconazole (Non-proprietary)
    Tioconazole 283 mg per 1 ml Tioconazole 283mg/ml medicated nail lacquer | 12 ml PoM £28.74 DT = £28.74
  - Trosyl (Pfizer Ltd)
    Tioconazole 283 mg per 1 ml Trosyl 283mg/ml nail solution | 12 ml PoM £27.38 DT = £28.74

ANTIFUNGALS > OTHER

Amorolfine

06-Oct-2020

- **INDICATIONS AND DOSE**
  Fungal nail infections
  - BY TRANSUNGUAL APPLICATION
  - Child 12–17 years: Apply 1–2 times a week for 6 months to treat finger nails and for toe nails 9–12 months (review at intervals of 3 months), apply to infected nails after filing and cleansing, allow to dry for approximately 3 minutes
  - Adult: Apply 1–2 times a week for 6 months to treat finger nails and for toe nails 9–12 months (review at intervals of 3 months), apply to infected nails after filing and cleansing, allow to dry for approximately 3 minutes

- **CAUTIONS** Avoid contact with ears · avoid contact with eyes and mucous membranes · use with caution in child likely to suck affected digits
- **SIDE-EFFECTS**
- **Rare or very rare** Nail discolouration · skin reactions
- **PATIENT AND CARER ADVICE** Cosmetic nail varnish may be applied at least 10 minutes after amorolfine nail lacquer; the nail varnish should be removed before repeat application of amorolfine. Avoid artificial nails during treatment.
- **EXCEPTIONS TO LEGAL CATEGORY**
  - In adults Amorolfine nail lacquer can be sold to the public if supplied for the treatment of mild cases of distal and lateral subungual onychomycoses caused by dermatophytes, yeasts and moulds; subject to treatment of max. 2 nails, max. strength of nail lacquer amorolfine 5% and a pack size of 3 mL.

- **MEDICINAL FORMS** There can be variation in the licensing of different medicines containing the same drug.
  Medicated nail lacquer
  CAUTIONARY AND ADVISORY LABELS 10
  - Amorolfine (Non-proprietary)
    Amorolfine (as Amorolfine hydrochloride) 50 mg per 1 ml Amorolfine 5% medicated nail lacquer | 5 ml PoM £16.21 DT = £7.96
  - Loceryl (Galderma (UK) Ltd)
    Amorolfine (as Amorolfine hydrochloride) 50 mg per 1 ml Loceryl 5% medicated nail lacquer | 5 ml PoM £9.08 DT = £7.96
  - Omicur (Morningside Healthcare Ltd)
    Amorolfine (as Amorolfine hydrochloride) 50 mg per 1 ml Omicur 5% medicated nail lacquer | 2.5 ml PoM £9.09 | 5 ml PoM £9.09 DT = £7.96

Griseofulvin

16-Jan-2020

- **INDICATIONS AND DOSE**
  Tinea pedis
  - TO THE SKIN
  - Adult: Apply 400 micrograms once daily, apply to an area approximately 13 cm^2; increased if necessary to 1.2 mg once daily for maximum treatment duration of 4 weeks, allow each spray to dry between application

- **CAUTIONS** Avoid contact with eyes and mucous membranes
- **INTERACTIONS** → Appendix 1: griseofulvin
- **SIDE-EFFECTS** Paraesthesia · skin irritation
- **PREGNANCY** Manufacturer advises avoid unless potential benefit outweighs risk.
- **BREAST FEEDING** Manufacturer advises avoid unless potential benefit outweighs risk.

» MEDICINAL FORMS There can be variation in the licensing of different medicines containing the same drug.

Spray

CAUTIONARY AND ADVISORY LABELS 15
EXCIPIENTS: May contain Benzyl alcohol
▸ Grisol (Transdermal Ltd)
Griseofulvin 10 mg per 1 gram Grisol 1% spray | 20 ml GSL £9.60
DT = £4.50

Terbinafine

12-May-2020

● INDICATIONS AND DOSE

Tinea pedis
▸ TO THE SKIN USING CREAM
▸ Adult: Apply 1–2 times a day for up to 1 week, to be applied thinly
▸ BY MOUTH USING TABLETS
▸ Adult: 250 mg once daily for 2-6 weeks

Tinea corporis
▸ TO THE SKIN USING CREAM
▸ Adult: Apply 1–2 times a day for up to 1–2 weeks, to be applied thinly, review treatment after 2 weeks
▸ BY MOUTH USING TABLETS
▸ Adult: 250 mg once daily for 4 weeks

Tinea cruris
▸ TO THE SKIN USING CREAM
▸ Adult: Apply 1–2 times a day for up to 1–2 weeks, to be applied thinly, review treatment after 2 weeks
▸ BY MOUTH USING TABLETS
▸ Adult: 250 mg once daily for 2-4 weeks

Dermatophyte infections of the nails
▸ BY MOUTH USING TABLETS
▸ Adult: 250 mg once daily for 6 weeks-3 months (occasionally longer in toenail infections)

Cutaneous candidiasis | Pityriasis versicolor
▸ TO THE SKIN USING CREAM
▸ Adult: Apply 1–2 times a day for 2 weeks, to be applied thinly, review treatment after 2 weeks

● CAUTIONS
▸ With oral use Psoriasis (risk of exacerbation) · risk of lupus erythematosus
▸ With topical use contact with eyes and mucous membranes should be avoided

● INTERACTIONS → Appendix 1: terbinafine

● SIDE-EFFECTS

GENERAL SIDE-EFFECTS
▸ **Common or very common** Skin reactions

SPECIFIC SIDE-EFFECTS
▸ **Common or very common**
▸ With oral use Appetite decreased · arthralgia · diarrhoea · gastrointestinal discomfort · gastrointestinal disorder · headache · myalgia · nausea
▸ **Uncommon**
▸ With oral use Taste altered
▸ With topical use Pain
▸ **Rare or very rare**
▸ With oral use Agranulocytosis · alopecia · cutaneous lupus erythematosus · dizziness · hepatic disorders · malaise · neutropenia · photosensitivity reaction · sensation abnormal · severe cutaneous adverse reactions (SCARs) · systemic lupus erythematosus (SLE) · thrombocytopenia · vertigo
▸ **Frequency not known**
▸ With oral use Anaemia · anxiety · depressive symptom · fatigue · fever · hearing impairment · influenza like illness · pancreatitis · pancytopenia · rhabdomyolysis · serum sickness-like reaction · smell altered · tinnitus · vasculitis · vision disorders
▸ With topical use Hypersensitivity

SIDE-EFFECTS, FURTHER INFORMATION
Liver toxicity With oral use; discontinue treatment if liver toxicity develops (including jaundice, cholestasis and hepatitis).
 Serious skin reactions With oral use; discontinue treatment in progressive skin rash (including Stevens-Johnson syndrome and toxic epidermal necrolysis).

● PREGNANCY
▸ With topical use Manufacturer advises use only if potential benefit outweighs risk— *animal* studies suggest no adverse effects.
▸ With oral use Manufacturer advises use only if potential benefit outweighs risk—no information available.

● BREAST FEEDING
▸ With topical use Manufacturer advises avoid—present in milk. Less than 5% of the dose is absorbed after topical application of terbinafine; avoid application to mother's chest.
▸ With oral use Avoid—present in milk.

● HEPATIC IMPAIRMENT
▸ With oral use Manufacturer advises avoid (risk of increased exposure).

● RENAL IMPAIRMENT
Dose adjustments ▸ With oral use Use half normal dose if eGFR less than 50 mL/minute/1.73 m^2 and no suitable alternative available.

● MONITORING REQUIREMENTS
▸ With oral use Monitor hepatic function before treatment and then periodically after 4–6 weeks of treatment—discontinue if abnormalities in liver function tests.

● PATIENT AND CARER ADVICE
▸ With oral use Manufacturer advises that patients should immediately report any signs or symptoms suggestive of liver dysfunction such as pruritus, unexplained persistent nausea, decreased appetite, anorexia, jaundice, vomiting, fatigue, right upper abdominal pain, dark urine, or pale stools. Patients with these symptoms should discontinue taking terbinafine and the patient's liver function should be immediately evaluated.

● EXCEPTIONS TO LEGAL CATEGORY
▸ With topical use Preparations of terbinafine hydrochloride (maximum 1%) can be sold to the public for use in those over 16 years for external use for the treatment of tinea pedis as a cream in a pack containing maximum 15 g, or for the treatment of tinea pedis and cruris as a cream in a pack containing maximum 15 g, or for the treatment of tinea pedis, cruris, and corporis as a spray in a pack containing maximum 30 mL spray or as a gel in a pack containing maximum 30 g gel.

● MEDICINAL FORMS There can be variation in the licensing of different medicines containing the same drug.

Tablet

CAUTIONARY AND ADVISORY LABELS 9
▸ Terbinafine (Non-proprietary)
Terbinafine (as Terbinafine hydrochloride) 250 mg Terbinafine 250mg tablets | 14 tablet PoM £18.11 DT = £1.54 | 28 tablet PoM £3.08–£34.93
▸ Lamisil (Novartis Pharmaceuticals UK Ltd)
Terbinafine (as Terbinafine hydrochloride) 250 mg Lamisil 250mg tablets | 14 tablet PoM £21.30 DT = £1.54 | 28 tablet PoM £41.09

Cream

EXCIPIENTS: May contain Benzyl alcohol, cetostearyl alcohol (including cetyl and stearyl alcohol), polysorbates
▸ Terbinafine (Non-proprietary)
Terbinafine hydrochloride 10 mg per 1 gram Terbinafine 1% cream | 15 gram PoM £3.17 DT = £1.81 | 30 gram PoM £6.33 DT = £3.62
▸ Lamisil (GlaxoSmithKline Consumer Healthcare)
Terbinafine hydrochloride 10 mg per 1 gram Lamisil 1% cream | 30 gram PoM £8.76 DT = £3.62

13

Skin

ANTISEPTICS AND DISINFECTANTS ›
UNDECENOATES

Undecenoic acid with zinc undecenoate

- **INDICATIONS AND DOSE**
Treatment of athletes foot
▸ TO THE SKIN
- Child: Apply twice daily, continue use for 7 days after lesions have healed
- Adult: Apply twice daily, continue use for 7 days after lesions have healed

Prevention of athletes foot
▸ TO THE SKIN
- Child: Apply once daily
- Adult: Apply once daily

- **UNLICENSED USE**
▸ In children *Mycota*® licensed for use in children (age range not specified by manufacturer).
- **CAUTIONS** Avoid broken skin · contact with eyes should be avoided · contact with mucous membranes should be avoided
- **SIDE-EFFECTS**
▸ **Rare or very rare** Skin irritation
SIDE-EFFECTS, FURTHER INFORMATION Treatment should be discontinued if irritation is severe.

- **MEDICINAL FORMS** There can be variation in the licensing of different medicines containing the same drug.
Cream
EXCIPIENTS: May contain Cetostearyl alcohol (including cetyl and stearyl alcohol), fragrances
▸ Mycota (zinc undecenoate / undecenoic acid) (Thornton & Ross Ltd)
Undecenoic acid 50 mg per 1 gram, Zinc undecenoate 200 mg per 1 gram Mycota cream | 25 gram [GSL] £2.01
Powder
EXCIPIENTS: May contain Fragrances
▸ Mycota (zinc undecenoate / undecenoic acid) (Thornton & Ross Ltd)
Undecenoic acid 20 mg per 1 gram, Zinc undecenoate 200 mg per 1 gram Mycota powder | 70 gram [GSL] £3.04 DT = £3.04

ANTISEPTICS AND DISINFECTANTS › OTHER

Chlorhexidine with nystatin

- **INDICATIONS AND DOSE**
Skin infections due to Candida spp.
▸ TO THE SKIN
- Child: Apply 2–3 times a day, continuing for 7 days after lesions have healed
- Adult: Apply 2–3 times a day, continuing for 7 days after lesions have healed

- **UNLICENSED USE**
▸ In children Licensed for use in children (age range not specified by manufacturer).
- **CAUTIONS** Avoid contact with eyes and mucous membranes
- **SIDE-EFFECTS** Hypersensitivity · skin reactions

- **MEDICINAL FORMS** There can be variation in the licensing of different medicines containing the same drug.
Cream
EXCIPIENTS: May contain Benzyl alcohol, cetostearyl alcohol (including cetyl and stearyl alcohol), polysorbates
▸ Chlorhexidine with nystatin (Non-proprietary)
Chlorhexidine hydrochloride 10 mg per 1 gram, Nystatin 100000 unit per 1 gram Nystatin 100,000units/g / Chlorhexidine hydrochloride 1% cream | 30 gram [PoM] £4.99 DT = £4.99

BENZOATES

Benzoic acid with salicylic acid
22-Nov-202

- **INDICATIONS AND DOSE**
Ringworm (tinea)
▸ TO THE SKIN
- Child: Apply twice daily
- Adult: Apply twice daily

- **UNLICENSED USE**
▸ In children Licensed for use in children (age range not specified by manufacturer).
- **CAUTIONS** Avoid broken or inflamed skin · avoid contact with eyes · avoid contact with mucous membranes
CAUTIONS, FURTHER INFORMATION
▸ Salicylate toxicity Salicylate toxicity may occur particularly if applied on large areas of skin.
- **SIDE-EFFECTS** Drug toxicity · eye irritation · mucosal irritation · skin reactions
- **PRESCRIBING AND DISPENSING INFORMATION** Benzoic Acid Ointment, Compound, BP has also been referred to as Whitfield's ointment.

- **MEDICINAL FORMS** Forms available from special-order manufacturers include: cream, ointment

2.3 Parasitic skin infections

Other drugs used for Parasitic skin infections Ivermectin, p. 643

PARASITICIDES

Benzyl benzoate
19-May-2020

- **INDICATIONS AND DOSE**
Scabies
▸ TO THE SKIN
- Adult: Apply over the whole body; repeat without bathing on the following day and wash off 24 hours later; a third application may be required in some cases

- **CAUTIONS** Avoid contact with eyes and mucous membranes · do not use on broken or secondarily infected skin
- **SIDE-EFFECTS** Eye irritation · mucosal irritation · skin irritation
- **BREAST FEEDING** Suspend feeding until product has been washed off.
- **PRESCRIBING AND DISPENSING INFORMATION** When prepared extemporaneously, the BP states Benzyl Benzoate Application, BP consists of benzyl benzoate 25% in an emulsion basis.
  Some manufacturers recommend application to the body but to exclude the head and neck. However, application should be extended to the scalp, neck, face, and ears. Note—dilution to reduce irritant effect also reduces efficacy.
- **LESS SUITABLE FOR PRESCRIBING** Benzyl benzoate is less suitable for prescribing.

- **MEDICINAL FORMS** Forms available from special-order manufacturers include: liquid

Dimeticone

04-Feb-2020

● **INDICATIONS AND DOSE**

Head lice

▸ TO THE SKIN

▸ Child: Apply once weekly for 2 doses, rub into dry hair and scalp, allow to dry naturally, shampoo after minimum 8 hours (or overnight)

▸ Adult: Apply once weekly for 2 doses, rub into dry hair and scalp, allow to dry naturally, shampoo after minimum 8 hours (or overnight)

● **UNLICENSED USE**
In children Not licensed for use in children under 6 months except under medical supervision.

> **IMPORTANT SAFETY INFORMATION**
> MHRA/CHM ADVICE: HEAD LICE ERADICATION PRODUCTS: RISK OF SERIOUS BURNS IF TREATED HAIR IS EXPOSED TO OPEN FLAMES OR OTHER SOURCES OF IGNITION (MARCH 2018)
> See Skin infections p. 1272.

● **CAUTIONS** Avoid contact with eyes · children under 6 months, medical supervision required

● **SIDE-EFFECTS** Alopecia · dyspnoea · eye irritation · hypersensitivity · scalp changes · skin reactions

● **MEDICINAL FORMS** There can be variation in the licensing of different medicines containing the same drug.

Liquid

▸ Hedrin (Thornton & Ross Ltd)
Dimeticone 40 mg per 1 gram Hedrin 4% lotion | 50 ml ℗ £3.28
DT = £3.28 | 150 ml ℗ £7.62 DT = £7.62

Cutaneous spray solution

▸ Hedrin (Thornton & Ross Ltd)
Dimeticone 40 mg per 1 gram Hedrin 4% spray | 120 ml ℗ £7.85
DT = £7.85

Malathion

04-Feb-2020

● **INDICATIONS AND DOSE**

Head lice

▸ TO THE SKIN

▸ Child: Apply once weekly for 2 doses, rub preparation into dry hair and scalp, allow to dry naturally, remove by washing after 12 hours

▸ Adult: Apply once weekly for 2 doses, rub preparation into dry hair and scalp, allow to dry naturally, remove by washing after 12 hours

Crab lice

▸ TO THE SKIN

▸ Child: Apply once weekly for 2 doses, apply preparation over whole body, allow to dry naturally, wash off after 12 hours or overnight

▸ Adult: Apply once weekly for 2 doses, apply preparation over whole body, allow to dry naturally, wash off after 12 hours or overnight

Scabies

▸ TO THE SKIN

▸ Child: Apply once weekly for 2 doses, apply preparation over whole body, and wash off after 24 hours, if hands are washed with soap within 24 hours, they should be retreated

▸ Adult: Apply once weekly for 2 doses, apply preparation over whole body, and wash off after 24 hours, if hands are washed with soap within 24 hours, they should be retreated

● **UNLICENSED USE**
▸ In children Not licensed for use in children under 6 months except under medical supervision.

> **IMPORTANT SAFETY INFORMATION**
> MHRA/CHM ADVICE: HEAD LICE ERADICATION PRODUCTS: RISK OF SERIOUS BURNS IF TREATED HAIR IS EXPOSED TO OPEN FLAMES OR OTHER SOURCES OF IGNITION (MARCH 2018)
> See Skin infections p. 1272.

● **CAUTIONS** Alcoholic lotions **not** recommended for head lice in children with severe eczema or asthma, or for scabies or crab lice · avoid contact with eyes · children under 6 months, medical supervision required · do not use lotion more than once a week for 3 consecutive weeks · do not use on broken or secondarily infected skin

● **SIDE-EFFECTS** Angioedema · eye swelling · hypersensitivity · skin reactions

● **PRESCRIBING AND DISPENSING INFORMATION** For scabies, manufacturer recommends application to the body but not necessarily to the head and neck. However, application should be extended to the scalp, neck, face, and ears.

● **MEDICINAL FORMS** There can be variation in the licensing of different medicines containing the same drug.

Liquid
EXCIPIENTS: May contain Cetostearyl alcohol (including cetyl and stearyl alcohol), fragrances, hydroxybenzoates (parabens)

▸ Derbac-M (G.R. Lane Health Products Ltd)
Malathion 5 mg per 1 gram Derbac-M 0.5% liquid | 150 ml ℗ £9.74

Permethrin

04-Feb-2020

● **INDICATIONS AND DOSE**

Scabies

▸ TO THE SKIN

▸ Child: Apply once weekly for 2 doses, apply 5% preparation over whole body including face, neck, scalp and ears then wash off after 8–12 hours. If hands are washed with soap within 8 hours of application, they should be treated again with cream

▸ Adult: Apply once weekly for 2 doses, apply 5% preparation over whole body including face, neck, scalp and ears then wash off after 8–12 hours. If hands are washed with soap within 8 hours of application, they should be treated again with cream

Crab lice

▸ TO THE SKIN

▸ Adult: Apply once weekly for 2 doses, apply 5% cream over whole body, allow to dry naturally and wash off after 12 hours or after leaving on overnight

Head lice

▸ TO THE SKIN

▸ Adult: Not recommended; no information given

● **UNLICENSED USE**
▸ In children *Dermal Cream* (scabies), not licensed for use in children under 2 months; not licensed for treatment of crab lice in children under 18 years. *Creme Rinse* (head lice) not licensed for use in children under 6 months except under medical supervision.

> **IMPORTANT SAFETY INFORMATION**
> MHRA/CHM ADVICE: HEAD LICE ERADICATION PRODUCTS: RISK OF SERIOUS BURNS IF TREATED HAIR IS EXPOSED TO OPEN FLAMES OR OTHER SOURCES OF IGNITION (MARCH 2018)
> See Skin infections p. 1272.

● **CAUTIONS** Avoid contact with eyes · children aged 2 months–2 years, medical supervision required for dermal cream (scabies) · children under 6 months, medical

13

Skin

supervision required for cream rinse (head lice) · do not use on broken or secondarily infected skin

- SIDE-EFFECTS Scalp irritation · skin reactions
- PRESCRIBING AND DISPENSING INFORMATION Manufacturer recommends application to the body but to exclude head and neck. However, application should be extended to the scalp, neck, face, and ears.
  Larger patients may require up to two 30-g packs for adequate treatment.
- LESS SUITABLE FOR PRESCRIBING Lyclear ® Creme Rinse is less suitable for prescribing.

- MEDICINAL FORMS There can be variation in the licensing of different medicines containing the same drug.
  Cream
  CAUTIONARY AND ADVISORY LABELS 10 (Dermal cream only)
  EXCIPIENTS: May contain Butylated hydroxytoluene, woolfat and related substances (including lanolin)
  ‣ Permethrin (Non-proprietary)
    Permethrin 50 mg per 1 gram Permethrin 5% cream | 30 gram P
    £7.46 DT = £7.46
  ‣ Lyclear (Omega Pharma Ltd)
    Permethrin 50 mg per 1 gram Lyclear 5% dermal cream |
    30 gram P £5.71 DT = £7.46
  Liquid
  EXCIPIENTS: May contain Cetostearyl alcohol (including cetyl and stearyl alcohol)
  ‣ Lyclear (Omega Pharma Ltd)
    Permethrin 10 mg per 1 gram Lyclear 1% creme rinse | 118 ml P
    £7.11 DT = £7.11

2.4 Viral skin infections

ANTIVIRALS > NUCLEOSIDE ANALOGUES

Aciclovir

09-Jun-2020

(Acyclovir)

- ● INDICATIONS AND DOSE

Herpes simplex infection (local treatment)
▶ TO THE SKIN
- ‣ Child: Apply 5 times a day for 5–10 days, to be applied to lesions approximately every 4 hours, starting at first sign of attack
- ‣ Adult: Apply 5 times a day for 5–10 days, to be applied to lesions approximately every 4 hours, starting at first sign of attack

- ● UNLICENSED USE
- ‣ In children Cream licensed for use in children (age range not specified by manufacturer).
- ● CAUTIONS Avoid cream coming in to contact with eyes and mucous membranes
- ● INTERACTIONS → Appendix 1: aciclovir
- ● SIDE-EFFECTS
- ‣ Uncommon Skin reactions
- ● PREGNANCY Limited absorption from topical aciclovir preparations.
- ● PATIENT AND CARER ADVICE
  Medicines for Children leaflet: Aciclovir cream for herpes
  www.medicinesforchildren.org.uk/aciclovir-cream-herpes-0
- ● PROFESSION SPECIFIC INFORMATION
  Dental practitioners' formulary
  Aciclovir Cream may be prescribed.
- ● EXCEPTIONS TO LEGAL CATEGORY A 2-g tube and a pump pack are on sale to the public for the treatment of cold sores.

- MEDICINAL FORMS There can be variation in the licensing of different medicines containing the same drug.
  Cream
  EXCIPIENTS: May contain Cetostearyl alcohol (including cetyl and stearyl alcohol), propylene glycol
  ‣ Aciclovir (Non-proprietary)
    Aciclovir 50 mg per 1 gram Aciclovir 5% cream | 2 gram PoM
    £1.34 DT = £1.34 | 10 gram PoM £7.05 DT = £6.66
  ‣ Zovirax (GlaxoSmithKline UK Ltd, GlaxoSmithKline Consumer Healthcare)
    Aciclovir 50 mg per 1 gram Zovirax 5% cream | 2 gram PoM £4.63
    DT = £1.34 | 10 gram PoM £13.96 DT = £6.66
    Zovirax Cold Sore 5% cream | 2 gram GSL £4.20–£4.49 DT = £1.34

3 Inflammatory skin conditions

3.1 Eczema and psoriasis

Eczema

02-Sep-2020

Types and management

Eczema (dermatitis) refers to a variety of skin conditions characterised by epidermal inflammation and itching. The main types of eczema are irritant, allergic contact, atopic, venous and discoid. Lichenification, due to scratching and rubbing, often presents in chronic eczema. *Atopic eczema* is one of the most common types and it usually involves itchy, red, dry skin which can become infected and lichenified.

EvGr Management of eczema involves the removal or treatment of contributory factors including occupational and domestic irritants. Known or suspected contact allergens should be avoided. ⚠ Rarely, ingredients in topical medicinal products may sensitise the skin; the BNF lists active ingredients together with excipients that have been associated with skin sensitisation.

EvGr Frequent and liberal use of emollients is advised for dry skin and itching associated with eczema. The choice of emollient is dependent on the dryness of the skin, and patient preference; this can be supplemented with bath or shower emollients. Emollients increase the efficacy of topical corticosteroids and have a steroid sparing action. The use of emollients should continue even if the eczema improves or if other treatment is being used. Aqueous cream is generally not recommended due to the high risk of developing skin reactions.

Topical corticosteroids are also often required in the management of eczema; the potency of the corticosteroid should be used in accordance to the severity and site of the condition. For eczema on the face, genitals, or axillae, consider a mild potency topical corticosteroid and only increase to a moderate potency topical corticosteroid if necessary. Moderate to potent topical corticosteroids are generally required for use in adults with moderate or severe eczema on the scalp, limbs, and trunk. Treatment should be reviewed regularly, especially if a potent topical corticosteroid is required. In patients with frequent flares, a topical corticosteroid can be applied to prevent further flares using various regimens (e.g. on 2 consecutive days each week). Emollient therapy should be continued during treatment with topical corticosteroids.

Under the care of a specialist, bandages (including those containing ichthammol with zinc oxide p. 1296) are sometimes applied over topical corticosteroids or emollients to treat eczema of the limbs. Dry-wrap dressings can be used to provide a physical barrier to help prevent scratching and improve retention of emollients. ⚠ See Wound management products and elasticated garments p. 1659 for details of elasticated viscose stockinette tubular bandages and garments, and silk clothing.

Topical pimecrolimus p. 1299 is licensed for the treatment of mild to moderate atopic eczema. Tacrolimus p. 1299 is licensed for topical use in the treatment of moderate to severe atopic eczema. EvGr Both are calcineurin inhibitors and should be considered as a second-line treatment option only, unless there is a specific reason to avoid or reduce the use of topical corticosteroids. Treatment of atopic eczema with topical pimecrolimus or topical tacrolimus should be initiated by a specialist.

Antihistamines are not recommended for routine use in the management of atopic eczema. However, if there is severe itching or urticaria, consider a non-sedating antihistamine. A sedating antihistamine can be considered if itching causes sleep disturbance. ⟨A⟩

Infection

EvGr Bacterial infection (commonly with *Staphylococcus aureus* and occasionally with *Streptococcus pyogenes*) can exacerbate eczema and may require treatment with topical or systemic antibacterial drugs. If the infected area is extensive, offer a short course of oral flucloxacillin p. 589 as first-line treatment; oral erythromycin p. 572 is an alternative if the patient is allergic or resistant to penicillin. Associated eczema is treated simultaneously with a topical corticosteroid which can be combined with a topical antimicrobial if the infection is localised. If infected eczema has not responded to treatment within 2 weeks, urgently refer to a specialist.

Immediate referral to secondary care is required in patients presenting with eczema herpeticum. ⟨A⟩

Severe refractory eczema

EvGr Systemic drugs acting on the immune system (such as ciclosporin p. 884, azathioprine p. 882 [unlicensed indication], and mycophenolate mofetil p. 891 [unlicensed indication]) and phototherapy are available for the management of some cases of severe refractory eczema; they are used under specialist supervision. ⟨A⟩ Dupilumab p. 1301 is licensed for the treatment of moderate to severe atopic eczema in patients requiring systemic therapy.

Alitretinoin p. 1305 is licensed for the treatment of severe chronic hand eczema refractory to potent topical corticosteroids; patients with hyperkeratotic features are more likely to respond to alitretinoin than those with pompholyx.

Seborrhoeic dermatitis

Seborrhoeic dermatitis (seborrhoeic eczema) is associated with species of the yeast *Malassezia* and affects the scalp, paranasal areas, and eyebrows. EvGr Shampoos active against the yeast (including those containing ketoconazole p. 1277 or coal tar p. 1297) and combinations of mild topical corticosteroids with suitable antimicrobials are used. ⟨A⟩

Psoriasis

01-Sep-2020

Overview

Psoriasis is an inflammatory skin disease that usually follows a relapsing and remitting course and may have nail or joint involvement. Different forms of psoriasis exist; chronic plaque psoriasis is the most common, and is characterised by epidermal thickening and scaling, usually affecting extensor surfaces and the scalp.

Occasionally, psoriasis is provoked or exacerbated by drugs such as lithium, chloroquine and hydroxychloroquine, beta-blockers, non-steroidal anti-inflammatory drugs, and ACE inhibitors. Psoriasis may not be seen until the drug has been taken for weeks or months.

Treatment

EvGr Offer topical treatment first-line to all patients with psoriasis. Topical treatment options include emollients, topical corticosteroids, coal tar preparations, and topical vitamin D and vitamin D analogues. When choosing topical treatment, consider patient preference, practical aspects of application, extent of psoriasis, and the variety of preparation forms available. ⟨A⟩

Emollients are widely used in psoriasis; they moisturise dry skin, reduce scaling, and relieve itching. They also soften cracked areas and help other topical treatments absorb through the skin to work more effectively. Some cases of mild psoriasis may settle with the use of emollients alone. EvGr Emollients may also be useful adjuncts to other more specific treatment. ⟨A⟩

Continuous long-term use of potent or very potent topical corticosteroids may cause psoriasis to become unstable, and lead to irreversible skin atrophy and striae. Widespread use (greater than 10% of body surface area affected) can also lead to systemic and local side-effects. EvGr Patients who have been on intermittent or short courses of potent or very potent topical corticosteroids should be offered a review of treatment at least annually.

Consecutive use of potent topical corticosteroids should not be used for more than 8 weeks at any one site; 4 weeks for very potent topical corticosteroids. Application may be restarted after a 4-week 'treatment break'; non-steroid treatments, such as topical vitamin D and vitamin D analogues, may be continued during this time. ⟨A⟩

Coal tar p. 1297 has anti-inflammatory, antipruritic, and anti-scaling properties and is often combined with other topical treatments for psoriasis. Several coal tar preparations are available including ointments, shampoos, and bath additives. EvGr Newer products are preferred to older products containing crude coal tar (coal tar BP), which is malodorous and usually messier to apply. ⟨A⟩

Topical vitamin D and vitamin D analogue preparations are available as ointments, gels, scalp solutions, and lotions. Tacalcitol p. 1307 and calcitriol p. 1307 may be less irritating than calcipotriol p. 1306.

Psoriasis of the trunk and limbs

EvGr Offer a potent topical corticosteroid and a topical vitamin D or vitamin D analogue applied once daily (at different times of the day) for up to 4 weeks as initial treatment. If satisfactory control is not achieved after a maximum of 8 weeks, offer a topical vitamin D or vitamin D analogue alone applied twice daily. If satisfactory control is not achieved after 8–12 weeks of twice-daily topical vitamin D or vitamin D analogue, offer either a potent topical corticosteroid applied twice daily for up to 4 weeks, or a coal tar preparation. A combination product containing calcipotriol with betamethasone p. 1288 for up to 4 weeks is an alternative in patients unable to use twice-daily potent topical corticosteroids, a coal tar preparation, or in patients where a once-daily application would improve adherence. A *very* potent topical corticosteroid can be offered under specialist supervision for a maximum of 4 weeks when other topical treatments have failed.

In patients with treatment-resistant psoriasis of the trunk or limbs, consider treatment with short-contact dithranol p. 1297. Treatment should be given in a specialist setting or the patient should be provided with educational support for self-use. ⟨A⟩

Scalp psoriasis

EvGr Offer a potent topical corticosteroid applied once daily for up to 4 weeks as initial treatment. If satisfactory control is not achieved after 4 weeks, consider a different formulation of the potent topical corticosteroid (e.g. a shampoo or mousse) and/or topical agents to remove or soften adherent scale (e.g. agents containing salicylic acid, emollients, oils). These agents should be used prior to applying the potent topical corticosteroid to allow effective penetration. If response to potent topical corticosteroid treatment remains unsatisfactory after a further 4 weeks of treatment, offer a combination product containing calcipotriol with betamethasone for up to 4 weeks. If treatment with calcipotriol with betamethasone for up to 4 weeks does not give a satisfactory response, offer either a very potent corticosteroid applied twice daily for 2 weeks, or a coal tar preparation, or refer the patient to a specialist.

In patients with mild to moderate scalp psoriasis who cannot use topical corticosteroids, offer treatment with a topical vitamin D or vitamin D analogue only. If treatment with a vitamin D or vitamin D analogue for up to 8 weeks does not give a satisfactory response, either offer a coal tar preparation or refer the patient to a specialist. The use of coal tar-based shampoos alone for the treatment of severe scalp psoriasis is not recommended. ⒶⒼ

Facial, flexural, and genital psoriasis
EvGr Offer a mild or moderate potency topical corticosteroid as initial treatment. The face, flexures, and genitals are particularly vulnerable to steroid atrophy therefore topical corticosteroids should only be used short-term (e.g. 1–2 weeks per month). If response to a moderate potency topical corticosteroid is inadequate, or there is serious risk of side-effects from continuous use, offer a topical calcineurin inhibitor, such as pimecrolimus p. 1299 or tacrolimus p. 1299 [unlicensed indications], for up to 4 weeks (initiated under specialist supervision). ⒶⒼ

Pustular or erythrodermic psoriasis
EvGr Widespread unstable psoriasis of erythrodermic or generalised pustular types requires urgent same-day specialist assessment and should be managed as a medical emergency. ⒶⒼ

Phototherapy
Phototherapy is available under the supervision of an appropriately trained healthcare professional. EvGr Narrowband ultraviolet B (UVB) phototherapy can be offered to patients with plaque or guttate psoriasis in whom topical treatment has failed to achieve control. ⒶⒼ

Photochemotherapy combining psoralen with ultraviolet A (PUVA) is available in specialist centres, given under the supervision of an appropriately trained healthcare professional. EvGr Psoralen enhances the effects of UVA and is administered either by mouth or topically. EvGr PUVA irradiation can be considered for the treatment of localised palmoplantar pustulosis and plaque-type psoriasis. ⒶⒼ Cumulative doses increase the risk of dysplastic and neoplastic skin lesions, especially squamous cell cancer.

EvGr Topical adjunctive therapy may be considered in patients receiving broadband or narrowband UVB phototherapy who have plaques that are resistant, or show an inadequate response to phototherapy alone, or are at difficult-to-treat sites, or in patients unable to take systemic treatment. Concomitant treatment of acitretin and PUVA is not routinely recommended. ⒶⒼ

Systemic treatment
Non-biological treatment
EvGr Under the supervision of a specialist, systemic non-biological treatment with methotrexate p. 957 or ciclosporin p. 884 may be offered to some patients with psoriasis that cannot be controlled with topical treatment *and* if the psoriasis has a significant impact on physical, psychological or social well-being. In addition, the psoriasis would have to be extensive, or localised with significant distress or functional impairment, or have failed phototherapy treatment.

Ciclosporin can be considered first-line in patients who need rapid or short-term disease control, have palmoplantar pustulosis, or who are considering conception (both men and women).

Only consider acitretin p. 1304 in patients where methotrexate and ciclosporin are not appropriate or have failed, or in patients with pustular forms of psoriasis. ⒶⒼ

Apremilast p. 1164 is licensed for the treatment of moderate to severe chronic plaque psoriasis in patients who failed to respond to other systemic treatments including ciclosporin, methotrexate, or PUVA, or in those who have contra-indications to or intolerance to these treatments. ⒶⒼ

Biological treatment
EvGr Biological drugs (e.g. adalimumab p. 1157, brodalumab p. 1300, etanercept p. 1159, guselkumab p. 1301, infliximab p. 1162, ixekizumab p. 1302, secukinumab p. 1149, ustekinumab p. 1151) should be initiated and supervised only by specialists experienced in the diagnosis and management of psoriasis. ⒶⒼ

> **Other drugs used for Eczema and psoriasis** Certolizumab pegol, p. 1158 · Dimethyl fumarate, p. 898

CORTICOSTEROIDS

Topical corticosteroids
18-Sep-2020

Overview
Topical corticosteroids are used for the treatment of inflammatory conditions of the skin (other than those arising from an infection), in particular eczema, contact dermatitis, insect stings, and eczema of scabies. Corticosteroids suppress the inflammatory reaction during use; they are not curative and on discontinuation a rebound exacerbation of the condition may occur. They are generally used to relieve symptoms and suppress signs of the disorder when other measures such as emollients are ineffective.

Topical corticosteroids are not recommended in the routine treatment of urticaria; treatment should only be initiated and supervised by a specialist. They should not be used indiscriminately in pruritus (where they will only benefit if inflammation is causing the itch) and are **not** recommended for acne vulgaris.

Systemic or very potent topical corticosteroids should be avoided or given only under specialist supervision in *psoriasis* because, although they may suppress psoriasis in the short term, relapse or vigorous rebound occurs on withdrawal (sometimes precipitating severe pustular psoriasis). See the role of topical corticosteroids in the treatment of psoriasis.

In general, the most potent topical corticosteroids should be reserved for recalcitrant dermatoses such as *chronic discoid lupus erythematosus, lichen simplex chronicus, hypertrophic lichen planus,* and *palmoplantar pustulosis*. Potent corticosteroids should generally be avoided on the face and skin flexures, but specialists occasionally prescribe them for use on these areas in certain circumstances.

When topical treatment has failed, intralesional corticosteroid injections may be used. These are more effective than the very potent topical corticosteroid preparations and should be reserved for severe cases where there are localised lesions such as *keloid scars, hypertrophic lichen planus,* or *localised alopecia areata*.

Perioral lesions
Hydrocortisone cream 1% p. 1291 can be used for up to 7 days to treat uninfected inflammatory lesions on the lips. Hydrocortisone with miconazole cream or ointment p. 1296 is useful where infection by susceptible organisms and inflammation co-exist, particularly for initial treatment (up to 7 days) e.g. in angular cheilitis. Organisms susceptible to miconazole include *Candida* spp. and many Gram-positive bacteria including streptococci and staphylococci.

Choice of formulation

Water-miscible corticosteroid *creams* are suitable for moist or weeping lesions whereas *ointments* are generally chosen for dry, lichenified or scaly lesions or where a more occlusive effect is required. *Lotions* may be useful when minimal application to a large or hair-bearing area is required or for the treatment of exudative lesions. *Occlusive polythene* or *hydrocolloid dressings* increase absorption, but also increase the risk of side-effects; they are therefore used only under supervision on a short-term basis for areas of very thick skin (such as the palms and soles). The inclusion of urea or salicylic acid also increases the penetration of the corticosteroid.

In the BNF publications topical corticosteroids for the skin are categorised as 'mild', 'moderately potent', 'potent' or 'very potent'; the **least potent** preparation which is effective should be chosen but dilution should be avoided whenever possible.

Absorption through the skin

Mild and *moderately potent* topical corticosteroids are associated with few side-effects but care is required in the use of *potent* and *very potent* corticosteroids. Absorption through the skin can rarely cause adrenal suppression and even Cushing's syndrome, depending on the area of the body being treated and the duration of treatment. Absorption is greatest where the skin is thin or raw, and from intertriginous areas; it is increased by occlusion.

For further information on side-effects that may occur from absorption through the skin, see Corticosteroids, general use p. 709.

Suitable quantities of corticosteroid preparations to be prescribed for specific areas of the body

Area of body	Creams and Ointments
Face and neck	15 to 30 g
Both hands	15 to 30 g
Scalp	15 to 30 g
Both arms	30 to 60g
Both legs	100 g
Trunk	100 g
Groins and genitalia	15 to 30 g

These amounts are usually suitable for an adult for a single daily application for 2 weeks

Compound preparations

The advantages of including other substances (such as antibacterials or antifungals) with corticosteroids in topical preparations are uncertain, but such combinations may have a place where inflammatory skin conditions are associated with bacterial or fungal infection, such as infected eczema. In these cases the antimicrobial drug should be chosen according to the sensitivity of the infecting organism and used regularly for a short period (typically twice daily for 1 week). Longer use increases the likelihood of resistance and of sensitisation.

The keratolytic effect of salicylic acid p. 1330 facilitates the absorption of topical corticosteroids; however, excessive and prolonged use of topical preparations containing salicylic acid may cause salicylism.

Topical corticosteroid preparation potencies

Potency of a topical corticosteroid preparation is a result of the formulation as well as the corticosteroid. Therefore, proprietary names are shown.

Mild
- Hydrocortisone 0.1–2.5%
- Dioderm
- Mildison
- Synalar 1 in 10 dilution

Mild with antimicrobials
- Canesten HC
- Daktacort
- Econacort
- Fucidin H
- Hydrocortisone with chlorhexidine hydrochloride and nystatin
- Terra-Cortril
- Timodine

Moderate
- Betnovate-RD
- Eumovate
- Haelan
- Modrasone
- Synalar 1 in 4 Dilution
- Ultralanum Plain

Moderate with antimicrobials
- Trimovate

Moderate with urea:
- Alphaderm

Potent
- Beclometasone dipropionate 0.025%
- Betamethasone valerate 0.1%
- Betacap
- Betesil
- Bettamousse
- Betnovate
- Cutivate
- Diprosone
- Elocon
- Hydrocortisone butyrate
- Locoid
- Locoid Crelo
- Metosyn
- Mometasone furoate 0.1%
- Nerisone
- Synalar

Potent with antimicrobials
- Aureocort
- Betamethasone and clioquinol
- Betamethasone and neomycin
- Fucibet
- Lotriderm
- Synalar C
- Synalar N

Potent with salicylic acid
- Diprosalic

Very potent
- Clarelux
- Dermovate
- Etrivex
- Nerisone Forte

Very potent with antimicrobials
- Clobetasol with neomycin and nystatin

Use in children

Children, especially infants, are particularly susceptible to side-effects. However, concern about the safety of topical corticosteroids in children should not result in the child being undertreated. The aim is to control the condition as well as possible; inadequate treatment will perpetuate the condition. A mild corticosteroid such as hydrocortisone 0.5% or 1% is useful for treating nappy rash and hydrocortisone 1% for atopic eczema in childhood. A moderately potent or potent corticosteroid may be appropriate for severe atopic eczema on the limbs, for 1–2 weeks only, switching to a less potent preparation as the condition improves. In an acute flare-up of atopic eczema, it may be appropriate to use more potent formulations of topical corticosteroids for a short period to regain control of the condition. A very potent corticosteroid should be initiated under the supervision of a specialist. Carers of young children should be advised that treatment should **not** necessarily be reserved to 'treat only the worst areas' and they may need to be advised that patient information leaflets may contain inappropriate advice for the patient's condition.

Corticosteroids (topical)

IMPORTANT SAFETY INFORMATION

MHRA/CHM ADVICE: CORTICOSTEROIDS: RARE RISK OF CENTRAL SEROUS CHORIORETINOPATHY WITH LOCAL AS WELL AS SYSTEMIC ADMINISTRATION (AUGUST 2017)

Central serous chorioretinopathy is a retinal disorder that has been linked to the systemic use of corticosteroids. Recently, it has also been reported after local administration of corticosteroids via inhaled and intranasal, epidural, intra-articular, topical dermal, and periocular routes. The MHRA recommends that patients should be advised to report any blurred vision or other visual disturbances with corticosteroid treatment given by any route; consider referral to an ophthalmologist for evaluation of possible causes if a patient presents with vision problems.

NHS IMPROVEMENT PATIENT SAFETY ALERT: STEROID EMERGENCY CARD TO SUPPORT EARLY RECOGNITION AND TREATMENT OF ADRENAL CRISIS IN ADULTS (AUGUST 2020)

A patient-held **Steroid Emergency Card** has been developed for patients with adrenal insufficiency and steroid dependence who are at risk of adrenal crisis. It aims to support healthcare staff with the early recognition of patients at risk of adrenal crisis and the emergency treatment of adrenal crisis. All eligible patients should be issued a Steroid Emergency Card. Providers that treat patients with acute physical illness or trauma, or who may require emergency treatment, elective surgery, or other invasive procedures, should establish processes to check for risk of adrenal crisis and confirm if the patient has a Steroid Emergency Card.

* CONTRA-INDICATIONS Acne · perioral dermatitis · potent corticosteroids in widespread plaque psoriasis · rosacea · untreated bacterial, fungal or viral skin lesions
* CAUTIONS Avoid prolonged use (particularly on the face) · cautions applicable to systemic corticosteroids may also apply if absorption occurs following topical and local use · dermatoses of infancy, including nappy rash (extreme caution required—treatment should be limited to 5–7 days) (in children) · infection · keep away from eyes · use potent or very potent topical corticosteroids under specialist supervision (in children) · use potent or very potent topical corticosteroids under specialist supervision in psoriasis (can result in rebound relapse, development of generalised pustular psoriasis, and local and systemic toxicity) (in adults)
* SIDE-EFFECTS
  * **Common or very common** Skin reactions · telangiectasia
  * **Rare or very rare** Adrenal suppression · hypertrichosis · skin depigmentation (may be reversible)
  * **Frequency not known** Local reaction · vasodilation

  SIDE-EFFECTS, FURTHER INFORMATION Side-effects applicable to systemic corticosteroids may also apply if absorption occurs following topical and local use. In order to minimise the side-effects of a topical corticosteroid, it is

important to apply it thinly to affected areas only, no more frequently than twice daily, and to use the least potent formulation which is fully effective.

* DIRECTIONS FOR ADMINISTRATION [EvGr] Topical corticosteroid preparations should be applied no more frequently than twice daily; once daily is often sufficient. ⒶTopical corticosteroids should be applied in sufficient quantity to cover the affected areas. The length of cream or ointment expelled from a tube may be used to specify the quantity to be applied to a given area of skin. This length can be measured in terms of a *fingertip unit* (the distance from the tip of the adult index finger to the first crease). One fingertip unit (approximately 500 mg from a tube with a standard 5 mm diameter nozzle) is sufficient to cover an area that is twice that of the flat adult handprint (palm and fingers). [EvGr] Several minutes should elapse between application of topical corticosteroids and emollients. Ⓐ
  * In children 'Wet-wrap bandaging' increases absorption into the skin, but should be initiated under the supervision of a trained healthcare professional.
* PRESCRIBING AND DISPENSING INFORMATION The potency of each topical corticosteroid should be included on the label with the directions for use. The label should be attached to the container (for example, the tube) rather than the outer packaging.
* PATIENT AND CARER ADVICE Patients or carers should be given advice on how to administer corticosteroid creams and ointments. If a patient is using topical corticosteroids of different potencies, the patient should be told when to use each corticosteroid. Patients and their carers should be reassured that side effects such as skin thinning and systemic effects rarely occur when topical corticosteroids are used appropriately.

F above

Alclometasone dipropionate

24-Sep-2020

* INDICATIONS AND DOSE

Inflammatory skin disorders such as eczemas
  * TO THE SKIN
  * Child: Apply 1–2 times a day, to be applied thinly
  * Adult: Apply 1–2 times a day, to be applied thinly

POTENCY
  * Alclometasone dipropionate cream 0.05%: moderate

* UNLICENSED USE
  * In children Licensed for use in children (age range not specified by manufacturer).
* PATIENT AND CARER ADVICE Patients or carers should be counselled on the application of alclometasone dipropionate cream.

* MEDICINAL FORMS There can be variation in the licensing of different medicines containing the same drug.

Cream

CAUTIONARY AND ADVISORY LABELS 28
EXCIPIENTS: May contain Cetostearyl alcohol (including cetyl and stearyl alcohol), chlorocresol, propylene glycol
  * Alclometasone dipropionate (Non-proprietary)
    Alclometasone dipropionate 500 microgram per 1 gram Alclometasone 0.05% cream | 50 gram [PoM] £12.99-£17.31

Beclometasone dipropionate

⚑ 1286

25-Sep-2020

(Beclomethasone dipropionate)

● **INDICATIONS AND DOSE**

Severe inflammatory skin disorders such as eczemas unresponsive to less potent corticosteroids | Psoriasis

▶ TO THE SKIN

▸ **Child:** Apply 1–2 times a day, to be applied thinly

▸ **Adult:** Apply 1–2 times a day, to be applied thinly

POTENCY

▸ Beclometasone dipropionate cream and ointment 0.025%: potent.

● **UNLICENSED USE**

In children   Not licensed for use in children under 1 year.

● **INTERACTIONS** → Appendix 1: corticosteroids

● **SIDE-EFFECTS** Vision blurred

● **MEDICINAL FORMS** There can be variation in the licensing of different medicines containing the same drug. Forms available from special-order manufacturers include: cream, ointment

Cream

CAUTIONARY AND ADVISORY LABELS 28

▸ Beclometasone dipropionate (Non-proprietary)
Beclometasone dipropionate 250 microgram per 1 gram   Beclometasone 0.025% cream | 30 gram [PoM] £68.00 DT = £68.00

Ointment

CAUTIONARY AND ADVISORY LABELS 28

▸ Beclometasone dipropionate (Non-proprietary)
Beclometasone dipropionate 250 microgram per 1 gram   Beclometasone 0.025% ointment | 30 gram [PoM] £68.00 DT = £68.00

Betamethasone

⚑ 1286

07-Dec-2020

● **DRUG ACTION** Betamethasone has very high glucocorticoid activity and insignificant mineralocorticoid activity.

● **INDICATIONS AND DOSE**

Severe inflammatory skin disorders such as eczemas unresponsive to less potent corticosteroids | Psoriasis

▶ TO THE SKIN

▸ **Child:** Apply 1–2 times a day, to be applied thinly

▸ **Adult:** Apply 1–2 times a day, to be applied thinly

POTENCY

▸ Betamethasone valerate 0.025% cream and ointment: moderate. Betamethasone valerate 0.1% cream, lotion, ointment, and scalp application: potent. Betamethasone valerate 0.12% foam: potent. Betamethasone dipropionate 0.05% cream, lotion, and ointment: potent.

BETESIL ®

Inflammatory skin disorders [unresponsive to less potent corticosteroids]

▶ TO THE SKIN

▸ **Adult:** Apply every 24 hours for up to 30 days, wait at least 30 minutes between applications, up to 6 medicated plasters may be used per day

● **UNLICENSED USE**

▸ With topical use in children *Betacap* ®, *Betnovate* ® and *Betnovate-RD* ® are not licensed for use in children under 1 year. *Bettamousse* ® is not licensed for use in children under 6 years.

● **CAUTIONS** Use of more than 100 g per week of 0.1% preparation likely to cause adrenal suppression

● **INTERACTIONS** → Appendix 1: corticosteroids

● **DIRECTIONS FOR ADMINISTRATION**

BETESIL ® Manufacturer advises cleanse and dry skin prior to plaster application. Plaster may be cut to fit area to be treated.

● **PATIENT AND CARER ADVICE** Patient counselling is advised for betamethasone cream, ointment, scalp application and foam (application).

BETESIL ® Manufacturer advises avoid contact with water after plaster applied.

● **MEDICINAL FORMS** There can be variation in the licensing of different medicines containing the same drug. Forms available from special-order manufacturers include: cream, ointment

Foam

CAUTIONARY AND ADVISORY LABELS 15, 28

EXCIPIENTS: May contain Cetostearyl alcohol (including cetyl and stearyl alcohol), polysorbates, propylene glycol

▸ Bettamousse (RPH Pharmaceuticals AB)
Betamethasone (as Betamethasone valerate) 1 mg per 1 gram   Bettamousse 0.1% cutaneous foam | 100 gram [PoM] £9.75 DT = £9.75

Medicated plaster

▸ Betesil (Derma UK Ltd)
Betamethasone valerate 2.25 mg   Betesil 2.25mg medicated plasters | 4 plaster [PoM] £13.98 DT = £13.98

Cream

CAUTIONARY AND ADVISORY LABELS 28

EXCIPIENTS: May contain Cetostearyl alcohol (including cetyl and stearyl alcohol), chlorocresol

▸ Betamethasone (Non-proprietary)
Betamethasone (as Betamethasone valerate) 1 mg per 1 gram   Betamethasone valerate 0.1% cream | 15 gram [PoM] £3.00 | 30 gram [PoM] £2.42 DT = £1.86 | 100 gram [PoM] £6.20 DT = £6.20

▸ Audavate (Accord Healthcare Ltd)
Betamethasone (as Betamethasone valerate) 250 microgram per 1 gram   Audavate RD 0.025% cream | 100 gram [PoM] £2.99 DT = £3.15
Betamethasone (as Betamethasone valerate) 1 mg per 1 gram   Audavate 0.1% cream | 30 gram [PoM] £1.14 DT = £1.86 | 100 gram [PoM] £3.24 DT = £6.20

▸ Betnovate (GlaxoSmithKline UK Ltd)
Betamethasone (as Betamethasone valerate) 250 microgram per 1 gram   Betnovate RD 0.025% cream | 100 gram [PoM] £3.15 DT = £3.15
Betamethasone (as Betamethasone valerate) 1 mg per 1 gram   Betnovate 0.1% cream | 30 gram [PoM] £1.43 DT = £1.86 | 100 gram [PoM] £4.05 DT = £6.20

▸ Diprosone (Merck Sharp & Dohme Ltd)
Betamethasone (as Betamethasone dipropionate) 500 microgram per 1 gram   Diprosone 0.05% cream | 30 gram [PoM] £2.16 DT = £2.16 | 100 gram [PoM] £6.12 DT = £6.12

Ointment

CAUTIONARY AND ADVISORY LABELS 28

▸ Betamethasone (Non-proprietary)
Betamethasone (as Betamethasone valerate) 1 mg per 1 gram   Betamethasone valerate 0.1% ointment | 30 gram [PoM] £1.94 DT = £1.94 | 100 gram [PoM] £6.47 DT = £6.47

▸ Audavate (Accord Healthcare Ltd)
Betamethasone (as Betamethasone valerate) 250 microgram per 1 gram   Audavate RD 0.025% ointment | 100 gram [PoM] £2.99 DT = £3.15
Betamethasone (as Betamethasone valerate) 1 mg per 1 gram   Audavate 0.1% ointment | 30 gram [PoM] £1.36 DT = £1.94 | 100 gram [PoM] £3.85 DT = £6.47

▸ Betnovate (GlaxoSmithKline UK Ltd)
Betamethasone (as Betamethasone valerate) 250 microgram per 1 gram   Betnovate RD 0.025% ointment | 100 gram [PoM] £3.15 DT = £3.15
Betamethasone (as Betamethasone valerate) 1 mg per 1 gram   Betnovate 0.1% ointment | 30 gram [PoM] £1.43 DT = £1.94 | 100 gram [PoM] £4.05 DT = £6.47

▸ Diprosone (Merck Sharp & Dohme Ltd)
Betamethasone (as Betamethasone dipropionate) 500 microgram per 1 gram   Diprosone 0.05% ointment | 30 gram [PoM] £2.16 DT = £2.16 | 100 gram [PoM] £6.12 DT = £6.12

13

Skin

Liquid

CAUTIONARY AND ADVISORY LABELS 15 (scalp lotion only), 28
EXCIPIENTS: May contain Cetostearyl alcohol (including cetyl and stearyl alcohol), hydroxybenzoates (parabens)

▸ Betacap (Dermal Laboratories Ltd)

Betamethasone (as Betamethasone valerate) 1 mg per 1 gram Betacap 0.1% scalp application | 100 ml [PoM] £3.75 DT = £3.75

▸ Betnovate (GlaxoSmithKline UK Ltd)

Betamethasone (as Betamethasone valerate) 1 mg per 1 gram Betnovate 0.1% scalp application | 100 ml [PoM] £4.99 DT = £3.75

Betnovate 0.1% lotion | 100 ml [PoM] £4.58 DT = £4.58

▸ Diprosone (Merck Sharp & Dohme Ltd)

Betamethasone (as Betamethasone dipropionate) 500 microgram per 1 ml Diprosone 0.05% lotion | 100 ml [PoM] £7.80 DT = £7.80

Combinations available: *Betamethasone with clioquinol,* p. 1292 · *Betamethasone with clotrimazole,* p. 1292 · *Betamethasone with fusidic acid,* p. 1293 · *Betamethasone with neomycin,* p. 1293 · *Betamethasone with salicylic acid,* p. 1293

Calcipotriol with betamethasone

04-Nov-2020

The properties listed below are those particular to the combination only. For the properties of the components please consider, calcipotriol p. 1306, betamethasone p. 1287.

● **INDICATIONS AND DOSE**

DOVOBET ® GEL

Scalp psoriasis

▸ TO THE SKIN

▸ Adult: Apply 1–4 g once daily usual duration of therapy 4 weeks; if necessary, treatment may be continued beyond 4 weeks or repeated, on the advice of a specialist, shampoo off after leaving on scalp overnight or during day, when different preparations containing calcipotriol used together, maximum total calcipotriol 5 mg in any one week

Mild to moderate plaque psoriasis

▸ TO THE SKIN

▸ Adult: Apply once daily for 8 weeks; if necessary, treatment may be continued beyond 8 weeks or repeated, on the advice of a specialist, apply to maximum 30% of body surface, when different preparations containing calcipotriol used together, max. total calcipotriol 5 mg in any one week; maximum 15 g per day

DOVOBET ® OINTMENT

Stable plaque psoriasis

▸ TO THE SKIN

▸ Adult: Apply once daily for 4 weeks; if necessary, treatment may be continued beyond 4 weeks or repeated, on the advice of a specialist, apply to a maximum 30% of body surface, when different preparations containing calcipotriol used together, max. total calcipotriol 5 mg in any one week; maximum 15 g per day

ENSTILAR ®

Psoriasis

▸ TO THE SKIN

▸ Adult: Apply once daily to be applied to the affected area for up to 4 weeks—consult product literature for further information; maximum 15 g per day

● CONTRA-INDICATIONS Erythrodermic psoriasis · pustular psoriasis

● INTERACTIONS → Appendix 1: corticosteroids · vitamin D substances

● NATIONAL FUNDING/ACCESS DECISIONS

ENSTILAR ® For full details see funding body website

Scottish Medicines Consortium (SMC) decisions

▸ Calcipotriol and betamethasone cutaneous foam (*Enstilar*®) for the topical treatment of psoriasis vulgaris in adults (September 2016) SMC No. 1182/16 Recommended

● MEDICINAL FORMS There can be variation in the licensing of different medicines containing the same drug.

Ointment

CAUTIONARY AND ADVISORY LABELS 28
EXCIPIENTS: May contain Butylated hydroxytoluene

▸ Dovobet (LEO Pharma)

Calcipotriol (as Calcipotriol hydrate) 50 microgram per 1 gram, Betamethasone (as Betamethasone dipropionate) 500 microgram per 1 gram Dovobet ointment | 30 gram [PoM] £19.84 DT = £19.84 | 60 gram [PoM] £39.68 | 120 gram [PoM] £73.86

Gel

CAUTIONARY AND ADVISORY LABELS 28
EXCIPIENTS: May contain Butylated hydroxytoluene

▸ Dovobet (LEO Pharma)

Calcipotriol (as Calcipotriol monohydrate) 50 microgram per 1 gram, Betamethasone (as Betamethasone dipropionate) 500 microgram per 1 gram Dovobet gel | 60 gram [PoM] £37.21 DT = £37.21 | 120 gram [PoM] £69.11

Foam

▸ Enstilar (LEO Pharma)

Calcipotriol (as Calcipotriol monohydrate) 50 microgram per 1 gram, Betamethasone (as Betamethasone dipropionate) 500 microgram per 1 gram Enstilar 50micrograms/g / 0.5 mg/g cutaneous foam | 60 gram [PoM] £39.68 DT = £39.68 | 120 gram [PoM] £79.36

F 1286

Clobetasol propionate

25-Sep-2020

● **INDICATIONS AND DOSE**

Short-term treatment only of severe resistant inflammatory skin disorders such as recalcitrant eczemas unresponsive to less potent corticosteroids | Psoriasis

▸ TO THE SKIN

▸ Child 1-17 years: Apply 1–2 times a day for up to 4 weeks, to be applied thinly

▸ Adult: Apply 1–2 times a day for up to 4 weeks, to be applied thinly, maximum 50 g of 0.05% preparation per week

POTENCY

▸ Clobetasol propionate 0.05% cream, foam, ointment, scalp application, and shampoo: very potent.

ETRIVEX ®

Moderate scalp psoriasis

▸ TO THE SKIN

▸ Adult: Apply once daily maximum duration of treatment 4 weeks, to be applied thinly then rinsed off after 15 minutes; frequency of application should be reduced after clinical improvement

● PATIENT AND CARER ADVICE Patients or carers should be given advice on how to administer clobetasol propionate foam, liquid (scalp application), cream, ointment and shampoo.

Scalp application Patients or carers should be advised to apply foam directly to scalp lesions (foam begins to subside immediately on contact with skin).

MEDICINAL FORMS There can be variation in the licensing of different medicines containing the same drug. Forms available from special-order manufacturers include: cream, ointment, paste

Shampoo
CAUTIONARY AND ADVISORY LABELS 28
▸ Etrivex (Galderma (UK) Ltd)
　Clobetasol propionate 500 microgram per 1 gram Etrivex
　500micrograms/g shampoo | 125 ml PoM £9.15 DT = £9.15

Cream
CAUTIONARY AND ADVISORY LABELS 28
EXCIPIENTS: May contain Beeswax, cetostearyl alcohol (including cetyl and stearyl alcohol), chlorocresol, propylene glycol
▸ ClobaDerm (Accord Healthcare Ltd)
　Clobetasol propionate 500 microgram per 1 gram ClobaDerm
　0.05% cream | 30 gram PoM £2.56 DT = £2.69 | 100 gram PoM
　£7.51 DT = £7.90
▸ Dermovate (GlaxoSmithKline UK Ltd)
　Clobetasol propionate 500 microgram per 1 gram Dermovate
　0.05% cream | 30 gram PoM £2.69 DT = £2.69 | 100 gram PoM
　£7.90 DT = £7.90

Ointment
CAUTIONARY AND ADVISORY LABELS 28
EXCIPIENTS: May contain Propylene glycol
▸ ClobaDerm (Accord Healthcare Ltd)
　Clobetasol propionate 500 microgram per 1 gram ClobaDerm
　0.05% ointment | 30 gram PoM £2.56 DT = £2.69 | 100 gram PoM
　£7.51 DT = £7.90
▸ Dermovate (GlaxoSmithKline UK Ltd)
　Clobetasol propionate 500 microgram per 1 gram Dermovate
　0.05% ointment | 30 gram PoM £2.69 DT = £2.69 | 100 gram PoM
　£7.90 DT = £7.90

Liquid
CAUTIONARY AND ADVISORY LABELS 15, 28
▸ Dermovate (GlaxoSmithKline UK Ltd)
　Clobetasol propionate 500 microgram per 1 gram Dermovate
　0.05% scalp application | 30 ml PoM £3.07 DT = £3.07 |
　100 ml PoM £10.42 DT = £10.42

Combinations available: *Clobetasol propionate with neomycin sulfate and nystatin,* p. 1294

⚑ 1286

Clobetasone butyrate
25-Sep-2020

● **INDICATIONS AND DOSE**

Eczemas and dermatitis of all types | Maintenance between courses of more potent corticosteroids
▸ TO THE SKIN
▸ Child: Apply 1–2 times a day, to be applied thinly
▸ Adult: Apply 1–2 times a day, to be applied thinly
POTENCY
▸ Clobetasone butyrate 0.05% cream and ointment: moderate.

● **UNLICENSED USE**
▸ In children Licensed for use in children (age range not specified by manufacturer).

● **PATIENT AND CARER ADVICE** Patients or carers should be advised on the application of clobetasone butyrate containing preparations.

● **EXCEPTIONS TO LEGAL CATEGORY** Cream can be sold to the public for short-term symptomatic treatment and control of patches of eczema and dermatitis (but not seborrhoeic dermatitis) in adults and children over 12 years provided pack does not contain more than 15 g.

● **MEDICINAL FORMS** There can be variation in the licensing of different medicines containing the same drug. Forms available from special-order manufacturers include: cream, ointment

Ointment
CAUTIONARY AND ADVISORY LABELS 28
▸ Clobavate (Teva UK Ltd)
　Clobetasone butyrate 500 microgram per 1 gram Clobavate
　0.05% ointment | 30 gram PoM £1.49 DT = £1.86 | 100 gram PoM
　£4.35 DT = £5.44

▸ Eumovate (GlaxoSmithKline UK Ltd)
　Clobetasone butyrate 500 microgram per 1 gram Eumovate
　0.05% ointment | 30 gram PoM £1.86 DT = £1.86 | 100 gram PoM
　£5.44 DT = £5.44

Cream
CAUTIONARY AND ADVISORY LABELS 28
EXCIPIENTS: May contain Cetostearyl alcohol (including cetyl and stearyl alcohol), chlorocresol
▸ Eumovate (GlaxoSmithKline Consumer Healthcare, GlaxoSmithKline UK Ltd)
　Clobetasone butyrate 500 microgram per 1 gram Eumovate
　Eczema and Dermatitis 0.05% cream | 15 gram P £4.60 DT = £4.60
　Eumovate 0.05% cream | 30 gram PoM £1.86 DT = £1.86 |
　100 gram PoM £5.44 DT = £5.44

Combinations available: *Clobetasone butyrate with nystatin and oxytetracycline,* p. 1294

⚑ 1286

Diflucortolone valerate
25-Sep-2020

13

Skin

● **INDICATIONS AND DOSE**

Severe inflammatory skin disorders such as eczemas unresponsive to less potent corticosteroids (using 0.3% diflucortolone valerate) | Short-term treatment of severe exacerbations (using 0.3% diflucortolone valerate) | Psoriasis (using 0.3% diflucortolone valerate)
▸ TO THE SKIN
▸ Child 4–17 years: Apply 1–2 times a day for up to 2 weeks, reducing strength as condition responds, to be applied thinly; maximum 60 g per week
▸ Adult: Apply 1–2 times a day for up to 2 weeks, reducing strength as condition responds, to be applied thinly; maximum 60 g per week

Severe inflammatory skin disorders such as eczemas unresponsive to less potent corticosteroids (using 0.1% diflucortolone valerate) | Psoriasis (using 0.1% diflucortolone valerate)
▸ TO THE SKIN
▸ Child: Apply 1–2 times a day for up to 4 weeks, to be applied thinly
▸ Adult: Apply 1–2 times a day for up to 4 weeks, to be applied thinly
POTENCY
▸ Diflucortolone valerate 0.1% cream and ointment: potent.
▸ Diflucortolone valerate 0.3% cream and ointment: very potent.

● **UNLICENSED USE**
▸ In children *Nerisone*® licensed for use in children (age range not specified by manufacturer); *Nerisone Forte*® not licensed for use in children under 4 years.

● **PRESCRIBING AND DISPENSING INFORMATION** Patients or carers should be advised on application of diflucortolone valerate containing preparations.

● **MEDICINAL FORMS** There can be variation in the licensing of different medicines containing the same drug.

Ointment
CAUTIONARY AND ADVISORY LABELS 28
▸ Nerisone (Meadow Laboratories Ltd)
　Diflucortolone valerate 1 mg per 1 gram Nerisone 0.1% ointment |
　30 gram PoM £3.98 DT = £3.98
　Diflucortolone valerate 3 mg per 1 gram Nerisone Forte 0.3%
　ointment | 15 gram PoM £4.70 DT = £4.70

Cream
CAUTIONARY AND ADVISORY LABELS 28
EXCIPIENTS: May contain Beeswax, cetostearyl alcohol (including cetyl and stearyl alcohol), disodium edetate, hydroxybenzoates (parabens)
▸ Nerisone (Meadow Laboratories Ltd)
　Diflucortolone valerate 1 mg per 1 gram Nerisone 0.1% cream |
　30 gram PoM £3.98 DT = £3.98
　Nerisone 0.1% oily cream | 30 gram PoM £4.95 DT = £4.95
　Diflucortolone valerate 3 mg per 1 gram Nerisone Forte 0.3% oily
　cream | 15 gram PoM £4.70 DT = £4.70

Fludroxycortide

25-Sep-2020

(Flurandrenolone)

● **INDICATIONS AND DOSE**

Inflammatory skin disorders such as eczemas

▸ TO THE SKIN

▸ Child: Apply 1–2 times a day, to be applied thinly

▸ Adult: Apply 1–2 times a day, to be applied thinly

POTENCY

▸ Fludroxycortide 0.0125% cream and ointment: moderate

HAELAN ® TAPE

Chronic localised recalcitrant dermatoses (but not acute or weeping)

▸ TO THE SKIN

▸ Child: Cut tape to fit lesion, apply to clean, dry skin shorn of hair, usually for 12 hours daily

▸ Adult: Cut tape to fit lesion, apply to clean, dry skin shorn of hair, usually for 12 hours daily

● **UNLICENSED USE**

▸ In children Licensed for use in children (age range not specified by manufacturer).

● **SIDE-EFFECTS** Cushing's syndrome · increased risk of infection

● **PATIENT AND CARER ADVICE** Patients or carers should be counselled on application of fludroxycortide cream and ointment.

● **MEDICINAL FORMS** There can be variation in the licensing of different medicines containing the same drug.

Ointment

CAUTIONARY AND ADVISORY LABELS 28

EXCIPIENTS: May contain Beeswax, cetostearyl alcohol (including cetyl and stearyl alcohol), polysorbates

▸ Fludroxycortide (Non-proprietary)

Fludroxycortide 125 microgram per 1 gram Fludroxycortide 0.0125% ointment | 60 gram [PoM] £5.99

Cream

CAUTIONARY AND ADVISORY LABELS 28

EXCIPIENTS: May contain Cetostearyl alcohol (including cetyl and stearyl alcohol), propylene glycol

▸ Fludroxycortide (Non-proprietary)

Fludroxycortide 125 microgram per 1 gram Fludroxycortide 0.0125% cream | 60 gram [PoM] £5.99 DT = £5.99

Impregnated dressing

▸ Fludroxycortide (Non-proprietary)

Fludroxycortide 4 microgram per 1 square cm Fludroxycortide 4micrograms/square cm tape 7.5cm | 20 cm [PoM] £12.49–£13.67 DT = £13.67 | 50 cm [PoM] £18.75

Fluocinolone acetonide

05-Nov-2020

● **INDICATIONS AND DOSE**

Severe inflammatory skin disorders such as eczemas | Psoriasis

▸ TO THE SKIN

▸ Child 1-17 years: Apply 1–2 times a day, to be applied thinly, reduce strength as condition responds

▸ Adult: Apply 1–2 times a day, to be applied thinly, reduce strength as condition responds

POTENCY

▸ Fluocinolone acetonide 0.025% cream, gel, and ointment: potent.

▸ Fluocinolone acetonide 0.00625% cream and ointment: moderate.

▸ Fluocinolone acetonide 0.0025% cream: mild.

● **INTERACTIONS** → Appendix 1: fluocinolone

● **PRESCRIBING AND DISPENSING INFORMATION** Gel is useful for application to the scalp and other hairy areas.

● **PATIENT AND CARER ADVICE** Patient counselling is advised for fluocinolone acetonide cream, gel and ointment (application).

● **MEDICINAL FORMS** There can be variation in the licensing of different medicines containing the same drug.

Ointment

CAUTIONARY AND ADVISORY LABELS 28

EXCIPIENTS: May contain Propylene glycol, woolfat and related substances (including lanolin)

▸ Synalar (Reig Jofre UK Ltd)

Fluocinolone acetonide 62.5 microgram per 1 gram Synalar 1 in 4 Dilution 0.00625% ointment | 50 gram [PoM] £4.84 DT = £4.84

Fluocinolone acetonide 250 microgram per 1 gram Synalar 0.025% ointment | 30 gram [PoM] £4.14 DT = £4.14 | 100 gram [PoM] £11.75 DT = £11.75

Cream

CAUTIONARY AND ADVISORY LABELS 28

EXCIPIENTS: May contain Benzyl alcohol, cetostearyl alcohol (including cetyl and stearyl alcohol), polysorbates, propylene glycol

▸ Synalar (Reig Jofre UK Ltd)

Fluocinolone acetonide 62.5 microgram per 1 gram Synalar 1 in 4 Dilution 0.00625% cream | 50 gram [PoM] £4.84 DT = £4.84

Fluocinolone acetonide 250 microgram per 1 gram Synalar 0.025% cream | 30 gram [PoM] £4.14 DT = £4.14 | 100 gram [PoM] £11.75 DT = £11.75

Gel

CAUTIONARY AND ADVISORY LABELS 28

EXCIPIENTS: May contain Hydroxybenzoates (parabens), propylene glycol

▸ Synalar (Reig Jofre UK Ltd)

Fluocinolone acetonide 250 microgram per 1 gram Synalar 0.025% gel | 30 gram [PoM] £5.56 DT = £5.56 | 60 gram [PoM] £10.02 DT = £10.02

Combinations available: *Fluocinolone acetonide with clioquinol*, p. 1294 · *Fluocinolone acetonide with neomycin*, p. 1294

Fluocinonide

25-Sep-2020

● **INDICATIONS AND DOSE**

Severe inflammatory skin disorders such as eczemas unresponsive to less potent corticosteroids | Psoriasis

▸ TO THE SKIN

▸ Child: Apply 1–2 times a day, to be applied thinly

▸ Adult: Apply 1–2 times a day, to be applied thinly

POTENCY

▸ Fluocinonide 0.05% cream and ointment: potent.

● **UNLICENSED USE**

▸ In children Not licensed for use in children under 1 year.

● **PATIENT AND CARER ADVICE** Patients or carers should be advised on the application of fluocinonide preparations.

● **MEDICINAL FORMS** There can be variation in the licensing of different medicines containing the same drug. Forms available from special-order manufacturers include: ointment

Ointment

CAUTIONARY AND ADVISORY LABELS 28

EXCIPIENTS: May contain Propylene glycol, woolfat and related substances (including lanolin)

▸ Metosyn (Reig Jofre UK Ltd)

Fluocinonide 500 microgram per 1 gram Metosyn 0.05% ointment | 25 gram [PoM] £3.50 DT = £3.50 | 100 gram [PoM] £13.15 DT = £13.15

Cream

CAUTIONARY AND ADVISORY LABELS 28

EXCIPIENTS: May contain Propylene glycol

▸ Metosyn FAPG (Reig Jofre UK Ltd)

Fluocinonide 500 microgram per 1 gram Metosyn FAPG 0.05% cream | 25 gram [PoM] £3.96 DT = £3.96 | 100 gram [PoM] £13.34 DT = £13.34

Fluticasone

F 1286
25-Sep-2020

● **INDICATIONS AND DOSE**

Severe inflammatory skin disorders such as dermatitis and eczemas unresponsive to less potent corticosteroids | Psoriasis
▸ TO THE SKIN
▸ **Child 3 months-17 years:** Apply 1–2 times a day, to be applied thinly
▸ **Adult:** Apply 1–2 times a day, to be applied thinly
POTENCY
▸ Fluticasone cream 0.05%: potent.
▸ Fluticasone ointment 0.005%: potent.

● INTERACTIONS → Appendix 1: corticosteroids
● PATIENT AND CARER ADVICE Patients or carers should be given advice on application of fluticasone creams and ointments.

● MEDICINAL FORMS There can be variation in the licensing of different medicines containing the same drug.
Cream
CAUTIONARY AND ADVISORY LABELS 28
EXCIPIENTS: May contain Cetostearyl alcohol (including cetyl and stearyl alcohol), imidurea, propylene glycol
▸ Fluticasone (Non-proprietary)
  Fluticasone propionate 500 microgram per 1 gram Fluticasone 0.05% cream | 30 gram PoM £5.68 DT = £4.24
▸ Cutivate (GlaxoSmithKline UK Ltd)
  Fluticasone propionate 500 microgram per 1 gram Cutivate 0.05% cream | 15 gram PoM £2.27 DT = £2.27 | 30 gram PoM £4.24 DT = £4.24

Ointment
CAUTIONARY AND ADVISORY LABELS 28
EXCIPIENTS: May contain Propylene glycol
▸ Cutivate (GlaxoSmithKline UK Ltd)
  Fluticasone propionate 50 microgram per 1 gram Cutivate 0.005% ointment | 15 gram PoM £2.27 DT = £2.27 | 30 gram PoM £4.24 DT = £4.24

Hydrocortisone

F 1286
23-Nov-2020

● DRUG ACTION Hydrocortisone has equal glucocorticoid and mineralocorticoid activity.

● **INDICATIONS AND DOSE**

Mild inflammatory skin disorders such as eczemas
▸ TO THE SKIN
▸ **Child:** Apply 1–2 times a day, to be applied thinly
▸ **Adult:** Apply 1–2 times a day, to be applied thinly
Nappy rash
▸ TO THE SKIN
▸ **Child:** Apply 1–2 times a day for no longer than 1 week, discontinued as soon as the inflammation subsides
POTENCY
▸ Hydrocortisone cream and ointment 0.5 to 2.5%: mild

● INTERACTIONS → Appendix 1: corticosteroids
● PRESCRIBING AND DISPENSING INFORMATION When hydrocortisone cream or ointment is prescribed and no strength is stated, the 1% strength should be supplied. Although *Dioderm*® contains only 0.1% hydrocortisone, the formulation is designed to provide a clinical activity comparable to that of Hydrocortisone Cream 1% BP.
● PATIENT AND CARER ADVICE Patient counselling is advised for hydrocortisone cream and ointment (application).
● PROFESSION SPECIFIC INFORMATION
Dental practitioners' formulary Hydrocortisone Cream 1% 15 g may be prescribed.

● EXCEPTIONS TO LEGAL CATEGORY
Over-the-counter hydrocortisone preparations Skin creams and ointments containing hydrocortisone (alone or with other ingredients) can be sold to the public for the treatment of allergic contact dermatitis, irritant dermatitis, insect bite reactions and mild to moderate eczema in patients over 10 years, to be applied sparingly over the affected area 1–2 times daily for max. 1 week. Over-the-counter hydrocortisone preparations should not be sold without medical advice for children under 10 years or for pregnant women; they should **not** be sold for application to the face, anogenital region, broken or infected skin (including cold sores, acne, and athlete's foot).

● MEDICINAL FORMS There can be variation in the licensing of different medicines containing the same drug. Forms available from special-order manufacturers include: cream, ointment
Cream
CAUTIONARY AND ADVISORY LABELS 28
EXCIPIENTS: May contain Benzyl alcohol, cetostearyl alcohol (including cetyl and stearyl alcohol), hydroxybenzoates (parabens), propylene glycol
▸ Hydrocortisone (Non-proprietary)
  Hydrocortisone 5 mg per 1 gram Hydrocortisone 0.5% cream | 15 gram PoM £44.00 DT = £1.30 | 30 gram PoM £2.60–£88.00
  Hydrocortisone 10 mg per 1 gram Hydrocortisone 1% cream | 15 gram PoM £18.88 DT = £1.56 | 30 gram PoM £29.32 DT = £3.12 | 50 gram PoM £44.12 DT = £5.20
  Hydrocortisone 25 mg per 1 gram Hydrocortisone 2.5% cream | 15 gram PoM £44.00 DT = £5.30 | 30 gram PoM £88.00
▸ Dermacort (Marlborough Pharmaceuticals Ltd)
  Hydrocortisone 1 mg per 1 gram Dermacort hydrocortisone 0.1% cream | 15 gram P £2.83 DT = £2.83
▸ Mildison Lipocream (Karo Pharma)
  Hydrocortisone 10 mg per 1 gram Mildison Lipocream 1% cream | 30 gram PoM £1.71 DT = £3.12

Ointment
CAUTIONARY AND ADVISORY LABELS 28
▸ Hydrocortisone (Non-proprietary)
  Hydrocortisone 5 mg per 1 gram Hydrocortisone 0.5% ointment | 15 gram PoM £44.00 DT = £44.00 | 30 gram PoM £88.00
  Hydrocortisone 10 mg per 1 gram Hydrocortisone 1% ointment | 15 gram PoM £16.55 DT = £1.47 | 30 gram PoM £24.96 DT = £2.93 | 50 gram PoM £39.41 DT = £4.88
  Hydrocortisone 25 mg per 1 gram Hydrocortisone 2.5% ointment | 15 gram PoM £44.00 DT = £24.47 | 30 gram PoM £48.94–£88.00

Combinations available: *Hydrocortisone with benzalkonium chloride, dimeticone and nystatin*, p. 1295 · *Hydrocortisone with chlorhexidine hydrochloride and nystatin*, p. 1295 · *Hydrocortisone with clotrimazole*, p. 1295 · *Hydrocortisone with fusidic acid*, p. 1295 · *Hydrocortisone with miconazole*, p. 1296 · *Hydrocortisone with oxytetracycline*, p. 1296

Hydrocortisone butyrate

F 1286
25-Sep-2020

● **INDICATIONS AND DOSE**

Severe inflammatory skin disorders such as eczemas unresponsive to less potent corticosteroids | Psoriasis
▸ TO THE SKIN
▸ **Child 1-17 years:** Apply 1–2 times a day, to be applied thinly
▸ **Adult:** Apply 1–2 times a day, to be applied thinly
POTENCY
▸ Hydrocortisone butyrate 0.1% cream, liquid, and ointment: potent

● PATIENT AND CARER ADVICE Patients or carers should be given advice on how to administer hydrocortisone butyrate lotion, cream, ointment and scalp lotion.
Medicines for Children leaflet: Hydrocortisone (topical) for eczema
www.medicinesforchildren.org.uk/hydrocortisone-topical-eczema

13

Skin

● MEDICINAL FORMS There can be variation in the licensing of different medicines containing the same drug. Forms available from special-order manufacturers include: ointment

Ointment
CAUTIONARY AND ADVISORY LABELS 28
▸ Locoid (LEO Pharma)
    Hydrocortisone butyrate 1 mg per 1 gram Locoid 0.1% ointment | 100 gram [PoM] £4.93 DT = £4.93

Cream
CAUTIONARY AND ADVISORY LABELS 28
EXCIPIENTS: May contain Benzyl alcohol, cetostearyl alcohol (including cetyl and stearyl alcohol), hydroxybenzoates (parabens)
▸ Locoid (LEO Pharma)
    Hydrocortisone butyrate 1 mg per 1 gram Locoid 0.1% cream | 100 gram [PoM] £4.93 DT = £4.93
▸ Locoid Lipocream (LEO Pharma)
    Hydrocortisone butyrate 1 mg per 1 gram Locoid 0.1% Lipocream | 100 gram [PoM] £5.17 DT = £4.93

Liquid
CAUTIONARY AND ADVISORY LABELS 15(excluding Locoid Crelo topical emulsion), 28
EXCIPIENTS: May contain Butylated hydroxytoluene, cetostearyl alcohol (including cetyl and stearyl alcohol), hydroxybenzoates (parabens), propylene glycol
▸ Locoid (LEO Pharma)
    Hydrocortisone butyrate 1 mg per 1 ml Locoid 0.1% scalp lotion | 100 ml [PoM] £6.83 DT = £6.83
▸ Locoid Crelo (LEO Pharma)
    Hydrocortisone butyrate 1 mg per 1 gram Locoid Crelo 0.1% topical emulsion | 100 gram [PoM] £5.91 DT = £5.91

◤ 1286

Mometasone furoate

10-Nov-2020

● INDICATIONS AND DOSE

Severe inflammatory skin disorders such as eczemas unresponsive to less potent corticosteroids | Psoriasis
▸ TO THE SKIN
▸ Child 2–17 years: Apply once daily, to be applied thinly (to scalp in case of lotion)
▸ Adult: Apply once daily, to be applied thinly (to scalp in case of lotion)
POTENCY
▸ Mometasone furoate 0.1% cream, ointment, and scalp lotion: potent.

● INTERACTIONS → Appendix 1: corticosteroids

● MEDICINAL FORMS There can be variation in the licensing of different medicines containing the same drug. Forms available from special-order manufacturers include: ointment

Cream
CAUTIONARY AND ADVISORY LABELS 28
EXCIPIENTS: May contain Beeswax
▸ Mometasone furoate (Non-proprietary)
    Mometasone furoate 1 mg per 1 gram Mometasone 0.1% cream | 30 gram [PoM] £4.39 DT = £3.05 | 100 gram [PoM] £12.58 DT = £10.17
▸ Elocon (Merck Sharp & Dohme Ltd)
    Mometasone furoate 1 mg per 1 gram Elocon 0.1% cream | 30 gram [PoM] £4.80 DT = £3.05 | 100 gram [PoM] £15.10 DT = £10.17

Ointment
CAUTIONARY AND ADVISORY LABELS 28
EXCIPIENTS: May contain Beeswax, propylene glycol
▸ Mometasone furoate (Non-proprietary)
    Mometasone furoate 1 mg per 1 gram Mometasone 0.1% ointment | 15 gram [PoM] £4.32 | 30 gram [PoM] £4.45 DT = £3.17 | 50 gram [PoM] £12.44 | 100 gram [PoM] £12.82 DT = £10.57
▸ Elocon (Merck Sharp & Dohme Ltd)
    Mometasone furoate 1 mg per 1 gram Elocon 0.1% ointment | 30 gram [PoM] £4.32 DT = £3.17 | 100 gram [PoM] £12.44 DT = £10.57

Liquid
CAUTIONARY AND ADVISORY LABELS 28
EXCIPIENTS: May contain Propylene glycol
▸ Elocon (Merck Sharp & Dohme Ltd)
    Mometasone furoate 1 mg per 1 gram Elocon 0.1% scalp lotion | 30 ml [PoM] £4.36 DT = £4.36

CORTICOSTEROIDS 〉 CORTICOSTEROID COMBINATIONS WITH ANTI-INFECTIVES

Betamethasone with clioquinol

03-Sep-2020

The properties listed below are those particular to the combination only. For the properties of the components please consider, betamethasone p. 1287.

● INDICATIONS AND DOSE

Severe inflammatory skin disorders such as eczemas associated with infection and unresponsive to less potent corticosteroids | Psoriasis (excluding widespread plaque psoriasis)
▸ TO THE SKIN
▸ Child 1–17 years: (consult product literature)
▸ Adult: (consult product literature)
POTENCY
▸ Betamethasone (as valerate) 0.1% with clioquinol cream and ointment: potent.

● INTERACTIONS → Appendix 1: corticosteroids

● PATIENT AND CARER ADVICE Stains clothing. Patients or carers should be counselled on application of betamethasone with clioquinol preparations.

● MEDICINAL FORMS There can be variation in the licensing of different medicines containing the same drug.

Ointment
CAUTIONARY AND ADVISORY LABELS 28
▸ Betamethasone with clioquinol (Non-proprietary)
    Betamethasone (as Betamethasone valerate) 1 mg per 1 gram, Clioquinol 30 mg per 1 gram Betamethasone valerate 0.1% / Clioquinol 3% ointment | 30 gram [PoM] £38.88 DT = £38.88

Cream
CAUTIONARY AND ADVISORY LABELS 28
EXCIPIENTS: May contain Cetostearyl alcohol (including cetyl and stearyl alcohol), chlorocresol
▸ Betamethasone with clioquinol (Non-proprietary)
    Betamethasone (as Betamethasone valerate) 1 mg per 1 gram, Clioquinol 30 mg per 1 gram Betamethasone valerate 0.1% / Clioquinol 3% cream | 30 gram [PoM] £38.88 DT = £38.88

Betamethasone with clotrimazole

03-Sep-2020

The properties listed below are those particular to the combination only. For the properties of the components please consider, betamethasone p. 1287, clotrimazole p. 1276.

● INDICATIONS AND DOSE

Short-term treatment of tinea infections and candidiasis
▸ TO THE SKIN
▸ Child 12–17 years: Apply twice daily for 2 weeks for tinea cruris, tinea corporis or candidiasis, or for 4 weeks for tinea pedis
▸ Adult: Apply twice daily for 2 weeks for tinea cruris, tinea corporis or candidiasis, or for 4 weeks for tinea pedis
POTENCY
▸ Betamethasone dipropionate 0.064% (=betamethasone 0.05%) with clotrimazole cream: potent.

● INTERACTIONS → Appendix 1: antifungals, azoles · corticosteroids

● PATIENT AND CARER ADVICE Patients or carers should be given advice on how to administer betamethasone with clotrimazole cream.

● MEDICINAL FORMS There can be variation in the licensing of different medicines containing the same drug.

Cream
CAUTIONARY AND ADVISORY LABELS 28
EXCIPIENTS: May contain Benzyl alcohol, cetostearyl alcohol (including cetyl and stearyl alcohol), propylene glycol
▸ Lotriderm (Merck Sharp & Dohme Ltd)
  Betamethasone dipropionate 640 microgram per 1 gram, Clotrimazole 10 mg per 1 gram Lotriderm cream | 30 gram PoM
  £6.34 DT = £6.34

Betamethasone with fusidic acid
03-Sep-2020

The properties listed below are those particular to the combination only. For the properties of the components please consider, betamethasone p. 1287, fusidic acid p. 608.

● INDICATIONS AND DOSE

Severe inflammatory skin disorders such as eczemas associated with infection and unresponsive to less potent corticosteroids
▸ TO THE SKIN
▸ Child: (consult product literature)
▸ Adult: (consult product literature)
POTENCY
▸ Betamethasone (as valerate) 0.1% with fusidic acid cream: potent.

● UNLICENSED USE
▸ In children *Fucibet® Lipid Cream* is not licensed for use in children under 6 years.

● INTERACTIONS → Appendix 1: corticosteroids · fusidate

● PATIENT AND CARER ADVICE Patients or carers should be counselled on application of betamethasone with fusidic acid preparations.

● MEDICINAL FORMS There can be variation in the licensing of different medicines containing the same drug.

Cream
CAUTIONARY AND ADVISORY LABELS 28
EXCIPIENTS: May contain Cetostearyl alcohol (including cetyl and stearyl alcohol), chlorocresol, hydroxybenzoates (parabens)
▸ Fucibet (LEO Pharma)
  Betamethasone (as Betamethasone valerate) 1 mg per 1 gram, Fusidic acid 20 mg per 1 gram Fucibet cream | 30 gram PoM
  £6.38 DT = £6.38 | 60 gram PoM £12.76 DT = £12.76
  Fucibet Lipid cream | 30 gram PoM £6.74 DT = £6.38
▸ Xemacort (Mylan)
  Betamethasone (as Betamethasone valerate) 1 mg per 1 gram, Fusidic acid 20 mg per 1 gram Xemacort 20mg/g / 1mg/g cream |
  30 gram PoM £6.05 DT = £6.38 | 60 gram PoM £12.45 DT = £12.76

Betamethasone with neomycin   18-Nov-2020

The properties listed below are those particular to the combination only. For the properties of the components please consider, betamethasone p. 1287, neomycin sulfate p. 1274.

● INDICATIONS AND DOSE

Severe inflammatory skin disorders such as eczemas unresponsive to less potent corticosteroids | Psoriasis
▸ TO THE SKIN USING OINTMENT, OR TO THE SKIN USING CREAM
▸ Child 2-17 years: Apply 1–2 times a day, to be applied thinly
▸ Adult: Apply 1–2 times a day, to be applied thinly
POTENCY
▸ Betamethasone (as valerate) 0.1% with neomycin cream and ointment: potent.

● INTERACTIONS → Appendix 1: corticosteroids · neomycin

● PATIENT AND CARER ADVICE Patient counselling is advised for betamethasone with neomycin cream and ointment (application).

● MEDICINAL FORMS There can be variation in the licensing of different medicines containing the same drug.

Ointment
CAUTIONARY AND ADVISORY LABELS 28
▸ Betamethasone with neomycin (Non-proprietary)
  Betamethasone (as Betamethasone valerate) 1 mg per 1 gram, Neomycin sulfate 5 mg per 1 gram Betamethasone valerate 0.1% / Neomycin 0.5% ointment | 30 gram PoM £38.88 DT = £31.36 |
  100 gram PoM £97.00 DT = £104.52

Cream
CAUTIONARY AND ADVISORY LABELS 28
EXCIPIENTS: May contain Cetostearyl alcohol (including cetyl and stearyl alcohol), chlorocresol
▸ Betamethasone with neomycin (Non-proprietary)
  Betamethasone (as Betamethasone valerate) 1 mg per 1 gram, Neomycin sulfate 5 mg per 1 gram Betamethasone valerate 0.1% / Neomycin 0.5% cream | 30 gram PoM £38.88 DT = £31.36 |
  100 gram PoM £97.00 DT = £104.52

Betamethasone with salicylic acid
11-Mar-2020

The properties listed below are those particular to the combination only. For the properties of the components please consider, betamethasone p. 1287, salicylic acid p. 1330.

● INDICATIONS AND DOSE
DIPROSALIC® OINTMENT

Severe inflammatory skin disorders such as eczemas unresponsive to less potent corticosteroids | Psoriasis
▸ TO THE SKIN
▸ Child: Apply 1–2 times a day, max. 60 g per week
▸ Adult: Apply 1–2 times a day, max. 60 g per week
POTENCY
▸ Betamethasone (as dipropionate) 0.05% with salicylic acid 3%: potent.

DIPROSALIC® SCALP APPLICATION

Severe inflammatory skin disorders such as eczemas unresponsive to less potent corticosteroids | Psoriasis
▸ TO THE SKIN
▸ Child: Apply 1–2 times a day, apply a few drops
▸ Adult: Apply 1–2 times a day, apply a few drops
POTENCY
▸ Betamethasone (as dipropionate) 0.05% with salicylic acid 2%: potent.

● INTERACTIONS → Appendix 1: corticosteroids

● PATIENT AND CARER ADVICE
DIPROSALIC® OINTMENT Patients or carers should be counselled on application of betamethasone and salicylic acid preparations.

DIPROSALIC® SCALP APPLICATION Patients or carers should be counselled on application of betamethasone and salicylic acid scalp application.

● MEDICINAL FORMS There can be variation in the licensing of different medicines containing the same drug.

Ointment
CAUTIONARY AND ADVISORY LABELS 28
▸ Diprosalic (Merck Sharp & Dohme Ltd)
  Betamethasone (as Betamethasone dipropionate) 500 microgram per 1 gram, Salicylic acid 30 mg per 1 gram Diprosalic 0.05%/3% ointment | 30 gram PoM £3.18 DT =
  £3.18 | 100 gram PoM £9.14 DT = £9.14

13

Skin

Liquid

CAUTIONARY AND ADVISORY LABELS 28

EXCIPIENTS: May contain Disodium edetate

▸ Diprosalic (Merck Sharp & Dohme Ltd)
Betamethasone (as Betamethasone dipropionate)
500 microgram per 1 ml, Salicylic acid 20 mg per 1 ml Diprosalic
0.05%/2% scalp application | 100 ml [PoM] £10.10 DT = £10.10

Clobetasol propionate with neomycin sulfate and nystatin

The properties listed below are those particular to the combination only. For the properties of the components please consider, clobetasol propionate p. 1288, neomycin sulfate p. 1274.

● **INDICATIONS AND DOSE**

Short-term treatment only of severe resistant inflammatory skin disorders such as recalcitrant eczemas associated with infection and unresponsive to less potent corticosteroids | Psoriasis associated with infection

▸ TO THE SKIN

▸ Adult: (consult product literature)

POTENCY

▸ Clobetasol propionate 0.05% with neomycin sulfate and nystatin cream and ointment: very potent.

● INTERACTIONS → Appendix 1: neomycin

● PATIENT AND CARER ADVICE Patients or carers should be advised on application of clobetasol propionate, neomycin sulfate and nystatin containing preparations.

● MEDICINAL FORMS There can be variation in the licensing of different medicines containing the same drug.

Ointment

CAUTIONARY AND ADVISORY LABELS 28

▸ Clobetasol propionate with neomycin sulfate and nystatin (Non-proprietary)
Clobetasol propionate 500 microgram per 1 gram, Neomycin sulfate 5 mg per 1 gram, Nystatin 100000 unit per 1 gram Clobetasol 500microgram / Neomycin 5mg / Nystatin 100,000units/g ointment | 30 gram [PoM] £87.00 DT = £87.00

Cream

CAUTIONARY AND ADVISORY LABELS 28

▸ Clobetasol propionate with neomycin sulfate and nystatin (Non-proprietary)
Clobetasol propionate 500 microgram per 1 gram, Neomycin sulfate 5 mg per 1 gram, Nystatin 100000 unit per 1 gram Clobetasol 500microgram / Neomycin 5mg / Nystatin 100,000units/g cream | 30 gram [PoM] £87.00 DT = £87.00

Clobetasone butyrate with nystatin and oxytetracycline

01-Sep-2020

The properties listed below are those particular to the combination only. For the properties of the components please consider, clobetasone butyrate p. 1289, oxytetracycline p. 603.

● **INDICATIONS AND DOSE**

Steroid-responsive dermatoses where candidal or bacterial infection is present

▸ TO THE SKIN

▸ Adult: (consult product literature)

POTENCY

▸ Clobetasone butyrate 0.05% with nystatin and oxytetracyline cream: moderate.

● INTERACTIONS → Appendix 1: tetracyclines

● PATIENT AND CARER ADVICE Stains clothing.

● MEDICINAL FORMS There can be variation in the licensing of different medicines containing the same drug.

Cream

CAUTIONARY AND ADVISORY LABELS 28

EXCIPIENTS: May contain Cetostearyl alcohol (including cetyl and stearyl alcohol), chlorocresol, sodium metabisulfite

▸ Trimovate (Ennogen Healthcare Ltd)
Clobetasone butyrate 500 microgram per 1 gram, Oxytetracycline (as Oxytetracycline calcium) 30 mg per 1 gram, Nystatin 100000 unit per 1 gram Trimovate cream | 30 gram [PoM] £12.45 DT = £12.45

Fluocinolone acetonide with clioquinol

20-Mar-2020

The properties listed below are those particular to the combination only. For the properties of the components please consider, fluocinolone acetonide p. 1290.

● **INDICATIONS AND DOSE**

Inflammatory skin disorders such as eczemas associated with infection

▸ TO THE SKIN

▸ Adult: Apply 2–3 times a day, to be applied thinly

POTENCY

▸ Clioquinol 3% with fluocinolone acetonide 0.025% cream and ointment: potent

● INTERACTIONS → Appendix 1: fluocinolone

● PATIENT AND CARER ADVICE Patient counselling is advised for clioquinol with fluocinolone acetonide cream and ointment (application). Ointment stains clothing.

● MEDICINAL FORMS There can be variation in the licensing of different medicines containing the same drug.

Ointment

CAUTIONARY AND ADVISORY LABELS 28

EXCIPIENTS: May contain Propylene glycol, woolfat and related substances (including lanolin)

▸ Synalar C (Reig Jofre UK Ltd)
Fluocinolone acetonide 250 microgram per 1 gram, Clioquinol 30 mg per 1 gram Synalar C ointment | 15 gram [PoM] £2.66 DT = £2.66

Cream

CAUTIONARY AND ADVISORY LABELS 28

EXCIPIENTS: May contain Cetostearyl alcohol (including cetyl and stearyl alcohol), disodium edetate, hydroxybenzoates (parabens), polysorbates, propylene glycol

▸ Synalar C (Reig Jofre UK Ltd)
Fluocinolone acetonide 250 microgram per 1 gram, Clioquinol 30 mg per 1 gram Synalar C cream | 15 gram [PoM] £2.66 DT = £2.66

Fluocinolone acetonide with neomycin

The properties listed below are those particular to the combination only. For the properties of the components please consider, fluocinolone acetonide p. 1290, neomycin sulfate p. 1274.

● **INDICATIONS AND DOSE**

Inflammatory skin disorders such as eczemas associated with infection | Psoriasis associated with infection

▸ TO THE SKIN

▸ Child 1-17 years: Apply 1–2 times a day, to be applied thinly, reducing strength as condition responds

▸ Adult: Apply 1–2 times a day, to be applied thinly, reducing strength as condition responds

POTENCY

▸ Fluocinolone acetonide 0.025% with neomycin 0.5% cream and ointment: potent.

● INTERACTIONS → Appendix 1: fluocinolone · neomycin

13

Skin

- PATIENT AND CARER ADVICE Patients or carers should be counselled on the application of fluocinolone acetonide with neomycin preparations.

- MEDICINAL FORMS No licensed medicines listed.

Hydrocortisone with benzalkonium chloride, dimeticone and nystatin

06-Mar-2020

The properties listed below are those particular to the combination only. For the properties of the components please consider, hydrocortisone p. 1291, dimeticone p. 1281.

- INDICATIONS AND DOSE

Mild inflammatory skin disorders such as eczemas associated with infection
- TO THE SKIN
- Child: Apply 3 times a day until lesion has healed, to be applied thinly
- Adult: Apply 3 times a day until lesion has healed, to be applied thinly

POTENCY
- Benzalkonium with dimeticone, hydrocortisone acetate 0.5%, and nystatin cream: mild.

- INTERACTIONS → Appendix 1: corticosteroids
- PATIENT AND CARER ADVICE Patients or carers should be advised on application of benzalkonium with dimeticone and hydrocortisone and nystatin preparations.

- MEDICINAL FORMS There can be variation in the licensing of different medicines containing the same drug.
Cream
CAUTIONARY AND ADVISORY LABELS 28
EXCIPIENTS: May contain Butylated hydroxyanisole, cetostearyl alcohol (including cetyl and stearyl alcohol), hydroxybenzoates (parabens), sodium metabisulfite, sorbic acid
- Timodine (Alliance Pharmaceuticals Ltd)
  Benzalkonium chloride 1 mg per 1 gram, Hydrocortisone 5 mg per 1 gram, Dimeticone 350 100 mg per 1 gram, Nystatin 100000 unit per 1 gram Timodine cream | 30 gram [PoM] £3.37

Hydrocortisone with chlorhexidine hydrochloride and nystatin

10-Mar-2020

The properties listed below are those particular to the combination only. For the properties of the components please consider, hydrocortisone p. 1291, chlorhexidine p. 1321.

- INDICATIONS AND DOSE

Mild inflammatory skin disorders such as eczemas associated with infection
- TO THE SKIN
- Child: (consult product literature)
- Adult: (consult product literature)

POTENCY
- Hydrocortisone 0.5% with chlorhexidine hydrochloride 1% and nystatin cream: mild
- Hydrocortisone 1% with chlorhexidine hydrochloride 1% and nystatin ointment: mild

- INTERACTIONS → Appendix 1: corticosteroids
- PATIENT AND CARER ADVICE Patients or carers should be given advice on application of chlorhexidine hydrochloride with hydrocortisone and nystatin preparations.

- MEDICINAL FORMS There can be variation in the licensing of different medicines containing the same drug.
Ointment
CAUTIONARY AND ADVISORY LABELS 28
- Hydrocortisone with chlorhexidine hydrochloride and nystatin (Non-proprietary)
  Chlorhexidine acetate 10 mg per 1 gram, Hydrocortisone 10 mg per 1 gram, Nystatin 100000 unit per 1 gram Nystatin 100,000units/g / Chlorhexidine acetate 1% / Hydrocortisone 1% ointment | 30 gram [PoM] £5.29 DT = £5.29
Cream
CAUTIONARY AND ADVISORY LABELS 28
EXCIPIENTS: May contain Benzyl alcohol, cetostearyl alcohol (including cetyl and stearyl alcohol), polysorbates
- Hydrocortisone with chlorhexidine hydrochloride and nystatin (Non-proprietary)
  Hydrocortisone 5 mg per 1 gram, Chlorhexidine hydrochloride 10 mg per 1 gram, Nystatin 100000 unit per 1 gram Nystatin 100,000units/g / Chlorhexidine hydrochloride 1% / Hydrocortisone 0.5% cream | 30 gram [PoM] £5.29 DT = £5.29

Hydrocortisone with clotrimazole

17-Mar-2020

The properties listed below are those particular to the combination only. For the properties of the components please consider, hydrocortisone p. 1291, clotrimazole p. 1276.

- INDICATIONS AND DOSE

Mild inflammatory skin disorders such as eczemas (associated with fungal infection)
- TO THE SKIN
- Child: (consult product literature)
- Adult: (consult product literature)

POTENCY
- Clotrimazole with hydrocortisone 1% cream: mild

- INTERACTIONS → Appendix 1: antifungals, azoles · corticosteroids
- PATIENT AND CARER ADVICE Patients or carers should be given advice on how to administer clotrimazole with hydrocortisone cream.
- EXCEPTIONS TO LEGAL CATEGORY A 15-g tube is on sale to the public for the treatment of athlete's foot and fungal infection of skin folds with associated inflammation in patients 10 years and over.

- MEDICINAL FORMS There can be variation in the licensing of different medicines containing the same drug.
Cream
CAUTIONARY AND ADVISORY LABELS 28
EXCIPIENTS: May contain Benzyl alcohol, cetostearyl alcohol (including cetyl and stearyl alcohol)
- Canesten HC (Bayer Plc)
  Clotrimazole 10 mg per 1 gram, Hydrocortisone 10 mg per 1 gram Canesten HC cream | 30 gram [PoM] £2.42 DT = £2.42

Hydrocortisone with fusidic acid

13-Mar-2020

The properties listed below are those particular to the combination only. For the properties of the components please consider, hydrocortisone p. 1291, fusidic acid p. 608.

- INDICATIONS AND DOSE

Mild inflammatory skin disorders such as eczemas associated with infection
- TO THE SKIN
- Child: (consult product literature)
- Adult: (consult product literature)

POTENCY
- Hydrocortisone with fusidic acid cream: mild

13

Skin

- INTERACTIONS → Appendix 1: corticosteroids · fusidate
- PATIENT AND CARER ADVICE Patients or carers should be advised on application of hydrocortisone with fusidic acid preparations.

- MEDICINAL FORMS There can be variation in the licensing of different medicines containing the same drug.
Cream
CAUTIONARY AND ADVISORY LABELS 28
EXCIPIENTS: May contain Butylated hydroxyanisole, cetostearyl alcohol (including cetyl and stearyl alcohol), polysorbates, potassium sorbate
- Fucidin H (Fusidic acid / Hydrocortisone) (LEO Pharma)
   Hydrocortisone acetate 10 mg per 1 gram, Fusidic acid 20 mg per 1 gram Fucidin H cream | 30 gram PoM £6.02 DT = £6.02 | 60 gram PoM £12.05 DT = £12.05

Hydrocortisone with miconazole

17-Mar-2020

The properties listed below are those particular to the combination only. For the properties of the components please consider, hydrocortisone p. 1291, miconazole p. 1277.

- INDICATIONS AND DOSE
Mild inflammatory skin disorders such as eczemas associated with infections
- TO THE SKIN
- Adult: (consult product literature)
POTENCY
- Hydrocortisone 1% with miconazole cream and ointment: mild

- INTERACTIONS → Appendix 1: antifungals, azoles · corticosteroids
- PATIENT AND CARER ADVICE Patients or carers should be advised on application of hydrocortisone with miconazole preparations.
- PROFESSION SPECIFIC INFORMATION
Dental practitioners' formulary
May be prescribed as Miconazole and Hydrocortisone Cream or Ointment for max. 7 days.
- EXCEPTIONS TO LEGAL CATEGORY A 15-g tube of hydrocortisone with miconazole cream is on sale to the public for the treatment of athlete's foot and candidal intertrigo.

- MEDICINAL FORMS There can be variation in the licensing of different medicines containing the same drug.
Ointment
CAUTIONARY AND ADVISORY LABELS 28
- Daktacort (Janssen-Cilag Ltd)
   Hydrocortisone 10 mg per 1 gram, Miconazole nitrate 20 mg per 1 gram Daktacort ointment | 30 gram PoM £2.50 DT = £2.50
Cream
CAUTIONARY AND ADVISORY LABELS 28
EXCIPIENTS: May contain Butylated hydroxyanisole, disodium edetate
- Daktacort (McNeil Products Ltd, Janssen-Cilag Ltd)
   Hydrocortisone 10 mg per 1 gram, Miconazole nitrate 20 mg per 1 gram Daktacort 2%/1% cream | 30 gram PoM £2.49 DT = £2.49

Hydrocortisone with oxytetracycline

The properties listed below are those particular to the combination only. For the properties of the components please consider, hydrocortisone p. 1291, oxytetracycline p. 603.

- INDICATIONS AND DOSE
Mild inflammatory skin disorders such as eczemas
- TO THE SKIN
- Child 12-17 years: (consult product literature)

- Adult: (consult product literature)
POTENCY
- Hydrocortisone 1% with oxytetracycline ointment: mild.

- INTERACTIONS → Appendix 1: corticosteroids · tetracyclines
- PREGNANCY Tetracyclines should not be given to pregnant women. Effects on skeletal development have been documented when tetracyclines have been used in the first trimester in animal studies. Administration during the second or third trimester may cause discoloration of the child's teeth.
- BREAST FEEDING Tetracyclines should not be given to women who are breast-feeding (although absorption and therefore discoloration of teeth in the infant is probably usually prevented by chelation with calcium in milk).
- PATIENT AND CARER ADVICE Patients should be given advice on the application of hydrocortisone with oxytetracycline ointment.

- MEDICINAL FORMS There can be variation in the licensing of different medicines containing the same drug.
Ointment
CAUTIONARY AND ADVISORY LABELS 28
- Terra-Cortril (Intrapharm Laboratories Ltd)
   Hydrocortisone 10 mg per 1 gram, Oxytetracycline (as Oxytetracycline hydrochloride) 30 mg per 1 gram Terra-Cortril ointment | 30 gram PoM £5.01 DT = £5.01

DERMATOLOGICAL DRUGS > ANTI-INFECTIVES

Ichthammol

- INDICATIONS AND DOSE
Chronic lichenified eczema
- TO THE SKIN
- Child 1-17 years: Apply 1–3 times a day
- Adult: Apply 1–3 times a day

- UNLICENSED USE
- In children No information available.
- SIDE-EFFECTS Skin irritation

- MEDICINAL FORMS There can be variation in the licensing of different medicines containing the same drug. Forms available from special-order manufacturers include: ointment, paste
Liquid
- Ichthammol (Non-proprietary)
   Ichthammol 1 mg per 1 mg Ichthammol liquid | 100 gram GSL £12.99 DT = £12.99 | 500 gram GSL £41.88

Ichthammol with zinc oxide

The properties listed below are those particular to the combination only. For the properties of the components please consider, ichthammol above.

- INDICATIONS AND DOSE
Chronic lichenified eczema
- TO THE SKIN
- Adult: (consult product literature)

- MEDICINAL FORMS There can be variation in the licensing of different medicines containing the same drug. Forms available from special-order manufacturers include: cream, ointment
Impregnated dressing
- Ichthopaste (Evolan Pharma AB)
   Ichthopaste bandage 7.5cm × 6m | 1 bandage £3.87

13

Skin

DERMATOLOGICAL DRUGS > ANTRACEN DERIVATIVES

Dithranol

23-Nov-2020

(Anthralin)

● **INDICATIONS AND DOSE**

Subacute and chronic psoriasis
▶ TO THE SKIN
  ‣ Adult: (consult product literature)

DITHROCREAM ®

Subacute and chronic psoriasis
▶ TO THE SKIN
  ‣ Adult: For application to skin or scalp, 0.1–0.5% cream suitable for overnight treatment, 1–2% cream for maximum 1 hour (consult product literature)

● **CONTRA-INDICATIONS** Acute and pustular psoriasis · hypersensitivity
● **CAUTIONS** Avoid sensitive areas of skin · avoid use near eyes
● **SIDE-EFFECTS** Skin reactions
● **PREGNANCY** No adverse effects reported.
● **BREAST FEEDING** No adverse effects reported.
● **DIRECTIONS FOR ADMINISTRATION** When applying dithranol, manufacturer advises hands should be protected by gloves or they should be washed thoroughly afterwards. Dithranol should be applied to chronic extensor plaques only, carefully avoiding normal skin.
● **PRESCRIBING AND DISPENSING INFORMATION** Treatment should be started with a low concentration such as dithranol 0.1%, and the strength increased gradually every few days up to 3%, according to tolerance.
● **PATIENT AND CARER ADVICE** Dithranol can stain the skin, hair and fabrics.
● **EXCEPTIONS TO LEGAL CATEGORY** Prescription only medicine if dithranol content more than 1%, otherwise may be sold to the public.

● **MEDICINAL FORMS** There can be variation in the licensing of different medicines containing the same drug. Forms available from special-order manufacturers include: ointment

Cream
CAUTIONARY AND ADVISORY LABELS 28
EXCIPIENTS: May contain Cetostearyl alcohol (including cetyl and stearyl alcohol), chlorocresol
  ‣ Dithrocream (Dermal Laboratories Ltd)
    Dithranol 1 mg per 1 gram Dithrocream 0.1% cream | 50 gram P
    £3.77 DT = £3.77
    Dithranol 2.5 mg per 1 gram Dithrocream 0.25% cream |
    50 gram P £4.04 DT = £4.04
    Dithranol 5 mg per 1 gram Dithrocream 0.5% cream | 50 gram P
    £4.66 DT = £4.66
    Dithranol 10 mg per 1 gram Dithrocream 1% cream | 50 gram P
    £5.42 DT = £5.42
    Dithranol 20 mg per 1 gram Dithrocream 2% cream |
    50 gram PoM £6.79 DT = £6.79

Combinations available: *Coal tar with dithranol and salicylic acid*, p. 1298

Dithranol with salicylic acid and zinc oxide

The properties listed below are those particular to the combination only. For the properties of the components please consider, dithranol above, salicylic acid p. 1330.

● **INDICATIONS AND DOSE**

Subacute and chronic psoriasis
▶ TO THE SKIN
  ‣ Adult: (consult local protocol)

● **MEDICINAL FORMS** Forms available from special-order manufacturers include: ointment, paste

DERMATOLOGICAL DRUGS > TARS

Coal tar

01-Sep-2020

● **INDICATIONS AND DOSE**

Psoriasis | Scaly scalp disorders such as psoriasis, eczema, seborrhoeic dermatitis and dandruff
▶ TO THE SKIN
  ‣ Child: (consult product literature)
  ‣ Adult: (consult product literature)

● **CONTRA-INDICATIONS** Avoid broken or inflamed skin · avoid eye area · avoid genital area · avoid mucosal areas · avoid rectal area · infection · sore, acute, or pustular psoriasis
● **CAUTIONS**
GENERAL CAUTIONS Application to face
SPECIFIC CAUTIONS
  ‣ When used for scaly scalp disorders, using shampoo Children under 12 years (consult product literature)
● **SIDE-EFFECTS** Photosensitivity reaction · skin reactions
● **PRESCRIBING AND DISPENSING INFORMATION** Coal Tar Solution BP contains coal tar 20%, Strong Coal Tar Solution BP contains coal tar 40%.
● **HANDLING AND STORAGE** Use suitable chemical protection gloves for extemporaneous preparation. May stain skin, hair and fabric.
● **PATIENT AND CARER ADVICE** May stain skin, hair and fabric.

● **MEDICINAL FORMS** There can be variation in the licensing of different medicines containing the same drug. Forms available from special-order manufacturers include: cream, ointment, paste

Cutaneous emulsion
EXCIPIENTS: May contain Hydroxybenzoates (parabens)
  ‣ Exorex (Teva UK Ltd)
    Coal tar solution 50 mg per 1 gram Exorex lotion | 100 ml GSL
    £8.11 DT = £8.11 | 250 ml GSL £16.24 DT = £16.24

Shampoo
EXCIPIENTS: May contain Fragrances, hydroxybenzoates (parabens)
  ‣ Alphosyl 2 in 1 (Omega Pharma Ltd)
    Coal tar extract alcoholic 50 mg per 1 gram Alphosyl 2 in 1
    shampoo | 250 ml GSL £5.81 DT = £5.81
  ‣ Neutrogena T/Gel Therapeutic (Johnson & Johnson Ltd)
    Coal tar extract 20 mg per 1 gram Neutrogena T/Gel Therapeutic
    shampoo | 125 ml GSL £4.11 DT = £4.11 | 250 ml GSL £6.18 DT =
    £6.18
  ‣ Polytar Scalp (Thornton & Ross Ltd)
    Coal tar solution 40 mg per 1 ml Polytar Scalp shampoo |
    150 ml GSL £3.46 DT = £3.46
  ‣ Psoriderm (Dermal Laboratories Ltd)
    Coal tar distilled 25 mg per 1 ml Psoriderm scalp lotion |
    250 ml P £4.74 DT = £4.74

13

Skin

Cream

EXCIPIENTS: May contain Isopropyl palmitate, lecithin, propylene glycol
▸ Psoriderm (Dermal Laboratories Ltd)
   Coal tar distilled 60 mg per 1 gram Psoriderm cream | 225 ml P
   £9.42 DT = £9.42

Coal tar with calamine
15-Jan-2019

The properties listed below are those particular to the combination only. For the properties of the components please consider, coal tar p. 1297.

● INDICATIONS AND DOSE

Psoriasis | Chronic atopic eczema (occasionally)
▸ TO THE SKIN
   ▸ Adult: Apply 1–2 times a day

IMPORTANT SAFETY INFORMATION

MHRA/CHM ADVICE (UPDATED DECEMBER 2018): EMOLLIENTS: NEW INFORMATION ABOUT RISK OF SEVERE AND FATAL BURNS WITH PARAFFIN-CONTAINING AND PARAFFIN-FREE EMOLLIENTS
See Emollient and barrier preparations p. 1265.

● PRESCRIBING AND DISPENSING INFORMATION When prepared extemporaneously, the BP states Calamine and Coal Tar Ointment BP, consists of calamine 12.5 g, strong coal tar solution 2.5 g, zinc oxide 12.5 g, hydrous wool fat 25 g, white soft paraffin 47.5 g.

● MEDICINAL FORMS Forms available from special-order manufacturers include: ointment

Coal tar with coconut oil and salicylic acid
19-Mar-2020

The properties listed below are those particular to the combination only. For the properties of the components please consider, coal tar p. 1297, salicylic acid p. 1330.

● INDICATIONS AND DOSE

Scaly scalp disorders | Psoriasis | Seborrhoeic dermatitis | Dandruff | Cradle cap
▸ TO THE SKIN USING SHAMPOO
   ▸ Child: Apply daily as required
   ▸ Adult: Apply daily as required

● MEDICINAL FORMS There can be variation in the licensing of different medicines containing the same drug.
Shampoo
▸ Capasal (Dermal Laboratories Ltd)
   Salicylic acid 5 mg per 1 gram, Coal tar distilled 10 mg per 1 gram, Coconut oil 10 mg per 1 gram Capasal Therapeutic shampoo | 250 ml P £4.69

Coal tar with dithranol and salicylic acid

The properties listed below are those particular to the combination only. For the properties of the components please consider, coal tar p. 1297, dithranol p. 1297, salicylic acid p. 1330.

● INDICATIONS AND DOSE

Subacute and chronic psoriasis
▸ TO THE SKIN
   ▸ Child: Apply up to twice daily
   ▸ Adult: Apply up to twice daily

● UNLICENSED USE
▸ In children *Psorin*® is licensed for use in children (age range not specified by manufacturer).

● MEDICINAL FORMS Forms available from special-order manufacturers include: ointment

Coal tar with salicylic acid
16-Jan-2019

The properties listed below are those particular to the combination only. For the properties of the components please consider, coal tar p. 1297, salicylic acid p. 1330.

● INDICATIONS AND DOSE

Psoriasis | Chronic atopic eczema
▸ TO THE SKIN USING OINTMENT
   ▸ Adult: Apply 1–2 times a day

IMPORTANT SAFETY INFORMATION

MHRA/CHM ADVICE (UPDATED DECEMBER 2018): EMOLLIENTS: NEW INFORMATION ABOUT RISK OF SEVERE AND FATAL BURNS WITH PARAFFIN-CONTAINING AND PARAFFIN-FREE EMOLLIENTS
See Emollient and barrier preparations p. 1265.

● PRESCRIBING AND DISPENSING INFORMATION When prepared extemporaneously, the BP states Coal Tar and Salicylic Acid Ointment, BP consists of coal tar 2 g, salicylic acid 2 g, emulsifying wax 11.4 g, white soft paraffin 19 g, coconut oil 54 g, polysorbate '80' 4 g, liquid paraffin 7.6 g.

● MEDICINAL FORMS Forms available from special-order manufacturers include: ointment

Coal tar with salicylic acid and precipitated sulfur
20-Mar-2020

The properties listed below are those particular to the combination only. For the properties of the components please consider, coal tar p. 1297, salicylic acid p. 1330.

● INDICATIONS AND DOSE

COCOIS® OINTMENT

Scaly scalp disorders including psoriasis, eczema, seborrhoeic dermatitis and dandruff
▸ TO THE SKIN USING SCALP OINTMENT
   ▸ Child 6–11 years: Medical supervision required
   ▸ Child 12–17 years: Apply once weekly as required, alternatively apply daily for the first 3–7 days (if severe), shampoo off after 1 hour
   ▸ Adult: Apply once weekly as required, alternatively apply daily for the first 3–7 days (if severe), shampoo off after 1 hour

SEBCO® OINTMENT

Scaly scalp disorders including psoriasis, eczema, seborrhoeic dermatitis and dandruff
▸ TO THE SKIN USING SCALP OINTMENT
   ▸ Child 6–11 years: Medical supervision required
   ▸ Child 12–17 years: Apply as required, alternatively apply daily for the first 3–7 days (if severe), shampoo off after 1 hour
   ▸ Adult: Apply as required, alternatively apply daily for the first 3–7 days (if severe), shampoo off after 1 hour

● MEDICINAL FORMS There can be variation in the licensing of different medicines containing the same drug.
Ointment
EXCIPIENTS: May contain Cetostearyl alcohol (including cetyl and stearyl alcohol)
▸ Cocois (RPH Pharmaceuticals AB)
   Salicylic acid 20 mg per 1 gram, Sulfur precipitated 40 mg per 1 gram, Coal tar solution 120 mg per 1 gram Cocois ointment | 40 gram GSL £6.22 | 100 gram GSL £11.69

▸ Sebco (Derma UK Ltd)
Salicylic acid 20 mg per 1 gram, Sulfur precipitated 40 mg per 1 gram, Coal tar solution 120 mg per 1 gram Sebco ointment | 40 gram [GSL] £7.91 | 100 gram [GSL] £13.38

Coal tar with zinc oxide
16-Jan-2019

The properties listed below are those particular to the combination only. For the properties of the components please consider, coal tar p. 1297.

● INDICATIONS AND DOSE

Psoriasis | Chronic atopic eczema
▸ TO THE SKIN
▸ Child: Apply 1–2 times a day
▸ Adult: Apply 1–2 times a day

IMPORTANT SAFETY INFORMATION
MHRA/CHM ADVICE (UPDATED DECEMBER 2018): EMOLLIENTS: NEW INFORMATION ABOUT RISK OF SEVERE AND FATAL BURNS WITH PARAFFIN-CONTAINING AND PARAFFIN-FREE EMOLLIENTS
See Emollient and barrier preparations p. 1265.

● PRESCRIBING AND DISPENSING INFORMATION No preparations available—when prepared extemporaneously, the BP states Zinc and Coal Tar Paste, BP consists of zinc oxide 6%, coal tar 6%, emulsifying wax 5%, starch 38%, yellow soft paraffin 45%.

● MEDICINAL FORMS Forms available from special-order manufacturers include: ointment, paste

IMMUNOSUPPRESSANTS > CALCINEURIN INHIBITORS AND RELATED DRUGS

Pimecrolimus
20-Oct-2020

● INDICATIONS AND DOSE

Short-term treatment of mild to moderate atopic eczema (including flares) when topical corticosteroids cannot be used (initiated by a specialist)
▸ TO THE SKIN
▸ Adult: Apply twice daily until symptoms resolve (stop treatment if eczema worsens or no response after 6 weeks)

Short-term treatment of facial, flexural, or genital psoriasis in patients unresponsive to, or intolerant of other topical therapy (initiated by a specialist)
▸ TO THE SKIN
▸ Adult: Apply twice daily until symptoms resolve (maximum duration of treatment 4 weeks)

● UNLICENSED USE Pimecrolimus is not licensed for short-term treatment of facial, flexural, or genital psoriasis in patients unresponsive to, or intolerant of other topical therapy.

● CONTRA-INDICATIONS Application to malignant or potentially malignant skin lesions · application under occlusion · congenital epidermal barrier defects · contact with eyes · contact with mucous membranes · generalised erythroderma · immunodeficiency · infection at treatment site

● CAUTIONS Alcohol consumption (risk of facial flushing and skin irritation) · avoid other topical treatments except emollients at treatment site · UV light (avoid excessive exposure to sunlight and sunlamps)

● INTERACTIONS → Appendix 1: pimecrolimus

● SIDE-EFFECTS
▸ **Common or very common** Increased risk of infection
▸ **Rare or very rare** Skin discolouration
▸ **Frequency not known** Skin papilloma

● PREGNANCY Manufacturer advises avoid; toxicity in *animal* studies following systemic administration.

● BREAST FEEDING Manufacturer advises caution; ensure infant does not come in contact with treated areas.

● NATIONAL FUNDING/ACCESS DECISIONS
For full details see funding body website
NICE decisions
▸ Tacrolimus and pimecrolimus for atopic eczema [for patients with mild atopic eczema or as first-line treatment for atopic eczema of any severity] (August 2004) NICE TA82 Not recommended

● MEDICINAL FORMS There can be variation in the licensing of different medicines containing the same drug.
Cream
CAUTIONARY AND ADVISORY LABELS 4, 11, 28
EXCIPIENTS: May contain Benzyl alcohol, cetostearyl alcohol (including cetyl and stearyl alcohol), propylene glycol
▸ Elidel (Mylan)
Pimecrolimus 10 mg per 1 gram Elidel 1% cream | 30 gram [PoM] £19.69 DT = £19.69 | 60 gram [PoM] £37.41 DT = £37.41 | 100 gram [PoM] £59.07 DT = £59.07

Tacrolimus
02-Dec-2020

● DRUG ACTION Tacrolimus is a calcineurin inhibitor.

● INDICATIONS AND DOSE

Short-term treatment of moderate to severe atopic eczema (including flares) in patients unresponsive to, or intolerant of conventional therapy (initiated by a specialist)
▸ TO THE SKIN
▸ Adult: Apply twice daily until lesion clears (consider other treatment if eczema worsens or no improvement after 2 weeks), initially 0.1% ointment to be applied thinly, reduce frequency to once daily or strength of ointment to 0.03% if condition allows

Prevention of flares in patients with moderate to severe atopic eczema and 4 or more flares a year who have responded to initial treatment with topical tacrolimus (initiated by a specialist)
▸ TO THE SKIN
▸ Adult: Apply twice weekly, 0.1% ointment to be applied thinly, with an interval of 2–3 days between applications, use short-term treatment regimen during an acute flare; review need for preventative therapy after 1 year

Short-term treatment of facial, flexural, or genital psoriasis in patients unresponsive to, or intolerant of other topical therapy (initiated under specialist supervision)
▸ TO THE SKIN
▸ Adult: Apply twice daily until symptoms resolve, 0.1% ointment to be applied thinly, reduce to once daily or switch to 0.03% ointment if condition allows, maximum duration of treatment 4 weeks

● UNLICENSED USE Short-term treatment of facial, flexural, or genital psoriasis is unlicensed.

● CONTRA-INDICATIONS Application to malignant or potentially malignant skin lesions · application under occlusion · avoid contact with eyes · avoid contact with mucous membranes · congenital epidermal barrier defects · generalised erythroderma · immunodeficiency · infection at treatment site

● CAUTIONS UV light (avoid excessive exposure to sunlight and sunlamps)

● INTERACTIONS → Appendix 1: tacrolimus

13

Skin

● SIDE-EFFECTS
▸ **Common or very common** Alcohol intolerance · increased risk of infection · sensation abnormal · skin reactions
▸ **Uncommon** Lymphadenopathy
▸ **Frequency not known** Malignancy · neoplasms
● ALLERGY AND CROSS-SENSITIVITY [EvGr] Contra-indicated if history of hypersensitivity to macrolides. ◈
● PREGNANCY Manufacturer advises avoid unless essential; toxicity in *animal* studies following systemic administration.
● BREAST FEEDING Avoid—present in breast milk (following systemic administration).
● HEPATIC IMPAIRMENT Manufacturer advises caution in hepatic failure.
● PATIENT AND CARER ADVICE Avoid excessive exposure to UV light including sunlight.
● NATIONAL FUNDING/ACCESS DECISIONS
For full details see funding body website
NICE decisions
▸ Tacrolimus and pimecrolimus for atopic eczema (August 2004) NICE TA82 Recommended
Scottish Medicines Consortium (SMC) decisions
▸ Tacrolimus 0.1% ointment (*Protopic*®) for moderate to severe atopic dermatitis in patients aged 16 years and over (April 2010) SMC No. 609/10 Recommended with restrictions

● MEDICINAL FORMS There can be variation in the licensing of different medicines containing the same drug.
Ointment
CAUTIONARY AND ADVISORY LABELS 4, 11, 28
EXCIPIENTS: May contain Beeswax
▸ Tacrolimus (Non-proprietary)
Tacrolimus (as Tacrolimus monohydrate) 1 mg per 1 gram Tacrolimus 0.1% ointment | 30 gram [PoM] £25.96 DT = £21.22 | 60 gram [PoM] £46.50 DT = £42.44
▸ Protopic (LEO Pharma)
Tacrolimus (as Tacrolimus monohydrate) 300 microgram per 1 gram Protopic 0.03% ointment | 30 gram [PoM] £23.33 DT = £23.33 | 60 gram [PoM] £42.55 DT = £42.55
Tacrolimus (as Tacrolimus monohydrate) 1 mg per 1 gram Protopic 0.1% ointment | 30 gram [PoM] £25.92 DT = £21.22 | 60 gram DT = £42.44

IMMUNOSUPPRESSANTS > INTERLEUKIN INHIBITORS

Brodalumab

03-Nov-2020

● DRUG ACTION Brodalumab is a recombinant human monoclonal antibody that binds with high affinity to interleukin-17RA and blocks the activity of pro-inflammatory cytokines.

● INDICATIONS AND DOSE
Moderate-to-severe plaque psoriasis (under expert supervision)
▸ BY SUBCUTANEOUS INJECTION
▸ **Adult:** 210 mg every week for 3 doses, followed by 210 mg every 2 weeks, consider discontinuing treatment if no response after 16 weeks

● CONTRA-INDICATIONS Active Crohn's disease · clinically significant active infection
● CAUTIONS Chronic infection · history of Crohn's disease (monitor for exacerbations) · history of depressive disorders (discontinue if new or worsening symptoms develop) · history of recurrent infection · history of suicidal ideation or behaviour (discontinue if new or worsening symptoms develop)

CAUTIONS, FURTHER INFORMATION
▸ Infection Manufacturer advises to consider anti-tuberculosis therapy for patients with latent tuberculosis before starting treatment with brodalumab.
Manufacturer advises patients should be brought up-to-date with current immunisation schedule before initiating treatment.
● INTERACTIONS → Appendix 1: monoclonal antibodies
● SIDE-EFFECTS
▸ **Common or very common** Arthralgia · diarrhoea · fatigue · headache · increased risk of infection · myalgia · nausea · oropharyngeal pain
▸ **Uncommon** Conjunctivitis
▸ **Frequency not known** Meningitis cryptococcal · suicidal behaviours
● CONCEPTION AND CONTRACEPTION Manufacturer advises that women of childbearing potential should use effective contraception during treatment and for at least 12 weeks after stopping treatment.
● PREGNANCY Manufacturer advises avoid—limited information available.
● BREAST FEEDING Manufacturer advises avoid—no information available.
● DIRECTIONS FOR ADMINISTRATION Manufacturer advises to take the syringe out of the refrigerator at least 30 minutes before administration, and to avoid injecting into areas of the skin that are tender, bruised, or affected by psoriasis. Patients may self-administer *Kyntheum*®, after appropriate training in subcutaneous injection technique.
● PRESCRIBING AND DISPENSING INFORMATION Brodalumab is a biological medicine. Biological medicines must be prescribed and dispensed by brand name, see *Biological medicines* and *Biosimilar medicines*, under Guidance on prescribing p. 1; manufacturer advises to record the brand name and batch number after each administration.
● HANDLING AND STORAGE Manufacturer advises store in a refrigerator (2–8°C) and protect from light—consult product literature for further information regarding storage outside refrigerator.
● PATIENT AND CARER ADVICE Manufacturer advises patients and their carers should be given training in subcutaneous injection technique. Manufacturer advises patients and their carers should seek medical advice if new or worsening symptoms of depression, suicidal ideation, or behaviour occur; they should also be advised to report signs and symptoms of infection.
● NATIONAL FUNDING/ACCESS DECISIONS
For full details see funding body website
NICE decisions
▸ Brodalumab for treating moderate to severe plaque psoriasis (March 2018) NICE TA511 Recommended with restrictions
Scottish Medicines Consortium (SMC) decisions
▸ Brodalumab (*Kyntheum*®) for the treatment of moderate-to-severe plaque psoriasis in adult patients who are candidates for systemic therapy (May 2018) SMC No. 1283/17 Recommended with restrictions

● MEDICINAL FORMS There can be variation in the licensing of different medicines containing the same drug.
Solution for injection
▸ Kyntheum (LEO Pharma) ▼
Brodalumab 140 mg per 1 ml Kyntheum 210mg/1.5ml solution for injection pre-filled syringes | 2 pre-filled disposable injection [PoM] £1,280.00

Dupilumab

23-Oct-2020

● DRUG ACTION Dupilumab is a recombinant human monoclonal antibody that inhibits interleukin-4 and interleukin-13 signaling.

● INDICATIONS AND DOSE

Moderate-to-severe atopic eczema (initiated by a specialist)
▸ BY SUBCUTANEOUS INJECTION
▸ Adult: Initially 600 mg, followed by 300 mg every 2 weeks, the initial dose should be administered as two consecutive 300 mg injections at different injection sites, review treatment if no response after 16 weeks

Severe asthma with type 2 inflammation [add-on maintenance therapy] (initiated by a specialist)
▸ BY SUBCUTANEOUS INJECTION
▸ Adult: Initially 400 mg, followed by 200 mg every 2 weeks, the initial dose should be administered as two consecutive 200 mg injections at different injection sites, review need for treatment yearly

Severe asthma with type 2 inflammation [add-on maintenance therapy for patients currently treated with oral corticosteroids or patients with co-morbid moderate-to-severe atopic dermatitis] (initiated by a specialist)
▸ BY SUBCUTANEOUS INJECTION
▸ Adult: Initially 600 mg, followed by 300 mg every 2 weeks, the initial dose should be administered as two consecutive 300 mg injections at different injection sites, review need for treatment yearly

● CAUTIONS Helminth infection
CAUTIONS, FURTHER INFORMATION
▸ Risk of infection Dupilumab may influence the immune response to helminth infections. Resolve pre-existing infection before initiating treatment; suspend treatment if resistant infection develops during therapy.
  Manufacturer advises patients should be brought up-to-date with live and live attenuated vaccines before initiating treatment.

● INTERACTIONS → Appendix 1: monoclonal antibodies

● SIDE-EFFECTS
▸ **Common or very common** Eosinophilia · eye inflammation · eye pruritus · headache · oral herpes
▸ **Rare or very rare** Hypersensitivity
▸ **Frequency not known** Pneumonia eosinophilic · vasculitis

SIDE-EFFECTS, FURTHER INFORMATION **Eosinophilic granulomatosis with polyangiitis (Churg-Strauss syndrome)** Churg-Strauss syndrome has occurred in patients given dupilumab; the reaction may be associated with the reduction of oral corticosteroid therapy. Churg-Strauss syndrome can present as vasculitic rash, cardiac complications, worsening pulmonary symptoms, or peripheral neuropathy in patients with eosinophilia.

● PREGNANCY Manufacturer advises use only if potential benefit outweighs risk—limited information available.

● BREAST FEEDING Manufacturer advises avoid—no information available.

● DIRECTIONS FOR ADMINISTRATION Manufacturer advises to inject into the thigh or abdomen (except for the 5 cm around the navel); or upper arm (if not self-administered); rotate injection site and avoid skin that is tender, damaged or scarred. Patients may self-administer *Dupixent®* after appropriate training in preparation and administration.

● PRESCRIBING AND DISPENSING INFORMATION Dupilumab is a biological medicine. Biological medicines must be prescribed and dispensed by brand name, see *Biological medicines* and *Biosimilar medicines*, under Guidance on prescribing p. 1; manufacturer advises to record the brand name and batch number after each administration.

● HANDLING AND STORAGE Manufacturer advises store in a refrigerator (2–8°C) and protect from light; pre-filled syringes may be kept at room temperature (max. 25°C) for max. 14 days.

● NATIONAL FUNDING/ACCESS DECISIONS
For full details see funding body website
NICE decisions
▸ **Dupilumab for treating moderate to severe atopic dermatitis (August 2018)** NICE TA534 Recommended with restrictions
Scottish Medicines Consortium (SMC) decisions
▸ **Dupilumab (*Dupixent®*) for treatment of moderate-to-severe atopic dermatitis (September 2018)** SMC No. SMC2011 Recommended with restrictions

● MEDICINAL FORMS There can be variation in the licensing of different medicines containing the same drug.
Solution for injection
EXCIPIENTS: May contain Polysorbates
▸ Dupixent (Sanofi) ▼
Dupilumab 150 mg per 1 ml Dupixent 300mg/2ml solution for injection pre-filled syringes | 2 pre-filled disposable injection [PoM] £1,264.89
Dupixent 300mg/2ml solution for injection pre-filled pens | 2 pre-filled disposable injection [PoM] £1,264.89
Dupilumab 175 mg per 1 ml Dupixent 200mg/1.14ml solution for injection pre-filled syringes | 2 pre-filled disposable injection [PoM] £1,264.89
Dupixent 200mg/1.14ml solution for injection pre-filled pens | 2 pre-filled disposable injection [PoM] £1,264.89

Guselkumab

06-Nov-2020

● DRUG ACTION Guselkumab is a recombinant human monoclonal antibody that binds selectively to interleukin-23 and blocks the activity of pro-inflammatory cytokines.

● INDICATIONS AND DOSE

Moderate-to-severe plaque psoriasis (specialist use only)
▸ BY SUBCUTANEOUS INJECTION
▸ Adult: Initially 100 mg, then 100 mg after 4 weeks, then maintenance 100 mg every 8 weeks, consider discontinuation if no response after 16 weeks

● CONTRA-INDICATIONS Clinically significant active infection

● CAUTIONS Risk of infection
CAUTIONS, FURTHER INFORMATION
▸ Risk of infection Manufacturer advises consider anti-tuberculosis therapy before initiation of guselkumab in patients with a past history of latent or active tuberculosis in whom an adequate course of treatment cannot be confirmed.
  Manufacturer advises consider completion of appropriate immunisations according to current guidelines before initiating treatment (consult product literature for appropriate interval between vaccination and administration of guselkumab).

● INTERACTIONS → Appendix 1: monoclonal antibodies

● SIDE-EFFECTS
▸ **Common or very common** Arthralgia · diarrhoea · headache · increased risk of infection · skin reactions

● CONCEPTION AND CONTRACEPTION Manufacturer advises effective contraception in women of childbearing potential during treatment and for at least 12 weeks after treatment.

● PREGNANCY Manufacturer advises avoid—no information available.

● BREAST FEEDING Manufacturer advises avoid during treatment and for up to 12 weeks after discontinuing treatment—no information available.

● PRE-TREATMENT SCREENING Manufacturer advises that patients should be evaluated for tuberculosis infection before treatment.

- MONITORING REQUIREMENTS Manufacturer advises monitor for signs and symptoms of active tuberculosis during and after treatment.
- DIRECTIONS FOR ADMINISTRATION Manufacturer advises to avoid injecting into areas of the skin that show psoriasis. Patients may self-administer *Tremfya®*, after appropriate training in subcutaneous injection technique.
- PRESCRIBING AND DISPENSING INFORMATION Manufacturer advises to record the brand name and batch number after each administration.
- HANDLING AND STORAGE Manufacturer advises store in a refrigerator (2–8°C) and protect from light.
- PATIENT AND CARER ADVICE Manufacturer advises patients and their carers should be advised to seek medical attention if signs or symptoms of infection occur (monitor closely and suspend treatment if infection is clinically significant or unresponsive to treatment).
  Self-administration Manufacturer advises patients may self-administer following training in subcutaneous injection technique.
- NATIONAL FUNDING/ACCESS DECISIONS
  For full details see funding body website
  NICE decisions
- ▸ **Guselkumab for treating moderate to severe plaque psoriasis (June 2018)** NICE TA521 Recommended with restrictions
  Scottish Medicines Consortium (SMC) decisions
- ▸ **Guselkumab (*Tremfya®*) for the treatment of moderate to severe plaque psoriasis in adults who are candidates for systemic therapy (June 2018)** SMC No. 1340/18 Recommended with restrictions

- MEDICINAL FORMS There can be variation in the licensing of different medicines containing the same drug.
  Solution for injection
  - ▸ Tremfya (Janssen-Cilag Ltd) ▼
    Guselkumab 100 mg per 1 ml Tremfya 100mg/1ml solution for injection pre-filled pens | 1 pre-filled disposable injection [PoM] £2,250.00

Ixekizumab

09-Nov-2020

- DRUG ACTION Ixekizumab is a human monoclonal antibody that binds to interleukin-17A and inhibits the release of pro-inflammatory cytokines and chemokines.

- INDICATIONS AND DOSE

Moderate-to-severe plaque psoriasis (under expert supervision) | Psoriatic arthritis with concomitant moderate-to-severe plaque psoriasis (under expert supervision)
  - ▸ BY SUBCUTANEOUS INJECTION
  - ▸ Adult: Initially 160 mg for 1 dose, followed by 80 mg after 2 weeks, then 80 mg every 2 weeks for 5 further doses (at weeks 4, 6, 8, 10 and 12), then maintenance 80 mg every 4 weeks, consider discontinuation of treatment if no response after 16–20 weeks

Psoriatic arthritis (under expert supervision)
  - ▸ BY SUBCUTANEOUS INJECTION
  - ▸ Adult: Initially 160 mg for 1 dose, then maintenance 80 mg every 4 weeks, consider discontinuation of treatment if no response after 16–20 weeks

- CONTRA-INDICATIONS Active infections (including active tuberculosis)
- CAUTIONS Chronic infection—monitor carefully and discontinue if serious, unresponsive infection develops · Crohn's disease · ulcerative colitis
  CAUTIONS, FURTHER INFORMATION
- ▸ Severe hypersensitivity reactions Severe hypersensitivity reactions have been reported—discontinue treatment immediately if symptoms occur.

- ▸ Latent tuberculosis Manufacturer advises that patients with latent tuberculosis should complete anti-tuberculosis therapy before starting ixekizumab.
- ▸ Inflammatory bowel disease Manufacturer advises to monitor closely for exacerbation.
- INTERACTIONS → Appendix 1: monoclonal antibodies
- SIDE-EFFECTS
- ▸ **Common or very common** Increased risk of infection · nausea · oropharyngeal pain
- ▸ **Uncommon** Conjunctivitis · neutropenia · skin reactions · thrombocytopenia
- ▸ **Frequency not known** Angioedema · dyspnoea · hypersensitivity (occasionally late-onset) · inflammatory bowel disease
- CONCEPTION AND CONTRACEPTION Manufacturer advises effective contraception during treatment and for at least 10 weeks after treatment in women of childbearing potential.
- PREGNANCY Manufacturer advises avoid—limited information available.
- BREAST FEEDING Manufacturer advises avoid—present in milk in *animal* studies.
- DIRECTIONS FOR ADMINISTRATION Manufacturer advises to avoid injecting into areas of the skin that show psoriasis; injection sites may be alternated. Patients may self-administer *Taltz®*, after appropriate training in subcutaneous injection technique.
- HANDLING AND STORAGE Manufacturer advises store in a refrigerator (2–8°C).
- PATIENT AND CARER ADVICE
  Self-administration If appropriate, patients and their carers should be given training in subcutaneous injection technique.
- NATIONAL FUNDING/ACCESS DECISIONS
  For full details see funding body website
  NICE decisions
- ▸ **Ixekizumab for treating moderate to severe plaque psoriasis (April 2017)** NICE TA442 Recommended with restrictions
- ▸ **Ixekizumab for treating active psoriatic arthritis after inadequate response to DMARDs (August 2018)** NICE TA537 Recommended with restrictions
  Scottish Medicines Consortium (SMC) decisions
- ▸ **Ixekizumab (*Taltz®*) for moderate to severe plaque psoriasis in adults who are candidates for systemic therapy (April 2017)** SMC No. 1223/17 Recommended with restrictions
- ▸ **Ixekizumab (*Taltz®*) alone or in combination with methotrexate for the treatment of active psoriatic arthritis in adult patients who have responded inadequately to, or who are intolerant to one or more disease-modifying anti-rheumatic drug therapies (October 2018)** SMC No. SMC2097 Recommended with restrictions

- MEDICINAL FORMS There can be variation in the licensing of different medicines containing the same drug.
  Solution for injection
  EXCIPIENTS: May contain Polysorbates
  - ▸ Taltz (Eli Lilly and Company Ltd) ▼
    Ixekizumab 80 mg per 1 ml Taltz 80mg/1ml solution for injection pre-filled pens | 1 pre-filled disposable injection [PoM] £1,125.00 (Hospital only)
    Taltz 80mg/1ml solution for injection pre-filled syringes | 1 pre-filled disposable injection [PoM] £1,125.00 (Hospital only)

Risankizumab

12-Nov-2020

- DRUG ACTION Risankizumab is a humanised monoclonal antibody that binds selectively to interleukin-23 and blocks the activity of pro-inflammatory cytokines.

- **INDICATIONS AND DOSE**

Moderate-to-severe plaque psoriasis (specialist use only)
▸ BY SUBCUTANEOUS INJECTION
▸ **Adult:** Initially 150 mg, then 150 mg after 4 weeks, then maintenance 150 mg every 12 weeks, consider discontinuation if no response after 16 weeks

- CONTRA-INDICATIONS Clinically significant active infection

- CAUTIONS Chronic infection · history of recurrent infection · risk of infection

CAUTIONS, FURTHER INFORMATION
▸ Risk of infection Manufacturer advises consider anti-tuberculosis therapy before initiation of risankizumab in patients with a history of latent or active tuberculosis in whom an adequate course of treatment cannot be confirmed.

Manufacturer advises consider completion of immunisations according to current guidelines before initiating treatment (consult product literature for appropriate interval between vaccination and administration of risankizumab).

- INTERACTIONS → Appendix 1: monoclonal antibodies

- SIDE-EFFECTS
▸ **Common or very common** Asthenia · headaches · increased risk of infection · pruritus

- CONCEPTION AND CONTRACEPTION Manufacturer advises effective contraception in women of childbearing potential during treatment and for at least 21 weeks after treatment.

- PREGNANCY Manufacturer advises avoid (limited information available).

- BREAST FEEDING Manufacturer advises avoid (no information available).

- PRE-TREATMENT SCREENING Manufacturer advises patients should be evaluated for tuberculosis infection before treatment.

- MONITORING REQUIREMENTS Manufacturer advises monitor for signs and symptoms of active tuberculosis during treatment.

- DIRECTIONS FOR ADMINISTRATION Manufacturer advises to take carton out of the refrigerator at least 15 minutes before administration, and to avoid injecting into areas of the skin that are show psoriasis. Patients may self-administer *Skyrizi*® after appropriate training in subcutaneous injection technique.

- PRESCRIBING AND DISPENSING INFORMATION Risankizumab is a biological medicine. Biological medicines must be prescribed and dispensed by brand name, see *Biological medicines* and *Biosimilar medicines*, under Guidance on prescribing p. 1; manufacturer advises to record the brand name and batch number after each administration.

- HANDLING AND STORAGE Manufacturer advises store in a refrigerator (2–8°C) and protect from light.

- PATIENT AND CARER ADVICE Manufacturer advises patients and their carers should be advised to seek medical attention if signs or symptoms of infection occur.

- NATIONAL FUNDING/ACCESS DECISIONS
For full details see funding body website
NICE decisions
▸ **Risankizumab for treating moderate to severe plaque psoriasis (August 2019)** NICE TA596 Recommended with restrictions

Scottish Medicines Consortium (SMC) decisions
▸ **Risankizumab (*Skyrizi*®) for the treatment of moderate to severe plaque psoriasis in adults who are candidates for systemic therapy (October 2019)** SMC No. SMC2196 Recommended with restrictions

- MEDICINAL FORMS There can be variation in the licensing of different medicines containing the same drug.
Solution for injection
EXCIPIENTS: May contain Polysorbates, sorbitol
▸ Skyrizi (AbbVie Ltd) ▼
Risankizumab 90.36 mg per 1 ml Skyrizi 75mg/0.83ml solution for injection pre-filled syringes | 2 pre-filled disposable injection PoM £3,326.09

Tildrakizumab

16-Nov-2020

- DRUG ACTION Tildrakizumab is a recombinant human monoclonal antibody that specifically binds to interleukin-23 and inhibits the release of pro-inflammatory cytokines and chemokines.

- **INDICATIONS AND DOSE**

Moderate-to-severe plaque psoriasis (under expert supervision)
▸ BY SUBCUTANEOUS INJECTION
▸ **Adult:** Initially 100 mg, then 100 mg after 4 weeks, then maintenance 100 mg every 12 weeks, consider discontinuation if no response after 28 weeks, in patients with a high disease burden, or with a body weight ≥ 90kg, a dose of 200 mg may provide greater efficacy

- CONTRA-INDICATIONS Clinically significant active infection

- CAUTIONS Chronic infection · history of recurrent infection · recent serious infection

CAUTIONS, FURTHER INFORMATION
▸ Risk of infection Manufacturer advises consider anti-tuberculosis therapy before initiation of tildrakizumab in patients with a history of tuberculosis, in whom an adequate course of treatment cannot be confirmed.

Manufacturer advises consider completion of immunisations according to current guidelines before initiating treatment (consult product literature for appropriate interval between vaccination and administration of tildrakizumab).

- INTERACTIONS → Appendix 1: monoclonal antibodies

- SIDE-EFFECTS
▸ **Common or very common** Back pain · diarrhoea · headache · increased risk of infection · nausea

- CONCEPTION AND CONTRACEPTION Manufacturer advises that women of childbearing potential should use effective contraception during treatment and for at least 17 weeks after stopping treatment.

- PREGNANCY Manufacturer advises avoid—limited information available.

- BREAST FEEDING Manufacturer advises avoid—limited information available.

- PRE-TREATMENT SCREENING Manufacturer advises patients should be evaluated for tuberculosis infection before treatment.

- MONITORING REQUIREMENTS Manufacturer advises monitor for signs and symptoms of active tuberculosis during and after treatment

- DIRECTIONS FOR ADMINISTRATION Manufacturer advises to take the syringe out of the refrigerator at least 30 minutes before administration, and to avoid injecting into areas of the skin that are affected by psoriasis or are tender, bruised, red, hard, thick, or scaly. Patients may

13

Skin

self-administer *Ilumetri*®, after appropriate training in subcutaneous injection technique.

- **PRESCRIBING AND DISPENSING INFORMATION** Tildrakizumab is a biological medicine. Biological medicines must be prescribed and dispensed by brand name, see *Biological medicines* and *Biosimilar medicines*, under Guidance on prescribing p. 1; manufacturer advises to record the brand name and batch number after each administration.
- **HANDLING AND STORAGE** Manufacturer advises store in a refrigerator (2–8°C) and protect from light—consult product literature for further information regarding storage outside refrigerator.
- **PATIENT AND CARER ADVICE** Manufacturer advises patients and their carers should be advised to seek medical advice if signs or symptoms of infection occur.
- **NATIONAL FUNDING/ACCESS DECISIONS** For full details see funding body website

  NICE decisions
  ▸ Tildrakizumab for treating moderate to severe plaque psoriasis (April 2019) NICE TA575 Recommended with restrictions

  Scottish Medicines Consortium (SMC) decisions
  ▸ Tildrakizumab (*Ilumetri*®) for the treatment of adults with moderate to severe plaque psoriasis who are candidates for systemic therapy (August 2019) SMC No. SMC2167 Recommended with restrictions

- **MEDICINAL FORMS** There can be variation in the licensing of different medicines containing the same drug.

  Solution for injection
  EXCIPIENTS: May contain Polysorbates
  ▸ Ilumetri (Almirall Ltd) ▼
  Tildrakizumab 100 mg per 1 ml Ilumetri 100mg/1ml solution for injection pre-filled syringes | 1 pre-filled disposable injection [PoM] £3,241.00 | 2 pre-filled disposable injection [PoM] £3,241.00

RETINOID AND RELATED DRUGS

Acitretin

28-Jan-2020

- **DRUG ACTION** Acitretin is a metabolite of etretinate.

INDICATIONS AND DOSE

Severe extensive psoriasis resistant to other forms of therapy (under expert supervision) | Palmoplantar pustular psoriasis (under expert supervision) | Severe congenital ichthyosis (under expert supervision)
▸ BY MOUTH
▸ Adult: Initially 25–30 mg daily for 2–4 weeks, then adjusted according to response to 25–50 mg daily, increased to up to 75 mg daily, dose only increased to 75 mg daily for short periods in psoriasis

Severe Darier's disease (keratosis follicularis) (under expert supervision)
▸ BY MOUTH
▸ Adult: Initially 10 mg daily for 2–4 weeks, then adjusted according to response to 25–50 mg daily

---

IMPORTANT SAFETY INFORMATION
MHRA/CHM ADVICE: ORAL RETINOID MEDICINES: REVISED AND SIMPLIFIED PREGNANCY PREVENTION EDUCATIONAL MATERIALS FOR HEALTHCARE PROFESSIONALS AND WOMEN (JUNE 2019)
New prescriber checklists, patient reminder cards, and pharmacy checklists are available to support the Pregnancy Prevention Programme in women and girls of childbearing potential taking oral acitretin, alitretinoin, or isotretinoin. Healthcare professionals are reminded that the use of oral retinoids is contra-indicated in pregnancy due to a high risk of serious congenital malformations, and any use in females must be within the conditions of the Pregnancy Prevention Programme

(see *Conception and contraception* and *Prescribing and dispensing information*).
Neuropsychiatric reactions have been reported in patients taking oral retinoids. Healthcare professionals are advised to monitor patients for signs of depression or suicidal ideation and refer for appropriate treatment, if necessary; particular care is needed in those with a history of depression. Patients should be advised to speak to their doctor if they experience any changes in mood or behaviour, and encouraged to ask family and friends to look out for any change in mood.

- **CONTRA-INDICATIONS** Hyperlipidaemia
- **CAUTIONS** Avoid excessive exposure to sunlight and unsupervised use of sunlamps · diabetes (can alter glucose tolerance—initial frequent blood glucose checks) · do not donate blood during and for 3 years after stopping therapy (teratogenic risk) · history of depression (risk of neuropsychiatric reactions) · in children use only in exceptional circumstances and monitor growth parameters and bone development (premature epiphyseal closure reported) · investigate atypical musculoskeletal symptoms
- **INTERACTIONS** → Appendix 1: retinoids
- **SIDE-EFFECTS**
  ▸ **Common or very common** Abdominal pain · arthralgia · brittle nails · conjunctivitis · diarrhoea · dry mouth · gastrointestinal disorder · haemorrhage · hair texture abnormal · headache · increased risk of infection · mucosal abnormalities · myalgia · nausea · oral disorders · peripheral oedema · skin reactions · thirst · vomiting · xerophthalmia
  ▸ **Uncommon** Dizziness · hepatic disorders · photosensitivity reaction · vision disorders
  ▸ **Rare or very rare** Bone pain · exostosis · idiopathic intracranial hypertension · peripheral neuropathy
  ▸ **Frequency not known** Angioedema · capillary leak syndrome · drowsiness · dysphonia · flushing · glucose tolerance impaired · granuloma · hearing impairment · hyperhidrosis · malaise · pyogenic granuloma · retinoic acid syndrome · taste altered · tinnitus

  SIDE-EFFECTS, FURTHER INFORMATION **Exostosis** Skeletal hyperostosis and extra-osseous calcification reported following long-term treatment with etretinate (of which acitretin is a metabolite) and premature epiphyseal closure in children.

  Benign intracranial hypertension Discontinue if severe headache, nausea, vomiting, or visual disturbances occur.

- **CONCEPTION AND CONTRACEPTION** The MHRA advises that women and girls of childbearing potential being treated with the oral retinoids acitretin, alitretinoin, or isotretinoin must be supported on a Pregnancy Prevention Programme with regular follow-up and pregnancy testing. Pregnancy prevention Effective contraception must be used.
  In females of childbearing potential (including those with a history of infertility), exclude pregnancy up to 3 days before treatment, every month during treatment, and every 1–3 months for 3 years after stopping treatment. Treatment should be started on day 2 or 3 of menstrual cycle. Females of childbearing age must practise effective contraception for at least 1 month before starting treatment, during treatment, and for at least 3 years after stopping treatment. Females should be advised to use at least 1 method of contraception, but ideally they should use 2 methods of contraception. Oral progestogen-only contraceptives are not considered effective. Barrier methods should not be used alone but can be used in conjunction with other contraceptive methods. Females should be advised to seek medical attention immediately if they become pregnant during treatment or within 3 years of stopping treatment. They should also be advised to

avoid alcohol during treatment and for 2 months after stopping treatment.

PREGNANCY Manufacturer advises avoid—teratogenic.

BREAST FEEDING Avoid.

HEPATIC IMPAIRMENT Manufacturer advises avoid in severe impairment.

RENAL IMPAIRMENT Avoid in severe impairment; increased risk of toxicity.

MONITORING REQUIREMENTS
Monitor serum-triglyceride and serum-cholesterol concentrations before treatment, 1 month after starting, then every 3 months.
Check liver function at start, then every 2–4 weeks for first 2 months and then every 3 months.

PRESCRIBING AND DISPENSING INFORMATION
Prescribing for females of childbearing potential The Pregnancy Prevention Programme is supported by the following materials provided by the manufacturer: *Checklists for prescribers and pharmacists*, and *Patient reminder cards*.

Each prescription for oral acitretin should be limited to a supply of up to 30 days' treatment. Pregnancy testing should ideally be carried out on the same day as prescription issuing and dispensing.

PATIENT AND CARER ADVICE
Risk of neuropsychiatric reactions The MHRA advises patients and carers to seek medical attention if changes in mood or behaviour occur.
Pregnancy Prevention Programme Pharmacists must ensure that female patients have a patient card—see also *Important safety information*.

MEDICINAL FORMS There can be variation in the licensing of different medicines containing the same drug. Forms available from special-order manufacturers include: oral suspension, oral solution

Capsule
CAUTIONARY AND ADVISORY LABELS 10, 11, 21
▸ Acitretin (Non-proprietary)
Acitretin 10 mg Acitretin 10mg capsules | 60 capsule PoM £26.65
DT = £26.64
Acitretin 25 mg Acitretin 25mg capsules | 60 capsule PoM £55.24
DT = £43.75
▸ Neotigason (Teva UK Ltd)
Acitretin 10 mg Neotigason 10mg capsules | 60 capsule PoM
£17.30 DT = £26.64
Acitretin 25 mg Neotigason 25mg capsules | 60 capsule PoM
£43.00 DT = £43.75

Alitretinoin

15-Jan-2020

INDICATIONS AND DOSE
Severe chronic hand eczema refractory to potent topical corticosteroids
▸ BY MOUTH
▸ Adult (prescribed by or under supervision of a consultant dermatologist): 30 mg once daily; reduced if not tolerated to 10 mg once daily for 12–24 weeks total duration of treatment, discontinue if no response after 12 weeks, course may be repeated in those who relapse

DOSE ADJUSTMENTS DUE TO INTERACTIONS
▸ Manufacturer advises reduce dose to 10 mg once daily with concurrent use of potent inhibitors of CYP3A4, CYP2C8 and moderate inhibitors of CYP2C9.

IMPORTANT SAFETY INFORMATION
MHRA/CHM ADVICE: ORAL RETINOID MEDICINES: REVISED AND SIMPLIFIED PREGNANCY PREVENTION EDUCATIONAL MATERIALS FOR HEALTHCARE PROFESSIONALS AND WOMEN (JUNE 2019)
New prescriber checklists, patient reminder cards, and pharmacy checklists are available to support the Pregnancy Prevention Programme in women and girls of

childbearing potential taking oral acitretin, alitretinoin, or isotretinoin. Healthcare professionals are reminded that the use of oral retinoids is contra-indicated in pregnancy due to a high risk of serious congenital malformations, and any use in females must be within the conditions of the Pregnancy Prevention Programme (see *Conception and contraception* and *Prescribing and dispensing information*).

Neuropsychiatric reactions have been reported in patients taking oral retinoids. Healthcare professionals are advised to monitor patients for signs of depression or suicidal ideation and refer for appropriate treatment, if necessary; particular care is needed in those with a history of depression. Patients should be advised to speak to their doctor if they experience any changes in mood or behaviour, and encouraged to ask family and friends to look out for any change in mood.

CONTRA-INDICATIONS Hypervitaminosis A · uncontrolled hyperlipidaemia · uncontrolled hypothyroidism

CAUTIONS Avoid blood donation during treatment and for at least 1 month after stopping treatment · dry eye syndrome · history of depression (risk of neuropsychiatric reactions)

INTERACTIONS → Appendix 1: retinoids

SIDE-EFFECTS
▸ **Common or very common** Alopecia · anaemia · conjunctivitis · dizziness · dry eye · dry mouth · eye irritation · fatigue · flushing · headache · hypercholesterolaemia · hypertension · hypertriglyceridaemia (risk of pancreatitis if triglycerides above 9 mmol/litre) · joint disorders · myalgia · nausea · oral disorders · skin reactions · tinnitus · vomiting
▸ **Uncommon** Bone disorders · cataract · dyspepsia · epistaxis · vision disorders
▸ **Rare or very rare** Anxiety · behaviour abnormal · depression · hair texture abnormal · idiopathic intracranial hypertension · mood altered · nail disorder · photosensitivity reaction · psychotic disorder · suicidal behaviours · vasculitis
▸ **Frequency not known** Inflammatory bowel disease · peripheral oedema

SIDE-EFFECTS, FURTHER INFORMATION Dry eyes may respond to lubricating eye ointment or tear replacement therapy.

Discontinue treatment if signs or symptoms of idiopathic intracranial hypertension such as headache, nausea, vomiting, papilloedema, or visual disturbances occur.

Risk of pancreatitis if triglycerides above 9 mmol/litre—discontinue if uncontrolled hypertriglyceridaemia or pancreatitis.

CONCEPTION AND CONTRACEPTION The MHRA advises that women and girls of childbearing potential being treated with the oral retinoids acitretin, alitretinoin, or isotretinoin must be supported on a Pregnancy Prevention Programme with regular follow-up and pregnancy testing.
Pregnancy prevention Effective contraception must be used.

In females of childbearing potential, exclude pregnancy a few days before treatment, every month during treatment (unless there are compelling reasons to indicate that there is no risk of pregnancy), and 4 weeks after stopping treatment. Females must practise effective contraception for at least 1 month before starting treatment, during treatment, and for at least 1 month after stopping treatment. They should be advised to use at least 1 method of contraception but ideally they should use 2 methods of contraception. Oral progestogen-only contraceptives are not considered effective. Barrier methods should not be used alone but can be used in conjunction with other contraceptive methods. Females

13

Skin

should be advised to discontinue treatment and to seek prompt medical attention if they become pregnant during treatment or within 1 month of stopping treatment.

- PREGNANCY Manufacturer advises avoid—teratogenic.
- BREAST FEEDING Manufacturer advises avoid.
- HEPATIC IMPAIRMENT Manufacturer advises avoid— limited information available.
- RENAL IMPAIRMENT Manufacturer advises avoid in severe impairment—no information available.
- MONITORING REQUIREMENTS Monitor serum lipids (more frequently in those with diabetes, history of hyperlipidaemia, or risk factors for cardiovascular disease)—discontinue if uncontrolled hyperlipidaemia.
- PRESCRIBING AND DISPENSING INFORMATION
Prescribing for females of childbearing potential The Pregnancy Prevention Programme is supported by the following materials provided by the manufacturer: *Checklists for prescribers and pharmacists*, and *Patient reminder cards*.

  Each prescription for oral alitretinoin should be limited to a supply of up to 30 days' treatment. Pregnancy testing should ideally be carried out on the same day as prescription issuing and dispensing.
- PATIENT AND CARER ADVICE
Risk of neuropsychiatric reactions The MHRA advises patients and carers to seek medical attention if changes in mood or behaviour occur.
UV light Manufacturer advises patients to avoid excessive exposure to UV light (including sunlight, solariums)— sunscreen with a high protection factor should be applied.
Pregnancy Prevention Programme Pharmacists must ensure that female patients have a patient card—see also *Important safety information*.
- NATIONAL FUNDING/ACCESS DECISIONS
For full details see funding body website
NICE decisions
  ‣ Alitretinoin for the treatment of severe chronic hand eczema (August 2009) NICE TA177 Recommended
- MEDICINAL FORMS There can be variation in the licensing of different medicines containing the same drug.
Capsule
CAUTIONARY AND ADVISORY LABELS 10, 11, 21
EXCIPIENTS: May contain Sorbitol
  ‣ Alitretinoin (Non-proprietary)
    Alitretinoin 10 mg Alitretinoin 10mg capsules | 30 capsule PoM £493.72–£592.50 DT = £493.72
    Alitretinoin 30 mg Alitretinoin 30mg capsules | 30 capsule PoM £493.72–£592.50 DT = £493.72
  ‣ Toctino (Stiefel Laboratories (UK) Ltd)
    Alitretinoin 10 mg Toctino 10mg capsules | 30 capsule PoM £493.72 DT = £493.72
    Alitretinoin 30 mg Toctino 30mg capsules | 30 capsule PoM £493.72 DT = £493.72

Tazarotene

14-Feb-2020

- INDICATIONS AND DOSE
Mild to moderate plaque psoriasis affecting up to 10% of skin area
  ‣ TO THE SKIN
  ‣ Adult: Apply once daily usually for up to 12 weeks, apply in the evening

- CAUTIONS Avoid contact with eczematous skin · avoid contact with eyes · avoid contact with face · avoid contact with hair-covered scalp · avoid contact with inflamed skin · avoid contact with intertriginous areas
- INTERACTIONS → Appendix 1: retinoids
- SIDE-EFFECTS
  ‣ Common or very common Paraesthesia · skin reactions

SIDE-EFFECTS, FURTHER INFORMATION Local irritation is more common with higher concentration and may require treatment interruption.

- CONCEPTION AND CONTRACEPTION Effective contraception required (oral progestogen-only contraceptives not considered effective).
- PREGNANCY Avoid.
- BREAST FEEDING Manufacturer advises avoid—present in milk in *animal* studies.
- PATIENT AND CARER ADVICE Avoid excessive exposure to UV light (including sunlight, solariums, PUVA or UVB treatment). Do not apply emollients or cosmetics within 1 hour of application. Wash hands immediately after use.

- MEDICINAL FORMS There can be variation in the licensing of different medicines containing the same drug.
Gel
EXCIPIENTS: May contain Benzyl alcohol, butylated hydroxyanisole, butylated hydroxytoluene, disodium edetate, polysorbates
  ‣ Zorac (Allergan Ltd)
    Tazarotene 500 microgram per 1 gram Zorac 0.05% gel | 30 gram PoM £14.09 DT = £14.09
    Tazarotene 1 mg per 1 gram Zorac 0.1% gel | 30 gram PoM £14.80 DT = £14.80

SALICYLIC ACID AND DERIVATIVES

Salicylic acid with zinc oxide

23-Nov-2020

- INDICATIONS AND DOSE
Hyperkeratotic skin disorders
  ‣ TO THE SKIN
  ‣ Adult: Apply twice daily

- CAUTIONS Avoid broken skin · avoid inflamed skin
CAUTIONS, FURTHER INFORMATION
  ‣ Salicylate toxicity Salicylate toxicity may occur particularly if applied on large areas of skin or neonatal skin.
- SIDE-EFFECTS Skin irritation
- PRESCRIBING AND DISPENSING INFORMATION Zinc and Salicylic Acid Paste BP is also referred to as Lassar's Paste. When prepared extemporaneously, the BP states Zinc and Salicylic Acid Paste, BP (Lassar's Paste) consists of zinc oxide 24%, salicylic acid 2%, starch 24%, white soft paraffin 50%.

- MEDICINAL FORMS Forms available from special-order manufacturers include: paste

VITAMINS AND TRACE ELEMENTS 〉 VITAMIN D AND ANALOGUES

Calcipotriol

02-Sep-2020

- INDICATIONS AND DOSE
Plaque psoriasis
  ‣ TO THE SKIN USING OINTMENT
  ‣ Adult: Apply 1–2 times a day, when preparations are used together maximum total calcipotriol 5 mg in any one week (e.g. scalp solution 60 mL with ointment 30 g or scalp solution 30 mL with ointment 60 g); maximum 100 g per week
Scalp psoriasis
  ‣ TO THE SKIN USING SCALP LOTION
  ‣ Adult: Apply twice daily, when preparations are used together maximum total calcipotriol 5 mg in any one week (e.g. scalp solution 60 mL with ointment 30 g or scalp solution 30 mL with ointment 60 g); maximum 60 mL per week

- CONTRA-INDICATIONS Calcium metabolism disorders

- CAUTIONS Avoid excessive exposure to sunlight and sunlamps · avoid use on face · erythrodermic exfoliative psoriasis (enhanced risk of hypercalcaemia) · generalised pustular psoriasis (enhanced risk of hypercalcaemia)
- INTERACTIONS → Appendix 1: vitamin D substances
- SIDE-EFFECTS
- ▸ **Common or very common** Skin reactions
- ▸ **Uncommon** Increased risk of infection
- ▸ **Rare or very rare** Hypercalcaemia · hypercalciuria · photosensitivity reaction
- PREGNANCY Manufacturers advise avoid unless essential.
- BREAST FEEDING No information available.
- HEPATIC IMPAIRMENT Manufacturers advise avoid in severe impairment (no information available).
- PATIENT AND CARER ADVICE
  Advice on application Patient information leaflet for *Dovonex*® ointment advises liberal application. However, patients should be advised of maximum recommended weekly dose.
  Hands should be washed thoroughly after application to avoid inadvertent transfer to other body areas.

- MEDICINAL FORMS There can be variation in the licensing of different medicines containing the same drug. Forms available from special-order manufacturers include: ointment

Ointment
EXCIPIENTS: May contain Disodium edetate, propylene glycol
 ▸ Calcipotriol (Non-proprietary)
  Calcipotriol 50 microgram per 1 gram Calcipotriol 50micrograms/g ointment | 30 gram PoM £7.43 DT = £7.43 | 60 gram PoM £11.56–£14.86 | 120 gram PoM £23.10–£29.72
 ▸ Dovonex (LEO Pharma)
  Calcipotriol 50 microgram per 1 gram Dovonex 50micrograms/g ointment | 30 gram PoM £5.78 DT = £7.43 | 60 gram PoM £11.56

Liquid
 ▸ Calcipotriol (Non-proprietary)
  Calcipotriol (as Calcipotriol hydrate) 50 microgram per 1 ml Calcipotriol 50micrograms/ml scalp solution | 60 ml PoM £72.60 DT = £70.65 | 120 ml PoM £141.29 DT = £141.29

Combinations available: *Calcipotriol with betamethasone*, p. 1288

⚐ 1132

Calcitriol

12-Oct-2020

(1,25-Dihydroxycholecalciferol)

- **INDICATIONS AND DOSE**
Mild to moderate plaque psoriasis
 ▸ TO THE SKIN
 ▸ **Adult:** Apply twice daily, not more than 35% of body surface to be treated daily; maximum 30 g per day

- CONTRA-INDICATIONS Do not apply under occlusion · patients with calcium metabolism disorders
- CAUTIONS Erythrodermic exfoliative psoriasis (enhanced risk of hypercalcaemia) · generalised pustular psoriasis (enhanced risk of hypercalcaemia)
- INTERACTIONS → Appendix 1: vitamin D substances
- PREGNANCY Manufacturer advises use in restricted amounts only if clearly necessary.
  Monitoring Monitor urine- and serum-calcium concentration in pregnancy.
- BREAST FEEDING Manufacturer advises avoid.
- HEPATIC IMPAIRMENT Manufacturer advises avoid.
- RENAL IMPAIRMENT Manufacturer advises avoid—no information available.
- HANDLING AND STORAGE Hands should be washed thoroughly after application to avoid inadvertent transfer to other body areas.

- MEDICINAL FORMS There can be variation in the licensing of different medicines containing the same drug.
Ointment
 ▸ Silkis (Galderma (UK) Ltd)
  Calcitriol 3 microgram per 1 gram Silkis ointment | 100 gram PoM £18.06 DT = £18.06

Tacalcitol

18-Feb-2020

- **INDICATIONS AND DOSE**
Plaque psoriasis
 ▸ TO THE SKIN
 ▸ **Adult:** Apply once daily, preferably at bedtime, maximum 10 g ointment or 10 mL lotion daily, when lotion and ointment used together, maximum total tacalcitol 280 micrograms in any one week (e.g. lotion 30 mL with ointment 40 g)

- CONTRA-INDICATIONS Calcium metabolism disorders
- CAUTIONS Avoid eyes · erythrodermic exfoliative psoriasis (enhanced risk of hypercalcaemia) · generalised pustular psoriasis (enhanced risk of hypercalcaemia) · if used in conjunction with UV treatment
  CAUTIONS, FURTHER INFORMATION
 ▸ UV treatment If tacalcitol is used in conjunction with UV treatment, UV radiation should be given in the morning and tacalcitol applied at bedtime.
- INTERACTIONS → Appendix 1: vitamin D substances
- SIDE-EFFECTS
- ▸ **Uncommon** Skin reactions
- ▸ **Frequency not known** Hypercalcaemia
- PREGNANCY Manufacturer advises avoid unless no safer alternative—no information available.
- BREAST FEEDING Manufacturer advises avoid application to breast area; no information available on presence in milk.
- MONITORING REQUIREMENTS Monitor serum calcium if risk of hypercalcaemia.
- PATIENT AND CARER ADVICE Hands should be washed thoroughly after application to avoid inadvertent transfer to other body areas.

- MEDICINAL FORMS There can be variation in the licensing of different medicines containing the same drug.
Ointment
 ▸ Curatoderm (Almirall Ltd)
  Tacalcitol (as Tacalcitol monohydrate) 4 microgram per 1 gram Curatoderm 4micrograms/g ointment | 30 gram PoM £13.40 DT = £13.40 | 100 gram PoM £30.86 DT = £30.86
Liquid
EXCIPIENTS: May contain Disodium edetate, propylene glycol
 ▸ Curatoderm (Almirall Ltd)
  Tacalcitol (as Tacalcitol monohydrate) 4 microgram per 1 gram Curatoderm 4micrograms/g lotion | 30 ml PoM £12.73 DT = £12.73

4   Perspiration
4.1   Hyperhidrosis

Hyperhidrosis

16-Jun-2020

Overview

Hyperhidrosis is defined as sweating in excess of normal body temperature regulation. It can be localised (focal) or affect the entire skin area, and can be classified by the absence (primary) or presence (secondary) of an underlying cause.

13

Skin

[EvGr] Patients with primary focal hyperhidrosis affecting axillae, palmar, or plantar areas, should be offered a topical preparation containing 20% aluminium chloride hexahydrate below. ⟨A⟩ This is a more potent antiperspirant compared to commercially available preparations and is available as a spray, roll-on, or solution. [EvGr] If the response to treatment is inadequate or not tolerated after 6 weeks, consider referral to a specialist.

Specialist management may also be appropriate in more severe cases of hyperhidrosis. Topical glycopyrronium bromide p. 1308 as a 0.05% solution, may be used in the iontophoretic treatment of hyperhidrosis of plantar and palmar areas. Botox ® contains botulinum toxin type A complex p. 428 and is licensed for intradermal use for severe hyperhidrosis of the axillae unresponsive to topical antiperspirant or other antihidrotic treatment. Oxybutynin hydrochloride p. 822 [unlicensed indication] can cause a reduction in sweat secretion through its effects on muscarinic receptors near the sweat glands; its use is limited due to antimuscarinic adverse effects. ⟨A⟩

ANTIMUSCARINICS

`F 821`

Glycopyrronium bromide

06-Nov-2020

(Glycopyrrolate)

- **INDICATIONS AND DOSE**
Iontophoretic treatment of hyperhidrosis
  ▸ TO THE SKIN
  ▸ Adult: Only 1 site to be treated at a time, maximum 2 sites treated in any 24 hours, treatment not to be repeated within 7 days (consult product literature)

- **CONTRA-INDICATIONS** Infections affecting the treatment site
  CONTRA-INDICATIONS, FURTHER INFORMATION Contra-indications applicable to systemic use should be considered; however, glycopyrronium is poorly absorbed and systemic effects unlikely with topical use.
- **CAUTIONS** Cautions applicable to systemic use should be considered; however, glycopyrronium is poorly absorbed and systemic effects unlikely with topical use.
- **INTERACTIONS** → Appendix 1: glycopyrronium
- **SIDE-EFFECTS** Abdominal discomfort · eating disorder · pain · paraesthesia
  SIDE-EFFECTS, FURTHER INFORMATION The possibility of systemic side-effects should be considered; however, glycopyrronium is poorly absorbed and systemic effects are unlikely with topical use.

- **MEDICINAL FORMS** There can be variation in the licensing of different medicines containing the same drug.
  Powder for solution for iontophoresis
  ▸ Glycopyrronium bromide (Non-proprietary)
    Glycopyrronium bromide 1 mg per 1 mg Glycopyrronium bromide powder for solution for iontophoresis | 3 gram [PoM] £327.00 DT = £327.00

DERMATOLOGICAL DRUGS ＞ ASTRINGENTS

Aluminium chloride hexahydrate

21-Nov-2020

- **INDICATIONS AND DOSE**
Hyperhidrosis affecting axillae, hands or feet
  ▸ TO THE SKIN
  ▸ Adult: Apply once daily, apply liquid formulation at night to dry skin, wash off the following morning, reduce frequency as condition improves—do not bathe immediately before use

Hyperhidrosis | Bromidrosis | Intertrigo | Prevention of tinea pedis and related conditions
  ▸ TO THE SKIN
  ▸ Adult: Apply powder to dry skin

- **CAUTIONS** Avoid contact with eyes · avoid contact with mucous membranes · avoid use on broken or irritated skin · do not shave axillae or use depilatories within 12 hours of application
- **SIDE-EFFECTS** Skin reactions
- **PATIENT AND CARER ADVICE** Avoid contact with clothing.
- **EXCEPTIONS TO LEGAL CATEGORY** A 30 mL pack of aluminium chloride hexahydrate 20% is on sale to the public.

- **MEDICINAL FORMS** There can be variation in the licensing of different medicines containing the same drug.
  Liquid
  CAUTIONARY AND ADVISORY LABELS 15
  ▸ Anhydrol (Dermal Laboratories Ltd)
    Aluminium chloride hexahydrate 200 mg per 1 ml Anhydrol Forte 20% solution | 60 ml [P] £2.51 DT = £2.51
  ▸ Driclor (GlaxoSmithKline Consumer Healthcare)
    Aluminium chloride hexahydrate 200 mg per 1 ml Driclor 20% solution | 60 ml [P] £5.41 DT = £2.51

5 Pruritus

Topical local antipruritics

Overview

Pruritus may be caused by systemic disease (such as obstructive jaundice, endocrine disease, chronic renal disease, iron deficiency, and certain malignant diseases), skin disease (e.g. psoriasis, eczema, urticaria, and scabies), drug hypersensitivity, or as a side-effect of opioid analgesics. Where possible, the underlying causes should be treated. An **emollient** may be of value where the pruritus is associated with dry skin. Pruritus that occurs in otherwise healthy elderly people can also be treated with an emollient. Levomenthol **cream** p. 1309 can be used to relieve pruritus; it exerts a cooling effect on the skin. Local antipruritics have a role in the treatment of pruritus in palliative care.

Preparations containing crotamiton p. 1309 are sometimes used but are of uncertain value. Preparations containing calamine are often ineffective.

A topical preparation containing doxepin 5% p. 1309 is licensed for the relief of pruritus in eczema; it can cause drowsiness and there may be a risk of sensitisation.

Pruritus is common in biliary obstruction, especially in primary biliary cirrhosis and drug-induced cholestasis. Oral administration of colestyramine p. 212 is the treatment of choice.

Topical antihistamines and local anaesthetics are only marginally effective and occasionally cause hypersensitivity. For *insect stings* and *insect bites*, a short course of a topical corticosteroid is appropriate. Short-term treatment with a **sedating antihistamine** may help in insect stings and in intractable pruritus where sedation is desirable. Calamine preparations are of little value for the treatment of insect stings or bites.

Topical local anaesthetics are indicated for the relief of local pain. Preparations may be absorbed, especially through mucosal surfaces, therefore excessive application should be avoided and they should preferably not be used for more than 3 days; not generally suitable for young children and are less suitable for prescribing.

Topical antihistamines should be avoided in eczema and are not recommended for longer than 3 days. They are less suitable for prescribing.

> **Other drugs used for Pruritus** Alimemazine tartrate, p. 298 · Cetirizine hydrochloride, p. 295 · Chlorphenamine maleate, p. 299 · Coal tar with calamine, p. 1298 · Hydroxyzine hydrochloride, p. 300 · Levocetirizine hydrochloride, p. 296

ANTIPRURITICS

| Calamine with zinc oxide

11-Mar-2020

● **INDICATIONS AND DOSE**

Minor skin conditions

▸ TO THE SKIN
▸ Child: (consult product literature)
▸ Adult: (consult product literature)

> **IMPORTANT SAFETY INFORMATION**
> MHRA/CHM ADVICE (UPDATED DECEMBER 2018): EMOLLIENTS: NEW INFORMATION ABOUT RISK OF SEVERE AND FATAL BURNS WITH PARAFFIN-CONTAINING AND PARAFFIN-FREE EMOLLIENTS
> See Emollient and barrier preparations p. 1265.

● CONTRA-INDICATIONS Avoid application of preparations containing zinc oxide prior to x-ray (zinc oxide may affect outcome of x-ray)
● LESS SUITABLE FOR PRESCRIBING Less suitable for prescribing.
● MEDICINAL FORMS There can be variation in the licensing of different medicines containing the same drug.

Cream
CAUTIONARY AND ADVISORY LABELS 15
▸ Calamine with zinc oxide (Non-proprietary)
Phenoxyethanol 5 mg per 1 gram, Zinc oxide 30 mg per 1 gram, Calamine 40 mg per 1 gram, Cetomacrogol emulsifying wax 50 mg per 1 gram, Self-emulsifying glyceryl monostearate 50 mg per 1 gram, Liquid paraffin 200 mg per 1 gram Aqueous calamine cream | 100 gram GSL £1.43 DT = £1.43

Liquid
▸ Calamine with zinc oxide (Non-proprietary)
Phenol liquefied 5 mg per 1 ml, Sodium citrate 5 mg per 1 ml, Bentonite 30 mg per 1 ml, Glycerol 50 mg per 1 ml, Zinc oxide 50 mg per 1 ml, Calamine 150 mg per 1 ml Calamine lotion | 200 ml GSL £0.94–£1.09 DT = £1.09

| Crotamiton

29-Apr-2020

● **INDICATIONS AND DOSE**

Pruritus (including pruritus after scabies)

▸ TO THE SKIN
▸ Child 1 month-2 years (on doctor's advice only): Apply once daily
▸ Child 3-17 years: Apply 2–3 times a day
▸ Adult: Apply 2–3 times a day

● CONTRA-INDICATIONS Acute exudative dermatoses
● CAUTIONS Avoid use in buccal mucosa · avoid use near eyes · avoid use on broken skin · avoid use on very inflamed skin · use on doctor's advice for children under 3 years
● PREGNANCY Manufacturer advises avoid, especially during the first trimester—no information available.
● BREAST FEEDING No information available; avoid application to nipple area.

● MEDICINAL FORMS There can be variation in the licensing of different medicines containing the same drug.

Cream
EXCIPIENTS: May contain Beeswax, cetostearyl alcohol (including cetyl and stearyl alcohol), fragrances, hydroxybenzoates (parabens)
▸ Eurax (Thornton & Ross Ltd)
Crotamiton 100 mg per 1 gram Eurax 10% cream | 30 gram GSL £2.50 DT = £2.50 | 100 gram GSL £4.35 DT = £4.35

| Doxepin

02-Sep-2020

● **INDICATIONS AND DOSE**

Pruritus in eczema

▸ TO THE SKIN
▸ Child 12-17 years: Apply up to 3 g 3–4 times a day, apply thinly; coverage should be less than 10% of body surface area; maximum 12 g per day
▸ Adult: Apply up to 3 g 3–4 times a day, apply thinly; coverage should be less than 10% of body surface area; maximum 12 g per day

● CAUTIONS Arrhythmias · avoid application to large areas · mania · severe heart disease · susceptibility to angle-closure glaucoma · urinary retention
● INTERACTIONS → Appendix 1: tricyclic antidepressants
● SIDE-EFFECTS Constipation · diarrhoea · dizziness · drowsiness · dry eye · dry mouth · dyspepsia · fever · headache · nausea · paraesthesia · skin reactions · suicidal behaviours · taste altered · urinary retention · vision blurred · vomiting
● PREGNANCY Manufacturer advises use only if potential benefit outweighs risk.
● BREAST FEEDING Manufacturer advises use only if potential benefit outweighs risk.
● HEPATIC IMPAIRMENT Manufacturer advises caution in severe impairment.
● PATIENT AND CARER ADVICE A patient information leaflet should be provided.
Driving and skilled tasks Drowsiness may affect performance of skilled tasks (e.g. driving).
Effects of alcohol enhanced.

● MEDICINAL FORMS There can be variation in the licensing of different medicines containing the same drug. Forms available from special-order manufacturers include: cream

Cream
CAUTIONARY AND ADVISORY LABELS 2, 10
EXCIPIENTS: May contain Benzyl alcohol
▸ Xepin (Cambridge Healthcare Supplies Ltd)
Doxepin hydrochloride 50 mg per 1 gram Xepin 5% cream | 30 gram PoM £13.66 DT = £13.66

MENTHOL AND DERIVATIVES

| Levomenthol

● **INDICATIONS AND DOSE**

Pruritus

▸ TO THE SKIN
▸ Adult: Apply 1–2 times a day

● MEDICINAL FORMS There can be variation in the licensing of different medicines containing the same drug. Forms available from special-order manufacturers include: cream

Cream
▸ AquaSoothe (Ennogen Healthcare Ltd)
Menthol 10 mg per 1 gram AquaSoothe 1% cream | 100 gram £3.70 DT = £3.97 | 500 gram £15.43 DT = £16.59
Menthol 20 mg per 1 gram AquaSoothe 2% cream | 50 gram £1.86 | 500 gram £15.43 DT = £16.97

13

Skin

13

Skin

▸ Arjun (Arjun Products Ltd)
Menthol 5 mg per 1 gram Arjun 0.5% cream | 500 gram £15.30 DT = £16.07
Menthol 10 mg per 1 gram Arjun 1% cream | 100 gram £3.25 DT = £3.97 | 500 gram £15.30 DT = £16.59
Menthol 20 mg per 1 gram Arjun 2% cream | 500 gram £15.30 DT = £16.97

▸ Dermacool (Pern Consumer Products Ltd)
Menthol 5 mg per 1 gram Dermacool 0.5% cream | 100 gram £3.85 | 500 gram £16.07 DT = £16.07
Menthol 10 mg per 1 gram Dermacool 1% cream | 100 gram £3.97 DT = £3.97 | 500 gram £16.59 DT = £16.59
Menthol 20 mg per 1 gram Dermacool 2% cream | 100 gram £4.07 | 500 gram £16.97 DT = £16.97
Menthol 50 mg per 1 gram Dermacool 5% cream | 100 gram £4.69 | 500 gram £17.48

▸ Menthoderm (Derma UK Ltd)
Menthol 5 mg per 1 gram Menthoderm 0.5% cream | 100 gram £3.12 | 500 gram £14.59 DT = £16.07
Menthol 10 mg per 1 gram Menthoderm 1% cream | 100 gram £3.20 DT = £3.97 | 500 gram £14.79 DT = £16.59
Menthol 20 mg per 1 gram Menthoderm 2% cream | 100 gram £3.85 | 500 gram £14.99 DT = £16.97

6 Rosacea and acne

Rosacea and Acne

29-Sep-2020

Acne

Treatment of acne should be commenced early to prevent scarring. Patients should be counselled that an improvement may not be seen for at least a couple of months. The choice of treatment depends on whether the acne is predominantly inflammatory or comedonal and its severity.

Mild to moderate acne is generally treated with topical preparations. Systemic treatment with oral antibacterials is generally used for *moderate to severe acne* or where topical preparations are not tolerated or are ineffective or where application to the site is difficult. Another oral preparation used for acne is the hormone treatment co-cyprindiol p. 1311 (cyproterone acetate with ethinylestradiol); it is for women only.

Severe acne (such as nodular or conglobate acne or acne at risk of permanent scarring) resistant to adequate courses of standard therapy with systemic antibacterials and topical therapy calls for early referral to a consultant dermatologist who may prescribe isotretinoin p. 1314 for administration by mouth.

Acne: topical preparations

In mild to moderate acne, comedones and inflamed lesions respond well to benzoyl peroxide p. 1312 or to a topical retinoid. Alternatively, topical application of an antibacterial such as erythromycin p. 572 or clindamycin p. 1312 may be effective for inflammatory acne. If topical preparations prove inadequate, oral preparations may be needed.

Benzoyl peroxide and azelaic acid

Benzoyl peroxide is effective in mild to moderate acne. Both comedones and inflamed lesions respond well to benzoyl peroxide. The lower concentrations seem to be as effective as higher concentrations in reducing inflammation. It is usual to start with a lower strength and to increase the concentration of benzoyl peroxide gradually. Adverse effects include local skin irritation, particularly when therapy is initiated, but the scaling and redness often subside with treatment continued at a reduced frequency of application. If the acne does not respond after 2 months then use of a topical antibacterial should be considered.

Azelaic acid p. 1313 has antimicrobial and anticomedonal properties. It may be an alternative to benzoyl peroxide or to a topical retinoid for treating mild to moderate comedonal

acne, particularly of the face. Some patients prefer azelaic acid because it is less likely to cause local irritation than benzoyl peroxide.

Topical antibacterials for acne

For many patients with mild to moderate inflammatory acne, topical antibacterials may be no more effective than topical benzoyl peroxide or tretinoin. Topical antibacterials are probably best reserved for patients who wish to avoid oral antibacterials or who cannot tolerate them. Topical preparations of erythromycin and clindamycin are effective for inflammatory acne. Topical antibacterials can produce mild irritation of the skin, and on rare occasions cause sensitisation; gastro-intestinal disturbances have been reported with topical clindamycin.

Antibacterial resistance of *Propionibacterium acnes* is increasing; there is cross-resistance between erythromycin and clindamycin. To avoid development of resistance:

- when possible use non-antibiotic antimicrobials (such as benzoyl peroxide or azelaic acid);
- avoid concomitant treatment with different oral and topical antibacterials;
- if a particular antibacterial is effective, use it for repeat courses if needed (short intervening courses of benzoyl peroxide or azelaic acid may eliminate any resistant propionibacteria);
- do not continue treatment for longer than necessary (however, treatment with a topical preparation should be continued for at least 6 months).

Some manufacturers of topical antibacterial preparations for acne advise that preparations containing alcohol are not suitable for use with benzoyl peroxide.

Topical retinoids and related preparations for acne

Topical tretinoin (available from 'special-order' manufacturers), its isomer isotretinoin, and adapalene (a retinoid-like drug) p. 1313, are useful for treating comedones and inflammatory lesions in mild to moderate acne. Several months of treatment may be needed to achieve an optimal response and the treatment should be continued until no new lesions develop. Isotretinoin is given by mouth in severe acne.

Other topical preparations for acne

Preparations containing aluminium oxide are not considered beneficial in acne.

A topical preparation of nicotinamide p. 1316 is available for inflammatory acne.

Acne: oral preparations

Systemic antibacterial treatment is useful for inflammatory acne if topical treatment is not adequately effective or if it is inappropriate. Anticomedonal treatment (e.g. with topical benzoyl peroxide) may also be required.

Either oxytetracycline p. 603 or tetracycline p. 604 is usually given for acne. If there is no improvement after the first 3 months another oral antibacterial should be used. Maximum improvement usually occurs after 4 to 6 months but in more severe cases treatment may need to be continued for 2 years or longer.

Doxycycline p. 601 and lymecycline p. 602 are alternatives to tetracycline.

Although minocycline p. 603 is as effective as other tetracyclines for acne, it is associated with a greater risk of lupus erythematosus-like syndrome. Minocycline sometimes causes irreversible pigmentation; it is given in a once or twice daily dose.

Erythromycin in a twice daily dose is an alternative for the management of acne but *propionibacteria* strains resistant to erythromycin are becoming widespread and this may explain poor response.

Trimethoprim p. 610 may be used for acne resistant to other antibacterials [unlicensed indication]. Prolonged treatment with trimethoprim may depress haematopoiesis; it should generally be initiated by specialists.

Concomitant use of different topical and systemic antibacterials is undesirable owing to the increased likelihood of the development of bacterial resistance.

Hormone treatment for acne

Co-cyprindiol (cyproterone acetate with ethinylestradiol) contains an anti-androgen. It is licensed for use in women with moderate to severe acne that has not responded to topical therapy or oral antibacterials, and for moderately severe hirsutism. Although it is an effective hormonal contraceptive, it should not be used solely for contraception.

Improvement of acne with co-cyprindiol probably occurs because of decreased sebum secretion which is under androgen control. Some women with moderately severe hirsutism may also benefit because hair growth is also androgen-dependent.

The MHRA/CHM have released important safety information regarding the use of cyproterone acetate and the risk of meningioma. For further information, see *Important safety information* for co-cyprindiol. The Faculty of Sexual and Reproductive Healthcare have released a statement in response to the MHRA/CHM information (available at: www.fsrh.org/standards-and-guidance/documents/fsrh-ceu-statement-new-advice-from-the-mhra-regarding/).

Oral retinoid for acne

The retinoid isotretinoin reduces sebum secretion. It is used for the systemic treatment of severe acne (such as nodular or conglobate acne or acne at risk of permanent scarring) resistant to adequate courses of standard therapy with systemic antibacterials and topical therapy.

Isotretinoin is a toxic drug that should be prescribed **only** by, or under the supervision of, a consultant dermatologist. It is given for at least 16 weeks; repeat courses are not normally required.

Side-effects of isotretinoin p. 1314 include severe dryness of the skin and mucous membranes, nose bleeds, and joint pains. The drug is **teratogenic** and must **not** be given to women of child-bearing age unless they practise effective contraception (oral progestogen-only contraceptives not considered effective) and then only after detailed assessment and explanation by the physician. Women must also be registered with a pregnancy prevention programme.

Although a causal link between isotretinoin use and psychiatric changes (including suicidal ideation) has not been established, the possibility should be considered before initiating treatment; if psychiatric changes occur during treatment, isotretinoin should be stopped, the prescriber informed, and specialist psychiatric advice should be sought.

The MHRA/CHM have released important safety information on the risks and precautions for the use of isotretinoin. For further information, see *Important safety information* for isotretinoin.

Rosacea

Rosacea is not comedonal (but may exist with acne which may be comedonal). Brimonidine tartrate p. 1317 is licensed for the treatment of facial erythema in rosacea. The pustules and papules of rosacea respond to topical azelaic acid p. 1313, topical ivermectin p. 1316 or to topical metronidazole p. 1275. Alternatively oral administration of oxytetracycline p. 603 or tetracycline p. 604, or erythromycin p. 572, can be used; courses usually last 6–12 weeks and are repeated intermittently. Doxycycline p. 601 can be used [unlicensed indication] if oxytetracycline or tetracycline is inappropriate (e.g. in renal impairment). A modified-release preparation of doxycycline is licensed in low daily doses for the treatment of facial rosacea. Camouflagers may be required for the redness.

6.1 Acne

ANTI-ANDROGENS

Co-cyprindiol

18-Aug-2020

● **INDICATIONS AND DOSE**

Moderate to severe acne in females of child-bearing age refractory to topical therapy or oral antibacterials | Moderately severe hirsutism

▸ BY MOUTH
▸ Females of childbearing potential: 1 tablet daily for 21 days, to be started on day 1 of menstrual cycle; subsequent courses repeated after a 7-day interval (during which withdrawal bleeding occurs), time to symptom remission, at least 3 months; review need for treatment regularly

IMPORTANT SAFETY INFORMATION

MHRA/CHM ADVICE: CYPROTERONE ACETATE: NEW ADVICE TO MINIMISE RISK OF MENINGIOMA (JUNE 2020)

Cyproterone acetate has been associated with an overall rare, but cumulative dose-dependent, increased risk of meningioma (single and multiple), mainly at doses of 25 mg/day and higher. Healthcare professionals are advised to monitor patients for meningiomas, and to permanently discontinue treatment if diagnosed. Use of cyproterone acetate, including co-cyprindiol, for all indications, is contra-indicated in those with meningioma or a history of meningioma.

● CONTRA-INDICATIONS Acute porphyrias p. 1107 · current breast cancer · heart disease associated with pulmonary hypertension or risk of embolus · history of stroke (including transient ischaemic attack) · ischaemic heart disease · known thrombogenic mutations (e.g. factor V Leiden, prothrombin mutation, protein S, protein C and antithrombin deficiencies) · medical treatment for varicose veins · migraine with aura · positive antiphospholipid antibodies · presence or history of liver tumours · previous or current venous or arterial thrombosis · severe or multiple risk factors for arterial or venous thromboembolism · systemic lupus erythematosus with antiphospholipid antibodies

● CAUTIONS Cardiac disease · cervical cancer · cholestasis with previous use of combined oral contraception—seek specialist advice before use · gallbladder disease—seek specialist advice before use · gene mutations associated with breast cancer (e.g. BRCA 1)—seek specialist advice before use · history of breast cancer—seek specialist advice before use · history of cholestasis during pregnancy · history of depression · hyperprolactinaemia—seek specialist advice before use · inflammatory bowel disease including Crohn's disease · migraine · personal or family history of hypertriglyceridaemia (increased risk of pancreatitis) · risk factors for arterial thromboembolism · risk factors for venous thromboembolism · sickle-cell disease · systemic lupus erythematosus · undiagnosed breast mass—seek specialist advice before use · undiagnosed vaginal bleeding

CAUTIONS, FURTHER INFORMATION

▸ Venous thromboembolism There is an increased risk of venous thromboembolism in women taking co-cyprindiol, particularly during the first year of use. The incidence of venous thromboembolism is 1.5–2 times higher in women using co-cyprindiol than in women using combined oral contraceptives containing levonorgestrel, but the risk may be similar to that associated with use of combined oral contraceptives containing third generation progestogens (desogestrel and gestodene) or drospirenone. Women requiring co-cyprindiol may have an inherently increased risk of cardiovascular disease.

For more information about the risk factors for venous thromboembolism, see combined hormonal contraceptive p. 841.

- INTERACTIONS → Appendix 1: anti-androgens
- SIDE-EFFECTS
- ▶ **Common or very common** Abdominal pain · breast abnormalities · depression · headaches · mood altered · nausea · weight changes
- ▶ **Uncommon** Diarrhoea · fluid retention · sexual dysfunction · skin reactions · vomiting
- ▶ **Rare or very rare** Contact lens intolerance · erythema nodosum · thromboembolism · vaginal discharge
- ▶ **Frequency not known** Amenorrhoea (on discontinuation) · angioedema aggravated · chorea exacerbated · hepatic function abnormal · hepatic neoplasm · hypertension · hypertriglyceridaemia · inflammatory bowel disease · menstrual cycle irregularities · suicidal behaviours
- PREGNANCY Avoid—risk of feminisation of male fetus with cyproterone.
- BREAST FEEDING Manufacturer advises avoid; possibility of anti-androgen effects in neonate with cyproterone.
- HEPATIC IMPAIRMENT Manufacturer advises caution; avoid in severe or active disease
- PRESCRIBING AND DISPENSING INFORMATION A mixture of cyproterone acetate and ethinylestradiol in the mass proportions 2000 parts to 35 parts, respectively.

- MEDICINAL FORMS There can be variation in the licensing of different medicines containing the same drug.

Tablet
- ▶ Co-cyprindiol (Non-proprietary)
  Ethinylestradiol 35 microgram, Cyproterone acetate 2 mg Co-cyprindiol 2000microgram/35microgram tablets | 63 tablet [PoM] £16.65 DT = £10.78
- ▶ Clairette (Stragen UK Ltd)
  Ethinylestradiol 35 microgram, Cyproterone acetate 2 mg Clairette 2000/35 tablets | 63 tablet [PoM] £5.90 DT = £10.78
- ▶ Dianette (Bayer Plc)
  Ethinylestradiol 35 microgram, Cyproterone acetate 2 mg Dianette tablets | 63 tablet [PoM] £7.71 DT = £10.78
- ▶ Teragezza (Morningside Healthcare Ltd)
  Ethinylestradiol 35 microgram, Cyproterone acetate 2 mg Teragezza 2000microgram/35microgram tablets | 63 tablet [PoM] £11.10 DT = £10.78

ANTIBACTERIALS > LINCOSAMIDES

Clindamycin

25-Nov-2020

- **INDICATIONS AND DOSE**

DALACIN T ® LOTION

Acne vulgaris
- ▶ TO THE SKIN
- ▶ Child: Apply twice daily, to be applied thinly
- ▶ Adult: Apply twice daily, to be applied thinly

DALACIN T ® SOLUTION

Acne vulgaris
- ▶ TO THE SKIN
- ▶ Child: Apply twice daily, to be applied thinly
- ▶ Adult: Apply twice daily, to be applied thinly

ZINDACLIN ® GEL

Acne vulgaris
- ▶ TO THE SKIN
- ▶ Child 12-17 years: Apply once daily, to be applied thinly
- ▶ Adult: Apply once daily, to be applied thinly

- INTERACTIONS → Appendix 1: clindamycin
- SIDE-EFFECTS
- ▶ **Common or very common** Skin reactions

- ▶ **Frequency not known** Abdominal pain · antibiotic associated colitis · folliculitis gram-negative · gastrointestinal disorder
- PATIENT AND CARER ADVICE Patients and their carers should be advised to discontinue and contact a doctor immediately if severe, prolonged or bloody diarrhoea develops.

- MEDICINAL FORMS There can be variation in the licensing of different medicines containing the same drug.
Gel
EXCIPIENTS: May contain Propylene glycol
- ▶ Zindaclin (Crawford Healthcare Ltd)
  Clindamycin (as Clindamycin phosphate) 10 mg per 1 gram Zindaclin 1% gel | 30 gram [PoM] £8.66 DT = £8.66
Liquid
EXCIPIENTS: May contain Cetostearyl alcohol (including cetyl and stearyl alcohol), hydroxybenzoates (parabens), propylene glycol
- ▶ Dalacin T (Pfizer Ltd)
  Clindamycin (as Clindamycin phosphate) 10 mg per 1 ml Dalacin T 1% topical lotion | 30 ml [PoM] £5.08 DT = £5.08 | 60 ml [PoM] £10.16
  Dalacin T 1% topical solution | 30 ml [PoM] £4.34 DT = £4.34 | 50 ml [PoM] £7.23

Combinations available: *Benzoyl peroxide with clindamycin*, p. 1313 · *Tretinoin with clindamycin*, p. 1315

ANTIBACTERIALS > MACROLIDES

Erythromycin with zinc acetate

20-Apr-2020

The properties listed below are those particular to the combination only. For the properties of the components please consider, erythromycin p. 572.

- **INDICATIONS AND DOSE**

Acne vulgaris
- ▶ TO THE SKIN
- ▶ Child: Apply twice daily
- ▶ Adult: Apply twice daily

- INTERACTIONS → Appendix 1: macrolides

- MEDICINAL FORMS There can be variation in the licensing of different medicines containing the same drug.
Liquid
- ▶ Zineryt (LEO Pharma)
  Zinc acetate 12 mg per 1 ml, Erythromycin 40 mg per 1 ml Zineryt lotion | 30 ml [PoM] £9.25 DT = £9.25 | 90 ml [PoM] £20.02 DT = £20.02

ANTISEPTICS AND DISINFECTANTS > PEROXIDES

Benzoyl peroxide

01-Sep-2020

- **INDICATIONS AND DOSE**

Acne vulgaris
- ▶ TO THE SKIN
- ▶ Child 12-17 years: Apply 1-2 times a day, preferably apply after washing with soap and water, start treatment with lower-strength preparations
- ▶ Adult: Apply 1-2 times a day, preferably apply after washing with soap and water, start treatment with lower-strength preparations

- CAUTIONS Avoid contact with broken skin · avoid contact with eyes · avoid contact with mouth · avoid contact with mucous membranes · avoid excessive exposure to sunlight
- SIDE-EFFECTS
- ▶ **Common or very common** Skin reactions
- ▶ **Frequency not known** Facial swelling

  SIDE-EFFECTS, FURTHER INFORMATION Reduce frequency or suspend use until skin irritation subsides and re-introduce at reduced frequency.

- PATIENT AND CARER ADVICE May bleach fabrics and hair.

- MEDICINAL FORMS There can be variation in the licensing of different medicines containing the same drug.

Gel

EXCIPIENTS: May contain Fragrances, propylene glycol
▸ Acnecide (Galderma (UK) Ltd)
    Benzoyl peroxide 50 mg per 1 gram Acnecide 5% gel | 30 gram P
    £5.44 DT = £5.44 | 60 gram P £10.68 DT = £10.68
    Acnecide Wash 5% gel | 100 gram P £8.81

Combinations available: *Adapalene with benzoyl peroxide,* p. 1314

Benzoyl peroxide with clindamycin

09-Mar-2020

The properties listed below are those particular to the combination only. For the properties of the components please consider, benzoyl peroxide p. 1312, clindamycin p. 1312.

- **INDICATIONS AND DOSE**

Acne vulgaris
▸ TO THE SKIN
▸ Child 12–17 years: Apply once daily, dose to be applied in the evening
▸ Adult: Apply once daily, dose to be applied in the evening

- INTERACTIONS → Appendix 1: clindamycin

- MEDICINAL FORMS There can be variation in the licensing of different medicines containing the same drug.

Gel

EXCIPIENTS: May contain Disodium edetate
▸ Duac (Stiefel Laboratories (UK) Ltd)
    Clindamycin (as Clindamycin phosphate) 10 mg per 1 gram, Benzoyl peroxide 30 mg per 1 gram Duac Once Daily gel (3% and 1%) | 30 gram PoM £13.14 DT = £13.14 | 60 gram PoM £26.28
    Clindamycin (as Clindamycin phosphate) 10 mg per 1 gram, Benzoyl peroxide 50 mg per 1 gram Duac Once Daily gel (5% and 1%) | 30 gram PoM £13.14 DT = £13.14 | 60 gram PoM £26.28 DT = £26.28

DERMATOLOGICAL DRUGS > ANTICOMEDONALS

Azelaic acid

21-Nov-2020

- **INDICATIONS AND DOSE**

FINACEA ®

Facial acne vulgaris
▸ TO THE SKIN
▸ Child 12–17 years: Apply twice daily, discontinue if no improvement after 1 month
▸ Adult: Apply twice daily, discontinue if no improvement after 1 month

Papulopustular rosacea
▸ TO THE SKIN
▸ Adult: Apply twice daily, discontinue if no improvement after 2 months

SKINOREN ®

Acne vulgaris
▸ TO THE SKIN
▸ Child 12–17 years: Apply twice daily
▸ Adult: Apply twice daily

Acne vulgaris in patients with sensitive skin
▸ TO THE SKIN
▸ Child 12–17 years: Apply once daily for 1 week, then apply twice daily
▸ Adult: Apply once daily for 1 week, then apply twice daily

- CAUTIONS Avoid contact with eyes · avoid contact with mouth · avoid contact with mucous membranes
- SIDE-EFFECTS
▸ **Uncommon** Skin reactions
▸ **Rare or very rare** Asthma exacerbated · cheilitis
▸ **Frequency not known** Angioedema · eye swelling

- MEDICINAL FORMS There can be variation in the licensing of different medicines containing the same drug.

Cream

EXCIPIENTS: May contain Propylene glycol
▸ Skinoren (LEO Pharma)
    Azelaic acid 200 mg per 1 gram Skinoren 20% cream | 30 gram PoM £4.49 DT = £4.49

Gel

EXCIPIENTS: May contain Disodium edetate, polysorbates, propylene glycol
▸ Finacea (LEO Pharma)
    Azelaic acid 150 mg per 1 gram Finacea 15% gel | 30 gram PoM £7.48 DT = £7.48

RETINOID AND RELATED DRUGS

Adapalene

28-Aug-2020

- **INDICATIONS AND DOSE**

Mild to moderate acne vulgaris
▸ TO THE SKIN
▸ Child 12–17 years: Apply once daily, apply thinly in the evening
▸ Adult: Apply once daily, apply thinly in the evening

- CAUTIONS Avoid accumulation in angles of the nose · avoid contact with eyes, nostrils, mouth and mucous membranes, eczematous, broken or sunburned skin · avoid exposure to UV light (including sunlight, solariums) · avoid in severe acne involving large areas · caution in sensitive areas such as the neck
- INTERACTIONS → Appendix 1: retinoids
- CONCEPTION AND CONTRACEPTION Females of child-bearing age must use effective contraception (oral progestogen-only contraceptives not considered effective).
- PREGNANCY Avoid.
- BREAST FEEDING Amount of drug in milk probably too small to be harmful; ensure infant does not come in contact with treated areas.
- PATIENT AND CARER ADVICE If sun exposure is unavoidable, an appropriate sunscreen or protective clothing should be used.

- MEDICINAL FORMS There can be variation in the licensing of different medicines containing the same drug.

Cream

CAUTIONARY AND ADVISORY LABELS 11
EXCIPIENTS: May contain Disodium edetate, hydroxybenzoates (parabens)
▸ Differin (Galderma (UK) Ltd)
    Adapalene 1 mg per 1 gram Differin 0.1% cream | 45 gram PoM £16.43 DT = £16.43

Gel

CAUTIONARY AND ADVISORY LABELS 11
EXCIPIENTS: May contain Disodium edetate, hydroxybenzoates (parabens), propylene glycol
▸ Differin (Galderma (UK) Ltd)
    Adapalene 1 mg per 1 gram Differin 0.1% gel | 45 gram PoM £16.43 DT = £16.43

13

Skin

Adapalene with benzoyl peroxide

02-Nov-2020

The properties listed below are those particular to the combination only. For the properties of the components please consider, adapalene p. 1313, benzoyl peroxide p. 1312.

- ● **INDICATIONS AND DOSE**

  Acne vulgaris
  - ▶ TO THE SKIN
  - ▶ Child 9–17 years: Apply once daily, to be applied thinly in the evening
  - ▶ Adult: Apply once daily, to be applied thinly in the evening

- ● INTERACTIONS → Appendix 1: retinoids
- ● CONCEPTION AND CONTRACEPTION Females of child-bearing age must use effective contraception (oral progestogen-only contraceptives not considered effective).
- ● PATIENT AND CARER ADVICE Gel may bleach clothing and hair.
- ● NATIONAL FUNDING/ACCESS DECISIONS
  For full details see funding body website
  Scottish Medicines Consortium (SMC) decisions
  - ▶ Adapalene 0.1% with benzoyl peroxide 2.5% gel (*Epiduo®*) for the cutaneous treatment of acne vulgaris when comedones, papules and pustules are present (April 2014) SMC No. 682/11 Recommended with restrictions

- ● MEDICINAL FORMS There can be variation in the licensing of different medicines containing the same drug.

  Gel
  CAUTIONARY AND ADVISORY LABELS 11
  EXCIPIENTS: May contain Disodium edetate, polysorbates, propylene glycol
  - ▶ Adapalene with benzoyl peroxide (Non-proprietary)
    Adapalene 3 mg per 1 gram, Benzoyl peroxide 25 mg per 1 gram Epiduo 0.3%/2.5% gel | 45 gram [PoM] £19.53 DT = £19.53
  - ▶ Epiduo (Galderma (UK) Ltd)
    Adapalene 1 mg per 1 gram, Benzoyl peroxide 25 mg per 1 gram Epiduo 0.1%/2.5% gel | 45 gram [PoM] £19.53 DT = £19.53

Isotretinoin

24-Sep-2020

- ● **INDICATIONS AND DOSE**

  Severe acne [(such as nodular or conglobate acne or acne at risk of permanent scarring) resistant to adequate courses of standard therapy with systemic antibacterials and topical therapy] (under expert supervision)
  - ▶ BY MOUTH
  - ▶ Adult: Initially 500 micrograms/kg daily in 1–2 divided doses, increased if necessary to 1 mg/kg daily for 16–24 weeks, repeat treatment course after a period of at least 8 weeks if relapse after first course; maximum 150 mg/kg per course

  IMPORTANT SAFETY INFORMATION

  MHRA/CHM ADVICE: ISOTRETINOIN (*ROACCUTANE®*): RARE REPORTS OF ERECTILE DYSFUNCTION AND DECREASED LIBIDO (OCTOBER 2017)
  An EU-wide review has concluded that on rare occasions, oral isotretinoin, indicated for severe acne, may cause sexual side-effects, including erectile dysfunction and decreased libido.

  MHRA/CHM ADVICE: ORAL RETINOID MEDICINES: REVISED AND SIMPLIFIED PREGNANCY PREVENTION EDUCATIONAL MATERIALS FOR HEALTHCARE PROFESSIONALS AND WOMEN (JUNE 2019)
  New prescriber checklists, patient reminder cards, and pharmacy checklists are available to support the

Pregnancy Prevention Programme in women and girls of childbearing potential taking oral acitretin, alitretinoin, or isotretinoin. Healthcare professionals are reminded that the use of oral retinoids is contra-indicated in pregnancy due to a high risk of serious congenital malformations, and any use in females must be within the conditions of the Pregnancy Prevention Programme (see *Conception and contraception* and *Prescribing and dispensing information*).

Neuropsychiatric reactions have been reported in patients taking oral retinoids. Healthcare professionals are advised to monitor patients for signs of depression or suicidal ideation and refer for appropriate treatment, if necessary; particular care is needed in those with a history of depression. Patients should be advised to speak to their doctor if they experience any changes in mood or behaviour, and encouraged to ask family and friends to look out for any change in mood.

MHRA/CHM ADVICE: ISOTRETINOIN (*ROACCUTANE®*): REMINDER OF IMPORTANT RISKS AND PRECAUTIONS (AUGUST 2020)
The MHRA reminds healthcare professionals that isotretinoin should only be prescribed for the treatment of severe forms of acne resistant to adequate courses of standard therapy with systemic antibacterials and topical therapy. Isotretinoin should be given under the supervision of physicians with expertise in the use of systemic retinoids, and a complete understanding of the risks of therapy and monitoring requirements (including signs of depression).

Healthcare professionals are also advised to counsel patients on the potential risks of isotretinoin, including neuropsychiatric reactions and sexual dysfunction.

The MHRA further reminds healthcare professionals that isotretinoin is a powerful teratogen associated with a high frequency of severe and life-threatening birth defects if there is exposure in utero; females of childbearing potential must meet the conditions of the Pregnancy Prevention Programme (see *Conception and contraception* and *Prescribing and dispensing information*).

- ● CONTRA-INDICATIONS Hyperlipidaemia · hypervitaminosis A
- ● CAUTIONS Avoid blood donation during treatment and for at least 1 month after treatment · diabetes · dry eye syndrome (associated with risk of keratitis) · history of depression (risk of neuropsychiatric reactions)
- ● INTERACTIONS → Appendix 1: retinoids
- ● SIDE-EFFECTS
  - ▶ Common or very common Alopecia · anaemia · arthralgia · back pain · cheilitis · dry eye · eye discomfort · eye inflammation · haemorrhage · headache · increased risk of infection · myalgia · nasal dryness · neutropenia · proteinuria · skin fragility (trauma may cause blistering) · skin reactions · thrombocytopenia · thrombocytosis
  - ▶ Rare or very rare Anxiety · arthritis · behaviour abnormal · bone disorders · bronchospasm · cataract · corneal opacity · depression · diabetes mellitus · dizziness · drowsiness · dry throat · gastrointestinal disorders · glomerulonephritis · hair changes · hearing impairment · hepatitis · hoarseness · hyperhidrosis · hyperuricaemia · idiopathic intracranial hypertension · inflammatory bowel disease · lymphadenopathy · malaise · mood altered · nail dystrophy · nausea · pancreatitis · photosensitivity reaction · psychotic disorder · pyogenic granuloma · seizure · suicidal behaviours · tendinitis · vasculitis · vision disorders
  - ▶ Frequency not known Psychiatric disorder · rhabdomyolysis · severe cutaneous adverse reactions (SCARs) · sexual dysfunction · vulvovaginal dryness

  SIDE-EFFECTS, FURTHER INFORMATION Risk of pancreatitis if triglycerides above 9 mmol/litre—discontinue if uncontrolled hypertriglyceridaemia or pancreatitis.

Discontinue treatment if skin peeling severe or haemorrhagic diarrhoea develops.

Visual disturbances require expert referral and possible withdrawal.

Psychiatric side-effects could require expert referral.

- CONCEPTION AND CONTRACEPTION The MHRA advises that women and girls of childbearing potential being treated with the oral retinoids acitretin, alitretinoin, or isotretinoin must be supported on a Pregnancy Prevention Programme with regular follow-up and pregnancy testing. Pregnancy prevention Effective contraception must be used.

In females of childbearing potential, exclude pregnancy a few days before treatment, every month during treatment (unless there are compelling reasons to indicate that there is no risk of pregnancy), and 4 weeks after stopping treatment. Females must practise effective contraception for at least 1 month before starting treatment, during treatment, and for at least 1 month after stopping treatment. They should be advised to use at least 1 method of contraception, but ideally they should use 2 methods of contraception. Oral progestogen-only contraceptives are not considered effective. Barrier methods should not be used alone, but can be used in conjunction with other contraceptive methods. Females should be advised to discontinue treatment and to seek prompt medical attention if they become pregnant during treatment or within 1 month of stopping treatment.

- PREGNANCY Manufacturer advises avoid—teratogenic.
- BREAST FEEDING Avoid.
- HEPATIC IMPAIRMENT Manufacturer advises avoid— limited information available.
- RENAL IMPAIRMENT

Dose adjustments In severe impairment, reduce initial dose (e.g. 10 mg daily) and increase gradually up to 1 mg/kg daily as tolerated.

- MONITORING REQUIREMENTS Measure hepatic function and serum lipids before treatment, 1 month after starting and then every 3 months (reduce dose or discontinue if transaminase or serum lipids persistently raised).
- PRESCRIBING AND DISPENSING INFORMATION Isotretinoin is an isomer of tretinoin.

Prescribing for females of childbearing potential The Pregnancy Prevention Programme is supported by the following materials provided by the manufacturer: *Checklists for prescribers and pharmacists*, and *Patient reminder cards.*

Each prescription for oral isotretinoin should be limited to a supply of up to 30 days' treatment. Pregnancy testing should ideally be carried out on the same day as prescription issuing and dispensing.

- PATIENT AND CARER ADVICE Warn patient to avoid wax epilation (risk of epidermal stripping), dermabrasion, and laser skin treatments (risk of scarring) during treatment and for at least 6 months after stopping; patient should avoid exposure to UV light (including sunlight) and use sunscreen and emollient (including lip balm) preparations from the start of treatment.

Risk of neuropsychiatric reactions The MHRA advises patients and carers to seek medical attention if changes in mood or behaviour occur.

Pregnancy Prevention Programme Pharmacists must ensure that female patients have a patient card—see also *Important safety information.*

- MEDICINAL FORMS There can be variation in the licensing of different medicines containing the same drug.

Capsule

CAUTIONARY AND ADVISORY LABELS 10, 11, 21
▸ Isotretinoin (Non-proprietary)
 Isotretinoin 5 mg Isotretinoin 5mg capsules | 30 capsule PoM
 £10.10–£10.15 | 56 capsule PoM £14.79 DT = £14.79
 Isotretinoin 10 mg Isotretinoin 10mg capsules | 30 capsule PoM
 £14.54 DT = £14.53

Isotretinoin 20 mg Isotretinoin 20mg capsules | 30 capsule PoM
 £20.00 DT = £16.66 | 56 capsule PoM £31.10–£37.85
 Isotretinoin 40 mg Isotretinoin 40mg capsules | 30 capsule PoM
 £38.98 DT = £38.98
▸ Roaccutane (Roche Products Ltd)
 Isotretinoin 10 mg Roaccutane 10mg capsules | 30 capsule PoM
 £14.54 DT = £14.53
 Isotretinoin 20 mg Roaccutane 20mg capsules | 30 capsule PoM
 £20.02 DT = £16.66

Tretinoin with clindamycin   10-Mar-2020

The properties listed below are those particular to the combination only. For the properties of the components please consider, tretinoin p. 982, clindamycin p. 1312.

- **INDICATIONS AND DOSE**

Facial acne
▸ TO THE SKIN
▸ Child 12–17 years: Apply daily, (to be applied thinly at bedtime)
▸ Adult: Apply daily, (to be applied thinly at bedtime)

- CONTRA-INDICATIONS Perioral dermatitis · personal or familial history of skin cancer · rosacea
- CAUTIONS Allow peeling (resulting from other irritant treatments) to subside before using a topical retinoid · avoid accumulation in angles of the nose · avoid contact with eyes, nostrils, mouth and mucous membranes, eczematous, broken or sunburned skin · avoid exposure to UV light (including sunlight, solariums) · avoid use of topical retinoids with keratolytic agents, abrasive cleaners, comedogenic or astringent cosmetics · caution in sensitive areas such as the neck · severe acne
- INTERACTIONS → Appendix 1: clindamycin · retinoids
- SIDE-EFFECTS Dry skin (discontinue if severe) · eye irritation · oedema · photosensitivity reaction · skin pigmentation change (transient) · skin reactions
- CONCEPTION AND CONTRACEPTION Females of child-bearing age must use effective contraception (oral progestogen-only contraceptives not considered effective).
- PREGNANCY Contra-indicated in pregnancy.
- BREAST FEEDING Amount of drug in milk after topical application probably too small to be harmful; ensure infant does not come in contact with treated areas.
- PATIENT AND CARER ADVICE If sun exposure is unavoidable, an appropriate sunscreen or protective clothing should be used.

Patients and carers should be warned that some redness and skin peeling can occur initially but settles with time. If undue irritation occurs, the frequency of application should be reduced or treatment suspended until the reaction subsides; if irritation persists, discontinue treatment. Several months of treatment may be needed to achieve an optimal response and the treatment should be continued until no new lesions develop.

- MEDICINAL FORMS There can be variation in the licensing of different medicines containing the same drug.

Gel
CAUTIONARY AND ADVISORY LABELS 11
EXCIPIENTS: May contain Butylated hydroxytoluene, hydroxybenzoates (parabens), polysorbates
▸ Treclin (Mylan)
 Tretinoin 250 microgram per 1 gram, Clindamycin (as Clindamycin phosphate) 10 mg per 1 gram Treclin 1%/0.025% gel | 30 gram PoM £11.94 DT = £11.94

13

Skin

Tretinoin with erythromycin   03-Apr-2020

The properties listed below are those particular to the combination only. For the properties of the components please consider, tretinoin p. 982, erythromycin p. 572.

- **INDICATIONS AND DOSE**

Acne
▶ TO THE SKIN
  ‣ Child: Apply 1–2 times a day, apply thinly
  ‣ Adult: Apply 1–2 times a day, apply thinly

- CONTRA-INDICATIONS Perioral dermatitis · personal or familial history of skin cancer · rosacea
- CAUTIONS Allow peeling (resulting from other irritant treatments) to subside before using a topical retinoid · avoid accumulation in angles of the nose · avoid contact with eyes, nostrils, mouth and mucous membranes, eczematous, broken or sunburned skin · avoid exposure to UV light (including sunlight, solariums) · avoid use of topical retinoids with keratolytic agents, abrasive cleaners, comedogenic or astringent cosmetics · caution in sensitive areas such as the neck · severe acne
- INTERACTIONS → Appendix 1: macrolides · retinoids
- SIDE-EFFECTS Dry skin (discontinue if severe) · eye irritation · oedema · photosensitivity reaction · skin eruption · skin pigmentation change (transient)
- CONCEPTION AND CONTRACEPTION Females of child-bearing age must use effective contraception (oral progestogen-only contraceptives not considered effective).
- PREGNANCY Contra-indicated in pregnancy.
- BREAST FEEDING Amount of drug in milk after topical application probably too small to be harmful; ensure infant does not come in contact with treated areas.
- PATIENT AND CARER ADVICE Patients and carers should be warned that some redness and skin peeling can occur initially but settles with time. If undue irritation occurs, the frequency of application should be reduced or treatment suspended until the reaction subsides; if irritation persists, discontinue treatment. Several months of treatment may be needed to achieve an optimal response and the treatment should be continued until no new lesions develop. If sun exposure is unavoidable, an appropriate sunscreen or protective clothing should be used.

- MEDICINAL FORMS There can be variation in the licensing of different medicines containing the same drug.
Liquid
CAUTIONARY AND ADVISORY LABELS 11
  ‣ Aknemycin Plus (Almirall Ltd)
    Tretinoin 250 microgram per 1 gram, Erythromycin 40 mg per 1 gram Aknemycin Plus solution | 25 ml PoM £7.05 DT = £7.05

VITAMINS AND TRACE ELEMENTS > VITAMIN B GROUP

Nicotinamide   06-May-2020

- **INDICATIONS AND DOSE**

Inflammatory acne vulgaris
▶ TO THE SKIN
  ‣ Adult: Apply twice daily, reduced to once daily or on alternate days, dose reduced if irritation occurs

- CAUTIONS Avoid contact with eyes · avoid contact with mucous membranes (including nose and mouth) · reduce frequency of application if excessive dryness, irritation or peeling
- SIDE-EFFECTS Paraesthesia · skin reactions

- MEDICINAL FORMS There can be variation in the licensing of different medicines containing the same drug.
Gel
  ‣ Freederm (Dendron Ltd)
    Nicotinamide 40 mg per 1 gram Freederm Treatment 4% gel | 25 gram P £5.56 DT = £5.56
  ‣ Nicam (Dermal Laboratories Ltd)
    Nicotinamide 40 mg per 1 gram Nicam 4% gel | 60 gram P £7.10 DT = £7.10

6.2 Rosacea

> **Other drugs used for Rosacea** Azelaic acid, p. 1313

ANTHELMINTICS

Ivermectin   20-Aug-2020

- **INDICATIONS AND DOSE**

Papulopustular rosacea
▶ TO THE SKIN
  ‣ Adult: Apply daily for up to 4 months, the treatment course may be repeated; discontinue if no improvement after 3 months

- INTERACTIONS → Appendix 1: ivermectin
- SIDE-EFFECTS
  ▶ Common or very common Skin reactions
- PREGNANCY Manufacturer advises avoid—limited information but toxicity following *oral* use in *animal* studies.
- BREAST FEEDING Manufacturer advises avoid—limited information but present in milk following *oral* use.
- HEPATIC IMPAIRMENT Manufacturer advises caution in severe impairment (no information available).
- DIRECTIONS FOR ADMINISTRATION Manufacturer advises apply thinly to the face only, avoiding contact with eyes, lips and mucosa.
- PATIENT AND CARER ADVICE Wash hands immediately after use.
- NATIONAL FUNDING/ACCESS DECISIONS
  For full details see funding body website
  Scottish Medicines Consortium (SMC) decisions
  ‣ Ivermectin (*Soolantra*®) for topical treatment of inflammatory lesions of rosacea (papulopustular) in adult patients (December 2015) SMC No. 1104/15 Recommended with restrictions
  All Wales Medicines Strategy Group (AWMSG) decisions
  ‣ Ivermectin (*Soolantra*®) for treatment of inflammatory lesions of rosacea (papulopustular) in adult patients (April 2016) AWMSG No. 1627 Recommended

- MEDICINAL FORMS There can be variation in the licensing of different medicines containing the same drug.
Cream
CAUTIONARY AND ADVISORY LABELS 28
EXCIPIENTS: May contain Cetostearyl alcohol (including cetyl and stearyl alcohol), disodium edetate, isopropyl palmitate, propylene glycol
  ‣ Soolantra (Galderma (UK) Ltd)
    Ivermectin 10 mg per 1 gram Soolantra 10mg/g cream | 30 gram PoM £18.29 DT = £18.29

SYMPATHOMIMETICS > ALPHA₂-ADRENOCEPTOR AGONISTS

Brimonidine tartrate

19-Nov-2020

- **DRUG ACTION** Brimonidine, an alpha₂-adrenoceptor agonist, is used to reduce erythema in rosacea by cutaneous vasoconstriction.

- **INDICATIONS AND DOSE**

Facial erythema in rosacea

▶ **TO THE SKIN**
▶ **Adult:** Apply once daily until erythema subsides, apply thinly, divide dose over forehead, chin, nose, and cheeks, max. 1 g of gel per day

DOSE EQUIVALENCE AND CONVERSION
▶ 1 g of gel contains 5 mg of brimonidine tartrate (equivalent to 3.3 mg of brimonidine).

IMPORTANT SAFETY INFORMATION
MHRA/CHM ADVICE: BRIMONIDINE GEL (*MIRVASO*®): RISK OF SYSTEMIC CARDIOVASCULAR EFFECTS (JUNE 2017)
Systemic cardiovascular effects including bradycardia, hypotension, and dizziness have been reported after application of brimonidine gel. To minimise the possibility of systemic absorption, it is important to avoid application to irritated or damaged skin, including after laser therapy.

MHRA/CHM ADVICE: BRIMONIDINE GEL (*MIRVASO*®): RISK OF EXACERBATION OF ROSACEA (NOVEMBER 2016)
Symptom exacerbation has been reported very commonly in patients treated with brimonidine gel. Treatment should be initiated with a small amount of gel (less than the maximum dose) for at least 1 week, then increased gradually, based on tolerability and response. Patients should be counselled on the importance of not exceeding the maximum daily dose, and advised to stop treatment and seek medical advice if symptoms worsen during treatment.

- **CAUTIONS** Cerebral insufficiency · coronary insufficiency · depression · postural hypotension · Raynaud's syndrome · severe cardiovascular disease · thromboangiitis obliterans
- **INTERACTIONS** → Appendix 1: brimonidine
- **SIDE-EFFECTS**
▶ **Common or very common** Dizziness · dry mouth · flushing · headache · skin reactions
▶ **Uncommon** Angioedema · eyelid oedema · feeling hot · nasal congestion · paraesthesia · peripheral coldness
▶ **Rare or very rare** Bradycardia · hypotension
- **PREGNANCY** Manufacturer advises avoid—limited information available.
- **BREAST FEEDING** Manufacturer advises avoid—no information available.
- **HEPATIC IMPAIRMENT** Manufacturer advises caution (no information available).
- **RENAL IMPAIRMENT** Manufacturer advises use with caution.
- **DIRECTIONS FOR ADMINISTRATION** Manufacturer advises avoid contact with eyes, mouth, and mucous membranes; avoid use on irritated or damaged skin or open wounds; apply other topical preparations (including cosmetics) only after brimonidine gel has dried on skin.
- **PATIENT AND CARER ADVICE** Patients should be advised on administration of gel.
- **NATIONAL FUNDING/ACCESS DECISIONS**
For full details see funding body website

Scottish Medicines Consortium (SMC) decisions
▶ Brimonidine (*Mirvaso*®) for the symptomatic treatment of facial erythema of rosacea in adult patients (January 2015) SMC No. 1016/14 Recommended with restrictions
All Wales Medicines Strategy Group (AWMSG) decisions
▶ Brimonidine (*Mirvaso*®) for the symptomatic treatment of facial erythema of rosacea in adult patients (September 2015) AWMSG No. 2168 Recommended with restrictions

- **MEDICINAL FORMS** There can be variation in the licensing of different medicines containing the same drug.

Gel
CAUTIONARY AND ADVISORY LABELS 28
EXCIPIENTS: May contain Hydroxybenzoates (parabens), propylene glycol
▶ Mirvaso (Galderma (UK) Ltd)
Brimonidine (as Brimonidine tartrate) 3 mg per 1 gram Mirvaso 3mg/g gel | 30 gram [PoM] £33.69 DT = £33.69

---

7 Scalp and hair conditions

Scalp and hair conditions

14-Aug-2020

Overview

Dandruff is considered to be a mild form of seborrhoeic dermatitis. Shampoos containing antimicrobial agents such as **pyrithione zinc** (which are widely available) and selenium p. 1318 may have beneficial effects. Shampoos containing **tar** extracts may be useful and they are also used in *psoriasis*. Ketoconazole shampoo p. 1277 should be considered for more persistent or severe dandruff or for seborrhoeic dermatitis of the scalp.

Corticosteroid gels and lotions can also be used.
Shampoos containing coal tar with salicylic acid p. 1298 may also be useful. A cream or an ointment containing coal tar with salicylic acid is very helpful in Psoriasis p. 1283 that affects the scalp. Patients who do not respond to these treatments may need to be referred to exclude the possibility of other skin conditions.

Cradle cap in infants may be treated with **coconut oil** or **olive oil** applications followed by shampooing.

Hirsutism

Hirsutism may result from hormonal disorders or as a side-effect of drugs such as minoxidil p. 1318, corticosteroids, anabolic steroids, androgens, danazol p. 783, and progestogens.

Weight loss can reduce hirsutism in obese women.
Women should be advised about local methods of hair removal, and in the mildest cases this may be all that is required.

Eflornithine p. 1319 an antiprotozoal drug, inhibits the enzyme ornithine decarboxylase in hair follicles. Topical eflornithine can be used as an adjunct to laser therapy for facial hirsutism in women.

Co-cyprindiol p. 1311 (cyproterone acetate with ethinylestradiol) may be effective for moderately severe hirsutism. Metformin hydrochloride p. 732 is an alternative in women with polycystic ovary syndrome [unlicensed indication]. Systemic treatment is required for 6–12 months before benefit is seen. The MHRA/CHM have released important safety information regarding the use of cyproterone acetate and the risk of meningioma. For further information, see *Important safety information* for co-cyprindiol. The Faculty of Sexual and Reproductive Healthcare have released a statement in response to the MHRA/CHM information (available at: www.fsrh.org/standards-and-guidance/documents/fsrh-ceu-statement-new-advice-from-the-mhra-regarding/).

13

Skin

Skin

13

Androgenetic alopecia

Finasteride p. 832 is licensed for the treatment of androgenetic alopecia in men. Continuous use for 3–6 months is required before benefit is seen, and effects are reversed 6–12 months after treatment is discontinued.

Topical application of minoxidil may stimulate limited hair growth in a small proportion of adults but only for as long as it is used.

> **Other drugs used for Scalp and hair conditions** Coal tar, p. 1297 · Coal tar with salicylic acid and precipitated sulfur, p. 1298

ANTISEPTICS AND DISINFECTANTS ›
UNDECENOATES

Cetrimide with undecenoic acid

- **INDICATIONS AND DOSE**

Scalp psoriasis | Seborrhoeic dermatitis | Dandruff
▸ TO THE SKIN
  ▸ Child: Apply 3 times a week for 1 week, then apply twice weekly
  ▸ Adult: Apply 3 times a week for 1 week, then apply twice weekly

- **MEDICINAL FORMS** No licensed medicines listed.

ANTISEPTICS AND DISINFECTANTS › OTHER

Benzalkonium chloride   26-Mar-2020

- **INDICATIONS AND DOSE**

Seborrhoeic scalp conditions associated with dandruff and scaling
▸ TO THE SKIN
  ▸ Child: Apply as required
  ▸ Adult: Apply as required

- **MEDICINAL FORMS** There can be variation in the licensing of different medicines containing the same drug.
Shampoo
  ▸ Dermax (Dermal Laboratories Ltd)
    Benzalkonium chloride **5 mg per 1 ml** Dermax Therapeutic 0.5% shampoo | 250 ml Ⓟ £5.69 DT = £5.69

VITAMINS AND TRACE ELEMENTS

Selenium

- **INDICATIONS AND DOSE**

Seborrhoeic dermatitis | Dandruff
▸ TO THE SKIN USING SHAMPOO
  ▸ Child 5-17 years: Apply twice weekly for 2 weeks, then apply once weekly for 2 weeks, then apply as required
  ▸ Adult: Apply twice weekly for 2 weeks, then apply once weekly for 2 weeks, then apply as required

Pityriasis versicolor
▸ TO THE SKIN USING SHAMPOO
  ▸ Adult: Apply once daily for 7 days, apply to the affected area and leave on for 10 minutes before rinsing off. The course may be repeated if necessary. Diluting with a small amount of water prior to application can reduce irritation

- **UNLICENSED USE** The use of selenium sulfide shampoo as a lotion for the treatment of pityriasis (tinea) versicolor is an unlicensed indication.

- **INTERACTIONS** → Appendix 1: selenium

- **PATIENT AND CARER ADVICE** Avoid using 48 hours before or after applying hair colouring, straightening or waving preparations.

- **MEDICINAL FORMS** There can be variation in the licensing of different medicines containing the same drug. Forms available from special-order manufacturers include: solution for infusion
Shampoo
  EXCIPIENTS: May contain Fragrances
  ▸ Selsun (Chattem (U.K.) Ltd)
    Selenium sulfide **25 mg per 1 ml** Selsun 2.5% shampoo | 50 ml Ⓟ £1.61 DT = £1.61 | 100 ml Ⓟ £2.15 DT = £2.15 | 150 ml Ⓟ £3.06 DT = £3.06

7.1 Alopecia

> **Other drugs used for Alopecia** Finasteride, p. 832

VASODILATORS › VASODILATOR ANTIHYPERTENSIVES

Minoxidil   07-Sep-2020

- **INDICATIONS AND DOSE**
REGAINE® FOR MEN EXTRA STRENGTH FOAM
Androgenetic alopecia
▸ TO THE SKIN
  ▸ Adult: Apply 0.5 capful twice daily, to be applied to the affected areas of scalp; discontinue if no improvement after 16 weeks
REGAINE® FOR MEN EXTRA STRENGTH SOLUTION
Androgenetic alopecia
▸ TO THE SKIN
  ▸ Adult: Apply 1 mL twice daily, to be applied to the affected areas of scalp; discontinue if no improvement after 1 year
REGAINE® FOR WOMEN REGULAR STRENGTH
Androgenetic alopecia
▸ TO THE SKIN
  ▸ Adult: Apply 1 mL twice daily, to be applied to the affected areas of scalp; discontinue if no improvement after 1 year

- **CONTRA-INDICATIONS** Phaeochromocytoma
- **CAUTIONS** Avoid contact with broken, infected, shaved, or inflamed skin · avoid contact with eyes · avoid contact with mouth · avoid contact with mucous membranes · avoid inhalation of spray mist · avoid occlusive dressings
- **INTERACTIONS** → Appendix 1: minoxidil
- **SIDE-EFFECTS**
  ▸ **Common or very common** Hair changes
  ▸ **Uncommon** Hypotension
  SIDE-EFFECTS, FURTHER INFORMATION When used topically systemic effects unlikely; only about 1–2% absorbed (greater absorption may occur with use on inflamed skin).
- **PREGNANCY** Avoid—possible toxicity including reduced placental perfusion. Neonatal hirsutism reported.
- **BREAST FEEDING** Present in milk but not known to be harmful.
- **PATIENT AND CARER ADVICE** Ensure hair and scalp dry before application. Patients and their carers should be advised to wash hands after application of liquid or foam.

● MEDICINAL FORMS There can be variation in the licensing of different medicines containing the same drug.

Liquid

CAUTIONARY AND ADVISORY LABELS 15

EXCIPIENTS: May contain Propylene glycol

▸ Regaine (McNeil Products Ltd, Johnson & Johnson Ltd)

Minoxidil 20 mg per 1 ml Regaine for Women Regular Strength 2% solution | 60 ml (GSL) £15.43

Minoxidil 50 mg per 1 ml Regaine for Men Extra Strength 5% scalp solution | 60 ml (GSL) £21.63 | 180 ml (GSL) £43.28

Foam

CAUTIONARY AND ADVISORY LABELS 15

EXCIPIENTS: May contain Butylated hydroxytoluene, cetostearyl alcohol (including cetyl and stearyl alcohol), polysorbates

▸ Regaine (McNeil Products Ltd)

Minoxidil 50 mg per 1 gram Regaine for Men Extra Strength 5% scalp foam | 60 gram (GSL) £23.33 DT = £23.33 | 180 gram (GSL) £50.01 DT = £50.01

7.2　Hirsutism

> **Other drugs used for Hirsutism** Co-cyprindiol, p. 1311

ANTIPROTOZOALS

▌Eflornithine

04-Nov-2020

● DRUG ACTION An antiprotozoal drug that inhibits the enzyme ornithine decarboxylase in hair follicles.

● INDICATIONS AND DOSE

Adjunct in the treatment of facial hirsutism in women

▸ TO THE SKIN

▸ Adult: Apply twice daily, to be applied thinly, discontinue use if no improvement after 4 months of treatment

● SIDE-EFFECTS

▸ **Common or very common** Alopecia · increased risk of infection · paraesthesia · skin reactions

▸ **Uncommon** Face oedema · flushing · hair changes · oral disorders · skin haemorrhage

▸ **Rare or very rare** Skin neoplasm

● PREGNANCY Toxicity in *animal* studies—manufacturer advises avoid.

● BREAST FEEDING Manufacturer advises avoid—no information available.

● PATIENT AND CARER ADVICE Medicines must be rubbed in thoroughly. Cosmetics may be applied over treated area 5 minutes after eflornithine, do not wash treated area for 4 hours after application.

● NATIONAL FUNDING/ACCESS DECISIONS For full details see funding body website

Scottish Medicines Consortium (SMC) decisions

▸ Eflornithine (*Vaniqa*®) for facial hirsutism in women (September 2005) SMC No. 159/05 Recommended with restrictions

● MEDICINAL FORMS There can be variation in the licensing of different medicines containing the same drug.

Cream

EXCIPIENTS: May contain Cetostearyl alcohol (including cetyl and stearyl alcohol), hydroxybenzoates (parabens)

▸ Vaniqa (Almirall Ltd)

Eflornithine (as Eflornithine hydrochloride monohydrate) 115 mg per 1 gram Vaniqa 11.5% cream | 60 gram (PoM) £56.87 DT = £56.87

8　Skin cleansers, antiseptics and desloughing agents

Skin cleansers, antiseptics and desloughing agents

Skin cleansers and antiseptics

Soap or detergent is used with water to cleanse intact skin; emollient preparations such as aqueous cream or emulsifying ointment can be used in place of soap or detergent for cleansing dry skin.

An antiseptic is used for skin that is infected or that is susceptible to recurrent infection. Detergent preparations containing chlorhexidine p. 1321 or povidone-iodine p. 1320, which should be thoroughly rinsed off, are used. Emollients may also contain antiseptics.

Antiseptics such as chlorhexidine or povidone-iodine are used on intact skin before surgical procedures; their antiseptic effect is enhanced by an alcoholic solvent. Antiseptic solutions containing cetrimide can be used if a detergent effect is also required.

Hydrogen peroxide p. 1322, an oxidising agent, can be used in solutions of up to 6% for skin disinfection, such as cleansing and deodorising wounds and ulcers. Hydrogen peroxide is also available as a cream for superficial bacterial skin infections.

For irrigating ulcers or wounds, lukewarm sterile sodium chloride 0.9% solution is used, but tap water is often appropriate.

Potassium permanganate below solution 1 in 10 000, a mild antiseptic with astringent properties, can be used for exudative eczematous areas; treatment should be stopped when the skin becomes dry.

Desloughing agents

Alginate, hydrogel and hydrocolloid dressings are effective at wound debridement. Sterile larvae (maggots) (available from BioMonde) are also used for managing sloughing wounds and are prescribable on the NHS.

Desloughing solutions and creams are of little clinical value. Substances applied to an open area are easily absorbed and perilesional skin is easily sensitised. Gravitational dermatitis may be complicated by superimposed contact sensitivity to substances such as neomycin sulfate p. 1274 or lanolin.

ANTISEPTICS AND DISINFECTANTS

▌Potassium permanganate

16-Dec-2020

● INDICATIONS AND DOSE

Cleansing and deodorising suppurating eczematous reactions and wounds

▸ TO THE SKIN

▸ Adult: For wet dressings or baths, use approximately 0.01% (1 in 10 000) solution

> IMPORTANT SAFETY INFORMATION
>
> NHS IMPROVEMENT PATIENT SAFETY ALERT: RISK OF DEATH OR SERIOUS HARM FROM ACCIDENTAL INGESTION OF POTASSIUM PERMANGANATE PREPARATIONS (DECEMBER 2014)
>
> Potassium permanganate is for external use only. Oral ingestion can cause fatality due to local inflammatory reactions that block the airways or cause perforations of the gastrointestinal tract, or through toxicity and organ failure. Following a number of reports of ingestion, NHS England advises that healthcare professionals should

13

Skin

consider whether action needs to be taken locally to reduce the risk of accidental ingestion occurring. Potassium permanganate is subject to the requirements of Control of Substances Hazardous to Health including: separate storage, additional hazard labelling, and issue only to staff and patients who have been educated to understand its safe use. Accidental ingestion should be treated as a medical emergency.

- CAUTIONS Irritant to mucous membranes
- DIRECTIONS FOR ADMINISTRATION With potassium permanganate tablets for solution, 1 tablet dissolved in 4 litres of water provides a 0.01% (1 in 10 000) solution.
- PATIENT AND CARER ADVICE Can stain clothing, skin and nails (especially with prolonged use).
- MEDICINAL FORMS There can be variation in the licensing of different medicines containing the same drug. Forms available from special-order manufacturers include: liquid

Tablet for cutaneous solution
- Permitabs (Alliance Pharmaceuticals Ltd)
  Potassium permanganate 400 mg Permitabs 400mg tablets for cutaneous solution | 30 tablet £19.92 DT = £19.92

ANTISEPTICS AND DISINFECTANTS > ALCOHOL DISINFECTANTS

Alcohol

(Industrial methylated spirit)

- **INDICATIONS AND DOSE**

Skin preparation before injection
- TO THE SKIN
- Child: Apply as required
- Adult: Apply as required

- CONTRA-INDICATIONS Neonates
- CAUTIONS Avoid broken skin · flammable · patients have suffered severe burns when diathermy has been preceded by application of alcoholic skin disinfectants
- INTERACTIONS → Appendix 1: alcohol
- SIDE-EFFECTS

  Overdose Features of acute alcohol intoxication include ataxia, dysarthria, nystagmus, and drowsiness, which may progress to coma, with hypotension and acidosis.
  For details on the management of poisoning, see Alcohol, under **Emergency treatment of poisoning p. 1413**.
- PRESCRIBING AND DISPENSING INFORMATION Industrial methylated spirits defined by the BP as a mixture of 19 volumes of ethyl alcohol of an appropriate strength with 1 volume of approved wood naphtha.
- MEDICINAL FORMS There can be variation in the licensing of different medicines containing the same drug.

  Liquid
  - Alcohol (Non-proprietary)
    Industrial methylated spirit 70% | 600 ml £6.56

ANTISEPTICS AND DISINFECTANTS > IODINE PRODUCTS

Povidone-iodine

- **INDICATIONS AND DOSE**

Skin disinfection
- TO THE SKIN
- Child: (consult product literature)
- Adult: (consult product literature)

BETADINE ® DRY POWDER SPRAY

Skin disinfection, particularly minor wounds and infections
- TO THE SKIN
- Adult: Not for use in serous cavities (consult product literature)

VIDENE ® SOLUTION

Skin disinfection
- TO THE SKIN
- Child: Apply undiluted in pre-operative skin disinfection and general antisepsis
- Adult: Apply undiluted in pre-operative skin disinfection and general antisepsis

VIDENE ® SURGICAL SCRUB ®

Skin disinfection
- TO THE SKIN
- Child: Use as a pre-operative scrub for hand and skin disinfection
- Adult: Use as a pre-operative scrub for hand and skin disinfection

VIDENE ® TINCTURE

Skin disinfection
- TO THE SKIN
- Adult: Apply undiluted in pre-operative skin disinfection

- CONTRA-INDICATIONS Avoid regular use in patients with thyroid disorders (in adults) · concomitant use of lithium · corrected gestational age under 32 weeks · infants body-weight under 1.5 kg · regular use in neonates
- CAUTIONS Broken skin · large open wounds

  CAUTIONS, FURTHER INFORMATION
  - Large open wounds The application of povidone–iodine to large wounds or severe burns may produce systemic adverse effects such as metabolic acidosis, hypernatraemia and impairment of renal function.

    VIDENE ® TINCTURE Procedures involving hot wire cautery and diathermy
- SIDE-EFFECTS Acute kidney injury · goitre · hyperthyroidism · hypothyroidism · metabolic acidosis · skin burning sensation
- PREGNANCY Sufficient iodine may be absorbed to affect the fetal thyroid in the second and third trimester.
- BREAST FEEDING Avoid regular or excessive use.
- RENAL IMPAIRMENT Avoid regular application to inflamed or broken skin or mucosa.
- EFFECT ON LABORATORY TESTS May interfere with thyroid function tests.

- MEDICINAL FORMS There can be variation in the licensing of different medicines containing the same drug. Forms available from special-order manufacturers include: liquid

  Spray
  - Betadine (Aspire Pharma Ltd)
    Povidone-Iodine 25 mg per 1 gram Betadine 2.5% dry powder spray | 100 ml GSL £9.95 DT = £9.95

  Liquid
  CAUTIONARY AND ADVISORY LABELS 15 (Only for use with alcoholic solutions)
  - Videne (Ecolab Healthcare Division)
    Povidone-Iodine 75 mg per 1 ml Videne 7.5% surgical scrub solution | 500 ml P £7.97 DT = £7.97
    Povidone-Iodine 100 mg per 1 ml Videne 10% antiseptic solution | 500 ml P £7.97 DT = £7.97

ANTISEPTICS AND DISINFECTANTS > OTHER

Chlorhexidine
01-Sep-2020

● **INDICATIONS AND DOSE**

CEPTON® LOTION

For skin disinfection in acne
▸ TO THE SKIN
▸ Child: (consult product literature)
▸ Adult: (consult product literature)

CEPTON® SKIN WASH

For use as skin wash in acne
▸ TO THE SKIN
▸ Child: (consult product literature)
▸ Adult: (consult product literature)

HIBITANE® PLUS 5% CONCENTRATE SOLUTION

General and pre-operative skin disinfection
▸ TO THE SKIN
▸ Child: (consult product literature)

HIBISCRUB®

Pre-operative hand and skin disinfection | General hand and skin disinfection
▸ TO THE SKIN
▸ Child: Use as alternative to soap (consult product literature)
▸ Adult: Use as alternative to soap (consult product literature)

HIBITANE OBSTETRIC®

For use in obstetrics and gynaecology as an antiseptic and lubricant
▸ TO THE SKIN
▸ Adult: To be applied to skin around vulva and perineum and to hands of midwife or doctor

HIBI® LIQUID HAND RUB+

Hand and skin disinfection
▸ TO THE SKIN
▸ Child: To be used undiluted (consult product literature)
▸ Adult: To be used undiluted (consult product literature)

HYDREX® SOLUTION

For pre-operative skin disinfection
▸ TO THE SKIN
▸ Child: (consult product literature)
▸ Adult: (consult product literature)

HYDREX® SURGICAL SCRUB

For pre-operative hand and skin disinfection | General hand disinfection
▸ TO THE SKIN
▸ Child: (consult product literature)
▸ Adult: (consult product literature)

UNISEPT®

For cleansing and disinfecting wounds and burns and swabbing in obstetrics
▸ TO THE SKIN
▸ Child: (consult product literature)
▸ Adult: (consult product literature)

IMPORTANT SAFETY INFORMATION

MHRA/CHM ADVICE: CHLORHEXIDINE SOLUTIONS: REMINDER OF THE RISK OF CHEMICAL BURNS IN PREMATURE INFANTS (NOVEMBER 2014)

In premature infants, use sparingly, monitor for skin reactions, and do not allow solution to pool—risk of severe chemical burns.

● CONTRA-INDICATIONS Not for use in body cavities

● CAUTIONS Avoid contact with brain · avoid contact with eyes · avoid contact with meninges · avoid contact with middle ear · use prior to diathermy (alcohol containing skin disinfectants)

● SIDE-EFFECTS Skin reactions

● DIRECTIONS FOR ADMINISTRATION

HIBITANE® PLUS 5% CONCENTRATE SOLUTION For pre-operative skin preparation, dilute 1 in 10 (0.5%) with alcohol 70%. For general skin disinfection, dilute 1 in 100 (0.05%) with water. Alcoholic solutions not suitable for use before diathermy or on neonatal skin.

● MEDICINAL FORMS There can be variation in the licensing of different medicines containing the same drug.

Cream
▸ Hibitane Obstetric (Derma UK Ltd)
  Chlorhexidine gluconate 10 mg per 1 gram Hibitane Obstetric 1% cream | 250 ml [GSL] £19.23 DT = £19.23

Liquid
CAUTIONARY AND ADVISORY LABELS 15 (For ethanolic solutions e.g. ChloraPrep® and Hydrex® only)
EXCIPIENTS: May contain Fragrances
▸ Cepton (Boston Healthcare Ltd)
  Chlorhexidine gluconate 10 mg per 1 ml Cepton 1% medicated skin wash | 150 ml [GSL] £34.75 DT = £34.75
▸ Hibi (Molnlycke Health Care Ltd)
  Chlorhexidine gluconate 5 mg per 1 ml HiBi Liquid Hand Rub+ 0.5% solution | 500 ml [GSL] £5.46 DT = £5.46
▸ Hibiscrub (Molnlycke Health Care Ltd)
  Chlorhexidine gluconate 40 mg per 1 ml HiBiScrub 4% solution | 125 ml [GSL] £1.56 | 250 ml [GSL] £4.42 DT = £4.42 | 500 ml £5.46 DT = £5.46 | 5000 ml [GSL] £24.96 DT = £24.96
▸ Hydrex (Ecolab Health Care Division)
  Chlorhexidine gluconate 5 mg per 1 ml Hydrex pink chlorhexidine gluconate 0.5% solution | 600 ml [GSL] £4.91 DT = £4.91 Hydrex clear chlorhexidine gluconate 0.5% solution | 600 ml [GSL] £4.91 DT = £4.91
  Chlorhexidine gluconate 40 mg per 1 ml Hydrex 4% Surgical Scrub | 250 ml [GSL] £4.47 DT = £4.42 | 500 ml [GSL] £4.96 DT = £5.46
▸ Sterets Unisept (Molnlycke Health Care Ltd)
  Chlorhexidine gluconate 500 microgram per 1 ml Sterets Unisept 0.05% solution 25ml sachets | 25 sachet [P] £5.54 DT = £5.54 Sterets Unisept 0.05% solution 100ml sachets | 10 sachet [P] £6.83 DT = £6.83

Chlorhexidine gluconate with isopropyl alcohol

The properties listed below are those particular to the combination only. For the properties of the components please consider, chlorhexidine above.

● **INDICATIONS AND DOSE**

Skin disinfection before invasive procedures
▸ TO THE SKIN
▸ Child 2 months–17 years: (consult product literature)
▸ Adult: (consult product literature)

● MEDICINAL FORMS There can be variation in the licensing of different medicines containing the same drug. Forms available from special-order manufacturers include: liquid

Liquid
CAUTIONARY AND ADVISORY LABELS 15
▸ ChloraPrep (Becton, Dickinson Ltd)
  Chlorhexidine gluconate 20 mg per 1 ml, Isopropyl alcohol 700 ml per 1 litre ChloraPrep with Tint solution 10.5ml applicators | 25 applicator [GSL] £76.65 DT = £73.00 ChloraPrep with Tint solution 26ml applicators | 25 applicator [GSL] £170.75 DT = £162.50 ChloraPrep solution 3ml applicators | 25 applicator [GSL] £21.25 DT = £21.25 ChloraPrep solution 1.5ml applicators | 20 applicator [GSL] £11.00 DT = £11.00 ChloraPrep with Tint solution 3ml applicators | 25 applicator [GSL] £22.31 DT = £21.25

13

Skin

ChloraPrep solution 0.67ml applicators | 200 applicator [GSL] £60.00
DT = £60.00
ChloraPrep solution 10.5ml applicators | 25 applicator [GSL] £73.00
DT = £73.00
ChloraPrep solution 26ml applicators | 25 applicator [GSL] £162.50
DT = £162.50

Chlorhexidine with cetrimide

The properties listed below are those particular to the combination only. For the properties of the components please consider, chlorhexidine p. 1321.

- **INDICATIONS AND DOSE**

Skin disinfection such as wound cleansing and obstetrics
▸ TO THE SKIN
▸ Child: To be used undiluted
▸ Adult: To be used undiluted

- **MEDICINAL FORMS** There can be variation in the licensing of different medicines containing the same drug.
Cream
▸ Savlon (Thornton & Ross Ltd)
  Chlorhexidine gluconate 1 mg per 1 gram, Cetrimide 5 mg per
  1 gram Savlon antiseptic cream | 15 gram [GSL] £0.90 DT = £0.90 |
  30 gram [GSL] £1.19 DT = £1.19 | 60 gram [GSL] £1.91 DT = £1.91 |
  100 gram [GSL] £2.78 DT = £2.78
Irrigation solution
▸ Chlorhexidine with cetrimide (Non-proprietary)
  Chlorhexidine acetate 150 microgram per 1 ml, Cetrimide 1.5 mg
  per 1 ml Chlorhexidine acetate 0.015% / Cetrimide 0.15% irrigation
  solution 1litre bottles | 1 bottle [P] [S]
Liquid
▸ Sterets Tisept (Molnlycke Health Care Ltd)
  Chlorhexidine gluconate 150 microgram per 1 ml, Cetrimide
  1.5 mg per 1 ml Sterets Tisept solution 25ml sachets | 25 sachet [P]
  £5.33 DT = £5.33
  Sterets Tisept solution 100ml sachets | 10 sachet [P] £6.85 DT = £6.85

Diethyl phthalate with methyl salicylate

- **INDICATIONS AND DOSE**

Skin preparation before injection
▸ TO THE SKIN
▸ Adult: Apply to the area to be disinfected

- **MEDICINAL FORMS** There can be variation in the licensing of different medicines containing the same drug.
Liquid
CAUTIONARY AND ADVISORY LABELS 15
▸ Diethyl phthalate with methyl salicylate (Non-proprietary)
  Methyl salicylate 5 ml per 1 litre, Diethyl phthalate 20 ml per
  1 litre, Castor oil 25 ml per 1 litre, Industrial methylated spirit
  950 ml per 1 litre Surgical spirit | 200 ml [GSL] £1.17 DT = £1.17 |
  1000 ml [GSL] £4.03

Hydrogen peroxide

29-Apr-2020

- **DRUG ACTION** Hydrogen peroxide is an oxidising agent.

- **INDICATIONS AND DOSE**

For skin disinfection, particularly cleansing and deodorising wounds and ulcers
▸ TO THE SKIN
▸ Adult: Use 3% and 6% solutions (consult product literature)

CRYSTACIDE ®

Superficial bacterial skin infection
▸ TO THE SKIN
▸ Child: Apply 2–3 times a day for up to 3 weeks
▸ Adult: Apply 2–3 times a day for up to 3 weeks
Localised non-bullous impetigo [in patients who are not systemically unwell or at high risk of complications]
▸ TO THE SKIN
▸ Child: Apply 2–3 times a day for 5–7 days
▸ Adult: Apply 2–3 times a day for 5–7 days

- **UNLICENSED USE**
▸ In children Licensed for use in children (age range not specified by manufacturer).

- **CONTRA-INDICATIONS** Closed body cavities (in adults) · deep wounds · large wounds · use as disinfection agent for surgical instruments (in adults) · use as enema (in adults) · use during surgery (in adults)

- **CAUTIONS** Avoid on eyes · avoid on healthy skin · incompatible with products containing iodine or potassium permanganate

- **PRESCRIBING AND DISPENSING INFORMATION** The BP directs that when hydrogen peroxide is prescribed, hydrogen peroxide solution 6% (20 vols) should be dispensed.
  Strong solutions of hydrogen peroxide which contain 27% (90 vols) and 30% (100 vols) are only for the preparation of weaker solutions.
  CRYSTACIDE ® For choice of therapy, see Skin infections, antibacterial therapy p. 541.

- **HANDLING AND STORAGE** Hydrogen peroxide bleaches fabric.

- **MEDICINAL FORMS** There can be variation in the licensing of different medicines containing the same drug. Forms available from special-order manufacturers include: liquid
Cream
EXCIPIENTS: May contain Edetic acid (edta), propylene glycol
▸ Crystacide (Reig Jofre UK Ltd)
  Hydrogen peroxide 10 mg per 1 gram Crystacide 1% cream |
  25 gram [P] £8.07 DT = £8.07 | 40 gram [P] £11.62
Liquid
▸ Hydrogen peroxide (Non-proprietary)
  Hydrogen peroxide 60 mg per 1 ml Hydrogen peroxide 6% solution
  | 200 ml [GSL] £0.67 DT = £0.67 | 500 ml [GSL] £3.28 |
  2000 ml [GSL] £9.59
  Hydrogen peroxide 90 mg per 1 ml Hydrogen peroxide 9% solution
  | 200 ml [GSL] £0.72 DT = £0.72
  Hydrogen peroxide 30 ml per 1 litre Hydrogen peroxide 3%
  solution | 200 ml [GSL] £0.63 DT = £0.63

Proflavine

- **INDICATIONS AND DOSE**

Infected wounds | Infected burns
▸ TO THE SKIN
▸ Adult: (consult product literature)

- **PATIENT AND CARER ADVICE** Stains clothing.

- **MEDICINAL FORMS** Forms available from special-order manufacturers include: liquid

Irrigation solutions

- **INDICATIONS AND DOSE**

Skin cleansing
▸ TO THE SKIN
▸ Child: Use for topical irrigation of wounds
▸ Adult: Use for topical irrigation of wounds

● IRRIGATION SOLUTIONS

Flowfusor sodium chloride 0.9% irrigation solution 120ml bottles (Fresenius Kabi Ltd) Sodium chloride 9 mg per 1 ml 1 bottle · NHS indicative price = £1.71 · Drug Tariff (Part IXa)

Irriclens sodium chloride 0.9% irrigation solution aerosol spray (ConvaTec Ltd) Sodium chloride 9 mg per 1 ml 240 ml · NHS indicative price = £3.69 · Drug Tariff (Part IXa)

Normasol sodium chloride 0.9% irrigation solution 100ml sachets (Molnlycke Health Care Ltd) Sodium chloride 9 mg per 1 ml 10 unit dose · NHS indicative price = £8.17 · Drug Tariff (Part IXa)

Normasol sodium chloride 0.9% irrigation solution 25ml sachets (Molnlycke Health Care Ltd) Sodium chloride 9 mg per 1 ml 25 unit dose · NHS indicative price = £6.62 · Drug Tariff (Part IXa)

Sodium chloride 0.9% irrigation solution 1litre bottles (Fresenius Kabi Ltd) Sodium chloride 9 mg per 1 ml 1 bottle · NHS indicative price = £1.09 · Drug Tariff (Part IXa)

Sodium chloride 0.9% irrigation solution 20ml Clinipod unit dose (Mayors Healthcare Ltd) Sodium chloride 9 mg per 1 ml 25 unit dose · NHS indicative price = £4.80 · Drug Tariff (Part IXa)

Sodium chloride 0.9% irrigation solution 20ml ISO-POD unit dose (St Georges Medical Ltd) Sodium chloride 9 mg per 1 ml 25 unit dose · NHS indicative price = £4.95 · Drug Tariff (Part IXa)

Sodium chloride 0.9% irrigation solution 20ml Irripod unit dose (C D Medical Ltd) Sodium chloride 9 mg per 1 ml 25 unit dose · NHS indicative price = £5.90 · Drug Tariff (Part IXa)

Sodium chloride 0.9% irrigation solution 20ml Sal-e Pods unit dose (Ennogen Healthcare Ltd) Sodium chloride 9 mg per 1 ml 25 unit dose · NHS indicative price = £4.80 · Drug Tariff (Part IXa)

Sodium chloride 0.9% irrigation solution 20ml Salipod unit dose (Sai-Meds Ltd) Sodium chloride 9 mg per 1 ml 25 unit dose · NHS indicative price = £4.99 · Drug Tariff (Part IXa)

Sodium chloride 0.9% irrigation solution 20ml Steripod unit dose (Molnlycke Health Care Ltd) Sodium chloride 9 mg per 1 ml 25 unit dose · NHS indicative price = £5.07 · Drug Tariff (Part IXa)

Sodium chloride 0.9% irrigation solution 20ml Sterowash unit dose (Steroplast Healthcare Ltd) Sodium chloride 9 mg per 1 ml 25 unit dose · NHS indicative price = £5.40 · Drug Tariff (Part IXa)

Sodium chloride 0.9% irrigation solution 20ml unit dose (Alissa Healthcare Research Ltd) Sodium chloride 9 mg per 1 ml 25 unit dose · NHS indicative price = £7.36 · Drug Tariff (Part IXa)

Sodium chloride 0.9% irrigation solution 20ml unit dose (Bell, Sons & Co (Druggists) Ltd) Sodium chloride 9 mg per 1 ml 25 unit dose · NHS indicative price = £6.76 · Drug Tariff (Part IXa)

Sodium chloride 0.9% irrigation solution 20ml unit dose (Crest Medical Ltd) Sodium chloride 9 mg per 1 ml 25 unit dose · NHS indicative price = £4.99 · Drug Tariff (Part IXa)

Sodium chloride 0.9% irrigation solution 20ml unit dose (Mylan) Sodium chloride 9 mg per 1 ml 25 unit dose · NHS indicative price = £5.50 · Drug Tariff (Part IXa)

Stericlens sodium chloride 0.9% irrigation solution aerosol spray (C D Medical Ltd) Sodium chloride 9 mg per 1 ml 100 ml · NHS indicative price = £2.07 · Drug Tariff (Part IXa)240 ml · NHS indicative price = £3.15 · Drug Tariff (Part IXa)

8.1 Minor cuts and abrasions

Minor cuts and abrasions

Management

Many preparations traditionally used to manage minor burns, and abrasions have fallen out of favour. Preparations containing camphor and sulfonamides should be avoided. Preparations such as magnesium sulfate paste are now rarely used to treat carbuncles and boils as these are best treated with antibiotics.

Cetrimide is used to treat minor cuts and abrasions and proflavine p. 1322 may be used to treat infected wounds or burns, but its use has now been largely superseded by other antiseptics or suitable antibacterials. The effervescent effect

of hydrogen peroxide p. 1322 is used to clean minor cuts and abrasions.

Flexible collodion (see castor oil with collodion and colophony below) may be used to seal minor cuts and wounds that have partially healed; skin tissue adhesives are used similarly, and also for additional suture support.

ANTISEPTICS AND DISINFECTANTS 〉 OTHER

Glycerol with magnesium sulfate and phenol

14-Dec-2020

● INDICATIONS AND DOSE

Treat carbuncles and boils

▶ TO THE SKIN
▹ Adult: To be applied under dressing

● DIRECTIONS FOR ADMINISTRATION Manufacturer advises paste should be stirred before use.

● MEDICINAL FORMS There can be variation in the licensing of different medicines containing the same drug.

Paste

▹ Glycerol with magnesium sulfate and phenol (Non-proprietary)
Phenol 5 mg per 1 gram, Magnesium sulfate dried 450 mg per 1 gram, Glycerol 550 mg per 1 gram Magnesium sulfate paste | 25 gram GSL £0.79-£1.97 | 50 gram GSL £1.03-£3.13 DT = £3.13

DERMATOLOGICAL DRUGS 〉 COLLODIONS

Castor oil with collodion and colophony

16-Dec-2020

● INDICATIONS AND DOSE

Used to seal minor cuts and wounds that have partially healed

▶ TO THE SKIN
▹ Child: (consult product literature)
▹ Adult: (consult product literature)

● ALLERGY AND CROSS-SENSITIVITY EvGr Contra-indicated if patient has an allergy to colophony in elastic adhesive plasters and tape. ⒨

● MEDICINAL FORMS There can be variation in the licensing of different medicines containing the same drug.

Liquid

▹ Castor oil with collodion and colophony (Non-proprietary)
Castor oil 25 mg per 1 ml, Colophony 25 mg per 1 ml, Collodion methylated 950 microlitre per 1 ml Flexible collodion methylated | 100 ml £14.37 | 500 ml £29.91

Skin adhesives

● SKIN ADHESIVES

Derma+Flex skin adhesive (Chemence Ltd)
0.5 ml · NHS indicative price = £5.36 · Drug Tariff (Part IXa)

Dermabond ProPen skin adhesive (Ethicon Ltd)
0.5 ml · NHS indicative price = £19.46 · Drug Tariff (Part IXa)

Histoacryl L skin adhesive (B.Braun Medical Ltd)
0.5 ml · NHS indicative price = £6.72 · Drug Tariff (Part IXa)

Histoacryl skin adhesive (B.Braun Medical Ltd)
0.5 ml · NHS indicative price = £6.50 · Drug Tariff (Part IXa)

Indermil skin adhesive (Covidien (UK) Commercial Ltd)
0.5 gram · NHS indicative price = £6.50 · Drug Tariff (Part IXa)

LiquiBand flow control tissue adhesive (Advanced Medical Solutions Ltd)
0.5 gram · NHS indicative price = £5.50 · Drug Tariff (Part IXa)

LiquiBand tissue adhesive (Advanced Medical Solutions Ltd)
0.5 gram · NHS indicative price = £5.50 · Drug Tariff (Part IXa)

13

Skin

9 Skin disfigurement

Camouflagers

Overview

Disfigurement of the skin can be very distressing to patients and may have a marked psychological effect. In skilled hands, or with experience, camouflage cosmetics can be very effective in concealing scars and birthmarks. The depigmented patches in vitiligo are also very disfiguring and camouflage creams are of great cosmetic value.

Opaque cover foundation or cream is used to mask skin pigment abnormalities; careful application using a combination of dark- and light-coloured cover creams set with powder helps to minimise the appearance of skin deformities.

Borderline substances

The preparations marked 'ACBS' can be prescribed on the NHS for postoperative scars and other deformities and as adjunctive therapy in the relief of emotional disturbances due to disfiguring skin disease, such as vitiligo.

Camouflages

- CAMOUFLAGES

Covermark classic foundation (Derma UK Ltd)
15 ml(ACBS) · NHS indicative price = £11.86

Covermark finishing powder (Derma UK Ltd)
25 gram(ACBS) · NHS indicative price = £11.86

Covermark removing cream (Derma UK Ltd)
200 ml · No NHS indicative price available

Deep Skin Cleanser (SkinKind Ltd)
100 ml · NHS indicative price = £19.50

Dermablend Dermasmooth Corrective Foundation (Vichy)
30 ml · No NHS indicative price available

Dermacolor Creme Effectiv (Kryolan UK Ltd)
50 ml · NHS indicative price = £5.73

Dermacolor body camouflage (Kryolan UK Ltd)
50 ml · NHS indicative price = £8.94

Dermacolor camouflage creme (Kryolan UK Ltd)
30 gram · NHS indicative price = £11.00

Dermacolor cleansing cream (Kryolan UK Ltd)
75 gram · No NHS indicative price available

Dermacolor fixing powder (Kryolan UK Ltd)
60 gram(ACBS) · NHS indicative price = £9.85

Keromask finishing powder (Bellava Ltd)
20 gram(ACBS) · NHS indicative price = £6.62

Keromask masking cream (Bellava Ltd)
15 ml(ACBS) · NHS indicative price = £6.62

Veil cleansing cream (Thomas Blake Cosmetic Creams Ltd)
50 gram · NHS indicative price = £2.45100 gram · NHS indicative price = £3.90

Veil cover cream (Thomas Blake Cosmetic Creams Ltd)
19 gram(ACBS) · NHS indicative price = £22.4244 gram(ACBS) · NHS indicative price = £33.3570 gram(ACBS) · NHS indicative price = £42.10

Veil finishing powder (Thomas Blake Cosmetic Creams Ltd)
35 gram(ACBS) · NHS indicative price = £24.58

10 Sun protection and photodamage

Sunscreen

05-Feb-2020

Sunscreen preparations

Solar ultraviolet irradiation can be harmful to the skin. It is responsible for disorders such as *polymorphic light eruption, solar urticaria,* and it provokes the various *cutaneous porphyrias*. It also provokes (or at least aggravates) skin lesions of *lupus erythematosus* and may aggravate *rosacea* and some other *dermatoses*. Certain drugs, such as demeclocycline, phenothiazines, or amiodarone, can cause photosensitivity. All these conditions (as well as *sunburn*) may occur after relatively short periods of exposure to the sun. Solar ultraviolet irradiation may provoke attacks of recurrent herpes labialis (but it is not known whether the effect of sunlight exposure is local or systemic).

The effects of exposure over longer periods include *ageing changes* and more importantly the initiation of *skin cancer*.

Solar ultraviolet radiation is approximately 200–400 nm in wavelength. The medium wavelengths (290–320 nm, known as UVB) cause *sunburn*. The long wavelengths (320–400 nm, known as UVA) are responsible for many *photosensitivity reactions* and *photodermatoses*. Both UVA and UVB contribute to long-term *photodamage* and to the changes responsible for *skin cancer* and ageing.

Sunscreen preparations contain substances that protect the skin against UVA and UVB radiation, but they are no substitute for covering the skin and avoiding sunlight. The sun protection factor (SPF, usually indicated in the preparation title) provides guidance on the degree of protection offered against UVB; it indicates the multiples of protection provided against burning, compared with unprotected skin; for example, an SPF of 8 should enable a person to remain 8 times longer in the sun without burning. However, in practice, users do not apply sufficient sunscreen product and the protection is lower than that found in experimental studies.

Some manufacturers use a star rating system to indicate the protection against UVA relative to protection against UVB for sunscreen products. However, the usefulness of the star rating system remains controversial. The EU Commission (September 2006) has recommended that the UVA protection factor for a sunscreen should be at least one-third of the sun protection factor (SPF); products that achieve this requirement will be labelled with a UVA logo alongside the SPF classification. Preparations that also contain reflective substances, such as titanium dioxide, provide the most effective protection against UVA.

Sunscreen preparations may rarely cause allergic reactions.

For optimum photoprotection, sunscreen preparations should be applied **thickly** and **frequently** (approximately 2 hourly). In photodermatoses, they should be used from spring to autumn. As maximum protection from sunlight is desirable, preparations with the highest SPF should be prescribed.

Ingredient nomenclature in sunscreen preparations

rINN	INCI
amiloxate	isoamyl *p*-methoxycinnamate
avobenzone	butyl methoxydibenzoylmethane
bemotrizinol	bis-ethylhexyloxyphenol methoxyphenyl triazine
bisoctrizole	methylene bis-benzotriazolyl tetramethylbutylphenol
ecamsule	terephthalylidene dicamphor sulfonic acid
ensulizole	phenylbenzimidazole sulfonic acid
enzacamene	4-methylbenzylidene camphor
octinoxate	octyl (or ethylhexyl) methoxycinnamate
octocrilene	octocrylene
oxybenzone	benzophenone-3

The European Commission Cosmetic Products Regulation (EC) 1223/2009 requires the use of INCI (International Nomenclature of Cosmetic Ingredients) for cosmetics and sunscreens. This table includes the rINN and the INCI synonym for the active ingredients of sunscreen preparations in the BNF

Borderline substances

LA Roche-Posay Anthelios ® XL SPF 50+ Cream; *Sunsense* ® Ultra (Ego) SPF 50+; *Uvistat* ® Lipscreen SPF 50; and *Uvistat* ® Suncream SPF 30 and 50 (see *About Borderline Substances*) are regarded as drugs when prescribed for skin protection against ultraviolet radiation and/or visible light in abnormal cutaneous photosensitivity causing severe cutaneous reactions in genetic disorders (including xeroderma pigmentosum and porphyrias), severe photodermatoses (both idiopathic and acquired) and in those with increased risk of ultraviolet radiation causing adverse effects due to chronic disease (such as haematological malignancies), medical therapies and/or procedures.

Photodamage

18-Nov-2020

Overview

EvGr Patients should be advised on the harms of prolonged sunlight exposure and how to adequately protect their skin from strong sunlight (e.g. use of topical sun protection preparations).

Topical treatments can be used for actinic (solar) keratoses. An emollient can be used as part of the management regimen for dry, sun-damaged elderly skin although the direct effect of emollient treatment is unclear; addition of urea or salicylic acid may provide benefit. Diclofenac sodium gel below may be suitable for the treatment of superficial lesions in mild disease. Fluorouracil cream p. 1326 is effective against most types of non-hypertrophic actinic keratosis; a solution containing fluorouracil with salicylic acid p. 1326 can be used for the treatment of low or moderately thick hyperkeratotic actinic keratosis. Imiquimod p. 1329 can be used for lesions on the face and scalp when cryotherapy or other topical treatments cannot be used. Fluorouracil and imiquimod produce a more marked inflammatory reaction than diclofenac sodium but lesions resolve faster. Photodynamic therapy in combination with methyl-5-aminolevulinate cream (Metvix ®) or 5-aminolaevulinic acid gel (Ameluz ®) is used in specialist centres for treating superficial and confluent, non-hypertrophic actinic keratosis when other treatments are inadequate or unsuitable; it is particularly suitable for

multiple and large-area lesions, cosmetically sensitive sites, lesions located at sites of poor healing, or where pain is likely to be an issue. Ⓐ

Imiquimod and topical fluorouracil are licensed for treating superficial basal cell carcinoma. EvGr Patients with skin lesions suspected to be a basal cell carcinoma should be considered for routine referral; a suspected cancer pathway referral should only be considered if there are concerns that delay may have a significant impact (due to factors such as lesion size and site). Photodynamic therapy in combination with methyl-5-aminolevulinate cream is used in specialist centres for treating thin nodular basal cell carcinomas when other treatments are unsuitable. It may also be used for superficial basal cell carcinomas, particularly for multiple and large-area lesions, cosmetically sensitive sites, and lesions located at sites of poor healing. Ⓐ

ANALGESICS > NON-STEROIDAL ANTI-INFLAMMATORY DRUGS

Diclofenac sodium

18-Nov-2020

● INDICATIONS AND DOSE

SOLARAZE ®

Actinic keratosis

▶ TO THE SKIN
  ▹ Adult: Apply twice daily for 60–90 days, to be applied thinly; maximum 8 g per day

● CAUTIONS Avoid contact with eyes · avoid contact with inflamed or broken skin · avoid contact with mucous membranes · not for use with occlusive dressings · topical application of large amounts can result in systemic effects, including hypersensitivity and asthma (renal disease has also been reported)

● INTERACTIONS → Appendix 1: NSAIDs

● SIDE-EFFECTS
▶ **Common or very common** Conjunctivitis · muscle tone increased · oedema · rash (discontinue) · sensation abnormal · skin reactions · skin ulcer
▶ **Uncommon** Abdominal pain · alopecia · diarrhoea · eye pain · haemorrhage · lacrimation disorder · nausea · seborrhoea
▶ **Rare or very rare** Acute kidney injury · angioedema · asthma · hypersensitivity · photosensitivity reaction · rash pustular
▶ **Frequency not known** Hair colour changes

SIDE-EFFECTS, FURTHER INFORMATION Topical application of large amounts of diclofenac can result in systemic effects.

● ALLERGY AND CROSS-SENSITIVITY EvGr Contra-indicated in patients with a history of hypersensitivity to aspirin or any other NSAID—which includes those in whom attacks of asthma, angioedema, urticaria or rhinitis have been precipitated by aspirin or any other NSAID. Ⓜ

● PREGNANCY Patient packs for topical preparations carry a warning to avoid during pregnancy.

● BREAST FEEDING Patient packs for topical preparations carry a warning to avoid during breast-feeding.

● DIRECTIONS FOR ADMINISTRATION For topical preparations, apply with gentle massage only.

● PRESCRIBING AND DISPENSING INFORMATION Caution—topical preparations not generally suitable for children.

● PATIENT AND CARER ADVICE For topical preparations, patients and their carers should be advised to wash hands immediately after use.

Photosensitivity Patients should be advised against excessive exposure to sunlight of area treated in order to avoid possibility of photosensitivity.

● MEDICINAL FORMS There can be variation in the licensing of different medicines containing the same drug.

Gel

EXCIPIENTS: May contain Benzyl alcohol, fragrances, propylene glycol

▸ Solaraze (Almirall Ltd)

Diclofenac sodium 30 mg per 1 gram Solaraze 3% gel | 50 gram [PoM] £38.30 DT = £38.30 | 100 gram [PoM] £76.60

ANTINEOPLASTIC DRUGS > ANTIMETABOLITES

Fluorouracil

11-Aug-2020

● INDICATIONS AND DOSE

Superficial malignant and pre-malignant skin lesions

▸ TO THE SKIN USING CREAM

▸ Adult: Apply 1–2 times a day for 3–4 weeks (usual duration of initial therapy), apply thinly to the affected area, maximum area of skin 500 cm^2 (e.g. 23 cm × 23 cm) treated at one time, alternative regimens may be used in some settings

● CAUTIONS Avoid contact with eyes and mucous membranes · dihydropyrimidine dehydrogenase deficiency · do not apply to bleeding lesions

● INTERACTIONS → Appendix 1: fluorouracil

● SIDE-EFFECTS

▸ **Common or very common** Alopecia · diarrhoea · mucositis · nausea · neutropenia · skin reactions · stomatitis · thrombocytopenia · vomiting

▸ **Uncommon** Dizziness · headache

▸ **Rare or very rare** Abdominal pain · chills · diarrhoea haemorrhagic · leucocytosis · pancytopenia · skin irritation (use a topical corticosteroid for severe discomfort associated with inflammatory reactions) · skin ulcer

▸ **Frequency not known** Conjunctival irritation · excessive tearing · keratitis · taste altered

● CONCEPTION AND CONTRACEPTION Contraceptive advice required, see *Pregnancy and reproductive function* in Cytotoxic drugs p. 932.

● PREGNANCY Manufacturers advise avoid (teratogenic).

● BREAST FEEDING Manufacturers advise avoid.

● HANDLING AND STORAGE Caution in handling—irritant to tissues.

● MEDICINAL FORMS There can be variation in the licensing of different medicines containing the same drug.

Cream

EXCIPIENTS: May contain Cetostearyl alcohol (including cetyl and stearyl alcohol), hydroxybenzoates (parabens), polysorbates, propylene glycol

▸ Efudix (Mylan)

Fluorouracil 50 mg per 1 gram Efudix 5% cream | 40 gram [PoM] £32.90 DT = £32.90

Fluorouracil with salicylic acid

The properties listed below are those particular to the combination only. For the properties of the components please consider, fluorouracil above, salicylic acid p. 1330.

● INDICATIONS AND DOSE

Low or moderately thick hyperkeratotic actinic keratosis

▸ TO THE SKIN

▸ Adult: Apply once daily for up to 12 weeks, reduced to 3 times a week if severe side effects occur and until side-effects improve, to be applied to the affected area, if treating area with thin epidermis, reduce frequency of application and monitor response more often; maximum area of skin treated at one time, 25 cm^2 (e.g. 5 cm × 5 cm)

● INTERACTIONS → Appendix 1: fluorouracil

● MEDICINAL FORMS There can be variation in the licensing of different medicines containing the same drug.

Cutaneous solution

CAUTIONARY AND ADVISORY LABELS 15

▸ Actikerall (Almirall Ltd)

Fluorouracil 5 mg/g, Salicylic acid 100 mg/g Actikerall 5mg/g / 100mg/g cutaneous solution | 25 ml [PoM] £38.30 DT = £38.30

PROTEIN KINASE C ACTIVATORS

Ingenol mebutate

09-Mar-2020

● INDICATIONS AND DOSE

Actinic keratosis on face and scalp

▸ TO THE SKIN

▸ Adult: Apply once daily for 3 days, use the 150 microgram/g gel

Actinic keratosis on trunk and extremities

▸ TO THE SKIN

▸ Adult: Apply once daily for 2 days, use the 500 microgram/g gel

---

IMPORTANT SAFETY INFORMATION

MHRA/CHM ADVICE (UPDATED FEBRUARY 2020): INGENOL MEBUTATE GEL (*PICATO*®): SUSPENSION OF THE LICENCE DUE TO RISK OF SKIN MALIGNANCY

Clinical studies have shown an increased incidence of benign and malignant skin tumours (such as basal and squamous cell carcinoma, Bowen's disease, and keratoacanthoma) in patients using ingenol mebutate gel; cases of neuroendocrine carcinoma of the skin, and atypical fibroxanthoma have also been reported. Healthcare professionals are advised to stop prescribing ingenol mebutate gel and consider alternative treatment options for actinic keratosis. The licence of ingenol mebutate has been suspended as a precautionary measure while investigations are carried out. Healthcare professionals should advise patients to be vigilant for the development of any new skin lesions within the treatment area and to seek immediate medical advice if any occur.

● CAUTIONS Avoid contact with broken skin · avoid contact with eyes · avoid contact with inside of ears · avoid contact with inside of nostrils · avoid contact with lips · avoid occlusive dressings on treated area

● SIDE-EFFECTS

▸ **Common or very common** Headache

▸ **Frequency not known** Neoplasms · skin eruption localised

● PREGNANCY Not absorbed from skin, but manufacturer advises avoid.

● BREAST FEEDING Not absorbed from skin; ensure infant does not come in contact with treated area for 6 hours after application.

● DIRECTIONS FOR ADMINISTRATION One tube covers skin area of 25 cm^2. Allow gel to dry on treatment area for 15 minutes. Avoid washing or touching the treated area for 6 hours after application; after this time, area may be washed with mild soap and water. Avoid use immediately after shower or less than 2 hours before bedtime.

● MEDICINAL FORMS No licensed medicines listed.

1 Superficial soft-tissue injuries and superficial thrombophlebitis

opical circulatory preparations

verview

hese preparations are used to improve circulation in
onditions such as bruising, superficial thrombophlebitis,
hilblains and varicose veins but are of little value. Chilblains
re best managed by avoidance of exposure to cold; neither
ystemic nor topical vasodilator therapy is established as
eing effective.

EPARINOIDS

Heparinoid

● INDICATIONS AND DOSE
Superficial thrombophlebitis | Bruising | Haematoma
▶ TO THE SKIN
▶ **Adult:** Apply up to 4 times a day

● CONTRA-INDICATIONS Should not be used on large areas of
skin, broken or sensitive skin, or mucous membranes
● LESS SUITABLE FOR PRESCRIBING Hirudoid ® is less
suitable for prescribing.

● MEDICINAL FORMS There can be variation in the licensing of
different medicines containing the same drug.
Cream
EXCIPIENTS: May contain Cetostearyl alcohol (including cetyl and
stearyl alcohol), hydroxybenzoates (parabens)
▶ Hirudoid (Genus Pharmaceuticals Ltd)
Heparinoid 3 mg per 1 gram Hirudoid 0.3% cream | 50 gram Ⓟ
£3.99 DT = £3.99
Gel
EXCIPIENTS: May contain Fragrances, propylene glycol
▶ Hirudoid (Genus Pharmaceuticals Ltd)
Heparinoid 3 mg per 1 gram Hirudoid 0.3% gel | 50 gram Ⓟ £3.99
DT = £3.99

2 Warts and calluses

Warts and calluses

Overview

Warts (verrucas) are caused by a human papillomavirus,
which most frequently affects the hands, feet (plantar warts),
and the anogenital region; treatment usually relies on local
tissue destruction. Warts may regress on their own and
treatment is required only if the warts are painful, unsightly,
persistent, or cause distress.
   Preparations of salicylic acid p. 1330, formaldehyde
p. 1328, glutaraldehyde p. 1328 or silver nitrate p. 1329 are
available for purchase by the public; they are suitable for the
removal of warts on hands and feet. Salicylic acid is a useful
keratolytic which may be considered first-line; it is also
suitable for the removal of *corns and calluses*. Preparations of
salicylic acid in a collodion basis are available but some
patients may develop an allergy to colophony in the
formulation; collodion should be avoided in children allergic
to elastic adhesive plaster. Cryotherapy causes pain,
swelling, and blistering, and may be no more effective than
topical salicylic acid in the treatment of warts.

Anogenital warts

The treatment of anogenital warts (condylomata acuminata)
should be accompanied by screening for other sexually
transmitted infections. Podophyllotoxin (the major active
ingredient of podophyllum) p. 1328 may be used for *soft,
non-keratinised* external anogenital warts. Patients with a
limited number of external warts or *keratinised* lesions may
be better treated with cryotherapy or other forms of physical
ablation.
   Imiquimod cream p. 1329 is licensed for the treatment of
external anogenital warts; it may be used for both
keratinised and non-keratinised lesions. It is also licensed
for the treatment of superficial basal cell carcinoma and
actinic keratosis. Camellia sinensis ointment below is
licensed for the treatment of external anogenital warts.
   Inosine pranobex p. 672 is licensed for adjunctive
treatment of genital warts but it has been superseded by
more effective drugs.

ANTINEOPLASTIC DRUGS 〉 PLANT ALKALOIDS

▌ Camellia sinensis   20-Aug-2020

● DRUG ACTION Camellia sinensis is an extract from green
tea leaves. The exact mechanism of action is not known;
non-clinical studies have shown inhibition of the growth
of activated keratinocytes, and anti-oxidative effects at the
site of application.

● INDICATIONS AND DOSE
**Warts (external genital and perianal) in
immunocompetent patients**
▶ TO THE LESION
▶ **Adult:** Apply up to 250 mg 3 times a day until complete
clearance of warts (maximum 16 weeks), do not exceed
treatment period even if new warts develop; maximum
750 mg per day
DOSE EQUIVALENCE AND CONVERSION
▶ 250 mg is equivalent to 0.5 cm of ointment.

● CAUTIONS Avoid broken skin · avoid contact with eyes ·
avoid contact with lips · avoid contact with mouth · avoid
contact with nostrils · avoid inflamed skin · uncircumcised
males (risk of phimosis) · vulvar region
● SIDE-EFFECTS
▶ **Uncommon** Balanoposthitis · increased risk of infection ·
lymphatic abnormalities · necrosis · painful sexual
intercourse · phimosis · skin reactions · urinary disorders
▶ **Frequency not known** Urinary tract stenosis · vaginal
discharge
● CONCEPTION AND CONTRACEPTION Manufacturer advises
Catephen ® may weaken condoms and vaginal
diaphragms—alternative methods of contraception should
be considered.
● PREGNANCY Manufacturer advises avoid—toxicity in
animal studies.
● BREAST FEEDING Manufacturer advises risk to infant
cannot be excluded—no information available.
● HEPATIC IMPAIRMENT Manufacturer advises avoid in
severe impairment (limited information available).
● DIRECTIONS FOR ADMINISTRATION Manufacturer advises
apply to each wart, ensuring a thin layer is left on the wart.
It is not necessary to wash off the ointment from the area
before next application.
● PATIENT AND CARER ADVICE Manufacturer advises the
ointment should be washed off before sexual activity.
Manufacturer advises female patients using tampons
should insert tampon before applying the ointment.
● NATIONAL FUNDING/ACCESS DECISIONS
For full details see funding body website

13

Skin

Scottish Medicines Consortium (SMC) decisions

▸ Camellia sinensis (green tea leaf) (*Catephen*®) for the cutaneous treatment of external genital and perianal warts (condylomata acuminata) in immunocompetent patients from the age of 18 years (April 2016) SMC No. 1133/16 Recommended with restrictions

All Wales Medicines Strategy Group (AWMSG) decisions

▸ Green tea leaf extract (*Catephen*®) for cutaneous treatment of external genital and perianal warts (condylomata acuminata) in immunocompetent patients from the age of 18 years (October 2016) AWMSG No. 2739 Recommended with restrictions

● MEDICINAL FORMS There can be variation in the licensing of different medicines containing the same drug.

Ointment
▸ Catephen (KoRa Healthcare)
Camellia sinensis extract 100 mg per 1 gram Catephen 10% ointment | 15 gram [PoM] £39.00 DT = £39.00

Podophyllotoxin

28-Jul-2020

● INDICATIONS AND DOSE

CONDYLINE®

Condylomata acuminata affecting the penis or the female external genitalia
▸ TO THE LESION
▸ Adult: Apply twice daily for 3 consecutive days, treatment may be repeated at weekly intervals if necessary for a total of five 3-day treatment courses, direct medical supervision for lesions in the female and for lesions greater than 4 cm^2 in the male, maximum 50 single applications ('loops') per session (consult product literature)

WARTICON® CREAM

Condylomata acuminata affecting the penis or the female external genitalia
▸ TO THE LESION
▸ Adult: Apply twice daily for 3 consecutive days, treatment may be repeated at weekly intervals if necessary for a total of four 3-day treatment courses, direct medical supervision for lesions greater than 4 cm^2

WARTICON® LIQUID

Condylomata acuminata affecting the penis or the female external genitalia
▸ TO THE LESION
▸ Adult: Apply twice daily for 3 consecutive days, treatment may be repeated at weekly intervals if necessary for a total of four 3-day treatment courses, direct medical supervision for lesions greater than 4 cm^2, maximum 50 single applications ('loops') per session (consult product literature)

● CAUTIONS Avoid normal skin · avoid open wounds · keep away from face · very irritant to eyes
● SIDE-EFFECTS Balanoposthitis · skin irritation
● PREGNANCY Avoid.
● BREAST FEEDING Avoid.

● MEDICINAL FORMS There can be variation in the licensing of different medicines containing the same drug.

Cream
EXCIPIENTS: May contain Butylated hydroxyanisole, cetostearyl alcohol (including cetyl and stearyl alcohol), hydroxybenzoates (parabens), sorbic acid
▸ Warticon (Phoenix Labs Ltd)
Podophyllotoxin 1.5 mg per 1 gram Warticon 0.15% cream | 5 gram [PoM] £17.83 DT = £17.83

Liquid
CAUTIONARY AND ADVISORY LABELS 15
▸ Condyline (Takeda UK Ltd)
Podophyllotoxin 5 mg per 1 ml Condyline 0.5% solution | 3.5 ml [PoM] £14.49 DT = £14.49
▸ Warticon (Phoenix Labs Ltd)
Podophyllotoxin 5 mg per 1 ml Warticon 0.5% solution | 3 ml [PoM] £14.86 DT = £14.86

ANTISEPTICS AND DISINFECTANTS ›
ALDEHYDES AND DERIVATIVES

Formaldehyde

● INDICATIONS AND DOSE

Warts, particularly plantar warts
▸ TO THE LESION
▸ Child: Apply twice daily
▸ Adult: Apply twice daily

● UNLICENSED USE
▸ In children Licensed for use in children (age range not specified by manufacturer).
● CAUTIONS Impaired peripheral circulation · not suitable for application to anogenital region · not suitable for application to face · not suitable for application to large areas · patients with diabetes at risk of neuropathic ulcers · protect surrounding skin and avoid broken skin · significant peripheral neuropathy
● SIDE-EFFECTS Asthma · cough · dysphagia · eye irritation · increased risk of infection · laryngospasm · skin reactions

● MEDICINAL FORMS There can be variation in the licensing of different medicines containing the same drug. Forms available from special-order manufacturers include: liquid

Liquid
▸ Formaldehyde (Non-proprietary)
Formaldehyde 40 mg per 1 ml Formaldehyde (Buffered) 4% solution | 1000 ml £3.90-£4.91 DT = £4.41
Formaldehyde 350 mg per 1 gram Formaldehyde solution | 500 ml £7.31 DT = £7.31 | 2000 ml £18.72

Glutaraldehyde

● INDICATIONS AND DOSE

Warts, particularly plantar warts
▸ TO THE LESION
▸ Child: Apply twice daily
▸ Adult: Apply twice daily

● UNLICENSED USE
▸ In children Licensed for use in children (age range not specified by manufacturer).
● CAUTIONS Not for application to anogenital areas · not for application to face · not for application to mucosa · protect surrounding skin
● SIDE-EFFECTS
▸ Rare or very rare Severe cutaneous adverse reactions (SCARs)
▸ Frequency not known Rash · skin irritation (discontinue if severe)

● MEDICINAL FORMS There can be variation in the licensing of different medicines containing the same drug.

Paint
▸ Glutarol (Dermal Laboratories Ltd)
Glutaraldehyde 100 mg per 1 ml Glutarol 10% cutaneous solution | 10 ml [P] £2.07 DT = £2.07

13

Skin

Silver nitrate

● **INDICATIONS AND DOSE**

Common warts
▶ TO THE LESION
▶ Child: Apply every 24 hours for up to 3 applications, apply moistened caustic pencil tip for 1–2 minutes. Instructions in proprietary packs generally incorporate advice to remove dead skin before use by gentle filing and to cover with adhesive dressing after application
▶ Adult: Apply every 24 hours for up to 3 applications, apply moistened caustic pencil tip for 1–2 minutes. Instructions in proprietary packs generally incorporate advice to remove dead skin before use by gentle filing and to cover with adhesive dressing after application

Verrucas
▶ TO THE LESION
▶ Child: Apply every 24 hours for up to 6 applications, apply moistened caustic pencil tip for 1–2 minutes. Instructions in proprietary packs generally incorporate advice to remove dead skin before use by gentle filing and to cover with adhesive dressing after application
▶ Adult: Apply every 24 hours for up to 6 applications, apply moistened caustic pencil tip for 1–2 minutes. Instructions in proprietary packs generally incorporate advice to remove dead skin before use by gentle filing and to cover with adhesive dressing after application

Umbilical granulomas
▶ TO THE SKIN
▶ Child: Apply moistened caustic pencil tip (usually containing silver nitrate 40%) for 1–2 minutes, protect surrounding skin with soft paraffin
▶ Adult: Apply moistened caustic pencil tip (usually containing silver nitrate 40%) for 1–2 minutes, protect surrounding skin with soft paraffin

● **UNLICENSED USE**
In children No age range specified by manufacturer.

● **CAUTIONS** Avoid broken skin · not suitable for application to ano-genital region · not suitable for application to face · not suitable for application to large areas · protect surrounding skin

● **SIDE-EFFECTS**
▶ **Rare or very rare** Argyria · methaemoglobinaemia

● **PATIENT AND CARER ADVICE** Patients should be advised that silver nitrate may stain fabric.

● **MEDICINAL FORMS** There can be variation in the licensing of different medicines containing the same drug.

Stick
▶ Avoca (Bray Group Ltd)
  Silver nitrate 400 mg per 1 gram Avoca 40% silver nitrate pencils | 1 applicator Ⓟ £1.16 DT = £1.16
  Silver nitrate 750 mg per 1 gram Avoca 75% silver nitrate applicators | 100 applicator Ⓟ £49.16 DT = £49.16
  Avoca 75% silver nitrate applicators with thick handles | 50 applicator Ⓟ £48.51
  Silver nitrate 950 mg per 1 gram Avoca 95% silver nitrate applicators | 100 applicator Ⓟ £52.60 DT = £52.60
  Avoca 95% silver nitrate pencils | 1 applicator Ⓟ £2.63 DT = £3.08
  Avoca wart and verruca treatment set | 1 applicator Ⓟ £3.08 DT = £3.08

▌Imiquimod

09-Nov-2020

● **INDICATIONS AND DOSE**

ALDARA ®
Warts (external genital and perianal)
▶ TO THE LESION
▶ Adult: Apply 3 times a week until lesions resolve (maximum 16 weeks), to be applied thinly at night

Superficial basal cell carcinoma
▶ TO THE LESION
▶ Adult: Apply daily for 5 nights of each week for 6 weeks, to be applied to lesion and 1 cm beyond it, assess response 12 weeks after completing treatment

Actinic keratosis
▶ TO THE LESION
▶ Adult: Apply 3 times a week for 4 weeks, to be applied to lesion at night, assess response after a 4 week treatment-free interval; repeat 4-week course if lesions persist, maximum 2 courses

ZYCLARA ®
Actinic keratosis
▶ TO THE SKIN
▶ Adult: Apply once daily for 2 weeks, to be applied at bedtime to lesion on face or balding scalp, repeat course after a 2-week treatment-free interval, assess response 8 weeks after second course; maximum 2 sachets per day

● **CAUTIONS** Autoimmune disease · avoid broken skin · avoid contact with eyes · avoid contact with lips · avoid contact with nostrils · avoid open wounds · immunosuppressed patients · not suitable for internal genital warts · uncircumcised males (risk of phimosis or stricture of foreskin)

● **SIDE-EFFECTS**
▶ **Common or very common** Appetite decreased · arthralgia · asthenia · headaches · increased risk of infection · lymphadenopathy · myalgia · nausea · pain
▶ **Uncommon** Anorectal disorder · chills · conjunctival irritation · depression · diarrhoea · dizziness · drowsiness · dry mouth · dysuria · erectile dysfunction · eyelid oedema · face oedema · fever · flushing · gastrointestinal discomfort · genital pain · hyperhidrosis · inflammation · influenza like illness · insomnia · irritability · laryngeal pain · malaise · nasal congestion · painful sexual intercourse · paraesthesia · penis disorder · skin reactions · skin ulcer · tinnitus · uterovaginal prolapse · vomiting · vulvovaginal disorders
▶ **Rare or very rare** Autoimmune disorder exacerbated
▶ **Frequency not known** Alopecia · cutaneous lupus erythematosus · severe cutaneous adverse reactions (SCARs)

● **CONCEPTION AND CONTRACEPTION** May damage latex condoms and diaphragms.

● **PREGNANCY** No evidence of teratogenicity or toxicity in *animal* studies; manufacturer advises caution.

● **BREAST FEEDING** No information available.

● **DIRECTIONS FOR ADMINISTRATION**
ZYCLARA ® ▶ **Important** Manufacturer advises cream should be rubbed in and allowed to stay on the treated area for 8 hours, then washed off with mild soap and water.
ALDARA ® ▶ **Important** Manufacturer advises cream should be rubbed in and allowed to stay on the treated area for 6–10 hours for warts or for 8 hours for basal cell carcinoma and actinic keratosis, then washed off with mild soap and water (uncircumcised males treating warts under foreskin should wash the area daily). The cream should be washed off before sexual contact.

13

Skin

- PATIENT AND CARER ADVICE A patient information leaflet should be provided.
- NATIONAL FUNDING/ACCESS DECISIONS
  For full details see funding body website
  Scottish Medicines Consortium (SMC) decisions
  ▸ Imiquimod (*Zyclara* ®) for the topical treatment of clinically typical, nonhyperkeratotic, nonhypertrophic, visible or palpable actinic keratosis (AK) of the full face or balding scalp in immunocompetent adults when other topical treatment options are contra-indicated or less appropriate (November 2019) SMC No. SMC2211 Recommended with restrictions

- MEDICINAL FORMS There can be variation in the licensing of different medicines containing the same drug.
  Cream
  CAUTIONARY AND ADVISORY LABELS 10
  EXCIPIENTS: May contain Benzyl alcohol, cetostearyl alcohol (including cetyl and stearyl alcohol), hydroxybenzoates (parabens), polysorbates
  ▸ Aldara (Mylan)
    Imiquimod 50 mg per 1 gram Aldara 5% cream 250mg sachets | 12 sachet PoM £48.60 DT = £48.60
  ▸ Zyclara (Mylan)
    Imiquimod 37.5 mg per 1 gram Zyclara 3.75% cream 250mg sachets | 28 sachet PoM £54.75 DT = £54.75

SALICYLIC ACID AND DERIVATIVES

Salicylic acid

- INDICATIONS AND DOSE
  OCCLUSAL ®
  Common and plantar warts
  ▸ TO THE LESION
  ▸ Child: Apply daily, treatment may need to be continued for up to 3 months
  ▸ Adult: Apply daily, treatment may need to be continued for up to 3 months
  VERRUGON ®
  For plantar warts
  ▸ TO THE LESION
  ▸ Child: Apply daily, treatment may need to be continued for up to 3 months
  ▸ Adult: Apply daily, treatment may need to be continued for up to 3 months

- UNLICENSED USE
  ▸ In children Not licensed for use in children under 2 years.
- CAUTIONS Avoid broken skin · impaired peripheral circulation · not suitable for application to anogenital region · not suitable for application to face · not suitable for application to large areas · patients with diabetes at risk of neuropathic ulcers · significant peripheral neuropathy
- SIDE-EFFECTS Skin irritation
- PATIENT AND CARER ADVICE Advise patient to apply carefully to wart and to protect surrounding skin (e.g. with soft paraffin or specially designed plaster); rub wart surface gently with file or pumice stone once weekly.

- MEDICINAL FORMS There can be variation in the licensing of different medicines containing the same drug.
  Ointment
  ▸ Verrugon (Optima Consumer Health Ltd)
    Salicylic acid 500 mg per 1 gram Verrugon complete 50% ointment | 6 gram P £4.44 DT = £4.44
  Liquid
  CAUTIONARY AND ADVISORY LABELS 15
  ▸ Occlusal (Alliance Pharmaceuticals Ltd)
    Salicylic acid 260 mg per 1 ml Occlusal 26% solution | 10 ml P £3.56 DT = £3.56

Salicylic acid with lactic acid

The properties listed below are those particular to the combination only. For the properties of the components please consider, salicylic acid above.

- INDICATIONS AND DOSE
  DUOFILM ®
  Plantar and mosaic warts
  ▸ TO THE LESION
  ▸ Adult: Apply daily, treatment may need to be continued for up to 3 months
  SALACTOL ®
  Warts, particularly plantar warts | Verrucas | Corns | Calluses
  ▸ TO THE LESION
  ▸ Adult: Apply daily, treatment may need to be continued for up to 3 months
  SALATAC ®
  Warts | Verrucas | Corns | Calluses
  ▸ TO THE LESION
  ▸ Adult: Apply daily, treatment may need to be continued for up to 3 months

- PRESCRIBING AND DISPENSING INFORMATION Preparation of salicylic acid in a collodion basis (*Salactol* ®) is available but some patients may develop an allergy to colophony in the formulation.

- MEDICINAL FORMS There can be variation in the licensing of different medicines containing the same drug.
  Paint
  CAUTIONARY AND ADVISORY LABELS 15
  ▸ Duofilm (GlaxoSmithKline Consumer Healthcare)
    Lactic acid 150 mg per 1 gram, Salicylic acid 167 mg per 1 gram Duofilm paint | 15 ml P £2.78 DT = £2.78
  ▸ Salactol (Dermal Laboratories Ltd)
    Lactic acid 167 mg per 1 gram, Salicylic acid 167 mg per 1 gram Salactol paint | 10 ml P £1.71 DT = £1.71
  Gel
  CAUTIONARY AND ADVISORY LABELS 15
  ▸ Salatac (Dermal Laboratories Ltd)
    Lactic acid 40 mg per 1 gram, Salicylic acid 120 mg per 1 gram Salatac gel | 8 gram P £2.98 DT = £2.98

Chapter 14
Vaccines

CONTENTS

1   Immunoglobulin therapy

IMMUNE SERA AND IMMUNOGLOBULINS ›
IMMUNOGLOBULINS

Immunoglobulins   23-Sep-2020

Passive immunity

Immunity with protection against certain infective organisms can be obtained by injecting preparations made from the plasma of immune individuals with adequate levels of antibody to the disease for which protection is sought. The duration of this passive immunity varies according to the dose and the type of immunoglobulin. Passive immunity may last only a few weeks; when necessary, passive immunisation can be repeated. Antibodies of human origin are usually termed immunoglobulins. The term antiserum is applied to material prepared in animals. Because of serum sickness and other allergic-type reactions that may follow injections of antisera, this therapy has been replaced wherever possible by the use of immunoglobulins. Reactions are theoretically possible after injection of human immunoglobulins but reports of such reactions are very rare.

Two types of human immunoglobulin preparation are available, normal immunoglobulin p. 1335 and **disease-specific immunoglobulins**.

Human normal immunoglobulin (HNIG) is prepared from pooled plasma obtained from donors outside the UK, tested and found non-reactive for hepatitis B surface antigen and for antibodies against hepatitis C virus and human immunodeficiency virus (types 1 and 2). A global shortage of human immunoglobulin and the rapidly increasing range of clinical indications for treatment with immunoglobulins has resulted in the need for a Demand Management programme in the UK, for further information consult the Department of Health and Social Care's **National Demand Management Programme for Immunoglobulin** and **Clinical Guidelines for Immunoglobulin Use** (both available at: igd.mdsas.com/).

For further information on the use of immunoglobulins, see Public Health England (PHE) guidance:
Immunoglobulin: when to use (www.gov.uk/government/ publications/immunoglobulin-when-to-use) and **Immunisation against Infectious Disease** (www.gov.uk/government/ collections/immunisation-against-infectious-disease-the-green-book).

Availability

Human normal immunoglobulin for intramuscular administration is available from the Immunisation, Hepatitis and Blood Safety Department of PHE's Centre for Infectious Disease Surveillance and some regional PHE and NHS laboratories, for the protection of contacts and the control of outbreaks of hepatitis A, measles, and rubella only. For other indications, subcutaneous or intravenous normal immunoglobulin may be purchased from the manufacturer (see Index of manufacturers p. 1691).

Various **disease-specific immunoglobulins** for intramuscular use are available from either the Immunisation, Hepatitis and Blood Safety Department of PHE's Centre for Infectious Disease Surveillance; some regional PHE and NHS laboratories; PHE's Rabies and Immunoglobulin Service; and/or through Bio Products Laboratory (BPL). Tetanus immunoglobulin p. 1337 is available from BPL, hospital pharmacies,or blood transfusion departments. Hepatitis B immunoglobulin p. 1334 required by transplant centres should be obtained commercially.

In Scotland all immunoglobulins are available from the *Scottish National Blood Transfusion Service* (SNBTS).

In Wales all immunoglobulins are available from the *Welsh Blood Service* (WBS).

In Northern Ireland all immunoglobulins are available from the *Northern Ireland Blood Transfusion Service* (NIBTS).

Normal immunoglobulin

Human normal immunoglobulin is prepared from pools of at least 1000 donations of human plasma; it contains immunoglobulin G (IgG) and antibodies to hepatitis A, measles, mumps, rubella, varicella, and other viruses that are currently prevalent in the general population.

Uses

Normal immunoglobulin (containing 10%–18% protein) is administered by *intramuscular injection* for the protection of susceptible contacts against **hepatitis A** virus (infectious hepatitis), **measles** and, to a lesser extent, **rubella**. Injection of immunoglobulin produces immediate protection lasting several weeks.

Normal immunoglobulin (containing 3%–12% protein) for *intravenous administration* is used as *replacement therapy* for patients with congenital agammaglobulinaemia and hypogammaglobulinaemia, and for the short-term treatment of idiopathic thrombocytopenic purpura and Kawasaki disease; it is also used for the prophylaxis of infection following bone-marrow transplantation and in children with symptomatic HIV infection who have recurrent bacterial infections. Normal immunoglobulin for replacement therapy may also be given intramuscularly or subcutaneously, but intravenous formulations are normally preferred. Intravenous immunoglobulin is also used in the treatment of Guillain-Barré syndrome as an alternative to plasma exchange.

For information on the use of intravenous normal immunoglobulin and alternative therapies for certain conditions, see the Department of Health and Social Care guideline: **Immunoglobulin Use** (www.gov.uk/government/ publications/clinical-guidelines-for-immunoglobulin-use-second-edition-update).

Hepatitis A

For close contacts (of the index case) who have chronic liver disease (including chronic hepatitis B or C infection), HIV infection (with a CD4 count < 200 cells per microlitre), are immunosuppressed, or are aged 60 years or over, normal immunoglobulin in addition to the monovalent hepatitis A vaccine p. 1369 is recommended within 14 days of exposure to the index case (up to 28 days in those with chronic liver disease). Normal immunoglobulin and the monovalent hepatitis A vaccine can be given at the same time, but should be given at separate injection sites.

For further information on post-exposure prophylaxis and information on risk assessment, see Hepatitis A vaccine p. 1345.

Measles

Intravenous or subcutaneous normal immunoglobulin may be given to prevent or attenuate an attack of measles in individuals who do not have adequate immunity. Patients with compromised immunity who have come into contact with measles should receive intravenous or subcutaneous normal immunoglobulin as soon as possible after exposure. It is most effective if given within 72 hours but can be effective if given within 6 days.

Subcutaneous or intramuscular normal immunoglobulin should also be considered for the following individuals if they have been in contact with a confirmed case of measles or with a person associated with a local outbreak:

* non-immune pregnant women
* infants under 9 months

Further advice should be sought from the Centre for Infections, Public Health England (tel. (020) 8200 6868).

Individuals with normal immunity who are not in the above categories and who have not been fully immunised against measles, can be given measles, mumps and rubella vaccine, live p. 1375 for prophylaxis following exposure to measles.

Rubella

Intramuscular immunoglobulin after exposure to rubella does **not** prevent infection in non-immune contacts and is **not** recommended for protection of pregnant women exposed to rubella. It may, however, reduce the likelihood of a clinical attack which may possibly reduce the risk to the fetus. Risk of intra-uterine transmission is greatest in the first 11 weeks of pregnancy, between 16 and 20 weeks there is minimal risk of deafness only, after 20 weeks there is no increased risk. Intramuscular normal immunoglobulin should be used only if termination of pregnancy would be unacceptable to the pregnant woman—it should be given as soon as possible after exposure. Serological follow-up of recipients is essential to determine if the woman has become infected despite receiving immunoglobulin.

For routine prophylaxis against Rubella, see measles, mumps and rubella vaccine, live.

Disease-specific immunoglobulins

Specific immunoglobulins are prepared by pooling the plasma of selected human donors with high levels of the specific antibody required. For further information, see PHE guidance: **Immunoglobulin: when to use** (www.gov.uk/government/publications/immunoglobulin-when-to-use).

There are no specific immunoglobulins for hepatitis A, measles, or rubella— normal immunoglobulin p. 1335 is used in certain circumstances. There is no specific immunoglobulin for mumps; neither normal immunoglobulin nor measles, mumps and rubella vaccine, live p. 1375 is effective as post-exposure prophylaxis.

Hepatitis B immunoglobulin

Disease-specific hepatitis B immunoglobulin p. 1334 (HBIG) is available for use in association with hepatitis B vaccine p. 1370 for the prevention of infection in laboratory and other personnel who have been accidentally inoculated with hepatitis B virus, and in infants born to mothers who have become infected with this virus in pregnancy or who are high-risk carriers. Hepatitis B immunoglobulin will not

inhibit the antibody response when given at the same time as hepatitis B vaccine but should be given at different sites.

An intravenous and subcutaneous preparation of hepatitis B immunoglobulin is licensed for the prevention of hepatitis B recurrence in HBV-DNA negative patients who have undergone liver transplantation for liver failure caused by the virus.

Rabies immunoglobulin

Rabies immunoglobulin p. 1336 should be considered following high risk exposure to rabies to give rapid protection until rabies vaccine p. 1376 (administered at a separate site) becomes effective. When indicated for post-exposure treatment, rabies immunoglobulin should be injected around the site of the wound where possible, rather than intramuscularly, as it neutralises rabies virus before the immune system can respond. There is limited benefit of intramuscular administration away from the wound site. For information about dosing and administration, see rabies immunoglobulin.

Rabies immunoglobulin is not recommended if:

* an individual is already partially or previously immunised (unless immunocompromised);
* more than 7 days have passed since the first dose of rabies vaccine or more than 1 day since the second dose of rabies vaccine;
* the rabies exposure was more than 12 months prior.

For further information on risk assessment and post-exposure treatment, see Rabies vaccine p. 1355.

Tetanus immunoglobulin

For the management of tetanus-prone wounds, tetanus immunoglobulin p. 1337 should be used in addition to wound cleansing and, where appropriate, antibacterial prophylaxis and a tetanus-containing vaccine. Tetanus immunoglobulin, together with metronidazole p. 575 and wound cleansing, should also be used for the treatment of established cases of tetanus.

Varicella–zoster immunoglobulin

Varicella infection in immunosuppressed individuals and pregnant women can lead to severe and even life-threatening varicella disease. Post-exposure prophylaxis is recommended to attenuate disease and to reduce the risk of complications.

Varicella-zoster immunoglobulin p. 1337 (VZIG) is recommended for individuals who have:

* had a significant exposure to varicella (chickenpox) or herpes zoster (shingles)—this depends on the type of varicella-zoster infection in the index case, the timing of the exposure in relation to onset of rash in the index case, and/or closeness and duration of contact; **and**
* a clinical condition that increases the risk of severe chickenpox; **and**
* no antibodies to varicella-zoster virus.

Due to a significant shortage of varicella-zoster immunoglobulin, stock has been prioritised for the most vulnerable groups, such as susceptible women exposed in the first 20 weeks of pregnancy. For susceptible pregnant women exposed after 20 weeks (from 21 weeks to delivery), either varicella-zoster immunoglobulin or aciclovir p. 672 [unlicensed] is recommended; valaciclovir p. 675 [unlicensed] may be used as an alternative. Varicella-zoster immunoglobulin may also be considered in susceptible individuals with renal impairment or intestinal malabsorption (such as inflammatory bowel disease).

For susceptible immunosuppressed individuals, an antiviral [unlicensed] is recommended unless there are significant concerns about renal toxicity or malabsorption. Aciclovir [unlicensed] is recommended first-line; valaciclovir [unlicensed] may be used as an alternative. Immunosuppressed individuals on long term aciclovir or

alaciclovir prophylaxis, may require their dose to be
emporarily increased.

For further information on risk assessment and the use of
ZIG or an antiviral for post-exposure prophylaxis, see the
HE guidance: **Varicella-zoster immunoglobulin**
available at: www.gov.uk/government/publications/varicella-
oster-immunoglobulin). Refer to the British HIV Association
or use of VZIG in individuals with HIV infection. See
www.bhiva.org/guidelines for further information.

Individuals who develop chickenpox despite post-
xposure prophylaxis require treatment with an antiviral;
here is no evidence that VZIG is effective in the treatment
of disease. For information on the treatment of chickenpox
or shingles, see *Varicella-zoster infections* in Herpesvirus
infections p. 671.

Anti-D (Rh₀) immunoglobulin

Anti-D (Rh₀) immunoglobulin below is prepared from plasma
taken from rhesus-negative donors who have been
immunised against the anti-D-antigen. Anti-D (Rh₀)
immunoglobulin is used to prevent a rhesus-negative
mother from forming antibodies to fetal rhesus-positive cells
which may pass into the maternal circulation. The objective
is to protect any subsequent child from the hazard of
haemolytic disease of the newborn.

Anti-D (Rh₀) immunoglobulin should be administered to
the mother following any sensitising episode (e.g. abortion,
miscarriage and birth); it should be injected within 72 hours
of the episode but even if a longer period has elapsed it may
still give protection and should be administered. Anti-D
(Rh₀) immunoglobulin is also given when significant feto-
maternal haemorrhage occurs in rhesus-negative women
during delivery. The dose of anti-D (Rh₀) immunoglobulin is
determined according to the level of exposure to rhesus-
positive blood.

Use of routine *antenatal* anti-D prophylaxis should be
given irrespective of previous anti-D prophylaxis for a
sensitising event early in the same pregnancy. Similarly,
postpartum anti-D prophylaxis should be given irrespective
of previous routine antenatal anti-D prophylaxis or
antenatal anti-D prophylaxis for a sensitising event in the
same pregnancy.

Anti-D (Rh₀) immunoglobulin is also given to women of
child-bearing potential after the inadvertent transfusion of
rhesus-incompatible blood components and is used for the
treatment of idiopathic thrombocytopenia purpura.

MMR vaccine

Measles, mumps and rubella vaccine, live may be given in
the postpartum period with anti-D (Rh₀) immunoglobulin
injection provided that separate syringes are used and the
products are administered into different limbs. If blood is
transfused, the antibody response to the vaccine may be
inhibited—measure rubella antibodies after 6–8 weeks and
revaccinate if necessary.

Anti-D (Rh₀) immunoglobulin　　03-Mar-2020

● **INDICATIONS AND DOSE**

**To rhesus-negative woman for prevention of Rh₀(D)
sensitisation, following birth of rhesus-positive infant**

▸ BY DEEP INTRAMUSCULAR INJECTION

▸ Females of childbearing potential: 500 units, dose to be
administered immediately or within 72 hours; for
transplacental bleed of over 4 mL fetal red cells, extra
100–125 units per mL fetal red cells, subcutaneous
route used for patients with bleeding disorders

**To rhesus-negative woman for prevention of Rh₀(D)
sensitisation, following any potentially sensitising
episode (e.g. stillbirth, abortion, amniocentesis) up to
20 weeks' gestation**

▸ BY DEEP INTRAMUSCULAR INJECTION

▸ Females of childbearing potential: 250 units per episode,
dose to be administered immediately or within
72 hours, subcutaneous route used for patients with
bleeding disorders

**To rhesus-negative woman for prevention of Rh₀(D)
sensitisation, following any potentially sensitising
episode (e.g. stillbirth, abortion, amniocentesis) after
20 weeks' gestation**

▸ BY DEEP INTRAMUSCULAR INJECTION

▸ Females of childbearing potential: 500 units per episode,
dose to be administered immediately or within
72 hours, subcutaneous route used for patients with
bleeding disorders

**To rhesus-negative woman for prevention of Rh₀(D)
sensitisation, antenatal prophylaxis**

▸ BY DEEP INTRAMUSCULAR INJECTION

▸ Females of childbearing potential: 500 units, dose to be
given at weeks 28 and 34 of pregnancy, if infant rhesus-
positive, a further dose is still needed immediately or
within 72 hours of delivery, subcutaneous route used
for patients with bleeding disorders

**To rhesus-negative woman for prevention of Rh₀(D)
sensitisation, antenatal prophylaxis (alternative NICE
recommendation)**

▸ BY DEEP INTRAMUSCULAR INJECTION

▸ Females of childbearing potential: 1000–1650 units, dose
to be given at weeks 28 and 34 of pregnancy,
alternatively 1500 units for 1 dose, dose to be given
between 28 and 30 weeks gestation

**To rhesus-negative woman for prevention of Rh₀(D)
sensitisation, following Rh₀(D) incompatible blood
transfusion**

▸ BY DEEP INTRAMUSCULAR INJECTION

▸ Females of childbearing potential: 100–125 units per mL
of transfused rhesus-positive red cells, subcutaneous
route used for patients with bleeding disorders

RHOPHYLAC ®

**To rhesus-negative woman for prevention of Rh₀(D)
sensitisation, following birth of rhesus-positive infant**

▸ BY INTRAMUSCULAR INJECTION, OR BY INTRAVENOUS
INJECTION

▸ Females of childbearing potential: 1000–1500 units, dose
to administered immediately or within 72 hours; for
large transplacental bleed, extra 100 units per mL fetal
red cells (preferably by intravenous injection),
intravenous route recommended for patients with
bleeding disorders

**To rhesus-negative woman for prevention of Rh₀(D)
sensitisation, following any potentially sensitising
episode (e.g. abortion, amniocentesis, chorionic villous
sampling) up to 12 weeks' gestation**

▸ BY INTRAMUSCULAR INJECTION, OR BY INTRAVENOUS
INJECTION

▸ Females of childbearing potential: 1000 units per
episode, dose to be administered immediately or within
72 hours, intravenous route recommended for patients
with bleeding disorders, higher doses may be required
after 12 weeks gestation

**To rhesus-negative woman for prevention of Rh₀(D)
sensitisation, antenatal prophylaxis**

▸ BY INTRAMUSCULAR INJECTION, OR BY INTRAVENOUS
INJECTION

▸ Females of childbearing potential: 1500 units, dose to be
given between weeks 28–30 of pregnancy; if infant
rhesus-positive, a further dose is still　　continued →

14

Vaccines

needed immediately or within 72 hours of delivery, intravenous route recommended for patients with bleeding disorders

To rhesus-negative woman for prevention of Rh$_0$(D) sensitisation, following Rh$_0$(D) incompatible blood transfusion
▸ BY INTRAVENOUS INJECTION
▸ Females of childbearing potential: 50 units per mL of transfused rhesus-positive blood, alternatively 100 units per of mL of erythrocyte concentrate, intravenous route recommended for patients with bleeding disorders

● CAUTIONS Immunoglobulin A deficiency · possible interference with live virus vaccines
CAUTIONS, FURTHER INFORMATION
▸ MMR vaccine MMR vaccine may be given in the postpartum period with anti-D (Rh$_0$) immunoglobulin injection provided that separate syringes are used and the products are administered into different limbs. If blood is transfused, the antibody response to the vaccine may be inhibited—measure rubella antibodies after 6–8 weeks and revaccinate if necessary.
● INTERACTIONS → Appendix 1: immunoglobulins
● SIDE-EFFECTS
▸ Uncommon Chills · fever · headache · malaise · skin reactions
▸ Rare or very rare Arthralgia · dyspnoea · hypersensitivity · hypotension · nausea · tachycardia · vomiting
▸ Frequency not known Intravascular haemolysis
● HANDLING AND STORAGE Care must be taken to store all immunological products under the conditions recommended in the product literature, otherwise the preparation may become ineffective. **Refrigerated storage** is usually necessary; many immunoglobulins need to be stored at 2–8°C and not allowed to freeze. Immunoglobulins should be protected from light. Opened multidose vials must be used within the period recommended in the product literature.
● NATIONAL FUNDING/ACCESS DECISIONS
For full details see funding body website
NICE decisions
▸ Routine antenatal anti-D prophylaxis for rhesus-negative women (August 2008) NICE TA156 Recommended

● MEDICINAL FORMS There can be variation in the licensing of different medicines containing the same drug.
Solution for injection
▸ D-Gam (Bio Products Laboratory Ltd)
Anti-D (RHO) immunoglobulin 500 unit D-Gam Anti-D immunoglobulin 500unit solution for injection vials | 1 vial PoM £38.25
Anti-D (RHO) immunoglobulin 1500 unit D-Gam Anti-D immunoglobulin 1,500unit solution for injection vials | 1 vial PoM £58.00
▸ Rhophylac (CSL Behring UK Ltd)
Anti-D (RHO) immunoglobulin 750 unit per 1 ml Rhophylac 1,500units/2ml solution for injection pre-filled syringes | 1 pre-filled disposable injection PoM £76.50

Cytomegalovirus immunoglobulin

16-Apr-2020

● INDICATIONS AND DOSE
Prophylaxis of cytomegalovirus infection in patients taking immunosuppressants, particularly transplant recipients (specialist use only)
▸ BY INTRAVENOUS INFUSION
▸ Adult: (consult product literature)

● CONTRA-INDICATIONS Selective IgA deficiency with IgA antibodies
● CAUTIONS Interference with live virus vaccines
CAUTIONS, FURTHER INFORMATION
▸ Interference with live virus vaccines Cytomegalovirus immunoglobulin may impair the immune response to live virus vaccines; such vaccines should only be given 3 months after CMV immunoglobulin treatment. Patients receiving measles vaccines should have their antibody status checked as impairment of immune response may persist for up to 1 year.
● INTERACTIONS → Appendix 1: immunoglobulins
● SIDE-EFFECTS Arthralgia · back pain · chills · cutaneous lupus erythematosus · dizziness · embolism and thrombosis · fatigue · fever · haemolysis · haemolytic anaemia · headache · hypotension · infusion related reaction · meningitis aseptic · myocardial infarction · nausea · neutropenia · renal impairment · skin reactions · stroke · transfusion-related acute lung injury · vomiting
● MONITORING REQUIREMENTS
▸ Manufacturer advises monitor for signs of infusion-related reactions during and for at least one hour after each infusion in patients receiving cytomegalovirus immunoglobulin for the first time, or following a prolonged period between treatments, or when a different human immunoglobulin has been used previously; monitor all other patients for at least 20 minutes after each infusion—in case of reaction, reduce rate or stop infusion as clinically appropriate.
▸ Manufacturer advises monitor urine output and serum creatinine.
● HANDLING AND STORAGE Care must be taken to store all immunological products under the conditions recommended in the product literature, otherwise the preparation may become ineffective. **Refrigerated storage** is usually necessary; many immunoglobulins need to be stored at 2–8°C and not allowed to freeze. Immunoglobulins should be protected from light. Opened multidose vials must be used within the period recommended in the product literature.

● MEDICINAL FORMS There can be variation in the licensing of different medicines containing the same drug.
Solution for infusion
▸ Cytotect CP Biotest (Biotest (UK) Ltd)
Cytomegalovirus immunoglobulin human 100 unit per 1 ml Cytotect CP Biotest 5,000units/50ml solution for infusion vials | 1 vial PoM £917.70
Cytotect CP Biotest 1,000units/10ml solution for infusion vials | 1 vial PoM £183.54

Hepatitis B immunoglobulin

06-Mar-2020

● INDICATIONS AND DOSE
Prophylaxis against hepatitis B infection
▸ BY INTRAMUSCULAR INJECTION
▸ Adult: 500 units, dose to be administered as soon as possible after exposure; ideally within 12–48 hours, but no later than 7 days after exposure

Prophylaxis against hepatitis B infection, after exposure to hepatitis B virus-contaminated material
▸ BY INTRAVENOUS INFUSION
▸ Adult: Dose to be administered as soon as possible after exposure, but no later than 72 hours (consult product literature)

Prevention of hepatitis B in haemodialysed patients
▸ BY INTRAVENOUS INFUSION
▸ Adult: (consult product literature)

Prophylaxis against re-infection of transplanted liver
▶ BY INTRAVENOUS INFUSION
▶ Adult: (consult product literature)

Prevention of hepatitis B re-infection more than 6 months **after liver transplantation in stable HBV-DNA negative patients**
▶ BY SUBCUTANEOUS INJECTION
▶ Adult (body-weight up to 75 kg): 500 units once weekly, increased if necessary up to 1000 units once weekly, dose to be started 2–3 weeks after last dose of intravenous hepatitis B immunoglobulin
▶ Adult (body-weight 75 kg and above): 1000 units once weekly, dose to be started 2–3 weeks after last dose of intravenous hepatitis B immunoglobulin

● CAUTIONS IgA deficiency · interference with live virus vaccines

● INTERACTIONS → Appendix 1: immunoglobulins

● SIDE-EFFECTS
▶ **Uncommon** Abdominal pain upper · headache
▶ **Rare or very rare** Cardiac discomfort · fatigue · hypersensitivity · hypertension · hypotension · muscle spasms · nasopharyngitis · oropharyngeal pain · palpitations · skin reactions

● PRESCRIBING AND DISPENSING INFORMATION Vials containing 200 units or 500 units (for intramuscular injection), available from selected Public Health England and NHS laboratories (except for Transplant Centres), also available from BPL.

● HANDLING AND STORAGE Care must be taken to store all immunological products under the conditions recommended in the product literature, otherwise the preparation may become ineffective. **Refrigerated storage** is usually necessary; many immunoglobulins need to be stored at 2–8°C and not allowed to freeze. Immunoglobulins should be protected from light. Opened multidose vials must be used within the period recommended in the product literature.

● MEDICINAL FORMS There can be variation in the licensing of different medicines containing the same drug.

Solution for injection
▶ Hepatitis B immunoglobulin (Non-proprietary)
    Hepatitis B immunoglobulin human 200 unit Hepatitis B immunoglobulin human 200unit solution for injection vials | 1 vial [PoM] £200.00
    Hepatitis B immunoglobulin human 500 unit Hepatitis B immunoglobulin human 500unit solution for injection vials | 1 vial [PoM] £500.00
▶ Zutectra (Biotest (UK) Ltd)
    Zutectra 500units/1ml solution for injection pre-filled syringes | 5 syringe [PoM] £1,500.00

Solution for infusion
▶ Hepatect CP (Biotest (UK) Ltd)
    Hepatitis B immunoglobulin human 50 unit per 1 ml Hepatect CP 100units/2ml solution for infusion vials | 1 vial [PoM] £55.00
    Hepatect CP 2000units/40ml solution for infusion vials | 1 vial [PoM] £1,100.00
    Hepatect CP 500units/10ml solution for infusion vials | 1 vial [PoM] £275.00
    Hepatect CP 5000units/100ml solution for infusion vials | 1 vial [PoM] £2,750.00
▶ Omri-Hep-B (Imported (Israel))
    Hepatitis B immunoglobulin human 50 unit per 1 ml Omri-Hep-B 5000units/100ml solution for infusion vials | 1 vial [PoM] ▨

Normal immunoglobulin

16-Nov-2020

● INDICATIONS AND DOSE

To control outbreaks of hepatitis A
▶ BY DEEP INTRAMUSCULAR INJECTION
▶ Adult: 500 mg

Rubella in pregnancy, prevention of clinical attack
▶ BY DEEP INTRAMUSCULAR INJECTION
▶ Females of childbearing potential: 750 mg

Antibody deficiency syndromes
▶ BY SUBCUTANEOUS INFUSION
▶ Adult: (consult product literature)

SUBGAM ®

Hepatitis A prophylaxis [post-exposure]
▶ BY INTRAMUSCULAR INJECTION
▶ Adult: 1000 mg

● UNLICENSED USE
SUBGAM ® *Subgam* ® is not licensed for prophylactic use, but due to difficulty in obtaining suitable immunoglobulin products, Public Health England recommends intramuscular use for prophylaxis against Hepatitis A or rubella.

● CONTRA-INDICATIONS Patients with selective IgA deficiency who have known antibody against IgA
PRIVIGEN ® Hyperprolinaemia (contains L-proline)
FLEBOGAMMA ® DIF Hereditary fructose intolerance (contains sorbitol)
HIZENTRA ® Hyperprolinaemia (contains L-proline)
GAMMAPLEX ® Hereditary fructose intolerance (contains sorbitol)

● CAUTIONS Agammaglobulinaemia with or without IgA deficiency · hypogammaglobulinaemia with or without IgA deficiency · interference with live virus vaccines
CAUTIONS, FURTHER INFORMATION
▶ Interference with live virus vaccines Normal immunoglobulin may **interfere with the immune response to live virus vaccines** which should therefore only be given **at least 3 weeks before or 3 months after** an injection of normal immunoglobulin (this does not apply to yellow fever vaccine since normal immunoglobulin does not contain antibody to this virus).
OCTAGAM ® Falsely elevated results with blood glucose testing systems (contains maltose)

● INTERACTIONS → Appendix 1: immunoglobulins

● SIDE-EFFECTS
▶ **Common or very common**
▶ With intramuscular use Chills
▶ With subcutaneous use Diarrhoea · dizziness · drowsiness · fatigue · gastrointestinal discomfort · headaches · hypotension · local reaction · myalgia · nausea · pain · skin reactions
▶ **Uncommon**
▶ With intramuscular use Dizziness · fatigue · feeling hot · headache · nausea · pain · skin reactions
▶ With subcutaneous use Paraesthesia
▶ **Rare or very rare**
▶ With intramuscular use Abdominal pain · arthralgia · musculoskeletal stiffness · myalgia · peripheral coldness · tremor
▶ **Frequency not known**
▶ With intramuscular use Chest discomfort · dyspnoea · facial swelling · fever · flushing · hyperhidrosis · hypertension · hypotension · malaise · oral paraesthesia · pallor · paraesthesia · tachycardia · vomiting
SIDE-EFFECTS, FURTHER INFORMATION Adverse reactions are more likely to occur in patients receiving normal immunoglobulin for the first time, or following a prolonged period between treatments, or when a different brand of normal immunoglobulin is administered.

● MONITORING REQUIREMENTS Monitor for acute renal failure; consider discontinuation if renal function deteriorates. Intravenous preparations with added sucrose have been associated with cases of renal dysfunction and acute renal failure.

14

Vaccines

- **DIRECTIONS FOR ADMINISTRATION**
  Preparations for subcutaneous use May be administered by intramuscular injection if subcutaneous route not possible; intramuscular route **not** for patients with thrombocytopenia or other bleeding disorders.
  GAMUNEX ® Use Glucose 5% intravenous infusion if dilution prior to infusion is required.
  KIOVIG ® Use Glucose 5% intravenous infusion if dilution prior to infusion is required.

- **PRESCRIBING AND DISPENSING INFORMATION** Antibody titres can vary widely between normal immunoglobulin preparations from different manufacturers—formulations are **not interchangeable**; patients should be maintained on the same formulation throughout long-term treatment to avoid adverse effects.

  ‣ With intramuscular use Available from the Centre for Infections and other regional Public Health England offices (for contacts and control of outbreaks only).

- **HANDLING AND STORAGE** Care must be taken to store all immunological products under the conditions recommended in the product literature, otherwise the preparation may become ineffective. **Refrigerated storage** is usually necessary; many immunoglobulins need to be stored at 2–8°C and not allowed to freeze. Immunoglobulins should be protected from light. Opened multidose vials must be used within the period recommended in the product literature.

- **MEDICINAL FORMS** There can be variation in the licensing of different medicines containing the same drug.
  Solution for injection
  ELECTROLYTES: May contain Sodium
  ‣ Hizentra (CSL Behring UK Ltd)
  Normal immunoglobulin human 200 mg per 1 ml Hizentra 2g/10ml solution for injection pre-filled syringes | 1 pre-filled disposable injection PoM £138.00
  ‣ Subgam (Bio Products Laboratory Ltd)
  Normal immunoglobulin human 160 mg per 1 ml Subgam 1g/6.25ml solution for injection vials | 1 vial PoM £50.00
  Subgam 4g/25ml solution for injection vials | 1 vial PoM £200.00
  Subgam 2g/12.5ml solution for injection vials | 1 vial PoM £100.00
  Solution for infusion
  EXCIPIENTS: May contain Glucose, maltose, sorbitol, sucrose
  ‣ Normal immunoglobulin (Non-proprietary)
  Normal immunoglobulin human 100 mg per 1 ml Normal immunoglobulin human 5g/50ml solution for infusion vials | 1 vial PoM Ⓢ (Hospital only)
  Normal immunoglobulin human 2.5g/25ml solution for infusion vials | 1 vial PoM Ⓢ
  Normal immunoglobulin human 20g/200ml solution for infusion vials | 1 vial PoM Ⓢ (Hospital only)
  Normal immunoglobulin human 10g/100ml solution for infusion vials | 1 vial PoM Ⓢ (Hospital only)
  Normal immunoglobulin human 30g/300ml solution for infusion vials | 1 vial PoM Ⓢ
  ‣ Flebogammadif (Grifols UK Ltd)
  Normal immunoglobulin human 50 mg per 1 ml Flebogamma DIF 2.5g/50ml solution for infusion vials | 1 vial PoM £150.00
  Flebogamma DIF 10g/200ml solution for infusion vials | 1 vial PoM £600.00
  Flebogamma DIF 5g/100ml solution for infusion vials | 1 vial PoM £300.00
  Flebogamma DIF 20g/400ml solution for infusion vials | 1 vial PoM £1,200.00
  ‣ Gammaplex (Bio Products Laboratory Ltd)
  Normal immunoglobulin human 50 mg per 1 ml Gammaplex 10g/200ml solution for infusion vials | 1 vial PoM £418.00 (Hospital only)
  Gammaplex 5g/100ml solution for infusion vials | 1 vial PoM £209.00 (Hospital only)
  Gammaplex 20g/400ml solution for infusion vials | 1 vial PoM £836.00 (Hospital only)
  Normal immunoglobulin human 100 mg per 1 ml Gammaplex 5g/50ml solution for infusion vials | 1 vial PoM £325.00 (Hospital only)
  Gammaplex 10g/100ml solution for infusion vials | 1 vial PoM £650.00 (Hospital only)

Gammaplex 20g/200ml solution for infusion vials | 1 vial PoM £1,300.00 (Hospital only)
‣ Gamunex (Grifols UK Ltd)
Normal immunoglobulin human 100 mg per 1 ml Gamunex 10% 1g/10ml solution for infusion vials | 1 vial PoM £50.00
Gamunex 10% 10g/100ml solution for infusion vials | 1 vial PoM £500.00 (Hospital only)
Gamunex 10% 20g/200ml solution for infusion vials | 1 vial PoM £1,000.00 (Hospital only)
Gamunex 10% 5g/50ml solution for infusion vials | 1 vial PoM £250.00 (Hospital only)
‣ Hizentra (CSL Behring UK Ltd)
Normal immunoglobulin human 200 mg per 1 ml Hizentra 2g/10ml solution for infusion vials | 1 vial PoM £138.00
Hizentra 1g/5ml solution for infusion vials | 1 vial PoM £69.00
Hizentra 4g/20ml solution for infusion vials | 1 vial PoM £276.00
‣ Kiovig (Shire Pharmaceuticals Ltd)
Normal immunoglobulin human 100 mg per 1 ml Kiovig 5g/50ml solution for infusion vials | 1 vial PoM £245.00 (Hospital only)
Kiovig 20g/200ml solution for infusion vials | 1 vial PoM £980.00 (Hospital only)
Kiovig 10g/100ml solution for infusion vials | 1 vial PoM £490.00 (Hospital only)
Kiovig 30g/300ml solution for infusion vials | 1 vial PoM £1,470.00
Kiovig 2.5g/25ml solution for infusion vials | 1 vial PoM £122.50
Kiovig 1g/10ml solution for infusion vials | 1 vial PoM £49.00
‣ Octagam (Octapharma Ltd)
Normal immunoglobulin human 50 mg per 1 ml Octagam 5% 10g/200ml solution for infusion bottles | 1 bottle PoM £480.00 (Hospital only)
Octagam 5% 5g/100ml solution for infusion bottles | 1 bottle PoM £240.00 (Hospital only)
Normal immunoglobulin human 100 mg per 1 ml Octagam 10% 10g/100ml solution for infusion bottles | 1 bottle PoM £690.00 (Hospital only)
Octagam 10% 20g/200ml solution for infusion bottles | 1 bottle PoM £1,380.00 (Hospital only)
Octagam 10% 5g/50ml solution for infusion bottles | 1 bottle PoM £345.00 (Hospital only)
Octagam 10% 2g/20ml solution for infusion vials | 1 vial PoM £138.00 (Hospital only)
‣ Panzyga (Octapharma Ltd)
Normal immunoglobulin human 100 mg per 1 ml Panzyga 10g/100ml solution for infusion bottles | 1 bottle PoM £586.50 (Hospital only)
Panzyga 20g/200ml solution for infusion bottles | 1 bottle PoM £1,173.00 (Hospital only)
Panzyga 5g/50ml solution for infusion bottles | 1 bottle PoM £293.25 (Hospital only)
‣ Privigen (CSL Behring UK Ltd)
Normal immunoglobulin human 100 mg per 1 ml Privigen 5g/50ml solution for infusion vials | 1 vial PoM £270.00 (Hospital only)
Privigen 20g/200ml solution for infusion vials | 1 vial PoM £1,080.00 (Hospital only)
Privigen 10g/100ml solution for infusion vials | 1 vial PoM £540.00 (Hospital only)
Privigen 2.5g/25ml solution for infusion vials | 1 vial PoM £135.00

Rabies immunoglobulin

16-Mar-2020

- **INDICATIONS AND DOSE**
  Post-exposure treatment against rabies infection
  ▸ BY LOCAL INFILTRATION, OR BY INTRAMUSCULAR INJECTION
  ‣ Child: 20 units/kg, dose administered by infiltration in and around the cleansed wound; if wound not visible or healed or if infiltration of whole volume not possible, give remainder by intramuscular injection into anterolateral thigh (remote from vaccination site). If more than 2 mL to be given by intramuscular injection then give in divided doses at different sites, to be given in combination with rabies vaccine, not required if more than 7 days have elapsed after the first dose of vaccine, or more than 1 day after the second dose of vaccine
  ‣ Adult: 20 units/kg, dose administered by infiltration in and around the cleansed wound; if wound not visible or

healed or if infiltration of whole volume not possible, give remainder by intramuscular injection into anterolateral thigh (remote from vaccination site). If more than 5 mL to be given by intramuscular injection then give in divided doses at different sites, to be given in combination with rabies vaccine, not required if more than 7 days have elapsed after the first dose of vaccine, or more than 1 day after the second dose of vaccine

- **CAUTIONS** IgA deficiency · interference with live virus vaccines
- **INTERACTIONS** → Appendix 1: immunoglobulins
- **SIDE-EFFECTS**
- **Rare or very rare** Arthralgia · chills · fatigue · fever · headache · hypersensitivity · hypotension · influenza like illness · malaise · nausea · skin reactions · tachycardia · vomiting
- **PRESCRIBING AND DISPENSING INFORMATION** The potency of individual batches of rabies immunoglobulin from the manufacturer may vary; potency may also be described differently by different manufacturers. It is therefore critical to know the potency of the batch to be used and the weight of the patient in order to calculate the specific volume required to provide the necessary dose.

  Available from Specialist and Reference Microbiology Division, Public Health England (also from BPL).
- **HANDLING AND STORAGE** Care must be taken to store all immunological products under the conditions recommended in the product literature, otherwise the preparation may become ineffective. **Refrigerated storage** is usually necessary; many immunoglobulins need to be stored at 2–8°C and not allowed to freeze. Immunoglobulins should be protected from light. Opened multidose vials must be used within the period recommended in the product literature.
- **MEDICINAL FORMS** There can be variation in the licensing of different medicines containing the same drug.
  Solution for injection
  ▸ Rabies immunoglobulin (Non-proprietary)
    Rabies immunoglobulin human 500 unit Rabies immunoglobulin human 500unit solution for injection vials | 1 vial [PoM] £1,000.00

Tetanus immunoglobulin

16-Mar-2020

- **INDICATIONS AND DOSE**
  Post-exposure prophylaxis
  ▸ BY INTRAMUSCULAR INJECTION
  ▸ Child: Initially 250 units, then increased to 500 units, dose is only increased if more than 24 hours have elapsed or there is risk of heavy contamination or following burns
  ▸ Adult: Initially 250 units, then increased to 500 units, dose is only increased if more than 24 hours have elapsed or there is risk of heavy contamination or following burns
  Treatment of tetanus infection
  ▸ BY INTRAMUSCULAR INJECTION
  ▸ Child: 150 units/kg, dose may be given over multiple sites
  ▸ Adult: 150 units/kg, dose may be given over multiple sites

- **CAUTIONS** IgA deficiency · interference with live virus vaccines
- **INTERACTIONS** → Appendix 1: immunoglobulins
- **SIDE-EFFECTS**
- **Rare or very rare** Anaphylactic reaction · hypotension
- **Frequency not known** Arthralgia · chest pain · dizziness · dyspnoea · face oedema · oral disorders · tremor

- **HANDLING AND STORAGE** Care must be taken to store all immunological products under the conditions recommended in the product literature, otherwise the preparation may become ineffective. **Refrigerated storage** is usually necessary; many immunoglobulins need to be stored at 2–8°C and not allowed to freeze. Immunoglobulins should be protected from light. Opened multidose vials must be used within the period recommended in the product literature.
- **MEDICINAL FORMS** There can be variation in the licensing of different medicines containing the same drug.
  Solution for injection
  ▸ Tetanus immunoglobulin (Non-proprietary)
    Tetanus immunoglobulin human 250 unit Tetanus immunoglobulin human 250unit solution for injection vials | 1 vial [PoM] £250.00 DT = £170.00

Varicella-zoster immunoglobulin

16-Oct-2020

(Antivaricella-zoster Immunoglobulin)

- **INDICATIONS AND DOSE**
  Prophylaxis against varicella infection
  ▸ BY INTRAMUSCULAR INJECTION
  ▸ Adult: 1 g, to be administered as soon as possible—not later than 10 days after exposure, second dose to be given if further exposure occurs more than 3 weeks after first dose

- **CAUTIONS** IgA deficiency · interference with live virus vaccines
- **INTERACTIONS** → Appendix 1: immunoglobulins
- **SIDE-EFFECTS** Arthralgia · chills · fever · headache · hypersensitivity · hypotension · malaise · nausea · skin reactions · tachycardia · vomiting
- **DIRECTIONS FOR ADMINISTRATION** Public Health England advises normal immunoglobulin for intravenous use may be used in those unable to receive intramuscular injections.

  Manufacturer advises if a large volume (>5 mL) is to be given by intramuscular injection then administer in divided doses at different sites.
- **PRESCRIBING AND DISPENSING INFORMATION** Available from selected Public Health England and NHS laboratories (also from Bio Products Laboratory).
- **HANDLING AND STORAGE** Care must be taken to store all immunological products under the conditions recommended in the product literature, otherwise the preparation may become ineffective. **Refrigerated storage** is usually necessary; many immunoglobulins need to be stored at 2–8°C and not allowed to freeze. Immunoglobulins should be protected from light. Opened multidose vials must be used within the period recommended in the product literature.
- **MEDICINAL FORMS** There can be variation in the licensing of different medicines containing the same drug.
  Solution for injection
  ▸ Varicella-Zoster (Bio Products Laboratory Ltd)
    Varicella-Zoster immunoglobulin human 250 mg Varicella-Zoster immunoglobulin human 250mg solution for injection vials | 1 vial [PoM] £750.00 DT = £600.00

14

Vaccines

2 Post-exposure prophylaxis

IMMUNE SERA AND IMMUNOGLOBULINS >
ANTITOXINS

Bezlotoxumab

18-Aug-2017

- **DRUG ACTION** Bezlotoxumab is a human monoclonal antitoxin antibody; it binds to *Clostridioides difficile* toxin B and neutralises its activity, preventing recurrence of *Clostridioides difficile* infection.

- **INDICATIONS AND DOSE**
  Prevention of recurrence of *Clostridioides difficile* infection in patients at high risk of reinfection
  ▸ BY INTRAVENOUS INFUSION
  ▸ Adult: 10 mg/kg for 1 dose, to be administered during the course of antibacterial therapy for *Clostridioides difficile* infection

- **SIDE-EFFECTS**
  ▸ **Common or very common** Dizziness · dyspnoea · fatigue · fever · headache · hypertension · infusion related reaction · nausea

- **PREGNANCY** Manufacturer advises avoid unless essential—limited information available.

- **BREAST FEEDING** Manufacturer advises avoid—no information available.

- **DIRECTIONS FOR ADMINISTRATION** Manufacturer advises for *intravenous infusion* (*Zinplava®*), give intermittently in Glucose 5 % *or* Sodium Chloride 0.9 %; dilute requisite dose to a concentration of 1–10 mg/mL with infusion fluid; give over 60 minutes via a central venous catheter or peripheral catheter using a low-protein binding filter (0.2–5 micron).

- **HANDLING AND STORAGE** Manufacturer advises store in a refrigerator (2–8 °C)—consult product literature for further information regarding storage conditions outside refrigerator and after preparation of the infusion.

- **MEDICINAL FORMS** There can be variation in the licensing of different medicines containing the same drug.
  Solution for infusion
  EXCIPIENTS: May contain Polysorbates
  ELECTROLYTES: May contain Sodium
  ▸ Zinplava (Merck Sharp & Dohme Ltd) ▼
  Bezlotoxumab 25 mg per 1 ml Zinplava 1g/40ml concentrate for solution for infusion vials | 1 vial [PoM] £2,470.00 (Hospital only)

Botulism antitoxin

- **DRUG ACTION** A preparation containing the specific antitoxic globulins that have the power of neutralising the toxins formed by types A, B, and E of *Clostridium botulinum*.

- **INDICATIONS AND DOSE**
  Post exposure prophylaxis of botulism
  ▸ BY INTRAMUSCULAR INJECTION
  ▸ Adult: (consult product literature)

- **SIDE-EFFECTS** Hypersensitivity
  SIDE-EFFECTS, FURTHER INFORMATION It is essential to read the contra-indications, warnings, and details of sensitivity tests on the package insert. Prior to treatment checks should be made regarding previous administration of any antitoxin and history of any allergic condition, e.g. asthma, hay fever, etc.

- **PRE-TREATMENT SCREENING** All patients should be tested for sensitivity (diluting the antitoxin if history of allergy).

- **PRESCRIBING AND DISPENSING INFORMATION** Available from local designated centres, for details see TOXBASE (requires registration) www.toxbase.org. For supplies outside working hours apply to other designated centres or to the Public Health England Colindale duty doctor (Tel (020) 8200 6868). For major incidents, obtain supplies from the local blood bank.
  The BP title Botulinum Antitoxin is not used because the preparation currently in use may have a different specification.

- **MEDICINAL FORMS** No licensed medicines listed.

Diphtheria antitoxin
(Dip/Ser)

- **INDICATIONS AND DOSE**
  Passive immunisation in suspected cases of diphtheria
  ▸ BY INTRAVENOUS INFUSION
  ▸ Adult: Dose should be given without waiting for bacteriological confirmation (consult product literature)

- **CAUTIONS**
  CAUTIONS, FURTHER INFORMATION
  ▸ Hypersensitivity Hypersensitivity is common after administration; resuscitation facilities should be available. Diphtheria antitoxin is no longer used for prophylaxis because of the risk of hypersensitivity; unimmunised contacts should be promptly investigated and given antibacterial prophylaxis and vaccine.

- **SIDE-EFFECTS**
  ▸ **Common or very common** Hypersensitivity

- **PRE-TREATMENT SCREENING** Diphtheria antitoxin is derived from horse serum and reactions are common; tests for hypersensitivity should be carried out before use.

- **PRESCRIBING AND DISPENSING INFORMATION** Available from Centre for Infections (Tel (020) 8200 6868) or in Northern Ireland from Public Health Laboratory, Belfast City Hospital (Tel (028) 9032 9241).

- **MEDICINAL FORMS** There can be variation in the licensing of different medicines containing the same drug.
  Solution for injection
  ▸ Diphtheria antitoxin (Non-proprietary)
  Diphtheria antitoxin 1000 unit per 1 ml Antidiphtheria serum 10,000units/10ml solution for injection ampoules | 1 ampoule [PoM] [X]

3 Tuberculosis diagnostic test

DIAGNOSTIC AGENTS

Tuberculin purified protein derivative
(Tuberculin PPD)

- **INDICATIONS AND DOSE**
  Mantoux test
  ▸ BY INTRADERMAL INJECTION
  ▸ Child: 2 units for one dose
  ▸ Adult: 2 units for one dose
  Mantoux test (if first test is negative and a further test is considered appropriate)
  ▸ BY INTRADERMAL INJECTION
  ▸ Child: 10 units for 1 dose
  ▸ Adult: 10 units for 1 dose

DOSE EQUIVALENCE AND CONVERSION
‣ 2 units is equivalent to 0.1 mL of 20 units/mL strength.
‣ 10 units is equivalent to 0.1 mL of 100 units/mL strength.

● CAUTIONS Mantoux test Response to tuberculin may be suppressed by viral infection, sarcoidosis, corticosteroid therapy, or immunosuppression due to disease or treatment and the MMR vaccine. If a tuberculin skin test has already been initiated, then the MMR should be delayed until the skin test has been read unless protection against measles is required urgently. If a child has had a recent MMR, and requires a tuberculin test, then a 4 week interval should be observed. Apart from tuberculin and MMR, all other live vaccines can be administered at any time before or after tuberculin.

● PRESCRIBING AND DISPENSING INFORMATION Available from ImmForm (SSI brand).
The strength of tuberculin PPD in currently available products may be different to the strengths of products used previously for the Mantoux test; care is required to select the correct strength.

● MEDICINAL FORMS There can be variation in the licensing of different medicines containing the same drug. Forms available from special-order manufacturers include: solution for injection
Solution for injection
‣ Tuberculin purified protein derivative (Non-proprietary)
Tuberculin purified protein derivative 20 tuberculin unit per 1 ml Tuberculin PPD RT 23 SSI 20 tuberculin units/ml solution for injection 1.5ml vials | 1 vial 🅟
Tuberculin purified protein derivative 100 tuberculin unit per 1 ml Tuberculin PPD RT 23 SSI 100 tuberculin units/ml solution for injection 1.5ml vials | 1 vial 🅟

4 Vaccination

Vaccination, general principles

02-Sep-2020

Active immunity

Active immunity can be acquired by natural disease or by vaccination. Vaccines induce active immunity and provide immunological memory by stimulating the production of antibodies and cells involved in the immune response. As a result, the immune system is able to recognise and respond rapidly to natural infection at a later date. Antibodies can be detected in the patient's blood or serum, but even in the absence of detectable antibodies, immunological memory may still be present. Vaccines consist of either:

● a *live attenuated* form of the virus (e.g. measles, mumps and rubella vaccine) or bacteria (e.g. Bacillus Calmette-Guérin vaccine),
● *inactivated* preparations of the virus (e.g. tick-borne encephalitis vaccine) or bacteria (e.g. meningococcal vaccine),
● *inactivated toxins (toxoids)* produced by a micro-organism (e.g. tetanus and diphtheria vaccines), or
● *extracts of* a micro-organism which may be derived from the organism (e.g. pneumococcal vaccine) or produced by recombinant DNA technology (e.g. hepatitis B vaccine).

Live attenuated virus vaccines usually promote a full, long-lasting antibody response. In rare cases, a mild form of the disease may occur with some vaccines, such as a rash following a measles-containing vaccine.

Inactivated vaccines or toxoids produce an antibody response following a primary course, which may last for months or years. In most cases booster (reinforcing)

injections are required for long-term protection. To stimulate the immune system more broadly, some polysaccharide vaccines have been enhanced by conjugation (such as the *Haemophilus influenzae* type B and meningococcal group C vaccines), while some inactivated vaccines contain an adjuvant (such as aluminium hydroxide or aluminium phosphate) to enhance the antibody response. Inactivated vaccines cannot cause the disease that they are designed to prevent.

Passive immunity

Passive immunity is acquired through the transfer of antibodies from immune individuals either across the placenta, or from the transfusion of blood or blood products including immunoglobulins (for further information, see Immunoglobulins p. 1331). Protection provided by the cross-placental transfer of antibodies provides the infant with temporary protection (commonly for a few weeks to months), and is more effective against some infections (e.g. tetanus and measles) than others (e.g. polio and pertussis).

Vaccination during pregnancy

Live vaccines should not be administered routinely to pregnant females due to the theoretical risk of fetal infection; these should generally be delayed until after delivery. The Immunisation Department of Public Health England (PHE) run a UK-wide surveillance programme on the safety of certain vaccines (measles, mumps, rubella, varicella-zoster, and human papillomavirus) given inadvertently during pregnancy or shortly before conception. For advice on the reporting, risk assessment, and management of inadvertent vaccination in pregnancy, see PHE guidance: **Vaccination in pregnancy** (available at: www.gov.uk/guidance/vaccination-in-pregnancy-vip).

There is no evidence of risk from vaccinating pregnant females with inactivated vaccines; they do not replicate so cannot harm the fetus. Some inactivated vaccines are actively recommended to prevent severe complications during pregnancy or to the new-born infant, such as the influenza vaccine, and diphtheria with tetanus, pertussis and poliomyelitis vaccine.

For further information on vaccination in pregnancy, see individual vaccine treatment summaries.

Vaccines in immunosuppression and HIV infection

Almost all individuals can be safely vaccinated; in only a few individuals is vaccination either contra-indicated or should be deferred. Specialist advice should be sought when in doubt, if using live vaccines, or if there are queries about an individual's degree of immunosuppression. In some situations, the specialist may decide that the risk of a specific disease outweighs any potential risk from the vaccine. Antibody responses may be lower in immunosuppressed individuals, therefore additional vaccine doses may be required.

Live vaccines can cause severe or fatal infections in some immunosuppressed individuals due to extensive replication of the vaccine strain. Live vaccines are therefore not recommended for individuals with some types of severe primary or acquired immunodeficiency, or for those who are on or have recently received high doses of certain immunosuppressive or biological therapies.

Inactivated vaccines cannot replicate so may be given to immunosuppressed individuals.

Wherever possible, immunisation or additional booster doses for individuals with immunosuppression, should be carried out either before immunosuppression occurs or deferred until an improvement in immunity has been seen. The optimal timing for any vaccination should be based upon a judgement about the relative need for rapid protection and the likely response. For infants born to females taking immunosuppressive biological therapy during pregnancy, live vaccines should be delayed by 6 months; therefore, the infant will not be eligible to receive the rotavirus vaccine, and if indicated, will need to have their Bacillus Calmette-Guérin vaccine deferred.

Most live vaccines used in the UK immunisation schedule can be safely given to close contacts of an immunosuppressed individual. They carry a low risk of transmission (or the risk can be minimised with simple precautions) from a recently vaccinated close contact to an immunosuppressed individual. Close contacts of immunosuppressed individuals should be fully immunised according to the national Immunisation schedule p. 1341 to reduce the risk of exposure to vaccine preventable conditions, and they should also be offered the annual Influenza vaccine p. 1348.

For further information on vaccines in immunosuppresion, see Chapter 6, Contra-indications and special considerations, and Chapter 7, Immunisation of individuals with underlying medical conditions in *Immunisation against infectious disease*- 'The Green Book' (see *Useful resources*).

For further information on vaccines for individuals with HIV infection, see the British HIV Association guideline: **Use of vaccines in HIV-positive adults** (available at: www.bhiva. org/vaccination-guidelines), or the Children's HIV Association guidelines: **Vaccination of HIV infected children** and **Preparing HIV-infected children and adolescents for travel** (available at: www.chiva.org.uk).

Vaccines and asplenia, splenic dysfunction, or complement disorders

The following vaccines are recommended for individuals with asplenia, splenic dysfunction, or complement disorders (including those taking complement inhibitors) depending on the age at which their condition is diagnosed:

- Influenza vaccine p. 1373;
- Meningococcal groups A with C and W135 and Y vaccine p. 1366 and meningococcal group B vaccine (rDNA, component, adsorbed) p. 1365;
- 13-valent pneumococcal polysaccharide conjugate vaccine (adsorbed) p. 1366 and/or 23-valent pneumococcal polysaccharide vaccine p. 1367. Patients on complement inhibitor therapy with eculizumab p. 1064 are not at increased risk of pneumococcal disease and do not require 23-valent pneumococcal polysaccharide vaccine p. 1367 or additional doses of 13-valent pneumococcal polysaccharide conjugate vaccine (adsorbed) p. 1366.

Additional booster doses of other vaccines should be considered depending on the individual's underlying condition—specialist advice may be required. For information on specific indications for immunisation of vulnerable groups, see Chapter 7, Immunisation of individuals with underlying medical conditions, in *Immunisation against infectious disease*- 'The Green Book' (see *Useful resources*).

Children first diagnosed or presenting aged under 1 *year* should be immunised according to the Immunisation schedule p. 1341. During their first year they should also be given 2 doses of meningococcal groups A with C and W135 and Y vaccine p. 1366 at least 4 weeks apart, and a dose of 13-valent pneumococcal polysaccharide conjugate vaccine (adsorbed) p. 1366 (in order to have received a total of 2 doses of 13-valent *pneumococcal polysaccharide conjugate vaccine (adsorbed)* with an 8 week interval). 8 weeks following their routine 1 year booster vaccines, they should receive a booster dose of meningococcal groups A with C and W135 and Y vaccine. An additional dose of 13-valent pneumococcal polysaccharide conjugate vaccine (adsorbed) p. 1366 should be given at least 8 weeks after the routine 13-valent pneumococcal polysaccharide conjugate vaccine (adsorbed) p. 1366 booster scheduled at 1 year. After their second birthday, a dose of 23-valent pneumococcal polysaccharide vaccine p. 1367 should be given at least

8 weeks after the last dose of 13-valent pneumococcal polysaccharide conjugate vaccine (adsorbed) p. 1366. The influenza vaccine should be given annually in children aged 6 months or older.

Children first diagnosed or presenting aged 1 *year to under* 2 *years* should be immunised according to the Immunisation schedule p. 1341, including any routine vaccines due at 1 year of age if not yet administered. 8 weeks following the routine 1 year booster vaccines a dose of meningococcal groups A with C and W135 and Y vaccine should be given. An additional dose of 13-valent pneumococcal polysaccharide conjugate vaccine (adsorbed) p. 1366 should be given at least 8 weeks after the 1 year 13-valent pneumococcal polysaccharide conjugate vaccine (adsorbed) p. 1366 booster dose. After their second birthday, a dose of 23-valent pneumococcal polysaccharide vaccine p. 1367 should be given at least 8 weeks after the last dose of 13-valent pneumococcal polysaccharide conjugate vaccine (adsorbed) p. 1366. The influenza vaccine should be given annually.

Children first diagnosed or presenting aged 2 *years to under* 10 *years* should be immunised according to the Immunisation schedule p. 1341. Additionally, they should be given a dose of meningococcal groups A with C and W135 and Y vaccine and 23-valent pneumococcal polysaccharide vaccine p. 1367. For children who have not received the full routine immunisation for meningococcal group B vaccine (rDNA, component, adsorbed) p. 1365, ensure that 2 doses, 8 weeks apart have been given since their first birthday. For children who have not received any 13-valent pneumococcal polysaccharide conjugate vaccine (adsorbed) p. 1366 previously, a single dose should be given, followed by a dose of 23-valent pneumococcal polysaccharide vaccine p. 1367 at least 8 weeks later. The influenza vaccine should be given annually.

Individuals first diagnosed aged 10 *years and over* regardless of previous immunisations, should be given a dose of 23-valent pneumococcal polysaccharide vaccine p. 1367, meningococcal group B vaccine (rDNA, component, adsorbed) and meningococcal groups A with C and W135 and Y vaccine. After 4 weeks, an additional dose of meningococcal group B vaccine (rDNA, component, adsorbed) should be given. The influenza vaccine should be given annually.

Vaccines and antitoxins availability

For information on availability of vaccines and antitoxins, see individual monographs.

For antivenom, see Poisoning, emergency treatment p. 1413.

Enquiries for vaccines not available commercially can also be made to:

Vaccines and Countermeasures Response Department
Public Health England
vaccinesupply@phe.gov.uk

In Northern Ireland, enquiries for vaccines not available commercially should be directed to Northern Health and Social Care Trust's Pharmacy Services (www.northerntrust. hscni.net/services/pharmaceutical-services/).

In Scotland, information about availability of vaccines can be obtained from a Specialist in Pharmaceutical Public Health.

In Wales, enquiries for vaccines not available commercially should be directed to the Welsh Medicines Information Centre (www.wmic.wales.nhs.uk/about/contactus/).

Useful Resources

Recommendations reflect advice from *Immunisation against infectious disease*- 'The Green Book'. Public Health England, 2013. Chapters from the handbook (including updates since 2013) are available at: www.gov.uk/government/collections/immunisation-against-infectious-disease-the-green-book

Immunisation schedule

28-Sep-2020

Routine immunisations, sources of information

The Joint Committee on Vaccination and Immunisation (JCVI) have issued statements on immunisation prioritisation, and delivery of the routine human papillomavirus vaccination programme for children, during the COVID-19 pandemic, available at: tinyurl.com/yygw3ea4 and tinyurl.com/yylaflue

The following recommendations reflect advice produced by Public Health England. Recommendations specific to each vaccine can be found in *Immunisation against infectious disease*– 'The Green Book'. Public Health England at: www.gov.uk/government/collections/immunisation-against-infectious-disease-the-green-book

The immunisation schedule reflects advice from 'The complete routine immunisation schedule' produced by Public Health England (2019). For the most up to date immunisation schedule, see: www.gov.uk/government/publications/the-complete-routine-immunisation-schedule

The Influenza immunisation recommendations reflect advice from the 'National flu immunisation programme plan 2020/2021' produced by Public Health England, Department of Health and Social Care, and NHS England. For the most up-to-date letter, see: www.gov.uk/government/publications/national-flu-immunisation-programme-plan

Vaccines for the immunisation schedule should be obtained from ImmForm at: portal.immform.phe.gov.uk

Preterm birth

Babies born preterm should receive all routine immunisations based on their actual date of birth. The risk of apnoea following vaccination is increased in preterm babies, particularly in those born at or before 28 weeks gestational age. If babies at risk of apnoea are in hospital at the time of their first immunisation, they should be monitored for respiratory complications for 48–72 hours after immunisation. If a baby develops apnoea, bradycardia, or desaturation after the first immunisation, the second immunisation should also be given in hospital with similar monitoring.

Individuals with unknown or incomplete immunisation history

For children born in the UK who present with an inadequate or unknown immunisation history, investigation into immunisations received should be carried out. Outstanding doses should be administered where the routine childhood immunisation schedule has not been completed.

For advice on dosing schedules for missed vaccinations, and the immunisation of individuals coming to the UK, consult Chapter 11, The UK immunisation schedule, in *Immunisation against infectious disease*– 'The Green Book'. Public Health England, available at: www.gov.uk/government/publications/immunisation-schedule-the-green-book-chapter-11

Immunisations for healthcare and laboratory staff

Vaccine-preventable diseases that can be transmitted from person to person are a risk for staff and patients in healthcare environments, and staff in laboratory environments. Therefore, all staff must be up-to-date with their routine immunisations. In addition, specific immunisations are recommended for certain staff groups due to the risk of acquiring or passing on infection. For detailed recommendations, consult Chapter 12, Immunisation of healthcare and laboratory staff in *Immunisation against infectious disease*– 'The Green Book'. Public Health England, available at: www.gov.uk/government/publications/immunisation-of-healthcare-and-laboratory-staff-the-green-book-chapter-12

14

Vaccines

Routine immunisation schedule

When to immunise	Vaccine given and dose schedule (for details of dose, see under individual vaccines)
Neonates at risk only	▸ Bacillus Calmette-Guérin vaccine p. 1363 (at birth, see Bacillus Calmette-Guérin vaccine p. 1343). ▸ Hepatitis B vaccine p. 1370 (at birth, 4 weeks, and 1 year, see Hepatitis B vaccine p. 1347).
8 weeks	▸ Diphtheria with tetanus, pertussis, hepatitis B, poliomyelitis and haemophilus influenzae type b vaccine p. 1362 (*Infanrix hexa*®). First dose. ▸ Meningococcal group B vaccine (rDNA, component, adsorbed) p. 1365 (*Bexsero*®). First dose. ▸ Changes have been made to the immunisation schedule for children born on or after 1st January 2020, see *12 weeks*. **For children born on or before** 31st December 2019, give pneumococcal polysaccharide conjugate vaccine (adsorbed) p. 1366 (*Prevenar 13*®). First dose. ▸ Rotavirus vaccine p. 1377 (*Rotarix*®). First dose.
12 weeks	▸ Diphtheria with tetanus, pertussis, hepatitis B, poliomyelitis and haemophilus influenzae type b vaccine (*Infanrix hexa*®). Second dose. ▸ **For children born on or after 1st January 2020,** give pneumococcal polysaccharide conjugate vaccine (adsorbed) (*Prevenar 13*®). Single dose. ▸ Rotavirus vaccine (*Rotarix*®). Second dose.
16 weeks	▸ Diphtheria with tetanus, pertussis, hepatitis B, poliomyelitis and haemophilus influenzae type b vaccine (*Infanrix hexa*®). Third dose. ▸ Meningococcal group B vaccine (rDNA, component, adsorbed) (*Bexsero*®). Second dose. ▸ **For children born on or before** 31st December 2019, give pneumococcal polysaccharide conjugate vaccine (adsorbed) (*Prevenar 13*®). Second dose.
1 year (on or after first birthday)	▸ Measles, mumps and rubella vaccine, live p. 1375 (*MMR VaxPRO*® or *Priorix*®). First dose. ▸ Meningococcal group B vaccine (rDNA, component, adsorbed) (*Bexsero*®). Single booster dose. ▸ Pneumococcal polysaccharide conjugate vaccine (adsorbed) (*Prevenar 13*®). **Single booster dose regardless of birth date.** ▸ Haemophilus influenzae type b with meningococcal group C vaccine p. 1364 (*Menitorix*®). Single booster dose.

continued →

When to immunise	Vaccine given and dose schedule (for details of dose, see under individual vaccines)
2–11 years on 31st August 2020 (including children in reception class and school years 1, 2, 3, 4, 5, 6, and 7).	▸ Influenza vaccine p. 1373. Each year from September. **Note:** live attenuated influenza nasal spray is recommended (*Fluenz Tetra* ®). If contra-indicated and the child is in a clinical risk group, use the recommended alternative inactivated influenza vaccine (see Influenza vaccine p. 1348).
3 years and 4 months, or soon after	▸ Diphtheria with tetanus, pertussis and poliomyelitis vaccine p. 1362 (*Boostrix-IPV*® or *Repevax*®). Single booster dose. ▸ Measles, mumps and rubella vaccine, live (*MMR VaxPRO*® or *Priorix*®). Second dose.
11–14 years. First dose of HPV vaccine will be offered to individuals aged 12–13 years in England, Wales, and Northern Ireland, and those aged 11–13 years in Scotland. For individuals aged 15 years and over, see Human papillomavirus vaccine p. 1347.	▸ Human papillomavirus vaccines p. 1372 (*Gardasil*®). 2 dose schedule; second dose 6–24 months after first dose. Only *Gardasil*® is offered as part of the national immunisation programme. For individuals who started the schedule with *Cervarix*®, but did not complete the vaccination course, the course can be completed with *Gardasil*®. Ideally one vaccine should be used for the entire course.
13–15 years	▸ Meningococcal groups A with C and W135 and Y vaccine p. 1366 (*Nimenrix*® or *Menveo*®). Single booster dose.
13–18 years	▸ Diphtheria with tetanus and poliomyelitis vaccine p. 1361 (*Revaxis*®). Single booster dose. **Note:** Can be given at the same time as the dose of meningococcal groups A with C and W135 and Y vaccine at 13–15 years of age.
Females of child-bearing age susceptible to rubella	▸ Measles, mumps and rubella vaccine, live. Females of child-bearing age who have not received 2 doses of a rubella-containing vaccine or who do not have a positive antibody test for rubella should be offered rubella immunisation (using the MMR vaccine)—exclude pregnancy before immunisation, and avoid pregnancy for one month after vaccination.
Pregnant females	▸ Acellular pertussis-containing vaccine administered as diphtheria with tetanus, pertussis and poliomyelitis vaccine (*Boostrix-IPV*® or *Repevax*®). 1 dose from the 16th week of pregnancy, preferably after the fetal anomaly scan (weeks 18–20). ▸ Influenza vaccine (inactivated). Single dose administered from September, regardless of the stage of pregnancy (see Influenza vaccine p. 1348).

Routine immunisations during adult life

When to immunise	Vaccine given and dose schedule (for details of dose, see under individual vaccines)
Under 25 years, those entering university who are at risk of meningococcal disease	▸ Meningococcal groups A with C and W135 and Y vaccine (*Nimenrix*® or *Menveo*®). Single dose. **Note:** Should be offered to those aged under 25 years entering university who have not received the meningococcal groups A with C and W135 and Y vaccine over the age of 10 years.
During adult life, if not previously immunised or 5 dose course is incomplete	▸ Diphtheria with tetanus and poliomyelitis vaccine.
65 years	▸ Pneumococcal polysaccharide vaccine p. 1367.
From 65 years	▸ Influenza vaccine (inactivated). Each year from September (see Influenza vaccine p. 1348).
70 years	▸ Varicella-zoster vaccine p. 1378. Single dose.

Anthrax vaccine

31-Oct-2018

Overview

Anthrax vaccine p. 1363 is made from antigens from inactivated *Bacillus anthracis* adsorbed onto an adjuvant. Anthrax immunisation is indicated for individuals who handle infected animals or process infected animal products where there is a potential risk of occupational exposure to *B. anthracis*. It is also recommended for occupations where workers are at risk of one-off high level exposures to anthrax (e.g. following a deliberate or accidental release of spores).

A 4-dose regimen is used for primary immunisation; a single booster dose should be given at 10-year intervals on up to 3 occasions to workers at potential continuous low level risk of exposure to anthrax. In those with potential intermittent high level exposure, a single booster dose should be offered just before entering situations with a specific high exposure risk. If such opportunities do not arise, a single booster dose should be given at 10-year intervals on up to 3 occasions to sustain protection.

In the event of proven or high probability of exposure to anthrax spores, a single booster dose should be given, in addition to antibacterial prophylaxis, except when a dose has been given in the preceding 12 months.

Advice on the treatment of previously unvaccinated individuals with a proven or high probability of exposure to anthrax spores can be found at: www.gov.uk/government/publications/chemical-biological-radiological-and-nuclear-incidents-recognise-and-respond.

All suspected cases of anthrax must be notified to the local health protection unit. Where there is a community level outbreak, specialist advice should be sought from Public Health England (tel. 020 8200 4400) or, in Scotland, Health Protection Scotland (tel. 0140 300 1191).

Useful Resources

Recommendations reflect Chapter 13, Anthrax, in *Immunisation against infectious disease*– 'The 'Green Book'. Public Health England. February 2017.
www.gov.uk/government/publications/anthrax-the-green-book-chapter-13

Bacillus Calmette-Guérin vaccine

-Oct-2019

Overview

The Bacillus Calmette-Guérin vaccine p. 1363 (BCG vaccine) contains a live attenuated strain derived from *Mycobacterium bovis* which is indicated for the prevention of Tuberculosis p. 616.

BCG vaccine is recommended for the following individuals immunisation has not previously been carried out and they are tuberculin-negative:

all neonates and infants (aged 0–12 months) living in areas of the UK where the annual incidence of tuberculosis is 40 cases per 100 000 or greater;

all neonates and infants (aged 0–12 months) with a parent or grandparent born in a country where the annual incidence of tuberculosis is 40 cases per 100 000 or greater;

previously unvaccinated children (aged 1–5 years) with a parent or grandparent born in a country where the annual incidence of tuberculosis is 40 cases per 100 000 or greater (tuberculin testing is not usually required);

previously unvaccinated children (aged 6–15 years) with a parent or grandparent born in a country where the annual incidence of tuberculosis is 40 cases per 100 000 or greater;

previously unvaccinated children (aged under 16 years) with close contact to cases of sputum smear-positive pulmonary or laryngeal tuberculosis;

previously unvaccinated children (aged under 16 years) who were born in, or lived for at least 3 months in a country where the annual incidence of tuberculosis is 40 cases per 100 000 or greater;

previously unvaccinated individuals at occupational risk (irrespective of age). This includes healthcare workers or laboratory staff who have direct contact with patients with tuberculosis or potentially infectious clinical materials, and veterinary and abattoir staff handling animals or animal materials that could be infected with tuberculosis. BCG vaccination can also be considered for staff working with prisoners, homeless people, people with drug and alcohol misuse, and those who work with refugees and asylum seekers.

Although protection provided by BCG vaccine may decrease with time, there is no evidence that repeat vaccination offers significant additional protection and therefore repeat BCG vaccination is not recommended.

The Bacillus Calmette-Guérin vaccine is contra-indicated in all HIV-infected individuals. For advice on BCG vaccination in immunosuppressed individuals, consult Chapter 32: Tuberculosis - 'The Green Book', Public Health England (see *Useful resources*).

For advice on drug treatment, see Tuberculosis p. 616; for the treatment of infection following vaccination, seek expert advice.

Travel

The risk of a traveller acquiring tuberculosis infection depends on several factors including the incidence of tuberculosis in that country, the duration of travel, the degree of contact with the local population, the work setting of the traveller (if any), the reason for travel, and the susceptibility and age of the traveller.

BCG vaccine is recommended for previously unvaccinated, tuberculin-negative individuals aged under 16 years, or for healthcare workers at high risk of exposure to patients with tuberculosis, who intend to travel for 3 months or more in a country where the annual incidence of tuberculosis is 40 cases per 100 000 or greater, or where the risk of multi-drug resistant tuberculosis is high. The risk of tourists acquiring tuberculosis infection is low and BCG vaccine is not required if no other factors are present.

A list of countries where the annual incidence of tuberculosis is 40 cases per 100 000 or greater, is available at www.gov.uk/government/publications/tuberculosis-tb-by-country-rates-per-100000-people.

Tuberculin skin testing

The tuberculin skin test (*Mantoux test*) is used to assess an individual's sensitivity to tuberculin protein when BCG vaccination is being considered or as an aid to diagnosis of tuberculosis. A tuberculin skin test involves administration of tuberculin purified protein derivative p. 1338 by intradermal injection. It is necessary before BCG vaccination for:

- individuals aged 6 years and over;
- children aged under 6 years living in a country for more than 3 months with an annual tuberculosis incidence of 40 cases per 100 000 or greater;
- those who have had close contact with a person with known tuberculosis;
- those who have a family history of tuberculosis within the last 5 years.

BCG vaccination can be given up to three months following a negative tuberculin test.

The BCG vaccine should not be administered to an individual with a positive tuberculin test—it is unnecessary and may cause a more severe local reaction. Those with a *Mantoux test* induration of 5 mm and greater should be referred to a tuberculosis clinic for assessment of the need for further investigation and treatment.

All suspected cases of tuberculosis must be notified to the local health protection unit. Where there is a community level outbreak, specialist advice should be sought from Public Health England (tel. 020 8200 4400) or, in Scotland, Health Protection Scotland (tel. 0140 300 1191).

Useful Resources

Recommendations reflect Chapter 32, Tuberculosis, in *Immunisation against infectious disease*– 'The Green Book'. Public Health England, August 2018.
www.gov.uk/government/publications/tuberculosis-the-green-book-chapter-32

Botulism antitoxin

Overview

A polyvalent botulism antitoxin p. 1338 is available for the post-exposure prophylaxis of botulism and for the treatment of persons thought to be suffering from botulism. It specifically neutralises the toxins produced by *Clostridium botulinum* types A, B, and E. It is not effective against infantile botulism as the toxin (type A) is seldom, if ever, found in the blood in this type of infection.

Useful Resources

Advice reflects that in the handbook Immunisation against Infectious Disease (2013), which in turn reflects the guidance of the Joint Committee on Vaccination and Immunisation (JCVI). The advice also incorporates changes announced by the Chief Medical Officer and Health Department Updates. Chapters from the handbook (including updates since 2013) are available at:
www.gov.uk/government/collections/immunisation-against-infectious-disease-the-green-book

Cholera vaccine

07-Nov-2018

Overview

Oral cholera vaccine p. 1364 contains inactivated Inaba (including El-Tor biotype) and Ogawa strains of *Vibrio cholerae*, serotype O1 together with recombinant B-subunit

14

Vaccines

of the cholera toxin produced in Inaba strains of *V. cholerae*, serotype O1.

Oral cholera vaccine is licensed for adults and children from 2 years of age who are travelling to endemic or epidemic areas on the basis of current recommendations. Immunisation should be completed at least one week before potential exposure. However, there is no requirement for cholera vaccination for international travel. After a full risk assessment, immunisation can be considered for the following individuals:

- relief or disaster aid workers;
- persons with remote itineraries in areas where cholera epidemics are occurring and there is limited access to medical care;
- travellers to potential cholera risk areas, for whom vaccination is considered potentially beneficial;
- individuals at occupational risk, such as laboratory workers who may be regularly exposed to cholera.

For dosing schedule, see cholera vaccine.

Immunisation with cholera vaccine does not provide complete protection and all travellers to a country where cholera exists should be warned that scrupulous attention to food, water, and personal hygiene is essential.

All suspected cases of cholera must be notified to the local health protection unit. Where there is a community level outbreak, specialist advice should be sought from Public Health England (tel. 020 8200 4400) or, in Scotland, Health Protection Scotland (tel. 0140 300 1191).

Contacts

Contacts of patients with cholera should maintain high standards of personal hygiene to avoid becoming infected. Cholera vaccine should not be used in the management of contacts of cases or in controlling the spread of infection.

Useful Resources

Recommendations reflect Chapter 14, Cholera, in *Immunisation against infectious disease*– 'The Green Book'. Public Health England, December 2013.
www.gov.uk/government/publications/cholera-the-green-book-chapter-14

Diphtheria vaccine

Overview

Diphtheria-containing vaccines are prepared from the toxin of *Corynebacterium diphtheriae* and adsorption on aluminium hydroxide or aluminium phosphate improves antigenicity. The vaccine stimulates the production of the protective antibody. The quantity of diphtheria toxoid in a preparation determines whether the vaccine is defined as 'high dose' or 'low dose'. Vaccines containing the higher dose of diphtheria toxoid are used for primary immunisation of children under 10 years of age. Vaccines containing the lower dose of diphtheria toxoid are used for primary immunisation in adults and children over 10 years. Single-antigen diphtheria vaccine is not available and adsorbed diphtheria vaccine is given as a combination product containing other vaccines.

For primary immunisation *of children aged between 2 months and 10 years*, vaccination is recommended usually in the form of 3 doses (separated by 1-month intervals) of diphtheria with tetanus, pertussis, hepatitis B, poliomyelitis and haemophilus influenzae type b vaccine p. 1362 (*Infanrix hexa®*) (see Immunisation schedule). In unimmunised individuals aged *over 10 years* the primary course comprises of 3 doses of **adsorbed diphtheria** [low dose], **tetanus and poliomyelitis (inactivated) vaccine**.

A booster dose should be given 3 years after the primary course (this interval can be reduced to a minimum of 1 year if the primary course was delayed). Children *under 10 years* should receive *either* **adsorbed diphtheria, tetanus,** **pertussis (acellular, component) and poliomyelitis (inactivated) vaccine** *or* **adsorbed diphtheria** [low dose], **tetanus, pertussis (acellular, component) and poliomyelitis (inactivated) vaccine** . Individuals aged *over* 10 *years* should receive **adsorbed diphtheria** [low dose], **tetanus, and poliomyelitis (inactivated) vaccine**.

A second booster dose, of adsorbed diphtheria [low dose], tetanus and poliomyelitis (inactivated) vaccine, should be given 10 years after the previous booster dose (this interval can be reduced to a minimum of 5 years if previous doses were delayed).

Diphtheria-containing vaccines for children over 10 years and adults

A **low dose** of diphtheria toxoid is sufficient to recall immunity in individuals previously immunised against diphtheria but whose immunity may have diminished with time; it is insufficient to cause serious reactions in an individual who is already immune. Preparations containing low dose diphtheria should be used for adults and children *over* 10 *years*, for both primary immunisation and booster doses.

Travel

Those intending to travel to areas with a risk of diphtheria infection should be fully immunised according to the UK schedule. If more than 10 years have lapsed since completion of the UK schedule, a dose of **adsorbed diphtheria** [low dose], **tetanus and poliomyelitis (inactivated) vaccine** should be administered.

Contacts

Staff in contact with diphtheria patients or with potentially pathogenic clinical specimens or working directly with *C. diphtheriae* or *C. ulcerans* should receive a booster dose if fully immunised (with 5 doses of diphtheria-containing vaccine given at appropriate intervals); further doses should be given at 10-year intervals if risk persists. Individuals at risk who are not fully immunised should complete the primary course; a booster dose should be given after 5 years and then at 10-year intervals. **Adsorbed diphtheria** [low dose], **tetanus and poliomyelitis (inactivated) vaccine** is used for this purpose; immunity should be checked by antibody testing at least 3 months after completion of immunisation.

Advice on the management of cases, carriers, contacts and outbreaks must be sought from health protection units. The immunisation history of infected individuals and their contacts should be determined; those who have been incompletely immunised should complete their immunisation and fully immunised individuals should receive a reinforcing dose. See advice on antibacterial treatment to prevent a secondary case of diphtheria in a non-immune individual.

Useful Resources

Advice reflects that in the handbook Immunisation against Infectious Disease (2013), which in turn reflects the guidance of the Joint Committee on Vaccination and Immunisation (JCVI). The advice also incorporates changes announced by the Chief Medical Officer and Health Department Updates. Chapters from the handbook (including updates since 2013) are available at:
www.gov.uk/government/collections/immunisation-against-infectious-disease-the-green-book

Haemophilus influenzae type b conjugate vaccine

25-Nov-2020

Overview

Haemophilus influenzae type b (Hib) containing vaccines are inactivated, and are made from capsular polysaccharide xtracted from cultures of Hib bacteria. The polysaccharide conjugated with a protein (such as tetanus toxoid) to increase immunogenicity, especially in young children. The .ib conjugate vaccine is only available as a combination reparation containing other vaccines.

Hib vaccination is given as a component of the routine hildhood immunisation programme to provide protection gainst invasive Hib disease for children aged under 10 years see Immunisation schedule p. 1341). If the child's routine immunisation is delayed, children aged under 10 years hould be immunised at the earliest opportunity. Hib accination may also be given to individuals aged 10 years nd over who are considered to be at increased risk of nvasive Hib disease.

A primary course consists of 3 doses of the diphtheria with etanus, pertussis, hepatitis B, poliomyelitis and haemophilus influenzae type b vaccine p. 1362, given at weekly intervals.

Children aged under 1 year should be given a primary course, followed by a booster dose of the haemophilus influenzae type b with meningococcal group C vaccine p. 1364 at 1 year of age (usually on or after the child's first birthday). This should be given at least 4 weeks after the last .ose of Hib-containing vaccine, and where there has been a lelay, can be given up until 10 years of age. Early immunisation with a primary course may be considered for children from 6 weeks of age if required in certain circumstances, such as for travel reasons (immunisation may be given at an interval of 3 weeks for 1 dose only, with the other 2 doses completed at an interval of at least 4 weeks).

If the primary course was commenced with the pentavalent diphtheria with tetanus, poliomyelitis and haemophilus influenzae type b vaccine p. 1363, it can be completed with the diphtheria with tetanus, pertussis, hepatitis B, poliomyelitis and haemophilus influenzae type b vaccine. If interrupted, the primary course should be resumed but not repeated, allowing a 4 week interval between doses.

Children aged 1 year to under 10 years who have not been immunised against Hib need to only receive 1 dose of the haemophilus influenzae type b with meningococcal group C vaccine. However, children who have not completed a primary course of diphtheria, tetanus, pertussis and polio, should be given 3 doses of the diphtheria with tetanus, pertussis, hepatitis B, poliomyelitis and haemophilus influenzae type b vaccine at 4 weekly intervals, in order to be fully protected against diphtheria, tetanus, pertussis and polio.

For further information on vaccination of children with uncertain or incomplete immunisation status, see Chapter 11, The UK immunisation schedule, in *Immunisation against infectious disease*- 'The Green Book'.

For information on immunisation of individuals with neurological conditions, see Chapter 16, *Haemophilus influenzae* type b (Hib), in *Immunisation against infectious disease*- 'The Green Book'.

Children with immunosuppression and HIV infection (regardless of CD4 count) should be given Hib-containing vaccines according to the routine immunisation schedule (see Immunisation schedule p. 1341). Consider re-immunisation after treatment completion—specialist advice may be required. Refer to the British HIV Association and Children's HIV Association for further information on the use of Hib-containing vaccines in individuals with HIV infection. See www.bhiva.org/guidelines and www.chiva.org.uk/ for further information.

Post-exposure management of invasive *Haemophilus influenzae* type b disease

Acute meningitis caused by Hib is a notifiable disease in England, Northern Ireland and Wales. For further

information, see *Notifiable diseases* in Antibacterials, principles of therapy p. 527.

To reduce the risk of secondary invasive Hib disease in the index case and their close contacts (such as contacts in a household, or a pre-school or primary school setting), antibacterial prophylaxis and vaccination may be required. Individual risk is determined by factors such as age, health status, and immunisation history. For information on antibacterial prophylaxis, see *Haemophilus influenzae type b infection: prevention of secondary disease* in Antibacterials, use for prophylaxis p. 529.

Children aged under 10 years who are unimmunised or partially immunised against Hib disease and are either the index case, a household contact of the index case, or a contact of the index case in a pre-school or primary school setting, should complete their primary immunisation. Vaccination of the index case should occur after recovery from invasive Hib infection. For further information on primary immunisation, see *Overview*. Children aged under 10 years who have completed their age-specific primary immunisation, and individuals of any age with asplenia or splenic dysfunction, may need an additional dose of a Hib-containing vaccine. For further information on vaccination following a case of invasive Hib disease, see Public Health England guidance: **Haemophilus influenzae type b** (see *Useful resources*).

Useful Resources

Recommendations reflect Chapter 16, *Haemophilus influenzae* type b (Hib), in *Immunisation against infectious disease*- 'The Green Book'. Public Health England. March 2011.
www.gov.uk/government/publications/haemophilus-influenzae-type-hib-the-green-book-chapter-16

Revised recommendations for the prevention of secondary *Haemophilus influenzae* type b (Hib) disease. Public Health England. 2009, updated July 2013.
www.gov.uk/government/publications/haemophilus-influenzae-type-b-hib-revised-recommendations-for-the-prevention-of-secondary-cases

Hepatitis A vaccine　　　　　22-Sep-2020

Overview

The hepatitis A vaccine p. 1369 is prepared from different strains of the virus grown in human diploid cells. The inactivated vaccine is available as a monovalent vaccine (different monovalent vaccines can be used interchangeably), or in combination with hepatitis B or typhoid—vaccine choice is dependent on which infection(s) the individual requires protection from. Immunisation with normal immunoglobulin p. 1335 can be used to provide immediate protection against hepatitis A.

Pre-exposure prophylaxis

Immunisation against hepatitis A is recommended for individuals at high risk of hepatitis A exposure, those with certain underlying medical conditions, and those at risk of complications, as listed:

- laboratory staff who may be exposed to the virus;
- staff and residents of homes for those with severe learning difficulties, or where personal hygiene among patients may be poor;
- workers at risk of repeated exposure to untreated sewage;
- individuals who work with primates;
- patients with haemophilia being treated with plasma-derived clotting factors;
- patients with severe liver disease regardless of the cause (consider for those with chronic hepatitis B or C infection and for patients with milder liver disease);

- individuals travelling to or going to reside in areas of intermediate or high prevalence, see *Travel* below;
- individuals who are at risk due to their sexual behaviour (such as men who have sex with men);
- parenteral drug misusers.

Immunisation may be considered under certain circumstances for:

- food packagers and handlers where a case or outbreak occurs—advice should be sought from the local Health Protection Team;
- staff in day-care facilities where there is a community outbreak—advice should be sought from the local Health Protection Team;
- healthcare workers.

Immunisation against hepatitis A infection requires a primary pre-exposure course. The immunisation regimens for monovalent hepatitis A vaccine and hepatitis A with typhoid vaccine p. 1370 consist of a single dose. For immunisation using the combined hepatitis A and B vaccine, the dosing regimen depends on the product used, see hepatitis A and B vaccine p. 1368 for dosing schedules (including accelerated course information).

Individuals with immunosuppression and HIV infection can be given hepatitis A-containing vaccines. Consider re-immunisation—specialist advice may be required. Refer to the British HIV Association or Children's HIV Association for further information on the use of hepatitis A vaccine in HIV-positive individuals. See www.bhiva.org or www.chiva.org.uk for further information.

Boosters

A booster dose is usually given 6–12 months after the initial dose of hepatitis A-containing vaccine, and ensures immunity beyond 10 years; however, successful boosting can occur even if the second dose is delayed by several years. A further booster dose 25 years after full primary immunisation is only considered necessary if the risk of hepatits A infection is still present.

Travel

Pre-exposure immunisation is recommended for individuals travelling to or going to reside in areas of high or intermediate prevalence. Immunisation should ideally be given 2 weeks prior to departure, but can be given up to the day of departure; the use of normal immunoglobulin for travel prophylaxis is no longer recommended. Care should also be taken to avoid hepatitis A exposure through food and water. Further information on country-specific hepatitis A risk is available from the National Travel Health Network and Centre (travelhealthpro.org.uk/) and Health Protection Scotland (www.travax.nhs.uk).

Post-exposure prophylaxis

Hepatitis A (acute infectious hepatitis) is a notifiable disease in the UK. For further information, see *Notifiable diseases* in Antibacterials, principles of therapy p. 527.

A risk assessment should be carried out for the index case (particularly if infection occurs in a non-household setting), and the national standard questionnaire also completed for all probable and confirmed cases. Verbal and written guidance on the importance of good hygiene practices (such as hand washing after using the toilet, changing nappies, and before preparing food) should be given to the index case, their family and other close contacts. If sexual transmission is the likely route (particularly between men who have sex with men), advice on prevention of hepatitis A spread during sex should also be given. For further information on the management of index cases and link to the national standard questionnaire, see Public Health England (PHE) guidance: **Public Health control and management of hepatitis A** (see *Useful resources*).

Close contacts of the index case(s) should have a risk assessment as soon as possible within 14 days of exposure.

Prophylactic treatment choice for close contacts depends on susceptibility (determined by age and health status) and time since exposure. There should be a low threshold for considering someone a close contact.

Close contacts should be considered immune if they have documented history of either a completed primary course within the past 10 years, or a single dose of monovalent vaccine within the past year, or if they have previously had laboratory-confirmed hepatitis A.

Post-exposure prophylaxis is **not** required for healthy close contacts aged under 1 year not attending childcare; immunisation should be offered to all those who assist in the child's toileting to prevent tertiary infection. For close contacts aged 2–12 months attending childcare, a dose of monovalent hepatitis A vaccine [unlicensed use] should be given within 14 days of exposure. If the child contact cannot be immunised, appropriate advice should be given on enhanced hygiene in the childcare setting; if enhanced hygiene standards cannot be met, the child should be excluded from childcare for 30 days. If exclusion of the child is not possible, all carers and children aged 2 months and above in the childcare setting should be immunised. In these cases, any child that goes on to require long-term protection against hepatitis A after their first birthday, should be given the full course of 2 doses.

For healthy close contacts aged 1–59 years, a single dose of monovalent hepatitis A vaccine is recommended within 14 days of exposure. A risk assessment is required to determine any continued risk of hepatitis A infection. To ensure long term protection, a second dose should be given after 6–12 months.

For close contacts who have chronic liver disease (including chronic hepatitis B or C infection), HIV infection (with a CD4 count < 200 cells per microlitre), are immunosuppressed, or are aged 60 years or over, normal immunoglobulin in addition to monovalent hepatitis A vaccine is recommended within 14 days of exposure (up to 28 days in those with chronic liver disease). To provide long term protection, a second dose should be given after 6–12 months.

Refer to the British HIV Association or Children's HIV Association for further information on the use of hepatitis A vaccine p. 1369 in HIV-positive individuals. See www.bhiva.org or www.chiva.org.uk for further information.

In households with more than one close contact, all unvaccinated household contacts seen within 8 weeks of jaundice onset in the index case, should be given the monovalent hepatitis A vaccine to prevent tertiary spread within the household.

For further information on the management of susceptible close contacts and for information on outbreaks, see PHE guidance: **Public Health control and management of hepatitis A** (see *Useful resources*); and for further information on normal immunoglobulin, see Immunoglobulins p. 1331.

Useful Resources

Recommendations reflect Chapter 17, Hepatitis A, in *Immunisation against infectious disease*- 'The Green Book'. Public Health England. December 2013.
www.gov.uk/government/publications/hepatitis-a-the-green-book-chapter-17

Public health control and management of hepatitis A. Public Health England. June 2017.
www.gov.uk/government/publications/hepatitis-a-infection-prevention-and-control-guidance

Hepatitis B vaccine

Overview

Hepatitis B vaccine p. 1370 contains inactivated hepatitis B virus surface antigen (HBsAg) adsorbed onto an adjuvant. It is made biosynthetically using recombinant DNA technology.

From August 2017, vaccination against hepatitis B is recommended as part of the **routine immunisation schedule**. Primary immunisation (see *Routine immunisation schedule*) requires 3 doses, administered at intervals of 1 month from the age of 2 months, to be given as part of the combined diphtheria with tetanus, pertussis, hepatitis B, poliomyelitis and haemophilus influenzae type b vaccine p. 1362 (*Infanrix hexa®*).

As part of the **selective neonatal immunisation programme**, vaccination is recommended for neonates whose mothers have had acute hepatitis B during pregnancy or are positive for hepatitis B surface antigen (regardless of e-antigen markers). Hepatitis B vaccination is started immediately after birth with a dose of the monovalent hepatitis B vaccine (no later than 24 hours after delivery), followed by a second dose at 4 weeks; the routine immunisation combination vaccine (*Infanrix hexa®*) at weeks 8, 12 and 16; and a further dose of the monovalent hepatitis B vaccine at one year of age.

Neonates born to highly infectious mothers should also receive hepatitis B immunoglobulin p. 1334 at the same time as the first dose of monovalent hepatitis B vaccine, but administered at a different site—more detailed guidance is given in the handbook *Immunisation against Infectious Disease* (www.gov.uk/government/publications/hepatitis-b-the-green-book-chapter-18).

Following **significant exposure to hepatitis B** (e.g. through needle-stick injury or unprotected sex) and for **pre-exposure prophylaxis in high-risk groups**, an 'accelerated schedule' using the single, monovalent hepatitis B vaccine is recommended immediately, with the second dose given 1 month after the initial dose, and the third dose given 2 months after the initial dose. For those at continued high risk following exposure, a fourth dose should be given 12 months after the first dose. More detailed guidance is given in the handbook *Immunisation against Infectious Disease*.

Specific hepatitis B immunoglobulin can also be indicated for use with the vaccine in those accidentally inoculated and in neonates at special risk of infection. If hepatitis B immunoglobulin is indicated, it should be given as soon as possible, ideally at the same time or within 24 hours of the first dose of vaccine, but not after seven days have elapsed since exposure. See also *Hepatitis B immunoglobulin* in Immunoglobulins p. 1331.

In the UK, groups at high-risk of hepatitis B include:

- parenteral drug misusers, their sexual partners, and household contacts; other drug misusers who are likely to 'progress' to injecting;
- individuals who change sexual partners frequently;
- close family contacts of a case or individual with chronic hepatitis B infection;
- individuals with haemophilia, those receiving regular blood transfusions or blood products, and carers responsible for the administration of such products;
- patients with chronic renal failure including those on haemodialysis. Haemodialysis patients should be monitored for antibodies annually and re-immunised if necessary. Home carers (of dialysis patients) should be vaccinated;
- individuals with chronic liver disease;
- healthcare personnel (including trainees) who have direct contact with blood or blood-stained body fluids or with patients' tissues;
- laboratory staff who handle material that may contain the virus;
- other occupational risk groups such as morticians and embalmers;
- staff and patients of day-care or residential accommodation for those with severe learning difficulties;
- staff and inmates of custodial institutions;
- those travelling to areas of high or intermediate prevalence who are at increased risk or who plan to remain there for lengthy periods;
- families adopting children from countries with a high or intermediate prevalence of hepatitis B;
- foster carers and their families.

Following a primary course of immunisation, most people do not require a reinforcing dose of a hepatitis B-containing vaccine. A single booster dose should be offered to healthcare workers approximately five years after primary immunisation, to patients on renal dialysis with anti-HBs levels below 10mlU/mL, and at the time of a subsequent significant exposure.

Immunisation does not eliminate the need for commonsense precautions for avoiding the risk of infection from known carriers by the routes of infection which have been clearly established, consult *Guidance for Clinical Health Care Workers: Protection against Infection with Blood-borne Viruses* (available at www.dh.gov.uk/).

Accidental inoculation of hepatitis B virus-infected blood into a wound, incision, needle-prick, or abrasion may lead to infection, whereas it is unlikely that indirect exposure to a carrier will do so.

A combined hepatitis A and B vaccine p. 1368 is also available.

Useful Resources

Advice reflects that in the handbook Immunisation against Infectious Disease (2013), which in turn reflects the guidance of the Joint Committee on Vaccination and Immunisation (JCVI). The advice also incorporates changes announced by the Chief Medical Officer and Health Department Updates. Chapters from the handbook (including updates since 2013) are available at:
www.gov.uk/government/collections/immunisation-against-infectious-disease-the-green-book

Human papillomavirus vaccine

24-Jul-2020

Overview

The human papillomavirus vaccines p. 1372 consist of virus-like particles prepared from the major protein of the viral coat or capsid and mimic the structure of the native virus, but do not contain any viral DNA. The vaccines are available as a bivalent vaccine (*Cervarix®*, containing human papillomavirus (HPV) types 16 and 18), a quadrivalent vaccine (*Gardasil®*, containing HPV types 6, 11, 16 and 18), and a nine-valent vaccine (*Gardasil 9®*, containing HPV types 6, 11, 16, 18, 31, 33, 45, 52 and 58). All are adjuvanted and used for the prevention of cervical and anal cancers, and pre-cancerous genital (cervical, vulvar, and vaginal) and anal lesions associated with HPV types 16 and 18. *Gardasil®* and *Gardasil 9®* are also effective at preventing genital warts. The vaccines may also provide some cross-protection against infection caused by other high-risk HPV types.

Although there is emerging evidence on interchangeability of the HPV vaccines, the same vaccine product should be used for an entire course. Only *Gardasil®* is offered as part of the national HPV programme and is recommended for eligible individuals aged 11 to 25 years, and for men who have sex with men aged up to and including 45 years of age.

14

Vaccines

The Joint Committee on Vaccination and Immunisation have issued a statement on delivery of the routine HPV vaccination programme to eligible children during the COVID-19 pandemic, available at: tinyurl.com/yylaflue.

As the vaccines do not protect against all strains of HPV, safe sex precautions should always be practiced; and for all females, routine cervical screening should continue at the scheduled age.

Children aged 9 to 14 years
The human papillomavirus vaccines are licensed for individuals from 9 years of age, however, vaccination in children aged 9 to 10 years is not offered as part of the national programme. A 2 dose schedule is recommended for children who receive the first dose before the age of 15 years. The first dose is usually given to children from 11 years, with the second dose given 6–24 months after the first dose. See Immunisation schedule p. 1341 for guidance on immunisation in different countries within the UK.

2 doses given less than 6 months apart should not be considered adequate to provide long term protection. A third dose should be given according to human papillomavirus vaccines dosing schedule.

Children and adults aged 15 to 25 years
Under the national programme in England, individuals remain eligible to receive the HPV vaccine up to the age of 25 years if they did not receive the vaccine when scheduled. A 3 dose schedule is recommended, with the second and third dose given 1 month and 4–6 months after the first dose respectively. All 3 doses should be given within a 12-month period (see human papillomavirus vaccines).

In cases where the second dose is given late and there is a high likelihood that the individual will not return, or it is not practical for the third dose to be given after three months, then the third dose can be given at least one month after the second dose.

Where appropriate, immunisation with the HPV vaccine should be offered to individuals aged under 25 years coming into the UK, as they may not have been offered protection in their country of origin. If they are aged 25 years and over, and commenced, but did not complete their vaccination, it is reasonable to complete their vaccination in the UK.

Vaccination of men who have sex with men and other at risk individuals
Men aged 15 to 45 years, who have sex with other men and attend Specialist Sexual Health Services or HIV clinics are eligible for vaccination if they have not previously been vaccinated. Immunisation should still be offered to eligible men who have sex with men, regardless of CD4 cell count, antiretroviral therapy use, viral load, or if known to be immunocompromised at the time of immunisation. A 3 dose schedule of *Gardasil*® should be given, with administration of doses aligned with clinic appointments. All 3 doses should be given within a 24 month period, but if the course has not been completed before the age of 46, it can still be completed provided the first dose was given as part of the pilot or national programme.

There may be considerable benefit in offering the HPV vaccination to individuals who attend Sexual Health Services or HIV clinics, who are not eligible under the national programme and are deemed to have a similar risk profile to that seen in men who have sex with men. This includes some transgender individuals, sex workers, and men and women living with HIV infection. For these individuals a 3 dose schedule of *Gardasil*® is recommended.

Refer to the British HIV Association for further information on the use of human papillomavirus vaccines in individuals with HIV infection. See www.bhiva.org/guidelines for further information.

Booster doses
Protection from human papillomavirus vaccines is maintained for at least 10 years, although protection is expected to last longer. There is no recommendation for the need for booster doses.

Useful Resources
Recommendations reflect Chapter 18a, Human papillomavirus, in *Immunisation against infectious disease*-'The Green Book'. Public Health England, July 2019. www.gov.uk/government/publications/human-papillomavirus-hpv-the-green-book-chapter-18a

HPV vaccination programme for men who have sex with men (MSM) - Clinical and operational guidance. Public Health England, April 2018. www.gov.uk/government/collections/hpv-vaccination-for-men-who-have-sex-with-men-msm-programme

Influenza vaccine

20-Aug-2020

Overview
While most viruses are antigenically stable, the influenza viruses A and B (especially A) are constantly altering their antigenic structure as indicated by changes in the haemagglutinins (H) and neuraminidases (N) on the surface of the viruses. It is essential that influenza vaccine p. 1373 in use contain the H and N components of the prevalent strain or strains as recommended each year by the World Health Organization.

The influenza vaccines recommended for immunisation are the adjuvanted trivalent influenza vaccine (inactivated), high dose trivalent influenza vaccine (inactivated), cell-grown quadrivalent influenza vaccine (inactivated), egg-grown quadrivalent influenza vaccine (inactivated), and live attenuated influenza vaccine. The choice of vaccine is dependent on the person's age and contra-indications.

The ideal time for immunisation is between September and early November.

Immunisation is recommended *for individuals at high risk* of serious complications from influenza, and to reduce transmission of infection. In the national flu immunisation programme 2020/2021, influenza vaccination is recommended for the following eligible groups:

- Individuals aged 6 months and over in a clinical risk group, such as those with:
  ‣ chronic respiratory disease;
  ‣ chronic heart disease;
  ‣ chronic liver disease;
  ‣ chronic renal disease at stage 3, 4, or 5;
  ‣ chronic neurological disease;
  ‣ diabetes mellitus;
  ‣ splenic dysfunction or asplenia;
  ‣ immunosuppression because of disease or treatment (including prolonged systemic corticosteroid treatment [for over 1 month at dose equivalents of prednisolone p. 718: *adult and child over 20 kg*, 20 mg or more daily; *child under 20 kg*, 1 mg/kg or more daily], and chemotherapy);
  ‣ HIV infection (regardless of immune status);
  ‣ morbid obesity (BMI of 40 kg/m^2 and above);
  ‣ learning disability.
- All children aged 2–11 years on 31st August 2020 (including those in reception class and school years 1, 2, 3, 4, 5, 6, and 7).
- All pregnant females (including those who become pregnant during the flu season).
- All adults aged 65 years and over (including those who turn 65 by 31st March 2021).

Residents of long-stay residential homes or other specific long-stay facilities, where rapid spread is likely to follow introduction of infection and cause high morbidity and mortality (this does not include, for instance, prisons, young offender institutions, or university halls of residence).

Individuals who receive a carer's allowance, or who are the main carer of an older or disabled individual whose welfare may be at risk if the carer falls ill.

Household contacts of those on the *NHS Shielded Patient List* or of immunocompromised individuals.

Frontline health and social care workers.

In the national flu immunisation programme 2020/2021, vaccination may also be further extended in November and December to adults aged between 50–64 years subject to vaccine supply. The extension will be phased to allow prioritisation of individuals in at-risk groups.

Children aged 6 months to less than 2 years who are in clinical risk groups should be offered the egg-grown quadrivalent inactivated influenza vaccine.

Children aged 2–17 years (including those in a clinical risk group) should be offered the live attenuated influenza vaccine, administered as a nasal spray (*Fluenz tetra*®). The live attenuated vaccine is thought to provide broader protection than inactivated vaccines. Children aged 2–11 years *not* in a clinical risk group whose parent refuses the live attenuated vaccine being given, may be offered the egg-grown or cell-grown inactivated influenza vaccine as an alternative where possible. For children *not* in a clinical risk group who have a severely immunocompromised household contact, the egg-grown or cell-grown inactivated influenza vaccine should be offered. For children in a clinical risk group in whom the live attenuated vaccine is contra-indicated or otherwise unsuitable, offer the:

- egg-grown quadrivalent inactivated influenza vaccine in children aged less than 9 years;
- cell-grown quadrivalent inactivated influenza vaccine in children aged 9 years and over who are vaccinated in a GP practice—if unavailable, GPs should offer the egg-grown quadrivalent inactivated influenza vaccine;
- egg-grown quadrivalent inactivated influenza vaccine to the small number of children aged 9 years and over who are vaccinated in a primary school setting.

Children aged 6 months to less than 9 years in a clinical risk group who have not had the influenza vaccine previously, should be offered 2 doses of the appropriate influenza vaccine, at least 4 weeks apart.

Children aged less than 9 years *not* in a clinical risk group who have not had the influenza vaccine previously and in whom the inactivated influenza vaccine is indicated, should be offered 2 doses, at least 4 weeks apart.

Adults aged 18 to 64 years in a clinical risk group or other eligible groups, should be offered the cell-grown quadrivalent inactivated influenza vaccine or as an alternative, the egg-grown quadrivalent inactivated influenza vaccine.

Pregnant females should be offered either the cell-grown quadrivalent inactivated influenza vaccine or as an alternative, the egg-grown quadrivalent inactivated influenza vaccine.

Adults aged 65 years and over (including those who turn 65 by 31st March 2021) should be offered the adjuvanted trivalent inactivated influenza vaccine; if unavailable, the cell-grown quadrivalent inactivated influenza vaccine is a suitable alternative. The high dose trivalent inactivated influenza vaccine is equally suitable but is **not eligible for reimbursement under the NHS flu vaccination 2020/2021 programme**.

For further information on the annual influenza programme, see PHE collection: **Annual flu programme** (available at: www.gov.uk/government/collections/annual-flu-programme); and for information on pandemic influenza,

avian influenza, and swine influenza, see www.gov.uk/government/collections/pandemic-flu-public-health-response, www.gov.uk/guidance/avian-influenza-bird-flu, and www.gov.uk/guidance/swine-influenza.

For the management of influenza, see Influenza p. 699.

Useful Resources

Recommendations reflect Chapter 19, Influenza, in *Immunisation against infectious disease*- 'The Green Book'. Public Health England. April 2019.
www.gov.uk/government/publications/influenza-the-green-book-chapter-19

National flu immunisation programme plan 2020/2021—update. Public Health England, Department of Health and Social Care, and NHS England. August 2020.
www.gov.uk/government/publications/national-flu-immunisation-programme-plan

Japanese encephalitis vaccine 14-Nov-2018

Overview

Japanese encephalitis is a mosquito-borne viral encephalitis caused by a *Flavivirus*.

Japanese encephalitis vaccine p. 1374 (*IXIARO*)® is an inactivated vaccine adsorbed onto an adjuvant. It is recommended for individuals who are going to reside in an area where Japanese encephalitis is endemic or epidemic. Travellers to South and South-East Asia and the Far East should be immunised if staying for a month or longer in endemic areas during the transmission season. Other travellers with shorter exposure periods should also be immunised if the risk is considered sufficient. Immunisation is also recommended for laboratory staff at risk of exposure to the virus.

The primary immunisation course of 2 doses should be completed at least one week before potential exposure to Japanese encephalitis virus.

In adults (aged under 65 years) and children (aged 2 months and over) at ongoing risk (including laboratory staff and long-term travellers), a single booster dose should be given 12 months after the primary immunisation course. A booster dose can be considered in adults aged 65 years and over, but the immune response is lower than in younger adults. For other travellers, a single booster dose should be given within 12–24 months after primary immunisation, before potential re-exposure to the Japanese encephalitis virus. Travellers aged 18–64 years should be offered a second booster dose at 10 years if they remain at risk.

Cases of Japanese encephalitis should be managed with supportive treatment.

Up-to-date information on the risk of Japanese encephalitis in specific countries can be obtained from the National Travel Health Network and Centre.

Useful Resources

Recommendations reflect Chapter 20, Japanese encephalitis, in *Immunisation against infectious disease*– 'The Green book'. Public Health England, June 2018.
www.gov.uk/government/publications/japanese-encephalitis-the-green-book-chapter-20

National Travel Health Network and Centre
nathnac.net

14

Vaccines

Measles, Mumps and Rubella vaccine

Overview

Measles vaccine has been replaced by a combined measles, mumps and rubella vaccine, live p. 1375 (MMR vaccine).

Measles, mumps and rubella vaccine, live aims to eliminate measles, mumps, and rubella (German measles) and congenital rubella syndrome. Every child should receive two doses of measles, mumps and rubella vaccine, live by entry to primary school, unless there is a valid contra-indication. Measles, mumps and rubella vaccine, live should be given irrespective of previous measles, mumps, or rubella infection or vaccination.

The first dose of measles, mumps and rubella vaccine, live is given to children at 1 year of age, on or after their first birthday. A second dose is given before starting school at 3 years and 4 months of age, or soon after (see Immunisation Schedule).

Children presenting for pre-school booster who have not received the first dose of measles, mumps and rubella vaccine, live should be given a dose of measles, mumps and rubella vaccine, live followed 3 months later by a second dose.

At school-leaving age or at entry into further education, measles, mumps and rubella vaccine, live immunisation should be offered to individuals of both sexes who have not received 2 doses during childhood. In those who have received only a single dose of measles, mumps and rubella vaccine, live in childhood, a second dose is recommended to achieve full protection. If 2 doses of measles, mumps and rubella vaccine, live are required, the second dose should be given one month after the initial dose. The decision on whether to vaccinate adults should take into consideration their vaccination history, the likelihood of the individual remaining susceptible, and the future risk of exposure and disease.

Measles, mumps and rubella vaccine, live should be used to protect against rubella in *seronegative women of child-bearing age* (see Immunisation Schedule); unimmunised healthcare workers who might put pregnant women and other vulnerable groups at risk of rubella or measles should be vaccinated. Measles, mumps and rubella vaccine, live may also be offered to previously *unimmunised and seronegative post-partum women* (see measles, mumps and rubella vaccine, live)—vaccination a few days after delivery is important because about 60% of congenital abnormalities from rubella infection occur in babies of women who have borne more than one child. Immigrants arriving after the age of school immunisation are particularly likely to require immunisation.

Contacts

Measles, mumps and rubella vaccine, live may also be used in the control of outbreaks of measles and should be offered to susceptible children aged over 6 months who are contacts of a case, within 3 days of exposure to infection. Children immunised before 12 months of age should still receive two doses of measles, mumps and rubella vaccine, live at the recommended ages. If one dose of measles, mumps and rubella vaccine, live has already been given to a child, then the second dose may be brought forward to at least one month after the first, to ensure complete protection. If the child is under 18 months of age and the second dose is given within 3 months of the first, then the routine dose before starting school at 3 years and 4 months of age (or soon after) should still be given. Children aged under 9 months for whom avoidance of measles infection is particularly important (such as those with history of recent severe illness) can be given normal immunoglobulin after exposure to measles; routine measles, mumps and rubella vaccine, live

immunisation should then be given after at least 3 months at the appropriate age.

Measles, mumps and rubella vaccine, live is **not suitable** for prophylaxis following exposure to mumps or rubella since the antibody response to the mumps and rubella components is too slow for effective prophylaxis.

Children and adults with impaired immune response should not receive live vaccines (see advice on HIV). If they have been exposed to measles infection they should be given normal immunoglobulin.

Travel

Unimmunised travellers, including children over 6 months, to areas where measles is endemic or epidemic should receive measles, mumps and rubella vaccine, live. Children immunised before 12 months of age should still receive two doses of measles, mumps and rubella vaccine, live at the recommended ages. If one dose of measles, mumps and rubella vaccine, live has already been given to a child, then the second dose should be brought forward to at least one month after the first, to ensure complete protection. If the child is under 18 months of age and the second dose is given within 3 months of the first, then the routine dose before starting school at 3 years and 4 months of age (or soon after) should still be given.

Useful Resources

Advice reflects that in the handbook Immunisation against Infectious Disease (2013), which in turn reflects the guidance of the Joint Committee on Vaccination and Immunisation (JCVI). The advice also incorporates changes announced by the Chief Medical Officer and Health Department Updates. Chapters from the handbook (including updates since 2013) are available at:

www.gov.uk/government/collections/immunisation-against-infectious-disease-the-green-book

Meningococcal vaccine

Overview

Almost all childhood meningococcal disease in the UK is caused by *Neisseria meningitidis* serogroups B and C. **Meningococcal group C conjugate vaccine** protects only against infection by serogroup C and **Meningococcal group B vaccine** protects only against infection by serogroup B. The risk of meningococcal disease declines with age—immunisation is not generally recommended after the age of 25 years.

Tetravalent meningococcal vaccines that cover serogroups A, C, W135, and Y are available. Although the duration of protection has not been established, the **meningococcal groups A, C, W135, and Y conjugate vaccine** is likely to provide longer-lasting protection than the unconjugated meningococcal polysaccharide vaccine. The antibody response to serogroup C in unconjugated meningococcal polysaccharide vaccines in young children may be suboptimal [not currently available in the UK].

Meningococcal group B vaccines, *Bexsero*®, and *Trumenba*® are licensed in the UK against infection caused by *Neisseria meningitidis* serogroup B. The use of *Bexsero*® is recommended in the Immunisation Schedule. *Bexsero*® contains 3 recombinant *Neisseria meningitidis* serogroup B proteins and the outer membrane vesicles from the NZ 98/254 strain, in order to achieve broad protection against *Neisseria meningitidis* serogroup B. *Trumenba*® contains 2 recombinant *Neisseria meningitidis* serogroup B proteins. The proteins are adsorbed onto an aluminium compound to stimulate an enhanced immune response.

Childhood immunisation

Meningococcal group C conjugate vaccine provides long-term protection against infection by serogroup C of *Neisseria*

meningitidis. Immunisation consists of 1 dose given at 12 months of age (as the haemophilus influenzae type b with meningococcal group C vaccine p. 1364) and a second dose given at 13–15 years of age (as the meningococcal groups A with C and W135 and Y vaccine p. 1366) (see Immunisation Schedule).

Meningococcal group B vaccine provides protection against infection by serogroup B of *Neisseria meningitidis*. Immunisation consists of 1 dose given at 2 months of age, a second dose at 4 months of age, and a booster dose at 12 months of age (see *Immunisation Schedule* above).

Unimmunised children aged under 12 months should be given 1 dose of meningococcal group B vaccine (rDNA, component, adsorbed) p. 1365 followed by a second dose of meningococcal group B vaccine (rDNA, component, adsorbed) two months later. They should then be vaccinated according to the Immunisation Schedule (ensuring at least a two month interval between doses of meningococcal group B vaccines). Unimmunised children aged 12–23 months should be given 2 doses of meningococcal group B vaccine (rDNA, component, adsorbed) separated by an interval of two months if they have received less than 2 doses in the first year of life. Unimmunised children aged 2–9 years should be given a single dose of meningococcal group C vaccine (as the haemophilus influenzae type b with meningococcal group C vaccine) followed by a booster dose of meningococcal groups A with C and W135 and Y vaccine at 13–15 years of age.

From 2015, unimmunised individuals aged 10–25 years, including those aged under 25 years who are attending university for the first time, should be given a single dose of meningococcal groups A with C and W135 and Y vaccine; a booster dose is not required.

Patients under 25 years of age with confirmed serogroup C disease, who have previously been immunised with meningococcal group C vaccine, should be offered meningococcal group C conjugate vaccine before discharge from hospital.

Travel

Individuals travelling to countries of risk should be immunised with meningococcal groups A, C, W135, and Y conjugate vaccine, even if they have previously received meningococcal group C conjugate vaccine. If an individual has recently received meningococcal group C conjugate vaccine, an interval of at least 4 weeks should be allowed before administration of the tetravalent (meningococcal groups A, C, W135, and Y) vaccine.

Vaccination is particularly important for those living or working with local people or visiting an area of risk during outbreaks.

Immunisation recommendations and requirements for visa entry for individual countries should be checked before travelling, particularly to countries in Sub-Saharan Africa, Asia, and the Indian sub-continent where epidemics of meningococcal outbreaks and infection are reported. Country-by-country information is available from the National Travel Health Network and Centre (www.nathnac.org/).

Proof of vaccination with the tetravalent meningococcal groups A with C and W135 and Y vaccine is required for those travelling to Saudi Arabia during the Hajj and Umrah pilgrimages (where outbreaks of the W135 strain have occurred).

Contacts

For advice on the immunisation of *laboratory workers and close contacts* of cases of meningococcal disease in the UK and on the role of the vaccine in the control of *local outbreaks*, consult Guidance for Public Health Management of Meningococcal Disease in the UK at www.gov.uk/phe. Also see for antibacterial prophylaxis for prevention of secondary cases of meningococcal meningitis.

The need for immunisation of laboratory staff who work directly with *Neisseria meningitidis* should be considered.

Useful Resources

Advice reflects that in the handbook Immunisation against Infectious Disease (2013), which in turn reflects the guidance of the Joint Committee on Vaccination and Immunisation (JCVI). The advice also incorporates changes announced by the Chief Medical Officer and Health Department Updates. Chapters from the handbook (including updates since 2013) are available at:
www.gov.uk/government/collections/immunisation-against-infectious-disease-the-green-book

Pertussis vaccine

28-May-2020

Overview

Pertussis vaccine is given as a combination preparation containing other vaccines. Acellular vaccines are derived from highly purified components of *Bordetella pertussis*. Primary immunisation against pertussis (whooping cough) requires 3 doses of an acellular pertussis-containing vaccine (see Immunisation schedule), given at intervals of 1 month from the age of 2 months.

All children up to the age of 10 years should receive primary immunisation with a combination vaccine of diphtheria with tetanus, pertussis, hepatitis B, poliomyelitis and haemophilus influenzae type b vaccine p. 1362 (*Infanrix hexa*®).

A booster dose of an acellular pertussis-containing vaccine should ideally be given 3 years after the primary course, although, the interval can be reduced to 1 year if the primary course was delayed. Children aged 1–10 years who have not received a *pertussis-containing* vaccine as part of their primary immunisation should be offered 1 dose of a suitable pertussis-containing vaccine; after an interval of at least 1 year, a booster dose of a suitable pertussis-containing vaccine should be given. Immunisation against pertussis is not routinely recommended in individuals over 10 years of age.

Vaccination of pregnant women against pertussis

In response to the pertussis outbreak, the UK health departments introduced a temporary programme (October 2012) to vaccinate pregnant women against pertussis, and this programme will continue until further notice. The aim of the programme is to boost the levels of pertussis–specific antibodies that are transferred through the placenta, from the mother to the fetus, so that the newborn is protected before routine immunisation begins at 2 months of age.

Pregnant women should be offered a single dose of acellular pertussis-containing vaccine (as adsorbed diphtheria [low dose], tetanus, pertussis (acellular, component) and poliomyelitis (inactivated) vaccine; *Boostrix-IPV*® or *Repevax*®) between 16 and 32 weeks of pregnancy. Public Health England has advised (2016) that the vaccine is probably best offered after the fetal anomaly scan at around 18–20 weeks. Pregnant women should be offered a single dose of acellular pertussis-containing vaccine up to the onset of labour if they missed the opportunity for vaccination at 16–32 weeks of pregnancy. A single dose of acellular pertussis-containing vaccine may also be offered to new mothers, who have never previously been vaccinated against pertussis, until the child receives the first vaccination.

While this programme is in place, women who become pregnant again should be offered vaccination during each pregnancy to maximise transplacental transfer of antibody.

Contacts

Vaccination against pertussis should be considered for close contacts of cases with pertussis who have been offered antibacterial prophylaxis. Unimmunised or partially immunised contacts under 10 years of age should complete

14

Vaccines

their vaccination against pertussis. A booster dose of an acellular pertussis-containing vaccine is recommended for contacts aged over 10 years who have not received a pertussis-containing vaccine in the last 5 years and who have not received adsorbed diphtheria [low dose], tetanus, and poliomyelitis (inactivated) vaccine in the last month.

Side-effects
Local reactions do not contra-indicate further doses.

The vaccine should not be withheld from children with a history to a preceding dose of:

- fever, irrespective of severity;
- persistent crying or screaming for more than 3 hours;
- severe local reaction, irrespective of extent.

Useful Resources
Advice reflects that in the handbook Immunisation against Infectious Disease (2013), which in turn reflects the guidance of the Joint Committee on Vaccination and Immunisation (JCVI). The advice also incorporates changes announced by the Chief Medical Officer and Health Department Updates. Chapters from the handbook (including updates since 2013) are available at:
www.gov.uk/government/collections/immunisation-against-infectious-disease-the-green-book

---

Pneumococcal vaccine
11-Sep-2020

Overview
The pneumococcal polysaccharide conjugate vaccine (adsorbed) p. 1366 and the pneumococcal polysaccharide vaccine p. 1367 protect against infection with *Streptococcus pneumoniae* (pneumococcus). Both vaccines contain polysaccharide from capsular pneumococci. The pneumococcal polysaccharide vaccine contains purified polysaccharide from **23 capsular types** of pneumococcus, whereas the pneumococcal polysaccharide conjugate vaccine (adsorbed) contains polysaccharide from either **10 capsular types** (*Synflorix*®) or **13 capsular types** (*Prevenar* 13®). Both vaccines are inactivated.

Prevenar 13® is the 13-valent pneumococcal polysaccharide conjugate vaccine (adsorbed) used for childhood immunisation. For children born on or before December 31st 2019, the schedule consists of 3 doses given at separate intervals. For children born on or after January 1st 2020, the schedule consists of 2 doses given at separate intervals. For more information on the schedule, see Immunisation schedule p. 1341. Children who present late for vaccination should be immunised according to *Children with unknown or incomplete vaccination histories*.

For further information on the use of *Prevenar* 13® pneumococcal polysaccharide conjugate vaccine (adsorbed) (including guidance on early immunisation, or shortened dosing intervals; and the management of children given the incorrect dosing schedule or pneumococcal vaccine, or if vaccinated overseas), see Public Health England guidance: **Pneumococcal vaccination: guidance for health professionals** (available from: www.gov.uk/government/publications/pneumococcal-vaccination-guidance-for-health-professionals).

The 23-valent pneumococcal polysaccharide vaccine is recommended for all adults aged 65 years and over (including those immunised during the influenza season and who turn 65 by the 31st March), and for adults and children aged 2 years and over in the following at-risk groups:

- asplenia or splenic dysfunction (including homozygous sickle cell disease and coeliac syndrome which could lead to splenic dysfunction);
- chronic respiratory disease (including severe asthma treated with continuous or frequent use of a systemic corticosteroid);

- chronic heart disease;
- chronic renal disease;
- chronic liver disease;
- diabetes mellitus requiring insulin or anti-diabetic medication;
- immunosuppression because of disease (e.g. HIV infection and genetic disorders affecting the immune system) or treatment (including prolonged systemic corticosteroid treatment for over 1 month at dose equivalents of prednisolone: *adult and child 20 kg and over*, 20 mg or more daily; *child under 20 kg*, 1 mg/kg or more daily, and chemotherapy);
- presence of cochlear implant;
- conditions where leakage of cerebrospinal fluid may occur.

The 23-valent pneumococcal polysaccharide vaccine should also be considered for those at risk of occupational exposure to metal fume (e.g. welders).

Where possible, the vaccine should be given at least 2 weeks (ideally 4–6 weeks) before splenectomy, chemotherapy or radiotherapy; patients should be given advice about the increased risk of pneumococcal infection. If it is not possible to vaccinate at least 2 weeks before splenectomy, chemotherapy or radiotherapy, the vaccine should be given at least 2 weeks after the splenectomy, and at least 3 months after completion of chemotherapy or radiotherapy. Vaccination advice for patients with leukaemia or those who have had a bone marrow transplant, and information on patient cards and leaflets for individuals with apslenia, are available in Chapter 25, Pneumococcal, in *Immunisation against infectious disease*- 'The Green Book'.

Vaccination regimens may differ depending on the individual's age, risk of pneumococcal disease, vaccination history, and immune status. Individuals in at-risk groups may require additional protection.

For information on revaccination with 23-valent pneumococcal polysaccharide vaccine for individuals in whom the antibody concentration is likely to decline rapidly, see *Revaccination*.

Children with unknown or incomplete vaccination histories

Individuals born on or before December 31st 2019
Unimmunised or partially immunised children who present late for vaccination and before the age of 1 year should receive 2 doses of the 13-valent pneumococcal polysaccharide conjugate vaccine (adsorbed) 2 months apart, and a booster dose on or after their first birthday, at least 2 months after the previous dose (intervals can be reduced to 1 month to allow the immunisation schedule to be completed promptly).

Children aged 1 year to under 2 years who are unimmunised or partially immunised should receive a single dose of the 13-valent pneumococcal polysaccharide conjugate vaccine (adsorbed).

Individuals born on or after January 1st 2020
Unimmunised or partially immunised children who present late for vaccination and before the age of 1 year should receive a single dose of the 13-valent pneumococcal polysaccharide conjugate vaccine (adsorbed), and a booster dose on or after their first birthday, at least 4 weeks after the previous dose.

Children aged 1 year to under 2 years who are unimmunised or partially immunised should receive a single dose of the 13-valent pneumococcal polysaccharide conjugate vaccine (adsorbed).

For the management of children who received one or more doses of 10-valent pneumococcal polysaccharide conjugate vaccine (adsorbed) in another country, refer to Chapter 25 (for infants born on or after 1 January 2020), Pneumococcal, in *Immunisation against infectious disease*- 'The Green Book'.

●ndividuals with an at-risk condition born on or ●efore December 31st 2019

Children diagnosed with at-risk conditions aged under 2 years
Children diagnosed with an at-risk condition aged under
. year should receive the 13-valent pneumococcal
●olysaccharide conjugate vaccine (adsorbed) according to
the Immunisation schedule p. 1341. Those who present late
●or vaccination should be immunised according to *Children
●ith unknown or incomplete vaccination histories*. A single
●ose of the 23-valent pneumococcal polysaccharide vaccine
●hould then be given at 2 years of age, at least 2 months after
the last dose of 13-valent pneumococcal polysaccharide
●onjugate vaccine (adsorbed).

Children aged under 2 years who are severely
immunocompromised, or those with asplenia, splenic
●ysfunction or complement disorders, should have an
●dditional dose of the 13-valent pneumococcal
●olysaccharide conjugate vaccine (adsorbed), given at least
● months after the booster dose due on or after their first
●irthday (the interval can be reduced to 1 month to allow the
immunisation schedule to be completed promptly). A single
●ose of the 23-valent pneumococcal polysaccharide vaccine
should then be given at 2 years of age, at least 2 months after
the last dose of 13-valent pneumococcal polysaccharide
●onjugate vaccine (adsorbed).

For further information on vaccination in individuals with
asplenia, splenic dysfunction, or complement disorders, see
Vaccination, general principles p. 1339.

**Children diagnosed with at-risk conditions aged 2 years to
under 10 years**
Children diagnosed or first presenting with an at-risk
condition who have completed their routine immunisation
schedule should receive a single dose of 23-valent
pneumococcal polysaccharide vaccine, at least 2 months
after the last dose of 13-valent pneumococcal polysaccharide
conjugate vaccine (adsorbed).

Children previously unvaccinated or partially vaccinated
with the 13-valent pneumococcal polysaccharide conjugate
vaccine (adsorbed) should receive a single dose of the
13-valent pneumococcal polysaccharide conjugate vaccine
(adsorbed), followed by a single dose of the 23-valent
pneumococcal polysaccharide vaccine at least 2 months
later.

For further information on vaccination in individuals with
asplenia, splenic dysfunction, or complement disorders, see
Vaccination, general principles p. 1339.

Severely immunocompromised children may have a sub-
optimal immunological response to the vaccine and should
be given an additional dose of the 13-valent pneumococcal
polysaccharide conjugate vaccine (adsorbed) p. 1366, even if
they are fully vaccinated. This should be followed by a single
dose of the 23-valent pneumococcal polysaccharide vaccine
p. 1367, at least 2 months after the last dose of 13-valent
pneumococcal polysaccharide conjugate vaccine (adsorbed).
If the 23-valent pneumococcal polysaccharide vaccine has
already been given, the 13-valent pneumococcal
polysaccharide conjugate vaccine (adsorbed) should be given
at least 6 months after.

**Individuals diagnosed with at-risk conditions aged 10 years
and over**
Individuals diagnosed or first presenting with an at-risk
condition should be given a single dose of the 23-valent
pneumococcal polysaccharide vaccine; no additional
23-valent pneumococcal polysaccharide vaccine is required
at 65 years of age.

For further information on vaccination in individuals with
asplenia, splenic dysfunction, or complement disorders, see
Vaccination, general principles p. 1339.

Severely immunocompromised individuals should be given
a single dose of the 13-valent pneumococcal polysaccharide
conjugate vaccine (adsorbed) followed by the 23-valent

pneumococcal polysaccharide vaccine at least 2 months
after, irrespective of their previous pneumococcal
vaccinations. If the 23-valent pneumococcal polysaccharide
vaccine has already been given, the 13-valent pneumococcal
polysaccharide conjugate vaccine (adsorbed) should be given
at least 6 months after.

Individuals with an at-risk condition born on or after January 1st 2020

Children diagnosed with at-risk conditions aged under 1 year
Children in an at-risk group (excluding those with asplenia,
splenic dysfunction or complement disorder, or who are
severely immunocompromised) should receive the 13-valent
pneumococcal polysaccharide conjugate vaccine (adsorbed)
according to the Immunisation schedule p. 1341. Those who
present late for vaccination should be immunised according
to *Children with unknown or incomplete vaccination histories*. A
single dose of the 23-valent pneumococcal polysaccharide
vaccine should then be given at 2 years of age, at least
8 weeks after the last dose of 13-valent pneumococcal
polysaccharide conjugate vaccine (adsorbed).

Children who are severely immunocompromised, or those
with asplenia, splenic dysfunction or complement disorders,
should receive 2 doses of the 13-valent pneumococcal
polysaccharide conjugate vaccine (adsorbed) at least 8 weeks
apart (commencing no earlier than 6 weeks of age), followed
by a single booster dose given on or after their first birthday.
An additional dose of 13-valent pneumococcal
polysaccharide conjugate vaccine (adsorbed) should be given
at least 8 weeks after the booster dose. A single dose of the
23-valent pneumococcal polysaccharide vaccine should then
be given at 2 years of age, at least 8 weeks after the last dose
of 13-valent pneumococcal polysaccharide conjugate
vaccine (adsorbed).

For further information on vaccination in individuals with
asplenia, splenic dysfunction, or complement disorders, see
Vaccination, general principles p. 1339.

**Children diagnosed with at-risk conditions aged 1 year to
under 2 years**
Children in an at-risk group (excluding those with asplenia,
splenic dysfunction or complement disorder, or who are
severely immunocompromised) should receive their
13-valent pneumococcal polysaccharide conjugate vaccine
(adsorbed) booster dose according to the Immunisation
schedule p. 1341. Those who present late for vaccination
should be immunised according to *Children with unknown or
incomplete vaccination histories*. A single dose of the
23-valent pneumococcal polysaccharide vaccine should then
be given at 2 years of age, at least 8 weeks after the last dose
of 13-valent pneumococcal polysaccharide conjugate
vaccine (adsorbed).

Children who are severely immunocompromised, or those
with asplenia, splenic dysfunction or complement disorders,
should receive their 13-valent pneumococcal polysaccharide
conjugate vaccine (adsorbed) booster dose according to the
Immunisation schedule p. 1341. Those who present late for
vaccination should be immunised according to *Children with
unknown or incomplete vaccination histories*. An additional
dose of the 13-valent pneumococcal polysaccharide
conjugate vaccine (adsorbed) should be given at least
8 weeks after the booster dose. A single dose of the 23-valent
pneumococcal polysaccharide vaccine should then be given
at 2 years of age, at least 8 weeks after the last dose of
13-valent pneumococcal polysaccharide conjugate vaccine
(adsorbed).

For further information on vaccination in individuals with
asplenia, splenic dysfunction, or complement disorders, see
Vaccination, general principles p. 1339.

14

Vaccines

Children diagnosed with at-risk conditions aged 2 years to under 10 years

Children diagnosed or first presenting with an at-risk condition (excluding those severely immunocompromised) who have completed their routine immunisation schedule should receive a single dose of 23-valent pneumococcal polysaccharide vaccine, at least 8 weeks after the last dose of 13-valent pneumococcal polysaccharide conjugate vaccine (adsorbed).

Children diagnosed or first presenting with an at-risk condition (excluding those severely immunocompromised) who are previously unimmunised or partially immunised with the 13-valent pneumococcal polysaccharide conjugate vaccine (adsorbed), should receive a single dose of the 13-valent pneumococcal polysaccharide conjugate vaccine (adsorbed), followed by a single dose of the 23-valent pneumococcal polysaccharide vaccine at least 8 weeks later.

For further information on vaccination in individuals with asplenia, splenic dysfunction, or complement disorders, see Vaccination, general principles p. 1339.

Severely immunocompromised children should be given a single dose of the 13-valent pneumococcal polysaccharide conjugate vaccine (adsorbed), regardless of immunisation status. This should be followed by a single dose of the 23-valent pneumococcal polysaccharide vaccine, at least 8 weeks after the last dose of 13-valent pneumococcal polysaccharide conjugate vaccine (adsorbed).

Individuals diagnosed with at-risk conditions aged 10 years and over

Individuals diagnosed or first presenting with an at-risk condition (excluding those who are severely immunocompromised) should be given a single dose of the 23-valent pneumococcal polysaccharide vaccine. The 23-valent pneumococcal polysaccharide vaccine is not required for individuals with asplenia, splenic dysfunction or complement disorders if they have already received a dose within the previous 2 years (due to a theoretical risk of pneumococcal serotype-specific hypo-responsiveness with revaccination).

For further information on vaccination in individuals with asplenia, splenic dysfunction, or complement disorders, see Vaccination, general principles p. 1339.

Severely immunocompromised individuals should be given a single dose of the 13-valent pneumococcal polysaccharide conjugate vaccine (adsorbed), followed by a single dose of the 23-valent pneumococcal polysaccharide vaccine at least 8 weeks after. The 13-valent pneumococcal polysaccharide conjugate vaccine (adsorbed) or additional 23-valent pneumococcal polysaccharide vaccine are not required if a 23-valent pneumococcal polysaccharide vaccine has already been received within the previous 2 years, due to a theoretical risk of pneumococcal serotype-specific hypo-responsiveness with re-vaccination.

Revaccination

Revaccination is not recommended for any clinical risk groups or age groups, except for individuals in whom the antibody concentration is likely to decline rapidly (e.g. asplenia, splenic dysfunction, or chronic renal disease), where revaccination is recommended every 5 years.

Management of cases

For the management of cases, contacts and outbreaks, refer to Chapter 25, Pneumococcal, in *Immunisation against infectious disease*- 'The Green Book' (see *Useful resources*).

Useful Resources

Recommendations reflect Chapter 25 (for infants born up to and including 31 December 2019), Pneumococcal, in *Immunisation against infectious disease*- 'The Green Book'. Public Health England, January 2018.
www.gov.uk/government/publications/pneumococcal-the-green-book-chapter-25

Recommendations reflect Chapter 25 (for infants born on or after 1 January 2020), Pneumococcal, in *Immunisation against infectious disease*- 'The Green Book'. Public Health England, January 2020.
www.gov.uk/government/publications/pneumococcal-the-green-book-chapter-25

Poliomyelitis vaccine

Overview

Two types of poliomyelitis vaccines (containing strains of poliovirus types 1, 2, and 3) are available, inactivated poliomyelitis vaccine (for injection) and live (oral) poliomyelitis vaccine. **Inactivated** poliomyelitis vaccines, only available in combined preparation, is recommended for routine immunisation.

A course of primary immunisation consists of 3 doses of a combined preparation containing inactivated poliomyelitis vaccines, starting at 2 months of age with intervals of 1 month between doses (see Immunisation schedule). A course of 3 doses should also be given to all unimmunised adults; no adult should remain unimmunised against poliomyelitis.

Two booster doses of a preparation containing inactivated poliomyelitis vaccines are recommended, the first before school entry and the second before leaving school (see Immunisation schedule). Further booster doses are only necessary for adults at special risk, such as travellers to endemic areas, or laboratory staff likely to be exposed to the viruses, or healthcare workers in possible contact with cases; booster doses should be given to such individuals every 10 years.

Live (oral) poliomyelitis vaccine is no longer available for routine use; its use may be considered during large outbreaks, but advice should be sought from Public Health England. The live (oral) vaccine poses a very rare risk of vaccine-associated paralytic polio because the attenuated strain of the virus can revert to a virulent form. For this reason the live (oral) vaccine must **not** be used for immunosuppressed individuals or their household contacts. The use of inactivated poliomyelitis vaccines removes the risk of vaccine-associated paralytic polio altogether.

Travel

Unimmunised travellers to areas with a high incidence of poliomyelitis should receive a full 3-dose course of a preparation containing inactivated poliomyelitis vaccines. Those who have not been vaccinated in the last 10 years should receive a booster dose of **adsorbed diphtheria [low dose], tetanus and poliomyelitis (inactivated) vaccine** . Information about countries with a high incidence of poliomyelitis can be obtained from www.travax.nhs.uk/ or from the National Travel Health Network and Centre (www.nathnac.org/).

Useful Resources

Advice reflects that in the handbook Immunisation against Infectious Disease (2013), which in turn reflects the guidance of the Joint Committee on Vaccination and Immunisation (JCVI). The advice also incorporates changes announced by the Chief Medical Officer and Health Department Updates. Chapters from the handbook (including updates since 2013) are available at:
www.gov.uk/government/collections/immunisation-against-infectious-disease-the-green-book

Rabies vaccine

13-Nov-2019

Overview

The rabies vaccine p. 1376 contains inactivated rabies virus cultured in either human diploid cells or purified chick embryo cells; vaccines may be used interchangeably to provide protection for pre-exposure prophylaxis and post-exposure treatment.

Pre-exposure prophylaxis

Immunisation with the rabies vaccine should be offered to those considered to be at risk of exposure to rabies within the UK, as listed:

- laboratory staff who routinely handle the rabies virus;
- workers at Defra-authorised quarantine premises and carriers;
- those who regularly handle bats, including on a voluntary basis;
- veterinary and technical staff who, by reason of their employment, encounter enhanced risk.

Immunisation is also recommended for those considered to be at risk of exposure to rabies travelling outside the UK, including:

- animal control and wildlife workers, veterinary staff or zoologists who regularly work in rabies enzootic (high risk) areas;
- travellers to rabies enzootic areas, especially if:
  ‣ post-exposure medical care and rabies biologics at the destination are lacking or in short supply;
  ‣ they are undertaking higher risk activities such as cycling or running;
  ‣ they are living or staying there for more than 1 month.

Immunisation against rabies requires a primary pre-exposure course of 3 doses administered over 21 or 28 days (preferred schedule if time allows), or an accelerated course of 3 doses over 7 days with an additional dose at 1 year. For dosing schedules, see rabies vaccine.

For further information on pre-exposure prophylaxis in individuals with immunosuppresion and/or HIV infection, see *Immunosuppression and HIV infection*.

Boosters

The requirement for booster doses is dependent on an individual's indication for pre-exposure prophylaxis and the likely frequency of ongoing exposures.

For laboratory workers who handle lyssavirus containing material (includes the rabies virus) a single booster dose of rabies vaccine should be given 1 year after the primary course has been completed. Further booster doses should be given based on 6-monthly antibody levels.

For individuals who may have frequent unrecognised exposures to the virus (such as bat handlers) a single booster dose of rabies vaccine should be given 1 year after the primary course has been completed. Further booster doses should then be given every 3–5 years or based on antibody levels.

For individuals at infrequent risk of exposure, but who are likely to have an unrecognised exposure (such as recreational cavers, veterinarians investigating suspect rabies cases and non-compliant imported pets, engineers maintaining rabies laboratory equipment or those entering rabies laboratories), should be given booster doses of rabies vaccine based on antibody levels from at least 1 year after the primary course has been completed.

For further information on antibody testing and booster doses, see PHE guidance: **Guidelines on timing of rabies boosters based on antibody levels** (see *Useful resources*).

Travel

Routine booster doses are not recommended for most travellers. A single booster dose of rabies vaccine can be considered, following a risk assessment, in those who have completed a primary course over 1 year ago and are travelling again to an enzootic area. Only 1 booster is needed in a traveller's lifetime.

Further information on country-specific rabies travel risk is available from the National Travel Health Network and Centre (travelhealthpro.org.uk/) and, in Scotland, from Health Protection Scotland (www.hps.scot.nhs.uk).

Post-exposure management

Medical practitioners must notify the proper officer at their local council or local health protection team of all suspected cases of rabies. For further information, see *Notifiable diseases* in Antibacterials, principles of therapy p. 527.

Following potential exposure to rabies, the wound or site of exposure (e.g. mucous membrane) should be cleansed under running water and washed for several minutes with soapy water as soon as possible. Disinfectant and a simple dressing can be applied, but suturing should be delayed until post-exposure treatment has begun otherwise it may increase the risk of introducing rabies virus into the nerves.

A full, rapid post-exposure risk assessment (based on detailed information about the circumstances of the potential exposure) is required so that post-exposure treatment, if indicated, can be started promptly. When post-exposure treatment is indicated, this should always be started without delay, even in the presence of other illness. If the exposure occurred many months or years previously, a full risk assessment should always be done and treatment considered as the incubation period for rabies can be prolonged.

The regimen used for post-exposure management depends on the composite rabies risk (assessed as a green, amber, or red rating using a combination of the country where the incident occurred and the type of animal involved, and the category of exposure), and the individual's past medical history (including immune status). For further information on risk assessment (including composite rabies risk) and the management of potential rabies exposure, see PHE guidance: **Guidelines on managing rabies post-exposure** (see *Useful resources*).

For individuals arriving in the UK who started post-exposure treatment via the intradermal route, the remaining doses should be given intramuscularly. If the regimen started was different to the UK regimen—seek specialist advice.

For post-exposure management in individuals with immunosuppression, see *Immunosuppression and HIV infection*; and for country-specific specialist contact details in England, Wales, Scotland and Northern Ireland, see Chapter 27: Rabies, in *Immunisation against infectious disease*- 'The Green Book'.

Post-exposure treatment of individuals who are fully immunised

Fully immunised individuals are those who have received at least 3 documented doses of rabies vaccine (on at least two separate days either as a primary pre-exposure prophylaxis course or as part of a previous rabies post-exposure treatment course), or documented rabies virus neutralising antibody (VNA) titres of at least 0.5 IU/ml.

For *fully immunised* individuals with a *green* composite rabies risk or who have completed a rabies post-exposure treatment course in the last 3 months, no treatment is required.

For *fully immunised* individuals with an *amber* or *red* composite rabies risk, give 2 doses of rabies vaccine (first dose on day 0 and second dose between days 3–7). Rabies immunoglobulin is not needed for these individuals. If rabies immunoglobulin is inadvertently given, individuals will need to complete a 4 dose course of rabies vaccine (on days 0, 3, 7 and 21).

14

Vaccines

Post-exposure treatment of individuals who are partially immunised

Partially immunised individuals are those who have had an incomplete/inadequate primary pre-exposure prophylaxis course or documented rabies virus neutralising antibody titres consistently less than 0.5 IU/mL.

For *partially immunised* individuals with a *green* composite rabies risk, no treatment is required.

For *partially immunised* individuals with an *amber* or *red* composite rabies risk, give 4 doses in total of rabies vaccine p. 1376 (on days 0, 3, 7 and 21). If the 4th dose of rabies vaccine is given before day 21, a 5th dose of vaccine should be administered 2 weeks after the 4th dose. Rabies immunoglobulin is not needed for these individuals.

Post-exposure treatment of individuals who are non-immunised

Non-immunised individuals are those who have never received rabies pre- or post-exposure immunisation.

For *non-immunised* individuals with a *green* composite rabies risk, no treatment is required.

For *non-immunised* individuals, with an *amber* or *red* composite rabies risk, give 4 doses in total of rabies vaccine (on days 0, 3, 7 and 21). If the 4th dose of rabies vaccine is given before day 21, a 5th dose of vaccine should be administered 2 weeks after the 4th dose.

Individuals with a *red* composite rabies risk should also be given rabies immunoglobulin p. 1336. This is not required if more than 7 days has passed since the first dose of rabies vaccine or more than 1 day since the second dose, or if the exposure was more than 12 months ago.

Immunosuppression and HIV infection

Refer to the British HIV Association for further information on the use of *rabies vaccine* and *rabies immunoglobulin* in individuals with HIV infection. See www.bhiva.org/guidelines for further information.

Pre-exposure prophylaxis

Pre-exposure prophylaxis may be given to individuals with immunosuppression and HIV infection (regardless of CD4 count). These individuals may not develop a full antibody response so re-immunisation should be considered upon completion of treatment and recovery has occurred, or in those with HIV when there has been immune recovery following commencement of antiretroviral treatment (such as a CD4 count >200 per mm^3).

Individuals who become immunosuppressed after receiving a primary course of immunisation, or having an antibody test or booster should be advised to seek medical advice for review of testing/booster vaccination frequency. They may no longer be able to produce an effective immune response following a rabies virus exposure and should be informed about the potential risks of continuing with activities that might lead to rabies virus exposures.

Post-exposure management

For *immunosuppressed* individuals with a *green* composite rabies risk, no treatment is required.

For *immunosuppressed* individuals with an *amber* or *red* composite rabies risk, give 5 doses in total of rabies vaccine (on days 0, 3, 7, 14, and 28 or 30) and rabies immunoglobulin. Post-exposure treatment response should be confirmed using antibody testing at the same time as the 4th dose (day 14); further antibody tests may be required depending on the results. Rabies immunoglobulin is not indicated if more than 7 days have passed since the first dose of rabies vaccine or more than 1 day since the second dose, or if the exposure was more than 12 months previously.

Useful Resources

Recommendations reflect Chapter 27, Rabies, in *Immunisation against infectious disease*- 'The Green Book'. Public Health England, June 2018.
www.gov.uk/government/publications/rabies-the-green-book-chapter-27

Guidelines on managing rabies post-exposure. Public health England, October 2019.
www.gov.uk/government/publications/rabies-post-exposure-prophylaxis-management-guidelines

Guidelines on timing of rabies boosters based on antibody levels. Public Health England, January 2020.
www.gov.uk/government/publications/rabies-post-exposure-treatment-timing-of-vaccine-booster

Rotavirus vaccine

02-Aug-2019

Overview

Rotavirus vaccine p. 1377 is a live, oral vaccine that protects young children against gastro-enteritis caused by rotavirus infection. The recommended schedule consists of 2 doses, the first at 8 weeks of age, and the second at 12 weeks of age (see Immunisation schedule p. 1341). The first dose of rotavirus vaccine must be given between 6 weeks and under 15 weeks of age and the second dose should be given after an interval of at least 4 weeks; the vaccine should not be started in children 15 weeks of age or older. Ideally, the full course should be completed before 16 weeks of age to provide protection before the main burden of disease, and to avoid a temporal association between vaccination and intussusception; the course must be completed before 24 weeks of age.

Children who inadvertently receive the first dose of rotavirus vaccine at 15 weeks of age or older should still receive a second dose after at least 4 weeks, providing that they will still be under 24 weeks of age at the time.

The rotavirus vaccine virus is excreted in the stool and may be transmitted to close contacts; however, vaccination of children with *immunosuppressed* close contacts may protect the contacts from wild-type rotavirus disease and outweigh any risk from transmission of vaccine virus. Carers of a recently vaccinated child should be advised of the need to wash their hands after changing the child's nappies.

Useful Resources

Recommendations reflect Chapter 27b, Rotavirus, in *Immunisation against infectious disease*– 'The Green book'. Public Health England, August 2015.
www.gov.uk/government/publications/rotavirus-the-green-book-chapter-27b

Smallpox vaccine

25-Jun-2020

Overview

The smallpox vaccine is prepared from the live vaccinia virus (a pox virus similar to smallpox, but less harmful). Routine immunisation against smallpox is not indicated, but should be considered for workers in laboratories where pox viruses (such as monkeypox or genetically modified vaccinia) are handled, and for others whose work involves an identifiable risk of exposure to pox viruses. For further information on the need for smallpox immunisation and for information on contra-indications and supply, contact the Public Health England Virus Reference Department (contact details available at: www.gov.uk/government/collections/virus-reference-department-vrd). In Scotland, information can be obtained from Health Protection Scotland (contact details available at: www.hps.scot.nhs.uk/about-us/contact-us/).

Refer to the British HIV Association for information on the use of smallpox vaccine in individuals with HIV. See www.bhiva.org/guidelines for further information.

A 24 hour on-call service for urgent diagnosis of smallpox is available; contact the Colindale Duty Doctor (Tel: 020 8200 4400). Medical practitioners must notify the proper officer at their local council or local health protection team of all suspected cases of smallpox. For further information, see *Notifiable diseases* in Antibacterials, principles of therapy p. 527.

Useful Resources

Recommendations reflect Chapter 29, Smallpox and vaccinia, in Immunisation against infectious disease - 'The Green Book'. Public Health England, March 2013. www.gov.uk/government/publications/smallpox-and-vaccinia-the-green-book-chapter-29

Tetanus vaccine

Overview

Tetanus vaccine contains a cell-free purified toxin of *Clostridium tetani* adsorbed on aluminium hydroxide or aluminium phosphate to improve antigenicity.

Primary immunisation for children under 10 years consists of 3 doses of a combined preparation containing adsorbed tetanus vaccine, with an interval of 1 month between doses (see *Routine immunisation schedule*). Following routine childhood vaccination, 2 booster doses of a preparation containing adsorbed tetanus vaccine are recommended, the first before school entry and the second before leaving school.

The recommended schedule of tetanus vaccination not only gives protection against tetanus in childhood but also gives the basic immunity for subsequent booster doses. In most circumstances, a total of 5 doses of tetanus vaccine is considered sufficient for long term protection.

For primary immunisation of adults and children over 10 years previously unimmunised against tetanus, 3 doses of **adsorbed diphtheria [low dose], tetanus and poliomyelitis (inactivated) vaccine** are given with an interval of 1 month between doses (see *Diphtheria-containing vaccines for children over 10 years and adults*).

When an individual presents for a booster dose but has been vaccinated following a tetanus-prone wound, the vaccine preparation administered at the time of injury should be determined. If this is not possible, the booster should still be given to ensure adequate protection against all antigens in the booster dose.

Very rarely, tetanus has developed after abdominal surgery; patients awaiting elective surgery should be asked about tetanus immunisation and immunised if necessary.

Parenteral drug abuse is also associated with tetanus; those abusing drugs by injection should be vaccinated if unimmunised—booster doses should be given if there is any doubt about their immunisation status.

All laboratory staff should be offered a primary course if unimmunised.

Wounds

Wounds are considered to be tetanus-prone if they are sustained more than 6 hours before surgical treatment or at any interval after injury and are puncture-type (particularly if contaminated with soil or manure) *or* show much devitalised tissue *or* are septic *or* are compound fractures *or* contain foreign bodies. All wounds should receive thorough cleansing.

- For *clean wounds*: fully immunised individuals (those who have received a total of 5 doses of a tetanus-containing vaccine at appropriate intervals) and those whose primary immunisation is complete (with boosters up to date), do not require tetanus vaccine; individuals whose primary immunisation is incomplete or whose boosters are not up to date require a reinforcing dose of a tetanus-containing vaccine (followed by further doses as required to complete the schedule); non-immunised individuals (or those whose immunisation status is not known or who have been fully

immunised but are now immunocompromised) should be given a dose of the appropriate tetanus-containing vaccine immediately (followed by completion of the full course of the vaccine if records confirm the need)
- For *tetanus-prone wounds*: management is as for clean wounds with the addition of a dose of tetanus immunoglobulin given at a different site; in fully immunised individuals and those whose primary immunisation is complete (with boosters up to date) the immunoglobulin is needed only if the risk of infection is especially high (e.g. contamination with manure). Antibacterial prophylaxis (with benzylpenicillin, co-amoxiclav, or metronidazole) may also be required for tetanus-prone wounds.

Useful Resources

Advice reflects that in the handbook Immunisation against Infectious Disease (2013), which in turn reflects the guidance of the Joint Committee on Vaccination and Immunisation (JCVI). The advice also incorporates changes announced by the Chief Medical Officer and Health Department Updates. Chapters from the handbook (including updates since 2013) are available at:

www.gov.uk/government/collections/immunisation-against-infectious-disease-the-green-book

Tick-borne encephalitis vaccine

08-Jul-2020

Overview

The tick-borne encephalitis (TBE) vaccine contains inactivated TBE virus (Neudörfl strain) grown in chick embryo cells. It is recommended for the protection of individuals at high risk of exposure to the TBE virus through their work or travel.

Immunisation with the tick-borne encephalitis vaccine, inactivated p. 1377 is therefore recommended for:

- individuals who travel, particularly in spring and summer, to endemic forested areas where ticks are most prevalent (including those who hike, camp, hunt, and undertake fieldwork);
- individuals who will be residing in an area where TBE is endemic or epidemic, especially those working in forestry, woodcutting, farming, and the military;
- laboratory workers who may be exposed to the TBE virus.

A 3 dose schedule of the tick-borne encephalitis vaccine, inactivated is recommended for children aged 1 year and over, and for adults. Sufficient protection can be expected for the ongoing tick season after the first 2 doses, and for at least 3 years after the 3rd dose. Booster doses are required every 3–5 years for those still at risk of TBE exposure. For dosing schedules, see tick-borne encephalitis vaccine, inactivated.

Refer to the British HIV Association for information on the use of tick-borne encephalitis vaccine, inactivated in individuals with HIV infection. See www.bhiva.org/guidelines for further information.

Further information on preventing or reducing the risk of TBE is available from the National Travel Health Network and Centre (nathnac.net/) and Health Protection Scotland (www.travax.nhs.uk/).

Post-exposure management

Unvaccinated individuals bitten by ticks in endemic areas should seek local medical advice. No specific therapy is available following exposure to tick-borne encephalitis; supportive treatment can significantly reduce morbidity and mortality. If tick-borne encephalitis is suspected, the referring clinician should discuss the case with a clinician at the Public Health England Rare and Imported Pathogens

Laboratory (contact details are available at: www.gov.uk/
guidance/tick-borne-encephalitis-epidemiology-diagnosis-and-
prevention).

Medical practitioners must notify the proper officer at
their local council or local health protection team of all
suspected cases of acute encephalitis of any cause. For
further information, see *Notifiable diseases* in Antibacterials,
principles of therapy p. 527.

Useful Resources

Recommendations reflect Chapter 31, Tick-borne
encephalitis, in *Immunisation against infectious disease*- 'The
Green Book'. Public Health England, April 2013.
www.gov.uk/government/publications/tick-borne-encephalitis-
the-green-book-chapter-31

Typhoid vaccine

29-Jul-2019

Overview

Typhoid vaccine p. 1368 is available as a Vi capsular
polysaccharide (from *Salmonella typhi*) vaccine for injection
and a live, attenuated *Salmonella typhi* vaccine for oral use.
Typhoid immunisation is advised for:

- travellers to areas where typhoid is endemic and whose
  planned activities put them at higher risk (country-by-
  country information is available from the National Travel
  Health Network and Centre);
- travellers to endemic areas where frequent or prolonged
  exposure to poor sanitation and poor food hygiene is
  likely;
- laboratory personnel who, in the course of their work, may
  be exposed to *Salmonella typhi*.

Capsular polysaccharide typhoid vaccine is given as a single
dose, usually by intramuscular injection. Children under
2 years [unlicensed] may respond suboptimally to the
vaccine, but children aged between 1–2 years should be
immunised if the risk of typhoid fever is considered high
(immunisation is not recommended for infants under
12 months). A single booster dose should be given at 3-year
intervals in adults and children over 2 years of age who
remain at risk from typhoid fever.

Oral typhoid vaccine is a live, attenuated vaccine
contained in an enteric-coated capsule recommended in
individuals aged 5 years and over. One capsule taken on
alternate days for a total of 3 doses, provides protection
7–10 days after the last dose. If travelling from a non-
endemic area to an area where typhoid is endemic, a booster
consisting of 3 doses is recommended every 3 years. The oral
typhoid vaccine should be avoided in immunosuppressed
and HIV-infected individuals.

Prevention of typhoid primarily depends on improving
sanitation and water supplies in endemic areas and on
scrupulous personal, food and water hygiene.

All suspected cases of typhoid fever must be notified to the
local health protection unit. Where there is a community
level outbreak, specialist advice should be sought from
Public Health England (tel. 020 8200 4400) or, in Scotland,
Health Protection Scotland (tel. 0140 300 1191).

Useful Resources

Recommendations reflect Chapter 33, Typhoid, in
Immunisation against infectious disease– 'The Green Book'.
Public Health England, May 2019.
www.gov.uk/government/publications/typhoid-the-green-book-
chapter-33

National Travel Health Network and Centre
nathnac.net

Varicella-zoster vaccine

28-Sep-202(

Overview

The varicella-zoster vaccine p. 1378 preparations contain
live, attenuated virus derived from the Oka strain of
varicella-zoster virus. The *Varilrix®* and *Varivax®* vaccines
provide protection against varicella (chickenpox)—there is
no data on interchangeability between these 2 vaccines, but
it is likely that a course can be completed effectively with the
different vaccine. The *Zostavax®* vaccine has a significantly
higher antigen content than the chickenpox vaccines and is
used to provide protection against herpes zoster (shingles).

Pre-exposure prophylaxis against varicella (chickenpox)

Varicella immunisation aims to protect individuals who are
at most risk of serious illness from exposure to the varicella-
zoster virus, by vaccinating specific individuals who are in
regular or close contact with those at risk. Individuals with a
definite history of chickenpox or shingles can be considered
immune. However, for individuals born and raised overseas a
history of chickenpox is a less reliable predictor of immunity
and routine testing should be considered.

Vaccination with the chickenpox varicella-zoster vaccine
(*Varilrix®* or *Varivax®*) is recommended for:

- non-immune or varicella-zoster antibody-negative
  healthcare workers who have patient contact (including
  cleaners, catering staff, and receptionists);
- non-immune laboratory staff who may be exposed to
  varicella-zoster virus in the course of their work in virology
  laboratories and clinical infectious disease units;
- non-immune healthy susceptible contacts of
  immunocompromised patients where continuing close
  contact is unavoidable.

Children aged 1 year and over and adults, should receive
2 doses of the chickenpox varicella-zoster vaccine at least
4–8 weeks apart. Vaccination should be postponed in acutely
unwell individuals until they have fully recovered, unless
protection is urgently required.

Within 1 month of vaccination, some individuals may
develop a localised rash at the injection site or a generalised
rash (papular or vesicular). Healthcare workers who develop
a post-vaccine rash should consult their occupational health
department for assessment before commencing work. The
vaccine virus strain can also establish latent infection and
reactivate to cause shingles in some individuals (the risk is
substantially lower than with wild chickenpox infection)—
cases of shingles should be investigated. For further
information on vaccine-related cutaneous rashes, see
Cautions, further information in varicella-zoster vaccine, and
Chapter 34, Varicella, in *Immunisation against infectious
disease*- 'The Green Book' (see *Useful resources*).

The chickenpox vaccines are not recommended for
individuals with immunosuppression—seek specialist advice
for those who require protection against chickenpox. Refer
to the British HIV Association or Children's HIV Association
for information on the use of varicella-zoster vaccines in
individuals with HIV infection (available at: www.bhiva.org/
guidelines and www.chiva.org.uk).

For information on post-exposure management, see
Varicella-zoster immunoglobulin in Immunoglobulins p. 1331.
Chickenpox is only a notifiable disease in Northern Ireland.
For further information, see *Notifiable diseases* in
Antibacterials, principles of therapy p. 527.

Immunisation against herpes zoster (shingles)

The national shingles vaccination programme (launched on
1st September 2013) aims to lower the incidence and severity
of shingles in older people, in whom the risk and severity of
disease, and of subsequent post herpetic neuralgia (PHN) is
higher.

Although the shingles varicella-zoster vaccine is licensed for use in individuals aged 50 years and over, immunisation should only be offered to individuals aged 70–79 years as part of the national immunisation program. This is because the burden of shingles disease is generally not as severe in individuals aged 50–69 years, and because of the limited vaccine effectiveness in older individuals. Inadvertent vaccination with the shingles vaccine in individuals aged under 50 years is unlikely to result in serious adverse effects as they are likely to be immune to chickenpox.

Eligible individuals who missed the opportunity to be vaccinated (as a result of lockdown or when shielding was recommended) during the COVID-19 pandemic and who turned 80 years during that period, can still be offered the shingles varicella-zoster vaccine up until the 31st December 2020.

Individuals should be offered a single dose of the shingles varicella-zoster vaccine. This aims to boost immunity in individuals with pre-existing varicella-zoster virus immunity to prevent the development of shingles in later years and significantly reduce the incidence of PHN. Administration of the shingles vaccine should be delayed in individuals who are being treated with oral or intravenous antivirals (such as aciclovir) until 48 hours after cessation of treatment. The need for a booster dose has not been established.

The shingles vaccine is not recommended for the treatment of shingles or PHN, but it can be given to those with a previous history of shingles. For further information see, Chapter 28a, Shingles (herpes zoster), in *Immunisation against infectious disease-* 'The Green Book' (see *Useful resources*).

There is a theoretical risk that individuals who develop a rash following shingles vaccination could transmit the attenuated vaccine virus to a susceptible individual. Individuals who develop a vesicular rash or varicella-zoster virus-like rash after shingles vaccination, should take precautionary measures and be tested. For further information, see Public Health England guidance: **Shingles vaccination: guidance for healthcare professionals** (available at: www.gov.uk/government/publications/shingles-vaccination-guidance-for-healthcare-professionals), and Chapter 28a, Shingles (herpes zoster), in *Immunisation against infectious disease-* 'The Green Book' (see *Useful resources*).

Immunisation against shingles for individuals with immunosuppression should be based on clinical risk assessment—seek specialist advice for those who require protection against shingles. For further information, see Chapter 28a, Shingles (herpes zoster), in *Immunisation against infectious disease-* 'The Green Book' (see *Useful resources*). Refer to the British HIV Association for information on the use of varicella-zoster vaccines in individuals with HIV infection (available at: www.bhiva.org/guidelines).

For information on post-exposure management, see *Varicella-zoster immunoglobulin* in Immunoglobulins p. 1331.

Pregnancy

The varicella-zoster vaccines are not recommended during pregnancy, and pregnancy should be avoided for 1 month after the last dose of the chickenpox varicella-zoster vaccine.

All exposure to varicella-zoster vaccine from 3 months before conception to any time during pregnancy, should be reported to the Immunisation Department of Public Health England (PHE) who run UK-wide surveillance on the safety of vaccines given in pregnancy. For advice on the reporting, risk assessment, and management of inadvertent vaccination in pregnancy, see PHE guidance: **Vaccination in pregnancy (VIP)** (available at: www.gov.uk/guidance/vaccination-in-pregnancy-vip). Pregnant women should be advised to seek prompt medical advice if they develop a vesicular rash following inadvertent vaccination with a varicella-zoster vaccine.

Useful Resources

Recommendations reflect Chapter 28a, Shingles (herpes zoster), in *Immunisation against infectious disease-* 'The Green Book'. Public Health England, February 2016. www.gov.uk/government/publications/shingles-herpes-zoster-the-green-book-chapter-28a

Recommendations reflect Chapter 34, Varicella, in *Immunisation against infectious disease-* 'The Green Book'. Public Health England, August 2015. www.gov.uk/government/publications/varicella-the-green-book-chapter-34

Yellow fever vaccine   23-Jan-2020

MHRA/CHM advice: stronger precautions in people with weakened immunity and in those aged 60 years or older

The MHRA and CHM have released important safety information regarding the use of the live yellow fever vaccine in those with weakened immunity, and in those aged 60 years or older. For further information, see *Important safety information* for yellow fever vaccine, live p. 1379.

Overview

Yellow fever vaccine, live is an attenuated preparation of yellow fever virus grown in chick eggs. Yellow fever vaccine, live is recommended for:

- laboratory workers handling infected material;
- individuals aged 9 months or older who are travelling to, or living in areas or countries with a risk of yellow fever transmission;
- individuals aged 9 months or older who are travelling to, or living in countries that require an International Certificate of Vaccination or Prophylaxis (ICVP) for entry (information about countries at risk of yellow fever is available from the National Travel Health Network and Centre).

Children aged under 9 months are at higher risk of vaccine-associated encephalitis, with the risk being inversely proportional to age. Children aged under 6 months should **not** be vaccinated. Children aged 6–9 months should only be vaccinated following a detailed risk assessment, and vaccination is generally only recommended if the risk of yellow fever transmission is high (such as during epidemics/outbreaks). If travel is unavoidable, seek expert advice on whether to vaccinate.

Yellow fever vaccine, live should be avoided in individuals with primary or acquired immunodeficiency due to a congenital condition or disease process, and in individuals who are immunosuppressed as a result of treatment.

If the yellow fever risk is unavoidable in HIV-infected individuals, consult the British HIV Association (bhiva.org/vaccination-guidelines) or other specialist advice.

For additional guidance on the suitability of immunisation against yellow fever, standardised checklists are available from: National Travel Health Network and Centre (see *Useful resources*) or Health Protection Scotland (www.Travax.nhs.uk).

A single-dose of yellow fever vaccine, live confers life-long immunity against yellow fever disease. Immunisation should be performed at least 10 days before travelling to an endemic area to allow protective immunity to develop and for the ICVP (if required) to become valid.

Reinforcing immunisation is not needed, except for a small subset of individuals at continued risk who may not have developed long-term protection from their initial yellow fever vaccine, live vaccination—seek expert advice.

All suspected cases of yellow fever must be notified to the local health protection unit. Where there is a community level outbreak, specialist advice should be sought from

Public Health England (tel. 020 8200 4400) or, in Scotland, Health Protection Scotland (tel. 0140 300 1191).

Useful Resources

Recommendations reflect Chapter 35, Yellow fever, in *Immunisation against infectious disease*- 'The Green Book'. Public Health England, January 2020.
www.gov.uk/government/publications/yellow-fever-the-green-book-chapter-35

National Travel Health Network and Centre
travelhealthpro.org.uk

Travel vaccinations and precautions

25-Sep-2020

Immunisation for travel

The National Travel Health Network and Centre have issued guidance on how to manage interrupted vaccination schedules which includes general principles for consideration, such as keeping to the recommended schedules, lengthening and shortening schedules, off-label administration and re-starting courses. For further information, see travelhealthpro.org.uk/news/517/interrupted-vaccination-schedules-general-principles-for-travel-health-professionals.

No special immunisation is required for travellers to the United States, Europe, Australia, or New Zealand, although all travellers should have immunity to tetanus and poliomyelitis (and childhood immunisations should be up to date); the tick-borne encephalitis vaccine is recommended for immunisation of those working in, or visiting, high-risk areas. Certain special precautions are required in non-European areas surrounding the Mediterranean, in Africa, the Middle East, Asia, and South America.

Travellers to areas that have a high incidence of **poliomyelitis** should be immunised with the appropriate vaccine; previously immunised travellers may be given a booster dose of a preparation containing inactivated poliomyelitis vaccine.

Immunisation against **meningococcal meningitis** is recommended for a number of areas of the world.

Hepatitis B vaccine is recommended for those travelling to areas of high or intermediate prevalence who intend to seek employment as healthcare workers or who plan to remain there for lengthy periods and who may therefore be at increased risk of acquiring infection as the result of medical or dental procedures carried out in those countries. Short-term tourists or business travellers are not generally at increased risk of infection but may put themselves at risk by their sexual behaviour when abroad.

Travellers who have not had a tetanus booster in the last 10 years and are visiting areas where medical attention may not be accessible should receive a booster dose of adsorbed diphtheria [low dose], tetanus and poliomyelitis (inactivated) vaccine, even if they have received 5 doses of a tetanus-containing vaccine previously.

There is no requirement for cholera vaccination as a condition for entry into any country, but **oral cholera vaccine** should be considered for backpackers and those travelling to situations where the risk is greatest (e.g. refugee camps). Regardless of vaccination, travellers to areas where cholera is endemic should take special care with food hygiene.

Advice on **diphtheria** is available from the National Travel Health Network and Centre (see *Useful resources*).

For guidance on immunisation against the following infectious diseases, refer to the individual treatment summaries listed:

- Hepatitis A (see Hepatitis A vaccine p. 1345).

- Japanese encephalitis (see Japanese encephalitis vaccine p. 1349).
- Rabies (see Rabies vaccine p. 1355).
- Tick-borne encephalitis (see Tick-borne encephalitis vaccine p. 1357).
- Tuberculosis (see Bacillus Calmette-Guérin vaccine p. 1343).
- Typhoid (see Typhoid vaccine p. 1358).
- Yellow fever (see Yellow fever vaccine p. 1359).

Immunisation requirements change from time to time, and information on the current requirements for any particular country may be obtained from the embassy or legation of the appropriate country; or the National Travel Health Network and Centre, Health Protection Scotland, the Welsh Government, or the Department of Health Northern Ireland (see *Useful resources*).

Precautions for avoiding infectious disease

In areas where sanitation is poor, good food hygiene is important to help prevent hepatitis A, typhoid, cholera, and other diarrhoeal diseases (including travellers' diarrhoea). Food should be freshly prepared and hot, and uncooked vegetables (including green salads) should be avoided; only fruits which can be peeled should be eaten. Only suitable bottled water, or tap water that has been boiled or treated with sterilising tablets, should be used for drinking.

For guidance on malaria precautions, see Malaria, prophylaxis p. 646 and Malaria, treatment p. 652.

Further information on preventing or reducing the risk of infectious diseases when travelling, visiting, working, or living in high risk areas is available from the National Travel Health Network and Centre and Health Protection Scotland (see *Useful resources*).

Useful resources

Department of Health Northern Ireland.
www.health-ni.gov.uk/contact

Health Protection Scotland (free for NHS Scotland users (registration required); subscription fee may be payable for users outside NHS Scotland).
www.travax.nhs.uk/

National Travel Health Network and Centre.
nathnac.net/

Welsh Government.
www.gov.wales/contact-us

VACCINES

Vaccines   🔘

> **IMPORTANT SAFETY INFORMATION**
>
> MHRA/CHM ADVICE (UPDATED NOVEMBER 2017)
>
> Following reports of death in neonates who received a live attenuated vaccine after exposure to a tumor necrosis factor alpha (TNF-a) inhibitor in utero, the MHRA has issued the following advice:
>
> - any infant who has been exposed to immunosuppressive treatment from the mother either in utero during pregnancy or via breastfeeding should have any live attenuated vaccination deferred for as long as a postnatal influence on the immune status of the infant remains possible;
> - in the case of infants who have been exposed to TNF-a inhibitors and other immunosuppressive biological medicines in utero, PHE advise that any live attenuated vaccination (e.g. BCG vaccine) should be deferred until the infant is age 6 months;
> - PHE advise if there is any doubt as to whether an infant due to receive a live attenuated vaccine may be immunosuppressed due to the mother's therapy,

including exposure through breast-feeding, specialist advice should be sought.

● CONTRA-INDICATIONS ▸ Impaired immune response Public Health England advises severely immunosuppressed patients should not be given live vaccines (including those with severe primary immunodeficiency).

● CAUTIONS Acute illness · minor illnesses

CAUTIONS, FURTHER INFORMATION PHE advises vaccination may be postponed if the individual is suffering from an acute illness; however, it is not necessary to postpone immunisation in patients with minor illnesses without fever or systemic upset.

▸ Impaired immune response and drugs affecting immune response Immune response to vaccines may be reduced in immunosuppressed patients and there is also a risk of generalised infection with live vaccines.

PHE advises:

● specialist advice should be sought for immuno-suppressed patients, or those being treated with high doses of corticosteroids (dose equivalents of prednisolone: **adults**, at least 40 mg daily for more than 1 week or at least 20 mg daily for more than 14 days; **children**, 2 mg/kg (or more than 40 mg) daily for more than 1 week or 1 mg/kg (or more than 20 mg) daily for more than 14 days) or other immunosuppressive drugs, or those being treated for malignant or non-malignant conditions with chemotherapy or generalised radiotherapy. Live vaccines should be postponed until at least 3 months after stopping high-dose systemic corticosteroids or non-biological oral immune modulating drugs, and at least 6 months after stopping other immunosuppressive drugs or generalised radiotherapy (at least 12 months after discontinuing immunosuppressive biological therapy).

▸ Predisposition to neurological problems PHE advises:

● when there is a personal or family history of *febrile* convulsions, there is an increased risk of these occurring during fever from any cause including immunisation, but this is not a contra-indication to immunisation. In children who have had a seizure associated with fever without neurological deterioration, immunisation is *recommended*; advice on the *management of fever* should be given before immunisation. When a child has had a convulsion not associated with fever, and the neurological condition is not deteriorating, immunisation is *recommended*;

● children with stable neurological disorders (e.g. spina bifida, congenital brain abnormality, and peri-natal hypoxic-ischaemic encephalopathy) should be immunised according to the recommended schedule;

● when there is a *still evolving neurological problem*, including poorly controlled epilepsy, immunisation should be deferred and the child referred to a specialist. Immunisation is recommended if a cause for the neurological disorder is identified. If a cause is not identified, immunisation should be deferred until the condition is stable.

● SIDE-EFFECTS

▸ **Common or very common** Appetite decreased · arthralgia (frequency not known in elderly) · diarrhoea (uncommon in elderly) · dizziness (uncommon in elderly) · fatigue · fever · headache · irritability · lymphadenopathy (uncommon in elderly) · malaise · myalgia · nausea (uncommon in elderly) · skin reactions (rare in elderly) · vomiting (uncommon in elderly)

▸ **Uncommon** Hypersensitivity (frequency not known in elderly)

● ALLERGY AND CROSS-SENSITIVITY Contra-indicated in patients with a confirmed anaphylactic reaction to a preceding dose of a vaccine containing the same antigens

or vaccine component (such as antibacterials in viral vaccines).

● PREGNANCY Live vaccines should not be administered routinely to pregnant women because of the theoretical risk of fetal infection but where there is a significant risk of exposure to disease, the need for vaccination usually outweighs any possible risk to the fetus. Termination of pregnancy following inadvertent immunisation is not recommended. There is no evidence of risk from vaccinating pregnant women with inactivated viral or bacterial vaccines or toxoids.

● BREAST FEEDING Although there is a theoretical risk of live vaccine being present in breast milk, vaccination is not contra-indicated for women who are breast-feeding when there is significant risk of exposure to disease. There is no evidence of risk from vaccinating women who are breast-feeding, with inactivated viral or bacterial vaccines or toxoids.

● DIRECTIONS FOR ADMINISTRATION Manufacturer advises if alcohol or disinfectant is used for cleansing the skin it should be allowed to evaporate before vaccination to prevent possible inactivation of live vaccines.

Public Health England advises when 2 or more live vaccines are required (and are not available as a combined preparation), they can be administered at any time before or after each other at different sites, preferably in a different limb; if more than one injection is to be given in the same limb, they should be administered at least 2.5 cm apart. See also Cautions, further information in Bacillus Calmette-Guérin vaccine p. 1363 and in measles, mumps and rubella vaccine, live p. 1375.

Vaccines should not be given intravenously. Most vaccines are given by the intramuscular route, although some are given by either the intradermal, deep subcutaneous, or oral route. Public Health England advises the intramuscular route is usually avoided in patients with **bleeding disorders** such as haemophilia or thrombocytopenia; vaccines usually given by the intramuscular route can be given by deep subcutaneous injection instead.

Particular attention must be paid to instructions on the use of diluents. Vaccines which are liquid suspensions or are reconstituted before use should be adequately mixed to ensure uniformity of the material to be injected.

● HANDLING AND STORAGE Care must be taken to store all vaccines under the conditions recommended in the product literature, otherwise the preparation may become ineffective. **Refrigerated storage** is usually necessary; many vaccines need to be stored at 2–8°C and not allowed to freeze. Vaccines should be protected from light. Reconstituted vaccines and opened multidose vials must be used within the period recommended in the product literature. Unused vaccines should be disposed of by incineration at a registered disposal contractor.

14

Vaccines

VACCINES > BACTERIAL AND VIRAL VACCINES, COMBINED

◀ 1360

Diphtheria with tetanus and poliomyelitis vaccine

● INDICATIONS AND DOSE

Primary immunisation

▸ BY INTRAMUSCULAR INJECTION

▸ Child 10–17 years: 0.5 mL every month for 3 doses

▸ Adult: 0.5 mL every month for 3 doses

continued →

Booster doses

▶ BY INTRAMUSCULAR INJECTION

▶ Child 10-17 years: 0.5 mL for 1 dose, first booster dose—should be given 3 years after primary course (this interval can be reduced to a minimum of 1 year if the primary course was delayed), then 0.5 mL for 1 dose, second booster dose—should be given 10 years after first booster dose (this interval can be reduced to a minimum of 5 years if previous doses were delayed), second booster dose may also be used as first booster dose in those over 10 years who have received only 3 previous doses of a diphtheria-containing vaccine

▶ Adult: 0.5 mL for 1 dose, first booster dose—should be given 3 years after primary course (this interval can be reduced to a minimum of 1 year if the primary course was delayed), then 0.5 mL for 1 dose, second booster dose—should be given 10 years after first booster dose (this interval can be reduced to a minimum of 5 years if previous doses were delayed), second booster dose may also be used as first booster dose in those over 10 years who have received only 3 previous doses of a diphtheria-containing vaccine

● SIDE-EFFECTS

▶ **Common or very common** Vertigo

▶ **Frequency not known** Abdominal pain · asthenia · chills · face oedema · influenza like illness · nerve disorders · pallor · seizure · shock · syncope · vaccination reactions

● PRESCRIBING AND DISPENSING INFORMATION Available as part of childhood schedule from health organisations or ImmForm.

● MEDICINAL FORMS There can be variation in the licensing of different medicines containing the same drug.
Suspension for injection
EXCIPIENTS: May contain Neomycin, polymyxin b, streptomycin
▶ Revaxis (Sanofi Pasteur)
Revaxis vaccine suspension for injection 0.5ml pre-filled syringes | 1 pre-filled disposable injection [PoM] £7.80 DT = £7.80

Ⓕ 1360

Diphtheria with tetanus, pertussis and poliomyelitis vaccine
29-Jul-2020

● INDICATIONS AND DOSE
First booster dose
▶ BY INTRAMUSCULAR INJECTION
▶ Child 3-9 years: 0.5 mL, to be given 3 years after primary immunisation
Vaccination of pregnant women against pertussis (using low dose vaccines)
▶ BY INTRAMUSCULAR INJECTION
▶ Females of childbearing potential: 0.5 mL for 1 dose

● SIDE-EFFECTS

▶ **Common or very common** Abdominal pain

▶ **Uncommon** Apathy (in children) · asthma · chills · drowsiness (very common in children) · dry throat (in children) · extensive swelling of vaccinated limb (very common in children) · oral herpes · pain · paraesthesia · sleep disorder (in children)

▶ **Frequency not known** Angioedema · asthenia · hypotonic-hyporesponsiveness episode · seizure

SIDE-EFFECTS, FURTHER INFORMATION The incidence of local and systemic reactions is lower with acellular pertussis vaccines than with whole-cell pertussis vaccines used previously.

Compared with primary vaccination, injection site reactions are more common with booster doses of vaccines containing acellular pertussis.

Public Health England has advised (2016) that the vaccine should not be withheld from children with a

history to a preceding dose of: fever, irrespective of severity; hypotonic-hyporesonsive episodes; persistent crying or screaming for more than 3 hours; severe local reaction, irrespective of extent.

● PREGNANCY Contra-indicated in pregnant women with a history of encephalopathy of unknown origin within 7 days of previous immunisation with a pertussis-containing vaccine. Contra-indicated in pregnant women with a history of transient thrombocytopenia or neurological complications following previous immunisation against diphtheria or tetanus.

● PRESCRIBING AND DISPENSING INFORMATION Pregnant women should be vaccinated using low dose vaccines (brands may include *Boostrix-IPV*® or *Repevax*®).

Available as part of childhood immunisation schedule from health organisations or ImmForm.

Available for vaccination of pregnant women from ImmForm.

● MEDICINAL FORMS There can be variation in the licensing of different medicines containing the same drug.
Suspension for injection
EXCIPIENTS: May contain Neomycin, polymyxin b, streptomycin
▶ Boostrix-IPV (GlaxoSmithKline UK Ltd)
Boostrix-IPV suspension for injection 0.5ml pre-filled syringes | 1 pre-filled disposable injection [PoM] £22.74 DT = £20.00
▶ Repevax (Sanofi Pasteur)
Repevax vaccine suspension for injection 0.5ml pre-filled syringes | 1 pre-filled disposable injection [PoM] £20.00 DT = £20.00

Ⓕ 1360

Diphtheria with tetanus, pertussis, hepatitis B, poliomyelitis and haemophilus influenzae type b vaccine
12-Oct-2017

● INDICATIONS AND DOSE
Primary immunisation (first dose)
▶ BY DEEP INTRAMUSCULAR INJECTION
▶ Child 2 months: 0.5 mL for 1 dose
Primary immunisation (second dose)
▶ BY DEEP INTRAMUSCULAR INJECTION
▶ Child 3 months: 0.5 mL for 1 dose, preferably administer at a different injection site to that of first dose
Primary immunisation (third dose)
▶ BY DEEP INTRAMUSCULAR INJECTION
▶ Child 4 months: 0.5 mL for 1 dose, preferably administer at a different injection site to that of second dose

● SIDE-EFFECTS

▶ **Common or very common** Anxiety · crying abnormal

▶ **Uncommon** Cough · drowsiness · extensive swelling of vaccinated limb · increased risk of infection

▶ **Rare or very rare** Angioedema · apnoea · hypotonic-hyporesponsiveness episode · seizure · swelling · thrombocytopenia

● PRESCRIBING AND DISPENSING INFORMATION Available as part of childhood schedule from health organisations or ImmForm.

● MEDICINAL FORMS There can be variation in the licensing of different medicines containing the same drug.
Powder and suspension for suspension for injection
EXCIPIENTS: May contain Neomycin, polymyxin b
▶ Infanrix Hexa (GlaxoSmithKline UK Ltd)
Infanrix Hexa vaccine powder and suspension for suspension for injection 0.5ml pre-filled syringes | 1 pre-filled disposable injection [PoM] Ⓢ

F 1360

Diphtheria with tetanus, pertussis, poliomyelitis and haemophilus influenzae type b vaccine

- **INDICATIONS AND DOSE**
Primary immunisation
▸ BY INTRAMUSCULAR INJECTION
▸ Child 2 months–9 years: 0.5 mL every month for 3 doses

- UNLICENSED USE *Infanrix-IPV+ Hib* ® not licensed for use in children over 36 months; *Pediacel* ® not licensed in children over 4 years. However, the Department of Health recommends that these be used for children up to 10 years.

- SIDE-EFFECTS
▸ **Common or very common** Crying abnormal · drowsiness · restlessness
▸ **Uncommon** Cough · extensive swelling of vaccinated limb · increased risk of infection · rhinorrhoea
▸ **Frequency not known** Angioedema · apnoea · hypotonic-hyporesponsiveness episode · seizure

SIDE-EFFECTS, FURTHER INFORMATION The incidence of local and systemic reactions is lower with acellular pertussis vaccines than with whole-cell pertussis vaccines used previously.

Compared with primary vaccination, injection site reactions are more common with booster doses of vaccines containing acellular pertussis.

Public Health England has advised (2016) that the vaccine should not be withheld from children with a history to a preceding dose of: fever, irrespective of severity; hypotonic-hyporesonsive episodes; persistent crying or screaming for more than 3 hours; severe local reaction, irrespective of extent.

- PRESCRIBING AND DISPENSING INFORMATION Available as part of childhood schedule from health organisations or ImmForm.

- MEDICINAL FORMS There can be variation in the licensing of different medicines containing the same drug.
Powder and suspension for suspension for injection
▸ Infanrix-IPV + Hib (GlaxoSmithKline UK Ltd)
Infanrix-IPV + Hib vaccine powder and suspension for suspension for injection 0.5ml pre-filled syringes | 1 pre-filled disposable injection PoM £27.86

VACCINES > BACTERIAL VACCINES

F 1360

Anthrax vaccine

31-Jan-2019

- **INDICATIONS AND DOSE**
Immunisation against anthrax
▸ BY INTRAMUSCULAR INJECTION
▸ Adult: Initially 0.5 mL every 3 weeks for 3 doses, followed by 0.5 mL after 6 months, to be administered in the deltoid region
Booster
▸ BY INTRAMUSCULAR INJECTION
▸ Adult: 0.5 mL every 10 years for up to 3 doses, to be administered in deltoid region

- SIDE-EFFECTS
▸ **Common or very common** Febrile disorders · influenza like illness
▸ **Rare or very rare** Angioedema · asthenia · hyperhidrosis · paraesthesia
▸ **Frequency not known** Bronchospasm · circulatory collapse · hypotension

- PRESCRIBING AND DISPENSING INFORMATION Available from Public Health England's Centre for Emergency Preparedness and Response (Porton Down).

- MEDICINAL FORMS There can be variation in the licensing of different medicines containing the same drug.
Suspension for injection
EXCIPIENTS: May contain Thiomersal
▸ Anthrax vaccine (Non-proprietary)
Anthrax vaccine (alum precipitated sterile filtrate) suspension for injection 0.5ml ampoules | 5 ampoule PoM Ⓢ
▸ BioThrax (Secretary of State for Health) ▼
BioThrax suspension for injection 5ml multidose vials | 1 vial PoM £751.71 | 300 vial PoM £225,513.09

F 1360

Bacillus Calmette-Guérin vaccine

24-Sep-2020

(BCG Vaccine)

- DRUG ACTION BCG (Bacillus Calmette-Guérin) is a live attenuated strain derived from *Mycobacterium bovis* which stimulates the development of immunity to *M. tuberculosis*.

- **INDICATIONS AND DOSE**
Immunisation against tuberculosis
▸ BY INTRADERMAL INJECTION
▸ Child 1–11 months: 0.05 mL, to be injected at insertion of deltoid muscle onto humerus (keloid formation more likely with sites higher on arm); tip of shoulder should be **avoided**
▸ Child 1–17 years: 0.1 mL, to be injected at insertion of deltoid muscle onto humerus (keloid formation more likely with sites higher on arm); tip of shoulder should be **avoided**
▸ Adult: 0.1 mL, to be injected at insertion of deltoid muscle onto humerus (keloid formation more likely with sites higher on arm); tip of shoulder should be **avoided**

- CONTRA-INDICATIONS Children less than 2 years of age in household contact with known or suspected case of active tuberculosis (in children) · generalised septic skin conditions
CONTRA-INDICATIONS, FURTHER INFORMATION
Manufacturer advises using a lesion-free site to administer BCG vaccine to patients with eczema.

- CAUTIONS   When BCG is given to infants, there is no need to delay routine primary immunisations. No further vaccination should be given in the arm used for BCG vaccination for at least 3 months because of the risk of regional lymphadenitis.

- INTERACTIONS → Appendix 1: live vaccines

- SIDE-EFFECTS
▸ **Uncommon** Lymphadenitis suppurative
▸ **Rare or very rare** Osteitis · osteomyelitis
▸ **Frequency not known** Seizure · syncope

- PRE-TREATMENT SCREENING Apart from children under 6 years, any person being considered for BCG immunisation must first be given a skin test for hypersensitivity to tuberculoprotein (see tuberculin purified protein derivative p. 1338). A skin test is not necessary for a child under 6 years provided that the child has not stayed for longer than 3 months in a country with an incidence of tuberculosis greater than 40 per 100 000, the child has not had contact with a person with tuberculosis, and there is no family history of tuberculosis within the last 5 years.

- DIRECTIONS FOR ADMINISTRATION
Intradermal injection technique Public Health England advises skin is stretched between thumb and forefinger and needle

14

Vaccines

(size 26G) inserted (bevel upwards) for about 3 mm into superficial layers of dermis (almost parallel with surface). Needle should be short with short bevel (can usually be seen through epidermis during insertion). Tense raised blanched bleb is sign of correct injection; 7 mm bleb ≡ 0.1 mL injection, 3 mm bleb ≡ 0.05 mL injection; if considerable resistance not felt, needle too deep and should be removed and reinserted before giving more vaccine. Jet injectors and multiple puncture devices should not be used.

● PRESCRIBING AND DISPENSING INFORMATION Available from health organisations or direct from ImmForm portal. immform.phe.gov.uk (SSI brand, multidose vial with diluent).

● MEDICINAL FORMS There can be variation in the licensing of different medicines containing the same drug.
Powder for injection
▸ Bacillus calmette-guérin vaccine (Non-proprietary)
  BCG Vaccine AJV powder for suspension for injection 1ml vials |
  10 vial [PoM] Ⓢ

F 1360

Cholera vaccine

23-Sep-2020

● INDICATIONS AND DOSE

Immunisation against cholera (for travellers to endemic or epidemic areas on the basis of current recommendations)
▸ BY MOUTH
▸ Child 2-5 years: 1 dose every 1-6 weeks for 3 doses, if more than 6 weeks have elapsed between doses, the primary course should be restarted, immunisation should be completed at least one week before potential exposure
▸ Child 6-17 years: 1 dose every 1-6 weeks for 2 doses, if more than 6 weeks have elapsed between doses, the primary course should be restarted, immunisation should be completed at least one week before potential exposure
▸ Adult: 1 dose every 1-6 weeks for 2 doses, if more than 6 weeks have elapsed between doses, the primary course should be restarted, immunisation should be completed at least one week before potential exposure

Booster
▸ BY MOUTH
▸ Child 2-5 years: A single booster dose can be given within 6 months after primary course, if more than 6 months have elapsed since the last vaccination, the primary course should be repeated
▸ Child 6-17 years: A single booster dose can be given within 2 years after primary course, if more than 2 years have elapsed since the last vaccination, the primary course should be repeated
▸ Adult: A single booster dose can be given within 2 years after primary course, if more than 2 years have elapsed since the last vaccination, the primary course should be repeated

● CONTRA-INDICATIONS Acute gastro-intestinal illness
● INTERACTIONS → Appendix 1: cholera vaccine
● SIDE-EFFECTS
▸ **Uncommon** Gastrointestinal discomfort · gastrointestinal disorders
▸ **Rare or very rare** Chills · cough · dehydration · drowsiness · hyperhidrosis · increased risk of infection · insomnia · pulmonary reaction · syncope · taste altered · throat pain
▸ **Frequency not known** Angioedema · asthenia · dyspnoea · hypertension · influenza like illness · lymphadenitis · pain · paraesthesia · sputum increased

● DIRECTIONS FOR ADMINISTRATION
▸ In children Manufacturer advises dissolve effervescent sodium bicarbonate granules in a glassful of water *or* chlorinated water (approximately 150 mL). For children over 6 years, add vaccine suspension to make one dose. For child 2-5 years, discard half (approximately 75 mL) of the solution, then add vaccine suspension to make one dose. Drink within 2 hours. Food, drink, and other oral medicines should be avoided for 1 hour before and after vaccination.
▸ In adults Manufacturer advises dissolve effervescent sodium bicarbonate granules in a glassful of water *or* chlorinated water (approximately 150 mL). Add vaccine suspension to make one dose. Drink within 2 hours. Food, drink, and other oral medicines should be avoided for 1 hour before and after vaccination.

● PATIENT AND CARER ADVICE Counselling on administration advised. Immunisation with cholera vaccine does not provide complete protection and all travellers to a country where cholera exists should be warned that scrupulous attention to food, water, and personal hygiene is **essential**.

● MEDICINAL FORMS There can be variation in the licensing of different medicines containing the same drug.
Oral suspension
▸ Dukoral (Valneva UK Ltd)
  Dukoral cholera vaccine oral suspension | 2 dose [PoM] £26.35 DT = £26.35

F 1360

Haemophilus influenzae type b with meningococcal group C vaccine

● INDICATIONS AND DOSE

Booster dose (for infants who have received primary immunisation with a vaccine containing *Haemophilus influenzae* type b component) and primary immunisation against *Neisseria meningitidis*
▸ BY INTRAMUSCULAR INJECTION
▸ Child 12-13 months: 0.5 mL for 1 dose

Immunisation against *Neisseria meningitidis* in an unimmunised patient
▸ BY INTRAMUSCULAR INJECTION
▸ Child 1-9 years: 0.5 mL for 1 dose

Booster dose (for children who have not been immunised against *Haemophilus influenza* type b) | Booster dose after recovery from *Haemophilus influenzae* type b disease (for index cases previously vaccinated, with low Hib antibody concentration or if it is not possible to measure antibody concentration)
▸ BY INTRAMUSCULAR INJECTION
▸ Child 1-9 years: 0.5 mL for 1 dose

Booster dose after recovery from *Haemophilus influenzae* type b disease (for fully vaccinated index cases with asplenia or splenic dysfunction, if previous dose received over 1 year ago)
▸ BY INTRAMUSCULAR INJECTION
▸ Child 1-17 years: 0.5 mL for 1 dose
▸ Adult: 0.5 mL for 1 dose

Booster dose (for patients diagnosed with asplenia, splenic dysfunction or complement deficiency at under 2 years of age)
▸ BY INTRAMUSCULAR INJECTION
▸ Child 2-17 years: 0.5 mL for 1 dose, this booster dose should be given after the second birthday, this is the second dose of haemophilus influenzae type B vaccine combined with meningococcal group C conjugate vaccine (the first dose is given during the routine immunisation schedule)

Booster dose (for patients diagnosed with asplenia, splenic dysfunction or complement deficiency at over 2 years of age)
▸ BY INTRAMUSCULAR INJECTION
▸ Child 2-17 years: 0.5 mL for 1 dose, this booster dose should be followed 2 months later by one dose of meningococcal A, C, W135, and Y conjugate vaccine (in patients from 11 years of age, this interval can be reduced to one month)
▸ Adult: 0.5 mL for 1 dose, this booster dose should be followed 1 month later by one dose of meningococcal A, C, W135, and Y conjugate vaccine

● UNLICENSED USE Not licensed for use in patients over 2 years.

● SIDE-EFFECTS
▸ **Common or very common** Drowsiness
▸ **Uncommon** Crying
▸ **Rare or very rare** Abdominal pain · insomnia
▸ **Frequency not known** Febrile seizure · meningism (but no evidence that vaccine causes meningococcal C meningitis) · muscle tone decreased

● PRESCRIBING AND DISPENSING INFORMATION Available as part of the childhood immunisation schedule from ImmForm.

● MEDICINAL FORMS There can be variation in the licensing of different medicines containing the same drug.
Powder and solvent for solution for injection
▸ Menitorix (GlaxoSmithKline UK Ltd)
Menitorix vaccine powder and solvent for solution for injection 0.5ml vials | 1 vial [PoM] £37.76 DT = £37.76

⚑ 1360

Meningococcal group B vaccine (rDNA, component, adsorbed)
19-Oct-2017

● INDICATIONS AND DOSE
BEXSERO®
Immunisation against *Neisseria meningitidis*, primary immunisation
▸ BY DEEP INTRAMUSCULAR INJECTION
▸ Child 2 months: 0.5 mL for 1 dose, injected preferably into deltoid region (or anterolateral thigh in infants), for information about the use of paracetamol for prophylaxis of post-immunisation pyrexia, see paracetamol p. 464.
▸ Child 4 months: 0.5 mL for 1 dose, injected preferably into deltoid region (or anterolateral thigh in infants), for information about the use of paracetamol for prophylaxis of post-immunisation pyrexia, see paracetamol p. 464.
Immunisation against *Neisseria meningitidis*, primary immunisation booster dose
▸ BY DEEP INTRAMUSCULAR INJECTION
▸ Child 12-23 months: 0.5 mL for 1 dose, injected preferably into deltoid region (or anterolateral thigh in infants)
Immunisation against *Neisseria meningitidis*, primary immunisation (in unimmunised patients)
▸ BY DEEP INTRAMUSCULAR INJECTION
▸ Child 6-11 months: 0.5 mL for 2 doses, separated by an interval of at least 2 months; booster dose of 0.5 mL given between 1–2 years of age and at least 2 months after completion of primary immunisation, injected preferably into deltoid region (or anterolateral thigh in infants)
▸ Child 12-23 months: 0.5 mL for 2 doses, separated by an interval of at least 2 months; booster dose of 0.5 mL given 12–24 months after completion of primary

immunisation, injected preferably into deltoid region (or anterolateral thigh in infants)
▸ Child 2-10 years: 0.5 mL for 2 doses, separated by an interval of at least 2 months. Injected preferably into deltoid region (or anterolateral thigh in infants)
▸ Child 11-17 years: 0.5 mL for 2 doses, separated by an interval of at least 1 month. Injected preferably into deltoid region
▸ Adult: 0.5 mL for 2 doses, separated by an interval of at least 1 month. Injected preferably into deltoid region

TRUMENBA®
Immunisation against *Neisseria meningitidis*, primary immunisation
▸ BY INTRAMUSCULAR INJECTION
▸ Child 10-17 years: 0.5 mL for 2 doses, separated by an interval of 6 months, alternatively 0.5 mL for 2 doses, separated by an interval of at least 1 month, followed by 0.5 mL as a third dose, given at least 4 months after the second dose, injected preferably into deltoid region, a booster dose should be considered for individuals at continued risk—consult product literature
▸ Adult: 0.5 mL for 2 doses, separated by an interval of 6 months, alternatively 0.5 mL for 2 doses, separated by an interval of at least 1 month, followed by 0.5 mL as a third dose, given at least 4 months after the second dose, injected preferably into deltoid region, a booster dose should be considered for individuals at continued risk—consult product literature

● SIDE-EFFECTS
▸ **Common or very common** Crying abnormal (in children) · drowsiness (in children) · eating disorder (in children)
▸ **Uncommon** Seizures (in children) · vascular disorders (in children)
▸ **Frequency not known** Extensive swelling of vaccinated limb · hypotonic-hyporesponsiveness episode (in children)

● MEDICINAL FORMS There can be variation in the licensing of different medicines containing the same drug.
Suspension for injection
EXCIPIENTS: May contain Kanamycin
▸ Bexsero (GlaxoSmithKline UK Ltd)
Bexsero vaccine suspension for injection 0.5ml pre-filled syringes | 1 pre-filled disposable injection [PoM] £75.00
▸ Trumenba (Pfizer Ltd) ▼
Trumenba vaccine suspension for injection 0.5ml pre-filled syringes | 1 pre-filled disposable injection [PoM] £75.00

⚑ 1360

Meningococcal group C vaccine
24-Sep-2020

● INDICATIONS AND DOSE
Patients with confirmed serogroup C disease (who have previously been immunised)
▸ BY INTRAMUSCULAR INJECTION
▸ Child 1-17 years: 0.5 mL for 1 dose, dose to be given before discharge from hospital
▸ Adult 18-24 years: 0.5 mL for 1 dose, dose to be given before discharge from hospital

● SIDE-EFFECTS
▸ **Common or very common** Anxiety (in children) · cough (in children) · crying (in children) · drowsiness (in children) · gastrointestinal discomfort (in children) · hyperhidrosis (in children) · increased risk of infection (in children)
▸ **Uncommon** Chills · eyelid oedema (in children) · flushing (in children) · influenza like illness (rare in children) · joint stiffness (in children)
▸ **Rare or very rare** Circulatory collapse (in children)
▸ **Frequency not known** Angioedema · apnoea · asthenia (uncommon in children) · dyspnoea · hypotonic-hyporesponsiveness episode · immune thrombocytopenic

14

Vaccines

purpura · meningism (but no evidence that vaccine causes meningococcal C meningitis) · musculoskeletal stiffness (uncommon in children) · nasal congestion (uncommon in children) · oedema (uncommon in children) · pain (very common in children) · respiratory disorders (uncommon in children) · seizures (uncommon in children) · sensation abnormal (uncommon in children) · sleep disorders (very common in children) · Stevens-Johnson syndrome · syncope (uncommon in children)

● PRESCRIBING AND DISPENSING INFORMATION Available as part of childhood immunisation schedule from ImmForm portal.immform.phe.gov.uk.

● MEDICINAL FORMS There can be variation in the licensing of different medicines containing the same drug.

Suspension for injection
‣ NeisVac-C (Pfizer Ltd)
NeisVac-C vaccine suspension for injection 0.5ml pre-filled syringes | 10 pre-filled disposable injection [PoM] £187.50

Ⓕ 1360

Meningococcal groups A with C and W135 and Y vaccine

● INDICATIONS AND DOSE

MENVEO ®

Primary immunisation against *Neisseria meningitidis*
‣ BY INTRAMUSCULAR INJECTION
‣ Child 13-15 years: 0.5 mL for 1 dose, dose preferably injected into deltoid region

Immunisation against *Neisseria meningitidis* in an unimmunised patient
‣ BY INTRAMUSCULAR INJECTION
‣ Child 10-17 years: 0.5 mL for 1 dose, booster dose is not required
‣ Adult 18-24 years: 0.5 mL for 1 dose, booster dose is not required

Immunisation against *Neisseria meningitidis* in those at risk of exposure to prevent invasive disease
‣ BY INTRAMUSCULAR INJECTION
‣ Child 3-11 months: 0.5 mL every month for 2 doses, dose preferably injected into deltoid region
‣ Child 1-17 years: 0.5 mL for 1 dose, dose preferably injected into deltoid region
‣ Adult: 0.5 mL for 1 dose, dose preferably injected into deltoid region

Patients attending university for the first time (who have not received the routine meningococcal groups A with C and W135 and Y conjugate vaccine over the age of 10 years)
‣ BY INTRAMUSCULAR INJECTION
‣ Adult 18-24 years: 0.5 mL for 1 dose

NIMENRIX ®

Primary immunisation against *Neisseria meningitidis*
‣ BY INTRAMUSCULAR INJECTION
‣ Child 13-15 years: 0.5 mL for 1 dose, to be injected preferably into deltoid region

Immunisation against *Neisseria meningitidis* in an unimmunised patient
‣ BY INTRAMUSCULAR INJECTION
‣ Child 10-17 years: 0.5 mL for 1 dose, booster dose is not required
‣ Adult 18-24 years: 0.5 mL for 1 dose, booster dose is not required

Immunisation against *Neisseria meningitidis* in those at risk of exposure
‣ BY INTRAMUSCULAR INJECTION
‣ Child 1-17 years: 0.5 mL for 1 dose, to be injected preferably into deltoid region (or anterolateral thigh in child 12–23 months), then 0.5 mL after 1 year if required for 1 dose, second dose should be considered in those who continue to be at risk of *Neisseria meningitidis* serogroup A infection
‣ Adult: 0.5 mL for 1 dose, to be injected preferably into deltoid region, then 0.5 mL after 1 year if required for 1 dose, second dose should be considered in those who continue to be at risk of *Neisseria meningitidis* serogroup A infection

Patients attending university for the first time (who have not received the routine meningococcal groups A with C and W135 and Y conjugate vaccine over the age of 10 years)
‣ BY INTRAMUSCULAR INJECTION
‣ Adult 18-24 years: 0.5 mL for 1 dose

● UNLICENSED USE
MENVEO ®
‣ In children *Menveo* ® is not licensed for use in children under 2 years.

● SIDE-EFFECTS
‣ Common or very common Drowsiness
‣ Uncommon Crying · insomnia · numbness · pain in extremity
‣ Frequency not known Extensive swelling of vaccinated limb

● MEDICINAL FORMS There can be variation in the licensing of different medicines containing the same drug.

Powder and solvent for solution for injection
‣ Menveo (GlaxoSmithKline UK Ltd)
Menveo vaccine powder and solvent for solution for injection 0.5ml vials | 1 vial [PoM] £30.00 DT = £30.00
‣ Nimenrix (Pfizer Ltd)
Nimenrix vaccine powder and solvent for solution for injection 0.5ml pre-filled syringes | 1 pre-filled disposable injection [PoM] £30.00 DT = £30.00

Ⓕ 1360

Pneumococcal polysaccharide conjugate vaccine (adsorbed)

24-Sep-2020

● INDICATIONS AND DOSE

PREVENAR 13 ®

Primary immunisation against pneumococcal infection—first dose [infants born on or after 1 January 2020]
‣ BY INTRAMUSCULAR INJECTION
‣ Child 12 weeks: 0.5 mL for 1 dose, anterolateral thigh is preferred site of injection in infants under 1 year

Primary immunisation against pneumococcal infection—booster dose [infants born on or after 1 January 2020]
‣ BY INTRAMUSCULAR INJECTION
‣ Child 1 year: 0.5 mL for 1 dose, anterolateral thigh is preferred site of injection in infants under 1 year; deltoid muscle is preferred in older children

Primary immunisation against pneumococcal infection—in those with asplenia, splenic dysfunction, complement disorder or severe immunocompromise [infants born on or after 1 January 2020]
‣ BY INTRAMUSCULAR INJECTION
‣ Child 6 weeks-11 months: 0.5 mL for 4 doses, the first two doses to be given at least 8 weeks apart, the third dose to be given on or after their first birthday, and the fourth dose to be given at least 8 weeks later. Anterolateral thigh is preferred site of injection in infants under 1 year; deltoid muscle is preferred in children

Immunisation against pneumococcal infection—unimmunised or partially immunised patients [infants born on or after 1 January 2020]

▸ BY INTRAMUSCULAR INJECTION

▸ Child 3–11 months: 0.5 mL for 1 dose, followed by 0.5 mL for 1 dose on or after their first birthday, given at least 4 weeks after the first dose. Anterolateral thigh is preferred site of injection in infants under 1 year

▸ Child 12–23 months: 0.5 mL for 1 dose, deltoid muscle is preferred site of injection in children

Immunisation against pneumococcal infection—unimmunised or partially immunised patients at increased risk [born on or after 1 January 2020]

▸ BY INTRAMUSCULAR INJECTION

▸ Child 2–9 years: 0.5 mL for 1 dose, deltoid muscle is preferred site of injection in children

Immunisation against pneumococcal infection—immunised patients with severe immunocompromise [born on or after 1 January 2020]

▸ BY INTRAMUSCULAR INJECTION

▸ Child 2–17 years: 0.5 mL for 1 dose, deltoid muscle is preferred site of injection in children

▸ Adult: 0.5 mL for 1 dose, deltoid muscle is preferred site of injection in adults

Primary immunisation against pneumococcal infection—first dose [infants born on or before 31 December 2019]

▸ BY INTRAMUSCULAR INJECTION

▸ Child 8 weeks: 0.5 mL for 1 dose, anterolateral thigh is preferred site of injection in infants under 1 year

Primary immunisation against pneumococcal infection—second dose [infants born on or before 31 December 2019]

▸ BY INTRAMUSCULAR INJECTION

▸ Child 16 weeks: 0.5 mL for 1 dose, anterolateral thigh is preferred site of injection in infants under 1 year

Primary immunisation against pneumococcal infection—booster dose [infants born on or before 31 December 2019]

▸ BY INTRAMUSCULAR INJECTION

▸ Child 1 year: 0.5 mL for 1 dose, anterolateral thigh is preferred site of injection in infants under 1 year; deltoid muscle is preferred site of injection in older children

Immunisation against pneumococcal infection—unimmunised or partially immunised patients [infants born on or before 31 December 2019]

▸ BY INTRAMUSCULAR INJECTION

▸ Child 3–11 months: 0.5 mL for 2 doses, given 2 months apart (interval may be reduced to 1 month to ensure immunisation schedule is completed), followed by 0.5 mL for 1 dose on their first birthday, given at least 2 months after the last dose. Anterolateral thigh is preferred site of injection in infants under 1 year

▸ Child 12–23 months: 0.5 mL for 1 dose, deltoid muscle is preferred site of injection in children

Immunisation against pneumococcal infection—immunised patients at increased risk [born on or before 31 December 2019]

▸ BY INTRAMUSCULAR INJECTION

▸ Child 14 months–17 years: 0.5 mL for 1 dose, given at least 2 months after primary immunisation booster dose, deltoid muscle is preferred site of injection in children

▸ Adult: 0.5 mL for 1 dose, deltoid muscle is preferred site of injection in adults

Immunisation against pneumococcal infection—unimmunised or partially immunised patients at increased risk [born on or before 31 December 2019]

▸ BY INTRAMUSCULAR INJECTION

▸ Child 3–11 months: 0.5 mL for 2 doses, given 2 months apart (interval may be reduced to 1 month to ensure

immunisation schedule is completed), followed by 0.5 mL for 1 dose on their first birthday, given at least 2 months after the last dose, followed by 0.5 mL for 1 dose, given at least 2 months after the last dose. Anterolateral thigh is preferred site of injection in infants under 1 year

▸ Adult: 0.5 mL for 1 dose, deltoid muscle is preferred site of injection in adults

SYNFLORIX ®

Immunisation against pneumococcal infection

▸ BY INTRAMUSCULAR INJECTION

▸ Child 6 weeks–4 years: Deltoid muscle is preferred site of injection in young children; anterolateral thigh is preferred site in infants (consult product literature)

● UNLICENSED USE

PREVENAR 13 ® The dose in BNF publications may differ from that in product literature.

● SIDE-EFFECTS

▸ **Common or very common** Drowsiness

▸ **Uncommon** Apnoea · crying abnormal · extensive swelling of vaccinated limb

▸ **Rare or very rare** Angioedema · hypotonic-hyporesponsiveness episode · Kawasaki disease · seizure

● PRESCRIBING AND DISPENSING INFORMATION

PREVENAR 13 ® Available as part of childhood immunisation schedule from ImmForm portal.immform. phe.gov.uk.

● MEDICINAL FORMS There can be variation in the licensing of different medicines containing the same drug.

Suspension for injection

▸ Prevenar (Pfizer Ltd)
Prevenar 13 vaccine suspension for injection 0.5ml pre-filled syringes | 1 pre-filled disposable injection PoM £49.10 DT = £49.10 | 10 pre-filled disposable injection PoM £491.00

▰ 1360

Pneumococcal polysaccharide vaccine

01-May-2019

● INDICATIONS AND DOSE

Primary immunisation against pneumococcal infection

▸ BY INTRAMUSCULAR INJECTION

▸ Elderly: 0.5 mL for 1 dose, deltoid muscle is preferred site of injection in adults

Immunisation against pneumococcal infection [in patients at increased risk]

▸ BY INTRAMUSCULAR INJECTION

▸ Child 2–17 years: 0.5 mL for 1 dose, dose should be administered at least 2 months after the last dose of the 13-valent pneumococcal polysaccharide conjugate vaccine (adsorbed), deltoid muscle is preferred site of injection in children and adults

▸ Adult: 0.5 mL for 1 dose, deltoid muscle is preferred site of injection in adults, primary immunisation with the pneumococcal polysaccharide vaccine is not required when these patients reach 65 years of age

Immunisation against pneumococcal infection [revaccination; booster dose in patients with no spleen, splenic dysfunction or chronic kidney disease]

▸ BY INTRAMUSCULAR INJECTION

▸ Child 7–17 years: 0.5 mL every 5 years, deltoid muscle is preferred site of injection in children and adults

▸ Adult: 0.5 mL every 5 years, deltoid muscle is preferred site of injection in adults

● SIDE-EFFECTS Angioedema · arthritis · asthenia · chills · febrile seizure · haemolytic anaemia · injected limb mobility decreased · leucocytosis · lymphadenitis · nerve

14

Vaccines

disorders · paraesthesia · peripheral oedema · thrombocytopenia

- **MEDICINAL FORMS** There can be variation in the licensing of different medicines containing the same drug.
  Solution for injection
  ▸ Pneumococcal polysaccharide vaccine (Non-proprietary)
    Pneumococcal polysaccharide vaccine solution for injection 0.5ml vials | 1 vial PoM £8.32 DT = £8.32
  ▸ Pneumovax 23 (Merck Sharp & Dohme Ltd)
    Pneumovax 23 solution for injection 0.5ml pre-filled syringes | 1 pre-filled disposable injection PoM £16.80 DT = £16.80

⚑ 1360

Typhoid vaccine
23-Sep-2020

- **DRUG ACTION** Typhoid vaccine protects against typhoid fever caused by *Salmonella typhi* infection; it is available as an oral live attenuated vaccine and an injectable polysaccharide vaccine.

- **INDICATIONS AND DOSE**
  Immunisation against typhoid fever [in children at high risk of typhoid fever]
  ▸ BY INTRAMUSCULAR INJECTION
  ▸ Child 12–23 months: 0.5 mL for 1 dose, dose should be given at least 2 weeks before potential exposure to typhoid infection, response may be suboptimal
  Immunisation against typhoid fever
  ▸ BY INTRAMUSCULAR INJECTION
  ▸ Child 2–17 years: 0.5 mL for 1 dose, dose should be given at least 2 weeks before potential exposure to typhoid infection
  ▸ Adult: 0.5 mL for 1 dose, dose should be given at least 2 weeks before potential exposure to typhoid infection
  ▸ BY MOUTH
  ▸ Child 5–17 years: 1 capsule every 2 days for 3 doses (on days 1, 3, and 5), course should be completed at least 1 week before potential exposure to typhoid infection
  ▸ Adult: 1 capsule every 2 days for 3 doses (on days 1, 3, and 5), course should be completed at least 1 week before potential exposure to typhoid infection
  Booster
  ▸ BY INTRAMUSCULAR INJECTION
  ▸ Child 2–17 years: 0.5 mL for 1 dose every 3 years
  ▸ Adult: 0.5 mL for 1 dose every 3 years
  ▸ BY MOUTH
  ▸ Child 5–17 years: 1 capsule every 2 days for 3 doses (on days 1, 3, and 5) every 3 years
  ▸ Adult: 1 capsule every 2 days for 3 doses (on days 1, 3, and 5) every 3 years

- **UNLICENSED USE**
  ▸ With intramuscular use in children Not licensed for use in children under 2 years.
- **CONTRA-INDICATIONS**
  ▸ With oral use Acute gastro-intestinal illness
- **INTERACTIONS** → Appendix 1: live vaccines
- **SIDE-EFFECTS**
  GENERAL SIDE-EFFECTS
  Shock
  SPECIFIC SIDE-EFFECTS
  ▸ **Common or very common**
  ▸ With oral use Gastrointestinal discomfort
  ▸ **Frequency not known**
  ▸ With oral use Asthenia · back pain · chills · flatulence · influenza like illness · paraesthesia
  ▸ With parenteral use Abdominal pain · asthma · syncope
- **DIRECTIONS FOR ADMINISTRATION** Manufacturer advises capsule should be taken one hour before a meal. Swallow as soon as possible after placing in mouth with a cold or lukewarm drink.

- **HANDLING AND STORAGE**
  ▸ With oral use It is important to store capsules in a refrigerator.
- **PATIENT AND CARER ADVICE**
  ▸ With oral use Patients or carers should be given advice on how to administer and store typhoid vaccine capsules.

- **MEDICINAL FORMS** There can be variation in the licensing of different medicines containing the same drug.
  Solution for injection
  ▸ Typhim Vi (Sanofi Pasteur)
    Salmonella typhi Vi capsular polysaccharide 50 microgram per 1 ml Typhim Vi 25micrograms/0.5ml vaccine solution for injection pre-filled syringes | 1 pre-filled disposable injection PoM £11.16 DT = £11.16 | 10 pre-filled disposable injection PoM £111.60 DT = £111.60
  Gastro-resistant capsule
  CAUTIONARY AND ADVISORY LABELS 25
  ▸ Vivotif (Emergent BioSolutions UK)
    Vivotif vaccine gastro-resistant capsules | 3 capsule PoM £14.77 DT = £14.77

  Combinations available: *Hepatitis A with typhoid vaccine,* p. 1370

VACCINES > VIRAL VACCINES

Hepatitis A and B vaccine
16-Nov-2020

The properties listed below are those particular to the combination only. For the properties of the components please consider, hepatitis A vaccine p. 1369, hepatitis B vaccine p. 1370.

- **INDICATIONS AND DOSE**
  AMBIRIX ®
  Immunisation against hepatitis A and hepatitis B infection [primary course]
  ▸ BY INTRAMUSCULAR INJECTION
  ▸ Child 1–15 years: Initially 1 mL for 1 dose, then 1 mL after 6–12 months for 1 dose, the deltoid region is the preferred site of injection in older children; anterolateral thigh may be used in infants; not to be injected into the buttock (vaccine efficacy reduced), subcutaneous route used for patients with bleeding disorders (but immune response may be reduced)
  Post-exposure prophylaxis against hepatitis A infection [for rapid protection]
  ▸ BY INTRAMUSCULAR INJECTION
  ▸ Child 1–15 years: 1 mL for 1 dose, the deltoid region is the preferred site of injection in older children; anterolateral thigh may be used in infants; not to be injected into the buttock (vaccine efficacy reduced), subcutaneous route used for patients with bleeding disorders (but immune response may be reduced)
  TWINRIX ® ADULT
  Immunisation against hepatitis A and hepatitis B infection [primary course]
  ▸ BY INTRAMUSCULAR INJECTION
  ▸ Child 16–17 years: Initially 1 mL every month for 2 doses, then 1 mL after 5 months for 1 dose, the deltoid region is the preferred site of injection; not to be injected into the buttock (vaccine efficacy reduced), subcutaneous route used for patients with bleeding disorders (but immune response may be reduced)
  ▸ Adult: Initially 1 mL every month for 2 doses, then 1 mL after 5 months for 1 dose, the deltoid region is the preferred site of injection; not to be injected into the buttock (vaccine efficacy reduced), subcutaneous route used for patients with bleeding disorders (but immune response may be reduced)

Immunisation against hepatitis A and hepatitis B infection [accelerated schedule for travellers departing within 1 month]
▶ BY INTRAMUSCULAR INJECTION
▶ Child 16-17 years: Initially 1 mL for 1 dose, then 1 mL after 7 days for 1 dose, then 1 mL after 14 days for 1 dose, then 1 mL for 1 dose given 12 months after the first dose, the deltoid region is the preferred site of injection; not to be injected into the buttock (vaccine efficacy reduced), subcutaneous route used for patients with bleeding disorders (but immune response may be reduced)
▶ Adult: Initially 1 mL for 1 dose, then 1 mL after 7 days for 1 dose, then 1 mL after 14 days for 1 dose, then 1 mL for 1 dose given 12 months after the first dose, the deltoid region is the preferred site of injection; not to be injected into the buttock (vaccine efficacy reduced), subcutaneous route used for patients with bleeding disorders (but immune response may be reduced)

TWINRIX ® PAEDIATRIC

Immunisation against hepatitis A and hepatitis B infection [primary course]
▶ BY INTRAMUSCULAR INJECTION
▶ Child 1-15 years: Initially 0.5 mL every month for 2 doses, then 0.5 mL after 5 months for 1 dose, the deltoid region is the preferred site of injection in older children; anterolateral thigh is the preferred site in infants; not to be injected into the buttock (vaccine efficacy reduced), subcutaneous route used for patients with bleeding disorders (but immune response may be reduced)

● UNLICENSED USE

AMBIRIX ® Public Health England advises that *Ambirix* ® may be used for post-exposure prophylaxis against hepatitis A infection where rapid protection is required, but is not licensed for this indication.

> IMPORTANT SAFETY INFORMATION
> *Ambirix* ® and *Twinrix* ® are not recommended for post-exposure prophylaxis following percutaneous (needle-stick), ocular, or mucous membrane exposure to hepatitis B virus.

● PRESCRIBING AND DISPENSING INFORMATION

TWINRIX ® PAEDIATRIC Primary course should be completed with *Twinrix* ® (single component vaccines given at appropriate intervals may be used for booster dose).

TWINRIX ® ADULT Primary course should be completed with *Twinrix* ® (single component vaccines given at appropriate intervals may be used for booster dose).

AMBIRIX ® Primary course should be completed with *Ambirix* ® (single component vaccines given at appropriate intervals may be used for booster dose).

● MEDICINAL FORMS There can be variation in the licensing of different medicines containing the same drug.
Suspension for injection
EXCIPIENTS: May contain Neomycin
▶ Ambirix (GlaxoSmithKline UK Ltd)
Ambirix vaccine suspension for injection 1ml pre-filled syringes | 1 pre-filled disposable injection PoM £31.18 DT = £31.18
▶ Twinrix (GlaxoSmithKline UK Ltd)
Twinrix Paediatric vaccine suspension for injection 0.5ml pre-filled syringes | 1 pre-filled disposable injection PoM £20.79 DT = £20.79
Twinrix Adult vaccine suspension for injection 1ml pre-filled syringes | 1 pre-filled disposable injection PoM £33.31 DT = £31.18 | 10 pre-filled disposable injection PoM £333.13

⚑ 1360

Hepatitis A vaccine

17-Nov-2020

● INDICATIONS AND DOSE

AVAXIM ®

Immunisation against hepatitis A infection
▶ BY INTRAMUSCULAR INJECTION
▶ Child 16-17 years: Initially 0.5 mL for 1 dose, then 0.5 mL after 6–12 months, dose given as booster; booster dose may be delayed by up to 3 years if not given after recommended interval following primary dose, the deltoid region is the preferred site of injection. The subcutaneous route may be used for patients with bleeding disorders; not to be injected into the buttock (vaccine efficacy reduced)
▶ Adult: Initially 0.5 mL for 1 dose, then 0.5 mL after 6–12 months, dose given as booster; booster dose may be delayed by up to 3 years if not given after recommended interval following primary dose, the deltoid region is the preferred site of injection. The subcutaneous route may be used for patients with bleeding disorders; not to be injected into the buttock (vaccine efficacy reduced)

HAVRIX JUNIOR MONODOSE ®

Immunisation against hepatitis A infection
▶ BY INTRAMUSCULAR INJECTION
▶ Child 1-15 years: Initially 0.5 mL for 1 dose, then 0.5 mL after 6–12 months, dose given as booster; booster dose may be delayed by up to 3 years if not given after recommended interval following primary dose, deltoid muscle is preferred site of injection in older children; anterolateral thigh is preferred site in infants and young children; not to be injected into the gluteal region. The subcutaneous route may be used for patients with bleeding disorders

HAVRIX MONODOSE ®

Immunisation against hepatitis A infection
▶ BY INTRAMUSCULAR INJECTION
▶ Child 16-17 years: Initially 1 mL for 1 dose, then 1 mL after 6–12 months, dose given as booster; booster dose may be delayed by up to 3 years if not given after recommended interval following primary dose, the deltoid region is the preferred site of injection; not to be injected into the gluteal region. The subcutaneous route may be used for patients with bleeding disorders
▶ Adult: Initially 1 mL for 1 dose, then 1 mL after 6–12 months, dose given as booster; booster dose may be delayed by up to 3 years if not given after recommended interval following primary dose, the deltoid region is the preferred site of injection; not to be injected into the gluteal region. The subcutaneous route may be used for patients with bleeding disorders

VAQTA ® ADULT

Immunisation against hepatitis A infection
▶ BY INTRAMUSCULAR INJECTION
▶ Adult: Initially 1 mL for 1 dose, then 1 mL after 6–18 months, dose given as booster, the deltoid region is the preferred site of injection. The subcutaneous route may be used for patients with bleeding disorders (but immune response may be delayed)

VAQTA ® PAEDIATRIC

Immunisation against hepatitis A infection
▶ BY INTRAMUSCULAR INJECTION
▶ Child 1-17 years: Initially 0.5 mL for 1 dose, then 0.5 mL after 6–18 months, dose given as booster, the deltoid region is the preferred site of injection. The subcutaneous route may be used for patients with bleeding disorders (but immune response may be reduced)

14

Vaccines

● SIDE-EFFECTS
► **Common or very common** Asthenia (uncommon in children) · pain (uncommon in children)
► **Uncommon** Anxiety (in children) · chills (in adults) · cough · crying (in children) · ear pain (rare in children) · gastrointestinal discomfort · gastrointestinal disorders (rare in children) · increased risk of infection (in adults) · influenza like illness (rare in children) · muscle weakness (in adults) · musculoskeletal stiffness (rare in children) · nasal complaints · paraesthesia (rare in children) · respiratory disorders (rare in children) · sensation of tightness (rare in children) · temperature sensation altered (rare in children) · vasodilation (rare in children)
► **Rare or very rare** Allergic rhinitis (in children) · apathy (in adults) · asthma (in children) · ataxia (in children) · burping (in children) · chest pain · constipation (in children) · dehydration (in children) · drowsiness (uncommon in children) · dry mouth (in adults) · eye discomfort · gait abnormal (in children) · infantile spitting up (in children) · menstrual disorder (in adults) · migraine (in adults) · muscle complaints (in adults) · oral ulceration (in adults) · oropharyngeal pain (in children) · photophobia (in adults) · screaming (in children) · sleep disorders (uncommon in children) · sweat changes (in children) · synovitis (in children) · throat oedema (in adults) · tremor (in adults) · vertigo (in adults) · watering eye (in adults)
► **Frequency not known** Guillain-Barre syndrome · thrombocytopenia

● MEDICINAL FORMS There can be variation in the licensing of different medicines containing the same drug.
Suspension for injection
EXCIPIENTS: May contain Neomycin
► Avaxim (Sanofi Pasteur)
Avaxim vaccine suspension for injection 0.5ml pre-filled syringes | 1 pre-filled disposable injection [PoM] £21.72 | 10 pre-filled disposable injection [PoM] £217.20
► Havrix (GlaxoSmithKline UK Ltd)
Havrix Monodose vaccine suspension for injection 1ml pre-filled syringes | 1 pre-filled disposable injection [PoM] £22.14 DT = £22.14 | 10 pre-filled disposable injection [PoM] £221.43
Havrix Junior Monodose vaccine suspension for injection 0.5ml pre-filled syringes | 1 pre-filled disposable injection [PoM] £16.77 | 10 pre-filled disposable injection [PoM] £167.68
► VAQTA (Merck Sharp & Dohme Ltd)
VAQTA Adult vaccine suspension for injection 1ml pre-filled syringes | 1 pre-filled disposable injection [PoM] £18.10 DT = £22.14
VAQTA Paediatric vaccine suspension for injection 0.5ml pre-filled syringes | 1 pre-filled disposable injection [PoM] £14.74

Hepatitis A with typhoid vaccine

16-Nov-2020

The properties listed below are those particular to the combination only. For the properties of the components please consider, hepatitis A vaccine p. 1369, typhoid vaccine p. 1368.

● INDICATIONS AND DOSE
VIATIM ®
Immunisation against hepatitis A and typhoid infection [primary course]
► BY INTRAMUSCULAR INJECTION
► Child 16-17 years: 1 mL for 1 dose, the deltoid region is the preferred site of injection; not to be injected into the buttock (vaccine efficacy reduced). The subcutaneous route may be used for patients with bleeding disorders, booster dose may be given using single or multicomponent vaccines
► Adult: 1 mL for 1 dose, the deltoid region is the preferred site of injection; not to be injected into the buttock (vaccine efficacy reduced). The subcutaneous route may be used for patients with bleeding disorders,

booster dose may be given using single or multicomponent vaccines

Immunisation against hepatitis A [booster dose for individuals who have received primary immunisation with monovalent hepatitis A vaccine, where protection against typhoid is also required]
► BY INTRAMUSCULAR INJECTION
► Child 16-17 years: 1 mL for 1 dose, within 36 months (preferably 6–12 months) of primary immunisation, the deltoid region is the preferred site of injection; not to be injected into the buttock (vaccine efficacy reduced). The subcutaneous route may be used for patients with bleeding disorders
► Adult: 1 mL for 1 dose, within 36 months (preferably 6–12 months) of primary immunisation, the deltoid region is the preferred site of injection; not to be injected into the buttock (vaccine efficacy reduced). The subcutaneous route may be used for patients with bleeding disorders

Immunisation against typhoid [booster dose for individuals who have received primary immunisation with hepatitis A and typhoid vaccine, where continued protection against typhoid is required]
► BY INTRAMUSCULAR INJECTION
► Child 16-17 years: 1 mL for 1 dose, 36 months after primary immunisation, the deltoid region is the preferred site of injection; not to be injected into the buttock (vaccine efficacy reduced). The subcutaneous route may be used for patients with bleeding disorders
► Adult: 1 mL for 1 dose, 36 months after primary immunisation, the deltoid region is the preferred site of injection; not to be injected into the buttock (vaccine efficacy reduced). The subcutaneous route may be used for patients with bleeding disorders

● MEDICINAL FORMS There can be variation in the licensing of different medicines containing the same drug.
Suspension for injection
EXCIPIENTS: May contain Neomycin
► ViATIM (Sanofi Pasteur)
ViATIM vaccine suspension for injection 1ml pre-filled syringes | 1 pre-filled disposable injection [PoM] £35.76 DT = £35.76

F 1360

Hepatitis B vaccine

● INDICATIONS AND DOSE
ENGERIX B ®
Immunisation against hepatitis B infection
► BY INTRAMUSCULAR INJECTION
► Child 1 month-15 years: 10 micrograms for 1 dose, then 10 micrograms after 1 month for 1 dose, followed by 10 micrograms after 5 months for 1 dose, deltoid muscle is preferred site of injection in older children; anterolateral thigh is preferred site in infants and young children; not to be injected into the buttock (vaccine efficacy reduced)
► Child 16-17 years: 20 micrograms for 1 dose, then 20 micrograms after 1 month for 1 dose, followed by 20 micrograms after 5 months for 1 dose, deltoid muscle is preferred site of injection; not to be injected into the buttock (vaccine efficacy reduced)
► Adult: 20 micrograms for 1 dose, then 20 micrograms after 1 month for 1 dose, followed by 20 micrograms after 5 months for 1 dose, deltoid muscle is preferred site of injection; not to be injected into the buttock (vaccine efficacy reduced)

Immunisation against hepatitis B infection (accelerated schedule)

▸ BY INTRAMUSCULAR INJECTION

▸ Neonate: 10 micrograms every month for 3 doses, followed by 10 micrograms after 10 months for 1 dose, anterolateral thigh is preferred site in neonates; not to be injected into the buttock (vaccine efficacy reduced), this dose should not be given to neonates born to hepatitis B surface antigen positive mother.

▸ Child 1 month–15 years: 10 micrograms every month for 3 doses, followed by 10 micrograms after 10 months for 1 dose, deltoid muscle is preferred site of injection in older children; anterolateral thigh is preferred site in infants and young children; not to be injected into the buttock (vaccine efficacy reduced)

▸ Child 16–17 years: 20 micrograms every month for 3 doses, followed by 20 micrograms after 10 months for 1 dose, deltoid muscle is preferred site of injection; not to be injected into the buttock (vaccine efficacy reduced)

▸ Adult: 20 micrograms every month for 3 doses, followed by 20 micrograms after 10 months for 1 dose, deltoid muscle is preferred site of injection; not to be injected into the buttock (vaccine efficacy reduced)

Immunisation against hepatitis B infection, alternative accelerated schedule

▸ BY INTRAMUSCULAR INJECTION

▸ Child 11–15 years: 20 micrograms for 1 dose, followed by 20 micrograms after 6 months, this schedule is not suitable if high risk of infection between doses or if compliance with second dose uncertain, deltoid muscle is preferred site of injection; not to be injected into the buttock (vaccine efficacy reduced)

Immunisation against hepatitis B infection (accelerated schedule in exceptional cases, e.g. for travellers departing within 1 month)

▸ BY INTRAMUSCULAR INJECTION

▸ Adult: 20 micrograms for 1 dose, then 20 micrograms after 7 days for 1 dose, followed by 20 micrograms after 14 days for 1 dose, followed by 20 micrograms for 1 dose, to be given 12 months after the first dose, deltoid muscle is preferred site of injection; not to be injected into the buttock (vaccine efficacy reduced)

Immunisation against hepatitis B infection (in renal insufficiency, including haemodialysis patients)

▸ BY INTRAMUSCULAR INJECTION

▸ Child 1 month–15 years: 10 micrograms every month for 2 doses, followed by 10 micrograms after 5 months for 1 dose, immunisation schedule and booster doses may need to be adjusted in those with low antibody concentration, deltoid muscle is preferred site of injection in older children; anterolateral thigh is preferred site in infants and young children; not to be injected into the buttock (vaccine efficacy reduced)

▸ Child 16–17 years: 40 micrograms every month for 3 doses, followed by 40 micrograms after 4 months for 1 dose, immunisation schedule and booster doses may need to be adjusted in those with low antibody concentration, deltoid muscle is preferred site of injection; not to be injected into the buttock (vaccine efficacy reduced)

▸ Adult: 40 micrograms every month for 3 doses, followed by 40 micrograms after 4 months for 1 dose, immunisation schedule and booster doses may need to be adjusted in those with low antibody concentration, deltoid muscle is preferred site of injection; not to be injected into the buttock (vaccine efficacy reduced)

Immunisation against hepatitis B infection (in renal insufficiency, including haemodialysis patients (accelerated schedule))

▸ BY INTRAMUSCULAR INJECTION

▸ Child 1 month–15 years: 10 micrograms every month for 3 doses, followed by 10 micrograms after 10 months for 1 dose, immunisation schedule and booster doses may need to be adjusted in those with low antibody concentration, deltoid muscle is preferred site of injection in older children; anterolateral thigh is preferred site in infants and young children; not to be injected into the buttock (vaccine efficacy reduced)

FENDRIX ®

Immunisation against hepatitis B infection in renal insufficiency (including pre-haemodialysis and haemodialysis patients)

▸ BY INTRAMUSCULAR INJECTION

▸ Child 15–17 years: 20 micrograms every month for 3 doses, followed by 20 micrograms after 4 months for 1 dose, immunisation schedule and booster doses may need to be adjusted in those with low antibody concentration, deltoid muscle is preferred site of injection; not to be injected into the buttock (vaccine efficacy reduced)

▸ Adult: 20 micrograms every month for 3 doses, followed by 20 micrograms after 4 months for 1 dose, immunisation schedule and booster doses may need to be adjusted in those with low antibody concentration, deltoid muscle is preferred site of injection; not to be injected into the buttock (vaccine efficacy reduced)

HBVAXPRO ®

Immunisation against hepatitis B infection

▸ BY INTRAMUSCULAR INJECTION

▸ Neonate: 5 micrograms for 1 dose, followed by 5 micrograms after 1 month for 1 dose, then 5 micrograms after 5 months for 1 dose, booster doses may be required in immunocompromised patients with low antibody concentration, anterolateral thigh is preferred site in neonates; not to be injected into the buttock (vaccine efficacy reduced), dose not to be used for neonate born to hepatitis B surface antigen positive mother.

▸ Child 1 month–15 years: 5 micrograms for 1 dose, followed by 5 micrograms after 1 month for 1 dose, then 5 micrograms after 5 months for 1 dose, booster doses may be required in immunocompromised patients with low antibody concentration, deltoid muscle is preferred site of injection in adults and older children; anterolateral thigh is preferred site in infants; not to be injected into the buttock (vaccine efficacy reduced)

▸ Child 16–17 years: 10 micrograms for 1 dose, followed by 10 micrograms after 1 month for 1 dose, followed by 10 micrograms after 5 months for 1 dose, booster doses may be required in immunocompromised patients with low antibody concentration, deltoid muscle is preferred site of injection in adults and older children; not to be injected into the buttock (vaccine efficacy reduced)

▸ Adult: 10 micrograms for 1 dose, followed by 10 micrograms after 1 month for 1 dose, followed by 10 micrograms after 5 months for 1 dose, booster doses may be required in immunocompromised patients with low antibody concentration, deltoid muscle is preferred site of injection in adults and older children; not to be injected into the buttock (vaccine efficacy reduced)

continued →

14

Vaccines

Immunisation against hepatitis B infection (accelerated schedule)

▸ BY INTRAMUSCULAR INJECTION

▸ Neonate: 5 micrograms every month for 3 doses, followed by 5 micrograms after 10 months for 1 dose, booster doses may be required in immunocompromised patients with low antibody concentration, anterolateral thigh is preferred site in neonates; not to be injected into the buttock (vaccine efficacy reduced), dose not to be used for neonate born to hepatitis B surface antigen positive mother.

▸ Child 1 month–15 years: 5 micrograms every month for 3 doses, followed by 5 micrograms after 10 months for 1 dose, booster doses may be required in immunocompromised patients with low antibody concentration, deltoid muscle is preferred site of injection in older children; anterolateral thigh is preferred site in infants; not to be injected into the buttock (vaccine efficacy reduced)

▸ Child 16–17 years: 10 micrograms every month for 3 doses, followed by 10 micrograms after 10 months for 1 dose, booster doses may be required in immunocompromised patients with low antibody concentration, deltoid muscle is preferred site of injection in older children; not to be injected into the buttock (vaccine efficacy reduced)

▸ Adult: 10 micrograms every month for 3 doses, followed by 10 micrograms after 10 months for 1 dose, booster doses may be required in immunocompromised patients with low antibody concentration, deltoid muscle is preferred site of injection; not to be injected into the buttock (vaccine efficacy reduced)

Neonate born to hepatitis B surface antigen-positive mother

▸ BY INTRAMUSCULAR INJECTION

▸ Neonate: 5 micrograms every month for 3 doses, first dose given at birth with hepatitis B immunoglobulin injection (separate site), followed by 5 micrograms after 10 months for 1 dose, anterolateral thigh is preferred site in neonates; not to be injected into the buttock (vaccine efficacy reduced).

Chronic haemodialysis patients

▸ BY INTRAMUSCULAR INJECTION

▸ Child 16–17 years: 40 micrograms every month for 2 doses, followed by 40 micrograms after 5 months for 1 dose, booster doses may be required in those with low antibody concentration, deltoid muscle is preferred site of injection in older children; not to be injected into the buttock (vaccine efficacy reduced)

▸ Adult: 40 micrograms every month for 2 doses, followed by 40 micrograms after 5 months for 1 dose, booster doses may be required in those with low antibody concentration, deltoid muscle is preferred site of injection; not to be injected into the buttock (vaccine efficacy reduced)

● SIDE-EFFECTS

▸ **Common or very common** Drowsiness · gastrointestinal disorder

▸ **Uncommon** Influenza like illness

▸ **Rare or very rare** Sensation abnormal

▸ **Frequency not known** Angioedema · apnoea · arthritis · encephalitis · encephalopathy · hypotension · meningitis · multiple sclerosis · muscle weakness · nerve disorders · paralysis · seizure · thrombocytopenia · vasculitis

● MEDICINAL FORMS There can be variation in the licensing of different medicines containing the same drug.

Suspension for injection

EXCIPIENTS: May contain Thiomersal

▸ Engerix B (GlaxoSmithKline UK Ltd)
Hepatitis B virus surface antigen 20 microgram per 1 ml Engerix B 10micrograms/0.5ml vaccine suspension for injection pre-filled syringes | 1 pre-filled disposable injection [PoM] £9.67 DT = £9.67
Engerix B 20micrograms/1ml vaccine suspension for injection pre-filled syringes | 1 pre-filled disposable injection [PoM] £12.99 DT = £12.99 | 10 pre-filled disposable injection [PoM] £129.92

▸ Fendrix (GlaxoSmithKline UK Ltd)
Hepatitis B virus surface antigen 40 microgram per 1 ml Fendrix 20micrograms/0.5ml vaccine suspension for injection pre-filled syringes | 1 pre-filled disposable injection [PoM] £38.10 DT = £38.10

▸ HBVAXPRO (Merck Sharp & Dohme Ltd)
Hepatitis B virus surface antigen 10 microgram per 1 ml HBVAXPRO 10micrograms/1ml vaccine suspension for injection pre-filled syringes | 1 pre-filled disposable injection [PoM] £12.20
HBVAXPRO 5micrograms/0.5ml vaccine suspension for injection pre-filled syringes | 1 pre-filled disposable injection [PoM] £8.95 DT = £8.95
Hepatitis B virus surface antigen 40 microgram per 1 ml HBvaxPRO 40micrograms/1ml vaccine suspension for injection vials | 1 vial [PoM] £27.60 DT = £27.60

↑ 1360

Human papillomavirus vaccines
29-Oct-2019

● INDICATIONS AND DOSE

CERVARIX ®

Immunisation against HPV-related premalignant lesions and cancer (cervical, vulvar, vaginal, and anal) [2 dose schedule]

▸ BY INTRAMUSCULAR INJECTION

▸ Child 9–14 years: 0.5 mL for 1 dose, followed by 0.5 mL after 5–24 months for 1 dose, if second dose administered earlier than 5 months after the first, a third dose should be administered, to be administered into deltoid region, if the 2 dose schedule is interrupted, it should be resumed (using the same vaccine) but not repeated, even if more than 24 months have elapsed since the first dose or if the patient is now older than 14 years

Immunisation against HPV-related premalignant lesions and cancer (cervical, vulvar, vaginal, and anal) [3 dose schedule]

▸ BY INTRAMUSCULAR INJECTION

▸ Child 15–17 years: 0.5 mL for 1 dose, followed by 0.5 mL after 1–2.5 months for 1 dose, then 0.5 mL after 5–12 months from the first dose for 1 dose, to be administered into deltoid region, if the 3 dose schedule is interrupted, it should be resumed (using the same vaccine) but not repeated, allowing the appropriate interval between the remaining doses

▸ Adult: 0.5 mL for 1 dose, followed by 0.5 mL after 1–2.5 months for 1 dose, then 0.5 mL after 5–12 months from the first dose for 1 dose, to be administered into deltoid region, if the 3 dose schedule is interrupted, it should be resumed (using the same vaccine) but not repeated, allowing the appropriate interval between the remaining doses

GARDASIL 9 ®

Immunisation against HPV-related premalignant lesions and cancer (cervical, vulvar, vaginal, and anal) and genital warts [2 dose schedule]

▸ BY INTRAMUSCULAR INJECTION

▸ Child 9–14 years: 0.5 mL for 1 dose, followed by 0.5 mL after 5–24 months for 1 dose, to be administered preferably into deltoid region or higher anterolateral thigh, if the 2 dose schedule is interrupted, it should be resumed (using the same vaccine) but not repeated, even if more than 24 months have elapsed since the first dose or if the patient is now older than 14 years

Immunisation against HPV-related premalignant lesions and cancer (cervical, vulvar, vaginal, and anal) and genital warts [3 dose schedule]
▶ BY INTRAMUSCULAR INJECTION
▶ Child 9–17 years: 0.5 mL for 1 dose, followed by 0.5 mL for 1 dose, second dose to be given at least 1 month after the first dose, then 0.5 mL for 1 dose, third dose to be given at least 3 months after the second dose, to be administered preferably into deltoid region or higher anterolateral thigh, the 3 dose schedule should be completed within 12 months of the first dose. If the schedule is interrupted, it should be resumed (using the same vaccine) but not repeated, allowing the appropriate interval between the remaining doses
▶ Adult: 0.5 mL for 1 dose, followed by 0.5 mL for 1 dose, second dose to be given at least 1 month after the first dose, then 0.5 mL for 1 dose, third dose to be given at least 3 months after the second dose, to be administered preferably into deltoid region or higher anterolateral thigh, the 3 dose schedule should be completed within 12 months of the first dose. If the schedule is interrupted, it should be resumed (using the same vaccine) but not repeated, allowing the appropriate interval between the remaining doses

GARDASIL®

Immunisation against HPV-related premalignant lesions and cancer (cervical, vulvar, vaginal, and anal) and genital warts [2 dose schedule]
▶ BY INTRAMUSCULAR INJECTION
▶ Child 9–14 years: 0.5 mL for 1 dose, followed by 0.5 mL after 6–24 months for 1 dose, to be administered preferably into deltoid region or higher anterolateral thigh, if the 2 dose schedule is interrupted, it should be resumed (using the same vaccine) but not repeated, even if more than 24 months have elapsed since the first dose or if the patient is now older than 14 years

Immunisation against HPV-related premalignant lesions and cancer (cervical, vulvar, vaginal, and anal) and genital warts [3 dose schedule]
▶ BY INTRAMUSCULAR INJECTION
▶ Child 9–17 years: 0.5 mL for 1 dose, followed by 0.5 mL for 1 dose, second dose to be given at least 1 month after the first dose, then 0.5 mL for 1 dose, third dose to be given at least 3 months after the second dose, to be administered preferably into deltoid region or higher anterolateral thigh, the 3 dose schedule should be completed within 12 months of the first dose, if the schedule is interrupted, it should be resumed (using the same vaccine) but not repeated, allowing the appropriate interval between the remaining doses
▶ Adult: 0.5 mL for 1 dose, followed by 0.5 mL for 1 dose, second dose to be given at least 1 month after the first dose, then 0.5 mL for 1 dose, third dose to be given at least 3 months after the second dose, to be administered preferably into deltoid region or higher anterolateral thigh, the 3 dose schedule should be completed within 12 months of the first dose, if the schedule is interrupted, it should be resumed (using the same vaccine) but not repeated, allowing the appropriate interval between the remaining doses

● UNLICENSED USE EvGr Human papillomavirus vaccines are used in a 2 dose immunisation schedule, Ⓐ but the interval between doses may differ from licensing.
GARDASIL® EvGr The 2 dose schedule is not licensed for use in children aged 14 years. Ⓐ

● SIDE-EFFECTS
▶ **Common or very common** Abdominal pain · gastrointestinal disorder · pain in extremity
▶ **Uncommon** Upper respiratory tract infection
▶ **Frequency not known** Acute disseminated encephalomyelitis · angioedema · asthenia · bronchospasm · chills · Guillain-Barre syndrome · immune thrombocytopenic purpura · syncope

● PREGNANCY Not known to be harmful, but vaccination should be postponed until completion of pregnancy.

● PRESCRIBING AND DISPENSING INFORMATION To avoid confusion, prescribers should specify the brand to be dispensed.

● MEDICINAL FORMS There can be variation in the licensing of different medicines containing the same drug.
Suspension for injection
▶ Cervarix (GlaxoSmithKline UK Ltd)
Cervarix vaccine suspension for injection 0.5ml pre-filled syringes | 1 pre-filled disposable injection PoM £80.50
▶ Gardasil (Merck Sharp & Dohme Ltd)
Gardasil vaccine suspension for injection 0.5ml pre-filled syringes | 1 pre-filled disposable injection PoM £86.50 DT = £86.50
▶ Gardasil 9 (Merck Sharp & Dohme Ltd)
Gardasil 9 vaccine suspension for injection 0.5ml pre-filled syringes | 1 pre-filled disposable injection PoM £105.00 DT = £105.00

⏴ 1360

Influenza vaccine
21-Sep-2020

● DRUG ACTION Influenza vaccines protect people at high risk from influenza and reduce transmission of infection; the nasal spray contains live attenuated strains, all other vaccines are inactivated.

● INDICATIONS AND DOSE
Annual immunisation against seasonal influenza
▶ BY INTRAMUSCULAR INJECTION
▶ Child 6 months–8 years: 0.5 mL for 1 dose, for children who have not received seasonal influenza vaccine previously, repeat dose after at least 4 weeks
▶ Child 9–17 years: 0.5 mL for 1 dose
▶ Adult: 0.5 mL for 1 dose
▶ BY INTRANASAL ADMINISTRATION
▶ Child 2–17 years: 0.2 mL for 1 dose, to be administered as 0.1 mL into each nostril
Annual immunisation against seasonal influenza (for children in clinical risk groups who have not received seasonal influenza vaccine previously)
▶ BY INTRAMUSCULAR INJECTION
▶ Child 6 months–8 years: 0.5 mL for 1 dose, followed by 0.5 mL for 1 dose, after at least 4 weeks
▶ BY INTRANASAL ADMINISTRATION
▶ Child 2–8 years: 0.2 mL for 1 dose, followed by 0.2 mL for 1 dose, after at least 4 weeks. Dose to be administered as 0.1 mL into each nostril

● UNLICENSED USE
▶ With intranasal use in children The Joint Committee on Vaccination and Immunisation advises offering a second dose of vaccine for annual immunisation against seasonal influenza to children in clinical risk groups only, but this differs from licensed advice.

● CONTRA-INDICATIONS Preparations marketed by Pfizer, or CSL Biotherapies in child under 5 years—increased risk of febrile convulsions
FLUENZ TETRA® Active wheezing · concomitant use with antiviral therapy for influenza · severe asthma
CONTRA-INDICATIONS, FURTHER INFORMATION
▶ Concomitant use with antiviral therapy for influenza Public Health England advises avoid immunisation for at least 48 hours after stopping the influenza antiviral agent. Administration of influenza antiviral agents within

14

Vaccines

two weeks of Fluenz Tetra® administration may reduce the effectiveness of the vaccine.

- ● INTERACTIONS → Appendix 1: live vaccines
- ● SIDE-EFFECTS
- ▶ Common or very common
- ▸ With intramuscular use Chills (uncommon in elderly) · hyperhidrosis · induration · local reactions · pain (uncommon in elderly)
- ▸ With intranasal use Nasal complaints
- ▶ Uncommon
- ▸ With intramuscular use Cough (in adults)
- ▸ With intranasal use Epistaxis · face oedema
- ▶ Rare or very rare
- ▸ With intramuscular use Vasodilation (in adults)
- ▶ Frequency not known
- ▸ With intramuscular use Angioedema · asthenia (in adults) · chest pain (in adults) · dyspnoea (in adults) · extensive swelling of vaccinated limb · eye erythema (in adults) · increased risk of infection · nerve disorders · nervous system disorders · paraesthesia · seizures · shock · syncope · throat tightness (in adults) · thrombocytopenia · vasculitis · wheezing (in adults)
- ▸ With intranasal use Guillain-Barre syndrome
- ● ALLERGY AND CROSS-SENSITIVITY Individuals with a history of egg allergy can be immunised with either an egg free influenza vaccine, if available, or an influenza vaccine with an ovalbumin content less than 120 nanograms/mL (facilities should be available to treat anaphylaxis). Vaccines with an ovalbumin content more than 120 nanograms/mL or where content is not stated should not be used in individuals with egg allergy. If an influenza vaccine containing ovalbumin is being considered in those with a history of anaphylaxis to egg or egg allergy with uncontrolled asthma, these individuals should be referred to a specialist in hospital.
- ● PREGNANCY Inactivated vaccines not known to be harmful.
  FLUENZ TETRA ® Avoid in pregnancy.
- ● BREAST FEEDING Inactivated vaccines not known to be harmful.
  FLUENZ TETRA ® Avoid in breast-feeding.
- ● DIRECTIONS FOR ADMINISTRATION Public Health England advises that individuals with **bleeding disorders** may be vaccinated by the intramuscular route, on the advice of a doctor familiar with their bleeding risk. Patients treated with medicines to reduce bleeding (e.g. for haemophilia) are advised to administer their medicine shortly prior to intramuscular vaccination.
- ● PRESCRIBING AND DISPENSING INFORMATION The available preparations are not licensed for use in all age-groups—further information can be found in the product literature for the individual vaccines. For choice of vaccine, see Influenza vaccine p. 1348.
  FLUARIX TETRA ® Ovalbumin content less than 100 nanograms/mL.
- ● PATIENT AND CARER ADVICE
  FLUENZ TETRA ® Avoid close contact with severely immunocompromised patients for 1–2 weeks after vaccination.
- ● MEDICINAL FORMS There can be variation in the licensing of different medicines containing the same drug.
  Spray
  EXCIPIENTS: May contain Gelatin, gentamicin
  ▸ Fluenz Tetra (AstraZeneca UK Ltd)
  Fluenz Tetra vaccine nasal suspension 0.2ml unit dose | 10 unit dose [PoM] £180.00
  Suspension for injection
  EXCIPIENTS: May contain Gentamicin, kanamycin, neomycin, polymyxin b

- ▸ Influenza vaccine (non-proprietary) ▼
  Trivalent influenza vaccine (split virion, inactivated) High Dose suspension for injection 0.5ml pre-filled syringes | 5 pre-filled disposable injection [PoM] £100.00
  Influenza vaccine (split virion, inactivated) suspension for injection 0.5ml pre-filled syringes | 10 pre-filled disposable injection [PoM] £65.90
  Quadrivalent influenza vaccine (split virion, inactivated) suspension for injection 0.5ml pre-filled syringes | 1 pre-filled disposable injection [PoM] £8.00 | 10 pre-filled disposable injection [PoM] £80.00
  Influenza Tetra MYL vaccine suspension for injection 0.5ml pre-filled syringes | 1 pre-filled disposable injection [PoM] £8.00 | 10 pre-filled disposable injection [PoM] £80.00
  Adjuvanted trivalent influenza vaccine (surface antigen, inactivated) suspension for injection 0.5ml pre-filled syringes | 1 pre-filled disposable injection [PoM] £9.79 | 10 pre-filled disposable injection [PoM] £97.90
- ▸ Fluad Tetra (Seqirus Vaccines Ltd)
  Fluad Tetra vaccine suspension for injection 0.5ml pre-filled syringes | 1 pre-filled disposable injection [PoM] £11.88 | 10 pre-filled disposable injection [PoM] £118.80
- ▸ Fluarix Tetra (GlaxoSmithKline UK Ltd)
  Fluarix Tetra vaccine suspension for injection 0.5ml pre-filled syringes | 1 pre-filled disposable injection [PoM] £9.94
- ▸ Flucelvax Tetra (Seqirus Vaccines Ltd) ▼
  Flucelvax Tetra vaccine suspension for injection 0.5ml pre-filled syringes | 1 pre-filled disposable injection [PoM] £9.94 | 10 pre-filled disposable injection [PoM] £99.40
- ▸ Imuvac (Mylan)
  Imuvac vaccine suspension for injection 0.5ml pre-filled syringes | 1 pre-filled disposable injection [PoM] £6.59 | 10 pre-filled disposable injection [PoM] £65.90
- ▸ Influvac Sub-unit (Mylan) ▼
  Influvac sub-unit Tetra vaccine suspension for injection 0.5ml pre-filled syringes | 1 pre-filled disposable injection [PoM] £9.94 | 10 pre-filled disposable injection [PoM] £99.40

🡒 1360

Japanese encephalitis vaccine

22-Feb-2019

- ● INDICATIONS AND DOSE
  Immunisation against Japanese encephalitis
  ▸ BY INTRAMUSCULAR INJECTION
  - Child 2–35 months: 0.25 mL every 28 days for 2 doses, alternatively 0.25 mL every 7 days for 2 doses, anterolateral thigh may be used as the injection site in infants; deltoid muscle is preferred site in older children, immunisation should be completed at least 1 week before potential exposure
  - Child 3–17 years: 0.5 mL every 28 days for 2 doses, alternatively 0.5 mL every 7 days for 2 doses, deltoid muscle is preferred site in older children, immunisation should be completed at least 1 week before potential exposure
  - Adult: 0.5 mL every 28 days for 2 doses, alternatively 0.5 mL every 7 days for 2 doses, deltoid muscle is preferred site of injection, immunisation should be completed at least 1 week before potential exposure
  First booster
  ▸ BY INTRAMUSCULAR INJECTION
  - Adult: 0.5 mL after 1–2 years, deltoid muscle is preferred site of injection, for those at continued risk, the booster dose should be given 1 year after completing the primary course
  - Elderly: 0.5 mL after 1 year, for those at continued risk, deltoid muscle is preferred site of injection
  Second booster
  ▸ BY INTRAMUSCULAR INJECTION
  - Adult: 0.5 mL after 10 years, for those at continued risk, deltoid muscle is preferred site of injection
- ● UNLICENSED USE
  ▸ When used for Immunisation against Japanese encephalitis The rapid schedule administered at days 0 and 7 is not licensed in children or the elderly.

SIDE-EFFECTS
▶ **Common or very common** Influenza like illness (frequency not known in children)
▶ **Uncommon** Abdominal pain (frequency not known in children) · asthenia (in adults) · chills (in adults) · hyperhidrosis (in adults) · migraine (in adults) · musculoskeletal stiffness (in adults) · vertigo (in adults)
▶ **Rare or very rare** Dyspnoea (in adults) · eyelid oedema (in adults) · neuritis (in adults) · pain in extremity (in adults) · palpitations (in adults) · paraesthesia (in adults) · peripheral oedema (in adults) · tachycardia (in adults) · taste altered (in adults) · thrombocytopenia (in adults)
▶ **Frequency not known** Cough (in children)
● PREGNANCY Although manufacturer advises avoid because of limited information, miscarriage has been associated with Japanese encephalitis virus infection acquired during the first 2 trimesters of pregnancy.

● MEDICINAL FORMS There can be variation in the licensing of different medicines containing the same drug.
Solution for injection
▶ Japanese encephalitis vaccine (Non-proprietary)
 Japanese encephalitis GCVC vaccine solution for injection 1ml vials | 1 vial ⓢ
 Japanese encephalitis GCVC vaccine solution for injection 20ml vials | 1 vial ⓢ
 Japanese encephalitis GCVC vaccine solution for injection 10ml vials | 1 vial ⓢ
Suspension for injection
▶ Ixiaro (Valneva UK Ltd)
 Ixiaro vaccine suspension for injection 0.5ml pre-filled syringes | 1 pre-filled disposable injection PoM £59.50 DT = £59.50

⚑ 1360

Measles, mumps and rubella vaccine, live

24-Sep-2020

● INDICATIONS AND DOSE
Primary immunisation against measles, mumps, and rubella (first dose)
▶ BY INTRAMUSCULAR INJECTION, OR BY DEEP SUBCUTANEOUS INJECTION
▸ Child 12–13 months: 0.5 mL for 1 dose
Primary immunisation against measles, mumps, and rubella (second dose)
▶ BY INTRAMUSCULAR INJECTION, OR BY DEEP SUBCUTANEOUS INJECTION
▸ Child 40 months–5 years: 0.5 mL for 1 dose
Rubella immunisation (in seronegative women, susceptible to rubella and in unimmunised, seronegative women, post-partum)
▶ BY INTRAMUSCULAR INJECTION, OR BY DEEP SUBCUTANEOUS INJECTION
▸ Females of childbearing potential: (consult product literature or local protocols)
Children presenting for pre-school booster, who have not received the primary immunisation (first dose) | Immunisation for patients at school-leaving age or at entry into further education, who have not completed the primary immunisation course | Control of measles outbreak | Immunisation for patients travelling to areas where measles is endemic or epidemic, who have not completed the primary immunisation
▶ BY INTRAMUSCULAR INJECTION, OR BY DEEP SUBCUTANEOUS INJECTION
▸ Child 6 months–17 years: (consult product literature or local protocols)
▸ Adult: (consult product literature or local protocols)

● UNLICENSED USE Not licensed for use in children under 9 months.

┌───┐
│ IMPORTANT SAFETY INFORMATION   │
│ MMR VACCINATION AND BOWEL DISEASE OR AUTISM   │
│ Reviews undertaken on behalf of the CSM, the Medical │
│ Research Council, and the Cochrane Collaboration, have │
│ not found any evidence of a link between MMR │
│ vaccination and bowel disease or autism. Information │
│ (including fact sheets and a list of references) may be │
│ obtained from www.dh.gov.uk/immunisation.   │
└───┘

● CAUTIONS Antibody response to measles component may be reduced after immunoglobulin administration or blood transfusion–leave an interval of at least 3 months before MMR immunisation
CAUTIONS, FURTHER INFORMATION
▶ Administration with other vaccines Public Health England advises MMR and yellow fever vaccines should not be administered on the same day; there should be a 4-week minimum interval between the vaccines. When protection is rapidly required, the vaccines can be given at any interval; an additional dose of MMR should be considered and re-vaccination with the yellow fever vaccine can also be considered in those at on-going risk.
  Public Health England advises MMR and varicella-zoster vaccines can be given on the same day or separated by a 4-week minimum interval. When protection is rapidly required, the vaccines can be given at any interval and an additional dose of the vaccine given second may be considered.
● INTERACTIONS → Appendix 1: live vaccines
● SIDE-EFFECTS
▶ **Uncommon** Increased risk of infection · rhinorrhoea
▶ **Frequency not known** Angioedema · arthritis · ataxia · cough · encephalopathy · eye inflammation · meningitis aseptic · nerve deafness · nerve disorders · oculomotor nerve paralysis · oedema · panniculitis · papillitis · paraesthesia · regional lymphadenopathy · respiratory disorders · seizures · Stevens-Johnson syndrome · subacute sclerosing panencephalitis · syncope · throat pain · thrombocytopenia · vasculitis
SIDE-EFFECTS, FURTHER INFORMATION Malaise, fever, or a rash can occur after the first dose of MMR vaccine–most commonly about a week after vaccination and lasting about 2 to 3 days.
  Febrile seizures occur rarely 6 to 11 days after MMR vaccination (the incidence is lower than that following measles infection).
  Idiopathic thrombocytopenic purpura Idiopathic thrombocytopenic purpura has occurred rarely following MMR vaccination, usually within 6 weeks of the first dose. The risk of idiopathic thrombocytopenic purpura after MMR vaccine is much less than the risk after infection with wild measles or rubella virus. Children who develop idiopathic thrombocytopenic purpura within 6 weeks of the first dose of MMR should undergo serological testing before the second dose is due; if the results suggest incomplete immunity against measles, mumps or rubella then a second dose of MMR is recommended. Samples should be sent to the Virus Reference Laboratory of the Health Protection Agency.
  Frequency of side effects Adverse reactions are considerably less frequent after the second dose of MMR vaccine than after the first.
● ALLERGY AND CROSS-SENSITIVITY MMR vaccine can be given safely even when the child has had an anaphylactic reaction to food containing egg. Dislike of eggs, refusal to eat egg, or confirmed anaphylactic reactions to egg-containing food is not a contra-indication to MMR vaccination. Children with a confirmed anaphylactic

14

Vaccines

reaction to the MMR vaccine should be assessed by a specialist.

- CONCEPTION AND CONTRACEPTION Exclude pregnancy before immunisation. Avoid pregnancy for at least 1 month after vaccination.
- PRESCRIBING AND DISPENSING INFORMATION Available as part of childhood immunisation schedule from health organisations or ImmForm portal.immform.phe.gov.uk.

- MEDICINAL FORMS There can be variation in the licensing of different medicines containing the same drug.
Powder and solvent for suspension for injection
EXCIPIENTS: May contain Gelatin, neomycin
  - M-M-RVAXPRO (Merck Sharp & Dohme Ltd)
    M-M-RVAXPRO vaccine powder and solvent for suspension for injection
    0.5ml pre-filled syringes | 1 pre-filled disposable injection [PoM]
    £11.00 DT = £11.00
Powder and solvent for solution for injection
EXCIPIENTS: May contain Neomycin
  - Priorix (GlaxoSmithKline UK Ltd)
    Priorix vaccine powder and solvent for solution for injection 0.5ml pre-filled syringes | 1 pre-filled disposable injection [PoM] £7.64 DT = £7.64

⌨ 1360

Rabies vaccine

17-Jun-2020

- INDICATIONS AND DOSE
Primary pre-exposure immunisation against rabies infection
▶ BY INTRAMUSCULAR INJECTION
  - Child: 1 mL for 3 doses (on days 0, 7, and 28), to be administered into deltoid region; in infants anterolateral thigh is recommended, final dose may be given from day 21 if insufficient time before travel
  - Adult: 1 mL for 3 doses (on days 0, 7, and 28), to be administered into deltoid region, final dose may be given from day 21 if insufficient time before travel

Primary pre-exposure immunisation against rabies infection [accelerated course]
▶ BY INTRAMUSCULAR INJECTION
  - Child: 1 mL for 3 doses (on days 0, 3, and 7), followed by 1 mL for 1 dose at 1 year if continued travel to high-risk areas, to be administered into deltoid region; in infants anterolateral thigh is recommended
  - Adult: 1 mL for 3 doses (on days 0, 3, and 7), followed by 1 mL for 1 dose at 1 year if continued travel to high-risk areas, to be administered into deltoid region

Pre-exposure immunisation booster dose [patients at frequent risk of exposure e.g. laboratory workers who handle lyssavirus-containing material]
▶ BY INTRAMUSCULAR INJECTION
  - Child: 1 mL for 1 dose, to be given 1 year after primary course is completed, then 1 mL, repeated if necessary, based on six-monthly antibody levels. To be administered into deltoid region; in infants anterolateral thigh is recommended
  - Adult: 1 mL for 1 dose, to be given 1 year after primary course is completed, then 1 mL, repeated if necessary, based on six-monthly antibody levels. To be administered into deltoid region

Pre-exposure immunisation booster dose [patients who may have frequent, unrecognised exposures e.g. bat handlers]
▶ BY INTRAMUSCULAR INJECTION
  - Child: 1 mL for 1 dose, to be given 1 year after primary course is completed, then 1 mL every 3–5 years, to be administered into deltoid region; in infants anterolateral thigh is recommended, the frequency of booster doses may alternatively be based on antibody levels

- Adult: 1 mL for 1 dose, to be given 1 year after primary course is completed, then 1 mL every 3–5 years, repeated if necessary, to be administered into deltoid region, the frequency of booster doses may alternatively be based on antibody levels

Pre-exposure immunisation booster dose [patients at infrequent risk of exposure]
▶ BY INTRAMUSCULAR INJECTION
  - Child: 1 mL for 1 dose, to be given at least 1 year after primary course is completed based on antibody levels, to be administered into deltoid region; in infants anterolateral thigh is recommended
  - Adult: 1 mL for 1 dose, to be given at least 1 year after primary course is completed based on antibody levels, to be administered into deltoid region

Post-exposure treatment [fully immunised patients with amber or red composite rabies risk] (administered on expert advice)
▶ BY INTRAMUSCULAR INJECTION
  - Child: 1 mL for 1 dose, followed by 1 mL after 3–7 days for 1 dose, to be administered into deltoid region; in infants anterolateral thigh is recommened, rabies immunoglobulin is not necessary
  - Adult: 1 mL for 1 dose, followed by 1 mL after 3–7 days for 1 dose, to be administered into deltoid region, rabies immunoglobulin is not necessary

Post-exposure treatment [partially immunised patients with amber or red composite rabies risk] (administered on expert advice)
▶ BY INTRAMUSCULAR INJECTION
  - Child: 1 mL for 4 doses (on days 0, 3, 7, and 21), to be administered into deltoid region; in infants anterolateral thigh is recommended, rabies immunoglobulin is not necessary
  - Adult: 1 mL for 4 doses (on days 0, 3, 7, and 21), to be administered into deltoid region, rabies immunoglobulin is not necessary

Post-exposure treatment [non-immunised patients with amber or red composite rabies risk] (administered on expert advice)
▶ BY INTRAMUSCULAR INJECTION
  - Child: 1 mL for 4 doses (on days 0, 3, 7, and 21), to be administered into deltoid region; in infants anterolateral thigh is recommended, rabies immunoglobulin also to be given to patients with red composite rabies risk (but is not required if more than 7 days have elapsed after the first dose of vaccine, or more than 1 day after the second dose of vaccine)
  - Adult: 1 mL for 4 doses (on days 0, 3, 7, and 21), to be administered into deltoid region, rabies immunoglobulin also to be given to patients with red composite rabies risk (but is not required if more than 7 days have elapsed after the first dose of vaccine, or more than 1 day after the second dose of vaccine)

Post-exposure treatment [immunosuppressed patients with amber or red composite rabies risk, regardless of immunisation status] (administered on expert advice)
▶ BY INTRAMUSCULAR INJECTION
  - Child: 1 mL for 5 doses (on days 0, 3, 7, 14, and 28 or 30), to be administered into deltoid region; in infants anterolateral thigh is recommended, rabies immunoglobulin also to be given (but is not required if more than 7 days have elapsed after the first dose of vaccine, or more than 1 day after the second dose of vaccine)
  - Adult: 1 mL for 5 doses (on days 0, 3, 7, 14, and 28 or 30), to be administered into deltoid region, rabies immunoglobulin also to be given (but is not required if more than 7 days have elapsed after the first dose of vaccine, or more than 1 day after the second dose of vaccine)

▸ **UNLICENSED USE** Public Health England advises rabies vaccine may be used as detailed below, although these situations are considered unlicensed:
● dosing regimens for post-exposure treatment.
● **INTERACTIONS** → Appendix 1: rabies vaccine
● **SIDE-EFFECTS**
Common or very common Asthenia · gastrointestinal discomfort
Rare or very rare Angioedema · chills · encephalitis · Guillain-Barre syndrome · hyperhidrosis · paraesthesia · syncope · vertigo
● **PREGNANCY** Because of the potential consequences of untreated rabies exposure and because rabies vaccination has not been associated with fetal abnormalities, pregnancy is not considered a contra-indication to post-exposure prophylaxis. Immunisation against rabies is indicated during pregnancy if there is substantial risk of exposure to rabies and rapid access to post-exposure prophylaxis is likely to be limited.

● **MEDICINAL FORMS** There can be variation in the licensing of different medicines containing the same drug.
Powder and solvent for suspension for injection
EXCIPIENTS: May contain Neomycin
▸ **Rabies vaccine (Non-proprietary)**
Rabies vaccine powder and solvent for suspension for injection 1ml vials | 1 vial PoM £40.84
▸ **Verorab (Imported (France))**
Verorab powder and solvent for suspension for injection 0.5ml vials | 1 vial PoM Ⓢ

Powder and solvent for solution for injection
EXCIPIENTS: May contain Neomycin
▸ **Rabipur (GlaxoSmithKline UK Ltd)**
Rabipur vaccine powder and solvent for solution for injection 1ml pre-filled syringes | 1 pre-filled disposable injection PoM £34.56

🔖 1360

Rotavirus vaccine

27-Jul-2020

● **DRUG ACTION** Rotavirus vaccine is a live, oral vaccine that protects young children against gastro-enteritis caused by rotavirus infection.

● **INDICATIONS AND DOSE**
Immunisation against gastro-enteritis caused by rotavirus
▸ BY MOUTH
▸ Child 6-23 weeks: 1.5 mL for 2 doses separated by an interval of at least 4 weeks, first dose must be given between 6-14 weeks of age; course should be completed before 24 weeks of age (preferably before 16 weeks)

IMPORTANT SAFETY INFORMATION
PUBLIC HEALTH ENGLAND: UPDATE TO GREEN BOOK (OCTOBER 2017)
Public Health England advises that immunisation with live vaccines should be delayed until 6 months of age in children born to mothers who received immunosuppressive biological therapy during pregnancy. In practice, this means that children born to mothers who were on immunosuppressive biological therapy during pregnancy will not be eligible to receive rotavirus vaccine.

● **CONTRA-INDICATIONS** History of intussusception · predisposition to intussusception · severe combined immunodeficiency disorder
CONTRA-INDICATIONS, FURTHER INFORMATION
▸ Immunosuppression With the exception of severe combined immunodeficiency disorder (and children born to mothers who received immunosuppressive biological therapy during pregnancy, see *Important safety information*), rotavirus vaccine is not contra-indicated in

immunosuppressed patients—benefit from vaccination is likely to outweigh the risk, if there is any doubt, Public Health England recommends seek specialist advice.

● **CAUTIONS** Diarrhoea (postpone vaccination) · immunosuppressed close contacts · vomiting (postpone vaccination)
CAUTIONS, FURTHER INFORMATION The rotavirus vaccine virus is excreted in the stool and may be transmitted to close contacts; however, Public Health England advises vaccination of those with immunosuppressed close contacts may protect the contacts from wild-type rotavirus disease and outweigh any risk from transmission of vaccine virus.

● **INTERACTIONS** → Appendix 1: live vaccines
● **SIDE-EFFECTS**
▸ **Uncommon** Abdominal pain · gastrointestinal disorders
▸ **Frequency not known** Apnoea · haematochezia
● **PATIENT AND CARER ADVICE** The rotavirus vaccine virus is excreted in the stool and may be transmitted to close contacts; carers of a recently vaccinated baby should be advised of the need to wash their hands after changing the baby's nappies.

● **MEDICINAL FORMS** There can be variation in the licensing of different medicines containing the same drug.
Oral suspension
▸ **Rotarix (GlaxoSmithKline UK Ltd)**
Rotarix vaccine live oral suspension 1.5ml tube | 1 tube PoM £34.76
DT = £34.76

🔖 1360

Tick-borne encephalitis vaccine, inactivated

● **INDICATIONS AND DOSE**
Initial immunisation against tick-borne encephalitis
▸ BY INTRAMUSCULAR INJECTION
▸ Child 1-15 years: 0.25 mL for 1 dose, followed by 0.25 mL after 1-3 months for 1 dose, then 0.25 mL after further 5-12 months for 1 dose, to achieve more rapid protection, second dose may be given 14 days after first dose, dose to be administered in deltoid region or anterolateral thigh in infants, in immunocompromised patients (including those receiving immunosuppressants), antibody concentration may be measured 4 weeks after second dose and dose repeated if protective levels not achieved
▸ Child 16-17 years: 0.5 mL for 1 dose, followed by 0.5 mL after 1-3 months for 1 dose, then 0.5 mL after further 5-12 months for 1 dose, to achieve more rapid protection, second dose may be given 14 days after first dose, dose to be administered in deltoid region, in immunocompromised patients (including those receiving immunosuppressants), antibody concentration may be measured 4 weeks after second dose and dose repeated if protective levels not achieved
▸ Adult: 0.5 mL for 1 dose, followed by 0.5 mL after 1-3 months for 1 dose, then 0.5 mL after further 5-12 months for 1 dose, to achieve more rapid protection, second dose may be given 14 days after first dose, dose to be administered in deltoid region, in immunocompromised patients (including those receiving immunosuppressants), antibody concentration may be measured 4 weeks after second dose and dose repeated if protective levels not achieved
▸ Elderly: 0.5 mL for 1 dose, followed by 0.5 mL after 1-3 months for 1 dose, then 0.5 mL after further 5-12 months for 1 dose, to achieve more rapid protection, second dose may be given

continued →

14

Vaccines

14 days after first dose, dose to be administered in deltoid region, antibody concentration may be measured 4 weeks after second dose and dose repeated if protective levels not achieved

Immunisation against tick-borne encephalitis, booster doses
▶ BY INTRAMUSCULAR INJECTION
▶ **Child 1-17 years:** First dose to be given within 3 years after initial course completed and then every 3–5 years, dose to be administered in deltoid region or anterolateral thigh in infants (consult product literature)
▶ **Adult:** First dose to be given within 3 years after initial course completed and then every 3–5 years, dose to be administered in deltoid region (consult product literature)

● SIDE-EFFECTS
▶ **Common or very common** Restlessness (in children) · sleep disorder (in children)
▶ **Rare or very rare** Asthenia · autoimmune disorder (in adults) · chills (uncommon in children) · demyelination (in adults) · drowsiness (in adults) · dyspnoea · eye pain · gait abnormal · gastrointestinal discomfort (uncommon in children) · hyperhidrosis · increased risk of infection · influenza like illness · joint swelling (in adults) · meningism · meningitis aseptic (in adults) · motor dysfunction · musculoskeletal stiffness · nerve disorders · oedema · pain · seizures · sensory disorder · tachycardia (in adults) · tinnitus · vertigo · vision disorders

● ALLERGY AND CROSS-SENSITIVITY Individuals with evidence of previous anaphylactic reaction to egg should not be given tick-borne encephalitis vaccine.

● MEDICINAL FORMS There can be variation in the licensing of different medicines containing the same drug.
Suspension for injection
EXCIPIENTS: May contain Gentamicin, neomycin
▶ TicoVac (Pfizer Ltd)
TicoVac Junior vaccine suspension for injection 0.25ml pre-filled syringes | 1 pre-filled disposable injection [PoM] £28.00
TicoVac vaccine suspension for injection 0.5ml pre-filled syringes | 1 pre-filled disposable injection [PoM] £32.00

Ⴔ 1360

Varicella-zoster vaccine
16-Oct-2020

● DRUG ACTION *Varilrix* ® and *Varivax* ® are live attenuated vaccines that protect against varicella (chickenpox) caused by varicella-zoster virus infection. *Zostavax* ® is a live attenuated vaccine that protects against herpes zoster (shingles) caused by varicella-zoster virus infection.

● INDICATIONS AND DOSE

VARILRIX ®
Prevention of varicella infection (chickenpox)
▶ BY SUBCUTANEOUS INJECTION
▶ **Child 1-17 years:** 0.5 mL every 4–6 weeks for 2 doses, to be administered into the deltoid region or anterolateral thigh
▶ **Adult:** 0.5 mL every 4–6 weeks for 2 doses, to be administered into the deltoid region or anterolateral thigh

VARIVAX ®
Prevention of varicella infection (chickenpox)
▶ BY SUBCUTANEOUS INJECTION, OR BY INTRAMUSCULAR INJECTION
▶ **Child 1-12 years:** 0.5 mL for 2 doses, interval of at least 4 weeks between each dose, to be administered into the deltoid region (or higher anterolateral thigh in young children)

▶ **Child 13-17 years:** 0.5 mL for 2 doses, interval of 4–8 weeks between each dose, to be administered preferably into the deltoid region
▶ **Adult:** 0.5 mL for 2 doses, interval of 4–8 weeks between each dose, to be administered preferably into the deltoid region

Prevention of varicella infection (chickenpox) in children with asymptomatic HIV infection
▶ BY SUBCUTANEOUS INJECTION, OR BY INTRAMUSCULAR INJECTION
▶ **Child 1-12 years:** 0.5 mL for 2 doses, interval of 12 weeks between each dose, to be administered into the deltoid region (or higher anterolateral thigh in young children)

ZOSTAVAX ®
Prevention of herpes zoster (shingles)
▶ BY SUBCUTANEOUS INJECTION, OR BY INTRAMUSCULAR INJECTION
▶ **Adult 70-79 years:** 0.65 mL for 1 dose, intramuscular route preferred, to be administered preferably into the deltoid region

● CAUTIONS Post-vaccination close contact with susceptible individuals
CAUTIONS, FURTHER INFORMATION Rarely, the varicella–zoster vaccine virus has been transmitted from the vaccinated individual to close contacts. Therefore, manufacturer advises contact with the following should be avoided if a vaccine-related cutaneous rash develops within 4–6 weeks of the first or second dose:
● varicella-susceptible pregnant women;
● individuals at high risk of severe varicella, including those with immunodeficiency or those receiving immunosuppressive therapy.
Public Health England advises healthcare workers who develop a generalised papular or vesicular rash on vaccination should avoid contact with patients until the lesions have crusted. Those who develop a localised rash after vaccination should cover the lesions and be allowed to continue working unless in contact with patients at high risk of severe varicella.
▶ Administration with MMR vaccine Public Health England advises varicella–zoster and MMR vaccines can be given on the same day or separated by a 4-week minimum interval. Where protection is rapidly required, the vaccines can be given at any interval and an additional dose of the vaccine given second may be considered.

● INTERACTIONS → Appendix 1: live vaccines

● SIDE-EFFECTS
▶ **Uncommon** Cough · drowsiness · increased risk of infection
▶ **Rare or very rare** Abdominal pain · conjunctivitis · Kawasaki disease · seizure · stroke · thrombocytopenia · vasculitis

● CONCEPTION AND CONTRACEPTION Manufacturer advises avoid pregnancy for 1 month after vaccination.

● PRESCRIBING AND DISPENSING INFORMATION
ZOSTAVAX ® Advice in the BNF may differ from that in product literature.
VARIVAX ®
▶ In children Advice in the BNF may differ from that in product literature.
VARILRIX ®
▶ In children Advice in the BNF may differ from that in product literature.

● MEDICINAL FORMS There can be variation in the licensing of different medicines containing the same drug.
Powder and solvent for suspension for injection
EXCIPIENTS: May contain Gelatin, neomycin
▶ Varivax (Merck Sharp & Dohme Ltd)
Varivax vaccine powder and solvent for suspension for injection 0.5ml vials | 1 vial [PoM] £30.28 DT = £30.28

- Zostavax (Merck Sharp & Dohme Ltd)
  Zostavax vaccine powder and solvent for suspension for injection
  0.65ml pre-filled syringes | 1 pre-filled disposable injection PoM
  £99.96 DT = £99.96

Powder and solvent for solution for injection
EXCIPIENTS: May contain Neomycin
- Varilrix (GlaxoSmithKline UK Ltd)
  Varilrix vaccine powder and solvent for solution for injection 0.5ml
  vials | 1 vial PoM £27.31 DT = £27.31

F 1360

Yellow fever vaccine, live

29-Jul-2020

● **INDICATIONS AND DOSE**

Immunisation against yellow fever
▶ BY DEEP SUBCUTANEOUS INJECTION
▶ Child 6–8 months (administered on expert advice): Infants
  under 9 months should be vaccinated only if the risk of
  yellow fever is high and unavoidable (consult product
  literature or local protocols)
▶ Child 9 months–17 years: 0.5 mL for 1 dose
▶ Adult: 0.5 mL for 1 dose

IMPORTANT SAFETY INFORMATION
MHRA/CHM ADVICE (UPDATED NOVEMBER 2019): YELLOW FEVER
VACCINE: STRONGER PRECAUTIONS IN PEOPLE WITH WEAKENED
IMMUNITY AND IN THOSE AGED 60 YEARS OR OLDER
The yellow fever vaccine (*Stamaril®*) has been associated
with the very rare, life-threatening reactions
viscerotropic disease (YEL-AVD) and neurotropic disease
(YEL-AND), which both resemble yellow fever infection.
It must not be given to patients who have had a
thymectomy, who are taking immunosuppressive or
immunomodulating biological drugs, or who have a first-
degree family history of YEL-AVD or YEL-AND following
vaccination that was unrelated to a known medical risk
factor. In patients aged 60 years and older, the vaccine
should only be administered when there is a significant
and unavoidable risk of acquiring yellow fever infection.
It must only be administered by healthcare professionals
specifically trained in the benefit-risk evaluation of
yellow fever vaccine. Healthcare professionals must
inform patients and carers about the early signs and
symptoms of YEL-AVD and YEL-AND, and advise them
to seek urgent medical attention if they occur; the
manufacturer's patient information leaflet should also
be provided. Healthcare professionals administering
vaccines should consult information in the YF Vaccine
Centre code of practice and strengthen protocols and
checklists to avoid inappropriate administration.

● CONTRA-INDICATIONS Children under 6 months · history of
thymus dysfunction
● CAUTIONS Individuals over 60 years—greater risk of
vaccine-associated adverse effects

CAUTIONS, FURTHER INFORMATION
▶ Administration with MMR vaccine Public Health England
advises yellow fever and MMR vaccines should not be
administered on the same day; there should be a 4-week
minimum interval between the vaccines. When protection
is rapidly required, the vaccines can be given at any
interval; an additional dose of MMR should be considered
and re-vaccination with the yellow fever vaccine can also
be considered in those at on-going risk.

● INTERACTIONS → Appendix 1: live vaccines
● SIDE-EFFECTS
▶ **Common or very common** Asthenia · crying (in children) ·
drowsiness (in children)
▶ **Uncommon** Abdominal pain
▶ **Rare or very rare** Rhinitis · yellow fever-associated
neurotropic disease · yellow fever-associated
viscerotropic disease

▶ **Frequency not known** Angioedema · influenza like illness ·
paraesthesia

SIDE-EFFECTS, FURTHER INFORMATION Very rare vaccine-
associated adverse effects may occur, such as viscerotropic
disease (yellow-fever vaccine-associated viscerotropic
disease, YEL-AVD), a syndrome which may include
metabolic acidosis, muscle and liver cirrhosis, and multi-
organ failure. Neurological disorders (yellow fever vaccine-
associated neurotropic disease, YEL-AND) such as
encephalitis have also been reported. These very rare
adverse effects usually occur after the first dose of yellow
fever vaccine in those with no previous immunity.
Increased risk of fatal reactions reported in patients aged
60 years and older and those who are immunosuppressed.

● ALLERGY AND CROSS-SENSITIVITY Yellow fever vaccine
should only be considered under the guidance of a
specialist in individuals with evidence of previous
anaphylactic reaction to egg.

● PREGNANCY Live yellow fever vaccine should not be given
during pregnancy because there is a theoretical risk of fetal
infection. Pregnant women should be advised not to travel
to areas at high risk of yellow fever. If exposure cannot be
avoided during pregnancy, then the vaccine should be
given if the risk from disease in the mother outweighs the
risk to the fetus from vaccination.

● BREAST FEEDING Avoid; seek specialist advice if exposure
to virus cannot be avoided.

● MEDICINAL FORMS There can be variation in the licensing of
different medicines containing the same drug.

Powder and solvent for suspension for injection
▶ Stamaril (Sanofi Pasteur)
  Stamaril vaccine powder and solvent for suspension for injection 0.5ml
  vials | 1 vial PoM £39.72 DT = £39.72

14

Vaccines

Chapter 15
Anaesthesia

CONTENTS

General anaesthesia

Anaesthesia (general)

Overview

Several different types of drug are given together during general anaesthesia. Anaesthesia is induced with either a volatile drug given by inhalation or with an intravenously administered drug; anaesthesia is maintained with an intravenous or inhalational anaesthetic. Analgesics, usually short-acting opioids, are also used. The use of neuromuscular blocking drugs necessitates intermittent positive-pressure ventilation. Following surgery, anticholinesterases can be given to reverse the effects of neuromuscular blocking drugs; specific antagonists can be used to reverse central and respiratory depression caused by some drugs used in surgery. A local topical anaesthetic can be used to reduce pain at the injection site.

Individual requirements vary considerably and the recommended doses are only a guide. Smaller doses are indicated in ill, shocked, or debilitated patients and in significant hepatic impairment, while robust individuals may require larger doses. The required dose of induction agent may be less if the patient has been premedicated with a sedative agent or if an opioid analgesic has been used.

Intravenous anaesthetics

Intravenous anaesthetics may be used either to induce anaesthesia or for maintenance of anaesthesia throughout surgery. Intravenous anaesthetics nearly all produce their effect in one arm-brain circulation time. Extreme care is required in surgery of the mouth, pharynx, or larynx where the airway may be difficult to maintain (e.g. in the presence of a tumour in the pharynx or larynx).

To facilitate tracheal intubation, induction is usually followed by a neuromuscular blocking drug or a short-acting opioid.

The doses of all intravenous anaesthetic drugs should be titrated to effect (except when using 'rapid sequence induction'); lower doses may be required in premedicated patients.

Total intravenous anaesthesia

This is a technique in which major surgery is carried out with all drugs given intravenously. Respiration can be spontaneous, or controlled with oxygen-enriched air. Neuromuscular blocking drugs can be used to provide relaxation and prevent reflex muscle movements. The main problem to be overcome is the assessment of depth of anaesthesia. Target Controlled Infusion (TCI) systems can be used to titrate intravenous anaesthetic infusions to predicted plasma-drug concentrations in ventilated adult patients.

Drugs used for intravenous anaesthesia

Propofol p. 1382, the most widely used intravenous anaesthetic, can be used for induction or maintenance of anaesthesia in adults and children, but it is not commonly used in neonates. Propofol is associated with rapid recovery and less hangover effect than other intravenous anaesthetics. Propofol can also be used for sedation during diagnostic procedures and sedation in adults in intensive care.

Thiopental sodium p. 356 is a barbiturate that is used for induction of anaesthesia, but has no analgesic properties. Induction is generally smooth and rapid, but dose-related cardiovascular and respiratory depression can occur. Awakening from a moderate dose of thiopental sodium is rapid because the drug redistributes into other tissues, particularly fat. However, metabolism is slow and sedative effects can persist for 24 hours. Repeated doses have a cumulative effect and recovery is much slower.

Etomidate p. 1382 is an intravenous agent associated with rapid recovery without a hangover effect. Etomidate causes less hypotension than thiopental sodium and propofol during induction. It produces a high incidence of extraneous muscle movements, which can be minimised by an opioid analgesic or a short-acting benzodiazepine given just before induction.

Ketamine p. 1399 is used rarely. Ketamine causes less hypotension than thiopental sodium and propofol during induction. It is used mainly for paediatric anaesthesia, particularly when repeated administration is required (such as for serial burns dressings); recovery is relatively slow and there is a high incidence of extraneous muscle movements. The main disadvantage of ketamine is the high incidence of hallucinations, nightmares, and other transient psychotic effects; these can be reduced by a benzodiazepine such as diazepam p. 362 or midazolam p. 358.

Inhalational anaesthetics

Inhalational anaesthetics include gases and volatile liquids. *Gaseous anaesthetics* require suitable equipment for storage and administration. *Volatile liquid anaesthetics* are administered using calibrated vaporisers, using air, oxygen, or nitrous oxide-oxygen mixtures as the carrier gas. To prevent hypoxia, the inspired gas mixture should contain a minimum of 25% oxygen at all times. Higher concentrations of oxygen (greater than 30%) are usually required during inhalational anaesthesia when nitrous oxide p. 1384 is being administered.

Volatile liquid anaesthetics

Volatile liquid anaesthetics can be used for induction and maintenance of anaesthesia, and following induction with an intravenous anaesthetic.

Isoflurane p. 1384 is a volatile liquid anaesthetic. Heart rhythm is generally stable during isoflurane anaesthesia, but heart-rate can rise, particularly in younger patients. Systemic arterial pressure and cardiac output can fall, owing to a decrease in systemic vascular resistance. Muscle relaxation occurs and the effects of muscle relaxant drugs are potentiated. Isoflurane is the preferred inhalational anaesthetic for use in obstetrics.

Desflurane p. 1384 is a rapid acting volatile liquid anaesthetic; it is reported to have about one-fifth the potency of isoflurane. Emergence and recovery from anaesthesia are particularly rapid because of its low solubility. Desflurane is not recommended for induction of anaesthesia as it is irritant to the upper respiratory tract.

Sevoflurane p. 1385 is a rapid acting volatile liquid anaesthetic and is more potent than desflurane. Emergence and recovery are particularly rapid, but slower than desflurane. Sevoflurane is non-irritant and is therefore often used for inhalational induction of anaesthesia; it has little effect on heart rhythm compared with other volatile liquid anaesthetics.

Nitrous oxide

Nitrous oxide is used for maintenance of anaesthesia and, in sub-anaesthetic concentrations, for analgesia. For *anaesthesia*, nitrous oxide is commonly used in a concentration of 50 to 66% in oxygen as part of a balanced technique in association with other inhalational or intravenous agents. Nitrous oxide is unsatisfactory as a sole anaesthetic owing to lack of potency, but is useful as part of a combination of drugs since it allows a significant reduction in dosage.

For analgesia (without loss of consciousness), a mixture of nitrous oxide and oxygen containing 50% of each gas (Entonox ®, Equanox ®) is used. Self-administration using a demand valve is popular in obstetric practice, for changing painful dressings, as an aid to postoperative physiotherapy, and in emergency ambulances.

Nitrous oxide may have a deleterious effect if used in patients with an air-containing closed space since nitrous oxide diffuses into such a space with a resulting increase in pressure. This effect may be dangerous in conditions such as pneumothorax, which may enlarge to compromise respiration, or in the presence of intracranial air after head injury, entrapped air following recent underwater dive, or recent intra-ocular gas injection.

Malignant hyperthermia

Malignant hyperthermia is a rare but potentially lethal complication of anaesthesia. It is characterised by a rapid rise in temperature, increased muscle rigidity, tachycardia, and acidosis. The most common triggers of malignant hyperthermia are the volatile anaesthetics. Suxamethonium chloride p. 1389 has also been implicated, but malignant hyperthermia is more likely if it is given following a volatile anaesthetic. Volatile anaesthetics and suxamethonium chloride should be avoided during anaesthesia in patients at high risk of malignant hyperthermia.

Dantrolene sodium p. 1400 is used in the treatment of malignant hyperthermia.

Sedation, anaesthesia, and resuscitation in dental practice

Overview

Sedation for dental procedures should be limited to conscious sedation. Diazepam p. 362 and temazepam p. 509 are effective anxiolytics for dental treatment in adults.

For details of sedation, anaesthesia, and resuscitation in dental practice see *A Conscious Decision: A review of the use of general anaesthesia and conscious sedation in primary dental care*; report by a group chaired by the Chief Medical Officer and Chief Dental Officer, July 2000 and associated documents. Further details can also be found in *Standards for Conscious Sedation in the Provision of Dental Care*; report of an Intercollegiate Advisory Committee for Sedation in Dentistry, 2015 www.rcseng.ac.uk/-/media/files/rcs/library-and-publications/non-journal-publications/dental-sedation-report.pdf.

Surgery and long-term medication

Overview

The risk of losing disease control on stopping long-term medication before surgery is often greater than the risk posed by continuing it during surgery. It is vital that the anaesthetist knows about **all** drugs that a patient is (or has been) taking.

Patients with adrenal atrophy resulting from long-term corticosteroid use may suffer a precipitous fall in blood pressure unless corticosteroid cover is provided during anaesthesia and in the immediate postoperative period. Anaesthetists must therefore know whether a patient is, or has been, receiving corticosteroids (including high-dose inhaled corticosteroids).

Other drugs that should normally not be stopped before surgery include antiepileptics, antiparkinsonian drugs, antipsychotics, anxiolytics, bronchodilators, cardiovascular drugs (but see potassium-sparing diuretics, angiotensin-converting enzyme inhibitors, and angiotensin-II receptor antagonists), glaucoma drugs, immunosuppressants, drugs of dependence, and thyroid or antithyroid drugs. Expert advice is required for patients receiving antivirals for HIV infection. See general advice on surgery in diabetic patients in Diabetes, surgery and medical illness p. 729.

Patients taking antiplatelet medication or an oral anticoagulant present an increased risk for surgery. In these circumstances, the anaesthetist and surgeon should assess the relative risks and decide jointly whether the antiplatelet or the anticoagulant drug should be stopped or replaced with heparin (unfractionated) p. 145 or low molecular weight heparin therapy. EvGr In patients with stable angina, perioperative aspirin p. 132 should be only continued where there is a high thrombotic risk (e.g. patients with a recent acute coronary syndrome, coronary artery stents, or an ischaemic stroke). Ⓐ

Drugs that should be stopped before surgery include combined oral contraceptives, see Contraceptives, hormonal p. 836; for advice on hormone replacement therapy, see Sex hormones p. 790. MAOIs can have important interactions with some drugs used during surgery, such as pethidine hydrochloride p. 489. Tricyclic antidepressants need not be stopped, but there may be an increased risk of arrhythmias and hypotension (and dangerous interactions with vasopressor drugs); therefore, the anaesthetist should be informed if they are not stopped. Lithium should be stopped 24 hours before major surgery but the normal dose can be continued for minor surgery (with careful monitoring of fluids and electrolytes). Potassium-sparing diuretics may need to be withheld on the morning of surgery because hyperkalaemia may develop if renal perfusion is impaired or if there is tissue damage. Angiotensin-converting enzyme (ACE) inhibitors and angiotensin-II receptor antagonists can be associated with severe hypotension after induction of anaesthesia; these drugs may need to be discontinued 24 hours before surgery. Herbal medicines may be associated with adverse effects when given with anaesthetic drugs and consideration should be given to stopping them before surgery.

ANAESTHETICS, GENERAL > INTRAVENOUS ANAESTHETICS

Etomidate

04-Sep-2020

- **INDICATIONS AND DOSE**
Induction of anaesthesia
- ▸ BY SLOW INTRAVENOUS INJECTION
- ▸ Adult: 150–300 micrograms/kg (max. per dose 60 mg), to be administered over 30-60 seconds (60 seconds in patients in whom hypotension might be hazardous)
- ▸ Elderly: 150–200 micrograms/kg (max. per dose 60 mg), to be administered over 30-60 seconds (60 seconds in patients in whom hypotension might be hazardous)

> IMPORTANT SAFETY INFORMATION
> Etomidate should only be administered by, or under the direct supervision of, personnel experienced in its use, with adequate training in anaesthesia and airway management, and when resuscitation equipment is available.

- CAUTIONS Acute circulatory failure (shock) · adrenal insufficiency · Avoid in Acute porphyrias p. 1107 · cardiovascular disease · elderly · fixed cardiac output · hypovolaemia

CAUTIONS, FURTHER INFORMATION
- ▸ Adrenal insufficiency Etomidate suppresses adrenocortical function, particularly during continuous administration, and it should not be used for maintenance of anaesthesia. It should be used with caution in patients with underlying adrenal insufficiency, for example, those with sepsis.

- INTERACTIONS → Appendix 1: etomidate

- SIDE-EFFECTS
- ▸ **Common or very common** Apnoea · hypotension · movement disorders · nausea · respiratory disorders · skin reactions · vascular pain · vomiting
- ▸ **Uncommon** Arrhythmias · cough · hiccups · hypersalivation · hypertension · muscle rigidity · neuromuscular dysfunction · nystagmus · procedural complications
- ▸ **Frequency not known** Adrenal insufficiency · atrioventricular block · cardiac arrest · embolism and thrombosis · seizures · shock · Stevens-Johnson syndrome · trismus

SIDE-EFFECTS, FURTHER INFORMATION **Pain on injection** Can be reduced by injecting into a larger vein or by giving an opioid analgesic just before induction.
Extraneous muscle movements Extraneous muscle movements can be minimised by an opioid analgesic or a short-acting benzodiazepine given just before induction.

- PREGNANCY May depress neonatal respiration if used during delivery.

- BREAST FEEDING Breast-feeding can be resumed as soon as mother has recovered sufficiently from anaesthesia.

- HEPATIC IMPAIRMENT
Dose adjustments Manufacturer advises reduce dose in liver cirrhosis.

- DIRECTIONS FOR ADMINISTRATION Manufacturer advises give over 30–60 seconds (60 seconds in patients in whom hypotension might be hazardous).

- PATIENT AND CARER ADVICE
Driving and skilled tasks Patients given sedatives and analgesics during minor outpatient procedures should be very carefully warned about the risk of driving or undertaking skilled tasks afterwards. For a short general anaesthetic the risk extends to **at least 24 hours** after administration. Responsible persons should be available to take patients home. The dangers of taking **alcohol** should also be emphasised.

- MEDICINAL FORMS There can be variation in the licensing of different medicines containing the same drug.
Solution for injection
EXCIPIENTS: May contain Propylene glycol
- ▸ Hypnomidate (Piramal Critical Care Ltd)
Etomidate 2 mg per 1 ml Hypnomidate 20mg/10ml solution for injection ampoules | 5 ampoule [PoM] £6.90
Emulsion for injection
- ▸ Etomidate-Lipuro (B.Braun Medical Ltd)
Etomidate 2 mg per 1 ml Etomidate-Lipuro 20mg/10ml emulsion for injection ampoules | 10 ampoule [PoM] £16.09

Propofol

13-Aug-2020

- **INDICATIONS AND DOSE**
Induction of anaesthesia using 0.5% or 1% injection
- ▸ BY SLOW INTRAVENOUS INJECTION, OR BY INTRAVENOUS INFUSION
- ▸ Adult 18-54 years: Usual dose 1.5–2.5 mg/kg, to be administered at a rate of 20–40 mg every 10 seconds until response, for debilitated patients use dose for 55 years and over
- ▸ Adult 55 years and over: Usual dose 1–1.5 mg/kg, to be administered at a rate of 20 mg every 10 seconds until response

Induction of anaesthesia using 2% injection
- ▸ BY INTRAVENOUS INFUSION
- ▸ Adult 18-54 years: Usual dose 1.5–2.5 mg/kg, to be administered at a rate of 20–40 mg every 10 seconds until response. For debilitated patients use dose for 55 years and over
- ▸ Adult 55 years and over: Usual dose 1–1.5 mg/kg, to be administered at a rate of 20 mg every 10 seconds until response

Maintenance of anaesthesia using 1% injection
- ▸ INITIALLY BY INTRAVENOUS INFUSION
- ▸ Adult: Usual dose 4–12 mg/kg/hour, alternatively (by slow intravenous injection) 25–50 mg, dose may be repeated according to response, for debilitated patients use dose for elderly
- ▸ Elderly: Usual dose 3–6 mg/kg/hour, alternatively (by slow intravenous injection) 25–50 mg, dose may be repeated according to response

Maintenance of anaesthesia using 2% injection
- ▸ BY INTRAVENOUS INFUSION
- ▸ Adult: Usual dose 4–12 mg/kg/hour, for debilitated patients use dose for elderly
- ▸ Elderly: Usual dose 3–6 mg/kg/hour

Sedation of ventilated patients in intensive care using 1% or 2% injection
- ▸ BY CONTINUOUS INTRAVENOUS INFUSION
- ▸ Adult: Usual dose 0.3–4 mg/kg/hour, adjusted according to response

Induction of sedation for surgical and diagnostic procedures using 0.5% or 1% injection
- ▸ BY SLOW INTRAVENOUS INJECTION
- ▸ Adult: Initially 0.5–1 mg/kg, to be administered over 1–5 minutes, dose and rate of administration adjusted according to desired level of sedation and response

Maintenance of sedation for surgical and diagnostic procedures using 0.5% injection
▸ INITIALLY BY INTRAVENOUS INFUSION
▸ Adult: Initially 1.5–4.5 mg/kg/hour, dose and rate of administration adjusted according to desired level of sedation and response, followed by (by slow intravenous injection) 10–20 mg, (if rapid increase in sedation required), patients over 55 years or debilitated may require lower initial dose and rate of administration

Maintenance of sedation for surgical and diagnostic procedures using 1% injection
▸ INITIALLY BY INTRAVENOUS INFUSION
▸ Adult: Initially 1.5–4.5 mg/kg/hour, dose and rate of administration adjusted according to desired level of sedation and response, followed by (by slow intravenous injection) 10–20 mg, (if rapid increase in sedation required), patients over 55 years or debilitated may require lower initial dose and rate of administration

Maintenance of sedation for surgical and diagnostic procedures using 2% injection
▸ INITIALLY BY INTRAVENOUS INFUSION
▸ Adult: Initially 1.5–4.5 mg/kg/hour, dose and rate of administration adjusted according to desired level of sedation and response, followed by (by slow intravenous injection) 10–20 mg, using 0.5% or 1% injection (if rapid increase in sedation required), patients over 55 years or debilitated may require lower initial dose and rate of administration

---

IMPORTANT SAFETY INFORMATION
Propofol should only be administered by, or under the direct supervision of, personnel experienced in its use, with adequate training in anaesthesia and airway management, and when resuscitation equipment is available.

● CAUTIONS Acute circulatory failure (shock) · cardiac impairment · cardiovascular disease · elderly · epilepsy · fixed cardiac output · hypotension · hypovolaemia · raised intracranial pressure · respiratory impairment
● INTERACTIONS → Appendix 1: propofol
● SIDE-EFFECTS
▸ **Common or very common** Apnoea · arrhythmias · headache · hypotension · localised pain · nausea · vomiting
▸ **Uncommon** Thrombosis
▸ **Rare or very rare** Epileptiform seizure (may be delayed) · pancreatitis · post procedural complications · pulmonary oedema · sexual disinhibition · soft tissue necrosis · urine discolouration
▸ **Frequency not known** Drug use disorders · dyskinesia · euphoric mood · heart failure · hepatomegaly · hyperkalaemia · hyperlipidaemia · metabolic acidosis · renal failure · respiratory depression · rhabdomyolysis

SIDE-EFFECTS, FURTHER INFORMATION **Bradycardia** Bradycardia may be profound and may be treated with intravenous administration of an antimuscarinic drug.
  Pain on injection Pain on injection can be reduced by intravenous lidocaine.
  Propofol infusion syndrome Prolonged infusion of propofol doses exceeding 4mg/kg/hour may result in potentially fatal effects, including metabolic acidosis, arrhythmias, cardiac failure, rhabdomyolysis, hyperlipidaemia, hyperkalaemia, hepatomegaly, and renal failure.

● PREGNANCY May depress neonatal respiration if used during delivery.
Dose adjustments Max. dose for maintenance of anaesthesia 6 mg/kg/hour.

● BREAST FEEDING Breast-feeding can be resumed as soon as mother has recovered sufficiently from anaesthesia.
● HEPATIC IMPAIRMENT Manufacturer advises caution.
● RENAL IMPAIRMENT Use with caution.
● MONITORING REQUIREMENTS Monitor blood-lipid concentration if risk of fat overload or if sedation longer than 3 days.
● DIRECTIONS FOR ADMINISTRATION Manufacturer advises shake before use; microbiological filter not recommended; may be administered via a Y-piece close to injection site co-administered with Glucose 5% or Sodium chloride 0.9%. 0.5% **emulsion** for injection or intermittent infusion; manufacturer advises may be administered undiluted, or diluted with Glucose 5% or Sodium chloride 0.9%; dilute to a concentration not less than 1 mg/mL. 1% **emulsion** for injection or infusion; manufacturer advises may be administered undiluted, or diluted with Glucose 5% (*Diprivan*®) or (*Propofol-Lipuro*®) or Sodium chloride 0.9% (*Propofol-Lipuro*® only); dilute to a concentration not less than 2 mg/mL; use within 6 hours of preparation. 2% **emulsion** for infusion; manufacturer advises do not dilute.

● PATIENT AND CARER ADVICE
Driving and skilled tasks Patients given sedatives and analgesics during minor outpatient procedures should be very carefully warned about the risk of driving or undertaking skilled tasks afterwards. For a short general anaesthetic the risk extends to **at least 24 hours** after administration. Responsible persons should be available to take patients home. The dangers of taking **alcohol** should also be emphasised.

● MEDICINAL FORMS There can be variation in the licensing of different medicines containing the same drug.
Emulsion for infusion
▸ Propofol (Non-proprietary)
  Propofol 10 mg per 1 ml Propofol 500mg/50ml emulsion for infusion vials | 1 vial PoM £5.00–£15.00 (Hospital only)
  Propofol-Lipuro 1% emulsion for infusion 50ml vials | 10 vial PoM £97.56 (Hospital only)
  Propofol 1g/100ml emulsion for infusion vials | 1 vial PoM £15.00–£18.50 (Hospital only)
  Propofol-Lipuro 1% emulsion for infusion 100ml vials | 10 vial PoM £186.66 (Hospital only)
  Propofol 20 mg per 1 ml Propofol 1g/50ml emulsion for infusion vials | 1 vial PoM £9.50–£15.00 (Hospital only)
  Propofol-Lipuro 2% emulsion for infusion 50ml vials | 10 vial PoM £186.64 (Hospital only)
▸ Diprivan (Aspen Pharma Trading Ltd)
  Propofol 10 mg per 1 ml Diprivan 1% emulsion for infusion 50ml pre-filled syringes | 1 pre-filled disposable injection PoM £10.68
  Propofol 20 mg per 1 ml Diprivan 2% emulsion for infusion 50ml pre-filled syringes | 1 pre-filled disposable injection PoM £15.16
▸ Propoven (Fresenius Kabi Ltd)
  Propofol 10 mg per 1 ml Propoven 1% emulsion for infusion 50ml vials | 10 vial PoM £120.60 (Hospital only)
  Propoven 1% emulsion for infusion 100ml vials | 10 vial PoM £241.50 (Hospital only)
  Propofol 20 mg per 1 ml Propoven 2% emulsion for infusion 50ml vials | 10 vial PoM £241.50 (Hospital only)
Emulsion for injection
▸ Propofol (Non-proprietary)
  Propofol 10 mg per 1 ml Propofol 200mg/20ml emulsion for injection vials | 5 vial PoM £3.50–£20.00 (Hospital only)
  Propofol-Lipuro 1% emulsion for injection 20ml ampoules | 5 ampoule PoM £20.16 (Hospital only)
▸ Diprivan (Aspen Pharma Trading Ltd)
  Propofol 10 mg per 1 ml Diprivan 1% emulsion for injection 20ml ampoules | 5 ampoule PoM £15.36 (Hospital only)
▸ Propofol-Lipuro (B.Braun Melsungen AG)
  Propofol 5 mg per 1 ml Propofol-Lipuro 0.5% emulsion for injection 20ml ampoules | 5 ampoule PoM £15.15
▸ Propoven (Fresenius Kabi Ltd)
  Propofol 10 mg per 1 ml Propoven 1% emulsion for injection 20ml ampoules | 5 ampoule PoM £23.90 (Hospital only)

15

Anaesthesia

ANAESTHETICS, GENERAL > VOLATILE LIQUID
ANAESTHETICS

Volatile halogenated anaesthetics

> **IMPORTANT SAFETY INFORMATION**
> Should only be administered by, or under the direct supervision of, personnel experienced in their use, with adequate training in anaesthesia and airway management, and when resuscitation equipment is available.

- **CONTRA-INDICATIONS** Susceptibility to malignant hyperthermia
- **CAUTIONS** Can trigger malignant hyperthermia · raised intracranial pressure (can increase cerebrospinal pressure)
- **SIDE-EFFECTS**
  ‣ **Common or very common** Agitation · apnoea · arrhythmias · chills · cough · dizziness · headache · hypersalivation · hypertension · hypotension · nausea · respiratory disorders · vomiting
  ‣ **Uncommon** Hypoxia
  ‣ **Frequency not known** Breath holding · cardiac arrest · haemorrhage · hepatic disorders · hyperkalaemia · malignant hyperthermia · QT interval prolongation · rhabdomyolysis · seizure
- **ALLERGY AND CROSS-SENSITIVITY** Can cause hepatotoxicity in those sensitised to halogenated anaesthetics.
- **DIRECTIONS FOR ADMINISTRATION** Volatile liquid anaesthetics are administered using calibrated vaporisers, using oxygen, oxygen-enriched air, or nitrous oxide-oxygen mixtures as the carrier gas (consult product literature).
- **PATIENT AND CARER ADVICE**
  Driving and skilled tasks Patients given sedatives and analgesics during minor outpatient procedures should be very carefully warned about the risks of driving and undertaking skilled tasks afterwards. For a short general anaesthetic, the risk extends **to at least 24 hours** after administration. Responsible persons should be available to take patients home. The dangers of taking **alcohol** should also be emphasised.

◀ above

Desflurane

- **INDICATIONS AND DOSE**

Induction of anaesthesia (but not recommended)
  ‣ BY INHALATION
  ‣ Adult: 4–11 %, to be inhaled through specifically calibrated vaporiser

Maintenance of anaesthesia (in nitrous oxide–oxygen)
  ‣ BY INHALATION
  ‣ Adult: 2–6 %, to be inhaled through a specifically calibrated vaporiser

Maintenance of anaesthesia (in oxygen or oxygen-enriched air)
  ‣ BY INHALATION
  ‣ Adult: 2.5–8.5 %, to be inhaled through a specifically calibrated vaporiser

- **INTERACTIONS** → Appendix 1: volatile halogenated anaesthetics
- **SIDE-EFFECTS**
  ‣ **Common or very common** Coagulation disorder · conjunctivitis

  ‣ **Uncommon** Myalgia · myocardial infarction · myocardial ischaemia · vasodilation
  ‣ **Frequency not known** Abdominal pain · asthenia · heart failure · hypokalaemia · malaise · metabolic acidosis · pancreatitis acute · shock · skin reactions · ventricular dysfunction · visual acuity decreased
- **PREGNANCY** May depress neonatal respiration if used during delivery.
- **BREAST FEEDING** Breast-feeding can be resumed as soon as mother has recovered sufficiently from anaesthesia.

- **MEDICINAL FORMS** There can be variation in the licensing of different medicines containing the same drug.
  Inhalation vapour
  ‣ Desflurane (Non-proprietary)
    Desflurane 1 ml per 1 ml Desflurane volatile liquid | 240 ml PoM Ⓢ (Hospital only)

◀ above

Isoflurane

12-Dec-201

- **INDICATIONS AND DOSE**

Induction of anaesthesia (in oxygen or nitrous oxide-oxygen)
  ‣ BY INHALATION
  ‣ Adult: Initially 0.5 %, increased to 3 %, adjusted according to response, administered using specifically calibrated vaporiser

Maintenance of anaesthesia (in nitrous oxide–oxygen)
  ‣ BY INHALATION
  ‣ Adult: 1–2.5 %, to be administered using specifically calibrated vaporiser; an additional 0.5–1% may be required when given with oxygen alone

Maintenance of anaesthesia in caesarean section (in nitrous oxide–oxygen)
  ‣ BY INHALATION
  ‣ Adult: 0.5–0.75 %, to be administered using specifically calibrated vaporiser

- **INTERACTIONS** → Appendix 1: volatile halogenated anaesthetics
- **SIDE-EFFECTS** Carboxyhaemoglobinaemia · chest discomfort · cognitive impairment · delirium · dyspnoea · ileus · mood altered (that can last several days) · myoglobinuria · skin reactions
- **PREGNANCY** May depress neonatal respiration if used during delivery.
- **BREAST FEEDING** Breast-feeding can be resumed as soon as mother has recovered sufficiently from anaesthesia.

- **MEDICINAL FORMS** There can be variation in the licensing of different medicines containing the same drug.
  Inhalation vapour
  ‣ Isoflurane (Non-proprietary)
    Isoflurane 1 ml per 1 ml Isoflurane inhalation vapour | 250 ml PoM £35.29 (Hospital only)
  ‣ AErrane (Baxter Healthcare Ltd)
    Isoflurane 1 ml per 1 ml AErrane volatile liquid | 250 ml PoM Ⓢ (Hospital only)

Nitrous oxide

12-Aug-2020

- **INDICATIONS AND DOSE**

Maintenance of anaesthesia in conjunction with other anaesthetic agents
  ‣ BY INHALATION
  ‣ Adult: 50–66 %, to be administered using suitable anaesthetic apparatus in oxygen

Analgesia

▶ BY INHALATION

▶ Adult: Up to 50 %, to be administered using suitable anaesthetic apparatus in oxygen, adjusted according to the patient's needs

IMPORTANT SAFETY INFORMATION
Nitrous oxide should only be administered by, or under the direct supervision of, personnel experienced in its use, with adequate training in anaesthesia and airway management, and when resuscitation equipment is available.

● CAUTIONS Entrapped air following recent underwater dive · pneumothorax · presence of intracranial air after head injury · recent intra-ocular gas injection

CAUTIONS, FURTHER INFORMATION Nitrous oxide may have a deleterious effect if used in patients with an air-containing closed space since nitrous oxide diffuses into such a space with a resulting increase in pressure. This effect may be dangerous in conditions such as pneumothorax, which may enlarge to compromise respiration, or in the presence of intracranial air after head injury, entrapped air following recent underwater dive, or recent intra-ocular gas injection.

● INTERACTIONS → Appendix 1: nitrous oxide

● SIDE-EFFECTS Abdominal distension · addiction · agranulocytosis · disorientation · dizziness · euphoric mood · megaloblastic anaemia · middle ear damage · myeloneuropathy · nausea · paraesthesia · sedation · subacute combined cord degeneration · tympanic membrane perforation · vomiting

SIDE-EFFECTS, FURTHER INFORMATION Exposure of patients to nitrous oxide for prolonged periods, either by continuous or by intermittent administration, may result in megaloblastic anaemia owing to interference with the action of vitamin B_{12}; neurological toxic effects can occur without preceding overt haematological changes. Depression of white cell formation may also occur.

● PREGNANCY May depress neonatal respiration if used during delivery.

● BREAST FEEDING Breast-feeding can be resumed as soon as mother has recovered sufficiently from anaesthesia.

● MONITORING REQUIREMENTS
▶ Assessment of plasma-vitamin B_{12} concentration should be considered in those at risk of deficiency, including the elderly, those who have a poor, vegetarian, or vegan diet, and those with a history of anaemia.
▶ Nitrous oxide should **not** be given continuously for longer than 24 hours or more frequently than every 4 days without close supervision and haematological monitoring.

● DIRECTIONS FOR ADMINISTRATION For analgesia (without loss of consciousness), manufacturer advises a mixture of nitrous oxide and oxygen containing 50% of each gas (*Entonox*®) is used.

● HANDLING AND STORAGE Exposure of theatre staff to nitrous oxide should be minimised (risk of serious side-effects).

● MEDICINAL FORMS There can be variation in the licensing of different medicines containing the same drug.
Inhalation gas
▶ Nitrous oxide (Non-proprietary)
Nitrous oxide 1 ml per 1 ml Nitrous oxide cylinders size E | 1800 litre P 🅢
Medical Nitrous Oxide cylinders size D | 900 litre P 🅢
Medical Nitrous Oxide cylinders size G | 9000 litre P 🅢
Nitrous oxide cylinders size F | 3600 litre P 🅢
Nitrous oxide cylinders size J | 18000 litre P 🅢
Nitrous oxide cylinders size G | 9000 litre P 🅢
Medical Nitrous Oxide cylinders size F | 3600 litre P 🅢

Nitrous oxide cylinders size D | 900 litre P 🅢
Medical Nitrous Oxide cylinders size E | 1800 litre P 🅢

⟆ 1384

Sevoflurane

● INDICATIONS AND DOSE

Induction of anaesthesia (in oxygen or nitrous oxide-oxygen)
▶ BY INHALATION
▶ Adult: Initially 0.5–1 %, then increased to up to 8 %, increased gradually, according to response, to be administered using specifically calibrated vaporiser

Maintenance of anaesthesia (in oxygen or nitrous oxide-oxygen)
▶ BY INHALATION
▶ Adult: 0.5–3 %, adjusted according to response, to be administered using specifically calibrated vaporiser

● CAUTIONS Susceptibility to QT-interval prolongation

● INTERACTIONS → Appendix 1: volatile halogenated anaesthetics

● SIDE-EFFECTS
▶ **Common or very common** Drowsiness · fever · hypothermia
▶ **Uncommon** Asthma · atrioventricular block · confusion
▶ **Frequency not known** Dystonia · intracranial pressure increased · muscle rigidity · nephritis tubulointerstitial · oedema · pancreatitis

● PREGNANCY May depress neonatal respiration if used during delivery.

● BREAST FEEDING Breast-feeding can be resumed as soon as mother has recovered sufficiently from anaesthesia.

● RENAL IMPAIRMENT Use with caution.

● MEDICINAL FORMS There can be variation in the licensing of different medicines containing the same drug.
Inhalation vapour
▶ Sevoflurane (Non-proprietary)
Sevoflurane 1 ml per 1 ml Sevoflurane volatile liquid | 250 ml £123.00 (Hospital only) PoM

1 **Anaesthesia adjuvants**

Pre-medication and peri-operative drugs

01-Sep-2020

Drugs that affect gastric pH

Regurgitation and aspiration of gastric contents (Mendelson's syndrome) can be an important complication of general anaesthesia, particularly in obstetrics and during emergency surgery, and requires prophylaxis against acid aspiration. Prophylaxis is also needed in those with gastro-oesophageal reflux disease and in circumstances where gastric emptying may be delayed.

An **H_2-receptor antagonist** can be used before surgery to increase the pH and reduce the volume of gastric fluid. It does not affect the pH of fluid already in the stomach and this limits its value in emergency procedures; an oral H_2-receptor antagonist can be given 1–2 hours before the procedure. Antacids are frequently used to neutralise the acidity of the fluid already in the stomach; 'clear' (non-particulate) antacids such as sodium citrate p. 833 are preferred.

Antimuscarinic drugs

Antimuscarinic drugs are used (less commonly nowadays) as premedicants to dry bronchial and salivary secretions which are increased by intubation, upper airway surgery, or some inhalational anaesthetics. They are also used before or with neostigmine p. 1170 to prevent bradycardia, excessive salivation, and other muscarinic actions of neostigmine. They also prevent bradycardia and hypotension associated with drugs such as propofol p. 1382 and suxamethonium chloride p. 1389.

Atropine sulfate p. 1386 is now rarely used for premedication but still has an emergency role in the treatment of vagotonic side-effects. Atropine sulfate may have a role in acute arrhythmias after myocardial infarction.

Hyoscine hydrobromide p. 458 reduces secretions and also provides a degree of amnesia, sedation, and anti-emesis. Unlike atropine sulfate it may produce bradycardia rather than tachycardia.

Glycopyrronium bromide p. 1387 reduces salivary secretions. When given intravenously it produces less tachycardia than atropine sulfate. It is widely used with neostigmine for reversal of non-depolarising neuromuscular blocking drugs.

Phenothiazines do not effectively reduce secretions when used alone.

Sedative drugs

Fear and anxiety before a procedure (including the night before) can be minimised by using a sedative drug, usually a **benzodiazepine**. Premedication may also augment the action of anaesthetics and provide some degree of pre-operative amnesia. The choice of drug depends on the individual, the nature of the procedure, the anaesthetic to be used, and other prevailing circumstances such as outpatients, obstetrics, and availability of recovery facilities. The choice also varies between elective and emergency procedures.

Premedicants can be given the night before major surgery; a further, smaller dose may be required before surgery. Alternatively, the first dose may be given on the day of the procedure.

Benzodiazepines

Benzodiazepines possess useful properties for premedication including relief of anxiety, sedation, and amnesia; short-acting benzodiazepines taken by mouth are the most common premedicants. Benzodiazepines are also used in intensive care units for sedation, particularly in those receiving assisted ventilation. Flumazenil p. 1422 is used to antagonise the effects of benzodiazepines.

Diazepam p. 362 is used to produce mild sedation with amnesia. It is a long-acting drug with active metabolites and a second period of drowsiness can occur several hours after its administration. Peri-operative use of diazepam in children is not recommended; its effect and timing of response are unreliable and paradoxical effects may occur.

Diazepam is relatively insoluble in water and preparations formulated in organic solvents are painful on intravenous injection and give rise to a high incidence of venous thrombosis (which may not be noticed for several days after the injection). Intramuscular injection of diazepam is painful and absorption is erratic. An emulsion formulated for intravenous injection is less irritant and reduces the risk of venous thrombosis; it is not suitable for intramuscular injection.

Temazepam p. 509 is given by mouth for premedication and has a shorter duration of action and a more rapid onset than oral diazepam; anxiolytic and sedative effects last about 90 minutes although there may be residual drowsiness.

Lorazepam p. 357 produces more prolonged sedation than temazepam and it has marked amnesic effects.

Midazolam p. 358 is a water-soluble benzodiazepine that is often used in preference to intravenous diazepam; recovery is faster than from diazepam, but may be significantly longer in the elderly, in patients with a low cardiac output, or after repeated dosing. Midazolam is associated with profound sedation when high doses are given intravenously or when it is used with certain other drugs.

Other drugs for sedation

Dexmedetomidine p. 1400 and clonidine hydrochloride p. 159 are alpha$_2$-adrenergic agonists with sedative properties. Dexmedetomidine is licensed for the sedation of patients receiving intensive care who need to remain responsive to verbal stimulation. Clonidine hydrochloride [unlicensed indication] can be used by mouth or by intravenous injection as a sedative agent when adequate sedation cannot be achieved with standard treatment.

Analgesia

For guidance on the use of analgesics before, during, or after surgery, see Peri-operative analgesia p. 1392.

Antagonists for central and respiratory depression

Respiratory depression is a major concern with opioid analgesics and it may be treated by artificial ventilation or be reversed by naloxone hydrochloride p. 1424. Naloxone hydrochloride will immediately reverse opioid-induced respiratory depression but the dose may have to be repeated because of the short duration of action of naloxone hydrochloride; however, naloxone hydrochloride will also antagonise the analgesic effect.

Flumazenil is a benzodiazepine antagonist for the reversal of the central sedative effects of benzodiazepines after anaesthetic and similar procedures. Flumazenil has a shorter half-life and duration of action than diazepam or midazolam so patients may become resedated.

Doxapram hydrochloride p. 315 is a central and respiratory stimulant but is of limited value in anaesthesia.

ANTIMUSCARINICS

⌐ 821

Atropine sulfate

24-Jul-2020

● INDICATIONS AND DOSE

Bradycardia due to acute massive overdosage of beta-blockers

▸ BY INTRAVENOUS INJECTION
▹ Child: 40 micrograms/kg (max. per dose 3 mg)
▹ Adult: 3 mg

Treatment of poisoning by organophosphorus insecticide or nerve agent (in combination with pralidoxime chloride)

▸ BY INTRAVENOUS INJECTION
▹ Child: 20 micrograms/kg every 5–10 minutes (max. per dose 2 mg) until the skin becomes flushed and dry, the pupils dilate, and bradycardia is abolished, frequency of administration dependent on the severity of poisoning
▹ Adult: 2 mg every 5–10 minutes until the skin becomes flushed and dry, the pupils dilate, and bradycardia is abolished, frequency of administration dependent on the severity of poisoning

Symptomatic relief of gastro-intestinal disorders characterised by smooth muscle spasm

▸ BY MOUTH
▹ Adult: 0.6–1.2 mg daily, dose to be taken at night

Premedication

▸ BY INTRAVENOUS INJECTION
▹ Child 12–17 years: 300–600 micrograms, to be administered immediately before induction of anaesthesia
▹ Adult: 300–600 micrograms, to be administered immediately before induction of anaesthesia

► BY SUBCUTANEOUS INJECTION, OR BY INTRAMUSCULAR INJECTION
► Child 12–17 years: 300–600 micrograms, to be administered 30–60 minutes before induction of anaesthesia
► Adult: 300–600 micrograms, to be administered 30–60 minutes before induction of anaesthesia

Intra-operative bradycardia
► BY INTRAVENOUS INJECTION
► Child 12–17 years: 300–600 micrograms, larger doses may be used in emergencies
► Adult: 300–600 micrograms, larger doses may be used in emergencies

Control of muscarinic side-effects of neostigmine in reversal of competitive neuromuscular block
► BY INTRAVENOUS INJECTION
► Child 12–17 years: 0.6–1.2 mg
► Adult: 0.6–1.2 mg

Excessive bradycardia associated with beta-blocker use
► BY INTRAVENOUS INJECTION
► Adult: 0.6–2.4 mg in divided doses (max. per dose 600 micrograms)

Bradycardia following myocardial infarction (particularly if complicated by hypotension)
► BY INTRAVENOUS INJECTION
► Adult: 500 micrograms every 3–5 minutes; maximum 3 mg per course

---

IMPORTANT SAFETY INFORMATION
Antimuscarinic drugs used for premedication to general anaesthesia should only be administered by, or under the direct supervision of, personnel experienced in their use.

● INTERACTIONS → Appendix 1: atropine
● SIDE-EFFECTS
► **Common or very common**
► With intravenous use Abdominal distension · anhidrosis · anxiety · arrhythmias · bronchial secretion decreased · dysphagia · gastrointestinal disorders · hallucination · hyperthermia · movement disorders · mydriasis · speech disorder · taste loss · thirst
► **Uncommon**
► With intravenous use Psychotic disorder
► **Rare or very rare**
► With intravenous use Angina pectoris · hypertensive crisis · seizure
► **Frequency not known**
► With intravenous use Insomnia
► With oral use Angle closure glaucoma · arrhythmias · bronchial secretion altered · chest pain · dysphagia · fever · gastrointestinal disorders · mydriasis · staggering · thirst
● PREGNANCY Not known to be harmful; manufacturer advises caution.
● BREAST FEEDING May suppress lactation; small amount present in milk—manufacturer advises caution.
● MONITORING REQUIREMENTS
► Control of muscarinic side-effects of neostigmine in reversal of competitive neuromuscular block Since atropine has a shorter duration of action than neostigmine, late unopposed bradycardia may result; close monitoring of the patient is necessary.
● LESS SUITABLE FOR PRESCRIBING
► With oral use Atropine tablets less suitable for prescribing. Any clinical benefit as a gastro-intestinal antispasmodic is outweighed by atropinic side-effects.
● EXCEPTIONS TO LEGAL CATEGORY
► With intramuscular use or intravenous use or subcutaneous use Prescription only medicine restriction does not apply where administration is for saving life in emergency.

● MEDICINAL FORMS There can be variation in the licensing of different medicines containing the same drug. Forms available from special-order manufacturers include: oral suspension, oral solution, solution for injection, solution for infusion

Solution for injection
► Atropine sulfate (Non-proprietary)
Atropine sulfate 100 microgram per 1 ml Atropine 500micrograms/5ml solution for injection pre-filled syringes | 1 pre-filled disposable injection [PoM] £13.00 | 10 pre-filled disposable injection [PoM] £130.00
Atropine sulfate 200 microgram per 1 ml Atropine 1mg/5ml solution for injection pre-filled syringes | 1 pre-filled disposable injection [PoM] £13.00 | 10 pre-filled disposable injection [PoM] £130.00
Atropine sulfate 300 microgram per 1 ml Atropine 3mg/10ml solution for injection pre-filled syringes | 1 pre-filled disposable injection [PoM] £13.00 DT = £7.29 | 10 pre-filled disposable injection [PoM] £130.00
Atropine sulfate 600 microgram per 1 ml Atropine 600micrograms/1ml solution for injection ampoules | 10 ampoule [PoM] £11.71 DT = £11.71
Atropine sulfate 1 mg per 1 ml Atropine 1mg/1ml solution for injection ampoules | 10 ampoule [PoM] £109.35–£114.82 DT = £109.35

F 821

Glycopyrronium bromide
06-Nov-2020
(Glycopyrrolate)

● INDICATIONS AND DOSE
Premedication at induction
► BY INTRAMUSCULAR INJECTION, OR BY INTRAVENOUS INJECTION
► Adult: 200–400 micrograms, alternatively 4–5 micrograms/kg (max. per dose 400 micrograms)

Intra-operative bradycardia
► BY INTRAVENOUS INJECTION
► Adult: 200–400 micrograms, alternatively 4–5 micrograms/kg (max. per dose 400 micrograms), repeated if necessary

Control of muscarinic side-effects of neostigmine in reversal of non-depolarising neuromuscular block
► BY INTRAVENOUS INJECTION
► Adult: 10–15 micrograms/kg, alternatively 200 micrograms per 1 mg of neostigmine to be administered

Bowel colic in palliative care | Excessive respiratory secretions in palliative care
► BY SUBCUTANEOUS INJECTION
► Adult: 200 micrograms every 4 hours and when required, hourly use is occasionally necessary, particularly in excessive respiratory secretions
► BY SUBCUTANEOUS INFUSION
► Adult: 0.6–1.2 mg/24 hours

IMPORTANT SAFETY INFORMATION
Antimuscarinic drugs used for premedication to general anaesthesia should only be administered by, or under the direct supervision of, personnel experienced in their use.

● INTERACTIONS → Appendix 1: glycopyrronium
● SIDE-EFFECTS Anhidrosis · bronchial secretion decreased · mydriasis
● PRESCRIBING AND DISPENSING INFORMATION
Palliative care For further information on the use of glycopyrronium bromide in palliative care, see www.medicinescomplete.com/#/content/palliative/glycopyrronium.

● MEDICINAL FORMS There can be variation in the licensing of different medicines containing the same drug.

Solution for injection

▸ Glycopyrronium bromide (Non-proprietary)

Glycopyrronium bromide 200 microgram per 1 ml Glycopyrronium bromide 200micrograms/1ml solution for injection ampoules | 10 ampoule PoM £14.00 DT = £9.95 | 10 ampoule PoM £5.72 DT = £9.95 (Hospital only) Glycopyrronium bromide 600micrograms/3ml solution for injection ampoules | 3 ampoule PoM £8.00 | 10 ampoule PoM £9.61 DT = £14.99 (Hospital only) | 10 ampoule PoM £14.99 DT = £14.99

1.1 Neuromuscular blockade

Neuromuscular blockade

Neuromuscular blocking drugs

Neuromuscular blocking drugs used in anaesthesia are also known as **muscle relaxants**. By specific blockade of the neuromuscular junction they enable light anaesthesia to be used with adequate relaxation of the muscles of the abdomen and diaphragm. They also relax the vocal cords and allow the passage of a tracheal tube. Their action differs from the muscle relaxants used in musculoskeletal disorders that act on the spinal cord or brain.

Patients who have received a neuromuscular blocking drug should **always** have their respiration assisted or controlled until the drug has been inactivated or antagonised. They should also receive sufficient concomitant inhalational or intravenous anaesthetic or sedative drugs to prevent awareness.

Non-depolarising neuromuscular blocking drugs

Non-depolarising neuromuscular blocking drugs (also known as competitive muscle relaxants) compete with acetylcholine for receptor sites at the neuromuscular junction and their action can be reversed with anticholinesterases such as neostigmine p. 1170. Non-depolarising neuromuscular blocking drugs can be divided into the **aminosteroid** group, comprising pancuronium bromide p. 1391, rocuronium bromide p. 1391, and vecuronium bromide p. 1391, and the **benzylisoquinolinium** group, comprising atracurium besilate p. 1389, cisatracurium p. 1390, and mivacurium p. 1390.

Non-depolarising neuromuscular blocking drugs have a slower onset of action than suxamethonium chloride p. 1389. These drugs can be classified by their duration of action as short-acting (15–30 minutes), intermediate-acting (30–40 minutes), and long-acting (60–120 minutes), although duration of action is dose-dependent. Drugs with a shorter or intermediate duration of action, such as atracurium besilate and vecuronium bromide p. 1391, are more widely used than those with a longer duration of action, such as pancuronium bromide.

Non-depolarising neuromuscular blocking drugs have no sedative or analgesic effects and are not considered to trigger malignant hyperthermia.

For patients receiving intensive care and who require tracheal intubation and mechanical ventilation, a non-depolarising neuromuscular blocking drug is chosen according to its onset of effect, duration of action, and side-effects. Rocuronium bromide, with a rapid onset of effect, may facilitate intubation. Atracurium besilate or cisatracurium may be suitable for long-term neuromuscular blockade since their duration of action is not dependent on elimination by the liver or the kidneys.

Atracurium besilate, a mixture of 10 isomers, is a benzylisoquinolinium neuromuscular blocking drug with an intermediate duration of action. It undergoes non-enzymatic metabolism which is independent of liver and kidney

function, thus allowing its use in patients with hepatic or renal impairment. Cardiovascular effects are associated with significant histamine release; histamine release can be minimised by administering slowly or in divided doses over at least 1 minute.

Cisatracurium is a single isomer of atracurium besilate. It is more potent and has a slightly longer duration of action than atracurium besilate and provides greater cardiovascular stability because cisatracurium lacks histamine-releasing effects.

Mivacurium, a benzylisoquinolinium neuromuscular blocking drug, has a short duration of action. It is metabolised by plasma cholinesterase and muscle paralysis is prolonged in individuals deficient in this enzyme. It is not associated with vagolytic activity or ganglionic blockade although histamine release can occur, particularly with rapid injection.

Pancuronium bromide, an aminosteroid neuromuscular blocking drug, has a long duration of action and is often used in patients receiving long-term mechanical ventilation in intensive care units. It lacks a histamine-releasing effect, but vagolytic and sympathomimetic effects can cause tachycardia and hypertension.

Rocuronium bromide exerts an effect within 2 minutes and has the most rapid onset of any of the non-depolarising neuromuscular blocking drugs. It is an aminosteroid neuromuscular blocking drug with an intermediate duration of action. It is reported to have minimal cardiovascular effects; high doses produce mild vagolytic activity.

Vecuronium bromide p. 1391, an aminosteroid neuromuscular blocking drug, has an intermediate duration of action. It does not generally produce histamine release and lacks cardiovascular effects.

Depolarising neuromuscular blocking drugs

Suxamethonium chloride has the most rapid onset of action of any of the neuromuscular blocking drugs and is ideal if fast onset and brief duration of action are required, e.g. with tracheal intubation. Unlike the non-depolarising neuromuscular blocking drugs, its action cannot be reversed and recovery is spontaneous; anticholinesterases such as neostigmine potentiate the neuromuscular block.

Suxamethonium chloride should be given after anaesthetic induction because paralysis is usually preceded by painful muscle fasciculations. While tachycardia occurs with single use, bradycardia may occur with repeated doses in adults and with the first dose in children. Premedication with atropine reduces bradycardia as well as the excessive salivation associated with suxamethonium chloride use.

Prolonged paralysis may occur in **dual block**, which occurs with high or repeated doses of suxamethonium chloride and is caused by the development of a non-depolarising block following the initial depolarising block. Individuals with myasthenia gravis are resistant to suxamethonium chloride but can develop dual block resulting in delayed recovery. Prolonged paralysis may also occur in those with low or atypical plasma cholinesterase. Assisted ventilation should be continued until muscle function is restored.

Suxamethonium chloride 02-Dec-2020

(Succinylcholine chloride)

- **DRUG ACTION** Suxamethonium acts by mimicking acetylcholine at the neuromuscular junction but hydrolysis is much slower than for acetylcholine; depolarisation is therefore prolonged, resulting in neuromuscular blockade.

- **INDICATIONS AND DOSE**

Neuromuscular blockade (short duration) during surgery and intubation
▶ BY INTRAVENOUS INJECTION
▶ Adult: 1–1.5 mg/kg

- **UNLICENSED USE** Doses of suxamethonium in BNF may differ from those in product literature.

┌───┐
IMPORTANT SAFETY INFORMATION
Should only be administered by, or under the direct
supervision of, personnel experienced in its use.
└───┘

- **CONTRA-INDICATIONS** Hyperkalaemia · low plasma-cholinesterase activity (including severe liver disease) · major trauma · neurological disease involving acute wasting of major muscle · personal or family history of congenital myotonic disease · personal or family history of malignant hyperthermia · prolonged immobilisation (risk of hyperkalaemia) · severe burns · skeletal muscle myopathies (e.g. Duchenne muscular dystrophy)

- **CAUTIONS** Cardiac disease · neuromuscular disease · raised intra-ocular pressure (avoid in penetrating eye injury) · respiratory disease · severe sepsis (risk of hyperkalaemia)

- **INTERACTIONS** → Appendix 1: suxamethonium

- **SIDE-EFFECTS**
▶ Common or very common Arrhythmias · bradycardia (may occur with repeated doses) · flushing · muscle contractions involuntary · myoglobinaemia · myoglobinuria · post procedural muscle pain · rash
▶ Rare or very rare Apnoea · cardiac arrest · hypersensitivity · malignant hyperthermia · respiratory disorders · trismus
SIDE-EFFECTS, FURTHER INFORMATION Premedication with atropine reduces bradycardia associated with suxamethonium use.

- **ALLERGY AND CROSS-SENSITIVITY** EvGr Allergic cross-reactivity between neuromuscular blocking drugs has been reported; caution is advised in cases of hypersensitivity to these drugs. ⟨M⟩

- **PREGNANCY** Mildly prolonged maternal neuromuscular blockade may occur.

- **BREAST FEEDING** Unlikely to be present in breast milk in significant amounts (ionised at physiological pH). Breast-feeding may be resumed once the mother recovered from neuromuscular block.

- **HEPATIC IMPAIRMENT** Manufacturer advises caution, particularly in end stage hepatic failure (increased risk of prolonged apnoea due to reduced hepatic synthesis of plasma cholinesterase).

- **MEDICINAL FORMS** There can be variation in the licensing of different medicines containing the same drug. Forms available from special-order manufacturers include: solution for injection

Solution for injection
▶ Suxamethonium chloride (Non-proprietary)
Suxamethonium chloride 50 mg per 1 ml Suxamethonium chloride 100mg/2ml solution for injection ampoules | 10 ampoule [PoM] £28.80–£50.00

▶ Anectine (Aspen Pharma Trading Ltd)
Suxamethonium chloride 50 mg per 1 ml Anectine 100mg/2ml solution for injection ampoules | 5 ampoule [PoM] £3.57 (Hospital only)

Non-depolarising neuromuscular blocking drugs

┌───┐
IMPORTANT SAFETY INFORMATION
Non-depolarising neuromuscular blocking drugs should
only be administered by, or under direct supervision of,
personnel experienced in their use, with adequate
training in anaesthesia and airway management.
└───┘

- **CAUTIONS** Burns (resistance can develop, increased doses may be required) · cardiovascular disease (reduce rate of administration) · electrolyte disturbances (response unpredictable) · fluid disturbances (response unpredictable) · hypothermia (activity prolonged, lower doses required) · myasthenia gravis (activity prolonged, lower doses required) · neuromuscular disorders (response unpredictable)

- **SIDE-EFFECTS**
▶ Common or very common Flushing · hypotension
▶ Uncommon Bronchospasm · hypersensitivity · skin reactions · tachycardia
▶ Rare or very rare Circulatory collapse · muscle weakness (after prolonged use in intensive care) · myopathy (after prolonged use in intensive care) · shock

- **ALLERGY AND CROSS-SENSITIVITY** Allergic cross-reactivity between neuromuscular blocking drugs has been reported; caution is advised in cases of hypersensitivity to these drugs.

- **PREGNANCY** Non-depolarising neuromuscular blocking drugs are highly ionised at physiological pH and are therefore unlikely to cross the placenta in significant amounts.

- **BREAST FEEDING** Non-depolarising neuromuscular blocking drugs are ionised at physiological pH and are unlikely to be present in milk in significant amounts. Breast-feeding may be resumed once the mother has recovered from neuromuscular block.

☞ above

Atracurium besilate

(Atracurium besylate)

- **INDICATIONS AND DOSE**

Neuromuscular blockade (short to intermediate duration) for surgery and intubation
▶ INITIALLY BY INTRAVENOUS INJECTION
▶ Adult: Initially 300–600 micrograms/kg, then (by intravenous injection) 100–200 micrograms/kg as required, alternatively (by intravenous injection) initially 300–600 micrograms/kg, followed by (by intravenous infusion) 300–600 micrograms/kg/hour

Neuromuscular blockade during intensive care
▶ INITIALLY BY INTRAVENOUS INJECTION
▶ Adult: Initially 300–600 micrograms/kg, initial dose is optional, then (by intravenous infusion) 270–1770 micrograms/kg/hour; (by intravenous infusion) usual dose 650–780 micrograms/kg/hour

DOSES AT EXTREMES OF BODY-WEIGHT
▶ To avoid excessive dosage in obese patients, dose should be calculated on the basis of ideal body-weight.

15

Anaesthesia

- INTERACTIONS → Appendix 1: neuromuscular blocking drugs, non-depolarising
- SIDE-EFFECTS
▶ **Rare or very rare** Cardiac arrest
▶ **Frequency not known** Seizure

SIDE-EFFECTS, FURTHER INFORMATION Hypotension, skin flushing, and bronchospasm is associated with histamine release. Manufacturer advises minimising effects of histamine release by administering over 1 minute in patients with cardiovascular disease or sensitivity to hypotension.

- DIRECTIONS FOR ADMINISTRATION For *intravenous infusion* (*Tracrium*®; Atracurium besilate injection, Hospira; Atracurium injection/infusion, Genus), give continuously in Glucose 5% or Sodium Chloride 0.9%; stability varies with diluent; dilute requisite dose with infusion fluid to a concentration of 0.5–5 mg/mL.

- MEDICINAL FORMS There can be variation in the licensing of different medicines containing the same drug. Forms available from special-order manufacturers include: solution for injection

Solution for injection
▶ Atracurium besilate (Non-proprietary)
  Atracurium besilate 10 mg per 1 ml Atracurium besilate 250mg/25ml solution for injection vials | 1 vial [PoM] £16.50 (Hospital only)
  Atracurium besilate 25mg/2.5ml solution for injection ampoules | 5 ampoule [PoM] £9.25–£11.50 (Hospital only) | 10 ampoule [PoM] £16.56–£18.50 (Hospital only)
  Atracurium besilate 50mg/5ml solution for injection ampoules | 5 ampoule [PoM] £17.50 (Hospital only) | 10 ampoule [PoM] £30.04–£35.00 (Hospital only)
▶ Tracrium (Aspen Pharma Trading Ltd)
  Atracurium besilate 10 mg per 1 ml Tracrium 250mg/25ml solution for injection vials | 2 vial [PoM] £25.81 (Hospital only)
  Tracrium 25mg/2.5ml solution for injection ampoules | 5 ampoule [PoM] £8.28 (Hospital only)
  Tracrium 50mg/5ml solution for injection ampoules | 5 ampoule [PoM] £15.02 (Hospital only)

Cisatracurium

◥ 1389

24-Jul-2020

- INDICATIONS AND DOSE

Neuromuscular blockade (intermediate duration) during surgery and intubation
▶ INITIALLY BY INTRAVENOUS INJECTION
▶ **Adult:** Initially 150 micrograms/kg, then (by intravenous injection) maintenance 30 micrograms/kg every 20 minutes, alternatively (by intravenous infusion) initially 180 micrograms/kg/hour, then (by intravenous infusion) maintenance 60–120 micrograms/kg/hour, maintenance dose administered after stabilisation

Neuromuscular blockade (intermediate duration) during intensive care
▶ INITIALLY BY INTRAVENOUS INJECTION
▶ **Adult:** Initially 150 micrograms/kg, initial dose is optional, then (by intravenous infusion) 180 micrograms/kg/hour, adjusted according to response; (by intravenous infusion) usual dose 30–600 micrograms/kg/hour

DOSES AT EXTREMES OF BODY-WEIGHT
▶ To avoid excessive dosage in obese patients, dose should be calculated on the basis of ideal body-weight.

- INTERACTIONS → Appendix 1: neuromuscular blocking drugs, non-depolarising
- SIDE-EFFECTS
▶ **Common or very common** Bradycardia
- DIRECTIONS FOR ADMINISTRATION For *intravenous infusion* (*Nimbex*®, *Nimbex Forte*®), manufacturer advises give continuously in Glucose 5% or Sodium Chloride 0.9%;

solutions of 2 mg/mL and 5 mg/mL may be infused undiluted; alternatively dilute with infusion fluid to a concentration of 0.1–2 mg/mL.

- MEDICINAL FORMS There can be variation in the licensing of different medicines containing the same drug.
Solution for injection
▶ Cisatracurium (Non-proprietary)
  Cisatracurium (as Cisatracurium besilate) 2 mg per 1 ml Cisatracurium besilate 10mg/5ml solution for injection ampoules | 5 ampoule [PoM] Ⓢ (Hospital only)
  Cisatracurium besilate 20mg/10ml solution for injection ampoules | 5 ampoule [PoM] £32.09–£37.75 (Hospital only) | 10 ampoule [PoM] £75.50 (Hospital only)
  Cisatracurium besilate 20mg/10ml solution for injection vials | 5 vial [PoM] £37.75 (Hospital only)
  Cisatracurium (as Cisatracurium besilate) 5 mg per 1 ml Cisatracurium besilate 150mg/30ml solution for injection vials | 1 vial [PoM] £26.43–£45.00 (Hospital only)
▶ Nimbex (Aspen Pharma Trading Ltd)
  Cisatracurium (as Cisatracurium besilate) 2 mg per 1 ml Nimbex 20mg/10ml solution for injection ampoules | 5 ampoule [PoM] £37.75 (Hospital only)
  Cisatracurium (as Cisatracurium besilate) 5 mg per 1 ml Nimbex Forte 150mg/30ml solution for injection vials | 1 vial [PoM] £31.09 (Hospital only)

◥ 1389

Mivacurium

- INDICATIONS AND DOSE

Neuromuscular blockade (short duration) during surgery and intubation
▶ INITIALLY BY INTRAVENOUS INJECTION
▶ **Adult:** 70–250 micrograms/kg; (by intravenous injection) maintenance 100 micrograms/kg every 15 minutes, alternatively (by intravenous infusion) maintenance 8–10 micrograms/kg/minute, (by intravenous infusion) adjusted in steps of 1 microgram/kg/minute every 3 minutes if required; (by intravenous infusion) usual dose 6–7 micrograms/kg/minute

DOSES AT EXTREMES OF BODY-WEIGHT
▶ To avoid excessive dosage in obese patients, dose should be calculated on the basis of ideal body-weight.

- CAUTIONS Burns (low plasma cholinesterase activity; dose titration required) · elderly
- INTERACTIONS → Appendix 1: neuromuscular blocking drugs, non-depolarising
- HEPATIC IMPAIRMENT Manufacturer advises caution in hepatic failure (increased duration of action).
Dose adjustments Manufacturer advises dose reduction in hepatic failure.
- RENAL IMPAIRMENT
Dose adjustments Clinical effect prolonged in renal failure—reduce dose according to response.
- DIRECTIONS FOR ADMINISTRATION For *intravenous infusion*, give continuously in Glucose 5% or Sodium chloride 0.9%. Dilute to a concentration of 500 micrograms/mL; may also be given undiluted. Doses up to 150 micrograms/kg may be given over 5–15 seconds, higher doses should be given over 30 seconds. In asthma, cardiovascular disease or in those sensitive to reduced arterial blood pressure, give over 60 seconds.

- MEDICINAL FORMS There can be variation in the licensing of different medicines containing the same drug.
Solution for injection
▶ Mivacron (Aspen Pharma Trading Ltd)
  Mivacurium (as Mivacurium chloride) 2 mg per 1 ml Mivacron 10mg/5ml solution for injection ampoules | 5 ampoule [PoM] £13.95 (Hospital only)
  Mivacron 20mg/10ml solution for injection ampoules | 5 ampoule [PoM] £22.57 (Hospital only)

Pancuronium bromide

28-Jul-2020

⚑ 1389

● **INDICATIONS AND DOSE**

Neuromuscular blockade (long duration) during surgery and intubation

▸ BY INTRAVENOUS INJECTION

▸ **Adult:** Initially 100 micrograms/kg, then 20 micrograms/kg as required

Neuromuscular blockade (long duration) during intensive care

▸ BY INTRAVENOUS INJECTION

▸ **Adult:** Initially 100 micrograms/kg, initial dose is optional, then 60 micrograms/kg every 60–90 minutes

DOSES AT EXTREMES OF BODY-WEIGHT

▸ To avoid excessive dosage in obese patients, dose should be calculated on the basis of ideal body-weight.

● INTERACTIONS → Appendix 1: neuromuscular blocking drugs, non-depolarising

● SIDE-EFFECTS Apnoea · arrhythmia · hypersalivation · increased cardiac output · miosis

SIDE-EFFECTS, FURTHER INFORMATION Pancuronium lacks histamine-releasing effect, but vagolytic and sympathomimetic effects can cause tachycardia.

● HEPATIC IMPAIRMENT Manufacturer advises caution (possibly slower onset and higher dose requirements due to resistance to neuromuscular blocking action which may lead to a prolonged recovery time).

● RENAL IMPAIRMENT Use with caution; prolonged duration of block.

● MEDICINAL FORMS There can be variation in the licensing of different medicines containing the same drug.

Solution for injection

▸ Pancuronium bromide (Non-proprietary)
Pancuronium bromide 2 mg per 1 ml Pancuronium bromide 4mg/2ml solution for injection ampoules | 10 ampoule [PoM] £50.00 (Hospital only)

⚑ 1389

Rocuronium bromide

05-Nov-2020

● **INDICATIONS AND DOSE**

Neuromuscular blockade (intermediate duration) during surgery and intubation

▸ INITIALLY BY INTRAVENOUS INJECTION

▸ **Adult:** Initially 600 micrograms/kg; (by intravenous injection) maintenance 150 micrograms/kg, alternatively (by intravenous infusion) maintenance 300–600 micrograms/kg/hour, adjusted according to response

▸ **Elderly:** Initially 600 micrograms/kg; (by intravenous injection) maintenance 75–100 micrograms/kg, alternatively (by intravenous infusion) maintenance up to 400 micrograms/kg/hour, adjusted according to response

Neuromuscular blockade (intermediate duration) during intensive care

▸ INITIALLY BY INTRAVENOUS INJECTION

▸ **Adult:** Initially 600 micrograms/kg, initial dose is optional; (by intravenous infusion) maintenance 300–600 micrograms/kg/hour for first hour, then (by intravenous infusion), adjusted according to response

DOSES AT EXTREMES OF BODY-WEIGHT

▸ To avoid excessive dosage in obese patients, dose should be calculated on the basis of ideal body-weight.

● INTERACTIONS → Appendix 1: neuromuscular blocking drugs, non-depolarising

● SIDE-EFFECTS

▸ **Uncommon** Procedural complications

▸ **Rare or very rare** Angioedema · face oedema · malignant hyperthermia · paralysis

● HEPATIC IMPAIRMENT Manufacturer advises caution (may prolong duration of action).

Dose adjustments Manufacturer advises consider dose reduction—consult product literature.

● RENAL IMPAIRMENT

Dose adjustments Reduce maintenance dose; prolonged paralysis.

● DIRECTIONS FOR ADMINISTRATION [EvGr] For *continuous intravenous infusion* or via drip tubing, may be diluted with Glucose 5% or Sodium Chloride 0.9%. Ⓜ

● MEDICINAL FORMS There can be variation in the licensing of different medicines containing the same drug.

Solution for injection

▸ Rocuronium bromide (Non-proprietary)
Rocuronium bromide 10 mg per 1 ml Rocuronium bromide 50mg/5ml solution for injection ampoules | 10 ampoule [PoM] £24.00–£28.00
Rocuronium bromide 50mg/5ml solution for injection vials | 10 vial [PoM] £28.00–£38.30 (Hospital only)
Rocuronium bromide 100mg/10ml solution for injection vials | 10 vial [PoM] £57.00 | 10 vial [PoM] £57.00–£76.70 (Hospital only)
Rocuronium bromide 100mg/10ml solution for injection ampoules | 10 ampoule [PoM] £57.00

▸ Esmeron (Merck Sharp & Dohme Ltd)
Rocuronium bromide 10 mg per 1 ml Esmeron 50mg/5ml solution for injection vials | 10 vial [PoM] £28.92 (Hospital only)

⚑ 1389

Vecuronium bromide

29-Jul-2020

● **INDICATIONS AND DOSE**

Neuromuscular blockade (intermediate duration) during surgery and intubation

▸ INITIALLY BY INTRAVENOUS INJECTION

▸ **Adult:** 80–100 micrograms/kg; (by intravenous injection) maintenance 20–30 micrograms/kg, adjusted according to response, max. 100 micrograms/kg in caesarean section, alternatively (by intravenous infusion) maintenance 0.8–1.4 micrograms/kg/minute, adjusted according to response

DOSES AT EXTREMES OF BODY-WEIGHT

▸ To avoid excessive dosage in obese patients, dose should be calculated on the basis of ideal body-weight.

● INTERACTIONS → Appendix 1: neuromuscular blocking drugs, non-depolarising

● SIDE-EFFECTS

▸ **Uncommon** Procedural complications

▸ **Rare or very rare** Angioedema · face oedema · paralysis

● HEPATIC IMPAIRMENT Manufacturer advises caution in significant impairment.

● RENAL IMPAIRMENT Use with caution.

● DIRECTIONS FOR ADMINISTRATION Manufacturer advises reconstitute each vial with 5 mL Water for Injections to give 2 mg/mL solution; *alternatively* reconstitute with up to 10 mL Glucose 5% *or* Sodium Chloride 0.9% *or* Water for Injections—unsuitable for further dilution if not reconstituted with Water for Injections. For *continuous intravenous infusion*, manufacturer advises dilute reconstituted solution to a concentration up to 40 micrograms/mL with Glucose 5% or Sodium Chloride 0.9%; reconstituted solution can also be given via drip tubing.

● MEDICINAL FORMS There can be variation in the licensing of different medicines containing the same drug.

Powder for solution for injection

▸ Vecuronium bromide (Non-proprietary)
Vecuronium bromide 10 mg Vecuronium bromide 10mg powder for solution for injection vials | 10 vial [PoM] £57.85 (Hospital only)

15

Anaesthesia

1.2 Neuromuscular blockade reversal

Neuromuscular blockade reversal

Neuromuscular blockade reversal

Anticholinesterases

Anticholinesterases reverse the effects of the non-depolarising (competitive) neuromuscular blocking drugs such as pancuronium bromide p. 1391 but they prolong the action of the depolarising neuromuscular blocking drug suxamethonium chloride p. 1389.

Neostigmine p. 1170 is used specifically for reversal of non-depolarising (competitive) blockade. It acts within one minute of intravenous injection and its effects last for 20 to 30 minutes; a second dose may then be necessary. Glycopyrronium bromide p. 1387 or alternatively atropine sulfate p. 1386, given before or with neostigmine, prevent bradycardia, excessive salivation, and other muscarinic effects of neostigmine.

Other drugs for reversal of neuromuscular blockade

Sugammadex below is a modified gamma cyclodextrin that can be used for rapid reversal of neuromuscular blockade induced by rocuronium bromide p. 1391 or vecuronium bromide p. 1391. In practice, sugammadex is used mainly for rapid reversal of neuromuscular blockade in an emergency.

ANTICHOLINESTERASES

Neostigmine with glycopyrronium bromide
17-Jul-2020

The properties listed below are those particular to the combination only. For the properties of the components please consider, neostigmine p. 1170, glycopyrronium bromide p. 1387.

- ● **INDICATIONS AND DOSE**
  Reversal of non-depolarising neuromuscular blockade
  ▶ BY INTRAVENOUS INJECTION
  ▶ Adult: 1–2 mL, repeated if necessary, alternatively 0.02 mL/kilogram, repeated if necessary; maximum 2 mL per course

- ● INTERACTIONS → Appendix 1: glycopyrronium · neostigmine

- ● DIRECTIONS FOR ADMINISTRATION For *intravenous injection,* manufacturer advises give over 10–30 seconds.

- ● MEDICINAL FORMS There can be variation in the licensing of different medicines containing the same drug.
  Solution for injection
  ▶ Neostigmine with glycopyrronium bromide (Non-proprietary)
  Glycopyrronium bromide 500 microgram per 1 ml, Neostigmine metilsulfate 2.5 mg per 1 ml Neostigmine 2.5mg/1ml / Glycopyrronium bromide 500micrograms/1ml solution for injection ampoules | 10 ampoule [PoM] £11.50

ANTIDOTES AND CHELATORS

Sugammadex
06-Aug-202

- ● **INDICATIONS AND DOSE**
  Routine reversal of neuromuscular blockade induced by rocuronium or vecuronium
  ▶ BY INTRAVENOUS INJECTION
  ▶ Adult: Initially 2–4 mg/kg, then 4 mg/kg if required, administered if recurrence of neuromuscular blockade occurs; consult product literature for further details
  Immediate reversal of neuromuscular blockade induced by rocuronium
  ▶ BY INTRAVENOUS INJECTION
  ▶ Adult: 16 mg/kg (consult product literature)

IMPORTANT SAFETY INFORMATION
Should only be administered by, or under the direct supervision of, personnel experienced in its use.

- ● CAUTIONS Cardiovascular disease (recovery may be delayed) · elderly (recovery may be delayed) · pre-existing coagulation disorders · recurrence of neuromuscular blockade—monitor respiratory function until fully recovered · use of anticoagulants (unrelated to surgery) · wait 24 hours before re-administering rocuronium · wait 24 hours before re-administering vecuronium

- ● INTERACTIONS → Appendix 1: sugammadex

- ● SIDE-EFFECTS
  ▶ **Common or very common** Abdominal pain · arrhythmias · cough · dizziness · headache · nausea · procedural complications · skin reactions · taste altered · vomiting
  ▶ **Uncommon** Hypersensitivity
  ▶ **Frequency not known** Bronchospasm

- ● PREGNANCY Use with caution—no information available.

- ● RENAL IMPAIRMENT Avoid if eGFR less than 30 mL/minute/1.73 m^2.

- ● NATIONAL FUNDING/ACCESS DECISIONS
  For full details see funding body website
  Scottish Medicines Consortium (SMC) decisions
  ▶ Sugammadex (*Bridion*®) for the routine reversal of neuromuscular blockade induced by rocuronium or vecuronium in adults and rocuronium in paediatric patients (March 2013) SMC No. 527/09 Recommended with restrictions

- ● MEDICINAL FORMS There can be variation in the licensing of different medicines containing the same drug.
  Solution for injection
  ELECTROLYTES: May contain Sodium
  ▶ Bridion (Merck Sharp & Dohme Ltd)
  Sugammadex (as Sugammadex sodium) 100 mg per 1 ml Bridion 500mg/5ml solution for injection vials | 10 vial [PoM] £1,491.00 (Hospital only)
  Bridion 200mg/2ml solution for injection vials | 10 vial [PoM] £596.40 (Hospital only)

1.3 Peri-operative analgesia

Peri-operative analgesia
01-Sep-2020

Overview

[EvGr] Postoperative pain management options should be discussed with patients prior to surgery. Take into account the patient's clinical features and the type of surgery, and discuss the patient's pain history, preferences and expectations, likely impact of the procedure on their pain, potential benefits and risks of treatment, and discharge plan. A multimodal approach using a combination of analgesics

rom different classes to manage postoperative pain should
be offered.

Consider prescribing pre-emptive analgesia to ensure that
the patient's pain is managed when the effects of local
anaesthesia wears off. Ⓐ

Non-opioid analgesics

EvGr Oral paracetamol p. 464 should be offered before and
after surgery irrespective of pain severity, with intravenous
paracetamol reserved for patients unable to take oral
medication.

Offer oral ibuprofen p. 1186 to manage immediate
postoperative pain (pain during the first 24 hours after
surgery) of all severities, except for patients who have had
surgery for a hip fracture—see NICE guideline: **Hip
fractures: management** for guidance, available at:
www.nice.org.uk/guidance/cg124. Intravenous NSAIDs should
be reserved for patients unable to take oral medication; if
offering intravenous NSAIDs, choose a traditional NSAID
rather than a COX-2 (cyclo-oxygenase-2) inhibitor. Ⓐ

Intramuscular injections of diclofenac sodium p. 1181 and
ketoprofen p. 1190 are rarely used; they are given deep into
the gluteal muscle to minimise pain and tissue damage.
Ketorolac trometamol p. 1395 is less irritant on
intramuscular injection but pain has been reported; it can
also be given by intravenous injection. Suppositories of
diclofenac sodium and ketoprofen may be effective
alternatives to the parenteral use of these drugs.

Since non-steroidal anti-inflammatory drugs (NSAIDs) do
not depress respiration, do not impair gastro-intestinal
motility, and do not cause dependence, they may be useful
alternatives or adjuncts to opioids for the relief of
postoperative pain.

Opioid analgesics

Opioid analgesics are now rarely used as premedicants; they
are more likely to be administered at induction. Pre-
operative use of opioid analgesics is generally limited to
those patients who require control of existing pain.

EvGr An oral opioid should only be offered if immediate
postoperative pain is expected to be moderate to severe. It
should be given as soon as the patient can eat and drink after
surgery, and the dose adjusted to help achieve functional
recovery (such as coughing and mobilising) as soon as
possible. Patients unable to take oral opioids should be
offered either a patient-controlled analgesia (PCA) or
continuous epidural. The benefit of a continuous epidural
should be taken into consideration for patients who are
having major or complex open-torso surgery, are expected to
have severe pain, or those who have cognitive impairment. If
opioids are used, see NICE guideline: **Controlled drugs:
safe use and management** (available at: www.nice.org.uk/
guidance/ng46) for information on prescribing controlled
drugs. Ⓐ

For guidance on the management of opioid-induced
respiratory depression, see Pre-medication and peri-
operative drugs p. 1385.

Intra-operative analgesia

Opioid analgesics given in small doses before or with
induction reduce the dose requirement of some drugs used
during anaesthesia.

Alfentanil p. 1397, fentanyl p. 478, and remifentanil
p. 1398 are particularly useful because they act within
1–2 minutes and have short durations of action. The initial
doses of alfentanil or fentanyl are followed either by
successive intravenous injections or by an intravenous
infusion; prolonged infusions increase the duration of effect.
Repeated intra-operative doses of alfentanil or fentanyl
should be given with care since the resulting respiratory
depression can persist postoperatively and occasionally it
may become apparent for the first time postoperatively when
monitoring of the patient might be less intensive. Alfentanil,

fentanyl, and remifentanil can cause muscle rigidity,
particularly of the chest wall or jaw; this can be managed by
the use of neuromuscular blocking drugs.

In contrast to other opioids which are metabolised in the
liver, remifentanil undergoes rapid metabolism by
nonspecific blood and tissue esterases; its short duration of
action allows prolonged administration at high dosage,
without accumulation, and with little risk of residual
postoperative respiratory depression. Remifentanil should
not be given by intravenous injection intraoperatively, but it
is well suited to continuous infusion; a supplementary
analgesic is given before stopping the infusion of
remifentanil.

EvGr A single dose of intravenous ketamine p. 1399
[unlicensed] should be considered either during or
immediately after surgery to supplement other types of pain
relief if, the patient's pain is expected to be moderate to
severe and an intravenous opioid alone does not provide
adequate pain relief, or the patient has opioid sensitivity.
Ⓐ

Useful resources

Perioperative care in adults. National Institute for Health
and Care Excellence. NICE guideline 180. August 2020.
www.nice.org.uk/guidance/ng180

ANAESTHETICS, GENERAL › NMDA RECEPTOR ANTAGONISTS

Esketamine   05-Nov-2020

● **DRUG ACTION** Esketamine is an isomer of ketamine that
blocks N-methyl-D-aspartate (NMDA) receptors and
interrupts the association pathways of the brain, resulting
in dissociative anaesthesia and analgesia and in
restoration of neural pathways regulating mood and
emotional behaviour.

● **INDICATIONS AND DOSE**

**Induction and maintenance of anaesthesia (specialist use
only)**
▶ BY SLOW INTRAVENOUS INJECTION
▸ Adult: 0.5–1 mg/kg, then maintenance 0.25–0.5 mg/kg
every 10–15 minutes, adjusted according to response
▶ BY INTRAMUSCULAR INJECTION
▸ Adult: 2–4 mg/kg, then maintenance 1–2 mg/kg every
10–15 minutes, adjusted according to response
▶ BY CONTINUOUS INTRAVENOUS INFUSION
▸ Adult: 0.5–3 mg/kg/hour, adjusted according to
response

**Analgesic supplementation of regional and local
anaesthesia (specialist use only)**
▶ BY CONTINUOUS INTRAVENOUS INFUSION
▸ Adult: 0.125–0.25 mg/kg/hour, adjusted according to
response

Analgesia in emergency medicine (specialist use only)
▶ BY INTRAMUSCULAR INJECTION
▸ Adult: 0.25–0.5 mg/kg, adjusted according to response
▶ BY SLOW INTRAVENOUS INJECTION
▸ Adult: 0.125–0.25 mg/kg, adjusted according to
response

Major depressive disorder (specialist use only)
▶ BY INTRANASAL ADMINISTRATION
▸ Adult: Initially 56 mg on day 1, then 56–84 mg twice
weekly for weeks 1–4, then 56–84 mg once weekly for
weeks 5–8, then 56–84 mg every 1–2 weeks from week
9 onwards, review continued treatment periodically,
treatment is recommended for at least 6 months after
depressive symptoms improve, all dose adjustments to
be made in 28 mg increments   continued →

Anaesthesia

15

▶ BY INTRANASAL ADMINISTRATION

▶ Elderly: Initially 28 mg on day 1, then 28–84 mg twice weekly for weeks 1–4, then 28–84 mg once weekly for weeks 5–8, then 28–84 mg every 1–2 weeks from week 9 onwards, review continued treatment periodically, treatment is recommended for at least 6 months after depressive symptoms improve, all dose adjustments to be made in 28 mg increments

Major depressive disorder (patients of Japanese origin) (specialist use only)

▶ BY INTRANASAL ADMINISTRATION

▶ Adult: Initially 28 mg on day 1, then 28–84 mg twice weekly for weeks 1–4, then 28–84 mg once weekly for weeks 5–8, then 28–84 mg every 1–2 weeks from week 9 onwards, review continued treatment periodically, treatment is recommended for at least 6 months after depressive symptoms improve, all dose adjustments to be made in 28 mg increments

DOSE EQUIVALENCE AND CONVERSION

▶ With intranasal use

▶ 28 mg equivalent to 2 sprays (1 spray administered into each nostril).

IMPORTANT SAFETY INFORMATION

Esketamine should only be administered by, or under the direct supervision of, personnel experienced in its use, with adequate training in anaesthesia and airway management, and when resuscitation equipment is available.

● CONTRA-INDICATIONS

GENERAL CONTRA-INDICATIONS

Acute porphyrias p. 1107 · patients in whom hypertension or raised intracranial pressure forms a serious risk

SPECIFIC CONTRA-INDICATIONS

▶ When used for Analgesia in emergency medicine or Analgesic supplementation of regional and local anaesthesia or Induction and maintenance of anaesthesia Eclampsia · ischaemic cardiac disorders (when used as sole anaesthetic agent) · pre-eclampsia

▶ When used for Major depressive disorder Aneurysmal vascular disease · cardiovascular events, including myocardial infarction (within 6 weeks) · intracerebral haemorrhage

● CAUTIONS

GENERAL CAUTIONS Hypertension · raised intracranial pressure · thyroid dysfunction

SPECIFIC CAUTIONS

▶ When used for Analgesia in emergency medicine or Analgesic supplementation of regional and local anaesthesia or Induction and maintenance of anaesthesia Chronic or acute alcohol consumption · decompensated cardiac failure · increased cerebrospinal fluid pressure · patients with multiple injuries or in poor condition—consult product literature · prolapsed umbilical cord · raised intra-ocular pressure · severe psychotic disorders · unstable angina pectoris · uterine rupture

▶ When used for Major depressive disorder Bipolar disorder (active or previous history) · cardiovascular conditions (clinically significant or unstable) · mania (active or previous history) · psychosis (active or previous history) · respiratory conditions (clinically significant or unstable)

CAUTIONS, FURTHER INFORMATION

▶ Cardiovascular or respiratory conditions

▶ When used for Major depressive disorder Esketamine should be administered where appropriately trained staff and resuscitation facilities are available.

● INTERACTIONS → Appendix 1: esketamine

● SIDE-EFFECTS

GENERAL SIDE-EFFECTS

▶ **Common or very common** Anxiety · dizziness · nausea · vomiting

SPECIFIC SIDE-EFFECTS

▶ **Common or very common**

▶ With intranasal use Drowsiness · dry mouth · dysarthria · feeling abnormal · feeling of body temperature change · hallucinations · headache · hyperacusia · hyperhidrosis · hypertension · mood altered · nasal complaints · oral disorders · perception altered · psychiatric disorders · sensation abnormal · tachycardia · taste altered · tinnitus · tremor · urinary disorders · vertigo · vision blurred

▶ With parenteral use Arrhythmias · hypersalivation · movement disorders · respiratory disorders · respiratory secretion increased · sleep disorders · vision disorders

▶ **Uncommon**

▶ With parenteral use Muscle tone increased · nystagmus · skin reactions

▶ **Rare or very rare**

▶ With parenteral use Hypotension

▶ **Frequency not known**

▶ With intranasal use Cystitis

▶ With parenteral use Disorientation · drug-induced liver injury · dysphoria · hallucination

● PREGNANCY

▶ When used for Induction and maintenance of anaesthesia or Analgesic supplementation of regional and local anaesthesia or Analgesia in emergency medicine Manufacturer advises use only if potential benefit outweighs risk—may depress neonatal respiration if used during delivery.

▶ When used for Major depressive disorder Manufacturer advises avoid—no information available.

● BREAST FEEDING

▶ When used for Induction and maintenance of anaesthesia or Analgesic supplementation of regional and local anaesthesia or Analgesia in emergency medicine Manufacturer advises present in milk—not thought to be harmful at therapeutic doses.

▶ When used for Major depressive disorder Manufacturer advises avoid—present in milk in *animal* studies.

● HEPATIC IMPAIRMENT

▶ When used for Induction and maintenance of anaesthesia or Analgesic supplementation of regional and local anaesthesia or Analgesia in emergency medicine Manufacturer advises caution (risk of prolonged action).

▶ When used for Major depressive disorder Manufacturer advises caution in moderate impairment when using maximum dose (84 mg); avoid in severe impairment—no information available.

Dose adjustments

▶ When used for Induction and maintenance of anaesthesia or Analgesic supplementation of regional and local anaesthesia or Analgesia in emergency medicine Manufacturer advises consider dose reduction.

● MONITORING REQUIREMENTS

▶ When used for Major depressive disorder Manufacturer advises monitor blood pressure at baseline, approximately 40 minutes after treatment, and as clinically indicated thereafter. Manufacturer advises monitor for urinary tract and bladder symptoms during treatment and refer to an appropriate healthcare provider if symptoms persist.

● DIRECTIONS FOR ADMINISTRATION

▶ With intramuscular use or intravenous use Manufacturer advises solution can be diluted with Glucose 5% *or* Sodium Chloride 0.9%.

▶ With intranasal use Manufacturer advises dose is administered via a single-use device delivering 28 mg as 2 sprays (1 spray per nostril). A second device is required for a 56 mg dose, and a third device is required for an 84 mg dose. Allow a break of 5 minutes between use of each device.

● PRESCRIBING AND DISPENSING INFORMATION
▶ When used for Major depressive disorder The manufacturer of *Spravato*® has provided the following materials: *Guide for Healthcare Professionals, Checklist for Healthcare Professionals* and *Patient Guide.*

● PATIENT AND CARER ADVICE
▶ When used for Major depressive disorder Manufacturer advises patients should be informed not to eat for at least 2 hours before and not to drink liquids for at least 30 minutes before treatment. Manufacturer advises patients who require a nasal corticosteroid or nasal decongestant on a dosing day should be informed not to administer these within 1 hour prior to treatment. Manufacturer advises patients and carers should seek immediate medical advice if symptoms worsen, or if suicidal behaviour or thoughts and unusual changes in behaviour occur.
▶ When used for Major depressive disorder A patient guide should be provided.

Missed doses
▶ When used for Major depressive disorder Manufacturer advises if more than 2 treatment sessions are missed, adjustment of the dose or frequency of treatment may be clinically appropriate.

Driving and skilled tasks
▶ When used for Induction and maintenance of anaesthesia or Analgesic supplementation of regional and local anaesthesia or Analgesia in emergency medicine Patients given sedatives and analgesics during minor outpatient procedures should be very carefully warned about the risk of driving or undertaking skilled tasks afterwards. For a short general anaesthetic the risk extends to **at least 24 hours** after administration. Responsible persons should be available to take patients home. The dangers of taking **alcohol** should also be emphasised. For information on 2015 legislation regarding driving whilst taking certain controlled drugs, including ketamine which has similar pharmacokinetic properties to esketamine, see *Drugs and driving* under Guidance on prescribing p. 1.
▶ When used for Major depressive disorder Manufacturer advises patients and carers should be counselled on the effects on driving and performance of skilled tasks— increased risk of somnolence, sedation, dissociative symptoms, perception disturbances, dizziness, vertigo and anxiety. For information on 2015 legislation regarding driving whilst taking certain controlled drugs, including ketamine which has similar pharmacokinetic properties to esketamine, see *Drugs and driving* under Guidance on prescribing p. 1.

● NATIONAL FUNDING/ACCESS DECISIONS
For full details see funding body website
Scottish Medicines Consortium (SMC) decisions
▶ Esketamine nasal spray (*Spravato*®) in combination with a selective serotonin reuptake inhibitor (SSRI) or serotonin-norepinephrine reuptake inhibitor (SNRI), for adults with treatment-resistant Major Depressive Disorder, who have not responded to at least two different treatments with antidepressants in the current moderate to severe depressive episode (September 2020) SMC No. SMC2258 Recommended

● MEDICINAL FORMS There can be variation in the licensing of different medicines containing the same drug.
Solution for injection
▶ Vesierra (Pfizer Ltd)
Esketamine (as Esketamine hydrochloride) 5 mg per 1 ml Vesierra 25mg/5ml solution for injection ampoules | 10 ampoule PoM £18.98 (Hospital only) CD2
Esketamine (as Esketamine hydrochloride) 25 mg per 1 ml Vesierra 50mg/2ml solution for injection ampoules | 10 ampoule PoM £26.31 (Hospital only) CD2

Spray
CAUTIONARY AND ADVISORY LABELS 2, 10
▶ Esketamine (non-proprietary) ▼
Esketamine (as Esketamine hydrochloride) 140 mg per 1 ml Spravato 28mg/0.2ml nasal spray unit dose | 1 unit dose PoM £163.00 (Hospital only) CD2 | 2 unit dose PoM £326.00 (Hospital only) CD2 | 3 unit dose PoM £489.00 (Hospital only) CD2

ANAESTHETICS, LOCAL

Bupivacaine with fentanyl

The properties listed below are those particular to the combination only. For the properties of the components please consider, bupivacaine hydrochloride p. 1403, fentanyl p. 478.

● INDICATIONS AND DOSE
During labour (once epidural block established)
▶ BY CONTINUOUS LUMBAR EPIDURAL INFUSION
▶ Adult: 10–18.75 mg/hour, dose of bupivacaine to be administered, maximum 400 mg bupivacaine in 24 hours and 16–30 micrograms/hour, dose of fentanyl to be administered, maximum 720 micrograms fentanyl in 24 hours

Postoperative pain (once epidural block established)
▶ BY CONTINUOUS EPIDURAL INFUSION
▶ Adult: 4–18.75 mg/hour, dose of bupivacaine to be administered, maximum 400 mg bupivacaine in 24 hours and 8–30 micrograms/hour, dose of fentanyl to be administered, maximum 720 micrograms fentanyl in 24 hours, to be administered by thoracic, upper abdominal or lower abdominal epidural infusion

● INTERACTIONS → Appendix 1: anaesthetics, local · opioids

● MEDICINAL FORMS There can be variation in the licensing of different medicines containing the same drug. Forms available from special-order manufacturers include: infusion, solution for infusion
Solution for infusion
▶ Bufyl (Advanz Pharma)
Fentanyl 2 microgram per 1 ml, Bupivacaine hydrochloride 1 mg per 1 ml Bufyl 1mg/ml and 2micrograms/ml 500ml infusion bags | 5 bag PoM £46.00 (Hospital only) CD2
Bufyl 1mg/ml and 2micrograms/ml 250ml infusion bags | 5 bag PoM £42.50 (Hospital only) CD2
Fentanyl (as Fentanyl citrate) 2 microgram per 1 ml, Bupivacaine hydrochloride 1.25 mg per 1 ml Bufyl 1.25mg/ml and 2micrograms/ml 250ml infusion bags | 5 bag PoM £45.25 (Hospital only) CD2
Bufyl 1.25mg/ml and 2micrograms/ml 500ml infusion bags | 10 bag PoM £92.00 (Hospital only) CD2

ANALGESICS › NON-STEROIDAL ANTI-INFLAMMATORY DRUGS

Ketorolac trometamol   07-Dec-2020

● INDICATIONS AND DOSE
Short-term management of moderate to severe acute postoperative pain only
▶ BY INTRAMUSCULAR INJECTION, OR BY INTRAVENOUS INJECTION
▶ Adult (body-weight up to 50 kg): Initially 10 mg, then 10–30 mg every 4–6 hours as required for maximum duration of treatment 2 days, frequency may be increased to up to every 2 hours during initial postoperative period; maximum 60 mg per day
▶ Adult (body-weight 50 kg and above): Initially 10 mg, then 10–30 mg every 4–6 hours as required for maximum duration of treatment 2 days, frequency may be increased to up to every 2 hours during initial postoperative period; maximum 90 mg per day

continued →

▸ **Elderly:** Initially 10 mg, then 10–30 mg every 4–6 hours as required for maximum duration of treatment 2 days, frequency may be increased to up to every 2 hours during initial postoperative period; maximum 60 mg per day

● CONTRA-INDICATIONS Active or history of gastro-intestinal bleeding · active or history of gastro-intestinal ulceration · coagulation disorders · complete or partial syndrome of nasal polyps · confirmed or suspected cerebrovascular bleeding · dehydration · following operations with high risk of haemorrhage or incomplete haemostasis · haemorrhagic diatheses · history of gastro-intestinal bleeding related to previous NSAID therapy · history of gastro-intestinal perforation related to previous NSAID therapy · hypovolaemia · severe heart failure

● CAUTIONS Allergic disorders · cardiac impairment (NSAIDs may impair renal function) · cerebrovascular disease · connective-tissue disorders · elderly (risk of serious side-effects and fatalities) · heart failure · history of gastro-intestinal disorders (e.g. ulcerative colitis, Crohn's disease) · ischaemic heart disease · may mask symptoms of infection · peripheral arterial disease · risk factors for cardiovascular events · uncontrolled hypertension

● INTERACTIONS → Appendix 1: NSAIDs

● SIDE-EFFECTS Agranulocytosis · angioedema · anxiety · aplastic anaemia · appetite decreased · asthenia · asthma · azotaemia · bradycardia · burping · chest pain · concentration impaired · confusion · constipation · Crohn's disease aggravated · depression · diarrhoea · dizziness · drowsiness · dry mouth · dyspnoea · electrolyte imbalance · embolism and thrombosis · euphoric mood · fever · flank pain · fluid retention · flushing · gastrointestinal discomfort · gastrointestinal disorders · haemolytic anaemia · haemorrhage · hallucination · headache · hearing loss · heart failure · hepatic disorders · hyperhidrosis · hyperkinesia · hypersensitivity · hypertension · hypotension · infertility female · malaise · meningitis aseptic (patients with connective-tissue disorders such as systemic lupus erythematosus may be especially susceptible) · musculoskeletal disorder · myalgia · myocardial infarction · nausea · nephritis tubulointerstitial · nephropathy · neutropenia · oedema · optic neuritis · oral disorders · pallor · palpitations · pancreatitis · paraesthesia · perforation · photosensitivity reaction · platelet aggregation inhibition · psychotic disorder · pulmonary oedema · renal impairment · respiratory disorders · seizure · severe cutaneous adverse reactions (SCARs) · skin reactions · sleep disorders · stroke · taste altered · thinking abnormal · thirst · thrombocytopenia · tinnitus · ulcer · urinary disorders · vertigo · visual impairment · vomiting · weight increased · wound haemorrhage

SIDE-EFFECTS, FURTHER INFORMATION For information about cardiovascular and gastrointestinal side-effects, and a possible exacerbation of symptoms in asthma, see Non-steroidal anti-inflammatory drugs. p. 1176

● ALLERGY AND CROSS-SENSITIVITY EvGr Contra-indicated in patients with a history of hypersensitivity to aspirin or any other NSAID—which includes those in whom attacks of asthma, angioedema, urticaria or rhinitis have been precipitated by aspirin or any other NSAID. ⓜ

● CONCEPTION AND CONTRACEPTION Caution—long-term use of some NSAIDs is associated with reduced female fertility, which is reversible on stopping treatment.

● PREGNANCY Avoid unless the potential benefit outweighs the risk. Avoid during the third trimester (risk of closure of fetal ductus arteriosus *in utero* and possibly persistent pulmonary hypertension of the newborn); onset of labour may be delayed and duration may be increased.

● BREAST FEEDING Amount too small to be harmful.

● HEPATIC IMPAIRMENT Manufacturer advises caution—may increase risk of renal impairment; avoid in hepatic failure.

● RENAL IMPAIRMENT Avoid if possible or use with caution. Avoid if serum creatinine greater than 160 micromol/litre.
Dose adjustments The lowest effective dose should be used for the shortest possible duration. Max. 60 mg daily by intramuscular injection or intravenous injection.
Monitoring In renal impairment monitor renal function; sodium and water retention may occur and renal function may deteriorate, possibly leading to renal failure.

● DIRECTIONS FOR ADMINISTRATION For *intravenous injection*, manufacturer advises give over at least 15 seconds.

● MEDICINAL FORMS There can be variation in the licensing of different medicines containing the same drug.
Solution for injection
▸ Ketorolac trometamol (Non-proprietary)
Ketorolac trometamol 30 mg per 1 ml Ketorolac 30mg/1ml solution for injection ampoules | 5 ampoule [PoM] £6.80–£20.00 DT = £5.36 (Hospital only)
▸ Toradol (Atnahs Pharma UK Ltd)
Ketorolac trometamol 30 mg per 1 ml Toradol 30mg/1ml solution for injection ampoules | 5 ampoule [PoM] £5.36 DT = £5.36 (Hospital only)

Parecoxib

17-Nov-2020

● DRUG ACTION Parecoxib is a selective inhibitor of cyclo-oxygenase-2.

● **INDICATIONS AND DOSE**
Short-term management of acute postoperative pain
▸ BY DEEP INTRAMUSCULAR INJECTION, OR BY INTRAVENOUS INJECTION
▸ **Adult:** Initially 40 mg, then 20–40 mg every 6–12 hours as required for up to 3 days; maximum 80 mg per day
▸ **Elderly (body-weight up to 50 kg):** Initially 20 mg; maximum 40 mg per day

● CONTRA-INDICATIONS Active gastro-intestinal bleeding · active gastro-intestinal ulceration · cerebrovascular disease · following coronary artery bypass graft surgery · inflammatory bowel disease · ischaemic heart disease · mild to severe heart failure · peripheral arterial disease

● CAUTIONS Allergic disorders · cardiac impairment (NSAIDs may impair renal function) · coagulation defects · connective-tissue disorders · dehydration (risk of renal impairment) · elderly (risk of serious side-effects and fatalities) · history of cardiac failure · history of gastro-intestinal disorders · hypertension · may mask symptoms of infection · oedema · risk factors for cardiovascular events

● INTERACTIONS → Appendix 1: NSAIDs

● SIDE-EFFECTS
▸ **Common or very common** Agitation · back pain · constipation · dizziness · gastrointestinal discomfort · gastrointestinal disorders · hyperhidrosis · hypertension · hypokalaemia · hypotension · increased risk of infection · insomnia · nausea · numbness · peripheral oedema · post procedural complications · renal impairment · respiratory disorders · skin reactions · vomiting
▸ **Uncommon** Appetite decreased · arrhythmias · arthralgia · asthenia · cerebrovascular insufficiency · dry mouth · ear pain · embolism and thrombosis · hyperglycaemia · myocardial infarction · thrombocytopenia
▸ **Rare or very rare** Hypersensitivity · pancreatitis · perioral swelling
▸ **Frequency not known** Angioedema · cardiovascular event · circulatory collapse · congestive heart failure · dyspnoea · fluid retention · hepatitis · renal failure (more common in

patients with pre-existing renal impairment) · severe cutaneous adverse reactions (SCARs)

SIDE-EFFECTS, FURTHER INFORMATION For information about cardiovascular and gastrointestinal side-effects, and a possible exacerbation of symptoms in asthma, see Non-steroidal anti-inflammatory drugs. p. 1176

- ALLERGY AND CROSS-SENSITIVITY [EvGr] Contra-indicated in patients with a history of hypersensitivity to aspirin or any other NSAID—which includes those in whom attacks of asthma, angioedema, urticaria or rhinitis have been precipitated by aspirin or any other NSAID. Contra-indicated in patients with a history of allergic drug reactions including sulfonamide hypersensitivity. ⟨M⟩
- CONCEPTION AND CONTRACEPTION Caution—long-term use of some NSAIDs is associated with reduced female fertility, which is reversible on stopping treatment.
- PREGNANCY Avoid unless the potential benefit outweighs the risk. Avoid during the third trimester (risk of closure of fetal ductus arteriosus *in utero* and possibly persistent pulmonary hypertension of the newborn); onset of labour may be delayed and duration may be increased.
- BREAST FEEDING Avoid—present in milk.
- HEPATIC IMPAIRMENT Manufacturer advises caution in moderate impairment (risk of increased exposure); avoid in severe impairment (no information available).
  Dose adjustments Manufacturer advises dose reduction to half the usual recommended dose in moderate impairment; maximum 40 mg daily.
- RENAL IMPAIRMENT Avoid if possible or use with caution.
  Dose adjustments The lowest effective dose should be used for the shortest possible duration.
  Monitoring In renal impairment monitor renal function; sodium and water retention may occur and renal function may deteriorate, possibly leading to renal failure.
- NATIONAL FUNDING/ACCESS DECISIONS
  For full details see funding body website
  Scottish Medicines Consortium (SMC) decisions
  - **Parecoxib (*Dynastat*®) for the short-term treatment of postoperative pain (January 2003)** SMC No. 27/02 Not recommended

- MEDICINAL FORMS There can be variation in the licensing of different medicines containing the same drug.

Powder and solvent for solution for injection
- Dynastat (Pfizer Ltd)
  Parecoxib (as Parecoxib sodium) 40 mg Dynastat 40mg powder and solvent for solution for injection vials | 5 vial [PoM] £28.34 DT = £28.34

Powder for solution for injection
- Parecoxib (Non-proprietary)
  Parecoxib (as Parecoxib sodium) 40 mg Parecoxib 40mg powder for solution for injection vials | 10 vial [PoM] £49.60 DT = £49.60 (Hospital only)
- Dynastat (Pfizer Ltd)
  Parecoxib (as Parecoxib sodium) 40 mg Dynastat 40mg powder for solution for injection vials | 10 vial [PoM] £49.60 DT = £49.60

ANALGESICS > OPIOIDS

F 467

Alfentanil

13-Nov-2020

- **INDICATIONS AND DOSE**

Spontaneous respiration: analgesia and enhancement of anaesthesia for short procedures
- BY INTRAVENOUS INJECTION
  - Adult: Initially up to 500 micrograms, dose to be administered over 30 seconds; supplemental doses 250 micrograms

Assisted ventilation: analgesia and enhancement of anaesthesia for short procedures
- BY INTRAVENOUS INJECTION
  - Adult: Initially 30–50 micrograms/kg, supplemental doses 15 micrograms/kg

Assisted ventilation: analgesia and enhancement of anaesthesia during maintenance of anaesthesia for longer procedures
- BY INTRAVENOUS INFUSION
  - Adult: Initially 50–100 micrograms/kg, dose to be administered over 10 minutes or as a bolus, followed by maintenance 30–60 micrograms/kg/hour

Assisted ventilation: analgesia and suppression of respiratory activity during intensive care for up to 4 days
- BY INTRAVENOUS INFUSION
  - Adult: Initially 2 mg/hour, adjusted according to response; usual dose 0.5–10 mg/hour, alternatively initially 5 mg in divided doses, to be administered over 10 minutes; dose used for more rapid initial control, reduce rate of administration if hypotension or bradycardia occur; additional doses of 0.5–1 mg may be given by intravenous injection during short painful procedures

DOSES AT EXTREMES OF BODY-WEIGHT
- To avoid excessive dosage in obese patients, dose should be calculated on the basis of ideal body-weight.

- CAUTIONS [EvGr] Repeated intra-operative doses of alfentanil should be given with care since the resulting respiratory depression can persist postoperatively and occasionally it may become apparent for the first time postoperatively when monitoring of the patient might be less intensive. ⟨M⟩
- INTERACTIONS → Appendix 1: opioids
- SIDE-EFFECTS
  - **Common or very common** Apnoea · chills · fatigue · hypertension · movement disorders · muscle rigidity · procedural complications
  - **Uncommon** Coma · hiccups · hypercapnia · pain · post procedural complications · respiratory disorders
  - **Rare or very rare** Agitation · crying · epistaxis · vascular pain
  - **Frequency not known** Cardiac arrest · cough · fever · loss of consciousness · seizure

  SIDE-EFFECTS, FURTHER INFORMATION Alfentanil can cause muscle rigidity, particularly of the chest wall or jaw; this can be managed by the use of neuromuscular blocking drugs.
- BREAST FEEDING Present in milk—withhold breast-feeding for 24 hours.
- HEPATIC IMPAIRMENT Manufacturer advises caution.
  Dose adjustments Manufacturer advises dose reduction and cautious titration.
- RENAL IMPAIRMENT Avoid use or reduce dose; opioid effects increased and prolonged and increased cerebral sensitivity occurs.
- DIRECTIONS FOR ADMINISTRATION Manufacturer advises 5 mg/mL injection should be diluted in Glucose 5% *or* Sodium Chloride 0.9% before use.

- MEDICINAL FORMS There can be variation in the licensing of different medicines containing the same drug. Forms available from special-order manufacturers include: solution for injection

Solution for injection
- Alfentanil (Non-proprietary)
  Alfentanil (as Alfentanil hydrochloride) 500 microgram per 1 ml Alfentanil 1mg/2ml solution for injection ampoules | 10 ampoule [PoM] £27.80 DT = £6.34 (Hospital only) [CD2] | 10 ampoule [PoM] £5.95 DT = £6.34 [CD2]

Alfentanil 25mg/50ml solution for injection vials | 1 vial PoM
£14.90 CD2
Alfentanil 5mg/10ml solution for injection ampoules |
5 ampoule PoM £16.00 DT = £16.00 (Hospital only) CD2 |
10 ampoule PoM £27.80 DT = £27.80 CD2
Alfentanil (as Alfentanil hydrochloride) 5 mg per 1 ml Alfentanil
5mg/1ml solution for injection ampoules | 10 ampoule PoM £21.95
DT = £23.19 (Hospital only) CD2
▸ Rapifen (Piramal Critical Care Ltd)
**Alfentanil (as Alfentanil hydrochloride) 500 microgram per
1 ml** Rapifen 5mg/10ml solution for injection ampoules |
5 ampoule PoM £16.00 DT = £16.00 CD2
Rapifen 1mg/2ml solution for injection ampoules | 10 ampoule PoM
£6.34 DT = £6.34 CD2
Alfentanil (as Alfentanil hydrochloride) 5 mg per 1 ml Rapifen
Intensive Care 5mg/1ml solution for injection ampoules |
10 ampoule PoM £23.19 DT = £23.19 (Hospital only) CD2

F 467

Remifentanil

30-Jul-2020

● **INDICATIONS AND DOSE**

**Analgesia and enhancement of anaesthesia at induction
(initial bolus injection)**
▸ BY INTRAVENOUS INJECTION
▸ Adult: Initially 0.25–1 microgram/kg, dose to be
administered over at least 30 seconds, if patient is to be
intubated more than 8 minutes after start of
intravenous infusion, initial bolus intravenous
injection dose is not necessary

**Analgesia and enhancement of anaesthesia at induction
with or without initial bolus dose**
▸ BY INTRAVENOUS INFUSION
▸ Adult: 30–60 micrograms/kg/hour, if patient is to be
intubated more than 8 minutes after start of
intravenous infusion, initial bolus intravenous
injection dose is not necessary

**Assisted ventilation: analgesia and enhancement of
anaesthesia during maintenance of anaesthesia (initial
bolus injection)**
▸ BY INTRAVENOUS INJECTION
▸ Adult: Initially 0.25–1 microgram/kg, dose to be
administered over at least 30 seconds

**Assisted ventilation: analgesia and enhancement of
anaesthesia during maintenance of anaesthesia with or
without initial bolus dose**
▸ BY INTRAVENOUS INFUSION
▸ Adult: 3–120 micrograms/kg/hour, dose to be
administered according to anaesthetic technique and
adjusted according to response, in light anaesthesia
additional doses can be given by intravenous injection
every 2–5 minutes during the intravenous infusion

**Spontaneous respiration: analgesia and enhancement of
anaesthesia during maintenance of anaesthesia**
▸ BY INTRAVENOUS INFUSION
▸ Adult: Initially 2.4 micrograms/kg/hour, adjusted
according to response; usual dose
1.5–6 micrograms/kg/hour

**Assisted ventilation: analgesia and sedation in intensive-
care patients (for max 3 days)**
▸ BY INTRAVENOUS INFUSION
▸ Adult: Initially 6–9 micrograms/kg/hour, then adjusted
in steps of 1.5 micrograms/kg/hour, allow at least
5 minutes between dose adjustments; usual dose
0.36–44.4 micrograms/kg/hour, if an infusion rate of
12 micrograms/kg/hour does not produce adequate
sedation add another sedative (consult product
literature for details)

**Assisted ventilation: additional analgesia during
stimulating or painful procedures in intensive-care
patients**
▸ BY INTRAVENOUS INFUSION
▸ Adult: Usual dose 15–45 micrograms/kg/hour,
maintain infusion rate of at least 6 micrograms/kg/hour
for at least 5 minutes before procedure and adjust
every 2–5 minutes according to requirements

Cardiac surgery
▸ Adult: (consult product literature)

DOSES AT EXTREMES OF BODY-WEIGHT
▸ To avoid excessive dosage in obese patients, dose
should be calculated on the basis of ideal body-weight.

● UNLICENSED USE Remifentanil doses in BNF may differ
from those in product literature.

● CONTRA-INDICATIONS Analgesia in conscious patients

● INTERACTIONS → Appendix 1: opioids

● SIDE-EFFECTS
▸ **Common or very common** Apnoea · muscle rigidity · post
procedural complications
▸ **Uncommon** Hypoxia
▸ **Rare or very rare** Cardiac arrest
▸ **Frequency not known** Agitation · atrioventricular block ·
hypertension · seizure

SIDE-EFFECTS, FURTHER INFORMATION In contrast to other
opioids which are metabolised in the liver, remifentanil
undergoes rapid metabolism by plasma esterases; it has
short duration of action which is independent of dose and
duration of infusion.
Muscle rigidity Remifentanil can cause muscle rigidity
that can be managed by the use of neuromuscular blocking
drugs.

● PREGNANCY No information available.

● BREAST FEEDING Avoid breast-feeding for 24 hours after
administration—present in milk in *animal* studies.

● HEPATIC IMPAIRMENT Manufacturer advises caution in
severe impairment (limited information available).

● RENAL IMPAIRMENT
Dose adjustments No dose adjustment necessary in renal
impairment.

● DIRECTIONS FOR ADMINISTRATION For *intravenous infusion*
(*Ultiva* ®), manufacturer advises give continuously in
Glucose 5% or Sodium Chloride 0.9% or Water for
Injections; reconstitute with infusion fluid to a
concentration of 1 mg/mL then dilute further to a
concentration of 20–250 micrograms/mL
(50 micrograms/mL recommended for general anaesthesia,
20–50 micrograms/mL recommended when used with
target controlled infusion (TCI) device).

● PRESCRIBING AND DISPENSING INFORMATION
Remifentanil should not be given by intravenous injection
intra-operatively, but it is well suited to continuous
infusion; a supplementary analgesic is given before
stopping the infusion of remifentanil.

● MEDICINAL FORMS There can be variation in the licensing of
different medicines containing the same drug.
Powder for solution for injection
▸ Remifentanil (Non-proprietary)
Remifentanil (as Remifentanyl hydrochloride) 1 mg Remifentanil
1mg powder for concentrate for solution for injection vials |
5 vial PoM £25.60 (Hospital only) CD2
Remifentanil (as Remifentanyl hydrochloride) 2 mg Remifentanil
2mg powder for concentrate for solution for injection vials |
5 vial PoM £51.13 (Hospital only) CD2
Remifentanil (as Remifentanyl hydrochloride) 5 mg Remifentanil
5mg powder for concentrate for solution for injection vials |
5 vial PoM £127.90–£131.74 (Hospital only) CD2

► Ultiva (Aspen Pharma Trading Ltd)
Remifentanil (as Remifentanyl hydrochloride) 1 mg Ultiva 1mg powder for solution for injection vials | 5 vial [PoM] £25.58 (Hospital only) [CD2]
Remifentanil (as Remifentanyl hydrochloride) 2 mg Ultiva 2mg powder for solution for injection vials | 5 vial [PoM] £51.15 (Hospital only) [CD2]
Remifentanil (as Remifentanyl hydrochloride) 5 mg Ultiva 5mg powder for solution for injection vials | 5 vial [PoM] £127.88 (Hospital only) [CD2]

1.4 Peri-operative sedation

Conscious sedation for clinical procedures

Overview

Sedation of patients during diagnostic and therapeutic procedures is used to reduce fear and anxiety, to control pain, and to minimise excessive movement. The choice of sedative drug will depend upon the intended procedure; some procedures are safer and more successful under anaesthesia. The patient should be *monitored carefully*; monitoring should begin as soon as the sedative is given or when the patient becomes drowsy, and should be continued until the patient wakes up.

ANAESTHETICS, GENERAL > NMDA RECEPTOR ANTAGONISTS

Ketamine   04-Dec-2019

● **INDICATIONS AND DOSE**

Induction and maintenance of anaesthesia for short procedures
► BY INTRAMUSCULAR INJECTION
► Adult: Initially 6.5–13 mg/kg, adjusted according to response, a dose of 10 mg/kg usually produces 12–25 minutes of surgical anaesthesia
► BY INTRAVENOUS INJECTION
► Adult: Initially 1–4.5 mg/kg, adjusted according to response, to be administered over at least 60 seconds, a dose of 2 mg/kg usually produces 5–10 minutes of surgical anaesthesia

Diagnostic manoeuvres and procedures not involving intense pain
► BY INTRAMUSCULAR INJECTION
► Adult: Initially 4 mg/kg

Induction and maintenance of anaesthesia for long procedures
► BY INTRAVENOUS INFUSION
► Adult: Initially 0.5–2 mg/kg, using an infusion solution containing 1 mg/ml; maintenance 10–45 micrograms/kg/minute, adjusted according to response

IMPORTANT SAFETY INFORMATION
Ketamine should only be administered by, or under the direct supervision of, personnel experienced in its use, with adequate training in anaesthesia and airway management, and when resuscitation equipment is available.

● CONTRA-INDICATIONS Acute porphyrias p. 1107 · eclampsia · head trauma · hypertension · pre-eclampsia · raised intracranial pressure · severe cardiac disease · stroke
● CAUTIONS Acute circulatory failure (shock) · cardiovascular disease · dehydration · elderly · fixed cardiac output · hallucinations · head injury · hypertension ·

hypovolaemia · increased cerebrospinal fluid pressure · intracranial mass lesions · nightmares · predisposition to seizures · psychotic disorders · raised intra-ocular pressure · respiratory tract infection · thyroid dysfunction

● INTERACTIONS → Appendix 1: ketamine
● SIDE-EFFECTS
► **Common or very common** Anxiety · behaviour abnormal · confusion · diplopia · hallucination · muscle tone increased · nausea · nystagmus · skin reactions · sleep disorders · tonic clonic movements · vomiting
► **Uncommon** Appetite decreased · arrhythmias · hypotension · respiratory disorders
► **Rare or very rare** Apnoea · cystitis · cystitis haemorrhagic · delirium · dysphoria · flashback · hypersalivation
► **Frequency not known** Drug-induced liver injury
   SIDE-EFFECTS, FURTHER INFORMATION Incidence of hallucinations can be reduced by premedicaton with a benzodiazepine (such as midazolam).

● PREGNANCY May depress neonatal respiration if used during delivery.
● BREAST FEEDING Avoid for at least 12 hours after last dose.
● HEPATIC IMPAIRMENT Manufacturer advises caution (risk of prolonged duration of action).
   Dose adjustments Manufacturer advises consider dose reduction.
● DIRECTIONS FOR ADMINISTRATION For *continuous intravenous infusion*, dilute to a concentration of 1 mg/mL with Glucose 5% *or* Sodium Chloride 0.9%; use microdrip infusion for maintenance of anaesthesia. For *intravenous injection*, dilute 100 mg/mL strength to a concentration of not more than 50 mg/mL with Glucose 5% *or* Sodium Chloride 0.9% *or* Water for Injections.
● PATIENT AND CARER ADVICE
   Driving and skilled tasks Patients given sedatives and analgesics during minor outpatient procedures should be very carefully warned about the risk of driving or undertaking skilled tasks afterwards. For a short general anaesthetic the risk extends to **at least 24 hours** after administration. Responsible persons should be available to take patients home. The dangers of taking **alcohol** should also be emphasised.
   For information on 2015 legislation regarding driving whilst taking certain controlled drugs, including ketamine, see *Drugs and driving* under Guidance on prescribing p. 1.

● MEDICINAL FORMS There can be variation in the licensing of different medicines containing the same drug. Forms available from special-order manufacturers include: solution for injection
Solution for injection
► Ketamine (Non-proprietary)
   Ketamine (as Ketamine hydrochloride) 10 mg per 1 ml Ketamin 10 Curamed 50mg/5ml solution for injection ampoules | 10 ampoule [PoM] [℞] [CD2]
   Ketamine (as Ketamine hydrochloride) 50 mg per 1 ml Ketamine 500mg/10ml solution for injection vials | 10 vial [PoM] £70.00 (Hospital only) [CD2]
   Ketamine 100mg/2ml solution for injection ampoules | 10 ampoule [PoM] [℞] [CD2]
   Ketamine 500mg/10ml solution for injection ampoules | 10 ampoule [PoM] £70.00 (Hospital only) [CD2]
   Ketamine (as Ketamine hydrochloride) 100 mg per 1 ml Ketalar 200mg/2ml solution for injection vials | 5 vial [PoM] [℞] [CD2]
► Ketalar (Pfizer Ltd)
   Ketamine (as Ketamine hydrochloride) 10 mg per 1 ml Ketalar 200mg/20ml solution for injection vials | 1 vial [PoM] £5.06 DT = £5.06 (Hospital only) [CD2]
   Ketamine (as Ketamine hydrochloride) 50 mg per 1 ml Ketalar 500mg/10ml solution for injection vials | 1 vial [PoM] £8.77 DT = £8.77 (Hospital only) [CD2]

15

Anaesthesia

HYPNOTICS, SEDATIVES AND ANXIOLYTICS ›
NON-BENZODIAZEPINE HYPNOTICS AND
SEDATIVES

Dexmedetomidine

07-Aug-2020

● **INDICATIONS AND DOSE**

Maintenance of sedation during intensive care
▸ BY INTRAVENOUS INFUSION
▸ Adult: 0.7 microgram/kg/hour, adjusted according to
response; usual dose 0.2–1.4 micrograms/kg/hour

> **IMPORTANT SAFETY INFORMATION**
> Dexmedetomidine should only be administered by, or
> under the direct supervision of, personnel experienced
> in its use, with adequate training in anaesthesia and
> airway management.

● CONTRA-INDICATIONS Acute cerebrovascular disorders ·
second- or third-degree AV block (unless pacemaker
fitted) · uncontrolled hypotension

● CAUTIONS Abrupt withdrawal after prolonged use ·
bradycardia · elderly (risk of hypotension) · ischaemic heart
disease (especially at higher doses) · malignant
hyperthermia · severe cerebrovascular disease (especially
at higher doses) · severe neurological disorders · spinal
cord injury

● INTERACTIONS → Appendix 1: dexmedetomidine

● SIDE-EFFECTS
▸ **Common or very common** Agitation · arrhythmias · dry
mouth · hyperglycaemia · hypertension · hyperthermia ·
hypoglycaemia · hypotension · myocardial infarction ·
myocardial ischaemia · nausea · respiratory depression ·
vomiting
▸ **Uncommon** Abdominal distension · apnoea ·
atrioventricular block · dyspnoea · hallucination ·
hypoalbuminaemia · metabolic acidosis · thirst

● PREGNANCY Manufacturer advises avoid unless potential
benefit outweighs risk—toxicity in *animal* studies.

● BREAST FEEDING Manufacturer advises avoid unless
potential benefit outweighs risk—present in milk in *animal*
studies.

● HEPATIC IMPAIRMENT Manufacturer advises caution
(increased risk of toxicity due to decreased clearance).
Dose adjustments Manufacturer advises consider dose
reduction.

● MONITORING REQUIREMENTS
▸ Monitor cardiac function.
▸ Monitor respiratory function in non-intubated patients.

● DIRECTIONS FOR ADMINISTRATION Manufacturer advises
to be diluted before use. For *intravenous infusion* given
continuously in Glucose 5% or Sodium Chloride 0.9%,
dilute to a concentration of 4 micrograms/mL.

● MEDICINAL FORMS There can be variation in the licensing of
different medicines containing the same drug.
  Solution for infusion
  ▸ Dexmedetomidine (Non-proprietary)
    Dexmedetomidine (as Dexmedetomidine hydrochloride)
    100 microgram per 1 ml Dexmedetomidine 1mg/10ml concentrate
    for solution for infusion vials | 4 vial [PoM] £313.10 (Hospital only) |
    5 vial [PoM] £391.50 (Hospital only)
    Dexmedetomidine 400micrograms/4ml concentrate for solution for
    infusion vials | 4 vial [PoM] £125.30 (Hospital only)
    Dexmedetomidine 200micrograms/2ml concentrate for solution for
    infusion ampoules | 5 ampoule [PoM] £78.30 (Hospital only)
  ▸ Dexdor (Orion Pharma (UK) Ltd)
    Dexmedetomidine (as Dexmedetomidine hydrochloride)
    100 microgram per 1 ml Dexdor 1mg/10ml concentrate for solution
    for infusion vials | 4 vial [PoM] £313.20 (Hospital only)

Dexdor 400micrograms/4ml concentrate for solution for infusion vials
| 4 vial [PoM] £125.28 (Hospital only)
Dexdor 200micrograms/2ml concentrate for solution for infusion
ampoules | 5 ampoule [PoM] £78.30 (Hospital only)

2   Malignant hyperthermia

MUSCLE RELAXANTS › DIRECTLY ACTING

Dantrolene sodium

01-Sep-2020

● DRUG ACTION Acts on skeletal muscle cells by interfering
with calcium efflux, thereby stopping the contractile
process.

● **INDICATIONS AND DOSE**

Malignant hyperthermia
▸ BY RAPID INTRAVENOUS INJECTION
▸ Adult: Initially 2–3 mg/kg, then 1 mg/kg, repeated if
necessary; maximum 10 mg/kg per course

Chronic severe spasticity of voluntary muscle
▸ BY MOUTH
▸ Adult: Initially 25 mg daily, then increased to up to
100 mg 4 times a day, dose increased at weekly
intervals; usual dose 75 mg 3 times a day

**Muscle cramps in motor neurone disease (specialist use
only)**
▸ BY MOUTH
▸ Adult: Initially 25 mg daily, then increased to up to
100 mg 4 times a day, dose increased at weekly
intervals

● UNLICENSED USE
▸ With oral use [EvGr] Dantrolene sodium is used for the
treatment of muscle cramps in motor neurone disease,
but is not licensed for this indication. ⟨Ɛ⟩

> **IMPORTANT SAFETY INFORMATION**
> Should only be administered by, or under the direct
> supervision of, personnel experienced in the use of
> dantrolene when used for malignant hyperthermia.

● CONTRA-INDICATIONS
▸ With oral use Acute muscle spasm · avoid when spasticity is
useful, for example, locomotion

● CAUTIONS
▸ With intravenous use Avoid extravasation (risk of tissue
necrosis)
▸ With oral use Females (hepatotoxicity) · history of liver
disorders (hepatotoxicity) · if doses greater than 400 mg
daily (hepatotoxicity) · impaired cardiac function ·
impaired pulmonary function · patients over 30 years
(hepatotoxicity) · therapeutic effect may take a few weeks
to develop— discontinue if no response within 6–8 weeks

● INTERACTIONS → Appendix 1: dantrolene

● SIDE-EFFECTS

GENERAL SIDE-EFFECTS
▸ **Common or very common** Abdominal pain · hepatic
disorders · nausea · respiratory disorders · skin reactions ·
speech disorder · vomiting
▸ **Uncommon** Crystalluria · hyperhidrosis
▸ **Frequency not known** Arrhythmias · dizziness · drowsiness

SPECIFIC SIDE-EFFECTS
▸ **Common or very common**
▸ With oral use Appetite decreased · chills · confusion ·
depression · eosinophilia · fever · headache · insomnia ·
nervousness · pericarditis · visual impairment
▸ **Uncommon**
▸ With oral use Constipation · dysphagia · haemorrhage ·
heart failure aggravated · urinary disorders

Frequency not known

With intravenous use Gastrointestinal haemorrhage · heart failure · localised pain · pulmonary oedema · seizure · thrombophlebitis

With oral use Asthenia · diarrhoea · dyspnoea · hypertension · malaise

● PREGNANCY

With intravenous use Use only if potential benefit outweighs risk.

With oral use Although teratological studies in *animals* have proved satisfactory, dantrolene sodium does cross the placenta, therefore manufacturer advises avoid.

● BREAST FEEDING

With intravenous use Present in milk—use only if potential benefit outweighs risk.

With oral use Present in milk—manufacturer advises avoid.

● HEPATIC IMPAIRMENT

With oral use Manufacturer advises avoid in hepatic impairment.

● MONITORING REQUIREMENTS

With oral use Test liver function before and at intervals during therapy.

● PATIENT AND CARER ADVICE

Hepatotoxicity ► With oral use Patients should be told how to recognise signs of liver disorder and advised to seek prompt medical attention if symptoms such as anorexia, nausea, vomiting, fatigue, abdominal pain, dark urine, or pruritus develop.

Driving and skilled tasks ► With oral use Drowsiness may affect performance of skilled tasks (e.g. driving); effects of alcohol enhanced.

● MEDICINAL FORMS There can be variation in the licensing of different medicines containing the same drug. Forms available from special-order manufacturers include: oral suspension, oral solution

Powder for solution for injection
► Dantrium (Forum Health Products Ltd)
    Dantrolene sodium 20 mg Dantrium Intravenous 20mg powder for solution for injection vials | 12 vial PoM £612.00 (Hospital only) | 36 vial PoM £1,836.00 (Hospital only)

Capsule
CAUTIONARY AND ADVISORY LABELS 2
► Dantrium (Forum Health Products Ltd)
    Dantrolene sodium 25 mg Dantrium 25mg capsules | 100 capsule PoM £16.87 DT = £16.87
    Dantrolene sodium 100 mg Dantrium 100mg capsules | 100 capsule PoM £43.07 DT = £43.07

Local anaesthesia

Anaesthesia (local)

Local anaesthetic drugs

The use of local anaesthetics by injection or by application to mucous membranes to produce local analgesia is discussed in this section.

Local anaesthetic drugs act by causing a reversible block to conduction along nerve fibres. They vary widely in their potency, toxicity, duration of action, stability, solubility in water, and ability to penetrate mucous membranes. These factors determine their application, e.g. topical (surface), infiltration, peripheral nerve block, intravenous regional anaesthesia (Bier's block), plexus, epidural (extradural), or spinal (intrathecal or subarachnoid) block. Local anaesthetics may also be used for postoperative pain relief, thereby reducing the need for analgesics such as opioids.

Bupivacaine hydrochloride p. 1403 has a longer duration of action than other local anaesthetics. It has a slow onset of action, taking up to 30 minutes for full effect. It is often used

in lumbar epidural blockade and is particularly suitable for continuous epidural analgesia in labour, or for postoperative pain relief. It is the principal drug used for spinal anaesthesia. Hyperbaric solutions containing glucose may be used for spinal block.

Levobupivacaine p. 1405, an isomer of bupivacaine, has anaesthetic and analgesic properties similar to bupivacaine hydrochloride, but is thought to have fewer adverse effects.

Lidocaine hydrochloride p. 1406 is effectively absorbed from mucous membranes and is a useful surface anaesthetic in concentrations up to 10%. Except for surface anaesthesia and dental anaesthesia, solutions should **not** usually exceed 1% in strength. The duration of the block (with adrenaline/epinephrine p. 238) is about 90 minutes.

Prilocaine hydrochloride p. 1410 is a local anaesthetic of low toxicity which is similar to lidocaine hydrochloride. A hyperbaric solution of prilocaine hydrochloride (containing glucose) may be used for spinal anaesthesia.

Ropivacaine hydrochloride p. 1411 is an amide-type local anaesthetic agent similar to bupivacaine hydrochloride. It is less cardiotoxic than bupivacaine hydrochloride, but also less potent.

Tetracaine p. 1412, a para-aminobenzoic acid ester, is an effective local anaesthetic for topical application; a 4% gel is indicated for anaesthesia before venepuncture or venous cannulation. It is rapidly absorbed from mucous membranes and should **never** be applied to inflamed, traumatised, or highly vascular surfaces. It should never be used to provide anaesthesia for bronchoscopy or cystoscopy because lidocaine hydrochloride is a safer alternative.

Administration by injection

The dose of local anaesthetic depends on the injection site and the procedure used. In determining the safe dosage, it is important to take account of the rate of absorption and excretion, and of the potency. The patient's age, weight, physique, and clinical condition, and the vascularity of the administration site and the duration of administration, must also be considered.

Uptake of local anaesthetics into the systemic circulation determines their duration of action and produces toxicity.

NHS Improvement has advised (September 2016) that, prior to administration, all injectable medicines must be drawn directly from their original ampoule or container into a syringe and should **never** be decanted into gallipots or open containers. This is to avoid the risk of medicines being confused with other substances, e.g. skin disinfectants, and to reduce the risk of contamination.

Great care must be taken to avoid accidental intravascular injection; local anaesthetic injections should be given slowly in order to detect inadvertent intravascular administration. When prolonged analgesia is required, a long-acting local anaesthetic is preferred to minimise the likelihood of cumulative systemic toxicity. Local anaesthesia around the oral cavity may impair swallowing and therefore increases the risk of aspiration.

Epidural anaesthesia is commonly used during surgery, often combined with general anaesthesia, because of its protective effect against the stress response of surgery. It is often used when good postoperative pain relief is essential.

Vasoconstrictors in combination with local anaesthetics

Local anaesthetics cause dilatation of blood vessels. The addition of a vasoconstrictor such as adrenaline/epinephrine to the local anaesthetic preparation diminishes local blood flow, slowing the rate of absorption and thereby prolonging the anaesthetic effect. Great care should be taken to avoid inadvertent intravenous administration of a preparation containing adrenaline/epinephrine, and it is **not** advisable to give adrenaline/epinephrine with a local anaesthetic injection in digits or appendages because of the risk of ischaemic necrosis.

15

Anaesthesia

Adrenaline/epinephrine must be used in a low concentration when administered with a local anaesthetic. Care must also be taken to calculate a safe maximum dose of local anaesthetic when using combination products.

In patients with severe hypertension or unstable cardiac rhythm, the use of adrenaline/epinephrine with a local anaesthetic may be hazardous. For these patients an anaesthetic without adrenaline/epinephrine should be used.

Dental anaesthesia

Lidocaine hydrochloride is widely used in dental procedures; it is most often used in combination with adrenaline/epinephrine. Lidocaine hydrochloride 2% combined with adrenaline/epinephrine 1 in 80 000 (12.5 micrograms/mL) is a safe and effective preparation; there is no justification for using higher concentrations of adrenaline/epinephrine.

The amide-type local anaesthetics **articaine** and mepivacaine hydrochloride p. 1409 are also used in dentistry; they are available in cartridges suitable for dental use. Mepivacaine hydrochloride is available with or without adrenaline/epinephrine and articaine is available with adrenaline.

In patients with severe hypertension or unstable cardiac rhythm, mepivacaine hydrochloride without adrenaline/epinephrine may be used. Alternatively, prilocaine hydrochloride with or without felypressin can be used but there is no evidence that it is any safer. Felypressin can cause coronary vasoconstriction when used at high doses; limit dose in patients with coronary artery disease.

Toxicity induced by local anaesthesia

For management of toxicity see Severe local anaesthetic-induced cardiovascular toxicity below.

Severe local anaesthetic-induced cardiovascular toxicity

Overview

After injection of a bolus of local anaesthetic, toxicity may develop at any time in the following hour. In the event of signs of toxicity during injection, the administration of the local anaesthetic must be stopped immediately.

Cardiovascular status must be assessed and cardiopulmonary resuscitation procedures must be followed.

In the event of local anaesthetic-induced cardiac arrest, standard cardiopulmonary resuscitation should be initiated immediately. Lidocaine must not be used as anti-arrhythmic therapy.

If the patient does not respond rapidly to standard procedures, 20% lipid emulsion such as *Intralipid*®[unlicensed indication] should be given intravenously at an initial bolus dose of 1.5 mL/kg over 1 minute, followed by an infusion of 15 mL/kg/hour. After 5 minutes, if cardiovascular stability has not been restored or circulation deteriorates, give a maximum of two further bolus doses of 1.5 mL/kg over 1 minute, 5 minutes apart, and increase the infusion rate to 30 mL/kg/hour. Continue infusion until cardiovascular stability and adequate circulation are restored or maximum cumulative dose of 12 mL/kg is given.

Standard cardiopulmonary resuscitation must be maintained throughout lipid emulsion treatment.

Propofol is not a suitable alternative to lipid emulsion.

Further advice on ongoing treatment should be obtained from the National Poisons Information Service.

Detailed treatment algorithms and accompanying notes are available at www.toxbase.org *or* can be found in the Association of Anaesthetists of Great Britain and Ireland safety guideline, Management of Severe Local Anaesthetic Toxicity and Management of Severe Local Anaesthetic Toxicity – Accompanying notes.

ANAESTHETICS, LOCAL

Adrenaline with articaine hydrochloride

19-Dec-201

(Carticaine hydrochloride with epinephrine)

- ● **INDICATIONS AND DOSE**

Infiltration anaesthesia in dentistry
 ▸ BY REGIONAL ADMINISTRATION
 ▸ **Adult:** Consult expert dental sources

DOSES AT EXTREMES OF BODY-WEIGHT
 ▸ To avoid excessive dosage in obese patients, dose should be calculated on the basis of ideal body-weight.

> IMPORTANT SAFETY INFORMATION
> Should only be administered by, or under the direct supervision of, personnel experienced in their use, with adequate training in anaesthesia and airway management, and should not be administered parenterally unless adequate resuscitation equipment is available.

- ● CONTRA-INDICATIONS Injection into infected tissues · injection into inflamed tissues · preparations containing preservatives should not be used for caudal, epidural, or spinal block

 CONTRA-INDICATIONS, FURTHER INFORMATION
 ▸ Injection site Manufacturer advises the local anaesthetic effect may be reduced when injected into an inflamed or infected area, due to altered local pH. Increased absorption into the blood also increases the possibility of systemic side-effects.

- ● CAUTIONS Arrhythmias · arteriosclerosis · cardiovascular disease · cerebrovascular disease · cor pulmonale · debilitated patients (consider dose reduction) · diabetes mellitus · elderly (consider dose reduction) · epilepsy · hypercalcaemia · hyperreflexia · hypertension · hyperthyroidism · hypokalaemia · hypovolaemia · impaired cardiac conduction · impaired respiratory function · ischaemic heart disease · myasthenia gravis · obstructive cardiomyopathy · occlusive vascular disease · organic brain damage · phaeochromocytoma · prostate disorders · psychoneurosis · severe angina · shock · susceptibility to angle-closure glaucoma

 CAUTIONS, FURTHER INFORMATION
 ▸ Use of vasoconstrictors In patients with severe hypertension or unstable cardiac rhythm, the use of adrenaline with a local anaesthetic may be hazardous. For these patients an anaesthetic without adrenaline should be used.

- ● INTERACTIONS → Appendix 1: articaine · sympathomimetics, vasoconstrictor

- ● SIDE-EFFECTS Face oedema · gingivitis · headache · nausea · sensation abnormal

 SIDE-EFFECTS, FURTHER INFORMATION Toxic effects after administration of local anaesthetics are a result of excessively high plasma concentrations; severe toxicity usually results from inadvertent intravascular injection. The toxicity mainly involves the central nervous and cardiovascular systems. The onset of toxicity can be unpredictable and delayed. Monitor as per local protocol for at least 30 minutes after administration.

- ● ALLERGY AND CROSS-SENSITIVITY
 ▸ Hypersensitivity and cross-sensitivity Hypersensitivity reactions occur mainly with the ester-type local anaesthetics, such as tetracaine; reactions are less frequent with the amide types; such as articaine,

bupivacaine, levobupivacaine, lidocaine, mepivacaine, prilocaine, and ropivacaine. Cross-sensitivity reactions may be avoided by using the alternative chemical type.

▶ PREGNANCY Use only if potential benefit outweighs risk—no information available.

▶ BREAST FEEDING Avoid breast-feeding for 48 hours after administration.

▶ HEPATIC IMPAIRMENT Manufacturer advises caution (increased risk of toxicity in severe impairment).

▶ RENAL IMPAIRMENT Manufacturers advise use with caution in severe impairment.

▶ MONITORING REQUIREMENTS Consider monitoring blood pressure and ECG (advised with systemic adrenaline/epinephrine).

● MEDICINAL FORMS There can be variation in the licensing of different medicines containing the same drug.
Solution for injection
EXCIPIENTS: May contain Sulfites
▶ Septanest (Septodont Ltd)
Adrenaline (as Adrenaline acid tartrate) 10 microgram per 1 ml, Articaine hydrochloride 40 mg per 1 ml Septanest 1 in 100,000 solution for injection cartridges | 50 cartridge PoM £24.95
Adrenaline (as Adrenaline acid tartrate) 5 microgram per 1 ml, Articaine hydrochloride 40 mg per 1 ml Septanest 1 in 200,000 solution for injection cartridges | 50 cartridge PoM £24.95

Bupivacaine hydrochloride
09-Dec-2019

● **INDICATIONS AND DOSE**
Surgical anaesthesia, lumbar epidural block
▶ BY REGIONAL ADMINISTRATION
▶ Adult: 75–150 mg, dose administered using a 5 mg/mL (0.5%) solution
Surgical anaesthesia, field block
▶ BY REGIONAL ADMINISTRATION
▶ Adult: Up to 150 mg, dose administered using a 2.5 mg/mL (0.25%) or 5 mg/mL (0.5%) solution
Surgical anaesthesia, thoracic epidural block
▶ BY THORACIC EPIDURAL
▶ Adult: 12.5–50 mg, dose administered using a 2.5 mg/mL (0.25%) or 5 mg/mL (0.5%) solution
Surgical anaesthesia, caudal epidural block
▶ BY REGIONAL ADMINISTRATION
▶ Adult: 50–150 mg, dose administered using a 2.5 mg/mL (0.25%) or 5 mg/mL (0.5%) solution
Surgical anaesthesia, major nerve block
▶ BY REGIONAL ADMINISTRATION
▶ Adult: 50–175 mg, dose administered using 5 mg/mL (0.5%) solution
Acute pain, intra-articular block
▶ BY INTRA-ARTICULAR INJECTION
▶ Adult: Up to 100 mg, dose administered using a 2.5 mg/mL (0.25%) solution; when co-administered with bupivacaine by another route, total max. 150 mg
Acute pain, thoracic epidural block
▶ BY CONTINUOUS EPIDURAL INFUSION
▶ Adult: 6.3–18.8 mg/hour, dose administered using a 1.25 mg/mL (0.125%) or 2.5 mg/mL (0.25%) solution; maximum 400 mg per day
Acute pain, labour
▶ BY CONTINUOUS EPIDURAL INFUSION
▶ Adult: 6.25–12.5 mg/hour, dose administered using a 1.25 mg/mL (0.125%) solution; maximum 400 mg per day
Acute pain, lumbar epidural block
▶ INITIALLY BY LUMBAR EPIDURAL
▶ Adult: 15–37.5 mg, then (by lumbar epidural) 15–37.5 mg, repeated when required at intervals of at

least 30 minutes, dose administered by intermittent injection using a 2.5 mg/mL (0.25%) solution, alternatively (by continuous epidural infusion) 12.5–18.8 mg/hour, dose administered using a 1.25 mg/mL (0.125%) or 2.5 mg/mL (0.25%) solution; maximum 400 mg per day
Acute pain, field block
▶ BY REGIONAL ADMINISTRATION
▶ Adult: Up to 150 mg, dose administered using a 2.5 mg/mL (0.25%) solution
DOSES AT EXTREMES OF BODY-WEIGHT
▶ To avoid excessive dosage in obese patients, dose should be calculated on the basis of ideal body-weight.
MARCAIN HEAVY ®
Intrathecal anaesthesia for surgery
▶ BY INTRATHECAL INJECTION
▶ Adult: 10–20 mg

IMPORTANT SAFETY INFORMATION
The licensed doses stated may not be appropriate in some settings and expert advice should be sought.
  Should only be administered by, or under the direct supervision of, personnel experienced in their use, with adequate training in anaesthesia and airway management, and should not be administered parenterally unless adequate resuscitation equipment is available.

● CONTRA-INDICATIONS Avoid injection into infected tissues · avoid injection into inflamed tissues · intravenous regional anaesthesia (Bier's block) · preparations containing preservatives should not be used for caudal, epidural, or spinal block
  CONTRA-INDICATIONS, FURTHER INFORMATION
▶ Injection site Manufacturer advises local anaesthetics should not be injected into inflamed or infected tissues. Increased absorption into the blood increases the possibility of systemic side-effects, and the local anaesthetic effect may also be reduced by altered local pH.
● CAUTIONS Cardiovascular disease · cerebral atheroma · complete heart block · debilitated patients (consider dose reduction) · elderly (consider dose reduction) · epilepsy · hypertension · hypotension · hypovolaemia · impaired cardiac conduction · impaired respiratory function · myasthenia gravis · myocardial depression may be more severe and more resistant to treatment · shock
● INTERACTIONS → Appendix 1: anaesthetics, local
● SIDE-EFFECTS
▶ **Common or very common** Arrhythmias · dizziness · hypertension · hypotension · nausea · paraesthesia · urinary retention · vomiting
▶ **Uncommon** Neurotoxicity
▶ **Rare or very rare** Arachnoiditis · cardiac arrest · diplopia · nerve disorders · paraplegia · paresis · respiratory depression
  SIDE-EFFECTS, FURTHER INFORMATION Toxic effects after administration of local anaesthetics are a result of excessively high plasma concentrations; severe toxicity usually results from inadvertent intravascular injection. The systemic toxicity of local anaesthetics mainly involves the central nervous and cardiovascular systems. The onset of toxicity can be unpredictable and delayed. Monitor as per local protocol for at least 30 minutes after administration.
● ALLERGY AND CROSS-SENSITIVITY
▶ Hypersensitivity and cross-sensitivity Hypersensitivity reactions occur mainly with the ester-type local anaesthetics, such as tetracaine; reactions are less frequent with the amide types, such as articaine, bupivacaine, levobupivacaine, lidocaine, mepivacaine,

prilocaine, and ropivacaine. Cross-sensitivity reactions may be avoided by using the alternative chemical type.

- PREGNANCY Large doses during delivery can cause neonatal respiratory depression, hypotonia, and bradycardia after epidural block.
  Dose adjustments Use lower doses for intrathecal use during late pregnancy.
- BREAST FEEDING Amount too small to be harmful.
- HEPATIC IMPAIRMENT Manufacturer advises use with caution in advanced liver dysfunction.
- RENAL IMPAIRMENT Use with caution in severe impairment.

- MEDICINAL FORMS There can be variation in the licensing of different medicines containing the same drug. Forms available from special-order manufacturers include: solution for injection, infusion, solution for infusion

Solution for injection
‣ Bupivacaine hydrochloride (Non-proprietary)
  Bupivacaine hydrochloride 2.5 mg per 1 ml Bupivacaine 25mg/10ml (0.25%) solution for injection vials | 10 vial [PoM] 🛇
  Bupivacaine 0.25% solution for injection 10ml Sure-Amp ampoules | 20 ampoule [PoM] £17.50 DT = £17.50
  Bupivacaine hydrochloride 5 mg per 1 ml Bupivacaine 0.5% solution for injection 10ml Sure-Amp ampoules | 20 ampoule [PoM] £18.30 DT = £18.30 (Hospital only)
  Bupivacaine 100mg/20ml (0.5%) solution for injection vials | 10 vial [PoM] 🛇
  Bupivacaine 50mg/10ml (0.5%) solution for injection ampoules | 10 ampoule [PoM] £7.56–£17.58 DT = £7.56 (Hospital only)
  Bupivacaine hydrochloride anhydrous 40 mg per 1 ml Bupivacain Sintetica 40mg/ml (4%) solution for injection ampoules | 10 ampoule [PoM] 🛇
‣ Marcain (Aspen Pharma Trading Ltd)
  Bupivacaine hydrochloride 2.5 mg per 1 ml Marcain 0.25% solution for injection 10ml Polyamp Steripack ampoules | 5 ampoule [PoM] £7.92 DT = £7.92 (Hospital only)
  Bupivacaine hydrochloride 5 mg per 1 ml Marcain 0.5% solution for injection 10ml Polyamp Steripack ampoules | 5 ampoule [PoM] £9.25 DT = £9.25 (Hospital only)

Infusion
‣ Bupivacaine hydrochloride (Non-proprietary)
  Bupivacaine hydrochloride 1 mg per 1 ml Bupivacaine 100mg/100ml (0.1%) infusion bags | 20 bag [PoM] 🛇
  Bupivacaine 250mg/250ml (0.1%) infusion bags | 5 bag [PoM] £60.87 | 20 bag [PoM] £243.48
  Bupivacaine hydrochloride 1.25 mg per 1 ml Bupivacaine 312.5mg/250ml (0.125%) infusion bags | 5 bag [PoM] £62.12 | 20 bag [PoM] £248.47

Bupivacaine with adrenaline
19-Dec-2019

The properties listed below are those particular to the combination only. For the properties of the components please consider, bupivacaine hydrochloride p. 1403, adrenaline/epinephrine p. 238.

- INDICATIONS AND DOSE
Surgical anaesthesia
▸ BY LUMBAR EPIDURAL, OR BY LOCAL INFILTRATION, OR BY CAUDAL EPIDURAL
‣ Adult: (consult product literature)
Acute pain management
▸ BY LUMBAR EPIDURAL, OR BY LOCAL INFILTRATION
‣ Adult: (consult product literature)

- CAUTIONS In patients with severe hypertension or unstable cardiac rhythm, the use of adrenaline with a local anaesthetic may be hazardous. For these patients an anaesthetic without adrenaline should be used.
- INTERACTIONS → Appendix 1: anaesthetics, local · sympathomimetics, vasoconstrictor

- MEDICINAL FORMS There can be variation in the licensing of different medicines containing the same drug.

Solution for injection
‣ Bupivacaine with adrenaline (Non-proprietary)
  Adrenaline (as Adrenaline acid tartrate) 5 microgram per 1 ml, Bupivacaine hydrochloride 2.5 mg per 1 ml Bupivacaine 25mg/10ml (0.25%) / Adrenaline (base) 50micrograms/10ml (1 in 200,000) solution for injection ampoules | 10 ampoule [PoM] £46.00 DT = £46.00
  Adrenaline (as Adrenaline acid tartrate) 5 microgram per 1 ml, Bupivacaine hydrochloride anhydrous 2.5 mg per 1 ml Carbostesin-adrenaline 0.25% / 100micrograms/20ml (1 in 200,000) solution for injection ampoules | 1 ampoule [PoM] 🛇
  Carbostesin-adrenaline 0.25% / 25micrograms/5ml (1 in 200,000) solution for injection ampoules | 1 ampoule [PoM] 🛇
  Adrenaline (as Adrenaline acid tartrate) 5 microgram per 1 ml, Bupivacaine hydrochloride 5 mg per 1 ml Bupivacaine 50mg/10ml (0.5%) / Adrenaline (base) 50micrograms/10ml (1 in 200,000) solution for injection ampoules | 10 ampoule [PoM] £51.75 DT = £51.75
  Adrenaline (as Adrenaline acid tartrate) 5 microgram per 1 ml, Bupivacaine hydrochloride anhydrous 5 mg per 1 ml Carbostesin-adrenaline 0.5% / 25micrograms/5ml (1 in 200,000) solution for injection ampoules | 1 ampoule [PoM] 🛇
  Carbostesin-adrenaline 0.5% / 100micrograms/20ml (1 in 200,000) solution for injection ampoules | 1 ampoule [PoM] 🛇

Chloroprocaine hydrochloride
21-May-2020

- DRUG ACTION Chloroprocaine is an ester-type local anaesthetic that blocks the generation and conduction of nerve impulses.

- INDICATIONS AND DOSE
Spinal anaesthesia for surgical procedures lasting 40 minutes or less (using 10 mg/ml solution) (specialist use only)
▸ BY SLOW INTRATHECAL INJECTION
‣ Adult: 40–50 mg (max. per dose 50 mg), dose depends on desired length of block
Surgical anaesthesia for procedures lasting 60 minutes or less, peripheral nerve block (using 20 mg/ml solution) (specialist use only)
▸ BY REGIONAL ADMINISTRATION
‣ Adult: (consult product literature)

IMPORTANT SAFETY INFORMATION
The licensed doses stated above may not be appropriate in some settings and expert advice should be sought.
  Should only be administered by, or under the direct supervision of, personnel experienced in their use, with adequate training in anaesthesia and airway management, and should not be administered parenterally unless adequate resuscitation equipment is available.

- CONTRA-INDICATIONS Avoid injection into infected tissues · avoid injection into inflamed tissues · hypovolaemia · impaired cardiac conduction · intravenous regional anaesthesia (Bier's block) · severe anaemia
  CONTRA-INDICATIONS, FURTHER INFORMATION
‣ Injection site Local anaesthetics should not be injected into inflamed or infected tissues nor should they be applied to damaged skin. Increased absorption into the blood increases the possibility of systemic side-effects, and the local anaesthetic effect may also be reduced by altered local pH.
- CAUTIONS Acute porphyrias p. 1107 · cardiovascular disease · complete heart block · debilitated patients (consider dose reduction) · elderly (consider dose reduction) · low plasma-cholinesterase activity (including severe liver disease) · neurological disorders · neuromuscular disorders · partial heart block
- INTERACTIONS → Appendix 1: chloroprocaine

● SIDE-EFFECTS

GENERAL SIDE-EFFECTS

▸ **Common or very common** Anxiety · dizziness · hypotension · nausea · vomiting

▸ **Uncommon** Arrhythmias · hearing impairment · hypertension · loss of consciousness · neurotoxicity · oral disorders · seizure · speech disorder · tinnitus · tremor · vision disorders

▸ **Rare or very rare** Cardiac arrest · drowsiness · faecal incontinence · myocardial contractility decreased · nerve disorders · neurological injury · perineal numbness · sexual dysfunction · urinary incontinence

SPECIFIC SIDE-EFFECTS

▸ **Common or very common**

▸ With intrathecal use Sensation abnormal

▸ When used by regional administration Anaesthetic complication · paraesthesia

▸ **Uncommon**

▸ With intrathecal use Headache · pain

▸ **Rare or very rare**

▸ With intrathecal use Motor dysfunction · respiratory disorders · spinal block

▸ When used by regional administration Dyspnoea · respiratory arrest

SIDE-EFFECTS, FURTHER INFORMATION Toxic effects after administration of local anaesthetics are a result of excessively high plasma concentrations; severe toxicity usually results from inadvertent intravascular injection. The systemic toxicity of local anaesthetics mainly involves the central nervous and cardiovascular systems. The onset of toxicity can be unpredictable and delayed. Monitor as per local protocol for at least 30 minutes after administration.

● ALLERGY AND CROSS-SENSITIVITY

▸ Hypersensitivity and cross-sensitivity Hypersensitivity reactions occur mainly with the ester-type local anaesthetics, such as tetracaine and chloroprocaine; reactions are less frequent with the amide types, such as articaine, bupivacaine, levobupivacaine, lidocaine, mepivacaine, prilocaine, and ropivacaine. Cross-sensitivity reactions may be avoided by using the alternative chemical type.

● PREGNANCY Manufacturer advises use only if potential benefit outweighs risk (limited information available); this does not preclude use at term for obstetrical anaesthesia.

● HEPATIC IMPAIRMENT Manufacturer advises caution in severe impairment.

● RENAL IMPAIRMENT Manufacturer advises use with caution.

● HANDLING AND STORAGE Manufacturer advises protect from light.

● MEDICINAL FORMS There can be variation in the licensing of different medicines containing the same drug.

Solution for injection

▸ Chloroprocaine hydrochloride (Non-proprietary)
  Chloroprocaine hydrochloride 20 mg per 1 ml Ampres
  400mg/20ml solution for injection vials | 1 vial [PoM] £14.72

▸ Ampres (Sintetica Ltd)
  Chloroprocaine hydrochloride 10 mg per 1 ml Ampres 50mg/5ml
  solution for injection ampoules | 10 ampoule [PoM] £87.50

| Levobupivacaine   08-Sep-2020

● INDICATIONS AND DOSE

Acute postoperative pain

▸ BY CONTINUOUS EPIDURAL INFUSION

▸ Adult: 12.5–18.75 mg/hour, dose administered using a 1.25 mg/mL (0.125%) or 2.5 mg/mL (0.25%) solution; maximum 400 mg per day

---

Acute labour pain

▸ BY LUMBAR EPIDURAL

▸ Adult: 15–25 mg, repeated at intervals of at least 15 minutes, dose administered using a 2.5 mg/mL (0.25%) solution; maximum 400 mg per day

▸ BY CONTINUOUS EPIDURAL INFUSION

▸ Adult: 5–12.5 mg/hour, dose administered using a 1.25 mg/mL (0.125%) solution; maximum 400 mg per day

Surgical anaesthesia, peripheral nerve block

▸ BY REGIONAL ADMINISTRATION

▸ Adult: 2.5–150 mg, dose administered using a 2.5 mg/mL (0.25%) or 5 mg/mL (0.5%) solution

Surgical anaesthesia, peribulbular nerve block

▸ BY REGIONAL ADMINISTRATION

▸ Adult: 37.5–112.5 mg, dose administered using a 7.5 mg/mL (0.75%) solution

Surgical anaesthesia for caesarean section

▸ BY LUMBAR EPIDURAL

▸ Adult: 75–150 mg, to be given over 15–20 minutes, dose administered using a 5 mg/mL (0.5%) solution

Surgical anaesthesia

▸ BY LUMBAR EPIDURAL

▸ Adult: 50–150 mg, to be given over 5 minutes, dose administered using a 5 mg/mL (0.5%) or 7.5 mg/mL (0.75%) solution

▸ BY INTRATHECAL INJECTION

▸ Adult: 15 mg, dose administered using a 5 mg/mL (0.5%) solution

▸ BY LOCAL INFILTRATION

▸ Adult: 2.5–150 mg, dose administered using a 2.5 mg/mL (0.25%) solution

DOSES AT EXTREMES OF BODY-WEIGHT

▸ To avoid excessive dosage in obese patients, dose should be calculated on the basis of ideal body-weight.

┌───┐
│ IMPORTANT SAFETY INFORMATION   │
│ The licensed doses stated may not be appropriate in │
│ some settings and expert advice should be sought. │
│   Should only be administered by, or under the direct │
│ supervision of, personnel experienced in their use, with │
│ adequate training in anaesthesia and airway │
│ management, and should not be administered │
│ parenterally unless adequate resuscitation equipment is │
│ available. │
└───┘

● CONTRA-INDICATIONS Avoid injection into infected tissues · avoid injection into inflamed tissues · intravenous regional anaesthesia (Bier's block) · preparations containing preservatives should not be used for caudal, epidural, or spinal block

CONTRA-INDICATIONS, FURTHER INFORMATION

▸ Injection site Manufacturer advises local anaesthetics should not be injected into inflamed or infected tissues. Increased absorption into the blood increases the possibility of systemic side-effects, and the local anaesthetic effect may also be reduced by altered local pH.

● CAUTIONS Cardiovascular disease · complete heart block · debilitated patients (consider dose reduction) · elderly (consider dose reduction) · epilepsy · hypovolaemia · impaired cardiac conduction · impaired respiratory function · myasthenia gravis · shock

● INTERACTIONS → Appendix 1: anaesthetics, local

● SIDE-EFFECTS

▸ **Common or very common** Anaemia · back pain · dizziness · fever · headache · hypotension · nausea · procedural pain · vomiting

▸ **Frequency not known** Angioedema · apnoea · arrhythmias · asthenia · atrioventricular block · bladder disorder · cardiac arrest · drowsiness · eye disorders · faecal incontinence ·

flushing · loss of consciousness · muscle twitching · muscle weakness · nerve disorders · neurological injury · oral hypoaesthesia · paralysis · priapism · respiratory disorders · seizure · sensation abnormal · skin reactions · sneezing · sweat changes · syncope · vision blurred

SIDE-EFFECTS, FURTHER INFORMATION The systemic toxicity of local anaesthetics mainly involves the central nervous and cardiovascular systems. Systemic toxicity can occur due to inadvertent intravascular injection. The onset of toxicity can be unpredictable and delayed. Monitor as per local protocol for at least 30 minutes after administration.

- ALLERGY AND CROSS-SENSITIVITY
- Hypersensitivity and cross-sensitivity Hypersensitivity reactions occur mainly with the ester-type local anaesthetics, such as tetracaine; reactions are less frequent with the amide types, such as articaine, bupivacaine, levobupivacaine, lidocaine, mepivacaine, prilocaine, and ropivacaine. Cross-sensitivity reactions may be avoided by using the alternative chemical type.
- PREGNANCY Large doses during delivery can cause neonatal respiratory depression, hypotonia, and bradycardia after epidural block. Avoid if possible in the first trimester—toxicity in *animal* studies. May cause fetal distress syndrome. Do not use for paracervical block in obstetrics. Do not use 7.5 mg/mL strength in obstetrics.
- BREAST FEEDING Amount too small to be harmful.
- HEPATIC IMPAIRMENT Manufacturer advises caution in impairment or patients with reduced hepatic blood flow (no information available).
- PRESCRIBING AND DISPENSING INFORMATION Levobupivacaine is an isomer of bupivacaine.
- MEDICINAL FORMS There can be variation in the licensing of different medicines containing the same drug.

Solution for injection

- Levobupivacaine (Non-proprietary)

  Levobupivacaine (as Levobupivacaine hydrochloride) 2.5 mg per 1 ml Levobupivacaine 25mg/10ml solution for injection ampoules | 5 ampoule [PoM] £9.45 (Hospital only)

  Levobupivacaine (as Levobupivacaine hydrochloride) 5 mg per 1 ml Levobupivacaine 50mg/10ml solution for injection ampoules | 5 ampoule [PoM] £10.85 (Hospital only)

  Levobupivacaine (as Levobupivacaine hydrochloride) 7.5 mg per 1 ml Levobupivacaine 75mg/10ml solution for injection ampoules | 5 ampoule [PoM] £16.20 (Hospital only)

- Chirocaine (AbbVie Ltd)

  Levobupivacaine (as Levobupivacaine hydrochloride) 2.5 mg per 1 ml Chirocaine 25mg/10ml solution for injection ampoules | 10 ampoule [PoM] £14.11 (Hospital only)

  Levobupivacaine (as Levobupivacaine hydrochloride) 5 mg per 1 ml Chirocaine 50mg/10ml solution for injection ampoules | 10 ampoule [PoM] £16.15 (Hospital only)

  Levobupivacaine (as Levobupivacaine hydrochloride) 7.5 mg per 1 ml Chirocaine 75mg/10ml solution for injection ampoules | 10 ampoule [PoM] £24.23 (Hospital only)

Infusion

- Levobupivacaine (Non-proprietary)

  Levobupivacaine (as Levobupivacaine hydrochloride).625 mg per 1 ml Levobupivacaine 62.5mg/100ml infusion bags | 5 bag [PoM] [N] Levobupivacaine 125mg/200ml infusion bags | 5 bag [PoM] [N] Levobupivacaine (as Levobupivacaine hydrochloride) 1.25 mg per 1 ml Levobupivacaine 125mg/100ml infusion bags | 5 bag [PoM] [N]

- Chirocaine (AbbVie Ltd)

  Levobupivacaine (as Levobupivacaine hydrochloride) 1.25 mg per 1 ml Chirocaine 125mg/100ml infusion bags | 24 bag [PoM] £174.22 Chirocaine 250mg/200ml infusion bags | 12 bag [PoM] £124.44

Lidocaine hydrochloride

10-Nov-2020

(Lignocaine hydrochloride)

- ● INDICATIONS AND DOSE

Infiltration anaesthesia

- ▸ BY LOCAL INFILTRATION
- ▸ Adult: Dose to be given according to patient's weight and nature of procedure; max. 200 mg, maximum dose 500 mg if given in solutions containing adrenaline

DOSES AT EXTREMES OF BODY-WEIGHT

- ▸ When used by local infiltration To avoid excessive dosage in obese patients, weight-based doses for non-emergency indications may need to be calculated on the basis of ideal body-weight.

Intravenous regional anaesthesia and nerve block

- ▸ BY REGIONAL ADMINISTRATION
- ▸ Adult: Seek expert advice

Pain relief (in anal fissures, haemorrhoids, pruritus ani, pruritus vulvae, herpes zoster, or herpes labialis) | Lubricant in cystoscopy | Lubricant in proctoscopy

- ▸ TO THE SKIN USING OINTMENT
- ▸ Adult: Apply 1–2 mL as required, avoid long-term use

Sore nipples from breast-feeding

- ▸ TO THE SKIN USING OINTMENT
- ▸ Adult: Apply using gauze and wash off immediately before next feed

LMX 4 ®

Anaesthesia before venous cannulation or venepuncture

- ▸ TO THE SKIN
- ▸ Child 1-2 months: Apply up to 1 g, apply thick layer to small area (2.5 cm × 2.5 cm) of non-irritated skin at least 30 minutes before procedure; may be applied under an occlusive dressing; max. application time 60 minutes, remove cream with gauze and perform procedure after approximately 5 minutes
- ▸ Child 3-11 months: Apply up to 1 g, apply thick layer to small area (2.5 cm × 2.5 cm) of non-irritated skin at least 30 minutes before procedure; may be applied under an occlusive dressing; max. application time 4 hours, remove cream with gauze and perform procedure after approximately 5 minutes
- ▸ Child 1-17 years: Apply 1–2.5 g, apply thick layer to small area (2.5 cm × 2.5 cm) of non-irritated skin at least 30 minutes before procedure; may be applied under an occlusive dressing; max. application time 5 hours, remove cream with gauze and perform procedure after approximately 5 minutes
- ▸ Adult: Apply 1–2.5 g, apply thick layer to small area (2.5 cm × 2.5 cm) of non-irritated skin at least 30 minutes before procedure; may be applied under an occlusive dressing; max. application time 5 hours, remove cream with gauze and perform procedure after approximately 5 minutes

VERSATIS ®

Postherpetic neuralgia

- ▸ TO THE SKIN
- ▸ Adult: Apply once daily for up to 12 hours, followed by a 12-hour plaster-free period; discontinue if no response after 4 weeks, to be applied to intact, dry, non-hairy, non-irritated skin, up to 3 plasters may be used to cover large areas; plasters may be cut

XYLOCAINE ®
During delivery in obstetrics
▶ TO THE SKIN
▶ Adult: Up to 20 doses

IMPORTANT SAFETY INFORMATION
▶ When used by local infiltration
The licensed doses stated may not be appropriate in
some settings and expert advice should be sought.
Should only be administered by, or under the direct
supervision of, personnel experienced in their use, with
adequate training in anaesthesia and airway
management, and should not be administered
parenterally unless adequate resuscitation equipment is
available.

● CONTRA-INDICATIONS
When used by regional administration Avoid injection into
infected tissues · avoid injection into inflamed tissues ·
complete heart block · preparations containing
preservatives should not be used for caudal, epidural, or
spinal block, or for intravenous regional anaesthesia
(Bier's block)
With topical use Application to the middle ear (can cause
ototoxicity) · should not be applied to damaged skin
CONTRA-INDICATIONS, FURTHER INFORMATION
▶ With topical use or when used by regional
administration Manufacturer advises local anaesthetics
should not be injected into inflamed or infected tissues nor
should they be applied to damaged skin. Increased
absorption into the blood increases the possibility of
systemic side-effects, and the local anaesthetic effect may
also be reduced by altered local pH.

● CAUTIONS
When used by regional administration Acute porphyrias
p. 1107 (consider infusion with glucose for its anti-
porphyrinogenic effects) · congestive cardiac failure
(consider lower dose) · debilitated patients (consider dose
reduction) · elderly (consider dose reduction) · epilepsy ·
hypovolaemia · impaired cardiac conduction · impaired
respiratory function · myasthenia gravis · post cardiac
surgery (consider lower dose) · shock
● INTERACTIONS → Appendix 1: antiarrhythmics
● SIDE-EFFECTS
▶ With parenteral use Anxiety · arrhythmias · atrioventricular
block · cardiac arrest · circulatory collapse · confusion ·
dizziness · drowsiness · euphoric mood · headache ·
hypotension (may lead to cardiac arrest) · loss of
consciousness · methaemoglobinaemia · muscle twitching ·
myocardial contractility decreased · nausea · neurological
effects · nystagmus · pain · psychosis · respiratory disorders
· seizure · sensation abnormal · temperature sensation
altered · tinnitus · tremor · vision blurred · vomiting
SIDE-EFFECTS, FURTHER INFORMATION **Toxic effects** The
systemic toxicity of local anaesthetics mainly involves the
central nervous and cardiovascular systems.

Methaemoglobinaemia Methylthioninium chloride is
licensed for the acute symptomatic treatment of drug-
induced methaemoglobinaemia.

● ALLERGY AND CROSS-SENSITIVITY
▶ Hypersensitivity and cross-sensitivity Hypersensitivity
reactions occur mainly with the ester-type local
anaesthetics, such as tetracaine; reactions are less
frequent with the amide types, such as articaine,
bupivacaine, levobupivacaine, lidocaine, mepivacaine,
prilocaine, and ropivacaine. Cross-sensitivity reactions
may be avoided by using the alternative chemical type.
● PREGNANCY Crosses the placenta but not known to be
harmful in *animal* studies—use if benefit outweighs risk.
When used as a local anaesthetic, large doses can cause

fetal bradycardia; if given during delivery can also cause
neonatal respiratory depression, hypotonia, or bradycardia
after paracervical or epidural block.
● BREAST FEEDING Present in milk but amount too small to
be harmful.
● HEPATIC IMPAIRMENT Manufacturer advises caution (risk
of increased exposure).
● RENAL IMPAIRMENT Possible accumulation of lidocaine
and active metabolite; caution in severe impairment.
● MONITORING REQUIREMENTS
▶ With systemic use Monitor ECG and have resuscitation
facilities available.
● NATIONAL FUNDING/ACCESS DECISIONS
VERSATIS ® For full details see funding body website
Scottish Medicines Consortium (SMC) decisions
▶ Lidocaine hydrochloride (*Versatis®*) for the treatment of
neuropathic pain associated with previous herpes zoster
infection (post-herpetic neuralgia, PHN) (August 2008)
SMC No. 334/06 Recommended with restrictions

● MEDICINAL FORMS There can be variation in the licensing of
different medicines containing the same drug. Forms available
from special-order manufacturers include: solution for
injection, liquid, ointment
Solution for injection
▶ Lidocaine hydrochloride (Non-proprietary)
 Lidocaine hydrochloride 5 mg per 1 ml Lidocaine 50mg/10ml
 (0.5%) solution for injection ampoules | 10 ampoule [PoM] £7.00
 Lidocaine hydrochloride 10 mg per 1 ml Lidocaine 100mg/10ml
 (1%) solution for injection Mini-Plasco ampoules | 20 ampoule [PoM]
 £1.15–£11.21
 Lidocaine 100mg/10ml (1%) solution for injection ampoules |
 10 ampoule [PoM] £5.00 DT = £5.00
 Lidocaine 200mg/20ml (1%) solution for injection vials | 10 vial [PoM]
 £22.00 DT = £22.00
 Lidocaine 200mg/20ml (1%) solution for injection ampoules |
 10 ampoule [PoM] £10.00–£11.00 DT = £11.00
 Lidocaine 50mg/5ml (1%) solution for injection ampoules |
 10 ampoule [PoM] £3.00–£12.00 DT = £3.00
 Lidocaine 200mg/20ml (1%) solution for injection Mini-Plasco
 ampoules | 20 ampoule [PoM] [S]
 Lidocaine 20mg/2ml (1%) solution for injection ampoules |
 10 ampoule [PoM] £12.00 DT = £2.50
 Lidocaine 50mg/5ml (1%) solution for injection Mini-Plasco ampoules
 | 20 ampoule [PoM] £6.50
 Lidocaine 50mg/5ml (1%) solution for injection Sure-Amp ampoules |
 20 ampoule [PoM] £6.00
 Lidocaine hydrochloride 20 mg per 1 ml Lidocaine 100mg/5ml
 (2%) solution for injection ampoules | 10 ampoule [PoM] £3.20–
 £12.00 DT = £3.20
 Lidocaine 400mg/20ml (2%) solution for injection vials | 10 vial [PoM]
 £23.00 DT = £23.00
 Lidocaine 200mg/10ml (2%) solution for injection Mini-Plasco
 ampoules | 20 ampoule [PoM] £14.95 DT = £14.95
 Lidocaine 400mg/20ml (2%) solution for injection Mini-Plasco
 ampoules | 20 ampoule [PoM] [S]
 Lidocaine 40mg/2ml (2%) solution for injection ampoules |
 10 ampoule [PoM] £12.00 DT = £2.70
 Lidocaine 100mg/5ml (2%) solution for injection Mini-Plasco ampoules
 | 20 ampoule [PoM] £7.50
 Lidocaine 400mg/20ml (2%) solution for injection ampoules |
 10 ampoule [PoM] £11.00–£11.40 DT = £11.40
Medicated plaster
EXCIPIENTS: May contain Hydroxybenzoates (parabens), propylene
glycol
▶ Ralvo (Grunenthal Ltd)
 Lidocaine 50 mg per 1 gram Ralvo 700mg medicated plasters |
 30 plaster [PoM] £61.54 DT = £72.40
▶ Versatis (Grunenthal Ltd)
 Lidocaine 50 mg per 1 gram Versatis 700mg medicated plasters |
 30 plaster [PoM] £72.40 DT = £72.40
Cream
EXCIPIENTS: May contain Benzyl alcohol, propylene glycol
▶ LMX 4 (Ferndale Pharmaceuticals Ltd)
 Lidocaine 40 mg per 1 gram LMX 4 cream | 5 gram [P] £2.98 DT =
 £2.98 | 30 gram [P] £14.90 DT = £14.90

15

Anaesthesia

▸ Vagisil medicated (Combe International Ltd)
Lidocaine 20 mg per 1 gram Vagisil 2% medicated cream |
30 gram GSL £2.99 DT = £2.99

Ointment

▸ Lidocaine hydrochloride (Non-proprietary)
Lidocaine hydrochloride 50 mg per 1 gram Lidocaine 5% ointment
| 15 gram P £9.00 DT = £8.28

Spray

▸ Xylocaine (Aspen Pharma Trading Ltd)
Lidocaine 10 mg per 1 actuation Xylocaine 10mg/dose spray sugar-
free | 50 ml P £6.29 DT = £6.29

Lidocaine with adrenaline
19-Dec-2019

The properties listed below are those particular to the
combination only. For the properties of the components
please consider, lidocaine hydrochloride p. 1406,
adrenaline/epinephrine p. 238.

● **INDICATIONS AND DOSE**

Local anaesthesia

▸ BY LOCAL INFILTRATION

▸ **Adult:** Dosed according to the type of nerve block
required (consult product literature)

● INTERACTIONS → Appendix 1: antiarrhythmics ·
sympathomimetics, vasoconstrictor

● **PROFESSION SPECIFIC INFORMATION**

Dental information
A variety of lidocaine injections with adrenaline is
available in dental cartridges.
Consult expert dental sources for specific advice in
relation to dose of lidocaine for dental anaesthesia.

● MEDICINAL FORMS There can be variation in the licensing of
different medicines containing the same drug. Forms available
from special-order manufacturers include: solution for
injection

Solution for injection
EXCIPIENTS: May contain Sulfites

▸ Lignospan Special (Septodont Ltd)
**Adrenaline (as Adrenaline acid tartrate) 12.5 microgram per 1 ml,
Lidocaine hydrochloride 20 mg per 1 ml** Lignospan Special
20mg/ml / 12.5micrograms/ml solution for injection 2.2ml cartridges
| 50 cartridge PoM £21.95 DT = £21.95
Lignospan Special 20mg/ml / 12.5micrograms/ml solution for injection
1.8ml cartridges | 50 cartridge PoM £21.95

▸ Rexocaine (Henry Schein Ltd)
**Adrenaline (as Adrenaline acid tartrate) 12.5 microgram per 1 ml,
Lidocaine hydrochloride 20 mg per 1 ml** Rexocaine 2% injection
2.2ml cartridges | 50 cartridge PoM £23.29 DT = £21.95

▸ Xylocaine with Adrenaline (Aspen Pharma Trading Ltd)
**Adrenaline (as Adrenaline acid tartrate) 5 microgram per 1 ml,
Lidocaine hydrochloride 10 mg per 1 ml** Xylocaine 1% with
Adrenaline 100micrograms/20ml (1 in 200,000) solution for injection
vials | 5 vial PoM £9.66 DT = £9.66
**Adrenaline (as Adrenaline acid tartrate) 5 microgram per 1 ml,
Lidocaine hydrochloride 20 mg per 1 ml** Xylocaine 2% with
Adrenaline 100micrograms/20ml (1 in 200,000) solution for injection
vials | 5 vial PoM £8.85 DT = £8.85 (Hospital only)

Lidocaine with cetrimide
27-Apr-2018

The properties listed below are those particular to the
combination only. For the properties of the components
please consider, lidocaine hydrochloride p. 1258.

● **INDICATIONS AND DOSE**

Anaesthesia and disinfection in dental practice

▸ TO MUCOUS MEMBRANES USING OROMUCOSAL SPRAY

▸ **Adult:** 10–20 mg, no more than 30 mg should be
applied to the same quadrant of the buccal cavity—
consult product literature, dose expressed as lidocaine

Anaesthesia in dental practice

▸ TO MUCOUS MEMBRANES USING DENTAL GEL

▸ **Adult:** Apply 100–500 mg, use cotton pellet for
application to dried mucosa, dose expressed as weight
of gel

DOSE EQUIVALENCE AND CONVERSION

▸ 1 metered dose of *Xylonor*® spray is equivalent to 10 mg
of lidocaine.

▸ 2 millimetres of *Xylonor*® gel is approximately
equivalent to 100 mg of gel (approximately equivalent
to 5 mg of lidocaine).

● CAUTIONS Sepsis (risk of rapid systemic absorption) ·
traumatised mucosa (risk of rapid systemic absorption)

● INTERACTIONS → Appendix 1: antiarrhythmics

● MEDICINAL FORMS There can be variation in the licensing of
different medicines containing the same drug.

Oromucosal gel

▸ Xylonor (Septodont Ltd)
Cetrimide 1.5 mg per 1 gram, Lidocaine 50 mg per 1 gram Xylonor
50mg/g / 1.5mg/g gel sugar-free | 15 gram PoM £4.00

Spray

▸ Xylonor (Septodont Ltd)
**Cetrimide 100 microgram per 1 gram, Lidocaine 10 mg per
1 gram** Xylonor 150mg/g / 1.5mg/g oromucosal spray sugar-free |
36 gram PoM £20.15

Lidocaine with phenylephrine

The properties listed below are those particular to the
combination only. For the properties of the components
please consider, lidocaine hydrochloride p. 111,
phenylephrine hydrochloride p. 203.

● **INDICATIONS AND DOSE**

**Anaesthesia before nasal surgery, endoscopy,
laryngoscopy, or removal of foreign bodies from the nose**

▸ BY INTRANASAL ADMINISTRATION

▸ **Adult:** Up to 8 sprays

● INTERACTIONS → Appendix 1: antiarrhythmics ·
sympathomimetics, vasoconstrictor

● MEDICINAL FORMS There can be variation in the licensing of
different medicines containing the same drug.

Spray

▸ Lidocaine with phenylephrine (Non-proprietary)
**Phenylephrine hydrochloride 5 mg per 1 ml, Lidocaine
hydrochloride 50 mg per 1 ml** Lidocaine 5% / Phenylephrine 0.5%
nasal spray | 2.5 ml PoM £14.90 DT = £14.19

Lidocaine with prilocaine
10-Mar-2020

The properties listed below are those particular to the
combination only. For the properties of the components
please consider, lidocaine hydrochloride p. 1406, prilocaine
hydrochloride p. 1410.

● **INDICATIONS AND DOSE**

**Anaesthesia before minor skin procedures including
venepuncture**

▸ TO THE SKIN

▸ **Child 1-2 months:** Apply up to 1 g for maximum 1 hour
before procedure, to be applied under occlusive
dressing, shorter application time of 15–30 minutes is
recommended for children with atopic dermatitis
(30 minutes before removal of mollusca); maximum
1 dose per day

▸ **Child 3-11 months:** Apply up to 2 g for maximum 1 hour
before procedure, to be applied under occlusive
dressing, shorter application time of 15–30 minutes is

recommended for children with atopic dermatitis (30 minutes before removal of mollusca); maximum 2 doses per day
‣ Child 1-11 years: Apply 1–5 hours before procedure, a thick layer should be applied under occlusive dressing, shorter application time of 15–30 minutes is recommended for children with atopic dermatitis (30 minutes before removal of mollusca); maximum 2 doses per day
‣ Child 12-17 years: Apply 1–5 hours before procedure (2–5 hours before procedures on large areas e.g. split skin grafting), a thick layer should be applied under occlusive dressing, shorter application time of 15–30 minutes is recommended for children with atopic dermatitis (30 minutes before removal of mollusca)
‣ Adult: Apply 1–5 hours before procedure (2–5 hours before procedures on large areas e.g. split skin grafting), a thick layer should be applied under occlusive dressing

Anaesthesia on genital skin before injection of local anaesthetics
‣ TO THE SKIN
‣ Adult: Apply under occlusive dressing for 15 minutes (males) or 60 minutes (females) before procedure

Anaesthesia before surgical treatment of lesions on genital mucosa
‣ TO THE SKIN
‣ Adult: Apply up to 10 g, to be applied 5–10 minutes before procedure

Anaesthesia before cervical curettage
‣ TO THE SKIN
‣ Adult: Apply 10 g in lateral vaginal fornices for 10 minutes

Anaesthesia before mechanical cleansing or debridement of leg ulcer
‣ TO THE SKIN
‣ Adult: Apply up to 10 g for 30–60 minutes, to be applied under occlusive dressing

FORTACIN ®

Primary premature ejaculation
‣ TO THE SKIN
‣ Adult: 3 sprays every 4 hours as required, to be applied to cover the glans penis (excess spray should be removed after 5 minutes and before intercourse); maximum 9 sprays per day

DOSE EQUIVALENCE AND CONVERSION
‣ For *Fortacin* ®: each dose of 3 sprays is equivalent to lidocaine 22.5 mg and prilocaine 7.5 mg.

● CONTRA-INDICATIONS Use in child less than 37 weeks corrected gestational age
● CAUTIONS
FORTACIN ® Acquired methaemoglobinaemia · anaemia · congenital methaemoglobinaemia
● INTERACTIONS → Appendix 1: anaesthetics, local · antiarrhythmics
● SIDE-EFFECTS
‣ **Common or very common** Sexual dysfunction (in adults)
‣ **Uncommon** Fever (in adults) · headache (in adults) · penis disorder (in adults)
‣ **Rare or very rare** Methaemoglobinaemia · skin reactions
SIDE-EFFECTS, FURTHER INFORMATION When applied to the glans penis, side-effects for sexual partners should be considered. Side-effects reported in female partners include vaginal candidiasis and dysuria.
● CONCEPTION AND CONTRACEPTION
FORTACIN ® Deterioration of polyurethane-based female and male condoms has been observed. Manufacturer

advises avoid in patients planning to conceive, or if it is essential to achieve penetration, then the glans penis should be washed thoroughly 5 minutes after application but before intercourse.
● PREGNANCY
FORTACIN ® Manufacturer advises preferably avoid unless an effective male barrier contraceptive is used—limited information available.
● HEPATIC IMPAIRMENT
FORTACIN ® Manufacturer advises caution in severe impairment (no information available).
● DIRECTIONS FOR ADMINISTRATION
FORTACIN ® Manufacturer advises when using the spray for the first time, shake and prime the unit with 3 sprays, and before each subsequent use, shake and prime the unit with 1 spray.
● PATIENT AND CARER ADVICE
Medicines for Children leaflet: EMLA cream for local anaesthesia www.medicinesforchildren.org.uk/emla-cream-local-anaesthesia

● MEDICINAL FORMS There can be variation in the licensing of different medicines containing the same drug.
Cream
‣ Denela (Teva UK Ltd)
Lidocaine 25 mg per 1 gram, Prilocaine 25 mg per 1 gram Denela 5% cream | 5 gram P £3.29 | 25 gram P £12.99 | 30 gram P £14.75 DT = £12.30
‣ Emla (Aspen Pharma Trading Ltd)
Lidocaine 25 mg per 1 gram, Prilocaine 25 mg per 1 gram Emla 5% cream | 5 gram P £2.25-£2.99 | 25 gram P £11.70 | 30 gram P £12.30 DT = £12.30
‣ Nulbia (Glenmark Pharmaceuticals Europe Ltd)
Lidocaine 25 mg per 1 gram, Prilocaine 25 mg per 1 gram Nulbia 5% cream | 5 gram P £1.58 | 25 gram P £7.88 | 30 gram P £8.61 DT = £12.30

Cutaneous spray solution
‣ Fortacin (Recordati Pharmaceuticals Ltd)
Prilocaine 50 mg per 1 ml, Lidocaine 150 mg per 1 ml Fortacin 150mg/ml / 50mg/ml cutaneous spray | 5 ml PoM £59.99 DT = £59.99

Mepivacaine hydrochloride   04-Dec-2019

● INDICATIONS AND DOSE
Infiltration anaesthesia and nerve block in dentistry
‣ Child 3-17 years: Consult expert dental sources
‣ Adult: Consult expert dental sources
DOSES AT EXTREMES OF BODY-WEIGHT
‣ To avoid excessive dosage in obese patients, dose should be calculated on the basis of ideal body-weight.

> IMPORTANT SAFETY INFORMATION
> Should only be administered by, or under the direct supervision of, personnel experienced in their use, with adequate training in anaesthesia and airway management, and should not be administered parenterally unless adequate resuscitation equipment is available.

● CONTRA-INDICATIONS Avoid injection into infected tissues · avoid injection into inflamed tissues · intravenous regional anaesthesia (Bier's block) · preparations containing preservatives should not be used for caudal, epidural, or spinal block · severe atrio-ventricular conduction disorders not controlled by a pacemaker
CONTRA-INDICATIONS, FURTHER INFORMATION
‣ Injection site Manufacturer advises the local anaesthetic effect may be reduced when injected into an inflamed or infected area, due to altered local pH. Increased absorption

into the blood also increases the possibility of systemic side-effects.

- **CAUTIONS** Cardiovascular disease · children (consider dose reduction) · debilitated patients (consider dose reduction) · elderly (consider dose reduction) · epilepsy · hypovolaemia · impaired cardiac conduction · impaired respiratory function · myasthenia gravis · shock
- **INTERACTIONS** → Appendix 1: anaesthetics, local
- **SIDE-EFFECTS**
- **Common or very common** Arrhythmias · dizziness · hypertension · hypotension · nausea · paraesthesia · vomiting
- **Uncommon** Neurotoxicity
- **Rare or very rare** Arachnoiditis · cardiac arrest · diplopia · nerve disorders · respiratory depression

SIDE-EFFECTS, FURTHER INFORMATION Toxic effects after administration of local anaesthetics are a result of excessively high plasma concentrations; severe toxicity usually results from inadvertent intravascular injection or too rapid injection. The systemic toxicity of local anaesthetics mainly involves the central nervous and cardiovascular systems. The onset of toxicity can be unpredictable and delayed. Monitor as per local protocol for at least 30 minutes after administration.

- **ALLERGY AND CROSS-SENSITIVITY**
- Hypersensitivity and cross-sensitivity Hypersensitivity reactions occur mainly with the ester-type local anaesthetics, such as tetracaine; reactions are less frequent with the amide types, such as articaine, bupivacaine, levobupivacaine, lidocaine, mepivacaine, prilocaine, and ropivacaine. Cross-sensitivity reactions may be avoided by using the alternative chemical type.
- **PREGNANCY** Use with caution in early pregnancy.
- **BREAST FEEDING** Use with caution.
- **HEPATIC IMPAIRMENT** Manufacturer advises caution; increased risk of toxic plasma concentrations in severe impairment.
- **RENAL IMPAIRMENT** Use with caution; increased risk of side-effects.
- **MEDICINAL FORMS** There can be variation in the licensing of different medicines containing the same drug.
  Solution for injection
  - Scandonest plain (Septodont Ltd)
    Mepivacaine hydrochloride 30 mg per 1 ml Scandonest plain 3% solution for injection 2.2ml cartridges | 50 cartridge [PoM] £21.95

Mepivacaine with adrenaline   19-Dec-2019

The properties listed below are those particular to the combination only. For the properties of the components please consider, mepivacaine hydrochloride p. 1409, adrenaline/epinephrine p. 238.

- **INDICATIONS AND DOSE**
  Infiltration anaesthesia and nerve block in dentistry
  - BY LOCAL INFILTRATION
  - Adult: (consult product literature)
- **INTERACTIONS** → Appendix 1: anaesthetics, local · sympathomimetics, vasoconstrictor
- **MEDICINAL FORMS** There can be variation in the licensing of different medicines containing the same drug.
  Solution for injection
  EXCIPIENTS: May contain Sulfites
  - Scandonest special (Septodont Ltd)
    Adrenaline 10 microgram per 1 ml, Mepivacaine hydrochloride 20 mg per 1 ml Scandonest special 2% solution for injection 2.2ml cartridges | 50 cartridge [PoM] £21.95

Prilocaine hydrochloride   12-Nov-202

- **INDICATIONS AND DOSE**

CITANEST 1% ®

Infiltration anaesthesia | Nerve block
- BY REGIONAL ADMINISTRATION
- Adult: 100–200 mg/minute, alternatively may be given in incremental doses; dose adjusted according to site of administration and response, and in elderly and debilitated patients (smaller doses may be required); maximum 400 mg per course

PRILOTEKAL ®

Spinal anaesthesia
- BY INTRATHECAL INJECTION
- Adult: Usual dose 40–60 mg (max. per dose 80 mg), dose may need to be reduced in elderly or debilitated patients, or in late pregnancy

DOSES AT EXTREMES OF BODY-WEIGHT
- To avoid excessive dosage in obese patients, dose should be calculated on the basis of ideal body-weight.

> **IMPORTANT SAFETY INFORMATION**
> Should only be administered by, or under the direct supervision of, personnel experienced in their use, with adequate training in anaesthesia and airway management, and should not be administered parenterally unless adequate resuscitation equipment is available.

- **CONTRA-INDICATIONS**
  GENERAL CONTRA-INDICATIONS
  Acquired methaemoglobinaemia · anaemia · avoid injection into infected tissues · avoid injection into inflamed tissues · congenital methaemoglobinaemia · preparations containing preservatives should not be used for caudal, epidural, or spinal block
  SPECIFIC CONTRA-INDICATIONS
  - With intrathecal use Serious cardiac conduction disorders
  CONTRA-INDICATIONS, FURTHER INFORMATION
  - Injection site Manufacturer advises local anaesthetics should not be injected into inflamed or infected tissues. Increased absorption into the blood increases the possibility of systemic side-effects, and the local anaesthetic effect may also be reduced by altered local pH.
- **CAUTIONS** Cardiovascular disease · debilitated patients (consider dose reduction) · elderly (consider dose reduction) · epilepsy · hypovolaemia · impaired cardiac conduction · impaired respiratory function · myasthenia gravis · severe or untreated hypertension · shock
- **INTERACTIONS** → Appendix 1: anaesthetics, local
- **SIDE-EFFECTS**
- **Common or very common** Arrhythmias · dizziness · hypertension · hypotension · nausea · paraesthesia · vomiting
- **Uncommon** Neurotoxicity
- **Rare or very rare** Cardiac arrest · methaemoglobinaemia · nerve disorders
- **Frequency not known** Diplopia · respiratory depression
SIDE-EFFECTS, FURTHER INFORMATION Toxic effects after administration of local anaesthetics are a result of excessively high plasma concentrations; severe toxicity usually results from inadvertent intravascular injection or too rapid injection. The systemic toxicity of local anaesthetics mainly involves the central nervous and cardiovascular systems. The onset of toxicity can be unpredictable and delayed. Monitor as per local protocol for at least 30 minutes after administration.

Methaemoglobinaemia Methaemoglobinaemia can be treated with an intravenous injection of methylthioninium chloride.

● ALLERGY AND CROSS-SENSITIVITY
▶ Hypersensitivity and cross-sensitivity Hypersensitivity reactions occur mainly with the ester-type local anaesthetics, such as tetracaine; reactions are less frequent with the amide types, such as articaine, bupivacaine, levobupivacaine, lidocaine, mepivacaine, prilocaine, and ropivacaine. Cross-sensitivity reactions may be avoided by using the alternative chemical type.

● PREGNANCY Large doses during delivery can cause neonatal respiratory depression, hypotonia, and bradycardia after epidural block. Avoid paracervical or pudendal block in obstetrics (neonatal methaemoglobinaemia reported).
Dose adjustments Use lower doses for intrathecal use during late pregnancy.

● BREAST FEEDING Present in milk but not known to be harmful.

● HEPATIC IMPAIRMENT ▶ Manufacturer advises caution.
Dose adjustments ▶ With intrathecal use Manufacturer advises consider dose reduction.

● RENAL IMPAIRMENT Use with caution.
Dose adjustments Lower doses may be required for intrathecal anaesthesia.

● NATIONAL FUNDING/ACCESS DECISIONS
PRILOTEKAL ® For full details see funding body website
Scottish Medicines Consortium (SMC) decisions
▶ Prilocaine hydrochloride (*Prilotekal*®) for spinal anaesthesia (January 2011) SMC No. 665/10 Recommended with restrictions

● MEDICINAL FORMS There can be variation in the licensing of different medicines containing the same drug.
Solution for injection
▶ Citanest (Aspen Pharma Trading Ltd)
  Prilocaine hydrochloride 10 mg per 1 ml Citanest 1% solution for injection 50ml vials | 1 vial [PoM] £5.06
▶ Prilotekal (Sintetica Ltd)
  Prilocaine hydrochloride 20 mg per 1 ml Prilotekal 100mg/5ml solution for injection ampoules | 10 ampoule [PoM] £78.80 (Hospital only)

Prilocaine with felypressin

The properties listed below are those particular to the combination only. For the properties of the components please consider, prilocaine hydrochloride p. 1410.

● INDICATIONS AND DOSE
Dental anaesthesia
▶ BY REGIONAL ADMINISTRATION
▶ Adult: Consult expert dental sources for specific advice

● INTERACTIONS → Appendix 1: anaesthetics, local

● SIDE-EFFECTS Bradycardia · cardiac arrest · dizziness · drowsiness · hypotension · loss of consciousness · methaemoglobinaemia · myocardial contractility decreased · nervousness · respiratory arrest · seizure · tremor · vision blurred

● MEDICINAL FORMS There can be variation in the licensing of different medicines containing the same drug.
Solution for injection
▶ Citanest with Octapressin (Dentsply Ltd)
  Prilocaine hydrochloride 30 mg per 1 ml, Felypressin.03 unit per 1 ml Citanest 3% with Octapressin Dental 0.066units/2.2ml solution for injection self aspirating cartridges | 50 cartridge [PoM] [℞]

Ropivacaine hydrochloride   09-Dec-2019

● INDICATIONS AND DOSE
Acute pain, peripheral nerve block
▶ BY REGIONAL ADMINISTRATION
▶ Adult: 10–20 mg/hour, dose administered as a continuous infusion or by intermittent injection using a 2 mg/mL (0.2%) solution

Acute pain, field block
▶ BY REGIONAL ADMINISTRATION
▶ Adult: 2–200 mg, dose administered using a 2 mg/mL (0.2%) solution

Acute pain, lumbar epidural block
▶ BY LUMBAR EPIDURAL
▶ Adult: 20–40 mg, followed by 20–30 mg at least every 30 minutes, dose administered using a 2 mg/mL (0.2%) solution

Acute labour pain
▶ BY CONTINUOUS EPIDURAL INFUSION
▶ Adult: 12–20 mg/hour, dose administered using a 2 mg/mL (0.2%) solution

Acute postoperative pain
▶ BY CONTINUOUS EPIDURAL INFUSION
▶ Adult: Up to 28 mg/hour, dose administered using a 2 mg/mL (0.2%) solution

Postoperative pain, thoracic epidural block
▶ BY CONTINUOUS EPIDURAL INFUSION
▶ Adult: 12–28 mg/hour, dose administered using a 2 mg/mL (0.2%) solution

Surgical anaesthesia, field block
▶ BY REGIONAL ADMINISTRATION
▶ Adult: 7.5–225 mg, dose administered using a 7.5 mg/mL (0.75%) solution

Surgical anaesthesia, major nerve block (brachial plexus block)
▶ BY REGIONAL ADMINISTRATION
▶ Adult: 225–300 mg, dose administered using a 7.5 mg/mL (0.75%) solution

Surgical anaesthesia, thoracic epidural block (to establish block for postoperative pain)
▶ BY THORACIC EPIDURAL
▶ Adult: 38–113 mg, dose administered using a 7.5 mg/mL (0.75%) solution

Surgical anaesthesia for caesarean section
▶ BY LUMBAR EPIDURAL
▶ Adult: 113–150 mg, to be administered in incremental doses using a 7.5 mg/mL (0.75%) solution

Surgical anaesthesia, lumbar epidural block
▶ BY LUMBAR EPIDURAL
▶ Adult: 113–200 mg, dose administered using a 7.5 mg/mL (0.75%) or 10 mg/mL (1%) solution

DOSES AT EXTREMES OF BODY-WEIGHT
▶ To avoid excessive dosage in obese patients, dose may need to be calculated on the basis of ideal bodyweight.

IMPORTANT SAFETY INFORMATION
Should only be administered by, or under the direct supervision of, personnel experienced in their use, with adequate training in anaesthesia and airway management, and should not be administered parenterally unless adequate resuscitation equipment is available.

● CONTRA-INDICATIONS Avoid injection into infected tissues · avoid injection into inflamed tissues · intravenous regional anaesthesia (Bier's block) · preparations containing preservatives should not be used for caudal, epidural, or spinal block

CONTRA-INDICATIONS, FURTHER INFORMATION

▸ Injection site Manufacturer advises local anaesthetics should not be injected into inflamed or infected tissues. Increased absorption into the blood increases the possibility of systemic side-effects, and the local anaesthetic effect may also be reduced by altered local pH.

● CAUTIONS Acute porphyrias p. 1107 · cardiovascular disease · complete heart block · debilitated patients (consider dose reduction) · elderly (consider dose reduction) · epilepsy · hypovolaemia · impaired cardiac conduction · impaired respiratory function · myasthenia gravis · shock

● INTERACTIONS → Appendix 1: anaesthetics, local

● SIDE-EFFECTS

▸ Common or very common Arrhythmias · back pain · chills · dizziness · headache · hypertension · hypotension · nausea · sensation abnormal · urinary retention · vomiting

▸ Uncommon Anxiety · dyspnoea · hypothermia · neurotoxicity · syncope

▸ Rare or very rare Cardiac arrest

▸ Frequency not known Dyskinesia

SIDE-EFFECTS, FURTHER INFORMATION Toxic effects after administration of local anaesthetics are a result of excessively high plasma concentrations; severe toxicity usually results from inadvertent intravascular injection. The systemic toxicity of local anaesthetics mainly involves the central nervous and cardiovascular systems. The onset of toxicity can be unpredictable and delayed. Monitor as per local protocol for at least 30 minutes after administration.

● ALLERGY AND CROSS-SENSITIVITY

▸ Hypersensitivity and cross-sensitivity Hypersensitivity reactions occur mainly with the ester-type local anaesthetics, such as tetracaine; reactions are less frequent with the amide types, such as articaine, bupivacaine, levobupivacaine, lidocaine, mepivacaine, prilocaine, and ropivacaine. Cross-sensitivity reactions may be avoided by using the alternative chemical type.

● PREGNANCY Not known to be harmful. Do not use for paracervical block in obstetrics.

● BREAST FEEDING Not known to be harmful.

● HEPATIC IMPAIRMENT Manufacturer advises caution in severe impairment.
  Dose adjustments Manufacturer advises consider dose reduction for repeat doses in severe impairment.

● RENAL IMPAIRMENT Caution in severe impairment. Increased risk of systemic toxicity in chronic renal failure.

● MEDICINAL FORMS There can be variation in the licensing of different medicines containing the same drug.
  Solution for injection
  ELECTROLYTES: May contain Sodium
  ▸ Ropivacaine hydrochloride (Non-proprietary)
  Ropivacaine hydrochloride 2 mg per 1 ml Ropivacaine 20mg/10ml solution for injection ampoules | 10 ampoule [PoM] £16.50–£27.84 (Hospital only)
  Ropivacaine hydrochloride 7.5 mg per 1 ml Ropivacaine 75mg/10ml solution for injection ampoules | 10 ampoule [PoM] £25.00–£28.40 (Hospital only)
  Ropivacaine hydrochloride 10 mg per 1 ml Ropivacaine 100mg/10ml solution for injection ampoules | 10 ampoule [PoM] £30.00–£31.74 (Hospital only)
  ▸ Naropin (Aspen Pharma Trading Ltd)
  Ropivacaine hydrochloride 2 mg per 1 ml Naropin 20mg/10ml solution for injection ampoules | 5 ampoule [PoM] £12.79 (Hospital only)
  Ropivacaine hydrochloride 7.5 mg per 1 ml Naropin 75mg/10ml solution for injection ampoules | 5 ampoule [PoM] £15.90 (Hospital only)
  Ropivacaine hydrochloride 10 mg per 1 ml Naropin 100mg/10ml solution for injection ampoules | 5 ampoule [PoM] £19.22 (Hospital only)

Infusion
ELECTROLYTES: May contain Sodium
▸ Ropivacaine hydrochloride (Non-proprietary)
  Ropivacaine hydrochloride 2 mg per 1 ml Ropivacaine 400mg/200ml infusion bags | 5 bag [PoM] £79.35–£82.05 (Hospital only) | 10 bag [PoM] £137.00 (Hospital only)
▸ Naropin (Aspen Pharma Trading Ltd)
  Ropivacaine hydrochloride 2 mg per 1 ml Naropin 400mg/200ml infusion Polybags | 5 bag [PoM] £86.70 (Hospital only)

Tetracaine

(Amethocaine)

10-Mar-2020

● INDICATIONS AND DOSE

Anaesthesia before venepuncture or venous cannulation
▸ TO THE SKIN
▸ Child 1 month–4 years: Apply contents of up to 1 tube (applied at separate sites at a single time or appropriate proportion) to site of venepuncture or venous cannulation and cover with occlusive dressing; remove gel and dressing after 30 minutes for venepuncture and after 45 minutes for venous cannulation
▸ Child 5–17 years: Apply contents of up to 5 tubes (applied at separate sites at a single time or appropriate proportion) to site of venepuncture or venous cannulation and cover with occlusive dressing; remove gel and dressing after 30 minutes for venepuncture and after 45 minutes for venous cannulation
▸ Adult: Apply contents of up to 5 tubes (applied at separate sites at a single time or appropriate proportion) to site of venepuncture or venous cannulation and cover with occlusive dressing; remove gel and dressing after 30 minutes for venepuncture and after 45 minutes for venous cannulation

● CONTRA-INDICATIONS Should not be applied to damaged skin

● INTERACTIONS → Appendix 1: anaesthetics, local

● SIDE-EFFECTS Oedema · skin reactions
  SIDE-EFFECTS, FURTHER INFORMATION The systemic toxicity of local anaesthetics mainly involves the central nervous system; systemic side effects unlikely as minimal absorption following topical application.

● ALLERGY AND CROSS-SENSITIVITY

▸ Hypersensitivity and cross-sensitivity Hypersensitivity reactions occur mainly with the ester-type local anaesthetics, such as tetracaine; reactions are less frequent with the amide types, such as articaine, bupivacaine, levobupivacaine, lidocaine, mepivacaine, prilocaine, and ropivacaine. Cross-sensitivity reactions may be avoided by using the alternative chemical type.

● BREAST FEEDING Not known to be harmful.

● PATIENT AND CARER ADVICE
  Medicines for Children leaflet: Tetracaine gel for local anaesthesia www.medicinesforchildren.org.uk/tetracaine-gel-local-anaesthesia

● MEDICINAL FORMS There can be variation in the licensing of different medicines containing the same drug.
  Gel
  EXCIPIENTS: May contain Hydroxybenzoates (parabens)
  ▸ Ametop (Forum Health Products Ltd)
  Tetracaine 40 mg per 1 gram Ametop 4% gel | 1.5 gram [P] £1.08 DT = £1.08

Chapter 16
Emergency treatment of poisoning

CONTENTS

Poisoning, emergency treatment

22-Oct-2020

Overview

These notes provide only an overview of the treatment of poisoning, and it is strongly recommended that either **TOXBASE** or the **UK National Poisons Information Service** be consulted when there is doubt about the degree of risk or about management.

Hospital admission

Patients who have features of poisoning should generally be admitted to hospital. Patients who have taken poisons with delayed action should also be admitted, even if they appear well. Delayed-action poisons include aspirin p. 132, iron, paracetamol p. 464, tricyclic antidepressants, and co-phenotrope p. 71 (diphenoxylate with atropine, *Lomotil*®); the effects of modified-release preparations are also delayed. A note of all relevant information, including what treatment has been given, should accompany the patient to hospital.

Further information

TOXBASE, the primary clinical toxicology database of the National Poisons Information Service, is available on the internet to registered users at www.toxbase.org (a backup site is available at www.toxbasebackup.org if the main site cannot be accessed). It provides information about routine diagnosis, treatment, and management of patients exposed to drugs, household products, and industrial and agricultural chemicals.

Specialist information and advice on the treatment of poisoning is available day and night from the **UK National Poisons Information Service** on the following number: Tel: 0344 892 0111.

Advice on laboratory analytical services can be obtained from TOXBASE or from the National Poisons Information Service. Help with identifying capsules or tablets may be available from a regional medicines information centre or from the National Poisons Information Service (out of hours).

General care

It is often impossible to establish with certainty the identity of the poison and the size of the dose. This is not usually important because only a few poisons (such as opioids, paracetamol, and iron) have specific antidotes; few patients require active removal of the poison. In most patients, treatment is directed at managing symptoms as they arise. Nevertheless, knowledge of the type and timing of poisoning can help in anticipating the course of events. All relevant information should be sought from the poisoned individual and from carers or parents. However, such information should be interpreted with care because it may not be complete or entirely reliable. Sometimes symptoms arise from other illnesses and patients should be assessed carefully. Accidents may involve domestic and industrial products (the contents of which are not generally known). The **National Poisons Information Service** should be consulted when there is doubt about any aspect of suspected poisoning.

Respiration

Respiration is often impaired in unconscious patients. An obstructed airway requires immediate attention. In the absence of trauma, the airway should be opened with simple measures such as chin lift or jaw thrust. An oropharyngeal or nasopharyngeal airway may be useful in patients with reduced consciousness to prevent obstruction, provided ventilation is adequate. Intubation and ventilation should be considered in patients whose airway cannot be protected or who have respiratory acidosis because of inadequate ventilation; such patients should be monitored in a critical care area.

Most poisons that impair consciousness also depress respiration. Assisted ventilation (either mouth-to-mouth or using a bag-valve-mask device) may be needed. Oxygen is not a substitute for adequate ventilation, although it should be given in the highest concentration possible in poisoning with carbon monoxide and irritant gases.

Blood pressure

Hypotension is common in severe poisoning with central nervous system depressants. A systolic blood pressure of less than 70 mmHg may lead to irreversible brain damage or renal tubular necrosis. Hypotension should be corrected initially by raising the foot of the bed and administration of an infusion of either sodium chloride p. 1089 or a colloid. Vasoconstrictor sympathomimetics are rarely required and their use may be discussed with the National Poisons Information Service.

Fluid depletion without hypotension is common after prolonged coma and after aspirin poisoning due to vomiting, sweating, and hyperpnoea.

Hypertension, often transient, occurs less frequently than hypotension in poisoning; it may be associated with sympathomimetic drugs such as amfetamines, phencyclidine, and cocaine.

Heart

Cardiac conduction defects and arrhythmias can occur in acute poisoning, notably with tricyclic antidepressants, some antipsychotics, and some antihistamines. Arrhythmias often respond to correction of underlying hypoxia, acidosis, or other biochemical abnormalities, but ventricular arrhythmias that cause serious hypotension require treatment. If the QT interval is prolonged, specialist advice should be sought because the use of some anti-arrhythmic drugs may be inappropriate. Supraventricular arrhythmias are seldom life-threatening and drug treatment is best withheld until the patient reaches hospital.

Body temperature

Hypothermia may develop in patients of any age who have been deeply unconscious for some hours, particularly following overdose with barbiturates or phenothiazines. It may be missed unless core temperature is measured using a low-reading rectal thermometer or by some other means. Hypothermia should be managed by prevention of further heat loss and appropriate re-warming as clinically indicated.

Hyperthermia can develop in patients taking CNS stimulants; children and the elderly are also at risk when taking therapeutic doses of drugs with antimuscarinic properties. Hyperthermia is initially managed by removing all unnecessary clothing and using a fan. Sponging with **tepid** water will promote evaporation. Advice about the management of severe hyperthermia resulting from conditions such as the serotonin syndrome, should be sought from the National Poisons Information Service on the management of severe hyperthermia resulting from conditions such as the serotonin syndrome.

Both hypothermia and hyperthermia require **urgent** hospitalisation for assessment and supportive treatment.

Convulsions during poisoning

Single short-lived convulsions (lasting less than 5 minutes) do not require treatment. If convulsions are protracted or recur frequently, lorazepam p. 357 or diazepam p. 362 (preferably as emulsion) should be given by slow intravenous injection into a large vein. Benzodiazepines should not be given by the intramuscular route for convulsions. If the intravenous route is not readily available, midazolam oromucosal solution p. 358 [unlicensed use in adults and children under 3 months] can be given by the buccal route or diazepam can be administered as a rectal solution.

Methaemoglobinaemia

Drug- or chemical-induced methaemoglobinaemia should be treated with methylthioninium chloride p. 1426 if the methaemoglobin concentration is 30% or higher, or if symptoms of tissue hypoxia are present despite oxygen therapy. Methylthioninium chloride reduces the ferric iron of methaemoglobin back to the ferrous iron of haemoglobin; in high doses, methylthioninium chloride can itself cause methaemoglobinaemia.

Poison removal and elimination

Prevention of absorption

Given by mouth, charcoal, activated p. 1421 can bind many poisons in the gastro-intestinal system, thereby reducing their absorption. The **sooner** it is given the **more effective** it is, but it may still be effective up to 1 hour after ingestion of the poison—longer in the case of modified-release preparations or or of drugs with antimuscarinic (anticholinergic) properties. It is particularly useful for the prevention of absorption of poisons that are toxic in small amounts, such as antidepressants.

Active elimination techniques

Repeated doses of charcoal, activated by mouth *enhance the elimination* of some drugs after they have been absorbed; repeated doses are given after overdosage with:

- Carbamazepine
- Dapsone
- Phenobarbital
- Quinine
- Theophylline

If vomiting occurs after dosing it should be treated (e.g. with an antiemetic drug) since it may reduce the efficacy of charcoal treatment. In cases of intolerance, the dose may be reduced and the frequency increased but this may compromise efficacy.

Charcoal, activated should **not** be used for poisoning with petroleum distillates, corrosive substances, alcohols, malathion, cyanides and metal salts including iron and lithium salts.

Other techniques intended to enhance the elimination of poisons after absorption are only practicable in hospital and are only suitable for a small number of severely poisoned patients. Moreover, they only apply to a limited number of poisons. Examples include:

- haemodialysis for ethylene glycol, lithium, methanol, phenobarbital, salicylates, and sodium valproate;
- alkalinisation of the urine for salicylates.

Removal from the gastro-intestinal tract

Gastric lavage is rarely required; for substances that cannot be removed effectively by other means (e.g. iron), it should be considered only if a life-threatening amount has been ingested within the previous hour. It should be carried out only if the airway can be protected adequately. Gastric lavage is contra-indicated if a corrosive substance or a petroleum distillate has been ingested, but it may occasionally be considered in patients who have ingested drugs that are not adsorbed by charcoal, such as iron or lithium. Induction of *emesis* (e.g. with ipecacuanha) is **not** recommended because there is no evidence that it affects absorption and it may increase the risk of aspiration.

Whole bowel irrigation (by means of a bowel cleansing preparation) has been used in poisoning with certain modified-release or enteric-coated formulations, in severe poisoning with iron and lithium salts, and if illicit drugs are carried in the gastro-intestinal tract ('body-packing'). However, it is not clear that the procedure improves outcome and advice should be sought from the National Poisons Information Service.

Alcohol, acute intoxication

Acute intoxication with alcohol (ethanol) is common in adults but also occurs in children. The features include ataxia, dysarthria, nystagmus, and drowsiness, which may progress to coma, with hypotension and acidosis. Aspiration of vomit is a special hazard and hypoglycaemia may occur in children and some adults. Patients are managed supportively, with particular attention to maintaining a clear airway and measures to reduce the risk of aspiration of gastric contents. The blood glucose is measured and glucose given if indicated.

Aspirin poisoning

The main features of salicylate poisoning are hyperventilation, tinnitus, deafness, vasodilatation, and sweating. Coma is uncommon but indicates very severe poisoning. The associated acid-base disturbances are complex.

Treatment must be in hospital, where plasma salicylate, pH, and electrolytes can be measured; absorption of aspirin may be slow and the plasma-salicylate concentration may continue to rise for several hours, requiring repeated measurement. Plasma-salicylate concentration may not correlate with clinical severity in the young and the elderly, and clinical and biochemical assessment is necessary. Generally, the clinical severity of poisoning is less below a plasma-salicylate concentration of 500 mg/litre (3.6 mmol/litre), unless there is evidence of metabolic acidosis. Activated charcoal can be given within 1 hour of ingesting more than 125 mg/kg of aspirin. Fluid losses should be replaced and intravenous sodium bicarbonate may be given (ensuring plasma-potassium concentration is within

Paracetamol overdose treatment graph

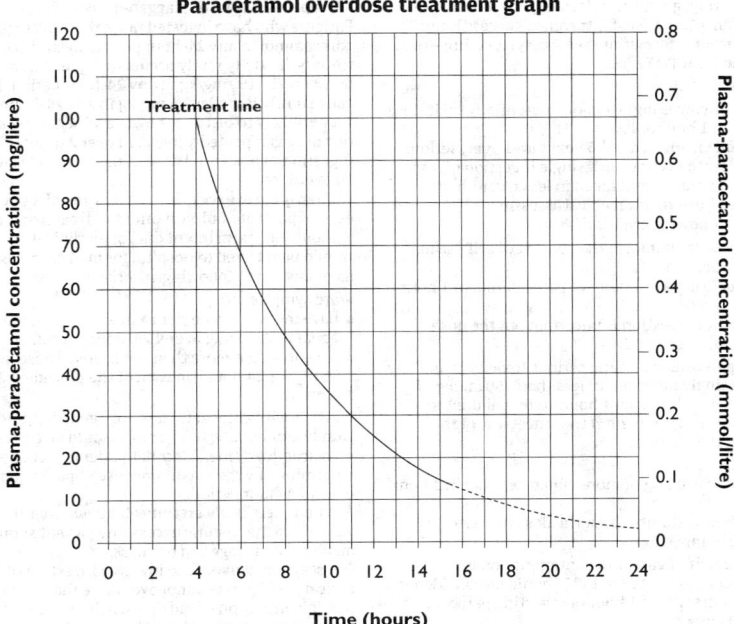

Patients whose plasma-paracetamol concentrations are on or above the **treatment line** should be treated with acetylcysteine by intravenous infusion.

The prognostic accuracy after 15 hours is uncertain, but a plasma-paracetamol concentration on or above the treatment line should be regarded as carrying a serious risk of liver damage.

Graph reproduced courtesy of Medicines and Healthcare products Regulatory Agency

the reference range) to enhance urinary salicylate excretion (optimum urinary pH 7.5–8.5).

Plasma-potassium concentration should be corrected before giving sodium bicarbonate as hypokalaemia may complicate alkalinisation of the urine.

Haemodialysis is the treatment of choice for severe salicylate poisoning and should be considered when the plasma-salicylate concentration exceeds 700 mg/litre (5.1 mmol/litre) or in the presence of severe metabolic acidosis.

Opioid poisoning

Opioids (narcotic analgesics) cause coma, respiratory depression, and pinpoint pupils. The specific antidote naloxone hydrochloride p. 1424 is indicated if there is coma or bradypnoea. Since naloxone has a shorter duration of action than many opioids, close monitoring and repeated injections are necessary according to the respiratory rate and depth of coma. When repeated administration of naloxone is required, it can be given by continuous intravenous infusion instead and the rate of infusion adjusted according to vital signs. The effects of some opioids, such as buprenorphine, are only partially reversed by naloxone.

Dextropropoxyphene and methadone have very long durations of action; patients may need to be monitored for long periods following large overdoses.

Naloxone reverses the opioid effects of dextropropoxyphene. The long duration of action of dextropropoxyphene calls for prolonged monitoring and further doses of naloxone may be required.

Norpropoxyphene, a metabolite of dextropropoxyphene,

also has cardiotoxic effects which may require treatment with sodium bicarbonate p. 1086 or magnesium sulfate p. 1099, or both. Arrhythmias may occur for up to 12 hours.

Paracetamol poisoning

In all cases of **intravenous paracetamol poisoning** clinicians are encouraged to contact the National Poisons Information Service for advice on risk assessment and management.

Toxic doses of paracetamol p. 464 may cause severe hepatocellular necrosis and, much less frequently, renal tubular necrosis. Nausea and vomiting, the early features of poisoning, usually settle within 24 hours. The recurrence of nausea and vomiting after 2–3 days, often associated with the onset of right subcostal pain and tenderness, usually indicates development of hepatic necrosis. Liver damage is maximal 3–4 days after paracetamol overdose and may lead to liver failure, encephalopathy, coma, and death.

The following guidance provides only an overview of the management of paracetamol overdosage from the *National Poisons Information Service TOXBASE* database.

To avoid underestimating the potentially toxic paracetamol dose ingested by obese patients who weigh more than 110 kg, use a body-weight of 110 kg (rather than their actual body-weight) when calculating the total dose of paracetamol ingested (in mg/kg).

Acetylcysteine p. 1425 prevents or reduces the severity of liver damage if given up to, and possibly beyond (in patients at risk of severe liver disease) 24 hours of ingesting paracetamol p. 464. It is most effective if given within 8 hours of paracetamol ingestion, after which effectiveness declines. Very rarely, giving acetylcysteine by mouth [unlicensed] is an alternative if intravenous access is not possible (for further information, see **Acetylcysteine—oral doses**, available from TOXBASE).

Acute overdose
Acute overdose involves ingestion of a potentially toxic dose of paracetamol in 1 hour or less.

For **adults and children aged 6 years and over**, serious toxicity is unlikely to occur from a single ingestion of less than 75 mg/kg of paracetamol taken in less than 1 hour. Refer patients to hospital for medical assessment if they meet any of the following criteria:
- have ingested paracetamol in the context of self-harm,
- are symptomatic,
- have ingested 75 mg/kg or more of paracetamol in 1 hour or less, or
- where the time of ingestion is uncertain but the dose ingested is 75 mg/kg or more.

For **children aged under 6 years**, serious toxicity is unlikely to occur from a single ingestion of less than 150 mg/kg of paracetamol taken in less than 1 hour. Refer children to hospital for medical assessment if they meet any of the following criteria:
- are symptomatic,
- have ingested 150 mg/kg or more of paracetamol in 1 hour or less, or
- where there is uncertainty about the dose ingested or circumstance of ingestion.

Although the benefit of gastric decontamination is uncertain, charcoal, activated p. 1421 should be considered if the patient presents within 1 hour of ingesting paracetamol in excess of 150 mg/kg.

Patients at risk of liver damage and therefore requiring acetylcysteine p. 1425, can be identified from a single measurement of the plasma-paracetamol concentration related to the time from ingestion, provided this time interval is not less than 4 hours; earlier samples cannot be interpreted. The concentration is plotted on a paracetamol treatment graph, with a reference line ('treatment line') joining plots of 100 mg/litre (0.66 mmol/litre) at 4 hours and 3.13 mg/litre (0.02 mmol/litre) at 24 hours, see *Paracetamol overdose treatment graph*.

Acetylcysteine treatment should commence in patients:
- whose plasma-paracetamol concentration falls on or above the *treatment line* on the paracetamol treatment graph;
- who present within 8 hours of ingestion of more than 150 mg/kg of paracetamol if there is going to be a delay of 8 hours or more in obtaining the paracetamol concentration after the overdose;
- who present 8–24 hours after ingestion of an acute overdose of more than 150 mg/kg of paracetamol even if the plasma-paracetamol concentration is not yet available;
- who present more than 24 hours after ingestion of an overdose if they are clearly jaundiced or have hepatic tenderness, their ALT is above the upper limit of normal (patients with chronically elevated ALT should be discussed with the National Poisons Information Service), their INR is greater than 1.3 (in the absence of another cause), or the paracetamol concentration is detectable.

Consider acetylcysteine treatment in patients who present within 24 hours of an overdose if biochemical tests suggest acute liver injury, even if the plasma paracetamol concentration is below the treatment line on the paracetamol treatment graph.

If the patient is not at risk of liver toxicity (i.e. the paracetamol concentration is below the treatment line or undetectable; the INR and ALT are normal; and the patient is asymptomatic) no treatment with an antidote is indicated; acetylcysteine may be discontinued if it has been started.

Where the time of ingestion is unknown, patients should be managed as a *staggered overdose*.

Therapeutic excess or staggered overdose
Patients who have ingested more than 150 mg/kg of paracetamol in any 24-hour period are at risk of serious toxicity. Toxicity rarely occurs with paracetamol doses between 75–150 mg/kg in any 24-hour period. Doses consistently less than 75 mg/kg in any 24-hour period are very unlikely to be toxic; however risk may be increased if this dose is repeatedly ingested over 2 or more days. Ingestion of a licensed dose of paracetamol is not considered an overdose.

Therapeutic excess is the ingestion of a potentially toxic dose of paracetamol with intent to treat pain or fever and without self-harm intent during its clinical use. All patients should be referred to hospital for medical assessment if they meet any of the following criteria:
- are symptomatic,
- have ingested more than a licensed dose and more than or equal to 75 mg/kg in any 24-hour period, or
- have ingested more than the licensed dose but less than 75 mg/kg/24 hours on each of the preceding 2 or more days.

Patients with clinical features of hepatic injury such as jaundice or hepatic tenderness should be treated urgently with acetylcysteine. For other patients, management is determined by the maximum dose of paracetamol ingested in any 24-hour period.

When there is uncertainty about whether the presentation was due to therapeutic excess, the patient should be managed as a *staggered overdose*.

A **staggered overdose** involves ingestion of a potentially toxic dose of paracetamol over more than 1 hour, with the possible intention of causing self-harm. All patients who have taken a staggered overdose should be referred to hospital for medical assessment. The MHRA advises that all patients who have ingested a staggered overdose should be treated with acetylcysteine without delay.

Clinically significant hepatotoxicity is unlikely and the patient is not considered to be at risk if, there has been at least 4 hours or more since the last paracetamol ingestion, the patient has no symptoms suggesting liver damage, the paracetamol concentration is less than 10 mg/L, their ALT is within the normal range, and their INR is 1.3 or less. Acetylcysteine can be discontinued in patients not considered to be at risk of clinically significant liver damage. If there is uncertainty about a patient's risk of toxicity after paracetamol overdose, advice should be sought from the National Poisons Information Service.

Acetylcysteine dose and administration
For paracetamol overdosage, there are two intravenous acetylcysteine regimens: the standard 21-hour regimen and the modified 12-hour regimen (also known as the Scottish and Newcastle Acetylcysteine Protocol (SNAP)). The SNAP regimen [unlicensed] is not endorsed by the MHRA, and its efficacy with regard to preventing liver toxicity is not fully established in all patterns of paracetamol overdose—it should only be used after discussion with a senior clinician. For further information, see **Acetylcysteine SNAP Doses—Adult** and **Acetylcysteine SNAP Doses—Children**, available from TOXBASE.

For the standard 21-hour regimen, acetylcysteine p. 1425 is given in a total dose that is divided into 3 consecutive intravenous infusions over a total of 21 hours. The tables below include the dose of acetylcysteine for adults and children of body-weight 40 kg and over, in terms of the volume of acetylcysteine Concentrate for Intravenous Infusion required for each of the 3 infusions. The requisite dose of acetylcysteine is added to glucose 5% p. 1090 or sodium chloride 0.9% Intravenous Infusion p. 1089. For information on dosing/administration for adults and children who weigh less than 40 kg, see **Acetylcysteine Doses—Children**, available from TOXBASE.

First infusion

Body-weight	Volume of Acetylcysteine Concentrate for Intravenous Infusion 200 mg/mL required to prepare first infusion
40–49 kg	34 mL
50–59 kg	42 mL
60–69 kg	49 mL
70–79 kg	57 mL
80–89 kg	64 mL
90–99 kg	72 mL
100–109 kg	79 mL
≥110 kg	83 mL (max. dose)

First infusion (based on an acetylcysteine dose of approx. 150 mg/kg)—add requisite volume of Acetylcysteine Concentrate for Intravenous Infusion to 200 mL Glucose 5% or sodium chloride 0.9% Intravenous Infusion; infuse over 1 hour.

Second infusion

Body-weight	Volume of Acetylcysteine Concentrate for Intravenous Infusion 200 mg/mL required to prepare second infusion
40–49 kg	12 mL
50–59 kg	14 mL
60–69 kg	17 mL
70–79 kg	19 mL
80–89 kg	22 mL
90–99 kg	24 mL
100–109 kg	27 mL
≥110 kg	28 mL (max. dose)

Second infusion (based on an acetylcysteine dose of approx. 50 mg/kg; start immediately after completion of first infusion)—add requisite volume of Acetylcysteine Concentrate for Intravenous Infusion to 500 mL Glucose 5% or sodium chloride 0.9% Intravenous Infusion; infuse over 4 hours.

Third infusion

Body-weight	Volume of Acetylcysteine Concentrate for Intravenous Infusion 200 mg/mL required to prepare third infusion
40–49 kg	23 mL
50–59 kg	28 mL
60–69 kg	33 mL
70–79 kg	38 mL
80–89 kg	43 mL
90–99 kg	48 mL
100–109 kg	53 mL
≥110 kg	55 mL (max. dose)

Third infusion (based on an acetylcysteine dose of approx. 100 mg/kg; start immediately after completion of second infusion)—add requisite volume of Acetylcysteine Concentrate for Intravenous Infusion to 1 litre Glucose 5% or sodium chloride 0.9% Intravenous Infusion; infuse over 16 hours.

Antidepressant poisoning

Tricyclic and related antidepressants

Tricyclic and related antidepressants cause dry mouth, coma of varying degree, hypotension, hypothermia, hyperreflexia, extensor plantar responses, convulsions, respiratory failure, cardiac conduction defects, and arrhythmias. Dilated pupils and urinary retention also occur. Metabolic acidosis may complicate severe poisoning; delirium with confusion, agitation, and visual and auditory hallucinations are common during recovery.

Assessment in hospital is strongly advised in case of poisoning by tricyclic and related antidepressants but symptomatic treatment can be given before transfer. Supportive measures to ensure a clear airway and adequate ventilation during transfer are mandatory. Intravenous lorazepam or intravenous diazepam (preferably in emulsion form) may be required to treat convulsions. Activated charcoal given within 1 hour of the overdose reduces absorption of the drug. Although arrhythmias are worrying, some will respond to correction of hypoxia and acidosis. The use of anti-arrhythmic drugs is best avoided, but intravenous infusion of sodium bicarbonate can arrest arrhythmias or prevent them in those with an extended QRS duration. Diazepam given by mouth is usually adequate to sedate delirious patients but large doses may be required.

Selective serotonin re-uptake inhibitors (SSRIs)

Symptoms of poisoning by selective serotonin re-uptake inhibitors include nausea, vomiting, agitation, tremor, nystagmus, drowsiness, and sinus tachycardia; convulsions may occur. Rarely, severe poisoning results in the serotonin syndrome, with marked neuropsychiatric effects, neuromuscular hyperactivity, and autonomic instability; hyperthermia, rhabdomyolysis, renal failure, and coagulopathies may develop.

Management of SSRI poisoning is supportive. Activated charcoal given within 1 hour of the overdose reduces absorption of the drug. Convulsions can be treated with lorazepam, diazepam, or midazolam oromucosal solution [unlicensed use in adults and children under 3 months] (see *Convulsions*). Contact the National Poisons Information Service for the management of hyperthermia or the serotonin syndrome.

Antimalarial poisoning

Overdosage with quinine, chloroquine, or hydroxychloroquine is extremely hazardous and difficult to treat. Urgent advice from the National Poisons Information Service is essential. Life-threatening features include arrhythmias (which can have a very rapid onset) and convulsions (which can be intractable).

Antipsychotic poisoning

Phenothiazines and related drugs

Phenothiazines cause less depression of consciousness and respiration than other sedatives. Hypotension, hypothermia, sinus tachycardia, and arrhythmias may complicate poisoning. Dystonic reactions can occur with therapeutic doses (particularly with prochlorperazine and trifluoperazine), and convulsions may occur in severe cases. Arrhythmias may respond to correction of hypoxia, acidosis, and other biochemical abnormalities, but specialist advice should be sought if arrhythmias result from a prolonged QT interval; the use of some anti-arrhythmic drugs can worsen such arrhythmias. Dystonic reactions are rapidly abolished by injection of drugs such as procyclidine hydrochloride p. 432 or diazepam p. 362 (emulsion preferred).

Second-generation antipsychotic drugs

Features of poisoning by second-generation antipsychotic drugs include drowsiness, convulsions, extrapyramidal symptoms, hypotension, and ECG abnormalities (including prolongation of the QT interval). Management is supportive.

Charcoal, activated p. 1421 can be given within 1 hour of ingesting a significant quantity of a second-generation antipsychotic drug.

Benzodiazepine poisoning

Benzodiazepines taken alone cause drowsiness, ataxia, dysarthria, nystagmus, and occasionally respiratory depression, and coma. Charcoal, activated can be given within 1 hour of ingesting a significant quantity of benzodiazepine, provided the patient is awake and the airway is protected. Benzodiazepines potentiate the effects of other central nervous system depressants taken concomitantly. Use of the benzodiazepine antagonist flumazenil p. 1422 [unlicensed indication] can be hazardous, particularly in mixed overdoses involving tricyclic antidepressants or in benzodiazepine-dependent patients. Flumazenil may prevent the need for ventilation, particularly in patients with severe respiratory disorders; it should be used on expert advice only and not as a diagnostic test in patients with a reduced level of consciousness.

Beta-blockers poisoning

Overdosages with beta-blockers may cause cardiac effects such as bradycardia, hypotension, syncope, conduction abnormalities, and heart failure. Bradycardia is the most common arrhythmia, but some beta-blockers may induce ventricular tachyarrhythmias secondary to prolongation of QT interval (e.g. sotalol) or QRS duration (e.g. propranolol). Although the predominant effects of beta-blocker overdose are on the heart, other features may also occur, such as central nervous system effects (including drowsiness, confusion, convulsions, hallucinations, and in severe cases coma), respiratory depression, and bronchospasm. The effects of overdosage can vary from one beta-blocker to another; propranolol overdosage in particular may cause coma and convulsions.

The following guidance provides only an overview of the management of beta-blocker overdosage from the *National Poisons Information Service TOXBASE database*.

All patients who have been exposed to beta-blockers as a result of self-harm should be referred for assessment. Medical assessment is recommended for all patients who are symptomatic or have ingested more than a toxic dose; and in those who are treatment naive or have taken more than their therapeutic dose, and have a significant cardiac history, asthma, chronic obstructive pulmonary disease, or are elderly. All patients who have exceeded their prescribed daily dose of 2 or more cardiotoxic agents should also be referred for medical assessment irrespective of the dose ingested. Hospital clinicians are encouraged to discuss all serious cases with the UK National Poisons Information Service.

For patients presenting with overdose, maintain a clear airway and adequate ventilation. Although the benefit of gastric decontamination is uncertain, charcoal, activated p. 1421 can be considered if the patient presents within 1 hour of ingestion of more than a potentially toxic dose.

For the management of hypotension, ensure adequate fluid resuscitation; in an emergency, vasopressors and inotropes can be initiated under the advice of an experienced physician. Intravenous glucagon p. 764 [unlicensed] is a treatment option for severe hypotension, heart failure, or cardiogenic shock. In severe cases, an insulin and glucose infusion can improve myocardial contractility and systemic perfusion, especially in the presence of acidosis. Consider intravenous sodium bicarbonate p. 1086 for correction of metabolic acidosis that persists despite correction of hypoxia and adequate fluid resuscitation—rapid correction is particularly important if QRS duration is prolonged. For symptomatic bradycardia, give intravenous atropine sulfate p. 1386; dobutamine p. 237 [unlicensed] or isoprenaline [unlicensed] (available from 'special-order' manufacturers or

specialist importing companies) may be considered if bradycardia is associated with hypotension. A temporary cardiac pacemaker can be used to increase the heart rate.

Treat bronchospasm with nebulised bronchodilators and corticosteroids.

If convulsions occur give oxygen, and correct acid-base and metabolic disturbances as required. Prolonged or frequent convulsions should be controlled with intravenous diazepam p. 362, lorazepam p. 357, or midazolam p. 358. If convulsions are unresponsive to treatment, the patient should be referred urgently to critical care.

Calcium-channel blockers poisoning

Features of calcium-channel blocker poisoning include nausea, vomiting, dizziness, agitation, confusion, and coma in severe poisoning. Metabolic acidosis and hyperglycaemia may occur. Verapamil and diltiazem have a profound cardiac depressant effect causing hypotension and arrhythmias, including complete heart block and asystole. The dihydropyridine calcium-channel blockers cause severe hypotension secondary to profound peripheral vasodilatation.

Charcoal, activated should be considered if the patient presents within 1 hour of overdosage with a calcium-channel blocker; repeated doses of activated charcoal are considered if a modified-release preparation is involved. In patients with significant features of poisoning, calcium chloride p. 1096 or calcium gluconate p. 1096 is given by injection; atropine sulfate is given to correct symptomatic bradycardia. In severe cases, an insulin and glucose infusion may be required in the management of hypotension and myocardial failure. For the management of hypotension, the choice of inotropic sympathomimetic depends on whether hypotension is secondary to vasodilatation or to myocardial depression—advice should be sought from the National Poisons Information Service.

Iron salts poisoning

Iron poisoning in childhood is usually accidental. The symptoms are nausea, vomiting, abdominal pain, diarrhoea, haematemesis, and rectal bleeding. Hypotension and hepatocellular necrosis can occur later. Coma, shock, and metabolic acidosis indicate severe poisoning.

Advice should be sought from the National Poisons Information Service if a significant quantity of iron has been ingested within the previous hour.

Mortality is reduced by intensive and specific therapy with desferrioxamine mesilate p. 1075, which chelates iron. The serum-iron concentration is measured as an emergency and intravenous desferrioxamine mesilate given to chelate absorbed iron in excess of the expected iron binding capacity. In severe toxicity intravenous desferrioxamine mesilate should be given immediately without waiting for the result of the serum-iron measurement.

Lithium poisoning

Most cases of lithium intoxication occur as a complication of long-term therapy and are caused by reduced excretion of the drug because of a variety of factors including dehydration, deterioration of renal function, infections, and co-administration of diuretics or NSAIDs (or other drugs that interact). Acute deliberate overdoses may also occur with delayed onset of symptoms (12 hours or more) owing to slow entry of lithium into the tissues and continuing absorption from modified-release formulations.

The early clinical features are non-specific and may include apathy and restlessness which could be confused with mental changes arising from the patient's depressive illness. Vomiting, diarrhoea, ataxia, weakness, dysarthria, muscle twitching, and tremor may follow. Severe poisoning is associated with convulsions, coma, renal failure, electrolyte imbalance, dehydration, and hypotension.

Therapeutic serum-lithium concentrations are within the range of 0.4–1 mmol/litre; concentrations in excess of mmol/litre are usually associated with serious toxicity and such cases may need treatment with haemodialysis if neurological symptoms or renal failure are present. In acute overdosage much higher serum-lithium concentrations may be present without features of toxicity and all that is usually necessary is to take measures to increase urine output (e.g. by increasing fluid intake but avoiding diuretics). Otherwise, treatment is supportive with special regard to electrolyte balance, renal function, and control of convulsions. Gastric lavage may be considered if it can be performed within 1 hour of ingesting significant quantities of lithium. Whole-bowel irrigation should be considered for significant ingestion, but advice should be sought from the National Poisons Information Service.

Stimulant-drug poisoning

Amfetamines cause wakefulness, excessive activity, paranoia, hallucinations, and hypertension followed by exhaustion, convulsions, hyperthermia, and coma. The early stages can be controlled by diazepam or lorazepam; advice should be sought from the National Poisons Information Service on the management of hypertension. Later, tepid sponging, anticonvulsants, and artificial respiration may be needed.

Cocaine

Cocaine stimulates the central nervous system, causing agitation, dilated pupils, tachycardia, hypertension, hallucinations, hyperthermia, hypertonia, and hyperreflexia; cardiac effects include chest pain, myocardial infarction, and arrhythmias.

Initial treatment of cocaine poisoning involves intravenous administration of diazepam to control agitation and cooling measures for hyperthermia (see Body temperature); hypertension and cardiac effects require specific treatment and expert advice should be sought.

Ecstasy

Ecstasy (methylenedioxymethamfetamine, MDMA) may cause severe reactions, even at doses that were previously tolerated. The most serious effects are delirium, coma, convulsions, ventricular arrhythmias, hyperthermia, rhabdomyolysis, acute renal failure, acute hepatitis, disseminated intravascular coagulation, adult respiratory distress syndrome, hyperreflexia, hypotension and intracerebral haemorrhage; hyponatraemia has also been associated with ecstasy use.

Treatment of methylenedioxymethamfetamine poisoning is supportive, with diazepam p. 362 to control severe agitation or persistent convulsions and close monitoring including ECG. Self-induced water intoxication should be considered in patients with ecstasy poisoning.

'Liquid ecstasy' is a term used for sodium oxybate (gamma-hydroxybutyrate, GHB), which is a sedative.

Theophylline poisoning

Theophylline and related drugs are often prescribed as modified-release formulations and toxicity can therefore be delayed. They cause vomiting (which may be severe and intractable), agitation, restlessness, dilated pupils, sinus tachycardia, and hyperglycaemia. More serious effects are haematemesis, convulsions, and supraventricular and ventricular arrhythmias. Severe hypokalaemia may develop rapidly.

Repeated doses of activated charcoal can be used to eliminate theophylline even if more than 1 hour has elapsed after ingestion and especially if a modified-release preparation has been taken (see also under Active Elimination Techniques). Ondansetron p. 454 may be effective for severe vomiting that is resistant to other antiemetics [unlicensed indication]. Hypokalaemia is corrected by intravenous infusion of potassium chloride

p. 1106 and may be so severe as to require 60 mmol/hour (high doses require ECG monitoring). Convulsions should be controlled by intravenous administration of lorazepam p. 357 or diazepam (see Convulsions). Sedation with diazepam may be necessary in agitated patients.

Provided the patient does not suffer from asthma, a short-acting beta-blocker can be administered intravenously to reverse severe tachycardia, hypokalaemia, and hyperglycaemia.

Cyanide poisoning

Oxygen should be administered to patients with cyanide poisoning. The choice of antidote depends on the severity of poisoning, certainty of diagnosis, and the cause. Dicobalt edetate p. 1421 is the antidote of choice when there is a strong clinical suspicion of severe cyanide poisoning, but it should **not** be used as a precautionary measure. Dicobalt edetate itself is toxic, associated with anaphylactoid reactions, and is potentially fatal if administered in the absence of cyanide poisoning. A regimen of sodium nitrite p. 1421 followed by sodium thiosulfate p. 1422 is an alternative if dicobalt edetate is not available.

Hydroxocobalamin p. 1072 (*Cyanokit*®—no other preparation of hydroxocobalamin is suitable) can be considered for use in victims of smoke inhalation who show signs of significant cyanide poisoning.

Ethylene glycol and methanol poisoning

Fomepizole (available from 'special-order' manufacturers or specialist importing companies) is the treatment of choice for ethylene glycol and methanol (methyl alcohol) poisoning. If necessary, **ethanol** (by mouth or by intravenous infusion) can be used, but with caution. Advice on the treatment of ethylene glycol and methanol poisoning should be obtained from the National Poisons Information Service. It is important to start antidote treatment promptly in cases of suspected poisoning with these agents.

Heavy metal poisoning

Heavy metal antidotes include succimer (DMSA) [unlicensed], unithiol (DMPS) [unlicensed], sodium calcium edetate [unlicensed], and dimercaprol. Dimercaprol in the management of heavy metal poisoning has been superseded by other chelating agents. In all cases of heavy metal poisoning, the advice of the National Poisons Information Service should be sought.

Noxious gases poisoning

Carbon monoxide

Carbon monoxide poisoning is usually due to inhalation of smoke, car exhaust, or fumes caused by blocked flues or incomplete combustion of fuel gases in confined spaces.

Immediate treatment of carbon monoxide poisoning is essential. The person should be moved to fresh air, the airway cleared, and high-flow **oxygen** 100% administered through a tight-fitting mask with an inflated face seal. Artificial respiration should be given as necessary and continued until adequate spontaneous breathing starts, or stopped only after persistent and efficient treatment of cardiac arrest has failed. The patient should be admitted to hospital because complications may arise after a delay of hours or days. Cerebral oedema may occur in severe poisoning and is treated with an intravenous infusion of mannitol p. 244. Referral for hyperbaric oxygen treatment should be discussed with the National Poisons Information Service if the patient is pregnant or in cases of severe poisoning, such as if the patient is or has been unconscious, or has psychiatric or neurological features other than a headache, or has myocardial ischaemia or an arrhythmia, or has a blood carboxyhaemoglobin concentration of more than 20%.

Sulfur dioxide, chlorine, phosgene, and ammonia

All of these gases can cause upper respiratory tract and conjunctival irritation. Pulmonary oedema, with severe breathlessness and cyanosis may develop suddenly up to 36 hours after exposure. Death may occur. Patients are kept under observation and those who develop pulmonary oedema are given oxygen. Assisted ventilation may be necessary in the most serious cases.

CS Spray poisoning

CS spray, which is used for riot control, irritates the eyes (hence 'tear gas') and the respiratory tract; symptoms normally settle spontaneously within 15 minutes. If symptoms persist, the patient should be removed to a well-ventilated area, and the exposed skin washed with soap and water after removal of contaminated clothing. Contact lenses should be removed and rigid ones washed (soft ones should be discarded). Eye symptoms should be treated by irrigating the eyes with physiological saline (or water if saline is not available) and advice sought from an ophthalmologist. Patients with features of severe poisoning, particularly respiratory complications, should be admitted to hospital for symptomatic treatment.

Nerve agent poisoning

Treatment of nerve agent poisoning is similar to organophosphorus insecticide poisoning, but advice must be sought from the National Poisons Information Service. The risk of cross-contamination is significant; adequate decontamination and protective clothing for healthcare personnel are essential. In emergencies involving the release of nerve agents, kits ('NAAS pods') containing pralidoxime chloride p. 1422 can be obtained through the Ambulance Service from the National Blood Service (or the Welsh Blood Service in South Wales or designated hospital pharmacies in Northern Ireland and Scotland—see TOXBASE for list of designated centres).

Pesticide poisoning

Organophosphorus insecticides

Organophosphorus insecticides are usually supplied as powders or dissolved in organic solvents. All are absorbed through the bronchi and intact skin as well as through the gut and inhibit cholinesterase activity, thereby prolonging and intensifying the effects of acetylcholine. Toxicity between different compounds varies considerably, and onset may be delayed after skin exposure.

Anxiety, restlessness, dizziness, headache, miosis, nausea, hypersalivation, vomiting, abdominal colic, diarrhoea, bradycardia, and sweating are common features of organophosphorus poisoning. Muscle weakness and fasciculation may develop and progress to generalised flaccid paralysis, including the ocular and respiratory muscles. Convulsions, coma, pulmonary oedema with copious bronchial secretions, hypoxia, and arrhythmias occur in severe cases. Hyperglycaemia and glycosuria without ketonuria may also be present.

Further absorption of the organophosphorus insecticide should be prevented by moving the patient to fresh air, removing soiled clothing, and washing contaminated skin. In severe poisoning it is vital to ensure a clear airway, frequent removal of bronchial secretions, and adequate ventilation and oxygenation; gastric lavage may be considered provided that the airway is protected. Atropine sulfate p. 1386 will reverse the muscarinic effects of acetylcholine and is given by intravenous injection until the skin becomes flushed and dry, the pupils dilate, and bradycardia is abolished.

Pralidoxime chloride p. 1422, a cholinesterase reactivator, is used as an adjunct to atropine sulfate in moderate or severe poisoning. It improves muscle tone within 30 minutes of administration. Pralidoxime chloride is continued until the patient has not required atropine sulfate for 12 hours.

Pralidoxime chloride can be obtained from designated centres, the names of which are held by the National Poisons Information Service.

Snake bites and animal stings

Snake bites

Envenoming from snake bite is uncommon in the UK. Many exotic snakes are kept, some illegally, but the only indigenous venomous snake is the adder (*Vipera berus*). The bite may cause local and systemic effects. Local effects include pain, swelling, bruising, and tender enlargement of regional lymph nodes. Systemic effects include early anaphylactic symptoms (transient hypotension with syncope, angioedema, urticaria, abdominal colic, diarrhoea, and vomiting), with later persistent or recurrent hypotension, ECG abnormalities, spontaneous systemic bleeding, coagulopathy, adult respiratory distress syndrome, and acute renal failure. Fatal envenoming is rare but the potential for severe envenoming must not be underestimated.

Early anaphylactic symptoms should be treated with **adrenaline/epinephrine p. 238**. Indications for european viper snake venom antiserum p. 1426 treatment include *systemic envenoming*, especially hypotension, ECG abnormalities, vomiting, haemostatic abnormalities, and marked local envenoming such that after bites on the hand or foot, swelling extends beyond the wrist or ankle within 4 hours of the bite. For those patients who present with clinical features of *severe envenoming* (e.g. shock, ECG abnormalities, or local swelling that has advanced from the foot to above the knee or from the hand to above the elbow within 2 hours of the bite), a higher initial dose of the european viper snake venom antiserum is recommended; if symptoms of *systemic envenoming* persist contact the National Poisons Information Service. Adrenaline/epinephrine injection must be immediately to hand for treatment of anaphylactic reactions to the european viper snake venom antiserum.

Antivenom is available for bites by certain foreign snakes and spiders, stings by scorpions and fish. For information on identification, management, and for supply in an emergency, telephone the National Poisons Information Service. Whenever possible the TOXBASE entry should be read, and relevant information collected, before telephoning the National Poisons Information Service.

Insect stings

Stings from ants, wasps, hornets, and bees cause local pain and swelling but seldom cause severe direct toxicity unless many stings are inflicted at the same time. If the sting is in the mouth or on the tongue local swelling may threaten the upper airway. The stings from these insects are usually treated by cleaning the area with a topical antiseptic. Bee stings should be removed as quickly as possible. Anaphylactic reactions require immediate treatment with intramuscular **adrenaline/epinephrine**; self-administered intramuscular adrenaline/epinephrine (e.g. *EpiPen®*) is the best first-aid treatment for patients with severe hypersensitivity. An inhaled bronchodilator should be used for asthmatic reactions, see also the management of anaphylaxis. A short course of an **oral antihistamine** or a **topical corticosteroid** may help to reduce inflammation and relieve itching. A vaccine containing extracts of bee and wasp venom can be used to reduce the risk of anaphylaxis and systemic reactions in patients with systemic hypersensitivity to bee or wasp stings.

Marine stings

The severe pain of weeverfish (*Trachinus vipera*) and Portuguese man-o'-war stings can be relieved by immersing the stung area immediately in uncomfortably hot, but not scalding, water (not more than 45°C). People stung by jellyfish and Portuguese man-o'-war around the UK coast should be removed from the sea as soon as possible.

dherent tentacles should be lifted off carefully (wearing
loves or using tweezers) or washed off with seawater.
lcoholic solutions, including suntan lotions, should **not** be
pplied because they can cause further discharge of stinging
airs. Ice packs can be used to reduce pain.

ther poisons

Consult either the National Poisons Information Service day
nd night or TOXBASE.

The **National Poisons Information Service** (Tel: 0344
92 0111) will provide specialist advice on all aspects of
oisoning day and night.

◄ Active elimination from the gastro-intestinal tract

ANTIDOTES AND CHELATORS > INTESTINAL
ADSORBENTS

Charcoal, activated   23-Jul-2020

- ● INDICATIONS AND DOSE
Reduction of absorption of poisons in the gastro-intestinal system
  ▸ BY MOUTH
  ▸ Neonate: 1 g/kg.

  ▸ Child 1 month–11 years: 1 g/kg (max. per dose 50 g)
  ▸ Child 12–17 years: 50 g
  ▸ Adult: 50 g
Active elimination of poisons
  ▸ BY MOUTH
  ▸ Neonate: 1 g/kg every 4 hours, dose may be reduced and the frequency increased if not tolerated, reduced dose may compromise efficacy

  ▸ Child 1 month–11 years: 1 g/kg every 4 hours (max. per dose 50 g), dose may be reduced and the frequency increased if not tolerated, reduced dose may compromise efficacy
  ▸ Child 12–17 years: Initially 50 g, then 50 g every 4 hours, reduced if not tolerated to 25 g every 2 hours, alternatively 12.5 g every 1 hour, reduced dose may compromise efficacy
  ▸ Adult: Initially 50 g, then 50 g every 4 hours, reduced if not tolerated to 25 g every 2 hours, alternatively 12.5 g every 1 hour, reduced dose may compromise efficacy
Accelerated elimination of teriflunomide
  ▸ BY MOUTH USING GRANULES
  ▸ Adult: 50 g every 12 hours for 11 days
Accelerated elimination of leflunomide (washout procedure)
  ▸ BY MOUTH USING GRANULES
  ▸ Adult: 50 g 4 times a day for 11 days

- ● UNLICENSED USE
  ▸ In adults Activated charcoal doses in BNF may differ from those in product literature.
- ● CAUTIONS Comatose patient (risk of aspiration—ensure airway is protected) · drowsy patient (risk of aspiration—ensure airway protected) · reduced gastrointestinal motility (risk of obstruction)
- ● SIDE-EFFECTS Bezoar · constipation · diarrhoea · gastrointestinal disorders
- ● DIRECTIONS FOR ADMINISTRATION TOXBASE advises suspension or reconstituted powder may be mixed with soft drinks (e.g. caffeine-free diet cola) or fruit juices to mask the taste.

- ● MEDICINAL FORMS There can be variation in the licensing of different medicines containing the same drug.
Oral suspension
  ▸ Charcodote (Teva UK Ltd)
    Activated charcoal 200 mg per 1 ml Charcodote 200mg/ml oral suspension sugar-free | 250 ml Ⓟ £11.88
Granules
  ▸ Carbomix (Kent Pharmaceuticals Ltd)
    Activated charcoal 813 mg per 1 gram Carbomix 81.3% granules sugar-free | 50 gram Ⓟ £11.90

2 Chemical toxicity

2.1 Cyanide toxicity

ANTIDOTES AND CHELATORS

Dicobalt edetate

- ● INDICATIONS AND DOSE
Severe poisoning with cyanides
  ▸ BY INTRAVENOUS INJECTION
  ▸ Child: Consult the National Poisons Information Service
  ▸ Adult: 300 mg, to be given over 1 minute (or 5 minutes if condition less serious), dose to be followed immediately by 50 mL of glucose intravenous infusion 50%; if response inadequate a second dose of both may be given, but risk of cobalt toxicity

- ● CAUTIONS Owing to toxicity to be used only for definite cyanide poisoning when patient tending to lose, or has lost, consciousness
- ● SIDE-EFFECTS Reflex tachycardia · vomiting
- ● EXCEPTIONS TO LEGAL CATEGORY Prescription only medicine restriction does not apply where administration is for saving life in emergency.
- ● MEDICINAL FORMS No licensed medicines listed.

Sodium nitrite   16-Mar-2018

- ● INDICATIONS AND DOSE
Poisoning with cyanides (used in conjunction with sodium thiosulfate)
  ▸ BY INTRAVENOUS INJECTION
  ▸ Child: Consult the National Poisons Information Service
  ▸ Adult: 300 mg

- ● SIDE-EFFECTS Arrhythmias · dizziness · headache · hypotension · palpitations
- ● EXCEPTIONS TO LEGAL CATEGORY Prescription only medicine restriction does not apply where administration is for saving life in emergency.
- ● MEDICINAL FORMS There can be variation in the licensing of different medicines containing the same drug.
Solution for injection
  ▸ Sodium nitrite (Non-proprietary)
    Sodium nitrite 30 mg per 1 ml Sodium nitrite 300mg/10ml solution for injection vials | 1 vial PoM Ⓢ (Hospital only)

16

Emergency treatment of poisoning

Sodium thiosulfate

16-Mar-2018

● **INDICATIONS AND DOSE**

Poisoning with cyanides

▸ BY INTRAVENOUS INJECTION

▸ **Child:** Consult the National Poisons Information Service

▸ **Adult:** 12.5 g, to be given over 10 minutes, dose may be repeated in severe cyanide poisoning

DOSE EQUIVALENCE AND CONVERSION

▸ 12.5 g equates to 50 mL of a 25% solution *or* 25 mL of a 50% solution.

● EXCEPTIONS TO LEGAL CATEGORY Prescription only medicine restriction does not apply where administration is for saving life in emergency.

● MEDICINAL FORMS There can be variation in the licensing of different medicines containing the same drug. Forms available from special-order manufacturers include: solution for injection

Solution for injection

▸ Sodium thiosulfate (Non-proprietary)
Sodium thiosulfate 250 mg per 1 ml Sodium thiosulfate 12.5g/50ml solution for injection vials | 1 vial [PoM] 🅢 (Hospital only)

2.2 Organophosphorus toxicity

Other drugs used for Organophosphorus toxicity Atropine sulfate, p. 1386

ANTIDOTES AND CHELATORS

Pralidoxime chloride

30-Jul-2020

● **INDICATIONS AND DOSE**

Adjunct to atropine in the treatment of poisoning by organophosphorus insecticide or nerve agent

▸ BY INTRAVENOUS INFUSION

▸ **Child:** Initially 30 mg/kg, to be given over 20 minutes, followed by 8 mg/kg/hour; maximum 12 g per day

▸ **Adult:** Initially 30 mg/kg, to be given over 20 minutes, followed by 8 mg/kg/hour; maximum 12 g per day

● UNLICENSED USE Pralidoxime chloride doses may differ from those in product literature.

▸ In children Licensed for use in children (age range not specified by manufacturer).

● CONTRA-INDICATIONS Poisoning with carbamates · poisoning with organophosphorus compounds without anticholinesterase activity

● CAUTIONS Myasthenia gravis

● SIDE-EFFECTS Dizziness · drowsiness · headache · hyperventilation · muscle weakness · nausea · tachycardia · vision disorders

● RENAL IMPAIRMENT Use with caution.

● DIRECTIONS FOR ADMINISTRATION Manufacturer advises the loading dose may be administered by intravenous injection (diluted to a concentration of 50 mg/mL with water for injections) over at least 5 minutes if pulmonary oedema is present or if it is not practical to administer an intravenous infusion.

▸ In children For *intravenous infusion*, manufacturer advises reconstitute each vial with 20 mL Water for Injections, then dilute to a concentration of 10–20 mg/mL with Sodium Chloride 0.9%.

● PRESCRIBING AND DISPENSING INFORMATION Available from designated centres for organophosphorus insecticide poisoning or from the National Blood Service (or Welsh

Ambulance Services for Mid West and South East Wales)—see TOXBASE for list of designated centres).

● EXCEPTIONS TO LEGAL CATEGORY Prescription only medicine restriction does not apply where administration is for saving life in emergency.

● MEDICINAL FORMS There can be variation in the licensing of different medicines containing the same drug.

Powder for solution for injection

▸ Protopam Chloride (Imported (United States))
Pralidoxime chloride 1 gram Protopam Chloride 1g powder for solution for injection vials | 6 vial [PoM] 🅢

3 Drug toxicity

3.1 Benzodiazepine toxicity

ANTIDOTES AND CHELATORS ›
BENZODIAZEPINE ANTAGONISTS

Flumazenil

24-Jul-2020

● **INDICATIONS AND DOSE**

Reversal of sedative effects of benzodiazepines in anaesthesia and clinical procedures

▸ BY INTRAVENOUS INJECTION

▸ **Adult:** 200 micrograms, dose to be administered over 15 seconds, then 100 micrograms every 1 minute if required; usual dose 300–600 micrograms; maximum 1 mg per course

Reversal of sedative effects of benzodiazepines in intensive care

▸ BY INTRAVENOUS INJECTION

▸ **Adult:** 300 micrograms, dose to be administered over 15 seconds, then 100 micrograms every 1 minute if required; maximum 2 mg per course

Reversal of sedative effects of benzodiazepines in intensive care (if drowsiness recurs after injection)

▸ INITIALLY BY INTRAVENOUS INFUSION

▸ **Adult:** 100–400 micrograms/hour, adjusted according to response, alternatively (by intravenous injection) 300 micrograms, adjusted according to response

---

IMPORTANT SAFETY INFORMATION
Flumazenil should only be administered by, or under the direct supervision of, personnel experienced in its use.

● CONTRA-INDICATIONS Life-threatening condition (e.g. raised intracranial pressure, status epilepticus) controlled by benzodiazepines

● CAUTIONS Avoid rapid injection following major surgery · avoid rapid injection in high-risk or anxious patients · benzodiazepine dependence (may precipitate withdrawal symptoms) · elderly · ensure neuromuscular blockade cleared before giving · head injury (rapid reversal of benzodiazepine sedation may cause convulsions) · history of panic disorders (risk of recurrence) · prolonged benzodiazepine therapy for epilepsy (risk of convulsions) · short-acting (repeat doses may be necessary—benzodiazepine effects may persist for at least 24 hours)

● SIDE-EFFECTS

▸ **Common or very common** Anxiety · diplopia · dry mouth · eye disorders · flushing · headache · hiccups · hyperhidrosis · hyperventilation · hypotension · insomnia · nausea · palpitations · paraesthesia · speech disorder · tremor · vertigo · vomiting

▸ **Uncommon** Abnormal hearing · arrhythmias · chest pain · chills · cough · dyspnoea · nasal congestion · seizure (more common in patients with epilepsy)

Frequency not known Withdrawal syndrome

▸ PREGNANCY Not known to be harmful.

▸ BREAST FEEDING Avoid breast-feeding for 24 hours.

▸ HEPATIC IMPAIRMENT Manufacturer advises caution (risk of increased half-life).
Dose adjustments Manufacturer advises cautious dose titration.

▸ DIRECTIONS FOR ADMINISTRATION For *continuous intravenous infusion*, manufacturer advises dilute with Glucose 5% or Sodium Chloride 0.9%.

▸ MEDICINAL FORMS There can be variation in the licensing of different medicines containing the same drug.
Solution for injection
▸ Flumazenil (Non-proprietary)
  Flumazenil 100 microgram per 1 ml Flumazenil 500micrograms/5ml solution for injection ampoules | 5 ampoule [PoM] £65.50–£72.46 (Hospital only) | 10 ampoule [PoM] £140.00 (Hospital only)

3.2 Digoxin toxicity

ANTIDOTES AND CHELATORS ⟩ ANTIBODIES

Digoxin-specific antibody
20-Jul-2020

● INDICATIONS AND DOSE

Treatment of known or strongly suspected life-threatening digoxin toxicity associated with ventricular arrhythmias or bradyarrhythmias unresponsive to atropine and when measures beyond the withdrawal of digoxin and correction of any electrolyte abnormalities are considered necessary
▸ BY INTRAVENOUS INFUSION
▸ Child: Serious cases of digoxin toxicity should be discussed with the National Poisons Information Service (consult product literature)
▸ Adult: Serious cases of digoxin toxicity should be discussed with the National Poisons Information Service (consult product literature)

● DIRECTIONS FOR ADMINISTRATION
▸ In adults For *intravenous infusion* (*DigiFab*®), manufacturer advises give intermittently in Sodium chloride 0.9%. Reconstitute with water for injections (4 mL/vial), then dilute with infusion fluid and give over 30 minutes.

● MEDICINAL FORMS There can be variation in the licensing of different medicines containing the same drug.
Powder for solution for infusion
▸ DigiFab (BTG International Ltd)
  Digoxin-specific antibody fragments 40 mg DigiFab 40mg powder for solution for infusion vials | 1 vial [PoM] £750.00 (Hospital only)

3.3 Heparin toxicity

ANTIDOTES AND CHELATORS

Protamine sulfate
02-Dec-2020

● INDICATIONS AND DOSE

Overdosage with intravenous injection of unfractionated heparin
▸ BY INTRAVENOUS INJECTION
▸ Adult: Dose to be administered at a rate not exceeding 5 mg/minute, 1 mg neutralises 80–100 units heparin when given within 15 minutes; if longer than 15 minute since heparin, less protamine required (consult product

literature for details) as heparin rapidly excreted; maximum 50 mg

Overdosage with intravenous infusion of unfractionated heparin
▸ BY INTRAVENOUS INJECTION
▸ Adult: 25–50 mg, to be administered once heparin infusion stopped at a rate not exceeding 5 mg/minute

Overdosage with subcutaneous injection of unfractionated heparin
▸ INITIALLY BY INTRAVENOUS INJECTION
▸ Adult: Initially 25–50 mg, to be administered at a rate not exceeding 5 mg/minute, 1 mg neutralises 100 units heparin, then (by intravenous infusion), any remaining dose to be administered over 8–16 hours; maximum 50 mg per course

Overdosage with subcutaneous injection of low molecular weight heparin
▸ BY INTRAVENOUS INJECTION, OR BY CONTINUOUS INTRAVENOUS INFUSION
▸ Adult: Dose to be administered by intermittent intravenous injection at a rate not exceeding 5 mg/minute, 1 mg neutralises approx. 100 units low molecular weight heparin (consult product literature of low molecular weight heparin for details); maximum 50 mg

● CAUTIONS Excessive doses can have an anticoagulant effect

● SIDE-EFFECTS
▸ **Rare or very rare** Hypertension · pulmonary oedema non-cardiogenic
▸ **Frequency not known** Acute pulmonary vasoconstriction · back pain · bradycardia · circulatory collapse · dyspnoea · fatigue · feeling hot · flushing · nausea · pulmonary hypertension · vomiting

● ALLERGY AND CROSS-SENSITIVITY [EvGr] Caution if increased risk of allergic reaction to protamine (includes previous treatment with protamine or protamine insulin, allergy to fish, men who are infertile or who have had a vasectomy and who may have antibodies to protamine). ◈Ⓜ

● MONITORING REQUIREMENTS Monitor activated partial thromboplastin time or other appropriate blood clotting parameters.

● PRESCRIBING AND DISPENSING INFORMATION The long half-life of low molecular weight heparins should be taken into consideration when determining the dose of protamine sulfate; the effects of low molecular weight heparins can persist for up to 24 hours after administration.

● MEDICINAL FORMS There can be variation in the licensing of different medicines containing the same drug.
Solution for injection
▸ Protamine sulfate (Non-proprietary)
  Protamine sulfate 10 mg per 1 ml Protamine sulfate 100mg/10ml solution for injection ampoules | 5 ampoule [PoM] [Ⓢ]
  Protamine sulfate 50mg/5ml solution for injection ampoules | 10 ampoule [PoM] £49.55

3.4 Opioid toxicity

OPIOID RECEPTOR ANTAGONISTS

| Naloxone hydrochloride   08-Jan-2020

- **INDICATIONS AND DOSE**

Overdosage with opioids
▶ **BY INTRAVENOUS INJECTION**
▸ **Child 1 month–11 years:** Initially 100 micrograms/kg
(max. per dose 2 mg), if no response, repeat at intervals
of 1 minute to a max. of 2 mg, then review diagnosis;
further doses may be required if respiratory function
deteriorates, doses can be given by subcutaneous or
intramuscular routes but only if intravenous route is
not feasible; intravenous administration has more
rapid onset of action
▸ **Child 12–17 years:** Initially 400 micrograms, then
800 micrograms for up to 2 doses at 1 minute intervals
if no response to preceding dose, then increased to
2 mg for 1 dose if still no response (4 mg dose may be
required in seriously poisoned patients), then review
diagnosis; further doses may be required if respiratory
function deteriorates, doses can be given by
subcutaneous or intramuscular routes but only if
intravenous route is not feasible; intravenous
administration has more rapid onset of action
▸ **Adult:** Initially 400 micrograms, then 800 micrograms
for up to 2 doses at 1 minute intervals if no response to
preceding dose, then increased to 2 mg for 1 dose if still
no response (4 mg dose may be required in seriously
poisoned patients), then review diagnosis; further
doses may be required if respiratory function
deteriorates, doses can be given by subcutaneous or
intramuscular routes but only if intravenous route is
not feasible; intravenous administration has more
rapid onset of action
▶ **BY CONTINUOUS INTRAVENOUS INFUSION**
▸ **Child:** Using an infusion pump, adjust rate according to
response (initially, rate may be set at 60% of the initial
resuscitative intravenous injection dose per hour). The
initial resuscitative *intravenous injection* dose is that
which maintained satisfactory ventilation for at least
15 minutes
▸ **Adult:** Using an infusion pump, adjust rate according to
response (initially, rate may be set at 60% of the initial
resuscitative intravenous injection dose per hour). The
initial resuscitative *intravenous injection* dose is that
which maintained satisfactory ventilation for at least
15 minutes
▶ **BY INTRANASAL ADMINISTRATION**
▸ **Child 14–17 years:** 1.8 mg, administered into one nostril,
if no response, give a second dose after 2–3 minutes. If
the patient responds to the first dose then relapses into
respiratory depression, give the second dose
immediately. Further doses should be administered
into alternate nostrils
▸ **Adult:** 1.8 mg, administered into one nostril, if no
response, give a second dose after 2–3 minutes. If the
patient responds to the first dose then relapses into
respiratory depression, give the second dose
immediately. Further doses should be administered
into alternate nostrils

Overdosage with opioids in a non-medical setting
▶ **BY INTRAMUSCULAR INJECTION**
▸ **Adult:** 400 micrograms every 2–3 minutes, each dose
given in subsequent resuscitation cycles if patient not
breathing normally, continue until consciousness
regained, breathing normally, medical assistance

available, or contents of syringe used up; to be injected
into deltoid region or anterolateral thigh
▶ **BY INTRANASAL ADMINISTRATION**
▸ **Child 14–17 years:** 1.8 mg, administered into one nostril,
if no response, give a second dose after 2–3 minutes. If
the patient responds to the first dose then relapses into
respiratory depression, give the second dose
immediately. Further doses should be administered
into alternate nostrils
▸ **Adult:** 1.8 mg, administered into one nostril, if no
response, give a second dose after 2–3 minutes. If the
patient responds to the first dose then relapses into
respiratory depression, give the second dose
immediately. Further doses should be administered
into alternate nostrils

Reversal of postoperative respiratory depression
▶ **INITIALLY BY INTRAVENOUS INJECTION**
▸ **Child 1 month–11 years:** 1 microgram/kg, repeated every
2–3 minutes if required
▸ **Child 12–17 years:** Initially 100–200 micrograms,
alternatively (by intravenous injection) initially
1.5–3 micrograms/kg, if response inadequate, give
subsequent doses, (by intravenous injection)
100 micrograms every 2 minutes, alternatively (by
intramuscular injection) 100 micrograms every
1–2 hours
▸ **Adult:** Initially 100–200 micrograms, alternatively (by
intravenous injection) initially 1.5–3 micrograms/kg, if
response inadequate, give subsequent doses, (by
intravenous injection) 100 micrograms every
2 minutes, alternatively (by intramuscular injection)
100 micrograms every 1–2 hours

DOSE EQUIVALENCE AND CONVERSION
▸ With intranasal use
▸ 1 spray equivalent to 1.8 mg.

PHARMACOKINETICS
▸ Naloxone has a short duration of action; repeated doses
or infusion may be necessary to reverse effects of
opioids with longer duration of action.

- **UNLICENSED USE** Naloxone doses in BNF may differ from
those in product literature.

> **IMPORTANT SAFETY INFORMATION**
> **SAFE PRACTICE**
> Doses used in acute opioid overdosage may not be
> appropriate for the management of opioid-induced
> respiratory depression and sedation in those receiving
> palliative care and in chronic opioid use.

- **CAUTIONS** Cardiovascular disease or those receiving
cardiotoxic drugs (serious adverse cardiovascular effects
reported) · maternal physical dependence on opioids (may
precipitate withdrawal in newborn) · pain · physical
dependence on opioids (precipitates withdrawal)
CAUTIONS, FURTHER INFORMATION
▸ Titration of dose In postoperative use, the dose should be
titrated for each patient in order to obtain sufficient
respiratory response; however, naloxone antagonises
analgesia.

- **SIDE-EFFECTS**
GENERAL SIDE-EFFECTS
▶ **Common or very common** Arrhythmias · dizziness ·
headache · hypertension · hypotension · nausea · vomiting
▶ **Uncommon** Diarrhoea · dry mouth · hyperhidrosis ·
hyperventilation · tremor
▶ **Rare or very rare** Cardiac arrest · erythema multiforme ·
pulmonary oedema

SPECIFIC SIDE-EFFECTS
Uncommon
With parenteral use Inflammation localised · pain · vascular irritation
Rare or very rare
With parenteral use Anxiety · seizure
Frequency not known
With parenteral use Analgesia reversed · asthenia · chills · death · dyspnoea · fever · irritability · nasal complaints · piloerection · yawning
PREGNANCY Use only if potential benefit outweighs risk.
BREAST FEEDING Not orally bioavailable.

DIRECTIONS FOR ADMINISTRATION
With intravenous use in children For *continuous intravenous infusion*, dilute to a concentration of up to 200 micrograms/mL with Glucose 5% or Sodium Chloride 0.9%.
With intravenous use in adults For *intravenous infusion* (*Minijet* ® Naloxone Hydrochloride), give continuously in Glucose 5% or Sodium Chloide 0.9%. Dilute to a concentration of up to 200 micrograms/mL and administer via an infusion pump.

▶ PRESCRIBING AND DISPENSING INFORMATION
With intranasal use The manufacturer has provided a *Healthcare Professional Guidance Document.*

▶ PATIENT AND CARER ADVICE Patients and carers should be given advice on how to administer naloxone nasal spray.
With intranasal use Patient training and information cards should be provided.

▶ MEDICINAL FORMS There can be variation in the licensing of different medicines containing the same drug.
Solution for injection
▶ Naloxone hydrochloride (Non-proprietary)
  Naloxone hydrochloride 20 microgram per 1 ml Naloxone 40micrograms/2ml solution for injection ampoules | 10 ampoule PoM £55.00
  Naloxone hydrochloride (as Naloxone hydrochloride dihydrate) 400 microgram per 1 ml Naloxone 400micrograms/1ml solution for injection ampoules | 10 ampoule PoM £36.00–£45.00 DT = £40.51
  Naloxone hydrochloride 1 mg per 1 ml Naloxone 2mg/2ml solution for injection pre-filled syringes | 1 pre-filled disposable injection PoM £16.80
▶ Prenoxad (Martindale Pharmaceuticals Ltd)
  Naloxone hydrochloride 1 mg per 1 ml Prenoxad 2mg/2ml solution for injection pre-filled syringes | 1 pre-filled disposable injection PoM £18.00
Spray
▶ Nyxoid (Napp Pharmaceuticals Ltd)
  Naloxone (as Naloxone hydrochloride dihydrate) 18 mg per 1 ml Nyxoid 1.8mg/0.1ml nasal spray 0.1ml unit dose | 2 unit dose PoM £26.00

3.5 Paracetamol toxicity

ANTIDOTES AND CHELATORS

Acetylcysteine   05-Oct-2020

● INDICATIONS AND DOSE
Paracetamol overdosage
▶ BY INTRAVENOUS INFUSION
▶ Child (body-weight up to 20 kg): Initially 150 mg/kg over 1 hour, dose to be administered in 3 mL/kg glucose 5%, followed by 50 mg/kg over 4 hours, dose to be administered in 7 mL/kg glucose 5%, then 100 mg/kg over 16 hours, dose to be administered in 14 mL/kg glucose 5%
▶ Child (body-weight 20-39 kg): Initially 150 mg/kg over 1 hour, dose to be administered in 100 mL glucose 5%, followed by 50 mg/kg over 4 hours, dose to be

administered in 250 mL glucose 5%, then 100 mg/kg over 16 hours, dose to be administered in 500 mL glucose 5%
▶ Child (body-weight 40 kg and above): 150 mg/kg over 1 hour, dose to be administered in 200 mL glucose 5%, then 50 mg/kg over 4 hours, to be started immediately after completion of first infusion, dose to be administered in 500 mL glucose 5%, then 100 mg/kg over 16 hours, to be started immediately after completion of second infusion, dose to be administered in 1 litre glucose 5%
▶ Adult (body-weight 40 kg and above): 150 mg/kg over 1 hour, dose to be administered in 200 mL glucose 5%, then 50 mg/kg over 4 hours, to be started immediately after completion of first infusion, dose to be administered in 500 mL glucose 5%, then 100 mg/kg over 16 hours, to be started immediately after completion of second infusion, dose to be administered in 1 litre glucose 5%

DOSES AT EXTREMES OF BODY-WEIGHT
▶ To avoid excessive dosage in obese patients, a ceiling weight of 110 kg should be used when calculating the dose for paracetamol overdosage.

┌───┐
│ IMPORTANT SAFETY INFORMATION   │
│ MHRA/CHM ADVICE: INTRAVENOUS ACETYLCYSTEINE FOR │
│ PARACETAMOL OVERDOSE: REMINDER OF AUTHORISED DOSE │
│ REGIMEN; POSSIBLE NEED FOR CONTINUED TREATMENT │
│ (JANUARY 2017)   │
│ The authorised dose regimen for acetylcysteine in │
│ paracetamol overdose is 3 consecutive intravenous │
│ infusions given over a total of 21 hours.   │
│   Continued treatment (given at the dose and rate as │
│ used in the third infusion) may be necessary depending │
│ on the clinical evaluation of the individual patient. │
└───┘

● CAUTIONS Asthma (see Side-effects for management of asthma but do not delay acetylcysteine treatment) · atopy · may slightly increase INR · may slightly increase prothrombin time

● SIDE-EFFECTS
▶ **Frequency not known** Acidosis · anaphylactoid reaction · angioedema · anxiety · arrhythmias · cardiac arrest · chest discomfort · cough · cyanosis · eye pain · eye swelling · generalised seizure · hyperhidrosis · hypertension · hypotension · joint disorders · malaise · nausea · pain facial · respiratory disorders · skin reactions · syncope · thrombocytopenia · vasodilation · vision blurred · vomiting

SIDE-EFFECTS, FURTHER INFORMATION Anaphylactoid reactions can be managed by suspending treatment and initiating appropriate management. Treatment may then be restarted at lower rate.

● DIRECTIONS FOR ADMINISTRATION For *intravenous infusion*, manufacturer advises Glucose 5% is preferred fluid; Sodium Chloride 0.9% is an alternative if Glucose 5% unsuitable.

● MEDICINAL FORMS There can be variation in the licensing of different medicines containing the same drug. Forms available from special-order manufacturers include: solution for infusion
Solution for infusion
ELECTROLYTES: May contain Sodium
▶ Acetylcysteine (Non-proprietary)
  Acetylcysteine 200 mg per 1 ml Acetylcysteine 2g/10ml solution for infusion ampoules | 10 ampoule PoM £21.26 DT = £21.26
▶ Parvolex (Phoenix Labs Ltd)
  Acetylcysteine 200 mg per 1 ml Parvolex 2g/10ml concentrate for solution for infusion ampoules | 10 ampoule PoM £22.50 DT = £21.26

16

Emergency treatment of poisoning

4 Methaemoglobinaemia

ANTIDOTES AND CHELATORS

Methylthioninium chloride

29-Jul-2020

(Methylene blue)

- **INDICATIONS AND DOSE**

Drug- or chemical-induced methaemoglobinaemia
▸ BY SLOW INTRAVENOUS INJECTION
▸ Child 3 months–17 years: Initially 1–2 mg/kg, then 1–2 mg/kg after 30–60 minutes if required, to be given over 5 minutes, seek advice from National Poisons Information Service if further repeat doses are required; maximum 7 mg/kg per course
▸ Adult: Initially 1–2 mg/kg, then 1–2 mg/kg after 30–60 minutes if required, to be given over 5 minutes, seek advice from National Poisons Information Service if further repeat doses are required; maximum 7 mg/kg per course

Aniline- or dapsone-induced methaemoglobinaemia
▸ BY SLOW INTRAVENOUS INJECTION
▸ Child 3 months–17 years: Initially 1–2 mg/kg, then 1–2 mg/kg after 30–60 minutes if required, to be given over 5 minutes, seek advice from National Poisons Information Service if further repeat doses are required; maximum 4 mg/kg per course
▸ Adult: Initially 1–2 mg/kg, then 1–2 mg/kg after 30–60 minutes if required, to be given over 5 minutes, seek advice from National Poisons Information Service if further repeat doses are required; maximum 4 mg/kg per course

- **CAUTIONS** Chlorate poisoning (reduces efficacy of methylthioninium) · G6PD deficiency (seek advice from National Poisons Information Service) · methaemoglobinaemia due to treatment of cyanide poisoning with sodium nitrite (seek advice from National Poisons Information Service) · pulse oximetry may give false estimation of oxygen saturation

- **INTERACTIONS** → Appendix 1: methylthioninium chloride

- **SIDE-EFFECTS**
▸ **Common or very common** Abdominal pain · anxiety · chest pain · dizziness · headache · hyperhidrosis · nausea · pain in extremity · paraesthesia · skin reactions · taste altered · urine discolouration · vomiting
▸ **Frequency not known** Aphasia · arrhythmias · confusion · faeces discoloured · fever · haemolytic anaemia · hyperbilirubinaemia (in infants) · hypertension · hypotension · injection site necrosis · mydriasis · tremor

- **PREGNANCY** No information available, but risk to fetus of untreated methaemoglobinaemia likely to be significantly higher than risk of treatment.

- **BREAST FEEDING** Manufacturer advises avoid breastfeeding for up to 6 days after administration—no information available.

- **RENAL IMPAIRMENT**
Dose adjustments Use with caution in severe impairment; dose reduction may be required.

- **DIRECTIONS FOR ADMINISTRATION**
▸ In children For *intravenous injection*, manufacturer advises may be diluted with Glucose 5% to minimise injection-site pain; not compatible with Sodium Chloride 0.9%.

- **MEDICINAL FORMS** There can be variation in the licensing of different medicines containing the same drug. Forms available from special-order manufacturers include: solution for injection

Solution for injection
▸ Methylthioninium chloride (Non-proprietary)
  Methylthioninium chloride 5 mg per 1 ml Methylthioninium chloride Proveblue 50mg/10ml solution for injection ampoules | 5 ampoule [PoM] £196.89
  Methylthioninium chloride 10 mg per 1 ml Methylthioninium chloride 50mg/5ml concentrate for solution for injection vials | 5 vial [PoM] £150.00 (Hospital only)

5 Snake bites

IMMUNE SERA AND IMMUNOGLOBULINS ⟩
ANTITOXINS

European viper snake venom antiserum

- **INDICATIONS AND DOSE**

Systemic envenoming from snake bites | Marked local envenoming
▸ BY INTRAVENOUS INJECTION, OR BY INTRAVENOUS INFUSION
▸ Child: Initially 10 mL for 1 dose, then 10 mL after 1–2 hours if required, the second dose should only be given if symptoms of systemic envenoming persist after the first dose, if symptoms of systemic envenoming persist contact the National Poisons Information Service
▸ Adult: Initially 10 mL for 1 dose, then 10 mL after 1–2 hours if required, the second dose should only be given if symptoms of systemic envenoming persist after the first dose, if symptoms of systemic envenoming persist contact the National Poisons Information Service

Severe systemic envenoming from snake bites in patients presenting with clinical features
▸ BY INTRAVENOUS INJECTION, OR BY INTRAVENOUS INFUSION
▸ Child: Initially 20 mL for 1 dose, if symptoms of systemic envenoming persist contact the National Poisons Information Service
▸ Adult: Initially 20 mL for 1 dose, if symptoms of systemic envenoming persist contact the National Poisons Information Service

- **DIRECTIONS FOR ADMINISTRATION** By *intravenous injection* given over 10–15 minutes or by *intravenous infusion* over 30 minutes after diluting in sodium chloride 0.9% (use 5 mL diluent/kg body-weight).

- **PRESCRIBING AND DISPENSING INFORMATION** To order, email immform@dh.gsi.gov.uk.

- **MEDICINAL FORMS** There can be variation in the licensing of different medicines containing the same drug.
Solution for injection
▸ Viper venom antiserum, European (equine) (Imported (Croatia))
  European viper snake venom antiserum 100 mg per 1 ml Viper venom antiserum, European (equine) 1g/10ml solution for injection vials | 1 vial [PoM] [℞]

Appendix 1
Interactions

Two or more drugs given at the same time can exert their effects independently or they can interact. Interactions may be beneficial and exploited therapeutically; this type of interaction is not within the scope of this appendix. Many interactions are harmless, and even those that are potentially harmful can often be managed, allowing the drugs to be used safely together. Nevertheless, adverse drug interactions should be reported to the Medicines and Healthcare products Regulatory Agency (MHRA), through the Yellow Card Scheme (see Adverse reactions to drugs p. 12), as for other adverse drug reactions.

Potentially harmful drug interactions may occur in only a small number of patients, but the true incidence is often hard to establish. Furthermore the severity of a harmful interaction is likely to vary from one patient to another. Patients at increased risk from drug interactions include the elderly and those with impaired renal or hepatic function.

Interactions can result in the potentiation or antagonism of one drug by another, or result in another effect, such as renal impairment. Drug interactions may develop either through pharmacokinetic or pharmacodynamic mechanisms.

Pharmacodynamic interactions

These are interactions between drugs which have similar or antagonistic pharmacological effects or side-effects. They might be due to competition at receptor sites, or occur between drugs acting on the same physiological system. They are usually predictable from a knowledge of the pharmacology of the interacting drugs; in general, those demonstrated with one drug are likely to occur with related drugs.

Pharmacokinetic interactions

These occur when one drug alters the absorption, distribution, metabolism, or excretion of another, thus increasing or decreasing the amount of drug available to produce its pharmacological effects. Pharmacokinetic interactions occurring with one drug do not necessarily occur uniformly across a group of related drugs.

Affecting absorption The rate of absorption and the total amount absorbed can both be altered by drug interactions. Delayed absorption is rarely of clinical importance unless a rapid effect is required (e.g. when giving an analgesic). Reduction in the total amount absorbed, however, can result in ineffective therapy.

Affecting distribution *Due to changes in protein binding*: To a variable extent most drugs are loosely bound to plasma proteins. Protein-binding sites are non-specific and one drug can displace another thereby increasing the proportion free to diffuse from plasma to its site of action. This only produces a detectable increase in effect if it is an extensively bound drug (more than 90%) that is not widely distributed throughout the body. Even so displacement rarely produces more than transient potentiation because this increased concentration of free drug will usually be eliminated.

Displacement from protein binding plays a part in the potentiation of warfarin by sulfonamides but these interactions become clinically relevant mainly because warfarin metabolism is also inhibited.

Induction or inhibition of drug transporter proteins: Drug transporter proteins, such as P-glycoprotein, actively transport drugs across biological membranes. Transporters can be induced or inhibited, resulting in changes in the concentrations of drugs that are substrates for the transporter. For example, rifampicin induces P-glycoprotein, particularly in the gut wall, resulting in decreased plasma concentrations of digoxin, a P-glycoprotein substrate.

Affecting metabolism Many drugs are metabolised in the liver. Drugs are either metabolised by phase I reactions (oxidation, reduction, or hydrolysis) or by phase II reactions (e.g. glucuronidation).

Phase I reactions are mainly carried out by the cytochrome P450 family of isoenzymes, of which CYP3A4 is the most important isoenzyme involved in the metabolism of drugs. Induction of cytochrome P450 isoenzymes by one drug can increase the rate of metabolism of another, resulting in lower plasma concentrations and a reduced effect. On withdrawal of the inducing drug, plasma concentrations increase and toxicity can occur.

Conversely when one drug inhibits cytochrome P450 isoenzymes, it can decrease the metabolism of another, leading to higher plasma concentrations, resulting in an increased effect with a risk of toxicity.

Isoenzymes of the hepatic cytochrome P450 system interact with a wide range of drugs. With knowledge of which isoenzymes are involved in a drug's metabolism, it is possible to predict whether certain pharmacokinetic interactions will occur. For example, carbamazepine is a potent inducer of CYP3A4, ketoconazole is potent inhibitor of CYP3A4, and midazolam is a substrate of CYP3A4. Carbamazepine reduces midazolam concentrations, and it is therefore likely that other drugs that are potent inducers of CYP3A4 will interact similarly with midazolam. Ketoconazole, however, increases midazolam concentrations, and it can be predicted that other drugs that are potent inhibitors of CYP3A4 will interact similarly.

Less is known about the enzymes involved in phase II reactions. These include UDP-glucuronyltransferases which, for example, might be induced by rifampicin, resulting in decreased metabolism of mycophenolate (a substrate for this enzyme) to its active form, mycophenolic acid.

Affecting renal excretion Drugs are eliminated through the kidney both by glomerular filtration and by active tubular secretion. Competition occurs between those which share active transport mechanisms in the proximal tubule. For example, salicylates and some other NSAIDs delay the excretion of methotrexate; serious methotrexate toxicity is possible. Changes in urinary pH can also affect the reabsorption of a small number of drugs, including methenamine.

A1

Interactions | Appendix 1

Relative importance of interactions

Levels of severity: Most interactions have been assigned a severity; this describes the likely effect of an unmanaged interaction on the patient.

Severe—the result may be a life-threatening event or have a permanent detrimental effect.

Moderate—the result could cause considerable distress or partially incapacitate a patient; they are unlikely to be life-threatening or result in long-term effects.

Mild—the result is unlikely to cause concern or incapacitate the majority of patients.

Unknown—used for those interactions that are predicted, but there is insufficient evidence to hazard a guess at the outcome.

Levels of evidence: Most interactions have been assigned a rating to indicate the weight of evidence behind the interaction.

Study—for interactions where the information is based on formal study including those for other drugs with same mechanism (e.g. known inducers, inhibitors, or substrates of cytochrome P450 isoenzymes or P-glycoprotein).

Anecdotal—interactions based on either a single case report or a limited number of case reports.

Theoretical—interactions that are predicted based on sound theoretical considerations. The information may have been derived from *in vitro* studies or based on the way other members in the same class act.

Action messages: Each interaction describes the effect that occurs, and the action to be taken, either based on manufacturer's advice from the relevant Summary of Product Characteristics or advice from a relevant authority (e.g. MHRA). An action message is only included where the combination is to be avoided, where a dose adjustment is required, or where specific administration requirements (e.g. timing of doses) are recommended. **Pharmacodynamic interactions**, with the exception of interactions with drugs that may prolong the QT interval, do not have an action message included as these will depend on individual patient circumstances.

Appendix 1 structure

❶ Drugs

Drugs are listed alphabetically. If a drug is a member of a drug class, all interactions for that drug will be listed under the drug class entry; in this case the drug entry provides direction to the relevant drug class where its interactions can be found.

Within a drug or drug class entry, interactions are listed alphabetically by the interacting drug or drug class. The interactions describe the effect that occurs, and the action to be taken, either based on manufacturer's advice from the relevant Summary of Product Characteristics or advice from a relevant authority (e.g. MHRA). An action message is only included where the combination is to be avoided, where a dose adjustment is required, or where specific administration requirements (e.g. timing of doses) are recommended. If two drugs have a pharmacodynamic effect in addition to a pharmacokinetic interaction, a cross-reference to the relevant pharmacodynamic effect table is included at the end of the pharmacokinetic message.

❷ Drug classes

The drugs that are members of a drug class are listed underneath the drug class entry in a blue box. Interactions for the class are then listed alphabetically by the interacting drug or drug class. If the interaction only applies to certain drugs in the class, these drugs will be shown in brackets after the drug class name.

❸ Supplementary information

If a drug has additional important information to be considered, this is shown in a blue box underneath the drug or drug class entry. This information might be food and lifestyle advice (including smoking and alcohol consumption), relate to the pharmacology of the drug or applicability of interactions to certain routes of administration, or it might be advice about separating administration times.

❹ Pharmacodynamic effects

Tables at the beginning of Appendix 1 cover pharmacodynamic effects. If a drug is included in one or more of these tables, this will be indicated at the top of the

---

❶ **Drug entry**
- ▸ Details of interaction between **drug entry** and another drug or drug class. Action statement. ⬚Severity Evidence
- ▸ Details of interaction between **drug entry** and another drug or drug class. Action statement. ⬚Severity Evidence
  → Also see **TABLE 1**

Drug entry → see Drug class entry

❷ **Drug class entry**

Drug A · Drug B · Drug C · Drug D

- ▸ Details of interaction between **drug class entry** and another drug or drug class. Action statement. ⬚Severity Evidence

❸ **Drug entry or Drug class entry**

Supplementary information

❹ **Drug entry or Drug class entry** → see **TABLE 1**

TABLE 1
Name of pharmacodynamic effect
Explanation of the effect

| Drug | Drug | Drug |
| Drug | Drug | Drug |

---

list of interactions for the drug or drug class. In addition to the list of interactions for a drug or drug class, these tables should always be consulted.

Each table describes the relevant pharmacodynamic effect and lists those drugs that are commonly associated with the effect. Concurrent use of two or more drugs from the same table is expected to increase the risk of the pharmacodynamic effect occurring. Please note these tables are not exhaustive.

TABLE 1
Drugs that cause hepatotoxicity

The following is a list of some drugs that cause hepatotoxicity (note that this list is not exhaustive). Concurrent use of two or more drugs from the list might increase this risk.

alcohol	dactinomycin	itraconazole	minocycline	streptozocin
alectinib	dantrolene	leflunomide	neratinib	sulfasalazine
asparaginase	demeclocycline	lenalidomide	oxytetracycline	teriflunomide
atorvastatin	doxycycline	lomitapide	paracetamol	tetracycline
bedaquiline	flucloxacillin	lymecycline	pegaspargase	tigecycline
carbamazepine	fluconazole	mercaptopurine	pravastatin	trabectedin
clavulanate	fluvastatin	methotrexate	rosuvastatin	valproate
crisantaspase	isoniazid	micafungin	simvastatin	vincristine

TABLE 2
Drugs that cause nephrotoxicity

The following is a list of some drugs that cause nephrotoxicity (note that this list is not exhaustive). Concurrent use of two or more drugs from the list might increase this risk.

aceclofenac	cefoxitin	dexketoprofen	methotrexate	tacrolimus
aciclovir	cefradine	diclofenac	nabumetone	telavancin
adefovir	ceftaroline	etodolac	naproxen	tenofovir disoproxil
amikacin	ceftazidime	etoricoxib	neomycin	tenoxicam
amphotericin B	ceftobiprole	flurbiprofen	oxaliplatin	tiaprofenic acid
bacitracin	ceftolozane	foscarnet	parecoxib	tobramycin
capreomycin	ceftriaxone	ganciclovir	pemetrexed	tolfenamic acid
carboplatin	cefuroxime	gentamicin	penicillamine	trimethoprim
cefaclor	celecoxib	ibuprofen	pentamidine	valaciclovir
cefadroxil	ciclosporin	ifosfamide	phenazone	valganciclovir
cefalexin	cidofovir	indometacin	piroxicam	vancomycin
cefazolin	cisplatin	ketoprofen	polymyxin b	zidovudine
cefepime	colistemethate (particularly	ketorolac	streptomycin	zoledronate
cefixime	intravenous)	mefenamic acid	streptozocin	
cefotaxime	dexibuprofen	meloxicam	sulindac	

TABLE 3
Drugs with anticoagulant effects

The following is a list of drugs that have anticoagulant effects. Concurrent use of two or more drugs from this list might increase the risk of bleeding; concurrent use of drugs with antiplatelet effects (see table of drugs with antiplatelet effects) might also increase this risk.

acenocoumarol	dabigatran	eptifibatide	phenindione	tirofiban
alteplase	dalteparin	fondaparinux	rivaroxaban	urokinase
apixaban	danaparoid	heparin	streptokinase	warfarin
argatroban	edoxaban	nicotinic acid	tenecteplase	
bivalirudin	enoxaparin	omega-3-acid ethyl esters	tinzaparin	

TABLE 4
Drugs with antiplatelet effects

The following is a list of drugs that have antiplatelet effects (note that this list is not exhaustive). Concurrent use of two or more drugs from this list might increase the risk of bleeding; concurrent use of drugs with anticoagulant effects (see table of drugs with anticoagulant effects) might also increase this risk.

aceclofenac	dasatinib	fluoxetine	mefenamic acid	sertraline
anagrelide	dexibuprofen	flurbiprofen	meloxicam	sulindac
aspirin	dexketoprofen	fluvoxamine	nabumetone	tenoxicam
bevacizumab	diclofenac	ibrutinib	naproxen	tiaprofenic acid
cangrelor	dipyridamole	ibuprofen	parecoxib	ticagrelor
celecoxib	duloxetine	iloprost	paroxetine	tolfenamic acid
cilostazol	epoprostenol	indometacin	phenazone	trastuzumab emtansine
citalopram	escitalopram	inotersen	piroxicam	venlafaxine
clopidogrel	etodolac	ketoprofen	prasugrel	vortioxetine
dapoxetine	etoricoxib	ketorolac	regorafenib	

TABLE 5
Drugs that cause thromboembolism

The following is a list of some drugs that cause thromboembolism (note that this list is not exhaustive). Concurrent use of two or more drugs from the list might increase this risk.

bleomycin	fluorouracil	necitumumab	tibolone	vinflunine
cyclophosphamide	fulvestrant	pentostatin	toremifene	vinorelbine
darbepoetin alfa	lenalidomide	pomalidomide	tranexamic acid	
doxorubicin	methotrexate	raloxifene	tretinoin	
epoetin alfa	methoxy polyethylene	strontium	vinblastine	
epoetin beta	glycol-epoetin beta	tamoxifen	vincristine	
epoetin zeta	mitomycin	thalidomide	vindesine	

TABLE 6
Drugs that cause bradycardia

The following is a list of drugs that cause bradycardia (note that this list is not exhaustive). Concurrent use of two or more drugs from the list might increase this risk.

acebutolol	carvedilol	fentanyl	nadolol	rivastigmine
alectinib	celiprolol	fingolimod	nebivolol	selegiline
alfentanil	cisatracurium	flecainide	neostigmine	siponimod
amiodarone	clonidine	galantamine	ozanimod	sotalol
apraclonidine	crizotinib	ivabradine	pasireotide	thalidomide
atenolol	digoxin	labetalol	pindolol	timolol
betaxolol	diltiazem	levobunolol	propranolol	tizanidine
bisoprolol	donepezil	methadone	pyridostigmine	verapamil
brimonidine	esmolol	metoprolol	remifentanil	

TABLE 7
Drugs that cause first dose hypotension

The following is a list of some drugs that can cause first-dose hypotension (note that this list is not exhaustive). Concurrent use of two or more drugs from the list might increase this risk.

alfuzosin	eprosartan	isosorbide dinitrate	prazosin	trandolapril
azilsartan	fosinopril	isosorbide mononitrate	quinapril	valsartan
candesartan	glyceryl trinitrate	lisinopril	ramipril	
captopril	imidapril	losartan	tamsulosin	
doxazosin	indoramin	olmesartan	telmisartan	
enalapril	irbesartan	perindopril	terazosin	

TABLE 8
Drugs that cause hypotension

The following is a list of some drugs that cause hypotension (note that this list is not exhaustive). Concurrent use of two or more drugs from the list might increase this risk.

acebutolol	chlorothiazide	haloperidol	minoxidil	risperidone
alcohol	chlorpromazine	hydralazine	moxisylyte	ropinirole
alfuzosin	chlortalidone	hydrochlorothiazide	moxonidine	rotigotine
aliskiren	clomipramine	hydroflumethiazide	nadolol	sacubitril
alprostadil	clonidine	iloprost	nebivolol	sapropterin
amantadine	clozapine	imidapril	nicardipine	selegiline
amitriptyline	dapagliflozin	imipramine	nicorandil	sevoflurane
amlodipine	desflurane	indapamide	nifedipine	sildenafil
apomorphine	diazoxide	indoramin	nimodipine	sodium oxybate
apraclonidine	diltiazem	irbesartan	nitroprusside	sotalol
aripiprazole	dipyridamole	isocarboxazid	nitrous oxide	spironolactone
asenapine	dosulepin	isoflurane	nortriptyline	sulpiride
atenolol	doxazosin	isosorbide dinitrate	olanzapine	tadalafil
avanafil	doxepin	isosorbide mononitrate	olmesartan	tamsulosin
azilsartan	droperidol	ketamine	paliperidone	telmisartan
baclofen	empagliflozin	labetalol	perindopril	terazosin
bendroflumethiazide	enalapril	lacidipine	pericyazine	thiopental
benperidol	eplerenone	lercanidipine	phenelzine	timolol
betaxolol	epoprostenol	levobunolol	pimozide	tizanidine
bisoprolol	eprosartan	levodopa	pindolol	torasemide
bortezomib	ertugliflozin	levomepromazine	pramipexole	trandolapril
brimonidine	esketamine	lisinopril	prazosin	tranylcypromine
bromocriptine	esmolol	lofepramine	prochlorperazine	trifluoperazine
bumetanide	etomidate	lofexidine	promazine	trimipramine
cabergoline	felodipine	losartan	propofol	valsartan
canagliflozin	flupentixol	loxapine	propranolol	vardenafil
candesartan	fluphenazine	lurasidone	quetiapine	verapamil
captopril	fosinopril	methoxyflurane	quinagolide	vernakalant
cariprazine	furosemide	methyldopa	quinapril	xipamide
carvedilol	glyceryl trinitrate	metolazone	ramipril	zuclopenthixol
celiprolol	guanfacine	metoprolol	riociguat	

TABLE 9
Drugs that prolong the QT interval

The following is a list of some drugs that prolong the QT-interval (note that this list is not exhaustive). In general, manufacturers advise that the use of two or more drugs that are associated with QT prolongation should be avoided. Increasing age, female sex, cardiac disease, and some metabolic disturbances (notably hypokalaemia) predispose to QT prolongation—concurrent use of drugs that reduce serum potassium might further increase this risk (see table of drugs that reduce serum potassium).

Drugs that are not known to prolong the QT interval but are predicted (by the manufacturer) to increase the risk of QT prolongation include: domperidone, fingolimod, granisetron, ivabradine, mefloquine, mizolastine, ozanimod, palonosetron, intravenous pentamidine, and siponimod. Most manufacturers advise avoiding concurrent use with drugs that prolong the QT interval.

amifampridine	clomipramine	glasdegib	panobinostat	tetrabenazine
amiodarone	crizotinib	haloperidol	pasireotide	tizanidine
amisulpride	dasatinib	hydroxyzine	pazopanib	tolterodine
anagrelide	delamanid	inotuzumab ozogamicin	pimozide	toremifene
apalutamide	desflurane	isoflurane	quinine	vandetanib
apomorphine	disopyramide	lapatinib	ranolazine	vardenafil
arsenic trioxide	dronedarone	lenvatinib	ribociclib	vemurafenib
artemether	droperidol	levomepromazine	risperidone	venlafaxine
artenimol	efavirenz	lithium	saquinavir	vernakalant
bedaquiline	encorafenib	lofexidine	sevoflurane	vinflunine
bosutinib	entrectinib	methadone	sildenafil	voriconazole
cabozantinib	eribulin	moxifloxacin	sorafenib	zuclopenthixol
ceritinib	erythromycin	nilotinib	sotalol	
chlorpromazine	escitalopram	ondansetron	sulpiride	
citalopram	flecainide	osimertinib	sunitinib	
clarithromycin	fluconazole	paliperidone	telavancin	

TABLE 10
Drugs with antimuscarinic effects

The following is a list of some drugs that have antimuscarinic effects (note that this list is not exhaustive). Concurrent use of two or more drugs from this list might increase the risk of these effects occurring.

aclidinium	cyclopentolate	haloperidol	orphenadrine	tiotropium
amantadine	cyproheptadine	homatropine	oxybutynin	tolterodine
amitriptyline	darifenacin	hydroxyzine	pimozide	trifluoperazine
atropine	dicycloverine	hyoscine	pridinol	trihexyphenidyl
baclofen	dimenhydrinate	imipramine	prochlorperazine	trimipramine
chlorphenamine	disopyramide	ipratropium	procyclidine	tropicamide
chlorpromazine	dosulepin	levomepromazine	promethazine	trospium
clemastine	doxepin	lofepramine	propafenone	umeclidinium
clomipramine	fesoterodine	loxapine	propantheline	
clozapine	flavoxate	nefopam	propiverine	
cyclizine	glycopyrronium	nortriptyline	solifenacin	

TABLE 11
Drugs with CNS depressant effects

The following is a list of some drugs with CNS depressant effects (note that this list is not exhaustive). Concurrent use of two or more drugs from this list might increase the risk of CNS depressant effects, such as drowsiness, which might affect the ability to perform skilled tasks (see 'Drugs and Driving' in Guidance on Prescribing p. 1).

agomelatine	clobazam	guanfacine	mianserin	propofol
alcohol	clomethiazole	haloperidol	midazolam	quetiapine
alfentanil	clomipramine	hydromorphone	mirtazapine	remifentanil
alimemazine	clonazepam	hydroxyzine	morphine	risperidone
alprazolam	clonidine	imipramine	moxonidine	ropivacaine
amisulpride	clozapine	isoflurane	nabilone	sevoflurane
amitriptyline	codeine	ketamine	nitrazepam	sodium oxybate
apraclonidine	cyclizine	ketotifen	nitrous oxide	sulpiride
aripiprazole	cyproheptadine	lamotrigine	nortriptyline	tapentadol
articaine	desflurane	levetiracetam	olanzapine	temazepam
asenapine	dexmedetomidine	levomepromazine	oxazepam	tetrabenazine
baclofen	diamorphine	lidocaine	oxycodone	tetracaine
benperidol	diazepam	lofepramine	paliperidone	thalidomide
brimonidine	dihydrocodeine	lofexidine	pentazocine	thiopental
buclizine	dipipanone	loprazolam	perampanel	tizanidine
bupivacaine	dosulepin	lorazepam	pericyazine	tramadol
buprenorphine	doxepin	lormetazepam	pethidine	trazodone
cannabidiol	dronabinol	loxapine	phenobarbital	trifluoperazine
cariprazine	droperidol	lurasidone	pimozide	trimipramine
chloral hydrate	esketamine	melatonin	pizotifen	venlafaxine
chlordiazepoxide	etomidate	mepivacaine	pregabalin	zolpidem
chloroprocaine	fentanyl	meprobamate	prilocaine	zopiclone
chlorphenamine	flupentixol	meptazinol	primidone	zuclopenthixol
chlorpromazine	fluphenazine	methadone	prochlorperazine	
cinnarizine	flurazepam	methocarbamol	promazine	
clemastine	gabapentin	methoxyflurane	promethazine	

TABLE 12

Drugs that cause peripheral neuropathy

The following is a list of some drugs that cause peripheral neuropathy (note that this list is not exhaustive). Concurrent use of two or more drugs from the list might increase this risk.

amiodarone	disulfiram	lamivudine	thalidomide	vinorelbine
bortezomib	docetaxel	metronidazole	vinblastine	
brentuximab vedotin	eribulin	nitrofurantoin	vincristine	
cabazitaxel	fosphenytoin	paclitaxel	vindesine	
cisplatin	isoniazid	phenytoin	vinflunine	

TABLE 13

Drugs that cause serotonin syndrome

The following is a list of some drugs that cause serotonin syndrome (note that this list is not exhaustive). See 'Serotonin Syndrome' and 'Monoamine-Oxidase Inhibitors' under Antidepressant drugs in BNF for more information and for specific advice on avoiding monoamine-oxidase inhibitors during and after administration of other serotonergic drugs.

almotriptan	fentanyl	methadone	phenelzine	tranylcypromine
bupropion	fluoxetine	methylthioninium chloride	procarbazine	trazodone
buspirone	fluvoxamine	mirtazapine	rasagiline	tryptophan
citalopram	frovatriptan	moclobemide	rizatriptan	venlafaxine
clomipramine	granisetron	naratriptan	safinamide	vortioxetine
dapoxetine	imipramine	ondansetron	selegiline	zolmitriptan
dexamfetamine	isocarboxazid	palonosetron	sertraline	
duloxetine	linezolid	paroxetine	St John's wort	
eletriptan	lisdexamfetamine	pentazocine	sumatriptan	
escitalopram	lithium	pethidine	tramadol	

TABLE 14

Antidiabetic drugs

The following is a list of antidiabetic drugs (note that this list is not exhaustive). Concurrent use of two or more drugs from the list might increase the risk of hypoglycaemia.

acarbose	empagliflozin	glimepiride	lixisenatide	saxagliptin
alogliptin	ertugliflozin	glipizide	metformin	semaglutide
canagliflozin	exenatide	insulin	nateglinide	sitagliptin
dapagliflozin	glibenclamide	linagliptin	pioglitazone	tolbutamide
dulaglutide	gliclazide	liraglutide	repaglinide	vildagliptin

TABLE 15

Drugs that cause myelosuppression

The following is a list of some drugs that cause myelosuppression (note that this list is not exhaustive). Concurrent use of two or more drugs from the list might increase this risk.

adalimumab	carmustine	fluorouracil	nelarabine	sorafenib
aldesleukin	ceritinib	ganciclovir	nilotinib	streptozocin
alemtuzumab	certolizumab pegol	gemcitabine	niraparib	sulfasalazine
amsacrine	chlorambucil	gemtuzumab ozogamicin	nivolumab	sunitinib
arsenic trioxide	cisplatin	golimumab	obinutuzumab	talazoparib
asparaginase	cladribine	hydroxycarbamide	olaparib	tegafur
axitinib	clofarabine	ibrutinib	oxaliplatin	temozolomide
azacitidine	crisantaspase	idarubicin	paclitaxel	temsirolimus
azathioprine	cyclophosphamide	ifosfamide	palbociclib	thalidomide
belatacept	cytarabine	imatinib	panobinostat	thiotepa
bendamustine	dacarbazine	infliximab	pegaspargase	tioguanine
bevacizumab	dactinomycin	inotuzumab ozogamicin	peginterferon alfa	topotecan
bexarotene	daratumumab	ipilimumab	pembrolizumab	trabectedin
bleomycin	dasatinib	irinotecan	pemetrexed	trastuzumab
blinatumomab	daunorubicin	leflunomide	pentostatin	trastuzumab emtansine
bortezomib	decitabine	lenalidomide	pixantrone	treosulfan
bosutinib	dexrazoxane	lomustine	pomalidomide	valganciclovir
brentuximab vedotin	dinutuximab	melphalan	procarbazine	vinblastine
busulfan	docetaxel	mercaptopurine	raltitrexed	vincristine
cabazitaxel	doxorubicin	methotrexate	ramucirumab	vindesine
cabozantinib	epirubicin	mifamurtide	regorafenib	vinflunine
canakinumab	eribulin	mitomycin	ribociclib	vinorelbine
capecitabine	estramustine	mitotane	rituximab	
carboplatin	etoposide	mitoxantrone	rucaparib	
carfilzomib	fludarabine	mogamulizumab	ruxolitinib	

TABLE 16
Drugs that increase serum potassium

The following is a list of some drugs that increase serum potassium concentrations (note that this list is not exhaustive). Concurrent use of two or more drugs from this list might increase the risk of hyperkalaemia (hyperkalaemia is particularly notable when ACE inhibitors or angiotensin-II receptor antagonists are given with spironolactone or eplerenone).

aceclofenac	diclofenac	heparin	naproxen	sulindac
aliskiren	drospirenone	ibuprofen	olmesartan	tacrolimus
amiloride	enalapril	imidapril	parecoxib	telmisartan
azilsartan	enoxaparin	indometacin	perindopril	tenoxicam
candesartan	eplerenone	irbesartan	phenazone	tiaprofenic acid
captopril	epoetin alfa	ketoprofen	piroxicam	tinzaparin
celecoxib	epoetin beta	ketorolac	potassium aminobenzoate	tolfenamic acid
ciclosporin	epoetin zeta	lisinopril	potassium canrenoate	tolvaptan
dalteparin	eprosartan	losartan	potassium chloride	trandolapril
darbepoetin alfa	etodolac	mefenamic acid	quinapril	triamterene
dexibuprofen	etoricoxib	meloxicam	ramipril	trimethoprim
dexketoprofen	flurbiprofen	nabumetone	spironolactone	valsartan

TABLE 17
Drugs that reduce serum potassium

The following is a list of some drugs that reduce serum potassium concentrations (note that this list is not exhaustive and that other drugs can cause hypokalaemia in overdose). Concurrent use of two or more drugs from this list might increase the risk of hypokalaemia. Hypokalaemia can increase the risk of torsade de pointes, which might be additive with the effects of drugs that prolong the QT interval (see table of drugs that prolong the QT interval).

aminophylline	bumetanide	furosemide	metolazone	torasemide
amphotericin B	chlorothiazide	hydrochlorothiazide	olodaterol	triamcinolone
bambuterol	chlortalidone	hydrocortisone	prednisolone	vilanterol
beclometasone	deflazacort	hydroflumethiazide	salbutamol	xipamide
bendroflumethiazide	dexamethasone	indacaterol	salmeterol	
betamethasone	fludrocortisone	indapamide	terbutaline	
budesonide	formoterol	methylprednisolone	theophylline	

TABLE 18
Drugs that cause hyponatraemia

The following is a list of some drugs that reduce sodium concentrations (note that this list is not exhaustive). Concurrent use of two or more drugs from this list might increase the risk of hyponatraemia.

aceclofenac	desmopressin	flurbiprofen	mefenamic acid	spironolactone
amiloride	dexibuprofen	fluvoxamine	meloxicam	sulindac
amitriptyline	dexketoprofen	furosemide	metolazone	tenoxicam
bendroflumethiazide	diclofenac	gabapentin	nabumetone	tiaprofenic acid
bumetanide	dosulepin	hydrochlorothiazide	naproxen	tolfenamic acid
carbamazepine	doxepin	hydroflumethiazide	nortriptyline	torasemide
celecoxib	duloxetine	ibuprofen	parecoxib	triamterene
chlorothiazide	eplerenone	imipramine	paroxetine	trimethoprim
chlortalidone	escitalopram	indapamide	phenazone	trimipramine
citalopram	etodolac	indometacin	piroxicam	xipamide
clomipramine	etoricoxib	ketoprofen	sertraline	
dapoxetine	fluoxetine	ketorolac	sodium picosulfate	

TABLE 19
Drugs that cause ototoxicity

The following is a list of some drugs that cause ototoxicity (note that this list is not exhaustive). Concurrent use of two or more drugs from the list might increase this risk.

amikacin	cisplatin	oxaliplatin	torasemide	vindesine
bumetanide	furosemide	streptomycin	vancomycin	vinflunine
capreomycin	gentamicin	telavancin	vinblastine	vinorelbine
carboplatin	neomycin	tobramycin	vincristine	

TABLE 20
Drugs with neuromuscular blocking effects

The following is a list of some drugs with neuromuscular blocking effects (note that this list is not exhaustive). Concurrent use of two or more drugs from the list might increase this risk.

amikacin	cisatracurium	neomycin	streptomycin
atracurium	colistimethate	pancuronium	suxamethonium
botulinum toxin type A	gentamicin	polymyxin b	tobramycin
botulinum toxin type B	mivacurium	rocuronium	vecuronium

List of drug interactions

The following is an alphabetical list of drugs and their interactions; to avoid excessive cross-referencing each drug or group is listed twice: in the alphabetical list and also against the drug or group with which it interacts.

5-HT3-receptor antagonists → see TABLE 13 p. 1432 (serotonin syndrome), TABLE 9 p. 1431 (QT-interval prolongation)

granisetron · ondansetron · palonosetron

▶ Anti-androgens (apalutamide, enzalutamide) are predicted to decrease the exposure to **ondansetron**. Moderate Study → Also see TABLE 9 p. 1431

▶ Antiepileptics (carbamazepine, fosphenytoin, phenobarbital, phenytoin, primidone) are predicted to decrease the exposure to **ondansetron**. Moderate Study

▶ Dopamine receptor agonists (apomorphine) increase the risk of severe hypotension when given with **ondansetron**. Avoid. Severe Study → Also see TABLE 9 p. 1431

▶ Dopamine receptor agonists (apomorphine) are predicted to increase the risk of severe hypotension when given with 5-HT3-receptor antagonists (granisetron, palonosetron). Severe Theoretical

▶ Mitotane is predicted to decrease the exposure to **ondansetron**. Moderate Study

▶ Rifamycins (rifampicin) are predicted to decrease the exposure to **ondansetron**. Moderate Study

Abacavir → see NRTIs

Abatacept

▶ Filgotinib is predicted to increase the risk of immunosuppression when given with **abatacept**. Avoid. Severe Theoretical

▶ Live vaccines are predicted to increase the risk of generalised infection (possibly life-threatening) when given with **abatacept**. Public Health England advises avoid (refer to Green Book). Severe Theoretical

▶ **Abatacept** is predicted to increase the risk of generalised infection (possibly life-threatening) when given with monoclonal antibodies (golimumab). Avoid. Severe Theoretical

Abemaciclib

▶ Anti-androgens (apalutamide, enzalutamide) are predicted to markedly decrease the exposure to **abemaciclib**. Avoid. Severe Study

▶ Antiarrhythmics (dronedarone) are predicted to increase the exposure to **abemaciclib**. Moderate Study

▶ Antiepileptics (carbamazepine, fosphenytoin, phenobarbital, phenytoin, primidone) are predicted to markedly decrease the exposure to **abemaciclib**. Severe Study

▶ Antifungals, azoles (fluconazole, isavuconazole, posaconazole) are predicted to increase the exposure to **abemaciclib**. Moderate Study

▶ Antifungals, azoles (itraconazole, ketoconazole, voriconazole) are predicted to increase the exposure to **abemaciclib**. Avoid or adjust **abemaciclib** dose, p. 1009. Severe Study

▶ Calcium channel blockers (diltiazem, verapamil) are predicted to increase the exposure to **abemaciclib**. Moderate Study

▶ Cobicistat is predicted to increase the exposure to **abemaciclib**. Avoid or adjust **abemaciclib** dose, p. 1009. Severe Study

▶ Crizotinib is predicted to increase the exposure to **abemaciclib**. Moderate Study

▶ Grapefruit juice is predicted to increase the exposure to **abemaciclib**. Avoid. Moderate Theoretical

▶ HIV-protease inhibitors are predicted to increase the exposure to **abemaciclib**. Avoid or adjust **abemaciclib** dose, p. 1009. Severe Study

▶ Idelalisib is predicted to increase the exposure to **abemaciclib**. Avoid or adjust **abemaciclib** dose, p. 1009. Severe Study

▶ Imatinib is predicted to increase the exposure to **abemaciclib**. Moderate Study

▶ Letermovir is predicted to increase the exposure to **abemaciclib**. Moderate Study

▶ Macrolides (clarithromycin) are predicted to increase the exposure to **abemaciclib**. Avoid or adjust **abemaciclib** dose, p. 1009. Severe Study

▶ Macrolides (erythromycin) are predicted to increase the exposure to **abemaciclib**. Moderate Study

▶ Mitotane is predicted to markedly decrease the exposure to **abemaciclib**. Avoid. Severe Study

▶ Neurokinin-1 receptor antagonists (aprepitant, netupitant) are predicted to increase the exposure to **abemaciclib**. Moderate Study

▶ Nilotinib is predicted to increase the exposure to **abemaciclib**. Moderate Study

▶ Rifamycins (rifampicin) are predicted to markedly decrease the exposure to **abemaciclib**. Avoid. Severe Study

▶ St John's wort is predicted to decrease the exposure to **abemaciclib**. Avoid. Severe Study

Abiraterone → see anti-androgens

Acalabrutinib

▶ Oral antacids is predicted to decrease the exposure to oral **acalabrutinib**. Separate administration by at least 2 hours. Moderate Theoretical

▶ Anti-androgens (apalutamide, enzalutamide) are predicted to decrease the exposure to **acalabrutinib**. Avoid. Severe Study

▶ Antiarrhythmics (dronedarone) are predicted to increase the exposure to **acalabrutinib**. Avoid or monitor. Severe Study

▶ Antiepileptics (carbamazepine, fosphenytoin, phenobarbital, phenytoin, primidone) are predicted to decrease the exposure to **acalabrutinib**. Avoid. Severe Study

▶ Antifungals, azoles (fluconazole, isavuconazole, posaconazole) are predicted to increase the exposure to **acalabrutinib**. Avoid or monitor. Severe Study

▶ Antifungals, azoles (itraconazole, ketoconazole, voriconazole) are predicted to increase the exposure to **acalabrutinib**. Avoid. Severe Study

▶ Calcium channel blockers (diltiazem, verapamil) are predicted to increase the exposure to **acalabrutinib**. Avoid or monitor. Severe Study

▶ Oral calcium salts (calcium carbonate) decrease the exposure to oral **acalabrutinib**. Separate administration by at least 2 hours. Moderate Study

▶ Cobicistat is predicted to increase the exposure to **acalabrutinib**. Avoid. Severe Study

▶ Crizotinib is predicted to increase the exposure to **acalabrutinib**. Avoid or monitor. Severe Study

▶ Endothelin receptor antagonists (bosentan) are predicted to decrease the exposure to **acalabrutinib**. Severe Theoretical

▶ H₂ receptor antagonists are predicted to decrease the exposure to **acalabrutinib**. **Acalabrutinib** should be taken 2 hours before or 10 hours after H₂ receptor antagonists. Moderate Theoretical

▶ HIV-protease inhibitors are predicted to increase the exposure to **acalabrutinib**. Avoid. Severe Study

▶ Idelalisib is predicted to increase the exposure to **acalabrutinib**. Avoid. Severe Study

▶ Imatinib is predicted to increase the exposure to **acalabrutinib**. Avoid or monitor. Severe Study

▶ Letermovir is predicted to increase the exposure to **acalabrutinib**. Avoid or monitor. Severe Study

▶ Macrolides (clarithromycin) are predicted to increase the exposure to **acalabrutinib**. Avoid. Severe Study

▶ Macrolides (erythromycin) are predicted to increase the exposure to **acalabrutinib**. Avoid or monitor. Severe Study

▶ Mitotane is predicted to decrease the exposure to **acalabrutinib**. Avoid. Severe Study

▶ Neurokinin-1 receptor antagonists (aprepitant, netupitant) are predicted to increase the exposure to **acalabrutinib**. Avoid or monitor. Severe Study

▶ Nilotinib is predicted to increase the exposure to **acalabrutinib**. Avoid or monitor. Severe Study

▶ NNRTIs (efavirenz, nevirapine) are predicted to decrease the exposure to **acalabrutinib**. Severe Theoretical

▶ Proton pump inhibitors are predicted to decrease the exposure to **acalabrutinib**. Avoid. Moderate Study

▶ Rifamycins (rifampicin) are predicted to decrease the exposure to **acalabrutinib**. Avoid. Severe Study

▶ Oral sodium bicarbonate is predicted to decrease the exposure to oral **acalabrutinib**. Separate administration by at least 2 hours. Moderate Theoretical

St John's wort is predicted to decrease the exposure to **acalabrutinib**. Avoid. [Severe] Theoretical

Acarbose → see TABLE 14 p. 1432 (antidiabetic drugs)
▶ **Acarbose** decreases the concentration of digoxin. [Moderate] Study
▶ Pancreatin is predicted to decrease the effects of **acarbose**. Avoid. [Moderate] Theoretical

ACE inhibitors → see TABLE 7 p. 1430 (first-dose hypotension), TABLE 8 p. 1430 (hypotension), TABLE 16 p. 1433 (increased serum potassium)

captopril · enalapril · fosinopril · imidapril · lisinopril · perindopril · quinapril · ramipril · trandolapril

▶ **ACE inhibitors** increase the risk of renal impairment when given with aliskiren. Use with caution or avoid **aliskiren** in selected patients, p. 193. [Severe] Study → Also see TABLE 8 p. 1430 → Also see TABLE 16 p. 1433
▶ **ACE inhibitors** are predicted to increase the risk of hypersensitivity and haematological reactions when given with allopurinol. [Severe] Anecdotal
▶ **ACE inhibitors** are predicted to increase the risk of anaemia and/or leucopenia when given with azathioprine. [Severe] Anecdotal
▶ Everolimus potentially increases the risk of angioedema when given with **ACE inhibitors**. [Severe] Anecdotal
▶ **ACE inhibitors** are predicted to increase the risk of hypersensitivity when given with gold. [Severe] Anecdotal
▶ **ACE inhibitors** are predicted to decrease the efficacy of icatibant and icatibant is predicted to decrease the efficacy of **ACE inhibitors**. Avoid. [Moderate] Theoretical
▶ **ACE inhibitors** are predicted to increase the concentration of lithium. Monitor and adjust dose. [Severe] Anecdotal
▶ **ACE inhibitors** are predicted to increase the risk of angioedema when given with temsirolimus. [Moderate] Theoretical
▶ **Quinapril** (tablet) decreases the absorption of oral tetracyclines (tetracycline). Avoid. [Moderate] Study

Acebutolol → see beta blockers, selective
Aceclofenac → see NSAIDs
Acenocoumarol → see coumarins
Acetazolamide
▶ **Acetazolamide** potentially increases the risk of toxicity when given with antiepileptics (valproate). [Severe] Study
▶ **Acetazolamide** potentially increases the risk of overheating and dehydration when given with antiepileptics (zonisamide). Avoid in children. [Severe] Theoretical
▶ **Acetazolamide** increases the risk of severe toxic reaction when given with aspirin (high-dose). [Severe] Study
▶ **Acetazolamide** alters the concentration of lithium. [Severe] Anecdotal
▶ **Acetazolamide** is predicted to decrease the efficacy of methenamine. Avoid. [Moderate] Theoretical
▶ **Acetazolamide** increases the urinary excretion of methotrexate. [Moderate] Study

Aciclovir → see TABLE 2 p. 1429 (nephrotoxicity)

ROUTE-SPECIFIC INFORMATION Since systemic absorption can follow topical application, the possibility of interactions should be borne in mind.

▶ Aciclovir increases the exposure to aminophylline. Monitor and adjust dose. [Severe] Anecdotal
▶ Mycophenolate is predicted to increase the risk of haematological toxicity when given with **aciclovir**. [Moderate] Theoretical
▶ Aciclovir is predicted to increase the exposure to theophylline. Monitor and adjust dose. [Severe] Theoretical

Acitretin → see retinoids
Aclidinium → see TABLE 10 p. 1431 (antimuscarinics)
Acrivastine → see antihistamines, non-sedating
Adalimumab → see monoclonal antibodies
Adapalene → see retinoids
Adefovir → see TABLE 2 p. 1429 (nephrotoxicity)
▶ Leflunomide is predicted to increase the exposure to **adefovir**. [Moderate] Theoretical
▶ Nitisinone is predicted to increase the exposure to **adefovir**. [Moderate] Study
▶ Teriflunomide is predicted to increase the exposure to **adefovir**. [Moderate] Study

Adenosine → see antiarrhythmics
Adrenaline/epinephrine → see sympathomimetics, vasoconstrictor
Afatinib
▶ Antiarrhythmics (amiodarone, dronedarone) are predicted to increase the exposure to **afatinib**. Separate administration by 12 hours. [Moderate] Study
▶ Antiepileptics (carbamazepine) are predicted to decrease the exposure to **afatinib**. [Moderate] Study
▶ Antifungals, azoles (itraconazole, ketoconazole) are predicted to increase the exposure to **afatinib**. Separate administration by 12 hours. [Moderate] Study
▶ Calcium channel blockers (verapamil) are predicted to increase the exposure to **afatinib**. Separate administration by 12 hours. [Moderate] Study
▶ Ciclosporin is predicted to increase the exposure to **afatinib**. Separate administration by 12 hours. [Moderate] Study
▶ HIV-protease inhibitors (lopinavir, ritonavir, saquinavir) are predicted to increase the exposure to **afatinib**. Separate administration by 12 hours. [Moderate] Study
▶ Lapatinib is predicted to increase the exposure to **afatinib**. Separate administration by 12 hours. [Moderate] Study
▶ Macrolides are predicted to increase the exposure to **afatinib**. Separate administration by 12 hours. [Moderate] Study
▶ Ranolazine is predicted to increase the exposure to **afatinib**. Separate administration by 12 hours. [Moderate] Study
▶ Rifamycins (rifampicin) are predicted to decrease the exposure to **afatinib**. [Moderate] Study
▶ St John's wort is predicted to decrease the exposure to **afatinib**. [Moderate] Study
▶ Vemurafenib is predicted to increase the exposure to **afatinib**. Separate administration by 12 hours. [Moderate] Study

Aflibercept

ROUTE-SPECIFIC INFORMATION Interactions do not generally apply to topical use unless specified.

Agalsidase alfa
▶ Aminoglycosides are predicted to decrease the effects of **agalsidase alfa**. Avoid. [Moderate] Theoretical
▶ Antiarrhythmics (amiodarone) are predicted to decrease the effects of **agalsidase alfa**. Avoid. [Moderate] Theoretical
▶ Antimalarials (chloroquine) are predicted to decrease the effects of **agalsidase alfa**. Avoid. [Moderate] Theoretical
▶ Hydroxychloroquine is predicted to decrease the effects of **agalsidase alfa**. Avoid. [Moderate] Theoretical

Agalsidase beta
▶ Aminoglycosides are predicted to decrease the effects of **agalsidase beta**. Avoid. [Moderate] Theoretical
▶ Antiarrhythmics (amiodarone) are predicted to decrease the effects of **agalsidase beta**. Avoid. [Moderate] Theoretical
▶ Antimalarials (chloroquine) are predicted to decrease the effects of **agalsidase beta**. Avoid. [Moderate] Theoretical
▶ Hydroxychloroquine is predicted to decrease the exposure to **agalsidase beta**. [Moderate] Theoretical

Agomelatine → see TABLE 11 p. 1431 (CNS depressant effects)

▶ Dose adjustment might be necessary if smoking started or stopped during treatment.
▶ Caution with concomitant use of drugs associated with hepatic injury.

▶ Antiepileptics (fosphenytoin, phenytoin) are predicted to decrease the exposure to **agomelatine**. [Moderate] Theoretical
▶ Combined hormonal contraceptives are predicted to increase the exposure to **agomelatine**. [Moderate] Study
▶ HIV-protease inhibitors (ritonavir) are predicted to decrease the exposure to **agomelatine**. [Moderate] Theoretical
▶ Leflunomide is predicted to decrease the exposure to **agomelatine**. [Moderate] Theoretical
▶ Mexiletine is predicted to increase the exposure to **agomelatine**. [Moderate] Study
▶ Quinolones (ciprofloxacin) are predicted to increase the exposure to **agomelatine**. [Moderate] Study
▶ Rifamycins (rifampicin) are predicted to decrease the exposure to **agomelatine**. [Moderate] Theoretical
▶ SSRIs (fluvoxamine) very markedly increase the exposure to **agomelatine**. Avoid. [Severe] Study

Agomelatine (continued)
▸ Teriflunomide is predicted to decrease the exposure to **agomelatine**. Moderate Theoretical
▸ Vemurafenib is predicted to increase the exposure to **agomelatine**. Use with caution or avoid. Moderate Theoretical

Albendazole
▸ Antiepileptics (carbamazepine, fosphenytoin, phenobarbital, phenytoin, primidone) decrease the concentration of **albendazole**. Moderate Study
▸ H₂ receptor antagonists (cimetidine) decrease the clearance of **albendazole**. Moderate Study
▸ HIV-protease inhibitors (ritonavir) decrease the exposure to **albendazole**. Moderate Study
▸ **Albendazole** slightly decreases the exposure to levamisole and levamisole moderately decreases the exposure to **albendazole**. Moderate Study

Alcohol → see TABLE 1 p. 1429 (hepatotoxicity), TABLE 8 p. 1430 (hypotension), TABLE 11 p. 1431 (CNS depressant effects)

ROUTE-SPECIFIC INFORMATION   Interactions do not generally apply to alcohol used for topical action unless specified.

▸ Alcohol potentially increases the risk of visual disturbances when given with antiepileptics (retigabine). Moderate Study
▸ Alcohol potentially causes a disulfiram-like reaction when given with antifungals, azoles (ketoconazole). Avoid. Moderate Anecdotal
▸ Alcohol causes serious, potentially fatal, CNS depression when given with clomethiazole. Avoid. Severe Study → Also see TABLE 11 p. 1431
▸ Alcohol (in those who drink heavily) potentially decreases the anticoagulant effect of coumarins. Severe Study
▸ Alcohol (excessive consumption) potentially increases the risk of gastrointestinal adverse effects when given with dimethyl fumarate. Avoid. Moderate Theoretical
▸ Alcohol causes an extremely unpleasant systemic reaction when given with disulfiram. Avoid for at least 24 hours before and up to 14 days after stopping treatment. Severe Study
▸ Alcohol potentially causes a disulfiram-like reaction when given with griseofulvin. Moderate Anecdotal
▸ Alcohol potentially causes a disulfiram-like reaction when given with levamisole. Moderate Study
▸ Alcohol (excessive consumption) potentially increases the risk of lactic acidosis when given with metformin. Avoid excessive alcohol consumption. Moderate Theoretical
▸ Alcohol potentially causes a disulfiram-like reaction when given with metronidazole. Avoid for at least 48 hours stopping treatment. Moderate Study
▸ Alcohol causes rapid release of opioids (hydromorphone, morphine) (from extended-release preparations). Avoid. Severe Study → Also see TABLE 11 p. 1431
▸ Alcohol (in those who drink heavily) causes severe liver damage when given with paracetamol. Severe Study → Also see TABLE 1 p. 1429
▸ Alcohol increases the risk of facial flushing and skin irritation when given with topical pimecrolimus. Moderate Study
▸ Alcohol potentially causes a disulfiram-like reaction when given with procarbazine. Moderate Anecdotal
▸ Alcohol potentially increases the concentration of retinoids (acitretin). Avoid and for 2 months after stopping **acitretin**. Moderate Study
▸ Alcohol increases the risk of facial flushing and skin irritation when given with topical tacrolimus. Moderate Study
▸ Alcohol potentially causes a disulfiram-like reaction when given with tinidazole. Avoid for 72 hours stopping treatment. Moderate Theoretical

Aldesleukin → see TABLE 15 p. 1432 (myelosuppression)
Aldosterone antagonists → see TABLE 18 p. 1433 (hyponatraemia), TABLE 8 p. 1430 (hypotension), TABLE 16 p. 1433 (increased serum potassium)

eplerenone · spironolactone

▸ Anti-androgens (apalutamide, enzalutamide) are predicted to decrease the exposure to **eplerenone**. Avoid. Moderate Theoretical
▸ Spironolactone is predicted to oppose the effects of anti-androgens (abiraterone). Avoid. Severe Theoretical

▸ Antiarrhythmics (amiodarone) are predicted to increase the exposure to **eplerenone**. Adjust **eplerenone** dose, p. 208. Severe Theoretical
▸ Antiarrhythmics (dronedarone) are predicted to increase the exposure to **eplerenone**. Adjust **eplerenone** dose, p. 208. Severe Study
▸ Antiepileptics (carbamazepine, fosphenytoin, phenobarbital, phenytoin, primidone) are predicted to decrease the exposure to **eplerenone**. Avoid. Moderate Theoretical → Also see TABLE 18 p. 1433
▸ Antifungals, azoles (fluconazole, isavuconazole, posaconazole) are predicted to increase the exposure to **eplerenone**. Adjust **eplerenone** dose, p. 208. Severe Study
▸ Antifungals, azoles (itraconazole, ketoconazole, voriconazole) are predicted to markedly increase the exposure to **eplerenone**. Avoid. Severe Study
▸ Calcium channel blockers (diltiazem, verapamil) are predicted to increase the exposure to **eplerenone**. Adjust **eplerenone** dose, p. 208. Severe Study → Also see TABLE 8 p. 1430
▸ Cobicistat is predicted to markedly increase the exposure to **eplerenone**. Avoid. Severe Study
▸ Crizotinib is predicted to increase the exposure to **eplerenone**. Adjust **eplerenone** dose, p. 208. Severe Study
▸ **Eplerenone** very slightly increases the exposure to digoxin. Mild Study
▸ **Spironolactone** increases the concentration of digoxin. Monitor and adjust dose. Moderate Study
▸ HIV-protease inhibitors are predicted to markedly increase the exposure to **eplerenone**. Avoid. Severe Study
▸ Idelalisib is predicted to markedly increase the exposure to **eplerenone**. Avoid. Severe Study
▸ Imatinib is predicted to increase the exposure to **eplerenone**. Adjust **eplerenone** dose, p. 208. Severe Study
▸ Letermovir is predicted to increase the exposure to **eplerenone**. Adjust **eplerenone** dose, p. 208. Severe Study
▸ **Eplerenone** potentially increases the concentration of lithium. Avoid. Moderate Theoretical
▸ **Spironolactone** potentially increases the concentration of lithium. Moderate Study
▸ Macrolides (clarithromycin) are predicted to markedly increase the exposure to **eplerenone**. Avoid. Severe Study
▸ Macrolides (erythromycin) are predicted to increase the exposure to **eplerenone**. Adjust **eplerenone** dose, p. 208. Severe Study
▸ Mitotane is predicted to decrease the exposure to **eplerenone**. Avoid. Moderate Theoretical
▸ **Spironolactone** is predicted to decrease the effects of mitotane. Avoid. Severe Anecdotal
▸ Neurokinin-1 receptor antagonists (aprepitant, netupitant) are predicted to increase the exposure to **eplerenone**. Adjust **eplerenone** dose, p. 208. Severe Study
▸ Nilotinib is predicted to increase the exposure to **eplerenone**. Adjust **eplerenone** dose, p. 208. Severe Study
▸ Rifamycins (rifampicin) are predicted to decrease the exposure to **eplerenone**. Avoid. Moderate Theoretical
▸ St John's wort is predicted to slightly decrease the exposure to **eplerenone**. Avoid. Moderate Study

Alectinib → see TABLE 6 p. 1430 (bradycardia), TABLE 1 p. 1429 (hepatotoxicity)
Alemtuzumab → see monoclonal antibodies
Alendronate → see bisphosphonates
Alfacalcidol → see vitamin D substances
Alfentanil → see opioids
Alfuzosin → see alpha blockers
Alimemazine → see antihistamines, sedating
Aliskiren → see TABLE 8 p. 1430 (hypotension), TABLE 16 p. 1433 (increased serum potassium)

FOOD AND LIFESTYLE   Avoid apple juice and orange juice as they greatly decrease aliskiren concentrations and plasma renin activity.

▸ ACE inhibitors increase the risk of renal impairment when given with **aliskiren**. Use with caution or avoid **aliskiren** in selected patients, p. 193. Severe Study → Also see TABLE 8 p. 1430 → Also see TABLE 16 p. 1433

Angiotensin-II receptor antagonists increase the risk of renal impairment when given with **aliskiren**. Use with caution or avoid **aliskiren** in selected patients, p. 193. Severe Study → Also see TABLE 8 p. 1430 → Also see TABLE 16 p. 1433

Antiarrhythmics (amiodarone, dronedarone) are predicted to increase the exposure to **aliskiren**. Severe Study

Antiepileptics (carbamazepine) decrease the exposure to **aliskiren**. Moderate Study

Antifungals, azoles (itraconazole) markedly increase the exposure to **aliskiren**. Avoid. Severe Study

Antifungals, azoles (ketoconazole) moderately increase the exposure to **aliskiren**. Moderate Study

Calcium channel blockers (verapamil) moderately increase the exposure to **aliskiren**. Moderate Study → Also see TABLE 8 p. 1430

Ceritinib is predicted to increase the exposure to **aliskiren**. Moderate Theoretical

Ciclosporin markedly increases the exposure to **aliskiren**. Avoid. Severe Study → Also see TABLE 16 p. 1433

Eliglustat is predicted to increase the exposure to **aliskiren**. Adjust dose. Moderate Study

Grapefruit juice moderately decreases the exposure to **aliskiren**. Avoid. Severe Study

HIV-protease inhibitors (ritonavir, saquinavir) are predicted to increase the exposure to **aliskiren**. Moderate Theoretical

Lapatinib is predicted to increase the exposure to **aliskiren**. Moderate Theoretical

Aliskiren slightly decreases the exposure to loop diuretics (furosemide). Moderate Study → Also see TABLE 8 p. 1430

Macrolides (azithromycin) are predicted to increase the exposure to **aliskiren**. Moderate Theoretical

Macrolides (clarithromycin, erythromycin) are predicted to increase the exposure to **aliskiren**. Moderate Study

Mirabegron is predicted to increase the exposure to **aliskiren**. Mild Theoretical

Paritaprevir (with ritonavir and ombitasvir) is predicted to increase the exposure to **aliskiren**. Moderate Study

Pibrentasvir (with glecaprevir) is predicted to increase the exposure to **aliskiren**. Moderate Study

Pitolisant is predicted to decrease the exposure to **aliskiren**. Mild Theoretical

Ranolazine is predicted to increase the exposure to **aliskiren**. Moderate Theoretical

Rifamycins (rifampicin) decrease the exposure to **aliskiren**. Moderate Study

St John's wort decreases the exposure to **aliskiren**. Moderate Study

Statins (atorvastatin) slightly to moderately increase the exposure to **aliskiren**. Moderate Study

Velpatasvir is predicted to increase the exposure to **aliskiren**. Severe Theoretical

Vemurafenib is predicted to increase the exposure to **aliskiren**. Use with caution and adjust dose. Moderate Theoretical

Alitretinoin → see retinoids

Alkylating agents → see TABLE 15 p. 1432 (myelosuppression), TABLE 2 p. 1429 (nephrotoxicity), TABLE 5 p. 1430 (thromboembolism)

bendamustine · busulfan · carmustine · chlorambucil · cyclophosphamide · dacarbazine · estramustine · ifosfamide · lomustine · melphalan · temozolomide · thiotepa · treosulfan

▸ Oral antacids are predicted to decrease the absorption of oral **estramustine**. Avoid. Moderate Study

▸ Antifungals, azoles (isavuconazole) are predicted to increase the exposure to **cyclophosphamide**. Moderate Study

▸ Antifungals, azoles (itraconazole) increase the risk of busulfan toxicity when given with **busulfan**. Monitor and adjust dose. Moderate Study

▸ Antifungals, azoles (miconazole) are predicted to increase the concentration of **busulfan**. Use with caution and adjust dose. Moderate Study

▸ Oral calcium salts decrease the absorption of **estramustine**. Severe Study

▸ Live vaccines are predicted to increase the risk of generalised infection (possibly life-threatening) when given with **alkylating agents**. Public Health England advises avoid (refer to Green Book). Severe Theoretical

▸ Metronidazole increases the risk of toxicity when given with **busulfan**. Severe Study

▸ Neurokinin-1 receptor antagonists (aprepitant, fosaprepitant) are predicted to increase the exposure to **ifosfamide**. Severe Theoretical

▸ Neurokinin-1 receptor antagonists (netupitant) very slightly increase the exposure to **cyclophosphamide**. Moderate Study

▸ Neurokinin-1 receptor antagonists (netupitant) are predicted to increase the exposure to **ifosfamide**. Moderate Study

▸ Paracetamol is predicted to decrease the clearance of **busulfan**. Moderate Theoretical

▸ Cyclophosphamide (high-dose) increases the risk of toxicity when given with **pentostatin**. Avoid. Severe Anecdotal → Also see TABLE 15 p. 1432 → Also see TABLE 5 p. 1430

▸ Cyclophosphamide increases the risk of prolonged neuromuscular blockade when given with suxamethonium. Moderate Study

Allopurinol

▸ ACE inhibitors are predicted to increase the risk of hypersensitivity and haematological reactions when given with **allopurinol**. Severe Anecdotal

▸ Allopurinol potentially increases the risk of haematological toxicity when given with azathioprine. Adjust **azathioprine** dose, p. 882. Severe Study

▸ Allopurinol is predicted to decrease the effects of capecitabine. Avoid. Severe Study

▸ Allopurinol potentially increases the risk of haematological toxicity when given with mercaptopurine. Adjust **mercaptopurine** dose, p. 956. Severe Study

▸ Allopurinol increases the risk of skin rash when given with penicillins (amoxicillin, ampicillin). Moderate Study

▸ Allopurinol is predicted to increase the risk of hyperuricaemia when given with pyrazinamide. Moderate Theoretical

▸ Thiazide diuretics are predicted to increase the risk of hypersensitivity reactions when given with **allopurinol**. Severe Theoretical

Almotriptan → see triptans

Alogliptin → see dipeptidylpeptidase-4 inhibitors

Alpelisib

▸ Alpelisib is predicted to decrease the efficacy of bupropion. Mild Theoretical

▸ Ciclosporin is predicted to increase the exposure to **alpelisib**. Moderate Theoretical

▸ Alpelisib is predicted to decrease the efficacy of coumarins (warfarin). Moderate Theoretical

▸ Eltrombopag is predicted to increase the exposure to **alpelisib**. Moderate Theoretical

▸ Lapatinib is predicted to increase the exposure to **alpelisib**. Moderate Theoretical

▸ Leflunomide is predicted to increase the exposure to **alpelisib**. Moderate Theoretical

▸ Proton pump inhibitors (pantoprazole) are predicted to increase the exposure to **alpelisib**. Moderate Theoretical

▸ Teriflunomide is predicted to increase the exposure to **alpelisib**. Moderate Theoretical

Alpha blockers → see TABLE 7 p. 1430 (first-dose hypotension), TABLE 8 p. 1430 (hypotension)

alfuzosin · doxazosin · indoramin · prazosin · tamsulosin · terazosin

▸ Antiarrhythmics (dronedarone) are predicted to increase the exposure to **tamsulosin**. Moderate Theoretical

▸ Antifungals, azoles (fluconazole, isavuconazole, posaconazole) are predicted to increase the exposure to **tamsulosin**. Moderate Theoretical

▸ Antifungals, azoles (itraconazole, ketoconazole, voriconazole) are predicted to increase the exposure to **doxazosin**. Moderate Study

▸ Antifungals, azoles (itraconazole, ketoconazole, voriconazole) are predicted to moderately increase the exposure to alpha blockers (alfuzosin, tamsulosin). Use with caution or avoid. Moderate Study

▸ Calcium channel blockers (diltiazem, verapamil) are predicted to increase the exposure to **tamsulosin**. Moderate Theoretical → Also see TABLE 8 p. 1430

Alpha blockers (continued)

▸ Cobicistat is predicted to moderately increase the exposure to alpha blockers (**alfuzosin, tamsulosin**). Use with caution or avoid. Moderate Study

▸ Cobicistat is predicted to increase the exposure to **doxazosin**. Moderate Study

▸ Crizotinib is predicted to increase the exposure to **tamsulosin**. Moderate Theoretical

▸ HIV-protease inhibitors are predicted to moderately increase the exposure to alpha blockers (**alfuzosin, tamsulosin**). Use with caution or avoid. Moderate Study

▸ HIV-protease inhibitors are predicted to increase the exposure to **doxazosin**. Moderate Study

▸ Idelalisib is predicted to moderately increase the exposure to alpha blockers (**alfuzosin, tamsulosin**). Use with caution or avoid. Moderate Study

▸ Idelalisib is predicted to increase the exposure to **doxazosin**. Moderate Study

▸ Imatinib is predicted to increase the exposure to **tamsulosin**. Moderate Theoretical

▸ Letermovir is predicted to increase the exposure to **tamsulosin**. Moderate Theoretical

▸ Macrolides (**clarithromycin**) are predicted to increase the exposure to **doxazosin**. Moderate Study

▸ Macrolides (**erythromycin**) are predicted to increase the exposure to **tamsulosin**. Moderate Theoretical

▸ Macrolides (**clarithromycin**) are predicted to moderately increase the exposure to alpha blockers (**alfuzosin, tamsulosin**). Use with caution or avoid. Moderate Study

▸ MAOIs, irreversible are predicted to increase the effects of **indoramin**. Avoid. Severe Theoretical → Also see TABLE 8 p. 1430

▸ Neurokinin-1 receptor antagonists (**aprepitant, netupitant**) are predicted to increase the exposure to **tamsulosin**. Moderate Theoretical

▸ Nilotinib is predicted to increase the exposure to **tamsulosin**. Moderate Theoretical

▸ **Alpha blockers** cause significant hypotensive effects when given with phosphodiesterase type-5 inhibitors. Patient should be stabilised on first drug then second drug should be added at the lowest recommended dose. Severe Study → Also see TABLE 8 p. 1430

▸ Ribociclib (high-dose) is predicted to increase the exposure to **alfuzosin**. Avoid. Moderate Theoretical

Alprazolam → see benzodiazepines

Alprostadil → see TABLE 8 p. 1430 (hypotension)

Alteplase → see TABLE 3 p. 1429 (anticoagulant effects)

Aluminium hydroxide

SEPARATION OF ADMINISTRATION **Aluminium-containing antacids** should preferably not be taken at the same time as other drugs since they might impair absorption. **Aluminium-containing antacids** might damage enteric coatings designed to prevent dissolution in the stomach.

▸ Oral **aluminium hydroxide** decreases the absorption of chenodeoxycholic acid. Moderate Study

▸ **Aluminium hydroxide** increases the risk of blocked enteral or nasogastric tubes when given with enteral feeds. Moderate Study

▸ **Aluminium hydroxide** is predicted to decrease the exposure to iron chelators (**deferasirox**). Avoid. Moderate Theoretical

▸ **Aluminium hydroxide** is predicted to decrease the absorption of iron chelators (**deferiprone**). Avoid. Moderate Theoretical

Amantadine → see dopamine receptor agonists

Ambrisentan → see endothelin receptor antagonists

Amfetamines → see TABLE 13 p. 1432 (serotonin syndrome)

dexamfetamine · lisdexamfetamine

▸ **Amfetamines** are predicted to decrease the effects of apraclonidine. Avoid. Severe Theoretical

▸ **Amfetamines** are predicted to increase the risk of adverse effects when given with atomoxetine. Severe Theoretical

▸ HIV-protease inhibitors (**ritonavir, tipranavir**) are predicted to increase the exposure to **amfetamines**. Severe Theoretical

▸ MAO-B inhibitors (**rasagiline, selegiline**) are predicted to increase the risk of severe hypertension when given with **amfetamines**. Avoid. Severe Theoretical → Also see TABLE 13 p. 1432

▸ MAO-B inhibitors (**safinamide**) are predicted to increase the risk of severe hypertension when given with **amfetamines**. Severe Theoretical → Also see TABLE 13 p. 1432

▸ **Amfetamines** are predicted to increase the risk of a hypertensive crisis when given with MAOIs, irreversible. Avoid and for 14 days after stopping the MAOI. Severe Anecdotal → Also see TABLE 13 p. 1432

▸ **Amfetamines** are predicted to increase the risk of a hypertensive crisis when given with moclobemide. Avoid. Severe Theoretical → Also see TABLE 13 p. 1432

▸ Nabilone is predicted to increase the risk of cardiovascular adverse effects when given with **amfetamines**. Severe Theoretical

▸ Phenothiazines are predicted to decrease the effects of **amfetamines** and **amfetamines** are predicted to decrease the effects of phenothiazines. Moderate Study

▸ SSRIs (**fluoxetine, paroxetine**) are predicted to increase the exposure to **amfetamines**. Severe Theoretical → Also see TABLE 13 p. 1432

Amifampridine → see TABLE 9 p. 1431 (QT-interval prolongation)

Amikacin → see aminoglycosides

Amiloride → see potassium-sparing diuretics

Aminoglycosides → see TABLE 2 p. 1429 (nephrotoxicity), TABLE 19 p. 1433 (ototoxicity), TABLE 20 p. 1433 (neuromuscular blocking effects)

amikacin · gentamicin · streptomycin · tobramycin

ROUTE-SPECIFIC INFORMATION Since systemic absorption can follow topical application, the possibility of interactions with topical **gentamicin** and **tobramycin** should be borne in mind.

▸ **Aminoglycosides** are predicted to decrease the effects of agalsidase alfa. Avoid. Moderate Theoretical

▸ **Aminoglycosides** are predicted to decrease the effects of agalsidase beta. Avoid. Moderate Theoretical

▸ Antifungals, azoles (**miconazole**) potentially decrease the exposure to **tobramycin**. Moderate Anecdotal

▸ Ataluren is predicted to increase the risk of nephrotoxicity when given with intravenous **aminoglycosides**. Avoid. Severe Study

▸ **Aminoglycosides** increase the risk of hypocalcaemia when given with bisphosphonates. Moderate Anecdotal → Also see TABLE 2 p. 1429

▸ **Aminoglycosides** potentially increase the concentration of digoxin. Monitor and adjust dose. Mild Study

▸ Loop diuretics increase the risk of nephrotoxicity when given with **aminoglycosides**. Avoid. Moderate Study → Also see TABLE 19 p. 1433

▸ **Aminoglycosides** are predicted to decrease the effects of neostigmine. Moderate Theoretical

▸ **Aminoglycosides** are predicted to decrease the effects of pyridostigmine. Moderate Theoretical

Aminophylline → see TABLE 17 p. 1433 (reduced serum potassium)

FOOD AND LIFESTYLE Smoking can increase aminophylline clearance and increased doses of aminophylline are therefore required; dose adjustments are likely to be necessary if smoking started or stopped during treatment.

▸ Aciclovir increases the exposure to **aminophylline**. Monitor and adjust dose. Severe Anecdotal

▸ **Aminophylline** is predicted to decrease the efficacy of antiarrhythmics (**adenosine**). Separate administration by 24 hours. Mild Theoretical

▸ Antiepileptics (**fosphenytoin**) are predicted to decrease the exposure to **aminophylline**. Adjust dose. Moderate Study

▸ Antiepileptics (**phenobarbital**) are predicted to decrease the exposure to **aminophylline**. Adjust dose. Moderate Theoretical

▸ Antiepileptics (**phenytoin**) decrease the exposure to **aminophylline**. Adjust dose. Moderate Study

▸ Antiepileptics (**primidone**) are predicted to increase the clearance of **aminophylline**. Adjust dose. Moderate Theoretical

▸ Antiepileptics (**stiripentol**) are predicted to increase the exposure to **aminophylline**. Avoid. Moderate Theoretical

▸ Beta blockers, non-selective are predicted to increase the risk of bronchospasm when given with **aminophylline**. Avoid. Severe Theoretical

Beta blockers, selective are predicted to increase the risk of bronchospasm when given with **aminophylline**. Avoid. Theoretical

Combined hormonal contraceptives are predicted to increase the exposure to **aminophylline**. Adjust dose. Moderate Theoretical

Aminophylline increases the risk of agitation when given with doxapram. Moderate Study

Esketamine is predicted to increase the risk of seizures when given with **aminophylline**. Avoid. Severe Theoretical

H_2 receptor antagonists (cimetidine) increase the concentration of **aminophylline**. Adjust dose. Severe Study

HIV-protease inhibitors (ritonavir) decrease the exposure to **aminophylline**. Adjust dose. Moderate Study

Interferons are predicted to slightly increase the exposure to **aminophylline**. Adjust dose. Moderate Theoretical

Iron chelators (deferasirox) are predicted to increase the exposure to **aminophylline**. Avoid. Moderate Theoretical

Isoniazid is predicted to affect the clearance of **aminophylline**. Severe Theoretical

Leflunomide decreases the exposure to **aminophylline**. Adjust dose. Moderate Study

Aminophylline is predicted to decrease the concentration of lithium. Moderate Theoretical

Macrolides (azithromycin) are predicted to increase the exposure to **aminophylline**. Moderate Theoretical

Macrolides (clarithromycin) are predicted to increase the exposure to **aminophylline**. Adjust dose. Moderate Theoretical

Aminophylline is predicted to decrease the exposure to macrolides (erythromycin). Adjust dose. Severe Study

▸ Methotrexate is predicted to decrease the clearance of **aminophylline**. Moderate Theoretical

Mexiletine is predicted to increase the exposure to **aminophylline**. Adjust dose. Moderate Theoretical

Monoclonal antibodies (blinatumomab) are predicted to transiently increase the exposure to **aminophylline**. Monitor and adjust dose. Moderate Theoretical

Monoclonal antibodies (sarilumab) potentially affect the exposure to **aminophylline**. Monitor and adjust dose. Moderate Theoretical

Monoclonal antibodies (tocilizumab) are predicted to decrease the exposure to **aminophylline**. Monitor and adjust dose. Moderate Theoretical

▸ Pentoxifylline is predicted to increase the concentration of **aminophylline**. Use with caution or avoid. Severe Theoretical

▸ **Aminophylline** is predicted to slightly increase the exposure to phosphodiesterase type-4 inhibitors (roflumilast). Avoid. Moderate Theoretical

▸ Quinolones (ciprofloxacin) are predicted to increase the exposure to **aminophylline**. Adjust dose. Moderate Theoretical

▸ Rifamycins (rifampicin) decrease the exposure to **aminophylline**. Adjust dose. Moderate Study

▸ Rucaparib is predicted to increase the exposure to **aminophylline**. Monitor and adjust dose. Moderate Study

▸ SSRIs (fluvoxamine) moderately to markedly increase the exposure to **aminophylline**. Avoid. Severe Study

▸ St John's wort is predicted to decrease the concentration of **aminophylline**. Severe Theoretical

▸ Sympathomimetics, vasoconstrictor (ephedrine) increase the risk of adverse effects when given with **aminophylline**. Avoid in children. Moderate Study

▸ Teriflunomide decreases the exposure to **aminophylline**. Adjust dose. Moderate Study

▸ Valaciclovir is predicted to increase the exposure to **aminophylline**. Severe Anecdotal

Aminosalicylic acid

▸ Aminosalicylic acid is predicted to increase the risk of methaemoglobinaemia when given with topical anaesthetics, local (prilocaine). Use with caution or avoid. Severe Theoretical

▸ Aminosalicylic acid is predicted to increase the risk of methaemoglobinaemia when given with dapsone. Severe Theoretical

Amiodarone → see antiarrhythmics
Amisulpride → see antipsychotics, second generation
Amitriptyline → see tricyclic antidepressants

Amlodipine → see calcium channel blockers
Amoxicillin → see penicillins
Amphotericin B → see TABLE 2 p. 1429 (nephrotoxicity), TABLE 17 p. 1433 (reduced serum potassium)

▸ Amphotericin B increases the risk of toxicity when given with flucytosine. Severe Study

▸ Micafungin slightly increases the exposure to **amphotericin B**. Avoid or monitor toxicity. Moderate Study

Ampicillin → see penicillins
Amsacrine → see TABLE 15 p. 1432 (myelosuppression)

▸ Live vaccines are predicted to increase the risk of generalised infection (possibly life-threatening) when given with amsacrine. Public Health England advises avoid (refer to Green Book). Severe Theoretical

Anaesthetics, local → see TABLE 11 p. 1431 (CNS depressant effects)

bupivacaine · levobupivacaine · mepivacaine · oxybuprocaine · prilocaine · proxymetacaine · ropivacaine · tetracaine

ROUTE-SPECIFIC INFORMATION Since systemic absorption can follow topical application, the possibility of interactions should be borne in mind.

▸ Aminosalicylic acid is predicted to increase the risk of methaemoglobinaemia when given with topical **prilocaine**. Use with caution or avoid. Severe Theoretical

▸ Anaesthetics, local are predicted to increase the risk of cardiodepression when given with antiarrhythmics. Severe Theoretical → Also see TABLE 11 p. 1431

▸ Antiepileptics (fosphenytoin, phenobarbital, phenytoin, primidone) are predicted to increase the risk of methaemoglobinaemia when given with topical **prilocaine**. Use with caution or avoid. Severe Theoretical → Also see TABLE 11 p. 1431

▸ Antiepileptics (phenytoin) are predicted to decrease the exposure to **ropivacaine**. Moderate Theoretical

▸ Antimalarials (chloroquine, primaquine) are predicted to increase the risk of methaemoglobinaemia when given with topical **prilocaine**. Use with caution or avoid. Severe Theoretical

▸ Dapsone is predicted to increase the risk of methaemoglobinaemia when given with topical **prilocaine**. Use with caution or avoid. Severe Theoretical

▸ HIV-protease inhibitors (ritonavir) are predicted to decrease the exposure to **ropivacaine**. Moderate Theoretical

▸ Leflunomide is predicted to decrease the exposure to **ropivacaine**. Moderate Theoretical

▸ Metoclopramide is predicted to increase the risk of methaemoglobinaemia when given with topical **prilocaine**. Avoid. Severe Theoretical

▸ Nitrates are predicted to increase the risk of methaemoglobinaemia when given with topical **prilocaine**. Avoid. Severe Theoretical

▸ Nitrofurantoin is predicted to increase the risk of methaemoglobinaemia when given with topical **prilocaine**. Use with caution or avoid. Severe Theoretical

▸ Nitroprusside is predicted to increase the risk of methaemoglobinaemia when given with **prilocaine**. Severe Theoretical

▸ Paracetamol is predicted to increase the risk of methaemoglobinaemia when given with topical **prilocaine**. Use with caution or avoid. Severe Theoretical

▸ Rifamycins (rifampicin) are predicted to decrease the exposure to **ropivacaine**. Moderate Theoretical

▸ SSRIs (fluvoxamine) decrease the clearance of **ropivacaine**. Avoid prolonged use. Moderate Study

▸ Sulfonamides potentially increase the risk of methaemoglobinaemia when given with topical **prilocaine**. Use with caution or avoid. Severe Anecdotal

▸ Teriflunomide is predicted to decrease the exposure to **ropivacaine**. Moderate Theoretical

Anagrelide → see TABLE 9 p. 1431 (QT-interval prolongation), TABLE 4 p. 1429 (antiplatelet effects)

▸ Combined hormonal contraceptives are predicted to increase the exposure to **anagrelide**. Moderate Theoretical

▸ Mexiletine is predicted to increase the exposure to **anagrelide**. Moderate Theoretical

Anagrelide (continued)
- Quinolones (ciprofloxacin) are predicted to increase the exposure to **anagrelide**. Moderate Theoretical
- SSRIs (fluvoxamine) are predicted to increase the exposure to **anagrelide**. Moderate Theoretical → Also see **TABLE 4** p. 1429

Anakinra
- **Anakinra** is predicted to increase the risk of generalised infection (possibly life-threatening) when given with etanercept. Avoid. Severe Theoretical
- Filgotinib is predicted to increase the risk of immunosuppression when given with **anakinra**. Avoid. Severe Theoretical
- Live vaccines are predicted to increase the risk of generalised infection (possibly life-threatening) when given with **anakinra**. Public Health England advises avoid (refer to Green Book). Severe Theoretical
- **Anakinra** is predicted to increase the risk of generalised infection (possibly life-threatening) when given with monoclonal antibodies (golimumab). Avoid. Severe Theoretical

Angiotensin-II receptor antagonists → see **TABLE 7** p. 1430 (first-dose hypotension), **TABLE 8** p. 1430 (hypotension), **TABLE 16** p. 1433 (increased serum potassium)

azilsartan · candesartan · eprosartan · irbesartan · losartan · olmesartan · telmisartan · valsartan

- **Angiotensin-II receptor antagonists** increase the risk of renal impairment when given with aliskiren. Use with caution or avoid **aliskiren** in selected patients, p. 193. Severe Study → Also see **TABLE 8** p. 1430 → Also see **TABLE 16** p. 1433
- Filgotinib is predicted to increase the exposure to **valsartan**. Avoid. Moderate Theoretical
- **Angiotensin-II receptor antagonists** potentially increase the concentration of lithium. Monitor concentration and adjust dose. Severe Anecdotal

Antacids

SEPARATION OF ADMINISTRATION Aluminium- and magnesium-containing antacids should preferably not be taken at the same time as other drugs since they might impair absorption. Aluminium- and magnesium-containing antacids might damage enteric coatings designed to prevent dissolution in the stomach.

- Oral **antacids** is predicted to decrease the exposure to oral acalabrutinib. Separate administration by at least 2 hours. Moderate Theoretical
- Oral **antacids** are predicted to decrease the absorption of oral alkylating agents (estramustine). Avoid. Moderate Study
- Oral **antacids** decrease the absorption of oral antiepileptics (gabapentin). **Gabapentin** should be taken 2 hours after antacids. Moderate Study
- Oral **antacids** decrease the absorption of oral antifungals, azoles (itraconazole) capsules. **Itraconazole** should be taken 2 hours before or 1 hour after antacids. Moderate Study
- Oral **antacids** decrease the absorption of oral antifungals, azoles (ketoconazole). Separate administration by at least 2 hours. Moderate Study
- Oral **antacids** decrease the absorption of oral antihistamines, non-sedating (fexofenadine). Separate administration by 2 hours. Mild Study
- Oral **antacids** decrease the absorption of oral antimalarials (chloroquine). Separate administration by at least 4 hours. Moderate Study
- Oral **antacids** are predicted to decrease the absorption of oral antimalarials (proguanil). Separate administration by at least 2 hours. Moderate Study
- Oral **antacids** decrease the absorption of oral aspirin (high-dose). Moderate Study
- Oral **antacids** decrease the exposure to oral bictegravir. Separate administration by at least 2 hours. Moderate Study
- Oral **antacids** decrease the absorption of oral bisphosphonates (alendronate). **Alendronate** should be taken at least 30 minutes before antacids. Moderate Study
- Oral **antacids** decrease the absorption of oral bisphosphonates (clodronate). Avoid antacids for 2 hours before or 1 hour after **clodronate**. Moderate Study

- Oral **antacids** are predicted to decrease the absorption of bisphosphonates (ibandronate). Avoid antacids for at least 6 hours before or 1 hour after **ibandronate**. Moderate Theoretical
- Oral **antacids** decrease the absorption of oral bisphosphonates (risedronate). Separate administration by at least 2 hours. Moderate Study
- Oral **antacids** are predicted to decrease the absorption of oral bosutinib. **Bosutinib** should be taken at least 12 hours before antacids. Moderate Theoretical
- Oral **antacids** are predicted to decrease the absorption of oral ceritinib. Separate administration by 2 hours. Moderate Theoretical
- Oral **antacids** are predicted to decrease the absorption of oral cholic acid. Separate administration by 5 hours. Mild Theoretical
- Oral **antacids** are predicted to decrease the absorption of oral corticosteroids (deflazacort). Separate administration by 2 hours. Moderate Theoretical
- Oral **antacids** decrease the absorption of oral corticosteroids (dexamethasone). Moderate Study
- Oral **antacids** decrease the absorption of oral dasatinib. Separate administration by at least 2 hours. Moderate Study
- Oral **antacids** are predicted to decrease the absorption of oral digoxin. Separate administration by 2 hours. Mild Study
- Oral **antacids** are predicted to decrease the absorption of oral dipyridamole (immediate release tablets). Moderate Theoretical
- Oral **antacids** decrease the exposure to oral dolutegravir. **Dolutegravir** should be taken 2 hours before or 6 hours after antacids. Moderate Study
- Oral **antacids** decrease the exposure to oral eltrombopag. **Eltrombopag** should be taken 2 hours before or 4 hours after antacids. Severe Study
- Oral **antacids** decrease the exposure to oral elvitegravir. Separate administration by at least 4 hours. Moderate Study
- Oral **antacids** are predicted to decrease the absorption of oral erlotinib. **Erlotinib** should be taken 2 hours before or 4 hours after antacids. Moderate Theoretical
- Oral **antacids** decrease the exposure to oral fibrates (gemfibrozil). Moderate Study
- Oral **antacids** are predicted to decrease the exposure to oral gefitinib. Moderate Theoretical
- Oral **antacids** are predicted to decrease the absorption of oral HIV-protease inhibitors (atazanavir). **Atazanavir** should be taken 2 hours before or 1 hour after antacids. Severe Theoretical
- Oral **antacids** are predicted to decrease the absorption of oral HIV-protease inhibitors (tipranavir). Separate administration by 2 hours. Moderate Study
- Oral **antacids** decrease the absorption of oral hydroxychloroquine. Separate administration by at least 4 hours. Moderate Study
- Oral **antacids** decrease the absorption of oral iron. Manufacturer advises iron should be taken 1 hour before or 2 hours after antacids. Moderate Study
- Oral **antacids** decrease the absorption of oral lapatinib. Avoid. Moderate Theoretical
- Oral **antacids** are predicted to decrease the exposure to oral ledipasvir. Separate administration by 4 hours. Moderate Theoretical
- Oral **antacids** decrease the exposure to oral mycophenolate. Moderate Study
- Oral **antacids** are predicted to decrease the exposure to oral neratinib. Separate administration by at least 3 hours. Mild Theoretical
- Oral **antacids** are predicted to decrease the absorption of oral nilotinib. Separate administration by at least 2 hours. Moderate Theoretical
- Oral **antacids** are predicted to decrease the exposure to oral NNRTIs (rilpivirine). **Rilpivirine** should be taken 4 hours before or 2 hours after antacids. Severe Theoretical
- Oral **antacids** are predicted to decrease the absorption of oral pazopanib. **Pazopanib** should be taken 1 hour before or 2 hours after antacids. Moderate Theoretical
- Oral **antacids** decrease the absorption of oral penicillamine. Separate administration by 2 hours. Mild Study
- Oral **antacids** decrease the absorption of oral phenothiazines. Moderate Anecdotal

Oral **antacids** increase the risk of metabolic alkalosis when given with oral polystyrene sulfonate. Severe Anecdotal

Oral **antacids** decrease the absorption of oral quinolones. **Quinolones** should be taken 2 hours before or 4 hours after antacids. Moderate Study

Oral **antacids** decrease the exposure to oral raltegravir. Avoid. Moderate Study

Oral **antacids** decrease the absorption of oral rifamycins (rifampicin). **Rifampicin** should be taken 1 hour before antacids. Moderate Study

Oral **antacids** decrease the exposure to oral riociguat. **Riociguat** should be taken 1 hour before or 2 hours after antacids. Mild Study

Oral **antacids** decrease the absorption of oral statins (rosuvastatin). Separate administration by 2 hours. Moderate Study

Oral **antacids** decrease the absorption of oral strontium. Separate administration by 2 hours. Moderate Study

Oral **antacids** decrease the absorption of oral sulpiride. Separate administration by 2 hours. Moderate Study

Oral **antacids** decrease the absorption of oral tetracyclines. Separate administration by 2 to 3 hours. Moderate Study

Oral **antacids** are predicted to decrease the absorption of oral thyroid hormones (levothyroxine). Separate administration by at least 4 hours. Moderate Anecdotal

Oral **antacids** are predicted to decrease the absorption of oral ursodeoxycholic acid. Separate administration by 2 hours. Moderate Theoretical

Oral **antacids** are predicted to decrease the concentration of oral velpatasvir. Separate administration by 4 hours. Moderate Theoretical

Antazoline → see antihistamines, sedating

Anthracyclines → see TABLE 15 p. 1432 (myelosuppression), TABLE 5 p. 1430 (thromboembolism)

daunorubicin · doxorubicin · epirubicin · idarubicin · mitoxantrone · pixantrone

GENERAL INFORMATION Caution is necessary with concurrent use of cardiotoxic drugs, or drugs that reduce cardiac contractility.

Calcium channel blockers (verapamil) moderately increase the exposure to **doxorubicin**. Moderate Study

Ciclosporin increases the concentration of anthracyclines (**daunorubicin, doxorubicin, epirubicin, idarubicin, mitoxantrone**). Severe Study

H_2 receptor antagonists (cimetidine) slightly increase the exposure to **epirubicin**. Avoid. Moderate Study

Leflunomide is predicted to increase the exposure to anthracyclines (**daunorubicin, doxorubicin, mitoxantrone**). Moderate Theoretical → Also see TABLE 15 p. 1432

Live vaccines are predicted to increase the risk of generalised infection (possibly life-threatening) when given with **anthracyclines**. Public Health England advises avoid (refer to Green Book). Severe Theoretical

Anthracyclines are predicted to increase the risk of cardiotoxicity when given with monoclonal antibodies (trastuzumab, trastuzumab emtansine). Avoid. Severe Theoretical → Also see TABLE 15 p. 1432

Teriflunomide is predicted to increase the exposure to anthracyclines (**daunorubicin, doxorubicin, mitoxantrone**). Moderate Study

Anti-androgens → see TABLE 9 p. 1431 (QT-interval prolongation)

abiraterone · apalutamide · bicalutamide · cyproterone · darolutamide · enzalutamide · flutamide

GENERAL INFORMATION Caution with concurrent chemotherapy—safety and efficacy with **abiraterone** and **enzalutamide** not established.

▸ Anti-androgens (**apalutamide, enzalutamide**) are predicted to decrease the exposure to 5-HT3-receptor antagonists (ondansetron). Moderate Study → Also see TABLE 9 p. 1431

▸ Anti-androgens (**apalutamide, enzalutamide**) are predicted to markedly decrease the exposure to abemaciclib. Avoid. Severe Study

▸ Anti-androgens (**apalutamide, enzalutamide**) are predicted to decrease the exposure to acalabrutinib. Avoid. Severe Study

▸ Aldosterone antagonists (spironolactone) are predicted to oppose the effects of **abiraterone**. Avoid. Severe Theoretical

▸ Anti-androgens (**apalutamide, enzalutamide**) are predicted to decrease the exposure to aldosterone antagonists (eplerenone). Avoid. Moderate Theoretical

▸ Anti-androgens (**apalutamide, enzalutamide**) are predicted to decrease the exposure to anti-androgens (abiraterone). Avoid. Severe Study

▸ Anti-androgens (**apalutamide**) are predicted to decrease the exposure to anti-androgens (darolutamide). Avoid. Moderate Study

▸ Anti-androgens (**enzalutamide**) are predicted to decrease the exposure to anti-androgens (darolutamide). Avoid. Moderate Study

▸ Anti-androgens (**apalutamide, enzalutamide**) are predicted to decrease the exposure to antiarrhythmics (disopyramide, dronedarone). Avoid. Severe Study → Also see TABLE 9 p. 1431

▸ Anti-androgens (**apalutamide, enzalutamide**) are predicted to decrease the efficacy of antiarrhythmics (propafenone). Moderate Study

▸ Anti-androgens (**apalutamide, enzalutamide**) are predicted to decrease the exposure to anticholinesterases, centrally acting (donepezil). Mild Study

▸ Antiepileptics (carbamazepine, fosphenytoin, phenobarbital, phenytoin, primidone) are predicted to decrease the exposure to **abiraterone**. Avoid. Severe Study

▸ Antiepileptics (carbamazepine, fosphenytoin, phenobarbital, phenytoin, primidone) are predicted to decrease the exposure to **darolutamide**. Avoid. Moderate Study

▸ **Enzalutamide** is predicted to slightly decrease the exposure to antiepileptics (brivaracetam). Moderate Theoretical

▸ Anti-androgens (**apalutamide, enzalutamide**) are predicted to decrease the exposure to antiepileptics (perampanel). Monitor and adjust dose. Moderate Study

▸ **Apalutamide** potentially decreases the exposure to antiepileptics (valproate). Mild Theoretical

▸ Antifungals, azoles (itraconazole) slightly increase the exposure to **darolutamide**. Monitor and adjust dose. Moderate Study

▸ Antifungals, azoles (itraconazole, ketoconazole, voriconazole) are predicted to increase the exposure to **apalutamide**. Mild Study → Also see TABLE 9 p. 1431

▸ Antifungals, azoles (ketoconazole) are predicted to increase the exposure to **darolutamide**. Monitor and adjust dose. Moderate Theoretical

▸ Anti-androgens (**apalutamide, enzalutamide**) are predicted to decrease the exposure to antifungals, azoles (isavuconazole). Avoid. Severe Study

▸ **Apalutamide** slightly decreases the exposure to antihistamines, non-sedating (fexofenadine). Mild Study

▸ **Darolutamide** is predicted to increase the concentration of antihistamines, non-sedating (fexofenadine). Moderate Theoretical

▸ Anti-androgens (**apalutamide, enzalutamide**) are predicted to decrease the exposure to antimalarials (artemether with lumefantrine). Avoid. Severe Study → Also see TABLE 9 p. 1431

▸ Anti-androgens (**apalutamide, enzalutamide**) are predicted to decrease the concentration of antimalarials (piperaquine). Avoid. Moderate Theoretical

▸ Anti-androgens (**apalutamide, enzalutamide**) are predicted to moderately decrease the exposure to antipsychotics, second generation (aripiprazole). Adjust **aripiprazole** dose, p. 415. Moderate Study

▸ Anti-androgens (**apalutamide, enzalutamide**) are predicted to decrease the exposure to antipsychotics, second generation (cariprazine). Avoid. Severe Theoretical

▸ **Enzalutamide** is predicted to decrease the exposure to antipsychotics, second generation (clozapine). Moderate Theoretical

▸ Anti-androgens (**apalutamide, enzalutamide**) are predicted to decrease the exposure to antipsychotics, second generation (lurasidone). Avoid. Moderate Study

▸ Anti-androgens (**apalutamide, enzalutamide**) are predicted to decrease the exposure to antipsychotics, second generation (paliperidone). Monitor and adjust dose. Severe Study → Also see TABLE 9 p. 1431

Anti-androgens (continued)

▸ Anti-androgens (**apalutamide, enzalutamide**) are predicted to decrease the exposure to antipsychotics, second generation (quetiapine). [Moderate] Study

▸ Anti-androgens (**apalutamide, enzalutamide**) are predicted to decrease the exposure to antipsychotics, second generation (risperidone). Adjust dose. [Moderate] Study →Also see TABLE 9 p. 1431

▸ Anti-androgens (**apalutamide, enzalutamide**) are predicted to decrease the exposure to avapritinib. Avoid. [Severe] Study

▸ Anti-androgens (**apalutamide, enzalutamide**) are predicted to decrease the exposure to axitinib. Avoid or adjust dose. [Moderate] Study

▸ Anti-androgens (**apalutamide, enzalutamide**) decrease the exposure to bedaquiline. Avoid. [Severe] Study →Also see TABLE 9 p. 1431

▸ Anti-androgens (**apalutamide, enzalutamide**) are predicted to decrease the exposure to benzodiazepines (alprazolam). Adjust dose. [Moderate] Theoretical

▸ **Apalutamide** is predicted to decrease the exposure to benzodiazepines (diazepam). Avoid or monitor. [Mild] Study

▸ Anti-androgens (**apalutamide, enzalutamide**) are predicted to decrease the exposure to benzodiazepines (midazolam). Monitor and adjust dose. [Moderate] Study

▸ **Abiraterone** is predicted to increase the exposure to beta blockers, selective (metoprolol). [Moderate] Study

▸ **Apalutamide** is predicted to decrease the exposure to beta$_2$ agonists (salmeterol). Avoid or monitor. [Moderate] Study

▸ Anti-androgens (**apalutamide, enzalutamide**) are predicted to decrease the exposure to bictegravir. Avoid. [Moderate] Study

▸ Anti-androgens (**apalutamide, enzalutamide**) slightly decrease the exposure to bortezomib. Avoid. [Severe] Study

▸ Anti-androgens (**apalutamide, enzalutamide**) are predicted to very markedly decrease the exposure to bosutinib. Avoid. [Severe] Study →Also see TABLE 9 p. 1431

▸ Anti-androgens (**apalutamide, enzalutamide**) are predicted to decrease the exposure to brigatinib. Avoid. [Severe] Study

▸ Anti-androgens (**apalutamide, enzalutamide**) are predicted to decrease the exposure to buspirone. Use with caution and adjust dose. [Severe] Study

▸ Anti-androgens (**apalutamide, enzalutamide**) moderately decrease the exposure to cabozantinib. Avoid. [Moderate] Study →Also see TABLE 9 p. 1431

▸ **Enzalutamide** is predicted to decrease the exposure to calcium channel blockers (amlodipine, felodipine, lacidipine, lercanidipine, nicardipine, nifedipine, nimodipine). Monitor and adjust dose. [Moderate] Study

▸ **Apalutamide** is predicted to decrease the exposure to calcium channel blockers (amlodipine, felodipine, lacidipine, lercanidipine, nicardipine, nimodipine). Monitor and adjust dose. [Moderate] Study

▸ **Enzalutamide** is predicted to decrease the exposure to calcium channel blockers (diltiazem, verapamil). [Severe] Study

▸ Anti-androgens (**apalutamide, enzalutamide**) are predicted to decrease the exposure to cannabidiol. Adjust dose. [Moderate] Study

▸ Anti-androgens (**apalutamide, enzalutamide**) are predicted to decrease the exposure to ceritinib. Avoid. [Severe] Study →Also see TABLE 9 p. 1431

▸ Anti-androgens (**apalutamide, enzalutamide**) decrease the concentration of ciclosporin. [Severe] Study

▸ Anti-androgens (**apalutamide, enzalutamide**) are predicted to alter the effects of cilostazol. [Moderate] Theoretical

▸ Anti-androgens (**apalutamide, enzalutamide**) are predicted to decrease the exposure to cinacalcet. Monitor and adjust dose. [Moderate] Study

▸ Anti-androgens (**apalutamide, enzalutamide**) decrease the exposure to clomethiazole. Monitor and adjust dose. [Moderate] Study

▸ **Clopidogrel** is predicted to increase the exposure to apalutamide. [Mild] Study

▸ **Clopidogrel** moderately increases the exposure to enzalutamide. Avoid or adjust enzalutamide dose, p. 991. [Severe] Study

▸ Anti-androgens (**apalutamide, enzalutamide**) are predicted to decrease the exposure to cobicistat. Avoid. [Severe] Theoretical

▸ **Cobicistat** is predicted to increase the exposure to apalutamide. [Mild] Study

▸ Anti-androgens (**apalutamide, enzalutamide**) are predicted to decrease the exposure to cobimetinib. Avoid. [Severe] Theoretica

▸ **Apalutamide** is predicted to decrease the exposure to colchicine. [Mild] Study

▸ Anti-androgens (**apalutamide, enzalutamide**) are predicted to decrease the exposure to corticosteroids (budesonide, deflazacort, dexamethasone, fludrocortisone, hydrocortisone, methylprednisolone, prednisolone, triamcinolone). Monitor an adjust dose. [Moderate] Study

▸ Anti-androgens (**apalutamide, enzalutamide**) are predicted to decrease the exposure to corticosteroids (fluticasone). [Unknown] Theoretical

▸ **Apalutamide** is predicted to decrease the exposure to coumarins. Avoid or monitor. [Mild] Study

▸ **Enzalutamide** potentially decreases the exposure to coumarins Avoid or adjust dose and monitor INR. [Severe] Study

▸ Anti-androgens (**apalutamide, enzalutamide**) are predicted to markedly decrease the exposure to crizotinib. Avoid. [Severe] Study →Also see TABLE 9 p. 1431

▸ Anti-androgens (**apalutamide, enzalutamide**) are predicted to decrease the exposure to dabrafenib. Avoid. [Moderate] Theoretical

▸ Anti-androgens (**apalutamide, enzalutamide**) are predicted to decrease the exposure to darifenacin. [Moderate] Theoretical

▸ **Enzalutamide** is predicted to decrease the exposure to dasabuvir. Avoid. [Severe] Theoretical

▸ Anti-androgens (**apalutamide, enzalutamide**) are predicted to markedly decrease the exposure to dasatinib. Avoid. [Severe] Study →Also see TABLE 9 p. 1431

▸ Anti-androgens (**apalutamide, enzalutamide**) are predicted to slightly decrease the exposure to delamanid. Avoid. [Moderate] Study →Also see TABLE 9 p. 1431

▸ Anti-androgens (**apalutamide, enzalutamide**) are predicted to markedly decrease the exposure to dienogest. [Severe] Study

▸ **Apalutamide** is predicted to decrease the exposure to digoxin. [Mild] Study

▸ Anti-androgens (**apalutamide, enzalutamide**) are predicted to decrease the exposure to dipeptidylpeptidase-4 inhibitors (linagliptin). [Moderate] Study

▸ Anti-androgens (**apalutamide, enzalutamide**) are predicted to moderately decrease the exposure to dipeptidylpeptidase-4 inhibitors (saxagliptin). [Moderate] Study

▸ Anti-androgens (**apalutamide, enzalutamide**) decrease the exposure to dolutegravir. Adjust dose. [Severe] Study

▸ Anti-androgens (**apalutamide, enzalutamide**) are predicted to decrease the exposure to dronabinol. Avoid or adjust dose. [Mild] Study

▸ Anti-androgens (**apalutamide, enzalutamide**) are predicted to decrease the exposure to elbasvir. Avoid. [Severe] Study

▸ Anti-androgens (**apalutamide, enzalutamide**) is predicted to decrease the exposure to elexacaftor. Avoid. [Severe] Theoretical

▸ **Abiraterone** is predicted to increase the exposure to eliglustat. Avoid or adjust dose—consult product literature. [Severe] Study

▸ Anti-androgens (**apalutamide, enzalutamide**) are predicted to decrease the exposure to eliglustat. Avoid. [Severe] Study

▸ Anti-androgens (**apalutamide, enzalutamide**) are predicted to decrease the concentration of elvitegravir. Avoid. [Severe] Theoretical

▸ Anti-androgens (**apalutamide, enzalutamide**) are predicted to decrease the exposure to encorafenib. [Severe] Theoretical →Also see TABLE 9 p. 1431

▸ Endothelin receptor antagonists (bosentan) are predicted to decrease the exposure to **darolutamide**. Avoid. [Moderate] Theoretical

▸ Anti-androgens (**apalutamide, enzalutamide**) affect the exposure to endothelin receptor antagonists (bosentan). Avoid. [Severe] Study

▸ Anti-androgens (**apalutamide, enzalutamide**) are predicted to decrease the exposure to endothelin receptor antagonists (macitentan). Avoid. [Severe] Study

Anti-androgens **(apalutamide, enzalutamide)** are predicted to decrease the exposure to entrectinib. Avoid. Severe Study → Also see **TABLE 9** p. 1431

Anti-androgens **(apalutamide, enzalutamide)** are predicted to decrease the effects of ergotamine. Moderate Theoretical

Anti-androgens **(apalutamide, enzalutamide)** are predicted to decrease the exposure to erlotinib. Avoid or adjust **erlotinib** dose, p. 1024. Severe Study

Anti-androgens **(apalutamide, enzalutamide)** are predicted to decrease the exposure to esketamine. Adjust dose. Moderate Theoretical

Anti-androgens **(apalutamide, enzalutamide)** are predicted to decrease the concentration of everolimus. Avoid or adjust dose. Severe Study

Anti-androgens **(apalutamide, enzalutamide)** moderately decrease the exposure to exemestane. Moderate Study

Anti-androgens **(apalutamide, enzalutamide)** are predicted to moderately decrease the exposure to factor XA inhibitors (apixaban). Use with caution or avoid. Severe Study

Anti-androgens **(apalutamide, enzalutamide)** are predicted to moderately decrease the exposure to factor XA inhibitors (rivaroxaban). Avoid unless patient can be monitored for signs of thrombosis. Severe Study

Anti-androgens **(apalutamide, enzalutamide)** are predicted to decrease the exposure to fesoterodine. Avoid. Moderate Study

Fibrates (gemfibrozil) are predicted to increase the exposure to **apalutamide**. Mild Study

Fibrates (gemfibrozil) moderately increase the exposure to **enzalutamide**. Avoid or adjust **enzalutamide** dose, p. 991. Severe Study

Anti-androgens **(apalutamide, enzalutamide)** are predicted to decrease the exposure to fingolimod. Moderate Study

Anti-androgens **(apalutamide, enzalutamide)** are predicted to decrease the exposure to fostamatinib. Avoid. Severe Study

Anti-androgens **(apalutamide, enzalutamide)** are predicted to decrease the exposure to gefitinib. Avoid. Severe Study

Anti-androgens **(apalutamide, enzalutamide)** are predicted to moderately decrease the exposure to glasdegib. Avoid. Severe Study → Also see **TABLE 9** p. 1431

Enzalutamide is predicted to greatly decrease the concentration of glecaprevir. Avoid. Severe Study

Anti-androgens **(apalutamide, enzalutamide)** are predicted to decrease the exposure to grazoprevir. Avoid. Severe Study

Anti-androgens **(apalutamide, enzalutamide)** are predicted to decrease the concentration of guanfacine. Adjust **guanfacine** dose, p. 372. Moderate Study

Anti-androgens **(apalutamide, enzalutamide)** decrease the concentration of haloperidol. Adjust dose. Moderate Study → Also see **TABLE 9** p. 1431

HIV-protease inhibitors are predicted to increase the exposure to **apalutamide**. Mild Study → Also see **TABLE 9** p. 1431

HIV-protease inhibitors (lopinavir, ritonavir, saquinavir) are predicted to increase the exposure to **darolutamide**. Monitor and adjust dose. Moderate Theoretical

Anti-androgens **(apalutamide, enzalutamide)** are predicted to decrease the exposure to ibrutinib. Avoid or adjust **ibrutinib** dose, p. 1027. Severe Study

Anti-androgens **(apalutamide, enzalutamide)** are predicted to decrease the exposure to idelalisib. Avoid. Severe Study

Idelalisib is predicted to increase the exposure to **apalutamide**. Mild Study

Anti-androgens **(apalutamide, enzalutamide)** are predicted to decrease the exposure to imatinib. Avoid. Moderate Study

Anti-androgens **(apalutamide, enzalutamide)** are predicted to decrease the exposure to irinotecan. Avoid. Severe Study

Anti-androgens **(apalutamide, enzalutamide)** are predicted to decrease the exposure to ivabradine. Adjust dose. Moderate Theoretical

Anti-androgens **(apalutamide, enzalutamide)** are predicted to moderately to markedly decrease the exposure to ivacaftor. Avoid. Severe Study

Anti-androgens **(apalutamide, enzalutamide)** are predicted to decrease the exposure to ixazomib. Avoid. Severe Study

▶ Anti-androgens **(apalutamide, enzalutamide)** are predicted to decrease the exposure to lapatinib. Avoid. Severe Study → Also see **TABLE 9** p. 1431

▶ Anti-androgens **(apalutamide, enzalutamide)** are predicted to moderately decrease the exposure to larotrectinib. Avoid. Moderate Study

▶ Anti-androgens **(apalutamide, enzalutamide)** are predicted to decrease the exposure to lomitapide. Monitor and adjust dose. Moderate Theoretical

▶ **Bicalutamide** is predicted to increase the exposure to lomitapide. Separate administration by 12 hours. Moderate Theoretical

▶ Anti-androgens **(apalutamide, enzalutamide)** are predicted to decrease the exposure to lorlatinib. Avoid. Severe Study

▶ Macrolides (clarithromycin) are predicted to increase the exposure to **apalutamide**. Mild Study → Also see **TABLE 9** p. 1431

▶ Macrolides (clarithromycin) are predicted to increase the exposure to **darolutamide**. Monitor and adjust dose. Moderate Theoretical

▶ Anti-androgens **(apalutamide, enzalutamide)** are predicted to decrease the exposure to maraviroc. Adjust dose. Severe Study

▶ Anti-androgens **(apalutamide, enzalutamide)** are predicted to slightly decrease the exposure to meglitinides (nateglinide). Mild Study

▶ **Darolutamide** is predicted to increase the concentration of meglitinides (repaglinide). Moderate Theoretical

▶ Anti-androgens **(apalutamide, enzalutamide)** are predicted to decrease the exposure to meglitinides (repaglinide). Monitor blood glucose and adjust dose. Moderate Study

▶ **Apalutamide** is predicted to decrease the exposure to methotrexate. Mild Study

▶ **Darolutamide** is predicted to increase the concentration of methotrexate. Moderate Theoretical

▶ Anti-androgens **(apalutamide, enzalutamide)** are predicted to decrease the exposure to midostaurin. Avoid. Severe Study

▶ Anti-androgens **(apalutamide, enzalutamide)** are predicted to decrease the exposure to mirtazapine. Adjust dose. Moderate Study

▶ Mitotane is predicted to decrease the exposure to **abiraterone**. Avoid. Severe Study

▶ Mitotane is predicted to decrease the exposure to **darolutamide**. Avoid. Moderate Study

▶ **Apalutamide** is predicted to decrease the exposure to moclobemide. Avoid or monitor. Mild Study

▶ Anti-androgens **(apalutamide, enzalutamide)** are predicted to decrease the exposure to monoclonal antibodies (polatuzumab vedotin). Moderate Theoretical

▶ Anti-androgens **(apalutamide, enzalutamide)** are predicted to decrease the exposure to montelukast. Mild Study

▶ Anti-androgens **(apalutamide, enzalutamide)** are predicted to markedly decrease the exposure to naldemedine. Avoid. Severe Study

▶ Anti-androgens **(apalutamide, enzalutamide)** are predicted to markedly decrease the exposure to naloxegol. Avoid. Moderate Study

▶ Anti-androgens **(apalutamide, enzalutamide)** are predicted to decrease the exposure to neratinib. Avoid. Severe Study

▶ Anti-androgens **(apalutamide, enzalutamide)** are predicted to markedly decrease the exposure to neurokinin-1 receptor antagonists (aprepitant). Avoid. Moderate Study

▶ Anti-androgens **(apalutamide, enzalutamide)** are predicted to decrease the exposure to neurokinin-1 receptor antagonists (fosaprepitant). Avoid. Moderate Theoretical

▶ Anti-androgens **(apalutamide, enzalutamide)** are predicted to decrease the exposure to neurokinin-1 receptor antagonists (netupitant). Avoid. Severe Study

▶ Anti-androgens **(apalutamide, enzalutamide)** are predicted to moderately decrease the exposure to nilotinib. Avoid. Severe Study → Also see **TABLE 9** p. 1431

▶ Anti-androgens **(apalutamide, enzalutamide)** are predicted to decrease the exposure to nitisinone. Adjust dose. Moderate Theoretical

▶ NNRTIs (efavirenz, nevirapine) are predicted to decrease the exposure to **darolutamide**. Avoid. Moderate Theoretical

Anti-androgens (continued)

‣ Anti-androgens **(apalutamide, enzalutamide)** are predicted to decrease the exposure to NNRTIs (doravirine). Avoid. Severe Study

‣ Anti-androgens **(apalutamide, enzalutamide)** are predicted to decrease the exposure to NNRTIs (etravirine). Avoid. Severe Theoretical

‣ **Enzalutamide** is predicted to decrease the exposure to NNRTIs (nevirapine). Severe Theoretical

‣ Anti-androgens **(apalutamide, enzalutamide)** markedly decrease the exposure to NNRTIs (rilpivirine). Avoid. Severe Study

‣ Anti-androgens **(apalutamide, enzalutamide)** are predicted to decrease the exposure to olaparib. Avoid. Moderate Theoretical

‣ **Enzalutamide** is predicted to decrease the exposure to ombitasvir. Avoid. Severe Theoretical

‣ Anti-androgens **(apalutamide, enzalutamide)** are predicted to decrease the exposure to opioids (alfentanil, fentanyl). Moderate Study

‣ Anti-androgens **(apalutamide, enzalutamide)** are predicted to decrease the exposure to opioids (buprenorphine). Monitor and adjust dose. Moderate Theoretical

‣ Anti-androgens **(apalutamide, enzalutamide)** decrease the exposure to opioids (methadone). Monitor and adjust dose. Severe Study → Also see TABLE 9 p. 1431

‣ Anti-androgens **(apalutamide, enzalutamide)** are predicted to decrease the exposure to opioids (oxycodone). Monitor and adjust dose. Moderate Study

‣ Anti-androgens **(apalutamide, enzalutamide)** are predicted to moderately decrease the exposure to osimertinib. Avoid. Moderate Study → Also see TABLE 9 p. 1431

‣ Anti-androgens **(apalutamide, enzalutamide)** are predicted to moderately decrease the exposure to ospemifene. Moderate Study

‣ Anti-androgens **(apalutamide, enzalutamide)** are predicted to decrease the exposure to palbociclib. Avoid. Severe Study

‣ Anti-androgens **(apalutamide, enzalutamide)** are predicted to decrease the exposure to panobinostat. Avoid. Moderate Theoretical → Also see TABLE 9 p. 1431

‣ Anti-androgens **(apalutamide, enzalutamide)** are predicted to decrease the exposure to paritaprevir (with ritonavir and ombitasvir). Avoid. Severe Study

‣ Anti-androgens **(apalutamide, enzalutamide)** are predicted to decrease the exposure to pazopanib. Avoid. Severe Theoretical → Also see TABLE 9 p. 1431

‣ Anti-androgens **(apalutamide, enzalutamide)** moderately decrease the exposure to phosphodiesterase type-4 inhibitors (apremilast). Avoid. Severe Study

‣ Anti-androgens **(apalutamide, enzalutamide)** are predicted to decrease the exposure to phosphodiesterase type-4 inhibitors (roflumilast). Avoid. Moderate Study

‣ Anti-androgens **(apalutamide, enzalutamide)** are predicted to decrease the exposure to phosphodiesterase type-5 inhibitors (avanafil, tadalafil). Avoid. Severe Study

‣ Anti-androgens **(apalutamide, enzalutamide)** are predicted to decrease the exposure to phosphodiesterase type-5 inhibitors (sildenafil, vardenafil). Moderate Theoretical → Also see TABLE 9 p. 1431

‣ Anti-androgens **(apalutamide, enzalutamide)** are predicted to moderately to markedly decrease the exposure to pibrentasvir. Avoid. Severe Study

‣ Anti-androgens **(apalutamide, enzalutamide)** are predicted to moderately decrease the exposure to pitolisant. Moderate Study

‣ Anti-androgens **(apalutamide, enzalutamide)** are predicted to decrease the exposure to ponatinib. Avoid. Moderate Theoretical

‣ Anti-androgens **(apalutamide, enzalutamide)** are predicted to markedly decrease the exposure to praziquantel. Avoid. Moderate Study

‣ **Apalutamide** is predicted to decrease the exposure to proton pump inhibitors (lansoprazole, rabeprazole). Avoid or monitor. Mild Study

‣ **Apalutamide** markedly decreases the exposure to proton pump inhibitors (omeprazole). Avoid or monitor. Moderate Study

‣ Anti-androgens **(apalutamide, enzalutamide)** are predicted to decrease the exposure to ranolazine. Avoid. Severe Study → Also see TABLE 9 p. 1431

‣ Anti-androgens **(apalutamide, enzalutamide)** are predicted to decrease the exposure to reboxetine. Moderate Anecdotal

‣ Anti-androgens **(apalutamide, enzalutamide)** are predicted to decrease the exposure to regorafenib. Avoid. Moderate Study

‣ Anti-androgens **(apalutamide, enzalutamide)** potentially decrease the exposure to remdesivir. Avoid. Moderate Theoretical

‣ Anti-androgens **(apalutamide, enzalutamide)** are predicted to markedly decrease the exposure to ribociclib. Avoid. Severe Study → Also see TABLE 9 p. 1431

‣ Rifamycins (rifampicin) are predicted to decrease the exposure to **abiraterone**. Avoid. Severe Study

‣ Rifamycins (rifampicin) are predicted to decrease the exposure to **darolutamide**. Avoid. Moderate Study

‣ Anti-androgens **(apalutamide, enzalutamide)** are predicted to decrease the exposure to ruxolitinib. Monitor and adjust dose. Moderate Study

‣ Anti-androgens **(apalutamide, enzalutamide)** are predicted to decrease the exposure to siponimod. Severe Study

‣ Anti-androgens **(apalutamide, enzalutamide)** are predicted to decrease the concentration of sirolimus. Avoid. Severe Study

‣ Anti-androgens **(apalutamide, enzalutamide)** are predicted to decrease the exposure to solifenacin. Moderate Theoretical

‣ Anti-androgens **(apalutamide, enzalutamide)** are predicted to decrease the exposure to sorafenib. Moderate Theoretical → Also see TABLE 9 p. 1431

‣ **Apalutamide** is predicted to decrease the exposure to SSRIs (citalopram). Avoid or monitor. Mild Study → Also see TABLE 9 p. 1431

‣ St John's wort is predicted to decrease the exposure to **darolutamide**. Avoid. Moderate Theoretical

‣ **Darolutamide** is predicted to increase the exposure to statins (atorvastatin, fluvastatin, rosuvastatin). Avoid. Severe Theoretical

‣ **Darolutamide** is predicted to increase the concentration of statins (pravastatin, simvastatin). Moderate Theoretical

‣ **Apalutamide** slightly decreases the exposure to statins (rosuvastatin). Mild Study

‣ **Apalutamide** is predicted to decrease the exposure to statins (simvastatin). Avoid or monitor. Moderate Study

‣ **Enzalutamide** is predicted to decrease the exposure to statins (simvastatin). Severe Study

‣ **Darolutamide** is predicted to increase the exposure to sulfasalazine. Avoid. Severe Theoretical

‣ **Darolutamide** is predicted to increase the concentration of sulfonylureas (glibenclamide). Moderate Theoretical

‣ Anti-androgens **(apalutamide, enzalutamide)** are predicted to decrease the exposure to sunitinib. Avoid or adjust sunitinib dose, p. 1044. Moderate Study → Also see TABLE 9 p. 1431

‣ Anti-androgens **(apalutamide, enzalutamide)** decrease the concentration of tacrolimus. Monitor and adjust dose. Severe Study

‣ Anti-androgens **(apalutamide, enzalutamide)** are predicted to decrease the exposure to taxanes (cabazitaxel, paclitaxel). Avoid. Severe Study

‣ Anti-androgens **(apalutamide, enzalutamide)** are predicted to decrease the exposure to taxanes (docetaxel). Severe Theoretical

‣ Anti-androgens **(apalutamide, enzalutamide)** are predicted to decrease the concentration of temsirolimus. Avoid. Severe Study

‣ Anti-androgens **(apalutamide, enzalutamide)** decrease the exposure to tetracyclines (doxycycline). Monitor and adjust dose. Moderate Study

‣ Anti-androgens **(apalutamide, enzalutamide)** are predicted to decrease the exposure to tezacaftor. Avoid. Severe Theoretical

‣ **Apalutamide** is predicted to decrease the exposure to thrombin inhibitors (dabigatran). Mild Study

‣ **Apalutamide** potentially decreases the exposure to thyroid hormones (levothyroxine). Mild Theoretical

‣ Anti-androgens **(apalutamide, enzalutamide)** are predicted to markedly decrease the exposure to ticagrelor. Avoid. Severe Study

‣ Anti-androgens **(apalutamide, enzalutamide)** are predicted to decrease the exposure to tivozanib. Severe Study

Anti-androgens **(apalutamide, enzalutamide)** are predicted to decrease the exposure to tofacitinib. Avoid. Severe Study

Anti-androgens **(apalutamide, enzalutamide)** are predicted to decrease the exposure to tolvaptan. Use with caution or avoid depending on indication. Severe Study

Darolutamide is predicted to increase the exposure to topotecan. Avoid. Severe Theoretical

Anti-androgens **(apalutamide, enzalutamide)** are predicted to decrease the exposure to toremifene. Adjust dose. Moderate Study → Also see TABLE 9 p. 1431

Anti-androgens **(apalutamide, enzalutamide)** are predicted to decrease the exposure to trabectedin. Avoid. Severe Theoretical

Enzalutamide is predicted to markedly decrease the exposure to ulipristal. Avoid and for 4 weeks after stopping **ulipristal**. Severe Theoretical

Anti-androgens **(apalutamide, enzalutamide)** are predicted to decrease the exposure to upadacitinib. Moderate Study

Anti-androgens **(apalutamide, enzalutamide)** are predicted to decrease the exposure to vandetanib. Avoid. Moderate Study → Also see TABLE 9 p. 1431

Anti-androgens **(apalutamide, enzalutamide)** are predicted to moderately decrease the exposure to velpatasvir. Avoid. Severe Study

Anti-androgens **(apalutamide, enzalutamide)** are predicted to decrease the exposure to vemurafenib. Avoid. Severe Theoretical → Also see TABLE 9 p. 1431

Anti-androgens **(apalutamide, enzalutamide)** are predicted to decrease the exposure to venetoclax. Avoid. Severe Study

Anti-androgens **(apalutamide, enzalutamide)** are predicted to decrease the exposure to vinca alkaloids (vinblastine, vincristine, vindesine). Severe Theoretical

Anti-androgens **(apalutamide, enzalutamide)** are predicted to decrease the exposure to vinca alkaloids (vinflunine). Avoid. Severe Theoretical → Also see TABLE 9 p. 1431

Anti-androgens **(apalutamide, enzalutamide)** are predicted to decrease the exposure to vinca alkaloids (vinorelbine). Use with caution or avoid. Severe Theoretical

Anti-androgens **(apalutamide, enzalutamide)** are predicted to decrease the exposure to vismodegib. Avoid. Moderate Theoretical

Anti-androgens **(apalutamide, enzalutamide)** are predicted to decrease the exposure to vortioxetine. Monitor and adjust dose. Moderate Study

Anti-androgens **(apalutamide, enzalutamide)** are predicted to decrease the concentration of voxilaprevir. Avoid. Severe Study

Anti-androgens **(apalutamide, enzalutamide)** are predicted to decrease the exposure to zopiclone. Adjust dose. Moderate Study

Anti-D (Rh₀) immunoglobulin → see immunoglobulins

Antiarrhythmics → see TABLE 6 p. 1430 (bradycardia), TABLE 8 p. 1430 (hypotension), TABLE 12 p. 1432 (peripheral neuropathy), TABLE 9 p. 1431 (QT-interval prolongation), TABLE 11 p. 1431 (CNS depressant effects), TABLE 10 p. 1431 (antimuscarinics)

adenosine · amiodarone · disopyramide · dronedarone · flecainide · lidocaine · propafenone · vernakalant

▸ **Amiodarone** has a long half-life; there is potential for drug interactions to occur for several weeks (or even months) after treatment with it has been stopped.

▸ Since systemic absorption can follow topical application of **lidocaine**, the possibility of interactions should be borne in mind.

▸ Avoid intravenous class I and class III antiarrhythmics for 4 hours before and after **vernakalant**.

▸ **Dronedarone** is predicted to increase the exposure to abemaciclib. Moderate Study

▸ **Dronedarone** is predicted to increase the exposure to acalabrutinib. Avoid or monitor. Severe Study

▸ Antiarrhythmics **(amiodarone, dronedarone)** are predicted to increase the exposure to afatinib. Separate administration by 12 hours. Moderate Study

▸ **Amiodarone** is predicted to decrease the effects of agalsidase alfa. Avoid. Moderate Theoretical

▸ **Amiodarone** is predicted to decrease the effects of agalsidase beta. Avoid. Moderate Theoretical

▸ **Amiodarone** is predicted to increase the exposure to aldosterone antagonists (eplerenone). Adjust **eplerenone** dose, p. 208. Severe Theoretical

▸ **Dronedarone** is predicted to increase the exposure to aldosterone antagonists (eplerenone). Adjust **eplerenone** dose, p. 208. Severe Study

▸ Antiarrhythmics **(amiodarone, dronedarone)** are predicted to increase the exposure to aliskiren. Severe Study

▸ **Dronedarone** is predicted to increase the exposure to alpha blockers (tamsulosin). Moderate Theoretical

▸ **Aminophylline** is predicted to decrease the efficacy of **adenosine**. Separate administration by 24 hours. Mild Theoretical

▸ Anaesthetics, local are predicted to increase the risk of cardiodepression when given with **antiarrhythmics**. Severe Theoretical → Also see TABLE 11 p. 1431

▸ Anti-androgens (apalutamide, enzalutamide) are predicted to decrease the efficacy of **propafenone**. Moderate Study

▸ Anti-androgens (apalutamide, enzalutamide) are predicted to decrease the exposure to antiarrhythmics (disopyramide, dronedarone). Avoid. Severe Study → Also see TABLE 9 p. 1431

▸ Antiarrhythmics **(propafenone)** are predicted to increase the risk of cardiodepression when given with antiarrhythmics **(amiodarone)**. Monitor and adjust dose. Severe Theoretical

▸ Antiarrhythmics **(amiodarone)** increase the concentration of antiarrhythmics **(flecainide)**. Adjust **flecainide** dose and monitor adverse effects. Severe Study → Also see TABLE 6 p. 1430 → Also see TABLE 9 p. 1431

▸ Antiarrhythmics **(propafenone)** are predicted to increase the risk of cardiodepression when given with antiarrhythmics **(lidocaine)**. Moderate Study

▸ Antiarrhythmics **(dronedarone)** are predicted to increase the exposure to antiarrhythmics **(propafenone)**. Monitor and adjust dose. Moderate Study

▸ Antiepileptics (carbamazepine, fosphenytoin, phenobarbital, phenytoin, primidone) are predicted to decrease the efficacy of **propafenone**. Moderate Study

▸ Antiepileptics (fosphenytoin, phenytoin) are predicted to decrease the exposure to **lidocaine**. Severe Anecdotal

▸ Antiepileptics (carbamazepine, fosphenytoin, phenobarbital, phenytoin, primidone) are predicted to decrease the exposure to antiarrhythmics **(disopyramide, dronedarone)**. Avoid. Severe Study

▸ **Amiodarone** is predicted to slightly increase the concentration of antiepileptics (fosphenytoin, phenytoin). Monitor and adjust dose. Severe Study → Also see TABLE 12 p. 1432

▸ Antifungals, azoles (fluconazole) are predicted to increase the exposure to **dronedarone**. Severe Theoretical → Also see TABLE 9 p. 1431

▸ Antifungals, azoles (fluconazole, isavuconazole, posaconazole) are predicted to increase the exposure to **propafenone**. Monitor and adjust dose. Moderate Study

▸ Antifungals, azoles (itraconazole, ketoconazole, voriconazole) are predicted to increase the exposure to **disopyramide**. Avoid. Severe Theoretical → Also see TABLE 9 p. 1431

▸ Antifungals, azoles (itraconazole, ketoconazole, voriconazole) very markedly increase the exposure to **dronedarone**. Avoid. Severe Study → Also see TABLE 9 p. 1431

▸ Antifungals, azoles (itraconazole, ketoconazole, voriconazole) are predicted to increase the exposure to **propafenone**. Monitor and adjust dose. Severe Study

▸ Antifungals, azoles (miconazole) are predicted to increase the exposure to **disopyramide**. Use with caution and adjust dose. Severe Theoretical

▸ Antifungals, azoles (posaconazole) are predicted to increase the exposure to antiarrhythmics **(disopyramide, dronedarone)**. Avoid. Severe Theoretical

▸ **Dronedarone** is predicted to increase the exposure to antihistamines, non-sedating (fexofenadine, mizolastine). Severe Theoretical

▸ **Dronedarone** is predicted to increase the exposure to antihistamines, non-sedating (rupatadine). Avoid. Moderate Study

▸ **Dronedarone** is predicted to increase the concentration of antimalarials (piperaquine). Severe Theoretical

Antiarrhythmics (continued)

▶ **Dronedarone** is predicted to increase the exposure to antipsychotics, second generation (cariprazine). Avoid. [Severe] Study

▶ **Dronedarone** is predicted to increase the exposure to antipsychotics, second generation (lurasidone). Adjust **lurasidone** dose. [Moderate] Study

▶ **Dronedarone** is predicted to increase the exposure to antipsychotics, second generation (quetiapine). Avoid. [Moderate] Study

▶ **Dronedarone** is predicted to increase the exposure to avapritinib. Avoid or adjust **avapritinib** dose, p. 1012. [Moderate] Study

▶ **Dronedarone** is predicted to increase the exposure to axitinib. [Moderate] Theoretical

▶ **Dronedarone** is predicted to increase the exposure to bedaquiline. Avoid prolonged use. [Mild] Theoretical → Also see **TABLE 9** p. 1431

▶ **Dronedarone** is predicted to increase the exposure to benzodiazepines (alprazolam). [Severe] Study

▶ **Dronedarone** is predicted to increase the exposure to benzodiazepines (midazolam). Monitor adverse effects and adjust dose. [Severe] Study

▶ Antiarrhythmics **(amiodarone, disopyramide, dronedarone, flecainide, lidocaine)** are predicted to increase the risk of cardiovascular adverse effects when given with beta blockers, non-selective. Use with caution or avoid. [Severe] Study → Also see **TABLE 6** p. 1430 → Also see **TABLE 9** p. 1431

▶ **Propafenone** is predicted to increase the risk of cardiovascular adverse effects when given with beta blockers, non-selective (labetalol, levobunolol, nadolol, pindolol, sotalol). Use with caution or avoid. [Severe] Study

▶ **Propafenone** increases the risk of cardiovascular adverse effects when given with beta blockers, non-selective (propranolol). Use with caution or avoid. [Severe] Study

▶ **Propafenone** is predicted to increase the exposure to beta blockers, non-selective **(timolol)** and beta blockers, non-selective **(timolol)** are predicted to increase the risk of cardiodepression when given with **propafenone**. [Severe] Anecdotal

▶ Antiarrhythmics **(amiodarone, disopyramide, dronedarone, flecainide, lidocaine)** are predicted to increase the risk of cardiovascular adverse effects when given with beta blockers, selective. Use with caution or avoid. [Severe] Study → Also see **TABLE 6** p. 1430

▶ **Propafenone** is predicted to increase the risk of cardiovascular adverse effects when given with beta blockers, selective (acebutolol, atenolol, betaxolol, bisoprolol, celiprolol, esmolol). Use with caution or avoid. [Severe] Study

▶ **Propafenone** is predicted to increase the exposure to beta blockers, selective **(metoprolol)**. [Moderate] Study

▶ **Propafenone** is predicted to increase the exposure to beta blockers, selective **(nebivolol)** and beta blockers, selective **(nebivolol)** are predicted to increase the risk of cardiodepression when given with **propafenone**. Avoid. [Severe] Theoretical

▶ Antiarrhythmics **(amiodarone, dronedarone)** are predicted to increase the exposure to bictegravir. Use with caution or avoid. [Moderate] Theoretical

▶ **Dronedarone** is predicted to increase the exposure to bosutinib. Avoid or adjust dose. [Severe] Theoretical → Also see **TABLE 9** p. 1431

▶ **Dronedarone** is predicted to increase the exposure to buspirone. Use with caution and adjust dose. [Moderate] Study

▶ **Dronedarone** is predicted to increase the exposure to cabozantinib. [Moderate] Theoretical → Also see **TABLE 9** p. 1431

▶ Caffeine citrate decreases the efficacy of **adenosine**. Separate administration by 24 hours. [Mild] Study

▶ Calcium channel blockers (diltiazem, verapamil) increase the exposure to **dronedarone** and dronedarone increases the exposure to calcium channel blockers (diltiazem, verapamil). [Moderate] Study

▶ Calcium channel blockers (diltiazem, verapamil) are predicted to increase the exposure to **propafenone**. Monitor and adjust dose. [Moderate] Study

▶ Calcium channel blockers (verapamil) increase the risk of cardiodepression when given with **flecainide**. [Severe] Anecdotal → Also see **TABLE 6** p. 1430

▶ **Dronedarone** is predicted to increase the exposure to calcium channel blockers (amlodipine, felodipine, lacidipine, lercanidipine, nicardipine, nifedipine, nimodipine). Monitor and adjust dose. [Moderate] Study

▶ **Amiodarone** is predicted to increase the risk of cardiodepression when given with calcium channel blockers (diltiazem, verapamil). Avoid. [Severe] Theoretical → Also see **TABLE 6** p. 1430

▶ **Disopyramide** is predicted to increase the risk of cardiodepression when given with calcium channel blockers (verapamil). [Severe] Theoretical

▶ **Amiodarone** is predicted to increase the exposure to ceritinib. [Moderate] Theoretical → Also see **TABLE 9** p. 1431

▶ Chloroprocaine is predicted to increase the risk of cardiovascular adverse effects when given with antiarrhythmics **(amiodarone, dronedarone, vernakalant)**. [Severe] Theoretical

▶ **Amiodarone** increases the concentration of ciclosporin. Monitor concentration and adjust dose. [Severe] Study

▶ **Dronedarone** is predicted to increase the concentration of ciclosporin. [Severe] Study

▶ Cobicistat potentially increases the concentration of antiarrhythmics **(amiodarone, disopyramide, flecainide, lidocaine)**. [Severe] Theoretical

▶ Cobicistat very markedly increases the exposure to **dronedarone**. Avoid. [Severe] Study

▶ Cobicistat is predicted to increase the exposure to **propafenone**. Monitor and adjust dose. [Severe] Study

▶ **Dronedarone** is predicted to increase the exposure to cobimetinib. [Severe] Theoretical

▶ **Amiodarone** is predicted to increase the exposure to colchicine. Avoid P-glycoprotein inhibitors or adjust **colchicine** dose, p. 1166. [Severe] Theoretical

▶ **Dronedarone** is predicted to increase the exposure to colchicine. Adjust **colchicine** dose with moderate CYP3A4 inhibitors, p. 1166. [Severe] Study

▶ **Dronedarone** is predicted to increase the exposure to corticosteroids (methylprednisolone). Monitor and adjust dose. [Moderate] Study

▶ **Amiodarone** increases the anticoagulant effect of coumarins. [Severe] Study

▶ **Propafenone** increases the anticoagulant effect of coumarins. Monitor INR and adjust dose. [Moderate] Study

▶ Crizotinib is predicted to increase the exposure to **propafenone**. Monitor and adjust dose. [Moderate] Study

▶ **Dronedarone** is predicted to slightly increase the exposure to darifenacin. [Moderate] Study

▶ Darifenacin is predicted to increase the concentration of **flecainide**. [Moderate] Theoretical

▶ **Dronedarone** is predicted to increase the exposure to dasatinib. [Severe] Study → Also see **TABLE 9** p. 1431

▶ **Dronedarone** is predicted to slightly increase the exposure to dienogest. [Moderate] Study

▶ Antiarrhythmics **(amiodarone, dronedarone)** are predicted to moderately increase the exposure to digoxin. Monitor and adjust **digoxin** dose, p. 117. [Severe] Study → Also see **TABLE 6** p. 1430

▶ **Propafenone** increases the concentration of digoxin. Monitor and adjust dose. [Severe] Study

▶ **Dronedarone** is predicted to increase the exposure to dipeptidylpeptidase-4 inhibitors (saxagliptin). [Mild] Study

▶ Dipyridamole increases the exposure to adenosine. Avoid or adjust dose. [Severe] Study

▶ **Dronedarone** increases the risk of QT-prolongation when given with domperidone. Avoid. [Severe] Study

▶ **Dronedarone** is predicted to increase the exposure to dopamine receptor agonists (bromocriptine). [Severe] Theoretical

▶ **Dronedarone** is predicted to increase the concentration of dopamine receptor agonists (cabergoline). [Severe] Anecdotal

▶ **Dronedarone** is predicted to moderately increase the exposure to dutasteride. [Mild] Study

▶ **Dronedarone** is predicted to increase the exposure to elexacaftor. Adjust tezacaftor with ivacaftor and elexacaftor p. 311 dose with moderate CYP3A4 inhibitors. [Severe] Theoretical

Antiarrhythmics **(dronedarone, propafenone)** are predicted to increase the exposure to eliglustat. Avoid or adjust dose—consult product literature. ⟨Severe⟩ Study

Dronedarone is predicted to moderately increase the exposure to encorafenib. ⟨Moderate⟩ Study → Also see TABLE 9 p. 1431

Endothelin receptor antagonists **(bosentan)** are predicted to decrease the exposure to **dronedarone**. ⟨Severe⟩ Theoretical

Dronedarone is predicted to increase the exposure to entrectinib. Avoid moderate CYP3A4 inhibitors or adjust **entrectinib** dose, p. 1023. ⟨Severe⟩ Theoretical → Also see TABLE 9 p. 1431

Dronedarone is predicted to increase the risk of ergotism when given with ergometrine. ⟨Severe⟩ Theoretical

Dronedarone is predicted to increase the risk of ergotism when given with ergotamine. ⟨Severe⟩ Theoretical

Antiarrhythmics **(amiodarone, dronedarone)** are predicted to increase the exposure to erlotinib. ⟨Moderate⟩ Theoretical

Dronedarone is predicted to increase the concentration of everolimus. Avoid or adjust dose. ⟨Moderate⟩ Study

Dronedarone is predicted to increase the exposure to factor XA inhibitors (apixaban). ⟨Moderate⟩ Theoretical

Dronedarone slightly increases the exposure to factor XA inhibitors (edoxaban). Adjust **edoxaban** dose, p. 137. ⟨Severe⟩ Study

Dronedarone is predicted to increase the exposure to factor XA inhibitors (rivaroxaban). Avoid. ⟨Moderate⟩ Theoretical

Dronedarone is predicted to increase the exposure to fesoterodine. Adjust **fesoterodine** dose with moderate CYP3A4 inhibitors in hepatic and renal impairment, p. 822. ⟨Mild⟩ Study

Antiarrhythmics **(amiodarone, dronedarone)** are predicted to increase the exposure to fidaxomicin. Avoid. ⟨Moderate⟩ Study

Dronedarone is predicted to increase the exposure to gefitinib. ⟨Moderate⟩ Theoretical

Dronedarone potentially increases the exposure to glecaprevir. ⟨Moderate⟩ Theoretical

Grapefruit juice increases the exposure to **amiodarone**. Avoid. ⟨Moderate⟩ Study

Grapefruit juice moderately increases the exposure to **dronedarone**. Avoid. ⟨Severe⟩ Study

Grapefruit juice increases the exposure to **propafenone**. Monitor and adjust dose. ⟨Moderate⟩ Study

Dronedarone is predicted to increase the concentration of guanfacine. Adjust **guanfacine** dose, p. 372. ⟨Moderate⟩ Theoretical

H₂ receptor antagonists (cimetidine) increase the exposure to **amiodarone**. ⟨Moderate⟩ Study

H₂ receptor antagonists (cimetidine) slightly increase the exposure to **flecainide**. Monitor and adjust dose. ⟨Mild⟩ Study

H₂ receptor antagonists (cimetidine) increase the exposure to **lidocaine**. Monitor and adjust dose. ⟨Moderate⟩ Study

H₂ receptor antagonists (cimetidine) are predicted to increase the exposure to **propafenone**. Monitor and adjust dose. ⟨Moderate⟩ Theoretical

HIV-protease inhibitors are predicted to increase the exposure to **amiodarone**. Avoid. ⟨Severe⟩ Theoretical → Also see TABLE 9 p. 1431

HIV-protease inhibitors are predicted to increase the exposure to **disopyramide**. ⟨Severe⟩ Theoretical → Also see TABLE 9 p. 1431

HIV-protease inhibitors very markedly increase the exposure to **dronedarone**. Avoid. ⟨Severe⟩ Study → Also see TABLE 9 p. 1431

HIV-protease inhibitors (ritonavir) are predicted to increase the exposure to **flecainide**. Avoid or monitor adverse effects. ⟨Severe⟩ Theoretical

HIV-protease inhibitors are predicted to increase the exposure to **lidocaine**. Avoid. ⟨Severe⟩ Study

HIV-protease inhibitors are predicted to increase the exposure to **propafenone**. Monitor and adjust dose. ⟨Severe⟩ Study

Amiodarone is predicted to increase the exposure to ibrutinib. Adjust **ibrutinib** dose, p. 1027. ⟨Severe⟩ Theoretical

Dronedarone is predicted to increase the exposure to ibrutinib. Adjust **ibrutinib** dose with moderate CYP3A4 inhibitors, p. 1027. ⟨Severe⟩ Study

Idelalisib is predicted to increase the exposure to **amiodarone**. Avoid. ⟨Moderate⟩ Theoretical

▶ Idelalisib very markedly increases the exposure to **dronedarone**. Avoid. ⟨Severe⟩ Study

▶ Idelalisib is predicted to increase the exposure to **propafenone**. Monitor and adjust dose. ⟨Severe⟩ Study

▶ Imatinib is predicted to increase the exposure to **dronedarone**. ⟨Severe⟩ Theoretical

▶ Imatinib is predicted to increase the exposure to **propafenone**. Monitor and adjust dose. ⟨Moderate⟩ Study

▶ **Dronedarone** is predicted to increase the exposure to ivabradine. Adjust **ivabradine** dose, p. 227. ⟨Severe⟩ Theoretical

▶ **Dronedarone** is predicted to increase the exposure to ivacaftor. Adjust ivacaftor p. 309 or tezacaftor with ivacaftor p. 311 or tezacaftor with ivacaftor and elexacftor p. 311 dose with moderate CYP3A4 inhibitors. ⟨Severe⟩ Study

▶ **Dronedarone** is predicted to increase the exposure to lapatinib. ⟨Moderate⟩ Study → Also see TABLE 9 p. 1431

▶ Antiarrhythmics **(amiodarone, dronedarone)** are predicted to increase the exposure to larotrectinib. ⟨Mild⟩ Theoretical

▶ Ledipasvir increases the risk of severe bradycardia or heart block when given with **amiodarone**. Refer to specialist literature. ⟨Severe⟩ Anecdotal

▶ Letermovir is predicted to increase the concentration of **amiodarone**. ⟨Moderate⟩ Theoretical

▶ Letermovir is predicted to increase the exposure to **propafenone**. Monitor and adjust dose. ⟨Moderate⟩ Study

▶ **Amiodarone** is predicted to increase the exposure to lomitapide. Separate administration by 12 hours. ⟨Moderate⟩ Theoretical

▶ **Dronedarone** is predicted to increase the exposure to lomitapide. Avoid. ⟨Moderate⟩ Theoretical

▶ **Dronedarone** is predicted to increase the exposure to loperamide. ⟨Severe⟩ Theoretical

▶ Macrolides (clarithromycin) very markedly increase the exposure to **dronedarone**. Avoid. ⟨Severe⟩ Study → Also see TABLE 9 p. 1431

▶ Macrolides (clarithromycin) are predicted to increase the exposure to **propafenone**. Monitor and adjust dose. ⟨Severe⟩ Study

▶ Macrolides (clarithromycin, erythromycin) are predicted to increase the exposure to **lidocaine**. ⟨Moderate⟩ Theoretical

▶ Macrolides (erythromycin) are predicted to moderately increase the exposure to **dronedarone**. Avoid. ⟨Severe⟩ Theoretical → Also see TABLE 9 p. 1431

▶ Macrolides (erythromycin) are predicted to increase the exposure to **propafenone**. Monitor and adjust dose. ⟨Moderate⟩ Study

▶ Mexiletine is predicted to increase the risk of torsade de pointes when given with **antiarrhythmics**. Avoid. ⟨Severe⟩ Theoretical

▶ **Dronedarone** is predicted to increase the exposure to midostaurin. ⟨Moderate⟩ Theoretical

▶ Mitotane is predicted to decrease the exposure to antiarrhythmics **(disopyramide, dronedarone)**. Avoid. ⟨Severe⟩ Study

▶ Mitotane is predicted to decrease the efficacy of **propafenone**. ⟨Moderate⟩ Study

▶ **Dronedarone** increases the risk of neutropenia when given with monoclonal antibodies (brentuximab vedotin). Monitor and adjust dose. ⟨Severe⟩ Theoretical

▶ Antiarrhythmics **(amiodarone, dronedarone)** are predicted to increase the exposure to naldemedine. ⟨Moderate⟩ Study

▶ **Dronedarone** is predicted to increase the exposure to naloxegol. Adjust **naloxegol** dose and monitor adverse effects, p. 70. ⟨Moderate⟩ Study

▶ **Dronedarone** is predicted to increase the exposure to neratinib. Avoid. ⟨Severe⟩ Study

▶ Neurokinin-1 receptor antagonists (aprepitant) increase the exposure to **dronedarone**. ⟨Severe⟩ Theoretical

▶ Neurokinin-1 receptor antagonists (aprepitant, netupitant) are predicted to increase the exposure to **propafenone**. Monitor and adjust dose. ⟨Moderate⟩ Study

▶ Nilotinib is predicted to increase the exposure to **propafenone**. Monitor and adjust dose. ⟨Moderate⟩ Study

▶ Antiarrhythmics **(amiodarone, dronedarone)** are predicted to increase the exposure to nintedanib. ⟨Moderate⟩ Study

Antiarrhythmics (continued)

▶ NNRTIs (efavirenz, nevirapine) are predicted to decrease the exposure to **dronedarone**. Severe Theoretical → Also see TABLE 9 p. 1431

▶ NSAIDs (celecoxib) are predicted to increase the exposure to antiarrhythmics (**flecainide, propafenone**). Monitor and adjust dose. Moderate Theoretical

▶ **Dronedarone** is predicted to increase the exposure to olaparib. Avoid moderate CYP3A4 inhibitors or adjust **olaparib** dose, p. 1051. Moderate Theoretical

▶ **Dronedarone** is predicted to increase the exposure to opioids (alfentanil, buprenorphine, fentanyl, oxycodone). Monitor and adjust dose. Moderate Study

▶ **Amiodarone** is predicted to increase the concentration of opioids (fentanyl). Moderate Theoretical → Also see TABLE 6 p. 1430

▶ **Dronedarone** is predicted to increase the exposure to opioids (methadone). Moderate Theoretical → Also see TABLE 9 p. 1431

▶ **Dronedarone** is predicted to increase the exposure to oxybutynin. Mild Theoretical

▶ Antiarrhythmics (**amiodarone, dronedarone**) are predicted to increase the exposure to panobinostat. Adjust dose. Moderate Theoretical → Also see TABLE 9 p. 1431

▶ **Dronedarone** is predicted to increase the exposure to pazopanib. Moderate Theoretical → Also see TABLE 9 p. 1431

▶ **Propafenone** is predicted to increase the anticoagulant effect of phenindione. Monitor and adjust dose. Moderate Theoretical

▶ **Dronedarone** is predicted to increase the exposure to phosphodiesterase type-5 inhibitors (avanafil). Adjust **avanafil** dose, p. 859. Moderate Theoretical

▶ **Dronedarone** is predicted to increase the exposure to phosphodiesterase type-5 inhibitors (sildenafil). Monitor or adjust **sildenafil** dose with moderate CYP3A4 inhibitors, p. 860. Moderate Study → Also see TABLE 9 p. 1431

▶ **Dronedarone** is predicted to increase the exposure to phosphodiesterase type-5 inhibitors (tadalafil). Severe Theoretical

▶ **Dronedarone** is predicted to increase the exposure to phosphodiesterase type-5 inhibitors (vardenafil). Adjust dose. Severe Theoretical → Also see TABLE 9 p. 1431

▶ **Amiodarone** is predicted to increase the exposure to pibrentasvir. Moderate Theoretical

▶ **Dronedarone** potentially increases the exposure to pibrentasvir. Moderate Theoretical

▶ **Dronedarone** is predicted to increase the exposure to pimozide. Avoid. Severe Theoretical → Also see TABLE 9 p. 1431

▶ Quinolones (ciprofloxacin) slightly increase the exposure to **lidocaine**. Mild Study

▶ **Dronedarone** is predicted to increase the exposure to ranolazine. Severe Study → Also see TABLE 9 p. 1431

▶ **Amiodarone** is predicted to increase the exposure to retinoids (alitretinoin). Adjust **alitretinoin** dose, p. 1305. Moderate Theoretical

▶ Ribociclib (high-dose) is predicted to increase the exposure to **amiodarone**. Avoid. Moderate Theoretical → Also see TABLE 9 p. 1431

▶ **Dronedarone** is predicted to increase the exposure to ribociclib. Moderate Study → Also see TABLE 9 p. 1431

▶ Rifamycins (rifampicin) are predicted to decrease the efficacy of **propafenone**. Moderate Study

▶ Rifamycins (rifampicin) are predicted to decrease the exposure to antiarrhythmics (**disopyramide, dronedarone**). Avoid. Severe Study

▶ **Dronedarone** is predicted to increase the exposure to ruxolitinib. Moderate Theoretical

▶ **Amiodarone** is predicted to increase the exposure to siponimod. Avoid depending on other drugs taken—consult product literature. Severe Study → Also see TABLE 6 p. 1430

▶ **Amiodarone** is predicted to increase the concentration of sirolimus. Severe Anecdotal

▶ **Dronedarone** increases the concentration of sirolimus. Monitor and adjust dose. Moderate Study

▶ Sofosbuvir is predicted to increase the risk of severe bradycardia or heart block when given with **amiodarone**. Refer to specialist literature. Severe Anecdotal

▶ SSRIs (fluvoxamine) are predicted to increase the exposure to **propafenone**. Monitor and adjust dose. Moderate Study

▶ **Dronedarone** is predicted to increase the exposure to SSRIs (citalopram, escitalopram, fluoxetine, fluvoxamine, paroxetine, sertraline). Severe Theoretical → Also see TABLE 9 p. 1431

▶ **Dronedarone** is predicted to increase the exposure to SSRIs (dapoxetine). Adjust **dapoxetine** dose with moderate CYP3A4 inhibitors, p. 867. Moderate Theoretical

▶ St John's wort is predicted to decrease the exposure to **dronedarone**. Avoid. Severe Theoretical

▶ **Amiodarone** is predicted to increase the risk of rhabdomyolysis when given with statins (atorvastatin). Monitor and adjust dose. Moderate Theoretical

▶ **Dronedarone** slightly increases the exposure to statins (atorvastatin). Monitor and adjust dose. Severe Study

▶ **Amiodarone** is predicted to increase the exposure to statins (fluvastatin). Severe Theoretical

▶ **Dronedarone** slightly increases the exposure to statins (rosuvastatin). Adjust dose. Severe Study

▶ **Amiodarone** increases the risk of rhabdomyolysis when given with statins (simvastatin). Adjust **simvastatin** dose, p. 219. Severe Study

▶ **Dronedarone** moderately increases the exposure to statins (simvastatin). Monitor and adjust dose. Severe Study

▶ **Amiodarone** is predicted to increase the exposure to sulfonylureas. Use with caution and adjust dose. Moderate Study

▶ **Dronedarone** is predicted to increase the exposure to sunitinib. Moderate Theoretical → Also see TABLE 9 p. 1431

▶ Lidocaine is predicted to increase the effects of suxamethonium. Moderate Study

▶ **Amiodarone** is predicted to increase the concentration of tacrolimus. Severe Anecdotal

▶ **Dronedarone** is predicted to increase the concentration of tacrolimus. Severe Study

▶ Antiarrhythmics (**amiodarone, dronedarone**) are predicted to slightly increase the exposure to talazoparib. Avoid or adjust **talazoparib** dose, p. 1052. Severe Study

▶ **Dronedarone** is predicted to increase the exposure to taxanes (cabazitaxel). Moderate Theoretical

▶ **Dronedarone** is predicted to increase the exposure to taxanes (paclitaxel). Severe Theoretical

▶ **Dronedarone** is predicted to increase the concentration of temsirolimus. Use with caution or avoid. Moderate Theoretical

▶ **Dronedarone** is predicted to increase the exposure to tezacaftor. Adjust tezacaftor with ivacaftor p. 311 or tezacaftor with ivacaftor and elexacftor p. 311 dose with moderate CYP3A4 inhibitors. Severe Study

▶ Theophylline decreases the efficacy of **adenosine**. Separate administration by 24 hours. Mild Study

▶ **Amiodarone** increases the exposure to thrombin inhibitors (dabigatran). Adjust **dabigatran** dose. Moderate Study

▶ **Dronedarone** slightly increases the exposure to thrombin inhibitors (dabigatran). Avoid. Severe Study

▶ **Amiodarone** is predicted to increase the risk of thyroid dysfunction when given with thyroid hormones. Avoid. Moderate Study

▶ **Amiodarone** is predicted to increase the exposure to ticagrelor. Use with caution or avoid. Severe Study

▶ **Dronedarone** given with a potent CYP2C19 inhibitor is predicted to increase the exposure to tofacitinib. Adjust **tofacitinib** dose, p. 1154. Moderate Study

▶ **Dronedarone** is predicted to increase the exposure to tolterodine. Mild Theoretical → Also see TABLE 9 p. 1431

▶ **Dronedarone** is predicted to increase the exposure to tolvaptan. Manufacturer advises caution or adjust **tolvaptan** dose with moderate CYP3A4 inhibitors, p. 708. Moderate Study

▶ Antiarrhythmics (**amiodarone, dronedarone**) are predicted to increase the exposure to topotecan. Severe Study

▶ Antiarrhythmics (**amiodarone, dronedarone**) are predicted to increase the concentration of trametinib. Moderate Theoretical

▶ **Dronedarone** is predicted to increase the exposure to trazodone. Moderate Theoretical

▶ **Dronedarone** is predicted to increase the exposure to tricyclic antidepressants. Avoid. Severe Theoretical → Also see TABLE 9 p. 1431

Propafenone is predicted to increase the concentration of tricyclic antidepressants. Moderate Theoretical → Also see TABLE 10 p. 1431

Amiodarone is predicted to increase the concentration of velpatasvir. Avoid or monitor. Moderate Theoretical

Amiodarone is predicted to increase the exposure to venetoclax. Avoid or monitor for toxicity. Severe Theoretical

Dronedarone is predicted to increase the exposure to venetoclax. Avoid or adjust dose—consult product literature. Severe Study

Dronedarone is predicted to increase the exposure to vinca alkaloids. Severe Theoretical → Also see TABLE 9 p. 1431

Dronedarone is predicted to increase the exposure to zopiclone. Adjust dose. Moderate Study

nticholinesterases, centrally acting → see TABLE 6 p. 1430 (bradycardia)

donepezil · galantamine · rivastigmine

Anti-androgens (apalutamide, enzalutamide) are predicted to decrease the exposure to **donepezil**. Mild Study

Antiepileptics (carbamazepine, fosphenytoin, phenytoin, primidone) are predicted to decrease the exposure to **donepezil**. Mild Study

Antifungals, azoles (itraconazole, ketoconazole, voriconazole) are predicted to increase the exposure to **galantamine**. Monitor and adjust dose. Moderate Study

Bupropion is predicted to increase the exposure to **galantamine**. Monitor and adjust dose. Moderate Study

Cinacalcet is predicted to increase the exposure to **galantamine**. Monitor and adjust dose. Moderate Study

Cobicistat is predicted to increase the exposure to **galantamine**. Monitor and adjust dose. Moderate Study

HIV-protease inhibitors are predicted to increase the exposure to **galantamine**. Monitor and adjust dose. Moderate Study

Idelalisib is predicted to increase the exposure to **galantamine**. Monitor and adjust dose. Moderate Study

Macrolides (clarithromycin) are predicted to increase the exposure to **galantamine**. Monitor and adjust dose. Moderate Study

Mitotane is predicted to decrease the exposure to **donepezil**. Mild Study

Anticholinesterases, centrally acting are predicted to decrease the effects of neuromuscular blocking drugs, non-depolarising. Moderate Theoretical → Also see TABLE 6 p. 1430

Rifamycins (rifampicin) are predicted to decrease the exposure to **donepezil**. Mild Study

SSRIs (fluoxetine, paroxetine) are predicted to increase the exposure to **galantamine**. Monitor and adjust dose. Moderate Study

Anticholinesterases, centrally acting increase the effects of suxamethonium. Moderate Theoretical

Terbinafine is predicted to increase the exposure to **galantamine**. Monitor and adjust dose. Moderate Study

Antiepileptics → see TABLE 1 p. 1429 (hepatotoxicity), TABLE 18 p. 1433 (hyponatraemia), TABLE 12 p. 1432 (peripheral neuropathy), TABLE 11 p. 1431 (CNS depressant effects)

brivaracetam · carbamazepine · eslicarbazepine · ethosuximide · fosphenytoin · gabapentin · lacosamide · lamotrigine · levetiracetam · oxcarbazepine · paraldehyde · perampanel · phenobarbital · phenytoin · pregabalin · primidone · retigabine · rufinamide · stiripentol · tiagabine · topiramate · valproate · vigabatrin · zonisamide

FOOD AND LIFESTYLE Avoid taking milk, dairy products, carbonated drinks, fruit juices, or caffeine-containing food and drinks at the same time as **stiripentol**.

▸ Antiepileptics (carbamazepine, fosphenytoin, phenobarbital, phenytoin, primidone) are predicted to decrease the exposure to 5-HT3-receptor antagonists (ondansetron). Moderate Study

▸ Antiepileptics (carbamazepine, fosphenytoin, phenobarbital, phenytoin, primidone) are predicted to markedly decrease the exposure to abemaciclib. Avoid. Severe Study

▸ Antiepileptics (carbamazepine, fosphenytoin, phenobarbital, phenytoin, primidone) are predicted to decrease the exposure to acalabrutinib. Avoid. Severe Study

▸ Acetazolamide potentially increases the risk of toxicity when given with **valproate**. Severe Study

▸ Acetazolamide potentially increases the risk of overheating and dehydration when given with **zonisamide**. Avoid in children. Severe Theoretical

▸ **Carbamazepine** is predicted to decrease the exposure to afatinib. Moderate Study

▸ Antiepileptics (fosphenytoin, phenytoin) are predicted to decrease the exposure to agomelatine. Moderate Theoretical

▸ Antiepileptics (carbamazepine, fosphenytoin, phenobarbital, phenytoin, primidone) decrease the concentration of albendazole. Moderate Study

▸ Alcohol potentially increases the risk of visual disturbances when given with **retigabine**. Moderate Study

▸ Antiepileptics (carbamazepine, fosphenytoin, phenobarbital, phenytoin, primidone) are predicted to decrease the exposure to aldosterone antagonists (eplerenone). Avoid. Moderate Theoretical → Also see TABLE 18 p. 1433

▸ **Carbamazepine** decreases the exposure to aliskiren. Moderate Study

▸ **Fosphenytoin** is predicted to decrease the exposure to aminophylline. Adjust dose. Moderate Study

▸ **Phenobarbital** is predicted to decrease the exposure to aminophylline. Adjust dose. Moderate Theoretical

▸ **Phenytoin** decreases the exposure to aminophylline. Adjust dose. Moderate Study

▸ **Primidone** is predicted to increase the clearance of aminophylline. Adjust dose. Moderate Study

▸ **Stiripentol** is predicted to increase the exposure to aminophylline. Avoid. Moderate Theoretical

▸ Antiepileptics (fosphenytoin, phenobarbital, phenytoin, primidone) are predicted to increase the risk of methaemoglobinaemia when given with topical anaesthetics, local (prilocaine). Use with caution or avoid. Severe Theoretical → Also see TABLE 11 p. 1431

▸ **Phenytoin** is predicted to decrease the exposure to anaesthetics, local (ropivacaine). Moderate Theoretical

▸ Oral antacids decrease the absorption of oral **gabapentin**. **Gabapentin** should be taken 2 hours after antacids. Moderate Study

▸ Anti-androgens (apalutamide) potentially decrease the exposure to **valproate**. Mild Theoretical

▸ Anti-androgens (apalutamide, enzalutamide) are predicted to decrease the exposure to **perampanel**. Monitor and adjust dose. Moderate Study

▸ Anti-androgens (enzalutamide) are predicted to slightly decrease the exposure to **brivaracetam**. Moderate Theoretical

▸ Antiepileptics (carbamazepine, fosphenytoin, phenobarbital, phenytoin, primidone) are predicted to decrease the exposure to anti-androgens (abiraterone). Avoid. Severe Study

▸ Antiepileptics (carbamazepine, fosphenytoin, phenobarbital, phenytoin, primidone) are predicted to decrease the exposure to anti-androgens (darolutamide). Avoid. Moderate Study

▸ Antiepileptics (carbamazepine, fosphenytoin, phenobarbital, phenytoin, primidone) are predicted to decrease the exposure to antiarrhythmics (disopyramide, dronedarone). Avoid. Severe Study

▸ Antiarrhythmics (amiodarone) are predicted to slightly increase the concentration of antiepileptics (fosphenytoin, phenytoin). Monitor and adjust dose. Severe Study → Also see TABLE 12 p. 1432

▸ Antiepileptics (fosphenytoin, phenytoin) are predicted to decrease the exposure to antiarrhythmics (lidocaine). Severe Anecdotal

▸ Antiepileptics (carbamazepine, fosphenytoin, phenobarbital, phenytoin, primidone) are predicted to decrease the efficacy of antiarrhythmics (propafenone). Moderate Study

▸ Antiepileptics (carbamazepine, fosphenytoin, phenobarbital, phenytoin, primidone) are predicted to decrease the exposure to anticholinesterases, centrally acting (donepezil). Mild Study

▸ Antiepileptics (carbamazepine) decrease the concentration of antiepileptics (brivaracetam). Moderate Study

▸ Antiepileptics (fosphenytoin, phenytoin) decrease the concentration of antiepileptics (brivaracetam). Moderate Study

▸ Antiepileptics (lamotrigine) potentially increase the concentration of antiepileptics (carbamazepine) and

A1

Interactions | Appendix 1

Antiepileptics (continued)

antiepileptics **(carbamazepine)** decrease the concentration of antiepileptics **(lamotrigine)**. Adjust **lamotrigine** dose and monitor **carbamazepine** concentration, p. 335, p. 327. Moderate Study

▸ Antiepileptics **(phenobarbital)** affect the concentration of antiepileptics **(carbamazepine)** and antiepileptics **(carbamazepine)** increase the concentration of antiepileptics **(phenobarbital)**. Adjust dose. Moderate Study

▸ Antiepileptics **(topiramate)** increase the risk of carbamazepine toxicity when given with antiepileptics **(carbamazepine)**. Moderate Study

▸ Antiepileptics **(stiripentol)** increase the concentration of antiepileptics **(carbamazepine, phenobarbital)**. Avoid in Dravet syndrome. Severe Study

▸ Antiepileptics **(carbamazepine)** slightly decrease the exposure to antiepileptics **(eslicarbazepine, oxcarbazepine)**. Monitor and adjust dose. Moderate Study

▸ Antiepileptics **(oxcarbazepine)** are predicted to increase the concentration of antiepileptics **(fosphenytoin)**. Monitor concentration and adjust dose. Moderate Study

▸ Antiepileptics **(stiripentol)** are predicted to increase the concentration of antiepileptics **(fosphenytoin)**. Severe Study

▸ Antiepileptics **(carbamazepine)** affect the concentration of antiepileptics **(fosphenytoin, phenytoin)** and antiepileptics **(fosphenytoin, phenytoin)** decrease the concentration of antiepileptics **(carbamazepine)**. Monitor and adjust dose. Severe Study

▸ Antiepileptics **(eslicarbazepine)** increase the exposure to antiepileptics **(fosphenytoin, phenytoin)** and antiepileptics **(fosphenytoin, phenytoin)** decrease the exposure to antiepileptics **(eslicarbazepine)**. Monitor and adjust dose. Moderate Study

▸ Antiepileptics **(valproate)** affect the concentration of antiepileptics **(fosphenytoin, phenytoin)** and antiepileptics **(fosphenytoin, phenytoin)** decrease the concentration of antiepileptics **(valproate)**. Severe Study

▸ Antiepileptics **(vigabatrin)** decrease the concentration of antiepileptics **(fosphenytoin, phenytoin)**. Mild Study

▸ Antiepileptics **(fosphenytoin)** decrease the concentration of antiepileptics **(lamotrigine)**. Monitor and adjust **lamotrigine** dose, p. 335. Moderate Study

▸ Antiepileptics **(phenobarbital, phenytoin, primidone)** decrease the concentration of antiepileptics **(lamotrigine)**. Monitor and adjust **lamotrigine** dose, p. 335. Moderate Study → Also see **TABLE 11** p. 1431

▸ Antiepileptics **(valproate)** increase the exposure to antiepileptics **(lamotrigine)**. Adjust **lamotrigine** dose and monitor rash, p. 335. Severe Study

▸ Antiepileptics **(lamotrigine)** are predicted to increase the concentration of antiepileptics **(oxcarbazepine)** and antiepileptics **(oxcarbazepine)** are predicted to decrease the concentration of antiepileptics **(lamotrigine)**. Monitor adverse effects and adjust dose. Moderate Study

▸ Antiepileptics **(carbamazepine, fosphenytoin)** are predicted to decrease the exposure to antiepileptics **(perampanel)**. Monitor and adjust dose. Moderate Study

▸ Antiepileptics **(oxcarbazepine)** decrease the concentration of antiepileptics **(perampanel)** and antiepileptics **(perampanel)** increase the concentration of antiepileptics **(oxcarbazepine)**. Monitor and adjust dose. Moderate Study

▸ Antiepileptics **(phenobarbital, phenytoin, primidone)** are predicted to decrease the exposure to antiepileptics **(perampanel)**. Monitor and adjust dose. Moderate Study → Also see **TABLE 11** p. 1431

▸ Antiepileptics **(phenytoin)** increase the concentration of antiepileptics **(phenobarbital)** and antiepileptics **(phenobarbital)** affect the concentration of antiepileptics **(phenytoin)**. Moderate Study

▸ Antiepileptics **(fosphenytoin)** increase the concentration of antiepileptics **(phenobarbital, primidone)** and antiepileptics **(phenobarbital, primidone)** affect the concentration of antiepileptics **(fosphenytoin)**. Moderate Study

▸ Antiepileptics **(oxcarbazepine)** are predicted to increase the concentration of antiepileptics **(phenytoin)**. Monitor concentration and adjust dose. Moderate Study

▸ Antiepileptics **(stiripentol)** are predicted to increase the concentration of antiepileptics **(phenytoin)**. Avoid in Dravet syndrome. Severe Study

▸ Antiepileptics **(carbamazepine)** potentially decrease the concentration of antiepileptics **(primidone)** and antiepileptics **(primidone)** potentially decrease the concentration of antiepileptics **(carbamazepine)**. Adjust dose. Moderate Anecdotal

▸ Antiepileptics **(phenytoin)** increase the concentration of antiepileptics **(primidone)** and antiepileptics **(primidone)** affect the concentration of antiepileptics **(phenytoin)**. Moderate Study

▸ Antiepileptics **(stiripentol)** are predicted to increase the concentration of antiepileptics **(primidone)**. Severe Theoretical

▸ Antiepileptics **(valproate)** affect the concentration of antiepileptics **(primidone)**. Monitor and adjust dose. Severe Study

▸ Antiepileptics **(carbamazepine)** slightly increase the clearance of antiepileptics **(retigabine)**. Moderate Study

▸ Antiepileptics **(fosphenytoin, phenytoin)** are predicted to slightly increase the clearance of antiepileptics **(retigabine)**. Moderate Study

▸ Antiepileptics **(valproate)** increase the exposure to antiepileptics **(rufinamide)**. Adjust **rufinamide** dose, p. 343. Moderate Study

▸ Antiepileptics **(carbamazepine, fosphenytoin, phenobarbital, phenytoin, primidone)** decrease the exposure to antiepileptics **(tiagabine)**. Monitor and adjust **tiagabine** dose, p. 348. Moderate Study

▸ Antiepileptics **(fosphenytoin, phenytoin)** decrease the concentration of antiepileptics **(topiramate)** and antiepileptics **(topiramate)** increase the concentration of antiepileptics **(fosphenytoin, phenytoin)**. Monitor and adjust dose. Moderate Study

▸ Antiepileptics **(phenobarbital, primidone)** are predicted to decrease the concentration of antiepileptics **(topiramate)**. Mild Study

▸ Antiepileptics **(phenobarbital)** decrease the concentration of antiepileptics **(valproate)** and antiepileptics **(valproate)** increase the concentration of antiepileptics **(phenobarbital)**. Monitor and adjust dose. Moderate Study

▸ Antiepileptics **(topiramate)** increase the risk of toxicity when given with antiepileptics **(valproate)**. Severe Study

▸ Antiepileptics **(carbamazepine)** slightly to moderately decrease the concentration of antiepileptics **(zonisamide)** and antiepileptics **(zonisamide)** affect the concentration of antiepileptics **(carbamazepine)**. Monitor and adjust dose. Moderate Study

▸ Antiepileptics **(fosphenytoin, phenytoin)** slightly to moderately decrease the concentration of antiepileptics **(zonisamide)**. Monitor and adjust dose. Moderate Study

▸ Antiepileptics **(phenobarbital, primidone)** are predicted to decrease the concentration of antiepileptics **(zonisamide)**. Monitor and adjust dose. Moderate Study

▸ Antiepileptics **(topiramate)** potentially increase the risk of overheating and dehydration when given with antiepileptics **(zonisamide)**. Avoid in children. Severe Theoretical

▸ Antifungals, azoles (itraconazole, ketoconazole, voriconazole) are predicted to very slightly increase the exposure to **perampanel**. Mild Study

▸ Antifungals, azoles (miconazole) increase the risk of carbamazepine toxicity when given with **carbamazepine**. Monitor and adjust dose. Severe Anecdotal

▸ Antifungals, azoles (miconazole) increase the risk of phenytoin toxicity when given with **fosphenytoin**. Monitor and adjust dose. Severe Anecdotal

▸ Antifungals, azoles (miconazole) increase the risk of phenytoin toxicity when given with **phenytoin**. Monitor and adjust dose. Severe Anecdotal

▸ **Carbamazepine** is predicted to decrease the efficacy of antifungals, azoles (fluconazole) and antifungals, azoles (fluconazole) increase the concentration of **carbamazepine**. Avoid or monitor **carbamazepine** concentration and adjust dose accordingly, p. 327. Severe Theoretical → Also see **TABLE 1** p. 1429

▸ Antifungals, azoles (fluconazole) increase the concentration of antiepileptics **(fosphenytoin, phenytoin)**. Monitor concentration and adjust dose. Moderate Study

▸ Antiepileptics **(carbamazepine, fosphenytoin, phenobarbital, phenytoin, primidone)** are predicted to decrease the exposure to antifungals, azoles (isavuconazole). Avoid. Severe Study

▸ **Fosphenytoin** very markedly decreases the exposure to antifungals, azoles (itraconazole). Avoid and for 14 days after stopping **fosphenytoin**. Moderate Study

▸ **Phenobarbital** decreases the concentration of antifungals, azoles (itraconazole). Avoid and for 14 days after stopping **phenobarbital**. Moderate Study

▸ **Phenytoin** very markedly decreases the exposure to antifungals, azoles (itraconazole). Avoid and for 14 days after stopping **phenytoin**. Moderate Study

▸ **Primidone** is predicted to decrease the concentration of antifungals, azoles (itraconazole). Moderate Theoretical

▸ **Carbamazepine** is predicted to decrease the efficacy of antifungals, azoles (itraconazole, voriconazole) and antifungals, azoles (itraconazole, voriconazole) increase the concentration of **carbamazepine**. Avoid or adjust dose. Moderate Theoretical → Also see TABLE 1 p. 1429

▸ **Carbamazepine** is predicted to decrease the efficacy of antifungals, azoles (ketoconazole) and antifungals, azoles (ketoconazole) slightly increase the concentration of **carbamazepine**. Avoid or monitor **carbamazepine** concentration and adjust dose accordingly, p. 327. Moderate Study

▸ **Phenobarbital** is predicted to decrease the concentration of antifungals, azoles (ketoconazole). Avoid. Moderate Study

▸ Antiepileptics **(fosphenytoin, phenytoin)** decrease the exposure to antifungals, azoles (ketoconazole). Avoid. Moderate Study

▸ **Primidone** is predicted to decrease the concentration of antifungals, azoles (ketoconazole, posaconazole). Avoid. Moderate Study

▸ **Carbamazepine** is predicted to decrease the efficacy of antifungals, azoles (posaconazole) and antifungals, azoles (posaconazole) increase the concentration of **carbamazepine**. Avoid. Moderate Theoretical

▸ **Phenobarbital** is predicted to decrease the concentration of antifungals, azoles (posaconazole). Avoid. Moderate Study

▸ Antiepileptics **(fosphenytoin, phenytoin)** are predicted to decrease the exposure to antifungals, azoles (posaconazole). Avoid. Moderate Study

▸ **Fosphenytoin** decreases the exposure to antifungals, azoles (voriconazole) and antifungals, azoles (voriconazole) increase the exposure to **fosphenytoin**. Avoid or adjust **voriconazole** dose and monitor phenytoin concentration, p. 638. Moderate Study

▸ **Phenytoin** decreases the exposure to antifungals, azoles (voriconazole) and antifungals, azoles (voriconazole) increase the exposure to **phenytoin**. Avoid or adjust **voriconazole** dose and monitor **phenytoin** concentration, p. 638, p. 340. Moderate Study

▸ Antiepileptics **(phenobarbital, primidone)** are predicted to decrease the concentration of antifungals, azoles (voriconazole). Avoid. Moderate Theoretical

▸ Antihistamines, sedating (hydroxyzine) potentially increase the risk of overheating and dehydration when given with **zonisamide**. Avoid in children. Severe Theoretical

▸ Antiepileptics **(carbamazepine, fosphenytoin, phenobarbital, phenytoin, primidone)** are predicted to decrease the exposure to antimalarials (artemether with lumefantrine). Avoid. Severe Study

▸ Antimalarials (pyrimethamine) increase the risk of haematological toxicity when given with antiepileptics **(fosphenytoin, phenytoin)**. Severe Study

▸ Antimalarials (pyrimethamine) are predicted to increase the risk of haematological toxicity when given with antiepileptics **(phenobarbital, primidone)**. Severe Theoretical

▸ Antiepileptics **(carbamazepine, fosphenytoin, phenobarbital, phenytoin, primidone)** are predicted to decrease the concentration of antimalarials (piperaquine). Avoid. Moderate Theoretical

▸ Antiepileptics **(carbamazepine, phenobarbital, primidone)** potentially increase the risk of toxicity when given with antimalarials (quinine). Unknown Study

▸ Antiepileptics **(carbamazepine, fosphenytoin, phenobarbital, phenytoin, primidone)** are predicted to moderately decrease the exposure to antipsychotics, second generation (aripiprazole). Adjust **aripiprazole** dose, p. 415. Moderate Study → Also see TABLE 11 p. 1431

▸ Antiepileptics **(carbamazepine, fosphenytoin, phenobarbital, phenytoin, primidone)** are predicted to decrease the exposure to antipsychotics, second generation (cariprazine). Avoid. Severe Theoretical → Also see TABLE 11 p. 1431

▸ **Carbamazepine** is predicted to increase the risk of myelosuppression when given with antipsychotics, second generation (clozapine). Avoid. Severe Anecdotal

▸ Antiepileptics **(fosphenytoin, phenobarbital, phenytoin, primidone)** are predicted to decrease the exposure to antipsychotics, second generation (clozapine). Moderate Anecdotal → Also see TABLE 11 p. 1431

▸ Antiepileptics **(carbamazepine, fosphenytoin, phenobarbital, phenytoin, primidone)** are predicted to decrease the exposure to antipsychotics, second generation (lurasidone). Avoid. Moderate Study → Also see TABLE 11 p. 1431

▸ **Carbamazepine** potentially decreases the exposure to antipsychotics, second generation (olanzapine). Monitor and adjust dose. Moderate Study

▸ **Phenytoin** is predicted to decrease the exposure to antipsychotics, second generation (olanzapine). Monitor and adjust dose. Moderate Study

▸ **Valproate** increases the risk of adverse effects when given with antipsychotics, second generation (olanzapine). Severe Study

▸ **Valproate** slightly increases the exposure to antipsychotics, second generation (paliperidone). Adjust dose. Moderate Study

▸ Antiepileptics **(carbamazepine, fosphenytoin, phenobarbital, phenytoin, primidone)** are predicted to decrease the exposure to antipsychotics, second generation (paliperidone). Monitor and adjust dose. Severe Study → Also see TABLE 11 p. 1431

▸ **Valproate** potentially increases the risk of neutropenia when given with antipsychotics, second generation (quetiapine). Moderate Study

▸ Antiepileptics **(carbamazepine, fosphenytoin, phenobarbital, phenytoin, primidone)** are predicted to decrease the exposure to antipsychotics, second generation (quetiapine). Moderate Study → Also see TABLE 11 p. 1431

▸ Antiepileptics **(carbamazepine, fosphenytoin, phenobarbital, phenytoin, primidone)** are predicted to decrease the exposure to antipsychotics, second generation (risperidone). Adjust dose. Moderate Study → Also see TABLE 11 p. 1431

▸ Antiepileptics **(carbamazepine, fosphenytoin, phenobarbital, phenytoin, primidone)** are predicted to decrease the exposure to avapritinib. Avoid. Severe Study

▸ Antiepileptics **(carbamazepine, fosphenytoin, phenobarbital, phenytoin, primidone)** are predicted to decrease the exposure to axitinib. Avoid or adjust dose. Moderate Study

▸ Antiepileptics **(carbamazepine, fosphenytoin, phenobarbital, phenytoin, primidone)** are predicted to decrease the exposure to bazedoxifene. Moderate Theoretical

▸ Antiepileptics **(carbamazepine, fosphenytoin, phenobarbital, phenytoin, primidone)** decrease the exposure to bedaquiline. Avoid. Severe Study → Also see TABLE 1 p. 1429

▸ Antiepileptics **(carbamazepine, fosphenytoin, phenobarbital, phenytoin, primidone)** are predicted to decrease the exposure to benzodiazepines (alprazolam). Adjust dose. Moderate Theoretical → Also see TABLE 11 p. 1431

▸ **Stiripentol** increases the concentration of benzodiazepines (clobazam). Severe Study

▸ Benzodiazepines (chlordiazepoxide) affect the concentration of antiepileptics **(fosphenytoin, phenytoin)**. Severe Study

▸ Benzodiazepines (clobazam, clonazepam) potentially affect the concentration of antiepileptics **(fosphenytoin, phenytoin)**. Severe Anecdotal

▸ Benzodiazepines (diazepam) potentially affect the concentration of antiepileptics **(fosphenytoin, phenytoin)**. Monitor concentration and adjust dose. Severe Study

Antiepileptics (continued)

▶ Antiepileptics **(carbamazepine, fosphenytoin, phenobarbital, phenytoin, primidone)** are predicted to decrease the exposure to benzodiazepines (midazolam). Monitor and adjust dose. Moderate Study → Also see TABLE 11 p. 1431

▶ Antiepileptics **(phenobarbital, primidone)** are predicted to decrease the exposure to beta blockers, non-selective (carvedilol, labetalol). Moderate Theoretical

▶ Antiepileptics **(phenobarbital, primidone)** are predicted to decrease the exposure to beta blockers, non-selective (propranolol). Moderate Study

▶ Antiepileptics **(phenobarbital, primidone)** are predicted to decrease the exposure to beta blockers, selective (acebutolol, bisoprolol, metoprolol, nebivolol). Moderate Study

▶ Antiepileptics **(carbamazepine, fosphenytoin, phenobarbital, phenytoin, primidone)** are predicted to decrease the exposure to bictegravir. Avoid. Moderate Study

▶ **Oxcarbazepine** is predicted to decrease the exposure to bictegravir. Avoid. Moderate Theoretical

▶ Antiepileptics **(carbamazepine, fosphenytoin, phenobarbital, phenytoin, primidone)** slightly decrease the exposure to bortezomib. Avoid. Severe Study → Also see TABLE 12 p. 1432

▶ Antiepileptics **(carbamazepine, fosphenytoin, phenobarbital, phenytoin, primidone)** are predicted to very markedly decrease the exposure to bosutinib. Avoid. Severe Study

▶ Antiepileptics **(carbamazepine, fosphenytoin, phenobarbital, phenytoin, primidone)** are predicted to decrease the exposure to brigatinib. Avoid. Severe Study

▶ Antiepileptics **(carbamazepine, fosphenytoin, phenobarbital, phenytoin, primidone)** are predicted to markedly decrease the exposure to bupropion. Severe Study

▶ **Valproate** increases the exposure to bupropion. Severe Study

▶ Antiepileptics **(carbamazepine, fosphenytoin, phenobarbital, phenytoin, primidone)** are predicted to decrease the exposure to buspirone. Use with caution and adjust dose. Severe Study

▶ Antiepileptics **(carbamazepine, fosphenytoin, phenobarbital, phenytoin, primidone)** moderately decrease the exposure to cabozantinib. Avoid. Moderate Study

▶ Antiepileptics **(fosphenytoin, phenytoin)** are predicted to moderately increase the clearance of caffeine citrate. Monitor and adjust dose. Moderate Study

▶ Calcium channel blockers (diltiazem) increase the concentration of **carbamazepine** and **carbamazepine** is predicted to decrease the exposure to calcium channel blockers (diltiazem). Monitor concentration and adjust dose. Severe Anecdotal

▶ Calcium channel blockers (verapamil) increase the concentration of **carbamazepine** and **carbamazepine** is predicted to decrease the exposure to calcium channel blockers (verapamil). Severe Anecdotal

▶ Antiepileptics **(carbamazepine, fosphenytoin, phenobarbital, phenytoin, primidone)** are predicted to decrease the exposure to calcium channel blockers (amlodipine, felodipine, lacidipine, lercanidipine, nicardipine, nifedipine, nimodipine). Monitor and adjust dose. Moderate Study

▶ Antiepileptics **(phenobarbital, primidone)** are predicted to decrease the exposure to calcium channel blockers (diltiazem, verapamil). Severe Study

▶ Calcium channel blockers (diltiazem, verapamil) potentially increase the concentration of antiepileptics **(fosphenytoin, phenytoin)** and antiepileptics **(fosphenytoin, phenytoin)** are predicted to decrease the exposure to calcium channel blockers (diltiazem, verapamil). Severe Study

▶ **Valproate** increases the exposure to calcium channel blockers (nimodipine). Adjust dose. Moderate Study

▶ Antiepileptics **(carbamazepine, fosphenytoin, phenobarbital, phenytoin, primidone)** are predicted to decrease the exposure to cannabidiol. Adjust dose. Moderate Study → Also see TABLE 11 p. 1431

▶ Cannabidiol increases the risk of increased ALT concentrations when given with **valproate**. Avoid or adjust dose. Severe Study

▶ Capecitabine increases the concentration of antiepileptics **(fosphenytoin, phenytoin)**. Severe Anecdotal

▶ Carbapenems decrease the concentration of **valproate**. Avoid. Severe Anecdotal

▶ Antiepileptics **(carbamazepine, fosphenytoin, phenytoin)** are predicted to decrease the concentration of caspofungin. Adjust caspofungin dose, p. 631. Moderate Theoretical

▶ Antiepileptics **(carbamazepine, fosphenytoin, phenobarbital, phenytoin, primidone)** are predicted to decrease the exposure to ceritinib. Avoid. Severe Study

▶ Antiepileptics **(phenobarbital, primidone)** are predicted to affect the efficacy of chenodeoxycholic acid. Monitor and adjust dose. Moderate Theoretical

▶ Antiepileptics **(phenobarbital, primidone)** decrease the concentration of chloramphenicol. Moderate Study

▶ Intravenous chloramphenicol increases the concentration of antiepileptics **(fosphenytoin, phenytoin)** and antiepileptics **(fosphenytoin, phenytoin)** affect the concentration of intravenous chloramphenicol. Monitor concentration and adjust dose. Severe Study

▶ **Phenobarbital** decreases the effects of cholic acid. Avoid. Moderate Study

▶ Antiepileptics **(carbamazepine, fosphenytoin, phenobarbital, phenytoin, primidone)** decrease the concentration of ciclosporin. Severe Study

▶ **Oxcarbazepine** decreases the concentration of ciclosporin. Severe Anecdotal

▶ Antiepileptics **(carbamazepine, fosphenytoin, phenobarbital, phenytoin, primidone)** are predicted to alter the effects of cilostazol. Moderate Theoretical

▶ Antiepileptics **(carbamazepine, fosphenytoin, phenobarbital, phenytoin, primidone)** are predicted to decrease the exposure to cinacalcet. Monitor and adjust dose. Moderate Study

▶ **Carbamazepine** is predicted to increase the risk of haematological toxicity when given with oral cladribine. Moderate Theoretical

▶ Antiepileptics **(carbamazepine, fosphenytoin, phenobarbital, phenytoin, primidone)** decrease the exposure to clomethiazole. Monitor and adjust dose. Moderate Study → Also see TABLE 11 p. 1431

▶ Antiepileptics **(carbamazepine, fosphenytoin, phenobarbital, phenytoin, primidone)** are predicted to decrease the exposure to cobicistat. Avoid. Severe Theoretical

▶ **Oxcarbazepine** is predicted to decrease the concentration of cobicistat. Severe Theoretical

▶ Cobicistat is predicted to very slightly increase the exposure to perampanel. Mild Study

▶ Antiepileptics **(carbamazepine, fosphenytoin, phenobarbital, phenytoin, primidone)** are predicted to decrease the exposure to cobimetinib. Avoid. Severe Theoretical

▶ Antiepileptics **(carbamazepine, eslicarbazepine, fosphenytoin, oxcarbazepine, perampanel, phenobarbital, phenytoin, primidone, rufinamide, topiramate)** are predicted to decrease the efficacy of combined hormonal contraceptives. For FSRH guidance, see Contraceptives, interactions p. 840. Severe Study

▶ Combined hormonal contraceptives alter the exposure to **lamotrigine**. Adjust dose. Moderate Study

▶ Antiepileptics **(carbamazepine, fosphenytoin, phenobarbital, phenytoin, primidone)** are predicted to decrease the exposure to corticosteroids (budesonide, deflazacort, dexamethasone, fludrocortisone, hydrocortisone, methylprednisolone, prednisolone, triamcinolone). Monitor and adjust dose. Moderate Study

▶ Antiepileptics **(carbamazepine, fosphenytoin, phenobarbital, phenytoin, primidone)** are predicted to decrease the exposure to corticosteroids (fluticasone). Unknown Theoretical

▶ Antiepileptics **(fosphenytoin, phenytoin)** are predicted to alter the anticoagulant effect of coumarins. Moderate Anecdotal

▶ Antiepileptics **(phenobarbital, primidone)** decrease the anticoagulant effect of coumarins. Monitor INR and adjust dose. Moderate Study

▶ **Carbamazepine** decreases the effects of coumarins. Monitor and adjust dose. Severe Study

▶ Antiepileptics **(carbamazepine, fosphenytoin, phenobarbital, phenytoin, primidone)** are predicted to markedly decrease the exposure to crizotinib. Avoid. Severe Study

▶ Antiepileptics **(carbamazepine, fosphenytoin, phenobarbital, phenytoin, primidone)** are predicted to decrease the exposure to dabrafenib. Avoid. Moderate Theoretical

▸ Danazol moderately increases the concentration of **carbamazepine**. Monitor and adjust dose. Severe Study

▸ Antiepileptics **(fosphenytoin, phenobarbital, phenytoin, primidone)** are predicted to increase the risk of methaemoglobinaemia when given with dapsone. Severe Theoretical

▸ Antiepileptics **(carbamazepine, fosphenytoin, phenobarbital, phenytoin, primidone)** are predicted to decrease the exposure to darifenacin. Moderate Theoretical

▸ Antiepileptics **(carbamazepine, fosphenytoin, phenobarbital, phenytoin, primidone)** are predicted to decrease the exposure to dasabuvir. Avoid. Severe Theoretical

▸ Antiepileptics **(carbamazepine, fosphenytoin, phenobarbital, phenytoin, primidone)** are predicted to markedly decrease the exposure to dasatinib. Avoid. Severe Study

▸ Antiepileptics **(carbamazepine, fosphenytoin, phenobarbital, phenytoin, primidone)** are predicted to slightly decrease the exposure to delamanid. Avoid. Moderate Study

▸ **Lamotrigine** is predicted to increase the risk of hyponatraemia when given with desmopressin. Severe Theoretical

▸ Antiepileptics **(carbamazepine, eslicarbazepine, fosphenytoin, oxcarbazepine, perampanel, phenobarbital, phenytoin, primidone, rufinamide, topiramate)** are predicted to decrease the efficacy of desogestrel. For FSRH guidance, see Contraceptives, interactions p. 840. Severe Theoretical

▸ **Desogestrel** is predicted to increase the exposure to **lamotrigine**. Moderate Study

▸ Diazoxide decreases the concentration of antiepileptics **(fosphenytoin, phenytoin)** and antiepileptics **(fosphenytoin, phenytoin)** are predicted to decrease the effects of diazoxide. Monitor concentration and adjust dose. Moderate Anecdotal

▸ Antiepileptics **(carbamazepine, fosphenytoin, phenobarbital, phenytoin, primidone)** are predicted to markedly decrease the exposure to dienogest. Severe Study

▸ Antiepileptics **(fosphenytoin, phenytoin)** are predicted to decrease the concentration of digoxin. Moderate Anecdotal

▸ Antiepileptics **(carbamazepine, fosphenytoin, phenobarbital, phenytoin, primidone)** are predicted to decrease the exposure to dipeptidylpeptidase-4 inhibitors (linagliptin). Moderate Study

▸ Antiepileptics **(carbamazepine, fosphenytoin, phenobarbital, phenytoin, primidone)** are predicted to moderately decrease the exposure to dipeptidylpeptidase-4 inhibitors (saxagliptin). Moderate Study

▸ Disulfiram increases the concentration of antiepileptics **(fosphenytoin, phenytoin)**. Monitor concentration and adjust dose. Severe Study → Also see **TABLE 12** p. 1432

▸ Antiepileptics **(carbamazepine, fosphenytoin, phenobarbital, phenytoin, primidone)** decrease the exposure to dolutegravir. Adjust dose. Severe Study

▸ **Oxcarbazepine** is predicted to decrease the exposure to dolutegravir. Adjust dose. Severe Theoretical

▸ Antiepileptics **(carbamazepine, fosphenytoin, phenobarbital, phenytoin, primidone)** are predicted to decrease the exposure to dronabinol. Avoid or adjust dose. Mild Study → Also see **TABLE 11** p. 1431

▸ **Phenytoin** is predicted to decrease the exposure to duloxetine. Moderate Theoretical

▸ Antiepileptics **(carbamazepine, fosphenytoin, phenobarbital, phenytoin, primidone)** are predicted to decrease the exposure to elbasvir. Avoid. Severe Study

▸ Antiepileptics **(carbamazepine, fosphenytoin, phenobarbital, phenytoin, primidone)** is predicted to decrease the exposure to elexacaftor. Avoid. Severe Theoretical

▸ Antiepileptics **(carbamazepine, fosphenytoin, phenobarbital, phenytoin, primidone)** are predicted to decrease the exposure to eliglustat. Avoid. Severe Study

▸ Antiepileptics **(carbamazepine, fosphenytoin, phenobarbital, phenytoin, primidone)** are predicted to decrease the concentration of elvitegravir. Avoid. Severe Theoretical

▸ Antiepileptics **(carbamazepine, fosphenytoin, phenobarbital, phenytoin, primidone)** are predicted to decrease the exposure to encorafenib. Severe Theoretical

▸ Antiepileptics **(carbamazepine, fosphenytoin, phenobarbital, phenytoin, primidone)** affect the exposure to endothelin receptor antagonists (bosentan). Avoid. Severe Study

▸ Antiepileptics **(carbamazepine, fosphenytoin, phenobarbital, phenytoin, primidone)** are predicted to decrease the exposure to endothelin receptor antagonists (macitentan). Avoid. Severe Study

▸ Enteral feeds decrease the absorption of **phenytoin**. Severe Study

▸ Antiepileptics **(carbamazepine, fosphenytoin, phenobarbital, phenytoin, primidone)** are predicted to decrease the exposure to entrectinib. Avoid. Severe Study

▸ Antiepileptics **(carbamazepine, fosphenytoin, phenobarbital, phenytoin, primidone)** are predicted to decrease the effects of ergotamine. Moderate Theoretical

▸ Antiepileptics **(carbamazepine, fosphenytoin, phenobarbital, phenytoin, primidone)** are predicted to decrease the exposure to erlotinib. Avoid or adjust **erlotinib** dose, p. 1024. Severe Study

▸ Antiepileptics **(carbamazepine, fosphenytoin, phenobarbital, phenytoin, primidone)** are predicted to decrease the exposure to esketamine. Adjust dose. Moderate Theoretical → Also see **TABLE 11** p. 1431

▸ Antiepileptics **(carbamazepine, eslicarbazepine, fosphenytoin, oxcarbazepine, perampanel, phenobarbital, phenytoin, primidone, rufinamide, topiramate)** are predicted to decrease the efficacy of etonogestrel. For FSRH guidance, see Contraceptives, interactions p. 840. Severe Theoretical

▸ Antiepileptics **(carbamazepine, fosphenytoin, phenobarbital, phenytoin, primidone)** are predicted to decrease the efficacy of etoposide. Moderate Study

▸ Antiepileptics **(carbamazepine, fosphenytoin, phenobarbital, phenytoin, primidone)** are predicted to decrease the concentration of everolimus. Avoid or adjust dose. Severe Study

▸ Antiepileptics **(carbamazepine, fosphenytoin, phenobarbital, phenytoin, primidone)** moderately decrease the exposure to exemestane. Moderate Study

▸ Antiepileptics **(carbamazepine, fosphenytoin, phenobarbital, phenytoin, primidone)** are predicted to moderately decrease the exposure to factor XA inhibitors (apixaban). Use with caution or avoid. Severe Study

▸ **Carbamazepine** is predicted to decrease the exposure to factor XA inhibitors (edoxaban). Moderate Study

▸ **Phenytoin** is predicted to decrease the exposure to factor XA inhibitors (edoxaban). Moderate Theoretical

▸ Antiepileptics **(carbamazepine, fosphenytoin, phenobarbital, phenytoin, primidone)** are predicted to moderately decrease the exposure to factor XA inhibitors (rivaroxaban). Avoid unless patient can be monitored for signs of thrombosis. Severe Study

▸ Antiepileptics **(carbamazepine, fosphenytoin, phenobarbital, phenytoin, primidone)** are predicted to decrease the exposure to fesoterodine. Avoid. Moderate Study

▸ Antiepileptics **(carbamazepine, fosphenytoin, phenobarbital, phenytoin, primidone)** are predicted to decrease the exposure to fingolimod. Moderate Study

▸ Fluorouracil increases the concentration of antiepileptics **(fosphenytoin, phenytoin)**. Monitor concentration and adjust dose. Severe Anecdotal

▸ Folates are predicted to decrease the concentration of antiepileptics **(fosphenytoin, phenobarbital, phenytoin, primidone)**. Monitor concentration and adjust dose. Severe Study

▸ Antiepileptics **(carbamazepine, fosphenytoin, phenobarbital, phenytoin, primidone)** are predicted to decrease the exposure to fostamatinib. Avoid. Severe Study

▸ Antiepileptics **(carbamazepine, fosphenytoin, phenobarbital, phenytoin, primidone)** are predicted to decrease the exposure to gefitinib. Avoid. Severe Study

▸ Antiepileptics **(carbamazepine, fosphenytoin, phenytoin)** are predicted to decrease the exposure to gilteritinib. Avoid. Severe Study

▸ Antiepileptics **(carbamazepine, fosphenytoin, phenobarbital, phenytoin, primidone)** are predicted to moderately decrease the exposure to glasdegib. Avoid. Severe Study

▸ Antiepileptics **(carbamazepine, fosphenytoin, phenobarbital, phenytoin, primidone)** are predicted to moderately decrease the exposure to glecaprevir. Avoid. Severe Study

▸ Antiepileptics **(eslicarbazepine, oxcarbazepine)** potentially decrease the exposure to glecaprevir. Avoid. Severe Theoretical

Antiepileptics (continued)

▶ **Valproate** potentially opposes the effects of glycerol phenylbutyrate. Moderate Theoretical

▶ Grapefruit juice slightly increases the exposure to **carbamazepine**. Monitor and adjust dose. Moderate Study

▶ Antiepileptics **(carbamazepine, fosphenytoin, phenobarbital, phenytoin, primidone)** are predicted to decrease the exposure to grazoprevir. Avoid. Severe Study

▶ Antiepileptics **(phenobarbital, primidone)** decrease the effects of griseofulvin. Moderate Study

▶ Antiepileptics **(carbamazepine, fosphenytoin, phenobarbital, phenytoin, primidone)** are predicted to decrease the concentration of guanfacine. Adjust **guanfacine** dose, p. 372. Moderate Study → Also see **TABLE 11** p. 1431

▶ **Oxcarbazepine** is predicted to decrease the concentration of guanfacine. Monitor and adjust **guanfacine** dose, p. 372. Moderate Theoretical

▶ Guanfacine increases the concentration of **valproate**. Monitor and adjust dose. Moderate Study

▶ H_2 receptor antagonists (cimetidine) transiently increase the concentration of **carbamazepine**. Monitor concentration and adjust dose. Moderate Study

▶ H_2 receptor antagonists (cimetidine) increase the concentration of antiepileptics **(fosphenytoin, phenytoin)**. Monitor concentration and adjust dose. Severe Study

▶ Antiepileptics **(carbamazepine, fosphenytoin, phenobarbital, phenytoin, primidone)** decrease the concentration of haloperidol. Adjust dose. Moderate Study → Also see **TABLE 11** p. 1431

▶ Haloperidol potentially increases the risk of overheating and dehydration when given with **zonisamide**. Avoid in children. Severe Theoretical

▶ HIV-protease inhibitors are predicted to affect the exposure to antiepileptics **(fosphenytoin, phenytoin)** and antiepileptics **(fosphenytoin, phenytoin)** decrease the concentration of HIV-protease inhibitors. Severe Theoretical

▶ HIV-protease inhibitors are predicted to affect the concentration of antiepileptics **(phenobarbital, primidone)** and antiepileptics **(phenobarbital, primidone)** are predicted to decrease the concentration of HIV-protease inhibitors. Severe Theoretical

▶ HIV-protease inhibitors are predicted to increase the exposure to **carbamazepine** and **carbamazepine** is predicted to decrease the exposure to HIV-protease inhibitors. Monitor and adjust dose. Severe Theoretical

▶ HIV-protease inhibitors (ritonavir) slightly decrease the exposure to **lamotrigine**. Severe Study

▶ HIV-protease inhibitors are predicted to very slightly increase the exposure to **perampanel**. Mild Study

▶ HIV-protease inhibitors (ritonavir) are predicted to decrease the concentration of **valproate**. Severe Anecdotal

▶ Antiepileptics **(carbamazepine, eslicarbazepine, fosphenytoin, oxcarbazepine, perampanel, phenobarbital, phenytoin, primidone, rufinamide, topiramate)** are predicted to decrease the effects of hormone replacement therapy. Moderate Anecdotal

▶ Hormone replacement therapy is predicted to alter the exposure to **lamotrigine**. Moderate Theoretical

▶ Antiepileptics **(carbamazepine, fosphenytoin, phenobarbital, phenytoin, primidone)** are predicted to decrease the exposure to ibrutinib. Avoid or adjust **ibrutinib** dose, p. 1027. Severe Study

▶ Antiepileptics **(carbamazepine, fosphenytoin, phenobarbital, phenytoin, primidone)** are predicted to decrease the exposure to idelalisib. Avoid. Severe Study

▶ Idelalisib is predicted to very slightly increase the exposure to **perampanel**. Mild Study

▶ Antiepileptics **(carbamazepine, fosphenytoin, phenobarbital, phenytoin, primidone)** are predicted to decrease the exposure to imatinib. Avoid. Moderate Study

▶ **Oxcarbazepine** decreases the exposure to imatinib. Avoid. Moderate Study

▶ Antiepileptics **(carbamazepine, fosphenytoin, phenobarbital, phenytoin, primidone)** are predicted to decrease the exposure to irinotecan. Avoid. Severe Study

▶ Antiepileptics **(carbamazepine, fosphenytoin, phenobarbital, phenytoin, primidone)** are predicted to decrease the exposure

to iron chelators (deferasirox). Monitor serum ferritin and adjust dose. Moderate Theoretical

▶ Isoniazid increases the concentration of antiepileptics **(fosphenytoin, phenytoin)**. Moderate Study → Also see **TABLE 12** p. 1432

▶ Isoniazid markedly increases the concentration of **carbamazepine** and **carbamazepine** increases the risk of hepatotoxicity when given with isoniazid. Monitor concentration and adjust dose. Severe Study → Also see **TABLE 1** p. 1429

▶ Antiepileptics **(carbamazepine, fosphenytoin, phenobarbital, phenytoin, primidone)** are predicted to decrease the exposure to ivabradine. Adjust dose. Moderate Theoretical

▶ Antiepileptics **(carbamazepine, fosphenytoin, phenobarbital, phenytoin, primidone)** are predicted to moderately to markedly decrease the exposure to ivacaftor. Avoid. Severe Study

▶ Antiepileptics **(carbamazepine, fosphenytoin, phenobarbital, phenytoin, primidone)** are predicted to decrease the exposure to ixazomib. Avoid. Severe Study

▶ Antiepileptics **(carbamazepine, fosphenytoin, phenobarbital, phenytoin, primidone)** are predicted to decrease the exposure to lapatinib. Avoid. Severe Study

▶ Antiepileptics **(carbamazepine, fosphenytoin, phenobarbital, phenytoin, primidone)** are predicted to moderately decrease the exposure to larotrectinib. Avoid. Moderate Study

▶ Antiepileptics **(fosphenytoin, oxcarbazepine, phenobarbital, phenytoin, primidone)** are predicted to decrease the exposure to ledipasvir. Avoid. Severe Theoretical

▶ **Carbamazepine** is predicted to decrease the exposure to ledipasvir. Avoid. Severe Study

▶ Antiepileptics **(carbamazepine, phenobarbital, primidone)** are predicted to decrease the concentration of letermovir. Moderate Theoretical

▶ Letermovir is predicted to decrease the concentration of antiepileptics **(fosphenytoin, phenytoin)** and antiepileptics **(fosphenytoin, phenytoin)** are predicted to decrease the concentration of letermovir. Moderate Theoretical

▶ Antiepileptics **(fosphenytoin, phenytoin)** decrease the effects of levodopa. Moderate Study

▶ Antiepileptics **(carbamazepine, eslicarbazepine, fosphenytoin, oxcarbazepine, perampanel, phenobarbital, phenytoin, primidone, rufinamide, topiramate)** are predicted to decrease the efficacy of levonorgestrel. For FSRH guidance, see Contraceptives, interactions p. 840. Severe Theoretical

▶ Antiepileptics **(carbamazepine, oxcarbazepine)** are predicted to increase the risk of neurotoxicity when given with lithium. Severe Anecdotal

▶ Antiepileptics **(carbamazepine, fosphenytoin, phenobarbital, phenytoin, primidone)** are predicted to decrease the exposure to lomitapide. Monitor and adjust dose. Moderate Theoretical → Also see **TABLE 1** p. 1429

▶ Antiepileptics **(fosphenytoin, phenytoin)** decrease the effects of loop diuretics (furosemide). Moderate Study

▶ Antiepileptics **(carbamazepine, fosphenytoin, phenobarbital, phenytoin, primidone)** are predicted to decrease the exposure to lorlatinib. Avoid. Severe Study

▶ Lumacaftor is predicted to decrease the exposure to antiepileptics **(carbamazepine, fosphenytoin, phenobarbital, phenytoin, primidone)**. Avoid. Severe Theoretical

▶ Macrolides (clarithromycin) slightly increase the concentration of **carbamazepine**. Monitor concentration and adjust dose. Severe Study

▶ Macrolides (clarithromycin) are predicted to very slightly increase the exposure to **perampanel**. Mild Study

▶ Macrolides (erythromycin) markedly increase the concentration of **carbamazepine**. Monitor concentration and adjust dose. Severe Study

▶ Antiepileptics **(phenobarbital, primidone)** are predicted to increase the effects of MAOIs, irreversible. Severe Theoretical

▶ **Carbamazepine** is predicted to increase the risk of severe toxic reaction when given with MAOIs, irreversible. Avoid and for 14 days after stopping the MAOI. Severe Theoretical

▶ Antiepileptics **(carbamazepine, fosphenytoin, phenobarbital, phenytoin, primidone)** are predicted to decrease the exposure to maraviroc. Adjust dose. Severe Study

Antiepileptics **(carbamazepine, fosphenytoin, phenobarbital, phenytoin, primidone)** are predicted to slightly decrease the exposure to meglitinides (nateglinide). [Mild] Study

Antiepileptics **(carbamazepine, fosphenytoin, phenobarbital, phenytoin, primidone)** are predicted to decrease the exposure to meglitinides (repaglinide). Monitor blood glucose and adjust dose. [Moderate] Study

Phenytoin is predicted to decrease the exposure to melatonin. [Moderate] Theoretical

Levetiracetam decreases the clearance of methotrexate. [Severe] Anecdotal

Antiepileptics **(phenobarbital, primidone)** are predicted to decrease the exposure to metronidazole. [Moderate] Study

Antiepileptics **(fosphenytoin, phenobarbital, phenytoin, primidone)** are predicted to decrease the effects of metyrapone. Avoid. [Moderate] Study

Phenytoin is predicted to increase the clearance of mexiletine. Monitor and adjust dose. [Moderate] Study

Antiepileptics **(phenobarbital, primidone)** are predicted to decrease the exposure to mianserin. [Moderate] Study → Also see **TABLE 11** p. 1431

▶ **Carbamazepine** markedly decreases the exposure to mianserin. Adjust dose. [Moderate] Study

▶ Antiepileptics **(carbamazepine, fosphenytoin, phenobarbital, phenytoin, primidone)** are predicted to decrease the exposure to midostaurin. Avoid. [Severe] Study

▶ Antiepileptics **(carbamazepine, fosphenytoin, phenobarbital, phenytoin, primidone)** are predicted to decrease the exposure to mirtazapine. Adjust dose. [Moderate] Study → Also see **TABLE 11** p. 1431

▶ Mitotane is predicted to decrease the exposure to **perampanel.** Monitor and adjust dose. [Moderate] Study

▶ Antiepileptics **(carbamazepine, phenobarbital, primidone)** are predicted to decrease the exposure to modafinil. [Mild] Theoretical

▶ Antiepileptics **(fosphenytoin, phenytoin)** are predicted to decrease the exposure to modafinil and modafinil is predicted to increase the concentration of antiepileptics **(fosphenytoin, phenytoin)**. Monitor concentration and adjust dose. [Moderate] Theoretical

▶ **Carbamazepine** is predicted to decrease the effects of monoclonal antibodies (brentuximab vedotin). [Severe] Theoretical

▶ Monoclonal antibodies (tocilizumab) are predicted to decrease the exposure to antiepileptics **(fosphenytoin, phenytoin)**. Monitor and adjust dose. [Moderate] Theoretical

▶ Antiepileptics **(carbamazepine, fosphenytoin, phenobarbital, phenytoin, primidone)** are predicted to decrease the exposure to monoclonal antibodies (polatuzumab vedotin). [Moderate] Theoretical

▶ Antiepileptics **(carbamazepine, fosphenytoin, phenobarbital, phenytoin, primidone)** are predicted to decrease the exposure to montelukast. [Mild] Study

▶ Antiepileptics **(carbamazepine, fosphenytoin, phenobarbital, phenytoin, primidone)** are predicted to markedly decrease the exposure to naldemedine. Avoid. [Severe] Study

▶ Antiepileptics **(carbamazepine, fosphenytoin, phenobarbital, phenytoin, primidone)** are predicted to markedly decrease the exposure to naloxegol. Avoid. [Moderate] Study

▶ Antiepileptics **(carbamazepine, fosphenytoin, phenobarbital, phenytoin, primidone)** are predicted to decrease the exposure to neratinib. Avoid. [Severe] Study → Also see **TABLE 1** p. 1429

▶ Antiepileptics **(carbamazepine, fosphenytoin, phenobarbital, phenytoin, primidone)** are predicted to markedly decrease the exposure to neurokinin-1 receptor antagonists (aprepitant). Avoid. [Moderate] Study

▶ Antiepileptics **(carbamazepine, fosphenytoin, phenobarbital, phenytoin, primidone)** are predicted to decrease the exposure to neurokinin-1 receptor antagonists (fosaprepitant). Avoid. [Moderate] Theoretical

▶ Antiepileptics **(carbamazepine, fosphenytoin, phenobarbital, phenytoin, primidone)** are predicted to decrease the exposure to neurokinin-1 receptor antagonists (netupitant). Avoid. [Severe] Study

▶ **Carbamazepine** is predicted to decrease the effects of (but acute use increases the effects of) neuromuscular blocking drugs,

non-depolarising (atracurium, cisatracurium, pancuronium, rocuronium, vecuronium). Monitor and adjust dose. [Moderate] Study

▶ Antiepileptics **(fosphenytoin, phenytoin)** decrease the effects of (but acute use increases the effects of) neuromuscular blocking drugs, non-depolarising (atracurium, cisatracurium, pancuronium, rocuronium, vecuronium). [Moderate] Study

▶ Antiepileptics **(carbamazepine, fosphenytoin, phenobarbital, phenytoin, primidone)** are predicted to moderately decrease the exposure to nilotinib. Avoid. [Severe] Study

▶ **Carbamazepine** is predicted to decrease the exposure to nintedanib. [Moderate] Study

▶ Antiepileptics **(carbamazepine, fosphenytoin, phenobarbital, phenytoin, primidone)** are predicted to decrease the exposure to nitisinone. Adjust dose. [Moderate] Theoretical

▶ NNRTIs (efavirenz) are predicted to affect the efficacy of **primidone** and **primidone** is predicted to slightly decrease the exposure to NNRTIs (efavirenz). [Severe] Theoretical

▶ NNRTIs (nevirapine) are predicted to decrease the concentration of antiepileptics **(carbamazepine, fosphenytoin, phenobarbital, phenytoin, primidone)** and antiepileptics **(carbamazepine, fosphenytoin, phenobarbital, phenytoin, primidone)** are predicted to decrease the concentration of NNRTIs (nevirapine). [Severe] Study

▶ **Oxcarbazepine** is predicted to decrease the exposure to NNRTIs (doravirine). Avoid. [Severe] Theoretical

▶ Antiepileptics **(carbamazepine, fosphenytoin, phenobarbital, phenytoin, primidone)** are predicted to decrease the exposure to NNRTIs (doravirine). Avoid. [Severe] Study

▶ **Carbamazepine** slightly decreases the exposure to NNRTIs (efavirenz) and NNRTIs (efavirenz) slightly decrease the exposure to **carbamazepine**. [Severe] Study

▶ **Phenobarbital** is predicted to decrease the exposure to NNRTIs (efavirenz) and NNRTIs (efavirenz) affect the concentration of **phenobarbital**. [Severe] Theoretical

▶ Antiepileptics **(fosphenytoin, phenytoin)** slightly decrease the exposure to NNRTIs (efavirenz) and NNRTIs (efavirenz) affect the concentration of antiepileptics **(fosphenytoin, phenytoin)**. [Severe] Theoretical

▶ Antiepileptics **(carbamazepine, fosphenytoin, phenobarbital, phenytoin, primidone)** are predicted to decrease the exposure to NNRTIs (etravirine). Avoid. [Severe] Theoretical

▶ **Oxcarbazepine** is predicted to decrease the concentration of NNRTIs (rilpivirine). Avoid. [Severe] Theoretical

▶ Antiepileptics **(carbamazepine, fosphenytoin, phenobarbital, phenytoin, primidone)** markedly decrease the exposure to NNRTIs (rilpivirine). Avoid. [Severe] Study

▶ Antiepileptics **(carbamazepine, eslicarbazepine, fosphenytoin, oxcarbazepine, perampanel, phenobarbital, phenytoin, primidone, rufinamide, topiramate)** are predicted to decrease the efficacy of norethisterone. For FSRH guidance, see Contraceptives, interactions p. 840. [Severe] Anecdotal

▶ Antiepileptics **(carbamazepine, fosphenytoin, phenobarbital, phenytoin, primidone)** are predicted to decrease the exposure to NRTIs (abacavir). [Moderate] Theoretical

▶ **Valproate** slightly increases the exposure to NRTIs (zidovudine). [Moderate] Study

▶ Antiepileptics **(carbamazepine, fosphenytoin, phenobarbital, phenytoin, primidone)** are predicted to decrease the exposure to olaparib. Avoid. [Moderate] Theoretical

▶ Antiepileptics **(carbamazepine, fosphenytoin, phenobarbital, phenytoin)** are predicted to decrease the exposure to ombitasvir. Avoid. [Severe] Theoretical

▶ Antiepileptics **(carbamazepine, fosphenytoin, phenobarbital, phenytoin, primidone)** are predicted to decrease the exposure to opioids (alfentanil, fentanyl). [Moderate] Study → Also see **TABLE 11** p. 1431

▶ Antiepileptics **(carbamazepine, fosphenytoin, phenobarbital, phenytoin, primidone)** are predicted to decrease the exposure to opioids (buprenorphine). Monitor and adjust dose. [Moderate] Theoretical → Also see **TABLE 11** p. 1431

▶ Antiepileptics **(carbamazepine, fosphenytoin, phenobarbital, phenytoin, primidone)** decrease the exposure to opioids (methadone). Monitor and adjust dose. [Severe] Study → Also see **TABLE 11** p. 1431

Antiepileptics (continued)

▶ Antiepileptics **(carbamazepine, fosphenytoin, phenobarbital, phenytoin, primidone)** are predicted to decrease the exposure to opioids (oxycodone). Monitor and adjust dose. Moderate Study → Also see TABLE 11 p. 1431

▶ **Carbamazepine** decreases the concentration of opioids (tramadol). Adjust dose. Severe Study

▶ Antiepileptics **(carbamazepine, fosphenytoin, phenobarbital, phenytoin, primidone)** are predicted to moderately decrease the exposure to osimertinib. Avoid. Moderate Study

▶ Antiepileptics **(carbamazepine, fosphenytoin, phenobarbital, phenytoin, primidone)** are predicted to moderately decrease the exposure to ospemifene. Moderate Study

▶ Oxybutynin potentially increases the risk of overheating and dehydration when given with **zonisamide**. Avoid in children. Severe Theoretical

▶ Antiepileptics **(carbamazepine, fosphenytoin, phenobarbital, phenytoin, primidone)** are predicted to decrease the exposure to palbociclib. Avoid. Severe Study

▶ Antiepileptics **(carbamazepine, fosphenytoin, phenobarbital, phenytoin, primidone)** are predicted to decrease the exposure to panobinostat. Avoid. Moderate Theoretical

▶ Antiepileptics **(carbamazepine, fosphenytoin, phenobarbital, phenytoin, primidone)** decrease the exposure to paracetamol. Moderate Study → Also see TABLE 1 p. 1429

▶ Antiepileptics **(carbamazepine, fosphenytoin, phenobarbital, phenytoin, primidone)** are predicted to decrease the exposure to paritaprevir (with ritonavir and ombitasvir). Avoid. Severe Study

▶ Antiepileptics **(carbamazepine, fosphenytoin, phenobarbital, phenytoin, primidone)** are predicted to decrease the exposure to pazopanib. Avoid. Severe Theoretical

▶ **Valproate** increases the risk of adverse effects when given with penicillins (pivmecillinam). Avoid. Severe Anecdotal

▶ Phenothiazines (chlorpromazine) decrease the concentration of antiepileptics **(phenobarbital, primidone)** and antiepleptics **(phenobarbital, primidone)** decrease the concentration of phenothiazines (chlorpromazine). Moderate Study → Also see TABLE 11 p. 1431

▶ Antiepileptics **(carbamazepine, fosphenytoin, phenobarbital, phenytoin, primidone)** moderately decrease the exposure to phosphodiesterase type-4 inhibitors (apremilast). Avoid. Severe Study

▶ Antiepileptics **(carbamazepine, fosphenytoin, phenobarbital, phenytoin, primidone)** are predicted to decrease the exposure to phosphodiesterase type-4 inhibitors (roflumilast). Avoid. Moderate Study

▶ Antiepileptics **(carbamazepine, fosphenytoin, phenobarbital, phenytoin, primidone)** are predicted to decrease the exposure to phosphodiesterase type-5 inhibitors (avanafil, tadalafil). Avoid. Severe Study

▶ Antiepileptics **(carbamazepine, fosphenytoin, phenobarbital, phenytoin, primidone)** are predicted to decrease the exposure to phosphodiesterase type-5 inhibitors (sildenafil, vardenafil). Moderate Theoretical

▶ Antiepileptics **(carbamazepine, fosphenytoin, phenobarbital, phenytoin, primidone)** are predicted to moderately to markedly decrease the exposure to pibrentasvir. Avoid. Severe Study

▶ Antiepileptics **(eslicarbazepine, oxcarbazepine)** potentially decrease the exposure to pibrentasvir. Avoid. Severe Theoretical

▶ Antiepileptics **(fosphenytoin, phenytoin)** are predicted to decrease the exposure to pirfenidone. Moderate Theoretical

▶ Antiepileptics **(carbamazepine, fosphenytoin, phenobarbital, phenytoin, primidone)** are predicted to moderately decrease the exposure to pitolisant. Moderate Study

▶ Antiepileptics **(carbamazepine, fosphenytoin, phenobarbital, phenytoin, primidone)** are predicted to decrease the exposure to ponatinib. Avoid. Moderate Theoretical

▶ Antiepileptics **(carbamazepine, fosphenytoin, phenobarbital, phenytoin, primidone)** are predicted to markedly decrease the exposure to praziquantel. Avoid. Moderate Study

▶ Antiepileptics **(carbamazepine, phenobarbital, phenytoin, primidone)** are predicted to increase the risk of hypersensitivity reactions when given with procarbazine. Severe Anecdotal

▶ **Fosphenytoin** is predicted to increase the risk of hypersensitivity when given with procarbazine. Severe Anecdotal

▶ **Valproate** potentially increases the concentration of propofol. Adjust dose. Severe Theoretical

▶ Quinolones (ciprofloxacin) affect the concentration of antiepileptics **(fosphenytoin, phenytoin)**. Monitor concentration and adjust dose. Severe Study

▶ Antiepileptics **(fosphenytoin, phenobarbital, phenytoin, primidone)** are predicted to affect the exposure to raltegravir. Use with caution or avoid. Moderate Theoretical

▶ **Carbamazepine** is predicted to affect the exposure to raltegravir. Moderate Theoretical

▶ Antiepileptics **(carbamazepine, fosphenytoin, phenobarbital, phenytoin, primidone)** are predicted to decrease the exposure to ranolazine. Severe Study

▶ Antiepileptics **(carbamazepine, fosphenytoin, phenobarbital, phenytoin, primidone)** are predicted to decrease the exposure to reboxetine. Moderate Anecdotal

▶ Antiepileptics **(carbamazepine, fosphenytoin, phenobarbital, phenytoin, primidone)** are predicted to decrease the exposure to regorafenib. Avoid. Moderate Study

▶ Antiepileptics **(carbamazepine, fosphenytoin, phenobarbital, phenytoin, primidone)** potentially decrease the exposure to remdesivir. Avoid. Moderate Theoretical

▶ Antiepileptics **(carbamazepine, fosphenytoin, phenobarbital, phenytoin, primidone)** are predicted to markedly decrease the exposure to ribociclib. Avoid. Severe Study

▶ Rifamycins (rifampicin) slightly decrease the exposure to brivaracetam. Adjust dose. Moderate Study

▶ Rifamycins (rifampicin) markedly increase the clearance of lamotrigine. Adjust **lamotrigine** dose, p. 335. Moderate Study

▶ Rifamycins (rifampicin) are predicted to decrease the exposure to perampanel. Monitor and adjust dose. Moderate Study

▶ Rifamycins (rifampicin) decrease the concentration of antiepileptics **(fosphenytoin, phenytoin)**. Use with caution and adjust dose. Moderate Study

▶ Antiepileptics **(phenobarbital, primidone)** are predicted to decrease the exposure to rifamycins (rifampicin) and rifamycins (rifampicin) are predicted to decrease the exposure to antiepileptics **(phenobarbital, primidone)**. Use with caution and adjust dose. Moderate Study

▶ **Rucaparib** is predicted to increase the exposure to **phenytoin**. Monitor and adjust dose. Moderate Study

▶ Antiepileptics **(carbamazepine, fosphenytoin, phenobarbital, phenytoin, primidone)** are predicted to decrease the exposure to ruxolitinib. Monitor and adjust dose. Moderate Study

▶ Antiepileptics **(carbamazepine, fosphenytoin, phenytoin)** are predicted to decrease the exposure to the active metabolite of selexipag. Adjust dose. Moderate Study

▶ **Valproate** is predicted to increase the exposure to selexipag. Unknown Theoretical

▶ Antiepileptics **(carbamazepine, fosphenytoin, phenobarbital, phenytoin, primidone)** are predicted to decrease the exposure to siponimod. Severe Study

▶ Antiepileptics **(carbamazepine, fosphenytoin, phenobarbital, phenytoin, primidone)** are predicted to decrease the concentration of sirolimus. Avoid. Severe Study

▶ **Valproate** increases the exposure to sodium oxybate. Adjust **sodium oxybate** dose, p. 512. Moderate Study

▶ **Valproate** potentially decreases the effects of sodium phenylbutyrate. Moderate Anecdotal

▶ Antiepileptics **(fosphenytoin, oxcarbazepine, phenobarbital, phenytoin, primidone)** are predicted to decrease the exposure to sofosbuvir. Avoid. Severe Theoretical

▶ **Carbamazepine** is predicted to decrease the exposure to sofosbuvir. Avoid. Severe Study

▶ Antiepileptics **(carbamazepine, fosphenytoin, phenobarbital, phenytoin, primidone)** are predicted to decrease the exposure to solifenacin. Moderate Theoretical

▶ Antiepileptics **(carbamazepine, fosphenytoin, phenobarbital, phenytoin, primidone)** are predicted to decrease the exposure to sorafenib. Moderate Theoretical

SSRIs (fluoxetine, fluvoxamine) are predicted to increase the concentration of antiepileptics **(fosphenytoin, phenytoin)**. Monitor and adjust dose. Severe Anecdotal

SSRIs (sertraline) potentially increase the risk of toxicity when given with antiepileptics **(fosphenytoin, phenytoin)**. Monitor concentration and adjust dose. Severe Anecdotal

Antiepileptics **(fosphenytoin, phenytoin)** decrease the concentration of SSRIs (paroxetine). Moderate Study

St John's wort is predicted to decrease the concentration of antiepileptics **(fosphenytoin, phenobarbital, phenytoin, primidone)**. Avoid. Severe Theoretical

St John's wort is predicted to decrease the exposure to **brivaracetam**. Moderate Theoretical

St John's wort is predicted to decrease the concentration of **carbamazepine**. Monitor and adjust dose. Moderate Theoretical

St John's wort is predicted to decrease the exposure to **perampanel**. Monitor and adjust dose. Moderate Theoretical

St John's wort is predicted to decrease the exposure to **tiagabine**. Avoid. Mild Theoretical

► Antiepileptics **(carbamazepine, eslicarbazepine)** are predicted to decrease the exposure to statins (atorvastatin). Monitor and adjust dose. Moderate Theoretical → Also see **TABLE 1** p. 1429

► Antiepileptics **(fosphenytoin, phenytoin)** potentially decrease the exposure to statins (atorvastatin, simvastatin). Moderate Anecdotal

► **Carbamazepine** moderately decreases the exposure to statins (simvastatin). Monitor and adjust dose. Severe Study → Also see **TABLE 1** p. 1429

► **Eslicarbazepine** moderately decreases the exposure to statins (simvastatin). Monitor and adjust dose. Moderate Study

► Sulfonamides (sulfadiazine) are predicted to increase the concentration of **fosphenytoin**. Monitor and adjust dose. Moderate Study

► Sulfonamides (sulfadiazine) increase the concentration of **phenytoin**. Monitor and adjust dose. Moderate Study

► Antiepileptics **(carbamazepine, fosphenytoin, phenobarbital, phenytoin, primidone)** are predicted to decrease the exposure to sunitinib. Avoid or adjust **sunitinib** dose, p. 1044. Moderate Study

► Antiepileptics **(fosphenytoin, phenytoin)** increase the effects of **suxamethonium**. Moderate Study

► **Carbamazepine** increases the risk of prolonged neuromuscular blockade when given with suxamethonium. Moderate Study

► Antiepileptics **(carbamazepine, fosphenytoin, phenobarbital, phenytoin, primidone)** decrease the concentration of **tacrolimus**. Monitor and adjust dose. Severe Study

► Antiepileptics **(carbamazepine, fosphenytoin, phenobarbital, phenytoin, primidone)** are predicted to decrease the exposure to taxanes (cabazitaxel, paclitaxel). Avoid. Severe Study → Also see **TABLE 12** p. 1432

► Antiepileptics **(carbamazepine, fosphenytoin, phenobarbital, phenytoin, primidone)** are predicted to decrease the exposure to taxanes (docetaxel). Severe Theoretical → Also see **TABLE 12** p. 1432

► **Tegafur** potentially increases the concentration of antiepileptics **(fosphenytoin, phenytoin)**. Monitor concentration and adjust dose. Severe Anecdotal

► Antiepileptics **(carbamazepine, fosphenytoin, phenobarbital, phenytoin, primidone)** are predicted to decrease the concentration of **temsirolimus**. Avoid. Severe Study

► Antiepileptics **(carbamazepine, fosphenytoin, oxcarbazepine, phenobarbital, phenytoin, primidone)** are predicted to decrease the exposure to tenofovir alafenamide. Avoid. Moderate Theoretical

► Antiepileptics **(carbamazepine, fosphenytoin, phenobarbital, phenytoin, primidone)** decrease the exposure to tetracyclines (doxycycline). Monitor and adjust dose. Moderate Study → Also see **TABLE 1** p. 1429

► Antiepileptics **(carbamazepine, fosphenytoin, phenobarbital, phenytoin, primidone)** are predicted to decrease the exposure to **tezacaftor**. Avoid. Severe Theoretical

► Antiepileptics **(fosphenytoin, phenytoin)** are predicted to decrease the exposure to theophylline. Adjust dose. Moderate Study

► Antiepileptics **(phenobarbital, primidone)** are predicted to increase the clearance of theophylline. Adjust dose. Moderate Theoretical

► **Carbamazepine** potentially increases the clearance of theophylline and theophylline decreases the exposure to **carbamazepine**. Adjust dose. Moderate Anecdotal

► **Stiripentol** is predicted to increase the exposure to theophylline. Avoid. Moderate Theoretical

► **Carbamazepine** is predicted to decrease the exposure to thrombin inhibitors (dabigatran). Avoid. Severe Study

► **Phenytoin** is predicted to decrease the exposure to thrombin inhibitors (dabigatran). Avoid. Severe Theoretical

► Antiepileptics **(fosphenytoin, phenytoin)** are predicted to increase the risk of hypothyroidism when given with thyroid hormones. Moderate Study

► Antiepileptics **(phenobarbital, primidone)** are predicted to decrease the effects of thyroid hormones. Moderate Theoretical

► **Carbamazepine** is predicted to increase the risk of hypothyroidism when given with thyroid hormones. Monitor and adjust dose. Moderate Study

► Antiepileptics **(carbamazepine, fosphenytoin, phenobarbital, phenytoin, primidone)** are predicted to markedly decrease the exposure to ticagrelor. Avoid. Severe Study

► Antiepileptics **(carbamazepine, fosphenytoin, phenobarbital, phenytoin, primidone)** are predicted to decrease the exposure to tivozanib. Severe Study

► Antiepileptics **(fosphenytoin, phenytoin)** moderately decrease the exposure to tizanidine. Mild Study

► Antiepileptics **(carbamazepine, fosphenytoin, phenobarbital, phenytoin, primidone)** are predicted to decrease the exposure to tofacitinib. Avoid. Severe Study

► Antiepileptics **(carbamazepine, fosphenytoin, phenobarbital, phenytoin, primidone)** are predicted to decrease the exposure to tolvaptan. Use with caution or avoid depending on indication. Severe Study

► Antiepileptics **(fosphenytoin, phenytoin)** increase the clearance of topotecan. Moderate Study

► Antiepileptics **(carbamazepine, fosphenytoin, phenobarbital, phenytoin, primidone)** are predicted to decrease the exposure to toremifene. Adjust dose. Moderate Study

► Antiepileptics **(carbamazepine, fosphenytoin, phenobarbital, phenytoin, primidone)** are predicted to decrease the exposure to trabectedin. Avoid. Severe Theoretical → Also see **TABLE 1** p. 1429

► **Carbamazepine** decreases the concentration of trazodone. Adjust dose. Moderate Anecdotal

► Tricyclic antidepressants (clomipramine, imipramine) potentially increase the risk of overheating and dehydration when given with zonisamide. Avoid in children. Severe Theoretical

► Antiepileptics **(phenobarbital, primidone)** are predicted to decrease the exposure to tricyclic antidepressants. Moderate Study → Also see **TABLE 11** p. 1431

► **Carbamazepine** decreases the exposure to tricyclic antidepressants. Adjust dose. Moderate Study → Also see **TABLE 18** p. 1433

► **Valproate** increases the concentration of tricyclic antidepressants (nortriptyline). Severe Study

► **Trimethoprim** increases the concentration of antiepileptics **(fosphenytoin, phenytoin)**. Moderate Study

► Antiepileptics **(carbamazepine, eslicarbazepine, fosphenytoin, oxcarbazepine, perampanel, phenobarbital, phenytoin, primidone, rufinamide, topiramate)** decrease the efficacy of ulipristal. For FSRH guidance, see Contraceptives, interactions p. 840. Severe Anecdotal

► Antiepileptics **(carbamazepine, fosphenytoin, phenobarbital, phenytoin, primidone)** are predicted to decrease the exposure to upadacitinib. Moderate Study

► Antiepileptics **(carbamazepine, fosphenytoin, phenobarbital, phenytoin, primidone)** are predicted to decrease the exposure to vandetanib. Moderate Study

► Antiepileptics **(carbamazepine, fosphenytoin, phenobarbital, phenytoin, primidone)** are predicted to moderately decrease the exposure to velpatasvir. Avoid. Severe Study

► **Oxcarbazepine** is predicted to decrease the exposure to velpatasvir. Avoid. Severe Theoretical

A1

Interactions | **Appendix 1**

Antiepileptics (continued)

▸ Antiepileptics **(carbamazepine, fosphenytoin, phenobarbital, phenytoin, primidone)** are predicted to decrease the exposure to vemurafenib. Avoid. Severe Theoretical

▸ Antiepileptics **(carbamazepine, fosphenytoin, phenobarbital, phenytoin, primidone)** are predicted to decrease the exposure to venetoclax. Avoid. Severe Study

▸ Antiepileptics **(carbamazepine, fosphenytoin, phenobarbital, phenytoin, primidone)** are predicted to decrease the exposure to vinca alkaloids (vinblastine, vincristine, vindesine). Severe Theoretical → Also see TABLE 1 p. 1429 → Also see TABLE 12 p. 1432

▸ Antiepileptics **(carbamazepine, fosphenytoin, phenobarbital, phenytoin, primidone)** are predicted to decrease the exposure to vinca alkaloids (vinflunine). Avoid. Severe Theoretical → Also see TABLE 12 p. 1432

▸ Antiepileptics **(carbamazepine, fosphenytoin, phenobarbital, phenytoin, primidone)** are predicted to decrease the exposure to vinca alkaloids (vinorelbine). Use with caution or avoid. Severe Theoretical → Also see TABLE 12 p. 1432

▸ Antiepileptics **(carbamazepine, fosphenytoin, phenobarbital, phenytoin, primidone)** are predicted to decrease the exposure to vismodegib. Avoid. Moderate Theoretical

▸ Antiepileptics **(fosphenytoin, phenytoin)** decrease the effects of vitamin D substances. Moderate Study

▸ Antiepileptics **(phenobarbital, primidone)** are predicted to decrease the effects of vitamin D substances. Moderate Theoretical

▸ **Carbamazepine** is predicted to decrease the effects of vitamin D substances. Moderate Study

▸ Antiepileptics **(phenobarbital, primidone)** potentially increase the risk of nephrotoxicity when given with volatile halogenated anaesthetics (methoxyflurane). Avoid. Severe Theoretical → Also see TABLE 11 p. 1431

▸ Antiepileptics **(carbamazepine, fosphenytoin, phenobarbital, phenytoin, primidone)** are predicted to decrease the exposure to vortioxetine. Monitor and adjust dose. Moderate Study

▸ Antiepileptics **(carbamazepine, fosphenytoin, phenobarbital, phenytoin, primidone)** are predicted to decrease the concentration of voxilaprevir. Avoid. Severe Study

▸ **Oxcarbazepine** is predicted to decrease the concentration of voxilaprevir. Avoid. Severe Theoretical

▸ **Carbamazepine** moderately decreases the exposure to zolpidem. Moderate Study

▸ Antiepileptics **(carbamazepine, fosphenytoin, phenobarbital, phenytoin, primidone)** are predicted to decrease the exposure to zopiclone. Adjust dose. Moderate Study → Also see TABLE 11 p. 1431

Antifungals, azoles → see TABLE 1 p. 1429 (hepatotoxicity), TABLE 9 p. 1431 (QT-interval prolongation)

clotrimazole · fluconazole · isavuconazole · itraconazole · ketoconazole · miconazole · posaconazole · voriconazole

▸ Since systemic absorption can follow topical application, the possibility of interactions with topical **clotrimazole** and **ketoconazole** should be borne in mind.

▸ In general, **fluconazole** interactions relate to multiple-dose treatment.

▸ The use of carbonated drinks, such as cola, improves **itraconazole, ketoconazole,** and **posaconazole** bioavailability.

▸ Interactions of **miconazole** apply to the oral gel formulation, as a sufficient quantity can be absorbed to cause systemic effects. Systemic absorption from intravaginal and topical formulations might also occur.

▸ Antifungals, azoles **(fluconazole, isavuconazole, posaconazole)** are predicted to increase the exposure to abemaciclib. Moderate Study

▸ Antifungals, azoles **(itraconazole, ketoconazole, voriconazole)** are predicted to increase the exposure to abemaciclib. Avoid or adjust **abemaciclib** dose, p. 1009. Severe Study

▸ Antifungals, azoles **(fluconazole, isavuconazole, posaconazole)** are predicted to increase the exposure to acalabrutinib. Avoid or monitor. Severe Study

▸ Antifungals, azoles **(itraconazole, ketoconazole, voriconazole)** are predicted to increase the exposure to acalabrutinib. Avoid. Severe Study

▸ Antifungals, azoles **(itraconazole, ketoconazole)** are predicted to increase the exposure to afatinib. Separate administration by 12 hours. Moderate Study

▸ Alcohol potentially causes a disulfiram-like reaction when given with **ketoconazole**. Avoid. Moderate Anecdotal

▸ Antifungals, azoles **(fluconazole, isavuconazole, posaconazole)** are predicted to increase the exposure to aldosterone antagonists (eplerenone). Adjust **eplerenone** dose, p. 208. Severe Study

▸ Antifungals, azoles **(itraconazole, ketoconazole, voriconazole)** are predicted to markedly increase the exposure to aldosterone antagonists (eplerenone). Avoid. Severe Study

▸ **Itraconazole** markedly increases the exposure to aliskiren. Avoid. Severe Study

▸ **Ketoconazole** moderately increases the exposure to aliskiren. Moderate Study

▸ **Itraconazole** increases the risk of busulfan toxicity when given with alkylating agents (busulfan). Monitor and adjust dose. Moderate Study

▸ **Miconazole** is predicted to increase the concentration of alkylating agents (busulfan). Use with caution and adjust dose. Moderate Theoretical

▸ **Isavuconazole** is predicted to increase the exposure to alkylating agents (cyclophosphamide). Moderate Study

▸ Antifungals, azoles **(itraconazole, ketoconazole, voriconazole)** are predicted to moderately increase the exposure to alpha blockers (alfuzosin, tamsulosin). Use with caution or avoid. Moderate Study

▸ Antifungals, azoles **(itraconazole, ketoconazole, voriconazole)** are predicted to increase the exposure to alpha blockers (doxazosin). Moderate Study

▸ Antifungals, azoles **(fluconazole, isavuconazole, posaconazole)** are predicted to increase the exposure to alpha blockers (tamsulosin). Moderate Theoretical

▸ **Miconazole** potentially decreases the exposure to aminoglycosides (tobramycin). Moderate Anecdotal

▸ Oral antacids decrease the absorption of oral **itraconazole** capsules. Itraconazole should be taken 2 hours before or 1 hour after antacids. Moderate Study

▸ Oral antacids decrease the absorption of oral **ketoconazole**. Separate administration by at least 2 hours. Moderate Study

▸ Anti-androgens (apalutamide, enzalutamide) are predicted to decrease the exposure to isavuconazole. Avoid. Severe Study

▸ Antifungals, azoles **(itraconazole, ketoconazole, voriconazole)** are predicted to increase the exposure to anti-androgens (apalutamide). Mild Study → Also see TABLE 9 p. 1431

▸ **Itraconazole** slightly increases the exposure to anti-androgens (darolutamide). Monitor and adjust dose. Moderate Study

▸ **Ketoconazole** is predicted to increase the exposure to anti-androgens (darolutamide). Monitor and adjust dose. Moderate Theoretical

▸ **Miconazole** is predicted to increase the exposure to antiarrhythmics (disopyramide). Use with caution and adjust dose. Severe Theoretical

▸ Antifungals, azoles **(itraconazole, ketoconazole, voriconazole)** are predicted to increase the exposure to antiarrhythmics (disopyramide). Avoid. Severe Theoretical → Also see TABLE 9 p. 1431

▸ **Posaconazole** is predicted to increase the exposure to antiarrhythmics (disopyramide, dronedarone). Avoid. Severe Theoretical

▸ **Fluconazole** is predicted to increase the exposure to antiarrhythmics (dronedarone). Severe Theoretical → Also see TABLE 9 p. 1431

▸ Antifungals, azoles **(itraconazole, ketoconazole, voriconazole)** very markedly increase the exposure to antiarrhythmics (dronedarone). Avoid. Severe Study → Also see TABLE 9 p. 1431

▸ Antifungals, azoles **(fluconazole, isavuconazole, posaconazole)** are predicted to increase the exposure to antiarrhythmics (propafenone). Monitor and adjust dose. Moderate Study

▸ Antifungals, azoles **(itraconazole, ketoconazole, voriconazole)** are predicted to increase the exposure to antiarrhythmics (propafenone). Monitor and adjust dose. [Severe] Study

▸ Antifungals, azoles **(itraconazole, ketoconazole, voriconazole)** are predicted to increase the exposure to anticholinesterases, centrally acting (galantamine). Monitor and adjust dose. [Moderate] Study

▸ Antiepileptics (carbamazepine) are predicted to decrease the efficacy of **fluconazole** and **fluconazole** increases the concentration of antiepileptics (carbamazepine). Avoid or monitor **carbamazepine** concentration and adjust dose accordingly, p. 327. [Severe] Theoretical → Also see TABLE 1 p. 1429

▸ Antiepileptics (carbamazepine) are predicted to decrease the efficacy of **ketoconazole** and **ketoconazole** slightly increases the concentration of antiepileptics (carbamazepine). Avoid or monitor **carbamazepine** concentration and adjust dose accordingly, p. 327. [Moderate] Study

▸ Antiepileptics (carbamazepine) are predicted to decrease the efficacy of **posaconazole** and **posaconazole** increases the concentration of antiepileptics (carbamazepine). Avoid. [Moderate] Theoretical

▸ Antiepileptics (carbamazepine, fosphenytoin, phenobarbital, phenytoin, primidone) are predicted to decrease the exposure to **isavuconazole**. Avoid. [Severe] Study

▸ Antiepileptics (fosphenytoin) very markedly decrease the exposure to **itraconazole**. Avoid and for 14 days after stopping **fosphenytoin**. [Moderate] Study

▸ Antiepileptics (fosphenytoin) decrease the exposure to **voriconazole** and **voriconazole** increases the exposure to antiepileptics (fosphenytoin). Avoid or adjust **voriconazole** dose and monitor phenytoin concentration, p. 638. [Moderate] Study

▸ Antiepileptics (fosphenytoin, phenytoin) decrease the exposure to **ketoconazole**. Avoid. [Moderate] Study

▸ Antiepileptics (fosphenytoin, phenytoin) are predicted to decrease the exposure to **posaconazole**. Avoid. [Moderate] Study

▸ Antiepileptics (phenobarbital) decrease the concentration of **itraconazole**. Avoid and for 14 days after stopping **phenobarbital**. [Moderate] Study

▸ Antiepileptics (phenobarbital) are predicted to decrease the concentration of **ketoconazole**. Avoid. [Moderate] Study

▸ Antiepileptics (phenobarbital) are predicted to decrease the concentration of **posaconazole**. Avoid. [Moderate] Study

▸ Antiepileptics (phenobarbital, primidone) are predicted to decrease the concentration of **voriconazole**. Avoid. [Moderate] Theoretical

▸ Antiepileptics (phenytoin) very markedly decrease the exposure to **itraconazole**. Avoid and for 14 days after stopping **phenytoin**. [Moderate] Study

▸ Antiepileptics (phenytoin) decrease the exposure to **voriconazole** and **voriconazole** increases the exposure to antiepileptics (phenytoin). Avoid or adjust **voriconazole** dose and monitor **phenytoin** concentration, p. 638, p. 340. [Moderate] Study

▸ Antiepileptics (primidone) are predicted to decrease the concentration of **itraconazole**. [Moderate] Theoretical

▸ **Miconazole** increases the concentration of antiepileptics (carbamazepine). Monitor and adjust dose. [Severe] Anecdotal

▸ **Miconazole** increases the risk of phenytoin toxicity when given with antiepileptics (fosphenytoin). Monitor and adjust dose. [Severe] Anecdotal

▸ **Fluconazole** increases the concentration of antiepileptics (fosphenytoin, phenytoin). Monitor concentration and adjust dose. [Moderate] Study

▸ Antiepileptics (carbamazepine) are predicted to decrease the efficacy of antifungals, azoles **(itraconazole, voriconazole)** and antifungals, azoles **(itraconazole, voriconazole)** increase the concentration of antiepileptics (carbamazepine). Avoid or adjust dose. [Moderate] Theoretical → Also see TABLE 1 p. 1429

▸ Antiepileptics (primidone) are predicted to decrease the concentration of antifungals, azoles **(ketoconazole, posaconazole)**. Avoid. [Moderate] Study

▸ Antifungals, azoles **(itraconazole, ketoconazole, voriconazole)** are predicted to very slightly increase the exposure to antiepileptics (perampanel). [Mild] Study

▸ **Miconazole** increases the risk of phenytoin toxicity when given with antiepileptics (phenytoin). Monitor and adjust dose. [Severe] Anecdotal

▸ Antifungals, azoles **(fluconazole)** are predicted to increase the exposure to antifungals, azoles **(isavuconazole)**. [Severe] Theoretical

▸ Antifungals, azoles **(itraconazole, ketoconazole, voriconazole)** are predicted to increase the exposure to antifungals, azoles **(isavuconazole)**. Avoid or monitor adverse effects. [Severe] Study

▸ Antifungals, azoles **(posaconazole)** are predicted to increase the exposure to antifungals, azoles **(isavuconazole)**. [Moderate] Theoretical

▸ **Miconazole** is predicted to increase the exposure to antihistamines, non-sedating (mizolastine). Avoid. [Moderate] Theoretical

▸ Antifungals, azoles **(fluconazole, isavuconazole, posaconazole)** are predicted to increase the exposure to antihistamines, non-sedating (mizolastine). [Severe] Theoretical

▸ Antifungals, azoles **(itraconazole, ketoconazole, voriconazole)** are predicted to increase the exposure to antihistamines, non-sedating (mizolastine). Avoid. [Severe] Study

▸ Antifungals, azoles **(fluconazole, isavuconazole, itraconazole, ketoconazole, posaconazole, voriconazole)** are predicted to increase the exposure to antihistamines, non-sedating (rupatadine). Avoid. [Moderate] Study

▸ **Ketoconazole** increases the exposure to antimalarials (mefloquine). [Moderate] Study

▸ Antifungals, azoles **(fluconazole, itraconazole, posaconazole, voriconazole)** are predicted to increase the exposure to antimalarials (mefloquine). [Moderate] Theoretical

▸ Antifungals, azoles **(fluconazole, isavuconazole, itraconazole, ketoconazole, posaconazole, voriconazole)** are predicted to increase the concentration of antimalarials (piperaquine). [Severe] Theoretical

▸ Antifungals, azoles **(itraconazole, ketoconazole, voriconazole)** are predicted to slightly increase the exposure to antipsychotics, second generation (aripiprazole). Adjust **aripiprazole** dose, p. 415. [Moderate] Study

▸ Antifungals, azoles **(fluconazole, isavuconazole, posaconazole)** are predicted to increase the exposure to antipsychotics, second generation (cariprazine). Avoid. [Severe] Study

▸ Antifungals, azoles **(itraconazole, ketoconazole, voriconazole)** are predicted to moderately increase the exposure to antipsychotics, second generation (cariprazine). Avoid. [Severe] Study

▸ **Posaconazole** moderately increases the exposure to antipsychotics, second generation (lurasidone). Avoid. [Severe] Study

▸ Antifungals, azoles **(fluconazole, isavuconazole)** are predicted to increase the exposure to antipsychotics, second generation (lurasidone). Adjust **lurasidone** dose. [Moderate] Study

▸ Antifungals, azoles **(itraconazole, ketoconazole, voriconazole)** are predicted to increase the exposure to antipsychotics, second generation (lurasidone, quetiapine). Avoid. [Severe] Study

▸ Antifungals, azoles **(fluconazole, isavuconazole, posaconazole)** are predicted to increase the exposure to antipsychotics, second generation (quetiapine). Avoid. [Moderate] Study

▸ Antifungals, azoles **(fluconazole, isavuconazole, posaconazole)** are predicted to increase the exposure to antipsychotics, second generation (risperidone). Adjust dose. [Moderate] Study → Also see TABLE 9 p. 1431

▸ Antifungals, azoles **(fluconazole, isavuconazole, posaconazole)** are predicted to increase the exposure to avapritinib. Avoid or adjust **avapritinib** dose, p. 1012. [Moderate] Study

▸ Antifungals, azoles **(itraconazole, ketoconazole, voriconazole)** are predicted to increase the exposure to avapritinib. Avoid. [Moderate] Study

▸ Antifungals, azoles **(fluconazole, isavuconazole, posaconazole)** are predicted to increase the exposure to axitinib. [Moderate] Theoretical

▸ Antifungals, azoles **(itraconazole, ketoconazole, voriconazole)** are predicted to increase the exposure to axitinib. Avoid or adjust dose. [Moderate] Study

▸ Antifungals, azoles **(fluconazole, isavuconazole, posaconazole)** are predicted to increase the exposure to bedaquiline. Avoid prolonged use. [Mild] Theoretical → Also see TABLE 1 p. 1429 → Also see TABLE 9 p. 1431

A1

Interactions | Appendix 1

Antifungals, azoles (continued)

▶ Antifungals, azoles **(itraconazole, ketoconazole, voriconazole)** are predicted to increase the exposure to bedaquiline. Avoid prolonged use. [Mild] Study → Also see **TABLE 1** p. 1429 → Also see **TABLE 9** p. 1431

▶ **Miconazole** is predicted to increase the exposure to benzodiazepines **(alprazolam)**. Use with caution and adjust dose. [Moderate] Theoretical

▶ Antifungals, azoles **(fluconazole, isavuconazole, posaconazole)** are predicted to increase the exposure to benzodiazepines **(alprazolam)**. [Severe] Study

▶ Antifungals, azoles **(itraconazole, ketoconazole, voriconazole)** moderately increase the exposure to benzodiazepines **(alprazolam)**. Avoid. [Moderate] Study

▶ Antifungals, azoles **(fluconazole, voriconazole)** potentially increase the exposure to benzodiazepines **(clobazam)**. Adjust dose. [Moderate] Theoretical

▶ Antifungals, azoles **(fluconazole, voriconazole)** moderately increase the exposure to benzodiazepines **(diazepam)**. Monitor and adjust dose. [Moderate] Study

▶ **Miconazole** is predicted to increase the exposure to intravenous benzodiazepines **(midazolam)**. Use with caution and adjust dose. [Moderate] Theoretical

▶ **Miconazole** is predicted to increase the exposure to oral benzodiazepines **(midazolam)**. Avoid. [Moderate] Theoretical

▶ Antifungals, azoles **(fluconazole, isavuconazole, posaconazole)** are predicted to increase the exposure to benzodiazepines **(midazolam)**. Monitor adverse effects and adjust dose. [Severe] Study

▶ Antifungals, azoles **(itraconazole, ketoconazole, voriconazole)** are predicted to markedly to very markedly increase the exposure to benzodiazepines **(midazolam)**. Avoid or adjust dose. [Severe] Study

▶ Antifungals, azoles **(itraconazole, ketoconazole)** are predicted to increase the exposure to beta blockers, non-selective **(nadolol)**. [Moderate] Study

▶ Antifungals, azoles **(itraconazole, ketoconazole, voriconazole)** are predicted to increase the exposure to beta$_2$ agonists **(salmeterol)**. Avoid. [Severe] Study

▶ Antifungals, azoles **(itraconazole, ketoconazole)** are predicted to increase the exposure to bictegravir. Use with caution or avoid. [Moderate] Theoretical

▶ **Posaconazole** is predicted to increase the exposure to bictegravir. [Moderate] Theoretical

▶ Antifungals, azoles **(itraconazole, ketoconazole, voriconazole)** slightly increase the exposure to bortezomib. [Moderate] Study

▶ Antifungals, azoles **(fluconazole, isavuconazole, posaconazole)** are predicted to increase the exposure to bosutinib. Avoid or adjust dose. [Severe] Theoretical → Also see **TABLE 9** p. 1431

▶ Antifungals, azoles **(itraconazole, ketoconazole, voriconazole)** are predicted to markedly increase the exposure to bosutinib. Avoid or adjust dose. [Severe] Study → Also see **TABLE 9** p. 1431

▶ Antifungals, azoles **(itraconazole, ketoconazole, voriconazole)** are predicted to increase the exposure to brigatinib. Adjust **brigatinib** dose, p. 1015. [Severe] Study

▶ **Isavuconazole** slightly increases the exposure to bupropion. Adjust dose. [Moderate] Study

▶ Antifungals, azoles **(fluconazole, isavuconazole, posaconazole)** are predicted to increase the exposure to buspirone. Use with caution and adjust dose. [Moderate] Study

▶ Antifungals, azoles **(itraconazole, ketoconazole, voriconazole)** are predicted to increase the exposure to buspirone. Adjust **buspirone** dose, p. 360. [Severe] Study

▶ **Miconazole** is predicted to increase the concentration of buspirone. Use with caution and adjust dose. [Moderate] Theoretical

▶ Antifungals, azoles **(fluconazole, isavuconazole, posaconazole)** are predicted to increase the exposure to cabozantinib. [Moderate] Theoretical → Also see **TABLE 9** p. 1431

▶ Antifungals, azoles **(itraconazole, ketoconazole, voriconazole)** slightly increase the exposure to cabozantinib. [Moderate] Study → Also see **TABLE 9** p. 1431

▶ Calcium channel blockers **(diltiazem, verapamil)** are predicted to increase the exposure to isavuconazole. [Moderate] Theoretical

▶ Antifungals, azoles **(fluconazole, isavuconazole, posaconazole)** are predicted to increase the exposure to calcium channel blockers **(amlodipine, felodipine, lacidipine, lercanidipine, nicardipine, nifedipine, nimodipine)**. Monitor and adjust dose. [Moderate] Study

▶ **Miconazole** is predicted to increase the exposure to calcium channel blockers **(amlodipine, felodipine, lacidipine, lercanidipine, nicardipine, nifedipine, nimodipine, verapamil)**. Use with caution and adjust dose. [Moderate] Theoretical

▶ Antifungals, azoles **(itraconazole, ketoconazole, voriconazole)** are predicted to increase the exposure to calcium channel blockers **(amlodipine, felodipine, lacidipine, nicardipine, nifedipine, nimodipine)**. Monitor and adjust dose. [Moderate] Study

▶ **Miconazole** is predicted to increase the exposure to calcium channel blockers **(diltiazem)**. [Moderate] Theoretical

▶ **Fluconazole** (high-dose) is predicted to increase the exposure to calcium channel blockers **(diltiazem, verapamil)**. [Moderate] Theoretical

▶ **Posaconazole** is predicted to increase the exposure to calcium channel blockers **(diltiazem, verapamil)**. [Moderate] Theoretical

▶ Antifungals, azoles **(itraconazole, ketoconazole, voriconazole)** are predicted to increase the exposure to calcium channel blockers **(diltiazem, verapamil)**. [Severe] Study

▶ Antifungals, azoles **(itraconazole, ketoconazole, voriconazole)** are predicted to markedly increase the exposure to calcium channel blockers **(lercanidipine)**. Avoid. [Severe] Study

▶ Antifungals, azoles **(itraconazole, ketoconazole, voriconazole)** are predicted to increase the exposure to cannabidiol. Avoid or adjust dose. [Mild] Study

▶ **Fluconazole** is predicted to increase the exposure to cannabidiol. [Moderate] Theoretical

▶ Antifungals, azoles **(itraconazole, ketoconazole, voriconazole)** are predicted to increase the exposure to ceritinib. Avoid or adjust **ceritinib** dose, p. 1017. [Severe] Study → Also see **TABLE 9** p. 1431

▶ Antifungals, azoles **(fluconazole, isavuconazole, posaconazole)** are predicted to increase the concentration of ciclosporin. [Severe] Study

▶ Antifungals, azoles **(itraconazole, ketoconazole, voriconazole)** increase the concentration of ciclosporin. [Severe] Study

▶ **Miconazole** increases the concentration of ciclosporin. Monitor and adjust dose. [Severe] Anecdotal

▶ Antifungals, azoles **(itraconazole, ketoconazole, voriconazole)** are predicted to moderately increase the exposure to cilostazol. Adjust **cilostazol** dose, p. 248. [Moderate] Study

▶ **Fluconazole** is predicted to increase the exposure to cilostazol. Adjust **cilostazol** dose, p. 248. [Moderate] Theoretical

▶ **Miconazole** is predicted to increase the exposure to cilostazol. Use with caution and adjust dose. [Moderate] Theoretical

▶ Antifungals, azoles **(itraconazole, ketoconazole, voriconazole)** are predicted to moderately increase the exposure to cinacalcet. Adjust dose. [Moderate] Study

▶ **Fluconazole** is predicted to decrease the efficacy of clopidogrel. Avoid. [Severe] Theoretical

▶ **Voriconazole** is predicted to decrease the efficacy of clopidogrel. Avoid. [Moderate] Study

▶ **Cobicistat** is predicted to increase the exposure to antifungals, azoles **(fluconazole, posaconazole)**. [Moderate] Theoretical

▶ **Cobicistat** is predicted to increase the exposure to antifungals, azoles **(itraconazole, ketoconazole)**. Adjust dose. [Moderate] Theoretical

▶ **Cobicistat** is predicted to increase the exposure to isavuconazole. Avoid or monitor adverse effects. [Severe] Study

▶ **Cobicistat** is predicted to affect the exposure to **voriconazole**. Avoid. [Moderate] Theoretical

▶ Antifungals, azoles **(fluconazole, isavuconazole, miconazole, posaconazole)** are predicted to increase the exposure to cobimetinib. [Severe] Theoretical

▶ Antifungals, azoles **(itraconazole, ketoconazole, voriconazole)** are predicted to markedly increase the exposure to cobimetinib. Avoid or monitor for toxicity. [Severe] Study

▶ Antifungals, azoles **(fluconazole, isavuconazole, posaconazole)** are predicted to increase the exposure to colchicine. Adjust **colchicine** dose with moderate CYP3A4 inhibitors, p. 1166. [Severe] Study

Antifungals, azoles (itraconazole, ketoconazole, voriconazole) are predicted to increase the exposure to colchicine. Avoid potent CYP3A4 inhibitors or adjust **colchicine** dose, p. 1166. Severe Study

▸ Antifungals, azoles (itraconazole, ketoconazole, voriconazole) are predicted to increase the exposure to corticosteroids (beclometasone) (risk with beclometasone is likely to be lower than with other corticosteroids). Moderate Theoretical

▸ Antifungals, azoles (itraconazole, ketoconazole, voriconazole) are predicted to increase the exposure to corticosteroids (betamethasone, budesonide, ciclesonide, deflazacort, dexamethasone, fludrocortisone, fluticasone, hydrocortisone, methylprednisolone, mometasone, prednisolone, triamcinolone). Avoid or monitor adverse effects. Severe Study

▸ **Miconazole** is predicted to increase the concentration of corticosteroids (methylprednisolone). Monitor and adjust dose. Moderate Theoretical

▸ Antifungals, azoles (fluconazole, isavuconazole, posaconazole) are predicted to increase the exposure to corticosteroids (methylprednisolone). Monitor and adjust dose. Moderate Study

▸ **Fluconazole** increases the anticoagulant effect of coumarins. Monitor INR and adjust dose. Severe Study

▸ **Itraconazole** potentially increases the anticoagulant effect of coumarins. Severe Anecdotal

▸ **Ketoconazole** potentially increases the anticoagulant effect of coumarins (warfarin). Monitor INR and adjust dose. Severe Anecdotal

▸ **Miconazole** greatly increases the anticoagulant effect of coumarins. MHRA advises avoid unless INR can be monitored closely; monitor for signs of bleeding. Severe Study

▸ **Voriconazole** increases the anticoagulant effect of coumarins. Monitor INR and adjust dose. Moderate Study

▸ Antifungals, azoles (itraconazole, ketoconazole, voriconazole) are predicted to moderately increase the exposure to crizotinib. Avoid. Moderate Study → Also see TABLE 9 p. 1431

▸ Antifungals, azoles (itraconazole, ketoconazole, voriconazole) are predicted to increase the exposure to dabrafenib. Use with caution or avoid. Moderate Study

▸ Antifungals, azoles (fluconazole, isavuconazole, posaconazole) are predicted to slightly increase the exposure to darifenacin. Moderate Study

▸ Antifungals, azoles (itraconazole, ketoconazole, voriconazole) are predicted to markedly to very markedly increase the exposure to darifenacin. Avoid. Severe Study

▸ Antifungals, azoles (fluconazole, isavuconazole, posaconazole) are predicted to increase the exposure to dasatinib. Severe Study → Also see TABLE 9 p. 1431

▸ Antifungals, azoles (itraconazole, ketoconazole, voriconazole) are predicted to markedly increase the exposure to dasatinib. Avoid or adjust dose—consult product literature. Severe Study → Also see TABLE 9 p. 1431

▸ Antifungals, azoles (itraconazole, ketoconazole, voriconazole) very slightly increase the exposure to delamanid. Severe Study → Also see TABLE 9 p. 1431

▸ Antifungals, azoles (fluconazole, isavuconazole, posaconazole) are predicted to slightly increase the exposure to dienogest. Moderate Study

▸ Antifungals, azoles (itraconazole, ketoconazole, voriconazole) are predicted to moderately increase the exposure to dienogest. Moderate Study

▸ **Isavuconazole** slightly increases the exposure to digoxin. Monitor and adjust dose. Moderate Study

▸ **Itraconazole** is predicted to markedly increase the concentration of digoxin. Monitor and adjust dose. Severe Study

▸ **Ketoconazole** is predicted to markedly increase the concentration of digoxin. Severe Study

▸ **Posaconazole** is predicted to increase the concentration of digoxin. Severe Study

▸ Antifungals, azoles (fluconazole, isavuconazole, posaconazole) are predicted to increase the exposure to dipeptidylpeptidase-4 inhibitors (saxagliptin). Mild Study

▸ Antifungals, azoles (itraconazole, ketoconazole, voriconazole) are predicted to increase the exposure to dipeptidylpeptidase-4 inhibitors (saxagliptin). Moderate Study

▸ Antifungals, azoles (fluconazole, isavuconazole, itraconazole, ketoconazole, posaconazole, voriconazole) increase the risk of QT-prolongation when given with domperidone. Avoid. Severe Study

▸ Antifungals, azoles (fluconazole, isavuconazole, posaconazole) are predicted to increase the exposure to dopamine receptor agonists (bromocriptine). Severe Theoretical

▸ Antifungals, azoles (itraconazole, ketoconazole, voriconazole) increase the exposure to dopamine receptor agonists (bromocriptine). Severe Study

▸ Antifungals, azoles (fluconazole, isavuconazole, itraconazole, ketoconazole, posaconazole, voriconazole) are predicted to increase the concentration of dopamine receptor agonists (cabergoline). Moderate Anecdotal

▸ **Isavuconazole** is predicted to increase the exposure to dopamine receptor agonists (pramipexole). Adjust dose. Moderate Study

▸ Antifungals, azoles (itraconazole, ketoconazole, voriconazole) are predicted to increase the exposure to dronabinol. Adjust dose. Mild Study

▸ **Ketoconazole** moderately increases the exposure to drospirenone. Severe Study

▸ Antifungals, azoles (fluconazole, isavuconazole, posaconazole) are predicted to moderately increase the exposure to dutasteride. Mild Study

▸ Antifungals, azoles (itraconazole, ketoconazole, voriconazole) are predicted to increase the exposure to dutasteride. Monitor adverse effects and adjust dose. Moderate Theoretical

▸ Antifungals, azoles (fluconazole, isavuconazole, posaconazole) is predicted to increase the exposure to elexacaftor. Adjust tezacaftor with ivacaftor and elexacftor p. 311 dose with moderate CYP3A4 inhibitors. Severe Theoretical

▸ Antifungals, azoles (itraconazole, ketoconazole, voriconazole) is predicted to increase the exposure to elexacaftor. Adjust tezacaftor with ivacaftor and elexacftor p. 311 dose with potent CYP3A4 inhibitors. Severe Study

▸ Antifungals, azoles (fluconazole, isavuconazole, itraconazole, ketoconazole, posaconazole, voriconazole) are predicted to increase the exposure to eliglustat. Avoid or adjust dose—consult product literature. Severe Study

▸ Antifungals, azoles (fluconazole, isavuconazole, posaconazole) are predicted to moderately increase the exposure to encorafenib. Moderate Study → Also see TABLE 9 p. 1431

▸ Antifungals, azoles (itraconazole, ketoconazole, voriconazole) are predicted to increase the exposure to encorafenib. Avoid or monitor. Severe Study → Also see TABLE 9 p. 1431

▸ Endothelin receptor antagonists (bosentan) are predicted to decrease the exposure to isavuconazole. Avoid. Severe Theoretical

▸ **Fluconazole** is predicted to increase the exposure to endothelin receptor antagonists (bosentan). Avoid. Severe Study

▸ **Itraconazole** is predicted to increase the exposure to endothelin receptor antagonists (bosentan). Moderate Theoretical

▸ **Ketoconazole** moderately increases the exposure to endothelin receptor antagonists (bosentan). Moderate Study

▸ **Voriconazole** is predicted to increase the exposure to endothelin receptor antagonists (bosentan). Avoid. Severe Theoretical

▸ Antifungals, azoles (itraconazole, ketoconazole, voriconazole) are predicted to increase the exposure to endothelin receptor antagonists (macitentan). Moderate Study

▸ Antifungals, azoles (fluconazole, isavuconazole, posaconazole) are predicted to increase the exposure to entrectinib. Avoid moderate CYP3A4 inhibitors or adjust **entrectinib** dose, p. 1023. Severe Theoretical → Also see TABLE 9 p. 1431

▸ Antifungals, azoles (itraconazole, ketoconazole, voriconazole) are predicted to increase the exposure to entrectinib. Avoid potent CYP3A4 inhibitors or adjust **entrectinib** dose, p. 1023. Severe Study → Also see TABLE 9 p. 1431

▸ Antifungals, azoles (fluconazole, isavuconazole, posaconazole) are predicted to increase the risk of ergotism when given with ergometrine. Severe Theoretical

Antifungals, azoles (continued)

▶ Antifungals, azoles **(itraconazole, ketoconazole, voriconazole)** are predicted to increase the risk of ergotism when given with ergometrine. Avoid. [Severe] Theoretical

▶ **Miconazole** is predicted to increase the exposure to ergometrine. Avoid. [Moderate] Theoretical

▶ Antifungals, azoles **(fluconazole, isavuconazole, posaconazole)** are predicted to increase the risk of ergotism when given with ergotamine. [Severe] Theoretical

▶ Antifungals, azoles **(itraconazole, ketoconazole, voriconazole)** are predicted to increase the risk of ergotism when given with ergotamine. Avoid. [Severe] Theoretical

▶ **Miconazole** is predicted to increase the exposure to ergotamine. Avoid. [Moderate] Theoretical

▶ Antifungals, azoles **(fluconazole, isavuconazole, posaconazole)** are predicted to increase the exposure to erlotinib. [Moderate] Theoretical

▶ Antifungals, azoles **(itraconazole, ketoconazole, voriconazole)** are predicted to slightly increase the exposure to erlotinib. Use with caution and adjust dose. [Moderate] Study

▶ Antifungals, azoles **(itraconazole, ketoconazole, voriconazole)** are predicted to increase the exposure to esketamine. Adjust dose. [Moderate] Study

▶ Antifungals, azoles **(fluconazole, isavuconazole, posaconazole)** are predicted to increase the concentration of everolimus. Avoid or adjust dose. [Moderate] Study

▶ Antifungals, azoles **(itraconazole, ketoconazole, voriconazole)** are predicted to increase the concentration of everolimus. Avoid. [Severe] Study

▶ **Itraconazole** is predicted to increase the exposure to factor XA inhibitors **(apixaban)**. Avoid. [Severe] Theoretical

▶ **Ketoconazole** slightly to moderately increases the exposure to factor XA inhibitors **(apixaban)**. Avoid. [Severe] Study

▶ **Voriconazole** is predicted to increase the exposure to factor XA inhibitors **(apixaban)**. Avoid. [Moderate] Theoretical

▶ **Itraconazole** is predicted to slightly increase the exposure to factor XA inhibitors **(edoxaban)**. [Severe] Theoretical

▶ **Ketoconazole** slightly increases the exposure to factor XA inhibitors **(edoxaban)**. Adjust **edoxaban** dose, p. 137. [Severe] Study

▶ Antifungals, azoles **(itraconazole, ketoconazole)** are predicted to moderately increase the exposure to factor XA inhibitors **(rivaroxaban)**. Avoid. [Severe] Study

▶ Antifungals, azoles **(fluconazole, isavuconazole, posaconazole)** are predicted to increase the exposure to fesoterodine. Adjust **fesoterodine** dose with moderate CYP3A4 inhibitors in hepatic and renal impairment, p. 822. [Mild] Study

▶ Antifungals, azoles **(itraconazole, ketoconazole, voriconazole)** are predicted to moderately increase the exposure to fesoterodine. Adjust **fesoterodine** dose with potent CYP3A4 inhibitors; avoid in hepatic and renal impairment, p. 822. [Severe] Study

▶ Antifungals, azoles **(itraconazole, ketoconazole)** are predicted to increase the exposure to fidaxomicin. Avoid. [Moderate] Study

▶ Antifungals, azoles **(itraconazole, ketoconazole, voriconazole)** are predicted to increase the exposure to fostamatinib. Monitor adverse effects and adjust dose. [Moderate] Study

▶ **Posaconazole** is predicted to increase the exposure to fostamatinib. Monitor adverse effects and adjust dose. [Moderate] Theoretical

▶ Antifungals, azoles **(fluconazole, isavuconazole, posaconazole)** are predicted to increase the exposure to gefitinib. [Moderate] Theoretical

▶ Antifungals, azoles **(itraconazole, ketoconazole, voriconazole)** are predicted to increase the exposure to gefitinib. [Moderate] Study

▶ Antifungals, azoles **(itraconazole, ketoconazole, voriconazole)** are predicted to increase the exposure to gilteritinib. [Moderate] Study

▶ Antifungals, azoles **(itraconazole, ketoconazole, voriconazole)** are predicted to moderately increase the exposure to glasdegib. Use with caution or avoid. [Moderate] Study → Also see **TABLE 9** p. 1431

▶ **Posaconazole** is predicted to increase the exposure to glasdegib. Use with caution or avoid. [Moderate] Theoretical

▶ Antifungals, azoles **(itraconazole, ketoconazole)** potentially increase the exposure to glecaprevir. [Moderate] Theoretical

▶ Antifungals, azoles **(itraconazole, ketoconazole, voriconazole)** are predicted to moderately to markedly increase the exposure to grazoprevir. Avoid. [Severe] Study

▶ Antifungals, azoles **(fluconazole, isavuconazole, posaconazole)** are predicted to increase the concentration of guanfacine. Adjust **guanfacine** dose, p. 372. [Moderate] Theoretical

▶ Antifungals, azoles **(itraconazole, ketoconazole, voriconazole)** are predicted to increase the exposure to guanfacine. Adjust **guanfacine** dose, p. 372. [Moderate] Study

▶ H_2 receptor antagonists are predicted to decrease the absorption of **itraconazole**. Administer **itraconazole** capsules with an acidic beverage, p. 636. [Moderate] Study

▶ H_2 receptor antagonists are predicted to decrease the absorption of **ketoconazole**. Administer **ketoconazole** with an acidic beverage, p. 720. [Moderate] Study

▶ H_2 receptor antagonists are predicted to decrease the exposure to **posaconazole**. Avoid use of posaconazole oral suspension. [Moderate] Study

▶ **Itraconazole** increases the concentration of haloperidol. [Moderate] Study

▶ **Fluconazole** slightly increases the exposure to HIV-protease inhibitors **(tipranavir)**. Avoid or adjust dose. [Moderate] Study

▶ HIV-protease inhibitors are predicted to increase the exposure to **isavuconazole**. Avoid or monitor adverse effects. [Severe] Study

▶ HIV-protease inhibitors are predicted to increase the exposure to **itraconazole**. Use with caution and adjust dose. [Severe] Study

▶ HIV-protease inhibitors are predicted to increase the exposure to **ketoconazole**. Use with caution and adjust dose. [Moderate] Study

▶ **Miconazole** is predicted to increase the concentration of HIV-protease inhibitors. Use with caution and adjust dose. [Moderate] Theoretical

▶ **Posaconazole** is predicted to increase the exposure to HIV-protease inhibitors. [Moderate] Study

▶ HIV-protease inhibitors are predicted to affect the exposure to **voriconazole** and **voriconazole** potentially affects the exposure to HIV-protease inhibitors. [Severe] Study → Also see **TABLE 9** p. 1431

▶ Antifungals, azoles **(fluconazole, isavuconazole, posaconazole)** are predicted to increase the exposure to ibrutinib. Adjust **ibrutinib** dose with moderate CYP3A4 inhibitors, p. 1027. [Severe] Study

▶ Antifungals, azoles **(itraconazole, ketoconazole, voriconazole)** are predicted to very markedly increase the exposure to ibrutinib. Avoid potent CYP3A4 inhibitors or adjust **ibrutinib** dose, p. 1027. [Severe] Study

▶ **Idelalisib** is predicted to increase the exposure to **isavuconazole**. Avoid or monitor adverse effects. [Severe] Study

▶ Antifungals, azoles **(fluconazole, posaconazole)** are predicted to increase the exposure to imatinib. [Moderate] Theoretical

▶ Antifungals, azoles **(itraconazole, ketoconazole, voriconazole)** are predicted to increase the exposure to imatinib. [Moderate] Study

▶ **Imatinib** is predicted to increase the exposure to **isavuconazole**. [Moderate] Theoretical

▶ Antifungals, azoles **(itraconazole, ketoconazole, voriconazole)** are predicted to increase the risk of toxicity when given with irinotecan. Avoid. [Moderate] Study

▶ Antifungals, azoles **(fluconazole, isavuconazole, posaconazole)** are predicted to increase the exposure to ivabradine. Adjust **ivabradine** dose, p. 227. [Severe] Theoretical

▶ Antifungals, azoles **(itraconazole, ketoconazole, voriconazole)** are predicted to increase the exposure to ivabradine. Avoid. [Severe] Study

▶ Antifungals, azoles **(fluconazole, isavuconazole, posaconazole)** are predicted to increase the exposure to ivacaftor. Adjust ivacaftor p. 309 or tezacaftor with ivacaftor p. 311 or tezacaftor with ivacaftor and elexacaftor p. 311 dose with moderate CYP3A4 inhibitors. [Severe] Study

▶ Antifungals, azoles **(itraconazole, ketoconazole, voriconazole)** are predicted to increase the exposure to ivacaftor. Adjust ivacaftor p. 309 or lumacaftor with ivacaftor p. 310 or tezacaftor with ivacaftor p. 311 or tezacaftor with ivacaftor and elexacftor p. 311 dose with potent CYP3A4 inhibitors. [Severe] Study

Lanthanum is predicted to decrease the absorption of **ketoconazole**. Separate administration by at least 2 hours. Moderate Theoretical

Antifungals, azoles **(fluconazole, isavuconazole, posaconazole)** are predicted to increase the exposure to lapatinib. Moderate Study → Also see TABLE 9 p. 1431

Antifungals, azoles **(itraconazole, ketoconazole, voriconazole)** are predicted to increase the exposure to lapatinib. Avoid. Moderate Study → Also see TABLE 9 p. 1431

Antifungals, azoles **(itraconazole, ketoconazole, voriconazole)** are predicted to moderately increase the exposure to larotrectinib. Avoid or adjust **larotrectinib** dose, p. 1031. Moderate Study

Letermovir slightly decreases the exposure to **voriconazole**. Moderate Study

Antifungals, azoles **(fluconazole, isavuconazole, posaconazole)** are predicted to increase the exposure to lomitapide. Avoid. Moderate Theoretical → Also see TABLE 1 p. 1429

Antifungals, azoles **(itraconazole, ketoconazole, voriconazole)** are predicted to markedly increase the exposure to lomitapide. Avoid. Severe Study → Also see TABLE 1 p. 1429

Clotrimazole is predicted to increase the exposure to lomitapide. Separate administration by 12 hours. Moderate Theoretical

Antifungals, azoles **(itraconazole, ketoconazole, voriconazole)** are predicted to increase the exposure to lorlatinib. Avoid or adjust **lorlatinib** dose, p. 1033. Severe Study

Lumacaftor is predicted to decrease the exposure to antifungals, azoles **(itraconazole, ketoconazole, posaconazole, voriconazole)**. Avoid or monitor efficacy. Moderate Theoretical

Lumacaftor is predicted to decrease the exposure to **fluconazole**. Adjust dose. Mild Theoretical

Macrolides (clarithromycin) are predicted to increase the exposure to **isavuconazole**. Avoid or monitor adverse effects. Severe Study

Macrolides (erythromycin) are predicted to increase the exposure to **isavuconazole**. Moderate Theoretical

Antifungals, azoles **(itraconazole, ketoconazole, voriconazole)** are predicted to markedly increase the exposure to maraviroc. Adjust dose. Severe Study

Antifungals, azoles **(itraconazole, ketoconazole, voriconazole)** are predicted to increase the exposure to meglitinides (repaglinide). Moderate Study

Metoclopramide potentially decreases the absorption of **posaconazole** (oral suspension). Moderate Study

Antifungals, azoles **(fluconazole, isavuconazole, posaconazole)** are predicted to increase the exposure to midostaurin. Moderate Theoretical

Antifungals, azoles **(itraconazole, ketoconazole, voriconazole)** are predicted to very markedly increase the exposure to midostaurin. Avoid or monitor for toxicity. Severe Study

Antifungals, azoles **(itraconazole, ketoconazole, voriconazole)** are predicted to increase the exposure to mirabegron. Adjust **mirabegron** dose in hepatic and renal impairment, p. 825. Moderate Study

Antifungals, azoles **(itraconazole, ketoconazole, voriconazole)** are predicted to increase the exposure to mirtazapine. Moderate Study

Mitotane is predicted to decrease the exposure to **isavuconazole**. Avoid. Severe Study

Antifungals, azoles **(itraconazole, ketoconazole, voriconazole)** are predicted to increase the exposure to modafinil. Mild Theoretical

Antifungals, azoles **(itraconazole, ketoconazole)** increase the risk of neutropenia when given with monoclonal antibodies (brentuximab vedotin). Monitor and adjust dose. Severe Study

Antifungals, azoles **(itraconazole, ketoconazole, voriconazole)** are predicted to increase the exposure to monoclonal antibodies (polatuzumab vedotin). Moderate Theoretical

Antifungals, azoles **(itraconazole, ketoconazole, voriconazole)** are predicted to increase the exposure to monoclonal antibodies (trastuzumab emtansine). Avoid. Severe Theoretical

Isavuconazole increases the exposure to mycophenolate. Moderate Study

Antifungals, azoles **(fluconazole, isavuconazole, posaconazole)** are predicted to increase the exposure to naldemedine. Moderate Study

Antifungals, azoles **(itraconazole, ketoconazole, voriconazole)** are predicted to increase the exposure to naldemedine. Avoid or monitor. Moderate Study

Antifungals, azoles **(fluconazole, isavuconazole, posaconazole)** are predicted to increase the exposure to naloxegol. Adjust **naloxegol** dose and monitor adverse effects, p. 70. Moderate Study

Antifungals, azoles **(itraconazole, ketoconazole, voriconazole)** are predicted to markedly increase the exposure to naloxegol. Avoid. Severe Study

Antifungals, azoles **(fluconazole, isavuconazole, posaconazole)** are predicted to increase the exposure to neratinib. Avoid. Severe Study → Also see TABLE 1 p. 1429

Antifungals, azoles **(itraconazole, ketoconazole, voriconazole)** are predicted to increase the exposure to neratinib. Avoid or adjust **neratinib** dose, p. 1034. Severe Study → Also see TABLE 1 p. 1429

Neurokinin-1 receptor antagonists (aprepitant) are predicted to increase the exposure to **isavuconazole**. Moderate Theoretical

Neurokinin-1 receptor antagonists (netupitant) are predicted to decrease the exposure to **isavuconazole**. Moderate Theoretical

Fluconazole is predicted to increase the exposure to neurokinin-1 receptor antagonists (aprepitant). Moderate Theoretical

Antifungals, azoles **(itraconazole, ketoconazole, voriconazole)** are predicted to markedly increase the exposure to neurokinin-1 receptor antagonists (aprepitant). Moderate Study

Posaconazole is predicted to increase the exposure to neurokinin-1 receptor antagonists (aprepitant, fosaprepitant). Moderate Study

Antifungals, azoles **(itraconazole, ketoconazole, voriconazole)** are predicted to increase the exposure to neurokinin-1 receptor antagonists (fosaprepitant). Moderate Theoretical

Antifungals, azoles **(itraconazole, ketoconazole, voriconazole)** are predicted to increase the exposure to neurokinin-1 receptor antagonists (netupitant). Moderate Study

Antifungals, azoles **(fluconazole, posaconazole)** are predicted to increase the exposure to nilotinib. Moderate Theoretical → Also see TABLE 9 p. 1431

Antifungals, azoles **(itraconazole, ketoconazole, voriconazole)** are predicted to moderately increase the exposure to nilotinib. Avoid. Severe Study → Also see TABLE 9 p. 1431

Antifungals, azoles **(itraconazole, ketoconazole)** are predicted to increase the exposure to nintedanib. Moderate Study

Antifungals, azoles **(itraconazole, ketoconazole, voriconazole)** are predicted to increase the exposure to nitisinone. Adjust dose. Moderate Theoretical

NNRTIs (efavirenz) slightly decrease the exposure to **itraconazole**. Avoid and for 14 days after stopping **efavirenz**. Moderate Study

NNRTIs (efavirenz) moderately decrease the exposure to **ketoconazole**. Severe Study

NNRTIs (efavirenz) slightly decrease the exposure to **posaconazole**. Avoid. Moderate Study

NNRTIs (efavirenz) moderately decrease the exposure to **voriconazole** and **voriconazole** slightly increases the exposure to NNRTIs (efavirenz). Adjust dose. Severe Study → Also see TABLE 9 p. 1431

NNRTIs (efavirenz, nevirapine) are predicted to decrease the exposure to **isavuconazole**. Avoid. Severe Theoretical

NNRTIs (nevirapine) moderately decrease the exposure to **itraconazole**. Avoid and for 14 days after stopping **nevirapine**. Moderate Study

NNRTIs (nevirapine) moderately decrease the exposure to **ketoconazole**. Avoid. Severe Study

NNRTIs (nevirapine) are predicted to decrease the exposure to **voriconazole** and **voriconazole** increases the exposure to NNRTIs (nevirapine). Monitor and adjust dose. Severe Theoretical

Antifungals, azoles **(itraconazole, ketoconazole, voriconazole)** are predicted to increase the exposure to NNRTIs (doravirine). Mild Study

Fluconazole slightly to moderately increases the exposure to NNRTIs (nevirapine). Moderate Study

Fluconazole slightly increases the exposure to NRTIs (zidovudine). Moderate Study

A1

Interactions | **Appendix 1**

Antifungals, azoles (continued)

▶ **Fluconazole** moderately increases the exposure to NSAIDs (celecoxib). Adjust **celecoxib** dose, p. 1178. Moderate Study

▶ **Voriconazole** slightly increases the exposure to NSAIDs (diclofenac). Monitor and adjust dose. Moderate Study

▶ **Voriconazole** moderately increases the exposure to NSAIDs (ibuprofen). Adjust dose. Moderate Study

▶ **Fluconazole** increases the exposure to NSAIDs (parecoxib). Monitor and adjust dose. Moderate Study

▶ Antifungals, azoles **(fluconazole, isavuconazole, posaconazole)** are predicted to increase the exposure to olaparib. Avoid moderate CYP3A4 inhibitors or adjust **olaparib** dose, p. 1051. Moderate Theoretical

▶ Antifungals, azoles **(itraconazole, ketoconazole, voriconazole)** are predicted to increase the exposure to olaparib. Avoid potent CYP3A4 inhibitors or adjust **olaparib** dose, p. 1051. Moderate Study

▶ **Miconazole** is predicted to increase the exposure to opioids (alfentanil). Use with caution and adjust dose. Moderate Theoretical

▶ Antifungals, azoles **(fluconazole, isavuconazole, posaconazole)** are predicted to increase the exposure to opioids (alfentanil, buprenorphine, fentanyl, oxycodone). Monitor and adjust dose. Moderate Study

▶ Antifungals, azoles **(itraconazole, ketoconazole, voriconazole)** are predicted to increase the exposure to opioids (alfentanil, buprenorphine, fentanyl, oxycodone). Monitor and adjust dose. Severe Study

▶ Antifungals, azoles **(fluconazole, isavuconazole, posaconazole)** are predicted to increase the exposure to opioids (methadone). Moderate Theoretical → Also see **TABLE 9** p. 1431

▶ Antifungals, azoles **(itraconazole, ketoconazole, voriconazole)** are predicted to increase the exposure to opioids (methadone). Adjust dose. Severe Theoretical → Also see **TABLE 9** p. 1431

▶ Antifungals, azoles **(itraconazole, ketoconazole, voriconazole)** are predicted to increase the exposure to ospemifene. Avoid in poor CYP2C9 metabolisers. Moderate Study

▶ **Fluconazole** increases the exposure to ospemifene. Use with caution or avoid. Moderate Study

▶ Antifungals, azoles **(fluconazole, isavuconazole, posaconazole)** are predicted to increase the exposure to oxybutynin. Mild Theoretical

▶ Antifungals, azoles **(itraconazole, ketoconazole, voriconazole)** are predicted to increase the exposure to oxybutynin. Mild Study

▶ Antifungals, azoles **(itraconazole, ketoconazole, voriconazole)** are predicted to increase the exposure to palbociclib. Avoid or adjust **palbociclib** dose, p. 1038. Severe Study

▶ Antifungals, azoles **(itraconazole, ketoconazole, voriconazole)** are predicted to increase the exposure to panobinostat. Adjust **panobinostat** dose; in hepatic impairment avoid, p. 979. Moderate Study → Also see **TABLE 9** p. 1431

▶ **Posaconazole** is predicted to increase the exposure to panobinostat. Adjust dose. Moderate Theoretical

▶ Antifungals, azoles **(itraconazole, ketoconazole, voriconazole)** are predicted to increase the exposure to paritaprevir. Avoid. Severe Study

▶ **Posaconazole** is predicted to increase the exposure to paritaprevir (with ritonavir and ombitasvir) and paritaprevir (with ritonavir and ombitasvir) is predicted to increase the exposure to **posaconazole**. Avoid. Severe Study

▶ Antifungals, azoles **(fluconazole, isavuconazole, posaconazole)** are predicted to increase the exposure to pazopanib. Moderate Theoretical → Also see **TABLE 9** p. 1431

▶ Antifungals, azoles **(itraconazole, ketoconazole, voriconazole)** are predicted to increase the exposure to pazopanib. Avoid or adjust **pazopanib** dose, p. 1039. Moderate Study → Also see **TABLE 9** p. 1431

▶ **Miconazole** greatly increases the anticoagulant effect of phenindione. Severe Theoretical

▶ Antifungals, azoles **(fluconazole, isavuconazole, posaconazole)** are predicted to increase the exposure to phosphodiesterase type-5 inhibitors (avanafil). Adjust **avanafil** dose, p. 859. Moderate Theoretical

▶ Antifungals, azoles **(itraconazole, ketoconazole, voriconazole)** are predicted to increase the exposure to phosphodiesterase type-5 inhibitors (avanafil, vardenafil). Avoid. Severe Study → Also see **TABLE 9** p. 1431

▶ **Miconazole** is predicted to increase the exposure to phosphodiesterase type-5 inhibitors (sildenafil). Use with caution and adjust dose. Severe Theoretical

▶ Antifungals, azoles **(fluconazole, isavuconazole, posaconazole)** are predicted to increase the exposure to phosphodiesterase type-5 inhibitors (sildenafil). Monitor or adjust **sildenafil** dose with moderate CYP3A4 inhibitors, p. 860. Moderate Study → Also see **TABLE 9** p. 1431

▶ Antifungals, azoles **(itraconazole, ketoconazole, voriconazole)** are predicted to increase the exposure to phosphodiesterase type-5 inhibitors (sildenafil). Avoid potent CYP3A4 inhibitors or adjust **sildenafil** dose, p. 860. Severe Study → Also see **TABLE 9** p. 1431

▶ Antifungals, azoles **(fluconazole, isavuconazole, posaconazole)** are predicted to increase the exposure to phosphodiesterase type-5 inhibitors (tadalafil). Severe Theoretical

▶ Antifungals, azoles **(itraconazole, ketoconazole, voriconazole)** are predicted to increase the exposure to phosphodiesterase type-5 inhibitors (tadalafil). Use with caution or avoid. Severe Study

▶ Antifungals, azoles **(fluconazole, isavuconazole, posaconazole)** are predicted to increase the exposure to phosphodiesterase type-5 inhibitors (vardenafil). Adjust dose. Severe Theoretical → Also see **TABLE 9** p. 1431

▶ Antifungals, azoles **(itraconazole, ketoconazole)** are predicted to increase the exposure to pibrentasvir. Moderate Theoretical

▶ Antifungals, azoles **(fluconazole, isavuconazole, posaconazole)** are predicted to increase the exposure to pimozide. Avoid. Severe Theoretical → Also see **TABLE 9** p. 1431

▶ Antifungals, azoles **(itraconazole, ketoconazole, voriconazole)** are predicted to increase the exposure to pimozide. Avoid. Severe Study → Also see **TABLE 9** p. 1431

▶ **Miconazole** is predicted to increase the exposure to pimozide. Avoid. Moderate Theoretical

▶ **Pioglitazone** potentially decreases the exposure to **isavuconazole**. Use with caution or avoid. Moderate Theoretical

▶ Antifungals, azoles **(itraconazole, ketoconazole, voriconazole)** are predicted to slightly increase the exposure to ponatinib. Monitor and adjust **ponatinib** dose, p. 1040. Moderate Study

▶ Antifungals, azoles **(itraconazole, ketoconazole, voriconazole)** are predicted to moderately increase the exposure to praziquantel. Mild Study

▶ Antifungals, azoles **(itraconazole, ketoconazole, voriconazole)** given with carbimazole are predicted to increase the exposure to propiverine. Adjust starting dose. Moderate Theoretical

▶ Proton pump inhibitors decrease the absorption of **itraconazole**. Administer itraconazole capsules with an acidic beverage. Moderate Study

▶ Proton pump inhibitors decrease the absorption of **ketoconazole**. Administer ketoconazole with an acidic beverage. Moderate Study

▶ Proton pump inhibitors decrease the absorption of **posaconazole** (oral suspension). Avoid. Moderate Study

▶ **Voriconazole** increases the exposure to proton pump inhibitors (esomeprazole, omeprazole). Adjust dose. Moderate Study

▶ Antifungals, azoles **(fluconazole, isavuconazole, posaconazole)** are predicted to increase the exposure to ranolazine. Severe Study → Also see **TABLE 9** p. 1431

▶ Antifungals, azoles **(itraconazole, ketoconazole, voriconazole)** are predicted to increase the exposure to ranolazine. Avoid. Severe Study → Also see **TABLE 9** p. 1431

▶ Antifungals, azoles **(itraconazole, ketoconazole, voriconazole)** are predicted to increase the exposure to reboxetine. Avoid. Moderate Study

▶ **Miconazole** is predicted to increase the concentration of reboxetine. Use with caution and adjust dose. Moderate Theoretical

▶ Antifungals, azoles **(itraconazole, ketoconazole, voriconazole)** are predicted to increase the exposure to regorafenib. Avoid. Moderate Study

▶ Antifungals, azoles **(fluconazole, itraconazole, ketoconazole, miconazole, voriconazole)** are predicted to increase the exposure to retinoids (alitretinoin). Adjust **alitretinoin** dose, p. 1305. Moderate Theoretical

Antifungals, azoles **(fluconazole, ketoconazole, voriconazole)** are predicted to increase the risk of tretinoin toxicity when given with retinoids (tretinoin). [Moderate] Study

Antifungals, azoles **(fluconazole, isavuconazole, posaconazole)** are predicted to increase the exposure to ribociclib. [Moderate] Study → Also see TABLE 9 p. 1431

Antifungals, azoles **(itraconazole, ketoconazole, voriconazole)** are predicted to increase the exposure to ribociclib. Avoid or adjust **ribociclib** dose, p. 1042. [Moderate] Study → Also see TABLE 9 p. 1431

Rifamycins (rifabutin) are predicted to decrease the exposure to **isavuconazole**. Avoid. [Severe] Theoretical

Rifamycins (rifabutin) decrease the concentration of **voriconazole** and voriconazole increases the concentration of rifamycins (rifabutin). Avoid or adjust **voriconazole** dose, p. 638. [Severe] Study

Rifamycins (rifampicin) slightly decrease the exposure to **fluconazole**. Adjust dose. [Moderate] Study

Rifamycins (rifampicin) are predicted to decrease the exposure to **isavuconazole**. Avoid. [Severe] Study

Rifamycins (rifampicin) markedly decrease the exposure to **itraconazole**. Avoid and for 14 days after stopping **rifampicin**. [Moderate] Study

Rifamycins (rifampicin) markedly decrease the exposure to **ketoconazole** and ketoconazole potentially decreases the exposure to rifamycins (rifampicin). Avoid. [Moderate] Study

Rifamycins (rifampicin) are predicted to decrease the exposure to **posaconazole**. Avoid. [Moderate] Anecdotal

Rifamycins (rifampicin) very markedly decrease the exposure to **voriconazole**. Avoid. [Moderate] Study

Fluconazole increases the risk of uveitis when given with rifamycins (rifabutin). Adjust dose. [Severe] Study

Ketoconazole is predicted to increase the concentration of rifamycins (rifabutin) and rifamycins (rifabutin) are predicted to decrease the concentration of **ketoconazole**. Avoid. [Severe] Theoretical

Miconazole is predicted to increase the concentration of rifamycins (rifabutin). Use with caution and adjust dose. [Moderate] Theoretical

Antifungals, azoles **(itraconazole, ketoconazole, posaconazole)** increase the concentration of rifamycins (rifabutin) and rifamycins (rifabutin) decrease the concentration of antifungals, azoles **(itraconazole, posaconazole)**. Avoid. [Severe] Study

Antifungals, azoles **(itraconazole, posaconazole)** are predicted to increase the exposure to riociguat. Adjust **riociguat** dose and monitor blood pressure, p. 198. [Moderate] Theoretical

Ketoconazole moderately increases the exposure to riociguat. Adjust **riociguat** dose and monitor blood pressure, p. 198. [Moderate] Study

Antifungals, azoles **(fluconazole, isavuconazole, posaconazole)** are predicted to increase the exposure to ruxolitinib. [Moderate] Theoretical

Antifungals, azoles **(itraconazole, ketoconazole, voriconazole)** are predicted to increase the exposure to ruxolitinib. Adjust dose and monitor adverse effects. [Moderate] Study

Fluconazole is predicted to increase the exposure to selexipag. [Unknown] Theoretical

Antifungals, azoles **(itraconazole, ketoconazole, voriconazole)** are predicted to increase the exposure to siponimod. Avoid depending on other drugs taken—consult product literature. [Severe] Theoretical

Miconazole is predicted to increase the exposure to siponimod. Avoid depending on other drugs taken—consult product literature. [Severe] Study

Antifungals, azoles **(fluconazole, isavuconazole, posaconazole)** increase the concentration of sirolimus. Monitor and adjust dose. [Moderate] Study

Antifungals, azoles **(itraconazole, ketoconazole, voriconazole)** are predicted to increase the exposure to sirolimus. Avoid. [Severe] Study

Miconazole is predicted to increase the concentration of sirolimus. Monitor and adjust dose. [Moderate] Study

Oral sodium bicarbonate decreases the absorption of **ketoconazole**. [Moderate] Study

▶ Sodium zirconium cyclosilicate is predicted to decrease the exposure to **antifungals, azoles**. Separate administration by at least 2 hours. [Moderate] Theoretical

▶ Antifungals, azoles **(itraconazole, ketoconazole, voriconazole)** are predicted to increase the exposure to solifenacin. Adjust solifenacin p. 824 or tamsulosin with solifenacin p. 830 dose; avoid in hepatic and renal impairment. [Severe] Study

▶ **Voriconazole** is predicted to increase the exposure to SSRIs (citalopram). [Severe] Theoretical → Also see TABLE 9 p. 1431

▶ Antifungals, azoles **(fluconazole, isavuconazole, posaconazole)** are predicted to increase the exposure to SSRIs (dapoxetine). Adjust **dapoxetine** dose with moderate CYP3A4 inhibitors, p. 867. [Moderate] Theoretical

▶ Antifungals, azoles **(itraconazole, ketoconazole, voriconazole)** are predicted to moderately increase the exposure to SSRIs (dapoxetine). Avoid potent CYP3A4 inhibitors or adjust **dapoxetine** dose, p. 867. [Severe] Study

▶ St John's wort is predicted to decrease the exposure to **isavuconazole**. Avoid. [Severe] Theoretical

▶ St John's wort moderately decreases the exposure to **voriconazole**. Avoid. [Moderate] Study

▶ **Fluconazole** potentially increases the risk of rhabdomyolysis when given with statins (atorvastatin). Monitor and adjust dose. [Severe] Anecdotal → Also see TABLE 1 p. 1429

▶ **Isavuconazole** slightly increases the exposure to statins (atorvastatin). [Moderate] Study

▶ **Miconazole** potentially increases the exposure to statins (atorvastatin). [Severe] Anecdotal

▶ **Posaconazole** is predicted to increase the exposure to statins (atorvastatin). Avoid. [Severe] Anecdotal

▶ Antifungals, azoles **(itraconazole, ketoconazole, voriconazole)** are predicted to increase the exposure to statins (atorvastatin). Avoid or adjust dose and monitor rhabdomyolysis. [Severe] Study → Also see TABLE 1 p. 1429

▶ Antifungals, azoles **(fluconazole, miconazole)** are predicted to increase the exposure to statins (fluvastatin). [Severe] Theoretical → Also see TABLE 1 p. 1429

▶ **Isavuconazole** is predicted to increase the exposure to statins (fluvastatin, rosuvastatin). [Moderate] Theoretical

▶ **Fluconazole** is predicted to increase the exposure to statins (simvastatin). Monitor and adjust dose. [Severe] Anecdotal → Also see TABLE 1 p. 1429

▶ **Isavuconazole** is predicted to increase the exposure to statins (simvastatin). Monitor and adjust dose. [Severe] Theoretical

▶ **Miconazole** is predicted to increase the exposure to statins (simvastatin). Avoid. [Severe] Theoretical

▶ **Posaconazole** markedly to very markedly increases the exposure to statins (simvastatin). Avoid. [Severe] Study

▶ Antifungals, azoles **(itraconazole, ketoconazole, voriconazole)** are predicted to increase the exposure to statins (simvastatin). Avoid. [Severe] Study → Also see TABLE 1 p. 1429

▶ **Isavuconazole** is predicted to increase the exposure to sulfasalazine. [Moderate] Theoretical

▶ Antifungals, azoles **(fluconazole, miconazole)** are predicted to increase the exposure to sulfonylureas. Use with caution and adjust dose. [Moderate] Study

▶ **Voriconazole** is predicted to increase the concentration of sulfonylureas. Use with caution and adjust dose. [Moderate] Study

▶ Antifungals, azoles **(fluconazole, isavuconazole, posaconazole)** are predicted to increase the exposure to sunitinib. [Moderate] Theoretical → Also see TABLE 9 p. 1431

▶ Antifungals, azoles **(itraconazole, ketoconazole, voriconazole)** are predicted to slightly increase the exposure to sunitinib. Avoid or adjust **sunitinib** dose, p. 1044. [Moderate] Study → Also see TABLE 9 p. 1431

▶ Antifungals, azoles **(fluconazole, isavuconazole, posaconazole)** are predicted to increase the concentration of tacrolimus. [Severe] Study

▶ Antifungals, azoles **(itraconazole, ketoconazole, voriconazole)** are predicted to increase the concentration of tacrolimus. Monitor and adjust dose. [Severe] Study

▶ **Miconazole** is predicted to increase the concentration of tacrolimus. Monitor and adjust dose. [Severe] Theoretical

Antifungals, azoles (continued)

▶ Antifungals, azoles **(itraconazole, ketoconazole)** are predicted to slightly increase the exposure to talazoparib. Avoid or adjust **talazoparib** dose, p. 1052. [Severe] Study

▶ Antifungals, azoles **(fluconazole, isavuconazole, posaconazole)** are predicted to increase the exposure to taxanes (cabazitaxel). [Moderate] Theoretical

▶ Antifungals, azoles **(itraconazole, ketoconazole, voriconazole)** are predicted to increase the exposure to taxanes (cabazitaxel). Avoid. [Severe] Study

▶ **Miconazole** is predicted to increase the concentration of taxanes (docetaxel). Use with caution and adjust dose. [Moderate] Theoretical

▶ Antifungals, azoles **(itraconazole, ketoconazole, voriconazole)** are predicted to moderately increase the exposure to taxanes (docetaxel). Avoid or adjust dose. [Severe] Study

▶ Antifungals, azoles **(itraconazole, ketoconazole, voriconazole)** are predicted to increase the exposure to taxanes (paclitaxel). [Severe] Theoretical

▶ Antifungals, azoles **(fluconazole, isavuconazole, posaconazole)** are predicted to increase the concentration of temsirolimus. Use with caution or avoid. [Moderate] Theoretical

▶ Antifungals, azoles **(itraconazole, ketoconazole, voriconazole)** are predicted to increase the concentration of temsirolimus. Avoid. [Severe] Theoretical

▶ Antifungals, azoles **(fluconazole, isavuconazole, posaconazole)** are predicted to increase the exposure to tezacaftor. Adjust tezacaftor with ivacaftor p. 311 or tezacaftor with ivacaftor and elexacftor p. 311 dose with moderate CYP3A4 inhibitors. [Severe] Study

▶ Antifungals, azoles **(itraconazole, ketoconazole, voriconazole)** are predicted to increase the exposure to tezacaftor. Adjust tezacaftor with ivacaftor p. 311 or tezacaftor with ivacaftor and elexacftor p. 311 dose with potent CYP3A4 inhibitors. [Severe] Study

▶ **Isavuconazole** is predicted to increase the exposure to thrombin inhibitors (dabigatran). Monitor and adjust dose. [Moderate] Study

▶ Antifungals, azoles **(itraconazole, ketoconazole)** are predicted to increase the exposure to thrombin inhibitors (dabigatran). Avoid. [Severe] Study

▶ Antifungals, azoles **(itraconazole, ketoconazole, voriconazole)** are predicted to markedly increase the exposure to ticagrelor. Avoid. [Severe] Study

▶ Antifungals, azoles **(itraconazole, ketoconazole, voriconazole)** are predicted to increase the exposure to tofacitinib. Adjust **tofacitinib** dose, p. 1154. [Moderate] Study

▶ **Fluconazole** increases the exposure to tofacitinib. Adjust **tofacitinib** dose, p. 1154. [Moderate] Study

▶ **Isavuconazole** given with a potent CYP2C19 inhibitor is predicted to increase the exposure to tofacitinib. Adjust **tofacitinib** dose, p. 1154. [Moderate] Study

▶ **Posaconazole** given with a potent CYP2C19 inhibitor is predicted to increase the exposure to tofacitinib. Adjust **tofacitinib** dose, p. 1154. [Moderate] Theoretical

▶ Antifungals, azoles **(fluconazole, isavuconazole, posaconazole)** are predicted to increase the exposure to tolterodine. [Mild] Theoretical → Also see **TABLE 9** p. 1431

▶ Antifungals, azoles **(itraconazole, ketoconazole, voriconazole)** are predicted to increase the exposure to tolterodine. Avoid. [Severe] Study → Also see **TABLE 9** p. 1431

▶ Antifungals, azoles **(fluconazole, isavuconazole, posaconazole)** are predicted to increase the exposure to tolvaptan. Manufacturer advises caution or adjust **tolvaptan** dose with moderate CYP3A4 inhibitors, p. 708. [Moderate] Study

▶ Antifungals, azoles **(itraconazole, ketoconazole, voriconazole)** are predicted to increase the exposure to tolvaptan. Manufacturer advises caution or adjust **tolvaptan** dose with potent CYP3A4 inhibitors, p. 708. [Severe] Study

▶ Antifungals, azoles **(itraconazole, ketoconazole)** are predicted to increase the exposure to topotecan. [Severe] Study

▶ **Isavuconazole** is predicted to increase the exposure to topotecan. [Moderate] Theoretical

▶ Antifungals, azoles **(itraconazole, ketoconazole, voriconazole)** predicted to increase the exposure to toremifene. [Moderate] Theoretical → Also see **TABLE 9** p. 1431

▶ Antifungals, azoles **(itraconazole, ketoconazole, voriconazole)** are predicted to increase the exposure to trabectedin. Avoid or adjust dose. [Severe] Theoretical → Also see **TABLE 1** p. 1429

▶ Antifungals, azoles **(itraconazole, ketoconazole, voriconazole)** are predicted to increase the concentration of trametinib. [Moderate] Theoretical

▶ Antifungals, azoles **(fluconazole, isavuconazole, posaconazole)** are predicted to increase the exposure to trazodone. [Moderate] Theoretical

▶ Antifungals, azoles **(itraconazole, ketoconazole, voriconazole)** are predicted to moderately increase the exposure to trazodone. Avoid or adjust dose. [Moderate] Study

▶ Antifungals, azoles **(itraconazole, ketoconazole, voriconazole)** increase the exposure to triptans (almotriptan). [Mild] Study

▶ Antifungals, azoles **(itraconazole, ketoconazole, voriconazole)** are predicted to markedly increase the exposure to triptans (eletriptan). Avoid. [Severe] Study

▶ Antifungals, azoles **(itraconazole, ketoconazole, voriconazole)** are predicted to increase the exposure to upadacitinib. Use with caution or avoid. [Severe] Study

▶ **Posaconazole** is predicted to increase the exposure to upadacitinib. Use with caution or avoid. [Moderate] Study

▶ Antifungals, azoles **(itraconazole, ketoconazole, voriconazole)** are predicted to increase the exposure to vemurafenib. [Severe] Theoretical → Also see **TABLE 9** p. 1431

▶ Antifungals, azoles **(fluconazole, isavuconazole, itraconazole, ketoconazole, posaconazole, voriconazole)** are predicted to increase the exposure to venetoclax. Avoid or adjust dose— consult product literature. [Severe] Study

▶ Antifungals, azoles **(itraconazole, ketoconazole, voriconazole)** are predicted to increase the exposure to venlafaxine. [Moderate] Study → Also see **TABLE 9** p. 1431

▶ Antifungals, azoles **(fluconazole, isavuconazole, itraconazole, ketoconazole, posaconazole, voriconazole)** are predicted to increase the exposure to vinca alkaloids. [Severe] Theoretical → Also see **TABLE 1** p. 1429 → Also see **TABLE 9** p. 1431

▶ **Miconazole** is predicted to increase the concentration of vinca alkaloids. Use with caution and adjust dose. [Moderate] Theoretical

▶ Antifungals, azoles **(clotrimazole, ketoconazole)** are predicted to decrease the exposure to vitamin D substances (colecalciferol). [Moderate] Theoretical

▶ Antifungals, azoles **(itraconazole, ketoconazole, voriconazole)** are predicted to increase the exposure to vitamin D substances (paricalcitol). [Moderate] Study

▶ Antifungals, azoles **(fluconazole, isavuconazole, posaconazole)** are predicted to increase the exposure to zopiclone. Adjust dose. [Moderate] Study

▶ Antifungals, azoles **(itraconazole, ketoconazole, voriconazole)** are predicted to increase the exposure to zopiclone. Adjust dose. [Moderate] Theoretical

Antihistamines, non-sedating → see **TABLE 9** p. 1431 (QT-interval prolongation)

acrivastine · azelastine · bilastine · cetirizine · desloratadine · fexofenadine · levocetirizine · loratadine · mizolastine · rupatadine

▶ Since systemic absorption can follow topical application, the possibility of interactions with topical **azelastine** should be borne in mind.

▶ Apple juice and orange juice decrease the exposure to **fexofenadine**.

▶ Oral antacids decrease the absorption of oral **fexofenadine**. Separate administration by 2 hours. [Mild] Study

▶ Anti-androgens (apalutamide) slightly decrease the exposure to **fexofenadine**. [Mild] Study

▶ Anti-androgens (darolutamide) are predicted to increase the concentration of **fexofenadine**. [Moderate] Theoretical

▶ Antiarrhythmics (dronedarone) are predicted to increase the exposure to **rupatadine**. Avoid. [Moderate] Study

▶ Antiarrhythmics (dronedarone) are predicted to increase the exposure to antihistamines, non-sedating **(fexofenadine, mizolastine)**. [Severe] Theoretical

▶ Antifungals, azoles (fluconazole, isavuconazole, itraconazole, ketoconazole, posaconazole, voriconazole) are predicted to increase the exposure to **rupatadine**. Avoid. [Moderate] Study

► Antifungals, azoles (fluconazole, isavuconazole, posaconazole) are predicted to increase the exposure to **mizolastine**. Theoretical

Antifungals, azoles (itraconazole, ketoconazole, voriconazole) are predicted to increase the exposure to **mizolastine**. Avoid. Severe Study

► Antifungals, azoles (miconazole) are predicted to increase the exposure to **mizolastine**. Avoid. Moderate Theoretical

► **Antihistamines, non-sedating** are predicted to decrease the effects of betahistine. Moderate Theoretical

► Calcium channel blockers (diltiazem, verapamil) are predicted to increase the exposure to **mizolastine**. Severe Theoretical

► Calcium channel blockers (diltiazem, verapamil) are predicted to increase the exposure to **rupatadine**. Avoid. Moderate Study

► Ceritinib is predicted to increase the exposure to **fexofenadine**. Moderate Theoretical

► Cobicistat is predicted to increase the exposure to **mizolastine**. Avoid. Severe Study

► Cobicistat is predicted to increase the exposure to **rupatadine**. Avoid. Moderate Study

► Crizotinib is predicted to increase the exposure to **mizolastine**. Severe Theoretical

► Crizotinib is predicted to increase the exposure to **rupatadine**. Avoid. Moderate Study

► Eliglustat is predicted to increase the exposure to **fexofenadine**. Adjust dose. Moderate Study

► Filgotinib is predicted to increase the exposure to **fexofenadine**. Avoid. Moderate Theoretical

► Grapefruit juice slightly decreases the exposure to **bilastine**. **Bilastine** should be taken 1 hour before or 2 hours after **grapefruit**. Moderate Study

► Grapefruit juice increases the exposure to **rupatadine**. Avoid. Moderate Study

► HIV-protease inhibitors are predicted to increase the exposure to **mizolastine**. Avoid. Severe Study

► HIV-protease inhibitors are predicted to increase the exposure to **rupatadine**. Avoid. Moderate Study

► Idelalisib is predicted to increase the exposure to **mizolastine**. Avoid. Severe Study

► Idelalisib is predicted to increase the exposure to **rupatadine**. Avoid. Moderate Study

► Imatinib is predicted to increase the exposure to **mizolastine**. Severe Theoretical

► Imatinib is predicted to increase the exposure to **rupatadine**. Avoid. Moderate Study

► Lapatinib is predicted to increase the exposure to **fexofenadine**. Moderate Theoretical

► Leflunomide is predicted to increase the exposure to **fexofenadine**. Moderate Study

► Letermovir is predicted to increase the concentration of **fexofenadine**. Moderate Theoretical

► Letermovir is predicted to increase the exposure to **mizolastine**. Severe Theoretical

► Letermovir is predicted to increase the exposure to **rupatadine**. Avoid. Moderate Study

► Macrolides (clarithromycin) are predicted to increase the exposure to **fexofenadine**. Avoid. Severe Study

► Macrolides (clarithromycin, erythromycin) are predicted to increase the exposure to **rupatadine**. Avoid. Moderate Study

► Macrolides (erythromycin) are predicted to increase the exposure to **mizolastine**. Severe Theoretical

► MAOIs, irreversible are predicted to increase the risk of antimuscarinic adverse effects when given with **antihistamines, non-sedating**. Avoid. Severe Theoretical

► Mirabegron is predicted to increase the exposure to **fexofenadine**. Mild Theoretical

► Neratinib is predicted to increase the exposure to **fexofenadine**. Moderate Study

► Neurokinin-1 receptor antagonists (aprepitant, netupitant) are predicted to increase the exposure to **mizolastine**. Severe Theoretical

► Neurokinin-1 receptor antagonists (aprepitant, netupitant) are predicted to increase the exposure to **rupatadine**. Avoid. Moderate Study

► Nilotinib is predicted to increase the exposure to **mizolastine**. Severe Theoretical

► Nilotinib is predicted to increase the exposure to **rupatadine**. Avoid. Moderate Study

► Pibrentasvir (with glecaprevir) is predicted to increase the exposure to **fexofenadine**. Moderate Study

► Pitolisant is predicted to decrease the exposure to **fexofenadine**. Mild Theoretical

► Rifamycins (rifampicin) are predicted to decrease the exposure to **bilastine**. Moderate Theoretical

► Rifamycins (rifampicin) increase the clearance of **fexofenadine**. Moderate Study

► Teriflunomide is predicted to increase the exposure to **fexofenadine**. Moderate Study

► Velpatasvir is predicted to increase the exposure to **fexofenadine**. Severe Theoretical

► Vemurafenib is predicted to increase the exposure to **fexofenadine**. Use with caution and adjust dose. Severe Theoretical

► Venetoclax is predicted to increase the exposure to **fexofenadine**. Moderate Theoretical

Antihistamines, sedating → see TABLE 9 p. 1431 (QT-interval prolongation), TABLE 11 p. 1431 (CNS depressant effects), TABLE 10 p. 1431 (antimuscarinics)

alimemazine · antazoline · buclizine · chlorphenamine · cinnarizine · clemastine · cyclizine · cyproheptadine · doxylamine · hydroxyzine · ketotifen · pizotifen · promethazine

ROUTE-SPECIFIC INFORMATION Since systemic absorption can follow topical application of **ketotifen**, the possibility of interactions should be borne in mind.

► **Hydroxyzine** potentially increases the risk of overheating and dehydration when given with antiepileptics (zonisamide). Avoid in children. Severe Theoretical

► **Antihistamines, sedating** are predicted to decrease the effects of betahistine. Moderate Theoretical

► MAOIs, irreversible are predicted to increase the risk of antimuscarinic adverse effects when given with **antihistamines, sedating**. Avoid. Severe Theoretical

► **Cyproheptadine** decreases the effects of metyrapone. Avoid. Moderate Study

► **Antihistamines, sedating** are predicted to decrease the efficacy of pitolisant. Moderate Theoretical

► **Cyproheptadine** potentially decreases the effects of SSRIs. Moderate Anecdotal

Antimalarials → see TABLE 9 p. 1431 (QT-interval prolongation)

artemether · artenimol · atovaquone · chloroquine · lumefantrine · mefloquine · piperaquine · primaquine · proguanil · pyrimethamine · quinine

PHARMACOLOGY Piperaquine has a long half-life; there is a potential for drug interactions to occur for up to 3 months after treatment has been stopped.

► **Chloroquine** is predicted to decrease the effects of agalsidase alfa. Moderate Theoretical

► **Chloroquine** is predicted to decrease the effects of agalsidase beta. Avoid. Moderate Theoretical

► Antimalarials (chloroquine, primaquine) are predicted to increase the risk of methaemoglobinaemia when given with topical anaesthetics, local (prilocaine). Use with caution or avoid. Severe Theoretical

► Oral antacids decrease the absorption of oral **chloroquine**. Separate administration by at least 4 hours. Moderate Study

► Oral antacids are predicted to decrease the absorption of oral **proguanil**. Separate administration by at least 2 hours. Moderate Study

► Anti-androgens (apalutamide, enzalutamide) are predicted to decrease the exposure to **artemether** (with lumefantrine). Avoid. Severe Study → Also see TABLE 9 p. 1431

► Anti-androgens (apalutamide, enzalutamide) are predicted to decrease the concentration of **piperaquine**. Avoid. Moderate Theoretical

► Antiarrhythmics (dronedarone) are predicted to increase the concentration of **piperaquine**. Severe Theoretical

A1

Interactions | Appendix 1

Antimalarials (continued)

▶ Antiepileptics (carbamazepine, fosphenytoin, phenobarbital, phenytoin, primidone) are predicted to decrease the exposure to **artemether** (with lumefantrine). Avoid. Severe Study

▶ Antiepileptics (carbamazepine, fosphenytoin, phenobarbital, phenytoin, primidone) are predicted to decrease the concentration of **piperaquine**. Avoid. Moderate Theoretical

▶ Antiepileptics (carbamazepine, phenobarbital, primidone) potentially increase the risk of toxicity when given with **quinine**. Unknown Study

▶ **Pyrimethamine** increases the risk of haematological toxicity when given with antiepileptics (fosphenytoin, phenytoin). Severe Study

▶ **Pyrimethamine** is predicted to increase the risk of haematological toxicity when given with antiepileptics (phenobarbital, primidone). Severe Theoretical

▶ Antifungals, azoles (fluconazole, isavuconazole, itraconazole, ketoconazole, posaconazole, voriconazole) are predicted to increase the concentration of **piperaquine**. Severe Theoretical

▶ Antifungals, azoles (fluconazole, itraconazole, posaconazole, voriconazole) are predicted to increase the exposure to **mefloquine**. Moderate Theoretical

▶ Antifungals, azoles (ketoconazole) increase the exposure to **mefloquine**. Moderate Study

▶ Antimalarials (**proguanil**) are predicted to increase the risk of adverse effects when given with antimalarials (**pyrimethamine**). Severe Theoretical

▶ **Mefloquine** is predicted to increase the risk of bradycardia when given with beta blockers, non-selective. Severe Theoretical

▶ **Mefloquine** is predicted to increase the risk of bradycardia when given with beta blockers, selective. Severe Theoretical

▶ **Mefloquine** is predicted to increase the risk of bradycardia when given with calcium channel blockers. Severe Theoretical

▶ Calcium channel blockers (diltiazem, verapamil) are predicted to increase the concentration of **piperaquine**. Severe Theoretical

▶ Calcium salts (calcium carbonate) decrease the absorption of **chloroquine**. Separate administration by at least 4 hours. Moderate Study

▶ Calcium salts (calcium carbonate) are predicted to decrease the absorption of **proguanil**. Separate administration by at least 2 hours. Moderate Study

▶ **Chloroquine** decreases the efficacy of oral cholera vaccine. Moderate Study

▶ Cobicistat is predicted to increase the concentration of **piperaquine**. Severe Theoretical

▶ Crizotinib is predicted to increase the concentration of **piperaquine**. Severe Theoretical

▶ Antimalarials (**chloroquine, primaquine**) are predicted to increase the risk of methaemoglobinaemia when given with dapsone. Severe Theoretical

▶ **Mefloquine** is predicted to increase the risk of bradycardia when given with digoxin. Severe Theoretical

▶ **Quinine** increases the concentration of digoxin. Monitor and adjust **digoxin** dose, p. 117. Severe Anecdotal

▶ Grapefruit juice increases the exposure to **artemether**. Unknown Study

▶ Grapefruit juice is predicted to increase the concentration of **piperaquine**. Avoid. Severe Theoretical

▶ H₂ receptor antagonists (cimetidine) decrease the clearance of **chloroquine**. Moderate Study

▶ H₂ receptor antagonists (cimetidine) slightly increase the exposure to **quinine**. Moderate Study

▶ HIV-protease inhibitors decrease the exposure to **atovaquone**. Avoid if boosted with ritonavir. Moderate Study

▶ HIV-protease inhibitors are predicted to increase the concentration of **piperaquine**. Severe Theoretical

▶ HIV-protease inhibitors are predicted to decrease the exposure to **proguanil**. Avoid. Moderate Study

▶ HIV-protease inhibitors are predicted to affect the exposure to **quinine**. Severe Study → Also see TABLE 9 p. 1431

▶ Idelalisib is predicted to increase the concentration of **piperaquine**. Severe Theoretical

▶ Imatinib is predicted to increase the concentration of **piperaquine**. Severe Theoretical

▶ Lanthanum is predicted to decrease the absorption of **chloroquine**. Separate administration by at least 2 hours. Moderate Theoretical

▶ **Chloroquine** is predicted to decrease the exposure to laronidase. Avoid simultaneous administration. Severe Theoretical

▶ Letermovir is predicted to increase the concentration of **piperaquine**. Severe Theoretical

▶ Macrolides (clarithromycin, erythromycin) are predicted to increase the concentration of **piperaquine**. Severe Theoretical

▶ Mepacrine is predicted to increase the concentration of **primaquine**. Avoid. Moderate Theoretical

▶ **Pyrimethamine** is predicted to increase the risk of adverse effects when given with methotrexate. Severe Theoretical

▶ Metoclopramide decreases the concentration of **atovaquone**. Avoid. Moderate Study

▶ Mitotane is predicted to decrease the exposure to **artemether** (with lumefantrine). Avoid. Severe Study

▶ Mitotane is predicted to decrease the concentration of **piperaquine**. Avoid. Moderate Theoretical

▶ Neurokinin-1 receptor antagonists (aprepitant, netupitant) are predicted to increase the concentration of **piperaquine**. Severe Theoretical

▶ Nilotinib is predicted to increase the concentration of **piperaquine**. Severe Theoretical

▶ NNRTIs (efavirenz) decrease the concentration of **artemether**. Severe Study → Also see TABLE 9 p. 1431

▶ NNRTIs (efavirenz) moderately decrease the exposure to **atovaquone**. Avoid. Moderate Study

▶ NNRTIs (efavirenz) affect the exposure to **proguanil**. Avoid. Moderate Study

▶ NNRTIs (etravirine) decrease the exposure to **artemether**. Moderate Study

▶ **Pyrimethamine** is predicted to increase the risk of adverse effects when given with NRTIs (zidovudine). Severe Theoretical

▶ **Pyrimethamine** is predicted to increase the risk of adverse effects when given with pemetrexed. Severe Theoretical

▶ **Chloroquine** is predicted to increase the risk of haematological toxicity when given with penicillamine. Avoid. Severe Theoretical

▶ **Chloroquine** moderately decreases the exposure to praziquantel. Use with caution and adjust dose. Moderate Study

▶ **Chloroquine** decreases the efficacy of rabies vaccine (intradermal). Avoid. Moderate Study

▶ **Chloroquine** potentially decrease the effects of remdesivir. Avoid. Moderate Theoretical

▶ Rifamycins (rifabutin) slightly decrease the exposure to **atovaquone**. Avoid. Moderate Study

▶ Rifamycins (rifampicin) are predicted to decrease the exposure to **artemether** (with lumefantrine). Avoid. Severe Study

▶ Rifamycins (rifampicin) moderately decrease the exposure to **atovaquone** and **atovaquone** slightly increases the exposure to rifamycins (rifampicin). Moderate Study

▶ Rifamycins (rifampicin) moderately decrease the exposure to **mefloquine**. Severe Study

▶ Rifamycins (rifampicin) are predicted to decrease the concentration of **piperaquine**. Avoid. Moderate Theoretical

▶ Rifamycins (rifampicin) decrease the exposure to **quinine**. Severe Study

▶ St John's wort is predicted to decrease the concentration of **piperaquine**. Avoid. Moderate Theoretical

▶ **Pyrimethamine** increases the risk of adverse effects when given with sulfonamides. Severe Study

▶ Tetracyclines (tetracycline) decrease the concentration of **atovaquone**. Moderate Study

▶ **Pyrimethamine** increases the risk of adverse effects when given with trimethoprim. Severe Study

Antipsychotics, second generation → see TABLE 8 p. 1430 (hypotension), TABLE 9 p. 1431 (QT-interval prolongation), TABLE 11 p. 1431 (CNS depressant effects), TABLE 10 p. 1431 (antimuscarinics)

amisulpride · aripiprazole · asenapine · cariprazine · clozapine · lurasidone · olanzapine · paliperidone · quetiapine · risperidone

▶ **Clozapine** and **olanzapine** dose adjustment might be necessary if smoking started or stopped during treatment.

▸ Avoid concomitant use of **clozapine** with drugs that have a substantial potential for causing agranulocytosis.

▸ Anti-androgens (apalutamide, enzalutamide) are predicted to moderately decrease the exposure to **aripiprazole**. Adjust **aripiprazole** dose, p. 415. Moderate Study

▸ Anti-androgens (apalutamide, enzalutamide) are predicted to decrease the exposure to **cariprazine**. Avoid. Severe Theoretical

▸ Anti-androgens (apalutamide, enzalutamide) are predicted to decrease the exposure to **lurasidone**. Avoid. Moderate Study

▸ Anti-androgens (apalutamide, enzalutamide) are predicted to decrease the exposure to **paliperidone**. Monitor and adjust dose. Severe Study → Also see TABLE 9 p. 1431

▸ Anti-androgens (apalutamide, enzalutamide) are predicted to decrease the exposure to **quetiapine**. Moderate Study

▸ Anti-androgens (apalutamide, enzalutamide) are predicted to decrease the exposure to **risperidone**. Adjust dose. Moderate Study → Also see TABLE 9 p. 1431

▸ Anti-androgens (enzalutamide) are predicted to decrease the exposure to **clozapine**. Moderate Theoretical

▸ Antiarrhythmics (dronedarone) are predicted to increase the exposure to **cariprazine**. Avoid. Severe Study

▸ Antiarrhythmics (dronedarone) are predicted to increase the exposure to **lurasidone**. Adjust **lurasidone** dose, p. 418. Moderate Study

▸ Antiarrhythmics (dronedarone) are predicted to increase the exposure to **quetiapine**. Avoid. Moderate Study

▸ Antiepileptics (carbamazepine) are predicted to increase the risk of myelosuppression when given with **clozapine**. Avoid. Severe Anecdotal

▸ Antiepileptics (carbamazepine) potentially decrease the exposure to **olanzapine**. Monitor and adjust dose. Moderate Study

▸ Antiepileptics (carbamazepine, fosphenytoin, phenobarbital, phenytoin, primidone) are predicted to moderately decrease the exposure to **aripiprazole**. Adjust **aripiprazole** dose, p. 415. Moderate Study → Also see TABLE 11 p. 1431

▸ Antiepileptics (carbamazepine, fosphenytoin, phenobarbital, phenytoin, primidone) are predicted to decrease the exposure to **cariprazine**. Avoid. Severe Theoretical → Also see TABLE 11 p. 1431

▸ Antiepileptics (carbamazepine, fosphenytoin, phenobarbital, phenytoin, primidone) are predicted to decrease the exposure to **lurasidone**. Avoid. Moderate Study → Also see TABLE 11 p. 1431

▸ Antiepileptics (carbamazepine, fosphenytoin, phenobarbital, phenytoin, primidone) are predicted to decrease the exposure to **paliperidone**. Monitor and adjust dose. Severe Study → Also see TABLE 11 p. 1431

▸ Antiepileptics (carbamazepine, fosphenytoin, phenobarbital, phenytoin, primidone) are predicted to decrease the exposure to **quetiapine**. Moderate Study → Also see TABLE 11 p. 1431

▸ Antiepileptics (carbamazepine, fosphenytoin, phenobarbital, phenytoin, primidone) are predicted to decrease the exposure to **risperidone**. Adjust dose. Moderate Study → Also see TABLE 11 p. 1431

▸ Antiepileptics (fosphenytoin, phenobarbital, phenytoin, primidone) are predicted to decrease the exposure to **clozapine**. Moderate Anecdotal → Also see TABLE 11 p. 1431

▸ Antiepileptics (phenytoin) are predicted to decrease the exposure to **olanzapine**. Monitor and adjust dose. Moderate Study

▸ Antiepileptics (valproate) increase the risk of adverse effects when given with **olanzapine**. Severe Study

▸ Antiepileptics (valproate) slightly increase the exposure to **paliperidone**. Adjust dose. Moderate Study

▸ Antiepileptics (valproate) potentially increase the risk of neutropenia when given with **quetiapine**. Moderate Study

▸ Antifungals, azoles (fluconazole, isavuconazole) are predicted to increase the exposure to **lurasidone**. Adjust **lurasidone** dose, p. 418. Moderate Study

▸ Antifungals, azoles (fluconazole, isavuconazole, posaconazole) are predicted to increase the exposure to **cariprazine**. Avoid. Severe Study

▸ Antifungals, azoles (fluconazole, isavuconazole, posaconazole) are predicted to increase the exposure to **quetiapine**. Avoid. Moderate Study

▸ Antifungals, azoles (itraconazole, ketoconazole, voriconazole) are predicted to slightly increase the exposure to **aripiprazole**. Adjust **aripiprazole** dose, p. 415. Moderate Study

▸ Antifungals, azoles (itraconazole, ketoconazole, voriconazole) are predicted to moderately increase the exposure to **cariprazine**. Avoid. Severe Study

▸ Antifungals, azoles (itraconazole, ketoconazole, voriconazole) are predicted to increase the exposure to **risperidone**. Adjust dose. Moderate Study → Also see TABLE 9 p. 1431

▸ Antifungals, azoles (posaconazole) moderately increase the exposure to **lurasidone**. Avoid. Severe Study

▸ Antifungals, azoles (itraconazole, ketoconazole, voriconazole) are predicted to increase the exposure to antipsychotics, second generation (**lurasidone, quetiapine**). Avoid. Severe Study

▸ Bupropion is predicted to moderately increase the exposure to **aripiprazole**. Adjust **aripiprazole** dose, p. 415. Moderate Study

▸ Bupropion is predicted to increase the exposure to **risperidone**. Adjust dose. Moderate Study

▸ Calcium channel blockers (diltiazem, verapamil) are predicted to increase the exposure to **cariprazine**. Avoid. Severe Study → Also see TABLE 8 p. 1430

▸ Calcium channel blockers (diltiazem, verapamil) are predicted to increase the exposure to **lurasidone**, p. 418. Moderate Study → Also see TABLE 8 p. 1430

▸ Calcium channel blockers (diltiazem, verapamil) are predicted to increase the exposure to **quetiapine**. Avoid. Moderate Study → Also see TABLE 8 p. 1430

▸ Cinacalcet is predicted to moderately increase the exposure to **aripiprazole**. Adjust **aripiprazole** dose, p. 415. Moderate Study

▸ Cinacalcet is predicted to increase the exposure to **risperidone**. Adjust dose. Moderate Study

▸ Cobicistat is predicted to increase the exposure to antipsychotics, second generation (**lurasidone, quetiapine**). Avoid. Severe Study

▸ Cobicistat is predicted to slightly increase the exposure to **aripiprazole**. Adjust **aripiprazole** dose, p. 415. Moderate Study

▸ Cobicistat is predicted to moderately increase the exposure to **cariprazine**. Avoid. Severe Study

▸ Cobicistat is predicted to increase the exposure to **risperidone**. Adjust dose. Moderate Study

▸ Combined hormonal contraceptives increase the concentration of **clozapine**. Monitor adverse effects and adjust dose. Severe Study

▸ Crizotinib is predicted to increase the exposure to **cariprazine**. Avoid. Severe Study

▸ Crizotinib is predicted to increase the exposure to **lurasidone**. Adjust **lurasidone** dose, p. 418. Moderate Study

▸ Crizotinib is predicted to increase the exposure to **quetiapine**. Avoid. Moderate Study

▸ Antipsychotics, second generation (amisulpride, olanzapine, paliperidone, quetiapine, risperidone) are predicted to decrease the effects of dopamine receptor agonists. Avoid. Moderate Theoretical → Also see TABLE 8 p. 1430 → Also see TABLE 9 p. 1431

▸ Antipsychotics, second generation (aripiprazole, clozapine) are predicted to decrease the effects of dopamine receptor agonists. Moderate Theoretical → Also see TABLE 8 p. 1430 → Also see TABLE 10 p. 1431

▸ **Asenapine** is predicted to decrease the effects of dopamine receptor agonists. Adjust dose. Moderate Theoretical → Also see TABLE 8 p. 1430

▸ Endothelin receptor antagonists (bosentan) are predicted to decrease the exposure to **cariprazine**. Avoid. Severe Theoretical

▸ Endothelin receptor antagonists (bosentan) are predicted to decrease the exposure to **lurasidone**. Monitor and adjust dose. Moderate Theoretical

▸ Endothelin receptor antagonists (bosentan) are predicted to decrease the exposure to **quetiapine**. Moderate Study

▸ Grapefruit juice is predicted to increase the exposure to antipsychotics, second generation (**lurasidone, quetiapine**). Avoid. Severe Theoretical

▸ Grapefruit juice is predicted to increase the exposure to **cariprazine**. Avoid. Moderate Study

▸ HIV-protease inhibitors are predicted to increase the exposure to antipsychotics, second generation (**lurasidone, quetiapine**). Avoid. Severe Study

A1

Antipsychotics, second generation (continued)

▶ HIV-protease inhibitors are predicted to slightly increase the exposure to **aripiprazole**. Adjust **aripiprazole** dose, p. 415. Moderate Study

▶ HIV-protease inhibitors are predicted to moderately increase the exposure to **cariprazine**. Avoid. Severe Study

▶ HIV-protease inhibitors (ritonavir) are predicted to affect the exposure to **clozapine**. Avoid. Severe Theoretical

▶ HIV-protease inhibitors (ritonavir) are predicted to decrease the exposure to **olanzapine**. Monitor and adjust dose. Moderate Study

▶ HIV-protease inhibitors are predicted to increase the exposure to **risperidone**. Adjust dose. Moderate Study → Also see TABLE 9 p. 1431

▶ Idelalisib is predicted to increase the exposure to antipsychotics, second generation (**lurasidone, quetiapine**). Avoid. Severe Study

▶ Idelalisib is predicted to slightly increase the exposure to **aripiprazole**. Adjust **aripiprazole** dose, p. 415. Moderate Study

▶ Idelalisib is predicted to moderately increase the exposure to **cariprazine**. Avoid. Severe Study

▶ Idelalisib is predicted to increase the exposure to **risperidone**. Adjust dose. Moderate Study

▶ Imatinib is predicted to increase the exposure to **cariprazine**. Avoid. Severe Study

▶ Imatinib is predicted to increase the exposure to **lurasidone**. Adjust **lurasidone** dose, p. 418. Moderate Study

▶ Imatinib is predicted to increase the exposure to **quetiapine**. Avoid. Severe Study

▶ Iron chelators (deferasirox) are predicted to increase the exposure to **clozapine**. Avoid. Moderate Theoretical

▶ Leflunomide is predicted to decrease the exposure to **clozapine**. Moderate Theoretical

▶ Leflunomide is predicted to decrease the exposure to **olanzapine**. Monitor and adjust dose. Moderate Study

▶ Letermovir is predicted to increase the exposure to **cariprazine**. Avoid. Severe Study

▶ Letermovir is predicted to increase the exposure to **quetiapine**. Avoid. Moderate Study

▶ Amisulpride is predicted to decrease the effects of levodopa. Avoid. Severe Theoretical

▶ Antipsychotics, second generation (**aripiprazole, clozapine, lurasidone, paliperidone**) are predicted to decrease the effects of levodopa. Severe Theoretical → Also see TABLE 8 p. 1430

▶ Asenapine is predicted to decrease the effects of levodopa. Adjust dose. Severe Theoretical → Also see TABLE 8 p. 1430

▶ Olanzapine decreases the effects of levodopa. Avoid or monitor worsening parkinsonian symptoms. Severe Anecdotal → Also see TABLE 8 p. 1430

▶ Quetiapine decreases the effects of levodopa. Severe Anecdotal → Also see TABLE 8 p. 1430

▶ Risperidone is predicted to decrease the effects of levodopa. Avoid or adjust dose. Severe Anecdotal → Also see TABLE 8 p. 1430

▶ Antipsychotics, second generation (**quetiapine, risperidone**) potentially increase the risk of neurotoxicity when given with lithium. Severe Anecdotal → Also see TABLE 9 p. 1431

▶ Macrolides (clarithromycin) are predicted to slightly increase the exposure to **aripiprazole**. Adjust **aripiprazole** dose, p. 415. Moderate Study

▶ Macrolides (clarithromycin) are predicted to moderately increase the exposure to **cariprazine**. Avoid. Severe Study

▶ Macrolides (clarithromycin) are predicted to increase the exposure to **risperidone**. Adjust dose. Moderate Study → Also see TABLE 9 p. 1431

▶ Macrolides (erythromycin) are predicted to increase the exposure to **cariprazine**. Avoid. Severe Study

▶ Macrolides (erythromycin) potentially increase the risk of toxicity when given with **clozapine**. Severe Anecdotal

▶ Macrolides (erythromycin) are predicted to increase the exposure to **lurasidone**. Adjust **lurasidone** dose, p. 418. Moderate Study

▶ Macrolides (erythromycin) are predicted to increase the exposure to **quetiapine**. Avoid. Moderate Study

▶ Macrolides (clarithromycin) are predicted to increase the exposure to antipsychotics, second generation (**lurasidone, quetiapine**). Avoid. Severe Study

▶ Methylphenidate increases the risk of dyskinesias when given with **paliperidone**. Severe Theoretical

▶ Risperidone increases the risk of dyskinesias when given with methylphenidate. Severe Anecdotal

▶ Mexiletine increases the concentration of **clozapine**. Monitor adverse effects and adjust dose. Severe Study

▶ Mexiletine is predicted to increase the exposure to **olanzapine**. Adjust dose. Moderate Anecdotal

▶ Mitotane is predicted to moderately decrease the exposure to **aripiprazole**. Adjust **aripiprazole** dose, p. 415. Moderate Study

▶ Mitotane is predicted to decrease the exposure to **cariprazine**. Avoid. Severe Theoretical

▶ Mitotane is predicted to decrease the exposure to **lurasidone**. Avoid. Moderate Study

▶ Mitotane is predicted to decrease the exposure to **paliperidone**. Monitor and adjust dose. Severe Study

▶ Mitotane is predicted to decrease the exposure to **quetiapine**. Moderate Study

▶ Mitotane is predicted to decrease the exposure to **risperidone**. Adjust dose. Moderate Study

▶ Neurokinin-1 receptor antagonists (aprepitant, netupitant) are predicted to increase the exposure to **cariprazine**. Avoid. Severe Study

▶ Neurokinin-1 receptor antagonists (aprepitant, netupitant) are predicted to increase the exposure to **lurasidone**. Adjust **lurasidone** dose, p. 418. Moderate Study

▶ Neurokinin-1 receptor antagonists (aprepitant, netupitant) are predicted to increase the exposure to **quetiapine**. Avoid. Moderate Study

▶ Nilotinib is predicted to increase the exposure to **cariprazine**. Avoid. Severe Study

▶ Nilotinib is predicted to increase the exposure to **lurasidone**. Adjust **lurasidone** dose, p. 418. Moderate Study

▶ Nilotinib is predicted to increase the exposure to **quetiapine**. Avoid. Moderate Study

▶ NNRTIs (efavirenz, nevirapine) are predicted to decrease the exposure to **cariprazine**. Avoid. Severe Theoretical

▶ NNRTIs (efavirenz, nevirapine) are predicted to decrease the exposure to **lurasidone**. Monitor and adjust dose. Moderate Theoretical

▶ NNRTIs (efavirenz, nevirapine) are predicted to decrease the exposure to **quetiapine**. Moderate Study

▶ Quinolones (ciprofloxacin) increase the concentration of **clozapine**. Monitor adverse effects and adjust dose. Severe Study

▶ Quinolones (ciprofloxacin) are predicted to increase the exposure to **olanzapine**. Adjust dose. Moderate Anecdotal

▶ Ribociclib (high-dose) is predicted to increase the exposure to **quetiapine**. Avoid. Moderate Theoretical

▶ Rifamycins (rifampicin) are predicted to moderately decrease the exposure to **aripiprazole**. Adjust **aripiprazole** dose, p. 415. Moderate Study

▶ Rifamycins (rifampicin) are predicted to decrease the exposure to **cariprazine**. Avoid. Severe Theoretical

▶ Rifamycins (rifampicin) decrease the exposure to **clozapine**. Severe Anecdotal

▶ Rifamycins (rifampicin) are predicted to decrease the exposure to **lurasidone**. Avoid. Moderate Study

▶ Rifamycins (rifampicin) are predicted to decrease the exposure to **olanzapine**. Monitor and adjust dose. Moderate Study

▶ Rifamycins (rifampicin) are predicted to decrease the exposure to **paliperidone**. Monitor and adjust dose. Severe Study

▶ Rifamycins (rifampicin) are predicted to decrease the exposure to **quetiapine**. Moderate Study

▶ Rifamycins (rifampicin) are predicted to decrease the exposure to **risperidone**. Adjust dose. Moderate Study

▶ SSRIs (fluoxetine, paroxetine) are predicted to moderately increase the exposure to **aripiprazole**. Adjust **aripiprazole** dose, p. 415. Moderate Study

▶ SSRIs (fluoxetine, paroxetine) are predicted to increase the exposure to **risperidone**. Adjust dose. Moderate Study

SSRIs (fluvoxamine) increase the exposure to **asenapine**. Moderate Study

SSRIs (fluvoxamine) increase the concentration of **clozapine**. Monitor adverse effects and adjust dose. Severe Study

SSRIs (fluvoxamine) moderately increase the exposure to **olanzapine**. Adjust dose. Severe Anecdotal

SSRIs (paroxetine) moderately increase the exposure to **asenapine**. Moderate Study

St John's wort is predicted to decrease the exposure to **cariprazine**. Avoid. Severe Theoretical

St John's wort is predicted to decrease the exposure to **lurasidone**. Monitor and adjust dose. Moderate Theoretical

St John's wort is predicted to decrease the exposure to **paliperidone**. Severe Theoretical

St John's wort is predicted to decrease the exposure to **quetiapine**. Moderate Study

Terbinafine is predicted to moderately increase the exposure to **aripiprazole**. Adjust **aripiprazole** dose, p. 415. Moderate Study

Terbinafine is predicted to increase the exposure to **risperidone**. Adjust dose. Moderate Study

Teriflunomide is predicted to decrease the exposure to **clozapine**. Moderate Theoretical

Teriflunomide is predicted to decrease the exposure to **olanzapine**. Monitor and adjust dose. Moderate Study

Antithymocyte immunoglobulin (rabbit) → see immunoglobulins

Apalutamide → see anti-androgens

Apixaban → see factor XA inhibitors

Apomorphine → see dopamine receptor agonists

Apraclonidine → see TABLE 6 p. 1430 (bradycardia), TABLE 8 p. 1430 (hypotension), TABLE 11 p. 1431 (CNS depressant effects)

▸ Amfetamines are predicted to decrease the effects of **apraclonidine**. Avoid. Severe Theoretical

▸ Methylphenidate is predicted to decrease the effects of **apraclonidine**. Avoid. Severe Theoretical

▸ Sympathomimetics, inotropic are predicted to decrease the effects of **apraclonidine**. Avoid. Severe Theoretical

▸ Sympathomimetics, vasoconstrictor are predicted to decrease the effects of **apraclonidine**. Avoid. Severe Theoretical

Apremilast → see phosphodiesterase type-4 inhibitors

Aprepitant → see neurokinin-1 receptor antagonists

Argatroban → see thrombin inhibitors

Aripiprazole → see antipsychotics, second generation

Arsenic trioxide → see TABLE 15 p. 1432 (myelosuppression), TABLE 9 p. 1431 (QT-interval prolongation)

Artemether → see antimalarials

Artenimol → see antimalarials

Articaine → see TABLE 11 p. 1431 (CNS depressant effects)

Ascorbic acid

▸ Ascorbic acid is predicted to increase the risk of cardiovascular adverse effects when given with iron chelators (deferiprone, desferrioxamine). Severe Theoretical

Asenapine → see antipsychotics, second generation

Asparaginase → see TABLE 1 p. 1429 (hepatotoxicity), TABLE 15 p. 1432 (myelosuppression)

▸ Asparaginase is predicted to increase the risk of hepatotoxicity when given with imatinib. Severe Theoretical → Also see TABLE 15 p. 1432

▸ Asparaginase affects the efficacy of methotrexate. Severe Anecdotal → Also see TABLE 1 p. 1429 → Also see TABLE 15 p. 1432

▸ Asparaginase potentially increases the risk of neurotoxicity when given with vinca alkaloids (vincristine). **Vincristine** should be taken 3 to 24 hours before asparaginase. Severe Anecdotal → Also see TABLE 1 p. 1429 → Also see TABLE 15 p. 1432

Aspirin → see TABLE 4 p. 1429 (antiplatelet effects)

▸ Acetazolamide increases the risk of severe toxic reaction when given with **aspirin** (high-dose). Severe Study

▸ Oral antacids decrease the absorption of oral **aspirin** (high-dose). Moderate Study

▸ Bismuth subsalicylate is predicted to increase the risk of adverse effects when given with **aspirin**. Avoid. Moderate Theoretical

▸ Aspirin (high-dose) is predicted to increase the risk of gastrointestinal irritation when given with bisphosphonates (alendronate, ibandronate). Moderate Study

▸ Aspirin (high-dose) is predicted to increase the risk of renal impairment when given with bisphosphonates (clodronate). Severe Theoretical

▸ Corticosteroids are predicted to decrease the concentration of aspirin (high-dose) and **aspirin** (high-dose) increases the risk of gastrointestinal bleeding when given with corticosteroids. Moderate Study

▸ Aspirin (high-dose) increases the risk of renal impairment when given with daptomycin. Moderate Study

▸ Erlotinib is predicted to increase the risk of gastrointestinal perforation when given with **aspirin** (high-dose). Severe Theoretical

▸ Aspirin (high-dose) is predicted to increase the risk of gastrointestinal bleeds when given with iron chelators (deferasirox). Severe Theoretical

▸ Aspirin (high-dose) is predicted to increase the risk of toxicity when given with methotrexate. Severe Study

▸ Aspirin is predicted to increase the risk of gastrointestinal perforation when given with nicorandil. Severe Theoretical

▸ NRTIs (zidovudine) increase the risk of haematological toxicity when given with **aspirin** (high-dose). Severe Study

▸ Aspirin (high-dose) potentially increases the exposure to pemetrexed. Use with caution or avoid. Severe Theoretical

▸ Aspirin (high-dose) increases the risk of acute renal failure when given with thiazide diuretics. Severe Theoretical

Ataluren

▸ Ataluren is predicted to increase the risk of nephrotoxicity when given with intravenous aminoglycosides. Avoid. Severe Study

▸ Rifamycins (rifampicin) decrease the exposure to **ataluren**. Moderate Study

Atazanavir → see HIV-protease inhibitors

Atenolol → see beta blockers, selective

Atezolizumab → see monoclonal antibodies

Atomoxetine

▸ Amfetamines are predicted to increase the risk of adverse effects when given with **atomoxetine**. Severe Theoretical

▸ Atomoxetine is predicted to increase the risk of cardiovascular adverse effects when given with beta$_2$ agonists (high-dose). Moderate Study

▸ Bupropion is predicted to markedly increase the exposure to atomoxetine. Adjust dose. Severe Study

▸ Cinacalcet is predicted to markedly increase the exposure to atomoxetine. Adjust dose. Severe Study

▸ Dacomitinib is predicted to markedly increase the exposure to atomoxetine. Avoid or adjust dose. Severe Study

▸ Eliglustat is predicted to increase the exposure to **atomoxetine**. Adjust dose. Moderate Theoretical

▸ MAOIs, irreversible are predicted to increase the risk of adverse effects when given with **atomoxetine**. Avoid and for 2 weeks after stopping the MAOI. Severe Theoretical

▸ Panobinostat is predicted to increase the exposure to atomoxetine. Monitor and adjust dose. Severe Theoretical

▸ SSRIs (fluoxetine, paroxetine) are predicted to markedly increase the exposure to atomoxetine. Adjust dose. Severe Study

▸ Terbinafine is predicted to markedly increase the exposure to atomoxetine. Adjust dose. Severe Study

Atorvastatin → see statins

Atovaquone → see antimalarials

Atracurium → see neuromuscular blocking drugs, non-depolarising

Atropine → see TABLE 10 p. 1431 (antimuscarinics)

ROUTE-SPECIFIC INFORMATION Since systemic absorption can follow topical application of **atropine**, the possibility of interactions should be borne in mind.

▸ Atropine increases the risk of severe hypertension when given with sympathomimetics, vasoconstrictor (phenylephrine). Severe Study

Avanafil → see phosphodiesterase type-5 inhibitors

Avapritinib

▸ Anti-androgens (apalutamide, enzalutamide) are predicted to decrease the exposure to **avapritinib**. Avoid. Severe Study

▸ Antiarrhythmics (dronedarone) are predicted to increase the exposure to **avapritinib**. Avoid or adjust **avapritinib** dose, p. 1012. Moderate Study

Avapritinib (continued)

▶ Antiepileptics (carbamazepine, fosphenytoin, phenobarbital, phenytoin, primidone) are predicted to decrease the exposure to **avapritinib**. Avoid. (Severe) Study

▶ Antifungals, azoles (fluconazole, isavuconazole, posaconazole) are predicted to increase the exposure to **avapritinib**. Avoid or adjust **avapritinib** dose, p. 1012. (Moderate) Study

▶ Antifungals, azoles (itraconazole, ketoconazole, voriconazole) are predicted to increase the exposure to **avapritinib**. Avoid. (Moderate) Study

▶ Calcium channel blockers (diltiazem, verapamil) are predicted to increase the exposure to **avapritinib**. Avoid or adjust **avapritinib** dose, p. 1012. (Moderate) Study

▶ Cobicistat is predicted to increase the exposure to **avapritinib**. Avoid. (Moderate) Study

▶ Corticosteroids (dexamethasone) are predicted to decrease the exposure to **avapritinib**. Avoid. (Severe) Theoretical

▶ Crizotinib is predicted to increase the exposure to **avapritinib**. Avoid or adjust **avapritinib** dose, p. 1012. (Moderate) Study

▶ Endothelin receptor antagonists (bosentan) are predicted to decrease the exposure to **avapritinib**. Avoid. (Severe) Study

▶ Grapefruit juice is predicted to increase the exposure to **avapritinib**. (Moderate) Theoretical

▶ HIV-protease inhibitors are predicted to increase the exposure to **avapritinib**. Avoid. (Moderate) Study

▶ Idelalisib is predicted to increase the exposure to **avapritinib**. Avoid. (Moderate) Study

▶ Imatinib is predicted to increase the exposure to **avapritinib**. Avoid or adjust **avapritinib** dose, p. 1012. (Moderate) Study

▶ Letermovir is predicted to increase the exposure to **avapritinib**. Avoid or adjust **avapritinib** dose, p. 1012. (Moderate) Study

▶ Macrolides (clarithromycin) are predicted to increase the exposure to **avapritinib**. Avoid. (Moderate) Study

▶ Macrolides (erythromycin) are predicted to increase the exposure to **avapritinib**. Avoid or adjust **avapritinib** dose, p. 1012. (Moderate) Study

▶ Mitotane is predicted to decrease the exposure to **avapritinib**. Avoid. (Severe) Study

▶ Neurokinin-1 receptor antagonists (aprepitant, netupitant) are predicted to increase the exposure to **avapritinib**. Avoid or adjust **avapritinib** dose, p. 1012. (Moderate) Study

▶ Nilotinib is predicted to increase the exposure to **avapritinib**. Avoid or adjust **avapritinib** dose, p. 1012. (Moderate) Study

▶ NNRTIs (efavirenz, nevirapine) are predicted to decrease the exposure to **avapritinib**. Avoid. (Severe) Study

▶ NNRTIs (etravirine) are predicted to decrease the exposure to **avapritinib**. Avoid. (Severe) Theoretical

▶ Rifamycins (rifampicin) are predicted to decrease the exposure to **avapritinib**. Avoid. (Severe) Study

▶ St John's wort is predicted to decrease the exposure to **avapritinib**. Avoid. (Severe) Study

Avelumab → see monoclonal antibodies

Axitinib → see TABLE 15 p. 1432 (myelosuppression)

▶ Anti-androgens (apalutamide, enzalutamide) are predicted to decrease the exposure to **axitinib**. Avoid or adjust dose. (Moderate) Study

▶ Antiarrhythmics (dronedarone) are predicted to increase the exposure to **axitinib**. (Moderate) Theoretical

▶ Antiepileptics (carbamazepine, fosphenytoin, phenobarbital, phenytoin, primidone) are predicted to decrease the exposure to **axitinib**. Avoid or adjust dose. (Moderate) Study

▶ Antifungals, azoles (fluconazole, isavuconazole, posaconazole) are predicted to increase the exposure to **axitinib**. (Moderate) Theoretical

▶ Antifungals, azoles (itraconazole, ketoconazole, voriconazole) are predicted to increase the exposure to **axitinib**. Avoid or adjust dose. (Moderate) Study

▶ Calcium channel blockers (diltiazem, verapamil) are predicted to increase the exposure to **axitinib**. (Moderate) Theoretical

▶ Cobicistat is predicted to increase the exposure to **axitinib**. Avoid or adjust dose. (Moderate) Study

▶ **Axitinib** is predicted to increase the risk of bleeding events when given with coumarins. (Severe) Theoretical

▶ Crizotinib is predicted to increase the exposure to **axitinib**. (Moderate) Theoretical

▶ Endothelin receptor antagonists (bosentan) are predicted to decrease the exposure to **axitinib**. (Moderate) Theoretical

▶ Grapefruit juice is predicted to increase the exposure to **axitinib**. (Moderate) Theoretical

▶ HIV-protease inhibitors are predicted to increase the exposure to **axitinib**. Avoid or adjust dose. (Moderate) Study

▶ Idelalisib is predicted to increase the exposure to **axitinib**. Avoid or adjust dose. (Moderate) Study

▶ Imatinib is predicted to increase the exposure to **axitinib**. (Moderate) Theoretical → Also see TABLE 15 p. 1432

▶ Letermovir is predicted to increase the exposure to **axitinib**. (Moderate) Theoretical

▶ Macrolides (clarithromycin) are predicted to increase the exposure to **axitinib**. Avoid or adjust dose. (Moderate) Study

▶ Macrolides (erythromycin) are predicted to increase the exposure to **axitinib**. (Moderate) Theoretical

▶ Mitotane is predicted to decrease the exposure to **axitinib**. Avoid or adjust dose. (Moderate) Study → Also see TABLE 15 p. 1432

▶ Neurokinin-1 receptor antagonists (aprepitant, netupitant) are predicted to increase the exposure to **axitinib**. (Moderate) Theoretical

▶ Nilotinib is predicted to increase the exposure to **axitinib**. (Moderate) Theoretical → Also see TABLE 15 p. 1432

▶ NNRTIs (efavirenz, nevirapine) are predicted to decrease the exposure to **axitinib**. (Moderate) Theoretical

▶ **Axitinib** is predicted to increase the risk of bleeding events when given with phenindione. (Severe) Theoretical

▶ Rifamycins (rifampicin) are predicted to decrease the exposure to **axitinib**. Avoid or adjust dose. (Moderate) Study

▶ St John's wort is predicted to decrease the exposure to **axitinib**. (Moderate) Theoretical

Azacitidine → see TABLE 15 p. 1432 (myelosuppression)

Azathioprine → see TABLE 15 p. 1432 (myelosuppression)

▶ ACE inhibitors are predicted to increase the risk of anaemia and/or leucopenia when given with **azathioprine**. (Severe) Anecdotal

▶ Allopurinol potentially increases the risk of haematological toxicity when given with **azathioprine**. Adjust **azathioprine** dose, p. 882. (Severe) Study

▶ **Azathioprine** decreases the anticoagulant effect of coumarins. (Moderate) Study

▶ Febuxostat is predicted to increase the exposure to **azathioprine**. Avoid. (Severe) Theoretical

▶ Filgotinib is predicted to increase the risk of immunosuppression when given with **azathioprine**. Avoid. (Severe) Theoretical

▶ Live vaccines are predicted to increase the risk of generalised infection (possibly life-threatening) when given with **azathioprine** (high-dose). Public Health England advises avoid (refer to Green Book). (Severe) Theoretical

Azelastine → see antihistamines, non-sedating

Azilsartan → see angiotensin-II receptor antagonists

Azithromycin → see macrolides

Bacillus Calmette-Guérin vaccine → see live vaccines

Bacitracin → see TABLE 2 p. 1429 (nephrotoxicity)

Baclofen → see TABLE 8 p. 1430 (hypotension), TABLE 11 p. 1431 (CNS depressant effects), TABLE 10 p. 1431 (antimuscarinics)

▶ **Baclofen** is predicted to increase the risk of adverse effects when given with levodopa. (Severe) Anecdotal → Also see TABLE 8 p. 1430

Balsalazide

▶ **Balsalazide** is predicted to decrease the concentration of digoxin. (Moderate) Theoretical

Bambuterol → see beta₂ agonists

Baricitinib

▶ Filgotinib is predicted to increase the risk of immunosuppression when given with **baricitinib**. Avoid. (Severe) Theoretical

▶ Leflunomide potentially increases the exposure to **baricitinib**. (Moderate) Theoretical

▶ Live vaccines are predicted to increase the risk of generalised infection (possibly life-threatening) when given with **baricitinib**. Avoid. (Severe) Theoretical

▶ Teriflunomide potentially increases the exposure to **baricitinib**. (Moderate) Theoretical

Basiliximab → see monoclonal antibodies

Bazedoxifene

  Antiepileptics (carbamazepine, fosphenytoin, phenobarbital, phenytoin, primidone) are predicted to decrease the exposure to bazedoxifene. Moderate Theoretical

  Rifamycins (rifampicin) are predicted to decrease the exposure to bazedoxifene. Moderate Theoretical

Beclometasone → see corticosteroids

Bedaquiline → see TABLE 1 p. 1429 (hepatotoxicity), TABLE 9 p. 1431 (QT-interval prolongation)

▸ Anti-androgens (apalutamide, enzalutamide) decrease the exposure to bedaquiline. Avoid. Study → Also see TABLE 9 p. 1431

▸ Antiarrhythmics (dronedarone) are predicted to increase the exposure to bedaquiline. Avoid prolonged use. Mild Theoretical → Also see TABLE 9 p. 1431

▸ Antiepileptics (carbamazepine, fosphenytoin, phenobarbital, phenytoin, primidone) decrease the exposure to bedaquiline. Avoid. Severe Study → Also see TABLE 1 p. 1429

▸ Antifungals, azoles (fluconazole, isavuconazole, posaconazole) are predicted to increase the exposure to bedaquiline. Avoid prolonged use. Mild Theoretical → Also see TABLE 1 p. 1429 → Also see TABLE 9 p. 1431

▸ Antifungals, azoles (itraconazole, ketoconazole, voriconazole) are predicted to increase the exposure to bedaquiline. Avoid prolonged use. Mild Study → Also see TABLE 1 p. 1429 → Also see TABLE 9 p. 1431

▸ Calcium channel blockers (diltiazem, verapamil) are predicted to increase the exposure to bedaquiline. Avoid prolonged use. Mild Theoretical

▸ Clofazimine potentially increases the risk of QT-prolongation when given with bedaquiline. Severe Study

▸ Cobicistat is predicted to increase the exposure to bedaquiline. Avoid prolonged use. Mild Study

▸ Crizotinib is predicted to increase the exposure to bedaquiline. Avoid prolonged use. Mild Theoretical → Also see TABLE 9 p. 1431

▸ Endothelin receptor antagonists (bosentan) are predicted to decrease the exposure to bedaquiline. Avoid. Severe Study

▸ HIV-protease inhibitors are predicted to increase the exposure to bedaquiline. Avoid prolonged use. Mild Study → Also see TABLE 9 p. 1431

▸ Idelalisib is predicted to increase the exposure to bedaquiline. Avoid prolonged use. Mild Study

▸ Imatinib is predicted to increase the exposure to bedaquiline. Avoid prolonged use. Mild Theoretical

▸ Letermovir is predicted to increase the exposure to bedaquiline. Avoid prolonged use. Mild Theoretical

▸ Macrolides (clarithromycin) are predicted to increase the exposure to bedaquiline. Avoid prolonged use. Mild Study → Also see TABLE 9 p. 1431

▸ Macrolides (erythromycin) are predicted to increase the exposure to bedaquiline. Avoid prolonged use. Mild Theoretical → Also see TABLE 9 p. 1431

▸ Mitotane decreases the exposure to bedaquiline. Avoid. Severe Study

▸ Neurokinin-1 receptor antagonists (aprepitant, netupitant) are predicted to increase the exposure to bedaquiline. Avoid prolonged use. Mild Theoretical

▸ Nilotinib is predicted to increase the exposure to bedaquiline. Avoid prolonged use. Mild Theoretical → Also see TABLE 9 p. 1431

▸ NNRTIs (efavirenz, nevirapine) are predicted to decrease the exposure to bedaquiline. Avoid. Severe Study → Also see TABLE 9 p. 1431

▸ NNRTIs (etravirine) are predicted to decrease the exposure to bedaquiline. Avoid. Severe Theoretical

▸ Rifamycins (rifampicin) decrease the exposure to bedaquiline. Avoid. Severe Study

▸ St John's wort is predicted to decrease the exposure to bedaquiline. Avoid. Severe Study

Bee venom extract

  GENERAL INFORMATION Desensitising vaccines should be avoided in patients taking beta-blockers (adrenaline might be ineffective in case of a hypersensitivity reaction) or ACE inhibitors (risk of severe anaphylactoid reactions).

Belatacept → see TABLE 15 p. 1432 (myelosuppression)

▸ Live vaccines are predicted to increase the risk of generalised infection (possibly life-threatening) when given with belatacept. Public Health England advises avoid (refer to Green Book). Severe Theoretical

Belimumab → see monoclonal antibodies

Bempedoic acid

▸ Bempedoic acid increases the exposure to statins (simvastatin). Adjust simvastatin dose, p. 219. Moderate Study

Bendamustine → see alkylating agents

Bendroflumethiazide → see thiazide diuretics

Benperidol → see TABLE 8 p. 1430 (hypotension), TABLE 11 p. 1431 (CNS depressant effects)

▸ Benperidol is predicted to decrease the effects of dopamine receptor agonists. Avoid. Moderate Theoretical → Also see TABLE 8 p. 1430

▸ Benperidol is predicted to decrease the effects of levodopa. Severe Study → Also see TABLE 8 p. 1430

Benzathine benzylpenicillin → see penicillins

Benzodiazepines → see TABLE 11 p. 1431 (CNS depressant effects)

> alprazolam · chlordiazepoxide · clobazam · clonazepam · diazepam · flurazepam · loprazolam · lorazepam · lormetazepam · midazolam · nitrazepam · oxazepam · temazepam

▸ Anti-androgens (apalutamide) are predicted to decrease the exposure to diazepam. Avoid or monitor. Mild Study

▸ Anti-androgens (apalutamide, enzalutamide) are predicted to decrease the exposure to alprazolam. Adjust dose. Moderate Theoretical

▸ Anti-androgens (apalutamide, enzalutamide) are predicted to decrease the exposure to midazolam. Monitor and adjust dose. Moderate Study

▸ Antiarrhythmics (dronedarone) are predicted to increase the exposure to alprazolam. Severe Study

▸ Antiarrhythmics (dronedarone) are predicted to increase the exposure to midazolam. Monitor adverse effects and adjust dose. Severe Study

▸ Antiepileptics (carbamazepine, fosphenytoin, phenobarbital, phenytoin, primidone) are predicted to decrease the exposure to alprazolam. Adjust dose. Moderate Theoretical → Also see TABLE 11 p. 1431

▸ Antiepileptics (carbamazepine, fosphenytoin, phenobarbital, phenytoin, primidone) are predicted to decrease the exposure to midazolam. Monitor and adjust dose. Moderate Study → Also see TABLE 11 p. 1431

▸ Antiepileptics (stiripentol) increase the concentration of clobazam. Severe Study

▸ Chlordiazepoxide affects the concentration of antiepileptics (fosphenytoin, phenytoin). Severe Study

▸ Diazepam potentially affects the concentration of antiepileptics (fosphenytoin, phenytoin). Monitor concentration and adjust dose. Severe Study

▸ Benzodiazepines (clobazam, clonazepam) potentially affect the concentration of antiepileptics (fosphenytoin, phenytoin). Severe Anecdotal

▸ Antifungals, azoles (fluconazole, isavuconazole, posaconazole) are predicted to increase the exposure to alprazolam. Severe Study

▸ Antifungals, azoles (fluconazole, isavuconazole, posaconazole) are predicted to increase the exposure to midazolam. Monitor adverse effects and adjust dose. Severe Study

▸ Antifungals, azoles (fluconazole, voriconazole) potentially increase the exposure to clobazam. Adjust dose. Moderate Theoretical

▸ Antifungals, azoles (fluconazole, voriconazole) moderately increase the exposure to diazepam. Monitor and adjust dose. Moderate Study

▸ Antifungals, azoles (itraconazole, ketoconazole, voriconazole) moderately increase the exposure to alprazolam. Avoid. Moderate Study

▸ Antifungals, azoles (itraconazole, ketoconazole, voriconazole) are predicted to markedly to very markedly increase the exposure to midazolam. Avoid or adjust dose. Severe Study

▸ Antifungals, azoles (miconazole) are predicted to increase the exposure to alprazolam. Use with caution and adjust dose. Moderate Theoretical

A1

Interactions | Appendix 1

Benzodiazepines (continued)

▸ Antifungals, azoles (miconazole) are predicted to increase the exposure to intravenous **midazolam**. Use with caution and adjust dose. Moderate Theoretical

▸ Antifungals, azoles (miconazole) are predicted to increase the exposure to oral **midazolam**. Avoid. Moderate Theoretical

▸ Calcium channel blockers (diltiazem, verapamil) are predicted to increase the exposure to **alprazolam**. Severe Study

▸ Calcium channel blockers (diltiazem, verapamil) are predicted to increase the exposure to **midazolam**. Monitor adverse effects and adjust dose. Severe Study

▸ Cannabidiol increases the exposure to the active metabolite of **clobazam** and **clobazam** increases the exposure to the active metabolite of cannabidiol. Adjust dose. Moderate Study → Also see **TABLE 11** p. 1431

▸ Cobicistat moderately increases the exposure to **alprazolam**. Avoid. Moderate Study

▸ Cobicistat is predicted to markedly to very markedly increase the exposure to **midazolam**. Avoid or adjust dose. Severe Study

▸ Crizotinib is predicted to increase the exposure to **alprazolam**. Severe Study

▸ Crizotinib is predicted to increase the exposure to **midazolam**. Monitor adverse effects and adjust dose. Severe Study

▸ Dabrafenib decreases the exposure to **midazolam**. Monitor and adjust dose. Moderate Study

▸ Endothelin receptor antagonists (bosentan) are predicted to decrease the concentration of **midazolam**. Monitor and adjust dose. Moderate Theoretical

▸ Entrectinib slightly increases the exposure to **midazolam**. Mild Study

▸ HIV-protease inhibitors moderately increase the exposure to **alprazolam**. Avoid. Moderate Study

▸ HIV-protease inhibitors (ritonavir) are predicted to increase the exposure to benzodiazepines (**diazepam, flurazepam**). Avoid. Moderate Theoretical

▸ HIV-protease inhibitors are predicted to markedly to very markedly increase the exposure to **midazolam**. Avoid or adjust dose. Severe Study

▸ Idelalisib moderately increases the exposure to **alprazolam**. Avoid. Moderate Study

▸ Idelalisib is predicted to markedly to very markedly increase the exposure to **midazolam**. Avoid or adjust dose. Severe Study

▸ Imatinib is predicted to increase the exposure to **alprazolam**. Severe Study

▸ Imatinib is predicted to increase the exposure to **midazolam**. Monitor adverse effects and adjust dose. Severe Study

▸ Larotrectinib slightly increases the exposure to **midazolam**. Use with caution and adjust dose. Mild Study

▸ Letermovir is predicted to increase the exposure to **alprazolam**. Severe Study

▸ Letermovir is predicted to increase the exposure to **midazolam**. Monitor adverse effects and adjust dose. Severe Study

▸ **Alprazolam** is predicted to increase the exposure to lomitapide. Separate administration by 12 hours. Moderate Theoretical

▸ Lorlatinib moderately decreases the exposure to **midazolam**. Avoid. Moderate Study

▸ Lumacaftor is predicted to decrease the exposure to **midazolam**. Avoid. Severe Theoretical

▸ Macrolides (clarithromycin) moderately increase the exposure to **alprazolam**. Avoid. Moderate Study

▸ Macrolides (clarithromycin) are predicted to markedly to very markedly increase the exposure to **midazolam**. Avoid or adjust dose. Severe Study

▸ Macrolides (erythromycin) are predicted to increase the exposure to **alprazolam**. Severe Study

▸ Macrolides (erythromycin) are predicted to increase the exposure to **midazolam**. Monitor adverse effects and adjust dose. Severe Study

▸ Mitotane is predicted to decrease the exposure to **alprazolam**. Adjust dose. Moderate Theoretical

▸ Mitotane is predicted to decrease the exposure to **midazolam**. Monitor and adjust dose. Moderate Study

▸ Moclobemide potentially increases the exposure to **clobazam**. Adjust dose. Moderate Theoretical

▸ Monoclonal antibodies (tocilizumab) are predicted to decrease the exposure to benzodiazepines (**alprazolam, diazepam, midazolam**). Monitor and adjust dose. Moderate Theoretical

▸ Neurokinin-1 receptor antagonists (aprepitant, netupitant) are predicted to increase the exposure to **alprazolam**. Severe Study

▸ Neurokinin-1 receptor antagonists (aprepitant, netupitant) are predicted to increase the exposure to **midazolam**. Monitor adverse effects and adjust dose. Severe Study

▸ Neurokinin-1 receptor antagonists (fosaprepitant) are predicted to increase the exposure to **alprazolam**. Moderate Study

▸ Neurokinin-1 receptor antagonists (fosaprepitant) slightly increase the exposure to **midazolam**. Moderate Study

▸ Nilotinib is predicted to increase the exposure to **alprazolam**. Severe Study

▸ Nilotinib is predicted to increase the exposure to **midazolam**. Monitor adverse effects and adjust dose. Severe Study

▸ NNRTIs (efavirenz) are predicted to alter the effects of **midazolam**. Avoid. Moderate Theoretical

▸ NNRTIs (nevirapine) decrease the concentration of **midazolam**. Monitor and adjust dose. Moderate Study

▸ Palbociclib increases the exposure to **midazolam**. Moderate Study

▸ Proton pump inhibitors (esomeprazole, omeprazole) potentially increase the exposure to **clobazam**. Adjust dose. Moderate Theoretical

▸ Ribociclib moderately increases the exposure to **midazolam**. Avoid. Moderate Study

▸ Rifamycins (rifampicin) are predicted to decrease the exposure to **alprazolam**. Adjust dose. Moderate Theoretical

▸ Rifamycins (rifampicin) are predicted to decrease the exposure to **chlordiazepoxide**. Moderate Theoretical

▸ Rifamycins (rifampicin) moderately decrease the exposure to **diazepam**. Avoid. Moderate Study

▸ Rifamycins (rifampicin) are predicted to decrease the exposure to **midazolam**. Monitor and adjust dose. Moderate Study

▸ Rifamycins (rifampicin) increase the clearance of benzodiazepines (**lorazepam, nitrazepam**). Moderate Study

▸ Rucaparib slightly increases the exposure to **midazolam**. Monitor and adjust dose. Severe Study

▸ SSRIs (fluoxetine, fluvoxamine) potentially increase the exposure to **clobazam**. Adjust dose. Moderate Theoretical

▸ SSRIs (fluvoxamine) moderately increase the exposure to **alprazolam**. Adjust dose. Moderate Study

▸ SSRIs (fluvoxamine) moderately increase the exposure to **diazepam**. Moderate Study

▸ St John's wort moderately decreases the exposure to **alprazolam**. Moderate Study

▸ St John's wort moderately decreases the exposure to **midazolam**. Monitor and adjust dose. Moderate Study

▸ Telotristat ethyl decreases the exposure to **midazolam**. Moderate Study

Benzydamine → see NSAIDs

Benzylpenicillin → see penicillins

Beta blockers, non-selective → see **TABLE 6** p. 1430 (bradycardia), **TABLE 8** p. 1430 (hypotension), **TABLE 9** p. 1431 (QT-interval prolongation)

carvedilol · labetalol · levobunolol · nadolol · pindolol · propranolol · sotalol · timolol

ROUTE-SPECIFIC INFORMATION Since systemic absorption can follow topical application of **levobunolol** and **timolol**, the possibility of interactions should be borne in mind.

▸ **Beta blockers, non-selective** are predicted to increase the risk of bronchospasm when given with aminophylline. Avoid. Severe Theoretical

▸ Antiarrhythmics (amiodarone, disopyramide, dronedarone, flecainide, lidocaine) are predicted to increase the risk of cardiovascular adverse effects when given with **beta blockers, non-selective**. Use with caution or avoid. Severe Study → Also see **TABLE 6** p. 1430 → Also see **TABLE 9** p. 1431

▸ Antiarrhythmics (propafenone) increase the risk of cardiovascular adverse effects when given with **propranolol**. Use with caution or avoid. Severe Study

▸ Antiarrhythmics (propafenone) are predicted to increase the exposure to **timolol** and **timolol** is predicted to increase the risk

of cardiodepression when given with antiarrhythmics (propafenone). [Severe] Anecdotal
▸ Antiarrhythmics (propafenone) are predicted to increase the risk of cardiovascular adverse effects when given with beta blockers, non-selective (**labetalol, levobunolol, nadolol, pindolol, sotalol**). Use with caution or avoid. [Severe] Study
▸ Antiepileptics (phenobarbital, primidone) are predicted to decrease the exposure to **propranolol**. [Moderate] Study
▸ Antiepileptics (phenobarbital, primidone) are predicted to decrease the exposure to beta blockers, non-selective (**carvedilol, labetalol**). [Moderate] Theoretical
▸ Antifungals, azoles (itraconazole, ketoconazole) are predicted to increase the exposure to **nadolol**. [Moderate] Study
▸ Antimalarials (mefloquine) are predicted to increase the risk of bradycardia when given with beta blockers, non-selective. [Severe] Theoretical
▸ Calcium channel blockers (diltiazem) are predicted to increase the risk of cardiodepression when given with **beta blockers, non-selective**. [Severe] Study → Also see **TABLE 6** p. 1430 → Also see **TABLE 8** p. 1430
▸ Calcium channel blockers (verapamil) increase the risk of cardiovascular adverse effects when given with **beta blockers, non-selective**. Avoid intravenous **verapamil**. [Severe] Study → Also see **TABLE 6** p. 1430 → Also see **TABLE 8** p. 1430
▸ Chloroprocaine is predicted to increase the risk of cardiovascular adverse effects when given with **sotalol**. [Severe] Theoretical
▸ Ciclosporin is predicted to increase the exposure to **nadolol**. [Moderate] Study
▸ Dacomitinib is predicted to markedly increase the exposure to **propranolol**. Avoid. [Severe] Study
▸ Eliglustat is predicted to increase the exposure to **propranolol**. Adjust dose. [Moderate] Study
▸ **Beta blockers, non-selective** are predicted to increase the risk of peripheral vasoconstriction when given with ergometrine. [Severe] Study
▸ **Beta blockers, non-selective** are predicted to increase the risk of peripheral vasoconstriction when given with ergotamine. [Severe] Study
▸ HIV-protease inhibitors (lopinavir, ritonavir, saquinavir) are predicted to increase the exposure to **nadolol**. [Moderate] Study
▸ **Beta blockers, non-selective** are predicted to increase the risk of bradycardia when given with lanreotide. [Moderate] Theoretical
▸ Lapatinib is predicted to increase the exposure to **nadolol**. [Moderate] Study
▸ Macrolides are predicted to increase the exposure to **nadolol**. [Moderate] Study
▸ Mexiletine potentially increases the risk of cardiovascular adverse effects when given with **beta blockers, non-selective**. Avoid or monitor. [Severe] Theoretical
▸ Ranolazine is predicted to increase the exposure to **nadolol**. [Moderate] Study
▸ Rifamycins (rifampicin) moderately decrease the exposure to **carvedilol**. [Moderate] Study
▸ Rifamycins (rifampicin) decrease the exposure to **propranolol**. Monitor and adjust dose. [Moderate] Study
▸ SSRIs (fluvoxamine) moderately increase the concentration of **propranolol**. [Moderate] Study
▸ **Beta blockers, non-selective** increase the risk of hypertension and bradycardia when given with sympathomimetics, inotropic (dobutamine). [Severe] Theoretical
▸ **Beta blockers, non-selective** are predicted to increase the risk of hypertension and bradycardia when given with sympathomimetics, vasoconstrictor (adrenaline/epinephrine, noradrenaline/norepinephrine). [Severe] Study
▸ **Beta blockers, non-selective** are predicted to increase the risk of bronchospasm when given with theophylline. Avoid. [Severe] Theoretical
▸ **Propranolol** slightly to moderately increases the exposure to triptans (rizatriptan). Adjust **rizatriptan** dose and separate administration by at least 2 hours, p. 501. [Moderate] Study
▸ Vemurafenib is predicted to increase the exposure to **nadolol**. [Moderate] Study

Beta blockers, selective → see **TABLE 6** p. 1430 (bradycardia), **TABLE 8** p. 1430 (hypotension)

acebutolol · atenolol · betaxolol · bisoprolol · celiprolol · esmolol · metoprolol · nebivolol

▸ Since systemic absorption can follow topical application of **betaxolol**, the possibility of interactions should be borne in mind.
▸ Orange juice greatly decreases the exposure to **celiprolol**.

▸ **Beta blockers, selective** are predicted to increase the risk of bronchospasm when given with aminophylline. Avoid. [Severe] Theoretical
▸ Anti-androgens (abiraterone) are predicted to increase the exposure to **metoprolol**. [Moderate] Study
▸ Antiarrhythmics (amiodarone, disopyramide, dronedarone, flecainide, lidocaine) are predicted to increase the risk of cardiovascular adverse effects when given with **beta blockers, selective**. Use with caution or avoid. [Severe] Study → Also see **TABLE 6** p. 1430
▸ Antiarrhythmics (propafenone) are predicted to increase the exposure to **metoprolol**. [Moderate] Study
▸ Antiarrhythmics (propafenone) are predicted to increase the exposure to **nebivolol** and **nebivolol** is predicted to increase the risk of cardiodepression when given with antiarrhythmics (propafenone). Avoid. [Severe] Theoretical
▸ Antiarrhythmics (propafenone) are predicted to increase the risk of cardiovascular adverse effects when given with beta blockers, selective (**acebutolol, atenolol, betaxolol, bisoprolol, celiprolol, esmolol**). Use with caution or avoid. [Severe] Study
▸ Antiepileptics (phenobarbital, primidone) are predicted to decrease the exposure to beta blockers, selective (**acebutolol, bisoprolol, metoprolol, nebivolol**). [Moderate] Study
▸ Antimalarials (mefloquine) are predicted to increase the risk of bradycardia when given with **beta blockers, selective**. [Severe] Theoretical
▸ Bupropion is predicted to increase the exposure to beta blockers, selective (**metoprolol, nebivolol**). [Moderate] Study
▸ Calcium channel blockers (diltiazem) are predicted to increase the risk of cardiodepression when given with **beta blockers, selective**. [Severe] Study → Also see **TABLE 6** p. 1430 → Also see **TABLE 8** p. 1430
▸ Calcium channel blockers (verapamil) increase the risk of cardiovascular adverse effects when given with **beta blockers, selective**. Avoid intravenous **verapamil**. [Severe] Study → Also see **TABLE 6** p. 1430 → Also see **TABLE 8** p. 1430
▸ Cinacalcet is predicted to increase the exposure to beta blockers, selective (**metoprolol, nebivolol**). [Moderate] Study
▸ Dacomitinib is predicted to markedly increase the exposure to beta blockers, selective (**metoprolol, nebivolol**). Avoid. [Severe] Study
▸ Duloxetine is predicted to increase the exposure to **metoprolol**. [Moderate] Study
▸ Eliglustat is predicted to increase the exposure to **metoprolol**. Adjust dose. [Moderate] Study
▸ **Beta blockers, selective** are predicted to increase the risk of peripheral vasoconstriction when given with ergometrine. [Severe] Study
▸ **Beta blockers, selective** are predicted to increase the risk of peripheral vasoconstriction when given with ergotamine. [Severe] Study
▸ Grapefruit juice greatly decreases the exposure to **celiprolol**. [Moderate] Study
▸ HIV-protease inhibitors (ritonavir) are predicted to increase the exposure to **metoprolol**. [Moderate] Study
▸ **Beta blockers, selective** are predicted to increase the risk of bradycardia when given with lanreotide. [Moderate] Theoretical
▸ Mexiletine potentially increases the risk of cardiovascular adverse effects when given with **beta blockers, selective**. Avoid or monitor. [Severe] Theoretical
▸ Mirabegron is predicted to increase the exposure to **metoprolol**. [Moderate] Study
▸ Panobinostat is predicted to increase the exposure to **metoprolol**. Monitor and adjust dose. [Moderate] Theoretical
▸ Panobinostat is predicted to increase the exposure to **nebivolol**. Monitor and adjust dose. [Mild] Theoretical
▸ Rifamycins (rifampicin) moderately decrease the exposure to **celiprolol**. [Moderate] Study

Beta blockers, selective (continued)
▸ Rifamycins (rifampicin) slightly decrease the exposure to beta blockers, selective (**bisoprolol, metoprolol**). [Mild] Study
▸ SSRIs (fluoxetine, paroxetine) are predicted to increase the exposure to beta blockers, selective (**metoprolol, nebivolol**). [Moderate] Study
▸ **Beta blockers, selective** increase the risk of hypertension and bradycardia when given with sympathomimetics, inotropic (dobutamine). [Moderate] Theoretical
▸ **Beta blockers, selective** are predicted to increase the risk of hypertension and bradycardia when given with sympathomimetics, vasoconstrictor (adrenaline/epinephrine, noradrenaline/norepinephrine). [Severe] Study
▸ Terbinafine is predicted to increase the exposure to beta blockers, selective (**metoprolol, nebivolol**). [Moderate] Study
▸ **Beta blockers, selective** are predicted to increase the risk of bronchospasm when given with theophylline. Avoid. [Severe] Theoretical
▸ Vaborbactam is predicted to increase the concentration of **metoprolol**. [Unknown] Theoretical
Beta₂ agonists → see TABLE 17 p. 1433 (reduced serum potassium)

bambuterol · formoterol · indacaterol · olodaterol · salbutamol · salmeterol · terbutaline · vilanterol

▸ Anti-androgens (apalutamide) are predicted to decrease the exposure to **salmeterol**. Avoid or monitor. [Moderate] Study
▸ Antifungals, azoles (itraconazole, ketoconazole, voriconazole) are predicted to increase the exposure to **salmeterol**. Avoid. [Severe] Study
▸ Atomoxetine is predicted to increase the risk of cardiovascular adverse effects when given with **beta₂ agonists** (high-dose). [Moderate] Study
▸ Cobicistat is predicted to increase the exposure to **salmeterol**. Avoid. [Severe] Study
▸ HIV-protease inhibitors are predicted to increase the exposure to **salmeterol**. Avoid. [Severe] Study
▸ Idelalisib is predicted to increase the exposure to **salmeterol**. Avoid. [Severe] Study
▸ **Beta₂ agonists** are predicted to increase the risk of glaucoma when given with ipratropium. [Moderate] Anecdotal
▸ **Beta₂ agonists** are predicted to increase the risk of elevated blood pressure when given with linezolid. Avoid. [Severe] Theoretical
▸ Macrolides (clarithromycin) are predicted to increase the exposure to **salmeterol**. Avoid. [Severe] Study
▸ MAO-B inhibitors (rasagiline, selegiline) are predicted to increase the risk of severe hypertension when given with **beta₂ agonists**. Avoid. [Severe] Theoretical
▸ MAO-B inhibitors (safinamide) are predicted to increase the risk of severe hypertension when given with **beta₂ agonists**. [Severe] Theoretical
▸ MAOIs, irreversible are predicted to increase the risk of cardiovascular adverse effects when given with **beta₂ agonists**. [Moderate] Anecdotal
▸ Neurokinin-1 receptor antagonists (aprepitant, netupitant) are predicted to increase the exposure to **salmeterol**. [Moderate] Study
Betahistine
▸ Antihistamines, non-sedating are predicted to decrease the effects of **betahistine**. [Moderate] Theoretical
▸ Antihistamines, sedating are predicted to decrease the effects of **betahistine**. [Moderate] Theoretical
Betamethasone → see corticosteroids
Betaxolol → see beta blockers, selective
Bevacizumab → see monoclonal antibodies
Bexarotene → see retinoids
Bezafibrate → see fibrates
Bicalutamide → see anti-androgens
Bictegravir
▸ Oral antacids decrease the exposure to oral **bictegravir**. Separate administration by 2 hours. [Moderate] Study
▸ Anti-androgens (apalutamide, enzalutamide) are predicted to decrease the exposure to **bictegravir**. Avoid. [Moderate] Study
▸ Antiarrhythmics (amiodarone, dronedarone) are predicted to increase the exposure to **bictegravir**. Use with caution or avoid. [Moderate] Theoretical

▸ Antiepileptics (carbamazepine, fosphenytoin, phenobarbital, phenytoin, primidone) are predicted to decrease the exposure to **bictegravir**. Avoid. [Moderate] Study
▸ Antiepileptics (oxcarbazepine) are predicted to decrease the exposure to **bictegravir**. Avoid. [Moderate] Theoretical
▸ Antifungals, azoles (itraconazole, ketoconazole) are predicted to increase the exposure to **bictegravir**. Use with caution or avoid. [Moderate] Theoretical
▸ Antifungals, azoles (posaconazole) are predicted to increase the exposure to **bictegravir**. [Moderate] Theoretical
▸ Calcium channel blockers (verapamil) are predicted to increase the exposure to **bictegravir**. Use with caution or avoid. [Moderate] Theoretical
▸ Ciclosporin is predicted to increase the exposure to **bictegravir**. Use with caution or avoid. [Moderate] Theoretical
▸ HIV-protease inhibitors (atazanavir) moderately increase the exposure to **bictegravir**. Avoid. [Severe] Study
▸ HIV-protease inhibitors (lopinavir, ritonavir, saquinavir) are predicted to increase the exposure to **bictegravir**. Use with caution or avoid. [Moderate] Theoretical
▸ Oral iron decreases the exposure to oral **bictegravir**. Manufacturer advises bictegravir should be taken 2 hours before iron. [Moderate] Study
▸ Lapatinib is predicted to increase the exposure to **bictegravir**. Use with caution or avoid. [Moderate] Theoretical
▸ Macrolides are predicted to increase the exposure to **bictegravir**. Use with caution or avoid. [Moderate] Theoretical
▸ **Bictegravir** slightly increases the exposure to metformin. [Moderate] Study
▸ Mitotane is predicted to decrease the exposure to **bictegravir**. Avoid. [Moderate] Study
▸ **Bictegravir** is predicted to increase the exposure to opioids (methadone). [Moderate] Theoretical
▸ Ranolazine is predicted to increase the exposure to **bictegravir**. Use with caution or avoid. [Moderate] Theoretical
▸ Rifamycins (rifabutin) slightly decrease the exposure to **bictegravir**. Avoid. [Moderate] Study
▸ Rifamycins (rifampicin) are predicted to decrease the exposure to **bictegravir**. Avoid. [Moderate] Study
▸ St John's wort is predicted to decrease the exposure to **bictegravir**. Avoid. [Moderate] Theoretical
▸ Sucralfate is predicted to decrease the exposure to **bictegravir**. Avoid. [Moderate] Theoretical
▸ Vemurafenib is predicted to increase the exposure to **bictegravir**. Use with caution or avoid. [Moderate] Theoretical
Bilastine → see antihistamines, non-sedating
Bismuth
▸ Bismuth subsalicylate is predicted to increase the risk of adverse effects when given with aspirin. Avoid. [Moderate] Theoretical
▸ Bismuth subsalicylate is predicted to increase the risk of bleeding events when given with drugs with anticoagulant effects (see TABLE 3 p. 1429). [Moderate] Theoretical
▸ Bismuth greatly decreases the efficacy of tetracyclines. Separate administration by 2 hours. [Moderate] Study
Bisoprolol → see beta blockers, selective
Bisphosphonates → see TABLE 2 p. 1429 (nephrotoxicity)

alendronate · clodronate · ibandronate · pamidronate · risedronate · zoledronate

▸ Aminoglycosides increase the risk of hypocalcaemia when given with **bisphosphonates**. [Moderate] Anecdotal → Also see TABLE 2 p. 1429
▸ Oral antacids decrease the absorption of oral **alendronate**. Alendronate should be taken at least 30 minutes before antacids. [Moderate] Study
▸ Oral antacids decrease the absorption of oral **clodronate**. Avoid antacids for 2 hours before or 1 hour after **clodronate**. [Moderate] Study
▸ Oral antacids are predicted to decrease the absorption of oral **ibandronate**. Avoid antacids for at least 6 hours before or 1 hour after **ibandronate**. [Moderate] Theoretical
▸ Oral antacids decrease the absorption of oral **risedronate**. Separate administration by at least 2 hours. [Moderate] Study

Aspirin (high-dose) is predicted to increase the risk of gastrointestinal irritation when given with bisphosphonates (**alendronate, ibandronate**). Moderate Study

Aspirin (high-dose) is predicted to increase the risk of renal impairment when given with **clodronate**. Severe Theoretical

Oral calcium salts decrease the absorption of **alendronate**. **Alendronate** should be taken at least 30 minutes before **calcium salts**. Moderate Study

Oral calcium salts decrease the absorption of **clodronate**. Avoid **calcium salts** for 2 hours before or 1 hour after **clodronate**. Moderate Study

Oral calcium salts are predicted to decrease the absorption of oral **ibandronate**. Avoid **calcium salts** for at least 6 hours before or 1 hour after **ibandronate**. Moderate Theoretical

Oral calcium salts decrease the absorption of **risedronate**. Separate administration by at least 2 hours. Moderate Study

Oral iron decreases the absorption of oral **clodronate**. **Clodronate** should be taken 1 hour before or 2 hours after iron. Moderate Study

Oral iron is predicted to decrease the absorption of oral **ibandronate**. **Ibandronate** should be taken 1 hour before or 6 hours after iron. Moderate Theoretical

Oral iron decreases the absorption of oral **risedronate**. Separate administration by at least 2 hours. Moderate Study

Bisphosphonates are predicted to increase the risk of gastrointestinal bleeding when given with iron chelators (deferasirox). Severe Theoretical

Oral magnesium decreases the absorption of oral **alendronate**. **Alendronate** should be taken at least 30 minutes before magnesium. Moderate Study

Oral magnesium decreases the absorption of oral **clodronate**. Avoid magnesium for 2 hours before or 1 hour after **clodronate**. Moderate Study

Oral magnesium is predicted to decrease the absorption of oral **ibandronate**. Avoid for at least 6 hours before or 1 hour after **ibandronate**. Moderate Theoretical

Oral magnesium decreases the absorption of oral **risedronate**. Separate administration by at least 2 hours. Moderate Study

NSAIDs are predicted to increase the risk of gastrointestinal irritation when given with bisphosphonates (**alendronate, ibandronate**). Moderate Study

NSAIDs are predicted to increase the risk of renal impairment when given with **clodronate**. Moderate Study

Bisphosphonates are predicted to decrease the effects of parathyroid hormone. Avoid. Moderate Study

Oral zinc decreases the absorption of oral **alendronate**. **Alendronate** should be taken at least 30 minutes before zinc . Moderate Study

Oral zinc decreases the absorption of oral **clodronate**. Avoid **zinc** for 2 hours before or 1 hour after **clodronate**. Moderate Study

Oral zinc is predicted to decrease the absorption of oral **ibandronate**. Avoid **zinc** for at least 6 hours before or 1 hour after **ibandronate**. Moderate Theoretical

Oral zinc decreases the absorption of oral **risedronate**. Separate administration by at least 2 hours. Moderate Study

Bivalirudin → see thrombin inhibitors

Bleomycin → see TABLE 15 p. 1432 (myelosuppression), TABLE 5 p. 1430 (thromboembolism)

▸ Live vaccines are predicted to increase the risk of generalised infection (possibly life-threatening) when given with **bleomycin**. Public Health England advises avoid (refer to Green Book). Severe Theoretical

▸ Monoclonal antibodies (brentuximab vedotin) increase the risk of pulmonary toxicity when given with **bleomycin**. Avoid. Severe Study → Also see TABLE 15 p. 1432

▸ Platinum compounds (cisplatin) increase the risk of pulmonary toxicity when given with **bleomycin**. Severe Study → Also see TABLE 15 p. 1432

Blinatumomab → see monoclonal antibodies

Bortezomib → see TABLE 8 p. 1430 (hypotension), TABLE 15 p. 1432 (myelosuppression), TABLE 12 p. 1432 (peripheral neuropathy)

▸ Anti-androgens (apalutamide, enzalutamide) slightly decrease the exposure to **bortezomib**. Avoid. Severe Study

▸ Antiepileptics (carbamazepine, fosphenytoin, phenobarbital, phenytoin, primidone) slightly decrease the exposure to **bortezomib**. Avoid. Severe Study → Also see TABLE 12 p. 1432

▸ Antifungals, azoles (itraconazole, ketoconazole, voriconazole) slightly increase the exposure to **bortezomib**. Severe Study

▸ Cobicistat slightly increases the exposure to **bortezomib**. Moderate Study

▸ HIV-protease inhibitors slightly increase the exposure to **bortezomib**. Moderate Study

▸ Idelalisib slightly increases the exposure to **bortezomib**. Moderate Study

▸ Macrolides (clarithromycin) slightly increase the exposure to **bortezomib**. Moderate Study

▸ Mitotane slightly decreases the exposure to **bortezomib**. Avoid. Severe Study → Also see TABLE 15 p. 1432

▸ Rifamycins (rifampicin) slightly decrease the exposure to **bortezomib**. Avoid. Severe Study

Bosentan → see endothelin receptor antagonists

Bosutinib → see TABLE 15 p. 1432 (myelosuppression), TABLE 9 p. 1431 (QT-interval prolongation)

▸ Oral antacids are predicted to decrease the absorption of oral **bosutinib**. **Bosutinib** should be taken at least 12 hours before antacids. Moderate Theoretical

▸ Anti-androgens (apalutamide, enzalutamide) are predicted to very markedly decrease the exposure to **bosutinib**. Avoid. Severe Study → Also see TABLE 9 p. 1431

▸ Antiarrhythmics (dronedarone) are predicted to increase the exposure to **bosutinib**. Avoid or adjust dose. Severe Theoretical → Also see TABLE 9 p. 1431

▸ Antiepileptics (carbamazepine, fosphenytoin, phenobarbital, phenytoin, primidone) are predicted to very markedly decrease the exposure to **bosutinib**. Avoid. Severe Study

▸ Antifungals, azoles (fluconazole, isavuconazole, posaconazole) are predicted to increase the exposure to **bosutinib**. Avoid or adjust dose. Severe Theoretical → Also see TABLE 9 p. 1431

▸ Antifungals, azoles (itraconazole, ketoconazole, voriconazole) are predicted to markedly increase the exposure to **bosutinib**. Avoid or adjust dose. Severe Study → Also see TABLE 9 p. 1431

▸ Calcium channel blockers (diltiazem, verapamil) are predicted to increase the exposure to **bosutinib**. Avoid or adjust dose. Severe Theoretical

▸ Cobicistat is predicted to markedly increase the exposure to **bosutinib**. Avoid or adjust dose. Severe Study

▸ **Bosutinib** is predicted to increase the risk of bleeding events when given with coumarins. Severe Theoretical

▸ Crizotinib is predicted to increase the exposure to **bosutinib**. Avoid or adjust dose. Severe Theoretical → Also see TABLE 9 p. 1431

▸ Endothelin receptor antagonists (bosentan) are predicted to decrease the exposure to **bosutinib**. Avoid. Severe Theoretical

▸ Grapefruit juice is predicted to increase the exposure to **bosutinib**. Moderate Theoretical

▸ H_2 receptor antagonists are predicted to decrease the absorption of **bosutinib**. Moderate Theoretical

▸ HIV-protease inhibitors are predicted to markedly increase the exposure to **bosutinib**. Avoid or adjust dose. Severe Study → Also see TABLE 9 p. 1431

▸ Idelalisib is predicted to markedly increase the exposure to **bosutinib**. Avoid or adjust dose. Severe Study

▸ Imatinib is predicted to increase the exposure to **bosutinib**. Avoid or adjust dose. Severe Theoretical → Also see TABLE 15 p. 1432

▸ Letermovir is predicted to increase the exposure to **bosutinib**. Avoid or adjust dose. Severe Theoretical

▸ Macrolides (clarithromycin) are predicted to markedly increase the exposure to **bosutinib**. Avoid or adjust dose. Severe Study → Also see TABLE 9 p. 1431

▸ Macrolides (erythromycin) are predicted to increase the exposure to **bosutinib**. Avoid or adjust dose. Severe Theoretical → Also see TABLE 9 p. 1431

▸ Mitotane is predicted to very markedly decrease the exposure to **bosutinib**. Avoid. Severe Study → Also see TABLE 15 p. 1432

▸ Modafinil is predicted to decrease the exposure to **bosutinib**. Avoid. Severe Theoretical

Bosutinib (continued)

▶ Neurokinin-1 receptor antagonists (aprepitant, netupitant) are predicted to increase the exposure to **bosutinib**. Avoid or adjust dose. Severe Theoretical
▶ Neurokinin-1 receptor antagonists (fosaprepitant) are predicted to increase the exposure to **bosutinib**. Severe Theoretical
▶ Nilotinib is predicted to increase the exposure to **bosutinib**. Avoid or adjust dose. Severe Theoretical → Also see TABLE 15 p. 1432 → Also see TABLE 9 p. 1431
▶ NNRTIs (efavirenz, etravirine, nevirapine) are predicted to decrease the exposure to **bosutinib**. Avoid. Severe Theoretical → Also see TABLE 9 p. 1431
▶ **Bosutinib** is predicted to increase the risk of bleeding events when given with phenindione. Severe Theoretical
▶ Pitolisant is predicted to decrease the exposure to **bosutinib**. Avoid. Severe Theoretical
▶ Proton pump inhibitors are predicted to decrease the absorption of **bosutinib**. Moderate Study
▶ Rifamycins (rifampicin) are predicted to very markedly decrease the exposure to **bosutinib**. Avoid. Severe Study
▶ St John's wort is predicted to decrease the exposure to **bosutinib**. Avoid. Severe Theoretical

Botulinum toxin type A → see botulinum toxins
Botulinum toxin type B → see botulinum toxins
Botulinum toxins → see TABLE 20 p. 1433 (neuromuscular blocking effects)

botulinum toxin type A · botulinum toxin type B

Bowel cleansing preparations

SEPARATION OF ADMINISTRATION Other oral drugs should not be taken 1 hour before, or after, administration of bowel cleansing preparations because absorption might be impaired. Consider withholding ACE inhibitors, angiotensin-II receptor antagonists, and NSAIDs on the day that bowel cleansing preparations are given and for up to 72 hours after the procedure. Also consider withholding diuretics on the day that bowel cleansing preparations are given.

Brentuximab vedotin → see monoclonal antibodies
Brigatinib

▶ Anti-androgens (apalutamide, enzalutamide) are predicted to decrease the exposure to **brigatinib**. Avoid. Severe Study
▶ Antiepileptics (carbamazepine, fosphenytoin, phenobarbital, phenytoin, primidone) are predicted to decrease the exposure to **brigatinib**. Avoid. Severe Study
▶ Antifungals, azoles (itraconazole, ketoconazole, voriconazole) are predicted to increase the exposure to **brigatinib**. Adjust **brigatinib** dose, p. 1015. Severe Study
▶ Cobicistat is predicted to increase the exposure to **brigatinib**. Adjust **brigatinib** dose, p. 1015. Severe Study
▶ **Brigatinib** decreases the exposure to combined hormonal contraceptives. Use additional contraceptive precautions. Severe Theoretical
▶ **Brigatinib** potentially increases the concentration of digoxin. Moderate Theoretical
▶ Endothelin receptor antagonists (bosentan) are predicted to decrease the exposure to **brigatinib**. Avoid. Severe Study
▶ Grapefruit juice is predicted to increase the concentration of **brigatinib**. Avoid. Severe Study
▶ HIV-protease inhibitors are predicted to increase the exposure to **brigatinib**. Adjust **brigatinib** dose, p. 1015. Severe Study
▶ Idelalisib is predicted to increase the exposure to **brigatinib**. Adjust **brigatinib** dose, p. 1015. Severe Study
▶ Macrolides (clarithromycin) are predicted to increase the exposure to **brigatinib**. Adjust **brigatinib** dose, p. 1015. Severe Study
▶ **Brigatinib** potentially increases the concentration of methotrexate. Moderate Theoretical
▶ Mitotane is predicted to decrease the exposure to **brigatinib**. Avoid. Severe Study
▶ NNRTIs (efavirenz, nevirapine) are predicted to decrease the exposure to **brigatinib**. Avoid. Severe Study
▶ NNRTIs (etravirine) are predicted to decrease the exposure to **brigatinib**. Avoid. Moderate Theoretical
▶ **Brigatinib** potentially decreases the concentration of opioids (alfentanil, fentanyl). Avoid. Moderate Theoretical

▶ Rifamycins (rifabutin) are predicted to decrease the exposure to **brigatinib**. Avoid. Moderate Theoretical
▶ Rifamycins (rifampicin) are predicted to decrease the exposure to **brigatinib**. Avoid. Severe Study
▶ **Brigatinib** potentially decreases the concentration of sirolimus. Avoid. Moderate Theoretical
▶ St John's wort is predicted to decrease the exposure to **brigatinib**. Avoid. Severe Study
▶ **Brigatinib** potentially decreases the concentration of tacrolimus. Avoid. Moderate Theoretical
▶ **Brigatinib** potentially increases the concentration of thrombin inhibitors (dabigatran). Moderate Theoretical

Brimonidine → see TABLE 6 p. 1430 (bradycardia), TABLE 8 p. 1430 (hypotension), TABLE 11 p. 1431 (CNS depressant effects)

Brinzolamide

ROUTE-SPECIFIC INFORMATION Since systemic absorption can follow topical application of **brinzolamide**, the possibility of interactions should be borne in mind.

Brivaracetam → see antiepileptics
Brodalumab → see monoclonal antibodies
Bromfenac → see NSAIDs
Bromocriptine → see dopamine receptor agonists
Buclizine → see antihistamines, sedating
Budesonide → see corticosteroids
Bumetanide → see loop diuretics
Bupivacaine → see anaesthetics, local
Buprenorphine → see opioids
Bupropion → see TABLE 13 p. 1432 (serotonin syndrome)

▶ Alpelisib is predicted to decrease the efficacy of **bupropion**. Mild Theoretical
▶ **Bupropion** is predicted to increase the exposure to anticholinesterases, centrally acting (galantamine). Monitor and adjust dose. Moderate Study
▶ Antiepileptics (carbamazepine, fosphenytoin, phenobarbital, phenytoin, primidone) are predicted to markedly decrease the exposure to **bupropion**. Severe Study
▶ Antiepileptics (valproate) increase the exposure to **bupropion**. Severe Study
▶ Antifungals, azoles (isavuconazole) slightly increase the exposure to **bupropion**. Adjust dose. Moderate Study
▶ **Bupropion** is predicted to moderately increase the exposure to antipsychotics, second generation (aripiprazole). Adjust **aripiprazole** dose, p. 415. Moderate Study
▶ **Bupropion** is predicted to increase the exposure to antipsychotics, second generation (risperidone). Adjust dose. Moderate Study
▶ **Bupropion** is predicted to markedly increase the exposure to atomoxetine. Adjust dose. Severe Study
▶ **Bupropion** is predicted to increase the exposure to beta blockers, selective (metoprolol, nebivolol). Moderate Study
▶ **Bupropion** is predicted to slightly increase the exposure to darifenacin. Mild Study
▶ **Bupropion** increases the risk of adverse effects when given with dopamine receptor agonists (amantadine). Moderate Study
▶ **Bupropion** is predicted to increase the exposure to eliglustat. Avoid or adjust dose—consult product literature. Severe Study
▶ HIV-protease inhibitors (ritonavir) are predicted to decrease the exposure to **bupropion**. Moderate Study
▶ **Bupropion** increases the risk of adverse effects when given with levodopa. Moderate Study
▶ **Bupropion** is predicted to increase the risk of intraoperative hypertension when given with linezolid. Severe Anecdotal → Also see TABLE 13 p. 1432
▶ **Bupropion** is predicted to increase the risk of severe hypertension when given with MAO-B inhibitors. Avoid. Moderate Theoretical → Also see TABLE 13 p. 1432
▶ **Bupropion** is predicted to increase the risk of severe hypertension when given with MAOIs, irreversible. Avoid and for 14 days after stopping the MAOI. Severe Theoretical → Also see TABLE 13 p. 1432
▶ Methylthioninium chloride is predicted to increase the risk of severe hypertension when given with **bupropion**. Avoid. Severe Theoretical → Also see TABLE 13 p. 1432
▶ **Bupropion** is predicted to increase the exposure to mexiletine. Moderate Study

Bupropion is predicted to increase the risk of severe hypertension when given with moclobemide. Avoid. [Severe] Theoretical → Also see TABLE 13 p. 1432

NNRTIs (efavirenz) are predicted to decrease the exposure to **bupropion**. [Moderate] Study

Bupropion is predicted to decrease the efficacy of opioids (codeine). [Moderate] Theoretical

Bupropion is predicted to decrease the efficacy of opioids (tramadol). [Severe] Study → Also see TABLE 13 p. 1432

Bupropion is predicted to moderately increase the exposure to pitolisant. Use with caution and adjust dose. [Moderate] Study

Rifamycins (rifampicin) are predicted to decrease the exposure to **bupropion**. [Moderate] Study

▸ **Bupropion** is predicted to increase the exposure to SSRIs (dapoxetine). [Moderate] Theoretical → Also see TABLE 13 p. 1432

▸ **Bupropion** is predicted to decrease the efficacy of tamoxifen. Avoid. [Severe] Study

▸ **Bupropion** is predicted to increase the exposure to the active metabolite of tetrabenazine. [Moderate] Study

▸ **Bupropion** is predicted to increase the exposure to tricyclic antidepressants. Monitor for toxicity and adjust dose. [Severe] Study → Also see TABLE 13 p. 1432

▸ **Bupropion** is predicted to increase the exposure to vortioxetine. Monitor and adjust dose. [Moderate] Study → Also see TABLE 13 p. 1432

Buspirone → see TABLE 13 p. 1432 (serotonin syndrome)

▸ Anti-androgens (apalutamide, enzalutamide) are predicted to decrease the exposure to **buspirone**. Use with caution and adjust dose. [Severe] Study

▸ Antiarrhythmics (dronedarone) are predicted to increase the exposure to **buspirone**. Use with caution and adjust dose. [Moderate] Study

▸ Antiepileptics (carbamazepine, fosphenytoin, phenobarbital, phenytoin, primidone) are predicted to decrease the exposure to **buspirone**. Use with caution and adjust dose. [Severe] Study

▸ Antifungals, azoles (fluconazole, isavuconazole, posaconazole) are predicted to increase the exposure to **buspirone**. Use with caution and adjust dose. [Moderate] Study

▸ Antifungals, azoles (itraconazole, ketoconazole, voriconazole) are predicted to increase the exposure to **buspirone**. Adjust **buspirone** dose, p. 360. [Severe] Study

▸ Antifungals, azoles (miconazole) are predicted to increase the concentration of **buspirone**. Use with caution and adjust dose. [Moderate] Theoretical

▸ Calcium channel blockers (diltiazem, verapamil) are predicted to increase the exposure to **buspirone**. Use with caution and adjust dose. [Moderate] Study

▸ Cobicistat is predicted to increase the exposure to **buspirone**. Adjust **buspirone** dose, p. 360. [Severe] Study

▸ Crizotinib is predicted to increase the exposure to **buspirone**. Use with caution and adjust dose. [Moderate] Study

▸ Grapefruit juice increases the exposure to **buspirone**. Avoid. [Mild] Study

▸ HIV-protease inhibitors are predicted to increase the exposure to **buspirone**. Adjust **buspirone** dose, p. 360. [Severe] Study

▸ Idelalisib is predicted to increase the exposure to **buspirone**. Adjust **buspirone** dose, p. 360. [Severe] Study

▸ Imatinib is predicted to increase the exposure to **buspirone**. Use with caution and adjust dose. [Moderate] Study

▸ Letermovir is predicted to increase the exposure to **buspirone**. Use with caution and adjust dose. [Moderate] Study

▸ **Buspirone** is predicted to increase the risk of elevated blood pressure when given with linezolid. Avoid. [Severe] Theoretical → Also see TABLE 13 p. 1432

▸ Macrolides (clarithromycin) are predicted to increase the exposure to **buspirone**. Adjust **buspirone** dose, p. 360. [Severe] Study

▸ Macrolides (erythromycin) are predicted to increase the exposure to **buspirone**. Use with caution and adjust dose. [Moderate] Study

▸ **Buspirone** is predicted to increase the risk of elevated blood pressure when given with MAOIs, irreversible. Avoid. [Severe] Anecdotal → Also see TABLE 13 p. 1432

▸ Mitotane is predicted to decrease the exposure to **buspirone**. Use with caution and adjust dose. [Severe] Study

▸ Neurokinin-1 receptor antagonists (aprepitant, netupitant) are predicted to increase the exposure to **buspirone**. Use with caution and adjust dose. [Moderate] Study

▸ Nilotinib is predicted to increase the exposure to **buspirone**. Use with caution and adjust dose. [Moderate] Study

▸ Rifamycins (rifampicin) are predicted to decrease the exposure to **buspirone**. Use with caution and adjust dose. [Severe] Study

Busulfan → see alkylating agents

Cabazitaxel → see taxanes

Cabergoline → see dopamine receptor agonists

Cabozantinib → see TABLE 15 p. 1432 (myelosuppression), TABLE 9 p. 1431 (QT-interval prolongation)

▸ Anti-androgens (apalutamide, enzalutamide) moderately decrease the exposure to **cabozantinib**. Avoid. [Moderate] Study → Also see TABLE 9 p. 1431

▸ Antiarrhythmics (dronedarone) are predicted to increase the exposure to **cabozantinib**. [Moderate] Theoretical → Also see TABLE 9 p. 1431

▸ Antiepileptics (carbamazepine, fosphenytoin, phenobarbital, phenytoin, primidone) moderately decrease the exposure to **cabozantinib**. [Moderate] Study

▸ Antifungals, azoles (fluconazole, isavuconazole, posaconazole) are predicted to increase the exposure to **cabozantinib**. [Moderate] Theoretical → Also see TABLE 9 p. 1431

▸ Antifungals, azoles (itraconazole, ketoconazole, voriconazole) slightly increase the exposure to **cabozantinib**. [Moderate] Study → Also see TABLE 9 p. 1431

▸ Calcium channel blockers (diltiazem, verapamil) are predicted to increase the exposure to **cabozantinib**. [Moderate] Theoretical

▸ Cobicistat slightly increases the exposure to **cabozantinib**. [Moderate] Study

▸ **Cabozantinib** is predicted to increase the risk of bleeding events when given with coumarins. [Severe] Theoretical

▸ Crizotinib is predicted to increase the exposure to **cabozantinib**. [Moderate] Theoretical → Also see TABLE 9 p. 1431

▸ Endothelin receptor antagonists (bosentan) are predicted to decrease the exposure to **cabozantinib**. [Moderate] Theoretical

▸ Grapefruit juice is predicted to increase the exposure to **cabozantinib**. [Moderate] Theoretical

▸ HIV-protease inhibitors slightly increase the exposure to **cabozantinib**. [Moderate] Study → Also see TABLE 9 p. 1431

▸ Idelalisib slightly increases the exposure to **cabozantinib**. [Moderate] Study

▸ Imatinib is predicted to increase the exposure to **cabozantinib**. [Moderate] Theoretical → Also see TABLE 15 p. 1432

▸ Letermovir is predicted to increase the exposure to **cabozantinib**. [Moderate] Theoretical

▸ Macrolides (clarithromycin) slightly increase the exposure to **cabozantinib**. [Moderate] Study → Also see TABLE 9 p. 1431

▸ Macrolides (erythromycin) are predicted to increase the exposure to **cabozantinib**. [Moderate] Theoretical → Also see TABLE 9 p. 1431

▸ Mitotane moderately decreases the exposure to **cabozantinib**. Avoid. [Moderate] Study → Also see TABLE 15 p. 1432

▸ Neurokinin-1 receptor antagonists (aprepitant, netupitant) are predicted to increase the exposure to **cabozantinib**. [Moderate] Theoretical

▸ Nilotinib is predicted to increase the exposure to **cabozantinib**. [Moderate] Theoretical → Also see TABLE 15 p. 1432 → Also see TABLE 9 p. 1431

▸ NNRTIs (efavirenz, nevirapine) are predicted to decrease the exposure to **cabozantinib**. [Moderate] Theoretical → Also see TABLE 9 p. 1431

▸ **Cabozantinib** is predicted to increase the risk of bleeding events when given with phenindione. [Severe] Theoretical

▸ Rifamycins (rifampicin) moderately decrease the exposure to **cabozantinib**. Avoid. [Moderate] Study

▸ St John's wort is predicted to decrease the exposure to **cabozantinib**. [Moderate] Theoretical

Caffeine citrate

▸ **Caffeine citrate** decreases the efficacy of antiarrhythmics (adenosine). Separate administration by 24 hours. [Mild] Study

▸ Antiepileptics (fosphenytoin, phenytoin) are predicted to moderately increase the clearance of **caffeine citrate**. Monitor and adjust dose. [Moderate] Study

Caffeine citrate (continued)

▸ HIV-protease inhibitors (ritonavir) are predicted to moderately increase the clearance of **caffeine citrate**. Monitor and adjust dose. [Moderate] Study

▸ Leflunomide is predicted to moderately increase the clearance of **caffeine citrate**. Monitor and adjust dose. [Moderate] Study

▸ Rifamycins (rifampicin) are predicted to moderately increase the clearance of **caffeine citrate**. Monitor and adjust dose. [Moderate] Study

▸ SSRIs (fluvoxamine) markedly decrease the clearance of **caffeine citrate**. Monitor and adjust dose. [Severe] Study

▸ Teriflunomide is predicted to moderately increase the clearance of **caffeine citrate**. Monitor and adjust dose. [Moderate] Study

▸ **Caffeine citrate** decreases the clearance of theophylline. [Moderate] Study

Calcipotriol → see vitamin D substances

Calcitonins

▸ **Calcitonins** decrease the concentration of lithium. Adjust dose. [Moderate] Study

Calcitriol → see vitamin D substances

Calcium acetate → see calcium salts

Calcium carbonate → see calcium salts

Calcium channel blockers → see TABLE 6 p. 1430 (bradycardia), TABLE 8 p. 1430 (hypotension)

amlodipine · diltiazem · felodipine · lacidipine · lercanidipine · nicardipine · nifedipine · nimodipine · verapamil

▸ Calcium channel blockers **(diltiazem, verapamil)** are predicted to increase the exposure to abemaciclib. [Moderate] Study

▸ Calcium channel blockers **(diltiazem, verapamil)** are predicted to increase the exposure to acalabrutinib. Avoid or monitor. [Severe] Study

▸ **Verapamil** is predicted to increase the exposure to afatinib. Separate administration by 12 hours. [Moderate] Study

▸ Calcium channel blockers **(diltiazem, verapamil)** are predicted to increase the exposure to aldosterone antagonists (eplerenone). Adjust **eplerenone** dose, p. 208. [Severe] Study → Also see TABLE 8 p. 1430

▸ **Verapamil** moderately increases the exposure to aliskiren. [Moderate] Study → Also see TABLE 8 p. 1430

▸ Calcium channel blockers **(diltiazem, verapamil)** are predicted to increase the exposure to alpha blockers (tamsulosin). [Moderate] Theoretical → Also see TABLE 8 p. 1430

▸ **Verapamil** moderately increases the exposure to anthracyclines (doxorubicin). [Moderate] Study

▸ Anti-androgens (enzalutamide) are predicted to decrease the exposure to calcium channel blockers **(amlodipine, felodipine, lacidipine, lercanidipine, nicardipine, nifedipine, nimodipine)**. Monitor and adjust dose. [Moderate] Study

▸ Anti-androgens (apalutamide) are predicted to decrease the exposure to calcium channel blockers **(amlodipine, felodipine, lacidipine, lercanidipine, nicardipine, nifedipine, nimodipine)**. Monitor and adjust dose. [Moderate] Study

▸ Anti-androgens (enzalutamide) are predicted to decrease the exposure to calcium channel blockers **(diltiazem, verapamil)**. [Severe] Study

▸ Antiarrhythmics (disopyramide) are predicted to increase the risk of cardiodepression when given with **verapamil**. [Severe] Theoretical

▸ Antiarrhythmics (dronedarone) are predicted to increase the exposure to calcium channel blockers **(amlodipine, felodipine, lacidipine, lercanidipine, nicardipine, nifedipine, nimodipine)**. Monitor and adjust dose. [Moderate] Study

▸ Antiarrhythmics (amiodarone) are predicted to increase the risk of cardiodepression when given with calcium channel blockers **(diltiazem, verapamil)**. Avoid. [Severe] Theoretical → Also see TABLE 6 p. 1430

▸ Calcium channel blockers **(diltiazem, verapamil)** increase the exposure to antiarrhythmics (dronedarone) and antiarrhythmics (dronedarone) increase the exposure to calcium channel blockers **(diltiazem, verapamil)**. [Moderate] Study

▸ **Verapamil** increases the risk of cardiodepression when given with antiarrhythmics (flecainide). [Severe] Anecdotal → Also see TABLE 6 p. 1430

▸ Calcium channel blockers **(diltiazem, verapamil)** are predicted to increase the exposure to antiarrhythmics (propafenone). Monitor and adjust dose. [Moderate] Study

▸ Antiepileptics (valproate) increase the exposure to **nimodipine**. Adjust dose. [Moderate] Study

▸ Antiepileptics (carbamazepine, fosphenytoin, phenobarbital, phenytoin, primidone) are predicted to decrease the exposure to calcium channel blockers **(amlodipine, felodipine, lacidipine, lercanidipine, nicardipine, nifedipine, nimodipine)**. Monitor and adjust dose. [Moderate] Study

▸ **Diltiazem** increases the concentration of antiepileptics (carbamazepine) and antiepileptics (carbamazepine) are predicted to decrease the exposure to **diltiazem**. Monitor concentration and adjust dose. [Severe] Anecdotal

▸ **Verapamil** increases the concentration of antiepileptics (carbamazepine) and antiepileptics (carbamazepine) are predicted to decrease the exposure to **verapamil**. [Severe] Anecdotal

▸ Antiepileptics (phenobarbital, primidone) are predicted to decrease the exposure to calcium channel blockers **(diltiazem, verapamil)**. [Severe] Study

▸ Calcium channel blockers **(diltiazem, verapamil)** potentially increase the concentration of antiepileptics (fosphenytoin, phenytoin) and antiepileptics (fosphenytoin, phenytoin) are predicted to decrease the exposure to calcium channel blockers **(diltiazem, verapamil)**. [Severe] Study

▸ Antifungals, azoles (itraconazole, ketoconazole, voriconazole) are predicted to markedly increase the exposure to **lercanidipine**. Avoid. [Severe] Study

▸ Antifungals, azoles (miconazole) are predicted to increase the exposure to **diltiazem**. [Moderate] Theoretical

▸ Antifungals, azoles (fluconazole, isavuconazole, posaconazole) are predicted to increase the exposure to calcium channel blockers **(amlodipine, felodipine, lacidipine, lercanidipine, nicardipine, nifedipine, nimodipine)**. Monitor and adjust dose. [Moderate] Study

▸ Antifungals, azoles (miconazole) are predicted to increase the exposure to calcium channel blockers **(amlodipine, felodipine, lacidipine, lercanidipine, nicardipine, nifedipine, nimodipine, verapamil)**. Use with caution and adjust dose. [Moderate] Theoretical

▸ Antifungals, azoles (itraconazole, ketoconazole, voriconazole) are predicted to increase the exposure to calcium channel blockers **(amlodipine, felodipine, lacidipine, nicardipine, nifedipine, nimodipine)**. Monitor and adjust dose. [Moderate] Study

▸ Antifungals, azoles (fluconazole) (high-dose) are predicted to increase the exposure to calcium channel blockers **(diltiazem, verapamil)**. [Moderate] Theoretical

▸ Antifungals, azoles (itraconazole, ketoconazole, voriconazole) are predicted to increase the exposure to calcium channel blockers **(diltiazem, verapamil)**. [Severe] Study

▸ Antifungals, azoles (posaconazole) are predicted to increase the exposure to calcium channel blockers **(diltiazem, verapamil)**. [Moderate] Theoretical

▸ Calcium channel blockers **(diltiazem, verapamil)** are predicted to increase the exposure to antifungals, azoles (isavuconazole). [Moderate] Theoretical

▸ Calcium channel blockers **(diltiazem, verapamil)** are predicted to increase the exposure to antihistamines, non-sedating (mizolastine). [Severe] Theoretical

▸ Calcium channel blockers **(diltiazem, verapamil)** are predicted to increase the exposure to antihistamines, non-sedating (rupatadine). Avoid. [Moderate] Study

▸ Antimalarials (mefloquine) are predicted to increase the risk of bradycardia when given with **calcium channel blockers**. [Severe] Theoretical

▸ Calcium channel blockers **(diltiazem, verapamil)** are predicted to increase the concentration of antimalarials (piperaquine). [Severe] Theoretical

▸ Calcium channel blockers **(diltiazem, verapamil)** are predicted to increase the exposure to antipsychotics, second generation (cariprazine). Avoid. [Severe] Study → Also see TABLE 8 p. 1430

▸ Calcium channel blockers **(diltiazem, verapamil)** are predicted to increase the exposure to antipsychotics, second generation (lurasidone). Adjust **lurasidone** dose. Moderate Study → Also see TABLE 8 p. 1430

Calcium channel blockers **(diltiazem, verapamil)** are predicted to increase the exposure to antipsychotics, second generation (quetiapine). Avoid. Moderate Study → Also see TABLE 8 p. 1430

Calcium channel blockers **(diltiazem, verapamil)** are predicted to increase the exposure to avapritinib. Avoid or adjust **avapritinib** dose, p. 1012. Moderate Study

Calcium channel blockers **(diltiazem, verapamil)** are predicted to increase the exposure to axitinib. Moderate Theoretical

Calcium channel blockers **(diltiazem, verapamil)** are predicted to increase the exposure to bedaquiline. Avoid prolonged use. Mild Theoretical

▸ Calcium channel blockers **(diltiazem, verapamil)** are predicted to increase the exposure to benzodiazepines **(alprazolam).** Severe Study

Calcium channel blockers **(diltiazem, verapamil)** are predicted to increase the exposure to benzodiazepines **(midazolam).** Monitor adverse effects and adjust dose. Severe Study

Diltiazem is predicted to increase the risk of cardiodepression when given with beta blockers, non-selective. Severe Study → Also see TABLE 6 p. 1430 → Also see TABLE 8 p. 1430

▸ **Verapamil** increases the risk of cardiovascular adverse effects when given with beta blockers, non-selective. Avoid intravenous **verapamil**, p. 178. Severe Study → Also see TABLE 6 p. 1430 → Also see TABLE 8 p. 1430

▸ **Diltiazem** is predicted to increase the risk of cardiodepression when given with beta blockers, selective. Severe Study → Also see TABLE 6 p. 1430 → Also see TABLE 8 p. 1430

▸ **Verapamil** increases the risk of cardiovascular adverse effects when given with beta blockers, selective. Avoid intravenous **verapamil**, p. 178. Severe Study → Also see TABLE 6 p. 1430 → Also see TABLE 8 p. 1430

▸ **Verapamil** is predicted to increase the exposure to bictegravir. Use with caution or avoid. Moderate Theoretical

▸ Calcium channel blockers **(diltiazem, verapamil)** are predicted to increase the exposure to bosutinib. Avoid or adjust dose. Severe Theoretical

▸ Calcium channel blockers **(diltiazem, verapamil)** are predicted to increase the exposure to buspirone. Use with caution and adjust dose. Moderate Study

▸ Calcium channel blockers **(diltiazem, verapamil)** are predicted to increase the exposure to cabozantinib. Moderate Theoretical

▸ Calcium channel blockers **(diltiazem)** are predicted to increase the exposure to calcium channel blockers **(amlodipine).** Monitor and adjust dose. Moderate Study → Also see TABLE 8 p. 1430

▸ Calcium channel blockers **(verapamil)** are predicted to increase the exposure to calcium channel blockers **(amlodipine, felodipine, lacidipine, lercanidipine, nicardipine, nifedipine, nimodipine).** Monitor and adjust dose. Moderate Study → Also see TABLE 8 p. 1430

▸ Calcium channel blockers **(diltiazem)** are predicted to increase the exposure to calcium channel blockers **(felodipine, lacidipine, lercanidipine, nicardipine, nifedipine, nimodipine).** Monitor and adjust dose. Moderate Study → Also see TABLE 8 p. 1430

▸ Calcium channel blockers **(diltiazem, verapamil)** are predicted to increase the concentration of ciclosporin. Severe Study

▸ Ciclosporin moderately increases the exposure to **lercanidipine**. Use with caution or avoid. Severe Study

▸ **Nicardipine** increases the concentration of ciclosporin. Severe Study

▸ Cobicistat is predicted to increase the exposure to calcium channel blockers **(amlodipine, felodipine, lacidipine, nicardipine, nifedipine, nimodipine).** Monitor and adjust dose. Moderate Study

▸ Cobicistat is predicted to increase the exposure to calcium channel blockers **(diltiazem, verapamil).** Severe Study

▸ Cobicistat is predicted to markedly increase the exposure to **lercanidipine**. Avoid. Severe Study

▸ Calcium channel blockers **(diltiazem, verapamil)** are predicted to increase the exposure to cobimetinib. Severe Theoretical

▸ Calcium channel blockers **(diltiazem, verapamil)** are predicted to increase the exposure to colchicine. Adjust **colchicine** dose with moderate CYP3A4 inhibitors, p. 1166. Severe Study

▸ Calcium channel blockers **(diltiazem, verapamil)** are predicted to increase the exposure to corticosteroids (methylprednisolone). Monitor and adjust dose. Moderate Study

▸ Crizotinib is predicted to increase the exposure to calcium channel blockers **(amlodipine, felodipine, lacidipine, lercanidipine, nicardipine, nifedipine, nimodipine).** Monitor and adjust dose. Moderate Study

▸ Intravenous dantrolene potentially increases the risk of acute hyperkalaemia and cardiovascular collapse when given with calcium channel blockers **(diltiazem, verapamil).** Avoid. Severe Anecdotal

▸ Calcium channel blockers **(diltiazem, verapamil)** are predicted to slightly increase the exposure to darifenacin. Moderate Study

▸ Calcium channel blockers **(diltiazem, verapamil)** are predicted to increase the exposure to dasatinib. Severe Study

▸ Calcium channel blockers **(diltiazem, verapamil)** are predicted to slightly increase the exposure to dienogest. Moderate Study

▸ Calcium channel blockers **(diltiazem, verapamil)** increase the concentration of digoxin. Monitor and adjust dose. Severe Study → Also see TABLE 6 p. 1430

▸ Calcium channel blockers **(diltiazem, verapamil)** are predicted to increase the exposure to dipeptidylpeptidase-4 inhibitors (saxagliptin). Mild Study

▸ Calcium channel blockers **(diltiazem, verapamil)** increase the risk of QT-prolongation when given with domperidone. Avoid. Severe Study

▸ Calcium channel blockers **(diltiazem, verapamil)** are predicted to increase the exposure to dopamine receptor agonists (bromocriptine). Severe Theoretical → Also see TABLE 8 p. 1430

▸ Calcium channel blockers **(diltiazem, verapamil)** are predicted to increase the concentration of dopamine receptor agonists (cabergoline). Moderate Anecdotal → Also see TABLE 8 p. 1430

▸ Calcium channel blockers **(diltiazem, verapamil)** are predicted to moderately increase the exposure to dutasteride. Mild Study

▸ Calcium channel blockers **(diltiazem, verapamil)** is predicted to increase the exposure to elexacaftor. Adjust tezacaftor with ivacaftor and elexacaftor p. 311 dose with moderate CYP3A4 inhibitors. Severe Theoretical

▸ Calcium channel blockers **(diltiazem, verapamil)** are predicted to increase the exposure to eliglustat. Avoid or adjust dose— consult product literature. Severe Study

▸ Calcium channel blockers **(diltiazem, verapamil)** are predicted to moderately increase the exposure to encorafenib. Moderate Study

▸ Endothelin receptor antagonists (bosentan) are predicted to decrease the exposure to calcium channel blockers **(amlodipine, felodipine, lacidipine, lercanidipine, nicardipine, nifedipine, nimodipine).** Monitor and adjust dose. Moderate Theoretical

▸ Endothelin receptor antagonists (bosentan) are predicted to decrease the exposure to calcium channel blockers **(diltiazem, verapamil).** Moderate Theoretical

▸ Calcium channel blockers **(diltiazem, verapamil)** are predicted to increase the exposure to entrectinib. Avoid moderate CYP3A4 inhibitors or adjust **entrectinib** dose, p. 1023. Severe Theoretical

▸ Calcium channel blockers **(diltiazem, verapamil)** are predicted to increase the risk of ergotism when given with ergometrine. Severe Theoretical

▸ Calcium channel blockers **(diltiazem, verapamil)** are predicted to increase the risk of ergotism when given with ergotamine. Severe Theoretical

▸ Calcium channel blockers **(diltiazem, verapamil)** are predicted to increase the exposure to erlotinib. Moderate Theoretical

▸ Calcium channel blockers **(diltiazem, verapamil)** are predicted to increase the concentration of everolimus. Avoid or adjust dose. Moderate Study

▸ **Verapamil** is predicted to increase the exposure to factor XA inhibitors (apixaban). Moderate Theoretical

▸ Calcium channel blockers **(diltiazem, verapamil)** are predicted to increase the exposure to fesoterodine. Adjust **fesoterodine** dose with moderate CYP3A4 inhibitors in hepatic and renal impairment, p. 822. Mild Study

▸ **Verapamil** is predicted to increase the exposure to fidaxomicin. Avoid. Moderate Study

A1

Interactions | Appendix 1

Calcium channel blockers (continued)

- Calcium channel blockers **(diltiazem, verapamil)** are predicted to increase the exposure to fingolimod. Avoid. Moderate Theoretical → Also see **TABLE 6** p. 1430
- **Diltiazem** is predicted to increase the exposure to fostamatinib. Monitor adverse effects and adjust dose. Moderate Theoretical
- Calcium channel blockers **(diltiazem, verapamil)** are predicted to increase the exposure to gefitinib. Moderate Theoretical
- Grapefruit juice very slightly increases the exposure to **amlodipine**. Avoid. Mild Study
- Grapefruit juice increases the exposure to calcium channel blockers **(nifedipine, verapamil)**. Avoid. Mild Study
- Grapefruit juice increases the exposure to **felodipine**. Avoid. Moderate Study
- Grapefruit juice is predicted to increase the exposure to **lercanidipine**. Avoid. Moderate Theoretical
- Grapefruit juice increases the exposure to **nicardipine**. Mild Study
- Grazoprevir is predicted to increase the concentration of **calcium channel blockers**. Moderate Theoretical
- Calcium channel blockers **(diltiazem, verapamil)** are predicted to increase the concentration of guanfacine. Adjust **guanfacine** dose, p. 372. Moderate Theoretical → Also see **TABLE 8** p. 1430
- H₂ receptor antagonists (cimetidine) (high-dose) are predicted to increase the exposure to **lercanidipine**. Moderate Theoretical
- H₂ receptor antagonists (cimetidine) moderately increase the exposure to **nifedipine**. Monitor and adjust dose. Severe Study
- H₂ receptor antagonists (cimetidine) increase the exposure to **verapamil**. Moderate Study
- H₂ receptor antagonists (cimetidine) slightly increase the exposure to calcium channel blockers **(diltiazem, nimodipine)**. Monitor and adjust dose. Moderate Study
- HIV-protease inhibitors are predicted to increase the exposure to calcium channel blockers **(amlodipine, felodipine, lacidipine, nicardipine, nifedipine, nimodipine)**. Monitor and adjust dose. Moderate Study
- HIV-protease inhibitors are predicted to increase the exposure to calcium channel blockers **(diltiazem, verapamil)**. Severe Study
- HIV-protease inhibitors are predicted to markedly increase the exposure to **lercanidipine**. Avoid. Severe Study
- Calcium channel blockers **(diltiazem, verapamil)** are predicted to increase the exposure to ibrutinib. Adjust **ibrutinib** dose with moderate CYP3A4 inhibitors, p. 1027. Severe Study
- Idelalisib is predicted to increase the exposure to calcium channel blockers **(amlodipine, felodipine, lacidipine, nicardipine, nifedipine, nimodipine)**. Monitor and adjust dose. Moderate Study
- Idelalisib is predicted to increase the exposure to calcium channel blockers **(diltiazem, verapamil)**. Severe Study
- Idelalisib is predicted to markedly increase the exposure to **lercanidipine**. Avoid. Severe Study
- Calcium channel blockers **(diltiazem, verapamil)** are predicted to increase the exposure to imatinib. Moderate Theoretical
- Imatinib is predicted to increase the exposure to calcium channel blockers **(amlodipine, felodipine, lacidipine, lercanidipine, nicardipine, nifedipine, nimodipine)**. Monitor and adjust dose. Moderate Study
- Calcium channel blockers **(diltiazem, verapamil)** are predicted to increase the exposure to ivabradine. Avoid. Moderate Study → Also see **TABLE 6** p. 1430
- Calcium channel blockers **(diltiazem, verapamil)** are predicted to increase the exposure to ivacaftor. Adjust ivacaftor p. 309 or tezacaftor with ivacaftor p. 311 or tezacaftor with ivacaftor and elexacaftor p. 311 dose with moderate CYP3A4 inhibitors. Severe Study
- Calcium channel blockers **(diltiazem, verapamil)** are predicted to increase the exposure to lapatinib. Moderate Study
- **Verapamil** is predicted to increase the exposure to larotrectinib. Mild Theoretical
- Letermovir is predicted to increase the exposure to calcium channel blockers **(amlodipine, felodipine, lacidipine, lercanidipine, nicardipine, nifedipine, nimodipine)**. Monitor and adjust dose. Moderate Study

- Calcium channel blockers **(diltiazem, verapamil)** are predicted to increase the risk of neurotoxicity when given with lithium. Severe Anecdotal
- Calcium channel blockers **(amlodipine, lacidipine)** are predicted to increase the exposure to lomitapide. Separate administration by 12 hours. Moderate Theoretical
- Calcium channel blockers **(diltiazem, verapamil)** are predicted to increase the exposure to lomitapide. Avoid. Moderate Theoretical
- Macrolides (clarithromycin) are predicted to markedly increase the exposure to **lercanidipine**. Avoid. Severe Study
- Macrolides (erythromycin) are predicted to increase the exposure to **diltiazem**. Severe Theoretical
- Macrolides (erythromycin) are predicted to increase the exposure to **verapamil**. Severe Study
- Macrolides (erythromycin) are predicted to increase the exposure to calcium channel blockers **(amlodipine, felodipine, lacidipine, lercanidipine, nicardipine, nifedipine, nimodipine)**. Monitor and adjust dose. Moderate Study
- Macrolides (clarithromycin) are predicted to increase the exposure to calcium channel blockers **(amlodipine, felodipine, lacidipine, nicardipine, nifedipine, nimodipine)**. Monitor and adjust dose. Moderate Study
- Macrolides (clarithromycin) are predicted to increase the exposure to calcium channel blockers **(diltiazem, verapamil)**. Severe Study
- Intravenous magnesium potentially increases the risk of hypotension when given with calcium channel blockers **(amlodipine, felodipine, lacidipine, lercanidipine, nicardipine, nifedipine, nimodipine, verapamil)** in pregnant women. Severe Anecdotal
- Mexiletine increases the risk of cardiovascular adverse effects when given with **diltiazem**. Avoid or monitor. Severe Theoretical
- Mexiletine potentially increases the risk of cardiovascular adverse effects when given with **verapamil**. Avoid or monitor. Severe Theoretical
- Calcium channel blockers **(diltiazem, verapamil)** are predicted to increase the exposure to midostaurin. Moderate Theoretical
- Mitotane is predicted to decrease the exposure to calcium channel blockers **(amlodipine, felodipine, lacidipine, lercanidipine, nicardipine, nifedipine, nimodipine)**. Monitor and adjust dose. Moderate Study
- Mitotane is predicted to decrease the exposure to **diltiazem**. Severe Study
- Monoclonal antibodies (tocilizumab) are predicted to decrease the exposure to **calcium channel blockers**. Monitor and adjust dose. Moderate Theoretical
- Calcium channel blockers **(diltiazem, verapamil)** are predicted to increase the exposure to naldemedine. Moderate Study
- Calcium channel blockers **(diltiazem, verapamil)** are predicted to increase the exposure to naloxegol. Adjust **naloxegol** dose and monitor adverse effects, p. 70. Moderate Study
- Calcium channel blockers **(diltiazem, verapamil)** are predicted to increase the exposure to neratinib. Severe Study
- Neurokinin-1 receptor antagonists (aprepitant, netupitant) are predicted to increase the exposure to calcium channel blockers **(amlodipine, felodipine, lacidipine, lercanidipine, nicardipine, nifedipine, nimodipine)**. Monitor and adjust dose. Moderate Study
- Calcium channel blockers **(diltiazem, verapamil)** are predicted to increase the exposure to neurokinin-1 receptor antagonists (aprepitant) and neurokinin-1 receptor antagonists (aprepitant) are predicted to increase the exposure to calcium channel blockers **(diltiazem, verapamil)**. Moderate Study
- Calcium channel blockers **(diltiazem, verapamil)** are predicted to increase the exposure to nilotinib. Moderate Theoretical
- Nilotinib is predicted to increase the exposure to calcium channel blockers **(amlodipine, felodipine, lacidipine, lercanidipine, nicardipine, nifedipine, nimodipine)**. Monitor and adjust dose. Moderate Study
- **Verapamil** is predicted to increase the exposure to nintedanib. Moderate Study
- NNRTIs (efavirenz, nevirapine) are predicted to decrease the exposure to calcium channel blockers **(amlodipine, felodipine, lacidipine, lercanidipine, nicardipine, nifedipine, nimodipine)**. Monitor and adjust dose. Moderate Theoretical

NNRTIs (efavirenz, nevirapine) are predicted to decrease the exposure to calcium channel blockers **(diltiazem, verapamil)**. Moderate Theoretical

Calcium channel blockers **(diltiazem, verapamil)** are predicted to increase the exposure to olaparib. Avoid moderate CYP3A4 inhibitors or adjust **olaparib** dose, p. 1051. Moderate Theoretical

Calcium channel blockers **(diltiazem, verapamil)** are predicted to increase the exposure to opioids (alfentanil, buprenorphine, fentanyl, oxycodone). Monitor and adjust dose. Moderate Study → Also see TABLE 6 p. 1430

Calcium channel blockers **(diltiazem, verapamil)** are predicted to increase the exposure to opioids (methadone). Moderate Theoretical → Also see TABLE 6 p. 1430

Calcium channel blockers **(diltiazem, verapamil)** are predicted to increase the exposure to oxybutynin. Mild Theoretical

▶ **Verapamil** is predicted to increase the exposure to panobinostat. Adjust dose. Moderate Theoretical

▶ Calcium channel blockers **(diltiazem, verapamil)** are predicted to increase the exposure to pazopanib. Moderate Theoretical

▶ Calcium channel blockers **(diltiazem, verapamil)** are predicted to increase the exposure to phosphodiesterase type-5 inhibitors (avanafil). Adjust **avanafil** dose, p. 859. Moderate Theoretical → Also see TABLE 8 p. 1430

▶ Calcium channel blockers **(diltiazem, verapamil)** are predicted to increase the exposure to phosphodiesterase type-5 inhibitors (sildenafil). Monitor or adjust **sildenafil** dose with moderate CYP3A4 inhibitors, p. 860. Moderate Study → Also see TABLE 8 p. 1430

▶ Calcium channel blockers **(diltiazem, verapamil)** are predicted to increase the exposure to phosphodiesterase type-5 inhibitors (tadalafil). Severe Theoretical → Also see TABLE 8 p. 1430

▶ Calcium channel blockers **(diltiazem, verapamil)** are predicted to increase the exposure to phosphodiesterase type-5 inhibitors (vardenafil). Adjust dose. Severe Theoretical → Also see TABLE 8 p. 1430

▶ **Verapamil** is predicted to increase the exposure to pibrentasvir. Moderate Theoretical

▶ Calcium channel blockers **(diltiazem, verapamil)** are predicted to increase the exposure to pimozide. Avoid. Severe Theoretical → Also see TABLE 8 p. 1430

▶ Calcium channel blockers **(diltiazem, verapamil)** are predicted to increase the exposure to ranolazine. Severe Study

▶ Calcium channel blockers **(diltiazem, verapamil)** are predicted to increase the exposure to ribociclib. Moderate Study

▶ Rifamycins (rifampicin) moderately decrease the exposure to **nifedipine**. Avoid. Severe Study

▶ Rifamycins (rifampicin) are predicted to decrease the exposure to calcium channel blockers **(amlodipine, felodipine, lacidipine, lercanidipine, nicardipine, nimodipine)**. Monitor and adjust dose. Moderate Study

▶ Rifamycins (rifampicin) greatly decrease the exposure to calcium channel blockers **(diltiazem, verapamil)**. Severe Study

▶ Calcium channel blockers **(diltiazem, verapamil)** are predicted to increase the exposure to ruxolitinib. Moderate Theoretical

▶ Calcium channel blockers **(diltiazem, verapamil)** increase the concentration of sirolimus. Monitor and adjust dose. Moderate Study

▶ Calcium channel blockers **(diltiazem, verapamil)** are predicted to increase the exposure to SSRIs (dapoxetine). Adjust **dapoxetine** dose with moderate CYP3A4 inhibitors, p. 867. Moderate Theoretical

▶ St John's wort is predicted to decrease the exposure to calcium channel blockers **(amlodipine, felodipine, lacidipine, lercanidipine, nicardipine, nifedipine, nimodipine)**. Monitor and adjust dose. Moderate Theoretical

▶ St John's wort is predicted to decrease the exposure to calcium channel blockers **(diltiazem, verapamil)**. Moderate Theoretical

▶ **Diltiazem** slightly to moderately increases the exposure to statins (atorvastatin). Monitor and adjust dose. Severe Anecdotal

▶ **Verapamil** is predicted to slightly to moderately increase the exposure to statins (atorvastatin). Monitor and adjust dose. Severe Theoretical

▶ **Amlodipine** slightly increases the exposure to statins (simvastatin). Adjust **simvastatin** dose, p. 219. Mild Study

▶ Calcium channel blockers **(diltiazem, verapamil)** moderately increase the exposure to statins (simvastatin). Monitor and adjust dose. Severe Study

▶ Calcium channel blockers **(diltiazem, verapamil)** are predicted to increase the exposure to sunitinib. Moderate Theoretical

▶ Calcium channel blockers **(diltiazem, verapamil)** are predicted to increase the concentration of tacrolimus. Severe Study

▶ **Nicardipine** potentially increases the concentration of tacrolimus. Monitor concentration and adjust dose. Severe Anecdotal

▶ **Verapamil** is predicted to slightly increase the exposure to talazoparib. Avoid or adjust **talazoparib** dose, p. 1052. Severe Study

▶ Calcium channel blockers **(diltiazem, verapamil)** are predicted to increase the exposure to taxanes (cabazitaxel). Moderate Theoretical

▶ Calcium channel blockers **(diltiazem, verapamil)** are predicted to increase the concentration of and the risk of angioedema when given with temsirolimus. Use with caution or avoid. Moderate Theoretical

▶ Temsirolimus is predicted to increase the risk of angioedema when given with calcium channel blockers **(amlodipine, felodipine, lacidipine, lercanidipine, nicardipine, nifedipine, nimodipine)**. Moderate Theoretical

▶ Calcium channel blockers **(diltiazem, verapamil)** are predicted to increase the exposure to tezacaftor. Adjust tezacaftor with ivacaftor p. 311 or tezacaftor with ivacaftor and elexacaftor p. 311 dose with moderate CYP3A4 inhibitors. Severe Study

▶ **Verapamil** increases the exposure to thrombin inhibitors (dabigatran). Adjust **dabigatran** dose. Severe Study

▶ Calcium channel blockers **(diltiazem, verapamil)** given with a potent CYP2C19 inhibitor are predicted to increase the exposure to tofacitinib. Adjust **tofacitinib** dose, p. 1154. Moderate Study

▶ Calcium channel blockers **(diltiazem, verapamil)** are predicted to increase the exposure to tolterodine. Mild Theoretical

▶ Calcium channel blockers **(diltiazem, verapamil)** are predicted to increase the exposure to tolvaptan. Manufacturer advises caution or adjust **tolvaptan** dose with moderate CYP3A4 inhibitors, p. 708. Moderate Study

▶ **Verapamil** is predicted to increase the exposure to topotecan. Severe Study

▶ **Verapamil** is predicted to increase the concentration of trametinib. Moderate Theoretical

▶ Calcium channel blockers **(diltiazem, verapamil)** are predicted to increase the exposure to trazodone. Moderate Theoretical

▶ Calcium channel blockers **(diltiazem, verapamil)** are predicted to increase the exposure to venetoclax. Avoid or adjust dose—consult product literature. Severe Study

▶ Calcium channel blockers **(diltiazem, verapamil)** are predicted to increase the exposure to vinca alkaloids. Severe Theoretical

▶ Calcium channel blockers **(diltiazem, verapamil)** are predicted to increase the exposure to zopiclone. Adjust dose. Moderate Study

Calcium chloride → see calcium salts
Calcium gluconate → see calcium salts
Calcium lactate → see calcium salts
Calcium phosphate → see calcium salts
Calcium salts

calcium acetate · calcium carbonate · calcium chloride · calcium gluconate · calcium lactate · calcium phosphate

SEPARATION OF ADMINISTRATION **Calcium carbonate-containing antacids** should preferably not be taken at the same time as other drugs since they might impair absorption. **Antacids** might damage enteric coatings designed to prevent dissolution in the stomach.

▶ Oral **calcium carbonate** decreases the exposure to oral acalabrutinib. Separate administration by at least 2 hours. Moderate Study

▶ Oral **calcium salts** decrease the absorption of alkylating agents (estramustine). Severe Study

▶ **Calcium carbonate** decreases the absorption of antimalarials (chloroquine). Separate administration by at least 4 hours. Moderate Study

A1

Interactions | Appendix 1

Calcium salts (continued)
▸ **Calcium carbonate** is predicted to decrease the absorption of antimalarials (proguanil). Separate administration by at least 2 hours. Moderate Study
▸ Oral **calcium salts** decrease the absorption of bisphosphonates (alendronate). **Alendronate** should be taken at least 30 minutes before **calcium salts**. Moderate Study
▸ Oral **calcium salts** decrease the absorption of bisphosphonates (clodronate). Avoid **calcium salts** for 2 hours before or 1 hour after **clodronate**. Moderate Study
▸ Oral **calcium salts** are predicted to decrease the absorption of oral bisphosphonates (ibandronate). Avoid **calcium salts** for at least 6 hours before or 1 hour after **ibandronate**. Moderate Theoretical
▸ Oral **calcium salts** decrease the absorption of bisphosphonates (risedronate). Separate administration by at least 2 hours. Moderate Study
▸ Cephalosporins (ceftriaxone) increase the risk of cardio-respiratory arrest when given with **calcium chloride**. Avoid. Severe Anecdotal
▸ Cephalosporins (ceftriaxone) increase the risk of cardio-respiratory arrest when given with intravenous **calcium gluconate**. Avoid. Severe Anecdotal
▸ Intravenous **calcium salts** increase the effects of digoxin. Avoid. Moderate Anecdotal
▸ Oral **calcium salts** decrease the absorption of dolutegravir. **Dolutegravir** should be taken 2 hours before or 6 hours after **calcium salts**. Moderate Study
▸ Oral **calcium salts** decrease the absorption of eltrombopag. **Eltrombopag** should be taken 2 hours before or 4 hours after **calcium salts**. Severe Study
▸ **Calcium carbonate** decreases the absorption of hydroxychloroquine. Separate administration by at least 4 hours. Moderate Study
▸ Oral **calcium carbonate** decreases the absorption of oral iron. **Calcium carbonate** should be taken 1 hour before or 2 hours after iron. Moderate Study
▸ **Calcium carbonate** is predicted to decrease the exposure to ledipasvir. Separate administration by 4 hours. Moderate Theoretical
▸ Oral **calcium carbonate** is predicted to decrease the exposure to oral neratinib. Separate administration by at least 3 hours. Mild Theoretical
▸ **Calcium carbonate** is predicted to slightly decrease the exposure to NNRTIs (rilpivirine). **Calcium carbonate** should be taken 2 hours before or 4 hours after **rilpivirine**. Severe Theoretical
▸ **Calcium carbonate** decreases the absorption of quinolones (ciprofloxacin). Separate administration by 2 hours. Moderate Study
▸ **Calcium carbonate** greatly decreases the exposure to raltegravir (high-dose). Avoid. Severe Study
▸ Oral **calcium salts** decrease the exposure to strontium. Separate administration by 2 hours. Moderate Study
▸ **Calcium carbonate** is predicted to decrease the absorption of tetracyclines. Separate administration by 2 to 3 hours. Moderate Theoretical
▸ Thiazide diuretics increase the risk of hypercalcaemia when given with **calcium salts**. Severe Anecdotal
▸ Oral **calcium salts** are predicted to decrease the absorption of thyroid hormones (levothyroxine). Separate administration by at least 4 hours. Moderate Anecdotal
▸ **Calcium carbonate** is predicted to decrease the concentration of velpatasvir. Separate administration by 4 hours. Moderate Anecdotal
▸ Oral **calcium salts** decrease the absorption of zinc. Moderate Study

Canagliflozin → see sodium glucose co-transporter 2 inhibitors
Canakinumab → see monoclonal antibodies
Candesartan → see angiotensin-II receptor antagonists
Cangrelor → see TABLE 4 p. 1429 (antiplatelet effects)
Cannabidiol → see TABLE 11 p. 1431 (CNS depressant effects)
▸ Anti-androgens (apalutamide, enzalutamide) are predicted to decrease the exposure to **cannabidiol**. Adjust dose. Moderate Study

▸ Antiepileptics (carbamazepine, fosphenytoin, phenobarbital, phenytoin, primidone) are predicted to decrease the exposure to **cannabidiol**. Adjust dose. Moderate Study → Also see TABLE 11 p. 1431
▸ **Cannabidiol** increases the risk of increased ALT concentration when given with antiepileptics (valproate). Avoid or adjust dose. Severe Study
▸ Antifungals, azoles (fluconazole) are predicted to increase the exposure to **cannabidiol**. Moderate Theoretical
▸ Antifungals, azoles (itraconazole, ketoconazole, voriconazole) are predicted to increase the exposure to **cannabidiol**. Avoid or adjust dose. Mild Study
▸ **Cannabidiol** increases the exposure to the active metabolite of benzodiazepines (clobazam) and benzodiazepines (clobazam) increase the exposure to the active metabolite of **cannabidiol**. Adjust dose. Moderate Study → Also see TABLE 11 p. 1431
▸ Cobicistat is predicted to increase the exposure to **cannabidiol**. Avoid or adjust dose. Mild Study
▸ HIV-protease inhibitors are predicted to increase the exposure to **cannabidiol**. Avoid or adjust dose. Mild Study
▸ Idelalisib is predicted to increase the exposure to **cannabidiol**. Avoid or adjust dose. Mild Study
▸ Macrolides (clarithromycin) are predicted to increase the exposure to **cannabidiol**. Avoid or adjust dose. Mild Study
▸ Mitotane is predicted to decrease the exposure to **cannabidiol**. Adjust dose. Moderate Study
▸ Moclobemide is predicted to increase the exposure to **cannabidiol**. Moderate Theoretical
▸ Proton pump inhibitors (esomeprazole) are predicted to increase the exposure to **cannabidiol**. Moderate Theoretical
▸ Rifamycins (rifampicin) are predicted to decrease the exposure to **cannabidiol**. Adjust dose. Moderate Study
▸ SSRIs (fluoxetine, fluvoxamine) are predicted to increase the exposure to **cannabidiol**. Moderate Theoretical
▸ St John's wort is predicted to decrease the exposure to **cannabidiol**. Adjust dose. Mild Study

Capecitabine → see TABLE 15 p. 1432 (myelosuppression)
▸ Allopurinol is predicted to decrease the effects of **capecitabine**. Avoid. Severe Study
▸ **Capecitabine** increases the concentration of antiepileptics (fosphenytoin, phenytoin). Severe Anecdotal
▸ **Capecitabine** increases the effects of coumarins. Monitor INR and adjust dose. Moderate Anecdotal
▸ Folates are predicted to increase the risk of toxicity when given with **capecitabine**. Severe Anecdotal
▸ H₂ receptor antagonists (cimetidine) are predicted to slightly increase the exposure to **capecitabine**. Severe Theoretical
▸ Live vaccines are predicted to increase the risk of generalised infection (possibly life-threatening) when given with **capecitabine**. Public Health England advises avoid (refer to Green Book). Severe Theoretical
▸ Metronidazole is predicted to increase the risk of capecitabine toxicity when given with **capecitabine**. Severe Theoretical

Caplacizumab
▸ **Caplacizumab** is predicted to increase the risk of bleeding events when given with drugs with anticoagulant effects (see TABLE 3 p. 1429). Severe Theoretical
▸ **Caplacizumab** is predicted to increase the risk of bleeding events when given with drugs with antiplatelet effects (see TABLE 4 p. 1429). Severe Theoretical

Capreomycin → see TABLE 2 p. 1429 (nephrotoxicity), TABLE 19 p. 1433 (ototoxicity)
Captopril → see ACE inhibitors
Carbamazepine → see antiepileptics
Carbapenems

ertapenem · imipenem · meropenem

▸ Carbapenems decrease the concentration of antiepileptics (valproate). Avoid. Severe Anecdotal
▸ Ganciclovir is predicted to increase the risk of seizures when given with **imipenem**. Avoid. Severe Anecdotal
▸ Valganciclovir is predicted to increase the risk of seizures when given with **imipenem**. Avoid. Severe Anecdotal

Carbidopa
▸ Oral iron is predicted to decrease the exposure to oral **carbidopa**. Moderate Theoretical

arbimazole

Carbimazole affects the concentration of digoxin. Monitor and adjust dose. Moderate Theoretical

Carbimazole decreases the effects of metyrapone. Avoid. Moderate Theoretical

Carbimazole given with a potent CYP3A4 inhibitor is predicted to increase the exposure to propiverine. Adjust starting dose. Moderate Theoretical

arboplatin → see platinum compounds

arfilzomib → see TABLE 15 p. 1432 (myelosuppression)

Carfilzomib potentially decreases the efficacy of combined hormonal contraceptives. Use additional contraceptive precautions. Severe Theoretical

ariprazine → see antipsychotics, second generation

armustine → see alkylating agents

arvedilol → see beta blockers, non-selective

aspofungin

▸ Antiepileptics (carbamazepine, fosphenytoin, phenytoin) are predicted to decrease the concentration of **caspofungin**. Adjust **caspofungin** dose, p. 631. Moderate Theoretical

Ciclosporin slightly increases the exposure to **caspofungin**. Severe Study

▸ Corticosteroids (dexamethasone) are predicted to decrease the concentration of **caspofungin**. Adjust **caspofungin** dose, p. 631. Moderate Theoretical

▸ NNRTIs (efavirenz) are predicted to decrease the concentration of **caspofungin**. Adjust dose. Moderate Study

▸ NNRTIs (nevirapine) are predicted to decrease the concentration of **caspofungin**. Adjust dose. Moderate Theoretical

▸ Rifamycins (rifampicin) decrease the concentration of **caspofungin**. Adjust **caspofungin** dose, p. 631. Moderate Study

Cefaclor → see cephalosporins
Cefadroxil → see cephalosporins
Cefalexin → see cephalosporins
Cefazolin → see cephalosporins
Cefepime → see cephalosporins
Cefiderocol → see cephalosporins
Cefixime → see cephalosporins
Cefotaxime → see cephalosporins
Cefoxitin → see cephalosporins
Cefradine → see cephalosporins
Ceftaroline → see cephalosporins
Ceftazidime → see cephalosporins
Ceftobiprole → see cephalosporins
Ceftolozane → see cephalosporins
Ceftriaxone → see cephalosporins
Cefuroxime → see cephalosporins
Celecoxib → see NSAIDs
Celiprolol → see beta blockers, selective
Cemiplimab → see monoclonal antibodies
Cephalosporins → see TABLE 2 p. 1429 (nephrotoxicity)

cefaclor · cefadroxil · cefalexin · cefazolin · cefepime · cefiderocol · cefixime · cefotaxime · cefoxitin · cefradine · ceftaroline · ceftazidime · ceftobiprole · ceftolozane · ceftriaxone · cefuroxime

ROUTE-SPECIFIC INFORMATION Interactions do not generally apply to topical use of **cefuroxime** unless specified.

▸ **Ceftriaxone** increases the risk of cardio-respiratory arrest when given with calcium salts (calcium chloride). Avoid. Severe Anecdotal

▸ **Ceftriaxone** increases the risk of cardio-respiratory arrest when given with intravenous calcium salts (calcium gluconate). Avoid. Severe Anecdotal

▸ Cephalosporins (cefazolin, ceftriaxone) potentially increase the risk of bleeding events when given with coumarins. Severe Anecdotal

▸ **Ceftobiprole** is predicted to increase the exposure to endothelin receptor antagonists (bosentan). Moderate Theoretical

▸ Leflunomide is predicted to increase the exposure to **cefaclor**. Moderate Theoretical

▸ Nitisinone is predicted to increase the exposure to **cefaclor**. Moderate Study

▸ Cephalosporins (cefazolin, ceftriaxone) potentially increase the risk of bleeding events when given with phenindione. Severe Anecdotal

▸ **Ceftobiprole** is predicted to increase the concentration of statins. Moderate Theoretical

▸ **Ceftobiprole** is predicted to increase the concentration of sulfonylureas (glibenclamide). Moderate Theoretical

▸ Teriflunomide is predicted to increase the exposure to **cefaclor**. Moderate Study

Ceritinib → see TABLE 15 p. 1432 (myelosuppression), TABLE 9 p. 1431 (QT-interval prolongation)

▸ **Ceritinib** is predicted to increase the exposure to aliskiren. Moderate Theoretical

▸ Oral antacids are predicted to decrease the absorption of oral **ceritinib**. Separate administration by 2 hours. Moderate Theoretical

▸ Anti-androgens (apalutamide, enzalutamide) are predicted to decrease the exposure to ceritinib. Avoid. Severe Study → Also see TABLE 9 p. 1431

▸ Antiarrhythmics (amiodarone) are predicted to increase the exposure to **ceritinib**. Moderate Theoretical → Also see TABLE 9 p. 1431

▸ Antiepileptics (carbamazepine, fosphenytoin, phenobarbital, phenytoin, primidone) are predicted to decrease the exposure to **ceritinib**. Avoid. Severe Study

▸ Antifungals, azoles (itraconazole, ketoconazole, voriconazole) are predicted to increase the exposure to **ceritinib**. Avoid or adjust **ceritinib** dose, p. 1017. Severe Study → Also see TABLE 9 p. 1431

▸ **Ceritinib** is predicted to increase the exposure to antihistamines, non-sedating (fexofenadine). Moderate Theoretical

▸ **Ceritinib** is predicted to increase the exposure to ciclosporin. Avoid. Severe Theoretical

▸ Cobicistat is predicted to increase the exposure to **ceritinib**. Avoid or adjust **ceritinib** dose, p. 1017. Severe Study

▸ **Ceritinib** is predicted to increase the exposure to colchicine. Moderate Theoretical

▸ **Ceritinib** is predicted to increase the exposure to coumarins (warfarin). Avoid. Severe Theoretical

▸ **Ceritinib** is predicted to increase the risk of bradycardia when given with digoxin. Avoid. Severe Theoretical

▸ **Ceritinib** is predicted to increase the exposure to ergotamine. Avoid. Severe Theoretical

▸ **Ceritinib** is predicted to increase the exposure to everolimus. Moderate Theoretical

▸ **Ceritinib** is predicted to increase the exposure to factor XA inhibitors (edoxaban). Moderate Theoretical

▸ Grapefruit juice is predicted to increase the exposure to **ceritinib**. Avoid. Severe Theoretical

▸ H_2 receptor antagonists are predicted to decrease the absorption of **ceritinib**. Moderate Theoretical

▸ HIV-protease inhibitors are predicted to increase the exposure to **ceritinib**. Avoid or adjust **ceritinib** dose, p. 1017. Severe Study → Also see TABLE 9 p. 1431

▸ Idelalisib is predicted to increase the exposure to **ceritinib**. Avoid or adjust **ceritinib** dose, p. 1017. Severe Study

▸ Lapatinib is predicted to increase the exposure to **ceritinib**. Moderate Theoretical → Also see TABLE 9 p. 1431

▸ **Ceritinib** is predicted to increase the exposure to loperamide. Moderate Theoretical

▸ Macrolides (azithromycin) are predicted to increase the exposure to **ceritinib**. Moderate Theoretical

▸ Macrolides (clarithromycin) are predicted to increase the exposure to **ceritinib**. Avoid or adjust **ceritinib** dose, p. 1017. Severe Study → Also see TABLE 9 p. 1431

▸ Mitotane is predicted to decrease the exposure to **ceritinib**. Avoid. Severe Study → Also see TABLE 15 p. 1432

▸ **Ceritinib** is predicted to increase the exposure to NSAIDs (celecoxib, diclofenac). Adjust dose. Moderate Theoretical

▸ **Ceritinib** is predicted to increase the exposure to opioids (alfentanil, fentanyl). Avoid. Severe Theoretical

▸ **Ceritinib** is predicted to increase the exposure to pimozide. Avoid. Severe Theoretical → Also see TABLE 9 p. 1431

▸ Proton pump inhibitors are predicted to decrease the absorption of **ceritinib**. Moderate Theoretical

▸ Ranolazine is predicted to increase the exposure to **ceritinib**. Moderate Theoretical → Also see TABLE 9 p. 1431

▸ Rifamycins (rifampicin) are predicted to decrease the exposure to **ceritinib**. Avoid. Severe Study

A1

Interactions | **Appendix 1**

Ceritinib (continued)

‣ **Ceritinib** is predicted to increase the exposure to sirolimus. Avoid. Severe Theoretical

‣ St John's wort is predicted to decrease the exposure to **ceritinib**. Avoid. Severe Theoretical

‣ **Ceritinib** is predicted to increase the exposure to sulfonylureas (glimepiride). Adjust dose. Moderate Theoretical

‣ **Ceritinib** is predicted to increase the exposure to tacrolimus. Avoid. Severe Theoretical

‣ **Ceritinib** is predicted to increase the exposure to taxanes (paclitaxel). Moderate Theoretical → Also see TABLE 15 p. 1432

‣ **Ceritinib** is predicted to increase the exposure to thrombin inhibitors (dabigatran). Moderate Theoretical

‣ **Ceritinib** is predicted to increase the exposure to topotecan. Moderate Theoretical → Also see TABLE 15 p. 1432

Certolizumab pegol → see monoclonal antibodies

Cetirizine → see antihistamines, non-sedating

Cetuximab → see monoclonal antibodies

Chenodeoxycholic acid

‣ Oral aluminium hydroxide decreases the absorption of chenodeoxycholic acid. Moderate Study

‣ Antiepileptics (phenobarbital, primidone) are predicted to affect the efficacy of **chenodeoxycholic acid**. Monitor and adjust dose. Moderate Theoretical

‣ Ciclosporin is predicted to affect the efficacy of **chenodeoxycholic acid**. Monitor and adjust dose. Moderate Theoretical

‣ Oral combined hormonal contraceptives potentially decrease the efficacy of oral **chenodeoxycholic acid**. Avoid. Moderate Theoretical

‣ Sirolimus is predicted to affect the efficacy of **chenodeoxycholic acid**. Monitor and adjust dose. Moderate Theoretical

Chloral hydrate → see TABLE 11 p. 1431 (CNS depressant effects)

‣ Intravenous loop diuretics (furosemide) potentially increase the risk of sweating, variable blood pressure, and tachycardia when given with **chloral hydrate**. Moderate Anecdotal

Chlorambucil → see alkylating agents

Chloramphenicol

ROUTE-SPECIFIC INFORMATION Since systemic absorption can follow topical application, the possibility of interactions should be borne in mind.

‣ Antiepileptics (phenobarbital, primidone) decrease the concentration of **chloramphenicol**. Moderate Study

‣ Intravenous **chloramphenicol** increases the concentration of antiepileptics (fosphenytoin, phenytoin) and antiepileptics (fosphenytoin, phenytoin) affect the concentration of intravenous **chloramphenicol**. Monitor concentration and adjust dose. Severe Study

‣ **Chloramphenicol** potentially increases the anticoagulant effect of coumarins. Moderate Anecdotal

‣ **Chloramphenicol** is predicted to increase the exposure to guanfacine. Adjust guanfacine dose, p. 372. Moderate Theoretical

‣ **Chloramphenicol** decreases the efficacy of iron. Moderate Anecdotal

‣ Rifamycins (rifampicin) decrease the concentration of **chloramphenicol**. Moderate Study

‣ **Chloramphenicol** is predicted to increase the exposure to sulfonylureas. Severe Study

‣ **Chloramphenicol** increases the concentration of tacrolimus. Severe Study

Chlordiazepoxide → see benzodiazepines

Chlormethine

ROUTE-SPECIFIC INFORMATION Since systemic absorption can follow topical application, the possibility of interactions should be borne in mind.

Chloroprocaine → see TABLE 11 p. 1431 (CNS depressant effects)

‣ **Chloroprocaine** is predicted to increase the risk of cardiovascular adverse effects when given with antiarrhythmics (amiodarone, dronedarone, vernakalant). Severe Theoretical

‣ **Chloroprocaine** is predicted to increase the risk of cardiovascular adverse effects when given with beta blockers, non-selective (sotalol). Severe Theoretical

‣ **Chloroprocaine** is predicted to decrease the effects of sulfonamides. Avoid. Severe Theoretical

Chloroquine → see antimalarials

Chlorothiazide → see thiazide diuretics

Chlorphenamine → see antihistamines, sedating

Chlorpromazine → see phenothiazines

Chlortalidone → see thiazide diuretics

Cholera vaccine

‣ Antimalarials (chloroquine) decrease the efficacy of oral **cholera vaccine**. Moderate Study

‣ Hydroxychloroquine is predicted to decrease the efficacy of oral **cholera vaccine**. Moderate Theoretical

Cholic acid

‣ Oral antacids are predicted to decrease the absorption of oral **cholic acid**. Separate administration by 5 hours. Mild Study

‣ Antiepileptics (phenobarbital) decrease the effects of **cholic acid**. Avoid. Moderate Study

‣ Ciclosporin affects the concentration of **cholic acid**. Avoid. Moderate Study

Choline salicylate

‣ Corticosteroids are predicted to decrease the concentration of **choline salicylate**. Moderate Study

Ciclesonide → see corticosteroids

Ciclosporin → see TABLE 2 p. 1429 (nephrotoxicity), TABLE 16 p. 1433 (increased serum potassium)

> ‣ Pomelo juice is predicted to increase ciclosporin exposure, and purple grape juice is predicted to decrease ciclosporin exposure.
> ‣ Since systemic absorption can follow topical application, the possibility of interactions should be borne in mind.

‣ **Ciclosporin** is predicted to increase the exposure to afatinib. Separate administration by 12 hours. Moderate Study

‣ **Ciclosporin** markedly increases the exposure to aliskiren. Avoid. Severe Study → Also see TABLE 16 p. 1433

‣ **Ciclosporin** is predicted to increase the exposure to alpelisib. Moderate Theoretical

‣ **Ciclosporin** increases the concentration of anthracyclines (daunorubicin, doxorubicin, epirubicin, idarubicin, mitoxantrone). Severe Study

‣ Anti-androgens (apalutamide, enzalutamide) decrease the concentration of **ciclosporin**. Severe Study

‣ Antiarrhythmics (amiodarone) increase the concentration of **ciclosporin**. Monitor concentration and adjust dose. Severe Study

‣ Antiarrhythmics (dronedarone) are predicted to increase the concentration of **ciclosporin**. Severe Study

‣ Antiepileptics (carbamazepine, fosphenytoin, phenobarbital, phenytoin, primidone) decrease the concentration of **ciclosporin**. Severe Study

‣ Antiepileptics (oxcarbazepine) decrease the concentration of **ciclosporin**. Severe Anecdotal

‣ Antifungals, azoles (fluconazole, isavuconazole, posaconazole) are predicted to increase the concentration of **ciclosporin**. Severe Study

‣ Antifungals, azoles (itraconazole, ketoconazole, voriconazole) increase the concentration of **ciclosporin**. Severe Study

‣ Antifungals, azoles (miconazole) increase the concentration of **ciclosporin**. Monitor and adjust dose. Severe Anecdotal

‣ **Ciclosporin** is predicted to increase the exposure to beta blockers, non-selective (nadolol). Moderate Study

‣ **Ciclosporin** is predicted to increase the exposure to bictegravir. Use with caution or avoid. Moderate Theoretical

‣ Calcium channel blockers (diltiazem, verapamil) are predicted to increase the concentration of **ciclosporin**. Severe Study

‣ Calcium channel blockers (nicardipine) increase the concentration of **ciclosporin**. Severe Study

‣ **Ciclosporin** moderately increases the exposure to calcium channel blockers (lercanidipine). Use with caution or avoid. Severe Study

‣ **Ciclosporin** slightly increases the exposure to caspofungin. Severe Study

‣ Ceritinib is predicted to increase the exposure to **ciclosporin**. Avoid. Severe Theoretical

‣ **Ciclosporin** is predicted to affect the efficacy of chenodeoxycholic acid. Monitor and adjust dose. Moderate Theoretical

Ciclosporin affects the concentration of cholic acid. Avoid. Moderate Study

Cobicistat increases the concentration of **ciclosporin**. Severe Study

Ciclosporin increases the exposure to colchicine. Avoid P-glycoprotein inhibitors or adjust **colchicine** dose, p. 1166. Severe Study

Crizotinib is predicted to increase the concentration of **ciclosporin**. Severe Study

Danazol increases the concentration of **ciclosporin**. Severe Study

Ciclosporin is predicted to increase the risk of rhabdomyolysis when given with daptomycin. Severe Theoretical

Ciclosporin is predicted to increase the exposure to darifenacin. Avoid. Moderate Theoretical

Ciclosporin increases the concentration of digoxin. Monitor and adjust dose. Severe Theoretical

Ciclosporin decreases the exposure to eltrombopag. Monitor and adjust dose. Moderate Study

Endothelin receptor antagonists (bosentan) moderately decrease the exposure to **ciclosporin** and **ciclosporin** moderately increases the exposure to endothelin receptor antagonists (bosentan). Avoid. Severe Study

Ciclosporin moderately increases the exposure to endothelin receptor antagonists (ambrisentan). Adjust **ambrisentan** dose, p. 197. Moderate Study

Entrectinib is predicted to increase the exposure to **ciclosporin**. Mild Theoretical

Ciclosporin is predicted to increase the exposure to erlotinib. Moderate Theoretical

Ciclosporin increases the exposure to etoposide. Monitor and adjust dose. Severe Study

Ciclosporin moderately increases the exposure to everolimus. Avoid or adjust dose. Severe Study

Ciclosporin moderately increases the exposure to ezetimibe and ezetimibe slightly increases the exposure to **ciclosporin**. Moderate Study

Ciclosporin slightly increases the exposure to factor XA inhibitors (edoxaban). Adjust **edoxaban** dose, p. 137. Severe Study

Fibrates (bezafibrate) are predicted to increase the risk of nephrotoxicity when given with **ciclosporin**. Severe Theoretical

Fibrates (fenofibrate) increase the risk of nephrotoxicity when given with **ciclosporin**. Severe Study

Ciclosporin is predicted to increase the exposure to fidaxomicin. Avoid. Moderate Study

Filgotinib is predicted to increase the risk of immunosuppression when given with **ciclosporin**. Avoid. Severe Theoretical

Ciclosporin increases the exposure to glecaprevir. Avoid or monitor. Severe Study

Grapefruit juice increases the concentration of **ciclosporin**. Avoid. Severe Study

Ciclosporin greatly increases the exposure to grazoprevir. Avoid. Severe Study

H₂ receptor antagonists (cimetidine) increase the concentration of **ciclosporin**. Mild Study

HIV-protease inhibitors increase the concentration of **ciclosporin**. Severe Study

Idelalisib increases the concentration of **ciclosporin**. Severe Study

Imatinib is predicted to increase the concentration of **ciclosporin**. Severe Study

Lanreotide is predicted to decrease the absorption of oral **ciclosporin**. Adjust dose. Severe Theoretical

Ciclosporin is predicted to increase the exposure to larotrectinib. Mild Study

Letermovir increases the exposure to **ciclosporin** and **ciclosporin** increases the exposure to letermovir. Monitor and adjust **letermovir** dose, p. 678. Severe Study

Live vaccines are predicted to increase the risk of generalised infection (possibly life-threatening) when given with **ciclosporin**. Public Health England advises avoid (refer to Green Book). Severe Theoretical

Ciclosporin is predicted to increase the exposure to lomitapide. Separate administration by 12 hours. Moderate Theoretical

Lorlatinib is predicted to decrease the exposure to **ciclosporin**. Avoid. Moderate Theoretical

Lumacaftor is predicted to decrease the exposure to **ciclosporin**. Avoid. Severe Theoretical

Macrolides (clarithromycin) increase the concentration of **ciclosporin**. Severe Study

Macrolides (erythromycin) are predicted to increase the concentration of **ciclosporin**. Severe Study

Ciclosporin moderately increases the exposure to meglitinides (repaglinide). Moderate Study

Ciclosporin is predicted to decrease the efficacy of mifamurtide. Avoid. Severe Theoretical

Mitotane decreases the concentration of **ciclosporin**. Severe Study

Monoclonal antibodies (blinatumomab) are predicted to transiently increase the exposure to **ciclosporin**. Monitor and adjust dose. Moderate Theoretical

Monoclonal antibodies (sarilumab) potentially affect the exposure to **ciclosporin**. Monitor and adjust dose. Moderate Theoretical

Monoclonal antibodies (tocilizumab) are predicted to decrease the exposure to **ciclosporin**. Monitor and adjust dose. Moderate Theoretical

Ciclosporin is predicted to increase the exposure to naldemedine. Moderate Study

Neurokinin-1 receptor antagonists (aprepitant, netupitant) are predicted to increase the concentration of **ciclosporin**. Severe Study

Nilotinib is predicted to increase the concentration of **ciclosporin**. Severe Study

Ciclosporin is predicted to increase the exposure to nintedanib. Moderate Study

NNRTIs (efavirenz) decrease the concentration of **ciclosporin**. Monitor concentration and adjust dose. Moderate Study

NNRTIs (nevirapine) are predicted to decrease the concentration of **ciclosporin**. Moderate Study

Ciclosporin increases the concentration of NSAIDs (diclofenac). Severe Study → Also see TABLE 2 p. 1429 → Also see TABLE 16 p. 1433

Octreotide decreases the absorption of oral **ciclosporin**. Adjust **ciclosporin** dose, p. 884. Severe Anecdotal

Ciclosporin is predicted to increase the exposure to the active metabolite of ozanimod. Avoid. Moderate Study

Palbociclib is predicted to increase the exposure to **ciclosporin**. Adjust dose. Moderate Theoretical

Ciclosporin is predicted to increase the exposure to panobinostat. Adjust dose. Moderate Theoretical

Pasireotide is predicted to decrease the absorption of oral **ciclosporin**. Adjust dose. Severe Theoretical

Pitolisant is predicted to decrease the exposure to **ciclosporin**. Avoid. Severe Theoretical

Ciclosporin is predicted to increase the concentration of ranolazine and ranolazine is predicted to increase the concentration of **ciclosporin**. Moderate Theoretical

Ribociclib is predicted to increase the exposure to **ciclosporin**. Use with caution and adjust dose. Moderate Theoretical

Rifamycins (rifampicin) decrease the concentration of **ciclosporin**. Severe Study

Ciclosporin very markedly increases the exposure to rifaximin. Severe Study

Ciclosporin is predicted to increase the exposure to riociguat. Moderate Theoretical

Rucaparib is predicted to increase the exposure to **ciclosporin**. Monitor and adjust dose. Moderate Study

Ciclosporin moderately increases the exposure to sirolimus. Separate administration by 4 hours. Severe Study

St John's wort decreases the concentration of **ciclosporin**. Avoid. Moderate Study

Ciclosporin very markedly increases the exposure to statins (atorvastatin). Avoid or adjust **atorvastatin** dose, p. 217. Severe Study

Ciclosporin moderately increases the exposure to statins (fluvastatin). Severe Study

Ciclosporin markedly to very markedly increases the exposure to statins (pravastatin). Adjust dose. Severe Study

Ciclosporin (continued)
▶ **Ciclosporin** markedly increases the exposure to statins (rosuvastatin, simvastatin). Avoid. Severe Study
▶ **Ciclosporin** increases the concentration of tacrolimus. Avoid. Severe Study → Also see TABLE 2 p. 1429 → Also see TABLE 16 p. 1433
▶ **Ciclosporin** is predicted to slightly increase the exposure to talazoparib. Avoid or adjust talazoparib dose, p. 1052. Severe Study
▶ **Ciclosporin** is predicted to increase the exposure to tenofovir alafenamide. Moderate Theoretical
▶ **Ciclosporin** is predicted to increase the exposure to tenofovir disoproxil. Moderate Theoretical → Also see TABLE 2 p. 1429
▶ **Ciclosporin** is predicted to increase the exposure to thrombin inhibitors (dabigatran). Avoid. Severe Theoretical
▶ **Ciclosporin** is predicted to increase the exposure to ticagrelor. Use with caution or avoid. Severe Study
▶ **Ciclosporin** increases the exposure to tofacitinib. Avoid. Severe Study
▶ **Ciclosporin** is predicted to increase the exposure to topotecan. Severe Study
▶ **Ciclosporin** is predicted to increase the concentration of trametinib. Moderate Theoretical
▶ Ursodeoxycholic acid affects the concentration of **ciclosporin**. Use with caution and adjust dose. Severe Anecdotal
▶ **Ciclosporin** is predicted to increase the exposure to venetoclax. Avoid or monitor for toxicity. Severe Theoretical
▶ Vitamin E substances affect the exposure to **ciclosporin**. Moderate Study
▶ **Ciclosporin** increases the concentration of voxilaprevir. Avoid. Severe Study

Cidofovir → see TABLE 2 p. 1429 (nephrotoxicity)

Cilostazol → see TABLE 4 p. 1429 (antiplatelet effects)

GENERAL INFORMATION Concurrent use with 2 or more antiplatelets or anticoagulants is contra-indicated.

▶ Anti-androgens (apalutamide, enzalutamide) are predicted to alter the effects of **cilostazol**. Moderate Theoretical
▶ Antiepileptics (carbamazepine, fosphenytoin, phenobarbital, phenytoin, primidone) are predicted to alter the effects of **cilostazol**. Moderate Theoretical
▶ Antifungals, azoles (fluconazole) are predicted to increase the exposure to **cilostazol**. Adjust cilostazol dose, p. 248. Moderate Theoretical
▶ Antifungals, azoles (itraconazole, ketoconazole, voriconazole) are predicted to moderately increase the exposure to **cilostazol**. Adjust cilostazol dose, p. 248. Moderate Study
▶ Antifungals, azoles (miconazole) are predicted to increase the exposure to **cilostazol**. Use with caution and adjust dose. Moderate Theoretical
▶ Cobicistat is predicted to moderately increase the exposure to **cilostazol**. Adjust cilostazol dose, p. 248. Moderate Study
▶ HIV-protease inhibitors are predicted to moderately increase the exposure to **cilostazol**. Adjust cilostazol dose, p. 248. Moderate Study
▶ Idelalisib is predicted to moderately increase the exposure to **cilostazol**. Adjust cilostazol dose, p. 248. Moderate Study
▶ **Cilostazol** is predicted to increase the exposure to lomitapide. Separate administration by 12 hours. Moderate Theoretical
▶ Macrolides (clarithromycin) are predicted to moderately increase the exposure to **cilostazol**. Adjust cilostazol dose, p. 248. Moderate Study
▶ Macrolides (erythromycin) slightly increase the exposure to **cilostazol**. Adjust cilostazol dose, p. 248. Moderate Study
▶ Mitotane is predicted to alter the effects of **cilostazol**. Moderate Theoretical
▶ Moclobemide is predicted to increase the exposure to **cilostazol**. Moderate Theoretical
▶ Proton pump inhibitors (esomeprazole) are predicted to increase the exposure to **cilostazol**. Moderate Theoretical
▶ Proton pump inhibitors (omeprazole) are predicted to increase the exposure to **cilostazol**. Adjust cilostazol dose, p. 248. Moderate Study
▶ Rifamycins (rifampicin) are predicted to alter the effects of **cilostazol**. Moderate Theoretical

▶ SSRIs (fluoxetine, fluvoxamine) are predicted to increase the exposure to **cilostazol**. Adjust cilostazol dose, p. 248. Moderate Theoretical → Also see TABLE 4 p. 1429
▶ St John's wort is predicted to alter the effects of **cilostazol**. Moderate Theoretical

Cimetidine → see H₂ receptor antagonists

Cinacalcet

FOOD AND LIFESTYLE Dose adjustment might be necessary if smoking started or stopped during treatment.

▶ Anti-androgens (apalutamide, enzalutamide) are predicted to decrease the exposure to **cinacalcet**. Monitor and adjust dose. Moderate Study
▶ **Cinacalcet** is predicted to increase the exposure to anticholinesterases, centrally acting (galantamine). Monitor and adjust dose. Moderate Study
▶ Antiepileptics (carbamazepine, fosphenytoin, phenobarbital, phenytoin, primidone) are predicted to decrease the exposure to **cinacalcet**. Monitor and adjust dose. Moderate Study
▶ Antifungals, azoles (itraconazole, ketoconazole, voriconazole) are predicted to moderately increase the exposure to **cinacalcet**. Adjust dose. Moderate Study
▶ **Cinacalcet** is predicted to moderately increase the exposure to antipsychotics, second generation (aripiprazole). Adjust aripiprazole dose, p. 415. Moderate Study
▶ **Cinacalcet** is predicted to increase the exposure to antipsychotics, second generation (risperidone). Adjust dose. Moderate Study
▶ **Cinacalcet** is predicted to markedly increase the exposure to atomoxetine. Adjust dose. Severe Study
▶ **Cinacalcet** is predicted to increase the exposure to beta blockers, selective (metoprolol, nebivolol). Moderate Study
▶ Cobicistat is predicted to moderately increase the exposure to **cinacalcet**. Adjust dose. Moderate Study
▶ **Cinacalcet** is predicted to slightly increase the exposure to darifenacin. Mild Study
▶ **Cinacalcet** is predicted to increase the exposure to eliglustat. Avoid or adjust dose—consult product literature. Severe Study
▶ **Cinacalcet** increases the risk of hypocalcaemia when given with etelcalcetide. Avoid. Severe Theoretical
▶ HIV-protease inhibitors are predicted to moderately increase the exposure to **cinacalcet**. Adjust dose. Moderate Study
▶ Idelalisib is predicted to moderately increase the exposure to **cinacalcet**. Adjust dose. Moderate Study
▶ Macrolides (clarithromycin) are predicted to moderately increase the exposure to **cinacalcet**. Adjust dose. Moderate Study
▶ **Cinacalcet** is predicted to increase the exposure to mexiletine. Moderate Study
▶ Mitotane is predicted to decrease the exposure to **cinacalcet**. Monitor and adjust dose. Moderate Study
▶ **Cinacalcet** is predicted to decrease the efficacy of opioids (codeine). Moderate Theoretical
▶ **Cinacalcet** is predicted to decrease the efficacy of opioids (tramadol). Severe Study
▶ **Cinacalcet** is predicted to moderately increase the exposure to pitolisant. Use with caution and adjust dose. Moderate Study
▶ Rifamycins (rifampicin) are predicted to decrease the exposure to **cinacalcet**. Monitor and adjust dose. Moderate Study
▶ SSRIs (fluvoxamine) are predicted to increase the exposure to **cinacalcet**. Adjust dose. Moderate Theoretical
▶ **Cinacalcet** is predicted to increase the exposure to SSRIs (dapoxetine). Moderate Theoretical
▶ **Cinacalcet** is predicted to decrease the efficacy of tamoxifen. Avoid. Severe Study
▶ **Cinacalcet** is predicted to increase the exposure to the active metabolite of tetrabenazine. Moderate Study
▶ **Cinacalcet** is predicted to increase the exposure to tricyclic antidepressants. Monitor for toxicity and adjust dose. Severe Study
▶ **Cinacalcet** is predicted to increase the exposure to vortioxetine. Monitor and adjust dose. Moderate Study

Cinnarizine → see antihistamines, sedating

Ciprofibrate → see fibrates

Ciprofloxacin → see quinolones

Cisatracurium → see neuromuscular blocking drugs, non-depolarising

isplatin → see platinum compounds

italopram → see SSRIs

ladribine → see TABLE 15 p. 1432 (myelosuppression)

SEPARATION OF ADMINISTRATION Oral cladribine might affect the absorption of concurrently administered drugs—consider separating administration by at least 3 hours.

Antiepileptics (carbamazepine) are predicted to increase the risk of haematological toxicity when given with oral **cladribine**. Moderate Theoretical

Live vaccines are predicted to increase the risk of generalised infection (possibly life-threatening) when given with **cladribine**. Public Health England advises avoid (refer to Green Book). Severe Theoretical

larithromycin → see macrolides

lavulanate → see TABLE 1 p. 1429 (hepatotoxicity)

lemastine → see antihistamines, sedating

lindamycin

ROUTE-SPECIFIC INFORMATION Since systemic absorption can follow topical application of **clindamycin**, the possibility of interactions should be borne in mind.

Clindamycin increases the effects of neuromuscular blocking drugs, non-depolarising. Severe Anecdotal

Clindamycin increases the effects of suxamethonium. Severe Anecdotal

:lobazam → see benzodiazepines

:lodronate → see bisphosphonates

:lofarabine → see TABLE 15 p. 1432 (myelosuppression)

Live vaccines are predicted to increase the risk of generalised infection (possibly life-threatening) when given with **clofarabine**. Public Health England advises avoid (refer to Green Book). Severe Theoretical

:lofazimine

▶ Clofazimine potentially increases the risk of QT-prolongation when given with bedaquiline. Severe Study

:lomethiazole → see TABLE 11 p. 1431 (CNS depressant effects)

▶ Alcohol causes serious, potentially fatal, CNS depression when given with **clomethiazole**. Avoid. Severe Study → Also see TABLE 11 p. 1431

▶ Anti-androgens (apalutamide, enzalutamide) decrease the exposure to **clomethiazole**. Monitor and adjust dose. Moderate Study

▶ Antiepileptics (carbamazepine, fosphenytoin, phenobarbital, phenytoin, primidone) decrease the exposure to **clomethiazole**. Monitor and adjust dose. Moderate Study → Also see TABLE 11 p. 1431

▶ Mitotane decreases the exposure to **clomethiazole**. Monitor and adjust dose. Moderate Study

▶ Rifamycins (rifampicin) decrease the exposure to **clomethiazole**. Monitor and adjust dose. Moderate Study

:lomipramine → see tricyclic antidepressants

:lonazepam → see benzodiazepines

:lonidine → see TABLE 6 p. 1430 (bradycardia), TABLE 8 p. 1430 (hypotension), TABLE 11 p. 1431 (CNS depressant effects)

▶ Tricyclic antidepressants decrease the antihypertensive effects of clonidine. Monitor and adjust dose. Moderate Anecdotal → Also see TABLE 8 p. 1430 → Also see TABLE 11 p. 1431

:lopidogrel → see TABLE 4 p. 1429 (antiplatelet effects)

▶ Clopidogrel is predicted to increase the exposure to anti-androgens (apalutamide). Mild Study

▶ Clopidogrel moderately increases the exposure to anti-androgens (enzalutamide). Avoid or adjust enzalutamide dose, p. 991. Severe Study

▶ Antifungals, azoles (fluconazole) are predicted to decrease the efficacy of **clopidogrel**. Avoid. Severe Theoretical

▶ Antifungals, azoles (voriconazole) are predicted to decrease the efficacy of **clopidogrel**. Avoid. Moderate Study

▶ Clopidogrel is predicted to increase the exposure to dabrafenib. Moderate Theoretical

▶ Clopidogrel is predicted to very markedly increase the exposure to dasabuvir. Avoid. Severe Study

▶ Grapefruit juice markedly decreases the exposure to **clopidogrel**. Severe Study

▶ Clopidogrel increases the exposure to meglitinides (repaglinide). Avoid. Severe Study

▶ Moclobemide is predicted to decrease the efficacy of **clopidogrel**. Avoid. Moderate Study

▶ Clopidogrel is predicted to moderately increase the exposure to montelukast. Moderate Study

▶ Clopidogrel is predicted to increase the exposure to the active metabolite of ozanimod. Severe Study

▶ Clopidogrel increases the exposure to pioglitazone. Monitor blood glucose and adjust dose. Severe Study

▶ Proton pump inhibitors (esomeprazole, omeprazole) are predicted to decrease the efficacy of **clopidogrel**. Avoid. Moderate Study

▶ Clopidogrel is predicted to increase the exposure to retinoids (alitretinoin). Adjust **alitretinoin** dose, p. 1305. Moderate Theoretical

▶ Clopidogrel is predicted to increase the exposure to selexipag. Adjust **selexipag** dose, p. 196. Moderate Study

▶ SSRIs (fluoxetine, fluvoxamine) are predicted to decrease the efficacy of **clopidogrel**. Avoid. Severe Theoretical → Also see TABLE 4 p. 1429

▶ Clopidogrel increases the exposure to statins (rosuvastatin). Adjust **rosuvastatin** dose, p. 218. Moderate Study

▶ Clopidogrel is predicted to increase the concentration of taxanes (paclitaxel). Severe Anecdotal

Clotrimazole → see antifungals, azoles

Clozapine → see antipsychotics, second generation

Cobicistat

▶ Cobicistat is predicted to increase the exposure to abemaciclib. Avoid or adjust **abemaciclib** dose, p. 1009. Severe Study

▶ Cobicistat is predicted to increase the exposure to acalabrutinib. Avoid. Severe Study

▶ Cobicistat is predicted to markedly increase the exposure to aldosterone antagonists (eplerenone). Avoid. Severe Study

▶ Cobicistat is predicted to moderately increase the exposure to alpha blockers (alfuzosin, tamsulosin). Use with caution or avoid. Moderate Study

▶ Cobicistat is predicted to increase the exposure to alpha blockers (doxazosin). Moderate Study

▶ Anti-androgens (apalutamide, enzalutamide) are predicted to decrease the exposure to cobicistat. Avoid. Severe Theoretical

▶ Cobicistat is predicted to increase the exposure to anti-androgens (apalutamide). Mild Study

▶ Cobicistat potentially increases the concentration of antiarrhythmics (amiodarone, disopyramide, flecainide, lidocaine). Severe Theoretical

▶ Cobicistat very markedly increases the exposure to antiarrhythmics (dronedarone). Avoid. Severe Study

▶ Cobicistat is predicted to increase the exposure to antiarrhythmics (propafenone). Monitor and adjust dose. Severe Study

▶ Cobicistat is predicted to increase the exposure to anticholinesterases, centrally acting (galantamine). Monitor and adjust dose. Moderate Study

▶ Antiepileptics (carbamazepine, fosphenytoin, phenobarbital, phenytoin, primidone) are predicted to decrease the exposure to cobicistat. Avoid. Severe Theoretical

▶ Antiepileptics (oxcarbazepine) are predicted to decrease the concentration of cobicistat. Severe Theoretical

▶ Cobicistat is predicted to very slightly increase the exposure to antiepileptics (perampanel). Mild Study

▶ Cobicistat is predicted to increase the exposure to antifungals, azoles (fluconazole, posaconazole). Moderate Theoretical

▶ Cobicistat is predicted to increase the exposure to antifungals, azoles (isavuconazole). Avoid or monitor adverse effects. Severe Study

▶ Cobicistat is predicted to increase the exposure to antifungals, azoles (itraconazole, ketoconazole). Adjust dose. Moderate Theoretical

▶ Cobicistat is predicted to affect the exposure to antifungals, azoles (voriconazole). Avoid. Moderate Theoretical

▶ Cobicistat is predicted to increase the exposure to antihistamines, non-sedating (mizolastine). Avoid. Severe Study

▶ Cobicistat is predicted to increase the exposure to antihistamines, non-sedating (rupatadine). Avoid. Moderate Study

▶ Cobicistat is predicted to increase the concentration of antimalarials (piperaquine). Severe Theoretical

A1

Interactions | Appendix 1

Cobicistat (continued)

▶ **Cobicistat** is predicted to slightly increase the exposure to antipsychotics, second generation (aripiprazole). Adjust **aripiprazole** dose, p. 415. Moderate Study

▶ **Cobicistat** is predicted to moderately increase the exposure to antipsychotics, second generation (cariprazine). Avoid. Severe Study

▶ **Cobicistat** is predicted to increase the exposure to antipsychotics, second generation (lurasidone, quetiapine). Avoid. Severe Study

▶ **Cobicistat** is predicted to increase the exposure to antipsychotics, second generation (risperidone). Adjust dose. Moderate Study

▶ **Cobicistat** is predicted to increase the exposure to avapritinib. Avoid. Moderate Study

▶ **Cobicistat** is predicted to increase the exposure to axitinib. Avoid or adjust dose. Moderate Study

▶ **Cobicistat** is predicted to increase the exposure to bedaquiline. Avoid prolonged use. Mild Study

▶ **Cobicistat** moderately increases the exposure to benzodiazepines (alprazolam). Avoid. Moderate Study

▶ **Cobicistat** is predicted to markedly to very markedly increase the exposure to benzodiazepines (midazolam). Avoid or adjust dose. Severe Study

▶ **Cobicistat** is predicted to increase the exposure to beta₂-agonists (salmeterol). Avoid. Severe Study

▶ **Cobicistat** slightly increases the exposure to bortezomib. Moderate Study

▶ **Cobicistat** is predicted to markedly increase the exposure to bosutinib. Avoid or adjust dose. Severe Study

▶ **Cobicistat** is predicted to increase the exposure to brigatinib. Adjust **brigatinib** dose, p. 1015. Severe Study

▶ **Cobicistat** is predicted to increase the exposure to buspirone. Adjust **buspirone** dose, p. 360. Severe Study

▶ **Cobicistat** slightly increases the exposure to cabozantinib. Moderate Study

▶ **Cobicistat** is predicted to increase the exposure to calcium channel blockers (amlodipine, felodipine, lacidipine, nicardipine, nifedipine, nimodipine). Monitor and adjust dose. Moderate Study

▶ **Cobicistat** is predicted to increase the exposure to calcium channel blockers (diltiazem, verapamil). Severe Study

▶ **Cobicistat** is predicted to markedly increase the exposure to calcium channel blockers (lercanidipine). Avoid. Severe Study

▶ **Cobicistat** is predicted to increase the exposure to cannabidiol. Avoid or adjust dose. Mild Study

▶ **Cobicistat** is predicted to increase the exposure to ceritinib. Avoid or adjust **ceritinib** dose, p. 1017. Severe Study

▶ **Cobicistat** increases the concentration of ciclosporin. Severe Study

▶ **Cobicistat** is predicted to moderately increase the exposure to cilostazol. Adjust **cilostazol** dose, p. 248. Moderate Study

▶ **Cobicistat** is predicted to moderately increase the exposure to cinacalcet. Adjust dose. Moderate Study

▶ **Cobicistat** is predicted to markedly increase the exposure to cobimetinib. Avoid or monitor for toxicity. Severe Study

▶ **Cobicistat** is predicted to increase the exposure to colchicine. Avoid potent CYP3A4 inhibitors or adjust **colchicine** dose, p. 1166. Severe Study

▶ **Cobicistat** is predicted to decrease the efficacy of combined hormonal contraceptives. Avoid. Severe Study

▶ **Cobicistat** is predicted to increase the exposure to corticosteroids (beclometasone) (risk with beclometasone is likely to be lower than with other corticosteroids). Moderate Theoretical

▶ **Cobicistat** is predicted to increase the exposure to corticosteroids (betamethasone, budesonide, ciclesonide, deflazacort, dexamethasone, fludrocortisone, fluticasone, hydrocortisone, methylprednisolone, mometasone, prednisolone, triamcinolone). Avoid or monitor adverse effects. Severe Study

▶ **Cobicistat** is predicted to moderately increase the exposure to crizotinib. Avoid. Moderate Study

▶ **Cobicistat** is predicted to increase the exposure to dabrafenib. Use with caution or avoid. Moderate Study

▶ **Cobicistat** is predicted to markedly to very markedly increase the exposure to darifenacin. Avoid. Severe Study

▶ **Cobicistat** is predicted to markedly increase the exposure to dasatinib. Avoid or adjust dose—consult product literature. Severe Study

▶ **Cobicistat** very slightly increases the exposure to delamanid. Severe Study

▶ **Cobicistat** is predicted to moderately increase the exposure to dienogest. Moderate Study

▶ **Cobicistat** is predicted to increase the exposure to dipeptidylpeptidase-4 inhibitors (saxagliptin). Moderate Study

▶ **Cobicistat** increases the risk of QT-prolongation when given with domperidone. Avoid. Severe Study

▶ **Cobicistat** increases the exposure to dopamine receptor agonists (bromocriptine). Severe Study

▶ **Cobicistat** is predicted to increase the concentration of dopamine receptor agonists (cabergoline). Moderate Anecdotal

▶ **Cobicistat** is predicted to increase the exposure to dronabinol. Adjust dose. Mild Study

▶ **Cobicistat** is predicted to increase the exposure to dutasteride. Monitor adverse effects and adjust dose. Moderate Theoretical

▶ **Cobicistat** is predicted to increase the exposure to elexacaftor. Adjust tezacaftor with ivacaftor and elexacftor p. 311 dose with potent CYP3A4 inhibitors. Severe Study

▶ **Cobicistat** is predicted to increase the exposure to eliglustat. Avoid or adjust dose—consult product literature. Severe Study

▶ **Cobicistat** is predicted to increase the exposure to encorafenib. Avoid or monitor. Severe Study

▶ Endothelin receptor antagonists (bosentan) are predicted to decrease the exposure to **cobicistat**. Avoid. Severe Theoretical

▶ **Cobicistat** is predicted to increase the exposure to endothelin receptor antagonists (macitentan). Moderate Study

▶ **Cobicistat** is predicted to increase the exposure to entrectinib. Avoid potent CYP3A4 inhibitors or adjust **entrectinib** dose, p. 1023. Severe Study

▶ **Cobicistat** is predicted to increase the risk of ergotism when given with ergometrine. Avoid. Severe Theoretical

▶ **Cobicistat** is predicted to increase the risk of ergotism when given with ergotamine. Avoid. Severe Theoretical

▶ **Cobicistat** is predicted to slightly increase the exposure to erlotinib. Use with caution and adjust dose. Moderate Study

▶ **Cobicistat** is predicted to increase the exposure to esketamine. Adjust dose. Moderate Study

▶ **Cobicistat** is predicted to increase the concentration of everolimus. Avoid. Severe Study

▶ **Cobicistat** is predicted to increase the exposure to factor XA inhibitors (apixaban, edoxaban, rivaroxaban). Avoid. Severe Theoretical

▶ **Cobicistat** is predicted to moderately increase the exposure to fesoterodine. Adjust **fesoterodine** dose with potent CYP3A4 inhibitors; avoid in hepatic and renal impairment, p. 822. Severe Study

▶ **Cobicistat** is predicted to increase the exposure to fostamatinib. Monitor adverse effects and adjust dose. Moderate Study

▶ **Cobicistat** is predicted to increase the exposure to gefitinib. Moderate Study

▶ **Cobicistat** is predicted to increase the exposure to gilteritinib. Moderate Study

▶ **Cobicistat** is predicted to moderately increase the exposure to glasdegib. Use with caution or avoid. Moderate Study

▶ **Cobicistat** potentially increases the exposure to glecaprevir. Moderate Theoretical

▶ **Cobicistat** is predicted to moderately to markedly increase the exposure to grazoprevir. Avoid. Severe Study

▶ **Cobicistat** is predicted to increase the exposure to guanfacine. Adjust **guanfacine** dose, p. 372. Moderate Study

▶ **Cobicistat** is predicted to very markedly increase the exposure to ibrutinib. Avoid potent CYP3A4 inhibitors or adjust **ibrutinib** dose, p. 1027. Severe Study

▶ **Cobicistat** is predicted to increase the exposure to imatinib. Moderate Study

▶ **Cobicistat** is predicted to increase the risk of toxicity when given with irinotecan. Avoid. Moderate Study

Cobicistat is predicted to increase the exposure to ivabradine. Avoid. Severe Study

Cobicistat is predicted to increase the exposure to ivacaftor. Adjust ivacaftor p. 309 or lumacaftor with ivacaftor p. 310 or tezacaftor with ivacaftor p. 311 or tezacaftor with ivacaftor and elexacftor p. 311 dose with potent CYP3A4 inhibitors. Severe Study

Cobicistat is predicted to increase the exposure to lapatinib. Avoid. Moderate Study

Cobicistat is predicted to moderately increase the exposure to larotrectinib. Avoid or adjust **larotrectinib** dose, p. 1031. Moderate Study

Cobicistat is predicted to markedly increase the exposure to lomitapide. Avoid. Severe Study

Cobicistat is predicted to increase the exposure to lorlatinib. Avoid or adjust **lorlatinib** dose, p. 1033. Severe Study

Cobicistat markedly increases the exposure to maraviroc. Refer to specialist literature. Severe Study

Cobicistat is predicted to increase the exposure to meglitinides (repaglinide). Moderate Study

Cobicistat potentially increases the exposure to mexiletine. Severe Theoretical

Cobicistat is predicted to very markedly increase the exposure to midostaurin. Avoid or monitor for toxicity. Severe Study

Cobicistat is predicted to increase the exposure to mirabegron. Adjust **mirabegron** dose in hepatic and renal impairment, p. 825. Moderate Study

Cobicistat is predicted to increase the exposure to mirtazapine. Moderate Study

Mitotane is predicted to decrease the exposure to **cobicistat**. Avoid. Severe Theoretical

Cobicistat is predicted to increase the exposure to modafinil. Mild Theoretical

Cobicistat is predicted to increase the exposure to monoclonal antibodies (polatuzumab vedotin). Moderate Theoretical

Cobicistat is predicted to increase the exposure to monoclonal antibodies (trastuzumab emtansine). Avoid. Severe Theoretical

Cobicistat is predicted to increase the exposure to naldemedine. Avoid or monitor. Moderate Study

Cobicistat is predicted to markedly increase the exposure to naloxegol. Avoid. Severe Study

Cobicistat is predicted to increase the exposure to neratinib. Avoid or adjust **neratinib** dose, p. 1034. Severe Study

Cobicistat is predicted to markedly increase the exposure to neurokinin-1 receptor antagonists (aprepitant). Moderate Study

Cobicistat is predicted to increase the exposure to neurokinin-1 receptor antagonists (fosaprepitant). Moderate Theoretical

Cobicistat is predicted to increase the exposure to neurokinin-1 receptor antagonists (netupitant). Moderate Study

Cobicistat is predicted to moderately increase the exposure to nilotinib. Avoid. Severe Study

Cobicistat is predicted to increase the exposure to nitisinone. Adjust dose. Moderate Theoretical

NNRTIs (efavirenz, nevirapine) are predicted to decrease the exposure to **cobicistat**. Avoid. Severe Theoretical

Cobicistat is predicted to increase the exposure to NNRTIs (doravirine). Mild Study

Cobicistat is predicted to increase the exposure to olaparib. Avoid potent CYP3A4 inhibitors or adjust **olaparib** dose, p. 1051. Moderate Study

Cobicistat is predicted to increase the exposure to opioids (alfentanil, buprenorphine, fentanyl, oxycodone). Monitor and adjust dose. Severe Study

Cobicistat is predicted to increase the exposure to ospemifene. Avoid in poor CYP2C9 metabolisers. Moderate Study

Cobicistat is predicted to increase the exposure to oxybutynin. Mild Study

Cobicistat is predicted to increase the exposure to palbociclib. Avoid or adjust **palbociclib** dose, p. 1038. Severe Study

Cobicistat is predicted to increase the exposure to panobinostat. Adjust **panobinostat** dose; in hepatic impairment avoid, p. 979. Moderate Study

Cobicistat is predicted to increase the exposure to paritaprevir. Avoid. Severe Study

Cobicistat is predicted to increase the exposure to pazopanib. Avoid or adjust **pazopanib** dose, p. 1039. Moderate Study

Cobicistat is predicted to increase the exposure to phosphodiesterase type-5 inhibitors (avanafil, vardenafil). Avoid. Severe Study

Cobicistat is predicted to increase the exposure to phosphodiesterase type-5 inhibitors (sildenafil). Avoid potent CYP3A4 inhibitors or adjust **sildenafil** dose, p. 860. Severe Study

Cobicistat is predicted to increase the exposure to phosphodiesterase type-5 inhibitors (tadalafil). Use with caution or avoid. Severe Study

Cobicistat is predicted to increase the exposure to pimozide. Avoid. Severe Study

Cobicistat is predicted to slightly increase the exposure to ponatinib. Monitor and adjust **ponatinib** dose, p. 1040. Moderate Study

Cobicistat is predicted to moderately increase the exposure to praziquantel. Mild Study

Cobicistat given with carbimazole is predicted to increase the exposure to propiverine. Adjust starting dose. Moderate Theoretical

Cobicistat is predicted to increase the exposure to ranolazine. Avoid. Moderate Study

Cobicistat is predicted to increase the exposure to reboxetine. Avoid. Moderate Study

Cobicistat is predicted to increase the exposure to regorafenib. Avoid. Moderate Study

Cobicistat is predicted to increase the exposure to retinoids (alitretinoin). Adjust **alitretinoin** dose, p. 1305. Moderate Theoretical

Cobicistat is predicted to increase the exposure to ribociclib. Avoid or adjust **ribociclib** dose, p. 1042. Moderate Study

Rifamycins (rifabutin) decrease the concentration of **cobicistat** and **cobicistat** increases the exposure to rifamycins (rifabutin). Avoid or adjust dose. Severe Study

Rifamycins (rifampicin) are predicted to decrease the exposure to **cobicistat**. Avoid. Severe Theoretical

Cobicistat is predicted to increase the exposure to ruxolitinib. Adjust dose and monitor adverse effects. Moderate Study

Cobicistat is predicted to increase the exposure to siponimod. Avoid depending on other drugs taken—consult product literature. Severe Theoretical

Cobicistat is predicted to increase the concentration of sirolimus. Avoid. Severe Study

Cobicistat is predicted to increase the exposure to solifenacin. Adjust solifenacin p. 824 or tamsulosin with solifenacin p. 830 dose; avoid in hepatic and renal impairment. Severe Study

Cobicistat is predicted to moderately increase the exposure to SSRIs (dapoxetine). Avoid potent CYP3A4 inhibitors or adjust **dapoxetine** dose, p. 867. Severe Study

St John's wort is predicted to decrease the exposure to **cobicistat**. Avoid. Severe Theoretical

Cobicistat is predicted to increase the exposure to statins (atorvastatin). Avoid or adjust dose and monitor rhabdomyolysis. Severe Study

Cobicistat is predicted to increase the exposure to statins (simvastatin). Avoid. Severe Study

Cobicistat is predicted to slightly increase the exposure to sunitinib. Avoid or adjust **sunitinib** dose, p. 1044. Moderate Study

Cobicistat is predicted to increase the concentration of tacrolimus. Monitor and adjust dose. Severe Study

Cobicistat is predicted to increase the exposure to taxanes (cabazitaxel). Avoid. Severe Study

Cobicistat is predicted to moderately increase the exposure to taxanes (docetaxel). Avoid or adjust dose. Severe Study

Cobicistat is predicted to increase the exposure to taxanes (paclitaxel). Severe Theoretical

Cobicistat is predicted to increase the concentration of temsirolimus. Avoid. Severe Theoretical

Cobicistat is predicted to increase the exposure to tezacaftor. Adjust tezacaftor with ivacaftor p. 311 or tezacaftor with ivacaftor and elexacftor p. 311 dose with potent CYP3A4 inhibitors. Severe Study

Cobicistat (continued)

▶ **Cobicistat** is predicted to increase the exposure to thrombin inhibitors (dabigatran). Avoid. Severe Theoretical

▶ **Cobicistat** is predicted to markedly increase the exposure to ticagrelor. Avoid. Severe Study

▶ **Cobicistat** is predicted to increase the exposure to tofacitinib. Adjust **tofacitinib** dose, p. 1154. Moderate Study

▶ **Cobicistat** is predicted to increase the exposure to tolterodine. Avoid. Severe Study

▶ **Cobicistat** is predicted to increase the exposure to tolvaptan. Manufacturer advises caution or adjust **tolvaptan** dose with potent CYP3A4 inhibitors, p. 708. Severe Study

▶ **Cobicistat** is predicted to increase the exposure to toremifene. Moderate Theoretical

▶ **Cobicistat** is predicted to increase the exposure to trabectedin. Avoid or adjust dose. Severe Theoretical

▶ **Cobicistat** is predicted to moderately increase the exposure to trazodone. Avoid or adjust dose. Moderate Study

▶ **Cobicistat** is predicted to slightly increase the exposure to tricyclic antidepressants. Mild Study

▶ **Cobicistat** increases the exposure to triptans (almotriptan). Mild Study

▶ **Cobicistat** is predicted to markedly increase the exposure to triptans (eletriptan). Avoid. Severe Study

▶ **Cobicistat** is predicted to increase the exposure to upadacitinib. Use with caution or avoid. Severe Study

▶ **Cobicistat** is predicted to increase the exposure to vemurafenib. Severe Theoretical

▶ **Cobicistat** is predicted to increase the exposure to venetoclax. Avoid or adjust dose—consult product literature. Severe Study

▶ **Cobicistat** is predicted to increase the exposure to venlafaxine. Moderate Study

▶ **Cobicistat** is predicted to increase the exposure to vinca alkaloids. Severe Theoretical

▶ **Cobicistat** is predicted to increase the exposure to vitamin D substances (paricalcitol). Moderate Study

▶ **Cobicistat** is predicted to increase the exposure to zopiclone. Adjust dose. Moderate Theoretical

Cobimetinib

▶ Anti-androgens (apalutamide, enzalutamide) are predicted to decrease the exposure to **cobimetinib**. Avoid. Severe Theoretical

▶ Antiarrhythmics (dronedarone) are predicted to increase the exposure to **cobimetinib**. Severe Theoretical

▶ Antiepileptics (carbamazepine, fosphenytoin, phenobarbital, phenytoin, primidone) are predicted to decrease the exposure to **cobimetinib**. Avoid. Severe Theoretical

▶ Antifungals, azoles (fluconazole, isavuconazole, miconazole, posaconazole) are predicted to increase the exposure to **cobimetinib**. Severe Theoretical

▶ Antifungals, azoles (itraconazole, ketoconazole, voriconazole) are predicted to markedly increase the exposure to **cobimetinib**. Avoid or monitor for toxicity. Severe Study

▶ Calcium channel blockers (diltiazem, verapamil) are predicted to increase the exposure to **cobimetinib**. Severe Theoretical

▶ Cobicistat is predicted to markedly increase the exposure to **cobimetinib**. Avoid or monitor for toxicity. Severe Study

▶ Crizotinib is predicted to increase the exposure to **cobimetinib**. Severe Theoretical

▶ Endothelin receptor antagonists (bosentan) are predicted to decrease the exposure to **cobimetinib**. Avoid. Severe Theoretical

▶ Grapefruit juice is predicted to increase the exposure to **cobimetinib**. Avoid. Severe Theoretical

▶ HIV-protease inhibitors are predicted to markedly increase the exposure to **cobimetinib**. Avoid or monitor for toxicity. Severe Study

▶ Idelalisib is predicted to markedly increase the exposure to **cobimetinib**. Avoid or monitor for toxicity. Severe Study

▶ Imatinib is predicted to increase the exposure to **cobimetinib**. Severe Theoretical

▶ Letermovir is predicted to increase the exposure to **cobimetinib**. Severe Theoretical

▶ Macrolides (clarithromycin) are predicted to markedly increase the exposure to **cobimetinib**. Avoid or monitor for toxicity. Severe Study

▶ Macrolides (erythromycin) are predicted to increase the exposure to **cobimetinib**. Severe Theoretical

▶ Mitotane is predicted to decrease the exposure to **cobimetinib**. Avoid. Severe Theoretical

▶ Neurokinin-1 receptor antagonists (aprepitant, netupitant) are predicted to increase the exposure to **cobimetinib**. Severe Theoretical

▶ Nilotinib is predicted to increase the exposure to **cobimetinib**. Severe Theoretical

▶ NNRTIs (efavirenz, nevirapine) are predicted to decrease the exposure to **cobimetinib**. Avoid. Severe Theoretical

▶ Rifamycins (rifampicin) are predicted to decrease the exposure to **cobimetinib**. Avoid. Severe Theoretical

▶ St John's wort is predicted to decrease the exposure to **cobimetinib**. Avoid. Severe Theoretical

Codeine → see opioids

Colchicine

▶ Anti-androgens (apalutamide) are predicted to decrease the exposure to **colchicine**. Mild Study

▶ Antiarrhythmics (amiodarone) are predicted to increase the exposure to **colchicine**. Avoid P-glycoprotein inhibitors or adjust **colchicine** dose, p. 1166. Severe Theoretical

▶ Antiarrhythmics (dronedarone) are predicted to increase the exposure to **colchicine**. Adjust **colchicine** dose with moderate CYP3A4 inhibitors, p. 1166. Severe Study

▶ Antifungals, azoles (fluconazole, isavuconazole, posaconazole) are predicted to increase the exposure to **colchicine**. Adjust **colchicine** dose with moderate CYP3A4 inhibitors, p. 1166. Severe Study

▶ Antifungals, azoles (itraconazole, ketoconazole, voriconazole) are predicted to increase the exposure to **colchicine**. Avoid potent CYP3A4 inhibitors or adjust **colchicine** dose, p. 1166. Severe Study

▶ Calcium channel blockers (diltiazem, verapamil) are predicted to increase the exposure to **colchicine**. Adjust **colchicine** dose with moderate CYP3A4 inhibitors, p. 1166. Severe Study

▶ Ceritinib is predicted to increase the exposure to **colchicine**. Moderate Theoretical

▶ Ciclosporin increases the exposure to **colchicine**. Avoid P-glycoprotein inhibitors or adjust **colchicine** dose, p. 1166. Severe Study

▶ Cobicistat is predicted to increase the exposure to **colchicine**. Avoid potent CYP3A4 inhibitors or adjust **colchicine** dose, p. 1166. Severe Study

▶ Crizotinib is predicted to increase the exposure to **colchicine**. Adjust **colchicine** dose with moderate CYP3A4 inhibitors, p. 1166. Severe Study

▶ Eliglustat is predicted to increase the exposure to **colchicine**. Avoid or adjust **colchicine** dose, p. 1166. Severe Theoretical

▶ **Colchicine** increases the risk of rhabdomyolysis when given with fibrates. Severe Anecdotal

▶ HIV-protease inhibitors are predicted to increase the exposure to **colchicine**. Avoid potent CYP3A4 inhibitors or adjust **colchicine** dose, p. 1166. Severe Study

▶ Idelalisib is predicted to increase the exposure to **colchicine**. Avoid potent CYP3A4 inhibitors or adjust **colchicine** dose, p. 1166. Severe Study

▶ Imatinib is predicted to increase the exposure to **colchicine**. Adjust **colchicine** dose with moderate CYP3A4 inhibitors, p. 1166. Severe Study

▶ Lapatinib is predicted to increase the exposure to **colchicine**. Avoid P-glycoprotein inhibitors or adjust **colchicine** dose, p. 1166. Moderate Theoretical

▶ Letermovir is predicted to increase the exposure to **colchicine**. Adjust **colchicine** dose with moderate CYP3A4 inhibitors, p. 1166. Severe Study

▶ Macrolides (azithromycin) are predicted to increase the exposure to **colchicine**. Avoid P-glycoprotein inhibitors or adjust **colchicine** dose, p. 1166. Severe Theoretical

▶ Macrolides (clarithromycin) are predicted to increase the exposure to **colchicine**. Avoid potent CYP3A4 inhibitors or adjust **colchicine** dose, p. 1166. Severe Study

▶ Macrolides (erythromycin) are predicted to increase the exposure to **colchicine**. Adjust **colchicine** dose with moderate CYP3A4 inhibitors, p. 1166. Severe Study

Mirabegron is predicted to increase the exposure to **colchicine**. [Mild] Theoretical

Neurokinin-1 receptor antagonists (aprepitant, netupitant) are predicted to increase the exposure to **colchicine**. Adjust **colchicine** dose with moderate CYP3A4 inhibitors, p. 1166. [Severe] Study

Nilotinib is predicted to increase the exposure to **colchicine**. Adjust **colchicine** dose with moderate CYP3A4 inhibitors, p. 1166. [Severe] Study

Pibrentasvir (with glecaprevir) is predicted to increase the exposure to **colchicine**. [Moderate] Study

Pitolisant is predicted to decrease the exposure to **colchicine**. [Mild] Theoretical

Ranolazine is predicted to increase the exposure to **colchicine**. Avoid P-glycoprotein inhibitors or adjust **colchicine** dose, p. 1166. [Severe] Theoretical

▸ **Colchicine** increases the risk of rhabdomyolysis when given with statins. [Severe] Anecdotal

Velpatasvir is predicted to increase the exposure to **colchicine**. [Severe] Theoretical

Vemurafenib is predicted to increase the exposure to **colchicine**. Avoid P-glycoprotein inhibitors or adjust **colchicine** dose, p. 1166. [Severe] Theoretical

Colecalciferol → see vitamin D substances

Colesevelam

SEPARATION OF ADMINISTRATION   Manufacturer advises take 4 hours before, or after, other drugs.

Colestipol

SEPARATION OF ADMINISTRATION   Manufacturer advises take other drugs at least 1 hour before, or 4 hours after, colestipol.

Colestyramine

SEPARATION OF ADMINISTRATION   Manufacturer advises take other drugs at least 1 hour before, or 4–6 hours after, colestyramine.

Colistimethate → see TABLE 2 p. 1429 (nephrotoxicity), **TABLE 20** p. 1433 (neuromuscular blocking effects)

Combined hormonal contraceptives

▸ **Combined hormonal contraceptives** are predicted to increase the exposure to agomelatine. [Moderate] Study

▸ **Combined hormonal contraceptives** are predicted to increase the exposure to aminophylline. Adjust dose. [Moderate] Theoretical

▸ **Combined hormonal contraceptives** are predicted to increase the exposure to anagrelide. [Moderate] Theoretical

▸ Antiepileptics (carbamazepine, eslicarbazepine, fosphenytoin, oxcarbazepine, perampanel, phenobarbital, phenytoin, primidone, rufinamide, topiramate) are predicted to decrease the efficacy of **combined hormonal contraceptives**. For FSRH guidance, see Contraceptives, interactions p. 840. [Severe] Study

▸ **Combined hormonal contraceptives** alter the exposure to antiepileptics (lamotrigine). Adjust dose. [Moderate] Study

▸ **Combined hormonal contraceptives** increase the concentration of antipsychotics, second generation (clozapine). Monitor adverse effects and adjust dose. [Severe] Study

▸ Brigatinib decreases the exposure to **combined hormonal contraceptives**. Use additional contraceptive precautions. [Severe] Theoretical

▸ Carfilzomib potentially decreases the efficacy of **combined hormonal contraceptives**. Use additional contraceptive precautions. [Severe] Theoretical

▸ Oral **combined hormonal contraceptives** potentially decrease the efficacy of oral chenodeoxycholic acid. Avoid. [Moderate] Theoretical

▸ Cobicistat is predicted to decrease the efficacy of **combined hormonal contraceptives**. Avoid. [Severe] Study

▸ **Combined hormonal contraceptives** (containing ethinylestradiol) increase the risk of increased ALT concentrations when given with dasabuvir. Avoid. [Severe] Study

▸ **Combined hormonal contraceptives** are predicted to increase the exposure to dopamine receptor agonists (ropinirole). Adjust dose. [Moderate] Study

▸ Encorafenib is predicted to affect the exposure to **combined hormonal contraceptives**. [Severe] Theoretical

▸ Endothelin receptor antagonists (bosentan) are predicted to decrease the efficacy of **combined hormonal contraceptives**. For FSRH guidance, see Contraceptives, interactions p. 840. [Severe] Study

▸ **Combined hormonal contraceptives** slightly increase the exposure to erlotinib. Monitor adverse effects and adjust dose. [Moderate] Study

▸ **Combined hormonal contraceptives** (containing ethinylestradiol) are predicted to increase the risk of increased ALT concentrations when given with glecaprevir. Avoid. [Severe] Study

▸ Griseofulvin potentially decreases the efficacy of **combined hormonal contraceptives**. For FSRH guidance, see Contraceptives, interactions p. 840. [Severe] Anecdotal

▸ HIV-protease inhibitors (atazanavir) (unboosted) increase the exposure to **combined hormonal contraceptives**. Adjust dose. [Severe] Study

▸ HIV-protease inhibitors (ritonavir) are predicted to decrease the efficacy of **combined hormonal contraceptives**. For FSRH guidance, see Contraceptives, interactions p. 840. [Severe] Study

▸ Larotrectinib potentially decreases the efficacy of **combined hormonal contraceptives**. Use additional contraceptive precautions. [Severe] Theoretical

▸ **Combined hormonal contraceptives** are predicted to increase the risk of venous thromboembolism when given with lenalidomide. Avoid. [Severe] Study

▸ Oral **combined hormonal contraceptives** slightly increase the exposure to lomitapide. Separate administration by 12 hours. [Moderate] Theoretical

▸ Lorlatinib is predicted to decrease the exposure to **combined hormonal contraceptives**. Avoid. [Moderate] Theoretical

▸ **Combined hormonal contraceptives** are predicted to increase the exposure to loxapine. Avoid. [Unknown] Theoretical

▸ Lumacaftor is predicted to decrease the efficacy of **combined hormonal contraceptives**. Use additional contraceptive precautions. [Severe] Theoretical

▸ **Combined hormonal contraceptives** slightly increase the exposure to MAO-B inhibitors (rasagiline). [Moderate] Study

▸ **Combined hormonal contraceptives** increase the exposure to MAO-B inhibitors (selegiline). Avoid. [Severe] Study

▸ **Combined hormonal contraceptives** are predicted to increase the exposure to melatonin. [Moderate] Theoretical

▸ **Combined hormonal contraceptives** decrease the effects of metyrapone. Avoid. [Moderate] Theoretical

▸ Modafinil is predicted to decrease the efficacy of **combined hormonal contraceptives**. For FSRH guidance, see Contraceptives, interactions p. 840. [Severe] Study

▸ Monoclonal antibodies (sarilumab) potentially decrease the exposure to **combined hormonal contraceptives**. [Severe] Theoretical

▸ Neurokinin-1 receptor antagonists (aprepitant, fosaprepitant) are predicted to decrease the efficacy of **combined hormonal contraceptives**. For FSRH guidance, see Contraceptives, interactions p. 840. [Severe] Study

▸ NNRTIs (efavirenz, nevirapine) are predicted to decrease the efficacy of **combined hormonal contraceptives**. For FSRH guidance, see Contraceptives, interactions p. 840. [Severe] Study

▸ NSAIDs (etoricoxib) increase the exposure to **combined hormonal contraceptives**. [Moderate] Study

▸ Olaparib potentially affects the efficacy of **combined hormonal contraceptives**. Use additional contraceptive precautions. [Moderate] Theoretical

▸ **Combined hormonal contraceptives** potentially oppose the effects of ospemifene. Avoid. [Severe] Theoretical

▸ **Combined hormonal contraceptives** (containing ethinylestradiol) are predicted to increase the risk of increased ALT concentrations when given with paritaprevir (with ritonavir and ombitasvir). Avoid. [Severe] Study

▸ **Combined hormonal contraceptives** are predicted to increase the exposure to phosphodiesterase type-4 inhibitors (roflumilast). [Moderate] Theoretical

▸ **Combined hormonal contraceptives** (containing ethinylestradiol) are predicted to increase the risk of increased ALT concentrations when given with pibrentasvir. Avoid. [Severe] Study

A1

Interactions | Appendix 1

Combined hormonal contraceptives (continued)

▸ **Combined hormonal contraceptives** are predicted to increase the exposure to pirfenidone. Use with caution and adjust dose. Moderate Study

▸ Pitolisant is predicted to decrease the efficacy of **combined hormonal contraceptives**. Avoid. Severe Theoretical

▸ **Combined hormonal contraceptives** are predicted to increase the risk of venous thromboembolism when given with pomalidomide. Avoid. Severe Theoretical

▸ **Combined hormonal contraceptives** potentially oppose the effects of raloxifene. Avoid. Severe Theoretical

▸ Rifamycins are predicted to decrease the efficacy of **combined hormonal contraceptives**. For FSRH guidance, see Contraceptives, interactions p. 840. Severe Study

▸ St John's wort decreases the efficacy of **combined hormonal contraceptives**. MHRA advises avoid. For FSRH guidance, see Contraceptives, interactions p. 840. Severe Anecdotal

▸ Sugammadex is predicted to decrease the exposure to **combined hormonal contraceptives**. Refer to patient information leaflet for missed pill advice. Severe Theoretical

▸ **Combined hormonal contraceptives** are predicted to increase the risk of venous thromboembolism when given with thalidomide. Avoid. Severe Study

▸ **Combined hormonal contraceptives** are predicted to increase the exposure to theophylline. Monitor and adjust dose. Moderate Theoretical

▸ **Combined hormonal contraceptives** increase the exposure to tizanidine. Avoid. Moderate Study

▸ **Combined hormonal contraceptives** are predicted to increase the exposure to triptans (zolmitriptan). Adjust **zolmitriptan** dose, p. 503. Moderate Theoretical

▸ Ulipristal is predicted to decrease the efficacy of **combined hormonal contraceptives**. Avoid. Severe Theoretical

▸ **Combined hormonal contraceptives** (containing ethinylestradiol) are predicted to increase the risk of increased ALT concentrations when given with voxilaprevir (with sofosbuvir and velpatasvir). Avoid. Severe Study

Corticosteroids → see TABLE 17 p. 1433 (reduced serum potassium)

beclometasone · betamethasone · budesonide · ciclesonide · deflazacort · dexamethasone · fludrocortisone · fluticasone · hydrocortisone · methylprednisolone · mometasone · prednisolone · triamcinolone

▸ With intravitreal use of **dexamethasone** in adults: caution with concurrent administration of anticoagulant or antiplatelet drugs—increased risk of haemorrhagic events.

▸ Interactions do not generally apply to corticosteroids used for topical action (including inhalation) unless specified. However, as systemic absorption might occur with **hydrocortisone** *eye drops*, the possibility of interactions should be borne in mind.

▸ Oral antacids are predicted to decrease the absorption of oral **deflazacort**. Separate administration by 2 hours. Moderate Theoretical

▸ Oral antacids decrease the absorption of oral **dexamethasone**. Moderate Study

▸ Anti-androgens (apalutamide, enzalutamide) are predicted to decrease the exposure to **fluticasone**. Unknown Theoretical

▸ Anti-androgens (apalutamide, enzalutamide) are predicted to decrease the exposure to corticosteroids (**budesonide, deflazacort, dexamethasone, fludrocortisone, hydrocortisone, methylprednisolone, prednisolone, triamcinolone**). Monitor and adjust dose. Moderate Study

▸ Antiarrhythmics (dronedarone) are predicted to increase the exposure to **methylprednisolone**. Monitor and adjust dose. Moderate Study

▸ Antiepileptics (carbamazepine, fosphenytoin, phenobarbital, phenytoin, primidone) are predicted to decrease the exposure to **fluticasone**. Unknown Theoretical

▸ Antiepileptics (carbamazepine, fosphenytoin, phenobarbital, phenytoin, primidone) are predicted to decrease the exposure to corticosteroids (**budesonide, deflazacort, dexamethasone, fludrocortisone, hydrocortisone, methylprednisolone, prednisolone, triamcinolone**). Monitor and adjust dose. Moderate Study

▸ Antifungals, azoles (fluconazole, isavuconazole, posaconazole) are predicted to increase the exposure to **methylprednisolone**. Monitor and adjust dose. Moderate Study

▸ Antifungals, azoles (itraconazole, ketoconazole, voriconazole) are predicted to increase the exposure to **beclometasone** (risk with beclometasone is likely to be lower than with other corticosteroids). Moderate Theoretical

▸ Antifungals, azoles (miconazole) are predicted to increase the concentration of **methylprednisolone**. Monitor and adjust dose. Moderate Theoretical

▸ Antifungals, azoles (itraconazole, ketoconazole, voriconazole) are predicted to increase the exposure to corticosteroids (**betamethasone, budesonide, ciclesonide, deflazacort, dexamethasone, fludrocortisone, fluticasone, hydrocortisone, methylprednisolone, mometasone, prednisolone, triamcinolone**). Avoid or monitor adverse effects. Severe Study

▸ **Corticosteroids** are predicted to decrease the concentration of aspirin (high-dose) and aspirin (high-dose) increases the risk of gastrointestinal bleeding when given with **corticosteroids**. Moderate Study

▸ **Dexamethasone** is predicted to decrease the exposure to avapritinib. Avoid. Severe Theoretical

▸ Calcium channel blockers (diltiazem, verapamil) are predicted to increase the exposure to **methylprednisolone**. Monitor and adjust dose. Moderate Study

▸ **Dexamethasone** is predicted to decrease the concentration of caspofungin. Adjust **caspofungin** dose, p. 631. Moderate Theoretical

▸ **Corticosteroids** are predicted to decrease the concentration of choline salicylate. Moderate Study

▸ Cobicistat is predicted to increase the exposure to **beclometasone** (risk with beclometasone is likely to be lower than with other corticosteroids). Moderate Theoretical

▸ Cobicistat is predicted to increase the exposure to corticosteroids (**betamethasone, budesonide, ciclesonide, deflazacort, dexamethasone, fludrocortisone, fluticasone, hydrocortisone, methylprednisolone, mometasone, prednisolone, triamcinolone**). Avoid or monitor adverse effects. Severe Study

▸ **Corticosteroids** are predicted to increase the effects of coumarins. Moderate Study

▸ Crizotinib is predicted to increase the exposure to **methylprednisolone**. Monitor and adjust dose. Moderate Study

▸ **Corticosteroids** increase the risk of gastrointestinal perforation when given with erlotinib. Severe Theoretical

▸ **Corticosteroids** potentially oppose the effects of glycerol phenylbutyrate. Moderate Theoretical

▸ Grapefruit juice moderately increases the exposure to oral **budesonide**. Avoid. Moderate Study

▸ HIV-protease inhibitors are predicted to increase the exposure to **beclometasone** (risk with beclometasone is likely to be lower than with other corticosteroids). Moderate Theoretical

▸ HIV-protease inhibitors are predicted to increase the exposure to corticosteroids (**betamethasone, budesonide, ciclesonide, deflazacort, dexamethasone, fludrocortisone, fluticasone, hydrocortisone, methylprednisolone, mometasone, prednisolone, triamcinolone**). Avoid or monitor adverse effects. Severe Study

▸ Idelalisib is predicted to increase the exposure to **beclometasone** (risk with beclometasone is likely to be lower than with other corticosteroids). Moderate Theoretical

▸ Idelalisib is predicted to increase the exposure to corticosteroids (**betamethasone, budesonide, ciclesonide, deflazacort, dexamethasone, fludrocortisone, fluticasone, hydrocortisone, methylprednisolone, mometasone, prednisolone, triamcinolone**). Avoid or monitor adverse effects. Severe Study

▸ Imatinib is predicted to increase the exposure to **methylprednisolone**. Monitor and adjust dose. Moderate Study

▸ **Corticosteroids** are predicted to increase the risk of gastrointestinal bleeding when given with iron chelators (deferasirox). Severe Theoretical

▸ Letermovir is predicted to increase the exposure to **methylprednisolone**. Monitor and adjust dose. Moderate Study

Live vaccines are predicted to increase the risk of generalised infection (possibly life-threatening) when given with **corticosteroids** (high-dose). Public Health England advises avoid (refer to Green Book). Severe Theoretical

Lumacaftor is predicted to decrease the exposure to **methylprednisolone**. Adjust dose. Severe Theoretical

Macrolides (clarithromycin) are predicted to increase the exposure to **beclometasone** (risk with beclometasone is likely to be lower than with other corticosteroids). Moderate Theoretical

Macrolides (erythromycin) are predicted to increase the exposure to **methylprednisolone**. Monitor and adjust dose. Moderate Study

Macrolides (clarithromycin) are predicted to increase the exposure to corticosteroids **(betamethasone, budesonide, ciclesonide, deflazacort, dexamethasone, fludrocortisone, fluticasone, hydrocortisone, methylprednisolone, mometasone, prednisolone, triamcinolone)**. Avoid or monitor adverse effects. Severe Study

Corticosteroids are predicted to decrease the efficacy of mifamurtide. Avoid. Severe Study

Mifepristone is predicted to decrease the efficacy of **corticosteroids**. Use with caution and adjust dose. Moderate Theoretical

Mitotane is predicted to decrease the exposure to corticosteroids **(budesonide, deflazacort, dexamethasone, fludrocortisone, hydrocortisone, methylprednisolone, prednisolone, triamcinolone)**. Monitor and adjust dose. Moderate Study

Mitotane is predicted to decrease the exposure to **fluticasone**. Unknown Theoretical

Corticosteroids **(betamethasone, deflazacort, dexamethasone, hydrocortisone, methylprednisolone, prednisolone)** are predicted to decrease the efficacy of monoclonal antibodies (atezolizumab, ipilimumab, nivolumab, pembrolizumab). Use with caution or avoid. Severe Theoretical

Monoclonal antibodies (tocilizumab) are predicted to decrease the exposure to corticosteroids **(dexamethasone, methylprednisolone)**. Monitor and adjust dose. Moderate Theoretical

► **Corticosteroids** are predicted to increase the risk of immunosuppression when given with monoclonal antibodies (dinutuximab). Avoid except in life-threatening situations. Severe Theoretical

Neurokinin-1 receptor antagonists (aprepitant) moderately increase the exposure to **dexamethasone**. Monitor and adjust dose. Moderate Study

Neurokinin-1 receptor antagonists (aprepitant, netupitant) are predicted to increase the exposure to oral **budesonide**. Moderate Study

Neurokinin-1 receptor antagonists (aprepitant, netupitant) are predicted to increase the exposure to **fluticasone**. Moderate Study

Neurokinin-1 receptor antagonists (aprepitant, netupitant) are predicted to increase the exposure to **methylprednisolone**. Monitor and adjust dose. Moderate Study

Neurokinin-1 receptor antagonists (netupitant) are predicted to increase the exposure to **dexamethasone**. Adjust dose. Moderate Study

► **Corticosteroids** are predicted to decrease the effects of neuromuscular blocking drugs, non-depolarising. Severe Anecdotal

► **Corticosteroids** increase the risk of gastrointestinal perforation when given with nicorandil. Severe Anecdotal

► Nilotinib is predicted to increase the exposure to **methylprednisolone**. Monitor and adjust dose. Moderate Study

► **Dexamethasone** is predicted to decrease the concentration of NNRTIs (rilpivirine). Avoid multiple-dose dexamethasone. Severe Theoretical

► NSAIDs increase the risk of gastrointestinal bleeding when given with **corticosteroids**. Severe Study

► **Corticosteroids** are predicted to increase the effects of phenindione. Moderate Anecdotal

► **Dexamethasone** decreases the exposure to praziquantel. Moderate Study

► Rifamycins (rifampicin) are predicted to decrease the exposure to **fluticasone**. Unknown Theoretical

► Rifamycins (rifampicin) are predicted to decrease the exposure to corticosteroids **(budesonide, deflazacort, dexamethasone, fludrocortisone, hydrocortisone, methylprednisolone, prednisolone, triamcinolone)**. Monitor and adjust dose. Moderate Study

► **Corticosteroids** potentially decrease the effects of sodium phenylbutyrate. Moderate Anecdotal

► **Corticosteroids** are predicted to decrease the effects of somatropin. Moderate Theoretical

► **Corticosteroids** are predicted to decrease the effects of suxamethonium. Severe Anecdotal

Coumarins → see TABLE 3 p. 1429 (anticoagulant effects)

acenocoumarol · warfarin

FOOD AND LIFESTYLE The effects of coumarins can be reduced or abolished by vitamin K, including that found in health foods, food supplements, enteral feeds, or large amounts of some green vegetables or green tea. Major changes in diet (especially involving salads and vegetables) and in alcohol consumption can affect anticoagulant control. Pomegranate juice is predicted to increase the INR in response to **acenocoumarol** and **warfarin**.

► Alcohol (in those who drink heavily) potentially decreases the anticoagulant effect of **coumarins**. Severe Study

► Alpelisib is predicted to decrease the efficacy of **warfarin**. Moderate Theoretical

► Anti-androgens (apalutamide) are predicted to decrease the exposure to **coumarins**. Avoid or monitor. Mild Study

► Anti-androgens (enzalutamide) potentially decrease the exposure to **coumarins**. Avoid or adjust dose and monitor INR. Severe Study

► Antiarrhythmics (amiodarone) increase the anticoagulant effect of **coumarins**. Severe Study

► Antiarrhythmics (propafenone) increase the anticoagulant effect of **coumarins**. Monitor INR and adjust dose. Moderate Study

► Antiepileptics (carbamazepine) decrease the effects of **coumarins**. Monitor and adjust dose. Severe Study

► Antiepileptics (fosphenytoin, phenytoin) are predicted to alter the anticoagulant effect of **coumarins**. Moderate Anecdotal

► Antiepileptics (phenobarbital, primidone) decrease the anticoagulant effect of **coumarins**. Monitor INR and adjust dose. Moderate Study

► Antifungals, azoles (fluconazole) increase the anticoagulant effect of **coumarins**. Monitor INR and adjust dose. Severe Study

► Antifungals, azoles (itraconazole) potentially increase the anticoagulant effect of **coumarins**. Severe Anecdotal

► Antifungals, azoles (ketoconazole) potentially increase the anticoagulant effect of **warfarin**. Monitor INR and adjust dose. Severe Anecdotal

► Antifungals, azoles (miconazole) greatly increase the anticoagulant effect of **coumarins**. MHRA advises avoid unless INR can be monitored closely; monitor for signs of bleeding. Severe Study

► Antifungals, azoles (voriconazole) increase the anticoagulant effect of **coumarins**. Monitor INR and adjust dose. Moderate Study

► Axitinib is predicted to increase the risk of bleeding events when given with **coumarins**. Severe Theoretical

► Azathioprine decreases the anticoagulant effect of **coumarins**. Moderate Study

► Bosutinib is predicted to increase the risk of bleeding events when given with **coumarins**. Severe Theoretical

► Cabozantinib is predicted to increase the risk of bleeding events when given with **coumarins**. Severe Theoretical

► Capecitabine increases the effects of **coumarins**. Monitor INR and adjust dose. Moderate Anecdotal

► Cephalosporins (cefazolin, ceftriaxone) potentially increase the risk of bleeding events when given with **coumarins**. Severe Anecdotal

► Ceritinib is predicted to increase the exposure to **warfarin**. Avoid. Severe Theoretical

Coumarins (continued)

‣ Chloramphenicol potentially increases the anticoagulant effect of **coumarins**. [Moderate] Anecdotal

‣ Corticosteroids are predicted to increase the effects of **coumarins**. [Moderate] Study

‣ Cranberry juice potentially increases the anticoagulant effect of **warfarin**. Avoid. [Severe] Anecdotal

‣ Crizotinib is predicted to increase the risk of bleeding events when given with **coumarins**. [Severe] Theoretical

‣ Dabrafenib is predicted to decrease the anticoagulant effect of **coumarins**. [Severe] Theoretical

‣ Danazol potentially increases the anticoagulant effect of **coumarins**. [Severe] Anecdotal

‣ Dasatinib is predicted to increase the risk of bleeding events when given with **coumarins**. [Severe] Theoretical

‣ Disulfiram increases the anticoagulant effect of **coumarins**. Monitor and adjust dose. [Severe] Study

‣ Elvitegravir is predicted to decrease the anticoagulant effect of **coumarins**. [Moderate] Theoretical

‣ Endothelin receptor antagonists (bosentan) decrease the anticoagulant effect of **coumarins**. [Moderate] Study

‣ Enteral feeds (vitamin-K containing) potentially decrease the anticoagulant effect of **coumarins**. [Severe] Anecdotal

‣ Erlotinib increases the anticoagulant effect of **coumarins**. [Severe] Anecdotal

‣ Fibrates are predicted to increase the anticoagulant effect of **coumarins**. Monitor INR and adjust dose. [Severe] Study

‣ Fluorouracil increases the anticoagulant effect of **coumarins**. [Severe] Anecdotal

‣ Fostamatinib potentially alters the anticoagulant effect of **warfarin**. [Moderate] Theoretical

‣ Gefitinib is predicted to increase the anticoagulant effect of **coumarins**. [Severe] Anecdotal

‣ Glucagon increases the anticoagulant effect of **warfarin**. [Severe] Study

‣ Glucosamine potentially decreases the anticoagulant effect of **acenocoumarol**. [Moderate] Anecdotal

‣ Glucosamine potentially increases the anticoagulant effect of **warfarin**. Avoid. [Moderate] Anecdotal

‣ Griseofulvin potentially decreases the anticoagulant effect of **coumarins**. [Moderate] Anecdotal

‣ H₂ receptor antagonists (cimetidine) increase the anticoagulant effect of **coumarins**. [Severe] Study

‣ HIV-protease inhibitors are predicted to affect the anticoagulant effect of **coumarins**. [Moderate] Study

‣ Imatinib is predicted to increase the risk of bleeding events when given with **coumarins**. [Severe] Theoretical

‣ Ivacaftor is predicted to increase the anticoagulant effect of **warfarin**. [Severe] Theoretical

‣ Ivermectin potentially increases the anticoagulant effect of **coumarins**. [Severe] Anecdotal

‣ Lapatinib is predicted to increase the risk of bleeding events when given with **coumarins**. [Severe] Theoretical

‣ Leflunomide increases the anticoagulant effect of **coumarins**. [Severe] Anecdotal

‣ Letermovir is predicted to decrease the concentration of **warfarin**. Monitor and adjust dose. [Moderate] Theoretical

‣ Lomitapide increases the exposure to **warfarin**. Monitor INR and adjust dose. [Severe] Study

‣ Macrolides (clarithromycin, erythromycin) increase the anticoagulant effect of **coumarins**. Monitor INR and adjust dose. [Severe] Anecdotal

‣ Mercaptopurine decreases the anticoagulant effect of **coumarins**. [Moderate] Anecdotal

‣ Metronidazole increases the anticoagulant effect of **coumarins**. Monitor INR and adjust dose. [Severe] Study

‣ Mexiletine potentially affects the exposure to **warfarin**. Avoid. [Unknown] Theoretical

‣ Monoclonal antibodies (blinatumomab) are predicted to transiently increase the exposure to **warfarin**. Monitor and adjust dose. [Moderate] Theoretical

‣ Monoclonal antibodies (sarilumab) potentially affect the exposure to **warfarin**. Monitor and adjust dose. [Severe] Theoretical

‣ Monoclonal antibodies (tocilizumab) are predicted to decrease the exposure to **warfarin**. Monitor and adjust dose. [Moderate] Theoretical

‣ Nandrolone is predicted to increase the anticoagulant effect of **coumarins**. Monitor and adjust dose. [Severe] Theoretical

‣ Neurokinin-1 receptor antagonists (aprepitant) decrease the anticoagulant effect of **coumarins**. [Moderate] Study

‣ Neurokinin-1 receptor antagonists (fosaprepitant) are predicted to decrease the anticoagulant effect of **coumarins**. [Moderate] Theoretical

‣ Nilotinib is predicted to increase the risk of bleeding events when given with **coumarins**. [Severe] Theoretical

‣ Nitisinone is predicted to increase the exposure to **warfarin**. [Moderate] Study

‣ NNRTIs (efavirenz) are predicted to affect the concentration of **coumarins**. Adjust dose. [Moderate] Theoretical

‣ NNRTIs (etravirine) increase the anticoagulant effect of **coumarins**. [Moderate] Theoretical

‣ NNRTIs (nevirapine) potentially alter the anticoagulant effect of **coumarins**. [Severe] Anecdotal

‣ Obeticholic acid decreases the anticoagulant effect of **warfarin**. [Severe] Study

‣ Oxymetholone increases the anticoagulant effect of **coumarins**. [Severe] Anecdotal

‣ Paracetamol increases the anticoagulant effect of **coumarins**. [Moderate] Study

‣ Paritaprevir (in fixed-dose combination with dasabuvir) decreases the anticoagulant effect of **acenocoumarol**. Monitor INR and adjust dose. [Severe] Anecdotal

‣ Paritaprevir (in fixed-dose combination) decreases the anticoagulant effect of **warfarin**. Monitor INR and adjust dose. [Severe] Anecdotal

‣ Pazopanib is predicted to increase the risk of bleeding events when given with **coumarins**. [Severe] Theoretical

‣ Penicillins potentially alter the anticoagulant effect of **coumarins**. Monitor INR and adjust dose. [Severe] Anecdotal

‣ Pitolisant is predicted to decrease the exposure to **warfarin**. [Mild] Theoretical

‣ Ponatinib is predicted to increase the risk of bleeding events when given with **coumarins**. [Severe] Theoretical

‣ Quinolones increase the anticoagulant effect of **coumarins**. [Severe] Anecdotal

‣ Ranibizumab increases the risk of bleeding events when given with **coumarins**. [Severe] Theoretical

‣ Regorafenib is predicted to increase the risk of bleeding events when given with **coumarins**. [Severe] Study

‣ Rifamycins (rifampicin) decrease the anticoagulant effect of **coumarins**. [Severe] Study

‣ Rucaparib slightly increases the exposure to **warfarin**. Monitor and adjust dose. [Severe] Study

‣ Ruxolitinib is predicted to increase the risk of bleeding events when given with **coumarins**. [Severe] Theoretical

‣ Sorafenib increases the anticoagulant effect of **coumarins**. [Severe] Anecdotal

‣ St John's wort decreases the anticoagulant effect of **coumarins**. Avoid. [Severe] Anecdotal

‣ Statins (fluvastatin, rosuvastatin) increase the anticoagulant effect of **coumarins**. Monitor INR and adjust dose. [Severe] Study

‣ Sucralfate potentially decreases the effects of **warfarin**. Separate administration by 2 hours. [Moderate] Anecdotal

‣ Sulfonamides (sulfadiazine) are predicted to increase the anticoagulant effect of **coumarins**. [Severe] Theoretical

‣ Sulfonamides (sulfamethoxazole) increase the anticoagulant effect of **coumarins**. [Severe] Study

‣ Sunitinib is predicted to increase the risk of bleeding events when given with **coumarins**. [Severe] Theoretical

‣ Tamoxifen increases the anticoagulant effect of **coumarins**. [Severe] Study

‣ Tegafur increases the anticoagulant effect of **coumarins**. [Moderate] Theoretical

‣ Teriflunomide affects the anticoagulant effect of **coumarins**. [Severe] Study

‣ Tetracyclines increase the risk of bleeding events when given with **coumarins**. [Moderate] Anecdotal

Tigecycline increases the risk of bleeding events when given with **coumarins**. [Moderate] Anecdotal

Tinidazole is predicted to increase the anticoagulant effect of **coumarins**. Monitor INR and adjust dose. [Severe] Theoretical

Toremifene is predicted to increase the anticoagulant effect of **coumarins**. [Severe] Theoretical

Trimethoprim is predicted to increase the anticoagulant effect of **coumarins**. [Severe] Study

Vandetanib is predicted to increase the risk of bleeding events when given with **coumarins**. [Severe] Theoretical

Venetoclax slightly increases the exposure to **warfarin**. [Moderate] Study

ranberry

Cranberry juice potentially increases the anticoagulant effect of coumarins (**warfarin**). [Severe] Anecdotal

risantaspase → see TABLE 1 p. 1429 (hepatotoxicity), TABLE 15 p. 1432 (myelosuppression)

Crisantaspase is predicted to increase the risk of hepatotoxicity when given with imatinib. [Severe] Theoretical → Also see TABLE 15 p. 1432

Crisantaspase affects the efficacy of methotrexate. [Severe] Anecdotal → Also see TABLE 1 p. 1429 → Also see TABLE 15 p. 1432

Crisantaspase potentially increases the risk of neurotoxicity when given with vinca alkaloids (vincristine). **Vincristine** should be taken 3 to 24 hours before **crisantaspase**. [Severe] Anecdotal → Also see TABLE 1 p. 1429 → Also see TABLE 15 p. 1432

rizotinib → see TABLE 6 p. 1430 (bradycardia), TABLE 9 p. 1431 (QT-interval prolongation)

GENERAL INFORMATION Caution with concurrent use of drugs that cause gastrointestinal perforation—discontinue treatment if gastrointestinal perforation occurs.

Crizotinib is predicted to increase the exposure to abemaciclib. [Moderate] Study

‣ **Crizotinib** is predicted to increase the exposure to acalabrutinib. Avoid or monitor. [Severe] Study

‣ **Crizotinib** is predicted to increase the exposure to aldosterone antagonists (eplerenone). Adjust **eplerenone** dose, p. 208. [Severe] Study

‣ **Crizotinib** is predicted to increase the exposure to alpha blockers (tamsulosin). [Moderate] Theoretical

‣ Anti-androgens (apalutamide, enzalutamide) are predicted to markedly decrease the exposure to **crizotinib**. Avoid. [Severe] Study → Also see TABLE 9 p. 1431

‣ **Crizotinib** is predicted to increase the exposure to antiarrhythmics (propafenone). Monitor and adjust dose. [Moderate] Study

‣ Antiepileptics (carbamazepine, fosphenytoin, phenobarbital, phenytoin, primidone) are predicted to markedly decrease the exposure to **crizotinib**. Avoid. [Severe] Study

‣ Antifungals, azoles (itraconazole, ketoconazole, voriconazole) are predicted to moderately increase the exposure to **crizotinib**. Avoid. [Moderate] Study → Also see TABLE 9 p. 1431

‣ **Crizotinib** is predicted to increase the exposure to antihistamines, non-sedating (mizolastine). [Severe] Theoretical

‣ **Crizotinib** is predicted to increase the exposure to antihistamines, non-sedating (rupatadine). Avoid. [Moderate] Study

‣ **Crizotinib** is predicted to increase the concentration of antimalarials (piperaquine). [Severe] Theoretical

‣ **Crizotinib** is predicted to increase the exposure to antipsychotics, second generation (cariprazine). Avoid. [Severe] Study

‣ **Crizotinib** is predicted to increase the exposure to antipsychotics, second generation (lurasidone). Adjust **lurasidone** dose. [Moderate] Study

‣ **Crizotinib** is predicted to increase the exposure to antipsychotics, second generation (quetiapine). Avoid. [Moderate] Study

‣ **Crizotinib** is predicted to increase the exposure to avapritinib. Avoid or adjust **avapritinib** dose, p. 1012. [Moderate] Study

‣ **Crizotinib** is predicted to increase the exposure to axitinib. [Moderate] Theoretical

‣ **Crizotinib** is predicted to increase the exposure to bedaquiline. Avoid prolonged use. [Mild] Theoretical → Also see TABLE 9 p. 1431

‣ **Crizotinib** is predicted to increase the exposure to benzodiazepines (alprazolam). [Severe] Study

‣ **Crizotinib** is predicted to increase the exposure to benzodiazepines (midazolam). Monitor adverse effects and adjust dose. [Severe] Study

‣ **Crizotinib** is predicted to increase the exposure to bosutinib. Avoid or adjust dose. [Severe] Theoretical → Also see TABLE 9 p. 1431

‣ **Crizotinib** is predicted to increase the exposure to buspirone. Use with caution and adjust dose. [Moderate] Study

‣ **Crizotinib** is predicted to increase the exposure to cabozantinib. [Moderate] Theoretical → Also see TABLE 9 p. 1431

‣ **Crizotinib** is predicted to increase the exposure to calcium channel blockers (amlodipine, felodipine, lacidipine, lercanidipine, nicardipine, nifedipine, nimodipine). Monitor and adjust dose. [Moderate] Study

‣ **Crizotinib** is predicted to increase the concentration of ciclosporin. [Severe] Study

‣ Cobicistat is predicted to moderately increase the exposure to **crizotinib**. Avoid. [Moderate] Study

‣ **Crizotinib** is predicted to increase the exposure to cobimetinib. [Severe] Theoretical

‣ **Crizotinib** is predicted to increase the exposure to colchicine. Adjust **colchicine** dose with moderate CYP3A4 inhibitors, p. 1166. [Severe] Study

‣ **Crizotinib** is predicted to increase the exposure to corticosteroids (methylprednisolone). Monitor and adjust dose. [Moderate] Study

‣ **Crizotinib** is predicted to increase the risk of bleeding events when given with coumarins. [Severe] Theoretical

‣ **Crizotinib** is predicted to slightly increase the exposure to darifenacin. [Moderate] Study

‣ **Crizotinib** is predicted to increase the exposure to dasatinib. [Severe] Study → Also see TABLE 9 p. 1431

‣ **Crizotinib** is predicted to slightly increase the exposure to dienogest. [Moderate] Study

‣ **Crizotinib** is predicted to increase the exposure to dipeptidylpeptidase-4 inhibitors (saxagliptin). [Mild] Study

‣ **Crizotinib** increases the risk of QT-prolongation when given with domperidone. Avoid. [Severe] Study

‣ **Crizotinib** is predicted to increase the exposure to dopamine receptor agonists (bromocriptine). [Severe] Theoretical

‣ **Crizotinib** is predicted to increase the concentration of dopamine receptor agonists (cabergoline). [Moderate] Anecdotal

‣ **Crizotinib** is predicted to moderately increase the exposure to dutasteride. [Mild] Study

‣ **Crizotinib** is predicted to increase the exposure to elexacaftor. Adjust tezacaftor with ivacaftor and elexacaftor p. 311 dose with moderate CYP3A4 inhibitors. [Severe] Theoretical

‣ **Crizotinib** is predicted to increase the exposure to eliglustat. Avoid or adjust dose—consult product literature. [Severe] Study

‣ **Crizotinib** is predicted to moderately increase the exposure to encorafenib. [Moderate] Study → Also see TABLE 9 p. 1431

‣ Endothelin receptor antagonists (bosentan) are predicted to decrease the exposure to **crizotinib**. Avoid. [Severe] Theoretical

‣ **Crizotinib** is predicted to increase the exposure to entrectinib. Avoid moderate CYP3A4 inhibitors or adjust **entrectinib** dose, p. 1023. [Severe] Theoretical → Also see TABLE 9 p. 1431

‣ **Crizotinib** is predicted to increase the risk of ergotism when given with ergometrine. [Severe] Theoretical

‣ **Crizotinib** is predicted to increase the risk of ergotism when given with ergotamine. [Severe] Theoretical

‣ **Crizotinib** is predicted to increase the exposure to erlotinib. [Moderate] Theoretical

‣ **Crizotinib** is predicted to increase the concentration of everolimus. Avoid or adjust dose. [Moderate] Study

‣ **Crizotinib** is predicted to increase the exposure to fesoterodine. Adjust **fesoterodine** dose with moderate CYP3A4 inhibitors in hepatic and renal impairment, p. 822. [Mild] Study

‣ **Crizotinib** is predicted to increase the exposure to gefitinib. [Moderate] Theoretical

‣ **Crizotinib** potentially decreases the exposure to glecaprevir. Avoid. [Severe] Theoretical

‣ Grapefruit juice is predicted to increase the exposure to **crizotinib**. Avoid. [Moderate] Theoretical

‣ **Crizotinib** is predicted to increase the concentration of guanfacine. Adjust **guanfacine** dose, p. 372. [Moderate] Theoretical

Crizotinib (continued)

▶ HIV-protease inhibitors are predicted to moderately increase the exposure to **crizotinib**. Avoid. Moderate Study → Also see TABLE 9 p. 1431

▶ **Crizotinib** is predicted to increase the exposure to ibrutinib. Adjust **ibrutinib** dose with moderate CYP3A4 inhibitors, p. 1027. Severe Study

▶ Idelalisib is predicted to moderately increase the exposure to **crizotinib**. Avoid. Moderate Study

▶ **Crizotinib** is predicted to increase the exposure to ivabradine. Adjust **ivabradine** dose, p. 227. Severe Theoretical → Also see TABLE 6 p. 1430

▶ **Crizotinib** is predicted to increase the exposure to ivacaftor. Adjust ivacaftor p. 309 or tezacaftor with ivacaftor p. 311 or tezacaftor with ivacaftor and elexacftor p. 311 dose with moderate CYP3A4 inhibitors. Severe Study

▶ **Crizotinib** is predicted to increase the exposure to lapatinib. Moderate Study → Also see TABLE 9 p. 1431

▶ **Crizotinib** is predicted to increase the exposure to lomitapide. Avoid. Moderate Theoretical

▶ Macrolides (clarithromycin) are predicted to moderately increase the exposure to **crizotinib**. Avoid. Moderate Study → Also see TABLE 9 p. 1431

▶ **Crizotinib** is predicted to increase the exposure to midostaurin. Moderate Theoretical

▶ Mitotane is predicted to markedly decrease the exposure to **crizotinib**. Avoid. Severe Study

▶ **Crizotinib** is predicted to increase the exposure to naldemedine. Moderate Study

▶ **Crizotinib** is predicted to increase the exposure to naloxegol. Adjust **naloxegol** dose and monitor adverse effects, p. 70. Moderate Study

▶ **Crizotinib** is predicted to increase the exposure to neratinib. Avoid. Severe Study

▶ NNRTIs (efavirenz, nevirapine) are predicted to decrease the exposure to **crizotinib**. Avoid. Severe Theoretical → Also see TABLE 9 p. 1431

▶ **Crizotinib** is predicted to increase the exposure to olaparib. Avoid moderate CYP3A4 inhibitors or adjust **olaparib** dose, p. 1051. Moderate Theoretical

▶ **Crizotinib** is predicted to increase the exposure to opioids (alfentanil, buprenorphine, fentanyl, oxycodone). Monitor and adjust dose. Moderate Study → Also see TABLE 6 p. 1430

▶ **Crizotinib** is predicted to increase the exposure to opioids (methadone). Moderate Theoretical → Also see TABLE 6 p. 1430 → Also see TABLE 9 p. 1431

▶ **Crizotinib** is predicted to increase the exposure to oxybutynin. Mild Theoretical

▶ **Crizotinib** is predicted to increase the exposure to pazopanib. Moderate Theoretical → Also see TABLE 9 p. 1431

▶ **Crizotinib** is predicted to increase the risk of bleeding events when given with phenindione. Severe Theoretical

▶ **Crizotinib** is predicted to increase the exposure to phosphodiesterase type-5 inhibitors (avanafil). Adjust **avanafil** dose, p. 859. Moderate Theoretical

▶ **Crizotinib** is predicted to increase the exposure to phosphodiesterase type-5 inhibitors (sildenafil). Monitor or adjust **sildenafil** dose with moderate CYP3A4 inhibitors, p. 860. Moderate Study → Also see TABLE 9 p. 1431

▶ **Crizotinib** is predicted to increase the exposure to phosphodiesterase type-5 inhibitors (tadalafil). Severe Theoretical

▶ **Crizotinib** is predicted to increase the exposure to phosphodiesterase type-5 inhibitors (vardenafil). Adjust dose. Severe Theoretical → Also see TABLE 9 p. 1431

▶ **Crizotinib** potentially decreases the exposure to pibrentasvir. Avoid. Severe Theoretical

▶ **Crizotinib** is predicted to increase the exposure to pimozide. Avoid. Severe Theoretical → Also see TABLE 9 p. 1431

▶ Pitolisant is predicted to decrease the exposure to **crizotinib**. Avoid. Severe Theoretical

▶ **Crizotinib** is predicted to increase the exposure to ranolazine. Severe Study → Also see TABLE 9 p. 1431

▶ **Crizotinib** is predicted to increase the exposure to ribociclib. Moderate Study → Also see TABLE 9 p. 1431

▶ Rifamycins (rifampicin) are predicted to markedly decrease the exposure to **crizotinib**. Avoid. Severe Study

▶ **Crizotinib** is predicted to increase the exposure to ruxolitinib. Moderate Theoretical

▶ **Crizotinib** increases the concentration of sirolimus. Monitor and adjust dose. Moderate Study

▶ **Crizotinib** is predicted to increase the exposure to SSRIs (dapoxetine). Adjust **dapoxetine** dose with moderate CYP3A4 inhibitors, p. 867. Moderate Theoretical

▶ St John's wort is predicted to decrease the exposure to **crizotinib**. Avoid. Severe Theoretical

▶ **Crizotinib** is predicted to increase the exposure to statins (atorvastatin, simvastatin). Monitor and adjust dose. Severe Theoretical

▶ **Crizotinib** is predicted to increase the exposure to sunitinib. Moderate Theoretical → Also see TABLE 9 p. 1431

▶ **Crizotinib** is predicted to increase the concentration of tacrolimus. Severe Study

▶ **Crizotinib** is predicted to increase the exposure to taxanes (cabazitaxel). Moderate Theoretical

▶ **Crizotinib** is predicted to increase the concentration of temsirolimus. Use with caution or avoid. Moderate Theoretical

▶ **Crizotinib** is predicted to increase the exposure to tezacaftor. Adjust tezacaftor with ivacaftor p. 311 or tezacaftor with ivacaftor and elexacftor p. 311 dose with moderate CYP3A4 inhibitors. Severe Study

▶ **Crizotinib** given with a potent CYP2C19 inhibitor is predicted to increase the exposure to tofacitinib. Adjust **tofacitinib** dose, p. 1154. Moderate Study

▶ **Crizotinib** is predicted to increase the exposure to tolterodine. Mild Theoretical → Also see TABLE 9 p. 1431

▶ **Crizotinib** is predicted to increase the exposure to tolvaptan. Manufacturer advises caution or adjust **tolvaptan** dose with moderate CYP3A4 inhibitors, p. 708. Moderate Study

▶ **Crizotinib** is predicted to increase the exposure to trazodone. Moderate Theoretical

▶ **Crizotinib** is predicted to increase the exposure to venetoclax. Avoid or adjust dose—consult product literature. Severe Study

▶ **Crizotinib** is predicted to increase the exposure to vinca alkaloids. Severe Theoretical → Also see TABLE 9 p. 1431

▶ **Crizotinib** is predicted to increase the exposure to zopiclone. Adjust dose. Moderate Study

Cyclizine → see antihistamines, sedating

Cyclopentolate → see TABLE 10 p. 1431 (antimuscarinics)

Cyclophosphamide → see alkylating agents

Cycloserine

▶ Cycloserine increases the risk of CNS toxicity when given with isoniazid. Monitor and adjust dose. Moderate Study

Cyproheptadine → see antihistamines, sedating

Cyproterone → see anti-androgens

Cytarabine → see TABLE 15 p. 1432 (myelosuppression)

▶ Cytarabine decreases the concentration of flucytosine. Avoid. Severe Study

▶ Live vaccines are predicted to increase the risk of generalised infection (possibly life-threatening) when given with cytarabine. Public Health England advises avoid (refer to Green Book). Severe Theoretical

Cytomegalovirus immunoglobulin → see immunoglobulins

Dabigatran → see thrombin inhibitors

Dabrafenib

▶ Anti-androgens (apalutamide, enzalutamide) are predicted to decrease the exposure to **dabrafenib**. Avoid. Moderate Theoretical

▶ Antiepileptics (carbamazepine, fosphenytoin, phenobarbital, phenytoin, primidone) are predicted to decrease the exposure to **dabrafenib**. Avoid. Moderate Theoretical

▶ Antifungals, azoles (itraconazole, ketoconazole, voriconazole) are predicted to increase the exposure to **dabrafenib**. Use with caution or avoid. Moderate Study

▶ **Dabrafenib** decreases the exposure to benzodiazepines (midazolam). Monitor and adjust dose. Moderate Study

▶ Clopidogrel is predicted to increase the exposure to **dabrafenib**. Moderate Theoretical

▶ Cobicistat is predicted to increase the exposure to **dabrafenib**. Use with caution or avoid. Moderate Study

Dabrafenib is predicted to decrease the anticoagulant effect of coumarins. [Severe] Theoretical

Fibrates (gemfibrozil) are predicted to increase the exposure to **dabrafenib**. [Moderate] Theoretical

HIV-protease inhibitors are predicted to increase the exposure to **dabrafenib**. Use with caution or avoid. [Moderate] Study

Idelalisib is predicted to increase the exposure to **dabrafenib**. Use with caution or avoid. [Moderate] Study

Macrolides (clarithromycin) are predicted to increase the exposure to **dabrafenib**. Use with caution or avoid. [Moderate] Study

Mitotane is predicted to decrease the exposure to **dabrafenib**. Avoid. [Moderate] Theoretical

Dabrafenib is predicted to decrease the exposure to NNRTIs (doravirine). Avoid or adjust doravirine p. 683 or lamivudine with tenofovir disoproxil and doravirine p. 692 dose. [Severe] Theoretical

▸ Rifamycins (rifampicin) are predicted to decrease the exposure to **dabrafenib**. Avoid. [Moderate] Theoretical

Dacarbazine → see alkylating agents

Dacomitinib

▸ **Dacomitinib** is predicted to markedly increase the exposure to atomoxetine. Avoid or adjust dose. [Severe] Study

▸ **Dacomitinib** is predicted to markedly increase the exposure to beta blockers, non-selective (propranolol). Avoid. [Severe] Study

▸ **Dacomitinib** is predicted to markedly increase the exposure to beta blockers, selective (metoprolol, nebivolol). Avoid. [Severe] Study

▸ **Dacomitinib** is predicted to markedly increase the exposure to eliglustat. Avoid or adjust dose—consult product literature. [Severe] Study

▸ H₂ receptor antagonists are predicted to decrease the concentration of **dacomitinib**. **Dacomitinib** should be taken 2 hours before or 10 hours after H₂ receptor antagonists. [Mild] Study

▸ Proton pump inhibitors are predicted to decrease the exposure to **dacomitinib**. Avoid. [Moderate] Study

▸ **Dacomitinib** is predicted to markedly increase the exposure to tolterodine. Avoid. [Severe] Study

▸ **Dacomitinib** is predicted to markedly increase the exposure to tricyclic antidepressants (imipramine, nortriptyline). Avoid. [Severe] Study

Dactinomycin → see TABLE 1 p. 1429 (hepatotoxicity), TABLE 15 p. 1432 (myelosuppression)

▸ Live vaccines are predicted to increase the risk of generalised infection (possibly life-threatening) when given with **dactinomycin**. Public Health England advises avoid (refer to Green Book). [Severe] Theoretical

Dalteparin → see low molecular-weight heparins

Danaparoid → see TABLE 3 p. 1429 (anticoagulant effects)

▸ Ranibizumab is predicted to increase the risk of bleeding events when given with **danaparoid**. [Severe] Theoretical

Danazol

▸ **Danazol** moderately increases the concentration of antiepileptics (carbamazepine). Monitor and adjust dose. [Severe] Study

▸ **Danazol** increases the concentration of ciclosporin. [Severe] Study

▸ **Danazol** potentially increases the anticoagulant effect of coumarins. [Severe] Anecdotal

▸ **Danazol** is predicted to increase the risk of rhabdomyolysis when given with statins (atorvastatin). [Severe] Theoretical

▸ **Danazol** increases the risk of rhabdomyolysis when given with statins (simvastatin). Avoid. [Severe] Anecdotal

▸ **Danazol** potentially increases the concentration of tacrolimus. [Severe] Anecdotal

Dantrolene → see TABLE 1 p. 1429 (hepatotoxicity)

▸ Intravenous **dantrolene** potentially increases the risk of acute hyperkalaemia and cardiovascular collapse when given with calcium channel blockers (diltiazem, verapamil). Avoid. [Severe] Anecdotal

Dapagliflozin → see sodium glucose co-transporter 2 inhibitors

Dapoxetine → see SSRIs

Dapsone

▸ Aminosalicylic acid is predicted to increase the risk of methaemoglobinaemia when given with **dapsone**. [Severe] Theoretical

▸ **Dapsone** is predicted to increase the risk of methaemoglobinaemia when given with topical anaesthetics, local (prilocaine). Use with caution or avoid. [Severe] Theoretical

▸ Antiepileptics (fosphenytoin, phenobarbital, phenytoin, primidone) are predicted to increase the risk of methaemoglobinaemia when given with **dapsone**. [Severe] Theoretical

▸ Antimalarials (chloroquine, primaquine) are predicted to increase the risk of methaemoglobinaemia when given with **dapsone**. [Severe] Theoretical

▸ Nitrates are predicted to increase the risk of methaemoglobinaemia when given with **dapsone**. [Severe] Theoretical

▸ Nitrofurantoin is predicted to increase the risk of methaemoglobinaemia when given with **dapsone**. [Severe] Theoretical

▸ Nitroprusside is predicted to increase the risk of methaemoglobinaemia when given with **dapsone**. [Severe] Theoretical

▸ Paracetamol is predicted to increase the risk of methaemoglobinaemia when given with **dapsone**. [Severe] Theoretical

▸ Rifamycins decrease the exposure to **dapsone**. [Moderate] Study

▸ Sulfonamides are predicted to increase the risk of methaemoglobinaemia when given with **dapsone**. [Severe] Theoretical

▸ **Dapsone** increases the exposure to trimethoprim and trimethoprim increases the exposure to **dapsone**. [Severe] Study

Daptomycin

▸ Aspirin (high-dose) increases the risk of renal impairment when given with **daptomycin**. [Moderate] Theoretical

▸ Ciclosporin is predicted to increase the risk of rhabdomyolysis when given with **daptomycin**. [Severe] Theoretical

▸ Fibrates are predicted to increase the risk of rhabdomyolysis when given with **daptomycin**. [Severe] Theoretical

▸ NSAIDs increase the risk of renal impairment when given with **daptomycin**. [Moderate] Theoretical

▸ Statins are predicted to increase the risk of rhabdomyolysis when given with **daptomycin**. [Severe] Theoretical

Daratumumab → see monoclonal antibodies

Darbepoetin alfa → see TABLE 5 p. 1430 (thromboembolism), TABLE 16 p. 1433 (increased serum potassium)

Darifenacin → see TABLE 10 p. 1431 (antimuscarinics)

▸ Anti-androgens (apalutamide, enzalutamide) are predicted to decrease the exposure to **darifenacin**. [Moderate] Theoretical

▸ Antiarrhythmics (dronedarone) are predicted to slightly increase the exposure to **darifenacin**. [Moderate] Study

▸ **Darifenacin** is predicted to increase the concentration of antiarrhythmics (flecainide). [Moderate] Theoretical

▸ Antiepileptics (carbamazepine, fosphenytoin, phenobarbital, phenytoin, primidone) are predicted to decrease the exposure to **darifenacin**. [Moderate] Theoretical

▸ Antifungals, azoles (fluconazole, isavuconazole, posaconazole) are predicted to slightly increase the exposure to **darifenacin**. [Moderate] Study

▸ Antifungals, azoles (itraconazole, ketoconazole, voriconazole) are predicted to markedly to very markedly increase the exposure to **darifenacin**. Avoid. [Severe] Study

▸ Bupropion is predicted to slightly increase the exposure to **darifenacin**. [Mild] Study

▸ Calcium channel blockers (diltiazem, verapamil) are predicted to slightly increase the exposure to **darifenacin**. [Moderate] Study

▸ Ciclosporin is predicted to increase the exposure to **darifenacin**. Avoid. [Moderate] Theoretical

▸ Cinacalcet is predicted to slightly increase the exposure to **darifenacin**. [Mild] Study

▸ Cobicistat is predicted to markedly to very markedly increase the exposure to **darifenacin**. Avoid. [Severe] Study

▸ Crizotinib is predicted to slightly increase the exposure to **darifenacin**. [Moderate] Study

Darifenacin (continued)

▸ Grapefruit juice is predicted to increase the exposure to **darifenacin**. Moderate Study
▸ HIV-protease inhibitors are predicted to markedly to very markedly increase the exposure to **darifenacin**. Avoid. Severe Study
▸ Idelalisib is predicted to markedly to very markedly increase the exposure to **darifenacin**. Avoid. Severe Study
▸ Imatinib is predicted to slightly increase the exposure to **darifenacin**. Moderate Study
▸ Letermovir is predicted to slightly increase the exposure to **darifenacin**. Moderate Study
▸ Macrolides (clarithromycin) are predicted to markedly to very markedly increase the exposure to **darifenacin**. Avoid. Severe Study
▸ Macrolides (erythromycin) are predicted to slightly increase the exposure to **darifenacin**. Moderate Study
▸ Mitotane is predicted to decrease the exposure to **darifenacin**. Moderate Theoretical
▸ Neurokinin-1 receptor antagonists (aprepitant, netupitant) are predicted to slightly increase the exposure to **darifenacin**. Moderate Study
▸ Nilotinib is predicted to slightly increase the exposure to **darifenacin**. Moderate Study
▸ Rifamycins (rifampicin) are predicted to decrease the exposure to **darifenacin**. Moderate Theoretical
▸ SSRIs (fluoxetine, paroxetine) are predicted to slightly increase the exposure to **darifenacin**. Mild Study
▸ St John's wort is predicted to decrease the exposure to **darifenacin**. Moderate Theoretical
▸ Terbinafine is predicted to slightly increase the exposure to **darifenacin**. Mild Study
▸ **Darifenacin** is predicted to increase the exposure to tricyclic antidepressants. Moderate Theoretical → Also see TABLE 10 p. 1431
Darolutamide → see anti-androgens
Darunavir → see HIV-protease inhibitors
Dasabuvir
▸ Anti-androgens (enzalutamide) are predicted to decrease the exposure to **dasabuvir**. Avoid. Severe Theoretical
▸ Antiepileptics (carbamazepine, fosphenytoin, phenobarbital, phenytoin, primidone) are predicted to decrease the exposure to **dasabuvir**. Avoid. Severe Theoretical
▸ Clopidogrel is predicted to very markedly increase the exposure to **dasabuvir**. Avoid. Severe Study
▸ Combined hormonal contraceptives (containing ethinylestradiol) increase the risk of increased ALT concentrations when given with **dasabuvir**. Avoid. Severe Study
▸ Fibrates (gemfibrozil) are predicted to very markedly increase the exposure to **dasabuvir**. Avoid. Severe Study
▸ **Dasabuvir** (with ombitasvir, paritaprevir, and ritonavir) decreases the concentration of HIV-protease inhibitors (darunavir). Avoid or adjust dose. Moderate Study
▸ **Dasabuvir** (with ombitasvir, paritaprevir, and ritonavir) increases the concentration of loop diuretics (furosemide). Adjust dose. Moderate Study
▸ Mitotane is predicted to decrease the exposure to **dasabuvir**. Avoid. Severe Theoretical
▸ NNRTIs (efavirenz) increase the risk of increased ALT concentrations when given with **dasabuvir**. Avoid. Severe Study
▸ NNRTIs (etravirine, nevirapine) are predicted to decrease the exposure to **dasabuvir**. Avoid. Severe Theoretical
▸ Rifamycins (rifampicin) are predicted to decrease the exposure to **dasabuvir**. Avoid. Severe Theoretical
▸ St John's wort is predicted to decrease the exposure to **dasabuvir**. Avoid. Severe Theoretical
▸ **Dasabuvir** increases the exposure to statins (rosuvastatin). Adjust rosuvastatin dose, p. 218. Moderate Study
Dasatinib → see TABLE 15 p. 1432 (myelosuppression), TABLE 9 p. 1431 (QT-interval prolongation), TABLE 4 p. 1429 (antiplatelet effects)
▸ Oral antacids decrease the absorption of oral **dasatinib**. Separate administration by at least 2 hours. Moderate Study
▸ Anti-androgens (apalutamide, enzalutamide) are predicted to markedly decrease the exposure to **dasatinib**. Avoid. Severe Study → Also see TABLE 9 p. 1431

▸ Antiarrhythmics (dronedarone) are predicted to increase the exposure to **dasatinib**. Severe Study → Also see TABLE 9 p. 1431
▸ Antiepileptics (carbamazepine, fosphenytoin, phenobarbital, phenytoin, primidone) are predicted to markedly decrease the exposure to **dasatinib**. Avoid. Severe Study
▸ Antifungals, azoles (fluconazole, isavuconazole, posaconazole) are predicted to increase the exposure to **dasatinib**. Severe Study → Also see TABLE 9 p. 1431
▸ Antifungals, azoles (itraconazole, ketoconazole, voriconazole) are predicted to markedly increase the exposure to **dasatinib**. Avoid or adjust dose—consult product literature. Severe Study → Also see TABLE 9 p. 1431
▸ Calcium channel blockers (diltiazem, verapamil) are predicted to increase the exposure to **dasatinib**. Severe Study
▸ Cobicistat is predicted to markedly increase the exposure to **dasatinib**. Avoid or adjust dose—consult product literature. Severe Study
▸ **Dasatinib** is predicted to increase the risk of bleeding events when given with coumarins. Severe Theoretical
▸ Crizotinib is predicted to increase the exposure to **dasatinib**. Severe Study → Also see TABLE 9 p. 1431
▸ Endothelin receptor antagonists (bosentan) are predicted to decrease the exposure to **dasatinib**. Severe Study
▸ Grapefruit juice is predicted to increase the exposure to **dasatinib**. Avoid. Moderate Theoretical
▸ H₂ receptor antagonists are predicted to decrease the exposure to **dasatinib**. Avoid. Moderate Study
▸ HIV-protease inhibitors are predicted to markedly increase the exposure to **dasatinib**. Avoid or adjust dose—consult product literature. Severe Study → Also see TABLE 9 p. 1431
▸ Idelalisib is predicted to markedly increase the exposure to **dasatinib**. Avoid or adjust dose—consult product literature. Severe Study
▸ Imatinib is predicted to increase the exposure to **dasatinib**. Severe Study → Also see TABLE 15 p. 1432
▸ Letermovir is predicted to increase the exposure to **dasatinib**. Severe Study
▸ Macrolides (clarithromycin) are predicted to markedly increase the exposure to **dasatinib**. Avoid or adjust dose—consult product literature. Severe Study → Also see TABLE 9 p. 1431
▸ Macrolides (erythromycin) are predicted to increase the exposure to **dasatinib**. Severe Study → Also see TABLE 9 p. 1431
▸ Mitotane is predicted to markedly decrease the exposure to **dasatinib**. Avoid. Severe Study → Also see TABLE 15 p. 1432
▸ Neurokinin-1 receptor antagonists (aprepitant, netupitant) are predicted to increase the exposure to **dasatinib**. Severe Study
▸ Nilotinib is predicted to increase the exposure to **dasatinib**. Severe Study → Also see TABLE 15 p. 1432 → Also see TABLE 9 p. 1431
▸ NNRTIs (efavirenz, nevirapine) are predicted to decrease the exposure to **dasatinib**. Severe Study → Also see TABLE 9 p. 1431
▸ **Dasatinib** is predicted to increase the risk of bleeding events when given with phenindione. Severe Theoretical
▸ Pitolisant is predicted to decrease the exposure to **dasatinib**. Avoid. Severe Theoretical
▸ Proton pump inhibitors are predicted to slightly to moderately decrease the exposure to **dasatinib**. Avoid. Severe Study
▸ Rifamycins (rifampicin) are predicted to markedly decrease the exposure to **dasatinib**. Severe Study
▸ Sodium zirconium cyclosilicate is predicted to decrease the exposure to **dasatinib**. Separate administration by at least 2 hours. Moderate Theoretical
▸ St John's wort is predicted to decrease the exposure to **dasatinib**. Severe Study
▸ **Dasatinib** is predicted to increase the exposure to statins (simvastatin). Moderate Theoretical
Daunorubicin → see anthracyclines
Decitabine → see TABLE 15 p. 1432 (myelosuppression)
Deferasirox → see iron chelators
Deferiprone → see iron chelators
Deflazacort → see corticosteroids
Delafloxacin → see quinolones
Delamanid → see TABLE 9 p. 1431 (QT-interval prolongation)
▸ Anti-androgens (apalutamide, enzalutamide) are predicted to slightly decrease the exposure to **delamanid**. Avoid. Moderate Study → Also see TABLE 9 p. 1431

Antiepileptics (carbamazepine, fosphenytoin, phenobarbital, phenytoin, primidone) are predicted to slightly decrease the exposure to **delamanid**. Avoid. [Moderate] Study

Antifungals, azoles (itraconazole, ketoconazole, voriconazole) very slightly increase the exposure to **delamanid**. [Severe] Study → Also see TABLE 9 p. 1431

Cobicistat very slightly increases the exposure to **delamanid**. [Severe] Study

HIV-protease inhibitors very slightly increase the exposure to **delamanid**. [Severe] Study → Also see TABLE 9 p. 1431

Idelalisib very slightly increases the exposure to **delamanid**. [Severe] Study

Macrolides (clarithromycin) very slightly increase the exposure to **delamanid**. [Severe] Study → Also see TABLE 9 p. 1431

Mitotane is predicted to slightly decrease the exposure to **delamanid**. Avoid. [Moderate] Study

Rifamycins (rifampicin) are predicted to slightly decrease the exposure to **delamanid**. Avoid. [Moderate] Study

Demeclocycline → see tetracyclines

Desferrioxamine → see iron chelators

Desflurane → see volatile halogenated anaesthetics

Desloratadine → see antihistamines, non-sedating

Desmopressin → see TABLE 18 p. 1433 (hyponatraemia)

Antiepileptics (lamotrigine) are predicted to increase the risk of hyponatraemia when given with **desmopressin**. [Severe] Theoretical

► Loperamide greatly increases the absorption of oral **desmopressin** (and possibly sublingual). [Moderate] Study

► Phenothiazines (chlorpromazine) are predicted to increase the risk of hyponatraemia when given with **desmopressin**. [Severe] Theoretical

Desogestrel

► Antiepileptics (carbamazepine, eslicarbazepine, fosphenytoin, oxcarbazepine, perampanel, phenobarbital, phenytoin, primidone, rufinamide, topiramate) are predicted to decrease the efficacy of **desogestrel**. For FSRH guidance, see Contraceptives, interactions p. 840. [Severe] Theoretical

► **Desogestrel** is predicted to increase the exposure to antiepileptics (lamotrigine). [Moderate] Study

► Endothelin receptor antagonists (bosentan) are predicted to decrease the efficacy of **desogestrel**. For FSRH guidance, see Contraceptives, interactions p. 840. [Severe] Theoretical

► Griseofulvin potentially decreases the efficacy of **desogestrel**. For FSRH guidance, see Contraceptives, interactions p. 840. [Severe] Anecdotal

► HIV-protease inhibitors (ritonavir) are predicted to decrease the efficacy of **desogestrel**. For FSRH guidance, see Contraceptives, interactions p. 840. [Severe] Theoretical

► Modafinil is predicted to decrease the efficacy of **desogestrel**. For FSRH guidance, see Contraceptives, interactions p. 840. [Severe] Theoretical

► Neurokinin-1 receptor antagonists (aprepitant, fosaprepitant) are predicted to decrease the efficacy of **desogestrel**. For FSRH guidance, see Contraceptives, interactions p. 840. [Severe] Theoretical

► NNRTIs (efavirenz, nevirapine) are predicted to decrease the efficacy of **desogestrel**. For FSRH guidance, see Contraceptives, interactions p. 840. [Severe] Theoretical

► Rifamycins are predicted to decrease the efficacy of **desogestrel**. For FSRH guidance, see Contraceptives, interactions p. 840. [Severe] Theoretical

► St John's wort is predicted to decrease the efficacy of **desogestrel**. MHRA advises avoid. For FSRH guidance, see Contraceptives, interactions p. 840. [Severe] Theoretical

► Sugammadex is predicted to decrease the exposure to **desogestrel**. Refer to patient information leaflet for missed pill advice. [Severe] Theoretical

► Ulipristal is predicted to decrease the efficacy of **desogestrel**. Avoid. [Severe] Theoretical

Dexamethasone → see corticosteroids

Dexamfetamine → see amfetamines

Dexibuprofen → see NSAIDs

Dexketoprofen → see NSAIDs

Dexmedetomidine → see TABLE 11 p. 1431 (CNS depressant effects)

Dexrazoxane → see iron chelators

Diamorphine → see opioids

Diazepam → see benzodiazepines

Diazoxide → see TABLE 8 p. 1430 (hypotension)

► **Diazoxide** decreases the concentration of antiepileptics (fosphenytoin, phenytoin) and antiepileptics (fosphenytoin, phenytoin) are predicted to decrease the effects of **diazoxide**. Monitor concentration and adjust dose. [Moderate] Anecdotal

► **Diazoxide** increases the risk of severe hypotension when given with hydralazine. [Severe] Study → Also see TABLE 8 p. 1430

Diclofenac → see NSAIDs

Dicycloverine → see TABLE 10 p. 1431 (antimuscarinics)

Dienogest

► Anti-androgens (apalutamide, enzalutamide) are predicted to markedly decrease the exposure to **dienogest**. [Severe] Study

► Antiarrhythmics (dronedarone) are predicted to slightly increase the exposure to **dienogest**. [Moderate] Study

► Antiepileptics (carbamazepine, fosphenytoin, phenobarbital, phenytoin, primidone) are predicted to markedly decrease the exposure to **dienogest**. [Severe] Study

► Antifungals, azoles (fluconazole, isavuconazole, posaconazole) are predicted to slightly increase the exposure to **dienogest**. [Moderate] Study

► Antifungals, azoles (itraconazole, ketoconazole, voriconazole) are predicted to moderately increase the exposure to **dienogest**. [Moderate] Study

► Calcium channel blockers (diltiazem, verapamil) are predicted to slightly increase the exposure to **dienogest**. [Moderate] Study

► Cobicistat is predicted to moderately increase the exposure to **dienogest**. [Moderate] Study

► Crizotinib is predicted to slightly increase the exposure to **dienogest**. [Moderate] Study

► HIV-protease inhibitors are predicted to moderately increase the exposure to **dienogest**. [Moderate] Study

► Idelalisib is predicted to moderately increase the exposure to **dienogest**. [Moderate] Study

► Imatinib is predicted to slightly increase the exposure to **dienogest**. [Moderate] Study

► Letermovir is predicted to slightly increase the exposure to **dienogest**. [Moderate] Study

► Macrolides (clarithromycin) are predicted to moderately increase the exposure to **dienogest**. [Moderate] Study

► Macrolides (erythromycin) are predicted to slightly increase the exposure to **dienogest**. [Moderate] Study

► Mitotane is predicted to markedly decrease the exposure to **dienogest**. [Severe] Study

► Neurokinin-1 receptor antagonists (aprepitant, netupitant) are predicted to slightly increase the exposure to **dienogest**. [Moderate] Study

► Nilotinib is predicted to slightly increase the exposure to **dienogest**. [Moderate] Study

► Rifamycins (rifampicin) are predicted to markedly decrease the exposure to **dienogest**. [Severe] Study

Digoxin → see TABLE 6 p. 1430 (bradycardia)

► Acarbose decreases the concentration of **digoxin**. [Moderate] Study

► Aldosterone antagonists (eplerenone) very slightly increase the exposure to **digoxin**. [Mild] Study

► Aldosterone antagonists (spironolactone) increase the concentration of **digoxin**. Monitor and adjust dose. [Moderate] Study

► Aminoglycosides potentially increase the concentration of **digoxin**. Monitor and adjust dose. [Mild] Study

► Oral antacids decrease the absorption of oral **digoxin**. Separate administration by 2 hours. [Mild] Study

► Anti-androgens (apalutamide) are predicted to decrease the exposure to **digoxin**. [Mild] Study

► Antiarrhythmics (amiodarone, dronedarone) are predicted to moderately increase the exposure to **digoxin**. Monitor and adjust **digoxin** dose, p. 117. [Severe] Study → Also see TABLE 6 p. 1430

► Antiarrhythmics (propafenone) increase the concentration of **digoxin**. Monitor and adjust dose. [Severe] Study

► Antiepileptics (fosphenytoin, phenytoin) are predicted to decrease the concentration of **digoxin**. [Moderate] Anecdotal

► Antifungals, azoles (isavuconazole) slightly increase the exposure to **digoxin**. Monitor and adjust dose. [Moderate] Study

Digoxin (continued)

▸ Antifungals, azoles (itraconazole) are predicted to markedly increase the concentration of **digoxin**. Monitor and adjust dose. Severe Study

▸ Antifungals, azoles (ketoconazole) are predicted to markedly increase the concentration of **digoxin**. Severe Study

▸ Antifungals, azoles (posaconazole) are predicted to increase the concentration of **digoxin**. Severe Study

▸ Antimalarials (mefloquine) are predicted to increase the risk of bradycardia when given with **digoxin**. Severe Theoretical

▸ Antimalarials (quinine) increase the concentration of **digoxin**. Monitor and adjust **digoxin** dose, p. 117. Severe Anecdotal

▸ Balsalazide is predicted to decrease the concentration of **digoxin**. Moderate Theoretical

▸ Brigatinib potentially increases the concentration of **digoxin**. Moderate Theoretical

▸ Calcium channel blockers (diltiazem, verapamil) increase the concentration of **digoxin**. Monitor and adjust dose. Severe Study → Also see TABLE 6 p. 1430

▸ Intravenous calcium salts increase the effects of **digoxin**. Avoid. Moderate Anecdotal

▸ Carbimazole affects the concentration of **digoxin**. Monitor and adjust dose. Moderate Theoretical

▸ Ceritinib is predicted to increase the risk of bradycardia when given with **digoxin**. Avoid. Severe Theoretical

▸ Ciclosporin increases the concentration of **digoxin**. Monitor and adjust dose. Severe Theoretical

▸ Drugs that reduce serum potassium are predicted to increase the risk of digoxin toxicity when given with **digoxin** (see TABLE 17 p. 1433). Severe Study

▸ Eliglustat increases the exposure to **digoxin**. Adjust dose. Moderate Study

▸ Fostamatinib slightly increases the exposure to **digoxin**. Monitor **digoxin** concentration and adjust dose, p. 117. Moderate Study

▸ Glecaprevir (with pibrentasvir) increases the exposure to **digoxin**. Moderate Study

▸ HIV-protease inhibitors (ritonavir) increase the concentration of **digoxin**. Adjust dose and monitor concentration. Severe Study

▸ Ivacaftor slightly increases the exposure to **digoxin**. Moderate Study

▸ Lapatinib is predicted to increase the exposure to **digoxin**. Moderate Theoretical

▸ Ledipasvir is predicted to increase the exposure to **digoxin**. Monitor and adjust dose. Moderate Theoretical

▸ Macrolides increase the concentration of **digoxin**. Severe Anecdotal

▸ Mirabegron slightly increases the exposure to **digoxin**. Monitor concentration and adjust dose. Severe Study

▸ Neomycin decreases the absorption of **digoxin**. Moderate Study

▸ Neratinib is predicted to slightly increase the exposure to **digoxin**. Moderate Theoretical

▸ Neuromuscular blocking drugs, non-depolarising (pancuronium) are predicted to increase the risk of cardiovascular adverse effects when given with **digoxin**. Severe Anecdotal

▸ NSAIDs (indometacin) increase the concentration of **digoxin**. Severe Study

▸ Paritaprevir (with ritonavir and ombitasvir) increases the exposure to **digoxin**. Monitor and adjust **digoxin** dose, p. 117. Moderate Study

▸ Penicillamine potentially decreases the concentration of **digoxin**. Separate administration by 2 hours. Severe Anecdotal

▸ Pibrentasvir (with glecaprevir) increases the exposure to **digoxin**. Moderate Study

▸ Pitolisant is predicted to decrease the exposure to **digoxin**. Mild Theoretical

▸ Ranolazine increases the concentration of **digoxin**. Moderate Study

▸ Ribociclib is predicted to increase the exposure to **digoxin**. Moderate Theoretical

▸ Rifamycins (rifampicin) decrease the concentration of **digoxin**. Moderate Study

▸ St John's wort decreases the concentration of **digoxin**. Avoid. Severe Anecdotal

▸ Sucralfate decreases the absorption of **digoxin**. Separate administration by 2 hours. Severe Anecdotal

▸ Sulfasalazine decreases the concentration of **digoxin**. Moderate Study

▸ Suxamethonium is predicted to increase the risk of cardiovascular adverse effects when given with **digoxin**. Severe Anecdotal

▸ Thyroid hormones are predicted to affect the concentration of **digoxin**. Monitor and adjust dose. Moderate Theoretical

▸ Ticagrelor increases the concentration of **digoxin**. Moderate Study

▸ Tolvaptan increases the concentration of **digoxin**. Mild Study

▸ Trimethoprim increases the concentration of **digoxin**. Moderate Study

▸ Vandetanib slightly increases the exposure to **digoxin**. Monitor ECG and adjust dose. Moderate Study

▸ Velpatasvir is predicted to increase the exposure to **digoxin**. Severe Study

▸ Vemurafenib slightly increases the exposure to **digoxin**. Use with caution and adjust dose. Severe Study

▸ Venetoclax increases the exposure to **digoxin**. Avoid or adjust dose. Severe Study

▸ Vitamin D substances are predicted to increase the risk of toxicity when given with **digoxin**. Severe Theoretical

▸ Voxilaprevir (with sofosbuvir and velpatasvir) is predicted to increase the exposure to **digoxin**. Monitor and adjust dose. Severe Theoretical

Dihydrocodeine → see opioids

Dihydrotachysterol → see vitamin D substances

Diltiazem → see calcium channel blockers

Dimenhydrinate → see TABLE 10 p. 1431 (antimuscarinics)

Dimethyl fumarate

▸ Alcohol (excessive consumption) potentially increases the risk of gastrointestinal adverse effects when given with **dimethyl fumarate**. Avoid. Moderate Theoretical

▸ Live vaccines are predicted to increase the risk of generalised infection (possibly life-threatening) when given with **dimethyl fumarate**. Public Health England advises avoid (refer to Green Book). Severe Theoretical

Dinutuximab → see monoclonal antibodies

Dipeptidylpeptidase-4 inhibitors → see TABLE 14 p. 1432 (antidiabetic drugs)

alogliptin · linagliptin · saxagliptin · sitagliptin · vildagliptin

▸ Anti-androgens (apalutamide, enzalutamide) are predicted to decrease the exposure to **linagliptin**. Moderate Study

▸ Anti-androgens (apalutamide, enzalutamide) are predicted to moderately decrease the exposure to **saxagliptin**. Moderate Study

▸ Antiarrhythmics (dronedarone) are predicted to increase the exposure to **saxagliptin**. Mild Study

▸ Antiepileptics (carbamazepine, fosphenytoin, phenobarbital, phenytoin, primidone) are predicted to decrease the exposure to **linagliptin**. Moderate Study

▸ Antiepileptics (carbamazepine, fosphenytoin, phenobarbital, phenytoin, primidone) are predicted to moderately decrease the exposure to **saxagliptin**. Moderate Study

▸ Antifungals, azoles (fluconazole, isavuconazole, posaconazole) are predicted to increase the exposure to **saxagliptin**. Mild Study

▸ Antifungals, azoles (itraconazole, ketoconazole, voriconazole) are predicted to increase the exposure to **saxagliptin**. Moderate Study

▸ Calcium channel blockers (diltiazem, verapamil) are predicted to increase the exposure to **saxagliptin**. Mild Study

▸ Cobicistat is predicted to increase the exposure to **saxagliptin**. Moderate Study

▸ Crizotinib is predicted to increase the exposure to **saxagliptin**. Mild Study

▸ Grapefruit juice is predicted to increase the exposure to **saxagliptin**. Mild Theoretical

▸ HIV-protease inhibitors are predicted to increase the exposure to **saxagliptin**. Moderate Study

▸ Idelalisib is predicted to increase the exposure to **saxagliptin**. Moderate Study

Imatinib is predicted to increase the exposure to **saxagliptin**. Mild Study

Letermovir is predicted to increase the exposure to **saxagliptin**. Mild Study

Linagliptin is predicted to increase the exposure to lomitapide. Separate administration by 12 hours. Moderate Theoretical

Macrolides (clarithromycin) are predicted to increase the exposure to **saxagliptin**. Moderate Study

Macrolides (erythromycin) are predicted to increase the exposure to **saxagliptin**. Mild Study

Mitotane is predicted to decrease the exposure to **linagliptin**. Moderate Study

Mitotane is predicted to moderately decrease the exposure to **saxagliptin**. Moderate Study

Neurokinin-1 receptor antagonists (aprepitant, netupitant) are predicted to increase the exposure to **saxagliptin**. Mild Study

Nilotinib is predicted to increase the exposure to **saxagliptin**. Mild Study

Rifamycins (rifampicin) are predicted to decrease the exposure to **linagliptin**. Moderate Study

Rifamycins (rifampicin) are predicted to moderately decrease the exposure to **saxagliptin**. Moderate Study

Diphenoxylate → see opioids

Dipipanone → see opioids

Dipyridamole → see TABLE 8 p. 1430 (hypotension), TABLE 4 p. 1429 (antiplatelet effects)

▸ Oral antacids are predicted to decrease the absorption of oral **dipyridamole** (immediate release tablets). Moderate Theoretical

▸ **Dipyridamole** increases the exposure to antiarrhythmics (adenosine). Avoid or adjust dose. Severe Study

▸ H_2 receptor antagonists are predicted to decrease the absorption of **dipyridamole** (immediate release tablets). Moderate Theoretical

▸ Proton pump inhibitors are predicted to decrease the absorption of **dipyridamole** (immediate release tablets). Moderate Theoretical

Disopyramide → see antiarrhythmics

Disulfiram → see TABLE 12 p. 1432 (peripheral neuropathy)

▸ Alcohol causes an extremely unpleasant systemic reaction when given with **disulfiram**. Avoid for at least 24 hours before and up to 14 days after stopping treatment. Severe Study

▸ **Disulfiram** increases the concentration of antiepileptics (fosphenytoin, phenytoin). Monitor concentration and adjust dose. Severe Study → Also see TABLE 12 p. 1432

▸ **Disulfiram** increases the anticoagulant effect of coumarins. Monitor and adjust dose. Severe Study

▸ **Disulfiram** increases the risk of acute psychoses when given with metronidazole. Severe Study → Also see TABLE 12 p. 1432

▸ **Disulfiram** is predicted to increase the anticoagulant effect of phenindione. Severe Theoretical

Dobutamine → see sympathomimetics, inotropic

Docetaxel → see taxanes

Docusate sodium

ROUTE-SPECIFIC INFORMATION Interactions do not generally apply to topical use of **docusate** unless specified.

Dolutegravir

▸ Oral antacids decrease the exposure to oral **dolutegravir**. **Dolutegravir** should be taken 2 hours before or 6 hours after antacids. Moderate Study

▸ Anti-androgens (apalutamide, enzalutamide) decrease the exposure to **dolutegravir**. Adjust dose. Severe Study

▸ Antiepileptics (carbamazepine, fosphenytoin, phenobarbital, phenytoin, primidone) decrease the exposure to **dolutegravir**. Adjust dose. Severe Study

▸ Antiepileptics (oxcarbazepine) are predicted to decrease the exposure to **dolutegravir**. Adjust dose. Severe Theoretical

▸ Oral calcium salts decrease the absorption of **dolutegravir**. **Dolutegravir** should be taken 2 hours before or 6 hours after calcium salts. Moderate Study

▸ **Dolutegravir** is predicted to increase the exposure to dopamine receptor agonists (pramipexole). Adjust dose. Moderate Study

▸ Encorafenib is predicted to increase the exposure to **dolutegravir**. Moderate Theoretical

▸ Endothelin receptor antagonists (bosentan) decrease the exposure to **dolutegravir**. Adjust dose. Severe Study

▸ HIV-protease inhibitors (fosamprenavir) boosted with ritonavir slightly decrease the exposure to **dolutegravir**. Avoid if resistant to HIV-integrase inhibitors. Severe Study

▸ HIV-protease inhibitors (tipranavir) moderately decrease the exposure to **dolutegravir**. Refer to specialist literature. Severe Study

▸ Oral iron decreases the absorption of oral **dolutegravir**. **Dolutegravir** should be taken 2 hours before or 6 hours after iron. Moderate Study

▸ **Dolutegravir** increases the exposure to metformin. Use with caution and adjust dose. Severe Study

▸ Mitotane decreases the exposure to **dolutegravir**. Adjust dose. Severe Study

▸ NNRTIs (efavirenz, nevirapine) decrease the exposure to **dolutegravir**. Adjust dose. Severe Study

▸ NNRTIs (etravirine) moderately decrease the exposure to **dolutegravir**. Avoid unless given with atazanavir, darunavir, or lopinavir (all boosted with ritonavir). Severe Study

▸ Rifamycins (rifampicin) decrease the exposure to **dolutegravir**. Adjust dose. Severe Study

▸ St John's wort decreases the exposure to **dolutegravir**. Adjust dose. Severe Study

▸ Sucralfate decreases the absorption of **dolutegravir**. Moderate Study

Domperidone → see TABLE 8 p. 1431 (QT-interval prolongation)

▸ Antiarrhythmics (dronedarone) increase the risk of QT-prolongation when given with **domperidone**. Avoid. Severe Study

▸ Antifungals, azoles (fluconazole, isavuconazole, itraconazole, ketoconazole, posaconazole, voriconazole) increase the risk of QT-prolongation when given with **domperidone**. Avoid. Severe Study

▸ Calcium channel blockers (diltiazem, verapamil) increase the risk of QT-prolongation when given with **domperidone**. Avoid. Severe Study

▸ Cobicistat increases the risk of QT-prolongation when given with **domperidone**. Avoid. Severe Study

▸ Crizotinib increases the risk of QT-prolongation when given with **domperidone**. Avoid. Severe Study

▸ **Domperidone** is predicted to decrease the prolactin-lowering effect of dopamine receptor agonists (bromocriptine, cabergoline). Moderate Theoretical

▸ HIV-protease inhibitors increase the risk of QT-prolongation when given with **domperidone**. Avoid. Severe Study

▸ Idelalisib increases the risk of QT-prolongation when given with **domperidone**. Avoid. Severe Study

▸ Imatinib increases the risk of QT-prolongation when given with **domperidone**. Avoid. Severe Study

▸ Letermovir increases the risk of QT-prolongation when given with **domperidone**. Avoid. Severe Study

▸ Macrolides (clarithromycin, erythromycin) increase the risk of QT-prolongation when given with **domperidone**. Avoid. Severe Study

▸ Neurokinin-1 receptor antagonists (aprepitant, netupitant) increase the risk of QT-prolongation when given with **domperidone**. Avoid. Severe Study

▸ Nilotinib increases the risk of QT-prolongation when given with **domperidone**. Avoid. Severe Study

Donepezil → see anticholinesterases, centrally acting

Dopamine → see sympathomimetics, inotropic

Dopamine receptor agonists → see TABLE 8 p. 1430 (hypotension), TABLE 9 p. 1431 (QT-interval prolongation), TABLE 10 p. 1431 (antimuscarinics)

amantadine · apomorphine · bromocriptine · cabergoline · pramipexole · quinagolide · ropinirole · rotigotine

FOOD AND LIFESTYLE Dose adjustment might be necessary if smoking started or stopped during treatment with **ropinirole**.

▸ **Apomorphine** is predicted to increase the risk of severe hypotension when given with 5-HT3-receptor antagonists (granisetron, palonosetron). Severe Theoretical

▸ **Apomorphine** increases the risk of severe hypotension when given with 5-HT3-receptor antagonists (ondansetron). Avoid. Severe Study → Also see TABLE 9 p. 1431

A1

Interactions | Appendix 1

Dopamine receptor agonists (continued)

▶ Antiarrhythmics (dronedarone) are predicted to increase the exposure to **bromocriptine**. Severe Theoretical

▶ Antiarrhythmics (dronedarone) are predicted to increase the concentration of **cabergoline**. Severe Anecdotal

▶ Antifungals, azoles (fluconazole, isavuconazole, itraconazole, ketoconazole, posaconazole, voriconazole) are predicted to increase the concentration of **cabergoline**. Moderate Anecdotal

▶ Antifungals, azoles (fluconazole, isavuconazole, posaconazole) are predicted to increase the exposure to **bromocriptine**. Severe Theoretical

▶ Antifungals, azoles (isavuconazole) are predicted to increase the exposure to **pramipexole**. Adjust dose. Moderate Study

▶ Antifungals, azoles (itraconazole, ketoconazole, voriconazole) increase the exposure to **bromocriptine**. Severe Study

▶ Antipsychotics, second generation (amisulpride, olanzapine, paliperidone, quetiapine, risperidone) are predicted to decrease the effects of **dopamine receptor agonists**. Avoid. Moderate Theoretical → Also see TABLE 8 p. 1430 → Also see TABLE 9 p. 1431

▶ Antipsychotics, second generation (aripiprazole, clozapine) are predicted to decrease the effects of **dopamine receptor agonists**. Moderate Theoretical → Also see TABLE 8 p. 1430 → Also see TABLE 10 p. 1431

▶ Antipsychotics, second generation (asenapine) are predicted to decrease the effects of **dopamine receptor agonists**. Adjust dose. Moderate Theoretical → Also see TABLE 8 p. 1430

▶ Benperidol is predicted to decrease the effects of **dopamine receptor agonists**. Avoid. Moderate Theoretical → Also see TABLE 8 p. 1430

▶ Bupropion increases the risk of adverse effects when given with **amantadine**. Moderate Study

▶ Calcium channel blockers (diltiazem, verapamil) are predicted to increase the exposure to **bromocriptine**. Severe Theoretical → Also see TABLE 8 p. 1430

▶ Calcium channel blockers (diltiazem, verapamil) are predicted to increase the concentration of **cabergoline**. Moderate Anecdotal → Also see TABLE 8 p. 1430

▶ Cobicistat increases the exposure to **bromocriptine**. Severe Study

▶ Cobicistat is predicted to increase the concentration of **cabergoline**. Moderate Anecdotal

▶ Combined hormonal contraceptives are predicted to increase the exposure to **ropinirole**. Adjust dose. Moderate Study

▶ Crizotinib is predicted to increase the exposure to **bromocriptine**. Severe Theoretical

▶ Crizotinib is predicted to increase the concentration of **cabergoline**. Moderate Anecdotal

▶ Dolutegravir is predicted to increase the exposure to **pramipexole**. Adjust dose. Moderate Study

▶ Domperidone is predicted to decrease the prolactin-lowering effect of dopamine receptor agonists (**bromocriptine, cabergoline**). Moderate Theoretical

▶ Dopamine receptor agonists (**cabergoline**) are predicted to increase the risk of ergotism when given with dopamine receptor agonists (**bromocriptine**). Avoid. Moderate Theoretical → Also see TABLE 8 p. 1430

▶ Dopamine receptor agonists (**amantadine**) are predicted to increase the exposure to dopamine receptor agonists (**pramipexole**). Adjust dose. Moderate Theoretical → Also see TABLE 8 p. 1430

▶ Droperidol is predicted to decrease the effects of **dopamine receptor agonists**. Avoid. Moderate Theoretical → Also see TABLE 8 p. 1430 → Also see TABLE 9 p. 1431

▶ Ergometrine is predicted to increase the risk of ergotism when given with **cabergoline**. Avoid. Moderate Theoretical

▶ Ergotamine is predicted to increase the risk of ergotism when given with dopamine receptor agonists (**bromocriptine, cabergoline**). Avoid. Moderate Theoretical

▶ Flupentixol is predicted to decrease the effects of **dopamine receptor agonists**. Avoid. Moderate Theoretical → Also see TABLE 8 p. 1430

▶ H₂ receptor antagonists (cimetidine) are predicted to increase the exposure to **pramipexole**. Adjust dose. Moderate Study

▶ Haloperidol is predicted to decrease the effects of **dopamine receptor agonists**. Avoid. Moderate Theoretical → Also see TABLE 8 p. 1430 → Also see TABLE 9 p. 1431 → Also see TABLE 10 p. 1431

▶ HIV-protease inhibitors increase the exposure to **bromocriptine**. Severe Study

▶ HIV-protease inhibitors are predicted to increase the concentration of **cabergoline**. Moderate Anecdotal

▶ Hormone replacement therapy decreases the clearance of **ropinirole**. Monitor and adjust dose. Moderate Study

▶ Idelalisib increases the exposure to **bromocriptine**. Severe Study

▶ Idelalisib is predicted to increase the concentration of **cabergoline**. Moderate Anecdotal

▶ Imatinib is predicted to increase the exposure to **bromocriptine**. Severe Theoretical

▶ Imatinib is predicted to increase the concentration of **cabergoline**. Moderate Anecdotal

▶ Letermovir is predicted to increase the exposure to **bromocriptine**. Severe Theoretical

▶ Loxapine is predicted to decrease the effects of **dopamine receptor agonists**. Moderate Theoretical → Also see TABLE 8 p. 1430 → Also see TABLE 10 p. 1431

▶ Macrolides (clarithromycin) increase the exposure to **bromocriptine**. Severe Study

▶ Macrolides (clarithromycin, erythromycin) are predicted to increase the concentration of **cabergoline**. Severe Study

▶ Macrolides (erythromycin) are predicted to increase the exposure to **bromocriptine**. Severe Theoretical

▶ Amantadine increases the risk of CNS toxicity when given with memantine. Use with caution or avoid. Severe Theoretical

▶ Memantine is predicted to increase the effects of dopamine receptor agonists (**apomorphine, bromocriptine, cabergoline, pramipexole, quinagolide, ropinirole, rotigotine**). Moderate Theoretical

▶ Metoclopramide is predicted to decrease the effects of dopamine receptor agonists (**apomorphine, bromocriptine, cabergoline, pramipexole, quinagolide, ropinirole, rotigotine**). Avoid. Moderate Study

▶ Mexiletine is predicted to increase the exposure to **ropinirole**. Adjust dose. Moderate Study

▶ Neurokinin-1 receptor antagonists (aprepitant, netupitant) are predicted to increase the exposure to **bromocriptine**. Severe Theoretical

▶ Neurokinin-1 receptor antagonists (aprepitant, netupitant) are predicted to increase the concentration of **cabergoline**. Moderate Anecdotal

▶ Nilotinib is predicted to increase the exposure to **bromocriptine**. Severe Theoretical

▶ Nilotinib is predicted to increase the concentration of **cabergoline**. Moderate Anecdotal

▶ Phenothiazines are predicted to decrease the effects of **dopamine receptor agonists**. Avoid. Moderate Theoretical → Also see TABLE 8 p. 1430 → Also see TABLE 9 p. 1431 → Also see TABLE 10 p. 1431

▶ Pimozide is predicted to decrease the effects of **dopamine receptor agonists**. Avoid. Moderate Theoretical → Also see TABLE 8 p. 1430 → Also see TABLE 9 p. 1431 → Also see TABLE 10 p. 1431

▶ Quinolones (ciprofloxacin) are predicted to increase the exposure to **ropinirole**. Adjust dose. Moderate Study

▶ Ranolazine is predicted to increase the exposure to **pramipexole**. Adjust dose. Moderate Study

▶ SSRIs (fluvoxamine) are predicted to increase the exposure to **ropinirole**. Adjust dose. Moderate Study

▶ Sulpiride is predicted to decrease the effects of **dopamine receptor agonists**. Avoid. Moderate Theoretical → Also see TABLE 8 p. 1430 → Also see TABLE 9 p. 1431

▶ Sympathomimetics, vasoconstrictor (isometheptene) potentially increase the risk of adverse effects when given with **bromocriptine**. Avoid. Severe Anecdotal

▶ Trimethoprim is predicted to increase the exposure to **pramipexole**. Adjust dose. Moderate Study

▶ Vandetanib is predicted to increase the exposure to **pramipexole**. Adjust dose. Moderate Study

▶ Zuclopenthixol is predicted to decrease the effects of **dopamine receptor agonists**. Avoid. Moderate Theoretical → Also see TABLE 8 p. 1430 → Also see TABLE 9 p. 1431

Doravirine → see NNRTIs

Dorzolamide

ROUTE-SPECIFIC INFORMATION Since systemic absorption can follow topical application of **dorzolamide**, the possibility of interactions should be borne in mind.

Dosulepin → see tricyclic antidepressants

Doxapram

Aminophylline increases the risk of agitation when given with **doxapram**. Moderate Study

MAOIs, irreversible are predicted to increase the effects of **doxapram**. Moderate Theoretical

Theophylline increases the risk of agitation when given with **doxapram**. Moderate Study

Doxazosin → see alpha blockers

Doxepin → see tricyclic antidepressants

Doxorubicin → see anthracyclines

Doxycycline → see tetracyclines

Doxylamine → see antihistamines, sedating

Dronabinol → see TABLE 11 p. 1431 (CNS depressant effects)

Anti-androgens (apalutamide, enzalutamide) are predicted to decrease the exposure to **dronabinol**. Avoid or adjust dose. Mild Study

Antiepileptics (carbamazepine, fosphenytoin, phenobarbital, phenytoin, primidone) are predicted to decrease the exposure to **dronabinol**. Avoid or adjust dose. Mild Study → Also see TABLE 11 p. 1431

Antifungals, azoles (itraconazole, ketoconazole, voriconazole) are predicted to increase the exposure to **dronabinol**. Adjust dose. Mild Study

Cobicistat is predicted to increase the exposure to **dronabinol**. Adjust dose. Mild Study

HIV-protease inhibitors are predicted to increase the exposure to **dronabinol**. Adjust dose. Mild Study

Idelalisib is predicted to increase the exposure to **dronabinol**. Adjust dose. Mild Study

Macrolides (clarithromycin) are predicted to increase the exposure to **dronabinol**. Adjust dose. Mild Study

Mitotane is predicted to decrease the exposure to **dronabinol**. Avoid or adjust dose. Mild Study

Rifamycins (rifampicin) are predicted to decrease the exposure to **dronabinol**. Avoid or adjust dose. Mild Study

St John's wort is predicted to decrease the exposure to **dronabinol**. Avoid or adjust dose. Mild Study

Dronedarone → see antiarrhythmics

Droperidol → see TABLE 8 p. 1430 (hypotension), TABLE 9 p. 1431 (QT-interval prolongation), TABLE 11 p. 1431 (CNS depressant effects)

Droperidol is predicted to decrease the effects of dopamine receptor agonists. Avoid. Moderate Theoretical → Also see TABLE 8 p. 1430 → Also see TABLE 9 p. 1431

Droperidol decreases the effects of levodopa. Severe Study → Also see TABLE 8 p. 1430

Drospirenone → see TABLE 16 p. 1433 (increased serum potassium)

Antifungals, azoles (ketoconazole) moderately increase the exposure to **drospirenone**. Severe Study

Drugs that cause serotonin syndrome

Opioids (tapentadol) are predicted to increase the risk of serotonin syndrome when given with **drugs that cause serotonin syndrome** (see TABLE 13 p. 1432). Severe Theoretical

Drugs that reduce serum potassium

Drugs that reduce serum potassium are predicted to increase the risk of digoxin toxicity when given with digoxin (see TABLE 17 p. 1433). Severe Study

Drugs with anticoagulant effects

▶ Bismuth subsalicylate is predicted to increase the risk of bleeding events when given with **drugs with anticoagulant effects** (see TABLE 3 p. 1429). Moderate Theoretical

▶ Caplacizumab is predicted to increase the risk of bleeding events when given with **drugs with anticoagulant effects** (see TABLE 3 p. 1429). Severe Theoretical

▶ Volanesorsen potentially increases the risk of bleeding events when given with **drugs with anticoagulant effects** (see TABLE 3 p. 1429). Avoid depending on platelet count—consult product literature. Severe Theoretical

Drugs with antimuscarinic effects

▶ Drugs with antimuscarinic effects decrease the absorption of levodopa (see TABLE 10 p. 1431). Moderate Theoretical

Drugs with antiplatelet effects

▶ Caplacizumab is predicted to increase the risk of bleeding events when given with **drugs with antiplatelet effects** (see TABLE 4 p. 1429). Severe Theoretical

▶ Volanesorsen potentially increases the risk of bleeding events when given with **drugs with antiplatelet effects** (see TABLE 4 p. 1429). Avoid depending on platelet count—consult product literature. Severe Theoretical

Dulaglutide → see glucagon-like peptide-1 receptor agonists

Duloxetine → see TABLE 18 p. 1433 (hyponatraemia), TABLE 13 p. 1432 (serotonin syndrome), TABLE 4 p. 1429 (antiplatelet effects)

▶ Antiepileptics (phenytoin) are predicted to decrease the exposure to **duloxetine**. Moderate Theoretical

▶ **Duloxetine** is predicted to increase the exposure to beta blockers, selective (metoprolol). Moderate Study

▶ **Duloxetine** is predicted to increase the exposure to eliglustat. Avoid or adjust dose—consult product literature. Severe Study

▶ HIV-protease inhibitors (ritonavir) are predicted to decrease the exposure to **duloxetine**. Moderate Theoretical

▶ Leflunomide is predicted to decrease the exposure to **duloxetine**. Moderate Theoretical

▶ **Duloxetine** is predicted to increase the exposure to pitolisant. Use with caution and adjust dose. Moderate Study

▶ Quinolones (ciprofloxacin) are predicted to increase the exposure to **duloxetine**. Avoid. Moderate Theoretical

▶ Rifamycins (rifampicin) are predicted to decrease the exposure to **duloxetine**. Moderate Theoretical

▶ SSRIs (fluvoxamine) markedly increase the exposure to **duloxetine**. Avoid. Severe Study → Also see TABLE 18 p. 1433 → Also see TABLE 13 p. 1432 → Also see TABLE 4 p. 1429

▶ Teriflunomide is predicted to decrease the exposure to **duloxetine**. Moderate Theoretical

▶ Vemurafenib is predicted to increase the exposure to **duloxetine**. Use with caution or avoid. Moderate Theoretical

Dupilumab → see monoclonal antibodies

Durvalumab → see monoclonal antibodies

Dutasteride

▶ Antiarrhythmics (dronedarone) are predicted to moderately increase the exposure to **dutasteride**. Mild Study

▶ Antifungals, azoles (fluconazole, isavuconazole, posaconazole) are predicted to moderately increase the exposure to **dutasteride**. Mild Study

▶ Antifungals, azoles (itraconazole, ketoconazole, voriconazole) are predicted to increase the exposure to **dutasteride**. Monitor adverse effects and adjust dose. Moderate Theoretical

▶ Calcium channel blockers (diltiazem, verapamil) are predicted to moderately increase the exposure to **dutasteride**. Mild Study

▶ Cobicistat is predicted to increase the exposure to **dutasteride**. Monitor adverse effects and adjust dose. Moderate Theoretical

▶ Crizotinib is predicted to moderately increase the exposure to **dutasteride**. Mild Study

▶ HIV-protease inhibitors are predicted to increase the exposure to **dutasteride**. Monitor adverse effects and adjust dose. Moderate Theoretical

▶ Idelalisib is predicted to increase the exposure to **dutasteride**. Monitor adverse effects and adjust dose. Moderate Theoretical

▶ Imatinib is predicted to moderately increase the exposure to **dutasteride**. Mild Study

▶ Letermovir is predicted to moderately increase the exposure to **dutasteride**. Mild Study

▶ Macrolides (clarithromycin) are predicted to increase the exposure to **dutasteride**. Monitor adverse effects and adjust dose. Moderate Theoretical

▶ Macrolides (erythromycin) are predicted to moderately increase the exposure to **dutasteride**. Mild Study

▶ Neurokinin-1 receptor antagonists (aprepitant, netupitant) are predicted to moderately increase the exposure to **dutasteride**. Mild Study

▶ Nilotinib is predicted to moderately increase the exposure to **dutasteride**. Mild Study

Eculizumab → see monoclonal antibodies

Edoxaban → see factor XA inhibitors

Efavirenz → see NNRTIs

Elbasvir

▸ Anti-androgens (apalutamide, enzalutamide) are predicted to decrease the exposure to **elbasvir**. Avoid. [Severe] Study
▸ Antiepileptics (carbamazepine, fosphenytoin, phenobarbital, phenytoin, primidone) are predicted to decrease the exposure to **elbasvir**. Avoid. [Severe] Study
▸ Endothelin receptor antagonists (bosentan) are predicted to moderately decrease the exposure to **elbasvir**. Avoid. [Severe] Study
▸ Mitotane is predicted to decrease the exposure to **elbasvir**. Avoid. [Severe] Study
▸ Modafinil is predicted to decrease the exposure to **elbasvir**. Avoid. [Unknown] Theoretical
▸ NNRTIs (efavirenz, nevirapine) are predicted to moderately decrease the exposure to **elbasvir**. Avoid. [Severe] Study
▸ NNRTIs (etravirine) are predicted to decrease the exposure to **elbasvir**. Avoid. [Unknown] Theoretical
▸ Rifamycins (rifampicin) are predicted to decrease the exposure to **elbasvir**. Avoid. [Severe] Study
▸ St John's wort is predicted to moderately decrease the exposure to **elbasvir**. Avoid. [Severe] Study
▸ **Elbasvir** increases the exposure to statins (atorvastatin). Adjust **atorvastatin** dose, p. 217. [Moderate] Study
▸ **Elbasvir** is predicted to increase the exposure to statins (fluvastatin). Adjust **fluvastatin** dose, p. 217. [Unknown] Theoretical
▸ **Elbasvir** increases the exposure to statins (rosuvastatin). Adjust **rosuvastatin** dose, p. 218. [Moderate] Study
▸ **Elbasvir** is predicted to increase the exposure to statins (simvastatin). Adjust **simvastatin** dose, p. 219. [Unknown] Theoretical
▸ **Elbasvir** is predicted to increase the concentration of sunitinib. Use with caution and adjust dose. [Moderate] Theoretical
▸ **Elbasvir** is predicted to increase the concentration of thrombin inhibitors (dabigatran). [Moderate] Theoretical

Eletriptan → see triptans

Elexacaftor

▸ Anti-androgens (apalutamide, enzalutamide) is predicted to decrease the exposure to **elexacaftor**. Avoid. [Severe] Theoretical
▸ Antiarrhythmics (dronedarone) is predicted to increase the exposure to **elexacaftor**. Adjust tezacaftor with ivacaftor and elexacftor p. 311 dose with moderate CYP3A4 inhibitors. [Severe] Theoretical
▸ Antiepileptics (carbamazepine, fosphenytoin, phenobarbital, phenytoin, primidone) is predicted to decrease the exposure to **elexacaftor**. Avoid. [Severe] Theoretical
▸ Antifungals, azoles (fluconazole, isavuconazole, posaconazole) is predicted to increase the exposure to **elexacaftor**. Adjust tezacaftor with ivacaftor and elexacftor p. 311 dose with moderate CYP3A4 inhibitors. [Severe] Theoretical
▸ Antifungals, azoles (itraconazole, ketoconazole, voriconazole) is predicted to increase the exposure to **elexacaftor**. Adjust tezacaftor with ivacaftor and elexacftor p. 311 dose with potent CYP3A4 inhibitors. [Severe] Theoretical
▸ Calcium channel blockers (diltiazem, verapamil) is predicted to increase the exposure to **elexacaftor**. Adjust tezacaftor with ivacaftor and elexacftor p. 311 dose with moderate CYP3A4 inhibitors. [Severe] Theoretical
▸ Cobicistat is predicted to increase the exposure to **elexacaftor**. Adjust tezacaftor with ivacaftor and elexacftor p. 311 dose with potent CYP3A4 inhibitors. [Severe] Study
▸ Crizotinib is predicted to increase the exposure to **elexacaftor**. Adjust tezacaftor with ivacaftor and elexacftor p. 311 dose with moderate CYP3A4 inhibitors. [Severe] Theoretical
▸ Grapefruit juice is predicted to increase the exposure to **elexacaftor**. Avoid. [Moderate] Theoretical
▸ HIV-protease inhibitors is predicted to increase the exposure to **elexacaftor**. Adjust tezacaftor with ivacaftor and elexacftor p. 311 dose with potent CYP3A4 inhibitors. [Severe] Study
▸ Idelalisib is predicted to increase the exposure to **elexacaftor**. Adjust tezacaftor with ivacaftor and elexacftor p. 311 dose with potent CYP3A4 inhibitors. [Severe] Study
▸ Imatinib is predicted to increase the exposure to **elexacaftor**. Adjust tezacaftor with ivacaftor and elexacftor p. 311 dose with moderate CYP3A4 inhibitors. [Severe] Theoretical

▸ Letermovir is predicted to increase the exposure to **elexacaftor**. Adjust tezacaftor with ivacaftor and elexacftor p. 311 dose with moderate CYP3A4 inhibitors. [Severe] Theoretical
▸ Macrolides (clarithromycin) is predicted to increase the exposure to **elexacaftor**. Adjust tezacaftor with ivacaftor and elexacftor p. 311 dose with potent CYP3A4 inhibitors. [Severe] Study
▸ Macrolides (erythromycin) is predicted to increase the exposure to **elexacaftor**. Adjust tezacaftor with ivacaftor and elexacftor p. 311 dose with moderate CYP3A4 inhibitors. [Severe] Theoretical
▸ Mitotane is predicted to decreases the exposure to **elexacaftor**. Avoid. [Severe] Theoretical
▸ Neurokinin-1 receptor antagonists (aprepitant, netupitant) is predicted to increase the exposure to **elexacaftor**. Adjust tezacaftor with ivacaftor and elexacftor p. 311 dose with moderate CYP3A4 inhibitors. [Severe] Theoretical
▸ Nilotinib is predicted to increase the exposure to **elexacaftor**. Adjust tezacaftor with ivacaftor and elexacftor p. 311 dose with moderate CYP3A4 inhibitors. [Severe] Theoretical
▸ Rifamycins (rifabutin) are predicted to decrease the exposure to **elexacaftor**. Avoid. [Severe] Theoretical
▸ Rifamycins (rifampicin) is predicted to decrease the exposure to **elexacaftor**. Avoid. [Severe] Theoretical
▸ St John's wort is predicted to decrease the exposure to **elexacaftor**. Avoid. [Severe] Theoretical

Eliglustat

▸ **Eliglustat** is predicted to increase the exposure to aliskiren. Adjust dose. [Moderate] Study
▸ Anti-androgens (abiraterone) are predicted to increase the exposure to **eliglustat**. Avoid or adjust dose—consult product literature. [Severe] Study
▸ Anti-androgens (apalutamide, enzalutamide) are predicted to decrease the exposure to **eliglustat**. [Severe] Study
▸ Antiarrhythmics (dronedarone, propafenone) are predicted to increase the exposure to **eliglustat**. Avoid or adjust dose—consult product literature. [Severe] Study
▸ Antiepileptics (carbamazepine, fosphenytoin, phenobarbital, phenytoin, primidone) are predicted to decrease the exposure to **eliglustat**. Avoid. [Severe] Study
▸ Antifungals, azoles (fluconazole, isavuconazole, itraconazole, ketoconazole, posaconazole, voriconazole) are predicted to increase the exposure to **eliglustat**. Avoid or adjust dose—consult product literature. [Severe] Study
▸ **Eliglustat** is predicted to increase the exposure to antihistamines, non-sedating (fexofenadine). Adjust dose. [Moderate] Study
▸ **Eliglustat** is predicted to increase the exposure to atomoxetine. Adjust dose. [Moderate] Theoretical
▸ **Eliglustat** is predicted to increase the exposure to beta blockers, non-selective (propranolol). Adjust dose. [Moderate] Study
▸ **Eliglustat** is predicted to increase the exposure to beta blockers, selective (metoprolol). Adjust dose. [Moderate] Study
▸ Bupropion is predicted to increase the exposure to **eliglustat**. Avoid or adjust dose—consult product literature. [Severe] Study
▸ Calcium channel blockers (diltiazem, verapamil) are predicted to increase the exposure to **eliglustat**. Avoid or adjust dose—consult product literature. [Severe] Study
▸ Cinacalcet is predicted to increase the exposure to **eliglustat**. Avoid or adjust dose—consult product literature. [Severe] Study
▸ Cobicistat is predicted to increase the exposure to **eliglustat**. Avoid or adjust dose—consult product literature. [Severe] Study
▸ **Eliglustat** is predicted to increase the exposure to colchicine. Avoid or adjust **colchicine** dose, p. 1166. [Severe] Theoretical
▸ Crizotinib is predicted to increase the exposure to **eliglustat**. Avoid or adjust dose—consult product literature. [Severe] Study
▸ Dacomitinib is predicted to markedly increase the exposure to **eliglustat**. Avoid or adjust dose—consult product literature. [Severe] Study
▸ **Eliglustat** increases the exposure to digoxin. Adjust dose. [Moderate] Study
▸ Duloxetine is predicted to increase the exposure to **eliglustat**. Avoid or adjust dose—consult product literature. [Severe] Study
▸ Endothelin receptor antagonists (bosentan) are predicted to decrease the exposure to **eliglustat**. [Moderate] Theoretical

Eliglustat is predicted to increase the exposure to everolimus. Adjust dose. [Moderate] Study

Eliglustat is predicted to increase the exposure to factor XA inhibitors (edoxaban). Adjust dose. [Moderate] Study

Grapefruit juice is predicted to increase the exposure to **eliglustat**. Avoid. [Severe] Theoretical

HIV-protease inhibitors are predicted to increase the exposure to **eliglustat**. Avoid or adjust dose—consult product literature. [Severe] Study

Idelalisib is predicted to increase the exposure to **eliglustat**. Avoid or adjust dose—consult product literature. [Severe] Study

Imatinib is predicted to increase the exposure to **eliglustat**. Avoid or adjust dose—consult product literature. [Severe] Study

Letermovir is predicted to increase the exposure to **eliglustat**. Avoid or adjust dose—consult product literature. [Severe] Study

Eliglustat is predicted to increase the exposure to loperamide. Adjust dose. [Moderate] Study

Macrolides (clarithromycin, erythromycin) are predicted to increase the exposure to **eliglustat**. Avoid or adjust dose—consult product literature. [Severe] Study

Mirabegron is predicted to increase the exposure to **eliglustat**. Avoid or adjust dose—consult product literature. [Severe] Study

Mitotane is predicted to decrease the exposure to **eliglustat**. Avoid. [Severe] Study

Moclobemide is predicted to increase the exposure to **eliglustat**. Avoid or adjust dose—consult product literature. [Severe] Theoretical

Neurokinin-1 receptor antagonists (aprepitant, netupitant) are predicted to increase the exposure to **eliglustat**. Avoid or adjust dose—consult product literature. [Severe] Study

Nilotinib is predicted to increase the exposure to **eliglustat**. Avoid or adjust dose—consult product literature. [Severe] Study

NNRTIs (efavirenz, nevirapine) are predicted to decrease the exposure to **eliglustat**. [Moderate] Theoretical

Quinolones (ciprofloxacin) are predicted to increase the exposure to **eliglustat**. Avoid or adjust dose—consult product literature. [Severe] Theoretical

Rifamycins (rifampicin) are predicted to decrease the exposure to **eliglustat**. Avoid. [Severe] Study

Eliglustat is predicted to increase the exposure to sirolimus. Adjust dose. [Moderate] Study

SSRIs (fluoxetine, paroxetine) are predicted to increase the exposure to **eliglustat**. Avoid or adjust dose—consult product literature. [Severe] Study

St John's wort is predicted to decrease the exposure to **eliglustat**. Avoid. [Severe] Study

Eliglustat is predicted to increase the exposure to taxanes (paclitaxel). Adjust dose. [Moderate] Study

Terbinafine is predicted to increase the exposure to **eliglustat**. Avoid or adjust dose—consult product literature. [Severe] Study

Eliglustat is predicted to increase the exposure to thrombin inhibitors (dabigatran). Adjust dose. [Moderate] Study

Eliglustat is predicted to increase the exposure to tolterodine. Adjust dose. [Moderate] Theoretical

Eliglustat is predicted to increase the exposure to topotecan. Adjust dose. [Moderate] Study

Eliglustat is predicted to increase the exposure to tricyclic antidepressants (nortriptyline). Adjust dose. [Moderate] Theoretical

Elotuzumab → see monoclonal antibodies

Eltrombopag

▸ **Eltrombopag** is predicted to increase the exposure to alpelisib. [Moderate] Theoretical

▸ Oral antacids decrease the absorption of oral **eltrombopag**. **Eltrombopag** should be taken 2 hours before or 4 hours after antacids. [Severe] Study

▸ Oral calcium salts decrease the absorption of **eltrombopag**. **Eltrombopag** should be taken 2 hours before or 4 hours after calcium salts. [Severe] Study

▸ Ciclosporin decreases the exposure to **eltrombopag**. Monitor and adjust dose. [Moderate] Study

▸ Oral iron is predicted to decrease the absorption of oral **eltrombopag**. **Eltrombopag** should be taken 2 hours before or 4 hours after iron. [Severe] Theoretical

▸ **Eltrombopag** is predicted to increase the exposure to larotrectinib. [Mild] Study

▸ **Eltrombopag** is predicted to increase the concentration of letermovir. [Moderate] Study

▸ **Eltrombopag** is predicted to increase the concentration of methotrexate. [Moderate] Theoretical

▸ **Eltrombopag** is predicted to increase the exposure to the active metabolite of ozanimod. Avoid. [Moderate] Study

▸ Rifamycins (rifampicin) are predicted to decrease the exposure to **eltrombopag** and **eltrombopag** is predicted to increase the concentration of rifamycins (rifampicin). [Moderate] Theoretical

▸ Oral selenium is predicted to decrease the absorption of **eltrombopag**. **Eltrombopag** should be taken 2 hours before or 4 hours after **selenium**. [Severe] Theoretical

▸ SSRIs (fluvoxamine) are predicted to increase the exposure to **eltrombopag**. [Moderate] Theoretical

▸ **Eltrombopag** is predicted to increase the exposure to statins. Monitor and adjust dose. [Moderate] Study

▸ **Eltrombopag** potentially increases the exposure to talazoparib. Avoid or monitor. [Moderate] Theoretical

▸ **Eltrombopag** is predicted to increase the exposure to tenofovir alafenamide. [Moderate] Theoretical

▸ **Eltrombopag** is predicted to increase the exposure to tenofovir disoproxil. [Moderate] Theoretical

▸ Oral zinc is predicted to decrease the absorption of **eltrombopag**. **Eltrombopag** should be taken 2 hours before or 4 hours after **zinc**. [Severe] Theoretical

Elvitegravir

▸ Oral antacids decrease the exposure to oral **elvitegravir**. Separate administration by at least 4 hours. [Moderate] Study

▸ Anti-androgens (apalutamide, enzalutamide) are predicted to decrease the concentration of **elvitegravir**. Avoid. [Severe] Theoretical

▸ Antiepileptics (carbamazepine, fosphenytoin, phenobarbital, phenytoin, primidone) are predicted to decrease the concentration of **elvitegravir**. Avoid. [Severe] Theoretical

▸ **Elvitegravir** is predicted to decrease the anticoagulant effect of coumarins. [Moderate] Theoretical

▸ Endothelin receptor antagonists (bosentan) are predicted to decrease the concentration of **elvitegravir**. Avoid. [Severe] Theoretical

▸ **Elvitegravir** markedly increases the exposure to grazoprevir. Avoid. [Severe] Study

▸ HIV-protease inhibitors (atazanavir, lopinavir) boosted with ritonavir increase the concentration of **elvitegravir**. Refer to specialist literature. [Moderate] Study

▸ Mitotane is predicted to decrease the concentration of **elvitegravir**. Avoid. [Severe] Theoretical

▸ NNRTIs (efavirenz, nevirapine) are predicted to decrease the concentration of **elvitegravir**. Avoid. [Severe] Theoretical

▸ Rifamycins (rifampicin) are predicted to decrease the concentration of **elvitegravir**. Avoid. [Severe] Theoretical

▸ St John's wort is predicted to decrease the concentration of **elvitegravir**. Avoid. [Severe] Theoretical

Empagliflozin → see sodium glucose co-transporter 2 inhibitors

Emtricitabine → see NRTIs

Enalapril → see ACE inhibitors

Encorafenib → see TABLE 9 p. 1431 (QT-interval prolongation)

▸ Anti-androgens (apalutamide, enzalutamide) are predicted to decrease the exposure to **encorafenib**. [Severe] Theoretical → Also see TABLE 9 p. 1431

▸ Antiarrhythmics (dronedarone) are predicted to moderately increase the exposure to **encorafenib**. [Moderate] Study → Also see TABLE 9 p. 1431

▸ Antiepileptics (carbamazepine, fosphenytoin, phenobarbital, phenytoin, primidone) are predicted to decrease the exposure to **encorafenib**. [Severe] Theoretical

▸ Antifungals, azoles (fluconazole, isavuconazole, posaconazole) are predicted to moderately increase the exposure to **encorafenib**. [Moderate] Study → Also see TABLE 9 p. 1431

▸ Antifungals, azoles (itraconazole, ketoconazole, voriconazole) are predicted to increase the exposure to **encorafenib**. Avoid or monitor. [Severe] Study → Also see TABLE 9 p. 1431

▸ Calcium channel blockers (diltiazem, verapamil) are predicted to moderately increase the exposure to **encorafenib**. [Moderate] Study

A1

Interactions | **Appendix 1**

Encorafenib (continued)
▸ Cobicistat is predicted to increase the exposure to **encorafenib**. Avoid or monitor. Severe Study
▸ **Encorafenib** is predicted to affect the exposure to combined hormonal contraceptives. Severe Theoretical
▸ Crizotinib is predicted to moderately increase the exposure to **encorafenib**. Moderate Study →Also see TABLE 9 p. 1431
▸ **Encorafenib** is predicted to increase the exposure to dolutegravir. Moderate Theoretical
▸ Grapefruit juice is predicted to increase the exposure to **encorafenib**. Avoid. Moderate Study
▸ HIV-protease inhibitors are predicted to increase the exposure to **encorafenib**. Avoid or monitor. Severe Study →Also see TABLE 9 p. 1431
▸ Idelalisib is predicted to increase the exposure to **encorafenib**. Avoid or monitor. Severe Study
▸ Imatinib is predicted to moderately increase the exposure to **encorafenib**. Moderate Study
▸ Letermovir is predicted to moderately increase the exposure to **encorafenib**. Moderate Study
▸ Macrolides (clarithromycin) are predicted to increase the exposure to **encorafenib**. Avoid or monitor. Severe Study →Also see TABLE 9 p. 1431
▸ Macrolides (erythromycin) are predicted to moderately increase the exposure to **encorafenib**. Moderate Study →Also see TABLE 9 p. 1431
▸ Mitotane is predicted to decrease the exposure to **encorafenib**. Severe Theoretical
▸ Neurokinin-1 receptor antagonists (aprepitant, netupitant) are predicted to moderately increase the exposure to **encorafenib**. Moderate Study
▸ Nilotinib is predicted to moderately increase the exposure to **encorafenib**. Moderate Study →Also see TABLE 9 p. 1431
▸ **Encorafenib** is predicted to increase the exposure to raltegravir. Moderate Theoretical
▸ Rifamycins (rifampicin) are predicted to decrease the exposure to **encorafenib**. Severe Theoretical
▸ St John's wort is predicted to decrease the exposure to **encorafenib**. Severe Theoretical

Endothelin receptor antagonists

ambrisentan · bosentan · macitentan

▸ **Bosentan** is predicted to decrease the exposure to acalabrutinib. Severe Theoretical
▸ Anti-androgens (apalutamide, enzalutamide) affect the exposure to **bosentan**. Avoid. Severe Study
▸ Anti-androgens (apalutamide, enzalutamide) are predicted to decrease the exposure to **macitentan**. Avoid. Severe Study
▸ **Bosentan** is predicted to decrease the exposure to anti-androgens (darolutamide). Avoid. Moderate Theoretical
▸ **Bosentan** is predicted to decrease the exposure to antiarrhythmics (dronedarone). Severe Theoretical
▸ Antiepileptics (carbamazepine, fosphenytoin, phenobarbital, phenytoin, primidone) affect the exposure to **bosentan**. Avoid. Severe Study
▸ Antiepileptics (carbamazepine, fosphenytoin, phenobarbital, phenytoin, primidone) are predicted to decrease the exposure to **macitentan**. Avoid. Severe Study
▸ Antifungals, azoles (fluconazole) are predicted to increase the exposure to **bosentan**. Avoid. Severe Study
▸ Antifungals, azoles (itraconazole) are predicted to increase the exposure to **bosentan**. Moderate Theoretical
▸ Antifungals, azoles (itraconazole, ketoconazole, voriconazole) are predicted to increase the exposure to **macitentan**. Moderate Study
▸ Antifungals, azoles (ketoconazole) moderately increase the exposure to **bosentan**. Moderate Study
▸ Antifungals, azoles (voriconazole) are predicted to increase the exposure to **bosentan**. Severe Theoretical
▸ **Bosentan** is predicted to decrease the exposure to antifungals, azoles (isavuconazole). Avoid. Severe Theoretical
▸ **Bosentan** is predicted to decrease the exposure to antipsychotics, second generation (cariprazine). Avoid. Severe Theoretical

▸ **Bosentan** is predicted to decrease the exposure to antipsychotics, second generation (lurasidone). Monitor and adjust dose. Moderate Theoretical
▸ **Bosentan** is predicted to decrease the exposure to antipsychotics, second generation (quetiapine). Moderate Study
▸ **Bosentan** is predicted to decrease the exposure to avapritinib. Avoid. Severe Study
▸ **Bosentan** is predicted to decrease the exposure to axitinib. Moderate Theoretical
▸ **Bosentan** is predicted to decrease the exposure to bedaquiline. Avoid. Severe Study
▸ **Bosentan** is predicted to decrease the concentration of benzodiazepines (midazolam). Monitor and adjust dose. Moderate Study
▸ **Bosentan** is predicted to decrease the exposure to bosutinib. Avoid. Severe Theoretical
▸ **Bosentan** is predicted to decrease the exposure to brigatinib. Avoid. Severe Study
▸ **Bosentan** is predicted to decrease the exposure to cabozantinib. Moderate Theoretical
▸ **Bosentan** is predicted to decrease the exposure to calcium channel blockers (amlodipine, felodipine, lacidipine, lercanidipine, nicardipine, nifedipine, nimodipine). Monitor and adjust dose. Moderate Theoretical
▸ **Bosentan** is predicted to decrease the exposure to calcium channel blockers (diltiazem, verapamil). Moderate Theoretical
▸ Cephalosporins (ceftobiprole) are predicted to increase the exposure to **bosentan**. Moderate Theoretical
▸ Ciclosporin moderately increases the exposure to **ambrisentan**. Adjust **ambrisentan** dose, p. 197. Moderate Study
▸ **Bosentan** moderately decreases the exposure to ciclosporin and ciclosporin moderately increases the exposure to **bosentan**. Avoid. Severe Study
▸ **Bosentan** is predicted to decrease the exposure to cobicistat. Avoid. Severe Theoretical
▸ Cobicistat is predicted to increase the exposure to **macitentan**. Moderate Study
▸ **Bosentan** is predicted to decrease the exposure to cobimetinib. Avoid. Severe Theoretical
▸ **Bosentan** is predicted to decrease the efficacy of combined hormonal contraceptives. For FSRH guidance, see Contraceptives, interactions p. 840. Severe Study
▸ **Bosentan** decreases the anticoagulant effect of coumarins. Moderate Study
▸ **Bosentan** is predicted to decrease the exposure to crizotinib. Avoid. Severe Theoretical
▸ **Bosentan** is predicted to decrease the exposure to dasatinib. Severe Study
▸ **Bosentan** is predicted to decrease the efficacy of desogestrel. For FSRH guidance, see Contraceptives, interactions p. 840. Severe Theoretical
▸ **Bosentan** decreases the exposure to dolutegravir. Adjust dose. Severe Study
▸ **Bosentan** is predicted to moderately decrease the exposure to elbasvir. Avoid. Severe Study
▸ **Bosentan** is predicted to decrease the exposure to eliglustat. Moderate Theoretical
▸ **Bosentan** is predicted to decrease the concentration of elvitegravir. Avoid. Severe Theoretical
▸ **Bosentan** is predicted to decrease the exposure to entrectinib. Avoid. Severe Theoretical
▸ **Bosentan** is predicted to decrease the effects of ergotamine. Moderate Theoretical
▸ **Bosentan** is predicted to decrease the exposure to erlotinib. Severe Theoretical
▸ **Bosentan** is predicted to decrease the efficacy of etonogestrel. For FSRH guidance, see Contraceptives, interactions p. 840. Severe Theoretical
▸ **Bosentan** is predicted to decrease the concentration of everolimus. Avoid or adjust dose. Severe Study
▸ Filgotinib is predicted to increase the exposure to **bosentan**. Avoid. Moderate Theoretical
▸ **Bosentan** is predicted to decrease the exposure to gefitinib. Avoid. Severe Theoretical

Bosentan is predicted to decrease the exposure to glasdegib. Avoid or adjust glasdegib dose, p. 1049. Severe Theoretical

Bosentan is predicted to decrease the exposure to glecaprevir. Avoid. Severe Study

Bosentan is predicted to markedly decrease the exposure to grazoprevir. Avoid. Severe Study

Bosentan is predicted to decrease the concentration of guanfacine. Adjust dose. Moderate Theoretical

HIV-protease inhibitors are predicted to increase the exposure to **bosentan**. Severe Study

HIV-protease inhibitors are predicted to increase the exposure to **macitentan**. Moderate Study

Bosentan is predicted to decrease the effects of hormone replacement therapy. Moderate Anecdotal

Bosentan is predicted to decrease the exposure to idelalisib. Avoid. Moderate Theoretical

Idelalisib is predicted to increase the exposure to **macitentan**. Moderate Study

Bosentan is predicted to decrease the exposure to imatinib. Moderate Study

Bosentan is predicted to decrease the exposure to ivacaftor. Moderate Study

Bosentan is predicted to decrease the exposure to lapatinib. Avoid. Severe Study

Bosentan is predicted to decrease the exposure to larotrectinib. Avoid. Moderate Study

Leflunomide is predicted to increase the exposure to **bosentan**. Moderate Study

Letermovir is predicted to increase the concentration of **bosentan**. Moderate Theoretical

Bosentan is predicted to decrease the efficacy of levonorgestrel. For FSRH guidance, see Contraceptives, interactions p. 840. Severe Theoretical

Bosentan is predicted to decrease the exposure to lorlatinib. Avoid. Severe Theoretical

Macrolides (clarithromycin) are predicted to increase the exposure to **bosentan**. Moderate Theoretical

Macrolides (clarithromycin) are predicted to increase the exposure to **macitentan**. Moderate Study

Bosentan is predicted to decrease the exposure to maraviroc. Avoid. Moderate Theoretical

Mitotane affects the exposure to **bosentan**. Avoid. Severe Study

Mitotane is predicted to decrease the exposure to **macitentan**. Avoid. Severe Study

Bosentan is predicted to decrease the exposure to neratinib. Severe Study

Bosentan is predicted to decrease the exposure to neurokinin-1 receptor antagonists (aprepitant). Moderate Study

Bosentan is predicted to decrease the exposure to neurokinin-1 receptor antagonists (fosaprepitant, netupitant). Moderate Theoretical

Bosentan is predicted to decrease the exposure to nilotinib. Avoid. Severe Theoretical

Bosentan is predicted to decrease the exposure to NNRTIs (doravirine). Avoid or adjust doravirine p. 683 or lamivudine with tenofovir disoproxil and doravirine p. 692 dose. Severe Theoretical

Bosentan is predicted to decrease the exposure to NNRTIs (etravirine). Avoid. Severe Study

Bosentan is predicted to decrease the exposure to NNRTIs (nevirapine). Severe Theoretical

Bosentan is predicted to decrease the exposure to NNRTIs (rilpivirine). Avoid. Severe Theoretical

Bosentan is predicted to decrease the efficacy of norethisterone. For FSRH guidance, see Contraceptives, interactions p. 840. Severe Anecdotal

Bosentan is predicted to decrease the exposure to olaparib. Avoid. Moderate Theoretical

Bosentan decreases the exposure to opioids (methadone). Monitor and adjust dose. Severe Study

Bosentan is predicted to decrease the exposure to osimertinib. Moderate Theoretical

Bosentan is predicted to decrease the exposure to ospemifene. Moderate Study

▸ **Bosentan** is predicted to decrease the exposure to paritaprevir (with ritonavir and ombitasvir). Avoid. Severe Study

▸ **Bosentan** decreases the exposure to phosphodiesterase type-5 inhibitors. Moderate Study

▸ **Bosentan** is predicted to decrease the exposure to pibrentasvir. Avoid. Severe Study

▸ **Bosentan** is predicted to decrease the exposure to ribociclib. Moderate Study

▸ Rifamycins (rifampicin) transiently increase the exposure to ambrisentan. Moderate Study

▸ Rifamycins (rifampicin) affect the exposure to **bosentan**. Avoid. Severe Study

▸ Rifamycins (rifampicin) are predicted to decrease the exposure to **macitentan**. Avoid. Severe Study

▸ **Bosentan** is predicted to decrease the exposure to ruxolitinib. Monitor and adjust dose. Moderate Theoretical

▸ **Bosentan** is predicted to decrease the exposure to siponimod. Manufacturer advises caution depending on genotype— consult product literature. Severe Theoretical

▸ **Bosentan** is predicted to decrease the concentration of sirolimus and sirolimus potentially increases the concentration of **bosentan**. Avoid. Severe Theoretical

▸ St John's wort is predicted to decrease the exposure to **bosentan**. Avoid. Moderate Theoretical

▸ St John's wort is predicted to decrease the exposure to **macitentan**. Avoid. Severe Theoretical

▸ **Bosentan** slightly decreases the exposure to statins (atorvastatin). Mild Study

▸ **Bosentan** moderately decreases the exposure to statins (simvastatin). Moderate Study

▸ **Bosentan** increases the risk of hepatotoxicity when given with sulfonylureas (glibenclamide). Avoid. Severe Study

▸ **Bosentan** is predicted to decrease the concentration of tacrolimus and tacrolimus potentially increases the concentration of **bosentan**. Avoid. Severe Theoretical

▸ **Bosentan** is predicted to decrease the exposure to taxanes (cabazitaxel). Avoid. Severe Study

▸ **Bosentan** is predicted to decrease the concentration of temsirolimus. Avoid. Severe Theoretical

▸ Teriflunomide is predicted to increase the exposure to **bosentan**. Moderate Study

▸ **Bosentan** is predicted to decrease the exposure to ticagrelor. Moderate Theoretical

▸ **Bosentan** is predicted to decrease the exposure to tofacitinib. Moderate Study

▸ **Bosentan** decreases the efficacy of ulipristal. For FSRH guidance, see Contraceptives, interactions p. 840. Severe Anecdotal

▸ **Bosentan** is predicted to decrease the exposure to velpatasvir. Avoid. Moderate Theoretical

▸ **Bosentan** is predicted to decrease the exposure to venetoclax. Avoid. Severe Study

▸ Venetoclax is predicted to increase the exposure to **bosentan**. Moderate Theoretical

▸ **Bosentan** is predicted to decrease the concentration of voxilaprevir. Avoid. Severe Theoretical

Enoxaparin → see low molecular-weight heparins

Entacapone

▸ Oral **entacapone** is predicted to decrease the absorption of oral iron. Separate administration by at least 2 hours. Moderate Theoretical

▸ **Entacapone** increases the exposure to levodopa. Monitor adverse effects and adjust dose. Moderate Study

▸ **Entacapone** is predicted to increase the risk of elevated blood pressure when given with MAOIs, irreversible. Avoid. Severe Theoretical

▸ **Entacapone** is predicted to increase the exposure to methyldopa. Moderate Theoretical

▸ **Entacapone** is predicted to increase the risk of cardiovascular adverse effects when given with sympathomimetics, inotropic. Moderate Theoretical

▸ **Entacapone** is predicted to increase the risk of cardiovascular adverse effects when given with sympathomimetics, vasoconstrictor (adrenaline/epinephrine, noradrenaline/norepinephrine). Moderate Study

A1

Interactions | Appendix 1

Enteral feeds

► Aluminium hydroxide increases the risk of blocked enteral or nasogastric tubes when given with **enteral feeds**. Moderate Study

► **Enteral feeds** decrease the absorption of antiepileptics (phenytoin). Severe Study

► **Enteral feeds** (vitamin-K containing) potentially decrease the anticoagulant effect of coumarins. Severe Anecdotal

► **Enteral feeds** (vitamin-K containing) potentially decrease the effects of phenindione. Severe Theoretical

► **Enteral feeds** decrease the exposure to quinolones (ciprofloxacin). Moderate Study

► Sucralfate increases the risk of blocked enteral or nasogastric tubes when given with **enteral feeds**. Separate administration by 1 hour. Moderate Study

► **Enteral feeds** decrease the exposure to theophylline. Moderate Study

Entrectinib → see TABLE 9 p. 1431 (QT-interval prolongation)

► Anti-androgens (apalutamide, enzalutamide) are predicted to decrease the exposure to **entrectinib**. Avoid. Severe Study → Also see TABLE 9 p. 1431

► Antiarrhythmics (dronedarone) are predicted to increase the exposure to **entrectinib**. Avoid moderate CYP3A4 inhibitors or adjust **entrectinib** dose, p. 1023. Severe Theoretical → Also see TABLE 9 p. 1431

► Antiepileptics (carbamazepine, fosphenytoin, phenobarbital, phenytoin, primidone) are predicted to decrease the exposure to **entrectinib**. Avoid. Severe Study

► Antifungals, azoles (fluconazole, isavuconazole, posaconazole) are predicted to increase the exposure to **entrectinib**. Avoid moderate CYP3A4 inhibitors or adjust **entrectinib** dose, p. 1023. Severe Theoretical → Also see TABLE 9 p. 1431

► Antifungals, azoles (itraconazole, ketoconazole, voriconazole) are predicted to increase the exposure to **entrectinib**. Avoid potent CYP3A4 inhibitors or adjust **entrectinib** dose, p. 1023. Severe Study → Also see TABLE 9 p. 1431

► **Entrectinib** slightly increases the exposure to benzodiazepines (midazolam). Mild Study

► Calcium channel blockers (diltiazem, verapamil) are predicted to increase the exposure to **entrectinib**. Avoid moderate CYP3A4 inhibitors or adjust **entrectinib** dose, p. 1023. Severe Theoretical

► **Entrectinib** is predicted to increase the exposure to ciclosporin. Mild Theoretical

► Cobicistat is predicted to increase the exposure to **entrectinib**. Avoid potent CYP3A4 inhibitors or adjust **entrectinib** dose, p. 1023. Severe Study

► Crizotinib is predicted to increase the exposure to **entrectinib**. Avoid moderate CYP3A4 inhibitors or adjust **entrectinib** dose, p. 1023. Severe Theoretical → Also see TABLE 9 p. 1431

► Endothelin receptor antagonists (bosentan) are predicted to decrease the exposure to **entrectinib**. Avoid. Severe Theoretical

► **Entrectinib** is predicted to increase the exposure to ergotamine. Mild Theoretical

► **Entrectinib** is predicted to increase the exposure to everolimus. Mild Theoretical

► Grapefruit is predicted to increase the exposure to **entrectinib**. Avoid. Severe Theoretical

► HIV-protease inhibitors are predicted to increase the exposure to **entrectinib**. Avoid potent CYP3A4 inhibitors or adjust **entrectinib** dose, p. 1023. Severe Study → Also see TABLE 9 p. 1431

► Idelalisib is predicted to increase the exposure to **entrectinib**. Avoid potent CYP3A4 inhibitors or adjust **entrectinib** dose, p. 1023. Severe Study

► Imatinib is predicted to increase the exposure to **entrectinib**. Avoid moderate CYP3A4 inhibitors or adjust **entrectinib** dose, p. 1023. Severe Theoretical

► Letermovir is predicted to increase the exposure to **entrectinib**. Avoid moderate CYP3A4 inhibitors or adjust **entrectinib** dose, p. 1023. Severe Theoretical

► Macrolides (clarithromycin) are predicted to increase the exposure to **entrectinib**. Avoid potent CYP3A4 inhibitors or adjust **entrectinib** dose, p. 1023. Severe Study → Also see TABLE 9 p. 1431

► Macrolides (erythromycin) are predicted to increase the exposure to **entrectinib**. Avoid moderate CYP3A4 inhibitors or

adjust **entrectinib** dose, p. 1023. Severe Theoretical → Also see TABLE 9 p. 1431

► Mitotane is predicted to decrease the exposure to **entrectinib**. Avoid. Severe Study

► Neurokinin-1 receptor antagonists (aprepitant, netupitant) are predicted to increase the exposure to **entrectinib**. Avoid moderate CYP3A4 inhibitors or adjust **entrectinib** dose, p. 1023. Severe Theoretical

► Nilotinib is predicted to increase the exposure to **entrectinib**. Avoid moderate CYP3A4 inhibitors or adjust **entrectinib** dose, p. 1023. Severe Theoretical → Also see TABLE 9 p. 1431

► NNRTIs (efavirenz, nevirapine) are predicted to decrease the exposure to **entrectinib**. Avoid. Severe Theoretical → Also see TABLE 9 p. 1431

► **Entrectinib** is predicted to increase the exposure to opioids (alfentanil, fentanyl). Mild Theoretical

► Rifamycins (rifampicin) are predicted to decrease the exposure to **entrectinib**. Avoid. Severe Study

► **Entrectinib** is predicted to increase the exposure to sirolimus. Mild Theoretical

► St John's wort is predicted to decrease the exposure to **entrectinib**. Avoid. Severe Theoretical

► **Entrectinib** is predicted to increase the exposure to temsirolimus. Mild Theoretical

Enzalutamide → see anti-androgens

Ephedrine → see sympathomimetics, vasoconstrictor

Epirubicin → see anthracyclines

Eplerenone → see aldosterone antagonists

Epoetin alfa → see TABLE 5 p. 1430 (thromboembolism), TABLE 16 p. 1433 (increased serum potassium)

Epoetin beta → see TABLE 5 p. 1430 (thromboembolism), TABLE 16 p. 1433 (increased serum potassium)

Epoetin zeta → see TABLE 5 p. 1430 (thromboembolism), TABLE 16 p. 1433 (increased serum potassium)

Epoprostenol → see TABLE 8 p. 1430 (hypotension), TABLE 4 p. 1429 (antiplatelet effects)

Eprosartan → see angiotensin-II receptor antagonists

Eptifibatide → see TABLE 3 p. 1429 (anticoagulant effects)

Ergocalciferol → see vitamin D substances

Ergometrine

► Antiarrhythmics (dronedarone) are predicted to increase the risk of ergotism when given with **ergometrine**. Severe Theoretical

► Antifungals, azoles (fluconazole, isavuconazole, posaconazole) are predicted to increase the risk of ergotism when given with **ergometrine**. Severe Theoretical

► Antifungals, azoles (itraconazole, ketoconazole, voriconazole) are predicted to increase the risk of ergotism when given with **ergometrine**. Avoid. Severe Theoretical

► Antifungals, azoles (miconazole) are predicted to increase the exposure to **ergometrine**. Moderate Theoretical

► Beta blockers, non-selective are predicted to increase the risk of peripheral vasoconstriction when given with **ergometrine**. Severe Study

► Beta blockers, selective are predicted to increase the risk of peripheral vasoconstriction when given with **ergometrine**. Severe Study

► Calcium channel blockers (diltiazem, verapamil) are predicted to increase the risk of ergotism when given with **ergometrine**. Severe Theoretical

► Cobicistat is predicted to increase the risk of ergotism when given with **ergometrine**. Avoid. Severe Theoretical

► Crizotinib is predicted to increase the risk of ergotism when given with **ergometrine**. Severe Theoretical

► **Ergometrine** is predicted to increase the risk of ergotism when given with dopamine receptor agonists (cabergoline). Avoid. Moderate Theoretical

► Esketamine is predicted to increase the risk of elevated blood pressure when given with **ergometrine**. Avoid. Severe Theoretical

► Grapefruit juice is predicted to increase the exposure to **ergometrine**. Severe Theoretical

► HIV-protease inhibitors are predicted to increase the risk of ergotism when given with **ergometrine**. Avoid. Severe Theoretical

◀ Idelalisib is predicted to increase the risk of ergotism when given with **ergometrine**. Avoid. Severe Theoretical

◀ Imatinib is predicted to increase the risk of ergotism when given with **ergometrine**. Severe Theoretical

◀ Ketamine is predicted to increase the risk of elevated blood pressure when given with **ergometrine**. Severe Theoretical

◀ Letermovir is predicted to increase the risk of ergotism when given with **ergometrine**. Severe Theoretical

◀ Macrolides (clarithromycin) are predicted to increase the risk of ergotism when given with **ergometrine**. Avoid. Severe Theoretical

◀ Macrolides (erythromycin) are predicted to increase the risk of ergotism when given with **ergometrine**. Severe Theoretical

◀ Neurokinin-1 receptor antagonists (aprepitant, netupitant) are predicted to increase the risk of ergotism when given with **ergometrine**. Severe Theoretical

◀ Nilotinib is predicted to increase the risk of ergotism when given with **ergometrine**. Severe Theoretical

Ergometrine potentially increases the risk of peripheral vasoconstriction when given with sympathomimetics, inotropic (dopamine). Avoid. Severe Anecdotal

Ergometrine is predicted to increase the risk of peripheral vasoconstriction when given with sympathomimetics, vasoconstrictor (noradrenaline/norepinephrine). Severe Anecdotal

Ergotamine

◀ Anti-androgens (apalutamide, enzalutamide) are predicted to decrease the effects of **ergotamine**. Moderate Theoretical

◀ Antiarrhythmics (dronedarone) are predicted to increase the risk of ergotism when given with **ergotamine**. Severe Theoretical

◀ Antiepileptics (carbamazepine, fosphenytoin, phenobarbital, phenytoin, primidone) are predicted to decrease the effects of **ergotamine**. Moderate Theoretical

◀ Antifungals, azoles (fluconazole, isavuconazole, posaconazole) are predicted to increase the risk of ergotism when given with **ergotamine**. Severe Theoretical

◀ Antifungals, azoles (itraconazole, ketoconazole, voriconazole) are predicted to increase the risk of ergotism when given with **ergotamine**. Avoid. Severe Theoretical

◀ Antifungals, azoles (miconazole) are predicted to increase the exposure to **ergotamine**. Avoid. Moderate Theoretical

◀ Beta blockers, non-selective are predicted to increase the risk of peripheral vasoconstriction when given with **ergotamine**. Severe Study

◀ Beta blockers, selective are predicted to increase the risk of peripheral vasoconstriction when given with **ergotamine**. Severe Study

◀ Calcium channel blockers (diltiazem, verapamil) are predicted to increase the risk of ergotism when given with **ergotamine**. Severe Theoretical

◀ Ceritinib is predicted to increase the exposure to **ergotamine**. Avoid. Severe Theoretical

◀ Cobicistat is predicted to increase the risk of ergotism when given with **ergotamine**. Avoid. Severe Theoretical

◀ Crizotinib is predicted to increase the risk of ergotism when given with **ergotamine**. Severe Theoretical

◀ **Ergotamine** is predicted to increase the risk of ergotism when given with dopamine receptor agonists (bromocriptine, cabergoline). Avoid. Moderate Theoretical

◀ Endothelin receptor antagonists (bosentan) are predicted to decrease the effects of **ergotamine**. Moderate Theoretical

◀ Entrectinib is predicted to increase the exposure to **ergotamine**. Mild Theoretical

◀ Grapefruit juice is predicted to increase the exposure to **ergotamine**. Severe Theoretical

◀ HIV-protease inhibitors are predicted to increase the risk of ergotism when given with **ergotamine**. Avoid. Severe Theoretical

◀ Idelalisib is predicted to increase the risk of ergotism when given with **ergotamine**. Avoid. Severe Theoretical

◀ Imatinib is predicted to increase the risk of ergotism when given with **ergotamine**. Severe Theoretical

◀ Larotrectinib is predicted to increase the exposure to **ergotamine**. Use with caution and adjust dose. Mild Theoretical

◀ Letermovir is predicted to increase the risk of ergotism when given with **ergotamine**. Severe Theoretical

▶ Lorlatinib is predicted to decrease the exposure to **ergotamine**. Avoid. Moderate Theoretical

▶ Macrolides (clarithromycin) are predicted to increase the risk of ergotism when given with **ergotamine**. Avoid. Severe Theoretical

▶ Macrolides (erythromycin) are predicted to increase the risk of ergotism when given with **ergotamine**. Severe Theoretical

▶ Mitotane is predicted to decrease the effects of **ergotamine**. Moderate Theoretical

▶ Neurokinin-1 receptor antagonists (aprepitant, netupitant) are predicted to increase the risk of ergotism when given with **ergotamine**. Severe Theoretical

▶ Nilotinib is predicted to increase the risk of ergotism when given with **ergotamine**. Severe Theoretical

▷ NNRTIs (efavirenz, nevirapine) are predicted to decrease the effects of **ergotamine**. Moderate Theoretical

▶ Palbociclib is predicted to increase the exposure to **ergotamine**. Adjust dose. Moderate Theoretical

▶ Ribociclib (high-dose) is predicted to increase the exposure to **ergotamine**. Avoid. Moderate Theoretical

▶ Rifamycins (rifampicin) are predicted to decrease the effects of **ergotamine**. Moderate Theoretical

▶ Rucaparib is predicted to increase the exposure to **ergotamine**. Monitor and adjust dose. Moderate Study

▷ St John's wort is predicted to decrease the effects of **ergotamine**. Moderate Theoretical

▶ Ticagrelor is predicted to increase the exposure to **ergotamine**. Avoid. Severe Theoretical

▷ Triptans (almotriptan) are predicted to increase the risk of vasoconstriction when given with **ergotamine**. **Ergotamine** should be taken at least 24 hours before or 6 hours after **almotriptan**. Severe Theoretical

▶ Triptans (eletriptan) increase the risk of vasoconstriction when given with **ergotamine**. Separate administration by 24 hours. Severe Study

▷ Triptans (frovatriptan, naratriptan) are predicted to increase the risk of vasoconstriction when given with **ergotamine**. Separate administration by 24 hours. Severe Theoretical

▷ Triptans (rizatriptan) are predicted to increase the risk of vasoconstriction when given with **ergotamine**. **Ergotamine** should be taken at least 24 hours before or 6 hours after **rizatriptan**. Severe Theoretical

▷ Triptans (sumatriptan) increase the risk of vasoconstriction when given with **ergotamine**. **Ergotamine** should be taken at least 24 hours before or 6 hours after **sumatriptan**. Severe Study

▷ Triptans (zolmitriptan) are predicted to increase the risk of vasoconstriction when given with **ergotamine**. **Ergotamine** should be taken at least 24 hours before or 6 hours after **zolmitriptan**. Severe Theoretical

Eribulin → see TABLE 15 p. 1432 (myelosuppression), TABLE 12 p. 1432 (peripheral neuropathy), TABLE 9 p. 1431 (QT-interval prolongation)

Erlotinib

FOOD AND LIFESTYLE Dose adjustment may be necessary if smoking started or stopped during treatment.

▶ Oral antacids are predicted to decrease the absorption of oral **erlotinib**. **Erlotinib** should be taken 2 hours before or 4 hours after antacids. Moderate Theoretical

▷ Anti-androgens (apalutamide, enzalutamide) are predicted to decrease the exposure to **erlotinib**. Avoid or adjust **erlotinib** dose, p. 1024. Severe Study

▷ Antiarrhythmics (amiodarone, dronedarone) are predicted to increase the exposure to **erlotinib**. Moderate Theoretical

▷ Antiepileptics (carbamazepine, fosphenytoin, phenobarbital, phenytoin, primidone) are predicted to decrease the exposure to **erlotinib**. Avoid or adjust **erlotinib** dose, p. 1024. Severe Study

▷ Antifungals, azoles (fluconazole, isavuconazole, posaconazole) are predicted to increase the exposure to **erlotinib**. Moderate Theoretical

▷ Antifungals, azoles (itraconazole, ketoconazole, voriconazole) are predicted to slightly increase the exposure to **erlotinib**. Use with caution and adjust dose. Moderate Study

▶ **Erlotinib** is predicted to increase the risk of gastrointestinal perforation when given with aspirin (high-dose). Severe Theoretical

▷ Calcium channel blockers (diltiazem, verapamil) are predicted to increase the exposure to **erlotinib**. Moderate Theoretical

Erlotinib (continued)

▸ Ciclosporin is predicted to increase the exposure to **erlotinib**. Moderate Theoretical

▸ Cobicistat is predicted to slightly increase the exposure to **erlotinib**. Use with caution and adjust dose. Moderate Study

▸ Combined hormonal contraceptives slightly increase the exposure to **erlotinib**. Monitor adverse effects and adjust dose. Moderate Study

▸ Corticosteroids increase the risk of gastrointestinal perforation when given with **erlotinib**. Severe Theoretical

▸ **Erlotinib** increases the anticoagulant effect of coumarins. Severe Anecdotal

▸ Crizotinib is predicted to increase the exposure to **erlotinib**. Moderate Theoretical

▸ Endothelin receptor antagonists (bosentan) are predicted to decrease the exposure to **erlotinib**. Severe Theoretical

▸ Grapefruit juice is predicted to increase the exposure to **erlotinib**. Moderate Theoretical

▸ H$_2$ receptor antagonists are predicted to decrease the exposure to **erlotinib**. **Erlotinib** should be taken 2 hours before or 10 hours after H$_2$ receptor antagonists. Moderate Study

▸ HIV-protease inhibitors are predicted to slightly increase the exposure to **erlotinib**. Use with caution and adjust dose. Moderate Study

▸ Idelalisib is predicted to slightly increase the exposure to **erlotinib**. Use with caution and adjust dose. Moderate Study

▸ Imatinib is predicted to increase the exposure to **erlotinib**. Moderate Theoretical

▸ Lapatinib is predicted to increase the exposure to **erlotinib**. Moderate Theoretical

▸ Letermovir is predicted to increase the exposure to **erlotinib**. Moderate Theoretical

▸ Macrolides (azithromycin, erythromycin) are predicted to increase the exposure to **erlotinib**. Moderate Theoretical

▸ Macrolides (clarithromycin) are predicted to slightly increase the exposure to **erlotinib**. Use with caution and adjust dose. Moderate Study

▸ Mexiletine slightly increases the exposure to **erlotinib**. Monitor adverse effects and adjust dose. Moderate Study

▸ Mitotane is predicted to decrease the exposure to **erlotinib**. Avoid or adjust **erlotinib** dose, p. 1024. Severe Study

▸ Neurokinin-1 receptor antagonists (aprepitant, netupitant) are predicted to increase the exposure to **erlotinib**. Moderate Theoretical

▸ Nilotinib is predicted to increase the exposure to **erlotinib**. Moderate Theoretical

▸ NNRTIs (efavirenz, nevirapine) are predicted to decrease the exposure to **erlotinib**. Severe Theoretical

▸ **Erlotinib** is predicted to increase the risk of gastrointestinal perforation when given with NSAIDs. Severe Theoretical

▸ **Erlotinib** is predicted to increase the risk of bleeding events when given with phenindione. Severe Theoretical

▸ Proton pump inhibitors are predicted to slightly decrease the exposure to **erlotinib**. Avoid. Moderate Study

▸ Quinolones (ciprofloxacin) slightly increase the exposure to **erlotinib**. Monitor adverse effects and adjust dose. Moderate Study

▸ Ranolazine is predicted to increase the exposure to **erlotinib**. Moderate Theoretical

▸ Rifamycins (rifampicin) are predicted to decrease the exposure to **erlotinib**. Avoid or adjust **erlotinib** dose, p. 1024. Severe Study

▸ Sodium zirconium cyclosilicate is predicted to decrease the exposure to **erlotinib**. Separate administration by at least 2 hours. Moderate Theoretical

▸ SSRIs (fluvoxamine) are predicted to increase the exposure to **erlotinib**. Monitor adverse effects and adjust dose. Moderate Theoretical

▸ St John's wort is predicted to decrease the exposure to **erlotinib**. Severe Theoretical

▸ Vemurafenib is predicted to increase the exposure to **erlotinib**. Moderate Theoretical

Ertapenem → see carbapenems

Ertugliflozin → see sodium glucose co-transporter 2 inhibitors

Erythromycin → see macrolides

Escitalopram → see SSRIs

Esketamine → see TABLE 8 p. 1430 (hypotension), TABLE 11 p. 1431 (CNS depressant effects)

▸ **Esketamine** is predicted to increase the risk of seizures when given with aminophylline. Avoid. Severe Theoretical

▸ Anti-androgens (apalutamide, enzalutamide) are predicted to decrease the exposure to **esketamine**. Adjust dose. Moderate Theoretical

▸ Antiepileptics (carbamazepine, fosphenytoin, phenobarbital, phenytoin, primidone) are predicted to decrease the exposure to **esketamine**. Adjust dose. Moderate Theoretical → Also see TABLE 11 p. 1431

▸ Antifungals, azoles (itraconazole, ketoconazole, voriconazole) are predicted to increase the exposure to **esketamine**. Adjust dose. Moderate Study

▸ Cobicistat is predicted to increase the exposure to **esketamine**. Adjust dose. Moderate Study

▸ **Esketamine** is predicted to increase the risk of elevated blood pressure when given with ergometrine. Avoid. Severe Theoretical

▸ HIV-protease inhibitors are predicted to increase the exposure to **esketamine**. Adjust dose. Moderate Study

▸ Idelalisib is predicted to increase the exposure to **esketamine**. Adjust dose. Moderate Study

▸ Macrolides (clarithromycin) are predicted to increase the exposure to **esketamine**. Adjust dose. Moderate Study

▸ Mitotane is predicted to decrease the exposure to **esketamine**. Adjust dose. Moderate Theoretical

▸ Rifamycins (rifampicin) are predicted to decrease the exposure to **esketamine**. Adjust dose. Moderate Theoretical

▸ **Esketamine** is predicted to increase the risk of seizures when given with theophylline. Avoid. Severe Theoretical

Eslicarbazepine → see antiepileptics

Esmolol → see beta blockers, selective

Esomeprazole → see proton pump inhibitors

Estramustine → see alkylating agents

Etanercept

▸ Anakinra is predicted to increase the risk of generalised infection (possibly life-threatening) when given with **etanercept**. Avoid. Severe Theoretical

▸ Filgotinib is predicted to increase the risk of immunosuppression when given with **etanercept**. Avoid. Severe Theoretical

▸ Live vaccines are predicted to increase the risk of generalised infection (possibly life-threatening) when given with **etanercept**. Public Health England advises avoid (refer to Green Book). Severe Theoretical

Etelcalcetide

▸ Cinacalcet increases the risk of hypocalcaemia when given with **etelcalcetide**. Avoid. Severe Theoretical

Ethambutol

▸ Isoniazid increases the risk of optic neuropathy when given with **ethambutol**. Severe Anecdotal

Ethosuximide → see antiepileptics

Etodolac → see NSAIDs

Etomidate → see TABLE 8 p. 1430 (hypotension), TABLE 11 p. 1431 (CNS depressant effects)

Etonogestrel

▸ Antiepileptics (carbamazepine, eslicarbazepine, fosphenytoin, oxcarbazepine, perampanel, phenobarbital, phenytoin, primidone, rufinamide, topiramate) are predicted to decrease the efficacy of **etonogestrel**. For FSRH guidance, see Contraceptives, interactions p. 840. Severe Theoretical

▸ Endothelin receptor antagonists (bosentan) are predicted to decrease the efficacy of **etonogestrel**. For FSRH guidance, see Contraceptives, interactions p. 840. Severe Theoretical

▸ Griseofulvin decreases the efficacy of **etonogestrel**. For FSRH guidance, see Contraceptives, interactions p. 840. Severe Anecdotal

▸ HIV-protease inhibitors (ritonavir) are predicted to decrease the efficacy of **etonogestrel**. For FSRH guidance, see Contraceptives, interactions p. 840. Severe Theoretical

▸ Modafinil is predicted to decrease the efficacy of **etonogestrel**. For FSRH guidance, see Contraceptives, interactions p. 840. Severe Theoretical

Neurokinin-1 receptor antagonists (**aprepitant, fosaprepitant**) are predicted to decrease the efficacy of **etonogestrel**. For FSRH guidance, see Contraceptives, interactions p. 840. Severe Theoretical

NNRTIs (**efavirenz, nevirapine**) are predicted to decrease the efficacy of **etonogestrel**. For FSRH guidance, see Contraceptives, interactions p. 840. Severe Theoretical

Rifamycins are predicted to decrease the efficacy of **etonogestrel**. For FSRH guidance, see Contraceptives, interactions p. 840. Severe Theoretical

St John's wort is predicted to decrease the efficacy of **etonogestrel**. MHRA advises avoid. For FSRH guidance, see Contraceptives, interactions p. 840. Severe Theoretical

Sugammadex is predicted to decrease the efficacy of **etonogestrel**. Use additional contraceptive precautions. Severe Theoretical

Ulipristal is predicted to decrease the efficacy of **etonogestrel**. Avoid. Severe Theoretical

toposide → see TABLE 15 p. 1432 (myelosuppression)

Antiepileptics (**carbamazepine, fosphenytoin, phenobarbital, phenytoin, primidone**) are predicted to decrease the efficacy of **etoposide**. Moderate Study

Ciclosporin increases the exposure to **etoposide**. Monitor and adjust dose. Severe Study

Live vaccines are predicted to increase the risk of generalised infection (possibly life-threatening) when given with **etoposide**. Public Health England advises avoid (refer to Green Book). Severe Theoretical

Neurokinin-1 receptor antagonists (**netupitant**) slightly increase the exposure to **etoposide**. Moderate Study

toricoxib → see NSAIDs

travirine → see NNRTIs

verolimus

Everolimus potentially increases the risk of angioedema when given with ACE inhibitors. Severe Anecdotal

Anti-androgens (**apalutamide, enzalutamide**) are predicted to decrease the concentration of **everolimus**. Avoid or adjust dose. Severe Study

Antiarrhythmics (**dronedarone**) are predicted to increase the concentration of **everolimus**. Avoid or adjust dose. Moderate Study

Antiepileptics (**carbamazepine, fosphenytoin, phenobarbital, phenytoin, primidone**) are predicted to decrease the concentration of **everolimus**. Avoid or adjust dose. Severe Study

Antifungals, azoles (**fluconazole, isavuconazole, posaconazole**) are predicted to increase the concentration of **everolimus**. Avoid or adjust dose. Moderate Study

Antifungals, azoles (**itraconazole, ketoconazole, voriconazole**) are predicted to increase the concentration of **everolimus**. Avoid. Severe Study

Calcium channel blockers (**diltiazem, verapamil**) are predicted to increase the concentration of **everolimus**. Avoid or adjust dose. Moderate Study

Ceritinib is predicted to increase the exposure to **everolimus**. Moderate Theoretical

Ciclosporin moderately increases the exposure to **everolimus**. Avoid or adjust dose. Severe Study

Cobicistat is predicted to increase the concentration of **everolimus**. Avoid. Severe Study

Crizotinib is predicted to increase the concentration of **everolimus**. Avoid or adjust dose. Moderate Study

Eliglustat is predicted to increase the exposure to **everolimus**. Adjust dose. Moderate Study

Endothelin receptor antagonists (**bosentan**) are predicted to decrease the concentration of **everolimus**. Avoid or adjust dose. Severe Study

Entrectinib is predicted to increase the exposure to **everolimus**. Mild Theoretical

Grapefruit juice is predicted to increase the exposure to **everolimus**. Avoid. Severe Theoretical

HIV-protease inhibitors are predicted to increase the concentration of **everolimus**. Avoid. Severe Study

Idelalisib is predicted to increase the concentration of **everolimus**. Avoid. Severe Study

▶ Imatinib is predicted to increase the concentration of **everolimus**. Avoid or adjust dose. Moderate Study

▶ Lapatinib is predicted to increase the exposure to **everolimus**. Moderate Theoretical

▶ Letermovir is predicted to increase the concentration of **everolimus**. Avoid or adjust dose. Moderate Study

▶ Live vaccines are predicted to increase the risk of generalised infection (possibly life-threatening) when given with **everolimus**. Public Health England advises avoid (refer to Green Book). Severe Theoretical

▶ **Everolimus** is predicted to increase the exposure to lomitapide. Separate administration by 12 hours. Mild Theoretical

▶ Lumacaftor is predicted to decrease the exposure to **everolimus**. Avoid. Severe Theoretical

▶ Macrolides (**clarithromycin**) are predicted to increase the concentration of **everolimus**. Avoid. Severe Study

▶ Macrolides (**erythromycin**) are predicted to increase the concentration of **everolimus**. Avoid or adjust dose. Moderate Study

▶ Mirabegron is predicted to increase the exposure to **everolimus**. Mild Theoretical

▶ Mitotane is predicted to decrease the concentration of **everolimus**. Avoid or adjust dose. Severe Study

▶ Neratinib is predicted to increase the exposure to **everolimus**. Moderate Study

▶ Neurokinin-1 receptor antagonists (**aprepitant, netupitant**) are predicted to increase the concentration of **everolimus**. Avoid or adjust dose. Moderate Study

▶ Nilotinib is predicted to increase the concentration of **everolimus**. Avoid or adjust dose. Moderate Study

▶ NNRTIs (**efavirenz, nevirapine**) are predicted to decrease the concentration of **everolimus**. Avoid or adjust dose. Severe Study

▶ Palbociclib is predicted to increase the exposure to **everolimus**. Adjust dose. Moderate Theoretical

▶ Pibrentasvir (with glecaprevir) is predicted to increase the exposure to **everolimus**. Moderate Study

▶ Pitolisant is predicted to decrease the exposure to **everolimus**. Avoid. Severe Theoretical

▶ Ribociclib is predicted to increase the exposure to **everolimus**. Use with caution and adjust dose. Moderate Theoretical

▶ Rifamycins (**rifampicin**) are predicted to decrease the concentration of **everolimus**. Avoid or adjust dose. Severe Study

▶ St John's wort is predicted to decrease the concentration of **everolimus**. Avoid or adjust dose. Severe Study

▶ Velpatasvir is predicted to increase the exposure to **everolimus**. Severe Study

▶ Vemurafenib is predicted to increase the exposure to **everolimus**. Use with caution and adjust dose. Severe Theoretical

▶ Venetoclax is predicted to increase the exposure to **everolimus**. Avoid or adjust dose. Severe Study

Exemestane

▶ Anti-androgens (**apalutamide, enzalutamide**) moderately decrease the exposure to **exemestane**. Moderate Study

▶ Antiepileptics (**carbamazepine, fosphenytoin, phenobarbital, phenytoin, primidone**) moderately decrease the exposure to **exemestane**. Moderate Study

▶ Mitotane moderately decreases the exposure to **exemestane**. Moderate Study

▶ Rifamycins (**rifampicin**) moderately decrease the exposure to **exemestane**. Moderate Study

▶ St John's wort is predicted to decrease the exposure to **exemestane**. Moderate Theoretical

Exenatide → see glucagon-like peptide-1 receptor agonists

Ezetimibe

▶ Ciclosporin moderately increases the exposure to **ezetimibe** and **ezetimibe** slightly increases the exposure to ciclosporin. Moderate Study

▶ Fibrates are predicted to increase the risk of gallstones when given with **ezetimibe**. Severe Theoretical

▶ **Ezetimibe** potentially increases the risk of rhabdomyolysis when given with statins. Severe Anecdotal

Factor XA inhibitors → see TABLE 3 p. 1429 (anticoagulant effects)

apixaban · edoxaban · fondaparinux · rivaroxaban

▸ Anti-androgens (apalutamide, enzalutamide) are predicted to moderately decrease the exposure to **apixaban**. Use with caution or avoid. [Severe] Study

▸ Anti-androgens (apalutamide, enzalutamide) are predicted to moderately decrease the exposure to **rivaroxaban**. Avoid unless patient can be monitored for signs of thrombosis. [Severe] Study

▸ Antiarrhythmics (dronedarone) are predicted to increase the exposure to **apixaban**. [Moderate] Theoretical

▸ Antiarrhythmics (dronedarone) slightly increase the exposure to **edoxaban**. Adjust **edoxaban** dose, p. 137. [Severe] Study

▸ Antiarrhythmics (dronedarone) are predicted to increase the exposure to **rivaroxaban**. Avoid. [Moderate] Theoretical

▸ Antiepileptics (carbamazepine) are predicted to decrease the exposure to **edoxaban**. [Moderate] Study

▸ Antiepileptics (carbamazepine, fosphenytoin, phenobarbital, phenytoin, primidone) are predicted to moderately decrease the exposure to **apixaban**. Use with caution or avoid. [Severe] Study

▸ Antiepileptics (carbamazepine, fosphenytoin, phenobarbital, phenytoin, primidone) are predicted to moderately decrease the exposure to **rivaroxaban**. Avoid unless patient can be monitored for signs of thrombosis. [Severe] Study

▸ Antiepileptics (phenytoin) are predicted to decrease the exposure to **edoxaban**. [Moderate] Study

▸ Antifungals, azoles (itraconazole) are predicted to increase the exposure to **apixaban**. Avoid. [Severe] Theoretical

▸ Antifungals, azoles (itraconazole) are predicted to slightly increase the exposure to **edoxaban**. [Severe] Theoretical

▸ Antifungals, azoles (itraconazole, ketoconazole) are predicted to moderately increase the exposure to **rivaroxaban**. Avoid. [Severe] Study

▸ Antifungals, azoles (ketoconazole) slightly to moderately increase the exposure to **apixaban**. Avoid. [Severe] Study

▸ Antifungals, azoles (ketoconazole) slightly increase the exposure to **edoxaban**. Adjust **edoxaban** dose, p. 137. [Severe] Study

▸ Antifungals, azoles (voriconazole) are predicted to increase the exposure to **apixaban**. Avoid. [Moderate] Theoretical

▸ Calcium channel blockers (verapamil) are predicted to increase the exposure to **apixaban**. [Moderate] Theoretical

▸ Ceritinib is predicted to increase the exposure to **edoxaban**. [Moderate] Theoretical

▸ Ciclosporin slightly increases the exposure to **edoxaban**. Adjust **edoxaban** dose, p. 137. [Severe] Study

▸ Cobicistat is predicted to increase the exposure to factor XA inhibitors (**apixaban, edoxaban, rivaroxaban**). Avoid. [Severe] Theoretical

▸ Eliglustat is predicted to increase the exposure to **edoxaban**. Adjust dose. [Moderate] Study

▸ HIV-protease inhibitors (lopinavir, ritonavir, saquinavir) are predicted to slightly increase the exposure to **edoxaban**. [Severe] Theoretical

▸ HIV-protease inhibitors (ritonavir) are predicted to increase the exposure to **apixaban**. Avoid. [Severe] Theoretical

▸ HIV-protease inhibitors (ritonavir) moderately increase the exposure to **rivaroxaban**. Avoid. [Severe] Study

▸ Lapatinib is predicted to slightly increase the exposure to **edoxaban**. [Severe] Theoretical

▸ Macrolides (azithromycin, clarithromycin) are predicted to slightly increase the exposure to **edoxaban**. [Severe] Theoretical

▸ Macrolides (erythromycin) are predicted to increase the exposure to **apixaban**. [Moderate] Theoretical

▸ Macrolides (erythromycin) slightly increase the exposure to **edoxaban**. Adjust **edoxaban** dose, p. 137. [Severe] Study

▸ Mirabegron is predicted to increase the exposure to **edoxaban**. [Mild] Theoretical

▸ Mitotane is predicted to moderately decrease the exposure to **apixaban**. Use with caution or avoid. [Severe] Study

▸ Mitotane is predicted to moderately decrease the exposure to **rivaroxaban**. Avoid unless patient can be monitored for signs of thrombosis. [Severe] Study

▸ Neratinib is predicted to increase the exposure to **edoxaban**. [Moderate] Study

▸ Paritaprevir (with ritonavir and ombitasvir) is predicted to increase the exposure to **edoxaban**. [Severe] Study

▸ Pibrentasvir (with glecaprevir) is predicted to increase the exposure to **edoxaban**. [Moderate] Study

▸ Pitolisant is predicted to decrease the exposure to **edoxaban**. [Mild] Theoretical

▸ Ranolazine is predicted to slightly increase the exposure to **edoxaban**. [Severe] Theoretical

▸ Rifamycins (rifampicin) are predicted to moderately decrease the exposure to **apixaban**. Use with caution or avoid. [Severe] Study

▸ Rifamycins (rifampicin) are predicted to decrease the exposure to **edoxaban**. [Moderate] Study

▸ Rifamycins (rifampicin) are predicted to moderately decrease the exposure to **rivaroxaban**. Avoid unless patient can be monitored for signs of thrombosis. [Severe] Study

▸ St John's wort is predicted to decrease the exposure to **apixaban**. Use with caution or avoid. [Moderate] Theoretical

▸ St John's wort is predicted to decrease the exposure to **edoxaban**. [Moderate] Study

▸ Velpatasvir is predicted to increase the exposure to **edoxaban**. [Severe] Theoretical

▸ Vemurafenib is predicted to slightly increase the exposure to **edoxaban**. [Moderate] Study

▸ Voxilaprevir (with sofosbuvir and velpatasvir) is predicted to increase the concentration of **edoxaban**. Avoid. [Severe] Theoretical

Famotidine → see H₂ receptor antagonists

Fampridine

▸ H₂ receptor antagonists (cimetidine) increase the concentration of **fampridine**. Avoid. [Severe] Theoretical

Febuxostat

▸ Febuxostat is predicted to increase the exposure to azathioprine. Avoid. [Severe] Theoretical

▸ Febuxostat is predicted to increase the exposure to mercaptopurine. Avoid. [Severe] Theoretical

Felbinac → see NSAIDs

Felodipine → see calcium channel blockers

Fenofibrate → see fibrates

Fentanyl → see opioids

Fesoterodine → see TABLE 10 p. 1431 (antimuscarinics)

▸ Anti-androgens (apalutamide, enzalutamide) are predicted to decrease the exposure to **fesoterodine**. Avoid. [Moderate] Study

▸ Antiarrhythmics (dronedarone) are predicted to increase the exposure to **fesoterodine**. Adjust **fesoterodine** dose with moderate CYP3A4 inhibitors in hepatic and renal impairment p. 822. [Mild] Study

▸ Antiepileptics (carbamazepine, fosphenytoin, phenobarbital, phenytoin, primidone) are predicted to decrease the exposure to **fesoterodine**. Avoid. [Moderate] Study

▸ Antifungals, azoles (fluconazole, isavuconazole, posaconazole) are predicted to increase the exposure to **fesoterodine**. Adjust **fesoterodine** dose with moderate CYP3A4 inhibitors in hepatic and renal impairment, p. 822. [Mild] Study

▸ Antifungals, azoles (itraconazole, ketoconazole, voriconazole) are predicted to moderately increase the exposure to **fesoterodine**. Adjust **fesoterodine** dose with potent CYP3A4 inhibitors; avoid in hepatic and renal impairment, p. 822. [Severe] Study

▸ Calcium channel blockers (diltiazem, verapamil) are predicted to increase the exposure to **fesoterodine**. Adjust **fesoterodine** dose with moderate CYP3A4 inhibitors in hepatic and renal impairment, p. 822. [Mild] Study

▸ Cobicistat is predicted to moderately increase the exposure to **fesoterodine**. Adjust **fesoterodine** dose with potent CYP3A4 inhibitors; avoid in hepatic and renal impairment, p. 822. [Severe] Study

▸ Crizotinib is predicted to increase the exposure to **fesoterodine**. Adjust **fesoterodine** dose with moderate CYP3A4 inhibitors in hepatic and renal impairment, p. 822. [Mild] Study

▸ HIV-protease inhibitors are predicted to moderately increase the exposure to **fesoterodine**. Adjust **fesoterodine** dose with potent CYP3A4 inhibitors; avoid in hepatic and renal impairment, p. 822. [Severe] Study

▸ Idelalisib is predicted to moderately increase the exposure to **fesoterodine**. Adjust **fesoterodine** dose with potent CYP3A4 inhibitors; avoid in hepatic and renal impairment, p. 822. [Severe] Study

Imatinib is predicted to increase the exposure to **fesoterodine**. Adjust **fesoterodine** dose with moderate CYP3A4 inhibitors in hepatic and renal impairment, p. 822. [Mild] Study

Letermovir is predicted to increase the exposure to **fesoterodine**. Adjust **fesoterodine** dose with moderate CYP3A4 inhibitors in hepatic and renal impairment, p. 822. [Mild] Study

Macrolides (clarithromycin) are predicted to moderately increase the exposure to **fesoterodine**. Adjust **fesoterodine** dose with potent CYP3A4 inhibitors; avoid in hepatic and renal impairment, p. 822. [Severe] Study

Macrolides (erythromycin) are predicted to increase the exposure to **fesoterodine**. Adjust **fesoterodine** dose with moderate CYP3A4 inhibitors in hepatic and renal impairment, p. 822. [Mild] Study

▸ Mitotane is predicted to decrease the exposure to **fesoterodine**. Avoid. [Severe] Study

▸ Neurokinin-1 receptor antagonists (aprepitant, netupitant) are predicted to increase the exposure to **fesoterodine**. Adjust **fesoterodine** dose with moderate CYP3A4 inhibitors in hepatic and renal impairment, p. 822. [Mild] Study

▸ Nilotinib is predicted to increase the exposure to **fesoterodine**. Adjust **fesoterodine** dose with moderate CYP3A4 inhibitors in hepatic and renal impairment, p. 822. [Mild] Study

▸ Rifamycins (rifampicin) are predicted to decrease the exposure to **fesoterodine**. Avoid. [Moderate] Study

▸ St John's wort is predicted to decrease the exposure to **fesoterodine**. Avoid. [Severe] Theoretical

Fexofenadine → see antihistamines, non-sedating

Fibrates

bezafibrate · ciprofibrate · fenofibrate · gemfibrozil

▸ Oral antacids decrease the exposure to oral **gemfibrozil**. [Moderate] Study

▸ **Gemfibrozil** is predicted to increase the exposure to anti-androgens (apalutamide). [Mild] Study

▸ **Gemfibrozil** moderately increases the exposure to anti-androgens (enzalutamide). Avoid or adjust **enzalutamide** dose, p. 991. [Severe] Study

▸ **Bezafibrate** is predicted to increase the risk of nephrotoxicity when given with ciclosporin. [Severe] Theoretical

▸ **Fenofibrate** increases the risk of nephrotoxicity when given with ciclosporin. [Severe] Study

▸ Colchicine increases the risk of rhabdomyolysis when given with **fibrates**. [Severe] Anecdotal

▸ **Fibrates** are predicted to increase the anticoagulant effect of coumarins. Monitor INR and adjust dose. [Severe] Study

▸ **Gemfibrozil** is predicted to increase the exposure to dabrafenib. [Moderate] Theoretical

▸ **Fibrates** are predicted to increase the risk of rhabdomyolysis when given with daptomycin. [Severe] Theoretical

▸ **Gemfibrozil** is predicted to very markedly increase the exposure to dasabuvir. Avoid. [Severe] Study

▸ **Fibrates** are predicted to increase the risk of gallstones when given with ezetimibe. [Severe] Theoretical

▸ **Fibrates** are predicted to increase the risk of hypoglycaemia when given with insulin. [Moderate] Theoretical

▸ **Gemfibrozil** is predicted to increase the exposure to irinotecan. Avoid. [Moderate] Theoretical

▸ **Gemfibrozil** is predicted to increase the concentration of letermovir. [Moderate] Study

▸ **Gemfibrozil** increases the exposure to meglitinides (repaglinide). Avoid. [Severe] Study

▸ **Gemfibrozil** is predicted to moderately increase the exposure to montelukast. [Moderate] Study

▸ **Gemfibrozil** is predicted to increase the exposure to the active metabolite of ozanimod. [Severe] Study

▸ **Fibrates** are predicted to increase the anticoagulant effect of phenindione. Monitor INR and adjust dose. [Severe] Study

▸ **Gemfibrozil** increases the exposure to pioglitazone. Monitor blood glucose and adjust dose. [Severe] Study

▸ **Gemfibrozil** is predicted to increase the exposure to retinoids (alitretinoin). Adjust **alitretinoin** dose, p. 1305. [Moderate] Theoretical

▸ **Gemfibrozil** increases the concentration of retinoids (bexarotene). Avoid. [Severe] Study

▸ **Gemfibrozil** increases the exposure to selexipag. Avoid. [Severe] Study

▸ **Ciprofibrate** increases the risk of rhabdomyolysis when given with statins (atorvastatin). Avoid or adjust dose. [Severe] Study

▸ **Bezafibrate** increases the risk of rhabdomyolysis when given with statins (atorvastatin, fluvastatin). [Severe] Study

▸ **Fenofibrate** increases the risk of rhabdomyolysis when given with statins (atorvastatin, simvastatin). Adjust **fenofibrate** dose, p. 214. [Severe] Anecdotal

▸ **Ciprofibrate** increases the risk of rhabdomyolysis when given with statins (fluvastatin). [Severe] Study

▸ **Fenofibrate** is predicted to increase the risk of rhabdomyolysis when given with statins (fluvastatin). Adjust **fenofibrate** dose, p. 214. [Severe] Theoretical

▸ **Fenofibrate** is predicted to increase the risk of rhabdomyolysis when given with statins (pravastatin). Avoid. [Severe] Theoretical

▸ Fibrates **(bezafibrate, ciprofibrate)** increase the risk of rhabdomyolysis when given with statins (pravastatin). Avoid. [Severe] Study

▸ **Fenofibrate** increases the risk of rhabdomyolysis when given with statins (rosuvastatin). Adjust **fenofibrate** and **rosuvastatin** doses, p. 214, p. 218. [Severe] Anecdotal

▸ Fibrates **(bezafibrate, ciprofibrate)** increase the risk of rhabdomyolysis when given with statins (rosuvastatin). Adjust **rosuvastatin** dose, p. 218. [Severe] Study

▸ Fibrates **(bezafibrate, ciprofibrate)** increase the risk of rhabdomyolysis when given with statins (simvastatin). Adjust **simvastatin** dose, p. 219. [Severe] Study

▸ **Gemfibrozil** increases the risk of rhabdomyolysis when given with statins. [Severe] Anecdotal

▸ **Fibrates** are predicted to increase the risk of hypoglycaemia when given with sulfonylureas. [Moderate] Theoretical

▸ **Gemfibrozil** is predicted to increase the concentration of taxanes (paclitaxel). [Severe] Anecdotal

▸ **Fibrates** are predicted to decrease the efficacy of ursodeoxycholic acid. Avoid. [Severe] Theoretical

Fidaxomicin

▸ Antiarrhythmics (amiodarone, dronedarone) are predicted to increase the exposure to **fidaxomicin**. [Moderate] Study

▸ Antifungals, azoles (itraconazole, ketoconazole) are predicted to increase the exposure to **fidaxomicin**. Avoid. [Moderate] Study

▸ Calcium channel blockers (verapamil) are predicted to increase the exposure to **fidaxomicin**. Avoid. [Moderate] Study

▸ Ciclosporin is predicted to increase the exposure to **fidaxomicin**. Avoid. [Moderate] Study

▸ HIV-protease inhibitors (lopinavir, ritonavir, saquinavir) are predicted to increase the exposure to **fidaxomicin**. Avoid. [Moderate] Study

▸ Lapatinib is predicted to increase the exposure to **fidaxomicin**. Avoid. [Moderate] Study

▸ Macrolides are predicted to increase the exposure to **fidaxomicin**. Avoid. [Moderate] Study

▸ Ranolazine is predicted to increase the exposure to **fidaxomicin**. Avoid. [Moderate] Study

▸ Vemurafenib is predicted to increase the exposure to **fidaxomicin**. Avoid. [Moderate] Study

Filgotinib

▸ **Filgotinib** is predicted to increase the risk of immunosuppression when given with abatacept. Avoid. [Severe] Theoretical

▸ **Filgotinib** is predicted to increase the risk of immunosuppression when given with anakinra. Avoid. [Severe] Theoretical

▸ **Filgotinib** is predicted to increase the exposure to angiotensin-II receptor antagonists (valsartan). Avoid. [Moderate] Theoretical

▸ **Filgotinib** is predicted to increase the exposure to antihistamines, non-sedating (fexofenadine). Avoid. [Moderate] Theoretical

▸ **Filgotinib** is predicted to increase the risk of immunosuppression when given with azathioprine. Avoid. [Severe] Theoretical

▸ **Filgotinib** is predicted to increase the risk of immunosuppression when given with baricitinib. Avoid. [Severe] Theoretical

Filgotinib (continued)
▶ **Filgotinib** is predicted to increase the risk of immunosuppression when given with ciclosporin. Avoid. Severe Theoretical
▶ **Filgotinib** is predicted to increase the exposure to endothelin receptor antagonists (bosentan). Avoid. Moderate Theoretical
▶ **Filgotinib** is predicted to increase the risk of immunosuppression when given with etanercept. Avoid. Severe Theoretical
▶ **Filgotinib** is predicted to increase the risk of immunosuppression when given with leflunomide. Avoid. Severe Theoretical
▶ Live vaccines are predicted to increase the risk of generalised infection (possibly life-threatening) when given with **filgotinib**. Avoid. Severe Theoretical
▶ **Filgotinib** is predicted to increase the exposure to meglitinides (repaglinide). Avoid. Moderate Theoretical
▶ **Filgotinib** is predicted to increase the risk of immunosuppression when given with monoclonal antibodies (adalimumab, certolizumab pegol, golimumab, infliximab, rituximab, sarilumab, secukinumab, tocilizumab). Avoid. Severe Theoretical
▶ **Filgotinib** is predicted to increase the exposure to statins (atorvastatin, pravastatin, rosuvastatin, simvastatin). Avoid. Moderate Theoretical
▶ **Filgotinib** is predicted to increase the exposure to sulfonylureas (glibenclamide). Avoid. Moderate Theoretical
▶ **Filgotinib** is predicted to increase the risk of immunosuppression when given with tacrolimus. Avoid. Severe Theoretical
▶ **Filgotinib** is predicted to increase the risk of immunosuppression when given with teriflunomide. Avoid. Severe Theoretical
▶ **Filgotinib** is predicted to increase the risk of immunosuppression when given with tofacitinib. Avoid. Severe Theoretical
Fingolimod → see TABLE 6 p. 1430 (bradycardia), TABLE 9 p. 1431 (QT-interval prolongation)
▶ Anti-androgens (apalutamide, enzalutamide) are predicted to decrease the exposure to **fingolimod**. Moderate Study
▶ Antiepileptics (carbamazepine, fosphenytoin, phenobarbital, phenytoin, primidone) are predicted to decrease the exposure to **fingolimod**. Moderate Study
▶ Calcium channel blockers (diltiazem, verapamil) are predicted to increase the exposure to **fingolimod**. Avoid. Moderate Theoretical → Also see TABLE 6 p. 1430
▶ Live vaccines are predicted to increase the risk of generalised infection (possibly life-threatening) when given with **fingolimod**. Public Health England advises avoid (refer to Green Book). Severe Theoretical
▶ Mitotane is predicted to decrease the exposure to **fingolimod**. Moderate Study
▶ Rifamycins (rifampicin) are predicted to decrease the exposure to **fingolimod**. Moderate Study
▶ St John's wort is predicted to decrease the exposure to **fingolimod**. Avoid. Moderate Theoretical
Flavoxate → see TABLE 10 p. 1431 (antimuscarinics)
Flecainide → see antiarrhythmics
Flucloxacillin → see penicillins
Fluconazole → see antifungals, azoles
Flucytosine
▶ Amphotericin B increases the risk of toxicity when given with **flucytosine**. Severe Study
▶ Cytarabine decreases the concentration of **flucytosine**. Avoid. Severe Study
▶ NRTIs (zidovudine) increase the risk of haematological toxicity when given with **flucytosine**. Monitor and adjust dose. Severe Theoretical
Fludarabine → see TABLE 15 p. 1432 (myelosuppression)
▶ Live vaccines are predicted to increase the risk of generalised infection (possibly life-threatening) when given with **fludarabine**. Public Health England advises avoid (refer to Green Book). Severe Theoretical

▶ **Fludarabine** increases the risk of pulmonary toxicity when given with pentostatin. Avoid. Severe Study → Also see TABLE 15 p. 1432
Fludrocortisone → see corticosteroids
Fluocinolone

▶ With intravitreal use of **fluocinolone** in adults: caution with concurrent administration of anticoagulant or antiplatelet drugs (higher incidence of conjunctival haemorrhage).
▶ Interactions do not generally apply to corticosteroids used for topical action unless specified.

Fluorouracil → see TABLE 15 p. 1432 (myelosuppression), TABLE 5 p. 1430 (thromboembolism)

ROUTE-SPECIFIC INFORMATION Since systemic absorption can follow topical application of **fluorouracil**, the possibility of interactions should be borne in mind.

▶ **Fluorouracil** increases the concentration of antiepileptics (fosphenytoin, phenytoin). Monitor concentration and adjust dose. Severe Anecdotal
▶ **Fluorouracil** increases the anticoagulant effect of coumarins. Severe Anecdotal
▶ Folates (folic acid) are predicted to increase the risk of toxicity when given with **fluorouracil**. Avoid. Severe Theoretical
▶ Folates (folinic acid) are predicted to increase the risk of toxicity when given with **fluorouracil**. Monitor and adjust dose. Severe Theoretical
▶ H₂ receptor antagonists (cimetidine) slightly increase the exposure to **fluorouracil**. Severe Study
▶ Live vaccines are predicted to increase the risk of generalised infection (possibly life-threatening) when given with **fluorouracil**. Public Health England advises avoid (refer to Green Book). Severe Theoretical
▶ Methotrexate potentially increases the risk of severe skin reaction when given with topical **fluorouracil**. Severe Anecdotal → Also see TABLE 15 p. 1432 → Also see TABLE 5 p. 1430
▶ Metronidazole increases the risk of toxicity when given with **fluorouracil**. Severe Study
Fluoxetine → see SSRIs
Flupentixol → see TABLE 8 p. 1430 (hypotension), TABLE 11 p. 1431 (CNS depressant effects)
▶ **Flupentixol** is predicted to decrease the effects of dopamine receptor agonists. Avoid. Moderate Theoretical → Also see TABLE 8 p. 1430
▶ **Flupentixol** decreases the effects of levodopa. Avoid or monitor worsening parkinsonian symptoms. Severe Theoretical → Also see TABLE 8 p. 1430
Fluphenazine → see phenothiazines
Flurazepam → see benzodiazepines
Flurbiprofen → see NSAIDs
Flutamide → see anti-androgens
Fluticasone → see corticosteroids
Fluvastatin → see statins
Fluvoxamine → see SSRIs
Folates

folic acid · folinic acid · levofolinic acid

▶ **Folates** are predicted to decrease the concentration of antiepileptics (fosphenytoin, phenobarbital, phenytoin, primidone). Monitor concentration and adjust dose. Severe Study
▶ **Folates** are predicted to increase the risk of toxicity when given with capecitabine. Severe Anecdotal
▶ **Folic acid** is predicted to increase the risk of toxicity when given with fluorouracil. Avoid. Severe Theoretical
▶ **Folinic acid** is predicted to increase the risk of toxicity when given with fluorouracil. Monitor and adjust dose. Severe Theoretical
▶ **Folates** are predicted to alter the effects of raltitrexed. Avoid. Moderate Study
▶ Sulfasalazine is predicted to decrease the absorption of **folates**. Moderate Study
▶ **Folates** are predicted to increase the risk of toxicity when given with tegafur. Severe Theoretical
Folic acid → see folates

Folinic acid → see folates

Fondaparinux → see factor XA inhibitors

Formoterol → see beta$_2$ agonists

Fosamprenavir → see HIV-protease inhibitors

Fosaprepitant → see neurokinin-1 receptor antagonists

Foscarnet → see TABLE 2 p. 1429 (nephrotoxicity)

▸ Foscarnet increases the risk of hypocalcaemia when given with pentamidine. Severe Anecdotal → Also see TABLE 2 p. 1429

Fosinopril → see ACE inhibitors

Fosphenytoin → see antiepileptics

Fostamatinib

▸ Anti-androgens (apalutamide, enzalutamide) are predicted to decrease the exposure to **fostamatinib**. Avoid. Severe Study

▸ Antiepileptics (carbamazepine, fosphenytoin, phenobarbital, phenytoin, primidone) are predicted to decrease the exposure to **fostamatinib**. Avoid. Severe Study

▸ Antifungals, azoles (itraconazole, ketoconazole, voriconazole) are predicted to increase the exposure to **fostamatinib**. Monitor adverse effects and adjust dose. Moderate Study

▸ Antifungals, azoles (posaconazole) are predicted to increase the exposure to **fostamatinib**. Monitor adverse effects and adjust dose. Moderate Theoretical

▸ Calcium channel blockers (diltiazem) are predicted to increase the exposure to **fostamatinib**. Monitor adverse effects and adjust dose. Moderate Theoretical

▸ Cobicistat is predicted to increase the exposure to **fostamatinib**. Monitor adverse effects and adjust dose. Moderate Study

▸ **Fostamatinib** potentially alters the anticoagulant effect of coumarins (warfarin). Moderate Theoretical

▸ **Fostamatinib** slightly increases the exposure to digoxin. Monitor **digoxin** concentration and adjust dose, p. 117. Moderate Study

▸ Grapefruit juice is predicted to increase the exposure to **fostamatinib**. Monitor adverse effects and adjust dose. Moderate Theoretical

▸ HIV-protease inhibitors are predicted to increase the exposure to **fostamatinib**. Monitor adverse effects and adjust dose. Moderate Study

▸ Idelalisib is predicted to increase the exposure to **fostamatinib**. Monitor adverse effects and adjust dose. Moderate Study

▸ Macrolides (clarithromycin) are predicted to increase the exposure to **fostamatinib**. Monitor adverse effects and adjust dose. Moderate Study

▸ Mitotane is predicted to decrease the exposure to **fostamatinib**. Avoid. Severe Study

▸ Rifamycins (rifampicin) are predicted to decrease the exposure to **fostamatinib**. Avoid. Severe Study

▸ **Fostamatinib** slightly increases the exposure to statins (rosuvastatin). Moderate Study

▸ **Fostamatinib** slightly increases the exposure to statins (simvastatin). Monitor adverse effects and adjust dose. Moderate Study

Frovatriptan → see triptans

Fulvestrant → see TABLE 5 p. 1430 (thromboembolism)

Furosemide → see loop diuretics

Fusidate

▸ **Fusidate** increases the risk of rhabdomyolysis when given with statins. Avoid. Severe Anecdotal

Gabapentin → see antiepileptics

Galantamine → see anticholinesterases, centrally acting

Ganciclovir → see TABLE 15 p. 1432 (myelosuppression), TABLE 2 p. 1429 (nephrotoxicity)

ROUTE-SPECIFIC INFORMATION Since systemic absorption can follow topical application, the possibility of interactions should be borne in mind.

▸ **Ganciclovir** is predicted to increase the risk of seizures when given with carbapenems (imipenem). Avoid. Severe Anecdotal

▸ Leflunomide is predicted to increase the exposure to **ganciclovir**. Moderate Theoretical → Also see TABLE 15 p. 1432

▸ Mycophenolate is predicted to increase the risk of haematological toxicity when given with **ganciclovir**. Moderate Theoretical

▸ Nitisinone is predicted to increase the exposure to **ganciclovir**. Moderate Study

▸ Teriflunomide is predicted to increase the exposure to **ganciclovir**. Moderate Study

Gefitinib

▸ Oral antacids are predicted to decrease the exposure to oral **gefitinib**. Moderate Theoretical

▸ Anti-androgens (apalutamide, enzalutamide) are predicted to decrease the exposure to **gefitinib**. Avoid. Severe Study

▸ Antiarrhythmics (dronedarone) are predicted to increase the exposure to **gefitinib**. Moderate Theoretical

▸ Antiepileptics (carbamazepine, fosphenytoin, phenobarbital, phenytoin, primidone) are predicted to decrease the exposure to **gefitinib**. Avoid. Severe Study

▸ Antifungals, azoles (fluconazole, isavuconazole, posaconazole) are predicted to increase the exposure to **gefitinib**. Moderate Theoretical

▸ Antifungals, azoles (itraconazole, ketoconazole, voriconazole) are predicted to increase the exposure to **gefitinib**. Moderate Study

▸ Calcium channel blockers (diltiazem, verapamil) are predicted to increase the exposure to **gefitinib**. Moderate Theoretical

▸ Cobicistat is predicted to increase the exposure to **gefitinib**. Moderate Study

▸ **Gefitinib** is predicted to increase the anticoagulant effect of coumarins. Severe Anecdotal

▸ Crizotinib is predicted to increase the exposure to **gefitinib**. Moderate Theoretical

▸ Endothelin receptor antagonists (bosentan) are predicted to decrease the exposure to **gefitinib**. Avoid. Severe Theoretical

▸ H$_2$ receptor antagonists are predicted to slightly to moderately decrease the exposure to **gefitinib**. Moderate Study

▸ HIV-protease inhibitors are predicted to increase the exposure to **gefitinib**. Moderate Study

▸ Idelalisib is predicted to increase the exposure to **gefitinib**. Moderate Study

▸ Imatinib is predicted to increase the exposure to **gefitinib**. Moderate Theoretical

▸ Letermovir is predicted to increase the exposure to **gefitinib**. Moderate Theoretical

▸ Macrolides (clarithromycin) are predicted to increase the exposure to **gefitinib**. Moderate Study

▸ Macrolides (erythromycin) are predicted to increase the exposure to **gefitinib**. Moderate Theoretical

▸ Mitotane is predicted to decrease the exposure to **gefitinib**. Avoid. Severe Study

▸ Neurokinin-1 receptor antagonists (aprepitant, netupitant) are predicted to increase the exposure to **gefitinib**. Moderate Theoretical

▸ Nilotinib is predicted to increase the exposure to **gefitinib**. Moderate Theoretical

▸ NNRTIs (efavirenz, nevirapine) are predicted to decrease the exposure to **gefitinib**. Avoid. Severe Theoretical

▸ **Gefitinib** is predicted to increase the risk of bleeding events when given with phenindione. Severe Theoretical

▸ Proton pump inhibitors are predicted to decrease the exposure to **gefitinib**. Severe Study

▸ Rifamycins (rifampicin) are predicted to decrease the exposure to **gefitinib**. Avoid. Severe Study

▸ St John's wort is predicted to decrease the exposure to **gefitinib**. Avoid. Severe Theoretical

Gemcitabine → see TABLE 15 p. 1432 (myelosuppression)

▸ Live vaccines are predicted to increase the risk of generalised infection (possibly life-threatening) when given with **gemcitabine**. Public Health England advises avoid (refer to Green Book). Severe Theoretical

Gemfibrozil → see fibrates

Gemtuzumab ozogamicin → see TABLE 15 p. 1432 (myelosuppression)

Gentamicin → see aminoglycosides

Gilteritinib

▸ Antiepileptics (carbamazepine, fosphenytoin, phenytoin) are predicted to decrease the exposure to **gilteritinib**. Avoid. Severe Study

▸ Antifungals, azoles (itraconazole, ketoconazole, voriconazole) are predicted to increase the exposure to **gilteritinib**. Moderate Study

▸ Cobicistat is predicted to increase the exposure to **gilteritinib**. Moderate Study

Gilteritinib (continued)

▸ HIV-protease inhibitors are predicted to increase the exposure to **gilteritinib**. Moderate Study
▸ Idelalisib is predicted to increase the exposure to **gilteritinib**. Moderate Study
▸ Macrolides (azithromycin, erythromycin) are predicted to increase the exposure to **gilteritinib**. Moderate Theoretical
▸ Macrolides (clarithromycin) are predicted to increase the exposure to **gilteritinib**. Moderate Study
▸ Rifamycins (rifampicin) moderately decrease the exposure to **gilteritinib**. Avoid. Severe Study
▸ **Gilteritinib** is predicted to decrease the efficacy of SSRIs (escitalopram, fluoxetine, sertraline). Avoid. Moderate Theoretical
▸ St John's wort is predicted to decrease the exposure to **gilteritinib**. Severe Study

Glasdegib → see TABLE 9 p. 1431 (QT-interval prolongation)

▸ Anti-androgens (apalutamide, enzalutamide) are predicted to moderately decrease the exposure to **glasdegib**. Avoid. Severe Study → Also see TABLE 9 p. 1431
▸ Antiepileptics (carbamazepine, fosphenytoin, phenobarbital, phenytoin, primidone) are predicted to moderately decrease the exposure to **glasdegib**. Avoid. Severe Study
▸ Antifungals, azoles (itraconazole, ketoconazole, voriconazole) are predicted to moderately increase the exposure to **glasdegib**. Use with caution or avoid. Moderate Study → Also see TABLE 9 p. 1431
▸ Antifungals, azoles (posaconazole) are predicted to increase the exposure to **glasdegib**. Use with caution or avoid. Moderate Theoretical
▸ Cobicistat is predicted to moderately increase the exposure to **glasdegib**. Use with caution or avoid. Moderate Study
▸ Endothelin receptor antagonists (bosentan) are predicted to decrease the exposure to **glasdegib**. Avoid or adjust **glasdegib** dose, p. 1049. Severe Theoretical
▸ Grapefruit is predicted to increase the exposure to **glasdegib**. Use with caution or avoid. Moderate Theoretical
▸ HIV-protease inhibitors are predicted to moderately increase the exposure to **glasdegib**. Use with caution or avoid. Moderate Study → Also see TABLE 9 p. 1431
▸ Idelalisib is predicted to moderately increase the exposure to **glasdegib**. Use with caution or avoid. Moderate Study
▸ Macrolides (clarithromycin) are predicted to moderately increase the exposure to **glasdegib**. Use with caution or avoid. Moderate Study → Also see TABLE 9 p. 1431
▸ Mitotane is predicted to moderately decrease the exposure to **glasdegib**. Avoid. Severe Study
▸ Modafinil is predicted to decrease the exposure to **glasdegib**. Avoid or adjust **glasdegib** dose, p. 1049. Moderate Theoretical
▸ NNRTIs (efavirenz, nevirapine) are predicted to decrease the exposure to **glasdegib**. Avoid or adjust **glasdegib** dose, p. 1049. Severe Theoretical → Also see TABLE 9 p. 1431
▸ NNRTIs (etravirine) are predicted to decrease the exposure to **glasdegib**. Avoid or adjust **glasdegib** dose, p. 1049. Moderate Theoretical
▸ Rifamycins (rifampicin) are predicted to moderately decrease the exposure to **glasdegib**. Avoid. Severe Study
▸ St John's wort is predicted to decrease the exposure to **glasdegib**. Avoid or adjust **glasdegib** dose, p. 1049. Severe Theoretical

Glecaprevir

▸ Anti-androgens (enzalutamide) are predicted to greatly decrease the concentration of **glecaprevir**. Avoid. Severe Study
▸ Antiarrhythmics (dronedarone) potentially increase the exposure to **glecaprevir**. Moderate Theoretical
▸ Antiepileptics (carbamazepine, fosphenytoin, phenobarbital, phenytoin, primidone) are predicted to moderately decrease the exposure to **glecaprevir**. Avoid. Severe Study
▸ Antiepileptics (eslicarbazepine, oxcarbazepine) potentially decrease the exposure to **glecaprevir**. Avoid. Severe Theoretical
▸ Antifungals, azoles (itraconazole, ketoconazole) potentially increase the exposure to **glecaprevir**. Moderate Theoretical
▸ Ciclosporin increases the exposure to **glecaprevir**. Avoid or monitor. Severe Study

▸ Cobicistat potentially increases the exposure to **glecaprevir**. Moderate Theoretical
▸ Combined hormonal contraceptives (containing ethinylestradiol) are predicted to increase the risk of increased ALT concentrations when given with **glecaprevir**. Avoid. Severe Study
▸ Crizotinib potentially decreases the exposure to **glecaprevir**. Avoid. Severe Theoretical
▸ **Glecaprevir** (with pibrentasvir) increases the exposure to digoxin. Moderate Study
▸ Endothelin receptor antagonists (bosentan) are predicted to decrease the exposure to **glecaprevir**. Avoid. Severe Study
▸ HIV-protease inhibitors (atazanavir, darunavir, lopinavir) boosted with ritonavir increase the exposure to **glecaprevir**. Avoid. Severe Study
▸ HIV-protease inhibitors (ritonavir) increase the exposure to **glecaprevir**. Avoid. Severe Study
▸ Lumacaftor potentially decreases the exposure to **glecaprevir**. Avoid. Severe Theoretical
▸ Mitotane is predicted to greatly decrease the concentration of **glecaprevir**. Avoid. Severe Study
▸ NNRTIs (efavirenz, nevirapine) are predicted to decrease the exposure to **glecaprevir**. Avoid. Severe Study
▸ Rifamycins (rifampicin) markedly affect the exposure to **glecaprevir**. Avoid. Severe Study
▸ St John's wort is predicted to decrease the exposure to **glecaprevir**. Avoid. Severe Study
▸ **Glecaprevir** (with pibrentasvir) markedly increases the exposure to statins (atorvastatin). Avoid. Severe Study
▸ **Glecaprevir** (with pibrentasvir) is predicted to increase the exposure to statins (fluvastatin). Moderate Theoretical
▸ **Glecaprevir** (with pibrentasvir) increases the exposure to statins (pravastatin). Use with caution and adjust **pravastatin** dose. Moderate Study
▸ **Glecaprevir** (with pibrentasvir) increases the exposure to statins (rosuvastatin). Use with caution and adjust **rosuvastatin** dose, p. 218. Moderate Study
▸ **Glecaprevir** (with pibrentasvir) increases the exposure to statins (simvastatin). Avoid. Moderate Study
▸ **Glecaprevir** (with pibrentasvir) slightly increases the exposure to tacrolimus. Monitor and adjust dose. Mild Study
▸ **Glecaprevir** (with pibrentasvir) increases the exposure to thrombin inhibitors (dabigatran). Avoid. Moderate Study

Glibenclamide → see sulfonylureas
Gliclazide → see sulfonylureas
Glimepiride → see sulfonylureas
Glipizide → see sulfonylureas

Glucagon

▸ **Glucagon** increases the anticoagulant effect of coumarins (warfarin). Severe Study

Glucagon-like peptide-1 receptor agonists → see TABLE 14 p. 1432 (antidiabetic drugs)

dulaglutide · exenatide · liraglutide · lixisenatide · semaglutide

▸ With standard-release **exenatide**: some orally administered drugs should be taken at least 1 hour before, or 4 hours after, exenatide injection.
▸ Some orally administered drugs should be taken at least 1 hour before, or 4 hours after, **lixisenatide** injection.

Glucosamine

▸ **Glucosamine** potentially decreases the anticoagulant effect of coumarins (acenocoumarol). Moderate Anecdotal
▸ **Glucosamine** potentially increases the anticoagulant effect of coumarins (warfarin). Avoid. Moderate Anecdotal

Glycerol phenylbutyrate

▸ Antiepileptics (valproate) potentially oppose the effects of glycerol phenylbutyrate. Moderate Theoretical
▸ Corticosteroids potentially oppose the effects of **glycerol phenylbutyrate**. Moderate Theoretical
▸ Haloperidol potentially opposes the effects of **glycerol phenylbutyrate**. Moderate Theoretical

Glyceryl trinitrate → see nitrates

Glycopyrronium → see TABLE 10 p. 1431 (antimuscarinics)

ROUTE-SPECIFIC INFORMATION　Since systemic absorption can follow topical application of **glycopyrronium**, the possibility of interactions should be borne in mind.

Gold
ACE inhibitors are predicted to increase the risk of hypersensitivity when given with **gold**. [Severe] Anecdotal
Gold potentially increases the risk of adverse effects when given with penicillamine (in those who have had previous adverse reactions to gold). Avoid. [Severe] Study

Golimumab → see monoclonal antibodies

Granisetron → see 5-HT3-receptor antagonists

Grapefruit
▸ **Grapefruit** juice is predicted to increase the exposure to abemaciclib. Avoid. [Moderate] Theoretical
▸ **Grapefruit** juice moderately decreases the exposure to aliskiren. Avoid. [Severe] Study
▸ **Grapefruit** juice increases the exposure to antiarrhythmics (amiodarone). Avoid. [Moderate] Study
▸ **Grapefruit** juice moderately increases the exposure to antiarrhythmics (dronedarone). Avoid. [Severe] Study
▸ **Grapefruit** juice increases the exposure to antiarrhythmics (propafenone). Monitor and adjust dose. [Moderate] Study
▸ **Grapefruit** juice slightly increases the exposure to antiepileptics (carbamazepine). Monitor and adjust dose. [Moderate] Study
▸ **Grapefruit** juice slightly decreases the exposure to antihistamines, non-sedating (bilastine). **Bilastine should be taken 1 hour before or 2 hours after grapefruit.** [Moderate] Study
▸ **Grapefruit** juice increases the exposure to antihistamines, non-sedating (rupatadine). Avoid. [Moderate] Study
▸ **Grapefruit** juice increases the exposure to antimalarials (artemether). [Unknown] Study
▸ **Grapefruit** juice is predicted to increase the concentration of antimalarials (piperaquine). Avoid. [Severe] Theoretical
▸ **Grapefruit** juice is predicted to increase the exposure to antipsychotics, second generation (cariprazine). Avoid. [Moderate] Study
▸ **Grapefruit** juice is predicted to increase the exposure to antipsychotics, second generation (lurasidone, quetiapine). Avoid. [Severe] Theoretical
▸ **Grapefruit** juice is predicted to increase the exposure to avapritinib. Avoid. [Moderate] Theoretical
▸ **Grapefruit** juice is predicted to increase the exposure to axitinib. [Moderate] Theoretical
▸ **Grapefruit** juice greatly decreases the exposure to beta blockers, selective (celiprolol). [Moderate] Study
▸ **Grapefruit** juice is predicted to increase the exposure to bosutinib. Avoid. [Moderate] Theoretical
▸ **Grapefruit** juice is predicted to increase the concentration of brigatinib. Avoid. [Severe] Study
▸ **Grapefruit** juice increases the exposure to buspirone. Avoid. [Mild] Study
▸ **Grapefruit** juice is predicted to increase the exposure to cabozantinib. [Moderate] Theoretical
▸ **Grapefruit** juice very slightly increases the exposure to calcium channel blockers (amlodipine). Avoid. [Mild] Study
▸ **Grapefruit** juice increases the exposure to calcium channel blockers (felodipine). Avoid. [Moderate] Study
▸ **Grapefruit** juice is predicted to increase the exposure to calcium channel blockers (lercanidipine). Avoid. [Moderate] Theoretical
▸ **Grapefruit** juice increases the exposure to calcium channel blockers (nicardipine). [Mild] Study
▸ **Grapefruit** juice increases the exposure to calcium channel blockers (nifedipine, verapamil). Avoid. [Mild] Study
▸ **Grapefruit** juice is predicted to increase the exposure to ceritinib. Avoid. [Severe] Theoretical
▸ **Grapefruit** juice increases the concentration of ciclosporin. Avoid. [Severe] Study
▸ **Grapefruit** juice markedly decreases the exposure to clopidogrel. [Severe] Study
▸ **Grapefruit** juice is predicted to increase the exposure to cobimetinib. Avoid. [Severe] Theoretical
▸ **Grapefruit** juice moderately increases the exposure to oral corticosteroids (budesonide). Avoid. [Moderate] Study

▸ **Grapefruit** juice is predicted to increase the exposure to crizotinib. Avoid. [Moderate] Theoretical
▸ **Grapefruit** juice is predicted to increase the exposure to darifenacin. [Moderate] Study
▸ **Grapefruit** juice is predicted to increase the exposure to dasatinib. Avoid. [Moderate] Theoretical
▸ **Grapefruit** juice is predicted to increase the exposure to dipeptidylpeptidase-4 inhibitors (saxagliptin). [Mild] Theoretical
▸ **Grapefruit** juice is predicted to increase the exposure to elexacaftor. Avoid. [Moderate] Theoretical
▸ **Grapefruit** juice is predicted to increase the exposure to eliglustat. Avoid. [Severe] Theoretical
▸ **Grapefruit** juice is predicted to increase the exposure to encorafenib. Avoid. [Moderate] Study
▸ **Grapefruit** is predicted to increase the exposure to entrectinib. Avoid. [Severe] Theoretical
▸ **Grapefruit** juice is predicted to increase the exposure to ergometrine. [Severe] Theoretical
▸ **Grapefruit** juice is predicted to increase the exposure to ergotamine. [Severe] Theoretical
▸ **Grapefruit** juice is predicted to increase the exposure to erlotinib. [Moderate] Theoretical
▸ **Grapefruit** juice is predicted to increase the exposure to everolimus. Avoid. [Severe] Theoretical
▸ **Grapefruit** juice is predicted to increase the exposure to fostamatinib. Monitor adverse effects and adjust dose. [Moderate] Theoretical
▸ **Grapefruit** is predicted to increase the exposure to glasdegib. Use with caution or avoid. [Moderate] Theoretical
▸ **Grapefruit** juice is predicted to increase the exposure to guanfacine. Avoid. [Moderate] Theoretical
▸ **Grapefruit** juice is predicted to increase the exposure to ibrutinib. Avoid. [Moderate] Theoretical
▸ **Grapefruit** juice is predicted to increase the exposure to imatinib. [Moderate] Theoretical
▸ **Grapefruit** juice is predicted to increase the exposure to ivabradine. Avoid. [Moderate] Study
▸ **Grapefruit** juice is predicted to increase the exposure to ivacaftor. Avoid. [Moderate] Theoretical
▸ **Grapefruit** juice is predicted to increase the exposure to lapatinib. Avoid. [Moderate] Theoretical
▸ **Grapefruit** juice is predicted to increase the exposure to larotrectinib. Avoid. [Moderate] Theoretical
▸ **Grapefruit** juice is predicted to increase the exposure to lomitapide. Avoid. [Mild] Theoretical
▸ **Grapefruit** juice is predicted to increase the concentration of lorlatinib. Avoid. [Moderate] Theoretical
▸ **Grapefruit** juice is predicted to increase the exposure to naldemedine. Avoid or monitor. [Moderate] Theoretical
▸ **Grapefruit** juice is predicted to increase the exposure to naloxegol. Avoid. [Moderate] Theoretical
▸ **Grapefruit** juice is predicted to increase the exposure to neratinib. Avoid. [Severe] Theoretical
▸ **Grapefruit** juice is predicted to increase the exposure to nilotinib. Avoid. [Severe] Theoretical
▸ **Grapefruit** juice is predicted to increase the exposure to olaparib. Avoid. [Moderate] Theoretical
▸ **Grapefruit** juice is predicted to increase the exposure to palbociclib. Avoid. [Severe] Theoretical
▸ **Grapefruit** juice is predicted to increase the exposure to pazopanib. Avoid. [Severe] Theoretical
▸ **Grapefruit** juice is predicted to increase the exposure to phosphodiesterase type-5 inhibitors. Use with caution or avoid. [Moderate] Study
▸ **Grapefruit** juice increases the exposure to pimozide. Avoid. [Severe] Theoretical
▸ **Grapefruit** juice is predicted to increase the exposure to ponatinib. [Moderate] Theoretical
▸ **Grapefruit** juice is predicted to increase the exposure to praziquantel. [Moderate] Study
▸ **Grapefruit** juice is predicted to increase the concentration of ranolazine. Avoid. [Severe] Theoretical
▸ **Grapefruit** juice is predicted to increase the exposure to regorafenib. Avoid. [Moderate] Theoretical

Grapefruit (continued)
▸ **Grapefruit** juice is predicted to increase the exposure to ribociclib. Avoid. Moderate Theoretical
▸ **Grapefruit** juice is predicted to increase the exposure to ruxolitinib. Severe Theoretical
▸ **Grapefruit** juice increases the concentration of sirolimus. Avoid. Moderate Study
▸ **Grapefruit** juice moderately increases the exposure to SSRIs (sertraline). Avoid. Moderate Study
▸ **Grapefruit** juice increases the exposure to statins (atorvastatin). Mild Study
▸ **Grapefruit** juice increases the exposure to statins (simvastatin). Avoid. Severe Study
▸ **Grapefruit** juice is predicted to increase the exposure to sunitinib. Avoid. Moderate Theoretical
▸ **Grapefruit** juice greatly increases the concentration of tacrolimus. Avoid. Severe Study
▸ **Grapefruit** juice is predicted to increase the concentration of temsirolimus. Use with caution or avoid. Moderate Theoretical
▸ **Grapefruit** juice is predicted to increase the exposure to tezacaftor. Avoid. Severe Study
▸ **Grapefruit** juice moderately increases the exposure to ticagrelor. Moderate Study
▸ **Grapefruit** juice increases the exposure to tolvaptan. Avoid. Moderate Study
▸ **Grapefruit** juice is predicted to increase the exposure to venetoclax. Avoid. Severe Theoretical

Grass pollen extract
GENERAL INFORMATION Desensitising vaccines should be avoided in patients taking beta-blockers (adrenaline might be ineffective in case of a hypersensitivity reaction) or ACE inhibitors (risk of severe anaphylactoid reactions).

Grazoprevir
▸ Anti-androgens (apalutamide, enzalutamide) are predicted to decrease the exposure to **grazoprevir**. Avoid. Severe Study
▸ Antiepileptics (carbamazepine, fosphenytoin, phenobarbital, phenytoin, primidone) are predicted to decrease the exposure to **grazoprevir**. Avoid. Severe Study
▸ Antifungals, azoles (itraconazole, ketoconazole, voriconazole) are predicted to moderately to markedly increase the exposure to **grazoprevir**. Avoid. Severe Study
▸ **Grazoprevir** is predicted to increase the concentration of calcium channel blockers. Moderate Theoretical
▸ Ciclosporin greatly increases the exposure to **grazoprevir**. Avoid. Severe Study
▸ Cobicistat is predicted to moderately to markedly increase the exposure to **grazoprevir**. Avoid. Severe Study
▸ Elvitegravir markedly increases the exposure to **grazoprevir**. Avoid. Severe Study
▸ Endothelin receptor antagonists (bosentan) are predicted to markedly decrease the exposure to **grazoprevir**. Avoid. Severe Study
▸ HIV-protease inhibitors are predicted to moderately to markedly increase the exposure to **grazoprevir**. Avoid. Severe Study
▸ Idelalisib is predicted to moderately to markedly increase the exposure to **grazoprevir**. Avoid. Severe Study
▸ Macrolides (clarithromycin) are predicted to moderately to markedly increase the exposure to **grazoprevir**. Avoid. Severe Study
▸ Mitotane is predicted to decrease the exposure to **grazoprevir**. Avoid. Severe Study
▸ Modafinil is predicted to decrease the exposure to **grazoprevir**. Avoid. Severe Study
▸ NNRTIs (efavirenz, nevirapine) are predicted to markedly decrease the exposure to **grazoprevir**. Avoid. Severe Study
▸ NNRTIs (etravirine) are predicted to decrease the exposure to **grazoprevir**. Avoid. Mild Theoretical
▸ Rifamycins (rifampicin) are predicted to decrease the exposure to **grazoprevir**. Avoid. Severe Study
▸ St John's wort is predicted to markedly decrease the exposure to **grazoprevir**. Avoid. Severe Study
▸ **Grazoprevir** increases the exposure to statins (atorvastatin). Adjust **atorvastatin** dose, p. 217. Moderate Study

▸ **Grazoprevir** is predicted to increase the exposure to statins (fluvastatin). Adjust **fluvastatin** dose, p. 217. Unknown Theoretical
▸ **Grazoprevir** increases the exposure to statins (rosuvastatin). Adjust **rosuvastatin** dose, p. 218. Moderate Study
▸ **Grazoprevir** is predicted to increase the exposure to statins (simvastatin). Adjust **simvastatin** dose, p. 219. Unknown Theoretical
▸ **Grazoprevir** is predicted to increase the concentration of sunitinib. Use with caution and adjust dose. Moderate Theoretical
▸ **Grazoprevir** increases the exposure to tacrolimus. Moderate Study

Griseofulvin
ROUTE-SPECIFIC INFORMATION Interactions do not generally apply to topical use unless specified.
▸ Alcohol potentially causes a disulfiram-like reaction when given with **griseofulvin**. Moderate Anecdotal
▸ Antiepileptics (phenobarbital, primidone) decrease the effects of **griseofulvin**. Moderate Study
▸ **Griseofulvin** potentially decreases the efficacy of combined hormonal contraceptives. For FSRH guidance, see Contraceptives, interactions p. 840. Severe Anecdotal
▸ **Griseofulvin** potentially decreases the anticoagulant effect of coumarins. Moderate Anecdotal
▸ **Griseofulvin** potentially decreases the efficacy of desogestrel. For FSRH guidance, see Contraceptives, interactions p. 840. Severe Anecdotal
▸ **Griseofulvin** decreases the efficacy of etonogestrel. For FSRH guidance, see Contraceptives, interactions p. 840. Severe Anecdotal
▸ **Griseofulvin** potentially decreases the efficacy of oral levonorgestrel. For FSRH guidance, see Contraceptives, interactions p. 840. Severe Anecdotal
▸ **Griseofulvin** potentially decreases the efficacy of norethisterone. For FSRH guidance, see Contraceptives, interactions p. 840. Severe Anecdotal
▸ **Griseofulvin** potentially decreases the efficacy of ulipristal. For FSRH guidance, see Contraceptives, interactions p. 840. Severe Anecdotal

Guanfacine → see TABLE 8 p. 1430 (hypotension), TABLE 11 p. 1431 (CNS depressant effects)
▸ Anti-androgens (apalutamide, enzalutamide) are predicted to decrease the concentration of **guanfacine**. Adjust **guanfacine** dose, p. 372. Moderate Study
▸ Antiarrhythmics (dronedarone) are predicted to increase the concentration of **guanfacine**. Adjust **guanfacine** dose, p. 372. Moderate Theoretical
▸ Antiepileptics (carbamazepine, fosphenytoin, phenobarbital, phenytoin, primidone) are predicted to decrease the concentration of **guanfacine**. Adjust **guanfacine** dose, p. 372. Moderate Study → Also see TABLE 11 p. 1431
▸ Antiepileptics (oxcarbazepine) are predicted to decrease the concentration of **guanfacine**. Monitor and adjust **guanfacine** dose, p. 372. Moderate Theoretical
▸ **Guanfacine** increases the concentration of antiepileptics (valproate). Monitor and adjust dose. Moderate Study
▸ Antifungals, azoles (fluconazole, isavuconazole, posaconazole) are predicted to increase the concentration of **guanfacine**. Adjust **guanfacine** dose, p. 372. Moderate Theoretical
▸ Antifungals, azoles (itraconazole, ketoconazole, voriconazole) are predicted to increase the exposure to **guanfacine**. Adjust **guanfacine** dose, p. 372. Moderate Study
▸ Calcium channel blockers (diltiazem, verapamil) are predicted to increase the concentration of **guanfacine**. Adjust **guanfacine** dose, p. 372. Moderate Theoretical → Also see TABLE 8 p. 1430
▸ Chloramphenicol is predicted to increase the exposure to **guanfacine**. Adjust **guanfacine** dose, p. 372. Moderate Study
▸ Cobicistat is predicted to increase the exposure to **guanfacine**. Adjust **guanfacine** dose, p. 372. Moderate Study
▸ Crizotinib is predicted to increase the concentration of **guanfacine**. Adjust **guanfacine** dose, p. 372. Moderate Theoretical
▸ Endothelin receptor antagonists (bosentan) are predicted to decrease the concentration of **guanfacine**. Adjust dose. Moderate Theoretical

Grapefruit juice is predicted to increase the exposure to **guanfacine**. Avoid. Moderate Theoretical

▸ HIV-protease inhibitors are predicted to increase the exposure to **guanfacine**. Adjust **guanfacine** dose, p. 372. Moderate Study
Idelalisib is predicted to increase the exposure to **guanfacine**. Adjust **guanfacine** dose, p. 372. Moderate Study

▸ Imatinib is predicted to increase the concentration of **guanfacine**. Adjust **guanfacine** dose, p. 372. Moderate Theoretical

▸ Letermovir is predicted to increase the concentration of **guanfacine**. Adjust **guanfacine** dose, p. 372. Moderate Theoretical
Macrolides (clarithromycin) are predicted to increase the exposure to **guanfacine**. Adjust **guanfacine** dose, p. 372. Moderate Study
Macrolides (erythromycin) are predicted to increase the concentration of **guanfacine**. Adjust **guanfacine** dose, p. 372. Moderate Theoretical

▸ **Guanfacine** is predicted to increase the concentration of metformin. Moderate Theoretical

▸ Mitotane is predicted to decrease the concentration of **guanfacine**. Adjust **guanfacine** dose, p. 372. Moderate Study

▸ Neurokinin-1 receptor antagonists (aprepitant, netupitant) are predicted to increase the concentration of **guanfacine**. Adjust **guanfacine** dose, p. 372. Moderate Theoretical

▸ Neurokinin-1 receptor antagonists (fosaprepitant) are predicted to increase the concentration of **guanfacine**. Moderate Theoretical

▸ Nilotinib is predicted to increase the concentration of **guanfacine**. Adjust **guanfacine** dose, p. 372. Moderate Theoretical

▸ NNRTIs (efavirenz, nevirapine) are predicted to decrease the concentration of **guanfacine**. Adjust dose. Moderate Theoretical

▸ Rifamycins (rifampicin) are predicted to decrease the concentration of **guanfacine**. Adjust **guanfacine** dose, p. 372. Moderate Study

▸ St John's wort is predicted to decrease the concentration of **guanfacine**. Adjust dose. Moderate Theoretical

Guselkumab → see monoclonal antibodies

H$_2$ receptor antagonists

cimetidine · famotidine · nizatidine · ranitidine

▸ **H$_2$ receptor antagonists** are predicted to decrease the exposure to acalabrutinib. **Acalabrutinib** should be taken 2 hours before or 10 hours after **H$_2$ receptor antagonists**. Moderate Theoretical

▸ **Cimetidine** decreases the clearance of albendazole. Moderate Study

▸ **Cimetidine** increases the concentration of aminophylline. Adjust dose. Severe Study

▸ **Cimetidine** slightly increases the exposure to anthracyclines (epirubicin). Avoid. Moderate Study

▸ **Cimetidine** increases the exposure to antiarrhythmics (amiodarone). Moderate Study

▸ **Cimetidine** slightly increases the exposure to antiarrhythmics (flecainide). Monitor and adjust dose. Mild Study

▸ **Cimetidine** increases the exposure to antiarrhythmics (lidocaine). Monitor and adjust dose. Moderate Study

▸ **Cimetidine** is predicted to increase the exposure to antiarrhythmics (propafenone). Monitor and adjust dose. Moderate Theoretical

▸ **Cimetidine** transiently increases the concentration of antiepileptics (carbamazepine). Monitor concentration and adjust dose. Moderate Study

▸ **Cimetidine** increases the concentration of antiepileptics (fosphenytoin, phenytoin). Monitor concentration and adjust dose. Severe Study

▸ **H$_2$ receptor antagonists** are predicted to decrease the absorption of antifungals, azoles (itraconazole). Administer **itraconazole** capsules with an acidic beverage, p. 636. Moderate Study

▸ **H$_2$ receptor antagonists** are predicted to decrease the absorption of antifungals, azoles (ketoconazole). Administer **ketoconazole** with an acidic beverage, p. 720. Moderate Study

▸ **H$_2$ receptor antagonists** are predicted to decrease the exposure to antifungals, azoles (posaconazole). Avoid use of posaconazole oral suspension. Moderate Study

▸ **Cimetidine** decreases the clearance of antimalarials (chloroquine). Moderate Study

▸ **Cimetidine** slightly increases the exposure to antimalarials (quinine). Moderate Study

▸ **H$_2$ receptor antagonists** are predicted to decrease the absorption of bosutinib. Moderate Theoretical

▸ **Cimetidine** slightly increases the exposure to calcium channel blockers (diltiazem, nimodipine). Monitor and adjust dose. Moderate Study

▸ **Cimetidine** (high-dose) is predicted to increase the exposure to calcium channel blockers (lercanidipine). Moderate Theoretical

▸ **Cimetidine** moderately increases the exposure to calcium channel blockers (nifedipine). Monitor and adjust dose. Severe Study

▸ **Cimetidine** increases the exposure to calcium channel blockers (verapamil). Moderate Study

▸ **Cimetidine** is predicted to slightly increase the exposure to capecitabine. Severe Theoretical

▸ **H$_2$ receptor antagonists** are predicted to decrease the absorption of ceritinib. Moderate Theoretical

▸ **Cimetidine** increases the concentration of ciclosporin. Mild Study

▸ **Cimetidine** increases the anticoagulant effect of coumarins. Severe Study

▸ **H$_2$ receptor antagonists** are predicted to decrease the concentration of dacomitinib. **Dacomitinib** should be taken 2 hours before or 10 hours after **H$_2$ receptor antagonists**. Mild Study

▸ **H$_2$ receptor antagonists** are predicted to decrease the exposure to dasatinib. Avoid. Moderate Study

▸ **H$_2$ receptor antagonists** are predicted to decrease the absorption of dipyridamole (immediate release tablets). Moderate Theoretical

▸ **Cimetidine** is predicted to increase the exposure to dopamine receptor agonists (pramipexole). Adjust dose. Moderate Study

▸ **H$_2$ receptor antagonists** are predicted to decrease the exposure to erlotinib. **Erlotinib** should be taken 2 hours before or 10 hours after **H$_2$ receptor antagonists**. Moderate Study

▸ **Cimetidine** increases the concentration of fampridine. Avoid. Severe Theoretical

▸ **Cimetidine** slightly increases the exposure to fluorouracil. Severe Study

▸ **H$_2$ receptor antagonists** are predicted to slightly to moderately decrease the exposure to gefitinib. Moderate Study

▸ **H$_2$ receptor antagonists** decrease the exposure to HIV-protease inhibitors (atazanavir). Monitor and adjust dose. Moderate Study

▸ **Cimetidine** is predicted to decrease the clearance of hydroxychloroquine. Moderate Theoretical

▸ **H$_2$ receptor antagonists** are predicted to decrease the absorption of lapatinib. Avoid. Moderate Theoretical

▸ **H$_2$ receptor antagonists** are predicted to decrease the exposure to ledipasvir. Adjust dose, see ledipasvir with sofosbuvir p. 668. Moderate Study

▸ Leflunomide is predicted to increase the exposure to H$_2$ receptor antagonists (cimetidine, famotidine). Moderate Theoretical

▸ **Cimetidine** is predicted to increase the exposure to lomitapide. Separate administration by 12 hours. Mild Theoretical

▸ **Ranitidine** is predicted to increase the exposure to lomitapide. Separate administration by 12 hours. Moderate Theoretical

▸ **Cimetidine** slightly increases the exposure to macrolides (erythromycin). Moderate Study

▸ **Cimetidine** increases the concentration of mebendazole. Moderate Study

▸ **Cimetidine** increases the exposure to metformin. Monitor and adjust dose. Moderate Study

▸ **Cimetidine** slightly increases the exposure to mirtazapine. Use with caution and adjust dose. Moderate Theoretical

▸ **Cimetidine** increases the exposure to moclobemide. Adjust **moclobemide** dose, p. 382. Mild Study

▸ **H$_2$ receptor antagonists** are predicted to decrease the exposure to neratinib. Avoid. Severe Theoretical

▸ **H$_2$ receptor antagonists** are predicted to decrease the absorption of nilotinib. **H$_2$ receptor antagonists** should be taken 10 hours before or 2 hours after **nilotinib**. Mild Theoretical

▸ Nitisinone is predicted to increase the exposure to H$_2$ receptor antagonists (cimetidine, famotidine). Moderate Study

A1

Interactions | Appendix 1

H₂ receptor antagonists (continued)

‣ **H₂ receptor antagonists** are predicted to decrease the exposure to NNRTIs (rilpivirine). **H₂ receptor antagonists** should be taken 12 hours before or 4 hours after **rilpivirine**. Severe Study

‣ **Cimetidine** increases the concentration of opioids (alfentanil). Use with caution and adjust dose. Severe Study

‣ **Cimetidine** increases the exposure to opioids (fentanyl). Moderate Study

‣ **H₂ receptor antagonists** are predicted to decrease the exposure to pazopanib. **H₂ receptor antagonists** should be taken 10 hours before or 2 hours after **pazopanib**. Moderate Theoretical

‣ **Cimetidine** increases the exposure to phenindione. Severe Anecdotal

‣ **Cimetidine** slightly increases the exposure to phosphodiesterase type-4 inhibitors (roflumilast). Moderate Study

‣ **Cimetidine** moderately increases the exposure to praziquantel. Moderate Study

‣ **H₂ receptor antagonists** potentially decrease the exposure to sofosbuvir. Adjust dose, see ledipasvir with sofosbuvir p. 668, sofosbuvir with velpatasvir p. 669, and sofosbuvir with velpatasvir and voxilaprevir p. 669. Moderate Study

‣ **Cimetidine** slightly increases the exposure to SSRIs (citalopram, escitalopram). Adjust dose. Moderate Study

‣ **Cimetidine** slightly increases the exposure to SSRIs (paroxetine, sertraline). Moderate Study

‣ **Cimetidine** is predicted to increase the risk of toxicity when given with tegafur. Severe Theoretical

‣ Teriflunomide is predicted to increase the exposure to H₂ receptor antagonists (**cimetidine, famotidine**). Moderate Study

‣ **Cimetidine** increases the concentration of theophylline. Adjust dose. Severe Study

‣ **Cimetidine** increases the exposure to tricyclic antidepressants. Moderate Study

‣ **Cimetidine** slightly increases the exposure to triptans (zolmitriptan). Adjust **zolmitriptan** dose, p. 503. Mild Study

‣ **H₂ receptor antagonists** are predicted to decrease the concentration of velpatasvir. Adjust dose, see sofosbuvir with velpatasvir p. 669. Moderate Study

‣ **Cimetidine** slightly increases the exposure to venlafaxine. Mild Study

Haloperidol → see TABLE 8 p. 1430 (hypotension), TABLE 9 p. 1431 (QT-interval prolongation), TABLE 11 p. 1431 (CNS depressant effects), TABLE 10 p. 1431 (antimuscarinics)

FOOD AND LIFESTYLE Dose adjustment might be necessary if smoking started or stopped during treatment.

‣ Anti-androgens (apalutamide, enzalutamide) decrease the concentration of **haloperidol**. Adjust dose. Moderate Study → Also see TABLE 9 p. 1431

‣ Antiepileptics (carbamazepine, fosphenytoin, phenobarbital, phenytoin, primidone) decrease the concentration of **haloperidol**. Adjust dose. Moderate Study → Also see TABLE 11 p. 1431

‣ **Haloperidol** potentially increases the risk of overheating and dehydration when given with antiepileptics (zonisamide). Avoid in children. Severe Theoretical

‣ Antifungals, azoles (itraconazole) increase the concentration of **haloperidol**. Moderate Study

‣ **Haloperidol** is predicted to decrease the effects of dopamine receptor agonists. Avoid. Moderate Theoretical → Also see TABLE 8 p. 1430 → Also see TABLE 9 p. 1431 → Also see TABLE 10 p. 1431

‣ **Haloperidol** potentially opposes the effects of glycerol phenylbutyrate. Moderate Theoretical

‣ HIV-protease inhibitors (ritonavir) are predicted to increase the exposure to **haloperidol**. Severe Theoretical

‣ **Haloperidol** decreases the effects of levodopa. Severe Study → Also see TABLE 8 p. 1430

‣ Mitotane decreases the concentration of **haloperidol**. Adjust dose. Moderate Study

‣ Rifamycins (rifampicin) decrease the concentration of **haloperidol**. Adjust dose. Moderate Study

‣ **Haloperidol** potentially decreases the effects of sodium phenylbutyrate. Moderate Anecdotal

‣ SSRIs (fluoxetine) increase the concentration of **haloperidol**. Adjust dose. Moderate Anecdotal

‣ SSRIs (fluvoxamine) increase the concentration of **haloperidol**. Adjust dose. Moderate Study

‣ Venlafaxine slightly increases the exposure to **haloperidol**. Severe Study → Also see TABLE 9 p. 1431 → Also see TABLE 11 p. 1431

Heparin → see TABLE 16 p. 1433 (increased serum potassium), TABLE 3 p. 1429 (anticoagulant effects)

‣ Ranibizumab increases the risk of bleeding events when given with **heparin**. Severe Theoretical

Hepatitis B immunoglobulin → see immunoglobulins

HIV-protease inhibitors → see TABLE 9 p. 1431 (QT-interval prolongation)

atazanavir · darunavir · fosamprenavir · lopinavir · ritonavir · saquinavir · tipranavir

‣ Caution on concurrent use of **atazanavir, lopinavir with ritonavir**, and **ritonavir** with drugs that prolong the PR interval.

‣ Concurrent use of **saquinavir** with drugs that prolong the PR interval is contra-indicated.

‣ Caution with concurrent use of **tipranavir** with drugs that increase risk of bleeding.

‣ **HIV-protease inhibitors** are predicted to increase the exposure to abemaciclib. Avoid or adjust **abemaciclib** dose, p. 1009. Severe Study

‣ **HIV-protease inhibitors** are predicted to increase the exposure to acalabrutinib. Avoid. Severe Study

‣ HIV-protease inhibitors (lopinavir, ritonavir, saquinavir) are predicted to increase the exposure to afatinib. Separate administration by 12 hours. Moderate Study

‣ **Ritonavir** is predicted to decrease the exposure to agomelatine. Moderate Theoretical

‣ **Ritonavir** decreases the exposure to albendazole. Moderate Study

‣ **HIV-protease inhibitors** are predicted to markedly increase the exposure to aldosterone antagonists (eplerenone). Avoid. Severe Study

‣ HIV-protease inhibitors (ritonavir, saquinavir) are predicted to increase the exposure to aliskiren. Moderate Theoretical

‣ **HIV-protease inhibitors** are predicted to moderately increase the exposure to alpha blockers (alfuzosin, tamsulosin). Use with caution or avoid. Moderate Study

‣ **HIV-protease inhibitors** are predicted to increase the exposure to alpha blockers (doxazosin). Moderate Study

‣ HIV-protease inhibitors (ritonavir, tipranavir) are predicted to increase the exposure to amfetamines. Severe Theoretical

‣ **Ritonavir** decreases the exposure to aminophylline. Adjust dose. Moderate Study

‣ **Ritonavir** is predicted to decrease the exposure to anaesthetics, local (ropivacaine). Moderate Theoretical

‣ Oral antacids are predicted to decrease the absorption of oral **atazanavir**. **Atazanavir** should be taken 2 hours before or 1 hour after antacids. Severe Theoretical

‣ Oral antacids are predicted to decrease the absorption of oral **tipranavir**. Separate administration by 2 hours. Moderate Study

‣ **HIV-protease inhibitors** are predicted to increase the exposure to anti-androgens (apalutamide). Mild Study → Also see TABLE 9 p. 1431

‣ HIV-protease inhibitors (lopinavir, ritonavir, saquinavir) are predicted to increase the exposure to anti-androgens (darolutamide). Monitor and adjust dose. Moderate Theoretical

‣ **HIV-protease inhibitors** are predicted to increase the exposure to antiarrhythmics (amiodarone). Avoid. Severe Theoretical → Also see TABLE 9 p. 1431

‣ **HIV-protease inhibitors** are predicted to increase the exposure to antiarrhythmics (disopyramide). Severe Theoretical → Also see TABLE 9 p. 1431

‣ **HIV-protease inhibitors** very markedly increase the exposure to antiarrhythmics (dronedarone). Avoid. Severe Study → Also see TABLE 9 p. 1431

‣ **Ritonavir** is predicted to increase the exposure to antiarrhythmics (flecainide). Avoid or monitor adverse effects. Severe Theoretical

‣ **HIV-protease inhibitors** are predicted to increase the exposure to antiarrhythmics (lidocaine). Avoid. Severe Study

▸ **HIV-protease inhibitors** are predicted to increase the exposure to antiarrhythmics (propafenone). Monitor and adjust dose. Severe Study

▸ **HIV-protease inhibitors** are predicted to increase the exposure to anticholinesterases, centrally acting (galantamine). Monitor and adjust dose. Moderate Study

▸ **HIV-protease inhibitors** are predicted to increase the exposure to antiepileptics (carbamazepine) and antiepileptics (carbamazepine) are predicted to decrease the exposure to **HIV-protease inhibitors**. Monitor and adjust dose. Severe Theoretical

▸ **HIV-protease inhibitors** are predicted to affect the exposure to antiepileptics (fosphenytoin, phenytoin) and antiepileptics (fosphenytoin, phenytoin) decrease the concentration of **HIV-protease inhibitors**. Severe Theoretical

▸ **Ritonavir** slightly decreases the exposure to antiepileptics (lamotrigine). Severe Study

▸ **HIV-protease inhibitors** are predicted to very slightly increase the exposure to antiepileptics (perampanel). Mild Study

▸ **HIV-protease inhibitors** are predicted to affect the concentration of antiepileptics (phenobarbital, primidone) and antiepileptics (phenobarbital, primidone) are predicted to decrease the concentration of **HIV-protease inhibitors**. Severe Theoretical

▸ **Ritonavir** is predicted to decrease the concentration of antiepileptics (valproate). Severe Anecdotal

▸ Antifungals, azoles (fluconazole) slightly increase the exposure to **tipranavir**. Avoid or adjust dose. Moderate Study

▸ Antifungals, azoles (miconazole) are predicted to increase the concentration of **HIV-protease inhibitors**. Use with caution and adjust dose. Moderate Theoretical

▸ Antifungals, azoles (posaconazole) are predicted to increase the exposure to **HIV-protease inhibitors**. Moderate Study

▸ **HIV-protease inhibitors** are predicted to increase the exposure to antifungals, azoles (isavuconazole). Avoid or monitor adverse effects. Severe Study

▸ **HIV-protease inhibitors** are predicted to increase the exposure to antifungals, azoles (itraconazole). Use with caution and adjust dose. Severe Study

▸ **HIV-protease inhibitors** are predicted to increase the exposure to antifungals, azoles (ketoconazole). Use with caution and adjust dose. Moderate Study

▸ **HIV-protease inhibitors** are predicted to affect the exposure to antifungals, azoles (voriconazole) and antifungals, azoles (voriconazole) potentially affect the exposure to **HIV-protease inhibitors**. Severe Study → Also see TABLE 9 p. 1431

▸ **HIV-protease inhibitors** are predicted to increase the exposure to antihistamines, non-sedating (mizolastine). Avoid. Severe Study

▸ **HIV-protease inhibitors** are predicted to increase the exposure to antihistamines, non-sedating (rupatadine). Avoid. Moderate Study

▸ **HIV-protease inhibitors** decrease the exposure to antimalarials (atovaquone). Avoid if boosted with ritonavir. Moderate Study

▸ **HIV-protease inhibitors** are predicted to increase the concentration of antimalarials (piperaquine). Severe Theoretical

▸ **HIV-protease inhibitors** are predicted to decrease the exposure to antimalarials (proguanil). Avoid. Moderate Study

▸ **HIV-protease inhibitors** are predicted to affect the exposure to antimalarials (quinine). Severe Study → Also see TABLE 9 p. 1431

▸ **HIV-protease inhibitors** are predicted to slightly increase the exposure to antipsychotics, second generation (aripiprazole). Adjust **aripiprazole** dose, p. 415. Moderate Study

▸ **HIV-protease inhibitors** are predicted to moderately increase the exposure to antipsychotics, second generation (cariprazine). Avoid. Severe Study

▸ **Ritonavir** is predicted to affect the exposure to antipsychotics, second generation (clozapine). Avoid. Severe Theoretical

▸ **HIV-protease inhibitors** are predicted to increase the exposure to antipsychotics, second generation (lurasidone, quetiapine). Avoid. Severe Study

▸ **Ritonavir** is predicted to decrease the exposure to antipsychotics, second generation (olanzapine). Monitor and adjust dose. Moderate Study

▸ **HIV-protease inhibitors** are predicted to increase the exposure to antipsychotics, second generation (risperidone). Adjust dose. Moderate Study → Also see TABLE 9 p. 1431

▸ **HIV-protease inhibitors** are predicted to increase the exposure to avapritinib. Avoid. Moderate Study

▸ **HIV-protease inhibitors** are predicted to increase the exposure to axitinib. Avoid or adjust dose. Moderate Study

▸ **HIV-protease inhibitors** are predicted to increase the exposure to bedaquiline. Avoid prolonged use. Mild Study → Also see TABLE 9 p. 1431

▸ **HIV-protease inhibitors** moderately increase the exposure to benzodiazepines (alprazolam). Avoid. Moderate Study

▸ **Ritonavir** is predicted to increase the exposure to benzodiazepines (diazepam, flurazepam). Avoid. Moderate Theoretical

▸ **HIV-protease inhibitors** are predicted to markedly to very markedly increase the exposure to benzodiazepines (midazolam). Avoid or adjust dose. Severe Study

▸ HIV-protease inhibitors **(lopinavir, ritonavir, saquinavir)** are predicted to increase the exposure to beta blockers, non-selective (nadolol). Moderate Study

▸ **Ritonavir** is predicted to increase the exposure to beta blockers, selective (metoprolol). Moderate Study

▸ **HIV-protease inhibitors** are predicted to increase the exposure to beta$_2$ agonists (salmeterol). Avoid. Severe Study

▸ **Atazanavir** moderately increases the exposure to bictegravir. Avoid. Severe Study

▸ HIV-protease inhibitors **(lopinavir, ritonavir, saquinavir)** are predicted to increase the exposure to bictegravir. Use with caution or avoid. Moderate Theoretical

▸ **HIV-protease inhibitors** slightly increase the exposure to bortezomib. Moderate Study

▸ **HIV-protease inhibitors** are predicted to markedly increase the exposure to bosutinib. Avoid or adjust dose. Severe Study → Also see TABLE 9 p. 1431

▸ **HIV-protease inhibitors** are predicted to increase the exposure to brigatinib. Adjust **brigatinib** dose, p. 1015. Severe Study

▸ **Ritonavir** is predicted to decrease the exposure to bupropion. Moderate Study

▸ **HIV-protease inhibitors** are predicted to increase the exposure to buspirone. Adjust **buspirone** dose, p. 360. Severe Study

▸ **HIV-protease inhibitors** slightly increase the exposure to cabozantinib. Moderate Study → Also see TABLE 9 p. 1431

▸ **Ritonavir** is predicted to moderately increase the clearance of caffeine citrate. Monitor and adjust dose. Moderate Study

▸ **HIV-protease inhibitors** are predicted to increase the exposure to calcium channel blockers (amlodipine, felodipine, lacidipine, nicardipine, nifedipine, nimodipine). Monitor and adjust dose. Moderate Study

▸ **HIV-protease inhibitors** are predicted to increase the exposure to calcium channel blockers (diltiazem, verapamil). Severe Study

▸ **HIV-protease inhibitors** are predicted to markedly increase the exposure to calcium channel blockers (lercanidipine). Avoid. Severe Study

▸ **HIV-protease inhibitors** are predicted to increase the exposure to cannabidiol. Avoid or adjust dose. Mild Study

▸ **HIV-protease inhibitors** are predicted to increase the exposure to ceritinib. Avoid or adjust **ceritinib** dose, p. 1017. Severe Study → Also see TABLE 9 p. 1431

▸ **HIV-protease inhibitors** increase the concentration of ciclosporin. Severe Study

▸ **HIV-protease inhibitors** are predicted to moderately increase the exposure to cilostazol. Adjust **cilostazol** dose, p. 248. Moderate Study

▸ **HIV-protease inhibitors** are predicted to moderately increase the exposure to cinacalcet. Adjust dose. Moderate Study

▸ **HIV-protease inhibitors** are predicted to markedly increase the exposure to cobimetinib. Avoid or monitor for toxicity. Severe Study

▸ **HIV-protease inhibitors** are predicted to increase the exposure to colchicine. Avoid potent CYP3A4 inhibitors or adjust **colchicine** dose, p. 1166. Severe Study

▸ **Atazanavir** (unboosted) increases the exposure to combined hormonal contraceptives. Adjust dose. Severe Study

HIV-protease inhibitors (continued)

▸ **Ritonavir** is predicted to decrease the efficacy of combined hormonal contraceptives. For FSRH guidance, see Contraceptives, interactions p. 840. Severe Study

▸ **HIV-protease inhibitors** are predicted to increase the exposure to corticosteroids (beclometasone) (risk with beclometasone is likely to be lower than with other corticosteroids). Moderate Theoretical

▸ **HIV-protease inhibitors** are predicted to increase the exposure to corticosteroids (betamethasone, budesonide, ciclesonide, deflazacort, dexamethasone, fludrocortisone, fluticasone, hydrocortisone, methylprednisolone, mometasone, prednisolone, triamcinolone). Avoid or monitor adverse effects. Severe Study

▸ **HIV-protease inhibitors** are predicted to affect the anticoagulant effect of coumarins. Moderate Study

▸ **HIV-protease inhibitors** are predicted to moderately increase the exposure to crizotinib. Avoid. Moderate Study → Also see TABLE 9 p. 1431

▸ **HIV-protease inhibitors** are predicted to increase the exposure to dabrafenib. Use with caution or avoid. Moderate Study

▸ **HIV-protease inhibitors** are predicted to markedly to very markedly increase the exposure to darifenacin. Avoid. Severe Study

▸ **Dasabuvir** (with ombitasvir, paritaprevir, and ritonavir) decreases the concentration of **darunavir**. Avoid or adjust dose. Moderate Study

▸ **HIV-protease inhibitors** are predicted to markedly increase the exposure to dasatinib. Avoid or adjust dose—consult product literature. Severe Study → Also see TABLE 9 p. 1431

▸ **HIV-protease inhibitors** very slightly increase the exposure to delamanid. Severe Study → Also see TABLE 9 p. 1431

▸ **Ritonavir** is predicted to decrease the efficacy of desogestrel. For FSRH guidance, see Contraceptives, interactions p. 840. Severe Theoretical

▸ **HIV-protease inhibitors** are predicted to moderately increase the exposure to dienogest. Moderate Study

▸ **Ritonavir** increases the concentration of digoxin. Adjust dose and monitor concentration. Severe Study

▸ **HIV-protease inhibitors** are predicted to increase the exposure to dipeptidylpeptidase-4 inhibitors (saxagliptin). Moderate Study

▸ **Fosamprenavir** boosted with ritonavir slightly decreases the exposure to dolutegravir. Avoid if resistant to HIV-integrase inhibitors. Severe Study

▸ **Tipranavir** moderately decreases the exposure to dolutegravir. Refer to specialist literature. Severe Study

▸ **HIV-protease inhibitors** increase the risk of QT-prolongation when given with domperidone. Avoid. Severe Study

▸ **HIV-protease inhibitors** increase the exposure to dopamine receptor agonists (bromocriptine). Severe Study

▸ **HIV-protease inhibitors** are predicted to increase the concentration of dopamine receptor agonists (cabergoline). Moderate Anecdotal

▸ **HIV-protease inhibitors** are predicted to increase the exposure to dronabinol. Adjust dose. Mild Study

▸ **Ritonavir** is predicted to decrease the exposure to duloxetine. Moderate Theoretical

▸ **HIV-protease inhibitors** are predicted to increase the exposure to dutasteride. Monitor adverse effects and adjust dose. Moderate Theoretical

▸ **HIV-protease inhibitors** is predicted to increase the exposure to elexacaftor. Adjust tezacaftor with ivacaftor and elexacaftor p. 311 dose with potent CYP3A4 inhibitors. Severe Study

▸ **HIV-protease inhibitors** are predicted to increase the exposure to eliglustat. Avoid or adjust dose—consult product literature. Severe Study

▸ **HIV-protease inhibitors** (atazanavir, lopinavir) boosted with ritonavir increase the concentration of elvitegravir. Refer to specialist literature. Moderate Study

▸ **HIV-protease inhibitors** are predicted to increase the exposure to encorafenib. Avoid or monitor. Severe Study → Also see TABLE 9 p. 1431

▸ **HIV-protease inhibitors** are predicted to increase the exposure to endothelin receptor antagonists (bosentan). Severe Study

▸ **HIV-protease inhibitors** are predicted to increase the exposure to endothelin receptor antagonists (macitentan). Moderate Study

▸ **HIV-protease inhibitors** are predicted to increase the exposure to entrectinib. Avoid potent CYP3A4 inhibitors or adjust entrectinib dose, p. 1023. Severe Study → Also see TABLE 9 p. 1431

▸ **HIV-protease inhibitors** are predicted to increase the risk of ergotism when given with ergometrine. Avoid. Severe Theoretical

▸ **HIV-protease inhibitors** are predicted to increase the risk of ergotism when given with ergotamine. Avoid. Severe Theoretical

▸ **HIV-protease inhibitors** are predicted to slightly increase the exposure to erlotinib. Use with caution and adjust dose. Moderate Study

▸ **HIV-protease inhibitors** are predicted to increase the exposure to esketamine. Adjust dose. Moderate Study

▸ **Ritonavir** is predicted to decrease the efficacy of etonogestrel. For FSRH guidance, see Contraceptives, interactions p. 840. Severe Theoretical

▸ **HIV-protease inhibitors** are predicted to increase the concentration of everolimus. Avoid. Severe Study

▸ **Ritonavir** is predicted to increase the exposure to factor XA inhibitors (apixaban). Avoid. Severe Theoretical

▸ **HIV-protease inhibitors** (lopinavir, ritonavir, saquinavir) are predicted to slightly increase the exposure to factor XA inhibitors (edoxaban). Severe Theoretical

▸ **Ritonavir** moderately increases the exposure to factor XA inhibitors (rivaroxaban). Avoid. Severe Study

▸ **HIV-protease inhibitors** are predicted to moderately increase the exposure to fesoterodine. Adjust fesoterodine dose with potent CYP3A4 inhibitors; avoid in hepatic and renal impairment, p. 822. Severe Study

▸ **HIV-protease inhibitors** (lopinavir, ritonavir, saquinavir) are predicted to increase the exposure to fidaxomicin. Avoid. Moderate Study

▸ **HIV-protease inhibitors** are predicted to moderately increase the exposure to fostamatinib. Monitor adverse effects and adjust dose. Moderate Study

▸ **HIV-protease inhibitors** are predicted to increase the exposure to gefitinib. Moderate Study

▸ **HIV-protease inhibitors** are predicted to increase the exposure to gilteritinib. Moderate Study

▸ **HIV-protease inhibitors** are predicted to moderately increase the exposure to glasdegib. Use with caution or avoid. Moderate Study → Also see TABLE 9 p. 1431

▸ **HIV-protease inhibitors** (atazanavir, darunavir, lopinavir) boosted with ritonavir increase the exposure to glecaprevir. Avoid. Severe Study

▸ **Ritonavir** increases the exposure to glecaprevir. Avoid. Severe Study

▸ **HIV-protease inhibitors** are predicted to moderately to markedly increase the exposure to grazoprevir. Avoid. Severe Study

▸ **HIV-protease inhibitors** are predicted to increase the exposure to guanfacine. Adjust guanfacine dose, p. 372. Moderate Study

▸ **H₂ receptor antagonists** decrease the exposure to **atazanavir**. Monitor and adjust dose. Moderate Study

▸ **Ritonavir** is predicted to increase the exposure to haloperidol. Severe Theoretical

▸ **Ritonavir** is predicted to decrease the effects of hormone replacement therapy. Moderate Anecdotal

▸ **HIV-protease inhibitors** are predicted to very markedly increase the exposure to ibrutinib. Avoid potent CYP3A4 inhibitors or adjust ibrutinib dose, p. 1027. Severe Study

▸ **HIV-protease inhibitors** are predicted to increase the exposure to imatinib. Moderate Study

▸ **HIV-protease inhibitors** are predicted to increase the risk of toxicity when given with irinotecan. Avoid. Moderate Study

▸ **Ritonavir** is predicted to decrease the exposure to iron chelators (deferasirox). Monitor serum ferritin and adjust dose. Moderate Theoretical

▸ **HIV-protease inhibitors** are predicted to increase the exposure to ivabradine. Avoid. Severe Study

▸ **HIV-protease inhibitors** are predicted to increase the exposure to ivacaftor. Adjust ivacaftor p. 309 or lumacaftor with ivacaftor p. 310 or tezacaftor with ivacaftor p. 311 or tezacaftor with ivacaftor and elexacftor p. 311 dose with potent CYP3A4 inhibitors. Severe Study

HIV-protease inhibitors are predicted to increase the exposure to lapatinib. Avoid. Moderate Study → Also see **TABLE 9** p. 1431

HIV-protease inhibitors are predicted to moderately increase the exposure to larotrectinib. Avoid or adjust **larotrectinib** dose, p. 1031. Moderate Study

Tipranavir boosted with ritonavir is predicted to decrease the exposure to ledipasvir. Avoid. Severe Theoretical

▸ HIV-protease inhibitors **(atazanavir, lopinavir)** boosted with ritonavir are predicted to increase the concentration of letermovir. Moderate Study

▸ **Ritonavir** is predicted to decrease the concentration of letermovir. Moderate Theoretical

▸ **Ritonavir** is predicted to decrease the efficacy of levonorgestrel. For FSRH guidance, see Contraceptives, interactions p. 840. Severe Theoretical

▸ **HIV-protease inhibitors** are predicted to markedly increase the exposure to lomitapide. Avoid. Severe Study

▸ **HIV-protease inhibitors** are predicted to increase the exposure to lorlatinib. Avoid or adjust **lorlatinib** dose, p. 1033. Severe Study

▸ Macrolides **(clarithromycin)** increase the exposure to **saquinavir** and **saquinavir** increases the exposure to macrolides **(clarithromycin)**. Avoid. Severe Study → Also see **TABLE 9** p. 1431

▸ Macrolides **(erythromycin)** are predicted to increase the exposure to **saquinavir**. Avoid. Severe Theoretical → Also see **TABLE 9** p. 1431

▸ **Atazanavir** is predicted to increase the exposure to macrolides **(clarithromycin)**. Adjust dose in renal impairment. Severe Study

▸ **Ritonavir** increases the exposure to macrolides **(clarithromycin)**. Adjust dose in renal impairment. Severe Study

▸ **Tipranavir** boosted with ritonavir increases the exposure to macrolides **(clarithromycin)** and macrolides **(clarithromycin)** increase the exposure to **tipranavir** boosted with ritonavir. Monitor; adjust dose in renal impairment. Severe Study

▸ HIV-protease inhibitors **(darunavir, fosamprenavir, lopinavir)** boosted with ritonavir are predicted to increase the exposure to macrolides **(clarithromycin)**. Adjust dose in renal impairment. Severe Study

▸ HIV-protease inhibitors **(atazanavir, darunavir, fosamprenavir, lopinavir, saquinavir, tipranavir)** are predicted to increase the exposure to macrolides **(erythromycin)**. Severe Theoretical

▸ **Darunavir** boosted with ritonavir markedly increases the exposure to maraviroc. Refer to specialist literature. Severe Study

▸ Maraviroc potentially decreases the exposure to **fosamprenavir** and **fosamprenavir** potentially decreases the exposure to maraviroc. Avoid. Severe Study

▸ HIV-protease inhibitors **(atazanavir, saquinavir)** moderately to markedly increase the exposure to maraviroc. Refer to specialist literature. Severe Study

▸ **Lopinavir** boosted with ritonavir moderately increases the exposure to maraviroc. Refer to specialist literature. Severe Study

▸ **Ritonavir** markedly increases the exposure to maraviroc. Refer to specialist literature. Severe Study

▸ **HIV-protease inhibitors** are predicted to increase the exposure to meglitinides **(repaglinide)**. Moderate Study

▸ **Ritonavir** is predicted to decrease the exposure to melatonin. Moderate Theoretical

▸ **Ritonavir** is predicted to increase the clearance of mexiletine. Monitor and adjust dose. Moderate Study

▸ **HIV-protease inhibitors** are predicted to very markedly increase the exposure to midostaurin. Avoid or monitor for toxicity. Severe Study

▸ **HIV-protease inhibitors** are predicted to increase the exposure to mirabegron. Adjust **mirabegron** dose in hepatic and renal impairment, p. 825. Moderate Study

▸ **HIV-protease inhibitors** are predicted to increase the exposure to mirtazapine. Moderate Study

▸ **HIV-protease inhibitors** are predicted to increase the exposure to modafinil. Mild Theoretical

▸ HIV-protease inhibitors **(lopinavir, ritonavir, saquinavir)** are predicted to increase the risk of neutropenia when given with

monoclonal antibodies **(brentuximab vedotin)**. Monitor and adjust dose. Severe Study

▸ **HIV-protease inhibitors** are predicted to increase the exposure to monoclonal antibodies **(polatuzumab vedotin)**. Moderate Study

▸ **HIV-protease inhibitors** are predicted to increase the exposure to monoclonal antibodies **(trastuzumab emtansine)**. Avoid. Severe Theoretical

▸ **HIV-protease inhibitors** are predicted to increase the exposure to naldemedine. Avoid or monitor. Moderate Study

▸ **HIV-protease inhibitors** are predicted to markedly increase the exposure to naloxegol. Avoid. Severe Study

▸ **HIV-protease inhibitors** are predicted to increase the exposure to neratinib. Avoid or adjust **neratinib** dose, p. 1034. Severe Study

▸ **HIV-protease inhibitors** are predicted to markedly increase the exposure to neurokinin-1 receptor antagonists **(aprepitant)**. Moderate Study

▸ **HIV-protease inhibitors** are predicted to increase the exposure to neurokinin-1 receptor antagonists **(fosaprepitant)**. Moderate Theoretical

▸ **HIV-protease inhibitors** are predicted to increase the exposure to neurokinin-1 receptor antagonists **(netupitant)**. Moderate Study

▸ **HIV-protease inhibitors** are predicted to moderately increase the exposure to nilotinib. Avoid. Severe Study → Also see **TABLE 9** p. 1431

▸ HIV-protease inhibitors **(lopinavir, ritonavir, saquinavir)** are predicted to increase the exposure to nintedanib. Moderate Study

▸ **HIV-protease inhibitors** are predicted to increase the exposure to nitisinone. Adjust dose. Moderate Theoretical

▸ NNRTIs **(efavirenz)** decrease the exposure to **HIV-protease inhibitors**. Refer to specialist literature. Severe Study → Also see **TABLE 9** p. 1431

▸ NNRTIs **(etravirine)** increase the exposure to **fosamprenavir** boosted with ritonavir. Refer to specialist literature. Moderate Study

▸ NNRTIs **(nevirapine)** decrease the exposure to **HIV-protease inhibitors**. Refer to specialist literature. Moderate Study

▸ **HIV-protease inhibitors** are predicted to increase the exposure to NNRTIs **(doravirine)**. Mild Study

▸ **Tipranavir** decreases the exposure to NNRTIs **(etravirine)**. Avoid. Severe Study

▸ **Ritonavir** is predicted to decrease the efficacy of norethisterone. For FSRH guidance, see Contraceptives, interactions p. 840. Severe Anecdotal

▸ **Tipranavir** slightly decreases the exposure to NRTIs **(abacavir)**. Avoid. Severe Study

▸ **Tipranavir** slightly decreases the exposure to NRTIs **(zidovudine)**. Avoid. Moderate Study

▸ **HIV-protease inhibitors** are predicted to increase the exposure to olaparib. Avoid potent CYP3A4 inhibitors or adjust **olaparib** dose, p. 1051. Moderate Study

▸ Ombitasvir (in fixed-dose combination with dasabuvir) decreases the concentration of **darunavir**. Avoid or adjust dose. Moderate Study

▸ **HIV-protease inhibitors** are predicted to increase the exposure to opioids **(alfentanil, buprenorphine, fentanyl, oxycodone)**. Monitor and adjust dose. Severe Study

▸ **HIV-protease inhibitors** boosted with ritonavir are predicted to decrease the exposure to opioids **(methadone)**. Moderate Study → Also see **TABLE 9** p. 1431

▸ **Ritonavir** is predicted to decrease the concentration of opioids **(morphine)**. Moderate Theoretical

▸ **Ritonavir** increases the risk of CNS toxicity when given with opioids **(pethidine)**. Avoid. Severe Study

▸ **HIV-protease inhibitors** are predicted to increase the exposure to ospemifene. Avoid in poor CYP2C9 metabolisers. Moderate Study

▸ **HIV-protease inhibitors** are predicted to increase the exposure to oxybutynin. Mild Study

▸ **HIV-protease inhibitors** are predicted to increase the exposure to palbociclib. Avoid or adjust **palbociclib** dose, p. 1038. Severe Study

▸ **HIV-protease inhibitors** are predicted to increase the exposure to panobinostat. Adjust **panobinostat** dose; in hepatic impairment avoid, p. 979. Moderate Study → Also see **TABLE 9** p. 1431

HIV-protease inhibitors (continued)

▸ **Atazanavir** boosted with ritonavir markedly increases the exposure to paritaprevir. Avoid or give unboosted. Moderate Study

▸ **Darunavir** boosted with ritonavir slightly decreases the exposure to paritaprevir. Avoid or give unboosted. Moderate Study

▸ HIV-protease inhibitors **(fosamprenavir, tipranavir)** boosted with ritonavir are predicted to increase the exposure to paritaprevir. Avoid. Severe Study

▸ **Lopinavir** boosted with ritonavir moderately to markedly increases the exposure to paritaprevir. Avoid. Severe Study

▸ **Saquinavir** is predicted to increase the exposure to paritaprevir (in fixed-dose combination). Avoid. Severe Study

▸ HIV-protease inhibitors are predicted to increase the exposure to pazopanib. Avoid or adjust **pazopanib** dose, p. 1039. Moderate Study → Also see TABLE 9 p. 1431

▸ HIV-protease inhibitors are predicted to increase the exposure to phosphodiesterase type-5 inhibitors **(avanafil, vardenafil).** Avoid. Severe Study → Also see TABLE 9 p. 1431

▸ HIV-protease inhibitors are predicted to increase the exposure to phosphodiesterase type-5 inhibitors **(sildenafil).** Avoid potent CYP3A4 inhibitors or adjust **sildenafil** dose, p. 860. Severe Study → Also see TABLE 9 p. 1431

▸ HIV-protease inhibitors are predicted to increase the exposure to phosphodiesterase type-5 inhibitors **(tadalafil).** Use with caution or avoid. Severe Study

▸ HIV-protease inhibitors **(atazanavir, lopinavir)** boosted with ritonavir increase the exposure to pibrentasvir. Avoid. Severe Study

▸ **Ritonavir** potentially increases the exposure to pibrentasvir. Severe Theoretical

▸ **Saquinavir** is predicted to increase the exposure to pibrentasvir. Moderate Theoretical

▸ HIV-protease inhibitors are predicted to increase the exposure to pimozide. Avoid. Severe Study → Also see TABLE 9 p. 1431

▸ **Ritonavir** is predicted to decrease the exposure to pirfenidone. Moderate Theoretical

▸ HIV-protease inhibitors are predicted to slightly increase the exposure to ponatinib. Monitor and adjust **ponatinib** dose, p. 1040. Moderate Study

▸ HIV-protease inhibitors are predicted to moderately increase the exposure to praziquantel. Mild Study

▸ HIV-protease inhibitors given with carbimazole are predicted to increase the exposure to propiverine. Adjust starting dose. Moderate Theoretical

▸ Proton pump inhibitors decrease the exposure to **atazanavir.** Avoid or adjust dose. Severe Study

▸ Proton pump inhibitors increase the exposure to **saquinavir.** Avoid. Severe Study

▸ **Tipranavir** decreases the exposure to proton pump inhibitors. Avoid. Severe Study

▸ **Atazanavir** increases the exposure to raltegravir (high-dose). Avoid. Moderate Study

▸ **Darunavir** increases the risk of rash when given with raltegravir. Moderate Study

▸ **Fosamprenavir** boosted with ritonavir decreases the exposure to raltegravir and raltegravir decreases the exposure to **fosamprenavir** boosted with ritonavir. Avoid. Severe Study

▸ **Tipranavir** boosted with ritonavir is predicted to decrease the exposure to raltegravir (high-dose). Avoid. Moderate Study

▸ HIV-protease inhibitors are predicted to increase the exposure to ranolazine. Avoid. Severe Study → Also see TABLE 9 p. 1431

▸ HIV-protease inhibitors are predicted to increase the exposure to reboxetine. Avoid. Moderate Study

▸ HIV-protease inhibitors are predicted to increase the exposure to regorafenib. Avoid. Moderate Study

▸ HIV-protease inhibitors are predicted to increase the exposure to retinoids (alitretinoin). Adjust **alitretinoin** dose, p. 1305. Moderate Theoretical

▸ HIV-protease inhibitors are predicted to increase the exposure to ribociclib. Avoid or adjust **ribociclib** dose, p. 1042. Moderate Study → Also see TABLE 9 p. 1431

▸ Rifamycins **(rifampicin)** slightly decrease the exposure to **ritonavir.** Severe Study

▸ Rifamycins **(rifampicin)** are predicted to decrease the exposure to **tipranavir.** Avoid. Severe Study

▸ Rifamycins **(rifampicin)** are predicted to moderately to markedly decrease the exposure to HIV-protease inhibitors **(atazanavir, darunavir, fosamprenavir, lopinavir, saquinavir).** Avoid. Severe Study

▸ **Ritonavir** markedly increases the exposure to rifamycins (rifabutin). Avoid or adjust dose. Severe Study

▸ HIV-protease inhibitors **(atazanavir, darunavir, fosamprenavir, lopinavir, saquinavir, tipranavir)** boosted with ritonavir increase the exposure to rifamycins **(rifabutin).** Monitor and adjust dose. Severe Study

▸ **Ritonavir** is predicted to increase the exposure to riociguat. Adjust dose and monitor blood pressure. Moderate Theoretical

▸ HIV-protease inhibitors are predicted to increase the exposure to ruxolitinib. Adjust dose and monitor adverse effects. Moderate Study

▸ HIV-protease inhibitors are predicted to increase the exposure to siponimod. Avoid depending on other drugs taken—consult product literature. Severe Study

▸ HIV-protease inhibitors are predicted to increase the concentration of sirolimus. Avoid. Severe Study

▸ Sodium zirconium cyclosilicate is predicted to decrease the exposure to **HIV-protease inhibitors.** Separate administration by at least 2 hours. Moderate Theoretical

▸ **Tipranavir** is predicted to decrease the exposure to sofosbuvir. Avoid. Severe Theoretical

▸ HIV-protease inhibitors are predicted to increase the exposure to solifenacin. Adjust solifenacin p. 824 or tamsulosin with solifenacin p. 830 dose; avoid in hepatic and renal impairment. Severe Study

▸ HIV-protease inhibitors are predicted to moderately increase the exposure to SSRIs (dapoxetine). Avoid potent CYP3A4 inhibitors or adjust **dapoxetine**, p. 867. Severe Study

▸ St John's wort is predicted to decrease the exposure to **HIV-protease inhibitors.** Avoid. Severe Study

▸ HIV-protease inhibitors are predicted to increase the exposure to statins (atorvastatin). Avoid or adjust dose and monitor rhabdomyolysis. Severe Study

▸ HIV-protease inhibitors slightly to moderately increase the exposure to statins (rosuvastatin). Avoid or adjust dose. Severe Study

▸ HIV-protease inhibitors are predicted to increase the exposure to statins (simvastatin). Avoid. Severe Study

▸ HIV-protease inhibitors are predicted to slightly increase the exposure to sunitinib. Avoid or adjust **sunitinib** dose, p. 1044. Moderate Study → Also see TABLE 9 p. 1431

▸ HIV-protease inhibitors are predicted to increase the concentration of tacrolimus. Monitor and adjust dose. Severe Study

▸ HIV-protease inhibitors **(lopinavir, ritonavir, saquinavir)** are predicted to slightly increase the exposure to talazoparib. Avoid or adjust **talazoparib** dose, p. 1052. Severe Study

▸ HIV-protease inhibitors are predicted to increase the exposure to taxanes (cabazitaxel). Avoid. Severe Study

▸ HIV-protease inhibitors are predicted to moderately increase the exposure to taxanes (docetaxel). Avoid or adjust dose. Severe Study

▸ HIV-protease inhibitors are predicted to increase the exposure to taxanes (paclitaxel). Severe Theoretical

▸ HIV-protease inhibitors are predicted to increase the concentration of temsirolimus. Avoid. Severe Theoretical

▸ HIV-protease inhibitors **(atazanavir, darunavir, lopinavir)** increase the exposure to tenofovir alafenamide. Avoid or adjust dose. Moderate Study

▸ **Tipranavir** is predicted to decrease the exposure to tenofovir alafenamide. Avoid. Moderate Theoretical

▸ HIV-protease inhibitors **(atazanavir, darunavir, lopinavir)** are predicted to increase the risk of renal impairment when given with tenofovir disoproxil. Severe Anecdotal

▸ HIV-protease inhibitors are predicted to increase the exposure to tezacaftor. Adjust tezacaftor with ivacaftor p. 311 or tezacaftor with ivacaftor and elexacftor p. 311 dose with potent CYP3A4 inhibitors. [Severe] Study

Ritonavir is predicted to decrease the exposure to theophylline. Adjust dose. [Moderate] Study

HIV-protease inhibitors **(lopinavir, ritonavir, saquinavir)** are predicted to increase the exposure to thrombin inhibitors **(dabigatran)**. Avoid. [Severe] Theoretical

Ritonavir decreases the concentration of thyroid hormones **(levothyroxine)**. MHRA advises monitor TSH for at least one month after starting or stopping ritonavir. [Moderate] Anecdotal

HIV-protease inhibitors are predicted to markedly increase the exposure to ticagrelor. Avoid. [Severe] Study

Ritonavir moderately decreases the exposure to tizanidine. [Mild] Study

HIV-protease inhibitors are predicted to increase the exposure to tofacitinib. Adjust **tofacitinib** dose, p. 1154. [Moderate] Study

HIV-protease inhibitors are predicted to increase the exposure to tolterodine. Avoid. [Severe] Study → Also see TABLE 9 p. 1431

HIV-protease inhibitors are predicted to increase the exposure to tolvaptan. Manufacturer advises caution or adjust **tolvaptan** dose with potent CYP3A4 inhibitors, p. 708. [Severe] Study

HIV-protease inhibitors **(lopinavir, ritonavir, saquinavir)** are predicted to increase the exposure to topotecan. [Severe] Study

HIV-protease inhibitors are predicted to increase the exposure to toremifene. [Moderate] Theoretical → Also see TABLE 9 p. 1431

HIV-protease inhibitors are predicted to increase the exposure to trabectedin. Avoid or adjust dose. [Severe] Theoretical

HIV-protease inhibitors **(lopinavir, ritonavir, saquinavir)** are predicted to increase the concentration of trametinib. [Moderate] Theoretical

HIV-protease inhibitors are predicted to moderately increase the exposure to trazodone. Avoid or adjust dose. [Moderate] Study

HIV-protease inhibitors **(ritonavir, tipranavir)** are predicted to increase the exposure to tricyclic antidepressants. [Moderate] Theoretical

HIV-protease inhibitors increase the exposure to triptans **(almotriptan)**. [Mild] Study

HIV-protease inhibitors are predicted to markedly increase the exposure to triptans **(eletriptan)**. Avoid. [Severe] Study

Lopinavir is predicted to increase the exposure to ulipristal. Avoid if used for uterine fibroids. [Severe] Study

Ritonavir decreases the efficacy of ulipristal. For FSRH guidance, see Contraceptives, interactions p. 840. [Severe] Anecdotal

HIV-protease inhibitors are predicted to increase the exposure to upadacitinib. Use with caution or avoid. [Severe] Study

Tipranavir is predicted to increase the exposure to velpatasvir. [Severe] Theoretical

HIV-protease inhibitors are predicted to increase the exposure to vemurafenib. [Severe] Theoretical → Also see TABLE 9 p. 1431

HIV-protease inhibitors are predicted to increase the exposure to venetoclax. Avoid or adjust dose—consult product literature. [Severe] Study

HIV-protease inhibitors are predicted to increase the exposure to venlafaxine. [Moderate] Study → Also see TABLE 9 p. 1431

HIV-protease inhibitors are predicted to increase the exposure to vinca alkaloids. [Severe] Theoretical → Also see TABLE 9 p. 1431

HIV-protease inhibitors are predicted to increase the exposure to vitamin D substances **(paricalcitol)**. [Moderate] Study

Atazanavir boosted with ritonavir increases the concentration of voxilaprevir. Avoid. [Severe] Study

Lopinavir boosted with ritonavir is predicted to increase the concentration of voxilaprevir. Avoid. [Severe] Theoretical

Tipranavir boosted with ritonavir is predicted to increase the concentration of voxilaprevir. [Severe] Theoretical

HIV-protease inhibitors are predicted to increase the exposure to zopiclone. Adjust dose. [Moderate] Theoretical

Homatropine → see TABLE 10 p. 1431 (antimuscarinics)

Hormone replacement therapy
▸ Antiepileptics **(carbamazepine, eslicarbazepine, fosphenytoin, oxcarbazepine, perampanel, phenobarbital, phenytoin, primidone, rufinamide, topiramate)** are predicted to decrease the effects of **hormone replacement therapy**. [Moderate] Anecdotal

▸ **Hormone replacement therapy** is predicted to alter the exposure to antiepileptics **(lamotrigine)**. [Moderate] Theoretical

▸ **Hormone replacement therapy** decreases the clearance of dopamine receptor agonists **(ropinirole)**. Monitor and adjust dose. [Moderate] Study

▸ Endothelin receptor antagonists **(bosentan)** are predicted to decrease the effects of **hormone replacement therapy**. [Moderate] Anecdotal

▸ HIV-protease inhibitors **(ritonavir)** are predicted to decrease the effects of **hormone replacement therapy**. [Moderate] Anecdotal

▸ **Hormone replacement therapy** is predicted to increase the risk of venous thromboembolism when given with lenalidomide. [Moderate] Theoretical

▸ **Hormone replacement therapy** is predicted to increase the exposure to MAO-B inhibitors **(selegiline)**. Avoid. [Moderate] Study

▸ Modafinil is predicted to decrease the effects of **hormone replacement therapy**. [Moderate] Anecdotal

▸ Neurokinin-1 receptor antagonists **(aprepitant, fosaprepitant)** are predicted to decrease the effects of **hormone replacement therapy**. [Moderate] Anecdotal

▸ NNRTIs **(efavirenz, nevirapine)** are predicted to decrease the effects of **hormone replacement therapy**. [Moderate] Anecdotal

▸ NSAIDs **(etoricoxib)** increase the exposure to **hormone replacement therapy**. [Moderate] Study

▸ **Hormone replacement therapy** potentially opposes the effects of ospemifene. Avoid. [Severe] Theoretical

▸ **Hormone replacement therapy** is predicted to increase the risk of venous thromboembolism when given with pomalidomide. [Severe] Theoretical

▸ **Hormone replacement therapy** potentially opposes the effects of raloxifene. Avoid. [Severe] Theoretical

▸ Rifamycins are predicted to decrease the effects of **hormone replacement therapy**. [Moderate] Anecdotal

▸ St John's wort is predicted to decrease the efficacy of **hormone replacement therapy**. [Moderate] Theoretical

▸ **Hormone replacement therapy** is predicted to increase the risk of venous thromboembolism when given with thalidomide. [Severe] Theoretical

▸ Oral **hormone replacement therapy** is predicted to decrease the effects of thyroid hormones. [Moderate] Theoretical

Hydralazine → see TABLE 8 p. 1430 (hypotension)
▸ Diazoxide increases the risk of severe hypotension when given with hydralazine. [Severe] Study → Also see TABLE 8 p. 1430

Hydrochlorothiazide → see thiazide diuretics

Hydrocortisone → see corticosteroids

Hydroflumethiazide → see thiazide diuretics

Hydromorphone → see opioids

Hydroxycarbamide → see TABLE 15 p. 1432 (myelosuppression)
▸ Live vaccines are predicted to increase the risk of generalised infection (possibly life-threatening) when given with hydroxycarbamide. Public Health England advises avoid (refer to Green Book). [Severe] Theoretical

Hydroxychloroquine
▸ **Hydroxychloroquine** is predicted to decrease the effects of agalsidase alfa. [Moderate] Theoretical

▸ **Hydroxychloroquine** is predicted to decrease the exposure to agalsidase beta. [Moderate] Theoretical

▸ Oral antacids decrease the absorption of oral **hydroxychloroquine**. Separate administration by at least 4 hours. [Moderate] Theoretical

▸ Calcium salts **(calcium carbonate)** decrease the absorption of **hydroxychloroquine**. Separate administration by at least 4 hours. [Moderate] Study

▸ **Hydroxychloroquine** is predicted to decrease the efficacy of oral cholera vaccine. [Moderate] Theoretical

▸ H₂ receptor antagonists **(cimetidine)** are predicted to decrease the clearance of **hydroxychloroquine**. [Moderate] Theoretical

▸ Lanthanum is predicted to decrease the absorption of **hydroxychloroquine**. Separate administration by at least 2 hours. [Moderate] Theoretical

▸ **Hydroxychloroquine** is predicted to decrease the exposure to laronidase. Avoid simultaneous administration. [Severe] Theoretical

A1

Interactions | Appendix 1

Interactions | Appendix 1

A1

Hydroxychloroquine (continued)
▶ **Hydroxychloroquine** is predicted to increase the risk of haematological toxicity when given with penicillamine. Avoid. Severe Theoretical
▶ **Hydroxychloroquine** is predicted to decrease efficacy rabies vaccine. Moderate Theoretical
▶ **Hydroxychloroquine** potentially decrease the effects of remdesivir. Avoid. Moderate Theoretical
Hydroxyzine → see antihistamines, sedating
Hyoscine → see TABLE 10 p. 1431 (antimuscarinics)
Ibandronate → see bisphosphonates
Ibrutinib → see TABLE 15 p. 1432 (myelosuppression), TABLE 4 p. 1429 (antiplatelet effects)

FOOD AND LIFESTYLE Avoid food or drink containing bitter (Seville) oranges as they are predicted to increase the exposure to ibrutinib.

▶ Anti-androgens (apalutamide, enzalutamide) are predicted to decrease the exposure to **ibrutinib**. Avoid or adjust **ibrutinib** dose, p. 1027. Severe Study
▶ Antiarrhythmics (amiodarone) are predicted to increase the exposure to **ibrutinib**. Adjust **ibrutinib** dose, p. 1027. Severe Theoretical
▶ Antiarrhythmics (dronedarone) are predicted to increase the exposure to **ibrutinib**. Adjust **ibrutinib** dose with moderate CYP3A4 inhibitors, p. 1027. Severe Study
▶ Antiepileptics (carbamazepine, fosphenytoin, phenobarbital, phenytoin, primidone) are predicted to decrease the exposure to **ibrutinib**. Avoid or adjust **ibrutinib** dose, p. 1027. Severe Study
▶ Antifungals, azoles (fluconazole, isavuconazole, posaconazole) are predicted to increase the exposure to **ibrutinib**. Adjust **ibrutinib** dose with moderate CYP3A4 inhibitors, p. 1027. Severe Study
▶ Antifungals, azoles (itraconazole, ketoconazole, voriconazole) are predicted to very markedly increase the exposure to **ibrutinib**. Avoid potent CYP3A4 inhibitors or adjust **ibrutinib** dose, p. 1027. Severe Study
▶ Calcium channel blockers (diltiazem, verapamil) are predicted to increase the exposure to **ibrutinib**. Adjust **ibrutinib** dose with moderate CYP3A4 inhibitors, p. 1027. Severe Study
▶ Cobicistat is predicted to very markedly increase the exposure to **ibrutinib**. Avoid potent CYP3A4 inhibitors or adjust **ibrutinib** dose, p. 1027. Severe Study
▶ Crizotinib is predicted to increase the exposure to **ibrutinib**. Adjust **ibrutinib** dose with moderate CYP3A4 inhibitors, p. 1027. Severe Study
▶ Grapefruit juice is predicted to increase the exposure to **ibrutinib**. Avoid. Moderate Theoretical
▶ HIV-protease inhibitors are predicted to very markedly increase the exposure to **ibrutinib**. Avoid potent CYP3A4 inhibitors or adjust **ibrutinib** dose, p. 1027. Severe Study
▶ Idelalisib is predicted to very markedly increase the exposure to **ibrutinib**. Avoid potent CYP3A4 inhibitors or adjust **ibrutinib** dose, p. 1027. Severe Study
▶ Imatinib is predicted to increase the exposure to **ibrutinib**. Adjust **ibrutinib** dose with moderate CYP3A4 inhibitors, p. 1027. Severe Study → Also see TABLE 15 p. 1432
▶ Letermovir is predicted to increase the exposure to **ibrutinib**. Adjust **ibrutinib** dose with moderate CYP3A4 inhibitors, p. 1027. Severe Study
▶ Macrolides (clarithromycin) are predicted to very markedly increase the exposure to **ibrutinib**. Avoid potent CYP3A4 inhibitors or adjust **ibrutinib** dose, p. 1027. Severe Study
▶ Macrolides (erythromycin) are predicted to increase the exposure to **ibrutinib**. Adjust **ibrutinib** dose with moderate CYP3A4 inhibitors, p. 1027. Severe Study
▶ Mitotane is predicted to decrease the exposure to **ibrutinib**. Avoid or adjust **ibrutinib** dose, p. 1027. Severe Study → Also see TABLE 15 p. 1432
▶ Neurokinin-1 receptor antagonists (aprepitant, netupitant) are predicted to increase the exposure to **ibrutinib**. Adjust **ibrutinib** dose with moderate CYP3A4 inhibitors, p. 1027. Severe Study
▶ Neurokinin-1 receptor antagonists (fosaprepitant) are predicted to slightly increase the exposure to **ibrutinib**. Moderate Theoretical

▶ Nilotinib is predicted to increase the exposure to **ibrutinib**. Adjust **ibrutinib** dose with moderate CYP3A4 inhibitors, p. 102? Severe Study → Also see TABLE 15 p. 1432
▶ Quinolones (ciprofloxacin) are predicted to increase the exposure to **ibrutinib**. Adjust **ibrutinib** dose, p. 1027. Severe Theoretical
▶ Rifamycins (rifampicin) are predicted to decrease the exposure to **ibrutinib**. Avoid or adjust **ibrutinib** dose, p. 1027. Severe Study
▶ St John's wort is predicted to decrease the exposure to **ibrutinib**. Avoid. Severe Theoretical
Ibuprofen → see NSAIDs
Icatibant
▶ ACE inhibitors are predicted to decrease the efficacy of **icatibant** and **icatibant** is predicted to decrease the efficacy of ACE inhibitors. Avoid. Moderate Theoretical
Idarubicin → see anthracyclines
Idelalisib
▶ **Idelalisib** is predicted to increase the exposure to abemaciclib. Avoid or adjust **abemaciclib** dose, p. 1009. Severe Study
▶ **Idelalisib** is predicted to increase the exposure to acalabrutinib. Avoid. Severe Study
▶ **Idelalisib** is predicted to markedly increase the exposure to aldosterone antagonists (eplerenone). Avoid. Severe Study
▶ **Idelalisib** is predicted to moderately increase the exposure to alpha blockers (alfuzosin, tamsulosin). Use with caution or avoid. Moderate Study
▶ **Idelalisib** is predicted to increase the exposure to alpha blockers (doxazosin). Moderate Study
▶ Anti-androgens (apalutamide, enzalutamide) are predicted to decrease the exposure to **idelalisib**. Avoid. Severe Study
▶ **Idelalisib** is predicted to increase the exposure to anti-androgens (apalutamide). Mild Study
▶ **Idelalisib** is predicted to increase the exposure to antiarrhythmics (amiodarone). Avoid. Moderate Theoretical
▶ **Idelalisib** very markedly increases the exposure to antiarrhythmics (dronedarone). Avoid. Severe Study
▶ **Idelalisib** is predicted to increase the exposure to antiarrhythmics (propafenone). Monitor and adjust dose. Severe Study
▶ **Idelalisib** is predicted to increase the exposure to anticholinesterases, centrally acting (galantamine). Monitor and adjust dose. Moderate Study
▶ Antiepileptics (carbamazepine, fosphenytoin, phenobarbital, phenytoin, primidone) are predicted to decrease the exposure to **idelalisib**. Avoid. Severe Study
▶ **Idelalisib** is predicted to very slightly increase the exposure to antiepileptics (perampanel). Mild Study
▶ **Idelalisib** is predicted to increase the exposure to antifungals, azoles (isavuconazole). Avoid or monitor adverse effects. Severe Study
▶ **Idelalisib** is predicted to increase the exposure to antihistamines, non-sedating (mizolastine). Avoid. Severe Study
▶ **Idelalisib** is predicted to increase the exposure to antihistamines, non-sedating (rupatadine). Avoid. Moderate Study
▶ **Idelalisib** is predicted to increase the concentration of antimalarials (piperaquine). Severe Theoretical
▶ **Idelalisib** is predicted to slightly increase the exposure to antipsychotics, second generation (aripiprazole). Adjust **aripiprazole** dose, p. 415. Moderate Study
▶ **Idelalisib** is predicted to moderately increase the exposure to antipsychotics, second generation (cariprazine). Avoid. Severe Study
▶ **Idelalisib** is predicted to increase the exposure to antipsychotics, second generation (lurasidone, quetiapine). Avoid. Severe Study
▶ **Idelalisib** is predicted to increase the exposure to antipsychotics, second generation (risperidone). Adjust dose. Moderate Study
▶ **Idelalisib** is predicted to increase the exposure to avapritinib. Avoid. Moderate Study
▶ **Idelalisib** is predicted to increase the exposure to axitinib. Avoid or adjust dose. Moderate Study
▶ **Idelalisib** is predicted to increase the exposure to bedaquiline. Avoid prolonged use. Mild Study

Idelalisib moderately increases the exposure to benzodiazepines (alprazolam). Avoid. Moderate Study

Idelalisib is predicted to markedly to very markedly increase the exposure to benzodiazepines (midazolam). Avoid or adjust dose. Severe Study

Idelalisib is predicted to increase the exposure to beta₂ agonists (salmeterol). Avoid. Severe Study

Idelalisib slightly increases the exposure to bortezomib. Moderate Study

Idelalisib is predicted to markedly increase the exposure to bosutinib. Avoid or adjust dose. Severe Study

Idelalisib is predicted to increase the exposure to brigatinib. Adjust **brigatinib** dose, p. 1015. Severe Study

Idelalisib is predicted to increase the exposure to buspirone. Adjust **buspirone** dose, p. 360. Severe Study

Idelalisib slightly increases the exposure to cabozantinib. Moderate Study

Idelalisib is predicted to increase the exposure to calcium channel blockers (amlodipine, felodipine, lacidipine, nicardipine, nifedipine, nimodipine). Monitor and adjust dose. Moderate Study

Idelalisib is predicted to increase the exposure to calcium channel blockers (diltiazem, verapamil). Severe Study

▶ **Idelalisib** is predicted to markedly increase the exposure to calcium channel blockers (lercanidipine). Avoid. Severe Study

▶ **Idelalisib** is predicted to increase the exposure to cannabidiol. Avoid or adjust dose. Mild Study

▶ **Idelalisib** is predicted to increase the exposure to ceritinib. Avoid or adjust **ceritinib** dose, p. 1017. Severe Study

▶ **Idelalisib** increases the concentration of ciclosporin. Severe Study

▶ **Idelalisib** is predicted to moderately increase the exposure to cilostazol. Adjust **cilostazol** dose, p. 248. Moderate Study

▶ **Idelalisib** is predicted to moderately increase the exposure to cinacalcet. Adjust dose. Moderate Study

▶ **Idelalisib** is predicted to markedly increase the exposure to cobimetinib. Avoid or monitor for toxicity. Severe Study

▶ **Idelalisib** is predicted to increase the exposure to colchicine. Avoid potent CYP3A4 inhibitors or adjust **colchicine** dose, p. 1166. Severe Study

▶ **Idelalisib** is predicted to increase the exposure to corticosteroids (beclometasone) (risk with beclometasone is likely to be lower than with other corticosteroids). Moderate Theoretical

▶ **Idelalisib** is predicted to increase the exposure to corticosteroids (betamethasone, budesonide, ciclesonide, deflazacort, dexamethasone, fludrocortisone, fluticasone, hydrocortisone, methylprednisolone, mometasone, prednisolone, triamcinolone). Avoid or monitor adverse effects. Severe Study

▶ **Idelalisib** is predicted to moderately increase the exposure to crizotinib. Avoid. Moderate Study

▶ **Idelalisib** is predicted to increase the exposure to dabrafenib. Use with caution or avoid. Moderate Study

▶ **Idelalisib** is predicted to markedly to very markedly increase the exposure to darifenacin. Avoid. Severe Study

▶ **Idelalisib** is predicted to markedly increase the exposure to dasatinib. Avoid or adjust dose—consult product literature. Severe Study

▶ **Idelalisib** very slightly increases the exposure to delamanid. Severe Study

▶ **Idelalisib** is predicted to moderately increase the exposure to dienogest. Moderate Study

▶ **Idelalisib** is predicted to increase the exposure to dipeptidylpeptidase-4 inhibitors (saxagliptin). Moderate Study

▶ **Idelalisib** increases the risk of QT-prolongation when given with domperidone. Avoid. Severe Study

▶ **Idelalisib** increases the exposure to dopamine receptor agonists (bromocriptine). Severe Study

▶ **Idelalisib** is predicted to increase the concentration of dopamine receptor agonists (cabergoline). Moderate Anecdotal

▶ **Idelalisib** is predicted to increase the exposure to dronabinol. Adjust dose. Mild Study

▶ **Idelalisib** is predicted to increase the exposure to dutasteride. Monitor adverse effects and adjust dose. Moderate Theoretical

▶ **Idelalisib** is predicted to increase the exposure to elexacaftor. Adjust tezacaftor with ivacaftor and elexacftor p. 311 dose with potent CYP3A4 inhibitors. Severe Study

▶ **Idelalisib** is predicted to increase the exposure to eliglustat. Avoid or adjust dose—consult product literature. Severe Study

▶ **Idelalisib** is predicted to increase the exposure to encorafenib. Avoid or monitor. Severe Study

▶ Endothelin receptor antagonists (bosentan) are predicted to decrease the exposure to **idelalisib**. Avoid. Moderate Theoretical

▶ **Idelalisib** is predicted to increase the exposure to endothelin receptor antagonists (macitentan). Moderate Study

▶ **Idelalisib** is predicted to increase the exposure to entrectinib. Avoid potent CYP3A4 inhibitors or adjust **entrectinib** dose, p. 1023. Severe Study

▶ **Idelalisib** is predicted to increase the risk of ergotism when given with ergometrine. Avoid. Severe Theoretical

▶ **Idelalisib** is predicted to increase the risk of ergotism when given with ergotamine. Avoid. Severe Theoretical

▶ **Idelalisib** is predicted to slightly increase the exposure to erlotinib. Use with caution and adjust dose. Moderate Study

▶ **Idelalisib** is predicted to increase the exposure to esketamine. Adjust dose. Moderate Study

▶ **Idelalisib** is predicted to increase the concentration of everolimus. Avoid. Severe Study

▶ **Idelalisib** is predicted to moderately increase the exposure to fesoterodine. Adjust **fesoterodine** dose with potent CYP3A4 inhibitors; avoid in hepatic and renal impairment, p. 822. Severe Study

▶ **Idelalisib** is predicted to moderately increase the exposure to fostamatinib. Monitor adverse effects and adjust dose. Moderate Study

▶ **Idelalisib** is predicted to increase the exposure to gefitinib. Moderate Study

▶ **Idelalisib** is predicted to increase the exposure to gilteritinib. Moderate Study

▶ **Idelalisib** is predicted to moderately increase the exposure to glasdegib. Use with caution or avoid. Moderate Study

▶ **Idelalisib** is predicted to moderately to markedly increase the exposure to grazoprevir. Avoid. Severe Study

▶ **Idelalisib** is predicted to increase the exposure to guanfacine. Adjust **guanfacine** dose, p. 372. Moderate Study

▶ **Idelalisib** is predicted to very markedly increase the exposure to ibrutinib. Avoid potent CYP3A4 inhibitors or adjust **ibrutinib** dose, p. 1027. Severe Study

▶ **Idelalisib** is predicted to increase the exposure to imatinib. Moderate Study

▶ **Idelalisib** is predicted to increase the risk of toxicity when given with irinotecan. Avoid. Moderate Study

▶ **Idelalisib** is predicted to increase the exposure to ivabradine. Avoid. Severe Study

▶ **Idelalisib** is predicted to increase the exposure to ivacaftor. Adjust ivacaftor p. 309 or lumacaftor with ivacaftor p. 310 or tezacaftor with ivacaftor p. 311 or tezacaftor with ivacaftor and elexacftor p. 311 dose with potent CYP3A4 inhibitors. Severe Study

▶ **Idelalisib** is predicted to increase the exposure to lapatinib. Avoid. Moderate Study

▶ **Idelalisib** is predicted to moderately increase the exposure to larotrectinib. Avoid or adjust **larotrectinib** dose, p. 1031. Moderate Study

▶ **Idelalisib** is predicted to markedly increase the exposure to lomitapide. Avoid. Severe Study

▶ **Idelalisib** is predicted to increase the exposure to lorlatinib. Avoid or adjust **lorlatinib** dose, p. 1033. Severe Study

▶ **Idelalisib** markedly increases the exposure to maraviroc. Adjust dose. Severe Theoretical

▶ **Idelalisib** is predicted to increase the exposure to meglitinides (repaglinide). Moderate Study

▶ **Idelalisib** is predicted to very markedly increase the exposure to midostaurin. Avoid or monitor for toxicity. Severe Study

▶ **Idelalisib** is predicted to increase the exposure to mirabegron. Adjust **mirabegron** dose in hepatic and renal impairment, p. 825. Moderate Study

▶ **Idelalisib** is predicted to increase the exposure to mirtazapine. Moderate Study

Idelalisib (continued)

▸ Mitotane is predicted to decrease the exposure to **idelalisib**. Avoid. Severe Study

▸ **Idelalisib** is predicted to increase the exposure to modafinil. Mild Theoretical

▸ **Idelalisib** is predicted to increase the exposure to monoclonal antibodies (polatuzumab vedotin). Moderate Theoretical

▸ **Idelalisib** is predicted to increase the exposure to monoclonal antibodies (trastuzumab emtansine). Avoid. Severe Theoretical

▸ **Idelalisib** is predicted to increase the exposure to naldemedine. Avoid or monitor. Moderate Study

▸ **Idelalisib** is predicted to markedly increase the exposure to naloxegol. Avoid. Severe Study

▸ **Idelalisib** is predicted to increase the exposure to neratinib. Avoid or adjust **neratinib** dose, p. 1034. Severe Study

▸ **Idelalisib** is predicted to markedly increase the exposure to neurokinin-1 receptor antagonists (aprepitant). Moderate Study

▸ **Idelalisib** is predicted to increase the exposure to neurokinin-1 receptor antagonists (fosaprepitant). Moderate Theoretical

▸ **Idelalisib** is predicted to increase the exposure to neurokinin-1 receptor antagonists (netupitant). Moderate Study

▸ **Idelalisib** is predicted to moderately increase the exposure to nilotinib. Avoid. Severe Study

▸ **Idelalisib** is predicted to increase the exposure to nitisinone. Adjust dose. Moderate Theoretical

▸ NNRTIs (efavirenz, nevirapine) are predicted to decrease the exposure to **idelalisib**. Avoid. Moderate Theoretical

▸ **Idelalisib** is predicted to increase the exposure to NNRTIs (doravirine). Mild Study

▸ **Idelalisib** is predicted to increase the exposure to olaparib. Avoid potent CYP3A4 inhibitors or adjust **olaparib** dose, p. 1051. Moderate Study

▸ **Idelalisib** is predicted to increase the exposure to opioids (alfentanil, buprenorphine, fentanyl, oxycodone). Monitor and adjust dose. Severe Study

▸ **Idelalisib** is predicted to increase the exposure to opioids (methadone). Severe Theoretical

▸ **Idelalisib** is predicted to increase the exposure to ospemifene. Avoid in poor CYP2C9 metabolisers. Moderate Study

▸ **Idelalisib** is predicted to increase the exposure to oxybutynin. Mild Study

▸ **Idelalisib** is predicted to increase the exposure to palbociclib. Avoid or adjust **palbociclib** dose, p. 1038. Severe Study

▸ **Idelalisib** is predicted to increase the exposure to panobinostat. Adjust **panobinostat** dose; in hepatic impairment avoid, p. 979. Moderate Study

▸ Paritaprevir is predicted to increase the exposure to **idelalisib**. Avoid. Severe Study

▸ **Idelalisib** is predicted to increase the exposure to pazopanib. Avoid or adjust **pazopanib** dose, p. 1039. Moderate Study

▸ **Idelalisib** is predicted to increase the exposure to phosphodiesterase type-5 inhibitors (avanafil, vardenafil). Avoid. Severe Study

▸ **Idelalisib** is predicted to increase the exposure to phosphodiesterase type-5 inhibitors (sildenafil). Avoid potent CYP3A4 inhibitors or adjust **sildenafil** dose, p. 860. Severe Study

▸ **Idelalisib** is predicted to increase the exposure to phosphodiesterase type-5 inhibitors (tadalafil). Use with caution or avoid. Severe Study

▸ **Idelalisib** is predicted to increase the exposure to pimozide. Avoid. Severe Study

▸ **Idelalisib** is predicted to slightly increase the exposure to ponatinib. Monitor and adjust **ponatinib** dose, p. 1040. Moderate Study

▸ **Idelalisib** is predicted to moderately increase the exposure to praziquantel. Mild Study

▸ **Idelalisib** given with carbimazole is predicted to increase the exposure to propiverine. Adjust starting dose. Moderate Theoretical

▸ **Idelalisib** is predicted to increase the exposure to ranolazine. Avoid. Severe Study

▸ **Idelalisib** is predicted to increase the exposure to reboxetine. Avoid. Moderate Study

▸ **Idelalisib** is predicted to increase the exposure to regorafenib. Avoid. Moderate Study

▸ **Idelalisib** is predicted to increase the exposure to retinoids (alitretinoin). Adjust **alitretinoin** dose, p. 1305. Moderate Theoretical

▸ **Idelalisib** is predicted to increase the exposure to ribociclib. Avoid or adjust **ribociclib** dose, p. 1042. Moderate Study

▸ Rifamycins (rifampicin) are predicted to decrease the exposure to **idelalisib**. Avoid. Severe Study

▸ **Idelalisib** is predicted to increase the exposure to ruxolitinib. Adjust dose and monitor adverse effects. Moderate Study

▸ **Idelalisib** is predicted to increase the exposure to siponimod. Avoid depending on other drugs taken—consult product literature. Severe Theoretical

▸ **Idelalisib** is predicted to increase the concentration of sirolimus. Avoid. Severe Study

▸ **Idelalisib** is predicted to increase the exposure to solifenacin. Adjust solifenacin p. 824 or tamsulosin with solifenacin p. 830 dose; avoid in hepatic and renal impairment. Severe Study

▸ **Idelalisib** is predicted to moderately increase the exposure to SSRIs (dapoxetine). Avoid potent CYP3A4 inhibitors or adjust **dapoxetine** dose, p. 867. Severe Study

▸ St John's wort is predicted to decrease the exposure to **idelalisib**. Avoid. Moderate Theoretical

▸ **Idelalisib** is predicted to increase the exposure to statins (atorvastatin). Avoid or adjust dose and monitor rhabdomyolysis. Severe Study

▸ **Idelalisib** is predicted to increase the exposure to statins (simvastatin). Avoid. Severe Study

▸ **Idelalisib** is predicted to slightly increase the exposure to sunitinib. Avoid or adjust **sunitinib** dose, p. 1044. Moderate Study

▸ **Idelalisib** is predicted to increase the concentration of tacrolimus. Monitor and adjust dose. Severe Study

▸ **Idelalisib** is predicted to increase the exposure to taxanes (cabazitaxel). Avoid. Severe Study

▸ **Idelalisib** is predicted to moderately increase the exposure to taxanes (docetaxel). Avoid or adjust dose. Severe Study

▸ **Idelalisib** is predicted to increase the exposure to taxanes (paclitaxel). Severe Theoretical

▸ **Idelalisib** is predicted to increase the concentration of temsirolimus. Avoid. Severe Theoretical

▸ **Idelalisib** is predicted to increase the exposure to tezacaftor. Adjust tezacaftor with ivacaftor p. 311 or tezacaftor with ivacaftor and elexacaftor p. 311 dose with potent CYP3A4 inhibitors. Severe Study

▸ **Idelalisib** is predicted to markedly increase the exposure to ticagrelor. Avoid. Severe Study

▸ **Idelalisib** is predicted to increase the exposure to tofacitinib. Adjust **tofacitinib** dose, p. 1154. Moderate Study

▸ **Idelalisib** is predicted to increase the exposure to tolterodine. Avoid. Severe Study

▸ **Idelalisib** is predicted to increase the exposure to tolvaptan. Manufacturer advises caution or adjust **tolvaptan** dose with potent CYP3A4 inhibitors, p. 708. Severe Study

▸ **Idelalisib** is predicted to increase the exposure to toremifene. Moderate Theoretical

▸ **Idelalisib** is predicted to increase the exposure to trabectedin. Avoid or adjust dose. Severe Theoretical

▸ **Idelalisib** is predicted to moderately increase the exposure to trazodone. Avoid or adjust dose. Moderate Study

▸ **Idelalisib** increases the exposure to triptans (almotriptan). Mild Study

▸ **Idelalisib** is predicted to markedly increase the exposure to triptans (eletriptan). Avoid. Severe Study

▸ **Idelalisib** is predicted to increase the exposure to upadacitinib. Use with caution or avoid. Severe Study

▸ **Idelalisib** is predicted to increase the exposure to vemurafenib. Severe Theoretical

▸ **Idelalisib** is predicted to increase the exposure to venetoclax. Avoid or adjust dose—consult product literature. Severe Study

▸ **Idelalisib** is predicted to increase the exposure to venlafaxine. Moderate Study

▸ **Idelalisib** is predicted to increase the exposure to vinca alkaloids. Severe Theoretical

▸ **Idelalisib** is predicted to increase the exposure to vitamin D substances (paricalcitol). Moderate Study

Idelalisib is predicted to increase the exposure to zopiclone. Adjust dose. [Moderate] Theoretical

Ifosfamide → see alkylating agents

Iloprost → see TABLE 8 p. 1430 (hypotension), TABLE 4 p. 1429 (antiplatelet effects)

Imatinib → see TABLE 15 p. 1432 (myelosuppression)

Imatinib is predicted to increase the exposure to abemaciclib. [Moderate] Study

Imatinib is predicted to increase the exposure to acalabrutinib. Avoid or monitor. [Severe] Study

Imatinib is predicted to increase the exposure to aldosterone antagonists (eplerenone). Adjust **eplerenone** dose, p. 208. [Severe] Study

Imatinib is predicted to increase the exposure to alpha blockers (tamsulosin). [Moderate] Theoretical

Anti-androgens (apalutamide, enzalutamide) are predicted to decrease the exposure to **imatinib**. Avoid. [Moderate] Study

Imatinib is predicted to increase the exposure to antiarrhythmics (dronedarone). [Severe] Theoretical

Imatinib is predicted to increase the exposure to antiarrhythmics (propafenone). Monitor and adjust dose. [Moderate] Study

Antiepileptics (carbamazepine, fosphenytoin, phenobarbital, phenytoin, primidone) are predicted to decrease the exposure to **imatinib**. Avoid. [Moderate] Study

Antiepileptics (oxcarbazepine) decrease the exposure to **imatinib**. Avoid. [Moderate] Study

Antifungals, azoles (fluconazole, posaconazole) are predicted to increase the exposure to **imatinib**. [Moderate] Theoretical

Antifungals, azoles (itraconazole, ketoconazole, voriconazole) are predicted to increase the exposure to **imatinib**. [Moderate] Study

Imatinib is predicted to increase the exposure to antifungals, azoles (isavuconazole). [Moderate] Theoretical

Imatinib is predicted to increase the exposure to antihistamines, non-sedating (mizolastine). [Severe] Theoretical

Imatinib is predicted to increase the exposure to antihistamines, non-sedating (rupatadine). Avoid. [Moderate] Study

Imatinib is predicted to increase the concentration of antimalarials (piperaquine). [Severe] Theoretical

Imatinib is predicted to increase the exposure to antipsychotics, second generation (cariprazine). Avoid. [Severe] Study

Imatinib is predicted to increase the exposure to antipsychotics, second generation (lurasidone). Adjust **lurasidone** dose. [Moderate] Study

Imatinib is predicted to increase the exposure to antipsychotics, second generation (quetiapine). Avoid. [Moderate] Study

Asparaginase is predicted to increase the risk of hepatotoxicity when given with **imatinib**. [Severe] Theoretical → Also see TABLE 15 p. 1432

Imatinib is predicted to increase the exposure to avapritinib. Avoid or adjust **avapritinib** dose, p. 1012. [Moderate] Study

Imatinib is predicted to increase the exposure to axitinib. [Moderate] Theoretical → Also see TABLE 15 p. 1432

Imatinib is predicted to increase the exposure to bedaquiline. Avoid prolonged use. [Mild] Theoretical

Imatinib is predicted to increase the exposure to benzodiazepines (alprazolam). [Severe] Study

Imatinib is predicted to increase the exposure to benzodiazepines (midazolam). Monitor adverse effects and adjust dose. [Severe] Study

Imatinib is predicted to increase the exposure to bosutinib. Avoid or adjust dose. [Severe] Theoretical → Also see TABLE 15 p. 1432

Imatinib is predicted to increase the exposure to buspirone. Use with caution and adjust dose. [Moderate] Study

Imatinib is predicted to increase the exposure to cabozantinib. [Moderate] Theoretical → Also see TABLE 15 p. 1432

Calcium channel blockers (diltiazem, verapamil) are predicted to increase the exposure to **imatinib**. [Moderate] Theoretical

Imatinib is predicted to increase the exposure to calcium channel blockers (amlodipine, felodipine, lacidipine, lercanidipine, nicardipine, nifedipine, nimodipine). Monitor and adjust dose. [Moderate] Study

Imatinib is predicted to increase the concentration of ciclosporin. [Severe] Study

▸ Cobicistat is predicted to increase the exposure to **imatinib**. [Moderate] Study

▸ **Imatinib** is predicted to increase the exposure to cobimetinib. [Severe] Theoretical

▸ **Imatinib** is predicted to increase the exposure to colchicine. Adjust **colchicine** dose with moderate CYP3A4 inhibitors, p. 1166. [Severe] Study

▸ **Imatinib** is predicted to increase the exposure to corticosteroids (methylprednisolone). Monitor and adjust dose. [Moderate] Study

▸ **Imatinib** is predicted to increase the risk of bleeding events when given with coumarins. [Severe] Theoretical

▸ Crisantaspase is predicted to increase the risk of hepatotoxicity when given with **imatinib**. [Severe] Theoretical → Also see TABLE 15 p. 1432

▸ **Imatinib** is predicted to slightly increase the exposure to darifenacin. [Moderate] Study

▸ **Imatinib** is predicted to increase the exposure to dasatinib. [Severe] Study → Also see TABLE 15 p. 1432

▸ **Imatinib** is predicted to slightly increase the exposure to dienogest. [Moderate] Study

▸ **Imatinib** is predicted to increase the exposure to dipeptidylpeptidase-4 inhibitors (saxagliptin). [Mild] Study

▸ **Imatinib** increases the risk of QT-prolongation when given with domperidone. Avoid. [Severe] Study

▸ **Imatinib** is predicted to increase the exposure to dopamine receptor agonists (bromocriptine). [Severe] Theoretical

▸ **Imatinib** is predicted to increase the concentration of dopamine receptor agonists (cabergoline). [Moderate] Anecdotal

▸ **Imatinib** is predicted to moderately increase the exposure to dutasteride. [Mild] Study

▸ **Imatinib** is predicted to increase the exposure to elexacaftor. Adjust tezacaftor with ivacaftor and elexacftor p. 311 dose with moderate CYP3A4 inhibitors. [Severe] Theoretical

▸ **Imatinib** is predicted to increase the exposure to eliglustat. Avoid or adjust dose—consult product literature. [Severe] Study

▸ **Imatinib** is predicted to moderately increase the exposure to encorafenib. [Moderate] Study

▸ Endothelin receptor antagonists (bosentan) are predicted to decrease the exposure to **imatinib**. [Moderate] Study

▸ **Imatinib** is predicted to increase the exposure to entrectinib. Avoid moderate CYP3A4 inhibitors or adjust **entrectinib** dose, p. 1023. [Severe] Theoretical

▸ **Imatinib** is predicted to increase the risk of ergotism when given with ergometrine. [Severe] Theoretical

▸ **Imatinib** is predicted to increase the risk of ergotism when given with ergotamine. [Severe] Theoretical

▸ **Imatinib** is predicted to increase the exposure to erlotinib. [Moderate] Theoretical

▸ **Imatinib** is predicted to increase the concentration of everolimus. Avoid or adjust dose. [Moderate] Study

▸ **Imatinib** is predicted to increase the exposure to fesoterodine. Adjust **fesoterodine** dose with moderate CYP3A4 inhibitors in hepatic and renal impairment, p. 822. [Mild] Study

▸ **Imatinib** is predicted to increase the exposure to gefitinib. [Moderate] Theoretical

▸ Grapefruit juice is predicted to increase the exposure to **imatinib**. [Moderate] Theoretical

▸ **Imatinib** is predicted to increase the concentration of guanfacine. Adjust **guanfacine** dose, p. 372. [Moderate] Theoretical

▸ HIV-protease inhibitors are predicted to increase the exposure to **imatinib**. [Moderate] Study

▸ **Imatinib** is predicted to increase the exposure to ibrutinib. Adjust **ibrutinib** dose with moderate CYP3A4 inhibitors, p. 1027. [Severe] Study → Also see TABLE 15 p. 1432

▸ Idelalisib is predicted to increase the exposure to **imatinib**. [Moderate] Study

▸ **Imatinib** is predicted to increase the exposure to ivabradine. Adjust **ivabradine** dose, p. 227. [Severe] Theoretical

▸ **Imatinib** is predicted to increase the exposure to ivacaftor. Adjust ivacaftor p. 309 or tezacaftor with ivacaftor p. 311 or tezacaftor with ivacaftor and elexacftor p. 311 dose with moderate CYP3A4 inhibitors. [Severe] Study

▸ **Imatinib** is predicted to increase the exposure to lapatinib. [Moderate] Study

Imatinib (continued)

▶ **Imatinib** is predicted to increase the exposure to lomitapide. Avoid. [Moderate] Theoretical

▶ Macrolides (clarithromycin) are predicted to increase the exposure to **imatinib**. [Moderate] Study

▶ Macrolides (erythromycin) are predicted to increase the exposure to **imatinib**. [Moderate] Theoretical

▶ **Imatinib** is predicted to increase the exposure to midostaurin. [Moderate] Theoretical

▶ Mitotane is predicted to decrease the exposure to **imatinib**. Avoid. [Moderate] Study → Also see TABLE 15 p. 1432

▶ **Imatinib** is predicted to increase the exposure to naldemedine. [Moderate] Study

▶ **Imatinib** is predicted to increase the exposure to naloxegol. Adjust **naloxegol** dose and monitor adverse effects, p. 70. [Moderate] Study

▶ **Imatinib** is predicted to increase the exposure to neratinib. Avoid. [Severe] Study

▶ Neurokinin-1 receptor antagonists (aprepitant, netupitant) are predicted to increase the exposure to **imatinib**. [Moderate] Theoretical

▶ NNRTIs (efavirenz, nevirapine) are predicted to decrease the exposure to **imatinib**. [Moderate] Study

▶ **Imatinib** is predicted to increase the exposure to olaparib. Avoid moderate CYP3A4 inhibitors or adjust **olaparib** dose, p. 1051. [Moderate] Theoretical → Also see TABLE 15 p. 1432

▶ **Imatinib** is predicted to increase the exposure to opioids (alfentanil, buprenorphine, fentanyl, oxycodone). Monitor and adjust dose. [Moderate] Study

▶ **Imatinib** is predicted to increase the exposure to opioids (methadone). [Moderate] Theoretical

▶ **Imatinib** is predicted to increase the exposure to oxybutynin. [Mild] Theoretical

▶ **Imatinib** increases the risk of hepatotoxicity when given with paracetamol. [Severe] Anecdotal

▶ **Imatinib** is predicted to increase the exposure to pazopanib. [Moderate] Theoretical

▶ Pegaspargase is predicted to increase the risk of hepatotoxicity when given with **imatinib**. [Severe] Theoretical → Also see TABLE 15 p. 1432

▶ **Imatinib** is predicted to increase the risk of bleeding events when given with phenindione. [Severe] Theoretical

▶ **Imatinib** is predicted to increase the exposure to phosphodiesterase type-5 inhibitors (avanafil). Adjust **avanafil** dose, p. 859. [Moderate] Theoretical

▶ **Imatinib** is predicted to increase the exposure to phosphodiesterase type-5 inhibitors (sildenafil). Monitor or adjust **sildenafil** dose with moderate CYP3A4 inhibitors, p. 860. [Moderate] Study

▶ **Imatinib** is predicted to increase the exposure to phosphodiesterase type-5 inhibitors (tadalafil). [Severe] Theoretical

▶ **Imatinib** is predicted to increase the exposure to phosphodiesterase type-5 inhibitors (vardenafil). Adjust dose. [Severe] Theoretical

▶ **Imatinib** is predicted to increase the exposure to pimozide. Avoid. [Severe] Theoretical

▶ **Imatinib** is predicted to increase the exposure to ranolazine. [Severe] Study

▶ **Imatinib** is predicted to increase the exposure to ribociclib. [Moderate] Study → Also see TABLE 15 p. 1432

▶ Rifamycins (rifampicin) are predicted to decrease the exposure to **imatinib**. Avoid. [Moderate] Study

▶ **Imatinib** is predicted to increase the exposure to ruxolitinib. [Moderate] Theoretical → Also see TABLE 15 p. 1432

▶ **Imatinib** increases the concentration of sirolimus. Monitor and adjust dose. [Moderate] Study

▶ **Imatinib** is predicted to increase the exposure to SSRIs (dapoxetine). Adjust **dapoxetine** dose with moderate CYP3A4 inhibitors, p. 867. [Moderate] Theoretical

▶ St John's wort is predicted to decrease the exposure to **imatinib**. [Moderate] Study

▶ **Imatinib** is predicted to increase the exposure to statins (atorvastatin). Monitor and adjust dose. [Severe] Theoretical

▶ **Imatinib** moderately increases the exposure to statins (simvastatin). Monitor and adjust dose. [Severe] Study

▶ **Imatinib** is predicted to increase the exposure to sunitinib. [Moderate] Theoretical → Also see TABLE 15 p. 1432

▶ **Imatinib** is predicted to increase the concentration of tacrolimus. [Severe] Study

▶ **Imatinib** is predicted to increase the exposure to taxanes (cabazitaxel). [Moderate] Theoretical → Also see TABLE 15 p. 1432

▶ Tedizolid is predicted to increase the exposure to **imatinib**. Avoid. [Moderate] Theoretical

▶ **Imatinib** is predicted to increase the concentration of temsirolimus. Use with caution or avoid. [Moderate] Theoretical → Also see TABLE 15 p. 1432

▶ **Imatinib** is predicted to increase the exposure to tezacaftor. Adjust tezacaftor with ivacaftor p. 311 or tezacaftor with ivacaftor and elexacaftor p. 311 dose with moderate CYP3A4 inhibitors. [Severe] Study

▶ **Imatinib** given with a potent CYP2C19 inhibitor is predicted to increase the exposure to tofacitinib. Adjust **tofacitinib** dose, p. 1154. [Moderate] Study

▶ **Imatinib** is predicted to increase the exposure to tolterodine. [Mild] Theoretical

▶ **Imatinib** is predicted to increase the exposure to tolvaptan. Manufacturer advises caution or adjust **tolvaptan** dose with moderate CYP3A4 inhibitors, p. 708. [Moderate] Study

▶ **Imatinib** is predicted to increase the exposure to trazodone. [Moderate] Theoretical

▶ **Imatinib** is predicted to increase the exposure to venetoclax. Avoid or adjust dose—consult product literature. [Severe] Study

▶ **Imatinib** is predicted to increase the exposure to vinca alkaloids. [Severe] Theoretical → Also see TABLE 15 p. 1432

▶ **Imatinib** is predicted to increase the exposure to zopiclone. Adjust dose. [Moderate] Study

Imidapril → see ACE inhibitors

Imipenem → see carbapenems

Imipramine → see tricyclic antidepressants

Immunoglobulins

Anti-D (Rh$_0$) immunoglobulin · antithymocyte immunoglobulin (rabbit) · cytomegalovirus immunoglobulin · hepatitis B immunoglobulin · normal immunoglobulin · rabies immunoglobulin · tetanus immunoglobulin · varicella-zoster immunoglobulin

▶ **Cytomegalovirus immunoglobulin** is predicted to decrease the efficacy of live vaccines. Avoid. [Severe] Theoretical

▶ **Cytomegalovirus immunoglobulin** is predicted to increase the risk of adverse effects when given with loop diuretics. Avoid. [Moderate] Theoretical

▶ **Normal immunoglobulin** is predicted to alter the effects of monoclonal antibodies (dinutuximab). Avoid. [Severe] Theoretical

Indacaterol → see beta$_2$ agonists

Indapamide → see thiazide diuretics

Indometacin → see NSAIDs

Indoramin → see alpha blockers

Infliximab → see monoclonal antibodies

Influenza vaccine (live) → see live vaccines

Inotersen → see TABLE 4 p. 1429 (antiplatelet effects)

Inotuzumab ozogamicin → see monoclonal antibodies

Insulin → see TABLE 14 p. 1432 (antidiabetic drugs)

▶ Fibrates are predicted to increase the risk of hypoglycaemia when given with **insulin**. [Moderate] Theoretical

Interferon beta → see interferons

Interferons → see TABLE 15 p. 1432 (myelosuppression)

interferon beta · peginterferon alfa

▶ **Interferons** are predicted to slightly increase the exposure to aminophylline. Adjust dose. [Moderate] Theoretical

▶ **Interferons** slightly increase the exposure to theophylline. Adjust dose. [Moderate] Study

Ipilimumab → see monoclonal antibodies

Ipratropium → see TABLE 10 p. 1431 (antimuscarinics)

▶ Beta$_2$ agonists are predicted to increase the risk of glaucoma when given with **ipratropium**. [Moderate] Anecdotal

Irbesartan → see angiotensin-II receptor antagonists

Irinotecan → see TABLE 15 p. 1432 (myelosuppression)

▶ Anti-androgens (apalutamide, enzalutamide) are predicted to decrease the exposure to **irinotecan**. Avoid. [Severe] Study

Antiepileptics (carbamazepine, fosphenytoin, phenobarbital, phenytoin, primidone) are predicted to decrease the exposure to **irinotecan**. Avoid. [Severe] Study

Antifungals, azoles (itraconazole, ketoconazole, voriconazole) are predicted to increase the risk of toxicity when given with **irinotecan**. Avoid. [Moderate] Study

Cobicistat is predicted to increase the risk of toxicity when given with **irinotecan**. Avoid. [Moderate] Study

Fibrates (gemfibrozil) are predicted to increase the exposure to **irinotecan**. Avoid. [Moderate] Theoretical

HIV-protease inhibitors are predicted to increase the risk of toxicity when given with **irinotecan**. Avoid. [Moderate] Study

▸ Idelalisib is predicted to increase the risk of toxicity when given with **irinotecan**. Avoid. [Moderate] Study

▸ Live vaccines are predicted to increase the risk of generalised infection (possibly life-threatening) when given with **irinotecan**. Public Health England advises avoid (refer to Green Book). [Severe] Theoretical

▸ Macrolides (clarithromycin) are predicted to increase the risk of toxicity when given with **irinotecan**. Avoid. [Moderate] Study

▸ Mitotane is predicted to decrease the exposure to **irinotecan**. Avoid. [Severe] Study → Also see **TABLE 15** p. 1432

▸ Neurokinin-1 receptor antagonists (aprepitant, fosaprepitant) are predicted to increase the exposure to intravenous **irinotecan**. [Severe] Theoretical

▸ Neurokinin-1 receptor antagonists (netupitant) are predicted to increase the exposure to **irinotecan**. [Moderate] Study

▸ **Irinotecan** is predicted to decrease the effects of neuromuscular blocking drugs, non-depolarising. [Moderate] Theoretical

▸ Pitolisant is predicted to decrease the exposure to **irinotecan**. [Mild] Theoretical

▸ Rifamycins (rifampicin) are predicted to decrease the exposure to **irinotecan**. Avoid. [Severe] Study

▸ St John's wort slightly decreases the exposure to **irinotecan**. Avoid. [Severe] Study

▸ **Irinotecan** is predicted to increase the risk of prolonged neuromuscular blockade when given with suxamethonium. [Moderate] Theoretical

Iron

▸ Oral antacids decrease the absorption of oral **iron**. Manufacturer advises iron should be taken 1 hour before or 2 hours after antacids. [Moderate] Study

▸ Oral **iron** decreases the exposure to oral bictegravir. Manufacturer advises bictegravir should be taken 2 hours before iron. [Moderate] Study

▸ Oral **iron** decreases the absorption of oral bisphosphonates (clodronate). Clodronate should be taken 1 hour before or 2 hours after iron. [Moderate] Study

▸ Oral **iron** is predicted to decrease the absorption of oral bisphosphonates (ibandronate). **Ibandronate** should be taken 1 hour before or 6 hours after iron. [Moderate] Theoretical

▸ Oral **iron** decreases the absorption of oral bisphosphonates (risedronate). Separate administration by at least 2 hours. [Moderate] Study

▸ Oral calcium salts (calcium carbonate) decrease the absorption of oral iron. **Calcium carbonate** should be taken 1 hour before or 2 hours after iron. [Moderate] Study

▸ Oral **iron** is predicted to decrease the exposure to oral carbidopa. [Moderate] Theoretical

▸ Chloramphenicol decreases the efficacy of oral **iron**. [Moderate] Anecdotal

▸ Oral **iron** decreases the absorption of oral dolutegravir. **Dolutegravir** should be taken 2 hours before or 6 hours after iron. [Moderate] Study

▸ Oral **iron** is predicted to decrease the absorption of oral eltrombopag. **Eltrombopag** should be taken 2 hours before or 4 hours after iron. [Severe] Theoretical

▸ Oral entacapone is predicted to decrease the absorption of oral **iron**. Separate administration by at least 2 hours. [Moderate] Theoretical

▸ Oral **iron** is predicted to decrease the absorption of oral iron chelators (deferiprone). [Moderate] Theoretical

▸ Oral **iron** decreases the absorption of oral levodopa. [Moderate] Study

▸ Oral **iron** decreases the effects of oral methyldopa. [Moderate] Study

▸ Oral **iron** is predicted to decrease the absorption of oral penicillamine. Separate administration by at least 2 hours. [Mild] Study

▸ Oral **iron** decreases the exposure to oral quinolones. Separate administration by at least 2 hours. [Moderate] Study

▸ Oral **iron** decreases the absorption of oral tetracyclines. **Tetracyclines** should be taken 2 to 3 hours after iron. [Moderate] Study

▸ Oral **iron** decreases the absorption of oral thyroid hormones (levothyroxine). Separate administration by at least 4 hours. [Moderate] Study

▸ Oral trientine potentially decreases the absorption of oral **iron**. [Moderate] Theoretical

▸ Oral zinc is predicted to decrease the efficacy of oral **iron** and oral **iron** is predicted to decrease the efficacy of oral zinc. [Moderate] Study

Iron chelators → see **TABLE 15** p. 1432 (myelosuppression)

deferasirox · deferiprone · desferrioxamine · dexrazoxane

▸ Aluminium hydroxide is predicted to decrease the exposure to **deferasirox**. Avoid. [Moderate] Theoretical

▸ Aluminium hydroxide is predicted to decrease the absorption of **deferiprone**. Avoid. [Moderate] Theoretical

▸ **Deferasirox** is predicted to increase the exposure to aminophylline. Avoid. [Moderate] Theoretical

▸ Antiepileptics (carbamazepine, fosphenytoin, phenobarbital, phenytoin, primidone) are predicted to decrease the exposure to **deferasirox**. Monitor serum ferritin and adjust dose. [Moderate] Theoretical

▸ **Deferasirox** is predicted to increase the exposure to antipsychotics, second generation (clozapine). Avoid. [Moderate] Theoretical

▸ Ascorbic acid is predicted to increase the risk of cardiovascular adverse effects when given with iron chelators (deferiprone, desferrioxamine). [Severe] Theoretical

▸ Aspirin (high-dose) is predicted to increase the risk of gastrointestinal bleeds when given with **deferasirox**. [Severe] Theoretical

▸ Bisphosphonates are predicted to increase the risk of gastrointestinal bleeding when given with **deferasirox**. [Severe] Theoretical

▸ Corticosteroids are predicted to increase the risk of gastrointestinal bleeding when given with **deferasirox**. [Severe] Theoretical

▸ HIV-protease inhibitors (ritonavir) are predicted to decrease the exposure to **deferasirox**. Monitor serum ferritin and adjust dose. [Moderate] Theoretical

▸ Oral iron is predicted to decrease the absorption of oral **deferiprone**. [Moderate] Theoretical

▸ Live vaccines are predicted to increase the risk of generalised infection (possibly life-threatening) when given with **dexrazoxane**. Avoid. [Severe] Theoretical

▸ **Deferasirox** moderately increases the exposure to meglitinides (repaglinide). Avoid. [Moderate] Study

▸ **Deferasirox** is predicted to increase the exposure to montelukast. [Moderate] Theoretical

▸ NSAIDs are predicted to increase the risk of gastrointestinal bleeding when given with **deferasirox**. [Severe] Theoretical

▸ NSAIDs (diclofenac) are predicted to increase the exposure to **deferiprone**. [Moderate] Theoretical

▸ **Deferasirox** is predicted to increase the exposure to pioglitazone. [Moderate] Study

▸ Rifamycins (rifampicin) are predicted to decrease the exposure to **deferasirox**. Monitor serum ferritin and adjust dose. [Moderate] Study

▸ **Deferasirox** is predicted to increase the exposure to selexipag. Adjust **selexipag** dose, p. 196. [Moderate] Study

▸ **Deferasirox** is predicted to increase the concentration of taxanes (paclitaxel). [Severe] Anecdotal

▸ **Deferasirox** increases the exposure to theophylline. Avoid. [Moderate] Study

▸ **Deferasirox** is predicted to increase the exposure to tizanidine. Avoid. [Moderate] Theoretical

A1

Interactions | Appendix 1

Iron chelators (continued)

▸ Oral zinc is predicted to decrease the absorption of oral deferiprone. [Moderate] Theoretical

Isavuconazole → see antifungals, azoles

Isocarboxazid → see MAOIs, irreversible

Isoflurane → see volatile halogenated anaesthetics

Isometheptene → see sympathomimetics, vasoconstrictor

Isoniazid → see TABLE 1 p. 1429 (hepatotoxicity), TABLE 12 p. 1432 (peripheral neuropathy)

FOOD AND LIFESTYLE Avoid tyramine-rich foods (such as mature cheeses, salami, pickled herring, *Bovril*®, *Oxo*®, *Marmite*® or any similar meat or yeast extract or fermented soya bean extract, and some beers, lagers or wines) or histamine-rich foods (such as very mature cheese or fish from the scromboid family (e.g. tuna, mackerel, salmon)) with **isoniazid**, as tachycardia, palpitation, hypotension, flushing, headache, dizziness, and sweating reported.

▸ **Isoniazid** is predicted to affect the clearance of aminophylline. [Severe] Theoretical

▸ **Isoniazid** markedly increases the concentration of antiepileptics (carbamazepine) and antiepileptics (carbamazepine) increase the risk of hepatotoxicity when given with **isoniazid**. Monitor concentration and adjust dose. [Severe] Study → Also see TABLE 1 p. 1429

▸ **Isoniazid** increases the concentration of antiepileptics (fosphenytoin, phenytoin). [Moderate] Study → Also see TABLE 12 p. 1432

▸ Cycloserine increases the risk of CNS toxicity when given with **isoniazid**. Monitor and adjust dose. [Moderate] Study

▸ **Isoniazid** increases the risk of optic neuropathy when given with ethambutol. [Severe] Anecdotal

▸ **Isoniazid** decreases the effects of levodopa. [Moderate] Study

▸ **Isoniazid** is predicted to increase the exposure to lomitapide. Separate administration by 12 hours. [Unknown] Theoretical → Also see TABLE 1 p. 1429

▸ **Isoniazid** is predicted to affect the clearance of theophylline. [Severe] Anecdotal

▸ **Isoniazid** potentially increases the risk of nephrotoxicity when given with volatile halogenated anaesthetics (methoxyflurane). Avoid. [Severe] Theoretical

Isosorbide dinitrate → see nitrates

Isosorbide mononitrate → see nitrates

Isotretinoin → see retinoids

Itraconazole → see antifungals, azoles

Ivabradine → see TABLE 6 p. 1430 (bradycardia), TABLE 9 p. 1431 (QT-interval prolongation)

▸ Anti-androgens (apalutamide, enzalutamide) are predicted to decrease the exposure to **ivabradine**. Adjust dose. [Moderate] Theoretical

▸ Antiarrhythmics (dronedarone) are predicted to increase the exposure to **ivabradine**. Adjust **ivabradine** dose, p. 227. [Severe] Theoretical

▸ Antiepileptics (carbamazepine, fosphenytoin, phenobarbital, phenytoin, primidone) are predicted to decrease the exposure to **ivabradine**. Adjust dose. [Moderate] Theoretical

▸ Antifungals, azoles (fluconazole, isavuconazole, posaconazole) are predicted to increase the exposure to **ivabradine**. Adjust **ivabradine** dose, p. 227. [Severe] Theoretical

▸ Antifungals, azoles (itraconazole, ketoconazole, voriconazole) are predicted to increase the exposure to **ivabradine**. Avoid. [Severe] Study

▸ Calcium channel blockers (diltiazem, verapamil) are predicted to increase the exposure to **ivabradine**. Avoid. [Moderate] Study → Also see TABLE 6 p. 1430

▸ Cobicistat is predicted to increase the exposure to **ivabradine**. Avoid. [Severe] Study

▸ Crizotinib is predicted to increase the exposure to **ivabradine**. Adjust **ivabradine** dose, p. 227. [Severe] Theoretical → Also see TABLE 6 p. 1430

▸ Grapefruit juice is predicted to increase the exposure to **ivabradine**. Avoid. [Moderate] Study

▸ HIV-protease inhibitors are predicted to increase the exposure to **ivabradine**. Avoid. [Severe] Study

▸ Idelalisib is predicted to increase the exposure to **ivabradine**. Avoid. [Severe] Study

▸ Imatinib is predicted to increase the exposure to **ivabradine**. Adjust **ivabradine** dose, p. 227. [Severe] Theoretical

▸ Macrolides (clarithromycin) are predicted to increase the exposure to **ivabradine**. Avoid. [Severe] Theoretical

▸ Macrolides (erythromycin) are predicted to increase the exposure to **ivabradine**. Avoid. [Severe] Theoretical

▸ Mitotane is predicted to decrease the exposure to **ivabradine**. Adjust dose. [Moderate] Theoretical

▸ Neurokinin-1 receptor antagonists (aprepitant, netupitant) are predicted to increase the exposure to **ivabradine**. Adjust **ivabradine** dose, p. 227. [Severe] Theoretical

▸ Nilotinib is predicted to increase the exposure to **ivabradine**. Adjust **ivabradine** dose, p. 227. [Severe] Theoretical

▸ Rifamycins (rifampicin) are predicted to decrease the exposure to **ivabradine**. Adjust dose. [Moderate] Theoretical

▸ St John's wort decreases the exposure to **ivabradine**. Avoid. [Moderate] Study

Ivacaftor

FOOD AND LIFESTYLE Avoid bitter (Seville) oranges as they are predicted to increase the exposure to ivacaftor.

▸ Anti-androgens (apalutamide, enzalutamide) are predicted to moderately to markedly decrease the exposure to **ivacaftor**. Avoid. [Severe] Study

▸ Antiarrhythmics (dronedarone) are predicted to increase the exposure to **ivacaftor**. Adjust ivacaftor p. 309 or tezacaftor with ivacaftor p. 311 or tezacaftor with ivacaftor and elexacftor p. 311 dose with moderate CYP3A4 inhibitors. [Severe] Study

▸ Antiepileptics (carbamazepine, fosphenytoin, phenobarbital, phenytoin, primidone) are predicted to moderately to markedly decrease the exposure to **ivacaftor**. Avoid. [Severe] Study

▸ Antifungals, azoles (fluconazole, isavuconazole, posaconazole) are predicted to increase the exposure to **ivacaftor**. Adjust ivacaftor p. 309 or tezacaftor with ivacaftor p. 311 or tezacaftor with ivacaftor and elexacftor p. 311 dose with moderate CYP3A4 inhibitors. [Severe] Study

▸ Antifungals, azoles (itraconazole, ketoconazole, voriconazole) are predicted to increase the exposure to **ivacaftor**. Adjust ivacaftor p. 309 or lumacaftor with ivacaftor p. 310 or tezacaftor with ivacaftor p. 311 or tezacaftor with ivacaftor and elexacftor p. 311 dose with potent CYP3A4 inhibitors. [Severe] Study

▸ Calcium channel blockers (diltiazem, verapamil) are predicted to increase the exposure to **ivacaftor**. Adjust ivacaftor p. 309 or tezacaftor with ivacaftor p. 311 or tezacaftor with ivacaftor and elexacftor p. 311 dose with moderate CYP3A4 inhibitors. [Severe] Study

▸ Cobicistat is predicted to increase the exposure to **ivacaftor**. Adjust ivacaftor p. 309 or lumacaftor with ivacaftor p. 310 or tezacaftor with ivacaftor p. 311 or tezacaftor with ivacaftor and elexacftor p. 311 dose with potent CYP3A4 inhibitors. [Severe] Study

▸ **Ivacaftor** is predicted to increase the anticoagulant effect of coumarins (warfarin). [Severe] Theoretical

▸ Crizotinib is predicted to increase the exposure to **ivacaftor**. Adjust ivacaftor p. 309 or tezacaftor with ivacaftor p. 311 or tezacaftor with ivacaftor and elexacftor p. 311 dose with moderate CYP3A4 inhibitors. [Severe] Study

▸ **Ivacaftor** slightly increases the exposure to digoxin. [Moderate] Study

▸ Endothelin receptor antagonists (bosentan) are predicted to decrease the exposure to **ivacaftor**. [Moderate] Study

▸ Grapefruit juice is predicted to increase the exposure to **ivacaftor**. Avoid. [Moderate] Study

▸ HIV-protease inhibitors are predicted to increase the exposure to **ivacaftor**. Adjust ivacaftor p. 309 or lumacaftor with ivacaftor p. 310 or tezacaftor with ivacaftor p. 311 or tezacaftor with ivacaftor and elexacftor p. 311 dose with potent CYP3A4 inhibitors. [Severe] Study

▸ Idelalisib is predicted to increase the exposure to **ivacaftor**. Adjust ivacaftor p. 309 or lumacaftor with ivacaftor p. 310 or tezacaftor with ivacaftor p. 311 or tezacaftor with ivacaftor and elexacftor p. 311 dose with potent CYP3A4 inhibitors. [Severe] Study

Imatinib is predicted to increase the exposure to **ivacaftor**. Adjust ivacaftor p. 309 or tezacaftor with ivacaftor p. 311 or tezacaftor with ivacaftor and elexacftor p. 311 dose with moderate CYP3A4 inhibitors. [Severe] Study

Letermovir is predicted to increase the exposure to **ivacaftor**. Adjust ivacaftor p. 309 or tezacaftor with ivacaftor p. 311 or tezacaftor with ivacaftor and elexacftor p. 311 dose with moderate CYP3A4 inhibitors. [Severe] Study

Ivacaftor is predicted to increase the exposure to lomitapide. Separate administration by 12 hours. [Moderate] Theoretical

Macrolides (clarithromycin) are predicted to increase the exposure to **ivacaftor**. Adjust ivacaftor p. 309 or lumacaftor with ivacaftor p. 310 or tezacaftor with ivacaftor p. 311 or tezacaftor with ivacaftor and elexacftor p. 311 dose with potent CYP3A4 inhibitors. [Severe] Study

Macrolides (erythromycin) are predicted to increase the exposure to **ivacaftor**. Adjust ivacaftor p. 309 or tezacaftor with ivacaftor p. 311 or tezacaftor with ivacaftor and elexacftor p. 311 dose with moderate CYP3A4 inhibitors. [Severe] Study

Mitotane is predicted to moderately to markedly decrease the exposure to **ivacaftor**. Avoid. [Severe] Study

Neurokinin-1 receptor antagonists (aprepitant, netupitant) are predicted to increase the exposure to **ivacaftor**. Adjust ivacaftor p. 309 or tezacaftor with ivacaftor p. 311 or tezacaftor with ivacaftor and elexacftor p. 311 dose with moderate CYP3A4 inhibitors. [Severe] Study

Nilotinib is predicted to increase the exposure to **ivacaftor**. Adjust ivacaftor p. 309 or tezacaftor with ivacaftor p. 311 or tezacaftor with ivacaftor and elexacftor p. 311 dose with moderate CYP3A4 inhibitors. [Severe] Study

NNRTIs (efavirenz, nevirapine) are predicted to decrease the exposure to **ivacaftor**. [Moderate] Study

Rifamycins (rifampicin) are predicted to moderately to markedly decrease the exposure to **ivacaftor**. Avoid. [Severe] Study

St John's wort is predicted to decrease the exposure to **ivacaftor**. Avoid. [Severe] Study

Ivermectin

ROUTE-SPECIFIC INFORMATION Since systemic absorption can follow topical application, the possibility of interactions should be borne in mind.

▸ **Ivermectin** potentially increases the anticoagulant effect of coumarins. [Severe] Anecdotal
▸ Levamisole increases the exposure to **ivermectin**. [Moderate] Study

Ixazomib

▸ Anti-androgens (apalutamide, enzalutamide) are predicted to decrease the exposure to **ixazomib**. Avoid. [Severe] Study
▸ Antiepileptics (carbamazepine, fosphenytoin, phenobarbital, phenytoin, primidone) are predicted to decrease the exposure to **ixazomib**. [Severe] Study
▸ Mitotane is predicted to decrease the exposure to **ixazomib**. Avoid. [Severe] Study
▸ Rifamycins (rifampicin) are predicted to decrease the exposure to **ixazomib**. Avoid. [Severe] Study
▸ St John's wort is predicted to decrease the exposure to **ixazomib**. [Severe] Theoretical

Ixekizumab → see monoclonal antibodies

Kaolin

▸ Kaolin is predicted to decrease the absorption of tetracyclines. [Moderate] Theoretical

Ketamine → see TABLE 8 p. 1430 (hypotension), TABLE 11 p. 1431 (CNS depressant effects)

▸ **Ketamine** is predicted to increase the risk of elevated blood pressure when given with ergometrine. [Severe] Theoretical
▸ Memantine is predicted to increase the risk of CNS adverse effects when given with **ketamine**. Avoid. [Severe] Theoretical

Ketoconazole → see antifungals, azoles
Ketoprofen → see NSAIDs
Ketorolac → see NSAIDs
Ketotifen → see antihistamines, sedating
Labetalol → see beta blockers, non-selective
Lacidipine → see calcium channel blockers
Lacosamide → see antiepileptics

Lamivudine → see NRTIs
Lamotrigine → see antiepileptics
Lanreotide
▸ Beta blockers, non-selective are predicted to increase the risk of bradycardia when given with **lanreotide**. [Moderate] Theoretical
▸ Beta blockers, selective are predicted to increase the risk of bradycardia when given with **lanreotide**. [Moderate] Theoretical
▸ **Lanreotide** is predicted to decrease the absorption of oral ciclosporin. Adjust dose. [Severe] Theoretical

Lansoprazole → see proton pump inhibitors

Lanthanum

▸ **Lanthanum** is predicted to decrease the absorption of antifungals, azoles (ketoconazole). Separate administration by at least 2 hours. [Moderate] Theoretical
▸ **Lanthanum** is predicted to decrease the absorption of antimalarials (chloroquine). Separate administration by at least 2 hours. [Moderate] Theoretical
▸ **Lanthanum** is predicted to decrease the absorption of hydroxychloroquine. Separate administration by at least 2 hours. [Moderate] Theoretical
▸ **Lanthanum** moderately decreases the exposure to quinolones. **Quinolones** should be taken 2 hours before or 4 hours after **lanthanum**. [Moderate] Study
▸ **Lanthanum** is predicted to decrease the absorption of tetracyclines. Separate administration by 2 hours. [Moderate] Theoretical
▸ **Lanthanum** decreases the absorption of thyroid hormones. Separate administration by 2 hours. [Moderate] Study

Lapatinib → see TABLE 9 p. 1431 (QT-interval prolongation)
▸ **Lapatinib** is predicted to increase the exposure to afatinib. Separate administration by 12 hours. [Moderate] Study
▸ **Lapatinib** is predicted to increase the exposure to aliskiren. [Moderate] Theoretical
▸ **Lapatinib** is predicted to increase the exposure to alpelisib. [Moderate] Theoretical
▸ Oral antacids decrease the absorption of oral **lapatinib**. Avoid. [Moderate] Theoretical
▸ Anti-androgens (apalutamide, enzalutamide) are predicted to decrease the exposure to **lapatinib**. [Severe] Study → Also see TABLE 9 p. 1431
▸ Antiarrhythmics (dronedarone) are predicted to increase the exposure to **lapatinib**. [Moderate] Study → Also see TABLE 9 p. 1431
▸ Antiepileptics (carbamazepine, fosphenytoin, phenobarbital, phenytoin, primidone) are predicted to decrease the exposure to **lapatinib**. [Severe] Study
▸ Antifungals, azoles (fluconazole, isavuconazole, posaconazole) are predicted to increase the exposure to **lapatinib**. [Moderate] Study → Also see TABLE 9 p. 1431
▸ Antifungals, azoles (itraconazole, ketoconazole, voriconazole) are predicted to increase the exposure to **lapatinib**. Avoid. [Moderate] Study → Also see TABLE 9 p. 1431
▸ **Lapatinib** is predicted to increase the exposure to antihistamines, non-sedating (fexofenadine). [Moderate] Theoretical
▸ **Lapatinib** is predicted to increase the exposure to beta blockers, non-selective (nadolol). [Moderate] Study
▸ **Lapatinib** is predicted to increase the exposure to bictegravir. Use with caution or avoid. [Moderate] Theoretical
▸ Calcium channel blockers (diltiazem, verapamil) are predicted to increase the exposure to **lapatinib**. [Moderate] Study
▸ **Lapatinib** is predicted to increase the exposure to ceritinib. [Moderate] Theoretical → Also see TABLE 9 p. 1431
▸ Cobicistat is predicted to increase the exposure to **lapatinib**. Avoid. [Moderate] Study
▸ **Lapatinib** is predicted to increase the exposure to colchicine. Avoid P-glycoprotein inhibitors or adjust **colchicine** dose, p. 1166. [Moderate] Theoretical
▸ **Lapatinib** is predicted to increase the risk of bleeding events when given with coumarins. [Severe] Theoretical
▸ Crizotinib is predicted to increase the exposure to **lapatinib**. [Moderate] Study → Also see TABLE 9 p. 1431
▸ **Lapatinib** is predicted to increase the exposure to digoxin. [Moderate] Theoretical
▸ Endothelin receptor antagonists (bosentan) are predicted to decrease the exposure to **lapatinib**. Avoid. [Severe] Study

Lapatinib (continued)

▶ **Lapatinib** is predicted to increase the exposure to erlotinib. Moderate Theoretical

▶ **Lapatinib** is predicted to increase the exposure to everolimus. Moderate Theoretical

▶ **Lapatinib** is predicted to slightly increase the exposure to factor XA inhibitors (edoxaban). Severe Theoretical

▶ **Lapatinib** is predicted to increase the exposure to fidaxomicin. Avoid. Moderate Study

▶ Grapefruit juice is predicted to increase the exposure to **lapatinib**. Avoid. Moderate Theoretical

▶ H_2 receptor antagonists are predicted to decrease the absorption of **lapatinib**. Avoid. Moderate Theoretical

▶ HIV-protease inhibitors are predicted to increase the exposure to **lapatinib**. Avoid. Moderate Study → Also see TABLE 9 p. 1431

▶ Idelalisib is predicted to increase the exposure to **lapatinib**. Avoid. Moderate Study

▶ Imatinib is predicted to increase the exposure to **lapatinib**. Moderate Study

▶ **Lapatinib** is predicted to increase the exposure to larotrectinib. Mild Theoretical

▶ Letermovir is predicted to increase the exposure to **lapatinib**. Moderate Study

▶ **Lapatinib** is predicted to increase the exposure to lomitapide. Separate administration by 12 hours. Mild Theoretical

▶ **Lapatinib** is predicted to increase the exposure to loperamide. Moderate Theoretical

▶ Macrolides (clarithromycin) are predicted to increase the exposure to **lapatinib**. Avoid. Moderate Study → Also see TABLE 9 p. 1431

▶ Macrolides (erythromycin) are predicted to increase the exposure to **lapatinib**. Moderate Study → Also see TABLE 9 p. 1431

▶ Mitotane is predicted to decrease the exposure to **lapatinib**. Avoid. Severe Study

▶ Neurokinin-1 receptor antagonists (aprepitant, netupitant) are predicted to increase the exposure to **lapatinib**. Moderate Study

▶ Nilotinib is predicted to increase the exposure to **lapatinib**. Moderate Study → Also see TABLE 9 p. 1431

▶ **Lapatinib** is predicted to increase the exposure to nintedanib. Moderate Study

▶ NNRTIs (efavirenz, nevirapine) are predicted to decrease the exposure to **lapatinib**. Avoid. Severe Study → Also see TABLE 9 p. 1431

▶ **Lapatinib** is predicted to increase the exposure to panobinostat. Adjust dose. Moderate Theoretical → Also see TABLE 9 p. 1431

▶ **Lapatinib** is predicted to increase the risk of bleeding events when given with phenindione. Severe Theoretical

▶ **Lapatinib** is predicted to increase the exposure to pibrentasvir. Moderate Theoretical

▶ Pitolisant is predicted to decrease the exposure to **lapatinib**. Avoid. Severe Theoretical

▶ Rifamycins (rifampicin) are predicted to decrease the exposure to **lapatinib**. Avoid. Severe Study

▶ **Lapatinib** is predicted to increase the exposure to sirolimus. Moderate Theoretical

▶ St John's wort is predicted to decrease the exposure to **lapatinib**. Avoid. Severe Study

▶ **Lapatinib** is predicted to slightly increase the exposure to talazoparib. Avoid or adjust talazoparib dose, p. 1052. Severe Study

▶ **Lapatinib** slightly increases the exposure to taxanes (paclitaxel). Severe Study

▶ Tedizolid is predicted to increase the exposure to **lapatinib**. Avoid. Moderate Theoretical

▶ **Lapatinib** is predicted to increase the exposure to thrombin inhibitors (dabigatran). Severe Theoretical

▶ **Lapatinib** is predicted to increase the exposure to topotecan. Severe Study

▶ **Lapatinib** is predicted to increase the concentration of trametinib. Moderate Theoretical

▶ **Lapatinib** is predicted to increase the exposure to venetoclax. Avoid or monitor for toxicity. Severe Theoretical

Laronidase

▶ Antimalarials (chloroquine) are predicted to decrease the exposure to **laronidase**. Avoid simultaneous administration. Severe Theoretical

▶ Hydroxychloroquine is predicted to decrease the exposure to **laronidase**. Avoid simultaneous administration. Severe Theoretical

Larotrectinib

▶ Anti-androgens (apalutamide, enzalutamide) are predicted to moderately decrease the exposure to **larotrectinib**. Avoid. Moderate Study

▶ Antiarrhythmics (amiodarone, dronedarone) are predicted to increase the exposure to **larotrectinib**. Mild Theoretical

▶ Antiepileptics (carbamazepine, fosphenytoin, phenobarbital, phenytoin, primidone) are predicted to moderately decrease the exposure to **larotrectinib**. Avoid. Moderate Study

▶ Antifungals, azoles (itraconazole, ketoconazole, voriconazole) are predicted to moderately increase the exposure to **larotrectinib**. Avoid or adjust **larotrectinib** dose, p. 1031. Moderate Study

▶ **Larotrectinib** slightly increases the exposure to benzodiazepines (midazolam). Use with caution and adjust dose. Mild Study

▶ Calcium channel blockers (verapamil) are predicted to increase the exposure to **larotrectinib**. Mild Theoretical

▶ Ciclosporin is predicted to increase the exposure to **larotrectinib**. Mild Study

▶ Cobicistat is predicted to moderately increase the exposure to **larotrectinib**. Avoid or adjust **larotrectinib** dose, p. 1031. Moderate Study

▶ **Larotrectinib** potentially decreases the efficacy of combined hormonal contraceptives. Use additional contraceptive precautions. Severe Theoretical

▶ Eltrombopag is predicted to increase the exposure to **larotrectinib**. Mild Study

▶ Endothelin receptor antagonists (bosentan) are predicted to decrease the exposure to **larotrectinib**. Avoid. Moderate Study

▶ **Larotrectinib** is predicted to increase the exposure to ergotamine. Use with caution and adjust dose. Mild Theoretical

▶ Grapefruit juice is predicted to increase the exposure to **larotrectinib**. Avoid. Moderate Theoretical

▶ HIV-protease inhibitors are predicted to moderately increase the exposure to **larotrectinib**. Avoid or adjust **larotrectinib** dose, p. 1031. Moderate Study

▶ Idelalisib is predicted to moderately increase the exposure to **larotrectinib**. Avoid or adjust **larotrectinib** dose, p. 1031. Moderate Study

▶ Lapatinib is predicted to increase the exposure to **larotrectinib**. Mild Theoretical

▶ Leflunomide is predicted to increase the exposure to **larotrectinib**. Mild Study

▶ Macrolides (azithromycin, erythromycin) are predicted to increase the exposure to **larotrectinib**. Mild Theoretical

▶ Macrolides (clarithromycin) are predicted to moderately increase the exposure to **larotrectinib**. Avoid or adjust **larotrectinib** dose, p. 1031. Moderate Study

▶ Mitotane is predicted to moderately decrease the exposure to **larotrectinib**. Avoid. Moderate Study

▶ NNRTIs (efavirenz, nevirapine) are predicted to decrease the exposure to **larotrectinib**. Avoid. Moderate Study

▶ **Larotrectinib** is predicted to increase the exposure to opioids (alfentanil, fentanyl). Use with caution and adjust dose. Mild Theoretical

▶ **Larotrectinib** is predicted to increase the exposure to pimozide. Use with caution and adjust dose. Mild Theoretical

▶ Ranolazine is predicted to increase the exposure to **larotrectinib**. Mild Theoretical

▶ Rifamycins (rifampicin) are predicted to moderately decrease the exposure to **larotrectinib**. Avoid. Moderate Study

▶ **Larotrectinib** is predicted to increase the exposure to sirolimus. Use with caution and adjust dose. Mild Theoretical

▶ St John's wort is predicted to decrease the exposure to **larotrectinib**. Avoid. Moderate Study

▶ **Larotrectinib** is predicted to increase the exposure to tacrolimus. Use with caution and adjust dose. Mild Theoretical

▶ Teriflunomide is predicted to increase the exposure to **larotrectinib**. Mild Study

Vemurafenib is predicted to increase the exposure to **larotrectinib**. Mild Theoretical

ledipasvir

Oral antacids are predicted to decrease the exposure to oral **ledipasvir**. Separate administration by 4 hours. Moderate Theoretical

- **Ledipasvir** increases the risk of severe bradycardia or heart block when given with antiarrhythmics (amiodarone). Refer to specialist literature. Severe Anecdotal

Antiepileptics (carbamazepine) are predicted to decrease the exposure to **ledipasvir**. Avoid. Severe Study

- Antiepileptics (fosphenytoin, oxcarbazepine, phenobarbital, phenytoin, primidone) are predicted to decrease the exposure to **ledipasvir**. Avoid. Severe Theoretical

- Calcium salts (calcium carbonate) are predicted to decrease the exposure to **ledipasvir**. Separate administration by 4 hours. Moderate Theoretical

- **Ledipasvir** is predicted to increase the exposure to digoxin. Monitor and adjust dose. Moderate Theoretical

- H₂ receptor antagonists are predicted to decrease the exposure to **ledipasvir**. Adjust dose, see ledipasvir with sofosbuvir p. 668. Moderate Study

- HIV-protease inhibitors (tipranavir) boosted with ritonavir are predicted to decrease the exposure to **ledipasvir**. Avoid. Severe Theoretical

- Proton pump inhibitors are predicted to decrease the exposure to **ledipasvir**. Adjust dose, see ledipasvir with sofosbuvir p. 668. Moderate Theoretical

- Rifamycins (rifabutin) are predicted to decrease the exposure to **ledipasvir**. Avoid. Severe Theoretical

- Rifamycins (rifampicin) are predicted to decrease the exposure to **ledipasvir**. Avoid. Severe Study

- Sodium zirconium cyclosilicate is predicted to decrease the exposure to **ledipasvir**. Separate administration by at least 2 hours. Moderate Theoretical

- St John's wort is predicted to decrease the exposure to **ledipasvir**. Avoid. Severe Study

- **Ledipasvir** is predicted to increase the exposure to statins (atorvastatin, fluvastatin, pravastatin, simvastatin). Monitor and adjust dose. Moderate Theoretical

- **Ledipasvir** is predicted to increase the exposure to statins (rosuvastatin). Avoid. Severe Theoretical

- **Ledipasvir** (with sofosbuvir) slightly increases the exposure to tenofovir disoproxil. Moderate Study

- **Ledipasvir** is predicted to increase the exposure to thrombin inhibitors (dabigatran). Moderate Theoretical

Leflunomide → see TABLE 1 p. 1429 (hepatotoxicity), TABLE 15 p. 1432 (myelosuppression)

PHARMACOLOGY Leflunomide has a long half-life; washout procedure recommended before switching to other DMARDs (consult product literature).

- **Leflunomide** is predicted to increase the exposure to adefovir. Moderate Theoretical

- **Leflunomide** is predicted to decrease the exposure to agomelatine. Moderate Theoretical

- **Leflunomide** is predicted to increase the exposure to alpelisib. Moderate Theoretical

- **Leflunomide** decreases the exposure to aminophylline. Adjust dose. Moderate Study

- **Leflunomide** is predicted to decrease the exposure to anaesthetics, local (ropivacaine). Moderate Theoretical

- **Leflunomide** is predicted to increase the exposure to anthracyclines (daunorubicin, doxorubicin, mitoxantrone). Moderate Theoretical → Also see TABLE 15 p. 1432

- **Leflunomide** is predicted to increase the exposure to antihistamines, non-sedating (fexofenadine). Moderate Study

- **Leflunomide** is predicted to decrease the exposure to antipsychotics, second generation (clozapine). Moderate Theoretical

- **Leflunomide** is predicted to decrease the exposure to antipsychotics, second generation (olanzapine). Monitor and adjust dose. Moderate Study

- **Leflunomide** potentially increases the exposure to baricitinib. Moderate Theoretical

- **Leflunomide** is predicted to moderately increase the clearance of caffeine citrate. Monitor and adjust dose. Moderate Study

- **Leflunomide** is predicted to increase the exposure to cephalosporins (cefaclor). Moderate Theoretical

- **Leflunomide** increases the anticoagulant effect of coumarins. Severe Anecdotal

- **Leflunomide** is predicted to decrease the exposure to duloxetine. Moderate Theoretical

- **Leflunomide** is predicted to increase the exposure to endothelin receptor antagonists (bosentan). Moderate Study

- Filgotinib is predicted to increase the risk of immunosuppression when given with **leflunomide**. Avoid. Severe Theoretical

- **Leflunomide** is predicted to increase the exposure to ganciclovir. Moderate Theoretical → Also see TABLE 15 p. 1432

- **Leflunomide** is predicted to increase the exposure to H₂ receptor antagonists (cimetidine, famotidine). Moderate Theoretical

- **Leflunomide** is predicted to increase the exposure to larotrectinib. Mild Study

- **Leflunomide** is predicted to increase the concentration of letermovir. Moderate Study

- Live vaccines are predicted to increase the risk of generalised infection (possibly life-threatening) when given with **leflunomide**. Public Health England advises avoid (refer to Green Book). Severe Theoretical

- **Leflunomide** is predicted to increase the exposure to loop diuretics (furosemide). Moderate Theoretical

- **Leflunomide** is predicted to increase the exposure to meglitinides (nateglinide). Moderate Theoretical

- **Leflunomide** is predicted to increase the exposure to meglitinides (repaglinide). Moderate Study

- **Leflunomide** is predicted to decrease the exposure to melatonin. Moderate Theoretical

- **Leflunomide** is predicted to increase the exposure to methotrexate. Moderate Theoretical → Also see TABLE 1 p. 1429 → Also see TABLE 15 p. 1432

- **Leflunomide** is predicted to increase the clearance of mexiletine. Monitor and adjust dose. Moderate Study

- **Leflunomide** is predicted to increase the exposure to montelukast. Moderate Theoretical

- **Leflunomide** is predicted to increase the exposure to NRTIs (zidovudine). Moderate Study

- **Leflunomide** is predicted to increase the exposure to NSAIDs (indometacin, ketoprofen). Moderate Theoretical

- **Leflunomide** is predicted to increase the exposure to oseltamivir. Moderate Theoretical

- **Leflunomide** is predicted to increase the exposure to the active metabolite of ozanimod. Avoid. Moderate Study

- **Leflunomide** is predicted to increase the exposure to penicillins (benzylpenicillin). Moderate Theoretical

- **Leflunomide** is predicted to increase the exposure to pioglitazone. Moderate Study

- **Leflunomide** is predicted to decrease the exposure to pirfenidone. Moderate Theoretical

- **Leflunomide** is predicted to increase the exposure to quinolones (ciprofloxacin). Moderate Theoretical

- **Leflunomide** is predicted to increase the exposure to rifamycins (rifampicin). Moderate Theoretical

- **Leflunomide** is predicted to increase the exposure to selexipag. Adjust **selexipag** dose, p. 196. Moderate Study

- **Leflunomide** is predicted to increase the exposure to statins (atorvastatin, fluvastatin, pravastatin, simvastatin). Moderate Study → Also see TABLE 1 p. 1429

- **Leflunomide** is predicted to increase the exposure to statins (rosuvastatin). Adjust dose. Moderate Study → Also see TABLE 1 p. 1429

- **Leflunomide** is predicted to increase the exposure to sulfasalazine. Moderate Study → Also see TABLE 1 p. 1429 → Also see TABLE 15 p. 1432

- **Leflunomide** is predicted to increase the exposure to sulfonylureas (glibenclamide). Moderate Study

- **Leflunomide** potentially increases the exposure to talazoparib. Avoid or monitor. Moderate Theoretical → Also see TABLE 15 p. 1432

- **Leflunomide** is predicted to increase the concentration of taxanes (paclitaxel). Severe Anecdotal → Also see TABLE 15 p. 1432

Leflunomide (continued)

▶ **Leflunomide** is predicted to increase the exposure to tenofovir alafenamide. Moderate Theoretical

▶ **Leflunomide** is predicted to increase the exposure to tenofovir disoproxil. Moderate Theoretical

▶ **Leflunomide** is predicted to decrease the exposure to theophylline. Adjust dose. Moderate Study

▶ **Leflunomide** moderately decreases the exposure to tizanidine. Mild Study

▶ **Leflunomide** is predicted to increase the exposure to topotecan. Moderate Study → Also see TABLE 15 p. 1432

Lenalidomide → see TABLE 1 p. 1429 (hepatotoxicity), TABLE 15 p. 1432 (myelosuppression), TABLE 5 p. 1430 (thromboembolism)

▶ Combined hormonal contraceptives are predicted to increase the risk of venous thromboembolism when given with **lenalidomide**. Avoid. Severe Theoretical

▶ Hormone replacement therapy is predicted to increase the risk of venous thromboembolism when given with **lenalidomide**. Moderate Theoretical

Lenvatinib → see TABLE 9 p. 1431 (QT-interval prolongation)

Lercanidipine → see calcium channel blockers

Letermovir

▶ **Letermovir** is predicted to increase the exposure to abemaciclib. Moderate Study

▶ **Letermovir** is predicted to increase the exposure to acalabrutinib. Avoid or monitor. Severe Study

▶ **Letermovir** is predicted to increase the exposure to aldosterone antagonists (eplerenone). Adjust **eplerenone** dose, p. 208. Severe Study

▶ **Letermovir** is predicted to increase the exposure to alpha blockers (tamsulosin). Moderate Theoretical

▶ **Letermovir** is predicted to increase the concentration of antiarrhythmics (amiodarone). Moderate Theoretical

▶ **Letermovir** is predicted to increase the exposure to antiarrhythmics (propafenone). Monitor and adjust dose. Moderate Study

▶ Antiepileptics (carbamazepine, phenobarbital, primidone) are predicted to decrease the concentration of **letermovir**. Moderate Theoretical

▶ **Letermovir** is predicted to decrease the concentration of antiepileptics (fosphenytoin, phenytoin) and antiepileptics (fosphenytoin, phenytoin) are predicted to decrease the concentration of **letermovir**. Moderate Theoretical

▶ **Letermovir** slightly decreases the exposure to antifungals, azoles (voriconazole). Moderate Study

▶ **Letermovir** is predicted to increase the concentration of antihistamines, non-sedating (fexofenadine). Moderate Theoretical

▶ **Letermovir** is predicted to increase the exposure to antihistamines, non-sedating (mizolastine). Severe Theoretical

▶ **Letermovir** is predicted to increase the exposure to antihistamines, non-sedating (rupatadine). Avoid. Moderate Study

▶ **Letermovir** is predicted to increase the concentration of antimalarials (piperaquine). Severe Theoretical

▶ **Letermovir** is predicted to increase the exposure to antipsychotics, second generation (cariprazine). Avoid. Severe Study

▶ **Letermovir** is predicted to increase the exposure to antipsychotics, second generation (quetiapine). Avoid. Moderate Study

▶ **Letermovir** is predicted to increase the exposure to avapritinib. Avoid or adjust **avapritinib** dose, p. 1012. Moderate Study

▶ **Letermovir** is predicted to increase the exposure to axitinib. Moderate Theoretical

▶ **Letermovir** is predicted to increase the exposure to bedaquiline. Avoid prolonged use. Mild Theoretical

▶ **Letermovir** is predicted to increase the exposure to benzodiazepines (alprazolam). Severe Study

▶ **Letermovir** is predicted to increase the exposure to benzodiazepines (midazolam). Monitor adverse effects and adjust dose. Severe Study

▶ **Letermovir** is predicted to increase the exposure to bosutinib. Avoid or adjust dose. Severe Theoretical

▶ **Letermovir** is predicted to increase the exposure to buspirone. Use with caution and adjust dose. Moderate Study

▶ **Letermovir** is predicted to increase the exposure to cabozantinib. Moderate Theoretical

▶ **Letermovir** is predicted to increase the exposure to calcium channel blockers (amlodipine, felodipine, lacidipine, lercanidipine, nicardipine, nifedipine, nimodipine). Monitor and adjust dose. Moderate Study

▶ **Letermovir** increases the exposure to ciclosporin and ciclosporin increases the exposure to **letermovir**. Monitor and adjust **letermovir** dose, p. 678. Severe Study

▶ **Letermovir** is predicted to increase the exposure to cobimetinib. Severe Theoretical

▶ **Letermovir** is predicted to increase the exposure to colchicine. Adjust **colchicine** dose with moderate CYP3A4 inhibitors, p. 1166. Severe Study

▶ **Letermovir** is predicted to increase the exposure to corticosteroids (methylprednisolone). Monitor and adjust dose. Moderate Study

▶ **Letermovir** is predicted to decrease the concentration of coumarins (warfarin). Monitor and adjust dose. Moderate Theoretical

▶ **Letermovir** is predicted to slightly increase the exposure to darifenacin. Moderate Study

▶ **Letermovir** is predicted to increase the exposure to dasatinib. Severe Study

▶ **Letermovir** is predicted to slightly increase the exposure to dienogest. Moderate Study

▶ **Letermovir** is predicted to increase the exposure to dipeptidylpeptidase-4 inhibitors (saxagliptin). Mild Study

▶ **Letermovir** increases the risk of QT-prolongation when given with domperidone. Avoid. Severe Study

▶ **Letermovir** is predicted to increase the exposure to dopamine receptor agonists (bromocriptine). Severe Theoretical

▶ **Letermovir** is predicted to moderately increase the exposure to dutasteride. Mild Study

▶ **Letermovir** is predicted to increase the exposure to elexacaftor. Adjust tezacaftor with ivacaftor and elexacftor p. 311 dose with moderate CYP3A4 inhibitors. Severe Theoretical

▶ **Letermovir** is predicted to increase the exposure to eliglustat. Avoid or adjust dose—consult product literature. Severe Study

▶ Eltrombopag is predicted to increase the concentration of **letermovir**. Moderate Study

▶ **Letermovir** is predicted to moderately increase the exposure to encorafenib. Moderate Study

▶ **Letermovir** is predicted to increase the concentration of endothelin receptor antagonists (bosentan). Moderate Theoretical

▶ **Letermovir** is predicted to increase the exposure to entrectinib. Avoid moderate CYP3A4 inhibitors or adjust **entrectinib** dose, p. 1023. Severe Theoretical

▶ **Letermovir** is predicted to increase the risk of ergotism when given with ergometrine. Severe Theoretical

▶ **Letermovir** is predicted to increase the risk of ergotism when given with ergotamine. Severe Theoretical

▶ **Letermovir** is predicted to increase the exposure to erlotinib. Moderate Theoretical

▶ **Letermovir** is predicted to increase the concentration of everolimus. Avoid or adjust dose. Moderate Study

▶ **Letermovir** is predicted to increase the exposure to fesoterodine. Adjust **fesoterodine** dose with moderate CYP3A4 inhibitors in hepatic and renal impairment, p. 822. Mild Study

▶ Fibrates (gemfibrozil) are predicted to increase the concentration of **letermovir**. Moderate Study

▶ **Letermovir** is predicted to increase the exposure to gefitinib. Moderate Theoretical

▶ **Letermovir** is predicted to increase the concentration of guanfacine. Adjust **guanfacine** dose, p. 372. Moderate Theoretical

▶ HIV-protease inhibitors (atazanavir, lopinavir) boosted with ritonavir are predicted to increase the concentration of **letermovir**. Moderate Study

▶ HIV-protease inhibitors (ritonavir) are predicted to decrease the concentration of **letermovir**. Moderate Theoretical

▶ **Letermovir** is predicted to increase the exposure to ibrutinib. Adjust **ibrutinib** dose with moderate CYP3A4 inhibitors, p. 1027. Severe Study

▶ **Letermovir** is predicted to increase the exposure to ivacaftor. Adjust ivacaftor p. 309 or tezacaftor with ivacaftor p. 311 or tezacaftor with ivacaftor and elexacftor p. 311 dose with moderate CYP3A4 inhibitors. Severe Study

▸ **Letermovir** is predicted to increase the exposure to lapatinib. Moderate Study

▸ **Leflunomide** is predicted to increase the concentration of **letermovir**. Moderate Study

▸ **Letermovir** is predicted to increase the exposure to lomitapide. Avoid. Moderate Theoretical

▸ **Macrolides** (clarithromycin, erythromycin) are predicted to increase the concentration of **letermovir**. Moderate Study

▸ **Letermovir** is predicted to increase the concentration of meglitinides (repaglinide). Avoid. Moderate Theoretical

▸ **Letermovir** is predicted to increase the exposure to midostaurin. Moderate Theoretical

▸ **Modafinil** is predicted to decrease the concentration of **letermovir**. Moderate Theoretical

▸ **Letermovir** is predicted to increase the exposure to naldemedine. Moderate Study

▸ **Letermovir** is predicted to increase the exposure to naloxegol. Adjust **naloxegol** dose and monitor adverse effects, p. 70. Moderate Study

▸ **Letermovir** is predicted to increase the exposure to neratinib. Avoid. Severe Study

▸ **NNRTIs** (efavirenz) are predicted to decrease the concentration of **letermovir**. Moderate Theoretical

▸ **NNRTIs** (etravirine) are predicted to decrease the exposure to **letermovir**. Moderate Theoretical

▸ **Letermovir** is predicted to increase the exposure to olaparib. Avoid moderate CYP3A4 inhibitors or adjust **olaparib** dose, p. 1051. Moderate Theoretical

▸ **Letermovir** is predicted to increase the exposure to opioids (alfentanil, buprenorphine, fentanyl, oxycodone). Monitor and adjust dose. Moderate Study

▸ **Letermovir** is predicted to increase the exposure to opioids (methadone). Moderate Theoretical

▸ **Letermovir** is predicted to increase the exposure to oxybutynin. Mild Theoretical

▸ **Letermovir** is predicted to increase the exposure to pazopanib. Moderate Theoretical

▸ **Letermovir** is predicted to increase the exposure to phosphodiesterase type-5 inhibitors (avanafil). Adjust **avanafil** dose, p. 859. Moderate Theoretical

▸ **Letermovir** is predicted to increase the exposure to phosphodiesterase type-5 inhibitors (sildenafil). Monitor or adjust **sildenafil** dose with moderate CYP3A4 inhibitors, p. 860. Moderate Study

▸ **Letermovir** is predicted to increase the exposure to phosphodiesterase type-5 inhibitors (tadalafil). Severe Theoretical

▸ **Letermovir** is predicted to increase the exposure to phosphodiesterase type-5 inhibitors (vardenafil). Adjust dose. Severe Theoretical

▸ **Letermovir** is predicted to increase the exposure to pimozide. Avoid. Severe Theoretical

▸ **Letermovir** is predicted to increase the exposure to ranolazine. Severe Study

▸ **Letermovir** is predicted to increase the exposure to ribociclib. Moderate Study

▸ **Rifamycins** (rifabutin) are predicted to decrease the concentration of **letermovir**. Moderate Theoretical

▸ **Rifamycins** (rifampicin) are predicted to affect the concentration of **letermovir**. Severe Theoretical

▸ **Letermovir** is predicted to increase the exposure to ruxolitinib. Moderate Theoretical

▸ **Letermovir** increases the concentration of sirolimus. Monitor and adjust dose. Moderate Study

▸ **Letermovir** is predicted to increase the exposure to SSRIs (dapoxetine). Adjust **dapoxetine** dose with moderate CYP3A4 inhibitors, p. 867. Moderate Theoretical

▸ **St John's wort** is predicted to decrease the concentration of **letermovir**. Moderate Theoretical

▸ **Letermovir** moderately increases the exposure to statins (atorvastatin). Avoid or adjust **atorvastatin** dose, p. 217. Severe Study

▸ **Letermovir** is predicted to increase the exposure to statins (fluvastatin). Monitor and adjust dose. Moderate Theoretical

▸ **Letermovir** is predicted to increase the exposure to statins (pravastatin). Avoid or adjust dose. Moderate Theoretical

▸ **Letermovir** is predicted to increase the exposure to statins (rosuvastatin, simvastatin). Avoid. Severe Study

▸ **Letermovir** is predicted to increase the concentration of sulfonylureas (glibenclamide). Moderate Theoretical

▸ **Letermovir** is predicted to increase the exposure to sunitinib. Moderate Theoretical

▸ **Letermovir** is predicted to increase the concentration of tacrolimus. Severe Study

▸ **Letermovir** is predicted to increase the exposure to taxanes (cabazitaxel). Moderate Theoretical

▸ **Teriflunomide** is predicted to increase the concentration of **letermovir**. Moderate Study

▸ **Letermovir** is predicted to increase the exposure to tezacaftor. Adjust tezacaftor with ivacaftor p. 311 or tezacaftor with ivacaftor and elexacftor p. 311 dose with moderate CYP3A4 inhibitors. Severe Study

▸ **Letermovir** is predicted to decrease the concentration of thrombin inhibitors (dabigatran). Avoid. Severe Theoretical

▸ **Letermovir** is predicted to increase the exposure to tolterodine. Mild Theoretical

▸ **Letermovir** is predicted to increase the exposure to tolvaptan. Manufacturer advises caution or adjust **tolvaptan** dose with moderate CYP3A4 inhibitors, p. 708. Moderate Study

▸ **Letermovir** is predicted to increase the exposure to trazodone. Moderate Theoretical

▸ **Letermovir** is predicted to increase the exposure to venetoclax. Avoid or adjust dose—consult product literature. Severe Study

▸ **Letermovir** is predicted to increase the exposure to vinca alkaloids. Severe Theoretical

▸ **Letermovir** is predicted to increase the exposure to zopiclone. Adjust dose. Moderate Study

Levamisole
▸ **Albendazole** slightly decreases the exposure to **levamisole** and **levamisole** moderately decreases the exposure to albendazole. Moderate Study

▸ **Alcohol** potentially causes a disulfiram-like reaction when given with **levamisole**. Moderate Study

▸ **Levamisole** increases the exposure to ivermectin. Moderate Study

Levetiracetam → see antiepileptics
Levobunolol → see beta blockers, non-selective
Levobupivacaine → see anaesthetics, local
Levocetirizine → see antihistamines, non-sedating
Levodopa → see TABLE 8 p. 1430 (hypotension)
▸ **Antiepileptics** (fosphenytoin, phenytoin) decrease the effects of **levodopa**. Severe Study

▸ **Antipsychotics, second generation** (amisulpride) are predicted to decrease the effects of **levodopa**. Avoid. Severe Theoretical

▸ **Antipsychotics, second generation** (aripiprazole, clozapine, lurasidone, paliperidone) are predicted to decrease the effects of **levodopa**. Severe Theoretical → Also see TABLE 8 p. 1430

▸ **Antipsychotics, second generation** (asenapine) are predicted to decrease the effects of **levodopa**. Adjust dose. Severe Theoretical → Also see TABLE 8 p. 1430

▸ **Antipsychotics, second generation** (olanzapine) decrease the effects of **levodopa**. Avoid or monitor worsening parkinsonian symptoms. Severe Anecdotal → Also see TABLE 8 p. 1430

▸ **Antipsychotics, second generation** (quetiapine) decrease the effects of **levodopa**. Severe Anecdotal → Also see TABLE 8 p. 1430

▸ **Antipsychotics, second generation** (risperidone) are predicted to decrease the effects of **levodopa**. Avoid or adjust dose. Severe Anecdotal → Also see TABLE 8 p. 1430

▸ **Baclofen** is predicted to increase the risk of adverse effects when given with **levodopa**. Severe Anecdotal → Also see TABLE 8 p. 1430

▸ **Benperidol** is predicted to decrease the effects of **levodopa**. Severe Study → Also see TABLE 8 p. 1430

▸ **Bupropion** increases the risk of adverse effects when given with **levodopa**. Moderate Study

▸ **Droperidol** decreases the effects of **levodopa**. Severe Study → Also see TABLE 8 p. 1430

▸ **Drugs with antimuscarinic effects** (see TABLE 10 p. 1431) decrease the absorption of **levodopa**. Moderate Theoretical

Levodopa (continued)

▸ Entacapone increases the exposure to **levodopa**. Monitor adverse effects and adjust dose. Moderate Study
▸ Flupentixol decreases the effects of **levodopa**. Avoid or monitor worsening parkinsonian symptoms. Severe Theoretical → Also see **TABLE 8** p. 1430
▸ Haloperidol decreases the effects of **levodopa**. Severe Study → Also see **TABLE 8** p. 1430
▸ Oral iron decreases the absorption of oral **levodopa**. Moderate Study
▸ Isoniazid decreases the effects of **levodopa**. Moderate Study
▸ **Levodopa** is predicted to increase the risk of elevated blood pressure when given with linezolid. Avoid. Severe Theoretical
▸ Loxapine is predicted to decrease the effects of **levodopa**. Severe Theoretical → Also see **TABLE 8** p. 1430
▸ MAO-B inhibitors are predicted to increase the effects of **levodopa**. Adjust dose. Mild Study → Also see **TABLE 8** p. 1430
▸ **Levodopa** increases the risk of a hypertensive crisis when given with MAOIs, irreversible. Avoid and for 14 days after stopping the MAOI. Severe Study → Also see **TABLE 8** p. 1430
▸ Memantine is predicted to increase the effects of **levodopa**. Moderate Theoretical
▸ Metoclopramide decreases the effects of **levodopa**. Avoid. Moderate Study
▸ **Levodopa** increases the risk of adverse effects when given with moclobemide. Moderate Study
▸ Opicapone increases the exposure to **levodopa**. Adjust dose. Moderate Study
▸ Phenothiazines decrease the effects of **levodopa**. Avoid or monitor worsening parkinsonian symptoms. Severe Study → Also see **TABLE 8** p. 1430
▸ Pimozide decreases the effects of **levodopa**. Severe Theoretical → Also see **TABLE 8** p. 1430
▸ Sulpiride is predicted to decrease the effects of **levodopa**. Avoid. Severe Theoretical → Also see **TABLE 8** p. 1430
▸ Tetrabenazine is predicted to decrease the effects of **levodopa**. Use with caution or avoid. Moderate Theoretical
▸ Tolcapone increases the exposure to **levodopa**. Monitor and adjust dose. Moderate Study
▸ Tryptophan greatly decreases the concentration of **levodopa**. Moderate Study
▸ Zuclopenthixol is predicted to decrease the effects of **levodopa**. Avoid or monitor worsening parkinsonian symptoms. Severe Theoretical → Also see **TABLE 8** p. 1430

Levofloxacin → see quinolones
Levofolinic acid → see folates
Levomepromazine → see phenothiazines
Levonorgestrel

▸ Antiepileptics (carbamazepine, eslicarbazepine, fosphenytoin, oxcarbazepine, perampanel, phenobarbital, phenytoin, primidone, rufinamide, topiramate) are predicted to decrease the efficacy of **levonorgestrel**. For FSRH guidance, see Contraceptives, interactions p. 840. Severe Theoretical
▸ Endothelin receptor antagonists (bosentan) are predicted to decrease the efficacy of **levonorgestrel**. For FSRH guidance, see Contraceptives, interactions p. 840. Severe Theoretical
▸ Griseofulvin potentially decreases the efficacy of oral **levonorgestrel**. For FSRH guidance, see Contraceptives, interactions p. 840. Severe Anecdotal
▸ HIV-protease inhibitors (ritonavir) are predicted to decrease the efficacy of **levonorgestrel**. For FSRH guidance, see Contraceptives, interactions p. 840. Severe Theoretical
▸ Lumacaftor is predicted to decrease the efficacy of **levonorgestrel**. Use additional contraceptive precautions. Severe Theoretical
▸ Modafinil is predicted to decrease the efficacy of **levonorgestrel**. For FSRH guidance, see Contraceptives, interactions p. 840. Severe Theoretical
▸ Neurokinin-1 receptor antagonists (aprepitant, fosaprepitant) are predicted to decrease the efficacy of **levonorgestrel**. For FSRH guidance, see Contraceptives, interactions p. 840. Severe Theoretical
▸ NNRTIs (efavirenz, nevirapine) are predicted to decrease the efficacy of **levonorgestrel**. For FSRH guidance, see Contraceptives, interactions p. 840. Severe Theoretical

▸ Rifamycins are predicted to decrease the efficacy of **levonorgestrel**. For FSRH guidance, see Contraceptives, interactions p. 840. Severe Theoretical
▸ St John's wort is predicted to decrease the efficacy of **levonorgestrel**. MHRA advises avoid. For FSRH guidance, see Contraceptives, interactions p. 840. Severe Theoretical
▸ Sugammadex is predicted to decrease the exposure to **levonorgestrel**. Use additional contraceptive precautions. Severe Theoretical
▸ Ulipristal is predicted to decrease the efficacy of **levonorgestrel**. Avoid. Severe Theoretical

Levothyroxine → see thyroid hormones
Lidocaine → see antiarrhythmics
Linagliptin → see dipeptidylpeptidase-4 inhibitors
Linezolid → see **TABLE 13** p. 1432 (serotonin syndrome)

FOOD AND LIFESTYLE Patients taking linezolid should avoid consuming large amounts of tyramine-rich foods (such as mature cheese, salami, pickled herring, *Bovril*®, *Oxo*®, *Marmite*® or any similar meat or yeast extract or fermented soya bean extract, and some beers, lagers or wines).

▸ Beta$_2$ agonists are predicted to increase the risk of elevated blood pressure when given with **linezolid**. Avoid. Severe Theoretical
▸ Bupropion is predicted to increase the risk of intraoperative hypertension when given with **linezolid**. Severe Anecdotal → Also see **TABLE 13** p. 1432
▸ Buspirone is predicted to increase the risk of elevated blood pressure when given with **linezolid**. Avoid. Severe Theoretical → Also see **TABLE 13** p. 1432
▸ Levodopa is predicted to increase the risk of elevated blood pressure when given with **linezolid**. Avoid. Severe Theoretical
▸ Macrolides (clarithromycin) increase the exposure to **linezolid**. Moderate Anecdotal
▸ MAO-B inhibitors (rasagiline, selegiline) are predicted to increase the risk of adverse effects when given with **linezolid**. Avoid and for 14 days after stopping the MAOI. Severe Theoretical → Also see **TABLE 13** p. 1432
▸ MAO-B inhibitors (safinamide) are predicted to increase the risk of adverse effects when given with **linezolid**. Avoid and for 1 week after stopping **safinamide**. Severe Theoretical → Also see **TABLE 13** p. 1432
▸ MAOIs, irreversible are predicted to increase the risk of adverse effects when given with **linezolid**. Avoid and for 14 days after stopping the MAOI. Severe Theoretical → Also see **TABLE 13** p. 1432
▸ Methylphenidate is predicted to increase the risk of elevated blood pressure when given with **linezolid**. Avoid. Severe Theoretical
▸ Moclobemide is predicted to increase the risk of adverse effects when given with **linezolid**. Avoid and for 14 days after stopping **moclobemide**, p. 382. Severe Theoretical → Also see **TABLE 13** p. 1432
▸ Ozanimod potentially increases the risk of a hypertensive crisis when given with **linezolid**. Avoid. Severe Theoretical
▸ Reboxetine is predicted to increase the risk of a hypertensive crisis when given with **linezolid**. Avoid. Severe Theoretical
▸ Rifamycins (rifampicin) slightly decrease the exposure to **linezolid**. Moderate Study
▸ Sympathomimetics, inotropic are predicted to increase the risk of elevated blood pressure when given with **linezolid**. Avoid. Severe Theoretical
▸ Sympathomimetics, vasoconstrictor (adrenaline/epinephrine, ephedrine, isometheptene, noradrenaline/norepinephrine, phenylephrine) are predicted to increase the risk of elevated blood pressure when given with **linezolid**. Avoid. Severe Theoretical
▸ Sympathomimetics, vasoconstrictor (pseudoephedrine) increase the risk of elevated blood pressure when given with **linezolid**. Avoid. Severe Study

Liothyronine → see thyroid hormones
Liraglutide → see glucagon-like peptide-1 receptor agonists
Lisdexamfetamine → see amfetamines
Lisinopril → see ACE inhibitors
Lithium → see **TABLE 13** p. 1432 (serotonin syndrome), **TABLE 9** p. 1431 (QT-interval prolongation)

ACE inhibitors are predicted to increase the concentration of **lithium**. Monitor and adjust dose. [Severe] Anecdotal

Acetazolamide alters the concentration of **lithium**. [Severe] Anecdotal

Aldosterone antagonists (eplerenone) potentially increase the concentration of **lithium**. Avoid. [Moderate] Theoretical

Aldosterone antagonists (spironolactone) potentially increase the concentration of **lithium**. [Moderate] Study

Aminophylline is predicted to decrease the concentration of **lithium**. [Moderate] Theoretical

Angiotensin-II receptor antagonists potentially increase the concentration of **lithium**. Monitor concentration and adjust dose. [Severe] Anecdotal

Antiepileptics (carbamazepine, oxcarbazepine) are predicted to increase the risk of neurotoxicity when given with **lithium**. [Severe] Anecdotal

Antipsychotics, second generation (quetiapine, risperidone) potentially increase the risk of neurotoxicity when given with **lithium**. [Severe] Anecdotal → Also see **TABLE 9** p. 1431

Calcitonins decrease the concentration of **lithium**. Adjust dose. [Moderate] Study

Calcium channel blockers (diltiazem, verapamil) are predicted to increase the risk of neurotoxicity when given with **lithium**. [Severe] Anecdotal

Loop diuretics increase the concentration of **lithium**. Monitor and adjust dose. [Severe] Study

Methyldopa increases the risk of neurotoxicity when given with **lithium**. [Severe] Anecdotal

Metronidazole is predicted to increase the concentration of **lithium**. Avoid or adjust dose. [Severe] Anecdotal

Mexiletine potentially affects the exposure to **lithium**. Avoid. [Unknown] Theoretical

NSAIDs increase the concentration of **lithium**. Monitor and adjust dose. [Severe] Study

Phenothiazines potentially increase the risk of neurotoxicity when given with **lithium**. [Severe] Anecdotal → Also see **TABLE 9** p. 1431

Potassium-sparing diuretics (triamterene) potentially increase the clearance of **lithium**. [Moderate] Study

Sodium bicarbonate decreases the concentration of **lithium**. [Severe] Anecdotal

Sulpiride potentially increases the risk of neurotoxicity when given with **lithium**. [Severe] Anecdotal → Also see **TABLE 9** p. 1431

Tetracyclines are predicted to increase the risk of lithium toxicity when given with **lithium**. Avoid or adjust dose. [Severe] Anecdotal

Theophylline is predicted to decrease the concentration of **lithium**. Monitor concentration and adjust dose. [Moderate] Anecdotal

Thiazide diuretics increase the concentration of **lithium**. Avoid or adjust dose and monitor concentration. [Severe] Study

Tricyclic antidepressants potentially increase the risk of neurotoxicity when given with **lithium**. [Severe] Anecdotal → Also see **TABLE 13** p. 1432 → Also see **TABLE 9** p. 1431

Zuclopenthixol potentially increases the risk of neurotoxicity when given with **lithium**. [Severe] Anecdotal → Also see **TABLE 9** p. 1431

Live vaccines

Bacillus Calmette-Guérin vaccine · influenza vaccine (live) · measles, mumps and rubella vaccine, live · rotavirus vaccine · typhoid vaccine, oral · varicella-zoster vaccine · yellow fever vaccine, live

GENERAL INFORMATION Oral typhoid vaccine is inactivated by concurrent administration of antibacterials or antimalarials: antibacterials should be avoided for 3 days before and after oral typhoid vaccination; *mefloquine* should be avoided for at least 12 hours before or after oral typhoid vaccination; for other antimalarials oral typhoid vaccine vaccination should be completed at least 3 days before the first dose of the antimalarial (except proguanil hydrochloride with atovaquone, which can be given concurrently).

▸ **Live vaccines** are predicted to increase the risk of generalised infection (possibly life-threatening) when given with abatacept. Public Health England advises avoid (refer to Green Book). [Severe] Theoretical

▸ **Live vaccines** are predicted to increase the risk of generalised infection (possibly life-threatening) when given with alkylating agents. Public Health England advises avoid (refer to Green Book). [Severe] Theoretical

▸ **Live vaccines** are predicted to increase the risk of generalised infection (possibly life-threatening) when given with amsacrine. Public Health England advises avoid (refer to Green Book). [Severe] Theoretical

▸ **Live vaccines** are predicted to increase the risk of generalised infection (possibly life-threatening) when given with anakinra. Public Health England advises avoid (refer to Green Book). [Severe] Theoretical

▸ **Live vaccines** are predicted to increase the risk of generalised infection (possibly life-threatening) when given with anthracyclines. Public Health England advises avoid (refer to Green Book). [Severe] Theoretical

▸ **Live vaccines** are predicted to increase the risk of generalised infection (possibly life-threatening) when given with azathioprine (high-dose). Public Health England advises avoid (refer to Green Book). [Severe] Theoretical

▸ **Live vaccines** are predicted to increase the risk of generalised infection (possibly life-threatening) when given with baricitinib. Avoid. [Severe] Theoretical

▸ **Live vaccines** are predicted to increase the risk of generalised infection (possibly life-threatening) when given with belatacept. Public Health England advises avoid (refer to Green Book). [Severe] Theoretical

▸ **Live vaccines** are predicted to increase the risk of generalised infection (possibly life-threatening) when given with bleomycin. Public Health England advises avoid (refer to Green Book). [Severe] Theoretical

▸ **Live vaccines** are predicted to increase the risk of generalised infection (possibly life-threatening) when given with capecitabine. Public Health England advises avoid (refer to Green Book). [Severe] Theoretical

▸ **Live vaccines** are predicted to increase the risk of generalised infection (possibly life-threatening) when given with ciclosporin. Public Health England advises avoid (refer to Green Book). [Severe] Theoretical

▸ **Live vaccines** are predicted to increase the risk of generalised infection (possibly life-threatening) when given with cladribine. Public Health England advises avoid (refer to Green Book). [Severe] Theoretical

▸ **Live vaccines** are predicted to increase the risk of generalised infection (possibly life-threatening) when given with clofarabine. Public Health England advises avoid (refer to Green Book). [Severe] Theoretical

▸ **Live vaccines** are predicted to increase the risk of generalised infection (possibly life-threatening) when given with corticosteroids (high-dose). Public Health England advises avoid (refer to Green Book). [Severe] Theoretical

▸ **Live vaccines** are predicted to increase the risk of generalised infection (possibly life-threatening) when given with cytarabine. Public Health England advises avoid (refer to Green Book). [Severe] Theoretical

▸ **Live vaccines** are predicted to increase the risk of generalised infection (possibly life-threatening) when given with dactinomycin. Public Health England advises avoid (refer to Green Book). [Severe] Theoretical

▸ **Live vaccines** are predicted to increase the risk of generalised infection (possibly life-threatening) when given with dimethyl fumarate. Public Health England advises avoid (refer to Green Book). [Severe] Theoretical

▸ **Live vaccines** are predicted to increase the risk of generalised infection (possibly life-threatening) when given with etanercept. Public Health England advises avoid (refer to Green Book). [Severe] Theoretical

▸ **Live vaccines** are predicted to increase the risk of generalised infection (possibly life-threatening) when given with etoposide. Public Health England advises avoid (refer to Green Book). [Severe] Theoretical

▸ **Live vaccines** are predicted to increase the risk of generalised infection (possibly life-threatening) when given with everolimus. Public Health England advises avoid (refer to Green Book). [Severe] Theoretical

Live vaccines (continued)

▸ **Live vaccines** are predicted to increase the risk of generalised infection (possibly life-threatening) when given with filgotinib. Avoid. [Severe] Theoretical

▸ **Live vaccines** are predicted to increase the risk of generalised infection (possibly life-threatening) when given with fingolimod. Public Health England advises avoid (refer to Green Book). [Severe] Theoretical

▸ **Live vaccines** are predicted to increase the risk of generalised infection (possibly life-threatening) when given with fludarabine. Public Health England advises avoid (refer to Green Book). [Severe] Theoretical

▸ **Live vaccines** are predicted to increase the risk of generalised infection (possibly life-threatening) when given with fluorouracil. Public Health England advises avoid (refer to Green Book). [Severe] Theoretical

▸ **Live vaccines** are predicted to increase the risk of generalised infection (possibly life-threatening) when given with gemcitabine. Public Health England advises avoid (refer to Green Book). [Severe] Theoretical

▸ **Live vaccines** are predicted to increase the risk of generalised infection (possibly life-threatening) when given with hydroxycarbamide. Public Health England advises avoid (refer to Green Book). [Severe] Theoretical

▸ Immunoglobulins (cytomegalovirus immunoglobulin) are predicted to decrease the efficacy of **live vaccines**. Avoid. [Severe] Theoretical

▸ **Live vaccines** are predicted to increase the risk of generalised infection (possibly life-threatening) when given with irinotecan. Public Health England advises avoid (refer to Green Book). [Severe] Theoretical

▸ **Live vaccines** are predicted to increase the risk of generalised infection (possibly life-threatening) when given with iron chelators (dexrazoxane). Avoid. [Severe] Theoretical

▸ **Live vaccines** are predicted to increase the risk of generalised infection (possibly life-threatening) when given with leflunomide. Public Health England advises avoid (refer to Green Book). [Severe] Theoretical

▸ **Live vaccines** are predicted to increase the risk of generalised infection (possibly life-threatening) when given with mercaptopurine (high-dose). Public Health England advises avoid (refer to Green Book). [Severe] Theoretical

▸ **Live vaccines** are predicted to increase the risk of generalised infection (possibly life-threatening) when given with methotrexate (high-dose). Public Health England advises avoid (refer to Green Book). [Severe] Theoretical

▸ **Live vaccines** are predicted to increase the risk of generalised infection (possibly life-threatening) when given with mitomycin. Public Health England advises avoid (refer to Green Book). [Severe] Theoretical

▸ **Live vaccines** are predicted to increase the risk of generalised infection (possibly life-threatening) when given with monoclonal antibodies. Public Health England advises avoid (refer to Green Book). [Severe] Theoretical

▸ **Live vaccines** are predicted to increase the risk of generalised infection (possibly life-threatening) when given with mycophenolate. Public Health England advises avoid (refer to Green Book). [Severe] Theoretical

▸ **Live vaccines** are predicted to increase the risk of generalised infection (possibly life-threatening) when given with ozanimod. Avoid and for 3 months after stopping ozanimod. [Severe] Theoretical

▸ **Live vaccines** are predicted to increase the risk of generalised infection (possibly life-threatening) when given with pemetrexed. Public Health England advises avoid (refer to Green Book). [Severe] Theoretical

▸ **Live vaccines** are predicted to increase the risk of generalised infection (possibly life-threatening) when given with platinum compounds. Public Health England advises avoid (refer to Green Book). [Severe] Theoretical

▸ **Live vaccines** are predicted to increase the risk of generalised infection (possibly life-threatening) when given with procarbazine. Public Health England advises avoid (refer to Green Book). [Severe] Theoretical

▸ **Live vaccines** are predicted to increase the risk of generalised infection (possibly life-threatening) when given with raltitrexed. Public Health England advises avoid (refer to Green Book). [Severe] Theoretical

▸ **Live vaccines** are predicted to increase the risk of generalised infection (possibly life-threatening) when given with siponimod. Avoid and for 4 weeks after stopping siponimod. [Severe] Theoretical

▸ **Live vaccines** are predicted to increase the risk of generalised infection (possibly life-threatening) when given with sirolimus. Public Health England advises avoid (refer to Green Book). [Severe] Theoretical

▸ **Live vaccines** are predicted to increase the risk of generalised infection (possibly life-threatening) when given with streptozocin. Public Health England advises avoid (refer to Green Book). [Severe] Theoretical

▸ **Live vaccines** are predicted to increase the risk of generalised infection (possibly life-threatening) when given with tacrolimus. Public Health England advises avoid (refer to Green Book). [Severe] Theoretical

▸ **Live vaccines** are predicted to increase the risk of generalised infection (possibly life-threatening) when given with taxanes (docetaxel, paclitaxel). Public Health England advises avoid (refer to Green Book). [Severe] Theoretical

▸ **Live vaccines** are predicted to increase the risk of generalised infection (possibly life-threatening) when given with tegafur. Public Health England advises avoid (refer to Green Book). [Severe] Theoretical

▸ **Live vaccines** are predicted to increase the risk of generalised infection (possibly life-threatening) when given with temsirolimus. Public Health England advises avoid (refer to Green Book). [Severe] Theoretical

▸ **Live vaccines** are predicted to increase the risk of generalised infection (possibly life-threatening) when given with teriflunomide. Public Health England advises avoid (refer to Green Book). [Severe] Theoretical

▸ **Live vaccines** are predicted to increase the risk of generalised infection (possibly life-threatening) when given with tioguanine. Public Health England advises avoid (refer to Green Book). [Severe] Theoretical

▸ **Live vaccines** potentially increase the risk of generalised infection (possibly life-threatening) when given with tofacitinib. Avoid. [Severe] Theoretical

▸ **Live vaccines** are predicted to increase the risk of generalised infection (possibly life-threatening) when given with topotecan. Public Health England advises avoid (refer to Green Book). [Severe] Theoretical

▸ **Live vaccines** are predicted to increase the risk of generalised infection (possibly life-threatening) when given with trabectedin. Public Health England advises avoid (refer to Green Book). [Severe] Theoretical

▸ **Live vaccines** are predicted to increase the risk of generalised infection (possibly life-threatening) when given with upadacitinib. Avoid. [Severe] Theoretical

▸ Venetoclax potentially decreases the efficacy of **live vaccines**. Avoid. [Severe] Theoretical

▸ **Live vaccines** are predicted to increase the risk of generalised infection (possibly life-threatening) when given with vinca alkaloids. Public Health England advises avoid (refer to Green Book). [Severe] Theoretical

Lixisenatide → see glucagon-like peptide-1 receptor agonists

Lofepramine → see tricyclic antidepressants

Lofexidine → see TABLE 8 p. 1430 (hypotension), TABLE 9 p. 1431 (QT-interval prolongation), TABLE 11 p. 1431 (CNS depressant effects)

Lomitapide → see TABLE 1 p. 1429 (hepatotoxicity)

FOOD AND LIFESTYLE Bitter (Seville) orange is predicted to increase the exposure to lomitapide; separate administration by 12 hours.

▸ Anti-androgens (apalutamide, enzalutamide) are predicted to decrease the exposure to **lomitapide**. Monitor and adjust dose. [Moderate] Theoretical

▸ Anti-androgens (bicalutamide) are predicted to increase the exposure to **lomitapide**. Separate administration by 12 hours. [Moderate] Theoretical

Antiarrhythmics (amiodarone) are predicted to increase the exposure to **lomitapide**. Separate administration by 12 hours. Moderate Theoretical

Antiarrhythmics (dronedarone) are predicted to increase the exposure to **lomitapide**. Avoid. Moderate Theoretical

Antiepileptics (carbamazepine, fosphenytoin, phenobarbital, phenytoin, primidone) are predicted to decrease the exposure to **lomitapide**. Monitor and adjust dose. Moderate Theoretical → Also see TABLE 1 p. 1429

Antifungals, azoles (clotrimazole) are predicted to increase the exposure to **lomitapide**. Separate administration by 12 hours. Moderate Theoretical

Antifungals, azoles (fluconazole, isavuconazole, posaconazole) are predicted to increase the exposure to **lomitapide**. Avoid. Moderate Theoretical → Also see TABLE 1 p. 1429

Antifungals, azoles (itraconazole, ketoconazole, voriconazole) are predicted to markedly increase the exposure to **lomitapide**. Avoid. Severe Study → Also see TABLE 1 p. 1429

Benzodiazepines (alprazolam) are predicted to increase the exposure to **lomitapide**. Separate administration by 12 hours. Moderate Theoretical

Calcium channel blockers (amlodipine, lacidipine) are predicted to increase the exposure to **lomitapide**. Separate administration by 12 hours. Moderate Theoretical

Calcium channel blockers (diltiazem, verapamil) are predicted to increase the exposure to **lomitapide**. Avoid. Moderate Theoretical

Ciclosporin is predicted to increase the exposure to **lomitapide**. Separate administration by 12 hours. Moderate Theoretical

Cilostazol is predicted to increase the exposure to **lomitapide**. Separate administration by 12 hours. Moderate Theoretical

Cobicistat is predicted to markedly increase the exposure to **lomitapide**. Avoid. Severe Study

Oral combined hormonal contraceptives slightly increase the exposure to **lomitapide**. Separate administration by 12 hours. Moderate Theoretical

Lomitapide increases the exposure to coumarins (warfarin). Monitor INR and adjust dose. Severe Study

Crizotinib is predicted to increase the exposure to **lomitapide**. Avoid. Moderate Theoretical

Dipeptidylpeptidase-4 inhibitors (linagliptin) are predicted to increase the exposure to **lomitapide**. Separate administration by 12 hours. Moderate Theoretical

Everolimus is predicted to increase the exposure to **lomitapide**. Separate administration by 12 hours. Mild Theoretical

Grapefruit juice is predicted to increase the exposure to **lomitapide**. Avoid. Mild Theoretical

H₂ receptor antagonists (cimetidine) are predicted to increase the exposure to **lomitapide**. Separate administration by 12 hours. Mild Theoretical

H₂ receptor antagonists (ranitidine) are predicted to increase the exposure to **lomitapide**. Separate administration by 12 hours. Moderate Theoretical

HIV-protease inhibitors are predicted to markedly increase the exposure to **lomitapide**. Avoid. Severe Study

Idelalisib is predicted to markedly increase the exposure to **lomitapide**. Avoid. Severe Study

Imatinib is predicted to increase the exposure to **lomitapide**. Avoid. Moderate Theoretical

Isoniazid is predicted to increase the exposure to **lomitapide**. Separate administration by 12 hours. Unknown Theoretical → Also see TABLE 1 p. 1429

Ivacaftor is predicted to increase the exposure to **lomitapide**. Separate administration by 12 hours. Moderate Theoretical

Lapatinib is predicted to increase the exposure to **lomitapide**. Separate administration by 12 hours. Mild Theoretical

Letermovir is predicted to increase the exposure to **lomitapide**. Avoid. Moderate Theoretical

Macrolides (azithromycin) are predicted to increase the exposure to **lomitapide**. Separate administration by 12 hours. Moderate Theoretical

Macrolides (clarithromycin) are predicted to markedly increase the exposure to **lomitapide**. Avoid. Severe Study

Macrolides (erythromycin) are predicted to increase the exposure to **lomitapide**. Avoid. Moderate Theoretical

▸ Mitotane is predicted to decrease the exposure to **lomitapide**. Monitor and adjust dose. Moderate Theoretical

▸ Neurokinin-1 receptor antagonists (aprepitant, netupitant) are predicted to increase the exposure to **lomitapide**. Avoid. Moderate Theoretical

▸ Neurokinin-1 receptor antagonists (fosaprepitant) are predicted to increase the exposure to **lomitapide**. Separate administration by 12 hours. Mild Theoretical

▸ Nilotinib is predicted to increase the exposure to **lomitapide**. Avoid. Moderate Theoretical

▸ Pazopanib is predicted to increase the exposure to **lomitapide**. Separate administration by 12 hours. Mild Theoretical

▸ Peppermint oil is predicted to increase the exposure to **lomitapide**. Separate administration by 12 hours. Moderate Theoretical

▸ Propiverine is predicted to increase the exposure to **lomitapide**. Separate administration by 12 hours. Moderate Theoretical

▸ Ranolazine is predicted to increase the exposure to **lomitapide**. Separate administration by 12 hours. Mild Theoretical

▸ Rifamycins (rifampicin) are predicted to decrease the exposure to **lomitapide**. Monitor and adjust dose. Moderate Theoretical

▸ SSRIs (fluoxetine) are predicted to increase the exposure to **lomitapide**. Separate administration by 12 hours. Unknown Theoretical

▸ SSRIs (fluvoxamine) are predicted to increase the exposure to **lomitapide**. Separate administration by 12 hours. Mild Theoretical

▸ **Lomitapide** increases the exposure to statins (atorvastatin). Adjust **lomitapide** dose or separate administration by 12 hours, p. 222. Mild Study → Also see TABLE 1 p. 1429

▸ **Lomitapide** increases the exposure to statins (simvastatin). Monitor and adjust **simvastatin** dose, p. 219. Moderate Study → Also see TABLE 1 p. 1429

▸ Tacrolimus is predicted to increase the exposure to **lomitapide**. Separate administration by 12 hours. Moderate Theoretical

▸ Ticagrelor is predicted to increase the exposure to **lomitapide**. Separate administration by 12 hours. Moderate Theoretical

▸ Tolvaptan is predicted to increase the exposure to **lomitapide**. Separate administration by 12 hours. Moderate Theoretical

Lomustine → see alkylating agents

Loop diuretics → see TABLE 18 p. 1433 (hyponatraemia), TABLE 8 p. 1430 (hypotension), TABLE 19 p. 1433 (ototoxicity), TABLE 17 p. 1433 (reduced serum potassium)

bumetanide · furosemide · torasemide

▸ Aliskiren slightly decreases the exposure to **furosemide**. Moderate Study → Also see TABLE 8 p. 1430

▸ **Loop diuretics** increase the risk of nephrotoxicity when given with aminoglycosides. Avoid. Moderate Study → Also see TABLE 19 p. 1433

▸ Antiepileptics (fosphenytoin, phenytoin) decrease the effects of **furosemide**. Moderate Study

▸ Intravenous **furosemide** potentially increases the risk of sweating, variable blood pressure, and tachycardia when given after chloral hydrate. Moderate Anecdotal

▸ Dasabuvir (with ombitasvir, paritaprevir, and ritonavir) increases the concentration of **furosemide**. Adjust dose. Moderate Study

▸ Immunoglobulins (cytomegalovirus immunoglobulin) are predicted to increase the risk of adverse effects when given with **loop diuretics**. Avoid. Moderate Theoretical

▸ Leflunomide is predicted to increase the exposure to **furosemide**. Moderate Theoretical

▸ **Loop diuretics** increase the concentration of lithium. Monitor and adjust dose. Severe Study

▸ Nitisinone is predicted to increase the exposure to **furosemide**. Moderate Study

▸ Paritaprevir (with ritonavir and ombitasvir) is predicted to increase the exposure to **furosemide**. Adjust dose. Moderate Theoretical

▸ Reboxetine is predicted to increase the risk of hypokalaemia when given with **loop diuretics**. Moderate Theoretical

▸ Teriflunomide is predicted to increase the exposure to **furosemide**. Moderate Study

A1

Interactions | Appendix 1

Loperamide

▸ Antiarrhythmics (dronedarone) are predicted to increase the exposure to **loperamide**. [Severe] Theoretical

▸ Ceritinib is predicted to increase the exposure to **loperamide**. [Moderate] Theoretical

▸ **Loperamide** greatly increases the absorption of oral desmopressin (and possibly sublingual). [Moderate] Study

▸ Eliglustat is predicted to increase the exposure to **loperamide**. Adjust dose. [Moderate] Study

▸ Lapatinib is predicted to increase the exposure to **loperamide**. [Moderate] Theoretical

▸ Mirabegron is predicted to increase the exposure to **loperamide**. [Mild] Theoretical

▸ Opicapone is predicted to increase the exposure to **loperamide**. Avoid. [Moderate] Study

▸ Paritaprevir (with ritonavir and ombitasvir) is predicted to increase the exposure to **loperamide**. [Moderate] Study

▸ Pibrentasvir (with glecaprevir) is predicted to increase the exposure to **loperamide**. [Moderate] Study

▸ Pitolisant is predicted to decrease the exposure to **loperamide**. [Mild] Theoretical

▸ Velpatasvir is predicted to increase the exposure to **loperamide**. [Severe] Theoretical

Lopinavir → see HIV-protease inhibitors

Loprazolam → see benzodiazepines

Loratadine → see antihistamines, non-sedating

Lorazepam → see benzodiazepines

Lorlatinib

▸ Anti-androgens (apalutamide, enzalutamide) are predicted to decrease the exposure to **lorlatinib**. [Severe] Study

▸ Antiepileptics (carbamazepine, fosphenytoin, phenobarbital, phenytoin, primidone) are predicted to decrease the exposure to **lorlatinib**. Avoid. [Severe] Study

▸ Antifungals, azoles (itraconazole, ketoconazole, voriconazole) are predicted to increase the exposure to **lorlatinib**. Avoid or adjust **lorlatinib** dose, p. 1033. [Severe] Study

▸ **Lorlatinib** moderately decreases the exposure to benzodiazepines (midazolam). Avoid. [Moderate] Study

▸ **Lorlatinib** is predicted to decrease the exposure to ciclosporin. Avoid. [Moderate] Theoretical

▸ Cobicistat is predicted to increase the exposure to **lorlatinib**. Avoid or adjust **lorlatinib** dose, p. 1033. [Severe] Study

▸ **Lorlatinib** is predicted to decrease the exposure to combined hormonal contraceptives. Avoid. [Moderate] Theoretical

▸ Endothelin receptor antagonists (bosentan) are predicted to decrease the exposure to **lorlatinib**. Avoid. [Severe] Theoretical

▸ **Lorlatinib** is predicted to decrease the exposure to ergotamine. Avoid. [Moderate] Theoretical

▸ Grapefruit juice is predicted to increase the concentration of **lorlatinib**. Avoid. [Moderate] Theoretical

▸ HIV-protease inhibitors are predicted to increase the exposure to **lorlatinib**. Avoid or adjust **lorlatinib** dose, p. 1033. [Severe] Study

▸ Idelalisib is predicted to increase the exposure to **lorlatinib**. Avoid or adjust **lorlatinib** dose, p. 1033. [Severe] Study

▸ Macrolides (clarithromycin) are predicted to increase the exposure to **lorlatinib**. Avoid or adjust **lorlatinib** dose, p. 1033. [Severe] Study

▸ Mitotane is predicted to decrease the exposure to **lorlatinib**. Avoid. [Severe] Study

▸ NNRTIs (efavirenz, nevirapine) are predicted to decrease the exposure to **lorlatinib**. Avoid. [Severe] Theoretical

▸ **Lorlatinib** is predicted to increase the exposure to opioids (alfentanil, fentanyl). Avoid. [Moderate] Theoretical

▸ **Lorlatinib** is predicted to decrease the exposure to pimozide. Avoid. [Moderate] Theoretical

▸ Rifamycins (rifampicin) are predicted to decrease the exposure to **lorlatinib**. Avoid. [Severe] Study

▸ **Lorlatinib** is predicted to decrease the exposure to sirolimus. Avoid. [Moderate] Theoretical

▸ St John's wort is predicted to decrease the exposure to **lorlatinib**. Avoid. [Severe] Theoretical

▸ **Lorlatinib** is predicted to decrease the exposure to tacrolimus. Avoid. [Moderate] Theoretical

Lormetazepam → see benzodiazepines

Losartan → see angiotensin-II receptor antagonists

Low molecular-weight heparins → see TABLE 16 p. 1433 (increased serum potassium), TABLE 3 p. 1429 (anticoagulant effects)

dalteparin · enoxaparin · tinzaparin

▸ Ranibizumab increases the risk of bleeding events when given with **low molecular-weight heparins**. [Severe] Theoretical

Loxapine → see TABLE 8 p. 1430 (hypotension), TABLE 11 p. 1431 (CNS depressant effects), TABLE 10 p. 1431 (antimuscarinics)

▸ Combined hormonal contraceptives are predicted to increase the exposure to **loxapine**. Avoid. [Unknown] Theoretical

▸ **Loxapine** is predicted to decrease the effects of dopamine receptor agonists. [Moderate] Theoretical → Also see TABLE 8 p. 1430 → Also see TABLE 10 p. 1431

▸ **Loxapine** is predicted to decrease the effects of levodopa. [Severe] Theoretical → Also see TABLE 8 p. 1430

▸ Mexiletine is predicted to increase the exposure to **loxapine**. Avoid. [Unknown] Theoretical

▸ Quinolones (ciprofloxacin) are predicted to increase the exposure to **loxapine**. Avoid. [Unknown] Theoretical

▸ SSRIs (fluvoxamine) are predicted to increase the exposure to **loxapine**. Avoid. [Unknown] Theoretical

Lumacaftor

▸ **Lumacaftor** is predicted to decrease the exposure to antiepileptics (carbamazepine, fosphenytoin, phenobarbital, phenytoin, primidone). Avoid. [Severe] Theoretical

▸ **Lumacaftor** is predicted to decrease the exposure to antifungals, azoles (fluconazole). Adjust dose. [Mild] Theoretical

▸ **Lumacaftor** is predicted to decrease the exposure to antifungals, azoles (itraconazole, ketoconazole, posaconazole, voriconazole). Avoid or monitor efficacy. [Moderate] Theoretical

▸ **Lumacaftor** is predicted to decrease the exposure to benzodiazepines (midazolam). Avoid. [Severe] Theoretical

▸ **Lumacaftor** is predicted to decrease the exposure to ciclosporin. Avoid. [Severe] Theoretical

▸ **Lumacaftor** is predicted to decrease the efficacy of combined hormonal contraceptives. Use additional contraceptive precautions. [Severe] Theoretical

▸ **Lumacaftor** is predicted to decrease the exposure to corticosteroids (methylprednisolone). Adjust dose. [Severe] Theoretical

▸ **Lumacaftor** is predicted to decrease the exposure to everolimus. Avoid. [Severe] Theoretical

▸ **Lumacaftor** potentially decreases the exposure to glecaprevir. Avoid. [Severe] Theoretical

▸ **Lumacaftor** is predicted to decrease the efficacy of levonorgestrel. Use additional contraceptive precautions. [Severe] Theoretical

▸ **Lumacaftor** is predicted to decrease the exposure to macrolides (clarithromycin, erythromycin). [Moderate] Theoretical

▸ **Lumacaftor** is predicted to decrease the exposure to NNRTIs (doravirine). Avoid. [Severe] Theoretical

▸ **Lumacaftor** potentially decreases the exposure to pibrentasvir. Avoid. [Severe] Theoretical

▸ **Lumacaftor** is predicted to decrease the exposure to rifamycins (rifabutin). Adjust dose. [Moderate] Theoretical

▸ **Lumacaftor** is predicted to decrease the exposure to sirolimus. Avoid. [Severe] Theoretical

▸ **Lumacaftor** is predicted to decrease the exposure to tacrolimus. Avoid. [Severe] Theoretical

▸ **Lumacaftor** is predicted to decrease the exposure to temsirolimus. Avoid. [Severe] Theoretical

▸ **Lumacaftor** is predicted to decrease the efficacy of ulipristal. Use additional contraceptive precautions. [Severe] Theoretical

Lumefantrine → see antimalarials

Lurasidone → see antipsychotics, second generation

Lymecycline → see tetracyclines

Macitentan → see endothelin receptor antagonists

Macrolides → see TABLE 9 p. 1431 (QT-interval prolongation)

azithromycin · clarithromycin · erythromycin

▸ Interactions do not generally apply to topical use of **azithromycin** unless specified.

▸ Since systemic absorption can follow topical application of **erythromycin**, the possibility of interactions should be borne in mind.

Clarithromycin is predicted to increase the exposure to abemaciclib. Avoid or adjust **abemaciclib** dose, p. 1009. Severe Study

Erythromycin is predicted to increase the exposure to abemaciclib. Moderate Study

Clarithromycin is predicted to increase the exposure to acalabrutinib. Avoid. Severe Study

Erythromycin is predicted to increase the exposure to acalabrutinib. Avoid or monitor. Severe Study

Macrolides are predicted to increase the exposure to afatinib. Separate administration by 12 hours. Moderate Study

Clarithromycin is predicted to markedly increase the exposure to aldosterone antagonists (eplerenone). Avoid. Severe Study

Erythromycin is predicted to increase the exposure to aldosterone antagonists (eplerenone). Adjust **eplerenone** dose, p. 208. Severe Study

Azithromycin is predicted to increase the exposure to aliskiren. Moderate Theoretical

Macrolides (clarithromycin, erythromycin) are predicted to increase the exposure to aliskiren. Moderate Study

Clarithromycin is predicted to moderately increase the exposure to alpha blockers (alfuzosin, tamsulosin). Use with caution or avoid. Moderate Study

Clarithromycin is predicted to increase the exposure to alpha blockers (doxazosin). Moderate Study

Erythromycin is predicted to increase the exposure to alpha blockers (tamsulosin). Moderate Theoretical

Azithromycin is predicted to increase the exposure to aminophylline. Moderate Theoretical

Clarithromycin is predicted to increase the exposure to aminophylline. Adjust dose. Moderate Theoretical

Aminophylline is predicted to decrease the exposure to erythromycin. Adjust dose. Severe Study

Clarithromycin is predicted to increase the exposure to anti-androgens (apalutamide). Mild Study → Also see TABLE 9 p. 1431

Clarithromycin is predicted to increase the exposure to anti-androgens (darolutamide). Monitor and adjust dose. Moderate Theoretical

Clarithromycin very markedly increases the exposure to antiarrhythmics (dronedarone). Avoid. Severe Study → Also see TABLE 9 p. 1431

Erythromycin is predicted to moderately increase the exposure to antiarrhythmics (dronedarone). Avoid. Severe Theoretical → Also see TABLE 9 p. 1431

Macrolides (clarithromycin, erythromycin) are predicted to increase the exposure to antiarrhythmics (lidocaine). Moderate Theoretical

Clarithromycin is predicted to increase the exposure to antiarrhythmics (propafenone). Monitor and adjust dose. Severe Study

Erythromycin is predicted to increase the exposure to antiarrhythmics (propafenone). Monitor and adjust dose. Moderate Study

Clarithromycin is predicted to increase the exposure to anticholinesterases, centrally acting (galantamine). Monitor and adjust dose. Moderate Study

Clarithromycin slightly increases the concentration of antiepileptics (carbamazepine). Monitor concentration and adjust dose. Severe Study

Erythromycin markedly increases the concentration of antiepileptics (carbamazepine). Monitor concentration and adjust dose. Severe Study

Clarithromycin is predicted to very slightly increase the exposure to antiepileptics (perampanel). Mild Study

Clarithromycin is predicted to increase the exposure to antifungals, azoles (isavuconazole). Avoid or monitor adverse effects. Severe Study

Erythromycin is predicted to increase the exposure to antifungals, azoles (isavuconazole). Moderate Theoretical

Clarithromycin is predicted to increase the exposure to antihistamines, non-sedating (mizolastine). Avoid. Severe Study

Erythromycin is predicted to increase the exposure to antihistamines, non-sedating (mizolastine). Severe Theoretical

▶ **Macrolides (clarithromycin, erythromycin)** are predicted to increase the exposure to antihistamines, non-sedating (rupatadine). Avoid. Moderate Study

▶ **Macrolides (clarithromycin, erythromycin)** are predicted to increase the concentration of antimalarials (piperaquine). Severe Theoretical

▶ **Clarithromycin** is predicted to slightly increase the exposure to antipsychotics, second generation (aripiprazole). Adjust **aripiprazole** dose, p. 415. Moderate Study

▶ **Clarithromycin** is predicted to moderately increase the exposure to antipsychotics, second generation (cariprazine). Avoid. Severe Study

▶ **Erythromycin** is predicted to increase the exposure to antipsychotics, second generation (cariprazine). Avoid. Severe Study

▶ **Erythromycin** potentially increases the risk of toxicity when given with antipsychotics, second generation (clozapine). Severe Anecdotal

▶ **Erythromycin** is predicted to increase the exposure to antipsychotics, second generation (lurasidone). Adjust **lurasidone** dose. Moderate Study

▶ **Clarithromycin** is predicted to increase the exposure to antipsychotics, second generation (lurasidone, quetiapine). Avoid. Severe Study

▶ **Erythromycin** is predicted to increase the exposure to antipsychotics, second generation (quetiapine). Avoid. Moderate Study

▶ **Clarithromycin** is predicted to increase the exposure to antipsychotics, second generation (risperidone). Adjust dose. Moderate Study → Also see TABLE 9 p. 1431

▶ **Clarithromycin** is predicted to increase the exposure to avapritinib. Avoid. Moderate Study

▶ **Erythromycin** is predicted to increase the exposure to avapritinib. Avoid or adjust **avapritinib** dose, p. 1012. Moderate Study

▶ **Clarithromycin** is predicted to increase the exposure to axitinib. Avoid or adjust dose. Moderate Study

▶ **Erythromycin** is predicted to increase the exposure to axitinib. Moderate Theoretical

▶ **Clarithromycin** is predicted to increase the exposure to bedaquiline. Avoid prolonged use. Mild Study → Also see TABLE 9 p. 1431

▶ **Erythromycin** is predicted to increase the exposure to bedaquiline. Avoid prolonged use. Mild Theoretical → Also see TABLE 9 p. 1431

▶ **Clarithromycin** moderately increases the exposure to benzodiazepines (alprazolam). Avoid. Moderate Study

▶ **Erythromycin** is predicted to increase the exposure to benzodiazepines (alprazolam). Severe Study

▶ **Clarithromycin** is predicted to markedly to very markedly increase the exposure to benzodiazepines (midazolam). Avoid or adjust dose. Severe Study

▶ **Erythromycin** is predicted to increase the exposure to benzodiazepines (midazolam). Monitor adverse effects and adjust dose. Severe Study

▶ **Macrolides** are predicted to increase the exposure to beta blockers, non-selective (nadolol). Moderate Study

▶ **Clarithromycin** is predicted to increase the exposure to beta$_2$ agonists (salmeterol). Avoid. Severe Study

▶ **Macrolides** are predicted to increase the exposure to bictegravir. Use with caution or avoid. Moderate Theoretical

▶ **Clarithromycin** slightly increases the exposure to bortezomib. Moderate Study

▶ **Clarithromycin** is predicted to markedly increase the exposure to bosutinib. Avoid or adjust dose. Severe Study → Also see TABLE 9 p. 1431

▶ **Erythromycin** is predicted to increase the exposure to bosutinib. Avoid or adjust dose. Severe Theoretical → Also see TABLE 9 p. 1431

▶ **Clarithromycin** is predicted to increase the exposure to brigatinib. Adjust **brigatinib** dose, p. 1015. Severe Study

▶ **Clarithromycin** is predicted to increase the exposure to buspirone. Adjust **buspirone** dose, p. 360. Severe Study

▶ **Erythromycin** is predicted to increase the exposure to buspirone. Use with caution and adjust dose. Moderate Study

Macrolides (continued)

▶ **Clarithromycin** slightly increases the exposure to cabozantinib. Moderate Study → Also see **TABLE 9** p. 1431

▶ **Erythromycin** is predicted to increase the exposure to cabozantinib. Moderate Theoretical → Also see **TABLE 9** p. 1431

▶ **Erythromycin** is predicted to increase the exposure to calcium channel blockers (**amlodipine, felodipine, lacidipine, lercanidipine, nicardipine, nifedipine, nimodipine**). Monitor and adjust dose. Moderate Study

▶ **Clarithromycin** is predicted to increase the exposure to calcium channel blockers (**amlodipine, felodipine, lacidipine, nicardipine, nifedipine, nimodipine**). Monitor and adjust dose. Moderate Study

▶ **Erythromycin** is predicted to increase the exposure to calcium channel blockers (**diltiazem**). Severe Theoretical

▶ **Clarithromycin** is predicted to increase the exposure to calcium channel blockers (**diltiazem, verapamil**). Severe Study

▶ **Clarithromycin** is predicted to markedly increase the exposure to calcium channel blockers (**lercanidipine**). Avoid. Severe Study

▶ **Erythromycin** is predicted to increase the exposure to calcium channel blockers (**verapamil**). Severe Study

▶ **Clarithromycin** is predicted to increase the exposure to cannabidiol. Avoid or adjust dose. Mild Study

▶ **Azithromycin** is predicted to increase the exposure to ceritinib. Moderate Theoretical

▶ **Clarithromycin** is predicted to increase the exposure to ceritinib. Avoid or adjust **ceritinib** dose, p. 1017. Severe Study → Also see **TABLE 9** p. 1431

▶ **Clarithromycin** increases the concentration of ciclosporin. Severe Study

▶ **Erythromycin** is predicted to increase the concentration of ciclosporin. Severe Study

▶ **Clarithromycin** is predicted to moderately increase the exposure to cilostazol. Adjust **cilostazol** dose, p. 248. Moderate Study

▶ **Erythromycin** slightly increases the exposure to cilostazol. Adjust **cilostazol** dose, p. 248. Moderate Study

▶ **Clarithromycin** is predicted to moderately increase the exposure to cinacalcet. Adjust dose. Moderate Study

▶ **Clarithromycin** is predicted to markedly increase the exposure to cobimetinib. Avoid or monitor for toxicity. Severe Study

▶ **Erythromycin** is predicted to increase the exposure to cobimetinib. Severe Theoretical

▶ **Azithromycin** is predicted to increase the exposure to colchicine. Avoid P-glycoprotein inhibitors or adjust **colchicine** dose, p. 1166. Severe Theoretical

▶ **Clarithromycin** is predicted to increase the exposure to colchicine. Avoid potent CYP3A4 inhibitors or adjust **colchicine** dose, p. 1166. Severe Study

▶ **Erythromycin** is predicted to increase the exposure to colchicine. Adjust **colchicine** dose with moderate CYP3A4 inhibitors, p. 1166. Severe Study

▶ **Clarithromycin** is predicted to increase the exposure to corticosteroids (**beclometasone**) (risk with beclometasone is likely to be lower than with other corticosteroids). Moderate Theoretical

▶ **Clarithromycin** is predicted to increase the exposure to corticosteroids (**betamethasone, budesonide, ciclesonide, deflazacort, dexamethasone, fludrocortisone, fluticasone, hydrocortisone, methylprednisolone, mometasone, prednisolone, triamcinolone**). Avoid or monitor adverse effects. Severe Study

▶ **Erythromycin** is predicted to increase the exposure to corticosteroids (**methylprednisolone**). Monitor and adjust dose. Moderate Study

▶ **Macrolides** (**clarithromycin, erythromycin**) increase the anticoagulant effect of coumarins. Monitor INR and adjust dose. Severe Anecdotal

▶ **Clarithromycin** is predicted to moderately increase the exposure to crizotinib. Avoid. Moderate Study → Also see **TABLE 9** p. 1431

▶ **Clarithromycin** is predicted to increase the exposure to dabrafenib. Use with caution or avoid. Moderate Study

▶ **Clarithromycin** is predicted to markedly to very markedly increase the exposure to darifenacin. Avoid. Severe Study

▶ **Erythromycin** is predicted to slightly increase the exposure to darifenacin. Moderate Study

▶ **Clarithromycin** is predicted to markedly increase the exposure to dasatinib. Avoid or adjust dose—consult product literature. Severe Study → Also see **TABLE 9** p. 1431

▶ **Erythromycin** is predicted to increase the exposure to dasatinib. Severe Study → Also see **TABLE 9** p. 1431

▶ **Clarithromycin** very slightly increases the exposure to delamanid. Severe Study → Also see **TABLE 9** p. 1431

▶ **Clarithromycin** is predicted to moderately increase the exposure to dienogest. Moderate Study

▶ **Erythromycin** is predicted to slightly increase the exposure to dienogest. Moderate Study

▶ **Macrolides** increase the concentration of digoxin. Severe Anecdotal

▶ **Clarithromycin** is predicted to increase the exposure to dipeptidylpeptidase-4 inhibitors (**saxagliptin**). Moderate Study

▶ **Erythromycin** is predicted to increase the exposure to dipeptidylpeptidase-4 inhibitors (**saxagliptin**). Mild Study

▶ **Macrolides** (**clarithromycin, erythromycin**) increase the risk of QT-prolongation when given with domperidone. Avoid. Severe Study

▶ **Clarithromycin** increases the exposure to dopamine receptor agonists (**bromocriptine**). Severe Study

▶ **Erythromycin** is predicted to increase the exposure to dopamine receptor agonists (**bromocriptine**). Severe Theoretical

▶ **Macrolides** (**clarithromycin, erythromycin**) are predicted to increase the concentration of dopamine receptor agonists (**cabergoline**). Avoid. Severe Study

▶ **Clarithromycin** is predicted to increase the exposure to dronabinol. Adjust dose. Mild Study

▶ **Clarithromycin** is predicted to increase the exposure to dutasteride. Monitor adverse effects and adjust dose. Moderate Theoretical

▶ **Erythromycin** is predicted to moderately increase the exposure to dutasteride. Mild Study

▶ **Clarithromycin** is predicted to increase the exposure to elexacaftor. Adjust tezacaftor with ivacaftor and elexacftor p. 311 dose with potent CYP3A4 inhibitors. Severe Study

▶ **Erythromycin** is predicted to increase the exposure to elexacaftor. Adjust tezacaftor with ivacaftor and elexacftor p. 311 dose with moderate CYP3A4 inhibitors. Severe Theoretical

▶ **Macrolides** (**clarithromycin, erythromycin**) are predicted to increase the exposure to eliglustat. Avoid or adjust dose—consult product literature. Severe Study

▶ **Clarithromycin** is predicted to increase the exposure to encorafenib. Avoid or monitor. Severe Study → Also see **TABLE 9** p. 1431

▶ **Erythromycin** is predicted to moderately increase the exposure to encorafenib. Moderate Study → Also see **TABLE 9** p. 1431

▶ **Clarithromycin** is predicted to increase the exposure to endothelin receptor antagonists (**bosentan**). Moderate Theoretical

▶ **Clarithromycin** is predicted to increase the exposure to endothelin receptor antagonists (**macitentan**). Moderate Study

▶ **Clarithromycin** is predicted to increase the exposure to entrectinib. Avoid potent CYP3A4 inhibitors or adjust **entrectinib** dose, p. 1023. Severe Study → Also see **TABLE 9** p. 1431

▶ **Erythromycin** is predicted to increase the exposure to entrectinib. Avoid moderate CYP3A4 inhibitors or adjust **entrectinib** dose, p. 1023. Severe Theoretical → Also see **TABLE 9** p. 1431

▶ **Clarithromycin** is predicted to increase the risk of ergotism when given with ergometrine. Avoid. Severe Theoretical

▶ **Erythromycin** is predicted to increase the risk of ergotism when given with ergometrine. Severe Theoretical

▶ **Clarithromycin** is predicted to increase the risk of ergotism when given with ergotamine. Avoid. Severe Theoretical

▶ **Erythromycin** is predicted to increase the risk of ergotism when given with ergotamine. Severe Theoretical

▶ **Clarithromycin** is predicted to slightly increase the exposure to erlotinib. Use with caution and adjust dose. Moderate Study

▶ **Macrolides** (**azithromycin, erythromycin**) are predicted to increase the exposure to erlotinib. Moderate Theoretical

Clarithromycin is predicted to increase the exposure to esketamine. Adjust dose. Moderate Study

▸ **Clarithromycin** is predicted to increase the concentration of everolimus. Avoid. Severe Study

▸ **Erythromycin** is predicted to increase the concentration of everolimus. Avoid or adjust dose. Moderate Study

▸ **Erythromycin** is predicted to increase the exposure to factor XA inhibitors (apixaban). Moderate Theoretical

▸ **Erythromycin** slightly increases the exposure to factor XA inhibitors (edoxaban). Adjust **edoxaban** dose, p. 137. Severe Study

▸ Macrolides **(azithromycin, clarithromycin)** are predicted to slightly increase the exposure to factor XA inhibitors (edoxaban). Severe Theoretical

▸ **Clarithromycin** is predicted to moderately increase the exposure to **fesoterodine**. Adjust **fesoterodine** dose with potent CYP3A4 inhibitors; avoid in hepatic and renal impairment, p. 822. Severe Study

▸ **Erythromycin** is predicted to increase the exposure to fesoterodine. Adjust **fesoterodine** dose with moderate CYP3A4 inhibitors in hepatic and renal impairment, p. 822. Mild Study

▸ **Macrolides** are predicted to increase the exposure to fidaxomicin. Avoid. Moderate Study

▸ **Clarithromycin** is predicted to increase the exposure to fostamatinib. Monitor adverse effects and adjust dose. Moderate Study

▸ **Clarithromycin** is predicted to increase the exposure to gefitinib. Moderate Study

▸ **Erythromycin** is predicted to increase the exposure to gefitinib. Moderate Theoretical

▸ **Clarithromycin** is predicted to increase the exposure to gilteritinib. Moderate Study

▸ Macrolides **(azithromycin, erythromycin)** are predicted to increase the exposure to gilteritinib. Moderate Theoretical

▸ **Clarithromycin** is predicted to moderately increase the exposure to glasdegib. Use with caution or avoid. Moderate Study → Also see TABLE 9 p. 1431

▸ **Clarithromycin** is predicted to moderately to markedly increase the exposure to grazoprevir. Avoid. Severe Study

▸ **Clarithromycin** is predicted to increase the exposure to guanfacine. Adjust **guanfacine** dose, p. 372. Moderate Study

▸ **Erythromycin** is predicted to increase the concentration of guanfacine. Adjust **guanfacine** dose, p. 372. Moderate Theoretical

▸ H₂ receptor antagonists (cimetidine) slightly increase the exposure to **erythromycin**. Moderate Study

▸ HIV-protease inhibitors (atazanavir) are predicted to increase the exposure to **clarithromycin**. Adjust dose in renal impairment. Severe Study

▸ HIV-protease inhibitors (atazanavir, darunavir, fosamprenavir, lopinavir, ritonavir, tipranavir) are predicted to increase the exposure to **erythromycin**. Severe Theoretical

▸ HIV-protease inhibitors (darunavir, fosamprenavir, lopinavir) boosted with ritonavir are predicted to increase the exposure to **clarithromycin**. Adjust dose in renal impairment. Severe Study

▸ HIV-protease inhibitors (ritonavir) increase the exposure to **clarithromycin**. Adjust dose in renal impairment. Severe Study

▸ HIV-protease inhibitors (tipranavir) boosted with ritonavir increase the exposure to **clarithromycin** and **clarithromycin** increases the exposure to HIV-protease inhibitors (tipranavir) boosted with ritonavir. Monitor; adjust dose in renal impairment. Severe Study

▸ **Clarithromycin** increases the exposure to HIV-protease inhibitors (saquinavir) and HIV-protease inhibitors (saquinavir) increase the exposure to **clarithromycin**. Avoid. Severe Study → Also see TABLE 9 p. 1431

▸ **Erythromycin** is predicted to increase the exposure to HIV-protease inhibitors (saquinavir). Avoid. Severe Theoretical → Also see TABLE 9 p. 1431

▸ **Clarithromycin** is predicted to very markedly increase the exposure to ibrutinib. Avoid potent CYP3A4 inhibitors or adjust **ibrutinib** dose, p. 1027. Severe Study

▸ **Erythromycin** is predicted to increase the exposure to ibrutinib. Adjust **ibrutinib** dose with moderate CYP3A4 inhibitors, p. 1027. Severe Study

▸ **Clarithromycin** is predicted to increase the exposure to imatinib. Moderate Study

▸ **Erythromycin** is predicted to increase the exposure to imatinib. Moderate Theoretical

▸ **Clarithromycin** is predicted to increase the risk of toxicity when given with irinotecan. Avoid. Moderate Study

▸ **Clarithromycin** is predicted to increase the exposure to ivabradine. Avoid. Severe Study

▸ **Erythromycin** is predicted to increase the exposure to ivabradine. Severe Theoretical

▸ **Clarithromycin** is predicted to increase the exposure to ivacaftor. Adjust ivacaftor p. 309 or lumacaftor with ivacaftor p. 310 or tezacaftor with ivacaftor p. 311 or tezacaftor with ivacaftor and elexacftor p. 311 dose with potent CYP3A4 inhibitors. Severe Study

▸ **Erythromycin** is predicted to increase the exposure to ivacaftor. Adjust ivacaftor p. 309 or tezacaftor with ivacaftor p. 311 or tezacaftor with ivacaftor and elexacftor p. 311 dose with moderate CYP3A4 inhibitors. Severe Study

▸ **Clarithromycin** is predicted to increase the exposure to lapatinib. Avoid. Moderate Study → Also see TABLE 9 p. 1431

▸ **Erythromycin** is predicted to increase the exposure to lapatinib. Moderate Study → Also see TABLE 9 p. 1431

▸ **Clarithromycin** is predicted to moderately increase the exposure to larotrectinib. Avoid or adjust **larotrectinib** dose, p. 1031. Moderate Study

▸ Macrolides **(azithromycin, erythromycin)** are predicted to increase the exposure to larotrectinib. Mild Theoretical

▸ Macrolides **(clarithromycin, erythromycin)** are predicted to increase the concentration of letermovir. Moderate Study

▸ **Clarithromycin** increases the exposure to linezolid. Moderate Anecdotal

▸ **Azithromycin** is predicted to increase the exposure to lomitapide. Separate administration by 12 hours. Moderate Theoretical

▸ **Clarithromycin** is predicted to markedly increase the exposure to lomitapide. Avoid. Severe Study

▸ **Erythromycin** is predicted to increase the exposure to lomitapide. Avoid. Moderate Theoretical

▸ **Clarithromycin** is predicted to increase the exposure to lorlatinib. Avoid or adjust **lorlatinib** dose, p. 1033. Severe Study

▸ Lumacaftor is predicted to decrease the exposure to macrolides **(clarithromycin, erythromycin)**. Moderate Theoretical

▸ **Clarithromycin** is predicted to markedly increase the exposure to maraviroc. Adjust dose. Severe Study

▸ **Clarithromycin** is predicted to increase the exposure to meglitinides (repaglinide). Moderate Study

▸ **Clarithromycin** is predicted to very markedly increase the exposure to midostaurin. Avoid or monitor for toxicity. Severe Study

▸ **Erythromycin** is predicted to increase the exposure to midostaurin. Moderate Theoretical

▸ **Clarithromycin** is predicted to increase the exposure to mirabegron. Adjust **mirabegron** dose in hepatic and renal impairment, p. 825. Moderate Study

▸ **Clarithromycin** is predicted to increase the exposure to mirtazapine. Moderate Study

▸ **Clarithromycin** is predicted to increase the exposure to modafinil. Mild Theoretical

▸ **Clarithromycin** increases the risk of neutropenia when given with monoclonal antibodies (brentuximab vedotin). Monitor and adjust dose. Severe Theoretical

▸ **Clarithromycin** is predicted to increase the exposure to monoclonal antibodies (polatuzumab vedotin). Moderate Theoretical

▸ **Clarithromycin** is predicted to increase the exposure to monoclonal antibodies (trastuzumab emtansine). Avoid. Severe Theoretical

▸ **Clarithromycin** is predicted to increase the exposure to naldemedine. Avoid or monitor. Moderate Study

▸ Macrolides **(azithromycin, erythromycin)** are predicted to increase the exposure to naldemedine. Moderate Study

▸ **Clarithromycin** is predicted to markedly increase the exposure to naloxegol. Avoid. Severe Study

Macrolides (continued)

▶ **Erythromycin** is predicted to increase the exposure to naloxegol. Adjust **naloxegol** dose and monitor adverse effects, p. 70. Moderate Study

▶ **Clarithromycin** is predicted to increase the exposure to neratinib. Avoid or adjust **neratinib** dose, p. 1034. Severe Study

▶ **Erythromycin** is predicted to increase the exposure to neratinib. Avoid. Severe Study

▶ **Clarithromycin** is predicted to markedly increase the exposure to neurokinin-1 receptor antagonists (**aprepitant**). Moderate Study

▶ **Erythromycin** is predicted to increase the exposure to neurokinin-1 receptor antagonists (**aprepitant**). Moderate Study

▶ **Clarithromycin** is predicted to increase the exposure to neurokinin-1 receptor antagonists (**fosaprepitant**). Moderate Theoretical

▶ **Clarithromycin** is predicted to increase the exposure to neurokinin-1 receptor antagonists (**netupitant**). Moderate Study

▶ **Clarithromycin** is predicted to moderately increase the exposure to nilotinib. Avoid. Severe Study → Also see TABLE 9 p. 1431

▶ **Erythromycin** is predicted to increase the exposure to nilotinib. Moderate Theoretical → Also see TABLE 9 p. 1431

▶ **Macrolides** are predicted to increase the exposure to nintedanib. Moderate Study

▶ **Clarithromycin** is predicted to increase the exposure to nitisinone. Adjust dose. Moderate Theoretical

▶ NNRTIs (**efavirenz, nevirapine**) decrease the exposure to **clarithromycin**. Moderate Study → Also see TABLE 9 p. 1431

▶ NNRTIs (**etravirine**) decrease the exposure to **clarithromycin** and **clarithromycin** slightly increases the exposure to NNRTIs (**etravirine**). Severe Study

▶ **Clarithromycin** is predicted to increase the exposure to NNRTIs (**doravirine**). Mild Study

▶ **Clarithromycin** decreases the absorption of NRTIs (**zidovudine**). Separate administration by at least 2 hours. Moderate Study

▶ **Clarithromycin** is predicted to increase the exposure to olaparib. Avoid potent CYP3A4 inhibitors or adjust **olaparib** dose, p. 1051. Moderate Study

▶ **Erythromycin** is predicted to increase the exposure to olaparib. Avoid moderate CYP3A4 inhibitors or adjust **olaparib** dose, p. 1051. Moderate Theoretical

▶ **Clarithromycin** is predicted to increase the exposure to opioids (**alfentanil, buprenorphine, fentanyl, oxycodone**). Monitor and adjust dose. Severe Study

▶ **Erythromycin** is predicted to increase the exposure to opioids (**alfentanil, buprenorphine, fentanyl, oxycodone**). Monitor and adjust dose. Moderate Study

▶ **Clarithromycin** is predicted to increase the concentration of opioids (**methadone**). Severe Theoretical → Also see TABLE 9 p. 1431

▶ **Erythromycin** is predicted to increase the exposure to opioids (**methadone**). Moderate Theoretical → Also see TABLE 9 p. 1431

▶ **Clarithromycin** is predicted to increase the exposure to ospemifene. Avoid in poor CYP2C9 metabolisers. Moderate Study

▶ **Clarithromycin** is predicted to increase the exposure to oxybutynin. Mild Study

▶ **Erythromycin** is predicted to increase the exposure to oxybutynin. Mild Theoretical

▶ **Clarithromycin** is predicted to increase the exposure to palbociclib. Avoid or adjust **palbociclib** dose, p. 1038. Severe Study

▶ **Clarithromycin** is predicted to increase the exposure to panobinostat. Adjust **panobinostat** dose; in hepatic impairment avoid, p. 979. Moderate Study → Also see TABLE 9 p. 1431

▶ **Macrolides** (**azithromycin, erythromycin**) are predicted to increase the exposure to panobinostat. Adjust dose. Moderate Theoretical → Also see TABLE 9 p. 1431

▶ **Clarithromycin** is predicted to increase the exposure to paritaprevir. Avoid. Severe Study

▶ **Erythromycin** is predicted to increase the exposure to paritaprevir. Moderate Theoretical

▶ **Clarithromycin** is predicted to increase the exposure to pazopanib. Avoid or adjust **pazopanib** dose, p. 1039. Moderate Study → Also see TABLE 9 p. 1431

▶ **Erythromycin** is predicted to increase the exposure to pazopanib. Moderate Theoretical → Also see TABLE 9 p. 1431

▶ **Erythromycin** is predicted to increase the exposure to phosphodiesterase type-5 inhibitors (**avanafil**). Adjust **avanafil** dose, p. 859. Moderate Theoretical

▶ **Clarithromycin** is predicted to increase the exposure to phosphodiesterase type-5 inhibitors (**avanafil, vardenafil**). Avoid. Severe Study → Also see TABLE 9 p. 1431

▶ **Clarithromycin** is predicted to increase the exposure to phosphodiesterase type-5 inhibitors (**sildenafil**). Avoid potent CYP3A4 inhibitors or adjust **sildenafil** dose, p. 860. Severe Study → Also see TABLE 9 p. 1431

▶ **Erythromycin** is predicted to increase the exposure to phosphodiesterase type-5 inhibitors (**sildenafil**). Monitor or adjust **sildenafil** dose with moderate CYP3A4 inhibitors, p. 860. Moderate Study → Also see TABLE 9 p. 1431

▶ **Clarithromycin** is predicted to increase the exposure to phosphodiesterase type-5 inhibitors (**tadalafil**). Use with caution or avoid. Severe Study

▶ **Erythromycin** is predicted to increase the exposure to phosphodiesterase type-5 inhibitors (**tadalafil**). Severe Theoretical

▶ **Erythromycin** is predicted to increase the exposure to phosphodiesterase type-5 inhibitors (**vardenafil**). Adjust dose. Severe Theoretical → Also see TABLE 9 p. 1431

▶ **Macrolides** are predicted to increase the exposure to pibrentasvir. Moderate Theoretical

▶ **Clarithromycin** is predicted to increase the exposure to pimozide. Avoid. Severe Study → Also see TABLE 9 p. 1431

▶ **Erythromycin** is predicted to increase the exposure to pimozide. Avoid. Severe Theoretical → Also see TABLE 9 p. 1431

▶ **Clarithromycin** is predicted to slightly increase the exposure to ponatinib. Monitor and adjust **ponatinib** dose, p. 1040. Moderate Study

▶ **Clarithromycin** is predicted to moderately increase the exposure to praziquantel. Mild Study

▶ **Clarithromycin** given with carbimazole is predicted to increase the exposure to propiverine. Adjust starting dose. Moderate Theoretical

▶ **Clarithromycin** is predicted to increase the exposure to ranolazine. Avoid. Severe Study → Also see TABLE 9 p. 1431

▶ **Erythromycin** is predicted to increase the exposure to ranolazine. Severe Study → Also see TABLE 9 p. 1431

▶ **Clarithromycin** is predicted to increase the exposure to reboxetine. Avoid. Moderate Study

▶ **Clarithromycin** is predicted to increase the exposure to regorafenib. Avoid. Moderate Study

▶ **Clarithromycin** is predicted to increase the exposure to retinoids (**alitretinoin**). Adjust **alitretinoin** dose, p. 1305. Moderate Theoretical

▶ **Clarithromycin** is predicted to increase the exposure to ribociclib. Avoid or adjust **ribociclib** dose, p. 1042. Moderate Study → Also see TABLE 9 p. 1431

▶ **Erythromycin** is predicted to increase the exposure to ribociclib. Moderate Study → Also see TABLE 9 p. 1431

▶ Rifamycins (**rifampicin**) decrease the concentration of **clarithromycin**. Severe Study

▶ **Azithromycin** increases the risk of neutropenia when given with rifamycins (**rifabutin**). Severe Study

▶ **Clarithromycin** increases the risk of uveitis when given with rifamycins (**rifabutin**). Adjust dose. Severe Study

▶ **Erythromycin** is predicted to increase the risk of uveitis when given with rifamycins (**rifabutin**). Adjust dose. Severe Theoretical

▶ **Clarithromycin** is predicted to increase the exposure to ruxolitinib. Adjust dose and monitor adverse effects. Moderate Study

▶ **Erythromycin** is predicted to increase the exposure to ruxolitinib. Moderate Theoretical

▶ **Clarithromycin** is predicted to increase the exposure to siponimod. Avoid depending on other drugs taken—consult product literature. Severe Theoretical

▶ **Clarithromycin** is predicted to increase the concentration of sirolimus. Avoid. Severe Study

▶ **Erythromycin** increases the concentration of sirolimus. Monitor and adjust dose. Moderate Study

Clarithromycin is predicted to increase the exposure to solifenacin. Adjust solifenacin p. 824 or tamsulosin with solifenacin p. 830 dose; avoid in hepatic and renal impairment. Severe Study

Clarithromycin is predicted to moderately increase the exposure to SSRIs (dapoxetine). Avoid potent CYP3A4 inhibitors or adjust **dapoxetine** dose, p. 867. Severe Study

Erythromycin is predicted to increase the exposure to SSRIs (dapoxetine). Adjust **dapoxetine** dose with moderate CYP3A4 inhibitors, p. 867. Moderate Theoretical

▶ **Clarithromycin** is predicted to increase the exposure to statins (atorvastatin). Avoid or adjust dose and monitor rhabdomyolysis. Severe Study

Erythromycin slightly increases the exposure to statins (atorvastatin). Monitor and adjust dose. Severe Anecdotal

▶ **Clarithromycin** moderately increases the exposure to statins (pravastatin). Severe Study

▶ **Erythromycin** is predicted to increase the exposure to statins (pravastatin). Severe Study

▶ **Clarithromycin** is predicted to increase the exposure to statins (simvastatin). Avoid. Severe Study

▶ **Erythromycin** markedly increases the exposure to statins (simvastatin). Avoid. Severe Study

▶ **Clarithromycin** is predicted to slightly increase the exposure to sulfonylureas. Moderate Theoretical

▶ **Clarithromycin** is predicted to slightly increase the exposure to sunitinib. Avoid or adjust **sunitinib** dose, p. 1044. Moderate Study → Also see TABLE 9 p. 1431

▶ **Erythromycin** is predicted to increase the exposure to sunitinib. Moderate Theoretical → Also see TABLE 9 p. 1431

▶ **Clarithromycin** is predicted to increase the concentration of tacrolimus. Monitor and adjust dose. Severe Study

▶ **Erythromycin** is predicted to increase the concentration of tacrolimus. Severe Study

▶ **Macrolides** are predicted to slightly increase the exposure to talazoparib. Avoid or adjust **talazoparib** dose, p. 1052. Severe Study

▶ **Clarithromycin** is predicted to increase the exposure to taxanes (cabazitaxel). Avoid. Severe Study

▶ **Erythromycin** is predicted to increase the exposure to taxanes (cabazitaxel). Moderate Theoretical

▶ **Clarithromycin** is predicted to moderately increase the exposure to taxanes (docetaxel). Avoid or adjust dose. Severe Study

▶ **Clarithromycin** is predicted to increase the exposure to taxanes (paclitaxel). Severe Theoretical

▶ **Clarithromycin** is predicted to increase the concentration of temsirolimus. Avoid. Severe Theoretical

▶ **Erythromycin** is predicted to increase the concentration of temsirolimus. Use with caution or avoid. Moderate Theoretical

▶ **Clarithromycin** is predicted to increase the exposure to tezacaftor. Adjust tezacaftor with ivacaftor p. 311 or tezacaftor with ivacaftor and elexacftor p. 311 dose with potent CYP3A4 inhibitors. Severe Study

▶ **Erythromycin** is predicted to increase the exposure to tezacaftor. Adjust tezacaftor with ivacaftor p. 311 or tezacaftor with ivacaftor and elexacftor p. 311 dose with moderate CYP3A4 inhibitors. Severe Study

▶ **Erythromycin** decreases the clearance of theophylline and theophylline potentially increases the clearance of **erythromycin**. Adjust dose. Severe Study

▶ **Macrolides (azithromycin, clarithromycin)** are predicted to increase the exposure to theophylline. Adjust dose. Moderate Anecdotal

▶ **Macrolides** are predicted to increase the exposure to thrombin inhibitors (dabigatran). Moderate Theoretical

▶ **Azithromycin** is predicted to increase the exposure to ticagrelor. Use with caution or avoid. Severe Study

▶ **Clarithromycin** is predicted to markedly increase the exposure to ticagrelor. Avoid. Severe Study

▶ **Clarithromycin** is predicted to increase the exposure to tofacitinib. Adjust **tofacitinib** dose, p. 1154. Moderate Study

▶ **Erythromycin** given with a potent CYP2C19 inhibitor is predicted to increase the exposure to tofacitinib. Adjust **tofacitinib** dose, p. 1154. Moderate Study

▶ **Clarithromycin** is predicted to increase the exposure to tolterodine. Avoid. Severe Study → Also see TABLE 9 p. 1431

▶ **Erythromycin** is predicted to increase the exposure to tolterodine. Mild Theoretical → Also see TABLE 9 p. 1431

▶ **Clarithromycin** is predicted to increase the exposure to tolvaptan. Manufacturer advises caution or adjust **tolvaptan** dose with potent CYP3A4 inhibitors, p. 708. Severe Study

▶ **Erythromycin** is predicted to increase the exposure to tolvaptan. Manufacturer advises caution or adjust **tolvaptan** dose with moderate CYP3A4 inhibitors, p. 708. Moderate Study

▶ **Macrolides** are predicted to increase the exposure to topotecan. Severe Study

▶ **Clarithromycin** is predicted to increase the exposure to toremifene. Moderate Theoretical → Also see TABLE 9 p. 1431

▶ **Clarithromycin** is predicted to increase the exposure to trabectedin. Avoid or adjust dose. Severe Theoretical

▶ **Macrolides** are predicted to increase the concentration of trametinib. Moderate Theoretical

▶ **Clarithromycin** is predicted to moderately increase the exposure to trazodone. Avoid or adjust dose. Moderate Study

▶ **Erythromycin** is predicted to increase the exposure to trazodone. Moderate Theoretical

▶ **Clarithromycin** increases the exposure to triptans (almotriptan). Mild Study

▶ **Clarithromycin** is predicted to markedly increase the exposure to triptans (eletriptan). Avoid. Severe Study

▶ **Erythromycin** moderately increases the exposure to triptans (eletriptan). Avoid. Moderate Study

▶ **Clarithromycin** is predicted to increase the exposure to upadacitinib. Use with caution or avoid. Severe Study

▶ **Clarithromycin** is predicted to increase the exposure to vemurafenib. Severe Theoretical → Also see TABLE 9 p. 1431

▶ **Macrolides (clarithromycin, erythromycin)** are predicted to increase the exposure to venetoclax. Avoid or adjust dose—consult product literature. Severe Study

▶ **Clarithromycin** is predicted to increase the exposure to venlafaxine. Moderate Study → Also see TABLE 9 p. 1431

▶ **Macrolides (clarithromycin, erythromycin)** are predicted to increase the exposure to vinca alkaloids. Severe Theoretical → Also see TABLE 9 p. 1431

▶ **Clarithromycin** is predicted to increase the exposure to vitamin D substances (paricalcitol). Moderate Study

▶ **Clarithromycin** is predicted to increase the exposure to zopiclone. Adjust dose. Moderate Theoretical

▶ **Erythromycin** is predicted to increase the exposure to zopiclone. Adjust dose. Moderate Study

Magnesium

SEPARATION OF ADMINISTRATION **Magnesium-containing antacids** should preferably not be taken at the same time as other drugs since they might impair absorption. **Magnesium-containing antacids** might damage enteric coatings designed to prevent dissolution in the stomach.

▶ Oral **magnesium** decreases the absorption of oral bisphosphonates (alendronate). **Alendronate** should be taken at least 30 minutes before magnesium. Moderate Study

▶ Oral **magnesium** decreases the absorption of oral bisphosphonates (clodronate). Avoid magnesium for 2 hours before or 1 hour after **clodronate**. Moderate Study

▶ Oral **magnesium** is predicted to decrease the absorption of oral bisphosphonates (ibandronate). Avoid for at least 6 hours before or 1 hour after **ibandronate**. Moderate Theoretical

▶ Oral **magnesium** decreases the absorption of oral bisphosphonates (risedronate). Separate administration by at least 2 hours. Moderate Study

▶ Intravenous **magnesium** potentially increases the risk of hypotension when given with calcium channel blockers (amlodipine, felodipine, lacidipine, lercanidipine, nicardipine, nifedipine, nimodipine, verapamil) in pregnant women. Severe Anecdotal

▶ Intravenous **magnesium** increases the effects of neuromuscular blocking drugs, non-depolarising. Moderate Study

▶ Oral **magnesium** trisilicate decreases the absorption of oral nitrofurantoin. Moderate Study

▶ Intravenous **magnesium** is predicted to increase the effects of suxamethonium. Moderate Study

MAO-B inhibitors → see **TABLE 6** p. 1430 (bradycardia), **TABLE 8** p. 1430 (hypotension), **TABLE 13** p. 1432 (serotonin syndrome)

rasagiline · safinamide · selegiline

FOOD AND LIFESTYLE Hypertension is predicted to occur when high-dose **selegiline** is taken with tyramine-rich foods (such as mature cheese, salami, pickled herring, Bovril®, Oxo®, Marmite® or any similar meat or yeast extract or fermented soya bean extract, and some beers, lagers or wines).

‣ MAO-B inhibitors **(rasagiline, selegiline)** are predicted to increase the risk of severe hypertension when given with amfetamines. Avoid. Severe Theoretical → Also see **TABLE 13** p. 1432
‣ **Safinamide** is predicted to increase the risk of severe hypertension when given with amfetamines. Severe Theoretical → Also see **TABLE 13** p. 1432
‣ MAO-B inhibitors **(rasagiline, selegiline)** are predicted to increase the risk of severe hypertension when given with beta₂ agonists. Avoid. Severe Theoretical
‣ **Safinamide** is predicted to increase the risk of severe hypertension when given with beta₂ agonists. Severe Theoretical
‣ Bupropion is predicted to increase the risk of severe hypertension when given with **MAO-B inhibitors**. Avoid. Moderate Theoretical → Also see **TABLE 13** p. 1432
‣ Combined hormonal contraceptives slightly increase the exposure to **rasagiline**. Moderate Study
‣ Combined hormonal contraceptives increase the exposure to **selegiline**. Avoid. Severe Study
‣ Hormone replacement therapy is predicted to increase the exposure to **selegiline**. Avoid. Moderate Study
‣ **MAO-B inhibitors** are predicted to increase the effects of levodopa. Adjust dose. Mild Study → Also see **TABLE 8** p. 1430
‣ MAO-B inhibitors **(rasagiline, selegiline)** are predicted to increase the risk of adverse effects when given with linezolid. Avoid and for 14 days after stopping the MAOI. Severe Theoretical → Also see **TABLE 13** p. 1432
‣ **Safinamide** is predicted to increase the risk of adverse effects when given with linezolid. Avoid and for 1 week after stopping **safinamide**. Severe Theoretical → Also see **TABLE 13** p. 1432
‣ MAO-B inhibitors **(rasagiline, selegiline)** are predicted to increase the risk of adverse effects when given with MAOIs, irreversible. Avoid and for 14 days after stopping the MAOI. Severe Theoretical → Also see **TABLE 8** p. 1430 → Also see **TABLE 13** p. 1432
‣ **Safinamide** is predicted to increase the risk of adverse effects when given with MAOIs, irreversible. Avoid and for 1 week after stopping **safinamide**. Severe Theoretical → Also see **TABLE 13** p. 1432
‣ MAO-B inhibitors **(rasagiline, selegiline)** are predicted to increase the risk of a hypertensive crisis when given with methylphenidate. Avoid. Severe Theoretical
‣ Mexiletine slightly increases the exposure to **rasagiline**. Moderate Study
‣ Moclobemide is predicted to increase the effects of MAO-B inhibitors **(rasagiline, selegiline)**. Avoid. Severe Theoretical → Also see **TABLE 13** p. 1432
‣ Moclobemide is predicted to increase the risk of adverse effects when given with **safinamide**. Avoid and for 1 week after stopping **safinamide**. Severe Theoretical → Also see **TABLE 13** p. 1432
‣ **Rasagiline** is predicted to increase the risk of adverse effects when given with opioids (pethidine). Avoid and for 14 days after stopping **rasagiline**. Severe Theoretical → Also see **TABLE 13** p. 1432
‣ **Safinamide** is predicted to increase the risk of adverse effects when given with opioids (pethidine). Avoid and for 1 week after stopping **safinamide**. Severe Theoretical → Also see **TABLE 13** p. 1432
‣ **Selegiline** increases the risk of adverse effects when given with opioids (pethidine). Avoid. Severe Anecdotal → Also see **TABLE 13** p. 1432
‣ Ozanimod potentially increases the risk of a hypertensive crisis when given with **MAO-B inhibitors** and **MAO-B inhibitors** potentially decrease the exposure to the active metabolite of ozanimod. Avoid. Severe Theoretical → Also see **TABLE 6** p. 1430
‣ Quinolones (ciprofloxacin) slightly increase the exposure to **rasagiline**. Moderate Study

‣ Reboxetine is predicted to increase the risk of a hypertensive crisis when given with MAO-B inhibitors **(rasagiline, selegiline)**. Avoid. Severe Theoretical
‣ Solriamfetol is predicted to increase the risk of a hypertensive crisis when given with **MAO-B inhibitors**. Avoid and for 14 days after stopping **MAO-B inhibitors**. Severe Theoretical
‣ Sympathomimetics, inotropic are predicted to increase the risk of a hypertensive crisis when given with **MAO-B inhibitors**. Avoid. Severe Anecdotal
‣ Sympathomimetics, vasoconstrictor are predicted to increase the risk of a hypertensive crisis when given with **MAO-B inhibitors**. Avoid. Severe Anecdotal
‣ Tetrabenazine potentially increases the risk of CNS excitation and hypertension when given with **MAO-B inhibitors**. Severe Theoretical

MAOIs, irreversible → see **TABLE 8** p. 1430 (hypotension), **TABLE 13** p. 1432 (serotonin syndrome)

isocarboxazid · phenelzine · tranylcypromine

FOOD AND LIFESTYLE Potentially life-threatening hypertensive crisis can develop in those taking MAOIs who eat tyramine-rich food (such as mature cheese, salami, pickled herring, Bovril®, Oxo®, Marmite® or any similar meat or yeast extract or fermented soya bean extract, and some beers, lagers or wines) or foods containing dopa (such as broad bean pods). Avoid tyramine-rich or dopa-rich food or drinks with, or for 2 to 3 weeks after stopping, the MAOI.

‣ **MAOIs, irreversible** are predicted to increase the effects of alpha blockers (indoramin). Avoid. Severe Theoretical → Also see **TABLE 8** p. 1430
‣ Amfetamines are predicted to increase the risk of a hypertensive crisis when given with **MAOIs, irreversible**. Avoid and for 14 days after stopping the MAOI. Severe Anecdotal → Also see **TABLE 13** p. 1432
‣ Antiepileptics (carbamazepine) are predicted to increase the risk of severe toxic reaction when given with **MAOIs, irreversible**. Avoid and for 14 days after stopping the MAOI. Severe Theoretical
‣ Antiepileptics (phenobarbital, primidone) are predicted to increase the effects of **MAOIs, irreversible**. Severe Theoretical
‣ **MAOIs, irreversible** are predicted to increase the risk of antimuscarinic adverse effects when given with antihistamines, non-sedating. Avoid. Severe Theoretical
‣ **MAOIs, irreversible** are predicted to increase the risk of antimuscarinic adverse effects when given with antihistamines, sedating. Avoid. Severe Theoretical
‣ **MAOIs, irreversible** are predicted to increase the risk of adverse effects when given with atomoxetine. Avoid and for 2 weeks after stopping the MAOI. Severe Theoretical
‣ **MAOIs, irreversible** are predicted to increase the risk of cardiovascular adverse effects when given with beta₂ agonists. Moderate Anecdotal
‣ Bupropion is predicted to increase the risk of severe hypertension when given with **MAOIs, irreversible**. Avoid and for 14 days after stopping the MAOI. Severe Theoretical → Also see **TABLE 13** p. 1432
‣ Buspirone is predicted to increase the risk of elevated blood pressure when given with **MAOIs, irreversible**. Avoid. Severe Anecdotal → Also see **TABLE 13** p. 1432
‣ **MAOIs, irreversible** are predicted to increase the effects of doxapram. Moderate Theoretical
‣ Entacapone is predicted to increase the risk of elevated blood pressure when given with **MAOIs, irreversible**. Avoid. Severe Theoretical
‣ Levodopa increases the risk of a hypertensive crisis when given with **MAOIs, irreversible**. Avoid and for 14 days after stopping the MAOI. Severe Study → Also see **TABLE 8** p. 1430
‣ **MAOIs, irreversible** are predicted to increase the risk of adverse effects when given with linezolid. Avoid and for 14 days after stopping the MAOI. Severe Theoretical → Also see **TABLE 13** p. 1432
‣ MAO-B inhibitors (rasagiline, selegiline) are predicted to increase the risk of adverse effects when given with **MAOIs, irreversible**. Avoid and for 14 days after stopping the MAOI. Severe Theoretical → Also see **TABLE 8** p. 1430 → Also see **TABLE 13** p. 1432

MAO-B inhibitors (safinamide) are predicted to increase the risk of adverse effects when given with **MAOIs, irreversible**. Avoid and for 1 week after stopping **safinamide**. Severe Theoretical → Also see **TABLE 13** p. 1432

MAOIs, irreversible are predicted to alter the antihypertensive effects of methyldopa. Avoid. Severe Theoretical → Also see **TABLE 8** p. 1430

Methylphenidate is predicted to increase the risk of a hypertensive crisis when given with **MAOIs, irreversible**. Avoid and for 14 days after stopping the MAOI. Severe Theoretical

Mianserin is predicted to increase the risk of toxicity when given with **MAOIs, irreversible**. Avoid and for 14 days after stopping the MAOI. Severe Theoretical

Nefopam is predicted to increase the risk of serious elevations in blood pressure when given with **MAOIs, irreversible**. Avoid. Severe Theoretical

Opicapone is predicted to increase the risk of elevated blood pressure when given with **MAOIs, irreversible**. Avoid. Severe Theoretical

Opioids are predicted to increase the risk of CNS excitation or depression when given with **MAOIs, irreversible**. Avoid. Severe Study → Also see **TABLE 13** p. 1432

Ozanimod potentially increases the risk of a hypertensive crisis when given with **MAOIs, irreversible**. Avoid Severe Theoretical

▸ **MAOIs, irreversible** are predicted to increase the risk of neuroleptic malignant syndrome when given with phenothiazines. Severe Theoretical → Also see **TABLE 8** p. 1430

▸ Pholcodine is predicted to increase the risk of CNS excitation or depression when given with **MAOIs, irreversible**. Avoid and for 14 days after stopping the MAOI. Severe Theoretical

▸ Reboxetine is predicted to increase the risk of a hypertensive crisis when given with **MAOIs, irreversible**. Avoid. Severe Theoretical

▸ Solriamfetol is predicted to increase the risk of a hypertensive crisis when given with **MAOIs, irreversible**. Avoid and for 14 days after stopping the MAOI. Severe Theoretical

▸ Sympathomimetics, inotropic are predicted to increase the risk of a hypertensive crisis when given with **MAOIs, irreversible**. Avoid and for 14 days after stopping the MAOI. Severe Theoretical

▸ Sympathomimetics, vasoconstrictor are predicted to increase the risk of a hypertensive crisis when given with **MAOIs, irreversible**. Avoid and for 14 days after stopping the MAOI. Severe Study

▸ Tetrabenazine potentially increases the risk of CNS excitation and hypertension when given with **MAOIs, irreversible**. Avoid and for 14 days after stopping the MAOI. Severe Study

▸ Tolcapone is predicted to increase the effects of **MAOIs, irreversible**. Avoid. Severe Theoretical

▸ Tricyclic antidepressants are predicted to increase the risk of severe toxic reaction when given with **MAOIs, irreversible**. Avoid and for 14 days after stopping the MAOI. Severe Theoretical → Also see **TABLE 8** p. 1430 → Also see **TABLE 13** p. 1432

▸ **MAOIs, irreversible** are predicted to increase the exposure to triptans (rizatriptan, sumatriptan). Avoid and for 14 days after stopping the MAOI. Severe Theoretical → Also see **TABLE 13** p. 1432

▸ **MAOIs, irreversible** are predicted to increase the exposure to triptans (zolmitriptan). Severe Theoretical → Also see **TABLE 13** p. 1432

▸ Tryptophan increases the risk of adverse effects when given with **MAOIs, irreversible**. Severe Anecdotal → Also see **TABLE 13** p. 1432

Maraviroc
▸ Anti-androgens (apalutamide, enzalutamide) are predicted to decrease the exposure to **maraviroc**. Adjust dose. Severe Study

▸ Antiepileptics (carbamazepine, fosphenytoin, phenobarbital, phenytoin, primidone) are predicted to decrease the exposure to **maraviroc**. Adjust dose. Severe Study

▸ Antifungals, azoles (itraconazole, ketoconazole, voriconazole) are predicted to markedly increase the exposure to **maraviroc**. Adjust dose. Severe Study

▸ Cobicistat markedly increases the exposure to **maraviroc**. Refer to specialist literature. Severe Study

▸ Endothelin receptor antagonists (bosentan) are predicted to decrease the exposure to **maraviroc**. Avoid. Moderate Theoretical

▸ HIV-protease inhibitors (atazanavir, saquinavir) moderately to markedly increase the exposure to **maraviroc**. Refer to specialist literature. Severe Study

▸ HIV-protease inhibitors (darunavir) boosted with ritonavir markedly increase the exposure to **maraviroc**. Refer to specialist literature. Severe Study

▸ HIV-protease inhibitors (lopinavir) boosted with ritonavir moderately increase the exposure to **maraviroc**. Refer to specialist literature. Severe Study

▸ HIV-protease inhibitors (ritonavir) markedly increase the exposure to **maraviroc**. Refer to specialist literature. Severe Study

▸ **Maraviroc** potentially decreases the exposure to HIV-protease inhibitors (fosamprenavir) and HIV-protease inhibitors (fosamprenavir) potentially decrease the exposure to **maraviroc**. Avoid. Severe Study

▸ Idelalisib markedly increases the exposure to **maraviroc**. Adjust dose. Severe Theoretical

▸ Macrolides (clarithromycin) are predicted to markedly increase the exposure to **maraviroc**. Adjust dose. Severe Study

▸ Mitotane is predicted to decrease the exposure to **maraviroc**. Adjust dose. Severe Study

▸ Neurokinin-1 receptor antagonists (aprepitant, netupitant) are predicted to increase the exposure to **maraviroc**. Moderate Study

▸ NNRTIs (efavirenz) decrease the exposure to **maraviroc**. Refer to specialist literature. Severe Theoretical

▸ NNRTIs (etravirine) (with a boosted protease inhibitor) increase the exposure to **maraviroc**. Avoid or adjust dose. Moderate Study

▸ Rifamycins (rifampicin) are predicted to decrease the exposure to **maraviroc**. Adjust dose. Severe Study

▸ St John's wort is predicted to decrease the exposure to **maraviroc**. Avoid. Severe Theoretical

Measles, mumps and rubella vaccine, live → see live vaccines

Mebendazole
▸ H₂ receptor antagonists (cimetidine) increase the concentration of **mebendazole**. Moderate Study

Medroxyprogesterone
▸ Sugammadex is predicted to decrease the exposure to **medroxyprogesterone**. Use additional contraceptive precautions. Severe Theoretical

Mefenamic acid → see NSAIDs

Mefloquine → see antimalarials

Meglitinides → see **TABLE 14** p. 1432 (antidiabetic drugs)

nateglinide · repaglinide

▸ Anti-androgens (apalutamide, enzalutamide) are predicted to slightly decrease the exposure to **nateglinide**. Mild Study

▸ Anti-androgens (apalutamide, enzalutamide) are predicted to decrease the exposure to **repaglinide**. Monitor blood glucose and adjust dose. Moderate Study

▸ Anti-androgens (darolutamide) are predicted to increase the concentration of **repaglinide**. Moderate Theoretical

▸ Antiepileptics (carbamazepine, fosphenytoin, phenobarbital, phenytoin, primidone) are predicted to slightly decrease the exposure to **nateglinide**. Mild Study

▸ Antiepileptics (carbamazepine, fosphenytoin, phenobarbital, phenytoin, primidone) are predicted to decrease the exposure to **repaglinide**. Monitor blood glucose and adjust dose. Moderate Study

▸ Antifungals, azoles (itraconazole, ketoconazole, voriconazole) are predicted to increase the exposure to **repaglinide**. Moderate Study

▸ Ciclosporin moderately increases the exposure to **repaglinide**. Moderate Study

▸ Clopidogrel increases the exposure to **repaglinide**. Avoid. Severe Study

▸ Cobicistat is predicted to increase the exposure to **repaglinide**. Moderate Study

▸ Fibrates (gemfibrozil) increase the exposure to **repaglinide**. Avoid. Severe Study

▸ Filgotinib is predicted to increase the exposure to **repaglinide**. Avoid. Moderate Theoretical

Meglitinides (continued)
▶ HIV-protease inhibitors are predicted to increase the exposure to **repaglinide**. Moderate Study
▶ Idelalisib is predicted to increase the exposure to **repaglinide**. Moderate Study
▶ Iron chelators (deferasirox) moderately increase the exposure to **repaglinide**. Avoid. Moderate Study
▶ Leflunomide is predicted to increase the exposure to **nateglinide**. Moderate Theoretical
▶ Leflunomide is predicted to increase the exposure to **repaglinide**. Moderate Study
▶ Letermovir is predicted to increase the concentration of **repaglinide**. Avoid. Moderate Study
▶ Macrolides (clarithromycin) are predicted to increase the exposure to **repaglinide**. Moderate Study
▶ Mitotane is predicted to slightly decrease the exposure to **nateglinide**. Mild Study
▶ Mitotane is predicted to decrease the exposure to **repaglinide**. Monitor blood glucose and adjust dose. Moderate Study
▶ Opicapone is predicted to increase the exposure to **repaglinide**. Avoid. Moderate Study
▶ Pitolisant is predicted to decrease the exposure to **repaglinide**. Mild Theoretical
▶ Rifamycins (rifampicin) are predicted to slightly decrease the exposure to **nateglinide**. Mild Study
▶ Rifamycins (rifampicin) are predicted to decrease the exposure to **repaglinide**. Monitor blood glucose and adjust dose. Moderate Study
▶ Teriflunomide is predicted to increase the exposure to **nateglinide**. Moderate Theoretical
▶ Teriflunomide is predicted to increase the exposure to **repaglinide**. Moderate Study
▶ Trimethoprim slightly increases the exposure to **repaglinide**. Avoid or monitor blood glucose. Moderate Study
▶ Venetoclax is predicted to increase the exposure to **repaglinide**. Moderate Study

Melatonin → see TABLE 11 p. 1431 (CNS depressant effects)
▶ Antiepileptics (phenytoin) are predicted to decrease the exposure to **melatonin**. Moderate Theoretical
▶ Combined hormonal contraceptives are predicted to increase the exposure to **melatonin**. Moderate Theoretical
▶ HIV-protease inhibitors (ritonavir) are predicted to decrease the exposure to **melatonin**. Moderate Theoretical
▶ Leflunomide is predicted to decrease the exposure to **melatonin**. Moderate Theoretical
▶ Mexiletine is predicted to increase the exposure to **melatonin**. Moderate Theoretical
▶ Quinolones (ciprofloxacin) are predicted to increase the exposure to **melatonin**. Moderate Theoretical
▶ Rifamycins (rifampicin) are predicted to decrease the exposure to **melatonin**. Moderate Theoretical
▶ SSRIs (fluvoxamine) very markedly increase the exposure to **melatonin**. Avoid. Severe Study
▶ Teriflunomide is predicted to decrease the exposure to **melatonin**. Moderate Theoretical
▶ Vemurafenib is predicted to increase the exposure to **melatonin**. Use with caution or avoid. Moderate Theoretical

Melphalan → see NSAIDs
Melphalan → see alkylating agents
Memantine
▶ Dopamine receptor agonists (amantadine) increase the risk of CNS toxicity when given with **memantine**. Use with caution or avoid. Severe Theoretical
▶ Memantine is predicted to increase the effects of dopamine receptor agonists (apomorphine, bromocriptine, cabergoline, pramipexole, quinagolide, ropinirole, rotigotine). Moderate Theoretical
▶ Memantine is predicted to increase the risk of CNS adverse effects when given with ketamine. Avoid. Severe Theoretical
▶ Memantine is predicted to increase the effects of levodopa. Moderate Theoretical
Mepacrine
▶ Mepacrine is predicted to increase the concentration of antimalarials (primaquine). Avoid. Moderate Theoretical
Mepivacaine → see anaesthetics, local

Meprobamate → see TABLE 11 p. 1431 (CNS depressant effects)
Meptazinol → see opioids
Mercaptopurine → see TABLE 1 p. 1429 (hepatotoxicity), TABLE 15 p. 1432 (myelosuppression)
▶ Allopurinol potentially increases the risk of haematological toxicity when given with **mercaptopurine**. Adjust mercaptopurine dose, p. 956. Severe Study
▶ Mercaptopurine decreases the anticoagulant effect of coumarins. Moderate Anecdotal
▶ Febuxostat is predicted to increase the exposure to **mercaptopurine**. Avoid. Severe Theoretical
▶ Live vaccines are predicted to increase the risk of generalised infection (possibly life-threatening) when given with **mercaptopurine** (high-dose). Public Health England advises avoid (refer to Green Book). Severe Theoretical
Meropenem → see carbapenems
Mesalazine

ROUTE-SPECIFIC INFORMATION The manufacturers of some mesalazine gastro-resistant and modified-release medicines (*Asacol MR* tablets, *Ipocol*, *Salofalk* granules) suggest that preparations that lower stool pH (e.g. lactulose) might prevent the release of mesalazine.

Metaraminol → see sympathomimetics, vasoconstrictor
Metformin → see TABLE 14 p. 1432 (antidiabetic drugs)
▶ Alcohol (excessive consumption) potentially increases the risk of lactic acidosis when given with **metformin**. Avoid excessive alcohol consumption. Moderate Theoretical
▶ Bictegravir slightly increases the exposure to **metformin**. Moderate Study
▶ Dolutegravir increases the exposure to **metformin**. Use with caution and adjust dose. Severe Study
▶ Guanfacine is predicted to increase the concentration of **metformin**. Moderate Theoretical
▶ H$_2$ receptor antagonists (cimetidine) increase the exposure to **metformin**. Monitor and adjust dose. Moderate Study
▶ Mexiletine is predicted to affect the exposure to **metformin**. Unknown Theoretical
▶ Pitolisant is predicted to increase the exposure to **metformin**. Mild Theoretical
▶ Ribociclib is predicted to increase the exposure to **metformin**. Moderate Theoretical
▶ Vandetanib increases the exposure to **metformin**. Monitor and adjust dose. Moderate Study
Methadone → see opioids
Methenamine
▶ Acetazolamide is predicted to decrease the efficacy of **methenamine**. Avoid. Moderate Theoretical
▶ Potassium citrate is predicted to decrease the efficacy of **methenamine**. Avoid. Moderate Theoretical
▶ Sodium bicarbonate is predicted to decrease the efficacy of **methenamine**. Avoid. Moderate Theoretical
▶ Sodium citrate is predicted to decrease the efficacy of **methenamine**. Avoid. Moderate Theoretical
Methocarbamol → see TABLE 11 p. 1431 (CNS depressant effects)
Methotrexate → see TABLE 1 p. 1429 (hepatotoxicity), TABLE 15 p. 1432 (myelosuppression), TABLE 2 p. 1429 (nephrotoxicity), TABLE 5 p. 1430 (thromboembolism)
▶ Acetazolamide increases the urinary excretion of **methotrexate**. Moderate Study
▶ Methotrexate is predicted to decrease the clearance of aminophylline. Moderate Theoretical
▶ Anti-androgens (apalutamide) are predicted to decrease the exposure to **methotrexate**. Mild Study
▶ Anti-androgens (darolutamide) are predicted to increase the concentration of **methotrexate**. Moderate Theoretical
▶ Antiepileptics (levetiracetam) decrease the clearance of **methotrexate**. Severe Anecdotal
▶ Antimalarials (pyrimethamine) are predicted to increase the risk of adverse effects when given with **methotrexate**. Severe Theoretical
▶ Asparaginase affects the efficacy of **methotrexate**. Severe Anecdotal → Also see TABLE 1 p. 1429 → Also see TABLE 15 p. 1432
▶ Aspirin (high-dose) is predicted to increase the risk of toxicity when given with **methotrexate**. Severe Study

Brigatinib potentially increases the concentration of **methotrexate**. Moderate Theoretical

Crisantaspase affects the efficacy of **methotrexate**. Severe Anecdotal → Also see TABLE 1 p. 1429 → Also see TABLE 15 p. 1432

Eltrombopag is predicted to increase the concentration of **methotrexate**. Moderate Theoretical

Methotrexate potentially increases the risk of severe skin reaction when given with topical fluorouracil. Severe Anecdotal → Also see TABLE 15 p. 1432 → Also see TABLE 5 p. 1430

Leflunomide is predicted to increase the exposure to **methotrexate**. Moderate Theoretical → Also see TABLE 1 p. 1429 → Also see TABLE 15 p. 1432

Live vaccines are predicted to increase the risk of generalised infection (possibly life-threatening) when given with **methotrexate** (high-dose). Public Health England advises avoid (refer to Green Book). Severe Theoretical

Nitisinone is predicted to increase the exposure to **methotrexate**. Moderate Study

Nitrous oxide potentially increases the risk of methotrexate toxicity when given with **methotrexate**. Avoid. Severe Study

NSAIDs are predicted to increase the risk of toxicity when given with **methotrexate**. Severe Study → Also see TABLE 2 p. 1429

Pegaspargase affects the efficacy of **methotrexate**. Severe Anecdotal → Also see TABLE 1 p. 1429 → Also see TABLE 15 p. 1432

Penicillins are predicted to increase the risk of toxicity when given with **methotrexate**. Severe Anecdotal → Also see TABLE 1 p. 1429

Potassium aminobenzoate increases the concentration of **methotrexate**. Moderate Theoretical

Proton pump inhibitors decrease the clearance of **methotrexate** (high-dose). Use with caution or avoid. Severe Study

Quinolones (ciprofloxacin) potentially increase the risk of toxicity when given with **methotrexate**. Severe Anecdotal

Regorafenib is predicted to increase the exposure to **methotrexate**. Moderate Theoretical → Also see TABLE 15 p. 1432

Retinoids (acitretin) are predicted to increase the concentration of **methotrexate**. Avoid. Moderate Anecdotal

Methotrexate is predicted to decrease the efficacy of sapropterin. Moderate Theoretical

Sulfonamides are predicted to increase the exposure to **methotrexate**. Use with caution or avoid. Severe Theoretical

Tedizolid is predicted to increase the exposure to **methotrexate**. Avoid. Moderate Theoretical

Methotrexate is predicted to increase the risk of toxicity when given with tegafur. Severe Theoretical → Also see TABLE 15 p. 1432

Teriflunomide is predicted to increase the exposure to **methotrexate**. Moderate Study → Also see TABLE 1 p. 1429

Methotrexate decreases the clearance of theophylline. Moderate Study

Trimethoprim increases the risk of adverse effects when given with **methotrexate**. Avoid. Severe Anecdotal → Also see TABLE 2 p. 1429

Methoxy polyethylene glycol-epoetin beta → see TABLE 5 p. 1430 (thromboembolism)

Methoxyflurane → see volatile halogenated anaesthetics

Methyldopa → see TABLE 8 p. 1430 (hypotension)

▸ Entacapone is predicted to increase the exposure to **methyldopa**. Moderate Theoretical

▸ Oral iron decreases the effects of oral **methyldopa**. Moderate Study

▸ **Methyldopa** increases the risk of neurotoxicity when given with lithium. Severe Anecdotal

▸ MAOIs, irreversible are predicted to alter the antihypertensive effects of **methyldopa**. Avoid. Severe Theoretical → Also see TABLE 8 p. 1430

Methylphenidate

▸ Antipsychotics, second generation (risperidone) increase the risk of dyskinesias when given with **methylphenidate**. Severe Anecdotal

▸ **Methylphenidate** increases the risk of dyskinesias when given with antipsychotics, second generation (paliperidone). Severe Theoretical

▸ **Methylphenidate** is predicted to decrease the effects of apraclonidine. Avoid. Severe Theoretical

▸ **Methylphenidate** is predicted to increase the risk of elevated blood pressure when given with linezolid. Avoid. Severe Theoretical

▸ MAO-B inhibitors (rasagiline, selegiline) are predicted to increase the risk of a hypertensive crisis when given with **methylphenidate**. Avoid. Severe Theoretical

▸ **Methylphenidate** is predicted to increase the risk of a hypertensive crisis when given with MAOIs, irreversible. Avoid and for 14 days after stopping the MAOI. Severe Theoretical

▸ **Methylphenidate** is predicted to increase the risk of a hypertensive crisis when given with moclobemide. Severe Theoretical

Methylprednisolone → see corticosteroids

Methylthioninium chloride → see TABLE 13 p. 1432 (serotonin syndrome)

▸ **Methylthioninium chloride** is predicted to increase the risk of severe hypertension when given with bupropion. Avoid. Severe Theoretical → Also see TABLE 13 p. 1432

Metoclopramide

▸ **Metoclopramide** is predicted to increase the risk of methaemoglobinaemia when given with topical anaesthetics, local (prilocaine). Avoid. Severe Theoretical

▸ **Metoclopramide** potentially decreases the absorption of antifungals, azoles (posaconazole) (oral suspension). Moderate Study

▸ **Metoclopramide** decreases the concentration of antimalarials (atovaquone). Avoid. Moderate Study

▸ **Metoclopramide** is predicted to decrease the effects of dopamine receptor agonists (apomorphine, bromocriptine, cabergoline, pramipexole, quinagolide, ropinirole, rotigotine). Avoid. Moderate Study

▸ **Metoclopramide** decreases the effects of levodopa. Avoid. Moderate Study

▸ **Metoclopramide** is predicted to increase the effects of neuromuscular blocking drugs, non-depolarising. Moderate Theoretical

▸ **Metoclopramide** increases the effects of suxamethonium. Moderate Study

Metolazone → see thiazide diuretics

Metoprolol → see beta blockers, selective

Metronidazole → see TABLE 12 p. 1432 (peripheral neuropathy)

ROUTE-SPECIFIC INFORMATION Since systemic absorption can follow topical application, the possibility of interactions should be borne in mind.

▸ Alcohol potentially causes a disulfiram-like reaction when given with **metronidazole**. Avoid for at least 48 hours stopping treatment. Moderate Study

▸ **Metronidazole** increases the risk of toxicity when given with alkylating agents (busulfan). Severe Study

▸ Antiepileptics (phenobarbital, primidone) are predicted to decrease the exposure to **metronidazole**. Moderate Study

▸ **Metronidazole** is predicted to increase the risk of capecitabine toxicity when given with capecitabine. Severe Theoretical

▸ **Metronidazole** increases the anticoagulant effect of coumarins. Monitor INR and adjust dose. Severe Study

▸ Disulfiram increases the risk of acute psychoses when given with **metronidazole**. Severe Study → Also see TABLE 12 p. 1432

▸ **Metronidazole** increases the risk of toxicity when given with fluorouracil. Severe Study

▸ **Metronidazole** is predicted to increase the concentration of lithium. Avoid or adjust dose. Severe Anecdotal

Metyrapone

▸ Antiepileptics (fosphenytoin, phenobarbital, phenytoin, primidone) are predicted to decrease the effects of **metyrapone**. Avoid. Moderate Study

▸ Antihistamines, sedating (cyproheptadine) decrease the effects of **metyrapone**. Avoid. Moderate Study

▸ Carbimazole decreases the effects of **metyrapone**. Avoid. Moderate Theoretical

▸ Combined hormonal contraceptives decrease the effects of **metyrapone**. Avoid. Moderate Theoretical

▸ Phenothiazines (chlorpromazine) decrease the effects of **metyrapone**. Avoid. Moderate Theoretical

▸ Propylthiouracil is predicted to decrease the effects of **metyrapone**. Avoid. Moderate Theoretical

Metyrapone (continued)

▸ Tricyclic antidepressants (**amitriptyline**) decrease the effects of **metyrapone**. Avoid. Moderate Theoretical

Mexiletine

FOOD AND LIFESTYLE Dose adjustment might be necessary if smoking started or stopped during treatment.

▸ **Mexiletine** is predicted to increase the exposure to agomelatine. Moderate Study

▸ **Mexiletine** is predicted to increase the exposure to aminophylline. Adjust dose. Moderate Theoretical

▸ **Mexiletine** is predicted to increase the exposure to anagrelide. Moderate Theoretical

▸ **Mexiletine** is predicted to increase the risk of torsade de pointes when given with antiarrhythmics. Avoid. Severe Theoretical

▸ Antiepileptics (**phenytoin**) are predicted to increase the clearance of **mexiletine**. Monitor and adjust dose. Moderate Study

▸ **Mexiletine** increases the concentration of antipsychotics, second generation (**clozapine**). Monitor adverse effects and adjust dose. Severe Study

▸ **Mexiletine** is predicted to increase the exposure to antipsychotics, second generation (**olanzapine**). Adjust dose. Moderate Anecdotal

▸ **Mexiletine** potentially increases the risk of cardiovascular adverse effects when given with beta blockers, non-selective. Avoid or monitor. Severe Theoretical

▸ **Mexiletine** potentially increases the risk of cardiovascular adverse effects when given with beta blockers, selective. Avoid or monitor. Severe Theoretical

▸ Bupropion is predicted to increase the exposure to **mexiletine**. Moderate Study

▸ **Mexiletine** increases the risk of cardiovascular adverse effects when given with calcium channel blockers (**diltiazem**). Avoid or monitor. Severe Theoretical

▸ **Mexiletine** potentially increases the risk of cardiovascular adverse effects when given with calcium channel blockers (**verapamil**). Avoid or monitor. Severe Theoretical

▸ Cinacalcet is predicted to increase the exposure to **mexiletine**. Moderate Study

▸ Cobicistat potentially increases the exposure to **mexiletine**. Severe Theoretical

▸ **Mexiletine** potentially affects the exposure to coumarins (**warfarin**). Avoid. Unknown Theoretical

▸ **Mexiletine** is predicted to increase the exposure to dopamine receptor agonists (**ropinirole**). Adjust dose. Moderate Study

▸ **Mexiletine** slightly increases the exposure to erlotinib. Monitor adverse effects and adjust dose. Moderate Study

▸ HIV-protease inhibitors (**ritonavir**) are predicted to increase the clearance of **mexiletine**. Monitor and adjust dose. Moderate Study

▸ Leflunomide is predicted to increase the clearance of **mexiletine**. Monitor and adjust dose. Moderate Study

▸ **Mexiletine** potentially affects the exposure to lithium. Avoid. Unknown Theoretical

▸ **Mexiletine** is predicted to increase the exposure to loxapine. Avoid. Unknown Theoretical

▸ **Mexiletine** slightly increases the exposure to MAO-B inhibitors (**rasagiline**). Moderate Study

▸ **Mexiletine** is predicted to increase the exposure to melatonin. Moderate Theoretical

▸ **Mexiletine** is predicted to affect the exposure to metformin. Unknown Theoretical

▸ Opioids potentially decrease the absorption of oral **mexiletine**. Moderate Study

▸ **Mexiletine** is predicted to increase the exposure to phenothiazines (**chlorpromazine**). Moderate Theoretical

▸ **Mexiletine** is predicted to increase the exposure to phosphodiesterase type-4 inhibitors (**roflumilast**). Moderate Theoretical

▸ **Mexiletine** is predicted to increase the exposure to pirfenidone. Use with caution and adjust dose. Moderate Study

▸ Rifamycins (**rifampicin**) are predicted to increase the clearance of **mexiletine**. Monitor and adjust dose. Moderate Study

▸ **Mexiletine** is predicted to increase the exposure to riluzole. Moderate Theoretical

▸ SSRIs (**fluoxetine, fluvoxamine, paroxetine**) are predicted to increase the exposure to **mexiletine**. Moderate Study

▸ Terbinafine is predicted to increase the exposure to **mexiletine**. Moderate Study

▸ Teriflunomide is predicted to increase the clearance of **mexiletine**. Monitor and adjust dose. Moderate Study

▸ **Mexiletine** is predicted to increase the exposure to theophylline. Monitor and adjust dose. Moderate Theoretical

▸ **Mexiletine** increases the exposure to tizanidine. Avoid. Moderate Study

▸ **Mexiletine** is predicted to increase the exposure to triptans (**zolmitriptan**). Adjust **zolmitriptan** dose, p. 503. Moderate Theoretical

Mianserin → see TABLE 11 p. 1431 (CNS depressant effects)

▸ Antiepileptics (**carbamazepine**) markedly decrease the exposure to **mianserin**. Adjust dose. Moderate Study

▸ Antiepileptics (**phenobarbital, primidone**) are predicted to decrease the exposure to **mianserin**. Moderate Study → Also see TABLE 11 p. 1431

▸ **Mianserin** is predicted to increase the risk of toxicity when given with MAOIs, irreversible. Avoid and for 14 days after stopping the MAOI. Severe Theoretical

▸ **Mianserin** is predicted to increase the risk of toxicity when given with moclobemide. Avoid and for 1 week after stopping **mianserin**. Severe Theoretical

▸ **Mianserin** is predicted to decrease the efficacy of pitolisant. Moderate Theoretical

▸ **Mianserin** decreases the effects of sympathomimetics, vasoconstrictor (**ephedrine**). Severe Anecdotal

Micafungin → see TABLE 1 p. 1429 (hepatotoxicity)

▸ **Micafungin** slightly increases the exposure to amphotericin B. Avoid or monitor toxicity. Moderate Study

Miconazole → see antifungals, azoles

Midazolam → see benzodiazepines

Midodrine → see sympathomimetics, vasoconstrictor

Midostaurin

▸ Anti-androgens (**apalutamide, enzalutamide**) are predicted to decrease the exposure to **midostaurin**. Avoid. Severe Study

▸ Antiarrhythmics (**dronedarone**) are predicted to increase the exposure to **midostaurin**. Moderate Study

▸ Antiepileptics (**carbamazepine, fosphenytoin, phenobarbital, phenytoin, primidone**) are predicted to decrease the exposure to **midostaurin**. Avoid. Severe Study

▸ Antifungals, azoles (**fluconazole, isavuconazole, posaconazole**) are predicted to increase the exposure to **midostaurin**. Moderate Theoretical

▸ Antifungals, azoles (**itraconazole, ketoconazole, voriconazole**) are predicted to very markedly increase the exposure to **midostaurin**. Avoid or monitor for toxicity. Severe Study

▸ Calcium channel blockers (**diltiazem, verapamil**) are predicted to increase the exposure to **midostaurin**. Moderate Theoretical

▸ Cobicistat is predicted to very markedly increase the exposure to **midostaurin**. Avoid or monitor for toxicity. Severe Study

▸ Crizotinib is predicted to increase the exposure to **midostaurin**. Moderate Theoretical

▸ HIV-protease inhibitors are predicted to very markedly increase the exposure to **midostaurin**. Avoid or monitor for toxicity. Severe Study

▸ Idelalisib is predicted to very markedly increase the exposure to **midostaurin**. Avoid or monitor for toxicity. Severe Study

▸ Imatinib is predicted to increase the exposure to **midostaurin**. Moderate Theoretical

▸ Letermovir is predicted to increase the exposure to **midostaurin**. Moderate Theoretical

▸ Macrolides (**clarithromycin**) are predicted to very markedly increase the exposure to **midostaurin**. Avoid or monitor for toxicity. Severe Study

▸ Macrolides (**erythromycin**) are predicted to increase the exposure to **midostaurin**. Moderate Theoretical

▸ Mitotane is predicted to decrease the exposure to **midostaurin**. Avoid. Severe Study

Neurokinin-1 receptor antagonists (aprepitant, netupitant) are predicted to increase the exposure to **midostaurin**. Moderate Theoretical

Nilotinib is predicted to increase the exposure to **midostaurin**. Moderate Theoretical

Rifamycins (rifampicin) are predicted to decrease the exposure to **midostaurin**. Avoid. Severe Study

St John's wort is predicted to decrease the exposure to **midostaurin**. Avoid. Severe Theoretical

Mifamurtide → see TABLE 15 p. 1432 (myelosuppression)

Ciclosporin is predicted to decrease the efficacy of **mifamurtide**. Avoid. Severe Theoretical

Corticosteroids are predicted to decrease the efficacy of **mifamurtide**. Avoid. Severe Theoretical

NSAIDs (high-dose) are predicted to decrease the efficacy of **mifamurtide**. Avoid. Severe Theoretical

Pimecrolimus is predicted to decrease the efficacy of **mifamurtide**. Avoid. Severe Theoretical

Sirolimus is predicted to decrease the efficacy of **mifamurtide**. Avoid. Severe Theoretical

Tacrolimus is predicted to affect the efficacy of **mifamurtide**. Avoid. Severe Theoretical

Mifepristone

Mifepristone is predicted to decrease the efficacy of corticosteroids. Use with caution and adjust dose. Moderate Theoretical

Minocycline → see tetracyclines

Minoxidil → see TABLE 8 p. 1430 (hypotension)

ROUTE-SPECIFIC INFORMATION   Since systemic absorption can follow topical application, the possibility of interactions should be borne in mind.

Mirabegron

▸ **Mirabegron** is predicted to increase the exposure to aliskiren. Mild Theoretical

▸ Antifungals, azoles (itraconazole, ketoconazole, voriconazole) are predicted to increase the exposure to **mirabegron**. Adjust **mirabegron** dose in hepatic and renal impairment, p. 825. Moderate Study

▸ **Mirabegron** is predicted to increase the exposure to antihistamines, non-sedating (fexofenadine). Mild Theoretical

▸ **Mirabegron** is predicted to increase the exposure to beta blockers, selective (metoprolol). Moderate Study

▸ Cobicistat is predicted to increase the exposure to **mirabegron**. Adjust **mirabegron** dose in hepatic and renal impairment, p. 825. Moderate Study

▸ **Mirabegron** is predicted to increase the exposure to colchicine. Mild Theoretical

▸ **Mirabegron** slightly increases the exposure to digoxin. Monitor concentration and adjust dose. Severe Study

▸ **Mirabegron** is predicted to increase the exposure to eliglustat. Avoid or adjust dose—consult product literature. Severe Study

▸ **Mirabegron** is predicted to increase the exposure to everolimus. Mild Theoretical

▸ **Mirabegron** is predicted to increase the exposure to factor XA inhibitors (edoxaban). Mild Theoretical

▸ HIV-protease inhibitors are predicted to increase the exposure to **mirabegron**. Adjust **mirabegron** dose in hepatic and renal impairment, p. 825. Moderate Study

▸ Idelalisib is predicted to increase the exposure to **mirabegron**. Adjust **mirabegron** dose in hepatic and renal impairment, p. 825. Moderate Study

▸ **Mirabegron** is predicted to increase the exposure to loperamide. Mild Theoretical

▸ Macrolides (clarithromycin) are predicted to increase the exposure to **mirabegron**. Adjust **mirabegron** dose in hepatic and renal impairment, p. 825. Moderate Study

▸ **Mirabegron** is predicted to increase the exposure to sirolimus. Mild Theoretical

▸ **Mirabegron** is predicted to increase the exposure to taxanes (paclitaxel). Mild Theoretical

▸ **Mirabegron** is predicted to increase the exposure to thrombin inhibitors (dabigatran). Severe Theoretical

▸ **Mirabegron** is predicted to increase the exposure to topotecan. Mild Theoretical

Mirtazapine → see TABLE 13 p. 1432 (serotonin syndrome), TABLE 11 p. 1431 (CNS depressant effects)

▸ Anti-androgens (apalutamide, enzalutamide) are predicted to decrease the exposure to **mirtazapine**. Adjust dose. Moderate Study

▸ Antiepileptics (carbamazepine, fosphenytoin, phenobarbital, phenytoin, primidone) are predicted to decrease the exposure to **mirtazapine**. Adjust dose. Moderate Study → Also see TABLE 11 p. 1431

▸ Antifungals, azoles (itraconazole, ketoconazole, voriconazole) are predicted to increase the exposure to **mirtazapine**. Moderate Study

▸ Cobicistat is predicted to increase the exposure to **mirtazapine**. Moderate Study

▸ H₂ receptor antagonists (cimetidine) slightly increase the exposure to **mirtazapine**. Use with caution and adjust dose. Moderate Theoretical

▸ HIV-protease inhibitors are predicted to increase the exposure to **mirtazapine**. Moderate Study

▸ Idelalisib is predicted to increase the exposure to **mirtazapine**. Moderate Study

▸ Macrolides (clarithromycin) are predicted to increase the exposure to **mirtazapine**. Moderate Study

▸ Mirtazapine is predicted to increase the exposure to **mirtazapine**. Adjust dose. Moderate Study

▸ **Mirtazapine** is predicted to decrease the efficacy of pitolisant. Moderate Theoretical

▸ Rifamycins (rifampicin) are predicted to decrease the exposure to **mirtazapine**. Adjust dose. Moderate Study

Mitomycin → see TABLE 15 p. 1432 (myelosuppression), TABLE 5 p. 1430 (thromboembolism)

▸ Live vaccines are predicted to increase the risk of generalised infection (possibly life-threatening) when given with **mitomycin**. Public Health England advises avoid (refer to Green Book). Severe Theoretical

Mitotane → see TABLE 15 p. 1432 (myelosuppression)

▸ **Mitotane** is predicted to decrease the exposure to 5-HT3-receptor antagonists (ondansetron). Moderate Study

▸ **Mitotane** is predicted to markedly decrease the exposure to abemaciclib. Avoid. Severe Study

▸ **Mitotane** is predicted to decrease the exposure to acalabrutinib. Avoid. Severe Study

▸ Aldosterone antagonists (spironolactone) are predicted to decrease the effects of **mitotane**. Avoid. Severe Anecdotal

▸ **Mitotane** is predicted to decrease the exposure to aldosterone antagonists (eplerenone). Avoid. Moderate Theoretical

▸ **Mitotane** is predicted to decrease the exposure to anti-androgens (abiraterone). Avoid. Severe Study

▸ **Mitotane** is predicted to decrease the exposure to anti-androgens (darolutamide). Avoid. Moderate Study

▸ **Mitotane** is predicted to decrease the exposure to antiarrhythmics (disopyramide, dronedarone). Avoid. Severe Study

▸ **Mitotane** is predicted to decrease the efficacy of antiarrhythmics (propafenone). Moderate Study

▸ **Mitotane** is predicted to decrease the exposure to anticholinesterases, centrally acting (donepezil). Mild Study

▸ **Mitotane** is predicted to decrease the exposure to antiepileptics (perampanel). Monitor and adjust dose. Moderate Study

▸ **Mitotane** is predicted to decrease the exposure to antifungals, azoles (isavuconazole). Avoid. Severe Study

▸ **Mitotane** is predicted to decrease the exposure to antimalarials (artemether with lumefantrine). Avoid. Severe Study

▸ **Mitotane** is predicted to decrease the concentration of antimalarials (piperaquine). Avoid. Moderate Theoretical

▸ **Mitotane** is predicted to moderately decrease the exposure to antipsychotics, second generation (aripiprazole). Adjust **aripiprazole** dose, p. 415. Moderate Study

▸ **Mitotane** is predicted to decrease the exposure to antipsychotics, second generation (cariprazine). Avoid. Severe Theoretical

▸ **Mitotane** is predicted to decrease the exposure to antipsychotics, second generation (lurasidone). Avoid. Moderate Study

Mitotane (continued)

▶ **Mitotane** is predicted to decrease the exposure to antipsychotics, second generation (paliperidone). Monitor and adjust dose. Severe Study

▶ **Mitotane** is predicted to decrease the exposure to antipsychotics, second generation (quetiapine). Moderate Study

▶ **Mitotane** is predicted to decrease the exposure to antipsychotics, second generation (risperidone). Adjust dose. Moderate Study

▶ **Mitotane** is predicted to decrease the exposure to avapritinib. Avoid. Severe Study

▶ **Mitotane** is predicted to decrease the exposure to axitinib. Avoid or adjust dose. Moderate Study → Also see TABLE 15 p. 1432

▶ **Mitotane** decreases the exposure to bedaquiline. Avoid. Severe Study

▶ **Mitotane** is predicted to decrease the exposure to benzodiazepines (alprazolam). Adjust dose. Moderate Theoretical

▶ **Mitotane** is predicted to decrease the exposure to benzodiazepines (midazolam). Monitor and adjust dose. Moderate Study

▶ **Mitotane** is predicted to decrease the exposure to bictegravir. Avoid. Moderate Study

▶ **Mitotane** slightly decreases the exposure to bortezomib. Avoid. Severe Study → Also see TABLE 15 p. 1432

▶ **Mitotane** is predicted to very markedly decrease the exposure to bosutinib. Avoid. Severe Study → Also see TABLE 15 p. 1432

▶ **Mitotane** is predicted to decrease the exposure to brigatinib. Avoid. Severe Study

▶ **Mitotane** is predicted to decrease the exposure to buspirone. Use with caution and adjust dose. Severe Study

▶ **Mitotane** moderately decreases the exposure to cabozantinib. Avoid. Moderate Study → Also see TABLE 15 p. 1432

▶ **Mitotane** is predicted to decrease the exposure to calcium channel blockers (amlodipine, felodipine, lacidipine, lercanidipine, nicardipine, nifedipine, nimodipine). Monitor and adjust dose. Moderate Study

▶ **Mitotane** is predicted to decrease the exposure to calcium channel blockers (diltiazem). Severe Study

▶ **Mitotane** is predicted to decrease the exposure to cannabidiol. Adjust dose. Moderate Study

▶ **Mitotane** is predicted to decrease the exposure to ceritinib. Avoid. Severe Study → Also see TABLE 15 p. 1432

▶ **Mitotane** decreases the concentration of ciclosporin. Severe Study

▶ **Mitotane** is predicted to alter the effects of cilostazol. Moderate Theoretical

▶ **Mitotane** is predicted to decrease the exposure to cinacalcet. Monitor and adjust dose. Moderate Study

▶ **Mitotane** decreases the exposure to clomethiazole. Monitor and adjust dose. Moderate Study

▶ **Mitotane** is predicted to decrease the exposure to cobicistat. Avoid. Severe Theoretical

▶ **Mitotane** is predicted to decrease the exposure to cobimetinib. Avoid. Severe Theoretical

▶ **Mitotane** is predicted to decrease the exposure to corticosteroids (budesonide, deflazacort, dexamethasone, fludrocortisone, hydrocortisone, methylprednisolone, prednisolone, triamcinolone). Monitor and adjust dose. Moderate Study

▶ **Mitotane** is predicted to decrease the exposure to corticosteroids (fluticasone). Unknown Theoretical

▶ **Mitotane** is predicted to markedly decrease the exposure to crizotinib. Avoid. Severe Study

▶ **Mitotane** is predicted to decrease the exposure to dabrafenib. Avoid. Moderate Theoretical

▶ **Mitotane** is predicted to decrease the exposure to darifenacin. Moderate Theoretical

▶ **Mitotane** is predicted to decrease the exposure to dasabuvir. Avoid. Severe Theoretical

▶ **Mitotane** is predicted to markedly decrease the exposure to dasatinib. Avoid. Severe Study → Also see TABLE 15 p. 1432

▶ **Mitotane** is predicted to slightly decrease the exposure to delamanid. Avoid. Moderate Study

▶ **Mitotane** is predicted to markedly decrease the exposure to dienogest. Severe Study

▶ **Mitotane** is predicted to decrease the exposure to dipeptidylpeptidase-4 inhibitors (linagliptin). Moderate Study

▶ **Mitotane** is predicted to moderately decrease the exposure to dipeptidylpeptidase-4 inhibitors (saxagliptin). Moderate Study

▶ **Mitotane** decreases the exposure to dolutegravir. Adjust dose. Severe Study

▶ **Mitotane** is predicted to decrease the exposure to dronabinol. Avoid or adjust dose. Mild Study

▶ **Mitotane** is predicted to decrease the exposure to elbasvir. Avoid. Severe Study

▶ **Mitotane** is predicted to decreases the exposure to elexacaftor. Avoid. Severe Theoretical

▶ **Mitotane** is predicted to decrease the exposure to eliglustat. Avoid. Severe Study

▶ **Mitotane** is predicted to decrease the concentration of elvitegravir. Avoid. Severe Theoretical

▶ **Mitotane** is predicted to decrease the exposure to encorafenib. Severe Theoretical

▶ **Mitotane** affects the exposure to endothelin receptor antagonists (bosentan). Avoid. Severe Study

▶ **Mitotane** is predicted to decrease the exposure to endothelin receptor antagonists (macitentan). Avoid. Severe Study

▶ **Mitotane** is predicted to decrease the exposure to entrectinib. Avoid. Severe Study

▶ **Mitotane** is predicted to decrease the effects of ergotamine. Moderate Theoretical

▶ **Mitotane** is predicted to decrease the exposure to erlotinib. Avoid or adjust erlotinib dose, p. 1024. Severe Study

▶ **Mitotane** is predicted to decrease the exposure to esketamine. Adjust dose. Moderate Theoretical

▶ **Mitotane** is predicted to decrease the concentration of everolimus. Avoid or adjust dose. Severe Study

▶ **Mitotane** moderately decreases the exposure to exemestane. Moderate Study

▶ **Mitotane** is predicted to moderately decrease the exposure to factor XA inhibitors (apixaban). Use with caution or avoid. Severe Study

▶ **Mitotane** is predicted to moderately decrease the exposure to factor XA inhibitors (rivaroxaban). Avoid unless patient can be monitored for signs of thrombosis. Severe Study

▶ **Mitotane** is predicted to decrease the exposure to fesoterodine. Avoid. Moderate Study

▶ **Mitotane** is predicted to decrease the exposure to fingolimod. Moderate Study

▶ **Mitotane** is predicted to decrease the exposure to fostamatinib. Avoid. Severe Study

▶ **Mitotane** is predicted to decrease the exposure to gefitinib. Avoid. Severe Study

▶ **Mitotane** is predicted to moderately decrease the exposure to glasdegib. Avoid. Severe Study

▶ **Mitotane** is predicted to greatly decrease the concentration of glecaprevir. Avoid. Severe Study

▶ **Mitotane** is predicted to decrease the exposure to grazoprevir. Avoid. Severe Study

▶ **Mitotane** is predicted to decrease the concentration of guanfacine. Adjust guanfacine dose, p. 372. Moderate Study

▶ **Mitotane** decreases the concentration of haloperidol. Adjust dose. Moderate Study

▶ **Mitotane** is predicted to decrease the exposure to ibrutinib. Avoid or adjust ibrutinib dose, p. 1027. Severe Study → Also see TABLE 15 p. 1432

▶ **Mitotane** is predicted to decrease the exposure to idelalisib. Avoid. Severe Study

▶ **Mitotane** is predicted to decrease the exposure to imatinib. Avoid. Moderate Study → Also see TABLE 15 p. 1432

▶ **Mitotane** is predicted to decrease the exposure to irinotecan. Avoid. Severe Study → Also see TABLE 15 p. 1432

▶ **Mitotane** is predicted to decrease the exposure to ivabradine. Adjust dose. Moderate Theoretical

▶ **Mitotane** is predicted to moderately to markedly decrease the exposure to ivacaftor. Avoid. Severe Study

▶ **Mitotane** is predicted to decrease the exposure to ixazomib. Avoid. Severe Study

▶ **Mitotane** is predicted to decrease the exposure to lapatinib. Avoid. Severe Study

Mitotane is predicted to moderately decrease the exposure to larotrectinib. Avoid. Moderate Study

Mitotane is predicted to decrease the exposure to lomitapide. Monitor and adjust dose. Moderate Theoretical

Mitotane is predicted to decrease the exposure to lorlatinib. Avoid. Severe Study

Mitotane is predicted to decrease the exposure to maraviroc. Adjust dose. Severe Study

Mitotane is predicted to slightly decrease the exposure to meglitinides (nateglinide). Mild Study

Mitotane is predicted to decrease the exposure to meglitinides (repaglinide). Monitor blood glucose and adjust dose. Moderate Study

Mitotane is predicted to decrease the exposure to midostaurin. Avoid. Severe Study

Mitotane is predicted to decrease the exposure to mirtazapine. Adjust dose. Moderate Study

Mitotane is predicted to decrease the exposure to monoclonal antibodies (polatuzumab vedotin). Moderate Theoretical

Mitotane is predicted to decrease the exposure to montelukast. Mild Study

Mitotane is predicted to markedly decrease the exposure to naldemedine. Avoid. Severe Study

Mitotane is predicted to markedly decrease the exposure to naloxegol. Avoid. Moderate Study

Mitotane is predicted to decrease the exposure to neratinib. Avoid. Severe Study

Mitotane is predicted to markedly decrease the exposure to neurokinin-1 receptor antagonists (aprepitant). Avoid. Moderate Study

Mitotane is predicted to decrease the exposure to neurokinin-1 receptor antagonists (fosaprepitant). Avoid. Moderate Theoretical

Mitotane is predicted to decrease the exposure to neurokinin-1 receptor antagonists (netupitant). Avoid. Severe Study

Mitotane is predicted to moderately decrease the exposure to nilotinib. Avoid. Severe Study → Also see TABLE 15 p. 1432

Mitotane is predicted to decrease the exposure to nitisinone. Adjust dose. Moderate Theoretical

Mitotane is predicted to decrease the exposure to NNRTIs (doravirine). Avoid. Severe Study

Mitotane is predicted to decrease the exposure to NNRTIs (etravirine). Avoid. Severe Theoretical

Mitotane is predicted to decrease the exposure to NNRTIs (nevirapine). Avoid. Severe Theoretical

Mitotane markedly decreases the exposure to NNRTIs (rilpivirine). Avoid. Severe Study

Mitotane is predicted to decrease the exposure to olaparib. Avoid. Moderate Theoretical → Also see TABLE 15 p. 1432

Mitotane is predicted to decrease the exposure to ombitasvir. Avoid. Severe Theoretical

Mitotane is predicted to decrease the exposure to opioids (alfentanil, fentanyl). Moderate Study

Mitotane is predicted to decrease the exposure to opioids (buprenorphine). Monitor and adjust dose. Moderate Theoretical

Mitotane decreases the exposure to opioids (methadone). Monitor and adjust dose. Severe Study

Mitotane is predicted to decrease the exposure to opioids (oxycodone). Monitor and adjust dose. Moderate Study

Mitotane is predicted to moderately decrease the exposure to osimertinib. Avoid. Moderate Study

Mitotane is predicted to moderately decrease the exposure to ospemifene. Moderate Study

Mitotane is predicted to decrease the exposure to palbociclib. Avoid. Severe Study → Also see TABLE 15 p. 1432

Mitotane is predicted to decrease the exposure to panobinostat. Avoid. Moderate Theoretical → Also see TABLE 15 p. 1432

Mitotane is predicted to decrease the exposure to paritaprevir (with ritonavir and ombitasvir). Avoid. Severe Study

Mitotane is predicted to decrease the exposure to pazopanib. Avoid. Severe Theoretical

Mitotane moderately decreases the exposure to phosphodiesterase type-4 inhibitors (apremilast). Avoid. Severe Study

Mitotane is predicted to decrease the exposure to phosphodiesterase type-4 inhibitors (roflumilast). Avoid. Moderate Study

Mitotane is predicted to decrease the exposure to phosphodiesterase type-5 inhibitors (avanafil, tadalafil). Avoid. Severe Study

Mitotane is predicted to decrease the exposure to phosphodiesterase type-5 inhibitors (sildenafil, vardenafil). Moderate Theoretical

Mitotane is predicted to moderately to markedly decrease the exposure to pibrentasvir. Avoid. Severe Study

Mitotane is predicted to moderately decrease the exposure to pitolisant. Moderate Study

Mitotane is predicted to decrease the exposure to ponatinib. Avoid. Moderate Theoretical

Mitotane is predicted to markedly decrease the exposure to praziquantel. Avoid. Moderate Study

Mitotane is predicted to decrease the exposure to ranolazine. Avoid. Severe Study

Mitotane is predicted to decrease the exposure to reboxetine. Moderate Anecdotal

Mitotane is predicted to decrease the exposure to regorafenib. Avoid. Moderate Study → Also see TABLE 15 p. 1432

Mitotane potentially decreases the exposure to remdesivir. Avoid. Moderate Theoretical

Mitotane is predicted to markedly decrease the exposure to ribociclib. Avoid. Severe Study → Also see TABLE 15 p. 1432

Mitotane is predicted to decrease the exposure to ruxolitinib. Monitor and adjust dose. Moderate Study → Also see TABLE 15 p. 1432

Mitotane is predicted to decrease the exposure to siponimod. Severe Study

Mitotane is predicted to decrease the concentration of sirolimus. Avoid. Severe Study

Mitotane is predicted to decrease the exposure to solifenacin. Moderate Theoretical

Mitotane is predicted to decrease the exposure to sorafenib. Moderate Theoretical → Also see TABLE 15 p. 1432

Mitotane is predicted to decrease the exposure to statins (simvastatin). Severe Study

Mitotane is predicted to decrease the exposure to sunitinib. Avoid or adjust **sunitinib** dose, p. 1044. Moderate Study → Also see TABLE 15 p. 1432

Mitotane decreases the concentration of tacrolimus. Monitor and adjust dose. Severe Study

Mitotane is predicted to decrease the exposure to taxanes (cabazitaxel, paclitaxel). Avoid. Severe Study → Also see TABLE 15 p. 1432

Mitotane is predicted to decrease the exposure to taxanes (docetaxel). Severe Theoretical → Also see TABLE 15 p. 1432

Mitotane is predicted to decrease the concentration of temsirolimus. Avoid. Severe Study → Also see TABLE 15 p. 1432

Mitotane decreases the exposure to tetracyclines (doxycycline). Monitor and adjust dose. Moderate Study

Mitotane is predicted to decrease the exposure to tezacaftor. Avoid. Severe Theoretical

Mitotane is predicted to markedly decrease the exposure to ticagrelor. Avoid. Severe Study

Mitotane is predicted to decrease the exposure to tivozanib. Severe Study

Mitotane is predicted to decrease the exposure to tofacitinib. Avoid. Severe Study

Mitotane is predicted to decrease the exposure to tolvaptan. Use with caution or avoid depending on indication. Severe Study

Mitotane is predicted to decrease the exposure to toremifene. Adjust dose. Moderate Study

Mitotane is predicted to decrease the exposure to trabectedin. Avoid. Severe Theoretical → Also see TABLE 15 p. 1432

Mitotane is predicted to decrease the exposure to upadacitinib. Moderate Study

Mitotane is predicted to decrease the exposure to vandetanib. Avoid. Moderate Study

Mitotane is predicted to moderately decrease the exposure to velpatasvir. Avoid. Severe Study

Mitotane (continued)

▶ **Mitotane** is predicted to decrease the exposure to vemurafenib. Avoid. [Severe] Theoretical

▶ **Mitotane** is predicted to decrease the exposure to venetoclax. Avoid. [Severe] Study

▶ **Mitotane** is predicted to decrease the exposure to vinca alkaloids (vinblastine, vincristine, vindesine). [Severe] Theoretical → Also see TABLE 15 p. 1432

▶ **Mitotane** is predicted to decrease the exposure to vinca alkaloids (vinflunine). Avoid. [Severe] Theoretical → Also see TABLE 15 p. 1432

▶ **Mitotane** is predicted to decrease the exposure to vinca alkaloids (vinorelbine). Use with caution or avoid. [Severe] Theoretical → Also see TABLE 15 p. 1432

▶ **Mitotane** is predicted to decrease the exposure to vismodegib. Avoid. [Moderate] Theoretical

▶ **Mitotane** is predicted to decrease the exposure to vortioxetine. Monitor and adjust dose. [Moderate] Study

▶ **Mitotane** is predicted to decrease the concentration of voxilaprevir. Avoid. [Severe] Study

▶ **Mitotane** is predicted to decrease the exposure to zopiclone. Adjust dose. [Moderate] Study

Mitoxantrone → see anthracyclines

Mivacurium → see neuromuscular blocking drugs, non-depolarising

Mizolastine → see antihistamines, non-sedating

Moclobemide → see TABLE 13 p. 1432 (serotonin syndrome)

FOOD AND LIFESTYLE Moclobemide is claimed to cause less potentiation of the pressor effect of tyramine than the traditional (irreversible) MAOIs, but patients should avoid consuming large amounts of tyramine-rich foods (such as mature cheese, salami, pickled herring, *Bovril*®, *Oxo*®, *Marmite*® or any similar meat or yeast extract or fermented soya bean extract, and some beers, lagers or wines).

▶ Amfetamines are predicted to increase the risk of a hypertensive crisis when given with **moclobemide**. Avoid. [Severe] Theoretical → Also see TABLE 13 p. 1432

▶ Anti-androgens (apalutamide) are predicted to decrease the exposure to **moclobemide**. Avoid or monitor. [Mild] Study

▶ **Moclobemide** potentially increases the exposure to benzodiazepines (clobazam). Adjust dose. [Moderate] Theoretical

▶ Bupropion is predicted to increase the risk of severe hypertension when given with **moclobemide**. Avoid. [Severe] Theoretical → Also see TABLE 13 p. 1432

▶ **Moclobemide** is predicted to increase the exposure to cannabidiol. [Moderate] Theoretical

▶ **Moclobemide** is predicted to increase the exposure to cilostazol. [Moderate] Theoretical

▶ **Moclobemide** is predicted to decrease the efficacy of clopidogrel. Avoid. [Moderate] Study

▶ **Moclobemide** is predicted to increase the exposure to eliglustat. Avoid or adjust dose—consult product literature. [Severe] Theoretical

▶ H₂ receptor antagonists (cimetidine) increase the exposure to **moclobemide**. Adjust **moclobemide** dose, p. 382. [Mild] Study

▶ Levodopa increases the risk of adverse effects when given with **moclobemide**. [Moderate] Study

▶ **Moclobemide** is predicted to increase the risk of adverse effects when given with linezolid. Avoid and for 14 days after stopping **moclobemide**. [Severe] Theoretical → Also see TABLE 13 p. 1432

▶ **Moclobemide** is predicted to increase the effects of MAO-B inhibitors (rasagiline, selegiline). Avoid. [Severe] Theoretical → Also see TABLE 13 p. 1432

▶ **Moclobemide** is predicted to increase the risk of adverse effects when given with MAO-B inhibitors (safinamide). Avoid and for 1 week after stopping safinamide. [Severe] Theoretical → Also see TABLE 13 p. 1432

▶ Methylphenidate is predicted to increase the risk of a hypertensive crisis when given with **moclobemide**. [Severe] Theoretical

▶ Mianserin is predicted to increase the risk of toxicity when given with **moclobemide**. Avoid and for 1 week after stopping mianserin. [Severe] Theoretical

▶ Opicapone is predicted to increase the risk of elevated blood pressure when given with **moclobemide**. Avoid. [Severe] Theoretical

▶ Ozanimod potentially increases the risk of a hypertensive crisis when given with **moclobemide**. Avoid. [Severe] Theoretical

▶ **Moclobemide** increases the risk of adverse effects when given with phenothiazines (levomepromazine). [Moderate] Study

▶ Reboxetine is predicted to increase the risk of a hypertensive crisis when given with **moclobemide**. Avoid. [Severe] Theoretical

▶ Sympathomimetics, vasoconstrictor (ephedrine, isometheptene, phenylephrine, pseudoephedrine) are predicted to increase the risk of a hypertensive crisis when given with **moclobemide**. Avoid. [Severe] Study

▶ Tetrabenazine potentially increases the risk of CNS excitation and hypertension when given with **moclobemide**. [Severe] Theoretical

▶ Tricyclic antidepressants are predicted to increase the risk of severe toxic reaction when given with **moclobemide**. Avoid. [Severe] Theoretical → Also see TABLE 13 p. 1432

▶ **Moclobemide** moderately increases the exposure to triptans (rizatriptan, sumatriptan). Avoid. [Moderate] Study → Also see TABLE 13 p. 1432

▶ **Moclobemide** slightly increases the exposure to triptans (zolmitriptan). Adjust zolmitriptan dose, p. 503. [Moderate] Study → Also see TABLE 13 p. 1432

Modafinil

▶ Antiepileptics (carbamazepine, phenobarbital, primidone) are predicted to decrease the exposure to **modafinil**. [Mild] Theoretical

▶ Antiepileptics (fosphenytoin, phenytoin) are predicted to decrease the exposure to **modafinil** and **modafinil** is predicted to increase the concentration of antiepileptics (fosphenytoin, phenytoin). Monitor concentration and adjust dose. [Moderate] Theoretical

▶ Antifungals, azoles (itraconazole, ketoconazole, voriconazole) are predicted to increase the exposure to **modafinil**. [Mild] Theoretical

▶ **Modafinil** is predicted to decrease the exposure to bosutinib. Avoid. [Severe] Theoretical

▶ Cobicistat is predicted to increase the exposure to **modafinil**. [Mild] Theoretical

▶ **Modafinil** is predicted to decrease the efficacy of combined hormonal contraceptives. For FSRH guidance, see Contraceptives, interactions p. 840. [Severe] Study

▶ **Modafinil** is predicted to decrease the efficacy of desogestrel. For FSRH guidance, see Contraceptives, interactions p. 840. [Severe] Theoretical

▶ **Modafinil** is predicted to decrease the exposure to elbasvir. Avoid. [Unknown] Theoretical

▶ **Modafinil** is predicted to decrease the efficacy of etonogestrel. For FSRH guidance, see Contraceptives, interactions p. 840. [Severe] Theoretical

▶ **Modafinil** is predicted to decrease the exposure to glasdegib. Avoid or adjust glasdegib dose, p. 1049. [Moderate] Theoretical

▶ **Modafinil** is predicted to decrease the exposure to grazoprevir. Avoid. [Severe] Theoretical

▶ HIV-protease inhibitors are predicted to increase the exposure to **modafinil**. [Mild] Theoretical

▶ **Modafinil** is predicted to decrease the effects of hormone replacement therapy. [Moderate] Anecdotal

▶ Idelalisib is predicted to increase the exposure to **modafinil**. [Mild] Theoretical

▶ **Modafinil** is predicted to decrease the concentration of letermovir. [Moderate] Theoretical

▶ **Modafinil** is predicted to decrease the efficacy of levonorgestrel. For FSRH guidance, see Contraceptives, interactions p. 840. [Severe] Theoretical

▶ Macrolides (clarithromycin) are predicted to increase the exposure to **modafinil**. [Mild] Theoretical

▶ **Modafinil** is predicted to decrease the exposure to NNRTIs (doravirine). Avoid or adjust doravirine p. 683 or lamivudine with tenofovir disoproxil and doravirine p. 692 dose. [Severe] Theoretical

▶ **Modafinil** is predicted to decrease the efficacy of norethisterone. For FSRH guidance, see Contraceptives, interactions p. 840. [Severe] Anecdotal

Rifamycins (rifampicin) are predicted to decrease the exposure to **modafinil**. [Moderate] Theoretical

Modafinil is predicted to decrease the exposure to sofosbuvir. Avoid. [Severe] Theoretical

Modafinil decreases the efficacy of ulipristal. For FSRH guidance, see Contraceptives, interactions p. 840. [Severe] Anecdotal

Modafinil is predicted to decrease the exposure to velpatasvir. Avoid. [Severe] Theoretical

Modafinil is predicted to decrease the concentration of voxilaprevir. Avoid. [Severe] Theoretical

Mogamulizumab → see monoclonal antibodies

Mometasone → see corticosteroids

Monoclonal antibodies → see TABLE 15 p. 1432 (myelosuppression), TABLE 12 p. 1432 (peripheral neuropathy), TABLE 5 p. 1430 (thromboembolism), TABLE 9 p. 1431 (QT-interval prolongation), TABLE 4 p. 1429 (antiplatelet effects)

adalimumab · alemtuzumab · atezolizumab · avelumab · basiliximab · belimumab · bevacizumab · blinatumomab · brentuximab vedotin · brodalumab · canakinumab · cemiplimab · certolizumab pegol · cetuximab · daratumumab · dinutuximab · dupilumab · durvalumab · eculizumab · elotuzumab · golimumab · guselkumab · infliximab · inotuzumab ozogamicin · ipilimumab · ixekizumab · mogamulizumab · natalizumab · necitumumab · nivolumab · obinutuzumab · ocrelizumab · panitumumab · pembrolizumab · pertuzumab · polatuzumab vedotin · ramucirumab · risankizumab · rituximab · sarilumab · secukinumab · siltuximab · tildrakizumab · tocilizumab · trastuzumab · trastuzumab emtansine · ustekinumab · vedolizumab

▸ **Abatacept** is predicted to increase the risk of generalised infection (possibly life-threatening) when given with **golimumab**. Avoid. [Severe] Theoretical

▸ **Blinatumomab** is predicted to transiently increase the exposure to aminophylline. Monitor and adjust dose. [Moderate] Theoretical

▸ **Sarilumab** potentially affects the exposure to aminophylline. Monitor and adjust dose. [Moderate] Theoretical

▸ **Tocilizumab** is predicted to decrease the exposure to aminophylline. Monitor and adjust dose. [Moderate] Theoretical

▸ **Anakinra** is predicted to increase the risk of generalised infection (possibly life-threatening) when given with **golimumab**. Avoid. [Severe] Theoretical

▸ **Anthracyclines** are predicted to increase the risk of cardiotoxicity when given with monoclonal antibodies **(trastuzumab, trastuzumab emtansine)**. Avoid. [Severe] Theoretical → Also see TABLE 15 p. 1432

▸ **Anti-androgens** (apalutamide, enzalutamide) are predicted to decrease the exposure to **polatuzumab vedotin**. [Moderate] Theoretical

▸ **Antiarrhythmics** (dronedarone) increase the risk of neutropenia when given with **brentuximab vedotin**. Monitor and adjust dose. [Severe] Theoretical

▸ **Antiepileptics** (carbamazepine) are predicted to decrease the effects of **brentuximab vedotin**. [Severe] Theoretical

▸ **Antiepileptics** (carbamazepine, fosphenytoin, phenobarbital, phenytoin, primidone) are predicted to decrease the exposure to **polatuzumab vedotin**. [Moderate] Theoretical

▸ **Tocilizumab** is predicted to decrease the exposure to antiepileptics (fosphenytoin, phenytoin). Monitor and adjust dose. [Moderate] Theoretical

▸ **Antifungals, azoles** (itraconazole, ketoconazole) increase the risk of neutropenia when given with **brentuximab vedotin**. Monitor and adjust dose. [Severe] Study

▸ **Antifungals, azoles** (itraconazole, ketoconazole, voriconazole) are predicted to increase the exposure to **polatuzumab vedotin**. [Moderate] Theoretical

▸ **Antifungals, azoles** (itraconazole, ketoconazole, voriconazole) are predicted to increase the exposure to **trastuzumab emtansine**. Avoid. [Severe] Theoretical

▸ **Tocilizumab** is predicted to decrease the exposure to benzodiazepines (alprazolam, diazepam, midazolam). Monitor and adjust dose. [Moderate] Theoretical

▸ **Brentuximab vedotin** increases the risk of pulmonary toxicity when given with bleomycin. Avoid. [Severe] Study → Also see TABLE 15 p. 1432

▸ **Tocilizumab** is predicted to decrease the exposure to calcium channel blockers. Monitor and adjust dose. [Moderate] Theoretical

▸ **Blinatumomab** is predicted to transiently increase the exposure to ciclosporin. Monitor and adjust dose. [Moderate] Theoretical

▸ **Sarilumab** potentially affects the exposure to ciclosporin. Monitor and adjust dose. [Moderate] Theoretical

▸ **Tocilizumab** is predicted to decrease the exposure to ciclosporin. Monitor and adjust dose. [Moderate] Theoretical

▸ **Cobicistat** is predicted to increase the exposure to **polatuzumab vedotin**. [Moderate] Theoretical

▸ **Cobicistat** is predicted to increase the exposure to **trastuzumab emtansine**. Avoid. [Severe] Theoretical

▸ **Sarilumab** potentially decreases the exposure to combined hormonal contraceptives. [Severe] Theoretical

▸ **Corticosteroids** are predicted to increase the risk of immunosuppression when given with **dinutuximab**. Avoid except in life-threatening situations. [Severe] Theoretical

▸ Corticosteroids (betamethasone, deflazacort, dexamethasone, hydrocortisone, methylprednisolone, prednisolone) are predicted to decrease the efficacy of monoclonal antibodies **(atezolizumab, ipilimumab, nivolumab, pembrolizumab)**. Use with caution or avoid. [Severe] Theoretical

▸ **Tocilizumab** is predicted to decrease the exposure to corticosteroids (dexamethasone, methylprednisolone). Monitor and adjust dose. [Moderate] Theoretical

▸ **Blinatumomab** is predicted to transiently increase the exposure to coumarins (warfarin). Monitor and adjust dose. [Moderate] Theoretical

▸ **Sarilumab** potentially affects the exposure to coumarins (warfarin). Monitor and adjust dose. [Severe] Theoretical

▸ **Tocilizumab** is predicted to decrease the exposure to coumarins (warfarin). Monitor and adjust dose. [Moderate] Theoretical

▸ **Filgotinib** is predicted to increase the risk of immunosuppression when given with monoclonal antibodies **(adalimumab, certolizumab pegol, golimumab, infliximab, rituximab, sarilumab, secukinumab, tocilizumab)**. Avoid. [Severe] Theoretical

▸ HIV-protease inhibitors (lopinavir, ritonavir, saquinavir) are predicted to increase the risk of neutropenia when given with **brentuximab vedotin**. Monitor and adjust dose. [Severe] Study

▸ HIV-protease inhibitors are predicted to increase the exposure to **polatuzumab vedotin**. [Moderate] Theoretical

▸ HIV-protease inhibitors are predicted to increase the exposure to **trastuzumab emtansine**. Avoid. [Severe] Theoretical

▸ **Idelalisib** is predicted to increase the exposure to **polatuzumab vedotin**. [Moderate] Theoretical

▸ **Idelalisib** is predicted to increase the exposure to **trastuzumab emtansine**. Avoid. [Severe] Theoretical

▸ **Immunoglobulins** (normal immunoglobulin) are predicted to alter the effects of **dinutuximab**. Avoid. [Severe] Theoretical

▸ **Live vaccines** are predicted to increase the risk of generalised infection (possibly life-threatening) when given with **monoclonal antibodies**. Public Health England advises avoid (refer to Green Book). [Severe] Theoretical

▸ **Macrolides** (clarithromycin) increase the risk of neutropenia when given with **brentuximab vedotin**. Monitor and adjust dose. [Severe] Theoretical

▸ Macrolides (clarithromycin) are predicted to increase the exposure to **polatuzumab vedotin**. [Moderate] Theoretical

▸ Macrolides (clarithromycin) are predicted to increase the exposure to **trastuzumab emtansine**. Avoid. [Severe] Theoretical

▸ **Mitotane** is predicted to decrease the exposure to **polatuzumab vedotin**. [Moderate] Theoretical

▸ **Ozanimod** potentially increases the risk of immunosuppression when given with **alemtuzumab**. Avoid. [Severe] Theoretical

▸ Rifamycins (rifampicin) decrease the effects of **brentuximab vedotin**. [Severe] Study

▸ Rifamycins (rifampicin) are predicted to decrease the exposure to **polatuzumab vedotin**. [Moderate] Theoretical

▸ **Siponimod** potentially increases the risk of immunosuppression when given with **alemtuzumab**. Avoid. [Severe] Theoretical

A1

Interactions | Appendix 1

Monoclonal antibodies (continued)

▶ **Sarilumab** potentially affects the exposure to sirolimus. Monitor and adjust dose. Moderate Theoretical
▶ **Sarilumab** is predicted to decrease the exposure to statins (atorvastatin, simvastatin). Moderate Study
▶ **Tocilizumab** is predicted to decrease the exposure to statins (atorvastatin, simvastatin). Monitor and adjust dose. Moderate Study
▶ **Sarilumab** potentially affects the exposure to tacrolimus. Monitor and adjust dose. Moderate Theoretical
▶ **Blinatumomab** is predicted to transiently increase the exposure to theophylline. Monitor and adjust dose. Moderate Theoretical
▶ **Sarilumab** potentially affects the exposure to theophylline. Monitor and adjust dose. Moderate Theoretical
▶ **Tocilizumab** is predicted to decrease the exposure to theophylline. Monitor and adjust dose. Moderate Theoretical

Montelukast

▶ Anti-androgens (apalutamide, enzalutamide) are predicted to decrease the exposure to **montelukast**. Mild Study
▶ Antiepileptics (carbamazepine, fosphenytoin, phenobarbital, phenytoin, primidone) are predicted to decrease the exposure to **montelukast**. Mild Study
▶ Clopidogrel is predicted to moderately increase the exposure to **montelukast**. Moderate Study
▶ Fibrates (gemfibrozil) are predicted to moderately increase the exposure to **montelukast**. Moderate Study
▶ Iron chelators (deferasirox) are predicted to increase the exposure to **montelukast**. Moderate Theoretical
▶ Leflunomide is predicted to increase the exposure to **montelukast**. Moderate Theoretical
▶ Mitotane is predicted to decrease the exposure to **montelukast**. Mild Study
▶ Opicapone is predicted to increase the exposure to **montelukast**. Avoid. Moderate Study
▶ Rifamycins (rifampicin) are predicted to decrease the exposure to **montelukast**. Mild Study
▶ Teriflunomide is predicted to increase the exposure to **montelukast**. Moderate Theoretical

Morphine → see opioids
Moxifloxacin → see quinolones
Moxisylyte → see TABLE 8 p. 1430 (hypotension)
Moxonidine → see TABLE 8 p. 1430 (hypotension), TABLE 11 p. 1431 (CNS depressant effects)

▶ Tricyclic antidepressants are predicted to decrease the effects of moxonidine. Avoid. Moderate Theoretical → Also see TABLE 8 p. 1430 → Also see TABLE 11 p. 1431

Mycophenolate

▶ **Mycophenolate** is predicted to increase the risk of haematological toxicity when given with aciclovir. Moderate Theoretical
▶ Oral antacids decrease the exposure to oral **mycophenolate**. Moderate Study
▶ Antifungals, azoles (isavuconazole) increase the exposure to **mycophenolate**. Moderate Study
▶ **Mycophenolate** is predicted to increase the risk of haematological toxicity when given with ganciclovir. Moderate Theoretical
▶ Live vaccines are predicted to increase the risk of generalised infection (possibly life-threatening) when given with **mycophenolate**. Public Health England advises avoid (refer to Green Book). Severe Theoretical
▶ Rifamycins (rifampicin) decrease the concentration of **mycophenolate**. Monitor and adjust dose. Severe Study
▶ **Mycophenolate** is predicted to increase the risk of haematological toxicity when given with valaciclovir. Moderate Theoretical
▶ **Mycophenolate** is predicted to increase the risk of haematological toxicity when given with valganciclovir. Moderate Theoretical

Nabilone → see TABLE 11 p. 1431 (CNS depressant effects)

▶ **Nabilone** is predicted to increase the risk of cardiovascular adverse effects when given with amfetamines. Severe Theoretical

Nabumetone → see NSAIDs

Nadolol → see beta blockers, non-selective

Naldemedine

▶ Anti-androgens (apalutamide, enzalutamide) are predicted to markedly decrease the exposure to **naldemedine**. Avoid. Severe Study
▶ Antiarrhythmics (amiodarone, dronedarone) are predicted to increase the exposure to **naldemedine**. Moderate Study
▶ Antiepileptics (carbamazepine, fosphenytoin, phenobarbital, phenytoin, primidone) are predicted to markedly decrease the exposure to **naldemedine**. Avoid. Severe Study
▶ Antifungals, azoles (fluconazole, isavuconazole, posaconazole) are predicted to increase the exposure to **naldemedine**. Moderate Study
▶ Antifungals, azoles (itraconazole, ketoconazole, voriconazole) are predicted to increase the exposure to **naldemedine**. Avoid or monitor. Moderate Study
▶ Calcium channel blockers (diltiazem, verapamil) are predicted to increase the exposure to **naldemedine**. Moderate Study
▶ Ciclosporin is predicted to increase the exposure to **naldemedine**. Moderate Study
▶ Cobicistat is predicted to increase the exposure to **naldemedine**. Avoid or monitor. Moderate Study
▶ Crizotinib is predicted to increase the exposure to **naldemedine**. Moderate Study
▶ Grapefruit juice is predicted to increase the exposure to **naldemedine**. Avoid or monitor. Moderate Theoretical
▶ HIV-protease inhibitors are predicted to increase the exposure to **naldemedine**. Avoid or monitor. Moderate Study
▶ Idelalisib is predicted to increase the exposure to **naldemedine**. Avoid or monitor. Moderate Study
▶ Imatinib is predicted to increase the exposure to **naldemedine**. Moderate Study
▶ Letermovir is predicted to increase the exposure to **naldemedine**. Moderate Study
▶ Macrolides (azithromycin, erythromycin) are predicted to increase the exposure to **naldemedine**. Moderate Study
▶ Macrolides (clarithromycin) are predicted to increase the exposure to **naldemedine**. Avoid or monitor. Moderate Study
▶ Mitotane is predicted to markedly decrease the exposure to **naldemedine**. Avoid. Severe Study
▶ Neurokinin-1 receptor antagonists (aprepitant, netupitant) are predicted to increase the exposure to **naldemedine**. Moderate Study
▶ Nilotinib is predicted to increase the exposure to **naldemedine**. Moderate Study
▶ Ranolazine is predicted to increase the exposure to **naldemedine**. Moderate Study
▶ Rifamycins (rifampicin) are predicted to markedly decrease the exposure to **naldemedine**. Avoid. Severe Study
▶ St John's wort is predicted to decrease the exposure to **naldemedine**. Avoid. Severe Study
▶ Vemurafenib is predicted to increase the exposure to **naldemedine**. Moderate Study

Nalmefene

GENERAL INFORMATION Discontinue treatment 1 week before anticipated use of opioids; if emergency analgesia is required during treatment, an increased dose of opioid analgesic might be necessary (monitor for opioid intoxication).

▶ **Nalmefene** is predicted to decrease the efficacy of opioids. Avoid. Severe Theoretical

Naloxegol

▶ Anti-androgens (apalutamide, enzalutamide) are predicted to markedly decrease the exposure to **naloxegol**. Avoid. Moderate Study
▶ Antiarrhythmics (dronedarone) are predicted to increase the exposure to **naloxegol**. Adjust naloxegol dose and monitor adverse effects, p. 70. Moderate Study
▶ Antiepileptics (carbamazepine, fosphenytoin, phenobarbital, phenytoin, primidone) are predicted to markedly decrease the exposure to **naloxegol**. Avoid. Moderate Study
▶ Antifungals, azoles (fluconazole, isavuconazole, posaconazole) are predicted to increase the exposure to **naloxegol**. Adjust naloxegol dose and monitor adverse effects, p. 70. Moderate Study

Antifungals, azoles (itraconazole, ketoconazole, voriconazole) are predicted to markedly increase the exposure to **naloxegol**. Avoid. ⟨Severe⟩ Study

Calcium channel blockers (diltiazem, verapamil) are predicted to increase the exposure to **naloxegol**. Adjust **naloxegol** dose and monitor adverse effects, p. 70. ⟨Moderate⟩ Study

Cobicistat is predicted to markedly increase the exposure to **naloxegol**. Avoid. ⟨Severe⟩ Study

Crizotinib is predicted to increase the exposure to **naloxegol**. Adjust **naloxegol** dose and monitor adverse effects, p. 70. ⟨Moderate⟩ Study

Grapefruit juice is predicted to increase the exposure to **naloxegol**. ⟨Moderate⟩ Theoretical

HIV-protease inhibitors are predicted to markedly increase the exposure to **naloxegol**. Avoid. ⟨Severe⟩ Study

Idelalisib is predicted to markedly increase the exposure to **naloxegol**. Avoid. ⟨Severe⟩ Study

▸ Imatinib is predicted to increase the exposure to **naloxegol**. Adjust **naloxegol** dose and monitor adverse effects, p. 70. ⟨Moderate⟩ Study

▸ Letermovir is predicted to increase the exposure to **naloxegol**. Adjust **naloxegol** dose and monitor adverse effects, p. 70. ⟨Moderate⟩ Study

▸ Macrolides (clarithromycin) are predicted to markedly increase the exposure to **naloxegol**. Avoid. ⟨Severe⟩ Study

▸ Macrolides (erythromycin) are predicted to increase the exposure to **naloxegol**. Adjust **naloxegol** dose and monitor adverse effects, p. 70. ⟨Moderate⟩ Study

▸ Mitotane is predicted to markedly decrease the exposure to **naloxegol**. Avoid. ⟨Severe⟩ Study

▸ Neurokinin-1 receptor antagonists (aprepitant, netupitant) are predicted to increase the exposure to **naloxegol**. Adjust **naloxegol** dose and monitor adverse effects, p. 70. ⟨Moderate⟩ Study

▸ Nilotinib is predicted to increase the exposure to **naloxegol**. Adjust **naloxegol** dose and monitor adverse effects, p. 70. ⟨Moderate⟩ Study

▸ Rifamycins (rifampicin) are predicted to markedly decrease the exposure to **naloxegol**. Avoid. ⟨Moderate⟩ Study

▸ St John's wort is predicted to decrease the exposure to **naloxegol**. Avoid. ⟨Moderate⟩ Theoretical

Naltrexone

GENERAL INFORMATION Avoid concurrent use of opioids with **naltrexone**.

Nandrolone

▸ Nandrolone is predicted to increase the anticoagulant effect of coumarins. Monitor and adjust dose. ⟨Severe⟩ Theoretical

▸ Nandrolone is predicted to increase the anticoagulant effect of phenindione. Monitor and adjust dose. ⟨Severe⟩ Theoretical

Naproxen → see NSAIDs
Naratriptan → see triptans
Natalizumab → see monoclonal antibodies
Nateglinide → see meglitinides
Nebivolol → see beta blockers, selective
Necitumumab → see monoclonal antibodies
Nefopam → see TABLE 10 p. 1431 (antimuscarinics)
▸ Nefopam is predicted to increase the risk of serious elevations in blood pressure when given with MAOIs, irreversible. Avoid. ⟨Severe⟩ Theoretical

Nelarabine → see TABLE 15 p. 1432 (myelosuppression)
Neomycin → see TABLE 2 p. 1429 (nephrotoxicity), TABLE 19 p. 1433 (ototoxicity), TABLE 20 p. 1433 (neuromuscular blocking effects)

ROUTE-SPECIFIC INFORMATION Since systemic absorption can follow topical application of **neomycin**, the possibility of interactions should be borne in mind.

▸ Neomycin decreases the absorption of digoxin. ⟨Moderate⟩ Study
▸ Neomycin moderately decreases the exposure to sorafenib. ⟨Moderate⟩ Study

Neostigmine → see TABLE 6 p. 1430 (bradycardia)
▸ Aminoglycosides are predicted to decrease the effects of **neostigmine**. ⟨Moderate⟩ Theoretical

Nepafenac → see NSAIDs
Neratinib → see TABLE 1 p. 1429 (hepatotoxicity)

▸ Oral antacids are predicted to decrease the exposure to oral **neratinib**. Separate administration by at least 3 hours. ⟨Mild⟩ Theoretical

▸ Anti-androgens (apalutamide, enzalutamide) are predicted to decrease the exposure to **neratinib**. Avoid. ⟨Severe⟩ Study

▸ Antiarrhythmics (dronedarone) are predicted to increase the exposure to **neratinib**. Avoid. ⟨Severe⟩ Study

▸ Antiepileptics (carbamazepine, fosphenytoin, phenobarbital, phenytoin, primidone) are predicted to decrease the exposure to **neratinib**. Avoid. ⟨Severe⟩ Study → Also see TABLE 1 p. 1429

▸ Antifungals, azoles (fluconazole, isavuconazole, posaconazole) are predicted to increase the exposure to **neratinib**. Avoid. ⟨Severe⟩ Study → Also see TABLE 1 p. 1429

▸ Antifungals, azoles (itraconazole, ketoconazole, voriconazole) are predicted to increase the exposure to **neratinib**. Avoid or adjust **neratinib** dose, p. 1034. ⟨Severe⟩ Study → Also see TABLE 1 p. 1429

▸ **Neratinib** is predicted to increase the exposure to antihistamines, non-sedating (fexofenadine). ⟨Moderate⟩ Study

▸ Calcium channel blockers (diltiazem, verapamil) are predicted to increase the exposure to **neratinib**. Avoid. ⟨Severe⟩ Study

▸ Oral calcium salts (calcium carbonate) are predicted to decrease the exposure to oral **neratinib**. Separate administration by at least 3 hours. ⟨Mild⟩ Theoretical

▸ Cobicistat is predicted to increase the exposure to **neratinib**. Avoid or adjust **neratinib** dose, p. 1034. ⟨Severe⟩ Study

▸ Crizotinib is predicted to increase the exposure to **neratinib**. Avoid. ⟨Severe⟩ Study

▸ **Neratinib** is predicted to slightly increase the exposure to digoxin. ⟨Moderate⟩ Study

▸ Endothelin receptor antagonists (bosentan) are predicted to decrease the exposure to **neratinib**. ⟨Severe⟩ Study

▸ **Neratinib** is predicted to increase the exposure to everolimus. ⟨Moderate⟩ Study

▸ **Neratinib** is predicted to increase the exposure to factor XA inhibitors (edoxaban). ⟨Moderate⟩ Study

▸ Grapefruit juice is predicted to increase the exposure to **neratinib**. Avoid. ⟨Severe⟩ Theoretical

▸ H₂ receptor antagonists are predicted to decrease the exposure to **neratinib**. Avoid. ⟨Severe⟩ Theoretical

▸ HIV-protease inhibitors are predicted to increase the exposure to **neratinib**. Avoid or adjust **neratinib** dose, p. 1034. ⟨Severe⟩ Study

▸ Idelalisib is predicted to increase the exposure to **neratinib**. Avoid or adjust **neratinib** dose, p. 1034. ⟨Severe⟩ Study

▸ Imatinib is predicted to increase the exposure to **neratinib**. Avoid. ⟨Severe⟩ Study

▸ Letermovir is predicted to increase the exposure to **neratinib**. Avoid. ⟨Severe⟩ Study

▸ Macrolides (clarithromycin) are predicted to increase the exposure to **neratinib**. Avoid or adjust **neratinib** dose, p. 1034. ⟨Severe⟩ Study

▸ Macrolides (erythromycin) are predicted to increase the exposure to **neratinib**. Avoid. ⟨Severe⟩ Study

▸ Mitotane is predicted to decrease the exposure to **neratinib**. Avoid. ⟨Severe⟩ Study

▸ Neurokinin-1 receptor antagonists (aprepitant, netupitant) are predicted to increase the exposure to **neratinib**. Avoid. ⟨Severe⟩ Study

▸ Nilotinib is predicted to increase the exposure to **neratinib**. Avoid. ⟨Severe⟩ Study

▸ NNRTIs (efavirenz, nevirapine) are predicted to decrease the exposure to **neratinib**. ⟨Severe⟩ Study

▸ Proton pump inhibitors are predicted to decrease the exposure to **neratinib**. Avoid. ⟨Severe⟩ Study

▸ Rifamycins (rifampicin) are predicted to decrease the exposure to **neratinib**. Avoid. ⟨Severe⟩ Study

▸ **Neratinib** is predicted to increase the exposure to sirolimus. ⟨Moderate⟩ Study

▸ St John's wort is predicted to decrease the exposure to **neratinib**. Avoid. ⟨Severe⟩ Theoretical

▸ **Neratinib** is predicted to increase the exposure to thrombin inhibitors (dabigatran). ⟨Moderate⟩ Study

Netupitant → see neurokinin-1 receptor antagonists
Neurokinin-1 receptor antagonists

   aprepitant · fosaprepitant · netupitant

A1

Interactions | Appendix 1

Neurokinin-1 receptor antagonists (continued)

▸ Neurokinin-1 receptor antagonists **(aprepitant, netupitant)** are predicted to increase the exposure to abemaciclib. Moderate Study

▸ Neurokinin-1 receptor antagonists **(aprepitant, netupitant)** are predicted to increase the exposure to acalabrutinib. Avoid or monitor. Severe Study

▸ Neurokinin-1 receptor antagonists **(aprepitant, netupitant)** are predicted to increase the exposure to aldosterone antagonists (eplerenone). Adjust **eplerenone** dose, p. 208. Severe Study

▸ **Netupitant** very slightly increases the exposure to alkylating agents **(cyclophosphamide)**. Moderate Study

▸ **Netupitant** is predicted to increase the exposure to alkylating agents **(ifosfamide)**. Moderate Study

▸ Neurokinin-1 receptor antagonists **(aprepitant, fosaprepitant)** are predicted to increase the exposure to alkylating agents **(ifosfamide)**. Severe Theoretical

▸ Neurokinin-1 receptor antagonists **(aprepitant, netupitant)** are predicted to increase the exposure to alpha blockers **(tamsulosin)**. Moderate Theoretical

▸ Anti-androgens **(apalutamide, enzalutamide)** are predicted to markedly decrease the exposure to **aprepitant**. Avoid. Moderate Study

▸ Anti-androgens **(apalutamide, enzalutamide)** are predicted to decrease the exposure to **fosaprepitant**. Avoid. Moderate Theoretical

▸ Anti-androgens **(apalutamide, enzalutamide)** are predicted to decrease the exposure to **netupitant**. Avoid. Severe Study

▸ **Aprepitant** increases the exposure to antiarrhythmics **(dronedarone)**. Severe Theoretical

▸ Neurokinin-1 receptor antagonists **(aprepitant, netupitant)** are predicted to increase the exposure to antiarrhythmics **(propafenone)**. Monitor and adjust dose. Moderate Study

▸ Antiepileptics **(carbamazepine, fosphenytoin, phenobarbital, phenytoin, primidone)** are predicted to markedly decrease the exposure to **aprepitant**. Avoid. Moderate Study

▸ Antiepileptics **(carbamazepine, fosphenytoin, phenobarbital, phenytoin, primidone)** are predicted to decrease the exposure to **fosaprepitant**. Avoid. Moderate Theoretical

▸ Antiepileptics **(carbamazepine, fosphenytoin, phenobarbital, phenytoin, primidone)** are predicted to decrease the exposure to **netupitant**. Avoid. Severe Study

▸ Antifungals, azoles **(fluconazole)** are predicted to increase the exposure to **aprepitant**. Moderate Theoretical

▸ Antifungals, azoles **(itraconazole, ketoconazole, voriconazole)** are predicted to markedly increase the exposure to **aprepitant**. Moderate Study

▸ Antifungals, azoles **(itraconazole, ketoconazole, voriconazole)** are predicted to increase the exposure to **fosaprepitant**. Moderate Theoretical

▸ Antifungals, azoles **(itraconazole, ketoconazole, voriconazole)** are predicted to increase the exposure to **netupitant**. Moderate Study

▸ Antifungals, azoles **(posaconazole)** are predicted to increase the exposure to neurokinin-1 receptor antagonists **(aprepitant, fosaprepitant)**. Moderate Study

▸ **Aprepitant** is predicted to increase the exposure to antifungals, azoles **(isavuconazole)**. Moderate Theoretical

▸ **Netupitant** is predicted to decrease the exposure to antifungals, azoles **(isavuconazole)**. Moderate Theoretical

▸ Neurokinin-1 receptor antagonists **(aprepitant, netupitant)** are predicted to increase the exposure to antihistamines, non-sedating **(mizolastine)**. Severe Theoretical

▸ Neurokinin-1 receptor antagonists **(aprepitant, netupitant)** are predicted to increase the exposure to antihistamines, non-sedating **(rupatadine)**. Avoid. Moderate Study

▸ Neurokinin-1 receptor antagonists **(aprepitant, netupitant)** are predicted to increase the concentration of antimalarials **(piperaquine)**. Severe Theoretical

▸ Neurokinin-1 receptor antagonists **(aprepitant, netupitant)** are predicted to increase the exposure to antipsychotics, second generation **(cariprazine)**. Avoid. Severe Study

▸ Neurokinin-1 receptor antagonists **(aprepitant, netupitant)** are predicted to increase the exposure to antipsychotics, second generation **(lurasidone)**. Adjust **lurasidone** dose. Moderate Study

▸ Neurokinin-1 receptor antagonists **(aprepitant, netupitant)** are predicted to increase the exposure to antipsychotics, second generation **(quetiapine)**. Avoid. Moderate Study

▸ Neurokinin-1 receptor antagonists **(aprepitant, netupitant)** are predicted to increase the exposure to avapritinib. Avoid or adjust **avapritinib** dose, p. 1012. Moderate Study

▸ Neurokinin-1 receptor antagonists **(aprepitant, netupitant)** are predicted to increase the exposure to axitinib. Moderate Theoretical

▸ Neurokinin-1 receptor antagonists **(aprepitant, netupitant)** are predicted to increase the exposure to bedaquiline. Avoid prolonged use. Mild Theoretical

▸ **Fosaprepitant** is predicted to increase the exposure to benzodiazepines **(alprazolam)**. Moderate Study

▸ Neurokinin-1 receptor antagonists **(aprepitant, netupitant)** are predicted to increase the exposure to benzodiazepines **(alprazolam)**. Severe Study

▸ **Fosaprepitant** slightly increases the exposure to benzodiazepines **(midazolam)**. Moderate Study

▸ Neurokinin-1 receptor antagonists **(aprepitant, netupitant)** are predicted to increase the exposure to benzodiazepines **(midazolam)**. Monitor adverse effects and adjust dose. Severe Study

▸ Neurokinin-1 receptor antagonists **(aprepitant, netupitant)** are predicted to increase the exposure to beta₂ agonists **(salmeterol)**. Moderate Study

▸ **Fosaprepitant** is predicted to increase the exposure to bosutinib. Severe Theoretical

▸ Neurokinin-1 receptor antagonists **(aprepitant, netupitant)** are predicted to increase the exposure to bosutinib. Avoid or adjust dose. Severe Theoretical

▸ Neurokinin-1 receptor antagonists **(aprepitant, netupitant)** are predicted to increase the exposure to buspirone. Use with caution and adjust dose. Moderate Study

▸ Neurokinin-1 receptor antagonists **(aprepitant, netupitant)** are predicted to increase the exposure to cabozantinib. Moderate Theoretical

▸ Calcium channel blockers **(diltiazem, verapamil)** are predicted to increase the exposure to **aprepitant** and **aprepitant** is predicted to increase the exposure to calcium channel blockers **(diltiazem, verapamil)**. Moderate Study

▸ Neurokinin-1 receptor antagonists **(aprepitant, netupitant)** are predicted to increase the exposure to calcium channel blockers **(amlodipine, felodipine, lacidipine, lercanidipine, nicardipine, nifedipine, nimodipine)**. Monitor and adjust dose. Moderate Study

▸ Neurokinin-1 receptor antagonists **(aprepitant, netupitant)** are predicted to increase the concentration of ciclosporin. Severe Study

▸ Cobicistat is predicted to markedly increase the exposure to **aprepitant**. Moderate Study

▸ Cobicistat is predicted to increase the exposure to **fosaprepitant**. Moderate Theoretical

▸ Cobicistat is predicted to increase the exposure to **netupitant**. Moderate Study

▸ Neurokinin-1 receptor antagonists **(aprepitant, netupitant)** are predicted to increase the exposure to cobimetinib. Severe Theoretical

▸ Neurokinin-1 receptor antagonists **(aprepitant, netupitant)** are predicted to increase the exposure to colchicine. Adjust **colchicine** dose with moderate CYP3A4 inhibitors, p. 1166. Severe Study

▸ Neurokinin-1 receptor antagonists **(aprepitant, fosaprepitant)** are predicted to decrease the efficacy of combined hormonal contraceptives. For FSRH guidance, see Contraceptives, interactions p. 840. Severe Study

▸ Neurokinin-1 receptor antagonists **(aprepitant, netupitant)** are predicted to increase the exposure to oral corticosteroids **(budesonide)**. Moderate Study

▸ **Aprepitant** moderately increases the exposure to corticosteroids **(dexamethasone)**. Monitor and adjust dose. Moderate Study

▸ **Netupitant** is predicted to increase the exposure to corticosteroids **(dexamethasone)**. Adjust dose. Moderate Study

Neurokinin-1 receptor antagonists **(aprepitant, netupitant)** are predicted to increase the exposure to corticosteroids (fluticasone). [Moderate] Study

Neurokinin-1 receptor antagonists **(aprepitant, netupitant)** are predicted to increase the exposure to corticosteroids (methylprednisolone). Monitor and adjust dose. [Moderate] Study

▸ **Aprepitant** decreases the anticoagulant effect of coumarins. [Moderate] Study

Fosaprepitant is predicted to decrease the anticoagulant effect of coumarins. [Moderate] Theoretical

▸ Neurokinin-1 receptor antagonists **(aprepitant, netupitant)** are predicted to slightly increase the exposure to darifenacin. [Moderate] Study

▸ Neurokinin-1 receptor antagonists **(aprepitant, netupitant)** are predicted to increase the exposure to dasatinib. [Severe] Study

▸ Neurokinin-1 receptor antagonists **(aprepitant, netupitant)** are predicted to decrease the efficacy of desogestrel. For FSRH guidance, see Contraceptives, interactions p. 840. [Severe] Theoretical

▸ Neurokinin-1 receptor antagonists **(aprepitant, netupitant)** are predicted to slightly increase the exposure to dienogest. [Moderate] Study

▸ Neurokinin-1 receptor antagonists **(aprepitant, netupitant)** are predicted to increase the exposure to dipeptidylpeptidase-4 inhibitors (saxagliptin). [Mild] Study

▸ Neurokinin-1 receptor antagonists **(aprepitant, netupitant)** increase the risk of QT-prolongation when given with domperidone. Avoid. [Severe] Study

▸ Neurokinin-1 receptor antagonists **(aprepitant, netupitant)** are predicted to increase the exposure to dopamine receptor agonists (bromocriptine). [Severe] Theoretical

▸ Neurokinin-1 receptor antagonists **(aprepitant, netupitant)** are predicted to increase the concentration of dopamine receptor agonists (cabergoline). [Moderate] Anecdotal

▸ Neurokinin-1 receptor antagonists **(aprepitant, netupitant)** are predicted to moderately increase the exposure to dutasteride. [Mild] Study

▸ Neurokinin-1 receptor antagonists **(aprepitant, netupitant)** is predicted to increase the exposure to elexacaftor. Adjust tezacaftor with ivacaftor and elexacftor p. 311 dose with moderate CYP3A4 inhibitors. [Severe] Theoretical

▸ Neurokinin-1 receptor antagonists **(aprepitant, netupitant)** are predicted to increase the exposure to eliglustat. Avoid or adjust dose—consult product literature. [Severe] Study

▸ Neurokinin-1 receptor antagonists **(aprepitant, netupitant)** are predicted to moderately increase the exposure to encorafenib. [Moderate] Study

▸ Endothelin receptor antagonists (bosentan) are predicted to decrease the exposure to aprepitant. [Moderate] Study

▸ Endothelin receptor antagonists (bosentan) are predicted to decrease the exposure to neurokinin-1 receptor antagonists **(fosaprepitant, netupitant)**. [Moderate] Theoretical

▸ Neurokinin-1 receptor antagonists **(aprepitant, netupitant)** are predicted to increase the exposure to entrectinib. Avoid moderate CYP3A4 inhibitors or adjust **entrectinib** dose, p. 1023. [Severe] Theoretical

▸ Neurokinin-1 receptor antagonists **(aprepitant, netupitant)** are predicted to increase the risk of ergotism when given with ergometrine. [Severe] Theoretical

▸ Neurokinin-1 receptor antagonists **(aprepitant, netupitant)** are predicted to increase the risk of ergotism when given with ergotamine. [Severe] Theoretical

▸ Neurokinin-1 receptor antagonists **(aprepitant, netupitant)** are predicted to increase the exposure to erlotinib. [Moderate] Theoretical

▸ Neurokinin-1 receptor antagonists **(aprepitant, fosaprepitant)** are predicted to decrease the efficacy of etonogestrel. For FSRH guidance, see Contraceptives, interactions p. 840. [Severe] Theoretical

▸ **Netupitant** slightly increases the exposure to etoposide. [Moderate] Study

▸ Neurokinin-1 receptor antagonists **(aprepitant, netupitant)** are predicted to increase the concentration of everolimus. Avoid or adjust dose. [Moderate] Study

▸ Neurokinin-1 receptor antagonists **(aprepitant, netupitant)** are predicted to increase the exposure to fesoterodine. Adjust **fesoterodine** dose with moderate CYP3A4 inhibitors in hepatic and renal impairment, p. 822. [Mild] Study

▸ Neurokinin-1 receptor antagonists **(aprepitant, netupitant)** are predicted to increase the exposure to gefitinib. [Moderate] Theoretical

▸ **Fosaprepitant** is predicted to increase the concentration of guanfacine. [Moderate] Theoretical

▸ Neurokinin-1 receptor antagonists **(aprepitant, netupitant)** are predicted to increase the concentration of guanfacine. Adjust **guanfacine** dose, p. 372. [Moderate] Theoretical

▸ HIV-protease inhibitors are predicted to markedly increase the exposure to **aprepitant**. [Moderate] Study

▸ HIV-protease inhibitors are predicted to increase the exposure to **fosaprepitant**. [Moderate] Theoretical

▸ HIV-protease inhibitors are predicted to increase the exposure to **netupitant**. [Moderate] Study

▸ Neurokinin-1 receptor antagonists **(aprepitant, fosaprepitant)** are predicted to decrease the effects of hormone replacement therapy. [Moderate] Anecdotal

▸ **Fosaprepitant** is predicted to slightly increase the exposure to ibrutinib. [Moderate] Theoretical

▸ Neurokinin-1 receptor antagonists **(aprepitant, netupitant)** are predicted to increase the exposure to ibrutinib. Adjust **ibrutinib** dose with moderate CYP3A4 inhibitors, p. 1027. [Severe] Study

▸ Idelalisib is predicted to markedly increase the exposure to **aprepitant**. [Moderate] Study

▸ Idelalisib is predicted to increase the exposure to **fosaprepitant**. [Moderate] Theoretical

▸ Idelalisib is predicted to increase the exposure to **netupitant**. [Moderate] Study

▸ Neurokinin-1 receptor antagonists **(aprepitant, netupitant)** are predicted to increase the exposure to imatinib. [Moderate] Theoretical

▸ **Netupitant** is predicted to increase the exposure to irinotecan. [Moderate] Study

▸ Neurokinin-1 receptor antagonists **(aprepitant, fosaprepitant)** are predicted to increase the exposure to intravenous irinotecan. [Severe] Theoretical

▸ Neurokinin-1 receptor antagonists **(aprepitant, netupitant)** are predicted to increase the exposure to ivabradine. Adjust **ivabradine** dose, p. 227. [Severe] Theoretical

▸ Neurokinin-1 receptor antagonists **(aprepitant, netupitant)** are predicted to increase the exposure to ivacaftor. Adjust ivacaftor p. 309 or tezacaftor with ivacaftor p. 311 or tezacaftor with ivacaftor and elexacftor p. 311 dose with moderate CYP3A4 inhibitors. [Severe] Study

▸ Neurokinin-1 receptor antagonists **(aprepitant, netupitant)** are predicted to increase the exposure to lapatinib. [Moderate] Study

▸ Neurokinin-1 receptor antagonists **(aprepitant, fosaprepitant)** are predicted to decrease the efficacy of levonorgestrel. For FSRH guidance, see Contraceptives, interactions p. 840. [Severe] Theoretical

▸ **Fosaprepitant** is predicted to increase the exposure to lomitapide. Separate administration by 12 hours. [Mild] Theoretical

▸ Neurokinin-1 receptor antagonists **(aprepitant, netupitant)** are predicted to increase the exposure to lomitapide. Avoid. [Moderate] Theoretical

▸ Macrolides (clarithromycin) are predicted to markedly increase the exposure to **aprepitant**. [Moderate] Study

▸ Macrolides (clarithromycin) are predicted to increase the exposure to **fosaprepitant**. [Moderate] Theoretical

▸ Macrolides (clarithromycin) are predicted to increase the exposure to **netupitant**. [Moderate] Study

▸ Macrolides (erythromycin) are predicted to increase the exposure to **aprepitant**. [Moderate] Study

▸ Neurokinin-1 receptor antagonists **(aprepitant, netupitant)** are predicted to increase the exposure to maraviroc. [Moderate] Study

▸ Neurokinin-1 receptor antagonists **(aprepitant, netupitant)** are predicted to increase the exposure to midostaurin. [Moderate] Theoretical

Neurokinin-1 receptor antagonists (continued)

▶ Mitotane is predicted to markedly decrease the exposure to **aprepitant**. Avoid. Moderate Study

▶ Mitotane is predicted to decrease the exposure to **fosaprepitant**. Avoid. Moderate Theoretical

▶ Mitotane is predicted to decrease the exposure to **netupitant**. Avoid. Severe Study

▶ Neurokinin-1 receptor antagonists **(aprepitant, netupitant)** are predicted to increase the exposure to **naldemedine**. Moderate Study

▶ Neurokinin-1 receptor antagonists **(aprepitant, netupitant)** are predicted to increase the exposure to **naloxegol**. Adjust **naloxegol** dose and monitor adverse effects, p. 70. Moderate Study

▶ Neurokinin-1 receptor antagonists **(aprepitant, netupitant)** are predicted to increase the exposure to **neratinib**. Avoid. Severe Study

▶ Neurokinin-1 receptor antagonists **(aprepitant, netupitant)** are predicted to increase the exposure to **nilotinib**. Moderate Theoretical

▶ NNRTIs (efavirenz, nevirapine) are predicted to decrease the exposure to **aprepitant**. Moderate Study

▶ NNRTIs (efavirenz, nevirapine) are predicted to decrease the exposure to neurokinin-1 receptor antagonists **(fosaprepitant, netupitant)**. Moderate Theoretical

▶ Neurokinin-1 receptor antagonists **(aprepitant, fosaprepitant)** are predicted to decrease the efficacy of norethisterone. For FSRH guidance, see Contraceptives, interactions p. 840. Severe Anecdotal

▶ Neurokinin-1 receptor antagonists **(aprepitant, netupitant)** are predicted to increase the exposure to **olaparib**. Avoid moderate CYP3A4 inhibitors or adjust **olaparib** dose, p. 1051. Moderate Theoretical

▶ Neurokinin-1 receptor antagonists **(aprepitant, netupitant)** are predicted to increase the exposure to opioids (alfentanil, buprenorphine, fentanyl, oxycodone). Monitor and adjust dose. Moderate Study

▶ Neurokinin-1 receptor antagonists **(aprepitant, netupitant)** are predicted to increase the exposure to opioids (methadone). Moderate Theoretical

▶ Neurokinin-1 receptor antagonists **(aprepitant, netupitant)** are predicted to increase the exposure to **oxybutynin**. Mild Theoretical

▶ Neurokinin-1 receptor antagonists **(aprepitant, netupitant)** are predicted to increase the exposure to **pazopanib**. Moderate Theoretical

▶ Neurokinin-1 receptor antagonists **(aprepitant, netupitant)** are predicted to increase the exposure to phosphodiesterase type-5 inhibitors (avanafil). Adjust **avanafil** dose, p. 859. Moderate Theoretical

▶ Neurokinin-1 receptor antagonists **(aprepitant, netupitant)** are predicted to increase the exposure to phosphodiesterase type-5 inhibitors (sildenafil). Monitor or adjust **sildenafil** dose with moderate CYP3A4 inhibitors, p. 860. Moderate Study

▶ Neurokinin-1 receptor antagonists **(aprepitant, netupitant)** are predicted to increase the exposure to phosphodiesterase type-5 inhibitors (tadalafil). Severe Theoretical

▶ Neurokinin-1 receptor antagonists **(aprepitant, netupitant)** are predicted to increase the exposure to phosphodiesterase type-5 inhibitors (vardenafil). Adjust dose. Severe Theoretical

▶ **Neurokinin-1 receptor antagonists** are predicted to increase the exposure to pimozide. Avoid. Severe Theoretical

▶ Neurokinin-1 receptor antagonists **(aprepitant, netupitant)** are predicted to increase the exposure to **ranolazine**. Severe Study

▶ Neurokinin-1 receptor antagonists **(aprepitant, netupitant)** are predicted to increase the exposure to **ribociclib**. Moderate Study

▶ Rifamycins (rifampicin) are predicted to markedly decrease the exposure to **aprepitant**. Moderate Study

▶ Rifamycins (rifampicin) are predicted to decrease the exposure to **fosaprepitant**. Avoid. Moderate Theoretical

▶ Rifamycins (rifampicin) are predicted to decrease the exposure to **netupitant**. Avoid. Severe Study

▶ Neurokinin-1 receptor antagonists **(aprepitant, netupitant)** are predicted to increase the exposure to **ruxolitinib**. Moderate Theoretical

▶ Neurokinin-1 receptor antagonists **(aprepitant, netupitant)** increase the concentration of sirolimus. Monitor and adjust dose. Moderate Study

▶ Neurokinin-1 receptor antagonists **(aprepitant, netupitant)** are predicted to increase the exposure to SSRIs (dapoxetine). Adjust **dapoxetine** dose with moderate CYP3A4 inhibitors, p. 867. Moderate Theoretical

▶ St John's wort is predicted to decrease the exposure to **netupitant**. Moderate Theoretical

▶ St John's wort is predicted to decrease the exposure to neurokinin-1 receptor antagonists **(aprepitant, fosaprepitant)**. Avoid. Moderate Theoretical

▶ Neurokinin-1 receptor antagonists **(aprepitant, netupitant)** are predicted to increase the exposure to statins (atorvastatin, simvastatin). Monitor and adjust dose. Severe Theoretical

▶ Neurokinin-1 receptor antagonists **(aprepitant, netupitant)** are predicted to increase the exposure to sunitinib. Moderate Theoretical

▶ Neurokinin-1 receptor antagonists **(aprepitant, netupitant)** are predicted to increase the concentration of tacrolimus. Severe Study

▶ Neurokinin-1 receptor antagonists **(aprepitant, netupitant)** are predicted to increase the exposure to taxanes (cabazitaxel). Moderate Theoretical

▶ **Netupitant** slightly increases the exposure to taxanes (docetaxel). Moderate Study

▶ **Netupitant** is predicted to increase the exposure to taxanes (paclitaxel). Moderate Study

▶ Neurokinin-1 receptor antagonists **(aprepitant, netupitant)** are predicted to increase the concentration of temsirolimus. Use with caution or avoid. Moderate Theoretical

▶ Neurokinin-1 receptor antagonists **(aprepitant, netupitant)** are predicted to increase the exposure to tezacaftor. Adjust tezacaftor with ivacaftor p. 311 or tezacaftor with ivacaftor and elexacftor p. 311 dose with moderate CYP3A4 inhibitors. Severe Study

▶ Neurokinin-1 receptor antagonists **(aprepitant, netupitant)** given with a potent CYP2C19 inhibitor are predicted to increase the exposure to tofacitinib. Adjust **tofacitinib** dose, p. 1154. Moderate Study

▶ Neurokinin-1 receptor antagonists **(aprepitant, netupitant)** are predicted to increase the exposure to tolterodine. Mild Theoretical

▶ Neurokinin-1 receptor antagonists **(aprepitant, netupitant)** are predicted to increase the exposure to tolvaptan. Manufacturer advises caution or adjust **tolvaptan** dose with moderate CYP3A4 inhibitors, p. 708. Moderate Study

▶ Neurokinin-1 receptor antagonists **(aprepitant, netupitant)** are predicted to increase the exposure to trazodone. Moderate Theoretical

▶ Neurokinin-1 receptor antagonists **(aprepitant, netupitant)** are predicted to increase the exposure to triptans (eletriptan). Moderate Study

▶ Neurokinin-1 receptor antagonists **(aprepitant, fosaprepitant)** decrease the efficacy of ulipristal. For FSRH guidance, see Contraceptives, interactions p. 840. Severe Anecdotal

▶ Neurokinin-1 receptor antagonists **(aprepitant, netupitant)** are predicted to increase the exposure to venetoclax. Avoid or adjust dose—consult product literature. Severe Study

▶ **Neurokinin-1 receptor antagonists** are predicted to increase the exposure to vinca alkaloids. Severe Theoretical

▶ Neurokinin-1 receptor antagonists **(aprepitant, netupitant)** are predicted to increase the exposure to zopiclone. Adjust dose. Moderate Study

Neuromuscular blocking drugs, non-depolarising → see TABLE 6 p. 1430 (bradycardia), **TABLE 20** p. 1433 (neuromuscular blocking effects)

atracurium · cisatracurium · mivacurium · pancuronium · rocuronium · vecuronium

▶ Anticholinesterases, centrally acting are predicted to decrease the effects of **neuromuscular blocking drugs, non-depolarising**. Moderate Theoretical → Also see TABLE 6 p. 1430

▶ Antiepileptics (carbamazepine) are predicted to decrease the effects of (but acute use increases the effects of) neuromuscular blocking drugs, non-depolarising **(atracurium, cisatracurium,**

pancuronium, rocuronium, vecuronium). Monitor and adjust dose. Moderate Study

Antiepileptics (fosphenytoin, phenytoin) decrease the effects of (but acute use increases the effects of) neuromuscular blocking drugs, non-depolarising (**atracurium, cisatracurium, pancuronium, rocuronium, vecuronium**). Moderate Study

Clindamycin increases the effects of **neuromuscular blocking drugs, non-depolarising**. Severe Anecdotal

Corticosteroids are predicted to decrease the effects of **neuromuscular blocking drugs, non-depolarising**. Severe Anecdotal

Pancuronium is predicted to increase the risk of cardiovascular adverse effects when given with digoxin. Severe Anecdotal

Irinotecan is predicted to decrease the effects of **neuromuscular blocking drugs, non-depolarising**. Moderate Theoretical

Intravenous magnesium increases the effects of **neuromuscular blocking drugs, non-depolarising**. Moderate Study

Metoclopramide is predicted to increase the effects of **neuromuscular blocking drugs, non-depolarising**. Moderate Theoretical

Penicillins (piperacillin) increase the effects of **neuromuscular blocking drugs, non-depolarising**. Moderate Study

▸ SSRIs potentially increase the risk of prolonged neuromuscular blockade when given with **mivacurium**. Unknown Theoretical

Nevirapine → see NNRTIs

Nicardipine → see calcium channel blockers

Nicorandil → see TABLE 8 p. 1430 (hypotension)

▸ Aspirin is predicted to increase the risk of gastrointestinal perforation when given with **nicorandil**. Severe Theoretical

▸ Corticosteroids increase the risk of gastrointestinal perforation when given with **nicorandil**. Severe Anecdotal

▸ **Nicorandil** is predicted to increase the risk of gastrointestinal perforation when given with NSAIDs. Severe Theoretical

▸ **Nicorandil** is predicted to increase the risk of hypotension when given with phosphodiesterase type-5 inhibitors. Avoid. Severe Theoretical → Also see TABLE 8 p. 1430

Nicotinic acid → see TABLE 3 p. 1429 (anticoagulant effects)

▸ **Nicotinic acid** is predicted to increase the risk of rhabdomyolysis when given with statins. Severe Theoretical

Nifedipine → see calcium channel blockers

Nilotinib → see TABLE 15 p. 1432 (myelosuppression), TABLE 9 p. 1431 (QT-interval prolongation)

▸ **Nilotinib** is predicted to increase the exposure to abemaciclib. Moderate Study

▸ **Nilotinib** is predicted to increase the exposure to acalabrutinib. Avoid or monitor. Severe Study

▸ **Nilotinib** is predicted to increase the exposure to aldosterone antagonists (eplerenone). Adjust **eplerenone** dose, p. 208. Severe Study

▸ **Nilotinib** is predicted to increase the exposure to alpha blockers (tamsulosin). Moderate Theoretical

▸ Oral antacids are predicted to decrease the absorption of oral **nilotinib**. Separate administration by at least 2 hours. Moderate Theoretical

▸ Anti-androgens (apalutamide, enzalutamide) are predicted to moderately decrease the exposure to **nilotinib**. Avoid. Severe Study → Also see TABLE 9 p. 1431

▸ **Nilotinib** is predicted to increase the exposure to antiarrhythmics (propafenone). Monitor and adjust dose. Moderate Study

▸ Antiepileptics (carbamazepine, fosphenytoin, phenobarbital, phenytoin, primidone) are predicted to moderately decrease the exposure to **nilotinib**. Avoid. Severe Study

▸ Antifungals, azoles (fluconazole, posaconazole) are predicted to increase the exposure to **nilotinib**. Moderate Theoretical → Also see TABLE 9 p. 1431

▸ Antifungals, azoles (itraconazole, ketoconazole, voriconazole) are predicted to moderately increase the exposure to **nilotinib**. Avoid. Severe Study → Also see TABLE 9 p. 1431

▸ **Nilotinib** is predicted to increase the exposure to antihistamines, non-sedating (mizolastine). Severe Theoretical

▸ **Nilotinib** is predicted to increase the exposure to antihistamines, non-sedating (rupatadine). Avoid. Moderate Study

▸ **Nilotinib** is predicted to increase the concentration of antimalarials (piperaquine). Severe Theoretical

▸ **Nilotinib** is predicted to increase the exposure to antipsychotics, second generation (cariprazine). Avoid. Severe Study

▸ **Nilotinib** is predicted to increase the exposure to antipsychotics, second generation (lurasidone). Adjust **lurasidone** dose. Moderate Study

▸ **Nilotinib** is predicted to increase the exposure to antipsychotics, second generation (quetiapine). Avoid. Moderate Study

▸ **Nilotinib** is predicted to increase the exposure to avapritinib. Avoid or adjust **avapritinib** dose, p. 1012. Moderate Study

▸ **Nilotinib** is predicted to increase the exposure to axitinib. Moderate Theoretical → Also see TABLE 15 p. 1432

▸ **Nilotinib** is predicted to increase the exposure to bedaquiline. Avoid prolonged use. Mild Theoretical → Also see TABLE 9 p. 1431

▸ **Nilotinib** is predicted to increase the exposure to benzodiazepines (alprazolam). Severe Study

▸ **Nilotinib** is predicted to increase the exposure to benzodiazepines (midazolam). Monitor adverse effects and adjust dose. Severe Study

▸ **Nilotinib** is predicted to increase the exposure to bosutinib. Avoid or adjust dose. Severe Theoretical → Also see TABLE 15 p. 1432 → Also see TABLE 9 p. 1431

▸ **Nilotinib** is predicted to increase the exposure to buspirone. Use with caution and adjust dose. Moderate Study

▸ **Nilotinib** is predicted to increase the exposure to cabozantinib. Moderate Theoretical → Also see TABLE 15 p. 1432 → Also see TABLE 9 p. 1431

▸ Calcium channel blockers (diltiazem, verapamil) are predicted to increase the exposure to **nilotinib**. Moderate Theoretical

▸ **Nilotinib** is predicted to increase the exposure to calcium channel blockers (amlodipine, felodipine, lacidipine, lercanidipine, nicardipine, nifedipine, nimodipine). Monitor and adjust dose. Moderate Study

▸ **Nilotinib** is predicted to increase the concentration of ciclosporin. Severe Study

▸ Cobicistat is predicted to moderately increase the exposure to **nilotinib**. Avoid. Severe Study

▸ **Nilotinib** is predicted to increase the exposure to cobimetinib. Severe Theoretical

▸ **Nilotinib** is predicted to increase the exposure to colchicine. Adjust **colchicine** dose with moderate CYP3A4 inhibitors, p. 1166. Severe Study

▸ **Nilotinib** is predicted to increase the exposure to corticosteroids (methylprednisolone). Monitor and adjust dose. Moderate Study

▸ **Nilotinib** is predicted to increase the risk of bleeding events when given with coumarins. Severe Theoretical

▸ **Nilotinib** is predicted to slightly increase the exposure to darifenacin. Moderate Study

▸ **Nilotinib** is predicted to increase the exposure to dasatinib. Severe Study → Also see TABLE 15 p. 1432 → Also see TABLE 9 p. 1431

▸ **Nilotinib** is predicted to slightly increase the exposure to dienogest. Moderate Study

▸ **Nilotinib** is predicted to increase the exposure to dipeptidylpeptidase-4 inhibitors (saxagliptin). Mild Study

▸ **Nilotinib** increases the risk of QT-prolongation when given with domperidone. Avoid. Severe Study

▸ **Nilotinib** is predicted to increase the exposure to dopamine receptor agonists (bromocriptine). Severe Theoretical

▸ **Nilotinib** is predicted to increase the concentration of dopamine receptor agonists (cabergoline). Moderate Anecdotal

▸ **Nilotinib** is predicted to moderately increase the exposure to dutasteride. Mild Study

▸ **Nilotinib** is predicted to increase the exposure to elexacaftor. Adjust tezacaftor with ivacaftor and elexacftor p. 311 dose with moderate CYP3A4 inhibitors. Severe Theoretical

▸ **Nilotinib** is predicted to increase the exposure to eliglustat. Avoid or adjust dose—consult product literature. Severe Study

▸ **Nilotinib** is predicted to moderately increase the exposure to encorafenib. Moderate Study → Also see TABLE 9 p. 1431

▸ Endothelin receptor antagonists (bosentan) are predicted to decrease the exposure to **nilotinib**. Avoid. Severe Theoretical

▸ **Nilotinib** is predicted to increase the exposure to entrectinib. Avoid moderate CYP3A4 inhibitors or adjust **entrectinib** dose, p. 1023. Severe Theoretical → Also see TABLE 9 p. 1431

Nilotinib (continued)

▸ **Nilotinib** is predicted to increase the risk of ergotism when given with ergometrine. [Severe] Theoretical

▸ **Nilotinib** is predicted to increase the risk of ergotism when given with ergotamine. [Severe] Theoretical

▸ **Nilotinib** is predicted to increase the exposure to erlotinib. [Moderate] Theoretical

▸ **Nilotinib** is predicted to increase the concentration of everolimus. Avoid or adjust dose. [Moderate] Study

▸ **Nilotinib** is predicted to increase the exposure to fesoterodine. Adjust **fesoterodine** dose with moderate CYP3A4 inhibitors in hepatic and renal impairment, p. 822. [Mild] Study

▸ **Nilotinib** is predicted to increase the exposure to gefitinib. [Moderate] Theoretical

▸ Grapefruit juice is predicted to increase the exposure to **nilotinib**. Avoid. [Severe] Theoretical

▸ **Nilotinib** is predicted to increase the concentration of guanfacine. Adjust **guanfacine** dose, p. 372. [Moderate] Theoretical

▸ H_2 receptor antagonists are predicted to decrease the absorption of **nilotinib**. H_2 **receptor antagonists** should be taken 10 hours before or 2 hours after **nilotinib**. [Mild] Theoretical

▸ HIV-protease inhibitors are predicted to moderately increase the exposure to **nilotinib**. Avoid. [Severe] Study → Also see TABLE 9 p. 1431

▸ **Nilotinib** is predicted to increase the exposure to ibrutinib. Adjust **ibrutinib** dose with moderate CYP3A4 inhibitors, p. 1027. [Severe] Study → Also see TABLE 15 p. 1432

▸ Idelalisib is predicted to moderately increase the exposure to **nilotinib**. Avoid. [Severe] Study

▸ **Nilotinib** is predicted to increase the exposure to ivabradine. Adjust **ivabradine** dose, p. 227. [Severe] Theoretical

▸ **Nilotinib** is predicted to increase the exposure to ivacaftor. Adjust ivacaftor p. 309 or tezacaftor with ivacaftor p. 311 or tezacaftor with ivacaftor and elexacftor p. 311 dose with moderate CYP3A4 inhibitors. [Severe] Study

▸ **Nilotinib** is predicted to increase the exposure to lapatinib. [Moderate] Study → Also see TABLE 9 p. 1431

▸ **Nilotinib** is predicted to increase the exposure to lomitapide. Avoid. [Moderate] Theoretical

▸ Macrolides (clarithromycin) are predicted to moderately increase the exposure to **nilotinib**. Avoid. [Severe] Study → Also see TABLE 9 p. 1431

▸ Macrolides (erythromycin) are predicted to increase the exposure to **nilotinib**. [Moderate] Theoretical → Also see TABLE 9 p. 1431

▸ **Nilotinib** is predicted to increase the exposure to midostaurin. [Moderate] Theoretical

▸ Mitotane is predicted to moderately decrease the exposure to **nilotinib**. Avoid. [Severe] Study → Also see TABLE 15 p. 1432

▸ **Nilotinib** is predicted to increase the exposure to naldemedine. [Moderate] Study

▸ **Nilotinib** is predicted to increase the exposure to naloxegol. Adjust **naloxegol** dose and monitor adverse effects, p. 70. [Moderate] Study

▸ **Nilotinib** is predicted to increase the exposure to neratinib. Avoid. [Severe] Study

▸ Neurokinin-1 receptor antagonists (aprepitant, netupitant) are predicted to increase the exposure to **nilotinib**. [Moderate] Theoretical

▸ NNRTIs (efavirenz, nevirapine) are predicted to decrease the exposure to **nilotinib**. Avoid. [Severe] Theoretical → Also see TABLE 9 p. 1431

▸ **Nilotinib** is predicted to increase the exposure to olaparib. Avoid moderate CYP3A4 inhibitors or adjust **olaparib** dose, p. 1051. [Moderate] Theoretical → Also see TABLE 15 p. 1432

▸ **Nilotinib** is predicted to increase the exposure to opioids (alfentanil, buprenorphine, fentanyl, oxycodone). Monitor and adjust dose. [Moderate] Study

▸ **Nilotinib** is predicted to increase the exposure to opioids (methadone). [Moderate] Theoretical → Also see TABLE 9 p. 1431

▸ **Nilotinib** is predicted to increase the exposure to oxybutynin. [Mild] Theoretical

▸ **Nilotinib** is predicted to increase the exposure to pazopanib. [Moderate] Theoretical → Also see TABLE 9 p. 1431

▸ **Nilotinib** is predicted to increase the risk of bleeding events when given with phenindione. [Severe] Theoretical

▸ **Nilotinib** is predicted to increase the exposure to phosphodiesterase type-5 inhibitors (avanafil). Adjust **avanafil** dose, p. 859. [Moderate] Theoretical

▸ **Nilotinib** is predicted to increase the exposure to phosphodiesterase type-5 inhibitors (sildenafil). Monitor or adjust sildenafil dose with moderate CYP3A4 inhibitors, p. 860. [Moderate] Study → Also see TABLE 9 p. 1431

▸ **Nilotinib** is predicted to increase the exposure to phosphodiesterase type-5 inhibitors (tadalafil). [Severe] Theoretical

▸ **Nilotinib** is predicted to increase the exposure to phosphodiesterase type-5 inhibitors (vardenafil). Adjust dose. [Severe] Theoretical → Also see TABLE 9 p. 1431

▸ **Nilotinib** is predicted to increase the exposure to pimozide. Avoid. [Severe] Theoretical → Also see TABLE 9 p. 1431

▸ Pitolisant is predicted to decrease the exposure to **nilotinib**. Avoid. [Severe] Theoretical

▸ **Nilotinib** is predicted to increase the exposure to ranolazine. [Severe] Study → Also see TABLE 9 p. 1431

▸ **Nilotinib** is predicted to increase the exposure to ribociclib. [Moderate] Study → Also see TABLE 15 p. 1432 → Also see TABLE 9 p. 1431

▸ Rifamycins (rifampicin) are predicted to moderately decrease the exposure to **nilotinib**. Avoid. [Severe] Study

▸ **Nilotinib** is predicted to increase the exposure to ruxolitinib. [Moderate] Theoretical → Also see TABLE 15 p. 1432

▸ **Nilotinib** increases the concentration of sirolimus. Monitor and adjust dose. [Moderate] Study

▸ Sodium zirconium cyclosilicate is predicted to decrease the exposure to **nilotinib**. Separate administration by at least 2 hours. [Moderate] Theoretical

▸ **Nilotinib** is predicted to increase the exposure to SSRIs (dapoxetine). Adjust **dapoxetine** dose with moderate CYP3A4 inhibitors, p. 867. [Moderate] Theoretical

▸ St John's wort is predicted to decrease the exposure to **nilotinib**. Avoid. [Severe] Theoretical

▸ **Nilotinib** is predicted to slightly increase the exposure to statins (atorvastatin). Monitor and adjust dose. [Severe] Theoretical

▸ **Nilotinib** is predicted to increase the exposure to statins (simvastatin). Monitor and adjust dose. [Severe] Theoretical

▸ **Nilotinib** is predicted to increase the exposure to sunitinib. [Moderate] Theoretical → Also see TABLE 15 p. 1432 → Also see TABLE 9 p. 1431

▸ **Nilotinib** is predicted to increase the concentration of tacrolimus. [Severe] Study

▸ **Nilotinib** is predicted to increase the exposure to taxanes (cabazitaxel). [Moderate] Theoretical → Also see TABLE 15 p. 1432

▸ **Nilotinib** is predicted to increase the concentration of temsirolimus. Use with caution or avoid. [Moderate] Theoretical → Also see TABLE 15 p. 1432

▸ **Nilotinib** is predicted to increase the exposure to tezacaftor. Adjust tezacaftor with ivacaftor p. 311 or tezacaftor with ivacaftor and elexacftor p. 311 dose with moderate CYP3A4 inhibitors. [Severe] Study

▸ **Nilotinib** given with a potent CYP2C19 inhibitor is predicted to increase the exposure to tofacitinib. Adjust **tofacitinib** dose, p. 1154. [Moderate] Study

▸ **Nilotinib** is predicted to increase the exposure to tolterodine. [Mild] Theoretical → Also see TABLE 9 p. 1431

▸ **Nilotinib** is predicted to increase the exposure to tolvaptan. Manufacturer advises caution or adjust **tolvaptan** dose with moderate CYP3A4 inhibitors, p. 708. [Moderate] Study

▸ **Nilotinib** is predicted to increase the exposure to trazodone. [Moderate] Theoretical

▸ **Nilotinib** is predicted to increase the exposure to venetoclax. Avoid or adjust dose—consult product literature. [Severe] Study

▸ **Nilotinib** is predicted to increase the exposure to vinca alkaloids. [Severe] Theoretical → Also see TABLE 15 p. 1432 → Also see TABLE 9 p. 1431

▸ **Nilotinib** is predicted to increase the exposure to zopiclone. Adjust dose. [Moderate] Study

Nimodipine → see calcium channel blockers

Nintedanib

Antiarrhythmics (amiodarone, dronedarone) are predicted to increase the exposure to **nintedanib**. Moderate Study

Antiepileptics (carbamazepine) are predicted to decrease the exposure to **nintedanib**. Moderate Study

Antifungals, azoles (itraconazole, ketoconazole) are predicted to increase the exposure to **nintedanib**. Moderate Study

Calcium channel blockers (verapamil) are predicted to increase the exposure to **nintedanib**. Moderate Study

Ciclosporin is predicted to increase the exposure to **nintedanib**. Moderate Study

HIV-protease inhibitors (lopinavir, ritonavir, saquinavir) are predicted to increase the exposure to **nintedanib**. Moderate Study

Lapatinib is predicted to increase the exposure to **nintedanib**. Moderate Study

Macrolides are predicted to increase the exposure to **nintedanib**. Moderate Study

Ranolazine is predicted to increase the exposure to **nintedanib**. Moderate Study

Rifamycins (rifampicin) are predicted to decrease the exposure to **nintedanib**. Moderate Study

St John's wort is predicted to decrease the exposure to **nintedanib**. Moderate Study

Vemurafenib is predicted to increase the exposure to **nintedanib**. Moderate Study

Niraparib → see TABLE 15 p. 1432 (myelosuppression)

Nitisinone
▶ **Nitisinone** is predicted to increase the exposure to adefovir. Moderate Study

▶ Anti-androgens (apalutamide, enzalutamide) are predicted to decrease the exposure to **nitisinone**. Adjust dose. Moderate Theoretical

▶ Antiepileptics (carbamazepine, fosphenytoin, phenobarbital, phenytoin, primidone) are predicted to decrease the exposure to **nitisinone**. Adjust dose. Moderate Theoretical

▶ Antifungals, azoles (itraconazole, ketoconazole, voriconazole) are predicted to increase the exposure to **nitisinone**. Adjust dose. Moderate Theoretical

▶ **Nitisinone** is predicted to increase the exposure to cephalosporins (cefaclor). Moderate Study

▶ Cobicistat is predicted to increase the exposure to **nitisinone**. Adjust dose. Moderate Theoretical

▶ **Nitisinone** is predicted to increase the exposure to coumarins (warfarin). Moderate Study

▶ **Nitisinone** is predicted to increase the exposure to ganciclovir. Moderate Study

▶ **Nitisinone** is predicted to increase the exposure to H_2 receptor antagonists (cimetidine, famotidine). Moderate Study

▶ HIV-protease inhibitors are predicted to increase the exposure to **nitisinone**. Adjust dose. Moderate Theoretical

▶ Idelalisib is predicted to increase the exposure to **nitisinone**. Adjust dose. Moderate Theoretical

▶ **Nitisinone** is predicted to increase the exposure to loop diuretics (furosemide). Moderate Study

▶ Macrolides (clarithromycin) are predicted to increase the exposure to **nitisinone**. Adjust dose. Moderate Theoretical

▶ **Nitisinone** is predicted to increase the exposure to methotrexate. Moderate Study

▶ Mitotane is predicted to decrease the exposure to **nitisinone**. Adjust dose. Moderate Theoretical

▶ **Nitisinone** is predicted to increase the exposure to NSAIDs (celecoxib). Moderate Study

▶ **Nitisinone** is predicted to increase the exposure to oseltamivir. Moderate Study

▶ **Nitisinone** is predicted to increase the exposure to penicillins (benzylpenicillin). Moderate Study

▶ Rifamycins (rifampicin) are predicted to decrease the exposure to **nitisinone**. Adjust dose. Moderate Theoretical

▶ **Nitisinone** is predicted to increase the exposure to sulfonylureas (glimepiride, tolbutamide). Moderate Study

Nitrates → see TABLE 7 p. 1430 (first-dose hypotension), TABLE 8 p. 1430 (hypotension)

glyceryl trinitrate · isosorbide dinitrate · isosorbide mononitrate

PHARMACOLOGY Drugs with antimuscarinic effects can cause dry mouth, which can reduce the effectiveness of sublingual glyceryl trinitrate tablets.

▶ **Nitrates** are predicted to increase the risk of methaemoglobinaemia when given with topical anaesthetics, local (prilocaine). Avoid. Severe Theoretical

▶ **Nitrates** are predicted to increase the risk of methaemoglobinaemia when given with dapsone. Severe Theoretical

▶ **Nitrates** potentially increase the risk of hypotension when given with phosphodiesterase type-5 inhibitors. Avoid. Severe Study → Also see TABLE 8 p. 1430

Nitrazepam → see benzodiazepines

Nitrofurantoin → see TABLE 12 p. 1432 (peripheral neuropathy)
▶ **Nitrofurantoin** is predicted to increase the risk of methaemoglobinaemia when given with topical anaesthetics, local (prilocaine). Use with caution or avoid. Severe Theoretical

▶ **Nitrofurantoin** is predicted to increase the risk of methaemoglobinaemia when given with dapsone. Severe Theoretical

▶ Oral magnesium trisilicate decreases the absorption of oral nitrofurantoin. Moderate Study

Nitroprusside → see TABLE 8 p. 1430 (hypotension)
▶ **Nitroprusside** is predicted to increase the risk of methaemoglobinaemia when given with anaesthetics, local (prilocaine). Severe Theoretical

▶ **Nitroprusside** is predicted to increase the risk of methaemoglobinaemia when given with dapsone. Severe Theoretical

Nitrous oxide → see TABLE 8 p. 1430 (hypotension), TABLE 11 p. 1431 (CNS depressant effects)
▶ **Nitrous oxide** potentially increases the risk of methotrexate toxicity when given with methotrexate. Avoid. Severe Study

Nivolumab → see monoclonal antibodies

Nizatidine → see H_2 receptor antagonists

NNRTIs → see TABLE 9 p. 1431 (QT-interval prolongation)

doravirine · efavirenz · etravirine · nevirapine · rilpivirine

▶ NNRTIs (efavirenz, nevirapine) are predicted to decrease the exposure to acalabrutinib. Severe Theoretical

▶ Oral antacids are predicted to decrease the exposure to oral rilpivirine. Rilpivirine should be taken 4 hours before or 2 hours after antacids. Severe Theoretical

▶ Anti-androgens (apalutamide, enzalutamide) are predicted to decrease the exposure to **doravirine**. Avoid. Severe Study

▶ Anti-androgens (apalutamide, enzalutamide) are predicted to decrease the exposure to **etravirine**. Avoid. Severe Theoretical

▶ Anti-androgens (apalutamide, enzalutamide) markedly decrease the exposure to **rilpivirine**. Avoid. Severe Study

▶ Anti-androgens (enzalutamide) are predicted to decrease the exposure to **nevirapine**. Severe Theoretical

▶ NNRTIs (efavirenz, nevirapine) are predicted to decrease the exposure to anti-androgens (darolutamide). Avoid. Moderate Theoretical

▶ NNRTIs (efavirenz, nevirapine) are predicted to decrease the exposure to antiarrhythmics (dronedarone). Severe Theoretical → Also see TABLE 9 p. 1431

▶ Antiepileptics (carbamazepine) slightly decrease the exposure to **efavirenz** and **efavirenz** slightly decreases the exposure to antiepileptics (carbamazepine). Severe Study

▶ Antiepileptics (carbamazepine, fosphenytoin, phenobarbital, phenytoin, primidone) are predicted to decrease the exposure to **doravirine**. Avoid. Severe Study

▶ Antiepileptics (carbamazepine, fosphenytoin, phenobarbital, phenytoin, primidone) are predicted to decrease the exposure to **etravirine**. Avoid. Severe Theoretical

▶ Antiepileptics (carbamazepine, fosphenytoin, phenobarbital, phenytoin, primidone) markedly decrease the exposure to **rilpivirine**. Avoid. Severe Study

▶ Antiepileptics (fosphenytoin, phenytoin) slightly decrease the exposure to **efavirenz** and **efavirenz** affects the concentration of antiepileptics (fosphenytoin, phenytoin). Severe Theoretical

NNRTIs (continued)

▶ Antiepileptics (oxcarbazepine) are predicted to decrease the exposure to **doravirine**. Avoid. Severe Theoretical

▶ Antiepileptics (oxcarbazepine) are predicted to decrease the concentration of **rilpivirine**. Avoid. Severe Theoretical

▶ Antiepileptics (phenobarbital) are predicted to decrease the exposure to **efavirenz** and **efavirenz** affects the concentration of antiepileptics (phenobarbital). Severe Theoretical

▶ **Nevirapine** is predicted to decrease the concentration of antiepileptics (carbamazepine, fosphenytoin, phenobarbital, phenytoin, primidone) and antiepileptics (carbamazepine, fosphenytoin, phenobarbital, phenytoin, primidone) are predicted to decrease the concentration of **nevirapine**. Severe Study

▶ **Efavirenz** is predicted to affect the efficacy of antiepileptics (primidone) and antiepileptics (primidone) are predicted to slightly decrease the exposure to **efavirenz**. Severe Theoretical

▶ Antifungals, azoles (fluconazole) slightly to moderately increase the exposure to **nevirapine**. Moderate Study

▶ Antifungals, azoles (itraconazole, ketoconazole, voriconazole) are predicted to increase the exposure to **doravirine**. Mild Study

▶ NNRTIs **(efavirenz, nevirapine)** are predicted to decrease the exposure to antifungals, azoles (isavuconazole). Avoid. Severe Theoretical

▶ **Efavirenz** slightly decreases the exposure to antifungals, azoles (itraconazole). Avoid and for 14 days after stopping **efavirenz**, p. 683. Moderate Study

▶ **Nevirapine** moderately decreases the exposure to antifungals, azoles (itraconazole). Avoid and for 14 days after stopping **nevirapine**. Moderate Study

▶ **Efavirenz** moderately decreases the exposure to antifungals, azoles (ketoconazole). Severe Study

▶ **Nevirapine** moderately decreases the exposure to antifungals, azoles (ketoconazole). Avoid. Severe Study

▶ **Efavirenz** slightly decreases the exposure to antifungals, azoles (posaconazole). Avoid. Moderate Study

▶ **Efavirenz** moderately decreases the exposure to antifungals, azoles (voriconazole) and antifungals, azoles (voriconazole) slightly increase the exposure to **efavirenz**. Adjust dose. Severe Study → Also see TABLE 9 p. 1431

▶ **Nevirapine** is predicted to decrease the exposure to antifungals, azoles (voriconazole) and antifungals, azoles (voriconazole) increase the exposure to **nevirapine**. Monitor and adjust dose. Severe Theoretical

▶ **Efavirenz** decreases the concentration of antimalarials (artemether). Severe Study → Also see TABLE 9 p. 1431

▶ **Etravirine** decreases the exposure to antimalarials (artemether). Moderate Study

▶ **Efavirenz** moderately decreases the exposure to antimalarials (atovaquone). Avoid. Moderate Study

▶ **Efavirenz** affects the exposure to antimalarials (proguanil). Avoid. Moderate Study

▶ NNRTIs **(efavirenz, nevirapine)** are predicted to decrease the exposure to antipsychotics, second generation (cariprazine). Avoid. Severe Theoretical

▶ NNRTIs **(efavirenz, nevirapine)** are predicted to decrease the exposure to antipsychotics, second generation (lurasidone). Monitor and adjust dose. Moderate Theoretical

▶ NNRTIs **(efavirenz, nevirapine)** are predicted to decrease the exposure to antipsychotics, second generation (quetiapine). Moderate Study

▶ **Etravirine** is predicted to decrease the exposure to avapritinib. Avoid. Severe Theoretical

▶ NNRTIs **(efavirenz, nevirapine)** are predicted to decrease the exposure to avapritinib. Avoid. Severe Study

▶ NNRTIs **(efavirenz, nevirapine)** are predicted to decrease the exposure to axitinib. Moderate Theoretical

▶ **Etravirine** is predicted to decrease the exposure to bedaquiline. Avoid. Severe Theoretical

▶ NNRTIs **(efavirenz, nevirapine)** are predicted to decrease the exposure to bedaquiline. Avoid. Severe Study → Also see TABLE 9 p. 1431

▶ **Efavirenz** is predicted to alter the effects of benzodiazepines (midazolam). Avoid. Moderate Theoretical

▶ **Nevirapine** decreases the concentration of benzodiazepines (midazolam). Monitor and adjust dose. Moderate Study

▶ NNRTIs **(efavirenz, etravirine, nevirapine)** are predicted to decrease the exposure to bosutinib. Avoid. Severe Theoretical → Also see TABLE 9 p. 1431

▶ **Etravirine** is predicted to decrease the exposure to brigatinib. Avoid. Moderate Theoretical

▶ NNRTIs **(efavirenz, nevirapine)** are predicted to decrease the exposure to brigatinib. Avoid. Severe Study

▶ **Efavirenz** is predicted to decrease the exposure to bupropion. Moderate Study

▶ NNRTIs **(efavirenz, nevirapine)** are predicted to decrease the exposure to cabozantinib. Moderate Theoretical → Also see TABLE p. 1431

▶ NNRTIs **(efavirenz, nevirapine)** are predicted to decrease the exposure to calcium channel blockers (amlodipine, felodipine, lacidipine, lercanidipine, nicardipine, nifedipine, nimodipine). Monitor and adjust dose. Moderate Theoretical

▶ NNRTIs **(efavirenz, nevirapine)** are predicted to decrease the exposure to calcium channel blockers (diltiazem, verapamil). Moderate Theoretical

▶ Calcium salts (calcium carbonate) are predicted to slightly decrease the exposure to **rilpivirine**. **Calcium carbonate** should be taken 2 hours before or 4 hours after **rilpivirine**. Severe Theoretical

▶ **Efavirenz** is predicted to decrease the concentration of caspofungin. Adjust dose. Moderate Study

▶ **Nevirapine** is predicted to decrease the concentration of caspofungin. Adjust dose. Moderate Theoretical

▶ **Efavirenz** decreases the concentration of ciclosporin. Monitor concentration and adjust dose. Moderate Study

▶ **Nevirapine** is predicted to decrease the concentration of ciclosporin. Moderate Study

▶ Cobicistat is predicted to increase the exposure to **doravirine**. Mild Study

▶ NNRTIs **(efavirenz, nevirapine)** are predicted to decrease the exposure to cobicistat. Avoid. Severe Theoretical

▶ NNRTIs **(efavirenz, nevirapine)** are predicted to decrease the exposure to cobimetinib. Avoid. Severe Theoretical

▶ NNRTIs **(efavirenz, nevirapine)** are predicted to decrease the efficacy of combined hormonal contraceptives. For FSRH guidance, see Contraceptives, interactions p. 840. Severe Study

▶ Corticosteroids (dexamethasone) are predicted to decrease the concentration of **rilpivirine**. Avoid multiple-dose dexamethasone. Severe Theoretical

▶ **Efavirenz** is predicted to affect the concentration of coumarins. Adjust dose. Moderate Theoretical

▶ **Etravirine** increases the anticoagulant effect of coumarins. Moderate Theoretical

▶ **Nevirapine** potentially alters the anticoagulant effect of coumarins. Severe Anecdotal

▶ NNRTIs **(efavirenz, nevirapine)** are predicted to decrease the exposure to crizotinib. Avoid. Severe Theoretical → Also see TABLE 9 p. 1431

▶ Dabrafenib is predicted to decrease the exposure to **doravirine**. Avoid or adjust doravirine p. 683 or lamivudine with tenofovir disoproxil and doravirine p. 692 dose. Severe Theoretical

▶ **Efavirenz** increases the risk of increased ALT concentrations when given with dasabuvir. Avoid. Severe Study

▶ NNRTIs **(etravirine, nevirapine)** are predicted to decrease the exposure to dasabuvir. Avoid. Severe Theoretical

▶ NNRTIs **(efavirenz, nevirapine)** are predicted to decrease the exposure to dasatinib. Severe Study → Also see TABLE 9 p. 1431

▶ NNRTIs **(efavirenz, nevirapine)** are predicted to decrease the efficacy of desogestrel. For FSRH guidance, see Contraceptives, interactions p. 840. Severe Theoretical

▶ **Etravirine** moderately decreases the exposure to dolutegravir. Avoid unless given with atazanavir, darunavir, or lopinavir (all boosted with ritonavir). Severe Study

▶ NNRTIs **(efavirenz, nevirapine)** decrease the exposure to dolutegravir. Adjust dose. Severe Study

▶ **Etravirine** is predicted to decrease the exposure to elbasvir. Avoid. Unknown Theoretical

▶ NNRTIs **(efavirenz, nevirapine)** are predicted to moderately decrease the exposure to elbasvir. Avoid. Severe Study

NNRTIs **(efavirenz, nevirapine)** are predicted to decrease the exposure to eliglustat. Moderate Theoretical

NNRTIs **(efavirenz, nevirapine)** are predicted to decrease the concentration of elvitegravir. Avoid. Severe Theoretical

Endothelin receptor antagonists **(bosentan)** are predicted to decrease the exposure to **doravirine**. Avoid or adjust doravirine p. 683 or lamivudine with tenofovir disoproxil and doravirine p. 692 dose. Severe Theoretical

Endothelin receptor antagonists **(bosentan)** are predicted to decrease the exposure to **etravirine**. Avoid. Severe Study

Endothelin receptor antagonists **(bosentan)** are predicted to decrease the exposure to **nevirapine**. Severe Theoretical

Endothelin receptor antagonists **(bosentan)** are predicted to decrease the exposure to **rilpivirine**. Avoid. Severe Theoretical

NNRTIs **(efavirenz, nevirapine)** are predicted to decrease the exposure to entrectinib. Avoid. Severe Theoretical → Also see **TABLE 9** p. 1431

NNRTIs **(efavirenz, nevirapine)** are predicted to decrease the effects of ergotamine. Moderate Theoretical

NNRTIs **(efavirenz, nevirapine)** are predicted to decrease the exposure to erlotinib. Severe Theoretical

NNRTIs **(efavirenz, nevirapine)** are predicted to decrease the efficacy of etonogestrel. For FSRH guidance, see Contraceptives, interactions p. 840. Severe Theoretical

NNRTIs **(efavirenz, nevirapine)** are predicted to decrease the concentration of everolimus. Avoid or adjust dose. Severe Study

NNRTIs **(efavirenz, nevirapine)** are predicted to decrease the exposure to gefitinib. Avoid. Severe Theoretical

Etravirine is predicted to decrease the exposure to glasdegib. Avoid or adjust **glasdegib** dose, p. 1049. Moderate Theoretical

NNRTIs **(efavirenz, nevirapine)** are predicted to decrease the exposure to glasdegib. Avoid or adjust **glasdegib** dose, p. 1049. Severe Theoretical → Also see **TABLE 9** p. 1431

NNRTIs **(efavirenz, nevirapine)** are predicted to decrease the exposure to glecaprevir. Avoid. Severe Study

Etravirine is predicted to decrease the exposure to grazoprevir. Avoid. Mild Theoretical

NNRTIs **(efavirenz, nevirapine)** are predicted to markedly decrease the exposure to grazoprevir. Avoid. Severe Study

NNRTIs **(efavirenz, nevirapine)** are predicted to decrease the concentration of guanfacine. Adjust dose. Moderate Theoretical

H₂ receptor antagonists are predicted to decrease the exposure to rilpivirine. **H₂ receptor antagonists** should be taken 12 hours before or 4 hours after **rilpivirine**. Severe Study

HIV-protease inhibitors are predicted to increase the exposure to **doravirine**. Mild Study

Efavirenz decreases the exposure to HIV-protease inhibitors. Refer to specialist literature. Severe Study → Also see **TABLE 9** p. 1431

HIV-protease inhibitors **(tipranavir)** decrease the exposure to **etravirine**. Avoid. Severe Study

Etravirine increases the exposure to HIV-protease inhibitors **(fosamprenavir)** boosted with ritonavir. Refer to specialist literature. Moderate Study

Nevirapine decreases the exposure to HIV-protease inhibitors. Refer to specialist literature. Moderate Study

NNRTIs **(efavirenz, nevirapine)** are predicted to decrease the effects of hormone replacement therapy. Moderate Anecdotal

Idelalisib is predicted to increase the exposure to **doravirine**. Mild Study

NNRTIs **(efavirenz, nevirapine)** are predicted to decrease the exposure to idelalisib. Avoid. Moderate Theoretical

NNRTIs **(efavirenz, nevirapine)** are predicted to decrease the exposure to imatinib. Moderate Study

NNRTIs **(efavirenz, nevirapine)** are predicted to decrease the exposure to ivacaftor. Moderate Study

NNRTIs **(efavirenz, nevirapine)** are predicted to decrease the exposure to lapatinib. Avoid. Severe Study → Also see **TABLE 9** p. 1431

NNRTIs **(efavirenz, nevirapine)** are predicted to decrease the exposure to larotrectinib. Avoid. Moderate Study

Efavirenz is predicted to decrease the concentration of letermovir. Moderate Theoretical

Etravirine is predicted to decrease the exposure to letermovir. Moderate Theoretical

► NNRTIs **(efavirenz, nevirapine)** are predicted to decrease the efficacy of levonorgestrel. For FSRH guidance, see Contraceptives, interactions p. 840. Severe Theoretical

► NNRTIs **(efavirenz, nevirapine)** are predicted to decrease the exposure to lorlatinib. Avoid. Severe Theoretical

► Lumacaftor is predicted to decrease the exposure to **doravirine**. Avoid. Severe Theoretical

► Macrolides **(clarithromycin)** are predicted to increase the exposure to **doravirine**. Mild Study

► **Etravirine** decreases the exposure to macrolides **(clarithromycin)** and macrolides **(clarithromycin)** slightly increase the exposure to **etravirine**. Severe Study

► NNRTIs **(efavirenz, nevirapine)** decrease the exposure to macrolides **(clarithromycin)**. Moderate Study → Also see **TABLE 9** p. 1431

► **Efavirenz** decreases the exposure to maraviroc. Refer to specialist literature. Severe Theoretical

► **Etravirine** (with a boosted protease inhibitor) increases the exposure to maraviroc. Avoid or adjust dose. Moderate Study

► Mitotane is predicted to decrease the exposure to **doravirine**. Avoid. Severe Study

► Mitotane is predicted to decrease the exposure to **etravirine**. Avoid. Severe Theoretical

► Mitotane is predicted to decrease the exposure to **nevirapine**. Severe Theoretical

► Mitotane markedly decreases the exposure to **rilpivirine**. Avoid. Severe Study

► Modafinil is predicted to decrease the exposure to **doravirine**. Avoid or adjust doravirine p. 683 or lamivudine with tenofovir disoproxil and doravirine p. 692 dose. Severe Theoretical

► NNRTIs **(efavirenz, nevirapine)** are predicted to decrease the exposure to neratinib. Severe Study

► NNRTIs **(efavirenz, nevirapine)** are predicted to decrease the exposure to neurokinin-1 receptor antagonists **(aprepitant)**. Moderate Study

► NNRTIs **(efavirenz, nevirapine)** are predicted to decrease the exposure to neurokinin-1 receptor antagonists **(fosaprepitant, netupitant)**. Moderate Theoretical

► NNRTIs **(efavirenz, nevirapine)** are predicted to decrease the exposure to nilotinib. Avoid. Severe Theoretical → Also see **TABLE 9** p. 1431

► NNRTIs **(efavirenz, nevirapine)** are predicted to decrease the exposure to NNRTIs **(doravirine)**. Avoid or adjust doravirine p. 683 or lamivudine with tenofovir disoproxil and doravirine p. 692 dose. Severe Theoretical

► NNRTIs **(nevirapine)** decrease the concentration of NNRTIs **(efavirenz)**. Avoid. Severe Study

► NNRTIs **(efavirenz)** are predicted to decrease the exposure to NNRTIs **(etravirine)**. Avoid. Severe Study

► NNRTIs **(nevirapine)** are predicted to decrease the exposure to NNRTIs **(etravirine)**. Avoid. Severe Study

► NNRTIs **(efavirenz, etravirine, nevirapine)** are predicted to decrease the exposure to NNRTIs **(rilpivirine)**. Avoid. Severe Theoretical

► NNRTIs **(efavirenz, nevirapine)** are predicted to decrease the efficacy of norethisterone. For FSRH guidance, see Contraceptives, interactions p. 840. Severe Anecdotal

► **Nevirapine** is predicted to decrease the concentration of NRTIs **(zidovudine)**. Refer to specialist literature. Severe Theoretical

► NNRTIs **(efavirenz, nevirapine)** are predicted to decrease the exposure to olaparib. Avoid. Moderate Theoretical

► NNRTIs **(efavirenz, etravirine, nevirapine)** are predicted to decrease the exposure to ombitasvir. Avoid. Severe Theoretical

► NNRTIs **(efavirenz, nevirapine)** decrease the exposure to opioids **(methadone)**. Monitor and adjust dose. Severe Study → Also see **TABLE 9** p. 1431

► **Efavirenz** is predicted to decrease the exposure to osimertinib. Moderate Theoretical → Also see **TABLE 9** p. 1431

► **Nevirapine** is predicted to decrease the exposure to osimertinib. Severe Theoretical

► NNRTIs **(efavirenz, nevirapine)** are predicted to decrease the exposure to ospemifene. Moderate Study

► **Etravirine** is predicted to decrease the exposure to paritaprevir. Avoid. Severe Theoretical

NNRTIs (continued)

▸ NNRTIs **(efavirenz, nevirapine)** are predicted to decrease the exposure to paritaprevir (with ritonavir and ombitasvir). Avoid. [Severe] Study

▸ **Etravirine** moderately decreases the exposure to phosphodiesterase type-5 inhibitors. Adjust dose. [Moderate] Study

▸ NNRTIs **(efavirenz, nevirapine)** are predicted to decrease the exposure to phosphodiesterase type-5 inhibitors. [Moderate] Theoretical → Also see **TABLE 9** p. 1431

▸ NNRTIs **(efavirenz, nevirapine)** are predicted to decrease the exposure to pibrentasvir. Avoid. [Severe] Study

▸ Pitolisant is predicted to decrease the exposure to **efavirenz**. [Mild] Theoretical

▸ Proton pump inhibitors are predicted to decrease the exposure to **rilpivirine**. Avoid. [Severe] Study

▸ NNRTIs **(efavirenz, nevirapine)** are predicted to decrease the exposure to ribociclib. [Moderate] Study → Also see **TABLE 9** p. 1431

▸ Rifamycins **(rifabutin)** moderately decrease the exposure to **doravirine**. Adjust doravirine p. 683 or lamivudine with tenofovir disoproxil and doravirine p. 692 dose. [Moderate] Study

▸ Rifamycins **(rifabutin)** decrease the exposure to **etravirine**. [Moderate] Study

▸ Rifamycins **(rifabutin)** slightly decrease the exposure to **rilpivirine**. Adjust dose. [Severe] Study

▸ Rifamycins **(rifampicin)** are predicted to decrease the exposure to **doravirine**. Avoid. [Severe] Study

▸ Rifamycins **(rifampicin)** slightly decrease the exposure to **efavirenz**. Adjust dose. [Severe] Study

▸ Rifamycins **(rifampicin)** are predicted to decrease the exposure to **etravirine**. Avoid. [Severe] Theoretical

▸ Rifamycins **(rifampicin)** decrease the concentration of **nevirapine**. Avoid. [Severe] Study

▸ Rifamycins **(rifampicin)** markedly decrease the exposure to **rilpivirine**. Avoid. [Severe] Study

▸ **Efavirenz** slightly decreases the exposure to rifamycins (rifabutin). Adjust dose. [Severe] Study

▸ NNRTIs **(efavirenz, nevirapine)** are predicted to decrease the exposure to ruxolitinib. Monitor and adjust dose. [Moderate] Theoretical

▸ NNRTIs **(efavirenz, nevirapine)** are predicted to decrease the exposure to siponimod. Manufacturer advises caution depending on genotype—consult product literature. [Severe] Theoretical

▸ **Doravirine** is predicted to decrease the exposure to sirolimus. Monitor **sirolimus** concentration and adjust dose, p. 886. [Moderate] Theoretical

▸ NNRTIs **(efavirenz, nevirapine)** are predicted to decrease the concentration of sirolimus. Monitor and adjust dose. [Moderate] Theoretical

▸ Sodium zirconium cyclosilicate is predicted to decrease the exposure to **rilpivirine**. Separate administration by at least 2 hours. [Moderate] Theoretical

▸ St John's wort is predicted to decrease the exposure to **etravirine**. Avoid. [Severe] Study

▸ St John's wort is predicted to decrease the exposure to NNRTIs **(doravirine, rilpivirine)**. Avoid. [Severe] Theoretical

▸ St John's wort is predicted to decrease the concentration of NNRTIs **(efavirenz, nevirapine)**. Avoid. [Severe] Theoretical

▸ NNRTIs **(efavirenz, nevirapine)** slightly decrease the exposure to statins (atorvastatin). [Mild] Study

▸ NNRTIs **(efavirenz, nevirapine)** moderately decrease the exposure to statins (simvastatin). [Moderate] Study

▸ **Doravirine** is predicted to decrease the exposure to tacrolimus. Monitor **tacrolimus** concentration and adjust dose, p. 887. [Moderate] Theoretical

▸ NNRTIs **(efavirenz, nevirapine)** are predicted to decrease the concentration of tacrolimus. Monitor and adjust dose. [Moderate] Theoretical

▸ NNRTIs **(efavirenz, nevirapine)** are predicted to decrease the exposure to taxanes (cabazitaxel). Avoid. [Severe] Study

▸ Telotristat ethyl is predicted to decrease the exposure to **doravirine**. Avoid or adjust doravirine p. 683 or lamivudine with tenofovir disoproxil and doravirine p. 692 dose. [Severe] Theoretical

▸ NNRTIs **(efavirenz, nevirapine)** are predicted to decrease the concentration of temsirolimus. Avoid. [Severe] Theoretical

▸ NNRTIs **(efavirenz, nevirapine)** are predicted to decrease the exposure to ticagrelor. [Moderate] Theoretical

▸ NNRTIs **(efavirenz, nevirapine)** are predicted to decrease the exposure to tofacitinib. [Moderate] Study

▸ NNRTIs **(efavirenz, nevirapine)** decrease the efficacy of ulipristal. For FSRH guidance, see Contraceptives, interactions p. 840. [Severe] Anecdotal

▸ NNRTIs **(efavirenz, nevirapine)** are predicted to decrease the exposure to velpatasvir. Avoid. [Moderate] Theoretical

▸ NNRTIs **(efavirenz, nevirapine)** are predicted to decrease the exposure to venetoclax. Avoid. [Severe] Study

▸ NNRTIs **(efavirenz, nevirapine)** are predicted to decrease the concentration of voxilaprevir. Avoid. [Severe] Theoretical

Noradrenaline/norepinephrine → see sympathomimetics, vasoconstrictor

Norethisterone

▸ Antiepileptics (carbamazepine, eslicarbazepine, fosphenytoin, oxcarbazepine, perampanel, phenobarbital, phenytoin, primidone, rufinamide, topiramate) are predicted to decrease the efficacy of **norethisterone**. For FSRH guidance, see Contraceptives, interactions p. 840. [Severe] Anecdotal

▸ Endothelin receptor antagonists (bosentan) are predicted to decrease the efficacy of **norethisterone**. For FSRH guidance, see Contraceptives, interactions p. 840. [Severe] Anecdotal

▸ Griseofulvin potentially decreases the efficacy of **norethisterone**. For FSRH guidance, see Contraceptives, interactions p. 840. [Severe] Anecdotal

▸ HIV-protease inhibitors (ritonavir) are predicted to decrease the efficacy of **norethisterone**. For FSRH guidance, see Contraceptives, interactions p. 840. [Severe] Anecdotal

▸ Modafinil is predicted to decrease the efficacy of **norethisterone**. For FSRH guidance, see Contraceptives, interactions p. 840. [Severe] Anecdotal

▸ Neurokinin-1 receptor antagonists (aprepitant, fosaprepitant) are predicted to decrease the efficacy of **norethisterone**. For FSRH guidance, see Contraceptives, interactions p. 840. [Severe] Anecdotal

▸ NNRTIs (efavirenz, nevirapine) are predicted to decrease the efficacy of **norethisterone**. For FSRH guidance, see Contraceptives, interactions p. 840. [Severe] Anecdotal

▸ Rifamycins are predicted to decrease the efficacy of **norethisterone**. For FSRH guidance, see Contraceptives, interactions p. 840. [Severe] Anecdotal

▸ St John's wort is predicted to decrease the efficacy of **norethisterone**. MHRA advises avoid. For FSRH guidance, see Contraceptives, interactions p. 840. [Severe] Anecdotal

▸ Sugammadex is predicted to decrease the exposure to **norethisterone**. Use additional contraceptive precautions. [Severe] Theoretical

▸ Ulipristal is predicted to decrease the efficacy of **norethisterone**. Avoid. [Severe] Theoretical

Normal immunoglobulin → see immunoglobulins
Nortriptyline → see tricyclic antidepressants
NRTIs → see **TABLE 2** p. 1429 (nephrotoxicity), **TABLE 12** p. 1432 (peripheral neuropathy)

abacavir · emtricitabine · lamivudine · zidovudine

▸ Antiepileptics (carbamazepine, fosphenytoin, phenobarbital, phenytoin, primidone) are predicted to decrease the exposure to **abacavir**. [Moderate] Theoretical

▸ Antiepileptics (valproate) slightly increase the exposure to **zidovudine**. [Moderate] Study

▸ Antifungals, azoles (fluconazole) slightly increase the exposure to **zidovudine**. [Moderate] Study

▸ Antimalarials (pyrimethamine) are predicted to increase the risk of adverse effects when given with **zidovudine**. [Severe] Theoretical

▸ **Zidovudine** increases the risk of haematological toxicity when given with aspirin (high-dose). [Severe] Study

▸ **Zidovudine** increases the risk of haematological toxicity when given with flucytosine. Monitor and adjust dose. [Severe] Theoretical

▸ HIV-protease inhibitors (tipranavir) slightly decrease the exposure to **abacavir**. Avoid. [Severe] Study

HIV-protease inhibitors (tipranavir) slightly decrease the exposure to **zidovudine**. Avoid. Moderate Study

Leflunomide is predicted to increase the exposure to **zidovudine**. Moderate Theoretical

Macrolides (clarithromycin) decrease the absorption of **zidovudine**. Separate administration by at least 2 hours. Moderate Study

NNRTIs (nevirapine) are predicted to decrease the concentration of **zidovudine**. Refer to specialist literature. Severe Theoretical

NRTIs **(zidovudine)** increase the risk of toxicity when given with NRTIs **(lamivudine)**. Severe Anecdotal

Zidovudine increases the risk of haematological toxicity when given with NSAIDs. Severe Study → Also see **TABLE 2** p. 1429

Ribavirin increases the risk of anaemia and/or leucopenia when given with **zidovudine**. Avoid. Severe Study

Teriflunomide is predicted to increase the exposure to **zidovudine**. Moderate Theoretical

Trimethoprim slightly increases the exposure to **lamivudine**. Moderate Study

SAIDs → see **TABLE 18** p. 1433 (hyponatraemia), **TABLE 2** p. 1429 (nephrotoxicity), **TABLE 16** p. 1433 (increased serum potassium), **TABLE 4** p. 1429 (antiplatelet effects)

aceclofenac · benzydamine · bromfenac · celecoxib · dexibuprofen · dexketoprofen · diclofenac · etodolac · etoricoxib · felbinac · flurbiprofen · ibuprofen · indometacin · ketoprofen · ketorolac · mefenamic acid · meloxicam · nabumetone · naproxen · nepafenac · parecoxib · phenazone · piroxicam · sulindac · tenoxicam · tiaprofenic acid · tolfenamic acid

ROUTE-SPECIFIC INFORMATION Since systemic absorption can follow topical application, the possibility of interactions should be borne in mind.

▸ **Celecoxib** is predicted to increase the exposure to antiarrhythmics (flecainide, propafenone). Monitor and adjust dose. Moderate Theoretical

Antifungals, azoles (fluconazole) moderately increase the exposure to **celecoxib**. Adjust **celecoxib** dose, p. 1178. Moderate Study

▸ Antifungals, azoles (fluconazole) increase the exposure to **parecoxib**. Monitor and adjust dose. Moderate Study

▸ Antifungals, azoles (voriconazole) slightly increase the exposure to **diclofenac**. Monitor and adjust dose. Moderate Study

▸ Antifungals, azoles (voriconazole) moderately increase the exposure to **ibuprofen**. Adjust dose. Moderate Study

▸ **NSAIDs** are predicted to increase the risk of gastrointestinal irritation when given with bisphosphonates (alendronate, ibandronate). Moderate Study

▸ **NSAIDs** are predicted to increase the risk of renal impairment when given with bisphosphonates (clodronate). Moderate Study

▸ Ceritinib is predicted to increase the exposure to NSAIDs **(celecoxib, diclofenac)**. Adjust dose. Moderate Study

▸ Ciclosporin increases the concentration of **diclofenac**. Severe Study → Also see **TABLE 2** p. 1429 → Also see **TABLE 16** p. 1433

▸ **Etoricoxib** increases the exposure to combined hormonal contraceptives. Moderate Study

▸ **NSAIDs** increase the risk of gastrointestinal bleeding when given with corticosteroids. Severe Study

▸ **NSAIDs** increase the risk of renal impairment when given with daptomycin. Moderate Theoretical

▸ **Indometacin** increases the concentration of digoxin. Severe Study

▸ Erlotinib is predicted to increase the risk of gastrointestinal perforation when given with **NSAIDs**. Severe Theoretical

▸ **Etoricoxib** increases the exposure to hormone replacement therapy. Moderate Study

▸ **NSAIDs** are predicted to increase the risk of gastrointestinal bleeding when given with iron chelators (deferasirox). Severe Theoretical

▸ **Diclofenac** is predicted to increase the exposure to iron chelators (deferiprone). Moderate Theoretical

▸ Leflunomide is predicted to increase the exposure to NSAIDs **(indometacin, ketoprofen)**. Moderate Theoretical

▸ **NSAIDs** increase the concentration of lithium. Monitor and adjust dose. Severe Study

▸ **NSAIDs** are predicted to increase the risk of toxicity when given with methotrexate. Severe Study → Also see **TABLE 2** p. 1429

▸ **NSAIDs** (high-dose) are predicted to decrease the efficacy of mifamurtide. Severe Theoretical

▸ Nicorandil is predicted to increase the risk of gastrointestinal perforation when given with **NSAIDs**. Severe Theoretical

▸ Nitisinone is predicted to increase the exposure to **celecoxib**. Moderate Study

▸ NRTIs (zidovudine) increase the risk of haematological toxicity when given with **NSAIDs**. Severe Study → Also see **TABLE 2** p. 1429

▸ **NSAIDs** are predicted to increase the exposure to pemetrexed. Use with caution or avoid. Severe Theoretical → Also see **TABLE 2** p. 1429

▸ **NSAIDs** potentially increase the risk of seizures when given with quinolones. Severe Theoretical

▸ Regorafenib is predicted to increase the exposure to **mefenamic acid**. Avoid. Moderate Theoretical → Also see **TABLE 4** p. 1429

▸ Rifamycins (rifampicin) moderately decrease the exposure to NSAIDs **(celecoxib, diclofenac, etoricoxib)**. Moderate Study

▸ Teriflunomide is predicted to increase the exposure to NSAIDs **(indometacin, ketoprofen)**. Moderate Theoretical

▸ **NSAIDs** increase the risk of acute renal failure when given with thiazide diuretics. Severe Theoretical → Also see **TABLE 18** p. 1433

Obeticholic acid

▸ **Obeticholic acid** decreases the anticoagulant effect of coumarins (warfarin). Severe Study

▸ **Obeticholic acid** is predicted to increase the exposure to theophylline. Severe Theoretical

▸ **Obeticholic acid** is predicted to increase the exposure to tizanidine. Severe Theoretical

Obinutuzumab → see monoclonal antibodies

Ocrelizumab → see monoclonal antibodies

Octreotide

▸ **Octreotide** decreases the absorption of oral ciclosporin. Adjust ciclosporin dose, p. 884. Severe Anecdotal

▸ **Octreotide** (short-acting) decreases the exposure to telotristat ethyl. **Telotristat ethyl** should be taken at least 30 minutes before **octreotide**. Moderate Study

Ofloxacin → see quinolones

Olanzapine → see antipsychotics, second generation

Olaparib → see **TABLE 15** p. 1432 (myelosuppression)

FOOD AND LIFESTYLE Bitter (Seville) orange is predicted to increase the exposure to olaparib.

▸ Anti-androgens (apalutamide, enzalutamide) are predicted to decrease the exposure to **olaparib**. Avoid. Moderate Theoretical

▸ Antiarrhythmics (dronedarone) are predicted to increase the exposure to **olaparib**. Avoid moderate CYP3A4 inhibitors or adjust **olaparib** dose, p. 1051. Moderate Theoretical

▸ Antiepileptics (carbamazepine, fosphenytoin, phenobarbital, phenytoin, primidone) are predicted to decrease the exposure to **olaparib**. Avoid. Moderate Theoretical

▸ Antifungals, azoles (fluconazole, isavuconazole, posaconazole) are predicted to increase the exposure to **olaparib**. Avoid moderate CYP3A4 inhibitors or adjust **olaparib** dose, p. 1051. Moderate Theoretical

▸ Antifungals, azoles (itraconazole, ketoconazole, voriconazole) are predicted to increase the exposure to **olaparib**. Avoid potent CYP3A4 inhibitors or adjust **olaparib** dose, p. 1051. Moderate Study

▸ Calcium channel blockers (diltiazem, verapamil) are predicted to increase the exposure to **olaparib**. Avoid moderate CYP3A4 inhibitors or adjust **olaparib** dose, p. 1051. Moderate Theoretical

▸ Cobicistat is predicted to increase the exposure to **olaparib**. Avoid potent CYP3A4 inhibitors or adjust **olaparib** dose, p. 1051. Moderate Study

▸ **Olaparib** potentially affects the efficacy of combined hormonal contraceptives. Use additional contraceptive precautions. Moderate Theoretical

▸ Crizotinib is predicted to increase the exposure to **olaparib**. Avoid moderate CYP3A4 inhibitors or adjust **olaparib** dose, p. 1051. Moderate Theoretical

▸ Endothelin receptor antagonists (bosentan) are predicted to decrease the exposure to **olaparib**. Avoid. Moderate Theoretical

A1

Interactions | Appendix 1

Olaparib (continued)
- Grapefruit juice is predicted to increase the exposure to **olaparib**. Avoid. Moderate Theoretical
- HIV-protease inhibitors are predicted to increase the exposure to **olaparib**. Avoid potent CYP3A4 inhibitors or adjust **olaparib** dose, p. 1051. Moderate Study
- Idelalisib is predicted to increase the exposure to **olaparib**. Avoid potent CYP3A4 inhibitors or adjust **olaparib** dose, p. 1051. Moderate Study
- Imatinib is predicted to increase the exposure to **olaparib**. Avoid moderate CYP3A4 inhibitors or adjust **olaparib** dose, p. 1051. Moderate Theoretical → Also see TABLE 15 p. 1432
- Letermovir is predicted to increase the exposure to **olaparib**. Avoid moderate CYP3A4 inhibitors or adjust **olaparib** dose, p. 1051. Moderate Theoretical
- Macrolides (clarithromycin) are predicted to increase the exposure to **olaparib**. Avoid potent CYP3A4 inhibitors or adjust **olaparib** dose, p. 1051. Moderate Study
- Macrolides (erythromycin) are predicted to increase the exposure to **olaparib**. Avoid moderate CYP3A4 inhibitors or adjust **olaparib** dose, p. 1051. Moderate Theoretical
- Mitotane is predicted to decrease the exposure to **olaparib**. Avoid. Moderate Theoretical → Also see TABLE 15 p. 1432
- Neurokinin-1 receptor antagonists (aprepitant, netupitant) are predicted to increase the exposure to **olaparib**. Avoid moderate CYP3A4 inhibitors or adjust **olaparib** dose, p. 1051. Moderate Theoretical
- Nilotinib is predicted to increase the exposure to **olaparib**. Avoid moderate CYP3A4 inhibitors or adjust **olaparib** dose, p. 1051. Moderate Theoretical → Also see TABLE 15 p. 1432
- NNRTIs (efavirenz, nevirapine) are predicted to decrease the exposure to **olaparib**. Avoid. Moderate Theoretical
- Rifamycins (rifampicin) are predicted to decrease the exposure to **olaparib**. Avoid. Moderate Theoretical
- St John's wort is predicted to decrease the exposure to **olaparib**. Avoid. Moderate Theoretical

Olmesartan → see angiotensin-II receptor antagonists

Olodaterol → see beta₂ agonists

Ombitasvir
- Anti-androgens (enzalutamide) are predicted to decrease the exposure to **ombitasvir**. Avoid. Severe Theoretical
- Antiepileptics (carbamazepine, fosphenytoin, phenobarbital, phenytoin) are predicted to decrease the exposure to **ombitasvir**. Severe Theoretical
- **Ombitasvir** (in fixed-dose combination with dasabuvir) decreases the concentration of HIV-protease inhibitors (darunavir). Avoid or adjust dose. Moderate Study
- Mitotane is predicted to decrease the exposure to **ombitasvir**. Avoid. Severe Theoretical
- NNRTIs (efavirenz, etravirine, nevirapine) are predicted to decrease the exposure to **ombitasvir**. Avoid. Severe Theoretical
- Rifamycins (rifampicin) are predicted to decrease the exposure to **ombitasvir**. Avoid. Severe Theoretical
- St John's wort is predicted to decrease the exposure to **ombitasvir**. Avoid. Severe Theoretical

Omega-3-acid ethyl esters → see TABLE 3 p. 1429 (anticoagulant effects)

Omeprazole → see proton pump inhibitors

Ondansetron → see 5-HT3-receptor antagonists

Opicapone
- **Opicapone** increases the exposure to levodopa. Adjust dose. Moderate Study
- **Opicapone** is predicted to increase the exposure to loperamide. Avoid. Moderate Study
- **Opicapone** is predicted to increase the risk of elevated blood pressure when given with MAOIs, irreversible. Avoid. Severe Theoretical
- **Opicapone** is predicted to increase the exposure to meglitinides (repaglinide). Avoid. Moderate Study
- **Opicapone** is predicted to increase the risk of elevated blood pressure when given with moclobemide. Avoid. Severe Theoretical
- **Opicapone** is predicted to increase the exposure to montelukast. Avoid. Moderate Study

- **Opicapone** is predicted to increase the exposure to pioglitazone. Avoid. Moderate Study
- **Opicapone** is predicted to increase the risk of cardiovascular adverse effects when given with sympathomimetics, inotropic. Severe Theoretical
- **Opicapone** is predicted to increase the risk of cardiovascular adverse effects when given with sympathomimetics, vasoconstrictor (adrenaline/epinephrine, noradrenaline/norepinephrine). Severe Theoretical

Opioids → see TABLE 6 p. 1430 (bradycardia), TABLE 13 p. 1432 (serotonin syndrome), TABLE 9 p. 1431 (QT-interval prolongation), TABLE 11 p. 1431 (CNS depressant effects)

> alfentanil · buprenorphine · codeine · diamorphine · dihydrocodeine · diphenoxylate · dipipanone · fentanyl · hydromorphone · meptazinol · methadone · morphine · oxycodone · pentazocine · pethidine · remifentanil · tapentadol · tramadol

- Alcohol causes rapid release of opioids (hydromorphone, morphine) (from extended-release preparations). Avoid. Severe Study → Also see TABLE 11 p. 1431
- Anti-androgens (apalutamide, enzalutamide) are predicted to decrease the exposure to **buprenorphine**. Monitor and adjust dose. Moderate Theoretical
- Anti-androgens (apalutamide, enzalutamide) decrease the exposure to **methadone**. Monitor and adjust dose. Severe Study → Also see TABLE 9 p. 1431
- Anti-androgens (apalutamide, enzalutamide) are predicted to decrease the exposure to **oxycodone**. Monitor and adjust dose. Moderate Study
- Anti-androgens (apalutamide, enzalutamide) are predicted to decrease the exposure to opioids (alfentanil, fentanyl). Moderate Study
- Antiarrhythmics (amiodarone) are predicted to increase the concentration of **fentanyl**. Moderate Theoretical → Also see TABLE 6 p. 1430
- Antiarrhythmics (dronedarone) are predicted to increase the exposure to **methadone**. Moderate Theoretical → Also see TABLE 9 p. 1431
- Antiarrhythmics (dronedarone) are predicted to increase the exposure to opioids (alfentanil, buprenorphine, fentanyl, oxycodone). Monitor and adjust dose. Moderate Study
- Antiepileptics (carbamazepine) decrease the concentration of **tramadol**. Adjust dose. Severe Study
- Antiepileptics (carbamazepine, fosphenytoin, phenobarbital, phenytoin, primidone) are predicted to decrease the exposure to **buprenorphine**. Monitor and adjust dose. Moderate Theoretical → Also see TABLE 11 p. 1431
- Antiepileptics (carbamazepine, fosphenytoin, phenobarbital, phenytoin, primidone) decrease the exposure to **methadone**. Monitor and adjust dose. Severe Study → Also see TABLE 11 p. 1431
- Antiepileptics (carbamazepine, fosphenytoin, phenobarbital, phenytoin, primidone) are predicted to decrease the exposure to **oxycodone**. Monitor and adjust dose. Moderate Study → Also see TABLE 11 p. 1431
- Antiepileptics (carbamazepine, fosphenytoin, phenobarbital, phenytoin, primidone) are predicted to decrease the exposure to opioids (alfentanil, fentanyl). Moderate Study → Also see TABLE 11 p. 1431
- Antifungals, azoles (fluconazole, isavuconazole, posaconazole) are predicted to increase the exposure to **methadone**. Moderate Theoretical → Also see TABLE 9 p. 1431
- Antifungals, azoles (itraconazole, ketoconazole, voriconazole) are predicted to increase the exposure to **methadone**. Adjust dose. Severe Theoretical → Also see TABLE 9 p. 1431
- Antifungals, azoles (miconazole) are predicted to increase the exposure to **alfentanil**. Use with caution and adjust dose. Moderate Theoretical
- Antifungals, azoles (fluconazole, isavuconazole, posaconazole) are predicted to increase the exposure to opioids (alfentanil, buprenorphine, fentanyl, oxycodone). Monitor and adjust dose. Moderate Study
- Antifungals, azoles (itraconazole, ketoconazole, voriconazole) are predicted to increase the exposure to opioids (alfentanil, buprenorphine, fentanyl, oxycodone). Monitor and adjust dose. Severe Study

Bictegravir is predicted to increase the exposure to **methadone**. Moderate Theoretical

Brigatinib potentially decreases the concentration of opioids **(alfentanil, fentanyl)**. Avoid. Moderate Theoretical

Bupropion is predicted to decrease the efficacy of **codeine**. Moderate Theoretical

Bupropion is predicted to decrease the efficacy of **tramadol**. Severe Study → Also see **TABLE 13** p. 1432

Calcium channel blockers (diltiazem, verapamil) are predicted to increase the exposure to **methadone**. Moderate Theoretical → Also see **TABLE 6** p. 1430

Calcium channel blockers (diltiazem, verapamil) are predicted to increase the exposure to opioids **(alfentanil, buprenorphine, fentanyl, oxycodone)**. Monitor and adjust dose. Moderate Study → Also see **TABLE 6** p. 1430

Ceritinib is predicted to increase the exposure to opioids **(alfentanil, fentanyl)**. Avoid. Severe Theoretical

Cinacalcet is predicted to increase the exposure to **codeine**. Moderate Theoretical

Cinacalcet is predicted to decrease the efficacy of **tramadol**. Severe Study

Cobicistat is predicted to increase the exposure to opioids **(alfentanil, buprenorphine, fentanyl, oxycodone)**. Monitor and adjust dose. Severe Study

Crizotinib is predicted to increase the exposure to **methadone**. Moderate Theoretical → Also see **TABLE 6** p. 1430 → Also see **TABLE 9** p. 1431

Crizotinib is predicted to increase the exposure to opioids **(alfentanil, buprenorphine, fentanyl, oxycodone)**. Monitor and adjust dose. Moderate Study → Also see **TABLE 6** p. 1430

► **Tapentadol** is predicted to increase the risk of serotonin syndrome when given with drugs that cause serotonin syndrome (see **TABLE 3** p. 1429). Severe Theoretical

► Endothelin receptor antagonists (bosentan) decrease the exposure to **methadone**. Monitor and adjust dose. Severe Study

► Entrectinib is predicted to increase the exposure to opioids **(alfentanil, fentanyl)**. Mild Theoretical

► H₂ receptor antagonists (cimetidine) increase the concentration of **alfentanil**. Use with caution and adjust dose. Severe Study

► H₂ receptor antagonists (cimetidine) increase the exposure to **fentanyl**. Moderate Study

► HIV-protease inhibitors boosted with ritonavir are predicted to decrease the exposure to **methadone**. Moderate Study → Also see **TABLE 9** p. 1431

► HIV-protease inhibitors (ritonavir) are predicted to decrease the concentration of **morphine**. Moderate Theoretical

► HIV-protease inhibitors (ritonavir) increase the risk of CNS toxicity when given with **pethidine**. Avoid. Severe Study

► HIV-protease inhibitors are predicted to increase the exposure to opioids **(alfentanil, buprenorphine, fentanyl, oxycodone)**. Monitor and adjust dose. Severe Study

► Idelalisib is predicted to increase the exposure to **methadone**. Severe Theoretical

► Idelalisib is predicted to increase the exposure to opioids **(alfentanil, buprenorphine, fentanyl, oxycodone)**. Monitor and adjust dose. Severe Study

► Imatinib is predicted to increase the exposure to **methadone**. Moderate Theoretical

► Imatinib is predicted to increase the exposure to opioids **(alfentanil, buprenorphine, fentanyl, oxycodone)**. Monitor and adjust dose. Moderate Study

► Larotrectinib is predicted to increase the exposure to opioids **(alfentanil, fentanyl)**. Use with caution and adjust dose. Mild Theoretical

► Letermovir is predicted to increase the exposure to **methadone**. Moderate Theoretical

► Letermovir is predicted to increase the exposure to opioids **(alfentanil, buprenorphine, fentanyl, oxycodone)**. Monitor and adjust dose. Moderate Study

► Lorlatinib is predicted to decrease the exposure to opioids **(alfentanil, fentanyl)**. Avoid. Moderate Theoretical

► Macrolides (clarithromycin) are predicted to increase the concentration of **methadone**. Severe Theoretical → Also see **TABLE 9** p. 1431

► Macrolides (erythromycin) are predicted to increase the exposure to **methadone**. Moderate Theoretical → Also see **TABLE 9** p. 1431

► Macrolides (clarithromycin) are predicted to increase the exposure to opioids **(alfentanil, buprenorphine, fentanyl, oxycodone)**. Monitor and adjust dose. Severe Study

► Macrolides (erythromycin) are predicted to increase the exposure to opioids **(alfentanil, buprenorphine, fentanyl, oxycodone)**. Monitor and adjust dose. Moderate Study

► MAO-B inhibitors (rasagiline) are predicted to increase the risk of adverse effects when given with **pethidine**. Avoid and for 14 days after stopping **rasagiline**. Severe Theoretical → Also see **TABLE 13** p. 1432

► MAO-B inhibitors (safinamide) are predicted to increase the risk of adverse effects when given with **pethidine**. Avoid and for 1 week after stopping **safinamide**. Severe Theoretical → Also see **TABLE 13** p. 1432

► MAO-B inhibitors (selegiline) increase the risk of adverse effects when given with **pethidine**. Avoid. Severe Anecdotal → Also see **TABLE 13** p. 1432

► **Opioids** are predicted to increase the risk of CNS excitation or depression when given with MAOIs, irreversible. Avoid. Severe Study → Also see **TABLE 13** p. 1432

► **Opioids** potentially decrease the absorption of oral mexiletine. Moderate Study

► Mitotane is predicted to decrease the exposure to **buprenorphine**. Monitor and adjust dose. Moderate Theoretical

► Mitotane decreases the exposure to **methadone**. Monitor and adjust dose. Severe Study

► Mitotane is predicted to decrease the exposure to opioids **(alfentanil, fentanyl)**. Moderate Study

► Mitotane is predicted to decrease the exposure to **oxycodone**. Monitor and adjust dose. Moderate Study

► Nalmefene is predicted to decrease the efficacy of **opioids**. Avoid. Severe Theoretical

► Neurokinin-1 receptor antagonists (aprepitant, netupitant) are predicted to increase the exposure to **methadone**. Moderate Theoretical

► Neurokinin-1 receptor antagonists (aprepitant, netupitant) are predicted to increase the exposure to opioids **(alfentanil, buprenorphine, fentanyl, oxycodone)**. Monitor and adjust dose. Moderate Study

► Nilotinib is predicted to increase the exposure to **methadone**. Moderate Theoretical → Also see **TABLE 9** p. 1431

► Nilotinib is predicted to increase the exposure to opioids **(alfentanil, buprenorphine, fentanyl, oxycodone)**. Monitor and adjust dose. Moderate Study

► NNRTIs (efavirenz, nevirapine) decrease the exposure to **methadone**. Monitor and adjust dose. Severe Study → Also see **TABLE 9** p. 1431

► **Opioids (buprenorphine)** are predicted to increase the risk of opiate withdrawal when given with opioids **(alfentanil)**. Severe Theoretical → Also see **TABLE 11** p. 1431

► **Opioids (pentazocine)** are predicted to increase the risk of opiate withdrawal when given with opioids **(alfentanil, codeine, diamorphine, dihydrocodeine, dipipanone, fentanyl, hydromorphone, meptazinol, methadone, morphine, oxycodone)**. Severe Theoretical → Also see **TABLE 13** p. 1432 → Also see **TABLE 11** p. 1431

► **Opioids (buprenorphine)** are predicted to increase the risk of opiate withdrawal when given with opioids **(codeine, diamorphine, dihydrocodeine, dipipanone, fentanyl, hydromorphone, meptazinol, methadone, morphine, oxycodone, pentazocine, pethidine, remifentanil, tapentadol, tramadol)**. Severe Theoretical → Also see **TABLE 11** p. 1431

► **Opioids (pentazocine)** are predicted to increase the risk of opiate withdrawal when given with opioids **(pethidine, remifentanil, tapentadol, tramadol)**. Severe Theoretical → Also see **TABLE 13** p. 1432 → Also see **TABLE 11** p. 1431

► **Opioids** potentially increase the risk of adverse effects when given with ozanimod. Severe Theoretical → Also see **TABLE 6** p. 1430

► Palbociclib is predicted to increase the exposure to opioids **(alfentanil, fentanyl)**. Adjust dose. Moderate Theoretical

► Pitolisant is predicted to decrease the exposure to **morphine**. Mild Theoretical

Opioids (continued)

▶ Ribociclib is predicted to increase the exposure to opioids (**alfentanil, fentanyl**). Use with caution and adjust dose. Moderate Theoretical

▶ Rifamycins (**rifampicin**) are predicted to decrease the exposure to **buprenorphine**. Monitor and adjust dose. Moderate Theoretical

▶ Rifamycins (**rifampicin**) decrease the exposure to **methadone**. Monitor and adjust dose. Severe Study

▶ Rifamycins (**rifampicin**) are predicted to decrease the exposure to **oxycodone**. Monitor and adjust dose. Moderate Study

▶ Rifamycins (**rifampicin**) are predicted to decrease the exposure to opioids (**alfentanil, fentanyl**). Moderate Study

▶ Rifamycins (**rifampicin**) decrease the exposure to opioids (**codeine, morphine**). Moderate Study

▶ Rucaparib is predicted to increase the exposure to opioids (**alfentanil, fentanyl**). Monitor and adjust dose. Moderate Study

▶ SSRIs (**fluoxetine, paroxetine**) are predicted to decrease the efficacy of **codeine**. Moderate Theoretical

▶ SSRIs (**fluoxetine, paroxetine**) are predicted to decrease the efficacy of **tramadol**. Severe Study → Also see TABLE 13 p. 1432

▶ St John's wort increase the exposure to **methadone**. Monitor and adjust dose. Severe Study → Also see TABLE 13 p. 1432

▶ St John's wort moderately decreases the exposure to **oxycodone**. Adjust dose. Moderate Study

▶ Terbinafine is predicted to decrease the efficacy of **codeine**. Moderate Theoretical

▶ Terbinafine is predicted to decrease the efficacy of **tramadol**. Severe Study

Orlistat

SEPARATION OF ADMINISTRATION Orlistat might affect the absorption of concurrently administered drugs—consider separating administration. Particular care should be taken with antiepileptics, antiretrovirals, and drugs that have a narrow therapeutic index.

Orphenadrine → see TABLE 10 p. 1431 (antimuscarinics)

Oseltamivir

▶ Leflunomide is predicted to increase the exposure to **oseltamivir**. Moderate Theoretical

▶ Nitisinone is predicted to increase the exposure to **oseltamivir**. Moderate Study

▶ Teriflunomide is predicted to increase the exposure to **oseltamivir**. Moderate Study

Osimertinib → see TABLE 9 p. 1431 (QT-interval prolongation)

▶ Anti-androgens (**apalutamide, enzalutamide**) are predicted to moderately decrease the exposure to **osimertinib**. Avoid. Moderate Study → Also see TABLE 9 p. 1431

▶ Antiepileptics (**carbamazepine, fosphenytoin, phenobarbital, phenytoin, primidone**) are predicted to moderately decrease the exposure to **osimertinib**. Avoid. Moderate Study

▶ Endothelin receptor antagonists (**bosentan**) are predicted to decrease the exposure to **osimertinib**. Moderate Theoretical

▶ Mitotane is predicted to moderately decrease the exposure to **osimertinib**. Avoid. Moderate Study

▶ NNRTIs (**efavirenz**) are predicted to decrease the exposure to **osimertinib**. Moderate Theoretical → Also see TABLE 9 p. 1431

▶ NNRTIs (**nevirapine**) are predicted to decrease the exposure to **osimertinib**. Severe Theoretical

▶ Rifamycins (**rifampicin**) are predicted to moderately decrease the exposure to **osimertinib**. Avoid. Moderate Study

▶ St John's wort is predicted to decrease the exposure to **osimertinib**. Avoid. Moderate Theoretical

▶ Osimertinib slightly increases the exposure to statins (**rosuvastatin**). Moderate Study

Ospemifene

▶ Anti-androgens (**apalutamide, enzalutamide**) are predicted to moderately decrease the exposure to **ospemifene**. Moderate Study

▶ Antiepileptics (**carbamazepine, fosphenytoin, phenobarbital, phenytoin, primidone**) are predicted to moderately decrease the exposure to **ospemifene**. Moderate Study

▶ Antifungals, azoles (**fluconazole**) increase the exposure to **ospemifene**. Use with caution or avoid. Moderate Study

▶ Antifungals, azoles (**itraconazole, ketoconazole, voriconazole**) are predicted to increase the exposure to **ospemifene**. Avoid in poor CYP2C9 metabolisers. Moderate Study

▶ Cobicistat is predicted to increase the exposure to **ospemifene**. Avoid in poor CYP2C9 metabolisers. Moderate Study

▶ Combined hormonal contraceptives potentially oppose the effects of **ospemifene**. Severe Theoretical

▶ Endothelin receptor antagonists (**bosentan**) are predicted to decrease the exposure to **ospemifene**. Moderate Study

▶ HIV-protease inhibitors are predicted to increase the exposure to **ospemifene**. Avoid in poor CYP2C9 metabolisers. Moderate Study

▶ Hormone replacement therapy potentially opposes the effects of **ospemifene**. Avoid. Severe Theoretical

▶ Idelalisib is predicted to increase the exposure to **ospemifene**. Avoid in poor CYP2C9 metabolisers. Moderate Study

▶ Macrolides (**clarithromycin**) are predicted to increase the exposure to **ospemifene**. Avoid in poor CYP2C9 metabolisers. Moderate Study

▶ Mitotane is predicted to moderately decrease the exposure to **ospemifene**. Moderate Study

▶ NNRTIs (**efavirenz, nevirapine**) are predicted to decrease the exposure to **ospemifene**. Moderate Study

▶ Rifamycins (**rifampicin**) are predicted to moderately decrease the exposure to **ospemifene**. Moderate Study

▶ St John's wort is predicted to decrease the exposure to **ospemifene**. Moderate Study

Oxaliplatin → see platinum compounds

Oxazepam → see benzodiazepines

Oxcarbazepine → see antiepileptics

Oxybuprocaine → see anaesthetics, local

Oxybutynin → see TABLE 10 p. 1431 (antimuscarinics)

▶ Antiarrhythmics (**dronedarone**) are predicted to increase the exposure to **oxybutynin**. Mild Theoretical

▶ Oxybutynin potentially increases the risk of overheating and dehydration when given with antiepileptics (**zonisamide**). Avoid in children. Severe Theoretical

▶ Antifungals, azoles (**fluconazole, isavuconazole, posaconazole**) are predicted to increase the exposure to **oxybutynin**. Mild Theoretical

▶ Antifungals, azoles (**itraconazole, ketoconazole, voriconazole**) are predicted to increase the exposure to **oxybutynin**. Mild Study

▶ Calcium channel blockers (**diltiazem, verapamil**) are predicted to increase the exposure to **oxybutynin**. Mild Theoretical

▶ Cobicistat is predicted to increase the exposure to **oxybutynin**. Mild Study

▶ Crizotinib is predicted to increase the exposure to **oxybutynin**. Mild Theoretical

▶ HIV-protease inhibitors are predicted to increase the exposure to **oxybutynin**. Mild Study

▶ Idelalisib is predicted to increase the exposure to **oxybutynin**. Mild Study

▶ Imatinib is predicted to increase the exposure to **oxybutynin**. Mild Theoretical

▶ Letermovir is predicted to increase the exposure to **oxybutynin**. Mild Theoretical

▶ Macrolides (**clarithromycin**) are predicted to increase the exposure to **oxybutynin**. Mild Study

▶ Macrolides (**erythromycin**) are predicted to increase the exposure to **oxybutynin**. Mild Study

▶ Neurokinin-1 receptor antagonists (**aprepitant, netupitant**) are predicted to increase the exposure to **oxybutynin**. Mild Theoretical

▶ Nilotinib is predicted to increase the exposure to **oxybutynin**. Mild Theoretical

Oxycodone → see opioids

Oxymetholone

▶ Oxymetholone increases the anticoagulant effect of coumarins. Severe Anecdotal

▶ Oxymetholone increases the anticoagulant effect of phenindione. Severe Anecdotal

Oxytetracycline → see tetracyclines

Ozanimod → see TABLE 6 p. 1430 (bradycardia), TABLE 9 p. 1431 (QT-interval prolongation)

FOOD AND LIFESTYLE Tyramine-rich foods might increase the risk of hypertensive crisis when given ozanimod.

▸ Ciclosporin is predicted to increase the exposure to the active metabolite of **ozanimod**. Avoid. Moderate Study

▸ Clopidogrel is predicted to increase the exposure to the active metabolite of **ozanimod**. Severe Study

▸ Eltrombopag is predicted to increase the exposure to the active metabolite of **ozanimod**. Avoid. Moderate Study

▸ Fibrates (gemfibrozil) are predicted to increase the exposure to the active metabolite of **ozanimod**. Severe Study

▸ Leflunomide is predicted to increase the exposure to the active metabolite of **ozanimod**. Avoid. Moderate Study

▸ **Ozanimod** potentially increases the risk of a hypertensive crisis when given with linezolid. Avoid. Severe Theoretical

▸ Live vaccines are predicted to increase the risk of generalised infection (possibly life-threatening) when given with **ozanimod**. Avoid and for 3 months after stopping **ozanimod**. Severe Theoretical

▸ **Ozanimod** potentially increases the risk of a hypertensive crisis when given with MAO-B inhibitors and MAO-B inhibitors potentially decrease the exposure to the active metabolite of **ozanimod**. Avoid. Severe Theoretical → Also see TABLE 6 p. 1430

▸ **Ozanimod** potentially increases the risk of a hypertensive crisis when given with MAOIs, irreversible. Avoid. Severe Theoretical

▸ **Ozanimod** potentially increases the risk of a hypertensive crisis when given with moclobemide. Avoid. Severe Theoretical

▸ **Ozanimod** potentially increases the risk of immunosuppression when given with monoclonal antibodies (alemtuzumab). Avoid. Severe Theoretical

▸ Opioids potentially increase the risk of adverse effects when given with **ozanimod**. Severe Theoretical → Also see TABLE 6 p. 1430

▸ Rifamycins (rifampicin) moderately decrease the exposure to the active metabolite of **ozanimod**. Moderate Study

▸ SSRIs potentially increase the risk of adverse effects when given with **ozanimod**. Severe Theoretical

▸ Sympathomimetics, vasoconstrictor potentially increase the risk of a hypertensive crisis when given with **ozanimod**. Severe Theoretical

▸ Teriflunomide is predicted to increase the exposure to the active metabolite of **ozanimod**. Avoid. Moderate Study

▸ Tricyclic antidepressants potentially increase the risk of adverse effects when given with **ozanimod**. Severe Theoretical

Paclitaxel → see taxanes

Palbociclib → see TABLE 15 p. 1432 (myelosuppression)

▸ Anti-androgens (apalutamide, enzalutamide) are predicted to decrease the exposure to **palbociclib**. Avoid. Severe Study

▸ Antiepileptics (carbamazepine, fosphenytoin, phenobarbital, phenytoin, primidone) are predicted to decrease the exposure to **palbociclib**. Avoid. Severe Study

▸ Antifungals, azoles (itraconazole, ketoconazole, voriconazole) are predicted to increase the exposure to **palbociclib**. Avoid or adjust **palbociclib** dose, p. 1038. Severe Study

▸ **Palbociclib** increases the exposure to benzodiazepines (midazolam). Moderate Study

▸ **Palbociclib** is predicted to increase the exposure to ciclosporin. Adjust dose. Moderate Theoretical

▸ Cobicistat is predicted to increase the exposure to **palbociclib**. Avoid or adjust **palbociclib** dose, p. 1038. Severe Study

▸ **Palbociclib** is predicted to increase the exposure to ergotamine. Adjust dose. Moderate Theoretical

▸ **Palbociclib** is predicted to increase the exposure to everolimus. Adjust dose. Moderate Theoretical

▸ Grapefruit juice is predicted to increase the exposure to **palbociclib**. Avoid. Severe Theoretical

▸ HIV-protease inhibitors are predicted to increase the exposure to **palbociclib**. Avoid or adjust **palbociclib** dose, p. 1038. Severe Study

▸ Idelalisib is predicted to increase the exposure to **palbociclib**. Avoid or adjust **palbociclib** dose, p. 1038. Severe Study

▸ Macrolides (clarithromycin) are predicted to increase the exposure to **palbociclib**. Avoid or adjust **palbociclib** dose, p. 1038. Severe Study

▸ Mitotane is predicted to decrease the exposure to **palbociclib**. Avoid. Severe Study → Also see TABLE 15 p. 1432

▸ **Palbociclib** is predicted to increase the exposure to opioids (alfentanil, fentanyl). Adjust dose. Moderate Theoretical

▸ **Palbociclib** is predicted to increase the exposure to pimozide. Adjust dose. Moderate Theoretical

▸ Rifamycins (rifampicin) are predicted to decrease the exposure to **palbociclib**. Avoid. Severe Study

▸ **Palbociclib** is predicted to increase the exposure to sirolimus. Adjust dose. Moderate Theoretical

▸ St John's wort is predicted to decrease the exposure to **palbociclib**. Avoid. Severe Theoretical

▸ **Palbociclib** is predicted to increase the exposure to tacrolimus. Adjust dose. Moderate Theoretical

Paliperidone → see antipsychotics, second generation

Palonosetron → see 5-HT3-receptor antagonists

Pamidronate → see bisphosphonates

Pancreatin

▸ **Pancreatin** is predicted to decrease the effects of acarbose. Avoid. Moderate Theoretical

Pancuronium → see neuromuscular blocking drugs, non-depolarising

Panitumumab → see monoclonal antibodies

Panobinostat → see TABLE 15 p. 1432 (myelosuppression), TABLE 9 p. 1431 (QT-interval prolongation)

FOOD AND LIFESTYLE Avoid pomegranate, pomegranate juice, and star fruit as they are predicted to increase panobinostat exposure.

▸ Anti-androgens (apalutamide, enzalutamide) are predicted to decrease the exposure to **panobinostat**. Avoid. Moderate Theoretical → Also see TABLE 9 p. 1431

▸ Antiarrhythmics (amiodarone, dronedarone) are predicted to increase the exposure to **panobinostat**. Adjust dose. Moderate Theoretical → Also see TABLE 9 p. 1431

▸ Antiepileptics (carbamazepine, fosphenytoin, phenobarbital, phenytoin, primidone) are predicted to decrease the exposure to **panobinostat**. Avoid. Moderate Theoretical

▸ Antifungals, azoles (itraconazole, ketoconazole, voriconazole) are predicted to increase the exposure to **panobinostat**. Adjust **panobinostat** dose; in hepatic impairment avoid, p. 979. Moderate Study → Also see TABLE 9 p. 1431

▸ Antifungals, azoles (posaconazole) are predicted to increase the exposure to **panobinostat**. Adjust dose. Moderate Theoretical

▸ **Panobinostat** is predicted to increase the exposure to atomoxetine. Monitor and adjust dose. Severe Theoretical

▸ **Panobinostat** is predicted to increase the exposure to beta blockers, selective (metoprolol). Monitor and adjust dose. Moderate Theoretical

▸ **Panobinostat** is predicted to increase the exposure to beta blockers, selective (nebivolol). Monitor and adjust dose. Mild Theoretical

▸ Calcium channel blockers (verapamil) are predicted to increase the exposure to **panobinostat**. Adjust dose. Moderate Theoretical

▸ Ciclosporin is predicted to increase the exposure to **panobinostat**. Adjust dose. Moderate Theoretical

▸ Cobicistat is predicted to increase the exposure to **panobinostat**. Adjust **panobinostat** dose; in hepatic impairment avoid, p. 979. Moderate Study

▸ HIV-protease inhibitors are predicted to increase the exposure to **panobinostat**. Adjust **panobinostat** dose; in hepatic impairment avoid, p. 979. Moderate Study → Also see TABLE 9 p. 1431

▸ Idelalisib is predicted to increase the exposure to **panobinostat**. Adjust **panobinostat** dose; in hepatic impairment avoid, p. 979. Moderate Study

▸ Lapatinib is predicted to increase the exposure to **panobinostat**. Adjust dose. Moderate Theoretical → Also see TABLE 9 p. 1431

▸ Macrolides (azithromycin, erythromycin) are predicted to increase the exposure to **panobinostat**. Adjust dose. Moderate Theoretical → Also see TABLE 9 p. 1431

▸ Macrolides (clarithromycin) are predicted to increase the exposure to **panobinostat**. Adjust **panobinostat** dose; in hepatic impairment avoid, p. 979. Moderate Study → Also see TABLE 9 p. 1431

▸ Mitotane is predicted to decrease the exposure to **panobinostat**. Avoid. Moderate Theoretical → Also see TABLE 15 p. 1432

Panobinostat (continued)
▸ **Panobinostat** is predicted to increase the exposure to pimozide. Avoid. Severe Theoretical → Also see TABLE 9 p. 1431
▸ Ranolazine is predicted to increase the exposure to **panobinostat**. Adjust dose. Moderate Theoretical → Also see TABLE 9 p. 1431
▸ Rifamycins (rifampicin) are predicted to decrease the exposure to **panobinostat**. Avoid. Moderate Theoretical
▸ St John's wort is predicted to decrease the exposure to **panobinostat**. Avoid. Moderate Theoretical
▸ Vemurafenib is predicted to increase the exposure to **panobinostat**. Adjust dose. Moderate Theoretical → Also see TABLE 9 p. 1431

Pantoprazole → see proton pump inhibitors
Paracetamol → see TABLE 1 p. 1429 (hepatotoxicity)
▸ Alcohol (in those who drink heavily) causes severe liver damage when given with **paracetamol**. Severe Study → Also see TABLE 1 p. 1429
▸ **Paracetamol** is predicted to decrease the clearance of alkylating agents (busulfan). Moderate Theoretical
▸ **Paracetamol** is predicted to increase the risk of methaemoglobinaemia when given with topical anaesthetics, local (prilocaine). Use with caution or avoid. Severe Theoretical
▸ Antiepileptics (carbamazepine, fosphenytoin, phenobarbital, phenytoin, primidone) decrease the exposure to **paracetamol**. Moderate Study → Also see TABLE 1 p. 1429
▸ **Paracetamol** increases the anticoagulant effect of coumarins. Moderate Study
▸ **Paracetamol** is predicted to increase the risk of methaemoglobinaemia when given with dapsone. Severe Theoretical
▸ Imatinib increases the risk of hepatotoxicity when given with **paracetamol**. Severe Anecdotal
▸ **Paracetamol** potentially increases the risk of high anion gap metabolic acidosis when given with penicillins (flucloxacillin). Severe Theoretical → Also see TABLE 1 p. 1429
▸ **Paracetamol** is predicted to increase the anticoagulant effect of phenindione. Severe Theoretical
▸ Pitolisant is predicted to decrease the exposure to **paracetamol**. Mild Theoretical
▸ Rifamycins (rifampicin) decrease the exposure to **paracetamol**. Moderate Study

Paraldehyde → see antiepileptics
Parathyroid hormone
▸ Bisphosphonates are predicted to decrease the effects of **parathyroid hormone**. Avoid. Moderate Study

Parecoxib → see NSAIDs
Paricalcitol → see vitamin D substances
Paritaprevir
▸ **Paritaprevir** (with ritonavir and ombitasvir) is predicted to increase the exposure to aliskiren. Moderate Study
▸ Anti-androgens (apalutamide, enzalutamide) are predicted to decrease the exposure to **paritaprevir** (with ritonavir and ombitasvir). Avoid. Severe Study
▸ Antiepileptics (carbamazepine, fosphenytoin, phenobarbital, phenytoin, primidone) are predicted to decrease the exposure to **paritaprevir** (with ritonavir and ombitasvir). Avoid. Severe Study
▸ Antifungals, azoles (itraconazole, ketoconazole, voriconazole) are predicted to increase the exposure to **paritaprevir**. Avoid. Severe Study
▸ Antifungals, azoles (posaconazole) are predicted to increase the exposure to **paritaprevir** (with ritonavir and ombitasvir) and **paritaprevir** (with ritonavir and ombitasvir) is predicted to increase the exposure to antifungals, azoles (posaconazole). Avoid. Severe Study
▸ Cobicistat is predicted to increase the exposure to **paritaprevir**. Avoid. Severe Study
▸ Combined hormonal contraceptives (containing ethinylestradiol) are predicted to increase the risk of increased ALT concentrations when given with **paritaprevir** (with ritonavir and ombitasvir). Avoid. Severe Study
▸ **Paritaprevir** (in fixed-dose combination with dasabuvir) decreases the anticoagulant effect of coumarins

(acenocoumarol). Monitor INR and adjust dose. Severe Anecdotal
▸ **Paritaprevir** (in fixed-dose combination) decreases the anticoagulant effect of coumarins (warfarin). Monitor INR and adjust dose. Severe Anecdotal
▸ **Paritaprevir** (with ritonavir and ombitasvir) increases the exposure to digoxin. Monitor and adjust **digoxin** dose, p. 117. Moderate Study
▸ Endothelin receptor antagonists (bosentan) are predicted to decrease the exposure to **paritaprevir** (with ritonavir and ombitasvir). Avoid. Severe Study
▸ **Paritaprevir** (with ritonavir and ombitasvir) is predicted to increase the exposure to factor XA inhibitors (edoxaban). Severe Study
▸ HIV-protease inhibitors (atazanavir) boosted with ritonavir markedly increase the exposure to **paritaprevir**. Avoid or give unboosted. Moderate Study
▸ HIV-protease inhibitors (darunavir) boosted with ritonavir slightly decrease the exposure to **paritaprevir**. Avoid or give unboosted. Moderate Study
▸ HIV-protease inhibitors (fosamprenavir, tipranavir) boosted with ritonavir are predicted to increase the exposure to **paritaprevir**. Avoid. Severe Study
▸ HIV-protease inhibitors (lopinavir) boosted with ritonavir moderately to markedly increase the exposure to **paritaprevir**. Avoid. Severe Study
▸ HIV-protease inhibitors (saquinavir) are predicted to increase the exposure to **paritaprevir** (in fixed-dose combination). Avoid. Severe Study
▸ **Paritaprevir** is predicted to increase the exposure to idelalisib. Avoid. Severe Study
▸ **Paritaprevir** (with ritonavir and ombitasvir) is predicted to increase the exposure to loop diuretics (furosemide). Adjust dose. Moderate Theoretical
▸ **Paritaprevir** (with ritonavir and ombitasvir) is predicted to increase the exposure to loperamide. Moderate Study
▸ Macrolides (clarithromycin) are predicted to increase the exposure to **paritaprevir**. Avoid. Severe Study
▸ Macrolides (erythromycin) are predicted to increase the exposure to **paritaprevir**. Moderate Theoretical
▸ Mitotane is predicted to decrease the exposure to **paritaprevir** (with ritonavir and ombitasvir). Avoid. Severe Study
▸ NNRTIs (efavirenz, nevirapine) are predicted to decrease the exposure to **paritaprevir** (with ritonavir and ombitasvir). Avoid. Severe Study
▸ NNRTIs (etravirine) are predicted to decrease the exposure to **paritaprevir**. Avoid. Severe Theoretical
▸ Rifamycins (rifampicin) are predicted to decrease the exposure to **paritaprevir** (with ritonavir and ombitasvir). Avoid. Severe Study
▸ St John's wort is predicted to decrease the exposure to **paritaprevir** (with ritonavir and ombitasvir). Avoid. Severe Study
▸ **Paritaprevir** (in fixed-dose combination) is predicted to increase the risk of rhabdomyolysis when given with statins (atorvastatin). Avoid. Severe Theoretical
▸ **Paritaprevir** (with ritonavir and ombitasvir) is predicted to increase the exposure to statins (fluvastatin). Avoid. Moderate Theoretical
▸ **Paritaprevir** (with ritonavir and ombitasvir) increases the exposure to statins (pravastatin). Adjust **pravastatin** dose. Moderate Study
▸ **Paritaprevir** (with ritonavir and ombitasvir) slightly to moderately increases the exposure to statins (rosuvastatin). Adjust **rosuvastatin** dose, p. 218. Moderate Study
▸ **Paritaprevir** (in fixed-dose combination) is predicted to increase the risk of rhabdomyolysis when given with statins (simvastatin). Avoid. Severe Theoretical
▸ **Paritaprevir** (with ritonavir and ombitasvir) is predicted to increase the exposure to taxanes (paclitaxel). Moderate Study
▸ **Paritaprevir** (with ritonavir and ombitasvir) is predicted to increase the exposure to thrombin inhibitors (dabigatran). Severe Study

Paritaprevir (with ritonavir and ombitasvir) is predicted to increase the exposure to thyroid hormones (levothyroxine). Monitor and adjust dose. Moderate Theoretical

Paritaprevir (with ritonavir and ombitasvir) is predicted to increase the exposure to topotecan. Moderate Study

paroxetine → see SSRIs

pasireotide → see TABLE 6 p. 1430 (bradycardia), TABLE 9 p. 1431 (QT-interval prolongation)

Pasireotide is predicted to decrease the absorption of oral ciclosporin. Adjust dose. Severe Theoretical

patiromer

SEPARATION OF ADMINISTRATION Manufacturer advises take 3 hours before, or after, other drugs.

pazopanib → see TABLE 9 p. 1431 (QT-interval prolongation)

Oral antacids are predicted to decrease the absorption of oral **pazopanib**. **Pazopanib** should be taken 1 hour before or 2 hours after antacids. Moderate Theoretical

Anti-androgens (apalutamide, enzalutamide) are predicted to decrease the exposure to **pazopanib**. Avoid. Severe Theoretical → Also see TABLE 9 p. 1431

Antiarrhythmics (dronedarone) are predicted to increase the exposure to **pazopanib**. Moderate Theoretical → Also see TABLE 9 p. 1431

Antiepileptics (carbamazepine, fosphenytoin, phenobarbital, phenytoin, primidone) are predicted to decrease the exposure to **pazopanib**. Avoid. Severe Theoretical

Antifungals, azoles (fluconazole, isavuconazole, posaconazole) are predicted to increase the exposure to **pazopanib**. Moderate Theoretical → Also see TABLE 9 p. 1431

Antifungals, azoles (itraconazole, ketoconazole, voriconazole) are predicted to increase the exposure to **pazopanib**. Avoid or adjust **pazopanib** dose, p. 1039. Moderate Study → Also see TABLE 9 p. 1431

Calcium channel blockers (diltiazem, verapamil) are predicted to increase the exposure to **pazopanib**. Moderate Theoretical

Cobicistat is predicted to increase the exposure to **pazopanib**. Avoid or adjust **pazopanib** dose, p. 1039. Moderate Study

Pazopanib is predicted to increase the risk of bleeding events when given with coumarins. Severe Theoretical

Crizotinib is predicted to increase the exposure to **pazopanib**. Moderate Theoretical → Also see TABLE 9 p. 1431

Grapefruit juice is predicted to increase the exposure to **pazopanib**. Severe Theoretical

H$_2$ receptor antagonists are predicted to decrease the exposure to **pazopanib**. H$_2$ receptor antagonists should be taken 10 hours before or 2 hours after **pazopanib**. Moderate Theoretical

HIV-protease inhibitors are predicted to increase the exposure to **pazopanib**. Avoid or adjust **pazopanib** dose, p. 1039. Moderate Study → Also see TABLE 9 p. 1431

Idelalisib is predicted to increase the exposure to **pazopanib**. Avoid or adjust **pazopanib** dose, p. 1039. Moderate Study

Imatinib is predicted to increase the exposure to **pazopanib**. Moderate Theoretical

Letermovir is predicted to increase the exposure to **pazopanib**. Moderate Theoretical

Pazopanib is predicted to increase the exposure to lomitapide. Separate administration by 12 hours. Mild Theoretical

Macrolides (clarithromycin) are predicted to increase the exposure to **pazopanib**. Avoid or adjust **pazopanib** dose, p. 1039. Moderate Study → Also see TABLE 9 p. 1431

Macrolides (erythromycin) are predicted to increase the exposure to **pazopanib**. Moderate Theoretical → Also see TABLE 9 p. 1431

Mitotane is predicted to decrease the exposure to **pazopanib**. Avoid. Severe Theoretical

Neurokinin-1 receptor antagonists (aprepitant, netupitant) are predicted to increase the exposure to **pazopanib**. Moderate Theoretical

Nilotinib is predicted to increase the exposure to **pazopanib**. Moderate Theoretical → Also see TABLE 9 p. 1431

Pazopanib is predicted to increase the risk of bleeding events when given with phenindione. Severe Theoretical

Proton pump inhibitors are predicted to decrease the exposure to **pazopanib**. Avoid or administer concurrently without food. Moderate Study

▶ Rifamycins (rifampicin) are predicted to decrease the exposure to **pazopanib**. Avoid. Severe Theoretical

▶ **Pazopanib** is predicted to affect the exposure to statins (atorvastatin). Moderate Anecdotal

▶ **Pazopanib** is predicted to affect the exposure to statins (pravastatin, rosuvastatin, simvastatin). Moderate Theoretical

Pegaspargase → see TABLE 1 p. 1429 (hepatotoxicity), TABLE 15 p. 1432 (myelosuppression)

▶ Pegaspargase is predicted to increase the risk of hepatotoxicity when given with imatinib. Severe Theoretical → Also see TABLE 15 p. 1432

▶ Pegaspargase affects the efficacy of methotrexate. Severe Anecdotal → Also see TABLE 1 p. 1429 → Also see TABLE 15 p. 1432

▶ Pegaspargase potentially increases the risk of neurotoxicity when given with vinca alkaloids (vincristine). Vincristine should be taken 3 to 24 hours before **pegaspargase**. Severe Anecdotal → Also see TABLE 1 p. 1429 → Also see TABLE 15 p. 1432

Peginterferon alfa → see interferons

Pembrolizumab → see monoclonal antibodies

Pemetrexed → see TABLE 15 p. 1432 (myelosuppression), TABLE 2 p. 1429 (nephrotoxicity)

▶ Antimalarials (pyrimethamine) are predicted to increase the risk of adverse effects when given with **pemetrexed**. Severe Theoretical

▶ Aspirin (high-dose) potentially increases the exposure to **pemetrexed**. Use with caution or avoid. Severe Theoretical

▶ Live vaccines are predicted to increase the risk of generalised infection (possibly life-threatening) when given with **pemetrexed**. Public Health England advises avoid (refer to Green Book). Severe Theoretical

▶ NSAIDs are predicted to increase the exposure to **pemetrexed**. Use with caution or avoid. Severe Theoretical → Also see TABLE 2 p. 1429

Penicillamine → see TABLE 2 p. 1429 (nephrotoxicity)

▶ Oral antacids decrease the absorption of oral **penicillamine**. Separate administration by 2 hours. Mild Study

▶ Antimalarials (chloroquine) are predicted to increase the risk of haematological toxicity when given with **penicillamine**. Avoid. Severe Theoretical

▶ **Penicillamine** potentially decreases the concentration of digoxin. Separate administration by 2 hours. Severe Anecdotal

▶ Gold potentially increases the risk of adverse effects when given with **penicillamine** (in those who have had previous adverse reactions to gold). Avoid. Severe Study

▶ Hydroxychloroquine is predicted to increase the risk of haematological toxicity when given with **penicillamine**. Avoid. Severe Theoretical

▶ Oral iron is predicted to decrease the absorption of oral **penicillamine**. Separate administration by at least 2 hours. Mild Study

▶ Zinc is predicted to decrease the absorption of **penicillamine**. Mild Theoretical

Penicillins → see TABLE 1 p. 1429 (hepatotoxicity)

amoxicillin · ampicillin · benzathine benzylpenicillin · benzylpenicillin · flucloxacillin · phenoxymethylpenicillin · piperacillin · pivmecillinam · temocillin

▶ Allopurinol increases the risk of skin rash when given with penicillins (amoxicillin, ampicillin). Moderate Study

▶ Antiepileptics (valproate) increase the risk of adverse effects when given with **pivmecillinam**. Avoid. Severe Anecdotal

▶ Penicillins potentially alter the anticoagulant effect of coumarins. Monitor INR and adjust dose. Severe Anecdotal

▶ Leflunomide is predicted to increase the exposure to **benzylpenicillin**. Moderate Theoretical

▶ Penicillins are predicted to increase the risk of toxicity when given with methotrexate. Severe Anecdotal → Also see TABLE 1 p. 1429

▶ Piperacillin increases the effects of neuromuscular blocking drugs, non-depolarising. Moderate Study

▶ Nitisinone is predicted to increase the exposure to **benzylpenicillin**. Moderate Study

▶ Paracetamol potentially increases the risk of high anion gap metabolic acidosis when given with **flucloxacillin**. Severe Theoretical → Also see TABLE 1 p. 1429

A1

Interactions | Appendix 1

A1

Interactions | **Appendix 1**

Penicillins (continued)
- **Penicillins** are predicted to increase the risk of bleeding events when given with phenindione. [Severe] Theoretical
- **Piperacillin** increases the effects of suxamethonium. [Moderate] Study
- **Teriflunomide** is predicted to increase the exposure to **benzylpenicillin**. [Moderate] Study

Pentamidine → see TABLE 2 p. 1429 (nephrotoxicity), TABLE 9 p. 1431 (QT-interval prolongation)
- **Foscarnet** increases the risk of hypocalcaemia when given with **pentamidine**. [Severe] Anecdotal → Also see TABLE 2 p. 1429

Pentazocine → see opioids

Pentostatin → see TABLE 15 p. 1432 (myelosuppression), TABLE 5 p. 1430 (thromboembolism)
- **Alkylating agents** (cyclophosphamide) (high-dose) increase the risk of toxicity when given with **pentostatin**. Avoid. [Severe] Anecdotal → Also see TABLE 15 p. 1432 → Also see TABLE 5 p. 1430
- **Fludarabine** increases the risk of pulmonary toxicity when given with **pentostatin**. Avoid. [Severe] Study → Also see TABLE 15 p. 1432

Pentoxifylline
- **Pentoxifylline** is predicted to increase the concentration of aminophylline. Use with caution or avoid. [Severe] Theoretical
- **Quinolones** (ciprofloxacin) very slightly increase the exposure to **pentoxifylline**. [Moderate] Study
- **SSRIs** (fluvoxamine) are predicted to increase the exposure to **pentoxifylline**. [Moderate] Theoretical
- **Pentoxifylline** increases the concentration of theophylline. Monitor and adjust dose. [Severe] Study

Peppermint
- **Peppermint** oil is predicted to increase the exposure to lomitapide. Separate administration by 12 hours. [Moderate] Theoretical

Perampanel → see antiepileptics
Pericyazine → see phenothiazines
Perindopril → see ACE inhibitors
Pertuzumab → see monoclonal antibodies
Pethidine → see opioids
Phenazone → see NSAIDs
Phenelzine → see MAOIs, irreversible
Phenindione → see TABLE 3 p. 1429 (anticoagulant effects)

FOOD AND LIFESTYLE The effects of phenindione can be reduced or abolished by vitamin K, including that found in health foods, food supplements, enteral feeds, or large amounts of some green vegetables or green tea. Major changes in diet (especially involving salads and vegetables) and in alcohol consumption can affect anticoagulant control.

- **Antiarrhythmics** (propafenone) are predicted to increase the anticoagulant effect of **phenindione**. Monitor and adjust dose. [Moderate] Theoretical
- **Antifungals, azoles** (miconazole) greatly increase the anticoagulant effect of **phenindione**. [Severe] Theoretical
- **Axitinib** is predicted to increase the risk of bleeding events when given with **phenindione**. [Severe] Theoretical
- **Bosutinib** is predicted to increase the risk of bleeding events when given with **phenindione**. [Severe] Theoretical
- **Cabozantinib** is predicted to increase the risk of bleeding events when given with **phenindione**. [Severe] Theoretical
- **Cephalosporins** (cefazolin, ceftriaxone) potentially increase the risk of bleeding events when given with **phenindione**. [Severe] Anecdotal
- **Corticosteroids** are predicted to increase the effects of **phenindione**. [Moderate] Anecdotal
- **Crizotinib** is predicted to increase the risk of bleeding events when given with **phenindione**. [Severe] Theoretical
- **Dasatinib** is predicted to increase the risk of bleeding events when given with **phenindione**. [Severe] Theoretical
- **Disulfiram** is predicted to increase the anticoagulant effect of **phenindione**. [Severe] Theoretical
- **Enteral feeds** (vitamin-K containing) potentially decrease the effects of **phenindione**. [Severe] Theoretical
- **Erlotinib** is predicted to increase the risk of bleeding events when given with **phenindione**. [Severe] Theoretical
- **Fibrates** are predicted to increase the anticoagulant effect of **phenindione**. Monitor INR and adjust dose. [Severe] Study

- **Gefitinib** is predicted to increase the risk of bleeding events when given with **phenindione**. [Severe] Theoretical
- **H₂ receptor antagonists** (cimetidine) increase the exposure to **phenindione**. [Severe] Anecdotal
- **Imatinib** is predicted to increase the risk of bleeding events when given with **phenindione**. [Severe] Theoretical
- **Lapatinib** is predicted to increase the risk of bleeding events when given with **phenindione**. [Severe] Theoretical
- **Nandrolone** is predicted to increase the anticoagulant effect of **phenindione**. Monitor and adjust dose. [Severe] Theoretical
- **Nilotinib** is predicted to increase the risk of bleeding events when given with **phenindione**. [Severe] Theoretical
- **Oxymetholone** increases the anticoagulant effect of **phenindione**. [Severe] Anecdotal
- **Paracetamol** is predicted to increase the anticoagulant effect of **phenindione**. [Severe] Theoretical
- **Pazopanib** is predicted to increase the risk of bleeding events when given with **phenindione**. [Severe] Theoretical
- **Penicillins** are predicted to increase the risk of bleeding events when given with **phenindione**. [Severe] Theoretical
- **Ponatinib** is predicted to increase the risk of bleeding events when given with **phenindione**. [Severe] Theoretical
- **Ranibizumab** is predicted to increase the risk of bleeding events when given with **phenindione**. [Severe] Theoretical
- **Regorafenib** is predicted to increase the risk of bleeding events when given with **phenindione**. [Severe] Theoretical
- **Ruxolitinib** is predicted to increase the risk of bleeding events when given with **phenindione**. [Severe] Theoretical
- **Sorafenib** is predicted to increase the risk of bleeding events when given with **phenindione**. [Severe] Theoretical
- **Statins** (rosuvastatin) are predicted to increase the anticoagulant effect of **phenindione**. Monitor INR and adjust dose. [Severe] Theoretical
- **Sunitinib** is predicted to increase the risk of bleeding events when given with **phenindione**. [Severe] Theoretical
- **Vandetanib** is predicted to increase the risk of bleeding events when given with **phenindione**. [Severe] Theoretical

Phenobarbital → see antiepileptics
Phenothiazines → see TABLE 8 p. 1430 (hypotension), TABLE 9 p. 1431 (QT-interval prolongation), TABLE 11 p. 1431 (CNS depressant effects), TABLE 10 p. 1431 (antimuscarinics)

chlorpromazine · fluphenazine · levomepromazine · pericyazine · prochlorperazine · promazine · trifluoperazine

FOOD AND LIFESTYLE **Chlorpromazine** and **fluphenazine** dose adjustment might be necessary if smoking started or stopped during treatment.

- **Phenothiazines** are predicted to decrease the effects of amfetamines and amfetamines are predicted to decrease the effects of **phenothiazines**. [Moderate] Study
- **Oral antacids** decrease the absorption of oral **phenothiazines**. [Moderate] Anecdotal
- **Chlorpromazine** decreases the concentration of antiepileptics (phenobarbital, primidone) and antiepileptics (phenobarbital, primidone) decrease the concentration of **chlorpromazine**. [Moderate] Study → Also see TABLE 11 p. 1431
- **Chlorpromazine** is predicted to increase the risk of hyponatraemia when given with desmopressin. [Severe] Theoretical
- **Phenothiazines** are predicted to decrease the effects of dopamine receptor agonists. Avoid. [Moderate] Theoretical → Also see TABLE 8 p. 1430 → Also see TABLE 9 p. 1431 → Also see TABLE 10 p. 1431
- **Phenothiazines** decrease the effects of levodopa. Avoid or monitor worsening parkinsonian symptoms. [Severe] Study → Also see TABLE 8 p. 1430
- **Phenothiazines** potentially increase the risk of neurotoxicity when given with lithium. [Severe] Anecdotal → Also see TABLE 9 p. 1431
- **MAOIs, irreversible** are predicted to increase the risk of neuroleptic malignant syndrome when given with **phenothiazines**. [Severe] Theoretical → Also see TABLE 8 p. 1430
- **Chlorpromazine** decreases the effects of metyrapone. Avoid. [Moderate] Theoretical

Mexiletine is predicted to increase the exposure to **chlorpromazine**. Moderate Theoretical

Moclobemide increases the risk of adverse effects when given with **levomepromazine**. Moderate Study

Quinolones (ciprofloxacin) are predicted to increase the exposure to **chlorpromazine**. Moderate Theoretical

SSRIs (fluvoxamine) are predicted to increase the exposure to **chlorpromazine**. Moderate Theoretical

henoxymethylpenicillin → see penicillins

henylephrine → see sympathomimetics, vasoconstrictor

henytoin → see antiepileptics

holcodine

Pholcodine is predicted to increase the risk of CNS excitation or depression when given with MAOIs, irreversible. Avoid and for 14 days after stopping the MAOI. Severe Theoretical

hosphodiesterase type-4 inhibitors

apremilast · roflumilast

Aminophylline is predicted to slightly increase the exposure to **roflumilast**. Avoid. Moderate Theoretical

Anti-androgens (apalutamide, enzalutamide) moderately decrease the exposure to **apremilast**. Avoid. Severe Study

Anti-androgens (apalutamide, enzalutamide) are predicted to decrease the exposure to **roflumilast**. Avoid. Moderate Study

Antiepileptics (carbamazepine, fosphenytoin, phenobarbital, phenytoin, primidone) moderately decrease the exposure to **apremilast**. Avoid. Severe Study

Antiepileptics (carbamazepine, fosphenytoin, phenobarbital, phenytoin, primidone) are predicted to decrease the exposure to **roflumilast**. Avoid. Moderate Study

► Combined hormonal contraceptives are predicted to increase the exposure to **roflumilast**. Moderate Theoretical

► H₂ receptor antagonists (cimetidine) slightly increase the exposure to **roflumilast**. Moderate Study

► Mexiletine is predicted to increase the exposure to **roflumilast**. Moderate Theoretical

► Mitotane moderately decreases the exposure to **apremilast**. Avoid. Severe Study

► Mitotane is predicted to decrease the exposure to **roflumilast**. Avoid. Moderate Study

► Quinolones (ciprofloxacin) are predicted to increase the exposure to **roflumilast**. Moderate Theoretical

► Rifamycins (rifampicin) moderately decrease the exposure to **apremilast**. Avoid. Severe Study

► Rifamycins (rifampicin) are predicted to decrease the exposure to **roflumilast**. Avoid. Moderate Study

► SSRIs (fluvoxamine) are predicted to increase the exposure to **roflumilast**. Moderate Study

► St John's wort is predicted to decrease the exposure to **apremilast**. Avoid. Severe Theoretical

► Theophylline is predicted to slightly increase the exposure to **roflumilast**. Avoid. Moderate Theoretical

Phosphodiesterase type-5 inhibitors → see TABLE 8 p. 1430 (hypotension), TABLE 9 p. 1431 (QT-interval prolongation)

avanafil · sildenafil · tadalafil · vardenafil

► Alpha blockers cause significant hypotensive effects when given with **phosphodiesterase type-5 inhibitors**. Patient should be stabilised on first drug then second drug should be added at the lowest recommended dose. Severe Study → Also see TABLE 8 p. 1430

► Anti-androgens (apalutamide, enzalutamide) are predicted to decrease the exposure to phosphodiesterase type-5 inhibitors **(avanafil, tadalafil)**. Avoid. Severe Study

► Anti-androgens (apalutamide, enzalutamide) are predicted to decrease the exposure to phosphodiesterase type-5 inhibitors **(sildenafil, vardenafil)**. Moderate Theoretical → Also see TABLE 9 p. 1431

► Antiarrhythmics (dronedarone) are predicted to increase the exposure to **avanafil**. Adjust **avanafil** dose, p. 859. Moderate Theoretical

► Antiarrhythmics (dronedarone) are predicted to increase the exposure to **sildenafil**. Monitor or adjust **sildenafil** dose with moderate CYP3A4 inhibitors, p. 860. Moderate Study → Also see TABLE 9 p. 1431

► Antiarrhythmics (dronedarone) are predicted to increase the exposure to **tadalafil**. Severe Theoretical

► Antiarrhythmics (dronedarone) are predicted to increase the exposure to **vardenafil**. Adjust dose. Severe Theoretical → Also see TABLE 9 p. 1431

► Antiepileptics (carbamazepine, fosphenytoin, phenobarbital, phenytoin, primidone) are predicted to decrease the exposure to phosphodiesterase type-5 inhibitors **(avanafil, tadalafil)**. Avoid. Severe Study

► Antiepileptics (carbamazepine, fosphenytoin, phenobarbital, phenytoin, primidone) are predicted to decrease the exposure to phosphodiesterase type-5 inhibitors **(sildenafil, vardenafil)**. Moderate Theoretical

► Antifungals, azoles (fluconazole, isavuconazole, posaconazole) are predicted to increase the exposure to **avanafil**. Adjust **avanafil** dose, p. 859. Moderate Theoretical

► Antifungals, azoles (fluconazole, isavuconazole, posaconazole) are predicted to increase the exposure to **sildenafil**. Monitor or adjust **sildenafil** dose with moderate CYP3A4 inhibitors, p. 860. Moderate Study → Also see TABLE 9 p. 1431

► Antifungals, azoles (fluconazole, isavuconazole, posaconazole) are predicted to increase the exposure to **tadalafil**. Severe Theoretical

► Antifungals, azoles (fluconazole, isavuconazole, posaconazole) are predicted to increase the exposure to **vardenafil**. Adjust dose. Severe Theoretical → Also see TABLE 9 p. 1431

► Antifungals, azoles (itraconazole, ketoconazole, voriconazole) are predicted to increase the exposure to **sildenafil**. Avoid potent CYP3A4 inhibitors or adjust **sildenafil** dose, p. 860. Severe Study → Also see TABLE 9 p. 1431

► Antifungals, azoles (itraconazole, ketoconazole, voriconazole) are predicted to increase the exposure to **tadalafil**. Use with caution or avoid. Severe Study

► Antifungals, azoles (miconazole) are predicted to increase the exposure to **sildenafil**. Use with caution and adjust dose. Severe Theoretical

► Antifungals, azoles (itraconazole, ketoconazole, voriconazole) are predicted to increase the exposure to phosphodiesterase type-5 inhibitors **(avanafil, vardenafil)**. Avoid. Severe Study → Also see TABLE 9 p. 1431

► Calcium channel blockers (diltiazem, verapamil) are predicted to increase the exposure to **avanafil**. Adjust **avanafil** dose, p. 859. Moderate Theoretical → Also see TABLE 8 p. 1430

► Calcium channel blockers (diltiazem, verapamil) are predicted to increase the exposure to **sildenafil**. Monitor or adjust **sildenafil** dose with moderate CYP3A4 inhibitors, p. 860. Moderate Study → Also see TABLE 8 p. 1430

► Calcium channel blockers (diltiazem, verapamil) are predicted to increase the exposure to **tadalafil**. Severe Theoretical → Also see TABLE 8 p. 1430

► Calcium channel blockers (diltiazem, verapamil) are predicted to increase the exposure to **vardenafil**. Adjust dose. Severe Theoretical → Also see TABLE 8 p. 1430

● Cobicistat is predicted to increase the exposure to phosphodiesterase type-5 inhibitors **(avanafil, vardenafil)**. Avoid. Severe Study

● Cobicistat is predicted to increase the exposure to **sildenafil**. Avoid potent CYP3A4 inhibitors or adjust **sildenafil** dose, p. 860. Severe Study

● Cobicistat is predicted to increase the exposure to **tadalafil**. Use with caution or avoid. Severe Study

● Crizotinib is predicted to increase the exposure to **avanafil**. Adjust **avanafil** dose, p. 859. Moderate Theoretical

● Crizotinib is predicted to increase the exposure to **sildenafil**. Monitor or adjust **sildenafil** dose with moderate CYP3A4 inhibitors, p. 860. Moderate Study → Also see TABLE 9 p. 1431

● Crizotinib is predicted to increase the exposure to **tadalafil**. Severe Theoretical

● Crizotinib is predicted to increase the exposure to **vardenafil**. Adjust dose. Severe Theoretical → Also see TABLE 9 p. 1431

● Endothelin receptor antagonists (bosentan) decrease the exposure to **phosphodiesterase type-5 inhibitors**. Moderate Study

Phosphodiesterase type-5 inhibitors (continued)

▸ Grapefruit juice is predicted to increase the exposure to **phosphodiesterase type-5 inhibitors**. Use with caution or avoid. Moderate Study

▸ HIV-protease inhibitors are predicted to increase the exposure to phosphodiesterase type-5 inhibitors (**avanafil, vardenafil**). Avoid. Severe Study → Also see TABLE 9 p. 1431

▸ HIV-protease inhibitors are predicted to increase the exposure to **sildenafil**. Avoid potent CYP3A4 inhibitors or adjust **sildenafil** dose, p. 860. Severe Study → Also see TABLE 9 p. 1431

▸ HIV-protease inhibitors are predicted to increase the exposure to **tadalafil**. Use with caution or avoid. Severe Study

▸ Idelalisib is predicted to increase the exposure to phosphodiesterase type-5 inhibitors (**avanafil, vardenafil**). Avoid. Severe Study

▸ Idelalisib is predicted to increase the exposure to **sildenafil**. Avoid potent CYP3A4 inhibitors or adjust **sildenafil** dose, p. 860. Severe Study

▸ Idelalisib is predicted to increase the exposure to **tadalafil**. Use with caution or avoid. Severe Study

▸ Imatinib is predicted to increase the exposure to **avanafil**. Adjust **avanafil** dose, p. 859. Moderate Theoretical

▸ Imatinib is predicted to increase the exposure to **sildenafil**. Monitor or adjust **sildenafil** dose with moderate CYP3A4 inhibitors, p. 860. Moderate Study

▸ Imatinib is predicted to increase the exposure to **tadalafil**. Severe Theoretical

▸ Imatinib is predicted to increase the exposure to **vardenafil**. Adjust dose. Severe Theoretical

▸ Letermovir is predicted to increase the exposure to **avanafil**. Adjust **avanafil** dose, p. 859. Moderate Theoretical

▸ Letermovir is predicted to increase the exposure to **sildenafil**. Monitor or adjust **sildenafil** dose with moderate CYP3A4 inhibitors, p. 860. Moderate Study

▸ Letermovir is predicted to increase the exposure to **tadalafil**. Severe Theoretical

▸ Letermovir is predicted to increase the exposure to **vardenafil**. Adjust dose. Severe Theoretical

▸ Macrolides (clarithromycin) are predicted to increase the exposure to **sildenafil**. Avoid potent CYP3A4 inhibitors or adjust **sildenafil** dose, p. 860. Severe Study → Also see TABLE 9 p. 1431

▸ Macrolides (clarithromycin) are predicted to increase the exposure to **tadalafil**. Use with caution or avoid. Severe Study

▸ Macrolides (erythromycin) are predicted to increase the exposure to **avanafil**. Adjust **avanafil** dose, p. 859. Moderate Theoretical

▸ Macrolides (erythromycin) are predicted to increase the exposure to **sildenafil**. Monitor or adjust **sildenafil** dose with moderate CYP3A4 inhibitors, p. 860. Moderate Study → Also see TABLE 9 p. 1431

▸ Macrolides (erythromycin) are predicted to increase the exposure to **tadalafil**. Severe Theoretical

▸ Macrolides (erythromycin) are predicted to increase the exposure to **vardenafil**. Adjust dose. Severe Theoretical → Also see TABLE 9 p. 1431

▸ Macrolides (clarithromycin) are predicted to increase the exposure to phosphodiesterase type-5 inhibitors (**avanafil, vardenafil**). Avoid. Severe Study → Also see TABLE 9 p. 1431

▸ Mitotane is predicted to decrease the exposure to phosphodiesterase type-5 inhibitors (**avanafil, tadalafil**). Avoid. Severe Study

▸ Mitotane is predicted to decrease the exposure to phosphodiesterase type-5 inhibitors (**sildenafil, vardenafil**). Moderate Theoretical

▸ Neurokinin-1 receptor antagonists (aprepitant, netupitant) are predicted to increase the exposure to **avanafil**. Adjust **avanafil** dose, p. 859. Moderate Theoretical

▸ Neurokinin-1 receptor antagonists (aprepitant, netupitant) are predicted to increase the exposure to **sildenafil**. Monitor or adjust **sildenafil** dose with moderate CYP3A4 inhibitors, p. 860. Moderate Study

▸ Neurokinin-1 receptor antagonists (aprepitant, netupitant) are predicted to increase the exposure to **tadalafil**. Severe Theoretical

▸ Neurokinin-1 receptor antagonists (aprepitant, netupitant) are predicted to increase the exposure to **vardenafil**. Adjust dose. Severe Theoretical

▸ Nicorandil is predicted to increase the risk of hypotension when given with **phosphodiesterase type-5 inhibitors**. Avoid. Severe Theoretical → Also see TABLE 8 p. 1430

▸ Nilotinib is predicted to increase the exposure to **avanafil**. Adjust **avanafil** dose, p. 859. Moderate Theoretical

▸ Nilotinib is predicted to increase the exposure to **sildenafil**. Monitor or adjust **sildenafil** dose with moderate CYP3A4 inhibitors, p. 860. Moderate Study → Also see TABLE 9 p. 1431

▸ Nilotinib is predicted to increase the exposure to **tadalafil**. Severe Theoretical

▸ Nilotinib is predicted to increase the exposure to **vardenafil**. Adjust dose. Severe Theoretical → Also see TABLE 9 p. 1431

▸ Nitrates potentially increase the risk of hypotension when given with **phosphodiesterase type-5 inhibitors**. Avoid. Severe Study → Also see TABLE 8 p. 1430

▸ NNRTIs (efavirenz, nevirapine) are predicted to decrease the exposure to **phosphodiesterase type-5 inhibitors**. Moderate Theoretical → Also see TABLE 9 p. 1431

▸ NNRTIs (etravirine) moderately decrease the exposure to **phosphodiesterase type-5 inhibitors**. Adjust dose. Moderate Study

▸ Ribociclib is predicted to increase the exposure to **sildenafil**. Avoid. Moderate Theoretical → Also see TABLE 9 p. 1431

▸ Rifamycins (rifampicin) are predicted to decrease the exposure to phosphodiesterase type-5 inhibitors (**avanafil, tadalafil**). Avoid. Severe Study

▸ Rifamycins (rifampicin) are predicted to decrease the exposure to phosphodiesterase type-5 inhibitors (**sildenafil, vardenafil**). Moderate Theoretical

▸ Riociguat is predicted to increase the risk of hypotension when given with **phosphodiesterase type-5 inhibitors**. Avoid. Severe Theoretical → Also see TABLE 8 p. 1430

▸ **Phosphodiesterase type-5 inhibitors** are predicted to increase the risk of hypotension when given with sapropterin. Moderate Theoretical → Also see TABLE 8 p. 1430

▸ St John's wort is predicted to decrease the exposure to **phosphodiesterase type-5 inhibitors**. Moderate Theoretical

Pibrentasvir

▸ **Pibrentasvir** (with glecaprevir) is predicted to increase the exposure to aliskiren. Moderate Study

▸ Anti-androgens (apalutamide, enzalutamide) are predicted to moderately to markedly decrease the exposure to **pibrentasvir**. Avoid. Severe Study

▸ Antiarrhythmics (amiodarone) are predicted to increase the exposure to **pibrentasvir**. Moderate Theoretical

▸ Antiarrhythmics (dronedarone) potentially increase the exposure to **pibrentasvir**. Moderate Theoretical

▸ Antiepileptics (carbamazepine, fosphenytoin, phenobarbital, phenytoin, primidone) are predicted to moderately to markedly decrease the exposure to **pibrentasvir**. Avoid. Severe Study

▸ Antiepileptics (eslicarbazepine, oxcarbazepine) potentially decrease the exposure to **pibrentasvir**. Avoid. Severe Theoretical

▸ Antifungals, azoles (itraconazole, ketoconazole) are predicted to increase the exposure to **pibrentasvir**. Moderate Theoretical

▸ **Pibrentasvir** (with glecaprevir) is predicted to increase the exposure to antihistamines, non-sedating (fexofenadine). Moderate Study

▸ Calcium channel blockers (verapamil) are predicted to increase the exposure to **pibrentasvir**. Moderate Theoretical

▸ **Pibrentasvir** (with glecaprevir) is predicted to increase the exposure to colchicine. Moderate Study

▸ Combined hormonal contraceptives (containing ethinylestradiol) are predicted to increase the risk of increased ALT concentrations when given with **pibrentasvir**. Avoid. Severe Study

▸ Crizotinib potentially decreases the exposure to **pibrentasvir**. Avoid. Severe Theoretical

▸ **Pibrentasvir** (with glecaprevir) increases the exposure to digoxin. Moderate Study

▸ Endothelin receptor antagonists (bosentan) are predicted to decrease the exposure to **pibrentasvir**. Avoid. Severe Study

Pibrentasvir (with glecaprevir) is predicted to increase the exposure to everolimus. Moderate Study

Pibrentasvir (with glecaprevir) is predicted to increase the exposure to factor XA inhibitors (edoxaban). Moderate Study

HIV-protease inhibitors (atazanavir, lopinavir) boosted with ritonavir increase the exposure to **pibrentasvir**. Avoid. Severe Study

HIV-protease inhibitors (ritonavir) potentially increase the exposure to **pibrentasvir**. Severe Theoretical

HIV-protease inhibitors (saquinavir) are predicted to increase the exposure to **pibrentasvir**. Moderate Theoretical

Lapatinib is predicted to increase the exposure to **pibrentasvir**. Moderate Theoretical

Pibrentasvir (with glecaprevir) is predicted to increase the exposure to loperamide. Moderate Study

Lumacaftor potentially decreases the exposure to **pibrentasvir**. Avoid. Severe Theoretical

Macrolides are predicted to increase the exposure to **pibrentasvir**. Moderate Theoretical

Mitotane is predicted to moderately to markedly decrease the exposure to **pibrentasvir**. Avoid. Severe Study

NNRTIs (efavirenz, nevirapine) are predicted to decrease the exposure to **pibrentasvir**. Avoid. Severe Study

Ranolazine is predicted to increase the exposure to **pibrentasvir**. Moderate Theoretical

Rifamycins (rifampicin) are predicted to moderately to markedly decrease the exposure to **pibrentasvir**. Avoid. Severe Study

Pibrentasvir (with glecaprevir) is predicted to increase the exposure to sirolimus. Moderate Study

St John's wort is predicted to decrease the exposure to **pibrentasvir**. Avoid. Severe Study

Pibrentasvir (with glecaprevir) markedly increases the exposure to statins (atorvastatin). Avoid. Severe Study

Pibrentasvir (with glecaprevir) is predicted to increase the exposure to statins (fluvastatin). Moderate Theoretical

Pibrentasvir (with glecaprevir) increases the exposure to statins (pravastatin). Use with caution and adjust **pravastatin** dose. Moderate Study

Pibrentasvir (with glecaprevir) increases the exposure to statins (rosuvastatin). Use with caution and adjust **rosuvastatin** dose, p. 218. Moderate Study

Pibrentasvir (with glecaprevir) increases the exposure to statins (simvastatin). Avoid. Moderate Study

Pibrentasvir (with glecaprevir) slightly increases the exposure to tacrolimus. Monitor and adjust dose. Mild Study

Pibrentasvir (with glecaprevir) is predicted to increase the exposure to taxanes (paclitaxel). Moderate Study

Pibrentasvir (with glecaprevir) increases the exposure to thrombin inhibitors (dabigatran). Avoid. Moderate Study

Pibrentasvir (with glecaprevir) is predicted to increase the exposure to topotecan. Moderate Study

Vemurafenib is predicted to increase the exposure to **pibrentasvir**. Moderate Theoretical

Pilocarpine

ROUTE-SPECIFIC INFORMATION Since systemic absorption can follow topical application, the possibility of interactions should be borne in mind.

Pimecrolimus

▸ Alcohol increases the risk of facial flushing and skin irritation when given with topical **pimecrolimus**. Moderate Study

▸ Pimecrolimus is predicted to decrease the efficacy of mifamurtide. Avoid. Severe Theoretical

Pimozide → see TABLE 8 p. 1430 (hypotension), TABLE 9 p. 1431 (QT-interval prolongation), TABLE 11 p. 1431 (CNS depressant effects), TABLE 10 p. 1431 (antimuscarinics)

▸ Antiarrhythmics (dronedarone) are predicted to increase the exposure to **pimozide**. Avoid. Severe Theoretical → Also see TABLE 9 p. 1431

▸ Antifungals, azoles (fluconazole, isavuconazole, posaconazole) are predicted to increase the exposure to **pimozide**. Avoid. Severe Theoretical → Also see TABLE 9 p. 1431

▸ Antifungals, azoles (itraconazole, ketoconazole, voriconazole) are predicted to increase the exposure to **pimozide**. Avoid. Severe Study → Also see TABLE 9 p. 1431

▸ Antifungals, azoles (miconazole) are predicted to increase the exposure to **pimozide**. Avoid. Moderate Theoretical

▸ Calcium channel blockers (diltiazem, verapamil) are predicted to increase the exposure to **pimozide**. Avoid. Severe Theoretical → Also see TABLE 8 p. 1430

▸ Ceritinib is predicted to increase the exposure to **pimozide**. Avoid. Severe Theoretical → Also see TABLE 9 p. 1431

▸ Cobicistat is predicted to increase the exposure to **pimozide**. Avoid. Severe Study

▸ Crizotinib is predicted to increase the exposure to **pimozide**. Avoid. Severe Theoretical → Also see TABLE 9 p. 1431

▸ **Pimozide** is predicted to decrease the effects of dopamine receptor agonists. Avoid. Moderate Theoretical → Also see TABLE 8 p. 1430 → Also see TABLE 9 p. 1431 → Also see TABLE 10 p. 1431

▸ Grapefruit juice increases the exposure to **pimozide**. Avoid. Severe Study

▸ HIV-protease inhibitors are predicted to increase the exposure to **pimozide**. Avoid. Severe Study → Also see TABLE 9 p. 1431

▸ Idelalisib is predicted to increase the exposure to **pimozide**. Avoid. Severe Study

▸ Imatinib is predicted to increase the exposure to **pimozide**. Avoid. Severe Theoretical

▸ Larotrectinib is predicted to increase the exposure to **pimozide**. Use with caution and adjust dose. Mild Theoretical

▸ Letermovir is predicted to increase the exposure to **pimozide**. Avoid. Severe Theoretical

▸ **Pimozide** decreases the effects of levodopa. Severe Theoretical → Also see TABLE 8 p. 1430

▸ Lorlatinib is predicted to decrease the exposure to **pimozide**. Avoid. Severe Theoretical

▸ Macrolides (clarithromycin) are predicted to increase the exposure to **pimozide**. Avoid. Severe Study → Also see TABLE 9 p. 1431

▸ Macrolides (erythromycin) are predicted to increase the exposure to **pimozide**. Avoid. Severe Theoretical → Also see TABLE 9 p. 1431

▸ Neurokinin-1 receptor antagonists are predicted to increase the exposure to **pimozide**. Avoid. Severe Theoretical

▸ Nilotinib is predicted to increase the exposure to **pimozide**. Avoid. Severe Theoretical → Also see TABLE 9 p. 1431

▸ Palbociclib is predicted to increase the exposure to **pimozide**. Adjust dose. Moderate Theoretical

▸ Panobinostat is predicted to increase the exposure to **pimozide**. Avoid. Severe Theoretical → Also see TABLE 9 p. 1431

▸ Pitolisant is predicted to decrease the exposure to **pimozide**. Avoid. Severe Theoretical

▸ Ribociclib (high-dose) is predicted to increase the exposure to **pimozide**. Avoid. Moderate Theoretical → Also see TABLE 9 p. 1431

▸ Rucaparib is predicted to increase the exposure to **pimozide**. Monitor and adjust dose. Moderate Study

Pindolol → see beta blockers, non-selective

Pioglitazone → see TABLE 14 p. 1432 (antidiabetic drugs)

▸ Pioglitazone potentially decreases the exposure to antifungals, azoles (isavuconazole). Use with caution or avoid. Moderate Theoretical

▸ Clopidogrel increases the exposure to **pioglitazone**. Monitor blood glucose and adjust dose. Severe Study

▸ Fibrates (gemfibrozil) increase the exposure to **pioglitazone**. Monitor blood glucose and adjust dose. Severe Study

▸ Iron chelators (deferasirox) are predicted to increase the exposure to **pioglitazone**. Moderate Study

▸ Leflunomide is predicted to increase the exposure to **pioglitazone**. Moderate Study

▸ Opicapone is predicted to increase the exposure to **pioglitazone**. Avoid. Moderate Study

▸ Rifamycins (rifampicin) moderately decrease the exposure to **pioglitazone**. Monitor and adjust dose. Moderate Study

▸ St John's wort slightly decreases the exposure to **pioglitazone**. Mild Study

▸ Teriflunomide is predicted to increase the exposure to **pioglitazone**. Moderate Study

Piperacillin → see penicillins

Piperaquine → see antimalarials

Pirfenidone

FOOD AND LIFESTYLE Smoking increases pirfenidone clearance; patients should be encouraged to stop smoking before and during treatment with pirfenidone.

‣ Antiepileptics (fosphenytoin, phenytoin) are predicted to decrease the exposure to **pirfenidone**. Moderate Theoretical
‣ Combined hormonal contraceptives are predicted to increase the exposure to **pirfenidone**. Use with caution and adjust dose. Moderate Study
‣ HIV-protease inhibitors (ritonavir) are predicted to decrease the exposure to **pirfenidone**. Moderate Theoretical
‣ Leflunomide is predicted to decrease the exposure to **pirfenidone**. Moderate Theoretical
‣ Mexiletine is predicted to increase the exposure to **pirfenidone**. Use with caution and adjust dose. Moderate Study
‣ Quinolones (ciprofloxacin) are predicted to increase the exposure to **pirfenidone**. Use with caution and adjust dose. Moderate Study
‣ Rifamycins (rifampicin) are predicted to decrease the exposure to **pirfenidone**. Avoid. Moderate Theoretical
‣ SSRIs (fluvoxamine) are predicted to moderately increase the exposure to **pirfenidone**. Avoid. Moderate Study
‣ Teriflunomide is predicted to decrease the exposure to **pirfenidone**. Moderate Theoretical

Piroxicam → see NSAIDs

Pitolisant

‣ **Pitolisant** is predicted to decrease the exposure to aliskiren. Mild Theoretical
‣ Anti-androgens (apalutamide, enzalutamide) are predicted to moderately decrease the exposure to **pitolisant**. Moderate Study
‣ Antiepileptics (carbamazepine, fosphenytoin, phenobarbital, phenytoin, primidone) are predicted to moderately decrease the exposure to **pitolisant**. Moderate Study
‣ **Pitolisant** is predicted to decrease the exposure to antihistamines, non-sedating (fexofenadine). Mild Theoretical
‣ Antihistamines, sedating are predicted to decrease the efficacy of **pitolisant**. Moderate Theoretical
‣ **Pitolisant** is predicted to decrease the exposure to bosutinib. Avoid. Severe Theoretical
‣ Bupropion is predicted to moderately increase the exposure to **pitolisant**. Use with caution and adjust dose. Moderate Study
‣ **Pitolisant** is predicted to decrease the exposure to ciclosporin. Avoid. Severe Theoretical
‣ Cinacalcet is predicted to moderately increase the exposure to **pitolisant**. Use with caution and adjust dose. Moderate Study
‣ **Pitolisant** is predicted to decrease the exposure to colchicine. Mild Theoretical
‣ **Pitolisant** is predicted to decrease the efficacy of combined hormonal contraceptives. Avoid. Severe Theoretical
‣ **Pitolisant** is predicted to decrease the exposure to coumarins (warfarin). Mild Theoretical
‣ **Pitolisant** is predicted to decrease the exposure to crizotinib. Avoid. Severe Theoretical
‣ **Pitolisant** is predicted to decrease the exposure to dasatinib. Avoid. Severe Theoretical
‣ **Pitolisant** is predicted to decrease the exposure to digoxin. Mild Theoretical
‣ Duloxetine is predicted to increase the exposure to **pitolisant**. Use with caution and adjust dose. Moderate Study
‣ **Pitolisant** is predicted to decrease the exposure to everolimus. Avoid. Severe Theoretical
‣ **Pitolisant** is predicted to decrease the exposure to factor XA inhibitors (edoxaban). Mild Theoretical
‣ **Pitolisant** is predicted to decrease the exposure to irinotecan. Mild Theoretical
‣ **Pitolisant** is predicted to decrease the exposure to lapatinib. Avoid. Severe Theoretical
‣ **Pitolisant** is predicted to decrease the exposure to loperamide. Mild Theoretical
‣ **Pitolisant** is predicted to decrease the exposure to meglitinides (repaglinide). Mild Theoretical
‣ **Pitolisant** is predicted to increase the exposure to metformin. Mild Theoretical
‣ Mianserin is predicted to decrease the efficacy of **pitolisant**. Moderate Theoretical

‣ Mirtazapine is predicted to decrease the efficacy of **pitolisant**. Moderate Theoretical
‣ Mitotane is predicted to moderately decrease the exposure to **pitolisant**. Moderate Study
‣ **Pitolisant** is predicted to decrease the exposure to nilotinib. Avoid. Severe Theoretical
‣ **Pitolisant** is predicted to decrease the exposure to NNRTIs (efavirenz). Mild Theoretical
‣ **Pitolisant** is predicted to decrease the exposure to opioids (morphine). Mild Theoretical
‣ **Pitolisant** is predicted to decrease the exposure to paracetamol. Mild Theoretical
‣ **Pitolisant** is predicted to decrease the exposure to pimozide. Avoid. Severe Theoretical
‣ Rifamycins (rifampicin) are predicted to moderately decrease the exposure to **pitolisant**. Moderate Study
‣ **Pitolisant** is predicted to decrease the exposure to sirolimus. Avoid. Severe Theoretical
‣ SSRIs (fluoxetine, paroxetine) are predicted to moderately increase the exposure to **pitolisant**. Use with caution and adjust dose. Moderate Study
‣ St John's wort is predicted to decrease the exposure to **pitolisant**. Monitor and adjust dose. Moderate Theoretical
‣ **Pitolisant** is predicted to decrease the exposure to tacrolimus. Avoid. Severe Theoretical
‣ **Pitolisant** is predicted to decrease the exposure to taxanes (docetaxel). Avoid. Severe Theoretical
‣ **Pitolisant** is predicted to decrease the exposure to taxanes (paclitaxel). Mild Theoretical
‣ **Pitolisant** is predicted to decrease the exposure to temsirolimus. Avoid. Severe Theoretical
‣ Terbinafine is predicted to moderately increase the exposure to **pitolisant**. Use with caution and adjust dose. Moderate Study
‣ **Pitolisant** is predicted to decrease the exposure to thrombin inhibitors (dabigatran). Mild Theoretical
‣ **Pitolisant** is predicted to decrease the exposure to topotecan. Mild Theoretical
‣ Tricyclic antidepressants are predicted to decrease the efficacy of **pitolisant**. Mild Theoretical
‣ Venlafaxine is predicted to increase the exposure to **pitolisant**. Use with caution and adjust dose. Mild Theoretical

Pivmecillinam → see penicillins

Pixantrone → see anthracyclines

Pizotifen → see antihistamines, sedating

Platinum compounds → see TABLE 15 p. 1432 (myelosuppression), TABLE 2 p. 1429 (nephrotoxicity), TABLE 19 p. 1433 (ototoxicity), TABLE 12 p. 1432 (peripheral neuropathy)

carboplatin · cisplatin · oxaliplatin

‣ Cisplatin increases the risk of pulmonary toxicity when given with bleomycin. Severe Study → Also see TABLE 15 p. 1432
‣ Live vaccines are predicted to increase the risk of generalised infection (possibly life-threatening) when given with **platinum compounds**. Public Health England advises avoid (refer to Green Book). Severe Theoretical

Polatuzumab vedotin → see monoclonal antibodies

Polymyxin b → see TABLE 2 p. 1429 (nephrotoxicity), TABLE 20 p. 1433 (neuromuscular blocking effects)

ROUTE-SPECIFIC INFORMATION Since systemic absorption can follow topical application of **polymyxin B**, the possibility of interactions should be borne in mind.

Polystyrene sulfonate

SEPARATION OF ADMINISTRATION Manufacturers advise take other drugs at least 3 hours before or after calcium- or sodium-polystyrene sulfonate; a 6-hour separation should be considered in gastroparesis.

‣ Oral antacids increase the risk of metabolic alkalosis when given with oral **polystyrene sulfonate**. Severe Anecdotal

Pomalidomide → see TABLE 15 p. 1432 (myelosuppression), TABLE 5 p. 1430 (thromboembolism)

‣ Combined hormonal contraceptives are predicted to increase the risk of venous thromboembolism when given with **pomalidomide**. Avoid. Severe Theoretical

Hormone replacement therapy is predicted to increase the risk of venous thromboembolism when given with **pomalidomide**. [Severe] Theoretical

Quinolones (ciprofloxacin) are predicted to increase the exposure to **pomalidomide**. Adjust **pomalidomide** dose, p. 1003. [Moderate] Theoretical

SSRIs (fluvoxamine) moderately increase the exposure to **pomalidomide**. Adjust **pomalidomide** dose, p. 1003. [Moderate] Study

Ponatinib

▸ Anti-androgens (apalutamide, enzalutamide) are predicted to decrease the exposure to **ponatinib**. Avoid. [Moderate] Theoretical

▸ Antiepileptics (carbamazepine, fosphenytoin, phenobarbital, phenytoin, primidone) are predicted to decrease the exposure to **ponatinib**. Avoid. [Moderate] Theoretical

▸ Antifungals, azoles (itraconazole, ketoconazole, voriconazole) are predicted to slightly increase the exposure to **ponatinib**. Monitor and adjust **ponatinib** dose, p. 1040. [Moderate] Study

▸ Cobicistat is predicted to slightly increase the exposure to **ponatinib**. Monitor and adjust **ponatinib** dose, p. 1040. [Moderate] Study

▸ **Ponatinib** is predicted to increase the risk of bleeding events when given with coumarins. [Severe] Theoretical

▸ Grapefruit juice is predicted to increase the exposure to **ponatinib**. [Moderate] Theoretical

▸ HIV-protease inhibitors are predicted to slightly increase the exposure to **ponatinib**. Monitor and adjust **ponatinib** dose, p. 1040. [Moderate] Study

▸ Idelalisib is predicted to slightly increase the exposure to **ponatinib**. Monitor and adjust **ponatinib** dose, p. 1040. [Moderate] Study

▸ Macrolides (clarithromycin) are predicted to slightly increase the exposure to **ponatinib**. Monitor and adjust **ponatinib** dose, p. 1040. [Moderate] Study

▸ Mitotane is predicted to decrease the exposure to **ponatinib**. Avoid. [Moderate] Theoretical

▸ **Ponatinib** is predicted to increase the risk of bleeding events when given with phenindione. [Severe] Theoretical

▸ Rifamycins (rifampicin) are predicted to decrease the exposure to **ponatinib**. Avoid. [Moderate] Theoretical

▸ St John's wort is predicted to decrease the exposure to **ponatinib**. Avoid. [Severe] Theoretical

Posaconazole → see antifungals, azoles

Potassium aminobenzoate → see TABLE 16 p. 1433 (increased serum potassium)

▸ **Potassium aminobenzoate** increases the concentration of methotrexate. [Moderate] Theoretical

▸ **Potassium aminobenzoate** is predicted to affect the efficacy of sulfonamides. Avoid. [Severe] Theoretical

Potassium canrenoate → see TABLE 16 p. 1433 (increased serum potassium)

Potassium chloride → see TABLE 16 p. 1433 (increased serum potassium)

Potassium citrate

▸ **Potassium citrate** is predicted to decrease the efficacy of methenamine. Avoid. [Moderate] Theoretical

▸ **Potassium citrate** increases the risk of adverse effects when given with sucralfate. Avoid. [Moderate] Theoretical

Potassium-sparing diuretics → see TABLE 18 p. 1433 (hyponatraemia), TABLE 16 p. 1433 (increased serum potassium)

amiloride · triamterene

▸ Triamterene potentially increases the clearance of lithium. [Moderate] Study

Pramipexole → see dopamine receptor agonists

Prasugrel → see TABLE 4 p. 1429 (antiplatelet effects)

Pravastatin → see statins

Praziquantel

▸ Anti-androgens (apalutamide, enzalutamide) are predicted to markedly decrease the exposure to **praziquantel**. Avoid. [Moderate] Study

▸ Antiepileptics (carbamazepine, fosphenytoin, phenobarbital, phenytoin, primidone) are predicted to markedly decrease the exposure to **praziquantel**. Avoid. [Moderate] Study

▸ Antifungals, azoles (itraconazole, ketoconazole, voriconazole) are predicted to moderately increase the exposure to **praziquantel**. [Mild] Study

▸ Antimalarials (chloroquine) moderately decrease the exposure to **praziquantel**. Use with caution and adjust dose. [Moderate] Study

▸ Cobicistat is predicted to moderately increase the exposure to **praziquantel**. [Mild] Study

▸ Corticosteroids (dexamethasone) decrease the exposure to **praziquantel**. [Moderate] Study

▸ Grapefruit juice is predicted to increase the exposure to **praziquantel**. [Moderate] Study

▸ H₂ receptor antagonists (cimetidine) moderately increase the exposure to **praziquantel**. [Moderate] Study

▸ HIV-protease inhibitors are predicted to moderately increase the exposure to **praziquantel**. [Mild] Study

▸ Idelalisib is predicted to moderately increase the exposure to **praziquantel**. [Mild] Study

▸ Macrolides (clarithromycin) are predicted to moderately increase the exposure to **praziquantel**. [Mild] Study

▸ Mitotane is predicted to markedly decrease the exposure to **praziquantel**. Avoid. [Moderate] Study

▸ Rifamycins (rifampicin) are predicted to markedly decrease the exposure to **praziquantel**. Avoid. [Moderate] Study

Prazosin → see alpha blockers

Prednisolone → see corticosteroids

Pregabalin → see antiepileptics

Pridinol → see TABLE 10 p. 1431 (antimuscarinics)

Prilocaine → see anaesthetics, local

Primaquine → see antimalarials

Primidone → see antiepileptics

Procarbazine → see TABLE 15 p. 1432 (myelosuppression), TABLE 13 p. 1432 (serotonin syndrome)

FOOD AND LIFESTYLE Procarbazine is a mild monoamine-oxidase inhibitor and might rarely interact with tyramine-rich foods (such as mature cheese, salami, pickled herring, *Bovril*®, *Oxo*®, *Marmite*® or any similar meat or yeast extract or fermented soya bean extract, and some beers, lagers or wines).

▸ Alcohol potentially causes a disulfiram-like reaction when given with **procarbazine**. [Moderate] Anecdotal

▸ Antiepileptics (carbamazepine, phenobarbital, phenytoin, primidone) are predicted to increase the risk of hypersensitivity reactions when given with **procarbazine**. [Severe] Anecdotal

▸ Antiepileptics (fosphenytoin) are predicted to increase the risk of hypersensitivity when given with **procarbazine**. [Severe] Anecdotal

▸ Live vaccines are predicted to increase the risk of generalised infection (possibly life-threatening) when given with **procarbazine**. Public Health England advises avoid (refer to Green Book). [Severe] Theoretical

Prochlorperazine → see phenothiazines

Procyclidine → see TABLE 10 p. 1431 (antimuscarinics)

▸ SSRIs (paroxetine) slightly increase the exposure to **procyclidine**. Monitor and adjust dose. [Moderate] Study

Proguanil → see antimalarials

Promazine → see phenothiazines

Promethazine → see antihistamines, sedating

Propafenone → see antiarrhythmics

Propantheline → see TABLE 10 p. 1431 (antimuscarinics)

Propiverine → see TABLE 10 p. 1431 (antimuscarinics)

▸ Antifungals, azoles (itraconazole, ketoconazole, voriconazole) given with carbimazole are predicted to increase the exposure to **propiverine**. Adjust starting dose. [Moderate] Theoretical

▸ Carbimazole given with a potent CYP3A4 inhibitor is predicted to increase the exposure to **propiverine**. Adjust starting dose. [Moderate] Theoretical

▸ Cobicistat given with carbimazole is predicted to increase the exposure to **propiverine**. Adjust starting dose. [Moderate] Theoretical

▸ HIV-protease inhibitors given with carbimazole are predicted to increase the exposure to **propiverine**. Adjust starting dose. [Moderate] Theoretical

Propiverine (continued)
▸ Idelalisib given with carbimazole is predicted to increase the exposure to **propiverine**. Adjust starting dose. Moderate Theoretical
▸ **Propiverine** is predicted to increase the exposure to lomitapide. Separate administration by 12 hours. Moderate Theoretical
▸ Macrolides (clarithromycin) given with carbimazole are predicted to increase the exposure to **propiverine**. Adjust starting dose. Moderate Theoretical
Propofol → see TABLE 8 p. 1430 (hypotension), TABLE 11 p. 1431 (CNS depressant effects)
▸ Antiepileptics (valproate) potentially increase the concentration of **propofol**. Adjust dose. Severe Theoretical
Propranolol → see beta blockers, non-selective
Propylthiouracil
▸ **Propylthiouracil** is predicted to decrease the effects of metyrapone. Avoid. Moderate Theoretical
Proton pump inhibitors

esomeprazole · lansoprazole · omeprazole · pantoprazole · rabeprazole

▸ **Proton pump inhibitors** are predicted to decrease the exposure to acalabrutinib. Avoid. Moderate Study
▸ **Pantoprazole** is predicted to increase the exposure to alpelisib. Moderate Theoretical
▸ Anti-androgens (apalutamide) markedly decrease the exposure to **omeprazole**. Avoid or monitor. Moderate Study
▸ Anti-androgens (apalutamide) are predicted to decrease the exposure to proton pump inhibitors **(lansoprazole, rabeprazole)**. Avoid or monitor. Mild Study
▸ Antifungals, azoles (voriconazole) increase the exposure to proton pump inhibitors **(esomeprazole, omeprazole)**. Adjust dose. Moderate Study
▸ **Proton pump inhibitors** decrease the absorption of antifungals, azoles (itraconazole). Administer itraconazole capsules with an acidic beverage. Moderate Study
▸ **Proton pump inhibitors** decrease the absorption of antifungals, azoles (ketoconazole). Administer ketoconazole with an acidic beverage. Moderate Study
▸ **Proton pump inhibitors** decrease the absorption of antifungals, azoles (posaconazole) (oral suspension). Avoid. Moderate Study
▸ Proton pump inhibitors **(esomeprazole, omeprazole)** potentially increase the exposure to benzodiazepines (clobazam). Adjust dose. Moderate Theoretical
▸ **Proton pump inhibitors** are predicted to decrease the absorption of bosutinib. Moderate Study
▸ **Esomeprazole** is predicted to increase the exposure to cannabidiol. Moderate Theoretical
▸ **Proton pump inhibitors** are predicted to decrease the absorption of ceritinib. Moderate Theoretical
▸ **Esomeprazole** is predicted to increase the exposure to cilostazol. Moderate Theoretical
▸ **Omeprazole** is predicted to increase the exposure to cilostazol. Adjust **cilostazol** dose, p. 248. Moderate Study
▸ Proton pump inhibitors **(esomeprazole, omeprazole)** are predicted to decrease the efficacy of clopidogrel. Avoid. Moderate Study
▸ **Proton pump inhibitors** are predicted to decrease the exposure to dacomitinib. Avoid. Moderate Study
▸ **Proton pump inhibitors** are predicted to slightly to moderately decrease the exposure to dasatinib. Avoid. Severe Study
▸ **Proton pump inhibitors** are predicted to decrease the absorption of dipyridamole (immediate release tablets). Moderate Theoretical
▸ **Proton pump inhibitors** are predicted to slightly decrease the exposure to erlotinib. Avoid. Moderate Study
▸ **Proton pump inhibitors** are predicted to decrease the exposure to gefitinib. Severe Theoretical
▸ HIV-protease inhibitors (tipranavir) decrease the exposure to proton pump inhibitors. Avoid. Severe Study
▸ **Proton pump inhibitors** decrease the exposure to HIV-protease inhibitors (atazanavir). Avoid or adjust dose. Severe Study
▸ **Proton pump inhibitors** increase the exposure to HIV-protease inhibitors (saquinavir). Avoid. Severe Study

▸ **Proton pump inhibitors** are predicted to decrease the exposure to ledipasvir. Adjust dose, see ledipasvir with sofosbuvir p. 668. Moderate Theoretical
▸ **Proton pump inhibitors** decrease the clearance of methotrexate (high-dose). Use with caution or avoid. Severe Study
▸ **Proton pump inhibitors** are predicted to decrease the exposure to neratinib. Avoid. Severe Study
▸ **Proton pump inhibitors** are predicted to decrease the exposure to NNRTIs (rilpivirine). Avoid. Severe Study
▸ **Proton pump inhibitors** are predicted to decrease the exposure to pazopanib. Avoid or administer concurrently without food. Moderate Study
▸ **Proton pump inhibitors** potentially decrease the exposure to sofosbuvir. Adjust dose, see ledipasvir with sofosbuvir p. 668, sofosbuvir with velpatasvir p. 669, and sofosbuvir with velpatasvir and voxilaprevir p. 669. Moderate Study
▸ **Esomeprazole** is predicted to slightly to moderately increase the exposure to SSRIs (citalopram, escitalopram). Monitor and adjust dose. Severe Theoretical
▸ **Omeprazole** slightly to moderately increases the exposure to SSRIs (citalopram, escitalopram). Monitor and adjust dose. Severe Study
▸ **Proton pump inhibitors** are predicted to decrease the concentration of velpatasvir. Adjust dose, see sofosbuvir with velpatasvir p. 669. Moderate Study
▸ **Proton pump inhibitors** are predicted to decrease the exposure to voxilaprevir. Adjust dose, see sofosbuvir with velpatasvir and voxilaprevir p. 669. Moderate Study
Proxymetacaine → see anaesthetics, local
Pseudoephedrine → see sympathomimetics, vasoconstrictor
Pyrazinamide
▸ Allopurinol is predicted to increase the risk of hyperuricaemia when given with **pyrazinamide**. Moderate Theoretical
Pyridostigmine → see TABLE 6 p. 1430 (bradycardia)
▸ Aminoglycosides are predicted to decrease the effects of **pyridostigmine**. Moderate Theoretical
Pyrimethamine → see antimalarials
Quetiapine → see antipsychotics, second generation
Quinagolide → see dopamine receptor agonists
Quinapril → see ACE inhibitors
Quinine → see antimalarials
Quinolones → see TABLE 9 p. 1431 (QT-interval prolongation)

ciprofloxacin · delafloxacin · levofloxacin · moxifloxacin · ofloxacin

▸ Avoid concurrent administration of dairy products and mineral-fortified drinks with *oral* **ciprofloxacin** due to reduced exposure.
▸ Since systemic absorption can follow topical application of **ciprofloxacin**, **levofloxacin**, and **ofloxacin**, the possibility of interactions should be borne in mind.
▸ Interactions do not generally apply to topical use of **moxifloxacin** unless specified.

▸ **Ciprofloxacin** is predicted to increase the exposure to agomelatine. Moderate Study
▸ **Ciprofloxacin** is predicted to increase the exposure to aminophylline. Adjust dose. Moderate Theoretical
▸ **Ciprofloxacin** is predicted to increase the exposure to anagrelide. Moderate Theoretical
▸ Oral antacids decrease the absorption of oral **quinolones**. **Quinolones** should be taken 2 hours before or 4 hours after antacids. Moderate Study
▸ **Ciprofloxacin** slightly increases the exposure to antiarrhythmics (lidocaine). Mild Study
▸ **Ciprofloxacin** affects the concentration of antiepileptics (fosphenytoin, phenytoin). Monitor concentration and adjust dose. Severe Study
▸ **Ciprofloxacin** increases the concentration of antipsychotics, second generation (clozapine). Monitor adverse effects and adjust dose. Severe Study
▸ **Ciprofloxacin** is predicted to increase the exposure to antipsychotics, second generation (olanzapine). Adjust dose. Moderate Anecdotal
▸ Calcium salts (calcium carbonate) decrease the absorption of **ciprofloxacin**. Separate administration by 2 hours. Moderate Study

Quinolones increase the anticoagulant effect of coumarins. Severe Anecdotal

Ciprofloxacin is predicted to increase the exposure to dopamine receptor agonists (ropinirole). Adjust dose. Moderate Study

Ciprofloxacin is predicted to increase the exposure to duloxetine. Avoid. Moderate Theoretical

Ciprofloxacin is predicted to increase the exposure to eliglustat. Avoid or adjust dose—consult product literature. Severe Theoretical

▸ Enteral feeds decrease the exposure to **ciprofloxacin**. Moderate Study

▸ **Ciprofloxacin** slightly increases the exposure to erlotinib. Monitor adverse effects and adjust dose. Moderate Study

▸ **Ciprofloxacin** is predicted to increase the exposure to ibrutinib. Adjust **ibrutinib** dose, p. 1027. Severe Theoretical

▸ Oral iron decreases the exposure to oral **quinolones**. Separate administration by at least 2 hours. Moderate Study

▸ Lanthanum moderately decreases the exposure to **quinolones**. **Quinolones** should be taken 2 hours before or 4 hours after **lanthanum**. Moderate Study

▸ Leflunomide is predicted to increase the exposure to **ciprofloxacin**. Moderate Theoretical

▸ **Ciprofloxacin** is predicted to increase the exposure to loxapine. Avoid. Unknown Theoretical

▸ **Ciprofloxacin** slightly increases the exposure to MAO-B inhibitors (rasagiline). Moderate Study

▸ **Ciprofloxacin** is predicted to increase the exposure to melatonin. Moderate Theoretical

▸ **Ciprofloxacin** potentially increases the risk of toxicity when given with methotrexate. Severe Anecdotal

▸ NSAIDs potentially increase the risk of seizures when given with **quinolones**. Severe Theoretical

▸ **Ciprofloxacin** very slightly increases the exposure to pentoxifylline. Moderate Study

▸ **Ciprofloxacin** is predicted to increase the exposure to phenothiazines (chlorpromazine). Moderate Theoretical

▸ **Ciprofloxacin** is predicted to increase the exposure to phosphodiesterase type-4 inhibitors (roflumilast). Moderate Theoretical

▸ **Ciprofloxacin** is predicted to increase the exposure to pirfenidone. Use with caution and adjust dose. Moderate Study

▸ **Ciprofloxacin** is predicted to increase the exposure to pomalidomide. Adjust **pomalidomide** dose, p. 1003. Moderate Theoretical

▸ **Ciprofloxacin** is predicted to increase the exposure to riluzole. Moderate Theoretical

▸ Strontium is predicted to decrease the absorption of **quinolones**. Avoid. Moderate Theoretical

▸ Sucralfate decreases the exposure to **quinolones**. Separate administration by 2 hours. Moderate Study

▸ Teriflunomide is predicted to increase the exposure to **ciprofloxacin**. Moderate Theoretical

▸ **Ciprofloxacin** is predicted to increase the exposure to theophylline. Monitor and adjust dose. Moderate Theoretical

▸ **Ciprofloxacin** increases the exposure to tizanidine. Avoid. Moderate Study

▸ **Ciprofloxacin** is predicted to increase the exposure to tolvaptan. Use with caution and adjust **tolvaptan** dose, p. 708. Moderate Theoretical

▸ **Ciprofloxacin** is predicted to increase the exposure to triptans (zolmitriptan). Adjust **zolmitriptan** dose, p. 503. Moderate Theoretical

▸ **Ciprofloxacin** is predicted to increase the exposure to venetoclax. Avoid or adjust dose—consult product literature. Severe Theoretical

▸ Zinc is predicted to decrease the exposure to **quinolones**. Separate administration by 2 hours. Moderate Study

Rabeprazole → see proton pump inhibitors

Rabies immunoglobulin → see immunoglobulins

Rabies vaccine

▸ Antimalarials (chloroquine) decrease the efficacy of **rabies vaccine** (intradermal). Moderate Study

▸ Hydroxychloroquine is predicted to decrease efficacy **rabies vaccine**. Moderate Theoretical

Raloxifene → see TABLE 5 p. 1430 (thromboembolism)

▸ Combined hormonal contraceptives potentially oppose the effects of **raloxifene**. Avoid. Severe Theoretical

▸ Hormone replacement therapy potentially opposes the effects of **raloxifene**. Avoid. Severe Theoretical

Raltegravir

▸ Oral antacids decrease the exposure to oral **raltegravir**. Avoid. Moderate Study

▸ Antiepileptics (carbamazepine) are predicted to affect the exposure to **raltegravir**. Moderate Theoretical

▸ Antiepileptics (fosphenytoin, phenobarbital, phenytoin, primidone) are predicted to affect the exposure to **raltegravir**. Use with caution or avoid. Moderate Theoretical

▸ Calcium salts (calcium carbonate) greatly decrease the exposure to **raltegravir** (high-dose). Avoid. Severe Study

▸ Encorafenib is predicted to increase the exposure to **raltegravir**. Moderate Theoretical

▸ HIV-protease inhibitors (atazanavir) increase the exposure to **raltegravir** (high-dose). Avoid. Moderate Study

▸ HIV-protease inhibitors (darunavir) increase the risk of rash when given with **raltegravir**. Moderate Study

▸ HIV-protease inhibitors (fosamprenavir) boosted with ritonavir decrease the exposure to **raltegravir** and **raltegravir** decreases the exposure to HIV-protease inhibitors (fosamprenavir) boosted with ritonavir. Avoid. Severe Study

▸ HIV-protease inhibitors (tipranavir) boosted with ritonavir are predicted to decrease the exposure to **raltegravir** (high-dose). Avoid. Moderate Study

▸ Rifamycins (rifampicin) slightly decrease the exposure to **raltegravir**. Avoid or adjust dose—consult product literature. Moderate Study

▸ Sodium zirconium cyclosilicate is predicted to decrease the exposure to **raltegravir**. Separate administration by at least 2 hours. Moderate Theoretical

Raltitrexed → see TABLE 15 p. 1432 (myelosuppression)

▸ Folates are predicted to alter the effects of **raltitrexed**. Avoid. Moderate Study

▸ Live vaccines are predicted to increase the risk of generalised infection (possibly life-threatening) when given with **raltitrexed**. Public Health England advises avoid (refer to Green Book). Severe Theoretical

Ramipril → see ACE inhibitors

Ramucirumab → see monoclonal antibodies

Ranibizumab

▸ **Ranibizumab** increases the risk of bleeding events when given with coumarins. Severe Theoretical

▸ **Ranibizumab** is predicted to increase the risk of bleeding events when given with danaparoid. Severe Theoretical

▸ **Ranibizumab** increases the risk of bleeding events when given with heparin. Severe Theoretical

▸ **Ranibizumab** increases the risk of bleeding events when given with low molecular-weight heparins. Severe Theoretical

▸ **Ranibizumab** is predicted to increase the risk of bleeding events when given with phenindione. Severe Theoretical

▸ **Ranibizumab** is predicted to increase the risk of bleeding events when given with thrombin inhibitors (argatroban). Severe Theoretical

▸ **Ranibizumab** is predicted to increase the risk of bleeding events when given with thrombin inhibitors (bivalirudin). Moderate Theoretical

Ranitidine → see H$_2$ receptor antagonists

Ranolazine → see TABLE 9 p. 1431 (QT-interval prolongation)

▸ **Ranolazine** is predicted to increase the exposure to afatinib. Separate administration by 12 hours. Moderate Study

▸ **Ranolazine** is predicted to increase the exposure to aliskiren. Moderate Theoretical

▸ Anti-androgens (apalutamide, enzalutamide) are predicted to decrease the exposure to **ranolazine**. Avoid. Severe Study → Also see TABLE 9 p. 1431

▸ Antiarrhythmics (dronedarone) are predicted to increase the exposure to **ranolazine**. Severe Study → Also see TABLE 9 p. 1431

▸ Antiepileptics (carbamazepine, fosphenytoin, phenobarbital, phenytoin, primidone) are predicted to decrease the exposure to **ranolazine**. Avoid. Severe Study

Ranolazine (continued)

▶ Antifungals, azoles (fluconazole, isavuconazole, posaconazole) are predicted to increase the exposure to **ranolazine**. Severe Study → Also see TABLE 9 p. 1431

▶ Antifungals, azoles (itraconazole, ketoconazole, voriconazole) are predicted to increase the exposure to **ranolazine**. Avoid. Severe Study → Also see TABLE 9 p. 1431

▶ **Ranolazine** is predicted to increase the exposure to beta blockers, non-selective (nadolol). Moderate Study

▶ **Ranolazine** is predicted to increase the exposure to bictegravir. Use with caution or avoid. Moderate Theoretical

▶ Calcium channel blockers (diltiazem, verapamil) are predicted to increase the exposure to **ranolazine**. Severe Study

▶ **Ranolazine** is predicted to increase the exposure to ceritinib. Moderate Theoretical → Also see TABLE 9 p. 1431

▶ Ciclosporin is predicted to increase the concentration of **ranolazine** and **ranolazine** is predicted to increase the concentration of ciclosporin. Moderate Theoretical

▶ Cobicistat is predicted to increase the exposure to **ranolazine**. Avoid. Severe Study

▶ **Ranolazine** is predicted to increase the exposure to colchicine. Avoid P-glycoprotein inhibitors or adjust **colchicine** dose, p. 1166. Severe Theoretical

▶ Crizotinib is predicted to increase the exposure to **ranolazine**. Severe Study → Also see TABLE 9 p. 1431

▶ **Ranolazine** increases the concentration of digoxin. Moderate Study

▶ **Ranolazine** is predicted to increase the exposure to dopamine receptor agonists (pramipexole). Adjust dose. Moderate Study

▶ **Ranolazine** is predicted to increase the exposure to erlotinib. Moderate Theoretical

▶ **Ranolazine** is predicted to slightly increase the exposure to factor XA inhibitors (edoxaban). Severe Theoretical

▶ **Ranolazine** is predicted to increase the exposure to fidaxomicin. Avoid. Moderate Study

▶ Grapefruit juice is predicted to increase the concentration of **ranolazine**. Avoid. Severe Theoretical

▶ HIV-protease inhibitors are predicted to increase the exposure to **ranolazine**. Avoid. Severe Study → Also see TABLE 9 p. 1431

▶ Idelalisib is predicted to increase the exposure to **ranolazine**. Avoid. Severe Study

▶ Imatinib is predicted to increase the exposure to **ranolazine**. Severe Study

▶ **Ranolazine** is predicted to increase the exposure to larotrectinib. Mild Theoretical

▶ Letermovir is predicted to increase the exposure to **ranolazine**. Severe Study

▶ **Ranolazine** is predicted to increase the exposure to lomitapide. Separate administration by 12 hours. Mild Theoretical

▶ Macrolides (clarithromycin) are predicted to increase the exposure to **ranolazine**. Avoid. Severe Study → Also see TABLE 9 p. 1431

▶ Macrolides (erythromycin) are predicted to increase the exposure to **ranolazine**. Severe Study → Also see TABLE 9 p. 1431

▶ Mitotane is predicted to decrease the exposure to **ranolazine**. Avoid. Severe Study

▶ **Ranolazine** is predicted to increase the exposure to naldemedine. Moderate Study

▶ Neurokinin-1 receptor antagonists (aprepitant, netupitant) are predicted to increase the exposure to **ranolazine**. Severe Study

▶ Nilotinib is predicted to increase the exposure to **ranolazine**. Severe Study → Also see TABLE 9 p. 1431

▶ **Ranolazine** is predicted to increase the exposure to nintedanib. Moderate Study

▶ **Ranolazine** is predicted to increase the exposure to panobinostat. Adjust dose. Moderate Theoretical → Also see TABLE 9 p. 1431

▶ **Ranolazine** is predicted to increase the exposure to pibrentasvir. Moderate Theoretical

▶ Rifamycins (rifampicin) are predicted to decrease the exposure to **ranolazine**. Avoid. Severe Study

▶ St John's wort is predicted to decrease the exposure to **ranolazine**. Avoid. Severe Study

▶ **Ranolazine** is predicted to increase the exposure to statins (atorvastatin). Moderate Theoretical

▶ **Ranolazine** slightly increases the exposure to statins (simvastatin). Adjust **simvastatin** dose, p. 219. Moderate Study

▶ **Ranolazine** increases the concentration of tacrolimus. Adjust dose. Severe Anecdotal

▶ **Ranolazine** is predicted to slightly increase the exposure to talazoparib. Avoid or adjust **talazoparib** dose, p. 1052. Severe Study

▶ **Ranolazine** is predicted to increase the exposure to thrombin inhibitors (dabigatran). Severe Theoretical

▶ **Ranolazine** is predicted to increase the exposure to ticagrelor. Use with caution or avoid. Severe Study

▶ **Ranolazine** is predicted to increase the exposure to topotecan. Severe Study

▶ **Ranolazine** is predicted to increase the concentration of trametinib. Moderate Theoretical

▶ **Ranolazine** is predicted to increase the exposure to venetoclax. Avoid or monitor for toxicity. Severe Theoretical

Rasagiline → see MAO-B inhibitors

Reboxetine

▶ Anti-androgens (apalutamide, enzalutamide) are predicted to decrease the exposure to **reboxetine**. Moderate Anecdotal

▶ Antiepileptics (carbamazepine, fosphenytoin, phenobarbital, phenytoin, primidone) are predicted to decrease the exposure to **reboxetine**. Moderate Anecdotal

▶ Antifungals, azoles (itraconazole, ketoconazole, voriconazole) are predicted to increase the exposure to **reboxetine**. Avoid. Moderate Study

▶ Antifungals, azoles (miconazole) are predicted to increase the concentration of **reboxetine**. Use with caution and adjust dose. Moderate Theoretical

▶ Cobicistat is predicted to increase the exposure to **reboxetine**. Avoid. Moderate Study

▶ HIV-protease inhibitors are predicted to increase the exposure to **reboxetine**. Avoid. Moderate Study

▶ Idelalisib is predicted to increase the exposure to **reboxetine**. Avoid. Moderate Study

▶ **Reboxetine** is predicted to increase the risk of a hypertensive crisis when given with linezolid. Avoid. Severe Theoretical

▶ **Reboxetine** is predicted to increase the risk of hypokalaemia when given with loop diuretics. Moderate Theoretical

▶ Macrolides (clarithromycin) are predicted to increase the exposure to **reboxetine**. Avoid. Moderate Study

▶ **Reboxetine** is predicted to increase the risk of a hypertensive crisis when given with MAO-B inhibitors (rasagiline, selegiline). Avoid. Severe Theoretical

▶ **Reboxetine** is predicted to increase the risk of a hypertensive crisis when given with MAOIs, irreversible. Avoid. Severe Theoretical

▶ Mitotane is predicted to decrease the exposure to **reboxetine**. Moderate Anecdotal

▶ **Reboxetine** is predicted to increase the risk of a hypertensive crisis when given with moclobemide. Avoid. Severe Theoretical

▶ Rifamycins (rifampicin) are predicted to decrease the exposure to **reboxetine**. Moderate Anecdotal

▶ **Reboxetine** is predicted to increase the risk of hypokalaemia when given with thiazide diuretics. Moderate Anecdotal

Regorafenib → see TABLE 15 p. 1432 (myelosuppression), TABLE 4 p. 1429 (antiplatelet effects)

▶ Anti-androgens (apalutamide, enzalutamide) are predicted to decrease the exposure to **regorafenib**. Avoid. Moderate Study

▶ Antiepileptics (carbamazepine, fosphenytoin, phenobarbital, phenytoin, primidone) are predicted to decrease the exposure to **regorafenib**. Avoid. Moderate Study

▶ Antifungals, azoles (itraconazole, ketoconazole, voriconazole) are predicted to increase the exposure to **regorafenib**. Avoid. Moderate Study

▶ Cobicistat is predicted to increase the exposure to **regorafenib**. Avoid. Moderate Study

▶ **Regorafenib** is predicted to increase the risk of bleeding events when given with coumarins. Severe Study

▶ Grapefruit juice is predicted to increase the exposure to **regorafenib**. Avoid. Moderate Theoretical

▶ HIV-protease inhibitors are predicted to increase the exposure to **regorafenib**. Avoid. Moderate Study

Idelalisib is predicted to increase the exposure to **regorafenib**. Avoid. Moderate Study

▸ Macrolides (clarithromycin) are predicted to increase the exposure to **regorafenib**. Avoid. Moderate Study

▸ **Regorafenib** is predicted to increase the exposure to methotrexate. Moderate Theoretical → Also see **TABLE 15** p. 1432

▸ Mitotane is predicted to decrease the exposure to **regorafenib**. Avoid. Moderate Study → Also see **TABLE 15** p. 1432

▸ **Regorafenib** is predicted to increase the exposure to NSAIDs (mefenamic acid). Avoid. Moderate Theoretical → Also see **TABLE 4** p. 1429

▸ **Regorafenib** is predicted to increase the risk of bleeding events when given with phenindione. Severe Theoretical

▸ Rifamycins (rifampicin) are predicted to decrease the exposure to **regorafenib**. Avoid. Moderate Study

▸ **Regorafenib** is predicted to increase the exposure to statins (atorvastatin, fluvastatin, rosuvastatin). Moderate Study

▸ **Regorafenib** is predicted to increase the exposure to sulfasalazine. Moderate Study → Also see **TABLE 15** p. 1432

▸ **Regorafenib** is predicted to increase the exposure to topotecan. Moderate Study → Also see **TABLE 15** p. 1432

Remdesivir

▸ Anti-androgens (apalutamide, enzalutamide) potentially decrease the exposure to **remdesivir**. Avoid. Moderate Theoretical

▸ Antiepileptics (carbamazepine, fosphenytoin, phenobarbital, phenytoin, primidone) potentially decrease the exposure to **remdesivir**. Avoid. Moderate Theoretical

▸ Antimalarials (chloroquine) potentially decrease the effects of **remdesivir**. Avoid. Moderate Theoretical

▸ Hydroxychloroquine potentially decrease the effects of **remdesivir**. Avoid. Moderate Theoretical

▸ Mitotane potentially decreases the exposure to **remdesivir**. Moderate Theoretical

▸ Rifamycins (rifampicin) potentially decrease the exposure to **remdesivir**. Avoid. Moderate Theoretical

Remifentanil → see opioids

Repaglinide → see meglitinides

Retigabine → see antiepileptics

Retinoids → see **TABLE 15** p. 1432 (myelosuppression), **TABLE 5** p. 1430 (thromboembolism)

acitretin · adapalene · alitretinoin · bexarotene · isotretinoin · tazarotene · tretinoin

▸ Avoid concomitant use of keratolytics in patients taking **acitretin** and **isotretinoin**.

▸ Since systemic absorption can follow topical application of **isotretinoin** and **tretinoin**, the possibility of interactions should be borne in mind.

▸ Alcohol potentially increases the concentration of acitretin. Avoid and for 2 months after stopping acitretin. Moderate Study

▸ Antiarrhythmics (amiodarone) are predicted to increase the exposure to **alitretinoin**. Adjust **alitretinoin** dose, p. 1305. Moderate Theoretical

▸ Antifungals, azoles (fluconazole, itraconazole, ketoconazole, miconazole, voriconazole) are predicted to increase the exposure to **alitretinoin**. Adjust **alitretinoin** dose, p. 1305. Moderate Theoretical

▸ Antifungals, azoles (fluconazole, ketoconazole, voriconazole) are predicted to increase the risk of tretinoin toxicity when given with **tretinoin**. Moderate Study

▸ Clopidogrel is predicted to increase the exposure to **alitretinoin**. Adjust **alitretinoin** dose, p. 1305. Moderate Theoretical

▸ Cobicistat is predicted to increase the exposure to **alitretinoin**. Adjust **alitretinoin** dose, p. 1305. Moderate Theoretical

▸ Fibrates (gemfibrozil) are predicted to increase the exposure to **alitretinoin**. Adjust **alitretinoin** dose, p. 1305. Moderate Theoretical

▸ Fibrates (gemfibrozil) increase the concentration of **bexarotene**. Avoid. Severe Study

▸ HIV-protease inhibitors are predicted to increase the exposure to **alitretinoin**. Adjust **alitretinoin** dose, p. 1305. Moderate Theoretical

▸ Idelalisib is predicted to increase the exposure to **alitretinoin**. Adjust **alitretinoin** dose, p. 1305. Moderate Theoretical

▸ Macrolides (clarithromycin) are predicted to increase the exposure to **alitretinoin**. Adjust **alitretinoin** dose, p. 1305. Moderate Theoretical

▸ **Acitretin** is predicted to increase the concentration of methotrexate. Avoid. Moderate Anecdotal

▸ Retinoids **(acitretin, alitretinoin, isotretinoin, tretinoin)** increase the risk of benign intracranial hypertension when given with tetracyclines. Avoid. Severe Anecdotal

▸ Retinoids **(acitretin, alitretinoin, isotretinoin, tretinoin)** increase the risk of benign intracranial hypertension when given with tigecycline. Avoid. Severe Anecdotal

▸ **Bexarotene** is predicted to increase the risk of toxicity when given with vitamin A. Adjust dose. Moderate Theoretical

▸ Retinoids **(acitretin, alitretinoin, isotretinoin)** are predicted to increase the risk of vitamin A toxicity when given with vitamin A. Moderate Theoretical

▸ **Tretinoin** is predicted to increase the risk of vitamin A toxicity when given with vitamin A. Avoid. Severe Study

Ribavirin

▸ **Ribavirin** increases the risk of anaemia and/or leucopenia when given with NRTIs (zidovudine). Avoid. Severe Study

Ribociclib → see **TABLE 15** p. 1432 (myelosuppression), **TABLE 9** p. 1431 (QT-interval prolongation)

FOOD AND LIFESTYLE Avoid concomitant use of pomegranate or pomegranate juice as it is predicted to increase ribociclib exposure.

▸ **Ribociclib** (high-dose) is predicted to increase the exposure to alpha blockers (alfuzosin). Avoid. Moderate Theoretical

▸ Anti-androgens (apalutamide, enzalutamide) are predicted to markedly decrease the exposure to **ribociclib**. Avoid. Severe Study → Also see **TABLE 9** p. 1431

▸ Antiarrhythmics (dronedarone) are predicted to increase the exposure to **ribociclib**. Moderate Study → Also see **TABLE 9** p. 1431

▸ **Ribociclib** (high-dose) is predicted to increase the exposure to antiarrhythmics (amiodarone). Avoid. Moderate Theoretical → Also see **TABLE 9** p. 1431

▸ Antiepileptics (carbamazepine, fosphenytoin, phenobarbital, phenytoin, primidone) are predicted to markedly decrease the exposure to **ribociclib**. Avoid. Severe Study

▸ Antifungals, azoles (fluconazole, isavuconazole, posaconazole) are predicted to increase the exposure to **ribociclib**. Moderate Study → Also see **TABLE 9** p. 1431

▸ Antifungals, azoles (itraconazole, ketoconazole, voriconazole) are predicted to increase the exposure to **ribociclib**. Avoid or adjust **ribociclib** dose, p. 1042. Moderate Study → Also see **TABLE 9** p. 1431

▸ **Ribociclib** (high-dose) is predicted to increase the exposure to antipsychotics, second generation (quetiapine). Avoid. Moderate Theoretical

▸ **Ribociclib** moderately increases the exposure to benzodiazepines (midazolam). Avoid. Moderate Study

▸ Calcium channel blockers (diltiazem, verapamil) are predicted to increase the exposure to **ribociclib**. Moderate Study

▸ **Ribociclib** is predicted to increase the exposure to ciclosporin. Use with caution and adjust dose. Moderate Theoretical

▸ Cobicistat is predicted to increase the exposure to **ribociclib**. Avoid or adjust **ribociclib** dose, p. 1042. Moderate Study

▸ Crizotinib is predicted to increase the exposure to **ribociclib**. Moderate Study → Also see **TABLE 9** p. 1431

▸ **Ribociclib** is predicted to increase the exposure to digoxin. Moderate Theoretical

▸ Endothelin receptor antagonists (bosentan) are predicted to decrease the exposure to **ribociclib**. Moderate Study

▸ **Ribociclib** (high-dose) is predicted to increase the exposure to ergotamine. Avoid. Moderate Theoretical

▸ **Ribociclib** is predicted to increase the exposure to everolimus. Use with caution and adjust dose. Moderate Theoretical

▸ Grapefruit juice is predicted to increase the exposure to **ribociclib**. Avoid. Moderate Theoretical

▸ HIV-protease inhibitors are predicted to increase the exposure to **ribociclib**. Avoid or adjust **ribociclib** dose, p. 1042. Moderate Study → Also see **TABLE 9** p. 1431

▸ Idelalisib is predicted to increase the exposure to **ribociclib**. Avoid or adjust **ribociclib** dose, p. 1042. Moderate Study

A1

Interactions | Appendix 1

Ribociclib (continued)

‣ Imatinib is predicted to increase the exposure to **ribociclib**. Moderate Study → Also see TABLE 15 p. 1432
‣ Letermovir is predicted to increase the exposure to **ribociclib**. Moderate Study
‣ Macrolides (clarithromycin) are predicted to increase the exposure to **ribociclib**. Avoid or adjust **ribociclib** dose, p. 1042. Moderate Study → Also see TABLE 9 p. 1431
‣ Macrolides (erythromycin) are predicted to increase the exposure to **ribociclib**. Moderate Study → Also see TABLE 9 p. 1431
‣ **Ribociclib** is predicted to increase the exposure to metformin. Moderate Theoretical
‣ Mitotane is predicted to markedly decrease the exposure to **ribociclib**. Avoid. Severe Study → Also see TABLE 15 p. 1432
‣ Neurokinin-1 receptor antagonists (aprepitant, netupitant) are predicted to increase the exposure to **ribociclib**. Moderate Study
‣ Nilotinib is predicted to increase the exposure to **ribociclib**. Moderate Study → Also see TABLE 15 p. 1432 → Also see TABLE 9 p. 1431
‣ NNRTIs (efavirenz, nevirapine) are predicted to decrease the exposure to **ribociclib**. Moderate Study → Also see TABLE 9 p. 1431
‣ **Ribociclib** is predicted to increase the exposure to opioids (alfentanil, fentanyl). Use with caution and adjust dose. Moderate Theoretical
‣ **Ribociclib** is predicted to increase the exposure to phosphodiesterase type-5 inhibitors (sildenafil). Avoid. Moderate Theoretical → Also see TABLE 9 p. 1431
‣ **Ribociclib** (high-dose) is predicted to increase the exposure to pimozide. Avoid. Moderate Theoretical → Also see TABLE 9 p. 1431
‣ Rifamycins (rifampicin) are predicted to markedly decrease the exposure to **ribociclib**. Avoid. Severe Study
‣ **Ribociclib** is predicted to increase the exposure to sirolimus. Use with caution and adjust dose. Moderate Theoretical
‣ St John's wort is predicted to decrease the exposure to **ribociclib**. Avoid. Severe Study
‣ **Ribociclib** is predicted to increase the exposure to statins (pravastatin, rosuvastatin). Moderate Theoretical
‣ **Ribociclib** (high-dose) is predicted to increase the exposure to statins (simvastatin). Avoid. Moderate Theoretical
‣ **Ribociclib** is predicted to increase the exposure to tacrolimus. Use with caution and adjust dose. Moderate Theoretical

Rifabutin → see rifamycins

Rifampicin → see rifamycins

Rifamycins

rifabutin · rifampicin

GENERAL INFORMATION Although some manufacturers class rifabutin as a potent inducer of CYP3A4, clinical data suggests it is potentially a weak inducer, and therefore the BNF does not extrapolate the interactions of potent CYP3A4 inducers to rifabutin. For those who wish to err on the side of caution, see the interactions of rifampicin but bear in mind other mechanisms might be involved.

‣ **Rifampicin** is predicted to decrease the exposure to 5-HT3-receptor antagonists (ondansetron). Moderate Study
‣ **Rifampicin** is predicted to markedly decrease the exposure to abemaciclib. Avoid. Severe Study
‣ **Rifampicin** is predicted to decrease the exposure to acalabrutinib. Avoid. Severe Study
‣ **Rifampicin** is predicted to decrease the exposure to afatinib. Moderate Study
‣ **Rifampicin** is predicted to decrease the exposure to agomelatine. Moderate Theoretical
‣ **Rifampicin** is predicted to decrease the exposure to aldosterone antagonists (eplerenone). Avoid. Moderate Theoretical
‣ **Rifampicin** decreases the exposure to aliskiren. Moderate Study
‣ **Rifampicin** decreases the exposure to aminophylline. Adjust dose. Moderate Study
‣ **Rifampicin** is predicted to decrease the exposure to anaesthetics, local (ropivacaine). Moderate Study
‣ Oral antacids decrease the absorption of oral **rifampicin**. **Rifampicin** should be taken 1 hour before antacids. Moderate Study
‣ **Rifampicin** is predicted to decrease the exposure to anti-androgens (abiraterone). Avoid. Severe Study

‣ **Rifampicin** is predicted to decrease the exposure to anti-androgens (darolutamide). Avoid. Moderate Study
‣ **Rifampicin** is predicted to decrease the exposure to antiarrhythmics (disopyramide, dronedarone). Avoid. Severe Study
‣ **Rifampicin** is predicted to decrease the efficacy of antiarrhythmics (propafenone). Moderate Study
‣ **Rifampicin** is predicted to decrease the exposure to anticholinesterases, centrally acting (donepezil). Mild Study
‣ Antiepileptics (phenobarbital, primidone) are predicted to decrease the exposure to **rifampicin** and **rifampicin** is predicted to decrease the exposure to antiepileptics (phenobarbital, primidone). Use with caution and adjust dose. Moderate Study
‣ **Rifampicin** slightly decreases the exposure to antiepileptics (brivaracetam). Adjust dose. Moderate Study
‣ **Rifampicin** decreases the concentration of antiepileptics (fosphenytoin, phenytoin). Use with caution and adjust dose. Moderate Study
‣ **Rifampicin** markedly increases the clearance of antiepileptics (lamotrigine). Adjust **lamotrigine** dose, p. 335. Moderate Study
‣ **Rifampicin** is predicted to decrease the exposure to antiepileptics (perampanel). Monitor and adjust dose. Moderate Study
‣ Antifungals, azoles (fluconazole) increase the risk of uveitis when given with **rifabutin**. Severe Study
‣ Antifungals, azoles (itraconazole, posaconazole) increase the concentration of **rifabutin** and **rifabutin** decreases the concentration of antifungals, azoles (itraconazole, posaconazole). Avoid. Severe Study
‣ Antifungals, azoles (ketoconazole) are predicted to increase the concentration of **rifabutin** and **rifabutin** is predicted to decrease the concentration of antifungals, azoles (ketoconazole). Avoid. Severe Theoretical
‣ Antifungals, azoles (miconazole) are predicted to increase the concentration of **rifabutin**. Use with caution and adjust dose. Moderate Theoretical
‣ **Rifabutin** slightly decreases the exposure to antifungals, azoles (fluconazole). Adjust dose. Moderate Study
‣ **Rifabutin** is predicted to decrease the exposure to antifungals, azoles (isavuconazole). Avoid. Severe Theoretical
‣ **Rifampicin** is predicted to decrease the exposure to antifungals, azoles (isavuconazole). Avoid. Severe Study
‣ **Rifampicin** markedly decreases the exposure to antifungals, azoles (itraconazole). Avoid and for 14 days after stopping **rifampicin**. Moderate Study
‣ **Rifampicin** markedly decreases the exposure to antifungals, azoles (ketoconazole) and antifungals, azoles (ketoconazole) potentially decrease the exposure to **rifampicin**. Avoid. Moderate Study
‣ **Rifampicin** is predicted to decrease the exposure to antifungals, azoles (posaconazole). Avoid. Moderate Anecdotal
‣ **Rifabutin** decreases the concentration of antifungals, azoles (voriconazole) and antifungals, azoles (voriconazole) increase the concentration of **rifabutin**. Avoid or adjust **voriconazole** dose, p. 638. Severe Study
‣ **Rifampicin** very markedly decreases the exposure to antifungals, azoles (voriconazole). Avoid. Moderate Study
‣ **Rifampicin** is predicted to decrease the exposure to antihistamines, non-sedating (bilastine). Moderate Theoretical
‣ **Rifampicin** increases the clearance of antihistamines, non-sedating (fexofenadine). Moderate Study
‣ **Rifampicin** is predicted to decrease the exposure to antimalarials (artemether with lumefantrine). Avoid. Severe Study
‣ **Rifabutin** slightly decreases the exposure to antimalarials (atovaquone). Avoid. Moderate Study
‣ **Rifampicin** moderately decreases the exposure to antimalarials (atovaquone) and antimalarials (atovaquone) slightly increase the exposure to **rifampicin**. Avoid. Moderate Study
‣ **Rifampicin** moderately decreases the exposure to antimalarials (mefloquine). Severe Study
‣ **Rifampicin** is predicted to decrease the concentration of antimalarials (piperaquine). Avoid. Moderate Theoretical
‣ **Rifampicin** decreases the exposure to antimalarials (quinine). Severe Study

Rifampicin is predicted to moderately decrease the exposure to antipsychotics, second generation (aripiprazole). Adjust **aripiprazole** dose, p. 415. [Moderate] Study

Rifampicin is predicted to decrease the exposure to antipsychotics, second generation (cariprazine). Avoid. [Severe] Theoretical

Rifampicin decreases the exposure to antipsychotics, second generation (clozapine). [Severe] Anecdotal

Rifampicin is predicted to decrease the exposure to antipsychotics, second generation (lurasidone). Avoid. [Moderate] Study

Rifampicin is predicted to decrease the exposure to antipsychotics, second generation (olanzapine). Monitor and adjust dose. [Moderate] Study

Rifampicin is predicted to decrease the exposure to antipsychotics, second generation (paliperidone). Monitor and adjust dose. [Severe] Study

Rifampicin is predicted to decrease the exposure to antipsychotics, second generation (quetiapine). [Moderate] Study

Rifampicin is predicted to decrease the exposure to antipsychotics, second generation (risperidone). Adjust dose. [Moderate] Study

Rifampicin decreases the exposure to ataluren. [Moderate] Study

Rifampicin is predicted to decrease the exposure to avapritinib. Avoid. [Severe] Study

Rifampicin is predicted to decrease the exposure to axitinib. Avoid or adjust dose. [Moderate] Study

Rifampicin is predicted to decrease the exposure to bazedoxifene. [Moderate] Theoretical

Rifampicin decreases the exposure to bedaquiline. Avoid. [Severe] Study

Rifampicin is predicted to decrease the exposure to benzodiazepines (alprazolam). Adjust dose. [Moderate] Theoretical

Rifampicin is predicted to decrease the exposure to benzodiazepines (chlordiazepoxide). [Moderate] Theoretical

Rifampicin moderately decreases the exposure to benzodiazepines (diazepam). Avoid. [Moderate] Study

Rifampicin increases the clearance of benzodiazepines (lorazepam, nitrazepam). [Moderate] Study

Rifampicin is predicted to decrease the exposure to benzodiazepines (midazolam). Monitor and adjust dose. [Moderate] Study

Rifampicin moderately decreases the exposure to beta blockers, non-selective (carvedilol). [Moderate] Study

Rifampicin decreases the exposure to beta blockers, non-selective (propranolol). Monitor and adjust dose. [Moderate] Study

Rifampicin slightly decreases the exposure to beta blockers, selective (bisoprolol, metoprolol). [Mild] Study

Rifampicin moderately decreases the exposure to beta blockers, selective (celiprolol). [Moderate] Study

Rifabutin slightly decreases the exposure to bictegravir. Avoid. [Moderate] Study

Rifampicin is predicted to decrease the exposure to bictegravir. Avoid. [Moderate] Study

Rifampicin slightly decreases the exposure to bortezomib. Avoid. [Severe] Study

Rifampicin is predicted to very markedly decrease the exposure to bosutinib. Avoid. [Severe] Study

Rifabutin is predicted to decrease the exposure to brigatinib. Avoid. [Moderate] Theoretical

Rifampicin is predicted to decrease the exposure to brigatinib. Avoid. [Severe] Study

Rifampicin is predicted to decrease the exposure to bupropion. [Moderate] Study

Rifampicin is predicted to decrease the exposure to buspirone. Use with caution and adjust dose. [Severe] Study

Rifampicin moderately decreases the exposure to cabozantinib. Avoid. [Moderate] Study

Rifampicin is predicted to moderately increase the clearance of caffeine citrate. Monitor and adjust dose. [Moderate] Study

Rifampicin is predicted to decrease the exposure to calcium channel blockers (amlodipine, felodipine, lacidipine, lercanidipine, nicardipine, nimodipine). Monitor and adjust dose. [Moderate] Study

Rifampicin greatly decreases the exposure to calcium channel blockers (diltiazem, verapamil). [Severe] Study

Rifampicin moderately decreases the exposure to calcium channel blockers (nifedipine). Avoid. [Severe] Study

Rifampicin is predicted to decrease the exposure to cannabidiol. Adjust dose. [Moderate] Study

Rifampicin decreases the concentration of caspofungin. Adjust **caspofungin** dose, p. 631. [Moderate] Study

Rifampicin is predicted to decrease the exposure to ceritinib. Avoid. [Severe] Study

Rifampicin decreases the concentration of chloramphenicol. [Moderate] Study

Rifampicin decreases the concentration of ciclosporin. [Severe] Study

Rifampicin is predicted to alter the effects of cilostazol. [Moderate] Theoretical

Rifampicin is predicted to decrease the exposure to cinacalcet. Monitor and adjust dose. [Moderate] Study

Rifampicin decreases the exposure to clomethiazole. Monitor and adjust dose. [Moderate] Study

Rifabutin decreases the concentration of cobicistat and cobicistat increases the exposure to **rifabutin**. Avoid or adjust dose. [Severe] Study

Rifampicin is predicted to decrease the exposure to cobicistat. Avoid. [Severe] Theoretical

Rifampicin is predicted to decrease the exposure to cobimetinib. Avoid. [Severe] Theoretical

Rifamycins are predicted to decrease the efficacy of combined hormonal contraceptives. For FSRH guidance, see Contraceptives, interactions p. 840. [Severe] Study

Rifampicin is predicted to decrease the exposure to corticosteroids (budesonide, deflazacort, dexamethasone, fludrocortisone, hydrocortisone, methylprednisolone, prednisolone, triamcinolone). Monitor and adjust dose. [Moderate] Study

Rifampicin is predicted to decrease the exposure to corticosteroids (fluticasone). [Unknown] Theoretical

Rifampicin decreases the anticoagulant effect of coumarins. [Severe] Study

Rifampicin is predicted to markedly decrease the exposure to crizotinib. Avoid. [Severe] Study

Rifampicin is predicted to decrease the exposure to dabrafenib. Avoid. [Moderate] Theoretical

Rifamycins decrease the exposure to dapsone. [Moderate] Study

Rifampicin is predicted to decrease the exposure to darifenacin. [Moderate] Theoretical

Rifampicin is predicted to decrease the exposure to dasabuvir. Avoid. [Severe] Theoretical

Rifampicin is predicted to markedly decrease the exposure to dasatinib. Avoid. [Severe] Study

Rifampicin is predicted to slightly decrease the exposure to delamanid. Avoid. [Moderate] Study

Rifamycins are predicted to decrease the efficacy of desogestrel. For FSRH guidance, see Contraceptives, interactions p. 840. [Severe] Theoretical

Rifampicin is predicted to markedly decrease the exposure to dienogest. [Severe] Study

Rifampicin decreases the concentration of digoxin. [Moderate] Study

Rifampicin is predicted to decrease the exposure to dipeptidylpeptidase-4 inhibitors (linagliptin). [Moderate] Study

Rifampicin is predicted to moderately decrease the exposure to dipeptidylpeptidase-4 inhibitors (saxagliptin). [Moderate] Study

Rifampicin decreases the exposure to dolutegravir. Adjust dose. [Severe] Study

Rifampicin is predicted to decrease the exposure to dronabinol. Avoid or adjust dose. [Mild] Study

Rifampicin is predicted to decrease the exposure to duloxetine. [Moderate] Theoretical

Rifampicin is predicted to decrease the exposure to elbasvir. Avoid. [Severe] Study

Rifabutin is predicted to decrease the exposure to elexacaftor. Avoid. [Severe] Theoretical

Rifampicin is predicted to decreases the exposure to elexacaftor. Avoid. [Severe] Theoretical

Rifamycins (continued)

▸ **Rifampicin** is predicted to decrease the exposure to eliglustat. Avoid. [Severe] Study

▸ **Rifampicin** is predicted to decrease the exposure to eltrombopag and eltrombopag is predicted to increase the concentration of **rifampicin**. [Moderate] Theoretical

▸ **Rifampicin** is predicted to decrease the concentration of elvitegravir. Avoid. [Severe] Theoretical

▸ **Rifampicin** is predicted to decrease the exposure to encorafenib. [Severe] Theoretical

▸ **Rifampicin** transiently increases the exposure to endothelin receptor antagonists (ambrisentan). [Moderate] Study

▸ **Rifampicin** affects the exposure to endothelin receptor antagonists (bosentan). Avoid. [Severe] Study

▸ **Rifampicin** is predicted to decrease the exposure to endothelin receptor antagonists (macitentan). Avoid. [Severe] Study

▸ **Rifampicin** is predicted to decrease the exposure to entrectinib. Avoid. [Severe] Study

▸ **Rifampicin** is predicted to decrease the effects of ergotamine. [Moderate] Theoretical

▸ **Rifampicin** is predicted to decrease the exposure to erlotinib. Avoid or adjust **erlotinib** dose, p. 1024. [Severe] Study

▸ **Rifampicin** is predicted to decrease the exposure to esketamine. Adjust dose. [Moderate] Theoretical

▸ **Rifamycins** are predicted to decrease the efficacy of etonogestrel. For FSRH guidance, see Contraceptives, interactions p. 840. [Severe] Theoretical

▸ **Rifampicin** is predicted to decrease the concentration of everolimus. Avoid or adjust dose. [Severe] Study

▸ **Rifampicin** moderately decreases the exposure to exemestane. [Moderate] Study

▸ **Rifampicin** is predicted to moderately decrease the exposure to factor XA inhibitors (apixaban). Use with caution or avoid. [Severe] Study

▸ **Rifampicin** is predicted to decrease the exposure to factor XA inhibitors (edoxaban). [Moderate] Study

▸ **Rifampicin** is predicted to moderately decrease the exposure to factor XA inhibitors (rivaroxaban). Avoid unless patient can be monitored for signs of thrombosis. [Severe] Study

▸ **Rifampicin** is predicted to decrease the exposure to fesoterodine. Avoid. [Moderate] Study

▸ **Rifampicin** is predicted to decrease the exposure to fingolimod. [Moderate] Study

▸ **Rifampicin** is predicted to decrease the exposure to fostamatinib. Avoid. [Severe] Study

▸ **Rifampicin** is predicted to decrease the exposure to gefitinib. Avoid. [Severe] Study

▸ **Rifampicin** moderately decreases the exposure to gilteritinib. Avoid. [Severe] Study

▸ **Rifampicin** is predicted to moderately decrease the exposure to glasdegib. Avoid. [Severe] Study

▸ **Rifampicin** markedly affects the exposure to glecaprevir. Avoid. [Severe] Study

▸ **Rifampicin** is predicted to decrease the exposure to grazoprevir. Avoid. [Severe] Study

▸ **Rifampicin** is predicted to decrease the concentration of guanfacine. Adjust **guanfacine** dose, p. 372. [Moderate] Study

▸ **Rifampicin** decreases the concentration of haloperidol. Adjust dose. [Moderate] Study

▸ HIV-protease inhibitors (atazanavir, darunavir, fosamprenavir, lopinavir, saquinavir, tipranavir) boosted with ritonavir increase the exposure to **rifabutin**. Monitor and adjust dose. [Severe] Study

▸ HIV-protease inhibitors (ritonavir) markedly increase the exposure to **rifabutin**. Avoid or adjust dose. [Severe] Study

▸ **Rifampicin** is predicted to moderately to markedly decrease the exposure to HIV-protease inhibitors (atazanavir, darunavir, fosamprenavir, lopinavir, saquinavir). Avoid. [Severe] Study

▸ **Rifampicin** slightly decreases the exposure to HIV-protease inhibitors (ritonavir). [Severe] Study

▸ **Rifampicin** is predicted to decrease the exposure to HIV-protease inhibitors (tipranavir). Avoid. [Severe] Study

▸ **Rifamycins** are predicted to decrease the effects of hormone replacement therapy. [Moderate] Anecdotal

▸ **Rifampicin** is predicted to decrease the exposure to ibrutinib. Avoid or adjust **ibrutinib** dose, p. 1027. [Severe] Study

▸ **Rifampicin** is predicted to decrease the exposure to idelalisib. Avoid. [Severe] Study

▸ **Rifampicin** is predicted to decrease the exposure to imatinib. Avoid. [Moderate] Study

▸ **Rifampicin** is predicted to decrease the exposure to irinotecan. Avoid. [Severe] Study

▸ **Rifampicin** is predicted to decrease the exposure to iron chelators (deferasirox). Monitor serum ferritin and adjust dose. [Moderate] Study

▸ **Rifampicin** is predicted to decrease the exposure to ivabradine. Adjust dose. [Moderate] Theoretical

▸ **Rifampicin** is predicted to moderately to markedly decrease the exposure to ivacaftor. Avoid. [Severe] Study

▸ **Rifampicin** is predicted to decrease the exposure to ixazomib. Avoid. [Severe] Study

▸ **Rifampicin** is predicted to decrease the exposure to lapatinib. Avoid. [Severe] Study

▸ **Rifampicin** is predicted to moderately decrease the exposure to larotrectinib. Avoid. [Moderate] Study

▸ **Rifabutin** is predicted to decrease the exposure to ledipasvir. Avoid. [Severe] Theoretical

▸ **Rifampicin** is predicted to decrease the exposure to ledipasvir. Avoid. [Severe] Study

▸ Leflunomide is predicted to increase the exposure to **rifampicin**. [Moderate] Theoretical

▸ **Rifabutin** is predicted to decrease the concentration of letermovir. [Moderate] Theoretical

▸ **Rifampicin** is predicted to affect the concentration of letermovir. [Severe] Theoretical

▸ **Rifamycins** are predicted to decrease the efficacy of levonorgestrel. For FSRH guidance, see Contraceptives, interactions p. 840. [Severe] Theoretical

▸ **Rifampicin** slightly decreases the exposure to linezolid. [Moderate] Study

▸ **Rifampicin** is predicted to decrease the exposure to lomitapide. Monitor and adjust dose. [Moderate] Theoretical

▸ **Rifampicin** is predicted to decrease the exposure to lorlatinib. Avoid. [Severe] Study

▸ Lumacaftor is predicted to decrease the exposure to **rifabutin**. Adjust dose. [Moderate] Theoretical

▸ Macrolides (azithromycin) increase the risk of neutropenia when given with **rifabutin**. [Severe] Study

▸ Macrolides (clarithromycin) increase the risk of uveitis when given with **rifabutin**. Adjust dose. [Severe] Study

▸ Macrolides (erythromycin) are predicted to increase the risk of uveitis when given with **rifabutin**. Adjust dose. [Severe] Theoretical

▸ **Rifampicin** decreases the concentration of macrolides (clarithromycin). [Severe] Study

▸ **Rifampicin** is predicted to decrease the exposure to maraviroc. Adjust dose. [Severe] Study

▸ **Rifampicin** is predicted to slightly decrease the exposure to meglitinides (nateglinide). [Mild] Study

▸ **Rifampicin** is predicted to decrease the exposure to meglitinides (repaglinide). Monitor blood glucose and adjust dose. [Moderate] Study

▸ **Rifampicin** is predicted to decrease the exposure to melatonin. [Moderate] Theoretical

▸ **Rifampicin** is predicted to increase the clearance of mexiletine. Monitor and adjust dose. [Moderate] Study

▸ **Rifampicin** is predicted to decrease the exposure to midostaurin. Avoid. [Severe] Study

▸ **Rifampicin** is predicted to decrease the exposure to mirtazapine. Adjust dose. [Moderate] Study

▸ **Rifampicin** is predicted to decrease the exposure to modafinil. [Moderate] Theoretical

▸ **Rifampicin** decreases the effects of monoclonal antibodies (brentuximab vedotin). [Severe] Study

▸ **Rifampicin** is predicted to decrease the exposure to monoclonal antibodies (polatuzumab vedotin). [Moderate] Theoretical

▸ **Rifampicin** is predicted to decrease the exposure to montelukast. [Mild] Study

Rifampicin decreases the concentration of mycophenolate. Monitor and adjust dose. Severe Study

Rifampicin is predicted to markedly decrease the exposure to naldemedine. Avoid. Severe Study

Rifampicin is predicted to markedly decrease the exposure to naloxegol. Avoid. Moderate Study

Rifampicin is predicted to decrease the exposure to neratinib. Avoid. Severe Study

Rifampicin is predicted to markedly decrease the exposure to neurokinin-1 receptor antagonists (aprepitant). Avoid. Moderate Study

Rifampicin is predicted to decrease the exposure to neurokinin-1 receptor antagonists (fosaprepitant). Avoid. Moderate Theoretical

Rifampicin is predicted to decrease the exposure to neurokinin-1 receptor antagonists (netupitant). Avoid. Severe Study

Rifampicin is predicted to moderately decrease the exposure to nilotinib. Avoid. Severe Study

Rifampicin is predicted to decrease the exposure to nintedanib. Moderate Study

Rifampicin is predicted to decrease the exposure to nitisinone. Adjust dose. Moderate Theoretical

NNRTIs (efavirenz) slightly decrease the exposure to rifabutin. Adjust dose. Severe Study

Rifabutin moderately decreases the exposure to NNRTIs (doravirine). Adjust doravirine p. 683 or lamivudine with tenofovir disoproxil and doravirine p. 692 dose. Moderate Study

Rifampicin is predicted to decrease the exposure to NNRTIs (doravirine). Avoid. Severe Study

Rifampicin slightly decreases the exposure to NNRTIs (efavirenz). Adjust dose. Severe Study

Rifabutin decreases the exposure to NNRTIs (etravirine). Moderate Study

Rifampicin is predicted to decrease the exposure to NNRTIs (etravirine). Avoid. Severe Theoretical

Rifampicin decreases the concentration of NNRTIs (nevirapine). Avoid. Severe Study

Rifabutin slightly decreases the exposure to NNRTIs (rilpivirine). Adjust dose. Severe Study

Rifampicin markedly decreases the exposure to NNRTIs (rilpivirine). Avoid. Severe Study

Rifamycins are predicted to decrease the efficacy of norethisterone. For FSRH guidance, see Contraceptives, interactions p. 840. Severe Anecdotal

Rifampicin moderately decreases the exposure to NSAIDs (celecoxib, diclofenac, etoricoxib). Moderate Study

Rifampicin is predicted to decrease the exposure to olaparib. Avoid. Moderate Theoretical

Rifampicin is predicted to decrease the exposure to ombitasvir. Avoid. Severe Theoretical

Rifampicin is predicted to decrease the exposure to opioids (alfentanil, fentanyl). Moderate Study

Rifampicin is predicted to decrease the exposure to opioids (buprenorphine). Monitor and adjust dose. Moderate Theoretical

Rifampicin decreases the exposure to opioids (codeine, morphine). Moderate Study

Rifampicin decreases the exposure to opioids (methadone). Monitor and adjust dose. Severe Study

Rifampicin is predicted to decrease the exposure to opioids (oxycodone). Monitor and adjust dose. Moderate Study

Rifampicin is predicted to moderately decrease the exposure to osimertinib. Avoid. Moderate Study

Rifampicin is predicted to moderately decrease the exposure to ospemifene. Moderate Study

Rifampicin moderately decreases the exposure to the active metabolite of ozanimod. Avoid. Moderate Study

Rifampicin is predicted to decrease the exposure to palbociclib. Avoid. Severe Study

Rifampicin is predicted to decrease the exposure to panobinostat. Avoid. Moderate Theoretical

Rifampicin decreases the exposure to paracetamol. Moderate Study

Rifampicin is predicted to decrease the exposure to paritaprevir (with ritonavir and ombitasvir). Avoid. Severe Study

▸ **Rifampicin** is predicted to decrease the exposure to pazopanib. Avoid. Severe Theoretical

▸ **Rifampicin** moderately decreases the exposure to phosphodiesterase type-4 inhibitors (apremilast). Avoid. Severe Study

▸ **Rifampicin** is predicted to decrease the exposure to phosphodiesterase type-4 inhibitors (roflumilast). Avoid. Moderate Study

▸ **Rifampicin** is predicted to decrease the exposure to phosphodiesterase type-5 inhibitors (avanafil, tadalafil). Avoid. Severe Study

▸ **Rifampicin** is predicted to decrease the exposure to phosphodiesterase type-5 inhibitors (sildenafil, vardenafil). Moderate Theoretical

▸ **Rifampicin** is predicted to moderately to markedly decrease the exposure to pibrentasvir. Avoid. Severe Study

▸ **Rifampicin** moderately decreases the exposure to pioglitazone. Monitor and adjust dose. Moderate Study

▸ **Rifampicin** is predicted to decrease the exposure to pirfenidone. Avoid. Moderate Theoretical

▸ **Rifampicin** is predicted to moderately decrease the exposure to pitolisant. Moderate Study

▸ **Rifampicin** is predicted to decrease the exposure to ponatinib. Avoid. Moderate Theoretical

▸ **Rifampicin** is predicted to markedly decrease the exposure to praziquantel. Avoid. Moderate Study

▸ **Rifampicin** slightly decreases the exposure to raltegravir. Avoid or adjust dose—consult product literature. Moderate Study

▸ **Rifampicin** is predicted to decrease the exposure to ranolazine. Avoid. Severe Study

▸ **Rifampicin** is predicted to decrease the exposure to reboxetine. Moderate Anecdotal

▸ **Rifampicin** is predicted to decrease the exposure to regorafenib. Avoid. Moderate Study

▸ **Rifampicin** potentially decreases the exposure to remdesivir. Avoid. Moderate Theoretical

▸ **Rifampicin** is predicted to markedly decrease the exposure to ribociclib. Avoid. Severe Study

▸ **Rifampicin** is predicted to decrease the exposure to ruxolitinib. Monitor and adjust dose. Moderate Study

▸ **Rifampicin** moderately decreases the exposure to the active metabolite of selexipag. Adjust dose. Moderate Study

▸ **Rifampicin** is predicted to decrease the exposure to siponimod. Severe Study

▸ **Rifampicin** is predicted to decrease the concentration of sirolimus. Avoid. Severe Study

▸ **Rifampicin** moderately decreases the exposure to sodium glucose co-transporter 2 inhibitors (canagliflozin). Adjust **canagliflozin** dose, p. 743. Moderate Study

▸ **Rifampicin** is predicted to decrease the exposure to sofosbuvir. Avoid. Severe Study

▸ **Rifampicin** is predicted to decrease the exposure to solifenacin. Moderate Theoretical

▸ **Rifampicin** is predicted to decrease the exposure to sorafenib. Moderate Theoretical

▸ **Rifampicin** markedly decreases the exposure to statins (atorvastatin). Manufacturer advises take both drugs at the same time. Moderate Study

▸ **Rifampicin** moderately decreases the exposure to statins (fluvastatin). Monitor and adjust dose. Moderate Study

▸ **Rifampicin** very markedly decreases the exposure to statins (simvastatin). Moderate Study

▸ **Rifampicin** is predicted to decrease the exposure to sulfonylureas. Moderate Study

▸ **Rifampicin** is predicted to decrease the exposure to sunitinib. Avoid or adjust **sunitinib** dose, p. 1044. Moderate Study

▸ **Rifampicin** decreases the concentration of tacrolimus. Monitor and adjust dose. Severe Study

▸ **Rifampicin** markedly decreases the exposure to tamoxifen. Unknown Study

▸ **Rifampicin** is predicted to decrease the exposure to taxanes (cabazitaxel, paclitaxel). Avoid. Severe Study

▸ **Rifampicin** is predicted to decrease the exposure to taxanes (docetaxel). Severe Theoretical

Rifamycins (continued)

▸ **Rifampicin** is predicted to decrease the concentration of temsirolimus. Avoid. Severe Study
▸ **Rifampicin** are predicted to decrease the exposure to tenofovir alafenamide. Avoid. Moderate Theoretical
▸ **Rifampicin** decreases the exposure to terbinafine. Adjust dose. Moderate Study
▸ Teriflunomide is predicted to increase the exposure to **rifampicin**. Moderate Theoretical
▸ **Rifampicin** decreases the exposure to tetracyclines (doxycycline). Monitor and adjust dose. Moderate Study
▸ **Rifamycins** are predicted to decrease the exposure to tezacaftor. Avoid. Severe Theoretical
▸ **Rifampicin** is predicted to decrease the exposure to theophylline. Adjust dose. Moderate Study
▸ **Rifampicin** is predicted to decrease the exposure to thrombin inhibitors (dabigatran). Avoid. Severe Study
▸ **Rifampicin** is predicted to markedly decrease the exposure to ticagrelor. Avoid. Severe Study
▸ **Rifampicin** is predicted to decrease the exposure to tivozanib. Severe Study
▸ **Rifampicin** moderately decreases the exposure to tizanidine. Mild Study
▸ **Rifampicin** is predicted to decrease the exposure to tofacitinib. Avoid. Severe Study
▸ **Rifampicin** is predicted to decrease the exposure to tolvaptan. Use with caution or avoid depending on indication. Severe Study
▸ **Rifampicin** is predicted to decrease the exposure to toremifene. Adjust dose. Moderate Study
▸ **Rifampicin** is predicted to decrease the exposure to trabectedin. Avoid. Severe Theoretical
▸ **Rifampicin** decreases the exposure to trimethoprim. Moderate Study
▸ **Rifamycins** decrease the efficacy of ulipristal. For FSRH guidance, see Contraceptives, interactions p. 840. Severe Anecdotal
▸ **Rifampicin** is predicted to decrease the exposure to upadacitinib. Moderate Study
▸ **Rifampicin** is predicted to decrease the exposure to vandetanib. Avoid. Moderate Study
▸ **Rifampicin** is predicted to moderately decrease the exposure to velpatasvir. Avoid. Severe Study
▸ **Rifampicin** is predicted to decrease the exposure to vemurafenib. Avoid. Severe Theoretical
▸ **Rifampicin** is predicted to decrease the exposure to venetoclax. Avoid. Severe Study
▸ **Rifampicin** is predicted to decrease the exposure to vinca alkaloids (vinblastine, vincristine, vindesine). Severe Theoretical
▸ **Rifampicin** is predicted to decrease the exposure to vinca alkaloids (vinflunine). Avoid. Severe Theoretical
▸ **Rifampicin** is predicted to decrease the exposure to vinca alkaloids (vinorelbine). Use with caution or avoid. Severe Theoretical
▸ **Rifampicin** is predicted to decrease the exposure to vismodegib. Avoid. Moderate Theoretical
▸ **Rifampicin** potentially increases the risk of nephrotoxicity when given with volatile halogenated anaesthetics (methoxyflurane). Avoid. Severe Theoretical
▸ **Rifampicin** is predicted to decrease the exposure to vortioxetine. Monitor and adjust dose. Moderate Study
▸ **Rifabutin** is predicted to decrease the concentration of voxilaprevir. Avoid. Severe Theoretical
▸ **Rifampicin** is predicted to decrease the concentration of voxilaprevir. Avoid. Severe Study
▸ **Rifampicin** moderately decreases the exposure to zolpidem. Moderate Study
▸ **Rifampicin** is predicted to decrease the exposure to zopiclone. Adjust dose. Moderate Study

Rifaximin

▸ Ciclosporin very markedly increases the exposure to **rifaximin**. Severe Study

Rilpivirine → see NNRTIs

Riluzole

FOOD AND LIFESTYLE Charcoal-grilled foods are predicted to decrease the exposure to riluzole.

▸ Mexiletine is predicted to increase the exposure to **riluzole**. Moderate Theoretical
▸ Quinolones (ciprofloxacin) are predicted to increase the exposure to **riluzole**. Moderate Theoretical
▸ SSRIs (fluvoxamine) are predicted to increase the exposure to **riluzole**. Moderate Theoretical

Riociguat → see TABLE 8 p. 1430 (hypotension)

FOOD AND LIFESTYLE Dose adjustment might be necessary if smoking is started or stopped during treatment.

▸ Oral antacids decrease the exposure to oral **riociguat**. Riociguat should be taken 1 hour before or 2 hours after antacids. Mild Study
▸ Antifungals, azoles (itraconazole, posaconazole) are predicted to increase the exposure to **riociguat**. Adjust riociguat dose and monitor blood pressure, p. 198. Moderate Theoretical
▸ Antifungals, azoles (ketoconazole) moderately increase the exposure to **riociguat**. Adjust riociguat dose and monitor blood pressure, p. 198. Moderate Study
▸ Ciclosporin is predicted to increase the exposure to **riociguat**. Moderate Theoretical
▸ HIV-protease inhibitors (ritonavir) are predicted to increase the exposure to **riociguat**. Adjust dose and monitor blood pressure. Moderate Theoretical
▸ Riociguat is predicted to increase the risk of hypotension when given with phosphodiesterase type-5 inhibitors. Avoid. Severe Theoretical → Also see TABLE 8 p. 1430

Risankizumab → see monoclonal antibodies
Risedronate → see bisphosphonates
Risperidone → see antipsychotics, second generation
Ritonavir → see HIV-protease inhibitors
Rituximab → see monoclonal antibodies
Rivaroxaban → see factor XA inhibitors
Rivastigmine → see anticholinesterases, centrally acting
Rizatriptan → see triptans
Rocuronium → see neuromuscular blocking drugs, non-depolarising
Roflumilast → see phosphodiesterase type-4 inhibitors
Ropinirole → see dopamine receptor agonists
Ropivacaine → see anaesthetics, local
Rosuvastatin → see statins
Rotavirus vaccine → see live vaccines
Rotigotine → see dopamine receptor agonists
Rucaparib → see TABLE 15 p. 1432 (myelosuppression)

▸ **Rucaparib** is predicted to increase the exposure to aminophylline. Monitor and adjust dose. Moderate Study
▸ **Rucaparib** is predicted to increase the exposure to antiepileptics (phenytoin). Monitor and adjust dose. Moderate Study
▸ **Rucaparib** slightly increases the exposure to benzodiazepines (midazolam). Monitor and adjust dose. Severe Study
▸ **Rucaparib** is predicted to increase the exposure to ciclosporin. Monitor and adjust dose. Moderate Study
▸ **Rucaparib** slightly increases the exposure to coumarins (warfarin). Monitor and adjust dose. Severe Study
▸ **Rucaparib** is predicted to increase the exposure to ergotamine. Monitor and adjust dose. Moderate Study
▸ **Rucaparib** is predicted to increase the exposure to opioids (alfentanil, fentanyl). Monitor and adjust dose. Moderate Study
▸ **Rucaparib** is predicted to increase the exposure to pimozide. Monitor and adjust dose. Moderate Study
▸ **Rucaparib** is predicted to increase the exposure to sirolimus. Monitor and adjust dose. Moderate Study
▸ **Rucaparib** is predicted to increase the exposure to tacrolimus. Monitor and adjust dose. Moderate Study
▸ **Rucaparib** is predicted to increase the exposure to theophylline. Monitor and adjust dose. Moderate Study
▸ **Rucaparib** is predicted to increase the exposure to tizanidine. Monitor and adjust dose. Moderate Study

Rufinamide → see antiepileptics
Rupatadine → see antihistamines, non-sedating
Ruxolitinib → see TABLE 15 p. 1432 (myelosuppression)

Anti-androgens (apalutamide, enzalutamide) are predicted to decrease the exposure to **ruxolitinib**. Monitor and adjust dose. Moderate Study

Antiarrhythmics (dronedarone) are predicted to increase the exposure to **ruxolitinib**. Moderate Theoretical

Antiepileptics (carbamazepine, fosphenytoin, phenobarbital, phenytoin, primidone) are predicted to decrease the exposure to **ruxolitinib**. Monitor and adjust dose. Moderate Study

Antifungals, azoles (fluconazole, isavuconazole, posaconazole) are predicted to increase the exposure to **ruxolitinib**. Moderate Theoretical

Antifungals, azoles (itraconazole, ketoconazole, voriconazole) are predicted to increase the exposure to **ruxolitinib**. Adjust dose and monitor adverse effects. Moderate Study

Calcium channel blockers (diltiazem, verapamil) are predicted to increase the exposure to **ruxolitinib**. Moderate Theoretical

Cobicistat is predicted to increase the exposure to **ruxolitinib**. Adjust dose and monitor adverse effects. Moderate Study

Ruxolitinib is predicted to increase the risk of bleeding events when given with coumarins. Severe Theoretical

Crizotinib is predicted to increase the exposure to **ruxolitinib**. Moderate Theoretical

Endothelin receptor antagonists (bosentan) are predicted to decrease the exposure to **ruxolitinib**. Monitor and adjust dose. Moderate Theoretical

Grapefruit juice is predicted to increase the exposure to **ruxolitinib**. Severe Theoretical

HIV-protease inhibitors are predicted to increase the exposure to **ruxolitinib**. Adjust dose and monitor adverse effects. Moderate Study

Idelalisib is predicted to increase the exposure to **ruxolitinib**. Adjust dose and monitor adverse effects. Moderate Study

Imatinib is predicted to increase the exposure to **ruxolitinib**. Moderate Theoretical → Also see TABLE 15 p. 1432

Letermovir is predicted to increase the exposure to **ruxolitinib**. Moderate Theoretical

Macrolides (clarithromycin) are predicted to increase the exposure to **ruxolitinib**. Adjust dose and monitor adverse effects. Moderate Study

Macrolides (erythromycin) are predicted to increase the exposure to **ruxolitinib**. Moderate Theoretical

Mitotane is predicted to decrease the exposure to **ruxolitinib**. Monitor and adjust dose. Moderate Study → Also see TABLE 15 p. 1432

Neurokinin-1 receptor antagonists (aprepitant, netupitant) are predicted to increase the exposure to **ruxolitinib**. Moderate Theoretical

Nilotinib is predicted to increase the exposure to **ruxolitinib**. Moderate Theoretical → Also see TABLE 15 p. 1432

NNRTIs (efavirenz, nevirapine) are predicted to decrease the exposure to **ruxolitinib**. Monitor and adjust dose. Moderate Theoretical

▶ **Ruxolitinib** is predicted to increase the risk of bleeding events when given with phenindione. Severe Theoretical

Rifamycins (rifampicin) are predicted to decrease the exposure to **ruxolitinib**. Monitor and adjust dose. Moderate Study

▶ St John's wort is predicted to decrease the exposure to **ruxolitinib**. Monitor and adjust dose. Moderate Theoretical

Sacubitril → see TABLE 8 p. 1430 (hypotension)

▶ Sacubitril is predicted to increase the exposure to statins. Severe Study

Safinamide → see MAO-B inhibitors
Salbutamol → see beta₂ agonists
Salmeterol → see beta₂ agonists
Sapropterin → see TABLE 8 p. 1430 (hypotension)

▶ Methotrexate is predicted to decrease the efficacy of **sapropterin**. Moderate Theoretical

▶ Phosphodiesterase type-5 inhibitors are predicted to increase the risk of hypotension when given with **sapropterin**. Moderate Theoretical → Also see TABLE 8 p. 1430

▶ Trimethoprim is predicted to decrease the efficacy of **sapropterin**. Moderate Theoretical

Saquinavir → see HIV-protease inhibitors
Sarilumab → see monoclonal antibodies
Saxagliptin → see dipeptidylpeptidase-4 inhibitors

Secukinumab → see monoclonal antibodies
Selegiline → see MAO-B inhibitors
Selenium

ROUTE-SPECIFIC INFORMATION Interactions do not generally apply to topical use unless specified.

▶ Oral **selenium** is predicted to decrease the absorption of eltrombopag. **Eltrombopag** should be taken 2 hours before or 4 hours after **selenium**. Severe Theoretical

Selexipag

▶ Antiepileptics (carbamazepine, fosphenytoin, phenytoin) are predicted to decrease the exposure to the active metabolite of **selexipag**. Adjust dose. Moderate Study

▶ Antiepileptics (valproate) are predicted to increase the exposure to **selexipag**. Unknown Theoretical

▶ Antifungals, azoles (fluconazole) are predicted to increase the exposure to **selexipag**. Unknown Theoretical

▶ Clopidogrel is predicted to increase the exposure to **selexipag**. Adjust **selexipag** dose, p. 196. Moderate Study

▶ Fibrates (gemfibrozil) increase the exposure to **selexipag**. Avoid. Severe Study

▶ Iron chelators (deferasirox) are predicted to increase the exposure to **selexipag**. Adjust **selexipag** dose, p. 196. Moderate Study

▶ Leflunomide is predicted to increase the exposure to **selexipag**. Adjust **selexipag** dose, p. 196. Moderate Study

▶ Rifamycins (rifampicin) moderately decrease the exposure to the active metabolite of **selexipag**. Adjust dose. Moderate Study

▶ Teriflunomide is predicted to increase the exposure to **selexipag**. Adjust **selexipag** dose, p. 196. Moderate Study

Semaglutide → see glucagon-like peptide-1 receptor agonists
Sertraline → see SSRIs
Sevelamer

SEPARATION OF ADMINISTRATION Drugs for which a reduction in bioavailability could be clinically important should be administered at least 1 hour before, or 3 hours after, sevelamer; alternatively consider monitoring blood concentrations.

Sevoflurane → see volatile halogenated anaesthetics
Sildenafil → see phosphodiesterase type-5 inhibitors
Siltuximab → see monoclonal antibodies
Silver sulfadiazine

PHARMACOLOGY Silver might inactivate enzymatic debriding agents—concurrent use might not be appropriate.

Simvastatin → see statins
Siponimod → see TABLE 6 p. 1430 (bradycardia), TABLE 9 p. 1431 (QT-interval prolongation)

▶ Anti-androgens (apalutamide, enzalutamide) are predicted to decrease the exposure to **siponimod**. Severe Study

▶ Antiarrhythmics (amiodarone) are predicted to increase the exposure to **siponimod**. Avoid depending on other drugs taken—consult product literature. Severe Study → Also see TABLE 6 p. 1430

▶ Antiepileptics (carbamazepine, fosphenytoin, phenobarbital, phenytoin, primidone) are predicted to decrease the exposure to **siponimod**. Severe Study

▶ Antifungals, azoles (itraconazole, ketoconazole, voriconazole) are predicted to increase the exposure to **siponimod**. Avoid depending on other drugs taken—consult product literature. Severe Theoretical

▶ Antifungals, azoles (miconazole) are predicted to increase the exposure to **siponimod**. Avoid depending on other drugs taken—consult product literature. Severe Study

▶ Cobicistat is predicted to increase the exposure to **siponimod**. Avoid depending on other drugs taken—consult product literature. Severe Theoretical

▶ Endothelin receptor antagonists (bosentan) are predicted to decrease the exposure to **siponimod**. Manufacturer advises caution depending on genotype—consult product literature. Severe Theoretical

▶ HIV-protease inhibitors are predicted to increase the exposure to **siponimod**. Avoid depending on other drugs taken—consult product literature. Severe Theoretical

A1

Interactions | Appendix 1

Siponimod (continued)

▶ Idelalisib is predicted to increase the exposure to **siponimod**. Avoid depending on other drugs taken—consult product literature. Severe Theoretical

▶ Live vaccines are predicted to increase the risk of generalised infection (possibly life-threatening) when given with **siponimod**. Avoid and for 4 weeks after stopping **siponimod**. Severe Theoretical

▶ Macrolides (clarithromycin) are predicted to increase the exposure to **siponimod**. Avoid depending on other drugs taken—consult product literature. Severe Theoretical

▶ Mitotane is predicted to decrease the exposure to **siponimod**. Severe Study

▶ **Siponimod** potentially increases the risk of immunosuppression when given with monoclonal antibodies (alemtuzumab). Avoid. Severe Theoretical

▶ NNRTIs (efavirenz, nevirapine) are predicted to decrease the exposure to **siponimod**. Manufacturer advises caution depending on genotype—consult product literature. Severe Theoretical

▶ Rifamycins (rifampicin) are predicted to decrease the exposure to **siponimod**. Severe Study

▶ St John's wort is predicted to decrease the exposure to **siponimod**. Manufacturer advises caution depending on genotype—consult product literature. Severe Theoretical

Sirolimus

▶ Anti-androgens (apalutamide, enzalutamide) are predicted to decrease the concentration of **sirolimus**. Avoid. Severe Study

▶ Antiarrhythmics (amiodarone) are predicted to increase the concentration of **sirolimus**. Severe Anecdotal

▶ Antiarrhythmics (dronedarone) increase the concentration of **sirolimus**. Monitor and adjust dose. Moderate Study

▶ Antiepileptics (carbamazepine, fosphenytoin, phenobarbital, phenytoin, primidone) are predicted to decrease the concentration of **sirolimus**. Avoid. Severe Study

▶ Antifungals, azoles (fluconazole, isavuconazole, posaconazole) increase the concentration of **sirolimus**. Monitor and adjust dose. Moderate Study

▶ Antifungals, azoles (itraconazole, ketoconazole, voriconazole) are predicted to increase the concentration of **sirolimus**. Avoid. Severe Study

▶ Antifungals, azoles (miconazole) are predicted to increase the concentration of **sirolimus**. Monitor and adjust dose. Moderate Study

▶ Brigatinib potentially decreases the concentration of **sirolimus**. Avoid. Moderate Theoretical

▶ Calcium channel blockers (diltiazem, verapamil) increase the concentration of **sirolimus**. Monitor and adjust dose. Moderate Study

▶ Ceritinib is predicted to increase the exposure to **sirolimus**. Avoid. Severe Theoretical

▶ **Sirolimus** is predicted to affect the efficacy of chenodeoxycholic acid. Monitor and adjust dose. Moderate Theoretical

▶ Ciclosporin moderately increases the exposure to **sirolimus**. Separate administration by 4 hours. Severe Study

▶ Cobicistat is predicted to increase the concentration of **sirolimus**. Avoid. Severe Study

▶ Crizotinib increases the concentration of **sirolimus**. Monitor and adjust dose. Moderate Study

▶ Eliglustat is predicted to increase the exposure to **sirolimus**. Adjust dose. Moderate Study

▶ Endothelin receptor antagonists (bosentan) are predicted to decrease the concentration of **sirolimus** and **sirolimus** potentially increases the concentration of endothelin receptor antagonists (bosentan). Avoid. Severe Theoretical

▶ Entrectinib is predicted to increase the exposure to **sirolimus**. Mild Theoretical

▶ Grapefruit juice increases the concentration of **sirolimus**. Avoid. Moderate Study

▶ HIV-protease inhibitors are predicted to increase the concentration of **sirolimus**. Avoid. Severe Study

▶ Idelalisib is predicted to increase the concentration of **sirolimus**. Avoid. Severe Study

▶ Imatinib increases the concentration of **sirolimus**. Monitor and adjust dose. Moderate Study

▶ Lapatinib is predicted to increase the exposure to **sirolimus**. Moderate Theoretical

▶ Larotrectinib is predicted to increase the exposure to **sirolimus**. Use with caution and adjust dose. Mild Theoretical

▶ Letermovir increases the concentration of **sirolimus**. Monitor and adjust dose. Moderate Study

▶ Live vaccines are predicted to increase the risk of generalised infection (possibly life-threatening) when given with **sirolimus**. Public Health England advises avoid (refer to Green Book). Severe Theoretical

▶ Lorlatinib is predicted to decrease the exposure to **sirolimus**. Avoid. Moderate Theoretical

▶ Lumacaftor is predicted to decrease the exposure to **sirolimus**. Avoid. Severe Theoretical

▶ Macrolides (clarithromycin) are predicted to increase the concentration of **sirolimus**. Avoid. Severe Study

▶ Macrolides (erythromycin) increase the concentration of **sirolimus**. Monitor and adjust dose. Moderate Study

▶ **Sirolimus** is predicted to decrease the efficacy of mifamurtide. Avoid. Severe Theoretical

▶ Mirabegron is predicted to increase the exposure to **sirolimus**. Mild Theoretical

▶ Mitotane is predicted to decrease the concentration of **sirolimus**. Avoid. Severe Study

▶ Monoclonal antibodies (sarilumab) potentially affect the exposure to **sirolimus**. Monitor and adjust dose. Moderate Theoretical

▶ Neratinib is predicted to increase the exposure to **sirolimus**. Moderate Study

▶ Neurokinin-1 receptor antagonists (aprepitant, netupitant) increase the concentration of **sirolimus**. Monitor and adjust dose. Moderate Study

▶ Nilotinib increases the concentration of **sirolimus**. Monitor and adjust dose. Moderate Study

▶ NNRTIs (doravirine) are predicted to decrease the exposure to **sirolimus**. Monitor **sirolimus** concentration and adjust dose, p. 886. Moderate Theoretical

▶ NNRTIs (efavirenz, nevirapine) are predicted to decrease the concentration of **sirolimus**. Monitor and adjust dose. Moderate Theoretical

▶ Palbociclib is predicted to increase the exposure to **sirolimus**. Adjust dose. Moderate Theoretical

▶ Pibrentasvir (with glecaprevir) is predicted to increase the exposure to **sirolimus**. Moderate Study

▶ Pitolisant is predicted to decrease the exposure to **sirolimus**. Avoid. Severe Theoretical

▶ Ribociclib is predicted to increase the exposure to **sirolimus**. Use with caution and adjust dose. Moderate Theoretical

▶ Rifamycins (rifampicin) are predicted to decrease the concentration of **sirolimus**. Avoid. Severe Study

▶ Rucaparib is predicted to increase the exposure to **sirolimus**. Monitor and adjust dose. Moderate Study

▶ St John's wort is predicted to decrease the concentration of **sirolimus**. Monitor and adjust dose. Severe Theoretical

▶ **Sirolimus** is predicted to decrease the concentration of tacrolimus and tacrolimus increases the exposure to **sirolimus**. Severe Study

▶ Velpatasvir is predicted to increase the exposure to **sirolimus**. Severe Theoretical

▶ Vemurafenib is predicted to increase the exposure to **sirolimus**. Use with caution and adjust dose. Severe Theoretical

▶ Venetoclax is predicted to increase the exposure to **sirolimus**. Avoid or adjust dose. Severe Study

Sitagliptin → see dipeptidylpeptidase-4 inhibitors

Sodium bicarbonate

ROUTE-SPECIFIC INFORMATION Interactions do not generally apply to topical use of **sodium bicarbonate** unless specified.

▶ Oral **sodium bicarbonate** is predicted to decrease the exposure to oral acalabrutinib. Separate administration by at least 2 hours. Moderate Theoretical

▶ Oral **sodium bicarbonate** decreases the absorption of antifungals, azoles (ketoconazole). Moderate Study

▶ **Sodium bicarbonate** decreases the concentration of lithium. Severe Anecdotal

Sodium bicarbonate is predicted to decrease the efficacy of methenamine. Avoid. Moderate Theoretical

Sodium citrate

Sodium citrate is predicted to decrease the efficacy of methenamine. Avoid. Moderate Theoretical

Sodium citrate is predicted to increase the risk of adverse effects when given with sucralfate. Avoid. Moderate Theoretical

Sodium glucose co-transporter 2 inhibitors → see TABLE 14 p. 1432 (antidiabetic drugs), TABLE 8 p. 1430 (hypotension)

canagliflozin · dapagliflozin · empagliflozin · ertugliflozin

Rifamycins (rifampin) moderately decrease the exposure to **canagliflozin**. Adjust **canagliflozin** dose, p. 743. Moderate Study

Sodium oxybate → see TABLE 8 p. 1430 (hypotension), TABLE 11 p. 1431 (CNS depressant effects)

Antiepileptics (valproate) increase the exposure to **sodium oxybate**. Adjust **sodium oxybate** dose, p. 512. Moderate Study

Sodium phenylbutyrate

Antiepileptics (valproate) potentially decrease the effects of **sodium phenylbutyrate**. Moderate Anecdotal

Corticosteroids potentially decrease the effects of **sodium phenylbutyrate**. Moderate Anecdotal

Haloperidol potentially decreases the effects of **sodium phenylbutyrate**. Moderate Anecdotal

Sodium picosulfate → see TABLE 18 p. 1433 (hyponatraemia)

Sodium zirconium cyclosilicate

▸ **Sodium zirconium cyclosilicate** is predicted to decrease the exposure to antifungals, azoles. Separate administration by at least 2 hours. Moderate Theoretical

▸ **Sodium zirconium cyclosilicate** is predicted to decrease the exposure to dasatinib. Separate administration by at least 2 hours. Moderate Theoretical

▸ **Sodium zirconium cyclosilicate** is predicted to decrease the exposure to erlotinib. Separate administration by at least 2 hours. Moderate Theoretical

▸ **Sodium zirconium cyclosilicate** is predicted to decrease the exposure to HIV-protease inhibitors. Separate administration by at least 2 hours. Moderate Theoretical

▸ **Sodium zirconium cyclosilicate** is predicted to decrease the exposure to ledipasvir. Separate administration by at least 2 hours. Moderate Theoretical

▸ **Sodium zirconium cyclosilicate** is predicted to decrease the exposure to nilotinib. Separate administration by at least 2 hours. Moderate Theoretical

▸ **Sodium zirconium cyclosilicate** is predicted to decrease the exposure to NNRTIs (rilpivirine). Separate administration by at least 2 hours. Moderate Theoretical

▸ **Sodium zirconium cyclosilicate** is predicted to decrease the exposure to raltegravir. Separate administration by at least 2 hours. Moderate Theoretical

Sofosbuvir

▸ **Sofosbuvir** is predicted to increase the risk of severe bradycardia or heart block when given with antiarrhythmics (amiodarone). Refer to specialist literature. Severe Anecdotal

▸ Antiepileptics (carbamazepine) are predicted to decrease the exposure to **sofosbuvir**. Avoid. Severe Study

▸ Antiepileptics (fosphenytoin, oxcarbazepine, phenobarbital, phenytoin, primidone) are predicted to decrease the exposure to **sofosbuvir**. Severe Theoretical

▸ H₂ receptor antagonists potentially decrease the exposure to **sofosbuvir**. Adjust dose, see ledipasvir with sofosbuvir p. 668, sofosbuvir with velpatasvir p. 669, and sofosbuvir with velpatasvir and voxilaprevir p. 669. Moderate Study

▸ HIV-protease inhibitors (tipranavir) are predicted to decrease the exposure to **sofosbuvir**. Avoid. Severe Theoretical

▸ Modafinil is predicted to decrease the exposure to **sofosbuvir**. Avoid. Severe Theoretical

▸ Proton pump inhibitors potentially decrease the exposure to **sofosbuvir**. Adjust dose, see ledipasvir with sofosbuvir p. 668, sofosbuvir with velpatasvir p. 669, and sofosbuvir with velpatasvir and voxilaprevir p. 669. Moderate Study

▸ Rifamycins (rifampicin) are predicted to decrease the exposure to **sofosbuvir**. Avoid. Severe Study

▸ St John's wort is predicted to decrease the exposure to **sofosbuvir**. Avoid. Severe Study

Solifenacin → see TABLE 10 p. 1431 (antimuscarinics)

▸ Anti-androgens (apalutamide, enzalutamide) are predicted to decrease the exposure to **solifenacin**. Moderate Theoretical

▸ Antiepileptics (carbamazepine, fosphenytoin, phenobarbital, phenytoin, primidone) are predicted to decrease the exposure to **solifenacin**. Moderate Theoretical

▸ Antifungals, azoles (itraconazole, ketoconazole, voriconazole) are predicted to increase the exposure to **solifenacin**. Adjust solifenacin p. 824 or tamsulosin with solifenacin p. 830 dose; avoid in hepatic and renal impairment. Severe Study

▸ Cobicistat is predicted to increase the exposure to **solifenacin**. Adjust solifenacin p. 824 or tamsulosin with solifenacin p. 830 dose; avoid in hepatic and renal impairment. Severe Study

▸ HIV-protease inhibitors are predicted to increase the exposure to **solifenacin**. Adjust solifenacin p. 824 or tamsulosin with solifenacin p. 830 dose; avoid in hepatic and renal impairment. Severe Study

▸ Idelalisib is predicted to increase the exposure to **solifenacin**. Adjust solifenacin p. 824 or tamsulosin with solifenacin p. 830 dose; avoid in hepatic and renal impairment. Severe Study

▸ Macrolides (clarithromycin) are predicted to increase the exposure to **solifenacin**. Adjust solifenacin p. 824 or tamsulosin with solifenacin p. 830 dose; avoid in hepatic and renal impairment. Severe Study

▸ Mitotane is predicted to decrease the exposure to **solifenacin**. Moderate Theoretical

▸ Rifamycins (rifampicin) are predicted to decrease the exposure to **solifenacin**. Moderate Theoretical

Solriamfetol

▸ **Solriamfetol** is predicted to increase the risk of a hypertensive crisis when given with MAO-B inhibitors. Avoid and for 14 days after stopping **MAO-B inhibitors**. Severe Theoretical

▸ **Solriamfetol** is predicted to increase the risk of a hypertensive crisis when given with MAOIs, irreversible. Avoid and for 14 days after stopping the MAOI. Severe Theoretical

Somatropin

▸ Corticosteroids are predicted to decrease the effects of **somatropin**. Moderate Theoretical

Sorafenib → see TABLE 15 p. 1432 (myelosuppression), TABLE 9 p. 1431 (QT-interval prolongation)

▸ Anti-androgens (apalutamide, enzalutamide) are predicted to decrease the exposure to **sorafenib**. Moderate Theoretical → Also see TABLE 9 p. 1431

▸ Antiepileptics (carbamazepine, fosphenytoin, phenobarbital, phenytoin, primidone) are predicted to decrease the exposure to **sorafenib**. Moderate Theoretical

▸ **Sorafenib** increases the anticoagulant effect of coumarins. Severe Anecdotal

▸ Mitotane is predicted to decrease the exposure to **sorafenib**. Moderate Theoretical → Also see TABLE 15 p. 1432

▸ Neomycin moderately decreases the exposure to **sorafenib**. Moderate Study

▸ **Sorafenib** is predicted to increase the risk of bleeding events when given with phenindione. Severe Theoretical

▸ Rifamycins (rifampicin) are predicted to decrease the exposure to **sorafenib**. Moderate Theoretical

Sotalol → see beta blockers, non-selective

Spironolactone → see aldosterone antagonists

SSRIs → see TABLE 18 p. 1433 (hyponatraemia), TABLE 13 p. 1432 (serotonin syndrome), TABLE 9 p. 1431 (QT-interval prolongation), TABLE 4 p. 1429 (antiplatelet effects)

citalopram · dapoxetine · escitalopram · fluoxetine · fluvoxamine · paroxetine · sertraline

▸ **Fluvoxamine** very markedly increases the exposure to agomelatine. Avoid. Severe Study

▸ SSRIs (fluoxetine, paroxetine) are predicted to increase the exposure to amfetamines. Severe Theoretical → Also see TABLE 13 p. 1432

▸ **Fluvoxamine** moderately to markedly increases the exposure to aminophylline. Avoid. Severe Study

▸ **Fluvoxamine** decreases the clearance of anaesthetics, local (ropivacaine). Avoid prolonged use. Moderate Study

▸ **Fluvoxamine** is predicted to increase the exposure to anagrelide. Moderate Theoretical → Also see TABLE 4 p. 1429

SSRIs (continued)

▶ Anti-androgens (apalutamide) are predicted to decrease the exposure to **citalopram**. Avoid or monitor. Mild Study → Also see TABLE 9 p. 1431

▶ Antiarrhythmics (dronedarone) are predicted to increase the exposure to **dapoxetine**. Adjust **dapoxetine** dose with moderate CYP3A4 inhibitors, p. 867. Moderate Theoretical

▶ Antiarrhythmics (dronedarone) are predicted to increase the exposure to SSRIs **(citalopram, escitalopram, fluoxetine, fluvoxamine, paroxetine, sertraline)**. Severe Theoretical → Also see TABLE 9 p. 1431

▶ **Fluvoxamine** is predicted to increase the exposure to antiarrhythmics (propafenone). Monitor and adjust dose. Moderate Study

▶ SSRIs **(fluoxetine, paroxetine)** are predicted to increase the exposure to anticholinesterases, centrally acting (galantamine). Monitor and adjust dose. Moderate Study

▶ Antiepileptics (fosphenytoin, phenytoin) decrease the concentration of **paroxetine**. Moderate Study

▶ **Sertraline** potentially increases the risk of toxicity when given with antiepileptics (fosphenytoin, phenytoin). Monitor concentration and adjust dose. Severe Anecdotal

▶ SSRIs **(fluoxetine, fluvoxamine)** are predicted to increase the concentration of antiepileptics (fosphenytoin, phenytoin). Monitor and adjust dose. Severe Anecdotal

▶ Antifungals, azoles (fluconazole, isavuconazole, posaconazole) are predicted to increase the exposure to **dapoxetine**. Adjust **dapoxetine** dose with moderate CYP3A4 inhibitors, p. 867. Moderate Theoretical

▶ Antifungals, azoles (itraconazole, ketoconazole, voriconazole) are predicted to moderately increase the exposure to **dapoxetine**. Avoid potent CYP3A4 inhibitors or adjust **dapoxetine** dose, p. 867. Severe Study

▶ Antifungals, azoles (voriconazole) are predicted to increase the exposure to **citalopram**. Severe Theoretical → Also see TABLE 9 p. 1431

▶ Antihistamines, sedating (cyproheptadine) potentially decrease the effects of **SSRIs**. Moderate Anecdotal

▶ SSRIs **(fluoxetine, paroxetine)** are predicted to moderately increase the exposure to antipsychotics, second generation (aripiprazole). Adjust **aripiprazole** dose, p. 415. Moderate Study

▶ **Fluvoxamine** increases the exposure to antipsychotics, second generation **(asenapine)**. Moderate Study

▶ **Paroxetine** moderately increases the exposure to antipsychotics, second generation (asenapine). Moderate Study

▶ **Fluvoxamine** increases the concentration of antipsychotics, second generation (clozapine). Monitor adverse effects and adjust dose. Severe Study

▶ **Fluvoxamine** moderately increases the exposure to antipsychotics, second generation (olanzapine). Adjust dose. Severe Anecdotal

▶ SSRIs **(fluoxetine, paroxetine)** are predicted to increase the exposure to antipsychotics, second generation (risperidone). Adjust dose. Moderate Study

▶ SSRIs **(fluoxetine, paroxetine)** are predicted to markedly increase the exposure to atomoxetine. Adjust dose. Severe Study

▶ **Fluvoxamine** moderately increases the exposure to benzodiazepines (alprazolam). Adjust dose. Moderate Study

▶ SSRIs **(fluoxetine, fluvoxamine)** potentially increase the exposure to benzodiazepines (clobazam). Adjust dose. Moderate Theoretical

▶ **Fluvoxamine** moderately increases the exposure to benzodiazepines (diazepam). Moderate Study

▶ **Fluvoxamine** moderately increases the concentration of beta blockers, non-selective (propranolol). Moderate Study

▶ SSRIs **(fluoxetine, paroxetine)** are predicted to increase the exposure to beta blockers, selective (metoprolol, nebivolol). Moderate Study

▶ Bupropion is predicted to increase the exposure to **dapoxetine**. Moderate Theoretical → Also see TABLE 13 p. 1432

▶ **Fluvoxamine** markedly decreases the clearance of caffeine citrate. Monitor and adjust dose. Severe Study

▶ Calcium channel blockers (diltiazem, verapamil) are predicted to increase the exposure to **dapoxetine**. Adjust **dapoxetine** dose with moderate CYP3A4 inhibitors, p. 867. Moderate Theoretical

▶ SSRIs **(fluoxetine, fluvoxamine)** are predicted to increase the exposure to cannabidiol. Moderate Theoretical

▶ SSRIs **(fluoxetine, fluvoxamine)** are predicted to increase the exposure to cilostazol. Adjust **cilostazol** dose, p. 248. Moderate Theoretical → Also see TABLE 4 p. 1429

▶ Cinacalcet is predicted to increase the exposure to **dapoxetine**. Moderate Theoretical

▶ **Fluvoxamine** is predicted to increase the exposure to cinacalcet. Adjust dose. Moderate Theoretical

▶ SSRIs **(fluoxetine, fluvoxamine)** are predicted to decrease the efficacy of clopidogrel. Avoid. Severe Theoretical → Also see TABLE 4 p. 1429

▶ Cobicistat is predicted to moderately increase the exposure to **dapoxetine**. Avoid potent CYP3A4 inhibitors or adjust **dapoxetine** dose, p. 867. Severe Study

▶ Crizotinib is predicted to increase the exposure to **dapoxetine**. Adjust **dapoxetine** dose with moderate CYP3A4 inhibitors, p. 867. Moderate Theoretical

▶ SSRIs **(fluoxetine, paroxetine)** are predicted to slightly increase the exposure to darifenacin. Mild Study

▶ **Fluvoxamine** is predicted to increase the exposure to dopamine receptor agonists (ropinirole). Adjust dose. Moderate Study

▶ **Fluvoxamine** markedly increases the exposure to duloxetine. Avoid. Moderate Study → Also see TABLE 18 p. 1433 → Also see TABLE 13 p. 1432 → Also see TABLE 4 p. 1429

▶ SSRIs **(fluoxetine, paroxetine)** are predicted to increase the exposure to eliglustat. Avoid or adjust dose—consult product literature. Severe Study

▶ **Fluvoxamine** is predicted to increase the exposure to eltrombopag. Moderate Theoretical

▶ **Fluvoxamine** is predicted to increase the exposure to erlotinib. Monitor adverse effects and adjust dose. Moderate Theoretical

▶ Gilteritinib is predicted to decrease the efficacy of SSRIs **(escitalopram, fluoxetine, sertraline)**. Avoid. Moderate Theoretical

▶ Grapefruit juice moderately increases the exposure to **sertraline**. Avoid. Moderate Study

▶ H_2 receptor antagonists (cimetidine) slightly increase the exposure to SSRIs **(citalopram, escitalopram)**. Adjust dose. Moderate Study

▶ H_2 receptor antagonists (cimetidine) slightly increase the exposure to SSRIs **(paroxetine, sertraline)**. Moderate Study

▶ **Fluoxetine** increases the concentration of haloperidol. Adjust dose. Moderate Anecdotal

▶ **Fluvoxamine** increases the concentration of haloperidol. Adjust dose. Moderate Study

▶ HIV-protease inhibitors are predicted to moderately increase the exposure to **dapoxetine**. Avoid potent CYP3A4 inhibitors or adjust **dapoxetine** dose, p. 867. Severe Study

▶ Idelalisib is predicted to moderately increase the exposure to **dapoxetine**. Avoid potent CYP3A4 inhibitors or adjust **dapoxetine** dose, p. 867. Severe Study

▶ Imatinib is predicted to increase the exposure to **dapoxetine**. Adjust **dapoxetine** dose with moderate CYP3A4 inhibitors, p. 867. Moderate Theoretical

▶ Letermovir is predicted to increase the exposure to **dapoxetine**. Adjust **dapoxetine** dose with moderate CYP3A4 inhibitors, p. 867. Moderate Theoretical

▶ **Fluoxetine** is predicted to increase the exposure to lomitapide. Separate administration by 12 hours. Unknown Theoretical

▶ **Fluvoxamine** is predicted to increase the exposure to lomitapide. Separate administration by 12 hours. Mild Theoretical

▶ **Fluvoxamine** is predicted to increase the exposure to loxapine. Avoid. Unknown Theoretical

▶ Macrolides (clarithromycin) are predicted to moderately increase the exposure to **dapoxetine**. Avoid potent CYP3A4 inhibitors or adjust **dapoxetine** dose, p. 867. Severe Study

▶ Macrolides (erythromycin) are predicted to increase the exposure to **dapoxetine**. Adjust **dapoxetine** dose with moderate CYP3A4 inhibitors, p. 867. Moderate Theoretical

Fluvoxamine very markedly increases the exposure to melatonin. Avoid. [Severe] Study

SSRIs **(fluoxetine, fluvoxamine, paroxetine)** are predicted to increase the exposure to mexiletine. [Moderate] Study

Neurokinin-1 receptor antagonists **(aprepitant, netupitant)** are predicted to increase the exposure to **dapoxetine**. Adjust **dapoxetine** dose with moderate CYP3A4 inhibitors, p. 867. [Moderate] Theoretical

SSRIs potentially increase the risk of prolonged neuromuscular blockade when given with neuromuscular blocking drugs, non-depolarising **(mivacurium)**. [Unknown] Theoretical

Nilotinib is predicted to increase the exposure to **dapoxetine**. Adjust **dapoxetine** dose with moderate CYP3A4 inhibitors, p. 867. [Moderate] Theoretical

SSRIs **(fluoxetine, paroxetine)** are predicted to decrease the efficacy of opioids **(codeine)**. [Moderate] Theoretical

SSRIs **(fluoxetine, paroxetine)** are predicted to decrease the efficacy of opioids **(tramadol)**. [Severe] Study → Also see TABLE 13 p. 1432

▶ **SSRIs** potentially increase the risk of adverse effects when given with ozanimod. [Severe] Theoretical

▶ **Fluvoxamine** is predicted to increase the exposure to pentoxifylline. [Moderate] Theoretical

▶ **Fluvoxamine** is predicted to increase the exposure to phenothiazines **(chlorpromazine)**. [Moderate] Theoretical

▶ **Fluvoxamine** is predicted to increase the exposure to phosphodiesterase type-4 inhibitors **(roflumilast)**. [Moderate] Study

▶ **Fluvoxamine** is predicted to moderately increase the exposure to pirfenidone. Avoid. [Moderate] Study

▶ SSRIs **(fluoxetine, paroxetine)** are predicted to moderately increase the exposure to pitolisant. Use with caution and adjust dose. [Moderate] Study

▶ **Fluvoxamine** moderately increases the exposure to pomalidomide. Adjust **pomalidomide** dose, p. 1003. [Moderate] Study

▶ **Paroxetine** slightly increases the exposure to procyclidine. Monitor and adjust dose. [Moderate] Study

▶ Proton pump inhibitors **(esomeprazole)** are predicted to slightly to moderately increase the exposure to SSRIs **(citalopram, escitalopram)**. Monitor and adjust dose. [Severe] Theoretical

▶ Proton pump inhibitors **(omeprazole)** slightly to moderately increase the exposure to SSRIs **(citalopram, escitalopram)**. Monitor and adjust dose. [Severe] Study

▶ **Fluvoxamine** is predicted to increase the exposure to riluzole. [Moderate] Theoretical

▶ SSRIs **(fluoxetine, paroxetine)** are predicted to increase the exposure to SSRIs **(dapoxetine)**. [Moderate] Theoretical → Also see TABLE 18 p. 1433 → Also see TABLE 13 p. 1432 → Also see TABLE 4 p. 1429

▶ **SSRIs** potentially increase the risk of prolonged neuromuscular blockade when given with suxamethonium. [Unknown] Theoretical

▶ SSRIs **(fluoxetine, paroxetine)** are predicted to decrease the efficacy of tamoxifen. Avoid. [Severe] Study

▶ Terbinafine is predicted to increase the exposure to **fluoxetine**. Adjust dose. [Moderate] Theoretical

▶ Terbinafine moderately increases the exposure to **paroxetine**. [Moderate] Study

▶ Terbinafine is predicted to increase the exposure to SSRIs **(citalopram, dapoxetine, escitalopram, fluvoxamine, sertraline)**. [Moderate] Theoretical

▶ SSRIs **(fluoxetine, paroxetine)** are predicted to increase the exposure to the active metabolite of tetrabenazine. [Moderate] Study

▶ **Fluvoxamine** moderately to markedly increases the exposure to theophylline. Avoid. [Severe] Study

▶ **Fluvoxamine** very markedly increases the exposure to tizanidine. Avoid. [Severe] Study

▶ SSRIs **(fluoxetine, fluvoxamine)** given with a moderate CYP3A4 inhibitor are predicted to increase the exposure to tofacitinib. Adjust **tofacitinib** dose, p. 1154. [Moderate] Study

▶ SSRIs **(fluoxetine, paroxetine)** are predicted to increase the exposure to tricyclic antidepressants. Monitor for toxicity and

adjust dose. [Severe] Study → Also see TABLE 18 p. 1433 → Also see TABLE 13 p. 1432

▶ **Fluvoxamine** increases the exposure to tricyclic antidepressants **(amitriptyline, imipramine)**. Adjust dose. [Severe] Study → Also see TABLE 18 p. 1433 → Also see TABLE 13 p. 1432

▶ **Fluvoxamine** markedly increases the exposure to tricyclic antidepressants **(clomipramine)**. Adjust dose. [Severe] Study → Also see TABLE 18 p. 1433 → Also see TABLE 13 p. 1432

▶ **Fluvoxamine** increases the concentration of triptans **(frovatriptan)**. [Severe] Study → Also see TABLE 13 p. 1432

▶ **Fluvoxamine** is predicted to increase the exposure to triptans **(zolmitriptan)**. Adjust **zolmitriptan** dose, p. 503. [Severe] Theoretical → Also see TABLE 13 p. 1432

▶ SSRIs **(fluoxetine, paroxetine)** are predicted to increase the exposure to vortioxetine. Monitor and adjust dose. [Moderate] Study → Also see TABLE 13 p. 1432 → Also see TABLE 4 p. 1429

St John's wort → see TABLE 13 p. 1432 (serotonin syndrome)

▶ **St John's wort** is predicted to decrease the exposure to abemaciclib. Avoid. [Severe] Study

▶ **St John's wort** is predicted to decrease the exposure to acalabrutinib. Avoid. [Severe] Theoretical

▶ **St John's wort** is predicted to decrease the exposure to afatinib. [Moderate] Study

▶ **St John's wort** is predicted to slightly decrease the exposure to aldosterone antagonists **(eplerenone)**. Avoid. [Moderate] Study

▶ **St John's wort** decreases the exposure to aliskiren. [Moderate] Study

▶ **St John's wort** is predicted to decrease the concentration of aminophylline. [Severe] Theoretical

▶ **St John's wort** is predicted to decrease the exposure to anti-androgens **(darolutamide)**. Avoid. [Moderate] Theoretical

▶ **St John's wort** is predicted to decrease the exposure to antiarrhythmics **(dronedarone)**. Avoid. [Severe] Theoretical

▶ **St John's wort** is predicted to decrease the exposure to antiepileptics **(brivaracetam)**. [Moderate] Theoretical

▶ **St John's wort** is predicted to decrease the concentration of antiepileptics **(carbamazepine)**. Monitor and adjust dose. [Moderate] Theoretical

▶ **St John's wort** is predicted to decrease the concentration of antiepileptics **(fosphenytoin, phenobarbital, phenytoin, primidone)**. Avoid. [Severe] Theoretical

▶ **St John's wort** is predicted to decrease the exposure to antiepileptics **(perampanel)**. Monitor and adjust dose. [Moderate] Theoretical

▶ **St John's wort** is predicted to decrease the exposure to antiepileptics **(tiagabine)**. Avoid. [Mild] Theoretical

▶ **St John's wort** is predicted to decrease the exposure to antifungals, azoles **(isavuconazole)**. Avoid. [Severe] Theoretical

▶ **St John's wort** moderately decreases the exposure to antifungals, azoles **(voriconazole)**. Avoid. [Moderate] Study

▶ **St John's wort** is predicted to decrease the concentration of antimalarials **(piperaquine)**. Avoid. [Moderate] Theoretical

▶ **St John's wort** is predicted to decrease the exposure to antipsychotics, second generation **(cariprazine)**. Avoid. [Severe] Theoretical

▶ **St John's wort** is predicted to decrease the exposure to antipsychotics, second generation **(lurasidone)**. Monitor and adjust dose. [Moderate] Theoretical

▶ **St John's wort** is predicted to decrease the exposure to antipsychotics, second generation **(paliperidone)**. [Severe] Theoretical

▶ **St John's wort** is predicted to decrease the exposure to antipsychotics, second generation **(quetiapine)**. [Moderate] Study

▶ **St John's wort** is predicted to decrease the exposure to avapritinib. Avoid. [Severe] Study

▶ **St John's wort** is predicted to decrease the exposure to axitinib. [Moderate] Theoretical

▶ **St John's wort** is predicted to decrease the exposure to bedaquiline. Avoid. [Severe] Study

▶ **St John's wort** moderately decreases the exposure to benzodiazepines **(alprazolam)**. [Moderate] Study

▶ **St John's wort** moderately decreases the exposure to benzodiazepines **(midazolam)**. Monitor and adjust dose. [Moderate] Study

A1

Interactions | **Appendix 1**

St John's wort (continued)

▶ **St John's wort** is predicted to decrease the exposure to bictegravir. Avoid. [Moderate] Theoretical

▶ **St John's wort** is predicted to decrease the exposure to bosutinib. Avoid. [Severe] Theoretical

▶ **St John's wort** is predicted to decrease the exposure to brigatinib. Avoid. [Severe] Study

▶ **St John's wort** is predicted to decrease the exposure to cabozantinib. [Moderate] Theoretical

▶ **St John's wort** is predicted to decrease the exposure to calcium channel blockers (amlodipine, felodipine, lacidipine, lercanidipine, nicardipine, nifedipine, nimodipine). Monitor and adjust dose. [Moderate] Theoretical

▶ **St John's wort** is predicted to decrease the exposure to calcium channel blockers (diltiazem, verapamil). [Moderate] Theoretical

▶ **St John's wort** is predicted to decrease the exposure to cannabidiol. Adjust dose. [Mild] Study

▶ **St John's wort** is predicted to decrease the exposure to ceritinib. Avoid. [Severe] Theoretical

▶ **St John's wort** decreases the concentration of ciclosporin. Avoid. [Moderate] Study

▶ **St John's wort** is predicted to alter the effects of cilostazol. [Moderate] Theoretical

▶ **St John's wort** is predicted to decrease the exposure to cobicistat. Avoid. [Severe] Theoretical

▶ **St John's wort** is predicted to decrease the exposure to cobimetinib. Avoid. [Severe] Theoretical

▶ **St John's wort** decreases the efficacy of combined hormonal contraceptives. MHRA advises avoid. For FSRH guidance, see Contraceptives, interactions p. 840. [Severe] Anecdotal

▶ **St John's wort** decreases the anticoagulant effect of coumarins. Avoid. [Severe] Anecdotal

▶ **St John's wort** is predicted to decrease the exposure to crizotinib. Avoid. [Severe] Theoretical

▶ **St John's wort** is predicted to decrease the exposure to darifenacin. [Moderate] Theoretical

▶ **St John's wort** is predicted to decrease the exposure to dasabuvir. Avoid. [Severe] Theoretical

▶ **St John's wort** is predicted to decrease the exposure to dasatinib. [Severe] Study

▶ **St John's wort** is predicted to decrease the efficacy of desogestrel. MHRA advises avoid. For FSRH guidance, see Contraceptives, interactions p. 840. [Severe] Theoretical

▶ **St John's wort** decreases the concentration of digoxin. Avoid. [Severe] Anecdotal

▶ **St John's wort** decreases the exposure to dolutegravir. Adjust dose. [Severe] Study

▶ **St John's wort** is predicted to decrease the exposure to dronabinol. Avoid or adjust dose. [Mild] Study

▶ **St John's wort** is predicted to moderately decrease the exposure to elbasvir. Avoid. [Severe] Study

▶ **St John's wort** is predicted to decrease the exposure to elexacaftor. Avoid. [Severe] Theoretical

▶ **St John's wort** is predicted to increase the exposure to eliglustat. Avoid. [Severe] Study

▶ **St John's wort** is predicted to decrease the concentration of elvitegravir. Avoid. [Severe] Theoretical

▶ **St John's wort** is predicted to decrease the exposure to encorafenib. [Severe] Theoretical

▶ **St John's wort** is predicted to decrease the exposure to endothelin receptor antagonists (bosentan). Avoid. [Moderate] Theoretical

▶ **St John's wort** is predicted to decrease the exposure to endothelin receptor antagonists (macitentan). Avoid. [Severe] Theoretical

▶ **St John's wort** is predicted to decrease the exposure to entrectinib. Avoid. [Severe] Theoretical

▶ **St John's wort** is predicted to decrease the effects of ergotamine. [Moderate] Theoretical

▶ **St John's wort** is predicted to decrease the exposure to erlotinib. Avoid. [Severe] Theoretical

▶ **St John's wort** is predicted to decrease the efficacy of etonogestrel. MHRA advises avoid. For FSRH guidance, see Contraceptives, interactions p. 840. [Severe] Theoretical

▶ **St John's wort** is predicted to decrease the concentration of everolimus. Avoid or adjust dose. [Severe] Study

▶ **St John's wort** is predicted to decrease the exposure to exemestane. [Moderate] Theoretical

▶ **St John's wort** is predicted to decrease the exposure to factor XA inhibitors (apixaban). Use with caution or avoid. [Moderate] Theoretical

▶ **St John's wort** is predicted to decrease the exposure to factor XA inhibitors (edoxaban). [Moderate] Study

▶ **St John's wort** is predicted to decrease the exposure to fesoterodine. Avoid. [Severe] Theoretical

▶ **St John's wort** is predicted to decrease the exposure to fingolimod. Avoid. [Moderate] Theoretical

▶ **St John's wort** is predicted to decrease the exposure to gefitinib. Avoid. [Severe] Theoretical

▶ **St John's wort** is predicted to decrease the exposure to gilteritinib. Avoid. [Severe] Study

▶ **St John's wort** is predicted to decrease the exposure to glasdegib. Avoid or adjust **glasdegib** dose, p. 1049. [Severe] Theoretical

▶ **St John's wort** is predicted to decrease the exposure to glecaprevir. Avoid. [Severe] Study

▶ **St John's wort** is predicted to markedly decrease the exposure to grazoprevir. Avoid. [Severe] Study

▶ **St John's wort** is predicted to decrease the concentration of guanfacine. Adjust dose. [Moderate] Theoretical

▶ **St John's wort** is predicted to decrease the exposure to HIV-protease inhibitors. Avoid. [Severe] Study

▶ **St John's wort** is predicted to decrease the efficacy of hormone replacement therapy. [Moderate] Theoretical

▶ **St John's wort** is predicted to decrease the exposure to ibrutinib. Avoid. [Severe] Theoretical

▶ **St John's wort** is predicted to decrease the exposure to idelalisib. Avoid. [Moderate] Theoretical

▶ **St John's wort** is predicted to decrease the exposure to imatinib. [Moderate] Study

▶ **St John's wort** slightly decreases the exposure to irinotecan. Avoid. [Severe] Study

▶ **St John's wort** decreases the exposure to ivabradine. Avoid. [Moderate] Study

▶ **St John's wort** is predicted to decrease the exposure to ivacaftor. Avoid. [Severe] Study

▶ **St John's wort** is predicted to decrease the exposure to ixazomib. Avoid. [Severe] Theoretical

▶ **St John's wort** is predicted to decrease the exposure to lapatinib. Avoid. [Severe] Study

▶ **St John's wort** is predicted to decrease the exposure to larotrectinib. Avoid. [Moderate] Study

▶ **St John's wort** is predicted to decrease the exposure to ledipasvir. Avoid. [Severe] Study

▶ **St John's wort** is predicted to decrease the concentration of letermovir. [Moderate] Theoretical

▶ **St John's wort** is predicted to decrease the efficacy of levonorgestrel. MHRA advises avoid. For FSRH guidance, see Contraceptives, interactions p. 840. [Severe] Theoretical

▶ **St John's wort** is predicted to decrease the exposure to lorlatinib. Avoid. [Severe] Theoretical

▶ **St John's wort** is predicted to decrease the exposure to maraviroc. Avoid. [Severe] Theoretical

▶ **St John's wort** is predicted to decrease the exposure to midostaurin. Avoid. [Severe] Theoretical

▶ **St John's wort** is predicted to decrease the exposure to naldemedine. Avoid. [Severe] Study

▶ **St John's wort** is predicted to decrease the exposure to naloxegol. Avoid. [Moderate] Theoretical

▶ **St John's wort** is predicted to decrease the exposure to neratinib. Avoid. [Severe] Theoretical

▶ **St John's wort** is predicted to decrease the exposure to neurokinin-1 receptor antagonists (aprepitant, fosaprepitant). Avoid. [Moderate] Theoretical

▶ **St John's wort** is predicted to decrease the exposure to neurokinin-1 receptor antagonists (netupitant). [Moderate] Theoretical

▶ **St John's wort** is predicted to decrease the exposure to nilotinib. Avoid. [Severe] Theoretical

St John's wort is predicted to decrease the exposure to nintedanib. [Moderate] Study

St John's wort is predicted to decrease the exposure to NNRTIs (doravirine, rilpivirine). Avoid. [Severe] Theoretical

St John's wort is predicted to decrease the concentration of NNRTIs (efavirenz, nevirapine). Avoid. [Severe] Theoretical

St John's wort is predicted to decrease the exposure to NNRTIs (etravirine). Avoid. [Severe] Study

St John's wort is predicted to decrease the efficacy of norethisterone. MHRA advises avoid. For FSRH guidance, see Contraceptives, interactions p. 840. [Severe] Anecdotal

St John's wort is predicted to decrease the exposure to olaparib. Avoid. [Moderate] Theoretical

St John's wort is predicted to decrease the exposure to ombitasvir. Avoid. [Severe] Theoretical

▸ **St John's wort** decreases the exposure to opioids (methadone). Monitor and adjust dose. [Severe] Study → Also see TABLE 13 p. 1432

St John's wort moderately decreases the exposure to opioids (oxycodone). Adjust dose. [Moderate] Study

▸ **St John's wort** is predicted to decrease the exposure to osimertinib. Avoid. [Moderate] Theoretical

▸ **St John's wort** is predicted to decrease the exposure to ospemifene. [Moderate] Study

▸ **St John's wort** is predicted to decrease the exposure to palbociclib. Avoid. [Severe] Theoretical

▸ **St John's wort** is predicted to decrease the exposure to panobinostat. Avoid. [Moderate] Theoretical

▸ **St John's wort** is predicted to decrease the exposure to paritaprevir (with ritonavir and ombitasvir). Avoid. [Severe] Study

▸ **St John's wort** is predicted to decrease the exposure to phosphodiesterase type-4 inhibitors (apremilast). Avoid. [Severe] Theoretical

▸ **St John's wort** is predicted to decrease the exposure to phosphodiesterase type-5 inhibitors. [Moderate] Theoretical

▸ **St John's wort** is predicted to decrease the exposure to pibrentasvir. Avoid. [Severe] Study

▸ **St John's wort** slightly decreases the exposure to pioglitazone. [Mild] Study

▸ **St John's wort** is predicted to decrease the exposure to pitolisant. Monitor and adjust dose. [Moderate] Theoretical

▸ **St John's wort** is predicted to decrease the exposure to ponatinib. Avoid. [Severe] Theoretical

▸ **St John's wort** is predicted to decrease the exposure to ranolazine. Avoid. [Severe] Study

▸ **St John's wort** is predicted to decrease the exposure to ribociclib. Avoid. [Severe] Study

▸ **St John's wort** is predicted to decrease the exposure to ruxolitinib. Monitor and adjust dose. [Moderate] Theoretical

▸ **St John's wort** is predicted to decrease the exposure to siponimod. Manufacturer advises caution depending on genotype—consult product literature. [Severe] Theoretical

▸ **St John's wort** is predicted to decrease the concentration of sirolimus. Monitor and adjust dose. [Severe] Theoretical

▸ **St John's wort** is predicted to decrease the exposure to sofosbuvir. Avoid. [Severe] Study

▸ **St John's wort** slightly decreases the exposure to statins (atorvastatin). [Mild] Study

▸ **St John's wort** moderately decreases the exposure to statins (simvastatin). [Moderate] Study

▸ **St John's wort** decreases the concentration of tacrolimus. Avoid. [Severe] Study

▸ **St John's wort** is predicted to decrease the exposure to taxanes (cabazitaxel). Avoid. [Severe] Study

▸ **St John's wort** is predicted to decrease the concentration of temsirolimus. Avoid. [Severe] Theoretical

▸ **St John's wort** is predicted to decrease the exposure to tenofovir alafenamide. Avoid. [Moderate] Theoretical

▸ **St John's wort** is predicted to decrease the exposure to tezacaftor. Avoid. [Severe] Theoretical

▸ **St John's wort** potentially decreases the exposure to theophylline. [Severe] Anecdotal

▸ **St John's wort** is predicted to decrease the exposure to thrombin inhibitors (dabigatran). Avoid. [Severe] Study

▸ **St John's wort** is predicted to decrease the exposure to ticagrelor. [Moderate] Theoretical

▸ **St John's wort** is predicted to decrease the exposure to tivozanib. Avoid. [Severe] Study

▸ **St John's wort** is predicted to decrease the exposure to tofacitinib. [Moderate] Study

▸ **St John's wort** is predicted to decrease the exposure to tolvaptan. Avoid. [Moderate] Theoretical

▸ **St John's wort** is predicted to decrease the exposure to topotecan. [Severe] Theoretical

▸ **St John's wort** decreases the efficacy of ulipristal. For FSRH guidance, see Contraceptives, interactions p. 840. [Severe] Anecdotal

▸ **St John's wort** is predicted to decrease the exposure to velpatasvir. Avoid. [Moderate] Theoretical

▸ **St John's wort** is predicted to decrease the exposure to venetoclax. Avoid. [Severe] Study

▸ **St John's wort** is predicted to decrease the exposure to vismodegib. Avoid. [Moderate] Theoretical

▸ **St John's wort** is predicted to decrease the concentration of voxilaprevir. Avoid. [Severe] Theoretical

Statins → see TABLE 1 p. 1429 (hepatotoxicity)

atorvastatin · fluvastatin · pravastatin · rosuvastatin · simvastatin

▸ **Atorvastatin** slightly to moderately increases the exposure to aliskiren. [Moderate] Study

▸ Oral antacids decrease the absorption of oral **rosuvastatin**. Separate administration by 2 hours. [Moderate] Study

▸ Anti-androgens (apalutamide) slightly decrease the exposure to **rosuvastatin**. [Mild] Study

▸ Anti-androgens (apalutamide) are predicted to decrease the exposure to **simvastatin**. Avoid or monitor. [Moderate] Study

▸ Anti-androgens (enzalutamide) are predicted to decrease the exposure to **simvastatin**. [Severe] Study

▸ Anti-androgens (darolutamide) are predicted to increase the exposure to statins (**atorvastatin, fluvastatin, rosuvastatin**). Avoid. [Severe] Theoretical

▸ Anti-androgens (darolutamide) are predicted to increase the concentration of statins (**pravastatin, simvastatin**). [Moderate] Theoretical

▸ Antiarrhythmics (amiodarone) are predicted to increase the risk of rhabdomyolysis when given with **atorvastatin**. Monitor and adjust dose. [Moderate] Theoretical

▸ Antiarrhythmics (amiodarone) are predicted to increase the exposure to **fluvastatin**. [Severe] Theoretical

▸ Antiarrhythmics (amiodarone) increase the risk of rhabdomyolysis when given with **simvastatin**. Adjust **simvastatin** dose, p. 219. [Severe] Study

▸ Antiarrhythmics (dronedarone) slightly increase the exposure to **atorvastatin**. Monitor and adjust dose. [Severe] Study

▸ Antiarrhythmics (dronedarone) slightly increase the exposure to **rosuvastatin**. Adjust dose. [Severe] Study

▸ Antiarrhythmics (dronedarone) moderately increase the exposure to **simvastatin**. Monitor and adjust dose. [Severe] Study

▸ Antiepileptics (carbamazepine) moderately decrease the exposure to **simvastatin**. Monitor and adjust dose. [Severe] Study → Also see TABLE 1 p. 1429

▸ Antiepileptics (carbamazepine, eslicarbazepine) are predicted to decrease the exposure to **atorvastatin**. Monitor and adjust dose. [Moderate] Theoretical → Also see TABLE 1 p. 1429

▸ Antiepileptics (eslicarbazepine) moderately decrease the exposure to **simvastatin**. Monitor and adjust dose. [Moderate] Study

▸ Antiepileptics (fosphenytoin, phenytoin) potentially decrease the exposure to statins (**atorvastatin, simvastatin**). [Moderate] Anecdotal

▸ Antifungals, azoles (fluconazole) potentially increase the risk of rhabdomyolysis when given with **atorvastatin**. Monitor and adjust dose. [Severe] Anecdotal → Also see TABLE 1 p. 1429

▸ Antifungals, azoles (fluconazole) are predicted to increase the exposure to **simvastatin**. Monitor and adjust dose. [Severe] Anecdotal → Also see TABLE 1 p. 1429

▸ Antifungals, azoles (fluconazole, miconazole) are predicted to increase the exposure to **fluvastatin**. [Severe] Theoretical → Also see TABLE 1 p. 1429

A1

Interactions | Appendix 1

Statins (continued)

▶ Antifungals, azoles (isavuconazole) slightly increase the exposure to **atorvastatin**. Moderate Study
▶ Antifungals, azoles (isavuconazole) are predicted to increase the exposure to **simvastatin**. Monitor and adjust dose. Severe Theoretical
▶ Antifungals, azoles (itraconazole, ketoconazole, voriconazole) are predicted to increase the exposure to **atorvastatin**. Avoid or adjust dose and monitor rhabdomyolysis. Severe Study → Also see **TABLE 1** p. 1429
▶ Antifungals, azoles (itraconazole, ketoconazole, voriconazole) are predicted to increase the exposure to **simvastatin**. Avoid. Severe Study → Also see **TABLE 1** p. 1429
▶ Antifungals, azoles (miconazole) potentially increase the exposure to **atorvastatin**. Severe Anecdotal
▶ Antifungals, azoles (miconazole) are predicted to increase the exposure to **simvastatin**. Avoid. Severe Theoretical
▶ Antifungals, azoles (posaconazole) are predicted to increase the exposure to **atorvastatin**. Avoid. Severe Anecdotal
▶ Antifungals, azoles (posaconazole) markedly to very markedly increase the exposure to **simvastatin**. Avoid. Severe Study
▶ Antifungals, azoles (isavuconazole) are predicted to increase the exposure to statins **(fluvastatin, rosuvastatin)**. Moderate Theoretical
▶ Bempedoic acid increases the exposure to **simvastatin**. Adjust **simvastatin** dose, p. 219. Moderate Study
▶ Calcium channel blockers (amlodipine) slightly increase the exposure to **simvastatin**. Adjust **simvastatin** dose, p. 219. Mild Study
▶ Calcium channel blockers (diltiazem) slightly to moderately increase the exposure to **atorvastatin**. Monitor and adjust dose. Severe Anecdotal
▶ Calcium channel blockers (diltiazem, verapamil) moderately increase the exposure to **simvastatin**. Monitor and adjust dose. Severe Study
▶ Calcium channel blockers (verapamil) are predicted to slightly to moderately increase the exposure to **atorvastatin**. Monitor and adjust dose. Severe Theoretical
▶ Cephalosporins (ceftobiprole) are predicted to increase the concentration of **statins**. Moderate Theoretical
▶ Ciclosporin very markedly increases the exposure to **atorvastatin**. Avoid or adjust **atorvastatin** dose, p. 217. Severe Study
▶ Ciclosporin moderately increases the exposure to **fluvastatin**. Severe Study
▶ Ciclosporin markedly to very markedly increases the exposure to **pravastatin**. Adjust dose. Severe Study
▶ Ciclosporin markedly increases the exposure to statins **(rosuvastatin, simvastatin)**. Avoid. Severe Study
▶ Clopidogrel increases the exposure to **rosuvastatin**. Adjust **rosuvastatin** dose, p. 218. Moderate Study
▶ Cobicistat is predicted to increase the exposure to **atorvastatin**. Avoid or adjust dose and monitor rhabdomyolysis. Severe Study
▶ Cobicistat is predicted to increase the exposure to **simvastatin**. Avoid. Severe Study
▶ Colchicine increases the risk of rhabdomyolysis when given with **statins**. Severe Anecdotal
▶ Statins **(fluvastatin, rosuvastatin)** increase the anticoagulant effect of coumarins. Monitor INR and adjust dose. Severe Study
▶ Crizotinib is predicted to increase the exposure to statins **(atorvastatin, simvastatin)**. Monitor and adjust dose. Severe Theoretical
▶ Danazol is predicted to increase the risk of rhabdomyolysis when given with **atorvastatin**. Severe Theoretical
▶ Danazol increases the risk of rhabdomyolysis when given with **simvastatin**. Avoid. Severe Anecdotal
▶ Statins are predicted to increase the risk of rhabdomyolysis when given with daptomycin. Severe Theoretical
▶ Dasabuvir increases the exposure to **rosuvastatin**. Adjust **rosuvastatin** dose, p. 218. Moderate Study
▶ Dasatinib is predicted to increase the exposure to **simvastatin**. Moderate Theoretical
▶ Elbasvir increases the exposure to **atorvastatin**. Adjust **atorvastatin** dose, p. 217. Moderate Study

▶ Elbasvir is predicted to increase the exposure to **fluvastatin**. Adjust **fluvastatin** dose, p. 217. Unknown Theoretical
▶ Elbasvir increases the exposure to **rosuvastatin**. Adjust **rosuvastatin** dose, p. 218. Moderate Study
▶ Elbasvir is predicted to increase the exposure to **simvastatin**. Adjust **simvastatin** dose, p. 219. Unknown Theoretical
▶ Eltrombopag is predicted to increase the exposure to **statins**. Monitor and adjust dose. Moderate Study
▶ Endothelin receptor antagonists (bosentan) slightly decrease the exposure to **atorvastatin**. Mild Study
▶ Endothelin receptor antagonists (bosentan) moderately decrease the exposure to **simvastatin**. Moderate Study
▶ Ezetimibe potentially increases the risk of rhabdomyolysis when given with **statins**. Severe Anecdotal
▶ Fibrates (bezafibrate, ciprofibrate) increase the risk of rhabdomyolysis when given with **pravastatin**. Avoid. Severe Study
▶ Fibrates (bezafibrate, ciprofibrate) increase the risk of rhabdomyolysis when given with **rosuvastatin**. Adjust **rosuvastatin** dose, p. 218. Severe Study
▶ Fibrates (bezafibrate, ciprofibrate) increase the risk of rhabdomyolysis when given with **simvastatin**. Adjust **simvastatin** dose, p. 219. Severe Study
▶ Fibrates (ciprofibrate) increase the risk of rhabdomyolysis when given with **atorvastatin**. Avoid or adjust dose. Severe Study
▶ Fibrates (ciprofibrate) increase the risk of rhabdomyolysis when given with **fluvastatin**. Severe Study
▶ Fibrates (fenofibrate) are predicted to increase the risk of rhabdomyolysis when given with **fluvastatin**. Adjust **fenofibrate** dose, p. 214. Severe Theoretical
▶ Fibrates (fenofibrate) are predicted to increase the risk of rhabdomyolysis when given with **pravastatin**. Avoid. Severe Theoretical
▶ Fibrates (fenofibrate) increase the risk of rhabdomyolysis when given with **rosuvastatin**. Adjust **fenofibrate** and **rosuvastatin** doses, p. 214, p. 218. Severe Anecdotal
▶ Fibrates (gemfibrozil) increase the risk of rhabdomyolysis when given with **statins**. Avoid. Severe Anecdotal
▶ Fibrates (bezafibrate) increase the risk of rhabdomyolysis when given with statins **(atorvastatin, fluvastatin)**. Severe Study
▶ Fibrates (fenofibrate) increase the risk of rhabdomyolysis when given with statins **(atorvastatin, simvastatin)**. Adjust **fenofibrate** dose, p. 214. Severe Anecdotal
▶ Filgotinib is predicted to increase the exposure to statins **(atorvastatin, pravastatin, rosuvastatin, simvastatin)**. Avoid. Moderate Theoretical
▶ Fostamatinib slightly increases the exposure to **rosuvastatin**. Moderate Study
▶ Fostamatinib slightly increases the exposure to **simvastatin**. Monitor adverse effects and adjust dose. Moderate Study
▶ Fusidate increases the risk of rhabdomyolysis when given with **statins**. Avoid. Severe Anecdotal
▶ Glecaprevir (with pibrentasvir) markedly increases the exposure to **atorvastatin**. Avoid. Severe Study
▶ Glecaprevir (with pibrentasvir) is predicted to increase the exposure to **fluvastatin**. Moderate Theoretical
▶ Glecaprevir (with pibrentasvir) increases the exposure to **pravastatin**. Use with caution and adjust **pravastatin** dose, p. 218. Moderate Study
▶ Glecaprevir (with pibrentasvir) increases the exposure to **rosuvastatin**. Use with caution and adjust **rosuvastatin** dose, p. 218. Moderate Study
▶ Glecaprevir (with pibrentasvir) increases the exposure to **simvastatin**. Avoid. Moderate Study
▶ Grapefruit juice increases the exposure to **atorvastatin**. Mild Study
▶ Grapefruit juice increases the exposure to **simvastatin**. Avoid. Severe Study
▶ Grazoprevir increases the exposure to **atorvastatin**. Adjust **atorvastatin** dose, p. 217. Moderate Study
▶ Grazoprevir is predicted to increase the exposure to **fluvastatin**. Adjust **fluvastatin** dose, p. 217. Unknown Theoretical
▶ Grazoprevir increases the exposure to **rosuvastatin**. Adjust **rosuvastatin** dose, p. 218. Moderate Study

Grazoprevir is predicted to increase the exposure to **simvastatin**. Adjust **simvastatin** dose, p. 219. Unknown Theoretical
HIV-protease inhibitors are predicted to increase the exposure to **atorvastatin**. Avoid or adjust dose and monitor rhabdomyolysis. Severe Study
HIV-protease inhibitors slightly to moderately increase the exposure to **rosuvastatin**. Avoid or adjust dose. Severe Study
HIV-protease inhibitors are predicted to increase the exposure to **simvastatin**. Avoid. Severe Study
Idelalisib is predicted to increase the exposure to **atorvastatin**. Avoid or adjust dose and monitor rhabdomyolysis. Severe Study
Idelalisib is predicted to increase the exposure to **simvastatin**. Avoid. Severe Study
Imatinib is predicted to increase the exposure to **atorvastatin**. Monitor and adjust dose. Severe Theoretical
Imatinib moderately increases the exposure to **simvastatin**. Monitor and adjust dose. Severe Study
Ledipasvir is predicted to increase the exposure to **rosuvastatin**. Avoid. Severe Theoretical
Ledipasvir is predicted to increase the exposure to statins **(atorvastatin, fluvastatin, pravastatin, simvastatin)**. Monitor and adjust dose. Moderate Theoretical
Leflunomide is predicted to increase the exposure to **rosuvastatin**. Adjust dose. Moderate Study → Also see **TABLE 1** p. 1429
Leflunomide is predicted to increase the exposure to statins **(atorvastatin, fluvastatin, pravastatin, simvastatin)**. Moderate Study → Also see **TABLE 1** p. 1429
Letermovir moderately increases the exposure to **atorvastatin**. Avoid or adjust **atorvastatin** dose, p. 217. Severe Study
Letermovir is predicted to increase the exposure to **fluvastatin**. Monitor and adjust dose. Moderate Theoretical
Letermovir is predicted to increase the exposure to **pravastatin**. Avoid or adjust dose. Moderate Theoretical
Letermovir is predicted to increase the exposure to statins **(rosuvastatin, simvastatin)**. Avoid. Severe Study
Lomitapide increases the exposure to **atorvastatin**. Adjust **lomitapide** dose or separate administration by 12 hours, p. 222. Mild Study → Also see **TABLE 1** p. 1429
Lomitapide increases the exposure to **simvastatin**. Monitor and adjust **simvastatin** dose, p. 219. Moderate Study → Also see **TABLE 1** p. 1429
Macrolides (clarithromycin) are predicted to increase the exposure to **atorvastatin**. Avoid or adjust dose and monitor rhabdomyolysis. Severe Study
Macrolides (clarithromycin) moderately increase the exposure to **pravastatin**. Severe Study
Macrolides (clarithromycin) are predicted to increase the exposure to **simvastatin**. Avoid. Severe Study
Macrolides (erythromycin) slightly increase the exposure to **atorvastatin**. Monitor and adjust dose. Severe Anecdotal
Macrolides (erythromycin) are predicted to increase the exposure to **pravastatin**. Severe Study
Macrolides (erythromycin) markedly increase the exposure to **simvastatin**. Avoid. Severe Study
Mitotane is predicted to decrease the exposure to **simvastatin**. Severe Study
Monoclonal antibodies (sarilumab) are predicted to decrease the exposure to statins **(atorvastatin, simvastatin)**. Moderate Study
Monoclonal antibodies (tocilizumab) are predicted to decrease the exposure to statins **(atorvastatin, simvastatin)**. Monitor and adjust dose. Moderate Study
Neurokinin-1 receptor antagonists (aprepitant, netupitant) are predicted to increase the exposure to statins **(atorvastatin, simvastatin)**. Monitor and adjust dose. Severe Theoretical
Nicotinic acid is predicted to increase the risk of rhabdomyolysis when given with **statins**. Severe Theoretical
Nilotinib is predicted to slightly increase the exposure to **atorvastatin**. Monitor and adjust dose. Severe Theoretical
Nilotinib is predicted to increase the exposure to **simvastatin**. Monitor and adjust dose. Severe Theoretical
NNRTIs (efavirenz, nevirapine) slightly decrease the exposure to **atorvastatin**. Mild Study

NNRTIs (efavirenz, nevirapine) moderately decrease the exposure to **simvastatin**. Moderate Study
Osimertinib slightly increases the exposure to **rosuvastatin**. Moderate Study
Paritaprevir (in fixed-dose combination) is predicted to increase the risk of rhabdomyolysis when given with **atorvastatin**. Avoid. Severe Theoretical
Paritaprevir (with ritonavir and ombitasvir) is predicted to increase the exposure to **fluvastatin**. Avoid. Moderate Theoretical
Paritaprevir (with ritonavir and ombitasvir) increases the exposure to **pravastatin**. Adjust **pravastatin** dose, p. 218. Moderate Study
Paritaprevir (with ritonavir and ombitasvir) slightly to moderately increases the exposure to **rosuvastatin**. Adjust **rosuvastatin** dose, p. 218. Moderate Study
Paritaprevir (in fixed-dose combination) is predicted to increase the risk of rhabdomyolysis when given with **simvastatin**. Avoid. Severe Theoretical
Pazopanib is predicted to affect the exposure to **atorvastatin**. Moderate Anecdotal
Pazopanib is predicted to affect the exposure to statins **(pravastatin, rosuvastatin, simvastatin)**. Theoretical
Rosuvastatin is predicted to increase the anticoagulant effect of phenindione. Monitor INR and adjust dose. Severe Theoretical
Pibrentasvir (with glecaprevir) markedly increases the exposure to **atorvastatin**. Avoid. Severe Study
Pibrentasvir (with glecaprevir) is predicted to increase the exposure to **fluvastatin**. Moderate Theoretical
Pibrentasvir (with glecaprevir) increases the exposure to **pravastatin**. Use with caution and adjust **pravastatin** dose, p. 218. Moderate Study
Pibrentasvir (with glecaprevir) increases the exposure to **rosuvastatin**. Use with caution and adjust **rosuvastatin** dose, p. 218. Moderate Study
Pibrentasvir (with glecaprevir) increases the exposure to **simvastatin**. Avoid. Moderate Study
Ranolazine is predicted to increase the exposure to **atorvastatin**. Moderate Theoretical
Ranolazine slightly increases the exposure to **simvastatin**. Adjust **simvastatin** dose, p. 219. Moderate Study
Regorafenib is predicted to increase the exposure to statins **(atorvastatin, fluvastatin, rosuvastatin)**. Moderate Study
Ribociclib (high-dose) is predicted to increase the exposure to **simvastatin**. Avoid. Moderate Theoretical
Ribociclib is predicted to increase the exposure to statins **(pravastatin, rosuvastatin)**. Theoretical
Rifamycins (rifampicin) markedly decrease the exposure to **atorvastatin**. Manufacturer advises take both drugs at the same time. Moderate Study
Rifamycins (rifampicin) moderately decrease the exposure to **fluvastatin**. Monitor and adjust dose. Moderate Study
Rifamycins (rifampicin) very markedly decrease the exposure to **simvastatin**. Moderate Study
Sacubitril is predicted to increase the exposure to **statins**. Severe Study
St John's wort slightly decreases the exposure to **atorvastatin**. Mild Study
St John's wort moderately decreases the exposure to **simvastatin**. Moderate Study
Fluvastatin slightly increases the exposure to sulfonylureas (glibenclamide). Mild Study
Tedizolid is predicted to increase the exposure to statins **(atorvastatin, fluvastatin, rosuvastatin)**. Avoid. Moderate Study
Teriflunomide moderately increases the exposure to **rosuvastatin**. Adjust **rosuvastatin** dose, p. 218. Moderate Study → Also see **TABLE 1** p. 1429
Teriflunomide is predicted to increase the exposure to statins **(atorvastatin, fluvastatin, pravastatin, simvastatin)**. Moderate Study → Also see **TABLE 1** p. 1429
Ticagrelor slightly increases the exposure to **simvastatin**. Adjust **simvastatin** dose, p. 219. Moderate Study
Tivozanib is predicted to decrease the exposure to **rosuvastatin**. Moderate Theoretical

Statins (continued)

▸ Velpatasvir increases the exposure to **rosuvastatin**. Adjust rosuvastatin dose and monitor adverse effects, p. 218. Severe Study

▸ Velpatasvir is predicted to increase the exposure to **simvastatin**. Monitor adverse effects and adjust dose. Severe Theoretical

▸ Venetoclax is predicted to increase the exposure to **atorvastatin**. Moderate Study

▸ Venetoclax is predicted to increase the exposure to statins **(fluvastatin, pravastatin, rosuvastatin, simvastatin)**. Moderate Theoretical

▸ Voxilaprevir (with sofosbuvir and velpatasvir) is predicted to increase the exposure to **atorvastatin**. Adjust atorvastatin dose, p. 217. Moderate Theoretical

▸ Voxilaprevir (with sofosbuvir and velpatasvir) moderately increases the exposure to **pravastatin**. Monitor and adjust pravastatin dose, p. 218. Moderate Study

▸ Voxilaprevir (with sofosbuvir and velpatasvir) markedly increases the exposure to **rosuvastatin**. Avoid. Severe Study

▸ Voxilaprevir (with sofosbuvir and velpatasvir) is predicted to increase the exposure to statins **(fluvastatin, simvastatin)**. Avoid. Moderate Theoretical

Stiripentol → see antiepileptics

Streptokinase → see TABLE 3 p. 1429 (anticoagulant effects)

Streptomycin → see aminoglycosides

Streptozocin → see TABLE 1 p. 1429 (hepatotoxicity), TABLE 15 p. 1432 (myelosuppression), TABLE 2 p. 1429 (nephrotoxicity)

▸ Live vaccines are predicted to increase the risk of generalised infection (possibly life-threatening) when given with **streptozocin**. Public Health England advises avoid (refer to Green Book). Severe Theoretical

Strontium → see TABLE 5 p. 1430 (thromboembolism)

▸ Oral antacids decrease the absorption of oral **strontium**. Separate administration by 2 hours. Moderate Study

▸ Oral calcium salts decrease the exposure to **strontium**. Separate administration by 2 hours. Moderate Study

▸ **Strontium** is predicted to decrease the absorption of quinolones. Avoid. Moderate Theoretical

▸ **Strontium** is predicted to decrease the absorption of tetracyclines. Avoid. Moderate Theoretical

Sucralfate

▸ **Sucralfate** is predicted to decrease the exposure to bictegravir. Avoid. Moderate Theoretical

▸ **Sucralfate** potentially decreases the effects of coumarins (warfarin). Separate administration by 2 hours. Moderate Anecdotal

▸ **Sucralfate** decreases the absorption of digoxin. Separate administration by 2 hours. Severe Anecdotal

▸ **Sucralfate** decreases the absorption of dolutegravir. Moderate Study

▸ **Sucralfate** increases the risk of blocked enteral or nasogastric tubes when given with enteral feeds. Separate administration by 1 hour. Moderate Study

▸ Potassium citrate increases the risk of adverse effects when given with **sucralfate**. Avoid. Moderate Theoretical

▸ **Sucralfate** decreases the exposure to quinolones. Separate administration by 2 hours. Moderate Study

▸ Sodium citrate is predicted to increase the risk of adverse effects when given with **sucralfate**. Avoid. Moderate Theoretical

▸ **Sucralfate** decreases the absorption of sulpiride. Separate administration by 2 hours. Moderate Study

▸ **Sucralfate** potentially decreases the absorption of theophylline. Separate administration by at least 2 hours. Moderate Study

▸ **Sucralfate** decreases the absorption of thyroid hormones (levothyroxine). Separate administration by at least 4 hours. Moderate Study

▸ **Sucralfate** is predicted to decrease the absorption of tricyclic antidepressants. Moderate Study

Sugammadex

▸ **Sugammadex** is predicted to decrease the exposure to combined hormonal contraceptives. Refer to patient information leaflet for missed pill advice. Severe Theoretical

▸ **Sugammadex** is predicted to decrease the exposure to desogestrel. Refer to patient information leaflet for missed pill advice. Severe Theoretical

▸ **Sugammadex** is predicted to decrease the efficacy of etonogestrel. Use additional contraceptive precautions. Severe Theoretical

▸ **Sugammadex** is predicted to decrease the exposure to levonorgestrel. Use additional contraceptive precautions. Severe Theoretical

▸ **Sugammadex** is predicted to decrease the exposure to medroxyprogesterone. Use additional contraceptive precautions. Severe Theoretical

▸ **Sugammadex** is predicted to decrease the exposure to norethisterone. Use additional contraceptive precautions. Severe Theoretical

Sulfadiazine → see sulfonamides

Sulfadoxine → see sulfonamides

Sulfamethoxazole → see sulfonamides

Sulfasalazine → see TABLE 1 p. 1429 (hepatotoxicity), TABLE 15 p. 1432 (myelosuppression)

▸ Anti-androgens (darolutamide) are predicted to increase the exposure to **sulfasalazine**. Avoid. Severe Theoretical

▸ Antifungals, azoles (isavuconazole) are predicted to increase the exposure to **sulfasalazine**. Moderate Theoretical

▸ **Sulfasalazine** decreases the concentration of digoxin. Moderate Study

▸ **Sulfasalazine** is predicted to decrease the absorption of folates. Moderate Study

▸ Leflunomide is predicted to increase the exposure to **sulfasalazine**. Moderate Study → Also see TABLE 1 p. 1429 → Also see TABLE 15 p. 1432

▸ Regorafenib is predicted to increase the exposure to **sulfasalazine**. Moderate Study → Also see TABLE 15 p. 1432

▸ Tedizolid is predicted to increase the exposure to **sulfasalazine**. Avoid. Moderate Study

▸ Teriflunomide is predicted to increase the exposure to **sulfasalazine**. Moderate Study → Also see TABLE 1 p. 1429

▸ Velpatasvir is predicted to increase the exposure to **sulfasalazine**. Moderate Theoretical

▸ Venetoclax is predicted to increase the exposure to **sulfasalazine**. Moderate Theoretical

▸ Voxilaprevir is predicted to increase the concentration of **sulfasalazine**. Avoid. Severe Theoretical

Sulfonamides

sulfadiazine · sulfadoxine · sulfamethoxazole

▸ **Sulfonamides** potentially increase the risk of methaemoglobinaemia when given with topical anaesthetics, local (prilocaine). Use with caution or avoid. Severe Anecdotal

▸ **Sulfadiazine** is predicted to increase the concentration of antiepileptics (fosphenytoin). Monitor and adjust dose. Moderate Study

▸ **Sulfadiazine** increases the concentration of antiepileptics (phenytoin). Monitor and adjust dose. Moderate Study

▸ Antimalarials (pyrimethamine) increase the risk of adverse effects when given with **sulfonamides**. Severe Study

▸ Chloroprocaine is predicted to decrease the effects of **sulfonamides**. Avoid. Severe Theoretical

▸ **Sulfadiazine** is predicted to increase the anticoagulant effect of coumarins. Severe Theoretical

▸ **Sulfamethoxazole** increases the anticoagulant effect of coumarins. Severe Study

▸ **Sulfonamides** are predicted to increase the risk of methaemoglobinaemia when given with dapsone. Severe Theoretical

▸ **Sulfonamides** are predicted to increase the exposure to methotrexate. Use with caution or avoid. Severe Theoretical

▸ Potassium aminobenzoate is predicted to affect the efficacy of **sulfonamides**. Avoid. Severe Theoretical

▸ **Sulfonamides** are predicted to increase the exposure to sulfonylureas. Moderate Study

▸ **Sulfonamides** are predicted to increase the effects of thiopental. Moderate Theoretical

Sulfonylureas → see TABLE 14 p. 1432 (antidiabetic drugs)

glibenclamide · gliclazide · glimepiride · glipizide · tolbutamide

▸ Anti-androgens (darolutamide) are predicted to increase the concentration of **glibenclamide**. Moderate Theoretical

▸ Antiarrhythmics (amiodarone) are predicted to increase the exposure to **sulfonylureas**. Use with caution and adjust dose. Moderate Study

▸ Antifungals, azoles (fluconazole, miconazole) are predicted to increase the exposure to **sulfonylureas**. Use with caution and adjust dose. Moderate Study

▸ Antifungals, azoles (voriconazole) are predicted to increase the concentration of **sulfonylureas**. Use with caution and adjust dose. Moderate Study

▸ Cephalosporins (ceftobiprole) are predicted to increase the concentration of **glibenclamide**. Moderate Theoretical

▸ Ceritinib is predicted to increase the exposure to **glimepiride**. Adjust dose. Moderate Theoretical

▸ Chloramphenicol is predicted to increase the exposure to **sulfonylureas**. Severe Study

▸ Endothelin receptor antagonists (bosentan) increase the risk of hepatotoxicity when given with **glibenclamide**. Avoid. Severe Study

▸ Fibrates are predicted to increase the risk of hypoglycaemia when given with **sulfonylureas**. Moderate Theoretical

▸ Filgotinib is predicted to increase the exposure to **glibenclamide**. Avoid. Moderate Theoretical

▸ Leflunomide is predicted to increase the exposure to **glibenclamide**. Moderate Study

▸ Letermovir is predicted to increase the concentration of **glibenclamide**. Moderate Theoretical

▸ Macrolides (clarithromycin) are predicted to slightly increase the exposure to **sulfonylureas**. Moderate Theoretical

▸ Nitisinone is predicted to increase the exposure to sulfonylureas (**glimepiride, tolbutamide**). Moderate Study

▸ Rifamycins (rifampicin) are predicted to decrease the exposure to **sulfonylureas**. Moderate Study

▸ Statins (fluvastatin) slightly increase the exposure to **glibenclamide**. Mild Study

▸ Sulfonamides are predicted to increase the exposure to **sulfonylureas**. Moderate Study

▸ Teriflunomide is predicted to increase the exposure to **glibenclamide**. Moderate Study

▸ Venetoclax is predicted to increase the exposure to **glibenclamide**. Moderate Theoretical

Sulindac → see NSAIDs

Sulpiride → see TABLE 8 p. 1430 (hypotension), TABLE 9 p. 1431 (QT-interval prolongation), TABLE 11 p. 1431 (CNS depressant effects)

▸ Oral antacids decrease the absorption of oral **sulpiride**. Separate administration by 2 hours. Moderate Study

▸ **Sulpiride** is predicted to decrease the effects of dopamine receptor agonists. Avoid. Moderate Theoretical → Also see TABLE 8 p. 1430 → Also see TABLE 9 p. 1431

▸ **Sulpiride** is predicted to decrease the effects of levodopa. Avoid. Severe Theoretical → Also see TABLE 8 p. 1430

▸ **Sulpiride** potentially increases the risk of neurotoxicity when given with lithium. Severe Anecdotal → Also see TABLE 9 p. 1431

▸ Sucralfate decreases the absorption of **sulpiride**. Separate administration by 2 hours. Moderate Study

Sumatriptan → see triptans

Sunitinib → see TABLE 15 p. 1432 (myelosuppression), TABLE 9 p. 1431 (QT-interval prolongation)

▸ Anti-androgens (apalutamide, enzalutamide) are predicted to decrease the exposure to **sunitinib**. Avoid or adjust **sunitinib** dose, p. 1044. Moderate Study → Also see TABLE 9 p. 1431

▸ Antiarrhythmics (dronedarone) are predicted to increase the exposure to **sunitinib**. Moderate Theoretical → Also see TABLE 9 p. 1431

▸ Antiepileptics (carbamazepine, fosphenytoin, phenobarbital, phenytoin, primidone) are predicted to decrease the exposure to **sunitinib**. Avoid or adjust **sunitinib** dose, p. 1044. Moderate Study

▸ Antifungals, azoles (fluconazole, isavuconazole, posaconazole) are predicted to increase the exposure to **sunitinib**. Moderate Theoretical → Also see TABLE 9 p. 1431

▸ Antifungals, azoles (itraconazole, ketoconazole, voriconazole) are predicted to slightly increase the exposure to **sunitinib**. Avoid

or adjust **sunitinib** dose, p. 1044. Moderate Study → Also see TABLE 9 p. 1431

▸ Calcium channel blockers (diltiazem, verapamil) are predicted to increase the exposure to **sunitinib**. Moderate Theoretical

▸ Cobicistat is predicted to slightly increase the exposure to **sunitinib**. Avoid or adjust **sunitinib** dose, p. 1044. Moderate Study

▸ **Sunitinib** is predicted to increase the risk of bleeding events when given with coumarins. Severe Theoretical

▸ Crizotinib is predicted to increase the exposure to **sunitinib**. Moderate Theoretical → Also see TABLE 9 p. 1431

▸ Elbasvir is predicted to increase the concentration of **sunitinib**. Use with caution and adjust dose. Moderate Theoretical

▸ Grapefruit juice is predicted to increase the exposure to **sunitinib**. Avoid. Moderate Theoretical

▸ Grazoprevir is predicted to increase the concentration of **sunitinib**. Use with caution and adjust dose. Moderate Theoretical

▸ HIV-protease inhibitors are predicted to slightly increase the exposure to **sunitinib**. Avoid or adjust **sunitinib** dose, p. 1044. Moderate Study → Also see TABLE 9 p. 1431

▸ Idelalisib is predicted to slightly increase the exposure to **sunitinib**. Avoid or adjust **sunitinib** dose, p. 1044. Moderate Study

▸ Imatinib is predicted to increase the exposure to **sunitinib**. Moderate Theoretical → Also see TABLE 15 p. 1432

▸ Letermovir is predicted to increase the exposure to **sunitinib**. Moderate Theoretical

▸ Macrolides (clarithromycin) are predicted to slightly increase the exposure to **sunitinib**. Avoid or adjust **sunitinib** dose, p. 1044. Moderate Study → Also see TABLE 9 p. 1431

▸ Macrolides (erythromycin) are predicted to increase the exposure to **sunitinib**. Moderate Theoretical → Also see TABLE 9 p. 1431

▸ Mitotane is predicted to decrease the exposure to **sunitinib**. Avoid or adjust **sunitinib** dose, p. 1044. Moderate Study → Also see TABLE 15 p. 1432

▸ Neurokinin-1 receptor antagonists (aprepitant, netupitant) are predicted to increase the exposure to **sunitinib**. Moderate Theoretical

▸ Nilotinib is predicted to increase the exposure to **sunitinib**. Moderate Theoretical → Also see TABLE 15 p. 1432 → Also see TABLE 9 p. 1431

▸ **Sunitinib** is predicted to increase the risk of bleeding events when given with phenindione. Severe Theoretical

▸ Rifamycins (rifampicin) are predicted to decrease the exposure to **sunitinib**. Avoid or adjust **sunitinib** dose, p. 1044. Moderate Study

Suxamethonium → see TABLE 20 p. 1433 (neuromuscular blocking effects)

▸ Alkylating agents (cyclophosphamide) increase the risk of prolonged neuromuscular blockade when given with **suxamethonium**. Moderate Study

▸ Antiarrhythmics (lidocaine) are predicted to increase the effects of **suxamethonium**. Moderate Study

▸ Anticholinesterases, centrally acting increase the effects of **suxamethonium**. Moderate Theoretical

▸ Antiepileptics (carbamazepine) increase the risk of prolonged neuromuscular blockade when given with **suxamethonium**. Moderate Study

▸ Antiepileptics (fosphenytoin, phenytoin) increase the effects of **suxamethonium**. Moderate Study

▸ Clindamycin increases the effects of **suxamethonium**. Severe Anecdotal

▸ Corticosteroids are predicted to decrease the effects of **suxamethonium**. Severe Anecdotal

▸ **Suxamethonium** is predicted to increase the risk of cardiovascular adverse effects when given with digoxin. Severe Anecdotal

▸ Irinotecan is predicted to increase the risk of prolonged neuromuscular blockade when given with **suxamethonium**. Moderate Theoretical

▸ Intravenous magnesium is predicted to increase the effects of **suxamethonium**. Moderate Study

▸ Metoclopramide increases the effects of **suxamethonium**. Moderate Study

Suxamethonium (continued)

▸ Penicillins (piperacillin) increase the effects of **suxamethonium**. Moderate Study

▸ SSRIs potentially increase the risk of prolonged neuromuscular blockade when given with **suxamethonium**. Unknown Theoretical

Sympathomimetics, inotropic

dobutamine · dopamine

▸ **Sympathomimetics, inotropic** are predicted to decrease the effects of apraclonidine. Avoid. Severe Theoretical

▸ Beta blockers, non-selective increase the risk of hypertension and bradycardia when given with **dobutamine**. Severe Theoretical

▸ Beta blockers, selective increase the risk of hypertension and bradycardia when given with **dobutamine**. Moderate Theoretical

▸ Entacapone is predicted to increase the risk of cardiovascular adverse effects when given with **sympathomimetics, inotropic**. Moderate Theoretical

▸ Ergometrine potentially increases the risk of peripheral vasoconstriction when given with **dopamine**. Avoid. Severe Anecdotal

▸ **Sympathomimetics, inotropic** are predicted to increase the risk of elevated blood pressure when given with linezolid. Avoid. Severe Theoretical

▸ **Sympathomimetics, inotropic** are predicted to increase the risk of a hypertensive crisis when given with MAO-B inhibitors. Avoid. Severe Anecdotal

▸ **Sympathomimetics, inotropic** are predicted to increase the risk of a hypertensive crisis when given with MAOIs, irreversible. Avoid and for 14 days after stopping the MAOI. Severe Theoretical

▸ Opicapone is predicted to increase the risk of cardiovascular adverse effects when given with **sympathomimetics, inotropic**. Severe Theoretical

▸ Tolcapone is predicted to increase the risk of cardiovascular adverse effects when given with **sympathomimetics, inotropic**. Moderate Theoretical

Sympathomimetics, vasoconstrictor

adrenaline/epinephrine · ephedrine · isometheptene · metaraminol · midodrine · noradrenaline/norepinephrine · phenylephrine · pseudoephedrine · xylometazoline

ROUTE-SPECIFIC INFORMATION Since systemic absorption can follow topical application of **phenylephrine** and **xylometazoline**, the possibility of interactions should be borne in mind.

▸ Ephedrine increases the risk of adverse effects when given with aminophylline. Avoid in children. Moderate Study

▸ **Sympathomimetics, vasoconstrictor** are predicted to decrease the effects of apraclonidine. Avoid. Severe Theoretical

▸ Atropine increases the risk of severe hypertension when given with **phenylephrine**. Severe Study

▸ Beta blockers, non-selective are predicted to increase the risk of hypertension and bradycardia when given with sympathomimetics, vasoconstrictor **(adrenaline/epinephrine, noradrenaline/norepinephrine)**. Severe Study

▸ Beta blockers, selective are predicted to increase the risk of hypertension and bradycardia when given with sympathomimetics, vasoconstrictor **(adrenaline/epinephrine, noradrenaline/norepinephrine)**. Severe Study

▸ Isometheptene potentially increases the risk of adverse effects when given with dopamine receptor agonists **(bromocriptine)**. Avoid. Severe Anecdotal

▸ Entacapone is predicted to increase the risk of cardiovascular adverse effects when given with sympathomimetics, vasoconstrictor **(adrenaline/epinephrine, noradrenaline/norepinephrine)**. Moderate Study

▸ Ergometrine is predicted to increase the risk of peripheral vasoconstriction when given with noradrenaline/norepinephrine. Severe Anecdotal

▸ Pseudoephedrine increases the risk of elevated blood pressure when given with linezolid. Avoid. Severe Study

▸ Sympathomimetics, vasoconstrictor **(adrenaline/epinephrine, ephedrine, isometheptene, noradrenaline/norepinephrine,**

phenylephrine) are predicted to increase the risk of elevated blood pressure when given with linezolid. Avoid. Severe Theoretical

▸ **Sympathomimetics, vasoconstrictor** are predicted to increase the risk of a hypertensive crisis when given with MAO-B inhibitors. Avoid. Severe Anecdotal

▸ **Sympathomimetics, vasoconstrictor** are predicted to increase the risk of a hypertensive crisis when given with MAOIs, irreversible. Avoid and for 14 days after stopping the MAOI. Severe Study

▸ Mianserin decreases the effects of **ephedrine**. Severe Anecdotal

▸ Sympathomimetics, vasoconstrictor **(ephedrine, isometheptene, phenylephrine, pseudoephedrine)** are predicted to increase the risk of a hypertensive crisis when given with moclobemide. Avoid. Severe Study

▸ Opicapone is predicted to increase the risk of cardiovascular adverse effects when given with sympathomimetics, vasoconstrictor **(adrenaline/epinephrine, noradrenaline/norepinephrine)**. Severe Theoretical

▸ **Sympathomimetics, vasoconstrictor** potentially increase the risk of a hypertensive crisis when given with ozanimod. Severe Theoretical

▸ Ephedrine increases the risk of adverse effects when given with theophylline. Avoid in children. Moderate Study

▸ Tolcapone is predicted to increase the effects of sympathomimetics, vasoconstrictor **(adrenaline/epinephrine, noradrenaline/norepinephrine)**. Moderate Theoretical

▸ Tricyclic antidepressants are predicted to decrease the effects of **ephedrine**. Avoid. Severe Study

▸ Tricyclic antidepressants increase the effects of sympathomimetics, vasoconstrictor **(adrenaline/epinephrine, noradrenaline/norepinephrine, phenylephrine)**. Avoid. Severe Study

Tacalcitol → see vitamin D substances

Tacrolimus → see TABLE 2 p. 1429 (nephrotoxicity), TABLE 16 p. 1433 (increased serum potassium)

▸ Pomelo and pomegranate juices might greatly increase the concentration of tacrolimus.

▸ Since systemic absorption can follow topical application, the possibility of interactions should be borne in mind.

▸ Alcohol increases the risk of facial flushing and skin irritation when given with topical **tacrolimus**. Moderate Study

▸ Anti-androgens (apalutamide, enzalutamide) decrease the concentration of **tacrolimus**. Monitor and adjust dose. Severe Study

▸ Antiarrhythmics (amiodarone) are predicted to increase the concentration of **tacrolimus**. Severe Anecdotal

▸ Antiarrhythmics (dronedarone) are predicted to increase the concentration of **tacrolimus**. Severe Study

▸ Antiepileptics (carbamazepine, fosphenytoin, phenobarbital, phenytoin, primidone) decrease the concentration of **tacrolimus**. Monitor and adjust dose. Severe Study

▸ Antifungals, azoles (fluconazole, isavuconazole, posaconazole) are predicted to increase the concentration of **tacrolimus**. Severe Study

▸ Antifungals, azoles (itraconazole, ketoconazole, voriconazole) are predicted to increase the concentration of **tacrolimus**. Monitor and adjust dose. Severe Study

▸ Antifungals, azoles (miconazole) are predicted to increase the concentration of **tacrolimus**. Monitor and adjust dose. Severe Theoretical

▸ Brigatinib potentially decreases the concentration of **tacrolimus**. Avoid. Moderate Theoretical

▸ Calcium channel blockers (diltiazem, verapamil) are predicted to increase the concentration of **tacrolimus**. Severe Study

▸ Calcium channel blockers (nicardipine) potentially increase the concentration of **tacrolimus**. Monitor concentration and adjust dose. Severe Anecdotal

▸ Ceritinib is predicted to increase the exposure to **tacrolimus**. Avoid. Severe Theoretical

▸ Chloramphenicol increases the concentration of **tacrolimus**. Severe Study

▸ Ciclosporin increases the concentration of **tacrolimus**. Avoid. Severe Study → Also see TABLE 2 p. 1429 → Also see TABLE 16 p. 1433

Cobicistat is predicted to increase the concentration of **tacrolimus**. Monitor and adjust dose. Severe Study

Crizotinib is predicted to increase the concentration of **tacrolimus**. Severe Study

▸ Danazol potentially increases the concentration of **tacrolimus**. Severe Anecdotal

Endothelin receptor antagonists (bosentan) are predicted to decrease the concentration of **tacrolimus** and **tacrolimus** potentially increases the concentration of endothelin receptor antagonists (bosentan). Avoid. Severe Theoretical

▸ Filgotinib is predicted to increase the risk of immunosuppression when given with **tacrolimus**. Avoid. Severe Theoretical

▸ Glecaprevir (with pibrentasvir) slightly increases the exposure to **tacrolimus**. Monitor and adjust dose. Mild Study

▸ Grapefruit juice greatly increases the concentration of **tacrolimus**. Avoid. Severe Study

▸ Grazoprevir increases the exposure to **tacrolimus**. Moderate Study

▸ HIV-protease inhibitors are predicted to increase the concentration of **tacrolimus**. Monitor and adjust dose. Severe Study

▸ Idelalisib is predicted to increase the concentration of **tacrolimus**. Monitor and adjust dose. Severe Study

▸ Imatinib is predicted to increase the concentration of **tacrolimus**. Severe Study

▸ Larotrectinib is predicted to increase the exposure to **tacrolimus**. Use with caution and adjust dose. Mild Theoretical

▸ Letermovir is predicted to increase the concentration of **tacrolimus**. Severe Study

▸ Live vaccines are predicted to increase the risk of generalised infection (possibly life-threatening) when given with **tacrolimus**. Public Health England advises avoid (refer to Green Book). Severe Theoretical

▸ **Tacrolimus** is predicted to increase the exposure to lomitapide. Separate administration by 12 hours. Moderate Theoretical

▸ Lorlatinib is predicted to decrease the exposure to **tacrolimus**. Avoid. Moderate Theoretical

▸ Lumacaftor is predicted to decrease the exposure to **tacrolimus**. Avoid. Severe Theoretical

▸ Macrolides (clarithromycin) are predicted to increase the concentration of **tacrolimus**. Monitor and adjust dose. Severe Study

▸ Macrolides (erythromycin) are predicted to increase the concentration of **tacrolimus**. Severe Study

▸ **Tacrolimus** is predicted to affect the efficacy of mifamurtide. Avoid. Severe Theoretical

▸ Mitotane decreases the concentration of **tacrolimus**. Monitor and adjust dose. Severe Study

▸ Monoclonal antibodies (sarilumab) potentially affect the exposure to **tacrolimus**. Monitor and adjust dose. Moderate Theoretical

▸ Neurokinin-1 receptor antagonists (aprepitant, netupitant) are predicted to increase the concentration of **tacrolimus**. Severe Study

▸ Nilotinib is predicted to increase the concentration of **tacrolimus**. Severe Study

▸ NNRTIs (doravirine) are predicted to decrease the exposure to **tacrolimus**. Monitor **tacrolimus** concentration and adjust dose, p. 887. Moderate Study

▸ NNRTIs (efavirenz, nevirapine) are predicted to decrease the concentration of **tacrolimus**. Monitor and adjust dose. Moderate Theoretical

▸ Palbociclib is predicted to increase the exposure to **tacrolimus**. Adjust dose. Moderate Theoretical

▸ Pibrentasvir (with glecaprevir) slightly increases the exposure to **tacrolimus**. Monitor and adjust dose. Mild Study

▸ Pitolisant is predicted to decrease the exposure to **tacrolimus**. Avoid. Severe Theoretical

▸ Ranolazine increases the concentration of **tacrolimus**. Adjust dose. Severe Anecdotal

▸ Ribociclib is predicted to increase the exposure to **tacrolimus**. Use with caution and adjust dose. Moderate Theoretical

▸ Rifamycins (rifampicin) decrease the concentration of **tacrolimus**. Monitor and adjust dose. Severe Study

▸ Rucaparib is predicted to increase the exposure to **tacrolimus**. Monitor and adjust dose. Moderate Study

▸ Sirolimus is predicted to decrease the concentration of **tacrolimus** and **tacrolimus** increases the exposure to sirolimus. Severe Study

▸ St John's wort decreases the concentration of **tacrolimus**. Avoid. Severe Study

▸ **Tacrolimus** is predicted to increase the exposure to thrombin inhibitors (dabigatran). Avoid. Severe Theoretical

▸ **Tacrolimus** increases the exposure to tofacitinib. Avoid. Severe Study

▸ **Tacrolimus** potentially increases the risk of serotonin syndrome when given with venlafaxine. Severe Anecdotal

Tadalafil → see phosphodiesterase type-5 inhibitors

Talazoparib → see TABLE 15 p. 1432 (myelosuppression)

▸ Antiarrhythmics (amiodarone, dronedarone) are predicted to slightly increase the exposure to **talazoparib**. Avoid or adjust **talazoparib** dose, p. 1052. Severe Study

▸ Antifungals, azoles (itraconazole, ketoconazole) are predicted to slightly increase the exposure to **talazoparib**. Avoid or adjust **talazoparib** dose, p. 1052. Severe Study

▸ Calcium channel blockers (verapamil) are predicted to slightly increase the exposure to **talazoparib**. Avoid or adjust **talazoparib** dose, p. 1052. Severe Study

▸ Ciclosporin is predicted to slightly increase the exposure to **talazoparib**. Avoid or adjust **talazoparib** dose, p. 1052. Severe Study

▸ Eltrombopag potentially increases the exposure to **talazoparib**. Avoid or monitor. Moderate Theoretical

▸ HIV-protease inhibitors (lopinavir, ritonavir, saquinavir) are predicted to slightly increase the exposure to **talazoparib**. Avoid or adjust **talazoparib** dose, p. 1052. Severe Study

▸ Lapatinib is predicted to slightly increase the exposure to **talazoparib**. Avoid or adjust **talazoparib** dose, p. 1052. Severe Study

▸ Leflunomide potentially increases the exposure to **talazoparib**. Avoid or monitor. Moderate Theoretical → Also see TABLE 15 p. 1432

▸ Macrolides are predicted to slightly increase the exposure to **talazoparib**. Avoid or adjust **talazoparib** dose, p. 1052. Severe Study

▸ Ranolazine is predicted to slightly increase the exposure to **talazoparib**. Avoid or adjust **talazoparib** dose, p. 1052. Severe Study

▸ Teriflunomide potentially increases the exposure to **talazoparib**. Avoid or monitor. Moderate Theoretical

▸ Vemurafenib is predicted to slightly increase the exposure to **talazoparib**. Avoid or adjust **talazoparib** dose, p. 1052. Severe Study

Tamoxifen → see TABLE 5 p. 1430 (thromboembolism)

▸ Bupropion is predicted to decrease the efficacy of **tamoxifen**. Avoid. Severe Study

▸ Cinacalcet is predicted to decrease the efficacy of **tamoxifen**. Avoid. Severe Study

▸ **Tamoxifen** increases the anticoagulant effect of coumarins. Severe Study

▸ Rifamycins (rifampicin) markedly decrease the exposure to **tamoxifen**. Unknown Study

▸ SSRIs (fluoxetine, paroxetine) are predicted to decrease the efficacy of **tamoxifen**. Avoid. Severe Study

▸ Terbinafine is predicted to decrease the efficacy of **tamoxifen**. Avoid. Severe Study

Tamsulosin → see alpha blockers

Tapentadol → see opioids

Taxanes → see TABLE 15 p. 1432 (myelosuppression), TABLE 12 p. 1432 (peripheral neuropathy)

cabazitaxel · docetaxel · paclitaxel

▸ Anti-androgens (apalutamide, enzalutamide) are predicted to decrease the exposure to **docetaxel**. Severe Theoretical

▸ Anti-androgens (apalutamide, enzalutamide) are predicted to decrease the exposure to taxanes (**cabazitaxel, paclitaxel**). Avoid. Severe Study

▸ Antiarrhythmics (dronedarone) are predicted to increase the exposure to **cabazitaxel**. Moderate Theoretical

▸ Antiarrhythmics (dronedarone) are predicted to increase the exposure to **paclitaxel**. Severe Theoretical

Taxanes (continued)

▶ Antiepileptics (carbamazepine, fosphenytoin, phenobarbital, phenytoin, primidone) are predicted to decrease the exposure to docetaxel. Severe Theoretical → Also see TABLE 12 p. 1432

▶ Antiepileptics (carbamazepine, fosphenytoin, phenobarbital, phenytoin, primidone) are predicted to decrease the exposure to taxanes (cabazitaxel, paclitaxel). Avoid. Severe Study → Also see TABLE 12 p. 1432

▶ Antifungals, azoles (fluconazole, isavuconazole, posaconazole) are predicted to increase the exposure to cabazitaxel. Moderate Theoretical

▶ Antifungals, azoles (itraconazole, ketoconazole, voriconazole) are predicted to increase the exposure to cabazitaxel. Avoid. Severe Study

▶ Antifungals, azoles (itraconazole, ketoconazole, voriconazole) are predicted to moderately increase the exposure to docetaxel. Avoid or adjust dose. Severe Study

▶ Antifungals, azoles (itraconazole, ketoconazole, voriconazole) are predicted to increase the exposure to paclitaxel. Severe Theoretical

▶ Antifungals, azoles (miconazole) are predicted to increase the concentration of docetaxel. Use with caution and adjust dose. Moderate Theoretical

▶ Calcium channel blockers (diltiazem, verapamil) are predicted to increase the exposure to cabazitaxel. Moderate Theoretical

▶ Ceritinib is predicted to increase the exposure to paclitaxel. Moderate Theoretical → Also see TABLE 15 p. 1432

▶ Clopidogrel is predicted to increase the concentration of paclitaxel. Severe Anecdotal

▶ Cobicistat is predicted to increase the exposure to cabazitaxel. Avoid. Severe Study

▶ Cobicistat is predicted to moderately increase the exposure to docetaxel. Avoid or adjust dose. Severe Study

▶ Cobicistat is predicted to increase the exposure to paclitaxel. Severe Theoretical

▶ Crizotinib is predicted to increase the exposure to cabazitaxel. Moderate Theoretical

▶ Eliglustat is predicted to increase the exposure to paclitaxel. Adjust dose. Moderate Study

▶ Endothelin receptor antagonists (bosentan) are predicted to decrease the exposure to cabazitaxel. Avoid. Severe Study

▶ Fibrates (gemfibrozil) are predicted to increase the concentration of paclitaxel. Severe Anecdotal

▶ HIV-protease inhibitors are predicted to increase the exposure to cabazitaxel. Avoid. Severe Study

▶ HIV-protease inhibitors are predicted to moderately increase the exposure to docetaxel. Avoid or adjust dose. Severe Study

▶ HIV-protease inhibitors are predicted to increase the exposure to paclitaxel. Severe Theoretical

▶ Idelalisib is predicted to increase the exposure to cabazitaxel. Avoid. Severe Study

▶ Idelalisib is predicted to moderately increase the exposure to docetaxel. Avoid or adjust dose. Severe Study

▶ Idelalisib is predicted to increase the exposure to paclitaxel. Severe Theoretical

▶ Imatinib is predicted to increase the exposure to cabazitaxel. Moderate Theoretical → Also see TABLE 15 p. 1432

▶ Iron chelators (deferasirox) are predicted to increase the concentration of paclitaxel. Severe Anecdotal

▶ Lapatinib slightly increases the exposure to paclitaxel. Severe Study

▶ Leflunomide is predicted to increase the concentration of paclitaxel. Severe Anecdotal → Also see TABLE 15 p. 1432

▶ Letermovir is predicted to increase the exposure to cabazitaxel. Moderate Theoretical

▶ Live vaccines are predicted to increase the risk of generalised infection (possibly life-threatening) when given with taxanes (docetaxel, paclitaxel). Public Health England advises avoid (refer to Green Book). Severe Theoretical

▶ Macrolides (clarithromycin) are predicted to increase the exposure to cabazitaxel. Avoid. Severe Study

▶ Macrolides (clarithromycin) are predicted to moderately increase the exposure to docetaxel. Avoid or adjust dose. Severe Study

▶ Macrolides (clarithromycin) are predicted to increase the exposure to paclitaxel. Severe Theoretical

▶ Macrolides (erythromycin) are predicted to increase the exposure to cabazitaxel. Moderate Theoretical

▶ Mirabegron is predicted to increase the exposure to paclitaxel. Mild Theoretical

▶ Mitotane is predicted to decrease the exposure to docetaxel. Severe Theoretical → Also see TABLE 15 p. 1432

▶ Mitotane is predicted to decrease the exposure to taxanes (cabazitaxel, paclitaxel). Avoid. Severe Study → Also see TABLE 15 p. 1432

▶ Neurokinin-1 receptor antagonists (aprepitant, netupitant) are predicted to increase the exposure to cabazitaxel. Moderate Theoretical

▶ Neurokinin-1 receptor antagonists (netupitant) slightly increase the exposure to docetaxel. Moderate Study

▶ Neurokinin-1 receptor antagonists (netupitant) are predicted to increase the exposure to paclitaxel. Moderate Study

▶ Nilotinib is predicted to increase the exposure to cabazitaxel. Moderate Theoretical → Also see TABLE 15 p. 1432

▶ NNRTIs (efavirenz, nevirapine) are predicted to decrease the exposure to cabazitaxel. Severe Study

▶ Paritaprevir (with ritonavir and ombitasvir) is predicted to increase the exposure to cabazitaxel. Moderate Study

▶ Pibrentasvir (with glecaprevir) is predicted to increase the exposure to paclitaxel. Moderate Study

▶ Pitolisant is predicted to decrease the exposure to docetaxel. Avoid. Severe Theoretical

▶ Pitolisant is predicted to decrease the exposure to paclitaxel. Mild Theoretical

▶ Rifamycins (rifampicin) are predicted to decrease the exposure to docetaxel. Severe Theoretical

▶ Rifamycins (rifampicin) are predicted to decrease the exposure to taxanes (cabazitaxel, paclitaxel). Avoid. Severe Study

▶ St John's wort is predicted to decrease the exposure to cabazitaxel. Avoid. Severe Study

▶ Teriflunomide is predicted to increase the concentration of paclitaxel. Severe Anecdotal

▶ Velpatasvir is predicted to increase the exposure to paclitaxel. Severe Theoretical

▶ Vemurafenib is predicted to increase the exposure to paclitaxel. Use with caution and adjust dose. Severe Theoretical

Tazarotene → see retinoids

Tedizolid

▶ Tedizolid is predicted to increase the exposure to imatinib. Avoid. Moderate Theoretical

▶ Tedizolid is predicted to increase the exposure to lapatinib. Avoid. Moderate Theoretical

▶ Tedizolid is predicted to increase the exposure to methotrexate. Avoid. Moderate Theoretical

▶ Tedizolid is predicted to increase the exposure to statins (atorvastatin, fluvastatin, rosuvastatin). Avoid. Moderate Study

▶ Tedizolid is predicted to increase the exposure to sulfasalazine. Avoid. Moderate Study

▶ Tedizolid is predicted to increase the exposure to topotecan. Avoid. Moderate Study

Tegafur → see TABLE 15 p. 1432 (myelosuppression)

▶ Tegafur potentially increases the concentration of antiepileptics (fosphenytoin, phenytoin). Monitor concentration and adjust dose. Severe Study

▶ Tegafur increases the anticoagulant effect of coumarins. Moderate Theoretical

▶ Folates are predicted to increase the risk of toxicity when given with tegafur. Severe Theoretical

▶ H₂ receptor antagonists (cimetidine) are predicted to increase the risk of toxicity when given with tegafur. Severe Theoretical

▶ Live vaccines are predicted to increase the risk of generalised infection (possibly life-threatening) when given with tegafur. Public Health England advises avoid (refer to Green Book). Severe Theoretical

▶ Methotrexate is predicted to increase the risk of toxicity when given with tegafur. Severe Theoretical → Also see TABLE 15 p. 1432

Teicoplanin

GENERAL INFORMATION If other nephrotoxic or neurotoxic drugs are given, monitor renal and auditory function on prolonged administration.

Telavancin → see TABLE 2 p. 1429 (nephrotoxicity), TABLE 19 p. 1433 (ototoxicity), TABLE 9 p. 1431 (QT-interval prolongation)

Telmisartan → see angiotensin-II receptor antagonists

Telotristat ethyl

Telotristat ethyl decreases the exposure to benzodiazepines (midazolam). Moderate Study

Telotristat ethyl is predicted to decrease the exposure to NNRTIs (doravirine). Avoid or adjust doravirine p. 683 or lamivudine with tenofovir disoproxil and doravirine p. 692 dose.

Octreotide (short-acting) decreases the exposure to **telotristat ethyl**. Telotristat ethyl should be taken at least 30 minutes before octreotide. Moderate Study

Temazepam → see benzodiazepines

Temocillin → see penicillins

Temozolomide → see alkylating agents

Temsirolimus → see TABLE 15 p. 1432 (myelosuppression)

ACE inhibitors are predicted to increase the risk of angioedema when given with **temsirolimus**. Moderate Theoretical

Anti-androgens (apalutamide, enzalutamide) are predicted to decrease the concentration of **temsirolimus**. Avoid. Severe Study

Antiarrhythmics (dronedarone) are predicted to increase the concentration of **temsirolimus**. Use with caution or avoid. Moderate Theoretical

Antiepileptics (carbamazepine, fosphenytoin, phenobarbital, phenytoin, primidone) are predicted to decrease the concentration of **temsirolimus**. Avoid. Severe Study

Antifungals, azoles (fluconazole, isavuconazole, posaconazole) are predicted to increase the concentration of **temsirolimus**. Use with caution or avoid. Moderate Theoretical

Antifungals, azoles (itraconazole, ketoconazole, voriconazole) are predicted to increase the concentration of **temsirolimus**. Avoid. Severe Theoretical

Calcium channel blockers (diltiazem, verapamil) are predicted to increase the concentration of and the risk of angioedema when given with **temsirolimus**. Use with caution or avoid. Moderate Theoretical

Temsirolimus is predicted to increase the risk of angioedema when given with calcium channel blockers (amlodipine, felodipine, lacidipine, lercanidipine, nicardipine, nifedipine, nimodipine). Moderate Theoretical

Cobicistat is predicted to increase the concentration of **temsirolimus**. Avoid. Severe Theoretical

Crizotinib is predicted to increase the concentration of **temsirolimus**. Use with caution or avoid. Moderate Theoretical

Endothelin receptor antagonists (bosentan) are predicted to decrease the concentration of **temsirolimus**. Avoid. Severe Theoretical

Entrectinib is predicted to increase the exposure to **temsirolimus**. Mild Theoretical

Grapefruit juice is predicted to increase the concentration of **temsirolimus**. Use with caution or avoid. Moderate Theoretical

HIV-protease inhibitors are predicted to increase the concentration of **temsirolimus**. Avoid. Severe Theoretical

Idelalisib is predicted to increase the concentration of **temsirolimus**. Avoid. Severe Theoretical

Imatinib is predicted to increase the concentration of **temsirolimus**. Use with caution or avoid. Moderate Theoretical → Also see TABLE 15 p. 1432

Live vaccines are predicted to increase the risk of generalised infection (possibly life-threatening) when given with **temsirolimus**. Public Health England advises avoid (refer to Green Book). Severe Theoretical

Lumacaftor is predicted to decrease the exposure to **temsirolimus**. Avoid. Severe Theoretical

Macrolides (clarithromycin) are predicted to increase the concentration of **temsirolimus**. Avoid. Severe Theoretical

Macrolides (erythromycin) are predicted to increase the concentration of **temsirolimus**. Use with caution or avoid. Moderate Theoretical

Mitotane is predicted to decrease the concentration of **temsirolimus**. Avoid. Severe Study → Also see TABLE 15 p. 1432

Neurokinin-1 receptor antagonists (aprepitant, netupitant) are predicted to increase the concentration of **temsirolimus**. Use with caution or avoid. Moderate Theoretical

Nilotinib is predicted to increase the concentration of **temsirolimus**. Use with caution or avoid. Moderate Theoretical → Also see TABLE 15 p. 1432

NNRTIs (efavirenz, nevirapine) are predicted to decrease the concentration of **temsirolimus**. Avoid. Severe Theoretical

Pitolisant is predicted to decrease the exposure to **temsirolimus**. Avoid. Severe Theoretical

Rifamycins (rifampicin) are predicted to decrease the concentration of **temsirolimus**. Avoid. Severe Study

St John's wort is predicted to decrease the concentration of **temsirolimus**. Avoid. Severe Theoretical

Tenecteplase → see TABLE 3 p. 1429 (anticoagulant effects)

Tenofovir alafenamide

Antiepileptics (carbamazepine, fosphenytoin, oxcarbazepine, phenobarbital, phenytoin, primidone) are predicted to decrease the exposure to **tenofovir alafenamide**. Avoid. Moderate Theoretical

Ciclosporin is predicted to increase the exposure to **tenofovir alafenamide**. Moderate Theoretical

Eltrombopag is predicted to increase the exposure to **tenofovir alafenamide**. Moderate Theoretical

HIV-protease inhibitors (atazanavir, darunavir, lopinavir) increase the exposure to **tenofovir alafenamide**. Avoid or adjust dose. Moderate Study

HIV-protease inhibitors (tipranavir) are predicted to decrease the exposure to **tenofovir alafenamide**. Avoid. Moderate Theoretical

Leflunomide is predicted to increase the exposure to **tenofovir alafenamide**. Moderate Theoretical

Rifamycins are predicted to decrease the exposure to **tenofovir alafenamide**. Avoid. Moderate Theoretical

St John's wort is predicted to decrease the exposure to **tenofovir alafenamide**. Avoid. Moderate Theoretical

Teriflunomide is predicted to increase the exposure to **tenofovir alafenamide**. Moderate Theoretical

Tenofovir disoproxil → see TABLE 2 p. 1429 (nephrotoxicity)

Ciclosporin is predicted to increase the exposure to **tenofovir disoproxil**. Moderate Theoretical → Also see TABLE 2 p. 1429

Eltrombopag is predicted to increase the exposure to **tenofovir disoproxil**. Moderate Theoretical

HIV-protease inhibitors (atazanavir, darunavir, lopinavir) are predicted to increase the risk of renal impairment when given with **tenofovir disoproxil**. Severe Anecdotal

Ledipasvir (with sofosbuvir) slightly increases the exposure to **tenofovir disoproxil**. Moderate Study

Leflunomide is predicted to increase the exposure to **tenofovir disoproxil**. Moderate Theoretical

Teriflunomide is predicted to increase the exposure to **tenofovir disoproxil**. Moderate Theoretical

Velpatasvir is predicted to increase the exposure to **tenofovir disoproxil**. Severe Study

Voxilaprevir (with sofosbuvir and velpatasvir) potentially increases the concentration of **tenofovir disoproxil**. Severe Study

Tenoxicam → see NSAIDs

Terazosin → see alpha blockers

Terbinafine

ROUTE-SPECIFIC INFORMATION Since systemic absorption can follow topical application, the possibility of interactions should be borne in mind.

Terbinafine is predicted to increase the exposure to anticholinesterases, centrally acting (galantamine). Monitor and adjust dose. Moderate Study

Terbinafine is predicted to moderately increase the exposure to antipsychotics, second generation (aripiprazole). Adjust aripiprazole dose, p. 415. Moderate Study

Terbinafine is predicted to increase the exposure to antipsychotics, second generation (risperidone). Adjust dose. Moderate Study

Terbinafine is predicted to markedly increase the exposure to atomoxetine. Adjust dose. Severe Study

Terbinafine (continued)
▶ **Terbinafine** is predicted to increase the exposure to beta blockers, selective (metoprolol, nebivolol). Moderate Study
▶ **Terbinafine** is predicted to slightly increase the exposure to darifenacin. Mild Study
▶ **Terbinafine** is predicted to increase the exposure to eliglustat. Avoid or adjust dose—consult product literature. Severe Study
▶ **Terbinafine** is predicted to increase the exposure to mexiletine. Moderate Study
▶ **Terbinafine** is predicted to decrease the efficacy of opioids (codeine). Moderate Theoretical
▶ **Terbinafine** is predicted to decrease the efficacy of opioids (tramadol). Severe Study
▶ **Terbinafine** is predicted to moderately increase the exposure to pitolisant. Use with caution and adjust dose. Moderate Study
▶ Rifamycins (rifampicin) decrease the exposure to **terbinafine**. Adjust dose. Moderate Study
▶ **Terbinafine** is predicted to increase the exposure to SSRIs (citalopram, dapoxetine, escitalopram, fluvoxamine, sertraline). Moderate Theoretical
▶ **Terbinafine** is predicted to increase the exposure to SSRIs (fluoxetine). Adjust dose. Moderate Theoretical
▶ **Terbinafine** moderately increases the exposure to SSRIs (paroxetine). Moderate Study
▶ **Terbinafine** is predicted to decrease the efficacy of tamoxifen. Avoid. Severe Study
▶ **Terbinafine** is predicted to increase the exposure to the active metabolite of tetrabenazine. Moderate Study
▶ **Terbinafine** is predicted to increase the exposure to tricyclic antidepressants. Monitor for toxicity and adjust dose. Severe Study
▶ **Terbinafine** is predicted to increase the exposure to vortioxetine. Monitor and adjust dose. Moderate Study
Terbutaline → see beta₂ agonists
Teriflunomide → see TABLE 1 p. 1429 (hepatotoxicity)
▶ **Teriflunomide** is predicted to increase the exposure to adefovir. Moderate Study
▶ **Teriflunomide** is predicted to decrease the exposure to agomelatine. Moderate Theoretical
▶ **Teriflunomide** is predicted to increase the exposure to alpelisib. Moderate Theoretical
▶ **Teriflunomide** decreases the exposure to aminophylline. Adjust dose. Moderate Study
▶ **Teriflunomide** is predicted to decrease the exposure to anaesthetics, local (ropivacaine). Moderate Theoretical
▶ **Teriflunomide** is predicted to increase the exposure to anthracyclines (daunorubicin, doxorubicin, mitoxantrone). Moderate Theoretical
▶ **Teriflunomide** is predicted to increase the exposure to antihistamines, non-sedating (fexofenadine). Moderate Study
▶ **Teriflunomide** is predicted to decrease the exposure to antipsychotics, second generation (clozapine). Moderate Theoretical
▶ **Teriflunomide** is predicted to decrease the exposure to antipsychotics, second generation (olanzapine). Monitor and adjust dose. Moderate Study
▶ **Teriflunomide** potentially increases the exposure to baricitinib. Moderate Theoretical
▶ **Teriflunomide** is predicted to moderately increase the clearance of caffeine citrate. Monitor and adjust dose. Moderate Study
▶ **Teriflunomide** is predicted to increase the exposure to cephalosporins (cefaclor). Moderate Study
▶ **Teriflunomide** affects the anticoagulant effect of coumarins. Severe Study
▶ **Teriflunomide** is predicted to decrease the exposure to duloxetine. Moderate Theoretical
▶ **Teriflunomide** is predicted to increase the exposure to endothelin receptor antagonists (bosentan). Moderate Study
▶ Filgotinib is predicted to increase the risk of immunosuppression when given with **teriflunomide**. Avoid. Severe Theoretical
▶ **Teriflunomide** is predicted to increase the exposure to ganciclovir. Moderate Study
▶ **Teriflunomide** is predicted to increase the exposure to H₂ receptor antagonists (cimetidine, famotidine). Moderate Study

▶ **Teriflunomide** is predicted to increase the exposure to larotrectinib. Mild Study
▶ **Teriflunomide** is predicted to increase the concentration of letermovir. Moderate Study
▶ Live vaccines are predicted to increase the risk of generalised infection (possibly life-threatening) when given with **teriflunomide**. Public Health England advises avoid (refer to Green Book). Severe Theoretical
▶ **Teriflunomide** is predicted to increase the exposure to loop diuretics (furosemide). Moderate Study
▶ **Teriflunomide** is predicted to increase the exposure to meglitinides (nateglinide). Moderate Theoretical
▶ **Teriflunomide** is predicted to increase the exposure to meglitinides (repaglinide). Moderate Study
▶ **Teriflunomide** is predicted to decrease the exposure to melatonin. Moderate Theoretical
▶ **Teriflunomide** is predicted to increase the exposure to methotrexate. Moderate Study → Also see TABLE 1 p. 1429
▶ **Teriflunomide** is predicted to increase the clearance of mexiletine. Monitor and adjust dose. Moderate Study
▶ **Teriflunomide** is predicted to increase the exposure to montelukast. Moderate Theoretical
▶ **Teriflunomide** is predicted to increase the exposure to NRTIs (zidovudine). Moderate Theoretical
▶ **Teriflunomide** is predicted to increase the exposure to NSAIDs (indometacin, ketoprofen). Moderate Theoretical
▶ **Teriflunomide** is predicted to increase the exposure to oseltamivir. Moderate Study
▶ **Teriflunomide** is predicted to increase the exposure to the active metabolite of ozanimod. Avoid. Moderate Study
▶ **Teriflunomide** is predicted to increase the exposure to penicillins (benzylpenicillin). Moderate Study
▶ **Teriflunomide** is predicted to increase the exposure to pioglitazone. Moderate Study
▶ **Teriflunomide** is predicted to decrease the exposure to pirfenidone. Moderate Theoretical
▶ **Teriflunomide** is predicted to increase the exposure to quinolones (ciprofloxacin). Moderate Theoretical
▶ **Teriflunomide** is predicted to increase the exposure to rifamycins (rifampicin). Moderate Theoretical
▶ **Teriflunomide** is predicted to increase the exposure to selexipag. Adjust **selexipag** dose, p. 196. Moderate Study
▶ **Teriflunomide** is predicted to increase the exposure to statins (atorvastatin, fluvastatin, pravastatin, simvastatin). Moderate Study → Also see TABLE 1 p. 1429
▶ **Teriflunomide** moderately increases the exposure to statins (rosuvastatin). Adjust **rosuvastatin** dose, p. 218. Moderate Study → Also see TABLE 1 p. 1429
▶ **Teriflunomide** is predicted to increase the exposure to sulfasalazine. Moderate Study → Also see TABLE 1 p. 1429
▶ **Teriflunomide** is predicted to increase the exposure to sulfonylureas (glibenclamide). Moderate Study
▶ **Teriflunomide** potentially increases the exposure to talazoparib. Avoid or monitor. Moderate Theoretical
▶ **Teriflunomide** is predicted to increase the concentration of taxanes (paclitaxel). Severe Anecdotal
▶ **Teriflunomide** is predicted to increase the exposure to tenofovir alafenamide. Moderate Theoretical
▶ **Teriflunomide** is predicted to increase the exposure to tenofovir disoproxil. Moderate Theoretical
▶ **Teriflunomide** is predicted to decrease the exposure to theophylline. Adjust dose. Moderate Study
▶ **Teriflunomide** moderately decreases the exposure to tizanidine. Mild Study
▶ **Teriflunomide** is predicted to increase the exposure to topotecan. Moderate Study
Tetanus immunoglobulin → see immunoglobulins
Tetrabenazine → see TABLE 9 p. 1431 (QT-interval prolongation), TABLE 11 p. 1431 (CNS depressant effects)
▶ Bupropion is predicted to increase the exposure to the active metabolite of **tetrabenazine**. Moderate Study
▶ Cinacalcet is predicted to increase the exposure to the active metabolite of **tetrabenazine**. Moderate Study
▶ **Tetrabenazine** is predicted to decrease the effects of levodopa. Use with caution or avoid. Moderate Theoretical

Tetrabenazine potentially increases the risk of CNS excitation and hypertension when given with MAO-B inhibitors. [Severe] Theoretical

Tetrabenazine potentially increases the risk of CNS excitation and hypertension when given with MAOIs, irreversible. Avoid and for 14 days after stopping the MAOI. [Severe] Theoretical

Tetrabenazine potentially increases the risk of CNS excitation and hypertension when given with moclobemide. [Severe] Theoretical

SSRIs (fluoxetine, paroxetine) are predicted to increase the exposure to the active metabolite of **tetrabenazine**. [Moderate] Study

Terbinafine is predicted to increase the exposure to the active metabolite of **tetrabenazine**. [Moderate] Study

etracaine → see anaesthetics, local

etracycline → see tetracyclines

etracyclines → see TABLE 1 p. 1429 (hepatotoxicity)

demeclocycline · doxycycline · lymecycline · minocycline · oxytetracycline · tetracycline

▸ Dairy products decrease the absorption of **demeclocycline**.
▸ Dairy products decrease the exposure to **oxytetracycline**.
▸ Interactions do not generally apply to topical use of **oxytetracycline** unless specified.
▸ Dairy products decrease the exposure to **tetracycline**—manufacturer advises take 1 hour before or 2 hours after dairy products.

▸ ACE inhibitors (quinapril) (tablet) decrease the absorption of oral **tetracycline**. Avoid. [Moderate] Study
▸ Oral antacids decrease the absorption of oral **tetracyclines**. Separate administration by 2 to 3 hours. [Moderate] Study
▸ Anti-androgens (apalutamide, enzalutamide) decrease the exposure to **doxycycline**. Monitor and adjust dose. [Moderate] Study
▸ Antiepileptics (carbamazepine, fosphenytoin, phenobarbital, phenytoin, primidone) decrease the exposure to **doxycycline**. Monitor and adjust dose. [Moderate] Study → Also see TABLE 1 p. 1429
▸ **Tetracycline** decreases the concentration of antimalarials (atovaquone). [Moderate] Study
▸ Bismuth greatly decreases the efficacy of **tetracyclines**. Separate administration by 2 hours. [Moderate] Study
▸ Calcium salts (calcium carbonate) are predicted to decrease the absorption of **tetracyclines**. Separate administration by 2 to 3 hours. [Moderate] Theoretical
▸ **Tetracyclines** increase the risk of bleeding events when given with coumarins. [Moderate] Anecdotal
▸ Oral iron decreases the absorption of oral **tetracyclines**. **Tetracyclines** should be taken 2 to 3 hours after iron. [Moderate] Study
▸ Kaolin is predicted to decrease the absorption of **tetracyclines**. [Moderate] Theoretical
▸ Lanthanum is predicted to decrease the absorption of **tetracyclines**. Separate administration by 2 hours. [Moderate] Theoretical
▸ **Tetracyclines** are predicted to increase the risk of lithium toxicity when given with lithium. Avoid or adjust dose. [Severe] Anecdotal
▸ Mitotane decreases the exposure to **doxycycline**. Monitor and adjust dose. [Moderate] Study
▸ Retinoids (acitretin, alitretinoin, isotretinoin, tretinoin) increase the risk of benign intracranial hypertension when given with **tetracyclines**. Avoid. [Severe] Anecdotal
▸ Rifamycins (rifampicin) decrease the exposure to **doxycycline**. Monitor and adjust dose. [Moderate] Study
▸ Strontium is predicted to decrease the absorption of **tetracyclines**. Avoid. [Moderate] Theoretical
▸ Oral zinc is predicted to decrease the absorption of **tetracyclines**. Separate administration by 2 to 3 hours. [Moderate] Theoretical

Tezacaftor

FOOD AND LIFESTYLE Avoid bitter (Seville) oranges as they are predicted to increase the exposure to tezacaftor.

▸ Anti-androgens (apalutamide, enzalutamide) are predicted to decrease the exposure to **tezacaftor**. Avoid. [Severe] Theoretical
▸ Antiarrhythmics (dronedarone) are predicted to increase the exposure to **tezacaftor**. Adjust tezacaftor with ivacaftor p. 311 or tezacaftor with ivacaftor and elexacftor p. 311 dose with moderate CYP3A4 inhibitors. [Severe] Study
▸ Antiepileptics (carbamazepine, fosphenytoin, phenobarbital, phenytoin, primidone) are predicted to decrease the exposure to **tezacaftor**. Avoid. [Severe] Theoretical
▸ Antifungals, azoles (fluconazole, isavuconazole, posaconazole) are predicted to increase the exposure to **tezacaftor**. Adjust tezacaftor with ivacaftor p. 311 or tezacaftor with ivacaftor and elexacftor p. 311 dose with moderate CYP3A4 inhibitors. [Severe] Study
▸ Antifungals, azoles (itraconazole, ketoconazole, voriconazole) are predicted to increase the exposure to **tezacaftor**. Adjust tezacaftor with ivacaftor p. 311 or tezacaftor with ivacaftor and elexacftor p. 311 dose with potent CYP3A4 inhibitors. [Severe] Study
▸ Calcium channel blockers (diltiazem, verapamil) are predicted to increase the exposure to **tezacaftor**. Adjust tezacaftor with ivacaftor p. 311 or tezacaftor with ivacaftor and elexacftor p. 311 dose with moderate CYP3A4 inhibitors. [Severe] Study
▸ Cobicistat is predicted to increase the exposure to **tezacaftor**. Adjust tezacaftor with ivacaftor p. 311 or tezacaftor with ivacaftor and elexacftor p. 311 dose with potent CYP3A4 inhibitors. [Severe] Study
▸ Crizotinib is predicted to increase the exposure to **tezacaftor**. Adjust tezacaftor with ivacaftor p. 311 or tezacaftor with ivacaftor and elexacftor p. 311 dose with moderate CYP3A4 inhibitors. [Severe] Study
▸ Grapefruit juice is predicted to increase the exposure to **tezacaftor**. Avoid. [Severe] Study
▸ HIV-protease inhibitors are predicted to increase the exposure to **tezacaftor**. Adjust tezacaftor with ivacaftor p. 311 or tezacaftor with ivacaftor and elexacftor p. 311 dose with potent CYP3A4 inhibitors. [Severe] Study
▸ Idelalisib is predicted to increase the exposure to **tezacaftor**. Adjust tezacaftor with ivacaftor p. 311 or tezacaftor with ivacaftor and elexacftor p. 311 dose with potent CYP3A4 inhibitors. [Severe] Study
▸ Imatinib is predicted to increase the exposure to **tezacaftor**. Adjust tezacaftor with ivacaftor p. 311 or tezacaftor with ivacaftor and elexacftor p. 311 dose with moderate CYP3A4 inhibitors. [Severe] Study
▸ Letermovir is predicted to increase the exposure to **tezacaftor**. Adjust tezacaftor with ivacaftor p. 311 or tezacaftor with ivacaftor and elexacftor p. 311 dose with moderate CYP3A4 inhibitors. [Severe] Study
▸ Macrolides (clarithromycin) are predicted to increase the exposure to **tezacaftor**. Adjust tezacaftor with ivacaftor p. 311 or tezacaftor with ivacaftor and elexacftor p. 311 dose with potent CYP3A4 inhibitors. [Severe] Study
▸ Macrolides (erythromycin) are predicted to increase the exposure to **tezacaftor**. Adjust tezacaftor with ivacaftor p. 311 or tezacaftor with ivacaftor and elexacftor p. 311 dose with moderate CYP3A4 inhibitors. [Severe] Study
▸ Mitotane is predicted to decrease the exposure to **tezacaftor**. Avoid. [Severe] Theoretical
▸ Neurokinin-1 receptor antagonists (aprepitant, netupitant) are predicted to increase the exposure to **tezacaftor**. Adjust tezacaftor with ivacaftor p. 311 or tezacaftor with ivacaftor and elexacftor p. 311 dose with moderate CYP3A4 inhibitors. [Severe] Study
▸ Nilotinib is predicted to increase the exposure to **tezacaftor**. Adjust tezacaftor with ivacaftor p. 311 or tezacaftor with ivacaftor and elexacftor p. 311 dose with moderate CYP3A4 inhibitors. [Severe] Study
▸ Rifamycins are predicted to decrease the exposure to **tezacaftor**. Avoid. [Severe] Theoretical
▸ St John's wort is predicted to decrease the exposure to **tezacaftor**. Avoid. [Severe] Theoretical

Thalidomide → see TABLE 6 p. 1430 (bradycardia), TABLE 15 p. 1432 (myelosuppression), TABLE 12 p. 1432 (peripheral neuropathy), TABLE 5 p. 1430 (thromboembolism), TABLE 11 p. 1431 (CNS depressant effects)

A1

Interactions | Appendix 1

Thalidomide (continued)

▶ Combined hormonal contraceptives are predicted to increase the risk of venous thromboembolism when given with **thalidomide**. Avoid. [Severe] Study
▶ Hormone replacement therapy is predicted to increase the risk of venous thromboembolism when given with **thalidomide**. [Severe] Theoretical

Theophylline → see TABLE 17 p. 1433 (reduced serum potassium)

FOOD AND LIFESTYLE Smoking can increase theophylline clearance and increased doses of theophylline are therefore required; dose adjustments are likely to be necessary if smoking started or stopped during treatment.

▶ Aciclovir is predicted to increase the exposure to **theophylline**. Monitor and adjust dose. [Severe] Theoretical
▶ **Theophylline** decreases the efficacy of antiarrhythmics (adenosine). Separate administration by 24 hours. [Mild] Study
▶ Antiepileptics (carbamazepine) potentially increase the clearance of **theophylline** and **theophylline** decreases the exposure to antiepileptics (carbamazepine). Adjust dose. [Moderate] Anecdotal
▶ Antiepileptics (fosphenytoin, phenytoin) are predicted to decrease the exposure to **theophylline**. Adjust dose. [Moderate] Study
▶ Antiepileptics (phenobarbital, primidone) are predicted to increase the clearance of **theophylline**. Adjust dose. [Moderate] Theoretical
▶ Antiepileptics (stiripentol) are predicted to increase the exposure to **theophylline**. Avoid. [Moderate] Theoretical
▶ Beta blockers, non-selective are predicted to increase the risk of bronchospasm when given with **theophylline**. Avoid. [Severe] Theoretical
▶ Beta blockers, selective are predicted to increase the risk of bronchospasm when given with **theophylline**. Avoid. [Severe] Theoretical
▶ Caffeine citrate decreases the clearance of **theophylline**. [Moderate] Study
▶ Combined hormonal contraceptives are predicted to increase the exposure to **theophylline**. Monitor and adjust dose. [Moderate] Theoretical
▶ **Theophylline** increases the risk of agitation when given with doxapram. [Moderate] Study
▶ Enteral feeds decrease the exposure to **theophylline**. [Moderate] Study
▶ Esketamine is predicted to increase the risk of seizures when given with **theophylline**. Avoid. [Severe] Theoretical
▶ H_2 receptor antagonists (cimetidine) increase the concentration of **theophylline**. Adjust dose. [Severe] Study
▶ HIV-protease inhibitors (ritonavir) are predicted to decrease the exposure to **theophylline**. Adjust dose. [Moderate] Study
▶ Interferons slightly increase the exposure to **theophylline**. Adjust dose. [Moderate] Study
▶ Iron chelators (deferasirox) increase the exposure to **theophylline**. Avoid. [Moderate] Study
▶ Isoniazid is predicted to affect the clearance of **theophylline**. [Severe] Anecdotal
▶ Leflunomide is predicted to decrease the exposure to **theophylline**. Adjust dose. [Moderate] Study
▶ **Theophylline** is predicted to decrease the concentration of lithium. Monitor concentration and adjust dose. [Moderate] Anecdotal
▶ Macrolides (azithromycin, clarithromycin) are predicted to increase the exposure to **theophylline**. Adjust dose. [Moderate] Anecdotal
▶ Macrolides (erythromycin) decrease the clearance of **theophylline** and **theophylline** potentially decreases the clearance of macrolides (erythromycin). Adjust dose. [Severe] Study
▶ Methotrexate decreases the clearance of **theophylline**. [Moderate] Study
▶ Mexiletine is predicted to increase the exposure to **theophylline**. Monitor and adjust dose. [Moderate] Theoretical
▶ Monoclonal antibodies (blinatumomab) are predicted to transiently increase the exposure to **theophylline**. Monitor and adjust dose. [Moderate] Theoretical

▶ Monoclonal antibodies (sarilumab) potentially affect the exposure to **theophylline**. Monitor and adjust dose. [Moderate] Theoretical
▶ Monoclonal antibodies (tocilizumab) are predicted to decrease the exposure to **theophylline**. Monitor and adjust dose. [Moderate] Theoretical
▶ Obeticholic acid is predicted to increase the exposure to **theophylline**. [Severe] Theoretical
▶ Pentoxifylline increases the concentration of **theophylline**. Monitor and adjust dose. [Severe] Study
▶ **Theophylline** is predicted to slightly increase the exposure to phosphodiesterase type-4 inhibitors (roflumilast). Avoid. [Moderate] Theoretical
▶ Quinolones (ciprofloxacin) are predicted to increase the exposure to **theophylline**. Monitor and adjust dose. [Moderate] Theoretical
▶ Rifamycins (rifampicin) are predicted to decrease the exposure to **theophylline**. Adjust dose. [Moderate] Study
▶ Rucaparib is predicted to increase the exposure to **theophylline**. Monitor and adjust dose. [Moderate] Study
▶ SSRIs (fluvoxamine) moderately to markedly increase the exposure to **theophylline**. Avoid. [Severe] Study
▶ St John's wort potentially decreases the exposure to **theophylline**. [Severe] Anecdotal
▶ Sucralfate potentially decreases the absorption of **theophylline**. Separate administration by at least 2 hours. [Moderate] Study
▶ Sympathomimetics, vasoconstrictor (ephedrine) increase the risk of adverse effects when given with **theophylline**. Avoid in children. [Moderate] Study
▶ Teriflunomide is predicted to decrease the exposure to **theophylline**. Adjust dose. [Moderate] Study
▶ Valaciclovir is predicted to increase the exposure to **theophylline**. [Severe] Theoretical
▶ Vemurafenib is predicted to increase the exposure to **theophylline**. Use with caution or avoid. [Moderate] Theoretical

Thiazide diuretics → see TABLE 18 p. 1433 (hyponatraemia), TABLE 8 p. 1430 (hypotension), TABLE 17 p. 1433 (reduced serum potassium)

bendroflumethiazide · chlorothiazide · chlortalidone · hydroflumethiazide · hydrochlorothiazide · indapamide · metolazone · xipamide

▶ **Thiazide diuretics** are predicted to increase the risk of hypersensitivity reactions when given with allopurinol. [Severe] Theoretical
▶ Aspirin (high-dose) increases the risk of acute renal failure when given with **thiazide diuretics**. [Severe] Theoretical
▶ **Thiazide diuretics** increase the risk of hypercalcaemia when given with calcium salts. [Severe] Anecdotal
▶ **Thiazide diuretics** increase the concentration of lithium. Avoid or adjust dose and monitor concentration. [Severe] Study
▶ NSAIDs increase the risk of acute renal failure when given with **thiazide diuretics**. [Severe] Theoretical → Also see TABLE 18 p. 1433
▶ Reboxetine is predicted to increase the risk of hypokalaemia when given with **thiazide diuretics**. [Moderate] Anecdotal
▶ **Thiazide diuretics** are predicted to increase the risk of hypercalcaemia when given with toremifene. [Severe] Theoretical
▶ **Thiazide diuretics** increase the risk of hypercalcaemia when given with vitamin D substances. [Moderate] Theoretical

Thiopental → see TABLE 8 p. 1430 (hypotension), TABLE 11 p. 1431 (CNS depressant effects)

▶ Sulfonamides are predicted to increase the effects of **thiopental**. [Moderate] Theoretical
▶ Tricyclic antidepressants increase the risk of cardiac arrhythmias and hypotension when given with **thiopental**. [Moderate] Study → Also see TABLE 8 p. 1430 → Also see TABLE 11 p. 1431

Thiotepa → see alkylating agents

Thrombin inhibitors → see TABLE 3 p. 1429 (anticoagulant effects)

argatroban · bivalirudin · dabigatran

▶ Anti-androgens (apalutamide) are predicted to decrease the exposure to **dabigatran**. [Mild] Study
▶ Antiarrhythmics (amiodarone) increase the exposure to **dabigatran**. Adjust **dabigatran** dose, p. 148. [Moderate] Study

Antiarrhythmics (dronedarone) slightly increase the exposure to **dabigatran**. Avoid. Severe Study

Antiepileptics (carbamazepine) are predicted to decrease the exposure to **dabigatran**. Avoid. Severe Study

Antiepileptics (phenytoin) are predicted to decrease the exposure to **dabigatran**. Avoid. Severe Theoretical

Antifungals, azoles (isavuconazole) are predicted to increase the exposure to **dabigatran**. Monitor and adjust dose. Moderate Study

Antifungals, azoles (itraconazole, ketoconazole) are predicted to increase the exposure to **dabigatran**. Avoid. Severe Study

Brigatinib potentially increases the concentration of **dabigatran**. Moderate Theoretical

Calcium channel blockers (verapamil) increase the exposure to **dabigatran**. Adjust **dabigatran** dose, p. 148. Severe Study

Ceritinib is predicted to increase the exposure to **dabigatran**. Moderate Theoretical

Ciclosporin is predicted to increase the exposure to **dabigatran**. Avoid. Severe Theoretical

Cobicistat is predicted to increase the exposure to **dabigatran**. Avoid. Severe Theoretical

Elbasvir is predicted to increase the concentration of **dabigatran**. Moderate Theoretical

Eliglustat is predicted to increase the exposure to **dabigatran**. Adjust dose. Moderate Study

Glecaprevir (with pibrentasvir) increases the exposure to **dabigatran**. Avoid. Moderate Study

HIV-protease inhibitors (lopinavir, ritonavir, saquinavir) are predicted to increase the exposure to **dabigatran**. Avoid. Severe Theoretical

Lapatinib is predicted to increase the exposure to **dabigatran**. Moderate Theoretical

Ledipasvir is predicted to increase the exposure to **dabigatran**. Moderate Theoretical

Letermovir is predicted to decrease the concentration of **dabigatran**. Avoid. Severe Theoretical

Macrolides are predicted to increase the exposure to **dabigatran**. Moderate Theoretical

Mirabegron is predicted to increase the exposure to **dabigatran**. Severe Theoretical

Neratinib is predicted to increase the exposure to **dabigatran**. Moderate Study

Paritaprevir (with ritonavir and ombitasvir) is predicted to increase the exposure to **dabigatran**. Severe Study

Pibrentasvir (with glecaprevir) increases the exposure to **dabigatran**. Avoid. Moderate Study

Pitolisant is predicted to decrease the exposure to **dabigatran**. Mild Theoretical

Ranibizumab is predicted to increase the risk of bleeding events when given with **argatroban**. Severe Theoretical

Ranibizumab is predicted to increase the risk of bleeding events when given with **bivalirudin**. Moderate Theoretical

Ranolazine is predicted to increase the exposure to **dabigatran**. Severe Study

Rifamycins (rifampicin) are predicted to decrease the exposure to **dabigatran**. Avoid. Severe Study

St John's wort is predicted to decrease the exposure to **dabigatran**. Avoid. Severe Study

Tacrolimus is predicted to increase the exposure to **dabigatran**. Avoid. Severe Theoretical

Velpatasvir increases the exposure to **dabigatran**. Avoid. Severe Study

Vemurafenib increases the exposure to **dabigatran**. Use with caution and adjust dose. Severe Theoretical

Venetoclax is predicted to increase the exposure to **dabigatran**. Avoid or adjust dose. Severe Study

Voxilaprevir (with sofosbuvir and velpatasvir) increases the concentration of **dabigatran**. Avoid. Severe Study

Thyroid hormones

levothyroxine · liothyronine

Oral antacids are predicted to decrease the absorption of oral **levothyroxine**. Separate administration by at least 4 hours. Moderate Anecdotal

Anti-androgens (apalutamide) potentially decrease the exposure to **levothyroxine**. Mild Theoretical

Antiarrhythmics (amiodarone) are predicted to increase the risk of thyroid dysfunction when given with **thyroid hormones**. Avoid. Moderate Study

Antiepileptics (carbamazepine) are predicted to increase the risk of hypothyroidism when given with **thyroid hormones**. Monitor and adjust dose. Moderate Study

Antiepileptics (fosphenytoin, phenytoin) are predicted to increase the risk of hypothyroidism when given with **thyroid hormones**. Moderate Study

Antiepileptics (phenobarbital, primidone) are predicted to decrease the effects of **thyroid hormones**. Moderate Theoretical

Oral calcium salts are predicted to decrease the absorption of **levothyroxine**. Separate administration by at least 4 hours. Moderate Anecdotal

Thyroid hormones are predicted to affect the concentration of digoxin. Monitor and adjust dose. Moderate Theoretical

HIV-protease inhibitors (ritonavir) decrease the concentration of **levothyroxine**. MHRA advises monitor TSH for at least one month after starting or stopping ritonavir. Moderate Anecdotal

Oral hormone replacement therapy is predicted to decrease the effects of **thyroid hormones**. Moderate Theoretical

Oral iron decreases the absorption of oral **levothyroxine**. Separate administration by at least 4 hours. Moderate Study

Lanthanum decreases the absorption of **thyroid hormones**. Separate administration by 2 hours. Moderate Study

Paritaprevir (with ritonavir and ombitasvir) is predicted to increase the exposure to **levothyroxine**. Monitor and adjust dose. Moderate Theoretical

Sucralfate decreases the absorption of **levothyroxine**. Separate administration by at least 4 hours. Moderate Study

Tiagabine → see antiepileptics

Tiaprofenic acid → see NSAIDs

Tibolone → see TABLE 5 p. 1430 (thromboembolism)

Ticagrelor → see TABLE 4 p. 1429 (antiplatelet effects)

Anti-androgens (apalutamide, enzalutamide) are predicted to markedly decrease the exposure to **ticagrelor**. Avoid. Severe Study

Antiarrhythmics (amiodarone) are predicted to increase the exposure to **ticagrelor**. Use with caution or avoid. Severe Study

Antiepileptics (carbamazepine, fosphenytoin, phenobarbital, phenytoin, primidone) are predicted to markedly decrease the exposure to **ticagrelor**. Avoid. Severe Study

Antifungals, azoles (itraconazole, ketoconazole, voriconazole) are predicted to markedly increase the exposure to **ticagrelor**. Avoid. Severe Study

Ciclosporin is predicted to increase the exposure to **ticagrelor**. Use with caution or avoid. Severe Study

Cobicistat is predicted to markedly increase the exposure to **ticagrelor**. Avoid. Severe Study

Ticagrelor increases the concentration of digoxin. Moderate Study

Endothelin receptor antagonists (bosentan) are predicted to decrease the exposure to **ticagrelor**. Moderate Theoretical

Ticagrelor is predicted to increase the exposure to ergotamine. Avoid. Severe Theoretical

Grapefruit juice moderately increases the exposure to **ticagrelor**. Moderate Study

HIV-protease inhibitors are predicted to markedly increase the exposure to **ticagrelor**. Avoid. Severe Study

Idelalisib is predicted to markedly increase the exposure to **ticagrelor**. Avoid. Severe Study

Ticagrelor is predicted to increase the exposure to lomitapide. Separate administration by 12 hours. Moderate Theoretical

Macrolides (azithromycin) are predicted to increase the exposure to **ticagrelor**. Use with caution or avoid. Severe Study

Macrolides (clarithromycin) are predicted to markedly increase the exposure to **ticagrelor**. Avoid. Severe Study

Mitotane is predicted to markedly decrease the exposure to **ticagrelor**. Avoid. Severe Study

NNRTIs (efavirenz, nevirapine) are predicted to decrease the exposure to **ticagrelor**. Moderate Theoretical

Ranolazine is predicted to increase the exposure to **ticagrelor**. Use with caution or avoid. Severe Study

Rifamycins (rifampicin) are predicted to markedly decrease the exposure to **ticagrelor**. Avoid. Severe Study

Ticagrelor (continued)
▸ St John's wort is predicted to decrease the exposure to ticagrelor. [Moderate] Theoretical
▸ Ticagrelor slightly increases the exposure to statins (simvastatin). Adjust **simvastatin** dose, p. 219. [Moderate] Study
▸ Vemurafenib is predicted to increase the exposure to ticagrelor. Use with caution or avoid. [Severe] Study

Tigecycline → see TABLE 1 p. 1429 (hepatotoxicity)
▸ **Tigecycline** increases the risk of bleeding events when given with coumarins. [Moderate] Anecdotal
▸ Retinoids (acitretin, alitretinoin, isotretinoin, tretinoin) increase the risk of benign intracranial hypertension when given with tigecycline. Avoid. [Severe] Anecdotal

Tildrakizumab → see monoclonal antibodies
Timolol → see beta blockers, non-selective
Tinidazole
▸ Alcohol potentially causes a disulfiram-like reaction when given with **tinidazole**. Avoid for 72 hours stopping treatment. [Moderate] Theoretical
▸ **Tinidazole** is predicted to increase the anticoagulant effect of coumarins. Monitor INR and adjust dose. [Severe] Theoretical

Tinzaparin → see low molecular-weight heparins
Tioguanine → see TABLE 15 p. 1432 (myelosuppression)
▸ Live vaccines are predicted to increase the risk of generalised infection (possibly life-threatening) when given with **tioguanine**. Public Health England advises avoid (refer to Green Book). [Severe] Theoretical

Tiotropium → see TABLE 10 p. 1431 (antimuscarinics)
Tipranavir → see HIV-protease inhibitors
Tirofiban → see TABLE 3 p. 1429 (anticoagulant effects)
Tivozanib
▸ Anti-androgens (apalutamide, enzalutamide) are predicted to decrease the exposure to **tivozanib**. [Severe] Study
▸ Antiepileptics (carbamazepine, fosphenytoin, phenobarbital, phenytoin, primidone) are predicted to decrease the exposure to **tivozanib**. [Severe] Study
▸ Mitotane is predicted to decrease the exposure to **tivozanib**. [Severe] Study
▸ Rifamycins (rifampicin) are predicted to decrease the exposure to **tivozanib**. [Severe] Study
▸ St John's wort is predicted to decrease the exposure to **tivozanib**. Avoid. [Severe] Study
▸ **Tivozanib** is predicted to decrease the exposure to statins (rosuvastatin). [Moderate] Theoretical

Tizanidine → see TABLE 6 p. 1430 (bradycardia), TABLE 8 p. 1430 (hypotension), TABLE 9 p. 1431 (QT-interval prolongation), TABLE 11 p. 1431 (CNS depressant effects)
▸ Antiepileptics (fosphenytoin, phenytoin) moderately decrease the exposure to **tizanidine**. [Mild] Study
▸ Combined hormonal contraceptives increase the exposure to **tizanidine**. Avoid. [Moderate] Study
▸ HIV-protease inhibitors (ritonavir) moderately decrease the exposure to **tizanidine**. [Mild] Study
▸ Iron chelators (deferasirox) are predicted to increase the exposure to **tizanidine**. Avoid. [Moderate] Theoretical
▸ Leflunomide moderately decreases the exposure to **tizanidine**. [Mild] Study
▸ Mexiletine increases the exposure to **tizanidine**. Avoid. [Moderate] Study
▸ Obeticholic acid is predicted to increase the exposure to **tizanidine**. [Severe] Theoretical
▸ Quinolones (ciprofloxacin) increase the exposure to **tizanidine**. Avoid. [Moderate] Study
▸ Rifamycins (rifampicin) moderately decrease the exposure to **tizanidine**. [Mild] Study
▸ Rucaparib is predicted to increase the exposure to **tizanidine**. Monitor and adjust dose. [Moderate] Study
▸ SSRIs (fluvoxamine) very markedly increase the exposure to **tizanidine**. Avoid. [Severe] Study
▸ Teriflunomide moderately decreases the exposure to **tizanidine**. [Mild] Study
▸ Vemurafenib moderately increases the exposure to **tizanidine**. Use with caution or avoid. [Moderate] Theoretical → Also see TABLE 9 p. 1431

Tobramycin → see aminoglycosides

Tocilizumab → see monoclonal antibodies
Tofacitinib
▸ Anti-androgens (apalutamide, enzalutamide) are predicted to decrease the exposure to **tofacitinib**. Avoid. [Severe] Study
▸ Antiarrhythmics (dronedarone) given with a potent CYP2C19 inhibitor are predicted to increase the exposure to **tofacitinib**. Adjust **tofacitinib** dose, p. 1154. [Moderate] Study
▸ Antiepileptics (carbamazepine, fosphenytoin, phenobarbital, phenytoin, primidone) are predicted to decrease the exposure to **tofacitinib**. Avoid. [Severe] Study
▸ Antifungals, azoles (fluconazole) increase the exposure to **tofacitinib**. Adjust **tofacitinib** dose, p. 1154. [Moderate] Study
▸ Antifungals, azoles (isavuconazole) given with a potent CYP2C19 inhibitor are predicted to increase the exposure to **tofacitinib**. Adjust **tofacitinib** dose, p. 1154. [Moderate] Study
▸ Antifungals, azoles (itraconazole, ketoconazole, voriconazole) are predicted to increase the exposure to **tofacitinib**. Adjust **tofacitinib** dose, p. 1154. [Moderate] Study
▸ Antifungals, azoles (posaconazole) given with a potent CYP2C19 inhibitor are predicted to increase the exposure to **tofacitinib**. Adjust **tofacitinib** dose, p. 1154. [Moderate] Theoretical
▸ Calcium channel blockers (diltiazem, verapamil) given with a potent CYP2C19 inhibitor are predicted to increase the exposure to **tofacitinib**. Adjust **tofacitinib** dose, p. 1154. [Moderate] Study
▸ Ciclosporin increases the exposure to **tofacitinib**. Avoid. [Severe] Study
▸ Cobicistat is predicted to increase the exposure to **tofacitinib**. Adjust **tofacitinib** dose, p. 1154. [Moderate] Study
▸ Crizotinib given with a potent CYP2C19 inhibitor is predicted to increase the exposure to **tofacitinib**. Adjust **tofacitinib** dose, p. 1154. [Moderate] Study
▸ Endothelin receptor antagonists (bosentan) are predicted to decrease the exposure to **tofacitinib**. [Moderate] Study
▸ Filgotinib is predicted to increase the risk of immunosuppression when given with **tofacitinib**. Avoid. [Severe] Theoretical
▸ HIV-protease inhibitors are predicted to increase the exposure to **tofacitinib**. Adjust **tofacitinib** dose, p. 1154. [Moderate] Study
▸ Idelalisib is predicted to increase the exposure to **tofacitinib**. Adjust **tofacitinib** dose, p. 1154. [Moderate] Study
▸ Imatinib given with a potent CYP2C19 inhibitor is predicted to increase the exposure to **tofacitinib**. Adjust **tofacitinib** dose, p. 1154. [Moderate] Study
▸ Live vaccines potentially increase the risk of generalised infection (possibly life-threatening) when given with **tofacitinib**. Avoid. [Severe] Theoretical
▸ Macrolides (clarithromycin) are predicted to increase the exposure to **tofacitinib**. Adjust **tofacitinib** dose, p. 1154. [Moderate] Study
▸ Macrolides (erythromycin) given with a potent CYP2C19 inhibitor are predicted to increase the exposure to **tofacitinib**. Adjust **tofacitinib** dose, p. 1154. [Moderate] Study
▸ Mitotane is predicted to decrease the exposure to **tofacitinib**. Avoid. [Severe] Study
▸ Neurokinin-1 receptor antagonists (aprepitant, netupitant) given with a potent CYP2C19 inhibitor are predicted to increase the exposure to **tofacitinib**. Adjust **tofacitinib** dose, p. 1154. [Moderate] Study
▸ Nilotinib given with a potent CYP2C19 inhibitor is predicted to increase the exposure to **tofacitinib**. Adjust **tofacitinib** dose, p. 1154. [Moderate] Study
▸ NNRTIs (efavirenz, nevirapine) are predicted to decrease the exposure to **tofacitinib**. [Moderate] Study
▸ Rifamycins (rifampicin) are predicted to decrease the exposure to **tofacitinib**. Avoid. [Severe] Study
▸ SSRIs (fluoxetine, fluvoxamine) given with a moderate CYP3A4 inhibitor are predicted to increase the exposure to **tofacitinib**. Adjust **tofacitinib** dose, p. 1154. [Moderate] Study
▸ St John's wort is predicted to decrease the exposure to **tofacitinib**. [Moderate] Study
▸ Tacrolimus increases the exposure to **tofacitinib**. Avoid. [Severe] Study

Tolbutamide → see sulfonylureas

Tolcapone

Tolcapone increases the exposure to levodopa. Monitor and adjust dose. [Moderate] Study

Tolcapone is predicted to increase the effects of MAOIs, irreversible. Avoid. [Severe] Theoretical

Tolcapone is predicted to increase the risk of cardiovascular adverse effects when given with sympathomimetics, inotropic. [Moderate] Theoretical

Tolcapone is predicted to increase the effects of sympathomimetics, vasoconstrictor (adrenaline/epinephrine, noradrenaline/norepinephrine). [Moderate] Theoretical

Tolfenamic acid → see NSAIDs

Tolterodine → see TABLE 9 p. 1431 (QT-interval prolongation), TABLE 10 p. 1431 (antimuscarinics)

Antiarrhythmics (dronedarone) are predicted to increase the exposure to **tolterodine**. [Mild] Theoretical → Also see TABLE 9 p. 1431

▸ Antifungals, azoles (fluconazole, isavuconazole, posaconazole) are predicted to increase the exposure to **tolterodine**. [Mild] Theoretical → Also see TABLE 9 p. 1431

▸ Antifungals, azoles (itraconazole, ketoconazole, voriconazole) are predicted to increase the exposure to **tolterodine**. Avoid. [Severe] Study → Also see TABLE 9 p. 1431

▸ Calcium channel blockers (diltiazem, verapamil) are predicted to increase the exposure to **tolterodine**. [Mild] Theoretical

▸ Cobicistat is predicted to increase the exposure to **tolterodine**. Avoid. [Severe] Study

▸ Crizotinib is predicted to increase the exposure to **tolterodine**. [Mild] Theoretical → Also see TABLE 9 p. 1431

▸ Dacomitinib is predicted to markedly increase the exposure to **tolterodine**. Avoid. [Severe] Study

▸ Eliglustat is predicted to increase the exposure to **tolterodine**. Adjust dose. [Moderate] Study

▸ HIV-protease inhibitors are predicted to increase the exposure to **tolterodine**. Avoid. [Severe] Study → Also see TABLE 9 p. 1431

▸ Idelalisib is predicted to increase the exposure to **tolterodine**. Avoid. [Severe] Study

▸ Imatinib is predicted to increase the exposure to **tolterodine**. [Mild] Theoretical

▸ Letermovir is predicted to increase the exposure to **tolterodine**. [Mild] Theoretical

▸ Macrolides (clarithromycin) are predicted to increase the exposure to **tolterodine**. Avoid. [Severe] Study → Also see TABLE 9 p. 1431

▸ Macrolides (erythromycin) are predicted to increase the exposure to **tolterodine**. [Mild] Theoretical → Also see TABLE 9 p. 1431

▸ Neurokinin-1 receptor antagonists (aprepitant, netupitant) are predicted to increase the exposure to **tolterodine**. [Mild] Theoretical

▸ Nilotinib is predicted to increase the exposure to **tolterodine**. [Mild] Theoretical → Also see TABLE 9 p. 1431

Tolvaptan → see TABLE 16 p. 1433 (increased serum potassium)

GENERAL INFORMATION Avoid concurrent use of drugs that increase serum-sodium concentrations.

▸ Anti-androgens (apalutamide, enzalutamide) are predicted to decrease the exposure to **tolvaptan**. Use with caution or avoid depending on indication. [Severe] Study

▸ Antiarrhythmics (dronedarone) are predicted to increase the exposure to **tolvaptan**. Manufacturer advises caution or adjust **tolvaptan** dose with moderate CYP3A4 inhibitors, p. 708. [Moderate] Study

▸ Antiepileptics (carbamazepine, fosphenytoin, phenobarbital, phenytoin, primidone) are predicted to decrease the exposure to **tolvaptan**. Use with caution or avoid depending on indication. [Severe] Study

▸ Antifungals, azoles (fluconazole, isavuconazole, posaconazole) are predicted to increase the exposure to **tolvaptan**. Manufacturer advises caution or adjust **tolvaptan** dose with moderate CYP3A4 inhibitors, p. 708. [Moderate] Study

▸ Antifungals, azoles (itraconazole, ketoconazole, voriconazole) are predicted to increase the exposure to **tolvaptan**. Manufacturer advises caution or adjust **tolvaptan** dose with potent CYP3A4 inhibitors, p. 708. [Severe] Study

▸ Calcium channel blockers (diltiazem, verapamil) are predicted to increase the exposure to **tolvaptan**. Manufacturer advises caution or adjust **tolvaptan** dose with moderate CYP3A4 inhibitors, p. 708. [Moderate] Study

▸ Cobicistat is predicted to increase the exposure to **tolvaptan**. Manufacturer advises caution or adjust **tolvaptan** dose with potent CYP3A4 inhibitors, p. 708. [Severe] Study

▸ Crizotinib is predicted to increase the exposure to **tolvaptan**. Manufacturer advises caution or adjust **tolvaptan** dose with moderate CYP3A4 inhibitors, p. 708. [Moderate] Study

▸ **Tolvaptan** increases the concentration of digoxin. [Mild] Study

▸ Grapefruit juice increases the exposure to **tolvaptan**. Avoid. [Moderate] Study

▸ HIV-protease inhibitors are predicted to increase the exposure to **tolvaptan**. Manufacturer advises caution or adjust **tolvaptan** dose with potent CYP3A4 inhibitors, p. 708. [Severe] Study

▸ Idelalisib is predicted to increase the exposure to **tolvaptan**. Manufacturer advises caution or adjust **tolvaptan** dose with potent CYP3A4 inhibitors, p. 708. [Severe] Study

▸ Imatinib is predicted to increase the exposure to **tolvaptan**. Manufacturer advises caution or adjust **tolvaptan** dose with moderate CYP3A4 inhibitors, p. 708. [Moderate] Study

▸ Letermovir is predicted to increase the exposure to **tolvaptan**. Manufacturer advises caution or adjust **tolvaptan** dose with moderate CYP3A4 inhibitors, p. 708. [Moderate] Study

▸ **Tolvaptan** is predicted to increase the exposure to lomitapide. Separate administration by 12 hours. [Moderate] Theoretical

▸ Macrolides (clarithromycin) are predicted to increase the exposure to **tolvaptan**. Manufacturer advises caution or adjust **tolvaptan** dose with potent CYP3A4 inhibitors, p. 708. [Severe] Study

▸ Macrolides (erythromycin) are predicted to increase the exposure to **tolvaptan**. Manufacturer advises caution or adjust **tolvaptan** dose with moderate CYP3A4 inhibitors, p. 708. [Moderate] Study

▸ Mitotane is predicted to decrease the exposure to **tolvaptan**. Use with caution or avoid depending on indication. [Severe] Study

▸ Neurokinin-1 receptor antagonists (aprepitant, netupitant) are predicted to increase the exposure to **tolvaptan**. Manufacturer advises caution or adjust **tolvaptan** dose with moderate CYP3A4 inhibitors, p. 708. [Moderate] Study

▸ Nilotinib is predicted to increase the exposure to **tolvaptan**. Manufacturer advises caution or adjust **tolvaptan** dose with moderate CYP3A4 inhibitors, p. 708. [Moderate] Study

▸ Quinolones (ciprofloxacin) are predicted to increase the exposure to **tolvaptan**. Use with caution and adjust **tolvaptan** dose, p. 708. [Moderate] Theoretical

▸ Rifamycins (rifampicin) are predicted to decrease the exposure to **tolvaptan**. Use with caution or avoid depending on indication. [Severe] Study

▸ St John's wort is predicted to decrease the exposure to **tolvaptan**. Avoid. [Moderate] Theoretical

Topiramate → see antiepileptics

Topotecan → see TABLE 15 p. 1432 (myelosuppression)

▸ Anti-androgens (darolutamide) are predicted to increase the exposure to **topotecan**. Avoid. [Severe] Theoretical

▸ Antiarrhythmics (amiodarone, dronedarone) are predicted to increase the exposure to **topotecan**. [Severe] Study

▸ Antiepileptics (fosphenytoin, phenytoin) increase the clearance of **topotecan**. [Moderate] Study

▸ Antifungals, azoles (isavuconazole) are predicted to increase the exposure to **topotecan**. [Moderate] Theoretical

▸ Antifungals, azoles (itraconazole, ketoconazole) are predicted to increase the exposure to **topotecan**. [Severe] Study

▸ Calcium channel blockers (verapamil) are predicted to increase the exposure to **topotecan**. [Severe] Study

▸ Ceritinib is predicted to increase the exposure to **topotecan**. [Moderate] Theoretical → Also see TABLE 15 p. 1432

▸ Ciclosporin is predicted to increase the exposure to **topotecan**. [Severe] Study

▸ Eliglustat is predicted to increase the exposure to **topotecan**. Adjust dose. [Moderate] Study

▸ HIV-protease inhibitors (lopinavir, ritonavir, saquinavir) are predicted to increase the exposure to **topotecan**. [Severe] Study

Topotecan (continued)
▶ Lapatinib is predicted to increase the exposure to **topotecan**. Severe Study
▶ Leflunomide is predicted to increase the exposure to **topotecan**. Moderate Study → Also see TABLE 15 p. 1432
▶ Live vaccines are predicted to increase the risk of generalised infection (possibly life-threatening) when given with **topotecan**. Public Health England advises avoid (refer to Green Book). Severe Theoretical
▶ Macrolides are predicted to increase the exposure to **topotecan**. Severe Study
▶ Mirabegron is predicted to increase the exposure to **topotecan**. Mild
▶ Paritaprevir (with ritonavir and ombitasvir) is predicted to increase the exposure to **topotecan**. Moderate Study
▶ Pibrentasvir (with glecaprevir) is predicted to increase the exposure to **topotecan**. Moderate Study
▶ Pitolisant is predicted to decrease the exposure to **topotecan**. Mild Theoretical
▶ Ranolazine is predicted to increase the exposure to **topotecan**. Severe Study
▶ Regorafenib is predicted to increase the exposure to **topotecan**. Moderate Study → Also see TABLE 15 p. 1432
▶ St John's wort is predicted to decrease the exposure to **topotecan**. Severe Theoretical
▶ Tedizolid is predicted to increase the exposure to **topotecan**. Avoid. Moderate Study
▶ Teriflunomide is predicted to increase the exposure to **topotecan**. Moderate Study
▶ Velpatasvir is predicted to increase the exposure to **topotecan**. Severe Theoretical
▶ Vemurafenib is predicted to increase the exposure to **topotecan**. Severe Study
▶ Venetoclax is predicted to increase the exposure to **topotecan**. Moderate Theoretical
▶ Voxilaprevir is predicted to increase the concentration of **topotecan**. Avoid. Severe Theoretical

Torasemide → see loop diuretics

Toremifene → see TABLE 5 p. 1430 (thromboembolism), TABLE 9 p. 1431 (QT-interval prolongation)
▶ Anti-androgens (apalutamide, enzalutamide) are predicted to decrease the exposure to **toremifene**. Adjust dose. Moderate Study → Also see TABLE 9 p. 1431
▶ Antiepileptics (carbamazepine, fosphenytoin, phenobarbital, phenytoin, primidone) are predicted to decrease the exposure to **toremifene**. Adjust dose. Moderate Study
▶ Antifungals, azoles (itraconazole, ketoconazole, voriconazole) are predicted to increase the exposure to **toremifene**. Moderate Theoretical → Also see TABLE 9 p. 1431
▶ Cobicistat is predicted to increase the exposure to **toremifene**. Moderate Theoretical
▶ **Toremifene** is predicted to increase the anticoagulant effect of coumarins. Severe Theoretical
▶ HIV-protease inhibitors are predicted to increase the exposure to **toremifene**. Moderate Theoretical → Also see TABLE 9 p. 1431
▶ Idelalisib is predicted to increase the exposure to **toremifene**. Moderate Theoretical
▶ Macrolides (clarithromycin) are predicted to increase the exposure to **toremifene**. Moderate Theoretical → Also see TABLE 9 p. 1431
▶ Mitotane is predicted to decrease the exposure to **toremifene**. Adjust dose. Moderate Study
▶ Rifamycins (rifampicin) are predicted to decrease the exposure to **toremifene**. Adjust dose. Moderate Study
▶ Thiazide diuretics are predicted to increase the risk of hypercalcaemia when given with **toremifene**. Severe Theoretical

Trabectedin → see TABLE 1 p. 1429 (hepatotoxicity), TABLE 15 p. 1432 (myelosuppression)
▶ Anti-androgens (apalutamide, enzalutamide) are predicted to decrease the exposure to **trabectedin**. Avoid. Severe Theoretical
▶ Antiepileptics (carbamazepine, fosphenytoin, phenobarbital, phenytoin, primidone) are predicted to decrease the exposure to **trabectedin**. Avoid. Severe Theoretical → Also see TABLE 1 p. 1429

▶ Antifungals, azoles (itraconazole, ketoconazole, voriconazole) are predicted to increase the exposure to **trabectedin**. Avoid or adjust dose. Severe Theoretical → Also see TABLE 1 p. 1429
▶ Cobicistat is predicted to increase the exposure to **trabectedin**. Avoid or adjust dose. Severe Theoretical
▶ HIV-protease inhibitors are predicted to increase the exposure to **trabectedin**. Avoid or adjust dose. Severe Theoretical
▶ Idelalisib is predicted to increase the exposure to **trabectedin**. Avoid or adjust dose. Severe Theoretical
▶ Live vaccines are predicted to increase the risk of generalised infection (possibly life-threatening) when given with **trabectedin**. Public Health England advises avoid (refer to Green Book). Severe Theoretical
▶ Macrolides (clarithromycin) are predicted to increase the exposure to **trabectedin**. Avoid or adjust dose. Severe Theoretical
▶ Mitotane is predicted to decrease the exposure to **trabectedin**. Avoid. Severe Theoretical → Also see TABLE 15 p. 1432
▶ Rifamycins (rifampicin) are predicted to decrease the exposure to **trabectedin**. Avoid. Severe Theoretical

Tramadol → see opioids

Trametinib
▶ Antiarrhythmics (amiodarone, dronedarone) are predicted to increase the concentration of **trametinib**. Moderate Theoretical
▶ Antifungals, azoles (itraconazole, ketoconazole) are predicted to increase the concentration of **trametinib**. Moderate Theoretical
▶ Calcium channel blockers (verapamil) are predicted to increase the concentration of **trametinib**. Moderate Theoretical
▶ Ciclosporin is predicted to increase the concentration of **trametinib**. Moderate Theoretical
▶ HIV-protease inhibitors (lopinavir, ritonavir, saquinavir) are predicted to increase the concentration of **trametinib**. Moderate Theoretical
▶ Lapatinib is predicted to increase the concentration of **trametinib**. Moderate Theoretical
▶ Macrolides are predicted to increase the concentration of **trametinib**. Moderate Theoretical
▶ Ranolazine is predicted to increase the concentration of **trametinib**. Moderate Theoretical
▶ Vemurafenib is predicted to increase the concentration of **trametinib**. Moderate Theoretical

Trandolapril → see ACE inhibitors

Tranexamic acid → see TABLE 5 p. 1430 (thromboembolism)

Tranylcypromine → see MAOIs, irreversible

Trastuzumab → see monoclonal antibodies

Trastuzumab emtansine → see monoclonal antibodies

Trazodone → see TABLE 13 p. 1432 (serotonin syndrome), TABLE 11 p. 1431 (CNS depressant effects)
▶ Antiarrhythmics (dronedarone) are predicted to increase the exposure to **trazodone**. Moderate Theoretical
▶ Antiepileptics (carbamazepine) decrease the concentration of **trazodone**. Adjust dose. Moderate Anecdotal
▶ Antifungals, azoles (fluconazole, isavuconazole, posaconazole) are predicted to increase the exposure to **trazodone**. Moderate Theoretical
▶ Antifungals, azoles (itraconazole, ketoconazole, voriconazole) are predicted to moderately increase the exposure to **trazodone**. Avoid or adjust dose. Moderate Study
▶ Calcium channel blockers (diltiazem, verapamil) are predicted to increase the exposure to **trazodone**. Moderate Theoretical
▶ Cobicistat is predicted to moderately increase the exposure to **trazodone**. Avoid or adjust dose. Moderate Study
▶ Crizotinib is predicted to increase the exposure to **trazodone**. Moderate Theoretical
▶ HIV-protease inhibitors are predicted to moderately increase the exposure to **trazodone**. Avoid or adjust dose. Moderate Study
▶ Idelalisib is predicted to moderately increase the exposure to **trazodone**. Avoid or adjust dose. Moderate Study
▶ Imatinib is predicted to increase the exposure to **trazodone**. Moderate Theoretical
▶ Letermovir is predicted to increase the exposure to **trazodone**. Moderate Theoretical

Macrolides (clarithromycin) are predicted to moderately increase the exposure to **trazodone**. Avoid or adjust dose. Moderate Study

Macrolides (erythromycin) are predicted to increase the exposure to **trazodone**. Moderate Theoretical

Neurokinin-1 receptor antagonists (aprepitant, netupitant) are predicted to increase the exposure to **trazodone**. Moderate Theoretical

Nilotinib is predicted to increase the exposure to **trazodone**. Moderate Theoretical

‣ee pollen extract

GENERAL INFORMATION Desensitising vaccines should be avoided in patients taking beta-blockers (adrenaline might be ineffective in case of a hypersensitivity reaction) or ACE inhibitors (risk of severe anaphylactoid reactions).

‣reosulfan → see alkylating agents
‣retinoin → see retinoids
‣iamcinolone → see corticosteroids
‣riamterene → see potassium-sparing diuretics
‣ricyclic antidepressants → see TABLE 18 p. 1433 (hyponatraemia), TABLE 8 p. 1430 (hypotension), TABLE 13 p. 1432 (serotonin syndrome), TABLE 9 p. 1431 (QT-interval prolongation), TABLE 11 p. 1431 (CNS depressant effects), TABLE 10 p. 1431 (antimuscarinics)

amitriptyline · clomipramine · dosulepin · doxepin · imipramine · lofepramine · nortriptyline · trimipramine

ROUTE-SPECIFIC INFORMATION Since systemic absorption can follow topical application, the possibility of interactions of topical **doxepin** should be borne in mind.

Antiarrhythmics (dronedarone) are predicted to increase the exposure to **tricyclic antidepressants**. Avoid. Severe Theoretical → Also see TABLE 9 p. 1431

Antiarrhythmics (propafenone) are predicted to increase the concentration of **tricyclic antidepressants**. Moderate Theoretical → Also see TABLE 10 p. 1431

Antiepileptics (carbamazepine) decrease the exposure to **tricyclic antidepressants**. Adjust dose. Moderate Study → Also see TABLE 18 p. 1433

‣ Antiepileptics (phenobarbital, primidone) are predicted to decrease the exposure to **tricyclic antidepressants**. Moderate Study → Also see TABLE 11 p. 1431

‣ Antiepileptics (valproate) increase the concentration of **nortriptyline**. Severe Study

‣ Tricyclic antidepressants **(clomipramine, imipramine)** potentially increase the risk of overheating and dehydration when given with antiepileptics (zonisamide). Avoid in children. Severe Theoretical

‣ Bupropion is predicted to increase the exposure to **tricyclic antidepressants**. Monitor for toxicity and adjust dose. Severe Study → Also see TABLE 13 p. 1432

‣ Cinacalcet is predicted to increase the exposure to **tricyclic antidepressants**. Monitor for toxicity and adjust dose. Severe Study

‣ Tricyclic antidepressants decrease the antihypertensive effects of clonidine. Monitor and adjust dose. Moderate Anecdotal → Also see TABLE 8 p. 1430 → Also see TABLE 11 p. 1431

‣ Cobicistat is predicted to slightly increase the exposure to **tricyclic antidepressants**. Mild Study

‣ Dacomitinib is predicted to markedly increase the exposure to tricyclic antidepressants **(imipramine, nortriptyline)**. Avoid. Severe Study

‣ Darifenacin is predicted to increase the exposure to **tricyclic antidepressants**. Moderate Theoretical → Also see TABLE 10 p. 1431

‣ Eliglustat is predicted to increase the exposure to **nortriptyline**. Adjust dose. Moderate Theoretical

‣ H_2 receptor antagonists (cimetidine) increase the exposure to **tricyclic antidepressants**. Moderate Study

‣ HIV-protease inhibitors (ritonavir, tipranavir) are predicted to increase the exposure to **tricyclic antidepressants**. Moderate Theoretical

‣ Tricyclic antidepressants potentially increase the risk of neurotoxicity when given with lithium. Severe Anecdotal → Also see TABLE 13 p. 1432 → Also see TABLE 9 p. 1431

‣ Tricyclic antidepressants are predicted to increase the risk of severe toxic reaction when given with MAOIs, irreversible. Avoid and for 14 days after stopping the MAOI. Severe Theoretical → Also see TABLE 8 p. 1430 → Also see TABLE 13 p. 1432

‣ Amitriptyline decreases the effects of metyrapone. Avoid. Moderate Theoretical

‣ Tricyclic antidepressants are predicted to increase the risk of severe toxic reaction when given with moclobemide. Avoid. Severe Theoretical → Also see TABLE 13 p. 1432

‣ Tricyclic antidepressants are predicted to decrease the effects of moxonidine. Avoid. Moderate Theoretical → Also see TABLE 8 p. 1430 → Also see TABLE 11 p. 1431

‣ Tricyclic antidepressants potentially increase the risk of adverse effects when given with ozanimod. Severe Theoretical

‣ Tricyclic antidepressants are predicted to decrease the efficacy of pitolisant. Mild Theoretical

‣ SSRIs (fluoxetine, paroxetine) are predicted to increase the exposure to **tricyclic antidepressants**. Monitor for toxicity and adjust dose. Severe Study → Also see TABLE 18 p. 1433 → Also see TABLE 13 p. 1432

‣ SSRIs (fluvoxamine) markedly increase the exposure to **clomipramine**. Adjust dose. Severe Study → Also see TABLE 18 p. 1433 → Also see TABLE 13 p. 1432

‣ SSRIs (fluvoxamine) increase the exposure to tricyclic antidepressants **(amitriptyline, imipramine)**. Adjust dose. Severe Study → Also see TABLE 18 p. 1433 → Also see TABLE 13 p. 1432

‣ Sucralfate is predicted to decrease the absorption of **tricyclic antidepressants**. Moderate Study

‣ Tricyclic antidepressants increase the effects of sympathomimetics, vasoconstrictor (adrenaline/epinephrine, noradrenaline/norepinephrine, phenylephrine). Avoid. Severe Study

‣ Tricyclic antidepressants are predicted to decrease the effects of sympathomimetics, vasoconstrictor (ephedrine). Avoid. Severe Study

‣ Terbinafine is predicted to increase the exposure to **tricyclic antidepressants**. Monitor for toxicity and adjust dose. Severe Study

‣ Tricyclic antidepressants increase the risk of cardiac arrhythmias and hypotension when given with thiopental. Moderate Study → Also see TABLE 8 p. 1430 → Also see TABLE 11 p. 1431

Trientine
‣ Oral trientine potentially decreases the absorption of oral iron. Moderate Theoretical
‣ Trientine potentially decreases the absorption of zinc. Moderate Theoretical

Trifluoperazine → see phenothiazines
Trihexyphenidyl → see TABLE 10 p. 1431 (antimuscarinics)
Trimethoprim → see TABLE 18 p. 1433 (hyponatraemia), TABLE 2 p. 1429 (nephrotoxicity), TABLE 16 p. 1433 (increased serum potassium)
‣ Trimethoprim increases the concentration of antiepileptics (fosphenytoin, phenytoin). Moderate Study
‣ Antimalarials (pyrimethamine) increase the risk of adverse effects when given with **trimethoprim**. Severe Study
‣ Trimethoprim is predicted to increase the anticoagulant effect of coumarins. Severe Study
‣ Dapsone increases the exposure to trimethoprim and **trimethoprim** increases the exposure to dapsone. Severe Study
‣ Trimethoprim increases the concentration of digoxin. Moderate Study
‣ Trimethoprim is predicted to increase the exposure to dopamine receptor agonists (pramipexole). Adjust dose. Moderate Study
‣ Trimethoprim slightly increases the exposure to meglitinides (repaglinide). Avoid or monitor blood glucose. Moderate Study
‣ Trimethoprim increases the risk of adverse effects when given with methotrexate. Avoid. Severe Anecdotal → Also see TABLE 2 p. 1429
‣ Trimethoprim slightly increases the exposure to NRTIs (lamivudine). Moderate Study
‣ Rifamycins (rifampicin) decrease the exposure to **trimethoprim**. Moderate Study
‣ Trimethoprim is predicted to decrease the efficacy of sapropterin. Moderate Theoretical

Trimipramine → see tricyclic antidepressants
Triptans → see TABLE 13 p. 1432 (serotonin syndrome)

almotriptan · eletriptan · frovatriptan · naratriptan · rizatriptan · sumatriptan · zolmitriptan

▸ Antifungals, azoles (itraconazole, ketoconazole, voriconazole) increase the exposure to **almotriptan**. Mild Study
▸ Antifungals, azoles (itraconazole, ketoconazole, voriconazole) are predicted to markedly increase the exposure to **eletriptan**. Avoid. Severe Study
▸ Beta blockers, non-selective (propranolol) slightly to moderately increase the exposure to **rizatriptan**. Adjust **rizatriptan** dose and separate administration by at least 2 hours, p. 501. Moderate Study
▸ Cobicistat increases the exposure to **almotriptan**. Mild Study
▸ Cobicistat is predicted to markedly increase the exposure to **eletriptan**. Avoid. Severe Study
▸ Combined hormonal contraceptives are predicted to increase the exposure to **zolmitriptan**. Adjust **zolmitriptan** dose, p. 503. Moderate Theoretical
▸ **Almotriptan** is predicted to increase the risk of vasoconstriction when given with ergotamine. **Ergotamine** should be taken at least 24 hours before or 6 hours after **almotriptan**. Severe Theoretical
▸ **Eletriptan** increases the risk of vasoconstriction when given with ergotamine. Separate administration by 24 hours. Severe Study
▸ **Rizatriptan** is predicted to increase the risk of vasoconstriction when given with ergotamine. **Ergotamine** should be taken at least 24 hours before or 6 hours after **rizatriptan**. Severe Theoretical
▸ **Sumatriptan** increases the risk of vasoconstriction when given with ergotamine. **Ergotamine** should be taken at least 24 hours before or 6 hours after **sumatriptan**. Severe Study
▸ Triptans (**frovatriptan, naratriptan**) are predicted to increase the risk of vasoconstriction when given with ergotamine. Separate administration by 24 hours. Severe Theoretical
▸ **Zolmitriptan** is predicted to increase the risk of vasoconstriction when given with ergotamine. **Ergotamine** should be taken at least 24 hours before or 6 hours after **zolmitriptan**. Severe Theoretical
▸ H₂ receptor antagonists (cimetidine) slightly increase the exposure to **zolmitriptan**. Adjust **zolmitriptan** dose, p. 503. Mild Study
▸ HIV-protease inhibitors increase the exposure to **almotriptan**. Mild Study
▸ HIV-protease inhibitors are predicted to markedly increase the exposure to **eletriptan**. Avoid. Severe Study
▸ Idelalisib increases the exposure to **almotriptan**. Mild Study
▸ Idelalisib is predicted to markedly increase the exposure to **eletriptan**. Avoid. Severe Study
▸ Macrolides (clarithromycin) increase the exposure to **almotriptan**. Mild Study
▸ Macrolides (clarithromycin) are predicted to markedly increase the exposure to **eletriptan**. Avoid. Severe Study
▸ Macrolides (erythromycin) moderately increase the exposure to **eletriptan**. Avoid. Moderate Study
▸ MAOIs, irreversible are predicted to increase the exposure to triptans (**rizatriptan, sumatriptan**). Avoid and for 14 days after stopping the MAOI. Severe Theoretical → Also see TABLE 13 p. 1432
▸ MAOIs, irreversible are predicted to increase the exposure to **zolmitriptan**. Severe Theoretical → Also see TABLE 13 p. 1432
▸ Mexiletine is predicted to increase the exposure to **zolmitriptan**. Adjust **zolmitriptan** dose, p. 503. Moderate Theoretical
▸ Moclobemide moderately increases the exposure to triptans (**rizatriptan, sumatriptan**). Avoid. Moderate Study → Also see TABLE 13 p. 1432
▸ Moclobemide slightly increases the exposure to **zolmitriptan**. Adjust **zolmitriptan** dose, p. 503. Moderate Study → Also see TABLE 13 p. 1432
▸ Neurokinin-1 receptor antagonists (aprepitant, netupitant) are predicted to increase the exposure to **eletriptan**. Moderate Study

▸ Quinolones (ciprofloxacin) are predicted to increase the exposure to **zolmitriptan**. Adjust **zolmitriptan** dose, p. 503. Moderate Theoretical
▸ SSRIs (fluvoxamine) increase the concentration of **frovatriptan**. Severe Study → Also see TABLE 13 p. 1432
▸ SSRIs (fluvoxamine) are predicted to increase the exposure to **zolmitriptan**. Adjust **zolmitriptan** dose, p. 503. Severe Theoretical → Also see TABLE 13 p. 1432
Tropicamide → see TABLE 10 p. 1431 (antimuscarinics)
Trospium → see TABLE 10 p. 1431 (antimuscarinics)
Tryptophan → see TABLE 13 p. 1432 (serotonin syndrome)
▸ **Tryptophan** greatly decreases the concentration of levodopa. Moderate Study
▸ **Tryptophan** increases the risk of adverse effects when given with MAOIs, irreversible. Severe Anecdotal → Also see TABLE 13 p. 1432
Typhoid vaccine, oral → see live vaccines
Ulipristal
▸ Anti-androgens (enzalutamide) are predicted to markedly decrease the exposure to **ulipristal**. Avoid and for 4 weeks after stopping **ulipristal**. Severe Theoretical
▸ Antiepileptics (carbamazepine, eslicarbazepine, fosphenytoin, oxcarbazepine, perampanel, phenobarbital, phenytoin, primidone, rufinamide, topiramate) decrease the efficacy of **ulipristal**. For FSRH guidance, see Contraceptives, interactions p. 840. Severe Anecdotal
▸ **Ulipristal** is predicted to decrease the efficacy of combined hormonal contraceptives. Avoid. Severe Theoretical
▸ **Ulipristal** is predicted to decrease the efficacy of desogestrel. Avoid. Severe Theoretical
▸ Endothelin receptor antagonists (bosentan) decrease the efficacy of **ulipristal**. For FSRH guidance, see Contraceptives, interactions p. 840. Severe Anecdotal
▸ **Ulipristal** is predicted to decrease the efficacy of etonogestrel. Avoid. Severe Theoretical
▸ Griseofulvin potentially decreases the efficacy of **ulipristal**. For FSRH guidance, see Contraceptives, interactions p. 840. Severe Anecdotal
▸ HIV-protease inhibitors (lopinavir) are predicted to increase the exposure to **ulipristal**. Avoid if used for uterine fibroids. Severe Study
▸ HIV-protease inhibitors (ritonavir) decrease the efficacy of **ulipristal**. For FSRH guidance, see Contraceptives, interactions p. 840. Severe Anecdotal
▸ **Ulipristal** is predicted to decrease the efficacy of levonorgestrel. Avoid. Severe Theoretical
▸ Lumacaftor is predicted to decrease the efficacy of **ulipristal**. Use additional contraceptive precautions. Severe Theoretical
▸ Modafinil decreases the efficacy of **ulipristal**. For FSRH guidance, see Contraceptives, interactions p. 840. Severe Anecdotal
▸ Neurokinin-1 receptor antagonists (aprepitant, fosaprepitant) decrease the efficacy of **ulipristal**. For FSRH guidance, see Contraceptives, interactions p. 840. Severe Anecdotal
▸ NNRTIs (efavirenz, nevirapine) decrease the efficacy of **ulipristal**. For FSRH guidance, see Contraceptives, interactions p. 840. Severe Anecdotal
▸ **Ulipristal** is predicted to decrease the efficacy of norethisterone. Avoid. Severe Theoretical
▸ Rifamycins decrease the efficacy of **ulipristal**. For FSRH guidance, see Contraceptives, interactions p. 840. Severe Anecdotal
▸ St John's wort decreases the efficacy of **ulipristal**. For FSRH guidance, see Contraceptives, interactions p. 840. Severe Anecdotal
Umeclidinium → see TABLE 10 p. 1431 (antimuscarinics)
Upadacitinib
▸ Anti-androgens (apalutamide, enzalutamide) are predicted to decrease the exposure to **upadacitinib**. Moderate Study
▸ Antiepileptics (carbamazepine, fosphenytoin, phenobarbital, phenytoin, primidone) are predicted to decrease the exposure to **upadacitinib**. Moderate Study
▸ Antifungals, azoles (itraconazole, ketoconazole, voriconazole) are predicted to increase the exposure to **upadacitinib**. Use with caution or avoid. Severe Study

Antifungals, azoles (posaconazole) are predicted to increase the exposure to **upadacitinib**. Use with caution or avoid. Moderate Study

Cobicistat is predicted to increase the exposure to **upadacitinib**. Use with caution or avoid. Severe Study

HIV-protease inhibitors are predicted to increase the exposure to **upadacitinib**. Use with caution or avoid. Severe Study

Idelalisib is predicted to increase the exposure to **upadacitinib**. Use with caution or avoid. Severe Study

Live vaccines are predicted to increase the risk of generalised infection (possibly life-threatening) when given with **upadacitinib**. Avoid. Severe Theoretical

Macrolides (clarithromycin) are predicted to increase the exposure to **upadacitinib**. Use with caution or avoid. Severe Study

Mitotane is predicted to decrease the exposure to **upadacitinib**. Moderate Study

Rifamycins (rifampin) are predicted to decrease the exposure to **upadacitinib**. Moderate Study

rokinase → see TABLE 3 p. 1429 (anticoagulant effects)

rsodeoxycholic acid

Oral antacids are predicted to decrease the absorption of oral **ursodeoxycholic acid**. Separate administration by 2 hours. Moderate Theoretical

Ursodeoxycholic acid affects the concentration of ciclosporin. Use with caution and adjust dose. Severe Anecdotal

Fibrates are predicted to decrease the efficacy of **ursodeoxycholic acid**. Avoid. Severe Theoretical

stekinumab → see monoclonal antibodies

aborbactam

Vaborbactam is predicted to increase the concentration of beta blockers, selective (metoprolol). Unknown Theoretical

Vaborbactam is predicted to increase the concentration of venlafaxine. Unknown Theoretical

alaciclovir → see TABLE 2 p. 1429 (nephrotoxicity)

Valaciclovir is predicted to increase the exposure to aminophylline. Severe Anecdotal

Mycophenolate is predicted to increase the risk of haematological toxicity when given with **valaciclovir**. Moderate Theoretical

Valaciclovir is predicted to increase the exposure to theophylline. Severe Theoretical

alganciclovir → see TABLE 15 p. 1432 (myelosuppression), TABLE 2 p. 1429 (nephrotoxicity)

Valganciclovir is predicted to increase the risk of seizures when given with carbapenems (imipenem). Avoid. Severe Anecdotal

Mycophenolate is predicted to increase the risk of haematological toxicity when given with **valganciclovir**. Moderate Theoretical

Valproate → see antiepileptics

Valsartan → see angiotensin-II receptor antagonists

Vancomycin → see TABLE 2 p. 1429 (nephrotoxicity), TABLE 19 p. 1433 (ototoxicity)

Vandetanib → see TABLE 9 p. 1431 (QT-interval prolongation)

▶ Anti-androgens (apalutamide, enzalutamide) are predicted to decrease the exposure to **vandetanib**. Avoid. Moderate Study → Also see TABLE 9 p. 1431

▶ Antiepileptics (carbamazepine, fosphenytoin, phenobarbital, phenytoin, primidone) are predicted to decrease the exposure to **vandetanib**. Moderate Study

▶ **Vandetanib** is predicted to increase the risk of bleeding events when given with coumarins. Severe Theoretical

▶ **Vandetanib** slightly increases the exposure to digoxin. Monitor ECG and adjust dose. Moderate Study

▶ **Vandetanib** is predicted to increase the exposure to dopamine receptor agonists (pramipexole). Adjust dose. Moderate Study

▶ **Vandetanib** increases the exposure to metformin. Monitor and adjust dose. Moderate Study

▶ Mitotane is predicted to decrease the exposure to **vandetanib**. Avoid. Moderate Study

▶ **Vandetanib** is predicted to increase the risk of bleeding events when given with phenindione. Severe Theoretical

▶ Rifamycins (rifampin) are predicted to decrease the exposure to **vandetanib**. Avoid. Moderate Study

Vardenafil → see phosphodiesterase type-5 inhibitors

Varicella-zoster immunoglobulin → see immunoglobulins

Varicella-zoster vaccine → see live vaccines

Vecuronium → see neuromuscular blocking drugs, non-depolarising

Vedolizumab → see monoclonal antibodies

Velpatasvir

▶ **Velpatasvir** is predicted to increase the exposure to aliskiren. Severe Theoretical

▶ Oral antacids are predicted to decrease the concentration of oral **velpatasvir**. Separate administration by 4 hours. Moderate Theoretical

▶ Anti-androgens (apalutamide, enzalutamide) are predicted to moderately decrease the exposure to **velpatasvir**. Avoid. Severe Study

▶ Antiarrhythmics (amiodarone) are predicted to increase the concentration of **velpatasvir**. Avoid or monitor. Moderate Theoretical

▶ Antiepileptics (carbamazepine, fosphenytoin, phenobarbital, phenytoin, primidone) are predicted to moderately decrease the exposure to **velpatasvir**. Avoid. Severe Study

▶ Antiepileptics (oxcarbazepine) are predicted to decrease the exposure to **velpatasvir**. Severe Theoretical

▶ **Velpatasvir** is predicted to increase the exposure to antihistamines, non-sedating (fexofenadine). Severe Theoretical

▶ Calcium salts (calcium carbonate) are predicted to decrease the concentration of **velpatasvir**. Separate administration by 4 hours. Moderate Anecdotal

▶ **Velpatasvir** is predicted to increase the exposure to colchicine. Severe Theoretical

▶ **Velpatasvir** is predicted to increase the exposure to digoxin. Severe Study

▶ Endothelin receptor antagonists (bosentan) are predicted to decrease the exposure to **velpatasvir**. Avoid. Moderate Theoretical

▶ **Velpatasvir** is predicted to increase the exposure to everolimus. Severe Theoretical

▶ **Velpatasvir** is predicted to increase the exposure to factor XA inhibitors (edoxaban). Severe Theoretical

▶ H_2 receptor antagonists are predicted to decrease the concentration of **velpatasvir**. Adjust dose, see sofosbuvir with velpatasvir p. 669. Moderate Study

▶ HIV-protease inhibitors (tipranavir) are predicted to increase the exposure to **velpatasvir**. Severe Theoretical

▶ **Velpatasvir** is predicted to increase the exposure to loperamide. Severe Theoretical

▶ Mitotane is predicted to moderately decrease the exposure to **velpatasvir**. Avoid. Severe Study

▶ Modafinil is predicted to decrease the exposure to **velpatasvir**. Avoid. Severe Theoretical

▶ NNRTIs (efavirenz, nevirapine) are predicted to decrease the exposure to **velpatasvir**. Avoid. Moderate Theoretical

▶ Proton pump inhibitors are predicted to decrease the concentration of **velpatasvir**. Adjust dose, see sofosbuvir with velpatasvir p. 669. Moderate Study

▶ Rifamycins (rifampin) are predicted to moderately decrease the exposure to **velpatasvir**. Avoid. Severe Study

▶ **Velpatasvir** is predicted to increase the exposure to sirolimus. Severe Theoretical

▶ St John's wort is predicted to decrease the exposure to **velpatasvir**. Avoid. Moderate Theoretical

▶ **Velpatasvir** increases the exposure to statins (rosuvastatin). Adjust **rosuvastatin** dose and monitor adverse effects, p. 218. Severe Study

▶ **Velpatasvir** is predicted to increase the exposure to statins (simvastatin). Monitor adverse effects and adjust dose. Severe Theoretical

▶ **Velpatasvir** is predicted to increase the exposure to sulfasalazine. Moderate Theoretical

▶ **Velpatasvir** is predicted to increase the exposure to taxanes (paclitaxel). Severe Theoretical

▶ **Velpatasvir** is predicted to increase the exposure to tenofovir disoproxil. Severe Study

▶ **Velpatasvir** increases the exposure to thrombin inhibitors (dabigatran). Avoid. Severe Study

▶ **Velpatasvir** is predicted to increase the exposure to topotecan. Severe Theoretical

A1

Interactions | **Appendix 1**

Vemurafenib → see TABLE 9 p. 1431 (QT-interval prolongation)

▸ **Vemurafenib** is predicted to increase the exposure to afatinib. Separate administration by 12 hours. Moderate Study

▸ **Vemurafenib** is predicted to increase the exposure to agomelatine. Use with caution or avoid. Moderate Theoretical

▸ **Vemurafenib** is predicted to increase the exposure to aliskiren. Use with caution and adjust dose. Moderate Theoretical

▸ Anti-androgens (apalutamide, enzalutamide) are predicted to decrease the exposure to **vemurafenib**. Avoid. Severe Theoretical → Also see TABLE 9 p. 1431

▸ Antiepileptics (carbamazepine, fosphenytoin, phenobarbital, phenytoin, primidone) are predicted to decrease the exposure to **vemurafenib**. Avoid. Severe Theoretical

▸ Antifungals, azoles (itraconazole, ketoconazole, voriconazole) are predicted to increase the exposure to **vemurafenib**. Severe Theoretical → Also see TABLE 9 p. 1431

▸ **Vemurafenib** is predicted to increase the exposure to antihistamines, non-sedating (fexofenadine). Use with caution and adjust dose. Severe Theoretical

▸ **Vemurafenib** is predicted to increase the exposure to beta blockers, non-selective (nadolol). Moderate Study

▸ **Vemurafenib** is predicted to increase the exposure to bictegravir. Use with caution or avoid. Moderate Theoretical

▸ Cobicistat is predicted to increase the exposure to **vemurafenib**. Severe Theoretical

▸ **Vemurafenib** is predicted to increase the exposure to colchicine. Avoid P-glycoprotein inhibitors or adjust **colchicine** dose, p. 1166. Severe Theoretical

▸ **Vemurafenib** slightly increases the exposure to digoxin. Use with caution and adjust dose. Severe Study

▸ **Vemurafenib** is predicted to increase the exposure to duloxetine. Use with caution or avoid. Moderate Theoretical

▸ **Vemurafenib** is predicted to increase the exposure to erlotinib. Moderate Theoretical

▸ **Vemurafenib** is predicted to increase the exposure to everolimus. Use with caution and adjust dose. Severe Theoretical

▸ **Vemurafenib** is predicted to slightly increase the exposure to factor XA inhibitors (edoxaban). Severe Theoretical

▸ **Vemurafenib** is predicted to increase the exposure to fidaxomicin. Avoid. Moderate Study

▸ HIV-protease inhibitors are predicted to increase the exposure to **vemurafenib**. Severe Theoretical → Also see TABLE 9 p. 1431

▸ Idelalisib is predicted to increase the exposure to **vemurafenib**. Severe Theoretical

▸ **Vemurafenib** is predicted to increase the exposure to larotrectinib. Mild Theoretical

▸ Macrolides (clarithromycin) are predicted to increase the exposure to **vemurafenib**. Severe Theoretical → Also see TABLE 9 p. 1431

▸ **Vemurafenib** is predicted to increase the exposure to melatonin. Use with caution or avoid. Moderate Theoretical

▸ Mitotane is predicted to decrease the exposure to **vemurafenib**. Avoid. Severe Theoretical

▸ **Vemurafenib** is predicted to increase the exposure to naldemedine. Moderate Study

▸ **Vemurafenib** is predicted to increase the exposure to nintedanib. Moderate Study

▸ **Vemurafenib** is predicted to increase the exposure to panobinostat. Adjust dose. Moderate Theoretical → Also see TABLE 9 p. 1431

▸ **Vemurafenib** is predicted to increase the exposure to pibrentasvir. Moderate Theoretical

▸ Rifamycins (rifampicin) are predicted to decrease the exposure to **vemurafenib**. Avoid. Severe Theoretical

▸ **Vemurafenib** is predicted to increase the exposure to sirolimus. Use with caution and adjust dose. Severe Theoretical

▸ **Vemurafenib** is predicted to slightly increase the exposure to talazoparib. Avoid or adjust **talazoparib** dose, p. 1052. Severe Study

▸ **Vemurafenib** is predicted to increase the exposure to taxanes (paclitaxel). Use with caution and adjust dose. Severe Theoretical

▸ **Vemurafenib** is predicted to increase the exposure to theophylline. Use with caution or avoid. Moderate Theoretical

▸ **Vemurafenib** increases the exposure to thrombin inhibitors (dabigatran). Use with caution and adjust dose. Severe Theoretical

▸ **Vemurafenib** is predicted to increase the exposure to ticagrelor. Use with caution or avoid. Severe Study

▸ **Vemurafenib** moderately increases the exposure to tizanidine. Use with caution or avoid. Moderate Theoretical → Also see TABLE 9 p. 1431

▸ **Vemurafenib** is predicted to increase the exposure to topotecan. Severe Study

▸ **Vemurafenib** is predicted to increase the concentration of trametinib. Moderate Theoretical

▸ **Vemurafenib** is predicted to increase the exposure to venetoclax. Avoid or monitor for toxicity. Severe Theoretical

Venetoclax

FOOD AND LIFESTYLE Avoid Seville (bitter orange) and star fruit as they might increase the exposure to venetoclax.

▸ Anti-androgens (apalutamide, enzalutamide) are predicted to decrease the exposure to **venetoclax**. Avoid. Severe Study

▸ Antiarrhythmics (amiodarone) are predicted to increase the exposure to **venetoclax**. Avoid or monitor for toxicity. Severe Theoretical

▸ Antiarrhythmics (dronedarone) are predicted to increase the exposure to **venetoclax**. Avoid or adjust dose—consult product literature. Severe Study

▸ Antiepileptics (carbamazepine, fosphenytoin, phenobarbital, phenytoin, primidone) are predicted to decrease the exposure to **venetoclax**. Avoid. Severe Study

▸ Antifungals, azoles (fluconazole, isavuconazole, itraconazole, ketoconazole, posaconazole, voriconazole) are predicted to increase the exposure to **venetoclax**. Avoid or adjust dose—consult product literature. Severe Study

▸ **Venetoclax** is predicted to increase the exposure to antihistamines, non-sedating (fexofenadine). Moderate Theoretical

▸ Calcium channel blockers (diltiazem, verapamil) are predicted to increase the exposure to **venetoclax**. Avoid or adjust dose—consult product literature. Severe Study

▸ Ciclosporin is predicted to increase the exposure to **venetoclax**. Avoid or monitor for toxicity. Severe Theoretical

▸ Cobicistat is predicted to increase the exposure to **venetoclax**. Avoid or adjust dose—consult product literature. Severe Study

▸ **Venetoclax** slightly increases the exposure to coumarins (warfarin). Moderate Study

▸ Crizotinib is predicted to increase the exposure to **venetoclax**. Avoid or adjust dose—consult product literature. Severe Study

▸ **Venetoclax** increases the exposure to digoxin. Avoid or adjust dose. Severe Study

▸ Endothelin receptor antagonists (bosentan) are predicted to decrease the exposure to **venetoclax**. Avoid. Severe Study

▸ **Venetoclax** is predicted to increase the exposure to endothelin receptor antagonists (bosentan). Moderate Theoretical

▸ **Venetoclax** is predicted to increase the exposure to everolimus. Avoid or adjust dose. Severe Study

▸ Grapefruit juice is predicted to increase the exposure to **venetoclax**. Avoid. Severe Theoretical

▸ HIV-protease inhibitors are predicted to increase the exposure to **venetoclax**. Avoid or adjust dose—consult product literature. Severe Study

▸ Idelalisib is predicted to increase the exposure to **venetoclax**. Avoid or adjust dose—consult product literature. Severe Study

▸ Imatinib is predicted to increase the exposure to **venetoclax**. Avoid or adjust dose—consult product literature. Severe Study

▸ Lapatinib is predicted to increase the exposure to **venetoclax**. Avoid or monitor for toxicity. Severe Theoretical

▸ Letermovir is predicted to increase the exposure to **venetoclax**. Avoid or adjust dose—consult product literature. Severe Study

▸ **Venetoclax** potentially decreases the efficacy of live vaccines. Avoid. Severe Theoretical

▸ Macrolides (clarithromycin, erythromycin) are predicted to increase the exposure to **venetoclax**. Avoid or adjust dose—consult product literature. Severe Study

▸ **Venetoclax** is predicted to increase the exposure to meglitinides (repaglinide). Moderate Theoretical

▸ Mitotane is predicted to decrease the exposure to **venetoclax**. Avoid. Severe Study

Neurokinin-1 receptor antagonists (aprepitant, netupitant) are predicted to increase the exposure to **venetoclax**. Avoid or adjust dose—consult product literature. Severe Study

Nilotinib is predicted to increase the exposure to **venetoclax**. Avoid or adjust dose—consult product literature. Severe Study

NNRTIs (efavirenz, nevirapine) are predicted to decrease the exposure to **venetoclax**. Avoid. Severe Study

Quinolones (ciprofloxacin) are predicted to increase the exposure to **venetoclax**. Avoid or adjust dose—consult product literature. Severe Theoretical

Ranolazine is predicted to increase the exposure to **venetoclax**. Avoid or monitor for toxicity. Severe Theoretical

Rifamycins (rifampicin) are predicted to decrease the exposure to **venetoclax**. Avoid. Severe Study

Venetoclax is predicted to increase the exposure to sirolimus. Avoid or adjust dose. Severe Study

St John's wort is predicted to decrease the exposure to **venetoclax**. Avoid. Severe Study

Venetoclax is predicted to increase the exposure to statins (atorvastatin). Moderate Study

Venetoclax is predicted to increase the exposure to statins (fluvastatin, pravastatin, rosuvastatin, simvastatin). Moderate Theoretical

Venetoclax is predicted to increase the exposure to sulfasalazine. Moderate Theoretical

Venetoclax is predicted to increase the exposure to sulfonylureas (glibenclamide). Moderate Theoretical

Venetoclax is predicted to increase the exposure to thrombin inhibitors (dabigatran). Avoid or adjust dose. Severe Study

Venetoclax is predicted to increase the exposure to topotecan. Moderate Theoretical

Vemurafenib is predicted to increase the exposure to **venetoclax**. Avoid or monitor for toxicity. Severe Theoretical

Venlafaxine → see TABLE 13 p. 1432 (serotonin syndrome), TABLE 9 p. 1431 (QT-interval prolongation), TABLE 11 p. 1431 (CNS depressant effects), TABLE 4 p. 1429 (antiplatelet effects)

Antifungals, azoles (itraconazole, ketoconazole, voriconazole) are predicted to increase the exposure to **venlafaxine**. Moderate Study → Also see TABLE 9 p. 1431

Cobicistat is predicted to increase the exposure to **venlafaxine**. Moderate Study

H₂ receptor antagonists (cimetidine) slightly increase the exposure to **venlafaxine**. Mild Study

Venlafaxine slightly increases the exposure to haloperidol. Severe Study → Also see TABLE 9 p. 1431 → Also see TABLE 11 p. 1431

HIV-protease inhibitors are predicted to increase the exposure to **venlafaxine**. Moderate Study → Also see TABLE 9 p. 1431

Idelalisib is predicted to increase the exposure to **venlafaxine**. Moderate Study

Macrolides (clarithromycin) are predicted to increase the exposure to **venlafaxine**. Moderate Study → Also see TABLE 9 p. 1431

Venlafaxine is predicted to increase the exposure to pitolisant. Use with caution and adjust dose. Mild Theoretical

Tacrolimus potentially increases the risk of serotonin syndrome when given with **venlafaxine**. Severe Anecdotal

Vaborbactam is predicted to increase the concentration of **venlafaxine**. Unknown Theoretical

Verapamil → see calcium channel blockers

Vernakalant → see antiarrhythmics

Verteporfin

GENERAL INFORMATION Caution on concurrent use with other photosensitising drugs.

Vigabatrin → see antiepileptics

Vilanterol → see beta₂ agonists

Vildagliptin → see dipeptidylpeptidase-4 inhibitors

Vinblastine → see vinca alkaloids

Vinca alkaloids → see TABLE 1 p. 1429 (hepatotoxicity), TABLE 15 p. 1432 (myelosuppression), TABLE 19 p. 1433 (ototoxicity), TABLE 12 p. 1432 (peripheral neuropathy), TABLE 5 p. 1430 (thromboembolism), TABLE 9 p. 1431 (QT-interval prolongation)

vinblastine · vincristine · vindesine · vinflunine · vinorelbine

▸ Anti-androgens (apalutamide, enzalutamide) are predicted to decrease the exposure to **vinflunine**. Avoid. Severe Theoretical → Also see TABLE 9 p. 1431

▸ Anti-androgens (apalutamide, enzalutamide) are predicted to decrease the exposure to **vinorelbine**. Use with caution or avoid. Severe Theoretical

▸ Anti-androgens (apalutamide, enzalutamide) are predicted to decrease the exposure to vinca alkaloids (**vinblastine, vincristine, vindesine**). Severe Theoretical

▸ Antiarrhythmics (dronedarone) are predicted to increase the exposure to vinca alkaloids. Severe Theoretical → Also see TABLE 9 p. 1431

▸ Antiepileptics (carbamazepine, fosphenytoin, phenobarbital, phenytoin, primidone) are predicted to decrease the exposure to **vinflunine**. Avoid. Severe Theoretical → Also see TABLE 12 p. 1432

▸ Antiepileptics (carbamazepine, fosphenytoin, phenobarbital, phenytoin, primidone) are predicted to decrease the exposure to **vinorelbine**. Use with caution or avoid. Severe Theoretical → Also see TABLE 12 p. 1432

▸ Antiepileptics (carbamazepine, fosphenytoin, phenobarbital, phenytoin, primidone) are predicted to decrease the exposure to vinca alkaloids (**vinblastine, vincristine, vindesine**). Severe Theoretical → Also see TABLE 1 p. 1429 → Also see TABLE 12 p. 1432

▸ Antifungals, azoles (fluconazole, isavuconazole, itraconazole, ketoconazole, posaconazole, voriconazole) are predicted to increase the exposure to vinca alkaloids. Severe Theoretical → Also see TABLE 1 p. 1429 → Also see TABLE 9 p. 1431

▸ Antifungals, azoles (miconazole) are predicted to increase the concentration of vinca alkaloids. Use with caution and adjust dose. Severe Theoretical

▸ Asparaginase potentially increases the risk of neurotoxicity when given with **vincristine**. **Vincristine** should be taken 3 to 24 hours before asparaginase. Severe Anecdotal → Also see TABLE 1 p. 1429 → Also see TABLE 15 p. 1432

▸ Calcium channel blockers (diltiazem, verapamil) are predicted to increase the exposure to vinca alkaloids. Severe Theoretical

▸ Cobicistat is predicted to increase the exposure to vinca alkaloids. Severe Theoretical

▸ Crisantaspase potentially increases the risk of neurotoxicity when given with **vincristine**. **Vincristine** should be taken 3 to 24 hours before crisantaspase. Severe Anecdotal → Also see TABLE 1 p. 1429 → Also see TABLE 15 p. 1432

▸ Crizotinib is predicted to increase the exposure to vinca alkaloids. Severe Theoretical → Also see TABLE 9 p. 1431

▸ HIV-protease inhibitors are predicted to increase the exposure to vinca alkaloids. Severe Theoretical → Also see TABLE 9 p. 1431

▸ Idelalisib is predicted to increase the exposure to vinca alkaloids. Severe Theoretical

▸ Imatinib is predicted to increase the exposure to vinca alkaloids. Severe Theoretical → Also see TABLE 15 p. 1432

▸ Letermovir is predicted to increase the exposure to vinca alkaloids. Severe Theoretical

▸ Live vaccines are predicted to increase the risk of generalised infection (possibly life-threatening) when given with vinca alkaloids. Public Health England advises avoid (refer to Green Book). Severe Theoretical

▸ Macrolides (clarithromycin, erythromycin) are predicted to increase the exposure to vinca alkaloids. Severe Theoretical → Also see TABLE 9 p. 1431

▸ Mitotane is predicted to decrease the exposure to vinca alkaloids (**vinblastine, vincristine, vindesine**). Severe Theoretical → Also see TABLE 15 p. 1432

▸ Mitotane is predicted to decrease the exposure to **vinflunine**. Avoid. Severe Theoretical → Also see TABLE 15 p. 1432

▸ Mitotane is predicted to decrease the exposure to **vinorelbine**. Use with caution or avoid. Severe Theoretical → Also see TABLE 15 p. 1432

▸ Neurokinin-1 receptor antagonists are predicted to increase the exposure to vinca alkaloids. Severe Theoretical

▸ Nilotinib is predicted to increase the exposure to vinca alkaloids. Severe Theoretical → Also see TABLE 15 p. 1432 → Also see TABLE 9 p. 1431

▸ Pegaspargase potentially increases the risk of neurotoxicity when given with **vincristine**. **Vincristine** should be taken 3 to 24 hours before pegaspargase. Severe Anecdotal → Also see TABLE 1 p. 1429 → Also see TABLE 15 p. 1432

Vinca alkaloids (continued)

▸ Rifamycins (rifampicin) are predicted to decrease the exposure to **vinflunine**. Avoid. Severe Theoretical
▸ Rifamycins (rifampicin) are predicted to decrease the exposure to **vinorelbine**. Use with caution or avoid. Severe Theoretical
▸ Rifamycins (rifampicin) are predicted to decrease the exposure to vinca alkaloids (**vinblastine, vincristine, vindesine**). Severe Theoretical

Vincristine → see vinca alkaloids
Vindesine → see vinca alkaloids
Vinflunine → see vinca alkaloids
Vinorelbine → see vinca alkaloids
Vismodegib

▸ Anti-androgens (apalutamide, enzalutamide) are predicted to decrease the exposure to **vismodegib**. Avoid. Moderate Theoretical
▸ Antiepileptics (carbamazepine, fosphenytoin, phenobarbital, phenytoin, primidone) are predicted to decrease the exposure to **vismodegib**. Avoid. Moderate Theoretical
▸ Mitotane is predicted to decrease the exposure to **vismodegib**. Avoid. Moderate Theoretical
▸ Rifamycins (rifampicin) are predicted to decrease the exposure to **vismodegib**. Avoid. Moderate Theoretical
▸ St John's wort is predicted to decrease the exposure to **vismodegib**. Avoid. Moderate Theoretical

Vitamin A

▸ Retinoids (acitretin, alitretinoin, isotretinoin) are predicted to increase the risk of vitamin A toxicity when given with **vitamin A**. Avoid. Severe Theoretical
▸ Retinoids (bexarotene) are predicted to increase the risk of toxicity when given with **vitamin A**. Adjust dose. Moderate Theoretical
▸ Retinoids (tretinoin) are predicted to increase the risk of vitamin A toxicity when given with **vitamin A**. Avoid. Severe Study

Vitamin D substances

alfacalcidol · calcipotriol · calcitriol · colecalciferol · dihydrotachysterol · ergocalciferol · paricalcitol · tacalcitol

ROUTE-SPECIFIC INFORMATION Since systemic absorption can follow topical application, the possibility of interactions with topical **calcitriol** should be borne in mind.

▸ Antiepileptics (carbamazepine) are predicted to decrease the effects of **vitamin D substances**. Moderate Study
▸ Antiepileptics (fosphenytoin, phenytoin) decrease the effects of **vitamin D substances**. Moderate Study
▸ Antiepileptics (phenobarbital, primidone) are predicted to decrease the effects of **vitamin D substances**. Moderate Theoretical
▸ Antifungals, azoles (clotrimazole, ketoconazole) are predicted to decrease the exposure to **colecalciferol**. Moderate Theoretical
▸ Antifungals, azoles (itraconazole, ketoconazole, voriconazole) are predicted to increase the exposure to **paricalcitol**. Moderate Study
▸ Cobicistat is predicted to increase the exposure to **paricalcitol**. Moderate Study
▸ **Vitamin D substances** are predicted to increase the risk of toxicity when given with digoxin. Severe Theoretical
▸ HIV-protease inhibitors are predicted to increase the exposure to **paricalcitol**. Moderate Study
▸ Idelalisib is predicted to increase the exposure to **paricalcitol**. Moderate Study
▸ Macrolides (clarithromycin) are predicted to increase the exposure to **paricalcitol**. Moderate Study
▸ Thiazide diuretics increase the risk of hypercalcaemia when given with **vitamin D substances**. Moderate Theoretical

Vitamin E substances

▸ **Vitamin E substances** affect the exposure to ciclosporin. Moderate Study

Volanesorsen

▸ **Volanesorsen** potentially increases the risk of bleeding events when given with drugs with anticoagulant effects (see TABLE 3 p. 1429). Avoid depending on platelet count—consult product literature. Severe Theoretical

▸ **Volanesorsen** potentially increases the risk of bleeding events when given with drugs with antiplatelet effects (see TABLE 4 p. 1429). Avoid depending on platelet count—consult product literature. Severe Theoretical

Volatile halogenated anaesthetics → see TABLE 8 p. 1430 (hypotension), TABLE 9 p. 1431 (QT-interval prolongation), TABLE 11 p. 1431 (CNS depressant effects)

desflurane · isoflurane · methoxyflurane · sevoflurane

▸ Antiepileptics (phenobarbital, primidone) potentially increase the risk of nephrotoxicity when given with **methoxyflurane**. Avoid. Severe Theoretical → Also see TABLE 11 p. 1431
▸ Isoniazid potentially increases the risk of nephrotoxicity when given with **methoxyflurane**. Avoid. Severe Theoretical
▸ Rifamycins (rifampicin) potentially increase the risk of nephrotoxicity when given with **methoxyflurane**. Avoid. Severe Theoretical

Voriconazole → see antifungals, azoles
Vortioxetine → see TABLE 13 p. 1432 (serotonin syndrome), TABLE 4 p. 1429 (antiplatelet effects)

▸ Anti-androgens (apalutamide, enzalutamide) are predicted to decrease the exposure to **vortioxetine**. Monitor and adjust dose. Moderate Study
▸ Antiepileptics (carbamazepine, fosphenytoin, phenobarbital, phenytoin, primidone) are predicted to decrease the exposure to **vortioxetine**. Monitor and adjust dose. Moderate Study
▸ Bupropion is predicted to increase the exposure to **vortioxetine**. Monitor and adjust dose. Moderate Study → Also see TABLE 13 p. 1432
▸ Cinacalcet is predicted to increase the exposure to **vortioxetine**. Monitor and adjust dose. Moderate Study
▸ Mitotane is predicted to decrease the exposure to **vortioxetine**. Monitor and adjust dose. Moderate Study
▸ Rifamycins (rifampicin) are predicted to decrease the exposure to **vortioxetine**. Monitor and adjust dose. Moderate Study
▸ SSRIs (fluoxetine, paroxetine) are predicted to increase the exposure to **vortioxetine**. Monitor and adjust dose. Moderate Study → Also see TABLE 13 p. 1432 → Also see TABLE 4 p. 1429
▸ Terbinafine is predicted to increase the exposure to **vortioxetine**. Monitor and adjust dose. Moderate Study

Voxilaprevir

▸ Anti-androgens (apalutamide, enzalutamide) are predicted to decrease the concentration of **voxilaprevir**. Avoid. Severe Study
▸ Antiepileptics (carbamazepine, fosphenytoin, phenobarbital, phenytoin, primidone) are predicted to decrease the concentration of **voxilaprevir**. Avoid. Severe Study
▸ Antiepileptics (oxcarbazepine) are predicted to decrease the concentration of **voxilaprevir**. Avoid. Severe Theoretical
▸ Ciclosporin increases the concentration of **voxilaprevir**. Avoid. Severe Study
▸ Combined hormonal contraceptives (containing ethinylestradiol) are predicted to increase the risk of increased ALT concentrations when given with **voxilaprevir** (with sofosbuvir and velpatasvir). Avoid. Severe Study
▸ **Voxilaprevir** (with sofosbuvir and velpatasvir) is predicted to increase the exposure to digoxin. Monitor and adjust dose. Severe Theoretical
▸ Endothelin receptor antagonists (bosentan) are predicted to decrease the concentration of **voxilaprevir**. Avoid. Severe Theoretical
▸ **Voxilaprevir** (with sofosbuvir and velpatasvir) is predicted to increase the concentration of factor Xa inhibitors (edoxaban). Avoid. Severe Theoretical
▸ HIV-protease inhibitors (atazanavir) boosted with ritonavir increase the concentration of **voxilaprevir**. Severe Study
▸ HIV-protease inhibitors (lopinavir) boosted with ritonavir are predicted to increase the concentration of **voxilaprevir**. Avoid. Severe Theoretical
▸ HIV-protease inhibitors (tipranavir) boosted with ritonavir are predicted to increase the concentration of **voxilaprevir**. Severe Theoretical
▸ Mitotane is predicted to decrease the concentration of **voxilaprevir**. Avoid. Severe Study

Modafinil is predicted to decrease the concentration of **voxilaprevir**. Avoid. [Severe] Theoretical

NNRTIs (efavirenz, nevirapine) are predicted to decrease the concentration of **voxilaprevir**. Avoid. [Severe] Theoretical

Proton pump inhibitors are predicted to decrease the exposure to **voxilaprevir**. Adjust dose, see sofosbuvir with velpatasvir and voxilaprevir p. 669. [Moderate] Study

Rifamycins (rifabutin) are predicted to decrease the concentration of **voxilaprevir**. Avoid. [Severe] Theoretical

Rifamycins (rifampicin) are predicted to decrease the concentration of **voxilaprevir**. Avoid. [Severe] Study

St John's wort is predicted to decrease the concentration of **voxilaprevir**. Avoid. [Severe] Theoretical

Voxilaprevir (with sofosbuvir and velpatasvir) is predicted to increase the exposure to statins (atorvastatin). Adjust **atorvastatin** dose, p. 217. [Moderate] Theoretical

Voxilaprevir (with sofosbuvir and velpatasvir) is predicted to increase the exposure to statins (fluvastatin, simvastatin). Avoid. [Moderate] Theoretical

Voxilaprevir (with sofosbuvir and velpatasvir) moderately increases the exposure to statins (pravastatin). Monitor and adjust **pravastatin** dose. [Moderate] Study

Voxilaprevir (with sofosbuvir and velpatasvir) markedly increases the exposure to statins (rosuvastatin). Avoid. [Severe] Study

Voxilaprevir is predicted to increase the concentration of sulfasalazine. Avoid. [Severe] Theoretical

Voxilaprevir (with sofosbuvir and velpatasvir) potentially increases the concentration of tenofovir disoproxil. [Severe] Study

Voxilaprevir (with sofosbuvir and velpatasvir) increases the concentration of thrombin inhibitors (dabigatran). Avoid. [Severe] Study

Voxilaprevir is predicted to increase the concentration of topotecan. Avoid. [Severe] Theoretical

Warfarin → see coumarins

Wasp venom extract

> **GENERAL INFORMATION** Desensitising vaccines should be avoided in patients taking beta-blockers (adrenaline might be ineffective in case of a hypersensitivity reaction) or ACE inhibitors (risk of severe anaphylactoid reactions).

Xipamide → see thiazide diuretics

Xylometazoline → see sympathomimetics, vasoconstrictor

Yellow fever vaccine, live → see live vaccines

Zidovudine → see NRTIs

Zinc

> **ROUTE-SPECIFIC INFORMATION** Interactions do not generally apply to topical use unless specified.

▸ Oral **zinc** decreases the absorption of oral bisphosphonates (alendronate). Alendronate should be taken at least 30 minutes before **zinc** . [Moderate] Study

▸ Oral **zinc** decreases the absorption of oral bisphosphonates (clodronate). Avoid **zinc** for 2 hours before or 1 hour after **clodronate**. [Moderate] Study

▸ Oral **zinc** is predicted to decrease the absorption of oral bisphosphonates (ibandronate). Avoid **zinc** for at least 6 hours before or 1 hour after **ibandronate**. [Moderate] Theoretical

▸ Oral **zinc** decreases the absorption of oral bisphosphonates (risedronate). Separate administration by at least 2 hours. [Moderate] Study

▸ Oral calcium salts decrease the absorption of **zinc**. [Moderate] Study

▸ Oral **zinc** is predicted to decrease the absorption of eltrombopag. **Eltrombopag** should be taken 2 hours before or 4 hours after **zinc**. [Severe] Theoretical

▸ Oral **zinc** is predicted to decrease the efficacy of oral iron and oral iron is predicted to decrease the efficacy of oral **zinc**. [Moderate] Study

▸ Oral **zinc** is predicted to decrease the absorption of oral iron chelators (deferiprone). [Moderate] Theoretical

▸ **Zinc** is predicted to decrease the absorption of penicillamine. [Mild] Theoretical

▸ **Zinc** is predicted to decrease the exposure to quinolones. Separate administration by 2 hours. [Moderate] Study

▸ Oral **zinc** is predicted to decrease the absorption of tetracyclines. Separate administration by 2 to 3 hours. [Moderate] Theoretical

▸ Trientine potentially decreases the absorption of **zinc**. [Moderate] Theoretical

Zoledronate → see bisphosphonates

Zolmitriptan → see triptans

Zolpidem → see TABLE 11 p. 1431 (CNS depressant effects)

▸ Antiepileptics (carbamazepine) moderately decrease the exposure to **zolpidem**. [Moderate] Study

▸ Rifamycins (rifampicin) moderately decrease the exposure to **zolpidem**. [Moderate] Study

Zonisamide → see antiepileptics

Zopiclone → see TABLE 11 p. 1431 (CNS depressant effects)

▸ Anti-androgens (apalutamide, enzalutamide) are predicted to decrease the exposure to **zopiclone**. Adjust dose. [Moderate] Study

▸ Antiarrhythmics (dronedarone) are predicted to increase the exposure to **zopiclone**. Adjust dose. [Moderate] Study

▸ Antiepileptics (carbamazepine, fosphenytoin, phenobarbital, phenytoin, primidone) are predicted to decrease the exposure to **zopiclone**. Adjust dose. [Moderate] Study → Also see TABLE 11 p. 1431

▸ Antifungals, azoles (fluconazole, isavuconazole, posaconazole) are predicted to increase the exposure to **zopiclone**. Adjust dose. [Moderate] Study

▸ Antifungals, azoles (itraconazole, ketoconazole, voriconazole) are predicted to increase the exposure to **zopiclone**. Adjust dose. [Moderate] Theoretical

▸ Calcium channel blockers (diltiazem, verapamil) are predicted to increase the exposure to **zopiclone**. Adjust dose. [Moderate] Study

▸ Cobicistat is predicted to increase the exposure to **zopiclone**. Adjust dose. [Moderate] Theoretical

▸ Crizotinib is predicted to increase the exposure to **zopiclone**. Adjust dose. [Moderate] Study

▸ HIV-protease inhibitors are predicted to increase the exposure to **zopiclone**. Adjust dose. [Moderate] Theoretical

▸ Idelalisib is predicted to increase the exposure to **zopiclone**. Adjust dose. [Moderate] Theoretical

▸ Imatinib is predicted to increase the exposure to **zopiclone**. Adjust dose. [Moderate] Study

▸ Letermovir is predicted to increase the exposure to **zopiclone**. Adjust dose. [Moderate] Study

▸ Macrolides (clarithromycin) are predicted to increase the exposure to **zopiclone**. Adjust dose. [Moderate] Theoretical

▸ Macrolides (erythromycin) are predicted to increase the exposure to **zopiclone**. Adjust dose. [Moderate] Study

▸ Mitotane is predicted to decrease the exposure to **zopiclone**. Adjust dose. [Moderate] Study

▸ Neurokinin-1 receptor antagonists (aprepitant, netupitant) are predicted to increase the exposure to **zopiclone**. [Moderate] Study

▸ Nilotinib is predicted to increase the exposure to **zopiclone**. Adjust dose. [Moderate] Study

▸ Rifamycins (rifampicin) are predicted to decrease the exposure to **zopiclone**. Adjust dose. [Moderate] Study

Zuclopenthixol → see TABLE 8 p. 1430 (hypotension), TABLE 9 p. 1431 (QT-interval prolongation), TABLE 11 p. 1431 (CNS depressant effects)

▸ **Zuclopenthixol** is predicted to decrease the effects of dopamine receptor agonists. Avoid. [Moderate] Theoretical → Also see TABLE 8 p. 1430 → Also see TABLE 9 p. 1431

▸ **Zuclopenthixol** is predicted to decrease the effects of levodopa. Avoid or monitor worsening parkinsonian symptoms. [Severe] Theoretical → Also see TABLE 8 p. 1430

▸ **Zuclopenthixol** potentially increases the risk of neurotoxicity when given with lithium. [Severe] Anecdotal → Also see TABLE 9 p. 1431

A1

Interactions | Appendix 1

Appendix 2
Borderline substances

CONTENTS

In certain conditions some foods (and toilet preparations) have characteristics of drugs and the Advisory Committee on Borderline Substances (ACBS) advises as to the circumstances in which such substances may be regarded as drugs. Prescriptions issued in accordance with the Committee's advice and endorsed 'ACBS' will normally not be investigated.

Information

General Practitioners are reminded that the ACBS recommends products on the basis that they may be regarded as drugs for the management of specified conditions. Doctors should satisfy themselves that the products can safely be prescribed, that patients are adequately monitored and that, where necessary, expert hospital supervision is available.

Foods which may be prescribed on FP10, GP10 (Scotland), or WP10 (Wales)

All the food products listed in this appendix have ACBS approval. Some products may not be approved in all three countries. The clinical condition for which the product has been approved is included with each entry.
Note Foods included in this appendix may contain cariogenic sugars and patients should be advised to take appropriate oral hygiene measures.

Enteral feeds and supplements

For most enteral feeds and nutritional supplements, the main source of **carbohydrate** is either maltodextrin or glucose syrup; other carbohydrate sources are listed in the relevant table, below. Feeds containing residual lactose (less than 1 g lactose/100 mL formula) are described as 'clinically lactose-free' or 'lactose-free' by some manufacturers. The presence of lactose (including residual lactose) in feeds is indicated in the relevant table, below. The primary sources of **protein** or **amino acids** are included with each product entry. The **fat** or **oil** content is derived from a variety of sources such as vegetables, soya bean, corn, palm nuts, and seeds; where the fat content is derived from animal or fish sources, this information is included in the relevant table, below. The presence of medium chain triglycerides (MCT) is also noted where the quantity exceeds 30% of the fat content.

Enteral feeds and nutritional supplements can contain varying amounts of **vitamins**, **minerals**, and **trace elements**—the manufacturer's product literature should be consulted for more detailed information. Feeds containing vitamin K may affect the INR in patients receiving warfarin. The suitability of food products for patients requiring a vegan, kosher, halal, or other compliant diet should be confirmed with individual manufacturers.
Note Feeds containing more than 6 g/100 mL protein or 2 g/100 mL fibre should be avoided in children unless recommended by an appropriate specialist or dietician.

Nutritional values

Nutritional values of products vary with flavour and pack size—consult product literature.

Other conditions for which ACBS products can be prescribed

This is a list of clinical conditions for which the ACBS has approved toilet preparations.
Dermatitis, Eczema and Pruritus
Aveeno® Cream; *Aveeno*® Lotion; *E*45® Emollient Bath Oil; *E*45® Emollient Wash Cream
Disfiguring skin lesions (birthmarks, mutilating lesions, scars, vitiligo)
Covermark® classic foundation and finishing powder; *Dermacolor*® Camouflage cream and fixing powder; *Keromask*® finishing powder and masking cream; *Veil*® Cover cream and Finishing Powder. (Cleansing Creams, Cleansing Milks, and Cleansing Lotions are excluded).
Disinfectants (antiseptics)
May be prescribed on an FP10 only when ordered in such quantities and with such directions as are appropriate for the treatment of patients, but not if ordered for general hygienic purposes.
Dry mouth (xerostomia)
For patients suffering from dry mouth as a result of having (or having undergone) radiotherapy, or sicca syndrome. *AS Saliva Orthana*®; *Biotène Oralbalance*®; *Glandosane*®; *Saliveze*®
Photodermatoses (skin protection in)
LA Roche-Posay Anthelios® XL SPF 50+ cream; *Sunsense*® Ultra (Ego) SPF 50+; *Uvistat*® Lipscreen SPF 50, *Uvistat*® Suncream SPF 30 and 50

Standard ACBS indications: Disease-related malnutrition, intractable malabsorption, pre-operative preparation of malnourished patients, dysphagia, proven inflammatory bowel disease, following total gastrectomy, short-bowel syndrome, bowel fistula

Borderline substances | **Appendix 2**

A2

Table 1 Enteral feeds (non-disease specific)

Less than 5 g protein/100 mL

Enteral feeds: 1 kcal/mL and less than 5 g protein/100 mL

Not suitable for use in child under 3 years unless otherwise stated; not recommended for use in children unless otherwise stated

Product	Formulation	Energy	Protein	Carbohydrate	Fat	Fibre	Special Characteristics	ACBS Indications	Presentation & Flavour
Fresubin® 1500 Complete (Fresenius Kabi Ltd)	Liquid (tube feed) per 100 mL	420 kJ (100 kcal)	3.8 g milk, soya proteins	13 g (sugars 0.9 g)	3.4 g	1.5 g	Contains fish oil, residual lactose, soya. Gluten-free	Borderline substances standard ACBS indications p. 1623 except bowel fistula and pre-operative preparation of malnourished patients.	Fresubin 1500 Complete liquid: 1.5 litre = £15.00
Fresubin® Original (Fresenius Kabi Ltd)	Liquid (sip or tube feed) per 100 mL	420 kJ (100 kcal)	3.8 g cows' milk soya	13.8 g (sugars 3.5 g)	3.4 g	Nil	Gluten-free Residual lactose Contains milk gelatin Feed in flexible pack contains fish oil and fish gelatin	Borderline substances standard ACBS indications p. 1623	Fresubin Original drink: blackcurrant, chocolate, nut, peach, vanilla 200ml = £2.43; Fresubin Original tube feed liquid: 500 ml = £4.70; 1000 ml = £9.33; 1500 ml = £13.99
Fresubin® Original Fibre (Fresenius Kabi Ltd)	Liquid (tube feed) per 100 mL	420 kJ (100 kcal)	3.8 g milk, soya proteins	13.0 g (sugars 0.9 g)	3.4 g	1.5 g	Contains fish oil, residual lactose, soya. Gluten-free	Borderline substances standard ACBS indications p. 1623 except bowel fistula and pre-operative preparation of malnourished patients.	Fresubin Original Fibre liquid: 500 ml = £5.33; 1000 ml = £10.64
Jevity® (Abbott Laboratories Ltd)	Liquid (tube feed) per 100 mL	449 kJ (107 kcal)	4 g caseinates	14.1 g (sugars 0.25 g)	3.47 g	1.76 g	Contains residual lactose, soya. Gluten-free	Borderline substances standard ACBS indications p. 1623 except bowel fistula.	Jevity liquid: 500 ml = £5.98; 1000 ml = £11.28; 1500 ml = £16.89
Nutrison® (Nutricia Ltd)	Liquid (tube feed) per 100 mL	420 kJ (100 kcal)	4 g cow's milk, pea, soya, whey proteins	12.3 g (sugars 0.7 g)	3.9 g	Trace	Contains fish oil, residual lactose, soya. Gluten-free Residual lactose	Borderline substances standard ACBS indications p. 1623.	Nutrison liquid: 500 ml = £5.55; 1000 ml = £9.75; 1500 ml = £14.63
Nutrison® Multi Fibre (Nutricia Ltd)	Liquid (tube feed) per 100 mL	430 kJ (103 kcal)	4 g caseinate, pea, soya, whey proteins	12.3 g (sugars 0.8 g)	3.9 g	1.5 g	Contains fish oil, residual lactose, soya. Gluten-free	Borderline substances standard ACBS indications p. 1623.	Nutrison Multi Fibre liquid: 500 ml = £6.00; 1000 ml = £11.30; 1500 ml = £16.92
Osmolite® (Abbott Laboratories Ltd)	Liquid (tube feed) per 100 mL	424 kJ (101 kcal)	4 g caseinates, soya protein isolate	13.6 g (sugars 0.6 g)	3.4 g	Nil	Contains residual lactose, soya. Gluten-free	Borderline substances standard ACBS indications p. 1623.	Osmolite liquid: 500 ml = £5.54; 1000 ml = £9.73; 1500 ml = £14.60

SOYA PROTEIN FORMULA

Not suitable for use in child under 3 years unless otherwise stated; not recommended for child under 6 years

Product	Formulation	Energy	Protein	Carbohydrate	Fat	Fibre	Special Characteristics	ACBS Indications	Presentation & Flavour
Fresubin® Soya Fibre (Fresenius Kabi Ltd)	Liquid (tube feed) per 100 mL	420 kJ (100 kcal)	3.8g soya protein	12.1 g (sugars 4.1 g)	3.6 g	2 g	Contains fish oil, soya. Gluten-free. Lactose-free.	Borderline substances standard ACBS indications p. 1623 except dysphagia. Also cows' milk protein intolerance, lactose intolerance.	Fresubin Soya Fibre liquid: 500 ml = £5.51
Nutrison® Soya (Nutricia Ltd)	Liquid (tube feed) per 100 mL	420 kJ (100 kcal)	4 g soya protein isolate	12.3 g (sugars 1 g)	3.9 g	Nil	Contains residual lactose, soya. Gluten-free.	Borderline substances standard ACBS indications p. 1623; also cow's milk protein and lactose intolerance.	Nutrison Soya liquid: 500 ml = £5.99; 1000 ml = £12.01
Nutrison® Soya Multi Fibre (Nutricia Ltd)	Liquid (tube feed) per 100 mL	430 kJ (103 kcal)	4 g soya protein	12.3 g (sugars 0.7 g)	3.9 g	1.5 g	Contains residual lactose, soya. Gluten-free.	Borderline substances standard ACBS indications p. 1623; also cows' milk protein and lactose intolerance.	Nutrison Soya Multi Fibre liquid: 1.5 litre = £19.97

PEPTIDE-BASED FORMULA

Not suitable for use in child under 3 years unless otherwise stated; not recommended for child under 6 years

Product	Formulation	Energy	Protein	Carbohydrate	Fat	Fibre	Special Characteristics	ACBS Indications	Presentation & Flavour
Nutrison® Peptisorb (Nutricia Ltd)	Liquid (tube feed) per 100 mL	425 kJ (100 kcal)	4 g whey protein hydrolysate	17.6 g (sugars 1.7 g)	1.7 g (MCT 47 %)	Nil	Contains residual lactose, soya. Gluten-free	Borderline substances standard ACBS indications p. 1623; also growth failure.	Nutrison Peptisorb liquid: 500 ml = £8.74; 1000 ml = £15.76
Peptamen® (Nestle Health Science)	Liquid (sip or tube feed) per 100 mL	420 kJ (100 kcal)	4 g whey peptides	12.7 g (sugars 480 mg)	3.7 g (MCT 70 %)	Nil	Gluten-free. Residual lactose	Short bowel syndrome, intractable malabsorption, proven inflammatory bowel disease, bowel fistula	Peptamen liquid: unflavoured 500 ml = £7.52; 1000 ml = £14.12; vanilla 800 ml = £13.38
Survimed® OPD (Fresenius Kabi Ltd)	Liquid (sip or tube feed) per 100 mL	420 kJ (100 kcal)	4.5-4.7 g whey protein hydrolysate	14.1-14.3 g (sugars 1.1-5 g)	2.8 g (MCT 48-51%)	less than or equal to 0.1 g	Contains fish oil (tube feed only), residual lactose. Gluten-free	Borderline substances standard ACBS indications p. 1623; also growth failure.	Survimed OPD liquid: 500 ml = £7.86; 800 ml = £13.56; 1000 ml = £15.72

Enteral feeds (non-disease specific); 5 g (or more) protein/100 mL

Enteral feeds: 1.5 kcal/mL and 5 g (or more) protein/100 mL

Not suitable for use in child under 3 years unless otherwise stated; not recommended for use in children unless otherwise stated

Product	Formulation	Energy	Protein	Carbohydrate	Fat	Fibre	Special Characteristics	ACBS Indications	Presentation & Flavour
Fresubin® 2250 Complete (Fresenius Kabi Ltd)	Liquid (tube feed) per 100 mL	630 kJ (150 kcal)	5.6 g milk, soya proteins	18 g (sugars 1.2 g)	5.8 g	1.5 g	Contains fish oil, residual lactose, soya. Gluten-free	Borderline substances standard ACBS indications p. 1623	Fresubin 2250 Complete liquid: 1.5 litre = £16.75
Fresubin® Energy (Fresenius Kabi Ltd)	Liquid (sip or tube feed) per 100 mL	630 kJ (150 kcal)	5.6 g milk, whey proteins	18.8 g (sugars 1.1-6.3)	5.8 g	Nil	Contains fish oil, residual lactose, soya. Gluten-free	Borderline substances standard ACBS indications p. 1623.	Fresubin Energy liquid unflavoured: 200 ml = £1.40; 500 ml = £6.27; 1000 ml = £11.80; 1500 ml = £16.99
Fresubin® Energy Fibre Tube Feed (Fresenius Kabi Ltd)	Liquid (tube feed) per 100 mL	630 kJ (150 kcal)	5.6 g milk, soya proteins	18 g (sugars 1.2 g)	5.8 g	1.5 g	Contains fish oil, residual lactose, soya. Gluten-free	Borderline substances standard ACBS indications p. 1623.	Fresubin Energy Fibre liquid unflavoured: 500 ml = £6.97; 1000 ml = £13.14; 1500 ml = £15.68
Fresubin® HP Energy (Fresenius Kabi Ltd)	Liquid (tube feed) per 100 mL	630 kJ (150 kcal)	7.5 g milk protein	17 g (sugars 1 g)	5.8 g (MCT 57 %)	Nil	Contains fish oil, residual lactose, soya. Gluten-free	Borderline substances standard ACBS indications p. 1623; also CAPD and haemodialysis.	Fresubin HP Energy liquid: 500 ml = £6.45; 1000 ml = £12.16

Borderline substances | **Appendix 2**

Enteral feeds (non-disease specific); 5 g (or more) protein/100 mL (product list continued)

Enteral feeds: 1.5 kcal/mL and 5 g (or more) protein/100 mL

Not suitable for use in child under 3 years unless otherwise stated; not recommended for use in children unless otherwise stated

Product	Formulation	Energy	Protein	Carbohydrate	Fat	Fibre	Special Characteristics	ACBS Indications	Presentation & Flavour
Fresubin® HP Energy Fibre (Fresenius Kabi Ltd)	Liquid (tube feed) per 100 mL	630 kJ (150 kcal)	7.5 g milk protein	16.2 g (sugars 1.11 g)	5.8 g (MCT 57%)	1.5 g	Contains fish oil, residual lactose, soya. Gluten-free	Borderline substances standard ACBS indications p. 1623 except dysphagia. Also CAPD and haemodialysis.	Fresubin HP Energy Fibre liquid: 500 ml = £7.18; 1000 ml = £13.63
Jevity® 1.5kcal (Abbott Laboratories Ltd)	Liquid (tube feed) per 100 mL	649 kJ (154 kcal)	6.38 g caseinates, soya protein isolate	20.1 g (sugars 1.3 g)	4.9 g	2.2 g	Contains residual lactose, soya. Gluten-free	Borderline substances standard ACBS indications p. 1623.	Jevity 1.5kcal liquid: 500 ml = £7.16; 1000 ml = £13.50; 1500 ml = £20.83
Nutrison® Energy (Nutricia Ltd)	Liquid (tube feed) per 100 mL	630 kJ (150 kcal)	6 g caseinate, pea, soya, whey proteins	18.3 g (sugars 1.1 g)	5.8 g	Nil	Contains fish oil, residual lactose, soya. Gluten-free	Borderline substances standard ACBS indications p. 1623	Nutrison Energy liquid: 500 ml = £6.47; 1000 ml = £12.17; 1500 ml = £18.21
Nutrison® Energy Multi Fibre (Nutricia Ltd)	Liquid (tube feed) per 100 mL	640 kJ (153 kcal)	6 g caseinates, pea, soya, whey proteins	18.4 g (sugars 2.4 g)	5.8 g	1.5 g	Contains residual lactose, soya. Gluten-free	Borderline substances standard ACBS indications p. 1623.	Nutrison Energy Multi Fibre liquid: 500 ml = £7.18; 1000 ml = £13.51; 1500 ml = £20.86
Nutrison® Peptisorb Plus HEHP (Nutricia Ltd)	Liquid (tube feed) per 100 ml	631 kJ (150 kcal)	7.5 g whey protein hydrolysate	18.7 g (sugars 1.4 g)	5 g (MCT 60%)	Less than 0.5 g	Contains residual lactose, soya. Gluten-free	Borderline substances standard ACBS indications p. 1623 except dysphagia.	Nutrison Peptisorb Plus HEHP liquid: 500 ml = £8.93; 1000 ml = £16.81
Nutrison® Protein Plus Energy (Nutricia Ltd)	Liquid (tube feed) per 100 mL	630 kJ (150 kcal)	7.5 g caseinates, pea, soya, whey proteins	16.9 g (sugars 3.3)	5.8 g	Less than 0.1 g	Contains fish oil, residual lactose, soya. Gluten-free	Borderline substances standard ACBS indications p. 1623.	Nutrison Protein Plus Energy liquid: 500 ml = £6.47; 1000 ml = £12.18
Osmolite® 1.5kcal (Abbott Laboratories Ltd)	Liquid (tube feed) per 100 mL	634 kJ (151 kcal)	6.3 g caseinates, soya protein isolate	20.4 g (sugars 1.2 g)	4.9 g	Nil	Contains residual lactose, soya. Gluten-free	Borderline substances standard ACBS indications p. 1623; also continuous ambulatory peritoneal dialysis (CAPD), and haemodialysis.	Osmolite 1.5kcal tube feed liquid: 500 ml = £6.44; 1000 ml = £12.15; 1500 ml = £18.18
Vital 1.5 kcal (Abbott Laboratories Ltd)	Liquid (sip or tube feed) per 100 mL	631 kJ (150 kcal)	6.75 g caseinate whey protein hydrolysate	18.4 g (sugars 3.6 g)	5.5 g (MCT 64%)	Nil	Gluten-free Residual lactose	Borderline substances standard ACBS indications p. 1623; except proven inflammatory bowel disease and following total gastrectomy; not recommended for use in children	Vital 1.5kcal liquid vanilla: 200 ml = £3.37; 1000 ml = £17.26

Enteral feeds: Less than 1.5 kcal/mL and 5 g (or more) protein/100 mL

Not suitable for use in child under 6 years unless otherwise stated; not recommended for use in children unless otherwise stated

Product	Formulation	Energy	Protein	Carbohydrate	Fat	Fibre	Special Characteristics	ACBS Indications	Presentation & Flavour
Fresubin® 1000 Complete (Fresenius Kabi Ltd)	Liquid (tube feed) per 100 mL	418 kJ (100 kcal)	5.5 g milk protein	12.5 g (sugars 1.1 g)	2.7 g	2 g	Contains fish oil, residual lactose, soya. Gluten-free	Borderline substances standard ACBS indications p. 1623	Fresubin 1000 Complete liquid: 1 litre = £12.07
Fresubin® 1200 Complete (Fresenius Kabi Ltd)	Liquid (tube feed) per 100 mL	504 kJ (120 kcal)	6 g milk protein	14 g (sugars 1.17 g)	4.1 g	2 g	Contains fish oil, residual lactose, soya. Gluten-free	Borderline substances standard ACBS indications p. 1623 except dysphagia.	Fresubin 1200 Complete liquid: 1 litre = £15.36
Fresubin® 1800 Complete (Fresenius Kabi Ltd)	Liquid (tube feed) per 100 mL	504 kJ (120 kcal)	6 g milk protein	14 g (sugars 1.17 g)	4.1 g	2 g	Contains fish oil, residual lactose, soya. Gluten-free	Borderline substances standard ACBS indications p. 1623 except dysphagia.	Fresubin 1800 Complete liquid: 1.5 litre = £15.36
Jevity® Plus (Abbott Laboratories Ltd)	Liquid (tube feed) per 100 mL	514 kJ (122 kcal)	5.6 g caseinates, soya protein isolate	15.1 g (sugars 0.8 g)	3.9 g	2.2 g	Contains residual lactose, soya. Gluten-free	Borderline substances standard ACBS indications p. 1623.	Jevity Plus liquid: 500 ml = £7.17; 1000 ml = £13.07; 1500 ml = £19.54
Jevity® Plus HP (Abbott Laboratories Ltd)	Liquid (tube feed) per 100 mL	551 kJ (131 kcal)	8.1 g casinates, milk, soya protein isolates	14.2 g (sugars 0.7 g)	4.3 g	1.5 g	Contains residual lactose, soya. Gluten-free	Borderline substances standard ACBS Indications p. 1623; also CAPD, haemodialysis.	Jevity Plus HP gluten free liquid: 500 ml = £7.03
Jevity® Promote (Abbott Laboratories Ltd)	Liquid (tube feed) per 100 mL	434 kJ (103 kcal)	5.6 g caseinates, soya protein isolate	12.0 g (sugars 0.5 g)	3.3 g	1.7 g	Contains residual lactose, soya. Gluten-free	Borderline substances standard ACBS indications p. 1623.	Jevity Promote liquid: 1 litre = £12.50
Nutrison® 800 Complete Multi Fibre (Nutricia Ltd)	Liquid (tube feed) per 100 mL	345 kJ (83 kcal)	5.5 g caseinate, pea, soya, whey proteins	8.8 g (sugars 0.6 g)	2.5 g	1.5 g	Contains fish oil, residual lactose, soya. Gluten-free	Borderline substances standard ACBS indications p. 1623 except bowel fistula.	Nutrison 800 Complete Multi Fibre liquid: 1 litre = £11.81
Nutrison® 1000 Complete Multi Fibre (Nutricia Ltd)	Liquid (tube feed) per 100 mL	440 kJ (104 kcal)	5.5 g caseinate, pea, soya, whey proteins	11.3 g (sugars 0.8 g)	3.7 g	2 g	Contains fish oil, residual lactose, soya. Gluten-free	Disease related malnutrition in patients with low energy and/or low fluid requirements.	Nutrison 1000 Complete Multi Fibre liquid: 1 litre = £12.54
Nutrison® 1200 Complete Multi Fibre (Nutricia Ltd)	Liquid (tube feed) per 100 mL	525 kJ (124 kcal)	5.5 g caseinates, pea, soya, whey proteins	15 g (sugars 1 g)	4.3 g	2 g	Contains fish oil, residual lactose, soya. Gluten-free	Borderline substances standard ACBS indications p. 1623 except bowel fistula.	Nutrison 1200 Complete Multi Fibre liquid: 1000 ml = £13.26; 1500 ml = £19.91
Nutrison® MCT (Nutricia Ltd)	Liquid (tube feed) per 100 mL	420 kJ (100 kcal)	5 g caseinates	12.6 g (sugars 1 g)	3.3 g (MCT 61%)	Nil	Contains residual lactose, soya. Gluten-free	Borderline substances standard ACBS indications p. 1623.	Nutrison MCT liquid: 1000 ml = £11.29

A2

A2

Borderline substances | Appendix 2

Enteral feeds: Less than 1.5 kcal/mL and 5 g (or more) protein/100 mL (product list continued)

Not suitable for use in child under 6 years unless otherwise stated; not recommended for use in children unless otherwise stated

Product	Formulation	Energy	Protein	Carbohydrate	Fat	Fibre	Special Characteristics	ACBS Indications	Presentation & Flavour
Nutrison® Protein Plus (Nutricia Ltd)	Liquid (tube feed) per 100 mL	525 kJ (125 kcal)	6.3 g caseinates, pea, soya, whey proteins	14.2 g (sugars 0.9 g)	4.9 g	less than 0.1 g	Contains fish oil, residual lactose, soya. Gluten-free	Disease related malnutrition.	Nutrison Protein Plus liquid: 500 ml = £5.98; 1 litre = £11.59
Nutrison® Protein Plus Multifibre (Nutricia Ltd)	Liquid (tube feed) per 100 mL	535 kJ (128 kcal)	6.3 g caseinates, pea, soya, whey proteins	14.1 g (sugars 1 g)	4.9 g	1.5 g	Contains fish oil, residual lactose, soya. Gluten-free	Disease related malnutrition.	Nutrison Protein Plus Multifibre liquid: 500 ml = £6.66; 1 litre = £12.92
Osmolite® Plus (Abbott Laboratories Ltd)	Liquid (tube feed) per 100 mL	508 kJ (121 kcal)	5.6 g caseinates	15.8 g (sugars 0.4 g)	3.9 g	Nil	Contains residual lactose, soya. Gluten-free	Borderline substances standard ACBS indications p. 1623.	Osmolite Plus liquid: 500 ml = £6.02; 1000 ml = £10.95
Peptamen® HN (Nestle Health Science)	Liquid (tube feed) per 100 mL	556 kJ (133 kcal)	6.6 g whey protein hydrolysates	15.6 g (sugars 1.4 g)	4.9 g (MCT 70%)	Nil	Gluten-free Residual lactose Hydrolysed with pork trypsin	Short bowel syndrome, intractable malabsorption, proven inflammatory bowel disease, bowel fistula Not suitable for child under 3 years	Peptamen HN liquid: 500 ml = £8.09; 1000 ml = £15.20
Perative® (Abbott Laboratories Ltd)	Liquid (sip or tube feed) per 100 mL	552 kJ (131 kcal)	6.7 g caseinates, whey protein hydrolysate	17.7 g (sugars 0.5 g)	3.7 g (MCT 37%)	Nil	Contains residual lactose, soya. Gluten-free	Borderline substances standard ACBS indications p. 1623 except dysphagia.	Perative liquid: 500 ml = £8.52; 1000 ml = £15.73
Survimed® OPD HN (Fresenius Kabi Ltd)	Liquid (tube feed) per 100 mL	560 kJ (133 kcal)	6.7 g whey protein hydrolysate	18.3 g (sugars 1.3 g)	3.7 g (MCT 52%)	less than or equal to 0.1 g	Contains fish oil, residual lactose. Gluten-free	Borderline substances standard ACBS indications p. 1623; also haemodialysis and continuous ambulatory peritoneal dialysis.	Survimed OPD HN liquid: 500 ml = £7.57

Enteral feeds: More than 1.5 kcal/mL and 5 g (or more) protein/100 mL

Not suitable for use in child under 1 year; not recommended for use in children unless otherwise stated

Product	Formulation	Energy	Protein	Carbohydrate	Fat	Fibre	Special Characteristics	ACBS Indications	Presentation & Flavour
Fresubin® 2kcal HP (Fresenius Kabi Ltd)	Liquid (tube feed) per 100 mL	840 kJ (200 kcal)	10 g milk protein	17.5 g (sugars 2.5 g)	10 g	Nil	Contains fish oil, residual lactose, soya. Gluten-free	Borderline substances standard ACBS indications p. 1623.	Fresubin 2kcal HP tube liquid feed: 500 ml = £7.87
Fresubin® 2kcal HP Fibre (Fresenius Kabi Ltd)	Liquid per 100 mL	840 kJ (200 kcal)	10 g milk protein	16.7 g (sugars 2.5 g)	10 g	1.5 g	Contains fish oil, residual lactose, soya. Gluten-free	Borderline substances standard ACBS indications p. 1623.	Fresubin 2kcal HP Fibre tube feed liquid: 500 ml = £9.43
TwoCal® (Abbott Laboratories Ltd)	Liquid (tube feed) per 100 mL	837 kJ (200 kcal)	8.4 g casein, milk protein isolate	21 g hydrolysed corn starch (sugars 4.7 g)	8.9 g	1 g	Contains residual lactose, soya. Gluten-free	Adults with or at risk of disease-related malnutrition, catabolic or fluid-restricted patients, and other patients requiring a 2kcal/mL feed.	TwoCal liquid: 200 ml = £3.19; 1 litre = £17.66

Table 2 Nutritional supplements (non-disease specific)

Nutritional supplements: less than 5 g protein/100 mL

Nutritional supplements: 1 kcal/mL and less than 5 g protein/100 mL

Not suitable for use in child under 1 year; not recommended for use in children unless otherwise stated

Product	Formulation	Energy	Protein	Carbohydrate	Fat	Fibre	Special Characteristics	ACBS Indications	Presentation & Flavour
Elemental 028® Extra liquid (Nutricia Ltd)	Liquid (sip feed) per 100 mL	360 kJ (86 kcal)	2.5 g protein equivalent (essential and nonessential amino acids)	11 g (sugars 4.7 g)	3.5 g (MCT 35%)	Nil	Gluten free, lactose-free	Short bowel syndrome, intractable malabsorption, proven inflammatory bowel disease, bowel fistula.	Elemental 028 Extra liquid: grapefruit, orange & pineapple, summer fruits 250 ml = £4.21
Elemental 028® Extra powder (Nutricia Ltd)	Standard dilution (20% w/v) of powder per 100 mL	374 kJ (89 kcal)	2.5 g protein equivalent (essential and nonessential amino acids)	12 g (sugars 1.1 g)	3.5 g (MCT 35%)	Nil	Gluten-free, lactose-free	Short bowel syndrome, intractable malabsorption, proven inflammatory bowel disease, bowel fistula.	Elemental 028 Extra powder: banana, orange, plain 100 g = £8.19
Powder provides: protein 12.5 g, carbohydrate 59 g, fat 17.5 g, energy 1871 kJ (443 kcal)/100 g									
Emsogen® (Nutricia Ltd)	Standard dilution (20 % w/v) of powder per 100 mL	368 kJ (88 kcal)	2.5 g protein equivalent (essential and nonessential amino acids)	12.0 g (sugars 1.6 g)	3.3 g (MCT 83 %)	Nil		Short-bowel syndrome, intractable malabsorption, proven inflammatory bowel disease, bowel fistula.	Emsogen powder unflavoured: 100 gram = £8.43
Powder provides: protein 12.5 g, carbohydrate 60.0 g, fat 16.4 g, energy 1839 kJ (438 kcal)/100 g									
Ensure® (Abbott Laboratories Ltd)	Liquid (sip or tube feed) per 100 mL	423 kJ (100 kcal)	4 g caseinates, soya protein isolate	13.6 g (sugars 3.8 g)	3.4 g	Nil	Contains residual lactose, soya. Gluten-free.	Disease-related malnutrition, intractable malabsorption, total gastrectomy, proven inflammatory bowel disease, and pre-operative preparation of patients who are undernourished.	Ensure liquid: chocolate, coffee, vanilla 250 ml = £2.45

Borderline substances | **Appendix 2**

A2

Nutritional supplements: More than 1 kcal/mL and less than 5 g protein/100 mL

Not suitable for use in child under 3 years; not recommended for use in child under 6 years unless otherwise stated

Product	Formulation	Energy	Protein	Carbohydrate	Fat	Fibre	Special Characteristics	ACBS Indications	Presentation & Flavour
Aymes® Shake Extra (Aymes International Ltd)	Powder per 100 g	2090 kJ (499 kcal)	4.8 g milk protein	62.9 g (sugar 22.4 g)	25.3 g	0.4 g	Contains lactose, soya. Gluten-free	Borderline substances standard ACBS indications p. 1623 except dysphagia.	Aymes Shake Extra Starter Pack powder: 4 sachet = £8.96; Aymes Shake Extra powder 85g sachets: banana, chocolate, strawberry, vanilla 6 sachet = £11.76
									Powder 85 g reconstituted with 240 ml milk provides: protein 12.4 g, carbohydrate 64.8 g, fat 31.3 g, energy 2462 kJ (589 kcal)
Ensure® Plus Juce (Abbott Laboratories Ltd)	Liquid (sip feed) per 100 mL	638 kJ (150 kcal)	4.8 g whey protein isolate	32.7 g (sugars 9.4 g)	Nil	Nil	Gluten-free Residual lactose Non-milk taste	Borderline substances standard ACBS indications p. 1623	Ensure Plus Juce liquid: apple, fruit punch, lemon & lime, orange, peach, strawberry 220 ml = £1.97
Fortijuce® (Nutricia Ltd)	Liquid (sip feed) per 100 mL	635 kJ (150 kcal)	3.9 g milk protein	33.5 g (sugars 13.1 g)	Nil	Nil	Contains residual lactose. Gluten-free.	Borderline substances standard ACBS indications p. 1623.	Fortijuce Starter Pack liquid: 800 ml = £8.08; Fortisip Range Starter Pack liquid: 2 litre = £20.20. Fortijuce liquid: apple, blackcurrant, forest fruits, lemon, orange, strawberry, tropical 200 ml = £2.02
Fresubin® Jucy (Fresenius Kabi Ltd)	Liquid (sip feed) per 100 mL	630 kJ (150 kcal)	4 g whey protein	33.5 g (sugars 8 g)	Nil	Nil	Contains residual lactose. Gluten-free.	Borderline substances standard ACBS indications p. 1623; also CAPD and haemodialysis.	Fresubin Jucy drink: apple, blackcurrant, cherry, orange, pineapple 800 ml = £8.04

Nutritional supplements: 5 g (or more) protein/100 mL

Nutritional supplements: 1.5 kcal/mL and 5 g (or more) protein/100 mL

Not suitable for use in child under 3 years unless otherwise stated; not recommended for use in children unless otherwise stated

Product	Formulation	Energy	Protein	Carbohydrate	Fat	Fibre	Special Characteristics	ACBS Indications	Presentation & Flavour
Altraplen® Protein (Nualtra Ltd)	Liquid (sip feed) per 100 mL	632 kJ (150 kcal)	10 g milk, soya proteins	15 g (sugars 4.6 g)	5.6 g	Nil	Contains residual lactose, soya. Gluten-free	Borderline substances standard ACBS indications p. 1623.	Altraplen Protein Starter Pack liquid: 400 ml = £3.29; strawberry, vanilla 800 ml = £6.78
Aymes® ActaCal Creme (Aymes International Ltd)	Semi-solid per 100 g	632 kJ (150 kcal)	7.5 g caseinates, milk protein	19 g (sugars 8.1 g)	4.9 g	Nil	Contains residual lactose. Gluten-free.	Borderline substances standard ACBS indications p. 1623 except dysphagia.	Aymes ActaCal Creme dessert: chocolate, vanilla 500 gram = £4.68
Aymes® Complete (Aymes International Ltd)	Liquid per 100 mL	630 kJ (150 kcal)	6 g milk protein	18 g (sugars 6.8 g)	6 g	Nil	Contains residual lactose. Gluten-free.	Borderline substances standard ACBS indications p. 1623.	Aymes Complete Starter Pack liquid: 800 ml = £5.60; Aymes Complete liquid: banana, chocolate, strawberry, vanilla 800 ml = £4.20
Ensure® Plus Advance (Abbott Laboratories Ltd)	Liquid (sip or tube feed) per 100 mL	631 kJ (150 kcal)	9.1 g caseinates, milk protein isolate, soya protein isolate, whey protein.	16.8 g sucrose (sugars 6.8 g)	4.8 g	0.75 g	Contains soya. Gluten-free	Frail elderly people (this is defined as older than 65 years with BMI less than or equal to 23 kg/m2 where clinical assessment and nutritional screening show the individual to be at risk of undernutrition).	Ensure Plus Advance liquid: banana, chocolate, coffee, strawberry, vanilla 220 ml = £2.20

Product	Formulation	Energy	Protein	Carbohydrate	Fat	Fibre	Special characteristics	Borderline substances/ACBS indications	Flavours, pack size and price
Ensure® Plus Commence (Abbott Laboratories Ltd)	Starter pack (5–10 day's supply), contains Ensure® Plus Commence (assorted flavours), 1 pack (10 x 200 ml) = £11.10								
Ensure® Plus Milkshake style (Abbott Laboratories Ltd)	Liquid (sip or tube feed) per 100 mL	632 kJ (150 kcal)	6.25 g cows' milk soya protein isolate	20.2 g (sugars 6.89 g)	4.92 g	Nil	Gluten-free Residual lactose	Borderline substances standard ACBS indications p. 1623; also CAPD, haemodialysis	Ensure Plus milkshake style liquid: banana, chocolate, coffee, fruits of the forest, neutral, peach, raspberry, strawberry, vanilla 200 ml = £1.11
Ensure® Plus Yoghurt style (Abbott Laboratories Ltd)	Liquid (sip feed) per 100 mL	632 kJ (150 kcal)	6.25 g cows' milk	20.2 g (sugars 11.7 g)	4.92 g	Nil	Gluten-free Residual lactose	Borderline substances standard ACBS indications p. 1623; also CAPD, haemodialysis	Ensure Plus yoghurt style liquid: orchard peach, strawberry swirl 200 ml = £1.14
Fortisip® Bottle (Nutricia Ltd)	Liquid (sip feed) per 100 mL	625 kJ (150 kcal)	5.9 g milk proteins	18.4 g (sugars 6.7 g)	5.8 g	Nil	Contains residual lactose, soya. Gluten free	Borderline substances standard ACBS indications p. 1623	Fortisip Bottle: banana, caramel, chocolate, neutral, orange, strawberry, tropical, vanilla, 200 ml = £1.12; Fortisip Range Starter Pack liquid: 2 litre = £20.20
Fortisip® Yogurt Style (Nutricia Ltd)	Liquid (sip feed) per 100 mL	630 kJ (150 kcal)	5.9 g cow's milk, whey protein	18.7 g (sugars 10.8 g)	5.8 g	Nil	Contains lactose, soya. Gluten-free	Borderline substances standard ACBS indications p. 1623	Fortisip Range Starter Pack liquid: 2 litre = £20.20; Fortisip Yogurt Style liquid: peach & orange, raspberry, vanilla and lemon 200 ml = £2.28
Fresubin® Energy Drink (Fresenius Kabi Ltd)	Liquid (sip feed) per 100 mL	630 kJ (150 kcal)	5.6 g milk protein	18.8 g (sugars 3.9-6.3 g)	5.8 g	Nil	Contains residual lactose, soya. Gluten-free.	Borderline substances standard ACBS indications p. 1623.	Fresubin Energy liquid: banana, blackcurrant, cappuccino, chocolate, lemon, strawberry, tropical fruits, vanilla 200 ml = £1.40
Fresubin® Energy Fibre Drink (Fresenius Kabi Ltd)	Liquid (sip feed) per 100 mL	630 kJ (150 kcal)	5.6 g milk protein	17.8 g (sugars 5-6.4 g)	5.8 g	2 g	Contains residual lactose, soya. Gluten-free.	Borderline substances standard ACBS indications p. 1623.	Fresubin Energy Fibre liquid: banana, caramel, cherry, chocolate, strawberry, vanilla 200 ml = £2.23
Fresubin® Protein Energy (Fresenius Kabi Ltd)	Liquid (sip feed) per 100 mL	630 kJ (150 kcal)	10 g milk protein	12.1-12.4 g maltodextrin and sucrose (sugars 6.5-7.4 g)	6.7 g	Nil	Contains residual lactose, soya. Gluten-free	Borderline substances standard ACBS indications p. 1623; also CAPD, haemodialysis.	Fresubin Protein Energy drink: cappuccino, chocolate, tropical fruits, vanilla, wild strawberry 200 ml = £2.15
Fresubin® Thickened (Fresenius Kabi Ltd)	Liquid (sip feed) per 100 mL	630 kJ (150 kcal)	10 g milk protein	12 g sucrose (sugars 6.6-7.3 g)	6.7 g	0.83 g	Contains soya, residual lactose. Fresubin® Thickened Level 2 is gluten-free	Dysphagia or disease-related malnutrition.	Fresubin Thickened Level 2: vanilla, wild strawberry 800 ml = £9.40; Fresubin Thickened Level 3: vanilla, wild strawberry 800 ml = £9.40
Fresubin® YOcrème (Fresenius Kabi Ltd)	Semi-solid per 100 g	630 kJ (150 kcal)	7.5 g whey protein	19.5 g (sugars 16.8 g)	4.7 g	Nil	Gluten-free Contains lactose	Dysphagia, or presence or risk of malnutrition Not suitable for child under 3 years	Fresubin YOcrème dessert: apricot-peach, biscuit, lemon, raspberry 500 gram = £8.68
Resource® Energy (Nestlé Health Science)	Liquid (sip feed) per 100 mL	637 kJ (151 kcal)	5.6 g milk protein	21 g (sugars 5.7 g)	5 g	Nil	Contains residual lactose, soya. Gluten-free	Borderline substances standard ACBS indications p. 1623 except bowel fistula.	Resource Energy liquid: apricot, chocolate, coffee, strawberry & raspberry, vanilla 800 ml = £8.45

Borderline substances | **Appendix 2**

Nutritional supplements: Less than 1.5 kcal/mL and 5 g (or more) protein/100 mL

Not suitable for use in child under 3 years; not recommended for child under 6 years

Product	Formulation	Energy	Protein	Carbohydrate	Fat	Fibre	Special Characteristics	ACBS Indications	Presentation & Flavour
Ensure® Plus Crème (Abbott Laboratories Ltd)	Semi-solid per 100 g	574 kJ (137 kcal)	5.68 g cow's milk soy protein isolates	18.4 g (sugars 12.4 g)	4.47 g	Nil	Gluten-free Residual lactose Contains soya	Borderline substances standard ACBS indications p. 1623; also CAPD, haemodialysis. Not suitable for child under 3 years; use with caution in child 3–5 years.	Ensure Plus Creme: banana, chocolate, neutral, vanilla 500 gram = £8.20
Nutilis® Fruit Dessert Level 4 (Nutricia Ltd)	Semi-Solid per 100 g	575 kJ (137 kcal)	6.9 g whey protein isolate	17 g (sugars 11.5 g)	4 g	2.6 g	Contains residual lactose, soya. Gluten-free	Borderline substances standard ACBS indications p. 1623 except bowel fistula; also CAPD, haemodialysis.	Nutilis Fruit Dessert Level 4: apple, strawberry 450 gram = £7.56
Oral Impact® (Nestle Health Science)	Standard dilution of powder (74 g in 250 mL water) (sip feed) per 100 mL	425 kJ (101 kcal)	5.6 g cows' milk	13.4 g (sugars 7.4 g)	2.8 g	1 g	Residual lactose Contains fish oil	Pre-operative nutritional supplement for malnourished patients or patients at risk of malnourishment Not suitable for child under 3 years; use with caution in child 3–5 years.	Oral Impact oral powder 74g sachets tropical: 5 sachet = £18.20

Powder provides: protein 16.8 g, carbohydrate 40.2 g, fat 8.3 g, fibre 3 g, energy 1276 kJ (303 kcal)/74 g.

Nutritional supplements: More than 1.5 kcal/mL and 5 g (or more) protein/100 mL

Not suitable for use in child under 6 years unless otherwise stated; not recommended for use in children unless otherwise stated

Product	Formulation	Energy	Protein	Carbohydrate	Fat	Fibre	Special Characteristics	ACBS Indications	Presentation & Flavour
Altraplen® Compact (Nualtra Ltd)	Liquid (sip feed) per 100 mL	1008 kJ (240 kcal)	9.6 g milk, soya proteins	28.8 g (sugars 11.6 g)	9.6 g	Nil	Contains residual lactose, soya. Gluten-free	Borderline substances standard ACBS indications p. 1623.	Altraplen Compact Starter Pack liquid: 500 ml = £5.96; Altraplen Compact liquid: banana, hazel chocolate, strawberry, vanilla 500 ml = £5.32
Aymes® 2.0kcal (Aymes International Ltd)	Liquid per 100 ml	840 kJ (200 kcal)	8 g milk protein	24 g (sugars 10 g)	8 g	Nil	Contains residual lactose	Borderline substances standard ACBS indications p. 1623 except dysphagia.	Aymes 2.0kcal liquid: banana, strawberry, vanilla 800 ml = £6.40
Aymes® ActaGain 2.4 Complete Maxi (Aymes International Ltd)	Liquid per 100 mL	1008 kJ (240 kcal)	9.6 g milk protein	28.8 g (sugars 8 g)	9.6 g	Nil	Contains residual lactose. Gluten-free	Borderline substances standard ACBS indications p. 1623 except dysphagia.	Aymes ActaGain 2.4 Complete Maxi liquid: banana, strawberry, vanilla 800 ml = £5.32
Aymes® ActaSolve Delight (Aymes International Ltd)	Powder per 100 g	1857 kJ (441 kcal)	15.2 g milk protein	62 g (sugars 38.6 g)	14.5 g	0.9 g	Contains lactose, soya	Borderline substances standard ACBS indications p. 1623 except dysphagia.	Aymes ActaSolve Delight Starter Pack powder: 3 sachet = £3.60; Aymes ActaSolve Delight powder 57 g sachets: butterscotch, lemon, mixed berries 7 sachet = £6.93

Powder 57 g reconstituted with 75 ml milk provides: protein 11.2 g, carbohydrate 38.7 g, fat 11.3 g, energy 1270 kJ (302 kcal)

Product	Formulation	Energy	Protein	Carbohydrate	Fat	Fibre	Special characteristics	ACBS indications	Presentations
Aymes® ActaSolve Smoothie (Aymes International Ltd)	Powder per 100 g	1892 kJ (450 kcal)	16.2 g soya protein isolate	62.8 g (sugars 24.8 g)	14.6 g	0.7 g	Contains soya. Gluten-free	Borderline substances standard ACBS indications p. 1623 except dysphagia.	Aymes ActaSolve Smoothie ... Pack powder: 4 sachet = £5.15; Aymes ActaSolve Smoothie powder 66g sachets: mango, peach, pineapple, strawberry & cranberry 7 sachet = £7.00
Powder 66 g reconstituted with 150ml water provides: protein 10.7 g, carbohydrate 41.5 g, fat 9.7 g, energy 1249 kJ (297 kcal)									
Aymes® Savoury (Aymes International Ltd)	Powder per 100 g	1842 kJ (441 kcal)	16.3 g milk protein	60.3 g (sugars 10.9 g)	14.9 g	0.4 g	Contains celery, lactose, meat derivatives (chicken flavour only). Gluten-free.	Borderline substances standard ACBS indications p. 1623 except dysphagia.	Aymes Savoury powder 57g sachets: chicken, vegetable 7 sachet = £4.90
Powder 57 g reconstituted with 200 ml water provides: protein 9.2 g, carbohydrate 34.3 g, fat 8.5 g, energy 1050 kJ (251 kcal)									
Aymes® Shake (Aymes International Ltd)	Powder per 100 g	1853 kJ (440 kcal)	21 g milk protein	56.8 g (sugars 31.3 g)	14.3 g	0.2 g	Contains lactose, soya. Gluten-free. May contain celery, egg, mustard, sulphites	Borderline substances standard ACBS indications p. 1623	Aymes Shake Starter Pack powder: 6 sachet = £3.97; Aymes Shake powder 57 g sachets: banana, chocolate, neutral, strawberry, vanilla 7 sachet = £3.43; Aymes shake powder: banana, chocolate, neutral, strawberry, vanilla 1600 gram = £13.72
Powder 57 g reconstituted with 200 ml whole milk provides: protein 19 g, carbohydrate 41.9 g, fat 15.6 g, energy 1608 kJ (383 kcal)									
Complan® Shake (Nutricia Ltd)	Standard dilution (24% w/v) of powder per 100 mL	673 kJ (160 kcal)	6.5 g cow's milk	18.9 g (sugars 11.6 g)	6.6 g	less than 0.04 g	Contains lactose. Gluten-free	Borderline substances standard ACBS indications p. 1623.	Complan Shake Starter Pack sachets: 5 sachet = £4.39; Complan Shake oral powder 57g sachets: banana, chocolate, milk, strawberry, vanilla 4 sachet = £2.80
Powder provides: protein 15.4 g, carbohydrate 62.5 g, fat 14.8 g, energy 1870 kJ (445 kcal)/100 g									
Ensure® Compact (Abbott Laboratories Ltd)	Liquid (sip or tube feed) per 100 mL	1008 kJ (240 kcal)	10.2 g Cows' milk	28.8 g (sugars 6.2 g)	9.35 g	Nil	Gluten-free Contains lactose	As a sole source of nutrition or as a nutritional supplement for the dietary management of patients with, or at risk of developing, disease-related malnutrition.	Ensure Compact liquid: banana, cafe latte, strawberry, vanilla 500 ml = £5.32
Ensure® Plus Fibre (Abbott Laboratories Ltd)	Liquid (sip feed) per 100 mL	652 kJ (155 kcal)	6.25 g caseinates, milk protein isolate, soya protein isolate	20.2 g sucrose (sugars 4.9 g)	4.92 g	2.5 g	Contains residual lactose, soya. Gluten-free	Borderline substances standard ACBS indications p. 1623; also CAPD, haemodialysis.	Ensure Plus Fibre liquid: banana, chocolate, raspberry, strawberry, vanilla 200 ml = £2.19
Ensure® TwoCal (Abbott Laboratories Ltd)	Liquid (sip or tube feed) per 100 mL	837 kJ (200 kcal)	8.4 g caseinates, milk protein	21 g (sugars 5 g)	8.9 g	1 g	Contains soya. Gluten-free	Borderline substances standard ACBS indications p. 1623; also haemodialysis and CAPD.	Ensure TwoCal liquid: banana, neutral, strawberry, vanilla 200 ml = £2.22

A2

Borderline substances | **Appendix 2**

Nutritional supplements: More than 1.5 kcal/mL and 5 g (or more) protein/100 mL (product list continued)

Not suitable for use in child under 6 years unless otherwise stated, not recommended for use in children unless otherwise stated

Product	Formulation	Energy	Protein	Carbohydrate	Fat	Fibre	Special Characteristics	ACBS Indications	Presentation & Flavour
Foodlink® Complete (Nualtra Ltd)	Powder per 100 g	1869 kJ (444 kcal)	21 g milk protein	56 g (sugars 43 g)	15 g	Nil	Contains lactose, soya. Gluten-free	Borderline substances standard ACBS indications p. 1623	Foodlink Complete Starter Pack powder 5 sachet = £3.31; Foodlink Complete powder 57 g sachets: banana, chocolate, natural, strawberry, vanilla 7 sachet = £3.43; Foodlink Complete powder: banana, chocolate, natural, strawberry, vanilla 1596 gram = £13.72
Powder 57 g reconstituted with 200 ml whole milk provides: protein 19 g, carbohydrate 41 g, fat 16 g, energy 1611 kJ (383 kcal)									
Foodlink® Complete Compact (Nualtra Ltd)	Powder per 100 g	1869 kJ (444 kcal)	21 g milk protein	56 g (sugars 43 g)	15 g	Nil	Contains lactose, soya. Gluten-free	Disease-related malnutrition.	Foodlink Complete Compact Starter Pack 5 sachet = £3.31; Foodlink Complete Compact powder 57 g sachets: banana, chocolate, natural, strawberry, vanilla 7 sachet = £3.43
Powder 57 g reconstituted with 100 ml whole milk provides: protein 15 g, carbohydrate 37 g, fat 12 g, energy 1338 kJ (318 kcal)									
Foodlink® Complete with Fibre (Nualtra Ltd)	Powder per 100 g	1779 kJ (423 kcal)	19 g milk, soya proteins	52 g (sugars 40 g)	14 g	7.2 g	Contains lactose, soya. Gluten-free	Borderline substances standard ACBS indications p. 1623	Foodlink Complete powder with fibre Starter Pack. 5 sachet = £3.67; Foodlink Complete powder with fibre 63g sachets: banana, chocolate, natural, strawberry, vanilla 7 sachet = £4.97
Powder 63 g reconstituted with 200 ml whole milk provides: protein 19 g, carbohydrate 42 g, fat 16 g, energy 1667 kJ (397 kcal)									
Forticreme® Complete (Nutricia Ltd)	Semi-solid per 100 g	675 kJ (160 kcal)	9.5 g milk proteins	19.2 g (sugars 10.6 g)	5 g	less than 0.5 g	Contains residual lactose. Gluten-free	Borderline substances standard ACBS indications p. 1623; also continuous ambulatory peritoneal dialysis (CAPD), haemodialysis.	Forticreme Complete dessert: banana, chocolate, forest fruits, vanilla 500 gram = £8.04
Fortisip® 2kcal (Nutricia Ltd)	Liquid (sip feed) per 100 mL	845 kJ (201 kcal)	10.1 g milk proteins	21 g (sugars 15.6 g)	8.6 g	Nil	Contains residual lactose, soya. Gluten-free	Borderline substances standard ACBS indications p. 1623; also CAPD and haemodialysis.	Fortisip 2kcal liquid: chocolate-caramel, forest fruit, mocha, strawberry, vanilla 200 ml = £2.22
Fortisip® Compact (Nutricia Ltd)	Liquid (sip feed) per 100 mL	1010 kJ (240 kcal)	9.6 g milk proteins	29.7 g (sugars 15 g)	9.3 g	Nil	Contains residual lactose. soya. Gluten-free	Borderline substances standard ACBS indications p. 1623	Fortisip Compact Starter Pack liquid: 750 ml = £7.98; Fortisip Compact liquid: apricot, banana, chocolate, forest fruit, mocha, neutral, strawberry, vanilla 500 ml = £5.32
Fortisip® Compact Fibre (Nutricia Ltd)	Liquid (sip feed) per 100 mL	1005 kJ (240 kcal)	9.5 g milk proteins	25.2 g (sugars 14.1 g)	10.4 g	3.6 g	Contains residual lactose. soya. Gluten-free.	Borderline substances standard ACBS indications p. 1623	Fortisip Compact Fibre Starter Pack liquid: 500 ml = £8.60; Fortisip Compact Fibre liquid: mocha, strawberry, vanilla 500 ml = £8.60

Product	Presentation	Energy	Protein	Carbohydrate	Fat	Fibre	Special characteristics	Borderline substances	Flavours / presentations / prices
Fortisip® Compact Protein (Nutricia Ltd)	Liquid (sip feed) per 100 mL	1010 kJ (240 kcal)	14.4 g milk proteins	24.4 g (sugars 13.3 g)	9.4 g	Nil	Contains residual lactose, soya. Gluten-free	Borderline substances standard ACBS indications p. 1623	Fortisip Compact Protein Pack liquid: 1000 ml = £16.00; Fortisip Compact Protein liquid: banana, berries, cool red fruits, hot tropical ginger, mocha, neutral, peach & mango, strawberry, vanilla 500 ml = £8.00
Fortisip® Extra (Nutricia Ltd)	Liquid (sip feed) per 100 mL	670 kJ (159 kcal)	9.8 g milk proteins	18.1 g (sugars 9 g)	5.3 g	Nil	Contains lactose, soya. Gluten-free	Borderline substances standard ACBS indications p. 1623	Fortisip Extra liquid: strawberry, vanilla 200 ml = £2.37
Fresubin® 2kcal (Fresenius Kabi Ltd)	Liquid (sip feed) per 100 mL	840 kJ (200 kcal)	10 g milk protein	22.5 g (sugars 3.2-5.8 g)	7.8 g	Nil	Contains residual lactose, soya. Gluten-free	Borderline substances standard ACBS indications p. 1623; also CAPD, haemodialysis.	Fresubin 2kcal drink: apricot-peach, cappuccino, fruits of the forest, neutral, toffee, vanilla 200 ml = £2.23
Fresubin® 2kcal Fibre (Fresenius Kabi Ltd)	Liquid (sip feed) per 100 mL	840 kJ (200 kcal)	10 g milk protein	21.7-21.8 g (sugars 3.3-5.9 g)	7.8 g	1.5 g	Contains residual lactose, soya. Gluten-free	Borderline substances standard ACBS indications p. 1623; also CAPD, haemodialysis.	Fresubin 2kcal Fibre drink: apricot-peach, cappuccino, chocolate, lemon, neutral, vanilla 200 ml = £2.23
Fresubin® Powder Extra (Fresenius Kabi Ltd)	Powder per 100 g	1764 kJ (420 kcal)	17.5 g milk, whey proteins	63 g (sugars 18.6 g)	10.9 g	Nil	Contains lactose. Gluten-free	Borderline substances standard ACBS indications p. 1623.	Fresubin Powder Extra oral powder 62g sachets: chocolate, neutral, strawberry, vanilla 7 sachet = £4.90

Powder 62 g reconstituted with 200 ml whole milk provides: protein 17.7 g, carbohydrate 48.5, fat 14.8 g, energy 1658 kJ (397 kcal)

Product	Presentation	Energy	Protein	Carbohydrate	Fat	Fibre	Special characteristics	Borderline substances	Flavours / presentations / prices
Nutilis® Complete Creme Level 3 (Nutricia Ltd)	Semi-solid per 100 g	1030 kJ (245 kcal)	9.6 g milk protein	29.1 g (sugars 11.8 g)	9.4 g	3.2 g	Contains residual lactose, soya. Gluten-free	Borderline substances standard ACBS indications p. 1623.	Nutilis Complete Creme Level 3 custard: chocolate, strawberry, vanilla 500 gram = £9.08
Nutilis® Complete Drink Level 3 (Nutricia Ltd)	Liquid (sip feed) per 100 mL	1025 kJ (245 kcal)	9.6 g caseinates, milk proteins	29.1 g (sugars 5.4 g)	9.3 g	3.2 g	Contains residual lactose, soya. Gluten-free	Borderline substances standard ACBS indications p. 1623.	Nutilis Complete Drink Level 3 liquid: chocolate, lemon tea, mango & passionfruit, strawberry, vanilla 500 ml = £9.08
Nutricrem® (Nualtra Ltd)	Semi-solid per 100 g	756 kJ (180 kcal)	10 g caseinates, milk protein, soya protein	18.8 g (sugars 9.7 g)	7.2 g	Nil	Contains residual lactose, soya. Gluten-free	Borderline substances standard ACBS indications p. 1623.	Nutricrem Starter Pack dessert: 500 gram = £6.54; Nutricrem dessert: chocolate orange, mint chocolate, strawberry, vanilla 500 gram = £6.78
Nutrison® Energy Multi Fibre Vanilla (Nutricia Ltd)	Liquid per 100 mL	645 kJ (154 kcal)	6 g milk protein	18.4 g (sugars 6.8 g)	5.8 g	2.2 g	Contains residual lactose, soya. Gluten-free	Borderline substances standard ACBS indications p. 1623.	Nutrison Energy Multi Fibre Vanilla liquid: 200 ml = £2.42
Renilon® 7.5 (Nutricia Ltd)	Liquid (sip feed) per 100 mL	835 kJ (199 kcal)	7.3 g milk protein	20 g (sugars 4.8 g)	10 g	Nil	Contains residual lactose, soya	Borderline substances standard ACBS indications p. 1623 except dysphagia.	Renilon 7.5 liquid: apricot, caramel 500 ml = £9.72
Resource® 2.0 Fibre (Nestle Health Science)	Liquid (sip or tube feed) per 100 mL	835 kJ (200 kcal)	9 g milk protein	20 g (sugars 6 g)	8.7 g	2.5 g	Contains residual lactose	Borderline substances standard ACBS indications p. 1623.	Resource Fibre 2.0 liquid: apricot, coffee, neutral, strawberry, summer fruit, vanilla 200 ml £2.08

Table 3 Specialised formulas

Specialised formulas: Infant and child see *BNF for Children*

Specialised formulas for specific clinical conditions

Not suitable for use in child under 3 years unless otherwise stated; not recommended for use in children unless otherwise stated

Product	Formulation	Energy	Protein	Carbohydrate	Fat	Fibre	Special Characteristics	ACBS Indications	Presentation & Flavour
Forticare® (Nutricia Ltd)	Liquid (sip feed) per 100 mL	685 kJ (163 kcal)	8.8 g milk protein	19.1 g (sugars 13.6 g)	5.3 g	2.1 g	Contains fish oil, residual lactose, soya. Electrolytes/100 mL: Na 4.8 mmol, K 5.5 mmol, Ca^2 4.2 mmol, P 3.9 mmol, Gluten-free	Patients with pancreatic cancer and patients with lung cancer undergoing chemotherapy.	Forticare liquid: cappuccino, orange & lemon, peach & ginger 500 ml = £10.04
Galactomin 17® (Nutricia Ltd)	Standard dilution (12.8 % w/v) of powder per 100 mL	275 kJ (66 kcal)	1.3 g caseinates	7.3 g (sugars 1.1 g)	3.5 g	Nil	Contains fish oil, residual lactose, soya. Electrolytes/100 mL: Na 0.75 mmol, K 1.7 mmol, Ca^2 1.4 mmol, P 0.9 mmol	Proven lactose intolerance in pre-school children, galactosaemia, and galactokinase deficiency.	Galactomin 17 powder: 400 gram = £19.28

Powder provides: protein 10.3 g, carbohydrate 57.1 g, fat 27.3 g, energy 2150 kJ (514 kcal)/100 g

Product	Formulation	Energy	Protein	Carbohydrate	Fat	Fibre	Special Characteristics	ACBS Indications	Presentation & Flavour
KetoCal® 4:1 (Nutricia Ltd)	Standard dilution (14.2 % w/v) of powder per 100 mL	411 kJ (100 kcal)	2 g casein, protein equivalent (amino acids), whey protein	0.41 g (sugars 0.14 g)	9.8 g	0.75 g	Contains residual lactose, soya. Electrolytes/100 mL: Na^+ 3.3 mmol, K^+ 3.1 mmol, Ca^{2+} 2.7 mmol, P^+ 2.1 mmol	For use as part of the ketogenic diet in the management of epilepsy resistant to drug therapy. Only to be prescribed on the advice of a secondary care physician with experience of the ketogenic diet.	KetoCal 4:1 powder: unflavoured, vanilla 300 gram = £34.99
KetoCal® 4:1 LQ (Nutricia Ltd)	Liquid (sip or tube feed) per 100 mL	620 kJ (150 kcal)	3.1 g caseinates, whey protein	0.6 g (sugars 0.4 g)	14.8 g	1.1 g	Contains residual lactose, soya. Electrolytes/100 mL: Na^+ 4.9 mmol, K^+ 4.7 mmol, Ca^{2+} 2.4 mmol, P^+ 3.1 mmol	Drug resistant epilepsy or other conditions for which a ketogenic diet is indicated.	KetoCal 4:1 LQ liquid: unflavoured, vanilla 200 ml = £4.98

Powder provides: protein 14.4 g, carbohydrate 2.9 g, fat 69.2 g, energy 2897 kJ (703 kcal)/100 g

Product	Formulation	Energy	Protein	Carbohydrate	Fat	Fibre	Special Characteristics	ACBS Indications	Presentation & Flavour
KetoClassic 3:1 Meal (KetoCare Foods Ltd)	Semi-solid per 100 g	936-1182 kJ (224-287 kcal)	5.1-5.2 g	2-3.7 g (sugars 0.8-2.6 g)	21.7-26.7 g	0.4-2.1 g	Contains egg and mustard (bolognese flavour), lactose (chicken flavour), and meat	Intractable epilepsy, pyruvate dehydrogenase deficiency, glucose transporter type 1 deficiency and other conditions where a ketogenic diet is indicated.	KetoClassic 3:1 Meal: bolognese 126 g pouches 14 pouch = £76.02; chicken 135 g pouches 14 pouch = £76.95; 30 pouch = £162.90
KetoClassic® 3:1 Bar (KetoCare Foods Ltd)	Solid per 100 g	2082 kJ (498 kcal)	10.8 g soya protein	3.3 g (sugars 2.8 g)	43.6 g	28.7 g	Contains nuts, soya, sulphur dioxide	Intractable epilepsy, pyruvate dehydrogenase deficiency, glucose transporter type 1 deficiency and other conditions where a ketogenic diet is indicated.	KetoClassic 3:1 Bar: 420 gram = £21.88

Product	Preparation	Energy	Protein	Carbohydrate	Fat		Allergen information	Indication	Price
KetoClassic® 3:1 Breakfast Muesli (KetoCare Foods Ltd)	Solid per 100 g	2569 kJ (623 kcal)	11 g	7.5 g (sugars 3.8 g)	57.1 g	17.5 g	Contains lactose, nuts, soya, sulphur dioxide	Intractable epilepsy, pyruvate dehydrogenase deficiency, glucose transporter type 1 deficiency and other conditions where a ketogenic diet is indicated.	KetoClassic 3:1 Breakfast muesli: 600 gram = £34.98
KetoClassic® 3:1 Breakfast Porridge (KetoCare Foods Ltd)	Solid per 100 g	2649 kJ (643 kcal)	11.7 g	7.8 g (sugars 5.4 g)	59.1 g	16.7 g	Contains lactose, nuts, sulphur dioxide	Intractable epilepsy, pyruvate dehydrogenase deficiency, glucose transporter type 1 deficiency and other conditions where a ketogenic diet is indicated.	KetoClassic 3:1 Breakfast porridge: 600 gram = £34.98
KetoClassic® 3:1 Savoury (KetoCare Foods Ltd)	Solid per 100 g	2190 kJ (531 kcal)	9 g	7.3 g (sugars 1.2 g)	48.7 g	13.7 g	Contains egg, lactose, nuts	Intractable epilepsy, pyruvate dehydrogenase deficiency, glucose transporter type 1 deficiency and other conditions where a ketogenic diet is indicated.	KetoClassic 3:1 Savoury meal: 840 gram = £43.40
Liquigen® (Nutricia Ltd)	Liquid (sip or tube feed) per 100 mL	1865 kJ (454 kcal)	Nil	Nil	50.4 g (MCT 97.4 %)	Nil		Steatorrhoea associated with cystic fibrosis of the pancreas, intestinal lymphangiectasia, surgery of the intestine, chronic liver disease, liver cirrhosis, other proven malabsorption syndromes, a ketogenic diet in the management of epilepsy, and in type 1 hyperlipoproteinaemia.	Liquigen emulsion: 250 ml = £10.63
MCT Oil (Nutricia Ltd)	Liquid per 100 mL	3515 kJ (855 kcal)	Nil	Nil	95 g MCT 100 %	Nil		Steatorrhoea associated with cystic fibrosis of the pancreas, intestinal lymphangiectasia, surgery of the intestine, chronic liver disease, liver cirrhosis, other proven malabsorption syndromes, ketogenic diet in management of epilepsy, type 1 hyperlipoproteinaemia.	MCT oil: 500 ml = £16.86
Modulen IBD® (Nestlé Health Science)	Standard dilution (20%) of powder (sip or tube feed) per 100 mL	420 kJ (100 kcal)	3.6 g casein	11 g (sugars 3.98 g)	4.7 g	Nil	Gluten-free Residual lactose	Crohn's disease active phase, and in remission if malnourished	Modulen IBD powder: 400 gram = £16.19

Powder provides: protein 18 g, carbohydrate 54 g, fat 23 g, energy 2070 kJ (500 kcal)/100 g.

Product	Preparation	Energy	Protein	Carbohydrate	Fat		Allergen information	Indication	Price
Monogen® (Nutricia Ltd)	Standard dilution (16.8% w/v) of powder per 100 mL	312 kJ (74 kcal)	2.2 g caseinate, whey protein	11.5 g (sugars 2 g)	2.2 g (MCT 84%)	Nil	Contains lactose, nuts	For the dietary management of disorders requiring a low LCT, high MCT intake, such as long chain fatty acid oxidation defects (long-chain acyl-CoA dehydrogenase deficiency (LCAD), carnitine palmitoyl transferase deficiency (CPTD)), primary and secondary lipoprotein lipase deficiency (hyperlipoproteinaemia type 1) chylothorax, lymphangiectasia.	Monogen powder: 400 gram = £23.30

Powder provides: protein 12.8 g, carbohydrate 68.6 g, fat 12.9 g, energy 1859 kJ (441 kcal)/100 g

Table 3 Specialised formulas (product list continued)

Specialised formulas for specific clinical conditions

Not suitable for use in child under 3 years unless otherwise stated; not recommended for use in children unless otherwise stated

Product	Formulation	Energy	Protein	Carbohydrate	Fat	Fibre	Special Characteristics	ACBS Indications	Presentation & Flavour
Nepro® HP (Abbott Laboratories Ltd)	Liquid (sip or tube feed) **per 100 mL**	752 kJ (180 kcal)	8.1 g caseinates, milk protein isolate	14.7 g (sugars 3.2 g)	9.8 g	1.3 g	Contains meat derivatives, residual lactose, soya. Gluten-free Electrolytes/100 mL: Na⁺ 3 mmol K⁺ 2.7 mmol Ca²⁺ 2.6 mmol P⁺ 2.3 mmol	Patients with chronic renal failure who are on haemodialysis or complete ambulatory peritoneal dialysis (CAPD), or patients with cirrhosis or other conditions requiring a high energy, low fluid, low electrolyte diet.	Nepro HP liquid: strawberry, vanilla 220 ml = £3.60; strawberry 500 ml, = £8.24
ProSure® (Abbott Laboratories Ltd)	Liquid (sip or tube feed) **per 100 mL**	536 kJ (127 kcal)	6.7 g caseinates, milk protein isolate	18.3 g sucrose (sugars 6.5 g)	2.6 g	2.1 g	Contains fish oil, residual lactose, soya. Gluten-free	Pancreatic cancer, oesophageal cancer and patients with lung cancer who are undergoing chemotherapy.	ProSure liquid: 220 ml = £3.69
Renamil® (Stanningley Pharma Ltd)	Powder **per 100 g**	2012 kJ (479 kcal)	5 g milk protein, whey protein isolate	71.2 g (sugars 6.8 g)	19.3 g	Nil	Contains lactose, soya. Gluten-free Electrolytes/100 mL: Na⁺ 3 mmol K⁺ 0.1 mmol Ca²⁺ 3.7 mmol P⁺ 0.8 mmol	Chronic renal failure.	Renamil powder 100g sachets: 10 sachet = £25.40
Renapro® (Stanningley Pharma Ltd)	Powder **per 100 g**	1558 kJ (372 kcal)	90 g whey protein	3.4 g	1 g	Nil	Gluten-free Do not use in cow's milk allergy or where absorption and digestive problems are present Electrolytes/100 g: Na⁺ 15.65 mmol K⁺ 4.60 mmol Ca²⁺ 4.74 mmol Mg²⁺ 0.82 mmol P⁺ 3.55 mmol	Nutritional supplement for biochemically proven hypoproteinaemia and patients undergoing dialysis. Not suitable for child under 1 year.	Renapro powder 20g sachets: 30 sachet = £69.60
								Powder provides: protein 18 g, energy 312 kJ (74 kcal)/20-g sachet.	
Renastart® (Vitaflo International Ltd)	Standard dilution (20%) of powder **per 100 mL**	414 kJ (99 kcal)	1.5 g cow's milk soya	12.5 g (sugars 1.3 g)	4.8 g	Nil	Contains lactose Electrolytes/100 mL: Na⁺ 2.1 mmol K⁺ 0.6 mmol Ca²⁺ 0.6 mmol P⁺ 0.6 mmol	Dietary management of renal failure in child from birth to 10 years.	Renastart powder: 400 gram = £29.81
								Powder provides: protein 7.5 g, carbohydrate 62.5 g, fat 23.8 g, energy 2071 kJ (494 kcal)/100 g.	
Respifor® (Nutricia Ltd)	Liquid (sip feed) **per 100 mL**	635 kJ (150 kcal)	7.5 g milk protein	22.6 g (sugars 6 g)	3.3 g	Nil	Contains lactose, soya Electrolytes/100 mL: Na⁺ 2.4 mmol K⁺ 2.8 mmol Ca²⁺ 3.9 mmol P⁺ 3.2 mmol	Disease related malnutrition in patients with chronic obstructive pulmonary disease (COPD) with a body mass index (BMI) of less than 20.	Respifor milkshake style liquid: chocolate, strawberry, vanilla 500 ml = £9.56

Product	Formulation	Energy	Protein	Carbohydrate	Fat	Fibre	Special Characteristics	ACBS Indications	Presentation & Flavour
Supportan® (Fresenius Kabi Ltd)	Liquid (sip feed) per 100 mL	630 kJ (150 kcal)	10 g milk protein	11.6 g sucrose (sugars 7 g)	6.7 g	1.5 g	Contains fish oil, residual lactose, soya. Gluten-free Electrolytes/100 mL: Na+ 2.1mmol K+ 3.3mmol Ca2+ 5.1mmol P+ 3.9mmol	Patients with pancreatic cancer or patients with lung cancer undergoing chemotherapy.	supportan drinks cappuccino, tropical fruits 800 ml = £11.60

Table 4 Feed supplements
High-energy supplements

High-energy supplements: carbohydrate
Not suitable for use in child under 3 years unless otherwise stated; not recommended for child 3-6 years unless otherwise stated

Product	Formulation	Energy	Protein	Carbohydrate	Fat	Fibre	Special Characteristics	ACBS Indications	Presentation & Flavour
Maxijul® Super Soluble (Nutricia Ltd)	Powder per 100 g	1615 kJ (380 kcal)	Nil	95 g (sugars 8.6g)	Nil	Nil	Lactose-free, gluten-free	Disease-related malnutrition, malabsorption states or other conditions requiring fortification with a high or readily available carbohydrate supplement.	Maxijul Super Soluble: powder 132g sachets 4 sachet = £7.43; powder 200 gram = £2.98; 25000 gram = £178.69
Powder 75 g reconstituted with 150 ml water provides: protein nil, carbohydrate 31.4 g, fat nil, energy 533 kJ (125 kcal)/100 g									
Polycal® liquid	Liquid per 100 mL	1050 kJ (247 kcal)	Nil	61.9 g (sugars 12.2 g)	Nil	Nil		Disease related malnutrition, malabsorption states or other conditions requiring fortification with a high or readily available carbohydrate supplement.	Polycal liquid: neutral, orange 200 ml = £1.96
Polycal® powder (Nutricia Ltd)	Standard dilution (10% w/v) of powder per 100 mL	82 kJ (19 kcal)	Nil	4.8 g (sugars 0.3 g)	Nil	Nil		Disease-related malnutrition, malabsorption states or other conditions requiring fortification with a high or readily available carbohydrate supplement.	Polycal powder: 400 gram = £4.84
Powder provides: protein Nil g, carbohydrate 96 g, fat Nil g, energy 1630 kJ (384 kcal)/100 g									
S.O.S.® (Vitaflo International Ltd)	Powder per 100 g	1590 kJ (380 kcal)	Nil	95 g (sugars 9 g)	Nil	Nil		For use as an emergency regimen in the dietary management of inborn errors of metabolism in adults and children from birth.	S.O.S.10 oral powder 21g sachets: 30 sachet = £8.26; S.O.S.15 oral powder 31g sachets: 30 sachet = £12.19; S.O.S.20 oral powder 42g sachets: 30 sachet = £16.53; S.O.S.25 oral powder 52g sachets: 30 sachet = £20.44
Vitajoule® (Vitaflo International Ltd)	Powder per 100 g	1590 kJ (380 kcal)	Nil	95 g Dried glucose syrup (sugars 9 g)	Nil	Nil	Gluten-free Lactose-free	Disease-related malnutrition, malabsorption states or other conditions requiring fortification with a high or readily available carbohydrate supplement.	Vitajoule powder: 500 gram = £4.94

Borderline substances | **Appendix 2**

A2

High-energy supplements: fat

Product	Formulation	Energy	Protein	Carbohydrate	Fat	Fibre	Special Characteristics	ACBS Indications	Presentation & Flavour
Calogen® (Nutricia Ltd)	Liquid (sip or tube feed) per 100 mL	1850 kJ (450 kcal)	Nil	0.1 g (sugar nil)	50 g	Nil	Banana and strawberry flavours not suitable for child under 3 years. Gluten-free. Lactose-free	Disease-related malnutrition, malabsorption states, or other conditions requiring fortification with a high fat supplement, with or without fluid and electrolyte restrictions.	Calogen emulsion: neutral, strawberry 200 ml = £4.92; 500 ml = £12.11; banana 500 ml = £12.11
Fresubin® 5kcal Shot (Fresenius Kabi Ltd)	Liquid (emulsion) per 100 mL	2100 kJ (500 kcal)	Nil	4.0 g (sucrose)	53.8 g	0.4 g	Gluten-free Lactose-free	Disease-related malnutrition, malabsorption states, or other conditions requiring fortification with a high fat (or fat and carbohydrate) supplement. Not suitable for child under 3 years.	Fresubin 5kcal shot drink: lemon, neutral 480 ml = £11.96

FAT AND CARBOHYDRATE

Product	Formulation	Energy	Protein	Carbohydrate	Fat	Fibre	Special Characteristics	ACBS Indications	Presentation & Flavour
Duocal® Super Soluble (Nutricia Ltd)	Powder per 100 g	2061 kJ (492 kcal)	Nil	72.7 g (sugars 6.5 g)	22.3 g (MCT 35 %)	Nil		Disease-related malnutrition, malabsorption states, or other conditions requiring fortification with a high fat (or fat and carbohydrate) supplement.	Duocal Super Soluble powder: 400 gram = £20.76

High-energy supplements: protein

Not suitable for use in child under 1 year unless otherwise stated; not recommended for child under 3 years unless otherwise stated

Product	Formulation	Energy	Protein	Carbohydrate	Fat	Fibre	Special Characteristics	ACBS Indications	Presentation & Flavour
ProSource® jelly (Nutrinovo Ltd)	Semi-solid per 100 mL	315 kJ (75 kcal)	16.9 g collagen protein, whey protein isolate	Less than 1 g	Nil	Less than 1 g	Contains porcine derivatives, residual lactose. Gluten-free	Hypoproteinaemia.	ProSource jelly: blackcurrant, fruit punch, lime, orange 118 ml = £2.04
ProSource® TF (Nutrinovo Ltd)	Liquid (tube feed) per 100 ml	373 kJ (98 kcal)	24.4 g collagen protein, protein equivalent (amino acids)	2.2 g (sugars nil)	Less than 1 g	Less than 1 g	Contains bovine derivatives. Gluten-free, lactose-free	Hypoproteinaemia.	ProSource TF liquid 45ml sachets: 100 sachet = £133.75
Protifar® (Nutricia Ltd)	Powder per 100 g	1580 kJ (373 kcal)	88.5 g cows' milk	less than 1.5 g	1.6 g	Nil	Gluten-free Residual lactose Electrolytes/100 mL: Na^+ 1.3 mmol K^+ 1.28 mmol Ca^{2+} 33.75 mmol P^+ 22.58 mmol	Nutritional supplement for use in biochemically proven hypoproteinaemia.	Protifar powder: 225 gram = £9.84

Powder provides: protein 2.2 g per 2.5 g.

Product	Formulation	Energy	Protein	Carbohydrate	Fat	Fibre	Special Characteristics	ACBS Indications	Presentation & Flavour
Renapro Shot® (Stanningley Pharma Ltd)	Liquid (sip or tube feed) per 100ml	641 kJ (150 kcal)	33 g collagen protein	2 g (fructose 2 g)	less than 0.1 g	Nil	Contains beef derivatives. Gluten-free	Dialysis patients with biochemically proven hypoproteinaemia.	Renapro Shot 60ml bottles: peach, wild berry 30 bottle = £69.60

PROTEIN AND CARBOHYDRATE

Not suitable for use in child under 6 months unless otherwise stated; not recommended for child under 3 years unless otherwise stated

Product	Formulation	Energy	Protein	Carbohydrate	Fat	Fibre	Special Characteristics	ACBS Indications	Presentation & Flavour
Dialamine® (Nutricia Ltd)	Standard dilution (20% w/v) of powder per 100 mL	264 kJ (62 kcal)	4.3 g protein equivalent (amino acids)	11.2 g (sugars 10.2 g)	Nil	Nil	Lactose-free	Chronic renal failure, hypoproteinaemia, wound fistula leakage with excessive protein loss, haemodialysis and other conditions requiring a controlled nitrogen or amino acid supplements intake.	Dialamine powder: 400 gram = £84.34

Powder provides: protein 25 g, carbohydrate 65 g, fat Nil g energy 1530 kJ (360 kcal)/100 g

Product	Formulation	Energy	Protein	Carbohydrate	Fat	Fibre	Special Characteristics	ACBS Indications	Presentation & Flavour
ProSource® liquid (Nutrinovo Ltd)	Liquid (sip or tube feed) per 100 mL	1400 kJ (333 kcal)	33.3 g collagen protein, whey protein isolate	50 g (sugars 26.7 g)	Less than 1 g	Less than 1 g	Contains residual lactose, porcine derivatives. Gluten-free	Biochemically proven hypoproteinaemia.	ProSource liquid 30ml sachets: citrus berry, lemon, neutral, orange creme 100 sachet = £110.11
ProSource® Plus (Nutrinovo Ltd)	Liquid (sip and tube feed) per 100 mL	1400 kJ (333 kcal)	50 g collagen protein, whey protein isolate	36.7 g sucrose (sugars 33.3 g)	Less than 1 g	Less than 1 g	Contains porcine derivatives, residual lactose. Gluten-free	Hypoproteinaemia.	ProSource Plus liquid 30ml sachets: citrus berry, neutral, orange creme 50 sachet = £78.32; 100 sachet = £156.63

PROTEIN, FAT, AND CARBOHYDRATE

Not suitable for use in child under 3 years unless otherwise stated; not recommended for child under 6 years unless otherwise stated

Product	Formulation	Energy	Protein	Carbohydrate	Fat	Fibre	Special Characteristics	ACBS Indications	Presentation & Flavour
Calogen® Extra (Nutricia Ltd)	Liquid (sip or tube feed) per 100 mL	1650 kJ (400 kcal)	5 g caseinates, whey protein hydrolysate	4.5 g (sugars 3.5 g)	40.3 g	Nil	Contains residual lactose. Gluten-free.	Disease related malnutrition, malabsorption states or other conditions requiring fortification with a high fat supplement with or without fluid restriction.	Calogen Extra Shots emulsion: neutral, strawberry 240 ml = £5.88; Calogen Extra emulsion: neutral, strawberry 200 ml = £4.98
Calshake® (Fresenius Kabi Ltd)	Standard dilution (28% w/v) of powder per 100 ml	795 kJ (190 kcal)	3.8 g milk protein	22.2 g (sugars 7 g)	9.5 g	less than 0.15 g	Contains lactose. Gluten-free. Neutral flavour not suitable for use in child under 1 year	Disease related malnutrition, malabsorption states or other conditions requiring fortification with a fat/carbohydrate supplement.	Calshake powder 87 g sachets: banana, neutral, strawberry, vanilla 7 sachet = £18.41; Calshake powder 90g sachets: chocolate 7 sachet = £18.41

Powder provides: protein 4.3 g, carbohydrate 67.3 g, fat 24.1 g, energy 2100 kJ (500 kcal)/100 g

Product	Formulation	Energy	Protein	Carbohydrate	Fat	Fibre	Special Characteristics	ACBS Indications	Presentation & Flavour
Enshake® (Abbott Laboratories Ltd)	Standard dilution (31.1% w/v) of powder per 100 mL	815 kJ (194 kcal)	5.2 g caseinate, milk, soya protein isolates	25.5 g 24.7 g corn syrup (sugars 7.4 g)	8 g	Nil	Contains residual lactose, soya. Gluten-free	Disease-related malnutrition, malabsorption states or other conditions requiring fortification with a fat/carbohydrate supplement.	Enshake oral powder 96.5g sachets: banana, chocolate, strawberry, vanilla 6 sachet = £15.65

Powder provides: protein 8.4 g, carbohydrate 69.5 g, fat 15.6 g, energy 1902 kJ (452 kcal)/100 g

Borderline substances | **Appendix 2**

A2

PROTEIN, FAT, AND CARBOHYDRATE (product list continued)

Not suitable for use in child under 3 years unless otherwise stated; not recommended for child under 6 years unless otherwise stated

Product	Formulation	Energy	Protein	Carbohydrate	Fat	Fibre	Special Characteristics	ACBS Indications	Presentation & Flavour
MCT Procal® (Vitaflo International Ltd)	Powder per 100 g	2742 kJ (657 kcal)	12.5 g cows' milk	20.6 g (sugars 3.1 g)	63.1 g (MCT 99%)	Nil	Contains lactose	Dietary management of disorders of long-chain fatty acid oxidation, fat malabsorption, and other disorders requiring a low LCT, high MCT supplement. Not suitable for child under 1 year.	MCT procal oral powder 16g sachets: 30 sachet = £26.85
Powder 16 g provides: protein 2 g, carbohydrate 3.3 g, fat 10.1 g, energy 439 kJ (105 kcal).									
Pro-Cal® (Vitaflo International Ltd)	Powder per 100 g	2764 kJ (667 kcal)	13.6 g cows' milk	28.2 g (sugars 16 g)	55.5 g	Nil	Contains lactose Gluten-free	Disease-related malnutrition, malabsorption states or other conditions requiring fortification with a fat / carbohydrate supplement (with protein). Suitable from one year of age.	Pro-Cal powder: 510 gram = £16.58; 1500 gram = £33.78; 12500 gram = £240.16
Powder 15 g provides: protein 2 g, carbohydrate 4.2 g, fat 8.3 g, energy 415 kJ (100 kcal).									
Pro-Cal® Shot (Vitaflo International Ltd)	Liquid per 100 mL	1385 kJ (334 kcal)	6.7 g cows' milk	13.4 g (sugars 13.3 g)	28.2 g	Nil	Contains lactose Gluten-free Contains soya	Disease-related malnutrition, malabsorption states, or other conditions requiring fortification with a high fat or carbohydrate (with protein) supplement. Not suitable for child under 3 years.	Pro-Cal shot: starter pack 360 ml = £7.86; banana, neutral, strawberry 720 ml = £15.71
Scandishake® Mix (Nutricia Ltd)	Powder per 100 g	2099 kJ (500 kcal)	4.7 g cows' milk	65 g (sugars 14.3 g)	24.7 g	Nil	Gluten-free Contains lactose	Disease-related malnutrition, malabsorption states, or other conditions requiring fortification with a high fat or carbohydrate (with protein) supplement. Not suitable for child under 3 years.	Scandishake Mix oral powder 85g sachets: banana, caramel, chocolate, strawberry, unflavoured, vanilla 6 sachet = £15.96
Powder: 85 g reconstituted with 240 mL whole milk provides: protein 11.7 g, carbohydrate 66.8 g, fat 30.4 g, energy 2457 kJ (588 kcal).									
Vitasavoury® (Vitaflo International Ltd)	Powder per 100 g	2562 kJ (619 kcal)	12 g cows' milk	22.5 g (sugars 1.4 g Chicken/2.7 g Golden Vegetable)	52 g	6.4 g	Contains lactose Contains soya (chicken flavour) Contains gluten (wheat) (chicken flavour) Contains celery (golden vegetable flavour)	Disease-related malnutrition, malabsorption states, or other conditions requiring fortification with a high fat or carbohydrate (with protein) supplement. Not suitable for child under 3 years.	Vitasavoury powder 50g sachets: chicken, golden vegetable 10 sachet = £21.44

Fibre, vitamin, and mineral supplements

Vitamin and Mineral supplements

Not suitable for child under 4 years unless otherwise stated

Product	Formulation	Energy	Protein	Carbohydrate	Fat	Fibre	Special Characteristics	ACBS Indications	Presentation & Flavour
DEKAs® Essential (Alveolus Biomedical B.V.)	Capsule per 100 g	2642 kJ (631 kcal)	Nil	50 g	49 g	Nil	Contains fish gelatin	For the dietary management of patients with cystic fibrosis on the specific recommendation of a specialist in cystic fibrosis.	DEKAs Essential capsules: 60 capsule = £36.51
DEKAs® Plus (Alveolus Biomedical B.V.)	Solid per 100 g	1577 kJ (377 kcal)	2.5 g	88 g (sugars 70 g)	1.8 g	Nil		For the dietary management of patients with cystic fibrosis on the specific recommendation of a specialist in cystic fibrosis.	DEKAs Plus chewable tablets: 60 tablet = £42.58
	Liquid per 100 mL	400 kJ (100 kcal)	2 g	22 g	Nil	Nil		For the dietary management of patients with cystic fibrosis on the specific recommendation of a specialist in cystic fibrosis.	DEKAs Plus liquid: 60 ml = £33.24
	Solid per 100 g	2090 kJ (500 kcal)	25 g	22 g (sugars less than 100 mg)	43 g	Nil	Contains bovine gelatin Contains soy	For the dietary management of patients with cystic fibrosis on the specific recommendation of a specialist in cystic fibrosis.	DEKAs Plus softgels capsules: 60 capsule = £42.58
FruitiVits® (Vitaflo International Ltd)	Powder per 100 g	133 kJ (33 kcal)	Nil	8.3 g (sugars 400 mg)	0.1 g	3.3 g		Vitamin, mineral, and trace element supplement in children 3-10 years with restrictive therapeutic diets	FruitiVits oral powder 6g sachets: 30 sachet = £72.63
Renavit® (Stanningley Pharma Ltd)	Tablet per 450 mg	3.15 kJ (0.75 kcal)	Nil	0.17 g	Nil	Nil		Dietary management of water-soluble vitamin deficiency in adults with renal failure on dialysis	Renavit tablets: 100 tablet = £12.86

A2

Feed additives

Special additives for conditions of intolerance

Glucose

▸ (Dextrose monohydrate) For use as an energy supplement in sucrose-isomaltase deficiency

Glucose powder for oral use BP 1980 (Ennogen Healthcare Ltd)
500 gram (ACBS) · No NHS indicative price available · Drug Tariff (Part VIIIA Category C) price = £1.75

Glucose powder for oral use BP 1980 (Thornton & Ross Ltd)
500 gram (ACBS) · NHS indicative price = £1.75 · Drug Tariff (Part VIIIA Category C) price = £1.75

Feed thickeners and pre-thickened drinks

Instant Carobel ®

▸ For thickening of liquids or foods in the treatment of vomiting.
POWDER, contains residual lactose.

Instant Carobel powder (Cow & Gate Ltd)
135 gram (ACBS) · NHS indicative price = £2.98

Multi-thick ®

▸ For thickening of liquids and foods in dysphagia. Not suitable for child under 3 years.
POWDER, modified maize starch, gluten and lactose-free.

Multi-thick powder (Abbott Laboratories Ltd)
250 gram (ACBS) · NHS indicative price = £4.83

Nutilis ® **Clear**

▸ For thickening of liquids or foods in dysphagia. Not suitable for use in child under 3 years.
POWDER, contains guar gum, maltodextrin, xanthan gum. Gluten free,lactose-free.

Nutilis Clear powder (Nutricia Ltd)
175 gram (ACBS) · NHS indicative price = £8.46

Nutilis Clear powder 1.25g sachets (Nutricia Ltd)
50 sachet (ACBS) · NHS indicative price = £11.37

Nutilis ® **Powder**

▸ For thickening of liquids or foods in dysphagia. Not suitable for use in child under 3 years of age.
POWDER, gluten-free and lactose-free.

Nutilis powder (Nutricia Ltd)
300 gram (ACBS) · NHS indicative price = £5.66

Resource ® **Thickened Drink**

▸ For dysphagia. Not suitable for children under 3 years.
LIQUID, carbohydrate: orange 21 g; apple 23 g, energy: orange 376 kJ (89 kcal); apple 396 kJ (93 kcal)/100 mL.

Resource Thickened Drink custard apple (Nestle Health Science)
114 ml (ACBS) · NHS indicative price = £0.78

Resource Thickened Drink custard orange (Nestle Health Science)
114 ml (ACBS) · NHS indicative price = £0.78

Resource Thickened Drink syrup orange (Nestle Health Science)
114 ml (ACBS) · NHS indicative price = £0.78

Resource ® **ThickenUp** ®

▸ For thickening of liquids or foods in dysphagia. Not suitable for use in child under 3 years.
POWDER, contains modified food starch (maize).

Resource ThickenUp powder 4.5g sachets (Nestle Health Science)
75 sachet (ACBS) · NHS indicative price = £18.49

Resource ThickenUp powder (Nestle Health Science)
227 gram (ACBS) · NHS indicative price = £4.66

Resource ® **ThickenUp** ® **Clear**

▸ For thickening of liquids or foods in dysphagia. Not suitable for use in child under 3 years.
POWDER, contains maltodextrin (corn, potato), potassium chloride, residual lactose (tin only), xanthan gum. Gluten-free.

Resource ThickenUp Clear powder (Nestle Health Science)
127 gram (ACBS) · NHS indicative price = £8.46

Resource ThickenUp Clear powder 1.2g sachets (Nestle Health Science)
24 sachet (ACBS) · NHS indicative price = £5.28

SLO Drinks ®

▸ Nutritional supplement for patient hydration in the dietary management of dysphagia. Not suitable for children under 3 years.
POWDER, carbohydrate content varies with flavour and chosen consistency (3 consistencies available), see product literature.

SLO Drink Stage 1: IDDSI 2 Mildly Thick oral powder blackcurrant (SLO Drinks Ltd)
25 cup (ACBS) · NHS indicative price = £7.50

SLO Drink Stage 1: IDDSI 2 Mildly Thick oral powder orange (SLO Drinks Ltd)
25 cup (ACBS) · NHS indicative price = £7.50

SLO Drink Stage 2: IDDSI 3 Moderately Thick oral powder blackcurrant (SLO Drinks Ltd)
25 cup (ACBS) · NHS indicative price = £7.50

SLO Drink Stage 2: IDDSI 3 Moderately Thick oral powder orange (SLO Drinks Ltd)
25 cup (ACBS) · NHS indicative price = £7.50

Thick and Easy ®

▸ For thickening of foods in dysphagia. Not suitable for children under 1 year except in cases of failure to thrive.
POWDERModified maize starch

Thick & Easy Original powder (Fresenius Kabi Ltd)
225 gram (ACBS) · NHS indicative price = £5.57 | 4540 gram (ACBS) · NHS indicative price = £96.75

Thicken Aid ®

▸ For thickening of foods in dysphagia. Not suitable for child under 1 year; not recommended for child under 3 years
POWDER, contains maltodextrin, modified maize starch.

Thicken Aid powder (Aymes International Ltd)
225 gram (ACBS) · NHS indicative price = £3.71

Thixo-D ®

▸ For thickening of foods in dysphagia. Not suitable for children under 1 year except in cases of failure to thrive.
POWDER, modified maize starch, gluten-free.

Thixo-D Original powder (Ecogreen Technologies Ltd)
375 gram (ACBS) · NHS indicative price = £8.10

Thixo-D Cal-Free powder (Ecogreen Technologies Ltd)
30 gram · NHS indicative price = £3.00

Flavouring preparations

FlavourPac ®

▸ For use with Vitaflo's range of unflavoured protein substitutes for metabolic diseases; not suitable for child under 3 years.
POWDER

FlavourPac oral powder 4g sachets blackcurrant (Vitaflo International Ltd)
30 sachet (ACBS) · NHS indicative price = £15.58

FlavourPac oral powder 4g sachets orange (Vitaflo International Ltd)
30 sachet (ACBS) · NHS indicative price = £15.58

FlavourPac oral powder 4g sachets raspberry (Vitaflo International Ltd)
30 sachet (ACBS) · NHS indicative price = £15.58

FlavourPac oral powder 4g sachets tropical (Vitaflo International Ltd)
30 sachet (ACBS) · NHS indicative price = £15.58

Modjul ® **Flavour System**

▸ For use with unflavoured amino acid and peptide-based Nutricia products used for the dietary management of various conditions including metabolic disorders and gastrointestinal disease.
POWDER

Nutricia Flavour Modjul powder blackcurrant (Nutricia Ltd)
100 gram (ACBS) · NHS indicative price = £13.97

Nutricia Flavour Modjul powder orange (Nutricia Ltd)
100 gram (ACBS) · NHS indicative price = £13.97

Nutricia Flavour Modjul powder pineapple (Nutricia Ltd)
100 gram (ACBS) · NHS indicative price = £13.97

Foods for special diets

Gluten-free foods

ACBS indications: established gluten-sensitive enteropathies including steatorrhoea due to gluten sensitivity, coeliac disease, and dermatitis herpetiformis.

Bread

LOAVES

Barkat ® Loaf
GLUTEN-FREE

Barkat gluten free par baked white bread sliced (Gluten Free Foods Ltd)
500 gram (ACBS) · NHS indicative price = £4.21

Barkat gluten free wholemeal bread sliced (Gluten Free Foods Ltd)
500 gram (ACBS) · NHS indicative price = £4.05

Genius Gluten Free ® Loaf
GLUTEN-FREE

Genius gluten free brown sandwich bread sliced (Genius Foods Ltd)
535 gram (ACBS) · NHS indicative price = £3.80

Genius gluten free white sandwich bread sliced (Genius Foods Ltd)
535 gram (ACBS) · NHS indicative price = £3.80

Glutafin ® Loaves
GLUTEN-FREE

Glutafin gluten free fibre loaf sliced (Dr Schar UK Ltd)
300 gram (ACBS) · NHS indicative price = £2.89

Glutafin gluten free white loaf sliced (Dr Schar UK Ltd)
300 gram (ACBS) · NHS indicative price = £2.89

Glutafin ® Select Loaves
GLUTEN-FREE

Glutafin gluten free Select fibre loaf sliced (Dr Schar UK Ltd)
400 gram (ACBS) · NHS indicative price = £3.43

Glutafin gluten free Select fresh brown loaf sliced (Dr Schar UK Ltd)
400 gram (ACBS) · NHS indicative price = £3.43

Glutafin gluten free Select fresh white loaf sliced (Dr Schar UK Ltd)
400 gram (ACBS) · NHS indicative price = £3.43

Glutafin gluten free Select seeded loaf sliced (Dr Schar UK Ltd)
400 gram (ACBS) · NHS indicative price = £3.72

Glutafin gluten free Select white loaf sliced (Dr Schar UK Ltd)
400 gram (ACBS) · NHS indicative price = £3.43

Juvela ® Loaf
GLUTEN-FREE

Juvela gluten free fresh fibre loaf sliced (Hero UK Ltd)
400 gram (ACBS) · NHS indicative price = £3.39

Juvela gluten free fresh white loaf sliced (Hero UK Ltd)
400 gram (ACBS) · NHS indicative price = £3.69

Juvela gluten free fibre loaf sliced (Hero UK Ltd)
400 gram (ACBS) · NHS indicative price = £3.54

Juvela gluten free part baked loaf (Hero UK Ltd)
400 gram (ACBS) · NHS indicative price = £3.95

Juvela gluten free part baked fibre loaf (Hero UK Ltd)
400 gram (ACBS) · NHS indicative price = £3.80

Juvela gluten free loaf unsliced (Hero UK Ltd)
400 gram (ACBS) · NHS indicative price = £3.54

Juvela gluten free fibre loaf unsliced (Hero UK Ltd)
400 gram (ACBS) · NHS indicative price = £3.54

Lifestyle ® Loaf
GLUTEN-FREE

Lifestyle gluten free brown bread sliced (Ultrapharm Ltd)
400 gram (ACBS) · NHS indicative price = £2.82

Lifestyle gluten free high fibre bread sliced (Ultrapharm Ltd)
400 gram · NHS indicative price = £2.82

Lifestyle gluten free white bread sliced (Ultrapharm Ltd)
400 gram · NHS indicative price = £2.82

Warburtons ® Loaf
GLUTEN-FREE

Warburtons gluten free brown bread sliced (Warburtons Ltd)
400 gram (ACBS) · NHS indicative price = £3.06

Warburtons gluten free white bread sliced (Warburtons Ltd)
400 gram (ACBS) · NHS indicative price = £3.06

BAGUETTES, BUNS AND ROLLS

Barkat ® Baguettes and rolls
GLUTEN-FREE

Barkat gluten free par baked rolls (Gluten Free Foods Ltd)
200 gram (ACBS) · NHS indicative price = £4.05

Barkat gluten free par baked baguettes (Gluten Free Foods Ltd)
200 gram (ACBS) · NHS indicative price = £4.05

Glutafin ® Baguettes and rolls
GLUTEN-FREE

Glutafin gluten free baguettes (Dr Schar UK Ltd)
350 gram (ACBS) · NHS indicative price = £3.51

Glutafin gluten free 4 white rolls (Dr Schar UK Ltd)
200 gram (ACBS) · NHS indicative price = £3.68

Glutafin gluten free part baked 4 fibre rolls (Dr Schar UK Ltd)
200 gram (ACBS) · NHS indicative price = £3.68

Glutafin ® Select Rolls
GLUTEN-FREE

Glutafin gluten free part baked 4 white rolls (Dr Schar UK Ltd)
200 gram (ACBS) · NHS indicative price = £3.68

Glutafin gluten free part baked 2 long white rolls (Dr Schar UK Ltd)
150 gram (ACBS) · NHS indicative price = £2.81

Juvela ® Rolls
GLUTEN-FREE

Juvela gluten free fresh fibre rolls (Hero UK Ltd)
425 gram (ACBS) · NHS indicative price = £4.42

Juvela gluten free fresh white rolls (Hero UK Ltd)
425 gram (ACBS) · NHS indicative price = £4.42

Juvela gluten free fibre bread rolls (Hero UK Ltd)
425 gram (ACBS) · NHS indicative price = £4.77

Juvela gluten free bread rolls (Hero UK Ltd)
425 gram (ACBS) · NHS indicative price = £4.77

Juvela gluten free part baked fibre bread rolls (Hero UK Ltd)
375 gram (ACBS) · NHS indicative price = £4.94

Juvela gluten free part baked white bread rolls (Hero UK Ltd)
375 gram (ACBS) · NHS indicative price = £4.94

Lifestyle ® Rolls
GLUTEN-FREE

Lifestyle gluten free brown bread rolls (Ultrapharm Ltd)
400 gram (ACBS) · NHS indicative price = £2.82

Lifestyle gluten free high fibre bread rolls (Ultrapharm Ltd)
400 gram (ACBS) · NHS indicative price = £2.82

Lifestyle gluten free white bread rolls (Ultrapharm Ltd)
400 gram (ACBS) · NHS indicative price = £2.82

Proceli ® Baguettes, buns and rolls
GLUTEN-FREE

Proceli gluten free part baked baguettes (Ambe Ltd)
250 gram (ACBS) · NHS indicative price = £3.24

Warburtons ® Baguettes and rolls
GLUTEN-FREE

Warburtons gluten free brown rolls (Warburtons Ltd)
220 gram (ACBS) · NHS indicative price = £2.55

Warburtons gluten free white rolls (Warburtons Ltd)
220 gram (ACBS) · NHS indicative price = £2.55

Cereals

Juvela ® Fibre flakes and oats
GLUTEN-FREE

Juvela gluten free fibre flakes (Hero UK Ltd)
300 gram · NHS indicative price = £2.78

Juvela gluten free flakes (Hero UK Ltd)
300 gram · NHS indicative price = £2.78

Juvela gluten free pure oats (Hero UK Ltd)
500 gram · NHS indicative price = £2.78

Nairns ® Porridge
GLUTEN-FREE

Nairn's gluten free oat porridge (Nairn's Oatcakes Ltd)
500 gram · NHS indicative price = £3.05

Cookies and biscuits

Barkat ® Biscuits
GLUTEN-FREE

Barkat gluten free digestive biscuits (Gluten Free Foods Ltd)
175 gram · NHS indicative price = £2.66

Glutafin ® Cookies and biscuits
GLUTEN-FREE

Glutafin gluten free digestive biscuits (Dr Schar UK Ltd)
150 gram · NHS indicative price = £2.13

Glutafin gluten free shortbread biscuits (Dr Schar UK Ltd)
100 gram · NHS indicative price = £1.73

Juvela ® Biscuits
GLUTEN-FREE

Juvela gluten free digestive biscuits (Hero UK Ltd)
150 gram · NHS indicative price = £3.05

Juvela gluten free savoury biscuits (Hero UK Ltd)
150 gram · NHS indicative price = £3.82

Juvela gluten free sweet biscuits (Hero UK Ltd)
150 gram · NHS indicative price = £2.88

Juvela gluten free tea biscuits (Hero UK Ltd)
150 gram · NHS indicative price = £3.05

Crackers, crispbreads, and breadsticks

Barkat ® Crackers
GLUTEN-FREE

Barkat gluten free matzo crackers (Gluten Free Foods Ltd)
200 gram · NHS indicative price = £3.59

Glutafin ® Crackers
GLUTEN-FREE

Glutafin gluten free crackers (Dr Schar UK Ltd)
200 gram · NHS indicative price = £3.46

Glutafin gluten free mini crackers (Dr Schar UK Ltd)
175 gram · NHS indicative price = £2.96

Juvela ® Crispbread
GLUTEN-FREE

Juvela gluten free crispbread (Hero UK Ltd)
200 gram · NHS indicative price = £4.64

Flour mixes and xanthan gum

FLOUR MIXES

Barkat ® Flour mix
GLUTEN-FREE

Barkat gluten free all purpose flour mix (Gluten Free Foods Ltd)
500 gram (ACBS) · NHS indicative price = £4.74

Finax ® Flour mix
GLUTEN-FREE

Finax gluten free coarse flour mix (Drossa Ltd)
900 gram (ACBS) · NHS indicative price = £8.85

Finax gluten free fibre bread mix (Drossa Ltd)
1000 gram (ACBS) · NHS indicative price = £10.14

Finax gluten free flour mix (Drossa Ltd)
900 gram (ACBS) · NHS indicative price = £8.85

Glutafin ® Flour mix
GLUTEN-FREE

Glutafin gluten free multipurpose white mix (Dr Schar UK Ltd)
500 gram (ACBS) · NHS indicative price = £6.66

Glutafin Select ® Flour mix
GLUTEN-FREE

Glutafin gluten free Select bread mix (Dr Schar UK Ltd)
500 gram (ACBS) · NHS indicative price = £6.66

Glutafin gluten free Select fibre bread mix (Dr Schar UK Ltd)
500 gram (ACBS) · NHS indicative price = £6.66

Glutafin gluten free Select multipurpose fibre mix (Dr Schar UK Ltd)
500 gram (ACBS) · NHS indicative price = £6.66

Glutafin gluten free Select multipurpose white mix (Dr Schar UK Ltd)
500 gram (ACBS) · NHS indicative price = £6.66

Juvela ® Flour mix
GLUTEN-FREE

Juvela gluten free fibre mix (Hero UK Ltd)
500 gram (ACBS) · NHS indicative price = £7.35

Juvela gluten free harvest mix (Hero UK Ltd)
500 gram (ACBS) · NHS indicative price = £7.35

Juvela gluten free mix (Hero UK Ltd)
500 gram (ACBS) · NHS indicative price = £7.35

Orgran ® Flour mix
GLUTEN-FREE

Orgran gluten free self-raising flour (Naturally Good Food Ltd)
500 gram · NHS indicative price = £3.10

Orgran gluten free all purpose plain flour (Naturally Good Food Ltd)
500 gram · NHS indicative price = £3.10

Proceli ® Flour mix
GLUTEN-FREE

Proceli gluten free basic mix (Ambe Ltd)
1000 gram (ACBS) · NHS indicative price = £9.95

Innovative Solutions Pure gluten free bakery blend mix (Innovative Solutions (UK) Ltd)
1000 gram (ACBS) · NHS indicative price = £4.63

Innovative Solutions Pure gluten free brown rice flour (Innovative Solutions (UK) Ltd)
500 gram (ACBS) · NHS indicative price = £1.86

Innovative Solutions Pure gluten free white rice flour (Innovative Solutions (UK) Ltd)
500 gram (ACBS) · NHS indicative price = £1.97

Innovative Solutions Pure gluten free potato flour (Innovative Solutions (UK) Ltd)
500 gram (ACBS) · NHS indicative price = £1.97

Innovative Solutions Pure gluten free tapioca flour (Innovative Solutions (UK) Ltd)
500 gram (ACBS) · NHS indicative price = £2.66

Innovative Solutions Pure gluten free brown teff flour (Innovative Solutions (UK) Ltd)
1000 gram (ACBS) · NHS indicative price = £5.61

Innovative Solutions Pure gluten free white teff flour (Innovative Solutions (UK) Ltd)
1000 gram (ACBS) · NHS indicative price = £5.61

Tobia ® Flour mix
GLUTEN-FREE

Tobia Teff gluten free brown bread mix (Tobia Teff UK Ltd)
1000 gram (ACBS) · NHS indicative price = £3.85

Tobia Teff gluten free white bread mix (Tobia Teff UK Ltd)
1000 gram (ACBS) · NHS indicative price = £3.85

Tritamyl ® Flour mix
GLUTEN-FREE

Tritamyl gluten free brown bread mix (Gluten Free Foods Ltd)
1000 gram (ACBS) · NHS indicative price = £7.24

Tritamyl gluten free flour mix (Gluten Free Foods Ltd)
2000 gram (ACBS) · NHS indicative price = £14.54

Tritamyl gluten free white bread mix (Gluten Free Foods Ltd)
2000 gram (ACBS) · NHS indicative price = £14.54

XANTHAN GUM

Pure ® Xanthan gum
GLUTEN-FREE

Innovative Solutions Pure xanthan gum (Innovative Solutions (UK) Ltd)
100 gram · NHS indicative price = £7.82

Pasta

Barkat ® Pasta
GLUTEN-FREE

Barkat gluten free pasta macaroni (Gluten Free Foods Ltd)
500 gram · NHS indicative price = £5.99

arkat gluten free pasta spaghetti (Gluten Free Foods Ltd)
0 gram · NHS indicative price = £5.99

arkat gluten free pasta spirals (Gluten Free Foods Ltd)
0 gram · NHS indicative price = £5.99

arkat gluten free pasta buckwheat penne (Gluten Free Foods Ltd)
0 gram · NHS indicative price = £2.98

arkat gluten free pasta buckwheat spirals (Gluten Free Foods Ltd)
0 gram · NHS indicative price = £2.98

Alimenta ® **Pasta**
LUTEN-FREE

Alimenta gluten free pasta acini di pepe (Drossa Ltd)
0 gram · NHS indicative price = £6.11 | 1000 gram · No NHS
dicative price available

Alimenta gluten free pasta formati misti (Drossa Ltd)
000 gram · NHS indicative price = £36.63

Alimenta gluten free pasta penne (Drossa Ltd)
0 gram · NHS indicative price = £6.11 | 1000 gram · No NHS
dicative price available

iAlimenta gluten free pasta sagnette (Drossa Ltd)
0 gram · NHS indicative price = £6.11

iAlimenta gluten free pasta spirali (Drossa Ltd)
0 gram · NHS indicative price = £6.11

iAlimenta gluten free pasta tubetti (Drossa Ltd)
0 gram · NHS indicative price = £6.03

iAlimenta gluten free potato pasta gnocchi (Drossa Ltd)
0 gram · NHS indicative price = £5.71

iAlimenta gluten free potato pasta perle di gnocchi (Drossa Ltd)
0 gram · NHS indicative price = £5.72

lutafin ® **Pasta**
LUTEN-FREE

lutafin gluten free pasta macaroni penne (Dr Schar UK Ltd)
00 gram · NHS indicative price = £6.73

lutafin gluten free pasta spirals (Dr Schar UK Ltd)
00 gram · NHS indicative price = £6.73

lutafin gluten free pasta long-cut spaghetti (Dr Schar UK Ltd)
00 gram · NHS indicative price = £6.73

uvela ® **Pasta**
LUTEN-FREE

uvela gluten free fibre penne (Hero UK Ltd)
00 gram · NHS indicative price = £6.61

uvela gluten free pasta fusilli (Hero LK Ltd)
00 gram · NHS indicative price = £7.21

Juvela gluten free pasta lasagne (Hero UK Ltd)
250 gram · NHS indicative price = £3.68

Juvela gluten free pasta macaroni (Hero UK Ltd)
00 gram · NHS indicative price = £7.21

Juvela gluten free pasta spaghetti (Hero UK Ltd)
00 gram · NHS indicative price = £7.21

Juvela gluten free pasta tagliatelle (Hero UK Ltd)
250 gram · NHS indicative price = £3.47

Organ ® **Pasta**
GLUTEN-FREE

Organ gluten free pasta rice & corn lasagne (Naturally Good Food
Ltd)
200 gram · NHS indicative price = £3.13

Organ gluten free pasta rice & corn macaroni (Naturally Good Food
Ltd)
250 gram · NHS indicative price = £2.42

Organ gluten free pasta buckwheat spirals (Naturally Good Food
Ltd)
250 gram · NHS indicative price = £2.42

Organ gluten free pasta brown rice spirals (Naturally Good Food
Ltd)
250 gram · NHS indicative price = £2.42

Organ gluten free pasta rice & corn spirals (Naturally Good Food
Ltd)
250 gram · NHS indicative price = £2.42

Rizopia ® **Pasta**
GLUTEN-FREE

Rizopia gluten free organic brown rice pasta fusilli (PGR Health
Foods Ltd)
500 gram · NHS indicative price = £2.72

Rizopia gluten free organic brown rice pasta lasagne (PGR Health
Foods Ltd)
375 gram · NHS indicative price = £2.72

Rizopia gluten free organic brown rice pasta penne (PGR Health
Foods Ltd)
500 gram · NHS indicative price = £2.72

Rizopia gluten free organic brown rice pasta spaghetti (PGR Health
Foods Ltd)
500 gram · NHS indicative price = £2.72

Pizza bases

Glutafin ® **Pizza base**
GLUTEN-FREE

Glutafin gluten free pizza base (Dr Schar UK Ltd)
300 gram · NHS indicative price = £6.56

Juvela ® **Pizza base**
GLUTEN-FREE

Juvela gluten free pizza base (Hero UK Ltd)
300 gram · NHS indicative price = £6.50

Proceli ® **Pizza base**
GLUTEN-FREE

Proceli gluten free pizza base (Ambe Ltd)
250 gram · NHS indicative price = £3.90

Gluten- and wheat-free foods

ACBS indications: established gluten-sensitive
enteropathies with coexisting established wheat sensitivity
only.

Glutafin ® **Flour mix, fibre and crispbread**
GLUTEN-FREE, WHEAT-FREE

Glutafin gluten free crispbread (Dr Schar UK Ltd)
150 gram · NHS indicative price = £3.25

Glutafin gluten free bread mix (Dr Schar UK Ltd)
500 gram (ACBS) · NHS indicative price = £6.66

Glutafin gluten free fibre bread mix (Dr Schar UK Ltd)
500 gram (ACBS) · NHS indicative price = £6.66

Glutafin gluten free wheat free fibre mix (Dr Schar UK Ltd)
500 gram (ACBS) · NHS indicative price = £6.66

Low-protein foods

ACBS indications: inherited metabolic disorders, renal or
liver failure, requiring a low-protein diet.

Bread

Juvela ® **Loaf and rolls**
LOW PROTEIN

Juvela gluten free loaf sliced (Hero UK Ltd)
400 gram (ACBS) · NHS indicative price = £3.54

Juvela low protein bread rolls (Hero UK Ltd)
350 gram (ACBS) · NHS indicative price = £4.52

Juvela low protein loaf sliced (Hero UK Ltd)
400 gram (ACBS) · NHS indicative price = £3.64

Loprofin ® **Bread**
LOW-PROTEIN

Loprofin low protein part baked bread rolls (Nutricia Ltd)
260 gram (ACBS) · NHS indicative price = £4.48

Loprofin low protein part baked loaf sliced (Nutricia Ltd)
400 gram (ACBS) · NHS indicative price = £4.26

Mevalia ® **Bread**
LOW-PROTEIN

Mevalia low protein ciabattine (Dr Schar UK Ltd)
260 gram (ACBS) · NHS indicative price = £3.38

Mevalia low protein grissini (Dr Schar UK Ltd)
150 gram (ACBS) · NHS indicative price = £6.28

A2

Borderline substances | Appendix 2

Mevalia low protein mini baguette (Dr Schar UK Ltd)
200 gram (ACBS) · NHS indicative price = £2.58

Mevalia low protein pan carre (Dr Schar UK Ltd)
400 gram (ACBS) · NHS indicative price = £3.29

Mevalia low protein pan rustico (Dr Schar UK Ltd)
400 gram (ACBS) · NHS indicative price = £3.29

Mevalia low protein pane casereccio (Dr Schar UK Ltd)
220 gram (ACBS) · NHS indicative price = £2.19

PK Foods ® **Loaf**
LOW PROTEIN

PK Foods low protein white bread sliced (Gluten Free Foods Ltd)
300 gram · NHS indicative price = £4.84

Cake, biscuits, and snacks

Loprofin ® **Cake, biscuits and snacks**
LOW-PROTEIN

Loprofin low protein crackers (Nutricia Ltd)
150 gram (ACBS) · NHS indicative price = £3.91

Loprofin low protein herb crackers (Nutricia Ltd)
150 gram (ACBS) · NHS indicative price = £3.91

Mevalia cake, biscuits and snacks
LOW-PROTEIN

Mevalia Lattis low protein drink (Dr Schar UK Ltd)
500 ml (ACBS) · NHS indicative price = £3.15

Mevalia low protein chocotino bars (Dr Schar UK Ltd)
100 gram (ACBS) · NHS indicative price = £4.91

Mevalia low protein cookies (Dr Schar UK Ltd)
200 gram (ACBS) · NHS indicative price = £6.72

Mevalia low protein frollini biscuits (Dr Schar UK Ltd)
200 gram (ACBS) · NHS indicative price = £7.39

Mevalia low protein fruit bar (Dr Schar UK Ltd)
125 gram (ACBS) · NHS indicative price = £4.70

PK Foods ® **Biscuits**
LOW-PROTEIN

PK Foods Aminex low protein rusks (Gluten Free Foods Ltd)
200 gram (ACBS) · NHS indicative price = £5.14

PK Foods low protein crispbread (Gluten Free Foods Ltd)
75 gram (ACBS) · NHS indicative price = £2.46

Promin ® **Cooked and flavoured pasta snax**
LOW-PROTEIN

Promin low protein Snax salt & vinegar 25g sachets (Firstplay Dietary Foods Ltd)
3 sachet · No NHS indicative price available | 12 sachet (ACBS) · NHS indicative price = £11.25

Promin low protein Snax ready salted 25g sachets (Firstplay Dietary Foods Ltd)
3 sachet · No NHS indicative price available | 12 sachet (ACBS) · NHS indicative price = £11.25

Promin low protein Snax jalapeno 25g sachets (Firstplay Dietary Foods Ltd)
3 sachet · No NHS indicative price available | 12 sachet (ACBS) · NHS indicative price = £11.25

Promin low protein Snax cheese & onion 25g sachets (Firstplay Dietary Foods Ltd)
3 sachet · No NHS indicative price available | 12 sachet (ACBS) · NHS indicative price = £11.25

Taranis ® **Cake bars**
LOW-PROTEIN

Taranis low protein apricot cake (Lactalis Nutrition Sante)
240 gram (ACBS) · NHS indicative price = £6.24

Taranis low protein lemon cake (Lactalis Nutrition Sante)
240 gram (ACBS) · NHS indicative price = £6.24

Taranis low protein pear cake (Lactalis Nutrition Sante)
240 gram (ACBS) · NHS indicative price = £6.24

Vita Bite ®
▸ Not recommended for any child under 1 year.
LOW PROTEIN.
Bar, protein 30 mg (less than 2.5 mg phenylalanine), carbohydrate 15.35 g, fat 8.4 g, energy 572 kJ (137 kcal)/25 g.

VitaBite bar (Vitaflo International Ltd)
175 gram (ACBS) · NHS indicative price = £9.72

Vitaflo Choices ® **Mini crackers**
LOW-PROTEIN

Vitaflo Choices mini crackers (Vitaflo International Ltd)
40 gram (ACBS) · NHS indicative price = £0.96

Cereals

Loprofin ® **Cereals**
LOW-PROTEIN

Loprofin low protein breakfast cereal flakes chocolate (Nutricia Ltd)
375 gram (ACBS) · NHS indicative price = £8.65

Loprofin low protein breakfast cereal flakes strawberry (Nutricia Ltd)
375 gram (ACBS) · NHS indicative price = £8.65

Loprofin low protein breakfast cereal loops (Nutricia Ltd)
375 gram (ACBS) · NHS indicative price = £8.97

Promin ® **Hot breakfast**
LOW-PROTEIN

Promin low protein hot breakfast powder 56g sachets original (Firstplay Dietary Foods Ltd)
6 sachet (ACBS) · NHS indicative price = £8.55

Promin low protein hot breakfast powder 57g sachets apple & cinnamon (Firstplay Dietary Foods Ltd)
6 sachet (ACBS) · NHS indicative price = £8.55

Promin low protein hot breakfast powder 57g sachets banana (Firstplay Dietary Foods Ltd)
6 sachet (ACBS) · NHS indicative price = £8.55

Promin low protein hot breakfast powder 57g sachets chocolate (Firstplay Dietary Foods Ltd)
6 sachet (ACBS) · NHS indicative price = £8.55

Desserts

PK Foods ® **Jelly**
LOW-PROTEIN

PK Foods low protein jelly mix dessert cherry (Gluten Free Foods Ltd)
320 gram (ACBS) · NHS indicative price = £8.19

PK Foods low protein jelly mix dessert orange (Gluten Free Foods Ltd)
320 gram (ACBS) · NHS indicative price = £8.19

Promin ® **Desserts**
LOW-PROTEIN

Promin low protein dessert 36.5g sachets caramel (Firstplay Dietary Foods Ltd)
6 sachet (ACBS) · NHS indicative price = £6.72

Promin low protein dessert 36.5g sachets chocolate & banana (Firstplay Dietary Foods Ltd)
6 sachet (ACBS) · NHS indicative price = £6.72

Promin low protein dessert 36.5g sachets custard (Firstplay Dietary Foods Ltd)
6 sachet (ACBS) · NHS indicative price = £6.72

Promin low protein dessert 36.5g sachets strawberry & vanilla (Firstplay Dietary Foods Ltd)
6 sachet (ACBS) · NHS indicative price = £6.72

Flour mixes and egg substitutes

Fate ® **Flour mixes and egg substitutes**
LOW-PROTEIN

Fate low protein all purpose mix (Fate Special Foods)
500 gram (ACBS) · NHS indicative price = £6.97

Fate low protein chocolate cake mix (Fate Special Foods)
500 gram (ACBS) · NHS indicative price = £6.97

Fate low protein plain cake mix (Fate Special Foods)
500 gram (ACBS) · NHS indicative price = £6.97

Juvela ® **Mix**
LOW-PROTEIN

Juvela low protein mix (Hero UK Ltd)
500 gram (ACBS) · NHS indicative price = £7.79

oprofin ® Flour mixes and egg substitutes
OW-PROTEIN

oprofin low protein cake mix chocolate (Nutricia Ltd)
00 gram (ACBS) · NHS indicative price = £9.68

oprofin low protein egg replacer (Nutricia Ltd)
00 gram (ACBS) · NHS indicative price = £16.81

oprofin low protein egg white replacer (Nutricia Ltd)
00 gram (ACBS) · NHS indicative price = £10.81

oprofin low protein mix (Nutricia Ltd)
00 gram (ACBS) · NHS indicative price = £9.01

Mevalia ® low protein flour mixes and egg substitutes
OW-PROTEIN

Mevalia low protein bread mix (Dr Schar UK Ltd)
00 gram (ACBS) · NHS indicative price = £5.98

Mevalia low protein egg replacer (Dr Schar UK Ltd)
00 gram (ACBS) · NHS indicative price = £8.16

K Foods ® Flour mix and egg substitute
OW-PROTEIN

K Foods low protein egg replacer (Gluten Free Foods Ltd)
00 gram (ACBS) · NHS indicative price = £4.16

K Foods low protein flour mix (Gluten Free Foods Ltd)
50 gram (ACBS) · NHS indicative price = £10.92

Pasta

oprofin ® Pasta
OW-PROTEIN

oprofin low protein pasta animal shapes (Nutricia Ltd)
00 gram (ACBS) · NHS indicative price = £9.20

oprofin low protein pasta fusilli (Nutricia Ltd)
00 gram (ACBS) · NHS indicative price = £9.55

oprofin low protein pasta lasagne (Nutricia Ltd)
250 gram (ACBS) · NHS indicative price = £4.65

oprofin low protein pasta long cut spaghetti (Nutricia Ltd)
00 gram (ACBS) · NHS indicative price = £9.55

oprofin low protein pasta macaroni elbows (Nutricia Ltd)
250 gram (ACBS) · NHS indicative price = £4.60

oprofin low protein pasta penne (Nutricia Ltd)
00 gram (ACBS) · NHS indicative price = £9.55

oprofin low protein pasta tagliatelle (Nutricia Ltd)
250 gram (ACBS) · NHS indicative price = £4.60

Loprofin low protein rice (Nutricia Ltd)
500 gram (ACBS) · NHS indicative price = £9.28

Mevalia ® Pasta
LOW-PROTEIN

Mevalia low protein fusilli (Dr Schar UK Ltd)
500 gram (ACBS) · NHS indicative price = £6.29

Mevalia low protein pasta ditali (Dr Schar UK Ltd)
500 gram (ACBS) · NHS indicative price = £6.29

Mevalia low protein penne (Dr Schar UK Ltd)
500 gram (ACBS) · NHS indicative price = £6.29

Mevalia low protein rice replacer (Dr Schar UK Ltd)
400 gram (ACBS) · NHS indicative price = £5.18

Mevalia low protein spaghetti (Dr Schar UK Ltd)
500 gram (ACBS) · NHS indicative price = £6.29

Promin ® Pasta
LOW-PROTEIN

Promin low protein pasta alphabets (Firstplay Dietary Foods Ltd)
500 gram (ACBS) · NHS indicative price = £7.39

Promin Plus low protein pasta macaroni (Firstplay Dietary Foods Ltd)
500 gram (ACBS) · NHS indicative price = £7.39

Promin Plus low protein pasta flat noodles (Firstplay Dietary Foods Ltd)
500 gram (ACBS) · NHS indicative price = £7.39

Promin low protein pasta shells (Firstplay Dietary Foods Ltd)
500 gram (ACBS) · NHS indicative price = £7.39

Promin low protein pasta short cut spaghetti (Firstplay Dietary Foods Ltd)
500 gram (ACBS) · NHS indicative price = £7.39

Promin low protein tricolour pasta spirals (Firstplay Dietary Foods Ltd)
500 gram (ACBS) · NHS indicative price = £7.39

Promin low protein pasta spirals (Firstplay Dietary Foods Ltd)
500 gram (ACBS) · NHS indicative price = £7.39

Promin low protein imitation rice (Firstplay Dietary Foods Ltd)
500 gram (ACBS) · NHS indicative price = £7.43

Promin low protein tricolour pasta alphabets (Firstplay Dietary Foods Ltd)
500 gram (ACBS) · NHS indicative price = £7.39

Promin low protein tricolour pasta shells (Firstplay Dietary Foods Ltd)
500 gram (ACBS) · NHS indicative price = £7.39

Promin low protein lasagne sheets (Firstplay Dietary Foods Ltd)
200 gram (ACBS) · NHS indicative price = £3.22

Pizza bases

Juvela ® Pizza base
LOW-PROTEIN

Juvela low protein pizza base (Hero UK Ltd)
360 gram (ACBS) · NHS indicative price = £8.61

Mevalia low protein pizza base
LOW-PROTEIN

Mevalia low protein pizza base (Dr Schar UK Ltd)
300 gram (ACBS) · NHS indicative price = £5.94

Savoury meals and mixes

Mevalia ® low protein burger mix
LOW-PROTEIN

Mevalia low protein burger mix (Dr Schar UK Ltd)
350 gram (ACBS) · NHS indicative price = £7.05

Promin ® Savoury meals and mixes
LOW-PROTEIN

Promin low protein cous cous (Firstplay Dietary Foods Ltd)
500 gram (ACBS) · NHS indicative price = £7.43

Promin low protein pasta elbows (Firstplay Dietary Foods Ltd)
500 gram · NHS indicative price = £7.39

Promin low protein pastameal (Firstplay Dietary Foods Ltd)
500 gram (ACBS) · NHS indicative price = £7.43

Promin low protein pasta macaroni (Firstplay Dietary Foods Ltd)
500 gram (ACBS) · NHS indicative price = £7.39

Promin Plus low protein pasta spirals (Firstplay Dietary Foods Ltd)
500 gram (ACBS) · NHS indicative price = £7.39

Promin low protein potato pot with croutons onion (Firstplay Dietary Foods Ltd)
200 gram (ACBS) · NHS indicative price = £17.45

Promin low protein potato pot with croutons cabbage & bacon (Firstplay Dietary Foods Ltd)
200 gram (ACBS) · NHS indicative price = £17.45

Promin low protein potato pot with croutons sausage (Firstplay Dietary Foods Ltd)
200 gram (ACBS) · NHS indicative price = £17.45

Promin low protein X-Pot all day scramble (Firstplay Dietary Foods Ltd)
240 gram (ACBS) · NHS indicative price = £22.20

Promin low protein X-Pot beef & tomato (Firstplay Dietary Foods Ltd)
240 gram (ACBS) · NHS indicative price = £22.20

Promin low protein X-Pot chip shop curry (Firstplay Dietary Foods Ltd)
240 gram (ACBS) · NHS indicative price = £22.20

Promin low protein X-Pot rogan style curry (Firstplay Dietary Foods Ltd)
240 gram (ACBS) · NHS indicative price = £22.20

Spreads

Taranis ® Spread
LOW-PROTEIN

Taranis low protein hazelnut spread (Lactalis Nutrition Sante)
230 gram (ACBS) · NHS indicative price = £8.15

A2

Borderline substances | Appendix 2

Nutritional supplements for metabolic diseases

Glutaric aciduria (type 1)

GA Gel ®
▸ Nutritional supplement for dietary management of type 1 glutaric aciduria in children 6 months–10 years.
GEL, protein equivalent (essential and non-essential amino acids except lysine, and low tryptophan) 10 g, carbohydrate 10.3 g, fat trace, energy 339 kJ (81 kcal)/24 g, with vitamins, minerals, and trace elements. To flavour unflavoured products, see FlavourPac p. 1644.

GA gel oral powder 24g sachets (Vitaflo International Ltd)
30 sachet (ACBS) · NHS indicative price = £240.23

XLYS, TRY Glutaridon ®
▸ Nutritional supplement for the dietary management of type 1 glutaric aciduria in children and adults; requires additional source of vitamins, minerals, and trace elements.
POWDER, protein equivalent (essential and non-essential amino acids except lysine and tryptophan) 79 g, carbohydrate 4 g, energy 1411 kJ (332 kcal)/100 g. To flavour unflavoured products, see Modjul Flavour System p. 1644.

XLYS TRY Glutaridon powder (Nutricia Ltd)
500 gram (ACBS) · NHS indicative price = £213.65

Glycogen storage disease

Glycosade ®
▸ A nutritional supplement for use in the dietary management of glycogen storage disease and other metabolic conditions where a constant supply of glucose is essential. Not suitable for use in children under 2 years.
POWDER, protein 200 mg, carbohydrate (maize starch) 47.6 g, fat 100 mg, fibre less than 600 mg, energy 803 kJ (192 kcal)/60 g.

Glycosade oral powder 60g sachets unflavoured (Vitaflo International Ltd)
30 sachet (ACBS) · NHS indicative price = £126.25

Homocystinuria or hypermethioninaemia

HCU cooler ®
▸ Nutritional supplement for the dietary management of homocystinuria. Not suitable for use in child under 3 years. Includes added vitamins A, B, C, D, E and K.
LIQUID, protein equivalent 11.5 g, carbohydrate 5.1 g, fat 0.9 g, energy 316 kJ (75 kcal)/100 mL.

HCU orange cooler15 liquid (Vitaflo International Ltd)
130 ml (ACBS) · NHS indicative price = £12.68

HCU red cooler10 liquid (Vitaflo International Ltd)
87 ml (ACBS) · NHS indicative price = £8.12

HCU red cooler15 liquid (Vitaflo International Ltd)
130 ml (ACBS) · NHS indicative price = £12.68

HCU red cooler20 liquid (Vitaflo International Ltd)
174 ml (ACBS) · NHS indicative price = £16.97

HCU Express ® 15
▸ A methionine-free protein substitute for use as a nutritional supplement in children over 8 years with homocystinuria.
POWDER, protein (essential and non-essential amino acids except methionine) 15 g, carbohydrate 3.8 g, fat 30 mg, energy 315 kJ (75.3 kcal)/25 g with vitamins, minerals, and trace elements. To flavour unflavoured products, see FlavourPac p. 1644.

HCU express15 oral powder 25g sachets (Vitaflo International Ltd)
30 sachet (ACBS) · NHS indicative price = £373.05

HCU Express ® 20
▸ A methionine-free protein substitute for use as a nutritional supplement in children over 8 years with homocystinuria.
POWDER, protein (essential and non-essential amino acids except methionine) 20 g, carbohydrate 4.7 g, fat 70 mg, energy 416 kJ (99 kcal)/34 g with vitamins, minerals, and trace

elements. To flavour unflavoured products, see FlavourPac p. 1644.

HCU express20 oral powder 34g sachets (Vitaflo International Ltd)
30 sachet (ACBS) · NHS indicative price = £481.98

HCU gel ®
▸ A methionine-free protein substitute for use as a nutritional supplement for the dietary management of children 1–10 years with homocystinuria.
POWDER, protein (essential and non-essential amino acids except methionine) 10 g, carbohydrate 10.3 g, fat 20 mg, energy 339 kJ (81 kcal)/24 g with vitamins, minerals, and trace elements. To flavour unflavoured products, see FlavourPac p. 1644.

HCU gel oral powder 24g sachets (Vitaflo International Ltd)
30 sachet (ACBS) · NHS indicative price = £240.17

HCU Lophlex ® LQ
▸ Nutritional supplement for the dietary management of homocystinuria. Not suitable for use in child under 4 years. Includes added vitamins A, B, C, D, E and K.
LIQUID, protein 16 g, carbohydrate 7 g, fat 0.35 g, energy 407 kJ (96 kcal)/100 mL.

HCU Lophlex LQ 10 liquid (Nutricia Ltd)
62.5 ml (ACBS) · NHS indicative price = £8.92

HCU Lophlex LQ 20 liquid (Nutricia Ltd)
125 ml (ACBS) · NHS indicative price = £18.40

HCU Maxamum ®
▸ Nutritional supplement for the dietary management of hypermethioninaemia, homocystinuria. Not suitable for use in child under 8 years. Includes added vitamins A, C, D, E and K.
POWDER, protein 39 g, carbohydrate 34 g, fat <0.5 g, energy 1260 kJ (297 kcal)/100 g.

HCU Maxamum powder (Nutricia Ltd)
500 gram (ACBS) · NHS indicative price = £180.78

HCU-LV ®
▸ Nutritional supplement for the dietary management of hypermethioninaemia or vitamin B6 non-responsive homocystinuria. Not suitable for use in child under 8 years. Includes added vitamins A, C, D E and K.
POWDER, protein 72 g, carbohydrate 9 g, fat 0.7 g, energy 1403 kJ (330 kcal)/100 g.

HCU-LV oral powder 27.8g sachets tropical (Nutricia Ltd)
30 sachet (ACBS) · NHS indicative price = £566.04

HCU-LV oral powder 27.8g sachets unflavoured (Nutricia Ltd)
30 sachet (ACBS) · NHS indicative price = £566.04

XMET Homidon ®
▸ Nutritional supplement for the dietary management of hypermethioninaemia or homocystinuria in children and adults.
POWDER, protein equivalent (essential and non-essential amino acids, except methionine) 77 g, carbohydrate 4.5 g, fat nil, energy 1386 kJ (326 kcal)/100 g. To flavour unflavoured products, see Modjul Flavour System p. 1644.

XMET Homidon powder (Nutricia Ltd)
500 gram (ACBS) · NHS indicative price = £213.65

Maple syrup urine disease

MSUD Aid III ®
▸ Nutritional supplement for the dietary management of maple syrup urine disease (MSUD) and related conditions when it is necessary to limit the intake of branched chain amino acids.
POWDER, protein 77 g, carbohydrate 4.5 g, fat nil, energy 1386 kJ (326 kcal)/100 g.

MSUD Aid 111 powder (Nutricia Ltd)
500 gram (ACBS) · NHS indicative price = £213.65

MSUD cooler ®
▸ Nutritional supplement for the dietary management of maple syrup urine disease. Not recommended for child under 3 years. Includes added vitamins A, B, C, D, E and K.
LIQUID, protein equivalent 11.5 g, carbohydrate 5.1 g, fat 0.9 g, energy 316 kJ (75 kcal)/100 mL.

MSUD orange cooler15 liquid (Vitaflo International Ltd)
30 ml (ACBS) · NHS indicative price = £12.68

MSUD red cooler10 liquid (Vitaflo International Ltd)
7 ml (ACBS) · NHS indicative price = £8.12

MSUD red cooler15 liquid (Vitaflo International Ltd)
30 ml (ACBS) · NHS indicative price = £12.68

MSUD red cooler20 liquid (Vitaflo International Ltd)
.74 ml (ACBS) · NHS indicative price = £16.97

MSUD express ® 15
Nutritional supplement for the dietary management of maple syrup urine disease in children over 8 years and adults.
POWDER, protein equivalent (essential and non-essential amino acids except leucine, isoleucine, and valine) 15 g, carbohydrate 5.8 g, fat less than 100 mg, energy 315 kJ (75 kcal)/25 g, with vitamins, minerals, and trace elements. To flavour unflavoured products, see FlavourPac p. 1644.

MSUD express15 oral powder 25g sachets (Vitaflo International Ltd)
30 sachet (ACBS) · NHS indicative price = £373.05

MSUD express ® 20
Nutritional supplement for the dietary management of maple syrup urine disease in children over 8 years and adults.
POWDER, protein equivalent (essential and non-essential amino acids except leucine, isoleucine, and valine) 20 g, carbohydrate 4.7 g, fat less than 100 mg, energy 416 kJ (99 kcal)/34 g, with vitamins, minerals, and trace elements. To flavour unflavoured products, see FlavourPac p. 1644.

MSUD express20 oral powder 34g sachets (Vitaflo International Ltd)
30 sachet (ACBS) · NHS indicative price = £481.98

MSUD Gel ®
Nutritional supplement for the dietary management of maple syrup urine disease in children 1–10 years.
POWDER, protein equivalent (essential and non-essential amino acids except leucine, isoleucine, and valine) 10 g, carbohydrate 10.3 g, fat less than 100 mg, energy 339 kJ (81 kcal)/24 g, with vitamins, minerals, and trace elements. To flavour unflavoured products, see FlavourPac p. 1644.

MSUD gel 24g sachets (Vitaflo International Ltd)
30 sachet (ACBS) · NHS indicative price = £242.99

MSUD Lophlex ® LQ
Nutritional supplement for the dietary management of maple syrup urine disease. Not recommended for child under 4 years. Includes added vitamins A, C, D, E and K.
LIQUID, protein equivalent (essential and non-essential amino acids) 16 g, carbohydrate 7 g, fat 0.35 g, energy 407 kJ (96 kcal)/100 mL.

MSUD Lophlex LQ 10 liquid (Nutricia Ltd)
62.5 ml (ACBS) · NHS indicative price = £8.92

MSUD Lophlex LQ 20 liquid (Nutricia Ltd)
125 ml (ACBS) · NHS indicative price = £18.40

MSUD Maxamum ®
Nutritional supplement for the dietary management of maple syrup urine disease. Not recommended for child under 8 years. Includes added vitamins A, B, C, D, E and K.
POWDER, protein equivalent (essential and non-essential amino acids) 39 g, carbohydrate 34 g, fat less than 0.5 g, energy 1260 kJ (297 kcal)/100 g.

MSUD Maxamum powder orange (Nutricia Ltd)
500 gram (ACBS) · NHS indicative price = £180.78

MSUD Maxamum powder unflavoured (Nutricia Ltd)
500 gram (ACBS) · NHS indicative price = £180.78

Methylmalonic or propionic acidaemia

MMA/PA Anamix ® Infant
▸ Nutritional supplement for the dietary management of proven methylmalonic acidaemia or propionic acidaemia in children from birth to 3 years.
POWDER, protein equivalent (essential and non-essential amino acids except methionine, threonine, and valine, and low isoleucine) 13.1 g, carbohydrate 49.5 g, fat 23 g, fibre 5.3 g, energy 1915 kJ (457 kcal)/100 g, with vitamins, minerals, and

trace elements; standard dilution (15%) provides protein equivalent 2 g, carbohydrate 7.4 g, fat 3.5 g, fibre 800 mg, energy 287 kJ (69 kcal)/100 mL.

MMA / PA Anamix Infant powder (Nutricia Ltd)
400 gram (ACBS) · NHS indicative price = £43.52

MMA/PA Maxamum ®
▸ Nutritional supplement for the dietary management of methylmalonic acidaemia or propionic acidaemia.
POWDER, protein equivalent (essential and non-essential amino acids except methionine, threonine, and valine, and low isoleucine) 39 g, carbohydrate 34 g, fat less than 500 mg, energy 1260 kJ (297 kcal)/100 g, with vitamins, minerals, and trace elements. To flavour unflavoured products, see Modjul Flavour System p. 1644.
Maxamum products are generally intended for use in children over 8 years.

MMA/PA Maxamum powder (Nutricia Ltd)
500 gram (ACBS) · NHS indicative price = £180.78

XMTVI Asadon ®
▸ Nutritional supplement for the dietary management of methylmalonic acidaemia or propionic acidaemia in children and adults.
POWDER, protein equivalent (essential and non-essential amino acids except methionine, threonine, and valine, and low isoleucine) 77 g, carbohydrate 4.5 g, fat nil, energy 1386 kJ (326 kcal)/100 g. To flavour unflavoured products, see Modjul Flavour System p. 1644.

XMTVI Asadon powder (Nutricia Ltd)
200 gram (ACBS) · NHS indicative price = £85.46

Other inborn errors of metabolism

Cystine500 ®
▸ Nutritional supplement for the dietary management of inborn errors of amino acid metabolism in adults and children from 3 years.
POWDER, cystine 500 mg, carbohydrate 3.3 g, fat nil, energy 64 kJ (15 kcal)/4 g

Cystine500 oral powder sachets (Vitaflo International Ltd)
30 sachet (ACBS) · NHS indicative price = £61.02

DocOmega ®
▸ Nutritional supplement for the dietary management of inborn errors of metabolism for adults and children from birth.
POWDER, protein (cows' milk, soya) 100 mg, carbohydrate 3.2 g, fat 500 mg (of which docosahexaenoic acid 200 mg), fibre nil, energy 74 kJ (18 kcal)/4 g, with minerals

DocOmega oral powder 4g sachets (Vitaflo International Ltd)
30 sachet (ACBS) · NHS indicative price = £44.16

EAA ® Supplement
▸ Nutritional supplement for the dietary management of disorders of protein metabolism including urea cycle disorders in children over 3 years.
POWDER, protein equivalent (essential amino acids) 5 g, carbohydrate 4 g, fat nil, energy 151 kJ (36 kcal)/12.5 g, with vitamins, minerals, and trace elements.

EAA Supplement oral powder 12.5g sachets (Vitaflo International Ltd)
50 sachet (ACBS) · NHS indicative price = £230.27

Isoleucine50 ®
▸ Nutritional supplement for use in the dietary management of inborn errors of amino acid metabolism in adults and children from birth.
POWDER, isoleucine 50 mg, carbohydrate 3.8 g, fat nil, energy 63 kJ (15 kcal)/4 g

Isoleucine50 oral powder 4g sachets (Vitaflo International Ltd)
30 sachet (ACBS) · NHS indicative price = £61.02

KeyOmega ®
▸ Nutritional supplement for the dietary management of inborn errors of metabolism. Includes added vitamin C.
POWDER, protein 4.4 g, carbohydrate 70 g, fat 19 g, energy 1999 kJ (476 kcal)/100 g.

A2

Borderline substances | Appendix 2

KeyOmega oral powder 4g sachets (Vitaflo International Ltd)
30 sachet (ACBS) · NHS indicative price = £45.16

Leucine100 ®
▸ Nutritional supplement for the dietary management of inborn errors of amino acid metabolism in adults and children from birth.
POWDER, leucine 100 mg, carbohydrate 3.7 g, fat nil, energy 63 kJ (15 kcal)/4 g

Leucine100 oral powder sachets (Vitaflo International Ltd)
30 sachet (ACBS) · NHS indicative price = £61.02

Low protein drink
▸ Nutritional supplement for the dietary management of inborn errors of amino acid metabolism in adults and children over 1 year.
POWDER, protein (cows' milk) 4.5 g (phenylalanine 100 mg), carbohydrate 59.5 g, fat 29.9 g, fibre nil, energy 2194 kJ (528 kcal)/100 g, with vitamins, minerals, and trace elements. Contains lactose.
Termed *Milupa* ® *lp-drink* by manufacturer.

Milupa LP drink (Nutricia Ltd)
400 gram (ACBS) · NHS indicative price = £10.00

Phenylalanine50 ®
▸ Nutritional supplement for use in the dietary management of inborn errors of metabolism in adults and children from birth.
POWDER, phenylalanine 50 mg, carbohydrate 3.8 g, fat nil, energy 63 kJ (15 kcal)/4 g

Phenylalanine50 oral powder sachets (Vitaflo International Ltd)
30 sachet (ACBS) · NHS indicative price = £59.25

ProZero ®
▸ A protein-free nutritional supplement for the dietary management of inborn errors of metabolism in children over 6 months and adults.
LIQUID, carbohydrate 8.1 g (of which sugars 3.5 g), fat 3.8 g, energy 278 kJ (66 kcal)/100 mL. Contains lactose.

ProZero liquid (Vitaflo International Ltd)
250 ml (ACBS) · NHS indicative price = £1.62 | 1000 ml (ACBS) · NHS indicative price = £6.50

Tyrosine1000 ®
▸ Nutritional supplement for the dietary management of inborn errors of amino acid metabolism in adults and children from birth.
POWDER, tyrosine 1 g, carbohydrate 2.9 g, fat nil, energy 63 kJ (15 kcal)/4-g sachet.

Tyrosine1000 oral powder 4g sachets (Vitaflo International Ltd)
30 sachet (ACBS) · NHS indicative price = £5.57

Valine50 ®
▸ Nutritional supplement for the dietary management of inborn errors of amino acid metabolism in adults and children from birth.
POWDER, valine 50 mg, carbohydrate 3.8 g, fat nil, energy 63 kJ (15 kcal)/4 g

Valine50 oral powder 4g sachets (Vitaflo International Ltd)
30 sachet (ACBS) · NHS indicative price = £61.02

Phenylketonuria

Easiphen ®
▸ Nutritional supplement for the dietary management of phenylketonuria. Not suitable for use in child under 8 years. Includes added vitamins A, B, C, D, E and K.
LIQUID, protein equivalent 6.7 g, carbohydrate 5.1 g, fat 2 g, energy 275 kJ (65 kcal)/100 mL

Easiphen liquid (Nutricia Ltd)
250 ml (ACBS) · NHS indicative price = £10.73

Glytactin RTD Lite 15
▸ Nutritional supplement for the dietary management of phenylketonuria. Not suitable for use in child under 3 years. Includes added vitamins A, B, C, D, E and K.
LIQUID, protein 6 g, carbohydrate 3 g, fat 1.4 g, energy 201 kJ (48 kcal)/100 mL.

Glytactin RTD Lite 15 liquid coffee mocha (Cambrooke Therapeutics)
250 ml (ACBS) · NHS indicative price = £8.55

Glytactin RTD Lite 15 liquid vanilla (Cambrooke Therapeutics)
250 ml (ACBS) · NHS indicative price = £8.55

L-Tyrosine
▸ Nutritional supplement for the dietary management of maternal phenylketonuria in patients with low plasma tyrosine levels.
POWDER, protein 90.1 g, carbohydrate nil, fat nil, energy 1532 k (360 kcal)/100 g.

L-Tyrosine powder (Nutricia Ltd)
100 gram (ACBS) · NHS indicative price = £25.16

Lophlex ®
▸ Nutritional supplement for the dietary management of proven phenylketonuria in children over 8 years and adults including pregnant women.
POWDER, protein equivalent (essential and non-essential amino acids except phenylalanine) 20 g, carbohydrate 2.5 g, fat 60 mg, fibre 220 mg, energy 385 kJ (91 kcal)/27.8-g sachet, with vitamins, minerals, and trace elements.

Lophlex powder 27.8g sachets berry (Nutricia Ltd)
30 sachet (ACBS) · NHS indicative price = £314.10

Lophlex powder 27.8g sachets orange (Nutricia Ltd)
30 sachet (ACBS) · NHS indicative price = £314.10

Lophlex powder 27.8g sachets unflavoured (Nutricia Ltd)
30 sachet (ACBS) · NHS indicative price = £314.10

Loprofin ® **PKU Drink**
▸ Nutritional supplement for the dietary management of phenylketonuria. Not suitable for use under 1 year.
LIQUID, protein 0.4 g, carbohydrate 5.0 g, fat 2.0 g, energy 166 kJ (40 kcal)/100 mL.

Loprofin PKU drink (Nutricia Ltd)
200 ml (ACBS) · NHS indicative price = £0.81

Loprofin ® **SNO-PRO**
▸ Nutritional supplement for the dietary management of phenylketonuria, chronic renal failure and other inborn errors of metabolism. Not suitable for use in child under 6 months.
LIQUID, protein 0.16 g, carbohydrate 10.8 g, fat 4.7 g, energy 371 kJ (89 kcal)/100 mL.

Loprofin SNO-PRO drink (Nutricia Ltd)
200 ml (ACBS) · NHS indicative price = £1.35

Phlexy-10 ® **Exchange System**
▸ Nutritional supplement for the dietary management of phenylketonuria.
TABLETS, protein equivalent (essential and non-essential amino acids except phenylalanine) 833 mg tablet.

Phlexy-10 tablets (Nutricia Ltd)
75 tablet (ACBS) · NHS indicative price = £31.03
DRINK MIX, powder, protein equivalent (essential and non-essential amino acids except phenylalanine) 8.33 g, carbohydrate 8.8 g/20-g sachet.

Phlexy-10 drink mix 20g sachets apple & blackcurrant (Nutricia Ltd)
30 sachet (ACBS) · NHS indicative price = £142.82

Phlexy-10 drink mix 20g sachets citrus burst (Nutricia Ltd)
30 sachet (ACBS) · NHS indicative price = £142.82

Phlexy-10 drink mix 20g sachets tropical surprise (Nutricia Ltd)
30 sachet (ACBS) · NHS indicative price = £142.82

Phlexy-Vits ®
▸ For use as a vitamin and mineral component of restricted therapeutic diets in children over 11 years and adults with phenylketonuria and similar amino acid abnormalities.
POWDER, vitamins, minerals, and trace elements

Phlexy-Vits powder 7g sachets (Nutricia Ltd)
30 sachet (ACBS) · NHS indicative price = £79.10
TABLETS, vitamins, minerals, and trace elements

Phlexy-Vits tablets (Nutricia Ltd)
180 tablet (ACBS) · NHS indicative price = £90.81

K Aid 4 ®

utritional supplement for the dietary management of henylketonuria.

OWDER, protein 79 g, carbohydrate 4.5 g, fat nil, energy 1420 kJ 34 kcal)/100 g.

K Aid 4 powder (Nutricia Ltd)
00 gram (ACBS) · NHS indicative price = £159.10

KU Air ®

utritional supplement for the dietary management of henylketonuria. Not suitable for use in child under 3 years. ncludes added vitamins A, B, C, D, E and K.

IQUID, protein equivalent 11.5 g, carbohydrate 1.5 g, fat 0.6 g, nergy 243 kJ (57 kcal)/100 mL.

KU Air15 gold liquid (Vitaflo International Ltd)
30 ml (ACBS) · NHS indicative price = £7.41

KU Air15 green liquid (Vitaflo International Ltd)
30 ml (ACBS) · NHS indicative price = £7.41

KU Air15 red liquid (Vitaflo International Ltd)
30 ml (ACBS) · NHS indicative price = £7.41

KU Air15 white liquid (Vitaflo International Ltd)
30 ml (ACBS) · NHS indicative price = £7.41

KU Air15 yellow liquid (Vitaflo International Ltd)
30 ml (ACBS) · NHS indicative price = £7.41

KU Air20 gold liquid (Vitaflo International Ltd)
74 ml (ACBS) · NHS indicative price = £9.95

KU Air20 green liquid (Vitaflo International Ltd)
74 ml (ACBS) · NHS indicative price = £9.95

KU Air20 red liquid (Vitaflo International Ltd)
74 ml (ACBS) · NHS indicative price = £9.95

KU Air20 white liquid (Vitaflo International Ltd)
74 ml (ACBS) · NHS indicative price = £9.95

KU Air20 yellow liquid (Vitaflo International Ltd)
74 ml (ACBS) · NHS indicative price = £9.95

PKU cooler10 ®
Nutritional supplement for the dietary management of phenylketonuria in children over 3 years.

LIQUID, protein equivalent (essential and non-essential amino acids except phenylalanine) 10 g, carbohydrate 4.7 g, energy 258 kJ (62 kcal)/87-mL pouch, with vitamins, minerals, and trace elements.

PKU orange cooler10 liquid (Vitaflo International Ltd)
87 ml (ACBS) · NHS indicative price = £5.16

PKU purple cooler10 liquid (Vitaflo International Ltd)
87 ml (ACBS) · NHS indicative price = £5.16

PKU red cooler10 liquid (Vitaflo International Ltd)
87 ml (ACBS) · NHS indicative price = £5.16

PKU white cooler10 liquid (Vitaflo International Ltd)
87 ml (ACBS) · NHS indicative price = £5.16

PKU yellow cooler10 liquid (Vitaflo International Ltd)
87 ml (ACBS) · NHS indicative price = £5.16

PKU cooler15 ®
Nutritional supplement for the dietary management of phenylketonuria in children over 3 years.

LIQUID, protein equivalent (essential and non-essential amino acids except phenylalanine) 15 g, carbohydrate 7 g, energy 386 kJ (92 kcal)/130-mL pouch, with vitamins, minerals, and trace elements.

PKU orange cooler15 liquid (Vitaflo International Ltd)
130 ml (ACBS) · NHS indicative price = £7.68

PKU purple cooler15 liquid (Vitaflo International Ltd)
130 ml (ACBS) · NHS indicative price = £7.68

PKU red cooler15 liquid (Vitaflo International Ltd)
130 ml (ACBS) · NHS indicative price = £7.68

PKU white cooler15 liquid (Vitaflo International Ltd)
130 ml (ACBS) · NHS indicative price = £7.68

PKU yellow cooler15 liquid (Vitaflo International Ltd)
130 ml (ACBS) · NHS indicative price = £7.68

PKU cooler20 ®
► Nutritional supplement for the dietary management of phenylketonuria in children over 3 years.

LIQUID, protein equivalent (essential and non-essential amino acids except phenylalanine) 20 g, carbohydrate 9.4 g, energy 517 kJ (124 kcal)/174-mL pouch, with vitamins, minerals, and trace elements.

PKU orange cooler20 liquid (Vitaflo International Ltd)
174 ml (ACBS) · NHS indicative price = £10.32

PKU purple cooler20 liquid (Vitaflo International Ltd)
174 ml (ACBS) · NHS indicative price = £10.32

PKU red cooler20 liquid (Vitaflo International Ltd)
174 ml (ACBS) · NHS indicative price = £10.32

PKU white cooler20 liquid (Vitaflo International Ltd)
174 ml (ACBS) · NHS indicative price = £10.32

PKU yellow cooler20 liquid (Vitaflo International Ltd)
174 ml (ACBS) · NHS indicative price = £10.32

PKU Easy ® **liquid**
► Nutritional supplement for the dietary management of phenylketonuria. Not suitable for use in child under 3 years. Includes added vitamins A, B, C, D, E and K.

LIQUID, protein equivalent (essential and non-essential amino acids) 11.5 g, carbohydrate 4.2 g, fat 0.4 g, energy 282 kJ (67 kcal)/100 mL.

PKU Easy liquid mixed berry (POA Pharma Scandinavia AB)
130 ml (ACBS) · NHS indicative price = £6.92

PKU Easy liquid orange citrus (POA Pharma Scandinavia AB)
130 ml (ACBS) · NHS indicative price = £6.92

PKU Easy ® **Shake & Go**
► Nutritional supplement for the dietary management of phenylketonuria. Not suitable for use in child under 3 years. Includes added vitamins A, B, C, D, E and K.

POWDER, protein 45 g, carbohydrate 42 g, fat 0.4 g, energy 1559 kJ (367 kcal)/100 g.

PKU Easy Shake & Go oral powder 34g sachets (POA Pharma Scandinavia AB)
30 sachet (ACBS) · NHS indicative price = £213.90

PKU express15 ®
► Nutritional supplement for the dietary management of phenylketonuria. Not recommended for children under 3 years.

POWDER, protein equivalent (essential and non-essential amino acids except phenylalanine) 15 g, carbohydrate 3.4 g, energy 310 kJ (74 kcal)/25 g, with vitamins, minerals, and trace elements. To flavour unflavoured products, see FlavourPac p. 1644.

PKU express15 powder 25g sachets lemon (Vitaflo International Ltd)
30 sachet (ACBS) · NHS indicative price = £226.17

PKU express15 powder 25g sachets orange (Vitaflo International Ltd)
30 sachet (ACBS) · NHS indicative price = £226.17

PKU express15 powder 25g sachets tropical (Vitaflo International Ltd)
30 sachet (ACBS) · NHS indicative price = £226.17

PKU express15 powder 25g sachets unflavoured (Vitaflo International Ltd)
30 sachet (ACBS) · NHS indicative price = £226.17

PKU express20 ®
► Nutritional supplement for the dietary management of phenylketonuria. Not recommended for children under 3 years.

POWDER, protein equivalent (essential and non-essential amino acids except phenylalanine) 20 g, carbohydrate 4.7 g, energy 422 kJ (101 kcal)/34 g, with vitamins, minerals, and trace elements. To flavour unflavoured products, see FlavourPac p. 1644.

PKU express20 powder 34g sachets lemon (Vitaflo International Ltd)
30 sachet (ACBS) · NHS indicative price = £292.20

PKU express20 powder 34g sachets orange (Vitaflo International Ltd)
30 sachet (ACBS) · NHS indicative price = £292.20

PKU express20 powder 34g sachets tropical (Vitaflo International Ltd)
30 sachet (ACBS) · NHS indicative price = £292.20

A2

Borderline substances | **Appendix 2**

PKU express20 powder 34g sachets unflavoured (Vitaflo International Ltd)
30 sachet (ACBS) · NHS indicative price = £292.20

PKU gel ®
▸ For use as part of the low-protein dietary management of phenylketonuria in children 6 months–10 years (unflavoured), 1–10 years (flavoured).
POWDER, protein equivalent (essential and non-essential amino acids except phenylalanine) 10 g, carbohydrate 10.3 g (unflavoured)/8.9 g (flavoured), fat less than 100 mg, energy 346 kJ (81 kcal) (unflavoured)/322 kJ (76 kcal) (flavoured)/24 g, with vitamins, minerals, and trace elements. PKU Orange contains soya. To flavour unflavoured products, see FlavourPac p. 1644.

PKU gel powder 24g sachets orange (Vitaflo International Ltd)
30 sachet (ACBS) · NHS indicative price = £156.46

PKU gel powder 24g sachets raspberry (Vitaflo International Ltd)
30 sachet (ACBS) · NHS indicative price = £156.46

PKU gel powder 24g sachets unflavoured (Vitaflo International Ltd)
30 sachet (ACBS) · NHS indicative price = £156.46

PKU GMPro ®
▸ Nutritional supplement for the dietary management of phenylketonuria. Not suitable for use in child under 3 years; not recommended for child under 6 years. Includes added vitamins A, B, C, D, E and K.
POWDER, protein 30 g, carbohydrate 37.5 g, fat 11.7 g, energy 1616 kJ (384 kcal)/100 g.

PKU GMPro oral powder 33.3g sachets (Nutricia Ltd)
16 sachet (ACBS) · NHS indicative price = £93.57

PKU GMPro ® **LQ**
▸ Nutritional supplement for the dietary management of phenylketonuria. Not suitable for use in child under 3 years, not recommended in child under 6 years. Includes added vitamins A, B C, D, E and K.
LIQUID, protein equivalent 4 g, carbohydrate 3.4 g, fat 1.6 g, energy 188 kJ (45 kcal)/100 mL.

PKU GMPro LQ liquid (Nutricia Ltd)
250 mL (ACBS) · NHS indicative price = £5.84

PKU Lophlex ® **LQ**
▸ Nutritional supplement for the dietary management of phenylketonuria. Not suitable for use in child under 1 year; not recommended for child under 4 years. Includes added vitamins A, B, C, D, E and K.
LIQUID, protein 16 g, carbohydrate 7 g, fat 0-0.4 g, energy 391-407 kJ (92-96 kcal)/100 mL.

PKU Lophlex LQ 10 liquid berry (Nutricia Ltd)
62.5 ml (ACBS) · NHS indicative price = £5.61

PKU Lophlex LQ 10 liquid juicy berries (Nutricia Ltd)
62.5 ml (ACBS) · NHS indicative price = £5.61

PKU Lophlex LQ 10 liquid juicy citrus (Nutricia Ltd)
62.5 ml (ACBS) · NHS indicative price = £5.61

PKU Lophlex LQ 10 liquid juicy orange (Nutricia Ltd)
62.5 ml (ACBS) · NHS indicative price = £5.61

PKU Lophlex LQ 10 liquid juicy tropical (Nutricia Ltd)
62.5 ml (ACBS) · NHS indicative price = £5.61

PKU Lophlex LQ 20 liquid berry (Nutricia Ltd)
125 ml (ACBS) · NHS indicative price = £11.19

PKU Lophlex LQ 20 liquid orange (Nutricia Ltd)
125 ml (ACBS) · NHS indicative price = £11.19

PKU Lophlex LQ 20 liquid juicy berries (Nutricia Ltd)
125 ml (ACBS) · NHS indicative price = £11.19

PKU Lophlex LQ 20 liquid juicy citrus (Nutricia Ltd)
125 ml (ACBS) · NHS indicative price = £11.19

PKU Lophlex LQ 20 liquid juicy orange (Nutricia Ltd)
125 ml (ACBS) · NHS indicative price = £11.19

PKU Lophlex LQ 20 liquid juicy tropical (Nutricia Ltd)
125 ml (ACBS) · NHS indicative price = £11.19

PKU Lophlex ® **Sensation 20**
▸ Nutritional supplement for the dietary management of phenylketonuria. Not suitable for use in child under 4 years. Includes added vitamins A, B, C, D, E and K.
SEMI-SOLID, protein 18.3 g, carbohydrate 18.5 g, fat 0.3 g, energy 648 kJ (152 kcal)/100 g.

PKU Lophlex Sensation 20 berries (Nutricia Ltd)
327 gram (ACBS) · NHS indicative price = £35.76

PKU Maxamum ®
▸ Nutritional supplement for the dietary management of phenylketonuria. Not suitable for use in child under 8 years. Includes added vitamins A, B, C, D, E and K.
POWDER, protein 39 g, carbohydrate 34 g, fat less than 0.5 g, energy 1260 kJ (297 kcal)/100 g.

PKU Maxamum oral powder 50g sachets orange (Nutricia Ltd)
30 sachet (ACBS) · NHS indicative price = £299.79

PKU Maxamum oral powder 50g sachets unflavoured (Nutricia Ltd)
30 sachet (ACBS) · NHS indicative price = £299.79

PKU Maxamum powder orange (Nutricia Ltd)
500 gram (ACBS) · NHS indicative price = £99.97

PKU Maxamum powder unflavoured (Nutricia Ltd)
500 gram (ACBS) · NHS indicative price = £99.97

Tyrosinaemia

Methionine-free TYR Anamix ® **Infant**
▸ Nutritional supplement for the dietary management of proven tyrosinaemia type 1 in children from birth to 3 years.
POWDER, protein equivalent (essential and non-essential amino acids except methionine, phenylalanine, and tyrosine) 13.1 g, carbohydrate 49.5 g, fat 23 g, fibre 5.3 g, energy 1915 kJ (457 kcal)/100 g, with vitamins, minerals, and trace elements; standard dilution (15%) provides protein equivalent 2 g, carbohydrate 7.4 g, fat 3.5 g, fibre 800 mg, energy 287 kJ (69 kcal)/100 mL.

TYR Anamix Infant methionine free powder (Nutricia Ltd)
400 gram (ACBS) · NHS indicative price = £43.52

TYR Anamix ® **Infant**
▸ Nutritional supplement for the dietary management of proven tyrosinaemia where plasma-methionine concentrations are normal in children from birth to 3 years.
POWDER, protein equivalent (essential and non-essential amino acids except phenylalanine and tyrosine) 13.1 g, carbohydrate 49.5 g, fat 23 g, fibre 5.3 g, energy 1915 kJ (457 kcal)/100 g, with vitamins, minerals, and trace elements; standard dilution (15%) provides protein equivalent 2 g, carbohydrate 7.4 g, fat 3.5 g, fibre 800 mg, energy 287 kJ (69 kcal)/100 mL.

TYR Anamix Infant methionine free powder (Nutricia Ltd)
400 gram (ACBS) · NHS indicative price = £43.52

TYR Anamix Infant powder (Nutricia Ltd)
400 gram (ACBS) · NHS indicative price = £43.52

TYR Cooler ®
▸ Nutritional supplement for the dietary management of tyrosinaemia. Not suitable for use in child under 3 years. Includes added vitamins A, B, C, D, E and K.
LIQUID, protein equivalent 11.5 g, carbohydrate 5.1 g, fat 0.9 g, energy 316 kJ (75 kcal)/100 mL.

TYR orange cooler15 liquid (Vitaflo International Ltd)
130 mL (ACBS) · NHS indicative price = £12.68

TYR red cooler10 liquid (Vitaflo International Ltd)
87 ml (ACBS) · NHS indicative price = £8.12

TYR red cooler15 liquid (Vitaflo International Ltd)
130 mL (ACBS) · NHS indicative price = £12.68

TYR red cooler20 liquid (Vitaflo International Ltd)
174 mL (ACBS) · NHS indicative price = £16.97

TYR ® **Easy Shake & Go**
▸ Nutritional supplement for the dietary management of tyrosinaemia. Not suitable for use in child under 3 years. Includes added vitamins A, B, C, D, E and K.

POWDER, protein equivalent 45 g, carbohydrate 38 g, fat less than 0.5 g, energy 1542 kJ (363 kcal)/100 g.

TYR Easy Shake & Go oral powder 34g sachets (POA Pharma Scandinavia AB)
30 sachet (ACBS) · NHS indicative price = £362.00

TYR express ®
Nutritional supplement for the dietary management of tyrosinaemia. Not suitable for use in child under 8 years. Includes added vitamins A, B, C, D, E and K.
POWDER, protein equivalent 60 g, carbohydrate 13.7 g, fat 0.2 g, energy 1260 kJ (297 kcal)/100 g.

TYR express15 oral powder 25g sachets (Vitaflo International Ltd)
30 sachet (ACBS) · NHS indicative price = £373.05

TYR express20 oral powder 34g sachets (Vitaflo International Ltd)
30 sachet (ACBS) · NHS indicative price = £481.98

TYR Lophlex ® **LQ**
Nutritional supplement for the dietary management of tyrosinaemia. Includes added vitamins A, B, C, D, E and K.
LIQUID, protein 16 g, carbohydrate 7 g, fat 0.4 g, energy 407 kJ (96 kcal)/100 mL

TYR Lophlex LQ 10 liquid (Nutricia Ltd)
62.5 ml (ACBS) · NHS indicative price = £8.92

TYR Lophlex LQ 20 liquid (Nutricia Ltd)
125 ml (ACBS) · NHS indicative price = £18.40

XPHEN TYR Tyrosidon ®
Nutritional supplement for the management of tyrosinaemia in children and adults where plasma-methionine concentrations are normal.
POWDER, protein equivalent (essential and non-essential amino acids except phenylalanine and tyrosine) 77 g, carbohydrate 4.5 g, fat nil, energy 1386 kJ (326 kcal)/100 g. To flavour unflavoured products, see Modjul Flavour System p. 1644.

XPHEN TYR Tyrosidon Free AA Mix powder (Nutricia Ltd)
500 gram (ACBS) · NHS indicative price = £213.65

Appendix 3
Cautionary and advisory labels for dispensed medicines

Guidance for cautionary and advisory labels

Medicinal forms within BNF publications include code numbers of the cautionary labels that pharmacists are recommended to add when dispensing. It is also expected that pharmacists will counsel patients and carers when necessary.

Counselling needs to be related to the age, experience, background, and understanding of the individual patient or carer. The pharmacist should ensure understanding of how to take or use the medicine and how to follow the correct dosage schedule. Any effects of the medicine on co-ordination, performance of skilled tasks (e.g. driving or work), any foods or medicines to be avoided, and what to do if a dose is missed should also be explained. Other matters, such as the possibility of staining of the clothes or skin, or discolouration of urine or stools by a medicine should also be mentioned.

For some medicines there is a special need for counselling, such as an unusual method or time of administration or a potential interaction with a common food or domestic remedy, and this should be mentioned where necessary.

Original packs

Most preparations are dispensed in unbroken original packs that include further advice for the patient in the form of patient information leaflets. Label 10 may be of value where appropriate. More general leaflets advising on the administration of preparations such as eye drops, eye ointments, inhalers, and suppositories are also available.

Scope of labels

In general no label recommendations have been made for injections on the assumption that they will be administered by a healthcare professional or a well-instructed patient. The labelling is not exhaustive and pharmacists are recommended to use their professional discretion in labelling new preparations and those for which no labels are shown.

Individual labelling advice is not given on the administration of the large variety of antacids. In the absence of instructions from the prescriber, and if on enquiry the patient has had no verbal instructions, the directions given under 'Dose' should be used on the label.

It is recognised that there may be occasions when pharmacists will use their knowledge and professional discretion and decide to omit one or more of the recommended labels for a particular patient. In this case counselling is of the utmost importance. There may also be an occasion when a prescriber does not wish additional cautionary labels to be used, in which case the prescription should be endorsed 'NCL' (no cautionary labels). The exact wording that is required instead should then be specified on the prescription.

Pharmacists label medicines with various wordings in addition to those directions specified on the prescription. Such labels include 'Shake the bottle', 'For external use only', and 'Store in a cool place', as well as 'Discard.... days after opening' and 'Do not use after....', which apply particularly to antibiotic mixtures, diluted liquid and topical preparations, and to eye-drops. Although not listed in the BNF these labels should continue to be used when appropriate; indeed, 'For external use only' is a legal requirement on external liquid preparations, while 'Keep out of the reach of children' is a legal requirement on all dispensed medicines. Care should be taken not to obscure other relevant information with adhesive labelling.

It is the usual practice for patients to take standard tablets with water or other liquid and for this reason no separate label has been recommended.

The label wordings recommended by the BNF apply to medicines dispensed against a prescription. Patients should be aware that a dispensed medicine should never be taken by, or shared with, anyone other than for whom the prescriber intended it. Therefore, the BNF does not include warnings against the use of a dispensed medicine by persons other than for whom it was specifically prescribed.

The label or labels for each preparation are recommended after careful consideration of the information available. However, it is recognised that in some cases this information may be either incomplete or open to a different interpretation. The BNF will therefore be grateful to receive any constructive comments on the labelling suggested for any preparation.

Recommended label wordings

For BNF 61 (March 2011), a revised set of cautionary and advisory labels were introduced. All of the existing labels were user-tested, and the revised wording selected reflects terminology that is better understood by patients.

Wordings which can be given as separate warnings are labels 1–19, 29–30, and 32. Wordings which can be incorporated in an appropriate position in the directions for dosage or administration are labels 21–28. A label has been omitted for number 20; labels 31 and 33 no longer apply to any medicines in the BNF and have therefore been deleted.

If separate labels are used it is recommended that the wordings be used without modification. If changes are made to suit computer requirements, care should be taken to retain the sense of the original.

Welsh labels

Comprehensive Welsh translations are available for each cautionary and advisory label.

Labels

1 **Warning: This medicine may make you sleepy**

Rhybudd: Gall y feddyginiaeth hon eich gwneud yn gysglyd
To be used on *preparations for children* containing antihistamines, or other preparations given to children where the warnings of label 2 on driving or alcohol would not be appropriate.

2 **Warning: This medicine may make you sleepy. If this happens, do not drive or use tools or machines. Do not drink alcohol**

Rhybudd: Gall y feddyginiaeth hon eich gwneud yn gysglyd. Peidiwch â gyrru, defnyddio offer llaw neu beiriannau os yw hyn yn digwydd. Peidiwch ag yfed alcohol
To be used on *preparations for adults that can cause drowsiness*, thereby affecting coordination and the ability to drive and operate hazardous machinery; label 1 is more appropriate for children. *It is an offence to drive while under the influence of drink or drugs.*

Some of these preparations only cause drowsiness in the first few days of treatment and some only cause drowsiness in higher doses.

In such cases the patient should be told that the advice applies until the effects have worn off. However many of these preparations can produce a slowing of reaction time and a loss of mental concentration that can have the same effects as drowsiness.

Avoidance of alcoholic drink is recommended because the effects of CNS depressants are enhanced by alcohol. Strict prohibition however could lead to some patients not taking the medicine. Pharmacists should therefore explain the risk and encourage compliance, particularly in patients who may think they already tolerate the effects of alcohol (see also label 3). Queries from patients with epilepsy regarding fitness to drive should be referred back to the patient's doctor.

Side-effects unrelated to drowsiness that may affect a patient's ability to drive or operate machinery safely include *blurred vision, dizziness, or nausea*. In general, no label has been recommended to cover these cases, but the patient should be suitably counselled.

Warning: This medicine may make you sleepy. If this happens, do not drive or use tools or machines

Rhybudd: Gall y feddyginiaeth hon eich gwneud yn gysglyd. Peidiwch â gyrru, defnyddio offer llaw neu beiriannau os yw hyn yn digwydd
To be used on *preparations containing monoamine-oxidase inhibitors*; the warning to avoid alcohol and dealcoholised (low alcohol) drink is covered by the patient information leaflet.

Also to be used as for label 2 but where alcohol is not an issue.

Warning: Do not drink alcohol

Rhybudd: Peidiwch ag yfed alcohol
To be used on *preparations where a reaction such as flushing may occur if alcohol is taken* (e.g. metronidazole). Alcohol may also enhance the hypoglycaemia produced by some oral antidiabetic drugs but routine application of a warning label is not considered necessary.

Patients should be advised not to drink alcohol for as long as they are receiving/using a course of medication, and in some cases for a period of time after the course is finished.

5 Do not take indigestion remedies 2 hours before or after you take this medicine

Peidiwch â chymryd meddyginiaethau camdreuliad 2 awr cyn neu ar ôl y feddyginiaeth hon
To be used with label 25 on *preparations coated to resist gastric acid* (e.g. enteric-coated tablets). This is to avoid the possibility of premature dissolution of the coating in the presence of an alkaline pH.

Label 5 also applies to drugs such as gabapentin *where the absorption is significantly affected by antacids*. Pharmacists will be aware (from a knowledge of physiology) that the usual time during which indigestion remedies should be avoided is at least 2 hours before and after the majority of medicines have been taken; when a manufacturer advises a different time period, this can be followed, and should be explained to the patient.

6 Do not take indigestion remedies, or medicines containing iron or zinc, 2 hours before or after you take this medicine

Peidiwch â chymryd meddyginiaethau camdreuliad neu feddyginiaethau sy'n cynnwys haearn neu sinc, 2 awr cyn neu ar ôl y feddyginiaeth hon
To be used on *preparations containing ofloxacin and some other quinolones, doxycycline, lymecycline, minocycline, and penicillamine*. These drugs chelate calcium, iron, and zinc and are less well absorbed when taken with calcium-containing antacids or preparations containing iron or zinc. Pharmacists will be aware (from a knowledge of physiology) that these incompatible preparations should be taken at least 2 hours apart for the majority of medicines; when a manufacturer advises a different time period, this can be followed, and should be explained to the patient.

7 Do not take milk, indigestion remedies, or medicines containing iron or zinc, 2 hours before or after you take this medicine

Peidiwch â chymryd llaeth, meddyginiaethau camdreuliad, neu feddyginiaeth sy'n cynnwys haearn neu sinc, 2 awr cyn neu ar ôl cymryd y feddyginiaeth hon
To be used on *preparations containing ciprofloxacin, norfloxacin, or tetracyclines that chelate calcium, iron, magnesium, and zinc,* and are thus less available for absorption. Pharmacists will be aware (from a knowledge of

physiology) that these incompatible preparations should be taken at least 2 hours apart for the majority of medicines; when a manufacturer advises a different time period, this can be followed, and should be explained to the patient. Doxycycline, lymecycline, and minocycline are less liable to form chelates and therefore only require label 6 (see above).

8 Warning: Do not stop taking this medicine unless your doctor tells you to stop

Rhybudd: Peidiwch â stopio cymryd y feddyginiaeth hon, oni bai fod eich meddyg yn dweud wrthych am stopio
To be used on *preparations that contain a drug which is required to be taken over long periods without the patient necessarily perceiving any benefit* (e.g. antituberculous drugs).

Also to be used on *preparations that contain a drug whose withdrawal is likely to be a particular hazard* (e.g. clonidine for hypertension). Label 10 (see below) is more appropriate for corticosteroids.

9 Space the doses evenly throughout the day. Keep taking this medicine until the course is finished, unless you are told to stop

Gadewch yr un faint o amser rhwng pob dôs yn ystod y dydd. Parhewch i gymryd y feddyginiaeth nes bod y cyfan wedi'i orffen, oni bai eich bod yn cael cyngor i stopio
To be used on *preparations where a course of treatment should be completed* to reduce the incidence of relapse or failure of treatment.

The preparations are antimicrobial drugs given by mouth. Very occasionally, some may have serious side-effects (e.g. diarrhoea in patients receiving clindamycin) and in such cases the patient may need to be advised of reasons for stopping treatment quickly and returning to the doctor.

10 Warning: Read the additional information given with this medicine

Rhybudd: Darllenwch y wybodaeth ychwanegol gyda'r feddyginiaeth hon
To be used particularly on *preparations containing anticoagulants, lithium, and oral corticosteroids*. The appropriate treatment card should be given to the patient and any necessary explanations given.

This label may also be used on other preparations to remind the patient of the instructions that have been given.

11 Protect your skin from sunlight—even on a bright but cloudy day. Do not use sunbeds

Diogelwch eich croen rhag golau'r haul, hyd yn oed ar ddiwrnod braf ond cymylog. Peidiwch â defnyddio gwely haul
To be used on *preparations that may cause phototoxic or photoallergic reactions* if the patient is exposed to ultraviolet radiation. Exposure to high intensity ultraviolet radiation from sunray lamps and sunbeds is particularly likely to cause reactions.

12 Do not take anything containing aspirin while taking this medicine

Peidiwch â chymryd unrhyw beth sy'n cynnwys aspirin gyda'r feddyginiaeth hon
To be used on *preparations containing sulfinpyrazone* whose activity is reduced by aspirin.

Label 12 should not be used for anticoagulants since label 10 is more appropriate.

13 Dissolve or mix with water before taking

Gadewch i doddi mewn dŵr cyn ei gymryd
To be used on *preparations that are intended to be dissolved in water* (e.g. soluble tablets) or *mixed with water* (e.g. powders, granules) before use. In a few cases other liquids such as fruit juice or milk may be used.

14 This medicine may colour your urine. This is harmless

Gall y feddyginiaeth hon liwio eich dŵr. Nid yw hyn yn arwydd o ddrwg
To be used on *preparations that may cause the patient's urine to turn an unusual colour*. These include triamterene (blue under some lights), levodopa (dark reddish), and rifampicin (red).

A3

Cautionary and advisory labels | **Appendix 3**

15 Caution: flammable. Keep your body away from fire or flames after you have put on the medicine

Rhybudd: Fflamadwy. Ar ôl rhoi'r feddyginiaeth ymlaen, cadwch yn glir o dân neu fflamau

To be used on *preparations containing sufficient flammable solvent to render them flammable if exposed to a naked flame.*

16 Dissolve the tablet under your tongue—do not swallow. Store the tablets in this bottle with the cap tightly closed. Get a new supply 8 weeks after opening

Rhowch y dabled i doddi dan eich tafod - peidiwch â'i lyncu. Cadwch y tabledi yn y botel yma gyda'r caead wedi'i gau yn dynn. Gofynnwch am dabledi newydd 8 wythnos ar ôl ei hagor

To be used on *glyceryl trinitrate tablets* to remind the patient not to transfer the tablets to plastic or less suitable containers.

17 Do not take more than... in 24 hours

Peidiwch â chymryd mwy na... mewn 24 awr

To be used on *preparations for the treatment of acute migraine* except those containing ergotamine, for which label 18 is used. The dose form should be specified, e.g. tablets or capsules.

It may also be used on preparations for which no dose has been specified by the prescriber.

18 Do not take more than... in 24 hours. Also, do not take more than... in any one week

Peidiwch â chymryd mwy na... mewn 24 awr. Hefyd, peidiwch â chymryd mwy na... mewn wythnos

To be used on preparations containing ergotamine. The dose form should be specified, e.g. tablets or suppositories.

19 Warning: This medicine makes you sleepy. If you still feel sleepy the next day, do not drive or use tools or machines. Do not drink alcohol

Rhybudd: Bydd y feddyginiaeth hon yn eich gwneud yn gysglyd. Os ydych yn dal i deimlo'n gysglyd drannoeth, peidiwch â gyrru, defnyddio offer llaw neu beiriannau. Peidiwch ag yfed alcohol

To be used on *preparations containing hypnotics (or some other drugs with sedative effects) prescribed to be taken at night.* On the rare occasions when hypnotics are prescribed for daytime administration (e.g. nitrazepam in epilepsy), this label would clearly not be appropriate. Also to be used as an *alternative to the label 2 wording* (the choice being at the discretion of the pharmacist) *for anxiolytics prescribed to be taken at night.*

It is hoped that this wording will convey adequately the problem of residual morning sedation after taking 'sleeping tablets'.

21 Take with or just after food, or a meal

Cymerwch gyda neu ar ôl bwyd

To be used on *preparations that are liable to cause gastric irritation, or those that are better absorbed with food.*

Patients should be advised that a *small amount of food is sufficient.*

22 Take 30 to 60 minutes before food

Cymerwch 30 i 60 munud cyn bwyd

To be used on some preparations *whose absorption is thereby improved.*

Most oral antibacterials require label 23 instead (see below).

23 Take this medicine when your stomach is empty. This means an hour before food or 2 hours after food

Cymerwch y feddyginiaeth hon ar stumog wag. Mae hyn yn golygu awr cyn, neu 2 awr ar ôl bwyd

To be used on *oral antibacterials whose absorption may be reduced by the presence of food and acid in the stomach.*

24 Suck or chew this medicine

Bydd angen cnoi neu sugno'r feddyginiaeth hon

To be used on *preparations that should be sucked or chewed.*

The pharmacist should use discretion as to which of these words is appropriate.

25 Swallow this medicine whole. Do not chew or crush

Llyncwch yn gyfan. Peidiwch â chnoi neu falu'n fân

To be used on *preparations that are enteric-coated or designed for modified-release.*

Also to be used on *preparations that taste very unpleasant or may damage the mouth* if not swallowed whole.

Patients should be advised (where relevant) that some modified-release preparations can be broken in half, but that the halved tablet should still be swallowed whole, and not chewed or crushed.

26 Dissolve this medicine under your tongue

Gadewch i'r feddyginiaeth hon doddi o dan y tafod

To be used on *preparations designed for sublingual use.* Patients should be advised to hold under the tongue and avoid swallowing until dissolved. The buccal mucosa between the gum and cheek is occasionally specified by the prescriber.

27 Take with a full glass of water

Cymerwch gyda llond gwydr o ddŵr

To be used on *preparations that should be well diluted* (e.g. chloral hydrate), *where a high fluid intake is required* (e.g. sulfonamides), or *where water is required to aid the action* (e.g. methylcellulose). The patient should be advised that 'a full glass' means at least 150 mL. In most cases fruit juice, tea, or coffee may be used.

28 Spread thinly on the affected skin only

Taenwch yn denau ar y croen sydd wedi'i effeithio yn unig

To be used on *external preparations* that should be applied sparingly (e.g. corticosteroids, dithranol).

29 Do not take more than 2 at any one time. Do not take more than 8 in 24 hours

Peidiwch â chymryd mwy na 2 ar unrhyw un adeg. Peidiwch â chymryd mwy nag 8 mewn 24 awr

To be used on containers of dispensed *solid dose preparations containing paracetamol for adults when the instruction on the label indicates that the dose can be taken on an 'as required' basis.* The dose form should be specified, e.g. tablets or capsules.

This label has been introduced because of the serious consequences of overdosage with paracetamol.

30 Contains paracetamol. Do not take anything else containing paracetamol while taking this medicine. Talk to a doctor at once if you take too much of this medicine, even if you feel well

Yn cynnwys paracetamol. Peidiwch â chymryd unrhyw beth arall sy'n cynnwys paracetamol tra'n cymryd y feddyginiaeth hon. Siaradwch gyda'ch meddyg ar unwaith os ydych yn cymryd gormod, hyd yn oed os ydych yn teimlo'n iawn

To be used on all containers of dispensed *preparations containing paracetamol.*

32 Contains aspirin. Do not take anything else containing aspirin while taking this medicine

Yn cynnwys aspirin. Peidiwch â chymryd unrhyw beth arall sy'n cynnwys aspirin tra'n cymryd y feddyginiaeth hon

To be used on containers of dispensed *preparations containing aspirin when the name on the label does not include the word 'aspirin'.*

Appendix 4
Wound management products and elasticated garments

CONTENTS

A4

Wound management | Appendix 4

The correct dressing for wound management depends not only on the type of wound but also on the stage of the healing process. The principal stages of healing are: cleansing, removal of debris; granulation, vascularisation; epithelialisation. The ideal dressing for moist wound healing needs to ensure that the wound remains: moist with exudate, but not macerated; free of clinical infection and excessive slough; free of toxic chemicals, particles or fibres; at the optimum temperature for healing; undisturbed by the need for frequent changes; at the optimum pH value. As wound healing passes through its different stages, different types of dressings may be required to satisfy better one or other of these requirements. Under normal circumstances, a moist environment is a necessary part of the wound healing process; exudate provides a moist environment and promotes healing, but excessive exudate can cause maceration of the wound and surrounding healthy tissue. The volume and viscosity of exudate changes as the wound heals. There are certain circumstances where moist wound healing is not appropriate (e.g. gangrenous toes associated with vascular disease).

Advanced wound dressings are designed to control the environment for wound healing, for example to donate fluid (hydrogels), maintain hydration (hydrocolloids), or to absorb wound exudate (alginates, foams).

Practices such as the use of irritant cleansers and desloughing agents may be harmful and are largely obsolete; removal of debris and dressing remnants should need minimal irrigation with lukewarm sterile sodium chloride 0.9% solution or water.

Hydrogel, hydrocolloid, and medical grade honey dressings can be used to deslough wounds by promoting autolytic

debridement; there is insufficient evidence to support any particular method of debridement for difficult-to-heal surgical wounds. Sterile larvae (maggots) are also available for biosurgical removal of wound debris.

There have been few clinical trials able to establish a clear advantage for any particular product. The choice between different dressings depends not only on the type and stage of the wound, but also on patient preference or tolerance, site of the wound, and cost. For further information, see Buyers' Guide: Advanced wound dressings (October 2008); NHS Purchasing and Supply Agency, Centre for Evidence-based Purchasing.

Prices quoted in Appendix 4 are basic NHS net prices; for further information see Prices in the BNF under How to use the BNF.

The table below gives suggestions for choices of primary dressing depending on the type of wound (a secondary dressing may be needed in some cases).

Basic wound contact dressings

Low adherence dressing

Low adherence dressings are used as interface layers under secondary absorbent dressings. Placed directly on the wound bed, non-absorbent, low adherence dressings are suitable for clean, granulating, lightly exuding wounds without necrosis, and protect the wound bed from direct contact with secondary dressings. Care must be taken to avoid granulation tissue growing into the weave of these dressings. Tulle dressings are manufactured from cotton or viscose fibres which are impregnated with white or yellow soft paraffin to prevent the fibres from sticking, but this is only partly successful and it may be necessary to change the

Wound contact material for different types of wounds

Wound PINK (epithelialising)

Low Exudate	Moderate Exudate
Low adherence p. 1659	Soft ploymer p. 1664
Vapour-permeable film p. 1663	Foam, low absorbent p. 1667
Soft polymer p. 1664	Alginate p. 1668
Hydrocolloid p. 1666	

Wound RED (granulating)
Symptoms or signs of infection, see Wounds with signs of infection

Low Exudate	Moderate Exudate	Heavy Exudate
Low adherence p. 1659	Hydrocolloid-fibrous p. 1666	Foam with extra absorbency p. 1667
Soft polymer p. 1664	Foam p. 1667	Hydrocolloid-fibrous p. 1666
Hydrocolloid p. 1666	Alginate p. 1668	Alginate p. 1668
Foam, low absorbent p. 1667		

Wound YELLOW (Sloughy) (granulating)
Symptoms or signs of infection, see Wounds with signs of infection

Low Exudate	Moderate Exudate	Heavy Exudate
Hydrogel p. 1662	Hydrocolloid-fibrous p. 1666	Hydrocolloid-fibrous p. 1666
Hydrocolloid p. 1666	Alginate p. 1668	Alginate p. 1668
		Capillary-action p. 1669

Wound BLACK (Necrotic/ Eschar)
Consider mechanical debridement alongside autolytic debridement

Low Exudate	Moderate Exudate	Heavy Exudate
Hydrogel p. 1662	Hydrocolloid p. 1666	Seek advice from wound care specialist
Hydrocolloid p. 1666	Hydrocolloid-fibrous p. 1666	
	Foam p. 1667	

Wounds with signs of infection
Consider systemic antibacterials if appropriate; also consider odour-absorbent dressings. For malodourous wounds with slough or necrotic tissue, consider mechanical or autolytic debridement

Low Exudate	Moderate Exudate	Heavy Exudate
Low adherence with honey p. 1669	Hydrocolloid-fibrous with silver p. 1672	Hydrocolloid-fibrous with silver p. 1671
Low adherence with iodine p. 1670	Foam with silver p. 1671	Foam extra absorbent, with silver p. 1671
Low adherence with silver p. 1671	Alginate with silver p. 1671	Alginate with honey p. 1670
Hydrocolloid with silver p. 1671	Honey-topical p. 1670	Alginate with silver p. 1671
	Cadexomer-iodine p. 1670	

Note In each section of this table the dressings are listed in order of increasing absorbency.
Some wound contact (primary) dressings require a secondary dressing

dressings frequently. The paraffin reduces absorbency of the dressing. Dressings with a reduced content (light loading) of soft paraffin are less liable to interfere with absorption; dressings with 'normal loading' (such as Jelonet ®) have been used for skin graft transfer. Knitted viscose primary dressing is an alternative to tulle dressings for exuding wounds; it can be used as the initial layer of multi-layer compression bandaging in the treatment of venous leg ulcers.

Knitted polyester primary dressing
Atrauman
Non-adherent knitted polyester primary dressing impregnated with neutral triglycerides
Atrauman dressing (Paul Hartmann Ltd) 10cm × 20cm= £0.82, 20cm × 30cm= £2.25, 5cm × 5cm= £0.35, 7.5cm × 10cm= £0.36

Knitted viscose primary dressing
N-A Dressing
Warp knitted fabric manufactured from a bright viscose monofilament.
N-A dressing (Systagenix Wound Management Ltd) 19cm × 9.5cm= £0.67, 9.5cm × 9.5cm= £0.35

N-A Ultra
Warp knitted fabric manufactured from a bright viscose monofilament.
N-A Ultra dressing (Systagenix Wound Management Ltd) 19cm × 9.5cm= £0.64, 9.5cm × 9.5cm= £0.34

Profore
Warp knitted fabric manufactured from a bright viscose monofilament.
Profore (Smith & Nephew Healthcare Ltd) wound contact layer 14cm × 20cm= £0.33

Tricotex
Warp knitted fabric manufactured from a bright viscose monofilament.
Tricotex dressing (Smith & Nephew Healthcare Ltd) 9.5cm × 9.5cm= £0.36

Paraffin Gauze Dressing
Cuticell
(Tulle Gras). Fabric of leno weave, weft and warp threads of cotton and/or viscose yarn, impregnated with white or yellow soft paraffin; for light or normal loading
Cuticell (BSN medical Ltd) Classic dressing 10cm × 10cm= £0.30

Jelonet
(Tulle Gras). Fabric of leno weave, weft and warp threads of cotton and/or viscose yarn, impregnated with white or yellow soft paraffin; for light or normal loading
Jelonet (Smith & Nephew Healthcare Ltd) dressing 10cm × 10cm= £0.43

Neotulle
(Tulle Gras). Fabric of leno weave, weft and warp threads of cotton and/or viscose yarn, impregnated with white or yellow soft paraffin; for light or normal loading
Neotulle (Neomedic Ltd) dressing 10cm × 10cm= £0.29

Absorbent dressings

Perforated film absorbent dressings are suitable only for wounds with mild to moderate amounts of exudate; they are not appropriate for leg ulcers or for other lesions that produce large quantities of viscous exudate. Dressings with an absorbent cellulose or polymer wadding layer are suitable for use on moderately to heavily exuding wounds.

Absorbent cellulose dressing

CelluDress

Absorbent Cellulose Dressing with Fluid Repellent Backing

CelluDress dressing (Medicareplus International Ltd) 10cm × 10cm= £0.19, 10cm × 15cm= £0.20, 10cm × 20cm= £0.22, 15cm × 20cm= £0.30, 20cm × 25cm= £0.40, 20cm × 30cm= £0.85

Eclypse

Absorbent Cellulose Dressing with Fluid Repellent Backing

Eclypse (Advancis Medical) Boot dressing 60cm × 70cm= £14.24, dressing 15cm × 15cm= £1.00, 20cm × 30cm= £2.21, 60cm × 40cm= £8.42

Exu-Dry

Absorbent Cellulose Dressing with Fluid Repellent Backing

Exu-Dry dressing (Smith & Nephew Healthcare Ltd) 10cm × 15cm= £1.19, 15cm × 23cm= £2.42, 23cm × 38cm= £5.62

Mesorb

Cellulose wadding pad with gauze wound contact layer and non-woven repellent backing

Mesorb dressing (Molnlycke Health Care Ltd) 10cm × 10cm= £0.64, 10cm × 15cm= £0.84, 10cm × 20cm= £1.03, 15cm × 20cm= £1.47, 20cm × 25cm= £2.32, 20cm × 30cm= £2.63

Zetuvit E

Absorbent Cellulose Dressing with Fluid Repellent Backing; sterile or non-sterile

Zetuvit (Paul Hartmann Ltd) E non-sterile dressing 10cm × 10cm= £0.07, 10cm × 20cm= £0.09, 20cm × 20cm= £0.15, 20cm × 40cm= £0.29, sterile dressing 10cm × 10cm= £0.22, 10cm × 20cm= £0.26, 20cm × 20cm= £0.41, 20cm × 40cm= £1.15

Absorbent perforated dressing

Adpore

Low-adherence primary dressing consisting of viscose and rayon absorbent pad with adhesive border.

Adpore dressing (Medicareplus International Ltd) 10cm × 10cm= £0.10, 10cm × 15cm= £0.16, 10cm × 20cm= £0.30, 10cm × 25cm= £0.34, 10cm × 30cm= £0.42, 10cm × 35cm= £0.50, 7cm × 8cm= £0.08

Cosmopore E

Low-adherence primary dressing consisting of viscose and rayon absorbent pad with adhesive border.

Cosmopor E dressing (Paul Hartmann Ltd) 10cm × 20cm= £0.47, 10cm × 25cm= £0.58, 10cm × 35cm= £0.81, 5cm × 7.2cm= £0.08, 8cm × 10cm= £0.18, 8cm × 15cm= £0.29

Cutiplast Steril

Low-adherence primary dressing consisting of viscose and rayon absorbent pad with adhesive border.

Cutiplast Steril dressing (Smith & Nephew Healthcare Ltd) 10cm × 20cm= £0.32, 10cm × 25cm= £0.33, 10cm × 30cm= £0.45, 8cm × 10cm= £0.11, 8cm × 15cm= £0.26

Leukomed

Low-adherence primary dressing consisting of viscose and rayon absorbent pad with adhesive border.

Leukomed dressing (BSN medical Ltd) 10cm × 20cm= £0.45, 10cm × 25cm= £0.50, 10cm × 30cm= £0.65, 10cm × 35cm= £0.75, 5cm × 7.2cm= £0.09, 8cm × 10cm= £0.19, 8cm × 15cm= £0.34

Medipore + Pad

Low-adherence primary dressing consisting of viscose and rayon absorbent pad with adhesive border.

Medipore + Pads dressing (3M Health Care Ltd) 10cm × 10cm= £0.16, 10cm × 15cm= £0.25, 10cm × 20cm= £0.38, 10cm × 25cm= £0.47, 10cm × 35cm= £0.65, 5cm × 7.2cm= £0.08

Medisafe

Low-adherence primary dressing consisting of viscose and rayon absorbent pad with adhesive border.

Medisafe dressing (Neomedic Ltd) 6cm × 8cm= £0.08, 8cm × 10cm= £0.13, 8cm × 12cm= £0.23, 9cm × 15cm= £0.29, 9cm × 20cm= £0.34, 9cm × 25cm= £0.36

Mepore

Low-adherence primary dressing consisting of viscose and rayon absorbent pad with adhesive border.

Mepore dressing (Molnlycke Health Care Ltd) 10cm × 11cm= £0.22, 11cm × 15cm= £0.37, 7cm × 8cm= £0.11, 9cm × 20cm= £0.45, 9cm × 25cm= £0.62, 9cm × 30cm= £0.71, 9cm × 35cm= £0.78

PremierPore

Low-adherence primary dressing consisting of viscose and rayon absorbent pad with adhesive border.

PremierPore dressing (Shermond) 10cm × 10cm= £0.12, 10cm × 15cm= £0.18, 10cm × 20cm= £0.32, 10cm × 25cm= £0.36, 10cm × 30cm= £0.45, 10cm × 35cm= £0.52, 5cm × 7cm= £0.05

Primapore

Low-adherence primary dressing consisting of viscose and rayon absorbent pad with adhesive border.

Primapore dressing (Smith & Nephew Healthcare Ltd) 10cm × 20cm= £0.46, 10cm × 25cm= £0.52, 10cm × 30cm= £0.66, 10cm × 35cm= £1.01, 6cm × 8.3cm= £0.19, 8cm × 10cm= £0.20, 8cm × 15cm= £0.35

Softpore

Low-adherence primary dressing consisting of viscose and rayon absorbent pad with adhesive border.

Softpore dressing (Richardson Healthcare Ltd) 10cm × 10cm= £0.13, 10cm × 15cm= £0.20, 10cm × 20cm= £0.35, 10cm × 25cm= £0.40, 10cm × 35cm= £0.49, 10cm × 35cm= £0.58, 6cm × 7cm= £0.06

Telfa Island

Low-adherence primary dressing consisting of viscose and rayon absorbent pad with adhesive border.

Absorbent perforated plastic film faced dressing

Absopad

Low-adherence primary dressing consisting of 3 layers— perforated polyester film wound contact layer, absorbent cotton pad, and hydrophobic backing.

Absopad dressing (Medicareplus International Ltd) 10cm × 10cm= £0.13, 20cm × 10cm= £0.28

Askina Pad

Low-adherence primary dressing consisting of 3 layers— perforated polyester film wound contact layer, absorbent cotton pad, and hydrophobic backing.

Askina (B.Braun Medical Ltd) Pad dressing 10cm × 10cm= £0.22

Melolin

Low-adherence primary dressing consisting of 3 layers— perforated polyester film wound contact layer, absorbent cotton pad, and hydrophobic backing.

Melolin dressing (Smith & Nephew Healthcare Ltd) 10cm × 10cm= £0.29, 20cm × 10cm= £0.56, 5cm × 5cm= £0.18

Skintact

Low-adherence primary dressing consisting of 3 layers— perforated polyester film wound contact layer, absorbent cotton pad, and hydrophobic backing.

Skintact dressing (Robinson Healthcare) 10cm × 10cm= £0.17, 20cm × 10cm= £0.34, 5cm × 5cm= £0.10

Solvaline N

Low-adherence primary dressing consisting of 3 layers— perforated polyester film wound contact layer, absorbent cotton pad, and hydrophobic backing.

Solvaline N dressing (Lohmann & Rauscher) 10cm × 10cm= £0.19, 20cm × 10cm= £0.37, 5cm × 5cm= £0.10

Telfa

Low-adherence primary dressing consisting of 3 layers— perforated polyester film wound contact layer, absorbent cotton pad, and hydrophobic backing.

Telfa dressing (H & R Healthcare Ltd) 10cm × 7.5cm= £0.16, 15cm × 7.5cm= £0.18, 20cm × 7.5cm= £0.29, 7.5cm × 5cm= £0.12

A4

Wound management | Appendix 4

Super absorbent cellulose and polymer primary dressing
Curea P1
Super absorbent cellulose and polymer primary dressing.
Curea P1 dressing (Charles S. Bullen Stomacare Ltd) 10cm × 10cm
square= £2.17, 10cm × 20cm rectangular= £3.67, 10cm × 30cm
rectangular= £5.25, 12cm × 12cm square= £2.67, 20cm × 20cm
square= £6.95, 20cm × 30cm rectangular= £10.11, 7.5cm ×
7.5cm square= £1.73

Curea P2
Super absorbent cellulose and polymer primary dressing
(non-adherent)
Curea P2 dressing (Charles S. Bullen Stomacare Ltd) 10cm × 20cm
rectangular= £4.53, 11cm × 11cm square= £2.49, 20cm × 20cm
square= £7.88, 20cm × 30cm rectangular= £10.68

Cutisorb Ultra
Super absorbent cellulose and polymer primary dressing
Cutisorb Ultra dressing (BSN medical Ltd) 10cm × 10cm square=
£2.13, 10cm × 20cm rectangular= £3.56, 20cm × 20cm square=
£6.68, 20cm × 30cm rectangular= £10.06

DryMax Extra
Super absorbent cellulose and polymer primary dressing
DryMax Extra Soft dressing (Espere Healthcare Ltd) 10cm × 10cm
square= £0.87, 10cm × 20cm rectangular= £1.04, 20cm × 20cm
square= £1.84, 20cm × 30cm rectangular= £2.33

ELECT Superabsorber
Super absorbent cellulose and polymer primary dressing

Zetuvit Plus
Super absorbent cellulose primary dressing
Zetuvit Plus dressing (Paul Hartmann Ltd) 10cm × 10cm= £0.85,
10cm × 20cm= £1.17, 15cm × 20cm= £1.35, 20cm × 25cm=
£1.84, 20cm × 40cm= £2.84

Super absorbent hydroconductive dressing
Drawtex
Super absorbent hydroconductive dressing with absorbent,
cross-action structures of viscose, polyester and cotton
Drawtex dressing (Martindale Pharmaceuticals Ltd) 10cm × 1.3m=
£16.00, 10cm × 10cm= £2.24, 10cm × 1m= £16.00, 15cm ×
20cm= £6.00, 20cm × 1m= £25.00, 20cm × 20cm= £6.98, 5cm ×
5cm= £0.95, 7.5cm × 1m= £15.50, 7.5cm × 7.5cm= £1.77

Advanced wound dressings

Advanced wound dressings can be used for both acute and
chronic wounds. Categories for dressings in this section start
with the least absorptive, moisture-donating hydrogel
dressings, followed by increasingly more absorptive
dressings. These dressings are classified according to their
primary component; some dressings are comprised of several
components.

Hydrogel dressings

Hydrogel dressings are most commonly supplied as an
amorphous, cohesive topical application that can take up the
shape of a wound. A secondary, non-absorbent dressing is
needed. These dressings are generally used to donate liquid
to dry sloughy wounds and facilitate autolytic debridement
of necrotic tissue; some also have the ability to absorb very
small amounts of exudate. Hydrogel products that do not
contain propylene glycol should be used if the wound is to be
treated with larval therapy. Hydrogel dressings have a fixed
structure and limited fluid-handling capacity; hydrogel sheet
dressings are best avoided in the presence of infection, and
are unsuitable for heavily exuding wounds.

Hydrogel application (amorphous)
ActivHeal Hydrogel
Hydrogel containing guar gum and propylene glycol
ActivHeal (Advanced Medical Solutions Ltd) Hydrogel dressing= £1.41

Aquaform
Hydrogel containing modified starch copolymer

Askina Gel
Hydrogel containing modified starch and glycerol

Cutimed
Hydrogel
Cutimed (BSN medical Ltd) Gel dressing= £3.13

Flexigran
Hydrogel containing modified starch and glycerol
Flexigran (A1 Pharmaceuticals) Gel dressing= £1.90

GranuGel
Hydrogel containing carboxymethylcellulose, pectin and
propylene glycol
GranuGEL (ConvaTec Ltd) Hydrocolloid Gel dressing= £2.45

Intrasite Gel
Hydrogel containing modified carmellose polymer and
propylene glycol
IntraSite (Smith & Nephew Healthcare Ltd) Gel dressing= £3.78

Nu-Gel
Hydrogel containing alginate and propylene glycol
Nu-Gel (Systagenix Wound Management Ltd) dressing= £2.13

Purilon Gel
Hydrogel containing carboxymethylcellulose and calcium
alginate
Purilon (Coloplast Ltd) Gel dressing= £2.39

Hydrogel sheet dressings
ActiFormCool
Hydrogel dressing
ActiFormCool sheet (L&R Medical UK Ltd) 10cm × 10cm square=
£2.77, 10cm × 15cm rectangular= £3.98, 20cm × 20cm square=
£8.34, 5cm × 6.5cm rectangular= £1.89

Aquaflo
Hydrogel dressing
Aquaflo (Covidien (UK) Commercial Ltd) sheet 7.5cm discs= £2.60

Coolie
Hydrogel dressing (without adhesive border)
Coolie (Zeroderma Ltd) sheet 7cm discs= £1.96

Gel FX
Hydrogel dressing (without adhesive border)
Gel FX sheet (Synergy Health (UK) Ltd) 10cm × 10cm square= £1.60,
15cm × 15cm square= £3.20

Geliperm
Hydrogel sheets
Geliperm (Geistlich Sons Ltd) sheet 10cm × 10cm square= £2.53

Hydrosorb
Absorbent, transparent, hydrogel sheets containing
polyurethane polymers covered with a semi-permeable film
Hydrosorb sheet (Paul Hartmann Ltd) 10cm × 10cm square= £2.34,
20cm × 20cm square= £7.01, 5cm × 7.5cm rectangular= £1.64

Hydrosorb Comfort
Absorbent, transparent, hydrogel sheets containing
polyurethane polymers covered with a semi-permeable film
(with adhesive border, waterproof)
Hydrosorb Comfort sheet (Paul Hartmann Ltd) 12.5cm × 12.5cm
square= £3.74, 4.5cm × 6.5cm rectangular= £1.94, 7.5cm ×
10cm rectangular= £2.57

Intrasite Conformable
Soft non-woven dressing impregnated with Intrasite ® gel
IntraSite Conformable dressing (Smith & Nephew Healthcare Ltd)
10cm × 10cm square= £1.90, 10cm × 20cm rectangular= £2.56,
10cm × 40cm rectangular= £4.58

Novovel
Glycerol-based hydrogel sheets (standard or thin)
Novogel sheet (Ford Medical Associates Ltd) 10cm × 10cm square=
£3.18, 15cm × 20cm rectangular= £6.07, 20cm × 40cm
rectangular= £11.56, 30cm × 30cm (0.15cm thickness) square=
£12.71, (0.30cm thickness) square= £13.47, 5cm × 7.5cm
rectangular= £1.99, 7.5cm diameter circular= £5.84

SanoSkin NET
Hydrogel sheet (without adhesive border)
SanoSkin (Ideal Medical Solutions Ltd) NET sheet 8.5cm × 12cm
rectangular= £2.28

Vacunet
Non-adherent, hydrogel coated polyester net dressing

...cunet dressing (Protex Healthcare Ltd) 10cm × 10cm square= ...93, 10cm × 15cm rectangular= £2.86

...dium hyaluronate dressings

...e hydrating properties of sodium hyaluronate promote ...ound healing, and dressings can be applied directly to the ...ound, or to a primary dressing (a secondary dressing should ...so be applied). The iodine and potassium iodide in these ...ressings prevent the bacterial decay of sodium hyaluronate ... the wound.

...yiodine® should be used with caution in thyroid disorders.

...viodine

...odium hyaluronate 1.5%, potassium iodide 0.15%, iodine ...1%, in a viscous solution

...apour-permeable films and membranes

...apour-permeable films and membranes allow the passage ...f water vapour and oxygen but are impermeable to water ...nd micro-organisms, and are suitable for lightly exuding ...ounds. They are highly conformable, provide protection, ...nd a moist healing environment; transparent film dressings ...ermit constant observation of the wound. Water vapour ...oss can occur at a slower rate than exudate is generated, so ...hat fluid accumulates under the dressing, which can lead to ...ssue maceration and to wrinkling at the adhesive contact ...ite (with risk of bacterial entry). Newer versions of these ...ressings have increased moisture vapour permeability.

...espite these advances, vapour-permeable films and ...embranes are unsuitable for infected, large heavily ...xuding wounds, and chronic leg ulcers. Vapour-permeable ...lms and membranes are suitable for partial-thickness ...ounds with minimal exudate, or wounds with eschar. Most ...ommonly, they are used as a secondary dressing over ...lginates or hydrogels; film dressings can also be used to ...rotect the fragile skin of patients at risk of developing ...inor skin damage caused by friction or pressure.

...on-woven fabric dressing with viscose-rayon pad.

...iko Fix

...or intravenous and subcutaneous catheter sites

...iko (Unomedical Ltd) Fix dressing 7cm × 8.5cm= £0.20

...apour-permeable Adhesive Film Dressing (Semi-permeable ...dhesive Dressing)

...xtensible, waterproof, water vapour-permeable ...olyurethane film coated with synthetic adhesive mass; ...ransparent. Supplied in single-use pieces.

...skina Derm

Extensible, waterproof, water vapour-permeable ...olyurethane film coated with synthetic adhesive mass; ...ransparent. Supplied in single-use pieces

...skina Derm dressing (B.Braun Medical Ltd) 10cm × 12cm= £1.13, 10cm × 20cm= £2.14, 15cm × 20cm= £2.59, 20cm × 30cm= ...4.64, 6cm × 7cm= £0.39

C-View

Extensible, waterproof, water vapour-permeable polyurethane film coated with synthetic adhesive mass; transparent. Supplied in single-use pieces

Dressfilm

Extensible, waterproof, water vapour-permeable polyurethane film coated with synthetic adhesive mass; transparent. Supplied in single-use pieces

Dressfilm (St Georges Medical Ltd) dressing 15cm × 20cm= £1.90

Hydrofilm

Extensible, waterproof, water vapour-permeable polyurethane film coated with synthetic adhesive mass; transparent. Supplied in single-use pieces

Hydrofilm dressing (Paul Hartmann Ltd) 10cm × 12.5cm= £0.44, 10cm × 15cm= £0.55, 10cm × 25cm= £0.85, 12cm × 25cm= £0.90, 15cm × 20cm= £1.01, 20cm × 30cm= £1.67, 6cm × 7cm= £0.24

Hypafix Transparent

Extensible, waterproof, water vapour-permeable polyurethane film coated with synthetic adhesive mass; transparent. Supplied in single-use pieces

Hypafix Transparent (BSN medical Ltd) dressing 10cm × 2m= £9.03

Leukomed T

Extensible, waterproof, water vapour-permeable polyurethane film coated with synthetic adhesive mass; transparent. Supplied in single-use pieces

Leukomed T dressing (BSN medical Ltd) 10cm × 12.5cm= £1.06, 11cm × 14cm= £1.29, 15cm × 20cm= £2.46, 15cm × 25cm= £2.63, 7.2cm × 5cm= £0.39, 8cm × 10cm= £0.73

Mepitel Film

Extensible, waterproof, water vapour-permeable polyurethane film coated with synthetic adhesive mass; transparent. Supplied in single-use pieces

Mepitel Film dressing (Molnlycke Health Care Ltd) 10.5cm × 12cm= £1.36, 10.5cm × 25cm= £2.63, 15.5cm × 20cm= £3.34, 6.5cm × 7cm= £0.50

Mepore Film

Extensible, waterproof, water vapour-permeable polyurethane film coated with synthetic adhesive mass; transparent. Supplied in single-use pieces

Mepore Film dressing (Molnlycke Health Care Ltd) 10cm × 12cm= £1.27, 10cm × 25cm= £2.47, 15cm × 20cm= £3.14, 6cm × 7cm= £0.47

OpSite Flexifix

Extensible, waterproof, water vapour-permeable polyurethane film coated with synthetic adhesive mass; transparent. Supplied in single-use pieces

OpSite Flexifix dressing (Smith & Nephew Healthcare Ltd) 10cm × 1m= £6.94, 5cm × 1m= £4.12

OpSite Flexigrid

Extensible, waterproof, water vapour-permeable polyurethane film coated with synthetic adhesive mass; transparent. Supplied in single-use pieces

OpSite Flexigrid dressing (Smith & Nephew Healthcare Ltd) 12cm × 12cm= £1.19, 15cm × 20cm= £3.00, 6cm × 7cm= £0.42

Polyskin II

Extensible, waterproof, water vapour-permeable polyurethane film coated with synthetic adhesive mass; transparent. Supplied in single-use pieces

Kendall Film dressing (H & R Healthcare Ltd) 10cm × 12cm= £1.03, 10cm × 20cm= £2.04, 15cm × 20cm= £2.35, 20cm × 25cm= £4.11, 4cm × 4cm= £0.36, 5cm × 7cm= £0.40

ProtectFilm

Extensible, waterproof, water vapour-permeable polyurethane film coated with synthetic adhesive mass; transparent. Supplied in single-use pieces

ProtectFilm dressing (Wallace, Cameron & Company Ltd) 10cm × 12cm= £0.20, 15cm × 20cm= £0.40, 6cm × 7cm= £0.11

Suprasorb F

Extensible, waterproof, water vapour-permeable polyurethane film coated with synthetic adhesive mass; transparent. Supplied in single-use pieces

Suprasorb F dressing (Lohmann & Rauscher) 10cm × 12cm= £0.83, 15cm × 20cm= £2.58, 5cm × 7cm= £0.34

Tegaderm

Extensible, waterproof, water vapour-permeable polyurethane film coated with synthetic adhesive mass; transparent. Supplied in single-use pieces

Tegaderm Film dressing (3M Health Care Ltd) 12cm × 12cm= £1.13, 15cm × 20cm= £2.44, 6cm × 7cm= £0.39

Tegaderm diamond

Extensible, waterproof, water vapour-permeable polyurethane film coated with synthetic adhesive mass; transparent. Supplied in single-use pieces

Tegaderm Diamond dressing (3M Health Care Ltd) 10cm × 12cm= £1.23, 6cm × 7cm= £0.45

A4

Wound management | Appendix 4

Vellafilm

Extensible, waterproof, water vapour-permeable polyurethane film coated with synthetic adhesive mass; transparent. Supplied in single-use pieces

Vellafilm dressing (Advancis Medical) 12cm × 12cm= £1.14, 12cm × 35cm= £2.84, 15cm × 20cm= £2.17

Vapour-permeable Adhesive Film Dressing with absorbent pad
Adpore Ultra

Film dressing with adsorbent pad

Adpore Ultra dressing (Medicareplus International Ltd) 10cm × 10cm= £0.14, 10cm × 15cm= £0.22, 10cm × 20cm= £0.33, 10cm × 25cm= £0.35, 10cm × 30cm= £0.52, 7cm × 8cm= £0.12

Vapour-permeable Adhesive Film Dressing with adsorbent pad
Alldress

Film dressing with adsorbent pad

Alldress dressing (Molnlycke Health Care Ltd) 10cm × 10cm= £0.99, 15cm × 15cm= £2.17, 15cm × 20cm= £2.68

C-View Post-Op

Film dressing with adsorbent pad

Clearpore

Film dressing with adsorbent pad

Clearpore dressing (Richardson Healthcare Ltd) 10cm × 10cm= £0.20, 10cm × 15cm= £0.24, 10cm × 20cm= £0.36, 10cm × 25cm= £0.40, 10cm × 30cm= £0.65, 6cm × 10cm= £0.15, 6cm × 7cm= £0.12

Hydrofilm Plus

Film dressing with adsorbent pad

Hydrofilm Plus dressing (Paul Hartmann Ltd) 10cm × 20cm= £0.48, 10cm × 25cm= £0.63, 10cm × 30cm= £0.72, 7.2cm × 5cm= £0.18, 9cm × 10cm= £0.28, 9cm × 15cm= £0.31

Leukomed T Plus

Film dressing with adsorbent pad

Leukomed T plus dressing (BSN medical Ltd) 10cm × 20cm= £1.40, 10cm × 25cm= £1.57, 10cm × 30cm= £2.63, 10cm × 35cm= £3.19, 7.2cm × 5cm= £0.28, 8cm × 10cm= £0.56, 8cm × 15cm= £0.84

Mepore Film & Pad

Film dressing with adsorbent pad

Mepore Film & Pad dressing (Molnlycke Health Care Ltd) 4cm × 5cm= £0.25, 5cm × 7cm= £0.25, 9cm × 10cm= £0.64, 9cm × 15cm= £0.94, 9cm × 20cm= £1.41, 9cm × 25cm= £1.55, 9cm × 30cm= £2.08, 9cm × 35cm= £2.58

Mepore Ultra

Film dressing with adsorbent pad

Mepore Ultra dressing (Molnlycke Health Care Ltd) 10cm × 11cm= £0.83, 11cm × 15cm= £1.22, 7cm × 8cm= £0.42, 9cm × 20cm= £1.56, 9cm × 25cm= £1.72, 9cm × 30cm= £2.84

OpSite Plus

Film dressing with adsorbent pad

OpSite Plus dressing (Smith & Nephew Healthcare Ltd) 10cm × 12cm= £1.26, 10cm × 20cm= £2.12, 10cm × 35cm= £3.52, 6.5cm × 5cm= £0.34, 8.5cm × 9.5cm= £0.93

OpSite Post-op

Film dressing with adsorbent pad

OpSite Post-Op dressing (Smith & Nephew Healthcare Ltd) 10cm × 12cm= £1.24, 10cm × 20cm= £2.08, 10cm × 25cm= £2.62, 10cm × 30cm= £3.10, 10cm × 35cm= £3.45, 8.5cm × 15.5cm= £1.26, 8.5cm × 9.5cm= £0.91

Pharmapore-PU

Film dressing with adsorbent pad

Pharmapore-PU dressing (Wallace, Cameron & Company Ltd) 10cm × 25cm= £0.38, 10cm × 30cm= £0.58, 8.5cm × 15.5cm= £0.20

PremierPore VP

Film dressing with adsorbent pad

PremierPore VP dressing (Shermond) 10cm × 10cm= £0.16, 10cm × 15cm= £0.24, 10cm × 20cm= £0.36, 10cm × 25cm= £0.38, 10cm × 30cm= £0.57, 10cm × 35cm= £0.70, 5cm × 7cm= £0.13

Tegaderm

Film dressing with adsorbent pad

Tegaderm + Pad dressing (3M Health Care Ltd) 5cm × 7cm= £0.26, 9cm × 10cm= £0.66, 9cm × 15cm= £0.97, 9cm × 20cm= £1.42, 9cm × 25cm= £1.60, 9cm × 35cm= £2.65

Tegaderm Absorbent Clear

Film dressing with clear acrylic polymer oval-shaped pad or rectangular-shaped pad

Tegaderm Absorbent Clear Acrylic dressing (3M Health Care Ltd) 11.1cm × 12.7cm oval= £4.18, 14.2cm × 15.8cm oval= £5.89, 14.9cm × 15.2cm rectangular= £8.83, 20cm × 20.3cm rectangular= £14.17, 7.6cm × 9.5cm oval= £3.23

Vapour-permeable transparent film dressing with adhesive foam border.
Central Gard

For intravenous and subcutaneous catheter sites

Central Gard dressing (Unomedical Ltd) 16cm × 7cm= £0.99, 16cm × 8.8cm= £1.08

EasI-V

For intravenous and subcutaneous catheter sites

EasI-V (ConvaTec Ltd) dressing 7cm × 7.5cm= £0.38

Vapour-permeable transparent, adhesive film dressing.
Hydrofilm I.V. Control

For intravenous and subcutaneous catheter sites

Hydrofilm (Paul Hartmann Ltd) I.V. Control dressing 7cm × 9cm= £0.32

Vapour-permeable, transparent, adhesive film dressing.
IV3000

For intravenous and subcutaneous catheter sites

IV3000 dressing (Smith & Nephew Healthcare Ltd) 10cm × 12cm= £1.47, 5cm × 6cm= £0.44, 6cm × 7cm= £0.59, 7cm × 9cm= £0.77, 9cm × 12cm= £1.53

Mepore IV

For intravenous and subcutaneous catheter sites

Mepore IV dressing (Molnlycke Health Care Ltd) 10cm × 11cm= £1.11, 5cm × 5.5cm= £0.32, 8cm × 9cm= £0.41

Pharmapore-PU IV

For intravenous and subcutaneous catheter sites

Pharmapore-PU-I.V dressing (Wallace, Cameron & Company Ltd) 6cm × 7cm= £0.08, 7cm × 8.5cm= £0.07, 7cm × 9cm= £0.17

Tegaderm IV

For intravenous and subcutaneous catheter sites

Tegaderm IV Advanced dressing with securing tapes (3M Health Care Ltd) 10cm × 15.5cm= £1.68, 7cm × 8.5cm= £0.60

Soft polymer dressings

Dressings with soft polymer, often a soft silicone polymer, in a non-adherent or gently adherent layer are suitable for use on lightly to moderately exuding wounds. For moderately to heavily exuding wounds, an absorbent secondary dressing can be added, or a soft polymer dressing with an absorbent pad can be used. Wound contact dressings coated with soft silicone have gentle adhesive properties and can be used on fragile skin areas or where it is beneficial to reduce the frequency of primary dressing changes. Soft polymer dressings should not be used on heavily bleeding wounds; blood clots can cause the dressing to adhere to the wound surface. For silicone keloid dressings see under Specialised dressings.

Cellulose dressings
Sorbion Sachet Border

Absorbent polymers in cellulose matrix, hypoallergenic polypropylene envelope, with adhesive border

Cutimed Sorbion Sachet Border dressing (BSN medical Ltd) 10cm × 10cm square= £3.06, 15cm × 15cm square= £4.66, 25cm × 15cm rectangular= £7.26

Sorbion Sachet EXTRA

Absorbent polymers in cellulose matrix, hypoallergenic polypropylene envelope

Cutimed Sorbion Sachet Extra dressing (BSN medical Ltd) 10cm × 10cm= £2.34, 20cm × 10cm= £3.88, 20cm × 20cm= £7.27, 30cm × 20cm= £10.37, 5cm × 5cm= £1.51, 7.5cm × 7.5cm= £1.85

Sorbion Sachet Multi Star

Absorbent polymers in cellulose matrix, hypoallergenic polypropylene envelope

Cutimed Sorbion Sachet Multi Star dressing (BSN medical Ltd) 14cm × 14cm= £5.08, 8cm × 8cm= £3.10

Sorbion Sachet S Drainage

Absorbent polymers in cellulose matrix, hypoallergenic polypropylene envelope ('v' shaped dressing)

Cutimed (BSN medical Ltd) Sorbion Sachet S drainage dressing 10cm × 10cm= £2.74

Suprasorb X

Biosynthetic cellulose fibre dressing

Suprasorb X dressing (Lohmann & Rauscher) 14cm × 20cm rectangular= £8.77, 2cm × 21cm rope= £6.81, 5cm × 5cm square= £2.13, 9cm × 9cm square= £4.42

With absorbent pad

Advazorb Border

Soft silicone wound contact dressing with polyurethane foam film backing and adhesive border

Advazorb Border dressing (Advancis Medical) 10cm × 10cm= £2.17, 10cm × 20cm= £3.00, 10cm × 30cm= £4.39, 12.5cm × 12.5cm= £2.67, 15cm × 15cm= £3.26, 20cm × 20cm= £5.64, 7.5cm × 7.5cm= £1.23

Advazorb Border Lite

Soft silicone wound contact dressing with polyurethane foam film backing and adhesive border

Advazorb Border Lite dressing (Advancis Medical) 10cm × 10cm= £1.95, 10cm × 20cm= £2.70, 10cm × 30cm= £3.96, 12.5cm × 12.5cm= £2.40, 15cm × 15cm= £2.94, 20cm × 20cm= £5.08, 7.5cm × 7.5cm= £1.11

Advazorb Silfix

Soft silicone wound contact dressing with polyurethane foam film backing

Advazorb Silfix dressing (Advancis Medical) 10cm × 10cm= £1.91, 10cm × 20cm= £3.29, 12.5cm × 12.5cm= £2.68, 15cm × 15cm= £3.47, 20cm × 20cm= £5.15, 7.5cm × 7.5cm= £1.02

Advazorb Silfix Lite

Soft silicone wound contact dressing with polyurethane foam film backing

Advazorb Silfix Lite dressing (Advancis Medical) 10cm × 10cm= £1.73, 10cm × 20cm= £2.96, 12.5cm × 12.5cm= £2.41, 15cm × 15cm= £3.12, 20cm × 20cm= £4.63, 7.5cm × 7.5cm= £0.92

Allevyn Gentle

Soft gel wound contact dressing, with polyurethane foam film backing

Allevyn Gentle Border

Silicone gel wound contact dressing, with polyurethane foam film backing

Allevyn Gentle Border (Smith & Nephew Healthcare Ltd) Heel dressing 23cm × 23.2cm= £10.14, dressing 10cm × 10cm= £2.30, 12.5cm × 12.5cm= £2.82, 17.5cm × 17.5cm= £5.56, 7.5cm × 7.5cm= £1.57

Allevyn Gentle Border Lite

Silicone gel wound contact dressing, with polyurethane foam film backing

Allevyn Gentle Border Lite dressing (Smith & Nephew Healthcare Ltd) 10cm × 10cm= £2.27, 15cm × 15cm= £4.01, 5.5cm × 12cm= £1.94, 5cm × 5cm= £0.94, 8cm × 15cm= £3.61

Allevyn Life

Soft silicone wound contact dressing, with central mesh screen, polyurethane foam film backing and adhesive border

Allevyn Life dressing (Smith & Nephew Healthcare Ltd) 10.3cm × 10.3cm= £1.78, 12.9cm × 12.9cm= £2.61, 15.4cm × 15.4cm= £3.19, 21cm × 21cm= £6.29

Cutimed Siltec

Soft silicone wound contact dressing, with polyurethane foam film backing

Cutimed Siltec (BSN medical Ltd) Sacrum dressing 17.5cm × 17.5cm= £4.63, 23cm × 23cm= £6.32, dressing 10cm × 10cm= £2.30, 10cm × 20cm= £3.80, 15cm × 15cm= £4.30, 20cm × 20cm= £6.52, 5cm × 6cm= £1.23

Cutimed Siltec B

Soft silicone wound contact dressing, with polyurethane foam film backing, with adhesive border, for lightly to moderately exuding wounds

Cutimed Siltec B dressing (BSN medical Ltd) 12.5cm × 12.5cm= £2.34, 15cm × 15cm= £3.12, 17.5cm × 17.5cm= £5.04, 22.5cm × 22.5cm= £6.16, 7.5cm × 7.5cm= £1.38

Cutimed Siltec L

Soft silicone wound contact dressing, with polyurethane foam film backing, for lightly to moderately exuding wounds

Cutimed Siltec L dressing (BSN medical Ltd) 10cm × 10cm= £1.60, 15cm × 15cm= £3.52, 5cm × 6cm= £1.09

Eclypse Adherent

Soft silicone wound contact layer with absorbent pad and film backing

Eclypse Adherent dressing (Advancis Medical) 10cm × 10cm= £3.09, 10cm × 20cm= £3.88, 15cm × 15cm= £5.16, 20cm × 30cm= £10.33, 17cm × 19cm sacral= £3.89, 22cm × 23cm sacral= £6.44

Flivasorb

Absorbent polymer dressing with non-adherent wound contact layer

Flivasorb Adhesive

Absorbent polymer dressing with non-adherent wound contact layer and adhesive border

Vliwasorb Adhesive dressing (Lohmann & Rauscher) 12cm × 12cm square= £3.43, 15cm × 15cm square= £4.70

Mepilex

Absorbent soft silicone dressing with polyurethane foam film backing

Mepilex (Molnlycke Health Care Ltd) Heel dressing 13cm × 20cm= £5.63, 15cm × 22cm= £6.44, XT dressing 10cm × 11cm= £2.75, 11cm × 20cm= £4.54, 15cm × 16cm= £4.98, 20cm × 21cm= £7.52, dressing 5cm × 5cm= £1.25

Mepilex Border

Absorbent soft silicone dressing with polyurethane foam film backing and adhesive border

Mepilex Border (Molnlycke Health Care Ltd) Heel dressing 18.5cm × 24cm= £6.70, Sacrum dressing 18cm × 18cm= £4.97, 23cm × 23cm= £8.11, dressing 10cm × 12.5cm= £2.76, 10cm × 20cm= £3.77, 10cm × 30cm= £5.66, 15cm × 17.5cm= £4.24, 17cm × 20cm= £6.16

Mepilex Border Lite

Thin absorbent soft silicone dressing with polyurethane foam film backing and adhesive border

Mepilex Border Lite dressing (Molnlycke Health Care Ltd) 15cm × 15cm= £3.99, 4cm × 5cm= £0.94, 5cm × 12.5cm= £2.04, 7.5cm × 7.5cm= £1.37

Mepilex Lite

Thin absorbent soft silicone dressing with polyurethane foam film backing

Mepilex Lite dressing (Molnlycke Health Care Ltd) 10cm × 10cm= £2.23, 15cm × 15cm= £4.33, 20cm × 50cm= £27.32, 6cm × 8.5cm= £1.87

Mepilex Transfer

Soft silicone exudate transfer dressing

Mepilex Transfer dressing (Molnlycke Health Care Ltd) 10cm × 12cm= £3.63, 15cm × 20cm= £10.98, 20cm × 50cm= £28.07, 7.5cm × 8.5cm= £2.30

Sorbion Sana

Non-adherent polyethylene wound contact dressing with absorbent core

Cutimed Sorbion Sana Gentle dressing (BSN medical Ltd) 12cm × 12cm= £2.59, 12cm × 22cm= £4.66, 22cm × 22cm= £8.30, 8.5cm × 8.5cm= £2.07

UrgotulDuo

Non-adherent soft polymer wound contact dressing with absorbent pad

UrgotulDuo dressing (Urgo Ltd) 10cm × 12cm= £3.98, 15cm × 20cm= £9.25, 5cm × 10cm= £2.58

Without absorbent pad
Adaptic Touch
Non-adherent soft silicone wound contact dressing
Adaptic Touch dressing (Systagenix Wound Management Ltd) 12.7cm ×
15cm= £4.65, 20cm × 32cm= £12.50, 5cm × 7.6cm= £1.13, 7.6cm
× 11cm= £2.25

Askina SilNet
Soft silicone-coated wound contact dressing
Askina SilNet dressing (B.Braun Medical Ltd) 10cm × 18cm= £5.17,
20cm × 30cm= £12.66, 5cm × 7.5cm= £1.17, 7.5cm × 10cm=
£2.37

Mepitel
Soft silicone, semi-transparent wound contact dressing
Mepitel dressing (Molnlycke Health Care Ltd) 12cm × 15cm= £5.65,
5cm × 7cm= £1.41, 8cm × 10cm= £2.82

Mepitel One
Soft silicone, thin, transparent wound contact dressing
Mepitel One dressing (Molnlycke Health Care Ltd) 13cm × 15cm=
£4.98, 24cm × 27.5cm= £14.25, 6cm × 7cm= £1.22, 9cm ×
10cm= £2.41

Physiotulle
Non-adherent soft polymer wound contact dressing
Physiotulle dressing (Coloplast Ltd) 10cm × 10cm= £2.38, 15cm ×
20cm= £7.25

Silflex
Soft silicone-coated polyester wound contact dressing
Silflex dressing (Advancis Medical) 12cm × 15cm= £4.74, 20cm ×
30cm= £12.19, 35cm × 60cm= £40.88, 5cm × 7cm= £1.15, 8cm
× 10cm= £2.35

Silon-TSR
Soft silicone polymer wound contact dressing
Silon-TSR dressing (Bio Med Sciences) 13cm × 13cm= £3.52, 13cm
× 25cm= £5.47, 28cm × 30cm= £7.37

Sorbion Contact
Non-adherent soft polymer wound contact dressing
Cutimed Sorbion Contact dressing (BSN medical Ltd) 10cm × 10cm=
£2.07, 10cm × 20cm= £4.14, 20cm × 20cm= £7.26, 20cm ×
30cm= £10.37, 7.5cm × 7.5cm= £1.55

Tegaderm Contact
Non-adherent soft polymer wound contact dressing
Tegaderm Contact dressing (3M Health Care Ltd) 20cm × 25cm=
£11.06, 7.5cm × 10cm= £2.32

Urgotul
Non-adherent soft polymer wound contact dressing
Urgotul dressing (Urgo Ltd) 10cm × 10cm= £3.13, 10cm × 40cm=
£10.53, 15cm × 15cm= £6.66, 15cm × 20cm= £8.86, 20cm ×
30cm= £14.25, 5cm × 5cm= £1.57

Hydrocolloid dressings
Hydrocolloid dressings are usually presented as a
hydrocolloid layer on a vapour-permeable film or foam pad.
Semi-permeable to water vapour and oxygen, these
dressings form a gel in the presence of exudate to facilitate
rehydration in lightly to moderately exuding wounds and
promote autolytic debridement of dry, sloughy, or necrotic
wounds; they are also suitable for promoting granulation.
Hydrocolloid-fibrous dressings made from modified
carmellose fibres resemble alginate dressings; hydrocolloid-
fibrous dressings are more absorptive and suitable for
moderately to heavily exuding wounds.

Hydrocolloid-fibrous dressings
Aquacel
Soft non-woven pad containing hydrocolloid-fibres
Aquacel (ConvaTec Ltd) Ribbon dressing 1cm × 45cm= £1.91, 2cm
× 45cm= £2.58, dressing 10cm × 10cm square= £2.55, 15cm ×
15cm square= £4.79, 4cm × 10cm rectangular= £1.37, 4cm ×
20cm rectangular= £2.02, 4cm × 30cm rectangular= £3.04, 5cm
× 5cm square= £1.07

Aquacel Foam
Soft non-woven pad containing hydrocolloid-fibres with
foam layer; with or without adhesive border

Aquacel Foam dressing (adhesive) (ConvaTec Ltd) 10cm × 10cm=
£2.25, 12.5cm × 12.5cm= £2.79, 17.5cm × 17.5cm= £5.58, 19.8c
× 14cm heel= £5.71, 20cm × 16.9cm sacral= £5.12, 21cm ×
21cm= £8.17, 25cm × 30cm= £10.58, 8cm × 8cm= £1.45,
(non-adhesive) 10cm × 10cm= £2.66, 15cm × 15cm= £4.48,
15cm × 20cm= £6.12, 20cm × 20cm= £7.30

UrgoClean Pad
Pad, hydrocolloid fibres coated with soft-adherent lipo-
colloidal wound contact layer
UrgoClean Pad dressing (Urgo Ltd) 10cm × 10cm square= £2.21,
20cm × 15cm rectangular= £4.16, 6cm × 6cm square= £0.99

UrgoClean Rope
Rope, non-woven rope containing hydrocolloid fibres
UrgoClean rope dressing (Urgo Ltd) 2.5cm × 40cm= £2.49, 5cm ×
40cm= £3.29

Polyurethane matrix dressing
Cutinova Hydro
Polyurethane matrix with absorbent particles and
waterproof polyurethane film
Cutinova Hydro dressing (Smith & Nephew Healthcare Ltd) 10cm ×
10cm square= £2.68, 15cm × 20cm rectangular= £5.66, 5cm ×
6cm rectangular= £1.33

With adhesive border
Biatain Super
Semi-permeable hydrocolloid dressing; without adhesive
border
Biatain Super dressing (adhesive) (Coloplast Ltd) 10cm × 10cm
square= £2.26, 12.5cm × 12.5cm square= £3.73, 12cm × 20cm
rectangular= £3.74, 15cm × 15cm square= £4.50, 20cm × 20cm
square= £7.02

Granuflex Bordered
Hydrocolloid wound contact layer bonded to plastic foam
layer, with outer semi-permeable polyurethane film
Granuflex Bordered dressing (ConvaTec Ltd) 10cm × 10cm square=
£3.51, 10cm × 13cm triangular= £4.14, 15cm × 15cm square=
£6.69, 15cm × 18cm triangular= £6.45, 6cm × 6cm square=
£1.85

Hydrocoll Border
Hydrocolloid dressing with adhesive border and absorbent
wound contact pad
Hydrocoll Border (bevelled edge) dressing (Paul Hartmann Ltd) 10cm
× 10cm square= £2.52, 12cm × 18cm sacral= £3.77, 15cm ×
15cm square= £4.73, 5cm × 5cm square= £1.05, 7.5cm × 7.5cm
square= £1.73, 8cm × 12cm concave= £2.22

Tegaderm Hydrocolloid
Hydrocolloid dressing with adhesive border; normal or thin
Tegaderm Hydrocolloid (3M Health Care Ltd) Thin dressing 10cm ×
12cm oval= £1.58, 13cm × 15cm oval= £2.95, dressing 10cm ×
12cm oval= £2.37, 13cm × 15cm oval= £4.42, 17.1cm × 16.1cm
sacral= £4.94

Without adhesive border
ActivHeal Hydrocolloid
Semi-permeable polyurethane film backing, hydrocolloid
wound contact layer, with or without polyurethane foam
later
ActivHeal Hydrocolloid (Advanced Medical Solutions Ltd) dressing
10cm × 10cm square= £1.58, 15cm × 15cm square= £3.43, 15cm
× 18cm sacral= £3.98, 5cm × 7.5cm rectangular= £0.78, foam
backed dressing 10cm × 10cm square= £1.55, 15cm × 15cm
square= £2.91, 15cm × 18cm sacral= £3.36, 5cm × 7.5cm
rectangular= £0.97

Askina Biofilm Transparent
Semi-permeable, polyurethane film dressing with
hydrocolloid adhesive

Biatain Super
Semi-permeable, hydrocolloid film dressing without
adhesive border
Biatain Super dressing (non-adhesive) (Coloplast Ltd) 10cm × 10cm
square= £2.26, 12.5cm × 12.5cm square= £3.73, 12cm × 20cm
rectangular= £3.74, 15cm × 15cm square= £4.50, 20cm × 20cm
square= £7.02

omfeel Plus Contour
ydrocolloid dressings containing carmellose sodium and
alcium alginate
omfeel Plus Contour dressing (Coloplast Ltd) 6cm × 8cm= £2.29,
cm × 11cm= £3.98

omfeel Plus Pressure Relieving
ydrocolloid dressings containing carmellose sodium and
alcium alginate
omfeel Plus Pressure Relief dressing (Coloplast Ltd) 10cm diameter
ircular= £4.79, 15cm diameter circular= £7.22, 7cm diameter
ircular= £3.58

omfeel Plus Transparent
ydrocolloid dressings containing carmellose sodium and
alcium alginate
omfeel Plus Transparent dressing (Coloplast Ltd) 10cm × 10cm
quare= £1.32, 15cm × 15cm square= £3.44, 15cm × 20cm
ectangular= £3.49, 20cm × 20cm square= £3.52, 5cm × 15cm
ectangular= £1.64, 5cm × 25cm rectangular= £2.66, 5cm ×
cm rectangular= £0.69, 9cm × 14cm rectangular= £2.51, 9cm
× 25cm rectangular= £3.57

omfeel Plus Ulcer
ydrocolloid dressings containing carmellose sodium and
alcium alginate
omfeel Plus dressing (Coloplast Ltd) 10cm × 10cm square= £2.53,
0cm × 20cm square= £7.80, 4cm × 6cm rectangular= £0.99

DuoDERM Extra Thin
Semi-permeable hydrocolloid dressing
DuoDERM Extra Thin dressing (ConvaTec Ltd) 10cm × 10cm square=
£1.39, 15cm × 15cm square= £3.00, 5cm × 10cm rectangular=
£0.79, 7.5cm × 7.5cm square= £0.84, 9cm × 15cm rectangular=
£1.86, 9cm × 25cm rectangular= £2.97, 9cm × 35cm
rectangular= £4.15

DuoDERM Signal
Semi-permeable hydrocolloid dressing with 'Time to change'
indicator
DuoDERM Signal dressing (ConvaTec Ltd) 10cm × 10cm square=
£2.23, 11cm × 19cm oval= £3.37, 14cm × 14cm square= £3.91,
18.5cm × 19.5cm heel= £5.46, 20cm × 20cm square= £7.77,
22.5cm × 20cm sacral= £6.38

Flexigran
Semi-permeable hydrocolloid dressing without adhesive
border; normal or thin
Flexigran (A1 Pharmaceuticals) Thin dressing 10cm × 10cm
square= £1.08, dressing 10cm × 10cm square= £2.19

Granuflex
Hydrocolloid wound contact layer bonded to plastic foam
layer, with outer semi-permeable polyurethane film
Granuflex (modified) dressing (ConvaTec Ltd) 10cm × 10cm square=
£2.94, 15cm × 15cm square= £5.58, 15cm × 20cm rectangular=
£6.05, 20cm × 20cm square= £8.40

Hydrocoll Basic
Hydrocolloid dressing with absorbent wound contact pad
Hydrocoll (Paul Hartmann Ltd) Basic dressing 10cm × 10cm square=
£2.56

Hydrocoll Thin Film
Thin hydrocolloid dressing with absorbent wound contact
pad
Hydrocoll Thin Film dressing (Paul Hartmann Ltd) 10cm × 10cm
square= £1.20, 15cm × 15cm square= £2.71, 7.5cm × 7.5cm
square= £0.73

Nu-Derm
Semi-permeable hydrocolloid dressing (normal and thin)
Nu-Derm dressing (Systagenix Wound Management Ltd) 10cm × 10cm
square= £1.57, 15cm × 15cm square= £3.21, 15cm × 18cm
sacral= £4.49, 20cm × 20cm square= £6.41, 5cm × 5cm square=
£0.86, 8cm × 12cm heel/elbow= £3.21, thin 10cm × 10cm
square= £1.07

Tegaderm Hydrocolloid
Hydrocolloid dressing without adhesive border; normal and
thin

Tegaderm Hydrocolloid (3M Health Care Ltd) Thin dressing 10cm ×
10cm square= £1.58, dressing 10cm × 10cm square= £2.41

Foam dressings

Dressings containing hydrophilic polyurethane foam
(adhesive or non-adhesive), with or without plastic film-
backing, are suitable for all types of exuding wounds, but not
for dry wounds; some foam dressings have a moisture-
sensitive film backing with variable permeability dependant
on the level of exudate Foam dressings vary in their ability to
absorb exudate; some are suitable only for lightly to
moderately exuding wounds, others have greater fluid-
handing capacity and are suitable for heavily exuding
wounds. Saturated foam dressings can cause maceration of
healthy skin if left in contact with the wound. Foam
dressings can be used in combination with other primary
wound contact dressings. If used under compression
bandaging or compression garments, the fluid-handling
capacity of the foam dressing may be reduced. Foam
dressings can also be used to provide a protective cushion for
fragile skin. A foam dressing containing ibuprofen is
available and may be useful for treating painful exuding
wounds.

Cavi-Care
Soft, conforming cavity wound dressing prepared by mixing
thoroughly for 15 seconds immediately before use and
allowing to expand its volume within the cavity

Polyurethane Foam Dressing
Cutimed Cavity
Cutimed Cavity dressing (BSN medical Ltd) 10cm × 10cm= £3.24,
15cm × 15cm= £4.86, 5cm × 6cm= £1.95

Kendall
Kendall Foam dressing (H & R Healthcare Ltd) 10cm × 10cm square=
£1.07, 10cm × 20cm rectangular= £2.07, 12.5cm × 12.5cm
square= £1.82, 15cm × 15cm square= £2.63, 20cm × 20cm
square= £3.04, 5cm × 5cm square= £0.72, 7.5cm × 7.5cm
square= £1.23, 8.5cm × 7.5cm rectangular (fenestrated)= £0.92

Polyurethane Foam Film Dressing with Adhesive Border
ActivHeal Foam Adhesive
ActivHeal Foam Adhesive dressing (Advanced Medical Solutions Ltd)
10cm × 10cm square= £1.63, 12.5cm × 12.5cm square= £1.68,
15cm × 15cm square= £2.15, 20cm × 20cm square= £4.50, 7.5cm
× 7.5cm square= £1.18

Allevyn Adhesive
Allevyn Adhesive dressing (Smith & Nephew Healthcare Ltd) 10cm ×
10cm square= £2.30, 12.5cm × 12.5cm square= £2.81, 12.5cm ×
22.5cm rectangular= £4.37, 17.5cm × 17.5cm square= £5.55,
17cm × 17cm anatomically shaped sacral= £4.17, 22.5cm ×
22.5cm square= £8.08, 22cm × 22cm anatomically shaped
sacral= £6.00, 7.5cm × 7.5cm square= £1.57

Biatain Adhesive
Biatain Adhesive dressing (Coloplast Ltd) 10cm × 10cm square=
£1.84, 12.5cm × 12.5cm square= £2.69, 17cm diameter contour=
£5.22, 18cm × 18cm square= £5.42, 18cm × 28cm rectangular=
£8.03, 19cm × 20cm heel= £5.42, 23cm × 23cm sacral= £4.64

Biatain Silicone
Biatain Silicone dressing (Coloplast Ltd) 10cm × 10cm= £2.23,
12.5cm × 12.5cm= £2.72, 15cm × 15cm= £4.04, 17.5cm ×
17.5cm= £5.37, 7.5cm × 7.5cm= £1.51

Kendall Island
Kendall Foam Island dressing (H & R Healthcare Ltd) 10cm × 10cm
square= £1.54, 15cm × 15cm square= £2.90, 20cm × 20cm
square= £5.46

PolyMem
PolyMem dressing (H & R Healthcare Ltd) (adhesive) 5cm × 5cm
square= £0.52, 16.5cm × 20.9cm oval= £6.79, 18.4cm × 20cm
sacral= £4.56, 5cm × 7.6cm oval= £1.16, 8.8cm × 12.7cm oval=
£2.06

Tegaderm Foam Adhesive
Tegaderm Foam dressing (adhesive) (3M Health Care Ltd) 10cm ×
11cm oval= £2.42, 13.9cm × 13.9cm circular (heel)= £4.30,
14.3cm × 14.3cm square= £3.60, 14.3cm × 15.6cm oval= £4.32,

19cm × 22.2cm oval= £7.09, 6.9cm × 6.9cm soft cloth border= £1.74, 6.9cm × 7.6cm oval= £1.49

Tielle

Tielle (Systagenix Wound Management Ltd) Lite dressing 11cm × 11cm square= £2.33, dressing 15cm × 15cm square= £3.92, 15cm × 20cm rectangular= £4.90, 18cm × 18cm square= £4.99, 7cm × 9cm rectangular= £1.29

Tielle Lite

Tielle Lite dressing (Systagenix Wound Management Ltd) 11cm × 11cm square= £2.33, 7cm × 9cm rectangular= £1.23, 8cm × 15cm rectangular= £2.86, 8cm × 20cm rectangular= £3.03

Tielle Plus

Tielle Plus dressing (Systagenix Wound Management Ltd) 11cm × 11cm square= £2.66, 15cm × 15cm sacrum= £3.17, square= £4.34, 15cm × 20cm rectangular= £5.45, 20cm × 26.5cm heel= £4.50

Polyurethane Foam Film Dressing without Adhesive Border

ActivHeal Foam Non-Adhesive

ActivHeal Non-Adhesive Foam polyurethane dressing (Advanced Medical Solutions Ltd) 10cm × 10cm square= £1.13, 10cm × 20cm rectangular= £2.34, 20cm × 20cm square= £3.92, 5cm × 5cm square= £0.75

Advazorb

Advazorb (Advancis Medical) Heel dressing 17cm × 21cm=£4.91, dressing 10cm × 10cm square= £1.12, 10cm × 20cm rectangular= £3.46, 12.5cm × 12.5cm square= £1.64, 15cm × 15cm square= £2.17, 20cm × 20cm square= £3.88, 5cm × 5cm square= £0.67, 7.5cm × 7.5cm square= £0.81

Advazorb Lite

Advazorb Lite dressing (Advancis Medical) 10cm × 10cm square= £1.00, 10cm × 20cm rectangular= £3.12, 12.5cm × 12.5cm square= £1.48, 15cm × 15cm square= £1.95, 20cm × 20cm square= £3.49, 7.5cm × 7.5cm square= £0.72

Allevyn Non-Adhesive

Allevyn dressing (non-adhesive) (Smith & Nephew Healthcare Ltd) 10.5cm × 13.5cm heel (cup shaped)= £5.37, 10cm × 10cm square= £2.63, 10cm × 20cm rectangular= £4.22, 20cm × 20cm square= £7.05, 5cm × 5cm square= £1.33

Askina Foam

Askina (B.Braun Medical Ltd) Foam Cavity dressing 2.4cm × 40cm= £2.54, Foam dressing 10cm × 10cm square= £2.27, 10cm × 20cm rectangular= £3.59, 20cm × 20cm square= £5.99, Heel dressing 12cm × 20cm= £4.86

Biatain -Ibu Non-Adhesive

Biatain-Ibu Non-Adhesive dressing (Coloplast Ltd) 10cm × 12cm rectangular= £3.48, 10cm × 22.5cm rectangular= £5.48, 15cm × 15cm square= £5.48, 20cm × 20cm square= £9.31, 5cm × 7cm rectangular= £1.81

Biatain -Ibu Soft-Hold

Biatain-Ibu Soft-Hold dressing (Coloplast Ltd) 10cm × 12cm rectangular= £3.48, 10cm × 22.5cm rectangular= £5.48, 15cm × 15cm square= £5.48

Biatain Non-Adhesive

Biatain Non-Adhesive dressing (Coloplast Ltd) 10cm × 10cm square= £2.50, 10cm × 20cm rectangular= £4.13, 15cm × 15cm square= £4.61, 20cm × 20cm square= £6.84, 5cm × 7cm rectangular= £1.38

Biatain Soft-Hold

Biatain Soft-Hold dressing (Coloplast Ltd) 10cm × 10cm square= £2.72, 10cm × 20cm rectangular= £4.13, 15cm × 15cm square= £4.52, 5cm × 7cm rectangular= £1.38

Kendall Plus

Kendall Foam Plus dressing (H & R Healthcare Ltd) 10cm × 10cm square= £1.48, 10cm × 20cm rectangular= £2.72, 15cm × 15cm square= £3.42, 20cm × 20cm square= £4.08, 5cm × 5cm square= £0.82, 7.5cm × 7.5cm square= £1.43, 8.5cm × 7.5cm rectangular (fenestrated)= £1.26

Kerraheel

Kerraheel (Crawford Healthcare Ltd) dressing 12cm × 20cm heel= £4.78

Lyofoam Max

Lyofoam Max dressing (Molnlycke Health Care Ltd) 10cm × 10cm square= £1.18, 10cm × 20cm rectangular= £2.08, 15cm × 15cm square= £2.22, 15cm × 20cm rectangular= £2.80, 20cm × 20cm square= £4.11, 7.5cm × 8.5cm rectangular= £1.12

PermaFoam

PermaFoam (Paul Hartmann Ltd) Classic dressing (non-adhesive) 8cm × 8cm square (fenestrated) = £1.31

PolyMem

PolyMem dressing (H & R Healthcare Ltd) 7cm × 7cm tube= £1.73, 9cm × 9cm tube= £2.19, finger/toe size 1= £2.52, 2= £2.52, 3= £2.52

PolyMem

PolyMem dressing (non-adhesive) (H & R Healthcare Ltd) 10cm × 10cm square= £2.49, 10cm × 61cm roll= £13.20, 13cm × 13cm square= £4.15, 17cm × 19cm rectangular= £6.13, 20cm × 60cm roll= £31.13, 8cm × 8cm square= £1.60

PolyMem Max

PolyMem Max dressing (H & R Healthcare Ltd) 11cm × 11cm square= £2.99, 20cm × 20cm square= £11.77

PolyMem WIC

PolyMem (H & R Healthcare Ltd) WIC dressing 8cm × 8cm= £3.72

Tegaderm Foam

Tegaderm Foam dressing (3M Health Care Ltd) 10cm × 10cm square= £2.23, 10cm × 20cm rectangular= £3.78, 10cm × 60cm rectangular= £12.77, 20cm × 20cm square= £6.03, 8.8cm × 8.8cm square (fenestrated)= £2.27

Transorbent

Transorbent dressing (adhesive) (B.Braun Medical Ltd) 10cm × 10cm square= £2.04, 15cm × 15cm square= £3.75, 20cm × 20cm square= £5.99, 5cm × 7cm rectangular= £1.08

UrgoCell TLC

UrgoTul Absorb dressing (Urgo Ltd) 10cm × 10cm= £2.41, 15cm × 20cm= £4.26, 6cm × 6cm= £1.23, 12cm × 19cm heel= £4.86

Alginate dressings

Non-woven or fibrous, non-occlusive, alginate dressings, made from calcium alginate, or calcium sodium alginate, derived from brown seaweed, form a soft gel in contact with wound exudate. Alginate dressings are highly absorbent and suitable for use on exuding wounds, and for the promotion of autolytic debridement of debris in very moist wounds. Alginate dressings also act as a haemostatic, but caution is needed because blood clots can cause the dressing to adhere to the wound surface. Alginate dressings should not be used if bleeding is heavy and extreme caution is needed if used for tumours with friable tissue. Alginate sheets are suitable for use as a wound contact dressing for moderately to heavily exuding wounds and can be layered into deep wounds; alginate rope can be used in sinus and cavity wounds to improve absorption of exudate and prevent maceration. If the dressing does not have an adhesive border or integral adhesive plastic film backing, a secondary dressing will be required.

ActivHeal Alginate

Calcium sodium alginate dressing

ActivHeal Alginate dressing (Advanced Medical Solutions Ltd) 10cm × 10cm= £1.15, 10cm × 20cm= £2.83, 5cm × 5cm= £0.59

ActivHeal Aquafiber

Non-woven, calcium sodium alginate dressing

ActivHeal Aquafiber (Advanced Medical Solutions Ltd) Rope dressing 2cm × 42cm= £1.81, dressing 10cm × 10cm= £1.48, 15cm × 15cm= £2.79, 5cm × 5cm= £0.62

Algisite M

Calcium alginate fibre, non-woven dressing

Algisite M (Smith & Nephew Healthcare Ltd) Rope dressing 2cm × 30cm= £3.65, dressing 10cm × 10cm= £2.01, 15cm × 20cm= £5.41, 5cm × 5cm= £0.97

Biatain Alginate

Alginate and carboxymethylcellulose dressing, highly absorbent, gelling dressing

...atain Alginate dressing (Coloplast Ltd) 10cm × 10cm= £2.43,
...cm × 15cm= £4.61, 44cm= £2.86, 5cm × 5cm= £1.02

...timed Alginate
...alcium sodium alginate dressing
...timed Alginate dressing (BSN medical Ltd) 10cm × 10cm= £1.62,
...cm × 20cm= £3.05, 5cm × 5cm= £0.77

...altostat
...alcium alginate fibre, non-woven
...altostat dressing (ConvaTec Ltd) 10cm × 20cm= £4.29, 15cm ×
...5cm= £7.38, 2g= £4.02, 5cm × 5cm= £1.00, 7.5cm × 12cm=
£2.19

...endall
...alcium alginate dressing
...endall Calcium Alginate (H & R Healthcare Ltd) Rope dressing
...0cm= £2.89, 61cm= £5.07, 91cm= £5.46, dressing 10cm ×
...0cm= £1.52, 10cm × 14cm= £2.45, 10cm × 20cm= £2.98, 15cm
... 25cm= £5.25, 30cm × 61cm= £27.56, 5cm × 5cm= £0.72

...endall Plus
...alcium alginate dressing
...endall (H & R Healthcare Ltd) Foam Plus dressing 10cm × 10cm
...quare= £1.48

...elgisorb
...alcium sodium alginate fibre, highly absorbent, gelling
...ressing, non-woven
...elgisorb (Molnlycke Health Care Ltd) Cavity dressing 2.2cm ×
...2cm= £3.55, dressing 10cm × 10cm= £1.88, 10cm × 20cm=
£3.52, 5cm × 5cm= £0.90

...orbalgon
...alcium alginate dressing
...orbalgon (Paul Hartmann Ltd) T dressing 2g= £3.63, dressing 10cm
... 10cm= £1.78, 5cm × 5cm= £0.85

...orbsan Flat
...alcium alginate fibre, highly absorbent, flat non-woven
...ads
...orbsan Flat dressing (Aspen Medical Europe Ltd) 10cm × 10cm=
...1.72, 10cm × 20cm= £3.22, 5cm × 5cm= £0.82

...orbsan Plus
...lginate dressing bonded to a secondary absorbent viscose
...ad
...orbsan Plus dressing (Aspen Medical Europe Ltd) 10cm × 15cm=
...3.12, 10cm × 20cm= £3.98, 15cm × 20cm= £5.53, 7.5cm ×
...0cm= £1.77

...orbsan Ribbon
...lginate dressing bonded to a secondary absorbent viscose
...ad
...orbsan (Aspen Medical Europe Ltd) Ribbon dressing 40cm= £2.06

...orbsan Surgical Packing
...lginate dressing bonded to a secondary absorbent viscose
...ad
...orbsan (Aspen Medical Europe Ltd) Packing dressing 2g= £3.50

Suprasorb A
Calcium alginate dressing
Suprasorb A (Lohmann & Rauscher) alginate dressing 10cm ×
10cm= £1.28, 5cm × 5cm= £0.65, cavity dressing 2g= £2.37

Tegaderm Alginate
Calcium alginate dressing
Tegaderm Alginate dressing (3M Health Care Ltd) 10cm × 10cm=
£1.75, 2cm × 30.4cm= £2.92, 5cm × 5cm= £0.83

Urgosorb
Alginate and carboxymethylcellulose dressing without
adhesive border
Urgosorb (Urgo Ltd) Pad dressing 10cm × 10cm= £2.22, 10cm ×
20cm= £4.07, 5cm × 5cm= £0.92, Rope dressing 30cm= £2.91

Capillary-acting dressings
Vacutex
Low-adherent dressing consisting of two external polyester
wound contact layers with central wicking polyester/cotton
mix absorbent layer
Vacutex dressing (Haddenham Healthcare Ltd) 10cm × 10cm= £1.70,
10cm × 15cm= £2.29, 10cm × 20cm= £2.75, 5cm × 5cm= £0.96

Odour absorbent dressings
Dressings containing activated charcoal are used to absorb
odour from wounds. The underlying cause of wound odour
should be identified. Wound odour is most effectively
reduced by debridement of slough, reduction in bacterial
levels, and frequent dressing changes. Fungating wounds
and chronic infected wounds produce high volumes of
exudate which can reduce the effectiveness of odour
absorbent dressings. Many odour absorbent dressings are
intended for use in combination with other dressings; odour
absorbent dressings with a suitable wound contact layer can
be used as a primary dressing.

Askina Carbosorb
Activated charcoal and non-woven viscose rayon dressing
Askina Carbosorb dressing (B.Braun Medical Ltd) 10cm × 10cm=
£3.00, 10cm × 20cm= £5.79

CarboFLEX
Dressing in 5 layers: wound-facing absorbent layer
containing alginate and hydrocolloid; water-resistant second
layer; third layer containing activated charcoal; non-woven
absorbent fourth layer; water-resistant backing layer
CarboFlex dressing (ConvaTec Ltd) 10cm × 10cm= £3.33, 15cm ×
20cm= £7.58, 8cm × 15cm oval= £4.00

Carbopad VC
Activated charcoal non-absorbent dressing
Carbopad VC dressing (Synergy Health (UK) Ltd) 10cm × 10cm=
£1.62, 10cm × 20cm= £2.19

CliniSorb Odour Control Dressings
Activated charcoal cloth enclosed in viscose rayon with outer
polyamide coating
CliniSorb dressing (CliniMed Ltd) 10cm × 10cm= £1.99, 10cm ×
20cm= £2.64, 15cm × 25cm= £4.26

Antimicrobial dressings
Spreading infection at the wound site requires treatment
with systemic antibacterials. For local wound infection, a
topical antimicrobial dressing can be used to reduce the level
of bacteria at the wound surface but will not eliminate a
spreading infection. Some dressings are designed to release
the antimicrobial into the wound, others act upon the
bacteria after absorption from the wound. The amount of
exudate present and the level of infection should be taken
into account when selecting an antimicrobial dressing.
Medical grade honey has antimicrobial and anti-
inflammatory properties. Dressings impregnated with iodine
can be used to treat clinically infected wounds. Dressings
containing silver should be used only when clinical signs or
symptoms of infection are present. Dressings containing
other antimicrobials such as polihexanide
(polyhexamethylene biguanide) or dialkylcarbamoyl chloride
are available for use on infected wounds. Although
hypersensitivity is unlikely with chlorhexidine impregnated
tulle dressing, the antibacterial efficacy of these dressings
has not been established.

Honey dressings
Medical grade honey has antimicrobial and anti-
inflammatory properties and can be used for acute or chronic
wounds. Medical grade honey has osmotic properties,
producing an environment that promotes autolytic
debridement; it can help control wound malodour. Honey
dressings should not be used on patients with extreme
sensitivity to honey, bee stings or bee products. Patients
with diabetes should be monitored for changes in blood-
glucose concentrations during treatment with topical honey
or honey-impregnated dressings.
For *Activon Tulle*®, where no size is stated by the prescriber
the 5 cm size is to be supplied.
Medihoney® *Antimicrobial Wound Gel* is not recommended for
use in deep wounds or body cavities where removal of waxes
may be difficult.

A4

Wound management | Appendix 4

A4

Wound management | **Appendix 4**

Honey-based topical application

Activon Honey
Medical grade manuka honey
Activon (Advancis Medical) Medical Grade Manuka Honey dressing= £2.77

L-Mesitran SOFT ointment dressing
Honey (medical grade) 40%
L-Mesitran (H & R Healthcare Ltd) SOFT ointment dressing= £3.62

MANUKApli Honey
Medical grade manuka honey
MANUKApli (Manuka Medical Ltd) dressing= £5.90

Medihoney Antibacterial Medical Honey
Medical grade, Leptospermum sp.
Medihoney (Integra NeuroSciences Ltd) Antibacterial Medical Honey dressing= £4.03

Medihoney Antibacterial Wound Gel
Medical grade, Leptospermum sp. 80% in natural waxes and oils
Medihoney (Integra NeuroSciences Ltd) Antibacterial Wound Gel dressing= £4.09

Melladerm Plus Honey
Medical grade; Bulgarian (mountain flower) 45% in basis containing polyethylene glycol
Melladerm (SanoMed Manufacturing BV) Plus dressing= £8.50

Sheet dressing

Actilite
Knitted viscose impregnated with medical grade manuka honey and manuka oil
Actilite gauze dressing (Advancis Medical) 10cm × 10cm= £1.23, 10cm × 20cm= £2.38, 5cm × 5cm= £0.71

Activon Tulle
Knitted viscose impregnated with medical grade manuka honey
Activon Tulle gauze dressing (Advancis Medical) 10cm × 10cm= £3.71, 5cm × 5cm= £2.25

Algivon
Absorbent, non-adherent calcium alginate dressing impregnated with medical grade manuka honey
Algivon dressing (Advancis Medical) 10cm × 10cm= £4.25, 5cm × 5cm= £2.48

Algivon Plus
Reinforced calcium alginate dressing impregnated with medical grade manuka honey
Algivon Plus (Advancis Medical) Ribbon dressing 2.5cm × 20cm= £4.20, dressing 10cm × 10cm= £4.20, 5cm × 5cm= £2.45

L-Mesitran Border
Hydrogel, semi-permeable dressing impregnated with medical grade honey, with adhesive border
L-Mesitran (H & R Healthcare Ltd) Border sheet 10cm × 10cm square= £2.76

L-Mesitran Hydro
Hydrogel, semi-permeable dressing impregnated with medical grade honey, without adhesive border
L-Mesitran (H & R Healthcare Ltd) Hydro sheet 10cm × 10cm square= £2.65

L-Mesitran Net
Hydrogel, non-adherent wound contact layer, without adhesive border
L-Mesitran (H & R Healthcare Ltd) Net sheet 10cm × 10cm square= £2.55

Medihoney Antibacterial Honey Apinate
Non-adherent calcium alginate dressing, impregnated with medical grade honey
Medihoney Antibacterial Honey Apinate (Integra NeuroSciences Ltd) dressing 10cm × 10cm square= £3.46, 5cm × 5cm square= £2.04, rope dressing 1.9cm × 30cm= £4.28

Medihoney Antibacterial Honey Tulle
Woven fabric impregnated with medical grade manuka honey

Medihoney (Integra NeuroSciences Ltd) Tulle dressing 10cm x10cm= £3.03

Medihoney Gel sheet
Sodium alginate dressing impregnated with medical grade honey
Medihoney Gel Sheet dressing (Integra NeuroSciences Ltd) 10cm × 10cm= £4.28, 5cm × 5cm= £1.78

MelMax
Acetate wound contact layer impregnated with buckwheat honey 75% in ointment basis

Melladerm Plus Tulle
Knitted viscose impregnated with medical grade honey (Bulgarian, mountain flower) 45% in a basis containing polyethylene glycol
Melladerm (SanoMed Manufacturing BV) Plus Tulle dressing 10cm × 10cm= £2.10

Iodine dressings
Cadexomer–iodine, like povidone–iodine, releases free iodine when exposed to wound exudate. The free iodine acts as an antiseptic on the wound surface, the cadexomer absorbs wound exudate and encourages de-sloughing. Two-component hydrogel dressings containing glucose oxidase and iodide ions generate a low level of free iodine in the presence of moisture and oxygen. Povidone–iodine fabric dressing is a knitted viscose dressing with povidone–iodine incorporated in a hydrophilic polyethylene glycol basis; this facilitates diffusion of the iodine into the wound and permits removal of the dressing by irrigation. The iodine has a wide spectrum of antimicrobial activity but it is rapidly deactivated by wound exudate. Systemic absorption of iodine may occur, particularly from large wounds or with prolonged use.
Iodoflex® and *Iodosorb*® are used for the treatment of chronic exuding wounds; max. single application 50 g, max. weekly application 150 g; max. duration up to 3 months in any single course of treatment. They are contra-indicated in patients receiving lithium, in thyroid disorders, in pregnancy and breast feeding, and in children; they should be used with caution in patients with severe renal impairment or history of thyroid disorder.
Iodozyme® is an antimicrobial dressing used for lightly to moderately exuding wounds. It is contra-indicated in thyroid disorders and in patients receiving lithium; it should be used with caution in children and in women who are pregnant or breast-feeding.
Oxyzyme® is used for non-infected, dry to moderately exuding wounds. It is contra-indicated in thyroid disorders and in patients receiving lithium; it should be used with caution in children and in women who are pregnant or breast-feeding.
Povidone-iodine Fabric Dressing is used as a wound contact layer for abrasions and superficial burns. It is contra-indicated in patients with severe renal impairment and in women who are pregnant or breast-feeding; it should be used with caution in patients with thyroid disease and in children under 6 months.

Iodoflex Paste
Iodine 0.9% as cadexomer–iodine in a paste basis with gauze backing
Iodoflex paste (Smith & Nephew Healthcare Ltd) dressing= 5g = £4.28, 10g = £8.54, 17g = £13.54

Iodosorb Ointment
Iodine 0.9% as cadexomer–iodine in an ointment basis
Iodosorb (Smith & Nephew Healthcare Ltd) ointment dressing= £9.44

Iodosorb Powder
Iodine 0.9% as cadexomer–iodine microbeads, 3-g sachet
Iodosorb (Smith & Nephew Healthcare Ltd) powder dressing sachets= £2.02

ovidone-iodine fabric dressing

adine

rug Tariff specification 43). Knitted viscose primary
essing impregnated with povidone–iodine ointment 10%
adine dressing (Systagenix Wound Management Ltd) 5cm × 5cm=
0.33, 9.5cm × 9.5cm= £0.49

lver dressings

ntimicrobial dressings containing silver should be used
nly when infection is suspected as a result of clinical signs
r symptoms (see also notes above). Silver ions exert an
ntimicrobial effect in the presence of wound exudate; the
olume of wound exudate as well as the presence of infection
hould be considered when selecting a silver-containing
ressing. Silver-impregnated dressings should not be used
outinely for the management of uncomplicated ulcers. It is
ecommended that these dressings should not be used on
cute wounds as there is some evidence to suggest they
elay wound healing. Dressings impregnated with silver
ulfadiazine have broad antimicrobial activity; if silver
ulfadiazine is applied to large areas, or used for prolonged
eriods, there is a risk of blood disorders and skin
iscoloration. The use of silver sulfadiazine-impregnated
ressings is contra-indicated in neonates, in pregnancy, and
n patients with significant renal or hepatic impairment,
ensitivity to sulfonamides, or G6PD deficiency. Large
mounts of silver sulfadiazine applied topically may interact
vith other drugs—see Appendix 1 (sulfonamides).

Alginate dressings

Algisite Ag

Calcium alginate dressing, with silver

Algisite Ag dressing (Smith & Nephew Healthcare Ltd) 10cm × 10cm=
4.31, 10cm × 20cm= £7.94, 2g= £5.96, 5cm × 5cm= £1.73

Askina Calgitrol Ag

Calcium alginate and silver alginate dressing with
polyurethane foam backing

Askina Calgitrol Ag dressing (B.Braun Medical Ltd) 10cm × 10cm
square= £3.33, 15cm × 15cm square= £6.44, 20cm × 20cm
square= £15.02

Askina Calgitrol Thin

Calcium alginate and silver alginate matrix, for use with
absorptive secondary dressings

Askina Calgitrol Thin dressing (B.Braun Medical Ltd) 10cm × 10cm
square= £4.24, 15cm × 15cm square= £9.51, 20cm × 20cm
square= £16.80, 5cm × 5cm square= £2.04

Melgisorb Ag

Alginate and carboxymethylcellulose dressing, with ionic
silver

Melgisorb Ag (Molnlycke Health Care Ltd) Cavity dressing 3cm ×
44cm= £4.72, dressing 10cm × 10cm= £3.79, 15cm × 15cm=
£8.02, 5cm × 5cm= £1.89

Silvercel

Alginate and carboxymethylcellulose dressing impregnated
with silver

Silvercel dressing (Systagenix Wound Management Ltd) 10cm × 20cm
rectangular= £7.82, 11cm × 11cm square= £4.21, 2.5cm ×
30.5cm rectangular= £4.54, 5cm × 5cm square= £1.71

Silvercel Non-adherent

Alginate and carboxymethylcellulose dressing with film
wound contact layer, impregnated with silver

Silvercel Non-Adherent (Systagenix Wound Management Ltd) cavity
dressing 2.5cm × 30.5cm= £3.98, dressing 10cm × 20cm
rectangular= £7.33, 11cm × 11cm square= £3.93, 5cm × 5cm
square= £1.64

Sorbsan Silver Flat

Calcium alginate fibre, highly absorbent, flat non-woven
pads, with silver

Sorbsan Silver Flat dressing (Aspen Medical Europe Ltd) 10cm ×
10cm= £4.00, 10cm × 20cm= £7.31, 5cm × 5cm= £1.58

Sorbsan Silver Plus

Calcium alginate dressing with absorbent backing, with
silver

Sorbsan Silver Plus dressing (Aspen Medical Europe Ltd) 10cm ×
15cm= £5.60, 10cm × 20cm= £6.82, 15cm × 20cm= £9.15, 7.5cm
× 10cm= £3.37

Sorbsan Silver Ribbon

With silver

Sorbsan (Aspen Medical Europe Ltd) Silver Ribbon dressing 1g=
£4.18

Sorbsan Silver Surgical Packing

With silver

Sorbsan (Aspen Medical Europe Ltd) Silver Packing dressing 2g=
£5.80

Suprasorb A + Ag

Calcium alginate dressing, with silver

Suprasorb A + Ag (Lohmann & Rauscher) dressing 10cm × 10cm=
£4.26, 10cm × 20cm= £7.87, 5cm × 5cm= £1.69, rope dressing
2g= £6.30

Tegaderm Alginate Ag

Calcium alginate and carboxymethylcellulose dressing, with
silver

Tegaderm Alginate Ag dressing (3M Health Care Ltd) 10cm × 10cm=
£3.30, 3cm × 30cm= £3.77, 5cm × 5cm= £1.42

Urgosorb Silver

Alginate and carboxymethylcellulose dressing, impregnated
with silver

Urgosorb Silver (Urgo Ltd) Rope dressing 2.5cm × 30cm= £3.86,
dressing 10cm × 10cm= £3.84, 10cm × 20cm= £7.24, 5cm ×
5cm= £1.61

Foam dressings

Acticoat Moisture Control

Three layer polyurethane dressing consisting of a silver
coated layer, a foam layer, and a waterproof layer

Acticoat Moisture Control dressing (Smith & Nephew Healthcare Ltd)
10cm × 10cm square= £17.66, 10cm × 20cm rectangular=
£34.41, 5cm × 5cm square= £7.55

Allevyn Ag

Silver sulfadiazine impregnated polyurethane foam film
dressing with or without adhesive border

Allevyn Ag (Smith & Nephew Healthcare Ltd) Adhesive dressing 10cm
× 10cm square= £5.71, 12.5cm × 12.5cm square= £7.50, 17.5cm
× 17.5cm square= £14.43, 17cm × 17cm sacral= £11.26, 22cm ×
22cm sacral= £15.10, 7.5cm × 7.5cm square= £3.62, Heel Non-
Adhesive dressing 10.5cm × 13.5cm= £11.17, Non-Adhesive
dressing 10cm × 10cm square= £6.37, 15cm × 15cm square=
£12.08, 20cm × 20cm square= £17.70, 5cm × 5cm square= £3.38

Biatain Ag

Silver impregnated polyurethane foam film dressing, with or
without adhesive border

Biatain Ag (Coloplast Ltd) cavity dressing 5cm × 8cm= £4.23,
dressing 10cm × 10cm square= £8.50, 10cm × 20cm
rectangular= £15.61, 12.5cm × 12.5cm square= £9.72, 15cm ×
15cm square= £17.05, 18cm × 18cm square= £19.50, 19cm ×
20cm heel= £19.23, 20cm × 20cm square= £24.05, 23cm × 23cm
sacral= £20.44, 5cm × 7cm rectangular= £3.49

PolyMem Silver

Silver impregnated polyurethane foam film dressing, with or
without adhesive border

PolyMem Silver (H & R Healthcare Ltd) WIC dressing 8cm × 8cm=
£7.10, dressing 10.8cm × 10.8cm square= £8.93, 12.7cm × 8.8cm
oval= £5.64, 17cm × 19cm rectangular= £17.89, 5cm × 7.6cm
oval= £2.29

UrgoCell Silver

Non-adherent, polyurethane foam film dressing with silver
in wound contact layer

Hydrocolloid dressings

Aquacel Ag

Soft non-woven pad containing hydrocolloid fibres, (silver
impregnated)

Aquacel Ag (ConvaTec Ltd) Ribbon dressing 1cm × 45cm= £3.20,
2cm × 45cm= £4.96, dressing 10cm × 10cm square= £4.93, 15cm
× 15cm square= £9.28, 20cm × 30cm rectangular= £23.03, 4cm

A4

Wound management | Appendix 4

× 10cm rectangular= £3.00, 4cm × 20cm rectangular= £3.91, 4cm × 30cm rectangular= £5.86

Physiotulle Ag

Non-adherent polyester fabric with hydrocolloid and silver sulfadiazine

Physiotulle (Coloplast Ltd) dressing 10cm × 10cm= £2.38

Low adherence dressing

Acticoat

Three-layer antimicrobial barrier dressing consisting of a polyester core between low adherent silver-coated high density polyethylene mesh (for 3-day wear)

Acticoat dressing (Smith & Nephew Healthcare Ltd) 10cm × 10cm square= £9.01, 10cm × 20cm rectangular= £14.09, 20cm × 40cm rectangular= £48.21, 5cm × 5cm square= £3.69

Acticoat 7

Five-layer antimicrobial barrier dressing consisting of a polyester core between low adherent silver-coated high density polyethylene mesh (for 7-day wear)

Acticoat 7 dressing (Smith & Nephew Healthcare Ltd) 10cm × 12.5cm rectangular= £19.10, 15cm × 15cm square= £34.34, 5cm × 5cm square= £6.41

Acticoat Flex 3

Conformable antimicrobial barrier dressing consisting of a polyester core between low adherent silver-coated high density polyethylene mesh (for 3-day wear)

Acticoat Flex 3 dressing (Smith & Nephew Healthcare Ltd) 10cm × 10cm square= £8.99, 10cm × 20cm rectangular= £14.05, 20cm × 40cm rectangular= £48.08, 5cm × 5cm square= £3.68

Acticoat Flex 7

Conformable antimicrobial barrier dressing consisting of a polyester core between low adherent silver-coated high density polyethylene mesh (for 7-day wear)

Acticoat Flex 7 dressing (Smith & Nephew Healthcare Ltd) 10cm × 12.5cm rectangular= £19.05, 15cm × 15cm square= £34.26, 5cm × 5cm square= £6.40

Atrauman Ag

Non-adherent polyamide fabric impregnated with silver and neutral triglycerides

Atrauman Ag dressing (Paul Hartmann Ltd) 10cm × 10cm= £1.31, 10cm × 20cm= £2.56, 5cm × 5cm= £0.54

Soft polymer dressings

Allevyn Ag Gentle

Soft polymer wound contact dressing, with silver sulfadiazine impregnated polyurethane foam layer, with or without adhesive border

Allevyn Ag Gentle (Smith & Nephew Healthcare Ltd) Border dressing 10cm × 10cm= £6.69, 12.5cm × 12.5cm= £8.61, 17.5cm × 17.5cm= £16.40, 7.5cm × 7.5cm= £4.45, dressing 10cm × 10cm= £6.50, 10cm × 20cm= £10.74, 15cm × 15cm= £12.09, 20cm × 20cm= £17.91, 5cm × 5cm= £3.49

Mepilex Ag

Soft silicone wound contact dressing with polyurethane foam film backing, with silver, with or without adhesive border

Mepilex (Molnlycke Health Care Ltd) Ag dressing 10cm × 10cm= £6.37, 10cm × 20cm= £10.50, 15cm × 15cm= £11.82, 20cm × 20cm= £17.51, 20cm × 50cm= £65.72, Border Ag dressing 10cm × 12.5cm= £6.41, 10cm × 20cm= £9.33, 10cm × 30cm= £14.00, 15cm × 17.5cm= £11.76, 17cm × 20cm= £15.24, 7cm × 7.5cm= £3.54, Border Sacrum Ag dressing 18cm × 18cm= £12.30, 20cm × 20cm= £14.95, 23cm × 23cm= £19.64, Heel Ag dressing 13cm × 20cm= £13.29, 15cm × 22cm= £14.89

Urgotul Silver

Non-adherent soft polymer wound contact dressing, with silver

Urgotul Silver dressing (Urgo Ltd) 10cm × 12cm= £3.24, 15cm × 20cm= £9.18

With charcoal

Actisorb Silver 220

Knitted fabric of activated charcoal, with one-way stretch, with silver residues, within spun-bonded nylon sleeve

Actisorb Silver 220 dressing (Systagenix Wound Management Ltd) 10.5cm × 10.5cm= £2.63, 10.5cm × 19cm= £4.78, 6.5cm × 9.5cm= £1.68

Other antimicrobials

Cutimed Siltec Sorbact

Polyurethane foam dressing with acetate fabric coated with dialkylcarbamoyl chloride, with adhesive border

Cutimed Siltec Sorbact dressing (BSN medical Ltd) 12.5cm × 12.5cm= £6.69, 15cm × 15cm= £8.29, 17.5cm × 17.5cm= £11.60, 22.5cm × 22.5cm= £17.64, 7.5cm × 7.5cm= £2.61, 17.5cm × 17.5cm sacral= £8.38, 23cm × 23cm sacral= £12.60

Cutimed Sorbact

Low adherence acetate tissue impregnated with dialkylcarbamoyl chloride; dressing pad, swabs, round swab or ribbon gauze, cotton

Cutimed Sorbact (BSN medical Ltd) Ribbon dressing 2cm × 50cm= £4.19, 5cm × 200cm= £8.25, Round swab 3cm= £3.42, dressing pad 10cm × 10cm= £5.71, 10cm × 20cm= £8.90, 7cm × 9cm= £3.65, swab 4cm × 6cm= £1.71, 7cm × 9cm= £2.85

Cutimed Sorbact Gel

Hydrogel dressing impregnated with dialkylcarbamoyl chloride

Cutimed Sorbact Gel dressing (BSN medical Ltd) 7.5cm × 15cm rectangular= £4.65, 7.5cm × 7.5cm square= £2.75

Cutimed Sorbact Hydroactive

Non-adhesive gel dressing with hydropolymer matrix and acetate fabric coated with dialkylcarbamoyl chloride

Cutimed Sorbact Hydroactive dressing (BSN medical Ltd) 14cm × 14cm= £5.57, 14cm × 24cm= £8.93, 19cm × 19cm= £10.49, 24cm × 24cm= £15.90, 7cm × 8.5cm= £3.82

Cutimed Sorbact Hydroactive B

Gel dressing with hydropolymer matrix and acetate fabric coated with dialkylcarbamoyl chloride, with adhesive border

Cutimed Sorbact Hydroactive B dressing (BSN medical Ltd) 10cm × 10cm= £7.36, 10cm × 20cm= £11.78, 15cm × 15cm= £13.85, 5cm × 6.5cm= £4.13

Flaminal Forte gel

Alginate with glucose oxidase and lactoperoxidase, for moderately to heavily exuding wounds

Flaminal (Flen Health UK Ltd) Forte gel dressing= £7.95

Flaminal Hydro gel

Alginate with glucose oxidase and lactoperoxidase, for lightly to moderately exuding wounds

Flaminal (Flen Health UK Ltd) Hydro gel dressing= £7.95

Kendall AMD

Foam dressing with polihexanide, without adhesive border

Kendall AMD Antimicrobial foam dressing (H & R Healthcare Ltd) 10cm × 10cm square= £4.76, 10cm × 20cm rectangular= £9.02, 15cm × 15cm square= £9.02, 20cm × 20cm square= £13.21, 5cm × 5cm square= £2.53, 8.8cm × 7.5cm rectangular (fenestrated)= £4.28

Kendall AMD Plus

Foam dressing with polihexanide, without adhesive border

Kendall AMD Antimicrobial Plus foam dressing (H & R Healthcare Ltd) 10cm × 10cm square= £5.00, 8.8cm × 7.5cm rectangular (fenestrated)= £4.48

Octenilin Wound gel

Wound gel, hydroxyethylcellulose and propylene glycol, with octenidine hydrochloride

Octenilin (Schulke & Mayr UK Ltd) Wound Gel dressing= 20ml = £4.78, 250ml = £25.21

Prontosan Wound Gel

Hydrogel containing betaine surfactant and polihexanide

Prontosan (B.Braun Medical Ltd) Wound Gel gel dressing= £6.62

Suprasorb X + PHMB

Biosynthetic cellulose fibre dressing with polihexanide

Suprasorb X + PHMB dressing (Lohmann & Rauscher) 14cm × 20cm rectangular= £12.06, 2cm × 21cm rope= £7.51, 5cm × 5cm square= £2.66, 9cm × 9cm square= £5.30

Ilfa AMD
Low adherence absorbent perforated plastic film faced dressing with polihexanide
Ilfa AMD dressing (H & R Healthcare Ltd) 10cm × 7.5cm= £0.18, 10cm × 7.5cm= £0.28

Ilfa AMD Island
Low adherence dressing with adhesive border and absorbent pad, with polihexanide
Ilfa AMD Island dressing (H & R Healthcare Ltd) 10cm × 12.5cm= £0.59, 10cm × 20cm= £0.86, 10cm × 25.5cm= £0.98, 10cm × 35cm= £1.22

Chlorhexidine gauze dressing
Bactigras
Fabric of leno weave, weft and warp threads of cotton and/or viscose yarn, impregnated with ointment containing chlorhexidine acetate
Bactigras gauze dressing (Smith & Nephew Healthcare Ltd) 10cm × 10cm= no price available, 5cm × 5cm= no price available

Irrigation fluids
Octenilin Wound irrigation solution
Aqueous solution containing glycerol, ethylhexylglycerin and octenidine hydrochloride
Octenilin (Schulke & Mayr UK Ltd) irrigation solution 350ml bottles= £4.60

Prontosan Wound Irrigation Solution
Aqueous solution containing betaine surfactant and polihexanide
Prontosan irrigation solution (B.Braun Medical Ltd) 350ml bottles= £4.96, 40ml unit dose= £14.72

Specialised dressings

Protease-modulating matrix dressings
Cadesorb Ointment
Cadesorb (Smith & Nephew Healthcare Ltd) ointment= £9.71

Catrix
Catrix dressing (Cranage Healthcare Ltd) sachets= £3.80

Promogran
Collagen and oxidised regenerated cellulose matrix, applied directly to wound and covered with suitable dressing
Promogran dressing (Systagenix Wound Management Ltd) 123 square cm= £15.92, 28 square cm= £5.29

Promogran Prisma Matrix
Collagen, silver and oxidised regenerated cellulose matrix, applied directly to wound and covered with suitable dressing
Promogran Prisma dressing (Systagenix Wound Management Ltd) 123 square cm= £18.31, 28 square cm= £6.43

UrgoStart
Soft adherent polymer matrix containing nano-oligosaccharide factor (NOSF), with polyurethane foam film backing
UrgoStart dressing (Urgo Ltd) 10cm × 10cm= £6.42, 15cm × 20cm= £11.54, 6cm × 6cm= £4.64, 12cm × 19cm heel= £8.84

UrgoStart Contact
Non-adherent soft polymer wound contact dressing containing nano-oligosaccharide factor (NOSF)
UrgoStart (Urgo Ltd) Contact dressing 5cm × 7cm= £3.07

Silicone keloid dressings
Silicone gel and gel sheets are used to reduce or prevent hypertrophic and keloid scarring. They should not be used on open wounds. Application times should be increased gradually. Silicone sheets can be washed and reused.

Silicone gel
Bapscarcare
Silicone gel
Bapscarcare (Espere Healthcare Ltd) gel= £17.12

Ciltech
Silicone gel
Ciltech (Su-Med International (UK) Ltd) gel= £50.00

Dermatix
Silicone gel
Dermatix gel (Meda Pharmaceuticals Ltd) = £60.53

Kelo-cote UV
Silicone gel with SPF 30 UV protection
Kelo-cote (Alliance Pharmaceuticals Ltd) UV gel= £17.88

Kelo-cote gel
Silicone gel
Kelo-cote (Alliance Pharmaceuticals Ltd) gel= £51.00

Kelo-cote spray
Silicone spray
Kelo-cote (Alliance Pharmaceuticals Ltd) spray= £51.00

ScarSil
Silicone gel
ScarSil (Jobskin Ltd) gel= £15.19

Silgel STC-SE
Silicone gel
Silgel (Nagor Ltd) STC-SE gel= £19.00

Silicone sheets
Advasil Conform
Self-adhesive silicone gel sheet with polyurethane film backing
Advasil Conform sheet (Advancis Medical) 10cm × 10cm square= £5.38, 15cm × 10cm rectangular= £9.48

Bapscarcare T
Self-adhesive silicone gel sheet
Bapscarcare T sheet (Espere Healthcare Ltd) 10cm × 15cm rectangular= £9.07, 5cm × 30cm rectangular= £9.07, 5cm × 7cm rectangular= £3.17

Cica-Care
Soft, self-adhesive, semi-occlusive silicone gel sheet with backing
Cica-Care sheet (Smith & Nephew Healthcare Ltd) 15cm × 12cm rectangular= £30.02, 6cm × 12cm rectangular= £15.40

Ciltech
Silicone gel sheet
Ciltech sheet (Su-Med International (UK) Ltd) 10cm × 10cm square= £7.50, 10cm × 20cm rectangular= £12.50, 15cm × 15cm square= £14.00

Dermatix
Self-adhesive silicone gel sheet (clear- or fabric-backed)
Dermatix (Meda Pharmaceuticals Ltd) Clear sheet 13cm × 13cm square= £15.79, 13cm × 25cm rectangular= £28.53, 20cm × 30cm rectangular= £51.97, 4cm × 13cm rectangular= £6.88, Fabric sheet 13cm × 13cm square= £15.79, 13cm × 25cm rectangular= £28.53, 20cm × 30cm rectangular= £51.97, 4cm × 13cm rectangular= £6.88

Mepiform
Self-adhesive silicone gel sheet with polyurethane film backing
Mepiform sheet (Molnlycke Health Care Ltd) 4cm × 31cm rectangular= £11.32, 5cm × 7cm rectangular= £3.58, 9cm × 18cm rectangular= £14.01

Scar FX
Self-adhesive, transparent, silicone gel sheet
Scar Fx sheet (Jobskin Ltd) 10cm × 20cm rectangular= £16.00, 22.5cm × 14.5cm shaped= £12.00, 25.5cm × 30.5cm rectangular= £60.00, 3.75cm × 22.5cm rectangular= £12.00, 7.5cm diameter shaped= £8.50

Silgel
Silicone gel sheet
Silgel sheet (Nagor Ltd) 10cm × 10cm square= £13.50, 10cm × 30cm rectangular= £31.50, 10cm × 5cm rectangular= £7.50, 15cm × 10cm rectangular= £19.50, 20cm × 20cm square= £40.00, 25cm × 15cm shaped= £21.12, 30cm × 5cm rectangular= £19.50, 40cm × 40cm square= £144.00, 46cm × 8.5cm shaped= £39.46, 5.5cm diameter shaped= £4.00

Adjunct dressings and appliances

Surgical absorbents

Surgical absorbents applied directly to the wound have many disadvantages—dehydration of and adherence to the wound, shedding of fibres, and the leakage of exudate ('strike through') with an associated risk of infection. Gauze and cotton absorbent dressings can be used as secondary layers in the management of heavily exuding wounds (but see also Capillary-action dressings). Absorbent cotton gauze fabric can be used for swabbing and cleaning skin. Ribbon gauze can be used post-operatively to pack wound cavities, but adherence to the wound bed will cause bleeding and tissue damage on removal of the dressing—an advanced wound dressing (e.g. hydrocolloid-fibrous, foam, or alginate) layered into the cavity is often more suitable.

Cotton

Absorbent Cotton, BP

Carded cotton fibres of not less than 10 mm average staple length, available in rolls and balls
Absorbent (Robert Bailey & Son Plc) cotton BP 1988

Absorbent Cotton, Hospital Quality

As for absorbent cotton but lower quality materials, shorter staple length etc.
Absorbent (Robert Bailey & Son Plc) cotton hospital quality

Gauze and cotton tissue

Gamgee Tissue (blue)

Consists of absorbent cotton enclosed in absorbent cotton gauze type 12 or absorbent cotton and viscose gauze type 2
Gamgee (Robinson Healthcare) tissue blue label

Gamgee Tissue (pink)

Consists of absorbent cotton enclosed in absorbent cotton gauze type 12 or absorbent cotton and viscose gauze type 2
Gamgee (Robinson Healthcare) tissue pink label DT

Gauze and tissue

Absorbent Cotton Gauze, BP 1988

Cotton fabric of plain weave, in rolls and as swabs (see below), usually Type 13 light, sterile
Absorbent (Robert Bailey & Son Plc) cotton BP 1988
Alvita (Alliance Healthcare (Distribution) Ltd) absorbent cotton BP 1988
Clini (CliniSupplies Ltd) absorbent cotton BP 1988
Vernaid (Synergy Health (UK) Ltd) absorbent cotton BP 1988

Absorbent Cotton and Viscose Ribbon Gauze, BP 1988

Woven fabric in ribbon form with fast selvedge edges, warp threads of cotton, weft threads of viscose or combined cotton and viscose yarn, sterile
Vernaid Fast Edge ribbon gauze sterile (Synergy Health (UK) Ltd) 1.25cm, 2.5cm

Lint

Absorbent Lint, BPC

Cotton cloth of plain weave with nap raised on one side from warp yarns
Absorbent (Robinson Healthcare) lint
Alvita (Alliance Healthcare (Distribution) Ltd) absorbent lint BPC
Clini (CliniSupplies Ltd) absorbent lint BPC

Pads

Drisorb

Absorbent Dressing Pads, Sterile
Drisorb (Synergy Health (UK) Ltd) dressing pad 10cm × 20cm= £0.17

PremierPad

Absorbent Dressing Pads, Sterile
PremierPad dressing pad (Shermond) 10cm × 20cm= £0.18, 20cm × 20cm= £0.25

XuPad

Absorbent Dressing Pads, Sterile
Xupad dressing pad (Richardson Healthcare Ltd) 10cm × 20cm= £0.17, 20cm × 20cm= £0.28, 20cm × 40cm= £0.40

Wound drainage pouches

Wound drainage pouches can be used in the management of wounds and fistulas with significant levels of exudate.

Biotrol Draina S

Wound drainage pouch
Biotrol Draina S wound drainage bag (B.Braun Medical Ltd) large (Transparent)= £99.10, medium (Transparent)= £80.58, mini (Transparent)= £80.82

Biotrol Draina S Vision

Wound drainage pouch
Draina S Vision (B.Braun Medical Ltd) 50 wound drainage bag= £104.98, 75 wound drainage bag= £110.90

Eakin Access window

For use with Eakin® pouches
Eakin (Pelican Healthcare Ltd) access window large= £39.19

Eakin Wound pouch, bung closure

Wound pouch, bung closure
Eakin wound drainage bag with bung closure (Pelican Healthcare Ltd) large= £106.37, medium= £78.37, small= £55.98, and access window for horizontal wounds, extra large= £106.37, for horizontal wounds, extra large= £95.17, for vertical incision wounds, extra large= £95.17, wounds, extra large= £95.17

Eakin Wound pouch, fold and tuck closure

Wound pouch, fold and tuck closure
Eakin wound drainage bag with fold and tuck closure (Pelican Healthcare Ltd) large= £95.17, medium= £72.78, small= £50.38, extra large= £83.97

Option Wound Manager

Wound drainage bag
Option wound manager bag (Oakmed Ltd) large= £166.06, medium= £139.33, small= £136.30, square= £145.38, extra small= £122.54

Option Wound Manager with access port

Wound drainage bag, with access port
Option wound manager bag with access port (Oakmed Ltd) large= £177.51, medium= £145.38, small= £142.36, square= £151.44, extra small= £133.99

Option Wound Manager, cut to fit

Wound drainage bag, cut to fit
Option wound manager bag (Oakmed Ltd) large= £87.30, medium= £83.35, small= £75.24

Welland Fistula bag

Wound drainage bag, cut-to-fit
Welland (Welland Medical Ltd) Fistula wound drainage bag= £85.20

Physical debridement pads

DebriSoft® is a pad that is used for the debridement of superficial wounds containing loose slough and debris, and for the removal of hyperkeratosis from the skin. DebriSoft® must be fully moistened with a wound cleansing solution before use and is not appropriate for use as a wound dressing.

DebriSoft Pad

Polyester fibres with bound edges and knitted outer surface coated with polyacrylate
Debrisoft (Lohmann & Rauscher) pad 10cm × 10cm= £6.69

Complex adjunct therapies

Topical negative pressure therapy

Accessories

Renasys

Soft port and connector
Renasys (Smith & Nephew Healthcare Ltd) Soft Port= £11.62, connector for use with soft port= £3.42

V.A.C.

Drape, gel for canister, Sensa T.R.A.C. Pad
SensaT.R.A.C. (KCI Medical Ltd) pad= £11.31
T.R.A.C.(KCI Medical Ltd) connector= £3.23
V.A.C. (KCI Medical Ltd) drape= £9.70, gel strips= £3.88

Venturi

Gel patches, adhesive, and connector

Venturi (Talley Group Ltd) adhesive gel patch= £15.16, connector= £15.16

WoundASSIST gel strip
WoundASSIST (Huntleigh Healthcare Ltd) TNP gel strip= £3.37

Vacuum assisted closure products
Exsu-Fast kit 1
Dressing Kit
Exsu-Fast (Synergy Health (UK) Ltd) dressing kit 1= £28.04

Exsu-Fast kit 2
Dressing Kit
Exsu-Fast (Synergy Health (UK) Ltd) dressing kit 2= £35.83

Exsu-Fast kit 3
Dressing Kit
Exsu-Fast (Synergy Health (UK) Ltd) dressing kit 3= £35.83

Exsu-Fast kit 4
Dressing Kit
Exsu-Fast (Synergy Health (UK) Ltd) dressing kit 4= £28.04

V.A.C GranuFoam
Polyurethane foam dressing (with adhesive drapes and pad connector); with or without silver
V.A.C. GranuFoam (KCI Medical Ltd) Bridge dressing kit= £33.09, Silver with SensaT.R.A.C dressing kit medium= £39.28, small= £33.86, dressing kit large= £32.73, medium= £28.22, small= £23.70

V.A.C Simplace
Spiral-cut polyurethane foam dressings, vapour-permeable adhesive film dressings (with adhesive drapes and pad connector)
V.A.C. Simplace EX dressing kit (KCI Medical Ltd) medium= £31.58, small= £27.47

V.A.C WhiteFoam
Polyvinyl alcohol foam dressing or dressing kit
V.A.C. WhiteFoam dressing (KCI Medical Ltd) large= £17.60, small= £10.99, kit large= £34.64, small= £26.76

Venturi
Wound sealing kit, flat drain; with or without channel drain
Venturi wound sealing kit with flat drain (Talley Group Ltd) large= £17.69, standard= £15.16

WoundASSIST
Wound pack and channel drain
WoundASSIST TNP dressing pack (Huntleigh Healthcare Ltd) medium/large= £23.85, small/medium= £20.81, channel drain medium/large= £23.85, small/medium= £20.81, extra large= £34.05

Wound drainage collection devices
ActiV.A.C.
Canister with gel
ActiV.A.C (KCI Medical Ltd) canister with gel= £29.35

S-Canister
Canister kit
S-Canister (Smith & Nephew Healthcare Ltd) kit= £19.00

V.A.C Freedom
Canister with gel
V.A.C.(KCI Medical Ltd) Freedom Canister with gel= £29.80

Venturi
Canister kit with solidifier
Venturi (Talley Group Ltd) Compact canister kit= £12.64, canister kit= £12.64

WoundASSIST wound pack
Canister
WoundASSIST (Huntleigh Healthcare Ltd) TNP canister= £20.30

Wound care accessories

Dressing packs
The role of dressing packs is very limited. They are used to provide a clean or sterile working surface; some packs shown below include cotton wool balls, which are not recommended for use on wounds.

Multiple Pack Dressing No. 1
Contains absorbent cotton, absorbent cotton gauze type 13 light (sterile), open-wove bandages (banded)
Vernaid (Synergy Health (UK) Ltd) multiple pack dressing

Non-drug tariff specification sterile dressing packs
Dressit
Vitrex gloves, large apron, disposable bag, paper towel, softswabs, adsorbent pad, sterile field
Dressit sterile dressing pack (Richardson Healthcare Ltd) with medium/large gloves= £0.60, small/medium gloves= £0.60

Nurse It
Contains latex-free, powder-free nitrile gloves, sterile laminated paper sheet, large apron, non-woven swabs, paper towel, disposable bag, compartmented tray, disposable forceps, paper measuring tape
Nurse It sterile dressing pack (Medicareplus International Ltd) with medium/large gloves= £0.55, small/medium gloves= £0.55

Polyfield Nitrile Patient Pack
Contains powder-free nitrile gloves, laminate sheet, non-woven swabs, towel, polythene disposable bag, apron
Polyfield Nitrile Patient Pack (Shermond) with large gloves= £0.52, medium gloves= £0.52, small gloves= £0.52

Sterile Dressing Pack with Non-Woven Pads
Vernaid
(Drug Tariff specification 35). Contains non-woven fabric covered dressing pad, non-woven fabric swabs, absorbent cotton wool balls, absorbent paper towel, water repellent inner wrapper
Vernaid (Synergy Health (UK) Ltd) sterile dressing pack with non-woven pads

Sterile dressing packs
Vernaid
(Drug Tariff specification 10). Contains gauze and cotton tissue pad, gauze swabs, absorbent cotton wool balls, absorbent paper towel, water repellent inner wrapper
Vernaid (Synergy Health (UK) Ltd) sterile dressing pack

Woven and fabric swabs
Gauze Swab, PB 1988
Consists of absorbent cotton gauze type 13 light or absorbent cotton and viscose gauze type 1 folded into squares or rectangles of 8-ply with no cut edges exposed, sterile or non-sterile
Alvita gauze swab 8ply (Alliance Healthcare (Distribution) Ltd) non-sterile 10cm × 10cm, sterile 7.5cm × 7.5cm
CS (CliniSupplies Ltd) gauze swab 8ply non-sterile 10cm × 10cm
Clini gauze swab 8ply (CliniSupplies Ltd) non-sterile 10cm × 10cm, sterile 7.5cm × 7.5cm
Gauze (Robert Bailey & Son Plc) swab 8ply non-sterile 10cm × 10cm
MeCoBo gauze swab 8ply (MeCoBo Ltd) non-sterile 10cm × 10cm, sterile 7.5cm × 7.5cm
Propax gauze (BSN medical Ltd) swab 8ply sterile 7.5cm × 7.5cm
Sovereign (Waymade Healthcare Plc) gauze swab 8ply sterile 7.5cm × 7.5cm
Steraid (Robert Bailey & Son Plc) gauze swab 8ply sterile 7.5cm × 7.5cm
Vernaid gauze swab 8ply (Synergy Health (UK) Ltd) non-sterile 10cm × 10cm, sterile 7.5cm × 7.5cm

Non-woven Fabric Swab
(Drug Tariff specification 28). Consists of non-woven fabric folded 4-ply; alternative to gauze swabs, type 13 light, sterile or non-sterile
CS (CliniSupplies Ltd) non-woven fabric swab 4ply non-sterile 10cm × 10cm
Clini non-woven fabric swab 4ply (CliniSupplies Ltd) non-sterile 10cm × 10cm, sterile 7.5cm × 7.5cm
CliniMed (CliniMed Ltd) non-woven fabric swab 4ply non-sterile 10cm × 10cm
MeCoBo (MeCoBo Ltd) non-woven fabric swab 4ply non-sterile 10cm × 10cm
Multisorb (BSN medical Ltd) non-woven fabric swab 4ply sterile 7.5cm × 7.5cm

Sofsorb non-woven fabric swab 4ply (Synergy Health (UK) Ltd) non-sterile 10cm × 10cm, sterile 7.5cm × 7.5cm
Softswab non-woven fabric swab 4ply (Richardson Healthcare Ltd) non-sterile 10cm × 10cm, sterile 7.5cm × 7.5cm
Topper (Systagenix Wound Management Ltd) 8 non-woven fabric swab 4ply non-sterile 10cm × 10cm

Filmated non-woven Fabric Swab
Regal
(Drug Tariff specification 29). Film of viscose fibres enclosed within non-woven viscose fabric folded 8-ply, non-sterile
Regal (Systagenix Wound Management Ltd) filmated swab 8ply 10cm × 10cm

Surgical adhesive tapes

Adhesive tapes are useful for retaining dressings on joints or awkward body parts. These tapes, particularly those containing rubber, can cause irritant and allergic reactions in susceptible patients; synthetic adhesives have been developed to overcome this problem, but they, too, may sometimes be associated with reactions. Synthetic adhesive, or silicon adhesive, tapes can be used for patients with skin reactions to plasters and strapping containing rubber, or undergoing prolonged treatment.

Adhesive tapes that are occlusive may cause skin maceration. Care is needed not to apply these tapes under tension, to avoid creating a tourniquet effect. If applied over joints they need to be orientated so that the area of maximum extensibility of the fabric is in the direction of movement of the limb.

Occlusive adhesive tapes
Blenderm
(Impermeable Plastic Adhesive Tape, BP 1988). Extensible water-impermeable plastic film spread with a polymericadhesive mass
Blenderm tape (3M Health Care Ltd) 2.5cm= £1.80, 5cm= £3.43

Sleek
(Impermeable Plastic Adhesive Tape, BP 1988). Extensible water-impermeable plastic film spread with an adhesive mass
Leukoplast Sleek tape (BSN medical Ltd) 2.5cm, 5cm, 7.5cm

Permeable adhesive tapes
3m Kind Removal Silicone Tape
Soft silicone, water-resistant, knitted fabric, polyurethane film adhesive tape
3M Micropore Silicone tape (3M Health Care Ltd) 2.5cm= £3.65, 5cm= £6.60

Chemifix
(Permeable, Apertured Non-Woven Synthetic Adhesive Tape, BP 1988). Non-woven fabric with a polyacrylate adhesive
Chemifix tape (Medicareplus International Ltd) 10cm= £2.10, 2.5cm= £0.90, 5cm= £1.40

Chemipore
(Permeable Non-Woven Synthetic Adhesive Tape, BP 1988). Backing of paper-based or non-woven textile material spread with a polymeric adhesive mass
Chemipore tape (Medicareplus International Ltd) 1.25cm= £0.27, 2.5cm= £0.70, 5cm= £0.95

Clinipore
(Permeable Non-Woven Synthetic Adhesive Tape, BP 1988). Backing of paper-based or non-woven textile material spread with a polymeric adhesive mass
Clinipore tape (CliniSupplies Ltd) 1.25cm= £0.36, 2.5cm= £0.74, 5cm= £1.01

Elastoplast
(Elastic Adhesive Tape, BP 1988). Woven fabric, elastic in warp (crepe-twisted cotton threads), weft of cotton and/or viscose threads, spread with adhesive mass containing zinc oxide
Tensoplast (BSN medical Ltd) elastic adhesive tape 2.5cm

Hypafix
(Permeable, Apertured Non-Woven Synthetic Adhesive Tape, BP 1988). Non-woven fabric with a polyacrylate adhesive
Hypafix tape (BSN medical Ltd) 10cm= £4.80, 15cm= £7.11, 2.5cm= £1.73, 20cm= £9.43, 30cm= £13.63, 5cm= £2.75

Insil
Soft silicone, water-resistant, knitted fabric, polyurethane film adhesive tape
Insil tape (Insight Medical Products Ltd) 2cm= £5.77, 4cm= £5.77

Leukofix
(Permeable Non-Woven Synthetic Adhesive Tape, BP 1988). Backing of paper-based or non-woven textile material spread with a polymeric adhesive mass
Leukofix tape (BSN medical Ltd) 1.25cm= £0.57, 2.5cm= £0.92, 5cm= £1.61

Leukopor
(Permeable Non-Woven Synthetic Adhesive Tape, BP 1988). Backing of paper-based or non-woven textile material spread with a polymeric adhesive mass
Leukopor tape (BSN medical Ltd) 1.25cm= £0.51, 2.5cm= £0.79, 5cm= £1.39

Mediplast
(Permeable Non-Woven Synthetic Adhesive Tape, BP 1988). Backing of paper-based or non-woven textile material spread with a polymeric adhesive mass
Mediplast tape (Neomedic Ltd) 1.25cm= £0.30, 2.5cm= £0.50

Mediplast
Fabric, plain weave, warp and weft of cotton and /or viscose, spread with an adhesive containing zinc oxide
Mediplast Zinc Oxide plaster (Neomedic Ltd) 1.25cm= £0.82, 2.5cm= £1.19, 5cm= £1.99, 7.5cm= £2.99

Mefix
(Permeable, Apertured Non-Woven Synthetic Adhesive Tape, BP 1988). Non-woven fabric with a polyacrylate adhesive
Mefix tape (Molnlycke Health Care Ltd) 10cm= £3.00, 15cm= £4.08, 2.5cm= £1.06, 20cm= £5.23, 30cm= £7.50, 5cm= £1.87

Mepitac
Soft silicone, water-resistant, knitted fabric, polyurethane film adhesive tape
Mepitac tape (Molnlycke Health Care Ltd) 2cm= £7.19, 4cm= £7.19

Micropore
(Permeable Non-Woven Synthetic Adhesive Tape, BP 1988). Backing of paper-based or non-woven textile material spread with a polymeric adhesive mass
Micropore tape (3M Health Care Ltd) 1.25cm= £0.63, 2.5cm= £0.93, 5cm= £1.65

Omnifix
(Permeable, Apertured Non-Woven Synthetic Adhesive Tape, BP 1988). Non-woven fabric with a polyacrylate adhesive
Omnifix tape (Paul Hartmann Ltd) 10cm= £4.23, 15cm= £6.24, 5cm= £2.51

OpSite Flexifix Gentle
Soft silicone, water-resistant, knitted fabric, polyurethane film adhesive tape
OpSite Flexifix Gentle tape (Smith & Nephew Healthcare Ltd) 2.5cm= £10.71, 5cm= £20.09

Primafix
(Permeable, Apertured Non-Woven Synthetic Adhesive Tape, BP 1988). Non-woven fabric with a polyacrylate adhesive
Primafix tape (Smith & Nephew Healthcare Ltd) 10cm= £2.46, 15cm= £3.63, 20cm= £4.47, 5cm= £1.67

Scanpor
(Permeable Non-Woven Synthetic Adhesive Tape, BP 1988). Backing of paper-based or non-woven textile material spread with a polymeric adhesive mass
Scanpor tape (Bio-Diagnostics Ltd) 1.25cm= £0.57, 2.5cm= £0.93, 5cm= £1.78, 7.5cm= £2.61

Siltape

Soft silicone, water-resistant, knitted fabric, polyurethane film adhesive tape

Siltape (Advancis Medical) 2cm= £5.79, 4cm= £5.79

Strappal

Fabric, plain weave, warp and weft of cotton and /or viscose, spread with an adhesive containing zinc oxide

Strappal adhesive tape (BSN medical Ltd) 2.5cm= £1.44, 5cm= £2.43, 7.5cm= £3.66

Transpore

Permeable Non-Woven Synthetic Adhesive Tape, BP 1988). Backing of paper-based or non-woven textile material spread with a polymeric adhesive mass

Transpore tape (3M Health Care Ltd) 2.5cm= £0.86, 5cm= £1.51

Zinc Oxide Adhesive Tape, BP 1988

Fabric, plain weave, warp and weft of cotton and /or viscose, spread with an adhesive containing zinc oxide

Fast Aid zinc oxide adhesive tape (Robinson Healthcare) 1.25cm, 2.5cm, 5cm, 7.5cm

Skin closure dressings

Skin closure strips are used as an alternative to sutures for minor cuts and lacerations. Skin tissue adhesive can be used for closure of minor skin wounds and for additional suture support.

Skin closure strips, sterile

Leukostrip

Drug Tariff specifies that these are specifically for personal administration by the prescriber

Leukostrip (Smith & Nephew Healthcare Ltd) skin closure strips 6.4mm × 76mm= £6.64

Omnistrip

Drug Tariff specifies that these are specifically for personal administration by the prescriber

Omnistrip (Paul Hartmann Ltd) skin closure strips sterile 6mm × 76mm= £25.21

Steri-strip

Drug Tariff specifies that these are specifically for personal administration by the prescriber

Steri-strip (3M Health Care Ltd) skin closure strips 6mm × 75mm= £8.93

Bandages

Non-extensible bandages

Skin closure strips are used as an alternative to sutures for minor cuts and lacerations. Skin tissue adhesive can be used for closure of minor skin wounds and for additional suture support.

Open-wove Bandage, Type 1 BP 1988

Cotton cloth, plain weave, warp of cotton, weft of cotton, viscose, or combination, one continuous length

Clini open wove bandage Type 1 BP 1988 (CliniSupplies Ltd) 10cm × 5m, 2.5cm × 5m, 5cm × 5m, 7.5cm × 5m

Vernaid white open wove bandage (Synergy Health (UK) Ltd) 10cm × 5m, 2.5cm × 5m, 5cm × 5m, 7.5cm × 5m

White open wove bandage (Robert Bailey & Son Plc) 10cm × 5m, 2.5cm × 5m, 5cm × 5m, 7.5cm × 5m

Triangular Calico Bandage, BP 1980

Unbleached calico right-angled triangle

Clini (CliniSupplies Ltd) triangular calico bandage BP 1980 90cm × 127cm

Triangular (BSN medical Ltd) calico bandage 90cm × 127cm

Light-weight conforming bandages

Lightweight conforming bandages are used for dressing retention, with the aim of keeping the dressing close to the wound without inhibiting movement or restricting blood flow. The elasticity of conforming-stretch bandages (also termed contour bandages) is greater than that of cotton conforming bandages.

Acti-Wrap

Fabric, plain weave, warp of polyamide filament, weft of cotton or viscose, fast edges, one continuous length, 4 m stretched (all)

Acti-Wrap (cohesive/latex free) bandage (L&R Medical UK Ltd) 10cm × 4m= £0.85, 6cm × 4m= £0.49, 8cm × 4m= £0.72

Cotton Conforming Bandage, BP 1988

Cotton fabric, plain weave, treated to impart some elasticity to warp and weft

Easifix

Fabric, plain weave, warp of polyamide filament, weft of cotton or viscose, fast edges, one continuous length, 4 m stretched (all)

Easifix bandage (BSN medical Ltd) 10cm × 4m= £0.52, 15cm × 4m= £0.89, 5cm × 4m= £0.36, 7.5cm × 4m= £0.44

Easifix K

Fabric, knitted warp of polyamide filament, weft of cotton or viscose, fast edges, one continuous length. 4 m stretched

Easifix K bandage (BSN medical Ltd) 10cm × 4m= £0.19, 15cm × 4m= £0.33, 2.5cm × 4m= £0.10, 5cm × 4m= £0.11, 7.5cm × 4m= £0.17

Hospiform

Fabric, plain weave, warp of polyamide, weft of viscose

Hospiform bandage (Paul Hartmann Ltd) 10cm × 4m= £0.20, 12cm × 4m= £0.25, 6cm × 4m= £0.14, 8cm × 4m= £0.18

K-Band

Fabric, knitted warp of polyamide filament, weft of cotton or viscose, fast edges, one continuous length. 4 m stretched

K-Band bandage (Urgo Ltd) 10cm × 4m= £0.29, 15cm × 4m= £0.52, 5cm × 4m= £0.21, 7cm × 4m= £0.27

Knit Fix

Fabric, knitted warp of polyamide filament, weft of cotton or viscose, fast edges, one continuous length. 4 m stretched

Knit Fix bandage (Robert Bailey & Son Plc) 10cm × 4m= £0.17, 15cm × 4m= £0.33, 5cm × 4m= £0.12, 7cm × 4m= £0.17

Knit-Band

Fabric, knitted warp of polyamide filament, weft of cotton or viscose, fast edges, one continuous length. 4 m stretched

Knit-Band bandage (CliniSupplies Ltd) 10cm × 4m= £0.18, 15cm × 4m= £0.31, 5cm × 4m= £0.10, 7cm × 4m= £0.16

Kontour

Fabric, plain weave, warp of polyamide filament, weft of cotton or viscose, fast edges, one continuous length, 4 m stretched (all)

Kontour bandage (Easigrip Ltd) 10cm × 4m= £0.40, 15cm × 4m= £0.66, 5cm × 4m= £0.28, 7.5cm × 4m= £0.35

Mollelast

Fabric, plain weave, warp of polyamide filament, weft of cotton or viscose, fast edges, one continuous length, 4 m stretched (all)

Mollelast (Lohmann & Rauscher) bandage 4cm × 4m= £0.31

Peha-haft

Polyamide and Cellulose Contour Bandage, cohesive, latex-free

Peha-haft bandage (Paul Hartmann Ltd) 10cm × 4m= £0.80, 12cm × 4m= £0.94, 2.5cm × 4m= £0.76, 4cm × 4m= £0.49, 6cm × 4m= £0.58, 8cm × 4m= £0.69

PremierBand

Polyamide and Cellulose Contour Bandage

PremierBand bandage (Shermond) 10cm × 4m= £0.17, 15cm × 4m= £0.25, 5cm × 4m= £0.12, 7.5cm × 4m= £0.14

Slinky

Fabric, plain weave, warp of polyamide filament, weft of cotton or viscose, fast edges, one continuous length, 4 m stretched (all)

Slinky bandage (Molnlycke Health Care Ltd) 10cm × 4m= £0.72, 15cm × 4m= £1.05, 7.5cm × 4m= £0.60

A4

Wound management | Appendix 4

Stayform

Fabric, plain weave, warp of polyamide filament, weft of cotton or viscose, fast edges, one continuous length, 4 m stretched (all)

Stayform bandage (Robinson Healthcare) 10cm × 4m= £0.40, 15cm × 4m= £0.69, 5cm × 4m= £0.29, 7.5cm × 4m= £0.36

Tubular bandages and garments

Tubular bandages are available in different forms, according to the function required of them. Some are used under orthopaedic casts and some are suitable for protecting areas to which creams or ointments (other than those containing potent corticosteroids) have been applied. The conformability of the elasticated versions makes them particularly suitable for retaining dressings on difficult parts of the body or for soft tissue injury, but their use as the only means of applying pressure to an oedematous limb or to a varicose ulcer is not appropriate, since the pressure they exert is inadequate. Compression hosiery reduces the recurrence of venous leg ulcers and should be considered for use after wound healing. Silk clothing is available as an alternative to elasticated viscose stockinette garments, for use in the management of severe eczema and allergic skin conditions.

Elasticated Surgical Tubular Stockinette, Foam padded is used for relief of pressure and elimination of friction in relevant area; porosity of foam lining allows normal water loss from skin surface.

For *Elasticated Tubular Bandage, BP* 1993, where no size stated by the prescriber, the 50 cm length should be supplied and width endorsed.

Non-elasticated Cotton Stockinette, Bleached, BP 1988 1m lengths is used as basis (with wadding) for Plaster of Paris bandages etc.; 6 m length, compression bandage.

For *Non-elasticated Ribbed Cotton and Viscose Surgical Tubular Stockinette, BP* 1988, the Drug Tariff specifies various combinations of sizes to provide sufficient material for part or full body coverage. It is used as protective dressings with tar-based and other steroid ointments.

Elasticated

Acti-Fast

(Drug Tariff specification 46). Lightweight plain-knitted elasticated tubular bandage

Acti-Fast 2-way stretch stockinette (L&R Medical UK Ltd) 10.75cm= £5.80, 17.5cm= £1.87, 20cm= £3.26, 3.5cm= £0.57, 5cm= £0.59, 7.5cm= £0.78

Clinifast

(Drug Tariff specification 46). Lightweight plain-knitted elasticated tubular bandage; various colours and sizes

CliniFast stockinette (CliniSupplies Ltd) 10.75cm= £6.11, 17.5cm= £1.85, 3.5cm= £0.57, 5cm= £0.59, 7.5cm= £0.78, clava 5-14 years= £6.82, 6 months-5 years= £5.91, cycle shorts large adult= £16.55, medium adult= £14.51, small adult= £12.73, gloves large adult= £5.08, child/small adult= £5.08, gloves medium adult= £5.08, child= £5.08, gloves small child= £5.08, leggings (Blue, Pink, White) 11-14 years= £12.01, 2-5 years= £9.60, 5-8 years= £10.81, 8-11 years= £12.01, mittens 2-8 years= £3.00, 8-14 years= £3.00, up to 24 months= £3.00, socks 8-14 years= £3.02, up to 8 years= £3.00, tights (Blue, Pink, White) 6-24 months= £7.21, vest long sleeve (Blue, Pink, White) 11-14 years= £12.01, 2-5 years= £9.60, 5-8 years= £10.81, 6-24 months= £7.21, 8-11 years= £12.01, vest short sleeve large adult= £16.55, medium adult= £14.51, small adult= £12.73

Comfifast

(Drug Tariff specification 46). Lightweight plain-knitted elasticated tubular bandage; various colours and sizes

Comfifast stockinette (Vernacare Ltd) 10.75cm= £6.04, 17.5cm= £1.83, 3.5cm= £0.56, 5cm= £0.58, 7.5cm= £0.77

Comfifast Easywrap

(Drug Tariff specification 46). Lightweight plain-knitted elasticated tubular bandage; various colours and sizes

Comfifast Easywrap stockinette (Vernacare Ltd) clava 5-14 years= £6.75, 6 months-5 years= £5.85, leggings 11-14 years= £11.88, 2-5 years= £9.50, 5-8 years= £10.69, 8-11 years= £11.88, mittens 2-8 years= £2.97, 8-14 years= £2.97, up to 24 months= £2.97, socks 8-14 years= £2.97, up to 8 years= £2.97, tights 6-24 months= £7.13, vest long sleeve 11-14 years= £11.88, 2-5 years= £9.50, 5-8 years= £10.69, 6-24 months= £7.13, 8-11years= £11.88

Comfifast Multistretch

(Drug Tariff specification 46). Lightweight plain-knitted elasticated tubular bandage; various colours and sizes

Comfifast MultiStretch 2-way stretch stockinette (Vernacare Ltd) 10.75cm= £6.45, 17.5cm= £2.49, 3.5cm= £0.61, 5cm= £0.63, 7.5cm= £0.83

Coverflex

(Drug Tariff specification 46). Lightweight plain-knitted elasticated tubular bandage; various colours and sizes

Easifast

(Drug Tariff specification 46). Lightweight plain-knitted elasticated tubular bandage; various colours and sizes

Easifast stockinette (Easigrip Ltd) 10.75cm= £7.23, 17.5cm= £1.91, 3.5cm= £0.65, 5cm= £0.69, 7.5cm= £0.94

Elasticated Surgical Tubular Stockinette, Foam padded or Tupipad

(Drug Tariff specification 25). Fabric as for Elasticated Tubular Bandage with polyurethane foam lining.

Elasticated Tubular Bandage, BP 1993

(Drug Tariff specification 25). Fabric as for Elasticated Tubular Bandage with polyurethane foam lining; lengths 50 cm and 1 m

CLINIgrip bandage (CliniSupplies Ltd) 10cm size F= £0.75, 12cm size G= £0.78, 6.25cm size B= £0.62, 6.75cm size C= £0.66, 7.5cm size D= £0.67, 8.75cm size E= £0.75

Comfigrip bandage (Vernacare Ltd) 10cm size F= £0.74, 12cm size G= £0.77, 6.25cm size B= £0.61, 6.75cm size C= £0.65, 7.5cm size D= £0.66, 8.75cm size E= £0.74

Eesiban ESTS bandage (E Sallis Ltd) 10cm size F= £1.80, 12cm size G= £2.09, 6.25cm size B= £0.87, 6.75cm size C= £0.95, 7.5cm size D= £0.95, 8.75cm size E= £1.80

Tubigrip bandage (Molnlycke Health Care Ltd) 10cm size F= £2.10, 12cm size G= £2.43, 6.25cm size B= £1.84, 6.75cm size C= £1.94, 7.5cm size D= £1.94, 8.75cm size E= £2.10

easiGRIP bandage (Easigrip Ltd) 10cm size F= £0.75, 12cm size G= £0.78, 6.25cm size B= £0.62, 6.75cm size C= £0.66, 7.5cm size D= £0.68, 8.75cm size E= £0.75

Skinnies

(Drug Tariff specification 46). Lightweight plain-knitted elasticated tubular bandage; various colours and sizes

Skinnies Viscose stockinette (Dermacea Ltd) body suit (Blue, Ecru, Pink) 3-6 months= £16.97, 6-12 months= £19.11, up to 3 months= £16.97, clava (Blue, Ecru, Pink) 5-14 years= £8.11, 6 months-5 years= £7.07, gloves large (Beige, Blue, Ecru, Grey, Pink) adult= £5.60, child= £5.60, gloves medium (Beige, Blue, Ecru, Grey, Pink) adult= £5.60, child= £5.60, gloves small (Blue, Ecru, Grey, Pink) adult= £5.55, child= £5.55, knee socks extra (Black, Natural, White) large adult 11+= £14.62, knee socks large (Black, Natural, White) adult 8-11= £14.62, child 2-4= £14.62, knee socks medium (Black, Natural, White) adult 6-8= £14.62, child 1-2= £14.62, knee socks small (Black, Natural, White) adult 4-6= £14.62, child 0-1= £14.62, leggings (Beige, Blue, Ecru, Grey, Pink) 11-14 years= £18.04, 2-5 years= £14.41, 5-8 years= £16.28, 6-24 months= £10.99, 8-11 years= £18.04, large adult= £26.36, medium adult= £24.34, small adult= £22.31, mittens (Blue, Ecru, Pink) 2-8 years= £4.06, 8-14 years= £4.06, up to 24 months= £4.06, socks (Blue, Ecru, Pink) 6 months-8 years= £4.48, 8-14 years= £4.48, vest long sleeve (Beige, Blue, Ecru, Grey, Pink) 11-14 years= £18.04, 2-5 years= £14.41, 5-8 years= £16.28, 6-24 months= £10.99, 8-11 years= £18.04, large adult= £26.36, medium adult= £24.34, small adult= £22.31, vest short sleeve (White) 11-14 years= £17.93, 2-5 years= £14.30, 5-8 years= £16.12, 6-24 months= £10.89, 8-11 years= £17.93, large adult= £26.26, medium adult= £24.23, small adult= £22.20, vest sleeveless (White) 11-14 years= £17.93, 2-5 years= £14.30, 5-8 years= £16.17, 6-24 months= £10.89, 8-11 years= £17.93, large adult= £26.26, medium adult= £24.23, small adult= £22.20

ubifast 2-way stretch

Drug Tariff specification 46). Lightweight plain-knitted elasticated tubular bandage; various colours and sizes

ubifast 2-way stretch stockinette (Molnlycke Health Care Ltd) 0.75cm= £5.74, 20cm= £3.20, 3.5cm= £0.62, 5cm= £0.64, 7.5cm= £0.77, gloves extra small child= £5.88, medium/large adult= £5.88, small child= £5.88, small/medium adult, medium/large child= £5.88, leggings 2-5 years= £15.63, 5-8 years= £17.58, 8-11 years= £19.53, socks (one size)= £4.95, tights 6-24 months= £11.72, vest long sleeve 11-14 years= £19.53, 2-5 years= £15.63, 5-8 years= £17.58, 6-24 months= £11.72, 8-11 years= £19.53

Non-elasticated

Cotton Stockinette, Bleached, BP 1988

Knitted fabric, cotton yarn, tubular length, 1m

Cotton stockinette bleached heavyweight (E Sallis Ltd) 10cm, 2.5cm, 5cm, 7.5cm

Silk Clothing

DermaSilk

Knitted silk fabric, hypoallergenic, sericin-free

DermaSilk (Espere Healthcare Ltd) medium/large= £42.37, medium-large= £31.53, body suit 0-3 months= £38.81, 12-18 months= £41.12, 18-24 months= £42.16, 24-36 months= £42.24, 3-6 months= £38.90, 6-9 months= £40.01, 9-12 months= £41.04, boxer shorts male adult extra large/XX large= £42.37, small/small= £42.37, briefs female adult extra large-XX large= £31.53, small-small= £31.53, facial mask adult= £21.29, child= £16.69, infant= £16.69, teen= £21.29, gloves extra large adult= £21.05, gloves large adult= £21.09, gloves medium adult= £21.09, child= £15.02, gloves small adult= £21.09, child= £15.02, leggings 9-12 months= £27.71, leggings 12-18 months= £29.99, leggings 18-24 months= £31.05, leggings 3-4 years= £32.22, leggings 3-6 months= £27.77, leggings 6-9 months= £28.88, leggings 9-12 months= £29.93, leggings adult female XX large= £79.71, extra large= £79.71, large= £79.71, medium= £79.71, small= £79.71, leggings adult male XX large= £79.71, extra large= £79.71, large= £79.71, medium= £79.71, small= £79.71, pyjamas 10-12 years= £83.41, 3-4 years= £72.28, 5-6 years= £76.74, 7-8 years= £80.07, roll neck shirt 10-12 years= £55.40, 3-4 years= £47.93, 5-6 years= £51.13, 7-8 years= £53.26, round neck shirt adult female XX large= £78.78, extra large= £78.78, large= £78.78, medium= £78.78, small= £78.78, round neck shirt adult male XX large= £78.78, extra large= £78.78, large= £78.78, medium= £78.78, small= £78.78, tubular sleeves= £34.27, sleeves= £27.77, undersocks adult 11-13= £18.75, 5 1/2 - 6 1/2= £18.75, 7 - 8 1/2= £18.75, 9 - 10 1/2= £18.75, undersocks child 2-5= £18.75, 3-8= £18.75, 9-1= £18.75, unisex roll neck shirt adult XX large= £78.78, extra large= £78.78, large= £78.78, medium= £78.78, small= £78.78

DreamSkin

Knitted silk fabric, hypoallergenic, sericin-free, with methyacrylate copolymer and zinc-based antibacterial

DreamSkin (DreamSkin Health Ltd) baby leggings with foldaway feet 0-3 months= £25.92, 12-18 months= £28.89, 18-24 months= £29.43, 3-4 years= £31.04, 3-6 months= £26.44, 6-9 months= £27.82, 9-12 months= £28.36, body suit 0-3 months= £36.52, 12-18 months= £39.61, 18-24 months= £40.15, 3-4 years= £41.76, 3-6 months= £37.04, 6-9 months= £38.54, 9-12 months= £39.10, boxer shorts 11-12 years= £22.02, boxer shorts 3-4 years= £22.02, boxer shorts 5-6 years= £22.02, boxer shorts 7-8 years= £22.02, boxer shorts 9-10 years= £22.02, boxer shorts male adult XX large= £34.63, extra large= £34.63, large= £34.63, medium= £34.63, small= £34.63, briefs 11-12 years= £22.02, briefs 3-4 years= £22.02, briefs 5-6 years= £22.02, briefs 7-8 years= £22.02, briefs 9-10 years= £22.02, briefs female adult XX large= £32.53, extra large= £32.53, large= £32.53, medium= £32.53, small= £32.53, eye mask= £10.46, footless leggings 11-12 years= £34.15, footless leggings 3-4 years= £31.04, footless leggings 5-6 years= £32.57, footless leggings 7-8 years= £33.10, footless leggings 9-10 years= £33.62, footless leggings adult XX large= £78.55, extra large= £78.55, large= £78.55, medium= £78.55, small= £78.55, footless leggings adult male XX large= £78.55, extra large= £78.55, large= £78.55, medium= £78.55, small= £78.55, gloves extra large adult= £20.62, gloves large adult= £20.62, gloves medium adult= £20.62, child= £14.69, gloves

small adult= £20.62, child= £14.69, head mask child= £16.08, infant= £16.08, teenager= £20.98, heel-less undersocks= £24.30, liner socks adult female 4 - 5 1/2= £18.48, 6 - 8 1/2= £18.48, liner socks adult male 6 - 8 1/2= £18.48, 9 - 11= £18.48, liner socks child 12 1/2 - 3 1/2= £18.48, 3 - 5 1/2= £18.48, 4 - 5 1/2= £18.48, 6 - 8 1/2= £18.48, 9 - 12= £18.48, polo neck shirt 11-12 years= £54.59, polo neck shirt 3-4 years= £47.23, polo neck shirt 5-6 years= £50.39, polo neck shirt 7-8 years= £52.49, polo neck shirt 9-10 years= £53.54, polo neck shirt adult female XX large= £77.64, extra large= £77.64, large= £77.64, medium= £77.64, small= £77.64, polo neck shirt adult male XX large= £77.64, extra large= £77.64, large= £77.64, medium= £77.64, small= £77.64, pyjamas 11-12 years= £80.35, 3-4 years= £69.63, 5-6 years= £73.92, 7-8 years= £77.13, 9-10 years= £78.77, round neck shirt 3-4 years= £47.24, round neck shirt 5-6 years= £49.34, round neck shirt 7-8 years= £51.45, round neck shirt 9-10 years= £52.50, round neck shirt adult female XX large= £77.64, extra large= £77.64, large= £77.64, medium= £77.64, small= £77.64, round neck shirt adult male XX large= £77.64, extra large= £77.64, large= £77.64, medium= £77.64, small= £77.64, tubular sleeves= £33.77, sleeves= £27.15

Support bandages

Light support bandages, which include the various forms of crepe bandage, are used in the prevention of oedema; they are also used to provide support for mild sprains and joints but their effectiveness has not been proven for this purpose. Since they have limited extensibility, they are able to provide light support without exerting undue pressure. For a warning against injudicious compression see Compression bandages.

CliniLite

Knitted fabric, viscose and elastomer yarn. Type 2 (light support bandage)

CliniLite bandage (CliniSupplies Ltd) 10cm × 4.5m= £0.81, 15cm × 4.5m= £1.18, 5cm × 4.5m= £0.45, 7.5cm × 4.5m= £0.62

CliniPlus

Knitted fabric, viscose and elastomer yarn. Type 2 (light support bandage)

CliniPlus (CliniSupplies Ltd) bandage 10cm × 8.7m= £1.83

Cotton Crepe Bandage

Light support bandage, 4.5 m stretched (all)

Hospicrepe 239 bandage (Paul Hartmann Ltd) 10cm × 4.5m= £0.81, 15cm × 4.5m= £1.18, 5cm × 4.5m= £0.44, 7.5cm × 4.5m= £0.63

Cotton Crepe Bandage, BP 1988

Fabric, plain weave, warp of crepe-twisted cotton threads; weft of cotton and/or viscose threads; stretch bandage. 4.5 m stretched (both)

Elastocrepe bandage (BSN medical Ltd) 10cm × 4.5m, 7.5cm × 4.5m
Flexocrepe bandage (Robinson Healthcare) 10cm × 4.5m, 7.5cm × 4.5m
Sterocrepe bandage (Steroplast Healthcare Ltd) 10cm × 4.5m, 7.5cm × 4.5m

Cotton Suspensory Bandage

(Drug Tariff). Type 1: cotton net bag with draw tapes and webbing waistband; small, medium, and large (all)

Crepe Bandage, BP 1988

Fabric, plain weave, warp of wool threads and crepe-twisted cotton threads, weft of cotton threads; stretch bandage; 4.5 m stretched

Alvita crepe bandage (Alliance Healthcare (Distribution) Ltd) 10cm × 4.5m, 15cm × 4.5m, 5cm × 4.5m, 7.5cm × 4.5m
Clinicrepe bandage (CliniSupplies Ltd) 10cm × 4.5m, 15cm × 4.5m, 5cm × 4.5m, 7.5cm × 4.5m
Crepe bandage (Robert Bailey & Son Plc) 10cm × 4.5m, 15cm × 4.5m, 5cm × 4.5m, 7.5cm × 4.5m
Propax crepe bandage (BSN medical Ltd) 10cm × 4.5m, 15cm × 4.5m, 5cm × 4.5m, 7.5cm × 4.5m
Vernaid crepe bandage (Synergy Health (UK) Ltd) 10cm × 4.5m, 15cm × 4.5m, 5cm × 4.5m, 7.5cm × 4.5m

Elset

Knitted fabric, viscose and elastomer yarn. Type 2 (light support bandage)

Elset (Molnlycke Health Care Ltd) S bandage 15cm × 12m= £5.78, bandage 10cm × 6m= £2.69, 10cm × 8m= £3.45, 15cm × 6m= £2.89

Hospicrepe 233

Fabric, plain weave, warp of crepe-twisted cotton threads, weft of cotton threads; stretch bandage, lighter than cotton crepe, 4.5 m stretched (all)

Hospicrepe 233 bandage (Paul Hartmann Ltd) 10cm × 4.5m= £0.96, 15cm × 4.5m= £1.36, 5cm × 4.5m= £0.52, 7.5cm × 4.5m= £0.72

Hospilite

Fabric, cotton, polyamide, and elastane; light support bandage (Type 2), 4.5 m stretched (all)

Hospilite bandage (Paul Hartmann Ltd) 10cm × 4.5m= £0.64, 15cm × 4.5m= £0.94, 5cm × 4.5m= £0.38, 7.5cm × 4.5m= £0.53

K-Lite

Knitted fabric, viscose and elastomer yarn. Type 2 (light support bandage)

K-Lite (Urgo Ltd) Long bandage 10cm × 5.25m= £1.19, bandage 10cm × 4.5m= £1.04, 15cm × 4.5m= £1.51, 5cm × 4.5m= £0.57, 7cm × 4.5m= £0.80

K-Plus

Knitted fabric, viscose and elastomer yarn. Type 2 (light support bandage)

K-Plus (Urgo Ltd) Long bandage 10cm × 10.25m= £2.74, bandage 10cm × 8.7m= £2.37

Knit-Firm

Knitted fabric, viscose and elastomer yarn. Type 2 (light support bandage)

Knit-Firm bandage (Millpledge Healthcare) 10cm × 4.5m= £0.66, 15cm × 4.5m= £0.96, 5cm × 4.5m= £0.36, 7cm × 4.5m= £0.51

L3

Knitted fabric, viscose and elastomer yarn. Type 2 (light support bandage)

L3 (Smith & Nephew Healthcare Ltd) bandage 10cm × 8.6m= £2.31

Neosport

Fabric, cotton, polyamide, and elastane; light support bandage (Type 2), 4.5 m stretched (all)

Neosport bandage (Neomedic Ltd) 10cm × 4.5m= £0.91, 15cm × 4.5m= £1.12, 5cm × 4.5m= £0.54, 7.5cm × 4.5m= £0.73

PremierBand

Fabric, plain weave, warp of crepe-twisted cotton threads, weft of cotton threads; stretch bandage, lighter than cotton crepe, 4.5 m stretched (all)

PremierBand bandage (Shermond) 10cm × 4.5m= £0.79, 15cm × 4.5m= £1.18, 5cm × 4.5m= £0.45, 7.5cm × 4.5m= £0.63

Profore #2

Fabric, cotton, polyamide, and elastane; light support bandage (Type 2), 4.5 m stretched (all)

Profore #2 (Smith & Nephew Healthcare Ltd) bandage 10cm × 4.5m= £1.42, latex free bandage 10cm × 4.5m= £1.50

Profore #3

Knitted fabric, viscose and elastomer yarn. Type 2 (light support bandage)

Profore #3 (Smith & Nephew Healthcare Ltd) bandage 10cm × 8.7m= £4.13, latex free bandage 10cm × 8.7m= £4.49

Setocrepe

Fabric, cotton, polyamide, and elastane; light support bandage (Type 2), 4.5 m stretched (all)

Setocrepe (Molnlycke Health Care Ltd) bandage 10cm × 4.5m= £1.24

Soffcrepe

Fabric, cotton, polyamide, and elastane; light support bandage (Type 2), 4.5 m stretched (all)

Soffcrepe bandage (BSN medical Ltd) 10cm × 4.5m= £1.29, 15cm × 4.5m= £1.87, 5cm × 4.5m= £0.72, 7.5cm × 4.5m= £1.02

Adhesive bandages

Elastic adhesive bandages are used to provide compression in the treatment of varicose veins and for the support of injured joints; they should no longer be used for the support of fractured ribs and clavicles. They have also been used with zinc paste bandage in the treatment of venous ulcers, but they can cause skin reactions in susceptible patients and may not produce sufficient pressures for healing (significantly lower than those provided by other compression bandages).

Elastic Adhesive Bandage, BP 1993

Woven fabric, elastic in warp (crepe-twisted cotton threads), weft of cotton and/or viscose threads spread with adhesive mass containing zinc oxide. 4.5 m stretched

Tensoplast bandage (BSN medical Ltd) 10cm × 4.5m, 5cm × 4.5m, 7.5cm × 4.5m

Cohesive bandages

Cohesive bandages adhere to themselves, but not to the skin and are useful for providing support for sports use where ordinary stretch bandages might become displaced and adhesive bandages are inappropriate. Care is needed in their application, however, since the loss of ability for movement between turns of the bandage to equalise local areas of high tension carries the potential for creating a tourniquet effect. Cohesive bandages can be used to support sprained joints and as an outer layer for multi-layer compression bandaging; they should not be used if arterial disease is suspected.

Cohesive extensible bandages

Coban

Bandage

Coban (3M Health Care Ltd) self-adherent bandage 10cm × 6m= £2.98

K Press

Bandage

K Press bandage (Urgo Ltd) 10cm × 6.5m, 10cm × 7.5m, 12cm × 7.5m, 8cm × 7.5cm

Profore #4

Bandage

Profore #4 (Smith & Nephew Healthcare Ltd) bandage 10cm × 2.5m= £3.41, latex free bandage 10cm × 2.5m= £3.71

Ultra Fast

Bandage

Ultra (Robinson Healthcare) Fast cohesive bandage 10cm × 6.3m= £2.62

Compression bandages

High compression products are used to provide the high compression needed for the management of gross varices, post-thrombotic venous insufficiency, venous leg ulcers, and gross oedema in average-sized limbs. Their use calls for an expert knowledge of the elastic properties of the products and experience in the technique of providing careful graduated compression. Incorrect application can lead to uneven and inadequate pressures or to hazardous levels of pressure. In particular, injudicious use of compression in limbs with arterial disease has been reported to cause severe skin and tissue necrosis (in some instances calling for amputation). Doppler testing is required before treatment with compression. Oral pentoxifylline p. 249 can be used as adjunct therapy if a chronic venous leg ulcer does not respond to compression bandaging [unlicensed indication].

High compression bandages

High Compression Bandage

Cotton, viscose, nylon, and Lycra ® extensible bandage, 3 m (unstretched)

K-ThreeC (Urgo Ltd) bandage 10cm × 3m= £2.95
SurePress (ConvaTec Ltd) bandage 10cm × 3m= £3.80

PEC High Compression Bandages

Polyamide, elastane, and cotton compression (high) extensible bandage, 3.5 m unstretched

Setopress (Molnlycke Health Care Ltd) bandage 10cm × 3.5m= £3.66

VEC High Compression Bandages

Viscose, elastane, and cotton compression (high) extensible bandage, 3 m unstretched (both)

Tensopress bandage (BSN medical Ltd) 10cm × 3m= £3.63, 7.5cm × 3m= £2.82

hort stretch compression bandages

ctico
.andage
.ctico bandage (L&R Medical UK Ltd) 10cm × 6m= £3.47, 12cm × m= £4.43, 4cm × 6m= £2.48, 6cm × 6m= £2.91, 8cm × 6m= 3.34

omprilan
.andage
.omprilan bandage (BSN medical Ltd) 10cm × 5m= £3.55, 12cm × m= £4.32, 6cm × 5m= £2.81, 8cm × 5m= £3.30

.osidal K
.andage
.osidal K bandage (Lohmann & Rauscher) 10cm × 10m= £6.24, 10cm × 5m= £3.58, 12cm × 5m= £4.35, 6cm × 5m= £2.75, 8cm × .m= £3.28

.ub-compression wadding bandage

.ellona Undercast Padding
Padding
.ellona Undercast padding bandage (Lohmann & Rausche) 10cm × 2.75m= £0.49, 15cm × 2.75m= £0.63, 5cm × 2.75m= £0.32, 7.5cm × 2.75m= £0.39

.lexi-Ban
Padding
.lexi-Ban (L&R Medical UK Ltd) bandage 10cm × 3.5m= £0.52

.-Soft
Padding
.-Soft (Urgo Ltd) Long bandage 10cm × 4.5m= £0.59, bandage 10cm × 3.5m= £0.47

Ortho-Band Plus
Padding
Ortho-Band (Millpledge Healthcare) Plus bandage 10cm × 3.5m= £0.37

Profore #1
Padding
Profore #1 (Smith & Nephew Healthcare Ltd) bandage 10cm × 3.5m= £0.74, latex free bandage 10cm × 3.5m= £0.80

Softexe
Padding
Softexe (Molnlycke Health Care Ltd) bandage 10cm × 3.5m= £0.62

SurePress
Padding
SurePress (ConvaTec Ltd) bandage 10cm × 3m= £3.80

Ultra Soft
Padding
Ultra (Robinson Healthcare) Soft wadding bandage 10cm × 3.5m= £0.39

Velband
Padding
Velband (BSN medical Ltd) absorbent padding bandage 10cm × 4.5m= £0.75

Multi-layer compression bandaging

Multi-layer compression bandaging systems are an alternative to High Compression Bandages for the treatment of venous leg ulcers. Compression is achieved by the combined effects of two or three extensible bandages applied over a layer of orthopaedic wadding and a wound contact dressing.

Four layer systems
K-Four
Padding

K-Four
Multi-layer compression bandaging kit, four layer system
K-Four (Urgo Ltd) Reduced Compression multi-layer compression bandage kit 18cm+ ankle circumference = £4.66, multi-layer compression bandage kit 18cm-25cm ankle circumference= £7.13, 25cm-30cm ankle circumference= £7.13, greater than 30cm ankle circumference= £9.82, less than 18cm ankle circumference= £7.45

Profore
Wound contact layer

Profore
Multi-layer compression bandaging kit, four layer system
Profore (Smith & Nephew Healthcare Ltd) Lite latex free multi-layer compression bandage kit= £6.25, multi-layer compression bandage kit= £5.75, latex free multi-layer compression bandage kit 18cm-25cm ankle circumference = £10.64, multi-layer compression bandage kit 18cm-25cm ankle circumference= £9.96, 25cm-30cm ankle circumference= £8.27, above 30cm ankle circumference= £12.38, up to 18cm ankle circumference= £10.69

Ultra Four
Wound contact layer

Ultra Four
Multi-layer compression bandaging kit, four layer system
Ultra Four (Robinson Healthcare) Reduced Compression multi-layer compression bandage kit= £4.19, multi-layer compression bandage kit 18cm-25cm ankle circumference= £5.73, up to 18cm ankle circumference= £6.48

Two layer systems
Coban 2
Multi-layer compression bandaging kit, two layer system (latex-free, foam bandage and cohesive compression bandage)
Coban 2 (3M Health Care Ltd) Lite multi-layer compression bandage kit= £8.40, multi-layer compression bandage kit 10cm × 3.5m= £8.40

K Two
Multi-layer compression bandaging kit, two layer system
UrgoKTwo (Urgo Ltd) Reduced latex free multi-layer compression bandage kit (10cm) 18cm-25cm ankle circumference= £8.87, 25cm-32cm ankle circumference= £9.69, Reduced multi-layer compression bandage kit 18cm-25cm ankle circumference= £8.35, 25cm-32cm ankle circumference= £9.13, latex free multi-layer compression bandage kit (10cm) 18cm-25cm ankle circumference= £8.87, 25cm-32cm ankle circumference= £9.69, multi-layer compression bandage kit (10cm) 18cm-25cm ankle circumference= £8.35, 25cm-32cm ankle circumference= £9.13, multi-layer compression bandage kit (12cm) 18cm-25cm ankle circumference= £10.53, 25cm-32cm ankle circumference= £11.51, multi-layer compression bandage kit (8cm) 18cm-25cm ankle circumference= £7.88, 25cm-32cm ankle circumference= £8.57, multi-layer compression bandage kit size 0 short 18cm-25cm ankle circumference= £7.05, with UrgoStart multi-layer compression bandage kit 18cm-25cm ankle circumference= £10.41, 25cm-32cm ankle circumference= £11.10

Medicated bandages

Zinc Paste Bandage has been used with compression bandaging for the treatment of venous leg ulcers. However, paste bandages are associated with hypersensitivity reactions and should be used with caution. Zinc paste bandages are also used with coal tar or ichthammol in chronic lichenified skin conditions such as chronic eczema (ichthammol often being preferred since its action is considered to be milder). They are also used with calamine in milder eczematous skin conditions.
Zipzoc® can be used with appropriate compression bandages or hosiery in chronic venous insufficiency.

Zinc Paste Bandage, BP 1993
Cotton fabric, plain weave, impregnated with suitable paste containing zinc oxide; requires additional bandaging
Excipients: may include cetostearyl alcohol, hydroxybenzoates
Viscopaste (Evolan Pharma AB) PB7 bandage 7.5cm × 6m= £3.84

Zinc Paste and Ichthammol Bandage, BP 1993
Cotton fabric, plain weave, impregnated with suitable paste containing zinc oxide and ichthammol; requires additional bandaging
Excipients: may include cetostearyl alcohol
Ichthopaste (Evolan Pharma AB) bandage 7.5cm × 6m= £3.87

Zipzoc
Sterile rayon stocking impregnated with ointment containing zinc oxide 20%

Zipzoc (Evolan Pharma AB) stockings= £34.70

Compression hosiery and garments

Compression (elastic) hosiery is used to treat conditions associated with chronic venous insufficiency, to prevent recurrence of thrombosis, or to reduce the risk of further venous ulceration after treatment with compression bandaging. Doppler testing to confirm arterial sufficiency is required before recommending the use of compression hosiery.

Before elastic hosiery can be dispensed, the quantity (single or pair), article (including accessories), and compression class must be specified by the prescriber. There are different compression values for graduated compression hosiery and lymphoedema garments (see table below). All dispensed elastic hosiery articles must state on the packaging that they conform with Drug Tariff technical specification No. 40, for further details see Drug Tariff.

Graduated Compression hosiery, Class 1 Light Support is used for superficial or early varices, varicosis during pregnancy. *Graduated Compression hosiery, Class 2 Medium Support* is used for varices of medium severity, ulcer treatment and prophylaxis, mild oedema, varicosis during pregnancy. *Graduated Compression hosiery, Class 3 Strong Support* is used for gross varices, post thrombotic venous insufficiency, gross oedema, ulcer treatment and prophylaxis.

Compression values for hosiery and lymphoedema garments *Class* 1: Compression hosiery (British standard) 14–17 mmHg, lymphoedema garments (European classification) 18–21 mmHg; *Class* 2 Compression hosiery (British standard) 18–24 mmHg, lymphoedema garments (European classification) 23–32 mmHg; *Class* 3 Compression hosiery (British standard) 25–35 mmHg, lymphoedema garments (European classification) 34–46 mmHg; *Class* 4 Compression hosiery (British standard)—not available, lymphoedema garments (European classification) 49–70 mmHg; *Class* 4 *super* Compression hosiery (British standard)—not available, lymphoedema garments (European classification) 60–90 mmHg.

Graduated compression hosiery

Class 1 Light Support
Hosiery, compression at ankle 14–17 mmHg, thigh length or below knee with knitted in heel

Class 2 Light Support
Hosiery, compression at ankle 14–17 mmHg, thigh length or below knee with knitted in heel

Accessories
Suspender
Suspender, for thigh stockings

Anklets
Class 2 Medium Support
Anklets, compression 18–24 mmHg, circular knit (standard and made-to-measure)

Class 3 Strong Support
Anklets, compression 18–24 mmHg, circular knit (standard and made-to-measure)

Knee caps
Class 2 Medium Support
Kneecaps, compression 18–24 mmHg, circular knit (standard and made-to-measure)

Class 3 Strong Support
Kneecaps, compression 18–24 mmHg, circular knit (standard and made-to-measure)

Lymphoedema garments

Lymphoedema compression garments are used to maintain limb shape and prevent additional fluid retention. Either flat-bed or circular knitting methods are used in the manufacture of elasticated compression garments. Seamless, circular-knitted garments (in standard sizes) can be used to prevent swelling if the lymphoedema is well controlled and if the limb is in good shape and without skin folds. Flat-knitted garments (usually made-to-measure) with a seam, provide greater rigidity and stiffness to maintain reduction of lymphoedema following treatment with compression bandages. A standard range of light, medium, or high compression garments are available, as well as low compression (12–16 mmHg) armsleeves, made-to-measure garments up to compression 90 mmHg, and accessories—see Drug Tariff for details. Note, there are different compression values for lymphoedema garments and graduated compression hosiery, see Compression hosiery and garments above.

Dental Practitioners' Formulary

List of Dental Preparations

The following list has been approved by the appropriate Secretaries of State, and the preparations therein may be prescribed by dental practitioners on form FP10D (GP14 in Scotland, WP10D in Wales).

Licensed **sugar-free** versions, where available, are preferred.
Licensed **alcohol-free** mouthwashes, where available, are preferred.

Aciclovir Cream, BP
Aciclovir Oral Suspension, BP, 200 mg/5 mL
Aciclovir Tablets, BP, 200 mg
Aciclovir Tablets, BP, 800 mg
Amoxicillin Capsules, BP
Amoxicillin Oral Powder, DPF
Amoxicillin Oral Suspension, BP
Artificial Saliva Gel, DPF
Artificial Saliva Oral Spray, DPF
Artificial Saliva Pastilles, DPF
Artificial Saliva Protective Spray, DPF
Artificial Saliva Substitutes as listed below (to be prescribed only for indications approved by ACBS (patients suffering from dry mouth as a result of having or, having undergone, radiotherapy or sicca syndrome):
  BioXtra ® Gel Mouthspray
  BioXtra ® Moisturising Gel
  Glandosane ®
  Saliveze ®
Artificial Saliva Substitute Spray, DPF
Aspirin Tablets, Dispersible, BP
Azithromycin Capsules, 250 mg, DPF
Azithromycin Oral Suspension, 200 mg/5 mL, DPF
Azithromycin Tablets, 250 mg, DPF
Azithromycin Tablets, 500 mg, DPF
Beclometasone Pressurised Inhalation, BP, 50 micrograms/metered inhalation, CFC-free, as:
  Clenil Modulite ®
Benzydamine Mouthwash, BP 0.15%
Benzydamine Oromucosal Spray, BP 0.15%
Betamethasone Soluble Tablets, 500 micrograms, DPF
Carbamazepine Tablets, BP
Cefalexin Capsules, BP
Cefalexin Oral Suspension, BP
Cefalexin Tablets, BP
Cefradine Capsules, BP
Cetirizine Oral Solution, BP, 5 mg/5 mL
Cetirizine Tablets, BP, 10 mg
Chlorhexidine Gluconate Gel, BP
Chlorhexidine Mouthwash, BP
Chlorhexidine Oral Spray, DPF
Chlorphenamine Oral Solution, BP
Chlorphenamine Tablets, BP
Choline Salicylate Dental Gel, BP
Clarithromycin Oral Suspension, 125 mg/5 mL, DPF
Clarithromycin Oral Suspension, 250 mg/5 mL, DPF
Clarithromycin Tablets, BP
Clindamycin Capsules, BP
Co-amoxiclav Tablets, BP, 250/125 (amoxicillin 250 mg as trihydrate, clavulanic acid 125 mg as potassium salt)
Co-amoxiclav Oral Suspension, BP, 125/31 (amoxicillin 125 mg as trihydrate, clavulanic acid 31.25 mg as potassium salt)/5 mL
Co-amoxiclav Oral Suspension, BP, 250/62 (amoxicillin 250 mg as trihydrate, clavulanic acid 62.5 mg as potassium salt)/5 mL
Diazepam Oral Solution, BP, 2 mg/5 mL
Diazepam Tablets, BP

Diclofenac Sodium Tablets, Gastro-resistant, BP
Dihydrocodeine Tablets, BP, 30 mg
Doxycycline Tablets, Dispersible, BP
Doxycycline Capsules, BP, 100 mg
Doxycycline Tablets, 20 mg, DPF
Ephedrine Nasal Drops, BP
Erythromycin Ethyl Succinate Oral Suspension, BP
Erythromycin Ethyl Succinate Tablets, BP
Erythromycin Stearate Tablets, BP
Erythromycin Tablets, Gastro-resistant, BP
Fluconazole Capsules, 50 mg, DPF
Fluconazole Oral Suspension, 50 mg/5 mL, DPF
Hydrocortisone Cream, BP, 1%
Hydrocortisone Oromucosal Tablets, BP
Hydrogen Peroxide Mouthwash, BP, 6%
Ibuprofen Oral Suspension, BP, sugar-free
Ibuprofen Tablets, BP
Lansoprazole Capsules, Gastro-resistant, BP
Lidocaine Ointment, BP, 5%
Lidocaine Spray 10%, DPF
Loratadine Syrup, 5 mg/5 mL, DPF
Loratadine Tablets, BP, 10 mg
Menthol and Eucalyptus Inhalation, BP 1980
Metronidazole Oral Suspension, BP
Metronidazole Tablets, BP
Miconazole Cream, BP
Miconazole Oromucosal Gel, BP
Miconazole and Hydrocortisone Cream, BP
Miconazole and Hydrocortisone Ointment, BP
Nystatin Oral Suspension, BP
Omeprazole Capsules, Gastro-resistant, BP
Oxytetracycline Tablets, BP
Paracetamol Oral Suspension, BP
Paracetamol Tablets, BP
Paracetamol Tablets, Soluble, BP
Phenoxymethylpenicillin Oral Solution, BP
Phenoxymethylpenicillin Tablets, BP
Promethazine Hydrochloride Tablets, BP
Promethazine Oral Solution, BP
Saliva Stimulating Tablets, DPF
Sodium Chloride Mouthwash, Compound, BP
Sodium Fluoride Mouthwash, BP
Sodium Fluoride Oral Drops, BP
Sodium Fluoride Tablets, BP
Sodium Fluoride Toothpaste 0.619%, DPF
Sodium Fluoride Toothpaste 1.1%, DPF
Sodium Fusidate Ointment, BP
Temazepam Oral Solution, BP
Temazepam Tablets, BP
Tetracycline Tablets, BP

Preparations in this list which are not included in the BP or BPC are described under Details of DPF preparations.
For details of preparations that can be prescribed, see individual entries under the relevant drug monographs throughout the BNF publications.

Details of DPF preparations

Preparations on the List of Dental Preparations which are specified as DPF are described as follows in the DPF. Although brand names have sometimes been included for identification purposes preparations on the list should be prescribed by non-proprietary name.

Amoxicillin Oral Powder
amoxicillin (as trihydrate) 3 g sachet

Artificial Saliva Gel
consists of lactoperoxidase, lactoferrin, lysozyme, glucose oxidase, xylitol in a gel basis

Artificial Saliva Oral Spray
(proprietary product: *Xerotin*) consists of water, sorbitol, carmellose (carboxymethylcellulose), potassium chloride, sodium chloride, potassium phosphate, magnesium chloride, calcium chloride and other ingredients, pH neutral

Artificial Saliva Pastilles
(proprietary product: *Salivix*), consists of acacia, malic acid, and other ingredients

Artificial Saliva Protective Spray
(proprietary product: *Aequasyal*) consists of oxidised glycerol triesters, silicon dioxide, flavouring agents, aspartame

Artificial Saliva Substitute Spray
(proprietary product: *AS Saliva Orthana Spray*) consists of mucin, methylparaben, benzalkonium chloride, EDTA, xylitol, peppermint oil, spearmint oil, mineral salts

Azithromycin Capsules
azithromycin 250 mg

Azithromycin Oral Suspension 200 mg/5 mL
azithromycin 200 mg/5 mL when reconstituted with water

Azithromycin Tablets
azithromycin 250 mg and 500 mg

Betamethasone Soluble Tablets 500 micrograms
betamethasone (as sodium phosphate) 500 micrograms

Chlorhexidine Oral Spray
(proprietary product: *Corsodyl Oral Spray*), chlorhexidine gluconate 0.2%

Clarithromycin Oral Suspension 125 mg/5 mL
clarithromycin 125 mg/5 mL when reconstituted with water

Clarithromycin Oral Suspension 250 mg/5 mL
clarithromycin 250 mg/5 mL when reconstituted with water

Doxycycline Tablets 20 mg
(proprietary product: *Periostat*), doxycycline (as hyclate) 20 mg

Fluconazole Capsules 50 mg
fluconazole 50 mg

Fluconazole Oral Suspension 50 mg/5 mL
(proprietary product: *Diflucan*), fluconazole 50 mg/5 mL when reconstituted with water

Lidocaine Spray 10%
(proprietary product: *Xylocaine Spray*), lidocaine 10% supplying 10 mg lidocaine/spray

Loratadine Syrup 5 mg/5 mL
loratadine 5 mg/5 mL

Saliva Stimulating Tablets
(proprietary product: *SST*), citric acid, malic acid and other ingredients in a sorbitol base

Sodium Fluoride Toothpaste 0.619%
(proprietary product: *Duraphat '2800 ppm' Toothpaste*), sodium fluoride 0.619%

Sodium Fluoride Toothpaste 1.1%
(proprietary product: *Duraphat '5000 ppm' Toothpaste*), sodium fluoride 1.1%

Approved list for prescribing by Community Practitioner Nurse Prescribers (NPF)

Nurse Prescribers' Formulary for Community Practitioners

The Nurse Prescribers' Formulary for Community Practitioners is for use by District Nurses and Specialist Community Public Health Nurses (including Health Visitors) who have received nurse prescriber training. It provides a list of preparations approved by the Secretary of State that can be prescribed for patients receiving NHS treatment on form FP10P (form HS21(N) in Northern Ireland, form GP10(N) in Scotland, forms WP10CN and WP10PN in Wales). Community practitioner nurse prescribers should only prescribe items appearing in the nurse prescribers' list set out below (for the indications specified). Most medicinal preparations should be prescribed generically, except where this would not be clinically appropriate or where there is no approved generic name—see individual entries for further information.

The Nurse Prescribers' Advisory Group p. vii oversees the preparation of the NPF and advises UK health ministers on the list of preparations that may be prescribed by community practitioner nurse prescribers. Feedback from nurse prescribers is welcome and will be taken into account when reviewing this list; comments and constructive criticism should be sent to editor@bnf.org.

How to use the NPF

The list of medicinal preparations includes:
- Links to BNF monographs to allow full prescribing information for each preparation to be accessed;
- Details of the indications for which each medicinal preparation can be prescribed;
- Signposting to doses for community practitioner nurse prescribers where these differ from those in the BNF for the specified indications;
- Additional information that should be considered before prescribing certain preparations.

The NPF should be used in conjunction with BNF monographs to ensure that all relevant prescribing information is considered when prescribing decisions are made; links to the relevant BNF monographs allow quick access to this prescribing information. Most of the doses that can be prescribed by nurse prescribers for the specified indications are in line with those in BNF monographs, so the BNF doses for those indications can be used. If doses that can be prescribed by nurse prescribers differ from those in the BNF, specific indications and doses have been added to BNF monographs. These can be found towards the bottom of indication and dose sections of the relevant monographs with the statement "dose approved for use by community practitioner nurse prescribers" following the indication; individual preparation entries signpost to these doses.

General guidance for community practitioner nurse prescribers (Nurse Prescribers' Formulary—General guidance) includes information on prescribing for nurse prescribers and can be found in online versions of the BNF and the BNF app. Treatment summaries for nurse prescribers (e.g. Nurse Prescribers' Formulary—Analgesics) can also be found in online versions of the BNF and the BNF app; these provide an overview of the drug management or prophylaxis

of conditions that are commonly managed by nurse prescribers and/or information on the use of appliances, such as stoma appliances. In order to select safe and effective medicines for individual patients, information in the treatment summaries must be used in conjunction with other prescribing details about the drugs and knowledge of the patient's medical and drug history.

Medicinal Preparations

Preparations on this list which are not included in the BP or BPC are described under Details of NPF preparations.

Almond oil ear drops p. 1244, BP
Removal of ear wax

Arachis oil enema p. 64, NPF
To soften impacted faeces

Aspirin tablet, dispersible, 300 mgs p. 132, BP (max. 96 tablets; max. pack size 32 tablets)
Mild to moderate pain| Pyrexia (for both indications, see doses for community practitioner nurse prescribers)

Bisacodyl suppositories p. 65, BP (includes 5-mg and 10-mg strengths)
Constipation (see dose for community practitioner nurse prescribers)

Bisacodyl tablets p. 65, BP
Constipation (see dose for community practitioner nurse prescribers)

Catheter maintenance solutions, sodium chloride p. 836, NPF
For removal of clots and other debris, to be instilled as required

Catheter maintenance solutions, 'Solution G' p. 836, NPF
For prevention of catheter encrustation and crystallisation; in very severe cases use 'Solution R'

Catheter maintenance solutions, 'Solution R' p. 836, NPF
For prevention of catheter encrustation and dissolution of crystallisation if 'Solution G' unsuccessful

Chlorhexidine gluconate alcoholic solutions containing at least 0.05%, see chlorhexidine p. 1321 and chlorhexidine gluconate with isopropyl alcohol p. 1321
Skin disinfection

Chlorhexidine gluconate aqueous solutions p. 1687 containing at least 0.05%
Skin disinfection

Choline salicylate dental gel p. 1260, BP
Mild oral and perioral lesions

Clotrimazole cream 1% p. 1276, BP
Fungal skin infections

Co-danthramer capsules, NPF [discontinued]
Co-danthramer capsules, strong, NPF [discontinued]
Co-danthramer oral suspension p. 66, NPF
In consultation with doctor, constipation in palliative care

Co-danthramer oral suspension, strong p. 66, NPF
In consultation with doctor, constipation in palliative care

Co-danthrusate capsules, BP [discontinued]
Co-danthrusate oral suspension p. 66, NPF
In consultation with doctor, constipation in palliative care

Crotamiton cream p. 1309, BP
Pruritus (including pruritus after scabies)

Crotamiton lotion, BP [discontinued]

Dimeticone barrier creams containing at least 10%, see barrier creams and ointments p. 1266
For use as a barrier preparation
Dimeticone lotion p. 1281, NPF
Head lice
Docusate sodium capsules p. 64, BP
Chronic constipation
Docusate sodium enema p. 64, NPF
Chronic constipation
Docusate sodium oral solution p. 64, BP
Chronic constipation
Docusate sodium oral solution, paediatric p. 64, BP
Chronic constipation
Econazole nitrate cream 1% p. 1277, BP
Fungal skin infections
Emollient creams and ointments, paraffin-containing p. 1270 as listed below:
Dry skin conditions| Eczema| Psoriasis| Ichthyosis| Pruritus
Cetraben® emollient cream
Dermamist®
Diprobase® cream
Diprobase® ointment
Doublebase®
Doublebase® Dayleve gel
E45® cream
Emulsifying ointment, BP
Hydromol® cream
Hydrous ointment, BP
Lipobase®
Liquid and white soft paraffin ointment, NPF
Neutrogena® Norwegian Formula Dermatological cream [discontinued]
Oilatum® cream
Oilatum® Junior cream
Paraffin, white soft, BP
Paraffin, yellow soft, BP
Ultrabase®
Unguentum M®
Emollients, urea-containing p. 1271 as listed below:
Aquadrate® 10% w/w cream
Dry, scaling, and itching skin
Balneum® Plus cream
Dry, scaling, and itching skin
E45® Itch Relief cream
Dry, scaling, and itching skin
Eucerin® Intensive 10% w/w urea treatment cream
Dry skin conditions including eczema, ichthyosis, xeroderma, and hyperkeratosis
Eucerin® Intensive 10% w/w urea treatment lotion
Dry skin conditions including eczema, ichthyosis, xeroderma, and hyperkeratosis
Hydromol® Intensive
Dry, scaling, and itching skin
Nutraplus® cream
Dry, scaling, and itching skin
Emollient bath and shower products, paraffin-containing p. 1267 as listed below:
Aqueous cream, BP
Dry skin conditions
Cetraben® emollient bath additive
Dry skin conditions, including eczema
Dermalo® bath emollient
Dermatitis| Dry skin conditions, including ichthyosis| Pruritus of the elderly
Doublebase® emollient bath additive
Dry skin conditions, including dermatitis and ichthyosis| Pruritus of the elderly
Doublebase® emollient shower gel
Dry, chapped, or itchy skin conditions
Doublebase® emollient wash gel
Dry, chapped, or itchy skin conditions

Hydromol® bath and shower emollient
Dry skin conditions| Eczema| Ichthyosis| Pruritus of the elderly
Oilatum® emollient
Dry skin conditions including dermatitis and ichthyosis| Pruritus of the elderly
Oilatum® gel [discontinued]
Oilatum® Junior bath additive
Dry skin conditions including dermatitis and ichthyosis| Pruritus of the elderly
Zerolatum® emollient medicinal bath oil
Dry skin conditions| Dermatitis| Ichthyosis
Emollient bath and shower products, soya-bean oil-containing p. 1269 as listed below:
Balneum® (except pack sizes that are not to be prescribed under the NHS (see Part XVIIIA of the Drug Tariff, Part XI of the Northern Ireland Drug Tariff))
Dry skin conditions including those associated with dermatitis and eczema
Balneum Plus® bath oil (except pack sizes that are not to be prescribed under the NHS (see Part XVIIIA of the Drug Tariff, Part XI of the Northern Ireland Drug Tariff))
Dry skin conditions including those associated with dermatitis and eczema where pruritus also experienced
Folic acid tablets 400 micrograms p. 1071, BP
Prevention of neural tube defects (in those at a low risk of conceiving a child with a neural tube defect)
Glycerol suppositories p. 67, BP
Constipation
Ibuprofen oral suspension p. 1186, BP (except for indications and doses that are prescription-only)
Pain and inflammation in rheumatic disease and other musculoskeletal disorders| Mild to moderate pain including dysmenorrhoea| Migraine| Dental pain| Headache| Fever| Symptoms of colds and influenza| Neuralgia| Mild to moderate pain| Pain and inflammation of soft-tissue injuries| Pyrexia with discomfort| Post-immunisation pyrexia in infants (for all indications, see doses for community practitioner nurse prescribers)
Ibuprofen tablets p. 1186, BP (except for indications and doses that are prescription-only)
Pain and inflammation in rheumatic disease and other musculoskeletal disorders| Mild to moderate pain including dysmenorrhoea| Migraine| Dental pain| Headache| Fever| Symptoms of colds and influenza| Neuralgia| Mild to moderate pain| Pain and inflammation of soft-tissue injuries| Pyrexia with discomfort (for all indications, see doses for community practitioner nurse prescribers)
Ispaghula husk granules p. 58, BP
Constipation (see dose for community practitioner nurse prescribers)
Ispaghula husk granules, effervescent p. 58, BP
Constipation (see dose for community practitioner nurse prescribers)
Ispaghula husk oral powder, BP [discontinued]
Lactulose solution p. 60, BP
Constipation (see dose for community practitioner nurse prescribers)
Lidocaine hydrochloride ointment p. 1406, BP
Sore nipples from breast-feeding
Lidocaine and chlorhexidine gel, BP, see chlorhexidine with lidocaine p. 835
Surface anaesthesia (see dose for community practitioner nurse prescribers)
Macrogol oral liquid, compound, NPF, see macrogol 3350 with potassium chloride, sodium bicarbonate and sodium chloride p. 61
Chronic constipation

Macrogol oral powder, compound, NPF, see macrogol 3350 with potassium chloride, sodium bicarbonate and sodium chloride p. 61

Chronic constipation| Faecal impaction (important: initial assessment by doctor; usual max. duration of treatment 3 days)

Macrogol oral powder, compound, half-strength, NPF, see macrogol 3350 with potassium chloride, sodium bicarbonate and sodium chloride p. 61

Chronic constipation| Faecal impaction (important: initial assessment by doctor; usual max. duration of treatment 3 days)

Magnesium hydroxide mixture p. 62, BP
Constipation

Magnesium sulfate paste, BP
Adjunct in management of boils, apply under dressing; stir before use

Malathion aqueous lotions p. 1281 containing at least 0.5%
Head lice| Scabies

Mebendazole oral suspension p. 644, NPF
Threadworm infections (see dose for community practitioner nurse prescribers)

Mebendazole tablets p. 644, NPF
Threadworm infections (see dose for community practitioner nurse prescribers)

Methylcellulose tablets p. 59, BP
Constipation

Miconazole cream 2% p. 1277, BP
Fungal skin infections

Miconazole oromucosal gel p. 1262, BP
Prevention and treatment of oral candidiasis (see dose for community practitioner nurse prescribers)

Mouthwash solution-tablets, NPF

Nicotine inhalation cartridge for oromucosal use p. 521, NPF
Nicotine replacement therapy

Nicotine lozenge p. 521, NPF
Nicotine replacement therapy

Nicotine medicated chewing gum p. 521, NPF
Nicotine replacement therapy in individuals who smoke fewer than 20 cigarettes each day| Nicotine replacement therapy in individuals who smoke more than 20 cigarettes each day or who require more than 15 pieces of 2-mg strength gum each day

Nicotine nasal spray p. 521, NPF
Nicotine replacement therapy

Nicotine oral spray p. 521, NPF
Nicotine replacement therapy

Nicotine sublingual tablets p. 521, NPF
Nicotine replacement therapy in individuals who smoke fewer than 20 cigarettes each day| Nicotine replacement therapy in individuals who smoke more than 20 cigarettes each day

Nicotine transdermal patches p. 521, NPF
Nicotine replacement therapy

Nystatin oral suspension p. 1263, BP
Oral and perioral fungal infections (see dose for community practitioner nurse prescribers)

Olive oil ear drops p. 1244, BP
Removal of earwax (see dose for community practitioner nurse prescribers)

Paracetamol oral suspension p. 464, BP (includes 120 mg/5 mL and 250 mg/5 mL strengths—both of which are available as sugar-free formulations)
Mild to moderate pain (in adults)| Pyrexia (in adults)| Pain (in children)| Pyrexia with discomfort (in children)| Post-immunisation pyrexia in infants (refer to doctor if pyrexia persists)

Paracetamol tablets p. 464, BP (max. 96 tablets; max. pack size 32 tablets)
Mild to moderate pain (in adults)| Pyrexia (in adults)| Pain (in children)| Pyrexia with discomfort (in children)

Paracetamol tablets, soluble p. 464, BP (max. 96 tablets; max. pack size 32 tablets)
Mild to moderate pain (in adults)| Pyrexia (in adults)| Pain (in children)| Pyrexia with discomfort (in children)

Permethrin cream p. 1281, NPF
Scabies

Phosphates enema, BP, see sodium acid phosphate with sodium phosphate p. 63
Constipation, using Phosphates enema BP Formula B| Constipation, using Phosphates enema (Cleen Ready-to-Use) (for both indications, see doses for community practitioner nurse prescribers)

Povidone-iodine solution p. 1320, BP
Skin disinfection

Senna oral solution p. 67, NPF
Constipation (see dose for community practitioner nurse prescribers)

Senna tablets p. 67, BP
Constipation (see dose for community practitioner nurse prescribers)

Senna with ispaghula husk granules p. 68, NPF
Constipation

Sodium chloride solution, sterile, BP, see Irrigation solutions p. 1322
Skin cleansing

Sodium citrate compound enema p. 833, NPF
Constipation (see dose for community practitioner nurse prescribers)

Sodium picosulfate capsules, NPF [discontinued]

Sodium picosulfate elixir p. 68, NPF
Constipation (see dose for community practitioner nurse prescribers)

Spermicidal contraceptive: Gygel® contraceptive jelly, see nonoxinol p. 858
Spermicidal contraceptive in conjunction with barrier methods of contraception such as diaphragms or caps

Sterculia granules p. 59, NPF
Constipation

Sterculia with frangula granules p. 60, NPF
Constipation

Titanium ointment, BP, see barrier creams and ointments p. 1266
For use as a barrier preparation

Water for injections, BP; available as 2-mL ampoules, 5-mL ampoules, 10-mL ampoules, 10-mL vials, 20-mL ampoules, and 100-mL vials

Zinc and castor oil ointment, BP, see barrier creams and ointments p. 1266
For use as a barrier preparation

Zinc oxide and dimeticone spray, NPF, see barrier creams and ointments p. 1266
For use as a barrier preparation

Zinc oxide impregnated medicated bandage, NPF, see Medicated bandages p. 1681

Zinc oxide impregnated medicated stocking, NPF, see Medicated bandages p. 1681

Zinc paste bandage, BP 1993, see Medicated bandages p. 1681

Zinc paste and ichthammol bandage, BP 1993, see Medicated bandages p. 1681

Appliances and Reagents (including Wound Management Products)

Community Practitioner Nurse Prescribers in England, Wales and Northern Ireland can prescribe any appliance or reagent in the relevant Drug Tariff. In the Scottish Drug Tariff, Appliances and Reagents which may **not** be prescribed by Nurses are annotated **Nx**.

Appliances (including Contraceptive Devices) as listed in Part IXA of the Drug Tariff (Part III of the Northern Ireland Drug Tariff, Part 3 (Appliances) and Part 2 (Dressings) of the Scottish Drug Tariff). (Where it is not appropriate for nurse prescribers in family planning clinics to prescribe contraceptive devices using form FP10(P) (forms WP10CN and WP10PN in Wales), they may prescribe using the same system as doctors in the clinic.)

Incontinence Appliances as listed in Part IXB of the Drug Tariff (Part III of the Northern Ireland Drug Tariff, Part 5 of the Scottish Drug Tariff).

Stoma Appliances and Associated Products as listed in Part IXC of the Drug Tariff (Part III of the Northern Ireland Drug Tariff, Part 6 of the Scottish Drug Tariff).

Chemical Reagents as listed in Part IXR of the Drug Tariff (Part II of the Northern Ireland Drug Tariff, Part 9 of the Scottish Drug Tariff).

The Drug Tariffs can be accessed online at:

National Health Service Drug Tariff for England and Wales: www.nhsbsa.nhs.uk/pharmacies-gp-practices-and-appliance-contractors/drug-tariff

Health and Personal Social Services for Northern Ireland Drug Tariff: www.hscbusiness.hscni.net/services/2034.htm

Scottish Drug Tariff: www.isdscotland.org/Health-topics/Prescribing-and-Medicines/Scottish-Drug-Tariff/

Details of NPF preparations

Preparations on the Nurse Prescribers' Formulary which are not included in the BP or BPC are described as follows in the Nurse Prescribers' Formulary. Although brand names have sometimes been included for identification purposes, it is recommended that non-proprietary names should be used for prescribing medicinal preparations in the NPF except where a non-proprietary name is not available.

Arachis oil enema
arachis oil 100%

Catheter maintenance solution, sodium chloride
(proprietary products: *OptiFlo S; Uro-Tainer Sodium Chloride; Uriflex-S*), sodium chloride 0.9%

Catheter maintenance solution, 'Solution G'
(proprietary products: *OptiFlo G; Uro-Tainer Suby G; Uriflex G*), citric acid 3.23%, magnesium oxide 0.38%, sodium bicarbonate 0.7%, disodium edetate 0.01%

Catheter maintenance solution, 'Solution R'
(proprietary products: *OptiFlo R; Uro-Tainer Solutio R; Uriflex R*), citric acid 6%, gluconolactone 0.6%, magnesium carbonate 2.8%, disodium edetate 0.01%

Chlorhexidine gluconate alcoholic solutions
(proprietary products: *ChloraPrep; Hydrex Solution; Hydrex spray*), chlorhexidine gluconate in alcoholic solution

Chlorhexidine gluconate aqueous solutions
(proprietary product: *Unisept*), chlorhexidine gluconate in aqueous solution

Co-danthramer capsules PoM
co-danthramer 25/200 (dantron 25 mg, poloxamer '188' 200 mg)

Co-danthramer capsules, strong PoM
co-danthramer 37.5/500 (dantron 37.5 mg, poloxamer '188' 500 mg)

Co-danthramer oral suspension PoM
co-danthramer 25/200 in 5 mL (dantron 25 mg, poloxamer '188' 200 mg/5 mL)

Co-danthramer oral suspension, strong PoM
co-danthramer 75/1000 in 5 mL (dantron 75 mg, poloxamer '188' 1 g/5 mL)

Co-danthrusate oral suspension PoM
(proprietary product: *Normax*), co-danthrusate 50/60 (dantron 50 mg, docusate sodium 60 mg/5 mL)

Dimeticone barrier creams
(proprietary products *Conotrane Cream*, dimeticone '350' 22%; *Siopel Barrier Cream*, dimeticone '1000' 10%), dimeticone 10–22%

Dimeticone lotion
(proprietary product: *Hedrin*), dimeticone 4%

Docusate enema
(proprietary product: *Norgalax Micro-enema*), docusate sodium 120 mg in 10 g

Liquid and white soft paraffin ointment
liquid paraffin 50%, white soft paraffin 50%

Macrogol oral liquid, compound
(proprietary product: *Movicol Liquid*), macrogol '3350' (polyethylene glycol '3350') 13.125 g, sodium bicarbonate 178.5 mg, sodium chloride 350.7 mg, potassium chloride 46.6 mg/25 mL

Macrogol oral powder, compound
(proprietary products: *Laxido Orange, Molaxole, Movicol*), macrogol '3350' (polyethylene glycol '3350') 13.125 g, sodium bicarbonate 178.5 mg, sodium chloride 350.7 mg, potassium chloride 46.6 mg/sachet; (amount of potassium chloride varies according to flavour of *Movicol*® as follows: plain-flavour (sugar-free) = 50.2 mg/sachet; lime and lemon flavour = 46.6 mg/sachet; chocolate flavour = 31.7 mg/sachet 1 sachet when reconstituted with 125 mL water provides K$^+$ 5.4 mmol/litre)

Macrogol oral powder, compound, half-strength
(proprietary product: *Movicol-Half*), macrogol '3350' (polyethylene glycol '3350') 6.563 g, sodium bicarbonate 89.3 g, sodium chloride 175.4 mg, potassium chloride 23.3 mg/sachet

Malathion aqueous lotions
(proprietary products: *Derbac-M Liquid*), malathion 0.5% in an aqueous basis

Mebendazole oral suspension PoM
(proprietary product: *Vermox*), mebendazole 100 mg/5 mL

Mebendazole tablets PoM
(proprietary products: *Ovex, Vermox*), mebendazole 100 mg (can be supplied for oral use in the treatment of enterobiasis in adults and children over 2 years provided its container or package is labelled to show a max. single dose of 100 mg and it is supplied in a container or package containing not more than 800 mg)

Mouthwash solution-tablets
consist of tablets which may contain antimicrobial, colouring and flavouring agents in a suitable soluble effervescent basis to make a mouthwash

Nicotine inhalation cartridge for oromucosal use
(proprietary products: *NicAssist Inhalator, Nicorette Inhalator*), nicotine 15 mg (for use with inhalation mouthpiece; to be prescribed as either a starter pack (6 cartridges with inhalator device and holder) or refill pack (42 cartridges with inhalator device)

Nicotine lozenge
nicotine (as bitartrate) 1 mg or 2 mg (proprietary product: *Nicorette Mint Lozenge, Nicotinell Mint Lozenge*), or nicotine (as resinate) 1.5 mg, 2 mg, or 4 mg (proprietary product: *NiQuitin Lozenges, NiQuitin Minis, NiQuitin Pre-quit*)

Nicotine medicated chewing gum
(proprietary products: *NicAssist Gum, Nicorette Gum, Nicotinell Gum, NiQuitin Gum*), nicotine 2 mg or 4 mg

Nicotine nasal spray
(proprietary product: *NicAssist Nasal Spray, Nicorette Nasal Spray*), nicotine 500 micrograms/metered spray

Nicotine oral spray
(proprietary product: *Nicorette Quickmist*), nicotine 1 mg/metered spray

Nicotine sublingual tablets
(proprietary product: *NicAssist Microtab, Nicorette Microtab*), nicotine (as a cyclodextrin complex) 2 mg (to be prescribed as either a starter pack (2 × 15-tablet discs with dispenser) or refill pack (7 × 15-tablet discs)

Nicotine transdermal patches
releasing in each 16 hours, nicotine approx. 5 mg, 10 mg, or 15 mg (proprietary products: *Boots NicAssist Patch, Nicorette Patch*), or releasing in each 16 hours approx. 10 mg, 15 mg, or 25 mg (proprietary products: *NicAssist Translucent Patch, Nicorette Invisi Patch*), or releasing in each 24 hours nicotine

approx. 7 mg, 14 mg, or 21 mg (proprietary products:
Nicopatch, Nicotinell TTS, NiQuitin, NiQuitin Clear)
prescriber should specify the brand to be dispensed)

Permethrin cream
(proprietary product: *Lyclear Dermal Cream*), permethrin 5%

Senna oral solution
(proprietary product: *Senokot Syrup*), sennosides 7.5 mg/5 mL

Senna and ispaghula granules
(proprietary product: *Manevac Granules*), senna fruit 12.4%,
ispaghula 54.2%

Sodium citrate compound enema
(proprietary products: *Micolette Micro-enema; Micralax
Micro-enema; Relaxit Micro-enema*),sodium citrate 450 mg
with glycerol, sorbitol and an anionic surfactant

Sodium picosulfate capsules
(proprietary products: *Dulcolax Perles*), sodium picosulfate
2.5 mg

Sodium picosulfate elixir
(proprietary product: *Dulcolax Liquid*), sodium picosulfate
5 mg/5 mL

Sterculia granules
(proprietary product: *Normacol Granules*), sterculia 62%

Sterculia and frangula granules
(proprietary product: *Normacol Plus Granules*), sterculia 62%,
frangula (standardised) 8%

Zinc oxide and dimeticone spray
(proprietary product: *Sprilon*), dimeticone 1.04%, zinc oxide
12.5% in a pressurised aerosol unit

Zinc oxide impregnated medicated bandage
(proprietary product: *Steripaste*), sterile cotton bandage
impregnated with paste containing zinc oxide 15%

Zinc oxide impregnated medicated stocking
(proprietary product: *Zipzoc*), sterile rayon stocking
impregnated with ointment containing zinc oxide 20%

Non-medical prescribing

Overview

A range of non-medical healthcare professionals can prescribe medicines for patients as either Independent or Supplementary Prescribers.

Independent prescribers are practitioners responsible and accountable for the assessment of patients with previously undiagnosed or diagnosed conditions and for decisions about the clinical management required, including prescribing. They are recommended to prescribe generically, except where this would not be clinically appropriate or where there is no approved non-proprietary name.

Supplementary prescribing is a partnership between an independent prescriber (a doctor or a dentist) and a supplementary prescriber to implement an agreed Clinical Management Plan for an individual patient with that patient's agreement.

Independent and Supplementary Prescribers are identified by an annotation next to their name in the relevant professional register.

Information and guidance on non-medical prescribing is available on the Department of Health website at www.dh. gov.uk/health/2012/04/prescribing-change.

For information on the mixing of medicines by Independent and Supplementary Prescribers, see *Mixing of medicines prior to administration in clinical practice: medical and non-medical prescribing*, National Prescribing Centre, May 2010 (available at www.gov.uk/government/uploads/ system/uploads/attachment_data/file/213885/dh_116360.pdf).

For information on the supply and administration of medicines to groups of patients using Patient Group Directions see Guidance on prescribing p. 1.

In order to protect patient safety, the initial prescribing and supply of medicines prescribed should normally remain separate functions performed by separate healthcare professionals.

Nurses

Nurse Independent Prescribers (formerly known as Extended Formulary Nurse Prescribers) are able to prescribe any medicine for any medical condition. Unlicensed medicines are excluded from the Nurse Prescribing Formulary in Scotland.

Nurse Independent Prescribers are able to prescribe, administer, and give directions for the administration of Schedule 2, 3, 4, and 5 Controlled Drugs. This extends to diamorphine hydrochloride p. 476, dipipanone, or cocaine for treating organic disease or injury, but not for treating addiction.

Nurse Independent Prescribers must work within their own level of professional competence and expertise.

The Approved list for prescribing by Community Practitioner Nurse Prescribers (NPF) p. 1685 for Community Practitioners provides information on prescribing.

Pharmacists

Pharmacist Independent Prescribers can prescribe any medicine for any medical condition. This includes unlicensed medicines, subject to accepted clinical good practice.

They are also able to prescribe, administer, and give directions for the administration of Schedule 2, 3, 4, and 5 Controlled Drugs. This extends to diamorphine hydrochloride p. 476, dipipanone, or cocaine for treating organic disease or injury, but not for treating addiction.

Pharmacist Independent Prescribers must work within their own level of professional competence and expertise.

Physiotherapists

Physiotherapist Independent Prescribers can prescribe any medicine for any medical condition. This includes "off-label" medicines subject to accepted clinical good practice. They are also allowed to prescribe the following Controlled Drugs: oral or injectable morphine p. 483, transdermal fentanyl p. 478 and oral diazepam p. 362, dihydrocodeine tartrate p. 477, lorazepam p. 357, oxycodone hydrochloride p. 486 or temazepam p. 509.

Physiotherapist Independent Prescribers must work within their own level of professional competence and expertise.

Therapeutic radiographers

Therapeutic Radiographer Independent Prescribers can prescribe any medicine for any medical condition. This includes "off-label" medicines subject to accepted clinical good practice. Prescribing of Controlled Drugs is subject to legislative changes. Therapeutic Radiographer Independent Prescribers must work within their own level of professional competence and expertise.

Optometrists

Optometrist Independent Prescribers can prescribe any licensed medicine for ocular conditions affecting the eye and the tissues surrounding the eye, except Controlled Drugs or medicines for parenteral administration. Optometrist Independent Prescribers must work within their own level of professional competence and expertise.

Podiatrists

Podiatrist Independent Prescribers can prescribe any medicine for any medical condition. This includes "off-label" medicines subject to accepted clinical good practice. They are also allowed to prescribe the following Controlled Drugs for oral administration: diazepam p. 362, dihydrocodeine tartrate p. 477, lorazepam p. 357 and temazepam p. 509.

Podiatrist Independent Prescribers must work within their own level of professional competence and expertise.

Paramedics

Paramedic Independent Prescribers can prescribe any medicine for any medical condition. This includes "off-label" medicines subject to accepted clinical good practice. Prescribing of Controlled Drugs is subject to legislative changes. Paramedic Independent Prescribers must work within their own level of professional competence and expertise.

Further Information

For further details about the different types of prescribers, see *Medicines, Ethics and Practice*, London, Pharmaceutical Press (always consult latest edition).

Index of manufacturers

The following is an alphabetical list of manufacturers and other companies referenced in the BNF, with their medicines information or general contact details. For information on 'special-order' manufacturers and specialist importing companies see 'Special-order manufacturers'.

3M Health Care Ltd, Tel: 01509 611611

A. Menarini Farmaceutica Internazionale SRL, Tel: 0800 0858678, menarini@medinformation.co.uk

A S Pharma Ltd, Tel: 01264 332172, info@ccmed.co.uk

A1 Pharmaceuticals, Tel: 01708 528900, enquiries@a1plc.co.uk

Abbott Healthcare Products Ltd, Tel: 0800 4701177, ukabbottnutrition@abbott.com

AbbVie Ltd, Tel: 01628 561092, ukmedinfo@abbvie.com

Accord Healthcare Ltd, Tel: 01271 385257, medinfo@accord-healthcare.com

Actavis UK Ltd, Tel: 01271 385257, medinfo@accord-healthcare.com

Actelion Pharmaceuticals UK Ltd, Tel: 0208 9873333, medinfo_uk@its.jnj.com

Advanced Medical Solutions Ltd, Tel: 01606 863500

Advancis Medical, Tel: 01623 751500

Advanz Pharma, Tel: 08700 703033, medicalinformation@advanzpharma.com

AgaMatrix Europe Ltd, Tel: 0800 0931812, info@agamatrix.co.uk

Aguettant Ltd, Tel: 01275 463691, info@aguettant.co.uk

Alan Pharmaceuticals, Tel: 020 72842887, info@alanpharmaceuticals.com

Alcon Eye Care Ltd, Tel: 0345 2669363, gb.medicaldepartment@alcon.com

Alexion Pharma UK Ltd, Tel: 0800 6891592, MedicalInformation.UK@alexion.com

Alimera Sciences Ltd, Tel: 0800 0191253, medicalinformation@alimerasciences.com

Alissa Healthcare Research Ltd, Tel: 01489 564069, enquiries@alissahealthcare.com

ALK-Abello Ltd, Tel: 0118 9037940, info@uk.alk-abello.com

Allergan Ltd, Tel: 01628 494026, UK_MedInfo@Allergan.com

Allergy Therapeutics (UK) Ltd, Tel: 01903 844700, marketsupport@allergytherapeutics.com

Alliance Pharmaceuticals Ltd, Tel: 01249 466966, medinfo@alliancepharma.co.uk

Almirall Ltd, Tel: 0800 0087399, Almirall@EU.ProPharmaGroup.com

Almus Pharmaceuticals Ltd, Tel: 0800 9177983, med.info@almus.co.uk

Altacor Ltd, Tel: 01189 026766, info@altacor-pharma.com

Ambe Ltd, Tel: 01732 760900, info@ambemedical.com

Amgen Ltd, Tel: 01223 436441, gbinfoline@amgen.com

Amicus Therapeutics UK Ltd, Tel: 01753 888567

AMO UK Ltd, Tel: 01344 864042, crc@its.jnj.com

Amryt Pharma, Tel: 01604 549952, medinfo@amrytpharma.com

AOP Orphan Pharmaceuticals AG, Tel: 0121 2624119, anne.worrallo-hickman@aoporphan.com

Aristo Pharma Ltd, Tel: 01483 920754, medinfo@aristo-pharma.co.uk

Arjun Products Ltd, Tel: 0800 0157806, info@arjunproducts.co.uk

Ascot Laboratories Ltd, Tel: 01923 711971, specials@ascotpharma.com

Aspar Pharmaceuticals Ltd, Tel: 020 82059846, info@aspar.co.uk

Aspen Pharma Trading Ltd, Tel: 0800 0087392, aspenmedinfo@professionalinformation.co.uk

Aspire Pharma Ltd, Tel: 01730 231148, medinfo@aspirepharma.co.uk

Astellas Pharma Ltd, Tel: 0800 7835018, medinfo.gb@astellas.com

AstraZeneca UK Ltd, Tel: 0800 7830033, medical.informationuk@astrazeneca.com

Atlantic Pharma Ltd, Tel: 0845 5191609, enquiries@atlanticpharma.co.uk

Atnahs Pharma UK Ltd, Tel: 01279 406759, pvservices@diamondpharmaservices.com

Auden McKenzie (Pharma Division) Ltd, Tel: 01271 385257, Medinfo@accord-healthcare.com

Aurobindo Pharma Ltd, Tel: 0208 8458811, medinfo@aurobindo.com

AYMES International Ltd, Tel: 0845 6805496, info@aymes.com

B. Braun Medical Ltd, Tel: 0114 2259000, info.bbmuk@bbraun.com

B. Braun Melsungen AG, Tel: +49 5661 710, info@bbraun.com

Bard Ltd, Tel: 01293 527888, customer.services@crbard.com

Bausch & Lomb UK Ltd, Tel: 01748 828849, medicalinformationuk@bausch.com

Baxter Healthcare Ltd, Tel: 01635 206345, medinfo_uki@baxter.com

Bayer Plc, Tel: 0118 2063000, medical.information@bayer.co.uk

BBI Healthcare Ltd, Tel: 01656 868930, info@bbihealthcare.com

Beacon Pharmaceuticals Ltd, Tel: 01233 506574, medical@athlone-laboratories.com

Beiersdorf UK Ltd, Tel: 0121 329 8800

Bell, Sons & Co (Druggists) Ltd, Tel: 0151 4221200, Med-info@bells-healthcare.com

Besins Healthcare (UK) Ltd, Tel: 0203 8620920, BHUK@professionalinformation.co.uk

BHR Pharmaceuticals Ltd, Tel: 02476 377210

BIAL Pharma UK Ltd, Tel: 01753 916010, medinfo.uk@bial.com

Bio Med Sciences, Tel: +1 610 5303193, info@silon.com

Bio Products Laboratory Ltd, Tel: 020 89572622, medinfo@bpl.co.uk

Bio-Diagnostics Ltd, Tel: 01684 592262, enquiries@bio-diagnostics.co.uk

Biogen Idec Ltd, Tel: 0800 0087401, MedInfoUKI@biogen.com

Biolitec Pharma Ltd, Tel: +49 3641 5195330, medinfo@biolitecpharma.com

BioMarin Europe Ltd, Tel: 0845 0177013, medinfoeu@bmrn.com

Bio-Tech Pharmacal Inc, Tel: +1 800 3451199, customerservice@bio-tech-pharm.com

Biotest (UK) Ltd, Tel: 0121 7448444, medicinesinformation.uk@biotest.com

Blumont Pharma Ltd, Tel: 01476 978568

BOC Medical, Tel: 0800 136603, healthcare.home-uk@boc.com

Boehringer Ingelheim Ltd, Tel: 01344 742579, medinfo@bra.boehringer-ingelheim.com

Boston Healthcare Ltd, Tel: 01908 363499, medinfo@bostonhealthcare.co.uk

Brancaster Pharma Ltd, Tel: 01737 243407, safety@brancasterpharma.com

Bray Group Ltd, Tel: 01367 240736, info@bray-healthcare.com

Bristol Laboratories Ltd, Tel: 01442 200922, info@bristol-labs.co.uk

Bristol-Myers Squibb Pharmaceuticals Ltd, Tel: 0800 7311736, medical.information@bms.com

Britannia Pharmaceuticals Ltd, Tel: 01483 920763, enquiries@medinformation.co.uk

Brown & Burk UK Ltd, Tel: 0208 5778200, bbukqa@bbukltd.com

BSN Medical Ltd, Tel: 01482 670100, orders.uk@bsnmedical.com

BTG International Ltd, Tel: +1 877 6269989, medical.services@btgplc.com

C D Medical Ltd, Tel: 01942 813933

Cambridge Healthcare Supplies Ltd, Tel: 01908 363434, medinfo@cambridge-healthcare.co.uk

Cambridge Sensors Ltd, Tel: 0800 0883920, info@microdotcs.com

CareFusion UK Ltd, Tel: 0800 0437546, carefusionGB@professionalinformation.co.uk

Carinopharm GmbH, Tel: 01748 828812, carinopharm@professionalinformation.co.uk

Casen Recordati S.L., Tel: +34 91 3517964, info@casenrecordati.com

CD Pharma Srl, Tel: +39 02 43980539, info@cdpharmagroup.one

Celgene Ltd, Tel: 08448 010045, medinfo.uk.ire@celgene.com

Chanelle Medical UK Ltd, Tel: 0870 1923283, chanelle@medinformation.co.uk

Charles S. Bullen Stomacare Ltd, Tel: 0800 888501

Chattem UK Ltd, consumer.affairs@chattem.com

Chemidex Pharma Ltd, Tel: 01784 477167, info@chemidex.co.uk

Cheplapharm Arzneimittel GmbH, Tel: 0800 1455034, cheplapharm@redlinepv.co.uk

Orphan Europe (UK) Ltd, Tel: +1 888 5758344, medinfo@recordatiraerediseases.com

Otsuka Novel Products GmbH, Tel: +49 89 206020500, medical@otsuka-onpg.com

Otsuka Pharmaceuticals UK Ltd, Tel: 0203 7475300, medical.information@otsuka-europe.com

Owen Mumford Ltd, Tel: 01993 812021, info@owenmumford.com

Pari Medical Ltd, Tel: +49 89 742846832, verena.prusinovsky@pari.com

Paul Hartmann Ltd, Tel: 01706 363200, info@uk.hartmann.info

PaxVax Ltd, Tel: 0800 0885449, medinfo.paxvax@apcerls.com

Peckforton Pharmaceuticals Ltd, Tel: 01908 363498, medinfo@peckforton.com

Pelican Healthcare Ltd, Tel: 0800 318282, contactus@pelicanhealthcare.co.uk

Pern Consumer Products Ltd, Tel: 0800 5999022, business_support@pern-consumer.co.uk

Pfizer Consumer Healthcare Ltd, Tel: 0333 5552526, carelineuk@pfizer.com

Pfizer Ltd, Tel: 01304 616161, Medical.Information@Pfizer.com

PGR Health Foods Ltd, Tel: 01992 581715, info@pgrhealthfoods.co.uk

Pharma Mar, S.A., Tel: +34 91 8466000, pharmamar@pharmamar.com

Pharma Nord (UK) Ltd, Tel: 01670 534900, info@pharmanord.co.uk

Pharmacosmos UK Ltd, Tel: 01844 269007, medinfo@pharmacosmos.co.uk

Pharmasure Ltd, Tel: 01923 233466, customercare@pharmasure.co.uk

Pharming Group N.V., Tel: 0161 6961478, medicalinformation@pharming.com

Phoenix Labs, Tel: +353 1 4688917, medicalinformation@phoenixlabs.ie

Pierre Fabre Ltd, Tel: 0800 0855292, medicalinformation@pierre-fabre.co.uk

Pinewood Healthcare, Tel: 01978 661261, drug.safety@wockhardt.co.uk

Pinnacle Biologics BV, Tel: +1 866 2482039, productinfo@concordialaboratories.com

Piramal Critical Care Ltd, Tel: 0800 7563979, medical.information@piramal.com

Pound International Ltd, Tel: 020 79353735, info@poundinternational.net

Proceli, Tel: 902 364334, info@proceli.com

Profile Pharma Ltd, Tel: 0800 0288942, info.profilepharma@zambongroup.com

Protex Healthcare (UK) Ltd, Tel: +32 475 548581, info@protexhealthcare.com

Proveca Ltd, Tel: 0333 2001866, medinfo@proveca.com

PTC Therapeutics Ltd, Tel: 0345 0754864, medinfo@ptcbio.com

Qdem Pharmaceuticals Ltd, Tel: 01223 426929, medicalinformationUKQdem@qdem.co.uk

Ranbaxy (UK) Ltd, Tel: 0208 8485052, medinfoeurope@sunpharma.com

Rayner Pharmaceuticals Ltd, Tel: 01279 406759, feedback@rayner.com

Reckitt Benckiser Healthcare (UK) Ltd, Tel: 0333 2005345

Recordati Pharmaceuticals Ltd, Tel: 01491 576336, medinfo@recordati.co.uk

Recordati Rare Diseases UK Ltd, Tel: 01491 414333, infoRRDUK@recordati.com

Reig Jofre UK Ltd, Tel: +34 93 4806710, medinfouk@reigjofre.com

Relonchem Ltd, Tel: 0151 556 1860, info@relonchem.com

Respironics (UK) Ltd, Tel: 0870 6077677

R.F. Medical Supplies Ltd, Tel: 01744 882206, enquiries@rfmedicalsupplies.co.uk

Richardson Healthcare Ltd, Tel: 0800 1701126, info@richardsonhealthcare.com

R.I.S. Products Ltd, Tel: 01438 840135, info@risproducts.co.uk

Rivopharm (UK) Ltd, Tel: 01279 406759, PVServices@diamondpharmaservices.com

Robinson Healthcare Ltd, Tel: 01909 735000, orders@robinsonhealthcare.com

Roche Products Ltd, Tel: 0800 3281629, medinfo.uk@roche.com

Rosemont Pharmaceuticals Ltd, Tel: 0113 2441400, rosemont.infodesk@perrigouk.com

RPH Pharmaceuticals AB, Tel: 0207 8621716, safety@elc-group.com

Sai-Meds Ltd, Talk2me@saimeds.com

Sandoz Ltd, Tel: 01276 698101, sandoz@professionalinformation.co.uk

Sanochemia Diagnostics UK Ltd, Tel: 0117 9290287, info@sanochemia.co.uk

Sanofi, Tel: 0800 0352525, uk-medicalinformation@sanofi.com

SanoMed Manufacturing bv, Tel: +32 50 393627, info@naturalsales.nl

Santen UK Ltd, Tel: 0345 0754863, medinfo@santen.co.uk

Santhera (UK) Ltd, Tel: 01423 850733, santhera@pi-arm.co.uk

Scope Ophthalmics Ltd, Tel: 0800 2700253, info@scopeophthalmics.com

Septodont Ltd, Tel 01622 695520

Seqirus Vaccines Ltd, Tel: 01748 828816, Seqirus@eu.propharmagroup.com

SERB, Tel: 0033 173032000, medinfo.uk1@serb.eu

Servier Laboratories Ltd, Tel: 01753 666409, medical.information-uk@servier.com

Seven Seas Ltd, Tel: 08000 728777, info@sseas.com

Shermond, Tel: 01530 278111

Shield Therapeutics (UK) Ltd, Tel: 0207 1868500, info@shieldtx.com

Shire Pharmaceuticals Ltd, Tel: 0333 3000181, medinfoemea@takeda.com

Siemens Healthcare Diagnostics Ltd, Tel: 01276 696000, custcare-service.healthcare.gb@siemens.com

Sintetica Ltd, Tel: 01748 827269, SinteticaGB@EU.PropharmaGroup.com

Slô Drinks Ltd, Tel: 0345 2222205, support@slodrinks.com

Smith & Nephew Healthcare Ltd, Tel: 0800 590173, customer.services.uki@smith-nephew.com

Sovereign Medical Ltd, Tel: 01268 823049, medinfo@amdipharm.com

SpePharm UK Ltd, Tel: +31 20 5670900

Spirit Healthcare Ltd, Tel: 0116 2865000, info@spirit-healthcare.co.uk

SSL International Plc, Tel: 0333 2005345

Stanningley Pharma Ltd, Tel: 01159 124253, medinfo@stanningleypharma.co.uk

STD Pharmaceutical Products Ltd, Tel: 01432 373555, enquiries@stdpharm.co.uk

Steroplast Healthcare Ltd, Tel: 0161 9023030 enquiries@steroplast.co.uk

Stiefel Laboratories (UK) Ltd, Tel: 0800 7838881, customercontactuk@gsk.com

Stiletto Foods (UK) Ltd, Tel: 0345 6021519, info@mrscrimbles.com

Stirling Anglian Pharmaceuticals Ltd, Tel: 0141 5856352, medinfo@stirlinganglianpharmaceuticals.com

Stragen UK Ltd, Tel: 0173 7735029, info@stragenuk.com

Strides Pharma (UK) Ltd, Tel: +91 80 67840000, sadiq.basha@stridesshasun.com

Su-Med International UK Ltd, Tel: 01457 890980

Sun Pharmaceutical Industries Europe B.V., Tel: +46 40 354854, info.se@sunpharma.com

Sunovion Pharmaceuticals Europe Ltd, Tel: 0207 8212840, Med.InfoEU@sunovion.com

SunVit-D3 Ltd, Tel: 0844 4822193, customerservice@sunvitd3.co.uk

Supra Enterprises Ltd, Tel: 0116 2222555, info@supra.org.uk

Sutherland Health Ltd, Tel: 01635 874488, info@sutherlandhealth.com

Swedish Orphan Biovitrum Ltd, Tel: 01748 828863, sobi@professionalinformation.co.uk

Synergy Biologics Ltd, Tel: 01922 705102, info@synergybiologics.co.uk

Synergy Pharmaceuticals, Tel: +1 212 2970020, info@synergypharma.com

Syner-Med (Pharmaceutical Products) Ltd, Tel: 0208 6556380, medicalinformation@syner-med.com

Systagenix Wound Management, Tel: 02030 278716, customercareuk@systagenix.com

Takeda UK Ltd, Tel: 0333 3000181, medinfoemea@takeda.com

Talley Group Ltd, Tel: 01794 503500

Techdow Pharma England Ltd, Tel: 01271 334609, medinfouk@eu.techdow.com

Teofarma, servizioclienti@teofarma.it

Tesaro UK Ltd, Tel: 03303 328100, contact-ukinor@tesarobio.com

Teva UK Ltd, Tel: 0207 5407117, medinfo@tevauk.com

Thame Laboratories Ltd, Tel: 0208 5153700, medinfo@bnsthamelabs.co.uk

The Boots Company Plc, Tel: 01159 595165

Thea Pharmaceuticals Ltd, Tel: 0345 5211290, thea-pharma@medinformation.co.uk

Theramex HQ UK Ltd, Tel: 0333 0096795, medinfo.uk@theramex.com

Thomas Blake Cosmetic Creams Ltd, Tel: 01207 272311

Thornton & Ross Ltd, Tel: 01484 848164, thorntonross@medinformation.co.uk

Tillomed Laboratories Ltd, Tel: 01480 402400, medical.information@tillomed.co.uk

Tillotts Pharma Ltd, Tel: 01522 813500, ukmedinfo@tillotts.com

Tobia Teff UK Ltd, Tel: 0207 0181210, info@tobiateff.co.uk

TopRidge Pharma (Ireland) Ltd, Tel: 0800 443252, drugsafety@navamedic.com orbet Laboratories Ltd, Tel: 01953 607856, nquiries@torbetlaboratories.co.uk

ransdermal Ltd, Tel: 0148 3920749, ransdermal.mi@primevigilance.com

RB Chemidica (UK) Ltd, Tel: 0845 3307556, nfo@trbchemedica.co.uk

riOn Pharma Ltd, Tel: 02392 255770, info@ rionpharma.co.uk

rudell Medical UK Ltd, Tel: 01256 338400, nfo@trudellmedical.co.uk

ypharm Ltd, Tel: 02037 694160, medinfo@ ypharm.com

lCB Pharma Ltd, Tel: 01753 777100, lCBCares.UK@ucb.com

Jltrapharm Ltd, Tel: 01495 765570, info@ ltrapharm.eu

Jnilever UK Home & Personal Care, Tel:)1372 945001

Jnivar by, Tel: 0151 4226240

Jnomedical Ltd, Tel: 0800 289738, wound.webcare@convatec.com

Urgo Ltd, Tel: 01509 502051, woundcare@ uk.urgo.com

Valneva UK Ltd, Tel: 01506 446608, medinfo@ valneva.com

Vega Nutritionals Ltd, Tel: 01639 825107, info@vegavitamins.co.uk

Veriton Pharma Ltd, Tel: 01932 690325, centralmedicalinformation@ veritonpharma.com

Vertex Pharmaceuticals (UK) Ltd, Tel: 01923 437672, vertexmedicalinfo@vrtx.com

Vifor Pharma UK Ltd, Tel: 01276 853633, medicalinfo_UK@viforpharma.com

ViiV Healthcare UK Ltd, Tel: 020 83806200

Visufarma UK Ltd, Tel: 0113 4680661, UKMedicalinformation@VISUfarma.com

Vitaflo International Ltd, Tel: 0151 7099020, vitaflo@vitaflo.co.uk

Vitalograph Ltd, Tel: 01280 827110

Wallace, Cameron & Company Ltd, Tel: 01698 354600, sales@wallacecameron.com

Wallace Manufacturing Chemists Ltd, Tel: 01235 538700

Warburtons, Tel: 0800 243684, customercare@warburtons.co.uk

Warner Chilcott UK Ltd, Tel: 01271 385257, Medinfo@accord-healthcare.com

Waymade Healthcare Plc, Tel: 01268 535200, info@waymade.co.uk

Welland Medical Ltd, Tel: 01293 615455, info@ wellandmedical.com

Wellfoods Ltd, Tel: 01226 382877, salesforce@ fostersbakery.co.uk

Williams Medical Supplies Ltd, Tel: 01685 846666, medicalservices@wms.co.uk

Wockhardt UK Ltd, Tel: 01978 661261

Wyvern Medical Ltd, Tel: 01264 332172, info@ wyvernmedical.co.uk

Zentiva, Tel: 0800 0902408, UKMedInfo@ zentiva.com

Zeroderma Ltd, Tel: 01484 848164, thorntonross@medinformation.co.uk

Special-order manufacturers

Unlicensed medicines are available from 'special-order' manufacturers and specialist-importing companies; the MHRA maintains a register of these companies at tinyurl.com/cdslke.

Licensed **hospital manufacturing units** also manufacture 'special-order' products as unlicensed medicines, the principal NHS units are listed below. A database (*Pro-File*; www.pro-file.nhs.uk) provides information on medicines manufactured in the NHS; access is restricted to NHS pharmacy staff.

The Association of Pharmaceutical Specials Manufacturers may also be able to provide further information about commercial companies (www.apsm-uk.com).

The MHRA recommends that an unlicensed medicine should only be used when a patient has special requirements that cannot be met by use of a licensed medicine.

As well as being available direct from the hospital manufacturer(s) concerned, many NHS-manufactured Specials may be bought from the Oxford Pharmacy Store, owned and operated by Oxford Health NHS Foundation Trust.

England

London

Barts and the London NHS Trust
Mr J. A. Rickard, Head of Barts Health Pharmaceuticals
Barts Health NHS Trust
The Royal London Hospital
Pathology and Pharmacy Building
80 Newark St
Whitechapel
London
E1 2ES
(020) 3246 0394 (order/enquiry)
barts.pharmaceuticals@bartshealth.nhs.uk

Guy's and St. Thomas' NHS Foundation Trust
Mr P. Forsey, Associate Chief Pharmacist
Guy's and St. Thomas' NHS Foundation Trust
Guy's Hospital
Pharmacy Department
Great Maze Pond
London
SE1 9RT
(020) 7188 4992 (order)
(020) 7188 5003 (enquiry)
Fax: (020) 7188 5013
paul.forsey@gstt.nhs.uk

Moorfields Pharmaceuticals
Mr. T. Record, Technical Director
Moorfields Pharmaceuticals
25 Provost St
London
N1 7NH
(020) 7684 9090 (order/enquiry)
Fax: (020) 7502 2332

London North West Healthcare NHS Trust
Mr K. Wong,
London North West Healthcare NHS Trust
Northwick Park Hospital
Watford Rd
Harrow
Middlesex
HA1 3UJ
(020) 8869 2295 (order)
(020) 8869 2204/2223 (enquiry)
kwong@nhs.net

Royal Free London NHS Foundation Trust
Mr J. Singh, Principal Pharmacist Technical Services
Royal Free Hospital Pharmacy Technical Services
Pond St
Hampstead
London
NW3 2QG
(020) 7830 2424 (order)
(020) 7830 2282 (enquiry)
Fax: (020) 7794 1875
rf.specials@nhs.net
jasdeep.singh1@nhs.net

St George's Healthcare NHS Trust
Mr V. Kumar, Assistant Chief Pharmacist
St George's Hospital
Technical Services
Blackshaw Rd
Tooting
London
SW17 0QT
(020) 8725 1770/1768
Fax: (020) 8725 3947
vinodh.kumar@stgeorges.nhs.uk

University College Hospital NHS Foundation Trust
Mr T. Murphy, Production Manager
University College Hospital
235 Euston Rd
London
NW1 2BU
(020) 7380 9723 (order)
(020) 7380 9472 (enquiry)
Fax: (020) 7380 9726
tony.murphy@uclh.nhs.uk

Midlands and Eastern

Barking, Havering and Redbridge University Trust
Mr N. Fisher, Senior Principal Pharmacist
Queen's Hospital
Pharmacy Department
Romford
Essex
RM7 0AG
(01708) 435 463 (order)
(01708) 435 042 (enquiry)
neil.fisher@bhrhospitals.nhs.uk

Burton Hospitals NHS Foundation Trust
Mr D. Raynor, Head of Pharmacy Manufacturing Unit
Queens Hospital
Burton Hospitals NHS Foundation Trust
Pharmacy Manufacturing Unit
Belvedere Rd
Burton-on-Trent
DE13 0RB
(01283) 511 511 ext: 5275 (order/enquiry)
Fax: (01283) 593 036
david.raynor@burtonft.nhs.uk

Colchester Hospital University NHS Foundation Trust
Mr S. Pullen, Pharmacy Production Manager
Colchester General Hospital
Main Pharmacy
Turner Rd
Colchester
Essex
CO4 5JL
(01206) 742 007 (order)
(01206) 744 208 (enquiry)
Fax: (01206) 841 249
pharmacy.stores@colchesterhospital.nhs.uk (order)
psu.enquiries@colchesterhospital.nhs.uk (enquiry)

Ipswich Hospital NHS Trust
Dr J. Harwood, Production Manager
Ipswich Hospital NHS Trust
Pharmacy Manufacturing Unit
Heath Rd
Ipswich,
IP4 5PD
(01473) 703 440 (order)
(01473) 703 603 (enquiry)
Fax: (01473) 703 609
john.harwood@ipswichhospital.nhs.uk

Nottingham University Hospitals NHS Trust
Mr J. Graham, Senior Pharmacist, Production
Nottingham University Hospitals NHS Trust
Pharmacy Production Units
Queens Medical Centre Campus
Nottingham
NG7 2UH
(0115) 924 9924 ext: 66521 (enquiry/order)
Fax: (0115) 970 9780
jeff.graham@nuh.nhs.uk

University Hospital of North Midlands NHS Trust
Ms K. Milner, Chief Technician
Royal Stoke University Hospital
University Hospital of North Midlands NHS Trust
Pharmacy Technical Services
Newcastle Road
Stoke-on-Trent
Staffordshire
ST4 6QG
(01782) 674 568 (order)
(01782) 674 568 (enquiry)
pharmacymanu@uhnm.nhs.uk
kate.milner@uhnm.nhs.uk

North East

The Newcastle upon Tyne Hospitals NHS Foundation Trust
Mr Y. Hunter-Blair, Production Manager
Royal Victoria Infirmary
Newcastle Specials
Pharmacy Production Unit
Queen Victoria Rd
Newcastle-upon-Tyne
NE1 4LP
(0191) 282 0395 (order)
(0191) 282 0389 (enquiry)
Fax: (0191) 282 0469
yan.hunter-blair@nuth.nhs.uk

orth West

reston Pharmaceuticals

s A. Bolch, Deputy Chief Pharmacist (PMU)
eston Pharmaceuticals
oyal Preston Hospital
ulwood
reston
R2 9HT
1772) 523 617 (order)
1772) 522 593 (enquiry)
ax: (01772) 523 645
ngela.bolch@lthtr.nhs.uk

tockport Pharmaceuticals

r A. Singleton, Head of Production
epping Hill Hospital
tockport NHS Foundation Trust
tockport Pharmaceuticals
tockport
K2 7JE
0161) 419 5666 (order)
0161) 419 5657 (enquiry)
ax: (0161) 419 5426
ndrew.singleton@stockport.nhs.uk

outh

ortsmouth Hospitals NHS Trust

Mr R. Lucas, Product Development Manager
ortsmouth Hospitals NHS Trust
harmacy Manufacturing Unit
nit D2, Railway Triangle Industrial Estate
Walton Road
arlington
ortsmouth
PO6 1TF
02392) 389 078 (order)
02392) 316 312 (enquiry)
ax: (02392) 316 316
obert.lucas@porthosp.nhs.uk

South West

orbay Pharmaceuticals

Mr Leon Rudd, Commercial Strategy Director
Torbay and South Devon Healthcare NHS
Foundation Trust
Torbay Pharmaceuticals
Wilkins Drive
Paignton
TQ4 7FG
(01803) 664 707
Fax: (01803) 664 354
eon.rudd@nhs.net

Yorkshire

Calderdale and Huddersfield NHS Foundation Trust

Dr B. Grewal, Managing Director
Calderdale and Huddersfield NHS Foundation
Trust
Huddersfield Pharmacy Specials
Gate 2 - Acre Mills, School St West
Huddersfield
HD3 3ET
(01484) 355 388 (order/enquiry)
info.hps@cht.nhs.uk

Northern Ireland

Victoria Pharmaceuticals

Mr S. Cameron, Production Manager -
Pharmacy
Victoria Pharmaceuticals
Royal Hospitals
Plenum Building
Grosvenor Road
Belfast
BT12 6BA
(028) 9615 1000 (order/enquiry)
Fax: (028) 9063 5282 (order/enquiry)
samuel.cameron@belfasttrust.hscni.net

Scotland

Tayside Pharmaceuticals

Mr S. Bath, Production Manager
Ninewells Hospital
Tayside Pharmaceuticals
Dundee
DD1 9SY
(01382) 632 052 (order)
(01382) 632 273 (enquiry)
Fax: (01382) 632 060
sbath@nhs.net

Wales

Cardiff and Vale University Health Board

Ms A. Jones, Principal Pharmacist - Head of
Technical Services
Cardiff and Vale University Health Board
20 Fieldway
Cardiff
CF14 4HY
(029) 2184 8120
Fax: (029) 2184 8130
contact@smpu.co.uk

Index

BNF

YellowCard
COMMISSION ON HUMAN MEDICINES (CHM)

It's easy to report online at:
www.mhra.gov.uk/yellowcard

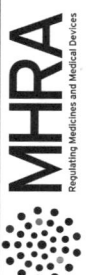

MHRA
Regulating Medicines and Medical Devices

REPORT OF SUSPECTED ADVERSE DRUG REACTIONS

If you suspect an adverse reaction may be related to one or more drugs/vaccines/complementary remedies, please complete this Yellow Card. See 'Adverse reactions to drugs' section in BNF or **www.mhra.gov.uk/yellowcard** for guidance. Do not be put off reporting because some details are not known.

PATIENT DETAILS   Patient Initials: _____   Sex: M / F   Is the patient pregnant? Y / N   Ethnicity: _____

Age (at time of reaction): _____   Weight (kg): _____   Identification number (e.g. Practice or Hospital Ref): _____

SUSPECTED DRUG(S)/VACCINE(S)

Drug/Vaccine (Brand if known)	Batch	Route	Dosage	Date started	Date stopped	Prescribed for

SUSPECTED REACTION(S)   Please describe the reaction(s) and any treatment given. (Please attach additional pages if necessary):

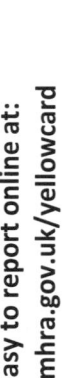

Outcome
☐ Recovered
☐ Recovering
☐ Continuing
☐ Other

Date reaction(s) started: _____   Date reaction(s) stopped: _____

Do you consider the reactions to be serious?   Yes / No

If yes, please indicate why the reaction is considered to be serious (please tick all that apply):

☐ Patient died due to reaction   ☐ Involved or prolonged inpatient hospitalisation
☐ Life threatening   ☐ Involved persistent or significant disability or incapacity
☐ Congenital abnormality   ☐ Medically significant; please give details: _____

If the reactions were not serious according to the categories above, how bad was the suspected reaction?

☐ Mild   ☐ Unpleasant, but did not affect everyday activities   ☐ Bad enough to affect everyday activities

It's easy to report online: www.mhra.gov.uk/yellowcard

OTHER DRUG(S) (including self-medication and complementary remedies)

Did the patient take any other medicines/vaccines/complementary remedies in the last 3 months prior to the reaction? Yes / No

If yes, please give the following information if known:

Drug/Vaccine (Brand if known)	Batch	Route	Dosage	Date started	Date stopped	Prescribed for

Additional relevant information e.g. medical history, test results, known allergies, rechallenge (if performed). For reactions relating to use of a medicine during pregnancy please state all other drugs taken during pregnancy, the last menstrual period, information on previous pregnancies, ultrasound scans, any delivery complications, birth defects or developmental concerns.

Please list any medicines obtained from the internet:

REPORTER DETAILS

Name and Professional Address:

Postcode: _____ Tel No: _____

Email:

Speciality:

Signature: _____ Date: _____

CLINICIAN (if not the reporter)

Name and Professional Address:

Postcode: _____ Tel No: _____

Email:

Speciality:

Date:

Information on adverse drug reactions received by the MHRA can be downloaded at **www.mhra.gov.uk/daps**

Stay up-to-date on the latest advice for the safe use of medicines with our monthly bulletin *Drug Safety Update* at: **www.mhra.gov.uk/drugsafetyupdate**

Please attach additional pages if necessary. Send to: FREEPOST YELLOW CARD (no other address details required)

BNF

YellowCard

COMMISSION ON HUMAN MEDICINES (CHM)

It's easy to report online at:
www.mhra.gov.uk/yellowcard

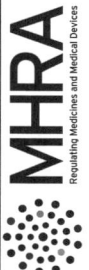

MHRA
Regulating Medicines and Medical Devices

REPORT OF SUSPECTED ADVERSE DRUG REACTIONS

If you suspect an adverse reaction may be related to one or more drugs/vaccines/complementary remedies, please complete this Yellow Card. See 'Adverse reactions to drugs' section in BNF or **www.mhra.gov.uk/yellowcard** for guidance. Do not be put off reporting because some details are not known.

PATIENT DETAILS

Patient Initials: _____   Sex: M / F   Is the patient pregnant? Y / N   Ethnicity: _____

Age (at time of reaction): _____   Weight (kg): _____   Identification number (e.g. Practice or Hospital Ref): _____

SUSPECTED DRUG(S)/VACCINE(S)

Drug/Vaccine (Brand if known)	Batch	Route	Dosage	Date started	Date stopped	Prescribed for

SUSPECTED REACTION(S)

Please describe the reaction(s) and any treatment given. (Please attach additional pages if necessary):

Outcome

Recovered ☐
Recovering ☐
Continuing ☐
Other ☐

Date reaction(s) started: _____   Date reaction(s) stopped: _____

Do you consider the reactions to be serious?   Yes / No

If yes, please indicate why the reaction is considered to be serious (please tick all that apply):

☐ Patient died due to reaction   ☐ Involved or prolonged inpatient hospitalisation
☐ Life threatening   ☐ Involved persistent or significant disability or incapacity
☐ Congenital abnormality   ☐ Medically significant; please give details: _____

If the reactions were not serious according to the categories above, how bad was the suspected reaction?

☐ Mild   ☐ Unpleasant, but did not affect everyday activities   ☐ Bad enough to affect everyday activities

It's easy to report online: www.mhra.gov.uk/yellowcard

OTHER DRUG(S) (including self-medication and complementary remedies)

Did the patient take any other medicines/vaccines/complementary remedies in the last 3 months prior to the reaction? Yes / No

If yes, please give the following information if known:

Drug/Vaccine (Brand if known)	Batch	Route	Dosage	Date started	Date stopped	Prescribed for

Additional relevant information e.g. medical history, test results, known allergies, rechallenge (if performed). For reactions relating to use of a medicine during pregnancy please state all other drugs taken during pregnancy, the last menstrual period, information on previous pregnancies, ultrasound scans, any delivery complications, birth defects or developmental concerns.

Please list any medicines obtained from the internet:

REPORTER DETAILS

Name and Professional Address:

Postcode: _____ Tel No: _____

Email:

Speciality:

Signature: _____ Date: _____

CLINICIAN (if not the reporter)

Name and Professional Address:

Postcode: _____ Tel No: _____

Email:

Speciality:

Date:

Information on adverse drug reactions received by the MHRA can be downloaded at **www.mhra.gov.uk/daps**

Stay up-to-date on the latest advice for the safe use of medicines with our monthly bulletin *Drug Safety Update* at: **www.mhra.gov.uk/drugsafetyupdate**

Please attach additional pages if necessary. Send to: FREEPOST YELLOW CARD (no other address details required)

Adult Advanced Life Support Algorithm

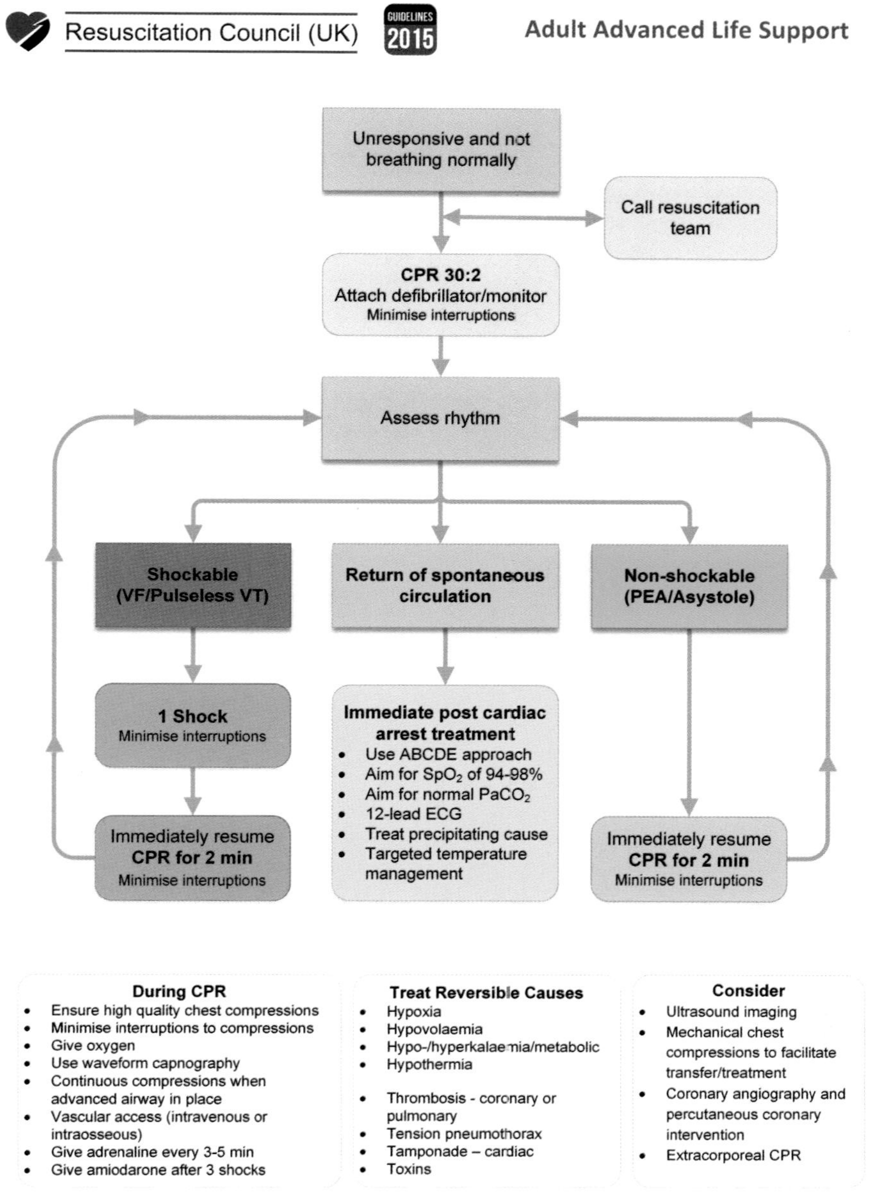

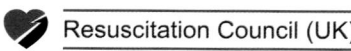 Resuscitation Council (UK) **Adult Advanced Life Support**

```
                Unresponsive and not
                breathing normally

                                          Call resuscitation
                                                team

                     CPR 30:2
               Attach defibrillator/monitor
                 Minimise interruptions

                   Assess rhythm
```

Shockable (VF/Pulseless VT)	Return of spontaneous circulation	Non-shockable (PEA/Asystole)

Shockable (VF/Pulseless VT)

1 Shock
Minimise interruptions

Immediately resume CPR for 2 min
Minimise interruptions

Return of spontaneous circulation

Immediate post cardiac arrest treatment
- Use ABCDE approach
- Aim for SpO$_2$ of 94-98%
- Aim for normal PaCO$_2$
- 12-lead ECG
- Treat precipitating cause
- Targeted temperature management

Non-shockable (PEA/Asystole)

Immediately resume CPR for 2 min
Minimise interruptions

During CPR
- Ensure high quality chest compressions
- Minimise interruptions to compressions
- Give oxygen
- Use waveform capnography
- Continuous compressions when advanced airway in place
- Vascular access (intravenous or intraosseous)
- Give adrenaline every 3-5 min
- Give amiodarone after 3 shocks

Treat Reversible Causes
- Hypoxia
- Hypovolaemia
- Hypo-/hyperkalaemia/metabolic
- Hypothermia

- Thrombosis - coronary or pulmonary
- Tension pneumothorax
- Tamponade – cardiac
- Toxins

Consider
- Ultrasound imaging
- Mechanical chest compressions to facilitate transfer/treatment
- Coronary angiography and percutaneous coronary intervention
- Extracorporeal CPR

Medical emergencies in the community

Overview

Drug treatment outlined below is intended for use by **appropriately qualified healthcare professionals** . Only drugs that are used for immediate relief are shown; advice on supporting care is not given. Where the patient's condition requires investigation and further treatment, the patient should be transferred to hospital promptly.

Acute coronary syndromes

▶ ANGINA: UNSTABLE
Aspirin dispersible tablets p. 132 (75 mg, 300 mg)
BY MOUTH (DISPERSED IN WATER OR CHEWED)
  ▶ Adult: 300 mg

▶ PLUS

▶ EITHER **Glyceryl trinitrate aerosol spray p. 233**
(400 micrograms/metered dose)
SUBLINGUALLY
  ▶ Adult: 1–2 sprays, repeated as required

▶ OR **Glyceryl trinitrate tablets** (300 micrograms, 500 micrograms, 600 micrograms)
SUBLINGUALLY
  ▶ Adult: 0.3–1 mg, repeated as required

▶ MYOCARDIAL INFARCTION: NON-ST-SEGMENT ELEVATION
Treat as for Angina: unstable

▶ MYOCARDIAL INFARCTION: ST-SEGMENT ELEVATION
Aspirin dispersible tablets (75 mg, 300 mg)
BY MOUTH (DISPERSED IN WATER OR CHEWED)
  ▶ Adult: 300 mg

Glyceryl trinitrate aerosol spray (400 micrograms/metered dose)
SUBLINGUALLY
  ▶ Adult: 1–2 sprays, repeated as required

▶ OR **Glyceryl trinitrate tablets** (300 micrograms, 500 micrograms, 600 micrograms)
SUBLINGUALLY
  ▶ Adult: 0.3–1 mg, repeated as required

Metoclopramide hydrochloride injection p. 451 (5 mg/mL)
BY INTRAVENOUS INJECTION
  ▶ Adult 18-19 years (body-weight up to 60 kg): 5 mg
  ▶ Adult 18-19 years (body-weight 60 kg and over): 10 mg
  ▶ Adult over 19 years: 10 mg

Diamorphine hydrochloride injection p. 476 (5 mg powder for reconstitution)
BY SLOW INTRAVENOUS INJECTION (1-2 MG/MINUTE)
  ▶ Adult: 5 mg followed by a further 2.5–5 mg if necessary
  ▶ Elderly or frail patients, reduce dose by half

▶ OR **Morphine sulfate injection p. 483** (10 mg/mL)
BY SLOW INTRAVENOUS INJECTION (1-2 MG/MINUTE)
  ▶ Adult: 5–10 mg followed by a further 5–10 mg if necessary
  ▶ Elderly or frail patients: reduce dose by half
Oxygen, if appropriate

Airways disease, obstructive

▶ ASTHMA: ACUTE
Regard each emergency consultation as being for **severe acute asthma** until shown otherwise; failure to respond adequately **at any time** requires immediate transfer to hospital

▶ EITHER **Salbutamol aerosol inhaler p. 269**
(100 micrograms/metered inhalation)
BY AEROSOL INHALATION VIA LARGE-VOLUME SPACER
(AND A CLOSE-FITTING FACE MASK IF CHILD UNDER 3 YEARS)
  ▶ Adult and child: 2–10 puffs each inhaled separately, repeated every 10–20 minutes or as necessary

▶ OR **Salbutamol nebuliser solution** (1 mg/mL, 2 mg/mL)
BY INHALATION OF NEBULISED SOLUTION (VIA OXYGEN-DRIVEN NEBULISER IF AVAILABLE)
  ▶ Child 4 years and below: 2.5 mg every 20–30 minutes or as necessary
  ▶ Child 5-11 years: 2.5–5 mg every 20–30 minutes or as necessary
  ▶ Child 12-17 years: 5 mg every 20–30 minutes or as necessary
  ▶ Adult: 5 mg every 20–30 minutes or as necessary

▶ OR **Terbutaline sulfate nebuliser solution p. 271** (2.5 mg/mL)
BY INHALATION OF NEBULISED SOLUTION (VIA OXYGEN-DRIVEN NEBULISER IF AVAILABLE)
  ▶ Child 4 years and below: 5 mg every 20–30 minutes or as necessary
  ▶ Child 5-11 years: 5–10 mg every 20–30 minutes or as necessary
  ▶ Child 12-17 years: 10 mg every 20–30 minutes or as necessary
  ▶ Adult: 10 mg every 20–30 minutes or as necessary

▶ PLUS **(in all cases)**

▶ EITHER **Prednisolone tablets p. 718 (or prednisolone soluble tablets)** (5 mg)
BY MOUTH
  ▶ Child 11 years and below: 1–2 mg/kg (max. 40 mg) once daily for up to 3 days or longer if necessary; if child has been taking an oral corticosteroid for more than a few days, give prednisolone 2 mg/kg (max. 60 mg) once daily
  ▶ Child 12-17 years: 40–50 mg once daily for at least 5 days
  ▶ Adult: 40–50 mg once daily for at least 5 days

▶ OR **Hydrocortisone p. 716 (preferably as sodium succinate)**
BY INTRAVENOUS INJECTION
  ▶ Child 17 years and below: 4 mg/kg (max. 100 mg) every 6 hours until conversion to oral prednisolone is possible; alternative dose if weight unavailable:
  ▶ Child 1 year and below: 25 mg
  ▶ Child 2-4 years: 50 mg
  ▶ Child 5-17 years: 100 mg
  ▶ Adult: 100 mg every 6 hours until conversion to oral prednisolone is possible

High-flow **oxygen** should be given if available (via face mask in children)

Monitor response 15 to 30 minutes after nebulisation; if any signs of acute asthma persist, arrange hospital admission. While awaiting ambulance, repeat **nebulised beta₂ agonist** (as above) and give with

ipratropium bromide nebuliser solution p. 262 (250 micrograms/mL)

BY INHALATION OF NEBULISED SOLUTION (VIA OXYGEN-DRIVEN NEBULISER IF AVAILABLE)

- Child 11 years and below: 250 micrograms, repeated every 20–30 minutes for the first 2 hours, then every 4–6 hours as necessary
- Child 12-17 years: 500 micrograms every 4–6 hours as necessary
- Adult: 500 micrograms every 4–6 hours as necessary

CROUP

Dexamethasone oral solution p. 714 (2 mg/5 mL)

BY MOUTH

- Child 1 month-2 years: 150 micrograms/kg as a single dose

Anaphylaxis

ANAPHYLAXIS

Adrenaline/epinephrine injection p. 238 (1 mg/mL (1 in 1000))

BY INTRAMUSCULAR INJECTION

- Child 5 years and below: 150 micrograms (0.15 mL), repeated every 5 minutes if necessary
- Child 6-11 years: 300 micrograms (0.3 mL), repeated every 5 minutes if necessary
- Child 12-17 years: 500 micrograms (0.5 mL), repeated every 5 minutes if necessary; 300 micrograms (0.3 mL) should be given if child is small or prepubertal
- Adult: 500 micrograms (0.5 mL), repeated every 5 minutes if necessary

High-flow **oxygen** and **intravenous fluids** should be given as soon as available.

Chlorphenamine maleate injection p. 299

BY INTRAMUSCULAR OR INTRAVENOUS INJECTION

May help counter histamine-mediated vasodilation and bronchoconstriction.

Hydrocortisone (preferably as sodium succinate)

BY INTRAVENOUS INJECTION

Has delayed action but should be given to severely affected patients to prevent further deterioration.

Bacterial infection

MENINGOCOCCAL DISEASE

Benzylpenicillin sodium injection p. 580 (600 mg, 1.2 g)

BY INTRAVENOUS INJECTION (OR BY INTRAMUSCULAR INJECTION IF VENOUS ACCESS NOT AVAILABLE)

- Neonate: 300 mg
- Child 1 month-11 months: 300 mg
- Child 1-9 years: 600 mg
- Child 10-17 years: 1.2 g
- Adult: 1.2 g

NOTE A single dose should be given before urgent transfer to hospital, so long as this does not delay the transfer.

- OR **if history of allergy to penicillin**

Cefotaxime injection p. 557 (1 g)

BY INTRAVENOUS INJECTION (OR BY INTRAMUSCULAR INJECTION IF VENOUS ACCESS NOT AVAILABLE)

- Neonate: 50 mg/kg
- Child 1 month-11 years: 50 mg/kg (max. 1 g)
- Child 12-17 years: 1 g
- Adult: 1 g

NOTE A single dose can be given before urgent transfer to hospital, so long as this does not delay the transfer.

- OR **if history of immediate hypersensitivity reaction (including anaphylaxis, angioedema, urticaria, or rash immediately after administration) to penicillin or to cephalosporins**

Chloramphenicol injection p. 605 (1 g)

BY INTRAVENOUS INJECTION

- Child: 12.5–25 mg/kg
- Adult: 12.5–25 mg/kg

NOTE A single dose can be given before urgent transfer to hospital, so long as this does not delay the transfer.

See also Central nervous system infections, antibacterial therapy p. 533.

Hypoglycaemia

- DIABETIC HYPOGLYCAEMIA

Glucose or sucrose

BY MOUTH

- Adult and child over 2 years: approx. 10–20 g (110–220 mL *Lucozade® Energy Original or* 100–200 mL *Coca-Cola®*—both non-diet versions *or* 2–4 teaspoonfuls of sugar *or* 3–6 sugar lumps) repeated after 10–15 minutes if necessary

- OR **if hypoglycaemia unresponsive *or* if oral route cannot be used**

Glucagon injection p. 764 (1 mg/mL)

BY SUBCUTANEOUS OR INTRAMUSCULAR INJECTION

- Child body-weight up to 25 kg: 500 micrograms (0.5 mL)
- Child body-weight 25 kg and over: 1 mg (1 mL)
- Adult: 1 mg (1 mL)

- OR **if hypoglycaemia prolonged *or* unresponsive to glucagon after 10 minutes**

Glucose intravenous infusion p. 1090 (10%)

BY INTRAVENOUS INJECTION INTO LARGE VEIN

- Child: 5 mL/kg (glucose 500 mg/kg)

Glucose intravenous infusion (20%)

BY INTRAVENOUS INJECTION INTO LARGE VEIN

- Adult: 50 mL

Seizures

- CONVULSIVE (INCLUDING FEBRILE) SEIZURES LASTING LONGER THAN 5 MINUTES

- EITHER **Diazepam rectal solution p. 362** (2 mg/mL, 4 mg/mL)

BY RECTUM

- Neonate: 1.25–2.5 mg, repeated once after 10–15 minutes if necessary
- Child 1 month-1 year: 5 mg, repeated once after 10–15 minutes if necessary
- Child 2-11 years: 5–10 mg, repeated once after 10–15 minutes if necessary
- Child 12-17 years: 10–20 mg, repeated once after 10–15 minutes if necessary
- Adult: 10–20 mg, repeated once after 10–15 minutes if necessary
- Elderly: 10 mg, repeated once after 10–15 minutes if necessary

- OR **Midazolam oromucosal solution p. 358**

BY BUCCAL ADMINISTRATION, REPEATED ONCE AFTER 10 MINUTES IF NECESSARY

- Neonate: 300 micrograms/kg [unlicensed]
- Child 1-2 months: 300 micrograms/kg (max. 2.5 mg) [unlicensed]
- Child 3 months-11 months: 2.5 mg
- Child 1-4 years: 5 mg
- Child 5-9 years: 7.5 mg
- Child 10-17 years: 10 mg
- Adult: 10 mg [unlicensed]

Approximate Conversions and Units

Conversion of pounds to kilograms

lb	kg
1	0.45
2	0.91
3	1.36
4	1.81
5	2.27
6	2.72
7	3.18
8	3.63
9	4.08
10	4.54
11	4.99
12	5.44
13	5.90
14	6.35

Conversion of stones to kilograms

stones	kg
1	6.35
2	12.70
3	19.05
4	25.40
5	31.75
6	38.10
7	44.45
8	50.80
9	57.15
10	63.50
11	69.85
12	76.20
13	82.55
14	88.90
15	95.25

Conversion from millilitres to fluid ounces

mL	fl oz
50	1.8
100	3.5
150	5.3
200	7.0
500	17.6
1000	35.2

Length

1 metre (m) = 1000 millimetres (mm)
1 centimetre (cm) = 10 mm
1 inch (in) = 25.4 mm
1 foot (ft) = 12 inches
12 inches = 304.8 mm

Mass

1 kilogram (kg) = 1000 grams (g)
1 gram (g) = 1000 milligrams (mg)
1 milligram (mg) = 1000 micrograms
1 microgram = 1000 nanograms
1 nanogram = 1000 picograms

Volume

1 litre = 1000 millilitres (mL)
1 millilitre (1 mL) = 1000 microlitres
1 pint ≈ 568 mL

Other units

1 kilocalorie (kcal) = 4186.8 joules (J)
1000 kilocalories (kcal) = 4.1868 megajoules (MJ)
1 megajoule (MJ) = 238.8 kilocalories (kcal)
1 millimetre of mercury (mmHg) = 133.3 pascals (Pa)
1 kilopascal (kPa) = 7.5 mmHg (pressure)

Plasma-drug concentrations

Plasma-drug concentrations in BNF publications are expressed in mass units per litre (e.g. mg/litre). The approximate equivalent in terms of amount of substance units (e.g. micromol/litre) is given in brackets.

Prescribing for children: weight, height, and gender

The table below shows the **mean values** for weight, height, and gender by age; these values have been derived from the UK-WHO growth charts 2009 and UK1990 standard centile charts, by extrapolating the 50th centile, and may be used to calculate doses in the absence of measurements. However, an individual's weight and height might vary considerably from the values in the table and it is important to ensure that the value chosen is appropriate. In most cases the actual measurement should be obtained as soon as possible and the dose re-calculated.

Age	Weight (kg)	Height (cm)
Full-term neonate	3.5	51
1 month	4.3	55
2 months	5.4	58
3 months	6.1	61
4 months	6.7	63
6 months	7.6	67
1 year	9	75
3 years	14	96
5 years	18	109
7 years	23	122
10 years	32	138
12 years	39	149
14 year old boy	49	163
14 year old girl	50	159
Adult male	68	176
Adult female	58	164

Recommended wording of cautionary and advisory labels

For details including Welsh Language translation see p. 1656

1. Warning: This medicine may make you sleepy

2. Warning: This medicine may make you sleepy. If this happens, do not drive or use tools or machines. Do not drink alcohol

3. Warning: This medicine may make you sleepy. If this happens, do not drive or use tools or machines

4. Warning: Do not drink alcohol

5. Do not take indigestion remedies 2 hours before or after you take this medicine

6. Do not take indigestion remedies, or medicines containing iron or zinc, 2 hours before or after you take this medicine

7. Do not take milk, indigestion remedies, or medicines containing iron or zinc, 2 hours before or after you take this medicine

8. Warning: Do not stop taking this medicine unless your doctor tells you to stop

9. Space the doses evenly throughout the day. Keep taking this medicine until the course is finished, unless you are told to stop

10. Warning: Read the additional information given with this medicine

11. Protect your skin from sunlight—even on a bright but cloudy day. Do not use sunbeds

12. Do not take anything containing aspirin while taking this medicine

13. Dissolve or mix with water before taking

14. This medicine may colour your urine. This is harmless

15. Caution: flammable. Keep your body away from fire or flames after you have put on the medicine

16. Dissolve the tablet under your tongue—do not swallow. Store the tablets in this bottle with the cap tightly closed. Get a new supply 8 weeks after opening

17. Do not take more than... in 24 hours

18. Do not take more than... in 24 hours. Also, do not take more than... in any one week

19. Warning: This medicine makes you sleepy. If you still feel sleepy the next day, do not drive or use tools or machines. Do not drink alcohol

21. Take with or just after food, or a meal

22. Take 30 to 60 minutes before food

23. Take this medicine when your stomach is empty. This means an hour before food or 2 hours after food

24. Suck or chew this medicine

25. Swallow this medicine whole. Do not chew or crush

26. Dissolve this medicine under your tongue

27. Take with a full glass of water

28. Spread thinly on the affected skin only

29. Do not take more than 2 at any one time. Do not take more than 8 in 24 hours

30. Contains paracetamol. Do not take anything else containing paracetamol while taking this medicine. Talk to a doctor at once if you take too much of this medicine, even if you feel well

32. Contains aspirin. Do not take anything else containing aspirin while taking this medicine

London Borough of
Barking & Dagenham

906000001642267		
A & H	19-Apr-2021	
615.134	£59.95	
BDBAR		

BNF 81
6459640